PEDIATRIC & NEONATAL DOSAGE HANDBOOK with INTERNATIONAL TRADE NAMES INDEX

A Universal Resource for Clinicians Treating Pediatric and Neonatal Patients

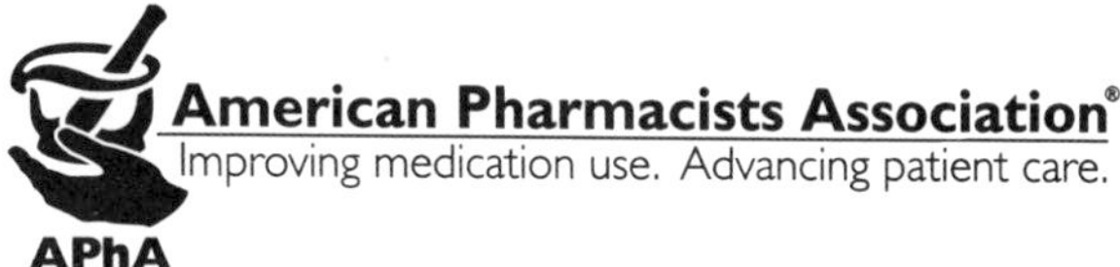

Lexicomp is the official drug reference for the American Pharmacists Association.

22nd Edition

Carol K. Taketomo, PharmD
Jane H. Hodding, PharmD
Donna M. Kraus, PharmD, FAPhA, FCCP

Lexicomp®

PEDIATRIC & NEONATAL DOSAGE HANDBOOK with INTERNATIONAL TRADE NAMES INDEX

A Universal Resource for Clinicians Treating Pediatric and Neonatal Patients

Carol K. Taketomo, PharmD
Director, Pharmacy and Nutritional Services
Children's Hospital Los Angeles
Los Angeles, California

Jane Hurlburt Hodding, PharmD
Executive Director, Pharmacy and Nutritional Services
Long Beach Memorial Medical Center and Miller Children's Hospital
Long Beach, California

Donna M. Kraus, PharmD, FAPhA, FPPAG, FCCP
Associate Professor of Pharmacy Practice
Departments of Pharmacy Practice and Pediatrics
Pediatric Clinical Pharmacist
University of Illinois at Chicago
Chicago, Illinois

Lexicomp®

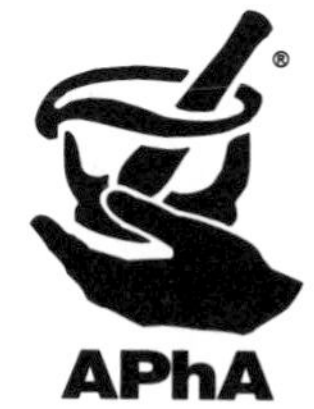

NOTICE

This data is intended to serve the user as a handy reference and not as a complete drug information resource. It does not include information on every therapeutic agent available. The publication covers 1,017 commonly used drugs and is specifically designed to present important aspects of drug data in a more concise format than is typically found in medical literature or product material supplied by manufacturers.

The nature of drug information is that it is constantly evolving because of ongoing research and clinical experience and is often subject to interpretation. While great care has been taken to ensure the accuracy of the information and recommendations presented, the reader is advised that the authors, editors, reviewers, contributors, and publishers cannot be responsible for the continued currency of the information or for any errors, omissions, or the application of this information, or for any consequences arising therefrom. Therefore, the author(s) and/or the publisher shall have no liability to any person or entity with regard to claims, loss, or damage caused, or alleged to be caused, directly or indirectly, by the use of information contained herein. Because of the dynamic nature of drug information, readers are advised that decisions regarding drug therapy must be based on the independent judgment of the clinician, changing information about a drug (eg, as reflected in the literature and manufacturer's most current product information), and changing medical practices. Therefore, this data is designed to be used in conjunction with other necessary information and is not designed to be solely relied upon by any user. The user of this data hereby and forever releases the authors and publishers from this data for any and all liability of any kind that might arise out of the use of this data. The editors are not responsible for any inaccuracy of quotation or for any false or misleading implication that may arise due to the text or formulas as used or due to the quotation of revisions no longer official.

Certain of the authors, editors, and contributors have written this book in their private capacities. No official support or endorsement by any federal or state agency or pharmaceutical company is intended or inferred.

The publishers have made every effort to trace any third party copyright holders, if any, for borrowed material. If they have inadvertently overlooked any, they will be pleased to make the necessary arrangements at the first opportunity.

If you have any suggestions or questions regarding any information presented in this data, please contact our drug information pharmacists at (855) 633-0577. Book revisions are available at our website at http://www.wolterskluwercdi.com/clinical-notices/revisions/.

This manual was produced using LIMS — A complete publishing service of Wolters Kluwer Clinical Drug Information, Inc.

Lexicomp®

ISBN 978-1-59195-349-4 (Domestic Edition)

ISBN 978-1-59195-350-0 (International Edition)

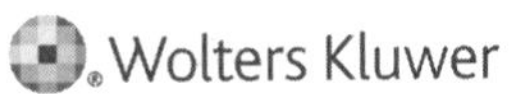

TABLE OF CONTENTS

PREFACE

This twenty-second edition of the *Pediatric & Neonatal Dosage Handbook* is designed to be a practical and convenient guide to the dosing and usage of medications in neonates, infants, children, and adolescents. The pediatric population is a dynamic group, with major changes in pharmacokinetics and pharmacodynamics taking place throughout infancy and childhood. Therefore, the need for the evaluation and establishment of medication dosing regimens in children of different ages is great.

Special considerations must be taken into account when dosing medications in pediatric and neonatal patients. Unfortunately, due to a lack of appropriate studies, most medications commonly used in neonates and children do not have FDA approved labeling for use in pediatric patients. Only 30% of drugs used in children in a 1988 survey carried FDA approval in their labeling. Seventy-five percent of medications listed in the *1990 Physicians' Desk Reference (PDR)* carried some type of precaution or disclaimer statement for use in children.[1] A more recent analysis of information in the 1998, 2002, and 2007 *PDR* found that although over 50% of prescription drug products carried FDA-approved labeling for use in pediatric patients, the percent of drugs with pediatric labeling actually **decreased** over time (1998: 55.9%; 2002: 54.3%; and 2007: 51.3%).[2] In addition, the number of drug entities with FDA-approved labeling for use in neonates decreased by 39% during this time frame. Another study found that 45% of parenteral medications used in the neonatal intensive care unit are not approved by the FDA for use in neonates.[3] Thus, further studies are needed to improve FDA drug labeling for pediatric patients, especially for neonates (and particularly preterm neonates). [4,5]

Investigations have also demonstrated the need for further improvement in FDA drug labeling for medications specifically used in critically ill children. One study found that 67% of medications used in a pediatric intensive care unit did not have FDA-approved labeling for use in pediatric patients or only had approval for use in limited age groups.[6] Of all drugs prescribed in a pediatric cardiac intensive care unit (CICU), 36% were prescribed "off-label" (ie, the drug did not have an FDA-approved labeled indication based on the patient's age); 94% of patients received one or more off-label medications; and the frequency of use of off-label drugs was higher in CICU patients who were younger, and in those with a higher severity of illness.[7] Considering the large number of medications without FDA-approved labeling that are used in critically ill neonates and children, further pediatric studies are clearly warranted to improve FDA drug labeling, and the safe and effective use of medications in these patients.

The FDA Modernization Act of 1997, the Children's Health Act of 2000, the Best Pharmaceuticals for Children Act of 2002, and the Pediatric Research Equity Act of 2003 have all helped to increase pediatric drug studies. The FDA Amendment Act of 2007, which was signed into law in September 2007, reauthorizes and amends the Pediatric Research Equity Act and the Best Pharmaceuticals for Children Act (Title IV and Title V, Public Law 110-85, 110th Congress). The Food and Drug Administration Safety and Innovation Act of 2012 renews and strengthens the Best Pharmaceuticals for Children Act and the Pediatric Research Equity Act by making these two laws permanent (and no longer subject to reauthorization every five years).

The FDA Modernization Act of 1997 (Section 111, Public Law 105-115, 105th Congress) **encouraged** pharmaceutical companies to conduct pediatric drug studies by allowing 6 months of market exclusivity to certain designated drugs. A list of drugs, for which additional pediatric information may produce pediatric health care benefits, was required by this law to be developed by the US Department of Health and Human Services (HHS), with input from the American Academy of Pediatrics, the Pediatric Pharmacology Research Unit Network,[8] and the US Pharmacopoeia. To date, the FDA has received 884 proposals from pharmaceutical companies to conduct pediatric drug studies under this Act (and subsequent acts) and has issued 470 written requests for studies. If these pediatric studies are completed as the FDA has specified, then these medications will qualify for the 6-month patent extension or additional market exclusivity. Two hundred eleven products have already had their marketing patents extended by this law and to date, 580 pediatric labeling changes have occurred.[9]

The pediatric section of the FDA Modernization Act was renewed by Congress and signed into law January 4, 2002. This new law, called the Best Pharmaceuticals for Children Act, reauthorized the use of the 6-month patent extension to **encourage** pharmaceutical companies to conduct pediatric drug research. This law called for the establishment of an Office of Pediatric Therapeutics within the FDA and established an FDA Pediatric Pharmacology Advisory Committee and a Pediatric Sub-committee of the Oncologic Drugs Advisory Committee. It also created a research fund for pediatric studies of drugs that are off patent, granted a special "priority status" to pediatric labeling changes, required the Department of Health and Human Services (along with the Institute of Medicine) to conduct a study to assess federally funded pediatric research, and called for the development of a Final Rule that required drug labeling to include a toll-free number to report adverse events.[10]

The Best Pharmaceuticals for Children Act was reauthorized, amended, and signed into law in September 2007, as part of the FDA Amendment Act of 2007.[9] This amended law establishes an internal review committee (the Pediatric Review Committee) within the FDA to review written requests that were issued and the submitted reports from drug manufacturers.[11] It also requires manufacturers who were granted a patent extension to revise pediatric labeling in a timely manner; reduces the patent extension from 6 months to 3 months for drugs with combined gross sales >1 billion dollars; prohibits the extension of market exclusivity for >9 months; requires manufacturers to explain why a pediatric formulation cannot be developed (when requested to perform pediatric studies); requires product labeling to include information about pediatric studies whether or not the studies demonstrate that the drug is safe and effective; requires the government to notify the public of pediatric drug formulations that were developed and studied and found to be safe and effective, but not introduced into the market within 1 year; and requires that a report be submitted to congress that assesses the use of patent extensions in making sure that medications used by pediatric patients are tested and properly labeled.[12]

The 1998 Pediatric Final Rule was an FDA regulation, titled "Regulations Requiring Manufacturers to Assess the Safety and Effectiveness of New Drugs and Biological Products in Pediatric Patients; Final Rule".[13] This important regulation **required** that manufacturers conduct pediatric studies for certain new and marketed drugs and biological products. This requirement was mandatory, and its scope included new drugs (ie, new chemical entities, new dosage forms, new indications, new routes of administration, and new dosing regimens) and certain marketed drugs (ie, where the drug product offered meaningful therapeutic benefit or had substantial use in pediatric patients, AND the absence of pediatric labeling posed a risk). This FDA regulation became effective April 1, 1999, but studies mandated under this rule were not required to be submitted to the FDA before December 2, 2000. The 1998 Pediatric Final Rule and the authority of the FDA to **require** manufacturers to conduct pediatric studies was challenged with a law suit. In March 2002, the FDA requested a 2-month stay on the lawsuit, so it could publish a notice and suspend the 1998 Pediatric Final Rule for 2 years. During the 2 year suspension of the Rule, the FDA planned to study whether the Best Pharmaceuticals for Children Act of 2002 made the 1998 Final Rule unnecessary. After multiple organizations lobbied Congress and the president, the Secretary of Health and Human Services announced in April 2002, that the FDA would continue to defend the Pediatric Final Rule of 1998 in court. However, on October 17, 2002, the US District Court for the District of Columbia barred the FDA from enforcing the Pediatric Final Rule. Fortunately, Congress passed the Pediatric Research Equity Act of 2003 (Public Law S.650, 108th Congress). This law essentially reinstates the Pediatric Final Rule and authorizes the FDA to **require** pharmaceutical manufacturers to conduct pediatric studies of certain drugs and biological products. It also establishes an FDA Pediatric Advisory Committee. The Pediatric Research Equity Act was reauthorized, amended, and signed into law in September 2007, as part of the FDA Amendment Act of 2007.

The Children's Health Act of 2000 was signed into law on October 17, 2000. This important law establishes a Pediatric Research Initiative (headed by the Director of the NIH) and provides funds to increase support for pediatric clinical research.

The Food and Drug Administration Safety and Innovation Act (FDASIA) was signed into law on July 9, 2012.[14] The pediatric provisions of this law renew and strengthen the Best Pharmaceuticals for Children Act and the Pediatric Research Equity Act. FDASIA makes both of these important Acts permanent and thus ensures that pediatric patients will have a permanent place in drug research and development. This new law requires a pediatric study plan to be submitted earlier by drug manufacturers subject to the Pediatric Research Equity Act. It also gives the FDA new authority to help ensure that requirements of the Pediatric Research Equity Act are met in a more timely fashion. These requirements should help increase pediatric drug development and generate pediatric drug information more quickly. FDASIA also addresses several neonatal concerns. It requires the Office of Pediatric Therapeutics to include a member with expertise in a pediatric subgroup that is less likely to be studied under other laws, and specifies that for five years after enactment, this should include an individual with expertise in neonatology. The Act also specifies that an FDA employee with expertise in neonatology should be a member of the Pediatric Review Committee. FDASIA also requires Best Pharmaceuticals for Children Act requests for pediatric drug studies to include a rationale for not including neonatal studies if none are requested. These requirements should help to increase neonatal drug information.

While these important laws, plus other FDA regulations such as the FDA labeling changes[15] that required expanded information in the Pediatric Use section of the package insert for all prescription drugs, will help to increase and disseminate pediatric and neonatal drug information, the practice of off-label prescribing in pediatric patients is a common occurrence. Off-label use is defined by The American Academy of Pediatrics (AAP) as: "The use of a drug that is not included in the package insert (approved labeling) for that drug and the purpose of off-label use is to benefit an individual patient". It is important to note that the term "off-label" does not imply an improper, illegal, contraindicated, or investigational use, nor does it necessarily signify a lack of data or clinical experience.[16] The content included within this handbook serves as a compilation of recommended pediatric and neonatal doses found in the literature, provides relevant clinical information regarding the use of drugs in all pediatric patients (neonates through adolescents), and is intended to assist pediatric health care professionals with evidence-based therapeutic decisions.

New in This Edition

This new edition incorporates additions and revisions in a format that we hope the user will find beneficial. Two **new** fields of information have been added. The Preparation for Administration field provides information regarding the preparation of drug products prior to administration, including dilution, reconstitution, etc. The second field added is Warnings: Additional Pediatric Considerations which provides further details for precautionary considerations that are specific to pediatric and neonatal patients.

As with each edition, hundreds of drug monographs have been updated and revised, including updates to many monographs based on new guideline recommendations. Thirty-one new monographs have been added: Acetic Acid, Propylene Glycol Diacetate, and Hydrocortisone; Amphotericin B Cholesteryl Sulfate Complex; Azacitidine; Azelastine and Fluticasone; Betaxolol (Ophthalmic); Botulism Antitoxin, Heptavalent; Brinzolamide and Brimonidine; Dexchlorpheniramine; Difluprednate; Dimethyl Sulfoxide; Doxylamine; Ecallantide; Eflornithine; Elosulfase Alfa; Ethiodized Oil; Flurandrenolide; Grass Pollen Allergen Extract (5 Grass Extract); Grass Pollen Allergen Extract (Timothy Grass); Papillomavirus (9-Valent) Vaccine (Human, Recombinant); Idursulfase; Levoleucovorin; Meningococcal Group B Vaccine; Oxymetholone; Peramivir; Perampanel; Raxibacumab; Retapamulin; Selenium; Sertaconazole; Tamsulosin; Travoprost. Also in this edition, the Bacitracin monograph was split into three monographs based on the route: Bacitracin (Ophthalmic), Bacitracin (Systemic), Bacitracin (Topical). This brings the total number of drug monographs to 1,017.

Two **new** appendices have been added: Fluoride Varnishes; Insulin Product Comparisons. Seven appendix pieces were revised and updated: Adult and Adolescent HIV; Carbohydrate Content of Medications; *H. pylori* Treatment in Pediatric Patients; Immunization Schedules; Pediatric HIV Treatment Guidelines; Prevention of Chemotherapy-Induced Nausea and Vomiting in Children; Safe Handling of Hazardous Drugs.

We hope this edition continues to be a valuable and practical source of clinical drug information for the pediatric health care professional. We welcome comments to further improve future editions.

References

1. Food and Drug Letter, Washington Business Information, Inc. November 23, 1990.
2. Young L, Lawes F, Tordoff J, Norris P, Reith D. Access to prescribing information for paediatric medicines in the USA: post-modernization. *Br J Clin Pharmacol*. 2009;67(3):341-346.
3. Kumar P, Walker JK, Hurt KM, Bennett KM, Grosshans N, Fotis MA. Medication use in the neonatal intensive care unit: current patterns and off-label use of parenteral medications. *J Pediatr*. 2008;152:412.
4. American Academy of Pediatrics, Committee on Drugs. Off-label use of drugs in children. *Pediatrics*. 2014;133:563-567.
5. Milne CP, Davis J. The pediatric studies initiative: after 15 years have we reached the limits of the law? *Clinical Therapeutics*. 2014:36:156-162.

6. Yang CP, Veltri MA, Anton B, Taster M, Berkowitz ID. Food and Drug Administration approval for medications used in the pediatric intensive care unit: a continuing conundrum. *Pediatr Crit Care Med*. 2011;12:e195-e199.

7. Maltz LA, Klugman D, Spaeder MC, Wessel DL. Off-label drug use in a single-center pediatric cardiac intensive care unit. *World J Pediatr Congenital Heart Surg*. 2013;4:262-266.

8. NIH funds network of centers for pediatric drug research. *Am J Hosp Pharm*. 1994;51:2546.

9. http://www.fda.gov/Drugs/DevelopmentApprovalProcess/DevelopmentResources/ucm049867.htm

10. Birenbaum D. Pediatric initiatives: a regulatory perspective of the US experience. 2002. Available at http://www.fda.gov/cder/pediatric/presentation/Ped_Init_2002_ DB/index.htm

11. Establishment of the Pediatric Review Committee, available at http://www.fda.gov/cder/pediatric/Pediatric_Review_Committee_Establishment%20_Memo.pdf

12. Ref B.S. 1156. The best pharmaceuticals for children amendments of 2007. Available at http://www.washingtonwatch.com/bills/show/110 SN 1156.html

13. "Department of Health and Human Services, Food and Drug Administration, 21CFR Parts 201, 312, 314, and 601, regulations requiring manufacturers to assess the safety and effectiveness of new drugs and biological products in pediatric patients; final rule. *Fed Regist*. 1998;63(231):66631-66672.

14. Food and Drug Administration Safety and Innovation Act (FDASIA), Title V – Pediatric Drugs and Devices, Public Law 112-144, 112th Congress, July 9, 2012. Available at http://www.gpo.gov/fdsys/pkg/PLAW-112publ144/pdf/PLAW-112publ144.pdf

15. "Pediatric use drug labeling NDA supplements due by December 1996 – FDA final rule; agency establishing pediatric subcommittee to track implementation. *F-D-C Reports – The Pink Sheet*. Wallace Werble Jr, Publisher; 1994.

16. American Academy of Pediatrics (AAP). Off-label use of drugs in children. *Pediatrics*. 2014; 33;563-567. Available at http://pediatrics.aappublications.org/content/133/3/563.full.pdf+html

ACKNOWLEDGMENTS

Special acknowledgement goes to all Lexicomp staff for their contributions to this handbook.

The authors wish to thank their families, friends, and colleagues who supported them in their efforts to complete this handbook.

Special thanks goes to Chris Lomax, PharmD, who played a significant role in bringing APhA and Lexicomp together.

In addition, Dr Taketomo would like to thank Robert Taketomo, PharmD, MBA for his professional guidance and continued support, Celeste Ewig, PharmD, BCPS, and the pharmacy staff at Children's Hospital, Los Angeles, for their assistance.

Dr Kraus would like to especially thank Keith A. Rodvold, PharmD, for his ongoing professional and personal support, and the pediatric and neonatal clinical pharmacists at the Children's Hospital University of Illinois for their assistance.

Dr Hodding would like to thank Glenn Hodding, PharmD; Neepa Rai, PharmD; and the pediatric pharmacists at Miller Children's Hospital for their continued professional and personal support.

Some of the material contained in this book was a result of pediatric pharmacy contributors throughout the United States and Canada. Lexicomp has assisted many pediatric medical institutions to develop hospital-specific formulary manuals that contain clinical drug information as well as dosing. Working with these pediatric clinical pharmacists, pediatric hospital pharmacy and therapeutics committees, and hospital drug information centers, Lexicomp has developed an evolutionary drug database that reflects the practice of pediatric pharmacy in these major pediatric institutions.

Special thanks to Jenny Campbell of Campbell and Co. Cartooning, Chagrin Falls, Ohio, who makes our *Pediatric & Neonatal Dosage Handbook* come alive with her wonderful cover illustrations.

NEONATAL EDITORIAL ADVISORY PANEL

DRUG INTERACTIONS EDITORIAL ADVISORY PANEL

Kay Burke, PharmD
Senior Clinical Editor
Wolters Kluwer

Jamie Hoffman, PharmD, BCPS
Senior Clinical Editor
Wolters Kluwer

Carrie Nemerovski, PharmD, BCPS
Pharmacotherapy Specialist
Wolters Kluwer

Steve Sklar, PharmD
Senior Clinical Manager
Wolters Kluwer

Stephen M. Stout, PharmD, MS, BCPS
Pharmacotherapy Specialist
Wolters Kluwer

Dan Streetman, PharmD, MS
Pharmacotherapy Specialist
Wolters Kluwer

David M. Weinstein, PhD, RPh
Senior Director, Clinical Content
Wolters Kluwer

EDITORIAL ADVISORY PANEL

M. Petrea Cober, PharmD, BCNSP
Clinical Pharmacy Coordinator
Neonatal Intensive Care Unit, Children's Hospital of Akron
Assistant Professor of Pharmacy Practice
Northeast Ohio Medical University (NEOMED)

Christine M. Cohn, PharmD, BCPS
Senior Clinical Editor
Wolters Kluwer

Jessica Connell, RN, BSN
Pharmacotherapy Contributor
Tifton, Georgia

Kim Connell, PharmD
Pharmacotherapy Contributor
Thomasville, Georgia

Amanda H. Corbett, PharmD, BCPS, FCCP, AAHIVE
Clinical Assistant Professor
Eshelman School of Pharmacy, University of North Carolina

Susan Cornell, PharmD, CDE, FAPhA, FAADE
Associate Professor
Department of Pharmacy Practice
Assistant Director of Experimental Education
Midwestern University, Chicago College of Pharmacy

Marilyn Cortell, RDH, MS, FAADH
Associate Professor
New York City College of Technology, City University of New York

Harold L. Crossley, DDS, MS, PhD
Professor Emeritus
Baltimore College of Dental Surgery, University of Maryland Baltimore

Melanie W. Cucchi, BS, PharmD, RPh
Clinical Manager
Wolters Kluwer

Laura Cummings, PharmD, BCPS
Pharmacotherapy Specialist
Wolters Kluwer

William J. Dana, PharmD, FASHP
Pharmacy Quality Assurance
Harris County Hospital District

Lacey Davis, PharmD, BCPS
Clinical Pharmacist – Hospice, Palliative Care, and Post-Acute Care
Aultman Hospital

Beth Deen, PharmD, BDNSP
Senior Pediatric Clinical Pharmacy Specialist
Cook Children's Medical Center

Jodi Dreiling, PharmD, BCPS
Pharmacotherapy Specialist in Critical Care
Akron General Medical Center

Kim S. Dufner, PharmD
Clinical Manager
Wolters Kluwer

Teri Dunsworth, PharmD, FCCP, BCPS
Pharmacotherapy Specialist
Wolters Kluwer

Michael S. Edwards, PharmD, MBA, BCOP
Chief, Oncology Pharmacy and *Director, Oncology Pharmacy Residency Program*
Walter Reed Army Medical Center

Vicki L. Ellingrod, PharmD, BCPP
Head, Clinical Pharmacogenomics Laboratory and *Associate Professor*
Department of Psychiatry, Colleges of Pharmacy and Medicine, University of Michigan

Kelley K. Engle, BSPharm
Pharmacotherapy Contributor
Stow, Ohio

Christopher Ensor, PharmD, BCPS (AQ-CV)
Clinical Pharmacy Specialist, Thoracic Transplantation
University of Pittsburgh Medical Center

Erin Fabian, PharmD, RPh, BCPS
Pharmacotherapy Specialist
Wolters Kluwer

Elizabeth A. Farrington, PharmD, FCCP, FCCM, FPPAG, BCPS
Pharmacist III - Pediatrics
New Hanover Regional Medical Center

Margaret A. Fitzgerald, MS, APRN, BC, NP-C, FAANP
President
Fitzgerald Health Education Associates, Inc.
Family Nurse Practitioner
Greater Lawrence Family Health Center

Matthew A. Fuller, PharmD, BCPS, BCPP, FASHP
Clinical Pharmacy Specialist, Psychiatry
Cleveland Department of Veterans Affairs Medical Center
Associate Clinical Professor of Psychiatry and *Clinical Instructor of Psychology*
Case Western Reserve University
Adjunct Associate Professor of Clinical Pharmacy
University of Toledo

Carole W. Fuseck, RN, MSN, VA-BC
Registered Nurse, Vascular Access
Fairview Hospital

Jason C. Gallagher, PharmD, BCPS
Clinical Pharmacy Specialist, Infectious Diseases and *Clinical Associate Professor*
Temple University Hospital

Joyce Generali, RPh, MS, FASHP
Director, Synthesized Referential Content
Wolters Kluwer

Heather L. Girand, PharmD
Professor of Pharmacy, Pediatrics
Pharmacy Practice, Ferris State University College of Pharmacy

Meredith D. Girard, MD, FACP
Medical Staff
Department of Internal Medicine, Summa Health Systems
Assistant Professor Internal Medicine
Northeast Ohio Medical University (NEOMED)

Morton P. Goldman, RPh, PharmD, BCPS, FCCP
Health Care Consultant
American Pharmacotherapy, Inc

Julie A. Golembiewski, PharmD
Clinical Associate Professor and *Clinical Pharmacist, Anesthesia/Pain*
Colleges of Pharmacy and Medicine, University of Illinois

Jeffrey P. Gonzales, PharmD, BCPS
Critical Care Clinical Pharmacy Specialist
University of Maryland Medical Center

Jennifer Fisher Lowe, PharmD, BCOP
Pharmacotherapy Contributor
Zionsville, Indiana

Sherry Luedtke, PharmD
Associate Professor
Department of Pharmacy Practice, Texas Tech University HSC School of Pharmacy

Shannon N. Lukez, RN, MSN, ANP-BC
Adult Nurse Practitioner – Orthopedics
Mountaineer Orthopedic Specialists

Janis MacKichan, PharmD, FAPhA
Professor and Vice Chair
Department of Pharmacy Practice, Northeast Ohio Medical University (NEOMED)

Jason Makii, PharmD, BCPS
Clinical Pharmacy Specialist, Neurosciences Critical Care
University Hospitals Case Medical Center

Melissa Makii, PharmD, BCPS
Clinical Pharmacy Specialist
Pediatric Oncology, Rainbow Babies & Children's Hospital

Vincent F. Mauro, BS, PharmD, FCCP
Professor of Clinical Pharmacy and *Adjunct Professor of Medicine*
Colleges of Pharmacy and Medicine, The University of Toledo

Joseph McGraw, PharmD, MPH, PhD, BCPS
Assistant Professor of Pharmaceutical Science and *Metabolism Laboratory Director*
Concordia University Wisconsin, School of Pharmacy

Ann Marie McMullin, MD
Associate Staff
Emergency Services Institute, Cleveland Clinic

Christopher McPherson, PharmD
Clinical Pharmacy Practice Manager
Neonatal Intensive Care Unit, Brigham and Women's Hospital
Instructor
Department of Pediatric Newborn Medicine, Harvard Medical School

Timothy F. Meiller, DDS, PhD
Professor
Oncology and Diagnostic Sciences, Baltimore College of Dental Surgery
Professor of Oncology
Marlene and Stewart Greenebaum Cancer Center, University of Maryland Medical System

Micheline Meiners, MSc, PhD
Pharmacotherapy Contributor
Lago Norte, Brazil

Cathy A. Meives, PharmD
Senior Clinical Manager
Wolters Kluwer

Megan Menon, PharmD, BCOP
Clinical Pharmacy Specialist
Roswell Park Cancer Institute

Charla E. Miller Nowak, RPh, PharmD
Neonatal Clinical Pharmacy Specialist
Wolfson Children's Hospital

Julie Miller, PharmD
Pharmacy Clinical Specialist, Cardiology
Columbus Children's Hospital

Katherine Mills, PharmD
Pharmacotherapy Contributor
Bristow, Virginia

Stephanie S. Minich, PharmD, BCOP
Pharmacotherapy Specialist
Wolters Kluwer

Kara M. Morris, DDS, MS
Pediatric Dentist
Olentangy Pediatric Dentistry

Kevin M. Mulieri, BS, PharmD
Pediatric Hematology/Oncology Clinical Specialist
Penn State Milton S. Hershey Medical Center
Instructor of Pharmacology
Penn State College of Medicine

Naoto Nakagawa, PharmD, PhD
Chief Pharmacist
Drug Information Center, Japan

Lynne Nakashima, PharmD
Professional Practice Leader, Clinical Professor
B.C. Cancer Agency, Vancouver Centre, University of BC

Carrie Nemerovski, PharmD, BCPS
Pharmacotherapy Specialist
Wolters Kluwer

Elizabeth A. Neuner, PharmD, BCPS
Infectious Diseases Clinical Specialist
Cleveland Clinic

Kimberly Novack, PharmD, BCPS
Clinical Pharmacy Specialist, Cystic Fibrosis and *Pharmacy Clinical Coordinator*
Nationwide Children's Hospital

Carlene N. Oliverio, PharmD, BCPS
Clinical Content Specialist
Wolters Kluwer

Neeta O'Mara, PharmD, BCPS
Clinical Pharmacist
Dialysis Clinic

Tom Palma, MS, RPh
Medical Science Pharmacist
Wolters Kluwer

Susie H. Park, PharmD, BCPP
Assistant Professor of Clinical Pharmacy
University of Southern California

Nicole Passerrello, PharmD, BCPS
Pharmacotherapy Specialist
Wolters Kluwer

Gayle Pearson, BSPharm, MSA
Drug Information Pharmacist
Peter Lougheed Centre, Alberta Health Services

Rebecca Pettit, PharmD, MBA, BCPS
Pediatric Pulmonary Clinical Pharmacy Specialist
Riley Hospital for Children, Indiana University Health, Department of Pharmacy

Jennifer L. Placencia, PharmD
Neonatal Clinical Pharmacy Specialist
Texas Children's Hospital

Geoffrey Wall, RPh, PharmD, FCCP, BCPS, CGP
Professor of Clinical Sciences and *Associate Professor of Pharmacy Practice*
Drake University

Kristin Watson, PharmD, BCPS
Assistant Professor, Cardiology and *Clinical Pharmacist, Cardiology Service*
Heart Failure Clinic, University of Maryland Medical Center

David M. Weinstein, PhD, RPh
Senior Director, Clinical Content
Wolters Kluwer

Sarah White, PharmD, BCPS
Pharmacotherapy Contributor
Medford, Oregon

Greg Wiggers, PharmD, PhD
Pharmacotherapy Specialist
Wolters Kluwer

Sherri J. Willard Argyres, MA, PharmD
Medical Science Pharmacist
Wolters Kluwer

John C. Williamson, PharmD, BCPS
Pharmacy Clinical Coordinator, Infectious Diseases
Wake Forest Baptist Health

Nathan Wirick, PharmD, BCPS
Clinical Specialist in Infectious Diseases and Antibiotic Management
Hillcrest Hospital

Wende Wood, RPh, BSPharm, BCPP
Pharmacotherapy Contributor
Toronto, Ontario, Canada

Richard L. Wynn, BSPharm, PhD
Professor of Pharmacology
Baltimore College of Dental Surgery, University of Maryland

Jessica Zatroch, DDS
Private Practice Dentist
Willoughby Hills, OH

ABOUT THE AUTHORS

Carol K. Taketomo, PharmD

Dr Taketomo received her doctorate from the University of Southern California School of Pharmacy. Subsequently, she completed a clinical pharmacy residency at the University of California Medical Center in San Diego. With over 35 years of clinical experience at one of the largest pediatric teaching hospitals in the nation, she is an acknowledged expert in the practical aspects of pediatric drug distribution and clinical pharmacy practice. She currently holds the appointment of Adjunct Assistant Professor of Pharmacy Practice at the University of Southern California School of Pharmacy.

In her current capacity as Director of Pharmacy and Nutritional Services at Children's Hospital of Los Angeles, Dr Taketomo plays an active role in the education and training of the medical, pharmacy, and nursing staff. She coordinates the Pharmacy Department's performance improvement and medication use evaluation programs, maintains the hospital's strict formulary program, and is the editor of the house staff manual. Her particular interests are strategies to influence physician prescribing patterns, introducing LEAN concepts into clinical practice and transitions of care, and methods to decrease medication errors in the pediatric setting. She has been the author of numerous publications and is an active presenter at professional meetings.

Dr Taketomo is a member of the American Pharmacists Association (APhA), American Society of Health-System Pharmacists (ASHP), California Society of Hospital Pharmacists (CSHP), and Southern California Pediatric Pharmacy Group.

Jane Hurlburt Hodding, PharmD

Dr Hodding earned a doctorate and completed her pharmacy residency at the University of California School of Pharmacy (UCSF) in San Francisco. She has held teaching positions as Assistant Clinical Professor of Pharmacy at UCSF as well as Assistant Clinical Professor of Pharmacy Practice at the University of Southern California in Los Angeles and now holds the position of Assistant Dean at UCSF School of Pharmacy. Currently, Dr Hodding is the Executive Director, Pharmacy and Nutritional Services at Long Beach Memorial and Miller Children's Hospital in Long Beach, California.

Throughout her 37 years of pediatric pharmacy practice, Dr Hodding has actively pursued methods to improve the safety of medication use in neonates, children, and adolescents. She has actively practiced as a clinical pharmacy specialist in neonatal intensive care, pediatric intensive care, and pediatric hematology/oncology. Parenteral nutrition is another area of focus. She has published numerous articles covering neonatal medication administration and aminoglycoside and theophylline clearance in premature infants.

Dr Hodding is a member of the American Pharmacists Association (APhA), American Society of Health-System Pharmacists (ASHP), and California Society of Hospital Pharmacists (CSHP). She is frequently an invited speaker on the topics of Medication Safety in Children, A Multidisciplinary Approach; Monitoring Drug Therapy in the NICU; Fluid and Electrolyte Therapy in Children; Drug Therapy Considerations in Children; and Parenteral Nutrition in the Premature Infant.

Donna M. Kraus, PharmD, FAPhA, FPPAG, FCCP

Dr Kraus received her Bachelor of Science in Pharmacy from the University of Illinois at Chicago (UIC). She worked for several years as a hospital pediatric/obstetric satellite pharmacist before earning her doctorate degree at the UIC. Dr Kraus then completed a postdoctoral pediatric specialty residency at the University of Texas Health Science Center in San Antonio. She served as a pediatric intensive care clinical pharmacist for 15 years and for the past 17 years has been an ambulatory care pediatric clinical pharmacist, specializing in pediatric HIV pharmacotherapy and patient/parent medication adherence. Dr Kraus has also served as a clinical pharmacist consultant to a pediatric long-term care facility for over 21 years. She currently holds the appointment of Associate Professor of Pharmacy Practice in both the Departments of Pharmacy Practice and Pediatrics at the University of Illinois in Chicago.

In her 38 years of active pharmacy experience, Dr Kraus has dealt with pediatric pharmacy issues and pharmacotherapy problems. She is an active educator and has been a guest lecturer in China, Thailand, and Hong Kong. Dr Kraus has played a leading role in the advanced training of postgraduate pharmacists and has been the Director of the UIC (ASHP accredited) Pediatric Residency and Fellowship Program for 28 years. Dr Kraus' research areas include pediatric drug dosing and developmental pharmacokinetics and pharmacodynamics. She has published a number of articles on various issues of pediatric pharmacy and pharmacotherapy.

Dr Kraus has been an active member of numerous professional associations including the American Pharmacists Association (APhA), American Society of Health-System Pharmacists (ASHP), Illinois Pharmacists Association (IPhA), American College of Clinical Pharmacy (ACCP), and Illinois College of Clinical Pharmacy (ICCP). She has served as Chairperson of the ASHP Commission on Therapeutics; member of the Board of Directors of the Pediatric Pharmacy Advocacy Group (PPAG); Member-at-Large of the Academy of Pharmaceutical Research and Science (APhA); member of the ASHP, Commission on Credentialing, Design/Writing Group, Educational Outcomes, Goals and Objectives for Postgraduate Year Two (PGY2) Pediatric Pharmacy Residency Programs (2007); member of the Alliance for Pediatric Quality, Improve First Measures Task Force; and member of the PPAG Advisory Board. Dr Kraus also served as an Editorial Board member of the *American Journal of Health-System Pharmacy* and the *Journal of Pediatric Pharmacy Practice*. Currently, she serves as an Editorial Board member of *The Journal of Pediatric Pharmacology and Therapeutics*. Dr Kraus was recently named by PPAG as the 2013 recipient of the Richard A. Helms Award of Excellence in Pediatric Pharmacy Practice. This award recognizes sustained and meritorious contributions to PPAG and to pediatric pharmacy practice; and contributions of importance to education, new knowledge, and outreach. Dr Kraus has been awarded Fellow status by the American Pharmacists Association, the Pediatric Pharmacy Advocacy Group, and the American College of Clinical Pharmacy. She is the APhA designated author for this handbook.

DESCRIPTIONS OF SECTIONS AND FIELDS USED IN THIS HANDBOOK

The *Pediatric & Neonatal Dosage Handbook, 22nd edition* is organized into a drug information section, an appendix, a therapeutic category & key word index, and an international trade names index.

Drug information is presented in a consistent format and provides the following:

Generic Name	US adopted name. "Tall Man" lettering appears for look-alike generic drug names as recommended by the FDA. See "FDA Differentiation Project: The Use of 'Tall Man' Letters" on page 30.
Pronunciation	Phonetic pronunciation guide
Medication Safety Issues	In an effort to promote the safe use of medications, this field is intended to highlight possible sources of medication errors such as sound-alike/look-alike drugs or highly concentrated formulations which require vigilance on the part of health care professionals. In addition, medications which have been associated with severe consequences in the event of a medication error are also identified in this field.
Related Information	Cross-reference to other pertinent drug information found in the Appendix.
Brand Names: US	Trade names (manufacturer-specific) found in the United States. The symbol [DSC] appears after trade names that have been recently discontinued.
Brand Names: Canada	Trade names found in Canada
Therapeutic Category	Unique systematic classification of medications
Generic Availability (US)	Indicates availability of generic products in the United States
Use	Information pertaining to appropriate indications or use of the drug. Labeled uses will be indicated in parentheses by "FDA-approved in", followed by the specific patient population. "FDA-approved in all ages" denotes ages day 0 through adult. This specific FDA approval information is currently being phased in to all monographs. Age-specific FDA approval may not be present in some monographs; product labeling should be consulted for additional detail. Uses mentioned at the end of the section without "FDA-approved" language are unique off-label pediatric uses.
Prescribing and Access Restrictions	Provides information on any special requirements regarding the prescribing, obtaining, or dispensing of drugs, including access restrictions pertaining to drugs with REMS elements and those drugs with access restrictions that are not REMS-related
Medication Guide Available	Identifies drugs that have an FDA-approved Medication Guide
Pregnancy Risk Factor	Five categories established by the FDA to indicate the potential of a systemically absorbed drug for causing risk to fetus
Pregnancy Considerations	A summary of human and/or animal information pertinent to or associated with the use of the drug as it relates to clinical effects on the fetus, newborn, or pregnant women
Breast-Feeding Considerations	A summary of available information pertinent to or associated with the human use of the drug as it relates to clinical effects on the nursing infant or postpartum woman
Contraindications	Information pertaining to inappropriate use of the drug as dictated by approved labeling
Warnings/Precautions	Precautionary considerations, hazardous conditions related to use of the drug, and disease states or patient populations in which the drug should be cautiously used. Boxed warnings, when present, are clearly identified and are adapted from the FDA-approved labeling. Consult the product labeling for the exact black box warning through the manufacturer's or the FDA website.
Warnings: Additional Pediatric Considerations	Provides further details for precautionary considerations that are specific to pediatric and neonatal patients
Adverse Reactions	Side effects are grouped by body system and include a listing of the more common and/or serious side effects. Due to space limitations, every reported side effect is not listed.
Drug Interactions	
Metabolism/Transport Effects	If a drug has demonstrated involvement with cytochrome P450 enzymes, or other metabolism or transport proteins, this field will identify the drug as an inhibitor, inducer, or substrate of the specific enzyme(s) (eg, CYP1A2 or UGT1A1). CYP450 isoenzymes are identified as substrates (minor or major), inhibitors (weak, moderate, or strong), and inducers (weak or strong).
Avoid Concomitant Use	Designates drug combinations which should not be used concomitantly, due to an unacceptable risk:benefit assessment. Frequently, the concurrent use of the agents is explicitly prohibited or contraindicated by the product labeling
Increased Effect/Toxicity	Drug combinations that result in a increased or toxic therapeutic effect between the drug listed in the monograph and other drugs or drug classes
Decreased Effect	Drug combinations that result in a decreased therapeutic effect between the drug listed in the monograph and other drugs or drug classes
Food Interactions	Possible important interactions between the drug listed in the monograph and food, alcohol, or other beverages
Storage/Stability	Information regarding storage and stability of commercially available products and products that have been reconstituted, diluted or otherwise prepared. Provides the time and conditions for which a solution or mixture will maintain potency.
Mechanism of Action	How the drug works in the body to elicit a response
Pharmacodynamics	Dose-response relationships including onset of action, time of peak action, and duration of action

Pharmacokinetics	Drug movement through the body over time. Pharmacokinetics deals with absorption, distribution, protein binding, metabolism, bioavailability, half-life, time to peak concentration, elimination, and clearance of drugs. Pharmacokinetic parameters help predict drug concentration and dosage requirements. Information is adult data unless noted.
Dosing: Neonatal	The amount of the drug to be typically administered during therapy; may also include dosing information for preterm neonates. Please note that dosages for neonates may be listed by variable parameters: Postnatal age (PNA) (eg, PNA ≤7 days), gestational age (GA), postmenstrual age (PMA), and/or by body weight (eg, 1,200 to 2,000 g or 1.2 to 2 kg). Neonatal-specific dosing adjustment in renal impairment for select drugs will be provided in this field if available. For additional information, consult **Dosing: Usual** field for suggested renal impairment adjustment.
Dosing: Usual	The amount of the drug to be typically given or taken during therapy; may include dosing information for infants, children, adolescents, and adults. Dosing information not from product labeling will have a citation. When both fixed-doses and weight-directed doses (eg, milligram per kilogram [mg/kg]) are listed, the preferred method is the weight-directed. When weight-directed (eg, mg/kg) and maximum doses are provided, use the weight-directed (mg/kg) dose to calculate the milligram dose for the patient, but do **not** exceed the maximum dose listed. Do **not** exceed adult maximum dosage for a given indication unless otherwise noted. If using fixed dosing based upon age, special care and lower doses should be used in children who have a low weight for their age. When ranges of doses are provided, initiate therapy at the lower end of the range and titrate the dose accordingly. For select drugs, the dosage adjustment in renal impairment (dose or interval) is given according to creatinine clearance (CrCl). Since most studies that recommend dosing guidelines in renal dysfunction are conducted in adult patients, CrCl is usually expressed in units of mL/minute. However, in order to extrapolate the adult information to the pediatric population, one must assume that the adults studied were of standard surface area (ie, 1.73 m^2). Therefore, although the value of CrCl listed for dosing adjustment in renal impairment or dosing interval in renal impairment may be expressed in mL/minute, it is assumed to be equal to the same value in mL/minute/1.73 m^2. To calculate the dose in a pediatric patient with renal dysfunction, first calculate the normal dose (ie, the dose for a patient without renal dysfunction), then use the guidelines to adjust the dose. For example, the normal piperacillin dose for a 20 kg child is 200 to 300 mg/kg/day divided every 4 to 6 hours. If one selected 300 mg/kg/day divided every 6 hours, the dose would be 1.5 g every 6 hours in normal renal function. If CrCl was 20 to 40 mL/minute/1.73 m^2, the dose would be 1.5 g every 8 hours and if CrCl was <20 mL/minute/1.73 m^2, the dose would be 1.5 g every 12 hours. Dosing adjustments in renal impairment are adult data, unless otherwise indicated.
Usual Infusion Concentrations: Neonatal	Information describing the usual concentrations of drugs for continuous infusion administration in the neonatal population, as appropriate. Concentrations are derived from the literature, manufacturer recommendation, or organizational recommendations (eg, the Institute for Safe Medication Practices [ISMP]) and are universally established. Institution-specific standard concentrations may differ from those listed.
Usual Infusion Concentrations: Pediatric	Information describing the usual concentrations of drugs for continuous infusion administration in pediatric population, as appropriate. Concentrations are derived from the literature, manufacturer recommendation, or organizational recommendations (eg, the Institute for Safe Medication Practices [ISMP]) and are universally established. Institution-specific standard concentrations may differ from those listed.
Preparation for Administration	Provides information regarding the preparation of drug products prior to administration, including dilution, reconstitution, etc.
Administration	Information regarding the recommended final concentration, and rates of administration of parenteral drugs, or other guidelines and relevant information to properly administer medications.
Vesicant/Extravasation Risk	Indicates whether the drug is considered to be a vesicant and likely to cause significant morbidity if the infusion infiltrates soft tissues.
Monitoring Parameters	Laboratory tests and patient physical parameters that should be monitored for safety and efficacy.
Reference Range	Therapeutic drug concentrations, such as specific target concentrations, timing of serum samples, etc; toxic serum concentrations are listed when appropriate
Test Interactions	Listing of assay interferences when relevant
Additional Information	Other data about the drug are offered when appropriate.
Product Availability	Provides availability information on products that have been approved by the FDA, but are not yet available for use. Estimates for when a product may be available are included, when this information is known. May also provide any unique or critical drug availability issues.
Controlled Substance	Contains controlled substance schedule information as assigned by the United States Drug Enforcement Administration (DEA) or Canadian Controlled Substance Act (CDSA). CDSA information is only provided for drugs available in Canada and not available in the US.
Dosage Forms Considerations	More specific information regarding product concentrations, ingredients, package sizes, amount of doses per container, and other important details pertaining to various formulations of medications
Dosage Forms	Information with regard to form, strength, and availability of the drug in the United States. **Note:** Additional formulation information (eg, excipients, preservatives) is included when available. Please consult labeling for further information.
Extemporaneous Preparations	Directions for preparing liquid formulations from solid drug products. May include stability information and references.

Appendix

The appendix offers a compilation of tables, guidelines, and conversion information which can often be helpful when considering patient care. This section is broken down into various sections for ease of use.

Therapeutic Category & Key Word Index

This index provides a useful listing of an easy-to-use therapeutic classification system. Also listed are controlled substances and preservative free, sugar free, dye free, and alcohol free medications.

International Trade Names Index

Alphabetical listing of international trade names covering over 100 countries.

DEFINITION OF AGE GROUP TERMINOLOGY

Information in this handbook is listed according to specific age or by age group. The following are definitions of age groups and age-related terminologies. These definitions should be used unless otherwise specified in the monograph.

Term	Definition
Gestational age (GA)[1]	The time from conception until birth. More specifically, gestational age is defined as the number of weeks from the first day of the mother's last menstrual period (LMP) until the birth of the baby. Gestational age at birth is assessed by the date of the LMP and by physical and neuromuscular examination (eg, New Ballard Score).
Postnatal age (PNA)[1]	Chronological age since birth
Postmenstrual age (PMA)[1]	Postmenstrual age is calculated as gestational age plus postnatal age (PMA = GA + PNA).
Neonate	A full-term newborn 0 to 28 days postnatal age. Some experts may also apply this terminology to a premature neonate who is >28 days but whose postmenstrual age (PMA) is ≤42 to 46 weeks.
Premature neonate[2]	Neonate born at <37 weeks gestational age
Term neonate[2]	Neonate born at 37 weeks 0 days to 41 weeks 6 days (average ~40 weeks) gestational age
Infant	1 month (>28 days) to 12 months of age
Child/Children	1 to 12 years of age
Adolescent	13 to 18 years of age
Adult	>18 years of age

[1]Engle WA; American Academy of Pediatrics Committee on Fetus and Newborn. Age terminology during the perinatal period. *Pediatrics.* 2004;114 (5):1362-1364.

[2]Fleischman AR, Oinuma M, Clark SL. Rethinking the definition of 'term pregnancy'. *Obstet Gynecol.* 2010;116(1):136-139.

PREGNANCY CATEGORIES

Pregnancy Categories (sometimes referred to as pregnancy risk factors) are a letter system presented under the *Teratogenic Effects* subsection of the product labeling. The system was initiated in 1979. The categories were required to be part of the package insert for prescription drugs that are systemically absorbed. The Food and Drug Administration (FDA) has updated prescribing labeling requirements and as of June 2015, the pregnancy categories will no longer be part of new product labeling. Prescription products which currently have a pregnancy category letter will be phasing this out of their product information.

The categories are defined as follows:

A Adequate and well-controlled studies in pregnant women have not shown that the drug increases the risk of fetal abnormalities.

B Animal reproduction studies show no evidence of impaired fertility or harm to the fetus; however, no adequate and well-controlled studies have been conducted in pregnant women.
or
Animal reproduction studies have shown adverse events; however, studies in pregnant women have not shown that the drug increases the risk of abnormalities.

C Animal reproduction studies have shown an adverse effect on the fetus. There are no adequate and well-controlled studies in humans and the benefits from the use of the drug in pregnant women may be acceptable, despite its potential risks.
or
Animal reproduction studies have not been conducted.

D Based on human data, the drug can cause fetal harm when administered to pregnant women, but the potential benefits from the use of the drug may be acceptable, despite its potential risks.

X Studies in animals or humans have demonstrated fetal abnormalities (or there is positive evidence of fetal risk based on reports and/or marketing experience) and the risk of using the drug in pregnant women clearly outweighs any possible benefit (for example, safer drugs or other forms of therapy are available).

In 2008, the Food and Drug Administration (FDA) proposed new labeling requirements which would eliminate the use of the pregnancy category system and replace it with scientific data and other information specific to the use of the drug in pregnant women. These proposed changes were suggested because the current category system may be misleading. For instance, some practitioners may believe that risk increases from category A to B to C to D to X, which is not the intent. In addition, practitioners may not be aware that some medications are categorized based on animal data, while others are based on human data. The new labeling requirements will contain pregnancy and lactation subsections, each describing a risk summary, clinical considerations, and section for specific data.

For full descriptions of the final rule, refer to the following website: http://www.fda.gov/Drugs/DevelopmentApprovalProcess/DevelopmentResources/Labeling/ucm093307.htm

ABBREVIATIONS, ACRONYMS, AND SYMBOLS

Abbreviations Which May Be Used in This Reference

Abbreviation	Meaning
½NS	0.45% sodium chloride
5-HT	5-hydroxytryptamine
AACT	American Academy of Clinical Toxicology
AAP	American Academy of Pediatrics
AAPC	antibiotic-associated pseudomembranous colitis
ABCB1	ATP-binding cassette sub-family B member 1 (also known as P-gP or MDR1)
ABCC2	ATP-binding cassette sub-family C member 2 (also known as MRP2)
ABCG2	ATP-binding cassette sub-family G member 2 (also known as BCRP)
ABG	arterial blood gases
ABMT	autologous bone marrow transplant
ABW	adjusted body weight
ACC	American College of Cardiology
ACE	angiotensin-converting enzyme
ACLS	advanced cardiac life support
ACOG	American College of Obstetricians and Gynecologists
ACTH	adrenocorticotrophic hormone
ADH	antidiuretic hormone
ADHD	attention-deficit/hyperactivity disorder
ADI	adequate daily intake
ADLs	activities of daily living
AED	antiepileptic drug
AHA	American Heart Association
AHCPR	Agency for Health Care Policy and Research
AIDS	acquired immunodeficiency syndrome
AIMS	Abnormal Involuntary Movement Scale
ALL	acute lymphoblastic leukemia
ALS	amyotrophic lateral sclerosis
ALT	alanine aminotransferase (formerly called SGPT)
AMA	American Medical Association
AML	acute myeloblastic leukemia
ANA	antinuclear antibodies
ANC	absolute neutrophil count
ANLL	acute nonlymphoblastic leukemia
APL	acute promyelocytic leukemia
aPTT	activated partial thromboplastin time
ARB	angiotensin receptor blocker
ARDS	acute respiratory distress syndrome
ASA-PS	American Society of Anesthesiologists – Physical Status P1: Normal, healthy patient P2: Patient having mild systemic disease P3: Patient having severe systemic disease P4: Patient having severe systemic disease which is a constant threat to life P5: Moribund patient; not expected to survive without the procedure P6: Patient declared brain-dead; organs being removed for donor purposes
AST	aspartate aminotransferase (formerly called SGOT)
ATP	adenosine triphosphate
AUC	area under the curve (area under the serum concentration-time curve)
A-V	atrial-ventricular
AVNRT	atrioventricular nodal reentrant tachycardia
AVRT	atrioventricular reentrant tachycardia
BCRP	breast cancer resistance protein
BDI	Beck Depression Inventory
BEC	blood ethanol concentration
BLS	basic life support
BMI	body mass index

Abbreviations Which May Be Used in This Reference *(continued)*

Abbreviation	Meaning
BMT	bone marrow transplant
BP	blood pressure
BPD	bronchopulmonary disease or dysplasia
BPH	benign prostatic hyperplasia
BPRS	Brief Psychiatric Rating Scale
BSA	body surface area
BSEP	bile salt export pump
BUN	blood urea nitrogen
CABG	coronary artery bypass graft
CAD	coronary artery disease
CADD	computer ambulatory drug delivery
cAMP	cyclic adenosine monophosphate
CAN	Canadian
CAPD	continuous ambulatory peritoneal dialysis
CAS	chemical abstract service
CBC	complete blood count
CBT	cognitive behavioral therapy
CDC	Centers for Disease Control and Prevention
CF	cystic fibrosis
CFC	chlorofluorocarbons
CGI	Clinical Global Impression
CHD	coronary heart disease
CHF	congestive heart failure; chronic heart failure
CI	cardiac index
CIE	chemotherapy-induced emesis
C-II	schedule two controlled substance
C-III	schedule three controlled substance
C-IV	schedule four controlled substance
C-V	schedule five controlled substance
CIV	continuous IV infusion
CLL	chronic lymphocytic leukemia
C_{max}	maximum plasma concentration
C_{min}	minimum plasma concentration
CML	chronic myelogenous leukemia
CMV	cytomegalovirus
CNS	central nervous system or coagulase negative staphylococcus
COLD	chronic obstructive lung disease
COMT	Catechol-*O*-methyltransferase
COPD	chronic obstructive pulmonary disease
COX	cyclooxygenase
CPK	creatine phosphokinase
CPR	cardiopulmonary resuscitation
CrCl	creatinine clearance
CRF	chronic renal failure
CRP	C-reactive protein
CRRT	continuous renal replacement therapy
CSF	cerebrospinal fluid
CSII	continuous subcutaneous insulin infusion
CT	computed tomography
CVA	cerebrovascular accident
CVP	central venous pressure
CVVH	continuous venovenous hemofiltration
CVVHD	continuous venovenous hemodialysis
CVVHDF	continuous venovenous hemodiafiltration
CYP	cytochrome
$D_5{}^1/_4NS$	dextrose 5% in sodium chloride 0.2%
$D_5{}^1/_2NS$	dextrose 5% in sodium chloride 0.45%

Abbreviations Which May Be Used in This Reference *(continued)*

Abbreviation	Meaning
D_5LR	dextrose 5% in lactated Ringer's
D_5NS	dextrose 5% in sodium chloride 0.9%
D_5W	dextrose 5% in water
$D_{10}W$	dextrose 10% in water
DBP	diastolic blood pressure
DEHP	di(3-ethylhexyl)phthalate
DIC	disseminated intravascular coagulation
DL_{co}	pulmonary diffusion capacity for carbon monoxide
DM	diabetes mellitus
DMARD	disease modifying antirheumatic drug
DNA	deoxyribonucleic acid
DSC	discontinued
DSM-IV	Diagnostic and Statistical Manual
DVT	deep vein thrombosis
EBV	Epstein-Barr virus
ECG	electrocardiogram
ECHO	echocardiogram
ECMO	extracorporeal membrane oxygenation
ECT	electroconvulsive therapy
ED	emergency department
EEG	electroencephalogram
EF	ejection fraction
EG	ethylene glycol
EGA	estimated gestational age
eGFR	estimated glomerular filtration rate
EIA	enzyme immunoassay
ELBW	extremely low birth weight
ELISA	enzyme-linked immunosorbent assay
EPS	extrapyramidal side effects
ESA	erythropoiesis-stimulating agent
ESR	erythrocyte sedimentation rate
ESRD	end stage renal disease
E.T.	endotracheal
EtOH	alcohol
FDA	Food and Drug Administration (United States)
FEV_1	forced expiratory volume exhaled after 1 second
FMO	Flavin-containing monooxygenase
FSH	follicle-stimulating hormone
FTT	failure to thrive
FVC	forced vital capacity
G-6-PD	glucose-6-phosphate dehydrogenase
GA	gestational age
GABA	gamma-aminobutyric acid
GAD	generalized anxiety disorder
GE	gastroesophageal
GERD	gastroesophageal reflux disease
GFR	glomerular filtration rate
GGT	gamma-glutamyltransferase
GI	gastrointestinal
GIST	gastrointestinal stromal tumor
GU	genitourinary
GVHD	graft versus host disease
HAM-A	Hamilton Anxiety Scale
HAM-D	Hamilton Depression Scale
HARS	HIV-associated adipose redistribution syndrome
HCAHPS	Hospital Consumer Assessment of Healthcare Providers and Systems
HCM	hypertrophic cardiomyopathy

Abbreviations Which May Be Used in This Reference *(continued)*

Abbreviation	Meaning
Hct	hematocrit
HCV	hepatitis C virus
HDL-C	high density lipoprotein cholesterol
HF	heart failure
HFA	hydrofluoroalkane
HFSA	Heart Failure Society of America
Hgb	hemoglobin
HIV	human immunodeficiency virus
HMG-CoA	3-hydroxy-3-methylglutaryl-coenzyme A
HOCM	hypertrophic obstructive cardiomyopathy
HPA	hypothalamic-pituitary-adrenal
HPLC	high performance liquid chromatography
HSV	herpes simplex virus
HTN	hypertension
HUS	hemolytic uremic syndrome
IBD	inflammatory bowel disease
IBS	irritable bowel syndrome
IBW	ideal body weight
ICD	implantable cardioverter defibrillator
ICH	intracranial hemorrhage
ICP	intracranial pressure
IDDM	insulin-dependent diabetes mellitus
IDSA	Infectious Diseases Society of America
IgG	immune globulin G
ILCOR	International Liaison Committee on Resuscitation
IM	intramuscular
INR	international normalized ration
Int. unit	international unit
I.O.	intraosseous
I & O	input and output
IOP	intraocular pressure
IQ	intelligence quotient
ITP	idiopathic thrombocytopenic purpura
IUGR	intrauterine growth retardation
IV	intravenous
IVH	intraventricular hemorrhage
IVP	intravenous push
IVPB	intravenous piggyback
JIA	juvenile idiopathic arthritis
JNC	Joint National Committee
JRA	juvenile rheumatoid arthritis
kg	kilogram
KIU	kallikrein inhibitor unit
KOH	potassium hydroxide
LAMM	L-α-acetyl methadol
LDH	lactate dehydrogenase
LDL-C	low density lipoprotein cholesterol
LE	lupus erythematosus
LFT	liver function test
LGA	large for gestational age
LH	luteinizing hormone
LP	lumbar posture
LR	lactated Ringer's
LV	left ventricular
LVEF	left ventricular ejection fraction
LVH	left ventricular hypertrophy
MAC	*Mycobacterium avium* complex

Abbreviations Which May Be Used in This Reference *(continued)*

Abbreviation	Meaning
MADRS	Montgomery Asbery Depression Rating Scale
MAO	monoamine oxidase
MAOIs	monamine oxidase inhibitors
MAP	mean arterial pressure
MDD	major depressive disorder
MDR1	multidrug resistence protein 1
MDRD	modification of diet in renal disease
MDRSP	multidrug resistant *streptococcus pneumoniae*
MI	myocardial infarction
MMSE	mini mental status examination
MOPP	mustargen (mechlorethamine), Oncovin® (vincristine), procarbazine, and prednisone
M/P	milk to plasma ratio
MPS I	mucopolysaccharidosis I
MRHD	maximum recommended human dose
MRI	magnetic resonance imaging
MRP2	multidrug resistance-associated protein 2
MRSA	methicillin-resistant *Staphylococcus aureus*
MUGA	multiple gated acquisition scan
NAEPP	National Asthma Education and Prevention Program
NAS	neonatal abstinence syndrome
NCI	National Cancer Institute
ND	nasoduodenal
NF	National Formulary
NFD	nephrogenic fibrosing dermopathy
NG	nasogastric
NHL	Non-Hodgkin lymphoma
NIDDM	noninsulin-dependent diabetes mellitus
NIH	National Institute of Health
NIOSH	National Institute for Occupational Safety and Health
NKA	no known allergies
NKDA	no known drug allergies
NMDA	n-methyl-d-aspartate
NMS	neuroleptic malignant syndrome
NNRTI	non-nucleoside reverse transcriptase inhibitor
NRTI	nucleoside reverse transcriptase inhibitor
NS	normal saline (0.9% sodium chloride)
NSAID	nonsteroidal anti-inflammatory drug
NSCLC	non-small cell lung cancer
NSF	nephrogenic systemic fibrosis
NSTEMI	Non-ST-elevation myocardial infarction
NYHA	New York Heart Association
OA	osteoarthritis
OAT	Organic anion transporter
OCD	obsessive-compulsive disorder
OCT	Organic cation transporter
OHSS	ovarian hyperstimulation syndrome
O.R.	operating room
OTC	over-the-counter (nonprescription)
PABA	para-aminobenzoic acid
PACTG	Pediatric AIDS Clinical Trials Group
PALS	pediatric advanced life support
PAT	paroxysmal atrial tachycardia
PCA	patient-controlled analgesia
PCI	percutaneous coronary intervention
PCP	*Pneumocystis jiroveci* pneumonia (also called *Pneumocystis carinii* pneumonia)
PCWP	pulmonary capillary wedge pressure
PD	Parkinson's disease; peritoneal dialysis

Abbreviations Which May Be Used in This Reference *(continued)*

Abbreviation	Meaning
PDA	patent ductus arteriosus
PDE-5	phosphodiesterase-5
PE	pulmonary embolism
PEG tube	percutaneous endoscopic gastrostomy tube
P-gP	P-glycoprotein
PHN	post-herpetic neuralgia
PICU	Pediatric Intensive Care Unit
PID	pelvic inflammatory disease
PIP	peak inspiratory pressure
PMA	postmenstrual age
PMDD	premenstrual dysphoric disorder
PNA	postnatal age
PONV	postoperative nausea and vomiting
PPHN	persistent pulmonary hypertension of the neonate
PPN	peripheral parenteral nutrition
PROM	premature rupture of membranes
PSVT	paroxysmal supraventricular tachycardia
PT	prothrombin time
PTH	parathyroid hormone
PTSD	post-traumatic stress disorder
PTT	partial thromboplastin time
PUD	peptic ulcer disease
PVC	premature ventricular contraction
PVD	peripheral vascular disease
PVR	peripheral vascular resistance
QTc	corrected QT interval
QTcF	corrected QT interval by Fridericia's formula
RA	rheumatoid arthritis
RAP	right arterial pressure
RDA	recommended daily allowance
REM	rapid eye movement
REMS	risk evaluation and mitigation strategies
RIA	radioimmunoassay
RNA	ribonucleic acid
RPLS	reversible posterior leukoencephalopathy syndrome
RSV	respiratory syncytial virus
SA	sinoatrial
SAD	seasonal affective disorder
SAH	subarachnoid hemorrhage
SBE	subacute bacterial endocarditis
SBP	systolic blood pressure
SCLC	small cell lung cancer
S_{cr}	serum creatinine
SERM	selective estrogen receptor modulator
SGA	small for gestational age
SGOT	serum glutamic oxaloacetic aminotransferase
SGPT	serum glutamic pyruvate transaminase
SI	International System of Units or Systeme international d'Unites
SIADH	syndrome of inappropriate antidiuretic hormone secretion
SIDS	sudden infant death syndrome
SLCO1B1	Solute carrier organic anion transporter family member 1B1
SLE	systemic lupus erythematosus
SLEDD	sustained low-efficiency daily diafiltration
SNRI	serotonin norepinephrine reuptake inhibitor
SSKI	saturated solution of potassium iodide
SSRIs	selective serotonin reuptake inhibitors
STD	sexually transmitted disease

Abbreviations Which May Be Used in This Reference *(continued)*

Abbreviation	Meaning
STEM I	ST-elevation myocardial infarction
SVR	systemic vascular resistance
SVT	supraventricular tachycardia
SWFI	sterile water for injection
SWI	sterile water for injection
$T_{1/2}$	half-life
T_3	triiodothyronine
T_4	thyroxine
TB	tuberculosis
TC	total cholesterol
TCA	tricyclic antidepressant
TD	tardive dyskinesia
TG	triglyceride
TIA	transient ischemic attack
TIBC	total iron binding capacity
TMA	thrombotic microangiopathy
T_{max}	time to maximum observed concentration, plasma
TNF	tumor necrosis factor
TPN	total parenteral nutrition
TSH	thyroid stimulating hormone
TT	thrombin time
TTP	thrombotic thrombocytopenic purpura
UA	urine analysis
UC	ulcerative colitis
UGT	UDP-glucuronosyltransferase
ULN	upper limits of normal
URI	upper respiratory infection
USAN	United States Adopted Names
USP	United States Pharmacopeia
UTI	urinary tract infection
UV	ultraviolet
V_d	volume of distribution
V_{dss}	volume of distribution at steady-state
VEGF	vascular endothelial growth factor
VF	ventricular fibrillation
VLBW	very low birth weight
VMA	vanillylmandelic acid
VT	ventricular tachycardia
VTE	venous thromboembolism
vWD	von Willebrand disease
VZV	varicella zoster virus
WHO	World Health Organization
w/v	weight for volume
w/w	weight for weight
YBOC	Yale Brown Obsessive-Compulsive Scale
YMRS	Young Mania Rating Scale

Common Weights, Measures, or Apothecary Abbreviations

Abbreviation	Meaning
<[1]	less than
>[1]	greater than
≤	less than or equal to
≥	greater than or equal to
ac	before meals or food
ad	to, up to

Common Weights, Measures, or Apothecary Abbreviations *(continued)*

Abbreviation	Meaning
ad lib	at pleasure
AM	morning
AMA	against medical advice
amp	ampul
amt	amount
aq	water
aq. dest.	distilled water
ASAP	as soon as possible
a.u.[1]	each ear
bid	twice daily
bm	bowel movement
C	Celsius, centigrade
cal	calorie
cap	capsule
cc[1]	cubic centimeter
cm	centimeter
comp	compound
cont	continue
d	day
d/c[1]	discharge
dil	dilute
disp	dispense
div	divide
dtd	give of such a dose
Dx	diagnosis
elix, el	elixir
emp	as directed
et	and
ex aq	in water
F	Fahrenheit
g	gram
gr	grain
gtt	a drop
h	hour
hs[1]	at bedtime
kcal	kilocalorie
kg	kilogram
L	liter
liq	a liquor, solution
M	molar
mcg	microgram
m. dict	as directed
mEq	milliequivalent
mg	milligram
microL	microliter
min	minute
mL	milliliter
mm	millimeter
mM	millimole
mm Hg	millimeters of mercury
mo	month
mOsm	milliosmoles
ng	nanogram
nmol	nanomole
no.	number
noc	in the night
non rep	do not repeat, no refills

Common Weights, Measures, or Apothecary Abbreviations *(continued)*

Abbreviation	Meaning
NPO	nothing by mouth
NV	nausea and vomiting
O, Oct	a pint
o.d.[1]	right eye
o.l.	left eye
o.s.[1]	left eye
o.u.[1]	each eye
pc, post cib	after meals
PM	afternoon or evening
PO	by mouth
P.R.	rectally
prn	as needed
pulv	a powder
q	every
qad	every other day
qh	every hour
qid	four times a day
qs	a sufficient quantity
qs ad	a sufficient quantity to make
Rx	take, a recipe
S.L.	sublingual
stat	at once, immediately
SubQ	subcutaneous
supp	suppository
syr	syrup
tab	tablet
tal	such
tid	three times a day
tr, tinct	tincture
trit	triturate
tsp	teaspoon
u.d.	as directed
ung	ointment
v.o.	verbal order
w.a.	while awake
x3	3 times
x4	4 times
y	year

[1]ISMP error-prone abbreviation

Additional abbreviations used and defined within a specific monograph or text piece may only apply to that text.

REFERENCES

The Institute for Safe Medication Practices (ISMP) list of Error-Prone Abbreviations, Symbols, and Dose Designations. Available at http://www.ismp.org/Tools/errorproneabbreviations.pdf

PREVENTING PRESCRIBING ERRORS

Prescribing errors account for the majority of reported medication errors and have prompted health care professionals to focus on the development of steps to make the prescribing process safer. Prescription legibility has been attributed to a portion of these errors and legislation has been enacted in several states to address prescription legibility. However, eliminating handwritten prescriptions and ordering medications through the use of technology [eg, computerized prescriber order entry (CPOE)] has been the primary recommendation. Whether a prescription is electronic, typed, or hand-printed, additional safe practices should be considered for implementation to maximize the safety of the prescribing process. Listed below are suggestions for safer prescribing:

- Ensure correct patient by using at least 2 patient identifiers on the prescription (eg, full name, birth date, or address). Review prescription with the patient or patient's caregiver.
- If pediatric patient, document patient's birth date or age and most recent weight. If geriatric patient, document patient's birth date or age.
- Prevent drug name confusion: For more information, see http://www.ismp.org/tools/confuseddrugnames.pdf.
  - Use TALLman lettering (eg, buPROPion, busPIRone, predniSONE, prednisoLONE). For more information, see http://www.fda.gov/drugs/drugsafety/medicationerrors/default.htm.
  - Avoid abbreviated drug names (eg, MSO_4, $MgSO_4$, MS, HCT, 6MP, MTX), as they may be misinterpreted and cause error.
  - Avoid investigational names for drugs with FDA approval (eg, FK-506, CBDCA).
  - Avoid chemical names such as 6-mercaptopurine or 6-thioguanine, as sixfold overdoses have been given when these were not recognized as chemical names. The proper names of these drugs are mercaptopurine or thioguanine.
  - Use care when prescribing drugs that look or sound similar (eg, look- alike, sound-alike drugs). Common examples include: Celebrex vs Celexa, hydroxyzine vs hydralazine, Zyprexa vs Zyrtec.
- Avoid dangerous, error-prone abbreviations (eg, regardless of letter-case: U, IU, QD, QOD, µg, cc, @). Do not use apothecary system or symbols. Additionally, text messaging abbreviations (eg, "2Day") should never be used.
  - For more information, see http://www.ismp.org/tools/errorproneabbreviations.pdf.
- Always use a leading zero for numbers <1 (0.5 mg is correct and .5 mg is **incorrect**) and never use a trailing zero for whole numbers (2 mg is correct and 2.0 mg is **incorrect**).
- Always use a space between a number and its units as it is easier to read. There should be no periods after the abbreviations mg or mL (10 mg is correct and 10mg is **incorrect**).
- For doses that are ≥1,000 dosing units, use properly placed commas to prevent 10-fold errors (100,000 units is correct and 100000 units is **incorrect**).
- Do not prescribe drug dosage by the type of container in which the drug is available (eg, do not prescribe "1 amp", "2 vials", etc).
- Do not write vague or ambiguous orders which have the potential for misinterpretation by other health care providers. Examples of vague orders to avoid: "Resume pre-op medications," "give drug per protocol," or "continue home medications."
- Review each prescription with patient (or patient's caregiver) including the medication name, indication, and directions for use.
- Take extra precautions when prescribing *high alert drugs* (drugs that can cause significant patient harm when prescribed in error). Common examples of these drugs include: Anticoagulants, chemotherapy, insulins, opioids, and sedatives.
  - For more information, see http://www.ismp.org/tools/institutionalhighalert.asp or http://www.ismp.org/communityRx/tools/ambulatoryhighalert.asp.

To Err Is Human: Building a Safer Health System, Kohn LT, Corrigan JM, Donaldson MS, eds. Washington, D.C.: National Academy Press. 2000.

A Complete Outpatient Prescription[1]

A complete outpatient prescription can prevent the prescriber, the pharmacist, and/or the patient from making a mistake and can eliminate the need for further clarification. The complete outpatient prescription should contain:

- Patient's full name
- Medication indication
- Allergies
- Prescriber name and telephone or pager number
- For pediatric patients: Their birth date or age and current weight
- For geriatric patients: Their birth date or age
- Drug name, dosage form and strength

- For pediatric patients: Intended daily weight-based dose so that calculations can be checked by the pharmacist (ie, mg/kg/day or units/kg/day)
- Number or amount to be dispensed
- Complete instructions for the patient or caregiver, including the purpose of the medication, directions for use (including dose), dosing frequency, route of administration, duration of therapy, and number of refills.
- Dose should be expressed in convenient units of measure.
- When there are recognized contraindications for a prescribed drug, the prescriber should indicate knowledge of this fact to the pharmacist (ie, when prescribing a potassium salt for a patient receiving an ACE inhibitor, the prescriber should write "K serum leveling being monitored").

Upon dispensing of the final product, the pharmacist should ensure that the patient or caregiver can effectively demonstrate the appropriate administration technique. An appropriate measuring device should be provided or recommended. Household teaspoons and tablespoons should not be used to measure liquid medications due to their variability and inaccuracies in measurement; oral medication syringes are recommended.

For additional information, see http://www.ismp.org/Newsletters/acutecare/articles/20020601.asp
[1]Levine SR, Cohen MR, Blanchard NR, et al. Guidelines for preventing medication errors in pediatrics. *J Pediatr Pharmacol Ther.* 2001;6:426-442.

FDA NAME DIFFERENTIATION PROJECT: THE USE OF "TALL MAN" LETTERS

Confusion between similar drug names is an important cause of medication errors. For years, The Institute For Safe Medication Practices (ISMP), has urged generic manufacturers to use a combination of large and small letters as well as bolding (ie, chlorpro**MAZINE** and chlorpro**PAMIDE**) to help distinguish drugs with look-alike names, especially when they share similar strengths. Recently the FDA's Division of Generic Drugs began to issue recommendation letters to manufacturers suggesting this novel way to label their products to help reduce this drug name confusion. Although this project has had marginal success, the method has successfully eliminated problems with products such as diphenhydr**AMINE** and dimenhy**DRINATE**. Hospitals should also follow suit by making similar changes in their own labels, preprinted order forms, computer screens and printouts, and drug storage location labels.

Lexi-Comp, Inc. Medical Publishing will use "Tall-Man" letters for the drugs suggested by the FDA or recommended by ISMP.

The following is a list of generic and brand name product names and recommended revisions.

Drug Product	Recommended Revision
acetazolamide	aceta**ZOLAMIDE**
alprazolam	**ALPRAZ**olam
amiloride	a**MIL**oride
amlodipine	am**LODIP**ine
aripiprazole	**ARIP**iprazole
atomoxetine	ato**MOX**etine
atorvastatin	atorva**STAT**in
Avinza	**AVIN**za
azacitidine	aza**CITID**ine
azathioprine	aza**THIO**prine
bupropion	bu**PROP**ion
buspirone	bus**PIR**one
carbamazepine	car**BAM**azepine
carboplatin	**CARBO**platin
cefazolin	ce**FAZ**olin
cefotetan	cefo**TE**tan
cefoxitin	cef**OX**itin
ceftazidime	cef**TAZ**idime
ceftriaxone	cef**TRIAX**one
Celebrex	Cele**BREX**
Celexa	Cele**XA**
chlordiazepoxide	chlordiaze**POXIDE**
chlorpromazine	chlorpro**MAZINE**
chlorpropamide	chlorpro**PAMIDE**
cisplatin	**CIS**platin
clobazam	clo**BAZ**am
clomiphene	clomi**PHENE**
clomipramine	clomi**PRAMINE**
clonazepam	clonaze**PAM**
clonidine	clo**NID**ine
clozapine	clo**ZAP**ine
cycloserine	cyclo**SERINE**
cyclosporine	cyclo**SPORINE**
dactinomycin	**DACTIN**omycin
daptomycin	**DAPTO**mycin
daunorubicin	**DAUNO**rubicin
dimenhydrinate	dimenhy**DRINATE**
diphenhydramine	diphenhydr**AMINE**
dobutamine	**DOBUT**amine
docetaxel	**DOCE**taxel
dopamine	**DOP**amine
doxorubicin	**DOXO**rubicin
duloxetine	**DUL**oxetine

Drug Product	Recommended Revision
ephedrine	e**PHED**rine
epinephrine	**EPINEPH**rine
epirubicin	**EPI**rubicin
eribulin	eri**BUL**in
fentanyl	fenta**NYL**
flavoxate	flavox**ATE**
fluoxetine	**FLU**oxetine
fluphenazine	flu**PHENAZ**ine
fluvoxamine	fluvoxa**MINE**
glipizide	glipi**ZIDE**
glyburide	gly**BURIDE**
guaifenesin	guai**FEN**esin
guanfacine	guan**FACINE**
Humalog	Huma**LOG**
Humulin	Humu**LIN**
hydralazine	hydr**ALAZINE**
hydrocodone	**HYDRO**codone
hydromorphone	**HYDRO**morphone
hydroxyzine	hydr**OXY**zine
idarubicin	**IDA**rubicin
infliximab	in**FLIX**imab
Invanz	**INV**anz
isotretinoin	**ISO**tretinoin
Klonopin	Klono**PIN**
Lamictal	La**MIC**tal
Lamisil	Lam**ISIL**
lamivudine	lami**VUD**ine
lamotrigine	lamo**TRI**gine
levetiracetam	Lev**ETIRA**cetam
levocarnitine	lev**OCARN**itine
lorazepam	**LOR**azepam
medroxyprogesterone	medroxy**PROGESTER**one
metformin	met**FORMIN**
methylprednisolone	methyl**PREDNIS**olone
methyltestosterone	methyl**TESTOSTER**one
metronidazole	metro**NIDAZOLE**
mitomycin	mito**MY**cin
mitoxantrone	Mito**XAN**trone
Nexavar	Nex**AVAR**
Nexium	Nex**IUM**
nicardipine	ni**CAR**dipine
nifedipine	**NIFE**dipine
nimodipine	ni**MOD**ipine
Novolin	Novo**LIN**
Novolog	Novo**LOG**
olanzapine	**OLANZ**apine
oxcarbazepine	**OX**carbazepine
oxycodone	oxy**CODONE**
Oxycontin	Oxy**CONTIN**
paclitaxel	**PACL**itaxel
paroxetine	**PAR**oxetine
pazopanib	**PAZOP**anib
pemetrexed	**PEME**trexed
penicillamine	penicill**AMINE**
pentobarbital	**PENT**obarbital
phenobarbital	**PHEN**obarbital
ponatinib	**PONAT**inib
pralatrexate	**PRALA**trexate

Drug Product	Recommended Revision
prednisolone	predniso**LONE**
prednisone	predni**SONE**
Prilosec	Pri**LOSEC**
Prozac	**PRO**zac
quetiapine	**QUE**tiapine
quinidine	qui**NID**ine
quinine	qui**NINE**
rabeprazole	**RABE**prazole
Risperdal	Risper**DAL**
risperidone	risperi**DONE**
rituximab	ri**TUX**imab
romidepsin	romi**DEP**sin
romiplostim	romi**PLOS**tim
ropinirole	r**OPINIR**ole
Sandimmune	sand**IMMUNE**
Sandostatin	Sando**STATIN**
Seroquel	**SERO**quel
Sinequan	**SINE**quan
sitagliptin	sita**GLIP**tin
Solu-Cortef	Solu-**CORTEF**
Solu-Medrol	Solu-**MEDROL**
sorafenib	**SORA**fenib
sufentanil	**SUF**entanil
sulfadiazine	sulf**ADIAZINE**
sulfasalazine	sulfa**SALA**zine
sumatriptan	**SUMA**triptan
sunitinib	**SUNI**tinib
Tegretol	**TEG**retol
tiagabine	tia**GAB**ine
tizanidine	ti**ZAN**idine
tolazamide	**TOLAZ**amide
tolbutamide	**TOLBUT**amide
tramadol	tra**MAD**ol
trazodone	tra**ZOD**one
Trental	**TREN**tal
valacyclovir	val**ACY**clovir
valganciclovir	val**GAN**ciclovir
vinblastine	vin**BLAS**tine
vincristine	vin**CRIS**tine
zolmitriptan	**ZOLM**itriptan
Zyprexa	Zy**PREXA**
Zyrtec	Zyr**TEC**

FDA and ISMP lists of look-alike drug names with recommended tall man letter. http://www.ismp.org/tools/tallmanletters.pdf. Accessed January 6, 2011.
Name differentiation project. http://www.fda.gov/Drugs/DrugSafety/MedicationErrors/ucm164587.htm. Accessed January 6, 2011.
U.S. Pharmacopeia. USP quality review: use caution – avoid confusion. March 2001, No. 76. http://www.usp.org

ALPHABETICAL LISTING OF DRUGS

◆ **A-25 [OTC]** *see* Vitamin A *on page 2186*

Abacavir (a BAK a veer)

Medication Safety Issues

High alert medication:

This medication is in a class the Institute for Safe Medication Practices (ISMP) includes among its list of drug classes that have a heightened risk of causing significant patient harm when used in error.

Related Information

Adult and Adolescent HIV *on page 2392*
Pediatric HIV *on page 2380*
Perinatal HIV *on page 2400*
Safe Handling of Hazardous Drugs *on page 2455*

Brand Names: US Ziagen

Brand Names: Canada Ziagen

Therapeutic Category Antiretroviral Agent; HIV Agents (Anti-HIV Agents); Nucleoside Reverse Transcriptase Inhibitor (NRTI)

Generic Availability (US) May be product dependent

Use Treatment of HIV-1 infection in combination with other antiretroviral agents (FDA approved in ages ≥3 months and adults); **Note:** HIV regimens consisting of **three** antiretroviral agents are strongly recommended.

Medication Guide Available Yes

Pregnancy Considerations Abacavir has a high level of transfer across the human placenta. No increased risk of overall birth defects has been observed following first trimester exposure according to data collected by the antiretroviral pregnancy registry. Cases of lactic acidosis/ hepatic steatosis syndrome related to mitochondrial toxicity have been reported in pregnant women with prolonged use of nucleoside analogues. It is not known if pregnancy itself potentiates this known side effect; however, women may be at increased risk of lactic acidosis and liver damage. In addition, these adverse events are similar to other rare but life-threatening syndromes which occur during pregnancy (eg, HELLP syndrome). Hepatic enzymes and electrolytes should be monitored in women receiving nucleoside analogues and clinicians should watch for early signs of the syndrome. In addition, mitochondrial dysfunction may develop in infants following in utero exposure. The pharmacokinetics of abacavir are not significantly changed by pregnancy and dose adjustment is not needed for pregnant women. The DHHS Perinatal HIV Guidelines consider abacavir in combination with lamivudine to be a preferred NRTI backbone for use in antiretroviral-naive pregnant women.

Regardless of CD4 count or HIV RNA copy number, all HIV-infected pregnant women should receive a combination antiretroviral (ARV) drug regimen. A combination of antepartum, intrapartum, and infant ARV prophylaxis is recommended. ARV therapy should be started as soon as possible in women with symptomatic infection. Although earlier initiation may be more effective in reducing the perinatal transmission of HIV, initiation may be delayed until after 12 weeks gestation in women who do not require immediate treatment after careful consideration of maternal conditions (eg, nausea and vomiting) and the potential risks of first trimester fetal exposure for specific agents. A scheduled cesarean delivery at 38 weeks gestation is recommended for all women with HIV RNA >1000 copies/mL or unknown concentrations near delivery in order to decrease transmission. If ARV therapy must be interrupted for <24 hours during the peripartum period, stop then restart all medications simultaneously in order to decrease the chance of developing resistance. Long-term follow-up is recommended for all infants exposed to ARV medications. In couples who want to conceive, the HIV-infected partner should attain maximum viral suppression prior to conception.

Healthcare providers are encouraged to enroll pregnant women exposed to antiretroviral medications in the Antiretroviral Pregnancy Registry (1-800-258-4263 or www.-APRegistry.com). Healthcare providers caring for HIV-infected women and their infants may contact the National Perinatal HIV Hotline (888-448-8765) for clinical consultation (HHS [perinatal] 2014).

Breast-Feeding Considerations Abacavir is excreted into breast milk. Maternal or infant antiretroviral therapy does not completely eliminate the risk of postnatal HIV transmission. In addition, multiclass-resistant virus has been detected in breast-feeding infants despite maternal therapy. Therefore, in the United States, where formula is accessible, affordable, safe, and sustainable, and the risk of infant mortality due to diarrhea and respiratory infections is low, complete avoidance of breast-feeding by HIV-infected women is recommended to decrease potential transmission of HIV (HHS [perinatal] 2014).

Contraindications Hypersensitivity to abacavir or any component of the formulation (do not rechallenge patients who have experienced hypersensitivity to abacavir regardless of *HLA-B*5701* status); moderate-to-severe hepatic impairment

Warnings/Precautions Hazardous agent; use appropriate precautions for handling and disposal (NIOSH 2014 [group 2]).

Abacavir should always be used as a component of a multidrug regimen; concomitant use with other abacavir-containing products is not recommended. Do not use abacavir/lamivudine (plus efavirenz or plus atazanavir/ ritonavir) in adolescent and adult HIV-1 patients with a pre-ART HIV RNA >100,000 copies/mL (HHS [adult] 2015). **[US Boxed Warning]: Serious and sometimes fatal hypersensitivity reactions have occurred.** Patients testing positive for the presence of the *HLA-B*5701* allele are at an increased risk for hypersensitivity reactions. Screening for *HLA-B*5701* allele status is recommended prior to initiating therapy or reinitiating therapy in patients of unknown status, including patients who previously tolerated therapy. Therapy is **not** recommended in patients testing positive for the *HLA-B*5701* allele. An allergy to abacavir should be documented in their medical record (HHS [adult] 2015). Reactions usually occur within 9 days of starting abacavir; ~90% occur within 6 weeks. Patients exhibiting symptoms from two or more of the following: Fever, skin rash, constitutional symptoms (malaise, fatigue, aches), respiratory symptoms (eg, pharyngitis, dyspnea, cough), and GI symptoms (eg, abdominal pain, diarrhea, nausea, vomiting) should discontinue therapy immediately and call for medical attention. Abacavir should be permanently discontinued if hypersensitivity cannot be ruled out, even when other diagnoses are possible and regardless of *HLA-B*5701* status. Abacavir SHOULD NOT be restarted because more severe symptoms may occur within hours, including LIFE-THREATENING HYPOTENSION AND DEATH. Fatal hypersensitivity reactions have occurred following the reintroduction of abacavir in patients whose therapy was interrupted (ie, interruption in drug supply, temporary discontinuation while treating other conditions). In some cases, signs of hypersensitivity may have been previously present, but attributed to other medical conditions (eg, acute onset respiratory diseases, gastroenteritis, reactions to other medications). If abacavir is restarted following an interruption in therapy, evaluate the patient for previously unsuspected symptoms of hypersensitivity. A higher incidence of severe hypersensitivity reactions may be associated with a 600 mg once daily dosing regimen.

[US Boxed Warning]: Lactic acidosis and severe hepatomegaly with steatosis (sometimes fatal) have occurred with antiretroviral nucleoside analogues. Female gender, prior liver disease, obesity, and prolonged treatment may increase the risk of hepatotoxicity. May be associated with fat redistribution. Immune reconstitution syndrome may develop, resulting in the occurrence of an inflammatory response to an indolent or residual opportunistic infection during initial HIV treatment or activation of autoimmune disorders (eg, Graves disease, polymyositis, Guillain-Barré syndrome) later in therapy; further evaluation and treatment may be required. Use with caution and adjust dosage in patients with mild hepatic dysfunction (contraindicated in moderate to severe dysfunction).

Use has been associated with an increased risk of myocardial infarction (MI) in observational studies; however, based on a meta-analysis of 26 randomized trials, the FDA has concluded there is not an increased risk. Consider using with caution in patients with risks for coronary heart disease and minimizing modifiable risk factors (eg, hypertension, hyperlipidemia, diabetes mellitus, and smoking) prior to use. Potentially significant interactions may exist, requiring dose or frequency adjustment, additional monitoring, and/or selection of alternative therapy. Some dosage forms may contain propylene glycol; large amounts are potentially toxic and have been associated with hyperosmolality, lactic acidosis, seizures and respiratory depression; use caution (AAP 1997; Zar 2007).

Warnings: Additional Pediatric Considerations May cause mild hyperglycemia; more common in pediatric patients. Some dosage forms may contain propylene glycol; in neonates large amounts of propylene glycol delivered orally, intravenously (eg, >3,000 mg/day), or topically have been associated with potentially fatal toxicities which can include metabolic acidosis, seizures, renal failure, and CNS depression; toxicities have also been reported in children and adults including hyperosmolality, lactic acidosis, seizures and respiratory depression; use caution (AAP, 1997; Shehab, 2009).

Adverse Reactions Hypersensitivity reactions (which may be fatal) occur in ~5% of patients. Symptoms may include abdominal pain, anaphylaxis, arthralgia, conjunctivitis, diarrhea, edema, fatigue, fever, headache, hepatic failure, lethargy, lymphadenopathy, malaise, mouth ulcerations, myalgia, myolysis, nausea, paresthesia, rash (including erythema multiforme), renal failure, respiratory symptoms (eg, adult respiratory distress syndrome, cough, dyspnea, pharyngitis, respiratory failure), vomiting.

Note: Rates of adverse reactions were defined during combination therapy with other antiretrovirals (lamivudine and efavirenz **or** lamivudine and zidovudine). Only reactions which occurred at a higher frequency in adults (except where noted) than in the comparator group are noted. Adverse reaction rates attributable to abacavir alone are not available.

Central nervous system: Abnormal dreams, anxiety, depression, dizziness, fatigue, fever/chills, headache, malaise

Dermatologic: Rash

Gastrointestinal: Abdominal pain, diarrhea, nausea, vomiting

Hematologic: Thrombocytopenia

Hepatic: AST increased

Neuromuscular & skeletal: Musculoskeletal pain

Miscellaneous: Hypersensitivity reactions, infection

Rare but important or life-threatening: Erythema multiforme, hepatotoxicity, immune reconstitution syndrome, lactic acidosis, MI, pancreatitis, Stevens-Johnson syndrome, toxic epidermal necrolysis

Drug Interactions

Metabolism/Transport Effects None known.

Avoid Concomitant Use There are no known interactions where it is recommended to avoid concomitant use.

Increased Effect/Toxicity

The levels/effects of Abacavir may be increased by: Ganciclovir-Valganciclovir; Ribavirin

Decreased Effect

Abacavir may decrease the levels/effects of: Methadone

The levels/effects of Abacavir may be decreased by: Methadone; Protease Inhibitors

Food Interactions Ethanol decreases the elimination of abacavir and may increase the risk of toxicity. Management: Monitor patients.

Storage/Stability Store at 20°C to 25°C (68°F to 77°F). Oral solution may be refrigerated; do not freeze.

Mechanism of Action Nucleoside reverse transcriptase inhibitor. Abacavir is a guanosine analogue which is phosphorylated to carbovir triphosphate which interferes with HIV viral RNA-dependent DNA polymerase resulting in inhibition of viral replication.

Pharmacokinetics (Adult data unless noted)

Absorption: Rapid and extensive

Distribution: Apparent V_d: 0.86 ± 0.15 L/kg

CSF to plasma AUC ratio: 27% to 33%

Protein binding: 50%

Metabolism: Hepatic via alcohol dehydrogenase and glucuronyl transferase to inactive carboxylate and glucuronide metabolites; not significantly metabolized by cytochrome P450 enzymes; intracellulary metabolized to carbovir triphosphate (active metabolite)

Bioavailability: Tablet: 83%; solution and tablet provide comparable AUCs

Half-life, elimination (serum):

Pediatric patients ≥3 months to ≤13 years: 1 to 1.5 hours (Hughes 1999; Kline 1999)

Adults: 1.54 ± 0.63 hours

Hepatic impairment (mild): Increases half-life by 58%

Half-life, intracellular: 12 to 26 hours

Time to peak serum concentration (Hughes 1999):

Pediatric patients ≥3 months to ≤13 years: Within 1.5 hours

Adults: 1 to 1.7 hours

Elimination: Urine: ~83% (1.2% as unchanged drug, 30% as 5'-carboxylic acid metabolite, 36% as the glucuronide, and 15% as other metabolites); feces (16% total dose)

Clearance (apparent): Single dose 8 mg/kg (Hughes 1999):

Pediatric patients ≥3 months to ≤13 years: 17.84 mL/minute/kg

Adults: 10.14 mL/minute/kg

Dosing: Usual

Pediatric: **HIV infection, treatment: Note:** Use in combination with other antiretroviral agents:

Infants <3 months: Not approved for use; safety, efficacy, and dosage not established

Infants ≥3 months, Children, and Adolescents <16 years:

Oral:

Twice-daily dosing:

Oral solution: 8 mg/kg/dose twice daily; maximum dose: 300 mg/dose

Oral tablet: Weight-band dosing for patients ≥14 kg who are able to swallow tablets (scored 300 mg tablets):

Manufacturer's labeling:

14 to < 20 kg: 150 mg (1/2 tablet) twice daily

20 to <25 kg: 150 mg (1/2 tablet) in the morning and 300 mg (1 tablet) in the evening

≥25 kg: 300 mg (1 tablet) twice daily

Alternate dosing (HHS [pediatric] 2015):

14 to 21 kg: 150 mg (1/2 tablet) twice daily

>21 to <30 kg: 150 mg (1/2 tablet) in the morning and 300 mg (1 tablet) in the evening

≥30 kg: 300 mg (1 tablet) twice daily

Once-daily dosing: **Note:** Not recommended as initial therapy. Efficacy of once daily dosing has only been demonstrated in patients who transitioned from twice daily dosing after 36 weeks of treatment. Some experts recommend reserving once daily therapy for use as a component of a once-daily regimen in clinically stable patients who have undetectable viral loads and stable CD4 counts for more than 6 months (HHS [pediatric] 2015).

Oral solution:

Manufacturer's labeling: 16 mg/kg/dose once daily; maximum dose: 600 mg/dose

Alternate dosing (HHS [pediatric] 2015): 16 to 20 mg/kg/dose once daily; maximum dose: 600 mg/dose

Oral tablet: Weight-band dosing for patients ≥14 kg who are able to swallow tablets (scored 300 mg tablets):

14 to < 20 kg: 300 mg (1 tablet) once daily

20 to <25 kg: 450 mg (1 + 1/2 tablet) once daily

≥25 kg: 600 mg (2 tablets) once daily

Adolescents ≥16 years: Oral: 300 mg twice daily or 600 mg once daily (HHS [pediatric], 2015)

Adult: **HIV infection, treatment:** Oral: Use in combination with other antiretroviral agents: 300 mg twice daily or 600 mg once daily

Dosing adjustment in renal impairment: There are no dosage adjustments provided in the manufacturer's labeling; however, renal is a minor route of elimination.

Dosing adjustment in hepatic impairment:

Mild hepatic impairment (Child-Pugh class A): Adults: 200 mg twice daily (using oral solution)

Moderate to severe hepatic impairment (Child-Pugh class B or C): All patients: Use is contraindicated

Administration Hazardous agent; use appropriate precautions for handling and disposal (NIOSH 2014 [group 2]).

Oral: May be administered without regard to food

Monitoring Parameters *HLA-B*5701* genotype status prior to initiating therapy or resuming therapy in patients of unknown *HLA-B*5701* status (including patients previously tolerating therapy); signs and symptoms of hypersensitivity reaction (in all patients, but especially in those untested for the *HLA-B*5701* allele)

Note: The absolute CD4 cell count is currently recommended to monitor immune status in children of all ages; CD4 percentage can be used as an alternative. This recommendation is based on the use of absolute CD4 cell counts in the current pediatric HIV infection stage classification and as thresholds for initiation of antiretroviral treatment (HHS [pediatric] 2015).

Prior to initiation of therapy: Genotypic resistance testing, CD4 and viral load (every 3 to 4 months), CBC with differential, LFTs, BUN, creatinine, electrolytes, glucose, urinalysis (every 6 to 12 months), and assessment of readiness for adherence with medication regimen. At initiation and with any change in treatment regimen: CBC with differential, electrolytes, calcium, phosphate, glucose, LFTs, bilirubin, urinalysis (at initiation), BUN, creatinine, albumin, total protein, lipid panel (at initiation), CD4, and viral load. After 1 to 2 weeks of therapy: Signs of medication toxicity and adherence. After 2 to 4 weeks of therapy: CBC with differential, viral load, signs of medication toxicity, and adherence; then every 3 to 4 months: CBC with differential, electrolytes, glucose, LFTs, bilirubin, BUN, creatinine, CD4, viral load, signs of medication toxicity, and adherence. Lipid panel and urinalysis every 6 to 12 months. CD4 monitoring frequency may be decreased to every 6 to 12 months in children who are adherent to therapy if the value is well above the threshold for opportunistic infections, viral suppression is sustained, and the clinical status is stable for more than 2 to 3 years (HHS [pediatric], 2015). Monitor for growth and development, signs of, HIV-specific physical conditions, HIV disease progression, opportunistic infections or lactic acidosis; serum creatine kinase.

Additional Information The patient Medication Guide, which includes written manufacturer information, should be dispensed to the patient with each new prescription and refill; the Warning Card describing the hypersensitivity reaction should be given to the patient to carry with them.

The development of the abacavir hypersensitivity reaction has been associated with certain HLA genotypes (eg, *HLA-B*5701*, *HLA-DR7*, *HLA-DQ3*) which may help predict which patients are at risk for developing the abacavir hypersensitivity reaction (Hetherington, 2002; Lucas, 2007; Mallal, 2002). Patients who test positive for the *HLA-B*5701* allele should have an abacavir allergy recorded in their medical record and should **not** receive abacavir. All patients who receive abacavir (and their caregivers) should be educated about the risk of abacavir hypersensitivity reactions (including patients who test negative for the *HLA-B*5701* allele, as the risk for the reaction is not completely eliminated). Approximately 4% of patients who test negative for the *HLA-B*5701* allele will experience a clinically suspected abacavir hypersensitivity reaction compared to 61% of those who test positive for the *HLA-B*5701* allele.

The prevalence of *HLA-B*5701* in the United States has been estimated to be 8% in Caucasians, 2.5% in African-Americans, 2% in Hispanics, 1% in Asians; in the sub-Saharan Africa it is <1%. Pretherapy identification of *HLA-B*5701*-positive patients and subsequent avoidance of abacavir therapy in these patients has been shown to significantly reduce the occurrence of abacavir-associated hypersensitivity reactions. A skin patch test is in development for clinical screening purposes; however, only PCR-mediated genotyping methods are currently in clinical practice use for documentation of this susceptibility marker. A familial predisposition to the abacavir hypersensitivity reaction has also been reported; use abacavir with great caution in children of parents who experience a hypersensitivity reaction to abacavir (Peyriére, 2001).

Reverse transcriptase mutations of K65R, L74V, Y115F, and M184V have been associated with abacavir resistance; at least 2-3 mutations are needed to decrease HIV susceptibility by 10-fold. The presence of a multiple number of these abacavir resistance-associated mutations, may confer cross-resistance for other nucleoside or nucleotide reverse transcriptase inhibitors (eg, didanosine, emtricitabine, lamivudine, zalcitabine, or tenofovir). A progressive decrease in abacavir susceptibility is associated with an increasing number of thymidine analogue mutations (TAMs; M41L, D67N, K70R, L210W, T215Y/F, K219E/R/H/Q/N).

Dosage Forms Excipient information presented when available (limited, particularly for generics); consult specific product labeling.

Solution, Oral:

Ziagen: 20 mg/mL (240 mL) [contains methylparaben, propylene glycol, propylparaben, saccharin sodium; strawberry-banana flavor]

Tablet, Oral:

Ziagen: 300 mg [scored]

Generic: 300 mg

Abacavir and Lamivudine

(a BAK a veer & la MI vyoo deen)

Medication Safety Issues

High alert medication:

This medication is in a class the Institute for Safe Medication Practices (ISMP) includes among its list of

drug classes that have a heightened risk of causing significant patient harm when used in error.

Related Information

Adult and Adolescent HIV *on page 2392*
Pediatric HIV *on page 2380*
Perinatal HIV *on page 2400*
Safe Handling of Hazardous Drugs *on page 2455*

Brand Names: US Epzicom

Brand Names: Canada Kivexa

Therapeutic Category Antiretroviral Agent; HIV Agents (Anti-HIV Agents); Nucleoside Analog Reverse Transcriptase Inhibitor (NRTI)

Generic Availability (US) No

Use Treatment of HIV-1 infection in combination with other antiretroviral agents (FDA approved in ages ≥18 years and adults); **Note:** HIV regimens consisting of **three** antiretroviral agents are strongly recommended.

Medication Guide Available Yes

Pregnancy Considerations The Department of Health and Human Services (HHS) Perinatal HIV Guidelines consider abacavir in combination with lamivudine to be a preferred nucleoside reverse transcriptase inhibitor (NRTI) backbone for use in antiretroviral-naive pregnant women (HHS [perinatal], 2014). See individual agents.

Breast-Feeding Considerations Abacavir and lamivudine are excreted into breast milk (HHS [perinatal], 2014). See individual agents.

Contraindications Hypersensitivity to abacavir, lamivudine, or any component of the formulation; hepatic impairment. Do not rechallenge patients who have experienced hypersensitivity to abacavir regardless of *HLA-B*5701* status.

Warnings/Precautions Hazardous agent (abacavir); use appropriate precautions for handling and disposal (NIOSH 2014 [group 2])

[US Boxed Warning]: This combination should only be used as part of a multidrug regimen for which the individual components are indicated. [US Boxed Warning]: Serious and sometimes fatal hypersensitivity reactions have occurred in patients taking abacavir (in Epzicom). Patients testing positive for the presence of the *HLA-B*5701* allele are at an increased risk for hypersensitivity reactions. Screening for *HLA-B*5701* allele status is recommended prior to initiating abacavir-containing therapy or reinitiating therapy in patients of unknown status, including patients who previously tolerated therapy. Epzicom is **not** recommended in patients testing positive for the *HLA-B*5701* allele. Additionally, *HLA-B*5701* allele-positive patients (including abacavir treatment naive) should have an allergy to abacavir documented in the patient's medical record (HHS [adult], 2014). Reactions usually occur within 9 days of starting abacavir; ~90% occur within 6 weeks Patients exhibiting symptoms from two or more of the following: Fever, skin rash, constitutional symptoms (eg, malaise, fatigue, aches), respiratory symptoms (eg, pharyngitis, dyspnea, cough), and GI symptoms (eg, abdominal pain, nausea, vomiting) should discontinue therapy immediately and seek medical attention. Epzicom should be permanently discontinued if hypersensitivity cannot be ruled out, even when other diagnoses are possible and regardless of *HLA-B*5701* status. Epzicom SHOULD NOT be restarted because more severe symptoms may occur within hours, including LIFE-THREATENING HYPOTENSION AND DEATH. Fatal hypersensitivity reactions have occurred following the reintroduction of abacavir in patients whose therapy was interrupted (ie, interruption in drug supply, temporary discontinuation while treating other conditions). Reactions occurred within hours. In some cases, signs of hypersensitivity may have been previously present, but attributed to other medical conditions (eg, acute onset respiratory diseases, gastroenteritis, reactions to other medications). If Epzicom is restarted following an interruption in therapy, evaluate the patient for previously unsuspected symptoms of hypersensitivity. Do not restart if hypersensitivity is suspected or if hypersensitivity cannot be ruled out regardless of *HLA-B*5701* status.

[US Boxed Warning]: Following discontinuation of lamivudine, severe acute exacerbations of hepatitis B in patients coinfected with HBV and HIV have been reported. Monitor patients closely for several months following discontinuation of therapy for chronic hepatitis B; clinical exacerbations may occur.

[US Boxed Warning]: Lactic acidosis and severe hepatomegaly with steatosis (sometimes fatal) have occurred with antiretroviral nucleoside analogues. Female gender, prior liver disease, obesity, and prolonged treatment may increase the risk of hepatotoxicity. Due to fixed dose of combination product, use is not recommended with renal impairment (CrCl <50 mL/minute). May be associated with fat redistribution. Patients may develop immune reconstitution syndrome resulting in the occurrence of an inflammatory response to an indolent or residual opportunistic infection during initial HIV treatment or activation of autoimmune disorders (eg, Graves' disease, polymyositis, Guillain-Barré syndrome) later in therapy; further evaluation and treatment may be required. Potentially significant drug-drug interactions may exist, requiring dose or frequency adjustment, additional monitoring, and/or selection of alternative therapy. Use with caution in combination with interferon alfa with or without ribavirin in HIV/HBV coinfected patients; monitor closely for hepatic decompensation, anemia, or neutropenia; dose reduction or discontinuation of interferon and/or ribavirin may be required if toxicity evident. Concomitant use of other abacavir or lamivudine-containing products with the fixed-dose combination product should be avoided. Concomitant use of emtricitabine-containing products should be avoided; cross-resistance may develop. Use has been associated with an increased risk of myocardial infarction (MI) in observational studies; however, based on a meta-analysis of 26 randomized trials, the FDA has concluded there is not an increased risk. Consider using with caution in patients with risks for coronary heart disease and minimizing modifiable risk factors (eg, hypertension, hyperlipidemia, diabetes mellitus, and smoking) prior to use.

Warnings: Additional Pediatric Considerations The major clinical toxicity of lamivudine in pediatric patients is pancreatitis; discontinue therapy if clinical signs, symptoms, or laboratory abnormalities suggestive of pancreatitis occur. Abacavir may cause mild hyperglycemia; more common in pediatric patients.

Adverse Reactions See individual agents.

Postmarketing and/or case reports: Alopecia, anaphylaxis, anemia, aplastic anemia, breath sounds abnormal, CPK increased, erythema multiforme, fat redistribution, hepatic steatosis, hepatitis B exacerbation, hyperglycemia, hypersensitivity reaction, immune reconstitution syndrome, lactic acidosis, lymphadenopathy, muscle weakness, pancreatitis, paresthesia, peripheral neuropathy, rhabdomyolysis, seizure, splenomegaly, Stevens-Johnson syndrome, stomatitis, urticaria, weakness, wheezing

Drug Interactions

Metabolism/Transport Effects None known.

Avoid Concomitant Use

Avoid concomitant use of Abacavir and Lamivudine with any of the following: Emtricitabine

Increased Effect/Toxicity

Abacavir and Lamivudine may increase the levels/effects of: Emtricitabine

The levels/effects of Abacavir and Lamivudine may be increased by: Ganciclovir-Valganciclovir; Ribavirin; Trimethoprim

Decreased Effect

Abacavir and Lamivudine may decrease the levels/effects of: Methadone

The levels/effects of Abacavir and Lamivudine may be decreased by: Methadone; Protease Inhibitors

Food Interactions Ethanol decreases the elimination of abacavir and may increase the risk of toxicity. Management: Monitor patients.

Storage/Stability Store at controlled room temperature of 15°C to 30°C (59°F to 86°F).

Mechanism of Action Nucleoside reverse transcriptase inhibitor combination.

Abacavir is a guanosine analogue which is phosphorylated to carbovir triphosphate which interferes with HIV viral RNA-dependent DNA polymerase resulting in inhibition of viral replication.

Lamivudine is a cytosine analog. After lamivudine is triphosphorylated, the principle mode of action is inhibition of HIV reverse transcription via viral DNA chain termination; inhibits RNA-dependent DNA polymerase activities of reverse transcriptase.

Pharmacokinetics (Adult data unless noted) One Epzicom tablet is bioequivalent, in the extent (AUC) of absorption and peak concentration, to two abacavir 300 mg tablets and two lamivudine 150 mg tablets; see individual agents

Dosing: Usual

Pediatric: **HIV infection, treatment:**

Children and Adolescents ≤50 kg: Not recommended; product is a fixed-dose combination.

Adolescents ≥16 years of age weighing >50 kg: Oral: 1 tablet daily (DHHS [pediatric], 2014)

Adult: **HIV infection, treatment:** Oral: 1 tablet daily

Dosing adjustment in renal impairment: CrCl ≤50 mL/minute: Use not recommended; use individual antiretroviral agents to reduce dosage

Dosing adjustment in hepatic impairment: Use is contraindicated; use individual antiretroviral agents to reduce dosage

Administration Hazardous agent (abacavir); use appropriate precautions for handling and disposal (NIOSH 2014 [group 2]). May be administered without regards to meals.

Monitoring Parameters *HLA-B*5701* genotype status prior to initiating therapy or resuming therapy in patients of unknown *HLA-B*5701* status (including patients previously tolerating therapy); signs and symptoms of abacavir hypersensitivity reaction (in all patients, but especially in those untested for the *HLA-B*5701* allele)

Note: Monitor CD4 percentage (if <5 years of age) or CD4 count (if ≥5 years of age) at least every 3 to 4 months (DHHS [pediatric], 2014).

Prior to initiation of therapy: Genotypic resistance testing, CD4 and viral load (every 3 to 4 months), CBC with differential, LFTs, BUN, creatinine, electrolytes, glucose, urinalysis (every 6 to 12 months), and assessment of readiness for adherence with medication regimen . At initiation and with any change in treatment regimen: CBC with differential, electrolytes, calcium, phosphate, glucose, LFTs, bilirubin, urinalysis (at initiation), BUN, creatinine, albumin, total protein, lipid panel (at initiation), CD4, and viral load. After 1 to 2 weeks of therapy: Signs of medication toxicity and adherence. After 2 to 4 weeks of therapy: CBC with differential, viral load, signs of medication toxicity, and adherence; then every 3 to 4 months: CBC with differential, electrolytes, glucose, LFTs, bilirubin, BUN, creatinine, CD4, viral load, signs of medication toxicity, and adherence. Every 6 to 12 months: Lipid panel and urinalysis. CD4 monitoring frequency may be decreased to every 6 to 12 months in children who are adherent to therapy if the value is well above the threshold for opportunistic infections, viral suppression is sustained, and the clinical status is stable for more than 2 to 3 years (DHHS [pediatric], 2014). Monitor for growth and development, signs of HIV-specific physical conditions, HIV disease progression, opportunistic infections, pancreatitis, or lactic acidosis; serum creatinine kinase.

Additional Information The development of the abacavir hypersensitivity reaction has been associated with certain HLA genotypes (eg, *HLA-B*5701*, *HLA-DR7*, *HLA-DQ3*) which may help predict which patients are at risk for developing the abacavir hypersensitivity reaction (Hetherington, 2002; Lucas, 2007; Mallal, 2002). Patients who test positive for the *HLA-B*5701* allele should have an abacavir allergy recorded in their medical record and should **not** receive abacavir. All patients who receive abacavir (and their caregivers) should be educated about the risk of abacavir hypersensitivity reactions (including patients who test negative for the *HLA-B*5701* allele, as the risk for the reaction is not completely eliminated). Approximately 4% of patients who test negative for the *HLA-B*5701* allele will experience a clinically suspected abacavir hypersensitivity reaction compared to 61% of those who test positive for the *HLA-B*5701* allele.

The prevalence of *HLA-B*5701* in the United States has been estimated to be 8% in Caucasians, 2.5% in African-Americans, 2% in Hispanics, <1% in Asians; in the sub-Saharan Africa it is 1%. Pretherapy identification of *HLA-B*5701*-positive patients and subsequent avoidance of abacavir therapy in these patients has been shown to significantly reduce the occurrence of abacavir-associated hypersensitivity reactions. A skin patch test is in development for clinical screening purposes; however, only PCR-mediated genotyping methods are currently in clinical practice use for documentation of this susceptibility marker. A familial predisposition to the abacavir hypersensitivity reaction has been reported; use abacavir with great caution in children of parents who experience a hypersensitivity reaction to abacavir (Peyriére, 2001).

Reverse transcriptase mutations of K65R, L74V, Y115F, and M184V have been associated with abacavir resistance; at least 2 to 3 mutations are needed to decrease HIV susceptibility by 10-fold. The presence of a multiple number of these abacavir resistance-associated mutations, may confer cross-resistance for other nucleoside or nucleotide reverse transcriptase inhibitors (eg, didanosine, emtricitabine, lamivudine, zalcitabine, or tenofovir). A progressive decrease in abacavir susceptibility is associated with an increasing number of thymidine analogue mutations (TAMs; M41L, D67N, K70R, L210W, T215Y/F, K219E/R/H/Q/N).

Dosage Forms Excipient information presented when available (limited, particularly for generics); consult specific product labeling.

Tablet, Oral:

Epzicom: Abacavir 600 mg and lamivudine 300 mg [contains fd&c yellow #6 (sunset yellow)]

Abacavir, Lamivudine, and Zidovudine

(a BAK a veer, la MI vyoo deen, & zye DOE vyoo deen)

Medication Safety Issues

High alert medication:

This medication is in a class the Institute for Safe Medication Practices (ISMP) includes among its list of drug classes that have a heightened risk of causing significant patient harm when used in error.

Related Information

Adult and Adolescent HIV *on page 2392*
Pediatric HIV *on page 2380*
Perinatal HIV *on page 2400*
Safe Handling of Hazardous Drugs *on page 2455*

Brand Names: US Trizivir

Brand Names: Canada Trizivir

Therapeutic Category Antiretroviral Agent; HIV Agents (Anti-HIV Agents); Nucleoside Analog Reverse Transcriptase Inhibitor (NRTI)

Generic Availability (US) Yes

Use Treatment of HIV-1 infection, either alone or in combination with other antiretroviral agents (FDA approved in adolescents ≥40 kg and adults); **Note:** HIV regimens consisting of **three** antiretroviral agents are strongly recommended; **Note:** Data on the use of this triple NRTI combination regimen in patients with baseline viral loads >100,000 copies/mL is limited.

Medication Guide Available Yes

Pregnancy Risk Factor C

Pregnancy Considerations Animal reproduction studies have not been conducted with this combination. The DHHS Perinatal HIV Guidelines generally do not recommend this combination in antiretroviral-naive pregnant women due to inferior virologic activity (HHS [Perinatal], 2014). See individual agents.

Breast-Feeding Considerations Abacavir, lamivudine, and zidovudine are excreted into breast milk. See individual agents.

Contraindications

Hypersensitivity to abacavir or any component of the formulation regardless of *HLA-B*5701* status; hepatic impairment.

Canadian labeling: Additional contraindications (not in US labeling): ANC <750 cells/mm^3; hemoglobin <7.5 g/dL or 4.65 mmol/L; patients screened positive for *HLA-B*5701* allele

Warnings/Precautions Hazardous agent (abacavir); use appropriate precautions for handling and disposal (NIOSH 2014 [group 2])

[U.S. Boxed Warning]: This combination should only be used as part of a multidrug regimen for which the individual components are indicated. [U.S. Boxed Warning]: Fatal hypersensitivity reactions have occurred in patients taking abacavir (in Trizivir). Patients testing positive for the presence of the *HLA-B*5701* allele are at an increased risk for hypersensitivity reactions. Screening for *HLA-B*5701* allele status is recommended prior to initiating abacavir-containing therapy or reinitiating therapy in patients of unknown status, including patients who previously tolerated abacavir therapy. Trizivir should **not** be used in patients testing positive for the *HLA-B*5701* allele. Additionally, allele-positive patients (including abacavir treatment naive) should have an allergy to abacavir documented in their medical record (HHS [adult], 2014). Reactions usually occur within 9 days of starting abacavir; ~90% occur within 6 weeks. Hypersensitivity is a multiorgan clinical syndrome characterized by a sign or symptom in 2 or more of the following groups; Group 1: Fevers; Group 2: Rash; Group 3: Gastrointestinal (eg, nausea, vomiting, diarrhea, abdominal pain); Group 4: Constitutional (eg, generalized malaise, fatigue, achiness); Group 5: Respiratory (eg, dyspnea, cough, pharyngitis).

Hypersensitivity to abacavir after a single sign or symptom has been reported infrequently. Less common signs of hypersensitivity include lethargy, myolysis, edema, abnormal chest radiograph findings (eg, diffuse or localized infiltrates), and paresthesia. Anaphylaxis, liver or renal failure and death have occurred in association with hypersensitivity. Physical findings of hypersensitivity to abacavir include lymphadenopathy, mucous membrane lesions (eg, conjunctivitis and mouth ulcerations), and rash (maculopapular, urticarial or variable in appearance), including erythema multiforme. Hypersensitivity reactions have occurred without rash. Laboratory abnormalities may include elevated liver function tests, elevated creatine phosphokinase, elevated serum creatinine and lymphopenia. If hypersensitivity is suspected, discontinue therapy immediately and obtain medical attention. Trizivir should be permanently discontinued if hypersensitivity cannot be ruled out, even when other diagnoses are possible and regardless of *HLA-B*5701* status. Trizivir SHOULD NOT be restarted because more severe symptoms may occur within hours, including LIFE-THREATENING HYPOTENSION AND DEATH. Fatal hypersensitivity reactions have occurred following the reintroduction of abacavir in patients whose therapy was interrupted (ie, interruption in drug supply, temporary discontinuation while treating other conditions). Reactions occurred within hours. In some cases, signs of hypersensitivity may have been previously present, but attributed to other medical conditions (eg, acute onset respiratory diseases, gastroenteritis, reactions to other medications). If Trizivir is to be restarted following an interruption in therapy, first evaluate the patient for previously unsuspected symptoms of hypersensitivity. Do not restart if hypersensitivity is suspected or if hypersensitivity cannot be ruled out regardless of *HLA-B*5701* status.

[U.S. Boxed Warning]: Lactic acidosis and severe hepatomegaly with steatosis have been reported with nucleoside analogues; risk factors may include prior liver disease, prolonged use, female gender and obesity. Pancreatitis has been observed with abacavir, lamivudine and zidovudine; rule out pancreatitis in patients who develop signs/symptoms (eg, nausea/vomiting, abdominal pain, elevated lipase and amylase) during therapy. Use with caution in patients with bone marrow compromise (eg, granulocyte count <1000 cells/mm^3 or hemoglobin <9.5 g/dL). Frequent complete blood counts are recommended in patients with advanced HIV-1 disease. Dosage interruption may be needed if anemia or neutropenia develops. **[U.S. Boxed Warnings]: Zidovudine has been associated with hematologic toxicities (eg, neutropenia, anemia) and myopathy (prolonged use); exacerbation of hepatitis B (including fatalities) has been reported with discontinuation of lamivudine in coinfected HIV/HBV patients;** monitor hepatic function (eg serum ALT) and HBV viral DNA closely for several months after discontinuing Trizivir in coinfected patients. Canadian labeling contraindicates use if ANC <750 cells/mm^3 or if hemoglobin <7.5 g/dL (4.65 mmol/L). May be associated with fat redistribution. Patients may develop immune reconstitution syndrome resulting in the occurrence of an inflammatory response to an indolent or residual opportunistic infection during initial HIV treatment or activation of autoimmune disorders (eg, Graves' disease, polymyositis, Guillain-Barré syndrome) later in therapy; further evaluation and treatment may be required. Use has been associated with an increased risk of myocardial infarction (MI) in observational studies; however, based on a meta-analysis of 26 randomized trials, the FDA has concluded there is not an increased risk. Consider using with caution in patients with risks for coronary heart disease and minimizing modifiable risk factors (eg, hypertension, hyperlipidemia, diabetes mellitus, and smoking) prior to use. Patients with prolonged prior nucleoside reverse transcriptase inhibitor (NRTI) exposure or presence of HIV-1 isolates containing multiple mutations conferring resistance to NRTIs have limited response to abacavir. The potential for cross resistance between abacavir and other NRTIs should be considered when evaluating new regimens in therapy experienced patients. Potentially significant drug-drug interactions may exist, requiring dose or frequency adjustment, additional monitoring, and/or selection of alternative therapy.

Trizivir, as a fixed-dose combination tablet, should not be used in patients <40 kg or those requiring dosage adjustment; should not be used in patients with CrCl <50 mL/minute.

Warnings: Additional Pediatric Considerations The major clinical toxicity of lamivudine in pediatric patients is pancreatitis; discontinue therapy if clinical signs, symptoms, or laboratory abnormalities suggestive of pancreatitis occur. Abacavir may cause mild hyperglycemia; more common in pediatric patients.

Adverse Reactions Fatal hypersensitivity reactions have occurred in patients taking abacavir (in Trizivir®). If Trizivir® is to be restarted following an interruption in therapy, first evaluate the patient for previously unsuspected symptoms of hypersensitivity. Do not restart if hypersensitivity is suspected or if hypersensitivity cannot be ruled out.

The following information is based on CNA3005 study data concerning effects noted in patients receiving abacavir, lamivudine, and zidovudine. See individual agents for additional information.

Central nervous system: Anxiety, depression, fatigue, fever/chills, headache, malaise
Dermatologic: Rash
Endocrine & metabolic: Triglycerides increased
Gastrointestinal: Amylase increased, diarrhea, GGT increased, nausea, pancreatitis, vomiting
Hematologic: Neutropenia
Hepatic: ALT increased
Neuromuscular & skeletal: CPK increased
Otic: Ear infection
Respiratory: Nose/throat infection
Miscellaneous: Hypersensitivity, viral infection

Drug Interactions

Metabolism/Transport Effects Refer to individual components.

Avoid Concomitant Use

Avoid concomitant use of Abacavir, Lamivudine, and Zidovudine with any of the following: Amodiaquine; BCG (Intravesical); CloZAPine; Dipyrone; Emtricitabine; Stavudine

Increased Effect/Toxicity

Abacavir, Lamivudine, and Zidovudine may increase the levels/effects of: Amodiaquine; CloZAPine; Emtricitabine; Ribavirin

The levels/effects of Abacavir, Lamivudine, and Zidovudine may be increased by: Acyclovir-Valacyclovir; Clarithromycin; Dexketoprofen; Dipyrone; DOXOrubicin (Conventional); DOXOrubicin (Liposomal); Fluconazole; Ganciclovir-Valganciclovir; Interferons; Methadone; Probenecid; Raltegravir; Teriflunomide; Trimethoprim; Valproic Acid and Derivatives

Decreased Effect

Abacavir, Lamivudine, and Zidovudine may decrease the levels/effects of: BCG (Intravesical); Methadone; Stavudine

The levels/effects of Abacavir, Lamivudine, and Zidovudine may be decreased by: Clarithromycin; DOXOrubicin (Conventional); DOXOrubicin (Liposomal); Methadone; Protease Inhibitors; Rifamycin Derivatives

Food Interactions Ethanol decreases the elimination of abacavir and may increase the risk of toxicity. Management: Monitor patients.

Storage/Stability Store at 15°C to 30°C (59°F to 86°F).

Mechanism of Action The combination of abacavir, lamivudine, and zidovudine is believed to act synergistically to inhibit reverse transcriptase via DNA chain termination after incorporation of the nucleoside analogue as well as to delay the emergence of mutations conferring resistance.

Pharmacokinetics (Adult data unless noted) One Trizivir tablet is bioequivalent, in the extent (AUC) and rate of absorption (peak concentration and time to peak concentration), to one abacavir 300 mg tablet, one lamivudine 150 mg tablet, plus one zidovudine 300 mg tablet; see individual agents

Dosing: Usual

Pediatric: **HIV infection, treatment:** May use alone or in combination with other antiretroviral agents:

Children and Adolescents <40 kg: Not recommended; product is a fixed-dose combination

Adolescents ≥40 kg: Oral: 1 tablet twice daily

Adult: **HIV infection, treatment:** Oral: 1 tablet twice daily

Dosing adjustment in renal impairment: CrCl <50 mL/minute: Use not recommended (use individual antiretroviral agents to reduce dosage).

Dosing adjustment in hepatic impairment: Use is contraindicated; use individual antiretroviral agents to reduce dosage.

Administration Hazardous agent (abacavir); use appropriate precautions for handling and disposal (NIOSH 2014 [group 2]). May be administered without regard to meals.

Monitoring Parameters *HLA-B*5701* genotype status prior to initiating therapy or resuming therapy in patients of unknown *HLA-B*5701* status (including patients previously tolerating therapy); signs and symptoms of abacavir hypersensitivity reaction (in all patients, but especially in those untested for the *HLA-B*5701* allele)

Note: Monitor CD4 percentage (if <5 years of age) or CD4 count (if ≥5 years of age) at least every 3 to 4 months (DHHS [pediatric], 2014)

Prior to initiation of therapy: Genotypic resistance testing, CD4 and viral load (every 3 to 4 months), CBC with differential, LFTs, BUN, creatinine, electrolytes, glucose, urinalysis (every 6 to 12 months), and assessment of readiness for adherence with medication regimen. At initiation and with any change in treatment regimen: CBC with differential, electrolytes, calcium, phosphate, glucose, LFTs, bilirubin, urinalysis (at initiation), BUN, creatinine, albumin, total protein, lipid panel (at initiation), CD4, and viral load. After 1 to 2 weeks of therapy: Signs of medication toxicity and adherence. After 2 to 4 weeks of therapy: CBC with differential, viral load, signs of medication toxicity and adherence; then every 3 to 4 months: CBC with differential, electrolytes, glucose, LFTs, bilirubin, BUN, creatinine, CD4, viral load, signs of medication toxicity, and adherence. Lipid panel and urinalysis every 6 to 12 months. CD4 monitoring frequency may be decreased to every 6 to 12 months in children who are adherent to therapy if the value is well above the threshold for opportunistic infections, viral suppression is sustained, and the clinical status is stable for more than 2 to 3 years (DHHS [pediatric], 2014). Monitor for growth and development, signs of HIV-specific physical conditions, HIV disease progression, opportunistic infections, hepatotoxicity, anemia, pancreatitis, or lactic acidosis; serum creatine kinase

Additional Information The development of the abacavir hypersensitivity reaction has been associated with certain HLA genotypes (eg, *HLA-B*5701*, *HLA-DR7*, *HLA-DQ3*) which may help predict which patients are at risk for developing the abacavir hypersensitivity reaction (Hetherington, 2002; Lucas, 2007; Mallal, 2002). Patients who test positive for the *HLA-B*5701* allele should have an abacavir allergy recorded in their medical record and should **not** receive abacavir. All patients who receive abacavir (and their caregivers) should be educated about the risk of abacavir hypersensitivity reactions (including patients who test negative for the *HLA-B*5701* allele, as the risk for the reaction is not completely eliminated). Approximately 4% of patients who test negative for the *HLA-B*5701* allele will experience a clinically suspected abacavir hypersensitivity reaction compared to 61% of those who test positive for the *HLA-B*5701* allele.

The prevalence of *HLA-B*5701* in the United States has been estimated to be 8% in Caucasians, 2.5% in African-Americans, 2% in Hispanics, 1% in Asians; in the sub-Saharan Africa it is <1%. Pretherapy identification of *HLA-B*5701*-positive patients and subsequent avoidance of abacavir therapy in these patients has been shown to significantly reduce the occurrence of abacavir-associated hypersensitivity reactions. A skin patch test is in development for clinical screening purposes; however, only PCR-mediated genotyping methods are currently in clinical practice use for documentation of this susceptibility marker. A familial predisposition to the abacavir hypersensitivity reaction has been reported; use abacavir with great caution in children of parents who experience a hypersensitivity reaction to abacavir (Peyriére, 2001).

Reverse transcriptase mutations of K65R, L74V, Y115F, and M184V have been associated with abacavir resistance; at least 2 to 3 mutations are needed to decrease HIV susceptibility by 10-fold. The presence of a multiple number of these abacavir resistance-associated mutations may confer cross-resistance for other nucleoside or nucleotide reverse transcriptase inhibitors (eg, didanosine, emtricitabine, lamivudine, zalcitabine, or tenofovir). A progressive decrease in abacavir susceptibility is associated with an increasing number of thymidine analogue mutations (TAMs; M41L, D67N, K70R, L210W, T215Y/F, K219E/R/H/Q/N).

Dosage Forms Excipient information presented when available (limited, particularly for generics); consult specific product labeling.

Tablet, Oral:

Trizivir: Abacavir sulfate 300 mg, lamivudine 150 mg, and zidovudine 300 mg [contains fd&c blue #2 (indigotine)]

Generic: Abacavir sulfate 300 mg, lamivudine 150 mg, and zidovudine 300 mg

◆ **Abacavir Sulfate** *see* Abacavir *on page 34*

◆ **Abacavir Sulfate and Lamivudine** *see* Abacavir and Lamivudine *on page 36*

Abatacept (ab a TA sept)

Medication Safety Issues

Sound-alike/look-alike issues:

Orencia may be confused with Oracea

Brand Names: US Orencia

Brand Names: Canada Orencia

Therapeutic Category Antirheumatic, Disease Modifying

Generic Availability (US) No

Use Treatment of moderately- to severely-active polyarticular juvenile idiopathic arthritis as monotherapy or concomitantly with methotrexate (IV: FDA approved in ages 6-17 years). Treatment of moderately- to severely-active rheumatoid arthritis as monotherapy or in combination with other DMARDs (IV; SubQ: FDA approved in adults). **Note:** Abatacept should not be used in combination with TNF antagonists or with other biologic rheumatoid arthritis drugs, such as anakinra.

Pregnancy Risk Factor C

Pregnancy Considerations Adverse effects were not observed in animal studies. Due to the potential risk for development of autoimmune disease in the fetus, use during pregnancy only if clearly needed. A pregnancy registry has been established to monitor outcomes of women exposed to abatacept during pregnancy (1-877-311-8972).

Breast-Feeding Considerations It is not known if abatacept is excreted into human milk. Due to the potential for serious adverse reactions in the nursing infant, a decision should be made to discontinue nursing or to discontinue the drug, taking into account the importance of treatment to the mother.

Contraindications There are no contraindications listed within the manufacturer's U.S. labeling.

Canadian labeling: Hypersensitivity to abatacept or any component of the formulation; patients with, or at risk of sepsis syndrome (eg, immunocompromised, HIV positive)

Warnings/Precautions Serious and potentially fatal infections (including tuberculosis and sepsis) have been reported, particularly in patients receiving concomitant immunosuppressive therapy. RA patients receiving a concomitant TNF antagonist experienced an even higher rate of serious infection. Caution should be exercised when considering the use of abatacept in any patient with a history of recurrent infections, with conditions that predispose them to infections, or with chronic, latent, or localized infections. Patients who develop a new infection while undergoing treatment should be monitored closely. If a patient develops a serious infection, abatacept should be discontinued. Screen patients for latent tuberculosis infection prior to initiating abatacept; safety in tuberculosis-positive patients has not been established. Treat patients testing positive according to standard therapy prior to initiating abatacept. Adult patients receiving abatacept in combination with TNF-blocking agents had higher rates of infections (including serious infections) than patients on TNF-blocking agents alone. Potentially significant drug-drug interactions may exist, requiring dose or frequency adjustment, additional monitoring, and/or selection of alternative therapy. The manufacturer does not recommend concurrent use with anakinra or TNF-blocking agents. Monitor for signs and symptoms of infection when transitioning from TNF-blocking agents to abatacept. Due to the effect of T-cell inhibition on host defenses, abatacept may affect immune responses against infections and malignancies; impact on the development and course of malignancies is not fully defined.

Use caution with chronic obstructive pulmonary disease (COPD), higher incidences of adverse effects (COPD exacerbation, cough, rhonchi, dyspnea) have been observed; monitor closely. Rare cases of hypersensitivity, anaphylaxis, or anaphylactoid reactions have been reported with intravenous administration; may occur with first infusion. Some reactions (hypotension, urticaria, dyspnea) occurred within 24 hours of infusion. Discontinue treatment if anaphylaxis or other serious allergic reaction occurs; medications for the treatment of hypersensitivity reactions should be available for immediate use. Patients should be screened for viral hepatitis prior to use; antirheumatic therapy may cause reactivation of hepatitis B. Patients should be brought up to date with all immunizations before initiating therapy. Live vaccines should not be given concurrently or within 3 months of discontinuation of therapy; there is no data available concerning secondary transmission of live vaccines in patients receiving therapy. Powder for injection may contain maltose, which may result in falsely-elevated serum glucose readings on the day of infusion. Higher incidences of infection and malignancy were observed in the elderly; use with caution.

Adverse Reactions Note: COPD patients experienced a higher frequency of COPD-related adverse reactions (COPD exacerbation, cough, dyspnea, pneumonia, rhonchi)

Cardiovascular: Hypertension

Central nervous system: Dizziness, headache

Dermatologic: Skin rash

Gastrointestinal: Abdominal pain, diarrhea, dyspepsia, nausea

Genitourinary: Urinary tract infection

Immunologic: Immunogenicity
Infection: Herpes simplex infection, influenza
Local: Injection site reaction
Neuromuscular & skeletal: Back pain, limb pain
Respiratory: Bronchitis, cough, nasopharyngitis, pneumonia, rhinitis, sinusitis, upper respiratory tract infection
Miscellaneous: Antibody development, fever, infection, infusion-related reaction
Rare but important or life-threatening: Acute lymphocytic leukemia, anaphylactoid reaction, anaphylaxis, cellulitis, diverticulitis, dyspnea, exacerbation of arthritis, exacerbation of chronic obstructive pulmonary disease, hypersensitivity, hypotension, joint wear, malignant lymphoma, malignant neoplasm (including malignant melanoma, malignant neoplasm of the bile duct, malignant neoplasm of bladder, malignant neoplasm of breast, malignant neoplasm of cervix, malignant neoplasm of kidney, malignant neoplasm of prostate, malignant neoplasm of skin, malignant neoplasm of thyroid, myelodysplastic syndrome, and uterine neoplasm), malignant neoplasm of lung, ovarian cyst, pruritus, pyelonephritis, rhonchi, urticaria, varicella, vasculitis (including hypersensitivity angiitis [cutaneous vasculitis and leukocytoclastic vasculitis]), wheezing

Drug Interactions

Metabolism/Transport Effects None known.

Avoid Concomitant Use

Avoid concomitant use of Abatacept with any of the following: Anakinra; Anti-TNF Agents; BCG; BCG (Intravesical); Belimumab; Natalizumab; Pimecrolimus; RiTUXimab; Tacrolimus (Topical); Tocilizumab; Tofacitinib; Vaccines (Live)

Increased Effect/Toxicity

Abatacept may increase the levels/effects of: Belimumab; Leflunomide; Natalizumab; Tofacitinib; Vaccines (Live)

The levels/effects of Abatacept may be increased by: Anakinra; Anti-TNF Agents; Denosumab; Pimecrolimus; RiTUXimab; Roflumilast; Tacrolimus (Topical); Tocilizumab; Trastuzumab

Decreased Effect

Abatacept may decrease the levels/effects of: BCG; BCG (Intravesical); Coccidioides immitis Skin Test; Sipuleucel-T; Vaccines (Inactivated); Vaccines (Live)

The levels/effects of Abatacept may be decreased by: Echinacea

Storage/Stability

Prefilled syringe: Store at 2°C to 8°C (36°F to 46°F); do not freeze. Protect from light.
Powder for injection: Prior to reconstitution, store at 2°C to 8°C (36°F to 46°F); do not freeze. Protect from light. After dilution, may be stored for up to 24 hours at room temperature or refrigerated at 2°C to 8°C (36°F to 46°F). Must be used within 24 hours of reconstitution.

Mechanism of Action Selective costimulation modulator; inhibits T-cell (T-lymphocyte) activation by binding to CD80 and CD86 on antigen presenting cells (APC), thus blocking the required CD28 interaction between APCs and T cells. Activated T lymphocytes are found in the synovium of rheumatoid arthritis patients.

Pharmacokinetics (Adult data unless noted)

Distribution: V_{dss}: 0.07 L/kg (range: 0.02 to 0.13 L/kg)
Bioavailability: SubQ: 78.6% (relative to IV administration)
Half-life elimination: RA: 13.1 days (range: 8 to 25 days)
Clearance: 0.22 to 0.23 mL/hour/kg
Children 6 to 17 years: JIA: 0.4 mL/hour/kg (increases with baseline body weight)

Dosing: Usual

Pediatric:

Juvenile idiopathic arthritis: Children and Adolescents 6 to 17 years: **Note:** Dose is based on body weight at each dose administration. IV: Following the initial IV infusion, repeat IV dose at 2 weeks and 4 weeks after the initial infusion, and every 4 weeks thereafter.
Patient weight:
<75 kg: 10 mg/kg
75 to 100 kg: 750 mg
>100 kg: 1000 mg

Rheumatoid arthritis: Adolescents ≥18 years:
IV: Weight-based dosing: Following the initial IV infusion (using the weight-based dosing), repeat IV infusion (using the same weight-based dosing) at 2 weeks and 4 weeks after the initial infusion, and every 4 weeks thereafter.
<60 kg: 500 mg
60 to 100 kg: 750 mg
>100 kg: 1000 mg
SubQ: 125 mg once weekly. **Note:** SubQ dosing may be initiated with or without an IV loading dose.
If initiating with an IV loading dose: Administer the initial IV infusion (using the weight-based dosing), then administer 125 mg SubQ within 24 hours of the infusion, followed by 125 mg SubQ once weekly thereafter.
If transitioning from IV therapy to SubQ therapy: Administer the first SubQ dose instead of the next scheduled IV dose.

Adult: **Rheumatoid arthritis:**
IV: Dosing is according to body weight. Following the initial IV infusion (using the weight-based dosing), repeat IV infusion (using the same weight-based dosing) at 2 weeks and 4 weeks after the initial infusion, and every 4 weeks thereafter.
<60 kg: 500 mg
60 to 100 kg: 750 mg
>100 kg: 1000 mg
SubQ: 125 mg once weekly. **Note:** SubQ dosing may be initiated with or without an IV loading dose.
If initiating with an IV loading dose: Administer the initial IV infusion (using the weight-based dosing), then administer 125 mg SubQ within 24 hours of the infusion, followed by 125 mg SubQ once weekly thereafter.
If transitioning from IV therapy to SubQ therapy: Administer the first SubQ dose instead of the next scheduled IV dose.

Dosing adjustment for renal impairment: There are no dosage adjustments provided in the manufacturer's labeling; not studied.

Dosing adjustment for hepatic impairment: There are no dosage adjustments provided in the manufacturer's labeling; not studied.

Preparation for Administration

IV: Prepare abatacept using only the silicone-free disposable syringe provided with each vial (for information on obtaining additional silicone-free disposable syringes contact Bristol-Myers Squibb at 1-800-ORENCIA). Reconstitute each vial with 10 mL SWFI using the provided silicone-free disposable syringe (discard solutions accidentally reconstituted with siliconized syringe as they may develop translucent particles). Inject SWFI down the side of the vial to avoid foaming. Gently rotate to dissolve; do not shake. The vial should be vented to allow any foam that is present to dissipate. The reconstituted solution contains 25 mg/mL abatacept. Further dilute (using a silicone-free syringe) in 100 mL NS to a final concentration of ≤10 mg/mL. Prior to adding abatacept to the 100 mL bag, the manufacturer recommends withdrawing a volume of NS equal to the abatacept volume required, resulting in a final volume of 100 mL. Mix gently; do not shake.
SubQ: Allow prefilled syringe to reach room temperature prior to administration by removing from refrigerator 30-60 minutes prior to administration.

Administration

IV: Administer through a 0.2 to 1.2 micron low protein-binding filter. Infuse over 30 minutes.

SubQ: Allow prefilled syringe to warm to room temperature for 30 to 60 minutes prior to administration. Inject into the front of the thigh (preferred), abdomen (except for 2-inch area around the navel), or the outer area of the upper arms (if administered by a caregiver). Rotate injection sites (≥1 inch apart); do not administer into tender, bruised, red, or hard skin.

Monitoring Parameters Monitor improvement of symptoms and physical function assessments (eg, joint swelling, pain, and tenderness; ESR or C-reactive protein level). Latent TB screening prior to initiating therapy; signs/symptoms of infection (prior to, during, and following therapy); CBC with differential; HBV screening prior to initiating signs and symptoms of hypersensitivity reaction; signs/symptoms of malignancy

Test Interactions Contains maltose; may result in falsely elevated blood glucose levels with dehydrogenase pyrroloquinolinequinone or glucose-dye-oxidoreductase testing methods on the day of infusion. Glucose monitoring methods which utilize glucose dehydrogenase nicotine adenine dinucleotide (GDH-NAD), glucose oxidase, or glucose hexokinase are recommended.

Dosage Forms Excipient information presented when available (limited, particularly for generics); consult specific product labeling.

Solution Prefilled Syringe, Subcutaneous [preservative free]:

Orencia: 125 mg/mL (1 mL)

Solution Reconstituted, Intravenous [preservative free]:

Orencia: 250 mg (1 ea)

- ◆ **Abbott-43818** *see* Leuprolide *on page 1229*
- ◆ **Abbott-Citalopram (Can)** *see* Citalopram *on page 476*
- ◆ **Abbott-Levetiracetam (Can)** *see* LevETIRAcetam *on page 1234*
- ◆ **Abbott-Olanzapine ODT (Can)** *see* OLANZapine *on page 1546*
- ◆ **Abbott-Pantoprazole (Can)** *see* Pantoprazole *on page 1618*
- ◆ **Abbott-Quetiapine (Can)** *see* QUEtiapine *on page 1815*
- ◆ **Abbott-Topiramate (Can)** *see* Topiramate *on page 2085*
- ◆ **ABC** *see* Abacavir *on page 34*
- ◆ **ABCD** *see* Amphotericin B Cholesteryl Sulfate Complex *on page 145*
- ◆ **Abelcet** *see* Amphotericin B (Lipid Complex) *on page 151*
- ◆ **Abelcet® (Can)** *see* Amphotericin B (Lipid Complex) *on page 151*
- ◆ **Abenol (Can)** *see* Acetaminophen *on page 44*
- ◆ **Abilify** *see* ARIPiprazole *on page 193*
- ◆ **Abilify Discmelt [DSC]** *see* ARIPiprazole *on page 193*
- ◆ **Abilify Maintena** *see* ARIPiprazole *on page 193*
- ◆ **ABLC** *see* Amphotericin B (Lipid Complex) *on page 151*
- ◆ **Absorica** *see* ISOtretinoin *on page 1171*
- ◆ **Abstral** *see* FentaNYL *on page 857*
- ◆ **ABthrax** *see* Raxibacumab *on page 1841*
- ◆ **Acanya** *see* Clindamycin and Benzoyl Peroxide *on page 493*

Acarbose (AY car bose)

Medication Safety Issues

Sound-alike/look-alike issues:

Precose may be confused with PreCare

High alert medication:

The Institute for Safe Medication Practices (ISMP) includes this medication among its list of drug classes which have a heightened risk of causing significant patient harm when used in error.

International issues:

Precose [US, Malaysia] may be confused with Precosa brand name for *Saccharomyces boulardii* [Finland, Sweden]

Brand Names: US Precose

Brand Names: Canada Glucobay

Therapeutic Category Antidiabetic Agent, Alpha-glucosidase Inhibitor; Antidiabetic Agent, Oral

Generic Availability (US) Yes

Use Management of type II diabetes mellitus (noninsulin-dependent, NIDDM) when hyperglycemia cannot be managed by diet alone; may be used concomitantly with metformin, a sulfonylurea, or insulin to improve glycemic control

Pregnancy Risk Factor B

Pregnancy Considerations Adverse events have not been observed in animal reproduction studies. Low amounts of acarbose are absorbed systemically which should limit fetal exposure.

In women with diabetes, maternal hyperglycemia can be associated with congenital malformations as well as adverse effects in the fetus, neonate, and the mother (ACOG 2005; ADA 2015; Kitzmiller 2008; Metzger 2007). To prevent adverse outcomes, prior to conception and throughout pregnancy maternal blood glucose and HbA_{1c} should be kept as close to target goals as possible but without causing significant hypoglycemia (ACOG 2013; ADA 2015; Blumer 2013; Kitzmiller 2008). Prior to pregnancy, effective contraception should be used until glycemic control is achieved (Kitzmiller 2008). Other agents are currently recommended to treat diabetes in pregnant women (ACOG 2013; Blumer 2013).

Breast-Feeding Considerations It is not known if acarbose is excreted in breast milk; however, low amounts of acarbose are absorbed systemically in adults, which may limit the amount that could distribute into breast milk. Breast-feeding is not recommended by the manufacturer.

Contraindications Hypersensitivity to acarbose or any component of the formulation; diabetic ketoacidosis; cirrhosis; inflammatory bowel disease, colonic ulceration, partial intestinal obstruction, patients predisposed to intestinal obstruction; chronic intestinal diseases associated with marked disorders of digestion or absorption conditions that may deteriorate as a result of increased gas formation in the intestine

Warnings/Precautions Treatment-emergent elevations of serum transaminases (AST and/or ALT) and hyperbilirubinemia may occur (dose-related). These elevations were asymptomatic, reversible, more common in females, and, in general, were not associated with other evidence of liver dysfunction. Fulminant hepatitis (may be fatal) has been reported. If elevations are observed, a reduction in dosage or withdrawal of therapy may be indicated, particularly if the elevations persist. Hypoglycemia is unlikely to occur with acarbose monotherapy but may occur with combination therapy (eg, sulfonylureas, insulin, metformin). In patients taking acarbose, oral glucose (dextrose) should be used instead of sucrose (cane sugar) in the treatment of mild-to-moderate hypoglycemia since the hydrolysis of sucrose to glucose and fructose is inhibited by acarbose. Use with caution in patients with hepatic impairment. Not ▶

recommended in patients with significant impairment (US labeling: serum creatinine >2 mg/dL; Canadian labeling: CrCl <25 mL/minute). It may be necessary to discontinue acarbose and administer insulin if the patient is exposed to stress (ie, fever, trauma, infection, surgery). Potentially significant interactions may exist, requiring dose or frequency adjustment, additional monitoring, and/or selection of alternative therapy. Increased intake of sucrose (cane sugar) and food that contains sucrose during treatment can lead to GI symptoms (eg, flatulence and bloating), loose stools, and occasionally diarrhea. If a diabetic diet is not followed, the GI side effects may be intensified. If severe symptoms develop in spite of adherence to a diabetic diet, temporarily or permanently reduce dose. Diabetes self-management education (DSME) is essential to maximize the effectiveness of therapy.

Adverse Reactions

Gastrointestinal: Diarrhea and abdominal pain tend to return to pretreatment levels over time; frequency and intensity of flatulence tend to abate with time

Hepatic: Transaminases increased

Rare but important or life-threatening: Edema, erythema, exanthema, hepatitis, ileus/subileus, jaundice, liver damage, pneumatosis cystoides intestinalis, rash, thrombocytopenia, urticaria

Drug Interactions

Metabolism/Transport Effects None known.

Avoid Concomitant Use There are no known interactions where it is recommended to avoid concomitant use.

Increased Effect/Toxicity

Acarbose may increase the levels/effects of: Hypoglycemia-Associated Agents

The levels/effects of Acarbose may be increased by: Alpha-Lipoic Acid; Androgens; MAO Inhibitors; Neomycin; Pegvisomant; Quinolone Antibiotics; Salicylates; Selective Serotonin Reuptake Inhibitors

Decreased Effect

Acarbose may decrease the levels/effects of: Digoxin

The levels/effects of Acarbose may be decreased by: Hyperglycemia-Associated Agents; Quinolone Antibiotics; Thiazide Diuretics

Storage/Stability

Store at <25°C (77°F). Protect from moisture.

Canadian labeling: Additional information (not in US labeling): Store tablets in foil pack until ready to use. At storage conditions up to 25°C and below 60% relative humidity, the unpacked tablets can be stored for up to two weeks (discoloration may occur at higher temperatures and/or humidity).

Mechanism of Action Competitive inhibitor of pancreatic α-amylase and intestinal brush border α-glucosidases, resulting in delayed hydrolysis of ingested complex carbohydrates and disaccharides and absorption of glucose; dose-dependent reduction in postprandial serum insulin and glucose peaks; inhibits the metabolism of sucrose to glucose and fructose

Pharmacodynamics Average decrease in fasting blood sugar: 20-30 mg/dL

Pharmacokinetics (Adult data unless noted)

Absorption: <2% absorbed as active drug

Metabolism: Metabolized exclusively within the GI tract, principally by intestinal bacteria and by digestive enzymes; 13 metabolites have been identified

Bioavailability: Low systemic bioavailability of parent compound

Elimination: Fraction absorbed as intact drug is almost completely excreted in urine

Dosing: Usual Oral:

Adolescents and Adults: Dosage must be individualized on the basis of effectiveness and tolerance; do not exceed the maximum recommended dose (use slow titration to prevent or minimize GI effects):

Initial: 25 mg 3 times/day; increase in 25 mg/day increments in 2-4 week intervals to maximum dose

Maximum dose:

Patients ≤60 kg: 50 mg 3 times/day

Patients >60 kg: 100 mg 3 times/day

Dosing adjustment in renal impairment:

Administration Oral: Administer with first bite of each main meal

Monitoring Parameters Fasting blood glucose; hemoglobin A_{1c}; liver enzymes every 3 months for the first year of therapy and periodically thereafter

Reference Range Target range:

Blood glucose: Fasting and preprandial: 80-120 mg/dL; bedtime: 100-140 mg/dL

Glycosylated hemoglobin (hemoglobin A_{1c}): <7%

Additional Information Acarbose has been used successfully to treat postprandial hypoglycemia in children with Nissen fundoplications. Six children (4-25 months) initially received 12.5 mg before each bolus feeding of formula containing complex carbohydrates. The dosage was increased in 12.5 mg increments (dosage range: 12.5-50 mg per dose) until postprandial serum glucose was stable ≥60 mg/dL. Most commonly reported side effects were flatulence, abdominal distension, and diarrhea (Ng, 2001).

Dosage Forms Excipient information presented when available (limited, particularly for generics); consult specific product labeling.

Tablet, Oral:

Precose: 25 mg, 50 mg, 100 mg

Generic: 25 mg, 50 mg, 100 mg

- **Accel-Amlodipine (Can)** *see* AmLODIPine *on page 133*
- **ACCEL-Celecoxib (Can)** *see* Celecoxib *on page 418*
- **Accel-Clarithromycin (Can)** *see* Clarithromycin *on page 482*
- **Accell-Citalopram (Can)** *see* Citalopram *on page 476*
- **Accel-Olanzapine (Can)** *see* OLANZapine *on page 1546*
- **Accolate** *see* Zafirlukast *on page 2203*
- **AccuNeb [DSC]** *see* Albuterol *on page 81*
- **Accupril** *see* Quinapril *on page 1820*
- **Accutane** *see* ISOtretinoin *on page 1171*
- **Acephen [OTC]** *see* Acetaminophen *on page 44*
- **Acerola C 500 [OTC]** *see* Ascorbic Acid *on page 202*
- **Acetadote** *see* Acetylcysteine *on page 57*

Acetaminophen (a seet a MIN oh fen)

Medication Safety Issues

Sound-alike/look-alike issues:

Acephen may be confused with AcipHex

FeverALL may be confused with Fiberall

Triaminic Children's Fever Reducer Pain Reliever may be confused with Triaminic cough and cold products

Tylenol may be confused with atenolol, timolol, Tylenol PM, Tylox

Infusion bottles of ropivacaine and IV acetaminophen look similar. Potentially fatal mix-ups have been reported in which a glass bottle of Naropin was mistaken for Ofirmev in perioperative areas.

Other safety concerns:

Duplicate therapy issues: This product contains acetaminophen, which may be a component of combination products. Do not exceed the maximum recommended daily dose of acetaminophen.

Infant concentration change: All children's and infant acetaminophen products are available as 160 mg/5 mL. Some remaining infant concentrated solutions of 80 mg/0.8 mL and 100 mg/mL may still be available on pharmacy shelves or in patient homes. Check concentrations closely prior to administering or dispensing and verify concentration available to patients prior to recommending a dose (November 2011).

Injection: Reports of 10-fold overdose errors using the parenteral product have occurred in the U.S. and Europe; calculation of doses in "mg" and subsequent administration of the dose in "mL" using the commercially available concentration of 10 mg/mL contributed to these errors. Expressing doses as mg **and** mL, as well as pharmacy preparation of doses, may decrease error potential (Dart, 2012; ISMP, 2012).

International issues:

Depon [Greece] may be confused with Depen brand name for penicillamine [U.S.]; Depin brand name for nifedipine [India]; Dipen brand name for diltiazem [Greece]

Duorol [Spain] may be confused with Diuril brand name for chlorothiazide [U.S., Canada]

Paralen [Czech Republic] may be confused with Aralen brand name for chloroquine [U.S., Mexico]

Related Information

Acetaminophen Serum Level Nomogram *on page 2449*

Oral Medications That Should Not Be Crushed or Altered *on page 2476*

Brand Names: US Acephen [OTC]; Aspirin Free Anacin Extra Strength [OTC]; Cetafen Extra [OTC]; Cetafen [OTC]; FeverAll Adult [OTC]; FeverAll Childrens [OTC]; FeverAll Infants [OTC]; FeverAll Junior Strength [OTC]; Little Fevers [OTC]; Mapap Arthritis Pain [OTC]; Mapap Children's [OTC]; Mapap Extra Strength [OTC]; Mapap Infant's [OTC]; Mapap [OTC]; Non-Aspirin Pain Reliever [OTC]; Nortemp Children's [OTC]; Ofirmev; Pain & Fever Children's [OTC]; Pain Eze [OTC]; Pharbetol Extra Strength [OTC]; Pharbetol [OTC]; Q-Pap Children's [OTC]; Q-Pap Extra Strength [OTC]; Q-Pap Infant's [OTC]; Q-Pap [OTC]; Silapap Children's [OTC]; Silapap Infant's [OTC]; Triaminic Children's Fever Reducer Pain Reliever [OTC]; Tylenol 8 Hour [OTC]; Tylenol Arthritis Pain [OTC]; Tylenol Children's Meltaways [OTC] [DSC]; Tylenol Children's [OTC]; Tylenol Extra Strength [OTC]; Tylenol Jr. Meltaways [OTC]; Tylenol [OTC]; Valorin Extra [OTC]; Valorin [OTC]

Brand Names: Canada Abenol; Apo-Acetaminophen; Atasol; Novo-Gesic; Pediatrix; Tempra; Tylenol

Therapeutic Category Analgesic, Non-narcotic; Antipyretic

Generic Availability (US) Yes: Excludes extended release products; injectable formulation

Use

Oral:

Immediate release:

Oral suspension, chewable tablets: Relief of minor aches and pains due to the common cold, flu, sore throat, headaches, and toothaches; reduction of fever (All indications: OTC products: FDA approved in infants and children <12 years; consult specific product formulations for appropriate age groups)

Caplet/tablet: Relief of minor aches and pains due to the common cold, headaches, minor pain of arthritis, backache, menstrual cramps, muscle aches, and toothaches (All indications: OTC products: FDA approved in ages ≥6 years and adults; consult specific product formulation for appropriate age group)

Extended release: Relief of minor aches and pains due to the common cold, headaches, backache, muscle aches, menstrual cramps, toothaches, and minor pain of arthritis; reduction of fever (All indications: OTC products: FDA approved in ages ≥12 or 18 years and adults; consult specific product formulations for appropriate age groups)

Parenteral: Treatment of mild to moderate pain and fever; treatment of moderate to severe pain when combined with opioid analgesia (All indications: FDA approved in ages ≥2 years and adults)

Rectal: Relief of minor aches, pains, and headaches; reduction of fever (All indications: OTC products: FDA approved in ages ≥6 months and adults; consult specific product formulation for appropriate age group); has also been used for management of postoperative pain

Pregnancy Risk Factor C

Pregnancy Considerations Adverse events were observed in some animal reproduction studies. Acetaminophen crosses the placenta and can be detected in cord blood, newborn serum, and urine immediately after delivery (Levy, 1975; Naga Rani, 1989; Wang, 1997). An increased risk of teratogenic effects has not been observed following maternal use of acetaminophen during pregnancy. Prenatal constriction of the ductus arteriosus has been noted in case reports following maternal use during the third trimester (Suhag, 2008; Wood, 2005). The use of acetaminophen in normal doses during pregnancy is not associated with an increased risk of miscarriage or still birth; however, an increase in fetal death or spontaneous abortion may be seen following maternal overdose if treatment is delayed (Li, 2003; Rebordosa, 2009; Riggs, 1989). Frequent maternal use of acetaminophen during pregnancy may be associated with wheezing and asthma in early childhood (Perzanowki, 2010).

Breast-Feeding Considerations Low concentrations of acetaminophen are excreted into breast milk and can be detected in the urine of nursing infants (Notarianni, 1987). Adverse reactions have generally not been observed; however, a rash caused by acetaminophen exposure was reported in one breast-feeding infant (Matheson, 1985). The manufacturer recommends that caution be used if administered to a nursing woman.

Contraindications

Injection: Hypersensitivity to acetaminophen or any component of the formulation; severe hepatic impairment or severe active liver disease

OTC labeling: When used for self-medication, do not use with other drug products containing acetaminophen or if allergic to acetaminophen or any of the inactive ingredients

Warnings/Precautions [Injection: U.S. Boxed Warning]: Acetaminophen has been associated with acute liver failure, at times resulting in liver transplant and death. Hepatotoxicity is usually associated with excessive acetaminophen intake and often involves more than one product that contains acetaminophen. Do not exceed the maximum recommended daily dose (>4 g daily in adults). In addition, chronic daily dosing may also result in liver damage in some patients. Limit acetaminophen dose from all sources (prescription, OTC, combination products) and all routes of administration (IV, oral, rectal) to ≤4 g/day (adults). Use with caution in patients with alcoholic liver disease; consuming ≥3 alcoholic drinks/day may increase the risk of liver damage. Use caution in patients with hepatic impairment or active liver disease; use of IV formulation is contraindicated in patients with severe hepatic impairment or severe active liver disease.

[Injection: U.S. Boxed Warning]: Take care to avoid dosing errors with acetaminophen injection, which could result in accidental overdose and death; ensure that the dose in mg is not confused with mL, dosing in patients <50 kg is based on body weight, infusion pumps are properly programmed, and total daily dose

of acetaminophen from all sources does not exceed the maximum daily limits.

Hypersensitivity and anaphylactic reactions have been reported including life-threatening anaphylaxis; discontinue immediately if symptoms occur. Serious and potentially fatal skin reactions, including acute generalized exanthematous pustulosis (AGEP), Stevens-Johnson syndrome (SJS), and toxic epidermal necrolysis (TEN), have occurred rarely with acetaminophen use. Discontinue therapy at the first appearance of skin rash.

Benzyl alcohol and derivatives: Some dosage forms may contain benzyl alcohol and/or sodium benzoate/benzoic acid; benzoic acid (benzoate) is a metabolite of benzyl alcohol; large amounts of benzyl alcohol (≥99 mg/kg/day) have been associated with a potentially fatal toxicity ("gasping syndrome") in neonates; the "gasping syndrome" consists of metabolic acidosis, respiratory distress, gasping respirations, CNS dysfunction (including convulsions, intracranial hemorrhage), hypotension and cardiovascular collapse (AAP, 1997; CDC, 1982); some data suggests that benzoate displaces bilirubin from protein binding sites (Ahlfors, 2001); avoid or use dosage forms containing benzyl alcohol and/or benzyl alcohol derivative with caution in neonates. See manufacturer's labeling.

Polysorbate 80: Some dosage forms may contain polysorbate 80 (also known as Tweens). Hypersensitivity reactions, usually a delayed reaction, have been reported following exposure to pharmaceutical products containing polysorbate 80 in certain individuals (Isaksson, 2002; Lucente 2000; Shelley, 1995). Thrombocytopenia, ascites, pulmonary deterioration, and renal and hepatic failure have been reported in premature neonates after receiving parenteral products containing polysorbate 80 (Alade, 1986; CDC, 1984). See manufacturer's labeling. Some products may contain aspartame which is metabolized to phenylalanine and must be avoided (or used with caution) in patients with phenylketonuria.

Propylene glycol: Some dosage forms may contain propylene glycol; large amounts are potentially toxic and have been associated hyperosmolality, lactic acidosis, seizures, and respiratory depression; use caution (AAP, 1997; Zar, 2007).

When used for self-medication (OTC), patients should be instructed to contact healthcare provider if symptoms get worse or new symptoms appear, redness or swelling is present in the painful area, fever lasts >3 days (all ages), or pain (excluding sore throat) lasts longer than: Adults: 10 days, Children and Adolescents: 5 days, Infants: 3 days. When treating children with sore throat, if sore throat is severe, persists for >2 days, or is followed by fever, rash, headache, nausea, or vomiting, consult health care provider immediately.

Use with caution in patients with chronic malnutrition or severe renal impairment; use intravenous formulation with caution in patients with severe hypovolemia. Use with caution in patients with known G6PD deficiency.

Warnings: Additional Pediatric Considerations Some dosage forms may contain propylene glycol; in neonates large amounts of propylene glycol delivered orally, intravenously (eg, >3,000 mg/day), or topically have been associated with potentially fatal toxicities which can include metabolic acidosis, seizures, renal failure, and CNS depression; toxicities have also been reported in children and adults including hyperosmolality, lactic acidosis, seizures and respiratory depression; use caution (AAP, 1997; Shehab, 2009).

Adverse Reactions Oral, Rectal:

Dermatologic: Skin rash

Endocrine & metabolic: Decreased serum bicarbonate, decreased serum calcium, decreased serum sodium, hyperchloremia, hyperuricemia, increased serum glucose

Genitourinary: Nephrotoxicity (with chronic overdose)

Hematologic & oncologic: Anemia, leukopenia, neutropenia, pancytopenia

Hepatic: Increased serum alkaline phosphatase, increased serum bilirubin

Hypersensitivity: Hypersensitivity reaction (rare)

Renal: Hyperammonemia, renal disease (analgesic)

IV:

Cardiovascular: Hypertension, hypotension, peripheral edema, tachycardia

Central nervous system: Agitation (children), anxiety, fatigue, headache (more common in adults), insomnia (more common in adults), trismus

Dermatologic: Pruritus (children), skin rash

Endocrine & metabolic: Hypervolemia, hypoalbuminemia, hypokalemia, hypomagnesemia, hypophosphatemia

Gastrointestinal: Abdominal pain, diarrhea, headache (more common in adults), insomnia (more common in adults), nausea (more common in adults), vomiting (more common in adults)

Genitourinary: Oliguria (children)

Hematologic & oncologic: Anemia

Hepatic: Increased serum transaminases

Local: Infusion site reaction (pain)

Neuromuscular & skeletal: Limb pain, muscle spasm

Ophthalmic: Periorbital edema

Respiratory: Abnormal breath sounds, atelectasis (children), dyspnea, hypoxia, pleural effusion, pulmonary edema, stridor, wheezing

Miscellaneous: Fever

Rare but important or life-threatening: Anaphylaxis, hepatic injury (dose-related), hypersensitivity reaction, severe dermatological reaction (acute generalized exanthematous pustulosis, Stevens-Johnson syndrome, toxic epidermal necrolysis)

Drug Interactions

Metabolism/Transport Effects Substrate of CYP1A2 (minor), CYP2A6 (minor), CYP2C9 (minor), CYP2D6 (minor), CYP2E1 (minor), CYP3A4 (minor); **Note** Assignment of Major/Minor substrate status based on clinically relevant drug interaction potential

Avoid Concomitant Use There are no known interactions where it is recommended to avoid concomitant use.

Increased Effect/Toxicity

Acetaminophen may increase the levels/effects of: Busulfan; Dasatinib; Imatinib; Mipomersen; Phenylephrine (Systemic); Prilocaine; Sodium Nitrite; SORAfenib; Vitamin K Antagonists

The levels/effects of Acetaminophen may be increased by: Alcohol (Ethyl); Dasatinib; Isoniazid; Metyrapone; Nitric Oxide; Probenecid; SORAfenib

Decreased Effect

The levels/effects of Acetaminophen may be decreased by: Barbiturates; CarBAMazepine; Cholestyramine Resin; Fosphenytoin-Phenytoin

Food Interactions Rate of absorption may be decreased when given with food. Management: Administer without regard to food.

Storage/Stability

Injection: Store intact vials at 20°C to 25°C (68°F to 77°F); do not refrigerate or freeze. Use within 6 hours of opening vial or transferring to another container. Discard any unused portion.

Oral formulations: Store at 20°C to 25°C (68°F to 77°F); avoid excessive heat (20°C [104°F]). Avoid high humidity (chewable tablets).

Suppositories: Store at 2°C to 27°C (25°F to 80°F); do not freeze.

Mechanism of Action Although not fully elucidated, believed to inhibit the synthesis of prostaglandins in the central nervous system and work peripherally to block pain impulse generation; produces antipyresis from inhibition of hypothalamic heat-regulating center

Pharmacodynamics

Onset of action:

- Oral: <1 hour
- IV: Analgesia: 5 to 10 minutes; Antipyretic: Within 30 minutes

Peak effect: IV: Analgesia: 1 hour

Duration:

- IV, Oral: Analgesia: 4 to 6 hours
- IV: Antipyretic: ≥6 hours

Pharmacokinetics (Adult data unless noted) Note: With the exception of half-life (see below), the pharmacokinetic profile in pediatric patients (0-18 years) is similar to adult patients.

Absorption: Primarily absorbed in small intestine (rate of absorption dependent upon gastric emptying); minimal absorption from stomach; varies by dosage form

Distribution: ~1 L/kg at therapeutic doses

Protein binding: 10% to 25% at therapeutic concentrations; 8% to 43% at toxic concentrations

Metabolism: At normal therapeutic dosages, primarily hepatic metabolism to sulfate and glucuronide conjugates, while a small amount is metabolized by CYP2E1 to a highly reactive intermediate N-acetyl-p-benzoquinone imine (NAPQI), which is conjugated rapidly with glutathione and inactivated to nontoxic cysteine and mercapturic acid conjugates. At toxic doses (as little as 4000 mg in a single day), glutathione conjugation becomes insufficient to meet the metabolic demand causing an increase in NAPQI concentrations, which may cause hepatic cell necrosis. Oral administration is subject to first-pass metabolism.

Half-life:

- Neonates: ~7 hours
- Infants: ~4 hours
- Children and Adolescents: ~3 hours
- Adults: ~2 hours; severe renal insufficiency (CrCl <30 mL/minute): 2 to 5.3 hours

Time to peak serum concentration:

- Oral: Immediate release: 10 to 60 minutes (may be delayed in acute overdoses)
- IV: 15 minutes

Elimination: Urine (<5% unchanged; 60% to 80% as glucuronide metabolites; 20% to 30% as sulfate metabolites; ~8% cysteine and mercapturic acid metabolites)

Dosing: Neonatal

Pain or fever:

Oral:

- GA 28 to 32 weeks: 10 to 12 mg/kg/dose every 6 to 8 hours; maximum daily dose: 40 mg/kg/**day** (Anand 2001; Anand 2002)
- GA 33 to 37 weeks or term neonates <10 days: 10 to 15 mg/kg/dose every 6 hours; maximum daily dose: 60 mg/kg/**day** (Anand 2001; Anand 2002)
- Term neonates ≥10 days: 10 to 15 mg/kg/dose every 4 to 6 hours (Anand 2001; Anand 2002); do not exceed 5 doses in 24 hours; maximum daily dose: 75 mg/kg/**day**

IV: Limited data available; dose not established; **Note:** Some experts do not recommend the use of IV acetaminophen in premature neonates <32 weeks PMA until pharmacokinetic and pharmacodynamic studies have been conducted in this age group (van den Anker 2011).

Loading dose (Allegaert 2007; Bartocci 2007): 20 mg/kg/dose

Maintenance dose (Allegaert 2007; Allegaert 2011; Bartocci 2007):

- PMA 28 to 32 weeks: 10 mg/kg/dose every 12 hours; some suggest 7.5 mg/kg/dose every 8 hours; maximum daily dose: 22.5 mg/kg/**day**
- PMA 33 to 36 weeks: 10 mg/kg/dose every 8 hours; some suggest 7.5 to 10 mg/kg/dose every 6 hours; maximum daily dose: 40 mg/kg/**day**
- PMA ≥37 weeks: 10 mg/kg/dose every 6 hours; maximum daily dose: 40 mg/kg/**day**
- **Note**: Manufacturer neonatal pharmacokinetic data suggests that 7.5 mg/kg/dose every 6 hours produces a similar pharmacokinetic exposure as standard dosing in children ≥2 years.

Rectal:

- GA 28 to 32 weeks: 20 mg/kg/dose every 12 hours; maximum daily dose: 40 mg/kg/**day** (Anand 2001; Anand 2002)
- GA 33 to 37 weeks or term neonates <10 days: Loading dose: 30 mg/kg; then 15 mg/kg/dose every 8 hours; maximum daily dose: 60 mg/kg/**day** (Anand 2001; Anand 2002)
- Term infants ≥10 days: Loading dose: 30 mg/kg; then 20 mg/kg/dose every 6 to 8 hours (Anand 2001; Anand 2002); do not exceed 5 doses in 24 hours; maximum daily dose: 75 mg/kg/**day**

Dosing: Usual Note: In 2011, McNeil Consumer Healthcare reduced the maximum daily doses and increased the dosing interval on the labeling of some of their acetaminophen OTC products used in older pediatric patients (usually children ≥12 years and adolescents) and adults in an attempt to protect consumers from inadvertent overdoses. For example, the maximum daily dose of Extra Strength Tylenol OTC and Regular Strength Tylenol OTC were decreased to 3000 mg/day and 3250 mg/day respectively, and the dosing interval for Extra Strength Tylenol OTC was increased. Health care professionals may still prescribe or recommend the 4 g adult daily maximum to patients ≥12 years of age (but are advised to use their own discretion and clinical judgment) (McNeil Consumer Healthcare 2014).

Pediatric:

Pain (mild to moderate) or fever: Note: Limit acetaminophen dose from all sources (prescription and OTC); maximum daily dose of acetaminophen should be limited to ≤75 mg/kg/day in ≤5 divided doses and not to exceed 4000 mg/day for most products although some formulations suggest lower maximum daily dosing (see dosing information for further detail):

Oral: **Note:** With OTC use, should not exceed recommended treatment duration unless directed by health care provider; for fever: 3 days (all ages); pain (excluding sore throat): Children ≥ 12 years and adolescents: 10 days, children: 5 days, or infants: 3 days; sore throat in children: 2 days

Weight-directed dosing: Infants, Children, and Adolescents: 10 to 15 mg/kg/dose every 4 to 6 hours as needed (American Pain Society 2008; Kliegman 2011; Sullivan 2011); do not exceed 5 doses in 24 hours; maximum daily dose: 75 mg/kg/**day** not to exceed 4,000 mg/**day**

Fixed dosing:

Oral suspension, chewable tablets: Infants and Children <12 years: Consult specific product formulations for appropriate age groups. See table; use of weight to select dose is preferred; if weight is not available, then use age; doses may be repeated every 4 hours; maximum: 5 doses/day

Acetaminophen Dosing (Oral)[1]

Weight (kg)	Weight (lbs)	Age	Dosage (mg)
2.7 to 5.3	6 to 11	0 to 3 mo	40
5.4 to 8.1	12 to 17	4 to 11 mo	80
8.2 to 10.8	18 to 23	1 to 2 y	120
10.9 to 16.3	24 to 35	2 to 3 y	160
16.4 to 21.7	36 to 47	4 to 5 y	240
21.8 to 27.2	48 to 59	6 to 8 y	320
27.3 to 32.6	60 to 71	9 to 10 y	400
32.7 to 43.2	72 to 95	11 y	480

[1]Manufacturer's recommendations are based on weight in pounds (OTC labeling); weight in kg listed here is derived from pounds and rounded; kg weight listed also is adjusted to allow for continuous weight ranges in kg. OTC labeling instructs consumer to consult with physician for dosing instructions in infants and children under 2 years of age.

Immediate release solid dosage formulations: **Note:** Actual OTC dosing recommendations may vary by product and/or manufacturer:

Children 6 to 11 years: 325 mg every 4 to 6 hours; maximum daily dose: 1,625 mg/**day**; **Note:** Do not use more than 5 days unless directed by a physician

Children ≥12 years and Adolescents:

Regular strength: 650 mg every 4 to 6 hours; maximum daily dose: 3,250 mg/**day** unless directed by a physician; under physician supervision daily doses ≤4,000 mg may be used

Extra strength: 1,000 mg every 6 hours; maximum daily dose: 3,000 mg/**day** unless directed by a physician; under physician supervision daily doses ≤4,000 mg may be used

Extended release: Children ≥12 years and Adolescents: 1,300 mg every 8 hours; maximum daily dose: 3,900 mg/**day**

IV:

Infants and Children <2 years: Limited data available: 7.5 to 15 mg/kg/dose every 6 hours; maximum daily dose: 60 mg/kg/**day** (Wilson-Smith, 2009)

Children ≥2 years and Adolescents:

<50 kg: 15 mg/kg/dose every 6 hours **or** 12.5 mg/kg/dose every 4 hours; maximum single dose: 15 mg/kg up to 750 mg; maximum daily dose: 75 mg/kg/**day** not to exceed 3,750 mg/**day**

≥50 kg: 1,000 mg every 6 hours **or** 650 mg every 4 hours; maximum single dose: 1,000 mg; maximum daily dose: 4,000 mg/**day**

Rectal:

Weight-directed dosing: Infants and Children <12 years: 10 to 20 mg/kg/dose every 4 to 6 hours as needed; **do not exceed 5 doses in 24 hours** (Kliegman 2011; Vernon 1979); maximum daily dose: 75 mg/kg/day

Fixed dosing:

Infants 6 to 11 months: 80 mg every 6 hours; maximum daily dose: 320 mg/**day**

Infants and Children 12 to 36 months: 80 mg every 4 to 6 hours; maximum daily dose: 400 mg/**day**

Children >3 to 6 years: 120 mg every 4 to 6 hours; maximum daily dose: 600 mg/**day**

Children >6 up to 12 years: 325 mg every 4 to 6 hours; maximum daily dose: 1,625 mg/**day**

Children ≥12 years and Adolescents: 650 mg every 4 to 6 hours; maximum daily dose: 3,900 mg/**day**

Pain; peri-/postoperative management; adjunct to opioid therapy:

IV:

Infants and Children <2 years: Limited data available: 7.5 to 15 mg/kg/dose every 6 hours; maximum daily dose: 60 mg/kg/**day** (Wilson-Smith, 2009)

Children ≥2 years and Adolescents:

<50 kg: 15 mg/kg/dose every 6 hours **or** 12.5 mg/kg/dose every 4 hours; maximum single dose: 15 mg/kg up to 750 mg; maximum daily dose: 75 mg/kg/**day** not to exceed 3,750 mg/**day**

≥50 kg: 1,000 mg every 6 hours or 650 mg every 4 hours; maximum single dose: 1,000 mg; maximum daily dose: 4,000 mg/day

Rectal: Limited data available: Children and Adolescents:

Loading dose: 40 mg/kg for 1 dose, in most trials, the dose was administered postoperatively (Birmingham 2001; Capici 2008; Hahn 2000; Mireskandari 2011; Prins 2008; Riad 2007; Viitanen 2003); a maximum dose of 1,000 mg was most frequently reported. However, in one trial evaluating 24 older pediatric patients (all patients ≥25 kg; mean age: ~13 years), the data suggested that a dose of 1,000 mg does not produce therapeutic serum concentrations (target for study: >10 mcg/mL) compared to a 40 mg/kg dose (up to ~2,000 mg); the resultant C_{max} was: 7.8 mcg/mL (1,000 mg dose group) vs 15.9 mcg/mL (40 mg/kg dose group). **Note:** Therapeutic serum concentrations for analgesia have not been well-established (Howell 2003).

Maintenance dose: 20 to 25 mg/kg/dose every 6 hours as needed for 2 to 3 days has been suggested if further pain control is needed postoperatively; maximum daily dose: 100 mg/kg/day; therapy longer than 5 days has not been evaluated (Birmingham 2001; Hahn 2000; Prins 2008).

Note: In the majority of trials, suppositories were not divided due to unequal distribution of drug within suppository; doses were rounded to the nearest mg amount using 1 or 2 suppositories of available product strengths.

Adult: **Note:** Limit acetaminophen dose from all sources (prescription and OTC) to <4 g/day. No dose adjustment required when converting between different acetaminophen formulations:

Pain or fever:

IV:

<50 kg: 15 mg/kg every 6 hours or 12.5 mg/kg every 4 hours; maximum single dose: 15 mg/kg up to 750 mg; maximum daily dose: 75 mg/kg/**day** (≤3,750 mg/day)

≥50 kg: 1,000 mg every 6 hours or 650 mg every 4 hours; maximum single dose: 1,000 mg/dose; maximum daily dose: 4,000 mg/**day**

Oral:

Immediate release: **Note:** Actual OTC dosing recommendations may vary by product and/or manufacturer: 325 to 650 mg every 4 to 6 hours or 1,000 mg 3 to 4 times/day; maximum daily dose: 4,000 mg/**day**

Extended release: 1,300 mg every 8 hours; maximum daily dose: 3,900 mg/**day**

Rectal: 325 to 650 mg every 4 to 6 hours or 1,000 mg 3 to 4 times daily; maximum daily dose: 4,000 mg/**day**

Dosing adjustment in renal impairment:

IV: Children ≥2 years, Adolescents, and Adults: CrCl ≤30 mL/minute: Use with caution; consider decreasing daily dose and extending dosing interval

Oral (Aronoff 2007):
Infants, Children, and Adolescents:
GFR ≥10 mL/minute/1.73 m^2: No adjustment required
GFR <10 mL/minute/1.73 m^2: Administer every 8 hours
Intermittent hemodialysis or peritoneal dialysis: Administer every 8 hours
CRRT: No adjustments necessary
Adults:
CrCl 10 to 50 mL/minute: Administer every 6 hours
CrCl <10 mL/minute: Administer every 8 hours
Intermittent hemodialysis or peritoneal dialysis: No adjustment necessary
CRRT: Administer every 8 hours

Dosing adjustment in hepatic impairment: Use with caution. Limited, low-dose therapy is usually well-tolerated in hepatic disease/cirrhosis; however, cases of hepatotoxicity at daily acetaminophen dosages <4,000 mg/day have been reported. Avoid chronic use in hepatic impairment.

Preparation for Administration
Parenteral: Injectable solution may be administered directly from the vial without further dilution. Use within 6 hours of opening vial or transferring to another container. Discard any unused portion; single-use vials only.
Doses <1,000 mg (<50 kg): Withdraw appropriate dose from vial and transfer to a separate sterile container (eg, glass bottle, plastic IV container, syringe) for administration. Small volume pediatric doses (up to 600 mg [60 mL]) may be placed in a syringe and infused over 15 minutes via syringe pump.
Doses of 1,000 mg (≥50 kg): Insert vented IV set through vial stopper.

Administration
Oral: Administer with food to decrease GI upset; shake drops and suspension well before use; do not crush or chew extended release products
Parenteral: For IV infusion only. May administer undiluted over 15 minutes. Use within 6 hours of opening vial or transferring to another container. Discard any unused portion; single-use vials only.
Rectal: Remove wrapper; insert suppository well up into the rectum.

Test Interactions Acetaminophen may cause false-positive urinary 5-hydroxyindoleacetic acid.

Additional Information 2 mg propacetamol (prodrug) = 1 mg paracetamol = 1 mg acetaminophen
Drops may contain saccharin.
Acetaminophen (15 mg/kg/dose given orally every 6 hours for 24 hours) did **not** relieve the intraoperative or the immediate postoperative pain associated with neonatal circumcision; some benefit was seen 6 hours after circumcision (Howard, 1994).
There is currently no scientific evidence to support alternating acetaminophen with ibuprofen in the treatment of fever (Mayoral, 2000).
Based on recommendations provided by the Food and Drug Administration (FDA), all over-the-counter (OTC) pediatric single-ingredient acetaminophen liquid products are noow only available as a single concentration of 160 mg/5 mL; the transition began in 2011. The concentration 80 mg/0.8 mL is no longer available in the US. The recommended mg/kg dose is unaffected.

Dosage Forms Excipient information presented when available (limited, particularly for generics); consult specific product labeling. [DSC] = Discontinued product
Caplet, oral: 500 mg
Cetafen Extra: 500 mg
Mapap Extra Strength: 500 mg
Mapap Extra Strength: 500 mg [scored]
Pain Eze: 650 mg
Tylenol: 325 mg
Tylenol Extra Strength: 500 mg
Caplet, extended release, oral:
Mapap Arthritis Pain: 650 mg
Tylenol 8 Hour: 650 mg
Tylenol Arthritis Pain: 650 mg
Capsule, oral:
Mapap Extra Strength: 500 mg
Elixir, oral:
Mapap Children's: 160 mg/5 mL (118 mL, 480 mL) [ethanol free; contains benzoic acid, propylene glycol, sodium benzoate; cherry flavor]
Injection, solution [preservative free]:
Ofirmev: 10 mg/mL (100 mL)
Liquid, oral: 160 mg/5 mL (120 mL, 473 mL); 500 mg/5 mL (240 mL)
Mapap Extra Strength: 500 mg/5 mL (237 mL) [contains propylene glycol, sodium 9 mg/15 mL, sodium benzoate; cherry flavor]
Q-Pap Children's: 160 mg/5 mL (118 mL, 473 mL) [ethanol free; contains propylene glycol, sodium 2 mg/5 mL, sodium benzoate; cherry flavor]
Q-Pap Children's: 160 mg/5 mL (118 mL) [ethanol free; contains propylene glycol, sodium 2 mg/5 mL, sodium benzoate; grape flavor]
Silapap Children's: 160 mg/5 mL (118 mL, 237 mL, 473 mL) [ethanol free, sugar free; contains propylene glycol, sodium benzoate; cherry flavor]
Tylenol Extra Strength: 500 mg/15 mL (240 mL) [ethanol free; contains propylene glycol, sodium benzoate; cherry flavor]
Solution, oral: 160 mg/5 mL (5 mL, 10 mL, 20 mL)
Pain & Fever Children's: 160 mg/5 mL (118 mL, 473 mL) [ethanol free, sugar free; contains propylene glycol, sodium 1 mg/5 mL, sodium benzoate; cherry flavor]
Solution, oral [drops]: 80 mg/0.8 mL (15 mL [DSC])
Little Fevers: 80 mg/mL (30 mL [DSC]) [dye free, ethanol free, gluten free; contains propylene glycol, sodium benzoate; berry flavor]
Q-Pap Infant's: 80 mg/0.8 mL (15 mL) [ethanol free; contains propylene glycol; fruit flavor]
Silapap Infant's: 80 mg/0.8 mL (15 mL, 30 mL) [ethanol free; contains propylene glycol, sodium benzoate; cherry flavor]
Suppository, rectal: 120 mg (12s); 325 mg (12s); 650 mg (12s)
Acephen: 120 mg (12s, 50s, 100s); 325 mg (6s, 12s, 50s, 100s); 650 mg (12s, 50s, 100s)
FeverAll Adults: 650 mg (50s)
FeverAll Childrens: 120 mg (6s, 50s)
FeverAll Infants: 80 mg (6s, 50s)
FeverAll Junior Strength: 325 mg (6s, 50s)
Suspension, oral: 160 mg/5 mL (5 mL, 10.15 mL, 20.3 mL)
Mapap Children's: 160 mg/5 mL (118 mL) [ethanol free; contains propylene glycol, sodium benzoate; cherry flavor]
Mapap Infant's: 160 mg/5 mL (59 mL) [dye free, ethanol free; contains propylene glycol, sodium benzoate; cherry flavor]
Nortemp Children's: 160 mg/5 mL (118 mL) [ethanol free; contains propylene glycol, sodium benzoate; cotton candy flavor]
Pain & Fever Children's: 160 mg/5 mL (60 mL) [ethanol free; contains propylene glycol, sodium benzoate; cherry flavor]
Q-Pap Children's: 160 mg/5 mL (118 mL) [ethanol free; contains sodium 2 mg/5 mL, sodium benzoate; bubblegum flavor]
Q-Pap Children's: 160 mg/5 mL (118 mL) [ethanol free; contains sodium 2 mg/5 mL, sodium benzoate; cherry flavor]
Q-Pap Children's: 160 mg/5 mL (118 mL) [ethanol free; contains sodium 2 mg/5 mL, sodium benzoate; grape flavor]

Tylenol Children's: 160 mg/5 mL (120 mL) [dye free, ethanol free; contains propylene glycol, sodium benzoate; cherry flavor]
Tylenol Children's: 160 mg/5 mL (120 mL) [ethanol free; contains propylene glycol, sodium 2 mg/5 mL, sodium benzoate; bubblegum flavor]
Tylenol Children's: 160 mg/5 mL (60 mL, 120 mL) [ethanol free; contains propylene glycol, sodium 2 mg/5 mL, sodium benzoate; cherry flavor]
Tylenol Children's: 160 mg/5 mL (120 mL) [ethanol free; contains propylene glycol, sodium 2 mg/5 mL, sodium benzoate; grape flavor]
Tylenol Children's: 160 mg/5 mL (120 mL) [ethanol free; contains propylene glycol, sodium 2 mg/5 mL, sodium benzoate; strawberry flavor]

Syrup, oral:
Triaminic Children's Fever Reducer Pain Reliever: 160 mg/5 mL (118 mL) [contains benzoic acid, sodium 6 mg/5 mL; bubblegum flavor]
Triaminic Children's Fever Reducer Pain Reliever: 160 mg/5 mL (118 mL) [contains sodium 5 mg/5 mL, sodium benzoate; grape flavor]

Tablet, oral: 325 mg, 500 mg
Aspirin Free Anacin Extra Strength: 500 mg
Cetafen: 325 mg
Mapap: 325 mg
Mapap Extra Strength: 500 mg
Non-Aspirin Pain Reliever: 325 mg
Pharbetol: 325 mg
Pharbetol Extra Strength: 500 mg
Q-Pap: 325 mg [scored]
Q-Pap Extra Strength: 500 mg [scored]
Tylenol: 325 mg
Tylenol Extra Strength: 500 mg
Valorin: 325 mg [sugar free]
Valorin Extra: 500 mg [sugar free]

Tablet, chewable, oral: 80 mg
Mapap Children's: 80 mg [fruit flavor]

Tablet, dipersible, oral: 80 mg, 160 mg
Mapap Children's: 80 mg [bubblegum flavor]
Mapap Children's: 80 mg [grape flavor]
Tylenol Children's Meltaways: 80 mg [scored; bubblegum flavor] [DSC]
Tylenol Children's Meltaways: 80 mg [scored; grape flavor] [DSC]
Tylenol Jr. Meltaways: 160 mg [bubblegum flavor]
Tylenol Jr. Meltaways: 160 mg [grape flavor]

Acetaminophen and Codeine

(a seet a MIN oh fen & KOE deen)

Medication Safety Issues

Sound-alike/look-alike issues:
Procet-30 may be confused with Percocet
Tylenol may be confused with atenolol, timolol, Tylox

High alert medication:
The Institute for Safe Medication Practices (ISMP) includes this medication among its list of drug classes which have a heightened risk of causing significant patient harm when used in error.

Other safety concerns:
Duplicate therapy issues: This product contains acetaminophen, which may be a component of other combination products. Do not exceed the maximum recommended daily dose of acetaminophen.
T3 is an error-prone abbreviation (mistaken as liothyronine)

International issues:
Codex: Brand name for acetaminophen/codeine [Brazil], but also the brand name for *saccharomyces boulardii* [Italy]
Codex [Brazil] may be confused with Cedax brand name for ceftibuten [US and multiple international markets]

Brand Names: US Capital/Codeine; Tylenol with Codeine #3; Tylenol with Codeine #4

Brand Names: Canada Acet-Codeine; PMS-Acetaminophen with Codeine Elixir; Procet-30; ratio-Emtec-30; ratio-Lenoltec; Triatec-30; Triatec-8; Triatec-8 Forte; Tylenol No. 1; Tylenol No. 1 Forte; Tylenol No. 2 with Codeine; Tylenol No. 3 with Codeine; Tylenol No. 4 with Codeine

Therapeutic Category Analgesic, Narcotic

Generic Availability (US) May be product dependent

Use Relief of mild to moderate pain (FDA approved in ages ≥3 years and adults)

Pregnancy Risk Factor C

Pregnancy Considerations Animal reproduction studies have not been conducted with this combination. Refer to individual monographs.

Breast-Feeding Considerations Acetaminophen and codeine are excreted in breast milk. Refer to individual monographs.

Contraindications
Hypersensitivity to acetaminophen, codeine, or any component of the formulation; postoperative pain management in children who have undergone tonsillectomy and/or adenoidectomy
Canadian labeling: Additional contraindications (not in US labeling): Use in pediatric patients <12 years. Some products may contraindicate use in patients <18 years (refer to specific product labeling).

Warnings/Precautions [US Boxed Warning]: Respiratory depression and death have occurred in children who received codeine following tonsillectomy and/or adenoidectomy and were found to have evidence of being ultrarapid metabolizers of codeine due to a CYP2D6 polymorphism. Deaths have also occurred in nursing infants after being exposed to high concentrations of morphine because the mothers were ultrarapid metabolizers. Use of codeine is contraindicated in the postoperative pain management of children who have undergone tonsillectomy and/or adenoidectomy. Health Canada does not recommend use of codeine containing products in children <12 years. After chronic maternal exposure to opioids, neonatal withdrawal syndrome may occur in the newborn; monitor neonate closely. Signs and symptoms include irritability, hyperactivity and abnormal sleep pattern, high pitched cry, tremor, vomiting, diarrhea and failure to gain weight. Onset, duration and severity depend on the drug used, duration of use, maternal dose, and rate of drug elimination by the newborn. Opioid withdrawal syndrome in the neonate, unlike in adults, may be life-threatening and should be treated according to protocols developed by neonatology experts.

Avoid use of codeine in patients with CNS depression or coma as these patients are susceptible to intracranial effects of CO_2 retention. Some products may contain metabisulfite which may cause allergic reactions. Use caution in patients with two or more copies of the variant CYP2D6*2 allele; may have extensive conversion to morphine and thus increased opioid-mediated effects. Avoid the use of codeine in these patients; consider alternative analgesics such as morphine or a nonopioid agent (Crews, 2012). The occurrence of this phenotype is seen in 0.5% to 1% of Chinese and Japanese, 0.5% to 1% of Hispanics, 1% to 10% of Caucasians, 3% of African-Americans, and 16% to 28% of North Africans, Ethiopians, and Arabs.

Rarely, acetaminophen may cause serious and potentially fatal skin reactions such as acute generalized exanthematous pustulosis, Stevens-Johnson syndrome (SJS), and toxic epidermal necrolysis (TEN). Discontinue treatment if severe skin reactions develop.

[US Boxed Warning]: Acetaminophen may cause severe hepatotoxicity, potentially requiring liver transplant or resulting in death; hepatotoxicity is usually

associated with excessive acetaminophen intake (>4 g/day in adults). Risk is increased with alcohol use, preexisting liver disease, and intake of more than one source of acetaminophen-containing medications. Chronic daily dosing in adults has also resulted in liver damage in some patients. Limit acetaminophen dose from all sources (prescription, OTC, combination products) and all routes of administration to <4 g/day in adults. Hypersensitivity and anaphylactic reactions have been reported with acetaminophen use; discontinue immediately if symptoms of allergic or hypersensitivity reactions occur. Use with caution in patients with hypersensitivity reactions to other phenanthrene-derivative opioid agonists (hydrocodone, hydromorphone, levorphanol, oxycodone, oxymorphone). Use acetaminophen caution in patients with known G6PD deficiency.

Codeine may cause CNS depression, which may impair physical or mental abilities; patients must be cautioned about performing tasks which require mental alertness (eg, operating machinery or driving). Use codeine with caution in patients with a history of drug abuse or acute alcoholism; potential for drug dependency exists. Tolerance, psychological and physical dependence may occur with prolonged use. Healthcare provider should be alert to the potential for abuse, misuse, and diversion of codeine. Concurrent use of agonist/antagonist analgesics may precipitate withdrawal symptoms and/or reduced analgesic efficacy in patients following prolonged therapy with mu opioid agonists. Abrupt discontinuation following prolonged use may also lead to withdrawal symptoms. Potentially significant interactions may exist, requiring dose or frequency adjustment, additional monitoring, and/or selection of alternative therapy. Consult drug interactions database for more detailed information.

This combination should be used with caution in elderly, debilitated, or morbidly obese patients; hypovolemia, or cardiovascular disease (including acute MI); adrenal insufficiency (including Addison disease); biliary tract impairment (including acute pancreatitis), severe renal or severe hepatic impairment; preexisting respiratory compromise (hypoxia and/or hypercapnia), COPD or other obstructive pulmonary disease, and kyphoscoliosis or other skeletal disorder which may alter respiratory function; thyroid disorders; prostatic hyperplasia nad/or urethral stricture; seizure disorder; head injury, intracranial lesions or increased intracranial pressure. Codeine may cause or aggravate constipation; chronic use may result in obstructive bowel disease, particularly in those with underlying intestinal motility disorders. May also be problematic in patients with unstable angina and patients post-myocardial infarction. Consider preventive measures (eg, stool softener, increased fiber) to reduce the potential for constipation. Codeine may cause dose-related respiratory depression. The risk is increased in elderly patients, debilitated patients, patients with conditions associated with hypoxia, hypercapnia, or upper airway obstruction, and patients who are CYP2D6 "ultrarapid metabolizers". Codeine may obscure diagnosis or clinical course of patients with acute abdominal conditions; may worsen gastrointestinal ileus due to reduced GI motility. Avoid use in patients with GI obstruction, particularly paralytic ileus; chronic use may result in obstructive bowel disease.

Note: Some non-US formulations (including most Canadian formulations) may contain caffeine as an additional ingredient. Caffeine may cause CNS and cardiovascular stimulation, as well as GI irritation in high doses. Use with caution in patients with a history of peptic ulcer or GERD; avoid in patients with symptomatic cardiac arrhythmias.

Some dosage forms may contain propylene glycol; large amounts are potentially toxic and have been associated hyperosmolality, lactic acidosis, seizures and respiratory depression; use caution (AAP, 1997; Zar, 2007).

Some dosage forms may contain sodium benzoate/benzoic acid; benzoic acid (benzoate) is a metabolite of benzyl alcohol; large amounts of benzyl alcohol (≥99 mg/kg/day) have been associated with a potentially fatal toxicity ("gasping syndrome") in neonates; the "gasping syndrome" consists of metabolic acidosis, respiratory distress, gasping respirations, CNS dysfunction (including convulsions, intracranial hemorrhage), hypotension, and cardiovascular collapse (AAP, 1997; CDC, 1982); some data suggests that benzoate displaces bilirubin from protein binding sites (Ahlfors, 2001); avoid or use dosage forms containing benzyl alcohol derivative with caution in neonates. See manufacturer's labeling.

Warnings: Additional Pediatric Considerations Some dosage forms may contain propylene glycol; in neonates large amounts of propylene glycol delivered orally, intravenously (eg, >3,000 mg/day), or topically have been associated with potentially fatal toxicities which can include metabolic acidosis, seizures, renal failure, and CNS depression; toxicities have also been reported in children and adults including hyperosmolality, lactic acidosis, seizures and respiratory depression; use caution (AAP, 1997; Shehab, 2009).

Adverse Reactions

Central nervous system: Dizziness, euphoria, sedation, voice disorder

Dermatologic: Pruritus

Gastrointestinal: Abdominal pain, constipation, nausea, vomiting

Hypersensitivity: Histamine release

Respiratory: Dyspnea

Rare but important or life-threatening: Antidiuretic hormone disease, biliary tract spasm, bradycardia, drug dependence, hypogonadism (Brennan, 2013; Debono, 2011), hypotension, increased intracranial pressure, miosis, palpitations, peripheral vasodilation, respiratory depression, urinary retention

Drug Interactions

Metabolism/Transport Effects Refer to individual components.

Avoid Concomitant Use

Avoid concomitant use of Acetaminophen and Codeine with any of the following: Azelastine (Nasal); Eluxadoline; Mixed Agonist / Antagonist Opioids; Orphenadrine; Paraldehyde; Thalidomide

Increased Effect/Toxicity

Acetaminophen and Codeine may increase the levels/effects of: Alvimopan; Azelastine (Nasal); Busulfan; CNS Depressants; Dasatinib; Desmopressin; Diuretics; Eluxadoline; Hydrocodone; Imatinib; Methotrimeprazine; Metyrosine; Mipomersen; Mirtazapine; Orphenadrine; Paraldehyde; Phenylephrine (Systemic); Pramipexole; Prilocaine; ROPINIRole; Rotigotine; Selective Serotonin Reuptake Inhibitors; Sodium Nitrite; SORAfenib; Suvorexant; Thalidomide; Vitamin K Antagonists; Zolpidem

The levels/effects of Acetaminophen and Codeine may be increased by: Alcohol (Ethyl); Amphetamines; Anticholinergic Agents; Antipsychotic Agents (Phenothiazines); Brimonidine (Topical); Cannabis; Dasatinib; Doxylamine; Dronabinol; Droperidol; HydrOXYzine; Isoniazid; Kava Kava; Magnesium Sulfate; Methotrimeprazine; Metyrapone; Nabilone; Nitric Oxide; Perampanel; Probenecid; Rufinamide; Sodium Oxybate; Somatostatin Analogs; SORAfenib; Succinylcholine; Tapentadol; Tetrahydrocannabinol

Decreased Effect

Acetaminophen and Codeine may decrease the levels/effects of: Pegvisomant

The levels/effects of Acetaminophen and Codeine may be decreased by: Ammonium Chloride; Barbiturates; CarBAMazepine; Cholestyramine Resin; CYP2D6 Inhibitors (Moderate); CYP2D6 Inhibitors (Strong); Fosphenytoin-Phenytoin; Mixed Agonist / Antagonist Opioids; Naltrexone

Storage/Stability Store at 20°C to 25°C (68°F to 77°F); protect from light.

Mechanism of Action

Acetaminophen: Although not fully elucidated, believed to inhibit the synthesis of prostaglandins in the central nervous system and peripherally block pain impulse generation; produces antipyresis from inhibition of hypothalamic heat-regulating center.

Codeine: Binds to opiate receptors in the CNS, causing inhibition of ascending pain pathways, altering the perception of and response to pain; causes cough suppression by direct central action in the medulla; produces generalized CNS depression.

Caffeine (contained in some non-US formulations) is a CNS stimulant; use with acetaminophen and codeine increases the level of analgesia provided by each agent.

Pharmacokinetics (Adult data unless noted) See individual agents.

Dosing: Usual Note: Doses should be titrated to appropriate analgesic effect:

Children and Adolescents: **Analgesia:** Oral:

Dosage for individual components:

Codeine: 0.5 to 1 mg/kg/dose every 4 to 6 hours; maximum dose: 60 mg/dose (APS, 2008); **Note:** Do not use for postoperative tonsillectomy and/or adenoidectomy pain management.

Acetaminophen: 10 to 15 mg/kg/dose every 4 to 6 hours; do **not** exceed 5 doses in 24 hours; maximum daily dose: 75 mg/kg/**day** not to exceed 4000 mg/**day**

Manufacturer's labeling: Oral solution: Dosage expressed as mL of formulation containing 120 mg acetaminophen and 12 mg codeine per 5 mL:

Children:

3 to 6 years: 5 mL 3 to 4 times daily as needed

7 to 12 years: 10 mL 3 to 4 times daily as needed

Adolescents: 15 mL every 4 hours as needed

Adults: **Analgesia:** Oral: 1 to 2 tablets every 4 hours; maximum total dose: 12 tablets/24 hours

Codeine: 30-60 mg/dose every 4-6 hours

Acetaminophen: Maximum total dose: 4000 mg/24 hours

Dosing adjustment in renal impairment: Children, Adolescents, and Adults: There are no specific dosage adjustments provided in the manufacturer's labeling; however, clearance may be reduced; active metabolites may accumulate. Use with caution; initiate at lower doses or longer dosing intervals followed by careful titration. See individual monographs for specific adjustments.

Dosing adjustment in hepatic impairment: Children, Adolescents, and Adults: There are no dosage adjustments provided in the manufacturer's labeling; however, product contains acetaminophen; use with caution. Cases of hepatotoxicity at daily acetaminophen dosages <4 g/day have been reported. See individual monographs.

Administration Oral: Administer with food to decrease GI upset; shake suspension well before use

Monitoring Parameters Pain relief, respiratory rate, mental status, blood pressure, bowel function; signs of misuse, abuse, and addiction

Test Interactions See individual agents.

Additional Information Tylenol® With Codeine elixir contains saccharin

Controlled Substance Liquid products: C-V; Tablet: C-III

Dosage Forms Excipient information presented when available (limited, particularly for generics); consult specific product labeling.

Solution, Oral:

Generic: Acetaminophen 120 mg and codeine phosphate 12 mg per 5 mL (5 mL, 12.5 mL, 118 mL, 120 mL, 473 mL)

Suspension, Oral:

Capital/Codeine: Acetaminophen 120 mg and codeine phosphate 12 mg per 5 mL (473 mL) [fruit punch flavor]

Tablet, Oral:

Tylenol with Codeine #3: Acetaminophen 300 mg and codeine phosphate 30 mg [contains sodium metabisulfite]

Tylenol with Codeine #4: Acetaminophen 300 mg and codeine phosphate 60 mg [contains sodium metabisulfite]

Generic: Acetaminophen 300 mg and codeine phosphate 15 mg, Acetaminophen 300 mg and codeine phosphate 30 mg, Acetaminophen 300 mg and codeine phosphate 60 mg

◆ **Acetaminophen and Hydrocodone** *see* Hydrocodone and Acetaminophen *on page* *1032*

◆ **Acetaminophen and Oxycodone** *see* Oxycodone and Acetaminophen *on page* *1594*

◆ **Acetasol HC** *see* Acetic Acid, Propylene Glycol Diacetate, and Hydrocortisone *on page* *56*

◆ **Acetazolam (Can)** *see* AcetaZOLAMIDE *on page* *52*

AcetaZOLAMIDE (a set a ZOLE a mide)

Medication Safety Issues

International issues:

Diamox [Canada and multiple international markets] may be confused with Diabinese brand name for chlorpropamide [Multiple international markets]; Dobutrex brand name for dobutamine [Multiple international markets]; Trimox brand name for amoxicillin [Brazil]; Zimox brand name for amoxicillin [Italy] and carbidopa/levodopa [Greece]

Related Information

Oral Medications That Should Not Be Crushed or Altered *on page* *2476*

Brand Names: US Diamox Sequels

Brand Names: Canada Acetazolam; Diamox®

Therapeutic Category Anticonvulsant, Miscellaneous; Carbonic Anhydrase Inhibitor; Diuretic, Carbonic Anhydrase Inhibitor

Generic Availability (US) Yes

Use

Oral:

Immediate release tablets: Adjunct treatment of edema due to congestive heart failure, drug-induced edema, centrencephalic epilepsies, chronic simple (open-angle) glaucoma, secondary glaucoma, and preoperatively in acute angle-closure glaucoma where delay of surgery is desired (FDA approved in adults); prevention or amelioration of symptoms associated with acute mountain sickness (FDA approved in adults)

Extended release capsules: Adjunctive treatment of chronic simple (open-angle) glaucoma, secondary glaucoma, and preoperatively in acute angle-closure glaucoma where delay of surgery is desired (FDA approved in adults); prevention or amelioration of symptoms associated with acute mountain sickness (FDA approved in adults)

Parenteral: Adjunct treatment of edema due to congestive heart failure, drug-induced edema, centrencephalic epilepsies, chronic simple (open-angle) glaucoma, secondary glaucoma, and preoperatively in acute angle-closure glaucoma where delay of surgery is desired (FDA approved in adults)

Pregnancy Risk Factor C

Pregnancy Considerations Adverse events have been observed in animal reproduction studies. Limited data is available following the use of acetazolamide in pregnant women for the treatment of idiopathic intracranial hypertension (Falardeau, 2013; Kesler, 2013).

Pregnant women exposed to acetazolamide during pregnancy for the treatment of seizure disorders are encouraged to enroll themselves into the AED Pregnancy Registry by calling 1-888-233-2334. Additional information is available at aedpregnancyregistry.org

Breast-Feeding Considerations Acetazolamide is excreted into breast milk. In a case report, low concentrations of acetazolamide were detected in the breast milk and the infant serum following a maternal dose of acetazolamide 500 mg twice daily. Acetazolamide concentrations in the breast milk were 1.3-2.1 mcg/mL, 1-9 hours after the dose. Acetazolamide concentrations in the infant serum were 0.2-0.6 mcg/mL, 2-12 hours after nursing. Maternal plasma concentrations were 5.2-6.4 mcg/mL, 1-7 hours after the dose. All levels were obtained on days 4-5 of therapy, 10 days after delivery (Söderman, 1984). Due to the potential for serious adverse reactions in the nursing infant, the manufacturer recommends a decision be made whether to discontinue nursing or to discontinue the drug, taking into account the importance of treatment to the mother.

Contraindications

Hypersensitivity to acetazolamide, sulfonamides, or any component of the formulation; hepatic disease or insufficiency; decreased sodium and/or potassium levels; adrenocortical insufficiency, cirrhosis; hyperchloremic acidosis, severe renal disease or dysfunction; long-term use in noncongestive angle-closure glaucoma

Note: Although the FDA approved product labeling states this medication is contraindicated with other sulfonamide-containing drug classes, the scientific basis of this statement has been challenged. See "Warnings/Precautions" for more detail.

Warnings/Precautions Use with caution in patients with hepatic dysfunction; in cirrhosis, avoid electrolyte and acid/base imbalances that might lead to hepatic encephalopathy. Use with caution in patients with respiratory acidosis and diabetes mellitus (may change glucose control). Use with caution or avoid in patients taking high-dose aspirin concurrently; may lead to severe adverse effects including tachypnea, anorexia, lethargy, coma, and death. Use with caution in the elderly; may be more sensitive to side effects. Impairment of mental alertness and/or physical coordination may occur. Increasing the dose does not increase diuresis and may increase the incidence of drowsiness and/or paresthesia; often results in a reduction of diuresis.

IM administration is painful because of the alkaline pH of the drug; use by this route is not recommended.

Sulfonamide ("sulfa") allergy: The FDA-approved product labeling for many medications containing a sulfonamide chemical group includes a broad contraindication in patients with a prior allergic reaction to sulfonamides. There is a potential for cross-reactivity between members of a specific class (eg, two antibiotic sulfonamides). However, concerns for cross-reactivity have previously extended to all compounds containing the sulfonamide structure (SO_2NH_2). An expanded understanding of allergic mechanisms indicates cross-reactivity between antibiotic sulfonamides and nonantibiotic sulfonamides may not occur or at the very least this potential is extremely low (Brackett 2004; Johnson 2005; Slatore 2004; Tornero 2004). In particular, mechanisms of cross-reaction due to antibody production (anaphylaxis) are unlikely to occur with nonantibiotic sulfonamides. T-cell-mediated (type IV) reactions (eg, maculopapular rash) are less well understood and it is not possible to completely exclude this potential based on current insights. In cases where prior reactions were severe (Stevens-Johnson syndrome/TEN), some clinicians choose to avoid exposure to these classes.

Warnings: Additional Pediatric Considerations Growth retardation has been reported in children receiving chronic therapy (possibly due to chronic acidosis).

Adverse Reactions Frequency not defined.

Cardiovascular: Flushing

Central nervous system: Ataxia, confusion, convulsions, depression, dizziness, drowsiness, excitement, fatigue, flaccid paralysis, headache, malaise, paresthesia

Dermatologic: Allergic skin reaction, skin photosensitivity, Stevens-Johnson syndrome, toxic epidermal necrolysis, urticaria

Endocrine & metabolic: Electrolyte imbalance, growth retardation (children), hyperglycemia, hypoglycemia, hypokalemia, hyponatremia, metabolic acidosis

Gastrointestinal: Decreased appetite, diarrhea, dysgeusia, glycosuria, melena, nausea, vomiting

Genitourinary: Crystalluria, hematuria

Hematologic and oncologic: Agranulocytosis, aplastic anemia, leukopenia, thrombocytopenia, thrombocytopenic purpura

Hepatic: Abnormal hepatic function tests, cholestatic jaundice, fulminant hepatic necrosis, hepatic insufficiency

Hypersensitivity: Anaphylaxis

Local: Pain at injection site

Ophthalmic: Myopia

Otic: Auditory disturbance, tinnitus

Renal: Polyuria, renal failure

Miscellaneous: Fever

Drug Interactions

Metabolism/Transport Effects None known.

Avoid Concomitant Use

Avoid concomitant use of AcetaZOLAMIDE with any of the following: Carbonic Anhydrase Inhibitors; Mecamylamine

Increased Effect/Toxicity

AcetaZOLAMIDE may increase the levels/effects of: Alpha-/Beta-Agonists (Indirect-Acting); Amphetamines; CarBAMazepine; Carbonic Anhydrase Inhibitors; CycloSPORINE (Systemic); DULoxetine; Flecainide; Fosphenytoin-Phenytoin; Hypotensive Agents; Levodopa; Mecamylamine; Memantine; MetFORMIN; Primidone; QuiNIDine; RisperiDONE; Sodium Bicarbonate; Sodium Phosphates

The levels/effects of AcetaZOLAMIDE may be increased by: Analgesics (Opioid); Barbiturates; Dexketoprofen; MAO Inhibitors; Nicorandil; Salicylates

Decreased Effect

AcetaZOLAMIDE may decrease the levels/effects of: Lithium; Methenamine; Primidone; Trientine

The levels/effects of AcetaZOLAMIDE may be decreased by: Mefloquine; Mianserin; Orlistat

Storage/Stability

Capsules, tablets: Store at controlled room temperature.

Injection: Store intact vials at 20°C to 25°C (68°F to 77°F). Store reconstituted solutions for 3 days under refrigeration at 2°C to 8°C (36°F to 46°F), or 12 hours at room temperature, 20°C to 25°C (68°F to 77°F).

Mechanism of Action Reversible inhibition of the enzyme carbonic anhydrase resulting in reduction of hydrogen ion secretion at renal tubule and an increased renal excretion of sodium, potassium, bicarbonate, and water. Decreases production of aqueous humor and inhibits carbonic anhydrase in central nervous system to retard abnormal and excessive discharge from CNS neurons.

Pharmacodynamics

Onset of action:
- Capsule, extended release: 2 hours
- Tablet: 1 to 1.5 hours
- IV: 2 minutes

Maximum effect:
- Capsule, extended release: 3 to 6 hours
- Tablet: 1 to 4 hours
- IV: 15 minutes

Duration:
- Capsule, extended release: 18 to 24 hours
- Tablet: 8 to 12 hours
- IV: 4 to 5 hours

Pharmacokinetics (Adult data unless noted)

Absorption: Appears to be dose dependent; erratic with daily doses >10 mg/kg

Distribution: Into erythrocytes and kidneys; crosses the blood-brain barrier

Protein binding: 95%

Half-life: 2.4 to 5.8 hours

Time to peak serum concentration: Immediate release tablet: 1 to 4 hours; extended release capsules: 3 to 6 hours

Elimination: 70% to 100% of an IV or tablet dose and 47% of an extended release capsule excreted unchanged in urine within 24 hours

Dosing: Usual

Pediatric:

Altitude illness, acute: Limited data available: Infants, Children, and Adolescents: Oral:

Prevention: 2.5 mg/kg/dose every 12 hours started either the day before (preferred) or on the day of ascent and may be discontinued after staying at the same elevation for 2 to 3 days or if descent initiated; maximum dose: 125 mg/dose (Luks 2010). **Note:** The International Society for Mountain Medicine does not recommend prophylaxis in children except in the rare circumstance of unavoidable rapid ascent or in children with known previous susceptibility to acute mountain sickness (Pollard 2001).

Treatment: Acute mountain sickness (AMS); moderate: 2.5 mg/kg/dose every 8 to 12 hours; maximum single dose: 250 mg. **Note:** With high altitude cerebral edema, dexamethasone is the primary treatment; however, acetazolamide may be used adjunctively with the same treatment dose (Luks 2010; Pollard 2001).

Glaucoma: Limited data available:

Children <12 years: Oral: Immediate release: 10 to 30 mg/kg/day divided every 6 to 8 hours; maximum daily dose: 1,000 mg/**day** (Portellos 1998; Sabri 2006)

Children ≥12 years and Adolescents: Oral: 15 to 30 mg/kg/day; maximum daily dose: 1,000 mg/**day**; dosing interval determined by dosage form: Immediate release tablet: Divided doses every 6 to 8 hours; Extended release capsules: Divided doses twice daily (Pagliaro 2002; Sabri 2006)

Edema: Limited data available: Infants, Children, and Adolescents: Oral, IV: Immediate release: 5 mg/kg/dose every other day in the morning (Pagliaro 2002)

Epilepsy, short-term management: Limited data available: Infants, Children, and Adolescents: Oral: Immediate release: Usual range: 4 to 16 mg/kg/day in 3 to 4 divided doses; may titrate; maximum daily dose: 30 mg/kg/**day** or 1,000 mg/**day** (whichever is less) (Reiss 1996); **Note:** Minimal additional benefit with doses >16 mg/kg/day; **extended release capsule is not recommended for treatment of epilepsy**

Pseudotumor cerebri: Limited data available:

Children: Usual reported dose: Initial: Oral: 15 to 25 mg/kg/day in 2 to 3 divided doses; may increase if needed to a maximum daily dose: 100 mg/kg/**day** or 2,000 mg/**day** (whichever is less); therapy continued until resolution of headache, disc swelling, and visual field abnormalities; usually several months (eg, 3 to months) (Distelmaier 2006; Hacifazlioglu 2012; K 2010; Per 2013; Rangwalla 2007; Soler 1998; Spennato 2011; Standridge 2010).

Adolescents: Initial: Oral: 500 mg twice daily; may increase if needed to a maximum daily dose 4,000 mg/**day** (Standridge 2010)

Adult:

Glaucoma: Oral, IV:

Chronic simple (open-angle): 250 mg 1 to 4 times/day or 500 mg extended release capsule twice daily

Secondary or acute (closed-angle): 250 to 500 mg; maintenance: 125 to 250 mg every 4 hours (250 mg every 12 hours has been effective in short-term treatment of some patients)

Edema: Oral, IV: 250 to 375 mg once daily

Epilepsy: Oral: 8 to 30 mg/kg/day in divided doses. A lower dosing range of 4 to 16 mg/kg/day in 1 to 4 divided doses has also been recommended; maximum daily dose: 30 mg/kg/**day** or 1,000 mg/**day** (Oles 1989; Reiss 1996). **Note:** Minimal additional benefit with doses >16 mg/kg/day; **extended release capsule is not recommended for treatment of epilepsy**

Altitude sickness: Oral: 500 to 1,000 mg daily in divided doses every 8 to 12 hours (immediate release tablets) or divided every 12 to 24 hours (extended release capsules). These doses are associated with more frequent and/or increased side effects. Alternative dosing has been recommended:

Prevention: 125 mg twice daily; beginning either the day before (preferred) or on the day of ascent; may be discontinued after staying at the same elevation for 2 to 3 days or if descent initiated (Basnyat 2006; Luks 2010). **Note:** In situations of rapid ascent (such as rescue or military operations), 1,000 mg/day is recommended by the manufacturer. The Wilderness Medical Society recommends consideration of using dexamethasone in addition to acetazolamide in these situations (Luks 2010).

Treatment: 250 mg twice daily. **Note:** With high altitude cerebral edema, dexamethasone is the primary treatment; however, acetazolamide may be used adjunctively with the same treatment dose (Luks 2010).

Dosing adjustment in renal impairment: There are no dosage adjustments provided in the manufacturer's labeling; acetazolamide is contraindicated in severe renal impairment. The following adjustments have been recommended (Aronoff 2007): Oral, IV: Adults: **Note:** Renally adjusted dose recommendations are based on doses of 250 mg every 6 hours:

- CrCl >50 mL/minute: No dosage adjustment recommended
- CrCl 10 to 50 mL/minute: Administer every 12 hours
- CrCl <10 mL/minute: Avoid use; contraindicated
- Hemodialysis: Moderately dialyzable (20% to 50%)
- Peritoneal dialysis: Supplemental dose is not necessary (Schwenk 1994)

Dosing adjustment in hepatic impairment: There are no dosage adjustments provided in the manufacturer's labeling; however, acetazolamide is contraindicated in patients with cirrhosis or severe liver impairment.

Preparation for Administration Parenteral: Reconstitute with at least 5 mL SWFI to provide a solution containing not more than 100 mg/mL; maximum concentration 100 mg/mL

Administration

Oral: Administer with food to decrease GI upset; tablet may be crushed and suspended in cherry or chocolate syrup to disguise the bitter taste of the drug

Parenteral:

IV: Direct IV injection is the preferred parenteral route of administration. Specific IV push rates are not provided in the manufacturer's labeling. Some have recommended a maximum rate of 500 mg/minute (Gahart 2014). Additionally, a study in adults to assess cerebrovascular reserve used a rapid IV push of up to 1 g over ≤1 minute (Piepgras 1990).

IM: Not recommended as the drug's alkaline pH makes it very painful

Monitoring Parameters Serum electrolytes, CBC and platelet counts; intraocular pressure in glaucoma patients; monitor growth in pediatric patients

Test Interactions May cause false-positive results for urinary protein with Albustix®, Labstix®, Albutest®, Bumintest®; interferes with HPLC theophylline assay and serum uric acid levels

Additional Information Sodium content of 500 mg injection: 2.049 mEq

Dosage Forms Excipient information presented when available (limited, particularly for generics); consult specific product labeling.

Capsule Extended Release 12 Hour, Oral:
- Diamox Sequels: 500 mg
- Generic: 500 mg

Solution Reconstituted, Injection [preservative free]:
- Generic: 500 mg (1 ea)

Tablet, Oral:
- Generic: 125 mg, 250 mg

Extemporaneous Preparations A 25 mg/mL oral suspension may be made with tablets and either a 1:1 mixture of Ora-Sweet® and Ora-Plus® or a 1:1 mixture of Ora-Sweet® SF and Ora-Plus®. Crush twelve 250 mg tablets in a mortar and reduce to a fine powder. Add small portions of chosen vehicle and mix to a uniform paste; mix while adding the vehicle in incremental proportions to **almost** 120 mL; transfer to a calibrated bottle, rinse mortar with vehicle, and add quantity of vehicle sufficient to make 120 mL. Label "shake well" and "refrigerate". Stable for 60 days (Allen, 1996). When diluted in 120 mL solution of cherry syrup concentrate diluted 1:4 with simple syrup, NF, it is stable 60 days refrigerated (preferred) or at room temperature (Nahata, 2004).

Allen LV Jr and Erickson MA 3rd, "Stability of Acetazolamide, Allopurinol, Azathioprine, Clonazepam, and Flucytosine in Extemporaneously Compounded Oral Liquids," *Am J Health Syst Pharm*, 1996, 53(16):1944-9.

Nahata MC, Pai VB, and Hipple TF, *Pediatric Drug Formulations*, 5th ed, Cincinnati, OH: Harvey Whitney Books Co, 2004.

◆ **Acet-Codeine (Can)** *see* Acetaminophen and Codeine *on page 50*

Acetic Acid (a SEE tik AS id)

Medication Safety Issues

Sound-alike/look-alike issues:

Acetic acid for irrigation may be confused with glacial acetic acid

VoSol® may be confused with Vexol®,VoSol® HC

Other safety concerns:

Glacial acetic acid (≥99%): Severe burns and permanent scarring have occurred after glacial acetic acid was accidently applied topically on patient's skin or mucous membranes. Care should be taken to ensure that diluted acetic acid solutions are used in patient care only and that there aren't mix-ups between these products and glacial acetic acid (ISMP, 2013).

Therapeutic Category Otic Agent, Anti-infective; Topical Skin Product

Generic Availability (US) Yes

Use

Otic solution: Treatment of superficial infections of the external auditory canal (FDA approved in ages ≥3 years and adults)

Irrigation solution: Irrigation of the bladder; periodic irrigation of indwelling catheters (FDA approved in adults)

Pregnancy Risk Factor C

Pregnancy Considerations Animal reproduction studies have not been conducted. Systemic absorption following bladder irrigation is not likely unless open lesions are present.

Breast-Feeding Considerations Use with caution in breast-feeding women.

Contraindications Hypersensitivity to acetic acid or any component of the formulation; during transurethral procedures (irrigation); perforated tympanic membrane (otic solution)

Warnings/Precautions Not for internal intake or IV infusion; topical use or irrigation use only. Use of irrigation in patients with mucosal lesions of urinary bladder may cause irritation. Open lesions of the bladder mucosa may result in systemic acidosis from absorption.

Adverse Reactions

Irrigation solution:
- Endocrine & Metabolic: Systemic acidosis
- Genitourinary: Urologic pain
- Local: Irritation
- Renal: Hematuria

Otic solution: Otic: Irritation, burning, stinging

Drug Interactions

Metabolism/Transport Effects None known.

Avoid Concomitant Use

Avoid concomitant use of Acetic Acid with any of the following: BCG; BCG (Intravesical)

Increased Effect/Toxicity There are no known significant interactions involving an increase in effect.

Decreased Effect

Acetic Acid may decrease the levels/effects of: BCG; BCG (Intravesical); BCG Vaccine (Immunization); Sodium Picosulfate

Storage/Stability

Irrigation solution: Store at room temperature at 20°C to 25°C (68°F to 77°F); avoid excessive heat; do not freeze.

Otic solution: Store at room temperature at 20°C to 25°C (68°F to 77°F).

Dosing: Usual

Pediatric: **Otitis externa, acute:** Children ≥3 years and Adolescents: Otic: Insert saturated wick of cotton; keep moist 24 hours by adding 3 to 5 drops every 4 to 6 hours; remove wick after 24 hours and instill 5 drops 3 to 4 times daily. **Note:** In children, 3 to 4 drops may be sufficient due to the smaller capacity of the ear canal.

Adult:

Irrigation, transurethral: Note: Dosage of an irrigating solution depends on the capacity or surface area of the structure being irrigated

Urinary bladder, continuous or intermittent irrigation: Transurethral: 0.25% irrigation solution: Usual volume: 500 to 1500 mL per 24 hours; the rate of administration will approximate the rate of urine flow

Indwelling urinary catheter, periodic irrigation to maintain patency: Transurethral: 0.25% irrigation solution: ~50 mL is required for each irrigation

Otitis externa, acute: Otic: Insert saturated wick of cotton; keep moist 24 hours by adding 3 to 5 drops every 4 to 6 hours; remove wick after 24 hours and instill 5 drops 3 to 4 times daily

Dosing adjustment in renal impairment: Children ≥3 years and Adolescents: There are no dosing adjustments provided in the manufacturer's labeling.

Dosing adjustment in renal impairment: Children ≥3 years and Adolescents: There are no dosing adjustments provided in the manufacturer's labeling.

Administration Not for internal intake or IV infusion; topical use or irrigation use only

Bladder irrigation: Urine pH should be checked at least 4 times daily and the irrigation rate adjusted to maintain a pH of 4.5 to 5; increasing the rate decreases the pH and vice versa

Dosage Forms Excipient information presented when available (limited, particularly for generics); consult specific product labeling.

Solution, Irrigation:

Generic: 0.25% (250 mL, 500 mL, 1000 mL)

Solution, Otic:

Generic: 2% (15 mL, 60 mL)

◆ **Acetic Acid, Hydrocortisone, and Propylene Glycol Diacetate** *see* Acetic Acid, Propylene Glycol Diacetate, and Hydrocortisone *on page* 56

Acetic Acid, Propylene Glycol Diacetate, and Hydrocortisone

(a SEE tik AS id, PRO pa leen GLY kole dye AS e tate, & hye droe KOR ti sone)

Medication Safety Issues

Sound-alike/look-alike issues:

VoSol may be confused with Vexol

Brand Names: US Acetasol HC; VoSolHC [DSC]

Therapeutic Category Otic Agent, Anti-infective

Generic Availability (US) Yes

Use Treatment of superficial infections of the external auditory canal (otitis externa) (FDA approved in ages ≥3 years and adults)

Contraindications Hypersensitivity to acetic acid, propylene glycol, hydrocortisone, or any component of the formulation; perforated tympanic membrane; herpes simplex; vaccinia, and varicella

Warnings/Precautions Transient stinging or burning may occur when first used in inflamed ear. Discontinue if sensitization or irritation occurs.

Adverse Reactions Otic: Transient burning or stinging may be noticed occasionally upon instillation

Drug Interactions

Metabolism/Transport Effects Refer to individual components.

Avoid Concomitant Use

Avoid concomitant use of Acetic Acid, Propylene Glycol Diacetate, and Hydrocortisone with any of the following: Aldesleukin; BCG; BCG (Intravesical)

Increased Effect/Toxicity

Acetic Acid, Propylene Glycol Diacetate, and Hydrocortisone may increase the levels/effects of: Ceritinib; Deferasirox

The levels/effects of Acetic Acid, Propylene Glycol Diacetate, and Hydrocortisone may be increased by: Telaprevir

Decreased Effect

Acetic Acid, Propylene Glycol Diacetate, and Hydrocortisone may decrease the levels/effects of: Aldesleukin; BCG; BCG (Intravesical); BCG Vaccine (Immunization); Corticorelin; Hyaluronidase; Sodium Picosulfate; Telaprevir

Storage/Stability Store at 20°C to 25°C (68°F to 77°F).

Dosing: Usual

Pediatric: **Otitis externa, acute:** Children ≥3 years and Adolescents: Otic: Insert saturated wick of cotton; keep moist 24 hours by adding 3 to 5 drops every 4 to 6 hours; remove wick after 24 hours and instill 5 drops 3 to 4 times daily. **Note:** In children, 3 to 4 drops may be sufficient due to the smaller capacity of the ear canal.

Adult: **Otitis externa, acute:** Otic: Insert saturated wick of cotton; keep moist 24 hours by adding 3 to 5 drops every 4 to 6 hours; remove wick after 24 hours and instill 5 drops 3 to 4 times daily

Dosing adjustment in renal impairment: Children ≥3 years and Adolescents: There are no dosing adjustments provided in the manufacturer's labeling.

Dosing adjustment in hepatic impairment: Children ≥3 years and Adolescents: There are no dosing adjustments provided in the manufacturer's labeling.

Administration Otic: Not for internal intake; topical use only; prior to use, warm suspension by holding bottle in hands; shake well before use; patient should lie with affected ear upward for instillation

Dosage Forms Excipient information presented when available (limited, particularly for generics); consult specific product labeling. [DSC] = Discontinued product

Solution, otic [drops]: Acetic acid 2%, propylene glycol diacetate 3%, and hydrocortisone 1% (10 mL)

Acetasol HC: Acetic acid 2%, propylene glycol diacetate 3%, and hydrocortisone 1% (10 mL) [contains benzethonium chloride]

VoSol HC: Acetic acid 2%, propylene glycol diacetate 3%, and hydrocortisone 1% (10 mL [DSC]) [contains benzethonium chloride]

◆ **Acetoxyl® (Can)** *see* Benzoyl Peroxide *on page* 270

◆ **Acetoxymethylprogesterone** *see* MedroxyPROGESTERone *on page* 1339

Acetylcholine (a se teel KOE leen)

Medication Safety Issues

Sound-alike/look-alike issues:

Acetylcholine may be confused with acetylcysteine

Brand Names: US Miochol-E

Brand Names: Canada Miochol®-E

Therapeutic Category Cholinergic Agent, Ophthalmic; Ophthalmic Agent, Miotic

Generic Availability (US) No

Use Produces complete miosis in cataract surgery, keratoplasty, iridectomy and other anterior segment surgery where rapid miosis is required (FDA approved in adults)

Contraindications Hypersensitivity to acetylcholine chloride or any component of the formulation

Warnings/Precautions During cataract surgery, use only after lens is in place. Open under aseptic conditions only; do not gas sterilize. Systemic effects rarely occur but can cause problems for patients with acute cardiac failure, bronchial asthma, peptic ulcer, hyperthyroidism, GI spasm, urinary tract obstruction, and Parkinson's disease.

Adverse Reactions

Cardiovascular: Bradycardia, flushing, hypotension

Ocular: Clouding, corneal edema, decompensation

Respiratory: Dyspnea

Miscellaneous: Diaphoresis

Drug Interactions

Metabolism/Transport Effects None known.

Avoid Concomitant Use There are no known interactions where it is recommended to avoid concomitant use.

Increased Effect/Toxicity

The levels/effects of Acetylcholine may be increased by: Acetylcholinesterase Inhibitors; Beta-Blockers

Decreased Effect There are no known significant interactions involving a decrease in effect.

Storage/Stability Store unopened vial at 4°C to 25°C (39°F to 77°F); prevent from freezing. Prepare solution immediately before use and discard unused portion. Acetylcholine solutions are unstable. Only use if solution is clear and colorless.

Mechanism of Action Causes contraction of the sphincter muscles of the iris, resulting in miosis and contraction of the ciliary muscle, leading to accommodation spasm

Pharmacodynamics

Onset of action: Miosis occurs promptly

Duration: ~20 minutes (Kanski, 1968); duration as long as 6 hours has been reported (Roszkowska, 1998)

Dosing: Usual Miosis; intraoperative: Adults: Intraocular: 0.5-2 mL of 1% injection (5-20 mg) instilled into anterior chamber before or after securing one or more sutures

Dosing adjustment in renal impairment: There are no dosage adjustments provided in the manufacturer's labeling.

Dosing adjustment in hepatic impairment: There are no dosage adjustments provided in the manufacturer's labeling.

Preparation for Administration Reconstitute in an aseptic environment immediately before use.

Administration Ophthalmic: Open under aseptic conditions only. Attach filter before irrigating eye. Instill into anterior chamber before or after securing one or more sutures; instillation should be gentle and parallel to the iris face and tangential to the pupil border; in cataract surgery, acetylcholine should be used only after delivery of the lens

Dosage Forms Excipient information presented when available (limited, particularly for generics); consult specific product labeling.

Solution Reconstituted, Intraocular, as chloride:

Miochol-E: 20 mg (1 ea) [contains mannitol]

◆ **Acetylcholine Chloride** *see* Acetylcholine *on page 56*

Acetylcysteine (a se teel SIS teen)

Medication Safety Issues

Sound-alike/look-alike issues:

Acetylcysteine may be confused with acetylcholine

Mucomyst may be confused with Mucinex

Related Information

Acetaminophen Serum Level Nomogram *on page 2449*

Brand Names: US Acetadote

Brand Names: Canada Acetylcysteine Injection; Acetylcysteine Solution; Mucomyst®; Parvolex®

Therapeutic Category Antidote, Acetaminophen; Mucolytic Agent

Generic Availability (US) Yes

Use

Inhalation: Adjunctive therapy in patients with abnormal or viscid mucous secretions in bronchopulmonary diseases, pulmonary complications of surgery, and cystic fibrosis; diagnostic bronchial studies [FDA approved in pediatric patients (age not specified) and adults]

Injection, Oral: Antidote for acute acetaminophen toxicity; prevention of radiocontrast-induced renal dysfunction [FDA approved in pediatric patients (age not specified) and adults]

Has also been used orally and rectally to treat distal intestinal obstruction syndrome (previously known as "meconium ileus or its equivalent")

Pregnancy Risk Factor B

Pregnancy Considerations Adverse events were not observed in animal reproduction studies. Based on limited reports using acetylcysteine to treat acetaminophen poisoning in pregnant women, acetylcysteine has been shown to cross the placenta and may provide protective levels in the fetus.

Acetylcysteine may be used to treat acetaminophen overdose in during pregnancy (Wilkes, 2005). In general, medications used as antidotes should take into consideration the health and prognosis of the mother; antidotes should be administered to pregnant women if there is a clear indication for use and should not be withheld because of fears of teratogenicity (Bailey, 2003).

Breast-Feeding Considerations It is not known if acetylcysteine is excreted in breast milk. The manufacturer recommends that caution be exercised when administering acetylcysteine to nursing women. Based on its pharmacokinetics, the drug should be nearly completely cleared 30 hours after administration; therefore, nursing women may consider resuming nursing 30 hours after dosing is complete.

Contraindications Hypersensitivity to acetylcysteine or any component of the formulation

Warnings/Precautions

Inhalation: Since increased bronchial secretions may develop after inhalation, percussion, postural drainage, and suctioning should follow. If bronchospasm occurs, administer a bronchodilator; discontinue acetylcysteine if bronchospasm progresses.

Intravenous: Acute flushing and erythema have been reported; usually occurs within 30-60 minutes and may resolve spontaneously. Serious anaphylactoid reactions have also been reported and are more commonly associated with IV administration, but may also occur with oral administration (Mroz, 1997). When used for acetaminophen poisoning, the incidence is reduced when the initial loading dose is administered over 60 minutes. The acetylcysteine infusion may be interrupted until treatment of allergic symptoms is initiated; the infusion can then be carefully restarted. Treatment for anaphylactoid reactions should be immediately available. Use caution in patients with asthma or history of bronchospasm as these patients may be at increased risk. Conversely, patients with high acetaminophen levels (>150 mg/dL) may be at a reduced risk for anaphylactoid reactions (Pakravan, 2008; Sandilands, 2009; Waring, 2008).

Acute acetaminophen poisoning: Acetylcysteine is indicated in patients with a serum acetaminophen level that indicates they are at "possible" risk or greater for hepatotoxicity when plotted on the Rumack-Matthew nomogram. There are several situations where the nomogram is of limited use. Serum acetaminophen levels obtained <4 hours postingestion are not interpretable; patients presenting late may have undetectable serum concentrations, despite having received a toxic dose. The nomogram is less predictive of hepatic injury following an acute overdose with an extended release acetaminophen product. The nomogram also does not take into account patients who may be at higher risk of acetaminophen toxicity (eg, alcoholics, malnourished patients, concurrent use of CYP2E1 enzyme-inducing agents [eg, isoniazid]). Nevertheless, acetylcysteine should be administered to any patient with signs of hepatotoxicity, even if the serum acetaminophen level is low or undetectable. Patients who present >24 hours after an acute ingestion or patients who present following an acute ingestion at an unknown time may be candidates for acetylcysteine therapy; consultation with a poison control center or clinical toxicologist is highly recommended.

Repeated supratherapeutic ingestion (RSTI) of acetaminophen: The Rumack-Matthew nomogram is not designed to be used following RSTIs. In general, an accurate past medical history, including a comprehensive acetaminophen ingestion history, in conjunction with AST concentrations and serum acetaminophen levels, may give the clinician insight as to the patient's risk of acetaminophen toxicity. Some experts recommend that acetylcysteine be administered to any patient with "higher than expected" serum acetaminophen levels or serum acetaminophen level >10 mcg/mL, even in the absence of hepatic injury; others recommend treatment for patients with laboratory evidence and/or signs and symptoms of hepatotoxicity (Hendrickson, 2006; Jones, 2000). Consultation with a poison control center or a clinical toxicologist is highly recommended.

Adverse Reactions

Inhalation:

Central nervous system: Chills, drowsiness, fever

Gastrointestinal: Nausea, stomatitis, vomiting

Local: Irritation, stickiness on face following nebulization

Respiratory: Bronchospasm, hemoptysis, rhinorrhea
Miscellaneous: Acquired sensitization (rare), clamminess, unpleasant odor during administration

Intravenous:
Cardiovascular: Edema, flushing, tachycardia
Dermatologic: Pruritus, rash, urticaria
Gastrointestinal: Nausea, vomiting
Respiratory: Pharyngitis, rhinorrhea, rhonchi, throat tightness
Miscellaneous: Anaphylactoid reaction
Rare but important or life-threatening: Anaphylaxis, angioedema, bronchospasm, chest tightness, cough, dizziness, dyspnea, headache, hypotension, respiratory distress, stridor, wheezing

Oral (Bebarta, 2010; Mroz, 1997):
Cardiovascular: Hypotension, tachycardia
Dermatologic: Angioedema, pruritus, urticaria
Gastrointestinal: Nausea, vomiting
Respiratory: Bronchospasm

Drug Interactions

Metabolism/Transport Effects None known.

Avoid Concomitant Use There are no known interactions where it is recommended to avoid concomitant use.

Increased Effect/Toxicity There are no known significant interactions involving an increase in effect.

Decreased Effect There are no known significant interactions involving a decrease in effect.

Storage/Stability

Solution for injection (Acetadote): Store unopened vials at room temperature, 20°C to 25°C (68°F to 77°F). Following reconstitution with D_5W, solution is stable for 24 hours at room temperature. A color change may occur in opened vials (light pink or purple) and does not affect the safety or efficacy.

Solution for inhalation: Store unopened vials at room temperature; once opened, store under refrigeration and use within 96 hours. A color change may occur in opened vials (light purple) and does not affect the safety or efficacy.

Mechanism of Action Exerts mucolytic action through its free sulfhydryl group which opens up the disulfide bonds in the mucoproteins thus lowering mucous viscosity.

In patients with acetaminophen toxicity, acetylcysteine acts as a hepatoprotective agent by restoring hepatic glutathione, serving as a glutathione substitute, and enhancing the nontoxic sulfate conjugation of acetaminophen.

The presumed mechanism in preventing contrast-induced nephropathy is its ability to scavenge oxygen-derived free radicals and improve endothelium-dependent vasodilation.

Pharmacodynamics

Onset of action: Inhalation: Mucus liquefaction occurs maximally within 5-10 minutes
Duration: Inhalation: Mucus liquefaction: More than 1 hour

Pharmacokinetics (Adult data unless noted)

Distribution: V_d: 0.47 L/kg
Protein binding: 83%
Half-life:
- Reduced acetylcysteine: 2 hours
- Total acetylcysteine:
  - Newborns: 11 hours
  - Adults: 5.6 hours

Time to peak serum concentration: Oral: 1 to 2 hours
Elimination: Urine

Dosing: Usual

Infants, Children, and Adolescents:

Acetaminophen poisoning: Infants, Children, and Adolescents: Begin treatment within 8 hours of ingestion to optimize therapy in patients whose serum acetaminophen levels fall above the "possible" toxicity line on the Rumack-Matthew nomogram. Treatment is also indicated in patients with a history of known or suspected acute acetaminophen ingestion of >150 mg/kg (child) or >7.5 g (adolescent) total dose when plasma levels are not available within 8-10 hours of ingestion or in patients presenting >24 hours after acute ingestion who have a measurable acetaminophen level.

Oral: 72-hour regimen: Consists of 18 doses; total dose delivered: 1330 mg/kg
- Loading dose: 140 mg/kg
- Maintenance dose: 70 mg/kg every 4 hours for 17 doses; repeat dose if emesis occurs within 1 hour of administration; **Note:** Consultation with a poison control center or clinical toxicologist is highly recommended when considering the discontinuation of oral acetylcysteine prior to the conclusion of a full 18-dose course of therapy.

IV (Acetadote): 21-hour regimen: Consists of 3 doses; total dose delivered: 300 mg/kg
- Loading dose: 150 mg/kg (maximum: 15 g) infused over 60 minutes
- Second dose: 50 mg/kg (maximum: 5000 mg) infused over 4 hours
- Third dose: 100 mg/kg (maximum: 10 g) infused over 16 hours

Respiratory conditions, adjuvant therapy: Note: Patients should receive an aerosolized bronchodilator 10-15 minutes prior to acetylcysteine:

Nebulized inhalation:

Face mask, mouth piece, tracheostomy:
- Infants: 1-2 mL of 20% solution (may be further diluted with sodium chloride or sterile water for inhalation) or 2-4 mL of 10% solution (undiluted); administer 3-4 times daily
- Children: 3-5 mL of 20% solution (may be further diluted with sodium chloride or sterile water for inhalation) or 6-10 mL of 10% solution (undiluted); administer 3-4 times daily
- Adolescents: 3-5 mL of 20% solution (may be further diluted with sodium chloride or sterile water for inhalation) or 6-10 mL of 10% solution (undiluted); administer 3-4 times daily; usual dosing range: 20% solution: 1-10 mL or 10% solution: 2-20 mL every 2-6 hours

Tent, croupette: 10% or 20% solution: Dose must be individualized; dose is volume of solution necessary to maintain a very heavy mist in tent or croupette; in some cases, may require up to 300 mL solution/treatment

Direct instillation: Children and Adolescents:
- Endotracheal: 1-2 mL of 10% to 20% solution every 1-4 hours as needed
- Percutaneous endotracheal catheter: 1-2 mL of 20% or 2-4 mL of 10% solution every 1-4 hours via syringe attached to catheter

Diagnostic bronchogram: Children and Adolescents: Nebulization or endotracheal: 1-2 mL of 20% solution or 2-4 mL of 10% solution administered 2-3 times prior to procedure

Distal intestinal obstruction syndrome (previously known as meconium ileus equivalent): Limited data available; dosing regimens variable (polyethylene glycol has become more widely used for this indication):

Oral:
- Children <10 years: 30 mL of 10% solution diluted in 30 mL juice or soda 3 times/day for 24 hours
- Children 10 years and Adolescents: 60 mL of 10% solution diluted in 60 mL juice or soda 3 times/day for 24 hours
- **Note:** Prior to treatment, administer a phosphosoda enema. A clear liquid diet should be used during the 24-hour acetylcysteine treatment

Rectal enema: Children: Varying dosages; 100-300 mL of 4% to 6% solution 2-4 times daily; 50 mL of 20% solution 1-4 times daily and 5-30 mL of 10% to 20% solution 3-4 times daily have been used; rectal enemas appear to have less favorable results than oral administration (Mascarenhas, 2003). **Note:** Higher concentrations (10% to 20%) appear to increase fluid in the bowel and lead to increased incidence of adverse effects (Perman 1975)

Adults:

Acetaminophen poisoning: Only the 72-hour oral and 21-hour IV regimens are FDA approved. Ideally, in patients with an acute acetaminophen ingestion, treatment should begin within 8 hours of ingestion or as soon as possible after ingestion. In patients who present following RSTI and treatment is deemed appropriate, acetylcysteine should be initiated immediately.

Oral: 72-hour regimen: Consists of 18 doses; total dose delivered: 1330 mg/kg

Loading dose: 140 mg/kg

Maintenance dose: 70 mg/kg every 4 hours; repeat dose if emesis occurs within 1 hour of administration; **Note:** Consultation with a poison control center or clinical toxicologist is highly recommended when considering the discontinuation of oral acetylcysteine prior to the conclusion of a full 18-dose course of therapy.

IV (Acetadote): 21-hour regimen: Consists of 3 doses; total dose delivered: 300 mg/kg

Loading dose: 150 mg/kg (maximum: 15 g) infused over 60 minutes

Second dose: 50 mg/kg (maximum: 5 g) infused over 4 hours

Third dose: 100 mg/kg (maximum: 10 g) infused over 16 hours

Respiratory conditions; adjuvant therapy: Note: Patients should receive an aerosolized bronchodilator 10-15 minutes prior to dose.

Inhalation, nebulization (face mask, mouth piece, tracheostomy): Acetylcysteine 10% and 20% solution (dilute 20% solution with sodium chloride or sterile water for inhalation); 10% solution may be used undiluted: 3-5 mL of 20% solution or 6-10 mL of 10% solution until nebulized given 3-4 times/day; dosing range: 1-10 mL of 20% solution or 2-20 mL of 10% solution every 2-6 hours

Inhalation, nebulization (tent, croupette): Dose must be individualized; may require up to 300 mL solution/ treatment

Direct instillation:

Into tracheostomy: 1-2 mL of 10% to 20% solution every 1-4 hours

Through percutaneous intratracheal catheter: 1-2 mL of 20% or 2-4 mL of 10% solution every 1-4 hours via syringe attached to catheter

Diagnostic bronchogram: Nebulization or intratracheal: 1-2 mL of 20% solution or 2-4 mL of 10% solution administered 2-3 times prior to procedure

Prevention of radiocontrast-induced renal dysfunction: Oral: 600 mg twice daily for 2 days (beginning the day before the procedure); hydrate patient concurrently

Preparation for Administration

Oral: Acetaminophen poisoning: Dilute the 20% solution 1:3 with a cola, orange juice, or other soft drink to prepare a 5% solution. Use within 1 hour of preparation.

Parenteral: IV (Acetadote): Acetaminophen poisoning: **Note:** Volume of diluent based on weight; compatible diluents include D_5W, ½NS, SWFI:

Patient weight 5 to 20 kg: Dilute dose in the following volumes of compatible diluents:

Loading dose: 3 mL/kg

Second dose: 7 mL/kg

Third dose: 200 mL

Patient weight 21 to 40 kg: Dilute dose in the following volumes of compatible diluents:

Loading dose: 100 mL

Second dose: 250 mL

Third dose: 500 mL

Patient weight: 41 to 100 kg: Dilute dose in the following volumes of compatible diluents. In patients requiring fluid restriction, decrease diluent volume by 50%.

Loading dose: 200 mL

Second dose: 500 mL

Third dose: 1,000 mL

Undiluted injection, solution (Acetadote) is hyperosmolar (2,600 mOsmol/L); when the diluent volume is decreased for patients <40 kg or requiring fluid restriction, the osmolarity of the solution may remain higher than desirable for intravenous infusion. To ensure tolerance of the infusion, osmolarity should be adjusted to a physiologically safe level (eg, ≥150 mOsmol/L in children).

Acetadote Concentration	Osmolarity in ½ NS	Osmolarity in D_5W	Osmolarity in Sterile Water for Injection
7 mg/mL	245 mOsmol/L	343 mOsmol/L	91 mOsmol/L
24 mg/mL	466 mOsmol/L	564 mOsmol/L	312 mOsmol/L

Solution for inhalation: The 20% solution may be diluted with sodium chloride or sterile water; the 10% solution may be used undiluted.

Rectal: Dilute the inhalation solution in NS to the desired final concentration of 4 to 6%; may also be given undiluted (Mascarenhas 2003; Perman 1975)

Administration

Oral: Acetaminophen poisoning: Administer as a 5% solution (see Preparation for Administration); use within 1 hour of preparation. If patient vomits within 1 hour of dose, readminister. **Note:** The unpleasant odor (sulfur-like) becomes less noticeable as treatment progresses. It is helpful to put the acetylcysteine on ice, in a cup with a cover, and drink through a straw; alternatively, administer via an NG tube.

Parenteral: IV (Acetadose): Acetaminophen poisoning:

Loading dose: Administer over 60 minutes

Second dose: Administer over 4 hours

Third dose: Administer over 16 hours

Inhalation solution: May be administered by nebulization either undiluted (both 10% and 20%) or diluted in NS

Rectal: Inhalation solution may be given undiluted (10% to 20%) or diluted to 4% to 6% solution and administer rectally (Mascarenhas 2003; Perman 1975)

Monitoring Parameters When used in acetaminophen overdose, determine acetaminophen level as soon as possible, but no sooner than 4 hours after ingestion of immediate release formulations or 2 hours after ingestion of liquid formulations (to ensure peak levels have been obtained); coingestion of acetaminophen with other medications which may delay GI peristalsis eg, antihistamines, opioids, may require repeated serum levels to determine the peak serum level; liver function tests

Dosage Forms Excipient information presented when available (limited, particularly for generics); consult specific product labeling.

Injection, solution [preservative free]: 20% (30 mL)

Acetadote: 20% [200 mg/mL] (30 mL)

Solution, for inhalation/oral: 10% [100 mg/mL] (10 mL, 30 mL); 20% [200 mg/mL] (10 mL, 30 mL)

Solution, for inhalation/oral [preservative free]: 10% [100 mg/mL] (4 mL, 10 mL, 30 mL); 20% [200 mg/mL] (4 mL, 10 mL, 30 mL)

◆ **Acetylcysteine Injection (Can)** *see* Acetylcysteine *on page 57*

◆ **Acetylcysteine Sodium** *see* Acetylcysteine *on page 57*

- ◆ **Acetylcysteine Solution (Can)** *see* Acetylcysteine *on page 57*
- ◆ **Acetylsalicylic Acid** *see* Aspirin *on page 206*
- ◆ **ACH Candesartan (Can)** *see* Candesartan *on page 358*
- ◆ **ACH-Ezetimibe (Can)** *see* Ezetimibe *on page 832*
- ◆ **ACH-Letrozole (Can)** *see* Letrozole *on page 1224*
- ◆ **ACH-Montelukast (Can)** *see* Montelukast *on page 1459*
- ◆ **Ach-Mycophenolate (Can)** *see* Mycophenolate *on page 1473*
- ◆ **Achromycin** *see* Tetracycline *on page 2035*
- ◆ **ACH-Temozolomide (Can)** *see* Temozolomide *on page 2012*
- ◆ **Aciclovir** *see* Acyclovir (Systemic) *on page 61*
- ◆ **Aciclovir** *see* Acyclovir (Topical) *on page 65*
- ◆ **Acid Control (Can)** *see* Famotidine *on page 847*
- ◆ **Acid Reducer [OTC]** *see* Famotidine *on page 847*
- ◆ **Acid Reducer [OTC]** *see* Ranitidine *on page 1836*
- ◆ **Acid Reducer (Can)** *see* Ranitidine *on page 1836*
- ◆ **Acid Reducer Maximum Strength [OTC]** *see* Famotidine *on page 847*
- ◆ **Acid Reducer Maximum Strength [OTC] [DSC]** *see* Ranitidine *on page 1836*
- ◆ **Acidulated Phosphate Fluoride** *see* Fluoride *on page 899*
- ◆ **Aciphex** *see* RABEprazole *on page 1828*
- ◆ **AcipHex Sprinkle** *see* RABEprazole *on page 1828*
- ◆ **Aclovate** *see* Alclometasone *on page 85*
- ◆ **Acne-Clear [OTC]** *see* Benzoyl Peroxide *on page 270*
- ◆ **AcneFree Severe Clearing Syst [OTC]** *see* Benzoyl Peroxide *on page 270*
- ◆ **Acne Medication [OTC] [DSC]** *see* Benzoyl Peroxide *on page 270*
- ◆ **Acne Medication 5 [OTC]** *see* Benzoyl Peroxide *on page 270*
- ◆ **Acne Medication 10 [OTC]** *see* Benzoyl Peroxide *on page 270*
- ◆ **Act [OTC]** *see* Fluoride *on page 899*
- ◆ **ACT-D** *see* DACTINomycin *on page 573*
- ◆ **ACT-Amlodipine (Can)** *see* AmLODIPine *on page 133*
- ◆ **ACT Atorvastatin (Can)** *see* AtorvaSTATin *on page 220*
- ◆ **ACT-Azithromycin (Can)** *see* Azithromycin (Systemic) *on page 242*
- ◆ **ACT Bosentan (Can)** *see* Bosentan *on page 294*
- ◆ **ACT Celecoxib (Can)** *see* Celecoxib *on page 418*
- ◆ **ACT Ciprofloxacin (Can)** *see* Ciprofloxacin (Systemic) *on page 463*
- ◆ **ACT Citalopram (Can)** *see* Citalopram *on page 476*
- ◆ **ACT Diltiazem CD (Can)** *see* Diltiazem *on page 661*
- ◆ **ACT Diltiazem T (Can)** *see* Diltiazem *on page 661*
- ◆ **Actemra** *see* Tocilizumab *on page 2079*
- ◆ **ACT-Enalapril (Can)** *see* Enalapril *on page 744*
- ◆ **ACT Escitalopram (Can)** *see* Escitalopram *on page 786*
- ◆ **ACT Etidronate (Can)** *see* Etidronate *on page 815*
- ◆ **ACT Ezetimibe (Can)** *see* Ezetimibe *on page 832*
- ◆ **ACT Fluconazole (Can)** *see* Fluconazole *on page 881*
- ◆ **ACT-Fluvoxamine (Can)** *see* FluvoxaMINE *on page 928*
- ◆ **ACTH** *see* Corticotropin *on page 536*
- ◆ **Acthar** *see* Corticotropin *on page 536*
- ◆ **ActHIB** *see Haemophilus* b Conjugate Vaccine *on page 998*
- ◆ **Acticin** *see* Permethrin *on page 1675*
- ◆ **Acticlate** *see* Doxycycline *on page 717*
- ◆ **Actidose-Aqua [OTC]** *see* Charcoal, Activated *on page 425*
- ◆ **Actidose/Sorbitol [OTC]** *see* Charcoal, Activated *on page 425*
- ◆ **Actifed (Can)** *see* Triprolidine and Pseudoephedrine *on page 2129*
- ◆ **Actigall** *see* Ursodiol *on page 2136*
- ◆ **ACT-Imatinib (Can)** *see* Imatinib *on page 1078*
- ◆ **Actinomycin** *see* DACTINomycin *on page 573*
- ◆ **Actinomycin D** *see* DACTINomycin *on page 573*
- ◆ **Actinomycin CI** *see* DACTINomycin *on page 573*
- ◆ **Actiq** *see* FentaNYL *on page 857*
- ◆ **ACT-Irbesartan (Can)** *see* Irbesartan *on page 1158*
- ◆ **Activase** *see* Alteplase *on page 105*
- ◆ **Activase rt-PA (Can)** *see* Alteplase *on page 105*
- ◆ **Activated Carbon** *see* Charcoal, Activated *on page 42*
- ◆ **Activated Charcoal** *see* Charcoal, Activated *on page 425*
- ◆ **Activated Dimethicone** *see* Simethicone *on page 192*
- ◆ **Activated Ergosterol** *see* Ergocalciferol *on page 772*
- ◆ **Activated Methylpolysiloxane** *see* Simethicone *on page 1927*
- ◆ **Activated PCC** *see* Anti-inhibitor Coagulant Comple (Human) *on page 176*
- ◆ **Active-Cyclobenzaprine** *see* Cyclobenzaprine *on page 548*
- ◆ **Active-Tramadol** *see* TraMADol *on page 2098*
- ◆ **Act Kids [OTC]** *see* Fluoride *on page 899*
- ◆ **ACT Levetiracetam (Can)** *see* LevETIRAcetam *on page 1234*
- ◆ **ACT Levofloxacin (Can)** *see* Levofloxacin (Systemic) *on page 1243*
- ◆ **ACT Losartan (Can)** *see* Losartan *on page 1302*
- ◆ **ACT-Metformin (Can)** *see* MetFORMIN *on page 1375*
- ◆ **ACT Nabilone (Can)** *see* Nabilone *on page 1478*
- ◆ **ACT Olanzapine (Can)** *see* OLANZapine *on page 154*
- ◆ **ACT Olanzapine ODT (Can)** *see* OLANZapine *on page 1546*
- ◆ **ACT Oxycodone CR (Can)** *see* OxyCODONE *on page 1590*
- ◆ **ACT Pantoprazole (Can)** *see* Pantoprazole *on page 1618*
- ◆ **ACT Pravastatin (Can)** *see* Pravastatin *on page 1749*
- ◆ **ACT-Quetiapine (Can)** *see* QUEtiapine *on page 1815*
- ◆ **ACT Ranitidine (Can)** *see* Ranitidine *on page 1836*
- ◆ **Act Restoring [OTC]** *see* Fluoride *on page 899*
- ◆ **ACT Risperidone (Can)** *see* RisperiDONE *on page 186*
- ◆ **ACT Rizatriptan (Can)** *see* Rizatriptan *on page 1879*
- ◆ **ACT Rizatriptan ODT (Can)** *see* Rizatriptan *on page 1879*
- ◆ **ACT Sertraline (Can)** *see* Sertraline *on page 1916*
- ◆ **ACT-Sildenafil (Can)** *see* Sildenafil *on page 1921*
- ◆ **ACT-Simvastatin (Can)** *see* Simvastatin *on page 1928*
- ◆ **ACT-Sumatriptan (Can)** *see* SUMAtriptan *on page 199*
- ◆ **ACT Temozolomide (Can)** *see* Temozolomide *on page 2012*
- ◆ **ACT Topiramate (Can)** *see* Topiramate *on page 2085*
- ◆ **Act Total Care [OTC]** *see* Fluoride *on page 899*

Acyclovir (Systemic) (ay SYE kloe veer)

Medication Safety Issues

Sound-alike/look-alike issues:

Acyclovir may be confused with ganciclovir, Retrovir, valacyclovir

Zovirax may be confused with Doribax, Valtrex, Zithromax, Zostrix, Zyloprim, Zyvox

Related Information

Management of Drug Extravasations *on page 2298*

Brand Names: US Zovirax

Brand Names: Canada Acyclovir Sodium for Injection; Acyclovir Sodium Injection; Apo-Acyclovir; Mylan-Acyclovir; ratio-Acyclovir; Teva-Acyclovir; Zovirax

Therapeutic Category Antiviral Agent, Oral; Antiviral Agent, Parenteral

Generic Availability (US) Yes

Use

Parenteral: Treatment of initial and prophylaxis of recurrent mucosal and cutaneous herpes simplex (HSV 1 and HSV 2) infections in immunocompromised patients (FDA approved in all ages); treatment of severe initial episodes of herpes genitalis in immunocompetent patients (FDA approved in ages ≥12 years and adults); treatment of herpes simplex encephalitis, including neonatal herpes simplex virus (FDA approved in all ages); treatment of varicella-zoster virus (VZV) infections in immunocompromised patients (FDA approved in all ages)

Oral: Treatment of chickenpox (varicella) in immunocompetent patients (FDA approved in ages ≥2 years and adults); treatment of initial episodes and prophylaxis of recurrent herpes simplex (HSV 2, genital herpes) and acute treatment of herpes zoster (shingles) (FDA approved in adults)

Has also been used for treatment of varicella-zoster infections in healthy, nonpregnant persons >13 years of age, children >12 months of age who have a chronic skin or lung disorder or are receiving long-term aspirin therapy, and immunocompromised patients; oral therapy has also been used for suppression following parenteral treatment of neonatal HSV infection

Pregnancy Risk Factor B

Pregnancy Considerations Teratogenic effects were not observed in animal reproduction studies. Acyclovir has been shown to cross the human placenta (Henderson, 1992). Results from a pregnancy registry, established in 1984 and closed in 1999, did not find an increase in the number of birth defects with exposure to acyclovir when compared to those expected in the general population. However, due to the small size of the registry and lack of long-term data, the manufacturer recommends using during pregnancy with caution and only when clearly needed. Acyclovir may be appropriate for the treatment of genital herpes in pregnant women (CDC, 2010).

Breast-Feeding Considerations Acyclovir is excreted in breast milk. The manufacturer recommends that caution be exercised when administering acyclovir to nursing women. Limited data suggest exposure to the nursing infant of ~0.3 mg/kg/day following oral administration of acyclovir to the mother. Nursing mothers with herpetic lesions near or on the breast should avoid breast-feeding (Gartner, 2005).

Contraindications Hypersensitivity to acyclovir, valacyclovir, or any component of the formulation

Warnings/Precautions Use with caution in immunocompromised patients; thrombocytopenic purpura/hemolytic uremic syndrome (TTP/HUS) has been reported. Use caution in the elderly, preexisting renal disease (may require dosage modification), or in those receiving other nephrotoxic drugs. Renal failure (sometimes fatal) has been reported. Maintain adequate hydration during oral or intravenous therapy. Use IV preparation with caution in patients with underlying neurologic abnormalities, serious hepatic or electrolyte abnormalities, or substantial hypoxia.

Varicella-zoster: Treatment should begin within 24 hours of appearance of rash; oral route not recommended for routine use in otherwise healthy children with varicella, but may be effective in patients at increased risk of moderate-to-severe infection (>12 years of age, chronic cutaneous or pulmonary disorders, long-term salicylate therapy, corticosteroid therapy).

Adverse Reactions

Oral:

Central nervous system: Headache, malaise

Gastrointestinal: Diarrhea, nausea, vomiting

Parenteral:

Dermatologic: Hives, itching, rash

Gastrointestinal: Nausea, vomiting

Hepatic: Liver function tests increased

Local: Inflammation at injection site, phlebitis

Renal: Acute renal failure, BUN increased, creatinine increased

All forms: Rare but important or life-threatening: Abdominal pain, aggression, agitation, anemia, anorexia, ataxia, coma, confusion, consciousness decreased, delirium, desquamation, disseminated intravascular coagulopathy (DIC), dizziness, dysarthria, encephalopathy, fatigue, fever, gastrointestinal distress, hallucinations, hematuria, hemolysis, hepatitis, hyperbilirubinemia, hypotension, insomnia, jaundice, leukocytoclastic vasculitis, leukocytosis, leukopenia, lymphadenopathy, mental depression, myalgia, neutrophilia, pain, psychosis, renal failure, renal pain, seizure, somnolence, sore throat, thrombocytopenia, thrombocytopenic purpura/hemolytic uremic syndrome (TTP/HUS), thrombocytosis, visual disturbances

Drug Interactions

Metabolism/Transport Effects None known.

Avoid Concomitant Use

Avoid concomitant use of Acyclovir (Systemic) with any of the following: Foscarnet; Varicella Virus Vaccine; Zoster Vaccine

Increased Effect/Toxicity

Acyclovir (Systemic) may increase the levels/effects of: Mycophenolate; Tenofovir; Zidovudine

The levels/effects of Acyclovir (Systemic) may be increased by: Foscarnet; Mycophenolate

Decreased Effect

Acyclovir (Systemic) may decrease the levels/effects of: Varicella Virus Vaccine; Zoster Vaccine

Food Interactions Food does not affect absorption of oral acyclovir.

Storage/Stability

Capsule, oral suspension, tablet: Store at controlled room temperature of 15°C to 25°C (59°F to 77°F); protect from capsule and tablet from moisture.

Injection: Store powder at controlled room temperature of 15°C to 25°C (59°F to 77°F). Reconstituted solutions remain stable for 12 hours at room temperature. Do not refrigerate reconstituted solutions or solutions diluted for infusion as they may precipitate. Once diluted for infusion, use within 24 hours.

Mechanism of Action Acyclovir is converted to acyclovir monophosphate by virus-specific thymidine kinase then further converted to acyclovir triphosphate by other cellular enzymes. Acyclovir triphosphate inhibits DNA synthesis and viral replication by competing with deoxyguanosine triphosphate for viral DNA polymerase and being incorporated into viral DNA.

Pharmacokinetics (Adult data unless noted)

Absorption: Oral: 15% to 30%

Distribution: Widely distributed throughout the body including brain, kidney, lungs, liver, spleen, muscle, uterus, vagina, and the CSF; CSF acyclovir concentration is 50% of serum concentration

V_d:

- Neonates to 3 months of age: 28.8 L/1.73 m^2
- Children 1 to 2 years: 31.6 L/1.73 m^2
- Children 2 to 7 years: 42 L/1.73 m^2

Protein binding: <9% to 33%

Metabolism: Converted by viral enzymes to acyclovir monophosphate, and further converted to diphosphate then triphosphate (active form) by cellular enzymes

Bioavailability: Oral: 10% to 20%; decreases with increasing dose

Half-life, terminal phase:

- Neonates: 4 hours
- Children 1 to 12 years: 2 to 3 hours
- Adults: 2 to 3.5 hours (with normal renal function); hemodialysis: ~5 hours

Time to peak serum concentration: Oral: Within 1.5 to 2 hours

Elimination: Primary route is the kidney with 60% to 90% of a dose excreted unchanged in the urine

Dosing: Neonatal

HSV infection, treatment: IV: 20 mg/kg/dose every 8 hours for 14 to 21 days; CNS and disseminated infections: 21 day treatment duration; skin and mucous membrane infections: 14 day treatment duration (CDC, 2010; Kimberlin, 2013; *Red Book* [AAP], 2012)

HSV, chronic suppression following disseminated or CNS infection: Limited data available: Oral:

AAP Recommendation (low dose, 6-month-course): 300 mg/m^2/dose every 8 hours; begin after completion of a 14- to 21-day-course of IV therapy dependent upon type of infection; duration of therapy: 6 months (Kimberlin, 2011; Kimberlin, 2013)

Alternate dosing (high-dose, 2-year-course) (Tiffany, 2005): Begin after completion of a 21-day-course of IV therapy; dosing based on a prospective trial of 16 consecutive neonates (GA: Premature: n=4; term= 12; age at treatment: Neonate: n=14; PNA >30 days: n=1); pharmacokinetic data were used to determine dosing regimen to maintain serum acyclovir concentration above target of 2 mcg/mL; treatment was continued for 2 years in 14 of 16 patients; results showed normal neurodevelopmental outcomes in 69% and normal motor development in 70%; no untoward effects were reported during the study duration.

Initial dosing: Approximate dose: 1200 to 1600 mg/m^2/dose twice daily

- Preterm neonate: Proportional decrease of full-term initial dose
- Full term or near term: 400 mg twice daily

Maintenance dosing: In the trial, serum acyclovir co centrations were evaluated to assess adequacy dosing to maintain serum concentrations above th target of 2 to 3 mcg/mL. Samples were collected hour after a witnessed dose; if the acyclovir seru concentration approached or was below the target; th dose was increased to the next greater 200 mg incr ment. Serum concentrations were evaluated every months; in order to limit the phlebotomy losses, follo up serum concentrations were not evaluated outsid of routine monitoring.

Varicella zoster (chickenpox), treatment: IV: 10 15 mg/kg/dose every 8 hours for 5 to 10 days; continu for ≥48 hours after the last new lesions have appeare (Ogilvie, 1998; Sauerbrei, 2007; Smith, 2009)

Dosing adjustment in renal impairment:

Manufacturer's labeling: IV:

- >50 mL/minute/1.73m^2: No adjustments necessary
- 25 to 50 mL/minute/1.73m^2: Administer every 12 hou
- 10 to 25mL/minute/1.73m^2: Administer every 24 hour
- 0 to 10 mL/minute/1.73m^2: Administer 50% of the dos every 24 hours

Alternate dosing: The following adjustments have bee recommended (Englund, 1991): IV:

- S_{cr} 0.8 to 1.1 mg/dL: Administer 20 mg/kg/dose eve 12 hours
- S_{cr} 1.2 to 1.5 mg/dL: Administer 20 mg/kg/dose eve 24 hours
- S_{cr} >1.5 mg/dL: Administer 10 mg/kg/dose every 2 hours

Dosing: Usual Note: Obese patients should be dose using ideal body weight.

Pediatric:

HSV neonatal infection, treatment and suppressiv therapy in very young infants (independent of H status):

Treatment (disseminated, CNS, or skin, eye, or mou disease): Infants 1 to 3 months: IV: 20 mg/kg/dos every 8 hours; treatment duration: For cutaneous ar mucous membrane infections (skin, eye, or mouth): 1 days; for CNS or disseminated infection: 21 day (CDC, 2010; Kimberlin, 2013; *Red Book* [AAP], 201

Chronic suppressive therapy: Limited data availabl Oral:

AAP Recommendation (low dose, 6-month-course Infants: 300 mg/**m^2**/dose every 8 hours; begin aft completion of a 14- to 21-day-course of IV thera dependent upon type of infection; duration of the apy: 6 months (Kimberlin, 2011; Kimberlin, 2013)

Alternate dosing (high dose, 2-year-course) (Tiffan 2005): Infants and Children <3 years: Begin aft completion of a 21-day course of IV therapy; dosin based on a prospective trial of 16 consecutive ne nates (GA: Premature: n=4; term= 12; age at trea ment: Neonate: n=14; PNA >30 days: n=1 pharmacokinetic data were used to determine dosin regimen to maintain serum acyclovir concentratio above target of 2 to 3 mcg/mL; treatment wa continued for 2 years in 14 of 16 patients; resul showed normal neurodevelopmental outcomes 69% and normal motor development in 70%; n untoward effects were reported during the stud duration.

Initial dosing: 400 mg twice daily; approximate dos 1200 to 1600 mg/m^2/dose twice daily

Maintenance dosing: **Note**: Approximate doses fo patients born at term:

- Infants 1 to <5 months: 400 mg twice daily
- Infants 5 to <9 months: 600 mg twice daily
- Infants and Children 9 to <15 months: 800 m twice daily
- Children 15 to 24 months: 1000 mg twice daily

Note: In the trial, serum acyclovir concentrations were evaluated to assess adequacy of dosing to maintain serum concentrations above the target of 2 to 3 mcg/mL. Samples were collected 1 hour after a witnessed dose; if the acyclovir serum concentration approached or was below the target; the dose was increased to the next greater 200 mg increment. Maximum dose: 1200 mg. Serum concentrations were evaluated every 3 months; in order to limit the phlebotomy losses, follow-up serum concentrations were not evaluated outside of routine monitoring.

HSV encephalitis, treatment: IV:

Infants and Children 3 months to <12 years:

Non-HIV-exposed/-positive: 10 to 15 mg/kg/dose every 8 hours for 14 to 21 days (*Red Book* [AAP], 2012)

HIV-exposed/-positive: 10 mg/kg/dose every 8 hours for 21 days; do not discontinue therapy until the repeat CSF HSV DNA PCR is negative (CDC, 2009)

Children ≥12 years and Adolescents (independent of HIV status): 10 mg/kg/dose every 8 hours for 14 to 21 days (*Red Book* [AAP], 2012)

HSV genital infection:

First infection, mild to moderate: Oral:

Non-HIV-exposed/-positive:

Children <12 years: 40 to 80 mg/kg/**day** divided in 3 to 4 doses per day for 5 to 10 days; maximum daily dose: 1000 mg/**day** (*Red Book* [AAP], 2012)

Children and Adolescents ≥12 years: 200 mg every 4 hours while awake (5 times daily) **or** 400 mg 3 times daily for 7 to 10 days; treatment can be extended beyond 10 days if healing is not complete (CDC, 2010; *Red Book* [AAP], 2012)

HIV-exposed/-positive:

Children <45 kg: 20 mg/kg/dose 3 times daily for 5 to 14 days; maximum dose: 400 mg (CDC, 2009)

Children ≥45 kg: 400 mg twice daily for 5 to 14 days (CDC, 2009)

Adolescents: 400 mg 3 times daily for 5 to 14 days (DHHS [adult], 2013)

First infection, severe (independent of HIV status): IV: Children and Adolescents ≥12 years: 5 mg/kg/dose every 8 hours for 5 to 7 days (*Red Book* [AAP], 2012)

Recurrent infection: Oral:

Children <12 years: 10 mg/kg/dose every 8 hours for up to 12 months; maximum daily dose: 1000 mg/**day**; re-evaluate after 12 months (*Red Book* [AAP], 2009)

Children and Adolescents ≥12 years:

Non-HIV-exposed/-positive: 200 mg every 4 hours while awake (5 times daily) for 5 days **or** 800 mg twice daily for 5 days **or** 800 mg 3 times daily for 2 days (CDC, 2010; *Red Book* [AAP], 2012)

HIV-exposed/-positive: Adolescents: 400 mg 3 times daily for 5 to 14 days (DHHS [adult], 2013)

Suppression, chronic: Oral:

Non-HIV-exposed/-positive:

Children <12 years: Limited data available: 20 to 25 mg/kg/dose twice daily; maximum dose: 400 mg (Bradley, 2011)

Children and Adolescents ≥12 years: 400 mg twice daily for up to 12 months (CDC, 2010; *Red Book* [AAP], 2012)

HIV-exposed/-positive:

Infants and Children: 20 mg/kg/dose twice daily; maximum dose: 400 mg (CDC, 2009)

Adolescents: 400 mg twice daily (DHHS [adult], 2013)

HSV gingivostomatitis:

Non-HIV-exposed/-positive: Primary infection: Oral:

AAP recommendations: Children and Adolescents: 20 mg/kg/dose 4 times daily for 7 days; usual maximum dose: 200 mg/dose, others have reported higher (400 mg/dose) (Bradley, 2014; Cernik, 2008; *Red Book* [AAP, 2012])

Alternate dosing: Infants ≥10 months, Children, and Adolescents: 15 mg/kg/dose five times daily for 7 days; maximum dose: 200 mg/dose (Amir, 1997; Balfour, 1999); dosing based on a placebo controlled trial in children 1 to 6 years of age (n=72, treatment group: n=31); results showed when treatment started within 72 hours of symptom onset a shorter duration of symptoms and viral shedding was observed (Amir, 1997)

HIV-exposed/-positive (CDC, 2009):

Mild, symptomatic: Oral: Infants and Children: 20 mg/kg/dose 3 times daily for 5 to 10 days; maximum dose: 400 mg

Moderate to severe, symptomatic: IV: Infants and Children: 5 to 10 mg/kg/dose every 8 hours; switch to oral therapy once lesions begin to regress

HSV, herpes labialis (cold sore) recurrent, chronic suppressive therapy: Oral: Children: 30 mg/kg/**day** in 3 divided doses for up to 12 months; maximum daily dose: 1000 mg/**day**; re-evaluate after 12 months (*Red Book* [AAP], 2012)

HSV mucosal or cutaneous infection:

Immunocompromised host:

Treatment:

IV: Infants, Children, and Adolescents: 10 mg/kg/dose every 8 hours for 7 to 14 days (*Red Book* [AAP], 2012)

Oral: Children ≥2 years and Adolescents: 1000 mg/**day** in 3 to 5 divided doses for 7 to 14 days; some suggest the maximum daily dose should not exceed 80 mg/kg/**day** (*Red Book*, 2009; *Red Book* [AAP], 2012)

Suppression, chronic (cutaneous, ocular) episodes: Oral:

Infants and Children (HIV-exposed/-positive): 20 mg/kg/dose twice daily for 5 to 14 days; maximum dose: 400 mg (CDC, 2009)

Children and Adolescents ≥12 years (independent of HIV status): 400 mg twice daily for up to 12 months (*Red Book* [AAP], 2012)

HSV orolabial (HIV-exposed/-positive): Adolescents: Oral: 400 mg 3 times daily for 5 to 10 days (DHHS [adult], 2013)

HSV progressive or disseminated infection, treatment (immunocompromised host) including HIV-exposed/-positive:

Non-HIV-exposed/-positive: Infants, Children, and Adolescents: IV: 10 mg/kg/dose every 8 hours for 7 to 21 days (*Red Book* [AAP], 2012)

HIV-exposed/-positive: Infants, Children, and Adolescents: IV: 10 mg/kg/dose every 8 hours for 21 days (CDC, 2009)

HSV prophylaxis; immunocompromised hosts, seropositive:

Hematopoietic stem cell transplant (HSCT) in seropositive recipient (Tomblyn, 2009):

Prevention of early reactivation: **Note:** Begin at conditioning and continue until engraftment or resolution of mucositis; whichever is longer (~30 days post-HSCT)

Infants, Children, and Adolescents <40 kg:

IV: 250 mg/$\mathbf{m^2}$/dose every 8 hours **or** 125 mg/$\mathbf{m^2}$/dose every 6 hours; maximum daily dose: 80 mg/kg/**day**

Oral: 60 to 90 mg/kg/**day** in 2 to 3 divided doses

Children and Adolescents ≥40 kg:

IV: 250 mg/$\mathbf{m^2}$/dose every 12 hours

Oral: 400 to 800 mg twice daily

Prevention of late reactivation: **Note:** Treatment during first year after HSCT.

Infants, Children, and Adolescents <40 kg: Oral: 60 to 90 mg/kg/**day** in 2 to 3 divided doses; maximum daily dose: 800 mg twice daily

Children and Adolescents ≥40 kg: Oral: 800 mg twice daily

HIV-exposed/-positive, prevention of HSV reactivation: Oral: Infants and Children: 20 mg/kg/dose twice daily, maximum dose: 400 mg (CDC, 2009)

Other immunocompromised hosts who are HSV seropositive:

IV: Infants, Children, and Adolescents: 5 mg/kg/dose every 8 hours during period of risk (*Red Book* [AAP], 2012)

Oral: Children ≥2 years and Adolescents: 200 mg every 4 hours while awake (5 doses daily) **or** 200 mg every 8 hours (*Red Book* [AAP], 2012)

Varicella zoster (chickenpox or shingles), prophylaxis (HIV-exposed/-positive): Oral: **Note:** Consider use if >96 hours postexposure or if VZV-immune globulin is not available; begin therapy 7 to 10 days after exposure

Infants and Children: 20 mg/kg/dose 4 times daily for 5 to 7 days; maximum dose: 800 mg (CDC, 2009)

Adolescents: 800 mg 5 times daily for 5 to 7 days (DHHS, 2013)

Varicella zoster (chickenpox), treatment:

Immunocompetent host:

Ambulatory therapy: Oral: Children ≥2 years and Adolescents: 20 mg/kg/dose 4 times daily for 5 days; maximum daily dose: 3200 mg/**day** (*Red Book* [AAP], 2012)

Hospitalized patient: IV: Children ≥2 years and Adolescents: 10 mg/kg/dose **or** 500 mg/**m²**/dose every 8 hours for 7 to 10 days (*Red Book* [AAP], 2012)

Immunocompromised host (non-HIV-exposed/-positive): IV:

Infants: 10 mg/kg/dose every 8 hours for 7 to 10 days (*Red Book* [AAP], 2012)

Children and Adolescents: 500 mg/**m²**/dose every 8 hours for 7 to 10 days; some experts recommend 10 mg/kg/dose every 8 hours (*Red Book* [AAP], 2012)

HIV-exposed/-positive:

Mild, uncomplicated disease and no or moderate immune suppression: Oral:

Infants and Children: 20 mg/kg/dose 4 times daily for 7 to 10 days or until no new lesions for 48 hours; maximum dose: 800 mg (CDC, 2009)

Adolescents: 800 mg 5 times daily for 5 to 7 days (DHHS [adult], 2013)

Severe, complicated disease or severe immune suppression: IV:

Infants: 10 mg/kg/dose every 8 hours for 7 to 10 days or until no new lesions for 48 hours (CDC, 2009)

Children: 10 mg/kg/dose **or** 500 mg/**m²**/dose every 8 hours for 7 to 10 days or until no new lesions for 48 hours (CDC, 2009)

Adolescents: 10 to 15 mg/kg/dose every 8 hours for 7 to 10 days; may convert to oral therapy after defervescence and if no evidence of visceral involvement is evident (DHHS [adult], 2013)

Varicella zoster (shingles; herpes zoster), treatment:

Immunocompetent host:

Ambulatory therapy: Oral: Children ≥12 years and Adolescents: 800 mg every 4 hours (5 doses per day) for 5 to 7 days (*Red Book* [AAP], 2012)

Hospitalized patient: IV:

Infants: 10 mg/kg/dose every 8 hours for 7 to 10 days (*Red Book* [AAP], 2012)

Children and Adolescents: 500 mg/**m²**/dose every 8 hours for 7 to 10 days; some experts recommend 10 mg/kg/dose every 8 hours (*Red Book* [AAP] 2012)

Immunocompromised host (non-HIV-exposed/-positive): IV: Infants, Children, and Adolescents 10 mg/kg/dose every 8 hours for 7 to 10 days (*Red Book* [AAP], 2012)

HIV-exposed/-positive:

Mild, uncomplicated disease and no or moderate immune suppression: Oral:

Infants and Children: 20 mg/kg/dose 4 times daily for 7 to 10 days; maximum dose: 800 mg; consider longer course if resolution of lesions is slow (CDC, 2009)

Adolescents: 800 mg 5 times daily for 7 to 10 days longer if lesions resolve slowly (DHHS [adult], 2013)

Severe immune suppression or complicated disease trigeminal nerve involvement, extensive multidermatomal zoster or extensive cutaneous lesions or visceral involvement: IV:

Infants: 10 mg/kg/dose every 8 hours until resolution of cutaneous lesions and visceral disease clearly begins, then convert to oral therapy to complete a 10 to 14 day total course of therapy (CDC, 2009)

Children: 10 mg/kg/dose **or** 500 mg/**m²**/dose every 8 hours until resolution of cutaneous lesions and visceral disease clearly begins, then convert to oral therapy to complete a 10 to 14 day total course of therapy (CDC, 2009)

Adolescents: 10 to 15 mg/kg/dose every 8 hours until clinical improvement is evident, then convert to oral therapy to complete a 10 to 14 day total course of therapy (DHHS [adult], 2013)

Varicella zoster, acute retinal necrosis, treatment (HIV-exposed/-positive):

Initial treatment: IV: **Note:** Follow up IV therapy with oral acyclovir or valacyclovir maintenance therapy.

Infants: 10 to 15 mg/kg/dose every 8 hours for 10 to 14 days (CDC, 2009)

Children: 10 to 15 mg/kg/dose **or** 500 mg/**m²**/dose every 8 hours for 10 to 14 days (CDC, 2009)

Adolescents: 10 to 15 mg/kg/dose every 8 hours for 10 to 14 days (DHHS, 2013)

Maintenance treatment; begin after 10 to 14 day course of IV acyclovir: Oral: Infants and Children: 20 mg/kg/dose every 8 hours for a total duration of therapy of 4 to 6 weeks (CDC, 2009)

Adult:

HSV encephalitis: IV: 10 mg/kg/dose every 8 hours for 10 days; 10 to 15 mg/kg/dose every 8 hours for 14 to 21 days has also been reported

HSV genital infection:

IV: Immunocompetent: Initial episode, severe: 5 mg/kg/dose every 8 hours for 5 to 7 days **or** 5 to 10 mg/kg/dose every 8 hours for 2 to 7 days, follow with oral therapy to complete at least 10 days of therapy (CDC, 2010)

Oral:

Initial episode: 200 mg every 4 hours while awake (5 times/day) **or** 400 mg 3 times daily for 7 to 10 days (CDC, 2010)

Recurrence: 200 mg every 4 hours while awake (5 times/day) for 5 days; begin at earliest signs of disease

Alternatively, the following regimens are also recommended by the CDC: 400 mg 3 times daily for 5 days; 800 mg twice daily for 5 days; 800 mg 3 times daily for 2 days (CDC, 2010)

Chronic suppression: 400 mg twice daily (CDC 2010) or 200 mg 3 to 5 times daily, for up to 12 months followed by re-evaluation

HSV mucocutaneous: Immunocompromised: Treatment: IV: 5 mg/kg/dose every 8 hours for 7 days (Leflore, 2000); dosing for up to 14 days also reported

Varicella Zoster (chickenpox): Begin treatment within the first 24 hours of rash onset:

Oral: >40 kg (immunocompetent): 800 mg/dose 4 times daily for 5 days

IV:

Manufacturer's labeling (immunocompromised): 10 mg/kg/dose every 8 hours for 7 days

AIDS*info* guidelines (immunocompromised): 10 to 15 mg/kg/dose every 8 hours for 7 to 10 days (DHHS, 2013)

Herpes zoster (shingles):

Immunocompetent: Oral: 800 mg every 4 hours (5 times daily) for 7 to 10 days

Immunocompromised: IV: 10 mg/kg/dose **or** 500 mg/m^2/dose every 8 hours for 7 days

Dosing adjustment in renal impairment:

Oral: Children, Adolescents, and Adults:

CrCl >25 mL/minute/1.73 m^2: No adjustment required

CrCl 10 to 25 mL/minute/1.73 m^2:

Normal dosing regimen 200 mg every 4 hours or 400 mg every 12 hours: No adjustment required

Normal dosing regimen 800 mg 5 times daily: Administer 800 mg every 8 hours

CrCl <10 mL/minute/1.73 m^2:

Normal dosing regimen 200 mg every 4 hours or 400 mg every 12 hours: Administer 200 mg every 12 hours

Normal dosing regimen 800 mg 5 times daily: Administer 800 mg every 12 hours

Intermittent hemodialysis (IHD): Dialyzable (60% reduction following a 6-hour session):

For a normal dosing regimen 200 mg 5 times daily or 400 mg every 12 hours: Administer 200 mg every 12 hours; administer after hemodialysis on dialysis days

For a normal dosing regimen 800 mg 5 times daily: Administer 800 mg every 12 hours; administer after hemodialysis on dialysis days

IV: Infants, Children, Adolescents, and Adults:

CrCl >50 mL/minute/1.73 m^2: No adjustment required

CrCl 25 to 50 mL/minute/1.73 m^2: Administer every 12 hours

CrCl 10 to 25 mL/minute/1.73 m^2: Administer every 24 hours

CrCl <10 mL/minute/1.73 m^2: Administer 50% of dose every 24 hours

Intermittent hemodialysis (IHD): Administer 50% of dose every 24 hours; administer after hemodialysis on dialysis days (Aronoff, 2007)

Peritoneal dialysis (PD): Administer 50% of normal dose every 24 hours; no supplemental dose needed (Aronoff, 2007)

Continuous renal replacement therapy (CRRT):

Infants, Children, and Adolescents: IV: 10 mg/kg/dose every 12 hours (Aronoff, 2007)

Adults: Drug clearance is highly dependent on the method of renal replacement, filter type, and flow rate. Appropriate dosing requires close monitoring of pharmacologic response, signs of adverse reactions due to drug accumulation, as well as drug concentrations in relation to target trough (if appropriate). The following are general recommendations only (based on dialysate flow/ultrafiltration rates of 1 to 2 L/hour and minimal residual renal function) and should not supersede clinical judgment (Heintz, 2009; Trotman, 2005):

CVVH: IV: 5 to 10 mg/kg every 24 hours

CVVHD/CVVHDF: IV: 5 to 10 mg/kg every 12 to 24 hours

Note: The higher end of dosage range (eg, 10 mg/kg every 12 hours for CVVHDF) is recommended for viral meningoencephalitis and varicella zoster virus infections.

Dosing adjustment in hepatic impairment: There are no dosage adjustments provided in the manufacturer's labeling.

Preparation for Administration Parenteral: Reconstitute vial for injection to 50 mg/mL with SWFI; do not use bacteriostatic water containing benzyl alcohol or parabens. For intravenous infusion, dilute in D_5W, D_5NS, $D_5\frac{1}{4}NS$, $D_5\frac{1}{2}NS$, LR, or NS to a final concentration ≤7 mg/mL. In fluid restricted patients, concentrations up to 10 mg/mL have been infused; concentrations >10 mg/mL increase the risk of phlebitis.

Administration

Oral: May administer with or without food; shake suspension well before use

Parenteral: Administer by slow IV infusion over at least 1 hour; rapid infusion is associated with nephrotoxicity due to crystalluria and renal tubular damage and should be avoided. Avoid IV push, IM, or SubQ administration.

Vesicant/Extravasation Risk Irritant at concentrations >7 mg/mL

Monitoring Parameters Urinalysis, BUN, serum creatinine, urine output; liver enzymes, CBC; neutrophil count at least twice weekly in neonates receiving acyclovir 60 mg/kg/day IV

Additional Information Sodium content of 1 g: 4.2 mEq

Dosage Forms Excipient information presented when available (limited, particularly for generics); consult specific product labeling.

Capsule, Oral:

Zovirax: 200 mg [contains fd&c blue #2 (indigotine), parabens]

Generic: 200 mg

Solution, Intravenous, as sodium [strength expressed as base]:

Generic: 50 mg/mL (10 mL, 20 mL)

Solution Reconstituted, Intravenous, as sodium [strength expressed as base]:

Generic: 500 mg (1 ea); 1000 mg (1 ea)

Suspension, Oral:

Zovirax: 200 mg/5 mL (473 mL) [contains methylparaben, propylparaben; banana flavor]

Generic: 200 mg/5 mL (473 mL)

Tablet, Oral:

Zovirax: 400 mg

Zovirax: 800 mg [contains fd&c blue #2 (indigotine)]

Generic: 400 mg, 800 mg

Acyclovir (Topical) (ay SYE kloe veer)

Medication Safety Issues

Sound-alike/look-alike issues:

Acyclovir may be confused with ganciclovir, Retrovir, valacyclovir

Zovirax may be confused with Doribax, Valtrex Zithromax, Zostrix, Zyloprim, Zyvox

International issues:

Opthavir [Mexico] may be confused with Optivar brand name for azelastine [U.S.]

Brand Names: US Sitavig; Zovirax

Brand Names: Canada Zovirax

Therapeutic Category Antiviral Agent, Topical

Generic Availability (US) May be product dependent

Use

Topical (cream): Treatment of recurrent herpes labialis (cold sores) (FDA approved in ages ≥12 years and adults)

Topical (ointment): Management of initial genital herpes and in limited, nonlife-threatening mucocutaneous HSV infections in immunocompromised patients (FDA approved in adults)

Pregnancy Risk Factor B

Pregnancy Considerations Teratogenic effects were not observed in animal studies. When administered orally, acyclovir crosses the placenta. Refer to the Acyclovir (Systemic) monograph for details. The amount of acyclovir available systemically following topical application of the cream or ointment is significantly less in comparison to oral doses.

Breast-Feeding Considerations When administered orally, acyclovir enters breast milk. Refer to the Acyclovir (Systemic) monograph for details. The amount of acyclovir available systemically following topical application of the cream or ointment is significantly less in comparison to oral doses. Nursing mothers with herpetic lesions near or on the breast should avoid breast-feeding.

Contraindications

Buccal tablet: Hypersensitivity to acyclovir, valacyclovir, milk protein concentrate or any component of the formulation

Cream, ointment: Hypersensitivity to acyclovir, valacyclovir, or any component of the formulation

Warnings/Precautions

Genital herpes: Physical contact should be avoided when lesions are present; transmission may also occur in the absence of symptoms. Treatment should begin with the first signs or symptoms. There are no data to support the use of acyclovir ointment to prevent transmission of infection to other persons or prevent recurrent infections if no signs or symptoms are present.

Herpes labialis: Treatment should begin with the first signs or symptoms. Cream is for external use only to the lips and face; do not apply to eye or inside the mouth or nose, or any mucous membranes. Ointment should also not be used in the eye and be used with caution in immunocompromised patients. Cream may be irritating and cause contact sensitization. Buccal tablets are applied to the area of the upper gum above the incisor tooth on the same side as the symptoms; do not apply to the inside of the lip or cheek. Some products may contain milk protein concentrate.

Warnings: Additional Pediatric Considerations Some dosage forms may contain propylene glycol; in neonates large amounts of propylene glycol delivered orally, intravenously (eg, >3,000 mg/day), or topically have been associated with potentially fatal toxicities which can include metabolic acidosis, seizures, renal failure, and CNS depression; toxicities have also been reported in children and adults including hyperosmolality, lactic acidosis, seizures and respiratory depression; use caution (AAP, 1997; Shehab, 2009).

Adverse Reactions

Central nervous system: Lethargy (buccal tablet)

Dermatologic: Erythema (buccal tablet), local pain (ointment; mild; includes transient burning and stinging), skin rash (buccal tablet)

Gastrointestinal: Aphthous stomatitis (buccal tablet), gingival pain (buccal tablet)

Local: Application site irritation (buccal tablet), application site reaction (cream; including dry lips, desquamation, dryness of skin, cracked lips, burning skin, pruritus, flakiness of skin, and stinging on skin)

Rare but important or life-threatening: Anaphylaxis, eczema

Drug Interactions

Metabolism/Transport Effects None known.

Avoid Concomitant Use There are no known interactions where it is recommended to avoid concomitant use.

Increased Effect/Toxicity There are no known significant interactions involving an increase in effect.

Decreased Effect There are no known significant interactions involving a decrease in effect.

Storage/Stability

Buccal tablet: Store at 20°C to 25°C (68°F to 77°F); excursions permitted between 15°C and 30°C (59°F and 86°F). Protect from moisture.

Cream: Store at or below 25°C (77°F); excursions permitted between 15°C and 30°C (59°F and 86°F).

Ointment: Store at controlled room temperature of 20°C to 25°C (68°F to 77°F) in a dry place.

Mechanism of Action Acyclovir is converted to acyclovir monophosphate by virus-specific thymidine kinase then further converted to acyclovir triphosphate by other cellular enzymes. Acyclovir triphosphate inhibits DNA synthesis and viral replication by competing with deoxyguanosine triphosphate for viral DNA polymerase and being incorporated into viral DNA.

Pharmacokinetics (Adult data unless noted) Absorption: Poorly absorbed

Dosing: Usual

Topical:

Cream: Herpes labialis (cold sores): Children ≥12 years and Adults: Apply 5 times/day for 4 days

Ointment:

Genital HSV, immunocompromised: Adults: Initial episode: 1/2" ribbon of ointment for a 4" square surface area every 3 hours (6 times/day) for 7 days

Mucocutaneous HSV, nonlife-threatening, immunocompromised: Adults: Ointment: 1/2" ribbon of ointment for a 4" square surface area every 3 hours (6 times/day) for 7 days

Administration For topical use only; do not apply to eye, inside the mouth or nose, or on unaffected skin.

Cream: Apply layer of cream to cover only the cold sore or cover the area with symptoms; rub cream in until it disappears.

Ointment: Use a fingercot or rubber glove when applying ointment to prevent autoinoculation of other body sites or transmission of infection to other persons.

Dosage Forms Excipient information presented when available (limited, particularly for generics); consult specific product labeling.

Cream, External:

Zovirax: 5% (5 g) [contains cetostearyl alcohol, propylene glycol]

Ointment, External:

Zovirax: 5% (30 g)

Generic: 5% (5 g, 15 g, 30 g)

Tablet, Buccal:

Sitavig: 50 mg [contains milk protein concentrate]

Acyclovir and Hydrocortisone

(ay SYE kloe veer & hye droe KOR ti sone)

Brand Names: US Xerese™

Therapeutic Category Antiviral Agent, Topical; Corticosteroid, Topical

Generic Availability (US) No

Use Early treatment of recurrent herpes labialis (cold sores) to shorten healing time and to reduce likelihood of ulceration (FDA approved in ages ≥6 years and adults)

Pregnancy Risk Factor B

Pregnancy Considerations Animal reproduction studies and studies in pregnant women have not been conducted with Xerese™. Systemic exposure of acyclovir and hydrocortisone after topical administration is minimal. See individual agents.

Breast-Feeding Considerations Systemic exposure of acyclovir and hydrocortisone after topical administration is minimal. See individual agents.

Contraindications There are no contraindications listed within the manufacturer's labeling.

Warnings/Precautions Treatment should begin with the first signs or symptoms. For external use only to the lip and around the mouth; do not apply to eye, inside the mouth or nose, or on the genitals. Contact healthcare provider if cold sore fails to heal in 2 weeks. Use with caution in immunocompromised patients. Use has been associated with local sensitization (irritation).

Warnings: Additional Pediatric Considerations Some dosage forms may contain propylene glycol; in neonates large amounts of propylene glycol delivered orally, intravenously (eg, >3,000 mg/day), or topically have been associated with potentially fatal toxicities which can include metabolic acidosis, seizures, renal failure, and CNS depression; toxicities have also been reported in children and adults including hyperosmolality, lactic acidosis, seizures, and respiratory depression; use caution (AAP 1997; Shehab 2009).

Adverse Reactions Rare but important or life-threatening:
Dermatologic: Burning, contact dermatitis, dryness, erythema, flaking, pigmentation changes, sensitization, signs/symptoms of inflammation, tingling

Drug Interactions

Metabolism/Transport Effects Refer to individual components.

Avoid Concomitant Use

Avoid concomitant use of Acyclovir and Hydrocortisone with any of the following: Aldesleukin

Increased Effect/Toxicity

Acyclovir and Hydrocortisone may increase the levels/effects of: Ceritinib; Deferasirox

The levels/effects of Acyclovir and Hydrocortisone may be increased by: Telaprevir

Decreased Effect

Acyclovir and Hydrocortisone may decrease the levels/effects of: Aldesleukin; Corticorelin; Hyaluronidase; Telaprevir

Storage/Stability Store at controlled room temperature of 20°C to 25°C (68°F to 77°F); excursions permitted to 15°C to 30°C (59°F to 86°F); do not freeze.

Mechanism of Action See individual agents.

Pharmacokinetics (Adult data unless noted) See individual agents.

Dosing: Usual

Pediatric: **Herpes labialis (cold sores):** Children ≥6 years and Adolescents: Topical: Apply 5 times daily for 5 days; initiate therapy at first sign of infection (ie, during the prodrome or when lesions appear)

Adult: **Herpes labialis (cold sores):** Topical: Apply 5 times daily for 5 days; initiate therapy at first sign of infection (ie, during the prodrome or when lesions appear)

Dosing adjustment in renal impairment: There are no dosage adjustments provided in the manufacturer's labeling.

Dosing adjustment in hepatic impairment: There are no dosage adjustments provided in the manufacturer's labeling.

Administration Topical: For external use only. Wash hands before and after use. Use sufficient amount to cover the affected area(s), including the outer margin of cold sore; do not rub affected area nor cover area with a bandage. Do not bathe or shower for 30 minutes following application. Not for use in the eye, inside the mouth or nose, or on the genitals.

Dosage Forms Excipient information presented when available (limited, particularly for generics); consult specific product labeling.

Cream, topical:

Xerese®: Acyclovir 5% and hydrocortisone 1% (5 g)

- **Acyclovir Sodium for Injection (Can)** *see* Acyclovir (Systemic) *on page 61*
- **Acyclovir Sodium Injection (Can)** *see* Acyclovir (Systemic) *on page 61*
- **ACZ885** *see* Canakinumab *on page 356*
- **Aczone** *see* Dapsone (Topical) *on page 581*
- **Adacel** *see* Diphtheria and Tetanus Toxoids, and Acellular Pertussis Vaccine *on page 681*
- **Adacel-Polio (Can)** *see* Diphtheria and Tetanus Toxoids, Acellular Pertussis, and Poliovirus Vaccine *on page 677*
- **Adalat XL (Can)** *see* NIFEdipine *on page 1516*
- **Adalat CC** *see* NIFEdipine *on page 1516*

Adalimumab (a da LIM yoo mab)

Medication Safety Issues

Sound-alike/look-alike issues:

Humira may be confused with Humulin, Humalog

Humira Pen may be confused with HumaPen Memoir (used with HumaLOG)

Brand Names: US Humira; Humira Pediatric Crohns Start; Humira Pen; Humira Pen-Crohns Starter; Humira Pen-Psoriasis Starter

Brand Names: Canada Humira

Therapeutic Category Antirheumatic, Disease Modifying; Gastrointestinal Agent, Miscellaneous; Monoclonal Antibody; Tumor Necrosis Factor (TNF) Blocking Agent

Generic Availability (US) No

Use Treatment of moderately to severely active polyarticular juvenile idiopathic arthritis (JIA) alone or in combination with methotrexate (FDA approved in ages 2 to 17 years weighing ≥10 kg); treatment and maintenance of remission in patients with moderately to severely active Crohn disease with inadequate response to conventional treatment or patients who have lost response to or are intolerant of infliximab (FDA approved ages ≥6 years and adults); moderately to severely active rheumatoid arthritis (RA) alone or in combination with methotrexate or other nonbiologic, disease-modifying antirheumatic drugs (DMARDs) (FDA approved in adults); active psoriatic arthritis alone or in combination with nonbiologic DMARDs (FDA approved in adults); active ankylosing spondylitis (FDA approved in adults); treatment of moderate to severe chronic plaque psoriasis when systemic therapy is required and other agents are less appropriate (FDA approved in adults); and treatment and maintenance of remission in patients with moderately to severely active ulcerative colitis unresponsive to immunosuppressants (FDA approved in adults). **Note:** Efficacy in ulcerative colitis patients who are intolerant or no longer responsive to other TNF blockers has not been established. Has also been used in children with idiopathic or JIA-associated uveitis and chronic uveitis.

Medication Guide Available Yes

Pregnancy Risk Factor B

Pregnancy Considerations Adverse events were not observed in animal reproduction studies. Adalimumab crosses the placenta and can be detected in cord blood at birth at concentrations higher than those in the maternal serum. In one study of pregnant women with inflammatory bowel disease, adalimumab was found to be measurable in a newborn for up to 11 weeks following delivery. Maternal doses of adalimumab were 40 mg every other week (n=9) or 40 mg weekly (n=1) and the last dose was administered 0.14-8 weeks prior to delivery (median 5.5 weeks) (Mahadevan, 2013). If therapy for inflammatory bowel disease is needed during pregnancy, adalimumab should be discontinued before 30 weeks gestation in order to decrease exposure to the newborn. In addition, the administration of live vaccines should be postponed until anti-TNF concentrations in the infant are negative (Habal, 2012; Mahadeven, 2013; Zelinkova, 2013).

Women exposed to adalimumab during pregnancy for the treatment of an autoimmune disease (eg, inflammatory bowel disease) may contact the OTIS Autoimmune Diseases Study at 877-311-8972.

Breast-Feeding Considerations Low concentrations of adalimumab may be detected in breast milk but are unlikely to be absorbed by a nursing infant. The manufacturer recommends caution be used if administered to a nursing woman.

Contraindications

There are no contraindications listed within the manufacturer's labeling.

Canadian labeling: Hypersensitivity to adalimumab or any component of the formulation; severe infection (eg, sepsis, tuberculosis, opportunistic infection); moderate-to-severe heart failure (NYHA class III/IV)

Warnings/Precautions [U.S. Boxed Warnings]: Patients should be evaluated for latent tuberculosis infection with a tuberculin skin test prior to therapy. Treatment of latent tuberculosis should be initiated before adalimumab is used. Tuberculosis (disseminated or extrapulmonary) has been reactivated while on adalimumab. Most cases have been reported within the first 8 months of treatment. **Patients with initial negative tuberculin skin tests should receive continued monitoring for tuberculosis throughout treatment; active tuberculosis has developed in this population during treatment.** Rare reactivation of hepatitis B virus (HBV) has occurred in chronic virus carriers; use with caution; evaluate prior to initiation and during treatment.

[U.S. Boxed Warning]: Patients receiving adalimumab are at increased risk for serious infections which may result in hospitalization and/or fatality; infections usually developed in patients receiving concomitant immunosuppressive agents (eg, methotrexate or corticosteroids) and may present as disseminated (rather than local) disease. Active tuberculosis (or reactivation of latent tuberculosis), invasive fungal (including aspergillosis, blastomycosis, candidiasis, coccidioidomycosis, histoplasmosis, and pneumocystosis) and bacterial, viral or other opportunistic infections (including legionellosis and listeriosis) have been reported in patients receiving TNF-blocking agents, including adalimumab. Monitor closely for signs/symptoms of infection. Discontinue for serious infection or sepsis. Consider risks versus benefits prior to use in patients with a history of chronic or recurrent infection. Consider empiric antifungal therapy in patients who are at risk for invasive fungal infection and develop severe systemic illness. Caution should be exercised when considering use in the elderly or in patients with conditions that predispose them to infections (eg, diabetes) or residence/travel from areas of endemic mycoses (blastomycosis, coccidioidomycosis, histoplasmosis), or with latent or localized infections. Do not initiate adalimumab therapy with clinically important active infection. Patients who develop a new infection while undergoing treatment should be monitored closely. There is limited experience with patients undergoing surgical procedures while on therapy; consider long half-life with planned procedures and monitor closely for infection.

[U.S. Boxed Warning]: Lymphoma and other malignancies (some fatal) have been reported in children and adolescent patients receiving TNF-blocking agents, including adalimumab. Half the cases are lymphomas (Hodgkin and non-Hodgkin) and the other cases are varied, but include malignancies not typically observed in this population. Most patients were receiving concomitant immunosuppressants. **[U.S. Boxed Warning]: Hepatosplenic T-cell lymphoma (HSTCL), a rare T-cell lymphoma, has also been reported primarily in patients with Crohn disease or ulcerative colitis treated with adalimumab and who received concomitant azathioprine or mercaptopurine; reports occurred predominantly in adolescent and young adult males.** Rare cases of lymphoma have also been reported in association with adalimumab. A higher incidence of nonmelanoma skin cancers was noted in adalimumab treated patients, when compared to the control group. Impact on the development and course of malignancies is not fully defined. May exacerbate preexisting or recent-onset central or peripheral nervous system demyelinating disorders. Consider discontinuing use in patients who develop peripheral or central nervous system demyelinating disorders during treatment.

May exacerbate preexisting or recent-onset demyelinating CNS disorders. Worsening and new-onset heart failure (HF) has been reported; use caution in patients with decreased left ventricular function. Use caution in patients with HF (Canadian labeling contraindicates use in NYHA III/IV). Patients should be brought up to date with all immunizations before initiating therapy. No data are available concerning the effects of adalimumab on vaccination. Live vaccines should not be given concurrently. No data are available concerning secondary transmission of live vaccines in patients receiving adalimumab. Rare cases of pancytopenia (including aplastic anemia) have been reported with TNF-blocking agents; with significant hematologic abnormalities, consider discontinuing therapy. Positive antinuclear antibody titers have been detected in patients (with negative baselines) treated with adalimumab. Rare cases of autoimmune disorder, including lupus-like syndrome, have been reported; monitor and discontinue adalimumab if symptoms develop. May cause hypersensitivity reactions, including anaphylaxis; monitor. Infection and malignancy has been reported at a higher incidence in elderly patients compared to younger adults; use caution in elderly patients. Potentially significant drug-drug interactions may exist, requiring dose or frequency adjustment, additional monitoring, and/or selection of alternative therapy.

The packaging (needle cover of prefilled syringe) may contain latex. Some dosage forms may contain polysorbate 80 (also known as Tweens). Hypersensitivity reactions, usually a delayed reaction, have been reported following exposure to pharmaceutical products containing polysorbate 80 in certain individuals (Isaksson, 2002; Lucente 2000; Shelley, 1995). Thrombocytopenia, ascites, pulmonary deterioration, and renal and hepatic failure have been reported in premature neonates after receiving parenteral products containing polysorbate 80 (Alade, 1986; CDC, 1984). See manufacturer's labeling. According to the Centers for Disease Control and Prevention (CDC), pen-shaped injection devices should never be used for more than one person (even when the needle is changed) because of the risk of infection. The injection device should be clearly labeled with individual patient information to ensure that the correct pen is used (CDC, 2012).

Warnings: Additional Pediatric Considerations Postmarketing reports of lymphomas and other malignancies were primarily in pediatric patients with Crohn disease or ulcerative colitis treated with adalimumab and who received concomitant azathioprine or mercaptopurine; reports occurred predominantly in adolescent and young adult males. As compared to the general population, an increased risk of lymphoma has been noted in clinical trials; however, rheumatoid arthritis has been previously associated with an increased rate of lymphoma. In an analysis of children and adolescents who had received TNF-blockers (etanercept and infliximab), the FDA identified 48 cases of malignancy. Of the 48 cases, ~50% were lymphomas (eg, Hodgkin and non-Hodgkin lymphoma). Other malignancies, such as leukemia, melanoma, and solid organ tumors were reported; malignancies rarely seen in children (eg, leiomyosarcoma, hepatic malignancies, and renal cell carcinoma) were also observed. Of note, most of these cases (88%) were receiving other immunosuppressive medications (eg, azathioprine and methotrexate). The role of TNF-blockers in the development of malignancies in children cannot be excluded. The FDA also reviewed 147 postmarketing reports of leukemia (including acute myeloid leukemia, chronic lymphocytic leukemia, and chronic myeloid leukemia) in patients (children and adults) using TNF-blockers. Average onset time to development of leukemia was within the first 1 to 2 years of TNF-blocker initiation.

Adverse Reactions

Cardiovascular: Atrial fibrillation, cardiac arrest, cardiac arrhythmia, cardiac failure, chest pain, coronary artery disease, deep vein thrombosis, hypertension, hypertensive encephalopathy, myocardial infarction, palpitations, pericardial effusion, pericarditis, peripheral edema, subdural hematoma, syncope, tachycardia, vascular disease

Central nervous system: Confusion, headache, myasthenia, paresthesia

Dermatologic: Alopecia, cellulitis, erysipelas, skin rash

Endocrine & metabolic: Dehydration, hypercholesterolemia, hyperlipidemia, ketosis, menstrual disease, parathyroid disease

Gastrointestinal: Abdominal pain, diverticulitis, esophagitis, gastroenteritis, gastrointestinal hemorrhage, nausea, vomiting

Genitourinary: Cholecystitis, cholelithiasis, cystitis, hematuria, pelvic pain, urinary tract infection

Hematologic & oncologic: Adenoma, agranulocytosis, carcinoma (including breast, gastrointestinal, skin, urogenital), granulocytopenia, leukopenia, malignant lymphoma, malignant melanoma, pancytopenia, paraproteinemia, polycythemia, positive ANA titer

Hepatic: Hepatic necrosis, increased serum alkaline phosphatase

Hypersensitivity: Hypersensitivity reaction (more common in children)

Immunologic: Antibody development (significance unknown)

Infection: Herpes zoster, sepsis, serious infection (more common in adults [Burmester, 2012])

Local: Injection site reaction

Neuromuscular & skeletal: Arthralgia, arthritis, arthropathy, back pain, bone fracture, increased creatine phosphokinase, limb pain, multiple sclerosis, muscle cramps, myasthenia, osteonecrosis, septic arthritis, synovitis, systemic lupus erythematosus, tendon disease, tremor

Ophthalmic: Cataract

Renal: Nephrolithiasis, pyelonephritis

Respiratory: Asthma, bronchospasm, dyspnea, flu-like symptoms, pleural effusion, pneumonia, respiratory depression, sinusitis, tuberculosis (including reactivation of latent infection; disseminated, miliary, lymphatic, peritoneal and pulmonary); upper respiratory tract infection

Miscellaneous: Abnormal healing, accidental injury, fever, postoperative complication (infection)

Rare but important or life-threatening: Abscess (limb, perianal), anal fissure, anaphylactoid reaction, anaphylaxis, angioedema, aplastic anemia, appendicitis, bacterial infection, basal cell carcinoma, cerebrovascular accident, cervical dysplasia, circulatory shock, cytopenia, dermal ulcer, endometrial hyperplasia, erythema multiforme, fixed drug eruption, fulminant necrotizing fasciitis, fungal infection, Guillain-Barre syndrome, hepatic failure, hepatitis B (reactivation), hepatosplenic T-cell lymphomas (children, adolescents, and young adults), hepatotoxicity (idiosyncratic) (Chalasani, 2014), herpes simplex infection, histoplasmosis, hypersensitivity angiitis, increased serum transaminases, interstitial pulmonary disease (eg, pulmonary fibrosis), intestinal obstruction, intestinal perforation, leukemia, liver metastases, lupus-like syndrome, lymphadenopathy, lymphocytosis, malignant neoplasm of ovary, meningitis (viral), Merkel cell carcinoma, mycobacterium avium complex, myositis (children and adolescents), neutropenia, optic neuritis, pancreatitis, pharyngitis (children and adolescents), protozoal infection, psoriasis (including new onset, palmoplantar, pustular, or exacerbation), pulmonary embolism, respiratory failure, sarcoidosis, septic shock, skin granuloma (annulare; children and adolescents), Stevens-Johnson syndrome, streptococcal pharyngitis (children and adolescents), testicular neoplasm, thrombocytopenia, vasculitis (systemic), viral infection

Drug Interactions

Metabolism/Transport Effects None known.

Avoid Concomitant Use

Avoid concomitant use of Adalimumab with any of the following: Abatacept; Anakinra; BCG; BCG (Intravesical); Belimumab; Canakinumab; Certolizumab Pegol; InFLIXimab; Natalizumab; Pimecrolimus; Rilonacept; Tacrolimus (Topical); Tocilizumab; Tofacitinib; Vaccines (Live); Vedolizumab

Increased Effect/Toxicity

Adalimumab may increase the levels/effects of: Abatacept; Anakinra; Belimumab; Canakinumab; Certolizumab Pegol; InFLIXimab; Leflunomide; Natalizumab; Rilonacept; Tofacitinib; Vaccines (Live); Vedolizumab

The levels/effects of Adalimumab may be increased by: Denosumab; Pimecrolimus; Roflumilast; Tacrolimus (Topical); Tocilizumab; Trastuzumab

Decreased Effect

Adalimumab may decrease the levels/effects of: BCG; BCG (Intravesical); Coccidioides immitis Skin Test; CycloSPORINE (Systemic); Sipuleucel-T; Theophylline Derivatives; Vaccines (Inactivated); Vaccines (Live); Warfarin

The levels/effects of Adalimumab may be decreased by: Echinacea

Storage/Stability Store under refrigeration at 2°C to 8°C (36°F to 46°F) in original container; do not freeze. Do not use if frozen even if it has been thawed. Protect from light. May be stored at room temperature up to a maximum of 25°C (77°F) for up to 14 days; discard if not used within 14 days.

Mechanism of Action Adalimumab is a recombinant monoclonal antibody that binds to human tumor necrosis factor alpha (TNF-alpha), thereby interfering with binding to TNFα receptor sites and subsequent cytokine-driven inflammatory processes. Elevated TNF levels in the synovial fluid are involved in the pathologic pain and joint destruction in immune-mediated arthritis. Adalimumab decreases signs and symptoms of psoriatic arthritis, rheumatoid arthritis, and ankylosing spondylitis. It inhibits progression of structural damage of rheumatoid and psoriatic arthritis. Reduces signs and symptoms and maintains clinical remission in Crohn disease and ulcerative colitis; reduces epidermal thickness and inflammatory cell infiltration in plaque psoriasis.

Pharmacokinetics (Adult data unless noted)

Distribution: V_d: 4.7-6 L; synovial fluid concentrations: 31% to 96% of serum

Bioavailability: Absolute: 64%

Half-life: ~2 weeks (range: 10-20 days)

Time to peak serum concentration: SubQ: 131 ± 56 hours

Elimination: Clearance increased in the presence of anti-adalimumab antibodies; decreased in patients ≥40 years

Dosing: Usual

Pediatric:

Crohn's disease; moderate to severe; refractory:

SubQ: Children ≥6 years and Adolescents:

17 kg to <40 kg: Initial: 80 mg divided into 2 injections (40 mg each) on day 1, then 40 mg administered 2 weeks later (day 15); and then on day 29, begin maintenance dose: 20 mg every other week

≥40 kg: Initial: 160 mg divided into 4 injections (40 mg each, administered on one day or as 2 injections per day over 2 consecutive days), then 80 mg (divided into 2 injections [40 mg each] administered on one day) 2 weeks later (day 15); and then on day 29 begin maintenance dose: 40 mg every other week

Juvenile idiopathic arthritis (JIA): SubQ: Children ≥2 years and Adolescents ≤17 years:

10 kg to <15 kg: 10 mg every other week

15 kg to <30 kg: 20 mg every other week

≥30 kg: 40 mg every other week

Ulcerative colitis; moderate to severe, refractory: Limited data available: SubQ: Children and Adolescents: Initial: 100 mg/m^2 (maximum dose: 160 mg/dose), then 50 mg/m^2 (maximum dose: 80 mg/dose) 2 weeks later; then on day 29, begin maintenance therapy: 25 mg/m^2 every other week (maximum dose: 40 mg/dose) (Turner 2012)

Uveitis: Limited data available; dosing regimens variable; SubQ:

Body surface area-directed dosing: Children ≥4 years and Adolescents: 24 or 40 mg/m^2 every 2 weeks; maximum dose 40 mg/dose (Gallagher, 2007; Simonini 2011). Dosing based on one prospective trial comparing 24 mg/m^2/dose every 2 weeks of adalimumab (n=16, ages 6 to 12 years) to infliximab (n=17, ages 5 to 13 years) and on a retrospective trial of biologic response modifiers, including five patients who received adalimumab at 40 mg/m^2/dose every 2 weeks.

Weight-directed dosing: Children ≥2 years and Adolescents (Biester 2007; Sens 2012; Tynjala 2008):

<30 kg: 20 mg every other week

>30 kg: 40 mg every other week

Adult:

Ankylosing spondylitis: SubQ: 40 mg every other week

Crohn's disease: SubQ: Initial: 160 mg divided into 4 doses (ie, given as 4 injections on day 1 or as 2 injections per day over 2 consecutive days), then 80 mg 2 weeks later (day 15); maintenance: 40 mg every other week beginning day 29; **Note:** Some patients may require 40 mg every week as maintenance therapy (Lichtenstein, 2009).

Plaque psoriasis: SubQ: Initial: 80 mg as a single dose; maintenance: 40 mg every other week beginning 1 week after initial dose

Psoriatic arthritis: SubQ: 40 mg every other week

Rheumatoid arthritis: SubQ: 40 mg every other week; may be administered with other DMARDs; patients not taking methotrexate may increase dose to 40 mg every week

Ulcerative colitis: SubQ:

Initial: 160 mg divided into 4 doses (given as 4 injections on day 1 or as 2 injections daily over 2 consecutive days), then 80 mg 2 weeks later (day 15)

Maintenance: 40 mg every other week beginning day 29. **Note:** Only continue maintenance dose in patients demonstrating clinical remission by 8 weeks (day 57) of therapy.

Dosing adjustment in renal impairment: Children, Adolescents, and Adults: There are no dosage adjustments provided in the manufacturer's labeling.

Dosing adjustment in hepatic impairment: Children, Adolescents, and Adults: There are no dosage adjustments provided in the manufacturer's labeling.

Administration For SubQ injection into thigh or lower abdomen (avoid areas within 2 inches of navel); rotate injection sites. May leave at room temperature for ~15 to 30 minutes prior to use; do not remove cap or cover while allowing product to reach room temperature. Do not use if solution is discolored or contains particulate matter. Do not administer to skin which is red, tender, bruised, or hard. Prefilled pens and syringes are available for use by patients (self-administration); the vial is intended for institutional use only. Vials do not contain a preservative; discard unused portion.

Monitoring Parameters Monitor improvement of symptoms and physical function assessments. Latent TB screening prior to initiating and during therapy; signs/symptoms of infection (prior to, during, and following therapy); CBC with differential; signs/symptoms/worsening of heart failure; HBV screening prior to initiating (all patients), HBV carriers (during and for several months following therapy); signs and symptoms of hypersensitivity reaction; symptoms of lupus-like syndrome; signs/symptoms of malignancy (eg, splenomegaly, hepatomegaly, abdominal pain, persistent fever, night sweats, weight loss), including periodic skin examination.

Dosage Forms Excipient information presented when available (limited, particularly for generics); consult specific product labeling.

Pen-injector Kit, Subcutaneous [preservative free]:

Humira Pen: 40 mg/0.8 mL (1 ea) [contains polysorbate 80]

Humira Pen-Crohns Starter: 40 mg/0.8 mL (1 ea) [contains polysorbate 80]

Humira Pen-Psoriasis Starter: 40 mg/0.8 mL (1 ea) [contains polysorbate 80]

Prefilled Syringe Kit, Subcutaneous [preservative free]:

Humira: 10 mg/0.2 mL (1 ea); 20 mg/0.4 mL (1 ea); 40 mg/0.8 mL (1 ea) [contains polysorbate 80]

Humira Pediatric Crohns Start: 40 mg/0.8 mL (1 ea) [contains polysorbate 80]

◆ **Adamantanamine Hydrochloride** *see* Amantadine *on page 112*

Adapalene (a DAP a leen)

Brand Names: US Differin

Brand Names: Canada Differin®; Differin® XP

Therapeutic Category Acne Products

Generic Availability (US) Yes

Use Topical treatment of acne vulgaris (FDA approved in ages ≥12 years and adults)

Pregnancy Risk Factor C

Pregnancy Considerations Adverse effects were observed in animal reproduction studies. Retinoids may cause harm when administered during pregnancy. A case report described maternal use of adapalene 1 month prior to pregnancy and through 13 weeks gestation; cerebral and ocular malformations were reported in the exposed fetus which resulted in termination of pregnancy (Autret 1997). In clinical trials, women of childbearing potential were required to have a negative pregnancy test prior to therapy.

Breast-Feeding Considerations It is not known if adapalene is excreted in breast milk. The manufacturer recommends that caution be exercised when administering adapalene to nursing women.

Contraindications Hypersensitivity to adapalene or any component of the formulation.

Lotion: There are no contraindications listed in the manufacturer's labeling.

Documentation of allergenic cross-reactivity for retinoids is limited. However, because of similarities in chemical structure and/or pharmacologic actions, the possibility of cross-sensitivity cannot be ruled out with certainty.

Warnings/Precautions Hypersensitivity reactions such as pruritus, face edema, eyelid edema, and swelling have been reported. Discontinue use immediately if allergic or anaphylactoid/anaphylactic reactions occur. Use is associated with increased susceptibility/sensitivity to UV light; avoid sunlamps or excessive sunlight exposure. Daily sunscreen use and other protective measures are recommended. Patients with sunburn should discontinue use until sunburn has healed. For external use only; avoid contact with abraded, broken, eczematous, or sunburned skin, mucous membranes, eyes, lips, and angles of the nose. Wax depilation is not recommended.

Certain cutaneous signs and symptoms such as erythema, dryness, scaling, stinging/burning, or pruritus may occur during treatment; these are most likely to occur during the first 2 to 4 weeks and will usually lessen with continued use. Treatment can increase skin sensitivity to weather extremes of wind or cold. Concomitant topical medications (eg, medicated or abrasive soaps and cleansers, or cosmetics with a strong drying effect, products with high concentrations of alcohol, astringents, spices or limes) should be avoided due to increased skin irritation. Depending on the severity of irritation, use moisturizer, reduce the frequency of application or discontinue use.

Warnings: Additional Pediatric Considerations May cause mild hyperglycemia; more common in pediatric patients. Some dosage forms may contain propylene glycol; in neonates large amounts of propylene glycol delivered orally, intravenously (eg, >3,000 mg/day), or topically have been associated with potentially fatal toxicities which can include metabolic acidosis, seizures, renal failure, and CNS depression; toxicities have also been reported in children and adults including hyperosmolality, lactic acidosis, seizures and respiratory depression; use caution (AAP, 1997; Shehab, 2009).

Adverse Reactions

Dermatologic: Burning/stinging, desquamation, dryness, erythema, pruritus, scaling, skin discomfort, skin irritation, sunburn

Rare but important or life-threatening: Acne flares, angioedema (gel), application site pain (gel), conjunctivitis, contact dermatitis, dermatitis, eczema, eyelid edema, facial edema (gel), lip swelling (gel), rash (cream/gel), skin discoloration

Drug Interactions

Metabolism/Transport Effects None known.

Avoid Concomitant Use

Avoid concomitant use of Adapalene with any of the following: Multivitamins/Fluoride (with ADE); Multivitamins/Minerals (with ADEK, Folate, Iron); Multivitamins/Minerals (with AE, No Iron)

Increased Effect/Toxicity

Adapalene may increase the levels/effects of: Porfimer; Verteporfin

The levels/effects of Adapalene may be increased by: Multivitamins/Fluoride (with ADE); Multivitamins/Minerals (with ADEK, Folate, Iron); Multivitamins/Minerals (with AE, No Iron)

Decreased Effect There are no known significant interactions involving a decrease in effect.

Storage/Stability Store at 20°C to 25°C (68°F to 77°F); excursions permitted to 15°C to 30°C (59°F to 86°F); do not freeze. Protect from light.

Lotion: Protect from light and heat; do not refrigerate.

Mechanism of Action Retinoid-like compound which is a modulator of cellular differentiation, keratinization, and inflammatory processes, all of which represent important features in the pathology of acne vulgaris

Pharmacodynamics Onset of action: 8-12 weeks

Pharmacokinetics (Adult data unless noted)

Absorption: Absorption through the skin is very low; only trace amounts have been measured in serum after chronic application

Elimination: Primarily in bile

Dosing: Usual Children ≥12 years, Adolescents, and Adults: **Acne, treatment:** Topical: Apply once daily in the evening

Dosing adjustment in renal impairment: There are no dosage adjustments provided in the manufacturer's labeling; however, dosage adjustment unlikely necessary due to low systemic absorption.

Dosing adjustment in hepatic impairment: There are no dosage adjustments provided in the manufacturer's labeling; however, dosage adjustment unlikely necessary due to low systemic absorption.

Administration Topical: For external use only. After cleansing the affected area with mild or soapless cleanser, apply a thin film of medication before retiring in the evening. Avoid contact with eyes, angles of the nose, lips and mucous membranes.

Monitoring Parameters Reduction in lesion size and/or inflammation; reduction in the number of lesions

Dosage Forms Excipient information presented when available (limited, particularly for generics); consult specific product labeling.

Cream, External:
- Differin: 0.1% (45 g)
- Generic: 0.1% (45 g)

Gel, External:
- Differin: 0.1% (45 g)
- Differin: 0.3% (45 g) [contains edetate disodium, methylparaben, propylene glycol]
- Generic: 0.1% (45 g); 0.3% (45 g)

Lotion, External:
- Differin: 0.1% (59 mL) [contains methylparaben, propylene glycol, propylparaben]
- Generic: 0.1% (59 mL)

Adapalene and Benzoyl Peroxide

(a DAP a leen & BEN zoe il peer OKS ide)

Brand Names: US Epiduo®

Brand Names: Canada Tactuo™

Therapeutic Category Acne Products; Topical Skin Product; Topical Skin Product, Acne

Generic Availability (US) No

Use Treatment of acne vulgaris (FDA approved in ages ≥9 years and adults)

Pregnancy Risk Factor C

Pregnancy Considerations There are no well-controlled studies in pregnant women. Use only if benefit outweighs the potential risk to fetus.

Contraindications There are no contraindications listed in the manufacturer's labeling.

Warnings/Precautions Avoid excessive exposure to sunlight and sunlamps. Certain cutaneous signs and symptoms (eg, erythema, dryness, scaling, burning/stinging) may occur during treatment; these are most likely to occur during the first 4 weeks and will usually lessen with continued use. Use concomitant topical acne therapy with caution. Avoid contact with abraded skin, eyes, and mucous membranes. May bleach hair or colored fabric. Concomitant use of benzoyl peroxide with sulfone products (eg, dapsone, sulfacetamide) may cause temporary discoloration (yellow/orange) of facial hair and skin. Application of products at separate times during the day or washing off benzoyl peroxide prior to application of other products may avoid skin discoloration (Dubina 2009).

Adverse Reactions

Dermatologic: Burning, contact dermatitis, dry skin, erythema, scaling, skin irritation, stinging

Rare but important or life-threatening: Blistering, conjunctivitis, eczema, eyelid edema, facial swelling, pain, photosensitivity, pruritus, rash, skin discoloration

Drug Interactions

Metabolism/Transport Effects None known.

Avoid Concomitant Use

Avoid concomitant use of Adapalene and Benzoyl Peroxide with any of the following: Multivitamins/Fluoride (with ADE); Multivitamins/Minerals (with ADEK, Folate, Iron); Multivitamins/Minerals (with AE, No Iron)

Increased Effect/Toxicity

Adapalene and Benzoyl Peroxide may increase the levels/effects of: Dapsone (Topical); Porfimer; Verteporfin

The levels/effects of Adapalene and Benzoyl Peroxide may be increased by: Multivitamins/Fluoride (with ADE); Multivitamins/Minerals (with ADEK, Folate, Iron); Multivitamins/Minerals (with AE, No Iron)

Decreased Effect There are no known significant interactions involving a decrease in effect.

Storage/Stability Store at 25°C (77°F); excursions permitted between 15°C to 30°C (59°F to 86°F). Protect from light and heat.

Mechanism of Action

Benzoyl peroxide releases free-radical oxygen which oxidizes bacterial proteins in the sebaceous follicles decreasing the number of anaerobic bacteria and decreasing irritating-type free fatty acids.

Adapalene is a retinoid-like compound which is a modulator of cellular differentiation, keratinization, and inflammatory processes, all of which represent important features in the pathology of acne vulgaris.

Pharmacodynamics Onset of action: ≥4-8 weeks (Eichenfield, 2013)

Pharmacokinetics (Adult data unless noted)

Metabolism: Benzoyl peroxide: Converted to benzoic acid in skin

Elimination: Adapalene: Primarily through bile; Benzoyl peroxide: Urine

Dosing: Usual Note: Application of more than recommended amount or more frequent administration does not result in quicker onset of action and is associated with more irritant effects.

Pediatric: **Acne vulgaris:** Children ≥7 years and Adolescents; limited data in children <9 years: Topical: Apply a thin film once daily to affected areas of cleansed and dried skin (Eichenfield, 2013)

Adult: **Acne vulgaris:** Topical: Apply a thin film once daily to affected areas of cleansed and dried skin

Administration Apply a pea-sized amount for each affected area of the face (eg, forehead, chin, each cheek). Skin should be clean and dry before applying. For external use only; avoid applying to eyes and mucous membranes.

Dosage Forms Excipient information presented when available (limited, particularly for generics); consult specific product labeling.

Gel, topical:

Epiduo®: Adapalene 0.1% and benzoyl peroxide 2.5% (45 g)

◆ **ADD 234037** *see* Lacosamide *on page 1200*

◆ **Addamel N** *see* Trace Elements *on page 2097*

◆ **Addaprin [OTC]** *see* Ibuprofen *on page 1064*

◆ **Adderall** *see* Dextroamphetamine and Amphetamine *on page 628*

◆ **Adderall XR** *see* Dextroamphetamine and Amphetamine *on page 628*

Adefovir (a DEF o veer)

Brand Names: US Hepsera

Brand Names: Canada Hepsera

Therapeutic Category Antiretroviral Agent, Reverse Transcriptase Inhibitor (Nucleotide)

Generic Availability (US) Yes

Use Treatment of chronic hepatitis B with evidence of active viral replication and either persistent elevations of ALT or AST or histologically active disease (FDA approved in ages ≥12 years and adults)

Pregnancy Risk Factor C

Pregnancy Considerations Adverse events were observed in some animal reproduction studies. Pregnant women exposed to adefovir should be registered with the pregnancy registry (800-258-4263).

Breast-Feeding Considerations It is not known if adefovir is excreted in breast milk. Due to the potential for serious adverse reactions in the nursing infant, a decision should be made whether to discontinue nursing or to discontinue the drug, taking into account the importance of treatment to the mother.

Contraindications Hypersensitivity to adefovir or any component of the formulation

Warnings/Precautions [U.S. Boxed Warning]: Use with caution in patients with renal dysfunction or in patients at risk of renal toxicity (including concurrent nephrotoxic agents or NSAIDs). Chronic administration may result in nephrotoxicity. Dosage adjustment is required in adult patients with renal dysfunction or in patients who develop renal dysfunction during therapy; no data available for use in children ≥12 years or adolescents with renal impairment. Not recommended as first line therapy of chronic HBV due to weak antiviral activity and high rate of resistance after first year. May be more appropriate as second-line agent in treatment-naïve patients. Combination therapy with lamivudine in nucleoside-naïve patients has not been shown to provide synergistic antiviral effects. In patients with lamivudine-resistant HBV, switching to adefovir monotherapy was associated with a higher risk of adefovir resistance compared to adding adefovir to lamivudine therapy (Lok, 2009).

Calculate creatinine clearance before initiation of therapy. Consider alternative therapy in patients who do not respond to adefovir monotherapy treatment. **[U.S. Boxed Warning]: May cause the development of HIV resistance in patients with unrecognized or untreated HIV infection.** Determine HIV status prior to initiating treatment with adefovir. **[U.S. Boxed Warning]: Fatal cases of lactic acidosis and severe hepatomegaly with steatosis have been reported with the use of nucleoside analogues alone or in combination with other antiretrovirals.** Female gender, obesity, and prolonged treatment may increase the risk of hepatotoxicity. Treatment should be discontinued in patients with lactic acidosis or signs/symptoms of hepatotoxicity (which may occur without marked transaminase elevations). **[U.S. Boxed Warning]: Acute exacerbations of hepatitis may occur (in up to 25% of patients) when antihepatitis therapy is discontinued.** Exacerbations typically occur within 12 weeks and may be self-limited or resolve upon resuming treatment; risk may be increased with advanced liver disease or cirrhosis. Monitor patients following discontinuation of therapy. Ethanol should be avoided in hepatitis B infection due to potential hepatic toxicity. Do not use concurrently with tenofovir (Viread®) or any product containing tenofovir (eg, Truvada®, Atripla®, Complera®).

Warnings: Additional Pediatric Considerations Efficacy in pediatric patients <12 years has not been reported; in clinical trials of children 2 to 12 years, positive responses to adefovir therapy were observed (13% to 17% of subjects evaluated); however, findings did not reach statistical significance (Jonas, 2008).

Adverse Reactions

Central nervous system: Headache

Dermatologic: Pruritus, rash

Endocrine & metabolic: Hypophosphatemia

Gastrointestinal: Abdominal pain, diarrhea, dyspepsia, flatulence, nausea, vomiting

Hepatic: Hepatitis exacerbation

Neuromuscular & skeletal: Back pain, weakness

Renal: Hematuria, renal failure, serum creatinine increased

Respiratory: Cough, rhinitis

Postmarketing and/or case reports: Fanconi syndrome, hepatitis, myopathy, nephrotoxicity, osteomalacia, pancreatitis, proximal renal tubulopathy

Drug Interactions

Metabolism/Transport Effects None known.

Avoid Concomitant Use

Avoid concomitant use of Adefovir with any of the following: Tenofovir

Increased Effect/Toxicity

Adefovir may increase the levels/effects of: Tenofovir

The levels/effects of Adefovir may be increased by: Ganciclovir-Valganciclovir; Ribavirin; Tenofovir

Decreased Effect

Adefovir may decrease the levels/effects of: Tenofovir

Food Interactions Food does not have a significant effect on adefovir absorption. Management: Administer without regard to meals.

Storage/Stability Store controlled room temperature of 25°C (77°F); excursions permitted between 15°C to 30°C (59°F to 86°F).

Mechanism of Action Acyclic nucleotide reverse transcriptase inhibitor (adenosine analog) which interferes with HBV viral RNA-dependent DNA polymerase resulting in inhibition of viral replication.

Pharmacokinetics (Adult data unless noted) Note: Pharmacokinetic data reported in pediatric patients (12-18 years) similar to reported adult data.

Distribution: 0.35-0.39 L/kg

Protein binding: ≤4%

Metabolism: Prodrug; rapidly converted to adefovir (active metabolite) in intestine

Bioavailability: 59%

Half-life elimination: 7.5 hours; prolonged in renal impairment

Time to peak serum concentration: Median: 1.75 hours (range: 0.58-4 hours)

Elimination: Urine (45% as active metabolite within 24 hours)

Dialysis: ~35% of dose (10 mg) removed during 4 hours hemodialysis session

Dosing: Usual

Children ≥2 years and Adolescents: **Hepatitis B infection, chronic: Note:** Optimal duration of treatment not established, continuation of therapy for at least 6 months after seroconversion has been suggested (Jonas, 2010). Prolonged therapy (4 years) has been reported to be safe and well-tolerated in pediatric patients (2 to 18 years). Patients not achieving a <2 log decrease in serum HBV DNA after at least 6 months of therapy should either receive additional treatment or be switched to an alternative therapy (Jonas, 2012; Lok, 2009).

Children 2 to <7 years: Limited data available; efficacy results variable: Oral: 0.3 mg/kg/dose once daily; maximum dose: 10 mg (Jonas, 2008; Jonas, 2012)

Children ≥7 to <12 years: Limited data available; efficacy results variable: Oral: 0.25 mg/kg/dose once daily; maximum dose: 10 mg (Jonas, 2008; Jonas, 2012)

Children ≥12 years and Adolescents: Oral: 10 mg once daily

Adults: **Hepatitis B infection, chronic:** Oral: 10 mg once daily

Treatment duration (AASLD practice guidelines):

Hepatitis Be antigen (HBeAg) positive chronic hepatitis: Treat ≥1 year until HBeAg seroconversion and undetectable serum HBV DNA; continue therapy for ≥6 months after HBeAg seroconversion

HBeAg negative chronic hepatitis: Treat >1 year until hepatitis B surface antigen (HBsAg) clearance

Note: Patients not achieving a <2 log decrease in serum HBV DNA after at least 6 months of therapy should either receive additional treatment or be switched to an alternative therapy (Lok, 2009).

Dosage adjustment in renal impairment:

Children ≥12 years and Adolescents: There are no dosage adjustments provided in manufacturer's labeling; no data available; consider dosage reduction.

Adults:

Manufacturer's labeling: Oral:

CrCl ≥50 mL/minute: No dosage adjustment necessary

CrCl 30 to 49 mL/minute: 10 mg every 48 hours

CrCl 10 to 29 mL/minute: 10 mg every 72 hours

CrCl <10 mL/minute: There are no dosage adjustments provided in manufacturer's labeling; no data available in nonhemodialysis patients.

Hemodialysis: 10 mg every 7 days (following dialysis)

The following guidelines have been used by some clinicians (Aronoff, 2007): Oral:

CrCl ≥50 mL/minute: No dosage adjustment necessary

CrCl 20 to 49 mL/minute: 10 mg every 48 hours

CrCl ≤19 mL/minute: 10 mg every 72 hours

Administration Oral: May be administered without regard to food.

Monitoring Parameters HIV status (prior to initiation of therapy); serum creatinine (prior to initiation and during therapy); LFTs for several months following discontinuation of adefovir; HBV DNA (every 3 to 6 months during therapy); HBeAg and anti-HBe

Dosage Forms Excipient information presented when available (limited, particularly for generics); consult specific product labeling.

Tablet, Oral, as dipivoxil:

Hepsera: 10 mg

Generic: 10 mg

◆ **Adefovir Dipivoxil** *see* Adefovir *on page 72*

◆ **Adenocard** *see* Adenosine *on page 73*

◆ **Adenoscan** *see* Adenosine *on page 73*

Adenosine (a DEN oh seen)

Medication Safety Issues

High alert medication:

This medication is in a class the Institute for Safe Medication Practices (ISMP) includes among its list of drug classes that have a heightened risk of causing significant patient harm when used in error.

Related Information

Adult ACLS Algorithms *on page 2236*

Pediatric ALS (PALS) Algorithms *on page 2233*

Brand Names: US Adenocard; Adenoscan

Brand Names: Canada Adenocard; Adenosine Injection, USP; PMS-Adenosine

Therapeutic Category Antiarrhythmic Agent, Miscellaneous

Generic Availability (US) Yes

Use Treatment of paroxysmal supraventricular tachycardia (PSVT), including that associated with accessory bypass tracts (eg, Wolff-Parkinson-White syndrome) (FDA approved in all ages); **Note:** When clinically advisable, appropriate vagal maneuvers should be attempted prior to adenosine administration; used in PALS algorithms for probable supraventricular tachycardia, stable regular monomorphic wide-complex tachycardia as a therapeutic (if arrhythmia supraventricular) and diagnostic maneuver; used in adult ACLS for stable narrow-complex regular tachycardias, unstable narrow-complex regular tachycardias while preparations are made for electrical cardioversion, stable regular monomorphic wide-complex tachycardia as a therapeutic (if arrhythmia supraventricular) and diagnostic maneuver; investigationally used as a continuous infusion for the treatment of primary pulmonary hypertension in adults and persistent pulmonary hypertension of the newborn (PPHN)

Pregnancy Risk Factor C

Pregnancy Considerations Animal reproduction studies have not been conducted. Adenosine is an endogenous substance and adverse fetal effects would not be anticipated. Case reports of administration during pregnancy have indicated no adverse effects on fetus or newborn attributable to adenosine (Blomström-Lundqvist, 2003). ACLS guidelines suggest use is safe and effective in pregnancy (ACLS [Neumar, 2010]).

Breast-Feeding Considerations Adenosine is endogenous in breast milk (Sugawara, 1995). Due to the potential for adverse reactions in the nursing infant, the manufacturer recommends a decision be made to interrupt nursing or not administer adenosine taking into account the importance of treatment to the mother.

Contraindications Hypersensitivity to adenosine or any component of the formulation; second- or third-degree AV block, sick sinus syndrome, or symptomatic bradycardia (except in patients with a functioning artificial pacemaker); known or suspected bronchoconstrictive or bronchospastic lung disease (Adenoscan), asthma (ACLS [Neumar, 2010]; Adenoscan prescribing information, 2014)

Warnings/Precautions ECG monitoring required during use. Equipment for resuscitation and trained personnel experienced in handling medical emergencies should always be immediately available. Adenosine decreases conduction through the AV node and may produce first-, second-, or third-degree heart block. Patients with preexisting S-A nodal dysfunction may experience prolonged sinus pauses after adenosine; use caution in patients with first-degree AV block or bundle branch block. Use is contraindicated in patients with high-grade AV block, sinus node dysfunction or symptomatic bradycardia (unless a functional artificial pacemaker is in place). Rare, prolonged episodes of asystole have been reported, with fatal outcomes in some cases. Discontinue adenosine in any patient who develops persistent or symptomatic high-grade AV block. Use caution in patients receiving other drugs which slow AV node conduction (eg, digoxin, verapamil). Potentially significant interactions may exist, requiring dose or frequency adjustment, additional monitoring, and/or selection of alternative therapy.

There have been reports of atrial fibrillation/flutter after adenosine administration in patients with PSVT associated with accessory conduction pathways; has also been reported in patients with or without a history of atrial fibrillation undergoing myocardial perfusion imaging with adenosine infusion. Adenosine may also produce profound vasodilation with subsequent hypotension. When used as a bolus dose (PSVT), effects are generally self-limiting (due to the short half-life of adenosine). However, when used as a continuous infusion (pharmacologic stress testing), effects may be more pronounced and persistent, corresponding to continued exposure; discontinue infusion in patients who develop persistent or symptomatic hypotension. Adenosine infusions should be used with caution in patients with autonomic dysfunction, stenotic valvular heart disease, pericarditis, pleural effusion, carotid stenosis (with cerebrovascular insufficiency), or uncorrected hypovolemia. Use caution in elderly patients; may be at increased risk of hemodynamic effects, bradycardia, and/or AV block.

Avoid use in patients with bronchoconstriction or bronchospasm (eg, asthma); dyspnea, bronchoconstriction, and respiratory compromise have occurred during use. Per the ACLS guidelines and the manufacturer of Adenoscan, use considered contraindicated in patients with asthma. Use caution in patients with obstructive lung disease not associated with bronchoconstriction (eg, emphysema, bronchitis). Immediately discontinue therapy if severe respiratory difficulty is observed. Appropriate measures for resuscitation should be available during use.

Adenocard: Transient AV block is expected. Administer as a rapid bolus, either directly into a vein or (if administered into an IV line), as close to the patient as possible (followed by saline flush). Dose reduction recommended when administered via central line (ACLS, 2010). When used in PSVT, at the time of conversion to normal sinus rhythm, a variety of new rhythms may appear on the ECG. Watch for proarrhythmic effects (eg, polymorphic ventricular tachycardia) during and shortly after administration/termination of arrhythmia. Benign transient occurrence of atrial and ventricular ectopy is common upon termination of arrhythmia. Adenosine does not convert atrial fibrillation/flutter to normal sinus rhythm; however, may be used diagnostically in these settings if the underlying rhythm is not apparent. Adenosine should not be used in patients with Wolff-Parkinson-White (WPW) syndrome and preexcited atrial fibrillation/flutter since ventricular fibrillation may result (AHA/ACC/HRS [January, 2014]). Use with extreme caution in heart transplant recipients; adenosine may cause prolonged asystole; reduction of initial adenosine dose is recommended (ACLS, 2010); considered by some to be contraindicated in this setting (Delacrétaz, 2006). Avoid use in irregular or polymorphic wide-complex tachycardias; may cause degeneration to ventricular fibrillation (ACLS, 2010). When used for PSVT, dosage reduction recommended when used with concomitant drugs which potentiate the effects of adenosine (carbamazepine, dipyridamole)

Adenoscan: Hypersensitivity reactions (including dyspnea, pharyngeal edema, erythema, flushing, rash, or chest discomfort) have been reported following Adenoscan administration. Seizures (new-onset or recurrent) have been reported following Adenoscan administration; risk may be increased with concurrent use of aminophylline. Use of any methylxanthine (eg aminophylline, caffeine, theophylline) is not recommended in patients experiencing seizures associated with Adenoscan administration. Drugs which antagonize adenosine (theophylline [includes aminophylline], caffeine) should be withheld for five half-lives prior to adenosine use. Avoid dietary caffeine for at least 12 hours prior to pharmacologic stress testing (Henzlova, 2006). Withhold dipyridamole-containing medications for at least 24 hours prior to pharmacologic stress testing (Henzlova, 2006).

Cardiovascular events: Cardiac arrest (fatal and nonfatal), myocardial infarction (MI), cerebrovascular accident (hemorrhagic and ischemic), and sustained ventricular tachycardia (requiring resuscitation) have occurred following Adenoscan use. Avoid use in patients with signs or symptoms of unstable angina, acute myocardial ischemia or cardiovascular instability due to possible increased risk of significant cardiovascular consequences. Appropriate measures for resuscitation should be available during use. In addition, systolic and diastolic pressure increases have been observed with Adenoscan infusion. In most instances, blood pressure increases resolved spontaneously within several minutes; occasionally, hypertension lasted for several hours.

Pulmonary artery hypertension: Acute vasodilator testing (not an approved use): Use with extreme caution in patients with concomitant heart failure (LV systolic dysfunction with significantly elevated left heart filling pressures) or pulmonary veno-occlusive disease/pulmonary capillary hemangiomatosis; significant decompensation has occurred with other highly selective pulmonary vasodilators resulting in acute pulmonary edema.

Adverse Reactions

Cardiovascular: Atrioventricular block, cardiac arrhythmia (transient and new arrhythmia after cardioversion; eg, atrial fibrillation, atrial premature contractions, premature ventricular contractions), chest pain, chest pressure (and discomfort), depression of ST segment on ECG, hypotension, palpitations

Central nervous system: Apprehension, dizziness, headache, nervousness, numbness, paresthesia

Dermatologic: Diaphoresis, facial flushing

Gastrointestinal: Gastrointestinal distress, Nausea

Neuromuscular & skeletal: Neck discomfort (includes throat, jaw), upper extremity discomfort

Respiratory: Dyspnea, hyperventilation

Rare but important or life-threatening: Atrial fibrillation, blurred vision, bradycardia, bronchospasm, cardiac arrest, increased intracranial pressure, injection site reaction, myocardial infarction, respiratory arrest, torsades de pointes, transient hypertension, ventricular arrhythmia, ventricular fibrillation, ventricular tachycardia

Drug Interactions

Metabolism/Transport Effects None known.

Avoid Concomitant Use There are no known interactions where it is recommended to avoid concomitant use.

Increased Effect/Toxicity

The levels/effects of Adenosine may be increased by: CarBAMazepine; Digoxin; Dipyridamole; Nicotine

Decreased Effect

The levels/effects of Adenosine may be decreased by: Caffeine and Caffeine Containing Products; Theophylline Derivatives

Storage/Stability Store between 15°C and 30°C (59°F and 86°F). Do **not** refrigerate; crystallization may occur (may dissolve by warming to room temperature).

Mechanism of Action

Antiarrhythmic actions: Slows conduction time through the AV node, interrupting the re-entry pathways through the AV node, restoring normal sinus rhythm

Myocardial perfusion scintigraphy: Adenosine also causes coronary vasodilation and increases blood flow in normal coronary arteries with little to no increase in stenotic coronary arteries; thallium-201 uptake into the stenotic coronary arteries will be less than that of normal coronary arteries revealing areas of insufficient blood flow.

Pharmacodynamics

Onset of action: Rapid

Duration: Very brief

Pharmacokinetics (Adult data unless noted)

Metabolism: Removed from systemic circulation primarily by vascular endothelial cells and erythrocytes (by cellular uptake); rapidly metabolized intracellularly; phosphorylated by adenosine kinase to adenosine monophosphate (AMP) which is then incorporated into high-energy pool; intracellular adenosine is also deaminated by adenosine deaminase to inosine; inosine can be metabolized to hypoxanthine, then xanthine and finally to uric acid.

Half-life: <10 seconds

Dosing: Neonatal Paroxysmal supraventricular tachycardia: Rapid IV: Initial dose: 0.05-0.1 mg/kg; if not effective within 1-2 minutes, increase dose by 0.05-0.1 mg/kg increments every 1-2 minutes to a maximum single dose of 0.3 mg/kg or until termination of PSVT

Dosing: Usual Paroxysmal supraventricular tachycardia:

PALS Guidelines, 2010: Infants and Children: Rapid IV; I.O.: Initial: 0.1 mg/kg (maximum: 6 mg); if not effective, give 0.2 mg/kg (maximum: 12 mg) (PALS, 2010)

Manufacturer's recommendations: Rapid IV:

Infants, Children, and Adolescents <50 kg: Initial dose: 0.05-0.1 mg/kg; if not effective within 1-2 minutes, increase dose by 0.05-0.1 mg/kg increments every 1-2 minutes to a maximum single dose of 0.3 mg/kg or until termination of PSVT

Children and Adolescents ≥50 kg and Adults: 6 mg, if not effective within 1-2 minutes, 12 mg may be given; may repeat 12 mg bolus if needed. **Note:** Initial dose of adenosine should be reduced to 3 mg if patient is currently receiving carbamazepine or dipyridamole, has a transplanted heart, or if adenosine is administered via central line (ACLS, 2010).

Preparation for Administration

Parenteral: IV:

Doses ≥600 mcg: Give undiluted

Doses <600 mcg: Further dilution of dose may be necessary to ensure complete and accurate administration; dilution with NS to a final concentration of 300 to 1,000 mcg/mL has been used; to prepare a 300 mcg/mL solution, add 3 mg of adenosine (1 mL) to 9 mL of NS; to prepare a 1,000 mcg/mL, add 3 mg of adenosine (1 mL) to 2 mL of NS

Administration Parenteral: For rapid bolus IV use, administer over 1 to 2 seconds at peripheral IV site closest to patient's heart (IV administration into lower extremities may result in therapeutic failure or requirement of higher doses); follow each bolus with NS flush (infants and children: 5 to 10 mL; adults: 20 mL); **Note:** The use of two syringes (one with adenosine dose and the other with NS flush) connected to a T-connector or stopcock is recommended for IV and I.O. administration (PALS 2010). If given IV peripherally in adults, elevate the extremity for 10 to 20 seconds after the NS flush. **Note:** Preliminary results in adults suggest adenosine may be administered via a central line at lower doses (eg, Adults: Initial dose: 3 mg); FDA approved labeling for pediatric patients weighing <50 kg states that doses listed may be administered either peripherally or centrally.

Monitoring Parameters Continuous ECG, heart rate, blood pressure, respirations

Additional Information Not effective in atrial flutter, atrial fibrillation, or ventricular tachycardia; short duration of action is an advantage as adverse effects are usually rapidly self-limiting; effects may be prolonged in patients with denervated transplanted hearts. Individualize treatment of prolonged adverse effects: Give IV fluids for hypotension, aminophylline/theophylline may antagonize effects.

Limited information is available regarding the use of adenosine for the treatment of persistent pulmonary hypertension of the newborn (PPHN); efficacy, optimal dose, and duration of therapy is not established; a randomized, masked, placebo-controlled pilot study of 18 term infants with PPHN used initial doses of 25 mcg/kg/minute (n=9); after 30 minutes, doses were increased to 50 mcg/kg/minute if no improvement in PaO_2 was observed; all patients received study drug via central line into the right atrium (inserted via the umbilical vein); significant improvement in oxygenation was observed in 4 of 9 newborns receiving 50 mcg/kg/minute; hypotension or tachycardia were not observed (Kondur, 1996).

Adenosine is also available as Adenoscan®, which is used in adults as an adjunct to thallium-201 myocardial perfusion scintigraphy; see package insert for further information on this use.

Dosage Forms Excipient information presented when available (limited, particularly for generics); consult specific product labeling.

Solution, Intravenous:

Adenocard: 6 mg/2 mL (2 mL); 12 mg/4 mL (4 mL)

Adenoscan: 3 mg/mL (20 mL, 30 mL)

Generic: 3 mg/mL (20 mL, 30 mL); 6 mg/2 mL (2 mL)

Solution, Intravenous [preservative free]:

Generic: 3 mg/mL (20 mL, 30 mL); 6 mg/2 mL (2 mL); 12 mg/4 mL (4 mL)

Agalsidase Beta (aye GAL si days BAY ta)

Medication Safety Issues

Sound-alike/look-alike issues:

Agalsidase beta may be confused with agalsidase alfa, alglucerase, alglucosidase alfa

Brand Names: US Fabrazyme

Brand Names: Canada Fabrazyme

Therapeutic Category Enzyme, α-galactosidase A; Fabry's Disease, Treatment Agent

Generic Availability (US) No

Use Treatment of Fabry disease (FDA approved in ages ≥8 years and adults)

Pregnancy Risk Factor B

Pregnancy Considerations Animal reproduction studies have not demonstrated adverse effects. There are no adequate and well-controlled studies in pregnant women. Women of childbearing potential are encouraged to enroll in Fabry registry (www.fabryregistry.com or 1-800-745-4447).

Breast-Feeding Considerations Nursing mothers are encouraged to enroll in Fabry registry.

Contraindications There are no contraindications listed within the manufacturer's labeling.

Warnings/Precautions Life-threatening anaphylactic and severe allergic reactions have been reported. Reactions may include angioedema, bronchospasm, chest discomfort, dysphagia, dyspnea, flushing, hypotension, nasal congestion, pruritus, rash, and urticaria. Stop infusion if severe reactions occur; immediate medical support should be readily available. Infusion-related reactions are common, and may be severe (chills, vomiting, hypotension, paresthesia); pretreatment with antipyretics and antihistamines is advised. Decrease infusion rate, temporarily discontinue infusion, and/or administer additional antipyretics, antihistamines, and/or steroids to manage infusion reactions. Immediate discontinuation of infusion should be considered for severe reactions. Appropriate medical support for the management of infusion reactions should be readily available. Infusion reactions have occurred despite premedication. Use with caution when readministering to patients with history of infusion reactions.

Use caution in patients with cardiovascular disease (may have increased risk of complications from infusion reactions; monitor closely). Most patients develop IgG antibodies to agalsidase beta within 3 months from the onset of therapy; skin test (IgE) reactivity has been observed. Rechallenge of patients with IgE-mediated reaction may be done with caution. A registry has been created to monitor therapeutic responses and adverse effects during long-term treatment, as well as effects on pregnant and breast-feeding women and their offspring; should be encouraged to register (www.fabryregistry.com or 1-800-745-4447).

Adverse Reactions Note: The most common and serious adverse reactions are infusion reactions (symptoms may include fever, tachycardia, hyper-/hypotension, throat tightness, dyspnea, chills, abdominal pain, paresthesia, pruritus, urticaria, vomiting).

Cardiovascular: Bradycardia, chest pain/discomfort, facial edema, flushing, hyper-/hypotension, pallor, peripheral edema, tachycardia, ventricular wall thickening

Central nervous system: Anxiety, chills, depression, dizziness, fatigue, fever, headache, hypoesthesia, pain

Dermatologic: Bruising, excoriation, pruritus, rash, urticaria

Gastrointestinal: Abdominal pain, diarrhea, nausea, toothache, vomiting, xerostomia

Local: Infusion site reactions, postprocedural complication, procedural pain, thermal burn

Neuromuscular & skeletal: Back pain, burning sensation, fall, muscle spasms, myalgia, pain in extremity, paresthesia

Otic: Hearing impairment, tinnitus

Renal: Creatinine increased

Respiratory: Congestion, cough, dyspnea, lower respiratory infection, nasal congestion, pharyngitis, sinusitis, throat tightness, upper respiratory tract infection, wheezing,

Miscellaneous: Feeling cold, fungal infection, IgG antibody formation, viral infection

Other reported severe reactions: Anaphylaxis, allergic reactions, arrhythmia, ataxia, cardiac arrest, cardiac output decreased, nephrotic syndrome, stroke, vertigo

Rare but important or life-threatening: Anaphylactic shock, angioedema (including dysphagia, edema of ears, edema of eye, edema of lips, edema of tongue, pharyngeal edema), arthralgia, bronchospasm, cerebrovascular accident, erythema, heart failure, hypoxia, hyperhidrosis, lacrimation increased, leukocytoclastic vasculitis, lymphadenopathy, MI, oxygen saturation decreased, palpitation, pneumonia, renal failure, respiratory failure, rhinorrhea, sepsis, weakness

Drug Interactions

Metabolism/Transport Effects None known.

Avoid Concomitant Use

Avoid concomitant use of Agalsidase Beta with any of the following: Amiodarone; Chloroquine; Gentamicin (Systemic)

Increased Effect/Toxicity There are no known significant interactions involving an increase in effect.

Decreased Effect

The levels/effects of Agalsidase Beta may be decreased by: Amiodarone; Chloroquine; Gentamicin (Systemic)

Storage/Stability Store intact vials between 2°C and 8°C (36°F and 46°F); do not freeze. Reconstituted solution is stable for 24 hours refrigerated.

Mechanism of Action Agalsidase beta is a recombinant form of the enzyme alpha-galactosidase-A, which is required for the hydrolysis of GL-3 and other glycosphingolipids. The compounds may accumulate (over many years) within the tissues of patients with Fabry disease, leading to renal and cardiovascular complications. In clinical trials of limited duration, agalsidase been noted to reduce tissue inclusions of a key sphingolipid (GL-3). It is believed that long-term enzyme replacement may reduce clinical manifestations of renal failure, cardiomyopathy, and stroke. However, the relationship to a reduction in clinical manifestations has not been established.

Pharmacokinetics (Adult data unless noted)

Distribution: V_d:

Children: 247-1097 mL/kg

Adults: 80-570 mL/kg

Half-life (dose dependent):

Children: 86-151 minutes

Adults: 45-102 minutes

Clearance:

Children: 1.1-5.8 mL/minute/kg

Adults: 0.8-4.9 mL/minute/kg

Dosing: Usual

Pediatric: **Fabry Disease:** Children ≥8 years and Adolescents: IV: 1 mg/kg/dose every 2 weeks

Adult: **Fabry Disease:** IV: 1 mg/kg/dose every 2 weeks

Preparation for Administration IV: Allow vials and diluent to reach room temperature prior to reconstitution (~30 minutes). Each 35 mg vial should be reconstituted with 7.2 mL SWFI; reconstitute 5 mg vials with 1.1 mL SWFI; inject down internal side wall of vial; roll and tilt gently; do not shake. Resulting solution contains 5 mg/mL. Do not use filter needle to prepare. To make final infusion solution, add the desired amount of reconstituted solution to NS to make a final volume based on patient weight (see table for dilution volumes). Prior to adding the volume of agalsidase beta dose to the NS, remove an equal volume of NS. Avoid vigorous shaking or agitation.

Recommended Minimum Volumes for Dilution

Patient Weight (kg)	Minimum Total Volume (mL)
<35	50
35.1-70	100
70.1-100	250
>100	500

Administration IV: Initial infusion not to exceed 15 mg/hour (0.25 mg/minute); after patient tolerance to initial infusion rate is established, the infusion rate may be increased in increments of 3 to 5 mg/hour (0.05- to 0.08 mg/minute) with subsequent infusions. Per the manufacturer's recommendation: For patients weighing <30 kg, the maximum infusion rate should remain at 0.25 mg/minute; for patients weighing >30 kg, the administration duration should not be less than 1.5 hours (based upon individual tolerability). An initial maximum infusion rate of 0.01 mg/minute should be used for rechallenge in patients with IgE antibodies; may increase infusion rate (doubling the infusion rate every 30 minutes) to a maximum rate of 0.25 mg/minute as tolerated. A 0.2 micron low protein-binding filter may be used during administration. Pretreatment with acetaminophen and an antihistamine is recommended to reduce infusion related side effects

Monitoring Parameters Vital signs during infusion; infusion-related reactions; globotriasylceramide (GL3) plasma levels; improvement in disease symptomatology

Reference Range
Normal endogenous activity of alpha-galactosidase A in plasma is approximately 170 nmol/hour/mL; in patients with Fabry's disease this activity is <1.5 nmol/hour/mL
Normal (goal) globotriasylceramide (GL3) <1.2 ng/microliter

Additional Information Agalsidase beta is an orphan drug; a Fabry Patient Support Group (800-745-4447) is available to assist patients in obtaining reimbursement from private insurers, Medicare, and Medicaid, and a Charitable Access Program sponsored by Genzyme provides the drug gratis to those patients in need. Detailed information regarding organizations and websites is also available in the Expert Panel Recommendations (Desnick, 2003)

Dosage Forms Excipient information presented when available (limited, particularly for generics); consult specific product labeling.
Solution Reconstituted, Intravenous:
Fabrazyme: 5 mg (1 ea); 35 mg (1 ea) [contains mouse protein (murine) (hamster)]

- ◆ **AG-Citalopram (Can)** *see* Citalopram *on page 476*
- ◆ **$AgNO_3$** *see* Silver Nitrate *on page 1926*
- ◆ **Agriflu (Can)** *see* Influenza Virus Vaccine (Inactivated) *on page 1108*
- ◆ **Agrylin** *see* Anagrelide *on page 163*
- ◆ **AHF (Human)** *see* Antihemophilic Factor (Human) *on page 167*
- ◆ **AHF (Human)** *see* Antihemophilic Factor/von Willebrand Factor Complex (Human) *on page 173*
- ◆ **AHF (Recombinant)** *see* Antihemophilic Factor (Recombinant) *on page 168*
- ◆ **A-hydroCort** *see* Hydrocortisone (Systemic) *on page 1038*
- ◆ **A-Hydrocort** *see* Hydrocortisone (Systemic) *on page 1038*
- ◆ **A-hydroCort** *see* Hydrocortisone (Topical) *on page 1041*
- ◆ **AICC** *see* Anti-inhibitor Coagulant Complex (Human) *on page 176*
- ◆ **Airomir (Can)** *see* Albuterol *on page 81*
- ◆ **AJ-PIP/TAZ (Can)** *see* Piperacillin and Tazobactam *on page 1706*
- ◆ **Akne-Mycin [DSC]** *see* Erythromycin (Topical) *on page 783*
- ◆ **AK Pentolate Oph Soln (Can)** *see* Cyclopentolate *on page 549*
- ◆ **AK-Poly-Bac™** *see* Bacitracin and Polymyxin B *on page 252*
- ◆ **AK Sulf Liq (Can)** *see* Sulfacetamide (Ophthalmic) *on page 1981*
- ◆ **Akten** *see* Lidocaine (Ophthalmic) *on page 1257*
- ◆ **Akwa Tears® [OTC]** *see* Ocular Lubricant *on page 1542*
- ◆ **Ala Cort** *see* Hydrocortisone (Topical) *on page 1041*
- ◆ **Ala Scalp** *see* Hydrocortisone (Topical) *on page 1041*
- ◆ **ala seb [OTC]** *see* Sulfur and Salicylic Acid *on page 1993*
- ◆ **Alavert [OTC]** *see* Loratadine *on page 1296*
- ◆ **Alavert™ Allergy and Sinus [OTC]** *see* Loratadine and Pseudoephedrine *on page 1298*
- ◆ **Alaway [OTC]** *see* Ketotifen (Ophthalmic) *on page 1196*
- ◆ **Alaway Childrens Allergy [OTC]** *see* Ketotifen (Ophthalmic) *on page 1196*

Albendazole (al BEN da zole)

Medication Safety Issues
Sound-alike/look-alike issues:
Albenza® may be confused with Aplenzin™, Relenza®
International issues:
Albenza [U.S.] may be confused with Avanza brand name for mirtazapine [Australia]

Brand Names: US Albenza

Therapeutic Category Anthelmintic

Generic Availability (US) No

Use Treatment of parenchymal neurocysticercosis due to active lesions caused by larval forms of *Taenia solium* (pork tapeworm) and treatment of cystic hydatid disease of the liver, lung, and peritoneum caused by the larval form of *Echinococcus granulosus* (dog tapeworm) [FDA approved in pediatric patients (age not specified) and adults]. Is also active against and has been used in the treatment of *Ascaris lumbricoides* (roundworm), *Ancylostoma caninum*, *Ancylostoma duodenale*, *Necator americanus* (hookworm), *Enterobius vermicularis* (pinworm), cutaneous larva migrans, *Gnathostoma spinigerum*, *Gongylonema* sp: *Mansonella perstans* (filariasis), *Opisthorchis sinensis* (liver fluke), visceral larva migrans (toxocariasis), *Echinococcus multilocularis*, *Clonorchis sinensis* (Chinese liver fluke), *Giardia lamblia*, *Cysticercus cellulosae*, *Trichuris trichiura* (whipworm), microsporidiosis, *Capillaria philippinensis*, *Baylisascaris procyonis*, and *Strongyloides stercoralis*.

Pregnancy Risk Factor C

Pregnancy Considerations Adverse events were observed in animal reproduction studies. Albendazole should not be used during pregnancy, if at all possible. The manufacturer recommends a pregnancy test prior to therapy in women of reproductive potential. Women should be advised to avoid pregnancy for at least 1 month following therapy. Discontinue if pregnancy occurs during treatment.

Breast-Feeding Considerations Albendazole excretion into breast milk was studied following a single oral 400 mg dose in breast-feeding women 2 weeks to 6 months postpartum (n=33). Mean albendazole concentrations 6 hours after the dose were 63.7 ± 11.9 ng/mL (maternal serum) and 31.9 ± 9.2 ng/mL (milk). An active and inactive metabolite was also detected in breast milk (Abdel-tawab, 2009). The manufacturer recommends that caution be exercised when administering albendazole to nursing women.

Contraindications Hypersensitivity to albendazole, benzimidazoles, or any component of the formulation

Warnings/Precautions Reversible elevations in hepatic enzymes have been reported; patients with abnormal LFTs and hepatic echinococcosis are at an increased risk of hepatotoxicity. Discontinue therapy if LFT elevations are >2 times the upper limit of normal; may consider restarting treatment with frequent monitoring of LFTs when hepatic enzymes return to pretreatment values. Agranulocytosis, aplastic anemia, granulocytopenia, leukopenia, and pancytopenia have occurred leading to fatalities (rare); use with caution in patients with hepatic impairment (more susceptible to hematologic toxicity). Discontinue therapy in all patients who develop clinically significant decreases in blood cell counts.

Neurocysticercosis: Corticosteroids (eg, dexamethasone or prednisolone) should be administered before or upon initiation of albendazole therapy to minimize inflammatory reactions and prevent cerebral hypertension. Anticonvulsant therapy should be used concurrently during the first week of therapy to prevent seizures. These measures are important to minimize neurological symptoms which may result from uncovering of preexisting neurocysticercosis when using albendazole to treat other conditions. If retinal lesions exist, weigh risk of further retinal damage due to albendazole-induced changes to the retinal lesion vs benefit of disease treatment.

Adverse Reactions

Central nervous system: Dizziness, fever, headache, intracranial pressure increased, meningeal signs, vertigo

Dermatologic: Alopecia

Gastrointestinal: Abdominal pain, nausea, vomiting

Hepatic: LFTs increased

Rare but important or life-threatening: Acute liver failure, acute renal failure, aplastic anemia, agranulocytosis, erythema multiforme, granulocytopenia, hepatitis, hypersensitivity reaction, leukopenia, neutropenia, pancytopenia, rash, Stevens-Johnson syndrome, thrombocytopenia, urticaria

Drug Interactions

Metabolism/Transport Effects **Substrate** of CYP1A2 (minor), CYP3A4 (minor); **Note:** Assignment of Major/Minor substrate status based on clinically relevant drug interaction potential

Avoid Concomitant Use There are no known interactions where it is recommended to avoid concomitant use.

Increased Effect/Toxicity

The levels/effects of Albendazole may be increased by: Grapefruit Juice

Decreased Effect

The levels/effects of Albendazole may be decreased by: Aminoquinolines (Antimalarial); CarBAMazepine; PHENobarbital; Phenytoin

Food Interactions Albendazole serum levels may be increased if taken with a fatty meal (increases the oral bioavailability by up to 5 times). Management: Should be administered with a high-fat meal (peanuts or ice cream).

Storage/Stability Store between 20°C and 25°C (68°F to 77°F)

Mechanism of Action Active metabolite, albendazole sulfoxide, causes selective degeneration of cytoplasmic microtubules in intestinal and tegmental cells of intestinal helminths and larvae; glycogen is depleted, glucose uptake and cholinesterase secretion are impaired, and desecratory substances accumulate intracellulary. ATP production decreases causing energy depletion, immobilization, and worm death.

Pharmacokinetics (Adult data unless noted) **Note:** In pediatric patients (6-13 years), pharmacokinetic values were reported to be similar to adult data.

Absorption: Poorly absorbed from the GI tract

Distribution: Widely distributed throughout the body including urine, bile, liver, cyst wall, cyst fluid, and CSF

Protein binding: 70%

Metabolism: Extensive first-pass metabolism; hepatic metabolism to albendazole sulfoxide, an active metabolite

Half-life: Albendazole sulfoxide: 8-12 hours

Time to peak serum concentration: 2-5 hours for the metabolite

Elimination: Biliary

Dosing: Usual Children and Adults: Oral:

Neurocysticercosis *(Taenia solium)*: **Note:** Patients should receive concurrent corticosteroid for the first week of albendazole therapy and anticonvulsant therapy as required.

<60 kg: 15 mg/kg/day in 2 divided doses (maximum: 800 mg/day) for 8-30 days

≥60 kg: 400 mg twice daily for 8-30 days

Hydatid disease *(Echinococcus granulosus)*:

<60 kg: 15 mg/kg/day in 2 divided doses (maximum: 800 mg/day); 28-day cycle followed by a 14-day albendazole-free interval, for a total of 3 cycles

≥60 kg: 400 mg twice daily; 28-day cycle followed by a 14-day albendazole-free interval, for a total of 3 cycles

Ancylostoma caninum, ascariasis (roundworm), hookworm, trichuriasis (whipworm): 400 mg as a single dose (*Red Book*, 2009)

Ascariasis: Children 12 months to 2 years: 200 mg as a single dose (World Health Organization Model Formulary for Children, 2010)

Baylisascaris procyonis: Children: 25 mg/kg/day for 20 days started as soon as possible (up to 3 days after possible infection) may prevent clinical disease and is recommended for children with known exposure (eg, ingestion of raccoon stool or contaminated soil). No drug has been demonstrated to be effective (*Red Book*, 2009).

Capillariasis: 400 mg once daily for 10 days (*Red Book*, 2009)

Clonorchis sinensis (Chinese liver fluke): 10 mg/kg/day once daily for 7 days (*Red Book*, 2009)

Cutaneous larva migrans: 400 mg once daily for 3 days (*Red Book*, 2009)

Enterobius vermicularis (pinworm): 400 mg as a single dose; repeat in 2 weeks (*Red Book*, 2009)

Filariasis (*Mansonella perstans*): 400 mg twice daily for 10 days (*Red Book*, 2009)

Filariasis (*Wuchereria Bancroft*, microfilaria reduction or suppression): 400 mg as a single dose (in combination with either ivermectin or diethylcarbamazine). **Note:** Albendazole/ivermectin combination does not kill all the adult worms (*Red Book*, 2009).

Giardiasis *(Giardia duodenalis)* (*Red Book*, 2009):

Children: 10 mg/kg/day once daily for 5 days

Adults: 400 mg once daily for 5 days

Gnathostoma spinigerum (Gnathostomiasis): 400 mg twice daily for 21 days (*Red Book*, 2009)

Gongylonema sp (Gongylonemiasis): 400 mg once daily for 3 days (*Red Book*, 2009)

Microsporidia infection (except *Enterocytozoon sp.* and *V. corneae*) in HIV-exposed/positive infants and children: 15 mg/kg/day in 2 divided doses (maximum: 800 mg/day) continued until immune reconstitution after HAART initiation

Microsporidiosis in non-HIV patients (*Red Book*, 2009):

Disseminated: 400 mg twice daily

Intestinal: 400 mg twice daily for 21 days

Ocular: 400 mg twice daily in combination with fumagillin

Strongyloidiasis (*Strongyloides stercoralis*): 400 mg twice daily for 7 days (*Red Book*, 2009)

Trichinellosis (*Trichinella spiralis*): 400 mg twice daily for 8-14 days (*Red Book*, 2009)

Visceral larva migrans (*Toxocariasis*): 400 mg twice daily for 5 days (*Red Book*, 2009)

Administration Oral: Administer with food. For children who have difficulty swallowing whole tablets, tablet may be crushed or chewed and swallowed with a drink of water.

Monitoring Parameters Monitor liver function tests, CBC at start of each cycle and every 2 weeks during therapy, fecal specimens for ova and parasites; pregnancy test

Dosage Forms Excipient information presented when available (limited, particularly for generics); consult specific product labeling.

Tablet, Oral:

Albenza: 200 mg [contains saccharin sodium]

◆ **Albenza** *see* Albendazole *on page 78*

◆ **Albuked 5** *see* Albumin *on page 79*

◆ **Albuked 25** *see* Albumin *on page 79*

Albumin (al BYOO min)

Medication Safety Issues

Sound-alike/look-alike issues:

Albuminar-25 (albumin) may be confused with Privigen (immune globulin) due to similar packaging

Albutein may be confused with albuterol

Buminate may be confused with bumetanide

Brand Names: US Albuked 25; Albuked 5; Albumin-ZLB; Albuminar-25; Albuminar-5; AlbuRx; Albutein; Buminate; Flexbumin; Human Albumin Grifols; Kedbumin; Plasbumin-25; Plasbumin-5

Brand Names: Canada Alburex 25; Alburex 5; Albutein 25%; Albutein 5%; Buminate-25%; Buminate-5%; Plasbumin-25; Plasbumin-5

Therapeutic Category Blood Product Derivative; Plasma Volume Expander

Generic Availability (US) Yes

Use Treatment of hypovolemia; plasma volume expansion and maintenance of cardiac output in the treatment of certain types of shock or impending shock; hypoproteinemia resulting in generalized edema or decreased intravascular volume (eg, hypoproteinemia associated with acute nephrotic syndrome, premature neonates)

Note: PALS and Neonatal Resuscitation 2000 Guidelines recommend isotonic crystalloid solutions (eg, NS or LR) as initial volume expansion; albumin is used less frequently due to limited supply, potential risk of infections, and an association with an increase in mortality (identified by meta-analyses); few studies in these analyses included children, so no firm conclusions in pediatric patients can be made

Pregnancy Risk Factor C

Pregnancy Considerations Animal reproduction studies have not been conducted. Albumin is used for the treatment of ovarian hyperstimulation syndrome (ASRM, 2008). Use for other indications may be considered in pregnant women when contraindications to nonprotein colloids exist (Liumbruno, 2009).

Breast-Feeding Considerations Endogenous albumin is found in breast milk. The manufacturer recommends that caution be exercised when administering albumin to nursing women.

Contraindications Hypersensitivity to albumin or any component of the formulation; severe anemia; cardiac failure; dilution with sterile water for injection

Warnings/Precautions Anaphylaxis may occur; discontinue immediately if allergic or anaphylactic reactions are suspected. Cardiac or respiratory failure, renal failure, or increasing intracranial pressure can occur; closely monitor hemodynamic parameters in all patients. Use with caution in conditions where hypervolemia and its consequences or hemodilution may increase the risk of adverse effects (eg, heart failure, pulmonary edema, hypertension, hemorrhagic diathesis, esophageal varices). Adjust rate of administration per hemodynamic status and solution concentration; monitor closely with rapid infusions. Avoid rapid infusions in patients with a history of cardiovascular disease (may cause circulatory overload and pulmonary edema). Discontinue at the first signs of cardiovascular overload (eg, headache, dyspnea, jugular venous distention, rales, abnormal elevations in systemic or central venous blood pressure). All patients should be observed for signs of hypervolemia such as pulmonary edema.

Use with caution in patients with hepatic or renal impairment because of added protein load. Use with caution in those patients for whom sodium restriction is necessary. The parenteral product may contain aluminum (Kelly, 1989); toxic aluminum concentrations may be seen with high doses, prolonged use, or renal dysfunction. Premature neonates are at higher risk due to immature renal function and aluminum intake from other parenteral sources. Parenteral aluminum exposure of >4 to 5 mcg/kg/day is associated with CNS and bone toxicity; tissue loading may occur at lower doses (Federal Register, 2002). See manufacturer's labeling. Albumin is a product of human plasma, may potentially contain infectious agents which could transmit disease. Screening of donors, as well as testing and/or inactivation or removal of certain viruses, reduces the risk. Infections thought to be transmitted by this product should be reported to the manufacturer. Packaging may contain natural latex rubber. Patients with chronic renal insufficiency receiving albumin solution may be at risk for accumulation of aluminum and potential toxicities (eg, hypercalcemia, vitamin D refractory osteodystrophy, anemia, and severe progressive encephalopathy). In patients with increased microvascular permeability (eg, sepsis, trauma, burn), the translocation of fluid from the interstitial compartment to the intravascular compartment may decrease due to increased albumin in the interstitial space. Furthermore, in extreme microvascular permeability states, administration of albumin (or other colloids) may increase the net flux of fluid into the interstitial space reducing intravascular volume and precipitating edematous states (eg, pulmonary edema) (Roberts, 1998).

Warnings: Additional Pediatric Considerations In neonates, use the 25% concentration with extreme caution due to risk of intraventricular hemorrhage (from rapid expansion of the intravascular volume); infuse slowly. May contain aluminum; toxic aluminum concentrations may be seen with high doses, prolonged use, or renal dysfunction. Premature neonates are at higher risk due to immature renal function and aluminum intake from other parenteral sources. Parenteral aluminum exposure of >4-5 mcg/kg/day is associated with CNS and bone toxicity and tissue loading may occur at lower doses.

Due to the occasional shortage of 5% human albumin, 5% solutions may at times be prepared by diluting 25% human albumin with NS or with D_5W (if sodium load is a concern); however, do not use sterile water to dilute albumin solutions, as this may result in hypotonic-associated hemolysis which can be fatal.

Adverse Reactions

Cardiovascular: Congestive heart failure (precipitation), edema, hypertension, hypotension, tachycardia

Central nervous system: Chills, headache

Dermatologic: Pruritus, skin rash, urticaria

Endocrine & metabolic: Hypervolemia

Gastrointestinal: Nausea, vomiting

Hypersensitivity: Anaphylaxis

Respiratory: Bronchospasm, pulmonary edema

Miscellaneous: Fever

Drug Interactions

Metabolism/Transport Effects None known.

Avoid Concomitant Use There are no known interactions where it is recommended to avoid concomitant use.

Increased Effect/Toxicity There are no known significant interactions involving an increase in effect.

Decreased Effect There are no known significant interactions involving a decrease in effect.

Storage/Stability Store at ≤30°C (86°F); do not freeze. Do not use solution if it is turbid or contains a deposit; use within 4 hours after opening vial; discard unused portion.

Mechanism of Action Provides increase in intravascular oncotic pressure and causes mobilization of fluids from interstitial into intravascular space

Pharmacodynamics Duration of volume expansion: ~24 hours

Pharmacokinetics (Adult data unless noted) Half-life: 21 days

Dosing: Neonatal IV: **Note:** Albumin **5%** should be used in hypovolemic or intravascularly depleted patients; albumin **25%** should be used in patients with fluid or sodium restrictions (eg, patients with hypoproteinemia and generalized edema, or nephrotic syndrome). Dose depends on condition of patient:

Hypoproteinemia: 0.5-1 g/kg/dose of 25% albumin; may repeat every 1-2 days

Hypovolemia, hypotension: Usual dose: 0.5 g/kg/dose of 5% albumin (10 mL/kg/dose); range: 0.25-0.5 g/kg/dose of 5% albumin (5-10 mL/kg/dose)

Dosing: Usual IV: **Note:** Albumin **5%** should be used in hypovolemic or intravascularly depleted patients; albumin **25%** should be used in patients with fluid or sodium restrictions (eg, patients with hypoproteinemia and generalized edema, or nephrotic syndrome). Dose depends on condition of patient:

Infants and Children:

Hypoproteinemia: 0.5-1 g/kg/dose of 25% albumin; may repeat every 1-2 days

Hypovolemia: 0.5-1 g/kg/dose (10-20 mL/kg/dose of 5% albumin); may repeat as needed; maximum dose: 6 g/kg/day (120 mL/kg/day of 5% albumin)

Nephrotic syndrome: 0.25-1 g/kg/dose of 25% albumin

Adults: 25 g; no more than 250 g should be administered within 48 hours

Nephrotic syndrome: 12.5-50 g/day in 3-4 divided doses

Preparation for Administration If 5% human albumin is unavailable, it may be prepared by diluting 25% human albumin with NS or D_5W (if sodium load is a concern). **Do not use sterile water** to dilute albumin solutions, as this has been associated with hypotonic-associated hemolysis.

Administration

Parenteral: IV: Too rapid infusion may result in vascular overload

Product-specific details:

Albuminar: May administer via the administration set provided (in-line 60 micron filter) or via any administration set; use of filter is optional; size of filter may vary according to institutional policy. Method of filter sterilization used by manufacturer includes 0.2 micron filter; however, aggregates may form under storage, shipping, and handling. Administration via very small filter will not damage product, but will slow flow rate.

Albutein: May administer via the administration set provided (in-line 50 micron filter) or via any administration set; use of filter is optional; size of filter may vary according to institutional policy. Method of production includes passage through 0.22 micron filter. May administer via filter as small as 0.22 microns.

Buminate: Administer via the administration set provided (in-line 15 micron filter) or via any filtered administration set; use ≥5 micron filter to ensure adequate flow rate

Plasbumin: May administer with or without an IV filter; filter as small as 0.22 microns may be used

Hypoproteinemia: Infuse over 2 to 4 hours; for neonates, dose may be added to parenteral nutrition solution and infused over 24 hours; **Note:** Parenteral nutrition solutions containing >25 g/L of albumin are more likely to occlude 0.22 micron in-line filters; but parenteral nutrition solutions containing albumin in concentrations as low as 10.8 g/L have also occluded 0.22 micron filters; use ≥5 micron filter to ensure adequate flow rate; addition of albumin to parenteral nutrition solutions may increase potential for growth of bacteria or fungi

Hypovolemia: Rate of infusion depends on severity of hypovolemia and patient's symptoms; usually infuse dose over 30 to 60 minutes (faster infusion rates may be clinically necessary)

Maximum rates of IV infusion after initial volume replacement:

5%: 2 to 4 mL/minute

25%: 1 mL/minute

Monitoring Parameters Observe for signs of hypervolemia, pulmonary edema, cardiac failure, vital signs, I & O, Hgb, Hct, urine specific gravity

Additional Information In certain conditions (eg, hypoproteinemia with generalized edema, nephrotic syndrome), doses of albumin may be followed with IV furosemide: 0.5-1 mg/kg/dose.

Both albumin 5% and 25% contain 130-160 mEq/L of sodium; albumin 5% is osmotically equivalent to an equal volume of plasma; albumin 25% is osmotically equivalent to 5 times its volume of plasma.

Dosage Forms Excipient information presented when available (limited, particularly for generics); consult specific product labeling. [DSC] = Discontinued product

Solution, Intravenous:

Albumin-ZLB: 5% (250 mL, 500 mL); 25% (50 mL, 100 mL)

Albuminar-5: 5% (250 mL, 500 mL)

Albuminar-25: 25% (50 mL, 100 mL)

AlbuRx: 5% (250 mL, 500 mL)

Albutein: 25% (50 mL, 100 mL)

Buminate: 5% (250 mL, 500 mL); 25% (20 mL)

Plasbumin-5: 5% (50 mL, 250 mL)

Plasbumin-25: 25% (20 mL, 50 mL, 100 mL)

Generic: 5% (50 mL [DSC]); 25% (50 mL, 100 mL)

Solution, Intravenous [preservative free]:

Albuked 5: 5% (250 mL)

Albuked 25: 25% (50 mL, 100 mL)

Albutein: 5% (250 mL, 500 mL); 25% (50 mL, 100 mL)

Flexbumin: 5% (250 mL); 25% (50 mL, 100 mL)

Human Albumin Grifols: 25% (50 mL, 100 mL)

Kedbumin: 25% (50 mL, 100 mL)

Plasbumin-5: 5% (50 mL, 250 mL)

Plasbumin-25: 25% (20 mL, 50 mL, 100 mL)

Generic: 5% (100 mL, 250 mL, 500 mL); 25% (50 mL, 100 mL)

◆ **Albuminar-5** *see* Albumin *on page 79*

◆ **Albuminar-25** *see* Albumin *on page 79*

◆ **Albumin (Human)** *see* Albumin *on page 79*

◆ **Albumin-ZLB** *see* Albumin *on page 79*

◆ **Alburex 5 (Can)** *see* Albumin *on page 79*

◆ **Alburex 25 (Can)** *see* Albumin *on page 79*

◆ **AlbuRx** *see* Albumin *on page 79*

◆ **Albutein** *see* Albumin *on page 79*

◆ **Albutein 5% (Can)** *see* Albumin *on page 79*

◆ **Albutein 25% (Can)** *see* Albumin *on page 79*

Albuterol (al BYOO ter ole)

Medication Safety Issues

Sound-alike/look-alike issues:

Albuterol may be confused with Albutein, atenolol

Proventil may be confused with Bentyl, PriLOSEC, Prinivil

Salbutamol may be confused with salmeterol

Ventolin may be confused with phentolamine, Benylin, Vantin

Related Information

Oral Medications That Should Not Be Crushed or Altered *on page 2476*

Brand Names: US AccuNeb [DSC]; ProAir HFA; ProAir RespiClick; Proventil HFA; Ventolin HFA; VoSpire ER

Brand Names: Canada Airomir; Apo-Salvent; Apo-Salvent AEM; Apo-Salvent CFC Free; Apo-Salvent Sterules; Dom-Salbutamol; Novo-Salbutamol HFA; PHL-Salbutamol; PMS-Salbutamol; ratio-Ipra-Sal; ratio-Salbutamol; Salbutamol HFA; Sandoz-Salbutamol; Teva-Salbutamol Sterinebs P.F.; Ventolin Diskus; Ventolin HFA; Ventolin I.V. Infusion; Ventolin Nebules P.F.; Ventolin Respirator

Therapeutic Category Adrenergic Agonist Agent; Antiasthmatic; $Beta_2$-Adrenergic Agonist; Bronchodilator; Sympathomimetic

Generic Availability (US) May be product dependent

Use

Oral: Treatment of bronchospasm in patients with reversible obstructive airway disease (Syrup: FDA approved in ages ≥2 years and adults; Immediate release and extended release tablets: FDA approved in ages ≥6 years and adults). **Note:** Although an FDA approved indication, the use of oral albuterol for management of acute asthma or long-term daily maintenance treatment is not recommended due to long onset of action and risk of side effects (GINA 2008; GINA 2012; NAEPP 2007)

Oral inhalation:

Inhalation aerosol (metered dose inhaler): Treatment or prevention of bronchospasm in patients with reversible obstructive airway disease; prevention of exercise-induced bronchospasm (All indications: FDA approved in ages ≥4 years and adults)

Nebulization solution: Treatment of bronchospasm in patients with reversible obstructive airway disease (FDA approved in ages ≥2 years and adults; Proventil: FDA approved in ages ≥12 years and adults); treatment of acute attacks of bronchospasm (FDA approved in ages ≥2 years and adults; Proventil: FDA approved in ages ≥12 years and adults). **Note:** Approval ages for generics may vary; consult prescribing information for details.

Pregnancy Risk Factor C

Pregnancy Considerations Adverse events have been observed in some animal reproduction studies. Albuterol crosses the placenta (Boulton, 1997). Congenital anomalies (cleft palate, limb defects) have rarely been reported following maternal use during pregnancy. Multiple medications were used in most cases, no specific pattern of defects has been reported, and no relationship to albuterol has been established. The amount of albuterol available systemically following inhalation is significantly less in comparison to oral doses.

Uncontrolled asthma is associated with adverse events on pregnancy (increased risk of perinatal mortality, preeclampsia, preterm birth, low birth weight infants). Albuterol is the preferred short acting beta agonist when treatment for asthma is needed during pregnancy (NAEPP, 2005; NAEPP, 2007).

Albuterol may affect uterine contractility. Maternal pulmonary edema and other adverse events have been reported when albuterol was used for tocolysis. Albuterol is not approved for use as a tocolytic; use caution when needed to treat bronchospasm in pregnant women. Use of the injection (Canadian product; not available in the U.S.) is specifically contraindicated in women during the first or second trimester who may be at risk of threatened abortion.

Breast-Feeding Considerations It is not known if albuterol is excreted in breast milk. The amount of albuterol available systemically following inhalation is significantly less in comparison to oral doses. According to the manufacturer, the decision to continue or discontinue breast-feeding during therapy should take into account the risk of exposure to the infant and the benefits of treatment to the mother. The use of beta-2-receptor agonists are not considered a contraindication to breast-feeding (NAEPP, 2005).

Contraindications Hypersensitivity to albuterol or any component of the formulation; severe hypersensitivity to milk proteins (powder for inhalation).

Injection formulation [Canadian product]: Hypersensitivity to albuterol or any component of the formulation; tachyarrhythmias; risk of abortion during first or second trimester

Warnings/Precautions Albuterol is a short-acting $beta_2$-agonist (SABA) that should be used as needed for quick relief of asthma symptoms. Based on a step-wise treatment approach using asthma guidelines, monotherapy without concurrent use of a long-term controller medication should only be reserved for patients with mild, intermittent forms of asthma without the presence of risk factors (Step 1 and/or exercise-induced) (GINA, 2015; NAEPP, 2007). Patient must be instructed to seek medical attention in cases where acute symptoms are not relieved or a previous level of response is diminished. The need to increase frequency of use may indicate deterioration of asthma, and treatment must not be delayed.

Use with caution in patients with cardiovascular disease (arrhythmia, coronary insufficiency, or hypertension, or HF heart failure); beta-agonists may produce ECG changes (flattening of the T wave, prolongation of the QTc interval, ST segment depression) and/or cause elevation in blood pressure, heart rate and result in CNS stimulation/excitation. $Beta_2$-agonists may increase risk of arrhythmia, increase serum glucose (and aggravate preexisting diabetes and ketoacidosis), or decrease serum potassium. Use with caution in patients with renal impairment.

Immediate hypersensitivity reactions (urticaria, angioedema, rash, bronchospasm), including anaphylaxis, have been reported. Do not exceed recommended dose; serious adverse events, including fatalities, have been associated with excessive use of inhaled sympathomimetics. Rarely, paradoxical bronchospasm may occur with use of inhaled bronchodilating agents (may be fatal); this should be distinguished from inadequate response. All patients should utilize a spacer device or valved holding chamber when using a metered-dose inhaler; in addition, use spacer for children <5 years of age and consider adding a face mask for infants and children <4 years of age. Powder for oral inhalation contains lactose; hypersensitivity reactions (eg, anaphylaxis, angioedema, pruritus, and rash) have been reported in patients with milk protein allergy. Potentially significant interactions may exist, requiring dose or frequency adjustment, additional monitoring, and/or selection of alternative therapy.

Warnings: Additional Pediatric Considerations CNS stimulation, hyperactivity, and insomnia occur more frequently in younger children than in adults. In children receiving oral albuterol therapy, erythema multiforme and Stevens-Johnson syndrome have been reported (rare). Outbreaks of lower respiratory tract colonization and infection have been attributed to contaminated multidose albuterol bottle.

Adverse Reactions Incidence of adverse effects is dependent upon age of patient, dose, and route of administration.

Cardiovascular: Chest discomfort, chest pain, edema, extrasystoles, flushing, hypertension, palpitations, tachycardia

Central nervous system: Anxiety, ataxia, depression, dizziness, drowsiness, emotional lability, excitement (children and adolescents 2 to 14 years), fatigue, headache, hyperactivity (children and adolescents 6 to 14 years), insomnia, malaise, migraine, nervousness, pain, restlessness, rigors, shakiness (children and adolescents 6 to 14 years), vertigo, voice disorder

Dermatologic: Diaphoresis, pallor (children 2 to 6 years), skin rash, urticaria

Endocrine & metabolic: Diabetes mellitus, increased serum glucose

Gastrointestinal: Anorexia (children 2 to 6 years), diarrhea, dyspepsia, eructation, flatulence, gastroenteritis, gastrointestinal symptoms (children 2 to 6 years), glossitis, increased appetite (children and adolescents 6 to 14 years), nausea, unpleasant taste (inhalation site), viral gastroenteritis, vomiting, xerostomia

Genitourinary: Difficulty in micturition, urinary tract infection

Hematologic & oncologic: Decreased hematocrit, decreased hemoglobin, decreased white blood cell count, lymphadenopathy

Hepatic: Increased serum ALT, increased serum AST
Hypersensitivity: Hypersensitivity reaction
Infection: Cold symptoms, infection
Local: Application site reaction (HFA inhaler)
Neuromuscular & skeletal: Back pain, hyperkinesia, leg cramps, muscle cramps, musculoskeletal pain, tremor
Ophthalmic: Conjunctivitis (children 2 to 6 years)
Otic: Otalgia, otitis media, ear disease, tinnitus
Respiratory: Bronchitis, bronchospasm (exacerbation of underlying pulmonary disease), cough, dyspnea, epistaxis (children and adolescents 6 to 14 years), exacerbation of asthma, flu-like symptoms, increased bronchial secretions, laryngitis, nasal congestion, nasopharyngitis, oropharyngeal edema, oropharyngeal pain, pharyngitis, pulmonary disease, respiratory tract disease, rhinitis, sinus headache, sinusitis, throat irritation, upper respiratory tract infection, upper respiratory tract inflammation, viral upper respiratory tract infection, wheezing
Miscellaneous: Accidental injury, fever
Rare but important or life-threatening: Anaphylaxis, atrial fibrillation, exacerbation of diabetes mellitus, gag reflex, glossitis, hyperglycemia, hypokalemia, hypotension, ketoacidosis, lactic acidosis, paradoxical bronchospasm, peripheral vasodilation, supraventricular tachycardia, tongue ulcer

Drug Interactions

Metabolism/Transport Effects None known.

Avoid Concomitant Use

Avoid concomitant use of Albuterol with any of the following: Beta-Blockers (Nonselective); Iobenguane I 123; Loxapine

Increased Effect/Toxicity

Albuterol may increase the levels/effects of: Atosiban; Highest Risk QTc-Prolonging Agents; Loop Diuretics; Loxapine; Moderate Risk QTc-Prolonging Agents; Sympathomimetics; Thiazide Diuretics

The levels/effects of Albuterol may be increased by: AtoMOXetine; Cannabinoid-Containing Products; Linezolid; MAO Inhibitors; Mifepristone; Tedizolid; Tricyclic Antidepressants

Decreased Effect

Albuterol may decrease the levels/effects of: Iobenguane I 123

The levels/effects of Albuterol may be decreased by: Beta-Blockers (Beta1 Selective); Beta-Blockers (Nonselective); Betahistine

Storage/Stability

HFA aerosols: Store at 15°C to 25°C (59°F to 77°F). Do not store at temperature >120°F. Do not puncture. Do not use or store near heat or open flame.
Ventolin HFA: Discard when counter reads 000 or 12 months after removal from protective pouch, whichever comes first. Store with mouthpiece down.
Infusion solution [Canadian product]: Ventolin IV: Store at 15°C to 30°C (59°F to 86°F). Protect from light. After dilution, discard unused portion after 24 hours.
Inhalation powder: Store between 15°C and 25°C (59°F and 77°F). Avoid exposure to extreme heat, cold, or humidity. Discard 13 months after opening the foil pouch, or when the counter displays 0, whichever comes first.
Solution for nebulization: Store at 2°C to 25°C (36°F to 77°F). Do not use if solution changes color or becomes cloudy. Products packaged in foil should be used within 1 week (or according to the manufacturer's recommendations) if removed from foil pouch.
Syrup: Store at 20°C to 25°C (68°F to 77°F).
Tablet: Store at 20°C to 25°C (68°F to 77°F).
Tablet, extended release: Store at 20°C to 25°C (68°F to 77°F)

Mechanism of Action Relaxes bronchial smooth muscle by action on beta$_2$-receptors with little effect on heart rate

Pharmacodynamics

Nebulization/oral inhalation:
Maximum effect: Peak bronchodilation: 0.5-2 hours
Duration: 2-5 hours
Oral:
Maximum effect: Peak bronchodilatation: Immediate release: 2-3 hours
Duration: Immediate release: 4-6 hours; extended release tablets: Up to 12 hours

Pharmacokinetics (Adult data unless noted)

Metabolism: By the liver to an inactive sulfate
Half-life:
Oral: 2.7-5 hours
Inhalation: 3.8 hours
Elimination: 30% appears in urine as unchanged drug

Dosing: Neonatal

Bronchodilation: Limited data available: Oral inhalation:
Nebulization: Usual reported dose: 1.25 to 2.5 mg/dose (Ballard 2002). In a retrospective report, 16 VLBW neonates (mean GA: 26.1 ± 1.2 weeks; mean birthweight: 817 ± 211 g) received 1.25 mg/dose every 8 hours for >2 weeks (Mhanna 2009)
Inhalation, aerosol (metered dose inhaler); mechanically ventilated patients: 90 mcg/spray: 1 to 2 puffs administered into the ventilator circuit was the most frequently reported dose in a survey of 68 neonatal intensive care units (Ballard 2002); typically used every 6 hours (Fok 1998); may consider more frequent use if clinically indicated

Dosing: Usual

Pediatric:
Asthma, acute exacerbation: Oral inhalation:
Outpatient: *Inhalation aerosol (metered dose inhaler):* 90 mcg/puff: Children and Adolescents: 2 to 6 puffs every 20 minutes (GINA 2014; NAEPP 2007); if good response after 2 doses then every 3 to 4 hours for 24 to 48 hours (NAEPP 2007); **Note:** GINA guideline dosing is based on the 100 mcg/puff salbutamol product (not available in U.S.) (GINA 2014)
Emergency care/hospital:
Inhalation aerosol (metered dose inhaler): 90 mcg/puff:
Children: Limited data available in ages <4 years: 4 to 8 puffs every 20 minutes for 3 doses then every 1 to 4 hours (NAEPP 2007)
Adolescents: 4 to 8 puffs every 20 minutes for up to 4 hours then every 1 to 4 hours (NAEPP 2007)
Nebulization:
Infants and Children: Limited data in ages <2 years:
Intermittent: 0.15 mg/kg (minimum dose: 2.5 mg) every 20 minutes for 3 doses then 0.15 to 0.3 mg/kg not to exceed 10 mg every 1 to 4 hours (NAEPP 2007)
Continuous: Dosing regimens variable; optimal dosage not established:
NIH Guidelines: 0.5 mg/kg/hour (NAEPP 2007)
Alternate dosing: Limited data available: 0.3 mg/kg/hour has also been used safely in the treatment of severe status asthmaticus in children (Papo 1993); higher doses of 3 mg/kg/hour ± 2.2 mg/kg/hour in children (n=19, mean age: 20.7 months ± 38 months) resulted in no cardiotoxicity (Katz 1993)
Adolescents:
Intermittent: 2.5 to 5 mg every 20 minutes for 3 doses then 2.5 to 10 mg every 1 to 4 hours as needed
Continuous: 10 to 15 mg/hour
Asthma, maintenance therapy (nonacute) (NAEPP 2007): Oral inhalation:
Inhalation, aerosol (metered dose inhaler): Infants, Children, and Adolescents: Limited data available in ages <4 years: 90 mcg/puff: 2 puffs every 4 to 6 hours as

needed. **Note:** Not recommended for long-term daily maintenance treatment; regular use exceeding 2 days/ week for symptom control (not prevention of exercise-induced bronchospasm) indicates the need for additional long-term control therapy.

Nebulization: Limited data in ages <2 years:

Albuterol Nebulization Dosage

Age	Dose (mg)	0.5% Solution (mL)	0.083% Solution (mL)	Frequency
Infants and Children <5 y	0.63 to 2.5 mg	0.13 to 0.5 mL	0.76 to 3 mL	Every 4 to 6 h
Children ≥5 y and Adolescents	1.25 to 5 mg	0.25 to 1 mL	1.5 to 6 mL	Every 4 to 8 h

Bronchospasm, treatment:

Oral inhalation:

Inhalation, aerosol (metered dose inhaler):

Manufacturer's labeling: Children ≥4 years and Adolescents: 90 mcg/puff: 1 to 2 puffs every 4 to 6 hours

Alternate dosing: Limited data available: Infants, Children, and Adolescents: 90 mcg/puff: 4 to 8 puffs every 15 to 20 minutes for 3 doses; then every 1 to 4 hours (Hegenbarth 2008)

Nebulization:

Manufacturer labeling: Children ≥2 years and Adolescents:

10 to 15 kg: 1.25 mg 3 to 4 times/day

>15 kg: 2.5 mg 3 to 4 times/day

Alternate dosing: Limited data available (Hegenbarth 2008): Infants, Children, and Adolescents:

Intermittent: 0.5% (5 mg/mL) solution: 2.5 mg every 20 minutes for 3 doses, then 0.15 to 0.3 mg/kg up to 10 mg every 1 to 4 hours

Continuous (prolonged nebulization): 0.5 mg/kg/ hour up to 10 to 15 mg/hour

Oral: **Note:** Not the preferred route for treatment of asthma; inhalation via nebulization or MDI is preferred (GINA 2014; GINA 2014a; NAEPP 2007)

Immediate release formulation (syrup, tablets):

Children 2 to 6 years: 0.1 to 0.2 mg/kg/dose 3 times daily; maximum dose: 4 mg

Children 6 to 12 years: 2 mg/dose 3 to 4 times daily

Adolescents: 2 to 4 mg/dose 3 to 4 times daily

Sustained release formulation (tablets):

Children ≥6 years: 0.3 to 0.6 mg/kg/**day** divided twice daily; maximum daily dose: 8 mg/**day**

Adolescents: 4 mg/dose twice daily; may increase to 8 mg/dose twice daily

Exercise-induced bronchospasm; prevention: (NAEPP 2007; Parsons 2013): Oral inhalation:

Inhalation, aerosol (metered dose inhaler): Limited data available in ages <4 years: 90 mcg/puff:

Infants and Children <5 years: 1 to 2 puffs 5 to 20 minutes before exercising

Children ≥5 years and Adolescents: 2 puffs 5 to 20 minutes before exercising

Hyperkalemia; adjunct therapy: Limited data available: Infants, Children, and Adolescents: Oral inhalation: *Nebulization:* 10 mg/dose or 0.3 to 0.5 mg/kg/dose has been used by some centers and based on experience that has shown the effective nebulization for hyperkalemia is 4 times more than the bronchodilatory dose (Furhman 2011; Weiner 1998; Weisburg 2008). **Note:** Albuterol should be not be used as the sole agent for treating severe hyperkalemia, especially in patients with renal failure.

Adult:

Bronchospasm:

Metered dose inhaler (90 mcg/puff): 2 puffs every 4 to 6 hours as needed (NAEPP 2007):

Acute treatment: 1 to 2 puffs; additional puffs may be necessary if inadequate relief; however, patients should be advised to promptly consult health care provider or seek medical attention if no relief from acute treatment

Maintenance: 1 to 2 puffs 3 to 4 times daily (maximum: 8 puffs daily)

Nebulization: 2.5 mg 3 to 4 times daily as needed; Quick relief: 1.25 to 5 mg every 4 to 8 hours as needed (NAEPP 2007)

Oral: **Note:** Oral is not the preferred route for treatment of asthma; inhalation via nebulization or MDI is preferred (NAEPP 2007).

Regular release: 2 to 4 mg/dose 3 to 4 times daily; maximum dose not to exceed 32 mg daily (divided doses)

Extended release: 8 mg every 12 hours; maximum dose not to exceed 32 mg/day (divided doses). A 4 mg dose every 12 hours may be sufficient in some patients, such as adults of low body weight.

Exacerbation of asthma (acute, severe) (NAEPP 2007):

Metered dose inhaler: 4 to 8 puffs every 20 minutes for up to 4 hours, then every 1 to 4 hours as needed

Nebulization solution: 2.5 to 5 mg every 20 minutes for 3 doses, then 2.5 to 10 mg every 1 to 4 hours as needed, or 10 to 15 mg/hour by continuous nebulization

Exercise-induced bronchospasm (prevention): *Metered dose inhaler (90 mcg/puff):* 2 puffs 5 to 30 minutes prior to exercise

Dosing adjustment in renal impairment: All patients: Use with caution in patients with renal impairment. No dosage adjustment required, including patients on hemodialysis, peritoneal dialysis, or CRRT (Aronoff 2007).

Dosing adjustment in hepatic impairment: There are no dosage adjustments provided in manufacturer's labeling.

Preparation for Administration Solution for nebulization: 0.5% solution: Dilute 0.25 mL (1.25 mg dose) or 0.5 mL (2.5 mg dose) of solution to a total of 3 mL with normal saline; also compatible with cromolyn or ipratropium nebulizer solutions

Administration

Oral inhalation: In infants and children <4 years, a face mask with either the metered dose inhaler or nebulizer is recommended (GINA 2014a; NAEPP 2007)

Inhalation, aerosol (metered dose inhaler): Prime the inhaler (before first use or if it has not been used for more than 2 weeks) by releasing 4 test sprays into the air away from the face (3 test sprays for ProAir HFA); shake well before use; use spacer for children <5 years of age and consider adding a face mask for infants and children <4 years of age. HFA inhalers should be cleaned with warm water at least once per week; allow to air dry completely prior to use.

Nebulization: Concentrated solutions (≥ 0.5%) should be diluted prior to use; adjust nebulizer flow to deliver dosage over 5 to 15 minutes; avoid contact of the dropper tip (multidose bottle) with any surface, including the nebulizer reservoir and associated ventilator equipment. For continuous nebulization, the total amount of fluid delivered is determined by nebulizer delivery device; usually 25 to 30 mL per 1 hour of nebulization, protocols may vary by institution (Hegenbarth 2008). Blow-by administration is not recommended; use a mask device if patient is unable to hold mouthpiece in mouth for administration.

Oral: Administer with food; do not crush or chew extended release tablets

Monitoring Parameters Serum potassium, oxygen saturation, heart rate, pulmonary function tests, respiratory rate, use of accessory muscles during respiration, suprasternal retractions; arterial or capillary blood gases (if patient's condition warrants)

Test Interactions Increased renin (S), increased aldosterone (S)

Dosage Forms Considerations

ProAir HFA 8.5 g canisters and Proventil HFA 6.7 g canisters contain 200 inhalations.

Ventolin HFA 18 g canisters contain 200 inhalations and the 8 g canisters contain 60 inhalations.

Dosage Forms Excipient information presented when available (limited, particularly for generics); consult specific product labeling. [DSC] = Discontinued product

Aerosol Powder Breath Activated, Inhalation:
- ProAir RespiClick: 90 mcg/actuation (1 ea) [contains milk protein]

Aerosol Solution, Inhalation:
- ProAir HFA: 90 mcg/actuation (8.5 g)
- Proventil HFA: 90 mcg/actuation (6.7 g)
- Ventolin HFA: 90 mcg/actuation (8 g, 18 g)

Nebulization Solution, Inhalation:
- Generic: 0.63 mg/3 mL (3 mL); 0.083% [2.5 mg/3 mL] (3 mL); 0.5% [2.5 mg/0.5 mL] (20 mL)

Nebulization Solution, Inhalation [preservative free]:
- AccuNeb: 0.63 mg/3 mL (3 mL [DSC]); 1.25 mg/3 mL (3 mL [DSC])
- Generic: 0.63 mg/3 mL (3 mL); 1.25 mg/3 mL (3 mL); 0.083% [2.5 mg/3 mL] (3 mL); 0.5% [2.5 mg/0.5 mL] (1 ea)

Syrup, Oral:
- Generic: 2 mg/5 mL (473 mL)

Tablet, Oral:
- Generic: 2 mg, 4 mg

Tablet Extended Release 12 Hour, Oral:
- VoSpire ER: 4 mg [contains fd&c blue #1 aluminum lake, fd&c yellow #10 aluminum lake]
- VoSpire ER: 8 mg
- Generic: 4 mg, 8 mg

◆ **Albuterol Sulfate** *see* Albuterol *on page* 81
◆ **Alcaine** *see* Proparacaine *on page* 1785
◆ **Alcaine® (Can)** *see* Proparacaine *on page* 1785
◆ **Alcalak [OTC]** *see* Calcium Carbonate *on page* 343

Alclometasone (al kloe MET a sone)

Medication Safety Issues

Sound-alike/look-alike issues:

Aclovate® may be confused with Accolate®

International issues:

Cloderm: Brand name for alclometasone [Indonesia], but also brand name for clobetasol [China, India, Malaysia, Singapore, Thailand]; clocortolone [U.S., Canada]; clotrimazole [Germany]

Related Information

Topical Corticosteroids *on page* 2262

Brand Names: US Aclovate

Therapeutic Category Adrenal Corticosteroid; Anti-inflammatory Agent; Corticosteroid, Topical; Glucocorticoid

Generic Availability (US) Yes

Use Treatment of inflammation and pruritic manifestations of corticosteroid-responsive dermatosis (low to medium potency topical corticosteroid) (FDA approved in ages ≥1 year and adults); **Note:** In pediatric patients, safety and efficacy ≥3 weeks have not been established.

Pregnancy Risk Factor C

Pregnancy Considerations Some corticosteroids were found to be teratogenic following topical application in animal reproduction studies. Topical products are not recommended for extensive use, in large quantities, or for long periods of time in pregnant women.

Breast-Feeding Considerations Systemic corticosteroids are excreted in human milk. It is not known if sufficient quantities of alclometasone are absorbed following topical administration to produce detectable amounts in breast milk.

Contraindications Hypersensitivity to alclometasone or any component of the formulation

Warnings/Precautions Topical corticosteroids may be absorbed percutaneously. Absorption may cause manifestations of Cushing's syndrome, hyperglycemia, or glycosuria. Absorption is increased by the use of occlusive dressings, application to denuded skin, or application to large surface areas. May cause hypercorticism or suppression of hypothalamic-pituitary-adrenal (HPA) axis, particularly in younger children or in patients receiving high doses for prolonged periods. HPA axis suppression may lead to adrenal crisis.

Prolonged treatment with corticosteroids has been associated with the development of Kaposi's sarcoma (case reports); if noted, discontinuation of therapy should be considered. Prolonged use may result in fungal or bacterial superinfection; discontinue if dermatological infection persists despite appropriate antimicrobial therapy. Local sensitization (redness, irritation) may occur; discontinue if sensitization is noted. Allergic contact dermatitis can occur, it is usually diagnosed by failure to heal rather than clinical exacerbation.

Safety and efficacy have not been established in children <1 year of age. Safety and efficacy for use >3 weeks has not been established. Children may absorb proportionally larger amounts after topical application and may be more prone to systemic effects. HPA axis suppression, intracranial hypertension, and Cushing's syndrome have been reported in children receiving topical corticosteroids. Prolonged use may affect growth velocity; growth should be routinely monitored in pediatric patients. Not for the treatment of diaper dermatitis.

Avoid use of topical preparations with occlusive dressings or on weeping or exudative lesions. If no improvement is seen within 2 weeks, reassessment of diagnosis may be necessary. Avoid contact with eyes. Generally not for routine use on the face, underarms, or groin area (including diapered area).

Warnings: Additional Pediatric Considerations The extent of percutaneous absorption is dependent on several factors, including epidermal integrity (intact vs abraded skin), formulation, age of the patient, prolonged duration of use, and the use of occlusive dressings. Percutaneous absorption of topical steroids is increased in neonates (especially preterm neonates), infants, and young children. Infants and small children may be more susceptible to HPA axis suppression, intracranial hypertension, Cushing syndrome, or other systemic toxicities due to larger skin surface area to body mass ratio.

Some dosage forms may contain propylene glycol; in neonates large amounts of propylene glycol delivered orally, intravenously (eg, >3,000 mg/day), or topically have been associated with potentially fatal toxicities which can include metabolic acidosis, seizures, renal failure, and CNS depression; toxicities have also been reported in children and adults including hyperosmolality, lactic acidosis, seizures and respiratory depression; use caution (AAP, 1997; Shehab, 2009).

Adverse Reactions

Dermatologic: Acne, allergic dermatitis, hypopigmentation, perioral dermatitis, skin atrophy, striae, miliaria

Endocrine & metabolic: HPA axis suppression, Cushing's syndrome, growth retardation

Local: Burning, erythema, itching, irritation, dryness, folliculitis, papular rash

Miscellaneous: Secondary infection

Drug Interactions

Metabolism/Transport Effects None known.

Avoid Concomitant Use

Avoid concomitant use of Alclometasone with any of the following: Aldesleukin

Increased Effect/Toxicity

Alclometasone may increase the levels/effects of: Ceritinib; Deferasirox

The levels/effects of Alclometasone may be increased by: Telaprevir

Decreased Effect

Alclometasone may decrease the levels/effects of: Aldesleukin; Corticorelin; Hyaluronidase; Telaprevir

Storage/Stability Store between 2°C and 30°C (36°F and 86°F).

Mechanism of Action Topical corticosteroids have anti-inflammatory, antipruritic, and vasoconstrictive properties. May depress the formation, release, and activity of endogenous chemical mediators of inflammation (kinins, histamine, liposomal enzymes, prostaglandins) through the induction of phospholipase A_2 inhibitory proteins (lipocortins) and sequential inhibition of the release of arachidonic acid. Alclometasone has low range potency.

Pharmacodynamics

Initial response (Ruthven, 1988):

Eczema: 5.3 days

Psoriasis: 6.7 days

Peak response (Ruthven, 1988):

Eczema: 13.9 days

Psoriasis: 14.8 days

Pharmacokinetics (Adult data unless noted) Absorption: Topical: 3% (when left on intact skin without an occlusive dressing for 8 hours). Percutaneous absorption varies and depends on many factors including vehicle used, integrity of epidermis, dose, and use of occlusive dressing; absorption is increased by occlusive dressings or with decreased integrity of skin (eg, inflammation or skin disease). Absorption also depends upon the anatomical site: Forearm 1%; scalp 4%; scrotum 36%

Dosing: Usual Children, Adolescents, and Adults: Topical: Apply to affected area 2-3 times daily. Therapy should be discontinued when control is achieved; if no improvement is seen within 2 weeks, reassessment of diagnosis may be necessary. Safety and efficacy have not been established for long term use (>3 weeks) in children. In general, the treated skin should not be covered due to potential increased absorption; however, occlusive dressings may be used when treating refractory lesions of psoriasis and other deep-seated dermatoses such as localized neurodermatitis (lichen simplex chronicus); monitor closely for toxicity.

Administration Topical: Apply sparingly in a thin film; rub in lightly; for external use only; avoid contact with the eyes; generally not for routine use on the face, underarms, or groin area (including diapered area). Do not use on open wounds or weeping lesions. The treated skin area should not be bandaged or covered unless directed by the prescriber. Wash hands thoroughly before and after use.

Monitoring Parameters Clinical signs and symptoms of improvement in condition; assessment of HPA suppression (eg, ACTH stimulation test, morning plasma cortisol test, urinary free cortisol test) if treatment for prolonged periods or if HPA axis suppression is suspected; growth in pediatric patients

Dosage Forms Excipient information presented when available (limited, particularly for generics); consult specific product labeling.

Cream, External, as dipropionate:

Aclovate: 0.05% (15 g, 60 g) [contains cetearyl alcoho[l], propylene glycol]

Generic: 0.05% (15 g, 45 g, 60 g)

Ointment, External, as dipropionate:

Generic: 0.05% (15 g, 45 g, 60 g)

◆ **Alclometasone Dipropionate** *see* Alclometasone *on page 85*

◆ **Alcohol, Absolute** *see* Alcohol (Ethyl) *on page 86*

◆ **Alcohol, Dehydrated** *see* Alcohol (Ethyl) *on page 86*

Alcohol (Ethyl) (AL koe hol, ETH il)

Medication Safety Issues

Sound-alike/look-alike issues:

Ethanol may be confused with Ethyol, Ethamolin

Brand Names: US Epi-Clenz [OTC]; Gel-Stat [OTC]; GelRite [OTC]; Isagel [OTC]; Lavacol [OTC]; Prevacar[e] [OTC]; Protection Plus [OTC]; Purell 2 in 1 [OTC]; Pure[ll] Lasting Care [OTC]; Purell Moisture Therapy [OTC]; Pure[ll] with Aloe [OTC]; Purell [OTC]

Brand Names: Canada Biobase; Biobase-G

Therapeutic Category Anti-infective Agent, Topical; Antidote, Ethylene Glycol Toxicity; Antidote, Methanol Toxicity; Fat Occlusion (Central Venous Catheter), Treatment Agent; Neurolytic

Generic Availability (US) Yes

Use

Injection: Therapeutic neurolysis of nerves or ganglia for the relief of intractable, chronic pain in such conditions as inoperable cancer and trigeminal neuralgia (dehydrated alcohol injection) (FDA approved in adults); epidural or individual motor nerve injections to control certain manifestations of cerebral palsy and spastic paraplegia, celiac plexus block to relieve pain of inoperable upper abdominal cancer, and intra- and subcutaneously for relief of intractable pruritis ani (diluted [40% to 50%] dehydrated alcohol injection: FDA approved in adults); has also been used as an antidote for the treatment of methanol and ethylene glycol intoxication, as a lock solution for the prevention and treatment of catheter-related infections, and for treatment of occluded central venous catheters due to lipid deposition from fat emulsion infusion (particularly 3-in-1 admixture)

Topical: Skin antiseptic (hand sanitizer gels, foams solutions and rubbing ethyl alcohol: FDA approved pediatric patients [age not specified] and adults)

Pregnancy Risk Factor C (injection)

Pregnancy Considerations Reproduction studies have not been conducted with alcohol injection. Ethanol crosses the placenta, enters the fetal circulation, and has teratogenic effects in humans. The following withdrawal symptoms have been noted in the neonate following maternal ethanol consumption during pregnancy: Crying, hyperactivity, irritability, poor suck, tremors, seizures, poor sleeping pattern, hyperphagia, and diaphoresis. Fetal alcohol syndrome (FAS) is a term referring to a combination of physical, behavioral, and cognitive abnormalities resulting from ethanol exposure during fetal development. Since a "safe" amount of ethanol consumption during pregnancy has not been determined, the AAP recommends those women who are pregnant or planning a pregnancy refrain from all ethanol intake. When used as an antidote during the second or third trimester, FAS is not likely to occur due to the short treatment period; use during the first trimester is controversial.

Breast-Feeding Considerations Ethanol is found in breast milk. Drowsiness, diaphoresis, deep sleep, weakness, decreased linear growth, and abnormal weight gain have been reported in infants following large amounts of ethanol ingestion by the mother. Ingestion >1 g/kg/day decreases milk ejection reflex. The actual clearance of ethanol from breast milk is dependent upon the mother's weight and amount of ethanol consumed.

Contraindications Hypersensitivity to ethyl alcohol or any component of the formulation; seizure disorder and diabetic coma; subarachnoid injection of dehydrated alcohol in patients receiving anticoagulants; pregnancy (prolonged use or high doses at term)

Warnings/Precautions Ethyl alcohol is a flammable liquid and should be kept cool and away from any heat source. Proper positioning of the patient for neurolytic administration is essential to control localization of the injection of dehydrated alcohol (which is hypobaric) into the subarachnoid space; avoid extravasation. Not for SubQ administration. Do not administer simultaneously with blood due to the possibility of pseudoagglutination or hemolysis; may potentiate severe hypoprothrombic bleeding. Clinical evaluation and periodic lab determinations, including serum ethanol levels, are necessary to monitor effectiveness, changes in electrolyte concentrations, and acid-base balance (when used as an antidote).

Use with caution in patients with diabetes (ethyl alcohol may decrease blood sugar), hepatic impairment, patients with gout, shock, following cranial surgery, and in anticipated postpartum hemorrhage. Monitor blood glucose closely, particularly in children as treatment of ingestions is associated with hypoglycemia. Avoid extravasation during IV administration. Ethyl alcohol passes freely into breast milk at a level approximately equivalent to maternal serum level; minimize dermal exposure of ethyl alcohol in infants as significant systemic absorption and toxicity can occur.

When used as a topical antiseptic, improper use may lead to product contamination. Although infrequent, product contamination has been associated with reports of localized and systemic infections. To reduce the risk of infection, ensure antiseptic products are used according to the labeled instructions; avoid diluting products after opening; and apply single-use containers only one time to one patient and discard any unused solution (FDA Drug Safety Communication, 2013).

Adverse Reactions

Cardiovascular: Flushing, hypotension

Central nervous system: Agitation, CNS depression, coma, disorientation, drowsiness, encephalopathy, headache, sedation, seizure (rare), vertigo

Endocrine & metabolic: Hypoglycemia

Gastrointestinal: Gastric irritation, nausea, vomiting

Genitourinary: Urinary retention

Local: Nerve and tissue destruction, phlebitis

Renal: Polyuria

Miscellaneous: Intoxication

Drug Interactions

Metabolism/Transport Effects None known.

Avoid Concomitant Use

Avoid concomitant use of Alcohol (Ethyl) with any of the following: Acitretin; Agomelatine; Alpha-Lipoic Acid; Amisulpride; Azelastine (Nasal); Bedaquiline; Cefminox; CycloSERINE; Dapoxetine; Didanosine; Disulfiram; Eluxadoline; Gabapentin Enacarbil; GuanFACINE; Hydrocodone; Lercanidipine; MAO Inhibitors; Mequitazine; MetFORMIN; Methadone; Methylphenidate; MetroNIDAZOLE (Systemic); Mianserin; Mirtazapine; Orphenadrine; Paraldehyde; Perampanel; Pipamperone [INT]; Sodium Oxybate; Stiripentol; Sulpiride; Suvorexant; Tapentadol; Tinidazole; Topiramate; Trabectedin; Zopiclone

Increased Effect/Toxicity

Alcohol (Ethyl) may increase the levels/effects of: Acetaminophen; Acetohydroxamic Acid; Acitretin; Agomelatine; Amantadine; Aminophylline; Azelastine (Nasal); Bedaquiline; Bromocriptine; Buprenorphine; BuPROPion; CloBAZam; CycloSERINE; Didanosine; Diethylpropion; Doxylamine; Eluxadoline; Ethionamide; Ezogabine; Fesoterodine; Fosphenytoin; Gabapentin Enacarbil; GuanFACINE; Hydrocodone; ISOtretinoin; Lercanidipine; Levomilnacipran; Lomitapide; MAO Inhibitors; Mequitazine; MetFORMIN; Methadone; Methylphenidate; Metyrosine; Mipomersen; Mirtazapine; Morniflumate; Niacin; Nicorandil; NIFEdipine; Orphenadrine; OXcarbazepine; Oxybutynin; Paraldehyde; Phendimetrazine; Phentermine; Phenytoin; Phosphodiesterase 5 Inhibitors; Pramipexole; Propranolol; ROPINIRole; Rotigotine; Rufinamide; Selective Serotonin Reuptake Inhibitors; Serotonin/Norepinephrine Reuptake Inhibitors; Sodium Oxybate; Sulpiride; Suvorexant; Tacrolimus (Systemic); Tapentadol; Theophylline; Thiazide Diuretics; Topiramate; Trabectedin; TraZODone; Treprostinil; Trimethobenzamide; Trospium; Vasodilators (Organic Nitrates); Zopiclone

The levels/effects of Alcohol (Ethyl) may be increased by: Amisulpride; Bromocriptine; BuPROPion; Cannabis; Cefminox; CefoTEtan; Chloramphenicol; Cisapride; CNS Depressants; Dapoxetine; Disulfiram; Dronabinol; Efavirenz; Griseofulvin; Ketoconazole (Systemic); MetroNIDAZOLE (Systemic); MetroNIDAZOLE (Topical); Mianserin; Nabilone; Perampanel; Pipamperone [INT]; Stiripentol; Sulfonylureas; Tacrolimus (Topical); Tetrahydrocannabinol; Tinidazole; Varenicline; Verapamil

Decreased Effect

Alcohol (Ethyl) may decrease the levels/effects of: Alpha-Lipoic Acid; Cyproterone; Fosphenytoin; Phenytoin; Propranolol; Vitamin K Antagonists

The levels/effects of Alcohol (Ethyl) may be decreased by: Efavirenz

Storage/Stability Store at room temperature; do not use unless solution is clear and container is intact.

Mechanism of Action When used to treat ethylene glycol or methanol toxicity, ethyl alcohol competitively inhibits alcohol dehydrogenase, an enzyme which catalyzes the metabolism of ethylene glycol and methanol to their toxic metabolites. In neurolysis, alcohol will destroy nerves at the site of injection.

Pharmacokinetics (Adult data unless noted)

Absorption: Oral: Rapid

Distribution: V_d: 0.6 to 0.7 L/kg; decreased in women

Metabolism: Hepatic (90% to 98%) to acetaldehyde or acetate by alcohol dehydrogenase

Half-life: Rate: 15 to 20 mg/dL/hour (range: 10 to 34 mg/dL/hour); increased in alcoholics

Elimination: Renal and lungs (~2% unchanged)

Dosing: Usual

Pediatric:

Antiseptic: Children and Adolescents: Ethyl rubbing alcohol: Topical: Apply 1 to 3 times daily as needed

Methanol or ethylene glycol ingestion: Limited data available (Barceloux 1999; Barceloux 2002): Infants, Children, and Adolescents: **Note:** IV administration is the preferred route; continue therapy until ethylene glycol and/or methanol is no longer detected or levels are <20 mg/dL **and** the patient is asymptomatic **and** metabolic acidosis has been corrected. If ethylene glycol and/or methanol levels are not available in a timely manner, continue therapy until the estimated time of clearance of ethylene glycol and/or methanol has elapsed **and** the patient is asymptomatic with a normal pH. If patient has coingested ethanol, measure the baseline serum ethanol concentration and adjust the ethyl alcohol loading dose based on results to achieve a serum ethanol level of ~100 mg/dL.

Absolute ethyl alcohol [98% (196 proof) = 77.4 g EtOH/dL]:

IV: **Note:** Contact the Poison Control Center for options related to compounding IV ethanol.

Initial: 600 to 700 mg/kg [equivalent to 7.6 to 8.9 mL/kg using a 10% solution]

Maintenance (not receiving hemodialysis): Goal of therapy is to maintain serum ethanol levels >100 mg/dL.

Nondrinker: 66 mg/kg/hour [equivalent to 0.83 mL/kg/hour using a **10% solution**]

Chronic drinker: 154 mg/kg/hour [equivalent to 1.96 mL/kg/hour using a **10% solution**]

Oral: **Note:** Solution must be diluted to a ≤20% concentration with water or juice and administered orally or via a nasogastric tube.

Initial: 600 to 700 mg/kg (equivalent to 0.78 to 0.9 mL/kg using a **98% solution**)

Maintenance (not receiving hemodialysis): Goal of therapy is to maintain serum ethanol levels >100 mg/dL

Nondrinker: 66 mg/kg/hour (equivalent to 0.09 mL/kg/hour using a **98% solution**)

Chronic drinker: 154 mg/kg/hour (equivalent to 0.20 mL/kg/hour using a **98% solution**)

Central venous catheter lock: Limited data available: Infants, Children, and Adolescents: See institution-based protocol: Dehydrated alcohol injection: I.V.:

Catheter-related blood stream infection (CRBSI):

Prophylaxis: **Note:** Use suggested in patients with long term catheters with a history of multiple CRBSI episode (IDSA [O'Grady 2011]); dosing regimens variable: 70% ethanol; instill a volume equal to the internal volume of the catheter once daily with a dwell time of 2 to 14 hours; withdraw ethanol at the end of the dwell time (Cober 2011; Mouw 2008; Wales 2011). Less frequent dosing (3 times per week) for a minimum 4 hour dwell time (Jones 2010) and once weekly dosing with a 2-hour dwell time (Pieroni 2013) have also shown to produce statistically significant reductions in infection rate and catheter loss; most study subjects were receiving long-term outpatient cyclic parenteral nutrition. However, a small case-series observed an increase in infection rate when the frequency of ethanol locks were decreased to less than daily (eg, twice weekly or once weekly; dwell times not specified) during an ethanol shortage; all patients in this study had tunneled silastic catheters (Ralls 2012)

Treatment: Dosing regimens variable: 70% ethanol; instill a volume equal to the internal volume of the catheter with a dwell time 4 to 25 hours; some protocols utilized single dose and others repeated the dose once daily for 3 to 5 days; dosing should be repeated for each lumen and used in combination with systemic antimicrobials (Danneberg 2003; McGrath 2011; Onland 2006; Valentine 2011). For fungal bloodstream infection, case-reports describe success using once daily with dwell times of 2 to 24 hours for 14 days following the patient's first negative blood culture (Blackwood 2011)

Fat occlusion of central venous catheters: Dehydrated alcohol injection: Up to 3 mL of 70% ethanol (maximum: 0.55 mL/kg); instill a volume equal to the internal volume of the catheter; may repeat if patency not restored after 30 to 60 minute dwell time; if dose repeated, reassess after 4-hour dwell time (Pennington 1987; Werlin 1995).

Adult:

Antiseptic: Ethyl rubbing alcohol: Topical: Apply 1 to 3 times daily as needed

Therapeutic neurolysis (nerve or ganglion block): Dehydrated alcohol injection 98%: Intraneural: Dosage variable depending upon the site of injection (eg, trigeminal neuralgia: 0.05 to 0.5 mL as a single injection per interspace vs subarachnoid injection: 0.5 to 1 mL as a single injection per interspace); single doses >1.5 mL are seldom required. **Note:** Administer when pain is from malignant origin only.

Replenishment of fluid and carbohydrate calories: Dehydrated alcohol infusion: Alcohol 5% and dextrose 5%: 1,000 to 2,000 mL/day by slow infusion

Dosing adjustment in renal impairment: There are no dosage adjustments provided in the manufacturer's labeling. Hemodialysis clearance: 300 to 400 mL/minute with an ethanol removal rate of 280 mg/minute.

Methanol or ethylene glycol ingestion: Infants, Children, Adolescents, and Adults: Absolute ethyl alcohol: Dosage adjustment for hemodialysis: Maintenance dose:

IV:

Nondrinker: 169 mg/kg/hour (equivalent to 2.13 mL/kg/hour using a **10% solution**)

Chronic drinker: 257 mg/kg/hour (equivalent to 3.26 mL/kg/hour using a **10% solution**)

Oral:

Nondrinker: 169 mg/kg/hour (equivalent to 0.22 mL/kg/hour using a **98% solution**)

Chronic drinker: 257 mg/kg/hour (equivalent to 0.33 mL/kg/hour using a **98% solution**)

Dosing adjustment in hepatic impairment: There are no dosage adjustments provided in the manufacturer's labeling.

Preparation for Administration

Oral: Ethylene glycol or methanol poisoning: Dilute ethyl alcohol (98% ethanol injection solution) to a ≤20% solution with water or juice.

Parenteral: IV:

Ethylene glycol or methanol poisoning: Dilute ethyl alcohol (98% ethanol injection solution) to a 10% solution in D_5W or $D_{10}W$.

Occluded central venous catheter/central venous catheter lock: To prepare 70% solution: Add 0.8 mL SWFI to 2 mL ethyl alcohol (98% ethanol injection solution) (Cober 2007)

Administration

Oral: Ethylene glycol or methanol poisoning: After diluting ethyl alcohol (98% ethanol injection solution) to ≤20% solution, administer hourly by mouth or via nasogastric tube. Out-of-hospital management with orally administered ethanol is not recommended.

Parenteral: Not for SubQ administration; IV:

Ethylene glycol or methanol poisoning: After diluting ethyl alcohol (98% ethanol injection solution) to 10% v/v solution, infuse initial dose over 60 minutes; central vein is the preferred route.

Occluded central venous catheter/central venous catheter lock: After diluting ethyl alcohol (98% ethanol injection solution) to 70% solution, instill with a volume equal to the internal volume of the catheter; assess patency at 30 to 60 minutes (or per institutional protocol); may repeat. Ensure adequate measurement of catheter volume to ensure adequate coverage of line and no excess ethanol is administered. Ethanol forms a visual precipitate with heparin or citrate, flush catheter well with normal saline before administration. (Cober 2007; Cober 2011)

Intraneural: Adult: Separate needles should be used for each of multiple injections or sites to prevent residual alcohol deposition at sites not intended for tissue destruction; inject slowly after determining proper placement of needle; since dehydrated alcohol is hypobaric when compared with spinal fluid, proper positioning of the patient is essential to control localization of injections into the subarachnoid space

Monitoring Parameters Antidotal therapy: Blood ethanol levels (at the end of the loading dose, every 1 to 2 hours until stabilized, and then every 2 to 4 hours thereafter); blood glucose, electrolytes (including serum magnesium), arterial pH, blood gases, methanol or ethylene glycol blood levels, heart rate, blood pressure

Reference Range

Symptoms associated with serum ethanol levels:

Nausea and vomiting: Serum level >100 mg/dL

Coma: Serum level >300 mg/dL

Antidote for methanol/ethylene glycol: Goal range: Blood ethanol level: 100-150 mg/dL (22-32 mmol/liter)

Dosage Forms Excipient information presented when available (limited, particularly for generics); consult specific product labeling.

Aerosol, foam, topical [instant hand sanitizer]:

Epi-Clenz™: 70% (240 mL) [contains aloe, vitamin E]

Gel, topical [foam/instant hand sanitizer]:

Epi-Clenz™: 70% (480 mL) [contains aloe, vitamin E]

Gel, topical [instant hand sanitizer]: 62% (1.5 mL, 118 mL, 354 mL, 473 mL)

Epi-Clenz™: 70% (45 mL, 120 mL, 480 mL) [contains aloe, vitamin E]

Gel-Stat™: 62% (120 mL, 480 mL) [contains aloe, vitamin E]

GelRite™: 67% (120 mL, 480 mL)

GelRite™: 67% (800 mL) [contains vitamin E]

Isagel®: 60% (59 mL, 118 mL, 621 mL, 800 mL)

Prevacare®: 60% (120 mL, 240 mL, 960 mL, 1200 mL, 1500 mL)

Purell®: 62% (60 mL, 360 mL, 1000 mL)

Purell®: 62% (15 mL, 30 mL, 59 mL, 60 mL, 120 mL, 236 mL, 240 mL, 250 mL, 360 mL, 500 mL, 800 mL, 1000 mL, 2000 mL) [contains moisturizers, vitamin E]

Purell®: 62% (15 mL, 60 mL, 360 mL, 800 mL, 1000 mL) [contains vitamin E]

Purell® Lasting Care: 62% (120 mL, 240 mL, 1000 mL) [contains moisturizers]

Purell® Moisture Therapy: 62% (75 mL)

Purell® with Aloe: 62% (60 mL, 120 mL, 354 mL, 800 mL, 1000 mL, 2000 mL) [contains aloe, moisturizers, tartrazine, vitamin E]

Purell® with Aloe: 62% (15 mL, 59 mL, 236 mL) [contains aloe, tartrazine, vitamin E]

Injection, solution [dehydrated, preservative free]: 98% (1 mL, 5 mL)

Liquid, topical [denatured]: 70% (480 mL, 3840 mL)

Liquid, topical [denatured/rubbing alcohol]:

Lavacol®: 70% (473 mL)

Lotion, topical [instant hand sanitizer]:

Purell® 2 in 1: 62% (60 mL, 360 mL, 1000 mL)

Pad, topical [instant hand sanitizer/towelette]:

Isagel®: 60% (50s, 300s)

Purell®: 62% (24s) [contains aloe, moisturizers, tartrazine, vitamin A, vitamin E]

Purell®: 62% (35s, 175s) [contains moisturizers, vitamin E]

Solution, topical [instant hand sanitizer]:

Protection Plus®: 62% (800 mL)

◆ **Aldactazide** *see* Hydrochlorothiazide and Spironolactone *on page 1030*

◆ **Aldactazide 25 (Can)** *see* Hydrochlorothiazide and Spironolactone *on page 1030*

◆ **Aldactazide 50 (Can)** *see* Hydrochlorothiazide and Spironolactone *on page 1030*

◆ **Aldactone** *see* Spironolactone *on page 1968*

Aldesleukin (al des LOO kin)

Medication Safety Issues

Sound-alike/look-alike issues:

Aldesleukin may be confused with oprelvekin

Proleukin may be confused with oprelvekin

High alert medication:

This medication is in a class the Institute for Safe Medication Practices (ISMP) includes among its list of drug classes which have a heightened risk of causing significant patient harm when used in error.

Related Information

Prevention of Chemotherapy-Induced Nausea and Vomiting in Children *on page 2368*

Brand Names: US Proleukin

Brand Names: Canada Proleukin

Therapeutic Category Antineoplastic Agent, Biologic Response Modulator; Antineoplastic Agent, Miscellaneous; Biological Response Modulator

Generic Availability (US) No

Use Treatment of metastatic renal cell carcinoma and metastatic melanoma (FDA approved in adults); has also been used in the treatment of high-risk neuroblastoma

Pregnancy Risk Factor C

Pregnancy Considerations Adverse events were observed in animal reproduction studies. Use during pregnancy only if benefits to the mother outweigh potential risk to the fetus. Effective contraception is recommended for fertile males and/or females using this medication.

Breast-Feeding Considerations It is not known if aldesleukin is excreted in breast milk. Due to the potential for serious adverse reactions in the breast-feeding infant, a decision should be made to discontinue breast-feeding or to discontinue the drug, taking into account the importance of treatment to the mother.

Contraindications Hypersensitivity to aldesleukin or any component of the formulation; patients with abnormal thallium stress or pulmonary function tests; patients who have had an organ allograft. **Re-treatment is contraindicated** in patients who have experienced sustained ventricular tachycardia (≥5 beats), uncontrolled or unresponsive cardiac arrhythmias, chest pain with ECG changes consistent with angina or MI, cardiac tamponade, intubation >72 hours, renal failure requiring dialysis for >72 hours, coma or toxic psychosis lasting >48 hours, repetitive or refractory seizures, bowel ischemia/perforation, or GI bleeding requiring surgery.

Warnings/Precautions [U.S. Boxed Warning]: Aldesleukin therapy has been associated with capillary leak syndrome (CLS), characterized by vascular tone loss and extravasation of plasma proteins and fluid into extravascular space. CLS results in hypotension and reduced organ perfusion, which may be severe and can result in death. Cardiac arrhythmia, angina, myocardial infarction, respiratory insufficiency (requiring intubation), gastrointestinal bleeding or infarction, renal insufficiency, edema and mental status changes are also associated with CLS. CLS onset is immediately after treatment initiation. Monitor fluid status and organ perfusion status carefully; consider fluids and/or pressor agents to maintain organ perfusion. **[U.S. Boxed Warning]: Therapy should be restricted to patients with normal cardiac and pulmonary functions as defined by thallium stress and formal pulmonary function testing. Extreme caution should be used in patients with a history of prior cardiac or pulmonary disease** and in patients who are fluid-restricted or where edema may be poorly tolerated. Withhold treatment for signs of organ hypoperfusion, including altered mental status, reduced urine output, systolic BP <90 mm Hg or cardiac arrhythmia. Once blood pressure is normalized, may consider diuretics for excessive weight gain/edema. Recovery from CLS generally begins soon after treatment cessation. Perform a thorough clinical evaluation prior to treatment initiation; exclude patients with significant cardiac, pulmonary, renal, hepatic, or central nervous system impairment from treatment. Patients with a more favorable performance status prior to treatment initiation are more likely to respond to aldesleukin treatment, with a higher response rate and generally lower toxicity.

[U.S. Boxed Warning]: Should be administered under the supervision of an experienced cancer chemotherapy physician in a facility with cardiopulmonary or intensive specialists and intensive care facilities available. Adverse effects are frequent and sometimes fatal. May exacerbate preexisting or initial presentation of autoimmune diseases and inflammatory disorders; exacerbation and/or new onset have been reported with aldesleukin and interferon alfa combination therapy. Thyroid disease (hypothyroidism, biphasic thyroiditis, and thyrotoxicosis) may occur; the onset of hypothyroidism is usually 4 to 17 weeks after treatment initiation; may be reversible upon treatment discontinuation (Hamnvik, 2011). Patients should be evaluated and treated for CNS metastases and have a negative scan prior to treatment; new neurologic symptoms and lesions have been reported in patients without preexisting evidence of CNS metastases (symptoms generally improve upon discontinuation, however, cases with permanent damage have been reported). Mental status changes (irritability, confusion, depression) can occur and may indicate bacteremia, sepsis, hypoperfusion, CNS malignancy, or CNS toxicity. May cause seizure; use with caution in patients with seizure disorder. Ethanol use may increase CNS adverse effects.

[U.S. Boxed Warning]: Impaired neutrophil function is associated with treatment; patients are at risk for disseminated infection (including sepsis and bacterial endocarditis), and central line-related gram-positive infections. Treat preexisting bacterial infection appropriately prior to treatment initiation. Antibiotic prophylaxis that has been associated with a reduced incidence of staphylococcal infections in aldesleukin studies includes the use of oxacillin, nafcillin, ciprofloxacin, or vancomycin. Monitor for signs of infection or sepsis during treatment.

[U.S. Boxed Warning]: Withhold treatment for patients developing moderate-to-severe lethargy or somnolence; continued treatment may result in coma. Standard prophylactic supportive care during high-dose aldesleukin treatment includes acetaminophen to relieve constitutional symptoms and an H_2 antagonist to reduce the risk of GI ulceration and/or bleeding. May impair renal or hepatic function; patients must have a serum creatinine ≤1.5 mg/dL prior to treatment. Concomitant nephrotoxic or hepatotoxic agents may increase the risk of renal or hepatic toxicity. Potentially significant drug-drug interactions may exist, requiring dose or frequency adjustment, additional monitoring, and/or selection of alternative therapy. Enhancement of cellular immune function may increase the risk of allograft rejection in transplant patients. An acute array of symptoms resembling aldesleukin adverse reactions (fever, chills, nausea, rash, pruritus, diarrhea, hypotension, edema, and oliguria) were observed within 1 to 4 hours after iodinated contrast media administration, usually when given within 4 weeks after aldesleukin treatment, although has been reported several months after aldesleukin treatment. The incidence of dyspnea and severe urogenital toxicities is potentially increased in elderly patients. Aldesleukin doses >12 to 15 million units/m^2 are associated with a moderate emetic potential; antiemetics are recommended to prevent nausea and vomiting (Dupuis, 2011).

Adverse Reactions

Cardiovascular: Arrhythmia, cardiac arrest, cardiovascular disorder (includes blood pressure and HF and ECG changes), edema, hypotension, MI, peripheral edema, supraventricular tachycardia, tachycardia, vasodilation, ventricular tachycardia

Central nervous system: Anxiety, chills, coma, confusion, dizziness, fever, malaise, pain, psychosis, somnolence, stupor

Dermatologic: Exfoliative dermatitis, pruritus, rash

Endocrine & metabolic: Acidosis, hypocalcemia, hypomagnesemia

Gastrointestinal: Abdomen enlarged, abdominal pain, anorexia, diarrhea, nausea, stomatitis, vomiting, weight gain

Hematologic: Anemia, coagulation disorder (includes intravascular coagulopathy), leukopenia, thrombocytopenia

Hepatic: Alkaline phosphatase increased, AST increased, hyperbilirubinemia

Neuromuscular & skeletal: Weakness

Renal: Acute renal failure, anuria, creatinine increased, oliguria

Respiratory: Apnea, cough, dyspnea; lung disorder (includes pulmonary congestion, rales, and rhonchi); respiratory disorder (includes acute respiratory distress syndrome, infiltrates and pulmonary changes); rhinitis

Miscellaneous: Antibody formation, infection, sepsis

Rare but important or life-threatening: Allergic interstitial nephritis, anaphylaxis, angioedema, asthma, atrial arrhythmia, AV block, blindness (transient or permanent), bowel infarction/necrosis/perforation, bradycardia, bullous pemphigoid, capillary leak syndrome, cardiomyopathy, cellulitis, cerebral edema, cerebral lesions, cerebral vasculitis, cholecystitis, colitis, crescentic IgA glomerulonephritis, Crohn's disease exacerbation, delirium, depression (severe; leading to suicide), diabetes mellitus, duodenal ulcer, encephalopathy, endocarditis, extrapyramidal syndrome, hemorrhage (including cerebral, gastrointestinal, retroperitoneal, subarachnoid, subdural), hepatic failure, hepatitis, hepatosplenomegaly, hypertension, hyperuricemia, hypothermia, hyperthyroidism, inflammatory arthritis, injection site necrosis, insomnia, intestinal obstruction, intestinal perforation, leukocytosis, malignant hyperthermia, meningitis, myocardial ischemia, myocarditis, myopathy, myositis, neuralgia, neuritis, neuropathy, neutropenia, NPN increased, oculobulbar myasthenia gravis, optic neuritis, organ perfusion decreased, pancreatitis, pericardial effusion, pericarditis, peripheral gangrene, phlebitis, pneumonia, pneumothorax, pulmonary edema, pulmonary embolus, respiratory acidosis, respiratory arrest, respiratory failure, rhabdomyolysis, scleroderma, seizure, Stevens-Johnson syndrome, stroke, syncope, thrombosis, thyroiditis, tracheoesophageal fistula, transient ischemic attack, tubular necrosis, ventricular extrasystoles

Drug Interactions

Metabolism/Transport Effects None known.

Avoid Concomitant Use

Avoid concomitant use of Aldesleukin with any of the following: BCG (Intravesical); CloZAPine; Corticosteroids; Dipyrone

Increased Effect/Toxicity

Aldesleukin may increase the levels/effects of: CloZAPine; DULoxetine; Hypotensive Agents; Iodinated Contrast Agents; Levodopa; RisperiDONE

The levels/effects of Aldesleukin may be increased by: Barbiturates; Dipyrone; Interferons (Alfa); Nicorandil

Decreased Effect

Aldesleukin may decrease the levels/effects of: BCG (Intravesical)

The levels/effects of Aldesleukin may be decreased by: Corticosteroids

Storage/Stability Store intact vials under refrigeration at 2°C to 8°C (36°F to 46°F). Protect from light. Plastic (polyvinyl chloride) bags result in more consistent drug delivery and are recommended. According to the manufacturer, reconstituted vials and solutions diluted for infusion are stable for 48 hours at room temperature or refrigerated although refrigeration is preferred because they do not contain preservatives. Do not freeze.

Mechanism of Action Aldesleukin is a human recombinant interleukin-2 product which promotes proliferation, differentiation, and recruitment of T and B cells, natural killer (NK) cells, and thymocytes; causes cytolytic activity in a subset of lymphocytes and subsequent interactions between the immune system and malignant cells; can stimulate lymphokine-activated killer (LAK) cells and tumor-infiltrating lymphocytes (TIL) cells.

Pharmacokinetics (Adult data unless noted)

Absorption: Oral: Not absorbed

Distribution: Primarily into plasma, lymphocytes, lungs, liver, kidney, and spleen

V_d: 6.3 to 7.9 L (Whittington 1993)

Metabolism: Renal (metabolized to amino acids in the cells lining the proximal convoluted tubules of the kidney)

Half-life:

Children:

Distribution: 14 ± 6 minutes

Elimination: 51 ± 11 minutes

Adults:

Distribution: 13 minutes

Elimination: 85 minutes

Elimination: Urine (primarily as metabolites)

Dosing: Usual

Pediatric: **Note:** Dosing and frequency may vary by indication, protocol, and/or treatment phase and hematologic response; refer to specific protocols. Consider premedication with an antipyretic to reduce fever, an H_2 antagonist for prophylaxis of gastrointestinal irritation/bleeding, antiemetics, and antidiarrheals; continue for 12 hours after the last aldesleukin dose. Antibiotic prophylaxis is recommended to reduce the incidence of infection. Aldesleukin doses >12 to 15 million units/m² are associated with a moderate emetic potential; antiemetics are recommended to prevent nausea and vomiting (Dupuis 2011):

Neuroblastoma: Limited data available: Children and Adolescents: IV: 3 million units/m²/day continuous infusion over 24 hours for 4 days during week 1 and 4.5 million units/m²/day continuous infusion over 24 hours for 4 days during week 2 of cycles 2 and 4 (regimen also includes isotretinoin, dinutuximab [an anti-GD2 antibody], and sargramostim) (Yu 2010).

Adult: **Note:** Consider premedication with an antipyretic to reduce fever, an H_2 antagonist for prophylaxis of gastrointestinal irritation/bleeding, antiemetics, and antidiarrheals; continue for 12 hours after the last aldesleukin dose. Antibiotic prophylaxis is recommended to reduce the incidence of infection. Aldesleukin doses >12 to 15 million units/m² are associated with a moderate emetic potential; antiemetics are recommended to prevent nausea and vomiting.

Metastatic renal cell carcinoma and metastatic melanoma: IV: Initial: 600,000 units/kg every 8 hours for a maximum of 14 doses; repeat after 9 days for a total of 28 doses per course; retreat if tumor shrinkage observed (and if no contraindications) at least 7 weeks after hospital discharge date

Dosing adjustment for toxicity: Withhold or interrupt a dose for toxicity; do not reduce the dose.

Cardiovascular toxicity:

Atrial fibrillation, supraventricular tachycardia, or bradycardia that is persistent, recurrent, or requires treatment: Withhold dose; may resume when asymptomatic with full recovery to normal sinus rhythm.

Systolic BP <90 mm Hg (with increasing pressor requirements): Withhold dose; may resume treatment when systolic BP ≥90 mm Hg and stable or pressor requirements improve.

Any ECG change consistent with MI, ischemia or myocarditis (with or without chest pain), or suspected cardiac ischemia: Withhold dose; may resume when asymptomatic, MI/myocarditis have been ruled out, suspicion of angina is low, or there is no evidence of ventricular hypokinesia.

CNS toxicity: Mental status change, including moderate confusion or agitation: Withhold dose; may resume when resolved completely.

Dermatologic toxicity: Bullous dermatitis or marked worsening of preexisting skin condition: Withhold dose; may treat with antihistamines or topical products (do not use topical steroids); may resume with resolution of all signs of bullous dermatitis.

Gastrointestinal: Stool guaiac repeatedly >3 to 4+: Withhold dose; may resume with negative stool guaiac.

Infection: Sepsis syndrome, clinically unstable: Withhold dose; may resume when sepsis syndrome has resolved, patient is clinically stable, and infection is under treatment.

Respiratory toxicity: Oxygen saturation <90%: Withhold dose; may resume when >90%.

Retreatment with aldesleukin is contraindicated with the following toxicities: Sustained ventricular tachycardia (≥5 beats), uncontrolled or unresponsive cardiac arrhythmias, chest pain with ECG changes consistent with angina or MI, cardiac tamponade, intubation >72 hours, renal failure requiring dialysis for >72 hours, coma or toxic psychosis lasting >48 hours, repetitive or refractory seizures, bowel ischemia/perforation, or GI bleeding requiring surgery

Dosing adjustment in renal impairment: Adults:

Preexisting renal impairment (prior to treatment initiation):

Serum creatinine ≤1.5 mg/dL: There are no dosage adjustments provided in the manufacturer's labeling.

Serum creatinine >1.5 mg/dL: Do not initiate treatment.

Renal toxicity during treatment:

Serum creatinine >4.5 mg/dL (or ≥4 mg/dL with severe volume overload, acidosis, or hyperkalemia): Withhold dose; may resume when <4 mg/dL and fluid/electrolyte status is stable.

Persistent oliguria or urine output <10 mL/hour for 16 to 24 hours with rising serum creatinine: Withhold dose; may resume when urine output >10 mL/hour with serum creatinine decrease of >1.5 mg/dL or normalization.

Hemodialysis: Retreatment is contraindicated in patients with renal failure requiring dialysis for >72 hours.

Dosing adjustment in hepatic impairment: Adults:

Hepatic impairment prior to treatment initiation: There are no dosage adjustments provided in the manufacturer's labeling.

Hepatotoxicity during treatment: Signs of hepatic failure (encephalopathy, increasing ascites, liver pain, hypoglycemia): Withhold dose and discontinue treatment for balance of cycle; may initiate a new course if indicated only after at least 7 weeks past resolution of all signs of hepatic failure (including hospital discharge).

Preparation for Administration Reconstitute vials with 1.2 mL SWFI (preservative free) to a concentration of 18 million [18 x 10^6 units (1.1 mg)]/1 mL; sterile water should be injected towards the side of the vial. Gently swirl; do not shake. Further dilute dosage in D_5W to a final concentration between 0.49 to 1.1 million units/mL (30 to 70 mcg/mL); final dilutions <0.49 million units/mL (30 mcg/mL) or >1.1 million units/mL (70 mcg/mL) have shown increased variability in drug stability and bioactivity and should be avoided; addition of 0.1% albumin has been used to increase stability and decrease the extent of sorption if low final concentrations cannot be avoided. Plastic (polyvinyl chloride) bags result in more consistent drug delivery and are recommended. Filtration may result in loss of bioactivity. Avoid bacteriostatic water for injection and NS for reconstitution or dilution; increased aggregation may occur.

For continuous IV infusion, dilute in D_5W maintaining the same final concentration.

Administration

Parenteral: Aldesleukin doses >12 to 15 million units/m^2 are associated with a moderate emetic potential; antiemetics are recommended to prevent nausea and vomiting (Dupuis 2011)

IV: Allow solution to reach room temperature prior to administration; infuse over 15 minutes; flush line before and after with D_5W, particularly if maintenance IV line contains sodium chloride. Some protocols infuse as a continuous infusion (Legha 1998; Yu 2010).

Monitoring Parameters Baseline and periodic: CBC with differential and platelets, blood chemistries including electrolytes, renal and hepatic function tests, and chest x-ray; pulmonary function tests and arterial blood gases (baseline), thallium stress test (prior to treatment). Monitor thyroid function tests (TSH at baseline then every 2 to 3 months during aldesleukin treatment [Hamnvik 2011]).

Monitoring during therapy should include daily (hourly if hypotensive) vital signs (temperature, pulse, blood pressure, and respiration rate), weight and fluid intake and output; in a patient with a decreased blood pressure, especially systolic BP <90 mm Hg, cardiac monitoring for rhythm should be conducted. If an abnormal complex or rhythm is seen, an ECG should be performed; vital signs in these hypotension patients should be taken hourly and central venous pressure (CVP) checked; monitor for change in mental status, and for signs of infection.

Additional Information 18 x 10^6 int. units = 1.1 mg protein

Dosage Forms Excipient information presented when available (limited, particularly for generics); consult specific product labeling.

Solution Reconstituted, Intravenous [preservative free]:
Proleukin: 22,000,000 units (1 ea)

- **Aldex AN [OTC]** *see* Doxylamine *on page 721*
- **Aldomet** *see* Methyldopa *on page 1399*
- **Aldurazyme** *see* Laronidase *on page 1222*
- **Aldurazyme® (Can)** *see* Laronidase *on page 1222*
- **Aler-Dryl [OTC]** *see* DiphenhydrAMINE (Systemic) *on page 668*
- **Alertec (Can)** *see* Modafinil *on page 1450*
- **Alevazol [OTC]** *see* Clotrimazole (Topical) *on page 518*
- **Aleve [OTC]** *see* Naproxen *on page 1489*
- **Aleve (Can)** *see* Naproxen *on page 1489*
- **Aleveer [OTC] [DSC]** *see* Capsaicin *on page 362*
- **Alfenta** *see* Alfentanil *on page 92*

Alfentanil (al FEN ta nil)

Medication Safety Issues

Sound-alike/look-alike issues:

Alfentanil may be confused with Anafranil, fentanyl, remifentanil, sufentanil

Alfenta may be confused with Sufenta

High alert medication:

The Institute for Safe Medication Practices (ISMP) includes this medication among its list of drug classes which have a heightened risk of causing significant patient harm when used in error.

Related Information

Opioid Conversion Table *on page 2285*

Brand Names: US Alfenta

Brand Names: Canada Alfenta; Alfentanil Injection, USP

Therapeutic Category Analgesic, Narcotic; General Anesthetic

Generic Availability (US) Yes

Use Analgesia; analgesia adjunct; anesthetic agent

Pregnancy Risk Factor C

Pregnancy Considerations Adverse events were observed in some animal reproduction studies. Alfentanil is known to cross the placenta, which may result in severe respiratory depression in the newborn (Mattingly, 2003). When used for pain relief during labor, opioids may temporarily affect the heart rate of the fetus (ACOG, 2002). Use during labor and delivery is not recommended by the manufacturer.

Breast-Feeding Considerations Alfentanil is excreted into breast milk. Significant concentrations were observed in breast milk following administration of alfentanil 60 mcg/kg to nine women who underwent postpartum tubal ligation; concentrations were undetectable after 28 hours. The manufacturer recommends that caution be used if administered to nursing women. Parenteral opioids used during labor have the potential to interfere with a newborn's natural reflex to nurse within the first few hours after birth. Nursing infants exposed to large doses of opioids should be monitored for apnea and sedation (Montgomery, 2012).

Contraindications Hypersensitivity to alfentanil or any component of the formulation or known intolerance to other opioid agonists

Warnings/Precautions Due to the high incidence of apnea, hypotension, tachycardia and muscle rigidity; alfentanil should be administered by individuals specifically trained in the use of anesthetic agents and should not be used in diagnostic or therapeutic procedures outside the monitored anesthesia setting; opioid antagonist, resuscitative and intubation equipment should be readily available. May cause hypotension; use with caution in patients with hypovolemia, cardiovascular disease (including acute MI), or drugs which may exaggerate hypotensive effects (including phenothiazines or general anesthetics). Shares the toxic potentials of opioid agonists, and precautions of opioid agonist therapy should be observed. Bradycardia has been observed in patients receiving alfentanil; use with caution when administering to patients with bradyarrhythmias. Degree of bradycardia may be more pronounced when administered with non-vagolytic skeletal muscle relaxants (eg, vecuronium, cisatracurium) or when anticholinergic agents (eg, atropine) are not used. Use with caution in patients with renal and/or hepatic impairment; duration of action may be prolonged.

Use with caution in patients with a history of drug abuse or acute alcoholism; potential for drug dependency exists. Tolerance, psychological and physical dependence may occur with prolonged use. Use with extreme caution in patients with head injury, intracranial lesions, or elevated intracranial pressure; exaggerated elevation of ICP may occur. Use with caution in patients who are morbidly obese, patients with pre-existing respiratory compromise (hypoxia and/or hypercapnia), COPD or other obstructive pulmonary disease, and kyphoscoliosis or other skeletal disorder which may alter respiratory function. Skeletal muscle rigidity is related to the dose and speed of administration. Inject slowly over 3 minutes; rapid IV infusion may result in skeletal muscle and chest wall rigidity, impaired ventilation, or respiratory distress/arrest. Initial doses up to 20 mcg/kg may cause skeletal muscle rigidity. Doses >130 mcg/kg will consistently cause muscle rigidity with an immediate onset; consider the concomitant use of a nondepolarizing skeletal muscle relaxant to decrease the incidence. Appropriately reduce the initial dose in elderly and debilitated patients; consider the effect of the initial dose in determining supplemental doses. Plasma clearance of alfentanil may be reduced and postoperative recovery may be prolonged.

Adverse Reactions

Cardiovascular: Bradycardia, cardiac arrhythmia, orthostatic hypotension, peripheral vasodilation

Central nervous system: CNS depression, confusion, drowsiness, intracranial pressure increased, sedation

Endocrine & metabolic: Antidiuretic hormone release
Gastrointestinal: Constipation, nausea, vomiting
Ocular: Blurred vision
Rare but important or life-threatening: Convulsions, mental depression, paradoxical CNS excitation or delirium, dizziness, dysesthesia, rash, urticaria, itching, biliary tract spasm, urinary tract spasm, respiratory depression, bronchospasm, laryngospasm, physical and psychological dependence with prolonged use; cold, clammy skin

Drug Interactions

Metabolism/Transport Effects **Substrate** of CYP3A4 (major); **Note:** Assignment of Major/Minor substrate status based on clinically relevant drug interaction potential

Avoid Concomitant Use

Avoid concomitant use of Alfentanil with any of the following: Azelastine (Nasal); Conivaptan; Crizotinib; Eluxadoline; Enzalutamide; Fusidic Acid (Systemic); Idelalisib; MAO Inhibitors; Mixed Agonist / Antagonist Opioids; Orphenadrine; Paraldehyde; Thalidomide

Increased Effect/Toxicity

Alfentanil may increase the levels/effects of: Alcohol (Ethyl); Alvimopan; Azelastine (Nasal); Beta-Blockers; Calcium Channel Blockers (Nondihydropyridine); CNS Depressants; Desmopressin; Diuretics; Eluxadoline; Hydrocodone; MAO Inhibitors; Methotrimeprazine; Metyrosine; Mirtazapine; Orphenadrine; Paraldehyde; Pramipexole; Propofol; ROPINIRole; Rotigotine; Selective Serotonin Reuptake Inhibitors; Suvorexant; Thalidomide; Zolpidem

The levels/effects of Alfentanil may be increased by: Amphetamines; Anticholinergic Agents; Antipsychotic Agents (Phenothiazines); Aprepitant; Brimonidine (Topical); Cannabis; Cimetidine; Conivaptan; Crizotinib; CYP3A4 Inhibitors (Moderate); CYP3A4 Inhibitors (Strong); Dasatinib; Diazepam; Diltiazem; Doxylamine; Dronabinol; Droperidol; Fluconazole; Fosaprepitant; Fusidic Acid (Systemic); HydrOXYzine; Idelalisib; Ivacaftor; Kava Kava; Luliconazole; Macrolide Antibiotics; Magnesium Sulfate; Methotrimeprazine; Mifepristone; Nabilone; Netupitant; Palbociclib; Perampanel; Rufinamide; Simeprevir; Sodium Oxybate; Stiripentol; Succinylcholine; Tapentadol; Tetrahydrocannabinol

Decreased Effect

Alfentanil may decrease the levels/effects of: Pegvisomant

The levels/effects of Alfentanil may be decreased by: Ammonium Chloride; Enzalutamide; Mixed Agonist / Antagonist Opioids; Naltrexone; Rifamycin Derivatives

Storage/Stability Undiluted injectable: Store at 20°C to 25°C (68°F to 77°F). Protect from light.

Mechanism of Action Binds with stereospecific receptors at many sites within the CNS, increases pain threshold, alters pain perception, inhibits ascending pain pathways; is an ultra short-acting opioid

Pharmacodynamics
Onset of action: Within 5 minutes
Duration: <15-20 minutes

Pharmacokinetics (Adult data unless noted) An early study of continuous infusion suggested nonlinear pharmacokinetics in neonates (Wiest, 1991).
Distribution: V_d beta:
Newborns, premature: 1 L/kg
Children: 0.163-0.48 L/kg
Adults: 0.46 L/kg
Protein binding:
Neonates: 67%
Adults: 88% to 92%
Bound to $alpha_1$-acid glycoprotein
Metabolism: Hepatic
Half-life, elimination:
Newborns, premature: 320-525 minutes
Children: 40-60 minutes
Adults: 83-97 minutes

Dosing: Neonatal IV: Doses should be titrated to appropriate effects; wide range of doses is dependent upon desired degree of analgesia/anesthesia

Dose not established; reported range: 9-20 mcg/kg/dose; a high percentage of neonates (GA: 30-40 weeks; PNA <3 days) receiving alfentanil (prior to procedures) at doses of 9-15 mcg/kg (mean dose: 11.7 mcg/kg) developed chest wall rigidity; 9 out of 20 (45%) developed mild or moderate rigidity that did not affect ventilation, while 4 out of 20 (20%) had severe rigidity interfering with respiration for ~5-10 minutes (Pokela, 1992). In a separate study, severe muscle rigidity developed in 5 out of 8 (63%) neonates (GA: 29-36 weeks; PNA 2-6 days) following a dose of 20 mcg/kg (Saarenmaa, 1996); use of a skeletal muscle relaxant to prevent chest wall rigidity is recommended; however, smaller alfentanil doses may be required in newborns.

Dosing: Usual IV: Doses should be titrated to appropriate effects; wide range of doses is dependent upon desired degree of analgesia/anesthesia
Children:
Pre-induction, emergence agitation prevention, analgesia in tonsillectomy, or dental procedure patients undergoing general anesthesia: 10-20 mcg/kg/dose (Annila, 1999; Bartolek, 2007; Kim, 2009; Kwak, 2010; Ng, 1999; Rahman Al-Refai, 2007)
Procedural analgesia for LP or bone marrow aspiration (in addition to propofol): Intermittent doses of 2-3 mcg/kg/dose (total dose: mean: 1.4 mcg/kg ± 2.4; range: 1.8-9.6 mcg/kg) were administered to 20 patients ages 2-16 years old (von Heijne, 2004)
Adults: Use lean body weight for patients who weigh >20% over ideal body weight; see table.

Alfentanil: Adult Dosing

Indication	Approximate Duration of Anesthesia (minute)	Induction Period (Initial Dose) (mcg/kg)	Maintenance Period (Increments/ Infusion)	Total Dose (mcg/kg)	Effects
Incremental injection	≤30	8-20	3-5 mcg/kg or 0.5-1 mcg/kg/minute	8-40	Spontaneously breathing or assisted ventilation when required.
	30-60	20-50	5-15 mcg/kg	Up to 75	Assisted or controlled ventilation required. Attenuation of response to laryngoscopy and intubation.
Continuous infusion	>45	50-75	0.5-3 mcg/kg/minute; average infusion rate: 1-1.5 mcg/kg/minute	Dependent on duration of procedure	Assisted or controlled ventilation required. Some attenuation of response to intubation and incision, with intraoperative stability.
Anesthetic induction	>45	130-245	0.5-1.5 mcg/kg/minute or general anesthetic	Dependent on duration of procedure	Assisted or controlled ventilation required. Administer slowly (over 3 minutes). Concentration of inhalation agents reduced by 30% to 50% for initial hour.

Preparation for Administration Parenteral:
IV: Dilute prior to administration with NS, D_5W, D_5NS or LR to a concentration of 25 to 80 mcg/mL
Continuous IV infusion: Further dilute in D_5W, NS D_5NS or LR to a concentration of 40 mcg/mL

Administration Parenteral: IV: Inject slowly over 3 to 5 minutes or by continuous IV infusion

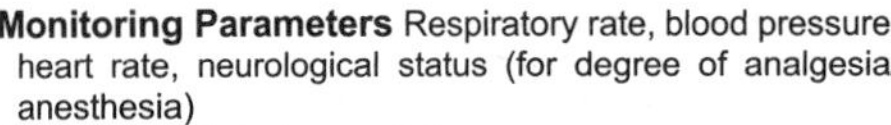

Monitoring Parameters Respiratory rate, blood pressure, heart rate, neurological status (for degree of analgesia/ anesthesia)

Controlled Substance C-II

Dosage Forms Excipient information presented when available (limited, particularly for generics); consult specific product labeling.

Injectable, Injection [preservative free]:
Alfenta: 500 mcg/mL (2 mL, 5 mL)
Generic: 500 mcg/mL (2 mL, 5 mL)

◆ **Alfentanil Hydrochloride** *see* Alfentanil *on page 92*

◆ **Alfentanil Injection, USP (Can)** *see* Alfentanil *on page 92*

◆ **Alglucosidase** *see* Alglucosidase Alfa *on page 94*

Alglucosidase Alfa (al gloo KOSE i dase AL fa)

Medication Safety Issues

Sound-alike/look-alike issues:

Alglucosidase alfa may be confused with agalsidase alfa, agalsidase beta, alglucerase

Brand Names: US Lumizyme; Myozyme

Brand Names: Canada Myozyme

Therapeutic Category Enzyme

Generic Availability (US) No

Use

Myozyme: Replacement therapy of alpha-glucosidase (GAA) for infantile-onset Pompe disease [FDA approved in pediatric patients (age not specified)]

Lumizyme: Replacement therapy of alpha-glucosidase (GAA) for Pompe disease (FDA approved in pediatrics patients [age not specified] and adults)

Prescribing and Access Restrictions Access to Myozyme is restricted by the manufacturer and allowed only to patients with infantile-onset Pompe disease. To obtain Myozyme, call 1-800-745-4447; no formal distribution program is established, but availability is controlled by Genzyme.

Pregnancy Risk Factor C

Pregnancy Considerations Adverse events were observed in some animal reproduction studies. Limited information is available related to use of alglucosidase alfa in pregnant women (deVries 2011).

A registry has been established for Pompe patients; women of childbearing potential are encouraged to enroll in the registry (www.pomperegistry.com or 1-800-745-4447).

Breast-Feeding Considerations Endogenous acid alfa-glucosidase can be detected in breast milk; concentrations are lower in women with Pompe disease. Following an infusion of alglucosidase alfa in one woman with Pompe disease, maximum enzyme activity was found in breast milk 2.5 hours after the dose and was ~0.3% of the maternal peak plasma value. Activity in breast milk returned to baseline values within 24 hours after the infusion (de Vries, 2011). The manufacturer recommends that caution be used if administered to breast-feeding women; exposure may be minimized by temporarily pumping and discarding breast milk for 24 hours after administration.

A registry has been established for Pompe patients; women who are breast-feeding are encouraged to enroll in the registry (www.pomperegistry.com or 1-800-745-4447)

Contraindications There are no contraindications listed in the manufacturer's labeling.

Warnings/Precautions **[U.S. Boxed Warning]: Life-threatening anaphylactic reactions and severe hypersensitivity reactions, some of which were IgE mediated, may occur. Severe immune-mediated reactions (eg, necrotizing skin lesions, nephrotic syndrome secondary to membranous glomerulonephritis, proteinuria, inflammatory arthropathy) may occur. Immediate medical support should be readily available.** Anaphylactic and severe hypersensitivity reactions may occur during and up to 3 hours after infusion. Patients who develop IgE antibodies to alglucosidase alfa may be at a higher risk; monitor these patients closely during administration. Immune-mediated reactions have occurred up to 3 years after initiation of therapy. Monitor urinalysis periodically. Monitor for immune-mediated reaction development. Consider testing for IgG titers in patients who develop allergic or immune-mediated reactions; may also test for IgE antibodies or other mediators of anaphylaxis. Consider risks/benefits of readministration following an anaphylactic or severe allergic reaction or an immune-mediated reaction; some patients have been successfully rechallenged under close clinical supervision; appropriate resuscitation measures should be available. Infusion-related reactions are common and may occur during and up to 2 hours after infusion; discontinue immediately for severe hypersensitivity or anaphylactic reaction; mild to moderate reactions may be managed by reducing the infusion rate and/or administering antihistamines and/or antipyretics. Appropriate medical support for the management of infusion reactions should be readily available. Use caution with subsequent infusions; infusion reactions have occurred despite premedication with antihistamines, antipyretics, and/or corticosteroids. Patients with acute underlying illness are at greater risk for infusion reactions, including cardiorespiratory failure; monitor closely during infusion. Although less common, delayed-onset (within 48 hours after administration) infusion reactions have also occurred. The presence of IgG antibodies has been observed within 3 months from the onset of therapy in the majority of patients. High and sustained IgG antibody titers may result in reduced efficacy of alglucosidase alfa (eg, loss of motor function, ventilator dependence, death). Regularly monitor all patients for development of IgG antibodies; consider testing for IgG titers in patients who develop hypersensitivity reactions, other immune-mediated reactions, or loss of clinical response. Patients with reduced clinical response may also be tested for inhibitory antibody activity.

[U.S. Boxed Warning]: Use caution in patients with compromised cardiac or respiratory function; risk of acute cardiorespiratory failure secondary to infusion-related reactions or fluid overload may be increased. Additional monitoring is warranted in this patient population. Cardiorespiratory failure has been observed in patients with cardiac hypertrophy up to 72 hours after infusion; arrhythmias have also been observed in patients with cardiac hypertrophy. Patients with sepsis may be at increased risk for cardiorespiratory failure during infusions. Some dosage forms may contain polysorbate 80 (also known as Tweens). Hypersensitivity reactions, usually a delayed reaction, have been reported following exposure to pharmaceutical products containing polysorbate 80 in certain individuals (Isaksson, 2002; Lucente 2000; Shelley 1995). Thrombocytopenia, ascites, pulmonary deterioration, and renal and hepatic failure have been reported in premature neonates after receiving parenteral products containing polysorbate 80 (Alade, 1986; CDC, 1984). See manufacturer's labeling. Use of general anesthesia for catheter placement for alglucosidase alfa infusions may be complicated by the presence of cardiac and skeletal (including respiratory) muscle weakness in patients with Pompe disease; use general anesthesia with caution. Monitor for development. A registry has been created to monitor therapeutic responses and adverse effects during long-term treatment; patients should be encouraged to register (www.pomperegistry.com or 1-800-745-4447).

Adverse Reactions

Cardiovascular: Bradycardia (infants and children), chest discomfort, chest pain, flushing, hypertension (infants and children), increased blood pressure, oxygen saturation decreased (infants and children), peripheral edema, tachycardia (infants and children)

Central nervous system: Agitation (infants and children), dizziness, drowsiness, fatigue, headache, malaise, pain, pain (postprocedural; more common in infants and children), paresthesia, rigors (infants and children), vertigo

Dermatologic: Diaper rash (infants and children), erythema (infants and children), hyperhidrosis, pallor (infants and children), papular rash, pruritus, skin rash (more common in infants and children), urticaria

Endocrine & metabolic: Hypokalemia

Gastrointestinal: Constipation (more common in infants and children), diarrhea (more common in infants and children), dyspepsia, gastroenteritis (more common in infants and children), gastroesophageal reflux disease (infants and children), nausea, oral candidiasis (infants and children), upper abdominal pain (children and adolescents), vomiting (more common in infants and children)

Hematologic & oncologic: Anemia (infants and children), lymphadenopathy

Hypersensitivity: Anaphylaxis, hypersensitivity reaction (infants and children)

Immunologic: Development of IgG antibodies (more common in adults; may affect efficacy)

Local: Catheter infection (infants and children), infusion site reaction, local swelling

Neuromuscular & skeletal: Muscle twitching, musculoskeletal pain, myalgia, stiffness, tremor

Ophthalmic: Blurred vision

Otic: Auditory impairment, otalgia, otitis media (infants and children)

Renal: Nephrolithiasis

Respiratory: Bronchiolitis (infants and children), cough (infants and children), cyanosis, dyspnea, epistaxis, nasopharyngitis (infants and children), pharyngeal edema, pharyngitis (more common in infants and children), pneumonia (infants and children), respiratory distress (infants and children), respiratory failure (infants and children), respiratory syncytial virus infection (infants and children), respiratory tract infection, rhinitis (children and adolescents), rhinorrhea (infants and children), tachypnea (infants and children), upper respiratory tract infection (more common in infants and children)

Miscellaneous: Fever (infants and children), infusion related reaction (infants and children)

Rare but important or life-threatening: Acute cardiorespiratory failure, aortic dissection, apnea, bronchospasm, cerebrovascular accident, convulsions, coronary artery disease, dehydration, flu-like symptoms, hemothorax, herniated disk, hyperparathyroidism, hypersensitivity, hypervolemia, livedo reticularis, muscle spasm, nephrotic syndrome (secondary to membranous glomerulonephritis), nodal arrhythmia, periorbital edema, pneumothorax, pulmonary infection, sepsis, skin necrosis, ventricular premature contractions

Drug Interactions

Metabolism/Transport Effects None known.

Avoid Concomitant Use There are no known interactions where it is recommended to avoid concomitant use.

Increased Effect/Toxicity There are no known significant interactions involving an increase in effect.

Decreased Effect There are no known significant interactions involving a decrease in effect.

Storage/Stability Store intact vials between 2°C and 8°C (36°F and 46°F). Final solutions for infusion should be used immediately if possible but may be stored for up to 24 hours between 2°C and 8°C (36°F and 46°F); do not freeze. Protect from light.

Mechanism of Action Alglucosidase alfa is a recombinant form of the enzyme acid alpha-glucosidase (GAA), which is required for glycogen cleavage. Due to an inherited GAA deficiency or absence, glycogen accumulates in the tissues of patients with Pompe disease, leading to progressive muscle weakness. In infantile-onset Pompe disease, glycogen accumulates in cardiac and skeletal muscles and hepatic tissue, leading to cardiomyopathy and respiratory failure. Juvenile- and adult-onset Pompe disease are limited to glycogen accumulation in skeletal muscle, leading to respiratory failure. Alglucosidase alfa binds to mannose-6-phosphate receptors on the cell surface, is internalized, and transported to lysosomes where it is activated for increased enzymatic glycogen cleavage.

Pharmacokinetics (Adult data unless noted)

Distribution: V_{ss}: Infants 1 to 7 months: 96 ± 16 mL/kg

Half-life elimination: Infants 1 to 7 months: 2.3 hours; Adults: 2.4 hours

Dosing: Usual

Pediatric:

Infantile-onset Pompe disease: Infants ≥1 month, Children, and Adolescents: Lumizyme, Myozyme: IV: 20 mg/kg every 2 weeks

Late-onset (noninfantile) Pompe disease: Infants ≥1 month, Children, and Adolescents: Lumizyme: IV: 20 mg/kg every 2 weeks

Adult: **Late-onset (noninfantile) Pompe disease:** Lumizyme: IV: 20 mg/kg every 2 weeks

Dosing adjustment in renal impairment: There are no dosage adjustments provided in the manufacturer's labeling.

Dosing adjustment in hepatic impairment: There are no dosage adjustments provided in the manufacturer's labeling.

Preparation for Administration Visually inspect the powder in the vial for particulate matter prior to reconstitution. After vial reaches room temperature, reconstitute each vial with 10.3 mL SWFI. Inject slowly down internal side wall of vial (do not inject into powder; avoid foaming). Roll and tilt gently; do not invert, swirl, or shake. Resulting solution contains 5 mg/mL. To make final infusion, add the desired amount of reconstituted solution (based on patient weight) to 50 to 1,000 mL NS (do not use filter needle to prepare) to a final concentration of 0.5 to 4 mg/mL. Remove airspace from infusion bag prior to admixture to minimize particle formation due to sensitivity of drug to air-liquid interfaces. Do not shake. Protect from light.

Administration Infuse through a low protein-binding, 0.2 micron in-line filter. Do not administer products with visualized particulate matter. Infuse over ~4 hours; initiate at 1 mg/kg/hour. If tolerated, increase by 2 mg/kg/hour every 30 minutes to a maximum rate of 7 mg/kg/hour. Decrease rate or temporarily hold for infusion reactions. Monitor vital signs prior to each rate increase. Protect from light.

Monitoring Parameters Liver enzymes (baseline and periodically; elevation may be due to disease process); vital signs during and following infusion; immune mediated reactions; volume overload; periodic urinalysis

The manufacturer recommends monitoring for IgG antibody formation every 3 months for 2 years, then annually. Consider testing if patient develops allergic or other suspected immune mediated reaction. No commercial tests are available; however, sampling kits can be obtained by contacting Genzyme Corporation at 1-800-745-4447.

Additional Information Patients with sustained positive IgG antibody titers (≥12,800) to alglucosidase alfa may have poorer clinical response. Most patients (89%) develop antibodies within the first 3 months of therapy; concern is with patients with sustained high (≥12,800) antibody titers. Patients developing a decreased motor function should be tested for neutralization of enzyme uptake or activity. Infusion reactions are more common in antibody-positive patients. Patients with moderate-to-severe or recurrent reactions with suspected mast-cell activation may be tested for alglucosidase alfa-specific IgE antibodies.

Dosage Forms Excipient information presented when available (limited, particularly for generics); consult specific product labeling.

Solution Reconstituted, Intravenous [preservative free]:
Lumizyme: 50 mg (1 ea) [contains polysorbate 80]
Myozyme: 50 mg (1 ea)

- **Alinia** *see* Nitazoxanide *on page 1519*
- **Alkeran** *see* Melphalan *on page 1348*
- **All Day Allergy [OTC]** *see* Cetirizine *on page 423*
- **All Day Allergy Childrens [OTC]** *see* Cetirizine *on page 423*
- **All Day Pain Relief [OTC]** *see* Naproxen *on page 1489*
- **All Day Relief [OTC]** *see* Naproxen *on page 1489*
- **Allegra 12 Hour (OTC) (Can)** *see* Fexofenadine *on page 874*
- **Allegra 24 Hour (OTC) (Can)** *see* Fexofenadine *on page 874*
- **Allegra Allergy [OTC]** *see* Fexofenadine *on page 874*
- **Allegra Allergy Childrens [OTC]** *see* Fexofenadine *on page 874*
- **Aller-Chlor [OTC]** *see* Chlorpheniramine *on page 441*
- **Allerdryl (Can)** *see* DiphenhydrAMINE (Systemic) *on page 668*
- **Allergy [OTC]** *see* Chlorpheniramine *on page 441*
- **Allergy [OTC]** *see* Loratadine *on page 1296*
- **Allergy 4 Hour [OTC] [DSC]** *see* Chlorpheniramine *on page 441*
- **Allergy Relief [OTC]** *see* Chlorpheniramine *on page 441*
- **Allergy Relief [OTC]** *see* DiphenhydrAMINE (Systemic) *on page 668*
- **Allergy Relief [OTC]** *see* Loratadine *on page 1296*
- **Allergy Relief Childrens [OTC]** *see* DiphenhydrAMINE (Systemic) *on page 668*
- **Allergy Relief For Kids [OTC]** *see* Loratadine *on page 1296*
- **Allergy-Time [OTC]** *see* Chlorpheniramine *on page 441*
- **Allerject (Can)** *see* EPINEPHrine (Systemic, Oral Inhalation) *on page 760*
- **Allernix (Can)** *see* DiphenhydrAMINE (Systemic) *on page 668*
- **Aller-Relief [OTC] (Can)** *see* Cetirizine *on page 423*
- **Allfen CD** *see* Guaifenesin and Codeine *on page 990*
- **Allfen CDX** *see* Guaifenesin and Codeine *on page 990*
- **Alloprin (Can)** *see* Allopurinol *on page 96*

Allopurinol (al oh PURE i nole)

Medication Safety Issues

Sound-alike/look-alike issues:

Allopurinol may be confused with Apresoline

Zyloprim may be confused with zolpidem, ZORprin, Zovirax

Related Information

Tumor Lysis Syndrome *on page 2371*

Brand Names: US Aloprim; Zyloprim

Brand Names: Canada Alloprin; Apo-Allopurinol; JAMP-Allopurinol; Mar-Allopurinol; Novo-Purol; Zyloprim

Therapeutic Category Antigout Agent; Uric Acid Lowering Agent

Generic Availability (US) May be product dependent

Use

Oral: Management of hyperuricemia associated with cancer treatment for leukemia, lymphoma, or solid tumor malignancies (FDA approved in pediatric patients [age not specified] and adults); management of primary or secondary gout (acute attack, tophi, joint destruction, uric acid lithiasis, and/or nephropathy) (FDA approved in adults); management of recurrent calcium oxalate calculi (with uric acid excretion >800 mg/day in men and >750 mg/day in women) (FDA approved in adults); has also been used for treatment of hyperuricemia associated with inborn errors of purine metabolism (Lesch-Nyhan syndrome) and recurrent calcium oxalate calculi associated with glycogen storage disease

IV: Management of hyperuricemia associated with cancer treatment for leukemia, lymphoma, or solid tumor malignancies who cannot tolerate oral therapy (FDA approved in children and adults)

Pregnancy Risk Factor C

Pregnancy Considerations Adverse events were observed in some animal reproduction studies. Allopurinol crosses the placenta (Torrance, 2009). An increased risk of adverse fetal events has not been observed (limited data) (Hoeltzenbein, 2013).

Breast-Feeding Considerations Allopurinol and its metabolite are excreted into breast milk; the metabolite was also detected in the serum of the nursing infant (Kamilli, 1993). The U.S. manufacturer recommends caution be used when administering allopurinol to nursing women. The Canadian labeling contraindicates use in nursing women except those with hyperuricemia secondary to malignancy.

Contraindications

Severe hypersensitivity reaction to allopurinol or any component of the formulation

Canadian labeling: Additional contraindications (not in U.S. labeling): Nursing mothers and children (except those with hyperuricemia secondary to malignancy or Lesch-Nyhan syndrome)

Warnings/Precautions Do not use to treat asymptomatic hyperuricemia. Has been associated with a number of hypersensitivity reactions, including severe reactions (vasculitis and Stevens-Johnson syndrome); discontinue at first sign of rash. Consider HLA-B*5801 testing in patients at a higher risk for allopurinol hypersensitivity syndrome (eg, Koreans with stage 3 or worse CKD and Han Chinese and Thai descent regardless of renal function) prior to initiation of therapy (ACR guidelines [Khanna, 2012]). Reversible hepatotoxicity has been reported; use with caution in patients with preexisting hepatic impairment. Bone marrow suppression has been reported; use caution with other drugs causing myelosuppression. Caution in renal impairment, dosage adjustments needed. Full effect on serum uric acid levels in chronic gout may take several weeks to become evident; gradual titration is recommended. Potentially significant drug-drug interactions may exist, requiring dose or frequency adjustment, additional monitoring, and/or selection of alternative therapy.

Adverse Reactions

Dermatologic: Skin rash

Endocrine & metabolic: Gout (acute)

Gastrointestinal: Diarrhea, nausea

Hepatic: Increased liver enzymes, increased serum alkaline phosphatase

Rare but important or life-threatening: Ageusia, agranulocytosis, alopecia, angioedema, aplastic anemia, cataract, cholestatic jaundice, ecchymoses, eczematoid dermatitis, eosinophilia, exfoliative dermatitis, hepatic necrosis, hepatitis, hepatomegaly, hepatotoxicity (idiosyncratic) (Chalasani, 2014), hyperbilirubinemia, hypersensitivity reaction, leukocytosis, leukopenia, lichen planus, macular retinitis, myopathy, necrotizing angiitis, nephritis, neuritis, neuropathy, onycholysis, pancreatitis, purpura, renal failure, skin granuloma (annulare), Stevens-Johnson syndrome, thrombocytopenia, toxic epidermal necrolysis, toxic pustuloderma, uremia, vasculitis, vesicobullous dermatitis

Drug Interactions

Metabolism/Transport Effects None known.

Avoid Concomitant Use

Avoid concomitant use of Allopurinol with any of the following: Didanosine; Pegloticase; Tegafur

Increased Effect/Toxicity

Allopurinol may increase the levels/effects of: Amoxicillin; Ampicillin; AzaTHIOprine; Bendamustine; CarBAMazepine; ChlorproPAMIDE; Cyclophosphamide; Didanosine; Mercaptopurine; Pegloticase; Theophylline Derivatives; Vitamin K Antagonists

The levels/effects of Allopurinol may be increased by: ACE Inhibitors; Loop Diuretics; Thiazide Diuretics

Decreased Effect

Allopurinol may decrease the levels/effects of: Tegafur

The levels/effects of Allopurinol may be decreased by: Antacids

Storage/Stability

Powder for injection: Store at controlled room temperature of 20°C to 25°C (68°F to 77°F). Following preparation, intravenous solutions should be stored at 20°C to 25°C (68°F to 77°F). Do not refrigerate reconstituted and/or diluted product. Must be administered within 10 hours of solution preparation.

Tablet: Store at controlled room temperature of 20°C to 25°C (68°F to 77°F). Protect from moisture and light.

Mechanism of Action Allopurinol inhibits xanthine oxidase, the enzyme responsible for the conversion of hypoxanthine to xanthine to uric acid. Allopurinol is metabolized to oxypurinol which is also an inhibitor of xanthine oxidase; allopurinol acts on purine catabolism, reducing the production of uric acid without disrupting the biosynthesis of vital purines.

Pharmacodynamics

Decrease in serum and urinary uric acid:

Gout: Onset of action: 2 to 3 days; maximum effect: ≥1 week

Hyperuricemia associated with chemotherapy: Maximum effect: 27 hours (Coiffier, 2008)

Pharmacokinetics (Adult data unless noted)

Absorption: Oral: ~90% from the GI tract

Distribution: V_{ss}: 0.87 L/kg

Protein binding: <1%

Metabolism: ~75% of drug metabolized to active metabolites, chiefly oxipurinol

Bioavailability: 53%

Half-life:

Allopurinol: 1 to 3 hours

Oxipurinol: ~15 hours

Time to peak serum concentration: Allopurinol: 1.54 hours; oxipurinol: 4.5 hours

Elimination: Urine (76% as oxypurinol; 12% unchanged drug); feces (20%)

Dosing: Usual

Pediatric: **Note:** Dosing presenting in multiple formats (mg/m²/dose, mg/m²/day, mg/kg/day, and a fixed mg dose); take extra precautions to ensure accuracy.

Hyperuricemia associated with chemotherapy management: Maintain adequate hydration; begin allopurinol 1 to 2 days before initiation of induction chemotherapy; may continue for 3 to 7 days after chemotherapy (Coiffier, 2008); daily doses >300 mg should be administered in divided doses:

Oral:

Manufacturer's labeling:

Children <6 years: 150 mg daily

Children 6 to 10 years: 300 mg daily

Children >10 years and Adolescents: 600 to 800 mg daily for 2 to 3 days in 2 to 3 divided doses

Alternate dosing: Tumor lysis syndrome; intermediate-risk: Limited data available (Coiffier, 2008): Infants, Children, and Adolescents:

Weight-directed dosing: 10 mg/kg/day divided every 8 hours; maximum daily dose: 800 mg/**day**

BSA-directed dosing: 50 to 100 mg/m²/**dose** every 8 hours; maximum daily dose: 300 mg/m²/**day**

IV: For patients unable to tolerate oral therapy (BSA-directed dosing):

Manufacturer's labeling: Children and Adolescents: Initial: 200 mg/m²/day administered once daily or in equally divided doses at 6-, 8-, or 12-hour intervals

Alternate dosing: Tumor lysis syndrome; intermediate-risk: Limited data available: Infants, Children, and Adolescents: 200 to 400 mg/m²/day in 1 to 3 divided doses; maximum daily dose: 600 mg/**day** (Coiffier, 2008)

Hyperuricemia associated with inborn errors of purine metabolism (Lesch-Nyhan syndrome): Oral: Infants, Children, and Adolescents: Initial: 5 to 10 mg/kg/day; adjust dose to maintain a high-normal serum uric acid concentration and a urinary uric acid/creatinine ratio <1; reported range: 3.7 to 9.7 mg/kg/day; usual maximum daily dose: 600 mg/**day** (Torres, 2007; Torres, 2007a).

Recurrent calcium oxalate renal stones (including glycogen storage disease): Limited data available: Oral: Children and Adolescents: 4 to 10 mg/kg/day in divided doses 3 to 4 times daily; maximum daily dose: 300 mg/**day** (Copelvitch, 2012; Santos-Victoriano, 1998)

Adult: **Note:** Oral doses >300 mg should be given in divided doses.

Gout (chronic): Oral: Initial: 100 mg once daily; increase at weekly intervals in increments of 100 mg/day as needed to achieve desired serum uric acid level. Usual dosage range: 200 to 300 mg/day in mild gout; 400 to 600 mg/day in moderate to severe tophaceous gout; maximum daily dose: 800 mg/day

Management of hyperuricemia associated with chemotherapy:

Oral: 600 to 800 mg daily in divided doses

IV: 200 to 400 mg/m²/day (maximum: 600 mg/day) beginning 1 to 2 days before chemotherapy

Note: Intravenous daily dose can be given as a single infusion or in equally divided doses at 6-, 8-, or 12-hour intervals. A fluid intake sufficient to yield a daily urinary output of at least 2 L in adults is desirable.

Recurrent calcium oxalate stones: Oral: 200 to 300 mg daily in single or divided doses; may adjust dose as needed to control hyperuricosuria

Dosing adjustment in renal impairment:

Infants, Children, and Adolescents: There are no dosage adjustments provided in the manufacturer's labeling; however, the following guidelines have been used by some clinicians:

Management of hyperuricemia associated with chemotherapy: Oral, IV:

Aronoff, 2007:

CrCl 30 to 50 mL/minute/1.73 m²: Administer 50% of normal dose

GFR 10 to 29 mL/minute/1.73 m²: Administer 50% of normal dose

GFR <10 mL/minute/1.73 m²: Administer 30% of normal dose

Intermittent hemodialysis: Administer 30% of normal dose

Peritoneal dialysis (PD): Administer 30% of normal dose

Continuous renal replacement therapy (CRRT): Administer 50% of normal dose

Coiffier, 2008: Dosage reduction of 50% is recommended in renal impairment

Adults:

Manufacturer's labeling: Oral, IV: Lower doses are required in renal impairment due to potential for accumulation of allopurinol and metabolites.

CrCl 10 to 20 mL/minute: 200 mg daily

CrCl 3 to 10 mL/minute: ≤100 mg daily

CrCl <3 mL/minute: ≤100 mg/dose at extended intervals

Alternate recommendations:

Management of hyperuricemia associated with chemotherapy: Oral, IV: Dosage reduction of 50% is recommended in renal impairment (Coiffier, 2008)

Gout: Oral:

Initiate therapy with 50 to 100 mg daily, and gradually increase to a maintenance dose to achieve a serum uric acid level of ≤6 mg/dL (with close monitoring of serum uric acid levels and for hypersensitivity) (Dalbeth, 2007).

or

In patients with stage 4 CKD or worse, initiate therapy at 50 mg/day, increasing the dose every 2 to 5 weeks to achieve desired uric acid levels of ≤6 mg/dL; doses >300 mg/day are permitted so long as they are accompanied by appropriate patient education and monitoring for toxicity (eg, pruritus, rash, elevated hepatic transaminases). Some patients may require therapy targeted at a serum uric acid level <5 mg/dL to control symptoms (ACR guidelines; Khanna, 2012).

Hemodialysis: Initial: 100 mg alternate days given postdialysis, increase cautiously to 300 mg based on response. If dialysis is on a daily basis, an additional 50% of the dose may be required postdialysis (Dalbeth, 2007)

Dosing adjustment in hepatic impairment: There are no dosage adjustments provided in the manufacturer's labeling.

Preparation for Administration Parenteral: Reconstitute 500 mg vial with 25 mL SWFI to prepare a 20 mg/mL solution; further dilute with D_5W or NS to final concentration not to exceed 6 mg/mL

Administration

Oral: Administer after meals with plenty of fluid; fluid intake should be administered to yield neutral or slightly alkaline urine and an output of ~2 L (in adults)

Parenteral: The rate of infusion is dependent upon the volume of the infusion; infuse maximum single daily doses (600 mg/day) over ≥30 minutes; whenever possible, therapy should be initiated at 12 to 24 hours (pediatric patients) **or** 24 to 48 hours (adults) before the start of chemotherapy known to cause tumor lysis (including adrenocorticosteroids) (Coiffier 2008). Intravenous daily therapy can be administered as a single infusion or in equally divided doses at 6-, 8-, or 12-hour interval.

Monitoring Parameters CBC, hepatic and renal function (especially at start of therapy), serum uric acid concentrations every 2 to 5 weeks during dose titration until desired level is achieved; every 6 months thereafter (ACR guidelines [Khanna, 2012]); 24-hour urinary urate (when treating calcium oxalate stones); signs and symptoms of hypersensitivity, hydration status (intake, urine output)

Reference Range

Children and Adolescents:

Uric Acid Normal Values

Age	Normal Serum Concentration
1 to 3 years	1.8 to 5 mg/dL
4 to 6 years	2.2 to 4.7 mg/dL
7 to 9 years	2 to 5 mg/dL
10 to 11 years Male Female	 2.3 to 5.4 mg/dL 3 to 4.7 mg/dL
12 to 13 years Male	 2.7 to 6.7 mg/dL
14 to 15 years Male	 2.4 to 7.8 mg/dL
12 to 15 years Female	 3 to 5.8 mg/dL
16 to 19 years Male Female	 4 to 8.6 mg/dL 3 to 5.9 mg/dL

Adult:

Males: 3.4 to 7 mg/dL or slightly more

Females: 2.4 to 6 mg/dL or slightly more

Target: ≤6 mg/dL

In adults, values >7 mg/dL are sometimes arbitrarily regarded as hyperuricemia, but there is no sharp line between normals on the one hand, and the serum uric acid of those with clinical gout. Normal ranges cannot be adjusted for purine ingestion, but high purine diet increases uric acid. Uric acid may be increased with body size, exercise, and stress.

Dosage Forms Excipient information presented when available (limited, particularly for generics); consult specific product labeling.

Solution Reconstituted, Intravenous, as sodium [strength expressed as base, preservative free]:

Aloprim: 500 mg (1 ea)

Tablet, Oral:

Zyloprim: 100 mg, 300 mg [scored]

Generic: 100 mg, 300 mg

Extemporaneous Preparations A 20 mg/mL oral suspension may be made with tablets and either a 1:1 mixture of Ora-Sweet® and Ora-Plus® or a 1:1 mixture of Ora-Sweet® SF and Ora-Plus® or a 1:4 mixture of cherry syrup concentrate and simple syrup, NF. Crush eight 300 mg tablets in a mortar and reduce to a fine powder. Add small portions of chosen vehicle and mix to a uniform paste; mix while adding the vehicle in incremental proportions to **almost** 120 mL; transfer to a calibrated bottle, rinse mortar with vehicle, and add quantity of vehicle sufficient to make 120 mL. Label "shake well". Stable for 60 days refrigerated or at room temperature (Allen, 1996; Nahata, 2004).

Allen LV Jr and Erickson MA 3rd, "Stability of Acetazolamide, Allopurinol, Azathioprine, Clonazepam, and Flucytosine in Extemporaneously Compounded Oral Liquids," *Am J Health Syst Pharm*, 1996, 53(16):1944-9.

Nahata MC, Pai VB, and Hipple TF, *Pediatric Drug Formulations*, 5th ed, Cincinnati, OH: Harvey Whitney Books Co, 2004.

◆ **Allopurinol Sodium** *see* Allopurinol *on page 96*

◆ **All-*trans* Retinoic Acid** *see* Tretinoin (Systemic) *on page 2108*

◆ **All-*trans* Vitamin A Acid** *see* Tretinoin (Systemic) *on page 2108*

Almotriptan (al moh TRIP tan)

Medication Safety Issues

Sound-alike/look-alike issues:

Axert may be confused with Antivert

Brand Names: US Axert

Brand Names: Canada Axert; Mylan-Almotriptan; Sandoz-Almotriptan

Therapeutic Category Antimigraine Agent; Serotonin 5-HT_{1D} Receptor Agonist

Generic Availability (US) Yes

Use Acute treatment of migraine with or without aura (FDA approved in ages 12-17 years and adults); **Note:** FDA labeled indication in adolescents is for patients with history of migraine lasting ≥4 hours when left untreated

Pregnancy Risk Factor C

Pregnancy Considerations Adverse events were observed in animal reproduction studies. Information related to almotriptan use in pregnancy is limited (Källén, 2011; Nezvalová-Henriksen, 2010; Nezvalová-Henriksen, 2012). Until additional information is available, other agents are preferred for the initial treatment of migraine in pregnancy (Da Silva, 2012; MacGregor, 2012; Williams, 2012).

Breast-Feeding Considerations It is not known if almotriptan is excreted in breast milk. The manufacturer recommends that caution be exercised when administering almotriptan to nursing women.

Contraindications Hypersensitivity to almotriptan or any component of the formulation; hemiplegic or basilar migraine; known or suspected ischemic heart disease (eg, angina pectoris, MI, documented silent ischemia, coronary artery vasospasm, Prinzmetal's variant angina); cerebrovascular syndromes (eg, stroke, transient ischemic attacks); peripheral vascular disease (eg, ischemic bowel disease); uncontrolled hypertension; use within 24 hours of another 5-HT_1 agonist; use within 24 hours of ergotamine derivatives and/or ergotamine-containing medications (eg, dihydroergotamine, ergotamine)

Warnings/Precautions Almotriptan is only indicated for the treatment of acute migraine headache; not indicated for migraine prophylaxis, or the treatment of cluster headaches, hemiplegic migraine, or basilar migraine. If a patient does not respond to the first dose, the diagnosis of acute migraine should be reconsidered.

Almotriptan should not be given to patients with documented ischemic or vasospastic CAD. Patients with risk factors for CAD (eg, hypertension, hypercholesterolemia, smoker, obesity, diabetes, strong family history of CAD, menopause, male >40 years of age) should undergo adequate cardiac evaluation prior to administration; if the cardiac evaluation is "satisfactory," the first dose of almotriptan should be given in the healthcare provider's office (consider ECG monitoring). All patients should undergo periodic evaluation of cardiovascular status during treatment. Cardiac events (coronary artery vasospasm, transient ischemia, myocardial infarction, ventricular tachycardia/fibrillation, cardiac arrest, and death), cerebral/subarachnoid hemorrhage, stroke, peripheral vascular ischemia, and colonic ischemia have been reported with 5-HT_1 agonist administration. Patients who experience sensations of chest pain/pressure/tightness or symptoms suggestive of angina following dosing should be evaluated for coronary artery disease or Prinzmetal's angina before receiving additional doses; if dosing is resumed and similar symptoms recur, monitor with ECG. Significant elevation in blood pressure, including hypertensive crisis, has also been reported on rare occasions following 5-HT_1 agonist administration in patients with and without a history of hypertension.

Acute migraine agents (eg, triptans, opioids, ergotamine, or a combination of the agents) used for 10 or more days per month may lead to worsening of headaches (medication overuse headache); withdrawal treatment may be necessary in the setting of overuse. Transient and permanent blindness and partial vision loss have been reported (rare) with 5-HT_1 agonist administration. Almotriptan contains a sulfonyl group which is structurally different from a sulfonamide. Cross-reactivity in patients with sulfonamide allergy has not been evaluated; however, the manufacturer recommends that caution be exercised in this patient population. Use with caution in liver or renal dysfunction. Symptoms of agitation, confusion, hallucinations, hyper-reflexia, myoclonus, shivering, and tachycardia (serotonin syndrome) may occur with concomitant proserotonergic drugs (ie, SSRIs/SNRIs or triptans) or agents which reduce almotriptan's metabolism. Concurrent use of serotonin precursors (eg, tryptophan) is not recommended. If concomitant administration with SSRIs is warranted, monitor closely, especially at initiation and with dose increases.

Adverse Reactions

Central nervous system: Dizziness, drowsiness, headache

Gastrointestinal: Nausea, vomiting, xerostomia

Neuromuscular & skeletal: Paresthesia

Rare but important or life-threatening: Anaphylactic shock, anaphylaxis, angina pectoris, angioedema, colitis, coronary artery vasospasm, hemiplegia, hypersensitivity reaction, hypertension, ischemic heart disease, mastalgia, myocardial infarction, neuropathy, seizure, skin rash, syncope, tachycardia, ventricular fibrillation, ventricular tachycardia

Drug Interactions

Metabolism/Transport Effects Substrate of CYP2D6 (minor), CYP3A4 (minor); **Note:** Assignment of Major/Minor substrate status based on clinically relevant drug interaction potential

Avoid Concomitant Use

Avoid concomitant use of Almotriptan with any of the following: Dapoxetine; Ergot Derivatives; MAO Inhibitors

Increased Effect/Toxicity

Almotriptan may increase the levels/effects of: Antipsychotic Agents; Droxidopa; Ergot Derivatives; Metoclopramide; Serotonin Modulators

The levels/effects of Almotriptan may be increased by: Antiemetics (5HT3 Antagonists); Antipsychotic Agents; CYP3A4 Inhibitors (Strong); Dapoxetine; Ergot Derivatives; MAO Inhibitors

Decreased Effect There are no known significant interactions involving a decrease in effect.

Storage/Stability Store at 25°C (77°F); excursions permitted to 15°C to 30°C (59°F to 86°F).

Mechanism of Action Selective agonist for serotonin (5-HT_{1B} and 5-HT_{1D} receptors) in cranial arteries; causes vasoconstriction and reduces sterile inflammation associated with antidromic neuronal transmission correlating with relief of migraine

Pharmacokinetics (Adult data unless noted)

Note: Reported values are similar between adolescent and adult patients (Baldwin, 2004).

Absorption: Well absorbed

Distribution: Apparent V_d: ~180-200 L

Protein binding: ~35%

Metabolism: MAO type A oxidative deamination (~27% of dose); via CYP3A4 and 2D6 (~12% of dose) to inactive metabolites

Bioavailability: ~70%

Half-life: Mean: 3-5 hours (Baldwin, 2004; McEnroe, 2005)

Time to peak serum concentration: 1-3 hours

Elimination: Urine (~75%; ~40% of total dose as unchanged drug); feces (~13% of total dose as unchanged drug and metabolites)

Dosing: Usual Adolescents 12-17 years and Adults: Oral: Initial: 6.25-12.5 mg in a single dose; if headache returns, may repeat the dose after 2 hours; no more than 2 doses (maximum daily dose: 25 mg). In clinical trials, 12.5 mg dose tended to be more effective in adults; individualize dose based on patient response.

Dosage adjustment in hepatic impairment: Adolescents and Adults: Initial: 6.25 mg in a single dose; maximum daily dose: 12.5 mg

Dosage adjustment in renal impairment: Adolescents and Adults: Severe renal impairment (CrCl ≤30 mL/minute): Initial: 6.25 mg in a single dose; maximum daily dose: 12.5 mg

Administration May administer without regard to meals.

Additional Information Safety of treating >4 headaches per month is not established; almotriptan is not indicated for migraine prophylaxis; safety and efficacy for cluster headaches have not been established.

Dosage Forms Excipient information presented when available (limited, particularly for generics); consult specific product labeling.

Tablet, Oral, as maleate:
- Axert: 6.25 mg
- Axert: 12.5 mg [contains fd&c blue #2 (indigotine)]
- Generic: 6.25 mg, 12.5 mg

◆ **Almotriptan Malate** *see* Almotriptan *on page 98*

◆ **Alocril** *see* Nedocromil *on page 1493*

◆ **Alocril® (Can)** *see* Nedocromil *on page 1493*

◆ **Alodox Convenience [DSC]** *see* Doxycycline *on page 717*

◆ **Aloe Vesta Antifungal [OTC]** *see* Miconazole (Topical) *on page 1431*

◆ **Aloprim** *see* Allopurinol *on page 96*

◆ **Alora** *see* Estradiol (Systemic) *on page 795*

◆ **Aloxi** *see* Palonosetron *on page 1609*

◆ **Alpha-Galactosidase-A (Recombinant)** *see* Agalsidase Beta *on page 76*

◆ **Alphagan (Can)** *see* Brimonidine (Ophthalmic) *on page 301*

◆ **Alphagan P** *see* Brimonidine (Ophthalmic) *on page 301*

◆ **Alphanate** *see* Antihemophilic Factor/von Willebrand Factor Complex (Human) *on page 173*

◆ **AlphaNine SD** *see* Factor IX (Human) *on page 838*

◆ **AlphaTrex** *see* Betamethasone (Topical) *on page 280*

◆ **Alph-E [OTC]** *see* Vitamin E *on page 2188*

◆ **Alph-E-Mixed [OTC]** *see* Vitamin E *on page 2188*

◆ **Alph-E-Mixed 1000 [OTC]** *see* Vitamin E *on page 2188*

ALPRAZolam (al PRAY zoe lam)

Medication Safety Issues

Sound-alike/look-alike issues:

ALPRAZolam may be confused with alprostadil, LORazepam, triazolam

Xanax may be confused with Fanapt, Lanoxin, Tenex, Tylox, Xopenex, Zantac, ZyrTEC

BEERS Criteria medication:

This drug may be potentially inappropriate for use in geriatric patients (Quality of evidence - high; Strength of recommendation - strong).

Related Information

Oral Medications That Should Not Be Crushed or Altered *on page 2476*

Brand Names: US ALPRAZolam Intensol; ALPRAZolam XR; Niravam; Xanax; Xanax XR

Brand Names: Canada Apo-Alpraz®; Apo-Alpraz® TS; Mylan-Alprazolam; NTP-Alprazolam; Nu-Alpraz; Teva-Alprazolam; Xanax TS™; Xanax®

Therapeutic Category Antianxiety Agent; Benzodiazepine

Generic Availability (US) May be product dependent

Use

Immediate release tablets and oral solution: Treatment of generalized anxiety disorder (GAD); anxiety associated with depression; short-term relief of symptoms of anxiety; treatment of panic disorder, with or without agoraphobia (All indications: FDA approved in ages ≥18 years and adults)

Extended release tablets: Treatment of panic disorder, with or without agoraphobia (FDA approved in ages ≥18 years and adults)

Oral disintegrating tablets (Niravam): Treatment of generalized anxiety disorder (GAD) and treatment of panic disorder, with or without agoraphobia (All indications: FDA approved in ages ≥18 years and adults)

Pregnancy Risk Factor D

Pregnancy Considerations Benzodiazepines have the potential to cause harm to the fetus. Alprazolam and its metabolites cross the human placenta. Teratogenic effects have been observed with some benzodiazepines; however, additional studies are needed. The incidence of premature birth and low birth weights may be increased following maternal use of benzodiazepines; hypoglycemia and respiratory problems in the neonate may occur following exposure late in pregnancy. Neonatal withdrawal symptoms may occur within days to weeks after birth and "floppy infant syndrome" (which also includes withdrawal symptoms) has been reported with some benzodiazepines (Bergman, 1992; Iqbal, 2002; Wikner, 2007).

Breast-Feeding Considerations Benzodiazepines are excreted into breast milk. In a study of eight postpartum women, peak concentrations of alprazolam were found in breast milk ~1 hour after the maternal dose and the half-life was ~14 hours. Samples were obtained over 36 hours following a single oral dose of alprazolam 0.5 mg. Metabolites were not detected in breast milk. In this study, the estimated exposure to the breast-feeding infant was ~3% of the weight-adjusted maternal dose (Oo, 1995). Drowsiness, lethargy, or weight loss in nursing infants have been observed in case reports following maternal use of some benzodiazepines (Iqbal, 2002). Breast-feeding is not recommended by the manufacturer.

Contraindications Hypersensitivity to alprazolam or any component of the formulation (cross-sensitivity with other benzodiazepines may exist); narrow-angle glaucoma; concurrent use with ketoconazole or itraconazole

Warnings/Precautions Rebound or withdrawal symptoms, including seizures, may occur following abrupt discontinuation or large decreases in dose (more common in adult patients receiving >4 mg/day or prolonged treatment); the risk of seizures appears to be greatest 24 to 72 hours following discontinuation of therapy. Breakthrough anxiety may occur at the end of dosing interval. Use with caution in patients receiving concurrent CYP3A4 inhibitors, moderate or strong CYP3A4 inducers, and major CYP3A4 substrates; consider alternative agents that avoid or lessen the potential for CYP-mediated interactions. Use with caution in renal impairment or predisposition to urate nephropathy; has weak uricosuric properties. In older adults, benzodiazepines increase the risk of impaired cognition, delirium, falls, fractures, and motor vehicle accidents. Due to increased sensitivity in this age group, avoid use for treatment of insomnia, agitation, or delirium (Beers Criteria). Use with caution in or debilitated patients, patients with hepatic disease (including alcoholics) or respiratory disease, or obese patients. Cigarette smoking may decrease alprazolam concentrations up to 50%.

Causes CNS depression (dose related) which may impair physical and mental capabilities. Patients must be cautioned about performing tasks that require mental alertness (eg, operating machinery or driving). Effects with other sedative drugs or ethanol may be potentiated

Benzodiazepines have been associated with falls and traumatic injury and should be used with extreme caution in patients who are at risk of these events.

Use caution in patients with depression, particularly if suicidal risk may be present. Episodes of mania or hypomania have occurred in depressed patients treated with alprazolam. May cause physical or psychological dependence. Acute withdrawal may be precipitated in patients after administration of flumazenil. Tolerance does not develop to the anxiolytic effects (Vinkers, 2012). Chronic use of this agent may increase the perioperative benzodiazepine dose needed to achieve desired effect.

Benzodiazepines have been associated with anterograde amnesia. Paradoxical reactions have been reported with benzodiazepines, particularly in adolescent/pediatric or psychiatric patients. Does not have analgesic, antidepressant, or antipsychotic properties.

Adverse Reactions

Central nervous system: Abnormal dreams, agitation, akathisia, altered mental status, ataxia, cognitive dysfunction, confusion, depersonalization, depression, derealization, disinhibition, disorientation, disturbance in attention, dizziness, drowsiness, dysarthria, dystonia, fatigue, fear, hallucination, headache, hypersomnia, hypoesthesia, insomnia, irritability, lethargy, malaise, memory impairment, nervousness, nightmares, paresthesia, restlessness, sedation, seizure, talkativeness, vertigo

Dermatologic: Dermatitis, diaphoresis, skin rash

Endocrine & metabolic: Decreased libido, Increased libido, menstrual disease, weight gain, weight loss

Gastrointestinal: Abdominal pain, anorexia, change in appetite, constipation, diarrhea, dyspepsia, nausea, sialorrhea, vomiting, xerostomia

Genitourinary: Difficulty in micturition, dysmenorrhea, sexual disorder, urinary incontinence

Hepatic: Increased liver enzymes, increased serum bilirubin, jaundice

Neuromuscular & skeletal: Arthralgia, back pain, dyskinesia, muscle cramps, muscle twitching, myalgia, tremor, weakness

Ophthalmic: Blurred vision

Respiratory: Allergic rhinitis, dyspnea, hyperventilation, nasal congestion, upper respiratory tract infection

Rare but important or life-threatening: Amnesia, angioedema, diplopia, falling, galactorrhea, gynecomastia, hepatic failure, hepatitis, homicidal ideation, hyperprolactinemia, hypomania, mania, peripheral edema, sleep apnea, Stevens-Johnson syndrome, suicidal ideation, tinnitus

Drug Interactions

Metabolism/Transport Effects **Substrate** of CYP3A4 (major); **Note:** Assignment of Major/Minor substrate status based on clinically relevant drug interaction potential; **Inhibits** CYP3A4 (weak)

Avoid Concomitant Use

Avoid concomitant use of ALPRAZolam with any of the following: Azelastine (Nasal); Conivaptan; Fusidic Acid (Systemic); Idelalisib; Indinavir; Itraconazole; Ketoconazole (Systemic); Methadone; OLANZapine; Orphenadrine; Paraldehyde; Pimozide; Sodium Oxybate; Thalidomide

Increased Effect/Toxicity

ALPRAZolam may increase the levels/effects of: Alcohol (Ethyl); ARIPiprazole; Azelastine (Nasal); Buprenorphine; CloZAPine; CNS Depressants; Dofetilide; Hydrocodone; Lomitapide; Methadone; Methotrimeprazine; Metyrosine; Mirtazapine; NiMODipine; Orphenadrine; Paraldehyde; Pimozide; Pramipexole; ROPINIRole; Rotigotine; Selective Serotonin Reuptake Inhibitors; Sodium Oxybate; Suvorexant; Thalidomide; Zolpidem

The levels/effects of ALPRAZolam may be increased by: Aprepitant; Boceprevir; Brimonidine (Topical); Cannabis; Conivaptan; CYP3A4 Inhibitors (Moderate); CYP3A4 Inhibitors (Strong); Dasatinib; Doxylamine; Dronabinol; Droperidol; FluvoxaMINE; Fosaprepitant; Fusidic Acid (Systemic); HydrOXYzine; Idelalisib; Indinavir; Itraconazole; Ivacaftor; Kava Kava; Ketoconazole (Systemic); Luliconazole; Macrolide Antibiotics; Magnesium Sulfate; Methotrimeprazine; Mifepristone; Nabilone; Netupitant; OLANZapine; Palbociclib; Perampanel; Protease Inhibitors; Rufinamide; Simeprevir; Stiripentol; Tapentadol; Teduglutide; Telaprevir; Tetrahydrocannabinol

Decreased Effect

The levels/effects of ALPRAZolam may be decreased by: Bosentan; CYP3A4 Inducers (Moderate); CYP3A4 Inducers (Strong); Dabrafenib; Deferasirox; Mitotane; Siltuximab; St Johns Wort; Theophylline Derivatives; Tocilizumab; Yohimbine

Food Interactions Alprazolam serum concentration is unlikely to be increased by grapefruit juice because of alprazolam's high oral bioavailability. The C_{max} of the extended release formulation is increased by 25% when a high-fat meal is given 2 hours before dosing. T_{max} is decreased 33% when food is given immediately prior to dose and increased by 33% when food is given ≥1 hour after dose. Management: Administer without regard to food.

Storage/Stability

Immediate release tablets: Store at 20°C to 25°C (68°F to 77°F).

Extended release tablets: Store at 25°C (77°F); excursions permitted to 15°C to 30°C (59°F to 86°F).

Orally-disintegrating tablet: Store at room temperature of 20°C to 25°C (68°F to 77°F). Protect from moisture. Seal bottle tightly and discard any cotton packaged inside bottle.

Mechanism of Action Binds to stereospecific benzodiazepine receptors on the postsynaptic GABA neuron at several sites within the central nervous system, including the limbic system, reticular formation. Enhancement of the inhibitory effect of GABA on neuronal excitability results by increased neuronal membrane permeability to chloride ions. This shift in chloride ions results in hyperpolarization (a less excitable state) and stabilization. Benzodiazepine receptors and effects appear to be linked to the GABA-A receptors. Benzodiazepines do not bind to GABA-B receptors.

Pharmacokinetics (Adult data unless noted)

Absorption: Oral:

- Immediate release: Rapidly and well absorbed
- Extended release tablet: Rate of absorption is increased following night time dosing (versus morning dosing)

Distribution: 0.9 to 1.2 L/kg

Protein binding: 80%, primarily to albumin

Metabolism: Hepatic, primarily via cytochrome P450 isoenzyme CYP3A; major metabolites: alpha-hydroxy-alprazolam (about half as active as alprazolam), 4-hydroxyalprazolam (active), and a benzophenone metabolite (inactive). **Note:** Active metabolites are not likely to contribute to pharmacologic effects due to low levels of activity and low concentrations.

Bioavailability: Similar for extended and immediate release tablets (~90%)

Half-life: **Note:** Half-life may be 25% longer in Asians compared to Caucasians.

- Immediate release tablet and oral solution: Mean: 11.2 hours (range: 6.3 to 26.9 hours)
- Extended release tablet: 10.7 to 15.8 hours
- Orally disintegrating tablet: Mean: 12.5 hours (range: 7.9 to 19.2 hours)
- Alcoholic liver disease: 19.7 hours (range: 5.8 to 65.3 hours)
- Obesity: 21.8 hours (range: 9.9 to 40.4 hours)

Time to peak serum concentration:

Immediate release table and oral solution: Within 1 to 2 hours

Extended release: Adolescents and Adults: ~9 hours, relatively steady from 4 to 12 hours (Glue, 2006); decreased by 1 hour when administered at nighttime (as compared to morning administration); decreased by 33% when administered with a high-fat meal; increased by 33% when administered ≥1 hour after a high-fat meal

Orally disintegrating tablet: 1.5-2 hours (if given with or without water); **Note:** Time to peak serum concentration occurs ~15 minutes earlier when taken with water (versus without); increased by 2 hours when administered with a high-fat meal

Elimination: Urine (as unchanged drug and metabolites)

Dosing: Usual Note: Titrate dose to effect; use lowest effective dose. The usefulness of this medication should be periodically reassessed.

Pediatric:

Anxiety: Oral:

Children ≥7 years and Adolescents <18 years: Limited data available: Immediate release: Dose not established; investigationally in children 7 to 16 years of age (n=13), initial doses of 0.005 mg/kg or 0.125 mg/dose were given 3 times/day for situational anxiety and increments of 0.125 to 0.25 mg/dose were used to increase doses to maximum of 0.02 mg/kg/dose or 0.06 mg/kg/day; a range of 0.375 to 3 mg/day was needed (Pfefferbaum, 1987). **Note:** A more recent study in 17 children (8 to 17 years of age) with overanxious disorder or avoidant disorders used initial daily doses of 0.25 mg for children <40 kg and 0.5 mg for those >40 kg. The dose was titrated at 2-day intervals to a maximum of 0.04 mg/kg/day. Required doses ranged from 0.5 to 3.5 mg/day with a mean of 1.6 mg/day. Based on clinical global ratings, alprazolam appeared to be better than placebo; however, this difference was **not** statistically significant (Simeon, 1992).

Adolescents ≥18 years: Immediate release: Initial: 0.25 to 0.5 mg 3 times daily; titrate dose upward as needed every 3 to 4 days; usual maximum daily dose: 4 mg/**day**. Patients requiring doses >4 mg/**day** should be increased cautiously. Periodic reassessment and consideration of dosage reduction is recommended.

Panic disorder: Adolescents ≥18 years: Oral:

Immediate release: Initial: 0.5 mg 3 times daily; titrate dose upward as needed every 3 to 4 days in increments ≤1 mg/day; mean dose used in controlled trials: 5 to 6 mg/**day**; maximum daily dose: 10 mg/**day** (rarely required)

Extended release: Initial: 0.5 to 1 mg once daily; titrate dose upward as needed every 3 to 4 days in increments ≤1 mg/day; usual dose: 3 to 6 mg/**day**; maximum daily dose: 10 mg/**day** (rarely required)

Switching from immediate release to extended release: Administer the same total daily dose, but give once daily; if effect is not adequate, titrate dose as above.

Premenstrual dysphoric disorder: Limited data available: Adolescents: Oral: Initial dose: 0.25 mg 3 times daily; titrate as needed. Usual daily dose: 1.25 to 2.25 mg/**day** (Kleigman, 2011)

Dose reduction: Abrupt discontinuation should be avoided. Daily dose must be gradually decreased no more frequently than every 3 days; however, some patients may require a slower reduction. If withdrawal symptoms occur, resume previous dose and discontinue on a less rapid schedule.

Adult:

Anxiety: Oral: Immediate release: Initial: 0.25 to 0.5 mg 3 times daily; titrate dose upward as needed every 3 to 4 days; usual maximum daily dose: 4 mg/**day**. Patients requiring doses >4 mg/day should be increased cautiously. Periodic reassessment and consideration of dosage reduction is recommended.

Panic disorder: Oral:

Immediate release: Initial: 0.5 mg 3 times daily; titrate dose upward as needed every 3 to 4 days in increments ≤1 mg/day; mean dose used in controlled trials: 5 to 6 mg/**day**; maximum daily dose: 10 mg/**day** (rarely required)

Extended release: Initial: 0.5 to 1 mg once daily; titrate dose upward as needed every 3 to 4 days in increments ≤1 mg/day; usual dose: 3 to 6 mg/**day**; maximum daily dose: 10 mg/**day** (rarely required)

Switching from immediate release to extended release: Administer the same total daily dose, but give once daily; if effect is not adequate, titrate dose as above

Dose reduction: Abrupt discontinuation should be avoided. Daily dose may be decreased by 0.5 mg every 3 days; however, some patients may require a slower reduction. If withdrawal symptoms occur, resume previous dose and discontinue on a less rapid schedule.

Dosing adjustment in renal impairment: There are no dosage adjustments provided in the manufacturer's labeling.

Dosing adjustment in hepatic impairment: Adults:

Advanced liver disease:

Immediate release: 0.25 mg twice daily to 3 times daily; titrate gradually if needed and tolerated.

Extended release: 0.5 mg once daily; titrate gradually if needed and tolerated

Administration Oral:

Immediate release tablet: Adults: May be administered sublingually if oral administration is not possible; absorption and onset of effect is comparable to oral administration (Scavone, 1987; Scavone, 1992)

Extended release tablet: Administer once daily, preferably in the morning; do not crush, chew, or break; swallow whole

Orally disintegrating tablet: Do not remove tablets from bottle until right before dose; using dry hands, place tablet on top of tongue. If using one-half of tablet, immediately discard remaining half (half tablet may not remain stable). Administration with water is not necessary.

Monitoring Parameters CNS and cardiovascular status, respiratory rate

Controlled Substance C-IV

Dosage Forms Excipient information presented when available (limited, particularly for generics); consult specific product labeling. [DSC] = Discontinued product

Concentrate, Oral:

ALPRAZolam Intensol: 1 mg/mL (30 mL) [unflavored flavor]

Tablet, Oral:

Xanax: 0.25 mg [scored]

Xanax: 0.5 mg [scored; contains fd&c yellow #6 (sunset yellow)]

Xanax: 1 mg [scored; contains fd&c blue #2 (indigotine)]

Xanax: 2 mg [scored]

Generic: 0.25 mg, 0.5 mg, 1 mg, 2 mg

Tablet Dispersible, Oral:

Niravam: 0.25 mg, 0.5 mg [DSC], 1 mg [DSC], 2 mg [DSC] [scored; orange flavor]

Generic: 0.25 mg, 0.5 mg, 1 mg, 2 mg

Tablet Extended Release 24 Hour, Oral:

ALPRAZolam XR: 0.5 mg

ALPRAZolam XR: 1 mg [contains fd&c yellow #10 (quinoline yellow)]

ALPRAZolam XR: 2 mg [contains fd&c blue #2 (indigotine)]

ALPRAZolam XR: 3 mg [contains fd&c blue #2 (indigotine), fd&c yellow #10 (quinoline yellow)]

Xanax XR: 0.5 mg

Xanax XR: 1 mg [contains fd&c yellow #10 (quinoline yellow)]
Xanax XR: 2 mg [contains fd&c blue #2 (indigotine)]
Xanax XR: 3 mg [contains fd&c blue #2 (indigotine), fd&c yellow #10 (quinoline yellow)]
Generic: 0.5 mg, 1 mg, 2 mg, 3 mg

Extemporaneous Preparations Note: Commercial oral solution is available (Alprazolam Intensol™: 1 mg/mL [dye free, ethanol free, sugar free; contains propylene glycol])

A 1 mg/mL oral suspension may be made with tablets and one of three different vehicles (a 1:1 mixture of Ora-Sweet® and Ora-Plus®, a 1:1 mixture of Ora-Sweet® SF and Ora-Plus®, or a 1:4 mixture of cherry syrup with Simple Syrup, NF). Crush sixty 2 mg tablets in a mortar and reduce to a fine powder. Add 40 mL of vehicle and mix to a uniform paste; mix while adding the vehicle in incremental proportions to **almost** 120 mL; transfer to a calibrated bottle, rinse mortar with vehicle, and add a quantity of vehicle sufficient to make 120 mL. Label "shake well" and "refrigerate". Stable for 60 days.

Nahata MC, Pai VB, and Hipple TF, *Pediatric Drug Formulations*, 5th ed, Cincinnati, OH: Harvey Whitney Books Co, 2004.

◆ **ALPRAZolam Intensol** *see* ALPRAZolam *on page 100*

◆ **ALPRAZolam XR** *see* ALPRAZolam *on page 100*

◆ **Alprolix** *see* Factor IX (Recombinant) *on page 842*

Alprostadil (al PROS ta dill)

Medication Safety Issues

Sound-alike/look-alike issues:

Alprostadil may be confused with alPRAZolam

Related Information

Emergency Drip Calculations *on page 2229*

Brand Names: US Caverject; Caverject Impulse; Edex; Muse; Prostin VR

Brand Names: Canada Alprostadil Injection USP; Caverject; Muse Pellet; Prostin VR

Therapeutic Category Prostaglandin

Generic Availability (US) May be product dependent

Use Temporary maintenance of patency of ductus arteriosus in neonates with ductal-dependent congenital heart disease until surgery can be performed. These defects include cyanotic (eg, pulmonary atresia, pulmonary stenosis, tricuspid atresia, Fallot's tetralogy, transposition of the great vessels) and acyanotic (eg, interruption of aortic arch, coarctation of aorta, hypoplastic left ventricle) heart disease.

Investigationally used for the treatment of pulmonary hypertension in infants and children with congenital heart defects with left-to-right shunts

Adult males: Diagnosis and treatment of erectile dysfunction

Pregnancy Risk Factor C (Muse)

Pregnancy Considerations Adverse events were observed in animal reproduction studies. Alprostadil is not indicated for use in women. The manufacturer of Muse recommends a condom barrier when being used during sexual intercourse with a pregnant woman.

Breast-Feeding Considerations Alprostadil is not indicated for use in women.

Contraindications

Alprostadil (intracavernous):

Conditions predisposing patients to priapism (eg, sickle cell anemia or trait, multiple myeloma, leukemia); patients with anatomical deformation or fibrotic conditions of the penis (eg, angulation, cavernosal fibrosis, or Peyronie disease); penile implants.

Caverject, Caverject impulse: Hypersensitivity to alprostadil or any component of the formulation; use in men for whom sexual activity is inadvisable or contraindicated. Intracavernosal alprostadil is intended for use in adult men only and is not indicated for use in women, children, or newborns.

Alprostadil (transurethral): Hypersensitivity to alprostadil, use in patients with urethral stricture, balanitis (inflammation/infection of the glans penis), severe hypospadias and curvature, and in patients with acute or chronic urethritis; in patients who are prone to venous thrombosis or who have a hyperviscosity syndrome (eg, sickle cell anemia or trait, thrombocythemia, polycythemia, multiple myeloma) and are therefore at increased risk of priapism (rigid erection lasting ≥6 hours). Should not be used in men for whom sexual activity is inadvisable or for sexual intercourse with a pregnant woman unless the couple uses a condom barrier.

Alprostadil (intravenous): There are no contraindications listed in the manufacturer's labeling.

Warnings/Precautions

Prostin VR Pediatric: Use cautiously in neonates with bleeding tendencies. **[U.S. Boxed Warning]: Apnea may occur in 10% to 12% of neonates with congenital heart defects, especially in those weighing <2 kg at birth.** Apnea usually appears during the first hour of drug infusion. When used for patency of ductus arteriosus infuse for the shortest time at the lowest dose consistent with good patient care. Use for >120 hours has been associated with antral hyperplasia and gastric outlet obstruction.

Caverject, Caverject Impulse, Edex, Muse: When used in erectile dysfunction, priapism may occur; treat prolonged priapism (erection persisting for >4 hours) immediately to avoid penile tissue damage and permanent loss of potency; discontinue therapy if signs of penile fibrosis develop (penile angulation, cavernosal fibrosis, or Peyronie disease). Underlying causes of erectile dysfunction should be evaluated and treated prior to therapy. Treatment for erectile dysfunction should not be used in men whom sexual activity is inadvisable because of underlying cardiovascular status. When used in erectile dysfunction (Muse), syncope occurring within 1 hour of administration has been reported. The potential for drug-drug interactions may occur when Muse is prescribed concomitantly with antihypertensives. Instruct patients to avoid ethanol consumption; may have vasodilating effect.

Benzyl alcohol and derivatives: Some dosage forms may contain benzyl alcohol; large amounts of benzyl alcohol (≥99 mg/kg/day) have been associated with a potentially fatal toxicity ("gasping syndrome") in neonates; the "gasping syndrome" consists of metabolic acidosis, respiratory distress, gasping respirations, CNS dysfunction (including convulsions, intracranial hemorrhage), hypotension, and cardiovascular collapse (AAP, 1997; CDC, 1982); some data suggests that benzoate displaces bilirubin from protein binding sites (Ahlfors 2001); avoid or use dosage forms containing benzyl alcohol with caution in neonates. See manufacturer's labeling.

Adverse Reactions

Intraurethral:

Central nervous system: Dizziness, headache, pain

Genitourinary: Penile pain, testicular pain, urethral bleeding (minor), urethral burning, vulvovaginal pruritus (female partner)

Rare but important or life-threatening: Tachycardia

Intracavernosal injection:

Cardiovascular: Hypertension

Central nervous system: Dizziness, headache

Genitourinary: Penile disease, penile pain, penile rash, penile swelling, prolonged erection (>4 hours), Peyronie's disease

Local: Bruising at injection site, hematoma at injection site

Rare but important or life-threatening: Balanitis, injection site hemorrhage, priapism

Intravenous:

Cardiovascular: Bradycardia, cardiac arrest, edema, flushing, hypertension, hypotension, tachycardia

Central nervous system: Dizziness, headache, seizure

Endocrine & metabolic: Hypokalemia

Gastrointestinal: Diarrhea

Hematologic & oncologic: Disseminated intravascular coagulation

Infection: Sepsis

Local: Local pain (in structures other than the injection site)

Neuromuscular & skeletal: Back pain

Respiratory: Apnea, cough, flu-like symptoms, nasal congestion, sinusitis, upper respiratory infection

Miscellaneous: Fever

Rare but important or life-threatening: Anemia, anuria, bradypnea, cardiac failure, cerebral hemorrhage, gastroesophageal reflux disease, hematuria, hemorrhage, hyperbilirubinemia, hyperemia, hyperirritability, hyperkalemia, hypoglycemia, hypothermia, neck hyperextension, peritonitis, second degree atrioventricular block, shock, supraventricular tachycardia, thrombocytopenia, ventricular fibrillation

Drug Interactions

Metabolism/Transport Effects None known.

Avoid Concomitant Use

Avoid concomitant use of Alprostadil with any of the following: Phosphodiesterase 5 Inhibitors

Increased Effect/Toxicity

The levels/effects of Alprostadil may be increased by: Phosphodiesterase 5 Inhibitors

Decreased Effect There are no known significant interactions involving a decrease in effect.

Storage/Stability

Caverject Impulse: Store at or below 25°C (77°F); excursions are permitted between 15°C and 30°C (59°F and 86°F). Following reconstitution, use within 24 hours and discard any unused solution; for single use only.

Caverject powder: The 5 mcg, 10 mcg, and 20 mcg vials should be stored at or below 25°C (77°F). The 40 mcg vial should be stored at 2°C to 8°C (36°F to 46°F) until dispensed. After dispensing, stable for up to 3 months at or below 25°C (77°F). Following reconstitution, all strengths should be stored at or below 25°C (77°F); do not refrigerate or freeze; use within 24 hours.

Edex: Store at 25°C (77°F); excursions are permitted between 15°C and 30°C (59°F and 86°F).

Muse: Refrigerate at 2°C to 8°C (36°F to 46°F); may be stored at room temperature for up to 14 days.

Prostin VR Pediatric: Refrigerate at 2°C to 8°C (36°F to 46°F). The following stability information has also been reported: May be stored at 20°C for up to 34 days or 30°C for up to 26 days (Cohen 2007). Prior to infusion, dilute with D_5W, $D_{10}W$, or NS; use within 24 hours.

Mechanism of Action Causes vasodilation by means of direct effect on vascular and ductus arteriosus smooth muscle; relaxes trabecular smooth muscle by dilation of cavernosal arteries when injected along the penile shaft, allowing blood flow to and entrapment in the lacunar spaces of the penis (ie, corporeal veno-occlusive mechanism)

Pharmacodynamics

Maximum effect:

Acyanotic congenital heart disease: Usual: 1.5-3 hours; range: 15 minutes to 11 hours

Cyanotic congenital heart disease: Usual: ~30 minutes

Duration: Ductus arteriosus will begin to close within 1-2 hours after drug is stopped

Pharmacokinetics (Adult data unless noted)

Metabolism: ~70% to 80% metabolized by oxidation during a single pass through the lungs; metabolite (13,14 dihydro-PGE_1) is active and has been identified in neonates

Half-life: 5-10 minutes; since the half-life is so short, the drug must be administered by continuous infusion

Elimination: Metabolites excreted in urine

Dosing: Neonatal Continuous IV infusion: 0.05-0.1 mcg/kg/minute; once therapeutic response is achieved, reduce rate to lowest effective dosage; with unsatisfactory response, increase rate gradually; maintenance: 0.01-0.4 mcg/kg/minute; higher doses may be required in patients receiving ECMO support (Stone, 2006); apnea may be less likely to occur at doses <0.015 mcg/kg/minute (Browning Carmo, 2007). **Note:** PGE_1 is usually given at an infusion rate of 0.1 mcg/kg/minute, but it is often possible to reduce the dosage to 1/2 or even 1/10 without losing the therapeutic effect.

Dosing: Usual Continuous IV infusion: Infants: 0.05-0.1 mcg/kg/minute; once therapeutic response is achieved, reduce rate to lowest effective dosage; with unsatisfactory response, increase rate gradually; maintenance: 0.01-0.4 mcg/kg/minute. **Note:** PGE_1 is usually given at an infusion rate of 0.1 mcg/kg/minute, but it is often possible to reduce the dosage to 1/2 or even 1/10 without losing the therapeutic effect.

Usual Infusion Concentrations: Neonatal IV infusion: 10 mcg/mL

Usual Infusion Concentrations: Pediatric IV infusion: 10 mcg/mL **or** 20 mcg/mL

Preparation for Administration

Continuous IV infusion: **Patent ductus arteriosus (PDA):** Prostin VR Pediatric: Dilute with D_5W, $D_{10}W$, or NS to a maximum concentration of 20 mcg/mL per the manufacturer. ISMP and Vermont Oxford Network recommend a standard concentration of 10 mcg/mL for neonates (ISMP 2011). Avoid direct contact of undiluted alprostadil with the plastic walls of volumetric infusion chambers because the drug will interact with the plastic and create a hazy solution; discard solution and volumetric chamber if this occurs.

Administration Continuous IV infusion: **Patent ductus arteriosus (PDA):** Prostin VR Pediatric: Administer into a large vein or alternatively through an umbilical artery catheter placed at the ductal opening; has also been administered via continuous infusion into the right pulmonary artery for treatment of pulmonary hypertension in infants and children with congenital heart defects with left-to-right shunts

Rate of infusion (mL/hour) = dose (mcg/kg/minute) x weight (kg) x 60 minutes/hour divided by concentration (mcg/mL)

Monitoring Parameters Arterial pressure, respiratory rate, heart rate, temperature, pO_2; monitor for gastric obstruction in patients receiving PGE_1 for longer than 120 hours; x-rays may be needed to assess cortical hyperostosis in patients receiving prolonged PGE_1 therapy

Additional Information Therapeutic response is indicated by an increase in systemic blood pressure and pH in those with restricted systemic blood flow and acidosis, or by an increase in oxygenation (pO_2) in those with restricted pulmonary blood flow. Most cases of bone changes occurred 4-6 weeks after starting alprostadil, but it has occurred as early as 9 days; cortical hyperostosis usually resolves over 6-12 months after stopping PGE_1 therapy

Other dosage forms of alprostadil [Caverject® injection, Caverject® Impulse™ injection, Edex® injection, and Muse® Pellet (urethral)] are indicated for the diagnosis and treatment of erectile dysfunction in adult males; see package inserts for further information for this use.

Dosage Forms Excipient information presented when available (limited, particularly for generics); consult specific product labeling.

Kit, Intracavernosal:
  Caverject Impulse: 10 mcg [contains benzyl alcohol]
  Caverject Impulse: 20 mcg
  Edex: 10 mcg, 20 mcg, 40 mcg
Pellet, Urethral:
  Muse: 125 mcg (1 ea, 6 ea); 250 mcg (1 ea, 6 ea); 500 mcg (1 ea, 6 ea); 1000 mcg (1 ea, 6 ea)
Solution, Injection:
  Prostin VR: 500 mcg/mL (1 mL) [contains benzyl alcohol]
  Generic: 500 mcg/mL (1 mL)
Solution Reconstituted, Intracavernosal:
  Caverject: 20 mcg (1 ea)
  Caverject: 20 mcg (1 ea); 40 mcg (1 ea) [contains benzyl alcohol]

- ◆ **Alprostadil Injection USP (Can)** *see* Alprostadil *on page 103*
- ◆ **Alsuma** *see* SUMAtriptan *on page 1995*
- ◆ **Altabax** *see* Retapamulin *on page 1846*
- ◆ **Altacaine** *see* Tetracaine (Ophthalmic) *on page 2034*
- ◆ **Altachlore [OTC]** *see* Sodium Chloride *on page 1938*
- ◆ **Altafrin** *see* Phenylephrine (Ophthalmic) *on page 1689*
- ◆ **Altalube [OTC]** *see* Artificial Tears *on page 201*
- ◆ **Altamist Spray [OTC]** *see* Sodium Chloride *on page 1938*
- ◆ **Altarussin [OTC]** *see* GuaiFENesin *on page 988*
- ◆ **Altaryl [OTC]** *see* DiphenhydrAMINE (Systemic) *on page 668*

Alteplase (AL te plase)

Medication Safety Issues

Sound-alike/look-alike issues:

Activase may be confused with Cathflo Activase, TNKase

Alteplase may be confused with Altace

"tPA" abbreviation should not be used when writing orders for this medication; has been misread as TNKase (tenecteplase)

High alert medication:

The Institute for Safe Medication Practices (ISMP) includes this medication (IV) among its list of drugs which have a heightened risk of causing significant patient harm when used in error.

Brand Names: US Activase; Cathflo Activase

Brand Names: Canada Activase rt-PA; Cathflo Activase

Therapeutic Category Thrombolytic Agent; Thrombotic Occlusion (Central Venous Catheter), Treatment Agent

Generic Availability (US) No

Use

Activase: Thrombolytic agent used in treatment of acute MI, acute ischemic stroke, and acute massive pulmonary embolism (All indications: FDA approved in adults)

CathFlo Activase: Treatment of occluded central venous access devices (catheters) to restore function (FDA approved in pediatric patients [age not specified] and adults)

Pregnancy Risk Factor C

Pregnancy Considerations Adverse events have been observed in animal reproduction studies. The risk of bleeding may be increased in pregnant women. Information related to alteplase use in pregnancy is limited (Leonhardt 2006; Li 2012) and most guidelines consider pregnancy to be a relative contraindication for its use (Jaff 2011; Jauch 2013; O'Gara 2013). Alteplase should not be withheld from pregnant women in life-threatening situations but should be avoided when safer alternatives are available (Bates 2012; Leonhardt 2006; Li 2012; Vanden Hoek 2010).

Breast-Feeding Considerations It is not known if alteplase is excreted in breast milk. The manufacturer recommends that caution be exercised when administering alteplase to nursing women.

Contraindications Hypersensitivity to alteplase or any component of the formulation

Treatment of STEMI or PE: Active internal bleeding; history of recent stroke; recent (within 3 months [ACCF/AHA: within 2 months]) intracranial or intraspinal surgery or serious head trauma; presence of intracranial conditions that may increase the risk of bleeding (eg, intracranial neoplasm, arteriovenous malformation, aneurysm); known bleeding diathesis; severe uncontrolled hypertension (ACCF/AHA: unresponsive to emergency therapy)

Additional contraindications according to the American Heart Association and American College of Cardiology Foundation (AHA [Jaff 2011]; ACCF/AHA [O'Gara 2013]): Active bleeding (excluding menses); any prior intracranial hemorrhage; suspected aortic dissection; ischemic stroke within 3 months **except** when within 4.5 hours; significant closed head or facial trauma within 3 months with radiographic evidence of bony fracture or brain injury

Treatment of AIS: Current intracranial hemorrhage; subarachnoid hemorrhage; active internal bleeding; recent (within 3 months) intracranial or intraspinal surgery or serious head trauma; presence of intracranial conditions that may increase the risk of bleeding (eg, intracranial neoplasm, arteriovenous malformation, aneurysm); known bleeding diathesis; severe uncontrolled hypertension

Additional contraindications according to the American Heart Association/American Stroke Association (AHA/ASA [Jauch 2013]): History of intracranial hemorrhage; suspicion of subarachnoid hemorrhage; stroke within 3 months; arterial puncture at a noncompressible site in previous 7 days; uncontrolled hypertension at time of treatment (eg, >185 mm Hg systolic or >110 mm Hg diastolic); multilobar cerebral infarction (hypodensity >1/3 cerebral hemisphere); known bleeding diathesis including but not limited to current use of oral anticoagulants with an INR >1.7 (or PT >15 seconds), current use of direct thrombin inhibitors or direct factor Xa inhibitors with elevated sensitive laboratory tests (eg, aPTT, INR, ECT, TT, or appropriate factor Xa activity assays) (See "**Note**"), administration of heparin within 48 hours preceding the onset of stroke with an elevated aPTT greater than the upper limit of normal, or platelet count <100,000/mm^3.

Note: The AHA/ASA guidelines do allow the use of alteplase in patients taking direct thrombin inhibitors (eg, dabigatran) or direct factor Xa inhibitors (eg, rivaroxaban) when sensitive laboratory tests (eg, aPTT, INR, ECT, TT, or appropriate direct factor Xa activity assays) are normal or the patient has not received a dose of these agents for >2 days (assuming normal renal function).

Additional exclusion criteria within clinical trials:

Presentation <3 hours after initial symptoms (NINDS, 1995): Time of symptom onset unknown, rapidly improving or minor symptoms, major surgery within 2 weeks, GI or urinary tract hemorrhage within 3 weeks, aggressive treatment required to lower blood pressure, glucose level <50 or >400 mg/dL, and lumbar puncture within 1 week.

Presentation 3 to 4.5 hours after initial symptoms (ECASS-III; Hacke 2008; AHA/ASA [Jauch 2013]): Age >80 years, time of symptom onset unknown, rapidly improving or minor symptoms, current use of oral anticoagulants regardless of INR, glucose level <50 or >400 mg/dL, aggressive intravenous treatment required to lower blood pressure, major surgery or severe trauma within 3 months, baseline National

Institutes of Health Stroke Scale (NIHSS) score >25 [ie, severe stroke], and history of both stroke and diabetes.

Warnings/Precautions Internal bleeding (intracranial, retroperitoneal, gastrointestinal, genitourinary, respiratory) or external bleeding, especially at arterial and venous puncture, sites may occur (may be fatal). The total dose should not exceed 90 mg for acute ischemic stroke or 100 mg for acute myocardial infarction or pulmonary embolism. Doses ≥150 mg associated with significantly increased risk of intracranial hemorrhage compared to doses ≤100 mg. Bleeding risk is low. Monitor all potential bleeding sites; if serious bleeding occurs, the infusion of alteplase and any other concurrent anticoagulants (eg, heparin) should be stopped. Concurrent heparin anticoagulation may contribute to bleeding. In the treatment of acute ischemic stroke, concurrent use of anticoagulants was not permitted during the initial 24 hours of the <3 hour window trial (NINDS 1995). The AHA/ASA does not recommend initiation of anticoagulant therapy within 24 hours of treatment with alteplase (Jauch 2013). Initiation of SubQ heparin (≤10,000 units) or equivalent doses of low molecular weight heparin for prevention of DVT during the first 24 hours of the 3 to 4.5 hour window trial was permitted and did not increase the incidence of intracerebral hemorrhage (Hacke 2008). For acute PE, withhold heparin during the 2-hour infusion period. Intramuscular injections and nonessential handling of the patient should be avoided. Venipunctures should be performed carefully and only when necessary. Avoid internal jugular and subclavian venous punctures. If arterial puncture is necessary, use an upper extremity vessel that can be manually compressed. Avoid aspirin for 24 hours following administration of alteplase; administration within 24 hours increases the risk of hemorrhagic transformation.

For the following conditions, the risk of bleeding is higher with use of thrombolytics and should be weighed against the benefits of therapy: Recent major surgery or procedure (eg, CABG, obstetrical delivery, organ biopsy, previous puncture of noncompressible vessels), traumatic or prolonged (>10 minutes) CPR (ACCF/AHA [O'Gara 2013]), lumbar puncture within 10 days (ASRA [Horlocker 2012]), cerebrovascular disease, recent intracranial hemorrhage, recent gastrointestinal or genitourinary bleeding, recent trauma, hypertension (adults with systolic BP >175 mm Hg and/or diastolic BP >110 mm Hg), high likelihood of left heart thrombus (eg, mitral stenosis with atrial fibrillation), acute pericarditis, subacute bacterial endocarditis, hemostatic defects including ones caused by severe renal or hepatic dysfunction, significant hepatic dysfunction, advanced age, diabetic hemorrhagic retinopathy or other hemorrhagic ophthalmic conditions, septic thrombophlebitis or occluded AV cannula at seriously infected site and/or any other condition in which bleeding constitutes a significant hazard or would be particularly difficult to manage because of location. Use with caution in patients receiving oral anticoagulants. In the treatment of acute ischemic stroke (AIS) within 3 hours of symptom onset, the current use of oral anticoagulants is a contraindication per the manufacturer. According to the AHA/ASA, the current use of oral anticoagulants producing an INR >1.7, direct thrombin inhibitors, or direct factor Xa inhibitors with elevated sensitive laboratory tests are contraindications. However, alteplase may be administered to patients with AIS having received direct thrombin inhibitors (eg, dabigatran) or direct factor Xa inhibitors (eg, rivaroxaban) when sensitive laboratory tests (eg, aPTT, INR, platelet count, ECT, TT, or appropriate direct factor Xa activity assays) are normal or the patient has not received a dose of these agents for >2 days (assuming normal renal function). When treating AIS 3 to 4.5 hours after symptom onset, the use of alteplase should be avoided with current use of any oral anticoagulant regardless of INR (Jauch 2013). In the treatment of STEMI, adjunctive use of parenteral anticoagulants (eg, enoxaparin, heparin, or fondaparinux) is recommended to improve vessel patency and prevent reocclusion and may also contribute to bleeding; monitor for bleeding (ACCF/AHA; O'Gara 2013). Alteplase has not been shown to treat adequately underlying deep vein thrombosis in patients with PE. Consider the possible risk of re-embolization due to the lysis of underlying deep venous thrombi in this setting.

Coronary thrombolysis may result in reperfusion arrhythmias (eg, accelerated idioventricular rhythm) (Miller 1986). Patients who present **within 3 hours** of stroke symptom onset should be treated with alteplase unless contraindications exist. A longer time window (**3 to 4.5 hours** after symptom onset) has been shown to be safe and efficacious for select individuals (Hacke 2008; AHA/ASA [Jauch 2013]). Treatment of patients with minor neurological deficit or with rapidly improving symptoms is not recommended. Follow standard management for STEMI while infusing alteplase.

Cholesterol embolization has been reported rarely in patients treated with thrombolytic agents. Although typically mild and transient, orolingual angioedema has occurred during and up to 2 hours after alteplase infusion in patients treated for AIS and STEMI. The use of concomitant ACE inhibitors and strokes involving the insular and frontal cortex are associated with an increased risk (Foster-Goldman 2013). The manufacturer recommends monitoring patients during and for several hours after infusion for orolingual angioedema. If angioedema develops, discontinue the infusion and promptly institute appropriate therapy.

Cathflo Activase: When used to restore catheter function, use Cathflo cautiously in those patients with known or suspected catheter infections. Evaluate catheter for other causes of dysfunction before use. Avoid excessive pressure when instilling into catheter.

Some dosage forms may contain polysorbate 80 (also known as Tweens). Hypersensitivity reactions, usually a delayed reaction, have been reported following exposure to pharmaceutical products containing polysorbate 80 in certain individuals (Isaksson 2002; Lucente 2000; Shelley 1995). Thrombocytopenia, ascites, pulmonary deterioration, and renal and hepatic failure have been reported in premature neonates after receiving parenteral products containing polysorbate 80 (Alade 1986; CDC 1984). See manufacturer's labeling.

Warnings: Additional Pediatric Considerations Significant bleeding complications including neonatal IVH and hemorrhage requiring PRBC transfusion have been reported in pediatric patients receiving systemic tPA therapy for thrombolysis (Monagle, 2012; Weiner, 1998).

Adverse Reactions As with all drugs which may affect hemostasis, bleeding is the major adverse effect associated with alteplase. Hemorrhage may occur at virtually any site. Risk is dependent on multiple variables, including the dosage administered, concurrent use of multiple agents which alter hemostasis, and patient predisposition. Rapid lysis of coronary artery thrombi by thrombolytic agents may be associated with reperfusion-related atrial and/or ventricular arrhythmia. **Note:** Lowest rate of bleeding complications expected with dose used to restore catheter function.

Cardiovascular: Hypotension
Central nervous system: Fever
Dermatologic: Bruising
Gastrointestinal: GI hemorrhage, nausea, vomiting
Genitourinary: GU hemorrhage
Hematologic: Bleeding

Local: Bleeding at catheter puncture site

Rare but important or life-threatening: Angioedema (orolingual), intracranial hemorrhage, retroperitoneal hemorrhage, pericardial hemorrhage, gingival hemorrhage, epistaxis, allergic reaction (anaphylaxis, anaphylactoid reactions, laryngeal edema, rash, and urticaria)

Additional cardiovascular events associated **with use in STEMI:** AV block, asystole, bradycardia, cardiac arrest, cardiac tamponade, cardiogenic shock, cholesterol crystal embolization, electromechanical dissociation, heart failure, hemorrhagic bursitis, mitral regurgitation, myocardial rupture, recurrent ischemia/infarction, pericardial effusion, pericarditis, pulmonary edema, ruptured intracranial AV malformation, seizure, thromboembolism, ventricular tachycardia

Additional events associated **with use in pulmonary embolism:** Pleural effusion, pulmonary re-embolization, pulmonary edema, thromboembolism

Additional events associated **with use in stroke:** Cerebral edema, cerebral herniation, new ischemic stroke, seizure

Drug Interactions

Metabolism/Transport Effects None known.

Avoid Concomitant Use There are no known interactions where it is recommended to avoid concomitant use.

Increased Effect/Toxicity

Alteplase may increase the levels/effects of: Anticoagulants; Dabigatran Etexilate; Prostacyclin Analogues

The levels/effects of Alteplase may be increased by: Agents with Antiplatelet Properties; Herbs (Anticoagulant/Antiplatelet Properties); Limaprost; Salicylates

Decreased Effect

The levels/effects of Alteplase may be decreased by: Aprotinin; Nitroglycerin

Storage/Stability

Activase: Store intact vials at room temperature (not to exceed 30°C [86°F]), or under refrigeration at 2°C to 8°C (36°F to 46°F); protect from light. Store reconstituted solution at 2°C to 30°C (36°F to 86°F) and use within 8 hours. Discard any unused solution

Cathflo Activase: Store intact vials at 2°C to 8°C (36°F to 46°F); protect from light. Store reconstituted solution at 2°C to 8°C (36°F to 46°F) and use within 8 hours. Discard any unused solution

Solutions of 0.5 mg/mL, 1 mg/mL, and 2 mg/mL in SWI retained ≥94% of fibrinolytic activity at 48 hours when stored at 2°C in plastic syringes; these solutions retained ≥90% of fibrinolytic activity when stored in plastic syringes at -25°C or -70°C for 7 or 14 days, thawed at room temperature and then stored at 2°C for 48 hours (Davis 2000). Solutions of 1 mg/mL in SWI were stable for 22 weeks in plastic syringes when stored at -30°C and for ~1 month in glass vials when stored at -20°C; bioactivity remained unchanged for 6 months in propylene containers when stored at -20°C and for 2 weeks in glass vials when stored at -70°C (Generali 2001).

Mechanism of Action Initiates local fibrinolysis by binding to fibrin in a thrombus (clot) and converts entrapped plasminogen to plasmin

Pharmacodynamics Duration: >50% present in plasma cleared ~5 minutes after infusion terminated, ~80% cleared within 10 minutes; fibrinolytic activity persists for up to 1 hour after infusion terminated (Semba 2000)

Pharmacokinetics (Adult data unless noted)

Distribution: V_d (initial): Approximates plasma volume

Half-life: Initial: 5 minutes

Elimination: Clearance: Rapidly from circulating plasma; 380 to 570 mL/minute; primarily hepatic; 80% of unbound drug is cleared within 10 minutes

Dosing: Neonatal

Occluded IV catheter: Intracatheter: **Dose listed is per lumen; for multilumen catheters, treat one lumen at a time; do not infuse into patient; dose should always be aspirated out of catheter after dwell.**

Manufacturer's labeling: Central venous catheter: Use a 1 mg/mL concentration; instill a volume equal to 110% of the internal lumen volume of the catheter; do not exceed 2 mg in 2 mL; leave in lumen for up to 2 hours, then aspirate out of catheter; may instill a second dose if catheter remains occluded after 2-hour dwell time

Alternate dosing:

Chest guidelines (Monagle 2008): Limited data available: Central venous catheter: 0.5 mg diluted in NS to a volume equal to the internal volume of the lumen; instill in lumen over 1 to 2 minutes; leave in lumen for 1 to 2 hours, then aspirate out of catheter; flush catheter with NS. **Note:** The most recent guidelines (2012) continue to recommend alteplase as a treatment option but specific dosage recommendation is not provided (Monagle 2012).

Soylu, 2010: Limited data available: Central venous catheter: 0.25 to 0.5 mg/mL solution; instill a volume to fill the catheter; leave in lumen for up to 2 hours, then aspirate out of catheter; dosing described in trial of 18 neonates including four patients with GA ≤32 weeks

Systemic thrombosis: Note: Dose must be titrated to effect. No pediatric studies have compared local to systemic thrombolytic therapy; therefore, there is no evidence to suggest that local infusions are superior. The pediatric patients' small vessel size may increase the chance of local damage to blood vessels and formation of a new thrombus; however, local infusion may be appropriate for catheter-related thrombosis if the catheter is already in place (Monagle 2012). Various "low-dose" regimens have been used, both with local (or regional) and systemic administration.

Standard dose infusion: IV: **Note:** The optimal dose for various thrombotic conditions is not established; most published papers consist of case reports and series; few prospective neonatal studies have been conducted; dose must be titrated to effect (eg, fibrinogen >100 to 150 mg/dL). Administration of FFP may be considered prior to dose infusion. Current *Chest* guidelines recommend use only when major vessel occlusion is causing critical compromise of organs or limbs in the neonate (Monagle, 2012).

Chest guidelines (Monagle 2012): Limited data available: Usual dose: 0.5 mg/kg/**hour** for 6 hours; reported range: 0.1 to 0.6 mg/kg/**hour**; some patients may require longer or shorter duration of therapy. Higher doses may be associated with an increased incidence of serious bleeding (Monagle 2008; Monagle 2012).

Additional reported standard dose regimens:

No loading dose regimens: Very limited data available: Seven neonates (GA: 24 to 38 weeks) with arterial thrombosis received a continuous IV infusion of 0.1 mg/kg/**hour** initially; infusion rate was titrated to maintain fibrinogen levels >100 mg/dL; dosage increases were made in 0.1 mg/kg/**hour** increments every 6 hours to a maximum of 0.4 mg/kg/**hour**; no heparin was used in these patients (Weiner, 1998). In case series of three neonates (GA: 26 to 36 weeks) with infective endocarditis and intracardiac thrombosis, a daily intermittent infusion of 0.2 mg/kg/**hour** over 6 hours for 5 days was used (Anderson, 2009).

Loading dose regimens: Limited data available; dosage reported varies widely: One trial of 16 neonates used a loading dose of 0.1 mg/kg over 10 minutes, followed by an intermittent infusion of 0.3 mg/kg/**hour** infusion for 3 hours every 12 to 24 hours as determined by response and monitoring parameters; a maximum of 4 additional intermittent doses were allowed; heparin was held during alteplase infusion (Farnoux, 1998). In another trial, a loading dose of 0.7 mg/kg bolus over 30 to 60 minutes was used followed by continuous IV infusion at an initial rate of 0.2 mg/kg/**hour** for 1 to 4 days in 13 neonates (GA: 27 to 42 weeks) with catheter-related thrombosis (used in conjunction with heparin infusion); reported effective range: 0.1 to 0.3 mg/kg/**hour** (Hartmann 2001).

Low dose infusion: Very limited data available: Initial dose: IV: 0.02 to 0.03 mg/kg/**hour**, titrate dose based on patient response, range reported 0.01 to 0.06 mg/kg/**hour**; duration of therapy based on patient response. A trial comparing standard-dose and low-dose alteplase in pediatric patients included five neonates (four preterm; PNA 1 to 14 days) with acute thrombus in low-dose group; dosing in neonates was initiated at 0.03 mg/kg/**hour**, in three neonates receiving systemic therapy, the effective dose was 0.03 mg/kg/**hour** in one patient and 0.06 mg/kg/**hour** in the other two patients; the remaining two neonates received local infusions and required a higher infusion rate (0.1 mg/kg/**hour** and 0.24 mg/kg/**hour**); duration of therapy ranged from 48 to 70 hours; complete clot resolution occurred in all patients. One preterm neonate with staphylococcal sepsis experienced a subdural bleed at the dose of 0.24 mg/kg/**hour** (Wang, 2003). One case series of four neonates and infants (PNA: 25 to 43 days, 2 preterm) with caval thrombosis due to central line reported using 0.02 to 0.1 mg/kg/**hour** with mixed results; resolution of clot occurred in only two patients (Anderson 1991).

Dosing: Usual

Pediatric:

Occluded IV catheters: Infants, Children, Adolescents: Intracatheter: **Dose listed is per lumen; for multilumen catheters, treat one lumen at a time; do not infuse into patient; dose should always be aspirated out of catheter after dwell.**

Manufacturer's labeling: Central venous catheter:

Patients <30 kg: Use a 1 mg/mL concentration; instill a volume equal to 110% of the internal lumen volume of the catheter; do not exceed 2 mg in 2 mL; may instill a second dose if catheter remains occluded after 2-hour dwell time

Patients ≥30 kg: 2 mg in 2 mL; may instill second dose if catheter remains occluded after 2-hour dwell time

Chest guidelines (Monagle 2008): **Note:** The most recent guidelines (2012) continue to recommend alteplase as a treatment option but specific dosage recommendation is not provided (Monagle 2012)

Central venous catheter: **Note:** Some institutions use lower doses (eg, 0.25 mg/0.5 mL) in infants 1 to <3 months

Patients ≤10 kg: 0.5 mg diluted in NS to a volume equal to the internal volume of the lumen; instill in lumen over 1 to 2 minutes; leave in lumen for 1 to 2 hours, then **aspirate out of catheter, do not infuse into patient;** flush catheter with NS.

Patients >10 kg: 1 mg in 1 mL of NS; use a volume equal to the internal volume of the lumen; maximum: 2 mg in 2 mL per lumen; instill in each lumen over 1 to 2 minutes; leave in lumen for 1 to 2 hours; then **aspirate out of catheter, do not infuse into patient;** flush catheter with NS

SubQ port:

Patients ≤10 kg: 0.5 mg diluted with NS to 3 mL

Patients >10 kg: 2 mg diluted with NS to 3 mL

Systemic thrombosis: Note: Dose must be titrated to effect. No pediatric studies have compared local to systemic thrombolytic therapy; therefore, there is no evidence to suggest that local infusions are superior. The pediatric patients' small vessel size may increase the chance of local damage to blood vessels and formation of a new thrombus; however, local infusion may be appropriate for catheter-related thromboses if the catheter is already in place (Monagle 2012).

Standard dose infusion: Limited data available; optimal dose not established; most published papers consist of case reports; few prospective pediatric studies have been conducted; several studies have used the following doses (Levy 1991; Weiner 1998): Infants, Children, and Adolescents: *Chest* 2012 and AHA 2013 recommendations: IV: Usual dose: 0.5 mg/kg/**hour** for 6 hours; range: 0.1 to 0.6 mg/kg/**hour**; some patients may require longer or shorter duration of therapy; higher doses may be associated with an increased incidence of serious bleeding (Giglia 2013; Monagle 2008; Monagle 2012).

Low-dose infusion: Limited data available. Various "low-dose" regimens have been used: Infants, Children, and Adolescents:

AHA 2013 recommendations: IV: 0.03 to 0.06 mg/kg/**hour** for 12 to 48 hours; maximum hourly dose: 2 mg/hour (Giglia 2013)

Additional reported regimens: IV:

Wang 2003: Initial: 0.01 to 0.03 mg/kg/**hour**; usual effective range: 0.015 to 0.03 mg/kg/**hour**; duration of therapy based on clinical response; in this study of 17 pediatric patients (1.5 to 18 years) with acute and chronic thrombus, dosing was titrated to effect up to 0.06 mg/kg/**hour** in children and adolescents; final effective range: 0.007 to 0.06 mg/kg/**hour**; administration included systemic therapy as well as local infusions directly at site of thrombus (n=4); duration of therapy ranged from 4 to 96 hours. A similar dosing range has been reported in pediatric case reports (Doyle 1992).

Leary 2010: Initial: 0.03 to 0.06 mg/kg/**hour** for 12 to 48 hours; doses were titrated as necessary up to 0.12 mg/kg/**hour**; dosing from a retrospective study of 23 patients (median age: 12 years, range: 6 months to 21.5 years) diagnosed with DVT; eight patients required a dose increase to 0.12 mg/kg/**hour**; overall response rate: 59%, with complete clot resolution in 18% and partial resolution in 41%

Bratincsák 2013: Initial: 0.05 mg/kg/**hour** for 30 minutes, if no signs of bleeding, rate increased to 0.1 mg/kg/**hour**; therapy used in 12 children with arterial or femoral vascular occlusions following cardiac catheterization

Catheter-directed infusion: Limited data available: Children and Adolescents: Intra-arterial, IV (administered through catheter or via catheter with tip placed at anatomic site of clot): 0.025 mg/kg/**hour** or 0.5 to 2 **mg/hour** for 12 to 24 hours (Giglia 2013)

Parapneumonic effusion: Limited data available: Infants >3 months, Children, and Adolescents: Intrapleural:

Fixed dose: 4 mg in 40 mL NS, first dose at time of chest tube placement with 1-hour dwell time, repeat every 24 hours for 3 days (total of 3 doses) (Bradley 2011; St. Peter 2009)

Weight-directed: 0.1 mg/kg (maximum: 3 mg) in 10 to 30 mL NS, first dose after chest tube placement, 0.75- to 1-hour dwell time, repeat every 8 hours for 3 days (total of 9 doses) (Bradley 2011; Hawkins 2004)

Adult:

ST-elevation myocardial infarction (STEMI): IV (Activase): **Note:** Manufacturer's labeling recommends 3-hour infusion regimen; however, accelerated regimen preferred by the ACCF/AHA (O'Gara 2013).

Accelerated regimen (weight-based):

Patients ≤67 kg: Infuse 15 mg IV bolus over 1 to 2 minutes followed by infusions of 0.75 mg/kg (not to exceed 50 mg) over 30 minutes then 0.5 mg/kg (not to exceed 35 mg) over 1 hour; maximum total dose: 100 mg

Patients >67 kg: Total dose: 100 mg over 1.5 hours; administered as a 15 mg IV bolus over 1 to 2 minutes followed by infusions of 50 mg over 30 minutes, then 35 mg over 1 hour; maximum total dose: 100 mg

Note: Thrombolytic should be administered within 30 minutes of hospital arrival. Generally, there is only a small trend for benefit of therapy after a delay of 12 to 24 hours from symptom onset, but thrombolysis may be considered for selected patients with ongoing ischemic pain and extensive ST elevation; however, primary PCI is preferred in these patients. Administer concurrent aspirin, clopidogrel, and anticoagulant therapy (ie, unfractionated heparin, enoxaparin, or fondaparinux) with alteplase (O'Gara 2013).

Acute massive or submassive pulmonary embolism (PE): IV (Activase): 100 mg over 2 hours; may be administered as a 10 mg bolus followed by 90 mg over 2 hours as was done in patients with submassive PE (Konstantinides 2002). **Note:** Not recommended for submassive PE with minor RV dysfunction, minor myocardial necrosis, and no clinical worsening or low-risk PE (ie, normotensive, no RV dysfunction, normal biomarkers) (Jaff 2011).

Acute ischemic stroke: IV (Activase): Within 3 hours of the onset of symptom onset **or** within 3 to 4.5 hours of symptom onset (Hacke 2008; Jauch 2013): **Note:** Perform noncontrast-enhanced CT or MRI prior to administration. Initiation of anticoagulants (eg, heparin) or antiplatelet agents (eg, aspirin) within 24 hours after starting alteplase is not recommended; however, initiation of aspirin within 24 to 48 hours after stroke onset is recommended (Jauch, 2013). Initiation of SubQ heparin (≤10,000 units) or equivalent doses of low molecular weight heparin for prevention of DVT during the first 24 hours of the 3 to 4.5 hour window trial did not increase incidence of intracerebral hemorrhage (Hacke 2008).

Recommended total dose: 0.9 mg/kg (maximum total dose: 90 mg)

Patients ≤100 kg: Load with 0.09 mg/kg (10% of 0.9 mg/kg dose) as an IV bolus over 1 minute, followed by 0.81 mg/kg (90% of 0.9 mg/kg dose) as a continuous infusion over 60 minutes

Patients >100 kg: Load with 9 mg (10% of 90 mg) as an IV bolus over 1 minute, followed by 81 mg (90% of 90 mg) as a continuous infusion over 60 minutes

Central venous catheter clearance: Intracatheter (Cathflo Activase 1 mg/mL):

Patients <30 kg: 110% of the internal lumen volume of the catheter, not to exceed 2 mg/2 mL; retain in catheter for 0.5 to 2 hours; may instill a second dose if catheter remains occluded

Patients ≥30 kg: 2 mg (2 mL); retain in catheter for 0.5 to 2 hours; may instill a second dose if catheter remains occluded

Dosing adjustment in renal impairment: There are no dosage adjustments provided in manufacturer's labeling.

Dosing adjustment in hepatic impairment: There are no dosage adjustments provided in manufacturer's labeling.

Usual Infusion Concentrations: Pediatric IV infusion: 0.5 mg/mL **or** 1 mg/mL

Preparation for Administration

Intracatheter: Cathflo Activase: Reconstitute with 2.2 mL SWFI; do not reconstitute with bacteriostatic water for injection; allow vial to stand undisturbed so large bubbles may dissipate; swirl gently, do not shake; complete dissolution occurs within 3 minutes. Final concentration: 1 mg/mL.

IV: Activase: Reconstitute vials with supplied diluent (SWFI); do not reconstitute with bacteriostatic water for injection; use large bore needle and syringe to reconstitute 50 mg vial (50 mg vial has a vacuum) and accompanying transfer device to reconstitute 100 mg vial (100 mg vial does not contain vacuum); swirl gently, do not shake; final concentration after reconstitution: 1 mg/mL. Reconstituted solution should be clear or pale yellow and transparent with a pH of 5 to 7.3. The 1 mg/mL solution may be administered or may be diluted further (immediately before use) with an equal volume of NS or D_5W to yield a final concentration of 0.5 mg/mL; swirl gently, do not shake; dilutions to concentrations <0.5 mg/mL are not recommended for routine clinical use; dilutions <0.5 mg/mL using D_5W or SWFI may result in a precipitate (Frazin 1990).

Administration

Parenteral:

Intracatheter: CathFlo Activase: Instill the appropriate dose into the occluded catheter; do not force solution into catheter; leave in lumen; evaluate catheter function (by attempting to aspirate blood) after 30 minutes; if catheter is functional, aspirate 4 to 5 mL of blood out of catheter in patients ≥10 kg or 3 mL in patients <10 kg to remove drug and residual clot, then gently flush catheter with NS; if catheter is still occluded, leave alteplase in lumen and evaluate catheter function after 120 minutes of dwell time; if catheter is functional, aspirate 4 to 5 mL of blood out of catheter in patients ≥10 kg or 3 mL in patients <10 kg and gently flush with NS; if catheter remains occluded after 120 minutes of dwell time, a second dose may be instilled by repeating the above administration procedure. Discard any unused solution (solution does not contain preservatives).

IV: Activase:

Bolus: Bolus dose may be readied using one of the following methods: 1) Remove bolus dose from reconstituted vial using syringe and needle; for 50 mg vial: Do not prime syringe with air, insert needle into vial stopper; for 100 mg vial, insert needle away from puncture mark created by transfer device; 2) Remove bolus dose from a port on the infusion line after priming; 3) Program an infusion pump to deliver the bolus at the beginning of the infusion. Administer over 1 minute followed by infusion.

Infusion: Remaining dose for STEMI, AIS, or total dose for acute pulmonary embolism may be administered as follows: Any quantity of drug not to be administered to the patient must be removed from vial(s) prior to administration of remaining dose.

50 mg vial: Use polyvinyl chloride IV bag or glass vial and infusion set

100 mg vial: Use same puncture site made by transfer device to insert spike end of infusion set and infuse from vial

May also be further diluted in NS or D_5W if desired.

Intrapleural: Instill dose into chest tube at time of chest tube placement and clamp drain. Although the optimum dwell time has not been determined, clinical trials more often have used either a 45 minute (Hawkins 2004) or 1 hour (Rahman 2011; St. Peter 2009) dwell time; after dwell period, release clamp and connect chest tube to continuous suction.

Monitoring Parameters

Systemic use: Blood pressure; CBC, reticulocyte, platelet count; fibrinogen level, plasminogen, fibrin/fibrinogen degradation products, PT, PTT, signs of bleeding

Intracatheter use: Catheter function (by attempting to aspirate blood); signs of sepsis, GI bleeding, bleeding at injection site, and venous thrombosis

Test Interactions Altered results of coagulation and fibrinolytic activity tests

Additional Information Activase and CathFlo Activase also contain L-arginine and phosphoric acid (for pH adjustment).

Advantages of alteplase include: Low immunogenicity, short half-life, direct activation of plasminogen, and a strong and specific affinity for fibrin. Failure of thrombolytic agents in newborns/neonates may occur due to the low plasminogen concentrations (~50% to 70% of adult levels); supplementing plasminogen (via administration of fresh frozen plasma) may possibly help. Osmolality of 1 mg/mL solution is ~215 mOsm/kg.

Dosage Forms Excipient information presented when available (limited, particularly for generics); consult specific product labeling.

Solution Reconstituted, Injection:
Cathflo Activase: 2 mg (1 ea)

Solution Reconstituted, Intravenous:
Activase: 50 mg (1 ea); 100 mg (1 ea)

- **Alteplase, Recombinant** *see* Alteplase *on page 105*
- **Alteplase, Tissue Plasminogen Activator, Recombinant** *see* Alteplase *on page 105*
- **Alti-Flurbiprofen (Can)** *see* Flurbiprofen (Systemic) *on page 915*
- **Alti-Ipratropium (Can)** *see* Ipratropium (Nasal) *on page 1157*
- **Alti-MPA (Can)** *see* MedroxyPROGESTERone *on page 1339*
- **Altoprev** *see* Lovastatin *on page 1305*

Aluminum Acetate (a LOO mi num AS e tate)

Brand Names: US Domeboro [OTC]; Gordon Boro-Packs [OTC]; Pedi-Boro [OTC]

Therapeutic Category Topical Skin Product

Generic Availability (US) Yes, may be product dependent

Use Astringent wet dressing for relief of inflammatory conditions of the skin and to reduce weeping that may occur in dermatitis; relieve minor skin irritations due to poison ivy, poison oak, poison sumac, insect bites, athlete's foot, and rashes caused by soaps, detergents, cosmetics, or jewelry

Pregnancy Considerations Animal reproduction studies have not been conducted. The amount of aluminum acetate available systemically following topical application is unknown.

Breast-Feeding Considerations It is not known if topically administered aluminum acetate is excreted in breast milk.

Warnings/Precautions For external use only; do not cover the treated area with plastic or other material to prevent evaporation. Avoid contact with eyes. Discontinue use if irritation occurs, condition worsens, or if symptoms persist more than 7 days; consult health care provider if irritation or sensitivity increases.

Drug Interactions

Metabolism/Transport Effects None known.

Avoid Concomitant Use

Avoid concomitant use of Aluminum Acetate with any of the following: BCG; BCG (Intravesical)

Increased Effect/Toxicity There are no known significant interactions involving an increase in effect.

Decreased Effect

Aluminum Acetate may decrease the levels/effects of: BCG; BCG (Intravesical); BCG Vaccine (Immunization); Sodium Picosulfate

Storage/Stability Store at room temperature. Protect from excessive heat.

Dosing: Usual Children and Adults: Topical: Soak the affected area in the solution 2-4 times/day for 15-30 minutes or apply wet dressing soaked in the solution 2-4 times/day for 30-minute treatment periods; rewet dressing with solution every few minutes to keep it moist

Preparation for Administration Dissolve 1 to 3 packets in 473 mL (16 oz) of cool or warm water; stir or shake until fully dissolved. Do not strain or filter. One powder packet dissolved in 16 oz of water makes a solution equivalent to a 1:40 dilution, 2 packets: 1:20 dilution, 3 packets: 1:13 dilution.

Administration Topical: Keep away from eyes; for external use only. When used as a compress or wet dressing, soak a clean soft cloth in the solution. Apply cloth loosely to affected area for 15 to 30 minutes.

Dosage Forms Excipient information presented when available (limited, particularly for generics); consult specific product labeling.

Powder, for solution, topical: Aluminum sulfate 1191 mg and calcium acetate 839 mg per packet (12s)
Domeboro: Aluminum sulfate tetradecahydrate 1347 mg and calcium acetate monohydrate 952 mg per packet (12s, 100s)
Gordon Boro-Packs: Aluminum sulfate 49% and calcium acetate 51% per packet (100s)
Pedi-Boro: Aluminum sulfate tetradecahydrate 1191 mg and calcium acetate monohydrate 839 mg per packet (12s, 100s)

Aluminum Hydroxide
(a LOO mi num hye DROKS ide)

Brand Names: US DermaMed [OTC]

Brand Names: Canada Amphojel; Basaljel

Therapeutic Category Antacid; Antidote; Gastrointestinal Agent, Gastric or Duodenal Ulcer Treatment; Protectant, Topical

Generic Availability (US) May be product dependent

Use

Oral: Adjunct for the relief of peptic ulcer pain and to promote healing of peptic ulcers; relief of sour stomach or stomach upset associated with hyperacidity; relief of heartburn; treatment of gastritis, esophagitis, and gastroesophageal reflux disease; reduce phosphate absorption in hyperphosphatemia

Topical: Temporary protection of minor cuts, scrapes, burns, and other skin irritations

Pregnancy Considerations Most aluminum-containing antacids are considered low risk during pregnancy (Mahadevan, 2006).

Warnings/Precautions Oral: Hypophosphatemia may occur with prolonged administration or large doses; aluminum intoxication and osteomalacia may occur in patients with uremia. Use with caution in patients with HF, renal failure, edema, cirrhosis, and low sodium diets, and patients who have recently suffered gastrointestinal hemorrhage; uremic patients not receiving dialysis may develop osteomalacia and osteoporosis due to phosphate depletion.

Elderly may be predisposed to constipation and fecal impaction. Careful evaluation of possible drug interactions must be done. When used as an antacid in ulcer treatment, consider buffer capacity (mEq/mL) to calculate dose.

Topical: Not for application over deep wounds, puncture wounds, infected areas, or lacerations. When used for self medication (OTC use), consult with healthcare provider if needed for >7 days

Adverse Reactions

Gastrointestinal: Constipation, discoloration of feces (white speckles), fecal impaction, nausea, stomach cramps, vomiting

Endocrine & metabolic: Hypomagnesemia, hypophosphatemia

Drug Interactions

Metabolism/Transport Effects None known.

Avoid Concomitant Use

Avoid concomitant use of Aluminum Hydroxide with any of the following: Deferasirox; QuiNINE; Raltegravir; Vitamin D Analogs

Increased Effect/Toxicity

Aluminum Hydroxide may increase the levels/effects of: Amphetamines; Dexmethylphenidate; Methylphenidate

The levels/effects of Aluminum Hydroxide may be increased by: Ascorbic Acid; Calcium Polystyrene Sulfonate; Citric Acid Derivatives; Multivitamins/Fluoride (with ADE); Multivitamins/Minerals (with ADEK, Folate, Iron); Multivitamins/Minerals (with AE, No Iron); Sodium Polystyrene Sulfonate; Vitamin D Analogs

Decreased Effect

Aluminum Hydroxide may decrease the levels/effects of: Allopurinol; Antipsychotic Agents (Phenothiazines); Atazanavir; Bisacodyl; Bismuth Subcitrate; Bisphosphonate Derivatives; Bosutinib; Captopril; Cefditoren; Cefpodoxime; Cefuroxime; Chenodiol; Chloroquine; Cholic Acid; Corticosteroids (Oral); Dabigatran Etexilate; Dabrafenib; Dasatinib; Deferasirox; Deferiprone; Delavirdine; Dolutegravir; Eltrombopag; Elvitegravir; Erlotinib; Ethambutol; Fexofenadine; Fosinopril; Gabapentin; HMG-CoA Reductase Inhibitors; Hyoscyamine; Iron Salts; Isoniazid; Itraconazole; Ketoconazole (Systemic); Ledipasvir; Levothyroxine; Mequitazine; Mesalamine; Methenamine; Multivitamins/Fluoride (with ADE); Mycophenolate; Nilotinib; PAZOPanib; PenicillAMINE; Phosphate Supplements; Potassium Acid Phosphate; QuiNINE; Quinolone Antibiotics; Raltegravir; Rilpivirine; Riociguat; Sotalol; Strontium Ranelate; Sulpiride; Tetracycline Derivatives; Trientine; Ursodiol

Storage/Stability Store at controlled room temperature. Avoid freezing.

Mechanism of Action As an antacid, aluminum hydroxide neutralizes hydrochloride in the stomach to form $Al(Cl)_3$ salt + H_2O, resulting in increased gastric pH and inhibition of pepsin activity (Weberg, 1998). As an agent for the short term treatment of hyperphosphatemia (off-label use), aluminum hydroxide binds phosphate in the gastrointestinal tract preventing absorption of phosphate (Schucker, 2005).

Pharmacodynamics

Duration: Dependent on gastric emptying time

Fasting state: 20-60 minutes

One hour after meals: Up to 3 hours

Pharmacokinetics (Adult data unless noted) Elimination: Excreted by the kidneys (normal renal function): 17% to 30%; combines with dietary phosphate in the intestine and is excreted in the feces

Dosing: Usual

Oral:

Antacid:

Children: 300-900 mg between meals and at bedtime

Adolescents and Adults: 600-1200 mg between meals and at bedtime; or 600 mg 5-6 times/day between meals; maximum daily dose: 3600 mg/day; do not use maximum daily dose for more than 2 weeks without physician consultation

Hyperphosphatemia associated with chronic renal failure:

Children: 30 mg/kg/day in divided doses 3 or 4 times/day; maximum daily dose: 3000 mg/day; titrate to normal serum phosphorus level

Adolescents and Adults: 300-600 mg 3 or 4 times/day; maximum daily dose: 3000 mg/day

Topical: Apply to affected area as needed; reapply at least every 12 hours

Administration

Oral: Shake suspension well before use; dose should be followed with water

Antacid: Administer 1-3 hours after meals

To decrease phosphorus: Administer within 20 minutes of a meal

Topical: For external use only

Monitoring Parameters Monitor for GI complaints, stool frequency; serum phosphate and serum aluminum concentrations in patients with chronic kidney disease

Reference Range Baseline serum aluminum level <20 mcg/L

Additional Information Sodium content of ALternaGel®: <0.11 mEq per 5 mL

Dosage Forms Excipient information presented when available (limited, particularly for generics); consult specific product labeling.

Ointment, External:

DermaMed: (113 g)

Suspension, Oral:

Generic: 320 mg/5 mL (473 mL)

Aluminum Hydroxide and Magnesium Hydroxide

(a LOO mi num hye DROKS ide & mag NEE zhum hye DROK side)

Brand Names: US Mag-Al [OTC]

Brand Names: Canada Diovol; Diovol Ex; Gelusil Extra Strength; Mylanta

Therapeutic Category Antacid; Gastrointestinal Agent, Gastric or Duodenal Ulcer Treatment

Generic Availability (US) No

Use Adjunct for the relief of heartburn, peptic ulcer pain, and to promote healing of peptic ulcers; relief of stomach upset associated with hyperacidity

Pregnancy Considerations Most aluminum- and magnesium-containing antacids are considered low risk during pregnancy (Mahadevan 2006).

Breast-Feeding Considerations Most aluminum- and magnesium-containing antacids are considered low risk in nursing women (Mahadevan 2006).

Contraindications OTC labeling: When used for self-medication, do not use if you have renal impairment

Warnings/Precautions Prolonged antacid therapy may result in hypophosphatemia; aluminum in antacid may form insoluble complexes with phosphate leading to decreased phosphate absorption in the GI tract. Rarely, severe hypophosphatemia can lead to anorexia, muscle weakness, malaise, and osteomalacia. Use with caution in patients with renal impairment; avoid use in severe renal impairment; hypermagnesemia or aluminum intoxication may occur in severe renal impairment, particularly with prolonged use. Aluminum intoxication may lead to osteomalacia or dialysis encephalopathy. Potentially significant interactions may exist, requiring dose or frequency adjustment, additional monitoring, and/or selection of alternative therapy. Some dosage forms may contain propylene glycol; large amounts are potentially toxic and have been associated hyperosmolality, lactic acidosis, seizures and respiratory depression; use caution (AAP 1997; Zar 2007).

Self-medication (OTC use): When used for self-medication, patients should be instructed to consult their healthcare prescriber prior to using if they are on a magnesium and/or sodium restricted diet. Do not take the maximum dose for >14 days.

Warnings: Additional Pediatric Considerations Some dosage forms may contain propylene glycol; in neonates large amounts of propylene glycol delivered orally, intravenously (eg, >3,000 mg/day), or topically have been associated with potentially fatal toxicities which can include metabolic acidosis, seizures, renal failure, and CNS depression; toxicities have also been reported in children and adults including hyperosmolality, lactic acidosis, seizures and respiratory depression; use caution (AAP, 1997; Shehab, 2009).

Adverse Reactions

Gastrointestinal: Constipation, chalky taste, cramping, fecal discoloration (white speckles), fecal impaction, nausea, vomiting

Endocrine & metabolic: Hypophosphatemia (rare), hypermagnesemia (rare)

Drug Interactions

Metabolism/Transport Effects None known.

Avoid Concomitant Use

Avoid concomitant use of Aluminum Hydroxide and Magnesium Hydroxide with any of the following: Calcium Polystyrene Sulfonate; Deferasirox; QuiNINE; Raltegravir; Sodium Polystyrene Sulfonate; Vitamin D Analogs

Increased Effect/Toxicity

Aluminum Hydroxide and Magnesium Hydroxide may increase the levels/effects of: Amphetamines; Calcium Channel Blockers; Calcium Polystyrene Sulfonate; Dexmethylphenidate; Gabapentin; Methylphenidate; Misoprostol; Neuromuscular-Blocking Agents; QuiNIDine; Sodium Polystyrene Sulfonate

The levels/effects of Aluminum Hydroxide and Magnesium Hydroxide may be increased by: Ascorbic Acid; Calcium Channel Blockers; Citric Acid Derivatives; Multivitamins/Fluoride (with ADE); Multivitamins/Minerals (with ADEK, Folate, Iron); Multivitamins/Minerals (with AE, No Iron); Vitamin D Analogs

Decreased Effect

Aluminum Hydroxide and Magnesium Hydroxide may decrease the levels/effects of: Allopurinol; Alpha-Lipoic Acid; Antipsychotic Agents (Phenothiazines); Atazanavir; Bisacodyl; Bismuth Subcitrate; Bisphosphonate Derivatives; Bosutinib; Captopril; Cefditoren; Cefpodoxime; Cefuroxime; Chenodiol; Chloroquine; Cholic Acid; Corticosteroids (Oral); Dabigatran Etexilate; Dabrafenib; Dasatinib; Deferasirox; Deferiprone; Delavirdine; Dolutegravir; Eltrombopag; Elvitegravir; Erlotinib; Ethambutol; Fexofenadine; Fosinopril; Gabapentin; HMG-CoA Reductase Inhibitors; Hyoscyamine; Iron Salts; Isoniazid; Itraconazole; Ketoconazole (Systemic); Ledipasvir; Levothyroxine; Mequitazine; Mesalamine; Methenamine; Multivitamins/Fluoride (with ADE); Mycophenolate; Nilotinib; PAZOPanib; PenicillAMINE; Phosphate Supplements; Potassium Acid Phosphate; QuiNINE; Quinolone Antibiotics; Raltegravir; Rilpivirine; Riociguat; Sotalol; Strontium Ranelate; Sulpiride; Tetracycline Derivatives; Trientine; Ursodiol

The levels/effects of Aluminum Hydroxide and Magnesium Hydroxide may be decreased by: Alpha-Lipoic Acid; Trientine

Storage/Stability Store at room temperature; avoid freezing.

Pharmacodynamics Duration: Dependent on gastric emptying time

Fasting state: 20-60 minutes

1 hour after meals: May be up to 3 hours

Dosing: Usual Note: Chronic administration is not recommended in children (Rudolph, 2001); dosing information for children is limited; very few published clinical trials are available. The following pediatric dosing represents suggestions from review articles (for children <12 years) or product labeling (children ≥12 years):

Liquid (aluminum hydroxide 200 mg and magnesium hydroxide 200 mg per 5 mL):

Children <12 years: 0.5-1 mL/kg/dose after meals and at bedtime (maximum dose: 15 mL) (Orenstein, 1988)

Children ≥12 years and Adults: 10-20 mL 4 times/day (maximum daily dose: 80 mL/day)

Suspension (aluminum hydroxide 500 mg and magnesium hydroxide 500 mg per 5 mL): Children ≥12 years and Adults: 10-20 mL 4 times/day, between meals and at bedtime (maximum daily dose: 45 mL/day)

Tablet (aluminum hydroxide 300 mg and magnesium hydroxide 150 mg):

Children 6-11 years: 1-2 tablets 4 times/day

Children ≥12 years and Adults: 1-2 tablets after meals and at bedtime, or as needed (maximum: 16 tablets/day)

Administration Oral:

Liquid, suspension: Shake suspensions well before use; administer 1-2 hours after meals when stomach acidity is highest

Tablet: Chew tablets thoroughly before swallowing or allow tablets to dissolve slowly in mouth; follow by a full glass of water

Monitoring Parameters GI complaints, stool frequency; serum phosphate concentrations in patients on hemodialysis receiving chronic aluminum-containing antacid therapy; serum electrolytes in patients with renal impairment receiving magnesium-containing antacids

Dosage Forms Excipient information presented when available (limited, particularly for generics); consult specific product labeling. [DSC] = Discontinued product

Liquid, oral:

Mag-Al: Aluminum hydroxide 200 mg and magnesium hydroxide 200 mg per 5 mL (30 mL) [dye free, ethanol free, sugar free; contains propylene glycol, sodium 4 mg/5 mL; peppermint flavor]

◆ **Aluminum Sucrose Sulfate, Basic** *see* Sucralfate *on page 1978*

◆ **Aluminum Sulfate and Calcium Acetate** *see* Aluminum Acetate *on page 110*

◆ **Aluminum Sulfate Tetradecahydrate and Calcium Acetate** *see* Aluminum Acetate *on page 110*

◆ **Alupent** *see* Metaproterenol *on page 1374*

◆ **Alvesco** *see* Ciclesonide (Oral Inhalation) *on page 456*

Amantadine (a MAN ta deen)

Medication Safety Issues

Sound-alike/look-alike issues:

Amantadine may be confused with amiodarone, ranitidine, rimantadine

Symmetrel may be confused with Synthroid®

Brand Names: Canada Dom-Amantadine; Mylan-Amantadine; PHL-Amantadine; PMS-Amantadine

Therapeutic Category Anti-Parkinson's Agent (Dopamine Agonist); Antiviral Agent; Antiviral Agent, Adamantane

Generic Availability (US) Yes

Use Prophylaxis and treatment of influenza A viral infection (FDA approved in ages ≥1 year and adults); **Note:** Due to high resistance rates, amantadine is no longer recommended by the CDC for the treatment or prophylaxis of influenza A (CDC, 2011); symptomatic and adjunct treatment of parkinsonism; treatment of drug-induced extrapyramidal reactions (FDA approved in adults); has also been used for attention-deficit/hyperactivity disorder (ADHD), autism, fatigue associated with multiple sclerosis, and in post-traumatic brain injury for behavior and cognition

Pregnancy Risk Factor C

Pregnancy Considerations Teratogenic effects were observed in animal studies and in case reports in humans.

Influenza infection may be more severe in pregnant women. Untreated influenza infection is associated with an increased risk of adverse events to the fetus and an increased risk of complications or death to the mother. Oseltamivir and zanamivir are currently recommended for the treatment or prophylaxis influenza in pregnant women and women up to 2 weeks postpartum. Antiviral agents are currently recommended as an adjunct to vaccination and should not be used as a substitute for vaccination in pregnant women (consult current CDC guidelines).

Healthcare providers are encouraged to refer women exposed to influenza vaccine, or who have taken an antiviral medication during pregnancy to the Vaccines and Medications in Pregnancy Surveillance System (VAMPSS) by contacting The Organization of Teratology Information Specialists (OTIS) at (877) 311-8972

Breast-Feeding Considerations The CDC recommends that women infected with the influenza virus follow general precautions (eg, frequent hand washing) to decrease viral transmission to the child. Mothers with influenza-like illnesses at delivery should consider avoiding close contact with the infant until they have received 48 hours of antiviral medication, fever has resolved, and cough and secretions can be controlled. These measures may help decrease (but not eliminate) the risk of transmitting influenza to the newborn during breast-feeding. During this time, breast milk can be expressed and bottle-fed to the infant by another person who is not infected. Protective measures, such as wearing a face mask, changing into a clean gown or clothing, and strict hand hygiene should be continued by the mother for ≥7 days after the onset of symptoms or until symptom-free for 24 hours. Infant care should be performed by a noninfected person when possible (consult current CDC guidelines).

Contraindications Hypersensitivity to amantadine or any component of the formulation

Warnings/Precautions May cause CNS depression, which may impair physical or mental abilities; patients must be cautioned about performing tasks which require mental alertness (eg, operating machinery or driving). Effects may be potentiated when used with other sedative drugs or ethanol. There have been reports of suicidal ideation/attempt in patients with and without a history of psychiatric illness. Use with caution in patients with liver disease, a history of recurrent and eczematoid dermatitis, uncontrolled psychosis or severe psychoneurosis, seizures and in those receiving CNS stimulant drugs; reduce dose in renal disease; when treating Parkinson's disease, do not discontinue abruptly. In many patients, the therapeutic benefits of amantadine are limited to a few months. Abrupt discontinuation may cause agitation, anxiety, delirium, delusions, depression, hallucinations, paranoia, parkinsonian crisis, slurred speech, or stupor. Upon discontinuation of amantadine therapy, gradually taper dose. Elderly patients may be more susceptible to the CNS effects (using 2 divided daily doses may minimize this effect); may require dosage reductions based on renal function. Use with caution in patients with HF, peripheral edema, or orthostatic hypotension; dosage reduction may be required. Avoid in untreated angle closure glaucoma.

Dopamine agonists have been associated with compulsive behaviors and/or loss of impulse control, which has manifested as pathological gambling, libido increases (hypersexuality), and/or binge eating. Causality has not been established, and controversy exists as to whether this phenomenon is related to the underlying disease, prior behaviors/addictions, and/or drug therapy. Dose reduction or discontinuation of therapy has been reported to reverse these behaviors in some, but not all cases. Risk for melanoma development is increased in Parkinson's disease patients; drug causation or factors contributing to risk have not been established. Patients should be monitored closely and periodic skin examinations should be performed. Tolerance has also been reported with long-term use (Zubenko, 1984).

Due to increased resistance, the ACIP has recommended that rimantadine and amantadine no longer be used for the treatment or prophylaxis of influenza A in the United States until susceptibility has been re-established; consult current guidelines.

Some dosage forms may contain propylene glycol; large amounts are potentially toxic and have been associated hyperosmolality, lactic acidosis, seizures and respiratory depression; use caution (AAP, 1997; Zar, 2007).

Adverse Reactions

Cardiovascular: Livedo reticularis, orthostatic hypotension, peripheral edema

Central nervous system: Abnormal dreams, agitation, anxiety, ataxia, confusion, delirium, depression, dizziness, drowsiness, fatigue, hallucination, headache, insomnia, irritability, nervousness

Gastrointestinal: Anorexia, constipation, diarrhea, nausea, xerostomia

Respiratory: Dry nose

Rare but important or life-threatening: Abnormal gait, acute respiratory tract failure, aggressive behavior, agranulocytosis, amnesia, anaphylaxis, cardiac arrest, cardiac arrhythmia, cardiac failure, coma, decreased libido, delusions, diaphoresis, dysphagia, dyspnea, eczema, EEG pattern changes, euphoria, fever, hyperkinesia, hypersensitivity reaction, hypertension, hypertonia, hypokinesia, hypotension, increased blood urea nitrogen, increased creatine phosphokinase, increased gamma-glutamyl transferase, increased lactate dehydrogenase, increased serum alkaline phosphatase, increased serum ALT, increased serum AST, increased serum bilirubin, increased serum creatinine, keratitis, leukocytosis, leukopenia, mania, muscle spasm, mydriasis, neuroleptic malignant syndrome (associated with dosage reduction or abrupt withdrawal of amantadine), neutropenia, oculogyric crisis, paranoia, paresthesia, pruritus, psychosis, pulmonary edema, seizure, skin photosensitivity, skin rash, slurred speech, stupor, suicidal ideation, suicide, suicide attempt, tachycardia, tachypnea, tremor, urinary retention, visual disturbance, vomiting, weakness

Drug Interactions

Metabolism/Transport Effects Substrate of OCT2

Avoid Concomitant Use

Avoid concomitant use of Amantadine with any of the following: Amisulpride

Increased Effect/Toxicity

Amantadine may increase the levels/effects of: BuPROPion; Glycopyrrolate; Highest Risk QTc-Prolonging Agents; Memantine; Moderate Risk QTc-Prolonging Agents; Trimethoprim

The levels/effects of Amantadine may be increased by: Alcohol (Ethyl); BuPROPion; MAO Inhibitors; Methylphenidate; Mifepristone; Trimethoprim

Decreased Effect

Amantadine may decrease the levels/effects of: Amisulpride; Antipsychotic Agents (First Generation [Typical]); Influenza Virus Vaccine (Live/Attenuated)

The levels/effects of Amantadine may be decreased by: Amisulpride; Antipsychotic Agents (First Generation [Typical]); Antipsychotic Agents (Second Generation [Atypical]); Metoclopramide

Storage/Stability Store at 25°C (77°F); excursions permitted to 15°C to 30°C (59°F to 86°F).

Mechanism of Action

Antiviral:

The mechanism of amantadine's antiviral activity has not been fully elucidated. It appears to primarily prevent the release of infectious viral nucleic acid into the host cell by interfering with the transmembrane domain of the viral M2 protein. Amantadine is also known to prevent viral assembly during replication. Amantadine inhibits the replication of influenza A virus isolates from each of the subtypes (ie, H1N1, H2N2 and H3N2), but has very little or no activity against influenza B virus isolates.

Parkinson disease:

The exact mechanism of amantadine in the treatment of Parkinson disease and drug-induced extrapyramidal reactions is not known. Data from early animal studies suggest that amantadine may have direct and indirect effects on dopamine neurons; however, recent studies have demonstrated that amantadine is a weak, noncompetitive NMDA receptor antagonist. Although amantadine has not been shown to possess direct anticholinergic activity, clinically, it exhibits anticholinergic-like side effects (dry mouth, urinary retention, and constipation).

Pharmacokinetics (Adult data unless noted)

Absorption: Well absorbed

Distribution: V_d: Normal: 1.5-6.1 L/kg; Renal failure: 5.1 ± 0.2 L/kg; in saliva, tear film, and nasal secretions; in animals, tissue (especially lung) concentrations higher than serum concentrations; crosses blood-brain barrier

Protein binding: Normal renal function: ~67%; Hemodialysis: ~59%

Metabolism: Not appreciable; small amounts of an acetyl metabolite identified

Bioavailability: 86% to 90%

Half-life: Normal renal function: 16 ± 6 hours (9-31 hours); Healthy, older (≥60 years) males: 29 hours (range: 20-41 hours); End-stage renal disease: 7-10 days

Time to peak serum concentration: 2-4 hours

Elimination: Urine (80% to 90% unchanged) by glomerular filtration and tubular secretion

Dialysis: Negligible amounts removed

Dosing: Usual

Pediatric:

Attention-deficit/hyperactivity disorder (ADHD): Limited data available: Oral: Children ≥5 years and Adolescents: Initial: 50 mg/**day**; titrate up at 4-7 day intervals in 50 mg increments to effect; reported range: 50-150 mg/**day** in divided doses 1-3 times daily (morning, noon, and 4 PM); maximum daily dose (weight-dependent): <30 kg: 100 mg/**day**; ≥30 kg: 150 mg/**day** (Donfrancecso, 2007; King, 2001; Mohammadi, 2010); dosing based on two small open-label trials (n=24, n=20; age range: 5-14 years) which suggested improvements in symptoms and ADHD outcome scores; a comparison trial with methylphenidate (n=40) did not detect differences in efficacy between the treatment groups (Mohammadi, 2010).

Autism (hyperactivity, irritability): Limited data available: Oral: Children ≥5 years and Adolescents: Initial: 2.5 mg/kg/dose once daily for 1 week, then increase to 2.5 mg/kg/dose twice daily; maximum daily dose: 200 mg/**day**; dosing based on short-term (4-week) double-blind, placebo-controlled trial of 39 pediatric patients (treatment group, n=19) which showed improvement in clinician-rated behavioral and hyperactivity ratings (King, 2001a).

Influenza A treatment/prophylaxis: Oral: **Note:** Due to issues of resistance, amantadine is no longer recommended for the treatment or prophylaxis of influenza A. Please refer to the current ACIP recommendations. The following is based on the manufacturer's labeling and ACIP recommendations:

Influenza A treatment:

1-9 years: 5 mg/kg/**day** in 2 divided doses (manufacturer's labeling: 4.4-8.8 mg/kg/**day**); maximum daily dose: 150 mg/**day**

≥10 years and <40 kg: 5 mg/kg/**day** in 2 divided doses (CDC, 2011)

≥10 years and ≥40 kg: 100 mg twice daily (CDC, 2011)

Note: Initiate within 24-48 hours after onset of symptoms; continue for 24-48 hours after symptom resolution (duration of therapy is generally 3-5 days)

Influenza A prophylaxis: Refer to "Influenza A treatment" dosing

Note: Continue prophylaxis throughout the peak influenza activity in the community or throughout the entire influenza season in patients who cannot be vaccinated. Development of immunity following vaccination takes ~2 weeks; amantadine therapy should be considered for high-risk patients from the time of vaccination until immunity has developed. For ages <9 years receiving influenza vaccine for the first time, amantadine prophylaxis should continue for 6 weeks (4 weeks after the first dose and 2 weeks after the second dose).

Multiple-sclerosis associated lassitude (fatigue): Limited data available (Pohl, 2007): Oral:

<10 years or weight <40 kg: 2.5 mg/kg/dose twice daily; maximum daily dose: 150 mg/**day**

≥10 years and weight ≥40 kg: 100 mg twice daily, may titrate dose to clinical response; maximum daily dose: 400 mg/**day**

Traumatic brain injury (TBI): Limited data available: Oral:

Children ≥6 years and Adolescents <16 years: 4-6 mg/kg/**day** in 2 divided doses; maximum daily dose (age or weight dependent): If <10 years or <40 kg: 150 mg/**day**; if ≥10 years or ≥40 kg: 200 mg/**day** (Beers, 2005; McMahon, 2009). While total daily dose similar in trials, the reported dosing approaches and efficacy results are variable (eg, timing of therapy initiation, duration of study, outcome measures) (Williams, 2007). In an open-label, case-controlled trial of 27 pediatric patients with TBI within the last 24 months prior to enrollment (n=17 amantadine treatment, n=10 controls), patients received 5 mg/kg/**day** for entire study period of 12 weeks; results showed improvement in behavior (parental report) and a subset analysis suggested therapy more effective on cognition for those with more recent injury (Beers, 2005). In a double-blind, placebo-controlled crossover trial of seven pediatric patients (mean age: 12.7 years) with TBI within last 12 weeks prior to enrollment, therapy was initiated at 4 mg/kg/**day** up to 300 mg/**day** for 1 week, and increased to 6 mg/kg/**day** up to 400 mg/**day** for Weeks 2 and 3 of the study duration; improved consciousness observed during treatment period of study (McMahon, 2009; Vargus-Adams, 2010).

Adolescents ≥16 years: Initial: 100 mg twice daily for 14 days; on Week 3 increase to 150 mg twice daily; may further increase to 200 mg twice daily on Week 4 if needed; dosing based on a multicenter, double-blind, placebo-controlled trial of 184 patients (age range: 16-65 years; treatment group, n= 87) which showed 4 weeks of amantadine therapy initiated at 4-16 weeks postinjury increased the rate of functional recovery (Giacino, 2012).

Adult:

Drug-induced extrapyramidal symptoms: Oral: 100 mg twice daily; may increase to 300 mg/day in divided doses, if needed

Parkinson's disease: Oral: Usual dose: 100 mg twice daily as monotherapy; may increase to 400 mg/day in divided doses, if needed, with close monitoring

Note: Patients with a serious concomitant illness or those receiving high doses of other antiparkinson drugs should be started at 100 mg/day; may increase to 100 mg twice daily, if needed, after one to several weeks

Influenza A treatment/prophylaxis: Oral: **Note:** Due to issues of resistance, amantadine is no longer recommended for the treatment or prophylaxis of influenza A. Please refer to the current ACIP recommendations. The following is based on the manufacturer's labeling:

Influenza A treatment: 200 mg once daily **or** 100 mg twice daily (may be preferred to reduce CNS effects)

Note: Initiate within 24-48 hours after onset of symptoms; continue for 24-48 hours after symptom resolution (duration of therapy is generally 3-5 days)

Influenza A prophylaxis: 200 mg once daily **or** 100 mg twice daily (may be preferred to reduce CNS effects)

Note: Continue prophylaxis throughout the peak influenza activity in the community or throughout the entire influenza season in patients who cannot be vaccinated. Development of immunity following vaccination takes ~2 weeks; amantadine therapy should be considered for high-risk patients from the time of vaccination until immunity has developed.

Dosing interval in renal impairment: Adults:

CrCl 30-50 mL/minute: Administer 200 mg on day 1, then 100 mg/day

CrCl 15-29 mL/minute: Administer 200 mg on day 1, then 100 mg on alternate days

CrCl <15 mL/minute: Administer 200 mg every 7 days

Hemodialysis: Administer 200 mg every 7 days

Peritoneal dialysis: No supplemental dose is needed

Continuous arteriovenous or venous-venous hemofiltration: No supplemental dose is needed

Administration Oral: May be taken without regard to food. For regimens with multiple daily dosing, timing of doses may vary based upon patient tolerance (eg, if insomnia develops, administer evening dose several hours before bedtime) and use [for ADHD, administer morning and noon; if thrice daily dosing, last dose should be given around 4 PM (Mohammadi, 2010)].

Monitoring Parameters Renal function; mental status, monitor for signs of neurotoxicity; periodic skin exam for melanoma, blood pressure

Test Interactions May interfere with urine detection of amphetamines/methamphetamines (false-positive).

Dosage Forms Excipient information presented when available (limited, particularly for generics); consult specific product labeling.

Capsule, Oral, as hydrochloride:
Generic: 100 mg

Syrup, Oral, as hydrochloride:
Generic: 50 mg/5 mL (10 mL, 473 mL)

Tablet, Oral, as hydrochloride:
Generic: 100 mg

- ◆ **Amantadine Hydrochloride** *see* Amantadine *on page 112*
- ◆ **Ambien** *see* Zolpidem *on page 2220*
- ◆ **Ambien CR** *see* Zolpidem *on page 2220*
- ◆ **AmBisome** *see* Amphotericin B (Liposomal) *on page 153*
- ◆ **AmBisome® (Can)** *see* Amphotericin B (Liposomal) *on page 153*
- ◆ **A-Methapred** *see* MethylPREDNISolone *on page 1409*
- ◆ **A-Methapred** *see* MethylPREDNISolone *on page 1409*
- ◆ **Amethocaine Hydrochloride** *see* Tetracaine (Ophthalmic) *on page 2034*
- ◆ **Amethocaine Hydrochloride** *see* Tetracaine (Systemic) *on page 2034*
- ◆ **Amethocaine Hydrochloride** *see* Tetracaine (Topical) *on page 2035*
- ◆ **Amethopterin** *see* Methotrexate *on page 1390*
- ◆ **Ametop (Can)** *see* Tetracaine (Topical) *on page 2035*
- ◆ **Amicar** *see* Aminocaproic Acid *on page 121*
- ◆ **Amidate** *see* Etomidate *on page 819*

Amifostine (am i FOS teen)

Medication Safety Issues

Sound-alike/look-alike issues:

Ethyol may be confused with ethanol

Related Information

Prevention of Chemotherapy-Induced Nausea and Vomiting in Children *on page 2368*

Brand Names: US Ethyol

Brand Names: Canada Ethyol

Therapeutic Category Antidote, Cisplatin; Cytoprotective Agent

Generic Availability (US) Yes

Use Reduction of cumulative renal toxicity associated with repeated administration of cisplatin in patients with advanced ovarian cancer (FDA approved in adults); reduction of moderate to severe xerostomia from radiation treatment of the head and neck where the radiation port includes a substantial portion of the parotid glands (FDA approved in adults); has also been used as a cytoprotective agent to selectively protect normal tissues against toxicity due to cytotoxic chemotherapy

Pregnancy Risk Factor C

Pregnancy Considerations Animal studies have demonstrated embryotoxicity. There are no adequate and well-controlled studies in pregnant women.

Breast-Feeding Considerations Due to the potential for adverse reactions in the nursing infant, breast-feeding should be discontinued.

Contraindications Hypersensitivity to aminothiol compounds or any component of the formulation

Warnings/Precautions Patients who are hypotensive or dehydrated should not receive amifostine. Interrupt antihypertensive therapy for 24 hours before treatment; patients who cannot safely stop their antihypertensives 24 hours before, should not receive amifostine. Adequately hydrated prior to treatment and keep in a supine position during infusion. Monitor blood pressure every 5 minutes during the infusion. If hypotension requiring interruption of therapy occurs, patients should be placed in the Trendelenburg position and given an infusion of normal saline using a separate IV line; subsequent infusions may require a dose reduction. Infusions >15 minutes are associated with a higher incidence of adverse effects. Use caution in patients with cardiovascular and cerebrovascular disease and any other patients in whom the adverse effects of hypotension may have serious adverse events.

Serious cutaneous reactions, including erythema multiforme, Stevens-Johnson syndrome, toxic epidermal necrolysis, toxoderma and exfoliative dermatitis have been reported with amifostine. May be delayed, developing up to weeks after treatment initiation. Cutaneous reactions have been reported more frequently when used as a radioprotectant. Discontinue treatment for severe/serious cutaneous reaction, or with fever. Withhold treatment and obtain dermatologic consultation for rash involving lips or mucosa (of unknown etiology outside of radiation port) and for bullous, edematous or erythematous lesions on hands, feet, or trunk; reinitiate only after careful evaluation.

Amifostine doses >300 mg/m^2 are associated with a moderate emetic potential (Dupuis, 2011). It is recommended that antiemetic medication, including dexamethasone 20 mg IV and a serotonin 5-HT$_3$ receptor antagonist be administered prior to and in conjunction with amifostine. Rare hypersensitivity reactions, including anaphylaxis and allergic reaction, have been reported; discontinue if allergic reaction occurs; do not rechallenge. Medications for the treatment of hypersensitivity reactions should be available.

Reports of clinically-relevant hypocalcemia are rare, but serum calcium levels should be monitored in patients at risk of hypocalcemia, such as those with nephrotic syndrome; may require calcium supplementation. Should not be used (in patients receiving chemotherapy for malignancies other than ovarian cancer) where chemotherapy is expected to provide significant survival benefit or in patients receiving definitive radiotherapy, unless within the context of a clinical trial.

Adverse Reactions

Cardiovascular: Hypotension

Endocrine & metabolic: Hypocalcemia

Gastrointestinal: Nausea/vomiting

Rare but important or life-threatening: Apnea, anaphylactoid reactions, anaphylaxis, arrhythmia, atrial fibrillation, atrial flutter, back pain, bradycardia, cardiac arrest, chest pain, chest tightness, chills, cutaneous eruptions, dizziness, erythema multiforme, exfoliative dermatitis, extrasystoles, dyspnea, fever, flushing, hiccups, hypersensitivity reactions (fever, rash, hypoxia, dyspnea, laryngeal edema), hypertension (transient), hypoxia, malaise, MI, myocardial ischemia, pruritus, rash (mild), renal failure, respiratory arrest, rigors, seizure, sneezing, somnolence, Stevens-Johnson syndrome, supraventricular tachycardia, syncope, tachycardia, toxic epidermal necrolysis, toxoderma, urticaria

Drug Interactions

Metabolism/Transport Effects None known.

Avoid Concomitant Use There are no known interactions where it is recommended to avoid concomitant use.

Increased Effect/Toxicity

The levels/effects of Amifostine may be increased by: Antihypertensives

Decreased Effect There are no known significant interactions involving a decrease in effect.

Storage/Stability Store intact vials of lyophilized powder at room temperature of 20°C to 25°C (68°F to 77°F). Reconstituted solutions (500 mg/10 mL) and solutions for infusion are chemically stable for up to 5 hours at room temperature (25°C) or up to 24 hours under refrigeration (2°C to 8°C).

Mechanism of Action Prodrug that is dephosphorylated by alkaline phosphatase in tissues to a pharmacologically-active free thiol metabolite. The free thiol is available to bind to, and detoxify, reactive metabolites of cisplatin; and can also act as a scavenger of free radicals that may be generated (by cisplatin or radiation therapy) in tissues.

Pharmacokinetics (Adult data unless noted)

Distribution: V_d: 6.4 L; unmetabolized prodrug is largely confined to the intravascular compartment; active metabolite is distributed into normal tissues with high concentrations in bone marrow, GI mucosa, skin, liver, and salivary glands

Protein binding: 4%

Metabolism: Amifostine (phosphorylated prodrug) is hydrolyzed by alkaline phosphatase to an active free sulfhydryl compound (WR-1065)

Half-life:

Children: 9.3 minutes (Fouladi, 2001)

Adults: 8 minutes

Elimination: Metabolites excreted in urine

Dosing: Usual Refer to individual protocols.

Pediatric:

Cytoprotective agent against cisplatin or high-dose alkylating agents: Limited data available: Efficacy results variable:

Gastrointestinal and hematologic toxicity reduction: Infants, Children, and Adolescents: IV: 740 mg/m^2/dose once daily prior to cytotoxic chemotherapy. In a study of patients (n=11, age range: 2.5 months to 17 years) receiving the same combination chemotherapy at the same doses (including cisplatin or high-dose alkylating agent) with or without amifostine, patients who received amifostine had significantly reduced incidences of mucositis and gastrointestinal toxicities and a significantly reduced requirement for erythrocyte transfusions. However, there was no difference in the number of platelet transfusions required (Cetingül, 2009). In another study in osteosarcoma patients treated with cisplatin or carboplatin as part of combination chemotherapy, there was a reduction in neutrophil and leukocyte toxicity in patients who received amifostine (n=17) compared to those who did not (n=19); however, amifostine did not protect against platelet effects (Petrilli, 2002). Other studies have not shown protection against myelosuppression (Adamson, 1995, Bernstein, 2006).

Nephrotoxicity reduction: Children and Adolescents: IV: 740 mg/m^2/dose given immediately prior to cisplatin. In a small study of intracavitary cisplatin therapy for solid tumors, three patients (ages: 2-6 years) received amifostine. Of these patients, only one experienced persistent renal dysfunction (Katzenstein, 2010).

Reduction of platinum-induced hearing loss: Children and Adolescents 3-20 years: IV: 600 mg/m^2/dose given immediately prior to and 3 hours into cisplatin administration has been shown to reduce cisplatin-induced hearing loss in patients with average-risk medulloblastoma. Amifostine did not protect against hearing loss in patients with high-risk medulloblastoma (Fouladi, 2008, Gurney, 2014). Other studies using a single dose of 740 mg/m^2 or 825 mg/m^2 immediately prior to cisplatin did not prevent ototoxicity (Katzenstein, 2009; Marina, 2005; Petrilli, 2002).

Xerostomia, moderate to severe from radiation of the head and neck, reduction: Limited data available: Children ≥7 years and Adolescents: SubQ: 200 mg once daily given 30 minutes prior to standard fraction radiation therapy. Dosing based on a small pilot study in pediatric patients who received subcutaneous amifostine (n=5, age range: 7-15 years) for a total of 129 injections. No grade 3 or 4 mucosal or skin reactions occurred (Anacak, 2007).

Adult: **Note:** Antiemetic medication, including dexamethasone 20 mg IV and a serotonin 5-HT_3 receptor antagonist, is recommended prior to and in conjunction with amifostine.

Cisplatin-induced renal toxicity, reduction: IV: 910 mg/m^2 once daily administered 30 minutes prior to cytotoxic chemotherapy

The infusion of amifostine should be interrupted if the systolic blood pressure decreases significantly from baseline, as defined below:

Decrease of 20 mm Hg if baseline systolic blood pressure <100

Decrease of 25 mm Hg if baseline systolic blood pressure 100-119

Decrease of 30 mm Hg if baseline systolic blood pressure 120-139

Decrease of 40 mm Hg if baseline systolic blood pressure 140-179

Decrease of 50 mm Hg if baseline systolic blood pressure ≥180

If blood pressure returns to normal within 5 minutes (assisted by fluid administration and postural management) and the patient is asymptomatic, the infusion may be restarted so that the full dose of amifostine may be administered. If the full dose of amifostine cannot be administered, the dose of amifostine for subsequent cycles should be 740 mg/m^2.

Xerostomia, moderate to severe from radiation of the head and neck, reduction: IV: 200 mg/m^2 once daily starting 15-30 minutes prior to standard fraction radiation therapy

Dosing adjustment in renal impairment: There are no dosage adjustments provided in the manufacturer's labeling.

Dosing adjustment in hepatic impairment: There are no dosage adjustments provided in the manufacturer's labeling.

Preparation for Administration Parenteral:

IV: Reconstitute 500 mg vials with 9.7 mL of NS to a concentration of 50 mg/mL; dose must be further diluted with NS to a final concentration of 5 to 40 mg/mL.

SubQ: Reconstitute with 2.5 mL NS or SWFI.

Administration Parenteral: IV: Administer amifostine doses ≥600 mg/m^2 as an IV intermittent infusion over 15 minutes since the 15-minute infusion is better tolerated than a more prolonged infusion. Administer 200 mg/m^2 dose as a 3-minute infusion. Patients should be kept in supine position during infusion and amifostine should be interrupted if the blood pressure decreases significantly from baseline or if the patient develops symptoms related to decreased cerebral or cardiovascular perfusion. Patients experiencing decreased blood pressure should receive a rapid infusion of NS and be kept supine or placed in the Trendelenburg position. Amifostine can be restarted if the blood pressure returns to the baseline level.

Monitoring Parameters Baseline blood pressure followed by a blood pressure reading every 5 minutes during the infusion and after administration if clinically indicated; monitor electrolytes, urinalysis, serum calcium, serum magnesium; monitor I & O; evaluate for cutaneous reactions prior to each dose

Dosage Forms Excipient information presented when available (limited, particularly for generics); consult specific product labeling.

Solution Reconstituted, Intravenous:

Ethyol: 500 mg (1 ea)

Generic: 500 mg (1 ea)

Solution Reconstituted, Intravenous [preservative free]:

Generic: 500 mg (1 ea)

Amikacin (am i KAY sin)

Medication Safety Issues

Sound-alike/look-alike issues:

Amikacin may be confused with Amicar, anakinra

Amikin may be confused with Amicar, Kineret

Brand Names: Canada Amikacin Sulfate Injection, USP; Amikin

Therapeutic Category Antibiotic, Aminoglycoside

Generic Availability (US) Yes

Use Treatment of serious infections (bone and respiratory infections, endocarditis, and septicemia) due to organisms resistant to gentamicin and tobramycin, including *Pseudomonas*, *Klebsiella*, *Enterobacter*, *Serratia*, *Proteus*, and *Providencia* species, and *E. coli* (FDA approved in all ages); has also been used for documented infection of susceptible mycobacterial organisms

Pregnancy Risk Factor D

Pregnancy Considerations Adverse events were not observed in the initial animal reproduction studies; however, renal toxicity has been reported in additional studies. Amikacin crosses the placenta, produces detectable serum levels in the fetus, and concentrates in the fetal kidneys. Because of several reports of total irreversible bilateral congenital deafness in children whose mothers received another aminoglycoside (streptomycin) during pregnancy, the manufacturer classifies amikacin as pregnancy risk factor D. Although serious side effects to the fetus have not been reported following maternal use of amikacin, a potential for harm exists.

Due to pregnancy-induced physiologic changes, some pharmacokinetic parameters of amikacin may be altered. Pregnant women have an average-to-larger volume of distribution which may result in lower peak serum levels than for the same dose in nonpregnant women. Serum half-life may also be shorter.

Breast-Feeding Considerations Amikacin is excreted into breast milk in trace amounts; however, it is not absorbed when taken orally. This limited oral absorption may minimize exposure to the nursing infant. Nondose-related effects could include modification of bowel flora. Breast-feeding is not recommended by the manufacturer.

Contraindications Hypersensitivity to amikacin sulfate or any component of the formulation; cross-sensitivity may exist with other aminoglycosides

Warnings/Precautions [U.S. Boxed Warning]: Amikacin may cause neurotoxicity, nephrotoxicity, and/or neuromuscular blockade and respiratory paralysis; usual risk factors include preexisting renal impairment, concomitant neuro-/nephrotoxic medications, advanced age and dehydration. Dose and/or frequency of administration must be monitored and modified in patients with renal impairment. Drug should be discontinued if signs of ototoxicity, nephrotoxicity, or hypersensitivity occur. Ototoxicity is proportional to the amount of drug given and the duration of treatment. Tinnitus or vertigo may be indications of vestibular injury and impending bilateral irreversible damage. Renal damage is usually reversible. Use with caution in patients with neuromuscular disorders, hearing loss and hypocalcemia. Prolonged use may result in fungal or bacterial superinfection, including *C. difficile*-associated diarrhea (CDAD) and pseudomembranous colitis; CDAD has been observed >2 months postantibiotic treatment. Solution contains sodium metabisulfate; use caution in patients with sulfite allergy.

Warnings: Additional Pediatric Considerations Use with caution in pediatric patients on extracorporeal membrane oxygenation (ECMO); pharmacokinetics of aminoglycosides may be altered; dosage adjustment and close monitoring necessary.

Adverse Reactions

Central nervous system: Neurotoxicity

Genitourinary: Nephrotoxicity

Otic: Auditory ototoxicity, vestibular ototoxicity

Rare but important or life-threatening: Dyspnea, eosinophilia, hypersensitivity reaction

Drug Interactions

Metabolism/Transport Effects None known.

Avoid Concomitant Use

Avoid concomitant use of Amikacin with any of the following: BCG; BCG (Intravesical); Foscarnet; Mannitol; Mecamylamine

Increased Effect/Toxicity

Amikacin may increase the levels/effects of: AbobotulinumtoxinA; Bisphosphonate Derivatives; CARBOplatin; Colistimethate; CycloSPORINE (Systemic); Mecamylamine; Neuromuscular-Blocking Agents; OnabotulinumtoxinA; RimabotulinumtoxinB; Tenofovir

The levels/effects of Amikacin may be increased by: Amphotericin B; Capreomycin; Cephalosporins (2nd Generation); Cephalosporins (3rd Generation); Cephalosporins (4th Generation); CISplatin; Foscarnet; Loop Diuretics; Mannitol; Nonsteroidal Anti-Inflammatory Agents; Tenofovir; Vancomycin

Decreased Effect

Amikacin may decrease the levels/effects of: BCG; BCG (Intravesical); BCG Vaccine (Immunization); Sodium Picosulfate; Typhoid Vaccine

The levels/effects of Amikacin may be decreased by: Penicillins

Storage/Stability Store intact vials at 20°C to 25°C (68°F to 77°F). Following admixture at concentrations of 0.25-5 mg/mL, amikacin is stable for 24 hours at room temperature, 60 days at 4°C (39°F), or 30 days at -15°C (5°F). Previously refrigerated or thawed frozen solutions are stable for 24 hours when stored at 25°C (77°F).

Mechanism of Action Inhibits protein synthesis in susceptible bacteria by binding to 30S ribosomal subunits

Pharmacodynamics Displays concentration-dependent killing; bacteriocidal

Pharmacokinetics (Adult data unless noted)

Absorption:
- IM: Rapid
- Oral: Poorly absorbed

Distribution: V_d: 0.25 L/kg; primarily into extracellular fluid (highly hydrophilic); 12% of serum concentration penetrates into bronchial secretions; poor penetration into the blood-brain barrier even when meninges are inflamed; V_d is increased in neonates and patients with edema, ascites, fluid overload; V_d is decreased in patients with dehydration

Protein-binding: ≤11%

Half-life:
- Infants:
  - Low birth weight, 1-3 days of age: 7 hours
  - Full-term >7 days: 4-5 hours
- Children: 1.6-2.5 hours
- Adolescents: 1.5 ± 1 hour
- Adults: Normal renal function: 1.4-2.3 hours
- Anuria: 28-86 hours; half-life and clearance are dependent on renal function

Time to peak serum concentration:
- IM: Within 45-120 minutes
- IV: Within 30 minutes following a 30-minute infusion

Elimination: Urine (94% to 98%); excreted unchanged via glomerular filtration within 24 hours

Dialysis: Dialyzable (50% to 100%); supplemental dose recommended after hemodialysis or peritoneal dialysis

Dosing: Neonatal Note: Dose not well-defined in premature infants; monitor closely. Dosage should be based on actual weight unless the patient has hydrops fetalis. Consider single-dose administration with serum concentration monitoring in patients with urine output <1 mL/kg/hour or serum creatinine >1.3 mg/dL rather than scheduled dosing. Consider prolongation of dosing interval when coadministered with ibuprofen or indomethacin or in neonates with history of the following: Birth depression, birth hypoxia/asphyxia, or cyanotic congenital heart disease.

General dosing; susceptible infection: IV:
- Age-directed dosing (Allegaert, 2006; Allegaert, 2008; Labaune, 2001; Sherwin, 2009):
  - PMA ≤27 weeks: 15-20 mg/kg/dose every 48 hours
  - PMA 28-33 weeks: 15-20 mg/kg/dose every 36 hours
  - PMA ≥34 weeks: 15 mg/kg/dose every 24 hours
- Weight-directed dosing (*Red Book*, 2012)
  - Body weight <1 kg:
    - PNA ≤14 days: 15 mg/kg/dose every 48 hours
    - PNA 15-28 days: 15 mg/kg/dose every 24-48 hours
  - Body weight 1-2 kg:
    - PNA ≤7 days: 15 mg/kg/dose every 48 hours
    - PNA 8-28 days: 15 mg/kg/dose every 24-48 hours
  - Body weight >2 kg:
    - PNA ≤7 days: 15 mg/kg/dose every 24 hours
    - PNA 8-28 days: 15 mg/kg/dose every 12-24 hours

Meningitis: IV: **Note:** Use smaller doses and longer intervals for neonates <2 kg (Tunkel, 2004):
- PNA ≤7 days and ≥2 kg: 15-20 mg/kg/**day** divided every 12 hours
- PNA >7 days and ≥2 kg: 30 mg/kg/**day** divided every 8 hours

Dosing: Usual Note: Dosage should be based on an estimate of ideal body weight. In morbidly obese children, adolescents, and adults, dosage requirement may best be estimated using a dosing weight of IBW + 0.4 (TBW - IBW). Dosage should be individualized based upon serum concentration monitoring.

Infants, Children, and Adolescents:

General dosing, severe, susceptible infections: IM, IV: 15-22.5 mg/kg/**day** divided every 8 hours (*Red Book*, 2012); some consultants recommend initial doses of 30 mg/kg/**day** divided every 8 hours in patients who may require larger doses

CNS infections:
- Meningitis (Tunkel, 2004):
  - Infants and Children: IV: 20-30 mg/kg/**day** divided every 8 hours
  - Adolescents: IV: 15 mg/kg/**day** divided every 8 hours
- VP-shunt infection, ventriculitis: Limited data available: Intraventricular/intrathecal **(use a preservative free preparation)**: 5-50 mg/**day**; usual dose: 30 mg/**day**

Cystic fibrosis, pulmonary infection:
- Traditional dosing: IV, IM: 10 mg/kg/dose every 8 hours
- Extended-interval dosing: IV: 30 mg/kg/dose every 24 hours (Flume, 2009); **Note:** The CF Foundation recommends extended-interval dosing as preferred over traditional dosing.

Intra-abdominal infection, complicated: IV: 15-22.5 mg/kg/day divided every 8-24 hours (Solomkin, 2010)

Mycobacterium, avium complex infection (MAC):
- Infants and Children: IV: 15-30 mg/kg/**day** divided every 12-24 hours as part of a multiple drug regimen; maximum daily dose: 1500 mg/**day** (DHHS, [pediatric], 2013)
- Adolescents: IV: 10-15 mg/kg/**day** every 24 hours as part of a multiple drug regimen; maximum daily dose: 1500 mg/**day** (DHHS [adult], 2013)

Tuberculosis, drug-resistant:
- Infants, Children, and Adolescents ≤14 years: IM, IV: 15-30 mg/kg/dose once daily as part of a multiple drug regimen; maximum daily dose: 1000 mg/**day** (ATS/CDC/IDSA, 2003; DHHS [pediatric], 2013)
- Adolescents ≥15 years, HIV-exposed/-positive: IM, IV: 15 mg/kg/dose once daily as part of a multiple drug regimen for the first 2-3 months; maximum daily dose: 1000 mg/**day** (ATS/CDC/IDSA, 2003; DHHS [adult], 2013)

Peritonitis (CAPD): Intraperitoneal: Continuous: Loading dose: 25 mg per liter of dialysate; maintenance dose: 12 mg per liter (Warady, 2012)

Adults: Individualization is critical because of the low therapeutic index

Initial and periodic peak and trough plasma drug levels should be determined, particularly in critically ill patients with serious infections or in disease states known to significantly alter aminoglycoside pharmacokinetics (eg, cystic fibrosis, burns, or major surgery). Manufacturer recommends a maximum daily dose of 15 mg/kg/**day** (or 1500 mg/**day** in heavier patients). Higher doses may be warranted based on therapeutic drug monitoring or susceptibility information.

Usual dosage range: IM, IV: 5-7.5 mg/kg/dose every 8 hours; **Note:** Some clinicians suggest a daily dose of 15-20 mg/kg for all patients with normal renal function. This dose is at least as efficacious with similar, if not less, toxicity than conventional dosing.

Hospital-acquired pneumonia (HAP): IV: 20 mg/kg/day with antipseudomonal beta-lactam or carbapenem (ATS guidelines, 2005)

Meningitis (susceptible gram-negative organisms): IV: 5 mg/kg every 8 hours (administered with another bacteriocidal drug)

***Mycobacterium fortuitum, M. chelonae, or M. abscessus*:** IV: 10-15 mg/kg daily for at least 2 weeks with high-dose cefoxitin

Dosing interval in renal impairment:

Infants, Children, and Adolescents: IM, IV:

The following adjustments have been recommended (Aronoff, 2007); **Note:** Renally adjusted dose recommendations are based on doses of 5-7.5 mg/kg/dose every 8 hours:
- GFR >50 mL/minute/1.73 m^2: No adjustment required

GFR 30-50 mL/minute/1.73 m^2: Administer every 12-18 hours
GFR 10-29 mL/minute/1.73 m^2: Administer every 18-24 hours
GFR <10 mL/minute/1.73 m^2: Administer every 48-72 hours
Intermittent hemodialysis: 5 mg/kg/dose; redose as indicated by serum concentrations
Peritoneal dialysis (PD): 5 mg/kg/dose; redose as indicated by serum concentrations
Continuous renal replacement therapy (CRRT): 7.5 mg/kg/dose every 12 hours, monitor serum concentrations

Adults: **Note:** Some patients may require larger or more frequent doses if serum levels document the need (ie, cystic fibrosis or febrile granulocytopenic patients):
CrCl ≥60 mL/minute: Administer every 8 hours
CrCl 40-60 mL/minute: Administer every 12 hours
CrCl 20-40 mL/minute: Administer every 24 hours
CrCl <20 mL/minute: Loading dose, then monitor levels
Intermittent hemodialysis (IHD) (administer after hemodialysis on dialysis days): Dialyzable (20%; variable; dependent on filter, duration, and type of HD): 5-7.5 mg/kg every 48-72 hours. Follow levels. Redose when pre-HD serum concentration <10 mg/L; redose when post-HD serum concentration <6-8 mcg/mL (Heintz, 2009). **Note:** Dosing dependent on the assumption of 3 times complete IHD sessions.
Peritoneal dialysis (PD): Dose as CrCl <20 mL/minute: Follow levels.
Continuous renal replacement therapy (CRRT) (Heintz, 2009; Trotman, 2005): Drug clearance is highly dependent on the method of renal replacement, filter type, and flow rate. Appropriate dosing requires close monitoring of pharmacologic response, signs of adverse reactions due to drug accumulation, as well as drug concentrations in relation to target trough (if appropriate). The following are general recommendations only (based on dialysate flow/ultrafiltration rates of 1-2 L/hour and minimal residual renal function) and should not supersede clinical judgment:
CVVH/CVVHD/CVVHDF: Loading dose of 10 mg/kg followed by maintenance dose of 7.5 mg/kg every 24-48 hours
Note: For severe gram-negative rod infections, target peak serum concentration of 15-30 mcg/mL; redose when serum concentration <10 mcg/mL (Heintz, 2009).

Preparation for Administration Parenteral: IV intermittent infusion: Dilute in a compatible solution (eg, NS, D_5W) to a final concentration of 0.25 to 5 mg/mL per the manufacturer; concentrations as high as 10 mg/mL have been reported (Murray 2014).

Administration
Parenteral: Administer other antibiotics, such as penicillins and cephalosporins, at least 1 hour before or after an amikacin dose; simultaneous administration may result in reduced antibacterial efficacy. Administer around-the-clock to promote less variation in peak and trough serum levels.
IM: Administer undiluted into a large muscle mass. Slower absorption and lower peak concentrations, probably due to poor circulation in the atrophic muscle, may occur following IM injection; in paralyzed patients, suggest IV route
Intermittent IV infusion: Infuse over 30 to 60 minutes; in infants infusion over 1 to 2 hours is recommended by the manufacturer.

Monitoring Parameters Urinalysis, urine output, BUN, serum creatinine, peak and trough serum amikacin concentrations; be alert to ototoxicity
With conventional dosing, typically obtain serum concentration after the third dose; exceptions for earlier monitoring may include neonates or patients with rapidly changing renal function. With extended-interval dosing, usually obtain serum concentration after first, second, or third dose.
Not all infants and children who receive aminoglycosides require monitoring of serum aminoglycoside concentrations. Indications for use of aminoglycoside serum concentration monitoring include:

- Treatment course >5 days
- Patients with decreased or changing renal function
- Patients with poor therapeutic response
- Neonates and Infants <3 months of age
- Atypical body constituency (obesity, expanded extracellular fluid volume)
- Clinical need for higher doses or shorter intervals (eg, cystic fibrosis, burns, endocarditis, meningitis, critically ill patients, relatively resistant organisms)
- Patients on hemodialysis or chronic ambulatory peritoneal dialysis
- Signs of nephrotoxicity or ototoxicity
- Concomitant use of other nephrotoxic agents

Reference Range Therapeutic levels:
Peak:
Life-threatening infections: 25-40 mcg/mL
Serious infections: 20-25 mcg/mL
Urinary tract infections: 15-20 mcg/mL
Trough: <8 mcg/mL; the American Thoracic Society (ATS) recommends trough levels of <4-5 mcg/mL for patients with hospital-acquired pneumonia
Timing of serum samples: Draw peak 30 minutes after completion of 30-minute infusion or at 1 hour following initiation of infusion or IM injection; draw trough within 30 minutes prior to next dose; aminoglycoside levels measured from blood taken from Silastic® central catheters can sometimes give falsely elevated readings

Test Interactions Some penicillin derivatives may accelerate the degradation of aminoglycosides *in vitro*, leading to a potential underestimation of aminoglycoside serum concentration.

Additional Information Some penicillins (eg, carbenicillin, ticarcillin, and piperacillin) have been shown to inactivate aminoglycosides *in vitro*. This has been observed to a greater extent with tobramycin and gentamicin, while amikacin has shown greater stability against inactivation. Concurrent use of these agents may pose a risk of reduced antibacterial efficacy *in vivo*, particularly in the setting of profound renal impairment; however, definitive clinical evidence is lacking. If combination penicillin/aminoglycoside therapy is desired in a patient with renal dysfunction, separation of doses (if feasible), and routine monitoring of aminoglycoside levels, CBC, and clinical response should be considered.

Dosage Forms Excipient information presented when available (limited, particularly for generics); consult specific product labeling.
Solution, Injection, as sulfate:
Generic: 500 mg/2 mL (2 mL); 1 g/4 mL (4 mL)
Solution, Injection, as sulfate [preservative free]:
Generic: 1 g/4 mL (4 mL)

◆ **Amikacin Sulfate** *see* Amikacin *on page 117*

◆ **Amikacin Sulfate Injection, USP (Can)** *see* Amikacin *on page 117*

◆ **Amikin (Can)** *see* Amikacin *on page 117*

AMILoride (a MIL oh ride)

Medication Safety Issues
Sound-alike/look-alike issues:
AMILoride may be confused with amiodarone, amLODIPine, inamrinone

Brand Names: Canada Midamor

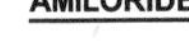

Therapeutic Category Antihypertensive Agent; Diuretic, Potassium Sparing

Generic Availability (US) Yes

Use Management of edema associated with CHF, hepatic cirrhosis, and hyperaldosteronism; hypertension; primary hyperaldosteronism; hypokalemia induced by kaliuretic diuretics

Pregnancy Risk Factor B

Pregnancy Considerations Adverse events were not observed in animal reproduction studies.

Breast-Feeding Considerations It is not known if amiloride is excreted in breast milk. Due to the potential for serious adverse reactions in the nursing infant, a decision should be made to discontinue nursing or to discontinue the drug, taking into account the importance of treatment to the mother.

Contraindications Hypersensitivity to amiloride or any component of the formulation; presence of elevated serum potassium levels (>5.5 mEq/L); if patient is receiving other potassium-conserving agents (eg, spironolactone, triamterene) or potassium supplementation (medicine, potassium-containing salt substitutes, potassium-rich diet) except in severe and/or refractory cases of hypokalemia; anuria; acute or chronic renal insufficiency; evidence of diabetic nephropathy. Patients with evidence of renal impairment (blood urea nitrogen [BUN] >30 mg/dL or serum creatinine >1.5 mg/dL) or diabetes mellitus should not receive amiloride without close, frequent monitoring of serum electrolytes and renal function.

Warnings/Precautions [US Boxed Warning]: Hyperkalemia (serum potassium levels >5.5 mEq/L) may occur, which can be fatal if not corrected; patients at higher risk include those with renal impairment, diabetes, and the elderly. Serum potassium levels must be monitored at frequent intervals especially when therapy is initiated, when dosages are changed or with any illness that may cause renal dysfunction. Risk of hyperkalemia may be increased when used concomitantly with other medications that may increase potassium (eg, angiotensin agents). Signs/symptoms of hyperkalemia include paresthesias, muscle weakness, fatigue, flaccid paralysis of limbs, bradycardia, shock, and ECG abnormalities. If hyperkalemia occurs, discontinue amiloride immediately and manage hyperkalemia as clinically appropriate. May decrease sodium and chloride and increase BUN, especially with concomitant diuretic therapy; close medical supervision and dose evaluation are required. Watch for and correct electrolyte disturbances; adjust dose to avoid dehydration.

In cirrhosis, avoid electrolyte and acid/base imbalances that might lead to hepatic encephalopathy. If possible, avoid use in patients with diabetes mellitus; if cannot be avoided, use with extreme caution and monitor electrolytes and renal function closely. Discontinue amiloride at least 3 days prior to glucose tolerance testing. Use with caution in patients who are at risk for metabolic or respiratory acidosis (eg, cardiopulmonary disease, poorly controlled diabetes); monitor acid base balance frequently. Amiloride is primarily eliminated renally; patients with renal impairment are at greater risk for toxicities.

Potentially significant drug-drug interactions may exist, requiring dose or frequency adjustment, additional monitoring, and/or selection of alternative therapy.

Adverse Reactions

Central nervous system: Dizziness, fatigue, headache
Endocrine & metabolic: Dehydration, gynecomastia, hyperchloremic metabolic acidosis, hyperkalemia, hyponatremia
Gastrointestinal: Abdominal pain, change in appetite, constipation, diarrhea, gas pain, nausea, vomiting
Genitourinary: Impotence
Neuromuscular & skeletal: Muscle cramps, weakness
Respiratory: Cough, dyspnea
Rare but important or life-threatening: Bladder spasm, cardiac arrhythmia, chest pain, dysuria, gastrointestinal hemorrhage, increased intraocular pressure, jaundice, orthostatic hypotension, palpitations, polyuria

Drug Interactions

Metabolism/Transport Effects Substrate of OCT2

Avoid Concomitant Use

Avoid concomitant use of AMILoride with any of the following: CycloSPORINE (Systemic); Spironolactone; Tacrolimus (Systemic)

Increased Effect/Toxicity

AMILoride may increase the levels/effects of: ACE Inhibitors; Amifostine; Ammonium Chloride; Antihypertensives; Cardiac Glycosides; CycloSPORINE (Systemic); Dofetilide; DULoxetine; Hypotensive Agents; Levodopa; Obinutuzumab; RisperiDONE; RiTUXimab; Sodium Phosphates; Spironolactone; Tacrolimus (Systemic)

The levels/effects of AMILoride may be increased by: Alfuzosin; Analgesics (Opioid); Angiotensin II Receptor Blockers; Barbiturates; Brimonidine (Topical); BuPROPion; Canagliflozin; Diazoxide; Drospirenone; Eplerenone; Heparin; Heparin (Low Molecular Weight); Herbs (Hypotensive Properties); MAO Inhibitors; Nicorandil; Nonsteroidal Anti-Inflammatory Agents; Pentoxifylline; Phosphodiesterase 5 Inhibitors; Potassium Salts; Prostacyclin Analogues; Tolvaptan

Decreased Effect

AMILoride may decrease the levels/effects of: Cardiac Glycosides; QuiNIDine

The levels/effects of AMILoride may be decreased by: Herbs (Hypertensive Properties); Methylphenidate; Nonsteroidal Anti-Inflammatory Agents; Yohimbine

Storage/Stability Store at 20°C to 25°C (68°F to 77°F). Avoid freezing or excessive heat. Protect from moisture.

Mechanism of Action Blocks epithelial sodium channels in the late distal convoluted tubule (DCT), and collecting duct which inhibits sodium reabsorption from the lumen. This effectively reduces intracellular sodium, decreasing the function of Na+/K+ATPase, leading to potassium retention and decreased calcium, magnesium, and hydrogen excretion. As sodium uptake capacity in the DCT/collecting duct is limited, the natriuretic, diuretic, and antihypertensive effects are generally considered weak.

Pharmacodynamics

Onset of action: 2 hours
Maximum effect: 6-10 hours
Duration: 24 hours

Pharmacokinetics (Adult data unless noted)

Absorption: 50%
Distribution: Adults: V_d: 350-380 L
Metabolism: No active metabolites
Half-life: Adults:
- Normal renal function: 6-9 hours
- End-stage renal disease: 21-144 hours

Elimination: Unchanged drug, equally in urine and feces

Dosing: Usual Oral:

Hypertension:
- Children: 0.4-0.625 mg/kg/day; maximum dose: 20 mg/day
- Adults: 5-10 mg/day in 1-2 divided doses (JNC 7)

Edema:
- Children 6-20 kg: 0.625 mg/kg/day in 1-2 divided doses; maximum dose: 10 mg/day
- Children >20 kg and Adults: 5-10 mg/day in 1-2 divided doses; maximum dose: 20 mg/day

Dosing adjustment in renal impairment:
- CrCl 10-50 mL/minute: Administer at 50% of normal dose
- CrCl <10 mL/minute: Avoid use

Administration Oral: Administer with food or milk

Monitoring Parameters Serum potassium, sodium, creatinine, BUN, blood pressure, fluid balance

Additional Information Studies utilizing aerosolized amiloride (5 mmol/L in 0.3% saline) in adult cystic fibrosis patients (Tomkiewicz, 1993) have suggested that inhaled amiloride is capable of improving the rheologic properties of the abnormally thickened mucus by increasing mucus sodium content

Dosage Forms Excipient information presented when available (limited, particularly for generics); consult specific product labeling.

Tablet, Oral, as hydrochloride:

Generic: 5 mg

Extemporaneous Preparations A 1 mg/mL oral suspension may be made with tablets. Crush ten 5 mg tablets in a mortar and reduce to a fine powder. Add small proportions up to 20 mL of Glycerin BP or Glycerin, USP and mix to uniform paste; mix while adding sterile water in incremental proportions to **almost** 50 mL; transfer to a calibrated bottle, rinse mortar with sterile water, and add quantity of sterile water sufficient to make 50 mL. Label "shake well" and "refrigerate". Stable for 21 days.

Nahata MC, Pai VB, and Hipple TF, *Pediatric Drug Formulations*, 5th ed, Cincinnati, OH: Harvey Whitney Books Co, 2004.

◆ **Amiloride HCl** *see* AMILoride *on page 119*

◆ **Amiloride Hydrochloride** *see* AMILoride *on page 119*

◆ **2-Amino-6-Mercaptopurine** *see* Thioguanine *on page 2049*

◆ **2-Amino-6-Methoxypurine Arabinoside** *see* Nelarabine *on page 1496*

◆ **Aminobenzylpenicillin** *see* Ampicillin *on page 156*

Aminocaproic Acid (a mee noe ka PROE ik AS id)

Medication Safety Issues

Sound-alike/look-alike issues:

Amicar® may be confused with amikacin, Amikin®

International issues:

Amicar [U.S.] may be confused with Omacor brand name for Omega-3-Acid Ethyl Esters [multiple international markets]

Brand Names: US Amicar

Therapeutic Category Hemostatic Agent

Generic Availability (US) Yes

Use To enhance hemostasis when fibrinolysis contributes to bleeding (causes may include cardiac surgery, hematologic disorders, neoplastic disorders, abruptio placentae, hepatic cirrhosis, and urinary fibrinolysis) (FDA approved in adults); has also been used for traumatic hyphema, prevention of perioperative bleeding, refractory hematuria, and prevention of bleeding associated with ECMO in high-risk patients

Pregnancy Risk Factor C

Pregnancy Considerations Animal reproduction studies have not been conducted.

Breast-Feeding Considerations It is not known if aminocaproic acid is excreted in breast milk. The manufacturer recommends that caution be exercised when administering aminocaproic acid to nursing women

Contraindications Disseminated intravascular coagulation (without heparin); evidence of an active intravascular clotting process

Warnings/Precautions Avoid rapid IV administration (may induce hypotension, bradycardia, or arrhythmia); rapid injection of undiluted solution is not recommended. Use with caution in patients with renal disease; aminocaproic acid may accumulate in patients with decreased renal function. Intrarenal obstruction may occur secondary to glomerular capillary thrombosis or clots in the renal pelvis and ureters. Do not use in hematuria of upper urinary tract origin unless possible benefits outweigh risks. Do not administer without a definite diagnosis of laboratory findings indicative of hyperfibrinolysis. Inhibition of fibrinolysis may promote clotting or thrombosis; more likely due to the presence of DIC. Skeletal muscle weakness ranging from mild myalgias and fatigue to severe myopathy with rhabdomyolysis and acute renal failure has been reported with prolonged use. Monitor CPK; discontinue treatment with a rise in CPK. Do not administer with factor IX complex concentrates or anti-inhibitor coagulant complexes; may increase risk for thrombosis.

Benzyl alcohol and derivatives: Some dosage forms may contain benzyl alcohol; large amounts of benzyl alcohol (≥99 mg/kg/day) have been associated with a potentially fatal toxicity ("gasping syndrome") in neonates; the "gasping syndrome" consists of metabolic acidosis, respiratory distress, gasping respirations, CNS dysfunction (including convulsions, intracranial hemorrhage), hypotension and cardiovascular collapse (AAP, 1997; CDC, 1982); some data suggests that benzoate displaces bilirubin from protein binding sites (Ahlfors, 2001); avoid or use dosage forms containing benzyl alcohol with caution in neonates. See manufacturer's labeling.

Adverse Reactions

Cardiovascular: Arrhythmia, bradycardia, edema, hypotension, intracranial hypertension, peripheral ischemia, syncope, thrombosis

Central nervous system: Confusion, delirium, dizziness, fatigue, hallucinations, headache, malaise, seizure, stroke

Dermatologic: Rash, pruritus

Gastrointestinal: Abdominal pain, anorexia, cramps, diarrhea, GI irritation, nausea, vomiting

Genitourinary: Dry ejaculation

Hematologic: Agranulocytosis, bleeding time increased, leukopenia, thrombocytopenia

Local: Injection site necrosis, injection site pain, injection site reactions

Neuromuscular & skeletal: CPK increased, myalgia, myositis, myopathy, rhabdomyolysis (rare), weakness

Ophthalmic: Vision decreased, watery eyes

Otic: Tinnitus

Renal: BUN increased, intrarenal obstruction (glomerular capillary thrombosis), myoglobinuria (rare), renal failure (rare)

Respiratory: Dyspnea, nasal congestion, pulmonary embolism

Miscellaneous: Allergic reaction, anaphylactoid reaction, anaphylaxis

Rare but important or life-threatening: Hepatic lesion, hyperkalemia, myocardial lesion

Drug Interactions

Metabolism/Transport Effects None known.

Avoid Concomitant Use

Avoid concomitant use of Aminocaproic Acid with any of the following: Anti-inhibitor Coagulant Complex (Human); Factor IX (Human); Factor IX (Recombinant); Factor IX Complex (Human) [(Factors II, IX, X)]

Increased Effect/Toxicity

Aminocaproic Acid may increase the levels/effects of: Anti-inhibitor Coagulant Complex (Human); Factor IX (Human); Factor IX (Recombinant); Factor IX Complex (Human) [(Factors II, IX, X)]; Fibrinogen Concentrate (Human)

The levels/effects of Aminocaproic Acid may be increased by: Fibrinogen Concentrate (Human); Tretinoin (Systemic)

Decreased Effect There are no known significant interactions involving a decrease in effect.

Storage/Stability Store intact vials, tablets, and syrup at 15°C to 30°C (59°F to 86°F). Do not freeze injection or syrup. Solutions diluted for IV use in D_5W or NS to concentrations of 10-100 mg/mL are stable at 4°C (39°F) and 23°C (73°F) for 7 days (Zhang, 1997).

Mechanism of Action Binds competitively to plasminogen; blocking the binding of plasminogen to fibrin and the subsequent conversion to plasmin, resulting in inhibition of fibrin degradation (fibrinolysis).

Pharmacodynamics Onset of action: Inhibition of fibrinolysis: Within 1-72 hours; onset shortened substantially with loading dose

Pharmacokinetics (Adult data unless noted)

Distribution: Widely distributes through intravascular and extravascular compartments

Metabolism: Hepatic metabolism is minimal

Bioavailability: Oral: 100%

Half-life: 1-2 hours

Time to peak serum concentration: Oral: 1.2 ± 0.45 hours

Elimination: Urine (65% as unchanged drug, 11% as metabolite)

Dosing: Neonatal

Prevention of bleeding associated with extracorporeal membrane oxygenation (ECMO), high-bleeding risk patients: Limited data available: IV: 100 mg/kg prior to or immediately after cannulation, followed by 25-30 mg/kg/hour for up to 72 hours; target activated clotting time (ACT) range during therapy of 180-200 seconds has been used (Downard, 2003; Horwitz, 1998; Wilson, 1993); variable results; patients requiring surgery just prior to or while on ECMO seem to benefit most

Prevention of perioperative bleeding associated with cardiac surgery: Limited data available: IV: 75 mg/kg administered at the beginning and end of cardiopulmonary bypass, along with 75 mg/100 mL added to the priming fluid for cardiopulmonary bypass (Martin, 2011)

Dosing: Usual

Pediatric:

Control of hemorrhage (oral, epistaxis, menorrhagia) in hemophilic patients, adjunct treatment: Limited data available: Infants, Children, and Adolescents: Oral: 50-100 mg/kg/dose every 6 hours; maximum daily dose: 24 **g/day** (Acharya, 2011)

Control of mucosal bleeding in thrombocytopenia/platelet dysfunction: Limited data available: Infants, Children, and Adolescents: Oral, IV: 50-100 mg/kg/dose every 6 hours; maximum daily dose: 24 **g/day** (Bussel, 2011; Lipton, 2011)

Hematuria (gross; upper tract), refractory: Limited data available: Children ≥11 years and Adolescents: Oral: 100 mg/kg/dose every 6 hours; continue for 2 days beyond resolution of hematuria; dosing based on case series (n=4) which showed hematuria resolution within 2-7 days; risks and benefits must be weighed prior to use (Kaye, 2010)

Prevention of bleeding associated with dental procedures in hemophilic patients: Limited data available: Infants, Children, and Adolescents: Oral: 50-100 mg/kg/dose every 6 hours; maximum daily dose: 24 **g/day**; used in conjunction with DDAVP or factor replacement therapy; continue for up to 7 days or until mucosal healing is complete (Acharya, 2011)

Prevention of bleeding associated with extracorporeal membrane oxygenation (ECMO), high-bleeding risk patients: Limited data available: Infants, Children, and Adolescents: IV: 100 mg/kg prior to or immediately after cannulation, followed by 25-30 mg/kg/hour for up to 72 hours; target activated clotting time (ACT) range during therapy of 180-200 seconds has been used (Downard, 2003; Horwitz, 1998; Wilson, 1993); variable results; patients requiring surgery just prior to or while on ECMO seem to benefit most

Prevention of perioperative bleeding associated with cardiac surgery: Limited data available:

Infants and Children <2 years: Dosing regimens variable: IV: In the largest trial (n=120, all patients <20 kg), a dose of 75 mg/kg was administered at the beginning and end of cardiopulmonary bypass (CPB), and 75 mg/100 mL was added to the CPB priming fluid (Martin, 2011a). Another study group in two separate trials (n=110, age range: 2 months to 14 years) used a 100 mg/kg dose after induction, during CPB pump priming, and when weaning CPB (over 3 hours) for a total of three doses (Chauhan, 2000; Chauhan, 2004).

Children ≥2 years and Adolescents: IV: 100 mg/kg after induction, during CPB pump priming, and when weaning CPB (over 3 hours) for a total of 3 doses; regimen used in two separate trials (n=110, age range: 2 months to 14 years) (Chauhan, 2000; Chauhan, 2004)

Prevention of perioperative bleeding associated with spinal surgery (eg, idiopathic scoliosis): Limited data available: Children ≥11 years and Adolescents: IV: 100 mg/kg (maximum dose: 5 **g**) administered over 15-20 minutes after induction, followed by a continuous IV infusion of 10 mg/kg/hour for the remainder of the surgery; discontinued at time of wound closure (Florentino-Pineda, 2001; Florentino-Pineda, 2004)

Traumatic hyphema: Limited data available: Infants, Children, and Adolescents: Oral: 50-100 mg/kg/dose every 4 hours for 5 days; maximum daily dose: 30 **g/day** (Brandt, 2001; Crouch, 1999; Teboul, 1995)

Adult: **Acute bleeding:** Oral, IV: Loading dose: 4-5 **g** during the first hour, followed by 1 **g**/hour for 8 hours (or 1.25 **g**/hour using oral solution) or until bleeding controlled (maximum daily dose: 30 **g**

Dosage adjustment in renal impairment: There are no dosage adjustments are provided in the manufacturer's labeling, but aminocaproic acid may accumulate in patients with decreased renal function; use with caution.

Dosage adjustment in hepatic impairment: There are no dosage adjustments are provided in the manufacturer's labeling (has not been studied).

Preparation for Administration Parenteral: Dilute IV solution in D_5W, NS, or LR to a maximum concentration of 20 mg/mL.

Administration

Oral: May administer without regard to food

Parenteral: Do not administer undiluted; rapid IV injection (IVP) of undiluted solution is not recommended due to possible hypotension, bradycardia, and arrhythmia.

Intermittent IV infusion: After further dilution, administer over 15 to 60 minutes (rate dependent upon use).

Continuous IV infusion: Must further dilute prior to administration.

Monitoring Parameters Fibrinogen, fibrin split products, serum creatinine kinase (long-term therapy); serum potassium, BUN, creatinine

Reference Range Therapeutic concentration: >130 mcg/mL (concentration necessary for inhibition of fibrinolysis)

Dosage Forms Excipient information presented when available (limited, particularly for generics); consult specific product labeling. [DSC] = Discontinued product

Solution, Intravenous:

Generic: 250 mg/mL (20 mL)

Syrup, Oral:

Amicar: 25% (473 mL) [raspberry flavor]

Generic: 25% (237 mL [DSC], 473 mL [DSC])

Tablet, Oral:

Amicar: 500 mg, 1000 mg [scored]

Generic: 500 mg [DSC], 1000 mg [DSC]

Aminophylline (am in OFF i lin)

Medication Safety Issues

Sound-alike/look-alike issues:

Aminophylline may be confused with amitriptyline, ampicillin

Related Information

Management of Drug Extravasations *on page 2298*
Theophylline *on page 2044*

Brand Names: Canada Aminophylline Injection; JAA-Aminophylline

Therapeutic Category Antiasthmatic; Bronchodilator; Respiratory Stimulant; Theophylline Derivative

Generic Availability (US) Yes

Use Treatment of symptoms and reversible airflow obstruction associated with asthma, COPD, or other chronic lung diseases [FDA approved in pediatric patients (age not specified) and adults]; has also been used for treatment of apnea of prematurity and to increase diaphragmatic contractility

Pregnancy Risk Factor C

Pregnancy Considerations Refer to Theophylline monograph.

Breast-Feeding Considerations Refer to Theophylline monograph.

Contraindications Hypersensitivity to theophylline, ethylenediamine, or any component of the formulation

Canadian labeling: Additional contraindications (not in U.S. labeling): Coronary artery disease where cardiac stimulation might prove harmful; patients with peptic ulcer disease

Warnings/Precautions If a patient develops signs and symptoms of theophylline toxicity, a serum level should be measured and subsequent doses held. Theophylline clearance may be decreased in patients with acute pulmonary edema, congestive heart failure, cor pulmonale, fever, hepatic disease, acute hepatitis, cirrhosis, hypothyroidism, sepsis with multiorgan failure, and shock; clearance may also be decreased in neonates, infants <3 months of age with decreased renal function, infants <1 year of age, the elderly >60 years of age, and patients following cessation of smoking. Due to potential saturation of theophylline clearance at serum levels within (or in some patients less than) the therapeutic range, dosage adjustment should be made in small increments (maximum: 25% dose increase). Due to wide interpatient variability, theophylline serum level measurements must be used to optimize therapy and prevent serious toxicity. Use caution with peptic ulcer (use is contraindicated in the Canadian labeling), hyperthyroidism, seizure disorder, hypertension, or tachyarrhythmias. Vesicant; ensure proper catheter or needle position prior to and during infusion; avoid extravasation.

Adverse Reactions Adverse events observed at therapeutic serum levels:

Cardiovascular: Flutter, tachycardia

Central nervous system: Behavior alterations (children), headache, insomnia, irritability, restlessness, seizures

Dermatologic: Allergic skin reactions, exfoliative dermatitis

Gastrointestinal: Diarrhea, nausea, vomiting

Neuromuscular & skeletal: Tremor

Renal: Diuresis (transient)

Drug Interactions

Metabolism/Transport Effects Substrate of CYP1A2 (major), CYP2C9 (minor), CYP2D6 (minor), CYP2E1 (major), CYP3A4 (major); **Note:** Assignment of Major/Minor substrate status based on clinically relevant drug interaction potential; **Inhibits** CYP1A2 (weak)

Avoid Concomitant Use

Avoid concomitant use of Aminophylline with any of the following: Conivaptan; Fusidic Acid (Systemic); Idelalisib; Iobenguane I 123; Riociguat

Increased Effect/Toxicity

Aminophylline may increase the levels/effects of: Formoterol; Indacaterol; Olodaterol; Pancuronium; Riociguat; Sympathomimetics; TiZANidine

The levels/effects of Aminophylline may be increased by: Abiraterone Acetate; Alcohol (Ethyl); Allopurinol; Antithyroid Agents; Aprepitant; AtoMOXetine; Cannabinoid-Containing Products; Cimetidine; Conivaptan; CYP1A2 Inhibitors (Moderate); CYP1A2 Inhibitors (Strong); CYP3A4 Inhibitors (Moderate); CYP3A4 Inhibitors (Strong); Dasatinib; Deferasirox; Disulfiram; Estrogen Derivatives; Febuxostat; FluvoxaMINE; Fosaprepitant; Fusidic Acid (Systemic); Idelalisib; Interferons; Isoniazid; Ivacaftor; Linezolid; Luliconazole; Macrolide Antibiotics; Methotrexate; Mexiletine; Mifepristone; Netupitant; Palbociclib; Peginterferon Alfa-2b; Pentoxifylline; Propafenone; QuiNINE; Quinolone Antibiotics; Simeprevir; Stiripentol; Tedizolid; Thiabendazole; Ticlopidine; Vemurafenib; Zafirlukast

Decreased Effect

Aminophylline may decrease the levels/effects of: Adenosine; Benzodiazepines; CarBAMazepine; Fosphenytoin; Iobenguane I 123; Lithium; Pancuronium; Phenytoin; Regadenoson; Thiopental; Zafirlukast

The levels/effects of Aminophylline may be decreased by: Adalimumab; Barbiturates; Beta-Blockers (Beta1 Selective); Beta-Blockers (Nonselective); Bosentan; Cannabis; CarBAMazepine; CYP1A2 Inducers (Strong); CYP3A4 Inducers (Moderate); CYP3A4 Inducers (Strong); Cyproterone; Dabrafenib; Deferasirox; Fosphenytoin; Isoproterenol; Mitotane; Phenytoin; Protease Inhibitors; Siltuximab; St Johns Wort; Teriflunomide; Thyroid Products; Tocilizumab

Food Interactions

Ethanol: Ethanol may decrease theophylline clearance. Management: Avoid or limit ethanol.

Food: Food does not appreciably affect absorption. Changes in diet may affect the elimination of theophylline; charcoal-broiled foods may increase elimination, reducing half-life by 50%. Management: Avoid extremes of dietary protein and carbohydrate intake.

Storage/Stability

Solution: Vials should be stored at room temperature of 20°C to 25°C (68°F to 77°F). Protect from light. Do not use solutions if discolored or if crystals are present.

Tablet: Store at room temperature of 20°C to 25°C (68°F to 77°F). Protect from light and moisture.

Mechanism of Action Causes bronchodilatation, diuresis, CNS and cardiac stimulation, and gastric acid secretion by blocking phosphodiesterase which increases tissue concentrations of cyclic adenine monophosphate (cAMP) which in turn promote catecholamine stimulation of lipolysis, glycogenolysis, and gluconeogenesis and induce release of epinephrine from adrenal medulla cells

Pharmacokinetics (Adult data unless noted) Aminophylline is the ethylenediamine salt of theophylline, pharmacokinetic parameters are those of **theophylline**; fraction available: 79% (eg, 100 mg aminophylline = 79 mg theophylline); refer to Theophylline monograph.

Dosing: Neonatal Note: All dosages expressed as aminophylline; dose should be individualized based on serum concentrations. Due to longer half-life than older patients, the time to achieve steady-state serum concentration is prolonged in neonates (see theophylline half-life table); obtain serum theophylline concentration after 48 to 72 hours of therapy (usually 72 hours in neonates); repeat values should be obtained 3 days after each change in dosage or weekly if on a stabilized dosage. If renal function decreased, consider dose reduction and additional monitoring.

Apnea of prematurity: IV:

Manufacturer's labeling:

Loading dose: 5.7 mg/kg/dose

Maintenance:

PNA ≤24 days: 1.27 mg/kg/dose every 12 hours to achieve a target concentration of 7.5 mcg/mL

PNA >24 days: 1.9 mg/kg/dose every 12 hours to achieve a target concentration of 7.5 mcg/mL

Alternate dosing:

Loading dose: 5 to 8 mg/kg/dose; in a prospective randomized controlled trial of 61 neonates (birth weight: <1500 g), a loading dose of 8 mg/kg/dose achieved targeted theophylline serum concentrations in more patients compared to a loading dose of 6 mg/kg/dose (Hochwald, 2002)

Maintenance: Initial: 2 to 6 mg/kg/day divided every 8 to 12 hours (Bhatt-Mehta, 2003; Hochwald, 2002); increased dosages may be indicated as liver metabolism increases; monitor serum concentrations to determine appropriate dosages

Dosing adjustment in renal impairment: Dose reduction and frequent monitoring of serum theophylline concentrations are required in neonates with decreased renal function; 50% of dose is excreted unchanged in the urine of neonates.

Dosing: Usual All dosages expressed as **aminophylline**; use ideal body weight to calculate dose; adjust dose based on steady-state serum concentrations.

Pediatric:

Obstructive airway disease, acute symptoms: Infants, Children, and Adolescents: **Note:** Not recommended for the treatment of asthma exacerbations (NAEPP, 2007).

Loading dose: IV:

Patients **not currently receiving** aminophylline or theophylline: 5.7 mg/kg/dose

Patients **currently receiving** aminophylline or theophylline: A loading dose is not recommended without first obtaining a serum theophylline concentration in patients who have received aminophylline or theophylline within the past 24 hours. The loading dose should be calculated as follows:

Dose = (C desired – C measured) (V_d)

C desired = desired serum theophylline concentration

C measured = measured serum theophylline concentration

Maintenance dose: Continuous IV infusion: **Note:** Dosing presented is to achieve a target concentration of 10 mcg/mL. Lower initial doses may be required in patients with reduced theophylline clearance. Dosage should be adjusted according to serum concentration measurements during the first 12- to 24-hour period.

Infants 4 to 6 weeks: 1.9 mg/kg/dose every 12 hours

Infants 6 to 52 weeks: Dose (mg/kg/**hour**) = [(0.008 X age in weeks) + 0.21] divided by 0.79

Children 1 to <9 years: 1.01 mg/kg/**hour**

Children 9 to <12 years: 0.89 mg/kg/**hour**

Adolescents 12 to <16 years (otherwise healthy, nonsmokers): 0.63 mg/kg/**hour**; maximum dose: 1139 mg/**day** unless serum concentrations indicate need for larger dose

Adolescents 12 to <16 years (cigarette or marijuana smokers): 0.89 mg/kg/**hour**

Adolescents ≥16 years (otherwise healthy, nonsmokers): 0.51 mg/kg/**hour**; maximum dose: 1139 mg/**day** unless serum concentrations indicate need for larger dose

Cardiac decompensation, cor pulmonale, hepatic dysfunction, sepsis with multiorgan failure, shock: Infants, Children, and Adolescents: Initial: 0.25 mg/kg/**hour**; maximum dose: 507 mg/**day** unless serum concentrations indicate need for larger dose.

Adult: **Obstructive airway disease, acute symptoms:**

Loading dose: IV:

Patients **not currently receiving** aminophylline or theophylline: 5.7 mg/kg/dose

Patients **currently receiving** aminophylline or theophylline: A loading dose is not recommended without first obtaining a serum theophylline concentration in patients who have received aminophylline or theophylline within the past 24 hours. The loading dose should be calculated as follows:

Dose = (desired serum theophylline concentration - measured serum theophylline concentration) (V_d)

Maintenance dose: IV: **Note:** Dosing presented is to achieve a target theophylline concentration of 10 mcg/mL unless otherwise noted. Lower initial doses may be required in patients with reduced theophylline clearance. Dosage should be adjusted according to serum level measurements during the first 12- to 24-hour period.

Adults ≤60 years (otherwise healthy, nonsmokers): 0.51 mg/kg/**hour**; maximum: 1139 mg/**day** unless serum levels indicate need for larger dose

Adults >60 years: 0.38 mg/kg/**hour**; maximum dose: 507 mg/**day** unless serum concentrations indicate need for larger dose

Cardiac decompensation, cor pulmonale, hepatic dysfunction, sepsis with multiorgan failure, shock: Initial: 0.25 mg/kg/**hour**; maximum dose: 507 mg/**day** unless serum concentrations indicate need for larger dose.

Dosage adjustment based on serum theophylline concentrations:

Infants, Children, Adolescents, and Adults: **Note:** Recheck serum theophylline concentrations 12 hours (children) or 24 hours (adults) after IV dose

<9.9 mcg/mL: If tolerated, but symptoms remain, increase dose by ~25%. Recheck serum theophylline concentrations.

10 to 14.9 mcg/mL: Maintain dosage if tolerated. Recheck serum concentrations at 24-hour intervals.

15 to 19.9 mcg/mL: Consider 10% dose reduction to improve safety margin even if dose is tolerated.

20 to 24.9 mcg/mL: Decrease dose by ~25%. Recheck serum concentrations.

25 to 30 mcg/mL: Stop infusion for 12 hours (children) or 24 hours (adults) and decrease subsequent doses by at least 25%. Recheck serum concentrations.

>30 mcg/mL: Stop dosing and treat overdose; if resumed, decrease subsequent doses by at least 50%. Recheck serum concentrations.

Dosing adjustment in renal impairment:

Infants 1 to 3 months: Consider dose reduction and frequent monitoring of serum theophylline concentrations

Infants >3 months, Children, Adolescents, and Adults: No adjustment necessary

Dosing adjustment in hepatic impairment: Infants, Children, Adolescents, and Adults: Initial: 0.25 mg/kg/**hour**; maximum dose: 507 mg/**day** unless serum concentrations indicate need for larger dose

Usual Infusion Concentrations: Pediatric IV infusion: 1 mg/mL

Preparation for Administration Parenteral: May administer undiluted at 25 mg/mL (Klaus 1989) or may further dilute to a concentration of ≥1 mg/mL.

Administration Parenteral: For IV administration only; IM use is not recommended; IM administration causes intense pain. Loading doses should be administered over 30 minutes; doses may be further diluted and infused over 20 to 30 minutes; maximum rate of infusion: 0.36 mg/kg/minute and should not exceed 25 mg/minute

Vesicant; ensure proper needle or catheter placement prior to and during IV infusion. Avoid extravasation. If extravasation occurs, stop infusion immediately and disconnect (leave needle/cannula in place); gently aspirate extravasated solution (do **NOT** flush the line); initiate hyaluronidase antidote (See Management of Drug Extravasations for more details); remove needle/cannula; apply dry cold compresses (Hurst, 2004); elevate extremity.

Vesicant/Extravasation Risk Vesicant

Monitoring Parameters Serum theophylline concentrations, heart rate, respiratory rate, number and severity of apnea spells (when used for apnea of prematurity); arterial or capillary blood gases (if applicable); pulmonary function tests

Reference Range Therapeutic concentrations:

Asthma: 5-15 mcg/mL

Apnea of prematurity: 6-12 mcg/mL; goal concentration is reduced due to decreased protein binding and higher free fraction

Guidelines for Drawing Theophylline Serum Concentrations

Dosage Form	When to Obtain Sample[A]
IV bolus	30 min after end of 30-min infusion
Continuous IV infusion	12-24 h after initiation of infusion

[A]The time to achieve steady-state serum concentration is prolonged in patients with longer half-lives (eg, infants and adults with cardiac or liver failure; see theophylline half-life table). In these patients, serum theophylline concentrations should be drawn after 48-72 hours of therapy; may need to obtain concentrations prior to steady-state to assess the patient's current progress or evaluate potential toxicity.

Test Interactions Plasma glucose, uric acid, free fatty acids, total cholesterol, HDL, HDL/LDL ratio, and urinary free cortisol excretion may be increased by theophylline. Theophylline may decrease triiodothyronine.

Additional Information Theophylline dose is 79% of aminophylline dose.

Each mg/kg of theophylline administered as a bolus will increase the serum theophylline concentration by an average of 2 mcg/mL.

Dosage Forms Excipient information presented when available (limited, particularly for generics); consult specific product labeling.

Solution, Intravenous, as dihydrate:

Generic: 25 mg/mL (10 mL, 20 mL)

- **Aminophylline Injection (Can)** *see* Aminophylline *on page 122*
- **5-Aminosalicylic Acid** *see* Mesalamine *on page 1368*

Amiodarone (a MEE oh da rone)

Medication Safety Issues

Sound-alike/look-alike issues:

Amiodarone may be confused with amantadine, aMILoride, inamrinone

Cordarone may be confused with Cardura, Cordran

High alert medication:

The Institute for Safe Medication Practices (ISMP) includes this medication among its list of drugs which have a heightened risk of causing significant patient harm when used in error.

BEERS Criteria medication:

This drug may be potentially inappropriate for use in geriatric patients (Quality of evidence - high; Strength of recommendation - strong).

Related Information

Adult ACLS Algorithms *on page 2236*

Pediatric ALS (PALS) Algorithms *on page 2233*

Brand Names: US Cordarone; Nexterone; Pacerone

Brand Names: Canada Amiodarone Hydrochloride For Injection; Apo-Amiodarone; Cordarone; Dom-Amiodarone; Mylan-Amiodarone; PHL-Amiodarone; PMS-Amiodarone; PRO-Amiodarone; Riva-Amiodarone; Sandoz-Amiodarone; Teva-Amiodarone

Therapeutic Category Antiarrhythmic Agent, Class III

Generic Availability (US) Yes

Use

Oral: Management of life-threatening recurrent ventricular arrhythmias [eg, recurrent ventricular fibrillation (VF) or recurrent hemodynamically unstable ventricular tachycardia (VT)] unresponsive to other therapy or in patients intolerant to other therapy (FDA approved in adults)

IV: Initiation of management and prophylaxis of frequently recurrent VF and hemodynamically unstable VT unresponsive to other therapy; VF and VT in patients requiring amiodarone who are not able to take oral therapy (All indications: FDA approved in adults)

Note: Also has been used to treat supraventricular arrhythmias unresponsive to other therapy. Amiodarone is recommended in the PALS guidelines for SVT (unresponsive to vagal maneuvers and adenosine). It is recommended in both the PALS and ACLS guidelines for cardiac arrest with pulseless VT or VF (unresponsive to defibrillation, CPR, and vasopressor administration) and control of hemodynamically-stable monomorphic VT or wide-complex tachycardia of uncertain origin. The drug is also recommended in the ACLS guidelines for re-entry SVT (unresponsive to vagal maneuvers and adenosine); control of rapid ventricular rate due to conduction via an accessory pathway in pre-excited atrial arrhythmias; control of stable narrow-complex tachycardia; and control of polymorphic VT with a normal QT interval.

Medication Guide Available Yes

Pregnancy Risk Factor D

Pregnancy Considerations Adverse events have been observed in some animal reproduction studies. Amiodarone crosses the placenta (~10% to 50%) and may cause fetal harm when administered to a pregnant woman, leading to congenital goiter, hypo- or hyperthyroidism, neurodevelopmental, or neurological effects in the neonate. Growth retardation and premature birth have also been noted (ESG, 2011). Amiodarone should be used in pregnant women only to treat arrhythmias that are life-threatening or refractory to other treatments (Blomström-Lundqvist, 2003; ESG, 2011).

Breast-Feeding Considerations Amiodarone and its active metabolite are excreted into human milk. Breast-feeding may lead to significant infant exposure and potential toxicity. Due to the long half-life, amiodarone may be present in breast milk for several days following discontinuation of maternal therapy (Hall, 2003). The manufacturer recommends that breast-feeding be discontinued if treatment is needed.

Contraindications Hypersensitivity to amiodarone, iodine, or any component of the formulation; severe sinus-node dysfunction causing marked sinus bradycardia; second- and third-degree heart block (except in patients with a functioning artificial pacemaker); bradycardia causing syncope (except in patients with a functioning artificial pacemaker); cardiogenic shock

Warnings/Precautions Note: Although the US Boxed Warnings pertain to the tablet prescribing information, these effects may also be seen with intravenous administration depending on duration of use.

[US Boxed Warning (tablet)]: Only indicated for patients with life-threatening arrhythmias because of risk of substantial toxicity. Alternative therapies should be tried first before using amiodarone. Patients should be hospitalized when amiodarone is initiated. The 2010 ACLS guidelines recommend IV amiodarone as the preferred antiarrhythmic for the treatment of pulseless VT/VF, both life-threatening arrhythmias. In patients with non-life-threatening arrhythmias (eg, atrial fibrillation), amiodarone should be used only if the use of other antiarrhythmics has proven ineffective or are contraindicated.

[US Boxed Warning (tablet)]: Pulmonary toxicity (hypersensitivity pneumonitis or interstitial/alveolar

pneumonitis and abnormal diffusion capacity without symptoms) may occur. Reports of acute-onset pulmonary injury (pulmonary infiltrates and/or mass on X-ray, pulmonary alveolar hemorrhage, pleural effusion, pulmonary fibrosis, bronchospasm, wheezing, fever, dyspnea, cough, hemoptysis, hypoxia) have occurred; some cases have progressed to respiratory failure and/or death. Fatalities due to pulmonary toxicity occur in ~10% of cases; most fatalities due to sudden cardiac death occurred when amiodarone was discontinued; rule out other causes of respiratory impairment before discontinuing amiodarone in patients with life-threatening arrhythmias; use extreme caution if dose is decreased or discontinued. If hypersensitivity pneumonitis occurs, discontinue amiodarone and institute steroid therapy; if interstitial/alveolar pneumonitis occurs, institute steroid therapy and reduce amiodarone dose or preferably, discontinue. Some cases of interstitial/alveolar pneumonitis may resolve following dosage reduction and steroid therapy; rechallenge at a lower dose has not resulted in return of interstitial/alveolar pneumonitis in some patients; however, in some patients the pulmonary lesions have not been reversible. Educate patients about monitoring for symptoms (eg, nonproductive cough, dyspnea, pleuritic pain, hemoptysis, wheezing, weight loss, fever, malaise). Evaluate new respiratory symptoms; preexisting pulmonary disease does not increase risk of developing pulmonary toxicity, but if pulmonary toxicity develops then the prognosis is worse. Use of lower doses may be associated with a decreased incidence, but pulmonary toxicity has been reported in patients treated with low doses. The lowest effective dose should be used as appropriate for the acuity/severity of the arrhythmia being treated. **[US Boxed Warning (tablet)]: Liver toxicity is common, but usually mild with evidence of only increased liver enzymes; severe liver toxicity can occur and has been fatal in a few cases.** Hepatic enzyme levels are frequently elevated in patients exposed to amiodarone; most cases are asymptomatic. If increases >3x ULN (or ≥2x baseline in patients with preexisting elevations), consider dose reduction or discontinuation. Monitor hepatic enzymes regularly in patients on relatively high maintenance doses. Elevated bilirubin levels have been reported have been reported in patients administered IV amiodarone.

[US Boxed Warning (tablet)]: Amiodarone can exacerbate arrhythmias, by making them more difficult to tolerate or reverse; other types of arrhythmias have occurred, including significant heart block, sinus bradycardia, new ventricular fibrillation, incessant ventricular tachycardia, increased resistance to cardioversion, and polymorphic ventricular tachycardia associated with QTc prolongation (torsades de pointes [TdP]). Risk may be increased with concomitant use of other antiarrhythmic agents or drugs that prolong the QTc interval. Proarrhythmic effects may be prolonged. Amiodarone should not be used in patients with Wolff-Parkinson-White (WPW) syndrome and preexcited atrial fibrillation/flutter since ventricular fibrillation may result (AHA/ACC/HRS [January, 2014]).

Monitor pacing or defibrillation thresholds in patients with implantable cardiac devices (eg, pacemakers, defibrillators). May cause hyper- or hypothyroidism; hyperthyroidism may result in thyrotoxicosis (including fatalities) and/or the possibility of arrhythmia breakthrough or aggravation. If any new signs of arrhythmia appear, consider the possibility of hyperthyroidism. Hypothyroidism (sometimes severe) may be primary or subsequent to resolution of preceding amiodarone-induced hyperthyroidism; myxedema (may be fatal) has been reported. If hyper- or hypothyroidism occurs, reduce dose or discontinue amiodarone. Thyroid nodules and/or thyroid cancer have also been reported. Use caution in patients with thyroid disease; thyroid function should be monitored prior to treatment and periodically thereafter, particularly in the elderly and in patients with underlying thyroid dysfunction. In acute myocardial infarction, beta-blocker therapy should still be initiated even though concomitant amiodarone therapy provides beta-blockade.

Regular ophthalmic examination (including slit lamp and fundoscopy) is recommended. May cause optic neuropathy and/or optic neuritis resulting in visual impairment (peripheral vision loss, changes in acuity) at any time during therapy; permanent blindness has occurred. If symptoms of optic neuropathy and/or optic neuritis occur, prompt ophthalmic evaluation is recommended. If diagnosis of optic neuropathy and/or optic neuritis is confirmed, reevaluate amiodarone therapy. Corneal microdeposits occur in a majority of adults and may cause visual disturbances in up to 10% of patients (blurred vision, halos); asymptomatic microdeposits may be reversible and are not generally considered a reason to discontinue treatment. Corneal refractive laser surgery is generally contraindicated in amiodarone users (from manufacturers of surgical devices).

Peripheral neuropathy has been reported rarely with chronic administration; may resolve when amiodarone is discontinued, but resolution may be slow and incomplete.

Amiodarone is a potent inhibitor of CYP enzymes and transport proteins (including p-glycoprotein), which may lead to increased serum concentrations/toxicity of a number of medications. Particular caution must be used when a drug with QTc-prolonging potential relies on metabolism via these enzymes, since the effect of elevated concentrations may be additive with the effect of amiodarone. Carefully assess risk:benefit of coadministration of other drugs which may prolong QTc interval. Additional potentially significant interactions may exist, requiring dose or frequency adjustment, additional monitoring, and/or selection of alternative therapy. Patients may still be at risk for amiodarone–related adverse reactions or drug interactions after the drug has been discontinued. The pharmacokinetics are complex (due to prolonged duration of action and half-life) and difficult to predict. Correct electrolyte disturbances, especially hypokalemia, hypomagnesemia, or hypocalcemia, prior to use and throughout therapy. Use caution when initiating amiodarone in patients on warfarin. Cases of increased INR with or without bleeding have occurred in patients treated with warfarin; monitor INR closely after initiating amiodarone in these patients.

In the treatment of atrial fibrillation in older adults, avoid antiarrhythmics as first-line treatment. In older adults, data suggests rate control may provide more benefits than risks compared to rhythm control for most patients (Beers Criteria).

May cause hypotension and bradycardia (infusion-rate related). May cause life-threatening or fatal cutaneous reactions, including Stevens-Johnson syndrome and toxic epidermal necrolysis (TEN). If symptoms or signs (eg, progressive skin rash often with blisters or mucosal lesions) occur, immediately discontinue. During long-term treatment, a blue-gray discoloration of exposed skin may occur; risk increased in patients with fair complexion or excessive sun exposure; may be related to cumulative dose and duration of therapy. There has been limited experience in patients receiving IV amiodarone for >3 weeks. Some dosage forms may contain polysorbate 80 (also known as Tweens). Hypersensitivity reactions, usually a delayed reaction, have been reported following exposure to pharmaceutical products containing polysorbate 80 in certain individuals (Isaksson, 2002; Lucente 2000; Shelley, 1995). Thrombocytopenia, ascites, pulmonary deterioration, and renal and hepatic failure have been reported in premature neonates after receiving parenteral products containing polysorbate 80 (Alade, 1986; CDC, 1984). See manufacturer's labeling.

Use caution and close perioperative monitoring in surgical patients; may enhance myocardial depressant and conduction effects of halogenated inhalational anesthetics; adult respiratory distress syndrome (ARDS) has been reported postoperatively (fatal in rare cases). Hypotension upon discontinuation of cardiopulmonary bypass during open-heart surgery have been reported (rare); relationship to amiodarone is unknown. Commercially-prepared premixed infusion contains the excipient cyclodextrin (sulfobutyl ether beta-cyclodextrin), which may accumulate in patients with renal insufficiency, although the clinical significance of this finding is uncertain (Luke, 2010).

Adverse Reactions

Cardiovascular: Asystole (IV), atrial fibrillation, atrioventricular block, atrioventricular dissociation, bradycardia, cardiac arrest, cardiac arrhythmia, cardiac conduction disturbance, cardiac failure, cardiogenic shock, edema, flushing, hypotension (IV, refractory in rare cases), peripheral thrombophlebitis (IV, with concentrations >3 mg/mL), pulseless electrical activity (PEA), torsades de pointes (rare), ventricular fibrillation, ventricular tachycardia

Central nervous system: Abnormal gait, altered sense of smell, ataxia, dizziness, fatigue, headache, insomnia, involuntary body movements, malaise, memory impairment, paresthesia, peripheral neuropathy, sleep disorder

Dermatologic: Blue-gray skin pigmentation (oral, with prolonged exposure to amiodarone), skin photosensitivity

Endocrine & metabolic: Decreased libido, hyperthyroidism, hypothyroidism

Gastrointestinal: Abdominal pain, altered salivation, anorexia, constipation, diarrhea, dysgeusia, nausea (more common in oral), vomiting

Hematologic & oncologic: Blood coagulation disorder

Hepatic: Abnormal hepatic function tests, hepatic disease, increased serum transaminases (more common in IV)

Neuromuscular & skeletal: Tremor

Ophthalmic: Corneal deposits (may cause visual disturbance), optic neuritis, photophobia, visual disturbance, visual halos

Respiratory: Hypersensitivity pneumonitis, interstitial pneumonitis, pulmonary edema (IV), pulmonary fibrosis, pulmonary toxicity

Miscellaneous: Fever

Rare but important or life-threatening: Acute renal failure, agranulocytosis, alopecia, anaphylactic shock, anaphylactoid reaction, anaphylaxis, aplastic anemia, bronchiolitis obliterans organizing pneumonia, bullous dermatitis, cholestatic hepatitis, cholestasis, delirium, demyelinating polyneuropathy, disorientation, DRESS syndrome, drug-induced Parkinson disease, eosinophilic pneumonia, epididymitis (noninfectious), erythema multiforme, exfoliation of skin, granuloma, hallucination, hemolytic anemia, hemoptysis, hepatic cirrhosis, hepatic failure, hepatitis, hepatotoxicity (idiosyncratic) (Chalasani 2014), hypoesthesia, hypotension, hypoxia, impotence, increased intracranial pressure, increased lactate dehydrogenase, increased serum alkaline phosphatase, increased serum creatinine, jaundice, leukocytoclastic vasculitis, malignant neoplasm of skin, mass (pulmonary), myopathy, optic neuropathy, pancreatitis, pancytopenia, pleural effusion, pleurisy, pseudotumor cerebri, pulmonary alveolar hemorrhage, pulmonary infiltrates, pulmonary phospholipidosis, prolonged Q-T interval on ECG (associated with worsening of arrhythmia), renal insufficiency, respiratory arrest, respiratory failure, rhabdomyolysis, SIADH, sinoatrial arrest, skin carcinoma, skin granuloma, skin sclerosis, spontaneous ecchymosis, Stevens-Johnson syndrome, superior vena cava syndrome, thrombocytopenia, thyroid cancer, thyroid nodule, thyrotoxicosis, tissue necrosis at injection site, toxic epidermal necrolysis, vasculitis, vortex keratopathy (Baden 2015)

Drug Interactions

Metabolism/Transport Effects **Substrate** of CYP1A2 (minor), CYP2C19 (minor), CYP2C8 (major), CYP2D6 (minor), CYP3A4 (major), P-glycoprotein; **Note:** Assignment of Major/Minor substrate status based on clinically relevant drug interaction potential; **Inhibits** CYP1A2 (weak), CYP2A6 (moderate), CYP2B6 (weak), CYP2C19 (weak), CYP2C9 (moderate), CYP2D6 (moderate), CYP3A4 (weak), OCT2, P-glycoprotein

Avoid Concomitant Use

Avoid concomitant use of Amiodarone with any of the following: Agalsidase Alfa; Agalsidase Beta; Antiarrhythmic Agents (Class Ia); Artesunate; Azithromycin (Systemic); Bosutinib; Ceritinib; Conivaptan; Fingolimod; Fusidic Acid (Systemic); Grapefruit Juice; Highest Risk QTc-Prolonging Agents; Idelalisib; Indinavir; Ivabradine; Lopinavir; Mifepristone; Moderate Risk QTc-Prolonging Agents; Nelfinavir; PAZOPanib; Pimozide; Propafenone; Ritonavir; Saquinavir; Silodosin; Sofosbuvir; Tegafur; Thioridazine; Tipranavir; Topotecan; VinCRIStine (Liposomal)

Increased Effect/Toxicity

Amiodarone may increase the levels/effects of: Afatinib; Antiarrhythmic Agents (Class Ia); Artesunate; Beta-Blockers; Bosentan; Bosutinib; Bradycardia-Causing Agents; Brentuximab Vedotin; Cannabis; Cardiac Glycosides; Carvedilol; Ceritinib; Colchicine; CycloSPORINE (Systemic); CYP2A6 Substrates; CYP2C9 Substrates; CYP2D6 Substrates; Dabigatran Etexilate; DOXOrubicin (Conventional); Dronabinol; Edoxaban; Everolimus; Fesoterodine; Flecainide; Fosphenytoin; Highest Risk QTc-Prolonging Agents; HMG-CoA Reductase Inhibitors; Hydrocodone; Lacosamide; Ledipasvir; Lidocaine (Systemic); Lidocaine (Topical); Lomitapide; Loratadine; Metoprolol; Mipomersen; Naloxegol; Nebivolol; NiMODipine; PAZOPanib; P-glycoprotein/ABCB1 Substrates; Phenytoin; Pimozide; Porfimer; Propafenone; Prucalopride; Rifaximin; Rivaroxaban; Silodosin; Tetrahydrocannabinol; Thioridazine; TiZANidine; Topotecan; Verteporfin; VinCRIStine (Liposomal); Vitamin K Antagonists

The levels/effects of Amiodarone may be increased by: Abiraterone Acetate; Aprepitant; Atazanavir; Azithromycin (Systemic); Boceprevir; Bretylium; Calcium Channel Blockers (Nondihydropyridine); Cimetidine; Cobicistat; Conivaptan; Cyclophosphamide; CYP2C8 Inhibitors (Moderate); CYP2C8 Inhibitors (Strong); CYP3A4 Inhibitors (Moderate); CYP3A4 Inhibitors (Strong); Darunavir; Deferasirox; Fingolimod; Fosamprenavir; Fosaprepitant; Fosphenytoin; Fusidic Acid (Systemic); Grapefruit Juice; Idelalisib; Indinavir; Ivabradine; Ivacaftor; Lidocaine (Topical); Lopinavir; Luliconazole; Mifepristone; Moderate Risk QTc-Prolonging Agents; Nelfinavir; Netupitant; Palbociclib; P-glycoprotein/ABCB1 Inhibitors; QTc-Prolonging Agents (Indeterminate Risk and Risk Modifying); Ritonavir; Ruxolitinib; Saquinavir; Simeprevir; Sofosbuvir; Stiripentol; Telaprevir; Tipranavir; Tofacitinib

Decreased Effect

Amiodarone may decrease the levels/effects of: Agalsidase Alfa; Agalsidase Beta; Artesunate; Clopidogrel; Codeine; Sodium Iodide I131; Tamoxifen; Tegafur; TraMADol

The levels/effects of Amiodarone may be decreased by: Bile Acid Sequestrants; Bosentan; CYP2C8 Inducers (Strong); CYP3A4 Inducers (Moderate); CYP3A4 Inducers (Strong); Dabrafenib; Deferasirox; Etravirine; Fosphenytoin; Grapefruit Juice; Mitotane; Orlistat; P-glycoprotein/ABCB1 Inducers; Phenytoin; Rifampin; Siltuximab; St Johns Wort; Tocilizumab

Food Interactions Food increases the rate and extent of absorption of amiodarone. Grapefruit juice increases bioavailability of oral amiodarone by 50% and decreases the conversion of amiodarone to N-DEA (active metabolite); altered effects are possible. Management: Take consistently with regard to meals; grapefruit juice should be avoided during therapy.

Storage/Stability

Tablets: Store at 20°C to 25°C (68°F to 77°F); protect from light.

Injection: Store undiluted vials and premixed solutions (Nexterone) at 20°C to 25°C (68°F to 77°F); excursions are permitted between 15°C and 30°C (59°F and 86°F). Protect from light during storage; protect from excessive heat. There is no need to protect solutions from light during administration. When vial contents are admixed in D_5W to a final concentration of 1-6 mg/mL, amiodarone is stable for 24 hours in glass or polyolefin bottles and for 2 hours in polyvinyl chloride (PVC) bags; do not use evacuated glass containers as buffer may cause precipitation. Nexterone is available as premixed solutions. Although amiodarone adsorbs to PVC tubing, all clinical studies used PVC tubing and the recommended doses account for adsorption; in adults, PVC tubing is recommended. Discard any unused portions of premixed solutions.

Mechanism of Action Class III antiarrhythmic agent which inhibits adrenergic stimulation (alpha- and beta-blocking properties), affects sodium, potassium, and calcium channels, prolongs the action potential and refractory period in myocardial tissue; decreases AV conduction and sinus node function

Pharmacodynamics

Onset of action: Oral: 2-3 days to 1-3 weeks after starting therapy; IV: (electrophysiologic effects) within hours; antiarrhythmic effects: 2-3 days to 1-3 weeks; mean onset of effect may be shorter in children vs adults and in patients receiving IV loading doses

Maximum effect: Oral: 1 week to 5 months

Duration of effects after discontinuation of oral therapy: Variable, 2 weeks to months: Children: less than a few weeks; adults: several months

Pharmacokinetics (Adult data unless noted)

Absorption: Oral: Slow and incomplete

Distribution:

- IV: Rapid redistribution with a decrease to 10% of peak values within 30-45 minutes after completion of infusion
  - V_{dss}: IV single dose: Mean range: 40-84 L/kg
- Oral: V_d: 66 L/kg: Range: 18-148 L/kg

Protein binding: >96%

Metabolism: Hepatic via CYP3A4 and CYP2C8 to active metabolite, N-desethylamiodarone; possible enterohepatic recirculation

Bioavailability: Oral: ~50% (range: 35% to 65%)

Half-life:

- Amiodarone:
  - Single dose: 58 days (range: 15-142 days)
  - Oral chronic therapy: Mean range: 40-55 days (range: 26-107 days)
  - IV single dose: Mean range: 9-36 days
  - Half-life is shortened in children vs adults
- N-desethylamiodarone (active metabolite):
  - Single dose: 36 days (range 14-75 days)
  - Oral chronic therapy: 61 days
  - IV single dose: Mean range: 9-30 days

Time to peak serum concentration: Oral: 3-7 hours

Elimination: Via biliary excretion; <1% excreted unchanged in urine

Dosing: Neonatal

Supraventricular tachycardia: Limited data available: Oral: Loading dose: 10-20 mg/kg/day in 2 divided doses for 7-10 days; dosage should then be reduced to 5-10 mg/kg/day once daily and continued for 2-7 months; dosing based on a study of 50 infants (<9 months of age) and neonates (as young as 1 day of life); **Note:** Patients who received a higher loading dose (20 mg/kg/day) were more likely to have a prolongation of the corrected QT interval (Etheridge, 2001).

Tachyarrhythmia, including junctional ectopic tachycardia (JET), paroxysmal supraventricular tachycardia (PSVT): Limited data available; the following dosing is based on studies that included neonates, infants, and children.

Loading dose: IV: 5 mg/kg given over 60 minutes; **Note:** Bolus infusion rates should generally not exceed 0.25 mg/kg/minute unless clinically indicated; most studies used bolus infusion time of 60 minutes to avoid hypotension; may repeat initial loading dose to a maximum total initial load: 10 mg/kg; do not exceed total daily bolus of 15 mg/kg/**day** (Etheridge, 2001; Figa, 1994; Haas, 2008; Raja, 1994; Soult, 1995).

Continuous IV infusion (if needed): **Note:** Reported dosing units for regimens are variable (mcg/kg/minute and mg/kg/day); use caution to ensure appropriate dose and dosing units are used; taper infusion as soon as clinically possible and switch to oral therapy if necessary.

- Dosing based on **mcg**/kg/**minute**: Initial: 5 **mcg**/kg/**minute**; increase incrementally as clinically needed; usual required dose: 10 **mcg**/kg/**minute**; range: 5-15 **mcg**/kg/**minute** (Figa, 1994; Kovacikova, 2009; Lane, 2010)
- Dosing based on **mg**/kg/**day**: Initial: 10 **mg**/kg/**day**; increase incrementally as clinically needed; range: 10-20 **mg**/kg/**day** (Haas, 2008; Lane, 2010; Raja, 1994; Soult, 1995)

Dosing: Usual

Pediatric:

Perfusing tachycardias: Infants, Children, and Adolescents: IV, I.O.: Loading dose: 5 mg/kg (maximum: 300 mg/dose) over 20-60 minutes; may repeat twice up to maximum total dose of 15 mg/kg during acute treatment (PALS, 2010)

Pulseless VT or VF: Infants, Children, and Adolescents: IV, I.O.: 5 mg/kg (maximum: 300 mg/dose) rapid bolus; may repeat twice up to a maximum total dose of 15 mg/kg during acute treatment (PALS, 2010)

Tachyarrhythmia, including junctional ectopic tachycardia (JET), paroxysmal supraventricular tachycardia (PSVT): Limited data available: Infants, Children, and Adolescents:

Oral: Loading dose: 10-15 mg/kg/day in 1-2 divided doses/day for 4-14 days or until adequate control of arrhythmia or prominent adverse effects occur; dosage should then be reduced to 5 mg/kg/day given once daily for several weeks; if arrhythmia does not recur, reduce to lowest effective dosage possible; usual daily minimal dose: 2.5 mg/kg/day; maintenance doses may be given for 5 of 7 days/week

Note: For infants, some have suggested BSA-directed dosing: Loading dose: 600-800 mg/**1.73 m²**/day in 1-2 divided doses (equivalent to 347-462 mg/m²/day); maintenance dose: 200-400 mg/**1.73 m²**/day once daily (equivalent to 116-231 mg/m²/day) (Bucknall, 1986; Coumel, 1980; Coumel, 1983; Paul, 1994)

Note: Prolongation of the corrected QT interval was more likely in infants <9 months of age who received higher loading doses (20 mg/kg/day vs 10 mg/kg/day in 2 divided doses) (n=50; mean age: 1 ± 1.5 months) (Etheridge, 2001)

IV: Loading dose: 5 mg/kg (maximum: 300 mg/dose) given over 60 minutes; **Note:** Bolus infusion rates should generally not exceed 0.25 mg/kg/minute unless clinically indicated; most studies used bolus infusion time of 60 minutes to avoid hypotension; may repeat initial loading dose to a maximum total initial load: 10 mg/kg; do not exceed total daily bolus of 15 mg/kg/**day** (Etheridge, 2001; Figa, 1994; Haas, 2008; Raja, 1994; Soult, 1995)

Note: Dividing the 5 mg/kg loading dose into 1 mg/kg aliquots (each administered over 5-10 minutes) has been used; an additional 1-5 mg/kg loading dose was given in the same manner, if needed, after 30 minutes (Perry, 1996)

Continuous IV infusion (if needed); **Note:** Reported dosing units for regimens are variable (mcg/kg/minute and mg/kg/day); use caution to ensure appropriate dose and dosing units are used; taper infusion as soon as clinically possible and switch to oral therapy if necessary.

Dosing based on **mcg**/kg/**minute**: Initial: 5 **mcg**/kg/**minute**; increase incrementally as clinically needed; usual required dose: 10 **mcg**/kg/**minute**; range: 5-15 **mcg**/kg/**minute**; maximum daily dose: 2200 mg/**day** (Figa, 1994; Kovacikova, 2009; Lane, 2010)

Dosing based on **mg**/kg/**day**: Initial: 10 **mg**/kg/**day**; increase incrementally as clinically needed; range: 10-20 **mg**/kg/**day**; maximum daily dose: 2200 mg/**day** (Lane, 2010; Perry, 1996; Raja, 1994; Soult, 1995)

Adult: **Note:** Lower loading and maintenance doses are preferable in women and all patients with low body weight.

Pulseless VT or VF (ACLS, 2010): IV push, I.O.: Initial: 300 mg; if pulseless VT or VF continues after subsequent defibrillation attempt or recurs, administer supplemental dose of 150 mg. **Note:** In this setting, administering **undiluted** is preferred (Dager, 2006; Skrifvars, 2004). *The Handbook of Emergency Cardiovascular Care* (Hazinski, 2010) and the 2010 ACLS guidelines (Neumar, 2010) do not make any specific recommendations regarding dilution of amiodarone in this setting. Experience is limited with I.O. administration of amiodarone (Neumar, 2010).

Upon return of spontaneous circulation, follow with an infusion of 1 mg/minute for 6 hours, then 0.5 mg/minute for 18 hours (mean daily doses >2100 mg/day have been associated with hypotension).

Perfusing tachycardias (ACLS, 2010): IV: Bolus doses for hemodynamically stable VT or wide QRS tachycardia of uncertain origin (regular rhythm): 150 mg given over 10 minutes; may repeat if necessary, followed by an infusion of 1 mg/minute for 6 hours, then 0.5 mg/minute; maximum daily dose: 2200 mg/**day** (Neumar, 2010)

Ventricular arrhythmias: Manufacturer's labeling:

Oral: Loading dose: 800-1600 mg/day in 1-2 divided doses for 1-3 weeks, then when adequate arrhythmia control is achieved, decrease to 600-800 mg/day in 1-2 divided doses for 1 month; maintenance: 400 mg daily; lower doses are recommended for supraventricular arrhythmias

IV: Loading dose: 1050 mg delivered over 24 hours as follows: 150 mg given over 10 minutes (at a rate of 15 mg/minute) followed by 360 mg given over 6 hours (at a rate of 1 mg/minute); follow with maintenance dose: 540 mg given over the next 18 hours (at a rate of 0.5 mg/minute); after the first 24 hours the maintenance dose is continued at 0.5 mg/minute; additional supplemental bolus doses of 150 mg infused over 10 minutes may be given for breakthrough VF or hemodynamically unstable VT; maintenance dose infusion may be increased to control arrhythmia; mean daily doses >2.1 g/day have been associated with hypotension

Atrial fibrillation: Pharmacologic cardioversion (ACC/AHA/ESC Practice Guidelines):

Oral:

Inpatient: 1200-1800 mg/day in divided doses until 10 **g** total, then 200-400 mg/day maintenance

Outpatient: 600-800 mg/day in divided doses until 10 **g** total, then 200-400 mg/day maintenance; although not supported by clinical evidence, a maintenance dose of 100 mg/day is commonly used especially for the elderly or patients with low body mass (Fuster, 2006; Zimetbaum, 2007). **Note:** Other regimens have been described and may be used clinically:

400 mg 3 times daily for 5-7 days, then 400 mg daily for 1 month, then 200 mg daily

or

10 mg/kg/day for 14 days, followed by 300 mg daily for 4 weeks, followed by maintenance dosage of 200 mg daily (Roy, 2000)

IV: 5-7 mg/kg over 30-60 minutes, then 1200-1800 mg/day continuous infusion until 10 **g** total; maintenance: See oral dosing.

Atrial fibrillation prophylaxis following open heart surgery: Note: A variety of regimens have been used in clinical trials, including oral and intravenous regimens:

Oral: Starting in postop recovery, 400 mg twice daily for up to 7 days. Alternative regimen of amiodarone: 600 mg/day for 7 days prior to surgery, followed by 200 mg/day until hospital discharge; has also been shown to decrease the risk of postoperative atrial fibrillation

IV: Starting at postop recovery, 1000 mg infused over 24 hours for 2 days has been shown to reduce the risk of postoperative atrial fibrillation

Atrial fibrillation, recurrent: No standard regimen defined; examples of regimens include: Oral: Initial: 10 mg/kg/day for 14 days; followed by 300 mg/day for 4 weeks, followed by maintenance dosage of 200 mg/day (Roy, 2000). Other regimens have been described and are used clinically (ie, 400 mg 3 times daily for 5-7 days, then 400 mg daily for 1 month, then 200 mg daily).

Transition from IV to oral therapy: Conversion from IV to oral therapy has not been formally evaluated. Some experts recommend a 1-2 day overlap when converting from IV to oral therapy especially when treating ventricular arrhythmias. Use the following as a guide assuming patient received 0.5 mg/minute for the listed duration of IV infusion:

<1 week infusion: 800-1600 mg/day

1-3 week infusion: 600-800 mg/day

>3 week infusion: 400 mg/day

Recommendations for conversion to intravenous amiodarone after oral administration: During long-term amiodarone therapy (ie, ≥4 months), the mean plasma-elimination half-life of the active metabolite of amiodarone in adults is 61 days. Replacement therapy may not be necessary in such patients if oral therapy is discontinued for a period <2 weeks, since any changes in serum amiodarone concentrations during this period may **not** be clinically significant.

Dosing adjustment in renal impairment: Adults: IV, Oral: No adjustment necessary; nondialyzable (parent and metabolite)

Dosing adjustment in hepatic impairment: Adults; IV Oral: No dosage adjustments are recommended in the manufacturer labeling; however, dosage adjustment may be necessary in substantial hepatic impairment; use with caution. If hepatic enzymes exceed 3 times normal or double in a patient with an elevated baseline, consider decreasing the dose or discontinuing amiodarone.

Usual Infusion Concentrations: Pediatric Note: Premixed solutions available.

IV infusion: 1.8 mg/mL

Preparation for Administration IV: **Perfusing arrhythmias:** Information based on adult data: Injection must be diluted before IV use. Maximum concentration for IV infusion: 6 mg/mL. Increased phlebitis may occur with peripheral infusions >3 mg/mL in D_5W, and concentrations ≤2.5 mg/mL may be less irritating. Solutions that will infuse for >2 hours must be prepared in a non-PVC container (eg, glass or polyolefin).

Infants, Children, and Adolescents: No data available regarding concentration for infusion; consider adult concentrations when diluting; commercially prepared premixed solutions in concentrations of 1.5 mg/mL and 1.8 mg/mL are available.

Adults: Usual dilutions: First loading infusion: 150 mg in 100 mL D_5W (1.5 mg/mL); then 900 mg in 500 mL D_5W (1.8 mg/mL) to deliver rest of dose

Administration

Oral: Administer at same time in relation to meals; do not administer with grapefruit juice. In adults, may administer in divided doses with meals if GI upset occurs or if taking large daily dose.

IV: Adjust administration rate to patient's clinical condition and urgency; give slowly to patients who have a pulse (ie, perfusing arrhythmia). With perfusing arrhythmias (eg, atrial fibrillation, stable ventricular tachycardia), do not exceed recommended IV concentrations or rates of infusion listed below (severe hepatic toxicity may occur). Slow the infusion rate if hypotension or bradycardia develops.

Pulseless VT or VF:

Infants, Children, and Adolescents: Administer via rapid IV bolus; adult data in this setting suggest administration of undiluted drug may be preferred (Dager 2006; Skrifvars 2004). **Note:** PALS guidelines (Kleinman 2010) do not specify dilution of bolus dose and *The Handbook of Emergency Cardiovascular Care* (Hazinski, 2010) and the ACLS guidelines (Neumar, 2010) do not make any specific recommendations regarding dilution of amiodarone in this setting.

Adults: May be administered rapidly and undiluted. **Note:** *The Handbook of Emergency Cardiovascular Care* (Hazinski 2010) and the 2010 ACLS guidelines (Neumar 2010) do not make any specific recommendations regarding dilution of amiodarone in this setting; however, in this setting, administering undiluted is preferred (Dager 2006; Skrifvars 2004).

Perfusing arrhythmias: Information based on adult data: Injection must be diluted before IV use. Administer via central venous catheter, if possible; increased phlebitis may occur with peripheral infusions >3 mg/mL in D_5W; the use of a central venous catheter with concentrations >2 mg/mL for infusions >1 hour is recommended. An in-line filter has been recommended during administration for continuous infusions to reduce the incidence of phlebitis. Must be infused via volumetric infusion device; drop size of IV solution may be reduced and underdosage may occur if drop counter-infusion sets are used. PVC tubing is recommended for administration regardless of infusion duration. **Incompatible** with heparin; flush with saline prior to and following infusion. **Note:** IV administration at lower flow rates (potentially associated with use in pediatrics) and higher concentrations than recommended may result in leaching of plasticizers (DEHP) from intravenous tubing. DEHP may adversely affect male reproductive tract development. Alternative means of dosing and administration (1 mg/kg aliquots) may need to be considered.

Infants, Children, and Adolescents: Administer loading dose over 20 to 60 minutes; may be followed by continuous IV infusion.

Monitoring Parameters Heart rate and rhythm, blood pressure, ECG, chest x-ray, pulmonary function tests, thyroid function tests; serum glucose, electrolytes (especially potassium and magnesium), triglycerides, liver enzymes; ophthalmologic exams including fundoscopy and slit-lamp examinations, physical signs and symptoms of thyroid dysfunction (lethargy, edema of hands and feet, weight gain or loss), and pulmonary toxicity (dyspnea, cough; oxygen saturation, blood gases). Monitor pacing or defibrillation thresholds in patients with implantable cardiac devices (eg, pacemakers, defibrillators) at initiation of therapy and periodically during treatment.

Reference Range Therapeutic: Chronic oral dosing: 1-2.5 mg/L (SI: 2-4 micromoles/L) (parent); desethyl metabolite (active) is present in equal concentration to parent drug; serum concentrations may not be of great value for predicting toxicity and efficacy; toxicity may occur even at therapeutic concentrations

Additional Information Intoxication with amiodarone necessitates ECG monitoring; bradycardia may be atropine resistant, IV isoproterenol or cardiac pacemaker may be required; hypotension, cardiogenic shock, heart block, QT prolongation and hepatotoxicity may also be seen; patients should be monitored for several days following overdose due to long half-life

IV product is used for acute treatment; the duration of IV treatment is usually 48-96 hours; however, in adults, infusions may be used cautiously for 2-3 weeks; there is limited experience with administering infusions for >3 weeks

Dosage Forms Considerations

Vials for injection contain benzyl alcohol which has been associated with "gasping syndrome" in neonates. Commercially-prepared premixed solutions do not contain benzyl alcohol.

Dosage Forms Excipient information presented when available (limited, particularly for generics); consult specific product labeling.

Solution, Intravenous, as hydrochloride:

Nexterone: 150 mg/100 mL (100 mL); 360 mg/200 mL (200 mL)

Generic: 150 mg/3 mL (3 mL); 450 mg/9 mL (9 mL); 900 mg/18 mL (18 mL)

Tablet, Oral, as hydrochloride:

Cordarone: 200 mg [scored]

Pacerone: 100 mg

Pacerone: 200 mg [scored; contains fd&c red #40, fd&c yellow #6 (sunset yellow)]

Pacerone: 400 mg [scored; contains fd&c yellow #10 aluminum lake]

Generic: 100 mg, 200 mg, 400 mg

Extemporaneous Preparations A 5 mg/mL oral suspension may be made with tablets and either a 1:1 mixture of Ora-Sweet® and Ora-Plus® or a 1:1 mixture of Ora-Sweet® SF and Ora-Plus® adjusted to a pH between 6-7 using a sodium bicarbonate solution (5 g/100 mL of distilled water). Crush five 200 mg tablets in a mortar and reduce to a fine powder. Add small portions of the chosen vehicle and mix to a uniform paste; mix while adding the vehicle in incremental proportions to **almost** 200 mL; transfer to a calibrated bottle, rinse mortar with vehicle, and add quantity of vehicle sufficient to make 200 mL. Label "shake well" and "protect from light". Stable for 42 days at room temperature or 91 days refrigerated (preferred) (Nahata, 2004).

Nahata MC, Pai VB, and Hipple TF, *Pediatric Drug Formulations*, 5th ed, Cincinnati, OH: Harvey Whitney Books Co, 2004.

◆ **Amiodarone Hydrochloride** *see* Amiodarone *on page 125*

◆ **Amiodarone Hydrochloride For Injection (Can)** *see* Amiodarone *on page 125*

Amitriptyline (a mee TRIP ti leen)

Medication Safety Issues

Sound-alike/look-alike issues:

Amitriptyline may be confused with aminophylline, imipramine, nortriptyline

Elavil may be confused with Aldoril, Eldepryl, enalapril, Equanil, Plavix

BEERS Criteria medication:

This drug may be potentially inappropriate for use in geriatric patients (Quality of evidence - high [moderate for SIADH]; Strength of recommendation - strong).

Related Information

Antidepressant Agents *on page 2257*

Brand Names: Canada Apo-Amitriptyline; Bio-Amitriptyline; Elavil; Levate; Novo-Triptyn; PMS-Amitriptyline

Therapeutic Category Antidepressant, Tricyclic (Tertiary Amine); Antimigraine Agent

Generic Availability (US) Yes

Use Treatment of various forms of depression, often in conjunction with psychotherapy; analgesic for certain chronic and neuropathic pain; migraine prophylaxis

Medication Guide Available Yes

Pregnancy Risk Factor C

Pregnancy Considerations Adverse events have been observed in some animal reproduction studies. Amitriptyline crosses the human placenta; CNS effects, limb deformities, and developmental delay have been noted in case reports (causal relationship not established). Tricyclic antidepressants may be associated with irritability, jitteriness, and convulsions (rare) in the neonate (Yonkers, 2009).

The ACOG recommends that therapy for depression during pregnancy be individualized; treatment should incorporate the clinical expertise of the mental health clinician, obstetrician, primary healthcare provider, and pediatrician (ACOG, 2008). According to the American Psychiatric Association (APA), the risks of medication treatment should be weighed against other treatment options and untreated depression. For women who discontinue antidepressant medications during pregnancy and who may be at high risk for postpartum depression, the medications can be restarted following delivery (APA, 2010). Treatment algorithms have been developed by the ACOG and the APA for the management of depression in women prior to conception and during pregnancy (Yonkers, 2009). Although not a first-line agent, amitriptyline may be used for the treatment of post-traumatic stress disorder in pregnant women (Bandelow, 2008). Migraine prophylaxis should be avoided during pregnancy; if needed, amitriptyline may be used if other agents are ineffective or contraindicated (Pringsheim, 2012).

Breast-Feeding Considerations Amitriptyline is excreted into breast milk. Based on information from six mother/infant pairs, following maternal use of amitriptyline 75-175 mg/day, the estimated exposure to the breast-feeding infant would be 0.2% to 1.9% of the weight-adjusted maternal dose. Adverse events have not been reported in nursing infants (four cases). Infants should be monitored for signs of adverse events; routine monitoring of infant serum concentrations is not recommended (Fortinguerra, 2009). Migraine prophylaxis should be avoided in women who are nursing; if needed, amitriptyline may be used if other agents are ineffective or contraindicated (Pringsheim, 2012). Due to the potential for serious adverse reactions in the nursing infant, the manufacturer recommends a decision be made whether to discontinue nursing or to discontinue the drug, taking into account the importance of treatment to the mother.

Contraindications Hypersensitivity to amitriptyline or any component of the formulation; coadministration with or within 14 days of MAOIs; coadministration with cisapride; acute recovery phase following myocardial infarction

Documentation of allergenic cross-reactivity for tricyclic antidepressants is limited. However, because of similarities in chemical structure and/or pharmacologic actions, the possibility of cross-sensitivity cannot be ruled out with certainty.

Warnings/Precautions [U.S. Boxed Warning]: Antidepressants increase the risk of suicidal thinking and behavior in children, adolescents, and young adults (18-24 years of age) with major depressive disorder (MDD) and other psychiatric disorders; consider risk prior to prescribing. Short-term studies did not show an increased risk in patients >24 years of age and showed a decreased risk in patients ≥65 years. Closely monitor for clinical worsening, suicidality, or unusual changes in behavior, particularly during the initial 1-2 months of therapy or during periods of dosage adjustments (increases or decreases); the patient's family or caregiver should be instructed to closely observe the patient and communicate condition with health care provider. A medication guide should be dispensed with each prescription. **Amitriptyline is not FDA-approved for use in children.**

The possibility of a suicide attempt is inherent in major depression and may persist until remission occurs. Worsening depression and severe abrupt suicidality that are not part of the presenting symptoms may require discontinuation or modification of drug therapy. The patient's family or caregiver should be alerted to monitor patients for the emergence of suicidality and associated behaviors (such as agitation, irritability, hostility, impulsivity, and hypomania) and notify healthcare provider.

May precipitate a shift to mania or hypomania in patients with bipolar disorder. Patients presenting with depressive symptoms should be screened for bipolar disorder. **Amitriptyline is not FDA approved for bipolar depression.**

The degree of sedation, anticholinergic effects, orthostasis, and conduction abnormalities are high relative to other antidepressants. Heart block may be precipitated in patients with preexisting conduction system disease and use is relatively contraindicated in patients with conduction abnormalities. May cause CNS depression, which may impair physical or mental abilities; patients must be cautioned about performing tasks that require mental alertness (eg, operating machinery or driving). Use with caution in patients with a history of cardiovascular disease (including previous MI, stroke, tachycardia, or conduction abnormalities). Use with caution in patients with urinary retention, benign prostatic hyperplasia, increased intraocular pressure (IOP), narrow-angle glaucoma, xerostomia, visual problems, constipation, or a history of bowel obstruction.

TCAs may rarely cause bone marrow suppression; monitor for any signs of infection and obtain CBC if symptoms (eg, fever, sore throat) evident. May alter glucose control - use with caution in patients with diabetes. Recommended by the manufacturer to discontinue prior to elective surgery; risks exist for drug interactions with anesthesia and for cardiac arrhythmias. However, definitive drug interactions have not been widely reported in the literature and continuation of tricyclic antidepressants is generally recommended as long as precautions are taken to reduce the significance of any adverse events that may occur (Pass, 2004). May lower seizure threshold - use caution in patients with a previous seizure disorder or condition predisposing to seizures such as brain damage, alcoholism, or concurrent therapy with other drugs which lower the seizure threshold. May increase the risks associated with electroconvulsive therapy. Bone fractures have been associated with antidepressant treatment. Consider the possibility of a fragility fracture if an antidepressant-treated patient presents with unexplained bone pain, point tenderness, swelling, or bruising (Rabenda, 2013; Rizzoli, 2012). Use with caution in patients with hepatic or renal dysfunction. May cause mild pupillary dilation which in susceptible individuals can lead to an episode of narrow-angle glaucoma. Consider evaluating patients who have not had an iridectomy for narrow-angle glaucoma risk factors. Avoid use in the elderly due to its potent anticholinergic and sedative properties, and potential to cause orthostatic hypotension. Therapy is relatively contraindicated in patients with symptomatic hypotension. In addition, may cause or exacerbate syndrome of inappropriate antidiuretic hormone secretion or hyponatremia; monitor sodium closely with initiation or dosage adjustments in older adults (Beers Criteria).

Abrupt discontinuation or interruption of antidepressant therapy has been associated with a discontinuation syndrome. Symptoms arising may vary with antidepressant however commonly include nausea, vomiting, diarrhea, headaches, light-headedness, dizziness, diminished appetite, sweating, chills, tremors, paresthesias, fatigue, somnolence, and sleep disturbances (eg, vivid dreams, insomnia). Greater risks for developing a discontinuation syndrome have been associated with antidepressants with shorter half-lives, longer durations of treatment, and abrupt discontinuation. For antidepressants of short or intermediate half-lives, symptoms may emerge within 2-5 days after treatment discontinuation and last 7-14 days (APA, 2010; Fava, 2006; Haddad, 2001; Shelton, 2001; Warner, 2006).

Adverse Reactions Anticholinergic effects may be pronounced; moderate to marked sedation can occur (tolerance to these effects usually occurs).

Cardiovascular: Atrioventricular conduction disturbance, cardiac arrhythmia, cardiomyopathy (rare), cerebrovascular accident, ECG changes (nonspecific), edema, facial edema, heart block, hypertension, myocardial infarction, orthostatic hypotension, palpitations, syncope, tachycardia

Central nervous system: Anxiety, ataxia, cognitive dysfunction, coma, confusion, delusions, disorientation, dizziness, drowsiness, drug withdrawal (nausea, headache, malaise, irritability, restlessness, dream and sleep disturbance, mania [rare], and hypomania [rare]), dysarthria, EEG pattern changes, excitement, extrapyramidal reaction (including abnormal involuntary movements and tardive dyskinesia), fatigue, hallucination, headache, hyperpyrexia, insomnia, lack of concentration, nightmares, numbness, paresthesia, peripheral neuropathy, restlessness, sedation, seizure, tingling of extremities

Dermatologic: Allergic skin rash, alopecia, diaphoresis, skin photosensitivity, urticaria

Endocrine & metabolic: Altered serum glucose, decreased libido, galactorrhea, gynecomastia, increased libido, SIADH, weight gain, weight loss

Gastrointestinal: Ageusia, anorexia, constipation, diarrhea, melanoglossia, nausea, paralytic ileus, parotid gland enlargement, stomatitis, unpleasant taste, vomiting, xerostomia

Genitourinary: Breast hypertrophy, impotence, testicular swelling, urinary frequency, urinary retention, urinary tract dilation

Hematologic & oncologic: Bone marrow depression (including agranulocytosis, leukopenia, and thrombocytopenia), eosinophilia, purpura

Hepatic: Hepatic failure, hepatitis (rare; including altered liver function and jaundice)

Hypersensitivity: Tongue edema

Neuromuscular & skeletal: Lupus-like syndrome, tremor, weakness

Ophthalmic: Accommodation disturbance, blurred vision, increased intraocular pressure, mydriasis

Otic: Tinnitus

Rare but important or life-threatening: Angle-closure glaucoma, neuroleptic malignant syndrome (rare; Stevens, 2008), serotonin syndrome (rare)

Drug Interactions

Metabolism/Transport Effects **Substrate** of CYP1A2 (minor), CYP2B6 (minor), CYP2C19 (minor), CYP2C9 (minor), CYP2D6 (major), CYP3A4 (minor); **Note:** Assignment of Major/Minor substrate status based on clinically relevant drug interaction potential; **Inhibits** CYP1A2 (weak), CYP2C19 (weak), CYP2C9 (weak), CYP2D6 (weak), CYP2E1 (weak)

Avoid Concomitant Use

Avoid concomitant use of Amitriptyline with any of the following: Aclidinium; Azelastine (Nasal); Cisapride; Dapoxetine; Eluxadoline; Glucagon; Iobenguane I 123; Ipratropium (Oral Inhalation); Linezolid; MAO Inhibitors; Methylene Blue; Moxonidine; Orphenadrine; Paraldehyde; Potassium Chloride; Thalidomide; Tiotropium; Umeclidinium

Increased Effect/Toxicity

Amitriptyline may increase the levels/effects of: AbobotulinumtoxinA; Alcohol (Ethyl); Alpha-/Beta-Agonists (Direct-Acting); Alpha1-Agonists; Amphetamines; Analgesics (Opioid); Anticholinergic Agents; Antipsychotic Agents; ARIPiprazole; Aspirin; Azelastine (Nasal); Beta2-Agonists; Buprenorphine; Cisapride; Citalopram; CNS Depressants; Desmopressin; Eluxadoline; Escitalopram; Fluconazole; Glucagon; Highest Risk QTc-Prolonging Agents; Hydrocodone; Methotrimeprazine; Methylene Blue; Metyrosine; Mirabegron; Moderate Risk QTc-Prolonging Agents; Nicorandil; NSAID (COX-2 Inhibitor); NSAID (Nonselective); OnabotulinumtoxinA; Orphenadrine; Paraldehyde; Potassium Chloride; Pramipexole; QuiNIDine; RimabotulinumtoxinB; ROPINIRole; Rotigotine; Serotonin Modulators; Sodium Phosphates; Sulfonylureas; Suvorexant; Thalidomide; Thiazide Diuretics; Tiotropium; TiZANidine; TraMADol; Vitamin K Antagonists; Yohimbine; Zolpidem

The levels/effects of Amitriptyline may be increased by: Abiraterone Acetate; Aclidinium; Altretamine; Antiemetics (5HT3 Antagonists); Antipsychotic Agents; Brimonidine (Topical); BuPROPion; Cannabis; Cimetidine; Cinacalcet; Citalopram; Cobicistat; CYP2D6 Inhibitors (Moderate); CYP2D6 Inhibitors (Strong); Dapoxetine; Darunavir; Dexmethylphenidate; Doxylamine; Dronabinol; Droperidol; DULoxetine; Escitalopram; Fluconazole; FLUoxetine; FluvoxaMINE; HydrOXYzine; Ipratropium (Oral Inhalation); Kava Kava; Linezolid; Lithium; Magnesium Sulfate; MAO Inhibitors; Methotrimeprazine; Methylphenidate; Metoclopramide; Metyrosine; Mianserin; Mifepristone; Nabilone; Panobinostat; PARoxetine; Peginterferon Alfa-2b; Perampanel; Pramlintide; Protease Inhibitors; QuiNIDine; Rufinamide; Sertraline; Sodium Oxybate; Tapentadol; Tedizolid; Terbinafine (Systemic); Tetrahydrocannabinol; Thyroid Products; Topiramate; TraMADol; Umeclidinium; Valproic Acid and Derivatives

Decreased Effect

Amitriptyline may decrease the levels/effects of: Acetylcholinesterase Inhibitors; Alpha1-Agonists; Alpha2-Agonists; Alpha2-Agonists (Ophthalmic); Iobenguane I 123; Itopride; Moxonidine; Secretin

The levels/effects of Amitriptyline may be decreased by: Acetylcholinesterase Inhibitors; Barbiturates; CarBAMazepine; Peginterferon Alfa-2b; St Johns Wort

Storage/Stability Store at 20°C to 25°C (68°F to 77°F). Protect from light.

Mechanism of Action Increases the synaptic concentration of serotonin and/or norepinephrine in the central nervous system by inhibition of their reuptake by the presynaptic neuronal membrane pump.

Pharmacodynamics Onset of action: Therapeutic antidepressant effects begin in 7-21 days; maximum effects may not occur for ≥2 weeks and as long as 4-6 weeks

Pharmacokinetics (Adult data unless noted)

Absorption: Oral: Rapid, well absorbed

Protein binding: >90%

Metabolism: In the liver to nortriptyline (active), hydroxy derivatives and conjugated derivatives

Half-life, adults: 9-25 hours (15-hour average)

Time to peak serum concentration: Within 4 hours

Elimination: Renal excretion of 18% as unchanged drug; small amounts eliminated in feces by bile

Dialysis: Nondialyzable

Dosing: Usual

Pediatric:

Chronic pain management: Limited data available: Children and Adolescents: Oral: Initial: 0.1 mg/kg at bedtime, may advance as tolerated over 2 to 3 weeks to 0.5 to 2 mg/kg at bedtime (APS 2008; Freidrichsdorf 2007; Kliegman 2011)

Depressive disorders: Note: Controlled clinical trials have not shown tricyclic antidepressants to be superior to placebo for the treatment of depression in children and adolescents (Dopheide 2006; Wagner 2005).

Children: Limited data available: Oral: Initial: 1 mg/kg/day given in 3 divided doses with increases to 1.5 mg/kg/day have been reported in a small number of children (n=9) 9 to 12 years of age; clinically, doses up to 3 mg/kg/day (5 mg/kg/day if monitored closely) have been proposed

Adolescents: Initial: 25 to 50 mg/day; may give in divided doses; increase gradually to 100 mg/day in divided doses; maximum dose: 200 mg/day

Migraine prophylaxis: Limited data available: Children: Oral: Initial: 0.25 mg/kg/day, given at bedtime; increase dose by 0.25 mg/kg/day every 2 weeks to 1 mg/kg/day. Reported dosing range: 0.2 to 1.7 mg/kg/day (Hershey 2000). Dosing based on a large open-label trial in 192 children (mean age 12 ± 3 years) with >3 headaches/month (61% with migraine, 8% with migraine with aura, and 10% with tension-type headaches) used an initial dose of 0.25 mg/kg/day given before bedtime; doses were increased every 2 weeks by 0.25 mg/kg/day to a final dose of 1 mg/kg/day; patients also used appropriate abortive medications and lifestyle adjustments; at initial reevaluation (mean: 67 days after initiation of therapy), the mean number of headaches per month significantly decreased from 17.1 to 9.2; the mean duration of headaches decreased from 11.5 to 6.3 hours; continued improvement was observed at follow-up visits; minimal adverse effects were reported. **Note:** Mean final dose was 0.99 ± 0.23 mg/kg; range: 0.16-1.7 mg/kg/day; ECGs were obtained on children receiving >1 mg/kg/day or in those describing a cardiac side effect (Hershey 2000).

Adult: **Depression:** Oral: Initial: 50 to 100 mg/day single dose at bedtime or in divided doses; dose may be gradually increased up to 300 mg/day; once symptoms are controlled, decrease gradually to lowest effective dose

Administration Oral: May administer with food to decrease GI upset

Monitoring Parameters Heart rate, blood pressure, mental status, weight. Monitor patient periodically for symptom resolution; monitor for worsening depression, suicidality, and associated behaviors (especially at the beginning of therapy or when doses are increased or decreased).

Reference Range Note: Plasma levels do not always correlate with clinical effectiveness

Therapeutic:

Amitriptyline plus nortriptyline (active metabolite): 100-250 ng/mL (SI: 360-900 nmol/L)

Nortriptyline 50-150 ng/mL (SI: 190-570 nmol/L)

Toxic: >500 ng/mL (SI: >1800 nmol/L)

Additional Information Due to promotion of weight gain with amitriptyline, other antidepressants (ie, imipramine or desipramine) may be preferred in heavy or obese children and adolescents

Dosage Forms Excipient information presented when available (limited, particularly for generics); consult specific product labeling.

Tablet, Oral, as hydrochloride:

Generic: 10 mg, 25 mg, 50 mg, 75 mg, 100 mg, 150 mg

- ◆ **Amitriptyline Hydrochloride** *see* Amitriptyline *on page 131*
- ◆ **AmLactin® [OTC]** *see* Lactic Acid and Ammonium Hydroxide *on page 1202*

AmLODIPine (am LOE di peen)

Medication Safety Issues

Sound-alike/look-alike issues:

AmLODIPine may be confused with aMILoride

Norvasc may be confused with Navane, Norvir, Vascor

International issues:

Norvasc [U.S., Canada, and multiple international markets] may be confused with Vascor brand name for imidapril [Philippines] and simvastatin [Malaysia, Singapore, and Thailand]

Brand Names: US Norvasc

Brand Names: Canada Accel-Amlodipine; ACT-Amlodipine; Amlodipine-Odan; Apo-Amlodipine; Auro-Amlodipine; Bio-Amlodipine; Dom-Amlodipine; GD-Amlodipine; JAMP-Amlodipine; Mar-Amlodipine; Mint-Amlodipine; Mylan-Amlodipine; Norvasc; PHL-Amlodipine; PMS-Amlodipine; Q-Amlodipine; RAN-Amlodipine; ratio-Amlodipine; Riva-Amlodipine; Sandoz Amlodipine; Septa-Amlodipine; Teva-Amlodipine

Therapeutic Category Antianginal Agent; Antihypertensive Agent; Calcium Channel Blocker; Calcium Channel Blocker, Dihydropyridine

Generic Availability (US) Yes

Use Treatment of hypertension (FDA approved in ages ≥6 years and adults); chronic stable angina (FDA approved in adults); vasospastic (Prinzmetal's) angina (FDA approved in adults); angiographically documented CAD [to decrease risk of hospitalization (due to angina) and coronary revascularization procedure] (FDA approved in adults)

Pregnancy Risk Factor C

Pregnancy Considerations Adverse events have been observed in some animal reproduction studies. Untreated chronic maternal hypertension is associated with adverse events in the fetus, infant, and mother. If treatment for hypertension during pregnancy is needed, other agents are preferred (ACOG 2013).

Breast-Feeding Considerations Amlodipine is excreted in breast milk. A study was conducted in 31 lactating women ~3 weeks postpartum. All women were administered amlodipine for pregnancy-induced hypertension (median daily dose 6.01 ± 2.31 mg). Sampling occurred ~10 days after dosing was initiated. The median predose amlodipine concentrations were 15.5 ng/mL (maternal serum) and 11.5 ng/mL (breast milk). The median estimated amlodipine exposure to the breastfeeding infant (relative infant dose) was 4.17 mcg/kg/day (median relative infant dose 4.18% based on the weight adjusted maternal dose). Variability was observed; the maximum relative infant dose calculated was 15.2% (Naito 2015). It is not known if amlodipine is excreted into breast milk. Breast-feeding is not recommended by the manufacturer.

Contraindications Hypersensitivity to amlodipine or any component of the formulation

Warnings/Precautions Increased angina and/or MI has occurred with initiation or dosage titration of calcium channel blockers. Symptomatic hypotension can occur; acute hypotension upon initiation is unlikely due to the gradual onset of action. Blood pressure must be lowered at a rate appropriate for the patient's clinical condition. Use caution in severe aortic stenosis and/or hypertrophic cardiomyopathy with outflow tract obstruction. Use caution in patients with hepatic impairment; may require lower starting dose; titrate slowly with severe hepatic impairment. The most common side effect is peripheral edema; occurs within 2 to 3 weeks of starting therapy. Reflex tachycardia may occur with use. Peak antihypertensive effect is delayed; dosage titration should occur after 7 to 14 days on a given dose. Initiate at a lower dose in the elderly.

Adverse Reactions

Cardiovascular: Flushing (more common in females), palpitations, peripheral edema (more common in females)

Central nervous system: Dizziness, drowsiness, fatigue, male sexual disorder

Dermatologic: Pruritus, skin rash

Gastrointestinal: Abdominal pain, nausea

Neuromuscular & skeletal: Muscle cramps, weakness

Respiratory: Dyspnea, pulmonary edema

Rare but important or life-threatening: Acute interstitial nephritis (Ejaz 2000), anorexia, atrial fibrillation, bradycardia, cholestasis, conjunctivitis, depression, diarrhea, difficulty in micturition, diplopia, dysphagia, epistaxis, erythema multiforme, exfoliative dermatitis, extrapyramidal reaction, eye pain, female sexual disorder, gingival hyperplasia, gynecomastia, hepatitis, hot flash, hyperglycemia, hypersensitivity angiitis, hypersensitivity reaction, hypoesthesia, increased serum transaminases, increased thirst, insomnia, leukopenia, maculopapular rash, myalgia, nocturia, orthostatic hypotension, osteoarthritis, pancreatitis, paresthesia, peripheral ischemia, peripheral neuropathy, phototoxicity, purpura, rigors, tachycardia, thrombocytopenia, tremor, vasculitis, ventricular tachycardia, weight gain

Drug Interactions

Metabolism/Transport Effects Substrate of CYP3A4 (major); **Note:** Assignment of Major/Minor substrate status based on clinically relevant drug interaction potential; **Inhibits** CYP1A2 (weak), CYP2A6 (weak), CYP2B6 (weak), CYP2C8 (weak), CYP2C9 (weak), CYP2D6 (weak), CYP3A4 (weak)

Avoid Concomitant Use

Avoid concomitant use of AmLODIPine with any of the following: Amodiaquine; Conivaptan; Fusidic Acid (Systemic); Idelalisib; Pimozide

Increased Effect/Toxicity

AmLODIPine may increase the levels/effects of: Amifostine; Amodiaquine; Antihypertensives; ARIPiprazole; Atosiban; Calcium Channel Blockers (Nondihydropyridine); Dofetilide; DULoxetine; Fosphenytoin; Hydrocodone; Hypotensive Agents; Levodopa; Lomitapide; Magnesium Salts; Neuromuscular-Blocking Agents (Nondepolarizing); NiMODipine; Nitroprusside; Obinutuzumab; Phenytoin; Pimozide; QuiNIDine; RisperiDONE; RiTUXimab; Simvastatin; Tacrolimus (Systemic); TiZANidine

The levels/effects of AmLODIPine may be increased by: Alfuzosin; Alpha1-Blockers; Antifungal Agents (Azole Derivatives, Systemic); Aprepitant; Barbiturates; Brimonidine (Topical); Calcium Channel Blockers (Nondihydropyridine); Conivaptan; CycloSPORINE (Systemic); CYP3A4 Inhibitors (Moderate); CYP3A4 Inhibitors (Strong); Dapoxetine; Dasatinib; Diazoxide; Fluconazole; Fosaprepitant; Fusidic Acid (Systemic); Grapefruit Juice; Herbs (Hypotensive Properties); Idelalisib; Ivacaftor; Luliconazole; Macrolide Antibiotics; Magnesium Salts; MAO Inhibitors; Mifepristone; Netupitant; Nicorandil; Palbociclib; Pentoxifylline; Phosphodiesterase 5 Inhibitors; Prostacyclin Analogues; Protease Inhibitors; QuiNIDine; Simeprevir; Stiripentol

Decreased Effect

AmLODIPine may decrease the levels/effects of: Clopidogrel; QuiNIDine

The levels/effects of AmLODIPine may be decreased by: Barbiturates; Bosentan; Calcium Salts; CarBAMazepine; CYP3A4 Inducers (Moderate); CYP3A4 Inducers (Strong); Dabrafenib; Deferasirox; Efavirenz; Herbs (Hypertensive Properties); Melatonin; Methylphenidate; Mitotane; Nafcillin; Rifamycin Derivatives; Siltuximab; St Johns Wort; Tocilizumab; Yohimbine

Food Interactions Grapefruit juice may modestly increase amlodipine levels. Management: Monitor closely with concurrent use.

Storage/Stability Store at 15°C to 30°C (59°F to 86°F).

Mechanism of Action Inhibits calcium ion from entering the "slow channels" or select voltage-sensitive areas of vascular smooth muscle and myocardium during depolarization, producing a relaxation of coronary vascular smooth muscle and coronary vasodilation; increases myocardial oxygen delivery in patients with vasospastic angina. Amlodipine directly acts on vascular smooth muscle to produce peripheral arterial vasodilation reducing peripheral vascular resistance and blood pressure.

Pharmacodynamics

Antihypertensive effects:

Onset of action: Adults: Significant reductions in blood pressure at 24 to 48 hours after first dose; slight increase in heart rate within 10 hours of administration may reflect some vasodilating activity (Donnelly 1993)

Duration: At least 24 hours. In adults, duration has been shown to extend to at least 72 hours when discontinued after 6 to 7 weeks of therapy (Biston 1999)

Pharmacokinetics (Adult data unless noted)

Absorption: Oral: Well absorbed

Distribution: Mean V_d:

Children >6 years: Similar to adults on a mg per kg basis; **Note:** Weight-adjusted V_d in younger children (<6 years of age) may be greater than in older children (Flynn 2006)

Adults: 21 L/kg (Scholz 1997)

Protein binding: ~93%

Metabolism: Hepatic (~90%) to inactive metabolites

Bioavailability: Oral: 64% to 90%

Half-life: Terminal: 30 to 50 hours; increased with hepatic dysfunction

Time to peak serum concentrations: 6 to 12 hours

Elimination: Urine (10% of total dose as unchanged drug, 60% of total dose as metabolites)

Clearance: May be decreased in patients with hepatic insufficiency or moderate to severe heart failure; weight-adjusted clearance in children >6 years of age is similar to adults; **Note:** Weight-adjusted clearance in younger children (<6 years of age) may be greater than in older children (Flynn 2006)

Dosing: Usual

Pediatric:

Hypertension: Oral: **Note:** For a summary of other pediatric studies see Additional Information

Children 1 to 5 years: Limited data available: **Note:** A population pharmacokinetic study found that children <6 years of age had weight-adjusted clearance and V_d of amlodipine that were significantly greater than children ≥6 years of age. This may suggest the need for higher mg/kg/day doses in younger children (<6 years of age); however, the study included only a small number of younger children (n=11) (Flynn 2006). One retrospective pediatric study (n=55) that included only eight patients 1-6 years of age used initial doses of 0.05-0.1 mg/kg/day; doses were titrated upwards as needed; mean required dose was significantly higher in patients 1-6 years of age (0.3 ± 0.16 mg/kg/day) compared to older children (6 to 12 years: 0.16 ± 0.12 mg/kg/day; 12 to 20 years: 0.14 ± 0.1 mg/kg/day) (Flynn 2000a).

Children and Adolescents 6 to 17 years: 2.5 to 5 mg once daily; doses >5 mg daily have not been fully studied. In a randomized, placebo-controlled trial of amlodipine in children (n=268; mean age: 12.1 years; range: 6 to 16 years), a significant reduction in systolic blood pressure (compared to placebo) was observed in both the 2.5 mg once daily and the 5 mg once daily amlodipine groups. The authors recommend an initial dose of 0.06 mg/kg/day with a maximum dose of 0.34 mg/kg/day (not to exceed 10 mg/day) (Flynn 2004).

Adult:

Coronary artery disease (CAD) (chronic stable angina, vasospastic angina, angiographically documented CAD [without heart failure or ejection fraction <40%]): Oral: 5 to 10 mg once daily

Hypertension: Oral: Initial: 5 mg once daily or 2.5 mg once daily in small or frail patients, or when adding amlodipine to other antihypertensive therapy; maximum daily dose: 10 mg/**day**. In general, titrate every 7 to 14 days. Titrate more rapidly, however, if clinically warranted, provided the patient is assessed frequently. Usual dosage range (ASH/ISH [Weber 2014]): 5 to 10 mg once daily. Target dose (JNC8 [James 2013]): 10 mg once daily

Dosing adjustment in renal impairment: Children ≥ 6 years, Adolescents, and Adults: No dosage adjustment necessary (Doyle 1989; Kungys 2003).

End-stage renal disease (ESRD) on dialysis: Adults: Hemodialysis and peritoneal dialysis do not enhance elimination; supplemental dose is not necessary (Kungys 2003).

Dosing adjustment in hepatic impairment: Adults:

Coronary artery disease (CAD) (chronic stable angina, vasospastic angina, angiographically documented CAD without heart failure or ejection fraction <40%): Initial: 5 mg once daily; titrate slowly in patients with severe hepatic impairment.

Hypertension: Initial: 2.5 mg once daily; titrate slowly in patients with severe hepatic impairment.

Administration Oral: May be administered without regard to food.

Monitoring Parameters Blood pressure, heart rate, liver enzymes

Additional Information Summary of additional pediatric studies:

In one prospective study, 21 hypertensive children (mean age: 13.1 years; range: 6-17 years) received the following initial daily doses of amlodipine based on weight groups: Children <50 kg: 0.05 mg/kg/day; children 50-70 kg: 2.5 mg daily; children >70 kg: 5 mg daily; mean initial dose: 0.07 ± 0.04 mg/kg/day; doses were increased by 25% to 50% (rounded to the nearest 2.5 mg) every 5-7 days to a maximum of 0.5 mg/kg/day, as needed to control blood pressure; the mean required dose was almost twice as high for children <13 years of age (0.29 ± 0.13 mg/kg/day) compared to children ≥13 years of age (0.16 ± 0.11 mg/kg/day) (Tallian 1999).

In a small randomized crossover trial, amlodipine was compared to nifedipine or felodipine in 11 hypertensive children (mean age: 16 years; range: 9-17 years); amlodipine was administered once daily as a liquid preparation (tablets dissolved in water immediately prior to administration); an initial daily dose of 0.1 mg/kg/day (maximum: 5 mg daily) was increased by 50% to 100% after 1 week to a maximum of 10 mg/day, as needed for blood pressure control; mean initial dose: 0.09 ± 0.01 mg/kg/day; mean required dose: 0.12 mg/kg/day (Rogan, 2000). A third prospective study used fixed mg doses, rather than dosing on a mg/kg basis (Pfammatter 1998).

A prospective study in 43 pediatric outpatients with chronic kidney disease (median age: 9 years; range: 1-19 years) used the following initial daily doses of amlodipine based on weight groups: Children 10-30 kg: 2.5 mg once daily; children ≥31 kg: 5 mg once daily. Doses were increased if needed to a maximum of 0.5 mg/kg/day (20 mg/day). Younger patients required significantly higher mg/kg/day doses of amlodipine compared to older children. This relationship was not observed when the dose was expressed as mg/m²/day. The authors recommend a dose of 7-10 mg/m² given once daily (von Vigier 2001).

Five retrospective studies used a variety of initial amlodipine doses ranging from 0.05-0.13 mg/kg/day; mean required dose after dosage titration (for all aged pediatric patients) ranged from 0.15-0.23 mg/kg/day (Andersen 2006; Flynn 2000a; Khattak 1998; Parker 2002; Silverstein 1999). Two of these studies noted a relationship between dose and age, with younger patients requiring higher mg/kg/day doses. Several retrospective studies used twice daily dosing in younger children, but it is unknown whether this reflects altered pharmacokinetics or physician prescribing habits. One population pharmacokinetic study suggests there is no justification for twice-daily dosing of amlodipine children (Flynn 2006). Further pediatric studies are needed.

Dosage Forms Excipient information presented when available (limited, particularly for generics); consult specific product labeling.

Tablet, Oral:

Norvasc: 2.5 mg, 5 mg, 10 mg

Generic: 2.5 mg, 5 mg, 10 mg

Extemporaneous Preparations A 1 mg/mL oral suspension may be made with tablets and either a 1:1 mixture of simple syrup and 1% methylcellulose or a 1:1 mixture of Ora-Plus® and Ora-Sweet®. Crush fifty 5 mg tablets in a mortar and reduce to a fine powder. Add small portions of the chosen vehicle and mix to a uniform paste; mix while adding the vehicle in incremental proportions to **almost** 250 mL; transfer to a calibrated bottle, rinse mortar with vehicle, and add quantity of vehicle sufficient to make 250 mL. Label "shake well" and "refrigerate". Stable for 56 days at room temperature or 91 days refrigerated.

Nahata MC, Morosco RS, and Hipple TF, "Stability of Amlodipine Besylate in Two Liquid Dosage Forms," *J Am Pharm Assoc (Wash)* 1999, 39(3):375-7.

- **Amlodipine Besylate** *see* AmLODIPine *on page 133*
- **Amlodipine-Odan (Can)** *see* AmLODIPine *on page 133*
- **Ammens® Original Medicated [OTC]** *see* Zinc Oxide *on page 2214*
- **Ammens® Shower Fresh [OTC]** *see* Zinc Oxide *on page 2214*
- **Ammonapse** *see* Sodium Phenylbutyrate *on page 1948*

Ammonium Chloride (a MOE nee um KLOR ide)

Therapeutic Category Metabolic Alkalosis Agent; Urinary Acidifying Agent

Generic Availability (US) Yes

Use Diuretic or systemic and urinary acidifying agent; treatment of hypochloremia

Pregnancy Risk Factor C

Pregnancy Considerations Animal reproduction studies have not been conducted.

Contraindications Severe hepatic or renal dysfunction; should not be administered when metabolic alkalosis due to vomiting of hydrochloric acid is accompanied by loss of sodium (excretion of sodium bicarbonate in the urine)

Warnings/Precautions Monitor closely for signs and symptoms of ammonia toxicity, including pallor, diaphoresis, altered breathing, bradycardia, arrhythmias, retching, twitching, seizure, and coma.

May result in increased ammonia concentrations leading to worsened encephalopathy (Adrogue 1998); use is contraindicated in severe hepatic impairment. May result in increased urea formation resulting in exacerbation of uremic symptoms (Devlin 2014); use is contraindicated in severe renal impairment. Use caution in patients with primary respiratory acidosis or pulmonary insufficiency.

Adverse Reactions

Central nervous system: Coma, drowsiness, EEG abnormalities, headache, mental confusion, seizure

Dermatologic: Rash

Endocrine & metabolic: Calcium-deficient tetany, hyperchloremia, hypokalemia, metabolic acidosis, potassium may be decreased, sodium may be decreased

Gastrointestinal: Abdominal pain, gastric irritation, nausea, vomiting

Hepatic: Ammonia may be increased

Local: Pain at site of injection

Neuromuscular & skeletal: Twitching

Respiratory: Hyperventilation

Drug Interactions

Metabolism/Transport Effects None known.

Avoid Concomitant Use There are no known interactions where it is recommended to avoid concomitant use.

Increased Effect/Toxicity

Ammonium Chloride may increase the levels/effects of: ChlorproPAMIDE; Salicylates

The levels/effects of Ammonium Chloride may be increased by: Potassium-Sparing Diuretics

Decreased Effect

Ammonium Chloride may decrease the levels/effects of: Alpha-/Beta-Agonists (Indirect-Acting); Amphetamines; Analgesics (Opioid); Mecamylamine

Storage/Stability Store intact vials at 20°C to 25°C (68°F to 77°F). Solution may crystallize if exposed to low temperatures. If crystals are observed, warm vial to room temperature in a water bath prior to use.

Mechanism of Action Increases acidity by increasing free hydrogen ion concentration

Pharmacokinetics (Adult data unless noted)

Metabolism: In the liver

Elimination: In urine

Dosing: Usual

Infants, Children, and Adolescents:

Metabolic alkalosis: IV: **Note:** Ammonium chloride is an alternative treatment and should be used only after sodium and potassium chloride supplementation has been optimized. The following equations represent different methods of chloride or alkalosis correction utilizing either the serum Cl^-, the serum HCO_3^-, or the base excess. These equations will yield different requirements of ammonium chloride. Initially, administer 1/2 to 2/3 of the calculated dose, and then re-evaluate.

Dosing of mEq NH_4Cl via the chloride-deficit method (hypochloremia):

mEq NH_4Cl = 0.2 L/kg x wt in kg x [103 - serum Cl^-] mEq/L

Dosing of mEq NH_4Cl via the bicarbonate-excess method (refractory hypochloremic metabolic alkalosis):

mEq NH_4Cl = 0.5 L/kg x wt in kg x [serum HCO_3^- - 24] mEq/L

Dosing of mEq NH^4Cl via the base excess method:

mEq NH_4Cl = 0.3 L/kg x wt in kg x base excess (mEq/L)

Urinary acidification: IV: 75 mg/kg/day in 4 divided doses; maximum daily dose: 6 g

Adults: **Metabolic alkalosis:** The following equations represent different methods of correction utilizing either the serum HCO_3^-, the serum chloride, or the base excess administer 50% of dose over 12 hours, then re-evaluate

Dosing of mEq NH_4Cl via the chloride-deficit method (hypochloremia):

Dose of mEq NH_4Cl = [0.2 L/kg x body weight (kg)] x [103 - observed serum chloride; **Note:** 0.2 L/kg is the estimated chloride volume of distribution and 103 is the average normal serum chloride concentration (mEq/L)

Dosing of mEq NH_4Cl via the bicarbonate-excess method (refractory hypochloremic metabolic alkalosis):

Dose of NH_4Cl = [0.5 L/kg x body weight (kg)] x (observed serum HCO_3^- - 24); **Note:** 0.5 L/kg is the estimated bicarbonate volume of distribution and 24 is the average normal serum bicarbonate concentration (mEq/L)

These equations will yield different requirements of ammonium chloride.

Preparation for Administration Parenteral: IV: Dilute prior to use to usual concentration of 0.2 mEq/mL; maximum concentration: 0.4 mEq/mL

Administration Parenteral: IV: Must be diluted prior to administration; administer by slow intravenous infusion to avoid local irritation and adverse effects. Infuse over 3 hours; maximum rate of infusion: 1 mEq/kg/hour; in adults rate of infusion should not exceed 5 mL/minute.

Monitoring Parameters Serum electrolytes, serum ammonia

Dosage Forms Excipient information presented when available (limited, particularly for generics); consult specific product labeling.

Injection, solution: Ammonium 5 mEq/mL and chloride 5 mEq/mL (20 mL) [equivalent to ammonium chloride 267.5 mg/mL]

- ◆ **Ammonium Hydroxide and Lactic Acid** *see* Lactic Acid and Ammonium Hydroxide *on page 1202*
- ◆ **Ammonium Lactate** *see* Lactic Acid and Ammonium Hydroxide *on page 1202*
- ◆ **Ammonul®** *see* Sodium Phenylacetate and Sodium Benzoate *on page 1947*
- ◆ **Amnesteem** *see* ISOtretinoin *on page 1171*

Amobarbital (am oh BAR bi tal)

Medication Safety Issues

BEERS Criteria medication:

This drug may be potentially inappropriate for use in geriatric patients (Quality of evidence - high; Strength of recommendation - strong).

Brand Names: US Amytal Sodium

Brand Names: Canada Amytal®

Therapeutic Category Anticonvulsant, Barbiturate; Barbiturate; General Anesthetic; Hypnotic; Sedative

Generic Availability (US) No

Use Hypnotic in short-term treatment of insomnia; to reduce anxiety and provide sedation preoperatively. Has been used as an alternative agent for treatment of refractory tonic-clonic seizures. See Additional Information for special uses.

Pregnancy Risk Factor D

Pregnancy Considerations Barbiturates cross the placenta and distribute in fetal tissue. Teratogenic effects have been reported with 1st trimester exposure. Exposure during the 3rd trimester may lead to symptoms of acute withdrawal following delivery; symptoms may be delayed up to 14 days.

Breast-Feeding Considerations Small amounts of barbiturates are excreted in breast milk; information specific for amobarbital is not available.

Contraindications Hypersensitivity to barbiturates or any component of the formulation; marked hepatic impairment; dyspnea or airway obstruction; porphyria

Warnings/Precautions Tolerance to hypnotic effect can occur; do not use for >2 weeks to treat insomnia. Potential for drug dependency exists, abrupt cessation may precipitate withdrawal, including status epilepticus in epileptic patients. Do not administer to patients in acute or chronic pain. Use caution in elderly, debilitated, renally impaired, hepatic dysfunction, or pediatric patients. May cause paradoxical responses, including agitation and hyperactivity, particularly in acute pain and pediatric patients. An increased risk for hazardous sleep-related activities such as sleep-driving; cooking and eating food, and making phone calls while asleep has been noted with sedative-hypnotic medications. Discontinue treatment in patients who report a sleep-driving episode. Use with caution in patients with depression or suicidal tendencies, or in patients with a history of drug abuse. Tolerance, psychological and physical dependence may occur with prolonged use.

May cause CNS depression, which may impair physical or mental abilities. Patients must be cautioned about performing tasks which require mental alertness (eg, operating machinery or driving). Effects with other sedative drugs or ethanol may be potentiated. Use of this agent as a hypnotic in the elderly is not recommended. Avoid use in the elderly due to risk of overdose with low dosages, tolerance to sleep effects, and increased risk of physical dependence (Beers Criteria).

May cause respiratory depression or hypotension, particularly when administered rapidly intravenously. Solution for injection is highly alkaline and extravasation may cause local tissue damage.

Warnings: Additional Pediatric Considerations Neonates may experience withdrawal symptoms with chronic maternal use; monitor for closely. In pediatric patients, barbiturates may produce paradoxical excitement.

Adverse Reactions Reported as barbiturate use (not specifically amobarbital).

Cardiovascular: Bradycardia, hypotension, syncope

Central nervous system: Agitation, anxiety, ataxia, confusion, CNS depression, dizziness, fever, hallucinations, headache, insomnia, nightmares, nervousness, psychiatric disturbances, somnolence, thinking abnormal

Gastrointestinal: Constipation, nausea, vomiting

Hematologic: Megaloblastic anemia (following chronic phenobarbital use)

Hepatic: Liver damage

Local: Injection site reaction

Neuromuscular & skeletal: Hyperkinesia

Respiratory: Apnea, atelectasis (postoperative), hypoventilation

Miscellaneous: Hypersensitivity reaction (including angioedema, rash, and exfoliative dermatitis)

Drug Interactions

Metabolism/Transport Effects Induces CYP2A6 (strong)

Avoid Concomitant Use

Avoid concomitant use of Amobarbital with any of the following: Azelastine (Nasal); Mianserin; Orphenadrine; Paraldehyde; Somatostatin Acetate; Thalidomide; Ulipristal; Voriconazole

Increased Effect/Toxicity

Amobarbital may increase the levels/effects of: Alcohol (Ethyl); Azelastine (Nasal); Buprenorphine; CNS Depressants; Hydrocodone; Hypotensive Agents; Meperidine; Methotrimeprazine; Metyrosine; Mirtazapine; Orphenadrine; Paraldehyde; Pramipexole; ROPINIRole; Rotigotine; Selective Serotonin Reuptake Inhibitors; Suvorexant; Thalidomide; Thiazide Diuretics; Zolpidem

The levels/effects of Amobarbital may be increased by: Brimonidine (Topical); Cannabis; Chloramphenicol; Doxylamine; Dronabinol; Droperidol; Felbamate; HydrOXYzine; Kava Kava; Magnesium Sulfate; Methotrimeprazine; Mianserin; Nabilone; Perampanel; Primidone; Rufinamide; Sodium Oxybate; Somatostatin Acetate; Tapentadol; Tetrahydrocannabinol; Valproic Acid and Derivatives

Decreased Effect

Amobarbital may decrease the levels/effects of: Acetaminophen; Beta-Blockers; Calcium Channel Blockers; Chloramphenicol; Contraceptives (Estrogens); Contraceptives (Progestins); CycloSPORINE (Systemic); CYP2A6 Substrates; Doxycycline; Etoposide; Etoposide Phosphate; Felbamate; Griseofulvin; LamoTRIgine; Mianserin; Teniposide; Theophylline Derivatives; Tricyclic Antidepressants; Ulipristal; Valproic Acid and Derivatives; Vitamin K Antagonists; Voriconazole

The levels/effects of Amobarbital may be decreased by: Mianserin; Multivitamins/Minerals (with ADEK, Folate, Iron); Pyridoxine; Rifamycin Derivatives

Storage/Stability Powder should be stored at 15°C to 30°C (59°F to 86°F). Following reconstitution, solution should be used within 30 minutes.

Mechanism of Action Interferes with transmission of impulses from the thalamus to the cortex of the brain resulting in an imbalance in central inhibitory and facilitatory mechanisms

Pharmacodynamics

Onset of action: Rapid, within minutes

Maximum effect: Hours

Duration: Variable

Pharmacokinetics (Adult data unless noted)

Distribution: Readily crosses placenta; small amounts enter breast milk

Metabolism: Primarily hepatic via microsomal enzymes

Half-life: Adults: 15-40 hours (mean: 25 hours)

Elimination: Metabolites are eliminated in the urine and feces; negligible amounts excreted unchanged in urine

Dosing: Usual Note: Dosage should be individualized with consideration of patient's age, weight, and medical condition.

Children:

Sedative: IM, IV: 6-12 years: Manufacturer's dosing range: 65-500 mg

Hypnotic: IM: 2-3 mg/kg/dose given before bedtime (maximum: 500 mg)

Adults:

Hypnotic: IM, IV: 65-200 mg at bedtime (mean range: IM: 65-500 mg; maximum single dose: 1000 mg)

Sedative: IM, IV: 30-50 mg 2-3 times/day

Dosing adjustment in renal/hepatic impairment: Dosing should be reduced; specific recommendations not available; drug is contraindicated in patients with marked hepatic impairment; avoid use in patients with premonitory signs of hepatic coma

Preparation for Administration

Parenteral: Following reconstitution, dose must be administered within 30 minutes.

IM: Reconstitute with 2.5 mL of SWFI to make a 20% solution. Rotate vial to dissolve, do not shake. Do not use unless a clear solution forms within 5 minutes.

IV: Reconstitute with 5 mL of SWFI to make a 10% IV solution; if other concentrations are necessary see manufacturer's labeling for detailed instructions. Rotate vial to dissolve, do not shake. Do not use unless a clear solution forms within 5 minutes.

Administration

Parenteral: Following reconstitution, dose must be administered within 30 minutes.

IM: Administer deeply into a large muscle. Do not use more than 5 mL at any single site (may cause tissue damage)

IV: Use only when IM administration is not feasible. Administer by slow IV injection (maximum rate: 50 mg/minute in adults)

Monitoring Parameters Vital signs should be monitored during injection and for several hours after administration. If using IV, monitor patency of IV access; extravasation may cause local tissue damage. Monitor hematologic, renal, and hepatic function with prolonged therapy.

Reference Range

Therapeutic: 1-5 mcg/mL (SI: 4-22 µmol/L)

Toxic: >10 mcg/mL (SI: >44 µmol/L)

Lethal: >50 mcg/mL

Additional Information Amobarbital has also been used for therapeutic or diagnostic "amobarbital interviewing" (Kavirajan, 1999) and the "Wada test" (ie, intracarotid amobarbital procedure) to lateralize speech and memory functions prior to brain surgery, in order to prevent or predict the degree of impact of the surgery (Breier, 2001; Grote, 2005; Hamer, 2000; Szabo, 1993).

Controlled Substance C-II

Dosage Forms Excipient information presented when available (limited, particularly for generics); consult specific product labeling.

Solution Reconstituted, Injection, as sodium:

Amytal Sodium: 500 mg (1 ea)

◆ **Amobarbital Sodium** *see* Amobarbital *on page 136*

◆ **Amoclan** *see* Amoxicillin and Clavulanate *on page 141*

Amoxicillin (a moks i SIL in)

Medication Safety Issues

Sound-alike/look-alike issues:

Amoxicillin may be confused with amoxapine, Augmentin

Amoxil may be confused with amoxapine

International issues:

Fisamox [Australia] may be confused with Fosamax brand name for alendronate [U.S., Canada, and multiple international markets] and Vigamox brand name for moxifloxacin [U.S., Canada, and multiple international markets]

Limoxin [Mexico] may be confused with Lanoxin brand name for digoxin [U.S., Canada, and multiple international markets]; Lincocin brand name for lincomycin [U.S., Canada, and multiple international markets]

Zimox: Brand name for amoxicillin [Italy], but also the brand name for carbidopa/levodopa [Greece]

Zimox [Italy] may be confused with Diamox which is the brand name for acetazolamide [Canada and multiple international markets]

Related Information

H. pylori Treatment in Pediatric Patients *on page 2358*

Oral Medications That Should Not Be Crushed or Altered *on page 2476*

Prevention of Infective Endocarditis *on page 2378*

Brand Names: US Moxatag

Brand Names: Canada Apo-Amoxi; Mylan-Amoxicillin; Novamoxin; NTP-Amoxicillin; Nu-Amoxi; PHL-Amoxicillin; PMS-Amoxicillin; Pro-Amox-250; Pro-Amox-500

Therapeutic Category Antibiotic, Penicillin

Generic Availability (US) Yes

Use

Immediate Release preparations (oral suspension, chewable tablets, tablets, and capsules): Treatment of infections of ear, nose, skin, and soft tissue, genitourinary tract, or upper or lower respiratory tract due to susceptible (beta-lactamase negative) organisms including *H. influenzae*, *N. gonorrhoeae*, *E. coli*, *P. mirabilis*, *E. faecalis*, streptococci, and nonpenicillinase-producing staphylococci (FDA approved in all ages); treatment of gonorrhea (FDA approved in ages ≥2 years and adults); combination therapy of *Helicobacter pylori* (FDA approved in adults); has also been used for the treatment of Lyme disease, prophylaxis of bacterial endocarditis, prophylaxis in sickle cell or asplenic patients, and post-exposure prophylaxis and treatment of anthrax

Extended release tablet (Moxatag®): Treatment of tonsillitis and/or pharyngitis secondary to *Streptococcus pyogenes* (FDA approved in ages ≥12 years and adults)

Pregnancy Risk Factor B

Pregnancy Considerations Adverse events have not been observed in animal reproduction studies. Maternal use of amoxicillin has generally not resulted in an increased risk of adverse fetal effects; however, an increased risk of cleft lip with cleft palate has been observed in some studies. It is the drug of choice for the treatment of chlamydial infections in pregnancy and for anthrax prophylaxis when penicillin susceptibility is documented. Amoxicillin may be used in certain situations prior to vaginal delivery in women at high risk for endocarditis.

Due to pregnancy-induced physiologic changes, oral amoxicillin clearance is increased during pregnancy resulting in lower concentrations and smaller AUCs. Oral ampicillin-class antibiotics are poorly absorbed during labor.

Breast-Feeding Considerations Very small amounts of amoxicillin are excreted in breast milk. The manufacturer recommends that caution be exercised when administering amoxicillin to nursing women. Nondose-related effects could include modification of bowel flora and allergic sensitization of the infant.

Contraindications Hypersensitivity to amoxicillin, penicillin, other beta-lactams, or any component of the formulation

Warnings/Precautions In patients with renal impairment, doses and/or frequency of administration should be modified in response to the degree of renal impairment; in addition, use of certain dosage forms (eg, extended release 775 mg tablet and immediate release 875 mg tablet) should be avoided in patients with CrCl <30 mL/minute or patients requiring hemodialysis. A high percentage of patients with infectious mononucleosis have developed rash during therapy with amoxicillin; ampicillin-class antibiotics not recommended in these patients. Serious and occasionally severe or fatal hypersensitivity (anaphylactoid) reactions have been reported in patients on penicillin therapy, especially with a history of beta-lactam hypersensitivity, history of sensitivity to multiple allergens, or previous IgE-mediated reactions (eg, anaphylaxis, angioedema, urticaria). Use with caution in asthmatic patients. Prolonged use may result in fungal or bacterial superinfection, including *C. difficile*-associated diarrhea (CDAD) and pseudomembranous colitis; CDAD has been observed >2 months postantibiotic treatment.

Chewable tablets contain phenylalanine.

Benzyl alcohol and derivatives: Some dosage forms may contain sodium benzoate/benzoic acid; benzoic acid (benzoate) is a metabolite of benzyl alcohol; large amounts of benzyl alcohol (≥99 mg/kg/day) have been associated with a potentially fatal toxicity ("gasping syndrome") in neonates; the "gasping syndrome" consists of metabolic acidosis, respiratory distress, gasping respirations, CNS dysfunction (including convulsions, intracranial hemorrhage), hypotension, and cardiovascular collapse (AAP 1997; CDC 1982); some data suggests that benzoate displaces bilirubin from protein binding sites (Ahlfors 2001); avoid or use dosage forms containing benzyl alcohol derivative with caution in neonates. See manufacturer's labeling.

Warnings: Additional Pediatric Considerations Epstein-Barr virus infection (infectious mononucleosis), acute lymphocytic leukemia, or cytomegalovirus infection increases risk for amoxicillin-induced maculopapular rash. Appearance of a rash should be carefully evaluated to differentiate a nonallergic amoxicillin rash from a hypersensitivity reaction. Amoxicillin rash occurs in 5% to 10% of children receiving amoxicillin and is a generalized dull, red, maculopapular rash, generally appearing 3 to 14 days after the start of therapy. It normally begins on the trunk and spreads over most of the body. It may be most intense at pressure areas, elbows, and knees. A high percentage (43% to 100%) of patients with infectious mononucleosis have developed rash during therapy; amoxicillin-class antibiotics are not recommended in these patients.

Adverse Reactions

Cardiovascular: Hypersensitivity angiitis

Central nervous system: Agitation, anxiety, behavioral changes, confusion, dizziness, headache, hyperactivity (reversible), insomnia, seizure

Dermatologic: Acute generalized exanthematous pustulosis, erythematous maculopapular rash, erythema multiforme, exfoliative dermatitis, Stevens-Johnson syndrome, toxic epidermal necrolysis, urticaria

Gastrointestinal: Dental discoloration (brown, yellow, or gray; rare), diarrhea, hemorrhagic colitis, melanoglossia, mucocutaneous candidiasis, nausea, pseudomembranous colitis, vomiting

Genitourinary: Crystalluria

Hematologic & oncologic: Agranulocytosis, anemia, eosinophilia, hemolytic anemia, leukopenia,thrombocytopenia, thrombocytopenia purpura

Hepatic: Cholestatic hepatitis, cholestatic jaundice, hepatitis (acute cytolytic), increased serum ALT, increased serum AST

Hypersensitivity: Anaphylaxis

Immunologic: Serum sickness-like reaction

Drug Interactions

Metabolism/Transport Effects None known.

Avoid Concomitant Use

Avoid concomitant use of Amoxicillin with any of the following: BCG; BCG (Intravesical); Probenecid

Increased Effect/Toxicity

Amoxicillin may increase the levels/effects of: Methotrexate; Vitamin K Antagonists

The levels/effects of Amoxicillin may be increased by: Allopurinol; Probenecid

Decreased Effect

Amoxicillin may decrease the levels/effects of: BCG; BCG (Intravesical); BCG Vaccine (Immunization); Mycophenolate; Sodium Picosulfate; Typhoid Vaccine

The levels/effects of Amoxicillin may be decreased by: Tetracycline Derivatives

Storage/Stability

Amoxil: Oral suspension remains stable for 14 days at room temperature or if refrigerated (refrigeration preferred). Unit-dose antibiotic oral syringes are stable at room temperature for at least 72 hours (Tu 1988).

Moxatag: Store at 25°C (77°F); excursions permitted to 15°C to 30°C (59°F to 86°F).

Mechanism of Action Inhibits bacterial cell wall synthesis by binding to one or more of the penicillin-binding proteins (PBPs) which in turn inhibits the final transpeptidation step of peptidoglycan synthesis in bacterial cell walls, thus inhibiting cell wall biosynthesis. Bacteria eventually lyse due to ongoing activity of cell wall autolytic enzymes (autolysins and murein hydrolases) while cell wall assembly is arrested.

Pharmacokinetics (Adult data unless noted)

Absorption: Oral: Rapid and nearly complete (74% to 92% of a single dose is absorbed)

Extended-release tablet: Rate of absorption is slower compared to immediate-release formulation

Distribution: Into liver, lungs, prostate, muscle, middle ear effusions, maxillary sinus secretions, bone, gallbladder, bile, and into ascitic and synovial fluids

Protein binding: 17% to 20%, lower in neonates

Metabolism: Partially hepatic

Half-life:

Neonates, full-term: 3.7 hours

Infants and children: 1-2 hours

Adults: Normal renal function: 0.7-1.4 hours

Patients with CrCl <10 mL/minute: 7-21 hours

Time to peak serum concentration:

Capsule: Within 2 hours

Extended release: 3.1 hours

Suspension: Neonates: 3-4.5 hours; children: 1 hour

Elimination: Renal excretion (60% unchanged drug)

Dosing: Neonatal Note: All neonatal dosing recommendations based on immediate release product formulations (ie, oral suspension).

General dosing, susceptible infection: Oral: 20 to 30 mg/kg/day in divided doses every 12 hours

Otitis media, acute (AOM): Oral: 30 to 40 mg/kg/day in divided doses every 8 hours (Bradley, 2014)

UTI, prophylaxis (hydronephrosis, vesicoureteral reflux): Oral: 10 to 15 mg/kg once daily (Belarmino, 2006; Greenbaum, 2006; Matoo, 2007)

Dosing: Usual

Pediatric: **Note:** Unless otherwise specified, all pediatric dosing recommendations based on immediate release product formulations (oral suspension, chewable tablet, tablet, and capsule).

General dosing, susceptible infection: Oral:

Mild to moderate infection:

Infants ≤3 months:

AAP recommendations (*Red Book*, 2012): 25 to 50 mg/kg/day in divided doses every 8 hours

Manufacturer labeling: 20 to 30 mg/kg/day in divided doses every 12 hours

Infants >3 months, Children, and Adolescents:

AAP recommendations (*Red Book*, 2012): 25 to 50 mg/kg/day in divided doses every 8 hours; maximum dose: 500 mg/dose

Manufacturer's labeling: 20 to 40 mg/kg/day in divided doses every 8 hours (maximum dose: 500 mg/dose) **or** 25 to 45 mg/kg/day in divided doses every 12 hours (maximum dose: 875 mg/dose)

Severe infection (as step-down therapy): Infants, Children, and Adolescents: Oral: 80 to 100 mg/kg/day in divided doses every 8 hours; maximum dose: 500 mg/dose for most indications (*Red Book*, 2012)

Anthrax: Oral:

Cutaneous, community-acquired or bioterrorism-related (Stevens, 2005):

Children <20 kg: 40 mg/kg/day in divided doses every 8 hours for 5 to 9 days

Children ≥20 kg: 500 mg every 8 hours for 5 to 9 days

Inhalational, postexposure prophylaxis (ACIP recommendations): **Note:** Use only if *B. anthracis* isolate is susceptible to amoxicillin (MIC ≤0.125 mcg/mL). Continue therapy for 30 to ≥60 days depending on vaccination status and for 14 days after the third vaccine dose (CDC, 2010); see Additional Information

Children <40 kg: Oral:

CDC recommendations: 45 mg/kg/day in divided doses every 8 hours; maximum dose: 500 mg/dose

AAP recommendations: 80 mg/kg/day in divided doses every 8 hours; maximum dose: 500 mg/dose. This higher dose is recommended due to the lack of data on lower amoxicillin dosages for treating anthrax and the high mortality rate (*Red Book*, 2012)

Children ≥40 kg: 500 mg every 8 hours

Endocarditis, prophylaxis: Infants, Children, and Adolescents: Oral: 50 mg/kg 1 hour before procedure; maximum dose: 2000 mg/dose (Wilson, 2007)

Lyme disease: Infants, Children, and Adolescents: Oral: 50 mg/kg/day in divided doses every 8 hours; maximum dose: 500 mg/dose (Halperin, 2007; Wormser, 2006)

Otitis media, acute (AOM): Infants ≥2 months and Children: Oral: 80 to 90 mg/kg/day in divided doses every 12 hours; variable duration of therapy, if <2 years of age or severe symptoms (any age): 10-day course; if 2 to 5 years of age with mild to moderate symptoms: 7-day course; ≥6 years of age with mild to moderate symptoms: 5- to 7-day course; some experts recommend initiating with 90 mg/kg/day (Bradley, 2014; Lieberthal, 2013; *Red Book*, 2012)

Peritonitis, prophylaxis (for patients receiving peritoneal dialysis who require dental procedures): Infants, Children, and Adolescents: Oral: 50 mg/kg administered 30 to 60 minutes before dental procedure; maximum dose: 2000 mg/dose (Warady, 2012)

Pneumonia, community-acquired: Infants ≥ 3 months, Children, and Adolescents: Oral:

Empiric therapy for presumed bacterial pneumonia: 90 mg/kg/day in divided doses every 12 hours; maximum daily dose: 4000 mg/**day**

Group A *Streptococcus*: 50 to 75 mg/kg/day in divided doses every 12 hours; maximum daily dose: 4000 mg/**day**

Haemophilus influenzae: 75 to 100 mg/kg/day in divided doses every 8 hours; maximum daily dose: 4000 mg/**day**

Streptococcus pneumonia (penicillin MIC ≤2 mcg/mL); mild infection or step-down therapy: 90 mg/kg/day in divided doses every 12 hours **or** 45 mg/kg/day in divided doses every 8 hours; maximum daily dose: 4000 mg/**day**

Pneumococcal infection prophylaxis for anatomic or functional asplenia [eg, sickle cell disease (SCD)] (Price, 2007; *Red Book*, 2012): Oral:

Before 2 months of age (or as soon as SCD is diagnosed or asplenia occurs) through 5 years of age: 20 mg/kg/day in divided doses every 12 hours; maximum dose: 250 mg/dose

≥6 years: 250 mg every 12 hours; **Note:** The decision to discontinue penicillin prophylaxis after 5 years of age in children who have not experienced invasive pneumococcal infection and have received recommended pneumococcal immunizations is patient and clinician dependent.

Rhinosinusitis, acute bacterial; uncomplicated: Oral: **Note:** AAP guidelines recommend amoxicillin as first-line empiric therapy for pediatric patients 1 to 18 years with uncomplicated cases and where resistance is not suspected; however, the IDSA guidelines consider amoxicillin/clavulanate as the preferred therapy (Chow, 2012; Wald, 2013): Children and Adolescents:

Low dose: 45 mg/kg/day in divided doses every 12 hours

High dose (use reserved for select patients; see **Note**): 80 to 90 mg/kg/day in divided doses every 12 hours; maximum dose: 1000 mg/dose; **Note:** Should only be used in the following: Mild to moderate infections in communities with a high prevalence of nonsusceptible *S. pneumoniae* resistance

Tonsillopharyngitis; Group A streptococcal infection, treatment and primary prevention of rheumatic fever: Oral:

Immediate release (oral suspension, chewable tablets, tablets, capsules): Children and Adolescents 3 to 18 years: 50 mg/kg once daily **or** 25 mg/kg twice daily for 10 days; maximum daily dose: 1000 mg/**day** (Gerber, 2009; Shulman, 2012)

Extended release tablets: Children ≥12 years and Adolescents: 775 mg once daily for 10 days; **Note:** Patient must be able to swallow tablet whole.

UTI, prophylaxis (hydronephrosis, vesicoureteral reflux): Oral: Infants ≤2 months: 10 to 15 mg/kg once daily; some suggest administration in the evening (drug resides in bladder longer); **Note:** Due to resistance, amoxicillin should not be used for prophylaxis after 2 months of age (Belarmino, 2006; Greenbaum, 2006; Mattoo, 2007).

Adult:

General dosing, susceptible infection: Oral: Immediate release: 250 to 500 mg every 8 hours **or** 500 to 875 mg tablets twice daily **or** extended release tablet 775 mg once daily

Chlamydial infection during pregnancy: Oral: 500 mg 3 times daily for 7 days (CDC, 2010)

Endocarditis prophylaxis: Oral: 2000 mg 30 to 60 minutes before procedure

***H. pylori* eradication:** Oral: 1000 mg twice daily for 14 days in combination with a proton pump inhibitor and at least one other antibiotic (clarithromycin)

Tonsillitis and/or pharyngitis: Oral: Extended release tablets: 775 mg once daily for 10 days

Dosing adjustment in renal impairment:

Infants, Children, and Adolescents: There are no dosage adjustments provided in the manufacturer's labeling; however, the following guidelines have been used by some clinicians (Aronoff, 2007): Oral:

Immediate release: Infants, Children, and Adolescents:

Mild to moderate infection: Dosing based on 25 to 50 mg/kg/day divided every 8 hours:

GFR >30 mL/minute/1.73 m^2: No adjustment required

GFR 10 to 29 mL/minute/1.73 m^2: 8 to 20 mg/kg/dose every 12 hours

GFR <10 mL/minute/1.73 m^2: 8 to 20 mg/kg/dose every 24 hours

Hemodialysis: Moderately dialyzable (20% to 50%); ~30% removed by 3-hour hemodialysis: 8 to 20 mg/kg/dose every 24 hours; give after dialysis

Peritoneal dialysis: 8 to 20 mg/kg/dose every 24 hours

Severe infection (high dose): Dosing based on 80 to 90 mg/kg/day divided every 12 hours:

GFR >30 mL/minute/1.73 m^2: No adjustment required

GFR 10 to 29 mL/minute/1.73 m^2: 20 mg/kg/dose every 12 hours; do not use the 875 mg tablet

GFR <10 mL/minute/1.73 m^2: 20 mg/kg/dose every 24 hours; do not use the 875 mg tablet

Hemodialysis: Moderately dialyzable (20% to 50%); ~30% removed by 3-hour hemodialysis: 20 mg/kg/dose every 24 hours; give after dialysis

Peritoneal dialysis: 20 mg/kg/dose every 24 hours

Extended release: Children ≥12 years and Adolescents: CrCl <30mL/minute: Do not use the 775 mg tablet

Adults: **Note:** The immediate release 875 mg tablet and the extended release 775 mg tablet should not be used in patients with a CrCl <30 mL/minute. Oral:

CrCl >30 mL/minute: No adjustment required.

CrCl 10-30 mL/minute: 250 to 500 mg every 12 hours depending on severity of infection

CrCl <10 mL/minute: 250 to 500 mg every 24 hours depending on severity of infection

Hemodialysis: Moderately dialyzable (20% to 50%); ~30% removed by 3-hour hemodialysis: Give dose after dialysis (Aronoff, 2007)

Peritoneal dialysis: 250 mg every 12 hours

Dosing adjustment in hepatic impairment: There are no dosage adjustments provided in the manufacturer's labeling.

Preparation for Administration Oral: Immediate release: Reconstitute powder for oral suspension with appropriate amount of water as specified on the bottle. Shake vigorously until suspended.

Administration Oral:

Immediate release: May be administered on an empty or full stomach; may be mixed with formula, milk, cold drink, or juice; administer dose immediately after mixing; shake suspension well before use.

Extended release: Take within 1 hour of finishing a meal; do not chew or crush tablet.

Monitoring Parameters With prolonged therapy, monitor renal, hepatic, and hematologic function periodically; observe for change in bowel frequency; monitor for signs of anaphylaxis during first dose

Test Interactions May interfere with urinary glucose tests using cupric sulfate (Benedict's solution, Clinitest)

Some penicillin derivatives may accelerate the degradation of aminoglycosides *in vitro*, leading to a potential underestimation of aminoglycoside serum concentration.

Additional Information Some penicillins (eg, carbenicillin, ticarcillin, and piperacillin) have been shown to inactivate aminoglycosides *in vitro*. This has been observed to a greater extent with tobramycin and gentamicin, while amikacin has shown greater stability against inactivation. Concurrent use of these agents may pose a risk of reduced antibacterial efficacy *in vivo*, particularly in the setting of profound renal impairment; however, definitive clinical evidence is lacking. If combination penicillin/aminoglycoside therapy is desired in a patient with renal dysfunction, separation of doses (if feasible), and routine monitoring of aminoglycoside levels, CBC, and clinical response should be considered.

Only use amoxicillin for postexposure inhalational anthrax prophylaxis if isolates of the specific *B. anthracis* are susceptible to amoxicillin (MIC ≤0.125 mcg/mL). Duration of antibiotic postexposure prophylaxis (PEP) is ≥60 days in a previously unvaccinated exposed person. Antimicrobial therapy should continue for 14 days after the third dose of PEP vaccine. Those who are partially or fully vaccinated should receive at least a 30-day course of antimicrobial PEP and continue with licensed vaccination regimen. Unvaccinated workers, even those wearing personal protective equipment with adequate respiratory protection, should receive antimicrobial PEP. Antimicrobial PEP is not required for fully vaccinated people (5-dose IM vaccination series with a yearly booster) who enter an anthrax area clothed in personal protective equipment. If respiratory protection is disrupted, a 30-day course of antimicrobial therapy is recommended (CDC, 2010).

Dosage Forms Excipient information presented when available (limited, particularly for generics); consult specific product labeling.

Capsule, Oral:
- Generic: 250 mg, 500 mg

Suspension Reconstituted, Oral:
- Generic: 125 mg/5 mL (80 mL, 100 mL, 150 mL); 200 mg/5 mL (50 mL, 75 mL, 100 mL); 250 mg/5 mL (80 mL, 100 mL, 150 mL); 400 mg/5 mL (50 mL, 75 mL, 100 mL)

Tablet, Oral:
- Generic: 500 mg, 875 mg

Tablet Chewable, Oral:
- Generic: 125 mg, 250 mg

Tablet Extended Release 24 Hour, Oral:
- Moxatag: 775 mg [contains cremophor el, fd&c blue #2 aluminum lake]
- Generic: 775 mg

Amoxicillin and Clavulanate

(a moks i SIL in & klav yoo LAN ate)

Medication Safety Issues

Sound-alike/look-alike issues:

Augmentin may be confused with amoxicillin, Azulfidine

Related Information

Oral Medications That Should Not Be Crushed or Altered *on page 2476*

Brand Names: US Amoclan; Augmentin; Augmentin ES-600; Augmentin XR

Brand Names: Canada Amoxi-Clav; Apo-Amoxi-Clav; Clavulin; Novo-Clavamoxin; ratio-Aclavulanate

Therapeutic Category Antibiotic, Beta-lactam and Beta-lactamase Combination; Antibiotic, Penicillin

Generic Availability (US) Yes

Use Infections caused by susceptible organisms involving the lower respiratory tract, otitis media, sinusitis, skin and skin structure, and urinary tract; spectrum same as amoxicillin in addition to beta-lactamase producing *M. catarrhalis*, *H. influenzae*, *N. gonorrhoeae*, and *S. aureus* (excluding MRSA) (FDA approved in all ages)

Pregnancy Risk Factor B

Pregnancy Considerations Adverse events have not been observed in animal reproduction studies. Both amoxicillin and clavulanic acid cross the placenta. Maternal use of amoxicillin/clavulanate has generally not resulted in an increased risk of birth defects. A possible increased risk of necrotizing enterocolitis in neonates or bowel disorders in children exposed to amoxicillin/clavulanate *in utero* has been observed. In women with acute infections during pregnancy, amoxicillin/clavulanate may be given if an antibiotic is required and appropriate based on bacterial sensitivity; however, use is not recommended in the management of preterm premature rupture of membranes. Oral ampicillin-class antibiotics are poorly absorbed during labor.

Breast-Feeding Considerations Amoxicillin is found in breast milk. The manufacturer recommends that caution be used if administered to breast-feeding women. The use of amoxicillin/clavulanate may be safe while breast-feeding. However, the risk of adverse events in the infant may be increased when compared to the use of amoxicillin alone and the risk may be related to maternal dose.

Contraindications

Hypersensitivity to amoxicillin, clavulanic acid, other beta-lactam antibacterial drugs (eg, penicillins, cephalosporins), or any component of the formulation; history of cholestatic jaundice or hepatic dysfunction with amoxicillin/clavulanate potassium therapy

Augmentin XR: Additional contraindications: Severe renal impairment (creatinine clearance <30 mL/minute) and hemodialysis patients

Canadian labeling: Additional contraindications (not in US labeling): Suspected or confirmed mononucleosis

Warnings/Precautions Hypersensitivity reactions, including anaphylaxis (some fatal), have been reported. Prolonged use may result in fungal or bacterial superinfection, including *C. difficile*-associated diarrhea (CDAD) and pseudomembranous colitis; CDAD has been observed >2 months postantibiotic treatment. Although rarely fatal, hepatic dysfunction (eg, cholestatic jaundice, hepatitis) has been reported. Patients at highest risk include those with serious underlying disease or concomitant medications. Hepatic toxicity is usually reversible. Monitor liver function tests at regular intervals in patients with hepatic impairment. High percentage of patients with infectious mononucleosis have developed rash during therapy; ampicillin class antibiotics not recommended in these patients. Incidence of diarrhea is higher than with amoxicillin alone. Due to differing content of clavulanic acid, not all formulations are interchangeable; use of an inappropriate product for a specific dosage could result in either diarrhea (which may be severe) or subtherapeutic clavulanic acid concentrations leading to decreased clinical efficacy. Low incidence of cross-allergy with cephalosporins exists. Monitor renal, hepatic, and hematopoietic function if therapy extends beyond approved duration times. Some products contain phenylalanine. Potentially significant drug-drug interactions may exist, requiring dose or frequency adjustment, additional monitoring, and/or selection of alternative therapy.

Warnings: Additional Pediatric Considerations Epstein-Barr virus infection (infectious mononucleosis), acute lymphocytic leukemia, or cytomegalovirus infection increase risk for penicillin-induced maculopapular rash. Appearance of a rash should be carefully evaluated to differentiate a nonallergic ampicillin rash from a hypersensitivity reaction; rash occurs in 5% to 10% of children and is a generalized dull red, maculopapular rash, generally appearing 3 to 14 days after the start of therapy. It normally begins on the trunk and spreads over most of the body. It may be most intense at pressure areas, elbows, and knees. A high percentage (43% to 100%) of patients with infectious mononucleosis have developed rash during therapy; ampicillin-class antibiotics are not recommended in these patients.

Adverse Reactions

Dermatologic: Diaper rash, skin rash, urticaria

Gastrointestinal: Abdominal distress, diarrhea, loose stools, nausea, vomiting

Genitourinary: Vaginitis

Infection: Candidiasis, vaginal mycosis

Rare but important or life-threatening: Cholestatic jaundice, flatulence, headache, hepatic insufficiency, hepatitis, hepatotoxicity (idiosyncratic) (Chalasani, 2014), increased liver enzymes, increased serum alkaline phosphatase, prolonged prothrombin time, thrombocythemia, vasculitis (hypersensitivity)

Additional adverse reactions seen with **ampicillin-class antibiotics:** Acute generalized exanthematous pustulosis, agitation, agranulocytosis, anaphylaxis, anemia, angioedema, anxiety, behavioral changes, confusion, convulsions, crystalluria, dental discoloration, dizziness, dyspepsia, enterocolitis, eosinophilia, erythema multiforme, exfoliative dermatitis, gastritis, glossitis, hematuria, hemolytic anemia, hemorrhagic colitis, hyperactivity, immune thrombocytopenia, increased serum bilirubin, increased serum transaminases, insomnia, interstitial nephritis, leukopenia, melanoglossia, mucocutaneous candidiasis, pruritus, pseudomembranous colitis, serum sickness-like reaction, Stevens-Johnson syndrome, stomatitis, thrombocytopenia, toxic epidermal necrolysis

Drug Interactions

Metabolism/Transport Effects None known.

Avoid Concomitant Use

Avoid concomitant use of Amoxicillin and Clavulanate with any of the following: BCG; BCG (Intravesical); Probenecid

Increased Effect/Toxicity

Amoxicillin and Clavulanate may increase the levels/effects of: Methotrexate; Vitamin K Antagonists

The levels/effects of Amoxicillin and Clavulanate may be increased by: Allopurinol; Probenecid

Decreased Effect

Amoxicillin and Clavulanate may decrease the levels/effects of: BCG; BCG (Intravesical); BCG Vaccine (Immunization); Mycophenolate; Sodium Picosulfate; Typhoid Vaccine

The levels/effects of Amoxicillin and Clavulanate may be decreased by: Tetracycline Derivatives

Storage/Stability

Powder for oral suspension: Store dry powder at or below 25°C (77°F). Reconstituted oral suspension should be kept in refrigerator. Discard unused suspension after 10 days (consult manufacturer labeling for specific recommendations). Unit-dose antibiotic oral syringes are stable under refrigeration for 24 hours (Tu, 1988).

Tablet: Store at or below 25°C (77°F). Dispense in original container.

Mechanism of Action Clavulanic acid binds and inhibits beta-lactamases that inactivate amoxicillin resulting in amoxicillin having an expanded spectrum of activity. Amoxicillin inhibits bacterial cell wall synthesis by binding to one or more of the penicillin-binding proteins (PBPs) which in turn inhibits the final transpeptidation step of peptidoglycan synthesis in bacterial cell walls, thus inhibiting cell wall biosynthesis. Bacteria eventually lyse due to ongoing activity of cell wall autolytic enzymes (autolysins and murein hydrolases) while cell wall assembly is arrested.

Pharmacokinetics (Adult data unless noted)

Absorption: Both amoxicillin and clavulanate are well absorbed

Distribution: Both widely distributed into lungs, pleural, peritoneal, synovial, and ascitic fluid as well as bone, gynecologic tissue, and middle ear fluid

Protein binding:
- Amoxicillin: 17% to 20%
- Clavulanate: 25%

Metabolism: Clavulanic acid: Hepatically metabolized

Half-life of both agents in adults with normal renal function: ~1 hour; amoxicillin pharmacokinetics are not affected by clavulanic acid

Time to peak serum concentration: Within 2 hours

Elimination: Urine (amoxicillin 50% to 70% unchanged drug; clavulanic acid 25% to 40% unchanged drug)

Dosing: Neonatal Note: Dosing based on amoxicillin component; dose and frequency are product specific; not all products are interchangeable, using a product with the incorrect amoxicillin:clavulanate ratio could result in subtherapeutic clavulanate concentrations or severe diarrhea.

General dosing, susceptible infection: Oral: 30 mg amoxicillin/kg/day divided every 12 hours using the 125 mg/5 mL suspension **only**

Dosing: Usual

Pediatric: **Note:** Dosing based on amoxicillin component; dose and frequency are product specific; not all products are interchangeable; using a product with the incorrect amoxicillin:clavulanate ratio could result in subtherapeutic clavulanic acid concentrations or severe diarrhea.

General dosing, susceptible infection: Oral:

Infants <3 months: 30 mg amoxicillin/kg/day divided every 12 hours using the 125 mg/5 mL oral suspension **only**

Infants ≥3 months, Children, and Adolescents:

Mild to moderate infection:

Patients weighing <40 kg: *Immediate release formulations:*

Twice daily dosing: 25 mg amoxicillin/kg/day in divided doses twice daily using the 200 mg/5 mL or 400 mg/5 mL oral suspension or the 200 mg or 400 mg chewable tablets; maximum single dose: 500 mg amoxicillin

Three times daily dosing: 20 mg amoxicillin/kg/day in divided doses 3 times daily using the 125 mg/5 mL or 250 mg/5 mL oral suspension; maximum single dose: 500 mg amoxicillin

Patients weighing ≥40 kg: *Immediate release formulations:*

Twice daily dosing: 500 mg amoxicillin every 12 hours using 500 mg tablet; or if difficulty swallowing, the 125 mg/5 mL or 250 mg/5mL oral suspension may be used

Three times daily dosing: 250 mg amoxicillin every 8 hours using the 250 mg tablet

More severe infection:

Patients weighing <40 kg: *Immediate release formulations:*

Twice daily dosing: 45 mg amoxicillin/kg/day in divided doses twice daily using the 200 mg/5 mL or 400 mg/5 mL oral suspension or the 200 mg or 400 mg **chewable** tablets; maximum single dose: 875 mg amoxicillin

Three times daily dosing: 40 mg amoxicillin/kg/day in divided doses 3 times daily using the 125 mg/5 mL or 250 mg/5 mL oral suspension; maximum single dose: 500 mg amoxicillin

Patients weighing ≥40 kg:

Immediate release formulations:

Twice daily dosing: 875 mg amoxicillin every 12 hours using the 875 mg tablet, or if difficulty swallowing, the 200 mg/5 mL or the 400 mg/5 mL oral suspension may be used

Three times daily dosing: 500 mg amoxicillin every 8 hours using the 500 mg tablet, or if difficulty swallowing, the 125 mg/5 mL or 250 mg/5mL oral suspension may be used

Extended release tablet: 2,000 mg amoxicillin every 12 hours.

Otitis media, acute: Infants ≥6 months and Children: Oral: 90 mg amoxicillin/kg/day divided every 12 hours for up to 10 days using the 600 mg/5 mL oral suspension **only** in children with severe illness, who have received amoxicillin in the past 30 days, who have treatment failure at 48 to 72 hours on first-line therapy, and when coverage for β-lactamase positive *H. influenzae* and *M. catarrhalis* is needed. Variable duration of therapy; the manufacturer suggests 10-day course in all patients, however new data suggests a shorter-course in some cases: If <2 years of age or severe symptoms (any age): 10-day course; if 2 to 5 years of age with mild to moderate symptoms: 7-day course; if ≥6 years of age with mild to moderate symptoms: 5- to 7-day course (AAP [Lieberthal 2013]). **Note:** Per the manufacturer, the 600 mg/5 mL formulation should only be used for patients weighing <40 kg.

Pneumonia, community-acquired: Infants ≥3 months, Children, and Adolescents: Oral:

Manufacturer's labeling:

Patients weighing <40 kg: *Immediate release formulations:*

Twice daily dosing: 45 mg amoxicillin/kg/day in divided doses twice daily using the 200 mg/5 mL or 400 mg/5 mL oral suspension or the 200 mg or 400 mg chewable tablets; maximum single dose: 875 mg amoxicillin

Three times daily dosing: 40 mg amoxicillin/kg/day in divided doses 3 times daily using the 125 mg/5 mL or 250 mg/5 mL oral suspension; maximum single dose: 500 mg amoxicillin

Patients weighing ≥40 kg:

Immediate release formulations:

Twice daily dosing: 875 mg amoxicillin every 12 hours using the 875 mg tablet or if difficulty swallowing, the 200 mg/5 mL or the 400 mg/5 mL oral suspension may be used

Three times daily dosing: 500 mg amoxicillin every 8 hours using the 500 mg tablet or if difficulty swallowing, the 125 mg/5 mL or 250 mg/5mL oral suspension may be used

Extended release tablet: 2,000 mg amoxicillin every 12 hours

Alternate dosing: IDSA guidelines; beta-lactamase positive *H. influenzae* strains (Bradley 2011): *Immediate release formulations:*

Standard dose: 45 mg amoxicillin/kg/day in divided doses 3 times daily using the 125 mg/5 mL or 250 mg/5 mL oral suspension formulation; if patient >40 kg, may also use 500 mg tablet; maximum single dose: 500 mg amoxicillin

High dose: 90 mg amoxicillin/kg/day in divided doses 2 times daily using the 600 mg/5 mL oral suspension formulation. A wider dosing range of 80 to 100 mg/kg/day divided every 8 hours has also been used (Bradley, 2002). **Note:** Per the manufacturer, the 600 mg/5 mL formulation should only be used for patients weighing <40 kg.

Rhinosinusitis, acute bacterial: Oral:

AAP recommendations (Wald 2013): Children and Adolescents: High-dose (use reserved for select patients; see **Note**): 80 to 90 mg amoxicillin/kg/day divided every 12 hours, using the 600 mg/5 mL oral suspension **only**; treatment duration variable: 10 to 28 days, some have suggested discontinuation of therapy 7 days after resolution of signs and symptoms of infection. **Note:** Recommended for patients with any of the following: Moderate to severe infection, age <2 years, childcare attendance, or recent antibiotic treatment. Per the manufacturer, the 600 mg/5 mL formulation should only be used for patients weighing <40 kg.

IDSA recommendations (Chow 2012): Infants ≥3 months, Children, and Adolescents:

Patients weighing <40 kg:

Standard dose: *Immediate release formulations:* 45 mg amoxicillin/kg/day divided every 12 hours for 10 to 14 days using the 200 mg/5 mL or 400 mg/5 mL oral suspension, or the 200 mg and 400 mg **chewable** tablets formulations **only**

High dose (use reserved for select patients; see **Note**): *Immediate release formulations:* 90 mg amoxicillin/kg/day divided every 12 hours for 10 to 14 days, using the 600 mg/5 mL oral suspension **only**; **Note:** Use recommended in the following: Areas with high endemic rates of penicillin-non-susceptible *S. pneumonia*, patients with severe infections, daycare attendance, age <2 years, recent hospitalization, antibiotic use within the past month, patients who are immunocompromised or if initial therapy fails (second-line therapy)

Patients weighing ≥40 kg:

Standard dose: *Immediate release formulations:* 500 mg amoxicillin every 8 hours using the 500 mg tablet only or 875 mg every 12 hours using the 875 mg tablet only for 5 to 7 days

High dose (use reserved for select patients; see **Note**): Extended release tablets: 2,000 mg (two 1,000 mg tablets) amoxicillin every 12 hours for 10 days; **Note:** Use recommended in the following: Areas with high endemic rates of penicillin-non-susceptible *S. pneumoniae*, patients with severe infections, recent hospitalization, antibiotic use within the past month, patients who are immunocompromised or if initial therapy fails (second-line therapy).

Skin and soft tissue infections, impetigo: Infants ≥3 months, Children, and Adolescents: Oral: 25 mg amoxicillin/kg/day in divided doses twice daily using the 200 mg/5 mL or 400 mg/5 mL oral suspension or the 200 mg or 400 mg **chewable** tablets; maximum single dose: 875 mg amoxicillin (Stevens 2005)

Streptococci, group A; chronic carrier treatment: Infants ≥3 months, Children, and Adolescents: Oral: 40 mg amoxicillin/kg/day in divided doses every 8 hours for 10 days using the 125 mg/5 mL or 250 mg/5 mL oral suspension or if patient weighs ≥40 kg, the 500 mg tablet; maximum single dose: 500 mg amoxicillin (Shulman 2012)

Urinary tract infections: Infants and Children 2 to 24 months: Oral: 20 to 40 mg amoxicillin/kg/day in divided doses 3 times daily using the 125 mg/5 mL or 250 mg/5 mL oral suspension; maximum single dose: 500 mg amoxicillin (AAP 2011)

Adult:

General dosing, susceptible infection: Oral:

Less severe infection: 250 mg every 8 hours using the 250 mg tablet **only**; **or** 500 mg every 12 hours using the 500 mg tablet, 125 mg/5 mL suspension, or 250 mg/5 mL suspension **only**

More severe infections and respiratory tract infections: 500 mg every 8 hours using the 500 mg tablet, 125 mg/5 mL suspension, or 250 mg/5 mL suspension **only**; **or** 875 mg every 12 hours using the 875 mg tablet, 200 mg/5 mL suspension, or 400 mg/5 mL suspension **only**

Rhinosinusitis, acute bacterial: Oral:

Immediate release tablet: 500 mg every 8 hours using the 500 mg tablet or 875 mg every 12 hours using the 875 mg tablet for 5 to 7 days

Extended release tablet: 2,000 mg (two 1,000 mg tablets) every 12 hours for 10 days

Note: May use high-dose therapy (extended release: 2,000 mg every 12 hours) if initial therapy fails, in areas with high endemic rates of penicillin-nonsusceptible *S. pneumoniae*, those with severe infections, age >65 years, recent hospitalization, antibiotic use within the past month, or who are immunocompromised (Chow 2012).

Bite wounds (animal/human) or erysipelas: Oral: 875 mg every 12 hours using the 875 mg tablet, 200 mg/5 mL suspension, or 400 mg/5 mL suspension **only**; **or** 500 mg every 8 hours using the 500 mg tablet, 125 mg/5 mL suspension, or 250 mg/5 mL suspension **only**

Pneumonia: Oral:

Aspiration: 875 mg every 12 hours using the 875 mg tablet, 200 mg/5 mL suspension, or 400 mg/5 mL suspension **only**

Community-acquired: 2,000 mg every 12 hours for 7 to 10 days using the 1,000 mg extended release tablet **only**

***Streptococci*, group A, chronic carrier treatment** (IDSA guidelines): Oral: 40 mg/kg/day divided every 8 hours (maximum daily dose: 2,000 mg/**day**) for 10 days (Shulman 2012)

Dosing adjustment in renal impairment:

Infants, Children, and Adolescents: There are no dosage adjustments provided in the manufacturer's labeling; however, the following guidelines have been used by some clinicians (Aronoff 2007): Oral:

Mild to moderate infection: Dosing based on 25 to 50 mg amoxicillin/kg/day divided every 8 hours:

GFR >30 mL/minute/1.73 m^2: No adjustment required

GFR 10 to 29 mL/minute/1.73 m^2: 8 to 20 mg amoxicillin/kg/dose every 12 hours

GFR <10 mL/minute/1.73 m^2: 8 to 20 mg amoxicillin/kg/dose every 24 hours

Hemodialysis: 8 to 20 mg amoxicillin/kg/dose every 24 hours; give after dialysis

Peritoneal dialysis: 8 to 20 mg amoxicillin/kg/dose every 24 hours

Severe infection (high dose): Dosing based on 80 to 90 mg amoxicillin/kg/day divided every 12 hours:

CrCl >30 mL/minute/1.73 m^2: No adjustment required

CrCl 10 to 29 mL/minute/1.73 m^2: 20 mg amoxicillin/kg/dose every 12 hours; do not use the 875 mg tablet

CrCl <10 mL/minute/1.73 m^2: 20 mg amoxicillin/kg/dose every 24 hours; do not use the 875 mg tablet

Hemodialysis: 20 mg amoxicillin/kg/dose every 24 hours; give after dialysis; do not use the 875 mg tablet

Peritoneal dialysis: 20 mg amoxicillin/kg/dose every 24 hours; do not use the 875 mg tablet

Adults:

CrCl ≥30 mL/minute: No adjustment required

CrCl <30 mL/minute: Do not use 875 mg tablet or extended release tablets

CrCl 10 to 30 mL/minute: 250 to 500 mg every 12 hours

CrCl <10 mL/minute: 250 to 500 mg every 24 hours

Hemodialysis: Moderately dialyzable (30%): 250 to 500 mg every 24 hours; administer an additional dose during and after dialysis. Do not use extended release tablets.

Peritoneal dialysis: Moderately dialyzable (20% to 50%):

Amoxicillin: Administer 250 mg every 12 hours

Clavulanic acid: Dose for CrCl <10 mL/minute

Dosing adjustment in hepatic impairment: There are no dosage adjustments provided in the manufacturer's labeling; use with caution. Use contraindicated in patients with a history of amoxicillin and clavulanate-associated hepatic dysfunction.

Preparation for Administration Reconstitute powder for oral suspension with appropriate amount of water as specified on the bottle. Shake vigorously until suspended.

Administration Oral: Can be given without regard to meals. Administer at the start of a meal to decrease the frequency or severity of GI side effects; may mix with milk, formula, or juice; shake suspension well before use

Monitoring Parameters With prolonged therapy, monitor renal, hepatic, and hematologic function periodically; monitor for signs of anaphylaxis during first dose

Test Interactions

May interfere with urinary glucose tests using cupric sulfate (Benedict's solution, Clinitest, Fehling's solution). Glucose tests based on enzymatic glucose oxidase reactions (eg, Clinistix) are recommended.

Ampicillin may transiently interfere with plasma concentrations of total conjugated estriol, estriol-glucuronide, conjugated estrone and estradiol in pregnant women.

Additional Information Products may not be interchangeable. Both the 250 mg and 500 mg tablets contain the same amount of clavulanic acid; two 250 mg tablets are not equivalent to one 500 mg tablet. Additionally, four 250 mg tablets or two 500 mg tablets are not equivalent to a single 1,000 mg extended release tablet. Based upon usual dosing in pediatric patients <40 kg, typical "TID" regimens provide 5 to 10 mg/kg/day of clavulanate and "BID" regimens 3.4 to 6.4 mg/kg/day.

Some penicillins (eg, carbenicillin, ticarcillin, piperacillin) have been shown to inactivate aminoglycosides *in vitro*. This has been observed to a greater extent with tobramycin and gentamicin, while amikacin has shown greater stability against inactivation. Concurrent use of these agents may pose a risk of reduced antibacterial efficacy *in vivo*, particularly in the setting of profound renal impairment. However, definitive clinical evidence is lacking. If combination penicillin/aminoglycoside therapy is desired in a patient with renal dysfunction, separation of doses (if feasible) and routine monitoring of aminoglycoside levels, CBC, and clinical response should be considered.

Dosage Forms Excipient information presented when available (limited, particularly for generics); consult specific product labeling. [DSC] = Discontinued product

Powder for suspension, oral:

Generic: 200: Amoxicillin 200 mg and clavulanate potassium 28.5 mg per 5 mL (50 mL, 75 mL, 100 mL); 250: Amoxicillin 250 mg and clavulanate potassium

62.5 mg per 5 mL (75 mL, 100 mL, 150 mL); 400: Amoxicillin 400 mg and clavulanate potassium 57 mg per 5 mL (50 mL, 75 mL, 100 mL); 600: Amoxicillin 600 mg and clavulanate potassium 42.9 mg per 5 mL (75 mL, 125 mL, 200 mL)

Amoclan:

200: Amoxicillin 200 mg and clavulanate potassium 28.5 mg per 5 mL (50 mL, 75 mL, 100 mL) [contains phenylalanine 7 mg/5 mL and potassium 0.14 mEq/5 mL; fruit flavor]

400: Amoxicillin 400 mg and clavulanate potassium 57 mg per 5 mL (50 mL, 75 mL, 100 mL) [contains phenylalanine 7 mg/5 mL and potassium 0.29 mEq/5 mL; fruit flavor]

600: Amoxicillin 600 mg and clavulanate potassium 42.9 mg per 5 mL (75 mL, 125 mL, 200 mL) [contains phenylalanine 7 mg/5 mL, potassium 0.248 mEq/5 mL; orange flavor]

Augmentin:

125: Amoxicillin 125 mg and clavulanate potassium 31.25 mg per 5 mL (75 mL, 100 mL, 150 mL) [contains potassium 0.16 mEq/5 mL; banana flavor]

200: Amoxicillin 200 mg and clavulanate potassium 28.5 mg per 5 mL (50 mL, 75 mL, 100 mL) [contains phenylalanine 7 mg/5 mL and potassium 0.14 mEq/5 mL; orange flavor] [DSC]

250: Amoxicillin 250 mg and clavulanate potassium 62.5 mg per 5 mL (75 mL, 100 mL, 150 mL) [contains potassium 0.32 mEq/5 mL; orange flavor]

400: Amoxicillin 400 mg and clavulanate potassium 57 mg per 5 mL (50 mL, 75 mL, 100 mL) [contains phenylalanine 7 mg/5 mL and potassium 0.29 mEq/5 mL; orange flavor] [DSC]

Augmentin ES-600:

600: Amoxicillin 600 mg and clavulanate potassium 42.9 mg per 5 mL (75 mL, 125 mL, 200 mL) [contains phenylalanine 7 mg/5 mL, potassium 0.23 mEq/5 mL; strawberry cream flavor]

Tablet, oral:

Generic: 250: Amoxicillin 250 mg and clavulanate potassium 125 mg; 500: Amoxicillin 500 mg and clavulanate potassium 125 mg; 875: Amoxicillin 875 mg and clavulanate potassium 125 mg

Augmentin:

250: Amoxicillin 250 mg and clavulanate potassium 125 mg [contains potassium 0.63 mEq/tablet] [DSC]

500: Amoxicillin 500 mg and clavulanate potassium 125 mg [contains potassium 0.63 mEq/tablet]

875: Amoxicillin 875 mg and clavulanate potassium 125 mg [contains potassium 0.63 mEq/tablet]

Tablet, chewable, oral:

Generic: 200: Amoxicillin 200 mg and clavulanate potassium 28.5 mg [contains phenylalanine]; 400: Amoxicillin 400 mg and clavulanate potassium 57 mg [contains phenylalanine]

Tablet, extended release, oral:

Generic: Amoxicillin 1000 mg and clavulanate acid 62.5 mg

Augmentin XR: 1000: Amoxicillin 1000 mg and clavulanate acid 62.5 mg [contains potassium 12.6 mg (0.32 mEq) and sodium 29.3 mg (1.27 mEq) per tablet; packaged in either a 7-day or 10-day package]

- ◆ **Amoxicillin and Clavulanate Potassium** *see* Amoxicillin and Clavulanate *on page 141*
- ◆ **Amoxicillin and Clavulanic Acid** *see* Amoxicillin and Clavulanate *on page 141*
- ◆ **Amoxicillin Trihydrate** *see* Amoxicillin *on page 138*
- ◆ **Amoxi-Clav (Can)** *see* Amoxicillin and Clavulanate *on page 141*
- ◆ **Amoxil** *see* Amoxicillin *on page 138*
- ◆ **Amoxycillin** *see* Amoxicillin *on page 138*
- ◆ **Amoxycillin and Clavulanate Potassium** *see* Amoxicillin and Clavulanate *on page 141*
- ◆ **Amoxycillin and Clavulanic Acid** *see* Amoxicillin and Clavulanate *on page 141*
- ◆ **Amphadase** *see* Hyaluronidase *on page 1025*
- ◆ **Amphetamine and Dextroamphetamine** *see* Dextroamphetamine and Amphetamine *on page 628*
- ◆ **Amphojel (Can)** *see* Aluminum Hydroxide *on page 110*
- ◆ **Amphotec** *see* Amphotericin B Cholesteryl Sulfate Complex *on page 145*
- ◆ **Amphotec® (Can)** *see* Amphotericin B Cholesteryl Sulfate Complex *on page 145*

Amphotericin B Cholesteryl Sulfate Complex

(am foe TER i sin bee kole LES te ril SUL fate KOM plecks)

Medication Safety Issues

High alert medication:

The Institute for Safe Medication Practices (ISMP) includes this medication among its list of drugs which have a heightened risk of causing significant patient harm when used in error.

Other safety concerns:

Lipid-based amphotericin formulations (Amphotec®) may be confused with conventional formulations (Amphocin®, Fungizone®)

Large overdoses have occurred when conventional formulations were dispensed inadvertently for lipid-based products. Single daily doses of conventional amphotericin formulation never exceed 1.5 mg/kg.

Brand Names: US Amphotec

Brand Names: Canada Amphotec®

Therapeutic Category Antifungal Agent, Parenteral

Generic Availability (US) No

Use Treatment of invasive aspergillosis in patients who have failed amphotericin B deoxycholate treatment, or who have renal impairment or unacceptable toxicity which precludes treatment with amphotericin B deoxycholate in effective doses (FDA approved in pediatric patients [age not specified] and adults)

Pregnancy Risk Factor B

Pregnancy Considerations Adverse events were not observed in animal reproduction studies. Amphotericin crosses the placenta and enters the fetal circulation. Amphotericin B is recommended for the treatment of serious systemic fungal diseases in pregnant women; refer to current guidelines (King, 1998).

Breast-Feeding Considerations It is not known if amphotericin is excreted into breast milk. Due to its poor oral absorption, systemic exposure to the nursing infant is expected to be decreased; however, because of the potential for toxicity, breast-feeding is not recommended (Mactal-Haaf, 2001).

Contraindications Hypersensitivity to amphotericin B or any component of the formulation (unless the benefits outweigh the possible risk to the patient)

Warnings/Precautions Anaphylaxis has been reported with amphotericin B-containing drugs. If severe respiratory distress occurs, the infusion should be immediately discontinued; the patient should not receive further infusions. During the initial dosing, the drug should be administered under close clinical observation. Acute infusion reactions, sometimes severe, may occur 1-3 hours after starting infusion. These reactions are usually more common with the first few doses and generally diminish with subsequent doses. Pretreatment with antihistamines/corticosteroids and/or decreasing the rate of infusion can be used to manage reactions. Avoid rapid infusion.

Warnings: Additional Pediatric Considerations In a multicenter study of pediatric patients (<16 years of age), amphotericin B cholestyrel sulfate complex (ABCD) use had a significantly lower incidence of renal toxicity (12%; 3/25 patients) than amphotericin B deoxycholate (52%; 11/21 patients).

Adverse Reactions

Cardiovascular: Chest pain, facial edema, hyper-/hypotension, tachycardia

Central nervous system: Abnormal thinking, chills, fever, headache, insomnia, somnolence, tremor

Dermatologic: Pruritus, rash, sweating

Endocrine & metabolic: Hyperglycemia, hypocalcemia, hypokalemia, hypomagnesemia, hypophosphatemia

Gastrointestinal: Abdominal enlargement, abdominal pain, diarrhea, dry mouth, hematemesis, jaundice, nausea, stomatitis, vomiting

Hematologic: Anemia, hemorrhage, thrombocytopenia

Hepatic: Alkaline phosphatase increased, hyperbilirubinemia, liver function test abnormal

Neuromuscular & skeletal: Back pain, rigor

Renal: Creatinine increased

Respiratory: Cough increased, dyspnea, epistaxis, hypoxia, rhinitis

Rare but important or life-threatening): Acidosis, arrhythmias (both atrial and ventricular), cardiac arrest, gastrointestinal hemorrhage, heart failure, injection site pain/ reaction, liver failure, oliguria, pleural effusion, renal failure, seizure, syncope

Note: Amphotericin B colloidal dispersion has an improved therapeutic index compared to conventional amphotericin B, and has been used safely in patients with amphotericin B-related nephrotoxicity; however, continued decline of renal function has occurred in some patients.

Drug Interactions

Metabolism/Transport Effects None known.

Avoid Concomitant Use

Avoid concomitant use of Amphotericin B Cholesteryl Sulfate Complex with any of the following: Foscarnet; Saccharomyces boulardii

Increased Effect/Toxicity

Amphotericin B Cholesteryl Sulfate Complex may increase the levels/effects of: Aminoglycosides; Cardiac Glycosides; Colistimethate; CycloSPORINE (Systemic); Flucytosine

The levels/effects of Amphotericin B Cholesteryl Sulfate Complex may be increased by: Corticosteroids (Orally Inhaled); Corticosteroids (Systemic); Foscarnet

Decreased Effect

Amphotericin B Cholesteryl Sulfate Complex may decrease the levels/effects of: Saccharomyces boulardii

The levels/effects of Amphotericin B Cholesteryl Sulfate Complex may be decreased by: Antifungal Agents (Azole Derivatives, Systemic)

Storage/Stability Store intact vials at 15°C to 30°C (59°F to 86°F). After reconstitution, the solution should be refrigerated at 2°C to 8°C (36°F to 46°F) and used within 24 hours. Concentrations of 0.1-2 mg/mL in D_5W are stable for 24 hours at 2°C to 8°C (36°F to 46°F).

Mechanism of Action Binds to ergosterol altering cell membrane permeability in susceptible fungi and causing leakage of cell components with subsequent cell death. Proposed mechanism suggests that amphotericin causes an oxidation-dependent stimulation of macrophages (Lyman, 1992).

Pharmacokinetics (Adult data unless noted)

Distribution: V_d: Total volume increases with higher doses, reflects increasing uptake by tissues (with 4 mg/kg/day = 4 L/kg); predominantly distributed in the liver; concentrations in kidneys and other tissues are lower than observed with conventional amphotericin B (Walsh 2008)

Half-life elimination: 28 to 29 hours; prolonged with higher doses

Dosing: Usual Note: Premedication for patients who experience fever, chills, hypotension, nausea, or other nonanaphylactic infusion-related immediate reactions may be given 30 to 60 minutes prior to drug administration: NSAIDs (with or without diphenhydramine) **or** acetaminophen with diphenhydramine **or** hydrocortisone may be given (Paterson 2008); if patient experiences rigors during infusion, meperidine may be administered. **Note:** A test dose immediately preceding the first dose is advisable when a new course of treatment occurs. A small amount of drug (eg, 10 mL of final preparation containing between 1.6 and 8.3 mg of drug) should be infused over 15 to 30 minutes and patient should be carefully observed for the next 30 minutes.

Pediatric: ***Aspergillosis*, invasive:** Infants, Children, and Adolescents: IV: Usual dose range: 3 to 4 mg/kg/day; doses as high as 6 mg/kg/day have been well tolerated in children ≥7 years and adolescents (Bowden 2002)

Adult: ***Aspergillosis*, invasive, treatment:** IV: Usual dosage range: 3 to 4 mg/kg/day. **Note:** 6 mg/kg/day has been used for treatment of life-threatening aspergillosis in immunocompromised patients (Bowden 2002)

Dosing adjustment in renal impairment:

Mild to moderate impairment: There are no dosage adjustments provided in manufacturer's labeling; however, no pharmacokinetic changes were noted in patients with mild to moderate impairment.

Severe impairment: There are no dosage adjustments provided in the manufacturer's labeling (has not been studied).

Dosing adjustment in hepatic impairment:

Mild to moderate impairment: There are no dosage adjustments provided in manufacturer's labeling; however, no pharmacokinetic changes were noted in patients with mild to moderate impairment.

Severe impairment: There are no dosage adjustments provided in the manufacturer's labeling (has not been studied).

Preparation for Administration Parenteral: IV: Reconstitute 50 mg and 100 mg vials with 10 mL and 20 mL of SWFI, respectively; resultant concentration: 5 mg/mL. Shake the vial gently by hand until all solid particles have dissolved. Further dilute amphotericin B colloidal dispersion with D_5W to a final concentration of ~0.6 mg/mL (range: 0.16 to 0.83 mg/mL).

Administration Parenteral: IV: Do not filter or use an inline filter for administration. Flush line with D_5W prior to infusion.

Initially infuse diluted solution at 1 mg/kg/hour. Rate of infusion may be increased with subsequent doses as patient tolerance allows (minimum infusion time: 2 hours).

For a patient who experiences chills, fever, hypotension, nausea, or other nonanaphylactic infusion-related reactions, premedicate with the following drugs, 30 to 60 minutes prior to drug administration: A nonsteroidal (eg, ibuprofen,) ± diphenhydramine **or** acetaminophen with diphenhydramine **or** hydrocortisone. If the patient experiences rigors during the infusion, meperidine may be administered. If severe respiratory distress occurs, the infusion should be immediately discontinued.

Monitoring Parameters Liver function tests, electrolytes, BUN, Cr, vital signs, CBC, I/O, prothrombin time, signs of hypokalemia (muscle weakness, cramping, drowsiness, ECG changes)

Additional Information The lipid portion of amphotericin B cholesteryl sulfate complex formulation does not contain phospholipids; for patients receiving parenteral nutrition, adjustment to the amount of lipids should not be needed (Sacks 1997).

Dosage Forms Excipient information presented when available (limited, particularly for generics); consult specific product labeling.

Suspension Reconstituted, Intravenous:

Amphotec: 50 mg (1 ea); 100 mg (1 ea) [contains edetate disodium, hydrochloric acid, lactose, sodium cholesteryl sulfate, tromethamine]

◆ **Amphotericin B Colloidal Dispersion** *see* Amphotericin B Cholesteryl Sulfate Complex *on page 145*

Amphotericin B (Conventional)

(am foe TER i sin bee con VEN sha nal)

Medication Safety Issues

High alert medication:

The Institute for Safe Medication Practices (ISMP) includes this medication (intrathecal administration) among its list of drugs which have a heightened risk of causing significant patient harm when used in error.

Other safety concerns:

Conventional amphotericin formulations (Amphocin, Fungizone) may be confused with lipid-based formulations (AmBisome, Abelcet, Amphotec).

Large overdoses have occurred when conventional formulations were dispensed inadvertently for lipid-based products. Single daily doses of conventional amphotericin formulation never exceed 1.5 mg/kg.

Brand Names: Canada Fungizone

Therapeutic Category Antifungal Agent, Systemic; Antifungal Agent, Topical

Generic Availability (US) Yes

Use Treatment of severe systemic infections and central nervous system infections caused by susceptible fungi, such as *Candida* species, *Histoplasma capsulatum*, *Cryptococcus neoformans*, *Aspergillus* species, *Blastomyces dermatitidis*, *Torulopsis glabrata*, and *Coccidioides immitis* [FDA approved in pediatric patients (age not specified) and adults]; has also been used for fungal peritonitis; irrigant for bladder fungal infections; used in fungal infection in patients with bone marrow transplantation, amebic meningoencephalitis, ocular aspergillosis (intraocular injection), and chemoprophylaxis (low-dose IV)

Pregnancy Risk Factor B

Pregnancy Considerations Adverse events were not observed in animal reproduction studies. Amphotericin crosses the placenta and enters the fetal circulation. No teratogenic or undue systemic toxicity (electrolyte imbalance or renal dysfunction) has been reported in the mother or fetus. Toxic maternal effects are to be expected and must be monitored (Perfect, 2010). Amphotericin B is recommended for the treatment of serious systemic fungal diseases in pregnant women. Refer to current guidelines (King, 1998).

Breast-Feeding Considerations It is not known if amphotericin is excreted into breast milk. Due to its poor oral absorption, systemic exposure to the nursing infant is expected to be decreased; however, because of the potential for toxicity, breast-feeding is not recommended (Mactal-Haaf, 2001).

Contraindications Hypersensitivity to amphotericin or any component of the formulation

Warnings/Precautions Anaphylaxis has been reported with amphotericin B-containing drugs. During the initial dosing, the drug should be administered under close clinical observation. May cause nephrotoxicity; usual risk factors include underlying renal disease, concomitant nephrotoxic medications and daily and/or cumulative dose of amphotericin. Avoid use with other nephrotoxic drugs; drug-induced renal toxicity usually improves with interrupting therapy, decreasing dosage, or increasing dosing interval. However permanent impairment may occur, especially in patients receiving large cumulative dose (eg, >5 g) and in those also receiving other nephrotoxic drugs. Hydration and sodium repletion prior to administration may reduce the risk of developing nephrotoxicity. Frequent monitoring of renal function is recommended. Acute reactions (eg, fever, shaking chills, hypotension, anorexia, nausea, vomiting, headache, tachypnea) are most common 1 to 3 hours after starting the infusion and diminish with continued therapy. Avoid rapid infusion to prevent hypotension, hypokalemia, arrhythmias, and shock. If therapy is stopped for >7 days, restart at the lowest dose recommended and increase gradually. Leukoencephalopathy has been reported following administration of amphotericin. Total body irradiation has been reported to be a possible predisposition.

[U.S. Boxed Warning]: Should be used primarily for treatment of progressive, potentially life-threatening fungal infections, not noninvasive forms of infection. [U.S. Boxed warning]: Verify the product name and dosage if dose exceeds 1.5 mg/kg.

Warnings: Additional Pediatric Considerations May premedicate patients who experience mild adverse reactions with acetaminophen and diphenhydramine 30 minutes prior to the amphotericin B infusion; meperidine and ibuprofen may help to reduce fevers and chills; hydrocortisone can be added to the infusion solution to reduce febrile and other systemic reactions. If therapy is stopped for >7 days, restart at the lowest dose recommended and increase gradually. Administer by slow IV infusion; rapid infusion has been associated with hypotension, hypokalemia, arrhythmias, and shock. Avoid extravasation; may cause chemical irritation; monitor infusion site; heparin 1 unit/1 mL of infusion solution can be added to reduce phlebitis. Use caution with intraperitoneal administration; use associated with irritation to the peritoneum and abdominal pain; not routinely used unless intolerance to other therapies (Warady, 2000).

Adverse Reactions

Systemic:

Cardiovascular: Flushing, hypertension, hypotension

Central nervous system: Arachnoiditis, chills, delirium, headache (less frequent with I.T), malaise, neuralgia (lumbar; especially with intrathecal therapy), pain (less frequent with I.T), paresthesia (especially with intrathecal therapy)

Endocrine & metabolic: Hypokalemia, hypomagnesemia

Gastrointestinal: Anorexia, diarrhea, epigastric pain, heartburn, nausea (less frequent with I.T), stomach cramps, vomiting (less frequent with I.T)

Genitourinary: Urinary retention

Hematologic & oncologic: Anemia (normochromic-normocytic), leukocytosis

Local: Pain at injection site (with or without phlebitis or thrombophlebitis [incidence may increase with peripheral infusion of admixtures])

Renal: Renal function abnormality (including azotemia, renal tubular acidosis, nephrocalcinosis [>0.1 mg/mL]), renal insufficiency

Respiratory: Tachypnea

Miscellaneous: Fever

Rare but important or life-threatening: Acute hepatic failure, agranulocytosis, anuria, blood coagulation disorder, bone marrow depression, bronchospasm, cardiac arrest, cardiac arrhythmia, cardiac failure, convulsions, diplopia, dyspnea, eosinophilia, exfoliation of skin, hearing loss, hemorrhagic gastroenteritis, hepatitis, hypersensitivity pneumonitis, increased liver enzymes, jaundice, leukoencephalopathy, leukopenia, maculopapular rash, melena, nephrogenic diabetes insipidus, oliguria, peripheral neuropathy, pruritus, pulmonary edema, renal failure, renal tubular acidosis, shock, Stevens-Johnson syndrome, thrombocytopenia, tinnitus, toxic epidermal necrolysis, ventricular fibrillation, vertigo (transient), visual disturbance, wheezing

Drug Interactions

Metabolism/Transport Effects None known.

Avoid Concomitant Use

Avoid concomitant use of Amphotericin B (Conventional) with any of the following: Foscarnet; Saccharomyces boulardii

Increased Effect/Toxicity

Amphotericin B (Conventional) may increase the levels/effects of: Aminoglycosides; Cardiac Glycosides; Colistimethate; CycloSPORINE (Systemic); Flucytosine

The levels/effects of Amphotericin B (Conventional) may be increased by: Corticosteroids (Orally Inhaled); Corticosteroids (Systemic); Foscarnet

Decreased Effect

Amphotericin B (Conventional) may decrease the levels/effects of: Saccharomyces boulardii

The levels/effects of Amphotericin B (Conventional) may be decreased by: Antifungal Agents (Azole Derivatives, Systemic)

Storage/Stability Store intact vials under refrigeration. Protect from light. Reconstituted vials are stable, protected from light, for 24 hours at room temperature and 1 week when refrigerated. Parenteral admixtures are stable, protected from light, for 24 hours at room temperature and 2 days under refrigeration. Short-term exposure (<24 hours) to light during IV infusion does **not** appreciably affect potency.

Mechanism of Action Binds to ergosterol altering cell membrane permeability in susceptible fungi and causing leakage of cell components with subsequent cell death. Proposed mechanism suggests that amphotericin causes an oxidation-dependent stimulation of macrophages (Lyman, 1992).

Pharmacokinetics (Adult data unless noted)

Absorption: Poor oral absorption

Distribution: Minimal amounts enter the aqueous humor, bile, pericardial fluid, pleural fluid, and synovial fluid

CNS penetration:

Preterm neonates (GA: 27.4 ± 5 weeks): High interpatient variability; 40% to 90% of serum concentrations (Baley, 1990)

Adults: Poor

V_d: Pediatric patients (0-18 years): Highly variable; reported range: 0.38-3.99 L/kg (Benson, 1989; Koren, 1988)

Protein binding: 90%

Half-life:

Premature neonates (GA: 27.4 ± 5 weeks): 14.8 hours (range: 5-82 hours) (Baley, 1990)

Infants and Children (4 months to 14 years): 18.1 ± 6.6 hours (range: 11.9-40.3 hours) (Benson, 1989)

Adult:

Initial: 15-48 hours

Terminal phase: 15 days

Elimination: Urine (2% to 5% unchanged); ~40% eliminated over 7-day period and may be detected in urine for up to 8 weeks after discontinued use

Clearance (Benson, 1989):

Infants and Children (8 months to 9 years): 0.57 ± 0.152 mL/minute/kg

Children and Adolescents (10-14 years): 0.24 ± 0.02 mL/minute/kg

Dialysis: Poorly dialyzed

Dosing: Neonatal Medication errors, including deaths, have resulted from confusion between lipid-based forms of amphotericin (Abelcet®, Amphotec®, AmBisome®) and conventional amphotericin B for injection; conventional amphotericin B for injection doses should not exceed 1.5 mg/kg/day

General dosing, susceptible infections:

IV: **Note:** Maintaining a sodium intake of >4 mEq/kg/day in premature neonates may reduce amphotericin B-associated nephrotoxicity (Turcu, 2009)

Initial: 0.5 mg/kg/dose once daily. The daily dose can then be gradually increased, usually in 0.25 mg/kg increments on each subsequent day until the desired daily dose is reached; maximum daily dose: 1.5 mg/kg/**day**; in critically ill patients, more rapid dosage acceleration (up to 0.5 mg/kg increments on each subsequent day) may be warranted

Maintenance dose: 0.25-1 mg/kg/dose once daily; infuse over 2-6 hours; rapidly progressing disease may require short-term use of doses up to 1.5 mg/kg/**day**; once therapy has been established, amphotericin B can be administered on an every-other-day basis at 1-1.5 mg/kg/dose

Irrigation, bladder: Limited data available: 50 **mcg**/mL solution, administered as either a continuous irrigation or as an intermittent irrigation 3 times per day with a dwell time of 60-90 minutes; dosing based on two case reports in neonates [PNA at treatment: 3 weeks; 3 months (PCA: 42 weeks)] (Ku, 2004; Martinez-Pajares, 2010)

Intrathecal, intraventricular, or intracisternal (preferably into the lateral ventricles through a cisternal Ommaya reservoir): Limited data available; some dosing based on experience in older pediatric patients: 25-100 **mcg** every 48-72 hours; increase to 500 **mcg** as tolerated (Chiou, 1994; Murphy; 2000; *Red Book*, 2012)

***Blastomycosis*, treatment:** IV: 1 mg/kg/dose once daily (Chapman, 2008)

Candidiasis:

Invasive, treatment: IV: 1 mg/kg/dose once daily for at least 3 weeks (Pappas, 2009)

Urinary tract infections, asymptomatic (high-risk patients); treatment: IV: 1 mg/kg/dose once daily (Pappas, 2009)

Urologic procedures; prophylaxis: IV: 0.3-0.6 mg/kg/dose once daily for several days before and after procedure (Pappas, 2009)

Dosing: Usual Medication errors, including deaths, have resulted from confusion between lipid-based forms of amphotericin (Abelcet®, Amphotec®, AmBisome®) and conventional amphotericin B for injection; conventional amphotericin B for injection doses should not exceed 1.5 mg/kg/day

Note: Premedication: For patients who experience infusion-related immediate reactions, premedicate with the following drugs 30-60 minutes prior to drug administration: NSAID (with or without diphenhydramine) **or** acetaminophen with diphenhydramine **or** hydrocortisone. If the patient experiences rigors during the infusion, meperidine may be administered.

Infants and Children:

Test dose: IV: 0.1 mg/kg/dose to a maximum of 1 mg; infuse over 20-60 minutes; an alternative method to the 0.1 mg/kg test dose is to initiate therapy with 0.25 mg/kg amphotericin administered over 6 hours; frequent observation of the patient and assessment of vital signs during the first several hours of the infusion is recommended; many clinicians believe a test dose is unnecessary

General dosing, susceptible infections:

IV:

Initial: 0.25-0.5 mg/kg/dose once daily; gradually increase daily, usually in 0.25 mg/kg increments until the desired daily dose is reached (maximum daily dose: 1.5 mg/kg/**day**); in critically ill patients, more rapid dosage acceleration may be warranted [eg, ≥0.5 mg/kg daily dose increase; others have initiated at target dose for life-threatening infection (DHHS [pediatric], 2013)

Maintenance dose: 0.25-1 mg/kg/dose once daily; rapidly progressing disease may require short-term use of doses to 1.5 mg/kg/**day**; once therapy has been established, amphotericin B may be administered on an every-other-day basis at 1-1.5 mg/kg/dose in some cases

Intrathecal, intraventricular, or intracisternal (preferably into the lateral ventricles through a cisternal Ommaya reservoir): Limited data available: 25-100 **mcg** every 72 hours; increase to 500 **mcg** as tolerated (Chiou, 1994; Murphy, 2000; *Red Book*, 2012)

Irrigation, bladder: Limited data available: 50 **mcg**/mL solution, administered as either a continuous irrigation or as an intermittent irrigation 3 times per day with a dwell time of 60-90 minutes (Fisher, 2011; Gubbins, 1999)

Aspergillosis:

Prophylaxis, immunocompromised: Limited data available: Intranasal: 7 mg amphotericin B in 7 mL sterile water was placed in a De Vilbiss atomizer and the aerosolized solution was instilled intranasally to each nostril 4 times daily delivering an average of 5 mg amphotericin/**day** to reduce the frequency of invasive aspergillosis in neutropenic patients (Jeffery, 1991)

Treatment, HIV-exposed/-positive: IV: 1-1.5 mg/kg/dose once daily for ≥12 weeks; duration should be individualized based upon clinical response (CDC, 2009)

***Blastomycosis* (independent of HIV status), moderately severe to severe disease:** IV: 0.7-1 mg/kg/dose once daily as initial therapy for 1-2 weeks, followed with oral itraconazole for a total of 12 months (Chapman, 2008)

Candidiasis; treatment:

Non-HIV-exposed/-positive (Pappas, 2009): IV:

Invasive: 0.5-1 mg/kg/dose once daily; duration of therapy dependent upon severity and site of infection

Urinary tract infections:

Prophylaxis, urologic procedures: 0.3-0.6 mg/kg daily for several days before and after procedure

Treatment:

Asymptomatic (high-risk patients): 1 mg/kg/dose once daily

Symptomatic: 0.3-0.6 mg/kg/dose once daily; duration for 1-7 days for symptomatic cystitis, 14 days for pyelonephritis

HIV-exposed/-positive: IV:

Invasive: 0.5-1.5 mg/kg/dose once daily; after fever resolution and stabilization, may decrease dose to 1.5 mg/kg once every other day; for candidemia, continue treatment for 2-3 weeks after last positive blood culture (CDC, 2009)

Esophageal: 0.3-0.7 mg/kg/dose once daily (DHHS [pediatric], 2013)

Oropharyngeal: 0.3-0.5 mg/kg/dose once daily (DHHS [pediatric], 2013)

Coccidioidomycosis:

Non-HIV-exposed/-positive (Galgiani, 2005):

Disseminated (non-CNS) disease: IV 0.5-1.5 mg/kg/dose every day or every other day; with or without concomitant azole antifungal; duration determined by clinical response

CNS disease: Intrathecal: 0.1-1.5 mg/dose; frequency ranging from daily to weekly (with or without concomitant azole therapy); initiate at a low dose and increase until intolerance (eg, severe vomiting, exhaustion, or transient dose-related mental status changes); duration determined by clinical response

Pulmonary disease, diffuse: IV 0.5-1.5 mg/kg/dose every day or every other day for several weeks, followed by an oral azole antifungal for a total length of therapy ≥12 months

HIV-exposed/-positive: Disseminated (non-CNS) disease, diffuse pulmonary disease; severely ill: IV: 0.5-1 mg/kg/dose once daily until clinical improvement; minimum of several weeks of therapy (DHHS [pediatric], 2013)

Cryptococcal disease:

CNS disease:

Non-HIV-exposed/-positive: IV: 0.7-1 mg/kg/dose once daily plus flucytosine; **Note:** Minimum 2-4-week induction, followed by consolidation and chronic suppressive therapy; may increase amphotericin dose to 1.5 mg/kg/day if flucytosine is not tolerated (Perfect, 2010)

HIV-exposed/-positive: IV: 1 mg/kg/day plus flucytosine or fluconazole; **Note:** Minimum 2-week induction, followed by consolidation and chronic suppressive therapy; a longer duration of induction therapy may be necessary if CSF is not negative or lack of clinical improvement; may increase amphotericin dose to 1.5 mg/kg/day alone or in combination with fluconazole if flucytosine is not tolerated (DHHS [pediatric], 2013)

Disseminated (non-CNS disease) or severe pulmonary disease: *Independent of HIV status:* IV: 0.7-1 mg/kg/dose once daily with or without flucytosine; duration of therapy depends on the site and severity of the infection and clinical response

Histoplasmosis:

Non-HIV-exposed/-positive: Severe disseminated (non-CNS) or pulmonary disease: IV: 0.7-1 mg/kg/dose once daily; **Note:** Minimum 1-2-week induction, followed by consolidation therapy (Wheat, 2007)

HIV-exposed/-positive: CNS or severe disseminated disease: IV: 0.7-1 mg/kg/dose once daily; **Note:** Conventional amphotericin B is an alternative therapy, lipid formulations are preferred (DHHS [pediatric], 2013)

Duration of induction:

Severe or moderately severe pulmonary disease: 1-2 week minimum

Disseminated or clinical improvement delayed: ≥2 weeks

CNS involvement: 4-6 weeks

Peritonitis (CAPD):

Intraperitoneal, dialysate: Children: 0.5-2 mg per liter of dialysate; either with or without low-dose IV amphotericin B therapy (Manley, 2000; Raajimakers, 2007; Warady, 2000)

IV: 1 mg/kg dose once daily (Warady, 2000)

Adolescents:

Test dose: IV: 0.1 mg/kg/dose to a maximum of 1 mg; infuse over 20-60 minutes; an alternative method to the 0.1 mg/kg test dose is to initiate therapy with 0.25 mg/kg amphotericin administered over 6 hours; frequent observation of the patient and assessment of vital signs during the first several hours of the infusion is recommended; many clinicians believe a test dose is unnecessary

General dosing, susceptible infections:

IV:

Initial: 0.25-0.5 mg/kg/dose once daily; gradually increase daily, usually in 0.25 mg/kg increments until the desired daily dose is reached (maximum daily dose: 1.5 mg/kg/**day**); in critically ill patients, more rapid dosage acceleration may be warranted (eg, ≥0.5 mg/kg daily dose increase)

Maintenance dose: 0.25-1 mg/kg/dose once daily; rapidly progressing disease may require short-term use of doses to 1.5 mg/kg/**day**; once therapy has been established, amphotericin B may be administered on an every-other-day basis at 1-1.5 mg/kg/dose in some cases

Intrathecal, intraventricular, or intracisternal (preferably into the lateral ventricles through a cisternal Ommaya reservoir): Limited data available; some dosing based on experience in older pediatric patients: 25-100 **mcg** every 48-72 hours; increase to 500 **mcg** as tolerated (*Red Book*, 2012)

Irrigation, bladder: Limited data available: 50 **mcg**/mL solution, administered as either a continuous irrigation or as an intermittent irrigation administered 3 times per day with a dwell time of 60-90 minutes (Fisher, 2011; Gubbins, 1999)

Aspergillosis:

Prophylaxis; immunocompromised: Limited data available: Intranasal: 7 mg amphotericin B in 7 mL sterile water was placed in a De Vilbiss atomizer and the aerosolized solution was instilled intranasally to each nostril 4 times daily delivering an average of 5 mg amphotericin/**day** to reduce the frequency of invasive aspergillosis in neutropenic patients (Jeffery, 1991)

Treatment; HIV-exposed/-positive: IV: 1 mg/kg/dose once daily until CD4 count is >200 cells/mm^3 and evidence of clinical response (DHHS [adult], 2013)

***Blastomycosis* (independant of HIV status), moderately severe to severe disease:** IV: 0.7-1 mg/kg/dose once daily as initial therapy for 1-2 weeks, followed with oral itraconazole for a total of 12 months (Chapman, 2008)

Candidiasis:

Non-HIV-exposed/-positive (Pappas 2009):

Invasive: IV: 0.5-1 mg/kg/dose once daily; duration of therapy dependent upon severity and site of infection

Urinary tract infections:

Prophylaxis, urologic procedures: IV: 0.3-0.6 mg/kg daily for several days before and after procedure

Treatment:

Asymptomatic (high-risk patients): IV: 1 mg/kg/dose once daily

Symptomatic: IV: 0.3-0.6 mg/kg/dose once daily; duration for 1-7 days for symptomatic cystitis, 14 days for pyelonephritis

HIV-exposed/-positive (DHHS [adult], 2013):

Esophageal: IV: 0.6 mg/kg/dose once daily for 14-21 days

Oropharyngeal, refractory: IV: 0.6 mg/kg/dose once daily for at least 7-14 days; depending upon response, a longer duration may be required

Coccidioidomycosis:

Non-HIV-exposed/-positive (Galgiani, 2005):

Disseminated (non-CNS) disease: IV: 0.5-1.5 mg/kg/dose every day or every other day; with or without concomitant azole antifungal; duration determined by clinical response

CNS disease: Intrathecal: 0.1-1.5 mg/dose; frequency ranging from daily to weekly (with or without concomitant azole therapy); initiate at a low dose and increase until intolerance is noted (eg, severe vomiting, exhaustion, or transient dose-related mental status changes); duration determined by clinical response

Pulmonary disease, diffuse: IV: 0.5-1.5 mg/kg/dose every day or every other day for several weeks, followed by an oral azole antifungal for a total length of therapy ≥12 months

HIV-exposed/-positive: Non-CNS disease: IV: 0.7-1 mg/kg/dose once daily until clinical improvement (DHHS [adult], 2013)

Cryptococcal disease (independent of HIV status):

CNS disease: IV: 0.7-1 mg/kg/dose once daily plus flucytosine or fluconazole; **Note:** Minimum 2-week induction, followed by consolidation and chronic suppressive therapy (DHHS [adult], 2013; Perfect, 2010)

Disseminated (non-CNS disease) or severe pulmonary disease: IV: 0.7-1 mg/kg/dose once daily with or without flucytosine; duration of therapy depends on the site and severity of infection and clinical response (Perfect, 2010)

Histoplasma: *Non-HIV-exposed/-positive:* Severe disseminated (non-CNS) or pulmonary disease: IV: 0.7-1 mg/kg/dose once daily; **Note:** Minimum 1-2-week induction, followed by consolidation therapy (Wheat, 2007)

Leishmaniasis, visceral (HIV-exposed/-positive): IV: 0.5-1 mg/kg/dose once daily for a total cumulative dose of 1500-2000 mg (DHHS [adult], 2013)

Peritonitis (CAPD):

Intraperitoneal, dialysate: 0.5-2 mg per liter of dialysate, either with or without low-dose IV amphotericin B therapy (Manley, 2000; Raajimakers, 2007; Warady, 2000)

IV: 1 mg/kg dose once daily (Warady, 2000)

Adults:

Test dose: IV: 1 mg infused over 20-30 minutes. Many clinicians believe a test dose is unnecessary.

Susceptible fungal infections: IV: 0.3-1.5 mg/kg/dose once daily; 1-1.5 mg/kg over 4-6 hours every other day may be given once therapy is established; aspergillosis, rhinocerebral mucormycosis, often require 1-1.5 mg/kg/day; maximum daily dose: 1.5 mg/kg/**day**

Peritoneal dialysis (PD): Administration in dialysate: 1-2 mg per liter of dialysate, either with or without low-dose IV amphotericin B (a total dose of 2-10 mg/kg given over 7-14 days). Precipitate may form in ionic dialysate solutions.

Dosing adjustment in renal impairment: Infants, Children, Adolescents, and Adults:

If renal dysfunction is due to the drug, the daily total can be decreased by 50% or the dose can be given every other day. IV therapy may take several months.

Renal replacement therapy: Poorly dialyzed; no supplemental dose or dosage adjustment necessary, including patients on intermittent hemodialysis or CRRT.

Dosing adjustment in hepatic impairment: There are no dosage adjustments provided in the manufacturer's labeling.

Preparation for Administration

IV: Add 10 mL of preservative-free SWFI to each vial of amphotericin B; **do not use bacteriostatic water**; benzyl alcohol, sodium chloride, or other electrolyte solutions may cause precipitation. Further dilute with D_5W, $D_{10}W$, up to $D_{20}W$ (Wiest 1991); final concentration should not exceed 0.1 mg/mL for peripheral administration. In patients unable to tolerate a large fluid volume, amphotericin B at a final concentration not to exceed 0.5 mg/mL in D_5W or $D_{10}W$ may be administered through a central venous catheter; an in-line filter (>1 micron mean pore diameter) may be used for administration (Kintzel 1992). Protect from light.

Intrathecal: Dilute dose in 0.5 to 2 mL of D_5W; use only preservative-free ingredients (Klaus 1989)

Irrigation solution (bladder): Further dilute reconstituted solution in sterile water to a final concentration of 50 mcg/mL (Fisher 2011; Gubbins 1999; Ku 2004; Martinez-Pajares 2010).

Administration

IV: Administer by IV infusion over 2 to 6 hours. For a patient who experiences chills, fever, hypotension, nausea, or other nonanaphylactic infusion-related reactions, premedicate with the following drugs 30 to 60 minutes prior to drug administration: A nonsteroidal (eg, ibuprofen,) ± diphenhydramine or acetaminophen with diphenhydramine or hydrocortisone. If the patient experiences rigors during the infusion, meperidine may be administered. Bolus infusion of normal saline immediately preceding, or immediately preceding and following amphotericin B may reduce drug-induced nephrotoxicity.

Risk of nephrotoxicity increases with amphotericin B doses >1 mg/kg/day.

Irrigation solution (bladder): Administer as a continuous irrigation or intermittently with a dwell time of 60 to 90 minutes (Fisher 2011; Gubbins 1999; Ku 2004; Martinez-Pajares 2010).

Monitoring Parameters Renal function (monitor frequently during therapy: Every other day during dose increases and at least weekly, thereafter), electrolytes (especially potassium and magnesium), liver function tests, temperature, PT/PTT, CBC; monitor input and output; monitor for signs of hypokalemia (muscle weakness, cramping, drowsiness, ECG changes, etc); blood pressure, temperature, pulse, respiration, IV site

Dosage Forms Excipient information presented when available (limited, particularly for generics); consult specific product labeling.

Solution Reconstituted, Injection, as desoxycholate:

Generic: 50 mg (1 ea)

◆ **Amphotericin B Deoxycholate** *see* Amphotericin B (Conventional) *on page 147*

◆ **Amphotericin B Desoxycholate** *see* Amphotericin B (Conventional) *on page 147*

Amphotericin B (Lipid Complex)

(am foe TER i sin bee LIP id KOM pleks)

Medication Safety Issues

High alert medication:

The Institute for Safe Medication Practices (ISMP) includes this medication among its list of drugs which have a heightened risk of causing significant patient harm when used in error.

Other safety concerns:

Lipid-based amphotericin formulations (Abelcet®) may be confused with conventional formulations (Fungizone®) or with other lipid-based amphotericin formulations (amphotericin B liposomal [AmBisome®]; amphotericin B cholesteryl sulfate complex [Amphotec®])

Large overdoses have occurred when conventional formulations were dispensed inadvertently for lipid-based products. Single daily doses of conventional amphotericin formulation never exceed 1.5 mg/kg.

Brand Names: US Abelcet

Brand Names: Canada Abelcet®

Therapeutic Category Antifungal Agent, Systemic

Generic Availability (US) No

Use Treatment of invasive fungal infections in patients who are refractory to or intolerant of conventional amphotericin B therapy (FDA approved in children and adults)

Pregnancy Risk Factor B

Pregnancy Considerations Adverse events were not observed in animal reproduction studies. Amphotericin crosses the placenta and enters the fetal circulation. Amphotericin B is recommended for the treatment of serious, systemic fungal diseases in pregnant women, refer to current guidelines (King, 1998).

Breast-Feeding Considerations It is not known if amphotericin is excreted into breast milk. Due to its poor oral absorption, systemic exposure to the nursing infant is expected to be decreased; however, because of the potential for toxicity, breast-feeding is not recommended (Mactal-Haaf, 2001).

Contraindications Hypersensitivity to amphotericin or any component of the formulation

Warnings/Precautions Anaphylaxis has been reported with amphotericin B-containing drugs. If severe respiratory distress occurs, the infusion should be immediately discontinued. During the initial dosing, the drug should be administered under close clinical observation. Acute reactions (including fever and chills) may occur 1-2 hours after starting an intravenous infusion. These reactions are usually more common with the first few doses and generally diminish with subsequent doses. Infusion has been rarely associated with hypotension, bronchospasm, arrhythmias, and shock. Acute pulmonary toxicity has been reported in patients receiving leukocyte transfusions and amphotericin B; amphotericin B lipid complex and concurrent leukocyte transfusions are not recommended. Concurrent use with antineoplastic agents may enhance the potential for renal toxicity, bronchospasm or hypotension; use with caution. Concurrent use of amphotericin B with other nephrotoxic drugs may enhance the potential for drug-induced renal toxicity.

Adverse Reactions Nephrotoxicity and infusion-related hyperpyrexia, rigor, and chilling are reduced relative to amphotericin deoxycholate.

Cardiovascular: Cardiac arrest, chest pain, hyper-/hypotension

Central nervous system: Chills, fever, headache, pain

Dermatologic: Rash

Endocrine & metabolic: Bilirubinemia, hypokalemia

Gastrointestinal: Abdominal pain, diarrhea, gastrointestinal hemorrhage, nausea, vomiting

Hematologic: Anemia, leukopenia, thrombocytopenia

Renal: Renal failure, serum creatinine increased

Respiratory: Dyspnea, respiratory disorder, respiratory failure

Miscellaneous: Infection, multiple organ failure, sepsis

Rare but important or life-threatening: Allergic reactions, anaphylactoid reactions, anuria, arrhythmias, asthma, blood dyscrasias, bronchospasm, BUN increased, cardiomyopathy, cerebral vascular accident, cholangitis, cholecystitis, coagulation abnormalities, deafness, dysuria, encephalopathy, eosinophilia, erythema multiforme, exfoliative dermatitis, extrapyramidal syndrome, hearing loss, hemoptysis, hepatic failure (acute), hepatitis, hepatomegaly, hepatotoxicity, hyper-/hypocalcemia, hyperkalemia, hypomagnesemia, injection site reaction, jaundice, leukocytosis, MI, myasthenia, oliguria, peripheral neuropathy, pleural effusion, pulmonary edema, pulmonary embolism, renal function decreased, renal tubular acidosis, seizures, shock, tachycardia, thrombophlebitis, transaminases increased, veno-occlusive liver disease, ventricular fibrillation, vertigo (transient), visual impairment

Drug Interactions

Metabolism/Transport Effects None known.

Avoid Concomitant Use

Avoid concomitant use of Amphotericin B (Lipid Complex) with any of the following: Foscarnet; Saccharomyces boulardii

Increased Effect/Toxicity

Amphotericin B (Lipid Complex) may increase the levels/effects of: Aminoglycosides; Cardiac Glycosides; Colistimethate; CycloSPORINE (Systemic); Flucytosine

The levels/effects of Amphotericin B (Lipid Complex) may be increased by: Corticosteroids (Orally Inhaled); Corticosteroids (Systemic); Foscarnet

Decreased Effect

Amphotericin B (Lipid Complex) may decrease the levels/effects of: Saccharomyces boulardii

The levels/effects of Amphotericin B (Lipid Complex) may be decreased by: Antifungal Agents (Azole Derivatives, Systemic)

Storage/Stability Intact vials should be stored at 2°C to 8°C (35°F to 46°F); do not freeze. Protect intact vials from exposure to light. Solutions for infusion are stable for 48 hours under refrigeration and for an additional 6 hours at room temperature.

Mechanism of Action Binds to ergosterol altering cell membrane permeability in susceptible fungi and causing leakage of cell components with subsequent cell death. Proposed mechanism suggests that amphotericin causes an oxidation-dependent stimulation of macrophages.

Pharmacokinetics (Adult data unless noted) Exhibits nonlinear kinetics; volume of distribution and clearance from blood increases with increasing dose

Distribution: High tissue concentration found in the liver, spleen, and lung

Half-life, terminal: 173 hours

Elimination: 0.9% of dose excreted in urine over 24 hours; effects of hepatic and renal impairment on drug disposition are unknown

Dialysis: Not hemodialyzable

Dosing: Neonatal Candidiasis, invasive: Limited data available: IV: 2.5-5 mg/kg/dose once daily; dosing based on experience reported in 28 neonates [median GA: 27 weeks; median weight: 1.06 kg (range: 0.48-4.9 kg)] (Würthwein, 2005); IDSA guidelines suggest an initial dose of 3 mg/kg (Pappas, 2009). Another report describes therapy initiation using a dose escalation approach with an initial dose of 1 mg/kg on day 1, followed by a daily increase of 1 mg/kg/day to a goal of 5 mg/kg/day (n=10; mean GA: 30.7 ± 3.9 weeks) (Cetin, 2005)

Dosing: Usual

Infants and Children: **Note:** For patients who experience infusion-related immediate reactions, premedicate with the following drugs 30-60 minutes prior to drug administration: NSAID (with or without diphenhydramine) or acetaminophen with diphenhydramine or hydrocortisone. If the patient experiences rigors during the infusion, meperidine may be administered.

General dosing, susceptible infections: IV: 5 mg/kg/dose once daily

***Aspergillosis*, invasive:**

Non-HIV-exposed/-infected: IV: 5 mg/kg/dose once daily; duration should be individualized based upon response (Walsh, 2008)

HIV-exposed/-infected: IV: 5 mg/kg/dose once daily for at least 12 weeks; duration should be individualized based on clinical response (CDC, 2009)

***Blastomycosis*, invasive:** IV: 3-5 mg/kg/day for initial therapy usually for 1-2 weeks, if CNS infection 4-6 weeks may be needed; follow with oral itraconazole for a total of 12 months (Chapman, 2008)

***Candidiasis*, invasive:**

Non-HIV-exposed/-infected: IV: 3-5 mg/kg/dose once daily; duration of therapy dependent upon severity and site of infection (Pappas, 2009)

HIV-exposed/-infected: IV: 5 mg/kg/dose once daily until 2-3 weeks after the last positive blood culture; may be used in combination with oral flucytosine for severe disease (eg, CNS involvement) (DHHS [pediatric], 2013)

***Coccidioidomycosis*, invasive:**

Non-HIV-exposed/-infected:

Disseminated infection, nonpulmonary: IV: 2-5 mg/kg/day with or without concomitant azole antifungal therapy (Galgiani, 2005)

Pulmonary infection, diffuse: IV: 2-5 mg/kg/day for several weeks, followed by an oral azole antifungal for a total length of therapy ≥12 months (Galgiani, 2005)

HIV-exposed/-infected: *Non-CNS infection:* IV: 5 mg/kg/dose once daily until clinical improvement; dose may be increased to as high as 10 mg/kg/dose once daily for life-threatening infection (DHHS [pediatric], 2013)

Cryptococcosis:

Disseminated (non-CNS or severe pulmonary disease) (independent of HIV status): IV: 5 mg/kg/dose once daily; for severe infection in HIV-exposed/-infected patients, may consider the addition of flucytosine (DHHS [pediatric], 2013; Perfect, 2010)

Meningitis: IV:

Non-HIV-exposed/-positive: 5 mg/kg/dose once daily with or without oral flucytosine for a minimum 2-week induction; combination with flucytosine is the preferred treatment (Perfect, 2010)

HIV-exposed/-positive: 5 mg/kg/day plus flucytosine or fluconazole; **Note:** Minimum 2 week induction followed by consolidation and chronic suppressive therapy; a longer duration of induction therapy may be necessary if CSF is not negative or lack of clinical improvement (DHHS [pediatric], 2013)

Histoplasmosis, acute pulmonary disease: IV: 3-5 mg/kg/day for 1-2 weeks followed by oral itraconazole for a total of 12 weeks; conventional amphotericin B typically preferred (Wheat, 2007)

Adolescents: **Note:** For patients who experience infusion-related immediate reactions, premedicate with the following drugs 30-60 minutes prior to drug administration: NSAID (with or without diphenhydramine) or acetaminophen with diphenhydramine or hydrocortisone 50-100 mg. If the patient experiences rigors during the infusion, meperidine may be administered.

General dosing, susceptible infection: IV: 5 mg/kg/dose once daily

***Aspergillosis*, invasive:**

Non-HIV-exposed/-infected: IV: 5 mg/kg/day; duration of treatment depends on site of infection, extent of disease, and level of immunosuppression (Walsh, 2008)

HIV-exposed/-infected: IV: 5 mg/kg/day treat until CD4 count >200 cells/mm^3 and evidence of clinical response (DHHS [adult], 2013)

***Blastomycosis*, invasive:** IV: 3-5 mg/kg/day for 1-2 weeks or until improvement, followed by oral itraconazole (Chapman, 2008)

***Candida* infection:**

General invasive candidal disease: IV: 3-5 mg/kg/day; duration of therapy dependent upon severity and site of infection. **Note:** In chronic disseminated candidiasis, transition to fluconazole after several weeks in stable patients is preferred (Pappas, 2009)

CNS infection: IV: 3-5 mg/kg/day (with or without flucytosine) for several weeks, followed by fluconazole (Pappas, 2009)

Endocarditis: IV: 3-5 mg/kg/dose once daily (with or without flucytosine); continue to treat for 4-6 weeks after device removal unless device cannot be removed then chronic suppression with fluconazole is recommended (Pappas, 2009)

Esophageal: HIV-exposed/-positive: IV: 3-4 mg/kg/dose once daily for 14-21 days (DHHS [adult], 2013)

Oropharyngeal, refractory: HIV-exposed/-positive: IV: 3-4 mg/kg/dose once daily for at least 7-14 days; depending upon response a longer duration may be required (DHHS [adult], 2013)

***Coccidioidomycosis*, invasive:**

Non-HIV-exposed/-infected:

Disseminated infection, nonpulmonary: IV: 2-5 mg/kg/day with or without concomitant azole antifungal therapy (Galgiani, 2005)

Pulmonary infection, diffuse: IV: 2-5 mg/kg/day for several weeks, followed by an oral azole antifungal for a total length of therapy ≥12 months (Galgiani, 2005)

HIV-exposed/-infected: *Non-CNS infection:* IV: 4-6 mg/kg/day until clinical improvement, then switch to fluconazole or itraconazole (DHHS [adult], 2013)

***Cryptococcosis* infection:**

Non-HIV-exposed/-infected:

Disseminated infection: IV: 5 mg/kg/day (with flucytosine if possible) for ≥4 weeks may be used for severe pulmonary cryptococcosis or for cryptococcemia with evidence of high fungal burden, followed by oral fluconazole. **Note:** If flucytosine is not given or treatment is interrupted, consider prolonging induction therapy for an additional 2 weeks (Perfect, 2010).

Meningitis, non-transplant patients: IV: Induction therapy: 5 mg/kg/day (with flucytosine if possible) for ≥4 weeks followed by oral fluconazole; should be used as an alternative to conventional amphotericin B in patients with renal concerns. **Note:** If flucytosine is not given or treatment is interrupted, consider prolonging induction therapy for an additional 2 weeks (Perfect, 2010).

Meningitis, transplant patients: IV: Induction therapy: 5 mg/kg/day (with flucytosine) for at least 2 weeks followed by oral fluconazole. **Note:** If flucytosine is not given, duration of therapy should be 4-6 weeks (Perfect, 2010).

HIV-exposed/-infected: *Cryptococcal meningitis or disseminated:* IV: Induction therapy: 5 mg/kg/day with flucytosine for at least 2 weeks, followed by oral fluconazole (DHHS [adult], 2013; Perfect, 2010); should be used as an alternative to conventional amphotericin B in patients with renal concerns. **Note:** If flucytosine is not given due to intolerance, duration of amphotericin B lipid complex therapy should be 4-6 weeks (Perfect, 2010).

Histoplasmosis:

Non-HIV-exposed/-positive: *Disseminated (non-CNS) or pulmonary disease:* IV: 5 mg/kg/dose once daily for 1-2 weeks followed by oral itraconazole (Wheat, 2007)

HIV-exposed/-positive: *Disseminated disease (moderately severe to severe):* Induction: IV: 3 mg/kg/dose once daily; **Note:** Minimum 2 week induction, longer if clinical improvement delayed; followed by oral itraconazole (DHHS [adult], 2013)

Leishmaniasis, visceral (HIV-exposed/-positive) (DHHS [adult], 2013):

Treatment: IV: 2-4 mg/kg/dose once daily **or** an interrupted schedule of 4 mg/kg/dose on days 1-5, and on days 10, 17, 24, 31, and 38 to achieve a total dose of 20-60 mg/kg

Chronic maintenance: IV: 3 mg/kg/dose every 21 days; **Note:** Use reserved for patients with visceral infection and CD4 count <200 cells/mm^3

***Sporotrichosis* infection:** IV:

Meningeal: 5 mg/kg/day for 4-6 weeks, followed by oral itraconazole (Kauffman, 2007)

Pulmonary, osteoarticular, and disseminated: 3-5 mg/kg/day, followed by oral itraconazole after a favorable response is seen with amphotericin initial therapy (Kauffman, 2007)

Adults: **Note:** For patients who experience infusion-related immediate reactions, premedicate with the following drugs 30-60 minutes prior to drug administration: NSAID (with or without diphenhydramine) or acetaminophen with diphenhydramine or hydrocortisone 50-100 mg. If the patient experiences rigors during the infusion, meperidine may be administered. **General dosing, susceptible infection:** IV: 5 mg/kg/dose once daily

Dosing adjustment in renal impairment: Infants, Children, Adolescents, and Adults:

Manufacturer's recommendations: There are no dosage adjustments provided in manufacturer's labeling (has not been studied).

Alternate recommendations: The following adjustments have been recommended (Aronoff, 2007):

Hemodialysis: No supplemental dosage necessary

Peritoneal dialysis: No supplemental dosage necessary

Continuous renal replacement therapy (CRRT): No supplemental dosage necessary

Dosing adjustment in hepatic impairment: There are no dosage adjustments provided in manufacturer's labeling (has not been studied).

Preparation for Administration Parenteral: IV: Shake the vial gently until there is no evidence of any yellow sediment at the bottom. Withdraw the appropriate dose from the vial using an 18-gauge needle. Remove the 18-gauge needle and attach the provided 5-micron filter needle to filter, and dilute the dose with D_5W to a final concentration of 1 mg/mL. Limited data suggests $D_{10}W$ and $D_{15}W$ may also be used for dilution (data on file [Sigma-Tau Pharmaceuticals, 2014]). Each filter needle may be used to filter up to four 100 mg vials. A final concentration of 2 mg/mL may be used for pediatric patients and patients with cardiovascular disease.

Do not dilute with saline solutions or mix with other drugs or electrolytes - compatibility has not been established

Administration Parenteral: IV: Prior to administration, amphotericin B lipid complex 5 mg/mL concentrated suspension must be diluted. Flush line with D_5W prior to infusion. Gently shake the IV container of diluted drug to insure that contents are thoroughly mixed then administer at a rate of 2.5 mg/kg/hour (over 2 hours). The manufacturer recommends that an in-line filter should **not** be used during administration of amphotericin B lipid complex. If infusion time exceeds 2 hours, mix the contents by gently rotating the infusion bag every 2 hours.

Monitoring Parameters BUN, serum creatinine, liver function tests, serum electrolytes, CBC; vital signs, I & O; monitor for signs of hypokalemia (muscle weakness, cramping, drowsiness, ECG changes, etc)

Additional Information The lipid portion of amphotericin B lipid complex formulation contains 0.045 kcal per 5 mg; for patients receiving parenteral nutrition, adjustment to the amount of lipids may be necessary (Sacks, 1997).

Dosage Forms Excipient information presented when available (limited, particularly for generics); consult specific product labeling.

Suspension, Intravenous:

Abelcet: 5 mg/mL (20 mL)

Amphotericin B (Liposomal)

(am foe TER i sin bee lye po SO mal)

Medication Safety Issues

High alert medication:

The Institute for Safe Medication Practices (ISMP) includes this medication among its list of drugs which have a heightened risk of causing significant patient harm when used in error.

Other safety concerns:

Lipid-based amphotericin formulations (AmBisome®) may be confused with conventional formulations (Amphocin, Fungizone) or with other lipid-based amphotericin formulations (Abelcet, Amphotec)

Large overdoses have occurred when conventional formulations were dispensed inadvertently for lipid-based products. Single daily doses of conventional amphotericin formulation never exceed 1.5 mg/kg.

Brand Names: US AmBisome

Brand Names: Canada AmBisome®

Therapeutic Category Antifungal Agent, Systemic

Generic Availability (US) No

Use Empirical therapy for presumed fungal infection in febrile, neutropenic patients; treatment of patients with *Aspergillus* species, *Candida* species, and/or *Cryptococcus* species infections refractory to amphotericin B desoxycholate (conventional amphotericin), or in patients where renal impairment or unacceptable toxicity precludes the use of amphotericin B desoxycholate; treatment of cryptococcal meningitis in HIV-infected patients; treatment of visceral leishmaniasis (all indications: FDA approved in ages ≥1 month and adults). Has also been used for treatment of systemic *Histoplasmosis* infection, blastomycosis, coccidioidomycosis, and mucormycosis

Pregnancy Risk Factor B

Pregnancy Considerations Adverse events were not observed in animal reproduction studies. Amphotericin crosses the placenta and enters the fetal circulation. Amphotericin B is recommended for the treatment of serious systemic fungal diseases in pregnant women; refer to current guidelines (King, 1998).

Breast-Feeding Considerations It is not known if amphotericin is excreted into breast milk. Due to its poor oral absorption, systemic exposure to the nursing infant is expected to be decreased; however, because of the potential for toxicity, breast-feeding is not recommended (Mactal-Haaf, 2001).

Contraindications Hypersensitivity to amphotericin B deoxycholate or any component of the formulation

Warnings/Precautions Patients should be under close clinical observation during initial dosing. As with other amphotericin B-containing products, anaphylaxis has been reported. Facilities for cardiopulmonary resuscitation should be available during administration. Acute infusion reactions (including fever and chills) may occur 1-2 hours after starting infusions; reactions are more common with the first few doses and generally diminish with subsequent doses. Immediately discontinue infusion if severe respiratory distress occurs; the patient should not receive further infusions. Concurrent use of amphotericin B with other nephrotoxic drugs may enhance the potential for drug-induced renal toxicity. Concurrent use with antineoplastic agents may enhance the potential for renal toxicity, bronchospasm or hypotension. Acute pulmonary toxicity has been reported in patients receiving simultaneous leukocyte transfusions and amphotericin B. Safety and efficacy have not been established in patients <1 month of age.

Adverse Reactions Nephrotoxicity and infusion-related hyperpyrexia, rigor, and chilling are reduced relative to amphotericin deoxycholate.

Cardiovascular: Atrial fibrillation, bradycardia, cardiac arrest, cardiac arrhythmia, cardiomegaly, chest pain, edema, facial edema, flushing, heart valve disease, hypertension, hypotension, localized phlebitis, orthostatic hypotension, peripheral edema, tachycardia, vascular disorder, vasodilatation

Central nervous system: Abnormality in thinking, agitation, anxiety, chills, coma, confusion, depression, dizziness, drowsiness, dysesthesia, dystonia, hallucination, headache, insomnia, malaise, nervousness, pain, paresthesia, rigors, seizure

Dermatologic: Alopecia, cellulitis, dermal ulcer, dermatological reaction, diaphoresis, maculopapular rash, pruritus, skin discoloration, skin rash, urticaria, vesiculobullous dermatitis, xeroderma

Endocrine & metabolic: Acidosis, hyperchloremia, hyperglycemia, hyperkalemia, hypermagnesemia, hypernatremia, hyperphosphatemia, hypervolemia, hypocalcemia, hypokalemia, hypomagnesemia, hyponatremia, hypophosphatemia, increased lactate dehydrogenase, increased nonprotein nitrogen

Gastrointestinal: Abdominal pain, anorexia, aphthous stomatitis, constipation, diarrhea, dyspepsia, dysphagia, enlargement of abdomen, eructation, fecal incontinence, flatulence, gastrointestinal hemorrhage, gingival hemorrhage, hematemesis, hemorrhoids, hiccups, increased serum amylase, intestinal obstruction, mucositis, nausea, rectal disease, stomatitis, vomiting, xerostomia

Genitourinary: Dysuria, hematuria, nephrotoxicity, toxic nephrosis, urinary incontence, vaginal hemorrhage

Hematologic & oncologic: Anemia, blood coagulation disorder, bruise, decreased prothrombin time, hemophthalmos, hemorrhage, hypoproteinemia, increased prothrombin time, leukopenia, oral hemorrhage, petechia, purpura, thrombocytopenia

Hepatic: Abnormal hepatic function tests (not specified), hepatic injury, hepatic veno-occlusive disease, hepatomegaly, hyperbilirubinemia, increased serum alkaline phosphatase, increased serum ALT, increased serum AST

Hypersensitivity: Delayed hypersensitivity, hypersensitivity reaction, transfusion reaction

Immunologic: Graft versus host disease

Infection: Infection, herpes simplex infection, sepsis

Local: Inflammation at injection site

Neuromuscular & skeletal: Arthralgia, back pain, myalgia, neck pain, ostealgia, tremor, weakness

Ophthalmic: Conjunctivitis, dry eyes

Renal: Acute renal failure, increased blood urea nitrogen, increased serum creatinine, renal failure, renal function abnormality

Respiratory: Asthma, atelectasis, cough, dry nose, dyspnea, epistaxis, flu-like symptoms, hemoptysis, hyperventilation, hypoxia, pharyngitis, pleural effusion, pneumonia, pulmonary disease, pulmonary edema, respiratory alkalosis, respiratory failure, respiratory insufficiency, rhinitis, sinusitis

Miscellaneous: Infusion related reactions (fever, chills, vomiting, nausea, dyspnea, tachycardia, hypertension, vasodilation, hypotension, hyperventilation, hypoxia), procedural complication

Rare but important or life-threatening: Agranulocytosis, angioedema, cyanosis, hemorrhagic cystitis, hypoventilation, rhabdomyolysis

Drug Interactions

Metabolism/Transport Effects None known.

Avoid Concomitant Use

Avoid concomitant use of Amphotericin B (Liposomal) with any of the following: Foscarnet; Saccharomyces boulardii

Increased Effect/Toxicity

Amphotericin B (Liposomal) may increase the levels/effects of: Aminoglycosides; Cardiac Glycosides; Colistimethate; CycloSPORINE (Systemic); Flucytosine

The levels/effects of Amphotericin B (Liposomal) may be increased by: Corticosteroids (Orally Inhaled); Corticosteroids (Systemic); Foscarnet

Decreased Effect

Amphotericin B (Liposomal) may decrease the levels/effects of: Saccharomyces boulardii

The levels/effects of Amphotericin B (Liposomal) may be decreased by: Antifungal Agents (Azole Derivatives, Systemic)

Storage/Stability Store intact vials at ≤25°C (≤77°F). Reconstituted vials are stable refrigerated at 2°C to 8°C (36°F to 46°F) for 24 hours. Do not freeze. Manufacturer's labeling states infusion should begin within 6 hours of dilution with D_5W; data on file with Astellas Pharma shows extended formulation stability when admixed in D_5W at 0.2-2 mg/mL (in polyolefin or PVC bags) for up to 11 days when stored refrigerated at 2°C to 8°C (36°F to 46°F).

Mechanism of Action Binds to ergosterol altering cell membrane permeability in susceptible fungi and causing leakage of cell components with subsequent cell death. Proposed mechanism suggests that amphotericin causes an oxidation-dependent stimulation of macrophages (Lyman, 1992).

Pharmacokinetics (Adult data unless noted) Exhibits nonlinear kinetics (greater than proportional increase in serum concentration with an increase in dose)

Distribution: V_d: 0.1-0.16 L/kg

Half-life (terminal): 100-153 hours

Dosing: Neonatal ***Candidiasis*, invasive:** Limited data available: IV: 3-5 mg/kg/dose once daily for ≥3 weeks

(Cetin, 2005; Juster-Reicher, 2003; Pappas, 2009; Queiroz-Telles, 2008); doses as high as 7 mg/kg/dose once daily have been used (Juster-Reicher, 2003); another report describes a dose escalation approach with dosing initiated with 1 mg/kg/dose on day 1 and increased by 1 mg/kg/dose once daily to a maximum of 5 mg/kg/dose once daily (preterm neonate: n=40; term neonate: n=4) (Scarcella, 1998)

Dosing: Usual

Infants and Children: **Note:** Premedication: For patients who experience infusion-related immediate reactions, premedicate with the following drugs 30-60 minutes prior to drug administration: NSAID (with or without diphenhydramine) **or** acetaminophen with diphenhydramine **or** hydrocortisone. If the patient experiences rigors during the infusion, meperidine may be administered.

General dosing:

Empiric therapy: IV: 3 mg/kg/dose once daily

Treatment, susceptible systemic infection: IV: 3-5 mg/kg/dose once daily

***Aspergillosis*, invasive:**

Non-HIV-exposed/-positive: IV: 3-5 mg/kg/dose once daily (Walsh, 2008)

HIV-exposed/-positive: IV: 5 mg/kg/dose once daily for at least 12 weeks; durations should be individualized based on clinical response (CDC, 2009); doses as high as 10 mg/kg/dose have been used in patients with documented *Aspergillus* infection

***Blastomycosis*, invasive:** IV: 3-5 mg/kg/day for initial therapy, if CNS infection 4-6 weeks may be needed; followed by oral itraconazole for a total of 12 months (Chapman, 2008)

***Candidiasis*, invasive:**

Non-HIV-exposed/-positive: IV: 3-5 mg/kg/dose once daily; duration of therapy dependent upon severity and site of infection (Filioti, 2007; Pappas, 2009)

HIV-exposed/-positive: IV: 5 mg/kg/dose once daily until 2-3 weeks after the last positive blood culture; may be used in combination with oral flucytosine for severe disease (eg, CNS involvement) (DHHS [pediatric], 2013)

***Coccidioidomycosis*, invasive:**

Non-HIV-exposed/-positive:

Disseminated infection, nonpulmonary: IV: 2-5 mg/kg/day with or without concomitant azole antifungal (Galgiani, 2005)

Pulmonary infection, diffuse: IV: 2-5 mg/kg/day for several weeks, followed by an oral azole antifungal for a total length of therapy ≥12 months (Galgiani, 2005)

HIV-exposed/-positive: *Non-CNS infection:* IV: 5 mg/kg/dose once daily until clinical improvement (minimum of several weeks of therapy); may be increased to as high as 10 mg/kg/dose once daily for life-threatening infection (DHHS [pediatric], 2013)

***Cryptococcosis*, invasive:**

Disseminated cryptococcosis (non-CNS or severe pulmonary disease) (independent of HIV status): IV: 3-5 mg/kg/dose once daily; may consider addition of oral flucytosine (DHHS [pediatric], 2013; Perfect, 2010)

Meningitis (HIV-exposed/-positive): IV: 6 mg/kg/dose once daily with or without oral flucytosine or fluconazole for a minimum 2-week induction; **Note:** Minimum 2 week induction, followed by consolidation and chronic suppressive therapy; a longer duration of induction therapy may be necessary if CSF is not negative or lack of clinical improvement (DHHS [pediatric], 2013)

Histoplasmosis:

Non-HIV-exposed/-positive: *Acute pulmonary disease:* IV: 3-5 mg/kg/day for 1-2 weeks followed by oral itraconazole for a total of 12 weeks; conventional amphotericin B typically preferred (Wheat, 2007)

HIV-exposed/-positive:

Disseminated infection (non-CNS disease): Treatment: IV: 3-5 mg/kg/dose once daily for at least 2 weeks for induction; if itraconazole not tolerated for consolidation therapy, may continue for 4-6 weeks (DHHS [pediatric], 2013)

CNS disease: Acute therapy: IV: 5 mg/kg/dose once daily for 4-6 weeks, followed by consolidation therapy (DHHS [pediatric], 2013)

Visceral leishmaniasis:

Immunocompetent patients: IV: Initial: 3 mg/kg/dose once daily on days 1-5; then repeat dose (3 mg/kg) on days 14 and 21. **Note:** Repeat course may be given to patients who do not achieve parasitic clearance.

Immunocompromised patients: IV: Initial: 4 mg/kg/dose once daily on days 1-5; then repeat dose (4 mg/kg) on days 10, 17, 24, 31, 38

Adolescents: **Note:** Premedication: For patients who experience nonanaphylactic infusion-related immediate reactions, premedicate with the following drugs 30-60 minutes prior to drug administration: NSAID (with or without diphenhydramine) **or** acetaminophen with diphenhydramine **or** hydrocortisone. If the patient experiences rigors during the infusion, meperidine may be administered.

General dosing: IV: 3-6 mg/kg/dose once daily; **Note:** Higher doses (15 mg/kg/day) have been used clinically (Walsh, 2001)

***Aspergillosis*, invasive:**

Non-HIV-exposed/-positive: IV: 3-5 mg/kg/dose once daily (Walsh, 2008)

HIV-exposed/-positive: IV: 5 mg/kg/dose once daily until CD4 count >200 cells/mm^3 and evidence of clinical response (DHHS [adult], 2013); doses as high as 10 mg/kg/dose have been used in patients with documented *Aspergillus* infection

***Blastomycosis*, invasive:** IV: 3-5 mg/kg/day for initial therapy, if CNS infection 4-6 weeks may be needed; followed by oral itraconazole for a total of 12 months (Chapman, 2008)

Candidiasis

Empiric therapy: IV: 3-5 mg/kg/dose once daily (Pappas, 2009)

Treatment:

General invasive Candidal disease (Independent of HIV status): IV: 3-5 mg/kg/dose once daily (Filioti, 2007; Pappas, 2009); **Note:** In HIV-exposed/-positive patients, doses at the higher end of the range may be considered (5 mg/kg/day); combination therapy with flucytosine may also be appropriate in some situations (DHHS [adult], 2013).

Endocarditis (Non-HIV-exposed/-positive): IV: 3-5 mg/kg/dose once daily (with or without flucytosine) for 6 weeks after valve replacement (Pappas, 2009)

Esophageal (HIV-exposed/-positive): IV: 3-4 mg/kg/dose once daily for 14-21 days (DHHS [adult], 2013)

Oropharyngeal, refractory (HIV-exposed/-positive): IV: 3-4 mg/kg/dose once daily for at least 7-14 days; depending upon response a longer duration may be required (DHHS [adult], 2013)

***Coccidioidomycosis*, invasive:**

Non-HIV-exposed/-positive:

Disseminated infection, nonpulmonary: IV: 2-5 mg/kg/day with or without concomitant azole antifungal (Galgiani, 2005)

Pulmonary infection, diffuse: IV: 2-5 mg/kg/day for several weeks, followed by an oral azole antifungal for a total length of therapy ≥12 months (Galgiani, 2005)

HIV-exposed/-positive: *Non-CNS infection:* IV: 4-6 mg/kg/dose once daily until clinical improvement (minimum of several weeks of therapy) (DHHS [adult], 2013)

***Cryptococcosis*, invasive:**

Disseminated cryptococcosis (non-CNS or severe pulmonary disease)

Non-HIV-exposed: IV: 3-4 mg/kg/dose once daily for at least 14 days; may consider addition of oral flucytosine (Perfect, 2010)

HIV-exposed/-positive: IV: 3-4 mg/kg/dose once daily with or without fluconazole (DHHS [adult], 2013)

Meningitis (HIV-exposed/-positive): IV: 3-4 mg/kg/dose once daily with or with fluconazole (DHHS [adult], 2013); doses up to 6 mg/kg/dose have been reported for treatment of meningoencephalitis and may be considered for treatment failure or high fungal burden disease (Perfect, 2010)

Histoplasmosis:

Non-HIV-exposed/-positive: IV: 3-5 mg/kg/day for 1-2 weeks followed with itraconazole (Wheat, 2007)

HIV-exposed/-positive (DHHS [adult], 2013): IV:

Non-CNS infection: 3 mg/kg/dose once daily

CNS infection: 5 mg/kg/dose once daily

Leishmaniasis:

Immunocompetent: Visceral infection: IV: 3 mg/kg/dose on days 1-5, and 3 mg/kg/dose on days 14 and 21; a repeat course may be given in patients who do not achieve parasitic clearance

HIV-exposed/-positive (DHHS [adult], 2013): IV:

Cutaneous or visceral infection, treatment:: IV: 2-4 mg/kg/dose once daily **or** an interrupted schedule of 4 mg/kg/dose on days 1-5, and on days 10, 17, 24, 31, and 38 to achieve a total dose of 20-60 mg/kg

Chronic maintenance therapy: IV: 4 mg/kg/dose every 2-4 weeks; **Note:** Use reserved for patients with visceral infection and CD4 count < 200 cells/mm^3:

***Sporotrichosis* infection:**

Disseminated, pulmonary, or osteoarticular disease: IV: 3-5 mg/kg/day, followed by oral itraconazole after a favorable response is seen with amphotericin initial therapy (Kauffman, 2007)

Meningeal: IV: 5 mg/kg/day for 4-6 weeks, followed by oral itraconazole (Kauffman, 2007)

Adults: **Note:** Premedication: For patients who experience nonanaphylactic infusion-related immediate reactions, premedicate with the following drugs 30-60 minutes prior to drug administration: NSAID (with or without diphenhydramine) **or** acetaminophen with diphenhydramine **or** hydrocortisone. If the patient experiences rigors during the infusion, meperidine may be administered. **General dosing, susceptible infection:** IV: 3-6 mg/kg/day; **Note:** Higher doses (15 mg/kg/day) have been used clinically (Walsh, 2001)

Dosing adjustment in renal impairment: Infants, Children, Adolescents, and Adults: No dosage adjustment provided in manufacturer's labeling (has not been studied).

Dosing adjustment in hepatic impairment: Infants, Children, Adolescents, and Adults: No dosage adjustment provided in manufacturer's labeling (has not been studied).

Preparation for Administration Parenteral: IV: Reconstitute with 12 mL SWFI to a concentration of 4 mg/mL; do not reconstitute with saline or add saline to the reconstituted solution or mix with other drugs; use of any solution other than those recommended, or the presence of a bacteriostatic agent in the solution, may cause precipitation. Shake vigorously for at least 30 seconds, until dispersed into a translucent yellow suspension; a 5-micron filter should be on the syringe used to inject the reconstituted product from the vial into the diluent. AmBisome may be diluted with D_5W, to a final concentration of 1 to 2 mg/mL; in infants and small children, a lower concentration of 0.2 to 0.5 mg/mL may be used to provide sufficient volume for infusion. Stability in $D_{10}W$, $D_{20}W$, or $D_{25}W$ has also been reported.

Administration Parenteral: IV: Do not use in-line filter less than 1 micron to administer AmBisome. Flush line with D_5W prior to infusion; infusion of diluted AmBisome should start within 6 hours of preparation; infuse over 2 hours; infusion time may be reduced to 1 hour in patients who tolerate the treatment. If the patient experiences discomfort during infusion, the duration of infusion may be increased. Discontinue if severe respiratory distress occurs.

For a patient who experiences chills, fever, hypotension, nausea, or other nonanaphylactic infusion-related reactions, premedicate with the following drugs, 30 to 60 minutes prior to drug administration: A nonsteroidal (eg, ibuprofen,) ± diphenhydramine or acetaminophen with diphenhydramine or hydrocortisone. If the patient experiences rigors during the infusion, meperidine may be administered.

Monitoring Parameters BUN, serum creatinine, liver function tests, serum electrolytes (particularly magnesium and potassium), CBC, vital signs, I & O; monitor for signs of hypokalemia (muscle weakness, cramping, drowsiness, ECG changes); monitor cardiac function if used concurrently with corticosteroids

Test Interactions Falsely-elevated serum phosphate may occur when using the PHOSm assay.

Additional Information The lipid portion of amphotericin B (liposomal) formulation contains 0.27 kcal per 5 mg; for patients receiving parenteral nutrition, adjustment to the amount of lipids may be necessary (Sacks, 1997).

Dosage Forms Excipient information presented when available (limited, particularly for generics); consult specific product labeling.

Suspension Reconstituted, Intravenous:

AmBisome: 50 mg (1 ea) [contains cholesterol, distearoyl phosphatidylglycerol, hydrogenated soy phosphatidylcholine, sodium succinate hexahydrate, sucrose, tocopherol, dl-alpha]

◆ **Amphotericin B Liposome** *see* Amphotericin B (Liposomal) *on page 153*

Ampicillin (am pi SIL in)

Medication Safety Issues

Sound-alike/look-alike issues:

Ampicillin may be confused with aminophylline

Related Information

Prevention of Infective Endocarditis *on page 2378*

Brand Names: Canada Ampicillin for Injection; Apo-Ampi; Novo-Ampicillin; Nu-Ampi

Therapeutic Category Antibiotic, Penicillin

Generic Availability (US) Yes

Use Treatment of susceptible respiratory, gastrointestinal, and urinary tract infections; bacterial meningitis, septicemia, and endocarditis [FDA approved in pediatric patients (age not specified) and adults]; susceptible organisms may include streptococci, pneumococci, enterococci, nonpenicillinase-producing staphylococci, *Listeria*, meningococci; some strains of *H. influenzae*, *P. mirabilis*, *Salmonella*, *Shigella*, *E. coli*, *Enterobacter*, and *Klebsiella*; has also been used as empiric therapy for neonatal sepsis or meningitis and endocarditis prophylaxis

Pregnancy Risk Factor B

Pregnancy Considerations Adverse events have not been observed in animal reproduction studies. Ampicillin crosses the placenta, providing detectable concentrations in the cord serum and amniotic fluid (Bolognese, 1968; Fisher, 1967; MacAulay, 1966). Maternal use of ampicillin has generally not resulted in an increased risk of birth defects (Aselton, 1985; Czeizel, 2001b; Heinonen, 1977; Jick, 1981; Puhó, 2007). Ampicillin is recommended for use in pregnant women for the management of preterm premature rupture of membranes (PPROM) and for the prevention of early-onset group B streptococcal (GBS) disease in newborns. Ampicillin may also be used in certain situations prior to vaginal delivery in women at high risk for endocarditis (ACOG, 2013; ACOG No. 120, 2011; ACOG No. 485, 2011; CDC [RR-10], 2010).

The volume of distribution of ampicillin is increased during pregnancy and the half-life is decreased. As a result, serum concentrations in pregnant patients are approximately 50% of those in nonpregnant patients receiving the same dose. Higher doses may be needed during pregnancy. Although oral absorption is not altered during pregnancy, oral ampicillin is poorly absorbed during labor (Philipson, 1977; Philipson, 1978; Wasz-Höckert, 1970).

Breast-Feeding Considerations Ampicillin is excreted in breast milk. The manufacturer recommends that caution be exercised when administering ampicillin to nursing women. Due to the low concentrations in human milk, minimal toxicity would be expected in the nursing infant. Nondose-related effects could include modification of bowel flora and allergic sensitization.

Contraindications Clinically significant hypersensitivity (eg, anaphylaxis) to ampicillin, any component of the formulation, or other penicillins; infections caused by penicillinase-producing organisms

Warnings/Precautions Dosage adjustment may be necessary in patients with renal impairment. Serious and occasionally severe or fatal hypersensitivity (anaphylactoid) reactions have been reported in patients on penicillin therapy, especially with a history of beta-lactam hypersensitivity, history of sensitivity to multiple allergens, or previous IgE-mediated reactions (eg, anaphylaxis, angioedema, urticaria). Serious anaphylactoid reactions require emergency treatment and airway management. Appropriate treatments must be readily available. Use with caution in asthmatic patients. Appearance of any rash should be carefully evaluated to differentiate a nonallergic ampicillin rash from a hypersensitivity reaction. High percentage of patients with infectious mononucleosis have developed rash during therapy with ampicillin; ampicillin-class antibiotics not recommended in these patients This rash (generalized maculopapular and pruritic) usually appears 7 to 10 days after initiation and usually resolves within a week of discontinuation. It is not known whether these patients are truly allergic to ampicillin. Ampicillin rash occurs in 5% to 10% of children receiving ampicillin and is a generalized dull red, maculopapular rash, generally appearing 3 to 14 days after the start of therapy. It normally begins on the trunk and spreads over most of the body. It may be most intense at pressure areas, elbows, and knees. Prolonged use may result in fungal or bacterial superinfection, including *Clostridium difficile*-associated diarrhea (CDAD) and pseudomembranous colitis; CDAD has been observed >2 months postantibiotic treatment.

Adverse Reactions

Central nervous system: Brain disease (penicillin-induced), glossalgia, seizure, sore mouth

Dermatologic: Erythema multiforme, exfoliative dermatitis, skin rash, urticaria

Note: Appearance of a rash should be carefully evaluated to differentiate (if possible) nonallergic ampicillin rash from hypersensitivity reaction. Incidence is higher in patients with viral infection, *Salmonella* infection, lymphocytic leukemia, or patients that have hyperuricemia.

Gastrointestinal: Diarrhea, enterocolitis, glossitis, melanoglossia, nausea, oral candidiasis, pseudomembranous colitis, stomatitis, vomiting

Hematologic & oncologic: Agranulocytosis, anemia, eosinophilia, hemolytic anemia, immune thrombocytopenia, leukopenia

Hepatic: Increased serum AST

Hypersensitivity: Anaphylaxis

Immunologic: Serum sickness-like reaction

Renal: Interstitial nephritis (rare)

Respiratory: Stridor

Miscellaneous: Fever

Drug Interactions

Metabolism/Transport Effects None known.

Avoid Concomitant Use

Avoid concomitant use of Ampicillin with any of the following: BCG; BCG (Intravesical); Probenecid

Increased Effect/Toxicity

Ampicillin may increase the levels/effects of: Methotrexate; Vitamin K Antagonists

The levels/effects of Ampicillin may be increased by: Allopurinol; Probenecid

Decreased Effect

Ampicillin may decrease the levels/effects of: Atenolol; BCG; BCG (Intravesical); BCG Vaccine (Immunization); Mycophenolate; Sodium Picosulfate; Typhoid Vaccine

The levels/effects of Ampicillin may be decreased by: Chloroquine; Lanthanum; Tetracycline Derivatives

Food Interactions Food decreases ampicillin absorption rate; may decrease ampicillin serum concentration. Management: Take at equal intervals around-the-clock, preferably on an empty stomach (30 minutes before or 2 hours after meals). Maintain adequate hydration, unless instructed to restrict fluid intake.

Storage/Stability

Oral:

- Capsules: Store at 20°C to 25°C (68°F to 77°F).
- Oral suspension: Store dry powder at 20°C to 25°C (68°F to 77°F). Once reconstituted, oral suspension is stable for 14 days under refrigeration.

IV:

- Solutions for IM or direct IV should be used within 1 hour.
- Stability of parenteral admixture (20 mg/mL) in NS at 25°C (77°F) is 8 hours and at 4°C (39°F) is 2 days.

Mechanism of Action Inhibits bacterial cell wall synthesis by binding to one or more of the penicillin-binding proteins (PBPs) which in turn inhibits the final transpeptidation step of peptidoglycan synthesis in bacterial cell walls, thus inhibiting cell wall biosynthesis. Bacteria eventually lyse due to ongoing activity of cell wall autolytic enzymes (autolysins and murein hydrolases) while cell wall assembly is arrested.

Pharmacokinetics (Adult data unless noted)

Absorption: Oral: 50%

Distribution: Into bile; penetration into CSF occurs with inflamed meninges only; low excretion into breast milk

Protein binding:

- Neonates: 10%
- Adults: 15% to 18%

Half-life:

- Neonates:
  - PNA 2-7 days: 4 hours
  - PNA 8-14 days: 2.8 hours
  - PNA 15-30 days: 1.7 hours
- Children and Adults: 1-1.8 hours
- Anuric patients: 8-20 hours

Time to peak serum concentration: Oral: Within 1-2 hours

Elimination: ~90% of drug excreted unchanged in urine within 24 hours; excreted in bile

Dosing: Neonatal

General dosing, susceptible infection (*Red Book*, 2012): IM, IV:

Body weight <1 kg:

PNA ≤14 days: 50 mg/kg/dose every 12 hours

PNA 15-28 days: 50 mg/kg/dose every 8 hours

Body weight 1-2 kg:

PNA ≤7 days: 50 mg/kg/dose every 12 hours

PNA 8-28 days: 50 mg/kg/dose every 8 hours

Body weight >2 kg:

PNA ≤7 days: 50 mg/kg/dose every 8 hours

PNA 8-28 days: 50 mg/kg/dose every 6 hours

Bacteremia, Group B streptococcal (presumed or proven) (*Red Book*, 2012): **Note:** Treatment of bacteremia without a defined focus should be for at least 10 days: IM, IV:

Body weight ≤2 kg:

PNA ≤7 days: 100 mg/kg/dose every 12 hours

PNA 8-28 days: 50 mg/kg/dose every 8 hours

Body weight >2 kg:

PNA ≤7 days: 100 mg/kg/dose every 12 hours

PNA 8-28 days: 50 mg/kg/dose every 6 hours

Meningitis, Group B streptococcal: IV:

PNA ≤7 days: 50-100 mg/kg/dose every 8 hours for at least 14 days if uncomplicated; some experts have also recommended 75 mg/kg/dose every 6 hours (*Red Book*, 2012; Tunkel, 2004)

PNA >7 days: 50-75 mg/kg/dose every 6 hours for at least 14 days if uncomplicated; some experts have also recommended 75 mg/kg/dose every 6 hours (*Red Book*, 2012; Tunkel, 2004)

Surgical prophylaxis: IV: 50 mg/kg as a single dose (*Red Book*, 2012)

Dosing: Usual

Infants, Children, and Adolescents:

General dosing, susceptible infection (*Red Book*, 2012):

Mild to moderate infection:

Oral: 50-100 mg/kg/day divided every 6 hours; maximum daily dose: 4000 mg/**day**

IM, IV: 100-150 mg/kg/day divided every 6 hours; maximum daily dose: 4000 mg/**day**

Severe infection: IM, IV: 200-400 mg/kg/day divided every 6 hours; maximum daily dose: 12 **g/day**

Community-acquired pneumonia (CAP) (IDSA/PIDS, 2011): Infants >3 months, Children, and Adolescents: **Note:** May consider addition of vancomycin or clindamycin to empiric therapy if community-acquired MRSA suspected. In children ≥5 years, a macrolide antibiotic should be added if atypical pneumonia cannot be ruled out.

Empiric treatment or *S. pneumoniae* (MICs for penicillin ≤2 mcg/mL) or *H. influenzae* (beta-lactamase negative) in fully immunized patients: IV: 150-200 mg/kg/day divided every 6 hours

Group A *Streptococcus*: IV: 200 mg/kg/day divided every 6 hours

S. pneumoniae (MICs for penicillin ≥4 mcg/mL): IV: 300-400 mg/kg/day divided every 6 hours

Endocarditis (Baddour, 2005)

Treatment: IV: 300 mg/kg/day divided every 4-6 hours in combination with other antibiotics for at least 4-6 weeks; some organisms may require longer duration (Baddour, 2005)

Prophylaxis:

Dental procedure or respiratory tract procedures (eg, tonsillectomy, adenoidectomy): IV, IM: 50 mg/kg within 30-60 minutes before procedure; maximum single dose: 2000 mg (Wilson, 2007)

Genitourinary and gastrointestinal tract procedures (high-risk patients): IV, IM: 50 mg/kg within 30 minutes prior to procedure; maximum dose: 2000 mg; followed by ampicillin 25 mg/kg (or amoxicillin 25 mg/kg orally) 6 hours later; must be used in combination with gentamicin. **Note:** As of April 2007, the American Heart Association guidelines now recommend prophylaxis only in patients undergoing invasive procedures and in whom underlying cardiac conditions may predispose to a higher risk of adverse outcomes should infection occur. Routine prophylaxis for GI/GU procedures is no longer recommended.

Intra-abdominal infection, complicated: IV: 200 mg/kg/**day** divided every 6 hours; maximum single dose: 2000 mg; maximize doses if undrained abdominal abscesses (Solomkin, 2010)

Meningitis: IV: 200-400 mg/kg/**day** divided every 6 hours; maximum daily dose: 12 **g/day** (*Red Book*, 2012; Tunkel, 2004)

Peritonitis (CAPD): Intraperitoneal: 125 mg per liter of dialysate for 2 weeks (Warady, 2012)

Surgical prophylaxis: IV: 50 mg/kg 30-60 minutes prior to procedure; may repeat in 2 hours; maximum single dose: 2000 mg (Bratzler, 2013; *Red Book*, 2012)

Adults:

Usual dosage range:

Oral: 250-500 mg every 6 hours

IM, IV: 1000-2000 mg every 4-6 hours or 50-250 mg/kg/**day** in divided doses (maximum daily dose: 12 **g/day**)

Cholangitis (acute): IV: 2000 mg every 4 hours with gentamicin

Diverticulitis: IM, IV: 2000 mg every 6 hours with metronidazole

Endocarditis:

Infective: IV: 12 **g/day** via continuous infusion or divided every 4 hours

Prophylaxis: Dental, oral, or respiratory tract procedures: IM, IV: 2000 mg within 30-60 minutes prior to procedure in patients not allergic to penicillin and unable to take oral amoxicillin. Intramuscular injections should be avoided in patients who are receiving anticoagulant therapy. In these circumstances, orally administered regimens should be given whenever possible. Intravenously administered antibiotics should be used for patients who are unable to tolerate or absorb oral medications. **Note:** American Heart Association (AHA) guidelines now recommend prophylaxis only in patients undergoing invasive procedures and in whom underlying cardiac conditions may predispose to a higher risk of adverse outcomes should infection occur.

Prophylaxis in total joint replacement patient: IM, IV: 2000 mg 1 hour prior to the procedure

Genitourinary and gastrointestinal tract procedures: IM, IV:

High-risk patients: 2000 mg within 30 minutes prior to procedure, followed by ampicillin 1000 mg (or amoxicillin 1000 mg orally) 6 hours later; must be used in combination with gentamicin. **Note:** As of April 2007, routine prophylaxis for GI/GU procedures is no longer recommended by the AHA.

Moderate-risk patients: 2000 mg within 30 minutes prior to procedure

Group B streptococcus (neonatal prophylaxis): IV: 2000 mg initial dose, then 1000 mg every 4 hours until delivery (CDC, 2010)

***Listeria* infections:** IV: 2000 mg every 4 hours (consider addition of aminoglycoside)

Mild to moderate infections: Oral: 250-500 mg every 6 hours

Prosthetic joint infection, *Enterococcus* spp (penicillin-susceptible): IV: 12 **g** continuous infusion every 24 hours **or** 2000 mg every 4 hours for 4-6 weeks; consider addition of aminoglycoside (Osmon, 2013)

Sepsis/meningitis: IV: 150-250 mg/kg/**day** divided every 3-4 hours (range: 6-12 **g/day**)

Urinary tract infections (*Enterococcus* suspected):
IV: 1000-2000 mg every 6 hours with gentamicin

Dosing adjustment in renal impairment:
Infants, Children, and Adolescents: The following adjustments have been recommended (Aronoff, 2007). **Note:** Renally adjusted dose recommendations are based on doses of 100-200 mg/kg/day divided every 6 hours: IM, IV:
- GFR 30-50 mL/minute/1.73 m^2: 35-50 mg/kg/dose every 6 hours
- GFR 10-29 mL/minute/1.73 m^2: 35-50 mg/kg/dose every 8-12 hours
- GFR <10 mL/minute/1.73 m^2: 35-50 mg/kg/dose every 12 hours
- Intermittent hemodialysis: 35-50 mg/kg/dose every 12 hours
- Peritoneal dialysis (PD): 35-50 mg/kg/dose every 12 hours
- Continuous renal replacement therapy (CRRT): 35-50 mg/kg/dose every 6 hours

Adults:
- CrCl >50 mL/minute: Administer every 6 hours
- CrCl 10-50 mL/minute: Administer every 6-12 hours
- CrCl <10 mL/minute: Administer every 12-24 hours
- Intermittent hemodialysis (IHD) (administer after hemodialysis on dialysis days): Dialyzable (20% to 50%): IV: 1-2 g every 12-24 hours (Heintz, 2009). **Note:** Dosing dependent on the assumption of 3 times/week, complete IHD sessions.
- Peritoneal dialysis (PD): 250 mg every 12 hours
- Continuous renal replacement therapy (CRRT) (Heintz, 2009): Drug clearance is highly dependent on the method of renal replacement, filter type, and flow rate. Appropriate dosing requires close monitoring of pharmacologic response, signs of adverse reactions due to drug accumulation, as well as drug concentrations in relation to target trough (if appropriate). The following are general recommendations only (based on dialysate flow/ultrafiltration rates of 1-2 L/hour and minimal residual renal function) and should not supersede clinical judgment:
  - CVVH: Loading dose of 2000 mg followed by 1000-2000 mg every 8-12 hours
  - CVVHD: Loading dose of 2000 mg followed by 1000-2000 mg every 8 hours
  - CVVHDF: Loading dose of 2000 mg followed by 1000-2000 mg every 6-8 hours

Preparation for Administration
Oral: Reconstitute powder for oral suspension with appropriate amount of water as specified on the bottle. Shake vigorously until suspended.
Parenteral:
IM: Reconstitute vial with SWFI to a final concentration of 125 to 250 mg/mL (see manufacturer's labeling for specific details).
IV:
IV push: Reconstitute vial with SWFI (see manufacturer labeling for specific details).
Intermittent IV infusion: Concentration should not exceed 30 mg/mL due to concentration-dependent stability restrictions.

Administration
Oral: Administer around-the-clock to promote less variation in peak and trough serum levels. Administer on an empty stomach (ie, 1 hour prior to or 2 hours after meals) to increase total absorption; shake suspension well before using
Parenteral:
IM: Inject deep IM into a large muscle mass
IV:
IV push: Doses ≤500 mg should be administered over 3 to 5 minutes; doses >500 mg should be administered over 10 to 15 minutes; rapid administration has been associated with seizures.
Intermittent IV infusion: Infuse over 10 to 15 minutes

Monitoring Parameters With prolonged therapy monitor renal, hepatic, and hematologic function periodically; observe for change in bowel frequency; observe for signs of anaphylaxis with first dose

Test Interactions May interfere with urinary glucose tests using cupric sulfate (Benedict's solution, Clinitest®)

Some penicillin derivatives may accelerate the degradation of aminoglycosides *in vitro*, leading to a potential underestimation of aminoglycoside serum concentration.

Additional Information Sodium content: Oral suspension (250 mg/5 mL, 5 mL): 10 mg (0.4 mEq); parenteral (1 g): 66.7 mg (3 mEq)

Some penicillins (eg, carbenicillin, ticarcillin, and piperacillin) have been shown to inactivate aminoglycosides *in vitro*. This has been observed to a greater extent with tobramycin and gentamicin, while amikacin has shown greater stability against inactivation. Concurrent use of these agents may pose a risk of reduced antibacterial efficacy *in vivo*, particularly in the setting of profound renal impairment; however, definitive clinical evidence is lacking. If combination penicillin/aminoglycoside therapy is desired in a patient with renal dysfunction, separation of doses (if feasible), and routine monitoring of aminoglycoside levels, CBC, and clinical response should be considered.

Dosage Forms Excipient information presented when available (limited, particularly for generics); consult specific product labeling.
Capsule, Oral:
Generic: 250 mg, 500 mg
Solution Reconstituted, Injection, as sodium [strength expressed as base]:
Generic: 125 mg (1 ea); 250 mg (1 ea); 500 mg (1 ea); 1 g (1 ea); 2 g (1 ea); 10 g (1 ea)
Solution Reconstituted, Injection, as sodium [strength expressed as base, preservative free]:
Generic: 250 mg (1 ea); 500 mg (1 ea)
Solution Reconstituted, Intravenous, as sodium [strength expressed as base]:
Generic: 1 g (1 ea); 2 g (1 ea); 10 g (1 ea)
Solution Reconstituted, Intravenous, as sodium [strength expressed as base, preservative free]:
Generic: 10 g (1 ea)
Suspension Reconstituted, Oral:
Generic: 125 mg/5 mL (100 mL, 200 mL); 250 mg/5 mL (100 mL, 200 mL)

Ampicillin and Sulbactam
(am pi SIL in & SUL bak tam)

Brand Names: US Unasyn
Brand Names: Canada Unasyn
Therapeutic Category Antibiotic, Beta-lactam and Beta-lactamase Combination; Antibiotic, Penicillin
Generic Availability (US) Yes
Use Treatment of susceptible bacterial infections involved with skin and skin structure (FDA approved in ages ≥1 year and adults); treatment of susceptible bacterial intra-abdominal infections and gynecological infections (FDA approved in adults); spectrum is that of ampicillin plus organisms producing beta-lactamases such as *Staphylococcus* sp, *Streptococcus* sp, *H. influenzae*, *E. coli*, *K. pneumonia*, *Proteus* sp (including *P. mirabilis*), *Acinetobacter calcoaceticus*, *Providencia rettgeri*, *Providencia stuartii*, *Morganella morganii*, *Neisseria gonorrhoeae*, *Enterobacter* sp, and anaerobes (including *B. fragilis*, *P. multocida*)
Pregnancy Risk Factor B

Pregnancy Considerations Adverse events have not been observed in animal reproduction studies. Both ampicillin and sulbactam cross the placenta. Maternal use of penicillins has generally not resulted in an increased risk of birth defects. When used during pregnancy, pharmacokinetic changes have been observed with ampicillin alone (refer to the Ampicillin monograph for details). Ampicillin/sulbactam may be considered for prophylactic use prior to cesarean delivery (consult current guidelines).

Breast-Feeding Considerations Ampicillin and sulbactam are both excreted into breast milk in low concentrations. The manufacturer recommends that caution be used if administering to lactating women. Nondose-related effects could include modification of bowel flora and allergic sensitization of the infant. The maternal dose of sulbactam does not need altered in the postpartum period. Also refer to the Ampicillin monograph.

Contraindications Hypersensitivity (eg, anaphylaxis or Stevens-Johnson syndrome) to ampicillin, sulbactam, or to other beta-lactam antibacterial drugs (eg, penicillins, cephalosporins), or any component of the formulations; history of cholestatic jaundice or hepatic dysfunction associated with ampicillin/sulbactam

Warnings/Precautions Dosage adjustment may be necessary in patients with renal impairment. Serious and occasionally severe or fatal hypersensitivity (anaphylactic) reactions have been reported in patients on penicillin therapy, especially with a history of beta-lactam hypersensitivity, history of sensitivity to multiple allergens. Patients with a history of penicillin hypersensitivity have experienced severe reactions when treated with cephalosporins. Before initiating therapy, carefully investigate previous penicillin, cephalosporin, or other allergen hypersensitivity. If an allergic reaction occurs, discontinue and institute appropriate therapy. Hepatitis and cholestatic jaundice have been reported (including fatalities). Toxicity is usually reversible. Monitor hepatic function at regular intervals in patients with hepatic impairment. High percentage of patients with infectious mononucleosis have developed rash during therapy with ampicillin; ampicillin-class antibacterials are not recommended in these patients. Appearance of a rash should be carefully evaluated to differentiate a nonallergic ampicillin rash from a hypersensitivity reaction. Prolonged use may result in fungal or bacterial superinfection, including *C. difficile*-associated diarrhea (CDAD) and pseudomembranous colitis; CDAD has been observed >2 months postantibiotic treatment.

Adverse Reactions Also see Ampicillin.

Cardiovascular: Thrombophlebitis

Dermatologic: Skin rash

Gastrointestinal: Diarrhea

Local: Pain at injection site (IM/IV)

Rare but important or life-threatening: Acute generalized exanthematous pustulosis, agranulocytosis, anemia, basophilia, candidiasis, casts in urine (hyaline), chest pain, chills, cholestasis, cholestatic hepatitis, *clostridium difficile* associated diarrhea, convulsions, decreased neutrophils, decreased serum albumin, decreased serum total protein, dysuria, edema, eosinophilia, erythema, erythema multiforme, erythrocyturia, exfoliative dermatitis, gastritis, glossitis, hairy tongue, headache, hemolytic anemia, hepatic insufficiency, hepatitis, hyperbilirubinemia, hypersensitivity reaction, immune thrombocytopenia, increased blood urea nitrogen, increased lactate dehydrogenase, increased liver enzymes, increased monocytes, increased serum creatinine, injection site reaction,interstitial nephritis, jaundice, leukopenia, lymphocytopenia, lymphocytosis (abnormal), nausea, positive direct Coombs test, pruritus, pseudomembranous colitis, Stevens-Johnson syndrome, stomatitis, thrombocythemia, thrombocytopenia, urinary retention, urticaria

Drug Interactions

Metabolism/Transport Effects None known.

Avoid Concomitant Use

Avoid concomitant use of Ampicillin and Sulbactam with any of the following: BCG; BCG (Intravesical); Probenecid

Increased Effect/Toxicity

Ampicillin and Sulbactam may increase the levels/effects of: Methotrexate; Vitamin K Antagonists

The levels/effects of Ampicillin and Sulbactam may be increased by: Allopurinol; Probenecid

Decreased Effect

Ampicillin and Sulbactam may decrease the levels/effects of: Atenolol; BCG; BCG (Intravesical); BCG Vaccine (Immunization); Mycophenolate; Sodium Picosulfate; Typhoid Vaccine

The levels/effects of Ampicillin and Sulbactam may be decreased by: Chloroquine; Lanthanum; Tetracycline Derivatives

Storage/Stability

Prior to reconstitution, store at 20°C to 25°C (68°F to 77°F).

IM: Concentration of 375 mg/mL (250 mg ampicillin/125 mg sulbacatam) should be used within 1 hour after reconstitution.

Intermittent IV infusion: Solutions made in NS are stable up to 72 hours when refrigerated whereas dextrose solutions (same concentration) are stable for only 4 hours. For stability related to specific concentrations and temperatures, see prescribing information.

Mechanism of Action Inhibits bacterial cell wall synthesis by binding to one or more of the penicillin-binding proteins (PBPs) which in turn inhibits the final transpeptidation step of peptidoglycan synthesis in bacterial cell walls, thus inhibiting cell wall biosynthesis. Bacteria eventually lyse due to ongoing activity of cell wall autolytic enzymes (autolysins and murein hydrolases) while cell wall assembly is arrested. The addition of sulbactam, a beta-lactamase inhibitor, to ampicillin extends the spectrum of ampicillin to include some beta-lactamase-producing organisms.

Pharmacokinetics (Adult data unless noted)

Ampicillin: See Ampicillin monograph

Sulbactam:

Distribution: Into bile, blister and tissue fluids; poor penetration into CSF with uninflamed meninges; higher concentrations attained with inflamed meninges; V_d (Nahata, 1999):

Children 1-12 years: ~0.35 L/kg

Adults: 0.25 L/kg

Protein binding: 38%

Half-life:

Children 1-12 years: Mean range: ~0.7-0.9 hours with normal renal function (Nahata, 1999)

Adults: 1-1.3 hours with normal renal function

Elimination: Urine (~75% to 85% as unchanged drug) within 8 hours

Dosing: Neonatal Note: Unasyn® (ampicillin/sulbactam) is a combination product formulated in a 2:1 ratio (eg, each 3 g vial contains 2 g of ampicillin and 1 g of sulbactam); review dosing units carefully. Dosage recommendations are expressed as mg of the **ampicillin** component.

Susceptible infection (non-CNS), treatment: IV:

Premature neonate: 100 mg/kg/day divided every 12 hours; dosing based on a pharmacokinetic analysis of 15 premature neonates using a 1:1 formulation of ampicillin to sulbactam (GA ≤28 weeks: n=6; GA >28 weeks: n=9) (Sutton, 1986)

Full-term neonate: 100 mg/kg/day divided every 8 hours for ≤8 days was used in 108 neonates (GA ≥37 weeks) (Manzoni, 2009)

Dosing: Usual Note: Unasyn® (ampicillin/sulbactam) is a combination product formulated in a 2:1 ratio (eg, each 3 g vial contains 2 g of ampicillin and 1 g of sulbactam); review dosing units carefully.

Infants, Children, and Adolescents <40 kg: **Note:** Dosage recommendations are expressed as mg of the **ampicillin** component.

General dosing, susceptible infection:

AAP dosing:

Mild to moderate infection: IV: 100-200 mg ampicillin/kg/day divided every 6 hours; maximum dose: 1000 mg ampicillin (*Red Book*, 2012); may also be administered IM (Bradley, 2012)

Severe infection: IV: 200 mg ampicillin/kg/day divided every 6 hours; maximum dose: 2000 mg (*Red Book*, 2012); higher doses up to 400 mg ampicillin/kg/day may be required for some infections (ie, meningitis)

Manufacturer's labeling: Children ≥1 year and Adolescents <40 kg: IV: 200 mg ampicillin/kg/day divided every 6 hours; maximum dose: 2000 mg ampicillin

Endocarditis, treatment: IV: 200 mg ampicillin/kg/day divided every 4-6 hours with gentamicin (optional; dependent upon organism) for at least 4-6 weeks; some organisms may require longer duration (Baddour, 2005)

Intra-abdominal infection: IV: 200 mg ampicillin/kg/day divided every 6 hours; **Note:** Due to high rates of *E. coli* resistance, not recommended for the treatment of community-acquired intra-abdominal infections (Solomkin, 2010)

Meningitis: IV: 200-400 mg ampicillin/kg/day divided every 6 hours (*Red Book*, 2009)

Rhinosinusitis, severe infection requiring hospitalization: Children and Adolescents: IV: 200-400 mg ampicillin/kg/day divided every 6 hours for 10-14 days; maximum dose: 2000 mg ampicillin (Chow, 2012)

Skin, soft tissue infection: IV: 200 mg ampicillin/kg/day divided every 6 hours

Children ≥40 kg and Adolescents ≥40 kg: **Note:** Doses expressed as total grams of the **ampicillin/sulbactam combination**.

General dosing, susceptible infection: IM, IV: 1.5-3 **g** every 6 hours (maximum daily dose: Unasyn® 12 **g/day**)

Amnionitis, cholangitis, diverticulitis, endometritis (with doxycycline), endophthalmitis, epididymitis/orchitis, liver abscess (with metronidazole), peritonitis: IV: 3 **g** every 6 hours; **Note:** Due to high rates of *E. coli* resistance, not recommended for the treatment of community-acquired intra-abdominal infections (Solomkin, 2010)

Bite (human, canine/feline): *Pasteurella multocida:* IV: 1.5-3 **g** every 6 hours (Stevens, 2005)

Endocarditis: IV: 3 **g** every 6 hours with gentamicin (optional; dependent upon organism) for 4-6 weeks (Baddour, 2005)

Pelvic inflammatory disease: IV: 3 **g** every 6 hours with doxycycline (CDC, 2010)

Rhinosinusitis, severe infection requiring hospitalization: IV: 1.5-3 **g** every 6 hours for 5-7 days (Chow, 2012)

Urinary tract infections, pyelonephritis: IV: 3 g every 6 hours for 14 days

Adults: **Note:** Doses expressed as total grams of the **ampicillin/sulbactam combination. General dosing, susceptible infection:** IM, IV: 1.5-3 **g** every 6 hours (maximum daily dose: Unasyn® 12 **g/day**)

Dosing interval in renal impairment: Children and Adults: **Note:** Doses expressed as **ampicillin/sulbactam combination**. IV:

CrCl ≥30 mL/minute/1.73 m^2: No dosage adjustment required.

CrCl 15-29 mL/minute/1.73 m^2: Administer every 12 hours.

CrCl 5-14 mL/minute/1.73 m^2: Administer every 24 hours.

Intermittent hemodialysis (IHD): Adults: 1.5-3 **g** every 12-24 hours (administer after hemodialysis on dialysis days) (Heintz, 2009). **Note:** Dosing dependent on the assumption of 3 times/week, complete IHD sessions.

Peritoneal dialysis (PD): Adults: 3 **g** every 24 hours

Continuous renal replacement therapy (CRRT): Adults: Drug clearance is highly dependent on the method of renal replacement, filter type, and flow rate. Appropriate dosing requires close monitoring of pharmacologic response, signs of adverse reactions due to drug accumulation, as well as drug concentrations in relation to target trough (if appropriate). The following are general recommendations only (based on dialysate flow/ultrafiltration rates of 1-2 L/hour and minimal residual renal function) and should not supersede clinical judgment (Heintz, 2009; Trotman, 2005):

CVVH: Initial: 3 **g**; maintenance: 1.5-3 **g** every 8-12 hours

CVVHD: Initial: 3 **g**; maintenance: 1.5-3 **g** every 8 hours

CVVHDF: Initial: 3 **g**; maintenance: 1.5-3 **g** every 6-8 hours

Preparation for Administration

IM: Reconstitute with SWFI or lidocaine (0.5% or 2%) to a final concentration of 375 mg/mL of Unasyn (ie, 250 mg/mL of ampicillin and 125 mg/mL of sulbactam)

IV: Use within several hours after preparation. Reconstitute with SWFI. Further dilute with a compatible solution; sodium chloride 0.9% (NS) is the diluent of choice for IV piggyback use; final concentration should not exceed 45 mg/mL Unasyn (30 mg/mL of ampicillin and 15 mg/mL of sulbactam)

Administration Parenteral:

IM: Administer by deep IM injection

IV: Administered by slow IV injection over 10 to 15 minutes or by intermittent IV infusion over 15 to 30 minutes

Monitoring Parameters With prolonged therapy monitor hematologic, renal, and hepatic function; observe for change in bowel frequency; monitor for signs of anaphylaxis during first dose

Test Interactions May interfere with urinary glucose tests using cupric sulfate (Benedict's solution, Fehling's solution, or Clinitest®).

Some penicillin derivatives may accelerate the degradation of aminoglycosides *in vitro*, leading to a potential underestimation of aminoglycoside serum concentration.

Additional Information Some penicillins (eg, carbenicillin, ticarcillin, and piperacillin) have been shown to inactivate aminoglycosides *in vitro*. This has been observed to a greater extent with tobramycin and gentamicin, while amikacin has shown greater stability against inactivation. Concomitant use of these agents may pose a risk of reduced antibacterial efficacy *in vivo*, particularly in the setting of profound renal impairment; however, definitive clinical evidence is lacking. If combination penicillin/aminoglycoside therapy is desired in a patient with renal dysfunction, separation of doses (if feasible), and routine monitoring of aminoglycoside concentrations, CBC, and clinical response should be considered.

Dosage Forms Excipient information presented when available (limited, particularly for generics); consult specific product labeling.

Injection, powder for reconstitution: 1.5 g: Ampicillin 1 g and sulbactam 0.5 g; 3 g: Ampicillin 2 g and sulbactam 1 g; 15 g: Ampicillin 10 g and sulbactam 5 g

Unasyn®:

1.5 g: Ampicillin 1 g and sulbactam 0.5 g [contains sodium 115 mg (5 mEq)/1.5 g)]

3 g: Ampicillin 2 g and sulbactam 1 g [contains sodium 115 mg (5 mEq)/1.5 g)]

15 g: Ampicillin 10 g and sulbactam 5 g [bulk package; contains sodium 115 mg (5 mEq)/1.5 g)]

- **Ampicillin for Injection (Can)** *see* Ampicillin *on page 156*
- **Ampicillin Sodium** *see* Ampicillin *on page 156*
- **Ampicillin Trihydrate** *see* Ampicillin *on page 156*
- **Amrix** *see* Cyclobenzaprine *on page 548*
- **Amylase, Lipase, and Protease** *see* Pancrelipase *on page 1614*

Amyl Nitrite (AM il NYE trite)

Therapeutic Category Antidote, Cyanide; Vasodilator, Coronary

Generic Availability (US) Yes

Use Treatment of angina pectoris (FDA approved in adults); has also been used as an adjunct treatment of cyanide toxicity

Note: Given the widespread use of newer nitrate compounds, the use of amyl nitrite for patients experiencing angina pectoris has fallen out of favor.

Pregnancy Risk Factor C

Pregnancy Considerations Animal reproduction studies have not been conducted. Because amyl nitrite significantly decreases systemic blood pressure and therefore blood flow to the fetus, use is contraindicated in pregnancy (per manufacturer). In addition, fetal hemoglobin may be more susceptible methemoglobin conversion (Valenzuela, 1986).

Breast-Feeding Considerations It is not known if amyl nitrite is excreted in breast milk. The manufacturer recommends that caution be exercised when administering amyl nitrite to nursing women.

Contraindications Glaucoma; recent head trauma or cerebral hemorrhage; pregnancy

Warnings/Precautions Use with caution in patients with increased intracranial pressure, low systolic blood pressure, and coronary artery disease. Transient episodes of dizziness, weakness, syncope, and cerebral ischemia secondary to postural hypotension may occur. Use with caution in patients with increased intracranial pressure; use is contraindicated in patient with recent head trauma or cerebral hemorrhage. Use with extreme caution or avoid in patients with severe aortic stenosis; may reduce coronary perfusion resulting in ischemia; considered by some to be a contraindication (Reagan, 2005).

Amyl nitrite may cause methemoglobin formation and severe hypotension resulting in diminished oxygen-carrying capacity; serious adverse effects may occur at doses less than the recommended therapeutic dose. Monitor for adequate perfusion and oxygenation; ensure patient is euvolemic. Use with caution in patients where the diagnosis of cyanide poisoning is uncertain, patients with preexisting diminished oxygen or cardiovascular reserve (eg, smoke inhalation victims, anemia, substantial blood loss, and cardiac or respiratory compromise), in patients at greater risk for developing methemoglobinemia (eg, congenital methemoglobin reductase deficiency), and in patients who may be susceptible to injury from vasodilation. The use of hydroxocobalamin is recommended in these patients. Use with caution with concomitant medications known to cause methemoglobinemia (eg, nitroglycerin, phenazopyridine). Collection of pretreatment blood cyanide concentrations does not preclude administration and should not delay administration in the emergency management of highly suspected or confirmed cyanide toxicity. Pretreatment levels may be useful as postinfusion levels may be inaccurate. Treatment of cyanide poisoning should include external decontamination and supportive therapy. Monitor patients for return of symptoms for 24-48 hours; repeat treatment should be administered if symptoms return. Fire victims and patients with cyanide poisoning related to smoke inhalation may present with both cyanide and carbon monoxide poisoning. In these patients, the induction of methemoglobinemia (due to amyl nitrite, sodium nitrite) is contraindicated until carbon monoxide levels return to normal due to the risk of tissue hypoxia. Methemoglobinemia decreases the oxygen carrying capacity of hemoglobin and the presence of carbon monoxide prevents hemoglobin from releasing oxygen to the tissues. In this scenario, sodium thiosulfate may be used alone to promote the clearance of cyanide. Hydroxocobalamin, however, should be considered to avoid the nitrite-related problems and because sodium thiosulfate has a slow onset of action. Consider consultation with a poison control center at 1-800-222-1222.

Methemoglobin reductase, which is responsible for converting methemoglobin back to hemoglobin, has reduced activity in pediatric patients. In addition, infants and young children have some proportion of fetal hemoglobin which forms methemoglobin more readily than adult hemoglobin. Therefore, pediatric patients (eg, neonates and infants <6 months) are more susceptible to excessive nitrite-induced methemoglobinemia. Nitrites should be avoided in pregnant patients due to fetal hemoglobin's susceptibility to oxidative stress. Hydroxocobalamin will circumvent this problem and may be a more effective and rapid alternative.

Adverse Reactions

Cardiovascular: Cerebral ischemia, facial flushing, hypotension, orthostatic hypotension, pallor, shock, syncope, tachycardia, vasodilation

Central nervous system: Dizziness, headache, intracranial pressure increased, restlessness

Dermatologic: Dermatitis, irritation

Gastrointestinal: Fecal incontinence, nausea, vomiting

Genitourinary: Urinary incontinence

Hematologic: Hemolytic anemia, methemoglobinemia

Neuromuscular & skeletal: Weakness

Ocular: Intraocular pressure increased, irritation

Miscellaneous: Diaphoresis

Drug Interactions

Metabolism/Transport Effects None known.

Avoid Concomitant Use

Avoid concomitant use of Amyl Nitrite with any of the following: Phosphodiesterase 5 Inhibitors; Riociguat

Increased Effect/Toxicity

Amyl Nitrite may increase the levels/effects of: DULoxetine; Hypotensive Agents; Levodopa; Prilocaine; Riociguat; RisperiDONE; Sodium Nitrite

The levels/effects of Amyl Nitrite may be increased by: Barbiturates; Nicorandil; Nitric Oxide; Phosphodiesterase 5 Inhibitors

Decreased Effect There are no known significant interactions involving a decrease in effect.

Storage/Stability Store in a cool place at 2°C to 8°C (36°F to 46°F). Protect from light. Contents are flammable; protect from open flame or spark.

Mechanism of Action Relaxes vascular smooth muscle; decreases venous ratios and arterial blood pressure; reduces left ventricular work; decreases myocardial O_2 consumption. When used for cyanide poisoning, amyl nitrite promotes the formation of methemoglobin which competes with cytochrome oxidase for the cyanide ion. Cyanide combines with methemoglobin to form cyanomethemoglobin, thereby freeing the cytochrome oxidase and allowing aerobic metabolism to continue.

Pharmacodynamics

Onset of action: Angina: Within 30 seconds

Duration: Angina: 3-5 minutes

Pharmacokinetics (Adult data unless noted)

Absorption: Inhalation: Readily absorbed through respiratory tract

Metabolism: In the liver to form inorganic nitrates (less potent)
Half-life:
Amyl nitrite: <1 hour
Methemoglobin: 1 hour
Elimination: Renal; ~33%

Dosing: Usual
Infants, Children and Adolescents:
Cyanide toxicity: Inhalation: 0.3 mL ampul crushed into a gauze pad and placed in front of the patient's mouth (or endotracheal tube if patient is intubated) to inhale over 15-30 seconds; repeat every minute until sodium nitrite can be administered. **Note:** Must separate administrations by at least 30 seconds to allow for adequate oxygenation; each ampul will last for ~3 minutes. Amyl nitrite is a temporary intervention that should only be used until IV sodium nitrite infusion is ready for administration (ATSDR).
Adults:
Cyanide toxicity: Inhalation: 0.3 mL ampul crushed into a gauze pad and placed in front of the patient's mouth (or endotracheal tube if patient is intubated) to inhale over 15-30 seconds; repeat every minute until sodium nitrite can be administered (Mokhlesi, 2003). **Note:** Must separate administrations by at least 30 seconds to allow for adequate oxygenation; each ampul will last for ~3 minutes. Amyl nitrite is a temporary intervention that should only be used until IV sodium nitrite infusion is ready for administration (ATSDR).
Angina: Inhalation: 2-6 nasal inhalations from 1 crushed ampul; may repeat in 3-5 minutes

Administration Administer nasally via inhalation. The patient should be lying down during administration. Crush the ampul in a gauze pad and place in front of patient's mouth (or endotracheal tube if intubated) and allow patient to inhale for 15-30 seconds; repeat every minute until sodium nitrite can be administered. One ampul lasts for ~3 minutes.

Monitoring Parameters Monitor blood pressure and heart rate during therapy
Cyanide toxicity: Monitor for at least 24-48 hours after administration; hemoglobin/hematocrit; co-oximetry; serum lactate levels; venous-arterial PO_2 gradient; serum methemoglobin and oxyhemoglobin. Pretreatment cyanide levels may be useful diagnostically.

Reference Range Symptoms associated with blood cyanide levels:
Flushing and tachycardia: 0.5-1 mcg/mL
Obtundation: 1-2.5 mcg/mL
Coma and respiratory depression: >2.5 mcg/mL
Death: >3 mcg/mL

Dosage Forms Excipient information presented when available (limited, particularly for generics); consult specific product labeling.
Liquid, for inhalation: USP: 85% to 103% (0.3 mL)

- ◆ **Amylobarbitone** *see* Amobarbital *on page* 136
- ◆ **Amytal® (Can)** *see* Amobarbital *on page* 136
- ◆ **Amytal Sodium** *see* Amobarbital *on page* 136
- ◆ **Anacaine** *see* Benzocaine *on page* 268
- ◆ **Anadrol-50** *see* Oxymetholone *on page* 1601
- ◆ **Anafranil** *see* ClomiPRAMINE *on page* 502
- ◆ **Anafranil® (Can)** *see* ClomiPRAMINE *on page* 502

Anagrelide (an AG gre lide)

Medication Safety Issues
Sound-alike/look-alike issues:
Anagrelide may be confused with anastrozole

Brand Names: US Agrylin

Brand Names: Canada Agrylin; Dom-Anagrelide; Mylan-Anagrelide; PMS-Anagrelide; Sandoz-Anagrelide

Therapeutic Category Antiplatelet Agent; Phosphodiesterase Enzyme Inhibitor; Phosphodiestrerase-3 Enzyme Inhibitor

Generic Availability (US) Yes

Use Treatment of thrombocythemia secondary to myeloproliferative disorders to decrease elevated platelet count and the associated risk of thrombosis and ameliorate symptoms including thrombo-hemorrhagic events (FDA approved in ages >6 years and adults)

Pregnancy Risk Factor C

Pregnancy Considerations Adverse events were observed in some animal reproduction studies. Data regarding use of anagrelide during pregnancy is limited. The manufacturer recommends effective contraception in women of childbearing potential.

Breast-Feeding Considerations It is not known if anagrelide is excreted in breast milk. Due to the potential for serious adverse reactions in the nursing infant, a decision should be made whether to discontinue nursing or to discontinue the drug, taking into account the importance of treatment to the mother.

Contraindications There are no contraindications listed in the manufacturer's labeling.

Warnings/Precautions Major hemorrhagic events have occurred when used concomitantly with aspirin. Monitor closely for bleeding, particularly when used concurrently with other agents known to increase bleeding risk (eg, anticoagulants, NSAIDs, antiplatelet agents, other phosphodiesterase 3 (PDE3) inhibitors, and selective serotonin reuptake inhibitors). Ventricular tachycardia and torsades de pointes have been reported. As with other PDE3 inhibitors, anagrelide may cause vasodilation, tachycardia, palpitations and heart failure. PDE3 inhibitors are associated with decreased survival (compared to placebo) in patients with class III or IV heart failure. Dose-related increases in heart rate and mean QTc interval have been observed in a clinical trial. The maximum change in mean heart rate was ~8 beats per minute (bpm) at a dose of 0.5 mg and ~29 bpm with a 2.5 mg dose. The maximum mean change in QTc I (individual subject correlation) from placebo was 7 ms and 13 ms with doses of 0.5 mg and 2.5 mg, respectively. Use is not recommended in patients with hypokalemia, congenital long QT syndrome, a known history of acquired QTc prolongation, or when using concomitant therapy which may prolong the QTc interval. Hypotension accompanied by dizziness may occur, particularly with higher doses. Use with caution in patients with cardiovascular disease (eg, heart failure, bradyarrhythmias, electrolyte abnormalities); consider periodic ECGs; benefits should outweigh risks. Pretreatment cardiovascular evaluation (including ECG) and careful monitoring during treatment is recommended. Interstitial lung disease (including allergic alveolitis, eosinophilic pneumonia, and interstitial pneumonitis) has been associated with use; onset is from 1 week to several years, usually presenting with progressive dyspnea with lung infiltrations; symptoms usually improve after discontinuation. Use caution in patients with mild to moderate hepatic dysfunction; dosage reduction and careful monitoring are required for moderate hepatic impairment; use has not been studied in patients with severe impairment. Hepatic impairment increases anagrelide exposure and may increase the risk of QTc prolongation. Monitor liver function prior to and during treatment. Renal abnormalities (including renal failure) have been observed with anagrelide use; may be associated with preexisting renal impairment, although dosage adjustment due to renal insufficiency was not required; monitor closely in patients with renal insufficiency. Potentially significant drug-drug interactions may exist, requiring dose or frequency adjustment, additional monitoring, and/or selection of alternative therapy.

Adverse Reactions

Cardiovascular: Angina pectoris, atrial fibrillation, cardiac arrhythmia, cardiac failure, cardiomegaly, cardiomyopathy, cerebrovascular accident, chest pain, complete atrioventricular block, decreased diastolic pressure (pediatric patients), edema, hypertension, increased heart rate (pediatric patients), myocardial infarction, orthostatic hypotension, palpitations, pericardial effusion, peripheral edema, syncope, systolic hypotension (pediatric patients), tachycardia, vasodilatation

Central nervous system: amnesia, chills, confusion, depression, dizziness, drowsiness, fatigue (pediatric patients), headache, insomnia, malaise, migraine, nervousness, pain, paresthesia

Dermatologic: Alopecia, pruritus, skin rash

Gastrointestinal: Abdominal pain, anorexia, constipation, diarrhea, dyspepsia, flatulence, gastritis, gastrointestinal hemorrhage, nausea, pancreatitis, vomiting

Hematologic & oncologic: Anemia, bruise, hemorrhage, thrombocytopenia

Hepatic: Increased liver enzymes

Neuromuscular & skeletal: Arthralgia, back pain, muscle cramps (pediatric patients), myalgia, weakness

Ophthalmic: Diplopia, visual field defect

Otic: Tinnitus

Renal: Hematuria, renal failure

Respiratory: cough, dyspnea, epistaxis, flu-like symptoms, pleural effusion, pneumonia, pulmonary fibrosis, pulmonary hypertension, pulmonary infiltrates

Miscellaneous: Fever

Rare but important or life-threatening: Eosinophilic pneumonitis, hepatotoxicity, hypersensitivity pneumonitis, interstitial nephritis, interstitial pneumonitis, leukocytosis, prolonged Q-T interval on ECG, skin photosensitivity (pediatric patients), torsades de pointes, ventricular tachycardia

Drug Interactions

Metabolism/Transport Effects None known.

Avoid Concomitant Use

Avoid concomitant use of Anagrelide with any of the following: Highest Risk QTc-Prolonging Agents; Ivabradine; Mifepristone; Moderate Risk QTc-Prolonging Agents; Urokinase

Increased Effect/Toxicity

Anagrelide may increase the levels/effects of: Agents with Antiplatelet Properties; Anticoagulants; Apixaban; Cilostazol; Collagenase (Systemic); Dabigatran Etexilate; Deoxycholic Acid; Highest Risk QTc-Prolonging Agents; Ibritumomab; Obinutuzumab; Riociguat; Rivaroxaban; Salicylates; Thrombolytic Agents; Tositumomab and Iodine I 131 Tositumomab; Urokinase

The levels/effects of Anagrelide may be increased by: Glucosamine; Herbs (Anticoagulant/Antiplatelet Properties); Ibrutinib; Ivabradine; Limaprost; MAO Inhibitors; Mifepristone; Moderate Risk QTc-Prolonging Agents; Multivitamins/Fluoride (with ADE); Multivitamins/Minerals (with ADEK, Folate, Iron); Multivitamins/Minerals (with AE, No Iron); Omega-3 Fatty Acids; Pentosan Polysulfate Sodium; Pentoxifylline; Prostacyclin Analogues; QTc-Prolonging Agents (Indeterminate Risk and Risk Modifying); Tipranavir; Vitamin E

Decreased Effect There are no known significant interactions involving a decrease in effect.

Storage/Stability Store at 25°C (77°F); excursions permitted to 15°C to 30°C (59°F to 86°F). Protect from light.

Mechanism of Action Anagrelide appears to inhibit cyclic nucleotide phosphodiesterase and the release of arachidonic acid from phospholipase, possibly by inhibiting phospholipase A_2. It also causes a dose-related reduction in platelet production, which results from decreased megakaryocyte hypermaturation (disrupts the postmitotic phase of maturation).

Pharmacodynamics

Onset of action: Initial: Within 7-14 days

Maximum effect: Complete response (platelets ≤600,000/mm^3): 4-12 weeks

Duration: 6-24 hours; upon discontinuation, platelet count begins to rise within 4 days

Pharmacokinetics (Adult data unless noted) Note: In pediatric patients 7-14 years; data has shown a decreased maximum serum concentration (48%) and AUC (55%) compared to adults when normalized to dose and bodyweight.

Metabolism: Hepatic, partially via CYP1A2; to two major metabolites, RL603 and 3-hydroxy anagrelide

Bioavailability: Food has no clinically significant effect

Half-life, elimination: 1.3 hours; similar data reported in pediatric patients 7-14 years

Time to peak, serum concentration: 1 hour; similar data reported in pediatric patients 7-14 years.

Elimination: Urine (<1% as unchanged drug)

Dosing: Usual

Pediatric:

Essential thrombocythemia: Very limited data available; several small case series: Children ≥6 years and Adolescents: Oral: Initial: 0.5 mg 2-3 times daily; increase at weekly intervals in 0.5 mg increments until platelet count begins to decrease; usual reported maintenance dose range: 1-2.5 mg/day; maximum daily dose: 10 mg/**day** (per manufacturer) although the maximum reported dose for essential thrombocythemia: 4 mg/**day**; once platelet count normalizes, further adjust dose to lowest effective dose; in some cases, discontinuation of therapy has been accomplished (Chintagumpala, 1995; Lackner, 1998; Lackner, 2006); **Note:** Essential thrombocytopenia is also considered a type myeloproliferative disorder.

Secondary thrombocythemia (associated with myeloproliferative disorders): Children >6 years and Adolescents: Oral: Initial: 0.5 mg once daily; usual range: 0.5 mg 1-4 times daily; median maintenance daily dose: Patient age 7-11 years: 1.75 mg/day; patient age: 11-14 years: 2 mg; **Note:** Maintain initial dose for ≥1 week, then adjust to the lowest effective dose to reduce and maintain platelet count <600,000/mm^3 ideally to the normal range; the dose must not be increased by >0.5 mg per day in any 1 week; maximum single dose: 2.5 mg; maximum daily dose: 10 mg/**day**

Adult: **Thrombocythemia:** Oral: Initial: 0.5 mg 4 times daily or 1 mg twice daily (most patients will experience adequate response at dose ranges of 1.5-3 mg/day); **Note:** Maintain initial dose for ≥1 week, then adjust to the lowest effective dose to reduce and maintain platelet count <600,000/mm^3 ideally to the normal range; the dose must not be increased by >0.5 mg per day in any 1 week; maximum single dose: 2.5 mg; maximum daily dose: 10 mg

Dosing adjustment in renal impairment: Children, Adolescents, and Adults: No adjustment required in renal insufficiency; monitor closely.

Dosing adjustment in hepatic impairment: Adults:

Moderate impairment: Initial: 0.5 mg once daily; maintain for at least 1 week with careful monitoring of cardiovascular status; the dose must not be increased by >0.5 mg/day in any 1 week

Severe impairment: Use is contraindicated

Administration May be administered without regard to food.

Monitoring Parameters Platelet count (every 2 days during the first week of treatment and at least weekly until the maintenance dose is reached; continue to monitor after cessation of treatment); CBC with differential (monitor closely during first 2 weeks of treatment), liver function (ALT and AST; baseline and during treatment), BUN, and serum creatinine (monitor closely during first weeks of treatment); serum electrolytes; blood pressure; heart rate; cardiovascular exam including ECG (pretreatment; monitor during therapy), signs/symptoms of interstitial lung disease. Monitor for thrombosis or bleeding.

Dosage Forms Excipient information presented when available (limited, particularly for generics); consult specific product labeling.

Capsule, Oral:

Agrylin: 0.5 mg

Generic: 0.5 mg, 1 mg

◆ **Anagrelide Hydrochloride** *see* Anagrelide *on page 163*

Anakinra (an a KIN ra)

Medication Safety Issues

Sound-alike/look-alike issues:

Anakinra may be confused with amikacin, Ampyra

Kineret may be confused with Amikin

High alert medication:

This medication is in a class the Institute for Safe Medication Practices (ISMP) includes among its list of drug classes that have a heightened risk of causing significant patient harm when used in error.

Brand Names: US Kineret

Brand Names: Canada Kineret

Therapeutic Category Antirheumatic, Disease Modifying; Interleukin-1 Receptor Antagonist

Generic Availability (US) No

Use Treatment of neonatal-onset multisystem inflammatory disease (NOMID), also known as chronic infantile neurological cutaneous and articular syndrome (CINCA), which is a cryopyrin-associated periodic syndrome (CAPS) [FDA approved in pediatric patients (age not specified) and adults]; treatment of moderately to severely active rheumatoid arthritis in patients who have failed one or more disease-modifying antirheumatic drugs (DMARDs); may be used alone or in combination with DMARDs that are not tumor necrosis factor (TNF)-blocking agents (eg, etanercept, adalimumab) (FDA approved in ages ≥18 years and adults); has also been used for reducing signs and symptoms of systemic juvenile idiopathic arthritic (SJIA) and polyarticular-course juvenile idiopathic arthritis (JIA)

Pregnancy Risk Factor B

Pregnancy Considerations Animal reproduction studies have not revealed any evidence of impaired fertility or harm to fetus. Women exposed to anakinra during pregnancy may contact the Organization of Teratology Information Services (OTIS), Rheumatoid Arthritis and Pregnancy Study at 1-877-311-8972.

Breast-Feeding Considerations Endogenous interleukin-1 receptor antagonist can be found in breast milk; although specific excretion of anakinra is not known. Use caution if administering to a nursing woman.

Contraindications Hypersensitivity to *E. coli*-derived proteins, anakinra, or any component of the formulation

Warnings/Precautions Anakinra is associated with an increased risk of infection in rheumatoid arthritis studies. Do not initiate in patients with an active infection. Patients who develop a new infection while undergoing treatment should be monitored closely. If a patient receiving anakinra for rheumatoid arthritis develops a serious infection, therapy should be discontinued; if a patient receiving anakinra for neonatal-onset multisystem inflammatory disease (NOMID) develop a serious infection, the risk of a NOMID flare should be weighed against the risks associated with continued treatment. Safety and efficacy have not been evaluated in immunosuppressed patients or patients with chronic infections; the impact on active or chronic infections has not been determined. Immunosuppressive therapy (including anakinra) may lead to reactivation of latent tuberculosis or other atypical or opportunistic infections; test patients for latent TB prior to initiation, and treat latent TB infection prior to use.

A decrease in neutrophil count may occur during treatment; assess neutrophil count at baseline, monthly for 3 months, then every 3 months for up to 1 year; in a limited number of patients with NOMID, neutropenia resolved over time with continued anakinra administration. May affect defenses against malignancies; impact on the development and course of malignancies is not fully defined; as compared to the general population, an increased risk of lymphoma has been noted in clinical trials; however, rheumatoid arthritis has been previously associated with an increased rate of lymphoma.

Potentially significant drug-drug interactions may exist, requiring dose or frequency adjustment, additional monitoring, and/or selection of alternative therapy. Use is not recommended in combination with tumor necrosis factor antagonists. Patients should be brought up to date with all immunizations before initiating therapy; live vaccines should not be given concurrently; there is no data available concerning the effects of therapy on vaccination or secondary transmission of live vaccines in patients receiving therapy. Hypersensitivity reactions, including anaphylactic reactions and angioedema have been reported; discontinue use if severe hypersensitivity occurs. Injection site reactions commonly occur and are generally mild with a duration of 14-28 days. Use caution in patients with renal impairment; extended dosing intervals (every other day) are recommended for severe renal insufficiency (CrCl <30 mL/minute) and ESRD. Use with caution in patients with asthma; may have increased risk of serious infection. Use caution in the elderly due to the potential for higher risk of infections. The packaging (needle cover) contains latex.

Some dosage forms may contain polysorbate 80 (also known as Tweens). Hypersensitivity reactions, usually a delayed reaction, have been reported following exposure to pharmaceutical products containing polysorbate 80 in certain individuals (Isaksson, 2002; Lucente 2000; Shelley, 1995). Thrombocytopenia, ascites, pulmonary deterioration, and renal and hepatic failure have been reported in premature neonates after receiving parenteral products containing polysorbate 80 (Alade, 1986; CDC, 1984). See manufacturer's labeling.

Adverse Reactions

Central nervous system: Fever, headache

Gastrointestinal: Diarrhea, nausea

Hematologic: Neutropenia

Local: Injection site reaction

Neuromuscular & skeletal: Arthralgia

Respiratory: Nasopharyngitis

Miscellaneous: Infection (including serious)

Rare but important or life-threatening: Cellulitis, hepatitis (noninfectious), hypersensitivity reactions (including anaphylaxis, angioedema, pruritus, rash, urticaria), increased serum transaminases, leukopenia, opportunistic infection, pneumonia (bacterial), pulmonary fibrosis, secondary malignancies (including lymphoma, melanoma), thrombocytopenia

Drug Interactions

Metabolism/Transport Effects None known.

Avoid Concomitant Use

Avoid concomitant use of Anakinra with any of the following: Abatacept; Anti-TNF Agents; BCG; BCG (Intravesical); Canakinumab; Natalizumab; Pimecrolimus; Tacrolimus (Topical); Tofacitinib; Vaccines (Live)

Increased Effect/Toxicity

Anakinra may increase the levels/effects of: Abatacept; Canakinumab; Leflunomide; Natalizumab; Tofacitinib; Vaccines (Live)

The levels/effects of Anakinra may be increased by: Anti-TNF Agents; Denosumab; Pimecrolimus; Roflumilast; Tacrolimus (Topical); Trastuzumab

Decreased Effect

Anakinra may decrease the levels/effects of: BCG; BCG (Intravesical); Coccidioides immitis Skin Test; Sipuleucel-T; Vaccines (Inactivated); Vaccines (Live)

The levels/effects of Anakinra may be decreased by: Echinacea

Storage/Stability Store in refrigerator at 2°C to 8°C (36°F to 46°F); do not freeze. Do not shake. Protect from light.

Mechanism of Action Antagonist of the interleukin-1 (IL-1) receptor. Endogenous IL-1 is induced by inflammatory stimuli and mediates a variety of immunological responses, including degradation of cartilage (loss of proteoglycans) and stimulation of bone resorption.

Pharmacokinetics (Adult data unless noted)

Bioavailability: SubQ: 95%

Half-life elimination: Terminal: 4-6 hours; severe renal impairment (CrCl <30 mL/minute): ~7 hours; ESRD: 9.7 hours (Yang, 2003)

Time to peak serum concentration: SubQ: 3-7 hours

Dosing: Usual

Pediatric:

Neonatal-onset multisystem inflammatory disease (NOMID) or chronic infantile neurological, cutaneous, and articular syndrome (CINCA) [cryopyrin-associated periodic syndromes (CAPS)]: Infants, Children, and Adolescents: SubQ: Initial: 1-2 mg/kg/day in 1-2 divided doses; adjust dose in 0.5-1 mg/kg increments as needed to control inflammation; usual maintenance dose: 3-4 mg/kg/day; maximum daily dose: 8 mg/kg/**day**. **Note:** Once-daily administration is preferred; however, the dose may also be divided and administered twice daily.

Juvenile idiopathic arthritis (JIA): Limited data available: SubQ:

Systemic-onset JIA (SOJIA): Children and Adolescents: Initial: 1-2 mg/kg/dose once daily; maximum initial dose: 100 mg; if no response, may titrate typically at 2-week intervals by doubling dose up to 4 mg/kg/dose once daily; maximum dose: 200 mg (Dewitt, 2012; Gattorno, 2006; Hedrich, 2012; Irigoyen, 2006; Lequerré, 2008; Nigrovi, 2011; Quartier, 2011)

Polyarticular course JIA: Children ≥2 years and Adolescents: 1 mg/kg once daily; maximum dose: 100 mg (Ilowite, 2009; Reiff, 2005)

Rheumatoid arthritis: Adolescents ≥18 years: SubQ: 100 mg once daily; administer at approximately the same time each day

Adult:

Neonatal-onset multisystem inflammatory disease (NOMID) or chronic infantile neurological, cutaneous, and articular syndrome (CINCA) [cryopyrin-associated periodic syndromes (CAPS)]: SubQ: Initial: 1-2 mg/kg daily in 1-2 divided doses; adjust dose in 0.5-1 mg/kg increments as needed; usual maintenance dose: 3-4 mg/kg daily; maximum daily dose: 8 mg/kg/**day**. **Note:** The prefilled syringe does not allow doses lower than 20 mg to be administered.

Rheumatoid arthritis: SubQ: 100 mg once daily; administer at approximately the same time each day

Dosing adjustment in renal impairment:

CrCl ≥30 mL/minute: No dosage adjustment necessary

CrCl <30 mL/minute:

NOMID: Infants, Children, Adolescents, and Adults: Decrease frequency of administration to every other day

Rheumatoid arthritis: Adolescents ≥18 years and Adults: Consider 100 mg every other day

ESRD: <2.5% of the dose is removed by hemodialysis or CAPD:

NOMID: Infants, Children, Adolescents, and Adults: Decrease frequency of administration to every other day

Rheumatoid arthritis: Adolescents ≥18 years and Adults: 100 mg every other day

Dosing adjustment in hepatic impairment: There are no dosage adjustments provided in the manufacturer's labeling (has not been studied).

Administration SubQ: Rotate injection sites: Outer area of upper arms, abdomen (do not use within 2 inches of belly button), front of middle thighs, or upper outer buttocks; injection should be given at least 1 inch away from previous injection site. Allow solution to warm to room temperature prior to use (30 minutes). Do not shake. Provided in single-use, preservative-free syringes with 27-gauge needles; discard any unused portion.

Monitoring Parameters CBC with differential (baseline, then monthly for 3 months, then every 3 months for a period up to 1 year); serum creatinine

Juvenile idiopathic arthritis: PPD screening (baseline and annually); CBC with differential and platelets, C-reactive protein, ESR, ferritin, and LDH [baseline, at follow-up visits (1-2 weeks, 1, 2, 6, and 9 months)] and with any treatment change (DeWitt, 2012)

Additional Information Anakinra is produced by recombinant DNA/*E. coli* technology.

Dosage Forms Excipient information presented when available (limited, particularly for generics); consult specific product labeling.

Solution Prefilled Syringe, Subcutaneous [preservative free]:

Kineret: 100 mg/0.67 mL (0.67 mL) [contains disodium edta, polysorbate 80]

- **Anapen (Can)** *see* EPINEPHrine (Systemic, Oral Inhalation) *on page 760*
- **Anapen Junior (Can)** *see* EPINEPHrine (Systemic, Oral Inhalation) *on page 760*
- **Anaprox** *see* Naproxen *on page 1489*
- **Anaprox DS** *see* Naproxen *on page 1489*
- **Anascorp** *see Centruroides* Immune F(ab')$_2$ (Equine) *on page 421*
- **Anaspaz** *see* Hyoscyamine *on page 1061*
- **Anbesol [OTC]** *see* Benzocaine *on page 268*
- **Anbesol® Baby (Can)** *see* Benzocaine *on page 268*
- **Anbesol Cold Sore Therapy [OTC]** *see* Benzocaine *on page 268*
- **Anbesol JR [OTC]** *see* Benzocaine *on page 268*
- **Anbesol Maximum Strength [OTC]** *see* Benzocaine *on page 268*
- **Ancef** *see* CeFAZolin *on page 388*
- **Anchoic Acid** *see* Azelaic Acid *on page 238*
- **Ancobon** *see* Flucytosine *on page 886*
- **Andriol (Can)** *see* Testosterone *on page 2025*
- **Androderm** *see* Testosterone *on page 2025*
- **AndroGel** *see* Testosterone *on page 2025*
- **AndroGel Pump** *see* Testosterone *on page 2025*
- **Andropository (Can)** *see* Testosterone *on page 2025*
- **Androxy [DSC]** *see* Fluoxymesterone *on page 910*
- **AneCream [OTC]** *see* Lidocaine (Topical) *on page 1258*
- **AneCream5 [OTC]** *see* Lidocaine (Topical) *on page 1258*
- **Anectine** *see* Succinylcholine *on page 1976*
- **Aneurine Hydrochloride** *see* Thiamine *on page 2048*
- **Anexate (Can)** *see* Flumazenil *on page 892*

- ◆ **Anhydrous Glucose** *see* Dextrose *on page 633*
- ◆ **Ansaid (Can)** *see* Flurbiprofen (Systemic) *on page 915*
- ◆ **Ansamycin** *see* Rifabutin *on page 1857*
- ◆ **Antacid [OTC]** *see* Calcium Carbonate *on page 343*
- ◆ **Antacid Calcium [OTC]** *see* Calcium Carbonate *on page 343*
- ◆ **Antacid Calcium Extra Strength [OTC]** *see* Calcium Carbonate *on page 343*
- ◆ **Antacid Extra Strength [OTC]** *see* Calcium Carbonate *on page 343*
- ◆ **Anti-D Immunoglobulin** *see* Rh_o(D) Immune Globulin *on page 1847*
- ◆ **Anti-CD20 Monoclonal Antibody** *see* RiTUXimab *on page 1875*
- ◆ **Anti-Dandruff [OTC]** *see* Selenium Sulfide *on page 1913*
- ◆ **Anti-Diarrheal [OTC]** *see* Loperamide *on page 1288*
- ◆ **Antidigoxin Fab Fragments, Ovine** *see* Digoxin Immune Fab *on page 657*
- ◆ **Antidiuretic Hormone** *see* Vasopressin *on page 2161*
- ◆ **Antifungal [OTC]** *see* Miconazole (Topical) *on page 1431*
- ◆ **Anti-Fungal [OTC]** *see* Tolnaftate *on page 2083*

Antihemophilic Factor (Human)

(an tee hee moe FIL ik FAK tor HYU man)

Medication Safety Issues

Sound-alike/look-alike issues:

Factor VIII may be confused with Factor XIII

Other safety concerns:

Confusion may occur due to the omitting of "Factor VIII" from some product labeling. Review product contents carefully prior to dispensing any antihemophilic factor.

Brand Names: US Hemofil M; Koate-DVI; Monoclate-P

Brand Names: Canada Hemofil M

Therapeutic Category Antihemophilic Agent; Blood Product Derivative

Generic Availability (US) No

Use Prevention and treatment of hemorrhagic episodes in patients with hemophilia A (classical hemophilia); perioperative management of patients with hemophilia A; can provide therapeutic effects in patients with acquired factor VIII inhibitors <10 Bethesda units/mL

Pregnancy Risk Factor C

Pregnancy Considerations Animal reproduction studies have not been conducted. Parvovirus B19 or hepatitis A, which may be present in plasma-derived products, may affect a pregnant woman more seriously than nonpregnant women.

Breast-Feeding Considerations It is not known if this product is excreted into breast milk.

Contraindications

Hemofil M and Monoclate-P: Hypersensitivity to any component of the formulation or mouse proteins

Koate-DVI: There are no contraindications listed in the manufacturer's labeling.

Warnings/Precautions Risk of viral transmission is not totally eradicated. Because antihemophilic factor is prepared from pooled plasma, it may contain the causative agent of viral hepatitis and other viral diseases. Hepatitis B vaccination is recommended for all patients. Hepatitis A vaccination is also recommended for seronegative patients. Antihemophilic factor contains trace amounts of blood groups A and B isohemagglutinins and when large or frequently repeated doses are given to individuals with blood groups A, B, and AB, the patient should be monitored for signs of progressive anemia and the possibility of intravascular hemolysis should be considered. Dosage requirements will vary in patients with factor VIII inhibitors; optimal treatment should be determined by clinical response. Frequency of use is determined by the severity of the disorder or bleeding pattern. Natural rubber latex is a component of Koate-DVI and Hemofil M packaging. Hemofil M and Monoclate-P contain trace amounts of mouse protein; use is contraindicated in patients with hypersensitivity to mouse protein. Some dosage forms may contain polysorbate 80 (also known as Tweens). Hypersensitivity reactions, usually a delayed reaction, have been reported following exposure to pharmaceutical products containing polysorbate 80 in certain individuals (Isaksson 2002; Lucente 2000; Shelley, 1995). Thrombocytopenia, ascites, pulmonary deterioration, and renal and hepatic failure have been reported in premature neonates after receiving parenteral products containing polysorbate 80 (Alade, 1986; CDC, 1984). See manufacturer's labeling. Products contain naturally occurring von Willebrand factor for stabilization, however efficacy has not been established for the treatment of von Willebrand disease. Products vary by preparation method; final formulations contain human albumin.

Warnings: Additional Pediatric Considerations Formation of factor VIII inhibitors (neutralizing antibodies to AHF human) may occur; reported incidence is 3% to 52%; an increase of inhibitor antibody concentration is seen at 2 to 7 days, with peak concentrations at 1 to 3 weeks after therapy; children <5 years of age are at greatest risk; higher doses of AHF may be needed if antibody is present; if antibody concentration is >10 Bethesda units/mL, patients may not respond to larger doses and alternative treatment modalities may be needed; monitor patients appropriately. Allergic-type hypersensitivity reactions, including anaphylaxis, may occur; discontinue therapy immediately if urticaria, hives, hypotension, tightness of the chest, wheezing, dyspnea, faintness, or anaphylaxis develop; emergency treatment and resuscitative measures (eg, epinephrine, oxygen) may be needed.

Adverse Reactions Rare but important or life-threatening: Acute hemolytic anemia, AHF inhibitor development, allergic reactions (rare), anaphylaxis (rare), bleeding tendency increased, blurred vision, chest tightness, chills, fever, headache, hyperfibrinogenemia, jittery feeling, lethargy, nausea, somnolence, stinging at the infusion site, stomach discomfort, tingling, urticaria, vasomotor reactions with rapid infusion, vomiting

Drug Interactions

Metabolism/Transport Effects None known.

Avoid Concomitant Use There are no known interactions where it is recommended to avoid concomitant use.

Increased Effect/Toxicity There are no known significant interactions involving an increase in effect.

Decreased Effect There are no known significant interactions involving a decrease in effect.

Storage/Stability Store under refrigeration, 2°C to 8°C (36°F to 46°F); avoid freezing. Use within 3 hours of reconstitution. Do not refrigerate after reconstitution, precipitation may occur.

Hemofil M: May also be stored at room temperature not to exceed 30°C (86°F).

Koate-DVI; Monoclate-P: May also be stored at room temperature of 25°C (77°F) for ≤6 months.

Mechanism of Action Protein (factor VIII) in normal plasma which is necessary for clot formation and maintenance of hemostasis; activates factor X in conjunction with activated factor IX; activated factor X converts prothrombin to thrombin, which converts fibrinogen to fibrin, and with factor XIII forms a stable clot

Pharmacodynamics Maximum effect: 1-2 hours

Pharmacokinetics (Adult data unless noted)

Distribution: Does not readily cross the placenta

Half-life: 4-24 hours; mean=12 hours (biphasic)

Dosing: Usual Children and Adults: IV: Individualize dosage based on coagulation studies performed prior to and during treatment at regular intervals:

Hemophilia A: For every 1 international unit per kg body weight of AHF (human) administered, factor VIII level should increase by 2%; calculated dosage should be adjusted to the actual vial size

Formula to calculate dosage required, based on desired increase in factor VIII (% of normal) (**Note:** This formula assumes that the patient's baseline AHF level is <1%): Units required = Body weight (kg) x 0.5 x desired increase in factor VIII (units/dL or % of normal)

Hospitalized patients: 20-50 units/kg/dose; may be higher for special circumstances. Dose can be given every 12-24 hours and more frequently in special circumstances.

Hemophilia A with high titer of inhibitor antibody: 50-75 units/kg/hour has been given

General dosing guidelines (consult individual product labeling for specific dosage recommendations):

Minor hemorrhage (required peak postinfusion AHF level: 20% to 40%): 10-20 units/kg; repeat every 12-24 hours for 1-3 days until bleeding is resolved or healing achieved; mild superficial or early hemorrhages may respond to a single dose

Moderate hemorrhage (required peak postinfusion AHF level: 30% to 60%): 15-30 units/kg; repeat every 12-24 hours for ≥3 days until pain and disability are resolved

Alternatively (to achieve peak postinfusion AHF level: 50%) Initial: 25 units/kg; maintenance: 10-15 units/kg every 8-12 hours

Severe/life-threatening hemorrhage (required peak postinfusion AHF level: 60% to 100%): 30-50 units/kg; repeat every 8-24 hours until threat is resolved

Alternatively (to achieve peak postinfusion AHF level: 80% to 100%): 40-50 units/kg; maintenance: 20-25 units/kg every 8-12 hours

Minor surgery (required peak postinfusion AHF level: Range 30% to 80%): 15-40 units/kg; dose is highly dependent upon procedure and specific product recommendations; for some procedures, a single dose plus oral antifibrinolytic therapy within 1 hour is sufficient; in other procedures, may repeat dose every 12-24 hours as needed

Major surgery (required peak pre- and postsurgery AHF level: 80% to 100%): 40-50 units/kg; repeat every 8-24 hours depending on state of healing

Prophylaxis: May also be given on a regular schedule to prevent bleeding

Preparation for Administration Parenteral: If refrigerated, the dried concentrate and diluent should be warmed to room temperature before reconstitution; see individual product labeling for specific reconstitution guidelines. Gently swirl or rotate vial after adding diluent; do not shake vigorously (**Note:** For Koate-DVI: Swirl vigorously without creating excessive foaming); use filter needle provided by manufacturer to draw product into syringe; use one filter needle per vial; do **not** refrigerate after reconstitution (precipitation may occur); administer within 3 hours after reconstitution; **Note:** Use plastic syringes, since AHF may stick to the surface of glass syringes.

Administration Parenteral: IV administration only. Administer through a separate line, do not mix with drugs or other IV fluids. Maximum rate of administration is product dependent:

Hemofil M: 10 mL/minute

Monoclate-P: 2 mL/minute

Koate-DVI: Total dose may be given over 5 to 10 minutes; adjust administration rate based on patient response

Monitoring Parameters Bleeding; heart rate and blood pressure (before and during IV administration); AHF levels prior to and during treatment; monitor for development of inhibitor antibodies by clinical observation (eg, inadequate control of bleeding with adequate doses) and laboratory tests (eg, inhibitor level, Bethesda assay). In patients with blood groups A, B, or AB who receive large or frequent doses, monitor Hct, direct Coombs' test, and signs of intravascular hemolysis

Reference Range

Plasma antihemophilic factor level:

Normal range: 50% to 150%

Level to prevent spontaneous hemorrhage: 5%

Required peak postinfusion AHF activity in blood (as % of normal or units/dL plasma):

Early hemarthrosis, muscle bleed, or oral bleed: 20% to 40%

More extensive hemarthrosis, muscle bleed, or hematoma: 30% to 60%

Life-threatening bleeds (such as head injury, throat bleed, severe abdominal pain): 80% to 100%

Minor surgery, including tooth extraction: 60% to 80%

Major surgery: 80% to 100% (pre- and postoperative)

Additional Information One unit of AHF is equal to the factor VIII activity present in 1 mL of normal human plasma. If bleeding is not controlled with adequate dose, test for the presence of factor VIII inhibitor; larger doses of AHF may be therapeutic with inhibitor titers <10 Bethesda units/mL; it may not be possible or practical to control bleeding if inhibitor titers >10 Bethesda units/mL (due to the very large AHF doses required); other treatments [eg, antihemophilic factor (porcine), factor IX complex concentrates, recombinant factor VIIa, or anti-inhibitor coagulant complex] may be needed in patients with inhibitor titers >10 Bethesda units/mL.

Dosage Forms Considerations

Strengths expressed with approximate values. Consult individual vial labels for exact potency within each vial.

Hemofil M packaged contents may contain natural rubber latex.

Dosage Forms Excipient information presented when available (limited, particularly for generics); consult specific product labeling. [DSC] = Discontinued product

Kit, Intravenous:

Monoclate-P: ~250 units, ~500 units, ~1000 units, ~1500 units [contains mouse protein (murine) (hamster)]

Solution Reconstituted, Intravenous:

Koate-DVI: ~500 units (1 ea) [contains albumin human, polyethylene glycol, polysorbate 80]

Solution Reconstituted, Intravenous [preservative free]:

Hemofil M: ~250 units (1 ea) [contains albumin human, mouse protein (murine) (hamster), polyethylene glycol]

Hemofil M: ~250 units (1 ea) [contains mouse protein (murine) (hamster), polyethylene glycol]

Hemofil M: ~500 units (1 ea) [contains albumin human, mouse protein (murine) (hamster), polyethylene glycol]

Hemofil M: ~500 units (1 ea) [contains mouse protein (murine) (hamster), polyethylene glycol]

Hemofil M: ~1000 units (1 ea); ~1700 units (1 ea) [contains albumin human, mouse protein (murine) (hamster), polyethylene glycol]

Koate-DVI: ~250 units (1 ea); ~500 units (1 ea [DSC]); ~1000 units (1 ea) [contains albumin human, polyethylene glycol, polysorbate 80]

Antihemophilic Factor (Recombinant)

(an tee hee moe FIL ik FAK tor ree KOM be nant)

Medication Safety Issues

Sound-alike/look-alike issues:

Factor VIII may be confused with Factor XIII

Other safety concerns:

Confusion may occur due to the omitting of "Factor VIII" from some product labeling. Review product contents carefully prior to dispensing any antihemophilic factor.

Brand Names: US Advate; Eloctate; Helixate FS; Kogenate FS; Kogenate FS Bio-Set; Novoeight; Recombinate; Xyntha; Xyntha Solofuse

Brand Names: Canada Advate; Helixate FS; Kogenate FS; Xyntha; Xyntha Solofuse

Therapeutic Category Antihemophilic Agent

Generic Availability (US) No

Use Note: Antihemophilic Factor (Recombinant) is not indicated for the treatment of von Willebrand disease.

Advate: Prevention and control of hemorrhagic episodes in patients with hemophilia A; perioperative management of patients with hemophilia A; routine prophylaxis to prevent or reduce the frequency of bleeding episodes in patients with hemophilia A (All indications: FDA approved in ages 0-16 years and adults)

Helixate FS, Kogenate FS: Prevention and control of hemorrhagic episodes in patients with hemophilia A; perioperative management of patients with hemophilia A; routine prophylaxis to reduce the frequency of bleeding episodes and reduce the risk of joint damage in children with hemophilia A with no pre-existing joint damage (All indications: FDA approved in ages 0-16 years)

Recombinate: Prevention and control of hemorrhagic episodes in patients with hemophilia A (FDA approved in all ages); perioperative management of patients with hemophilia A (FDA approved in all ages)

Xyntha: Prevention and control of hemorrhagic episodes in patients with hemophilia A (FDA approved in ages ≥12 years and adults); perioperative management of patients with hemophilia A (FDA approved in ages ≥12 years and adults)

Has also been used in patients with acquired factor VIII inhibitors <10 Bethesda units/mL

Pregnancy Risk Factor C

Pregnancy Considerations Animal reproduction studies have not been conducted.

Breast-Feeding Considerations It is not known if antihemophilic factor (recombinant) is excreted in breast milk. The manufacturer recommends that caution be exercised when administering antihemophilic factor (recombinant) to nursing women.

Contraindications Hypersensitivity (eg, anaphylaxis) to antihemophilic factor, mouse or hamster protein (Advate, Helixate FS, Novoeight, Kogenate FS, Recombinate, Xyntha), bovine protein (Recombinate only), or any component of the formulation

Warnings/Precautions Monitor for signs of formation of antibodies to factor VIII; may occur at any time but more common in young children with severe hemophilia. The dosage requirement will vary in patients with factor VIII inhibitors; optimal treatment should be determined by clinical response. Allergic hypersensitivity reactions (including anaphylaxis) may occur; discontinue if hypersensitivity symptoms occur and administer appropriate treatment. Products vary by preparation method. Recombinate is stabilized using human albumin. Eloctate, Helixate FS, Kogenate FS, and Xyntha are stabilized with sucrose. Advate, Helixate FS, Kogenate FS, Novoeight, and Xyntha may contain trace amounts of mouse or hamster protein. Some dosage forms may contain polysorbate 80 (also known as Tweens). Hypersensitivity reactions, usually a delayed reaction, have been reported following exposure to pharmaceutical products containing polysorbate 80 in certain individuals (Isaksson, 2002; Lucente 2000; Shelley, 1995). Thrombocytopenia, ascites, pulmonary deterioration, and renal and hepatic failure have been reported in premature neonates after receiving parenteral products containing polysorbate 80 (Alade, 1986; CDC, 1984). See manufacturer's labeling. Recombinate may contain mouse, hamster or bovine protein. Products may contain von Willebrand factor for stabilization; however, efficacy has not been established for the treatment of von Willebrand's disease.

Warnings: Additional Pediatric Considerations Allergic-type hypersensitivity reactions including anaphylaxis may occur; discontinue therapy immediately if urticaria, hives, hypotension, tightness of the chest, wheezing, or anaphylaxis develop; emergency treatment and resuscitative measures (eg, epinephrine, oxygen) may be needed. Clinical response to antihemophilic factor administration may vary; dosage must be individualized based on coagulation studies (performed prior to treatment and at regular intervals during treatment) and clinical response. If bleeding is not controlled with the recommended dose, determine plasma level of factor VIII and follow with a sufficient dose to achieve satisfactory clinical response. If plasma levels of factor VIII fail to increase as expected or bleeding continues, suspect the presence of an inhibitor; test as appropriate. Formation of factor VIII inhibitors (neutralizing antibodies to AHF recombinant) may occur at any time, but is more common in young children with severe hemophilia during the first years of therapy, or in patients at any age who received little prior therapy with factor VIII; monitor patients appropriately.

Adverse Reactions

Central nervous system: Chills, headache, malaise, pain, procedural pain (including angiopathy)

Dermatologic: Pruritus, skin rash, urticaria

Gastrointestinal: Diarrhea, nausea, vomiting

Hematologic & oncologic: Increased factor VIII inhibitors

Local: Catheter infection, injection site reaction

Neuromuscular & skeletal: Arthralgia, weakness

Otic: Otic infection

Respiratory: Cough, nasal congestion, nasopharyngitis, pharyngolaryngeal pain, rhinorrhea, upper respiratory tract infection

Miscellaneous: Fever (3% to 43%), limb injury (10%)

Rare but important or life-threatening: Anorexia, catheter complication (venous catheter access), chest pain, cyanosis, hematoma, hypersensitivity reaction, hypertension, hypotension, loss of consciousness, maculopapular rash, tachycardia, vasodilatation

Drug Interactions

Metabolism/Transport Effects None known.

Avoid Concomitant Use There are no known interactions where it is recommended to avoid concomitant use.

Increased Effect/Toxicity There are no known significant interactions involving an increase in effect.

Decreased Effect There are no known significant interactions involving a decrease in effect.

Storage/Stability Prior to reconstitution, store refrigerated at 2°C to 8°C (36°F to 46°F); do not freeze. Do not refrigerate after reconstitution.

Advate/Eloctate: May also be stored at room temperature for up to 6 months; do not return to refrigerator. Use within 3 hours of reconstitution.

Helixate FS: May also be stored at room temperature (not to exceed 25°C [77°F]) up to 12 months; do not return to refrigerator. Protect from extreme exposure to light during storage. Use within 3 hours of reconstitution.

Kogenate FS: May also be stored at room temperature (not to exceed 25°C [77°F]) up to 12 months; do not return to refrigerator. Protect from extreme exposure to light during storage. Use within 3 hours of reconstitution.

Novoeight: May also be stored at room temperature (not to exceed 30°C [86°F]) up to 12 months; do not return to refrigerator; after 12 months at room temperature, use immediately or discard. Store in original package to protect from light. Use within 4 hours of reconstitution.

Recombinate: May also be stored at room temperature, not to exceed 30°C (86°F). Use within 3 hours of reconstitution.

Xyntha: May also be stored at room temperature (not to exceed 25°C [77°F]) up to 3 months; after room temperature storage, product may be returned to the refrigerator until the expiration date; however, do not store at room temperature and return to refrigerator temperature more than once. Avoid prolonged exposure to light during storage. Use within 3 hours of reconstitution.

Xyntha Solofuse: May also be stored at room temperature not to exceed 25°C [77°F]) up to 3 months; do not return to refrigerator; after 3 months at room temperature, must use immediately or discard. Use within 3 hours of reconstitution.

Mechanism of Action Factor VIII replacement, necessary for clot formation and maintenance of hemostasis. It activates factor X in conjunction with activated factor IX; activated factor X converts prothrombin to thrombin, which converts fibrinogen to fibrin, and with factor XIII forms a stable clot.

Pharmacokinetics (Adult data unless noted) Half-life:

Children 4-18 years of age (mean age: 12 years): 10.7 hours (range: 7.8-15.3)

Adults: 11-15 hours

Dosing: Neonatal

Individualize dosage based on coagulation studies performed prior to treatment and at regular intervals during treatment; for every 1 international unit per kg body weight of rAHF administered, factor VIII level should increase by 2% (or 2 units/dL); calculated dosage should be adjusted to the actual vial size

Control or prevention of bleeding in patients with factor VIII deficiency (hemophilia A): IV: Dosage is expressed in units of factor VIII activity (ie, international units) and must be individualized based on formulation, severity of factor VIII deficiency, extent and location of bleed, and clinical situation of patient.

Formula for units required to raise blood level:

Number of Factor VIII Units required = body weight (in kg) x 0.5 units/kg per units/dL x desired factor VIII level increase (units/dL or %)

For example, for a desired 100% level in a 3 kg patient who has an actual level of 20%: Number of Factor VIII Units needed = 3 kg x 80% x 0.5 units/kg per units/dL = 120 units

Manufacturer's labeling: Advate, Helixate FS, Kogenate FS, Recombinate: Desired Factor VIII level, dosing interval, and duration based on hemorrhage type: IV:

Minor hemorrhage (early joint hemorrhage, mild muscle or oral bleed): 10-20 units/kg/dose

Desired factor VIII levels (% or units/dL): 20-40

Frequency of dosing: Every 8-24 hours

Duration of treatment: 1-3 days until bleeding is resolved or healing achieved; mild, superficial, or early hemorrhages may respond to a single dose

Moderate hemorrhage (intramuscular bleed, hematoma, moderate bleeding into oral cavity, definite joint bleed, and known trauma): 15-30 units/kg/dose

Desired factor VIII levels (% or units/dL): 30-60

Frequency of dosing: Every 8-24 hours

Duration of treatment: ≥3 days until bleeding, pain, and disability are resolved or healing is achieved

Severe/life-threatening hemorrhage (GI, intracranial, intra-abdominal, intrathoracic bleeding, retroperitoneal, retropharyngeal, illiopsoas, CNS bleeding or head trauma, fractures):

Helixate FS, Kogenate FS: Initial: 40-50 units/kg; maintenance: 20-25 units/kg/dose

Desired factor VIII levels (% or units/dL): 80-100

Frequency of dosing: Every 8-12 hours

Duration of treatment: Until bleeding is resolved (duration not specified)

Advate, Recombinate: 30-50 units/kg/dose

Desired factor VIII levels (% or units/dL): 60-100

Frequency of dosing: Every 6-12 hours (Advate) or every 8-24 hours (Recombinate)

Duration of treatment: Until bleeding is resolved (duration not specified)

Perioperative management: IV:

Minor surgery (including dental extractions):

Advate: 30-50 units/kg as bolus infusion beginning within 1 hour prior to surgery; for dental procedures, adjunctive therapy may be considered

Desired factor VIII levels (% or units/dL): 60-100

Frequency of dosing: Every 12-24 hours as needed to control bleeding

Duration of treatment: Until bleeding is resolved (duration not specified)

Helixate FS, Kogenate FS: 15-30 units/kg/dose

Desired factor VIII levels (% or units/dL): 30-60

Frequency of dosing: Every 12-24 hours

Duration of treatment: Until bleeding is resolved (duration not specified)

Recombinate:

Desired factor VIII levels (% or units/dL): 60-80

Frequency of dosing: Single dose plus oral antifibrinolytic therapy within 1 hour is sufficient for most cases

Major surgery (tonsillectomy, hernia repair, intracranial, intra-abdominal, or intrathoracic surgery; joint replacement, trauma):

Advate: 40-60 units/kg/dose

Desired factor VIII levels (% or units/dL): Pre- and postoperative levels: 80-120; verify 100% activity has been achieved prior to surgery

Frequency of dosing: Every 6-24 hours as needed

Duration of treatment: Based on desired level and state of healing

Helixate FS, Kogenate FS: 50 units/kg/dose

Desired factor VIII levels (% or units/dL): Pre- and postoperative levels: 100; verify 100% activity has been achieved prior to surgery

Frequency of dosing: Every 6-12 hours as needed

Duration of treatment: Until healing is complete (~10-14 days)

Recombinate:

Desired factor VIII levels (% or units/dL): Pre- and postoerative: 80-100

Frequency of dosing: Every 8-24 hours depending on state of healing

Routine prophylaxis: IV:

Advate: 20-40 units/kg/dose every other day (3-4 times weekly). Alternatively, an every-third-day dosing regimen may be used to target factor VIII trough levels of ≥1%

Helixate FS, Kogenate FS: **Note:** For use in patients with no pre-existing joint damage: 25 units/kg/dose given every other day.

Dosing: Usual

Pediatric:

Individualize dosage based on coagulation studies performed prior to treatment and at regular intervals during treatment; for every 1 international unit per kg body weight of rAHF administered, factor VIII level should increase by 2% (or 2 units/dL); calculated dosage should be adjusted to the actual vial size

Control or prevention of bleeding in patients with factor VIII deficiency (hemophilia A): IV: Infants, Children, and Adolescents: Dosage is expressed in units of factor VIII activity (ie, international units) and must be individualized based on formulation, severity of factor VIII deficiency, extent and location of bleed, and clinical situation of patient.

Formula for units required to raise blood level:
Number of Factor VIII Units required = body weight (in kg) x 0.5 units/kg per units/dL x desired VIII level increase (units/dL or %)
For example, for a desired 100% level in a 25 kg patient who has an actual level of 20%: Number of Factor VIII Units needed = 25 kg x 80% x 0.5 units/kg per units/dL = 1000 units

Manufacturer's labeling: Advate, Helixate FS, Kogenate FS, Recombinate, Xyntha: Desired factor VIII level, dosing interval, and duration based on hemorrhage type: IV:
Minor hemorrhage (early joint hemorrhage, mild muscle or oral bleed): 10-20 units/kg/dose
Desired factor VIII levels (% or units/dL): 20-40
Frequency of dosing: Every 8-24 hours (Advate: <6 years old) **or** every 12-24 hours (Advate: ≥6 years old; Helixate FS; Kogentae FS; Xyntha)
Duration of treatment: 1-3 days until bleeding is resolved or healing achieved; mild, superficial, or early hemorrhages may respond to a single dose
Moderate hemorrhage (intramuscular bleed, hematoma, moderate bleeding into oral cavity, definite joint bleed, and known trauma): 15-30 units/kg/dose
Desired factor VIII levels (% or units/dL): 30-60
Frequency of dosing: Every 8-24 hours (Advate: <6 years old) **or** every 12-24 hours (Advate: ≥6 years old; Helixate FS; Kogenate FS; Xyntha)
Duration of treatment: ≥3 days until bleeding, pain, and disability are resolved or healing is achieved
Severe/life-threatening hemorrhage (GI, intracranial, intra-abdominal, intrathoracic bleeding, retroperitoneal, retropharyngeal, illiopsoas, CNS bleeding or head trauma, fractures):
Helixate FS, Kogenate FS: Initial: 40-50 units/kg; maintenance: 20-25 units/kg/dose
Desired factor VIII levels (% or units/dL): 80-100
Frequency of dosing: Every 8-12 hours
Duration of treatment: Until bleeding is resolved (duration not specified)
Advate, Recombinate, Xyntha: 30-50 units/kg/dose
Desired factor VIII levels (% or units/dL): 60-100
Frequency of dosing: Every 6-12 hours (Advate: <6 years old) **or** 8-24 hours (Advate: ≥6 years old; Recombinate; Xyntha)
Duration of treatment: Until bleeding is resolved (duration not specified)

Alternative dosing: **Note:** The following recommendations reflect guideline recommendations for general dosing requirements; may vary from those found within prescribing information or practitioner preference:
IV: Infants, Children, and Adolescents: Desired factor VIII level to maintain and duration based on site of hemorrhage/clinical situation (when no significant resource constraints exist) [WFH guidelines (Srivastava, 2013)]. **Note:** Factor VIII level may either be expressed as units/dL or as %. Dosing frequency most commonly corresponds to the half-life of factor VIII but should be determined based on an assessment of factor VIII levels before the next dose.
Joint: 40-60 units/dL for 1-2 days; may be longer if response is inadequate
Superficial muscle (no neurovascular compromise): 40-60 units/dL for 2-3 days, sometimes longer if response is inadequate
Iliopsoas and deep muscle with neurovascular injury, or substantial blood loss: Initial: 80-100 units/dL for 1-2 days; Maintenance: 30-60 units/dL for 3-5 days, sometimes longer as secondary prophylaxis during physiotherapy
CNS/head: Initial: 80-100 units/dL for 1-7 days; Maintenance: 50 units/dL for 8-21 days
Throat and neck: Initial: 80-100 units/dL for 1-7 days; Maintenance: 50 units/dL for 8-14 days
Gastrointestinal: Initial: 80-100 units/dL for 7-14 days; Maintenance: 50 units/dL (duration not specified)
Renal: 50 units/dL for 3-5 days
Deep laceration: 50 units/dL for 5-7 days
Continuous IV infusion: Infants, Children, and Adolescents: Limited data available: **Note:** For patients who require prolonged periods of treatment (eg, intracranial hemorrhage or surgery) to avoid peaks and troughs associated with intermittent infusions [Batorova, 2002; Poon, 2012; WFH guidelines (Srivastava, 2013)]:
Following initial bolus to achieve the desired factor VIII level: Initial dosing: 2-4 units/kg/hour; adjust dose based on frequent factor VIII assays and calculation of factor VIII clearance at steady-state using the following equations:
Factor VIII clearance (mL/kg/hour) = (current infusion rate in units/kg/hour) / (plasma Factor level in units/**mL**)
New infusion rate (units/kg/hour) = (factor VIII clearance in mL/kg/hour) x (desired plasma level in units/**mL**)

Perioperative management: IV: Infants, Children, and Adolescents:
Manufacturer's labeling: Desired factor VIII level, dosing interval, and duration based on surgery type:
Minor surgery (including dental extractions):
Advate: 30-50 units/kg as bolus infusion beginning within 1 hour prior to surgery; for dental procedures, adjunctive therapy may be considered
Desired factor VIII levels (% or units/dL): 60-100
Frequency of dosing: Every 12-24 hours as needed to control bleeding
Duration of treatment: Until bleeding is resolved (duration not specified)
Helixate FS, Kogenate FS, Xyntha: 15-30 units/kg/dose; for dental procedures, a single dose plus oral antifibrinolytic therapy within 1 hour may be sufficient
Desired factor VIII levels (% or units/dL): 30-60
Frequency of dosing: Every 12-24 hours
Duration of treatment: 3-4 days or until bleeding is resolved
Recombinate:
Desired factor VIII levels (% or units/dL): 60-80
Frequency of dosing: Single dose plus oral antifibrinolytic therapy within 1 hour is sufficient for most cases
Major surgery (tonsillectomy, hernia repair, intracranial, intra-abdominal or intrahtoracic surgery; joint replacement, trauma):
Advate: 40-60 units/kg/dose
Desired factor VIII levels (% or units/dL): Pre- and postoperative levels: 80-120; verify 100% activity has been achieved prior to surgery
Frequency of dosing: Every 6-24 hours (<6 years old) **or** every 8-24 hours (≥6 years old) as needed
Duration of treatment: Based on desired level and state of healing
Helixate FS, Kogenate FS: 50 units/kg/dose
Desired factor VIII levels (% or units/dL): Pre- and postoperative levels: 100; verify 100% activity has been achieved prior to surgery
Frequency of dosing: Every 6-12 hours as needed
Duration of treatment: Until healing is complete (~10-14 days)
Recombinate: 40-50 units/kg/dose
Desired factor VIII levels (% or units/dL): Pre- and postoperative: 80-100
Frequency of dosing: Every 8-24 hours

Duration of treatment: Based on state of healing

Xyntha: Children ≥12 years and Adolescents:

Desired factor VIII levels (% or units/dL): 60-100

Frequency of dosing: Every 8-24 hours

Duration of treatment: Until bleeding is resolved and wound healing is achieved

Alternative dosing: **Note:** The following recommendations reflect guideline recommendations for general dosing requirements; may vary from those found within prescribing information or practitioner preference:

IV: Desired factor VIII level to maintain and duration based on site of hemorrhage/clinical situation (when no significant resource constraints exist) [WFH guidelines (Srivastava, 2013)]. **Note:** Factor VIII level may either be expressed as units/dL or as %. Dosing frequency most commonly corresponds to the half-life of factor VIII but should be determined based on an assessment of factor VIII levels before the next dose.

Surgery (major):

Preop: 80-100 units/dL

Postop: 60-80 units/dL for 1-3 days; then 40-60 units/dL for 4-6 days; then 30-50 units/dL for 7-14 days

Surgery (minor):

Preop: 50-80 units/dL

Postop: 30-80 units/dL for 1-5 days depending on procedure type

Continuous IV infusion: Infants, Children, and Adolescents: Limited data available: Initial: 25-50 units/kg prior to surgery, followed by continuous infusion at a rate of 3-5 units/kg/hour; regimen based on two studies evaluating use in pediatric surgery patients (age range: 0.9-17 years); rate was adjusted and additional boluses given as needed to maintain desired factor VIII level (Batorova, 2012; Dingli, 2002)

Routine prophylaxis: IV: Infants, Children, and Adolescents:

Manufacturer's labeling:

Advate: 20-40 units/kg/dose every other day (3-4 times weekly). Alternatively, an every-third-day dosing regimen may be used to target factor VIII trough levels of ≥1%

Helixate FS, Kogenate FS: **Note:** For use in patients with no pre-existing joint damage: 25 units/kg/dose given every other day

Alternative dosing: 15-30 units/kg/dose 3 times weekly (WFH guidelines [Srivastava, 2013] [Utrecht protocol]) **or** 25-40 units/kg/dose 3 times weekly (WFH guidelines [Srivastava, 2013] [Malmö protocol]) **or** 25-50 units/kg/dose administered 3 times weekly **or** every other day (National Hemophilia Foundation, MASAC recommendation, 2007); optimum regimen has yet to be defined.

Adults:

Hemophilia: IV: **Individualize dosage based on coagulation studies performed prior to treatment and at regular intervals during treatment.** In general, administration of factor VIII 1 unit/kg will increase circulating factor VIII levels by ~2 units/dL (or 2%). (General guidelines presented; consult individual product labeling for specific dosing recommendations.)

Dosage based on desired factor VIII increase (%):

To calculate dosage needed based on desired factor VIII increase (%):

Body weight (kg) x 0.5 units/kg x desired factor VIII increase (%) = units factor VIII required

For example: 50 kg x 0.5 units/kg x 30 (% increase) = 750 units factor VIII

Dosage based on expected factor VIII increase (%):

It is also possible to calculate the **expected** % factor VIII increase:

(# units administered x 2%/units/kg) divided by body weight (kg) = expected % factor VIII increase

For example: (1400 units x 2%/units/kg) divided by 70 kg = 40%

General guidelines (consult individual product labeling for specific dosage recommendations):

Minor hemorrhage: 10-20 units/kg as a single dose to achieve FVIII plasma level ~20% to 40% of normal. Mild superficial or early hemorrhages may respond to a single dose; may repeat dose every 12-24 hours for 1-3 days until bleeding is resolved or healing achieved.

Moderate hemorrhage/minor surgery: 15-30 units/kg to achieve FVIII plasma level 30% to 60% of normal. May repeat 1 dose at 12-24 hours if needed. Some products suggest continuing for ≥3 days until pain and disability are resolved.

Major to life-threatening hemorrhage: Initial dose 30-50 units/kg followed by a maintenance dose of 20-50 units/kg every 8-24 hours until threat is resolved, to achieve FVIII plasma level 60% to 100% of normal.

Minor surgery (including tooth extraction): 15-50 units/kg to raise factor VIII level to ~30% to 100% before procedure/surgery. May repeat every 12-24 hours until bleeding is resolved.

Major surgery: 40-60 units/kg given preoperatively to raise factor VIII level to ~60% to 120% before surgery begins. May repeat as necessary after 6-24 hours until wound healing. Intensity of therapy may depend on type of surgery and postoperative regimen.

If bleeding is not controlled with adequate dose, test for presence of inhibitor. It may not be possible or practical to control bleeding if inhibitor titers >10 Bethesda units/mL.

Preparation for Administration Parenteral: IV: If refrigerated, the dried concentrate and diluent should be warmed to room temperature before reconstitution; see individual product labeling for specific reconstitution guidelines. Gently agitate or rotate vial after adding diluent, do not shake vigorously. Use filter needle provided by manufacturer to draw product into syringe (all products except Xyntha); do not refrigerate after reconstitution; administer within 3 hours after reconstitution; **Note:** Use plastic syringes, since rAHF may stick to the surface of glass syringes.

Administration Parenteral: IV administration only; use administration sets/tubing provided by manufacturer (if provided). Adjust administration rate based on patient response.

Advate: Infuse over ≤5 minutes; maximum infusion rate: 10 mL/minute

Helixate FS, Kogenate FS: Infuse over 1 to 15 minutes; based on patient tolerability; use sterile administration set provided by manufacturer.

Recombinate:

Reconstitution with 5 mL of SWFI: Infuse at a maximum rate of 5 mL/minute

Reconstitution with 10 mL of SWFI: Infuse at a maximum rate of 10 mL/minute

Xyntha, Xyntha Solufuse: Infuse over several minutes; adjust based on patient comfort. Do not admix or administer in same tubing as other medications.

WFH recommendations: Infuse slowly with maximum rate determined by age: Young children: 100 **units**/minute; Adults: 3 mL/minute; may also administer as a continuous infusion in select patients (WFH guidelines [Srivastava 2013]).

Monitoring Parameters Bleeding; heart rate and blood pressure (before and during IV administration); factor VIII levels prior to and during treatment; monitor for the development of inhibitor antibodies by clinical observations (eg, inadequate control of bleeding with adequate doses) and laboratory tests (eg, inhibitor level, Bethesda assay)

Reference Range

Classification of hemophilia; normal is defined as 1 unit/mL of factor VIII

Severe: Factor level <1% of normal

Moderate: Factor level 1% to 5% of normal

Mild: Factor level >5% to <40% of normal

Additional Information One unit of rAHF is equal to the factor VIII activity present in 1 mL of fresh pooled human plasma. If bleeding is not controlled with adequate dose, test for the presence of factor VIII inhibitor; larger doses of rAHF may be therapeutic with inhibitor titers <10 Bethesda units/mL; it may not be possible or practical to control bleeding if inhibitor titers >10 Bethesda units/mL (due to the very large rAHF doses required); other treatments [eg, antihemophilic factor (porcine), factor IX complex concentrates, recombinant factor VIIa, or anti-inhibitor coagulant complex] may be needed in patients with inhibitor titers >10 Bethesda units/mL

Dosage Forms Considerations Strengths expressed with approximate values. Consult individual vial labels for exact potency within each vial.

Dosage Forms Excipient information presented when available (limited, particularly for generics); consult specific product labeling.

Kit, Intravenous:

Kogenate FS: 250 units, 500 units, 1000 units [contains mouse protein (murine) (hamster)]

Kit, Intravenous [preservative free]:

Helixate FS: 250 units, 500 units, 1000 units, 2000 units, 3000 units [contains polysorbate 80]

Kogenate FS: 2000 units, 3000 units [contains mouse protein (murine) (hamster)]

Kogenate FS Bio-Set: 250 units, 500 units, 1000 units, 2000 units, 3000 units

Xyntha: 250 units, 500 units, 1000 units, 2000 units [albumin free; contains mouse protein (murine) (hamster), polysorbate 80]

Xyntha Solofuse: 250 units, 500 units, 1000 units, 2000 units, 3000 units [albumin free; contains mouse protein (murine) (hamster), polysorbate 80]

Solution Reconstituted, Intravenous [preservative free]:

Advate: 250 units (1 ea); 500 units (1 ea); 1000 units (1 ea); 1500 units (1 ea); 2000 units (1 ea); 3000 units (1 ea); 4000 units (1 ea) [albumin free; contains polysorbate 80]

Eloctate: 250 units (1 ea); 500 units (1 ea); 750 units (1 ea); 1000 units (1 ea); 1500 units (1 ea); 2000 units (1 ea); 3000 units (1 ea)

Novoeight: 250 units (1 ea); 500 units (1 ea); 1000 units (1 ea); 1500 units (1 ea); 2000 units (1 ea); 3000 units (1 ea) [contains mouse protein (murine) (hamster), polysorbate 80]

Recombinate: 220-400 units (1 ea); 401-800 units (1 ea); 801-1240 units (1 ea); 1241-1800 units (1 ea); 1801-2400 units (1 ea) [contains albumin human, polyethylene glycol, polysorbate 80]

Antihemophilic Factor/von Willebrand Factor Complex (Human)

(an tee hee moe FIL ik FAK tor von WILL le brand FAK tor KOM plex HYU man)

Medication Safety Issues

Sound-alike/look-alike issues:

Factor VIII may be confused with Factor XIII

Brand Names: US Alphanate; Humate-P; Wilate

Brand Names: Canada Humate-P

Therapeutic Category Antihemophilic Agent; Blood Product Derivative

Generic Availability (US) No

Use

Hemophilia A (Factor VIII deficiency): Alphanate®, Humate-P®: Prevention and treatment of hemorrhagic episodes in hemophilia A (classic hemophilia) (Alphanate®: FDA approved in ages >16 years and adults; Humate-P®: FDA approved in adults); prevention and treatment of hemorrhagic episodes with acquired factor VIII deficiency (Alphanate®: FDA approved in ages >16 years and adults)

von Willebrand disease (VWD):

Alphanate®: Prophylaxis for surgical and/or invasive procedures in patients with VWD when desmopressin is either ineffective or contraindicated [FDA approved in pediatric patients (age not specified) and adults]. **Note:** Not indicated for patients with severe VWD undergoing major surgery.

Humante-P®: Treatment of spontaneous and trauma-induced hemorrhagic episodes and prevention of excessive perioperative bleeding in patients with mild to moderate and severe VWD where the use of desmopressin is suspected or known to be inadequate (FDA approved in ages ≥1 month and adults). **Note:** Not indicated for the prophylaxis of spontaneous bleeding episodes.

Wilate®: Treatment of spontaneous and trauma-induced bleeding in patients with severe VWD, including mild or moderate disease when use of desmopressin is known or suspected to be inadequate or contraindicated (FDA approved in ages ≥5 years and adults). **Note:** Not indicated for prophylaxis of spontaneous bleeding or prevention of excessive bleeding during and after surgery.

Pregnancy Risk Factor C

Pregnancy Considerations Animal reproduction studies have not been conducted. Parvovirus B19 or hepatitis A, which may be present in plasma-derived products, may affect a pregnant woman more seriously than nonpregnant women.

Breast-Feeding Considerations No human or animal data is available. Breast-feeding is not recommended by the manufacturer.

Contraindications History of anaphylactic or severe systemic response to antihemophilic factor or von Willebrand factor formulations; hypersensitivity to any component of the formulation

Warnings/Precautions Use caution when treating VWD in patients with risk factors for thrombosis; risk of thromboembolic events may be increased with ongoing use; monitor concentrations of von Willebrand factor and factor VIII closely; avoid excessive increases in factor VIII activity. Incidence of thrombosis may be increased in females. Allergic reactions, including anaphylaxis, have been observed; monitor patients closely during infusion; patients experiencing anaphylactic reactions should be evaluated for the presence of inhibitors. Risk of viral transmission is not totally eradicated. Because antihemophilic factor is prepared from pooled plasma, it may contain the causative agent of viral hepatitis and other viral diseases. Strongly consider hepatitis A and B vaccination. Neutralizing antibodies (inhibitors) may develop to factor VIII or von Willebrand factor, particularly in patients with type 3 (severe) von Willebrand disease. Patients who develop antibodies against von Willebrand factor will not have an effective clinical response to therapy and infusions may result in anaphylactic reactions; these patients should be managed by an experienced physician and alternatives to therapy should be considered. Any patient who has an inadequate response to therapy or a severe adverse reaction should be evaluated for the presence of inhibitors. the dosage requirement will vary in patients with factor VIII inhibitors; optimal treatment should be determined by clinical response. In patients with hemophilia A, the dosage requirement will vary in patients with factor VIII inhibitors; optimal treatment should be determined by clinical response.

Some dosage forms may contain polysorbate 80 (also known as Tweens). Hypersensitivity reactions, usually a delayed reaction, have been reported following exposure to pharmaceutical products containing polysorbate 80 in certain individuals (Isaksson, 2002; Lucente 2000; Shelley, 1995). Thrombocytopenia, ascites, pulmonary deterioration, and renal and hepatic failure have been reported in premature neonates after receiving parenteral products containing polysorbate 80 (Alade, 1986; CDC, 1984). See manufacturer's labeling.

Alphanate and Humate-P contain trace amounts of blood groups A and B isohemagglutinins. Use caution when large or frequently repeated doses are given to individuals with blood groups A, B, and AB; the patient should be monitored for signs of progressive anemia and the possibility of intravascular hemolysis should be considered.

Warnings: Additional Pediatric Considerations Formation of factor VIII inhibitors (neutralizing antibodies to AHF human) may occur, particularly in patients with Type 3 (severe) von Willebrand factor; reported overall incidence is 3% to 52%; an increase of inhibitor antibody concentration is seen at 2 to 7 days, with peak concentrations at 1 to 3 weeks after therapy; children <5 years of age may also be at greatest risk. Patients who develop antibodies (usually antibody concentration >10 Bethesda units/mL) against von Willebrand factor will not have an effective clinical response to therapy and infusions may result in anaphylactic reactions; these patients should be managed by an experienced physician and alternatives to therapy should be considered. Any patient who has an inadequate response to therapy or a severe adverse reaction should be evaluated for the presence of inhibitors.

Adverse Reactions

Cardiovascular: Cardiorespiratory arrest, chest tightness, edema, femoral venous thrombosis, flushing, hypervolemia, orthostatic hypotension, shock, thromboembolic events, vasodilation

Central nervous system: Chills, dizziness, fever, headache, lethargy, pain, seizure, somnolence

Dermatologic: Itching, pruritus, rash, urticaria

Endocrine & metabolic: Parotid gland swelling

Gastrointestinal: Nausea, vomiting

Hematologic: Hematocrit decreased (moderate), hemorrhage, hemolysis, pseudothrombocytopenia (severe)

Hepatic: ALT increased

Local: Injection site stinging, phlebitis

Neuromuscular & skeletal: Extremity pain, joint pain, paresthesia, rigors

Respiratory: Cough, dyspnea, pharyngitis, pulmonary embolus (large doses)

Miscellaneous: Allergic reactions, anaphylactic reactions, factor VIII inhibitor formation, hypersensitivity reactions, von Willebrand factor inhibitor formation

Drug Interactions

Metabolism/Transport Effects None known.

Avoid Concomitant Use There are no known interactions where it is recommended to avoid concomitant use.

Increased Effect/Toxicity There are no known significant interactions involving an increase in effect.

Decreased Effect There are no known significant interactions involving a decrease in effect.

Storage/Stability

Alphanate: Store intact vials at ≤25°C (77°F); do not freeze. May store reconstituted solution at room temperature (≤30°C). Use within 3 hours of reconstitution; do not refrigerate after reconstitution.

Humate-P®: Store unopened vials at ≤25°C (≤77°F) until expiration date on label; avoid freezing. Use within 3 hours of reconstitution. Do not refrigerate after reconstitution, precipitation may occur.

Wilate: Store intact vials for ≤36 months under refrigeration at 2°C to 8°C (36°F to 46°F); do not freeze. Protect from light. Intact vials may also be stored at room temperature (not to exceed 25°C/77°F) for ≤6 months. Once stored at room temperature, do not return to the refrigerator. Following reconstitution, use solution immediately.

Mechanism of Action Factor VIII and von Willebrand factor (VWF), obtained from pooled human plasma, are used to replace endogenous factor VIII and VWF in patients with hemophilia or VWD. Factor VIII in conjunction with activated factor IX, activates factor X which converts prothrombin to thrombin and fibrinogen to fibrin. VWF promotes platelet aggregation and adhesion to damaged vascular endothelium and acts as a stabilizing carrier protein for factor VIII. (Circulating levels of functional VWF are measured as ristocetin cofactor activity [VWF: RCo].)

Pharmacodynamics

Onset: Shortening of bleeding time: Immediate

Maximum effect: 1-2 hours

Duration: VWD: Shortening of bleeding time: <6 hours postinfusion; VWF multimers detected in the plasma: 24 hours after infusion

Pharmacokinetics (Adult data unless noted)

Distribution: V_{dss}: VWF:RCo: 53-72 mL/kg

Half-life, elimination:

FVIII coagulant activity (FVIII:C 8-28 hours in patients with hemophilia A

VWF:RCo: 3-34 hours in patients with VWD

Dosing: Usual Note: Individualize dosage based on coagulation studies performed prior to and during treatment at regular intervals:

Hemophilia A; Factor VIII deficiency: Alphanate®, Humate-P®: General guidelines provided (consult specific product labeling for Alphanate® or Humate-P®):

Infants, Children, Adolescents, and Adults: Limited data in pediatric patients <16 years: IV: In general, administration of 1 unit/kg of factor VIII will increase circulating factor VIII levels by ~2 units/dL (or 2%); calculated dosage should be adjusted to the actual vial size.

The formula to calculate required dosage based on desired increase in factor VIII (% of normal); **Note:** This formula assumes that the patient's baseline AHF level is <1%:

Units required = Body weight (kg) x 0.5 x desired increase in factor VIII (units or % of normal)

Minor hemorrhage: Loading dose: FVIII:C 15 units/kg to achieve FVIII:C plasma level ~30% of normal. One infusion may be adequate. If second infusion is needed, half the loading dose may be given once or twice daily for 1-2 days.

Moderate hemorrhage: Loading dose: FVIII:C 25 units/kg to achieve FVIII:C plasma level ~50% of normal. Maintenance: FVIII:C 15 units/kg every 8-12 hours for 1-2 days in order to maintain FVIII:C plasma levels at 30% of normal. Repeat the same dose once or twice daily for up to 7 days or until adequate wound healing.

Life-threatening hemorrhage: Loading dose: FVIII:C 40-50 units/kg. Maintenance: FVIII:C 20-25 units/kg every 8 hours to maintain FVIII:C plasma levels at 80% to 100% of normal for 7 days. Continue same dose once or twice daily for another 7 days in order to maintain FVIII:C levels at 30% to 50% of normal.

von Willebrand disease (VWD); treatment: Dosage is expressed in international units of von Willebrand factor: Ristocetin cofactor (VWF:RCo): Dose must be individualized based on type of VWD, extent and location of bleeding, clinical status of patient, and coagulation studies performed prior to and at regular intervals during treatment. Products are not identical and should not be used interchangeably (NHLBI, 2007).

Hemorrhage:

Humate P: Infants, Children, Adolescents, and Adults: IV: **Note:** In general, administration of 1 unit/kg of factor VIII would be expected to raise circulating VWF:RCo ~5 units/dL

Type 1, mild VWD: Major hemorrhage or minor hemorrhage (if desmopressin is not appropriate):

Loading dose: 40-60 units/kg

Maintenance dose: 40-50 units/kg/dose every 8-12 hours for 3 days, maintain VWF:RCo nadir >50%; follow with 40-50 units/kg once daily for up to 7 days

Type 1, moderate or severe VWD:

Minor hemorrhage: 40-50 units/kg/dose for 1-2 doses

Major hemorrhage:

Loading dose: 50-75 units/kg

Maintenance dose: 40-60 units/kg/dose every 8-12 hours for 3 days; maintain VWF:RCo nadir >50%; follow with 40-60 units/kg/dose once daily for up to 7 days

Types 2 and 3 VWD:

Minor hemorrhage: 40-50 units/kg/dose for 1-2 doses

Major hemorrhage:

Loading dose: 60-80 units/kg

Maintenance dose: 40-60 units/kg/dose every 8-12 hours for 3 days, maintain VWF:RCo nadir >50%; follow with 40-60 units/kg/dose once daily for up to 7 days

Wilate: Children ≥5 years, Adolescents, and Adults: IV:

Minor hemorrhage:

Loading dose: 20-40 units/kg

Maintenance dose: 20-30 units/kg/dose every 12-24 hours for ≤3 days, keeping the VWF:RCo nadir >30%

Major hemorrhage:

Loading dose: 40-60 units/kg

Maintenance dose: 20-40 units/kg/dose every 12-24 hours for 5-7 days, keeping the VWF:RCo nadir >50%

von Willebrand disease (VWD); surgical/procedural prophylaxis: Note: Not for patients with type 3 VWD undergoing major surgery

Alphanate:

Infants, Children, and Adolescents: IV:

Preoperative dose: 75 units/kg as a single dose 1 hour prior to surgery

Maintenance dose: 50-75 units/kg/dose every 8-12 hours as clinically needed. May reduce dose after third postoperative day; continue treatment until healing is complete. Goal is to keep the VWF:RCo nadir >50 units/dL at least for the first 3 days (NHLBI, 2007)

Adults (except patients with type 3 undergoing major surgery): IV:

Preoperative dose: 60 units/kg 1 hour prior to surgery

Maintenance dose: 40-60 units/kg/dose every 8-12 hours as clinically needed. May reduce dose after third postoperative day; continue treatment until healing is complete. For minor procedures, maintain VWF of 40% to 50% during postoperative days 1-3; for major procedures maintain VWF of 40% to 50% for ≥3-7 days postoperative.

Humate-P®: Infants, Children, Adolescents, and Adults: IV:

Emergency surgery: 50-60 units/kg; monitor trough coagulation factor levels for subsequent doses

Surgical management (nonemergency): **Note:** Whenever possible, the *in vivo* recovery (IVR) should be measured and baseline plasma VWF:RCo and FVIII activity should be assessed in all patients prior to surgery. The formula to calculate the IVR is as follows: Measure baseline plasma VWF:RCo; then infuse VWF:RCo 60 units/kg IV at time zero; measure VWF:RCo at 30 minutes after infusion. IVR = (plasma VWF:RCo at 30 minutes minus plasma VWF:RCof at baseline) divided by 60 units/kg.

Loading dose: Loading dose calculation based on baseline target VWF:RCo: (Target peak VWF:RCo - Baseline VWF:RCo) x weight (in kg) / IVR = units VWF:RCo required. Administer loading dose 1-2 hours prior to surgery. **Note:** If *in vivo* recovery (IVR) is not available, assume IVR of 2 units/dL for every one VWF:RCo unit/kg administered.

Target peak VWF:RCo concentrations following loading dose:

Major surgery/emergency: 100 units/dL

Minor/oral surgery: 50-60 units/dL

Note: Oral surgery is <2 extractions of nonmolars without bony involvement; extractions of ≥2 teeth or >1 impacted wisdom tooth is considered major surgery.

Maintenance dose: Initial: One-half loading dose followed by subsequent dosing determined by target trough concentrations, generally administered every 8-12 hours; patients with shorter half-lives may require dosing every 6 hours

Target maintenance trough VWF:RCo concentrations and minimum duration of treatment:

Major surgery: >50 units/dL for up to 3 days, followed by >30 units/dL; minimum duration of treatment: 72 hours

Minor surgery: ≥30 units/dL; minimum duration of treatment: 48 hours

Oral surgery: ≥30 units/dL; minimum duration of treatment: 8-12 hours

Preparation for Administration Parenteral: IV: If refrigerated, the dried concentrate and diluent should be warmed to room temperature before reconstitution; see product labeling for specific reconstitution guidelines. Gently swirl or rotate vial after adding diluent; do not shake vigorously. Use provided filter transfer set to withdraw solution from vial of Alphanate or Humate-P; remove filter spike prior to administration. Use provided transfer device to reconstitute Wilate. Use plastic syringes; AHF may stick to the surface of glass syringes.

Administration Parenteral: IV: Administer through a separate line, do not mix with drugs or other IV fluids

Alphanate: Infuse slowly; maximum rate: 10 mL/minute

Humate-P: Infuse slowly; maximum rate: 4 mL/minute

Wilate: Infuse slowly at a rate of 2 to 4 mL/minute

Monitoring Parameters Signs and symptoms of intravascular hemolysis or bleeding; heart rate and blood pressure (before and during IV administration). AHF levels prior to and during treatment; in patients with circulating inhibitors, the inhibitor level should be monitored; hematocrit; VWF activity (circulating levels of functional VWF are measured as ristocetin cofactor activity [VWF:RCo]). In surgical patients, monitor VWF:RCo at baseline and after surgery, trough VWF:RCo and FVIII:C at least daily.

Reference Range Hemophilia: Classification of hemophilia; normal is defined as 1 unit/mL of factor VIII:C

Severe: Factor level <1% of normal

Moderate: Factor level 1% to 5% of normal

Mild: Factor level >5% to 30% of normal

Additional Information One unit of AHF is equal to the factor VIII activity present in 1 mL of normal human plasma. If bleeding is not controlled with adequate dose, test for the presence of factor VIII inhibitor; larger doses of AHF may be therapeutic with inhibitor titers <10 Bethesda units/mL; it may not be possible or practical to control bleeding if inhibitor titers >10 Bethesda units/mL (due to the very large AHF doses required); other treatments [eg, antihemophilic factor (porcine), factor IX complex concentrates, recombinant factor VIIa, or anti-inhibitor coagulant complex] may be needed in patients with inhibitor titers >10 Bethesda units/mL.

Exact potency varies among products and between lots of the same product; each vial contains the exact labeled amount of VWF activity, as measured with the Ristocetin cofactor activity (VWF:RCo), and factor VIII (FVIII) activity and should be consulted prior to use. However, the average ratio between VWF:RCo and FVIII among available products is:

Alphanate®: Average ratio not provided by manufacturer or in available literature

Humate-P®: Average ratio of VWF:RCo to FVIII is 2.4:1

Wilate®: Average ratio of VWF:RCo to FVIII is ~1:1

Dosage Forms Considerations Strengths expressed with approximate values. Consult individual vial labels for exact potency within each vial.

Dosage Forms Excipient information presented when available (limited, particularly for generics); consult specific product labeling. [DSC] = Discontinued product

Injection, powder for reconstitution [human derived]:

Alphanate:

250 units [Factor VIII and VWF:RCo ratio varies by lot; contains albumin and polysorbate 80; packaged with diluent]

500 units [Factor VIII and VWF:RCo ratio varies by lot; contains albumin and polysorbate 80; packaged with diluent]

1000 units [Factor VIII and VWF:RCo ratio varies by lot; contains albumin and polysorbate 80; packaged with diluent]

1500 units [Factor VIII and VWF:RCo ratio varies by lot; contains albumin and polysorbate 80; packaged with diluent]

2000 units [Factor VIII and VWF:RCo ratio varies by lot; contains albumin and polysorbate 80; packaged with diluent]

Humate-P:

FVIII 250 units and VWF:RCo 600 units [contains albumin; packaged with diluent]

FVIII 500 units and VWF:RCo 1200 units [contains albumin; packaged with diluent]

FVIII 1000 units and VWF:RCo 2400 units [contains albumin; packaged with diluent]

Wilate:

FVIII 450 units and VWF:RCo 450 units [contains polysorbate 80 (in diluent); packaged with diluent] [DSC]

FVIII 500 units and VWF:RCo 500 units [contains polysorbate 80 (in diluent); packaged with diluent]

FVIII 900 units and VWF:RCo 900 units [contains polysorbate 80 (in diluent); packaged with diluent] [DSC]

FVIII 1000 units and VWF:RCo 1000 units [contains polysorbate 80 (in diluent); packaged with diluent]

◆ **Anti-Hist Allergy [OTC]** *see* DiphenhydrAMINE (Systemic) *on page 668*

Anti-inhibitor Coagulant Complex (Human)

(an TEE in HI bi tor coe AG yoo lant KOM pleks HYU man)

Brand Names: US FEIBA

Brand Names: Canada FEIBA NF

Therapeutic Category Antihemophilic Agent; Blood Product Derivative

Generic Availability (US) No

Use Control of spontaneous bleeding episodes or to cover surgical interventions in hemophilia A and hemophilia B patients [FDA approved in infants (>28 days of life), children, and adults]

Pregnancy Risk Factor C

Pregnancy Considerations Animal reproduction studies have not been conducted.

Breast-Feeding Considerations It is not known if this product is excreted in breast milk. The manufacturer recommends that caution be exercised when administering anti-inhibitor coagulant complex to nursing women.

Contraindications Known anaphylactic or severe hypersensitivity to anti-inhibitor coagulant complex or any component of the formulation, including factors of the kinin generating system; disseminated intravascular coagulation (DIC); acute thrombosis or embolism (including myocardial infarction)

Warnings/Precautions Allergic reactions (including severe anaphylactoid reactions) have been observed following administration. Discontinue immediately with signs/symptoms of hypersensitivity. Appropriate medication including epinephrine should be readily available.

[U.S. Boxed Warning]: Thrombotic and thromboembolic events (including venous thrombosis, pulmonary embolism, disseminated intravascular coagulation [DIC], myocardial infarction and stroke) have been reported following administration of anti-inhibitor coagulant complex, particularly with administration Monitor patients receiving anti-inhibitor coagulant complex for signs and symptoms of thromboembolic events especially if more than 100 units/kg is administered of high doses and/or in patients with thrombotic risk factors. Advanced atherosclerotic disease, crush injury, septicemia, or concomitant treatment with factor VIIa due to increased risk of developing thrombotic events due to circulating tissue factor or predisposing coagulopathy. Weigh the potential benefit of treatment with anti-inhibitor coagulant complex against the potential risk of these thromboembolic events. Thromboembolic events may be increased with concurrent use of an antifibrinolytic (tranexamic acid, aminocaproic acid); avoid or delay use of antifibrinolytic for at least 12 hours.

The manufacturer recommends that anti-inhibitor coagulant complex should only be used to control bleeding resulting from coagulation factor deficiencies in patients with inhibitors to coagulation factor VIII or coagulation factor IX. Tests used to monitor hemostatic activity, such as aPTT and thromboelastography (TEG), are **not** useful for monitoring responses with anti-inhibitor coagulant complex (Hoffman, 2012); dosing to normalize these values may result in DIC. Product of human plasma; may potentially contain infectious agents that could transmit disease. During the manufacturing process, screening of donors, as well as testing and/or inactivation or removal of certain viruses, reduces the risk. Infections thought to be transmitted by this product should be reported to the manufacturer and/or to FDA MedWatch. Patients with signs/symptoms of infection (eg, fever, chills, drowsiness) should be encouraged to consult health care provider. Product contains minute amounts of factor VIII, which may cause an anamnestic response; anamnestic rises were not associated with reduced efficacy.

Adverse Reactions

Cardiovascular: Blood pressure decreased, chest discomfort/pain, flushing, hyper-/hypotension, MI, tachycardia, thromboembolism

Central nervous system: Chills, dizziness, fever, headache, hypoesthesia (including facial), malaise, paresthesia, somnolence

Dermatologic: Angioedema, pruritus, rash, urticaria

Gastrointestinal: Abdominal discomfort, diarrhea, dysgeusia, nausea, vomiting

Hematologic: DIC, stroke (embolic/thrombotic), thrombosis (arterial/venous)
Local: Injection site pain
Respiratory: Bronchospasm, cough, dyspnea, pulmonary embolism, wheezing
Miscellaneous: Allergic reaction (including anaphylaxis), anamnestic response, hypersensitivity

Drug Interactions

Metabolism/Transport Effects None known.

Avoid Concomitant Use

Avoid concomitant use of Anti-inhibitor Coagulant Complex (Human) with any of the following: Antifibrinolytic Agents

Increased Effect/Toxicity

The levels/effects of Anti-inhibitor Coagulant Complex (Human) may be increased by: Antifibrinolytic Agents

Decreased Effect There are no known significant interactions involving a decrease in effect.

Storage/Stability Prior to reconstitution, store at room temperature (maximum of 25°C [77°F]); store in the original package to protect from light. Do **not** freeze. Following reconstitution, infusion must be completed within 3 hours.

Mechanism of Action Multiple interactions of the components in anti-inhibitor coagulant complex restore the impaired thrombin generation of hemophilia patients with inhibitors. *In vitro*, anti-inhibitor coagulant complex shortens the activated partial thromboplastin time of plasma containing factor VIII inhibitor.

Dosing: Usual Dosage is dependent upon the severity and location of bleeding, type and level of inhibitors, and whether the patient has a history of an anamnestic increase in antihemophilic inhibitor levels following use of preparations containing antihemophilic factor. Maximum dose should only be exceeded if bleeding severity warrants; monitor closely for DIC and/or coronary ischemia.

Infants, Children, and Adults: IV: **Note:** Considered a first-line treatment when factor VIII inhibitor titer is >5 Bethesda units (BU) (antihemophilic factor may be preferred when titer <5 BU)

General dosing: 50-100 units/kg (maximum: 200 units/kg/**day**); dosage may vary with the bleeding site and severity

Joint hemorrhage: 50 units/kg every 12 hours; may increase to 100 units/kg every 12 hours; (maximum: 200 units/kg/**day**)

Mucous membrane bleeding: 50 units/kg every 6 hours; may increase to 100 units/kg every 6 hours for up to two doses (maximum: 200 units/kg/**day**)

Soft tissue hemorrhage: 100 units/kg every 12 hours (maximum: 200 units/kg/**day**)

Other severe hemorrhages: 100 units/kg every 12 hours; may be given every 6 hours if needed (maximum: 200 units/kg/**day**)

Preparation for Administration IV: If refrigerated, allow the vials of anti-inhibitor coagulant complex (concentrate) and SWFI (diluent) to reach room temperature. Reconstitute with provided SWFI. Swirl to gently dissolve powder; do not shake. Do not refrigerate after reconstitution.

Administration IV: For IV injection or infusion only; maximum infusion rate: 2 units/kg/minute. Following reconstitution, complete infusion use within 3 hours.

Monitoring Parameters Monitor for control of bleeding; signs and symptoms of DIC (blood pressure changes, pulse rate changes, chest pain/cough, fibrinogen decreased, platelet count decreased, fibrin-fibrinogen degradation products, significantly-prolonged thrombin time, PT, or partial thromboplastin time); hemoglobin and hematocrit; hypotension; have epinephrine ready to treat hypersensitivity reactions. **Note:** Tests used to control efficacy such as aPTT, WBCT, and TEG do not correlate with clinical improvement. Dosing to normalize these values may result in DIC.

Additional Information Note: Dosage is expressed in units of factor VIII inhibitor bypassing activity. One unit of activity is defined as that amount of anti-inhibitor coagulant complex that shortens the activated partial thromboplastin time (aPTT) of a high titer factor VIII inhibitor reference plasma to 50% of the blank value.

Dosage Forms Considerations FEIBA strengths expressed in terms of Factor VIII inhibitor bypassing activity with nominal strength values. Consult individual vial labels for exact potency within each vial.

Dosage Forms Excipient information presented when available (limited, particularly for generics); consult specific product labeling.

Solution Reconstituted, Intravenous [preservative free]:
FEIBA: 500 units (1 ea); 1000 units (1 ea); 2500 units (1 ea)

◆ **Anti-Itch [OTC]** *see* DiphenhydrAMINE (Topical) *on page 672*

◆ **Anti-Itch Maximum Strength [OTC]** *see* DiphenhydrAMINE (Topical) *on page 672*

◆ **Anti-Itch Maximum Strength [OTC]** *see* Hydrocortisone (Topical) *on page 1041*

Antipyrine and Benzocaine

(an tee PYE reen & BEN zoe kane)

Brand Names: US Aurodex® [DSC]

Brand Names: Canada Auralgan®

Therapeutic Category Otic Agent, Analgesic; Otic Agent, Cerumenolytic

Generic Availability (US) Yes

Use Temporary relief of pain and reduction of inflammation associated with acute otitis media (congestive and serous stages); facilitates ear wax removal

Pregnancy Risk Factor C

Pregnancy Considerations Animal reproduction studies have not been conducted with this combination.

Contraindications Hypersensitivity to antipyrine, benzocaine, or any component of the formulation; perforated tympanic membrane; ear discharge

Warnings/Precautions Methemoglobinemia may occur (rare) with combination product; methemoglobinemia has been reported with some topical products containing higher concentrations (14% to 20%) of benzocaine. For otic use only, do not apply to eyes. Discontinue if sensitization or irritation occur.

Warnings: Additional Pediatric Considerations Methemoglobinemia has been reported with benzocaine topical products containing higher concentrations (14% to 20%) of benzocaine but is rare with combination products (concentration: 1.4%) (Rodriguez, 1994). Fatal methemoglobinemia was reported in a 4-month old infant who received 3 times the prescribed dose of ear drops containing benzocaine 0.25% and antipyrine 5.4%; causality was not proven (Logan, 2005). Use of otic anesthetics may mask symptoms of a fulminating middle ear infection (acute otitis media); not intended for prolonged use.

Adverse Reactions No adverse reactions are reported in the manufacturer's labeling. Refer to Benzocaine monograph.

Drug Interactions

Metabolism/Transport Effects None known.

Avoid Concomitant Use There are no known interactions where it is recommended to avoid concomitant use.

Increased Effect/Toxicity

Antipyrine and Benzocaine may increase the levels/effects of: Prilocaine; Sodium Nitrite

The levels/effects of Antipyrine and Benzocaine may be increased by: Nitric Oxide

Decreased Effect There are no known significant interactions involving a decrease in effect.

Storage/Stability Store at 15°C to 30°C (59°F to 86°F); protect from heat. Protect from light. Do not use if solution is brown or contains a precipitate. Discard 6 months after placing dropper into solution.

Mechanism of Action Antipyrine has analgesic properties; benzocaine is a local anesthetic; the glycerin base provides decreased middle ear pressure by osmosis.

Pharmacodynamics Onset of action: Pain relief: ~30 minutes (Hoberman, 1997)

Dosing: Usual Infants, Children, Adolescents, and Adults:

Acute otitis media, adjunct for associated pain and swelling: Otic: Fill ear canal, then moisten cotton pledget, place in external ear; repeat every 1-2 hours until pain and congestion are relieved

Ear wax removal; adjunct to loosen cerumen and to dry the ear canal or minimize associated discomfort: Otic: Instill drops 3 times daily for 2-3 days; moisten cotton pledget with antipyrine and benzocaine solution and place in external ear after solution instillation

Dosing adjustment in renal impairment: There are no dosage adjustments provided in the manufacturer's labeling.

Dosing adjustment in hepatic impairment: There are no dosage adjustments provided in the manufacturer's labeling.

Administration Otic: Patient should lie down with affected ear upward and medication instilled; remain in the position to allow penetration of solution. Avoid touching dropper to ears or fingers. Do not rinse dropper after use.

Acute otitis media: Fill ear canal with solution, then moisten cotton pledget with antipyrine and benzocaine solution and place in external ear

Ear wax removal: Moisten cotton pledget with antipyrine and benzocaine solution and place in external ear after solution instillation

Additional Information Product availability variable, some products previously on market (eg, Auralgan) are no longer available due to FDA regulations; see website for additional information at http://www.fda.gov/Drugs/GuidanceComplianceRegulatoryInformation/EnforcementActivitiesbyFDA/SelectedEnforcementActionsonUnapprovedDrugs/ucm238675.htm#ophthalmic

Dosage Forms Excipient information presented when available (limited, particularly for generics); consult specific product labeling.

Solution, otic [drops]: Antipyrine 5.4% and benzocaine 1.4% (10 mL, 15 mL), Antipyrine 5.5% and benzocaine 1.4% (14 mL)

Aurodex™: Antipyrine 5.4% and benzocaine 1.4% (10 mL) [DSC]

Antithymocyte Globulin (Equine)

(an te THY moe site GLOB yu lin, E kwine)

Medication Safety Issues

Sound-alike/look-alike issues:

Antithymocyte globulin equine (Atgam) may be confused with antithymocyte globulin rabbit (Thymoglobulin)

Atgam may be confused with Ativan

High alert medication:

This medication is in a class the Institute for Safe Medication Practices (ISMP) includes among its list of drug classes that have a heightened risk of causing significant patient harm when used in error.

Brand Names: US Atgam

Brand Names: Canada Atgam

Therapeutic Category Immunosuppressant Agent; Polyclonal Antibody

Generic Availability (US) No

Use Prevention and/or treatment of acute renal allograft rejection [FDA approved in pediatrics (age not specified) and adults]; treatment of moderate to severe aplastic anemia in patients not considered suitable candidates for bone marrow transplantation; [FDA approved in pediatrics (age not specified) and adults]; has also been used in prevention or treatment of graft-vs-host disease following allogenic stem cell transplantation; prevention and treatment of other solid organ (other than renal) allograft rejection; treatment of myelodysplastic syndrome (MDS)

Pregnancy Risk Factor C

Pregnancy Considerations Adverse events were observed in some animal reproduction studies. Women exposed to Atgam during pregnancy may be enrolled in the National Transplantation Pregnancy Registry (877-955-6877).

Breast-Feeding Considerations It is not known if antithymocyte globulin (equine) is excreted into breast milk. Due to the potential for serious adverse reactions in the nursing infant, the manufacturer recommends a decision be made whether to discontinue nursing or to discontinue the drug, taking into account the importance of treatment to the mother.

Contraindications History of severe systemic reaction (eg, anaphylactic reaction) to prior administration of antithymocyte globulin or other equine gamma globulins

Warnings/Precautions **[U.S. Boxed Warning]: Should only be used by physicians experienced in immunosuppressive therapy in the management of renal transplantation or aplastic anemia. Adequate laboratory and supportive medical resources must be readily available in the facility for patient management.** Hypersensitivity and anaphylactic reactions may occur; discontinue for symptoms of anaphylaxis; immediate treatment (including epinephrine 1:1000) should be available. Systemic reaction (rash, dyspnea, hypotension, tachycardia, or anaphylaxis) precludes further administration of antithymocyte globulin (equine; ATG). Respiratory distress, hypotension, or pain (chest, flank, or back) may indicate an anaphylactoid/anaphylactic reaction. Serious immune-mediated reactions have been reported (rare), including anaphylaxis, infusion reactions, and serum sickness. Skin testing is recommended prior to administration of the initial ATG dose. A positive skin test is suggestive of an increased risk for systemic allergic reactions with an infusion, although anaphylaxis may occur in patients who display negative skin tests. If ATG treatment is deemed appropriate following a positive skin test, the first infusion should be administered in a controlled environment with intensive life support immediately available.

Discontinue if severe and unremitting thrombocytopenia and/or leukopenia occur in solid organ transplant patients. Clinically significant hemolysis has been reported (rarely); severe and unremitting hemolysis may require treatment discontinuation; chest, flank or back pain may indicate hemolysis. Abnormal hepatic function tests have been observed in patients with aplastic anemia and other hematologic disorders receiving ATG. ATG is an immunosuppressant; monitor closely for signs of infection. An increased incidence of cytomegalovirus (CMV) infection has been reported in studies. Administer via central line due to chemical phlebitis that may occur with a peripheral vein. Dose must be administered over at least 4 hours. Patient may need to be pretreated with an antipyretic, antihistamine, and/or corticosteroid. Intradermal skin testing is recommended prior to first-dose administration. Product of equine and human plasma; may have a risk of transmitting disease, including a theoretical risk of Creutzfeldt-Jakob disease (CJD). Product potency and activity may vary from lot to lot. Potentially significant drug-drug interactions may exist, requiring dose or frequency adjustment, additional monitoring, and/or selection of alternative therapy. Live viral vaccines may not replicate and antibody response may be reduced if administered during ATG treatment. Patients should not be immunized with attenuated live viral vaccines for 6 months after treatment.

Adverse Reactions

Cardiovascular: Bradycardia, cardiac irregularity, chest pain, edema, heart failure, hyper-/hypotension, myocarditis

Central nervous system: Agitation, chills, fever, headache, lethargy, lightheadedness, listlessness, seizure, viral encephalopathy

Dermatologic: Pruritus, rash, urticaria

Gastrointestinal: Diarrhea, nausea, stomatitis, vomiting

Hematologic: Leukopenia, thrombocytopenia

Hepatic: Hepatosplenomegaly, liver function tests abnormal

Local: Burning soles/palms, injection site reactions (pain, redness, swelling), phlebitis, thrombophlebitis,

Neuromuscular & skeletal: Aches, arthralgia, back pain, joint stiffness, myalgia

Ocular: Periorbital edema

Renal: Proteinuria, renal function tests abnormal

Respiratory: Dyspnea, pleural effusion, respiratory distress

Miscellaneous: Anaphylactic reaction, diaphoresis, lymphadenopathy, night sweats, serum sickness, viral infection

Rare but important or life-threatening: Abdominal pain, acute renal failure, anaphylactoid reaction, anemia, aplasia, apnea, confusion, cough, deep vein thrombosis, disorientation, dizziness, eosinophilia, epigastric pain, epistaxis, erythema, faintness, flank pain, GI bleeding, GI perforation, granulocytopenia, hemolysis, hemolytic anemia, herpes simplex reactivation, hiccups, hyperglycemia, iliac vein obstruction, infection, involuntary movement, kidney enlarged/ruptured, laryngospasm, malaise, neutropenia, pancytopenia, paresthesia, pulmonary edema, renal artery thrombosis, rigidity, sore mouth/throat, tachycardia, toxic epidermal necrosis, tremor, vasculitis, viral hepatitis, weakness, wound dehiscence

Drug Interactions

Metabolism/Transport Effects None known.

Avoid Concomitant Use

Avoid concomitant use of Antithymocyte Globulin (Equine) with any of the following: BCG; BCG (Intravesical); Natalizumab; Pimecrolimus; Tacrolimus (Topical); Tofacitinib; Vaccines (Live)

Increased Effect/Toxicity

Antithymocyte Globulin (Equine) may increase the levels/effects of: Leflunomide; Natalizumab; Tofacitinib; Vaccines (Live)

The levels/effects of Antithymocyte Globulin (Equine) may be increased by: Denosumab; Pimecrolimus; Roflumilast; Tacrolimus (Topical); Trastuzumab

Decreased Effect

Antithymocyte Globulin (Equine) may decrease the levels/effects of: BCG; BCG (Intravesical); Coccidioides immitis Skin Test; Sipuleucel-T; Vaccines (Inactivated); Vaccines (Live)

The levels/effects of Antithymocyte Globulin (Equine) may be decreased by: Echinacea

Storage/Stability Refrigerate ampules at 2°C to 8°C (36°F to 46°F). Do not freeze. Do not shake. Solutions diluted for infusion are stable for 24 hours (including infusion time) under refrigeration. Allow infusion solution to reach room temperature prior to administration.

Mechanism of Action Immunosuppressant involved in the elimination of antigen-reactive T lymphocytes (killer cells) in peripheral blood or alteration in the function of T-lymphocytes, which are involved in humoral immunity and partly in cell-mediated immunity; induces complete or partial hematologic response in aplastic anemia

Pharmacokinetics (Adult data unless noted)

Distribution: Poor into lymphoid tissues; binds to circulating lymphocytes, granulocytes, platelets, bone marrow cells

Half-life, plasma: 1.5-12 days

Elimination: ~1% of dose excreted in urine

Dosing: Usual Intradermal skin test is recommended prior to administration of the initial dose of ATG; use 0.1 mL of a fresh 1:1000 dilution of ATG in NS; observe the skin test every 15 minutes for 1 hour; a local reaction ≥10 mm diameter with a wheal or erythema or both should be considered a positive skin test; if a positive skin test occurs, the first infusion should be administered in a controlled environment with intensive life support immediately available. A systemic reaction precludes further administration of the drug. The absence of a reaction does **not** preclude the possibility of an immediate sensitivity reaction.

IV: Children and Adults:

Aplastic anemia protocol: 10-20 mg/kg/day for 8-14 days; additional every other day therapy can be administered up to a total of 21 doses in 28 days. One study (Rosenfeld, 1995) used a dose of 40 mg/kg/day once daily over 4 hours for 4 days.

Renal allograft: Dosage range: Children: 5-25 mg/kg/day; Adults: 10-30 mg/kg/day

Induction dose (delaying the onset of allograft rejection): 15 mg/kg/day for 14 days, then every other day for 14 days for a total of 21 doses in 28 days. Initial dose should be administered within 24 hours before or after transplantation.

Treatment of rejection: 10-15 mg/kg/day for 14 days; additional every other day therapy can be administered up to a total of 21 doses

Acute GVHD treatment (off-label use): 30 mg/kg/dose every other day for 6 doses (MacMillan, 2007) or 15 mg/kg/dose twice daily for 10 doses (MacMillan, 2002)

Dosage adjustment for toxicity:

Anaphylaxis: Stop infusion immediately; administer epinephrine. May require corticosteroids, respiration assistance, and/or other resuscitative measures. Do not resume infusion.

Hemolysis (severe and unremitting): May require discontinuation of treatment

Preparation for Administration IV: Dilute into inverted bottle of sterile vehicle to ensure that undiluted lymphocyte immune globulin does not contact air. Gently rotate or swirl to mix; do not shake. Final concentration should be 4 mg/mL. May be diluted in NS, $D_5{}^{1/4}NS$, $D_5{}^{1/2}NS$ **(do not use D_5W; low salt concentrations may result in precipitation)**.

Administration IV: Infuse dose over at least 4 hours through a 0.2 to 1 micron in-line filter. Allow solution to reach room temperature prior to infusion. Infusion must be completed with 24 hours of preparation. May cause vein irritation (chemical phlebitis) if administered peripherally; infuse into a vascular shunt, arterial venous fistula, or high-flow central vein. Any severe systemic reaction to the skin test, such as generalized rash, tachycardia, dyspnea, hypotension, or anaphylaxis, should preclude further therapy. Epinephrine and resuscitative equipment should be nearby. Patient may need to be pretreated with an antipyretic, antihistamine, and/or corticosteroid. Mild itching and erythema can be treated with antihistamines.

First dose: Premedicate with diphenhydramine orally 30 minutes prior to and hydrocortisone IV 15 minutes prior to infusion and acetaminophen 2 hours after start of infusion.

Monitoring Parameters Lymphocyte profile; CBC with differential and platelet count, vital signs during administration, renal function test

Dosage Forms Excipient information presented when available (limited, particularly for generics); consult specific product labeling.

Injectable, Intravenous:

Atgam: 50 mg/mL (5 mL) [thimerosal free]

Antithymocyte Globulin (Rabbit)

(an te THY moe site GLOB yu lin RAB bit)

Medication Safety Issues

Sound-alike/look-alike issues:

Antithymocyte globulin rabbit (Thymoglobulin®) may be confused with antithymocyte globulin equine (Atgam®)

High alert medication:

This medication is in a class the Institute for Safe Medication Practices (ISMP) includes among its list of drug classes that have a heightened risk of causing significant patient harm when used in error.

Brand Names: US Thymoglobulin

Brand Names: Canada Thymoglobulin

Therapeutic Category Immunosuppressant Agent

Generic Availability (US) No

Use Treatment of acute rejection of renal transplant; used in conjunction with concomitant immunosuppression (FDA approved in adults); has also been used as induction therapy in renal transplant; treatment of myelodysplastic syndrome (MDS); prevention and/or treatment of acute rejection after bone marrow, heart/lung, liver, intestinal, or multivisceral transplantation in conjunction with other immunosuppressive agents

Pregnancy Risk Factor C

Pregnancy Considerations Animal reproduction studies have not been conducted. Women exposed to thymoglobulin during pregnancy may be enrolled in the National Transplantation Pregnancy Registry (877-955-6877).

Breast-Feeding Considerations This product has not been evaluated in nursing women; the manufacturer recommends that breast-feeding be discontinued if therapy is needed.

Contraindications Hypersensitivity to antithymocyte globulin, rabbit proteins, or any component of the formulation; acute or chronic infection

Warnings/Precautions [U.S. Boxed Warning]: Should only be used by physicians experienced in immunosuppressive therapy for the treatment of renal transplant patients. Medical surveillance is required during the infusion. Initial dose must be administered over at least 6 hours into a high flow vein; patient may need pretreatment with an antipyretic, antihistamine, and/or corticosteroid. Hypersensitivity and fatal anaphylactic reactions can occur; immediate treatment (including epinephrine 1:1000) should be available. An increased incidence of lymphoma, post-transplant lymphoproliferative disease (PTLD), other malignancies, or severe infections may develop following concomitant use of immunosuppressants and prolonged use or overdose of antithymocyte globulin. Appropriate antiviral, antibacterial, antiprotozoal, and/or antifungal prophylaxis is recommended. Reversible neutropenia or thrombocytopenia may result from the development of cross-reactive antibodies.

Release of cytokines by activated monocytes and lymphocytes may cause fatal cytokine release syndrome (CRS) during administration of antithymocyte globulin. Rapid infusion rates of have been associated with CRS in case reports. Symptoms range from a mild, self-limiting "flu-like reaction" to severe, life-threatening reactions. Severe or life-threatening symptoms include hypotension, acute respiratory distress syndrome, pulmonary edema, myocardial infarction, and tachycardia. Patients should not be immunized with attenuated live viral vaccines during or shortly after treatment; safety of immunization following therapy has not been studied. Potentially significant drug-drug interactions may exist, requiring dose or frequency adjustment, additional monitoring, and/or selection of alternative therapy.

Adverse Reactions

Cardiovascular: Hypertension, peripheral edema, tachycardia

Central nervous system: Chills, dizziness, fever, headache, malaise, pain

Endocrine & metabolic: Hyperkalemia

Gastrointestinal: Abdominal pain, diarrhea, gastritis, gastrointestinal moniliasis, nausea

Genitourinary: Urinary tract infection

Hematologic: Leukopenia, thrombocytopenia

Neuromuscular & skeletal: Weakness

Respiratory: Dyspnea

Miscellaneous: Antirabbit antibody development, cytomegalovirus infection, herpes simplex infection, oral moniliasis, sepsis, systemic infection

Rare but important or life-threatening: Anaphylaxis, cytokine release syndrome, PTLD, neutropenia, serum sickness (delayed)

Drug Interactions

Metabolism/Transport Effects None known.

Avoid Concomitant Use

Avoid concomitant use of Antithymocyte Globulin (Rabbit) with any of the following: BCG; BCG (Intravesical); Natalizumab; Pimecrolimus; Tacrolimus (Topical); Tofacitinib; Vaccines (Live)

Increased Effect/Toxicity

Antithymocyte Globulin (Rabbit) may increase the levels/effects of: Leflunomide; Natalizumab; Tofacitinib; Vaccines (Live)

The levels/effects of Antithymocyte Globulin (Rabbit) may be increased by: Denosumab; Pimecrolimus; Roflumilast; Tacrolimus (Topical); Trastuzumab

Decreased Effect

Antithymocyte Globulin (Rabbit) may decrease the levels/effects of: BCG; BCG (Intravesical); Coccidioides immitis Skin Test; Sipuleucel-T; Vaccines (Inactivated); Vaccines (Live)

The levels/effects of Antithymocyte Globulin (Rabbit) may be decreased by: Echinacea

Storage/Stability Store powder under refrigeration at 2°C to 8°C (36°F to 46°F); do not freeze. Protect from light. Reconstituted product is stable for up to 24 hours at room temperature; however, since it contains no preservatives, it should be used immediately following reconstitution.

Mechanism of Action Polyclonal antibody which appears to cause immunosuppression by acting on T-cell surface antigens and depleting CD4 lymphocytes

Pharmacodynamics Onset of action (T-cell depletion): Within one day

Pharmacokinetics (Adult data unless noted) Half-life: 2-3 days

Dosing: Usual IV: (refer to individual protocols):

Children:

Bone marrow transplantation: 1.5-3 mg/kg/day once daily for 4 consecutive days before transplantation

Treatment of graft-versus-host disease: 1.5 mg/kg/dose once daily or every other day

Renal transplantation:

Induction: 1-2 mg/kg/day once daily for 4-5 days initiated at time of transplant

Acute rejection: 1.5mg/kg/day once daily for 7-14 days

Heart/lung transplantation:

Induction: 1-2 mg/kg/day depending on baseline platelet count once daily for 5 days

Rejection: 2 mg/kg/day once daily for 5 days

Liver, intestinal, or multivisceral transplant:

Preconditioning/induction: Pretransplant: 2 mg/kg; postop day 1: 3 mg/kg

Rejection: 1.5 mg/kg/day once daily for 7-14 days based upon biopsy results; maximum dose: 2 mg/kg/dose

Adults: Acute renal transplant rejection: 1.5 mg/kg/day once daily for 7-14 days

Preparation for Administration Parenteral: Allow vials to reach room temperature, then reconstitute each vial with 5 mL SWFI. Rotate vial gently until dissolved; resulting concentration is 5 mg/mL of thymoglobulin. Further dilute dose to a final concentration of 0.5 mg/mL (eg, one vial (25 mg) in 50 mL saline or dextrose); in adults, total volume is usually 50 to 500 mL depending on total number of vials needed per dose. Mix by gently inverting infusion bag once or twice.

Administration Parenteral: Administer by slow IV infusion over 6 to 12 hours for the preconditioning/induction dose or over 6 hours for the initial acute rejection treatment dose; infuse over 4 hours for subsequent doses if first dose tolerated. Administer through an in-line filter with pore size of 0.22 microns via central line or high flow vein. Premedication with corticosteroids, acetaminophen, and/or an antihistamine may reduce infusion-related reactions.

Monitoring Parameters Platelet count, CBC with differential, lymphocyte count, vital signs during infusion

Test Interactions Potential interference with rabbit antibody-based immunoassays

Additional Information Antiviral therapy should be given prophylactically during antithymocyte globulin (rabbit) use.

Dosage Forms Excipient information presented when available (limited, particularly for generics); consult specific product labeling.

Solution Reconstituted, Intravenous:

Thymoglobulin: 25 mg (1 ea) [contains glycine, mannitol, sodium chloride]

◆ **Antithymocyte Immunoglobulin** *see* Antithymocyte Globulin (Equine) *on page 178*

◆ **Antithymocyte Immunoglobulin** *see* Antithymocyte Globulin (Rabbit) *on page 180*

◆ **Antitoxin** *see* Botulism Antitoxin, Heptavalent *on page 297*

◆ **Antitumor Necrosis Factor Alpha (Human)** *see* Adalimumab *on page 67*

◆ **Anti-VEGF Monoclonal Antibody** *see* Bevacizumab *on page 285*

◆ **Anti-VEGF rhuMAb** *see* Bevacizumab *on page 285*

◆ **Antivenin (*Centruroides*) Immune F(ab')$_2$ (Equine)** *see* *Centruroides* Immune F(ab')$_2$ (Equine) *on page 421*

◆ **Antivenin (Crotalidae) Polyvalent, FAB (Ovine)** *see* *Crotalidae* Polyvalent Immune Fab (Ovine) *on page 543*

Antivenin (*Latrodectus mactans*)

(an tee VEN in lak tro DUK tus MAK tans)

Therapeutic Category Antivenin

Generic Availability (US) Yes

Use Treatment of patients with symptoms (eg, cramping, intractable pain, hypertension) refractory to supportive measures due to *Latrodectus mactans* (black widow spider) envenomation (FDA approved in children and adults); has also been used for treatment of patients with symptoms (eg, cramping, intractable pain, hypertension) refractory to supportive measures due to other *Latrodectus* spp (including *L. bishopi*, *L. geometricus*, *L. hesperus*, and *L. variolus*) envenomation

Pregnancy Risk Factor C

Pregnancy Considerations Animal reproduction studies have not been conducted. Use during pregnancy (second and third trimester) has been described in case reports; all patients delivered healthy infants (Handel, 1994; Russell, 1979; Sherman, 2000). In general, medications used as antidotes should take into consideration the health and prognosis of the mother; antidotes should be administered to pregnant women if there is a clear indication for use and should not be withheld because of fears of teratogenicity (Bailey, 2003). Treatment of a pregnant patient with antivenom should be considered early in the course of an envenomation and in patients experiencing local, regional, or systemic effects refractory to opioids and/or benzodiazepines (Brown, 2013).

Breast-Feeding Considerations It is not known if antivenin (*Latrodectus mactans*) is excreted in breast milk. The manufacturer recommends that caution be exercised when administering antivenin (*Latrodectus mactans*) to nursing women.

Warnings/Precautions Carefully review allergies and history of exposure to products containing horse serum. History of atopic sensitivity to horses may increase risk of immediate sensitivity reactions. Use with caution in patients with asthma, hay fever, or urticaria; fatal anaphylaxis has been reported in patients with a history of asthma. All patients require close monitoring in a setting where resuscitation can be performed. Allergic reactions occur less frequently than described in initial studies (Clark, 2001; Offerman, 2011). One retrospective study reviewed 163 cases of black widow spider envenomation; 58 patients received antivenin therapy and only 1 case of anaphylaxis occurred (Clark, 1992). The risk of reaction appears to be greatest with bolus administration of undiluted antivenin (Clark, 2001). A skin or conjunctival test may be performed prior to use; however, the utility of skin and conjunctival tests to accurately identify patients at risk of early (anaphylactic) or late (serum sickness) hypersensitivity reactions to horse-derived antivenins has been questioned (WHO, 2005). Normal horse serum (1:10 dilution) is included for sensitivity testing. The absence of a skin or conjunctival hypersensitivity reaction does not exclude the possibility of anaphylaxis or hypersensitivity following antivenin administration. The false-negative rate for skin testing is 10% with similar agents. Conversely, hypersensitivity is not an absolute contraindication in a significantly envenomated patient. A desensitization protocol is available if sensitivity tests are mildly or questionably positive to reduce risk of immediate severe hypersensitivity reaction. According to the manufacturer, desensitization should be performed when antivenin administration would be lifesaving; however, the risk of anaphylaxis should be weighed against the risks associated with delayed antivenin administration (Rojnuckarin, 2009). Due to an increased risk for complications of envenomation, the administration of antivenin may be the preferred initial therapy in patients >60 years of age. Delayed serum sickness, albeit uncommon, may occur 1 to 2 weeks following administration, especially when large doses are used (Clark, 2001). Some products may contain thimerosal.

Adverse Reactions

Dermatologic: Rash (rare; associated with hypersensitivity reaction)

Neuromuscular & skeletal: Muscle cramps

Miscellaneous: Anaphylaxis, hypersensitivity reactions, serum sickness

Drug Interactions

Metabolism/Transport Effects None known.

Avoid Concomitant Use There are no known interactions where it is recommended to avoid concomitant use.

Increased Effect/Toxicity There are no known significant interactions involving an increase in effect.

Decreased Effect There are no known significant interactions involving a decrease in effect.

Storage/Stability Refrigerate at 2°C to 8°C (36°F to 46°F). Do not freeze.

Note: As of July 2014, the U.S. Food and Drug Administration (FDA) has granted extended expiration dating for antivenin lot 0672105 (contained in packaged lot H019984) until January 3, 2015. However, the extension does not apply to the manufacturer-supplied sterile diluent; do not use expired diluent. Further information may be found at http://www.fda.gov/BiologicsBloodVaccines/SafetyAvailability/ucm404162.htm.

Mechanism of Action Neutralizes the venom of *Latrodectus mactans* (black widow spiders), but may also be effective following envenomation by other *Latrodectus* species (including *L. bishopi, L. geometricus, L. hesperus,* and *L. variolus*) (Clark, 2001; Isbister, 2003).

Pharmacodynamics Onset of action: Within 30 minutes with envenomation symptoms subsiding after 1-3 hours

Dosing: Usual

Infants, Children, and Adolescents: **Note:** Limited data in infants (Monte 2011; Nordt, 2012). The initial dose of antivenin should be administered as soon as possible for prompt relief of symptoms. Delayed antivenin administration may still be effective in treating patients with prolonged or refractory symptoms resulting from black widow spider bites; a case report describes use of antivenin administration up to 90 hours after bite (O'Malley, 1999); however, delayed administration may decrease effectiveness (Edberg, 2009).

Sensitivity testing: Intradermal skin test or conjunctival test may be performed prior to antivenin administration:

Skin test: Intradermal: Up to 0.02 mL of a 1:10 dilution of normal horse serum (provided in kit) in NS; evaluate after 10 minutes against a control test (intradermal injection of 0.02 mL NS). **Note:** Positive reaction consists of an urticarial wheal surrounded by a zone of erythema.

Conjunctival test: Instill 1 drop of 1:100 dilution of normal horse serum into conjunctival sac; a positive reaction is indicated by itching of the eye and/or reddening of conjunctiva, usually occurring within 10 minutes

Desensitization: In separate vials or syringes, prepare 1:10 and 1:100 dilutions of antivenin in NS:

SubQ: Inject 0.1 mL, followed by 0.2 mL and 0.5 mL of a 1:100 dilution at 15- to 30-minute intervals. During desensitization procedure, proceed with the next dose only if a reaction has **not** occurred following the previous dose. Repeat procedure with a 1:10 dilution of antivenin; and then with undiluted antivenin. If no reaction has occurred following administration of 0.5 mL of undiluted antivenin, continue the dose at 15-minute intervals until the entire dose has been administered.

If a reaction occurs, apply a tourniquet proximal to the injection site and administer epinephrine (1:1000) SubQ or IV proximal to the tourniquet or into another extremity. Wait at least 30 minutes, then administer another antivenin injection at the previous dilution which did not evoke a reaction.

***Latrodectus mactans* (black widow spider) envenomation; other *Latrodectus* spp envenomation** (Clark, 2001): Limited data available for some types of envenomations. **Note:** If a positive reaction to a skin or conjunctival test occurs and antivenin therapy is necessary, pretreat the patient with intravenous diphenhydramine and an H_2-blocker while having a syringe of epinephrine (1:1000) at the bedside:

Infants and Children <12 years: IM; IV (preferred): One vial (2.5 mL); a second dose may be needed in some cases; more than 1 to 2 vials are rarely required

Children ≥12 years and Adolescents: IM, IV: One vial (2.5 mL); a second dose may be needed in some cases; more than 1 to 2 vials are rarely required

Adults: The initial dose of antivenin should be administered as soon as possible for prompt relief of symptoms. Delayed antivenin administration may still be effective in treating patients with prolonged or refractory symptoms resulting from black widow spider bites; case report of antivenin administration up to 90 hours after bite (O'Malley, 1999); however, delayed administration may decrease effectiveness (Edberg, 2009).

Sensitivity testing: Intradermal skin test or conjunctival test may be performed prior to antivenin administration:

Skin test: Intradermal: Up to 0.02 mL of a 1:10 dilution of normal horse serum in NS; evaluate after 10 minutes against a control test (intradermal injection of NS). **Note:** A positive reaction is an urticarial wheal surrounded by a zone of erythema.

Conjunctival test: Ophthalmic: Instill 1 drop of a 1:10 dilution of normal horse serum into the conjunctival sac; **Note:** Itching of the eye and/or reddening of conjunctiva indicates a positive reaction, usually occurring within 10 minutes.

Desensitization: In separate vials or syringes, prepare 1:10 and 1:100 dilutions of antivenin in NS.

SubQ: Inject 0.1 mL, 0.2 mL, and 0.5 mL of the 1:100 dilution at 15- to 30-minute intervals. During this procedure, proceed with the next dose only if a reaction has **not** occurred following the previous dose. Repeat procedure using the 1:10 dilution and then undiluted antivenin. If no reaction has occurred following administration of 0.5 mL of undiluted antivenin, continue the dose at 15-minute intervals until the entire dose has been administered.

If a reaction occurs, apply a tourniquet proximal to the injection site and administer epinephrine (1:1000) SubQ or IV proximal to the tourniquet or into another extremity. Wait at least 30 minutes; then administer another antivenin injection at the previous dilution which did not evoke a reaction.

Dosing adjustment for renal impairment: There are no dosage adjustments provided in the manufacturer's labeling.

Dosing adjustment for hepatic impairment: There are no dosage adjustments provided in the manufacturer's labeling.

Preparation for Administration Parenteral: Reconstitute vial with 2.5 mL of the provided diluent or SWFI. With needle still in rubber stopper, shake vial to dissolve. Excessive agitation or shaking of the reconstituted vial may cause foaming, which may lead to denaturation of the antivenin. When reconstituted, solution can range from a light straw to a dark tea color.

IV: Further dilute in 10 to 50 mL NS. When reconstituted, solution can range from a light straw to a dark tea color. **Note:** IV is the preferred route in severe cases with shock or in children <12 years of age.

Administration

IM: Administer into the anterolateral thigh. Apply tourniquet if an adverse reaction occurs.

IV: Infuse over 15 to 30 minutes (Clark 2001). IV administration preferred in severe cases, with shock, or in children <12 years of age. There appears to be no clinical difference in efficacy between the IM and IV route of administration (Isbister 2008). If an immediate hypersensitivity reaction occurs, immediately interrupt antivenin infusion and provide appropriate supportive therapy. If administration of antivenin can be resumed after control of the reaction, reinitiate at a slower infusion rate.

Monitoring Parameters Vital signs; hypersensitivity reactions; serum sickness (for 8-12 days following administration); worsening of symptoms due to envenomation

Additional Information The venom of the black widow spider is a neurotoxin that causes release of a presynaptic neurotransmitter. Within 1 hour of the bite, the clinical effects of black widow spider envenomation (BWSE) include sharp pain, muscle spasm, weakness, tremor, severe abdominal pain with rigidity, hypertension, respiratory distress, diaphoresis, and facial swelling. Priapism has been reported in pediatric patients following BWSE (Hoover, 2004; Quan, 2009).

Dosage Forms Excipient information presented when available (limited, particularly for generics); consult specific product labeling.

Kit, Injection:

Generic: 6000 Antivenin units

- **Apo-Modafinil (Can)** *see* Modafinil *on page 1450*
- **Apo-Mometasone (Can)** *see* Mometasone (Nasal) *on page 1454*
- **Apo-Montelukast (Can)** *see* Montelukast *on page 1459*
- **Apo-Mycophenolate (Can)** *see* Mycophenolate *on page 1473*
- **Apo-Nadol (Can)** *see* Nadolol *on page 1480*
- **Apo-Napro-Na (Can)** *see* Naproxen *on page 1489*
- **Apo-Napro-Na DS (Can)** *see* Naproxen *on page 1489*
- **Apo-Naproxen (Can)** *see* Naproxen *on page 1489*
- **Apo-Naproxen EC (Can)** *see* Naproxen *on page 1489*
- **Apo-Naproxen SR (Can)** *see* Naproxen *on page 1489*
- **Apo-Nifed PA (Can)** *see* NIFEdipine *on page 1516*
- **Apo-Nitrofurantoin (Can)** *see* Nitrofurantoin *on page 1521*
- **Apo-Nizatidine (Can)** *see* Nizatidine *on page 1528*
- **Apo-Nortriptyline (Can)** *see* Nortriptyline *on page 1532*
- **Apo-Oflox (Can)** *see* Ofloxacin (Systemic) *on page 1542*
- **Apo-Olanzapine (Can)** *see* OLANZapine *on page 1546*
- **Apo-Olanzapine ODT (Can)** *see* OLANZapine *on page 1546*
- **Apo-Omeprazole (Can)** *see* Omeprazole *on page 1555*
- **Apo-Ondansetron (Can)** *see* Ondansetron *on page 1564*
- **Apo-Orciprenaline® (Can)** *see* Metaproterenol *on page 1374*
- **Apo-Oxaprozin (Can)** *see* Oxaprozin *on page 1582*
- **Apo-Oxybutynin (Can)** *see* Oxybutynin *on page 1588*
- **Apo-Oxycodone/Acet (Can)** *see* Oxycodone and Acetaminophen *on page 1594*
- **Apo-Oxycodone CR (Can)** *see* OxyCODONE *on page 1590*
- **APOP [DSC]** *see* Sulfacetamide (Topical) *on page 1982*
- **Apo-Paclitaxel (Can)** *see* PACLitaxel (Conventional) *on page 1602*
- **Apo-Pantoprazole (Can)** *see* Pantoprazole *on page 1618*
- **Apo-Paroxetine (Can)** *see* PARoxetine *on page 1634*
- **Apo-Pen VK (Can)** *see* Penicillin V Potassium *on page 1660*
- **Apo-Perphenazine® (Can)** *see* Perphenazine *on page 1676*
- **Apo-Pimozide® (Can)** *see* Pimozide *on page 1704*
- **Apo-Piroxicam (Can)** *see* Piroxicam *on page 1710*
- **Apo-Pravastatin (Can)** *see* Pravastatin *on page 1749*
- **Apo-Prazo (Can)** *see* Prazosin *on page 1752*
- **Apo-Prednisone (Can)** *see* PredniSONE *on page 1760*
- **Apo-Primidone® (Can)** *see* Primidone *on page 1766*
- **Apo-Procainamide (Can)** *see* Procainamide *on page 1769*
- **Apo-Prochlorperazine (Can)** *see* Prochlorperazine *on page 1774*
- **Apo-Propranolol (Can)** *see* Propranolol *on page 1789*
- **Apo-Quetiapine (Can)** *see* QUEtiapine *on page 1815*
- **Apo-Quinapril (Can)** *see* Quinapril *on page 1820*
- **Apo-Quinidine (Can)** *see* QuiNIDine *on page 1822*
- **Apo-Quinine® (Can)** *see* QuiNINE *on page 1825*
- **Apo-Rabeprazole (Can)** *see* RABEprazole *on page 1828*
- **Apo-Ranitidine (Can)** *see* Ranitidine *on page 1836*
- **Apo-Risperidone (Can)** *see* RisperiDONE *on page 1866*
- **Apo-Rizatriptan (Can)** *see* Rizatriptan *on page 1879*
- **Apo-Rizatriptan RPD (Can)** *see* Rizatriptan *on page 1879*
- **Apo-Rosuvastatin (Can)** *see* Rosuvastatin *on page 1886*
- **Apo-Salvent (Can)** *see* Albuterol *on page 81*
- **Apo-Salvent AEM (Can)** *see* Albuterol *on page 81*
- **Apo-Salvent CFC Free (Can)** *see* Albuterol *on page 81*
- **Apo-Salvent Sterules (Can)** *see* Albuterol *on page 81*
- **Apo-Sertraline (Can)** *see* Sertraline *on page 1916*
- **Apo-Sildenafil (Can)** *see* Sildenafil *on page 1921*
- **Apo-Simvastatin (Can)** *see* Simvastatin *on page 1928*
- **Apo-Sotalol (Can)** *see* Sotalol *on page 1963*
- **Apo-Sucralfate (Can)** *see* Sucralfate *on page 1978*
- **Apo-Sulfasalazine (Can)** *see* SulfaSALAzine *on page 1990*
- **Apo-Sulfatrim (Can)** *see* Sulfamethoxazole and Trimethoprim *on page 1986*
- **Apo-Sulfatrim DS (Can)** *see* Sulfamethoxazole and Trimethoprim *on page 1986*
- **Apo-Sulfatrim Pediatric (Can)** *see* Sulfamethoxazole and Trimethoprim *on page 1986*
- **Apo-Sulin (Can)** *see* Sulindac *on page 1994*
- **Apo-Sumatriptan (Can)** *see* SUMAtriptan *on page 1995*
- **Apo-Tamox (Can)** *see* Tamoxifen *on page 2005*
- **Apo-Tamsulosin CR (Can)** *see* Tamsulosin *on page 2008*
- **Apo-Terazosin (Can)** *see* Terazosin *on page 2020*
- **Apo-Terbinafine (Can)** *see* Terbinafine (Systemic) *on page 2021*
- **Apo-Tetra (Can)** *see* Tetracycline *on page 2035*
- **Apo-Theo LA® (Can)** *see* Theophylline *on page 2044*
- **Apo-Timop® (Can)** *see* Timolol (Ophthalmic) *on page 2067*
- **Apo-Topiramate (Can)** *see* Topiramate *on page 2085*
- **Apo-Tramadol (Can)** *see* TraMADol *on page 2098*
- **Apo-Travoprost Z (Can)** *see* Travoprost *on page 2104*
- **Apo-Trazodone (Can)** *see* TraZODone *on page 2105*
- **Apo-Trazodone D (Can)** *see* TraZODone *on page 2105*
- **Apo-Trimethoprim® (Can)** *see* Trimethoprim *on page 2126*
- **Apo-Valacyclovir (Can)** *see* ValACYclovir *on page 2138*
- **Apo-Valganciclovir (Can)** *see* ValGANciclovir *on page 2139*
- **Apo-Valproic (Can)** *see* Valproic Acid and Derivatives *on page 2143*
- **Apo-Valsartan (Can)** *see* Valsartan *on page 2149*
- **Apo-Venlafaxine XR (Can)** *see* Venlafaxine *on page 2166*
- **Apo-Verap (Can)** *see* Verapamil *on page 2170*
- **Apo-Verap SR (Can)** *see* Verapamil *on page 2170*
- **Apo-Voriconazole (Can)** *see* Voriconazole *on page 2190*
- **Apo-Warfarin (Can)** *see* Warfarin *on page 2195*
- **Apo-Zidovudine (Can)** *see* Zidovudine *on page 2207*
- **APPG** *see* Penicillin G Procaine *on page 1659*
- **Apprilon (Can)** *see* Doxycycline *on page 717*

Aprepitant (ap RE pi tant)

Medication Safety Issues

Sound-alike/look-alike issues:

Aprepitant may be confused with fosaprepitant

Emend (aprepitant) oral capsule formulation may be confused with Emend for injection (fosaprepitant)

Related Information

Prevention of Chemotherapy-Induced Nausea and Vomiting in Children *on page* 2368

Brand Names: US Emend

Brand Names: Canada Emend

Therapeutic Category Antiemetic; Substance P/Neurokinin 1 Receptor Antagonist

Generic Availability (US) No

Use Prevention of acute and delayed nausea and vomiting associated with initial and repeat courses of moderate and highly emetogenic cancer chemotherapy (MEC & HEC) (in combination with other antiemetic agents); prevention of postoperative nausea and vomiting (PONV) (All indications: FDA approved in adults)

Pregnancy Risk Factor B

Pregnancy Considerations Adverse events were not observed in animal reproduction studies. Use during pregnancy only if clearly needed. Efficacy of hormonal contraceptive may be reduced; alternative or additional methods of contraception should be used both during treatment with fosaprepitant or aprepitant and for at least 1 month following the last fosaprepitant/aprepitant dose.

Breast-Feeding Considerations It is not known if aprepitant is excreted in breast milk. Due to the potential for adverse reactions in the nursing infant, the decision to discontinue aprepitant or to discontinue breast-feeding should take into account the benefits of treatment to the mother.

Contraindications Hypersensitivity to aprepitant or any component of the formulation; concurrent use with cisapride or pimozide

Warnings/Precautions Potentially significant drug-drug interactions may exist, requiring dose or frequency adjustment, additional monitoring, and/or selection of alternative therapy. Use caution with severe hepatic impairment (Child-Pugh class C); has not been studied. Not studied for treatment of existing nausea and vomiting. Chronic continuous administration is not recommended.

Adverse Reactions Note: Adverse reactions reported as part of a combination chemotherapy regimen or with general anesthesia.

Cardiovascular: Bradycardia, hypotension

Central nervous system: Dizziness, fatigue

Endocrine & metabolic: Dehydration

Gastrointestinal: Abdominal pain, constipation, diarrhea, dyspepsia, epigastric distress, gastritis, hiccups, nausea, stomatitis

Genitourinary Proteinuria

Hepatic: Increased serum ALT, increased serum AST

Neuromuscular & skeletal: Weakness

Renal: Increased blood urea nitrogen

Rare but important or life-threatening: Acid regurgitation, acne vulgaris, anaphylaxis, anemia, angioedema, anxiety, arthralgia, back pain, candidiasis, confusion, conjunctivitis, cough, decreased appetite, decreased serum albumin, decreased visual acuity, deep vein thrombosis, depression, diabetes mellitus, diaphoresis, disorientation, dysarthria, dysgeusia, dysphagia, dyspnea, dysuria, edema, enterocolitis, eructation, erythrocyturia, febrile neutropenia, flatulence, flushing, glycosuria, herpes simplex infection, hyperglycemia, hypersensitivity reaction, hypertension, hypoesthesia, hypokalemia, hyponatremia, hypothermia, hypovolemia, hypoxia, increased serum alkaline phosphatase, increased serum bilirubin, leukocytosis, leukocyturia, malaise, miosis, musculoskeletal pain, myalgia, myasthenia, myocardial infarction, neutropenic sepsis, obstipation, pain, palpitations, pelvic pain, perforated duodenal ulcer, peripheral neuropathy, peripheral sensory neuropathy, pharyngitis, pharyngolaryngeal pain, pneumonia, pneumonitis, pruritus, pulmonary embolism, renal insufficiency, respiratory insufficiency, respiratory tract infection, rhinorrhea, rigors, sensory disturbance, septic shock, sialorrhea, skin rash, Stevens-Johnson syndrome, syncope, tachycardia, thrombocytopenia, toxic epidermal necrolysis, tremor, urinary tract infection, urticaria, voice disorder, weight loss, wheezing, xerostomia

Drug Interactions

Metabolism/Transport Effects Substrate of CYP1A2 (minor), CYP2C19 (minor), CYP3A4 (major); **Note:** Assignment of Major/Minor substrate status based on clinically relevant drug interaction potential; **Inhibits** CYP2C19 (weak), CYP2C9 (weak), CYP3A4 (moderate); **Induces** CYP2C9 (strong), CYP3A4 (weak)

Avoid Concomitant Use

Avoid concomitant use of Aprepitant with any of the following: Bosutinib; Cisapride; Conivaptan; Domperidone; Fusidic Acid (Systemic); Ibrutinib; Idelalisib; Ivabradine; Lomitapide; Naloxegol; Olaparib; Pimozide; Simeprevir; Tolvaptan; Trabectedin; Ulipristal

Increased Effect/Toxicity

Aprepitant may increase the levels/effects of: Avanafil; Bosentan; Bosutinib; Budesonide (Systemic, Oral Inhalation); Budesonide (Topical); Cannabis; Cilostazol; Cisapride; Colchicine; Corticosteroids (Systemic); CYP3A4 Substrates; Dapoxetine; Diltiazem; Dofetilide; Domperidone; DOXOrubicin (Conventional); Dronabinol; Eliglustat; Eplerenone; Everolimus; FentaNYL; Halofantrine; Hydrocodone; Ibrutinib; Ifosfamide; Imatinib; Ivabradine; Ivacaftor; Lomitapide; Lurasidone; Naloxegol; NiMODipine; Olaparib; OxyCODONE; Pimecrolimus; Pimozide; Propafenone; Ranolazine; Rivaroxaban; Salmeterol; Saxagliptin; Simeprevir; Sirolimus; Suvorexant; Tetrahydrocannabinol; Tolvaptan; Trabectedin; Ulipristal; Vilazodone; Zopiclone; Zuclopenthixol

The levels/effects of Aprepitant may be increased by: Conivaptan; CYP3A4 Inhibitors (Moderate); CYP3A4 Inhibitors (Strong); Dasatinib; Diltiazem; Fosaprepitant; Fusidic Acid (Systemic); Idelalisib; Luliconazole; Mifepristone; Netupitant; Palbociclib; Stiripentol

Decreased Effect

Aprepitant may decrease the levels/effects of: ARIPiprazole; Contraceptives (Estrogens); Contraceptives (Progestins); CYP2C9 Substrates; Diclofenac (Systemic); Hydrocodone; NiMODipine; PARoxetine; Saxagliptin; TOLBUTamide; Warfarin

The levels/effects of Aprepitant may be decreased by: Bosentan; CYP3A4 Inducers (Moderate); CYP3A4 Inducers (Strong); Dabrafenib; Deferasirox; Mitotane; PARoxetine; Rifampin; Siltuximab; St Johns Wort; Tocilizumab

Food Interactions Aprepitant serum concentration may be increased when taken with grapefruit juice. Management: Avoid concurrent use.

Storage/Stability Store at room temperature of 20°C to 25°C (68°F to 77°F).

Mechanism of Action Prevents acute and delayed vomiting by inhibiting the substance P/neurokinin 1 (NK_1) receptor; augments the antiemetic activity of 5-HT_3 receptor antagonists and corticosteroids to inhibit acute and delayed phases of chemotherapy-induced emesis.

Pharmacokinetics (Adult data unless noted)

Distribution: V_d: ~70 L; crosses the blood-brain barrier

Protein binding: >95%

Metabolism: Extensively hepatic via CYP3A4 (major); CYP1A2 and CYP2C19 (minor); forms 7 metabolites (weakly active)
Bioavailability: 60% to 65%
Half-life: ~9-13 hours
Time to peak serum concentration: 3-4 hours
Elimination: Primarily via metabolism

Dosing: Usual

Pediatric:

Chemotherapy-induced nausea and vomiting (CINV), prevention: Limited data available:

Highly emetogenic chemotherapy: **Note:** Use in combination with 5-HT3 antagonist antiemetic ± dexamethasone

Children <12 years: Efficacy results variable; optimal dose not established; dosinog based on two small trials: Oral:

<10 kg: 40 mg on day 1, followed by 20 mg on days 2 and 3 (Bodge, 2014)

10 to <15 kg: 80 mg on day 1, followed by 40 mg on days 2 and 3 (Bodge, 2014; Choi, 2010).

15 to 20 kg: Dosing regimens variable: 80 mg once daily for 3 days has been described in a retrospective trial (n=7) (Choi, 2010); another small trial used 80 mg once on day 1, followed by 40 mg on days 2 and 3 (Bodge, 2014)

>20 kg: 125 mg 30 minutes prior to chemotherapy on day 1, followed by 80 mg once daily on days 2 and 3 has been described in a retrospective trial (n=24; mean age: 10 years) (Choi, 2010)

Children ≥12 years and Adolescents: POGO recommendations (Dupuis, 2013): Oral: 125 mg prior to chemotherapy on day 1, followed by 80 mg once daily on days 2 and 3

Moderately emetogenic chemotherapy: Efficacy results variable; optimal dose not established: Children and Adolescents: Oral:

<10 kg: 40 mg on day 1, followed by 20 mg on days 2 and 3 (Bodge, 2014)

10 to <15 kg: Dosing regimens variable: 80 mg on day 1, followed by 40 mg on days 2 and 3 (Bodge, 2014; Choi, 2010)

15 to 20 kg: Dosing regimens variable: 80 mg once daily for 3 days has been described in a retrospective trial (n=7) (Choi, 2010); another small trial used 80 mg once on day 1, followed by 40 mg on days 2 and 3 (Bodge, 2014)

>20 kg: 125 mg 30 minutes prior to chemotherapy on day 1, followed by 80 mg once daily on days 2 and 3 has been described in a retrospective trial (n=24; mean age: 10 years) (Choi, 2010)

Adult:

Chemotherapy-induced nausea and vomiting, prevention: Oral:

Highly emetogenic chemotherapy: 125 mg 1 hour prior to chemotherapy on day 1, followed by 80 mg once daily on days 2 and 3 (in combination with a 5-HT_3 antagonist antiemetic on day 1 and dexamethasone on days 1-4)

Moderately emetogenic chemotherapy: 125 mg 1 hour prior to chemotherapy on day 1, followed by 80 mg once daily on days 2 and 3 (in combination with a 5-HT_3 antagonist antiemetic and dexamethasone on day 1)

Postoperative nausea and vomiting (PONV), prevention: Oral: 40 mg within 3 hours prior to induction

Dosing adjustment in renal impairment: Adult:

Mild, moderate, or severe impairment: No dosage adjustment necessary.

Dialysis-dependent end-stage renal disease (ESRD): No dosage adjustment necessary.

Dosing adjustment in hepatic impairment: Adult:

Mild to moderate impairment (Child-Pugh class A or B): No dosage adjustment necessary.

Severe impairment (Child-Pugh class C): Use with caution; no data available

Administration Oral: May be administered without regard to food, 1 hour prior to chemotherapy on day 1 of treatment and in the morning on the subsequent next 2 days or within 3 hours prior to induction of anesthesia.

Dosage Forms Excipient information presented when available (limited, particularly for generics); consult specific product labeling.

Capsule, Oral:

Emend: 40 mg, 80 mg, 125 mg, 80 mg & 125 mg

Extemporaneous Preparations A 20 mg/mL oral aprepitant suspension may be prepared with capsules and a 1:1 combination of Ora-Sweet® and Ora-Plus® (or Ora-Blend®). Empty the contents of four 125 mg capsules into a mortar and reduce to a fine powder (process will take 10-15 minutes). Add small portions of vehicle and mix to a uniform paste. Add sufficient vehicle to form a liquid; transfer to a graduated cylinder, rinse mortar with vehicle, and add quantity of vehicle sufficient to make 25 mL. Label "shake well" and "refrigerate". Stable for 90 days refrigerated.

Dupuis LL, Lingertat-Walsh K, and Walker SE, "Stability of an Extemporaneous Oral Liquid Aprepitant Formulation," *Support Care Cancer*, 2009, 17(6):701-6.

- **Aprepitant Injection** *see* Fosaprepitant *on page 939*
- **Apresoline** *see* HydrALAZINE *on page 1027*
- **Apriso** *see* Mesalamine *on page 1368*
- **Aprodine [OTC]** *see* Triprolidine and Pseudoephedrine *on page 2129*
- **Aptensio XR** *see* Methylphenidate *on page 1402*
- **Aptivus** *see* Tipranavir *on page 2070*
- **Aquacort® (Can)** *see* Hydrocortisone (Topical) *on page 1041*
- **AquaMEPHYTON® (Can)** *see* Phytonadione *on page 1698*
- **Aquanil HC [OTC]** *see* Hydrocortisone (Topical) *on page 1041*
- **Aquasol A** *see* Vitamin A *on page 2186*
- **Aquasol E [OTC]** *see* Vitamin E *on page 2188*
- **Aquavit-E [OTC]** *see* Vitamin E *on page 2188*
- **Aqueous Procaine Penicillin G** *see* Penicillin G Procaine *on page 1659*
- **Aqueous Selenium [OTC]** *see* Selenium *on page 1912*
- **Aqueous Vitamin D [OTC]** *see* Cholecalciferol *on page 448*
- **Aqueous Vitamin E [OTC]** *see* Vitamin E *on page 2188*
- **Ara-C** *see* Cytarabine (Conventional) *on page 566*
- **Arabinosylcytosine** *see* Cytarabine (Conventional) *on page 566*
- **Aralen** *see* Chloroquine *on page 437*
- **Aranesp (Can)** *see* Darbepoetin Alfa *on page 585*
- **Aranesp (Albumin Free)** *see* Darbepoetin Alfa *on page 585*
- **Arbinoxa** *see* Carbinoxamine *on page 372*
- **Arcalyst** *see* Rilonacept *on page 1862*
- **Aredia (Can)** *see* Pamidronate *on page 1611*
- **Arestin Microspheres (Can)** *see* Minocycline *on page 1440*

Argatroban (ar GA troh ban)

Medication Safety Issues

Sound-alike/look-alike issues:

Argatroban may be confused with Aggrastat, Orgaran

High alert medication:

The Institute for Safe Medication Practices (ISMP) includes this medication among its list of drugs which have a heightened risk of causing significant patient harm when used in error.

Therapeutic Category Anticoagulant, Thrombin Inhibitor

Generic Availability (US) Yes

Use Prophylaxis or treatment of thrombosis in patients with heparin-induced thrombocytopenia (HIT) (FDA approved in adults); anticoagulant for percutaneous coronary intervention (PCI) in patients who have or are at risk for thrombosis associated HIT (FDA approved in adults). Has also been studied in children with HIT for procedural anticoagulation including cardiac catheterization, extracorporeal membrane oxygenation (ECMO), and hemodialysis/hemofiltration

Pregnancy Risk Factor B

Pregnancy Considerations Adverse events were not observed in animal studies. Information related to argatroban in pregnancy is limited. Use of parenteral direct thrombin inhibitors in pregnancy should be limited to those women who have severe allergic reactions to heparin, including heparin-induced thrombocytopenia, and who cannot receive danaparoid (Guyatt, 2012).

Breast-Feeding Considerations It is not known if argatroban is excreted in human milk. Because of the serious potential of adverse effects to the nursing infant, a decision to discontinue nursing or discontinue argatroban should be considered.

Contraindications Hypersensitivity to argatroban or any component of the formulation; major bleeding

Warnings/Precautions Hemorrhage can occur at any site in the body. Extreme caution should be used when there is an increased danger of hemorrhage, such as severe hypertension, immediately following lumbar puncture, spinal anesthesia, major surgery (including brain, spinal cord, or eye surgery), congenital or acquired bleeding disorders, and gastrointestinal ulcers. Use caution in critically-ill patients; reduced clearance may require dosage reduction. Use caution with hepatic dysfunction. Argatroban prolongs the PT/INR. Concomitant use with warfarin will cause increased prolongation of the PT and INR greater than that of warfarin alone. If warfarin is initiated concurrently with argatroban, initial PT/INR goals while on argatroban may require modification; alternative guidelines for monitoring therapy should be followed. Safety and efficacy for use with other thrombolytic agents has not been established. Discontinue all parenteral anticoagulants prior to starting therapy. Allow reversal of heparin's effects before initiation. Patients with hepatic dysfunction may require >4 hours to achieve full reversal of argatroban's anticoagulant effect following treatment. Avoid use during PCI in patients with clinically significant hepatic disease or elevations of ALT/AST (≥3 times ULN); use in these patients has not been evaluated. Limited pharmacokinetic and dosing information is available from use in critically-ill children with heparin-induced thrombocytopenia (HIT).

Warnings: Additional Pediatric Considerations The appropriate goals of anticoagulation and duration of treatment in pediatric patients have not been established. In pediatric trials, hypokalemia and abdominal pain were reported (Young, 2007).

Adverse Reactions As with all anticoagulants, bleeding is the major adverse effect of argatroban. Hemorrhage may occur at virtually any site. Risk is dependent on multiple variables, including the intensity of anticoagulation and patient susceptibility.

Cardiovascular: Angina pectoris, bradycardia, cardiac arrest, chest pain (PCI related), coronary occlusion, hypotension, ischemic heart disease, myocardial infarction (PCI), thrombosis, vasodilation, ventricular tachycardia

Central nervous system: Headache, intracranial hemorrhage, pain

Dermatologic: Dermatological reaction (bullous eruption, rash)

Gastrointestinal: Abdominal pain, diarrhea, gastrointestinal hemorrhage, nausea, vomiting

Genitourinary: Genitourinary tract hemorrhage (including hematuria)

Hematologic & oncologic: Brachial bleeding, decreased hematocrit, decreased hemoglobin, groin bleeding, minor hemorrhage (CABG related)

Neuromuscular & skeletal: Back pain (PCI related)

Respiratory: Cough, dyspnea, hemoptysis

Miscellaneous: Fever

Rare but important or life-threatening: Aortic valve stenosis, bleeding at injection site (or access site; minor), hypersensitivity reaction, local hemorrhage (limb and below-the-knee stump), pulmonary edema, retroperitoneal bleeding

Drug Interactions

Metabolism/Transport Effects None known.

Avoid Concomitant Use

Avoid concomitant use of Argatroban with any of the following: Apixaban; Dabigatran Etexilate; Edoxaban; Omacetaxine; Rivaroxaban; Urokinase; Vorapaxar

Increased Effect/Toxicity

Argatroban may increase the levels/effects of: Anticoagulants; Collagenase (Systemic); Deferasirox; Deoxycholic Acid; Ibritumomab; Nintedanib; Obinutuzumab; Omacetaxine; Rivaroxaban; Tositumomab and Iodine I 131 Tositumomab

The levels/effects of Argatroban may be increased by: Agents with Antiplatelet Properties; Apixaban; Dabigatran Etexilate; Dasatinib; Edoxaban; Herbs (Anticoagulant/Antiplatelet Properties); Ibrutinib; Limaprost; Nonsteroidal Anti-Inflammatory Agents; Omega-3 Fatty Acids; Pentosan Polysulfate Sodium; Prostacyclin Analogues; Salicylates; Sugammadex; Thrombolytic Agents; Tibolone; Tipranavir; Urokinase; Vitamin E; Vorapaxar

Decreased Effect

The levels/effects of Argatroban may be decreased by: Estrogen Derivatives; Progestins

Storage/Stability

Vials for injection, 2.5 mL (100 mg/mL) concentrate: Prior to use, store vial in original carton at 25°C (77°F); excursions permitted to 15ºC to 30º C (59ºF to 86°F). Do not freeze. Retain in the original carton to protect from light. The diluted, prepared solution is stable for 24 hours at 20°C to 25°C (68°F to 77°F) in ambient indoor light. Do not expose to direct sunlight. Prepared solutions that are protected from light and kept at 20°C to 25°C (68°F to 77°F) or under refrigeration at 2°C to 8°C (36°F to 46°F) are stable for up to 96 hours.

Premixed vials for infusion, 50 mL or 125 mL (1 mg/mL): Store at controlled room temperature of 20°C to 25°C (68°F to 77°F). Keep in original container to protect from light.

Mechanism of Action A direct, highly-selective thrombin inhibitor. Reversibly binds to the active thrombin site of free and clot-associated thrombin. Inhibits fibrin formation; activation of coagulation factors V, VIII, and XIII; activation of protein C; and platelet aggregation.

Pharmacodynamics Onset of action: Immediate

Pharmacokinetics (Adult data unless noted)

Distribution: Distributes primarily to intracellular fluid

V_d: 174 mL/kg

Protein binding: Total: 54%; Albumin: 20%; α_1-acid glycoprotein: 34%

Metabolism: Hepatic via hydroxylation and aromatization. Metabolism via CYP3A4/5 to four known metabolites plays a minor role. Unchanged argatroban is the major plasma component. Plasma concentration of primary metabolite (M1) is 0% to 20% of the parent drug; M1 is three- to fivefold weaker.

Half-life, terminal: 39-51 minutes; hepatic impairment: 181 minutes

Elimination: Feces via biliary secretion (65%; 14% unchanged); urine (22%; 16% unchanged)

Clearance:

Pediatric patients (seriously ill): 0.16 L/kg/hour; 50% lower than healthy adults

Pediatric patients (seriously ill with elevated bilirubin due to hepatic impairment or cardiac complications; n=4): 0.03 L/kg/hour; 80% lower than pediatric patients with normal bilirubin

Adult: 0.31 L/kg/hour (5.1 mL/kg/minute); hepatic impairment: 1.9 mL/kg/minute

Dialysis: Hemodialysis: 20% dialyzed

Dosing: Usual

Pediatric:

Heparin-induced thrombocytopenia: Limited data available: Infants and Children ≤16 years: **Note:** Titration of maintenance dose must consider multiple factors including current argatroban dose, current aPTT, target aPTT, and clinical status of the patient. For specific uses, required maintenance dose is highly variable between patients. Additionally, during the course of treatment, patient's dosing requirements may change as clinical status changes (eg, sicker patients require lower dose); frequent dosage adjustments may be required to maintain desired anticoagulant activity (Alsoufi 2004; Boshkov 2006). If argatroban therapy is used concurrently with or following FFP or a thrombolytic, some centers decrease dose by half (Alsoufi 2004).

Continuous IV infusion: Manufacturer's recommendations:

Initial dose: 0.75 mcg/kg/minute

Maintenance dose: Measure aPTT after 2 hours; adjust dose until the steady-state aPTT is 1.5 to 3 times the initial baseline value, not exceeding 100 seconds; adjust in increments of 0.1 to 0.25 mcg/kg/minute for normal hepatic function; reduce dose in hepatic impairment.

Note: A lower initial infusion rate may be needed in other pediatric patients with reduced clearance of argatroban (eg, patients with heart failure, multiple organ system failure, severe anasarca, or postcardiac surgery). This precaution is based on adult studies of patients with these disease states who had reduced argatroban clearance.

Conversion to oral anticoagulant: Because there may be a combined effect on the INR when argatroban is combined with warfarin, loading doses of warfarin should not be used. Warfarin therapy should be started at the expected daily dose. Once combined INR on warfarin and argatroban is >4, stop argatroban. Repeat INR measurement in 4 to 6 hours; if INR is below therapeutic level, argatroban therapy may be restarted. Repeat procedure daily until desired INR on warfarin alone is obtained. Another option is to use factor X levels to monitor the effect of warfarin anticoagulation. When factor X level is <0.3, warfarin is considered therapeutic and at which time argatroban can be discontinued (Alsoufi 2004; Boshkov 2006).

Adult: **Heparin-induced thrombocytopenia:** Continuous IV infusion:

Initial dose: 2 mcg/kg/minute; use actual body weight up to 130 kg (BMI up to 51 kg/m^2) (Rice, 2007)

Maintenance dose: Patient may not be at steady state but measure aPTT after 2 hours; adjust dose until the steady-state aPTT is 1.5-3.0 times the initial baseline value, not exceeding 100 seconds; dosage should not exceed 10 mcg/kg/minute

Note: Critically-ill patients with normal hepatic function became excessively anticoagulated with FDA approved or lower starting doses of argatroban. Doses between 0.15-1.3 mcg/kg/minute were required to maintain aPTTs in the target range (Reichert, 2003). In a prospective observational study of critically-ill patients with multiple organ dysfunction (MODS) and suspected or proven HIT, an initial infusion dose of 0.2 mcg/kg/minute was found to be sufficient and safe in this population (Beiderlinden, 2007). Consider reducing starting dose to 0.2 mcg/kg/minute in critically-ill patients with MODS defined as a minimum number of two organ failures. Another report of a cardiac patient with anasarca secondary to acute renal failure had a reduction in argatroban clearance similar to patients with hepatic dysfunction. Reduced clearance may have been due to reduced liver perfusion (de Denus, 2003). The American College of Chest Physicians has recommended an initial infusion rate of 0.5-1.2 mcg/kg/minute for patients with heart failure, MODS, severe anasarca, or postcardiac surgery (Hirsch, 2008).

Conversion to oral anticoagulant: Because there may be a combined effect on the INR when argatroban is combined with warfarin, loading doses of warfarin should not be used. Warfarin therapy should be started at the expected daily dose.

Patients receiving ≤2 mcg/kg/minute of argatroban: Argatroban therapy can be stopped when the combined INR on warfarin and argatroban is >4; repeat INR measurement in 4-6 hours; if INR is below therapeutic level, argatroban therapy may be restarted. Repeat procedure daily until desired INR on warfarin alone is obtained.

Patients receiving >2 mcg/kg/minute of argatroban: In order to predict the INR on warfarin alone, reduce dose of argatroban to 2 mcg/kg/minute; measure INR for argatroban and warfarin 4-6 hours after dose reduction; argatroban therapy can be stopped when the combined INR on warfarin and argatroban is >4. Repeat INR measurement in 4-6 hours; if INR is below therapeutic level, argatroban therapy may be restarted. Repeat procedure daily until desired INR on warfarin alone is obtained.

Note: The American College of Chest Physicians recommends monitoring chromogenic factor X assay when transitioning from argatroban to warfarin (Hirsh, 2008). Factor X levels <45% have been associated with INR values >2 after the effects of argatroban have been eliminated (Arpino, 2005).

Dosing adjustment in renal impairment: Dosage adjustment is not required.

Dosing adjustment in hepatic impairment: Decreased clearance is seen with hepatic impairment; dose should be reduced.

Infants and Children ≤16 years: Heparin-induced thrombocytopenia; IV continuous infusion:

Initial dose: 0.2 mcg/kg/minute

Maintenance dose: Measure aPTT after 2 hours; adjust dose until the steady-state aPTT is 1.5-3 times the initial baseline value, not exceeding 100 seconds; adjust in increments of ≤0.05 mcg/kg/minute.

Adults: Moderate hepatic impairment: IV continuous infusion: Initial dose: 0.5 mcg/kg/minute; monitor aPTT closely; adjust dose as clinically needed. **Note:** During

PCI, avoid use in patients with elevations of ALT/AST (>3 times ULN); the use of argatroban in these patients has not been evaluated.

Usual Infusion Concentrations: Pediatric Note: Premixed solutions available.

IV infusion: 1000 **mcg**/mL

Preparation for Administration IV: Vials for injection, 2.5 mL (100 mg/mL) concentrate: Dilute to a final concentration of 1 mg/mL. Solution may be mixed with NS, D_5W, or LR. Do not mix with other medications prior to dilution. Mix by repeated inversion for 1 minute. A slight but brief haziness may occur upon mixing; use of diluent at room temperature is recommended.

Premixed vials for infusion, 50 mL or 125 mL (1 mg/mL): No further dilution is required.

Administration IV: For IV use only. Administer bolus dose over 3 to 5 minutes through a large bore intravenous line.

Monitoring Parameters HIT: Obtain baseline aPTT prior to start of therapy. Check aPTT 2 hours after start of therapy and any dosage adjustment. Monitor hemoglobin, hematocrit, platelets, signs and symptoms of bleeding.

Test Interactions Argatroban may elevate PT/INR levels in the absence of warfarin. If warfarin is started, initial PT/INR goals while on argatroban may require modification. The American College of Chest Physicians suggests monitoring chromogenic factor X assay when transitioning from argatroban to warfarin (Garcia, 2012) or overlapping administration of warfarin for a minimum of 5 days until INR is within target range; recheck INR after anticoagulant effect of argatroban has dissipated (Guyatt, 2012). Factor Xa levels <45% have been associated with INR values >2 after the effects of argatroban have been eliminated (Arpino, 2005).

Additional Information Molecular weight: 526.66; argatroban is a synthetic anticoagulant (direct thrombin inhibitor) derived from L-arginine. Increases in aPTT, ACT, PT, INR, and TT occur in a dose-dependent fashion with increasing doses of argatroban. Adult studies have established the use of aPTT for patients with HIT and ACT for patients with PCI procedures. Therapeutic ranges for PT, INR, and TT have not been identified.

A reversal agent to argatroban is not available. Should life-threatening bleeding occur, discontinue argatroban immediately, obtain an aPTT and other coagulation tests, and provide symptomatic and supportive care.

Infants and Children ≤16 years: Doses reported in the literature for infants and children with HIT for procedural anticoagulation:

Cardiac Catheterization: Dose not established; the following doses have been used in limited reports: Initial IV bolus dose: 150-250 mcg/kg, followed by continuous IV infusion at an initial rate 5-15 mcg/kg/minute; one case series adjusted the continuous infusion dose to maintain target ACT >300 seconds (n=4). **Note:** Data is limited to an open-labeled study of a mixed population that included six pediatric cardiac catheterization patients and case reports/series (n=4 patients) [Alsoufi, 2004; GlaxoSmithKline Result Summary, 2007 (manufacturer unpublished data); Young, 2007]. Further studies are required before these doses can be recommended.

ECMO: Dose not established; data is limited to an open-labeled study of a mixed population that included one infant on ECMO, published and submitted abstracts, and case reports/series (n=16 patients) [Alsoufi, 2004; GlaxoSmithKline Result Summary, 2007 (manufacturer unpublished data); Hursting, 2006; Potter, 2007; Tcheng, 2004]. Further studies are required before these doses can be recommended.

The reported argatroban doses used to prime the ECMO circuit have varied widely; more recent reports utilize an ECMO priming dose between 30-50 mcg based upon patient's clinical status and ACT, followed by a continuous IV infusion at an initial rate of 0.5-2 mcg/kg/minute; continuous infusion doses were adjusted to maintain target ACT of at least 200 seconds; reported ACT target ranges varied from 160-300 seconds or aPTT 2 times initial baseline value. Dosing requirements ranging from 0.1-24 mcg/kg/minute have been reported. If patient not previously anticoagulated on heparin prior to starting argatroban, an initial bolus dose may be required.

Hemodialysis/Hemofiltration: Dose not established; clinical data limited to case series/reports (Alsoufi, 2004; Hursting, 2006; Young, 2007). Further studies are required before these doses can be recommended. The following doses have been used in limited reports: IV continuous infusion: Initial dose: 0.5-2 mcg/kg/minute; infusions were adjusted to maintain target ACT at least >160 seconds or aPTT >50 seconds; when reported, ACT target ranges were 160-200 seconds and aPTT 50-75 seconds. Reported dosing requirements were 0.1-2 mcg/kg/minute. If patient not previously anticoagulated on heparin prior to starting argatroban, an initial bolus dose may be required; initial bolus doses of 65 mcg/kg and 250 mcg/kg have each been reported.

Dosage Forms Excipient information presented when available (limited, particularly for generics); consult specific product labeling.

Solution, Intravenous:

Generic: 125 mg/125 mL (125 mL); 250 mg/250 mL (250 mL); 100 mg/mL (2.5 mL)

Solution, Intravenous [preservative free]:

Generic: 50 mg/50 mL (50 mL); 100 mg/mL (2.5 mL)

Arginine (AR ji neen)

Medication Safety Issues

Administration issues:

The Food and Drug Administration (FDA) has identified several cases of fatal arginine overdose in children and has recommended that healthcare professionals always recheck dosing calculations prior to administration of arginine. Doses used in children should not exceed usual adult doses.

Brand Names: US R-Gene 10

Therapeutic Category Diagnostic Agent, Growth Hormone Function; Metabolic Alkalosis Agent; Urea Cycle Disorder (UCD) Treatment Agent

Generic Availability (US) No

Use Diagnostic agent in pituitary function test (stimulant for the release of growth hormone) (FDA approved in pediatric patients [age not specified] and adults); has also been used for management of severe, uncompensated, metabolic alkalosis (pH ≥7.55) **after** optimizing therapy with sodium or potassium chloride supplements treatment; prevention of necrotizing enterocolitis in neonates; and for treatment/prevention of hyperammonemia associated with urea cycle disorders

Pregnancy Risk Factor B

Pregnancy Considerations Teratogenic effects were not observed in animal studies; however, the manufacturer does not recommend use of arginine during pregnancy.

Breast-Feeding Considerations Amino acids are excreted in breast milk, the amount following arginine administration is not known.

Contraindications Hypersensitivity to arginine or any component of the formulation

Warnings/Precautions Arginine infusion has been associated with acute electrolyte disturbances, including hyperkalemia, hyponatremia (following overdose), hypophosphatemia, and acidosis; risk is increased in patients with hepatic impairment, renal dysfunction, or diabetes mellitus. Severe reactions, including anaphylaxis, have been reported; appropriate medical treatment should be readily available. If extravasation occurs, local tissue damage may ensue. Use with caution in patients with diabetes mellitus, renal failure or hepatic failure; use may lead to life-threatening hyperkalemia. Use with caution in patients with electrolyte imbalance. Use with caution in children. Several cases of fatal arginine overdose in children have been reported; symptoms of overdose may be delayed; healthcare professionals should always recheck dosing calculations prior to administration of arginine.

Warnings: Additional Pediatric Considerations In neonates, infants, and children overdosage has resulted in hyperchloremic metabolic acidosis, cerebral edema, or possibly death; each 1 mEq chloride delivers 1 mEq hydrogen; monitor acid base balance closely, particularly in neonates. Arginine hydrochloride is metabolized to nitrogen-containing products for excretion; the temporary effect of a high nitrogen load on the kidneys should be evaluated. Accumulation of excess arginine may result in an overproduction of nitric oxide, leading to vasodilation and hypotension (Summar 2001).

Oral products available in the US are often marketed as dietary supplements. When using these products, patients should take care to ensure that they are receiving pharmaceutical grade supplements of L-arginine and verify the formulation (free base vs arginine HCl). The National Urea Cycle Disorders Foundation cautions against using oral dietary supplements of arginine HCL (National Urea Cycles Disorder Foundation).

Adverse Reactions

Cardiovascular: Flushing (with rapid IV infusion)

Central nervous system: Headache

Gastrointestinal: Nausea, vomiting

Local: Venous irritation

Neuromuscular & skeletal: Numbness

Rare but important or life-threatening: Anaphylaxis, cerebral edema, hematuria, hyperkalemia, hypersensitivity reaction, injection site reaction, skin burn/necrosis (due to extravasation), lethargy, loss of consciousness, perioral tingling

Drug Interactions

Metabolism/Transport Effects None known.

Avoid Concomitant Use There are no known interactions where it is recommended to avoid concomitant use.

Increased Effect/Toxicity There are no known significant interactions involving an increase in effect.

Decreased Effect There are no known significant interactions involving a decrease in effect.

Storage/Stability Store at room temperature of 25°C (77°F). Do not use if frozen.

Mechanism of Action Stimulates pituitary release of growth hormone and prolactin through origins in the hypothalamus; patients with impaired pituitary function have lower or no increase in plasma concentrations of growth hormone after administration of arginine. Arginine hydrochloride has been used for severe metabolic alkalosis due to its high chloride content. Arginine hydrochloride has been used investigationally to treat metabolic alkalosis. Arginine contains 475 mEq of hydrogen ions and 475 mEq of chloride ions/L. Arginine is metabolized by the liver to produce hydrogen ions. It may be used in patients with relative hepatic insufficiency because arginine combines with ammonia in the body to produce urea. Arginine is a precursor to nitric oxide and can produce vasodilation and inhibition of platelet aggregation.

Pharmacokinetics (Adult data unless noted)

Absorption: Oral: Well absorbed

Distribution: V_d: ~33 L/kg following a 30 g IV dose

Bioavailability: Oral: ~68%

Half-life: 0.7 to 1.3 hours

Time to peak serum concentration:

Oral: ~2 hours

IV: 20 to 30 minutes

Dosing: Neonatal

Hyperammonemia, acute (urea cycle disorders): Limited data available: **Note:** Administered concomitantly with sodium benzoate and sodium phenylacetate. Dosage based on specific enzyme deficiency; therapy should continue until ammonia levels are in normal range. Do not repeat loading dose unless severe disorder or receiving dialysis; if used, minimum 6 hour interval between loading doses (Summar 2001). **Note: Dosing based on arginine hydrochloride product.**

Weight-directed dosing:

Argininosuccinic acid lyase (ASL) or argininosuccinic acid synthetase (ASS, Citrullinemia) deficiency: IV: Loading dose: 600 mg/kg followed by a continuous IV infusion of 600 mg/kg/day (Batshaw 2001; NORD 2012; Summar 2001; UCD Conference group 2001)

Carbamyl phosphate synthetase (CPS), ornithine transcarbamylase (OTC) or N-acetylglutamate synthetase (NAGS) deficiency: IV: Loading dose: 200 mg/kg followed by a continuous IV infusion of 200 mg/kg/day (Batshaw 2001; NORD 2012; Summar 2001)

Comatose patients: IV: Loading dose: 600 mg/kg followed by a continuous IV infusion of 250 mg/kg/day (UCD Conference group 2001)

Noncomatose patients: IV: Loading dose: 200 mg/kg followed by a continuous IV infusion of 200 mg/kg/day (Batshaw 2001; NORD 2012)

Unconfirmed/pending diagnosis: IV: Loading dose: 600 mg/kg followed by a continuous IV infusion of 600 mg/kg/day (NORD 2012; Summar 2001). If ASS and ASL are excluded as diagnostic possibilities, reduce dose to 200 mg/kg/day.

BSA-directed dosing:

Argininosuccinic acid lyase (ASL) or argininosuccinic acid synthetase (ASS, citrullinemia) deficiency: IV: Loading dose: 12 **g/m²** followed by a continuous IV infusion of 12 **g/m²**/day (Batshaw 2001; Brusilow 1996)

Carbamyl phosphate synthetase (CPS) or ornithine transcarbamylase (OTC) deficiency: IV: Loading dose: 4 **g/m²** followed by a continuous IV infusion of 4 **g/m²**/day (Batshaw 2001; Brusilow 1996)

Urea cycle disorders, chronic therapy: Limited data available: **Note:** Dose should be individualized based on patient response; doses may need to be increased by ~50% as part of a sick-day routine (Berry 2001). **Note: Dosing based on arginine-free base powder product:**

Argininosuccinic acid lyase (ASL) or argininosuccinic acid synthetase (ASS, citrullinemia) deficiency (Batshaw 2001; Berry 2001; Brusilow 1996; NORD 2012; Summar 2001):

Weight-directed dosing: Oral: 400 to 700 mg/kg/day in 3 to 4 divided doses

BSA-directed dosing: Oral: 8.8 to 15.4 g/m²/day in 3 to 4 divided doses

Carbamyl phosphate synthetase (CPS), ornithine transcarbamylase (OTC) or N-acetylglutamate synthetase (NAGS) deficiency: **Note:** Citrulline may be preferred for some patients (Batshaw, 2001; Brusilow 1996; NORD 2012):

Weight-directed dosing: Oral: 170 mg/kg/day in 3 to 4 divided doses

BSA-directed dosing: Oral: 3.8 g/m²/day in 3 to 4 divided doses

Necrotizing enterocolitis (NEC), prevention: Limited data available: Oral, IV: 261 mg/kg/day added to enteral or parenteral nutrition beginning on day of life 2 to 5 and continued for 28 consecutive days. Dosing based on a single-center, prospective, double-blind, randomized, placebo-controlled trial of neonates (Treatment group: n=75, GA: <32 weeks; birth weight: <1,250 g) in Canada. Arginine supplementation decreased the NEC incidence when compared to placebo (6.7% vs 27%) (Amin 2002; Shah 2007). **Note:** The only commercial product available in the US is arginine HCl injection and it is not known whether the hydrochloride salt was used in the Canadian study. Increased administration of HCl in this patient population could result in hyperchloremic metabolic acidosis.

Dosing: Usual

Pediatric:

Pituitary function test: Note: Dosing based on arginine hydrochloride product: Infants, Children, and Adolescents: IV: 0.5 **g**/kg over 30 minutes; maximum dose: 30 **g** dose

Metabolic alkalosis: Limited data available: Infants, Children, and Adolescents: IV: **Note:** Arginine hydrochloride is an alternative treatment for uncompensated metabolic alkalosis after sodium chloride and potassium chloride supplementation have been optimized; it should not be used as initial therapy for chloride supplementation. Each 1 g of arginine hydrochloride provides 4.75 mEq chloride. **Note: Dosing based on arginine hydrochloride product.**

Arginine hydrochloride dose (mEq) = 0.5 x weight (kg) x [HCO_3^- - 24] where HCO_3^- = the patient's serum bicarbonate concentration in mEq/L (Martin 1982); give 1/2 to 2/3 of calculated dose and reevaluate.

To correct hypochloremia: Arginine hydrochloride dose (mEq) = 0.2 x weight (kg) x [103 - Cl^-] where Cl^- = the patient's serum chloride concentration in mEq/L (Martin 1982); give 1/2 to 2/3 of calculated dose and reevaluate.

Hyperammonemia, acute (urea cycle disorders): Limited data available: Infants, Children, and Adolescents: **Note:** Administered concomitantly with sodium benzoate and sodium phenylacetate. Dosage based on specific enzyme deficiency; therapy should continue until ammonia levels are in normal range. If patient already receiving arginine therapy, consider either a reduction in the loading dose or possible elimination (Batshaw 2001); if a loading dose is used, it should not be repeated (NORD 2012). **Note: Dosing based on arginine hydrochloride product.**

Weight-directed dosing:

Argininosuccinic acid lyase (ASL) or argininosuccinic acid synthetase (ASS, citrullinemia) deficiency: IV: Loading dose: 600 mg/kg followed by a continuous IV infusion of 600 mg/kg/day (Batshaw 2001; NORD 2012).

Carbamyl phosphate synthetase (CPS), ornithine transcarbamylase (OTC) or N-acetylglutamate synthetase (NAGS) deficiency: IV: Loading dose: 200 mg/kg followed by a continuous IV infusion of 200 mg/kg/day (Batshaw 2001; NORD 2012).

Unconfirmed/pending diagnosis: IV: Loading dose: 600 mg/kg followed by a continuous IV infusion of 600 mg/kg/day (NORD 2012). If ASS and ASL are excluded as diagnostic possibilities, reduce dose to 200 mg/kg/day.

BSA-directed dosing:

Argininosuccinic acid lyase (ASL) or argininosuccinic acid synthetase (ASS, citrullinemia) deficiency: IV: Loading dose: 12 g/**m²** followed by a continuous IV infusion of 12 g/**m²**/day (Batshaw 2001; Brusilow 1996)

Carbamyl phosphate synthetase (CPS) or ornithine transcarbamylase (OTC) disorder: IV: Loading dose: 4 g/**m²** followed by a continuous IV infusion of 4 g/**m²**/day (Batshaw 2001; Brusilow 1996)

Urea cycle disorders, chronic therapy: Limited data available: Infants, Children, and Adolescents: **Note:** Dose should be individualized based on patient response; doses may need to be increased by ~50% as part of a sick-day routine (Berry 2001): **Note: Dosing based on arginine-free base powder product:**

Argininosuccinic acid lyase (ASL) or argininosuccinic acid synthetase (ASS, citrullinemia) deficiency (Batshaw 2001; Berry 2001; Brusilow 1996; NORD 2012):

Weight-directed dosing: Oral: 400 to 700 mg/kg/day in 3 to 4 divided doses

BSA-directed dosing: Oral: 8.8 to 15.4 g/m²/day in 3 to 4 divided doses

Carbamyl phosphate synthetase (CPS), ornithine transcarbamylase (OTC) or N-acetylglutamate synthetase (NAGS) deficiency: **Note:** Citrulline may be preferred for some patients (Batshaw, 2001; Brusilow 1996; NORD 2012):

Weight-directed dosing: Oral: 170 mg/kg/day in 3 to 4 divided doses

BSA-directed dosing: Oral: 3.8 g/m²/day in 3 to 4 divided doses

Adult: **Pituitary function test: Note: Dosing based on arginine hydrochloride product:** IV: 30 g over 30 minutes

Dosing adjustment in renal impairment: There are no dosage adjustments provided in the manufacturer's labeling; use with caution; use may lead to life-threatening hyperkalemia.

Dosing adjustment in hepatic impairment: There are no dosage adjustments provided in the manufacturer's labeling; use with caution; use may lead to life-threatening hyperkalemia.

Preparation for Administration IV: Dependent upon use: Urea cycle disorders: May dilute in 25 to 35 mL of $D_{10}W$ (Summar 2001; UCD Conference group 2001)

Administration

IV: Arginine hydrochloride:

Pituitary function test: Administer undiluted over 30 minutes. For doses <30 g (<300 mL), the manufacturer recommends transferring the dose to a separate container prior to administration.

Urea cycle disorders: May be infused without further dilution; however, very irritating to tissues, dilution is recommended; central line preferred. Administer loading dose over 90 minutes (UCD conference 2001).

Oral, powder: Arginine-free base: Take with meals and space doses evenly throughout the day.

Monitoring Parameters Acid-base status (arterial or capillary blood gases), serum electrolytes, BUN, glucose, plasma growth hormone concentrations (when evaluating growth hormone reserve), plasma ammonia and amino acids (when treating urea cycle disorders), infusion site

Reference Range

Pituitary function test: If intact pituitary function, human growth hormone levels should rise after arginine administration to 10-30 ng/mL (control range: 0-6 ng/mL)

Urea cycle disorders: Goal arginine: 50 to 200 µmol/L (Leonard 2002)

Additional Information When treating urea cycle disorders, sodium bicarbonate use may be necessary to neutralize the acidifying effects of arginine HCl (UCD conference group 2001).

Equivalents (Haeberle 2012):

100 mg arginine free base = 0.574 mmols

100 mg arginine HCL = 0.475 mmol

Dosage Forms Considerations R-Gene 10 contains chloride 47.5 mEq per 100 mL

Dosage Forms Excipient information presented when available (limited, particularly for generics); consult specific product labeling.

Solution, Intravenous, as hydrochloride [preservative free]:

R-Gene 10: 10% (300 mL)

◆ **Arginine HCl** *see* Arginine *on page 190*
◆ **Arginine Hydrochloride** *see* Arginine *on page 190*
◆ **8-Arginine Vasopressin** *see* Vasopressin *on page 2161*
◆ **Aridol** *see* Mannitol *on page 1321*

ARIPiprazole (ay ri PIP ray zole)

Medication Safety Issues

Sound-alike/look-alike issues:

Abilify may be confused with Ambien

ARIPiprazole may be confused with proton pump inhibitors (dexlansoprazole, esomeprazole, lansoprazole, omeprazole, pantoprazole, RABEprazole)

BEERS Criteria medication:

This drug may be potentially inappropriate for use in geriatric patients (Quality of evidence - moderate; Strength of recommendation - strong).

Other safety issues:

There are two formulations available for intramuscular administration: Abilify is an immediate release short-acting formulation and Abilify Maintena is an extended-release formulation. These products are **not** interchangeable.

Brand Names: US Abilify; Abilify Discmelt [DSC]; Abilify Maintena

Brand Names: Canada Abilify; Abilify Maintena

Therapeutic Category Second Generation (Atypical) Antipsychotic

Generic Availability (US) May be product dependent

Use

Oral: Acute and maintenance treatment of schizophrenia (FDA approved in ages ≥13 years and adults); acute treatment of bipolar disorder (with acute manic or mixed episodes) (FDA approved in ages ≥10 years and adults); adjunctive therapy (to lithium or valproate) for acute treatment of bipolar disorder (with acute manic or mixed episodes) (FDA approved in ages ≥10 years and adults); treatment of irritability associated with autistic disorder (including symptoms of aggression, deliberate self-injurious behavior, temper tantrums, quickly changing moods) (FDA approved in ages 6 to 17 years); treatment of Tourette's disorder (FDA approved in ages 6 to 18 years); adjunctive treatment (to antidepressants) of major depressive disorder (FDA approved in adults). Has also been used in children and adolescents for treatment of ADHD, conduct disorders, and irritability associated with other pervasive developmental disorders.

Injection:

Immediate release: Abilify: Acute treatment of agitation associated with schizophrenia or bipolar disorder (manic or mixed) (FDA approved in adults)

Extended release: Abilify Maintena: Treatment of schizophrenia (FDA approved in adults)

Medication Guide Available Yes

Pregnancy Risk Factor C

Pregnancy Considerations Adverse events were observed in animal reproduction studies. Aripiprazole crosses the placenta; aripiprazole and dehydro-aripiprazole can be detected in the cord blood at delivery (Nguyen, 2011; Watanabe, 2011). Antipsychotic use during the third trimester of pregnancy has a risk for abnormal muscle movements (extrapyramidal symptoms [EPS]) and/or withdrawal symptoms in newborns following delivery. Symptoms in the newborn may include agitation, feeding disorder, hypertonia, hypotonia, respiratory distress, somnolence, and tremor; these effects may be self-limiting or require hospitalization.

Treatment algorithms have been developed by the ACOG and the APA for the management of depression in women prior to conception and during pregnancy (Yonkers, 2009). The ACOG recommends that therapy during pregnancy be individualized; treatment with psychiatric medications during pregnancy should incorporate the clinical expertise of the mental health clinician, obstetrician, primary healthcare provider, and pediatrician. Safety data related to atypical antipsychotics during pregnancy is limited and routine use is not recommended. However, if a woman is inadvertently exposed to an atypical antipsychotic while pregnant, continuing therapy may be preferable to switching to a typical antipsychotic that the fetus has not yet been exposed to; consider risk:benefit (ACOG, 2008).

Healthcare providers are encouraged to enroll women exposed to aripiprazole during pregnancy in the National Pregnancy Registry for Atypical Antipsychotics (866-961-2388 or http://www.womensmentalhealth.org/clinical-and-research-programs/pregnancyregistry/).

Breast-Feeding Considerations Aripiprazole is excreted in breast milk (Schlotterbeck, 2007; Watanabe, 2011). In one case report, milk concentrations were ~20% of the maternal plasma concentration (maternal dose: 15 mg/day; ~6 months postpartum) (Schlotterbeck, 2007); however, aripiprazole was not detected in the breast milk in a second case (limit of detection 10 ng/mL; maternal dose: 15 mg/day; ~1 month postpartum) (Lutz, 2010). Aripiprazole was also detected in the neonatal blood 6 days after delivery in a breast-fed infant also exposed during pregnancy. In this case report, the authors suggest *in utero* exposure could have contributed to the findings due to the long elimination half-life of aripiprazole (Watanabe, 2011). In one report, lactation was not able to be established, possibly due to changes in maternal prolactin potentially caused by aripiprazole (Mendhekar, 2006). The manufacturer recommends a decision be made whether to discontinue nursing or to discontinue the drug, taking into account the importance of treatment to the mother.

Contraindications Hypersensitivity (eg, anaphylaxis, pruritus, urticaria) to aripiprazole or any component of the formulation.

Warnings/Precautions [US Boxed Warning]: Elderly patients with dementia-related psychosis treated with antipsychotics are at an increased risk of death compared to placebo. Most deaths appeared to be either cardiovascular (eg, heart failure, sudden death) or infectious (eg, pneumonia) in nature. In addition, an increased incidence of cerebrovascular effects (eg, transient ischemic attack, cerebrovascular accidents) has been reported in studies of placebo-controlled trials of aripiprazole in elderly patients with dementia-related psychosis. Use with caution in dementia with Lewy bodies; antipsychotics may worsen dementia symptoms and patients with dementia with Lewy bodies are more sensitive to the extrapyramidal side effects (APA, [Rabins, 2007]). **Aripiprazole is not approved for the treatment of dementia-related psychosis.**

[US Boxed Warning]: Antidepressants increase the risk of suicidal thinking and behavior in children, adolescents, and young adults (18 to 24 years of age) with major depressive disorder (MDD) and other psychiatric disorders; consider risk prior to prescribing. The possibility of a suicide attempt is inherent in major depression and may persist until remission occurs. Patients treated with antidepressants should be observed for clinical worsening and suicidality, especially during the initial few months of a course of drug therapy, or at times of dose changes, either increases or decreases. Prescriptions should be written for the smallest quantity consistent with good patient care. The patient's family or caregiver should be alerted to monitor patients for the emergence of suicidality and associated behaviors; patients should be instructed to notify their healthcare provider if any of these symptoms or worsening depression or psychosis occur.

Leukopenia, neutropenia, and agranulocytosis (sometimes fatal) have been reported in clinical trials and postmarketing reports with antipsychotic use; presence of risk factors (eg, preexisting low WBC/ANC or history of drug-induced leuko-/neutropenia) should prompt periodic blood count assessment. Discontinue therapy at first signs of blood dyscrasias or if absolute neutrophil count <1,000/mm^3.

A medication guide concerning the use of antidepressants should be dispensed with each prescription. Aripiprazole is not FDA approved for adjunctive treatment of depression in children.

May cause extrapyramidal symptoms (EPS), including pseudoparkinsonism, acute dystonic reactions, akathisia, and tardive dyskinesia (risk of these reactions is very low relative to typical/conventional antipsychotics, frequencies reported are similar to placebo). Risk of dystonia (and probably other EPS) may be greater with increased doses, use of conventional antipsychotics, males, and younger patients. May be associated with neuroleptic malignant syndrome (NMS).

May cause CNS depression, which may impair physical or mental abilities; patients must be cautioned about performing tasks that require mental alertness (eg, operating machinery, driving). May cause orthostatic hypotension (although reported rates are similar to placebo); use caution in patients at risk of this effect or those who would not tolerate transient hypotensive episodes (cerebrovascular disease, cardiovascular disease, or other medications which may predispose).

Use caution in patients with Parkinson disease; antipsychotics may aggravate motor disturbances (APA [Lehman, 2004; Rabins, 2007]). Use with caution in patients with predisposition to seizures or severe cardiac disease. May alter cardiac conduction; life-threatening arrhythmias have occurred with therapeutic doses of antipsychotics. Esophageal dysmotility and aspiration have been associated with antipsychotic use; use caution in patients at risk for aspiration pneumonia (eg, Alzheimer dementia). May alter temperature regulation. Potentially significant interactions may exist, requiring dose or frequency adjustment, additional monitoring, and/or selection of alternative therapy.

Atypical antipsychotics have been associated with metabolic changes including loss of glucose control, lipid changes, and weight gain (risk profile varies with product). Development of hyperglycemia in some cases, may be extreme and associated with ketoacidosis, hyperosmolar coma, or death. Reports of hyperglycemia with aripiprazole therapy have been few and specific risk associated with this agent is not known. Use caution in patients with diabetes or other disorders of glucose regulation; monitor for worsening of glucose control.

Use in elderly patients with dementia-related psychosis is associated with an increased risk of mortality and cerebrovascular accidents; aripiprazole is not approved for the treatment of dementia-related psychosis; avoid antipsychotic use for behavioral problems associated with dementia unless alternative nonpharmacologic therapies have failed and patient may harm self or others. In addition, use may cause or exacerbate syndrome of inappropriate antidiuretic hormone secretion or hyponatremia; monitor sodium closely with initiation or dosage adjustments in older adults (Beers Criteria).

Tablets may contain lactose; avoid use in patients with galactose intolerance or glucose-galactose malabsorption.

Orally disintegrating tablets may contain phenylalanine.

There are two formulations available for intramuscular administration: Abilify is an immediate-release short-acting formulation and Abilify Maintena is an extended-release formulation. These products are **not** interchangeable.

Warnings: Additional Pediatric Considerations Aripiprazole may cause a higher than normal weight gain in children and adolescents; monitor growth (including weight, height, BMI, and waist circumference) in pediatric patients receiving aripiprazole; compare weight gain to standard growth curves. **Note:** A prospective, nonrandomized cohort study followed 338 antipsychotic naive pediatric patients (age: 4 to 19 years) for a median of 10.8 weeks (range: 10.5 to 11.2 weeks) and reported the following significant mean increases in weight in kg (and % change from baseline): Olanzapine: 8.5 kg (15.2%), quetiapine: 6.1 kg (10.4%), risperidone: 5.3 kg (10.4%), and aripiprazole: 4.4 kg (8.1%) compared to the control cohort: 0.2 kg (0.65%). Increases in metabolic indices (eg, serum cholesterol, triglycerides, glucose) were also reported; however, these changes were not significant in patients receiving aripiprazole (Correll, 2009); additionally, in clinical trials, lipid changes observed with aripiprazole monotherapy in pediatric patients were similar to those observed with placebo. Biannual monitoring of cardiometabolic indices after the first 3 months of therapy is suggested (Correll, 2009). Children and adolescents may experience a higher frequency of some adverse effects than adults, including EPS (20% vs 5%), fatigue (17% vs 8%), and somnolence (23% vs 6%).

Pediatric psychiatric disorders are frequently serious mental disorders which present with variable symptoms that do not always match adult diagnostic criteria. Conduct a thorough diagnostic evaluation and carefully consider risks of psychotropic medication before initiation in pediatric patients with schizophrenia, bipolar disorder, or irritability associated with autistic disorder. Medication therapy for pediatric patients with these disorders is indicated as part of a total treatment program that frequently includes educational, psychological, and social interventions.

Some dosage forms may contain propylene glycol; in neonates large amounts of propylene glycol delivered orally, intravenously (eg, >3,000 mg/day), or topically have been associated with potentially fatal toxicities which can include metabolic acidosis, seizures, renal failure, and CNS depression; toxicities have also been reported in children and adults including hyperosmolality, lactic acidosis, seizures and respiratory depression; use caution (AAP, 1997; Shehab, 2009).

Adverse Reactions

Cardiovascular: Hypertension, orthostatic hypotension, peripheral edema, tachycardia

Central nervous system: Agitation (more common in oral), akathisia (more common in adults), anxiety (more common in oral), ataxia, dizziness, drooling, drowsiness (more common in children & adolescents), dystonia, extrapyramidal reaction (more common in children & adolescents), fatigue (more common in children & adolescents), headache (more common in adults), hypersomnia, insomnia (less common in injection), irritability, lethargy, pain, restlessness, sedation (more common in children & adolescents)

Dermatologic: Skin rash

Endocrine & metabolic: Decreased HDL cholesterol (more common in injection), increased LDL cholesterol, increased serum cholesterol (more common in injection), increased serum glucose (more common in adults), increased serum triglycerides (more common in injection), increased thirst, weight gain (more common in children & adolescents), weight loss

Gastrointestinal: Abdominal distress, anorexia, constipation, decreased appetite, diarrhea, dyspepsia, gastric distress, increased appetite, nausea, sialorrhea, toothache, upper abdominal pain, vomiting (more common in oral), xerostomia

Genitourinary: Dysmenorrhea, urinary incontinence
Hematologic & oncologic: Neutropenia
Local: Injection site reaction, pain at injection site
Neuromuscular & skeletal: Arthralgia, back pain, dyskinesia, limb pain, muscle cramps, muscle rigidity, muscle spasm, musculoskeletal pain, myalgia, stiffness, tremor, weakness
Ophthalmic: Blurred vision
Respiratory: Aspiration pneumonia, cough, dyspnea, epistaxis, nasal congestion, nasopharyngitis, pharyngolaryngeal pain, rhinorrhea, upper respiratory tract infection
Miscellaneous: Fever
Rare but important or life-threatening: Abnormal bilirubin levels, abnormal gait, abnormal hepatic function tests, agranulocytosis, akinesia, alopecia, altered s erum glucose, amenorrhea, angina pectoris, anorgasmia, atrial fibrillation, atrial flutter, atrioventricular block, bradycardia, bruxism, cardiopulmonary arrest cardiorespiratory arrest, catatonia, cerebrovascular accident, chest discomfort, choreoathetosis, cogwheel rigidity, convulsions, decreased serum cholesterol, decreased serum triglycerides, delirium, depression, diabetes mellitus, diabetic ketoacidosis, diplopia, disruption of body temperature regulation, drug-induced Parkinson's disease, dry tongue, dysgeusia, dystonia (oromandibular), edema, erectile dysfunction, esophagitis, extrasystoles, eyelid edema, falling, gastroesophageal reflux disease, gynecomastia, hepatitis, hirsutism, homicidal ideation, hostility, hyperglycemia, hyperhidrosis, hyperinsulinism, hyperlipidemia, hypersensitivity, hypersexuality, hypertonia, hypoglycemia, hypokalemia, hypokinesia, hyponatremia, hypotension, hypotonia, increased blood urea nitrogen, increased creatinine clearance, increased creatine phosphokinase, increased gamma-glutamyl transferase, increased lactate dehydrogenase, increased serum prolactin, intentional injury, ischemic heart disease, jaundice, joint stiffness, leukopenia, mastalgia, memory impairment, mobility disorder, muscle twitching, myasthenia,myocardial infarction, myoclonus, neuroleptic malignant syndrome, obesity, oculogyric crisis, pancreatitis, panic attack, photopsia, pollakiuria presyncope, priapism, prolonged Q-T interval on ECG, psychosis, rhabdomyolysis, seizure (including injection), skin photosensitivity, sleep talking, somnambulism, suicidal ideation, suicidal tendencies, supraventricular tachycardia, syncope, tardive dyskinesia, thrombocytopenia, tics, tongue spasm, tonic-clonic seizures, transient ischemic attacks, urinary retention, ventricular tachycardia

Drug Interactions

Metabolism/Transport Effects Substrate of CYP2D6 (major), CYP3A4 (major); **Note:** Assignment of Major/Minor substrate status based on clinically relevant drug interaction potential

Avoid Concomitant Use

Avoid concomitant use of ARIPiprazole with any of the following: Amisulpride; Azelastine (Nasal); Conivaptan; Fusidic Acid (Systemic); Idelalisib; Metoclopramide; Orphenadrine; Paraldehyde; Sulpiride; Thalidomide

Increased Effect/Toxicity

ARIPiprazole may increase the levels/effects of: Alcohol (Ethyl); Amisulpride; Azelastine (Nasal); Buprenorphine; CNS Depressants; DULoxetine; FLUoxetine; Haloperidol; Highest Risk QTc-Prolonging Agents; Hydrocodone; Mequitazine; Methadone; Methotrimeprazine; Methylphenidate; Metyrosine; Mirtazapine; Moderate Risk QTc-Prolonging Agents; Orphenadrine; Paraldehyde; PARoxetine; Ritonavir; Selective Serotonin Reuptake Inhibitors; Serotonin Modulators; Sulpiride; Suvorexant; Thalidomide; Zolpidem

The levels/effects of ARIPiprazole may be increased by: Abiraterone Acetate; Acetylcholinesterase Inhibitors (Central); Brimonidine (Topical); Cannabis; Conivaptan; CYP2D6 Inhibitors (Moderate); CYP2D6 Inhibitors (Strong); CYP2D6 Inhibitors (Weak); CYP3A4 Inhibitors (Moderate); CYP3A4 Inhibitors (Strong); CYP3A4 Inhibitors (Weak); Dasatinib; Doxylamine; Dronabinol; Droperidol; DULoxetine; FLUoxetine; Fusidic Acid (Systemic); Haloperidol; HydrOXYzine; Idelalisib; Ivacaftor; Kava Kava; Lithium; Luliconazole; Magnesium Sulfate; Methadone; Methotrimeprazine; Methylphenidate; Metoclopramide; Metyrosine; Mifepristone; Nabilone; Netupitant; Palbociclib; Panobinostat; PARoxetine; Peginterferon Alfa-2b; Perampanel; Ritonavir; Serotonin Modulators; Sertraline; Simeprevir; Sodium Oxybate; Stiripentol; Tapentadol; Tetrahydrocannabinol

Decreased Effect

ARIPiprazole may decrease the levels/effects of: Amphetamines; Antidiabetic Agents; Anti-Parkinson's Agents (Dopamine Agonist); Haloperidol; Quinagolide

The levels/effects of ARIPiprazole may be decreased by: CYP3A4 Inducers; Dabrafenib; Lithium; Mitotane; Peginterferon Alfa-2b; Siltuximab; St Johns Wort; Tocilizumab

Food Interactions Ingestion with a high-fat meal delays time to peak plasma level. Management: Administer without regard to meals.

Storage/Stability

Injection, powder (extended release):

Prefilled syringe: Store below 30°C (86°F). Do not freeze. Protect from light and store in original package.

Vial for reconstitution: Store unused vials at 25°C (77°F); excursions permitted to 15°C to 30°C (59°F to 86°F). If the suspension is not administered immediately after reconstitution, store at room temperature in the vial (do not store in a syringe).

Injection, solution (immediate release): Store at 25°C (77°F); excursions permitted to 15°C to 30°C (59°F to 86°F). Protect from light. Retain in carton until time of use.

Oral solution and tablets: Store at 25°C (77°F); excursions permitted to 15°C to 30°C (59°F to 86°F). Use oral solution within 6 months after opening.

Mechanism of Action Aripiprazole is a quinolinone antipsychotic which exhibits high affinity for D_2, D_3, 5-HT_{1A}, and 5-HT_{2A} receptors; moderate affinity for D_4, 5-HT_{2C}, 5-HT_7, $alpha_1$ adrenergic, and H_1 receptors. It also possesses moderate affinity for the serotonin reuptake transporter; has no affinity for muscarinic (cholinergic) receptors. Aripiprazole functions as a partial agonist at the D_2 and 5-HT_{1A} receptors, and as an antagonist at the 5-HT_{2A} receptor.

Pharmacodynamics Onset: Initial: 1-3 weeks

Pharmacokinetics (Adult data unless noted) Note: In pediatric patients 10 to 17 years of age, the pharmacokinetic parameters of aripiprazole and dehydro-aripiprazole have been shown to be similar to adult values when adjusted for weight.

Absorption: Well absorbed

Distribution: V_{dss}: 4.9 L/kg

Protein binding: ≥99%, primarily to albumin

Metabolism: Hepatic, via CYP2D6 and CYP3A4; the dehydro-aripiprazole metabolite has affinity for D_2 receptors similar to the parent drug and represents 40% of the parent drug exposure in plasma

Bioavailability: IM: 100%; Oral: Tablet: 87%; **Note:** Orally disintegrating tablets are bioequivalent to tablets; oral solution to tablet ratio of geometric mean for peak concentration is 122% and for AUC is 114%.

Half-life elimination: Aripiprazole: 75 hours; dehydro-aripiprazole: 94 hours; IM: Extended release (terminal): ~30 days (with 300 mg once monthly dose) and 47 days (with 400 mg once monthly dose)

CYP2D6 poor metabolizers: Aripiprazole: 146 hours

Time to peak serum concentration:
IM: Immediate release: 1 to 3 hours; extended release (after multiple doses): 5 to 7 days
Oral: 3 to 5 hours; With high-fat meal: Aripiprazole: Delayed by 3 hours; dehydro-aripiprazole: Delayed by 12 hours

Elimination: Feces (55%, ~18% of dose as unchanged drug); urine (25%, <1% unchanged drug)

Dosing: Usual Note: Oral solution may be substituted for the oral tablet on a mg-per-mg basis, up to 25 mg. Patients receiving 30 mg tablets should be given 25 mg oral solution. Orally disintegrating tablets (Abilify Discmelt) are bioequivalent to the immediate release tablets (Abilify). Immediate release and extended release parenteral products are **not** interchangeable.

Pediatric:

Attention-deficit/hyperactivity disorder (ADHD): Limited data available: Children ≥8 years and Adolescents: Oral: Initial: 2.5 mg/day; may increase on a weekly basis by 2.5 mg/day increments as tolerated; maximum daily dose: 10 mg/day; dosing based on an open-label, pilot study (n=23, age: 8 to 12 years) which reported significant improvement in ADHD outcome scores without an impact on cognitive measures (positive or negative); mean final dose: 6.7 ± 2.4 mg/day (Findling 2008). Other aripiprazole published reports in pediatric and adolescent patients in which ADHD is a comorbid diagnosis within the study population exist; however, effectiveness in ADHD was not a reported primary outcome measure (Bastiaens 2009; Budman 2008; Findling 2009; Murphy 2009; Valicenti-McDermott 2006).

Autism; treatment of associated irritability (including aggression, deliberate self-injurious behavior, temper tantrums, and quickly changing moods): Children and Adolescents 6 to 17 years: Oral: Initial: 2 mg daily for 7 days, followed by 5 mg daily; subsequent dose increases may be made in 5 mg increments every ≥7 days, up to a maximum daily dose of 15 mg/**day**

Bipolar I disorder (acute manic or mixed episodes): Children and Adolescents 10 to 17 years: Oral: Initial: 2 mg daily for 2 days, followed by 5 mg daily for 2 days with a further increase to target dose of 10 mg daily; subsequent dose increases may be made in 5 mg increments, up to a maximum daily dose of 30 mg/**day**. **Note:** The safety of doses >30 mg/day has not been evaluated.

Conduct disorder (CD); aggression: Limited data available: Children ≥6 years and Adolescents: Oral: Initial: Patient weight <25 kg: 1 mg/day; 25 to 50 kg: 2 mg/day; 51 to 70 kg: 5 mg/day; >70 kg: 10 mg/day; may titrate after 2 weeks to clinical effectiveness; maximum daily dose: 15 mg/**day**. Dosing based on an open-label, prospective study (n=23; age: 6 to 17 years) which evaluated pharmacokinetics and effectiveness in patients with a primary diagnosis of CD (with or without comorbid ADHD); results showed improvement in CD symptom scores with only minor improvements in cognition (Findling 2009).

Pervasive Developmental Disorder Not Otherwise Specified (PDD-NOS) or Asperger's Disorder; treatment of associated irritability (aggression, self-injury, tantrums): Limited data available: Children ≥4 years and Adolescents: Oral:
Preschool age: Initial dose: 1.25 mg/day with titration every ≥5 days in 1.25 mg/day increments as tolerated or clinically indicated (Masi 2009)
Prepubertal children: Initial dose: 1.25 to 2.5 mg/day with titration every 3 to 5 days in 1.25 to 2.5 mg/day increments as tolerated or clinically indicated; maximum daily dose: 15 mg/**day** (Masi 2009; Stigler 2009)
Adolescents: Initial dose: 2.5 to 5 mg/day with titration every 5 days in 2.5 to 5 mg/day increments as tolerated or clinically indicated; doses >5 mg/day were divided twice daily; if sleep disorder was reported, the dose was given in morning and/or at lunchtime (Masi 2009); maximum daily dose: 15 mg/**day** (Stigler 2009)

An open-labeled, pilot study (n=25; mean age: 8.6 years; range: 5 to 17 years) reported an 88% response with a mean final dose of 7.8 mg/day (range: 2.5 to 15 mg/day) (Stigler 2009). A retrospective, non-controlled, open-label study of 34 PDD patients (mean age: 10.2 years; range: 4 to 15 years) included 10 patients with autistic disorder and 24 patients with PDD-NOS reported a mean final dose: 8.1 ± 4.9 mg/day and an overall response rate of 32.4% (29.2% in patients with PDD-NOS) (Masi 2009). In a retrospective chart review of children and adolescents with developmental disability and a wide range of psychiatric disorders (n=32; age: 5 to 19 years), a mean starting dose of aripiprazole of 7.1 ± 0.32 mg/day and a mean maintenance dose of 10.55 ± 6.9 mg/day was used; a response rate of 56% was reported for the overall population. However, a study population subset analysis in patients with mental retardation (n=18) showed a lower response rate in patients with mental retardation with PDD-NOS (38%) than in patients with mental retardation without PDD-NOS (100%) (Valicenti-McDermott 2006).

Schizophrenia: Adolescents 13 to 17 years: Oral: Initial: 2 mg daily for 2 days, followed by 5 mg daily for 2 days with a further increase to target dose of 10 mg daily; subsequent dose increases may be made in 5 mg increments up to a maximum daily dose of 30 mg/**day**. **Note:** 30 mg/day was **not** found to be more effective than the 10 mg/day dose.

Tourette's syndrome, tic disorders: Children ≥6 years and Adolescents: Oral:
Patient weight <50 kg: Initial: 2 mg daily for 2 days, then increase to target dose of 5 mg/day; in patients not achieving optimal control, dose may be further titrated at weekly intervals up to 10 mg/day
Patient weight ≥50 kg: Initial: 2 mg daily for 2 days, then increase to 5 mg/day for 5 days, then increase to target dose of 10 mg/day on day 8 of therapy; in patients not achieving optimal control, dose may be further titrated at weekly intervals in 5 mg/day increments up to 20 mg/day

Adult:

Acute agitation (schizophrenia/bipolar mania): IM: Immediate release: 9.75 mg as a single dose (range: 5.25 to 15 mg; a lower dose of 5.25 mg IM may be considered when clinical factors warrant); may repeat at ≥2-hour intervals to a maximum daily dose of 30 mg/day; **Note:** If ongoing therapy with aripiprazole is necessary, transition to oral therapy as soon as possible.

Bipolar I disorder (acute manic or mixed episodes):
Monotherapy: Initial: 15 mg once daily. May increase to 30 mg once daily if clinically indicated (maximum 30 mg/day); safety of doses >30 mg/day has not been evaluated
Adjunct to lithium or valproic acid: Initial: 10 to 15 mg once daily. May increase to 30 mg once daily if clinically indicated (maximum: 30 mg/day); safety of doses >30 mg/day has not been evaluated.

Depression (adjunctive with antidepressants): Oral: Initial: 2 to 5 mg/day (range: 2 to 15 mg/day); dosage adjustments of up to 5 mg/day may be made in intervals of ≥1 week up to a maximum of 15 mg/day; **Note:** Dosing based on patients already receiving antidepressant therapy.

Schizophrenia:
Oral: 10 to 15 mg once daily; may be increased to a maximum of 30 mg once daily (efficacy at dosages above 10 to 15 mg has not been shown to be

increased). Dosage titration should not be more frequent than every 2 weeks.

IM, extended release (Abilify Maintena): 400 mg once monthly (doses should be separated by ≥26 days); **Note:** Tolerability should be established using oral aripiprazole prior to initiation of parenteral therapy. Continue oral aripiprazole (or other oral antipsychotic) for 14 days during initiation of parenteral therapy.

Missed doses:

Second or third doses missed:

>4 weeks but <5 weeks since last dose: Administer next dose as soon as possible

>5 weeks since last dose: Administer oral aripiprazole for 14 days with next injection

Fourth or subsequent doses missed:

>4 weeks but <6 weeks since last dose: Administer next dose as soon as possible

>6 weeks since last dose: Administer oral aripiprazole for 14 days with next injection

Dosage adjustment for adverse effects: Consider reducing dose to 300 mg once monthly

Dosage adjustment with concurrent CYP450 inducer or inhibitor therapy:

Oral: Children, Adolescents, and Adults: IM (immediate release): Adults:

CYP3A4 inducers (eg, carbamazepine, rifampin): Aripiprazole dose should be doubled over 1 to 2 weeks; dose should be subsequently reduced if concurrent inducer agent discontinued.

Strong CYP3A4 inhibitors (eg, ketoconazole): Aripiprazole dose should be reduced to 50% of the usual dose, and proportionally increased upon discontinuation of the inhibitor agent.

CYP2D6 inhibitors (eg, fluoxetine, paroxetine): Aripiprazole dose should be reduced to 50% of the usual dose, and proportionally increased upon discontinuation of the inhibitor agent. **Note:** When aripiprazole is administered as adjunctive therapy to patients with MDD, the dose should **not** be adjusted, follow usual dosing recommendations.

CYP3A4 and CYP2D6 inhibitors: Aripiprazole dose should be reduced to 25% of the usual dose. In patients receiving inhibitors of differing (eg, moderate 3A4/strong 2D6) or same (eg, moderate 3A4/moderate 2D6) potencies (excluding concurrent strong inhibitors), further dosage adjustments can be made to achieve the desired clinical response. In patients receiving strong CYP3A4 and 2D6 inhibitors, aripiprazole dose is proportionally increased upon discontinuation of one or both inhibitor agents.

IM, extended release (Abilify Maintena): Adults: **Note:** Dosage adjustments are not recommended for concomitant use of CYP3A4 inhibitors, CYP2D6 inhibitors, or CYP3A4 inducers for <14 days. In patients who had their aripiprazole dose adjusted for concomitant therapy, the aripiprazole dose may need to be increased if the CYP3A4 and/or CYP2D6 inhibitor is withdrawn.

CYP3A4 inducers: Avoid use; aripiprazole serum concentrations may fall below effective levels.

Strong CYP3A4 **or** CYP2D6 inhibitors:

Current aripiprazole dose of 300 mg once monthly: Reduce aripiprazole dose to 200 mg once monthly

Current aripiprazole dose of 400 mg once monthly: Reduce aripiprazole dose to 300 mg once monthly

Strong CYP3A4 inhibitors **and** CYPD2D6 inhibitors:

Current aripiprazole dose of 300 mg once monthly: Reduce aripiprazole dose to 160 mg once monthly

Current aripiprazole dose of 400 mg once monthly: Reduce aripiprazole dose to 200 mg once monthly

Dosage adjustment based on CYP2D6 metabolizer status:

Oral: Children, Adolescents, and Adults: IM (Immediate release): Adults: Aripiprazole dose should be reduced to 50% of the usual dose in CYP2D6 poor metabolizers and to 25% of the usual dose in poor metabolizers receiving a concurrent strong CYP3A4 inhibitor; subsequently adjust dose for favorable clinical response.

IM, extended release (Abilify Maintena): Adults: Reduce aripiprazole dose to 300 mg once monthly in CYP2D6 poor metabolizers; reduce dose to 200 mg once monthly in CYP2D6 poor metabolizers receiving a concurrent CYP3A4 inhibitor for >14 days.

Dosing adjustment in renal impairment: No dosage adjustment required.

Dosing adjustment in hepatic impairment: No dosage adjustment required.

Preparation for Administration Injection, powder for reconstitution: Reconstitute using 1.5 mL sterile water for injection (SWFI) (provided) for the 300 mg vial or 1.9 mL SWFI (provided) for the 400 mg vial to a final concentration of 200 mg/mL; residual SWFI should be discarded after reconstitution. Shake vigorously for 30 seconds or until the suspension is uniform; the resulting suspension will be milky white and opaque. If the suspension is not administered immediately after reconstitution, shake vigorously for 60 seconds prior to administration.

Administration

Oral (all dosage forms): May be administered with or without food.

Orally-disintegrating tablet: Do not remove tablet from blister pack until ready to administer; do not push tablet through foil (tablet may become damaged); peel back foil to expose tablet; use dry hands to remove tablet and place immediately on tongue. Tablet dissolves rapidly in saliva and may be swallowed without liquid; if needed, tablet can be taken with liquid. Do not split tablet.

Injection: For IM use only; do not administer SubQ or IV; **Note:** Immediate release and extended release parenteral products are **not** interchangeable.

Immediate release (Abilify): Inject slowly into deep muscle mass

Extended release (Abilify Maintena): Inject slowly into gluteal muscle using the provided 1.5 inch (38 mm) needle for nonobese patients or the provided 2 inch (50 mm) needle for obese patients. Do not massage muscle after administration. Rotate injection sites between the two gluteal muscles. Administer monthly (doses should be separated by ≥26 days).

Monitoring Parameters Vital signs; CBC with differential; fasting lipid profile and fasting blood glucose/Hb A_{1c} (prior to treatment, at 3 months, then annually); weight, growth, BMI, and waist circumference (especially in children), personal/family history of diabetes, blood pressure, mental status, abnormal involuntary movement scale (AIMS), extrapyramidal symptoms (EPS). Weight should be assessed prior to treatment, at 4 weeks, 8 weeks, 12 weeks, and then at quarterly intervals. Consider titrating to a different antipsychotic agent for a weight gain ≥5% of the initial weight. Monitor patient periodically for symptom resolution; monitor for worsening depression, suicidality, and associated behaviors (especially at the beginning of therapy or when doses are increased or decreased)

Additional Information Long-term usefulness of aripiprazole should be periodically re-evaluated in patients receiving the drug for extended periods of time.

Dosage Forms Considerations Oral solution contains fructose 200 mg and sucrose 400 mg per mL.

Dosage Forms Excipient information presented when available (limited, particularly for generics); consult specific product labeling. [DSC] = Discontinued product

Solution, Intramuscular:

Abilify: 9.75 mg/1.3 mL (1.3 mL [DSC])

Solution, Oral:

Abilify: 1 mg/mL (150 mL [DSC]) [contains methylparaben, propylene glycol, propylparaben; orange cream flavor]

Suspension Reconstituted, Intramuscular:
Abilify Maintena: 300 mg (1 ea); 400 mg (1 ea)
Tablet, Oral:
Abilify: 2 mg, 5 mg, 10 mg, 15 mg, 20 mg, 30 mg
Generic: 2 mg, 5 mg, 10 mg, 15 mg, 20 mg, 30 mg
Tablet Dispersible, Oral:
Abilify Discmelt: 10 mg [DSC], 15 mg [DSC] [contains aspartame, fd&c blue #2 aluminum lake]

- ◆ **Aristospan (Can)** *see* Triamcinolone (Systemic) *on page 2112*
- ◆ **Aristospan Intra-Articular** *see* Triamcinolone (Systemic) *on page 2112*
- ◆ **Aristospan Intralesional** *see* Triamcinolone (Systemic) *on page 2112*
- ◆ **Armour Thyroid** *see* Thyroid, Desiccated *on page 2058*
- ◆ **Arnuity Ellipta** *see* Fluticasone (Oral Inhalation) *on page 919*
- ◆ **Arranon** *see* Nelarabine *on page 1496*
- ◆ **Arsenic (III) Oxide** *see* Arsenic Trioxide *on page 198*

Arsenic Trioxide (AR se nik tri OKS id)

Medication Safety Issues

High alert medication:

This medication is in a class the Institute for Safe Medication Practices (ISMP) includes among its list of drug classes which have a heightened risk of causing significant patient harm when used in error.

Related Information

Management of Drug Extravasations *on page 2298*
Prevention of Chemotherapy-Induced Nausea and Vomiting in Children *on page 2368*
Safe Handling of Hazardous Drugs *on page 2455*

Brand Names: US Trisenox

Brand Names: Canada Trisenox

Therapeutic Category Antineoplastic Agent, Miscellaneous

Generic Availability (US) No

Use Remission induction and consolidation in patients with relapsed or refractory acute promyelocytic leukemia (APL) characterized by t(15;17) translocation or PML/RAR-alpha gene expression (FDA approved in ages ≥4 years and adults); has also been used in the initial treatment of APL and the treatment of myelodysplastic syndrome (MDS)

Pregnancy Considerations Adverse events have been observed in animal reproduction studies. Arsenic crosses the human placenta. In studies of women exposed to high levels of arsenic from drinking water, cord blood levels were similar to maternal serum levels. Dimethylarsinic acid (DMA) was the form of arsenic found in the fetus. An increased risk of low birth weight and still births were observed in women who ingested high levels of dietary arsenic. Women of childbearing potential should avoid pregnancy; effective contraception should be used during and after therapy. The Canadian labeling contraindicates use in pregnant women. It also recommends that women of childbearing potential avoid pregnancy, and male patients wear condoms during intercourse with women who are pregnant or of childbearing potential during therapy and for 3 months following therapy discontinuation.

Breast-Feeding Considerations Arsenic is naturally found in breast milk; concentrations range from 0.2 to 6 mcg/kg. In studies of women exposed to high levels of arsenic from drinking water, breast milk concentrations were low (~3.1 mcg/kg) and did not correlate with maternal serum levels. The possible effect of maternal arsenic trioxide therapy on breast milk concentrations is not known. Due to the potential for serious adverse reactions in a nursing infant, the manufacturer recommends discontinuing breast-feeding during therapy. The Canadian labeling contraindicates use in nursing women and recommends avoiding nursing during treatment and for 3 months after therapy discontinuation.

Contraindications

Hypersensitivity to arsenic or any component of the formulation

Canadian labeling: Additional contraindications (not in US labeling): Pregnancy; breast-feeding

Warnings/Precautions Hazardous agent - use appropriate precautions for handling and disposal (NIOSH 2014 [group 1]). **[US Boxed Warnings]: May prolong the QT interval and lead to torsade de pointes or complete AV block, which may be fatal. Risk factors for torsade de pointes include extent of prolongation, HF, a history of torsade de pointes, preexisting QT interval prolongation, patients taking medications know to prolong the QT interval or potassium-wasting diuretics, and conditions which cause hypokalemia or hypomagnesemia. If possible, discontinue all medications known to prolong the QT interval. [US Boxed Warning]: A baseline 12-lead ECG, serum electrolytes (potassium, calcium, magnesium), and creatinine should be obtained prior to treatment.** QT prolongation was observed 1 to 5 weeks after infusion, and returned to baseline by 8 weeks after infusion. Monitor ECG at baseline and then weekly; more frequently if clinically indicated. If baseline QTc >500 msec, correct prior to treatment. If QTc >500 msec during treatment, reassess, correct contributing factors, and consider temporarily withholding treatment. If syncope or irregular heartbeat develop during therapy, hospitalize patient for monitoring; assess electrolytes and do not reinitiate until QTc <460 msec, electrolyte abnormalities are corrected and syncope/irregular heartbeat has resolved.

[US Boxed Warning]: May cause APL differentiation syndrome (formerly called retinoic-acid-APL [RA-APL] syndrome), which is characterized by dyspnea, fever, weight gain, pulmonary infiltrates, and pleural or pericardial effusions, with or without leukocytosis. May be fatal. High-dose steroids (dexamethasone 10 mg IV twice daily for at least 3 days or until signs/symptoms subside; initiate immediately if APL differentiation syndrome is suspected) have been used for treatment; in general, most patients may continue arsenic trioxide during treatment of APL differentiation syndrome. May lead to the development of hyperleukocytosis (leukocytes ≥10,000/mm^3); did not correlate with baseline WBC counts and generally was not as high during consolidation as observed during induction treatment. Use with caution in patients with hepatic impairment; in patients with severe hepatic impairment, monitor closely for toxicity. Use with caution in patients with severe renal impairment (dose reduction may be warranted); systemic exposure to metabolites may be higher; has not been studied in dialysis patients. Monitor electrolytes, CBC with differential, and coagulation parameters at least twice a week during induction and weekly during consolidation; more frequently if clinically indicated. Arsenic trioxide is associated with a moderate emetic potential; antiemetics are recommended to prevent nausea and vomiting (Dupuis 2011). Potentially significant interactions may exist, requiring dose or frequency adjustment, additional monitoring, and/or selection of alternative therapy.

Adverse Reactions

Cardiovascular: Abnormal ECG (not QT prolongation), atrial dysrhythmia, chest pain, edema, facial edema, flushing, hyper-/hypotension, pallor, palpitation, QT interval >500 msec, tachycardia, torsade de pointes

Central nervous system: Agitation, anxiety, coma, confusion, depression, dizziness, fatigue, fever, headache, insomnia, pain, seizure, somnolence

Dermatologic: Bruising, dermatitis, dry skin, erythema, hyperpigmentation, local exfoliation, petechia, pruritus, skin lesions, urticaria
Endocrine & metabolic: Acidosis, hyperglycemia, hyperkalemia, hypocalcemia, hypoglycemia, hypokalemia, hypomagnesemia, intermenstrual bleeding
Gastrointestinal: Abdominal distension, abdominal pain, abdominal tenderness, anorexia, appetite decreased, caecitis, constipation, diarrhea, dyspepsia, fecal incontinence, gastrointestinal hemorrhage, hemorrhagic diarrhea, loose stools, nausea, oral blistering, oral candidiasis, sore throat, vomiting, weight gain/loss, xerostomia
Genitourinary: Incontinence, vaginal hemorrhage
Hematologic: Anemia, APL differentiation syndrome, DIC, febrile neutropenia, hemorrhage, leukocytosis, neutropenia, thrombocytopenia
Hepatic: ALT increased, AST increased
Local: Injection site: Edema, erythema, pain
Neuromuscular & skeletal: Arthralgia, back pain, bone pain, limb pain, myalgia, neck pain, neuropathy, paresthesia, rigors, tremor, weakness
Ocular: Blurred vision, dry eye, eye irritation, eyelid edema, painful red eye
Otic: Earache, tinnitus
Renal: Renal failure, renal impairment, oliguria
Respiratory: Breath sounds decreased, cough, crepitations, dyspnea, epistaxis, hemoptysis, hypoxia, nasopharyngitis, pleural effusion, postnasal drip, pulmonary edema, rales, rhonchi, sinusitis, tachypnea, upper respiratory tract infection, wheezing
Miscellaneous: Bacterial infection, diaphoresis increased, herpes simplex, injection site edema, herpes zoster, hypersensitivity, lymphadenopathy, night sweats, sepsis
Rare but important or life-threatening: Acute respiratory distress syndrome, AV block, capillary leak syndrome, CHF, heart block, hypoalbuminemia, hyponatremia, hypophosphatemia, lipase increased, mitochondrial myopathy, pancytopenia, peripheral neuropathy, pneumonitis, pulmonary infiltrate, respiratory distress, stomatitis, ventricular extrasystoles, ventricular tachycardia

Drug Interactions

Metabolism/Transport Effects None known.

Avoid Concomitant Use

Avoid concomitant use of Arsenic Trioxide with any of the following: BCG (Intravesical); CloZAPine; Dipyrone; Highest Risk QTc-Prolonging Agents; Ivabradine; Mifepristone; Moderate Risk QTc-Prolonging Agents

Increased Effect/Toxicity

Arsenic Trioxide may increase the levels/effects of: CloZAPine; Highest Risk QTc-Prolonging Agents

The levels/effects of Arsenic Trioxide may be increased by: Dipyrone; Ivabradine; Mifepristone; Moderate Risk QTc-Prolonging Agents; QTc-Prolonging Agents (Indeterminate Risk and Risk Modifying)

Decreased Effect

Arsenic Trioxide may decrease the levels/effects of: Antidiabetic Agents; BCG (Intravesical)

Storage/Stability Store at 25°C (77°F); excursions permitted to 15°C to 30°C (59°F to 86°F); do not freeze. Following dilution, solution for infusion is stable for 24 hours at room temperature or 48 hours when refrigerated.

Mechanism of Action Induces apoptosis in APL cells via morphological changes and DNA fragmentation; also damages or degrades the fusion protein promyelocytic leukemia (PML)-retinoic acid receptor (RAR) alpha

Pharmacokinetics (Adult data unless noted)

Distribution: V_d: As^{III}: 562 L; widely distributed throughout body tissues; orally administered arsenic trioxide distributes into the CNS
Metabolism: Arsenic trioxide is immediately hydrolyzed to the active form, arsenious acid (As^{III}) which is methylated (hepatically) to the less active pentavalent metabolites, monomethylarsonic acid (MMA^V) and dimethylarsinic acid (DMA^V) by methyltransferases; As^{III} is also oxidized to the minor metabolite, arsenic acid (As^V)
Half-life elimination: AS^{III}: 10-14 hours; MMA^V: ~32 hours; DMA^V: ~72 hours
Time to peak serum concentrations: As^{III}: At the end of infusion; MMA^V and DMA^V; ~10-24 hours
Elimination: Urine (MMA^V, DMA^V, and 15% of a dose as unchanged As^{III})

Dosing: Usual IV:

Children and Adolescents:

Acute promyelocytic leukemia (APL), relapsed or refractory: Children ≥4 years and Adolescents:
Induction: 0.15 mg/kg/day; administer daily until bone marrow remission; maximum induction: 60 doses
Consolidation: 0.15 mg/kg/day starting 3-6 weeks after completion of induction therapy; maximum consolidation: 25 doses over a period of up to 5 weeks

APL initial treatment: Limited data available
Induction, consolidation, and maintenance (Mathews, 2006): Dosing based on experience available for children ≥3 years; however, age was not an exclusion criteria in clinical trial
Induction: 0.15 mg/kg/day (maximum dose: 10 mg); administer daily until bone marrow remission; maximum induction: 60 doses
Consolidation: 0.15 mg/kg/day (maximum dose: 10 mg) for 4 weeks, starting 4 weeks after completion of induction therapy
Maintenance: 0.15 mg/kg/dose (maximum dose: 10 mg) administered 10 days per month for 6 months, starting 4 weeks after completion of consolidation therapy
In combination with tretinoin (Ravandi, 2009): Dosing based on experience available for adolescents ≥14 years; however, age was not an exclusion criteria in clinical trial
Induction (beginning 10 days after initiation of tretinoin): 0.15 mg/kg/day until bone marrow remission; maximum induction: 75 doses
Consolidation: 0.15 mg/kg/day Monday through Friday for 4 weeks every 8 weeks for 4 cycles (weeks 1 to 4, 9 to 12, 17 to 20, and 25 to 28)

Adults:

APL, relapsed or refractory:
Induction: 0.15 mg/kg/day; administer daily until bone marrow remission; maximum induction: 60 doses
Consolidation: 0.15 mg/kg/day starting 3-6 weeks after completion of induction therapy; maximum consolidation: 25 doses over a period of up to 5 weeks

Dosage adjustment in renal impairment:
Severe renal impairment (CrCl <30 mL/minute): Use with caution (systemic exposure to metabolites may be higher); may require dosage reduction; monitor closely for toxicity
Dialysis patients: Has not been studied

Dosage adjustment in hepatic impairment: Use with caution; severe hepatic impairment (Child-Pugh class C): Monitor closely for toxicity

Preparation for Administration Hazardous agent; use appropriate precautions for handling and disposal (NIOSH 2014 [group1]). Dilute in 100 to 250 mL D_5W or NS. Discard unused portion of ampul.

Administration Hazardous agent; use appropriate precautions for handling and disposal (NIOSH 2014 [group 1]). Do not mix with other medications. Infuse over 1 to 2 hours. If acute vasomotor reactions occur, may infuse over a maximum of 4 hours. Does not require administration via a central venous catheter.

Vesicant/Extravasation Risk May be an irritant

Monitoring Parameters Baseline then weekly 12-lead ECG; monitor electrolytes, CBC with differential, and coagulation at baseline then at least twice weekly during induction and at least weekly during consolidation; more frequent monitoring may be necessary in unstable patients

Dosage Forms Excipient information presented when available (limited, particularly for generics); consult specific product labeling.

Solution, Intravenous:

Trisenox: 10 mg/10 mL (10 mL)

◆ **Artane** *see* Trihexyphenidyl *on page 2124*

◆ **Artemether and Benflumetol** *see* Artemether and Lumefantrine *on page 200*

Artemether and Lumefantrine

(ar TEM e ther & loo me FAN treen)

Brand Names: US Coartem

Therapeutic Category Antimalarial Agent

Generic Availability (US) No

Use Treatment of acute, uncomplicated malaria infections due to *Plasmodium falciparum*, including malaria in geographical regions where chloroquine resistance has been reported [FDA approved in children ≥2 months (and at least 5 kg) and adults]

Note: Not approved for treatment of severe or complicated *Plasmodium falciparum* malaria or prevention of malaria

Pregnancy Risk Factor C

Pregnancy Considerations Adverse events were observed in some animal reproduction studies. Safety data from an observational pregnancy study included 500 pregnant women exposed to artemether/lumefantrine and did not show an increased in adverse outcomes or teratogenic effects over background rate. Approximately one-third of these patients were in the third trimester. Efficacy has not been established in pregnant patients. Treatment failures with standard doses have been reported in pregnant women in areas where drug resistant parasites are prevalent. This may be attributed to lower serum concentration of both artemether and lumefantrine in this population (McGready 2008). Malaria infection in pregnant women may be more severe than in nonpregnant women. Because *P. falciparum* malaria can cause maternal death and fetal loss, pregnant women traveling to malaria-endemic areas must use personal protection against mosquito bites. Artemether and lumefantrine may be used as an alternative treatment of malaria in pregnant women but use in the first trimester is generally avoided; consult current CDC guidelines.

Breast-Feeding Considerations It is not known if artemether or lumefantrine are excreted into breast milk. According to the manufacturer, the decision to continue or discontinue breast-feeding during therapy should take into account the risk of exposure to the infant and the benefits of treatment to the mother.

Contraindications Hypersensitivity to artemether, lumefantrine, or any component of the formulation; concurrent use with strong CYP3A4 inducers (eg, rifampin, carbamazepine, phenytoin, St John's wort)

Warnings/Precautions Use associated with prolonging the QT interval; avoid use in patients at risk for QT prolongation, including patients with a history of long QT syndrome, family history of congenital QT prolongation or sudden death, symptomatic arrhythmias, clinically relevant bradycardia, severe heart disease, known hypokalemia, hypomagnesemia or concurrent administration of antiarrhythmics (eg, Class Ia or III), drugs metabolized by CYP2D6 known to have cardiac effects (eg, flecainide, tricyclic antidepressants), or other drugs known to prolong the QT interval (eg, antipsychotics, antidepressants, macrolides, fluoroquinolones, triazole antifungals, or cisapride). ECG monitoring is advised if concomitant use of agents that prolong the QT interval is medically required. In addition, do not use halofantrine (not available in the U.S.) and artemether/lumefantrine within 1 month of one another due to the potential additive effects on the QT interval. After discontinuation of artemether/lumefantrine, drugs that prolong the QT interval, including quinidine and quinine, should be used with caution. Other potentially significant drug-drug interactions may exist, requiring dose or frequency adjustment, additional monitoring, and/or selection of alternative therapy.

Not indicated for the treatment of severe or complicated malaria or for the prevention of malaria. In the event of disease reappearance after a quiescent period, patients should be treated with a different antimalarial drug. Use caution in patients with severe hepatic or renal impairment.

Adverse Reactions

Cardiovascular: Palpitation (adults)

Central nervous system: Chills (more common in adults), dizziness (more common in adults), fatigue (more common in adults), fever, headache (more common in adults), insomnia (adults), malaise (adults), sleep disorder (adults), vertigo (adults)

Dermatologic: Pruritus (adults), skin rash

Gastrointestinal: Abdominal pain, anorexia (more common in adults), diarrhea, increased serum aspartate aminotransferase, nausea (more common in adults), vomiting

Hematologic & oncologic: Anemia

Hepatic: Hepatomegaly

Infection: Malaria, plasmodium falciparum (exacerbation: children)

Neuromuscular & skeletal: Arthralgia (more common in adults), myalgia (more common in adults), weakness (more common in adults)

Respiratory: Cough (more common in children), nasopharyngitis, rhinitis

Miscellaneous: Fever

Rare but important or life-threatening: Abnormal gait, abnormal lymphocytes, abscess, agitation, asthma, ataxia, back pain, bullous dermatitis, conjunctivitis, decreased hematocirt, decreased platelet count, decreased white blood cell count, dysphagia, emotional lability, eosinophilia, fine motor control disorder, hematuria, hyper-reflexia, hypoesthesia, hypokalemia, impetigo, leukocytosis, nystagmus, oral herpes, otic infection, peptic ulcer, pneumonia, proteinuria, tinnitus, tremor, upper respiratory tract infection, urinary tract infection, urticaria

Drug Interactions

Metabolism/Transport Effects Refer to individual components.

Avoid Concomitant Use

Avoid concomitant use of Artemether and Lumefantrine with any of the following: Antimalarial Agents; Artemether; CYP3A4 Inducers (Strong); Halofantrine; Highest Risk QTc-Prolonging Agents; Ivabradine; Lumefantrine; Mifepristone; Moderate Risk QTc-Prolonging Agents; St Johns Wort; Thioridazine

Increased Effect/Toxicity

Artemether and Lumefantrine may increase the levels/effects of: Antimalarial Agents; Antipsychotic Agents (Phenothiazines); CYP2D6 Substrates; Dapsone (Systemic); Dapsone (Topical); DOXOrubicin (Conventional); Etravirine; Fesoterodine; Halofantrine; Highest Risk QTc-Prolonging Agents; Lumefantrine; Metoprolol; Nebivolol; Thioridazine

The levels/effects of Artemether and Lumefantrine may be increased by: Antimalarial Agents; Artemether; CYP3A4 Inhibitors (Strong); Dapsone (Systemic); Etravirine; Grapefruit Juice; Ivabradine; Mifepristone; Moderate Risk QTc-Prolonging Agents; QTc-Prolonging Agents (Indeterminate Risk and Risk Modifying)

Decreased Effect

Artemether and Lumefantrine may decrease the levels/effects of: ARIPiprazole; Codeine; Contraceptives (Estrogens); Contraceptives (Progestins); Hydrocodone; NiMODipine; Saxagliptin; Tamoxifen; TraMADol

The levels/effects of Artemether and Lumefantrine may be decreased by: Bosentan; CYP3A4 Inducers (Moderate); CYP3A4 Inducers (Strong); Dabrafenib; Deferasirox; Efavirenz; Etravirine; Nevirapine; Siltuximab; St Johns Wort; Tocilizumab

Food Interactions Absorption of artemether and lumefantrine is increased in the presence of food. The bioavailability of artemether increases two- to threefold and lumefantrine increases 16-fold (particularly a high-fat meal). Administration with grapefruit juice may result in increased concentrations of artemether and/or lumefantrine and potentiate QT prolongation. Management: Administer with a full meal for maximal absorption. Avoid grapefruit juice.

Storage/Stability Store at 25°C (77°F); excursions permitted to 15°C to 30°C (59°F to 86°F).

Mechanism of Action A coformulation of artemether and lumefantrine with activity against *Plasmodium falciparum.* Artemether and major metabolite dihydroartemisinin (DHA) are rapid schizontocides with activity attributed to the endoperoxide moiety common to each substance. Artemether inhibits an essential calcium adenosine triphosphatase. The exact mechanism of lumefantrine is unknown, but it may inhibit the formation of β-hematin by complexing with hemin. Both artemether and lumefantrine inhibit nucleic acid and protein synthesis. Artemether rapidly reduces parasite biomass and lumefantrine eliminates residual parasites.

Pharmacokinetics (Adult data unless noted)

Absorption:
- Artemether: Rapid; enhanced with food
- Lumefantrine: Initial absorption at 2 hours; enhanced with food

Protein binding:
- Artemether: 95%
- Dihydroartemisinin (DHA): 47% to 76%
- Lumefantrine: 99.7%

Metabolism: Artemether is hepatically metabolized to an active metabolite, dihydroartemisinin (DHA) catalyzed predominately by CYP3A4/5 and to a lesser extent by CYP2B6, CYP2C9, and CYP2C19. The artemether/DHA AUC ratio is 1.2 after one dose and 0.3 after six doses which may indicate autoinduction. Lumefantrine is hepatically metabolized to desbutyl-lumefantrine by CYP3A4.

Bioavailability: Absorption is increased in the presence of food. The bioavailability of artemether increases two- to threefold and lumefantrine increases 16-fold (particularly a high fat meal)

Half-life:
- Artemether: 1-2 hours
- DHA: 2 hours
- Lumefantrine: 72-144 hours

Time to peak serum concentration:
- Artemether: ~2 hours
- Lumefantrine: ~6-8 hours

Elimination: No excretion data exist for humans

Dosing: Usual Malaria, uncomplicated (due to *P. falciparum*, including chloroquine resistant *P. falciparum*): **Note:** Not for treatment of severe or complicated *Plasmodium falciparum* malaria or prevention of malaria

Infants ≥2 months, Children, and Adolescents ≤16 years: Oral:
- 5 kg to <15 kg: One tablet at hour 0 and at hour 8 on the first day and then one tablet twice daily (in the morning and evening) on days 2 and 3 (total of 6 tablets per treatment course)
- 15 kg to <25 kg: Two tablets at hour 0 and at hour 8 on the first day and then two tablets twice daily (in the morning and evening) on days 2 and 3 (total of 12 tablets per treatment course)
- 25 kg to <35 kg: Three tablets at hour 0 and at hour 8 on the first day and then three tablets twice daily (in the morning and evening) on day 2 and 3 (total of 18 tablets per treatment course)
- ≥35 kg: Four tablets at hour 0 and at hour 8 on the first day and then four tablets twice daily (in the morning and evening) on days 2 and 3 (total of 24 tablets per treatment course)

Adolescents >16 years and Adults (≥35 kg): Oral: Four tablets at hour 0 and at hour 8 on the first day and then four tablets twice daily (in the morning and evening) on days 2 and 3 (total of 24 tablets per treatment course). If patient is <35 kg, refer to dosing in children.

Administration Administer with a full meal for best absorption. For infants, children, and patients unable to swallow tablets: Crush tablet and mix with 5-10 mL of water in a clean container; administer; rinse container with water and administer remaining contents. The crushed mixture should be followed with food/milk, infant formula, pudding, porridge, or broth if possible. Repeat dose if vomiting occurs within 2 hours of administration; for persistent vomiting, explore alternative therapy.

Monitoring Parameters Monitor for adequate food consumption (to ensure absorption and efficacy); ECG monitoring is advised if concomitant use of other agents that prolong the QT interval is medically required.

Dosage Forms Excipient information presented when available (limited, particularly for generics); consult specific product labeling.

Tablet:
- Coartem: Artemether 20 mg and lumefantrine 120 mg

Artificial Tears (ar ti FISH il tears)

Medication Safety Issues

Sound-alike/look-alike issues:

Isopto® Tears may be confused with Isoptin®

Brand Names: US Advanced Eye Relief™ Dry Eye Environmental [OTC]; Advanced Eye Relief™ Dry Eye Rejuvenation [OTC]; Altalube [OTC]; Bion® Tears [OTC]; GenTeal PM [OTC]; HypoTears [OTC]; Murine Tears® [OTC]; Puralube [OTC]; Soothe® Hydration [OTC]; Soothe® [OTC]; Systane® Ultra [OTC]; Systane® [OTC]; Tears Again® [OTC]; Tears Naturale PM [OTC]; Tears Naturale® Forte [OTC]; Tears Naturale® Free [OTC]; Tears Naturale® II [OTC]; Viva-Drops® [OTC]

Brand Names: Canada Teardrops®

Therapeutic Category Ophthalmic Agent, Miscellaneous

Generic Availability (US) Yes

Use Ophthalmic lubricant; for relief of dry eyes and eye irritation; protectant against further irritation (OTC: FDA approved in adults; refer to product-specific information regarding FDA approval in pediatric patients); has also been used for symptomatic treatment of dry eye associated with conjunctivitis, blepharitis, and keratitis

Warnings/Precautions Ophthalmic solutions may contain benzalkonium chloride which may be absorbed by contact lenses. Remove contact lenses before using. Some dosage forms may contain polysorbate 80 (also known as Tweens). Hypersensitivity reactions, usually a delayed reaction, have been reported following exposure to pharmaceutical products containing polysorbate 80 in certain individuals (Isaksson, 2002; Lucente 2000; Shelley, 1995). Thrombocytopenia, ascites, pulmonary deterioration, and renal and hepatic failure have been reported in premature neonates after receiving parenteral products containing polysorbate 80 (Alade, 1986; CDC, 1984). See manufacturer's labeling. Preservative free formulations are preferred in patients with severe dry eye or patients on multiple eye drops for chronic disease. Once opened, single use containers should be discarded; do not reuse. When used for self-medication (OTC), stop use and contact healthcare provider if changes in vision, eye pain, continued redness or irritation occur, or if the condition worsens or persists for more than 72 hours. To avoid contamination, do not touch tip of container to any surface. Replace cap after using. Do not use if solution is cloudy or changes color.

Warnings: Additional Pediatric Considerations Some dosage forms may contain propylene glycol; in neonates large amounts of propylene glycol delivered orally, intravenously (eg, >3000 mg/day), or topically have been associated with potentially fatal toxicities which can include metabolic acidosis, seizures, renal failure, and CNS depression; toxicities have also been reported in children and adults including hyperosmolality, lactic acidosis, seizures and respiratory depression; use caution (AAP, 1997; Shehab, 2009).

Adverse Reactions Ocular: blurred vision, crusting of eyelids, mild stinging

Drug Interactions

Metabolism/Transport Effects None known.

Avoid Concomitant Use There are no known interactions where it is recommended to avoid concomitant use.

Increased Effect/Toxicity There are no known significant interactions involving an increase in effect.

Decreased Effect There are no known significant interactions involving a decrease in effect.

Storage/Stability Store at room temperature.

Mechanism of Action Products contain demulcents (ie, cellulose derivatives, dextran 70, gelatin, polyols, polyvinal alcohol, or povidone); usually a water-soluble polymer, applied topically to the eye to protect and lubricate mucous membrane surfaces and relieve dryness and irritation

Dosing: Neonatal Ophthalmic: **Ocular dryness/irritation:** 1 drop into eye(s) as needed to relieve symptoms; **Note:** Neonatal data are unavailable; dosage extrapolated from older pediatric patients.

Dosing: Usual Ophthalmic:

Infants, Children, and Adolescents:

Ocular dryness/irritation: 1-2 drops into eye(s) as needed to relieve symptoms

Dry eye associated with ocular inflammation (eg, blepharitis, conjunctivitis, keratitis): 1-2 drops into eye(s) at least twice daily or as needed to relieve symptoms (Sethuraman, 2009)

Adults: **Ocular dryness/irritation:** 1-2 drops into eye(s) as needed to relieve symptoms

Administration Wash hands thoroughly before administration; do not touch tip of container to the eye or any surface; replace cap after use. Some products should not be used with contact lenses; consult specific product information.

Dosage Forms Excipient information presented when available (limited, particularly for generics); consult specific product labeling.

Gel, ophthalmic:

Systane: Polyethylene glycol 400 0.4% and propylene glycol 0.3% (10 mL, 15 mL)

Ointment, ophthalmic:

Altalube: Petrolatum 85% and mineral oil 15% (3.5 g)

GenTeal PM: Petrolatum 85% and mineral oil 15% (3.5 g)

Puralube: Petrolatum 85% and mineral oil 15% (3.5 g)

Tears Naturale PM: Petrolatum 94% and mineral oil 3% (3.5 g) [contains lanolin]

Solution, ophthalmic:

Advanced Eye Relief™ Dry Eye Environmental: Glycerin 1% (15 mL) [contains benzalkonium chloride]

Advanced Eye Relief™ Dry Eye Rejuvenation: Glycerin 0.3% and propylene glycol 1% (30 mL) [contains benzalkonium chloride]

HypoTears: Polyvinyl alcohol 1% and polyethylene glycol 400 1% (30 mL) [contains benzalkonium chloride]

Murine Tears®: Polyvinyl alcohol 0.5% and povidone 0.6% (15 mL) [contains benzalkonium chloride]

Soothe® Hydration: Povidone 1.25% (15 mL)

Systane® Ultra: Polyethylene glycol 400 0.4% and propylene glycol 0.3% (5 mL, 10 mL)

Systane®: Polyethylene glycol 400 0.4% and propylene glycol 0.3% (5 mL, 15 mL, 30 mL)

Tears Again®: Polyvinyl alcohol 1.4% (30 mL) [contains benzalkonium chloride]

Tears Naturale® II: Dextran 70 0.1% and hydroxypropyl methylcellulose 2910 0.3% (30 mL)

Tears Naturale® Forte: Dextran 70 1%, glycerin 0.2%, and hydroxypropyl methylcellulose 2910 0.3% (30 mL)

Solution, ophthalmic [preservative free]:

Bion® Tears: Dextran 70 0.1% and hydroxypropyl methylcellulose 2910 0.3% per 0.4 mL (28s)

Soothe®: Glycerin 0.6% and propylene glycol 0.6% per 0.6 mL (28s)

Systane® Ultra: Polyethylene glycol 400 0.4% and propylene glycol 0.3% per 0.4 mL (24s)

Tears Naturale® Free: Dextran 70 0.1% and hydroxypropyl methylcellulose 2910 0.3% per 0.5 mL (36s, 60s)

Viva-Drops®: Polysorbate 80 1% (0.5 mL, 10 mL)

- **As_2O_3** *see* Arsenic Trioxide *on page 198*
- **ASA** *see* Aspirin *on page 206*
- **5-ASA** *see* Mesalamine *on page 1368*
- **Asacol (Can)** *see* Mesalamine *on page 1368*
- **Asacol 800 (Can)** *see* Mesalamine *on page 1368*
- **Asacol HD** *see* Mesalamine *on page 1368*
- **Asaphen (Can)** *see* Aspirin *on page 206*
- **Asaphen E.C. (Can)** *see* Aspirin *on page 206*
- **Ascocid [OTC]** *see* Ascorbic Acid *on page 202*
- **Ascocid-ISO-pH [OTC]** *see* Ascorbic Acid *on page 202*
- **Ascor L 500** *see* Ascorbic Acid *on page 202*
- **Ascor L NC** *see* Ascorbic Acid *on page 202*

Ascorbic Acid (a SKOR bik AS id)

Medication Safety Issues

International issues:

Rubex [Ireland] may be confused with Brivex brand name for brivudine [Switzerland]

Rubex: Brand name for ascorbic acid [Ireland], but also the brand name for doxorubicin [Brazil]

Brand Names: US Acerola C 500 [OTC]; Asco-Tabs-1000 [OTC]; Ascocid [OTC]; Ascocid-ISO-pH [OTC]; Ascor L 500; Ascor L NC; BProtected Vitamin C [OTC]; C-500 [OTC]; C-Time [OTC]; Cemill SR [OTC]; Cemill [OTC]; Chew-C [OTC]; Fruit C 500 [OTC]; Fruit C [OTC]; Fruity C [OTC]; Mega-C/A Plus; Ortho-CS 250; Vita-C [OTC]

Brand Names: Canada Ascor L 500; Vitamin C

Therapeutic Category Nutritional Supplement; Urinary Acidifying Agent; Vitamin, Water Soluble

Generic Availability (US) May be product dependent

Use

Oral: Dietary supplement of Vitamin C (OTC: FDA approved in adults); has also been used for urinary acidification

Parenteral: Prevention and treatment of scurvy (All indications: FDA approved in adults)

Pregnancy Risk Factor C

Pregnancy Considerations Animal reproduction studies have not been conducted. Maternal plasma concentrations of ascorbic acid decrease as pregnancy progresses due to hemodilution and increased transfer to the fetus. Some pregnant women (eg, smokers) may require supplementation greater than the RDA (IOM, 2000).

Breast-Feeding Considerations Ascorbic acid is excreted in breast milk; regulatory mechanisms prevent concentrations from exceeding a required amount (IOM, 2000). The manufacturer recommends that caution be exercised when administering ascorbic acid to nursing women.

Contraindications There are no contraindications listed in the manufacturer's labeling.

Warnings/Precautions Patients with diabetes mellitus should not take excessive doses for extended periods of time. Use large doses with caution in patients with renal disorders or patients prone to recurrent renal calculi, patients with glucose-6-phosphatase dehydrogenase (G6PD) deficiency, or patients with hemochromatosis; may have increased risk of adverse events (IOM, 2000).

Aluminum: The parenteral product may contain aluminum; toxic aluminum concentrations may be seen with high doses, prolonged use, or renal dysfunction. Premature neonates are at higher risk due to immature renal function and aluminum intake from other parenteral sources. Parenteral aluminum exposure of >4 to 5 mcg/kg/day is associated with CNS and bone toxicity; tissue loading may occur at lower doses (Federal Register, 2002). See manufacturer's labeling. Avoid rapid IV injection; may cause temporary faintness or dizziness. Some products may contain sodium; use with caution in sodium restricted patients.

Benzyl alcohol and derivatives: Some dosage forms may contain sodium benzoate/benzoic acid; benzoic acid (benzoate) is a metabolite of benzyl alcohol; large amounts of benzyl alcohol (≥99 mg/kg/day) have been associated with a potentially fatal toxicity ("gasping syndrome") in neonates; the "gasping syndrome" consists of metabolic acidosis, respiratory distress, gasping respirations, CNS dysfunction (including convulsions, intracranial hemorrhage), hypotension, and cardiovascular collapse (AAP, 1997; CDC, 1982); some data suggests that benzoate displaces bilirubin from protein binding sites (Ahlfors, 2001); avoid or use dosage forms containing benzyl alcohol derivative with caution in neonates. See manufacturer's labeling.

Warnings: Additional Pediatric Considerations Some dosage forms may contain propylene glycol; in neonates large amounts of propylene glycol delivered orally, intravenously (eg, >3,000 mg/day), or topically have been associated with potentially fatal toxicities which can include metabolic acidosis, seizures, renal failure, and CNS depression; toxicities have also been reported in children and adults including hyperosmolality, lactic acidosis, seizures and respiratory depression; use caution (AAP, 1997; Shehab, 2009).

Adverse Reactions

Endocrine & metabolic: Hyperoxaluria (with large doses)

Rare but important or life-threatening: Dizziness, fatigue, flank pain, headache

Drug Interactions

Metabolism/Transport Effects None known.

Avoid Concomitant Use There are no known interactions where it is recommended to avoid concomitant use.

Increased Effect/Toxicity

Ascorbic Acid may increase the levels/effects of: Aluminum Hydroxide; Deferoxamine; Estrogen Derivatives

Decreased Effect

Ascorbic Acid may decrease the levels/effects of: Amphetamines; Bortezomib; CycloSPORINE (Systemic)

The levels/effects of Ascorbic Acid may be decreased by: Copper

Storage/Stability

Injection: Store under refrigeration (2°C to 8°C); protect from light. Use within 4 hours of vial entry; discard remaining portion.

Oral: Store at room temperature.

Mechanism of Action Ascorbic acid is an essential water soluble vitamin that acts as a cofactor and antioxidant. Ascorbic acid is an electron donor used for collagen hydroxylation, carnitine biosynthesis, and hormone/amino acid biosynthesis. It is required for connective tissue synthesis as well as iron absorption and storage (IOM, 2000).

Pharmacodynamics Onset of action: Reversal of scurvy symptoms: 2 days to 3 weeks

Pharmacokinetics (Adult data unless noted)

Absorption: Oral: Readily absorbed; absorption is an active process and is thought to be dose-dependent

Distribution: Widely distributed

Protein binding: 25%

Metabolism: Hepatic, by oxidation and sulfation

Elimination: In urine; there is an individual specific renal threshold for ascorbic acid; when blood levels are high, ascorbic acid is excreted in urine, whereas when the levels are subthreshold (doses up to 80 mg/day) very little if any ascorbic acid is excreted into urine

Dosing: Neonatal

Adequate Intake (AI): Oral: 40 mg daily (~6 mg/kg/day)

Parenteral nutrition, maintenance requirement (Vanek, 2012): IV:

Preterm: 15-25 mg/kg/day

Term: 80 mg daily

Dosing: Usual

Infants, Children, and Adolescents:

Adequate Intake (AI): Oral:

1-6 months: 40 mg daily (~6 mg/kg/day)

7-12 months: 50 mg daily (~6 mg/kg/day)

Recommended daily allowance (RDA): Oral:

1-3 years: 15 mg daily

4-8 years: 25 mg daily

9-13 years: 45 mg daily

14-18 years: Males: 75 mg daily, females: 65 mg daily

Dietary supplement: Oral: 35-100 mg daily

Parenteral nutrition, maintenance requirement (Vanek, 2012): IV:

Infants: 15-25 mg/kg/day; maximum daily dose: 80 mg/**day**

Children and Adolescents: 80 mg daily

Scurvy: Oral, IM, IV, SubQ: Initial: 100 mg/dose 3 times daily for 1 week (300 mg/day) followed by 100 mg once daily until normalization of tissue saturation, usually 1-3 months (AAP, 2009; Weinstein, 2001)

Urinary acidification: Oral: 500 mg every 6-8 hours

Adults:

Recommended daily allowance (RDA): Oral: **Note:** Upper limit of intake should not exceed 2000 mg/day

Males: 90 mg daily

Females: 75 mg daily

Pregnant females:

≤18 years: 80 mg daily; upper limit of intake should not exceed 1800 mg/day

19-50 years: 85 mg daily; upper limit of intake should not exceed 2000 mg/day

Lactating females:

≤18 years: 115 mg daily; upper limit of intake should not exceed 1800 mg/day

19-50 years: 120 mg daily; upper limit of intake should not exceed 2000 mg/day

Adult smoker: Add an additional 35 mg daily

Dietary supplement (variable): Oral: 50-200 mg daily

Parenteral nutrition, maintenance requirement: IV: ASPEN Recommendations: 200 mg/day (Vanek, 2012)

Scurvy: Oral, IV, IM, SubQ: 100-250 mg 1-2 times daily for at least 2 weeks

Urinary acidification: Oral: 4-12 **grams** daily in 3-4 divided doses
Wound healing: IV: 300-500 mg daily for 7-10 days
Severe burns: IV: 1000-2000 mg daily

Preparation for Administration Parenteral: Prior to IV administration, dilute in a large volume parenteral solution (eg, NS, glucose). **Note:** Pressure may develop in the vial during storage.

Administration
Oral: May be administered without regard to meals
Parenteral: Use only in circumstances when the oral route is not possible; IM preferred parenteral route due to improved utilization; for IV use dilute and infuse over at least 10 minutes; rapid infusion may cause dizziness

Reference Range
Normal levels: 10-20 mcg/mL
Scurvy: <1-1.5 mcg/mL

Test Interactions False-negative urinary glucose test; false-negative stool occult blood 48 to 72 hours after ascorbic acid ingestion

Additional Information Sodium content of 1 g: ~5 mEq

Dosage Forms Excipient information presented when available (limited, particularly for generics); consult specific product labeling. [DSC] = Discontinued product
Capsule Extended Release, Oral:
C-Time: 500 mg
Generic: 500 mg
Capsule Extended Release, Oral [preservative free]:
Generic: 500 mg
Crystals, Oral:
Vita-C: (120 g, 480 g) [animal products free, gelatin free, gluten free, lactose free, no artificial color(s), no artificial flavor(s), starch free, sugar free, yeast free]
Liquid, Oral:
BProtected Vitamin C: 500 mg/5 mL (236 mL) [contains propylene glycol, saccharin sodium, sodium benzoate; citrus flavor]
Generic: 500 mg/5 mL (473 mL)
Powder, Oral:
Ascocid: (227 g)
Generic: (113 g, 120 g, 480 g)
Powder Effervescent, Oral:
Ascocid-ISO-pH: (150 g) [corn free, rye free, wheat free]
Solution, Injection:
Generic: 500 mg/mL (50 mL)
Solution, Injection [preservative free]:
Ascor L 500: 500 mg/mL (50 mL)
Ascor L NC: 500 mg/mL (50 mL) [corn free]
Mega-C/A Plus: 500 mg/mL (50 mL)
Solution, Injection, as sodium ascorbate [preservative free]:
Ortho-CS 250: 250 mg/mL (100 mL) [contains edetate disodium, water, sterile]
Generic: 250 mg/mL (30 mL)
Syrup, Oral:
Generic: 500 mg/5 mL (118 mL, 473 mL)
Tablet, Oral:
Asco-Tabs-1000: 1000 mg [color free, starch free, sugar free]
Generic: 100 mg, 250 mg, 500 mg, 1000 mg
Tablet, Oral [preservative free]:
Generic: 250 mg, 500 mg
Tablet Chewable, Oral:
Chew-C: 500 mg
Fruit C 500: 500 mg [animal products free, gelatin free, gluten free, kosher certified, lactose free, no artificial color(s), no artificial flavor(s), starch free, sugar free, yeast free]
Fruit C: 100 mg [animal products free, gelatin free, gluten free, lactose free, no artificial color(s), no artificial flavor(s), starch free, sugar free, yeast free]
Fruity C: 250 mg
Generic: 100 mg, 250 mg, 500 mg
Tablet Chewable, Oral [preservative free]:
C-500: 500 mg [animal products free, gluten free, soy free, starch free, yeast free]
Generic: 500 mg
Tablet Extended Release, Oral:
Cemill: 500 mg
Cemill SR: 1000 mg
Generic: 500 mg, 1000 mg, 1500 mg
Tablet Extended Release, Oral [preservative free]:
Generic: 1000 mg [DSC]
Wafer, Oral [preservative free]:
Acerola C 500: 500 mg (50 ea) [corn free, no artificial color(s), no artificial flavor(s), wheat free, yeast free; contains acerola (malpighia glabra)]

- **Asco-Tabs-1000 [OTC]** *see* Ascorbic Acid *on page 202*
- **Ascriptin Maximum Strength [OTC]** *see* Aspirin *on page 206*
- **Ascriptin Regular Strength [OTC]** *see* Aspirin *on page 206*
- **Asmanex 7 Metered Doses** *see* Mometasone (Oral Inhalation) *on page 1452*
- **Asmanex 14 Metered Doses** *see* Mometasone (Oral Inhalation) *on page 1452*
- **Asmanex 30 Metered Doses** *see* Mometasone (Oral Inhalation) *on page 1452*
- **Asmanex 60 Metered Doses** *see* Mometasone (Oral Inhalation) *on page 1452*
- **Asmanex 120 Metered Doses** *see* Mometasone (Oral Inhalation) *on page 1452*
- **Asmanex HFA** *see* Mometasone (Oral Inhalation) *on page 1452*
- **Asmanex Twisthaler (Can)** *see* Mometasone (Oral Inhalation) *on page 1452*

Asparaginase (*Erwinia*)
(a SPEAR a ji nase er WIN i ah)

Medication Safety Issues
Sound-alike/look-alike issues:
Asparaginase *(Erwinia)* may be confused with asparaginase *(E. coli)*, pegaspargase
Erwinaze may be confused with Elaprase, Elspar, Oncaspar
High alert medication:
This medication is in a class the Institute for Safe Medication Practices (ISMP) includes among its list of drug classes which have a heightened risk of causing significant patient harm when used in error.

Related Information
Prevention of Chemotherapy-Induced Nausea and Vomiting in Children *on page 2368*

Brand Names: US Erwinaze

Brand Names: Canada Erwinase

Therapeutic Category Antineoplastic Agent, Enzyme; Antineoplastic Agent, Miscellaneous

Generic Availability (US) No

Use Treatment (in combination with other chemotherapy agents) of acute lymphoblastic leukemia (ALL) in patients with hypersensitivity to *E. coli*-derived asparaginase (FDA approved in ages ≥2 years and adults)

Prescribing and Access Restrictions Erwinaze is distributed through Accredo Health Group, Inc. (1-877-900-9223).

Pregnancy Risk Factor C

Pregnancy Considerations Adverse events were observed in animal reproduction studies.

Breast-Feeding Considerations It is not known if asparaginase *Erwinia chrysanthemi* is excreted in breast milk. Due to the potential for serious adverse reactions in the nursing infant, the manufacturer recommends a decision be made to discontinue nursing or to discontinue the drug, taking into account the importance of treatment to the mother.

Contraindications

History of serious hypersensitivity reactions, including anaphylaxis to asparaginase (*Erwinia*) or any component of the formulation; history of serious pancreatitis, serious thrombosis, or serious hemorrhagic event with prior asparaginase treatment

Canadian labeling: Additional contraindications (not in the U.S. labeling): Women who are or may become pregnant

Warnings/Precautions Serious hypersensitivity reactions (grade 3 and 4), including anaphylaxis, have occurred in 5% of patients in clinical trials. Immediate treatment for hypersensitivity reactions should be available during treatment; discontinue for serious hypersensitivity reactions (and administer appropriate treatment).

Pancreatitis has been reported in 5% of patients in clinical trials; promptly evaluate with symptoms suggestive of pancreatitis. For mild pancreatitis, withhold treatment until signs and symptoms subside and amylase levels return to normal; may resume after resolution. Discontinue for severe or hemorrhagic pancreatitis characterized by abdominal pain >72 hours and amylase ≥2 x ULN. Further use is contraindicated if severe pancreatitis is diagnosed.

Serious thrombotic events, including sagittal sinus thrombosis and pulmonary embolism, have been reported with asparaginase formulations. Decreases in fibrinogen, protein C activity, protein S activity, and antithrombin III have been noted following a 2-week treatment course administered intramuscularly. Discontinue for hemorrhagic or thrombotic events; may resume treatment after resolution (contraindicated with history of serious thrombosis or hemorrhagic event with prior asparaginase treatment).

In clinical trials, 4% of patients experienced glucose intolerance; may be irreversible; monitor glucose levels (baseline and periodic) during treatment; may require insulin administration.

Do not interchange *Erwinia* asparaginase for *E. coli* asparaginase or pegaspargase; ensure the proper formulation, route of administration, and dose prior to administration.

Adverse Reactions

Hypersensitivity: Hypersensitivity reaction (includes anaphylaxis, urticaria)

Cardiovascular: Thrombosis (includes pulmonary embolism and cerebrovascular accident)

Endocrine & metabolic: Abnormal transaminase, decreased glucose tolerance, hyperglycemia (IV: more common)

Gastrointestinal: Abdominal pain, diarrhea, mucositis, nausea (IV: more common), pancreatitis, vomiting (IV: more common)

Local: Injection site reaction

Miscellaneous: Fever

Rare but important or life-threatening: Acute renal failure, anorexia, bone marrow depression (rare), changes in serum lipids, disseminated intravascular coagulation, hemorrhage, hepatomegaly, hyperammonemia, hyperbilirubinemia, malabsorption syndrome, seizure, transient ischemic attacks, weight loss

Drug Interactions

Metabolism/Transport Effects None known.

Avoid Concomitant Use There are no known interactions where it is recommended to avoid concomitant use.

Increased Effect/Toxicity

Asparaginase (Erwinia) may increase the levels/effects of: Dexamethasone (Systemic)

Decreased Effect There are no known significant interactions involving a decrease in effect.

Storage/Stability Store intact vials refrigerated at 2°C to 8°C (36°F to 46°F). Protect from light. Within 15 minutes of reconstitution, withdraw appropriate volume for dose into a polypropylene syringe. Do not freeze or refrigerate reconstituted solution; discard if not administered within 4 hours.

Mechanism of Action Asparaginase catalyzes the deamidation of asparagine to aspartic acid and ammonia, reducing circulating levels of asparagine. Leukemia cells lack asparagine synthetase and are unable to synthesize asparagine. Asparaginase reduces the exogenous asparagine source for the leukemic cells, resulting in cytotoxicity specific to leukemic cells.

Pharmacokinetics (Adult data unless noted) Half-life elimination: IM: ~16 hours (Asselin 1993; Avramis 2005); IV: ~7.5 hours

Dosing: Usual Note: If administering IV, consider monitoring nadir serum asparaginase activity (NSAA) levels; if desired levels are not achieved, change to IM administration.

Pediatric: **Acute lymphoblastic leukemia (ALL):** IM, IV: Children ≥2 year and Adolescents:

As a substitute for pegaspargase: 25,000 units/m^2/dose 3 times weekly (Mon, Wed, Fri) for 6 doses for each planned pegaspargase dose

As a substitute for asparaginase (E. coli): 25,000 units/m^2/dose for each scheduled asparaginase (*E. coli*) dose

Adult: **Acute lymphoblastic leukemia (ALL):** IM, IV:

As a substitute for pegaspargase: 25,000 units/m^2 3 times weekly (Mon, Wed, Fri) for 6 doses for each planned pegaspargase dose

As a substitute for asparaginase (*E. coli*): 25,000 units/m^2 for each scheduled asparaginase (*E. coli*) dose

Dosage adjustment for toxicity:

Hemorrhagic or thrombotic event: Discontinue treatment; may resume treatment upon symptom resolution.

Pancreatitis:

Mild pancreatitis: Withhold treatment until signs and symptoms subside and amylase returns to normal; may resume after resolution.

Severe or hemorrhagic pancreatitis (abdominal pain >72 hours and amylase ≥2 x ULN): Discontinue treatment; further use is contraindicated.

Serious hypersensitivity: Discontinue treatment.

Dosing adjustment in renal impairment: There are no dosage adjustments provided in the manufacturer's labeling.

Dosing adjustment in hepatic impairment: There are no dosage adjustments provided in the manufacturer's labeling.

Preparation for Administration Parenteral: Reconstitute each vial with 1 mL of preservative-free NS to obtain a concentration of 10,000 units/mL, or with 2 mL preservative free NS to obtain a concentration of 5,000 units/mL. Gently direct the NS down the wall of the vial (do not inject forcefully into or onto the powder). Dissolve by gently swirling or mixing; do not shake or invert the vial. Resulting reconstituted solution should be clear and colorless and free of visible particles or protein aggregates. Within 15 minutes of reconstitution, withdraw appropriate volume for dose into a polypropylene syringe. If administering intravenously, slowly inject the appropriate volume of reconstituted solution into 100 mL of NS; do not shake or squeeze the bag. Administer within 4 hours of reconstitution.

Administration Parenteral: Following administration observe patient for hypersensitivity reactions; have resuscitation equipment and medication available for treatment of anaphylaxis.

IM: The volume of each single injection site should be limited to 2 mL; use multiple injection sites for volumes >2 mL.

IV: Infuse over 1 hour; do not infuse other medications through the same IV line.

Monitoring Parameters CBC with differential, amylase, liver enzymes, blood glucose (baseline and periodically during treatment), coagulation parameters, for IV administration, consider monitoring nadir serum asparaginase activity (NSAA) levels. Monitor for symptoms of hypersensitivity; symptoms of pancreatitis, thrombosis, or hemorrhage

Dosage Forms Excipient information presented when available (limited, particularly for generics); consult specific product labeling.

Solution Reconstituted, Intramuscular:

Erwinaze: 10,000 units (1 ea)

- **Asparaginase *Erwinia chrysanthemi*** *see* Asparaginase (*Erwinia*) *on page 204*
- **Aspart Insulin** *see* Insulin Aspart *on page 1118*
- **Aspercin [OTC]** *see* Aspirin *on page 206*

Aspirin (AS pir in)

Medication Safety Issues

Sound-alike/look-alike issues:

Aspirin may be confused with Afrin
Ascriptin may be confused with Aricept
Ecotrin may be confused with Edecrin, Epogen
Halfprin may be confused with Haltran
ZORprin may be confused with Zyloprim

International issues:

Cartia [multiple international markets] may be confused with Cartia XT brand name for diltiazem [U.S.]

BEERS Criteria medication:

This drug may be potentially inappropriate for use in geriatric patients (Quality of evidence - moderate; Strength of recommendation - strong).

Related Information

Oral Medications That Should Not Be Crushed or Altered *on page 2476*

Brand Names: US Ascriptin Maximum Strength [OTC]; Ascriptin Regular Strength [OTC]; Aspercin [OTC]; Aspir-low [OTC]; Aspirtab [OTC]; Bayer Aspirin Extra Strength [OTC]; Bayer Aspirin Regimen Adult Low Strength [OTC]; Bayer Aspirin Regimen Children's [OTC]; Bayer Aspirin Regimen Regular Strength [OTC]; Bayer Genuine Aspirin [OTC]; Bayer Plus Extra Strength [OTC]; Bayer Women's Low Dose Aspirin [OTC]; Buffasal [OTC]; Bufferin Extra Strength [OTC]; Bufferin [OTC]; Buffinol [OTC]; Ecotrin Arthritis Strength [OTC]; Ecotrin Low Strength [OTC]; Ecotrin [OTC]; Halfprin [OTC]; St Joseph Adult Aspirin [OTC]; Tri-Buffered Aspirin [OTC]

Brand Names: Canada Asaphen; Asaphen E.C.; Entrophen; Novasen; Praxis ASA EC 81 Mg Daily Dose; Pro-AAS EC-80

Therapeutic Category Analgesic, Non-narcotic; Anti-inflammatory Agent; Antiplatelet Agent; Antipyretic; Nonsteroidal Anti-inflammatory Drug (NSAID), Oral; Salicylate

Generic Availability (US) Yes

Use Treatment of mild to moderate pain, inflammation, and fever (OTC: All products: FDA approved in adults; refer to product-specific information regarding FDA approval in pediatric patients, most products FDA approved in ages ≥12 years), has also been used for adjunctive treatment of Kawasaki disease; prevention of vascular mortality during suspected acute MI; prevention of recurrent MI; prevention of MI in patients with angina; prevention of recurrent stroke and mortality following TIA or stroke; management of rheumatoid arthritis, and rheumatic fever; adjunctive therapy in revascularization procedures (coronary artery bypass graft, percutaneous transluminal coronary angioplasty, carotid endarterectomy)

Pregnancy Considerations Salicylates have been noted to cross the placenta and enter fetal circulation. Adverse effects reported in the fetus include mortality, intrauterine growth retardation, salicylate intoxication, bleeding abnormalities, and neonatal acidosis. Use of aspirin close to delivery may cause premature closure of the ductus arteriosus. Adverse effects reported in the mother include anemia, hemorrhage, prolonged gestation, and prolonged labor (Østensen, 1998). Low-dose aspirin may be used to prevent preeclampsia in women with a history of early-onset preeclampsia and preterm delivery (<34 0/7 weeks), or preeclampsia in ≥1 prior pregnancy (ACOG, 2013). Low-dose aspirin is used to treat complications resulting from antiphospholipid syndrome in pregnancy (either primary or secondary to SLE) (ACCP [Guyatt, 2012]; Carp, 2004; Tincani, 2003). Low-dose aspirin to prevent thrombosis may also be used during the second and third trimesters in women with prosthetic valves (mechanical or bioprosthetic). The use of warfarin is recommended, along with low dose aspirin, in those with mechanical prosthetic valves (Nishimura, 2014). In general, low doses during pregnancy needed for the treatment of certain medical conditions have not been shown to cause fetal harm; however, discontinuing therapy prior to delivery is recommended (Østensen, 2006). Use of safer agents for routine management of pain or headache should be considered.

Breast-Feeding Considerations Low amounts of aspirin can be found in breast milk. Milk/plasma ratios ranging from 0.03 to 0.3 have been reported. Peak levels in breast milk are reported to be at ~9 hours after a dose. Metabolic acidosis was reported in one infant following an aspirin dose of 3.9 g/day in the mother. The WHO considers occasional doses of aspirin to be compatible with breast-feeding, but to avoid long-term therapy and consider monitoring the infant for adverse effects (WHO, 2002). Other sources suggest avoiding aspirin while breast-feeding due to the theoretical risk of Reye's syndrome (Bar-Oz, 2003; Spigset, 2000). When used for vascular indications, breast-feeding may be continued during low-dose aspirin therapy (ACCP [Guyatt, 2012]).

Contraindications OTC labeling: When used for self-medication, do not use if allergic to aspirin or other pain reliever/fever reducer or for at least 7 days after tonsillectomy or oral surgery.

Warnings/Precautions Use with caution in patients with platelet and bleeding disorders, renal dysfunction, dehydration, erosive gastritis, or peptic ulcer disease. Heavy ethanol use (>3 drinks/day) can increase bleeding risks. Avoid use in severe renal failure or in severe hepatic failure. Low-dose aspirin for cardioprotective effects is associated with a two- to fourfold increase in UGI events (eg, symptomatic or complicated ulcers); risks of these events increase with increasing aspirin dose; during the chronic phase of aspirin dosing, doses >81 mg are not recommended unless indicated (Bhatt, 2008). Use of safer agents for routine management of pain or headache throughout pregnancy should be considered. If possible, avoid use during the third trimester of pregnancy.

Discontinue use if tinnitus or impaired hearing occurs. Caution in mild-to-moderate renal failure (only at high dosages). Patients with sensitivity to tartrazine dyes, nasal polyps, and asthma may have an increased risk of salicylate sensitivity. In the treatment of acute ischemic stroke, avoid aspirin for 24 hours following administration of alteplase; administration within 24 hours increases the risk of hemorrhagic transformation (Jauch, 2013). Concurrent use of aspirin and clopidogrel is not recommended for secondary prevention of ischemic stroke or TIA in patients unable to take oral anticoagulants due to hemorrhagic risk (Furie, 2011). Surgical patients should avoid ASA if possible, for 1 to 2 weeks prior to surgery, to reduce the risk of excessive bleeding (except in patients with cardiac stents that have not completed their full course of dual antiplatelet therapy [aspirin, clopidogrel]; patient-specific situations need to be discussed with cardiologist; AHA/ACC/SCAI/ ACS/ADA Science Advisory provides recommendations). When used concomitantly with ≤325 mg of aspirin, NSAIDs (including selective COX-2 inhibitors) substantially increase the risk of gastrointestinal complications (eg, ulcer); concomitant gastroprotective therapy (eg, proton pump inhibitors) is recommended (Bhatt, 2008). Potentially significant drug-drug interactions may exist, requiring dose or frequency adjustment, additional monitoring, and/ or selection of alternative therapy.

Elderly: Avoid chronic use of doses >325 mg/day (unless alternative agents ineffective and patient can receive concomitant gastroprotective agent); nonselective oral NSAID use is associated with an increased risk of GI bleeding and peptic ulcer disease in older adults in high risk category (eg, >75 years or age or receiving concomitant oral/parenteral corticosteroids, anticoagulants, or antiplatelet agents) (Beers Criteria).

When used for self-medication (OTC labeling): Children and teenagers who have or are recovering from chickenpox or flu-like symptoms should not use this product. Changes in behavior (along with nausea and vomiting) may be an early sign of Reye's syndrome; patients should be instructed to contact their healthcare provider if these occur.

Some dosage forms may contain polysorbate 80 (also known as Tweens). Hypersensitivity reactions, usually a delayed reaction, have been reported following exposure to pharmaceutical products containing polysorbate 80 in certain individuals (Isaksson, 2002; Lucente 2000; Shelley, 1995). Thrombocytopenia, ascites, pulmonary deterioration, and renal and hepatic failure have been reported in premature neonates after receiving parenteral products containing polysorbate 80 (Alade, 1986; CDC, 1984). See manufacturer's labeling.

Aspirin resistance is defined as measurable, persistent platelet activation that occurs in patients prescribed a therapeutic dose of aspirin. Clinical aspirin resistance, the recurrence of some vascular event despite a regular therapeutic dose of aspirin, is considered aspirin treatment failure. Estimates of biochemical aspirin resistance range from 5.5% to 60% depending on the population studied and the assays used (Gasparyan, 2008). Patients with aspirin resistance may have a higher risk of cardiovascular events compared to those who are aspirin sensitive (Gum, 2003).

Warnings: Additional Pediatric Considerations Do not use aspirin in children <12 years (APS 2008) and adolescents (per manufacturer) who have or who are recovering from chickenpox or flu symptoms (due to the association with Reye's syndrome); when using aspirin, changes in behavior (along with nausea and vomiting) may be an early sign of Reye's syndrome; instruct patients and caregivers to contact their health care provider if these symptoms occur.

Adverse Reactions As with all drugs which may affect hemostasis, bleeding is associated with aspirin. Hemorrhage may occur at virtually any site. Risk is dependent on multiple variables including dosage, concurrent use of multiple agents which alter hemostasis, and patient susceptibility. Many adverse effects of aspirin are dose related, and are extremely rare at low dosages. Other serious reactions are idiosyncratic, related to allergy or individual sensitivity.

Cardiovascular: Cardiac arrhythmia, edema, hypotension, tachycardia

Central nervous system: Agitation, cerebral edema, coma, confusion, dizziness, fatigue, headache, hyperthermia, insomnia, lethargy, nervousness, Reye's syndrome

Dermatologic: Skin rash, urticaria

Endocrine & metabolic: Acidosis, dehydration, hyperglycemia, hyperkalemia, hypernatremia (buffered forms), hypoglycemia (children)

Gastrointestinal: Duodenal ulcer, dyspepsia, epigastric distress, gastritis, gastrointestinal erosion, gastrointestinal ulcer, heartburn, nausea, stomach pain, vomiting

Genitourinary: Postpartum hemorrhage, prolonged gestation, prolonged labor, proteinuria, stillborn infant

Hematologic & oncologic: Anemia, blood coagulation disorder, disseminated intravascular coagulation, hemolytic anemia, hemorrhage, iron deficiency anemia, prolonged prothrombin time, thrombocytopenia

Hepatic: Hepatitis (reversible), hepatotoxicity, increased serum transaminases

Hypersensitivity: Anaphylaxis, angioedema

Neuromuscular & skeletal: Acetabular bone destruction, rhabdomyolysis, weakness

Otic: Hearing loss, tinnitus

Renal: Increased blood urea nitrogen, increased serum creatinine, interstitial nephritis, renal failure (including cases caused by rhabdomyolysis), renal insufficiency, renal papillary necrosis

Respiratory: Asthma, bronchospasm, dyspnea, hyperventilation, laryngeal edema, noncardiogenic pulmonary edema, respiratory alkalosis, tachypnea

Miscellaneous: Low birth weight

Rare but important or life-threatening: Anorectal stenosis (suppository), atrial fibrillation (toxicity), cardiac conduction disturbance (toxicity), cerebral infarction (ischemic), cholestatic jaundice, colitis, colonic ulceration, coronary artery vasospasm, delirium, esophageal obstruction, esophagitis (with esophageal ulcer), hematoma (esophageal), macular degeneration (age-related) (Li 2014), oral mucosa ulcer (aspirin-containing chewing gum), periorbital edema, rhinosinusitis

Drug Interactions

Metabolism/Transport Effects Substrate of CYP2C9 (minor); **Note:** Assignment of Major/Minor substrate status based on clinically relevant drug interaction potential; **Induces** CYP2C19 (weak/moderate)

Avoid Concomitant Use

Avoid concomitant use of Aspirin with any of the following: Dexketoprofen; Floctafenine; Influenza Virus Vaccine (Live/Attenuated); Ketorolac (Nasal); Ketorolac (Systemic); Omacetaxine; Urokinase

Increased Effect/Toxicity

Aspirin may increase the levels/effects of: Agents with Antiplatelet Properties; Alendronate; Anticoagulants; Apixaban; Blood Glucose Lowering Agents; Carbonic Anhydrase Inhibitors; Carisoprodol; Collagenase (Systemic); Corticosteroids (Systemic); Dabigatran Etexilate; Deoxycholic Acid; Dexketoprofen; Heparin; Ibritumomab; Methotrexate; Nicorandil; NSAID (COX-2 Inhibitor); Obinutuzumab; Omacetaxine; PRALAtrexate; Rivaroxaban; Salicylates; Thrombolytic Agents; Ticagrelor; Tositumomab and Iodine I 131 Tositumomab; Urokinase; Valproic Acid and Derivatives; Varicella Virus-Containing Vaccines; Vitamin K Antagonists

The levels/effects of Aspirin may be increased by: Agents with Antiplatelet Properties; Ammonium Chloride; Antidepressants (Tricyclic, Tertiary Amine); Calcium Channel Blockers (Nondihydropyridine); Dasatinib; Floctafenine; Ginkgo Biloba; Glucosamine; Herbs (Anticoagulant/Antiplatelet Properties); Ibrutinib; Influenza Virus Vaccine (Live/Attenuated); Ketorolac (Nasal); Ketorolac (Systemic); Limaprost; Loop Diuretics; Multivitamins/Fluoride (with ADE); Multivitamins/Minerals (with ADEK, Folate, Iron); Multivitamins/Minerals (with AE, No Iron); NSAID

(Nonselective); Omega-3 Fatty Acids; Pentosan Polysulfate Sodium; Pentoxifylline; Potassium Acid Phosphate; Prostacyclin Analogues; Selective Serotonin Reuptake Inhibitors; Serotonin/Norepinephrine Reuptake Inhibitors; Tipranavir; Treprostinil; Vitamin E

Decreased Effect

Aspirin may decrease the levels/effects of: ACE Inhibitors; Carisoprodol; Dexketoprofen; Hyaluronidase; Loop Diuretics; Multivitamins/Fluoride (with ADE); Multivitamins/Minerals (with ADEK, Folate, Iron); Multivitamins/Minerals (with AE, No Iron); NSAID (Nonselective); Probenecid; Ticagrelor; Tiludronate

The levels/effects of Aspirin may be decreased by: Corticosteroids (Systemic); Dexketoprofen; Floctafenine; Ketorolac (Nasal); Ketorolac (Systemic); NSAID (Nonselective)

Food Interactions Food may decrease the rate but not the extent of oral absorption. Benedictine liqueur, prunes, raisins, tea, and gherkins have a potential to cause salicylate accumulation. Fresh fruits containing vitamin C may displace drug from binding sites, resulting in increased urinary excretion of aspirin. Curry powder, paprika, licorice; may cause salicylate accumulation. These foods contain 6 mg salicylate/100 g. An ordinary American diet contains 10-200 mg/day of salicylate. Management: Administer with food or large volume of water or milk to minimize GI upset. Limit curry powder, paprika, licorice.

Storage/Stability Store oral dosage forms (caplets, tablets) at room temperature; protect from moisture; see product-specific labeling for details. Keep suppositories in refrigerator; do not freeze. Hydrolysis of aspirin occurs upon exposure to water or moist air, resulting in salicylate and acetate, which possess a vinegar-like odor. Do not use if a strong odor is present.

Mechanism of Action Irreversibly inhibits cyclooxygenase-1 and 2 (COX-1 and 2) enzymes, via acetylation, which results in decreased formation of prostaglandin precursors; irreversibly inhibits formation of prostaglandin derivative, thromboxane A_2, via acetylation of platelet cyclooxygenase, thus inhibiting platelet aggregation; has antipyretic, analgesic, and anti-inflammatory properties

Pharmacokinetics (Adult data unless noted)

Absorption: From the stomach and small intestine

Distribution: Readily distributes into most body fluids and tissues; hydrolyzed to salicylate (active) by esterases in the GI mucosa, red blood cells, synovial fluid and blood

Metabolism: Primarily by hepatic microsomal enzymes

Half-life: 15 to 20 minutes; metabolic pathways are saturable such that salicylate half-life is dose-dependent ranging from 3 hours at lower doses (300-600 mg), 5 to 6 hours (after 1 g) and 10 hours with higher doses

Time to peak serum concentration: Salicylate: ~1 to 2 hours

Elimination: Renal as salicylate and conjugated metabolites

Dosing: Neonatal Full-term neonate: **Antiplatelet effects:** Postoperative congenital heart repair or recurrent arterial ischemic stroke: Oral: Adequate neonatal studies have not been performed; neonatal dosage is derived from clinical experience and is not well established; suggested doses: 1 to 5 mg/kg/dose once daily (Monagle 2012). Doses are typically rounded to a convenient amount (eg, 1/4 of 81 mg tablet)

Dosing: Usual

Infants, Children, and Adolescents: **Note:** Doses are typically rounded to a convenient amount (eg, 1/4 of 81 mg tablet):

Analgesic: Oral, rectal: **Note:** Do not use aspirin in children <12 years (APS, 2008) and adolescents (per manufacturer) who have or who are recovering from chickenpox or flu symptoms due to the association with Reye's syndrome (APS, 2008):

Infants, Children, and Adolescents weighing <50 kg: 10 to 15 mg/kg/dose every 4 to 6 hours; maximum daily dose: The lesser value of either 120 mg/kg/**day** or 4,000 mg/**day** (APS, 2008)

Children ≥12 years and Adolescents weighing ≥50 kg: 325 to 650 mg every 4 to 6 hours; maximum daily dose: 4,000 mg/**day**

Anti-inflammatory: Oral: Initial: 60 to 90 mg/kg/**day** in divided doses; usual maintenance: 80 to 100 mg/kg/**day** divided every 6 to 8 hours; monitor serum concentrations (Levy, 1978)

Antiplatelet effects: Limited data available: Oral: Adequate pediatric studies have not been performed; pediatric dosage is derived from adult studies and clinical experience and is not well established; suggested doses have ranged from 1 to 5 mg/kg/dose once daily (Monagle, 2012) to 5 to 10 mg/kg/dose once daily. Doses are typically rounded to a convenient amount (eg, 1/2 of 81 mg tablet).

Acute ischemic stroke (AIS):

Noncardioembolic: 1 to 5 mg/kg/dose once daily for ≥2 years; patients with recurrent AIS or TIAs should be transitioned to clopidogrel, LMWH, or warfarin (Monagle, 2012)

Secondary to Moyamoya and non-Moyamoya vasculopathy: 1 to 5 mg/kg/dose once daily; **Note:** In non-Moyamoya vasculopathy, continue aspirin for 3 months, with subsequent use guided by repeat cerebrovascular imaging (Monagle, 2012).

Prosthetic heart valve:

Bioprosthetic aortic valve (with normal sinus rhythm): 1 to 5 mg/kg/dose once daily for 3 months (Guyatt, 2012; Monagle, 2012)

Mechanical aortic and/or mitral valve: 1 to 5 mg/kg/dose once daily combined with vitamin K antagonist (eg, warfarin) is recommended as first-line antithrombotic therapy (Guyatt, 2012; Monagle, 2012). Alternative regimens: 6 to 20 mg/kg/dose once daily in combination with dipyridamole (Bradley, 1985; El Makhlouf, 1987; LeBlanc, 1993; Serra, 1987; Solymar, 1991)

Blalock-Taussig shunts; postoperative; primary prophylaxis: 1 to 5 mg/kg/dose once daily (Monagle, 2012)

Fontan surgery, postoperative; primary prophylaxis: 1 to 5 mg/kg/dose once daily (Monagle, 2012)

Ventricular assist device (VAD) placement: 1 to 5 mg/kg/dose once daily initiated within 72 hours of VAD placement; should be used with heparin (initiated between 8 to 48 hours following implantation) and with or without dipyridamole (Monagle, 2012)

Kawasaki disease: Limited data available: Oral: 80 to 100 mg/kg/**day** divided every 6 hours for up to 14 days until fever resolves for at least 48 hours; then decrease dose to 1 to 5 mg/kg/**day** once daily. In patients without coronary artery abnormalities, give lower dose (eg, 1 to 5 mg/kg/**day**; AHA suggests 3 to 5 mg/kg/**day**) for 6 to 8 weeks. In patients with coronary artery abnormalities, low-dose aspirin should be continued indefinitely (in addition to therapy with warfarin) (Monagle, 2012; Newburger, 2004; *Red Book*, 2012)

Rheumatic fever: Limited data available: Oral: Initial: 100 mg/kg/**day** divided into 4-5 doses; if response inadequate, may increase dose to 125 mg/kg/**day**; continue for 2 weeks; then decrease dose to 60-70 mg/kg/**day** in divided doses for an additional 3 to 6 weeks (WHO Guidelines, 2001)

Migratory polyarthritis, with carditis without cardiomegaly or congestive heart failure: Initial: 100 mg/kg/**day** in 4 divided doses for 3 to 5 days, followed by 75 mg/kg/**day** in 4 divided doses for 4 weeks

Carditis and cardiomegaly or congestive heart failure: At the beginning of the tapering of the prednisone dose, aspirin should be started at 75 mg/kg/**day** in 4 divided doses for 6 weeks

Adults:

Acute coronary syndrome (ST-segment elevation myocardial infarction [STEMI], unstable angina (UA)/non-ST-segment elevation myocardial infarction [NSTEMI]): Oral: Initial: 162 to 325 mg given on presentation (patient should chew nonenteric-coated aspirin especially if not taking before presentation); for patients unable to take oral, may use rectal suppository [300 to 600 mg (Antman, 2004; Maalouf, 2009)]. Maintenance (secondary prevention): 75 to 162 mg once daily indefinitely (Anderson, 2007) or 81 to 325 mg once daily; 81 mg once daily preferred (O'Gara, 2013). **Note:** When aspirin is used with ticagrelor, the recommended maintenance dose of aspirin is 81 mg/day (Jneid, 2012; O'Gara, 2013).

UA/NSTEMI: Concomitant antiplatelet therapy (Jneid, 2012):

If invasive strategy chosen: Aspirin is recommended in combination with either clopidogrel, ticagrelor (or prasugrel if at the time of PCI) or an IV GP IIb/IIIa inhibitor (if given before PCI, eptifibatide and tirofiban are preferred agents).

If noninvasive strategy chosen: Aspirin is recommended in combination with clopidogrel or ticagrelor.

Analgesic and antipyretic:

Oral: 325 to 650 mg every 4 to 6 hours; maximum daily dose: 4000 mg/**day**

Rectal: 300 to 600 mg every 4 to 6 hours; maximum daily dose: 4000 mg/**day**

Anti-inflammatory: Oral: Initial: 2400-3600 mg/day in divided doses; usual maintenance: 3600-5400 mg/day; monitor serum concentrations

CABG: Oral: 100 to 325 mg once daily initiated either preoperatively or within 6 hours postoperatively; continue indefinitely (ACCF/AHA [Hillis, 2011]). For secondary prevention in patients with prior CABG surgery, the American College of Chest Physicians recommends the use of 75 to 100 mg daily (ACCP [Vandvik, 2012]).

Coronary artery disease (CAD), established: Oral: 75 to 100 mg once daily (Guyatt, 2012)

PCI: Oral:

Nonemergent PCI: Preprocedure: 81 to 325 mg [325 mg (nonenteric coated) in aspirin-naive patients] starting at least 2 hours (preferably 24 hours) before procedure. Postprocedure: 81 mg once daily continued indefinitely [in combination with a $P2Y_{12}$ inhibitor (eg, clopidogrel, prasugrel, ticagrelor) up to 12 months] (Levine, 2011)

Primary PCI: Preprocedure: 162 to 325 mg as early as possible prior to procedure; 325 mg preferred followed by a maintenance dose of 81 mg once daily even when a stent is deployed (O'Gara, 2013)

Alternatively, in patients who have undergone elective PCI with either bare metal or drug-eluting stent placement: The American College of Chest Physicians recommends the use of 75 to 325 mg once daily (in combination with clopidogrel) for 1 month (BMS) or 3-6 months (dependent upon DES type) followed by 75 to 100 mg once daily (in combination with clopidogrel) for up to 12 months. For patients who underwent PCI but did not have stent placement, 75 to 325 mg once daily (in combination with clopidogrel) for 1 month is recommended. In either case, single antiplatelet therapy (either aspirin or clopidogrel) is recommended indefinitely (Guyatt, 2012).

Primary prevention: Oral:

American College of Cardiology/American Heart Association: Prevention of myocardial infarction: 75 to 162 mg once daily. **Note:** Patients are most likely to benefit if their 10-year coronary heart disease risk is ≥6% (Antman, 2004).

American College of Chest Physicians: Prevention of myocardial infarction and stroke: Select individuals ≥50 years of age (without symptomatic cardiovascular disease): 75 to 100 mg once daily (Guyatt, 2012; Grade 2B, weak recommendation)

Stroke/TIA: Oral:

Acute ischemic stroke/TIA: Initial: 160 to 325 mg within 48 hours of stroke/TIA onset, followed by 75 to 100 mg once daily (Guyatt, 2012). The AHA/ASA recommends an initial dose of 325 mg within 24 to 48 hours after stroke; do not administer aspirin within 24 hours after administration of alteplase (Jauch, 2013).

Cardioembolic, secondary prevention (oral anticoagulation unsuitable): 75 to 100 mg once daily (in combination with clopidogrel) (Guyatt, 2012)

Cryptogenic with patent foramen ovale (PFO) or atrial septal aneurysm: 50 to 100 mg once daily (Guyatt, 2012)

Noncardioembolic, secondary prevention: 75 to 325 mg once daily (Smith, 2011) **or** 75 to 100 mg once daily (Guyatt, 2012). **Note:** Combination aspirin/extended release dipyridamole or clopidogrel is preferred over aspirin alone (The ACTIVE Investigators, 2009; Guyatt, 2012).

Women at high risk, primary prevention: 81 mg once daily **or** 100 mg every other day (Goldstein, 2010)

Dosing adjustment in renal impairment:

Infants, Children, and Adolescents: The following the adjustments have been recommended (Aronoff, 2007):

GFR ≥10 mL/minute/1.73 m^2: No dosage adjustment necessary.

GFR <10 mL/minute/1.73 m^2: Avoid use.

Intermittent hemodialysis: Dialyzable: 50% to 100%; administer daily dose after dialysis session

Peritoneal dialysis: Avoid use

CRRT: No dosage adjustment necessary; monitor serum concentrations

Adults:

CrCl <10 mL/minute: Avoid use.

Dialyzable (50% to 100%)

Administration Oral: Administer with water, food, or milk to decrease GI upset. Do not crush or chew enteric coated tablets; these preparations should be swallowed whole. For acute myocardial infarction, have patient chew immediate release tablet.

Monitoring Parameters Serum salicylate concentration with chronic use; may not be necessary in Kawasaki disease; **Note:** Decreased aspirin absorption and increased salicylate clearance has been observed in children with acute Kawasaki disease; these patients rarely achieve therapeutic serum salicylate concentrations; thus, monitoring of serum salicylate concentrations is not necessary in most of these children.

Reference Range

Timing of serum samples: Peak concentrations usually occur 2 hours after normal doses but may occur 6-24 hours after acute toxic ingestion.

Salicylate serum concentrations correlate with the pharmacological actions and adverse effects observed. See table.

Serum Salicylate: Clinical Correlations

Serum Salicylate Concentration (mcg/mL)	Desired Effects	Adverse Effects / Intoxication
~100	Antiplatelet Antipyresis Analgesia	GI intolerance and bleeding, hypersensitivity, hemostatic defects
150 to 300	Anti-inflammatory	Mild salicylism
250 to 400	Treatment of rheumatic fever	Nausea/vomiting, hyperventilation, salicylism, flushing, sweating, thirst, headache, diarrhea, and tachycardia
>400 to 500		Respiratory alkalosis, hemorrhage, excitement, confusion, asterixis, pulmonary edema, convulsions, tetany, metabolic acidosis, fever, coma, cardiovascular collapse, renal and respiratory failure

Test Interactions False-negative results for glucose oxidase urinary glucose tests (Clinistix); false-positives using the cupric sulfate method (Clinitest); also, interferes with Gerhardt test, VMA determination; 5-HIAA, xylose tolerance test and T_3 and T_4

Dosage Forms Excipient information presented when available (limited, particularly for generics); consult specific product labeling.

Caplet, oral: 500 mg
- Bayer Aspirin Extra Strength: 500 mg
- Bayer Genuine Aspirin: 325 mg
- Bayer Women's Low Dose Aspirin: 81 mg [contains elemental calcium 300 mg]

Caplet, oral [buffered]:
- Ascriptin Maximum Strength: 500 mg [contains aluminum hydroxide, calcium carbonate, magnesium hydroxide]
- Bayer Plus Extra Strength: 500 mg [contains calcium carbonate]

Caplet, enteric coated, oral:
- Bayer Aspirin Regimen Regular Strength: 325 mg

Suppository, rectal: 300 mg (12s); 600 mg (12s)

Tablet, oral: 325 mg
- Aspercin: 325 mg
- Aspirtab: 325 mg
- Bayer Genuine Aspirin: 325 mg

Tablet, oral [buffered]: 325 mg
- Ascriptin Regular Strength: 325 mg [contains aluminum hydroxide, calcium carbonate, magnesium hydroxide]
- Buffasal: 325 mg [contains magnesium oxide]
- Bufferin: 325 mg [contains calcium carbonate, magnesium carbonate, magnesium oxide]
- Bufferin Extra Strength: 500 mg [contains calcium carbonate, magnesium carbonate, magnesium oxide]
- Buffinol: 324 mg [sugar free; contains magnesium oxide]
- Tri-Buffered Aspirin: 325 mg [contains calcium carbonate, magnesium carbonate, magnesium oxide]

Tablet, chewable, oral: 81 mg
- Bayer Aspirin Regimen Children's: 81 mg [cherry flavor]
- Bayer Aspirin Regimen Children's: 81 mg [orange flavor]
- St Joseph Adult Aspirin: 81 mg

Tablet, enteric coated, oral: 81 mg, 325 mg, 650 mg
- Aspir-low: 81 mg
- Bayer Aspirin Regimen Adult Low Strength: 81 mg
- Ecotrin: 325 mg
- Ecotrin Arthritis Strength: 500 mg
- Ecotrin Low Strength: 81 mg
- Halfprin: 81 mg
- St Joseph Adult Aspirin: 81 mg

- ◆ **Aspirin and Oxycodone** *see* Oxycodone and Aspirin *on page 1597*
- ◆ **Aspirin Free Anacin Extra Strength [OTC]** *see* Acetaminophen *on page 44*
- ◆ **Aspir-low [OTC]** *see* Aspirin *on page 206*
- ◆ **Aspirtab [OTC]** *see* Aspirin *on page 206*
- ◆ **Astagraf XL** *see* Tacrolimus (Systemic) *on page 1999*
- ◆ **Astelin [DSC]** *see* Azelastine (Nasal) *on page 239*
- ◆ **Astelin (Can)** *see* Azelastine (Nasal) *on page 239*
- ◆ **Astepro** *see* Azelastine (Nasal) *on page 239*
- ◆ **Asthmanefrin Refill [OTC]** *see* EPINEPHrine (Systemic, Oral Inhalation) *on page 760*
- ◆ **Asthmanefrin Starter Kit [OTC]** *see* EPINEPHrine (Systemic, Oral Inhalation) *on page 760*
- ◆ **Astramorph** *see* Morphine (Systemic) *on page 1461*
- ◆ **Atacand** *see* Candesartan *on page 358*
- ◆ **Atarax (Can)** *see* HydrOXYzine *on page 1058*
- ◆ **Atasol (Can)** *see* Acetaminophen *on page 44*

Atazanavir (at a za NA veer)

Medication Safety Issues

High alert medication:

This medication is in a class the Institute for Safe Medication Practices (ISMP) includes among its list of drug classes that have a heightened risk of causing significant patient harm when used in error.

Related Information

Adult and Adolescent HIV *on page 2392*

Pediatric HIV *on page 2380*

Perinatal HIV *on page 2400*

Brand Names: US Reyataz

Brand Names: Canada Reyataz

Therapeutic Category Antiretroviral Agent; HIV Agents (Anti-HIV Agents); Protease Inhibitor

Generic Availability (US) No

Use Treatment of HIV-1 infection in combination with other antiretroviral agents (Oral powder: FDA approved in ages ≥3 months weighing 10 to <25 kg; Oral capsule: FDA approved in ages ≥6 years and adults). **Note:** HIV regimens consisting of **three** antiretroviral agents are strongly recommended; low-dose ritonavir (booster dose) is recommended in combination with atazanavir in all patients <13 years of age and in antiretroviral-experienced patients with prior virologic failure.

Pregnancy Risk Factor B

Pregnancy Considerations Adverse events were not observed in animal reproduction studies. Atazanavir has a low level of transfer across the human placenta with cord blood concentrations reported as 13% to 21% of maternal serum concentrations at delivery. An increased risk of teratogenic effects has not been observed based on information collected by the antiretroviral pregnancy registry. A small increased risk of preterm birth has been associated with maternal use of protease inhibitor-based combination antiretroviral (ARV) therapy during pregnancy; however, the benefits of use generally outweigh this risk and protease inhibitors (PIs) should not be withheld if otherwise recommended. Hyperglycemia, new onset of diabetes mellitus, or diabetic ketoacidosis have been reported with PIs; it is not clear if pregnancy increases this risk. Hyperbilirubinemia or hypoglycemia may occur in neonates following *in utero* exposure to atazanavir, although data are conflicting.

The DHHS Perinatal HIV Guidelines recommend atazanavir as a preferred PI in antiretroviral-naive pregnant women when combined with low-dose ritonavir boosting. Pharmacokinetic studies suggest that standard dosing during pregnancy may provide decreased plasma concentrations and some experts recommend increased doses during the second and third trimesters. However, the manufacturer notes that dose adjustment is not required unless using concomitant H_2-receptor blockers or tenofovir or for ARV-naive pregnant women taking efavirenz. May give as once-daily dosing.

Regardless of CD4 count or HIV RNA copy number, all HIV-infected pregnant women should receive a combination antiretroviral (ARV) drug regimen. A combination of antepartum, intrapartum, and infant ARV prophylaxis is recommended. ARV therapy should be started as soon as possible in women with symptomatic infection. Although earlier initiation may be more effective in reducing the perinatal transmission of HIV, initiation may be delayed until after 12 weeks gestation in women who do not require immediate treatment after careful consideration of maternal conditions (eg, nausea and vomiting) and the potential risks of first trimester fetal exposure for specific agents. A scheduled cesarean delivery at 38 weeks gestation is recommended for all women with HIV RNA >1000 copies/mL or unknown concentrations near delivery in order to decrease transmission. If ARV therapy must be interrupted for <24 hours during the peripartum period, stop then restart all medications simultaneously in order to decrease the chance of developing resistance. Long-term follow-up is recommended for all infants exposed to ARV medications. In couples who want to conceive, the HIV-infected partner should attain maximum viral suppression prior to conception.

Healthcare providers are encouraged to enroll pregnant women exposed to antiretroviral medications in the Antiretroviral Pregnancy Registry (1-800-258-4263 or www.APRegistry.com). Healthcare providers caring for HIV-infected women and their infants may contact the National Perinatal HIV Hotline (888-448-8765) for clinical consultation (DHHS [perinatal], 2014).

Breast-Feeding Considerations Atazanavir is excreted into breast milk. Maternal or infant antiretroviral therapy does not completely eliminate the risk of postnatal HIV transmission. In addition, multiclass-resistant virus has been detected in breast-feeding infants despite maternal therapy. Therefore, in the United States, where formula is accessible, affordable, safe, and sustainable, and the risk of infant mortality due to diarrhea and respiratory infections is low, complete avoidance of breast-feeding by HIV-infected women is recommended to decrease potential transmission of HIV (DHHS [perinatal], 2014).

Contraindications

Hypersensitivity (eg, Stevens-Johnson syndrome, erythema multiforme, or toxic skin eruptions) to atazanavir or any component of the formulation; concurrent therapy with alfuzosin, cisapride, ergot derivatives (dihydroergotamine, ergonovine, ergotamine, methylergonovine), indinavir, irinotecan, lovastatin, midazolam (oral), nevirapine, pimozide, rifampin, sildenafil (when used for pulmonary artery hypertension [eg, Revatio]), simvastatin, St John's wort, or triazolam; coadministration with drugs that strongly induce CYP3A and may lead to lower atazanavir exposure and loss of efficacy.

Canadian labeling: Additional contraindications (not in U.S. labeling): Concomitant use of quinidine or bepridil (currently not marketed in Canada)

Warnings/Precautions Atazanavir may prolong PR interval; ECG monitoring should be considered in patients with preexisting conduction abnormalities or with medications which prolong AV conduction (dosage adjustment required with some agents); rare cases of second-degree AV block have been reported. May cause or exacerbate preexisting hepatic dysfunction; use caution in patients with transaminase elevations prior to therapy or underlying hepatic disease, such as hepatitis B or C or cirrhosis; monitor closely at baseline and during treatment. Not recommended in patients with severe hepatic impairment. In combination with ritonavir, is not recommended in patients with any degree of hepatic impairment.

Asymptomatic elevations in bilirubin (unconjugated) occur commonly during therapy with atazanavir; consider alternative therapy if bilirubin is >5 times ULN. Evaluate alternative etiologies if transaminase elevations also occur.

Cases of nephrolithiasis have been reported in postmarketing surveillance; temporary or permanent discontinuation of therapy should be considered if symptoms develop. Not recommended for use in treatment-experienced patients with end stage renal disease (ESRD) on hemodialysis.

Protease inhibitors have been associated with a variety of hypersensitivity events (some severe), including rash, anaphylaxis (rare), angioedema, bronchospasm, erythema multiforme, Stevens-Johnson syndrome (rare) and/or toxic skin eruptions (including DRESS [drug rash, eosinophilia and systemic symptoms] syndrome). It is generally recommended to discontinue treatment if severe rash or moderate symptoms accompanied by other systemic symptoms occur.

Use with caution in patients with hemophilia A or B; increased bleeding during protease inhibitor therapy has been reported. Changes in glucose tolerance, hyperglycemia, exacerbation of diabetes, DKA, and new-onset diabetes mellitus have been reported in patients receiving protease inhibitors. May be associated with fat redistribution (buffalo hump, increased abdominal girth, breast engorgement, facial atrophy). Immune reconstitution syndrome may develop resulting in the occurrence of an inflammatory response to an indolent or residual opportunistic infection during initial HIV treatment or activation of autoimmune disorders (eg, Graves' disease, polymyositis, Guillain-Barré syndrome) later in therapy; further evaluation and treatment may be required. Oral powder contains phenylalanine; avoid or use with caution in patients with phenylketonuria. Oral powder is not recommended for use in children <10 kg or ≥25 kg. Do not use in children <3 months of age due to potential for kernicterus. Potentially significant drug-drug interactions may exist, requiring dose or frequency adjustment, additional monitoring, and/or selection of alternative therapy.

Warnings: Additional Pediatric Considerations Skin rash may occur with atazanavir use, usually mild to moderate; maculopapular; reported incidence lower in pediatric patients (14% Grade 2 to 4) than adults (21% all grades); median onset: 7.3 weeks; treatment may be continued if rash is mild to moderate (rash may resolve; median duration: 1.4 weeks); discontinue therapy in cases of severe rash. May cause cough; reported incidence in children: 21%. May cause fever; higher incidence observed in children compared to adults (19% vs 2%).

Adverse Reactions Includes data from both treatment-naive and treatment-experienced patients; listed for adults unless otherwise specified.

Cardiovascular: First degree atrioventricular block, second degree atrioventricular block, peripheral edema

Central nervous system: Depression, dizziness, headache (more common in children), insomnia, peripheral neuropathy

Dermatologic: Skin rash (more common in adults)
Endocrine & metabolic: Hyperglycemia, hypoglycemia (children), increased amylase (children and adults), increased serum cholesterol (≥240 mg/dL), increased serum triglycerides
Gastrointestinal: Abdominal pain, diarrhea (more common in children), increased serum lipase (children and adults), nausea, vomiting (more common in children)
Hematologic & oncologic: Decreased hemoglobin (children and adults), neutropenia (more common in children), thrombocytopenia
Hepatic: Increased serum ALT (children and adults; more common in patients seropositive for hepatitis B and/or C), increased serum AST (more common in patients seropositive for hepatitis B and/or C), increased serum bilirubin (children and adults), jaundice
Neuromuscular & skeletal: Increased creatine phosphokinase, limb pain (children), myalgia
Respiratory: Cough (children), nasal congestion (children), oropharyngeal pain (children), rhinorrhea (children), wheezing (children)
Miscellaneous: Fever (more common in children)
Rare but important or life-threatening: Cholecystitis, cholelithiasis, cholestasis, complete atrioventricular block (rare), diabetes mellitus, DRESS syndrome, edema, erythema multiforme, immune reconstitution syndrome, interstitial nephritis, left bundle branch block, maculopapular rash, nephrolithiasis, pancreatitis, prolongation P-R interval on ECG, prolonged Q-T interval on ECG, Stevens-Johnson syndrome, torsades de pointes

Drug Interactions

Metabolism/Transport Effects **Substrate** of CYP3A4 (major); **Note:** Assignment of Major/Minor substrate status based on clinically relevant drug interaction potential; **Inhibits** CYP1A2 (weak), CYP2C8 (weak), CYP2C9 (weak), CYP3A4 (strong), SLCO1B1, UGT1A1

Avoid Concomitant Use

Avoid concomitant use of Atazanavir with any of the following: Ado-Trastuzumab Emtansine; Alfuzosin; Amodiaquine; Apixaban; Astemizole; Avanafil; Axitinib; Barnidipine; Belinostat; Bosutinib; Buprenorphine; Cabozantinib; Ceritinib; Cisapride; Conivaptan; Crizotinib; Dapoxetine; Domperidone; Dronedarone; Eplerenone; Ergot Derivatives; Everolimus; Fusidic Acid (Systemic); Halofantrine; Ibrutinib; Idelalisib; Indinavir; Irinotecan; Isavuconazonium Sulfate; Ivabradine; Lapatinib; Lercanidipine; Lomitapide; Lovastatin; Lurasidone; Macitentan; Midazolam; Naloxegol; Nevirapine; Nilotinib; NiMODipine; Nisoldipine; Olaparib; PACLitaxel (Conventional); Palbociclib; Pimozide; Ranolazine; Red Yeast Rice; Regorafenib; Repaglinide; Rifampin; Rivaroxaban; Salmeterol; Silodosin; Simeprevir; Simvastatin; St Johns Wort; Suvorexant; Tamsulosin; Terfenadine; Ticagrelor; Tipranavir; Tolvaptan; Toremifene; Trabectedin; Triazolam; Ulipristal; Vemurafenib; VinCRIStine (Liposomal); Vorapaxar; Voriconazole

Increased Effect/Toxicity

Atazanavir may increase the levels/effects of: Ado-Trastuzumab Emtansine; Alfuzosin; Almotriptan; Alosetron; ALPRAZolam; Amiodarone; Amodiaquine; Apixaban; ARIPiprazole; Astemizole; AtorvaSTATin; Avanafil; Axitinib; Barnidipine; Bedaquiline; Belinostat; Bortezomib; Bosentan; Bosutinib; Brentuximab Vedotin; Brinzolamide; Budesonide (Nasal); Budesonide (Systemic, Oral Inhalation); Budesonide (Topical); Buprenorphine; Cabazitaxel; Cabozantinib; Calcium Channel Blockers (Dihydropyridine); Calcium Channel Blockers (Nondihydropyridine); Cannabis; CarBAMazepine; Ceritinib; Cilostazol; Cisapride; Clarithromycin; Colchicine; Conivaptan; Contraceptives (Progestins); Corticosteroids (Orally Inhaled); Corticosteroids (Systemic); Crizotinib; Cyclophosphamide; CycloSPORINE (Systemic); CYP3A4 Substrates; Dapoxetine; Dasatinib; Digoxin; Domperidone; DOXOrubicin (Conventional); Dronabinol; Dronedarone; Dutasteride; Eliglustat; Eluxadoline; Elvitegravir; Enfuvirtide; Eplerenone; Ergot Derivatives; Erlotinib; Etizolam; Etravirine; Everolimus; FentaNYL; Fesoterodine; Fluticasone (Nasal); Fluticasone (Oral Inhalation); Fluvastatin; GuanFACINE; Halofantrine; Highest Risk QTc-Prolonging Agents; Hydrocodone; Ibrutinib; Iloperidone; Imatinib; Imidafenacin; Indinavir; Irinotecan; Isavuconazonium Sulfate; Ivabradine; Ivacaftor; Ixabepilone; Lacosamide; Lapatinib; Lercanidipine; Levobupivacaine; Levomilnacipran; Lomitapide; Lovastatin; Lurasidone; Macitentan; Maraviroc; Meperidine; MethylPREDNISolone; Midazolam; Mifepristone; Minoxidil (Systemic); Moderate Risk QTc-Prolonging Agents; Naloxegol; Nefazodone; Nevirapine; Nilotinib; NiMODipine; Nisoldipine; Olaparib; Ospemifene; Oxybutynin; OxyCODONE; PACLitaxel (Conventional); Palbociclib; Panobinostat; Parecoxib; Paricalcitol; PAZOPanib; Pimecrolimus; Pimozide; Pitavastatin; PONATinib; Pranlukast; PrednisoLONE (Systemic); PredniSONE; Propafenone; Protease Inhibitors; QUEtiapine; QuiNIDine; Ramelteon; Ranolazine; Red Yeast Rice; Regorafenib; Repaglinide; Retapamulin; Rifabutin; Rilpivirine; Riociguat; Rivaroxaban; RomiDEPsin; Rosiglitazone; Rosuvastatin; Ruxolitinib; Salmeterol; Saxagliptin; Sildenafil; Silodosin; Simeprevir; Simvastatin; SORAfenib; Suvorexant; Tacrolimus (Systemic); Tacrolimus (Topical); Tadalafil; Tamsulosin; Tasimelteon; Temsirolimus; Tenofovir; Terfenadine; Tetrahydrocannabinol; Ticagrelor; TiZANidine; Tofacitinib; Tolterodine; Tolvaptan; Toremifene; Trabectedin; TraMADol; TraZODone; Triazolam; Tricyclic Antidepressants; Ulipristal; Vardenafil; Vemurafenib; Vilazodone; VinCRIStine (Liposomal); Vorapaxar; Voriconazole; Warfarin; Zopiclone; Zuclopenthixol

The levels/effects of Atazanavir may be increased by: Clarithromycin; Conivaptan; CycloSPORINE (Systemic); CYP3A4 Inhibitors (Moderate); CYP3A4 Inhibitors (Strong); Delavirdine; Enfuvirtide; Fusidic Acid (Systemic); Idelalisib; Indinavir; Luliconazole; Mifepristone; Netupitant; Posaconazole; Simeprevir; Stiripentol; Telaprevir

Decreased Effect

Atazanavir may decrease the levels/effects of: Abacavir; Antidiabetic Agents; Boceprevir; Clarithromycin; Contraceptives (Estrogens); Delavirdine; Didanosine; Disulfiram; Ifosfamide; LamoTRIgine; Meperidine; Prasugrel; Telaprevir; Ticagrelor; Valproic Acid and Derivatives; Voriconazole; Zidovudine

The levels/effects of Atazanavir may be decreased by: Antacids; Boceprevir; Bosentan; Buprenorphine; CarBAMazepine; CYP3A4 Inducers (Moderate); CYP3A4 Inducers (Strong); Dabrafenib; Deferasirox; Didanosine; Efavirenz; Etravirine; Garlic; H2-Antagonists; Minocycline; Mitotane; Nevirapine; Proton Pump Inhibitors; Rifampin; Siltuximab; St Johns Wort; Tenofovir; Tipranavir; Tocilizumab; Voriconazole

Food Interactions Bioavailability of atazanavir increased when taken with food. Management: Administer with food.

Storage/Stability

Store capsules at 25°C (77°F); excursions are permitted between 15°C and 30°C (59°F and 86°F).
Store oral powder below 30°C (86°F). Store oral powder in the original packet and do not open until ready to use. Once the oral powder is mixed with food or beverage, it may be kept at 20°C to 30°C (68°F to 86°F) for up to 1 hour prior to administration.

Mechanism of Action Binds to the site of HIV-1 protease activity and inhibits cleavage of viral Gag-Pol polyprotein precursors into individual functional proteins required for infectious HIV. This results in the formation of immature, noninfectious viral particles.

Pharmacokinetics (Adult data unless noted)

Absorption: Rapid; enhanced with food

Distribution: CSF: Plasma concentration ratio (range): 0.0021 to 0.0226

Protein binding: 86%; binds to both $alpha_1$-acid glycoprotein and albumin (similar affinity)

Metabolism: Hepatic, primarily by cytochrome P450 isoenzyme CYP3A; also undergoes biliary elimination; major biotransformation pathways include mono-oxygenation and deoxygenation; minor pathways for parent drug or metabolites include glucuronidation, N-dealkylation, hydrolysis and oxygenation with dehydrogenation; 2 minor inactive metabolites have been identified

Half-life:

Adults: Unboosted: 7 to 8 hours, Boosted with ritonavir: 9 to 18 hours

Adults with hepatic impairment: 12 hours

Time to peak serum concentration: 2 to 3 hours

Elimination: 13% of the dose is excreted in the urine (7% as unchanged drug); 79% of the dose is excreted in feces (20% as unchanged drug)

Dosing: Neonatal Not recommended due to risk of kernicterus

Dosing: Usual

Pediatric: **HIV infection, treatment:** Use in combination with other antiretroviral agents. **Note:** Oral capsules and oral powder are not interchangeable. In adult studies, the bioavailability of oral capsules was higher than that of oral powder.

Infants 1 to <3 months: Not recommended due to risk of kernicterus

Infants ≥3 months, Children, and Adolescents <18 years: Oral:

Note: Pediatric patients <13 years of age must receive atazanavir **plus** ritonavir taken together once daily with food. Dosing recommendations do not exist for patients <40 kg who receive concomitant tenofovir. For all pediatric patients, follow the adult recommendations about timing of concomitant H_2-receptor blockers and proton pump inhibitors; do not exceed recommended adult maximum doses of these concurrent agents. Pediatric patients ≥13 years and ≥40 kg who receive concomitant tenofovir, H_2-receptor blockers, or proton pump inhibitors must take atazanavir **plus** ritonavir.

Ritonavir unboosted regimen: Antiretroviral-naïve patients ≥13 years and ≥40 kg who are not able to tolerate ritonavir: Oral capsule: Atazanavir 400 mg once daily (without ritonavir). **Note:** Ritonavir boosted atazanavir dosing regimen is preferred; data indicates that higher atazanavir dosing (ie, higher on a mg/kg or mg/m^2 basis than predicted by adult dosing guidelines) may be needed when atazanavir is used without ritonavir boosting in children and adolescents (DHHS [pediatric] 2015).

Ritonavir boosted regimen: Antiretroviral-naïve and experienced patients:

Oral powder: Infants and Children weighing 10 to <25 kg:

10 to <15 kg: 200 mg (4 packets) **plus** ritonavir 80 mg once daily

15 to <25 kg: 250 mg (5 packets) **plus** ritonavir 80 mg once daily

Note: For children weighing 25 to <35 kg who are unable to swallow a capsule, some experts recommend the investigational dose of 300 mg (6 packets) plus ritonavir 80 mg once daily (DHHS [pediatric] 2015)

Oral capsule: Children and Adolescents 6 to <18 years: **Note:** Some experts recommend switching to the capsule formulation for any child ≥25 kg (regardless of age) when they can swallow a capsule whole (DHHS [pediatric] 2015).

15 kg to <20 kg: Atazanavir 150 mg **plus** ritonavir 100 mg once daily

20 kg to <40 kg: Atazanavir 200 mg **plus** ritonavir 100 mg once daily; some experts would increase to 300 mg atazanavir for patients ≥35 kg, especially when given with tenofovir (DHHS [pediatric] 2015)

≥40 kg: Atazanavir 300 mg **plus** ritonavir 100 mg once daily

Adolescents ≥18 years and Adults: **HIV infection, treatment:** Oral:

Antiretroviral-naïve patients: Atazanavir 300 mg once daily **plus** ritonavir 100 mg once daily **or** atazanavir 400 mg once daily in patients unable to tolerate ritonavir.

Antiretroviral-experienced patients: Atazanavir 300 mg once daily **plus** ritonavir 100 mg once daily. **Note:** Atazanavir without ritonavir is not recommended in antiretroviral-experienced patients with prior virologic failure.

Pregnant patients (antiretroviral-naïve or experienced): Atazanavir 300 mg once daily **plus** ritonavir 100 mg once daily. **Note:** Preferred regimen for pregnant patients who are antiretroviral-naïve. Postpartum dosage adjustment not needed. Observe patient for adverse events, especially within 2 months after delivery. Dose adjustments required for treatment-experienced patients during their second and third trimester if concomitant tenofovir **or** H_2 antagonist use (insufficient information for dose adjustment if **both** tenofovir and an H_2 antagonist are used). Some experts recommend atazanavir 400 mg plus ritonavir 100 mg in all pregnant women during the second and third trimesters due to decreased plasma concentrations (DHHS [perinatal] 2014).

Dosing adjustments for concomitant therapy:

Coadministration with didanosine buffered or enteric-coated formulations: All patients: Administer atazanavir 2 hours before or 1 hour after didanosine buffered or enteric-coated formulations

Coadministration with efavirenz:

Antiretroviral-naïve patients: Adults: Atazanavir 400 mg **plus** ritonavir 100 mg with efavirenz 600 mg (all once daily but administered at different times; atazanavir and ritonavir with food and efavirenz on an empty stomach, preferably at bedtime)

Antiretroviral-experienced patients: Concurrent use not recommended due to decreased atazanavir exposure

Coadministration with H_2-receptor antagonists:

Antiretroviral-naïve patients: Daily dose of atazanavir **plus** ritonavir given simultaneously with, or at least 10 hours after, the H_2-receptor antagonist; dosage of H_2-receptor antagonist must be limited to the equivalent of 40 mg dose of famotidine twice daily in adults; administer with food

Patients unable to tolerate ritonavir: Adults: Atazanavir 400 mg once daily given at least 2 hours before or at least 10 hours after an H_2 antagonist; dosage of H_2-receptor antagonist must be limited to the equivalent daily dose of ≤40 mg famotidine (single dose: ≤20 mg)

Antiretroviral-experienced patients: Daily dose of atazanavir **plus** ritonavir given simultaneously with, or at least 10 hours after, the H_2-receptor antagonist; dosage of H_2-receptor antagonist must be limited to the equivalent of a 20 mg dose of famotidine twice daily in adults; administer with food

Antiretroviral-experienced pregnant patients in the second or third trimester: Adults: Atazanavir 400 mg plus ritonavir 100 mg simultaneously with, or at least 10 hours after an H_2 antagonist. **Note:** Insufficient information for dose adjustment if tenofovir **and** an H_2-antagonist are used.

Coadministration with proton pump inhibitor:
Antiretroviral-naïve patients: Daily dose of atazanavir **plus** ritonavir given 12 hours after the proton pump inhibitor; dosage of proton pump inhibitor must be limited to the equivalent of a 20 mg dose of omeprazole/day in adults; administer with food
Antiretroviral-experienced patients: Concurrent use **not** recommended
Coadministration with tenofovir: Adults:
Antiretroviral-naïve patients: Atazanavir 300 mg **plus** ritonavir 100 mg given with tenofovir 300 mg (all as a single daily dose); administer with food; do **not** use tenofovir and atazanavir without booster doses of ritonavir; if H_2-receptor antagonist is coadministered, increase atazanavir to 400 mg **plus** ritonavir 100 mg once daily (see Coadministration with H_2-receptor antagonist)
Antiretroviral-experienced patients: Atazanavir 300 mg plus ritonavir 100 mg given with tenofovir 300 mg (all as a single daily dose); if H_2 antagonist coadministered (not to exceed equivalent daily dose of ≤40 mg famotidine), increase atazanavir to 400 mg (plus ritonavir 100 mg) once daily
Antiretroviral-experienced pregnant patients in the second or third trimester: Atazanavir 400 mg plus ritonavir 100 mg. **Note:** Insufficient information for dose adjustment if tenofovir **and** an H_2 antagonist are used.

Dosing adjustment in renal impairment:
Patients with renal impairment, including severe renal impairment who are not managed with hemodialysis: Infants ≥3 months, Children, Adolescents, and Adults: No dosage adjustment required
Patients with end-stage renal disease managed with hemodialysis: Not appreciably removed during hemodialysis. Only 2.1% of the dose was removed during a 4-hour dialysis session; however, mean AUC, peak, and trough serum concentrations were 25% to 43% lower (versus adults with normal renal function) when atazanavir was administered either prior to, or after hemodialysis; mechanism of the decrease is not currently known.
Antiretroviral-naïve patients: Adults: Atazanavir 300 mg **plus** ritonavir 100 mg once daily
Antiretroviral-experienced patients: Do not use atazanavir; dosage is not known

Dosing adjustment in hepatic impairment:
Atazanavir:
Mild to moderate hepatic insufficiency: Adults: Use with caution; if moderate hepatic impairment (Child-Pugh class B) and no prior virologic failure, consider dose reduction of atazanavir to 300 mg once daily
Severe hepatic impairment (Child-Pugh Class C): Do not use
Note: Patients with underlying hepatitis B or C or those with marked elevations in transaminases prior to treatment may be at increased risk of hepatic decompensation or further increases in transaminases with atazanavir therapy (monitor patients closely).
Atazanavir and ritonavir: Combination therapy with ritonavir in patients with hepatic impairment is **not** recommended.

Preparation for Administration
Oral powder: It is preferable to mix oral powder with food, such as applesauce or yogurt; may also be mixed with a beverage (eg, milk, infant formula, water) for infants who can drink from a cup.
Determine the number of packets (4 or 5 packets) needed. Mix with a small amount (one tablespoon) of soft food (preferred [eg, applesauce, yogurt]) or beverage (milk, formula, water). Must be administered within 1 hour of preparation.

Administration Administer with food to enhance absorption. Administer atazanavir 2 hours before or 1 hour after didanosine buffered formulations, didanosine enteric-coated capsules, other buffered medications, or antacids. Administer atazanavir (with ritonavir) simultaneously with, or at least 10 hours after, H_2-receptor antagonists; administer atazanavir (without ritonavir) at least 2 hours before or at least 10 hours after H_2-receptor antagonist. Administer atazanavir (with ritonavir) 12 hours after proton pump inhibitor.
Additional formulation specific information:
Oral capsules: Swallow capsules whole, do not open.
Oral powder:
Mixing with food: Using a spoon, mix the recommended number of oral powder packets with a minimum of one tablespoon of food (such as applesauce or yogurt) in a small container. Feed the mixture to the infant or young child. Add an additional one tablespoon of food to the container, mix, and feed the child the residual mixture.
Mixing with a beverage such as milk or water in a small drinking cup: Using a spoon, mix the recommended number of oral powder packets with a minimum of 30 mL of the beverage in a drinking cup. Have the child drink the mixture. Add an additional 15 mL more of beverage to the cup, mix, and have the child drink the residual mixture. If water is used, food should also be taken at the same time.
Mixing with liquid infant formula using an oral dosing syringe and a small medicine cup: Using a spoon, mix the recommended number of oral powder packets with 10 mL of prepared liquid infant formula in the medicine cup. Draw up the full amount of the mixture into an oral syringe and administer into either right or left inner cheek of infant. Pour another 10 mL of formula into the medicine cup to rinse off remaining oral powder in cup. Draw up residual mixture into the syringe and administer into either right or left inner cheek of infant. Administration of atazanavir and infant formula using an infant bottle is not recommended because full dose may not be delivered.
Administer the entire dosage of oral powder (mixed in the food or beverage) within 1 hour of preparation (may leave the mixture at room temperature during this 1 hour period). Ensure that the patient eats or drinks all the food or beverage that contains the powder. Additional food may be given after consumption of the entire mixture. Administer ritonavir immediately following oral powder administration.

Monitoring Parameters Note: The absolute CD4 cell count is currently recommended to monitor immune status in children of all ages; CD4 percentage can be used as an alternative. This recommendation is based on the use of absolute CD4 cell counts in the current pediatric HIV infection stage classification and as thresholds for initiation of antiretroviral treatment (HHS [pediatric] 2015).

Prior to initiation of therapy: Genotypic resistance testing, CD4 and viral load (every 3 to 4 months), CBC with differential, LFTs, BUN, creatinine, electrolytes, glucose, urinalysis (every 6 to 12 months), and assessment of readiness for adherence with medication regimen. At initiation and with any change in treatment regimen: CBC with differential, electrolytes, calcium, phosphate, glucose, LFTs, bilirubin, urinalysis (at initiation), BUN, creatinine, albumin, total protein, lipid panel (at initiation), CD4, and viral load. After 1 to 2 weeks of therapy: Signs of medication toxicity and adherence. After 2 to 4 weeks of therapy: CBC with differential, viral load, signs of medication toxicity, and adherence; then every 3 to 4 months: CBC with differential, electrolytes, glucose, LFTs, bilirubin, BUN, creatinine, CD4, viral load, signs of medication toxicity, and adherence. Every 6 to 12 months: Lipid panel and urinalysis. CD4 monitoring frequency may be decreased to every 6 to 12 months in children who are adherent to therapy if the value is well above the threshold for opportunistic infections, viral suppression is sustained, and the clinical status is stable for more than 2 to 3 years (DHHS [pediatric] 2015). Monitor for growth and development, signs of HIV-specific physical conditions, HIV disease progression, opportunistic infections or pancreatitis.

Reference Range Plasma trough concentration ≥150 ng/mL (DHHS [pediatric] 2015)

Additional Information Preliminary studies have shown that appropriate atazanavir serum concentrations are difficult to achieve in pediatric patients even with higher doses (on a mg/kg or m^2 basis). Optimal dosing in children <6 years of age is under investigation; the addition of low-dose ritonavir (booster doses) to increase atazanavir serum concentrations may be required and is currently being evaluated. Results of a pediatric Phase II clinical trial (IMPAACT/PACTG 1020A) of atazanavir oral capsules suggest that when used **without** ritonavir boosting, children ≥6 and <13 years of age require atazanavir 520 mg/m^2/day and adolescents ≥13 years of age require atazanavir 620 mg/m^2/day (once daily doses of 600 to 900 mg/day). When used in combination **with** ritonavir, the study used atazanavir 205 mg/m^2/day (once daily doses of 250 to 375 mg/day) (DHHS [pediatric] 2015).

Dosage Forms Excipient information presented when available (limited, particularly for generics); consult specific product labeling.

Capsule, Oral, as sulfate:

Reyataz: 150 mg, 200 mg, 300 mg [contains fd&c blue #2 (indigotine)]

Packet, Oral, as sulfate:

Reyataz: 50 mg (30 ea) [contains aspartame; orange-vanilla flavor]

◆ **Atazanavir Sulfate** *see* Atazanavir *on page 210*

Atenolol (a TEN oh lole)

Medication Safety Issues

Sound-alike/look-alike issues:

Atenolol may be confused with albuterol, Altenol, timolol, Tylenol

Tenormin may be confused with Imuran, Norpramin, thiamine, Trovan

Brand Names: US Tenormin

Brand Names: Canada Apo-Atenol; Ava-Atenolol; CO Atenolol; Dom-Atenolol; JAMP-Atenolol; Mint-Atenolol; Mylan-Atenolol; Nu-Atenol; PMS-Atenolol; RAN-Atenolol; ratio-Atenolol; Riva-Atenolol; Sandoz-Atenolol; Septa-Atenolol; Tenormin; Teva-Atenolol

Therapeutic Category Antianginal Agent; Antihypertensive Agent; Beta-Adrenergic Blocker

Generic Availability (US) Yes

Use Treatment of hypertension, alone or in combination with other agents (FDA approved in adults); management of angina pectoris (FDA approved in adults); post-MI patients (to reduce cardiovascular mortality) (FDA approved in adults); has also been used for management of arrhythmias, infantile hemangioma, and thyrotoxicosis

Pregnancy Risk Factor D

Pregnancy Considerations Studies in pregnant women have demonstrated a risk to the fetus; therefore, the manufacturer classifies atenolol as pregnancy category D. Atenolol crosses the placenta and is found in cord blood. In a cohort study, an increased risk of cardiovascular defects was observed following maternal use of beta-blockers during pregnancy. Intrauterine growth restriction (IUGR), small placentas, as well as fetal/neonatal bradycardia, hypoglycemia, and/or respiratory depression have been observed following *in utero* exposure to beta-blockers as a class. Adequate facilities for monitoring infants at birth should be available. Untreated chronic maternal hypertension and pre-eclampsia are also associated with adverse events in the fetus, infant, and mother. The maternal pharmacokinetic parameters of atenolol during the second and third trimesters are within the ranges reported in nonpregnant patients. Although atenolol has shown efficacy in the treatment of hypertension in pregnancy, it is not the drug of choice due to potential IUGR in the infant.

Breast-Feeding Considerations Atenolol is excreted in breast milk and has been detected in the serum and urine of nursing infants. Peak concentrations in breast milk have been reported to occur between 2 to 8 hours after the maternal dose and in some cases are higher than the peak maternal serum concentration. Although most studies have not reported adverse events in nursing infants, avoiding maternal use while nursing infants with renal dysfunction or infants <44 weeks postconceptual age has been suggested. Beta-blockers with less distribution into breast milk may be preferred. The manufacturer recommends that caution be exercised when administering atenolol to nursing women.

Contraindications Hypersensitivity to atenolol or any component of the formulation; sinus bradycardia; sinus node dysfunction; heart block greater than first-degree (except in patients with a functioning artificial pacemaker); cardiogenic shock; uncompensated cardiac failure; pulmonary edema; pregnancy

Warnings/Precautions Consider preexisting conditions such as sick sinus syndrome before initiating. Administer cautiously in compensated heart failure and monitor for a worsening of the condition (efficacy of atenolol in heart failure has not been established). **[U.S. Boxed Warning]: Beta-blocker therapy should not be withdrawn abruptly (particularly in patients with CAD), but gradually tapered to avoid acute tachycardia, hypertension, and/or ischemia.** Beta-blockers without alpha1-adrenergic receptor blocking activity should be avoided in patients with Prinzmetal variant angina (Mayer, 1998). Chronic beta-blocker therapy should not be routinely withdrawn prior to major surgery. Beta-blockers should be avoided in patients with bronchospastic disease (asthma). Atenolol, with B_1 selectivity, has been used cautiously in bronchospastic disease with close monitoring. May precipitate or aggravate symptoms of arterial insufficiency in patients with PVD and Raynaud's disease; use with caution and monitor for progression of arterial obstruction. Use cautiously in patients with diabetes - may mask hypoglycemic symptoms. May mask signs of hyperthyroidism (eg, tachycardia); use caution if hyperthyroidism is suspected, abrupt withdrawal may precipitate thyroid storm. Alterations in thyroid function tests may be observed. Use cautiously in the renally impaired (dosage adjustment required). Caution in myasthenia gravis or psychiatric disease (may cause CNS depression). Bradycardia may be observed more frequently in elderly patients (>65 years of age); dosage reductions may be necessary. Adequate alpha-blockade is required prior to use of any beta-blocker for patients with untreated pheochromocytoma. May induce or exacerbate psoriasis. Use caution with history of severe anaphylaxis to allergens; patients taking beta-blockers may become more sensitive to repeated challenges. Treatment of anaphylaxis (eg, epinephrine) in patients taking beta-blockers may be ineffective or promote undesirable effects. Use with caution in patients on concurrent digoxin, verapamil, or diltiazem; bradycardia or heart block can occur. Use with caution in patients receiving inhaled anesthetic agents known to depress myocardial contractility.

Adverse Reactions

Cardiovascular: Bradycardia (persistent), cardiac failure, chest pain, cold extremities, complete atrioventricular block, edema, hypotension, Raynaud's phenomenon, second degree atrioventricular block

Central nervous system: Confusion, decreased mental acuity, depression, dizziness, fatigue, headache, insomnia, lethargy, nightmares

Gastrointestinal: Constipation, diarrhea, nausea

Genitourinary: Impotence

Rare but important or life-threatening: Alopecia, dyspnea (especially with large doses), hallucination, increased liver enzymes, lupus-like syndrome, Peyronie's disease, positive ANA titer, psoriasiform eruption, psychosis, thrombocytopenia, wheezing

Drug Interactions

Metabolism/Transport Effects None known.

Avoid Concomitant Use

Avoid concomitant use of Atenolol with any of the following: Ceritinib; Floctafenine; Methacholine; Rivastigmine

Increased Effect/Toxicity

Atenolol may increase the levels/effects of: Alpha-/Beta-Agonists (Direct-Acting); Alpha1-Blockers; Alpha2-Agonists; Amifostine; Antihypertensives; Bradycardia-Causing Agents; Bupivacaine; Cardiac Glycosides; Ceritinib; Cholinergic Agonists; Disopyramide; DULoxetine; Ergot Derivatives; Fingolimod; Grass Pollen Allergen Extract (5 Grass Extract); Hypotensive Agents; Insulin; Ivabradine; Lacosamide; Levodopa; Lidocaine (Systemic); Lidocaine (Topical); Mepivacaine; Methacholine; Midodrine; Obinutuzumab; RisperiDONE; RiTUXimab; Sulfonylureas

The levels/effects of Atenolol may be increased by: Acetylcholinesterase Inhibitors; Alpha2-Agonists; Amiodarone; Anilidopiperidine Opioids; Barbiturates; Bretylium; Brimonidine (Topical); Calcium Channel Blockers (Nondihydropyridine); Diazoxide; Dipyridamole; Disopyramide; Dronedarone; Floctafenine; Glycopyrrolate; Herbs (Hypotensive Properties); MAO Inhibitors; Nicorandil; NIFEdipine; Pentoxifylline; Phosphodiesterase 5 Inhibitors; Prostacyclin Analogues; Regorafenib; Reserpine; Rivastigmine; Ruxolitinib; Tofacitinib

Decreased Effect

Atenolol may decrease the levels/effects of: Beta2-Agonists; Theophylline Derivatives

The levels/effects of Atenolol may be decreased by: Ampicillin; Herbs (Hypertensive Properties); Methylphenidate; Nonsteroidal Anti-Inflammatory Agents; Yohimbine

Food Interactions Atenolol serum concentrations may be decreased if taken with food. Management: Administer without regard to meals.

Storage/Stability Store at 20°C to 25°C (68°F to 77°F).

Mechanism of Action Competitively blocks response to beta-adrenergic stimulation, selectively blocks $beta_1$-receptors with little or no effect on $beta_2$-receptors except at high doses

Pharmacodynamics

Beta-blocking effect:

Onset of action: Oral: ≤1 hour

Maximum effect: Oral: 2 to 4 hours

Duration: Oral: ≥24 hours

Antihypertensive effect:

Duration: Oral: 24 hours

Pharmacokinetics (Adult data unless noted)

Absorption: Oral: Rapid, but incomplete from the GI tract; ~50% absorbed

Distribution: Does not cross the blood-brain barrier; low lipophilicity

Protein binding: Low (6% to 16%)

Metabolism: Limited hepatic metabolism

Half-life, beta:

Newborns (<24 hours of age) born to mothers receiving atenolol: Mean: 16 hours; up to 35 hours (Rubin, 1983)

Children and Adolescents 5 to 16 years of age: Mean: 4.6 hours; range: 3.5 to 7 hours; patients >10 years of age may have longer half-life (>5 hours) compared to children 5 to 10 years of age (<5 hours) (Buck, 1989)

Adults: 6 to 7 hours

Prolonged half-life with renal dysfunction

Time to peak serum concentration: Oral: Within 2 to 4 hours

Elimination: 50% as unchanged drug in urine; 50% in feces

Dosing: Usual

Pediatric: **Note:** Dosage should be individualized based on patient response.

Arrhythmias: Limited data available: Infants, Children and Adolescents: Oral:

Long QT syndrome: Usual range: 0.5 to 1 mg/kg/day either once daily or in divided doses every 12 hours (Kliegman, 2011). In a retrospective trial (n=57; mean age: 9 ± 6 years) that titrated atenolol to achieve a maximum heart rate less than 150 bpm (Holter monitor and exercise treadmill), higher doses were reported mean effective dose: 1.4 ± 0.5 mg/kg/day in 2 divided doses (Moltedo, 2011)

Supraventricular tachycardia: Usual range: 0.3 to 1 mg/kg/day either once daily or in divided doses every 12 hours (Kliegman, 2011, Mehta, 1996; Trippel 1989). In two separate trials, titration of the dose to >1.4 mg/kg/day did not show additional treatment successes and potentially increased the risk of adverse effects (Mehta, 1996; Trippel, 1989).

Hemangioma, infantile: Limited data available: Infants and Children <2 years: Oral: 1 mg/kg/dose once daily for 6 months; dosing based on a randomized, controlled noninferiority trial compared to propranolol (n=23 total atenolol treatment group: n=13); atenolol was found to be as effective as propranolol; no significant adverse effects were reported in either group (Abarzua-Araya, 2014)

Hypertension: Oral: Children and Adolescents: Initial 0.5 to 1 mg/kg/day either once daily or divided in doses twice daily; titrate dose to effect; usual range: 0.5 to 1.5 mg/kg/day; maximum daily dose: 2 mg/kg/**day** not to exceed 100 mg/**day** (NHBPEP, 2004; NLHBI, 2011)

Thyrotoxicosis: Limited data available: Oral: Children and Adolescents: 1 to 2 mg/kg once daily; may increase to twice daily if needed; maximum dose: 100 mg/dose (Bahn 2011; Kliegman 2011)

Adult:

Angina pectoris: Oral: 50 mg once daily; may increase to 100 mg once daily. Some patients may require 200 mg daily.

Hypertension: Oral: Initial: 25 to 50 mg either once daily, after 1 to 2 weeks, may increase to 100 mg once daily. Usual dose (ASH/ISH [Weber, 2014]): 100 mg once daily; target dose (JNC 8 [James, 2013]): 100 mg once daily; doses >100 mg are unlikely to produce any further benefit.

Postmyocardial infarction: Oral: 100 mg once daily or 50 mg twice daily for 6 to 9 days postmyocardial infarction

Dosing in adjustment in renal impairment:

Children and Adolescents: There are no dosage adjustments provided in the manufacturer's labeling; however, the following guidelines have been used (Aronoff, 2007): **Note:** Renally adjusted dose recommendations are based on doses of 0.8 to 1.5 mg/kg/day:

GFR >50 mL/minute/1.73 m^2: No dosage adjustment necessary

CrCl 30 to 50 mL/minute/1.73 m^2: Maximum dose: 1 mg/kg/dose every 24 hours; maximum daily dose: 50 mg/**day**

CrCl <30 mL/minute/1.73 m^2: Maximum dose: 1 mg/kg/dose every 48 hours

Intermittent hemodialysis: Moderately dialyzable (20% to 50%); maximum dose: 1 mg/kg/dose every 48 hours; give after hemodialysis

Peritoneal dialysis: Maximum dose: 1 mg/kg/dose every 48 hours
Continuous renal replacement therapy: Maximum dose: 1 mg/kg/dose every 24 hours
Adults:
CrCl > 35 mL/minute: No dosage adjustment necessary
CrCl 15 to 35 mL/minute: Maximum dose: 50 mg daily
CrCl <15 mL/minute: Maximum dose: 25 mg daily
Hemodialysis: Moderately dialyzable (20% to 50%); administer dose postdialysis or administer 25 mg to 50 mg supplemental dose after each dialysis
Peritoneal dialysis: Elimination is not enhanced; supplemental dose is not necessary

Dosing adjustment in hepatic impairment: There are no dosage adjustments provided in the manufacturer's labeling; however, atenolol undergoes minimal hepatic metabolism.

Administration Oral: May be administered without regard to food

Monitoring Parameters Blood pressure, heart rate, ECG, fluid intake and output, daily weight, respiratory rate

Test Interactions Increased glucose; decreased HDL

Additional Information Limited data suggests that atenolol may have a shorter half-life and faster clearance in patients with Marfan syndrome. Higher doses (2 mg/kg/day divided every 12 hours) have been used in patients with Marfan syndrome (6 to 22 years of age) to decrease aortic root growth rate and prevent aortic dissection or rupture; further studies are needed (Reed, 1993).

Dosage Forms Excipient information presented when available (limited, particularly for generics); consult specific product labeling. [DSC] = Discontinued product
Tablet, Oral:
Tenormin: 25 mg, 50 mg
Tenormin: 50 mg [DSC] [scored]
Tenormin: 100 mg
Generic: 25 mg, 50 mg, 100 mg

Extemporaneous Preparations A 2 mg/mL oral suspension may be made with tablets. Crush four 50 mg tablets in a mortar and reduce to a fine powder. Add a small amount of glycerin and mix to a uniform paste. Mix while adding Ora-Sweet® SF vehicle in incremental proportions to **almost** 100 mL; transfer to a calibrated bottle, rinse mortar with vehicle, and add quantity of vehicle sufficient to make 100 mL. Label "shake well" and "refrigerate". Stable for 90 days.

Nahata MC, Pai VB, and Hipple TF, *Pediatric Drug Formulations*, 5th ed, Cincinnati, OH: Harvey Whitney Books Co, 2004.

- **ATG** *see* Antithymocyte Globulin (Equine) *on page 178*
- **Atgam** *see* Antithymocyte Globulin (Equine) *on page 178*
- **Athletes Foot Spray [OTC]** *see* Tolnaftate *on page 2083*
- **Ativan** *see* LORazepam *on page 1299*
- **Atlizumab** *see* Tocilizumab *on page 2079*
- **ATO** *see* Arsenic Trioxide *on page 198*

AtoMOXetine (AT oh mox e teen)

Medication Safety Issues
Sound-alike/look-alike issues:
AtoMOXetine may be confused with atorvaSTATin

Related Information
Oral Medications That Should Not Be Crushed or Altered *on page 2476*

Brand Names: US Strattera

Brand Names: Canada Apo-Atomoxetine; DOM-Atomoxetine; Mylan-Atomoxetine; PMS-Atomoxetine; RIVA-Atomoxetine; Sandoz-Atomoxetine; Strattera; Teva-Atomoxetine

Therapeutic Category Norepinephrine Reuptake Inhibitor, Selective

Generic Availability (US) No

Use Treatment of attention-deficit/hyperactivity disorder (ADHD) (FDA approved in ages ≥6 years and adults)

Medication Guide Available Yes

Pregnancy Risk Factor C

Pregnancy Considerations Adverse events have been observed in animal reproduction studies. Information related to atomoxetine use in pregnancy is limited; appropriate contraception is recommended for sexually active women of childbearing potential (Heiligenstein, 2003).

Breast-Feeding Considerations It is not known if atomoxetine is excreted in breast milk. The manufacturer recommends that caution be exercised when administering atomoxetine to nursing women.

Contraindications Hypersensitivity to atomoxetine or any component of the formulation; use with or within 14 days of MAO inhibitors; narrow-angle glaucoma; current or past history of pheochromocytoma; severe cardiac or vascular disorders in which the condition would be expected to deteriorate with clinically important increases in blood pressure (eg, 15 to 20 mm Hg) or heart rate (eg, 20 beats/minute).

Canadian labeling: Additional contraindications (not in U.S. labeling): Symptomatic cardiovascular diseases, moderate-to-severe hypertension; advanced arteriosclerosis; uncontrolled hyperthyroidism

Warnings/Precautions [US Boxed Warning]: Use caution in pediatric patients; may be an increased risk of suicidal ideation. Closely monitor for clinical worsening, suicidality, or unusual changes in behavior; especially during the initial few months of a course of drug therapy, or at times of dose changes, either increases or decreases. The family or caregiver should be instructed to closely observe the patient and communicate condition with healthcare provider. New or worsening symptoms of hostility or aggressive behaviors have been associated with atomoxetine, particularly with the initiation of therapy. Treatment-emergent psychotic or manic symptoms (eg, hallucinations, delusional thinking, mania) may occur in children and adolescents without a prior history of psychotic illness or mania; consider discontinuation of treatment if symptoms occur. Use caution in patients with comorbid bipolar disorder; therapy may induce mixed/manic episode. Atomoxetine is not approved for major depressive disorder. Patients presenting with depressive symptoms should be screened for bipolar disorder. Recommended to be used as part of a comprehensive treatment program for attention deficit disorders. Atomoxetine does not worsen anxiety in patients with existing anxiety disorders or tics related to Tourette's disorder.

Use caution with hepatic disease (dosage adjustments necessary in moderate and severe hepatic impairment). Use may be associated with rare but severe hepatotoxicity, including hepatic failure; discontinue and do not restart if signs or symptoms of hepatotoxic reaction (eg, jaundice, pruritus, flu-like symptoms, dark urine, right upper quadrant tenderness) or laboratory evidence of liver disease are noted. Use caution in patients who are poor metabolizers of CYP2D6 metabolized drugs ("poor metabolizers"), bioavailability increases; dosage adjustments are recommended in patients known to be CYP2D6 poor metabolizers. In clinical trials, at therapeutic doses, atomoxetine consistently did not prolong the QT/QTc interval; however, one placebo-controlled study in healthy CYP2D6 poor metabolizers demonstrated a statistically significant increase in QTc with increasing atomoxetine concentrations (Loghin 2012; Martinez-Raga 2013). Case reports suggest that atomoxetine overdose may increase the QT interval; however, this occurred when atomoxetine was combined with other agents known to have QT prolongation potential or inhibit CYP2D6 (Barker 2004; Sawant

2004). Atomoxetine, at high concentrations ex vivo, has demonstrated hERG channel block (Scherer 2009).

Orthostasis can occur; use caution in patients predisposed to hypotension or those with abrupt changes in heart rate or blood pressure. Atomoxetine has been associated with serious cardiovascular events including sudden death in patients with preexisting structural cardiac abnormalities or other serious heart problems (sudden death in children and adolescents; sudden death, stroke, and MI in adults). Atomoxetine should be avoided in patients with known serious structural cardiac abnormalities, cardiomyopathy, serious heart rhythm abnormalities, or other serious cardiac problems that could increase the risk of sudden death that these conditions alone carry. Patients should be carefully evaluated for cardiac disease prior to initiation of therapy. Perform a prompt cardiac evaluation in patients who develop symptoms of exertional chest pain, unexplained syncope, or other symptoms suggestive of cardiac disease during treatment. May cause increased heart rate or blood pressure; use caution with hypertension or other cardiovascular or cerebrovascular disease; CYP2D6 poor metabolizers may experience greater increases in blood pressure and heart rate effects. Use caution in patients with a history of urinary retention or bladder outlet obstruction; may cause urinary retention/hesitancy; use caution in patients with history of urinary retention or bladder outlet obstruction. Prolonged and painful erections (priapism), sometimes requiring surgical intervention, have been reported with stimulant and atomoxetine use in pediatric and adult patients. Priapism has been reported to develop after some time on the drug, often subsequent to an increase in dose and also during a period of drug withdrawal (drug holidays or discontinuation). Patients with certain hematological dyscrasias (eg, sickle cell disease), malignancies, perineal trauma, or concomitant use of alcohol, illicit drugs, or other medications associated with priapism may be at increased risk. Patients who develop abnormally sustained or frequent and painful erections should discontinue therapy and seek immediate medical attention. An emergent urological consultation should be obtained in severe cases. Use has been associated with different dosage forms and products; it is not known if rechallenge with a different formulation will risk recurrence. Avoidance of stimulants and atomoxetine may be preferred in patients with severe cases that were slow to resolve and/or required detumescence (Eiland, 2014). Allergic reactions (including anaphylactic reactions, angioneurotic edema, urticaria, and rash) may occur (rare).

Growth in pediatric patients should be monitored during treatment. Height and weight gain may be reduced during the first 9 to 12 months of treatment, but should recover by 3 years of therapy.

Warnings: Additional Pediatric Considerations Serious cardiovascular events, including sudden death, may occur in patients with preexisting structural cardiac abnormalities or other serious heart problems. Sudden death has been reported in children and adolescents; sudden death, stroke, and MI have been reported in adults. Avoid the use of atomoxetine in patients with known serious structural cardiac abnormalities, cardiomyopathy, serious heart rhythm abnormalities, coronary artery disease, or other serious cardiac problems that could place patients at an increased risk to the noradrenergic effects of atomoxetine. Patients should be carefully evaluated for cardiac disease prior to initiation of therapy. The American Heart Association recommends that all children diagnosed with ADHD who may be candidates for medication, such as atomoxetine, should have a thorough cardiovascular assessment prior to initiation of therapy. This assessment should include a combination of medical history, family history, and physical examination focusing on cardiovascular disease risk factors. An ECG is not mandatory but should be considered. If a child displays symptoms of cardiovascular disease, including chest pain, dyspnea, or fainting, parents should seek immediate medical care for the child. In a recent retrospective study on the possible association between stimulant medication use and sudden death in children, 564 previously healthy children who died suddenly in motor vehicle accidents were compared to a group of 564 previously healthy children who died suddenly. Two of the 564 (0.4%) children in motor vehicle accidents were taking stimulant medications compared to 10 of 564 (1.8%) children who died suddenly. While the authors of this study conclude there may be an association between stimulant use and sudden death in children, there were a number of limitations to the study and the FDA cannot conclude this information impacts the overall risk benefit profile of these medications (Gould, 2009). In a large retrospective cohort study involving 1,200,438 children and young adults (aged 2 to 24 years), none of the currently available stimulant medications or atomoxetine were shown to increase the risk of serious cardiovascular events (ie, acute MI, sudden cardiac death, or stroke) in current (adjusted hazard ratio: 0.75; 95% CI: 0.31 to 1.85) or former (adjusted hazard ratio: 1.03; 95% CI: 0.57 to 1.89) users compared to nonusers. It should be noted that due to the upper limit of the 95% CI, the study could not rule out a doubling of the risk, albeit low (Cooper, 2011).

May cause significant increases in blood pressure and heart rate; in pediatric clinical trials, incidences of maximum increases in SBP, DBP, and HR compared to placebo were as follows: SBP (≥20 mm Hg): 12.5% vs 8.7%; DBP (≥15 mm Hg): 21.5% vs 14.1%; and HR (≥20 bpm): 23.4% vs 11.5%; monitor blood pressure and pulse at baseline, with dosage increases, and periodically during therapy. Use caution in patients with underlying medical conditions which may be exacerbated by increases in blood pressure and/or heart rate, including hypertension, tachycardia, or other cardiovascular or cerebrovascular conditions; use is contraindicated in patients with severe cardiovascular disorders who may experience clinical deterioration of condition with clinical increases in blood pressure or heart rate.

In pediatric patients, suppression of growth (height and weight) has been reported during the initial 9 to 12 months of therapy and has been shown to recover to normative values by 3 years of therapy; this growth pattern has been observed to be independent of pubertal status and patient's metabolic profile (ie, poor or extensive metabolizer); growth should be monitored during treatment.

Adverse Reactions Some adverse reactions may be increased in "poor metabolizers" (CYP2D6).

Cardiovascular: Cold extremities, flushing, increased diastolic blood pressure (≥15 mm Hg), orthostatic hypotension, palpitations, prolonged Q-T interval on ECG, syncope, systolic hypertension, tachycardia

Central nervous system: Abnormal dreams, agitation, anxiety, chills, depression, disturbed sleep, dizziness, drowsiness, emotional lability, fatigue, headache (children and adolescents), hostility (children and adolescents), insomnia, irritability, jitteriness, paresthesia (adults; postmarketing observation in children), restlessness, sensation of cold

Dermatologic: Excoriation, hyperhidrosis, pruritus, skin rash, urticaria

Endocrine & metabolic: Decreased libido, hot flash, increased thirst, menstrual disease, weight loss

Gastrointestinal: Abdominal pain, anorexia, constipation, decreased appetite, dysgeusia, dyspepsia, flatulence, nausea, vomiting, xerostomia

Genitourinary: Dysmenorrhea, dysuria, ejaculatory disorder, erectile dysfunction, orgasm abnormal, pollakiuria, prostatitis, testicular pain, urinary frequency, urinary retention

Neuromuscular & skeletal: Muscle spasm, tremor, weakness
Ophthalmic: Blurred vision, conjunctivitis, mydriasis
Respiratory: Pharyngolaryngeal pain
Miscellaneous: Therapeutic response unexpected
Rare but important or life-threatening: Cerebrovascular accident, delusions, growth suppression (children), hallucination, hepatotoxicity, hypersensitivity reaction, hypomania, impulsivity, mania, myocardial infarction, panic attack, pelvic pain, priapism, Raynaud's phenomenon, rhabdomyolysis, seizure (including patients with no prior history or known risk factors for seizure), severe hepatic disease, suicidal ideation, tics

Drug Interactions

Metabolism/Transport Effects Substrate of CYP2C19 (minor), CYP2D6 (major); **Note:** Assignment of Major/ Minor substrate status based on clinically relevant drug interaction potential; **Inhibits** CYP2D6 (weak)

Avoid Concomitant Use

Avoid concomitant use of AtoMOXetine with any of the following: Iobenguane I 123; MAO Inhibitors

Increased Effect/Toxicity

AtoMOXetine may increase the levels/effects of: ARIPiprazole; Beta2-Agonists; Highest Risk QTc-Prolonging Agents; Moderate Risk QTc-Prolonging Agents; Sympathomimetics

The levels/effects of AtoMOXetine may be increased by: Abiraterone Acetate; Cobicistat; CYP2D6 Inhibitors (Moderate); CYP2D6 Inhibitors (Strong); Darunavir; MAO Inhibitors; Mifepristone; Panobinostat; Peginterferon Alfa-2b

Decreased Effect

AtoMOXetine may decrease the levels/effects of: Iobenguane I 123

The levels/effects of AtoMOXetine may be decreased by: Peginterferon Alfa-2b

Storage/Stability Store at 25°C (77°F); excursions are permitted between 15°C and 30°C (59°F and 86°F).

Mechanism of Action Selectively inhibits the reuptake of norepinephrine (Ki 4.5 nM) with little to no activity at the other neuronal reuptake pumps or receptor sites.

Pharmacokinetics (Adult data unless noted) The pharmacokinetics in pediatric patients ≥6 years of age have been shown to be similar to those of adult patients.
Absorption: Oral: Rapid
Distribution: V_d: IV: 0.85 L/kg
Protein binding: 98%, primarily albumin
Metabolism: Hepatic, primarily by oxidative metabolism via CYP2D6 to 4-hydroxyatomoxetine (major metabolite regardless of CYP2D6 status, active, equipotent to atomoxetine) with subsequent glucuronidation; also metabolized via CYP2C19 to N-desmethlyatomoxetine (active, minimal activity). **Note:** CYP2D6 poor metabolizers have atomoxetine AUCs that are ~10-fold higher and peak concentrations that are ~fivefold greater than extensive metabolizers; 4-hyroxyatomoxetine plasma concentrations are very low (extensive metabolizers: 1% of atomoxetine concentrations; poor metabolizers: 0.1% of atomoxetine concentrations
Bioavailability: Extensive metabolizers: 63%; poor metabolizers: 94%
Half-life:
Atomoxetine: Extensive metabolizers: 5.2 hours; poor metabolizers: 21.6 hours
4-hydroxyatomoxetine: Extensive metabolizers: 6-8 hours
N-desmethlyatomoxetine: Extensive metabolizers: 6-8 hours; poor metabolizers: 34-40 hours
Time to peak serum concentration: 1-2 hours; delayed 3 hours by high-fat meal
Elimination: Urine: <3% is excreted unchanged; 80% excreted as 4-hydroxyatomoxetine glucuronide; feces: <17%

Dosing: Usual Attention-deficit/hyperactivity disorder:
Children ≥6 years and Adolescents, weighing ≤70 kg: Oral: Initial: 0.5 mg/kg/day; increase after a minimum of 3 days to ~1.2 mg/kg/day; may administer once daily in the morning or divide into 2 doses and administer in the morning and late afternoon/early evening; maximum daily dose: 1.4 mg/kg/**day** or 100 mg/**day**, whichever is less. **Note:** Doses >1.2 mg/kg/day have not been shown to provide additional benefit.
Dosage adjustment with concurrent strong CYP2D6 inhibitors (eg, paroxetine, fluoxetine, quinidine) use or patients known to be CYP2D6 poor metabolizers: Oral: Initial: 0.5 mg/kg/day for 4 weeks; increase dose to 1.2 mg/kg/day only if clinically needed and the initial dose is well tolerated; do not exceed 1.2 mg/kg/**day**
Children ≥6 years and Adolescents, weighing >70 kg and Adults: Oral: Initial: 40 mg daily; increase after a minimum of 3 days to ~80 mg daily; may administer once daily in the morning or divide into 2 doses and administer in morning and late afternoon/early evening. After an additional 2-4 weeks, may increase (if needed) to maximum daily dose: 100 mg/**day**.
Dosage adjustment with concurrent strong CYP2D6 inhibitors (eg, paroxetine, fluoxetine, quinidine) use or patients known to be CYP2D6 poor metabolizers: Oral: Initial: 40 mg daily for 4 weeks; increase dose to 80 mg daily only if clinically needed and the initial dose is well tolerated; do not exceed 80 mg daily

Dosage adjustment in renal impairment: Children ≥6 years, Adolescents, and Adults: No dosage adjustments are recommended.

Dosage adjustment in hepatic impairment: Children ≥6 years, Adolescents, and Adults:
Moderate hepatic impairment (Child-Pugh class B): Administer 50% of normal dose
Severe hepatic impairment (Child-Pugh class C): Administer 25% of normal dose

Administration Oral: May be administered without regard to food. Do not crush, chew, or open capsule; swallow whole with water or other liquids. **Note:** Atomoxetine is an ocular irritant; if capsule is opened accidently and contents come into contact with eye, flush eye immediately with water and obtain medical advice; wash hands and any potentially contaminated surface as soon as possible.

Monitoring Parameters Family members and caregivers need to monitor patient daily for emergence of irritability, agitation, unusual changes in behavior, and suicide ideation. Pediatric patients should be monitored closely for suicidality, clinical worsening, or unusual changes in behavior, especially during the initial few months of therapy or at times of dose changes. Appearance of symptoms needs to be immediately reported to healthcare provider.

Evaluate for cardiac disease prior to initiation of therapy with thorough medical history, family history, and physical exam; consider ECG; perform ECG and echocardiogram if findings suggest cardiac disease; promptly conduct cardiac evaluation in patients who develop chest pain, unexplained syncope, or any other symptom of cardiac disease during treatment. Monitor body weight, BMI, height and growth rate (in children); CNS activity; blood pressure and heart rate and rhythm (baseline, following dose increases, and periodically during treatment); liver enzymes in patients with symptoms of liver dysfunction; sleep, appetite, abnormal movements. Patients should be re-evaluated at appropriate intervals to assess continued need of the medication. Monitor for new psychotic symptoms, appearance or worsening of aggressive behavior, or hostility.

Additional Information Atomoxetine hydrochloride is the R(-) isomer. Therapy may be discontinued without being tapered. Total daily doses >150 mg/day and single doses >120 mg/dose have not been systematically evaluated. Medications used to treat ADHD should be part of a total treatment program that may include other components such as psychological, educational, and social measures. If used for an extended period of time, long-term usefulness of atomoxetine should be periodically re-evaluated for the individual patient.

Dosage Forms Excipient information presented when available (limited, particularly for generics); consult specific product labeling.

Capsule, Oral:

Strattera: 10 mg, 18 mg, 25 mg, 40 mg, 60 mg

Strattera: 80 mg, 100 mg [contains fd&c blue #2 (indigotine)]

◆ **Atomoxetine Hydrochloride** *see* AtoMOXetine *on page 217*

AtorvaSTATin (a TORE va sta tin)

Medication Safety Issues

Sound-alike/look-alike issues:

AtorvaSTATin may be confused with atoMOXetine, lovastatin, nystatin, pitavastatin, pravastatin, rosuvastatin, simvastatin

Lipitor may be confused with labetalol, Levatol, lisinopril, Loniten, Lopid, Mevacor, Zocor, ZyrTEC

Related Information

Oral Medications That Should Not Be Crushed or Altered *on page 2476*

Brand Names: US Lipitor

Brand Names: Canada ACT Atorvastatin; Apo-Atorvastatin; Auro-Atorvastatin; Ava-Atorvastatin; Dom-Atorvastatin; GD-Atorvastatin; JAMP-Atorvastatin; Lipitor; Mylan-Atorvastatin; Novo-Atorvastatin; PMS-Atorvastatin; RAN-Atorvastatin; ratio-Atorvastatin; Riva-Atorvastatin; Sandoz-Atorvastatin

Therapeutic Category Antilipemic Agent; HMG-CoA Reductase Inhibitor

Generic Availability (US) Yes

Use Hyperlipidemia: Adjunct to dietary therapy in pediatric patients with heterozygous familial hypercholesterolemia if LDL-C remains ≥190 mg/dL, if ≥160 mg/dL with family history of premature CHD or presence of ≥2 cardiovascular risk factors (FDA approved in boys and postmenarchal girls 10-17 years). Adjunct to dietary therapy to decrease elevated serum total and low density lipoprotein cholesterol (LDL-C), apolipoprotein B (apo-B), and triglyceride levels, and to increase high density lipoprotein cholesterol (HDL-C) in patients with primary hypercholesterolemia (heterozygous, familial and nonfamilial) and mixed dyslipidemia (Fredrickson types IIa and IIb) (FDA approved in adults); treatment of homozygous familial hypercholesterolemia (FDA approved in adults); treatment of isolated hypertriglyceridemia (Fredrickson type IV); treatment of primary dysbetalipoproteinemia (Fredrickson Type III) (FDA approved in adults)

Primary prevention of cardiovascular disease in high risk patients (FDA approved in adults); risk factors include: Age ≥55 years, smoking, hypertension, low HDL-C, or family history of early coronary heart disease; secondary prevention of cardiovascular disease to reduce the risk of MI, stroke, revascularization procedures, and angina in patients with evidence of coronary heart disease and to reduce the risk of hospitalization for heart failure. Has also been used in prevention of graft coronary artery disease in heart transplant patients.

Pregnancy Risk Factor X

Pregnancy Considerations Adverse events were observed in animal reproductions studies. There are reports of congenital anomalies following maternal use of HMG-CoA reductase inhibitors in pregnancy; however, maternal disease, differences in specific agents used, and the low rates of exposure limit the interpretation of the available data (Godfrey 2012; Lecarpentier 2012). Cholesterol biosynthesis may be important in fetal development; serum cholesterol and triglycerides increase normally during pregnancy. The discontinuation of lipid lowering medications temporarily during pregnancy is not expected to have significant impact on the long term outcomes of primary hypercholesterolemia treatment.

Use of atorvastatin is contraindicated in pregnancy or those who may become pregnant. HMG-CoA reductase inhibitors should be discontinued prior to pregnancy (ADA 2013). If treatment of dyslipidemias is needed in pregnant women or in women of reproductive age, other agents are preferred (Berglund 2012; Stone 2013). The manufacturer recommends administration to women of childbearing potential only when conception is highly unlikely and patients have been informed of potential hazards.

Breast-Feeding Considerations It is not known if atorvastatin is excreted into breast milk. Due to the potential for serious adverse reactions in a nursing infant, use while breast-feeding is contraindicated by the manufacturer.

Contraindications Hypersensitivity to atorvastatin or any component of the formulation; active liver disease; unexplained persistent elevations of serum transaminases; pregnancy (or those who may become pregnant); breast-feeding

Note: Telaprevir Canadian product monograph contraindicates use with atorvastatin.

Warnings/Precautions Secondary causes of hyperlipidemia should be ruled out prior to therapy. Atorvastatin has not been studied when the primary lipid abnormality is chylomicron elevation (Fredrickson types I and V). Liver function tests must be obtained prior to initiating therapy, repeat if clinically indicated thereafter. May cause hepatic dysfunction. Use with caution in patients who consume large amounts of ethanol or have a history of liver disease; monitoring is recommended. Use is contraindicated in patients with active liver disease or unexplained persistent elevations of serum transaminases; monitoring is recommended. Use high-dose atorvastatin with caution in patients with prior stroke or TIA; the risk of hemorrhagic stroke may be increased.

Rhabdomyolysis with acute renal failure has occurred. Risk is dose related and is increased with concurrent use of lipid-lowering agents which may cause rhabdomyolysis (fibric acid derivatives or niacin at doses ≥1 g/day) or during concurrent use with potent CYP3A4 inhibitors (including amiodarone, clarithromycin, erythromycin, itraconazole, ketoconazole, nefazodone, grapefruit juice in large quantities, verapamil, or protease inhibitors such as indinavir, nelfinavir, or ritonavir). Ensure patient is on the lowest effective atorvastatin dose. If concurrent use of clarithromycin or combination protease inhibitors (eg, lopinavir/ritonavir or ritonavir/saquinavir) is warranted consider dose adjustment of atorvastatin. Do not use with cyclosporine, gemfibrozil, tipranavir plus ritonavir, or telaprevir. Monitor closely if used with other drugs associated with myopathy. Weigh the risk versus benefit when combining any of these drugs with atorvastatin. Discontinue in any patient in which CPK levels are markedly elevated (>10 times ULN) or if myopathy is suspected/diagnosed. The manufacturer recommends temporary discontinuation for elective major surgery, acute medical or surgical conditions, or in any patient experiencing an acute or serious condition predisposing to renal failure (eg, sepsis, hypotension, trauma, uncontrolled seizures). Based on current research and clinical guidelines (Fleisher 2009), HMG-CoA reductase inhibitors should be continued in the perioperative period. Use with caution in patients with advanced age, these patients are predisposed to myopathy. Immune-mediated necrotizing myopathy (IMNM), an autoimmune-mediated myopathy, has been reported (rarely) with HMG-CoA reductase inhibitor therapy. IMNM presents as proximal muscle weakness with elevated CPK levels, which persists despite discontinuation of HMG-CoA reductase inhibitor therapy; additionally, muscle biopsy may show necrotizing myopathy with limited inflammation; immunosuppressive therapy (eg, corticosteroids, azathioprine) may be used for treatment.

Some dosage forms may contain polysorbate 80 (also known as Tweens). Hypersensitivity reactions, usually a delayed reaction, have been reported following exposure to pharmaceutical products containing polysorbate 80 in certain individuals (Isaksson 2002; Lucente 2000; Shelley, 1995). Thrombocytopenia, ascites, pulmonary deterioration, and renal and hepatic failure have been reported in premature neonates after receiving parenteral products containing polysorbate 80 (Alade, 1986; CDC, 1984). See manufacturer's labeling.

Adverse Reactions

Cardiovascular: Hemorrhagic stroke

Central nervous system: Insomnia

Endocrine & metabolic: Diabetes mellitus

Gastrointestinal: Diarrhea, dyspepsia, nausea

Genitourinary: Urinary tract infection

Hepatic: Increased serum transaminases

Neuromuscular & skeletal: Arthralgia, limb pain, myalgia, muscle spasm, musculoskeletal pain

Respiratory: Nasopharyngitis, pharyngolaryngeal pain

Rare but important or life-threatening: Abdominal pain, abnormal hepatic function tests, alopecia, anaphylaxis, anemia, angioedema, anorexia, cholestasis, cholestatic jaundice, cognitive dysfunction (reversible), confusion (reversible), depression, elevated glycosylated hemoglobin (HbA_{1c}), epistaxis, eructation, erythema multiforme, gynecomastia, hematuria, hepatic failure, hepatitis, hyperglycemia, hypoesthesia, increased creatinine phosphokinase, increased serum alkaline phosphatase, increased serum glucose, jaundice, joint swelling, muscle fatigue, myasthenia, myopathy, myositis, neck stiffness, nightmares, pancreatitis, paresthesia, peripheral edema, peripheral neuropathy, rhabdomyolysis, rupture of tendon, Stevens-Johnson syndrome, thrombocytopenia, toxic epidermal necrolysis

Drug Interactions

Metabolism/Transport Effects Substrate of CYP3A4 (major), P-glycoprotein, SLCO1B1; **Note:** Assignment of Major/Minor substrate status based on clinically relevant drug interaction potential; **Inhibits** CYP3A4 (weak), P-glycoprotein

Avoid Concomitant Use

Avoid concomitant use of AtorvaSTATin with any of the following: Bosutinib; Conivaptan; CycloSPORINE (Systemic); Fusidic Acid (Systemic); Gemfibrozil; Idelalisib; PAZOPanib; Pimozide; Posaconazole; Red Yeast Rice; Silodosin; Telaprevir; Tipranavir; Topotecan; VinCRIStine (Liposomal)

Increased Effect/Toxicity

AtorvaSTATin may increase the levels/effects of: Afatinib; Aliskiren; ARIPiprazole; Bosutinib; Brentuximab Vedotin; Cimetidine; Colchicine; DAPTOmycin; Digoxin; Diltiazem; Dofetilide; DOXOrubicin (Conventional); Edoxaban; Everolimus; Hydrocodone; Ketoconazole (Systemic); Ledipasvir; Lomitapide; Midazolam; Naloxegol; NiMODipine; PAZOPanib; P-glycoprotein/ABCB1 Substrates; Pimozide; Prucalopride; Rifaximin; Rivaroxaban; Silodosin; Spironolactone; Topotecan; Trabectedin; Verapamil; VinCRIStine (Liposomal)

The levels/effects of AtorvaSTATin may be increased by: Acipimox; Amiodarone; Aprepitant; Azithromycin (Systemic); Bezafibrate; Boceprevir; Ciprofibrate; Clarithromycin; Cobicistat; Colchicine; Conivaptan; CycloSPORINE (Systemic); CYP3A4 Inhibitors (Moderate); CYP3A4 Inhibitors (Strong); Cyproterone; Danazol; Dasatinib; Diltiazem; Dronedarone; Eltrombopag; Erythromycin (Systemic); Fenofibrate and Derivatives; Fluconazole; Fosaprepitant; Fusidic Acid (Systemic); Gemfibrozil; Grapefruit Juice; Idelalisib; Itraconazole; Ivacaftor; Ketoconazole (Systemic); Luliconazole; Mifepristone; Netupitant; Niacin; Niacinamide; Palbociclib; P-glycoprotein/ABCB1 Inhibitors; Posaconazole; Protease Inhibitors; QuiNINE; Raltegravir; Ranolazine; Red Yeast Rice; Sildenafil; Simeprevir; Stiripentol; Telaprevir; Telithromycin; Teriflunomide; Ticagrelor; Tipranavir; Verapamil; Voriconazole

Decreased Effect

AtorvaSTATin may decrease the levels/effects of: Dabigatran Etexilate; Lanthanum

The levels/effects of AtorvaSTATin may be decreased by: Antacids; Bexarotene (Systemic); Bile Acid Sequestrants; Bosentan; CYP3A4 Inducers (Moderate); CYP3A4 Inducers (Strong); Dabrafenib; Deferasirox; Efavirenz; Etravirine; Fosphenytoin; Mitotane; P-glycoprotein/ABCB1 Inducers; Phenytoin; Rifamycin Derivatives; Siltuximab; St Johns Wort; Tocilizumab

Food Interactions Atorvastatin serum concentrations may be increased by grapefruit juice. Management: Avoid concurrent intake of large quantities of grapefruit juice (>1 quart/day).

Storage/Stability Store at controlled room temperature of 20°C to 25°C (68°F to 77°F).

Mechanism of Action Inhibitor of 3-hydroxy-3-methylglutaryl coenzyme A (HMG-CoA) reductase, the rate-limiting enzyme in cholesterol synthesis (reduces the production of mevalonic acid from HMG-CoA); this then results in a compensatory increase in the expression of LDL receptors on hepatocyte membranes and a stimulation of LDL catabolism. In addition to the ability of HMG-CoA reductase inhibitors to decrease levels of high-sensitivity C-reactive protein (hsCRP), they also possess pleiotropic properties including improved endothelial function, reduced inflammation at the site of the coronary plaque, inhibition of platelet aggregation, and anticoagulant effects (de Denus 2002; Ray 2005).

Pharmacodynamics

Onset of action: Within 2 weeks

Maximum effect: After 4 weeks

LDL reduction: 10 mg/day: 39% (for each doubling of this dose, LDL is lowered approximately 6%)

Pharmacokinetics (Adult data unless noted)

Absorption: Oral: Rapidly absorbed; extensive first-pass metabolism in GI mucosa and liver

Distribution: V_d: ~381 L

Protein binding: >98%

Metabolism: Extensive metabolism to ortho- and parahydroxylated derivatives and various beta-oxidation products with equivalent *in vitro* activity to atorvastatin; plasma concentrations are elevated in patients with chronic alcoholic liver disease and Childs-Pugh class A and B liver disease

Bioavailability: Absolute: 14%

Half-life: 14 hours (half-life of inhibitory activity due to active metabolites is 20-30 hours)

Time to peak serum concentration: 1-2 hours

Elimination: Primarily in bile following hepatic and/or extra-hepatic metabolism; does not appear to undergo enterohepatic recirculation; <2% excreted in urine

Dialysis: Due to the high protein binding, atorvastatin is not expected to be cleared by dialysis (not studied)

Dosing: Usual Dosage should be individualized according to the baseline LDL-C level, the recommended goal of therapy, and patient response; adjustments should be made at intervals of 4 weeks (adults: 2-4 weeks).

Children and Adolescents:

Heterozygous familial and nonfamilial hypercholesterolemia: Oral: **Note:** Begin treatment if after adequate trial of diet, the following are present: LDL-C ≥190 mg/dL or LDL-C remains ≥160 mg/dL and positive family history of premature cardiovascular disease or meets NCEP classification (NHLBI 2011). Therapy may be considered for children 8-9 years of age meeting the above criteria or for children with diabetes mellitus and LDL-C ≥130 mg/dL (Daniels, 2008).

Children 6-10 years of age (Tanner stage I): Limited data available: Initial: 5 mg once daily; if LDL-C target not achieved after 4 weeks may increase to maximum daily dose: 10 mg/**day**; dosing based on trial which included 13 patients as part of a larger study population (n=45); efficacy and tolerability were similar to a group of children age 10-17 years receiving 10-20 mg/day (Gandelman, 2011)

Children and Adolescents 10-17 years: Initial: 10 mg once daily; if LDL-C target not achieved after 4 weeks may increase to a maximum daily dose: 20 mg/**day**; doses >20 mg have not been studied

Hyperlipidemia: Oral: Children and Adolescents 10-17 years (males and postmenarchal females): Initial: 10 mg once daily; if LDL-C target not achieved after 1-3 months, may increase to a maximum daily dose: 20 mg/**day**; doses >20 mg have not been studied (McCrindle, 2007; NHLBI, 2011)

Prevention of graft coronary artery disease: Limited data available: Oral: Children and Adolescents: 0.2 mg/kg/day rounded to nearest 2.5 mg increment; not to exceed age-appropriate doses (Chin, 2002; Chin, 2008)

Adults:

Hypercholesterolemia (heterozygous familial and nonfamilial) and mixed hyperlipidemia (Fredrickson types IIa and IIb): Oral: Initial: 10-20 mg once daily; patients requiring >45% reduction in LDL-C may be started at 40 mg once daily; range: 10-80 mg once daily

Homozygous familial hypercholesterolemia: Oral: 10-80 mg once daily

Dosage adjustment for atorvastatin with concomitant medications: Adults:

Boceprevir, nelfinavir: Use lowest effective atorvastatin dose (not to exceed 40 mg daily)

Clarithromycin, itraconazole, fosamprenavir, ritonavir (plus darunavir, fosamprenavir, or saquinavir): Use lowest effective atorvastatin dose (not to exceed 20 mg daily)

Dosing adjustment in renal impairment: Children ≥10 years, Adolescents, and Adults: Because atorvastatin does not undergo significant renal excretion, dose modification is not necessary.

Dosing adjustment in hepatic impairment: There are no dosage adjustments provided in the manufacturer labeling; contraindicated in active liver disease or in patients with unexplained persistent elevations of serum transaminases.

Administration Oral: May be taken without regard to meals or time of day. Swallow whole; do not break, crush, or chew.

Monitoring Parameters

Pediatric patients: Baseline: ALT, AST, and creatine phosphokinase levels (CPK); fasting lipid panel (FLP) and repeat ALT and AST should be checked after 4 weeks of therapy; if no myopathy symptoms or laboratory abnormalities, then monitor FLP, ALT, and AST every 3 to 4 months during the first year and then every 6 months thereafter (NHLBI, 2011)

Adults:

2013 ACC/AHA Blood Cholesterol Guideline recommendations (Stone, 2013):

Lipid panel (total cholesterol, HDL, LDL, triglycerides): Baseline lipid panel; fasting lipid profile within 4 to 12 weeks after initiation or dose adjustment and every 3 to 12 months (as clinically indicated) thereafter. If 2 consecutive LDL levels are <40 mg/dL, consider decreasing the dose.

Hepatic transaminase levels: Baseline measurement of hepatic transaminase levels (ie, ALT); measure hepatic function if symptoms suggest hepatotoxicity (eg, unusual fatigue or weakness, loss of appetite, abdominal pain, dark-colored urine or yellowing of skin or sclera) during therapy.

CPK: CPK should not be routinely measured. Baseline CPK measurement is reasonable for some individuals (eg, family history of statin intolerance or muscle disease, clinical presentation, concomitant drug therapy that may increase risk of myopathy). May measure CPK in any patient with symptoms suggestive of myopathy (pain, tenderness, stiffness, cramping, weakness, or generalized fatigue).

Evaluate for new-onset diabetes mellitus during therapy; if diabetes develops, continue statin therapy and encourage adherence to a heart-healthy diet, physical activity, a healthy body weight, and tobacco cessation.

If patient develops a confusional state or memory impairment, may evaluate patient for nonstatin causes (eg, exposure to other drugs), systemic and neuropsychiatric causes, and the possibility of adverse effects associated with statin therapy.

Manufacturer recommendation: Liver enzyme tests at baseline and repeated when clinically indicated. Measure CPK when myopathy is being considered or may measure CPK periodically in high risk patients (eg, drug-drug interaction). Upon initiation or titration, lipid panel should be analyzed within 2 to 4 weeks.

Dosage Forms Excipient information presented when available (limited, particularly for generics); consult specific product labeling.

Tablet, Oral:

Lipitor: 10 mg, 20 mg, 40 mg, 80 mg

Generic: 10 mg, 20 mg, 40 mg, 80 mg

◆ **Atorvastatin Calcium** *see* AtorvaSTATin *on page 220*

Atovaquone (a TOE va kwone)

Brand Names: US Mepron

Brand Names: Canada Mepron

Therapeutic Category Antiprotozoal

Generic Availability (US) Yes

Use Prevention of *Pneumocystis jirovecii* pneumonia (PCP) and second-line treatment of mild to moderate PCP in patients intolerant of trimethoprim/sulfamethoxazole (TMP/SMX) (FDA approved in ages ≥13 years and adults); mild to moderate PCP is defined as an alveolar-arterial oxygen diffusion gradient ≤45 mm Hg and PaO_2 ≥60 mm Hg on room air; patients intolerant of TMP/SMX are defined as having a significant rash (ie, Stevens-Johnson-like syndrome), neutropenia, or hemolysis; has also been used for the treatment of babesiosis and the prevention of first episode of toxoplasmosis in HIV-infected children and adults

Pregnancy Risk Factor C

Pregnancy Considerations Adverse events were observed in animal reproduction studies. Diagnosis and treatment of *Pneumocystis jirovecii* pneumonia (PCP) in pregnant women is the same as in nonpregnant women; however, information specific to the use of atovaquone in pregnancy is limited (DHHS [OI] 2013).

Breast-Feeding Considerations It is not known if atovaquone is excreted in breast milk. The manufacturer recommends that caution be exercised when administering atovaquone to nursing women.

Contraindications Hypersensitivity to atovaquone or any component of the formulation

Warnings/Precautions Hypersensitivity reactions (eg, angioedema, bronchospasm, throat tightness, urticaria) have occurred. When used for *Pneumocystis jirovecii* pneumonia (PCP) treatment, has only been indicated in mild-to-moderate PCP; not studied for use in severe PCP; atovaquone has less adverse effects than trimethoprim-sulfamethoxazole ([TMP-SMZ], the treatment of choice for mild-to-moderate PCP), although atovaquone is less effective than TMP-SMZ (DHHS [OI] 2013). Use with caution in elderly patients. Absorption may be decreased in patients who have diarrhea or vomiting; monitor closely and consider use of an antiemetic; if severe, consider use of an alternative antiprotozoal. Consider parenteral therapy with alternative agents in patients who have difficulty taking atovaquone with food; gastrointestinal disorders may limit absorption of oral medications; may not achieve adequate plasma levels. Use with caution in patients with severe hepatic impairment; monitor closely; rare cases of cholestatic hepatitis, elevated liver function tests, and fatal liver failure have been reported. Potentially significant drug-drug interactions may exist, requiring dose or frequency adjustment, additional monitoring, and/or selection of alternative therapy.

Benzyl alcohol and derivatives: Some dosage forms may contain benzyl alcohol; large amounts of benzyl alcohol (≥99 mg/kg/day) have been associated with a potentially fatal toxicity ("gasping syndrome") in neonates; the "gasping syndrome" consists of metabolic acidosis, respiratory distress, gasping respirations, CNS dysfunction (including convulsions, intracranial hemorrhage), hypotension and cardiovascular collapse (AAP, 1997; CDC, 1982); some data suggests that benzoate displaces bilirubin from protein binding sites (Ahlfors 2001); avoid or use dosage forms containing benzyl alcohol with caution in neonates. See manufacturer's labeling.

Adverse Reactions

Cardiovascular: Hypotension
Central nervous system: Anxiety, depression, dizziness, headache, insomnia, pain
Dermatologic: Diaphoresis, pruritus, skin rash
Endocrine & metabolic: Hyperglycemia, hypoglycemia, hyponatremia, increased amylase
Gastrointestinal: Abdominal pain, amylase increased, anorexia, constipation, diarrhea, dysgeusia, dyspepsia, heartburn, nausea, oral candidiasis, vomiting
Hematologic & oncologic: Anemia, neutropenia
Hepatic: Increased liver enzymes
Infection: Infection
Neuromuscular & skeletal: Myalgia, weakness
Renal: Increased blood urea nitrogen, increased serum creatinine
Respiratory: Bronchospasm, cough, dyspnea, flu-like symptoms, rhinitis, sinusitis
Miscellaneous: Fever
Rare but important or life-threatening: Acute renal failure, angioedema, constriction of the pharynx, corneal disease (vortex keratopathy), desquamation, erythema multiforme, hepatic failure (rare), hepatitis (rare), hypersensitivity reaction, methemoglobinemia, pancreatitis, Stevens-Johnson syndrome, thrombocytopenia, urticaria

Drug Interactions

Metabolism/Transport Effects None known.

Avoid Concomitant Use

Avoid concomitant use of Atovaquone with any of the following: Efavirenz; Rifamycin Derivatives; Ritonavir

Increased Effect/Toxicity

Atovaquone may increase the levels/effects of: Etoposide

Decreased Effect

Atovaquone may decrease the levels/effects of: Indinavir

The levels/effects of Atovaquone may be decreased by: Efavirenz; Metoclopramide; Rifamycin Derivatives; Ritonavir; Tetracycline

Food Interactions Ingestion with a fatty meal increases absorption. Management: Administer with food, preferably high-fat meals (peanuts or ice cream).

Storage/Stability Store at 15°C to 25°C (59°F to 77°F). Do not freeze.

Mechanism of Action Inhibits electron transport in mitochondria resulting in the inhibition of key metabolic enzymes responsible for the synthesis of nucleic acids and ATP

Pharmacokinetics (Adult data unless noted)

Absorption: Oral:
Infants and Children <2 years of age: Decreased absorption
Adults: Oral suspension: Absorption is enhanced 1.4-fold with food; decreased absorption with single doses exceeding 750 mg
Distribution: V_{dss}: 0.6 L/kg; CSF concentration is <1% of the plasma concentration
Protein binding: >99%
Bioavailability: Suspension (administered with food): 47%
Half-life, elimination:
Children (4 months to 12 years): 60 hours (range: 31-163 hours)
Adults: 2.9 days
Adults with AIDS: 2.2 days
Time to peak serum concentration: Dual peak serum concentrations at 1 to 8 hours and at 24 to 96 hours after dose due to enterohepatic cycling
Elimination: ~94% is recovered as unchanged drug in feces; 0.6% excreted in urine

Dosing: Neonatal Oral: *Pneumocystis jirovecii* pneumonia (PCP) (CDC, 2009): Treatment: 30-40 mg/kg/day divided twice daily

Dosing: Usual Oral:

Infants and Children:
Pneumocystis jirovecii pneumonia (PCP) (CDC, 2009):
Treatment:
1 to <3 months: 30-40 mg/kg/day divided twice daily (maximum dose: 1500 mg/day)
3-23 months: 45 mg/kg/day divided twice daily (maximum dose: 1500 mg/day)
≥24 months: 30-40 mg/kg/day divided twice daily (maximum dose: 1500 mg/day)
Prophylaxis:
1-3 months: 30 mg/kg/day once daily (maximum dose: 1500 mg/day)
4-24 months: 45 mg/kg/day once daily (maximum dose: 1500 mg/day)
>24 months: 30 mg/kg/day once daily (maximum dose: 1500 mg/day)
Toxoplasma gondii, prophylaxis (CDC, 2009):
1-3 months: 30 mg/kg once daily (maximum dose: 1500 mg/day)
4-24 months: 45 mg/kg once daily (maximum dose: 1500 mg/day)
>24 months: 30 mg/kg once daily (maximum dose: 1500 mg/day)
Babesiosis: 40 mg/kg/day divided twice daily (maximum dose: 1500 mg/day) with azithromycin 12 mg/kg/day once daily for 7-10 days

Adolescents 13-16 years and Adults:
Pneumocystis jirovecii pneumonia (PCP):
Treatment: 750 mg/dose twice daily for 21 days
Prophylaxis: 1500 mg once daily
Toxoplasma gondii encephalitis (CDC, 2009):
Prophylaxis: 1500 mg once daily
Treatment: 750 mg 4 times daily or 1500 mg twice daily for at least 6 weeks after resolution of signs and symptoms
Suppression after treatment: 750 mg 2-4 times/day
Babesiosis: 750 mg/dose twice daily for 7-10 days with azithromycin; 600 mg once daily for 7-10 days (*Red Book*, 2009)

Administration Oral: Administer with food or a high-fat meal; gently shake suspension before using

Monitoring Parameters CBC with differential, liver enzymes, serum chemistries, serum amylase

Additional Information The suspension contains the inactive ingredient poloxamer 188

Dosage Forms Excipient information presented when available (limited, particularly for generics); consult specific product labeling.
Suspension, Oral:
Mepron: 750 mg/5 mL (5 mL, 210 mL) [contains benzyl alcohol; citrus flavor]
Generic: 750 mg/5 mL (210 mL)

Atovaquone and Proguanil
(a TOE va kwone & pro GWA nil)

Brand Names: US Malarone®

Brand Names: Canada Malarone®; Malarone® Pediatric

Therapeutic Category Antimalarial Agent

Generic Availability (US) Yes: Excludes pediatric strength tablet

Use Prevention (FDA approved in pediatric patients >11 kg and adults) or treatment (FDA approved in pediatric patients >5 kg and adults) of acute, uncomplicated *P. falciparum* malaria, including chloroquine-resistant *P. falciparum*

Pregnancy Risk Factor C

Pregnancy Considerations Teratogenic effects were not observed with the combination of atovaquone/proguanil in animal reproduction studies using concentrations similar to the estimated human exposure. The pharmacokinetics of atovaquone and proguanil are changed during pregnancy. Malaria infection in pregnant women may be more severe than in nonpregnant women. Because *P. falciparum* malaria can cause maternal death and fetal loss, pregnant women traveling to malaria-endemic areas must use personal protection against mosquito bites. Atovaquone/proguanil may be used as an alternative treatment of malaria in pregnant women; consult current CDC guidelines.

Breast-Feeding Considerations Small quantities of proguanil are found in breast milk. This combination is not recommended if nursing infants <5 kg (safety data is limited concerning therapeutic use in infants <5 kg)

Contraindications Hypersensitivity to atovaquone, proguanil, or any component of the formulation; prophylactic use in severe renal impairment (CrCl <30 mL/minute)

Warnings/Precautions Not indicated for cerebral malaria or other severe manifestations of complicated malaria. Delayed cases of *P. falciparum* malaria may occur after stopping prophylaxis; travelers returning from endemic areas who develop febrile illnesses should be evaluated for malaria. Recrudescent infections or infections following prophylaxis with this agent should be treated with alternative agent(s). Absorption of atovaquone may be decreased in patients who have diarrhea or vomiting; monitor closely and consider use of an antiemetic. If severe, consider use of an alternative antimalarial. Increased transaminase levels and hepatitis have been reported with prophylactic use; single case report of hepatic failure requiring transplantation documented. Monitor closely and use caution in patients with existing hepatic impairment. Elevations in AST/ALT may persist for up to 4 weeks following treatment (Looareesuwan, 1999). Administer with caution to patients with preexisting renal disease. May use with caution for treatment of malaria treatment in patients with severe renal impairment (CrCl <30 mL/minute) if benefit outweighs risk. Contraindicated for prophylactic use in severe renal impairment due to the risk of pancytopenia in patients with severe renal impairment treated with proguanil. Treatment failures have been reported in patients >100 kg (case reports); follow-up monitoring is recommended (Durand, 2008).

Adverse Reactions The following adverse reactions were reported in patients being treated for malaria. When used for prophylaxis, reactions are similar to those seen with placebo.

Central nervous system: Dizziness, headache
Dermatologic: Pruritus
Gastrointestinal: Abdominal pain, anorexia, diarrhea, nausea, vomiting
Hepatic: Transaminase increases (increased LFT values typically normalized after ~4 weeks)
Neuromuscular & skeletal: Weakness
Rare but important or life-threatening: Anaphylaxis (rare), anemia (rare), angioedema, cholestasis, erythema multiforme (rare), hallucinations, hepatitis (rare), hepatic failure (case report), neutropenia, pancytopenia (with severe renal impairment), photosensitivity, psychotic episodes (rare), rash, seizure (rare), Stevens-Johnson syndrome (rare), stomatitis, urticaria, vasculitis (rare)

Drug Interactions

Metabolism/Transport Effects None known.

Avoid Concomitant Use

Avoid concomitant use of Atovaquone and Proguanil with any of the following: Artemether; Efavirenz; Lumefantrine; Rifamycin Derivatives; Ritonavir

Increased Effect/Toxicity

Atovaquone and Proguanil may increase the levels/effects of: Antipsychotic Agents (Phenothiazines); Dapsone (Systemic); Dapsone (Topical); Etoposide; Lumefantrine; Warfarin

The levels/effects of Atovaquone and Proguanil may be increased by: Artemether; Dapsone (Systemic)

Decreased Effect

Atovaquone and Proguanil may decrease the levels/effects of: Indinavir; Typhoid Vaccine

The levels/effects of Atovaquone and Proguanil may be decreased by: Efavirenz; Metoclopramide; Rifamycin Derivatives; Ritonavir; Tetracycline

Food Interactions Atovaquone taken with dietary fat significantly increases the rate and extent of absorption; AUC is increased 2-3 times and C_{max} is increased 5 times as compared to administration during a fasted state. Management: Administer with food or milk-based drink at the same time each day.

Storage/Stability Store at 25°C (77°F); excursions permitted to 15°C to 30°C (59°F to 86°F).

Mechanism of Action
Atovaquone: Selectively inhibits parasite mitochondrial electron transport.
Proguanil: The metabolite cycloguanil inhibits dihydrofolate reductase, disrupting deoxythymidylate synthesis. Together, atovaquone/cycloguanil affect the erythrocytic and exoerythrocytic stages of development.

Pharmacokinetics (Adult data unless noted)

Atovaquone: See Atovaquone monograph.

Proguanil:
Absorption: Extensive
Distribution: V_d: Pediatric patients: 42 L/kg

Protein binding: 75%
Metabolism: Hepatic to active metabolites, cycloguanil (via CYP2C19) and 4-chlorophenylbiguanide
Half-life elimination: 12-21 hours
Elimination: Urine (40% to 60%)

Dosing: Usual Oral:
Children (dosage based on body weight):
Prevention of malaria: Start 1-2 days prior to entering a malaria-endemic area, continue throughout the stay and for 7 days after leaving area. Take as a single dose, once daily. **Note:** AAP (*Red Book*, 2009) states that atovaquone and proguanil can be used for prevention in a child ≥5 kg if travel cannot be avoided to areas where chloroquine-resistant *P. falciparum* exists.
5-8 kg: Atovaquone/proguanil: 31.25 mg/12.5 mg
9-10 kg: Atovaquone/proguanil: 46.88 mg/18.75 mg
Manufacturer's dosing:
11-20 kg: Atovaquone/proguanil 62.5 mg/25 mg
21-30 kg: Atovaquone/proguanil 125 mg/50 mg
31-40 kg: Atovaquone/proguanil 187.5 mg/75 mg
>40 kg: Atovaquone/proguanil 250 mg/100 mg
Treatment of acute malaria: Take as a single dose, once daily for 3 consecutive days.
5-8 kg: Atovaquone/proguanil 125 mg/50 mg
9-10 kg: Atovaquone/proguanil 187.5 mg/75 mg
11-20 kg: Atovaquone/proguanil 250 mg/100 mg
21-30 kg: Atovaquone/proguanil 500 mg/200 mg
31-40 kg: Atovaquone/proguanil 750 mg/300 mg
>40 kg: Atovaquone/proguanil 1 g/400 mg
Adults:
Prevention of malaria: Atovaquone/proguanil 250 mg/100 mg once daily; start 1-2 days prior to entering a malaria-endemic area, continue throughout the stay and for 7 days after leaving area
Treatment of acute malaria: Atovaquone/proguanil 1 g/400 mg as a single dose, once daily for 3 consecutive days. **Note:** Consultants recommend dividing the daily dose in 2 to decrease nausea and vomiting.

Dosage adjustment in renal impairment: Should not be used as prophylaxis in severe renal impairment (CrCl <30 mL/minute). For treatment of malaria, alternative regimens should be used in patients with CrCl <30 mL/minute unless benefits outweigh the risks. No dosage adjustment required in mild to moderate renal impairment.

Dosage adjustment in hepatic impairment: No dosage adjustment required in mild to moderate hepatic impairment. No data available for use in severe hepatic impairment.

Administration Administer with food or milk at the same time each day. If vomiting occurs within 1 hour of administration, repeat the dose. Tablets are not palatable if chewed due to bitter taste. For children who have difficulty swallowing tablets, tablets may be crushed and mixed with condensed milk just prior to administration.

Dosage Forms Excipient information presented when available (limited, particularly for generics); consult specific product labeling.
Tablet, oral: Atovaquone 250 mg and proguanil hydrochloride 100 mg
Malarone®: Atovaquone 250 mg and proguanil hydrochloride 100 mg
Tablet, oral [pediatric]:
Malarone®: Atovaquone 62.5 mg and proguanil hydrochloride 25 mg

◆ **Atovaquone and Proguanil Hydrochloride** *see* Atovaquone and Proguanil *on page 224*

◆ **ATRA** *see* Tretinoin (Systemic) *on page 2108*

Atracurium (a tra KYOO ree um)

Medication Safety Issues
High alert medication:
The Institute for Safe Medication Practices (ISMP) includes this medication among its list of drugs which have a heightened risk of causing significant patient harm when used in error.
Other safety concerns:
United States Pharmacopeia (USP) 2006: The Interdisciplinary Safe Medication Use Expert Committee of the USP has recommended the following:
- Hospitals, clinics, and other practice sites should institute special safeguards in the storage, labeling, and use of these agents and should include these safeguards in staff orientation and competency training.
- Healthcare professionals should be on **high alert** (especially vigilant) whenever a neuromuscular-blocking agent (NMBA) is stocked, ordered, prepared, or administered.

Brand Names: Canada Atracurium Besylate Injection

Therapeutic Category Neuromuscular Blocker Agent, Nondepolarizing; Skeletal Muscle Relaxant, Paralytic

Generic Availability (US) Yes

Use Adjunct to general anesthesia, to facilitate endotracheal intubation, and to provide skeletal muscle relaxation during surgery or mechanical ventilation (FDA approved in ages ≥1 month and adults)

Pregnancy Risk Factor C

Pregnancy Considerations Adverse events were observed in animal reproduction studies. Small amounts of atracurium have been shown to cross the placenta when given to women during cesarean section.

Breast-Feeding Considerations It is not known if atracurium is excreted in breast milk. The manufacturer recommends that caution be exercised when administering atracurium to nursing women.

Contraindications Hypersensitivity to atracurium besylate or any component of the formulation

Warnings/Precautions Reduce initial dosage and inject slowly (over 1 to 2 minutes) in patients in whom substantial histamine release would be potentially hazardous (eg, patients with clinically-important cardiovascular disease). Maintenance of an adequate airway and respiratory support is critical. Certain clinical conditions may result in potentiation or antagonism of neuromuscular blockade:
Antagonism: Respiratory alkalosis, hypercalcemia, demyelinating lesions, peripheral neuropathies, denervation, and muscle trauma
Potentiation: Electrolyte abnormalities (eg, severe hypocalcemia, severe hypokalemia, hypermagnesemia), neuromuscular diseases, metabolic acidosis, metabolic alkalosis, respiratory acidosis, Eaton-Lambert syndrome and myasthenia gravis

Resistance may occur in burn patients (≥20% of total body surface area), usually several days after the injury, and may persist for several months after wound healing. Resistance may occur in patients who are immobilized. Cross-sensitivity with other neuromuscular-blocking agents may occur; use extreme caution in patients with previous anaphylactic reactions. Use caution in the elderly. Bradycardia may be more common with atracurium than with other neuromuscular-blocking agents since it has no clinically-significant effects on heart rate to counteract the bradycardia produced by anesthetics. Should be administered by adequately trained individuals familiar with its use.

Benzyl alcohol and derivatives: Some dosage forms may contain benzyl alcohol; large amounts of benzyl alcohol (≥99 mg/kg/day) have been associated with a potentially fatal toxicity ("gasping syndrome") in neonates; the "gasping syndrome" consists of metabolic acidosis, respiratory distress, gasping respirations, CNS dysfunction (including convulsions, intracranial hemorrhage), hypotension and cardiovascular collapse (AAP, 1997; CDC, 1982); some data suggests that benzoate displaces bilirubin from protein binding sites (Ahlfors, 2001); avoid or use dosage forms containing benzyl alcohol with caution in neonates. See manufacturer's labeling.

Adverse Reactions Mild, rare, and generally suggestive of histamine release

Cardiovascular: Flushing

Rare but important or life-threatening: Bronchial secretions, erythema, hives, itching, wheezing

Postmarketing and/or case reports: Acute quadriplegic myopathy syndrome (prolonged use), allergic reaction, bradycardia, bronchospasm, dyspnea, hypotension, injection site reaction, laryngospasm, myositis ossificans (prolonged use), seizure, tachycardia, urticaria

Causes of prolonged neuromuscular blockade: Accumulation of active metabolites; cumulative drug effect, metabolism/excretion decreased (hepatic and/or renal impairment); electrolyte imbalance (hypokalemia, hypocalcemia, hypermagnesemia, hypernatremia); excessive drug administration; hypothermia

Drug Interactions

Metabolism/Transport Effects None known.

Avoid Concomitant Use

Avoid concomitant use of Atracurium with any of the following: QuiNINE

Increased Effect/Toxicity

Atracurium may increase the levels/effects of: Cardiac Glycosides; Corticosteroids (Systemic); OnabotulinumtoxinA; RimabotulinumtoxinB

The levels/effects of Atracurium may be increased by: AbobotulinumtoxinA; Aminoglycosides; Calcium Channel Blockers; Capreomycin; Clindamycin (Topical); Colistimethate; CycloSPORINE (Systemic); Fosphenytoin-Phenytoin; Inhalational Anesthetics; Ketorolac (Nasal); Ketorolac (Systemic); Lincosamide Antibiotics; Lithium; Loop Diuretics; Magnesium Salts; Polymyxin B; Procainamide; QuiNIDine; QuiNINE; Spironolactone; Tetracycline Derivatives; Vancomycin

Decreased Effect

The levels/effects of Atracurium may be decreased by: Acetylcholinesterase Inhibitors; Fosphenytoin-Phenytoin; Loop Diuretics

Storage/Stability Refrigerate intact vials at 2°C to 8°C (36°F to 46°F); protect from freezing. Use vials within 14 days upon removal from the refrigerator to room temperature of 25°C (77°F). Dilutions of 0.2 mg/mL or 0.5 mg/mL in 0.9% sodium chloride, dextrose 5% in water, or 5% dextrose in sodium chloride 0.9% are stable for up to 24 hours at room temperature or under refrigeration.

Mechanism of Action Blocks neural transmission at the myoneural junction by binding with cholinergic receptor sites

Pharmacodynamics

Onset of action: IV: 1-4 minutes

Maximum effect: Within 3-5 minutes

Duration: Recovery begins in 20-35 minutes when anesthesia is balanced

Pharmacokinetics (Adult data unless noted)

Distribution: V_d:
- Infants: 0.21 L/kg
- Children: 0.13 L/kg
- Adults: 0.1 L/kg

Metabolism: Some metabolites are active; undergoes rapid nonenzymatic degradation (Hofmann elimination) in the bloodstream; additional metabolism occurs via ester hydrolysis

Half-life: Elimination:
- Infants: 20 minutes
- Children: 17 minutes
- Adults: 16 minutes

Elimination: Clearance:
- Infants: 7.9 mL/kg/minute
- Children: 6.8 mL/kg/minute
- Adults: 5.3 mL/kg/minute

Dosing: Neonatal Paralysis/skeletal muscle relaxation: IV: 0.25-0.4 mg/kg initially followed by maintenance doses of 0.25 mg/kg as needed to maintain neuromuscular blockade **or** a continuous IV infusion 0.4 mg/kg/**hour** (Clarkson, 2001; Kalli, 1988); **Note:** Higher intermittent doses (eg, 0.5 mg/kg) have been associated with toxicity and fatal outcomes in premature neonates (Clarkson, 2001)

Dosing: Usual Paralysis/skeletal muscle relaxation:

Infants and Children ≤2 years:

IV: 0.3-0.4 mg/kg initially followed by maintenance doses of 0.3-0.4 mg/kg as needed to maintain neuromuscular blockade

Continuous IV infusion: 0.6-1.2 mg/kg/**hour** or 10-20 **mcg**/kg/minute

Children >2 years to Adults:

IV: 0.4-0.5 mg/kg then 0.08-0.1 mg/kg 20-45 minutes after initial dose to maintain neuromuscular block; repeat dose at 15- to 25-minute intervals

Continuous IV infusion: Initial: 0.54-0.6 mg/kg/**hour** or 9-10 **mcg**/kg/minute at initial signs of recovery from bolus dose; block is usually maintained by a rate of 0.3-0.54 mg/kg/**hour** or 5-9 **mcg**/kg/minute (range: 0.1-0.9 mg/kg/**hour** or 2-15 **mcg**/kg/minute).

Dosage adjustment in hepatic or renal impairment: Not necessary

Dosage adjustment with enflurane or isoflurane: Reduce dosage by 33%

Dosage adjustment with induced hypothermia (cardiobypass surgery): Reduce dosage by 50%

Preparation for Administration Parenteral: For continuous IV infusion, dilute in D_5W, NS or D_5NS to a maximum concentration of 0.5 mg/mL; more concentrated solutions have reduced stability (ie, <24 hours at room temperature). Atracurium should not be mixed with alkaline solutions.

Administration Parenteral: May be administered undiluted as a bolus injection; do not administer IM due to tissue irritation. For continuous IV infusions, further dilute and administer via an infusion pump; use infusion solutions within 24 hours of preparation.

Monitoring Parameters Muscle twitch response to peripheral nerve stimulation, heart rate, blood pressure, assisted ventilation status

Additional Information Neuromuscular blockade may be reversed with neostigmine; atropine or glycopyrrolate should be available to treat excessive cholinergic effects from neostigmine

Dosage Forms Excipient information presented when available (limited, particularly for generics); consult specific product labeling.

Solution, Intravenous, as besylate:

Generic: 50 mg/5 mL (5 mL); 100 mg/10 mL (10 mL)

Solution, Intravenous, as besylate [preservative free]:

Generic: 50 mg/5 mL (5 mL)

- ◆ **Atracurium Besylate** *see* Atracurium *on page 225*
- ◆ **Atracurium Besylate Injection (Can)** *see* Atracurium *on page 225*
- ◆ **Atralin** *see* Tretinoin (Topical) *on page 2111*
- ◆ **Atriance™ (Can)** *see* Nelarabine *on page 1496*
- ◆ **Atripla** *see* Efavirenz, Emtricitabine, and Tenofovir *on page 734*
- ◆ **AtroPen** *see* Atropine *on page 227*

Atropine (A troe peen)

Medication Safety Issues

BEERS Criteria medication:

This drug may be potentially inappropriate for use in geriatric patients (Quality of evidence - varies based on comorbidity; Strength of recommendation - varies based on comorbidity)

International issues:

Atropt [Australia and New Zealand] may be confused with Azopt brand name for brinzolamide [U.S., Canada, and multiple international markets]

Related Information

Adult ACLS Algorithms *on page 2236*

Pediatric ALS (PALS) Algorithms *on page 2233*

Brand Names: US AtroPen; Atropine-Care [DSC]; Isopto Atropine

Brand Names: Canada Dioptic's Atropine Solution; Isopto® Atropine

Therapeutic Category Antiasthmatic; Anticholinergic Agent; Anticholinergic Agent, Ophthalmic; Antidote, Organophosphate Poisoning; Antispasmodic Agent, Gastrointestinal; Bronchodilator; Ophthalmic Agent, Mydriatic

Generic Availability (US) May be product dependent

Use

Parenteral:

Auto-injector: Antidote for anticholinesterase poisoning (carbamate insecticides, nerve agents, organophosphate insecticides, muscarinic poisoning) (FDA approved in all ages)

Injection: Preoperative medication to inhibit salivation and secretions; treatment of symptomatic sinus bradycardia, AV block (nodal level) adjuvant use with anticholinesterases (eg, edrophonium, neostigmine) to decrease their side effects during reversal of neuromuscular blockade [All indications: FDA approved in pediatric patients (age not specified) and adults]; **Note:** Use is no longer recommended in the management of asystole or pulseless electrical activity (PEA) (ACLS, 2010)

Ophthalmic: Produce mydriasis and cycloplegia for examination of the retina and optic disc and accurate measurement of refractive errors; produce papillary dilation in inflammatory conditions (eg, uveitis) (All indications: FDA approved in adults; refer to product-specific information regarding FDA approval in pediatric patients)

Prescribing and Access Restrictions The AtroPen® formulation is available for use primarily by the Department of Defense.

Pregnancy Risk Factor B/C (manufacturer specific)

Pregnancy Considerations Animal reproduction studies have not been conducted. Atropine has been found to cross the human placenta.

Breast-Feeding Considerations Trace amounts of atropine are excreted into breast milk. Anticholinergic agents may suppress lactation.

Contraindications Hypersensitivity to atropine or any component of the formulation; narrow-angle glaucoma; adhesions between the iris and lens (ophthalmic product); pyloric stenosis; prostatic hypertrophy

Note: No contraindications exist in the treatment of life-threatening organophosphate or carbamate insecticide or nerve agent poisoning.

Warnings/Precautions Heat prostration may occur in the presence of high environmental temperatures. Psychosis may occur in sensitive individuals or following use of excessive doses. Avoid use if possible in patients with obstructive uropathy or in other conditions resulting in urinary retention; use is contraindicated in patients with prostatic hypertrophy. Avoid use in patients with paralytic ileus, intestinal atony of the elderly or debilitated patient, severe ulcerative colitis, and toxic megacolon complicating ulcerative colitis. Use with caution in patients with autonomic neuropathy, hyperthyroidism, renal or hepatic impairment, myocardial ischemia, HF, tachyarrhythmias (including sinus tachycardia), hypertension, and hiatal hernia associated with reflux esophagitis. Treatment-related blood pressure increases and tachycardia may lead to ischemia, precipitate an MI, or increase arrhythmogenic potential. In heart transplant recipients, atropine will likely be ineffective in treatment of bradycardia due to lack of vagal innervation of the transplanted heart; cholinergic reinnervation may occur over time (years), so atropine may be used cautiously; however, some may experience paradoxical slowing of the heart rate and high-degree AV block upon administration (ACLS, 2010; Bernheim, 2004).

Avoid relying on atropine for effective treatment of type II second-degree or third-degree AV block (with or without a new wide QRS complex). Asystole or bradycardic pulseless electrical activity (PEA): Although no evidence exists for significant detrimental effects, routine use is unlikely to have a therapeutic benefit and is no longer recommended (ACLS, 2010).

AtroPen®: There are no absolute contraindications for the use of atropine in severe organophosphate or carbamate insecticide or nerve agent poisonings; however in mild poisonings, use caution in those patients where the use of atropine would be otherwise contraindicated. Formulation for use by trained personnel only. Clinical symptoms consistent with highly-suspected organophosphate or carbamate insecticides or nerve agent poisoning should be treated with antidote immediately; administration should not be delayed for confirmatory laboratory tests. Signs of atropinization include flushing, mydriasis, tachycardia, and dryness of the mouth or nose. Monitor effects closely when administering subsequent injections as necessary. The presence of these effects is not indicative of the success of therapy; inappropriate use of mydriasis as an indicator of successful treatment has resulted in atropine toxicity. Reversal of bronchial secretions is the preferred indicator of success. Adjunct treatment with a cholinesterase reactivator (eg, pralidoxime) may be required in patients with toxicity secondary to organophosphorus insecticides or nerve agents. Treatment should always include proper evacuation and decontamination procedures; medical personnel should protect themselves from inadvertent contamination. Antidotal administration is intended only for initial management; definitive and more extensive medical care is required following administration. Individuals should not rely solely on antidote for treatment, as other supportive measures (eg, artificial respiration) may still be required. Atropine reverses the muscarinic but not the nicotinic effects associated with anticholinesterase toxicity.

Children may be more sensitive to the anticholinergic effects of atropine; use with caution in children with spastic paralysis. May be inappropriate in older adults depending on comorbidities (eg, dementia, delirium) due to its potent anticholinergic effects (Beers Criteria).

Warnings: Additional Pediatric Considerations Use with caution in children with spastic paralysis or brain damage; children are at increased risk for rapid rise in body temperature due to suppression of sweat gland activity. Paradoxical hyperexcitability may occur in children given large doses. Infants with Down syndrome have both increased sensitivity to cardiac effects and mydriasis.

Adverse Reactions Severity and frequency of adverse reactions are dose related and vary greatly; listed reactions are limited to significant and/or life-threatening.

Cardiovascular: Cardiac arrhythmia, flushing, hypotension, palpitations, tachycardia

Central nervous system: Ataxia, coma, delirium, disorientation, dizziness, drowsiness, excitement, hallucination, headache, insomnia, nervousness

Dermatologic: Anhidrosis, scarlatiniform rash, skin rash, urticaria

Gastrointestinal: Ageusia, bloating, constipation, delayed gastric emptying, nausea, paralytic ileus, vomiting, xerostomia

Genitourinary: Urinary hesitancy, urinary retention

Hypersensitivity: Anaphylaxis

Neuromuscular & skeletal: Laryngospasm, weakness

Ocular: Angle-closure glaucoma, blurred vision, cycloplegia, dry eye syndrome, increased intraocular pressure, mydriasis

Respiratory: Dry nose, dry throat, dyspnea, pulmonary edema

Miscellaneous: Fever

Drug Interactions

Metabolism/Transport Effects None known.

Avoid Concomitant Use

Avoid concomitant use of Atropine with any of the following: Aclidinium; Eluxadoline; Glucagon; Ipratropium (Oral Inhalation); Potassium Chloride; Tiotropium; Umeclidinium

Increased Effect/Toxicity

Atropine may increase the levels/effects of: AbobotulinumtoxinA; Analgesics (Opioid); Anticholinergic Agents; Cannabinoid-Containing Products; Eluxadoline; Glucagon; Mirabegron; OnabotulinumtoxinA; Potassium Chloride; RimabotulinumtoxinB; Thiazide Diuretics; Tiotropium; Topiramate

The levels/effects of Atropine may be increased by: Aclidinium; Ipratropium (Oral Inhalation); Mianserin; Pramlintide; Umeclidinium

Decreased Effect

Atropine may decrease the levels/effects of: Acetylcholinesterase Inhibitors; Itopride; Metoclopramide; Secretin

The levels/effects of Atropine may be decreased by: Acetylcholinesterase Inhibitors

Storage/Stability

Injection: Store injection at controlled room temperature of 15°C to 30°C (59°F to 86°F); avoid freezing. In addition, AtroPen® should be protected from light. Preparation of bulk atropine solution for mass chemical terrorism at a concentration of 1 mg/mL is stable for 72 hours at 4°C to 8°C (39°F to 46°F); 20°C to 25°C (68°F to 77°F); 32°C to 36°C (90°F to 97°F) (Dix, 2003).

Ophthalmic products: Store at 20°C to 25°C (68°F to 77°F); keep tightly closed.

Mechanism of Action Blocks the action of acetylcholine at parasympathetic sites in smooth muscle, secretory glands, and the CNS; increases cardiac output, dries secretions. Atropine reverses the muscarinic effects of cholinergic poisoning due to agents with acetylcholinesterase inhibitor activity by acting as a competitive antagonist of acetylcholine at muscarinic receptors. The primary goal in cholinergic poisonings is reversal of bronchorrhea and bronchoconstriction. Atropine has no effect on the nicotinic receptors responsible for muscle weakness, fasciculations, and paralysis.

Pharmacodynamics

Inhibition of salivation:

- Onset of action: IM: 30 minutes
- Maximum effect: IM: 1-1.6 hours
- Duration: IM: Up to 4 hours

Increased heart rate:

- Onset of action: IM: 5-40 minutes
- Maximum effect:
  - IM: 20 minutes to 1 hour
  - IV: 2-4 minutes

Pharmacokinetics (Adult data unless noted)

Absorption: Well absorbed from all dosage forms

Distribution: Widely distributes throughout the body; crosses the blood-brain barrier

Protein binding: 14% to 22%

Metabolism: Hepatic via enzymatic hydrolysis

Half-life:

- Children <2 years: 6.9 ± 3 hours
- Children >2 years: 2.5 ± 1.2 hours
- Adults: 3 ± 0.9 hours

Time to peak serum concentration: IM: Auto-injector: 3 minutes

Elimination: Urine (30% to 50% as unchanged drug and metabolites)

Dosing: Neonatal

Bradycardia: Note: Not part of neonatal resuscitation algorithm; some institutions have used the following:

IV, I.O.: 0.02 mg/kg/dose; use of a minimum dosage of 0.1 mg will result in dosages >0.02 mg/kg and is not recommended (Barrington, 2011); there is no documented minimum dosage in this age group; may repeat once in 3 to 5 minutes; reserve use for those patients unresponsive to improved oxygenation and epinephrine

Endotracheal: 0.04 to 0.06 mg/kg/dose; may repeat once if needed

Inhibit salivation and secretions (preanesthesia): IM, IV, SubQ: Patient weight <5 kg: 0.02 mg/kg/dose 30 to 60 minutes preoperatively then every 4 to 6 hours as needed; use of a minimum dosage of 0.1 mg will result in dosages >0.02 mg/kg and is not recommended (Barrington, 2011); there is no documented minimum dosage in this age group

Intubation, nonemergent (preferred vagolytic): IM, IV: 0.02 mg/kg/dose (Kumar, 2010)

Organophosphate or carbamate insecticide or nerve agent poisoning: Note: The dose of atropine required varies considerably with the severity of poisoning. The total amount of atropine used for carbamate poisoning is usually less than with organophosphate insecticide or nerve agent poisoning. Severely poisoned patients may exhibit significant tolerance to atropine; ≥2 times the suggested doses may be needed. Titrate to pulmonary status (decreased bronchial secretions); consider administration of atropine via continuous IV infusion in patients requiring large doses of atropine. Once patient is stable for a period of time, the dose/dosing frequency may be decreased. Pralidoxime is a component of the management of organophosphate insecticide and nerve agent toxicity; refer to pralidoxime for the specific route and dose.

IV, IM: Initial: 0.05 to 0.1 mg/kg; repeat every 5 to 10 minutes as needed, doubling the dose if previous dose did not induce atropinization (Hegenbarth, 2008; Reigart, 1999; Rotenberg, 2003). Maintain atropinization by administering repeat doses as needed for ≥2 to 12 hours based on recurrence of symptoms (Reigart, 1999).

Continuous IV infusion: Following atropinization (see above), administer 10% to 20% of the total loading dose required to induce atropinization as a continuous IV infusion per hour; adjust as needed to maintain adequate atropinization without atropine toxicity (Eddleston, 2004; Roberts, 2007)

IM: AtroPen: 0.25 mg (yellow pen):

Mild symptoms (≥2 mild symptoms): Administer one 0.25 mg (yellow pen) dose as soon as an exposure is known or strongly suspected. If severe symptoms develop after the first dose, 2 additional doses should be repeated in rapid succession 10 minutes after the first dose; do not administer more than 3 doses. If profound anticholinergic effects occur in the absence of excessive bronchial secretions, further doses of atropine should be withheld. Mild symptoms of insecticide or nerve agent poisoning, as provided by manufacturer in the AtroPen product labeling to guide therapy, include: Blurred vision, bradycardia, breathing difficulties, chest tightness, coughing, drooling, miosis, muscular twitching, nausea, runny nose, salivation increased, stomach cramps, tachycardia, teary eyes, tremor, vomiting, or wheezing.

Severe symptoms (≥1 severe symptom): Immediately administer **three** 0.25 mg (yellow pen) doses. Severe symptoms of insecticide or nerve agent poisoning, as provided by manufacturer in the AtroPen product labeling to guide therapy, include: Breathing difficulties (severe), confused/strange behavior, defecation (involuntary), muscular twitching/generalized weakness (severe), respiratory secretions (severe), seizure, unconsciousness, urination (involuntary); **Note:** Neonates and infants may become drowsy or unconscious with muscle floppiness as opposed to muscle twitching.

Endotracheal: Increase the dose by 2 to 3 times the usual IV dose. Mix with 3 to 5 mL of normal saline and administer. Flush with 3 to 5 mL of NS and follow with 5 assisted manual ventilations (Rotenberg, 2003)

Refraction: Ophthalmic: Instill 1 drop of 0.25% solution 3 times/day for 3 days before the procedure

Uveitis: Ophthalmic: Instill 1 drop of 0.5% solution 1 to 3 times daily

Dosing: Usual

Pediatric:

Bradycardia: Infants, Children, and Adolescents:

IV, I.O.: 0.02 mg/kg/dose; minimum dose recommended by PALS: 0.1 mg; however, use of a minimum dosage of 0.1 mg in patients <5 kg will result in dosages >0.02 mg/kg and is not recommended (Barrington, 2011); there is no documented minimum dosage in this age group; maximum single dose: 0.5 mg; may repeat once in 3 to 5 minutes; maximum total dose: 1 mg (PALS, 2010).

Endotracheal: 0.04 to 0.06 mg/kg/dose; may repeat once if needed (PALS, 2010)

Inhibit salivation and secretions (preanesthesia): Infants, Children, and Adolescents: IM, IV, SubQ: Administer dose 30 to 60 minutes preoperatively then every 4 to 6 hours as needed:

Weight-directed dosing (Nelson, 1996):

Infants weighing <5 kg: 0.02 mg/kg/dose; use of a fixed minimum dosage of 0.1 mg will result in dosages >0.02 mg/kg; there is no documented minimum dosage in this age group

Infants and Children weighing ≥5 kg: 0.01 to 0.02 mg/kg/dose; maximum single dose: 0.4 mg; minimum dose: 0.1 mg

Fixed dosing:

3 to 7 kg (7 to 16 lb): 0.1 mg
8 to 11 kg (17 to 24 lb): 0.15 mg
11 to 18 kg (24 to 40 lb): 0.2 mg
18 to 29 kg (40 to 65 lb): 0.3 mg
≥30 kg (≥65 lb): 0.4 mg

Organophosphate or carbamate insecticide or nerve agent poisoning: Infants, Children, and Adolescents: **Note:** The dose of atropine required varies considerably with the severity of poisoning. The total amount of atropine used for carbamate poisoning is usually less than with organophosphate insecticide or nerve agent poisoning. Severely poisoned patients may exhibit significant tolerance to atropine; ≥2 times the suggested doses may be needed. Titrate to pulmonary status (decreased bronchial secretions); consider administration of atropine via continuous IV infusion in patients requiring large doses of atropine. Once patient is stable for a period of time, the dose/dosing frequency may be decreased. Pralidoxime is a component of the management of organophosphate insecticide and nerve agent toxicity; refer to Pralidoxime monograph for the specific route and dose.

IV, IM: Initial: 0.05 to 0.1 mg/kg; repeat every 5 to 10 minutes as needed, doubling the dose if previous dose does not induce atropinization (Hegenbarth, 2008; Reigart, 1999; Rotenberg, 2003). Maintain atropinization by administering repeat doses as needed for ≥2 to 12 hours based on recurrence of symptoms (Reigart, 1999).

Continuous IV infusion: Following atropinization, administer 10% to 20% of the total loading dose required to induce atropinization as a continuous IV infusion per hour; adjust as needed to maintain adequate atropinization without atropine toxicity (Eddleston, 2004; Roberts, 2007)

IM (AtroPen): Number of doses dependent upon symptom severity:

Weight-directed dosing:

<6.8 kg (15 lb): 0.25 mg/dose (yellow pen)
6.8 to 18 kg (15 to 40 lb): 0.5 mg/dose (blue pen)
18 to 41 kg (40 to 90 lb): 1 mg/dose (dark red pen)
>41 kg (>90 lb): 2 mg/dose (green pen)

Mild symptoms (≥2 mild symptoms): Administer the weight-based dose listed above as soon as an exposure is known or strongly suspected. If severe symptoms develop after the first dose, 2 additional doses should be repeated in rapid succession 10 minutes after the first dose; do not administer more than 3 doses. If profound anticholinergic effects occur in the absence of excessive bronchial secretions, further doses of atropine should be withheld. Mild symptoms of insecticide or nerve agent poisoning, as provided by manufacturer in the AtroPen product labeling to guide therapy, include: Blurred vision, bradycardia, breathing difficulties, chest tightness, coughing, drooling, miosis, muscular twitching, nausea, runny nose, salivation increased, stomach cramps, tachycardia, teary eyes, tremor, vomiting, or wheezing.

Severe symptoms (≥1 severe symptom): Immediately administer **three** weight-based doses in rapid succession. Symptoms of insecticide or nerve agent poisoning, as provided by manufacturer in the AtroPen product labeling to guide therapy, include: Breathing difficulties (severe), confused/strange behavior, defecation (involuntary), muscular twitching/generalized weakness (severe), respiratory secretions (severe), seizure, unconsciousness, urination (involuntary); **Note:** Infants may become drowsy or unconscious with muscle floppiness as opposed to muscle twitching.

Endotracheal: Increase the dose by 2 to 3 times the usual IV dose. Mix with 3 to 5 mL of normal saline and administer. Flush with 3 to 5 mL of NS and follow with 5 assisted manual ventilations (Rotenberg, 2003).

Refraction: Ophthalmic:

Infants: Instill 1 drop of 0.25% solution 3 times/day for 3 days before the procedure

Children: 1 to 5 years: Instill 1 drop of 0.5% solution 3 times/day for 3 days before the procedure

Children and Adolescents >5 years or Children with dark irides: Instill 1 drop of 1% solution 3 times/day for 3 days before the procedure

Uveitis: Infants, Children, and Adolescents: Ophthalmic: Instill 1 drop of 0.5% solution 1 to 3 times daily

Adult: **Note:** Doses <0.5 mg have been associated with paradoxical bradycardia:

Bradycardia: IV: 0.5 mg every 3 to 5 minutes, not to exceed a total of 3 mg or 0.04 mg/kg (ACLS, 2010)

Neuromuscular blockade reversal: IV: 25 to 30 mcg/kg 30-60 seconds before neostigmine or 7 to 10 mcg/kg 30 to 60 seconds before edrophonium

Organophosphate or carbamate insecticide or nerve agent poisoning: Note: The dose of atropine required varies considerably with the severity of poisoning. The total amount of atropine used for carbamate poisoning is usually less than with organophosphate insecticide or nerve agent poisoning. Severely poisoned patients may exhibit significant tolerance to atropine; ≥2 times the suggested doses may be needed. Titrate to pulmonary status (decreased bronchial secretions); consider administration of atropine via continuous IV infusion in patients requiring large doses of atropine. Once patient is stable for a period of time, the dose/dosing frequency may be decreased. If atropinization occurs after 1 to 2 mg of atropine then re-evaluate working diagnosis (Reigart, 1999). Pralidoxime is a component of the management of organophosphate insecticide and nerve agent toxicity; refer to Pralidoxime monograph for the specific route and dose.

IM (AtroPen):

Mild symptoms (≥2 mild symptoms): Administer 2 mg as soon as an exposure is known or strongly suspected. If severe symptoms develop after the first dose, 2 additional doses should be repeated in rapid succession 10 minutes after the first dose; do not administer more than 3 doses. If profound anticholinergic effects occur in the absence of excessive bronchial secretions, further doses of atropine should be withheld. Mild symptoms of insecticide or nerve agent poisoning, as provided by manufacturer in the AtroPen® product labeling to guide therapy, include: Blurred vision, bradycardia, breathing difficulties, chest tightness, coughing, drooling, miosis, muscular twitching, nausea, runny nose, salivation increased, stomach cramps, tachycardia, teary eyes, tremor, vomiting, or wheezing.

Severe symptoms (≥1 severe symptom): Immediately administer **three** 2 mg doses in rapid succession. Severe symptoms of insecticide or nerve agent poisoning, as provided by manufacturer in the AtroPen product labeling to guide therapy include: Breathing difficulties (severe), confused/strange behavior, defecation (involuntary), muscular twitching/generalized weakness (severe), respiratory secretions (severe), seizure, unconsciousness, urination (involuntary)

Inhibit salivation and secretions (preanesthesia): IM, IV, SubQ: 0.4 to 0.6 mg 30 to 60 minutes preop and repeat every 4 to 6 hours as needed

Mydriasis, cycloplegia (preprocedure): Ophthalmic: Solution (1%): Instill 1 to 2 drops 1 hour before the procedure

Uveitis: Ophthalmic:

Solution (1%): Instill 1 to 2 drops up to 4 times/day

Ointment: Apply a small amount in the conjunctival sac up to 3 times/day. Compress the lacrimal sac by digital pressure for 1 to 3 minutes after instillation

Dosing adjustment in renal impairment: There are no dosage adjustments provided in the manufacturer's labeling.

Dosing adjustment in hepatic impairment: There are no dosage adjustments provided in the manufacturer's labeling.

Preparation for Administration Parenteral: **Mass chemical terrorism:** Preparation of bulk atropine solution: Add atropine sulfate powder to 100 mL NS in polyvinyl chloride bags to yield a final concentration of 1 mg/mL (Dix 2003).

Administration

Endotracheal: Administer and flush with 1 to 5 mL NS or SWFI based on patient size, followed by 5 manual ventilations. Absorption may be greater with sterile water. Stop compressions (if using for cardiac arrest), spray the drug quickly down the tube. Follow immediately with several quick insufflations and continue chest compressions.

Parenteral:

IV: Administer undiluted by rapid IV injection; slow injection may result in paradoxical bradycardia

IM: AtroPen: Administer to the outer thigh. Firmly grasp the autoinjector with the green tip (0.5 mg, 1 mg, and 2 mg autoinjector) or black tip (0.25 mg autoinjector) pointed down; remove the yellow safety release (0.5 mg, 1 mg, and 2 mg autoinjector) or gray safety release (0.25 autoinjector). Firmly jab the green tip at a 90° angle against the outer thigh; may be administered through clothing as long as pockets at the injection site are empty. In thin patients or patients <6.8 kg (15 lb), bunch up the thigh prior to injection. Hold the autoinjector in place for 10 seconds following the injection; remove the autoinjector and massage the injection site. After administration, the needle will be visible; if the needle is not visible, repeat the above steps with more pressure. After use, bend the needle against a hard surface (needle does not retract) to avoid accidental injury.

Ophthalmic: Instill solution into conjunctival sac of affected eye(s); compress lacrimal sac with digital pressure for 2 to 3 minutes after instillation; avoid contact of bottle tip with eye or skin

Monitoring Parameters Heart rate, blood pressure, pulse, mental status; intravenous administration requires a cardiac monitor

Organophosphate or carbamate insecticide or nerve agent poisoning: Heart rate, blood pressure, respiratory status, oxygenation secretions. Maintain atropinization with repeated dosing as indicated by clinical status. Crackles in lung bases, or continuation of cholinergic signs, may be signs of inadequate dosing. Pulmonary improvement may not parallel other signs of atropinization. Monitor for signs and symptoms of atropine toxicity (eg, fever, muscle fasciculations, delirium); if toxicity occurs, discontinue atropine and monitor closely.

Additional Information Due to the discontinuance of 0.5% ophthalmic solutions commercially, 0.5% and 0.25% solutions may be prepared under sterile conditions by dilution of 1% atropine ophthalmic solution with artificial tears; 0.5%: An equal part dilution (equal volume of 1% atropine with artificial tears) and 0.25%: Dilute 2.5 mL 1% atropine with 7.5 mL artificial tears

Dosage Forms Excipient information presented when available (limited, particularly for generics); consult specific product labeling. [DSC] = Discontinued product

Device, Intramuscular, as sulfate:

AtroPen: 0.25 mg/0.3 mL (0.3 mL) [pyrogen free]

AtroPen: 0.5 mg/0.7 mL (0.7 mL); 1 mg/0.7 mL (0.7 mL); 2 mg/0.7 mL (0.7 mL) [pyrogen free; contains phenol]

Ointment, Ophthalmic, as sulfate:

Generic: 1% (3.5 g)

Solution, Injection, as sulfate:

Generic: 0.05 mg/mL (5 mL); 0.1 mg/mL (5 mL, 10 mL); 0.4 mg/mL (1 mL, 20 mL); 1 mg/mL (1 mL)

Solution, Injection, as sulfate [preservative free]:

Generic: 0.4 mg/mL (1 mL); 0.8 mg/mL (0.5 mL); 1 mg/mL (1 mL)

Solution, Ophthalmic, as sulfate:

Atropine-Care: 1% (2 mL [DSC], 5 mL [DSC], 15 mL [DSC]) [contains benzalkonium chloride, edetate disodium]

Isopto Atropine: 1% (5 mL, 15 mL)

Generic: 1% (2 mL, 5 mL, 15 mL)

◆ **Atropine and Diphenoxylate** *see* Diphenoxylate and Atropine *on page 673*

◆ **Atropine-Care [DSC]** *see* Atropine *on page 227*

Auranofin (au RANE oh fin)

Medication Safety Issues

Sound-alike/look-alike issues:

Ridaura may be confused with Cardura

Brand Names: US Ridaura

Brand Names: Canada Ridaura®

Therapeutic Category Gold Compound

Generic Availability (US) No

Use Management of active stage of classic or definite rheumatoid arthritis in patients who do not respond to or tolerate other agents (FDA approved in adults)

Pregnancy Risk Factor C

Pregnancy Considerations Adverse events were observed in animal reproduction studies.

Breast-Feeding Considerations Injectable gold salts have been detected in breast milk.

Contraindications History of severe toxicity to gold compounds including anaphylaxis, bone marrow aplasia, severe hematologic disorders, exfoliative dermatitis, necrotizing enterocolitis, or pulmonary fibrosis.

Warnings/Precautions [U.S. Boxed Warning]: Signs of gold toxicity include pruritus, rash, and stomatitis. Dermatitis and lesions of the mucous membranes are common and may be serious; pruritus may precede the early development of a skin reaction and a metallic taste may precede oral mucous membrane reactions. Dermatitis may be aggravated by sun exposure. Use with caution in patients with skin rash; may increase risk and/or symptoms of gold toxicity and toxicity may be more difficult to detect.

[U.S. Boxed Warning]: Signs of gold toxicity include persistent diarrhea as well as nausea, vomiting, anorexia, abdominal cramps, and ulcerative enterocolitis (rare). Diarrhea may be managed with a dose reduction. Use with caution in patients with inflammatory bowel disease; may increase risk and/or symptoms of gold toxicity and toxicity may be more difficult to detect.

[U.S. Boxed Warning]: Signs of gold toxicity include hematologic depression (decreased hemoglobin, leukocytes (WBC <4000/mm^3), granulocytes (<1500/mm^3), or platelets (<150,000/mm^3). Symptoms of gold toxicity may be difficult to detect in patients with prior abnormalities. Therapy should be discontinued if signs and symptoms (eg, purpura, ecchymoses, petechiae) of thrombocytopenia develop or if platelet count falls to <100,000/mm^3; therapy should not be reinitiated until thrombocytopenia resolves and if thrombocytopenia was not caused by the gold therapy.

[U.S. Boxed Warning]: Signs of gold toxicity include proteinuria and hematuria. Renal toxicity ranges from mild proteinuria to nephrotic syndrome. Use with caution in patients with renal impairment; may increase risk and/or symptoms of gold toxicity and toxicity may be more difficult to detect. Therapy should be discontinued if proteinuria or microscopic hematuria develops.

[U.S. Boxed Warning]: Use is only indicated in select patients with active rheumatoid arthritis.

[U.S. Boxed Warning]: Physicians should be experienced with chrysotherapy and should be familiar with the risks and benefits of therapy.

[U.S. Boxed Warning]: Laboratory monitoring should be reviewed prior to each new prescription. The possibility of adverse reactions should be discussed with patients prior to initiation and patients should be advised to report any symptoms indicating toxicity. Disease states should be stable prior to initiating therapy. May be associated with the development of cholestatic jaundice. Use with caution in patients with hepatic impairment; may increase risk and/or symptoms of gold toxicity and toxicity may be more difficult to detect. Use may be associated with interstitial fibrosis; monitor closely.

Benzyl alcohol and derivatives: Some dosage forms may contain benzyl alcohol; large amounts of benzyl alcohol (≥99 mg/kg/day) have been associated with a potentially fatal toxicity ("gasping syndrome") in neonates; the "gasping syndrome" consists of metabolic acidosis, respiratory distress, gasping respirations, CNS dysfunction (including convulsions, intracranial hemorrhage), hypotension and cardiovascular collapse (AAP, 1997; CDC, 1982); some data suggests that benzoate displaces bilirubin from protein binding sites (Ahlfors, 2001); avoid or use dosage forms containing benzyl alcohol with caution in neonates. See manufacturer's labeling.

Warnings: Additional Pediatric Considerations In pediatric trials, diarrhea was the most common adverse effect (Giannini, 1990).

Adverse Reactions

Dermatologic: Alopecia, pruritus, rash, urticaria

Gastrointestinal: Abdominal pain, anorexia, constipation, diarrhea/loose stools, dysgeusia, dyspepsia, flatulence, glossitis, nausea, stomatitis, vomiting

Hematologic: Eosinophilia, leukopenia, thrombocytopenia

Hepatic: Transaminases increased

Ocular: Conjunctivitis

Renal: Hematuria, proteinuria

Rare but important or life-threatening: Agranulocytosis, aplastic anemia, angioedema, corneal deposits, dysphagia, enterocolitis (ulcerative), fever, GI hemorrhage, gingivitis, gold bronchitis, hepatotoxicity, interstitial pneumonitis, jaundice, metallic taste, melena, neutropenia, pancytopenia, peripheral neuropathy, pure red cell aplasia. **Note:** Exfoliative dermatitis has been reported with other gold compounds.

Drug Interactions

Metabolism/Transport Effects None known.

Avoid Concomitant Use There are no known interactions where it is recommended to avoid concomitant use.

Increased Effect/Toxicity There are no known significant interactions involving an increase in effect.

Decreased Effect There are no known significant interactions involving a decrease in effect.

Storage/Stability Store at 15°C to 30°C (59°F to 86°F). Protect from light.

Mechanism of Action The exact mechanism of action of gold is unknown; gold is taken up by macrophages which results in inhibition of phagocytosis and lysosomal membrane stabilization; other actions observed are decreased serum rheumatoid factor and alterations in immunoglobulins. Additionally, complement activation is decreased, prostaglandin synthesis is inhibited, and lysosomal enzyme activity is decreased.

Pharmacodynamics Onset of action: Therapeutic response may not be seen for 3-4 months after start of therapy, as long as 6 months in some patients

Pharmacokinetics (Adult data unless noted) Note: Due to rapid metabolism, the pharmacokinetics of auranofin are based on gold concentrations, not auranofin.

Absorption: Oral: 25%

Protein binding: 60%

Metabolism: Rapid; intact auranofin not detectable in the blood

Half-life: 21-31 days (half-life dependent upon single or multiple dosing)

Time to peak serum concentration: Within 2 hours

Elimination: 60% of absorbed gold is eliminated in urine while the remainder is eliminated in feces

Dosing: Usual

Children ≥18 months and Adolescents ≤17 years: **Juvenile idiopathic arthritis (rheumatoid):** Limited data available: Oral: Initial: 0.1-0.15 mg/kg/day in 1-2 divided doses; usual maintenance: 0.15 mg/kg/day in 1-2 divided doses; maximum daily dose: 0.2 mg/kg/**day** or 9 mg/**day**. **Note:** With current market availability, may not be able to replicate the exact dosing used in trials; in trials, doses were rounded to nearest whole mg using 1 mg tablet (no longer available) (Brewer, 1983; Giannini, 1990; Marcolongo, 1988)

Adults: **Rheumatoid arthritis:** Oral: 6 mg/day in 1-2 divided doses; after 6 months may be increased to 9 mg/day in 3 divided doses; if still no response after 3 months at 9 mg/day, discontinue drug

Dosage adjustment in renal impairment: Adults: There are no dosage adjustments provided in the manufacturer's labeling. The following guidelines have been used by some clinicians (Aronoff, 2007):

CrCl 50-80 mL/minute: Reduce dose to 50%

CrCl <50 mL/minute: Avoid use

Dosage adjustment in hepatic impairment: There are no dosage adjustments provided in the manufacturer's labeling.

Administration Take with or without food; some centers have recommended to administer with food if it causes GI upset.

Monitoring Parameters Baseline and periodic (at least monthly): CBC with differential, platelet count, urinalysis for protein; baseline renal and liver function tests; skin and oral mucosa examinations; specific questioning for symptoms of pruritus, rash, stomatitis, or metallic taste

Reference Range Gold: Normal: 0-0.1 mcg/mL (SI: 0-0.0064 micromoles/L); Therapeutic: 1-3 mcg/mL (SI: 0.06-0.18 micromoles/L); Urine <0.1 mcg/24 hours

Test Interactions May enhance the response to a tuberculin skin test

Additional Information Metallic taste may indicate stomatitis

Dosage Forms Excipient information presented when available (limited, particularly for generics); consult specific product labeling.

Capsule, Oral:

Ridaura: 3 mg [contains benzyl alcohol]

- ◆ **Auraphene-B [OTC]** *see* Carbamide Peroxide *on page 371*
- ◆ **Auro-Amlodipine (Can)** *see* AmLODIPine *on page 133*
- ◆ **Auro-Atorvastatin (Can)** *see* AtorvaSTATin *on page 220*
- ◆ **Auro-Carvedilol (Can)** *see* Carvedilol *on page 380*
- ◆ **Auro-Cefixime (Can)** *see* Cefixime *on page 395*
- ◆ **Auro-Cefprozil (Can)** *see* Cefprozil *on page 405*
- ◆ **Auro-Cefuroxime (Can)** *see* Cefuroxime *on page 414*
- ◆ **Auro-Ciprofloxacin (Can)** *see* Ciprofloxacin (Systemic) *on page 463*
- ◆ **Auro-Citalopram (Can)** *see* Citalopram *on page 476*
- ◆ **Auro-Clindamycin (Can)** *see* Clindamycin (Systemic) *on page 487*
- ◆ **Auro-Cyclobenzaprine (Can)** *see* Cyclobenzaprine *on page 548*
- ◆ **Aurodex® [DSC]** *see* Antipyrine and Benzocaine *on page 177*
- ◆ **Auro-Gabapentin (Can)** *see* Gabapentin *on page 954*
- ◆ **Auro-Irbesartan (Can)** *see* Irbesartan *on page 1158*
- ◆ **Auro-Lamotrigine (Can)** *see* LamoTRIgine *on page 1211*
- ◆ **Auro-Letrozole (Can)** *see* Letrozole *on page 1224*
- ◆ **Auro-Levetiracetam (Can)** *see* LevETIRAcetam *on page 1234*
- ◆ **Auro-Lisinopril (Can)** *see* Lisinopril *on page 1280*
- ◆ **Auro-Losartan (Can)** *see* Losartan *on page 1302*
- ◆ **Auro-Meloxicam (Can)** *see* Meloxicam *on page 1346*
- ◆ **Auro-Metformin (Can)** *see* MetFORMIN *on page 1375*
- ◆ **Auro-Montelukast (Can)** *see* Montelukast *on page 1459*
- ◆ **Auro-Montelukast Chewable Tablets (Can)** *see* Montelukast *on page 1459*
- ◆ **Auro-Nevirapine (Can)** *see* Nevirapine *on page 1507*
- ◆ **Auro-Omeprazole (Can)** *see* Omeprazole *on page 1555*
- ◆ **Auro-Paroxetine (Can)** *see* PARoxetine *on page 1634*
- ◆ **Auro-Quetiapine (Can)** *see* QUEtiapine *on page 1815*
- ◆ **Auro-Sertraline (Can)** *see* Sertraline *on page 1916*
- ◆ **Auro-Simvastatin (Can)** *see* Simvastatin *on page 1928*
- ◆ **Auro-Terbinafine (Can)** *see* Terbinafine (Systemic) *on page 2021*
- ◆ **AURO-Topiramate (Can)** *see* Topiramate *on page 2085*
- ◆ **Auro-Valsartan (Can)** *see* Valsartan *on page 2149*
- ◆ **Auvi-Q** *see* EPINEPHrine (Systemic, Oral Inhalation) *on page 760*
- ◆ **Ava-Atenolol (Can)** *see* Atenolol *on page 215*
- ◆ **Ava-Atorvastatin (Can)** *see* AtorvaSTATin *on page 220*
- ◆ **Ava-Cefprozil (Can)** *see* Cefprozil *on page 405*
- ◆ **Ava-Clindamycin (Can)** *see* Clindamycin (Systemic) *on page 487*
- ◆ **Ava-Cyclobenzaprine (Can)** *see* Cyclobenzaprine *on page 548*
- ◆ **Ava-Diltiazem (Can)** *see* Diltiazem *on page 661*
- ◆ **Ava-Famciclovir (Can)** *see* Famciclovir *on page 846*
- ◆ **Ava-Fluoxetine (Can)** *see* FLUoxetine *on page 906*
- ◆ **Ava-Fluvoxamine (Can)** *see* FluvoxaMINE *on page 928*
- ◆ **Ava-Fosinopril (Can)** *see* Fosinopril *on page 943*
- ◆ **AVA-Furosemide (Can)** *see* Furosemide *on page 951*
- ◆ **Avage** *see* Tazarotene *on page 2010*
- ◆ **Ava-Glyburide (Can)** *see* GlyBURIDE *on page 975*
- ◆ **Ava-Hydrochlorothiazide (Can)** *see* Hydrochlorothiazide *on page 1028*
- ◆ **Ava-Irbesartan (Can)** *see* Irbesartan *on page 1158*
- ◆ **Avakine** *see* InFLIXimab *on page 1104*
- ◆ **Ava-Lovastatin (Can)** *see* Lovastatin *on page 1305*
- ◆ **Ava-Meloxicam (Can)** *see* Meloxicam *on page 1346*
- ◆ **Ava-Metformin (Can)** *see* MetFORMIN *on page 1375*
- ◆ **Ava-Metoprolol (Can)** *see* Metoprolol *on page 1418*
- ◆ **Ava-Metoprolol (Type L) (Can)** *see* Metoprolol *on page 1418*
- ◆ **Avamys (Can)** *see* Fluticasone (Nasal) *on page 917*
- ◆ **Ava-Naproxen EC (Can)** *see* Naproxen *on page 1489*
- ◆ **Avandia** *see* Rosiglitazone *on page 1884*

- ◆ **Ava-Nortriptyline (Can)** *see* Nortriptyline *on page 1532*
- ◆ **Ava-Omeprazole (Can)** *see* Omeprazole *on page 1555*
- ◆ **Ava-Ondansetron (Can)** *see* Ondansetron *on page 1564*
- ◆ **Ava-Pantoprazole (Can)** *see* Pantoprazole *on page 1618*
- ◆ **Avapro** *see* Irbesartan *on page 1158*
- ◆ **Ava-Risperidone (Can)** *see* RisperiDONE *on page 1866*
- ◆ **Avastin** *see* Bevacizumab *on page 285*
- ◆ **Ava-Sumatriptan (Can)** *see* SUMAtriptan *on page 1995*
- ◆ **Ava-Valsartan (Can)** *see* Valsartan *on page 2149*
- ◆ **Avaxim (Can)** *see* Hepatitis A Vaccine *on page 1011*
- ◆ **Avaxim-Pediatric (Can)** *see* Hepatitis A Vaccine *on page 1011*
- ◆ **Aveed** *see* Testosterone *on page 2025*
- ◆ **Aventyl (Can)** *see* Nortriptyline *on page 1532*
- ◆ **Avidoxy** *see* Doxycycline *on page 717*
- ◆ **AVINza [DSC]** *see* Morphine (Systemic) *on page 1461*
- ◆ **Avita** *see* Tretinoin (Topical) *on page 2111*
- ◆ **AVP** *see* Vasopressin *on page 2161*
- ◆ **Axert** *see* Almotriptan *on page 98*
- ◆ **Axid** *see* Nizatidine *on page 1528*
- ◆ **Axid AR [OTC]** *see* Nizatidine *on page 1528*
- ◆ **Axiron** *see* Testosterone *on page 2025*
- ◆ **Aygestin** *see* Norethindrone *on page 1530*
- ◆ **Ayr [OTC]** *see* Sodium Chloride *on page 1938*
- ◆ **Ayr Nasal Mist Allergy/Sinus [OTC]** *see* Sodium Chloride *on page 1938*
- ◆ **Ayr Saline Nasal [OTC]** *see* Sodium Chloride *on page 1938*
- ◆ **Ayr Saline Nasal Drops [OTC]** *see* Sodium Chloride *on page 1938*
- ◆ **Ayr Saline Nasal Gel [OTC]** *see* Sodium Chloride *on page 1938*
- ◆ **Ayr Saline Nasal No-Drip [OTC]** *see* Sodium Chloride *on page 1938*
- ◆ **AYR Saline Nasal Rinse [OTC]** *see* Sodium Chloride *on page 1938*

AzaCITIDine (ay za SYE ti deen)

Medication Safety Issues

Sound-alike/look-alike issues:

AzaCITIDine may be confused with azaTHIOprine

High alert medication:

This medication is in a class the Institute for Safe Medication Practices (ISMP) includes among its list of drug classes which have a heightened risk of causing significant patient harm when used in error.

Related Information

Prevention of Chemotherapy-Induced Nausea and Vomiting in Children *on page 2368*

Safe Handling of Hazardous Drugs *on page 2455*

Brand Names: US Vidaza

Brand Names: Canada Vidaza

Therapeutic Category Antineoplastic Agent, Antimetabolite (Pyrimidine)

Generic Availability (US) Yes

Use Treatment of myelodysplastic syndrome (MDS) in patients with the following subtypes: Refractory anemia or refractory anemia with ringed sideroblasts (if accompanied by neutropenia or thrombocytopenia or requiring transfusions), refractory anemia with excess blasts, refractory anemia with excess blasts in transformation, and chronic myelomonocytic leukemia (FDA approved in adults)

Pregnancy Risk Factor D

Pregnancy Considerations Adverse events were observed in animal reproduction studies. Women of childbearing potential should be advised to avoid pregnancy during treatment. In addition, males should be advised to avoid fathering a child while on azacitidine therapy.

Breast-Feeding Considerations It is not known if azacitidine is excreted in breast milk. Due to the potential for serious adverse reactions in the nursing infant, a decision should be made to discontinue the drug or to discontinue breast-feeding, taking into account the importance of treatment to the mother.

Contraindications Hypersensitivity to azacitidine, mannitol, or any component of the formulation; advanced malignant hepatic tumors

Warnings/Precautions

Hazardous agent; use appropriate precautions for handling and disposal (NIOSH 2014 [group 1]). May cause hepatotoxicity in patients with preexisting hepatic impairment. Progressive hepatic coma leading to death has been reported in patients with extensive tumor burden due to metastatic disease, especially those with a baseline albumin <30 g/L. Patients with hepatic impairment were excluded from clinical studies for myelodysplastic syndrome (MDS). Use is contraindicated in patients with advanced malignant hepatic tumors. Renal toxicities, including serum creatinine elevations, renal tubular acidosis (serum bicarbonate decrease to <20 mEq/L associated with alkaline urine and serum potassium <3 mEq/L), and renal failure (some fatal), have been reported with intravenous azacitidine when used in combination with other chemotherapy agents. Withhold or reduce the dose with unexplained decreases in serum bicarbonate <20 mEq/L or if elevations in BUN or serum creatinine occur. Patients with renal impairment may be at increased risk for renal toxicity. Severe renal impairment did not have a major effect on azacitidine exposure after multiple subcutaneous administrations and no dosage adjustment is necessary for the first cycle, however, monitor closely for toxicity (azacitidine and metabolites are excreted renally).

Neutropenia, thrombocytopenia, and anemia are common; may cause therapy delays and/or dosage reductions; monitor blood counts prior to each cycle (at a minimum), and more frequently if clinically indicated. Azacitidine is associated with a moderate emetic potential (Basch, 2011; Dupuis, 2011; Roila, 2010); antiemetics are recommended to prevent nausea and vomiting. Injection site reactions commonly occurred with subcutaneous administration. Potentially significant drug-drug interactions may exist, requiring dose or frequency adjustment, additional monitoring, and/or selection of alternative therapy.

Some dosage forms may contain polysorbate 80 (also known as Tweens). Hypersensitivity reactions, usually a delayed reaction, have been reported following exposure to pharmaceutical products containing polysorbate 80 in certain individuals (Isaksson, 2002; Lucente 2000; Shelley, 1995). Thrombocytopenia, ascites, pulmonary deterioration, and renal and hepatic failure have been reported in premature neonates after receiving parenteral products containing polysorbate 80 (Alade, 1986; CDC, 1984). See manufacturer's labeling.

Adverse Reactions

Cardiovascular: Chest pain, chest wall pain, heart murmur, hypertension, hypotension Peripheral edema, syncope, tachycardia

Central nervous system: Anxiety, depression, dizziness, Fatigue, headache, hypoesthesia, insomnia, lethargy, malaise, pain, postoperative pain, rigors

Dermatologic: Cellulitis, diaphoresis, erythema, pallor, pruritus, night sweats, rash at injection site, skin lesion, skin nodules, skin rash, urticaria, xeroderma
Endocrine & metabolic: Hypokalemia, pitting edema, weight loss
Gastrointestinal: Abdominal distention, abdominal pain, abdominal tenderness, anorexia, constipation, diarrhea, dyspepsia, dysphagia, gingival hemorrhage, hemorrhoids, loose stools, nausea, stomatitis, tongue ulcer, vomiting
Genitourinary: Dysuria, hematuria, urinary tract infection
Hematologic & oncologic: Anemia, bone marrow depression (nadir: days 10 to 17; recovery: days 28 to 31), bruise, febrile neutropenia, hematoma, leukopenia, Lymphadenopathy, neutropenia, oral hemorrhage, oral mucosal petechiae, petechia, postprocedural hemorrhage, thrombocytopenia
Hypersensitivity: Transfusion reaction
Infection: Herpes simplex infection
Local: Bruising at injection site, erythema at injection site (more common with IV administration), hematoma at injection site, induration at injection site, injection site granuloma, injection site reaction, itching at injection site, pain at injection site (more common with IV administration), skin discoloration at injection site, swelling at injection site
Neuromuscular & skeletal: Arthralgia, back pain, limb pain, muscle cramps, myalgia, weakness
Respiratory: Abnormal breath sounds, atelectasis, cough, dyspnea, epistaxis, nasal congestion, nasopharyngitis, pharyngitis, pharyngolaryngeal pain, pleural effusion, pneumonia, post nasal drip, rales, rhinitis, rhinorrhea, rhonchi, sinusitis, upper respiratory infection, wheezing
Miscellaneous: Fever
Rare but important or life-threatening: Abscess (limb, perirectal), aggravated bone pain, agranulocytosis, anaphylactic shock, atrial fibrillation, azotemia, bacterial infection, blastomycosis, bone marrow failure, cardiac failure, cardiorespiratory arrest, catheter site hemorrhage, cellulitis, cerebral hemorrhage, cholecystectomy, cholecystitis, congestive cardiomyopathy, decreased serum bicarbonate, dehydration, diverticulitis, fibrosis (interstitial and alveolar), gastrointestinal hemorrhage, glycosuria, hemophthalmos, hemoptysis, hepatic coma, hypersensitivity reaction, hypophosphatemia, increased serum creatinine, injection site infection, interstitial pulmonary disease, intracranial hemorrhage, leukemia cutis, melena, neutropenic sepsis, orthostatic hypotension, pancytopenia, pneumonitis, polyuria, pulmonary infiltrates, pyoderma gangrenosum, renal failure, renal tubular acidosis, respiratory distress, seizure, sepsis, sepsis syndrome, septic shock, splenomegaly, Sweet's syndrome, tissue necrosis at injection site, toxoplasmosis, tumor lysis syndrome

Drug Interactions

Metabolism/Transport Effects None known.

Avoid Concomitant Use

Avoid concomitant use of AzaCITIDine with any of the following: BCG; BCG (Intravesical); CloZAPine; Dipyrone; Natalizumab; Pimecrolimus; Tacrolimus (Topical); Tofacitinib; Vaccines (Live)

Increased Effect/Toxicity

AzaCITIDine may increase the levels/effects of: CloZAPine; Leflunomide; Natalizumab; Tofacitinib; Vaccines (Live)

The levels/effects of AzaCITIDine may be increased by: Denosumab; Dipyrone; Pimecrolimus; Roflumilast; Tacrolimus (Topical); Trastuzumab

Decreased Effect

AzaCITIDine may decrease the levels/effects of: BCG; BCG (Intravesical); Coccidioides immitis Skin Test; Sipuleucel-T; Vaccines (Inactivated); Vaccines (Live)

The levels/effects of AzaCITIDine may be decreased by: Echinacea

Storage/Stability Prior to reconstitution, store intact vials at room temperature of 25°C (77°F); excursions permitted to 15°C to 30°C (59°F to 86°F).

SubQ suspension: Following reconstitution, suspension may be stored at room temperature for up to 1 hour prior to immediate administration (administer within 1 hour of reconstitution). If administration is delayed, refrigerate reconstituted suspension immediately (either in vial or syringe); may be stored for up to 8 hours (if reconstituted with room temperature SWFI) or up to 22 hours (if reconstituted with refrigerated SWFI). After removal from refrigerator, may be allowed up to 30 minutes to reach room temperature prior to administration.

IV solution: **Solutions for IV administration have very limited stability and must be prepared immediately prior to each dose.** Administration must be completed within 1 hour of (vial) reconstitution.

Mechanism of Action Antineoplastic effects may be a result of azacitidine's ability to promote hypomethylation of DNA, restoring normal gene differentiation and proliferation. Azacitidine also exerts direct toxicity to abnormal hematopoietic cells in the bone marrow.

Pharmacokinetics (Adult data unless noted)

Absorption: SubQ: Rapid and complete
Distribution: V_d: IV: 76 ± 26 L; does not cross blood-brain barrier
Metabolism: Hepatic; hydrolysis to several metabolites
Bioavailability: SubQ: ~89%
Half-life elimination: IV, SubQ: ~4 hours
Time to peak serum concentration: SubQ: 30 minutes
Elimination: Urine (50% to 85%); feces (<1%)

Dosing: Usual

Pediatric: **Note:** Dosing and frequency may vary by protocol and/or treatment phase; refer to specific protocol.
Acute myeloid leukemia (AML): Limited data available; efficacy results variable:
SubQ: Children ≥2 years and Adolescents: 75 mg/m^2/dose once daily for 7 days; dosing from a patient population (n=53) that included adults up to 84 years of age; the minimum age of subjects in the trial was 5 years of age although minimum inclusion criteria was 2 years of age; used in combination with tretinoin and valproic acid for refractory or relapsed cases with clinical activity observed (Soriano, 2007). Additional trials are in progress evaluating only pediatric patient study populations; one trial underway is a Phase I, dose-finding in relapsed or refractory AML or ALL; the dosing being evaluated is 50 or 75 mg/m^2/dose once daily for 5 days in combination with fludarabine and cytarabine; results pending (NCT01861002, 2014)
IV: Dosing regimens variable: Children and Adolescents: 300 mg/m^2/dose once daily for 2 consecutive days has been used for induction and intensive consolidation therapy in various combinations in newly diagnosed patients (Ravindranath, 2005; Ribiero, 2005). **Note:** Frequency of use of azacitidine therapy for AML (newly diagnosed) has decreased as newer therapies have replaced previous protocols.

Adult: **Myelodysplastic syndromes (MDS):** IV, SubQ: Initial Cycle: 75 mg/m^2/day for 7 days. Subsequent cycles: 75 mg/m^2/day for 7 days every 4 weeks; dose may be increased to 100 mg/m^2/day if no benefit is observed after 2 cycles and no toxicity other than nausea and vomiting have occurred. Patients should be treated for a minimum of 4 to 6 cycles; treatment may be continued as long as patient continues to benefit.

Note: Alternate schedules (which have produced hematologic response) have been used for convenience in community oncology centers (Lyons, 2009): SubQ:

75 mg/m²/day for 5 days (Mon to Fri), 2 days rest (Sat, Sun), then 75 mg/m²/day for 2 days (Mon, Tues); repeat cycle every 28 days **or**

50 mg/m²/day for 5 days (Mon to Fri), 2 days rest (Sat, Sun), then 50 mg/m²/day for 5 days (Mon to Fri); repeat cycle every 28 days **or**

75 mg/m²/day for 5 days (Mon to Fri), repeat cycle every 28 days

Dosing adjustment based on hematology: Adults: IV, SubQ:

For baseline WBC ≥3.0 x 109/L, ANC ≥1.5 x 109/L, and platelets ≥75 x 109/L:

Nadir count: ANC <0.5 x 109/L or platelets <25 x 109/L: Administer 50% of dose during next treatment course

Nadir count: ANC 0.5 to 1.5 x 109/L or platelets 25 to 50 x 109/L: Administer 67% of dose during next treatment course

Nadir count: ANC >1.5 x 109/L or platelets >50 x 109/L: Administer 100% of dose during next treatment course

For baseline WBC <3 x 109/L, ANC <1.5 x 109/L, or platelets <75 x 109/L: Adjust dose as follows based on nadir counts and bone marrow biopsy cellularity at the time of nadir, unless clear improvement in differentiation at the time of the next cycle:

WBC or platelet nadir decreased 50% to 75% from baseline and bone marrow biopsy cellularity at time of nadir 30% to 60%: Administer 100% of dose during next treatment course

WBC or platelet nadir decreased 50% to 75% from baseline and bone marrow biopsy cellularity at time of nadir 15% to 30%: Administer 50% of dose during next treatment course

WBC or platelet nadir decreased 50% to 75% from baseline and bone marrow biopsy cellularity at time of nadir <15%: Administer 33% of dose during next treatment course

WBC or platelet nadir decreased >75% from baseline and bone marrow biopsy cellularity at time of nadir 30% to 60%: Administer 75% of dose during next treatment course

WBC or platelet nadir decreased >75% from baseline and bone marrow biopsy cellularity at time of nadir 15% to 30%: Administer 50% of dose during next treatment course

WBC or platelet nadir decreased >75% from baseline and bone marrow biopsy cellularity at time of nadir <15%: Administer 33% of dose during next treatment course

Note: If a nadir defined above occurs, administer the next treatment course 28 days after the start of the preceding course as long as WBC and platelet counts are >25% above the nadir and rising. If a >25% increase above the nadir is not seen by day 28, reassess counts every 7 days. If a 25% increase is not seen by day 42, administer 50% of the scheduled dose.

Dosing adjustment based on serum electrolytes: If serum bicarbonate falls to <20 mEq/L (unexplained decrease): Reduce dose by 50% for next treatment course

Dosing adjustment in renal impairment: Adults:

Renal impairment at *baseline*:

Mild to moderate impairment (CrCl ≥30 mL/minute): No dosage adjustment necessary (Douvali, 2012)

Severe impairment (CrCl <30 mL/minute): No dosage adjustment necessary for cycle 1; due to renal excretion of azacitidine and metabolites, monitor closely for toxicity.

Renal toxicity *during* treatment: Unexplained increases in BUN or serum creatinine: Delay next cycle until values reach baseline or normal, then reduce dose by 50% for next treatment course.

Dosing adjustment in hepatic impairment: There are no dosage adjustments provided in the manufacturer's labeling (has not been studied); use is contraindicated in patients with advanced malignant hepatic tumors.

Preparation for Administration Hazardous agent; use appropriate precautions for handling and disposal (NIOSH 2014 [group 1]). If reconstituted solution comes in contact with skin, wash immediately and thoroughly with soap and water; if comes in contact with mucous membranes, flush thoroughly with water.

SubQ: Slowly add 4 mL SWFI to each vial, resulting in a concentration of 25 mg/mL. Vigorously shake or roll vial until a suspension is formed (suspension will be cloudy). The manufacturer recommends dividing doses >4 mL equally into 2 syringes. Do not filter after reconstitution (may remove active drug). Resuspend contents of syringe by vigorously rolling between palms immediately prior to administration.

IV: Reconstitute vial with 10 mL SWFI to form a 10 mg/mL solution; vigorously shake or roll vial until solution is dissolved and clear. Further dilute in 50 to 100 mL of NS or LR injection for infusion.

Discard unused portion (does not contain preservatives); do not save unused portions for later administration.

Administration Hazardous agent; use appropriate precautions for handling and disposal (NIOSH 2014 [group 1]). If azacitidine suspension comes in contact with the skin, immediately wash with soap and water; if it comes into contact with mucous membranes, flush thoroughly with water. Azacitidine is associated with a moderate emetic potential (Basch 2011; Dupuis 2011; Roila 2010); premedication to prevent nausea and vomiting is recommended.

SubQ: The manufacturer recommends equally dividing volumes >4 mL into 2 syringes and injecting into 2 separate sites; however, policies for maximum SubQ administration volume may vary by institution; interpatient variations may also apply. Rotate sites for each injection (thigh, abdomen, or upper arm). Administer subsequent injections at least 1 inch from previous injection sites and never into areas where the site is tender, bruise, red, or hard. Allow refrigerated suspensions to come to room temperature up to 30 minutes prior to administration. Resuspend by inverting the syringe 2 to 3 times and then rolling the syringe between the palms for 30 seconds.

IV: Infuse over 10 to 40 minutes; infusion must be completed within 1 hour of vial reconstitution.

Monitoring Parameters Liver function tests (baseline), electrolytes (baseline and prior to each cycle), CBC with differential and platelets (baseline and prior to each cycle, more frequently if indicated), renal function tests (BUN and serum creatinine at baseline and prior to each cycle); monitor for nausea/vomiting and injection site reactions.

Dosage Forms Excipient information presented when available (limited, particularly for generics); consult specific product labeling.

Suspension Reconstituted, Injection:

Generic: 100 mg (1 ea)

Suspension Reconstituted, Injection [preservative free]:

Vidaza: 100 mg (1 ea)

Generic: 100 mg (1 ea)

- ◆ **AZA-CR** *see* AzaCITIDine *on page* 233
- ◆ **Azactam** *see* Aztreonam *on page* 248
- ◆ **Azactam in Dextrose** *see* Aztreonam *on page* 248
- ◆ **Azacytidine** *see* AzaCITIDine *on page* 233
- ◆ **5-Azacytidine** *see* AzaCITIDine *on page* 233
- ◆ **Azasan** *see* AzaTHIOprine *on page* 236
- ◆ **AzaSite** *see* Azithromycin (Ophthalmic) *on page* 247

AzaTHIOprine (ay za THYE oh preen)

Medication Safety Issues

Sound-alike/look-alike issues:

AzaTHIOprine may be confused with azaCITIDine, azidothymidine, azithromycin, Azulfidine

Imuran may be confused with Elmiron, Enduron, Imdur, Inderal, Tenormin

High alert medication:

This medication is in a class the Institute for Safe Medication Practices (ISMP) includes among its list of drug classes that have a heightened risk of causing significant patient harm when used in error.

Other safety concerns:

Azathioprine is metabolized to mercaptopurine; concurrent use of these commercially-available products has resulted in profound myelosuppression.

Related Information

Safe Handling of Hazardous Drugs *on page 2455*

Brand Names: US Azasan; Imuran

Brand Names: Canada Apo-Azathioprine; Imuran; Mylan-Azathioprine; Teva-Azathioprine

Therapeutic Category Immunosuppressant Agent

Generic Availability (US) Yes

Use Adjunct with other agents in prevention of kidney transplant rejection (FDA approved in adults); management of active rheumatoid arthritis (FDA approved in adults); has also been used as an immunosuppressant in a variety of autoimmune diseases such as SLE, juvenile idiopathic arthritis (JIA), JIA-associated uveitis, myasthenia gravis, and autoimmune hepatitis, and as a steroid-sparing agent for inflammatory bowel disease

Pregnancy Risk Factor D

Pregnancy Considerations Adverse events have been observed in animal reproduction studies. Azathioprine crosses the placenta in humans; congenital anomalies, immunosuppression, hematologic toxicities (lymphopenia, pancytopenia), and intrauterine growth retardation have been reported. Azathioprine should not be used to treat rheumatoid arthritis during pregnancy. Women of child-bearing potential should avoid becoming pregnant during treatment.

The National Transplantation Pregnancy Registry (NTPR, Temple University) is a registry for pregnant women taking immunosuppressants following any solid organ transplant. The NTPR encourages reporting of all immunosuppressant exposures during pregnancy in transplant recipients at 877-955-6877.

Breast-Feeding Considerations Azathioprine is excreted in breast milk. Due to potential for serious adverse reactions in the nursing infant, breast-feeding is not recommended by the manufacturer.

Contraindications Hypersensitivity to azathioprine or any component of the formulation; pregnancy (in patients with rheumatoid arthritis); patients with rheumatoid arthritis and a history of treatment with alkylating agents (eg, cyclophosphamide, chlorambucil, melphalan) may have a prohibitive risk of malignancy with azathioprine treatment

Warnings/Precautions Hazardous agent - use appropriate precautions for handling and disposal (NIOSH 2014 [group 2]).

[U.S. Boxed Warning]: Immunosuppressive agents, including azathioprine, increase the risk of development of malignancy; lymphoma (in post-transplant patients) and hepatosplenic T-cell lymphoma (HSTCL) (in patients with inflammatory bowel disease) have been reported. Patients should be informed of the risk for malignancy development. HSTCL is a rare white blood cell cancer that is usually fatal and has predominantly occurred in adolescents and young adults treated for Crohn disease or ulcerative colitis and receiving TNF blockers (eg, adalimumab, certolizumab pegol, etanercept, golimumab), azathioprine, and/or mercaptopurine. Most cases of HSTCL have occurred in patients treated with a combination of immunosuppressant agents, although there have been reports of HSTCL in patients receiving azathioprine or mercaptopurine monotherapy. Renal transplant patients are also at increased risk for malignancy (eg, skin cancer, lymphoma); limit sun and ultraviolet light exposure and use appropriate sun protection.

Dose-related hematologic toxicities (leukopenia, thrombocytopenia, and anemias, including macrocytic anemia, or pancytopenia) may occur; may be severe and/or delayed. Patients with intermediate thiopurine methyltransferase (TPMT) activity may be at increased risk for hematologic toxicity at conventional azathioprine doses; patients with low or absent TPMT activity are at risk for severe, life-threatening myelotoxicity. Myelosuppression may be more severe with renal transplants undergoing rejection. Monitor CBC with differential and platelets weekly during the first month, then twice a month for 2 months, then monthly (or more frequently if clinically indicated). May require treatment interruption or dose reduction.

Chronic immunosuppression increases the risk of serious, sometimes fatal, infections (bacterial, viral, fungal, protozoal, and opportunistic). Progressive multifocal leukoencephalopathy (PML), an opportunistic CNS infection caused by reactivation of the JC virus, has been reported in patients receiving immunosuppressive therapy, including azathioprine; promptly evaluate any patient presenting with neurological changes. Consider decreasing the degree of immunosuppression with consideration to the risk of organ rejection in transplant patients.

Use with caution in patients with liver disease or renal impairment; monitor hematologic function closely. Azathioprine is metabolized to mercaptopurine; concomitant use may result in profound myelosuppression and should be avoided. Patients with genetic deficiency of thiopurine methyltransferase (TPMT) or concurrent therapy with drugs which may inhibit TPMT are more sensitive to myelosuppressive effects. Patients with intermediate TPMT activity may be at risk for increased myelosuppression; those with low or absent TPMT activity are at risk for developing severe myelotoxicity. TPMT genotyping or phenotyping may assist in identifying patients at risk for developing toxicity. Consider TPMT testing in patients with abnormally low CBC unresponsive to dose reduction. TPMT testing does not substitute for CBC monitoring. Potentially significant drug-drug interactions may exist, requiring dose or frequency adjustment, additional monitoring, and/or selection of alternative therapy. Xanthine oxidase inhibitors may increase risk for hematologic toxicity; reduce azathioprine dose when used concurrently with allopurinol; patients with low or absent TPMT activity may require further dose reductions or discontinuation.

Hepatotoxicity (transaminase, bilirubin, and alkaline phosphatase elevations) may occur, usually in renal transplant patients and generally within 6 months of transplant; normally reversible with discontinuation; monitor liver function periodically. Rarely, hepatic sinusoidal obstruction syndrome (SOS; formerly called veno-occlusive disease) has been reported; discontinue if hepatic SOS is suspected. Severe nausea, vomiting, diarrhea, rash, fever, malaise, myalgia, hypotension, and liver enzyme abnormalities may occur within the first several weeks of treatment and are generally reversible upon discontinuation. **[U.S. Boxed Warning]: Should be prescribed by physicians familiar with the risks, including hematologic toxicities and mutagenic potential.** Immune response to vaccines may be diminished.

Warnings: Additional Pediatric Considerations The development of secondary hemophagocytic lymphohistiocytosis (HLH), a rare and frequently fatal activation of macrophages which causes phagocytosis of all bone marrow blood cell lines, is increased (100-fold) in pediatric patients diagnosed with inflammatory bowel disease due to chronic inflammation; this risk is further increased with concomitant thiopurine (ie, azathioprine or mercaptopurine) therapy, Epstein-Barr virus, or possibly other infections; if patient on thiopurine therapy presents with fever for at least 5 days, cervical lymphadenopathy, and lymphopenia, discontinue immunosuppressive therapy and further diagnostic evaluation for HLH should be performed; delay in diagnosis has been associated with increased mortality (Biank, 2011).

Adverse Reactions

Central nervous system: Malaise

Gastrointestinal: Diarrhea, nausea and vomiting (rheumatoid arthritis)

Hematologic and oncologic: Leukopenia (more common in renal transplant), neoplasia (renal transplant), thrombocytopenia

Hepatic: Hepatotoxicity, increased serum alkaline phosphatase, increased serum bilirubin, increased serum transaminases

Infection: Increased susceptibility to infection (more common in renal transplant; includes bacterial, fungal, protozoal, viral, opportunistic, and reactivation of latent infections)

Neuromuscular & skeletal: Myalgia

Miscellaneous: Fever

Rare but important or life-threatening: Abdominal pain, acute myelocytic leukemia, alopecia, anemia, arthralgia, bone marrow depression, hemorrhage, hepatic veno-occlusive disease, hepatosplenic T-cell lymphomas, hepatotoxicity (idiosyncratic) (Chalasani, 2014), hypersensitivity, hypotension, interstitial pneumonitis (reversible), JC virus infection, macrocytic anemia, malignant lymphoma, malignant neoplasm of skin, negative nitrogen balance, pancreatitis, pancytopenia, progressive multifocal leukoencephalopathy, skin rash, steatorrhea, Sweet's syndrome (acute febrile neutrophilic dermatosis)

Drug Interactions

Metabolism/Transport Effects None known.

Avoid Concomitant Use

Avoid concomitant use of AzaTHIOprine with any of the following: BCG; BCG (Intravesical); Febuxostat; Mercaptopurine; Natalizumab; Pimecrolimus; Tacrolimus (Topical); Tofacitinib

Increased Effect/Toxicity

AzaTHIOprine may increase the levels/effects of: Cyclophosphamide; Leflunomide; Mercaptopurine; Natalizumab; Tofacitinib; Vaccines (Live)

The levels/effects of AzaTHIOprine may be increased by: 5-ASA Derivatives; ACE Inhibitors; Allopurinol; Denosumab; Febuxostat; Pimecrolimus; Ribavirin; Roflumilast; Sulfamethoxazole; Tacrolimus (Topical); Trastuzumab; Trimethoprim

Decreased Effect

AzaTHIOprine may decrease the levels/effects of: BCG; BCG (Intravesical); Coccidioides immitis Skin Test; Sipuleucel-T; Vaccines (Inactivated); Vaccines (Live); Vitamin K Antagonists

The levels/effects of AzaTHIOprine may be decreased by: Echinacea

Storage/Stability

Tablet: Store at 15°C to 25°C (59°F to 77°F). Protect from light and moisture.

Powder for injection [Canadian product]: Store intact vials at 15°C to 25°C (59°F to 77°F). Protect from light. Use immediately after preparation; discard unused portion.

Mechanism of Action Azathioprine is an imidazolyl derivative of mercaptopurine; metabolites are incorporated into replicating DNA and halt replication; also block the pathway for purine synthesis (Taylor, 2005). The 6-thioguanine nucleotide metabolites appear to mediate the majority of azathioprine's immunosuppressive and toxic effects.

Pharmacokinetics (Adult data unless noted)

Absorption: Oral: Well absorbed

Protein binding: ~30%

Metabolism: Hepatic; metabolized to 6-mercaptopurine via glutathione S-transferase (GST). Further metabolism in the liver and GI tract, via three major pathways: Hypoxanthine guanine phosphoribosyltransferase (to active metabolites: 6-thioguanine-nucleotides, or 6-TGNs), xanthine oxidase (to inactive metabolite: 6-thiouric acid), and thiopurine methyltransferase (TPMT) (to inactive metabolite: 6-methylmercaptopurine)

Time to peak serum concentration: Oral: 1 to 2 hours (including metabolites)

Half-life, elimination: Azathioprine and mercaptopurine: Variable: ~2 hours (Taylor, 2005)

Elimination: Urine (primarily as metabolites)

Dosing: Usual Note: Patients with intermediate TPMT activity may be at risk for increased myelosuppression; those with low or absent TPMT activity receiving conventional azathioprine doses are at risk for developing severe, life-threatening myelotoxicity. Dosage reductions are recommended for patients with reduced TPMT activity. **Note:** IV dose is equivalent to oral dose (dosing should be transitioned from IV to oral as soon as tolerated).

Pediatric:

Hepatitis, autoimmune: Limited data available: Children and Adolescents: Oral: Initial: 0.5 mg/kg/dose once daily; titrate as needed up to 2 mg/kg/dose once daily; for long-term therapy, a low-dose of 1 to 1.5 mg/kg/day may be effective in some patients (Della Corte, 2012; Vitfell-Pedersen, 2012)

Inflammatory bowel disease: Limited data available: Infants, Children, and Adolescents: Oral: 2 to 2.5 mg/kg/dose once daily; titrate to effect; usual reported range: 1 to 3 mg/kg/dose once daily; reported maximum daily dose: 4 mg/kg/day or 200 mg/day; may takes several weeks of therapy to be fully effective (Fuentes, 2003; Punati, 2011; Riello, 2011; Sandhu, 2010). Some data suggest that pediatric patients ≤6 years may require higher doses to achieve remission; a median dose of 3.51 mg/kg/day (maximum daily dose: 5 mg/kg/day) was reported to induce remission in 62% of patients ≤6 years of age vs 17% of those receiving lower doses (ie, <2 to 3 mg/kg/day study group; median dose: 2.46 mg/kg/day) (Grossman, 2008).

Immune thrombocytopenia (ITP), chronic refractory: Limited data available: Children ≥2 years and Adolescents: Oral: Maintenance: 2 to 2.5 mg/kg/day, rounded to the nearest 50 mg (Boruchov, 2007)

Juvenile-idiopathic arthritis (rheumatoid arthritis): Limited data available: Children and Adolescents: Oral: 2 to 2.5 mg/kg/dose once daily; data limited to single double-blind, placebo-controlled trial of pediatric patients (n=17 treatment group); efficacy results were not statistically significant (response rate: Treatment: 41% vs placebo: 27%); data suggested a minimum trial of 12 weeks to fully assess therapeutic response (AHRQ, 2011; Hashkes, 2005; Kvien, 1986)

Lupus nephritis, mild: Limited data available: Children and Adolescents: Oral: 2 to 2.5 mg/kg/dose once daily (Bertsias, 2012; Marks, 2010); **Note:** Some data suggest less effective in non-Caucasian pediatric patients; some centers recommend use for primary induction in Caucasian patients with less severe disease (Adams, 2006; Marks, 2010).

Myasthenia gravis, juvenile: Limited data available: Children and Adolescents: Oral: 1 to 3 mg/kg/dose once daily (Ashraf, 2006; Lindner, 1997)

Transplantation, solid organ: Limited data available: Infants, Children, and Adolescents: Oral: Initial: 3 to 5 mg/kg/dose once daily, beginning at the time of transplant; maintenance: 1 to 3 mg/kg/dose once daily (Denfield, 2010; Ford, 2006)

Uveitis, JIA-associated: Limited data available: Children and Adolescents: Oral: Initial mean dose: 2.4 mg/kg/dose once daily; reported range: 1.4 to 3.2 mg/kg/dose once daily; in a retrospective review of 41 children, a mean maintenance 2.1 mg/kg/dose (range: 1 to 2.8 mg/kg/dose) once daily was reported as monotherapy and/or in combination with other immunosuppressive agents; infectious etiology was excluded; the authors recommend doses of <3 mg/kg/day (Goebel, 2011)

Adult:

Renal transplantation (treatment usually started the day of transplant; however, has been initiated [rarely] 1 to 3 days prior to transplant): Oral: Initial: 3 to 5 mg/kg/day usually given as a single daily dose, then maintenance 1 to 3 mg/kg/day

Rheumatoid arthritis: Oral:

Initial: 1 mg/kg/day (50 to 100 mg) given once daily or divided twice daily for 6 to 8 weeks; may increase by 0.5 mg/kg every 4 weeks until response or up to a maximum daily dose of 2.5 mg/kg/**day**; an adequate trial should be a minimum of 12 weeks

Maintenance dose: Reduce dose by 0.5 mg/kg (~25 mg daily) every 4 weeks until lowest effective dose is reached; optimum duration of therapy not specified; may be discontinued abruptly

Dosage adjustment for concomitant use with allopurinol:

Infants, Children, and Adolescents: Limited data available

Adults: Reduce azathioprine dose to one-third or one-fourth the usual dose when used concurrently with allopurinol. Patients with low or absent TPMT activity may require further dose reductions or discontinuation.

Dosage adjustment for toxicity:

Infants, Children, and Adolescents: Limited data available

Adults:

Rapid WBC count decrease, persistently low WBC count, or serious infection: Reduce dose or temporarily withhold treatment.

Severe toxicity in renal transplantation: May require discontinuation.

Hepatic sinusoidal obstruction syndrome (SOS; veno-occlusive disease): Permanently discontinue.

Dosing adjustment in renal impairment:

Infants, Children, and Adolescents (Aronoff, 2007):

GFR >50 mL/minute/1.73m^2: No adjustment required.

GFR 10 to 50 mL/minute/1.73m^2: Administer 75% of dose once daily.

GFR <10 mL/minute/1.73m^2: Administer 50% of dose once daily.

Hemodialysis (dialyzable; ~45% removed in 8 hours): Administer 50% of normal dose once daily.

CAPD: Administer 50% of normal dose once daily.

CRRT: Administer 75% of normal dose once daily.

Adults: There are no specific dosage adjustments provided in manufacturer's labeling; however, oliguric patients, particularly those with tubular necrosis in the immediate post-transplant period (cadaveric transplant) may have delayed clearance and typically receive lower doses. The following adjustments have been recommended (Aronoff, 2007):

CrCl >50 mL/minute: No adjustment required.

CrCl 10 to 50 mL/minute: Administer 75% of normal dose.

CrCl <10 mL/minute: Administer 50% of normal dose.

Hemodialysis (dialyzable; ~45% removed in 8 hours): Administer 50% of normal dose; supplement: 0.25 mg/kg

CRRT: Administer 75% of normal dose.

Dosing adjustment in hepatic impairment: There are no dosage adjustments provided in the manufacturer's labeling.

Administration Hazardous agent; use appropriate precautions for handling and disposal (NIOSH 2014 [group 2]).

Oral: Administer with food or may administer in divided doses to decrease GI upset.

Monitoring Parameters CBC with differential and platelets (weekly during first month, twice monthly for months 2 and 3, then monthly; monitor more frequently with dosage modifications), total bilirubin, liver function tests, creatinine clearance, TPMT genotyping or phenotyping (consider TPMT testing in patients with abnormally low CBC unresponsive to dose reduction); monitor for symptoms of infection

For use as immunomodulatory therapy in inflammatory bowel disease (Crohn disease or ulcerative colitis), monitor CBC with differential weekly for 1 month, then biweekly for 1 month, followed by monitoring every 1-2 months throughout the course of therapy; monitor more frequently if symptomatic. LFTs should be assessed every 3 months. Monitor for signs/symptoms of malignancy (eg, splenomegaly, hepatomegaly, abdominal pain, persistent fever, night sweats, weight loss).

Test Interactions TPMT phenotyping results will not be accurate following recent blood transfusions.

Dosage Forms Excipient information presented when available (limited, particularly for generics); consult specific product labeling.

Tablet, Oral:

Azasan: 75 mg, 100 mg [scored]

Imuran: 50 mg [scored]

Generic: 50 mg

Extemporaneous Preparations Hazardous agent: Use appropriate precautions for handling and disposal (NIOSH 2014 [group 2]).

A 50 mg/mL oral suspension may be prepared with tablets. Crush one-hundred-twenty 50 mg tablets in a mortar and reduce to a fine powder. Add 40 mL of either cherry syrup (diluted 1:4 with Simple Syrup, USP); a 1:1 mixture of Ora-Sweet® and Ora-Plus®; or a 1:1 mixture of Ora-Sweet® SF and Ora-Plus®, and mix to a uniform paste. Mix while adding the vehicle in incremental proportions to **almost** 120 mL; transfer to a calibrated bottle, rinse mortar with vehicle, and add quantity of vehicle sufficient to make 120 mL. Label "shake well", "refrigerate", and "protect from light". Stable for 60 days refrigerated.

Allen LV Jr and Erickson MA 3rd, "Stability of Acetazolamide, Allopurinol, Azathioprine, Clonazepam, and Flucytosine in Extemporaneously Compounded Oral Liquids," *Am J Health Syst Pharm*, 1996, 53(16):1944-9.

◆ **Azathioprine Sodium** *see* AzaTHIOprine *on page* 236

◆ **5-AZC** *see* AzaCITIDine *on page* 233

Azelaic Acid (a zeh LAY ik AS id)

Brand Names: US Azelex; Finacea

Brand Names: Canada Finacea

Therapeutic Category Acne Products

Generic Availability (US) No

Use Topical:

Cream: Azelex: Treatment of mild to moderate inflammatory acne vulgaris (FDA approved in ages ≥12 years and adults)

Gel: Finacea: Treatment of inflammatory papules and pustules of mild to moderate rosacea (FDA approved in adults)

Pregnancy Risk Factor B

Pregnancy Considerations Adverse events have been observed in animal reproduction studies following oral administration. The amount of azelaic acid available systemically following topical administration is minimal (<4%).

Breast-Feeding Considerations It is not known if azelaic acid is excreted in breast milk. The amount of azelaic acid available systemically following topical administration is minimal (<4%); a significant change from baseline azelaic acid levels in the milk is not expected. The manufacturer of the cream recommends that caution be exercised when administering azelaic acid to nursing women. The manufacturer of the gel recommends a decision be made whether to discontinue nursing or to discontinue the drug, taking into account the importance of treatment to the mother.

Contraindications

Cream: Hypersensitivity to azelaic acid or any component of the formulation

Gel: There are no contraindications listed in the manufacturer's labeling

Warnings/Precautions For external use only; not for oral, ophthalmic, or vaginal use; avoid contact with the eyes, mouth, and other mucous membranes. Hypersensitivity reactions have been reported; discontinue use if signs/symptoms occur. A few cases of hypopigmentation after use have been reported; monitor for changes in skin color, especially in patients with dark complexions. Skin irritation (eg, pruritus, burning, stinging) may occur, usually during the first weeks of therapy. Discontinue use if severe skin irritation or sensitivity occurs. Use of occlusive dressings or wrappings should be avoided. Reassess use if no improvement is seen after 12 weeks of therapy.

Some dosage forms may contain polysorbate 80 (also known as Tweens). Hypersensitivity reactions, usually a delayed reaction, have been reported following exposure to pharmaceutical products containing polysorbate 80 in certain individuals (Isaksson, 2002; Lucente 2000; Shelley, 1995). Thrombocytopenia, ascites, pulmonary deterioration, and renal and hepatic failure have been reported in premature neonates after receiving parenteral products containing polysorbate 80 (Alade, 1986; CDC, 1984). See manufacturer's labeling.

Warnings: Additional Pediatric Considerations Some dosage forms may contain propylene glycol; in neonates large amounts of propylene glycol delivered orally, intravenously (eg, >3,000 mg/day), or topically have been associated with potentially fatal toxicities which can include metabolic acidosis, seizures, renal failure, and CNS depression; toxicities have also been reported in children and adults including hyperosmolality, lactic acidosis, seizures and respiratory depression; use caution (AAP, 1997; Shehab, 2009).

Adverse Reactions

Dermatologic: Acne (gel), burning sensation of skin, contact dermatitis, desquamation, erythema, pruritus, skin irritation, stinging of skin, tingling of skin, xeroderma, xerosis

Rare but important or life-threatening: Dermatitis, edema, exacerbation of asthma, exacerbation of herpes labialis, hypersensitivity reaction, hypertrichosis, hypopigmentation, iridocyclitis, skin depigmentation (small spots), skin rash, vitiligo

Drug Interactions

Metabolism/Transport Effects None known.

Avoid Concomitant Use There are no known interactions where it is recommended to avoid concomitant use.

Increased Effect/Toxicity There are no known significant interactions involving an increase in effect.

Decreased Effect There are no known significant interactions involving a decrease in effect.

Storage/Stability Store at 15°C to 30°C (59°F to 86°F); do not freeze. Store cream on its side.

Mechanism of Action Azelaic acid is a dietary constituent normally found in whole grain cereals; can be formed endogenously. Exact mechanism is not known. *In vitro*, azelaic acid possesses antimicrobial activity against *Propionibacterium acnes* and *Staphylococcus epidermidis*. May decrease microcomedo formation.

Pharmacodynamics Onset of action (cream): Within 4 weeks

Pharmacokinetics (Adult data unless noted)

Absorption (cream): ~3% to 5% penetrates stratum corneum; up to 10% found in epidermis and dermis; 4% systemic absorption

Half-life (elimination): Topical: 12 hours

Elimination: Primarily unchanged in the urine

Dosing: Usual Topical:

Children ≥12 years and Adolescents: **Acne vulgaris:** Cream (Azelex 20%): Apply twice daily in the morning and evening; may reduce to once daily if persistent skin irritation occurs.

Adults:

Acne vulgaris: Cream (Azelex 20%): Apply twice daily in the morning and evening; may reduce to once daily if persistent skin irritation occurs.

Rosacea: Gel (Finacea 15%): Apply to affected areas of the face twice daily in the morning and evening; reassess if no improvement after 12 weeks of therapy.

Administration Topical: Apply a thin film and gently massage into to clean, dry skin; wash hands following application. Avoid the use of occlusive dressings or wrappings. For gel formulation, cosmetics may be applied after the gel has dried. Use only mild soaps or soapless cleansing lotion for facial cleansing. Not intended for intravaginal, ophthalmic, or oral use.

Monitoring Parameters Reduction in lesion size and/or inflammation; reduction in the number of lesions

Dosage Forms Excipient information presented when available (limited, particularly for generics); consult specific product labeling.

Cream, External:

Azelex: 20% (30 g, 50 g)

Gel, External:

Finacea: 15% (50 g) [contains benzoic acid, disodium edta, polysorbate 80, propylene glycol]

Azelastine (Nasal) (a ZEL as teen)

Medication Safety Issues

Sound-alike/look-alike issues:

Astelin may be confused with Astepro

Brand Names: US Astelin [DSC]; Astepro

Brand Names: Canada Astelin

Therapeutic Category Antihistamine, Nasal

Generic Availability (US) Yes

Use

Astelin: Treatment of the symptoms of seasonal allergic rhinitis (FDA approved in ages ≥5 years and adults) and vasomotor rhinitis (FDA approved in ages ≥12 years and adults)

Astepro: Treatment of the symptoms of seasonal allergic rhinitis and perennial allergic rhinitis (FDA approved in ages ≥6 years and adults)

Pregnancy Risk Factor C

Pregnancy Considerations Adverse events have been observed in some animal reproduction studies. Azelastine is systemically absorbed following nasal inhalation and may have side effects similar to other antihistamines. However, data related to the use of azelastine in pregnancy is limited; if treatment for rhinitis in a pregnant woman is needed, other agents are preferred (Wallace 2008).

Breast-Feeding Considerations It is not known if azelastine (nasal) is excreted in breast milk. The manufacturer recommends that caution be exercised when administering azelastine (nasal) to nursing women.

Contraindications There are no contraindications listed in the manufacturer's labeling.

Warnings/Precautions May cause CNS depression, which may impair physical or mental abilities; patients must be cautioned about performing tasks that require mental alertness (eg, operating machinery or driving). Potentially significant interactions may exist, requiring dose or frequency adjustment, additional monitoring, and/or selection of alternative therapy.

Adverse Reactions Adverse reactions may be dose-, indication-, or product-dependent:

Cardiovascular: Flushing, hypertension, tachycardia

Central nervous system: Abnormality in thinking, anxiety, bitter taste, depersonalization, depression, dizziness, drowsiness, dysesthesia, fatigue, headache, hypoesthesia, malaise, nervousness, sleep disorder, vertigo

Dermatologic: Contact dermatitis, eczema, folliculitis, furunculosis

Endocrine & metabolic: Albuminuria, amenorrhea, weight gain

Gastrointestinal: Abdominal pain, ageusia, aphthous stomatitis, constipation, diarrhea, dysgeusia (children), gastroenteritis, glossitis, increased appetite, nausea, toothache, vomiting, xerostomia

Genitourinary: Hematuria, mastalgia

Hepatic: Increased serum ALT

Hypersensitivity: Hypersensitivity reaction

Infection: Cold symptoms (children), herpes simplex infection, upper respiratory tract infection (children), viral infection

Neuromuscular & skeletal: Back pain, dislocation of temporomandibular joint, hyperkinesia, limb pain, myalgia, rheumatoid arthritis

Ophthalmic: Conjunctivitis, eye pain, watery eyes

Otic: Otitis media (infants and children)

Renal: Polyuria

Respiratory: Asthma, bronchitis, bronchospasm, burning sensation of the nose, cough (more common in older children than infants and young children), epistaxis, laryngitis, nasal congestion, nasal discomfort, nasal mucosa ulcer, paranasal sinus hypersecretion, paroxysmal nocturnal dyspnea, pharyngolaryngeal pain, pharyngitis, postnasal drip, rhinitis (exacerbation), sinusitis, sneezing, sore nose (infants and children), sore throat

Miscellaneous: Fever, laceration

Rare but important or life-threatening: Altered sense of smell, anaphylactoid reaction, anosmia, atrial fibrillation, chest pain, confusion, drug tolerance, increased serum transaminases, insomnia, muscle spasm, urinary retention, xerophthalmia

Drug Interactions

Metabolism/Transport Effects Substrate of CYP1A2 (minor), CYP2C19 (minor), CYP2D6 (minor), CYP3A4 (minor); **Note:** Assignment of Major/Minor substrate status based on clinically relevant drug interaction potential; **Inhibits** CYP2B6 (weak), CYP2C19 (weak), CYP2C9 (weak), CYP2D6 (weak)

Avoid Concomitant Use

Avoid concomitant use of Azelastine (Nasal) with any of the following: Aclidinium; Alcohol (Ethyl); CNS Depressants; Eluxadoline; Glucagon; Ipratropium (Oral Inhalation); Orphenadrine; Paraldehyde; Potassium Chloride; Thalidomide; Tiotropium; Umeclidinium

Increased Effect/Toxicity

Azelastine (Nasal) may increase the levels/effects of: AbobotulinumtoxinA; Anticholinergic Agents; Eluxadoline; Glucagon; Metyrosine; Mirabegron; OnabotulinumtoxinA; Orphenadrine; Paraldehyde; Potassium Chloride; Pramipexole; RimabotulinumtoxinB; ROPINIRole; Rotigotine; Selective Serotonin Reuptake Inhibitors; Thalidomide; Thiazide Diuretics; Tiotropium

The levels/effects of Azelastine (Nasal) may be increased by: Aclidinium; Alcohol (Ethyl); Brimonidine (Topical); Cannabis; CNS Depressants; Dronabinol; Ipratropium (Oral Inhalation); Kava Kava; Magnesium Sulfate; Nabilone; Pramlintide; Rufinamide; Tetrahydrocannabinol; Umeclidinium

Decreased Effect

Azelastine (Nasal) may decrease the levels/effects of: Acetylcholinesterase Inhibitors; Benzylpenicilloyl Polylysine; Betahistine; Hyaluronidase; Itopride; Metoclopramide; Secretin

The levels/effects of Azelastine (Nasal) may be decreased by: Acetylcholinesterase Inhibitors; Amphetamines

Storage/Stability Store upright at 20°C to 25°C (68°F to 77°F); protect from freezing.

Mechanism of Action Competes with histamine for H_1-receptor sites on effector cells and inhibits the release of histamine and other mediators involved in the allergic response; when used intranasally, reduces hyper-reactivity of the airways; increases the motility of bronchial epithelial cilia, improving mucociliary transport

Pharmacodynamics

Onset of action: 30 minutes to 1 hour

Maximum effect: 3 hours

Duration: 12 hours

Pharmacokinetics (Adult data unless noted)

Protein binding: 88%; desmethylazelastine: 97%

Metabolism: Metabolized by cytochrome P450 enzyme system; active metabolite desmethylazelastine

Bioavailability: 40%

Half-life, elimination: Azelastine: 22-25 hours; desmethylazelastine: 52-57 hours

Time to peak serum concentration: 2-4 hours

Elimination: Clearance: 0.5 L/hour/kg

Dosing: Usual Note: Astepro and Astelin are not interchangeable; Astelin delivers 137 mcg/spray; Astepro 0.1% delivers 137 mcg/spray; Astepro 0.15% delivers 205.5 mcg/spray

Children and Adolescents:

Perennial allergic rhinitis: Intranasal:

Astepro 0.1%: Children 6-11 years: 1 spray **per nostril** twice daily

Astepro 0.15%:

Children 6-11 years: 1 spray **per nostril** twice daily

Children ≥12 years and Adolescents: 2 sprays **per nostril** twice daily

Seasonal allergic rhinitis: Intranasal:

Astelin:

Children 5-11 years: 1 spray **per nostril** twice daily

Children ≥12 years and Adolescents: 1-2 sprays **per nostril** twice daily

Astepro 0.1%:

Children 6-11 years: 1 spray **per nostril** twice daily

Children ≥12 years and Adolescents: 1-2 sprays **per nostril** twice daily

Astepro 0.15%: Children ≥12 years and Adolescents: 1-2 sprays **per nostril** twice daily **or** 2 sprays **per nostril** once daily

Vasomotor rhinitis: Intranasal: Astelin: Children ≥12 years and Adolescents: 2 sprays **per nostril** twice daily

Adults:

Perennial allergic rhinitis: (Astepro 0.15%): Intranasal: 2 sprays **per nostril** twice daily

Seasonal allergic rhinitis: Intranasal:

Astelin, Astepro 0.1%: 1-2 sprays **per nostril** twice daily

Astepro 0.15%: 1-2 sprays **per nostril** twice daily or 2 sprays **per nostril** once daily

Vasomotor rhinitis (Astelin): Intranasal: 2 sprays **per nostril** twice daily

Dosing adjustment in renal impairment: There are no dosage adjustments provided in the manufacturer's labeling.

Dosing adjustment in hepatic impairment: There are no dosage adjustments provided in the manufacturer's labeling.

Administration Before use, the delivery system should be primed with 4 sprays (Astelin), 6 sprays (Astepro), or until a fine mist appears; when 3 or more days have elapsed since the last use, the pump should be reprimed with 2 sprays or until a fine mist appears. Blow nose to clear nostrils. Remove the dust cover. Keep head tilted downward when spraying. Insert applicator into nostril, keeping bottle upright, and close off the other nostril. Breathe in through nose. While inhaling, press pump to release spray. Alternate sprays between nostrils. After each use, wipe the spray tip with a clean tissue or cloth. Avoid spraying in eyes or mouth.

Dosage Forms Considerations Astelin and Astepro 30 mL bottles contain 200 sprays each.

Dosage Forms Excipient information presented when available (limited, particularly for generics); consult specific product labeling. [DSC] = Discontinued product

Solution, Nasal, as hydrochloride:

Astelin: 137 mcg/spray (30 mL [DSC]) [contains benzalkonium chloride, edetate disodium]

Astepro: 0.15% (30 mL) [contains benzalkonium chloride, edetate disodium]

Generic: 0.1% (30 mL); 0.15% (30 mL)

Azelastine (Ophthalmic) (a ZEL as teen)

Medication Safety Issues

Sound-alike/look-alike issues:

Optivar® may be confused with Optiray®, Optive™

International issues:

Optivar [U.S.] may be confused with Opthavir brand name for acyclovir [Mexico]

Brand Names: US Optivar [DSC]

Therapeutic Category Antiallergic, Ophthalmic

Generic Availability (US) Yes

Use Treatment of itching of the eye associated with allergic conjunctivitis

Pregnancy Risk Factor C

Pregnancy Considerations Animal reproduction studies have shown toxic effects to the fetus at maternally toxic doses.

Breast-Feeding Considerations It is not known if azelastine (ophthalmic) is excreted in breast milk. The manufacturer recommends that caution be exercised when administering azelastine (ophthalmic) to nursing women.

Contraindications Hypersensitivity to azelastine or any component of the formulation

Warnings/Precautions Solution contains benzalkonium chloride; wait at least 10 minutes after instilling solution before inserting soft contact lenses. Do not use contact lenses if eyes are red.

Adverse Reactions

Central nervous system: Fatigue, headache

Dermatologic: Pruritus

Gastrointestinal: Bitter taste

Ocular: Blurred vision (temporary), conjunctivitis, eye pain, transient burning/stinging

Respiratory: Asthma, dyspnea, pharyngitis, rhinitis

Miscellaneous: Flu-like syndrome

Drug Interactions

Metabolism/Transport Effects None known.

Avoid Concomitant Use There are no known interactions where it is recommended to avoid concomitant use.

Increased Effect/Toxicity There are no known significant interactions involving an increase in effect.

Decreased Effect There are no known significant interactions involving a decrease in effect.

Storage/Stability Store upright at controlled room temperature of 2°C to 25°C (36°F to 77°F).

Mechanism of Action Competes with histamine for H_1-receptor sites on effector cells and inhibits the release of histamine and other mediators involved in the allergic response

Dosing: Usual Ophthalmic: Children ≥3 years and Adults: Instill 1 drop into each affected eye twice daily

Administration Apply finger pressure to lacrimal sac during and for 1-2 minutes after instillation to decrease risk of systemic effects; avoid contact of bottle tip with skin or eye.

Dosage Forms Excipient information presented when available (limited, particularly for generics); consult specific product labeling. [DSC] = Discontinued product

Solution, Ophthalmic, as hydrochloride:

Optivar: 0.05% (6 mL [DSC]) [contains benzalkonium chloride]

Generic: 0.05% (6 mL)

Azelastine and Fluticasone

(a ZEL as teen & floo TIK a sone)

Brand Names: US Dymista

Therapeutic Category Corticosteroid, Nasal; Histamine H_1 Antagonist, Second Generation

Generic Availability (US) No

Use Symptomatic relief of seasonal allergic rhinitis (FDA approved in ages ≥6 years and adults)

Pregnancy Risk Factor C

Pregnancy Considerations Adverse events have been observed in animal reproduction studies. Refer to individual monographs.

Breast-Feeding Considerations It is not known if azelastine or fluticasone are excreted in breast milk. The manufacturer recommends that caution be exercised when administering azelastine and fluticasone to nursing women. Refer to individual monographs.

Contraindications There are no contraindications listed in the manufacturers' labeling.

Warnings/Precautions See individual agents.

Warnings: Additional Pediatric Considerations In a small pediatric study of fluticasone use conducted over 1 year, no statistically significant effect on growth velocity or clinically relevant changes in bone mineral density or HPA axis function were observed in children 3 to 9 years of age receiving fluticasone propionate nasal spray (200 mcg/day; n=56) versus placebo (n=52); effects at higher doses or in susceptible pediatric patients cannot be ruled out.

Adverse Reactions Reactions reported with combination product; also see individual agents.

Central nervous system: Headache

Gastrointestinal: Dysgeusia

Respiratory: Epistaxis (frequency and severity may be increased in children)

Rare but important or life-threatening: Anosmia, anxiety, application site irritation, atrial fibrillation, blurred vision, bronchospasm, cataract, chest pain, confusion, conjunctivitis, dizziness, drowsiness, dry nose, dry throat, dyspnea, erythema, eye irritation, fatigue, generalized ache, glaucoma, hoarseness, hypersensitivity reaction, hypertension, increased heart rate, increased intraocular pressure, muscle spasm, nasal sores, nervousness, palpitations, paresthesia, pruritus, skin rash, sore throat, swelling of eye, drug tolerance, urinary retention, visual disturbance, xerophthalmia

Drug Interactions

Metabolism/Transport Effects Refer to individual components.

Avoid Concomitant Use

Avoid concomitant use of Azelastine and Fluticasone with any of the following: Aclidinium; Alcohol (Ethyl); CNS Depressants; Eluxadoline; Glucagon; Ipratropium (Oral Inhalation); Orphenadrine; Paraldehyde; Potassium Chloride; Ritonavir; Thalidomide; Tiotropium; Tipranavir; Umeclidinium

Increased Effect/Toxicity

Azelastine and Fluticasone may increase the levels/effects of: AbobotulinumtoxinA; Anticholinergic Agents; Ceritinib; Eluxadoline; Glucagon; Metyrosine; Mirabegron; OnabotulinumtoxinA; Orphenadrine; Paraldehyde; Potassium Chloride; Pramipexole; RimabotulinumtoxinB; ROPINIRole; Rotigotine; Selective Serotonin Reuptake Inhibitors; Thalidomide; Thiazide Diuretics; Tiotropium

The levels/effects of Azelastine and Fluticasone may be increased by: Aclidinium; Alcohol (Ethyl); Brimonidine (Topical); Cannabis; CNS Depressants; Cobicistat; CYP3A4 Inhibitors (Strong); Dronabinol; Ipratropium (Oral Inhalation); Kava Kava; Magnesium Sulfate; Nabilone; Pramlintide; Ritonavir; Rufinamide; Telaprevir; Tetrahydrocannabinol; Tipranavir; Umeclidinium

Decreased Effect

Azelastine and Fluticasone may decrease the levels/effects of: Acetylcholinesterase Inhibitors; Benzylpenicilloyl Polylysine; Betahistine; Hyaluronidase; Itopride; Metoclopramide; Secretin

The levels/effects of Azelastine and Fluticasone may be decreased by: Acetylcholinesterase Inhibitors; Amphetamines

Storage/Stability Store at 20°C to 25°C (68°F to 77°F); do not refrigerate or freeze. Protect from light. Store in upright position with cap on.

Mechanism of Action Azelastine competes with histamine for H_1receptor sites on effector cells and inhibits the release of histamine and other mediators involved in the allergic response; when used intranasally, reduces hyperreactivity of the airways; increases the motility of bronchial epithelial cilia, improving mucociliary transport.

Fluticasone belongs to a group of corticosteroids which utilizes a fluorocarbothioate ester linkage at the 17 carbon position; extremely potent vasoconstrictive and anti-inflammatory activity.

Pharmacodynamics See individual agents.

Pharmacokinetics (Adult data unless noted) See individual agents.

Dosing: Usual

Pediatric: **Seasonal allergic rhinitis:**

Children 4 to 5 years: Limited data available; efficacy not established: Intranasal: 1 spray (137 mcg azelastine/50 mcg fluticasone) **per nostril** twice daily was evaluated in 61 patients as part of a larger pediatric trial, data did not fully establish efficacy; safety profile similar to older children (NCT01915823, 2014)

Children ≥6 years and Adolescents: Intranasal: 1 spray (137 mcg azelastine/50 mcg fluticasone) **per nostril** twice daily

Adult: **Seasonal allergic rhinitis:** Intranasal: 1 spray (137 mcg azelastine/50 mcg fluticasone) **per nostril** twice daily

Dosing adjustment in renal impairment: There are no dosage adjustments provided in the manufacturer's labeling.

Dosing adjustment in hepatic impairment: There are no dosage adjustments provided in the manufacturer's labeling.

Administration For intranasal administration only. Prime pump (press 6 times or until fine spray appears) prior to first use. If 14 or more days have elapsed since last use, then reprime pump with 1 spray or until a fine mist appears. Shake bottle gently before using. Blow nose to clear nostrils. Keep head tilted downward when spraying. Insert applicator tip 1/4 to 1/2 inch into nostril, keeping bottle upright, and close off the other nostril. Breathe in through nose. While inhaling, press pump to release spray. After each use, wipe the spray tip with a clean tissue or cloth and replace cap. Avoid spraying directly into nasal septum, eyes or mouth. Discard after 120 medicated sprays have been used (do not count initial priming sprays), even if bottle is not completely empty.

Monitoring Parameters Mucous membranes for signs of fungal infection, growth (pediatric patients), signs/symptoms of HPA axis suppression/adrenal insufficiency; ocular changes; possible eosinophilic conditions (including Churg-Strauss syndrome)

Additional Information When used short term as adjunctive therapy in acute bacterial rhinosinusitis (ABRS), intranasal steroids show modest symptomatic improvement and few adverse effects, improvement is primarily due to increased sinus drainage. Use should be considered optional in ABRS; however, intranasal corticosteroids should be routinely prescribed to ABRS patients who have a history of or concurrent allergic rhinitis (Chow, 2012).

Dosage Forms Excipient information presented when available (limited, particularly for generics); consult specific product labeling.

Suspension, intranasal [spray]:

Dymista: Azelastine hydrochloride 0.1% [137 mcg/spray] and fluticasone propionate 0.037% [50 mcg/spray] (23 g) [contains benzalkonium chloride; 120 metered sprays]

◆ **Azelastine Hydrochloride** *see* Azelastine (Nasal) *on page 239*

◆ **Azelastine Hydrochloride** *see* Azelastine (Ophthalmic) *on page 241*

◆ **Azelex** *see* Azelaic Acid *on page 238*

◆ **Azidothymidine** *see* Zidovudine *on page 2207*

◆ **Azidothymidine, Abacavir, and Lamivudine** *see* Abacavir, Lamivudine, and Zidovudine *on page 38*

Azithromycin (Systemic) (az ith roe MYE sin)

Medication Safety Issues

Sound-alike/look-alike issues:

Azithromycin may be confused with azathioprine, erythromycin

Zithromax may be confused with Fosamax, Zinacef, Zovirax

Related Information

Prevention of Infective Endocarditis *on page 2378*

Brand Names: US Zithromax; Zithromax Tri-Pak; Zithromax Z-Pak; Zmax

Brand Names: Canada ACT-Azithromycin; Apo-Azithromycin; Apo-Azithromycin Z; Azithromycin for Injection; Azithromycin for Injection, USP; Dom-Azithromycin; GD-Azithromycin; Mylan-Azithromycin; Novo-Azithromycin; PHL-Azithromycin; PMS-Azithromycin; PRO-Azithromycine; Riva-Azithromycin; Sandoz-Azithromycin; Zithromax; Zithromax For Intravenous Injection; Zmax SR

Therapeutic Category Antibiotic, Macrolide

Generic Availability (US) Yes

Use

Oral:

Immediate release; oral suspension, tablets: Treatment of acute otitis media due to *H. influenzae*, *M. catarrhalis*, or *S. pneumoniae* (FDA approved in pediatric patient ages ≥6 months); treatment of pharyngitis/tonsillitis due to *S. pyogenes* (FDA approved in ages ≥2 years and adults); treatment of community-acquired pneumonia due to susceptible organisms, including *C. pneumoniae*, *M. pneumoniae*, *H. influenzae*, *S. pneumoniae*

(FDA approved in ages ≥6 months and adults). [Oral azithromycin is not indicated for use in patients with pneumonia who have moderate to severe disease and judged to be inappropriate for oral therapy or have any risk factors such as cystic fibrosis, nosocomial infection, known or suspected bacteremia, hospitalization, elderly or debilitated patients, or patients with significant underlying health problems that may compromise their ability to respond to their illness (including immunodeficiency or functional asplenia)]; treatment of sinusitis or COPD exacerbation due to *H. influenzae, M. catarrhalis*, or *S. pneumoniae* (FDA approved in adults); treatment of infections of the skin and skin structure, acute pelvic inflammatory disease, chancroid, and urethritis and cervicitis due to susceptible strains of *C. trachomatis, N. gonorrhoeae, M. catarrhalis, H. influenzae, S. aureus, S. pyogenes, S. pneumoniae, Mycoplasma pneumoniae, M. avium* complex, *C. psittaci*, and *C. pneumoniae* (FDA approved in adults). Has also been used for treatment of babesiosis, pertussis, endocarditis prophylaxis in penicillin allergic patients, and cystic fibrosis lung disease

Extended release (Zmax); oral suspension: Treatment of community-acquired pneumonia due to *C. pneumoniae, M. pneumoniae, H. influenzae, S. pneumonia* (FDA approved in ages ≥6 months and adults); treatment of acute bacterial sinusitis due to *H. influenzae, M. catarrhalis, or S. pneumoniae* (FDA approved in adults)

Parenteral: Treatment of community-acquired pneumonia due to susceptible *C. pneumoniae, L. pneumophilia, M. pneumoniae, H. influenzae, S. aureus, S. pneumoniae*; treatment of pelvic inflammatory disease due to susceptible *C. pneumonia, N. gonorrhoeae*, or *M. hominis* (FDA approved in adults)

Pregnancy Risk Factor B

Pregnancy Considerations Adverse events were not observed in animal reproduction studies. Azithromycin crosses the placenta (Ramsey, 2003). The maternal serum half-life of azithromycin is unchanged in early pregnancy and decreased at term; however, high concentrations of azithromycin are sustained in the myometrium and adipose tissue (Fischer, 2012; Ramsey, 2003). Azithromycin is recommended for the treatment of several infections, including chlamydia, gonococcal infections, and *Mycobacterium avium* complex (MAC) in pregnant patients (consult current guidelines) (CDC, 2010; DHHS, 2013).

Breast-Feeding Considerations Azithromycin is excreted in low amounts into breast milk (Kelsey, 1994). Decreased appetite, diarrhea, rash, and somnolence have been reported in nursing infants exposed to macrolide antibiotics (Goldstein, 2009). The manufacturer recommends that caution be exercised when administering azithromycin to breast-feeding women.

Contraindications Hypersensitivity to azithromycin, other macrolide (eg, azalide or ketolide) antibiotics, or any component of the formulation; history of cholestatic jaundice/hepatic dysfunction associated with prior azithromycin use

Note: The manufacturer does not list concurrent use of pimozide as a contraindication; however, azithromycin is listed as a contraindication in the manufacturer's labeling for pimozide.

Warnings/Precautions Use with caution in patients with preexisting liver disease; hepatocellular and/or cholestatic hepatitis, with or without jaundice, hepatic necrosis, failure and death have occurred. Discontinue immediately if symptoms of hepatitis occur (malaise, nausea, vomiting, abdominal colic, fever). Allergic reactions have been reported (rare); reappearance of allergic reaction may occur shortly after discontinuation without further azithromycin exposure. May mask or delay symptoms of incubating gonorrhea or syphilis, so appropriate culture and susceptibility tests should be performed prior to initiating a treatment regimen. Prolonged use may result in fungal or bacterial superinfection, including *C. difficile*-associated diarrhea (CDAD); CDAD has been observed >2 months postantibiotic treatment. Use caution with renal dysfunction. Macrolides (especially erythromycin) have been associated with rare QTc prolongation and ventricular arrhythmias, including torsade de pointes; consider avoiding use in patients with prolonged QT interval, congenital long QT syndrome, history of torsade de pointes, bradyarrhythmias, uncorrected hypokalemia or hypomagnesemia, clinically significant bradycardia, uncompensated heart failure, or concurrent use of Class IA (eg, quinidine, procainamide) or Class III (eg, amiodarone, dofetilide, sotalol) antiarrhythmic agents or other drugs known to prolong the QT interval. Use with caution in patients with myasthenia gravis.

Oral suspensions (immediate release and extended release) are not interchangeable.

Adverse Reactions

Dermatologic: Pruritus, skin rash

Gastrointestinal: Abdominal pain, anorexia, diarrhea, nausea, stomach cramps, vomiting

Genitourinary: Vaginitis

Local: (with IV administration): Local inflammation, pain at injection site

Rare but important or life-threatening: Acute renal failure, ageusia, aggressive behavior, anaphylaxis, anemia, angioedema, anosmia, auditory disturbance, candidiasis, cardiac arrhythmia (including ventricular tachycardia), chest pain, cholestatic jaundice, conjunctivitis (pediatric patients), deafness, DRESS syndrome, eczema, edema, enteritis, erythema multiforme (rare), fungal dermatitis, fungal infection, gastritis, hearing loss, hepatic failure, hepatic necrosis, hepatitis, hepatotoxicity (idiosyncratic) (Chalasani, 2014), hyperactivity, hyperkinesia, hypotension, increased liver enzymes, insomnia, interstitial nephritis, jaundice, leukopenia, melena, mucositis, nephritis, neutropenia (mild), oral candidiasis, pancreatitis, pharyngitis, pleural effusion, prolonged Q-T interval on ECG (rare), pseudomembranous colitis, pyloric stenosis, seizure, skin photosensitivity, Stevens-Johnson syndrome (rare), syncope, taste perversion, thrombocytopenia, tongue discoloration (rare), torsades de pointes (rare), toxic epidermal necrolysis (rare), vesiculobullous rash

Drug Interactions

Metabolism/Transport Effects Substrate of CYP3A4 (minor); **Note:** Assignment of Major/Minor substrate status based on clinically relevant drug interaction potential; **Inhibits** CYP1A2 (weak), P-glycoprotein

Avoid Concomitant Use

Avoid concomitant use of Azithromycin (Systemic) with any of the following: Amiodarone; BCG; BCG (Intravesical); Bosutinib; Highest Risk QTc-Prolonging Agents; Ivabradine; Mifepristone; PAZOPanib; Pimozide; QuiNINE; Silodosin; Terfenadine; Topotecan; VinCRIStine (Liposomal)

Increased Effect/Toxicity

Azithromycin (Systemic) may increase the levels/effects of: Afatinib; Amiodarone; AtorvaSTATin; Bosutinib; Brentuximab Vedotin; Cardiac Glycosides; Colchicine; CycloSPORINE (Systemic); Dabigatran Etexilate; DOXOrubicin (Conventional); Edoxaban; Everolimus; Highest Risk QTc-Prolonging Agents; Ivermectin (Systemic); Ledipasvir; Lovastatin; Moderate Risk QTc-Prolonging Agents; Naloxegol; PAZOPanib; P-glycoprotein/ABCB1 Substrates; Pimozide; Prucalopride; QuiNINE; Rifaximin; Rilpivirine; Rivaroxaban; Silodosin; Simvastatin; Tacrolimus (Systemic); Tacrolimus (Topical); Terfenadine; TiZANidine; Topotecan; VinCRIStine (Liposomal); Vitamin K Antagonists

The levels/effects of Azithromycin (Systemic) may be increased by: Ivabradine; Mifepristone; Nelfinavir; QTc-Prolonging Agents (Indeterminate Risk and Risk Modifying)

Decreased Effect

Azithromycin (Systemic) may decrease the levels/effects of: BCG; BCG (Intravesical); BCG Vaccine (Immunization); Sodium Picosulfate; Typhoid Vaccine

Food Interactions Rate and extent of GI absorption may be altered depending upon the formulation. Azithromycin suspension, not tablet form, has significantly increased absorption (46%) with food. Management: Immediate release suspension and tablet may be taken without regard to food; extended release suspension should be taken on an empty stomach (at least 1 hour before or 2 hours following a meal).

Storage/Stability

Injection (Zithromax): Store intact vials of injection at room temperature. Reconstituted solution is stable for 24 hours when stored below 30°C (86°F). The diluted solution is stable for 24 hours at or below room temperature (30°C [86°F]) and for 7 days if stored under refrigeration (5°C [41°F]).

Suspension, immediate release (Zithromax): Store dry powder below 30°C (86°F). Store reconstituted suspension at 5°C to 30°C (41°F to 86°F) and use within 10 days.

Suspension, extended release (Zmax): Store dry powder ≤30°C (86°F). Following reconstitution, store at 25°C (77°F); excursions permitted to 15°C to 30°C (59°F to 86°F); do not refrigerate or freeze. Should be consumed within 12 hours following reconstitution.

Tablet (Zithromax): Store between 15°C to 30°C (59°F to 86°F).

Mechanism of Action Inhibits RNA-dependent protein synthesis at the chain elongation step; binds to the 50S ribosomal subunit resulting in blockage of transpeptidation

Pharmacokinetics (Adult data unless noted)

Absorption: Oral: Rapid from the GI tract

Distribution: Extensive tissue distribution into skin, lungs, tonsils, bone, prostate, cervix; CSF concentrations are low

V_d: 31-33 L/kg

Protein binding: 7% to 51% (concentration-dependent and dependent on $alpha_1$-acid glycoprotein concentrations)

Metabolism: Hepatic to inactive metabolites

Bioavailability: Tablet, immediate release oral suspension: 34% to 52%; extended release oral suspension: 28% to 43%

Half-life, terminal:

Infants and Children 4 months to 15 years: 54.5 hours

Adults: Immediate release: 68-72 hours; Extended release: 59 hours

Time to peak serum concentration: Oral:

Immediate release: 2-3 hours

Extended release oral suspension: 3-5 hours

Elimination: 50% of dose is excreted unchanged in bile; 6% to 14% of dose is excreted unchanged in urine

Dosing: Neonatal Note: Extended release suspension (Zmax) is not interchangeable with immediate-release formulations. All oral doses are expressed as immediate release azithromycin unless otherwise specified.

General dosing, susceptible infection (*Red Book* [AAP], 2012):

Oral: 10-20 mg/kg once daily

IV: 10 mg/kg once daily

Bronchopulmonary dysplasia, prevention: Limited data available: Oral, IV: 10 mg/kg once daily for 7 days, followed by 5 mg/kg once daily for 5 weeks was used in 19 mechanically ventilated premature neonates (mean GA: 25.6 weeks; PNA: <72 hours; birth weight ≤1000 g) and decreased corticosteroid use and duration of mechanical ventilation compared to placebo (Ballard, 2007)

Chlamydial conjunctivitis or chlamydial pneumonia: Oral, IV: 20 mg/kg once daily for 3 days (*Red Book* [AAP], 2012)

Pertussis, treatment and postexposure prophylaxis: Oral, IV: 10 mg/kg once daily for 5 days (*Red Book* [AAP], 2012)

Dosing: Usual Note: Extended release suspension (Zmax) is not interchangeable with immediate-release formulations. All doses are expressed as immediate release azithromycin unless otherwise specified.

Pediatric:

General dosing, susceptible infection (*Red Book* [AAP], 2012): Infants, Children, and Adolescents:

Mild to moderate infection: Oral: 5 to 12 mg/kg/dose; typically administered as 10 to 12 mg/kg/dose on day 1 followed by 5 to 6 mg/kg once daily for remainder of treatment duration; usual maximum dose for the total course: 1500 to 2000 mg

Serious infection: IV: 10 mg/kg once daily; maximum dose: 500 mg/dose

Babesiosis: Infants, Children, and Adolescents: Oral: 10 mg/kg once on day 1 (maximum dose: 500 mg/dose), then 5 mg/kg once daily on days 2 to 10 (maximum dose: 250 mg/dose) in combination with atovaquone; longer duration of therapy may be necessary in some cases; in immunocompromised patients, higher doses (eg, adults: 600 to 1000 mg daily) may be required (*Red Book*, 2012; Wormser, 2006)

Bartonellosis: Oral:

Cat scratch disease (*B. henselae*) with extensive lymphadenopathy (IDSA [Stevens], 2014): *Non-HIV-exposed/-positive:*

Infants, Children, and Adolescents ≤45 kg: 10 mg/kg once on day 1 (maximum dose: 500 mg/dose), followed by 5 mg/kg once daily on days 2 to 5 (maximum dose: 250 mg/dose)

Children and Adolescents >45 kg: 500 mg as a single dose on day 1, then 250 mg once daily for 4 additional days

Cutaneous bacillary angiomatosis (*B. henselae* or *B. quintana*): *HIV- exposed/-positive:* Infants, Children, and Adolescents: 5 to 12 mg/kg once daily; maximum dose: 600 mg/dose; usual treatment duration: 3 months (CDC, 2009)

Chancroid (CDC, 2010; *Red Book*, 2012): Oral:

<45 kg: 20 mg/kg as a single dose; maximum dose: 1000 mg/dose

≥45 kg: 1000 mg as a single dose

Chlamydial infections:

Cervicitis, urethritis (*C. trachomatis*): Children and Adolescents ≥45 kg: Oral: 1000 mg as a single dose (CDC, 2010; *Red Book* [AAP], 2012)

Conjunctivitis: Infants: Oral, IV: 20 mg/kg once daily for 3 days (*Red Book* [AAP], 2012)

Pneumonia, community-acquired (Bradley, 2011): Infants >3 months, Children, and Adolescents:

Mild infection or step-down therapy: Oral: 10 mg/kg once on day 1 (maximum dose: 500 mg/dose) followed by 5 mg/kg once daily on days 2-5 (maximum dose: 250 mg/dose)

Severe infection: IV: 10 mg/ kg once daily for at least 2 days, then transition to oral route with a single daily dose of 5 mg/kg to complete course of therapy; maximum dose: 500 mg/dose

Cystic fibrosis; improve lung function, reduce exacerbation frequency: Limited data available; dosing regimen variable (Mogayzel, 2013; Saiman, 2003; Saiman; 2010): Children ≥6 years and Adolescents: Oral: 18 to 35.9 kg: 250 mg three times weekly (Monday, Wednesday, Friday)

≥36 kg: 500 mg three times weekly (Monday, Wednesday, Friday)

Diarrhea, infectious:

Campylobacter: Infants, Children, and Adolescents: Oral: 10 mg/kg once daily for 3 days; maximum dose: 500 mg/dose (*Red Book* [AAP], 2012)

Shigellosis: Infants, Children, and Adolescents: Oral:

AAP Recommendation: 12 mg/kg once on day 1 (maximum dose: 500 mg/dose), followed by 6 mg/kg once daily on days 2 to 5 (maximum dose: 250 mg/dose) (*Red Book* [AAP], 2012)

Alternate dosing: 10 mg/kg once daily for 3 days (Dupont, 2009; Mackell, 2005); WHO Guidelines recommend up to 20 mg/kg/dose and in some cases, a wider range of duration of therapy (eg, 1 to 5 days) (WHO, 2005)

Endocarditis; prophylaxis: Infants, Children, and Adolescents: Oral: 15 mg/kg/dose 30 to 60 minutes before procedure; maximum dose: 500 mg/dose (Wilson, 2007)

Gonococcal infection; uncomplicated (cervicitis, urethritis, anorectal): Oral:

Children <45 kg: 20 mg/kg as a single dose; maximum dose: 1000 mg/dose (*Red Book* [AAP], 2012)

Children > 8 years and ≥45 kg and Adolescents: 1000 mg as a single dose (CDC, 2012; *Red Book* [AAP], 2012)

Group A streptococcal infection; treatment of streptococcal tonsillopharyngitis:

Manufacturer's labeling and AHA/AAP recommendations: Infants, Children, and Adolescents: Oral: 12 mg/kg/dose once daily for 5 days; maximum dose: 500 mg/dose (Gerber, 2009; *Red Book* [AAP], 2012)

Alternate dosing:

IDSA reconmendations: **Note:** Recommended as an alternative agent for group A streptococcal pharyngitis in penicillin-allergic patients. Infants, Children, and Adolescents: Oral: 12 mg/kg (maximum: 500 mg/dose) on day 1 followed by 6 mg/kg/dose (maximum: 250 mg/dose) once daily on days 2 through 5 (Shulman, 2012); Recommended by the Infectious Disease Society of America (IDSA) as an alternative agent for group A streptococcal pharyngitis in penicillin-allergic patients (Shulman, 2012).

Three-day regimen: Limited data available: Children and Adolescents: Oral: 20 mg/kg/dose once daily for 3 days; maximum dose: 1000 mg/dose (Cohen, 2004; O'Doherty, 1996)

Meningococcal disease, chemoprophylaxis of high-risk contacts: Infants, Children, and Adolescents: Oral: 10 mg/kg as a single dose; maximum dose: 500 mg/dose; **Note:** Not routinely recommended; may consider if fluoroquinolone resistance detected (*Red Book* [AAP], 2012)

***Mycobacterium avium* complex (MAC) infection:**

HIV-exposed/-positive:

Infants and Children (DHHS [pediatric], 2013): Oral:

Treatment: 10 to 12 mg/kg once daily in combination with ethambutol, with or without rifabutin; maximum dose: 500 mg/dose; treatment duration at least 12 months; dependent upon clinical response

Primary prevention of first episode: Preferred: 20 mg/kg once **weekly** (maximum dose: 1200 mg/dose) **or** alternatively, 5 mg/kg once daily (maximum dose: 250 mg/dose)

Secondary prevention of recurring episodes: 5 mg/kg once daily in combination with ethambutol, with or without rifabutin; maximum dose: 250 mg/dose

Adolescents (DHHS [adult], 2013): Oral:

Treatment: 500 to 600 mg daily in combination with ethambutol

Primary prophylaxis: 1200 mg once weekly **or** alternatively, 600 mg twice weekly

Secondary prophylaxis: 500 to 600 mg daily in combination with ethambutol

Non-HIV-exposed/-positive (Bradley, 2011): Infants >3 months, Children, and Adolescents:

Mild infection or step-down therapy: Oral: 10 mg/kg once on day 1 (maximum dose: 500 mg/dose) followed by 5 mg/kg once daily on days 2 to 5 (maximum dose: 250 mg/dose)

Severe infection: IV: 10 mg/kg once daily for at least 2 days (maximum dose: 500 mg/dose), then transition to oral route with a single daily dose of 5 mg/kg to complete course of therapy (maximum dose: 250 mg/dose)

Otitis media, acute (AOM): Infants ≥6 months, Children, and Adolescents: Oral: **Note:** Due to increased *S pneumonia* and *H. influenzae* resistance, azithromycin is not routinely recommended as a treatment option (AAP, [Lieberthal, 2013])

Single dose regimen: 30 mg/kg as a single dose; maximum dose: 1500 mg/dose; if patient vomits within 30 minutes of dose, repeat dosing has been administered although limited data available on safety

Three-day regimen: 10 mg/kg once daily for 3 days; maximum dose: 500 mg/dose

Five-day regimen: 10 mg/kg once on day 1 (maximum dose: 500 mg/dose), followed by 5 mg/kg (maximum dose: 250 mg/dose) once daily on days 2 to 5

Peritonitis, prophylaxis for patients receiving peritoneal dialysis who require dental procedures: Infants, Children, and Adolescents: Oral: 15 mg/kg administered 30 to 60 minutes before dental procedure; maximum dose: 500 mg/dose (Warady, 2012)

Pertussis (CDC, 2005, *Red Book* [AAP], 2012): Oral, IV:

Infants 1 to 5 months: 10 mg/kg/dose once daily for 5 days

Infants ≥6 months, Children, and Adolescents: 10 mg/kg once on day 1 (maximum dose: 500 mg/dose), followed by 5 mg/kg once daily on days 2 to 5 (maximum dose: 250 mg/dose)

Pneumonia, community-acquired (excluding mycobacterial and chlamydial):

Oral:

Immediate release: Infants >3 months, Children, and Adolescents: 10 mg/kg once on day 1 (maximum dose: 500 mg/dose), followed by 5 mg/kg (maximum dose: 250 mg/dose) once daily on days 2 to 5 (Bradley, 2011)

Extended release oral suspension (Zmax): Infants ≥6 months, Children, and Adolescents: 60 mg/kg as a single dose; maximum dose: 2000 mg/dose

IV: Infants >3 months, Children, and Adolescents: 10 mg/kg once daily for at least 2 days, follow IV therapy by the oral route with a single daily dose of 5 mg/kg to complete a 5-day course of therapy; maximum dose: 500 mg/dose (Bradley, 2011)

Rhinosinusitis, bacterial: Oral: Infants ≥6 months, Children, and Adolescents: 10 mg/kg once daily for 3 days; maximum dose: 500 mg/dose; **Note:** Although FDA approved, macrolides are not recommended for empiric therapy due to high rates of resistance (Chow, 2012).

Sexual victimization, prophylaxis: Oral: **Note:** Use in combination with cefixime or ceftriaxone and completion of hepatitis B virus immunization; also consider prophylaxis for trichomoniasis and bacterial vaginosis (CDC, 2010; *Red Book* [AAP], 2012).

Children <45 kg: 20 mg/kg as a single dose

Children ≥45 kg and Adolescents: 1000 mg as a single dose

***Toxoplasma gondii*, encephalitis (HIV-exposed/-positive); treatment and prevention:** Oral: Adolescents: 900 to 1200 mg once daily in combination with pyrimethamine/leucovorin; treatment duration: 6 weeks or longer if extensive disease or incomplete response at 6 weeks (DHHS [adult], 2013)

Adult:

Rhinosinusitis, bacterial: Oral: 500 mg once daily for 3 days. **Note:** Although FDA approved, macrolides are not recommended for empiric therapy due to high rates of resistance (Chow, 2012).

Alternate regimen: Extended release suspension (Zmax): 2000 mg as a single dose

Chancroid due to *H. ducreyi*: Oral: 1000 mg as a single dose (CDC, 2010)

Cervicitis, urethritis: Nongonococcal *Chlamydia trachomatis*: Oral: 1000 mg as a single dose

Gonococcal infection, uncomplicated (cervix, rectum, urethra): Oral: 1000 mg as a single dose in combination with ceftriaxone (preferred) or cefixime (only if ceftriaxone unavailable); if cefixime is used, test-of-cure in 7 days is recommended (CDC, 2012). **Note:** Monotherapy with azithromycin single dose of 2000 mg has been associated with resistance and/or treatment failure; however, may be appropriate for treatment of a gonococcal infection in pregnant women who cannot tolerate a cephalosporin (CDC, 2010).

Patients with severe cephalosporin allergy: 2000 mg as a single dose and test-of-cure in 7 days (CDC, 2012)

Gonococcal infection, uncomplicated (pharynx): Oral: 1000 mg as a single dose in combination with ceftriaxone (CDC, 2012)

Gonococcal infection, expedited partner therapy: Oral: 1000 mg as a single dose in combination with cefixime (CDC, 2012). **Note:** Only used if a heterosexual partner cannot be linked to evaluation and treatment in a timely manner; dose delivered to partner by patient, collaborating pharmacy, or disease investigation specialist.

Granuloma inguinale (donovanosis): Oral: 1000 mg once a week for at least 3 weeks and until lesions have healed (CDC, 2010)

Endocarditis prophylaxis: Oral: 500 mg 30-60 minutes before procedure. **Note:** American Heart Association (AHA) guidelines now recommend prophylaxis only in patients undergoing invasive procedures and in whom underlying cardiac conditions may predispose to a higher risk of adverse outcomes should infection occur. As of April 2007, routine prophylaxis for GI/GU procedures is no longer recommended by the AHA (Wilson, 2007).

Mild to moderate respiratory tract, skin, and soft tissue infections: Oral: 500 mg in a single loading dose on day 1 followed by 250 mg daily as a single dose on days 2-5

Alternative regimen: Bacterial exacerbation of COPD: 500 mg daily for a total of 3 days

***Mycobacterium avium* complex disease, disseminated, in patients with advanced HIV infection:** Oral:

Treatment: 600 mg daily in combination with ethambutol

Primary prophylaxis: 1200 mg once weekly (preferred), with **or** without rifabutin or alternatively, 600 mg twice weekly (DHHS [adult], 2013)

Secondary prophylaxis: 500 to 600 mg daily in combination with ethambutol (DHHS [adult], 2013)

Pelvic inflammatory disease: IV: 500 mg as a single dose for 1 to 2 days, follow IV therapy by the oral route with a single daily dose of 250 mg to complete a 7-day course of therapy

Pharyngitis/tonsillitis, group A streptococci:

Manufacturer labeling: Oral: 500 mg on day 1 followed by 250 mg once daily on days 2 to 5

IDSA guidelines: Oral: 12 mg/kg (maximum: 500 mg) on day 1 followed by 6 mg/kg/dose (maximum: 250 mg) once daily days 2 to 5. **Note:** Recommended by the Infectious Disease Society of America (IDSA) as an alternative agent for group A streptococcal pharyngitis in penicillin-allergic patients (Shulman, 2012).

Pneumonia, community-acquired:

Oral: 500 mg on day 1 followed by 250 mg once daily on days 2 to 5

Alternate regimen: Extended release suspension (Zmax): 2000 mg as a single dose

IV: 500 mg as a single dose for at least 2 days; follow IV therapy by the oral route with a single daily dose of 500 mg to complete a 7- to 10-day course of therapy

Pertussis: Oral: 500 mg on day 1 followed by 250 mg once daily on days 2 to 5 (CDC, 2005)

Prophylaxis against sexually transmitted diseases following sexual assault: Oral: 1000 mg as a single dose (in combination with a cephalosporin and metronidazole) (CDC, 2010)

Dosing adjustment in renal impairment: Infants ≥6 months, Children, Adolescents, and Adults:

Use with caution in patients with GFR <10 mL/minute (AUC increased by 35% compared to patients with normal renal function); however, no dosage adjustment is provided in the manufacturer's labeling.

No supplemental dose or dosage adjustment necessary, including patients on intermittent hemodialysis, peritoneal dialysis, or continuous renal replacement therapy (eg, CVVHD) (Aronoff, 2007; Heintz, 2009).

Dosing adjustment in hepatic impairment: Azithromycin is predominantly hepatically eliminated; however, there is no dosage adjustment provided in the manufacturer's labeling. Use with caution due to potential for hepatotoxicity (rare); discontinue immediately for signs or symptoms of hepatitis.

Preparation for Administration

Oral:

Immediate release oral suspension: Reconstitute powder for oral suspension with appropriate amount of water as specified on the bottle. Shake vigorously until suspended.

Oral suspension 1,000 mg packet for a single dose: Prepare by mixing contents of 1 packet with approximately 60 mL of water.

Extended release oral suspension: Prepare 2,000 mg azithromycin suspension by reconstituting with 60 mL of water to a final concentration of 27 mg/mL

Parenteral: Prepare initial solution by adding 4.8 mL of SWFI to the 500 mg vial resulting in a concentration of 100 mg/mL. Use of a standard syringe is recommended due to the vacuum in the vial (which may draw additional solution through an automated syringe).

The initial solution should be further diluted to a concentration of 1 mg/mL to 2 mg/mL in NS, D_5W, or LR.

Administration

Oral:

Immediate release: May administer without regard to food; do not administer with antacids that contain aluminum or magnesium.

Oral suspension, multiple doses: Shake well before use.

Oral suspension 1,000 mg packet for a single dose: Administer the entire contents immediately after mixing; add an additional 60 mL of water, mix, and drink. Do not use to administer any other dose except 1,000 mg or 2,000 mg.

Extended release oral suspension: Shake suspension well before use; administer on an empty stomach 1 hour before or 2 hours after a meal; must be administered within 12 hours of reconstitution. May be administered without regard to antacids containing aluminum or magnesium.

Parenteral: **Do not give IM or by direct IV injection.** Administer IV infusion at a final concentration of 1 mg/mL over 3 hours; for a 2 mg/mL concentration, infuse over 1 hour; do not infuse over a period of less than 60 minutes.

Monitoring Parameters Liver function tests, WBC with differential; number and type of stools/day for diarrhea; monitor patients receiving azithromycin and drugs known to interact with erythromycin (ie, theophylline, digoxin, anticoagulants, triazolam) since there are still very few studies examining drug-drug interactions with azithromycin. When used as part of alternative treatment for gonococcal infection, test-of-cure 7 days after dose (CDC, 2012).

Dosage Forms Excipient information presented when available (limited, particularly for generics); consult specific product labeling.

Packet, Oral:
- Zithromax: 1 g (3 ea, 10 ea) [cherry-banana flavor]
- Generic: 1 g (3 ea, 10 ea)

Solution Reconstituted, Intravenous:
- Zithromax: 500 mg (1 ea)
- Generic: 500 mg (1 ea); 2.5 g (1 ea)

Solution Reconstituted, Intravenous [preservative free]:
- Generic: 500 mg (1 ea)

Suspension Reconstituted, Oral:
- Zithromax: 100 mg/5 mL (15 mL) [cherry-vanilla-banana flavor]
- Zithromax: 200 mg/5 mL (15 mL, 22.5 mL, 30 mL) [cherry flavor]
- Zmax: 2 g (1 ea) [cherry-banana flavor]
- Generic: 100 mg/5 mL (15 mL); 200 mg/5 mL (15 mL, 22.5 mL, 30 mL)

Tablet, Oral:
- Zithromax: 250 mg, 500 mg, 600 mg
- Zithromax Tri-Pak: 500 mg
- Zithromax Z-Pak: 250 mg
- Generic: 250 mg, 500 mg, 600 mg

Azithromycin (Ophthalmic) (az ith roe MYE sin)

Medication Safety Issues

Sound-alike/look-alike issues:

Azithromycin may be confused with azathioprine, erythromycin

Brand Names: US AzaSite

Therapeutic Category Antibiotic, Ophthalmic

Generic Availability (US) No

Use Treatment of bacterial conjunctivitis due to susceptible CDC coryneform group G, *H. influenzae*, *S. aureus*, *S. mitis* group, or *S. pneumoniae* (FDA approved in ages ≥1 year and adults); has also been used for *Ophthalmia neonatorum* prophylaxis

Pregnancy Risk Factor B

Pregnancy Considerations Adverse events were not observed in animal reproduction studies. The amount of azithromycin available systemically following topical application of the ophthalmic drops is estimated to be below quantifiable limits. Systemic absorption would be required in order for azithromycin to cross the placenta and reach the fetus. When administered orally or IV, azithromycin crosses the placenta. Refer to the Azithromycin (Systemic) monograph for details.

Breast-Feeding Considerations It is not known if azithromycin is excreted into breast milk following ophthalmic administration. The amount of azithromycin available systemically following topical application of the ophthalmic drops is estimated to be below quantifiable limits. Systemic absorption would be required in order for azithromycin to enter breast milk. The manufacturer recommends that caution be exercised when administering azithromycin eye drops to nursing women. When administered orally or IV, azithromycin enters breast milk. Refer to the Azithromycin (Systemic) monograph for details.

Contraindications Hypersensitivity to azithromycin or any component of the formulation

Warnings/Precautions For topical ophthalmic use only; do not inject subconjunctivally or introduce directly into the anterior chamber of the eye. Severe hypersensitivity reactions, including anaphylaxis, angioedema, and dermatologic reactions, have been reported with systemic use of azithromycin. Prolonged use may lead to overgrowth of nonsusceptible organisms, including fungi. Discontinue use and institute alternative therapy if superinfection is suspected. Contains benzalkonium chloride which may be absorbed by contact lenses; contact lens should not be worn during treatment.

Adverse Reactions

Ocular: Eye irritation

Rare but important or life-threatening: Abnormal taste, blurred vision, contact dermatitis, corneal erosion, dry eyes, eye pain, facial edema, hives, nasal congestion, ocular reactions (burning, discharge, irritation, itching, stinging), periocular swelling, punctate keratitis, rash, sinusitis, urticaria, visual acuity decreased

Drug Interactions

Metabolism/Transport Effects None known.

Avoid Concomitant Use There are no known interactions where it is recommended to avoid concomitant use.

Increased Effect/Toxicity There are no known significant interactions involving an increase in effect.

Decreased Effect There are no known significant interactions involving a decrease in effect.

Storage/Stability Prior to use, store unopened under refrigeration at 2°C to 8°C (36°F to 46°F). After opening, store at 2°C to 25°C (36°F to 77°F) for ≤14 days; discard any remaining solution after 14 days.

Mechanism of Action Inhibits RNA-dependent protein synthesis at the chain elongation step; binds to the 50S ribosomal subunit resulting in blockage of transpeptidation

Dosing: Neonatal Gonococcal ophthalmia or chlamydial ophthalmia, prophylaxis (*Ophthalmia neonatorum*): Limited data available: 1-2 drops in each conjunctival sac; efficacy studies are lacking; however, may consider use during shortages of erythromycin ophthalmic ointment (CDC, 2006)

Dosing: Usual Bacterial conjunctivitis: Children ≥1 year and Adults: Instill 1 drop in the affected eye(s) twice daily (8-12 hours apart) for 2 days, then 1 drop once daily for 5 days.

Administration For topical ophthalmic use only. Avoid contacting tip with skin or eye. Invert closed bottle and shake once before each use. Remove cap with bottle inverted. Tilt head back and gently squeeze inverted bottle to instill drop.

Dosage Forms Excipient information presented when available (limited, particularly for generics); consult specific product labeling.

Solution, Ophthalmic:
- AzaSite: 1% (2.5 mL) [contains benzalkonium chloride, disodium edta]

- ◆ **Azithromycin Dihydrate** *see* Azithromycin (Systemic) *on page 242*
- ◆ **Azithromycin for Injection (Can)** *see* Azithromycin (Systemic) *on page 242*
- ◆ **Azithromycin for Injection, USP (Can)** *see* Azithromycin (Systemic) *on page 242*
- ◆ **Azithromycin Monohydrate** *see* Azithromycin (Systemic) *on page 242*
- ◆ **Azo-Gesic [OTC]** *see* Phenazopyridine *on page 1678*
- ◆ **Azolen Tincture [OTC]** *see* Miconazole (Topical) *on page 1431*

Aztreonam (AZ tree oh nam)

Medication Safety Issues

Sound-alike/look-alike issues:

Aztreonam may be confused with azidothymidine

Brand Names: US Azactam; Azactam in Dextrose; Cayston

Brand Names: Canada Cayston

Therapeutic Category Antibiotic, Miscellaneous

Generic Availability (US) May be product dependent

Use

Injection: Treatment of patients with documented multidrug resistant aerobic gram-negative infection in which beta-lactam therapy is contraindicated; used for UTI, lower respiratory tract infections, intra-abdominal infections, and gynecological infections caused by susceptible organisms (FDA approved in ages ≥9 months and adults); treatment of susceptible skin and skin-structure infections and septicemia (FDA approved in adults)

Inhalation (nebulized, Cayston®): Improve respiratory symptoms in cystic fibrosis patients with *Pseudomonas aeruginosa* in the lungs (FDA approved in ages ≥7 years and adults)

Prescribing and Access Restrictions Cayston (aztreonam inhalation solution) is only available through a select group of specialty pharmacies and cannot be obtained through a retail pharmacy. Because Cayston® may only be used with the Altera Nebulizer System, it can only be obtained from the following specialty pharmacies: Cystic Fibrosis Services, Inc; IV Solutions; Foundation Care; and Pharmaceutical Specialties, Inc. This network of specialty pharmacies ensures proper access to both the drug and device. To obtain the medication and proper nebulizer, contact the Cayston Access Program at 1-877-7CAYSTON (1-877-722-9786) or at www.cayston.com.

Pregnancy Risk Factor B

Pregnancy Considerations Adverse events have not been observed in animal reproduction studies; therefore, the manufacturer classifies aztreonam as pregnancy category B. Aztreonam crosses the placenta and enters cord blood during middle and late pregnancy. Distribution to the fetus is minimal in early pregnancy. The amount of aztreonam available systemically following inhalation is significantly less in comparison to doses given by injection.

Breast-Feeding Considerations Very small amounts of aztreonam are excreted in breast milk. The poor oral absorption of aztreonam (<1%) may limit adverse effects to the infant. Nondose-related effects could include modification of bowel flora. Maternal use of aztreonam inhalation is not likely to pose a risk to breast-feeding infants.

Contraindications Hypersensitivity to aztreonam or any component of the formulation

Warnings/Precautions Rare cross-allergenicity to penicillins, cephalosporins, or carbapenems may occur; use with caution in patients with a history of hypersensitivity to beta-lactams. Use caution in renal impairment; dosing adjustment required for the injectable formulation. Prolonged use may result in fungal or bacterial superinfection, including *C. difficile*-associated diarrhea (CDAD) and pseudomembranous colitis; CDAD has been observed >2 months postantibiotic treatment. Use with caution in bone marrow transplant patients with multiple risk factors for toxic epidermal necrolysis (TEN) (eg, sepsis, radiation therapy, drugs known to cause TEN); rare cases of TEN in this population have been reported. Patients colonized with *Burkholderia cepacia* have not been studied. Potentially significant interactions may exist, requiring dose or frequency adjustment, additional monitoring, and/or selection of alternative therapy. Safety and efficacy has not been established in patients with FEV_1 <25% or >75% predicted. To reduce the development of resistant bacteria and maintain efficacy reserve use for CF patients with known *Pseudomonas aeruginosa*. Bronchospasm may occur occur following nebulization; administer a bronchodilator prior to treatment.

Adverse Reactions

Inhalation:

Cardiovascular: Chest discomfort

Dermatologic: Skin rash

Gastrointestinal: Abdominal pain, sore throat, vomiting

Respiratory: Bronchospasm, cough, nasal congestion, wheezing

Miscellaneous: Fever (more common in children)

Rare but important or life-threatening: Arthralgia, facial edema, hypersensitivity reaction, joint swelling, tightness in chest and throat

Injection:

Dermatologic: Rash (more common in children)

Gastrointestinal: Diarrhea, nausea, vomiting

Hematologic & oncologic: Eosinophilia (more common in children), neutropenia (more common in children), thrombocythemia (more common in children)

Hepatic: Increased serum transaminases (ALT/AST; children)

Local: Inflammation at injection site, injection site reaction (erythema, induration; more common in children), pain at injection site (more common in children)

Renal: Increased serum creatinine (children)

Miscellaneous: Fever

Rare but important or life-threatening: Anaphylaxis, anemia, angioedema, aphthous stomatitis, *Clostridium difficile* associated diarrhea, erythema multiforme, exfoliative dermatitis, gastrointestinal hemorrhage, hepatitis, leukocytosis, leukopenia, oral mucosa ulcer, pancytopenia, positive direct Coombs test, prolonged partial thromboplastin time, prolonged prothrombin time, pseudomembranous colitis, seizure, thrombocytopenia, toxic epidermal necrolysis, vaginitis, ventricular bigeminy (transient), ventricular premature contractions (transient), vulvovaginal candidiasis

Drug Interactions

Metabolism/Transport Effects None known.

Avoid Concomitant Use

Avoid concomitant use of Aztreonam with any of the following: BCG; BCG (Intravesical)

Increased Effect/Toxicity There are no known significant interactions involving an increase in effect.

Decreased Effect

Aztreonam may decrease the levels/effects of: BCG; BCG (Intravesical); BCG Vaccine (Immunization); Sodium Picosulfate; Typhoid Vaccine

Storage/Stability

Inhalation: Prior to reconstitution, store at 2°C to 8°C (36°F to 46°F). Once removed from refrigeration, aztreonam and the diluent may be stored at room temperature (up to 25°C [77°F]) for ≤28 days. Protect from light. Use immediately after reconstitution.

Vials: Prior to reconstitution, store at room temperature; avoid excessive heat. After reconstitution, solutions for infusion with a final concentration of ≤20 mg/mL should be used within 48 hours if stored at room temperature or within 7 days if refrigerated. Solutions for infusion with a final concentration of >20 mg/mL (if prepared with SWFI or NS **only**) should also be used within 48 hours if stored at room temperature or within 7 days if refrigerated; all other solutions for infusion with a final concentration >20 mg/mL must be used immediately after preparation (unless prepared with SWFI or NS).

Premixed frozen containers: Store unused container frozen at ≤-20°C (-4°F). Frozen container can be thawed at room temperature of 25°C (77°F) or in a refrigerator, 2°C to 8°C (36°F to 46°F). Thawed solution should be used within 48 hours if stored at room temperature or within 14 days if stored under refrigeration. **Do not freeze.**

Mechanism of Action Inhibits bacterial cell wall synthesis by binding to one or more of the penicillin-binding proteins (PBPs) which in turn inhibits the final transpeptidation step of peptidoglycan synthesis in bacterial cell walls, thus inhibiting cell wall biosynthesis. Bacteria eventually lyse due to ongoing activity of cell wall autolytic enzymes (autolysins and murein hydrolases) while cell wall assembly is arrested. Monobactam structure makes cross-allergenicity with beta-lactams unlikely.

Pharmacokinetics (Adult data unless noted)

Absorption: IM: Well absorbed; Oral inhalation: Poorly absorbed

Distribution: Injection: Widely distributed into body tissues, cerebrospinal fluid, bronchial secretions, peritoneal fluid, bile, and bone

V_d:

Neonates: 0.26-0.36 L/kg

Children: 0.2-0.29 L/kg

Adults: 0.2 L/kg

Protein binding: 56%

Half-life: Injection:

Neonates:

<7 days, ≤2.5 kg: 5.5-9.9 hours

<7 days, >2.5 kg: 2.6 hours

1 week to 1 month: 2.4 hours

Children 2 months to 12 years: 1.7 hours

Children with cystic fibrosis: 1.3 hours

Adults: 1.3-2.2 hours (half-life prolonged in renal failure)

Time to peak serum concentration: Within 60 minutes after an IM dose

Elimination:

Injection: 60% to 70% excreted unchanged in the urine by active tubular secretion and glomerular filtration; 12% excreted in feces

Inhalation: Urine (10% of the total dose)

Dialysis: Moderately dialyzable

Hemodialysis: 27% to 58% in 4 hours

Peritoneal dialysis: 10% with a 6-hour dwell time

Dosing: Neonatal General dosing, susceptible infection: IM, IV (*Red Book*, 2012):

Body weight <1 kg:

PNA ≤14 days: 30 mg/kg/dose every 12 hours

PNA 15-28 days: 30 mg/kg/dose every 8-12 hours

Body weight 1-2 kg:

PNA ≤7 days: 30 mg/kg/dose every 12 hours

PNA 8-28 days: 30 mg/kg/dose every 8-12 hours

Body weight >2 kg:

PNA ≤7 days: 30 mg/kg/dose every 8 hours

PNA 8-28 days: 30 mg/kg/dose every 6 hours

Dosing: Usual

Infants, Children, and Adolescents:

General dosing, susceptible infection: IM, IV (*Red Book*, 2012):

Mild to moderate infection: 30 mg/kg every 8 hours; maximum daily dose: 3000 mg/**day**

Severe infection: 30 mg/kg every 6-8 hours; maximum daily dose: 8 g/**day**

Cystic fibrosis *(Pseudomonas aeruginosa)*:

Inhalation (nebulizer): Children ≥7 years and Adolescents: 75 mg via nebulization 3 times daily (at least 4 hours apart) for 28 days; administer in repeated cycles of 28 days on drug, followed by 28 days off drug

IV: 150-200 mg/kg/day in divided doses every 6-8 hours; higher doses have been used: 200-300 mg/kg/day divided every 6 hours; maximum daily dose: 12 **g/day** (Zobell, 2012)

Intra-abdominal infections, complicated: IV: 90-120 mg/kg/day divided every 6-8 hours; maximum dose: 2000 mg (Solomkin, 2010)

Peritonitis (CAPD): Intraperitoneal: Continuous: Loading dose: 1000 mg per liter of dialysate; maintenance dose: 250 mg per liter (Warady, 2000)

Surgical prophylaxis: Children and Adolescents: IV: 30 mg/kg as a single dose; may repeat in 4 hours; maximum dose: 2000 mg (Bratzler, 2013)

Adults:

General dosing, susceptible infection:

Moderately severe systemic infections:

IM: 1000 mg every 8-12 hours

IV: 1000-2000 mg every 8-12 hours

Severe systemic or life-threatening infections (especially if caused by *Pseudomonas aeruginosa*): IV: 2000 mg every 6-8 hours; maximum daily dose: 8 **g/day**

Cystic fibrosis *(Pseudomonas aeruginosa)*: Inhalation (nebulizer): 75 mg via nebulization 3 times daily (at least 4 hours apart) for 28 days; administer in repeated cycles of 28 days on drug, followed by 28 days off drug

Meningitis (gram-negative): IV: 2000 mg every 6-8 hours

Urinary tract infection: IM, IV: 500-1000 mg every 8-12 hours

Dosing adjustment in renal impairment:

Infants, Children, and Adolescents: IM, IV: The following adjustments have been recommended (Aronoff, 2007). **Note:** Renally adjusted dose recommendations are based on doses of 90-120 mg/kg/**day** divided every 8 hours.

GFR ≥30 mL/minute/1.73 m^2: No adjustment required

GFR 10-29 mL/minute/1.73 m^2: 15-20 mg/kg every 8 hours

GFR <10 mL/minute/1.73 m^2: 7.5-10 mg/kg every 12 hours

Intermittent hemodialysis: 7.5-10 mg/kg every 12 hours

Peritoneal dialysis (PD): 7.5-10 mg/kg every 12 hours

Continuous renal replacement therapy (CRRT): No adjustment required.

Inhalation (nebulized): No adjustment required.

Adults:

IM, IV:

CrCl 10-30 mL/minute: Give 50% of the usual dose at the usual interval

CrCl <10 mL/minute: Give a full first dose, then give 25% of the dose at the usual interval

Hemodialysis: Give a full first dose, then give 25% of the dose at the usual interval; for serious infections give 12.5% of the initial dose after each dialysis session. Alternatively, may administer 500 mg every 12 hours (Heintz, 2009). **Note:** Dosing dependent on the assumption of 3 times weekly, complete IHD sessions.

Peritoneal dialysis: Give a full first dose, then give 25% of the dose at the usual interval

Continuous renal replacement therapy (CRRT) (Heintz, 2009; Trotman, 2005): Drug clearance is highly dependent on the method of renal replacement, filter type, and flow rate. Appropriate dosing requires close monitoring of pharmacologic response, signs of adverse reactions due to drug accumulation, as well as drug concentrations in relation to target trough (if appropriate). The following are general recommendations only (based on dialysate flow/ultrafiltration rates of 1-2 L/hour and minimal residual renal function) and should not supersede clinical judgment:

CVVH: Loading dose of 2000 mg followed by 1000-2000 mg every 12 hours

CVVHD/CVVHDF: Loading dose of 2000 mg followed by either 1000 mg every 8 hours **or** 2000 mg every 12 hours (Heintz, 2009)

Inhalation (nebulized): No adjustment required.

Dosing adjustment in hepatic impairment: There are no dosage adjustments provided in the manufacturer's labeling; however, minor hepatic elimination of aztreonam does occur. Use with caution in patients with impaired hepatic function; appropriate monitoring is recommended.

Preparation for Administration

Parenteral:

IM: Reconstitute vial with at least 3 mL SWFI, sterile bacteriostatic water for injection, NS, or bacteriostatic sodium chloride per gram of aztreonam to a final concentration of ≤333 mg/mL; immediately shake vigorously. Do **not** mix with any local anesthetic agent.

IV:

Bolus injection: Reconstitute vial with 6 to 10 mL SWFI; immediately shake vigorously; maximum concentration of 66 mg/mL.

Infusion: Reconstitute vial with at least 3 mL SWFI per gram of aztreonam; immediately shake vigorously. Reconstituted solutions are colorless to light yellow straw and may turn pink upon standing without affecting potency. Further dilute in an appropriate solution for infusion to a final concentration not to exceed 20 mg/mL.

Inhalation: Reconstitute immediately prior to use. Squeeze diluent into opened glass vial of Cayston. Replace rubber stopper and gently swirl vial until contents have completely dissolved.

Administration

Parenteral:

IV: IV route is preferred for doses >1,000 mg or in patients with severe life-threatening infections. Administer by IVP over 3 to 5 minutes or by intermittent infusion over 20 to 60 minute.

IM: Administer by deep IM injection into a large muscle mass such as the upper outer quadrant of the gluteus maximus or lateral part of the thigh. Doses >1,000 mg should be administered IV. Do **not** mix with any local anesthetic agent.

Inhalation: Administer only using an Altera nebulizer system; dose can be nebulized over 2 to 3 minutes. Administer alone; do not mix with other inhaled nebulizer medications. Administer doses ≥4 hours apart. Administer a bronchodilator before administration of aztreonam (short-acting 15 minutes to 4 hours before; long-acting: 30 minutes to 12 hours before). For patients on multiple inhaled therapies, administer bronchodilator first, then mucolytic, and lastly, aztreonam.

Monitoring Parameters

Injection: Periodic renal and hepatic function tests; monitor for stool frequency; monitor for signs of anaphylaxis during first dose

Inhalation: FEV_1

Test Interactions May interfere with urine glucose tests containing cupric sulfate (Benedict's solution, Clinitest); positive Coombs' test

Dosage Forms Excipient information presented when available (limited, particularly for generics); consult specific product labeling.

Solution, Intravenous:

Azactam in Dextrose: 1 g (50 mL); 2 g (50 mL) [sodium free]

Solution Reconstituted, Inhalation [preservative free]:

Cayston: 75 mg (84 mL) [arginine free]

Solution Reconstituted, Injection:

Azactam: 1 g (1 ea); 2 g (1 ea) [sodium free]

Generic: 1 g (1 ea); 2 g (1 ea)

- **Azulfidine** *see* SulfaSALAzine *on page 1990*
- **Azulfidine EN-tabs** *see* SulfaSALAzine *on page 1990*
- **B-2-400 [OTC]** *see* Riboflavin *on page 1856*
- **B6** *see* Pyridoxine *on page 1810*
- **Baby Anbesol [OTC]** *see* Benzocaine *on page 268*
- **Baby Aspirin** *see* Aspirin *on page 206*
- **Baby Ayr Saline [OTC]** *see* Sodium Chloride *on page 1938*
- **BabyBIG®** *see* Botulism Immune Globulin (Intravenous-Human) *on page 299*
- **Bacid® [OTC]** *see Lactobacillus on page 1203*
- **Bacid (Can)** *see Lactobacillus on page 1203*
- **BACiiM** *see* Bacitracin (Systemic) *on page 250*
- **BaciJect (Can)** *see* Bacitracin (Systemic) *on page 250*
- **Bacitin (Can)** *see* Bacitracin (Topical) *on page 252*

Bacitracin (Systemic) (bas i TRAY sin)

Medication Safety Issues

Sound-alike/look-alike issues:

Bacitracin may be confused with Bactrim, Bactroban

Brand Names: US BACiiM

Brand Names: Canada BaciJect

Therapeutic Category Antibiotic, Miscellaneous

Generic Availability (US) Yes

Use Treatment of pneumonia and empyema in infants caused by susceptible staphylococci (FDA approved in infants); **Note:** Due to toxicity risks, systemic use of bacitracin is rare and should be limited to situations where less toxic alternatives would not be effective.

Pregnancy Considerations This product is not indicated for use in women of reproductive age.

Breast-Feeding Considerations This product is not indicated for use in women of reproductive age.

Contraindications Hypersensitivity to bacitracin or any component of the formulation

Warnings/Precautions [U.S. Boxed Warning]: IM use may cause renal failure due to tubular and glomerular necrosis; monitor renal function daily. Avoid concurrent use with other nephrotoxic drugs; discontinue use if toxicity occurs. Maintain adequate fluid intake and hydration throughout therapy. Do not exceed recommended doses. Use with caution in patients who have been previously exposed to bacitracin; anaphylactic reactions have occurred on repeat exposure especially with irrigation use (Damm, 2011; Elsner, 1990; Farley, 1995). Prolonged use may result in fungal or bacterial superinfection, including *C. difficile*-associated diarrhea (CDAD) and pseudomembranous colitis; CDAD has been observed >2 months postantibiotic treatment. Do not administer intravenously because severe thrombophlebitis occurs. Should only be used when adequate laboratory facilities are available and constant patient supervision is available.

Warnings: Additional Pediatric Considerations Anaphylactic reactions may occur on repeat exposure; anaphylaxis and other hypersensitivity reactions have been reported with application of bacitracin ointment and with intraprocedure irrigation use; use with caution in patients who have been previously exposed to bacitracin (Damm, 2011; Elsner, 1990; Farley, 1995). Procaine is recommended in the preparation of solutions to lessen pain of injection; avoid use in patients with hypersensitivity to procaine.

Bacitracin is seldom used systemically; consider confirmation of use and route with prescriber prior to administration. Bacitracin is a mixture of antimicrobial polypeptides and should be dosed in "units".

Adverse Reactions

Dermatologic: Skin rash
Endocrine & metabolic: Albuminuria
Gastrointestinal: Nausea, vomiting
Genitourinary: Azotemia, casts in urine, nephrotoxicity
Local: Pain at injection site
Renal: Renal failure
Rare but important or life-threatening: Anaphylaxis (intraoperative exposure [Damm, 2011])

Drug Interactions

Metabolism/Transport Effects None known.

Avoid Concomitant Use

Avoid concomitant use of Bacitracin (Systemic) with any of the following: BCG; BCG (Intravesical); Colistimethate; Kanamycin; Neomycin; Polymyxin B; Streptomycin

Increased Effect/Toxicity

The levels/effects of Bacitracin (Systemic) may be increased by: Colistimethate; Kanamycin; Neomycin; Polymyxin B; Streptomycin

Decreased Effect

Bacitracin (Systemic) may decrease the levels/effects of: BCG; BCG (Intravesical); BCG Vaccine (Immunization); Sodium Picosulfate

Storage/Stability Solution for injection (IM use only): Store unreconstituted vials in the refrigerator at 2°C to 8°C (36°F to 46°F). Once reconstituted, bacitracin is stable for 1 week under refrigeration at 2°C to 8°C (36°F to 46°F).

Mechanism of Action Inhibits bacterial cell wall synthesis by preventing transfer of mucopeptides into the growing cell wall

Pharmacokinetics (Adult data unless noted)

Absorption: Infants: Rapidly following IM administration
Distribution: Infants: Widely distributed in all body organs and is demonstrable in ascitic and pleural fluids
Elimination: Infants: Urine

Dosing: Neonatal Pneumonia and empyema; staphylococcal: Note: Due to toxicity risks, systemic use of bacitracin should be limited to situations where less toxic alternatives would not be effective; systemic use in neonatal patients is rare. **Do not administer IV**:

Neonates: IM:
≤2.5 kg: 900 units/kg/day in 2 to 3 divided doses
>2.5 kg: 1000 units/kg/day in 2 to 3 divided doses

Dosing: Usual

Pediatric: **Pneumonia and empyema; staphylococcal: Note:** Due to toxicity risks, systemic use of bacitracin should be limited to situations where less toxic alternatives would not be effective; systemic use in pediatric patients is rare. **Do not administer IV**:
Infants: IM:
≤2.5 kg: 900 units/kg/day in 2 to 3 divided doses
>2.5 kg: 1000 units/kg/day in 2 to 3 divided doses

Preparation for Administration Parenteral: IM: Bacitracin sterile powder should be dissolved in NS containing 2% procaine hydrochloride; concentration after reconstitution should be between 5,000 to 10,000 units/mL. Do not use diluents containing parabens; cloudy solutions and precipitation have occurred.

Administration Parenteral: Bacitracin is seldom used systemically, consider confirmation of use and route with prescriber prior to administration. For IM administration only; administer to upper outer quadrant of the buttocks; rotate administration site. **Do not administer IV.**

Monitoring Parameters Renal function tests, fluid intake, urine output

Additional Information 1 unit is equivalent to 0.026 mg

Dosage Forms Excipient information presented when available (limited, particularly for generics); consult specific product labeling.

Solution Reconstituted, Intramuscular:
BACiiM: 50,000 units (1 ea)
Generic: 50,000 units (1 ea)
Solution Reconstituted, Intramuscular [preservative free]:
Generic: 50,000 units (1 ea)

Bacitracin (Ophthalmic) (bas i TRAY sin)

Medication Safety Issues

Sound-alike/look-alike issues:

Bacitracin may be confused with Bactrim, Bactroban

Therapeutic Category Antibiotic, Ophthalmic

Generic Availability (US) Yes

Use Treatment of superficial ocular infections involving the conjunctiva or cornea due to bacterial infections (has activity against gram-positive bacilli) (FDA approved in pediatric patients [age not specified] and adults)

Pregnancy Considerations Bacitracin is not absorbed systemically following ophthalmic administration (Robert, 2001). If ophthalmic agents are needed during pregnancy, the minimum effective dose should be used in combination with punctual occlusion to decrease potential exposure to the fetus (Samples, 1988).

Breast-Feeding Considerations Bacitracin is not absorbed systemically following ophthalmic administration (Robert, 2001).

Contraindications Hypersensitivity to bacitracin or any component of the formulation

Warnings/Precautions Use with caution in patients who have been previously exposed to bacitracin; anaphylactic reactions have occurred on repeat exposure (Elsner, 1990; Farley, 1995). Should not be used in deep seated ocular infections or if infection is likely to become systemic. Prolonged use may result in overgrowth of nonsusceptble organisms, particularly fungi; if new infection develops, initiate appropriate therapy.

Adverse Reactions

Hypersensitivity: Hypersensitivity reaction (Hätinen, 1985)
Rare but important or life-threatening: Contact dermatitis (Pichichero, 2011)

Drug Interactions

Metabolism/Transport Effects None known.

Avoid Concomitant Use There are no known interactions where it is recommended to avoid concomitant use.

Increased Effect/Toxicity There are no known significant interactions involving an increase in effect.

Decreased Effect There are no known significant interactions involving a decrease in effect.

Storage/Stability Store at 20°C to 25°C (68°F to 77°F).

Mechanism of Action Inhibits bacterial cell wall synthesis by preventing transfer of mucopeptides into the growing cell wall

Dosing: Usual

Pediatric: **Ophthalmic infection:** Infants, Children, and Adolescents: Ophthalmic: Apply ribbon 1 to 3 times daily
Adult: **Ophthalmic infection:** Ophthalmic: Apply 1 to 3 times daily

Administration Ophthalmic: For topical ophthalmic use only; apply directly to conjunctival sac; avoid gross contamination of ointment during application. For blepharitis;

after carefully removing all scales and crusts, apply uniformly over lid margins.

Additional Information 1 unit is equivalent to 0.026 mg

Dosage Forms Excipient information presented when available (limited, particularly for generics); consult specific product labeling.

Ointment, Ophthalmic:

Generic: 500 units/g (1 g, 3.5 g)

Bacitracin (Topical) (bas i TRAY sin)

Medication Safety Issues

Sound-alike/look-alike issues:

Bacitracin may be confused with Bactrim, Bactroban

Brand Names: Canada Bacitin

Therapeutic Category Antibiotic, Topical

Generic Availability (US) Yes

Use Prevention of infection in minor cuts, scrapes, or burns (FDA approved in pediatric patients [age not specified] and adults)

Pregnancy Considerations Although large studies have not been conducted, absorption is limited following topical application; use during pregnancy has not been associated with an increased risk of adverse fetal events (Leachman, 2006; Murase, 2014).

Breast-Feeding Considerations Absorption is limited following topical application (Murase, 2014). Although large studies have not been conducted, use of topical bacitracin in breast-feeding women has not been associated with an increased risk of adverse events in the nursing infant (Leachman, 2006).

Contraindications Hypersensitivity to bacitracin or any component of the formulation

Warnings/Precautions Use with caution in patients who have been previously exposed to bacitracin; anaphylactic reactions have occurred on repeat exposure (Elsner, 1990, Farley, 1995)

Topical anti-infective (self-medication, OTC use): Use longer than 1 week is not recommended unless directed by prescriber. Do not use in eyes or over large areas of the body. Seek advice from healthcare provider prior to use for deep puncture wounds, bites, or serious burns or if condition persists for longer than 1 week. Stop use and consult health care provider if allergic reaction or rash develops.

Adverse Reactions Rare but important or life-threatening: Anaphylaxis (Elsner, 1990; Farley, 1995)

Drug Interactions

Metabolism/Transport Effects None known.

Avoid Concomitant Use There are no known interactions where it is recommended to avoid concomitant use.

Increased Effect/Toxicity There are no known significant interactions involving an increase in effect.

Decreased Effect There are no known significant interactions involving a decrease in effect.

Storage/Stability Topical ointment (OTC): Store at 15°C to 30°C (59°F to 86°F).

Mechanism of Action Inhibits bacterial cell wall synthesis by preventing transfer of mucopeptides into the growing cell wall

Pharmacokinetics (Adult data unless noted) Absorption: Poor from mucous membranes and intact or denuded skin

Dosing: Usual

Pediatric: **Prevention of infection:** Topical: Children and Adolescents: Apply small amount 1 to 3 times daily; duration of therapy >7 days is not recommended, unless directed by health care provider.

Administration Clean the affected area. Apply a small amount of product (an amount equal to the surface area of the tip of a finger); may cover with sterile bandage.

Additional Information 1 unit is equivalent to 0.026 mg

Dosage Forms Excipient information presented when available (limited, particularly for generics); consult specific product labeling.

Ointment, External, as zinc [strength expressed as base]:

Generic: 500 units/g (1 ea, 1 g, 14 g, 14.2 g, 15 g, 28 g, 28.35 g, 28.4 g, 30 g, 120 g, 453.9 g, 454 g)

Bacitracin and Polymyxin B

(bas i TRAY sin & pol i MIKS in bee)

Medication Safety Issues

Sound-alike/look-alike issues:

Betadine® may be confused with Betagan®, betaine

Brand Names: US AK-Poly-Bac™; Polycin™; Polysporin® [OTC]

Brand Names: Canada LID-Pack®; Optimyxin®

Therapeutic Category Antibiotic, Ophthalmic; Antibiotic, Topical

Generic Availability (US) Yes

Use Treatment of superficial infections involving the conjunctiva and/or cornea caused by susceptible organisms; prevent infection in minor cuts, scrapes and burns

Pregnancy Risk Factor C

Pregnancy Considerations Animal reproduction studies have not been conducted with this combination.

Breast-Feeding Considerations It is not known if bacitracin or polymyxin B are excreted into breast milk. The manufacturer recommends that caution be exercised when administering to nursing women.

Contraindications Hypersensitivity to bacitracin, polymyxin B, or any component of the formulation

Adverse Reactions Local: Anaphylactoid reactions, burning, conjunctival erythema, itching, rash, swelling

Drug Interactions

Metabolism/Transport Effects None known.

Avoid Concomitant Use There are no known interactions where it is recommended to avoid concomitant use.

Increased Effect/Toxicity There are no known significant interactions involving an increase in effect.

Decreased Effect There are no known significant interactions involving a decrease in effect.

Mechanism of Action See individual agents.

Pharmacokinetics (Adult data unless noted) Absorption: Insignificant from intact skin or mucous membrane

Dosing: Usual Children and Adults:

Ophthalmic: Instill 1/4" to 1/2" directly into conjunctival sac(s) every 3-4 hours depending on severity of the infection

Topical: Apply a small amount of ointment or dusting of powder to the affected area 1-3 times/day

Administration Ophthalmic: Do not use topical ointment in the eyes; avoid contact of tube tip with skin or eye

Dosage Forms Excipient information presented when available (limited, particularly for generics); consult specific product labeling.

Ointment, ophthalmic: Bacitracin 500 units and polymyxin B 10,000 units per g (3.5 g)

AK-Poly-Bac™: Bacitracin 500 units and polymyxin B 10,000 units per g (3.5 g)

Polycin™: Bacitracin 500 units and polymyxin B 10,000 units per g (3.5 g)

Ointment, topical: Bacitracin 500 units and polymyxin B 10,000 units per g (15 g, 30 g)

Polysporin®: Bacitracin 500 units and polymyxin B 10,000 units per g (0.9 g, 15 g, 30 g)

Powder, topical:

Polysporin®: Bacitracin 500 units and polymyxin B 10,000 units per g (10 g)

Bacitracin, Neomycin, and Polymyxin B

(bas i TRAY sin, nee oh MYE sin, & pol i MIKS in bee)

Brand Names: US Neo-Polycin™; Neosporin® Neo To Go® [OTC]; Neosporin® Topical [OTC]

Therapeutic Category Antibiotic, Ophthalmic; Antibiotic, Topical

Generic Availability (US) Yes

Use Help prevent infection in minor cuts, scrapes and burns; short-term treatment of superficial external ocular infections caused by susceptible organisms

Pregnancy Risk Factor C

Pregnancy Considerations Animal reproduction studies have not been conducted with this combination.

Breast-Feeding Considerations It is not known if bacitracin, neomycin, or polymyxin B is excreted into breast milk. The manufacturer recommends that caution be exercised when administering to nursing women.

Contraindications Hypersensitivity to neomycin, polymyxin B, zinc bacitracin, or any component of the formulation; epithelial herpes simplex keratitis; mycobacterial or fungal infections; topical ointments for external use only

Warnings/Precautions

Topical ointment: When used for self-medication (OTC use), patients should notify healthcare provider if needed for >1 week. Should not be used for self-medication on deep or puncture wounds, animal bites, or serious burns. Not for application to large areas of the body.

Ophthalmic ointment: Bacterial keratitis has been reported with the use of topical ophthalmic products in multiple-dose containers. Care should be taken to not contaminate the container.

Adverse Reactions

Dermatologic: Allergic contact dermatitis, reddening

Local: Failure to heal, irritation, itching, swelling

Ophthalmic: Conjunctival edema

Miscellaneous: Anaphylaxis

Drug Interactions

Metabolism/Transport Effects None known.

Avoid Concomitant Use There are no known interactions where it is recommended to avoid concomitant use.

Increased Effect/Toxicity There are no known significant interactions involving an increase in effect.

Decreased Effect There are no known significant interactions involving a decrease in effect.

Mechanism of Action See individual agents.

Dosing: Usual Children and Adults:

Ophthalmic ointment: Instill into the conjunctival sac 1 or more times daily every 3-4 hours for 7-10 days

Topical: Apply 1-3 times/day

Administration

Ophthalmic: Avoid contamination of the tip of the ointment tube

Topical: Apply a thin layer to the cleansed affected area; may cover with a sterile bandage

Dosage Forms Excipient information presented when available (limited, particularly for generics); consult specific product labeling.

Ointment, ophthalmic: Bacitracin 400 units, neomycin 3.5 mg, and polymyxin B 10,000 units per g (3.5 g)

Neo-Polycin™: Bacitracin 400 units, neomycin 3.5 mg, and polymyxin B 10,000 units per g (3.5 g)

Ointment, topical: Bacitracin 400 units, neomycin 3.5 mg, and polymyxin B 5000 units per g (0.9 g, 15 g, 30 g, 454 g)

Neosporin®: Bacitracin 400 units, neomycin 3.5 mg, and polymyxin B 5000 units per g (15 g, 30 g)

Neosporin® Neo To Go®: Bacitracin 400 units, neomycin 3.5 mg, and polymyxin B 5000 units per g (0.9 g)

Bacitracin, Neomycin, Polymyxin B, and Hydrocortisone

(bas i TRAY sin, nee oh MYE sin, pol i MIKS in bee, & hye droe KOR ti sone)

Brand Names: US Cortisporin Ointment; Neo-Polycin HC

Brand Names: Canada Cortisporin Topical Ointment

Therapeutic Category Antibiotic, Ophthalmic; Antibiotic, Otic; Antibiotic, Topical; Corticosteroid, Ophthalmic; Corticosteroid, Otic; Corticosteroid, Topical

Generic Availability (US) Yes: Ophthalmic ointment

Use

Ophthalmic: Prevention and treatment of susceptible inflammatory conditions where bacterial infection (or risk of infection) is present (FDA approved in adults)

Topical: Treatment of corticosteroid-responsive dermatoses with secondary infection (FDA approved in adults)

Pregnancy Risk Factor C

Pregnancy Considerations Adverse events have been observed with topical corticosteroids in animal reproduction studies. If ophthalmic agents are needed during pregnancy, the minimum effective dose should be used in combination with punctual occlusion to decrease potential exposure to the fetus (Samples, 1988). Refer to individual agents.

Breast-Feeding Considerations It is not known if systemic absorption following topical administration results in detectable quantities in human milk. The manufacturers of the topical ointment recommend a decision be made whether to discontinue nursing or to discontinue the drug, taking into account the importance of treatment to the mother. The manufacturers of the ophthalmic ointment recommend that caution be exercised when administering to nursing women. Refer to individual agents.

Contraindications

Hypersensitivity to bacitracin, neomycin, polymyxin B, hydrocortisone, or any component of the formulation.

Ophthalmic ointment: Most viral diseases of the cornea and conjunctiva, including epithelial herpes simplex keratitis (dendritic keratitis), vaccinia and varicella; mycobacterial ophthalmic infection; fungal diseases of ocular structures.

Topical ointment: Ophthalmic administration; external ear canal administration (if eardrum is perforated); in tuberculous, fungal, or viral skin lesions.

Warnings/Precautions Topical corticosteroids may be absorbed percutaneously. Absorption of topical corticosteroids may cause manifestations of Cushing syndrome, hyperglycemia, or glycosuria. Absorption is increased by the use of occlusive dressings, application to denuded skin, or application to large surface areas. Systemic absorption of topical corticosteroids may cause hypercorticism or suppression of hypothalamic-pituitary-adrenal (HPA) axis, particularly in younger children or in patients receiving high doses for prolonged periods. HPA axis suppression may lead to adrenal crisis. Prolonged use may increase the incidence of secondary infection, mask acute infection (including fungal infections), prolong or exacerbate viral infections, or limit response to vaccines.

Children may absorb proportionally larger amounts of corticosteroids after topical application and may be more prone to systemic effects. HPA axis suppression, intracranial hypertension, and Cushing syndrome have been reported in children receiving topical corticosteroids. Prolonged use may affect growth velocity; growth should be routinely monitored in pediatric patients.

Neomycin may cause cutaneous sensitization. Symptoms of neomycin sensitization include itching, reddening, edema, and failure to heal. Discontinuation of product and avoidance of similar products should be considered. Neomycin can induce permanent sensorineural hearing loss due to cochlear damage; risk is greater with prolonged use. Prolonged treatment with corticosteroids has been associated with the development of Kaposi sarcoma (case reports); if noted, discontinuation of therapy should be considered (Goedert, 2012).

Ophthalmic ointment: Never directly introduce (eg, inject) into the anterior chamber. May retard corneal wound healing. Prolonged use may result in ocular hypertension and/or glaucoma (damage to the optic nerve, defects in visual acuity and fields of vision) and in posterior subcapsular cataract formation. Long-term use may cause corneal and scleral thinning; potentially resulting in perforation. Use with caution in glaucoma. Use following ocular cataract surgery may delay healing and increase the incidence of filtering blebs. Inadvertent contamination of multiple-dose ophthalmic tube tip has caused bacterial keratitis.

Topical ointment: Limit therapy to 7 days of treatment.

Adverse Reactions For additional information, see individual agents.

Ophthalmic ointment:

Dermatologic: Delayed wound healing, rash

Ocular: Cataracts, corneal thinning, glaucoma, irritation, keratitis (bacterial), intraocular pressure increase, optic nerve damage, scleral thinning

Miscellaneous: Hypersensitivity (including anaphylaxis), secondary infection, sensitization to kanamycin, paromomycin, streptomycin, and gentamicin

Topical ointment:

Dermatologic: Acneiform eruptions, allergic contact dermatitis, burning skin, dryness, folliculitis, hypertrichosis, hypopigmentation, irritation, maceration of skin, miliaria, ocular hypertension, perioral dermatitis, pruritus, skin atrophy, striae

Otic: Ototoxicity

Renal: Nephrotoxicity

Miscellaneous: Hypersensitivity (including anaphylaxis), secondary infection, sensitization to karamycin, paromycin, streptomycin, and gentamicin

Drug Interactions

Metabolism/Transport Effects None known.

Avoid Concomitant Use

Avoid concomitant use of Bacitracin, Neomycin, Polymyxin B, and Hydrocortisone with any of the following: Aldesleukin

Increased Effect/Toxicity

Bacitracin, Neomycin, Polymyxin B, and Hydrocortisone may increase the levels/effects of: Ceritinib; Deferasirox

The levels/effects of Bacitracin, Neomycin, Polymyxin B, and Hydrocortisone may be increased by: NSAID (Ophthalmic); Telaprevir

Decreased Effect

Bacitracin, Neomycin, Polymyxin B, and Hydrocortisone may decrease the levels/effects of: Aldesleukin; Corticorelin; Hyaluronidase; Telaprevir

Storage/Stability

Ophthalmic ointment: Store at 15°C to 30°C (59°F to 86°F).

Topical ointment: Store at 15°C to 25°C (59°F to 77°F).

Mechanism of Action See individual agents.

Pharmacokinetics (Adult data unless noted) See individual agents.

Dosing: Usual Children and Adults:

Ophthalmic: Ointment: Instill 1/2" ribbon to inside of lower lid every 3-4 hours until improvement occurs

Topical: Apply thin film sparingly 2-4 times/day for up to 7 days. Therapy should be discontinued when control is achieved or after a week; if no improvement is seen, reassessment of diagnosis may be necessary.

Monitoring Parameters If ophthalmic ointment is used >10 days or in patients with glaucoma, monitor intraocular pressure (IOP).

Dosage Forms Excipient information presented when available (limited, particularly for generics); consult specific product labeling.

Ointment, ophthalmic: Bacitracin 400 units, neomycin 3.5 mg, polymyxin B 10,000 units, and hydrocortisone 10 mg per g (3.5 g)

Neo-Polycin™ HC: Bacitracin 400 units, neomycin 3.5 mg, polymyxin B 10,000 units, and hydrocortisone 10 mg per g (3.5 g)

Ointment, topical:

Cortisporin®: Bacitracin 400 units, neomycin 3.5 mg, polymyxin B 5000 units, and hydrocortisone 10 mg per g (15 g)

Baclofen (BAK loe fen)

Medication Safety Issues

Sound-alike/look-alike issues:

Baclofen may be confused with Bactroban

Lioresal may be confused with lisinopril, Lotensin

High alert medication:

The Institute for Safe Medication Practices (ISMP) includes this medication (intrathecal administration) among its list of drugs which have a heightened risk of causing significant patient harm when used in error.

Brand Names: US EnovaRX-Baclofen; Equipto-Baclofen; Gablofen; Lioresal

Brand Names: Canada Apo-Baclofen; Dom-Baclofen; Lioresal; Lioresal D.S.; Lioresal Intrathecal; Mylan-Baclofen; Novo-Baclofen; PHL-Baclofen; PMS-Baclofen; ratio-Baclofen; Riva-Baclofen; VPI-Baclofen Intrathecal

Therapeutic Category Skeletal Muscle Relaxant, Nonparalytic

Generic Availability (US) May be product dependent

Use Treatment of cerebral spasticity, reversible spasticity associated with multiple sclerosis or spinal cord lesions; intrathecal use for the management of spasticity in patients who are unresponsive to oral baclofen or experience intolerable CNS side effects; treatment of trigeminal neuralgia; adjunctive treatment of tardive dyskinesia

Pregnancy Risk Factor C

Pregnancy Considerations Adverse events were observed in animal reproduction studies. Withdrawal symptoms in the neonate were noted in a case report following the maternal use of oral baclofen 20 mg 4 times/day throughout pregnancy (Ratnayaka, 2001). Plasma concentrations following administration of intrathecal baclofen are significantly less than those with oral doses; exposure to the fetus is expected to be limited (Morton, 2009).

Breast-Feeding Considerations Baclofen is excreted into breast milk. Very small amounts were found in the breast milk of a woman 14 days postpartum after oral use. Following a single oral dose of baclofen 20 mg, the total amount of baclofen excreted in breast milk within 26 hours was 22 mcg (Eriksson, 1981). Adverse events were not observed in a nursing infant following maternal use of intrathecal baclofen 200 mcg/day throughout pregnancy and while nursing (Morton, 2009). Due to the potential for adverse events in the nursing infant, breast-feeding is not recommended by the manufacturer.

Contraindications

Hypersensitivity to baclofen or any component of the formulation

Intrathecal: IV, IM, SubQ, or epidural administration

Warnings/Precautions **[US Boxed Warning]: Abrupt withdrawal of intrathecal baclofen has resulted in severe sequelae (hyperpyrexia, obtundation, rebound/exaggerated spasticity, muscle rigidity, and**

rhabdomyolysis), leading to organ failure and some fatalities. Prevention of abrupt discontinuation requires careful attention to programming and monitoring of infusion system, refill scheduling and procedures, and pump alarms. Risk may be higher in patients with injuries at T-6 or above, history of baclofen withdrawal, or limited ability to communicate. Abrupt withdrawal of oral therapy has been associated with hallucinations and seizures; gradual dose reductions (over ~1 to 2 weeks) are recommended in the absence of severe adverse reactions.

Patients receiving intrathecal baclofen should be infection-free prior to the test dose and pump implantation. Clinicians should be experienced with chronic intrathecal infusion therapy. Pump should only be implanted if patients' response to bolus intrathecal baclofen was adequately evaluated and found to be safe and effective. Resuscitative equipment should be readily available. Monitor closely during the initial phase of pump use and when adjusting the dosing rate and/or the concentration in the reservoir. Educate patients and caregivers on proper home care of the pump and insertion site; early symptoms of baclofen withdrawal (eg, return of baseline spasticity, hypotension, paresthesia, pruritus); signs/symptoms of overdose (eg, dizziness, somnolence, respiratory depression, seizures); and appropriate actions in the event of an overdose. Cases (most from pharmacy compounded preparations) of intrathecal mass formation at the implanted catheter tip have been reported; may lead to loss of clinical response, pain or new/worsening neurological effects. Neurosurgical evaluation and/or an appropriate imaging study should be considered if a mass is suspected. Use caution with history of autonomic dysreflexia; presence of nociceptive stimuli or abrupt baclofen withdrawal may cause an autonomic dysreflexia episode.

May cause CNS depression, which may impair physical or mental abilities; patients must be cautioned about performing tasks which require mental alertness (eg, operating machinery or driving). Elderly patients are more sensitive to the effects of baclofen and are more likely to experience adverse CNS effects at higher doses. Use with caution in patients with seizure disorder, renal impairment, respiratory disease, psychiatric disease, peptic ulcer disease, decreased GI motility, and/or gastrointestinal obstructive disorders.

Efficacy of oral baclofen has not been established in patients with stroke, Parkinson disease, or cerebral palsy; therefore, use is not recommended. Not indicated for spasticity associated with rheumatic disorders. Use with caution when spasticity is utilized to sustain upright posture and balance in locomotion, or when spasticity is necessary to obtain increased function. Adverse effects are more likely in patients with spastic states of cerebral origin; cautious dosing and careful monitoring are necessary.

Animal studies have shown an increased incidence in ovarian cysts; however, incidence observed in multiple sclerosis patients treated with baclofen for up to one year was similar to the estimated incidence in healthy females. Spontaneous resolution occurred in most of these MS patients while continuing treatment. May cause acute urinary retention (may be related to underlying disease); use with caution in patients with urinary obstruction. Potentially significant drug-drug interactions may exist, requiring dose or frequency adjustment, additional monitoring, and/or selection of alternative therapy.

Adverse Reactions

Cardiovascular: Hypotension, peripheral edema

Central nervous system: Abnormality in thinking, agitation, chills, coma, confusion, convulsions, depression, dizziness, drowsiness, headache, hypertonia, hypotonia, insomnia, pain, paresthesia, speech disturbance

Dermatologic: Pruritus, urticaria

Gastrointestinal: Constipation, diarrhea, nausea, sialorrhea, vomiting, xerostomia

Genitourinary: Difficulty in micturition, impotence, urinary frequency, urinary incontinence, urinary retention

Neuromuscular & skeletal: Back pain, tremor, weakness

Ophthalmic: Ambylopia

Respiratory: Dyspnea, hypoventilation, pneumonia

Miscellaneous: Accidental injury

Rare but important or life-threatening: Accommodation disturbance, akathisia, albuminuria, alopecia, amnesia, apnea, ataxia, blurred vision, bradycardia, bradypnea, carcinoma, chest pain, decreased appetite, deep vein thrombosis, dehydration, diaphoresis, diplopia, disorientation, dysarthria, dysautonomia, dysgeusia, dysphagia, dysphoria, dystonia, dysuria, epilepsy, facial edema, fecal incontinence, gastrointestinal hemorrhage, hyperglycemia, hyperhidrosis, hypertension, hyperventilation, hypothermia, hysteria, inhibited ejaculation, intestinal obstruction, lethargy, leukocytosis, loss of postural reflex, lower extremity weakness, malaise, miosis, muscle rigidity, myalgia, mydriasis, nephrolithiasis, nocturia, nystagmus, occult blood in stools, oliguria, opisthotonus, pallor, palpitations, petechial rash, pulmonary embolism, respiratory depression, sedation, slurred speech, strabismus, suicidal ideation, syncope, vasodilatation

Withdrawal reactions have occurred with abrupt discontinuation (particularly severe with intrathecal use).

Drug Interactions

Metabolism/Transport Effects None known.

Avoid Concomitant Use

Avoid concomitant use of Baclofen with any of the following: Azelastine (Nasal); Orphenadrine; Paraldehyde; Thalidomide

Increased Effect/Toxicity

Baclofen may increase the levels/effects of: Alcohol (Ethyl); Azelastine (Nasal); Buprenorphine; CNS Depressants; Hydrocodone; Lacidipine; Methotrimeprazine; Metyrosine; Mirtazapine; Orphenadrine; Paraldehyde; Pramipexole; ROPINIRole; Rotigotine; Selective Serotonin Reuptake Inhibitors; Suvorexant; Thalidomide; Zolpidem

The levels/effects of Baclofen may be increased by: Brimonidine (Topical); Cannabis; Doxylamine; Dronabinol; Droperidol; HydrOXYzine; Kava Kava; Magnesium Sulfate; Methotrimeprazine; Nabilone; Perampanel; Rufinamide; Sodium Oxybate; Tapentadol; Tetrahydrocannabinol

Decreased Effect There are no known significant interactions involving a decrease in effect.

Storage/Stability

Injection: Do not store above 30°C (86°F). Does not require refrigeration. Do not freeze or heat sterilize.

Tablets: Store at 20°C to 25°C (68°F to 77°F).

Mechanism of Action Inhibits the transmission of both monosynaptic and polysynaptic reflexes at the spinal cord level, possibly by hyperpolarization of primary afferent fiber terminals, with resultant relief of muscle spasticity

Pharmacodynamics

Oral: Muscle relaxation effects require 3-4 days and maximal clinical effects are not seen for 5-10 days

Intrathecal:

- Bolus:
  - Onset of action: 30 minutes to 1 hour
  - Maximum effect: 4 hours
  - Duration: 4-8 hours
- Continuous intrathecal infusion:
  - Onset of action: 6-8 hours
  - Maximum activity: 24-48 hours

Pharmacokinetics (Adult data unless noted)

Oral:

Absorption: Rapid; absorption from the GI tract is thought to be dose dependent

Protein binding: 30%

Metabolism: Minimal in the liver (15%)

Half-life: 2.5-4 hours

Time to peak serum concentration: Oral: Within 2-3 hours

Elimination: 85% of dose excreted in urine and feces as unchanged drug

Intrathecal:

Half-life, CSF elimination: 1.5 hours

Clearance, CSF: 30 mL/hour

Dosing: Usual

Oral: Dose-related side effects (eg, sedation) may be minimized by slow titration; lower initial doses than described below (2.5-5 mg **daily**) may be used with subsequent titration to 8 hourly doses.

Children: Limited published data in children; the following is a compilation of small prospective studies (Albright, 1996; Milla, 1977; Scheinberg, 2006) and one large retrospective analysis of baclofen use in children (Lubsch, 2006):

<2 years: 10-20 mg **daily** divided every 8 hours; titrate dose every 3 days in increments of 5-15 mg/day to a maximum of 40 mg **daily**

2-7 years: 20-30 mg **daily** divided every 8 hours; titrate dose every 3 days in increments of 5-15 mg/day to a maximum of 60 mg **daily**

≥8 years: 30-40 mg **daily** divided every 8 hours; titrate dosage as above to a maximum of 120 mg **daily**

Note: Lubsch retrospective analysis noted that higher daily dosages of baclofen were needed as the time increased from injury onset, as age increased, and as the number of concomitant antispasticity medications increased. Each of these variables may represent drug tolerance or progressive spasticity. In this review, doses as high as 200 mg **daily** were used.

Adults: 5 mg 3 times/day, may increase 5 mg/dose every 3 days to a maximum of 80 mg/day

Intrathecal: Children and Adults:

Screening dosage: 50 mcg for 1 dose and observe for 4-8 hours; very small children may receive 25 mcg; if ineffective, a repeat dosage increased by 50% (eg, 75 mcg) may be repeated in 24 hours; if still suboptimal, a third dose increased by 33% (eg, 100 mcg) may be repeated in 24 hours; patients who do not respond to 100 mcg intrathecally should not be considered for continuous chronic administration via an implantable pump

Maintenance dose: Continuous infusion: Initial: Depending upon the screening dosage and its duration:

If the screening dose duration >8 hours: Daily dose = effective screening dose

If the screening dose duration <8 hours: Daily dose = **twice** effective screening dose

Continuous infusion dose mcg/hour = daily dose divided by 24 hours

Note: Further adjustments in infusion rate may be done every 24 hours as needed; for spinal cord-related spasticity, increase in 10% to 30% increments/24 hours; for spasticity of cerebral origin, increase in 5% to 10% increments/24 hours

Average daily dose:

Children ≤12 years: 100-300 mcg/day (4.2-12.5 mcg/hour); doses as high as 1000 mcg/day have been used

Children >12 years and Adults: 300-800 mcg/day (12.5-33 mcg/hour); doses as high as 2000 mcg/day have been used

Dosing adjustment in renal impairment: Oral: There are no dosage adjustments provided in the manufacturer's labeling; however, baclofen is primarily renally eliminated; use with caution; dosage reduction may be necessary.

Dosing adjustment in hepatic impairment: Oral: There are no dosage adjustments provided in the manufacturer's labeling.

Preparation for Administration Parenteral: Intrathecal: For screening dosages, dilute with preservative-free sodium chloride to a final concentration of 50 mcg/mL. For maintenance infusions, concentrations of 500 to 2,000 mcg/mL may be used; if preparing a concentration that is not commercially available, preservative-free sodium chloride must be used.

Administration

Oral: Administer with food or milk

Parenteral: Intrathecal: Screening dosage: Administer as a bolus injection by barbotage into the subarachnoid space over at least 1 minute, followed by maintenance infusion via implantable infusion pump; do not abruptly discontinue intrathecal baclofen administration

Monitoring Parameters Muscle rigidity, spasticity (decrease in number and severity of spasms), modified Ashworth score

Dosage Forms Considerations EnovaRX-Baclofen and Equipto-Baclofen creams are compounded from kits. Refer to manufacturer's labeling for compounding instructions.

Dosage Forms Excipient information presented when available (limited, particularly for generics); consult specific product labeling.

Cream, External:

EnovaRX-Baclofen: 1% (60 g, 120 g) [contains cetyl alcohol]

Equipto-Baclofen: 2% (120 g)

Solution, Intrathecal [preservative free]:

Gablofen: 50 mcg/mL (1 mL); 10,000 mcg/20 mL (20 mL); 20,000 mcg/20 mL (20 mL); 40,000 mcg/20 mL (20 mL) [antioxidant free]

Lioresal: 0.05 mg/mL (1 mL); 10 mg/20 mL (20 mL); 10 mg/5 mL (5 mL); 40 mg/20 mL (20 mL) [antioxidant free]

Tablet, Oral:

Generic: 10 mg, 20 mg

Extemporaneous Preparations A 5 mg/mL oral suspension may be made with tablets. Crush thirty 20 mg tablets in a mortar and reduce to a fine powder. Add a small amount of glycerin and mix to a uniform paste. Mix while adding Simple Syrup, NF in incremental proportions to **almost** 120 mL; transfer to a calibrated bottle, rinse mortar with vehicle, and add a sufficient quantity of vehicle to make 120 mL. Label "shake well" and "refrigerate". Stable for 35 days (Johnson, 1993).

A 10 mg/mL oral suspension may be made with tablets. Crush one-hundred-twenty 10 mg tablets in a mortar and reduce to a fine powder. Add small portions (60 mL) of a 1:1 mixture of Ora-Sweet® and Ora-Plus® and mix to a uniform paste; mix while adding the vehicle in incremental proportions to **almost** 120 mL; transfer to a calibrated bottle, rinse mortar with vehicle, and add quantity of vehicle sufficient to make 120 mL. Label "shake well" and "refrigerate". Stable for 60 days (Allen, 1996).

Allen LV Jr and Erickson MA 3rd, "Stability of Baclofen, Captopril, Diltiazem Hydrochloride, Dipyridamole, and Flecainide Acetate in Extemporaneously Compounded Oral Liquids," *Am J Health Syst Pharm*, 1996, 53(18):2179-84.

Johnson CE and Hart SM, "Stability of an Extemporaneously Compounded Baclofen Oral Liquid," *Am J Hosp Pharm*, 1993, 50 (11):2353-5.

◆ **Bactocill in Dextrose** *see* Oxacillin *on page 1576*

◆ **Bactrim** *see* Sulfamethoxazole and Trimethoprim *on page 1986*

◆ **Bactrim DS** *see* Sulfamethoxazole and Trimethoprim *on page 1986*

◆ **Bactroban** *see* Mupirocin *on page 1471*

- ◆ **Bactroban Nasal** *see* Mupirocin *on page 1471*
- ◆ **Baking Soda** *see* Sodium Bicarbonate *on page 1936*
- ◆ **BAL** *see* Dimercaprol *on page 665*
- ◆ **Bal in Oil** *see* Dimercaprol *on page 665*
- ◆ **Balmex® [OTC]** *see* Zinc Oxide *on page 2214*
- ◆ **Balminil Decongestant (Can)** *see* Pseudoephedrine *on page 1801*
- ◆ **Balminil DM E (Can)** *see* Guaifenesin and Dextromethorphan *on page 992*
- ◆ **Balminil Expectorant (Can)** *see* GuaiFENesin *on page 988*
- ◆ **Balnetar [OTC]** *see* Coal Tar *on page 523*

Balsalazide (bal SAL a zide)

Medication Safety Issues

Sound-alike/look-alike issues:

Colazal may be confused with Clozaril

Brand Names: US Colazal; Giazo

Therapeutic Category 5-Aminosalicylic Acid Derivative; Anti-inflammatory Agent

Generic Availability (US) May be product dependent

Use

Capsules: Short-term treatment of mildly to moderately active ulcerative colitis (FDA approved in ages ≥5 years and adults); Pediatric patients (5-17 years): 8 weeks of therapy; Adult patients: 12 weeks of therapy

Tablets (Giazo™): Short-term treatment (8 weeks) of mildly to moderately active ulcerative colitis (FDA approved in males ≥18 years and adults)

Pregnancy Risk Factor B

Pregnancy Considerations Teratogenic effects were not observed in animal reproduction studies. Mesalamine (5-aminosalicylic acid) is the active metabolite of balsalazide; mesalamine is known to cross the placenta.

Breast-Feeding Considerations Mesalamine, 5-aminosalicylic acid, is the active metabolite of balsalazide. Low levels of mesalamine enter breast milk; a case of bloody diarrhea in a breast-fed infant has been reported.

Contraindications Hypersensitivity to balsalazide or its metabolites, salicylates, or any component of the formulation

Warnings/Precautions Pyloric stenosis may prolong gastric retention of balsalazide. Renal toxicity and hepatic failure have been observed with other mesalamine (5-aminosalicylic acid) products; use with caution in patients with known renal or hepatic disease. Symptomatic worsening of ulcerative colitis may occur following initiation of treatment. May cause an acute intolerance syndrome (cramping, acute abdominal pain, bloody diarrhea; sometimes fever, headache, rash); discontinue if this occurs. May cause staining of teeth or tongue if capsule is opened and sprinkled on food.

Warnings: Additional Pediatric Considerations May exacerbate symptoms of ulcerative colitis; reported incidence higher in children than adults (6% vs 1%). Children may experience a higher frequency of some adverse effects than adults, including: Headache (15% vs 8%), abdominal pain (~13% vs 6%), and vomiting (10% vs ≤4%).

Adverse Reactions

Central nervous system: Fatigue, fever, headache (more common in children than adults), insomnia

Endocrine & metabolic: Dysmenorrhea

Gastrointestinal: Abdominal pain (more common in children than adults), anorexia, cramps, constipation, diarrhea, dyspepsia, flatulence, hematochezia, nausea, stomatitis, ulcerative colitis exacerbation, vomiting, xerostomia

Genitourinary: Urinary tract infection

Hematologic: Anemia

Neuromuscular & skeletal: Arthralgia, musculoskeletal pain, myalgia

Respiratory: Cough, pharyngolaryngeal pain, pharyngitis, respiratory infection, rhinitis

Miscellaneous: Flu-like syndrome

Rare but important or life-threatening: Alopecia, alveolitis, AST increased, back pain, blood pressure increased, cholestatic jaundice, cirrhosis, defecation urgency, dizziness, dyspnea, edema, erythema nodosum, facial edema, fever, gastroenteritis, gastroesophageal reflux, hard stool, heart rate increased, hepatocellular damage, hepatotoxicity, hyperbilirubinemia, hypersensitivity, interstitial nephritis, jaundice, Kawasaki-like syndrome, lethargy, liver failure, liver necrosis, liver function tests increased, malaise, myocarditis, pain, pancreatitis, pericarditis, pleural effusion, pneumonia (with and without eosinophilia), pruritus, rash, renal failure, vasculitis

Drug Interactions

Metabolism/Transport Effects None known.

Avoid Concomitant Use There are no known interactions where it is recommended to avoid concomitant use.

Increased Effect/Toxicity

Balsalazide may increase the levels/effects of: Heparin; Heparin (Low Molecular Weight); Thiopurine Analogs; Varicella Virus-Containing Vaccines

The levels/effects of Balsalazide may be increased by: Nonsteroidal Anti-Inflammatory Agents

Decreased Effect

Balsalazide may decrease the levels/effects of: Cardiac Glycosides

Storage/Stability Store at controlled room temperature of 20°C to 25°C (68°F to 77°F); excursions permitted to 15°C to 30°C (59°F to 86°F).

Mechanism of Action Balsalazide is a prodrug, converted by bacterial azoreduction to 5-aminosalicylic acid (mesalamine, active), 4-aminobenzoyl-β-alanine (inert), and their metabolites. 5-aminosalicylic acid may decrease inflammation by blocking the production of arachidonic acid metabolites topically in the colon mucosa.

Pharmacodynamics Onset of action: Delayed; may require several days to weeks (2 weeks); similar in adults and children

Pharmacokinetics (Adult data unless noted)

Absorption: Very low and variable; in children, reported systemic absorption of 5-ASA (active) lower than adults (C_{max}: 67% lower, AUC: 64% lower)

Protein binding: ≥99%

Metabolism: Azoreduced in the colon to 5-aminosalicylic acid (active), 4-aminobenzoyl-β-alanine (inert), and N-acetylated metabolites

Half-life: Primary effect is topical (colonic mucosa); therapeutic effect appears not to be influenced by the systemic half-life of balsalazide (1.9 hours) or its metabolites (5-ASA [9.5 hours], N-Ac-5-ASA [10.4 hours])

Time to peak serum concentration: Capsule: 1-2 hours; Tablet: 0.5 hours

Elimination: Feces (65% as 5-aminosalicylic acid, 4-aminobenzoyl-β-alanine, and N-acetylated metabolites); urine (11.3% as N-acetylated metabolites); Parent drug: Urine or feces (<1%)

Dosing: Usual

Children ≥5 years and Adolescents ≤17 years: **Ulcerative colitis:** Oral: Capsules: 2.25 g/day or 6.75 g/day for up to 8 weeks administered as either:

2.25 g (three 750 mg capsules) 3 times daily (total daily dose: 6.75 g/day)

or

750 mg (one capsule) 3 times daily (total daily dose: 2.25 g/day)

Note: Limited blinded clinical trial in children did not demonstrate significant improvement between total daily doses of 6.75 g or 2.25 g (Quiros, 2009).

Adolescents ≥18 years and Adults: **Ulcerative colitis:**

Capsule: 2.25 g (three 750 mg capsules) 3 times daily for up to 8-12 weeks

Tablet (Giazo™): Males: 3.3 g (three 1.1 g tablets) twice daily for up to 8 weeks

Dosing adjustment in renal impairment: There are no dosage adjustments provided in manufacturer's labeling. Renal toxicity has been observed with other 5-aminosalicylic acid products; use with caution.

Dosing adjustment in hepatic impairment: There are no dosage adjustments provided in manufacturer's labeling.

Administration

Capsules: Should be swallowed whole or may be opened and sprinkled on applesauce. Applesauce mixture may be chewed; swallow immediately, do not store mixture for later use. When sprinkled on food, may cause staining of teeth or tongue. Color variation of powder inside capsule (ranging from orange to yellow) is expected.

Tablets: Administer with or without food.

Monitoring Parameters Improvement or worsening of symptoms; renal function (prior to initiation, then periodically); liver function tests

Additional Information Balsalazide 750 mg is equivalent to mesalamine 267 mg.

Dosage Forms Excipient information presented when available (limited, particularly for generics); consult specific product labeling.

Capsule, Oral, as disodium:

Colazal: 750 mg

Generic: 750 mg

Tablet, Oral, as disodium:

Giazo: 1.1 g

- ◆ **Balsalazide Disodium** *see* Balsalazide *on page 257*
- ◆ **Banophen [OTC]** *see* DiphenhydrAMINE (Systemic) *on page 668*
- ◆ **Banophen [OTC]** *see* DiphenhydrAMINE (Topical) *on page 672*
- ◆ **Banzel** *see* Rufinamide *on page 1891*
- ◆ **Baraclude** *see* Entecavir *on page 756*
- ◆ **Baridium [OTC]** *see* Phenazopyridine *on page 1678*
- ◆ **Basaljel (Can)** *see* Aluminum Hydroxide *on page 110*
- ◆ **Base Ointment** *see* Zinc Oxide *on page 2214*

Basiliximab (ba si LIK si mab)

Medication Safety Issues

High alert medication:

This medication is in a class the Institute for Safe Medication Practices (ISMP) includes among its list of drug classes that have a heightened risk of causing significant patient harm when used in error.

Brand Names: US Simulect

Brand Names: Canada Simulect

Therapeutic Category Monoclonal Antibody

Generic Availability (US) No

Use In combination with an immunosuppressive regimen (cyclosporine and corticosteroids), induction therapy for the prophylaxis of acute organ rejection in patients receiving renal transplants (FDA approved in pediatric patients [age not specified] and adults); basiliximab has also been used in liver and heart transplant patients

Pregnancy Risk Factor B

Pregnancy Considerations Adverse effects were not observed in animal reproduction studies. IL-2 receptors play an important role in the development of the immune system. Women of childbearing potential should use effective contraceptive measures before beginning treatment, during, and for 4 months after completion of basiliximab treatment. The National Transplantation Pregnancy Registry (NTPR, Temple University) is a registry for pregnant women taking immunosuppressants following any solid organ transplant. The NTPR encourages reporting of all immunosuppressant exposures during pregnancy in transplant recipients at 877-955-6877.

Breast-Feeding Considerations It is not known if basiliximab is excreted in human milk. Because many immunoglobulins are secreted in milk and the potential for serious adverse reactions exists, a decision should be made to discontinue nursing or discontinue the drug, taking into account the importance of the drug to the mother. The Canadian labeling recommends women avoid nursing for 4 months following the last dose.

Contraindications Known hypersensitivity to basiliximab or any component of the formulation

Warnings/Precautions To be used as a component of an immunosuppressive regimen which includes cyclosporine and corticosteroids. The incidence of lymphoproliferative disorders and/or opportunistic infections may be increased by immunosuppressive therapy. Severe hypersensitivity reactions, occurring within 24 hours, have been reported. Reactions, including anaphylaxis, have occurred both with the initial exposure and/or following re-exposure after several months. Use caution during re-exposure to a subsequent course of therapy in a patient who has previously received basiliximab; patients in whom concomitant immunosuppression was prematurely discontinued due to abandoned transplantation or early graft loss are at increased risk for developing a severe hypersensitivity reaction upon re-exposure. Discontinue permanently if a severe reaction occurs. Medications for the treatment of hypersensitivity reactions should be available for immediate use. Treatment may result in the development of human antimurine antibodies (HAMA); however, limited evidence suggesting the use of muromonab-CD3 or other murine products is not precluded. **[U.S. Boxed Warning]: Should be administered under the supervision of a physician experienced in immunosuppression therapy and organ transplant management.** In renal transplant patients receiving basiliximab plus prednisone, cyclosporine, and mycophenolate, new-onset diabetes, glucose intolerance, and impaired fasting glucose were observed at rates significantly higher than observed in patients receiving prednisone, cyclosporine, and mycophenolate without basiliximab (Aasebo, 2010). Potentially significant drug-drug interactions may exist, requiring dose or frequency adjustment, additional monitoring, and/or selection of alternative therapy.

Adverse Reactions

Cardiovascular: Abnormal heart sounds, angina, arrhythmia, atrial fibrillation, chest pain, generalized edema, heart failure, hyper-/hypotension,peripheral edema, tachycardia

Central nervous system: Agitation, anxiety, depression, dizziness, fatigue, fever, headache, hypoesthesia, insomnia, malaise, pain

Dermatologic: Acne, cyst, hypertrichosis, pruritus, rash, skin disorder, skin ulceration, wound complications

Endocrine & metabolic: Acidosis, dehydration, diabetes mellitus, fluid overload, glucocorticoids increased, hyper-/hypocalcemia, hypercholesterolemia, hyperglycemia, hyper-/hypokalemia, hyperlipemia, hypertriglyceridemia, hyperuricemia, hypoglycemia, hypomagnesemia, hyponatremia, hypophosphatemia, hypoproteinemia

Gastrointestinal: Abdomen enlarged, abdominal pain, constipation, diarrhea, dyspepsia esophagitis, flatulence, gastroenteritis, GI hemorrhage, gingival hyperplasia, melena, moniliasis, nausea, stomatitis (including ulcerative), vomiting, weight gain

Genitourinary: Bladder disorder, dysuria, genital edema (male), impotence, ureteral disorder, urinary frequency, urinary retention, urinary tract infection
Hematologic: Anemia, hematoma, hemorrhage, leukopenia, polycythemia, purpura, thrombocytopenia, thrombosis
Neuromuscular & skeletal: Arthralgia, arthropathy, back pain, cramps, fracture, hernia, leg pain, myalgia, neuropathy, paresthesia, rigors, tremor, weakness
Ocular: Abnormal vision, cataract, conjunctivitis
Renal: Albuminuria, hematuria, nonprotein nitrogen increased, oliguria, renal function abnormal, renal tubular necrosis
Respiratory: Bronchitis, bronchospasm, cough, dyspnea, infection (upper respiratory), pharyngitis, pneumonia, pulmonary edema, rhinitis, sinusitis
Miscellaneous: Accidental trauma, cytomegalovirus (CMV) infection, herpes infection (simplex and zoster), infection, sepsis
Rare but important or life-threatening: Anaphylaxis, capillary leak syndrome, cytokine release syndrome, diabetes (new onset), fasting glucose impaired, glucose intolerance, hypersensitivity reaction (including heart failure, hypotension, tachycardia, bronchospasm, dyspnea, pulmonary edema, respiratory failure, sneezing, pruritus, rash, urticaria), lymphoproliferative disease

Drug Interactions

Metabolism/Transport Effects None known.

Avoid Concomitant Use

Avoid concomitant use of Basiliximab with any of the following: BCG; BCG (Intravesical); Belimumab; Natalizumab; Pimecrolimus; Tacrolimus (Topical); Tofacitinib; Vaccines (Live)

Increased Effect/Toxicity

Basiliximab may increase the levels/effects of: Belimumab; Leflunomide; Natalizumab; Tofacitinib; Vaccines (Live)

The levels/effects of Basiliximab may be increased by: Denosumab; Pimecrolimus; Roflumilast; Tacrolimus (Topical); Trastuzumab

Decreased Effect

Basiliximab may decrease the levels/effects of: BCG; BCG (Intravesical); Coccidioides immitis Skin Test; Sipuleucel-T; Vaccines (Inactivated); Vaccines (Live)

The levels/effects of Basiliximab may be decreased by: Echinacea

Storage/Stability Store intact vials refrigerated at 2°C to 8°C (36°F to 46°F). Should be used immediately after reconstitution; however, if not used immediately, reconstituted solution may be stored at 2°C to 8°C for up to 24 hours or at room temperature for up to 4 hours. Discard the reconstituted solution if not used within 24 hours.

Mechanism of Action Chimeric (murine/human) immunosuppressant monoclonal antibody which blocks the alpha-chain of the interleukin-2 (IL-2) receptor complex; this receptor is expressed on activated T lymphocytes and is a critical pathway for activating cell-mediated allograft rejection

Pharmacodynamics Duration: 36 days ± 14 days (determined by IL-2R alpha saturation in patients also on cyclosporine and corticosteroids)

Pharmacokinetics (Adult data unless noted) Note: Values based on data from renal transplant patients
Distribution: V_{dss}:
Children 1-11 years: 4.8 ± 2.1 L
Adolescents 12-16 years: 7.8 ± 5.1 L
Adults: 8.6 ± 4.1 L
Half-life:
Children 1-11 years: 9.5 ± 4.5 days
Adolescents 12-16 years: 9.1 ± 3.9 days
Adults: 7.2 ± 3.2 days
Elimination: Clearance:
Children 1-11 years: 17 ± 6 mL/hour; in pediatric liver transplant patients, significant basiliximab loss through ascites fluid can increase total body clearance and reduce IL-2R (CD25) saturation duration; dosage adjustments may be necessary (Cintorino, 2006; Kovarik, 2002; Spada, 2006)
Adolescents 12-16 years: 31 ±19 mL/hour
Adults: 41 ± 19 mL/hour

Dosing: Usual Note: Patients previously administered basiliximab should only be re-exposed to a subsequent course of therapy with extreme caution.
Infants, Children, and Adolescents:
Renal transplantation: IV:
Patient weight <35 kg:
Initial dose: 10 mg administered within 2 hours prior to renal transplant surgery
Second dose: 10 mg administered 4 days after transplantation; hold second dose if complications occur (including severe hypersensitivity reactions or graft loss)
Patient weight ≥35 kg:
Initial dose: 20 mg administered within 2 hours prior to renal transplant surgery
Second dose: 20 mg administered 4 days after transplantation; hold second dose if complications occur (including severe hypersensitivity reactions or graft loss)
Liver transplantation: IV: Limited data available (Cintorino, 2006; Kovarik, 2002; Spada, 2006):
Patient weight <35 kg:
Initial dose: 10 mg administered within 6 hours of organ perfusion
Second dose: 10 mg administered 4 days after transplantation; hold second dose if complications occur (including severe hypersensitivity reactions or graft loss)
Third dose: 10 mg has been repeated on postoperative days 8-10 if ascites fluid loss exceeds 70 mL/kg or >5 L
Patient weight ≥35 kg:
Initial dose: 20 mg administered within 6 hours of organ perfusion
Second dose: 20 mg administered 4 days after transplantation; hold second dose if complications occur (including severe hypersensitivity reactions or graft loss)
Third dose: 20 mg has been repeated on postoperative days 8-10 if ascites fluid loss exceeds 70 mL/kg or if total ascites volume ≥5 L
Heart transplantation: IV: Limited data available (Ford, 2005; Grundy, 2009):
Patient weight <35 kg:
Initial dose: 10 mg administered immediately before cardiopulmonary by-pass started or within 6 hours of organ perfusion
Second dose: 10 mg administered 4 days after transplantation; hold second dose if complications occur (including severe hypersensitivity reactions or graft loss)
Patient weight ≥35 kg:
Initial dose: 20 mg administered immediately before cardiopulmonary by-pass started or within 6 hours of organ perfusion
Second dose: 20 mg administered 4 days after transplantation; hold second dose if complications occur (including severe hypersensitivity reactions or graft loss)
Adults: **Renal transplantation:** IV:
Initial dose: 20 mg administered within 2 hours prior to renal transplant surgery
Second dose: 20 mg administered 4 days after transplantation; hold second dose if complications occur

(including severe hypersensitivity reactions or graft loss)

Dosing adjustment in renal impairment: There are no dosage adjustments provided in manufacturer's labeling.

Dosing adjustment in hepatic impairment: There are no dosage adjustments provided in manufacturer's labeling.

Preparation for Administration IV: Reconstitute with preservative-free SWFI (reconstitute 10 mg vial with 2.5 mL, 20 mg vial with 5 mL). Shake gently to dissolve. May further dilute reconstituted solution with 25 mL (10 mg) or 50 mL (20 mg) NS or D_5W. When mixing the solution, gently invert the bag to avoid foaming. Do not shake solutions diluted for infusion.

Administration For IV administration only. Administer only after assurance that patient will receive renal graft and immunosuppression. Reconstituted basiliximab solution may be administered without further dilution as a bolus injection over 10 minutes or further diluted and infused over 20 to 30 minutes. Bolus injection is associated with nausea, vomiting, and local pain at the injection site.

Monitoring Parameters CBC with differential, vital signs, immunologic monitoring of T cells, renal function, serum glucose, signs or symptoms of hypersensitivity, infection

Reference Range Serum concentration >0.2 mcg/mL

Dosage Forms Excipient information presented when available (limited, particularly for generics); consult specific product labeling.

Solution Reconstituted, Intravenous [preservative free]:
Simulect: 10 mg (1 ea); 20 mg (1 ea)

- ◆ **BAT** *see* Botulism Antitoxin, Heptavalent *on page 297*
- ◆ **Baycadron [DSC]** *see* Dexamethasone (Systemic) *on page 610*
- ◆ **Bayer Aspirin Extra Strength [OTC]** *see* Aspirin *on page 206*
- ◆ **Bayer Aspirin Regimen Adult Low Strength [OTC]** *see* Aspirin *on page 206*
- ◆ **Bayer Aspirin Regimen Children's [OTC]** *see* Aspirin *on page 206*
- ◆ **Bayer Aspirin Regimen Regular Strength [OTC]** *see* Aspirin *on page 206*
- ◆ **Bayer Genuine Aspirin [OTC]** *see* Aspirin *on page 206*
- ◆ **Bayer Plus Extra Strength [OTC]** *see* Aspirin *on page 206*
- ◆ **Bayer Women's Low Dose Aspirin [OTC]** *see* Aspirin *on page 206*
- ◆ **Baza Antifungal [OTC]** *see* Miconazole (Topical) *on page 1431*
- ◆ **BCNU** *see* Carmustine *on page 377*
- ◆ **BCX-1812** *see* Peramivir *on page 1672*
- ◆ **Bebulin** *see* Factor IX Complex (Human) [(Factors II, IX, X)] *on page 836*
- ◆ **Bebulin VH** *see* Factor IX Complex (Human) [(Factors II, IX, X)] *on page 836*
- ◆ **Becenum** *see* Carmustine *on page 377*

Beclomethasone (Nasal) (be kloe METH a sone)

Brand Names: US Beconase AQ; Qnasl; Qnasl Childrens

Brand Names: Canada Apo-Beclomethasone; Mylan-Beclo AQ; Rivanase AQ

Therapeutic Category Corticosteroid, Intranasal

Generic Availability (US) No

Use

Beconase® AQ: Management of nasal symptoms associated with seasonal or perennial allergic and non-allergic (vasomotor) rhinitis and prevention of recurrence of nasal polyps following surgical removal (FDA approved in ages ≥6 years and adults)

Qnasl™: Management of nasal symptoms associated with seasonal and perennial allergic rhinitis (FDA approved in ages ≥12 years and adults)

Intranasal corticosteroids have also been used as an adjunct to antibiotics in empiric treatment of acute bacterial rhinosinusitis primarily in patients with history of allergic rhinitis (Chow, 2012), in pediatric patients with mild obstructive sleep apnea syndrome who cannot undergo adenotonsillectomy or who still have symptoms after surgery (Marcus, 2012), and for children with nasal obstruction caused by adenoidal hypertrophy.

Pregnancy Risk Factor C

Pregnancy Considerations Adverse events have been observed in some animal reproduction studies. Hypoadrenalism may occur in newborns following maternal use of corticosteroids in pregnancy; monitor. Intranasal corticosteroids are recommended for the treatment of rhinitis during pregnancy; the lowest effective dose should be used (NAEPP, 2005; Wallace, 2008).

Breast-Feeding Considerations It is not known if beclomethasone is excreted in breast milk. The manufacturer recommends that caution be exercised when administering to nursing women. Use of inhaled corticosteroids is not a contraindication to breast-feeding (NAEPP, 2005).

Contraindications

Hypersensitivity to beclomethasone or any component of the formulation

Documentation of allergenic cross-reactivity for intranasal steroids is limited. However, the possibility of cross-sensitivity cannot be ruled out with certainty because of similarities in chemical structure and/or pharmacologic actions.

Canadian labeling: Additional contraindications (not in U.S. labeling): Active or quiescent tuberculosis or untreated fungal, bacterial and viral infections.

Warnings/Precautions Hypersensitivity reactions (including anaphylaxis, angioedema, rash, urticaria, and wheezing) have been reported; discontinue for severe reactions. May cause hypercorticism or suppression of hypothalamic-pituitary-adrenal (HPA) axis, particularly in younger children or in patients receiving high doses for prolonged periods. HPA axis suppression may lead to adrenal crisis. Withdrawal and discontinuation of a corticosteroid should be done slowly and carefully. Particular care is required when patients are transferred from systemic corticosteroids to inhaled products due to possible adrenal insufficiency or withdrawal from steroids, including an increase in allergic symptoms. Patients receiving >20 mg per day of prednisone (or equivalent) may be most susceptible. Fatalities have occurred due to adrenal insufficiency in asthmatic patients during and after transfer from systemic corticosteroids to aerosol steroids; aerosol steroids do not provide the systemic steroid needed to treat patients having trauma, surgery, or infections.

Hypersensitivity reactions, including anaphylaxis, angioedema, rash and urticaria have been reported; discontinue for severe reactions. Avoid nasal corticosteroid use in patients with recent nasal septal ulcers, nasal surgery or nasal trauma until healing has occurred. Nasal septal perforation and localized Candida albicans infections of the nose and/or pharynx may occur. Nasal discomfort, epistaxis, and nasal ulceration may also occur; periodically examine nasal mucosa in patients on long-term therapy. Monitor patients for adverse nasal effects; discontinuation of therapy may be necessary if an infection occurs.

Increased intraocular pressure, open-angle glaucoma, and cataracts have occurred with intranasal corticosteroid use; use with caution in patients with a history of increased intraocular pressure, cataracts and/or glaucoma. Consider routine eye exams in chronic users or in patients who report visual changes.

Prolonged use of corticosteroids may increase the incidence of secondary infections, mask an acute infection (including fungal infections), prolong or exacerbate viral infections, or limit response to vaccines; avoid exposure to chickenpox and/or measles, especially if not immunized. Avoid use or use with caution in patients with latent/active tuberculosis, untreated bacterial or fungal infections (local or systemic), viral or parasitic infections, or ocular herpes simplex.

Avoid using higher than recommended dosages; suppression of linear growth (ie, reduction of growth velocity), reduced bone mineral density, or hypercorticism (Cushing syndrome) may occur; titrate to lowest effective dose. Reduction in growth velocity may occur when corticosteroids are administered to pediatric patients, even at recommended doses via intranasal route (monitor growth). There have been reports of systemic corticosteroid withdrawal symptoms (eg, joint/muscle pain, lassitude, depression) when withdrawing oral inhalation therapy.

For rhinitis, do not use in the presence of untreated localized infection involving the nasal mucosa; do not continue use beyond 3 weeks in the absence of significant symptomatic improvement. For nasal polyps, treatment may need to be continued for several weeks or more before a therapeutic result can be fully assessed; recurrence can occur after stopping treatment.

Adverse Reactions

Central nervous system: Altered sense of smell, anosmia, dizziness, headache

Dermatologic: Skin rash, urticaria

Endocrine & metabolic: Adrenal suppression (at high doses or in susceptible individuals), hypercorticoidism (at high doses or in susceptible individuals)

Gastrointestinal: Ageusia, nausea, oral candidiasis (rare; more likely with aqueous solution), unpleasant taste

Hypersensitivity: Anaphylactoid reaction, anaphylaxis, angioedema

Immunologic: Immunosuppression

Neuromuscular & skeletal: Decreased linear skeletal growth rate

Ophthalmic: Cataract, glaucoma, intraocular pressure increased, lacrimation

Respiratory: Bronchospasm, dry nose, epistaxis, nasal congestion, nasal candidiasis (rare; more likely with aqueous solution), nasal mucosa irritation (erosion), pharyngeal candidiasis (rare; more likely with aqueous solution), rhinorrhea, sneezing, upper respiratory tract infection (children), wheezing

Respiratory: Nasopharyngitis (more commin in adults)

Miscellaneous: Fever (children), wound healing impairment

Rare but important or life-threatening: Nasal mucosa ulcer, nasal septum perforation

Drug Interactions

Metabolism/Transport Effects None known.

Avoid Concomitant Use There are no known interactions where it is recommended to avoid concomitant use.

Increased Effect/Toxicity

Beclomethasone (Nasal) may increase the levels/effects of: Ceritinib

Decreased Effect There are no known significant interactions involving a decrease in effect.

Storage/Stability

Beconase AQ: Store between 15°C to 30°C (59°F to 86°F).

Qnasl: Store at 25°C (77°F), excursions permitted to 15°C to 30°C (59°F to 86°F). Do not puncture. Do not store near heat or open flame. Do not expose to temperatures higher than 49°C (120°F).

Mechanism of Action Controls the rate of protein synthesis; depresses the migration of polymorphonuclear leukocytes, fibroblasts; reverses capillary permeability and lysosomal stabilization at the cellular level to prevent or control inflammation

Pharmacodynamics Onset of action: Within a few days up to 2 weeks

Pharmacokinetics (Adult data unless noted)

Distribution: V_d: Beclomethasone dipropionate (BDP): 20 L; 17-BMP: 424 L

Protein binding: BDP 87%; 17-BMP: 94% to 96%

Metabolism: BDP is a prodrug (inactive) which undergoes rapid hydrolysis to 17-BMP (active monoester) during absorption; BDP is also metabolized in the liver via cytochrome P450 isoenzyme CYP3A4 to 17-BMP and two other less active metabolites: Beclomethasone-21-monopropionate (21-BMP) and beclomethasone (BOH)

Bioavailability: Beconase AQ®: 17-BMP: 44% (43% from swallowed portion)

Half-life, elimination: BDP: 0.5 hours; 17-BMP: 2.7 hours

Elimination: Feces (60%), urine (12%; as free and conjugated metabolites)

Dosing: Usual Note: Product formulations are not interchangeable: Beconase® AQ: One spray delivers 42 mcg; Qnasl®: One spray delivers 80 mcg

Children and Adolescents:

Nasal airway obstruction/adenoidal hypertrophy: Limited data available; dosing regimens variable: Intranasal: Beconase AQ®: Children 5-12 years: Initial: 168 mcg twice daily delivered as 84 mcg (2 sprays) **per nostril** twice daily for 4 weeks, followed by 84 mcg twice daily delivered as 42 mcg (1 spray) **per nostril** twice daily. Dosing based on a double-blind, placebo-controlled crossover study (n=17, age range: 5-11 years); results showed significant reduction in adenoid hypertrophy and related obstructive nasal symptoms following 4 weeks of beclomethasone therapy vs placebo (Demain, 1995). Positive efficacy findings were also observed in a single-blind, placebo-controlled crossover study of 53 children (mean age: 3.8 ± 1.3 years) using a total daily dose of 400 mcg/day [200 mcg twice daily (using 50 mcg/spray formulation, not available in U.S.)] delivered as 100 mcg (2 sprays) **per nostril** twice daily (Criscuoli, 2003). Lower daily dosage (200 mcg/day) have not been found effective (Lepcha, 2002).

Allergic rhinitis: Intranasal:

Beconase® AQ:

Children 6-12 years: Initial: 84 mcg twice daily delivered as 42 mcg (1 spray) **per nostril** twice daily; may increase if needed to 168 mcg twice daily delivered as 84 mcg (2 sprays) **per nostril** twice daily; once symptoms are adequately controlled, decrease dose to 84 mcg twice daily delivered as 42 mcg (1 spray) **per nostril** twice daily.

Children and Adolescents ≥12 years: 84 or 168 mcg twice daily delivered as 42 mcg (1 spray) or 84 mcg (2 sprays) **per nostril** twice daily.

Qnasl™: Children and Adolescents ≥12 years: 320 mcg once daily delivered as 160 mcg (2 sprays) **per nostril** once daily

Nasal polyps (postsurgical prophylaxis), vasomotor rhinitis: Intranasal: Beconase® AQ:

Children 6-12 years: Initial: 84 mcg twice daily delivered as 42 mcg (1 spray) **per nostril** twice daily; may increase if needed to 168 mcg twice daily delivered as 84 mcg (2 sprays) **per nostril** twice daily; once symptoms are adequately controlled, decrease dose to 84 mcg twice daily delivered as 42 mcg (1 spray) **per nostril** twice daily

Children and Adolescents ≥12 years: 84 or 168 mcg twice daily delivered as 42 mcg (1 spray) or 84 mcg (2 sprays) **per nostril** twice daily

Adults:

Allergic rhinitis: Intranasal:

Beconase® AQ: 84 or 168 mcg twice daily delivered as 42 mcg (1 spray) or 84 mcg (2 sprays) **per nostril** twice daily

Qnasl™: 320 mcg once daily delivered as 160 mcg (2 sprays) **per nostril** once daily

Nasal polyps (postsurgical prophylaxis), vasomotor rhinitis: Intranasal: Beconase AQ®: 84 or 168 mcg twice daily delivered as 42 mcg (1 spray) or 84 mcg (2 sprays) **per nostril** twice daily

Dosing adjustment in renal impairment: There are no dosage adjustments provided in the manufacturer's labeling.

Dosing adjustment in hepatic impairment: There are no dosage adjustments provided in the manufacturer's labeling.

Administration Shake well prior to each use. Blow nose to clear nostrils. Insert applicator into nostril, keeping bottle upright, and close off the other nostril. Breathe in through nose. While inhaling, press pump to release spray. Avoid spraying directly onto the nasal septum or into eyes. Discard after the "discard by" date or after labeled number of doses has been used, even if bottle is not completely empty.

Beconase® AQ: Prior to initial use, prime pump 6 times (or until fine spray appears); repeat priming if product not used for ≥7 days. Nasal applicator and dust cap may be washed in warm water and dry thoroughly.

Qnasl™: Prior to initial use, prime pump 4 times. If product not used for ≥7 days, prime pump 2 times.

Monitoring Parameters Mucous membranes for signs of fungal infection, growth (pediatric patients), signs/symptoms of HPA axis suppression/adrenal insufficiency; ocular changes

Additional Information When used short term as adjunctive therapy in acute bacterial rhinosinusitis (ABRS), intranasal steroids show modest symptomatic improvement and few adverse effects; improvement is primarily due to increased sinus drainage. Use should be considered optional in ABRS; however, intranasal corticosteroids should be routinely prescribed to ABRS patients who have a history of or concurrent allergic rhinitis (Chow 2012).

Dosage Forms Considerations

Beconase AQ 25 g bottles contain 180 sprays.

Qnasl 8.7 g bottles contain 120 actuations.

Dosage Forms Excipient information presented when available (limited, particularly for generics); consult specific product labeling.

Aerosol Solution, Nasal, as dipropionate:

Qnasl: 80 mcg/actuation (8.7 g)

Qnasl Childrens: 40 mcg/actuation (4.9 g)

Suspension, Nasal, as dipropionate:

Beconase AQ: 42 mcg/spray (25 g) [contains benzalkonium chloride]

Beclomethasone (Oral Inhalation)

(be kloe METH a sone)

Related Information

Inhaled Corticosteroids *on page 2261*

Brand Names: US Qvar

Brand Names: Canada QVAR

Therapeutic Category Adrenal Corticosteroid; Anti-inflammatory Agent; Antiasthmatic; Corticosteroid, Inhalant (Oral); Glucocorticoid

Generic Availability (US) No

Use Long-term (chronic) control of persistent bronchial asthma (FDA approved in ages ≥5 years and adults); **not** indicated for the relief of acute bronchospasm. Also used to help reduce or discontinue oral corticosteroid therapy for asthma.

Pregnancy Risk Factor C

Pregnancy Considerations Adverse events have been observed in animal reproduction studies. Hypoadrenalism may occur in newborns following maternal use of corticosteroids in pregnancy. Based on available data, an overall increased risk of congenital malformations or a decrease in fetal growth has not been associated with maternal use of inhaled corticosteroids during pregnancy (Bakhireva, 2005; NAEPP, 2005; Namazy, 2004). Uncontrolled asthma is associated with adverse events in pregnancy (increased risk of perinatal mortality, pre-eclampsia, preterm birth, low birth weight infants). Inhaled corticosteroids are recommended for the treatment of asthma during pregnancy (most information available using budesonide) (ACOG, 2008; NAEPP, 2005).

Breast-Feeding Considerations Other corticosteroids have been found in breast milk; however, information for beclomethasone is not available. Due to the potential for serious adverse reactions in the nursing infant, the manufacturer recommends a decision be made whether to discontinue nursing or to discontinue the drug, taking into account the importance of treatment to the mother. Use of inhaled corticosteroids is not a contraindication to breast-feeding (NAEPP, 2005).

Contraindications

Hypersensitivity to beclomethasone or any component of the formulation; status asthmaticus, or other acute asthma episodes requiring intensive measures

Documentation of allergenic cross-reactivity for corticosteroids is limited. However, because of similarities in chemical structure and/or pharmacologic actions, the possibility of cross-sensitivity cannot be ruled out with certainty.

Canadian labeling: Additional contraindications (not in US labeling): Moderate to severe bronchiectasis requiring intensive measures; untreated fungal, bacterial, or tubercular infections of the respiratory tract

Warnings/Precautions May cause hypercorticism or suppression of hypothalamic-pituitary-adrenal (HPA) axis, particularly in younger children or in patients receiving high doses for prolonged periods. HPA axis suppression may lead to adrenal crisis. Withdrawal and discontinuation of a corticosteroid should be done slowly and carefully. Particular care is required when patients are transferred from systemic corticosteroids to inhaled products due to possible adrenal insufficiency or withdrawal from steroids, including an increase in allergic symptoms. Patients receiving >20 mg per day of prednisone (or equivalent) may be most susceptible. Fatalities have occurred due to adrenal insufficiency in asthmatic patients during and after transfer from systemic corticosteroids to aerosol steroids; aerosol steroids do **not** provide the systemic steroid needed to treat patients having trauma, surgery, or infections (particularly gastroenteritis), or other conditions with severe electrolyte loss. Select surgical patients on long-term, high-dose, inhaled corticosteroid (ICS), should be given stress doses of hydrocortisone intravenously during the surgical period and the dose reduced rapidly within 24 hours after surgery (Expert Panel Report 3, 2007).

Bronchospasm may occur with wheezing after inhalation (possibly life-threatening); if bronchospasm occurs, discontinue steroid and treat with a fast-acting bronchodilator. Supplemental steroids (oral or parenteral) may be needed during stress or severe asthma attacks. Not to be used in status asthmaticus or for the relief of acute bronchospasm. Immediate hypersensitivity reactions may occur, including angioedema, bronchospasm, rash, and urticaria; discontinue use if reaction occurs. Corticosteroid use may cause psychiatric disturbances, including depression, euphoria, insomnia, mood swings, and personality changes. Preexisting psychiatric conditions may be exacerbated by corticosteroid use. Prolonged use of corticosteroids may also increase the incidence of secondary infection, mask acute infection (including fungal infections), prolong or exacerbate viral infections, or limit response to vaccines. Avoid use, if possible, in patients with ocular herpes, active or quiescent respiratory or untreated viral, fungal, parasitic or bacterial systemic infections (Canadian labeling contraindicates use with untreated respiratory infections). Exposure to chickenpox or measles should be avoided. Close observation is required in patients with latent tuberculosis and/or TB reactivity; restrict use in active TB. Prolonged treatment with corticosteroids has been associated with the development of Kaposi sarcoma (case reports); if noted, discontinuation of therapy should be considered. *Candida albicans* infections may occur in the mouth and pharynx; rinsing (and spitting) with water after inhaler use may decrease risk. Rare cases of vasculitis (Churg-Strauss syndrome) or other systemic eosinophilic conditions can occur; often associated with decrease and/or withdrawal of oral corticosteroid therapy following initiation of inhaled corticosteroid.

Use with caution in patients with major risk factors for decreased bone mineral count. Use with caution in patients with thyroid disease, hepatic impairment, renal impairment, cardiovascular disease, diabetes, glaucoma, cataracts, myasthenia gravis, patients at risk for seizures, or GI diseases (diverticulitis, peptic ulcer, ulcerative colitis). Use caution following acute MI (corticosteroids have been associated with myocardial rupture). Because of the risk of adverse effects, systemic corticosteroids should be used cautiously in elderly patients in the smallest possible effective dose for the shortest duration.

Orally inhaled corticosteroids may cause a reduction in growth velocity in pediatric patients (~1 centimeter per year [range: 0.3 to 1.8 cm per year] and related to dose and duration of exposure). To minimize the systemic effects of orally inhaled corticosteroids, each patient should be titrated to the lowest effective dose. Growth should be routinely monitored in pediatric patients. A gradual tapering of dose may be required prior to discontinuing therapy; there have been reports of systemic corticosteroid withdrawal symptoms (eg, joint/muscle pain, lassitude, depression) when withdrawing oral inhalation therapy. When transferring to oral inhalation therapy from systemic corticosteroid therapy; previously suppressed allergic conditions (rhinitis, conjunctivitis, eczema, arthritis, and eosinophilic conditions) may be unmasked; during transition monitor pulmonary function tests (FEV_1 or PEF), beta-agonist use, and asthma symptoms and observe for signs and symptoms of adrenal insufficiency.

Warnings: Additional Pediatric Considerations Reduction in growth velocity may occur when corticosteroids are administered to pediatric patients, even at recommended doses via inhaled route; reduction in growth velocity is related to dose and duration of exposure; monitor growth. With beclomethasone-HFA (Qvar), the mean reduction in growth velocity was 0.5 cm/year less than that with the previous beclomethasone CFC inhaler formulation. Use of Qvar with a spacer device is not recommended in children<5 years of age due to the decreased amount of medication that is delivered with increasing wait times; patients should be instructed to inhale immediately if using a spacer device.

Adverse Reactions

Central nervous system: Headache, pain, voice disorder

Gastrointestinal: Nausea

Genitourinary: Dysmenorrhea

Neuromuscular & skeletal: Back pain

Respiratory: Cough, pharyngitis, rhinitis, sinusitis, upper respiratory tract infection

Rare but important or life-threatening: Anaphylactoid reaction, anaphylaxis, behavioral changes (such as aggressiveness, depression, sleep disturbances, psychomotor hyperactivity, suicidal ideation; more common in children), decreased linear skeletal growth rate (in children/adolescents), hypersensitivity reaction (immediate and delayed; including angioedema, bronchospasm, rash, urticaria), HPA-axis suppression; rarely glaucoma, increased intraocular pressure, and cataracts have been reported with inhaled corticosteroids

Drug Interactions

Metabolism/Transport Effects None known.

Avoid Concomitant Use

Avoid concomitant use of Beclomethasone (Oral Inhalation) with any of the following: Aldesleukin; BCG; BCG (Intravesical); Loxapine; Natalizumab; Pimecrolimus; Tacrolimus (Topical); Tofacitinib

Increased Effect/Toxicity

Beclomethasone (Oral Inhalation) may increase the levels/effects of: Amphotericin B; Ceritinib; Deferasirox; Leflunomide; Loop Diuretics; Loxapine; Natalizumab; Thiazide Diuretics; Tofacitinib

The levels/effects of Beclomethasone (Oral Inhalation) may be increased by: Denosumab; Pimecrolimus; Tacrolimus (Topical); Telaprevir; Trastuzumab

Decreased Effect

Beclomethasone (Oral Inhalation) may decrease the levels/effects of: Aldesleukin; BCG; BCG (Intravesical); Coccidioides immitis Skin Test; Corticorelin; Hyaluronidase; Sipuleucel-T; Telaprevir; Vaccines (Inactivated)

The levels/effects of Beclomethasone (Oral Inhalation) may be decreased by: Echinacea

Storage/Stability Store at 25°C (77°F); excursions are permitted between 15°C and 30°C (59°F and 86°F). Do not use or store near heat or open flame. Do not puncture canisters. Store on concave end of canister with actuator on top.

Mechanism of Action Controls the rate of protein synthesis; depresses the migration of polymorphonuclear leukocytes, fibroblasts; reverses capillary permeability and lysosomal stabilization at the cellular level to prevent or control inflammation

Pharmacodynamics Onset of action: Within 1-2 days in some patients; usually within 1-2 weeks; Maximum effect: 3-4 weeks

Pharmacokinetics (Adult data unless noted)

Absorption: Readily absorbed; quickly hydrolyzed by pulmonary esterases to active metabolite, beclomethasone-17-monoproprionate (17-BMP), prior to absorption

Distribution: V_d: Beclomethasone dipropionate (BDP): 20 L; 17-BMP: 424 L

Protein binding: BDP 87%; 17-BMP: 94% to 96%

Metabolism: BDP is a prodrug (inactive) which undergoes rapid hydrolysis to 17-BMP (active monoester) during absorption; BDP is also metabolized in the liver via cytochrome P450 isoenzyme CYP3A4 to 17-BMP and two other less active metabolites: Beclomethasone-21-monopropionate (21-BMP) and beclomethasone (BOH)

Half-life, elimination: BDP: 0.5 hours; 17-BMP: 2.7 hours

Time to peak serum concentration: BDP: 0.5 hours; 17-BMP: 0.7 hours

Elimination: Primary route of excretion is via feces (~60%); <10% to 12% of oral dose excreted in urine as metabolites

Dosing: Usual

Pediatric: **Note:** Doses should be titrated to the lowest effective dose once asthma is controlled: **Asthma, maintenance therapy:** Children ≥5 years and Adolescents: Inhalation, oral:

Manufacturer's labeling (Qvar):

Children 5-11 years: Initial: 40 mcg twice daily; maximum dose: 80 mcg twice daily

Children ≥12 years and Adolescents:
No previous inhaled corticosteroids: Initial: 40-80 mcg twice daily; maximum dose: 320 mcg twice daily
Previous inhaled corticosteroid use: Initial: 40-160 mcg twice daily; maximum dose: 320 mcg twice daily
Note: Therapeutic ratio between Qvar and other beclomethasone inhalers (eg, CFC formulations; however, none are currently available in U.S.) has not been established.

Alternate dosing: NIH Asthma Guidelines (NAEPP, 2007): HFA formulation (Qvar):
Children 5-11 years: Administer in divided doses:
"Low" dose: 80-160 mcg/day (40 mcg/puff: 2-4 puffs/day or 80 mcg/puff: 1-2 puffs/day)
"Medium" dose: >160-320 mcg/day (40 mcg/puff: 4-8 puffs/day or 80 mcg/puff: 2-4 puffs/day)
"High" dose: >320 mcg/day (40 mcg/puff: >8 puffs/day or 80 mcg/puff: >4 puff/day)
Children ≥12 years and Adolescents:
"Low" dose: 80-240 mcg/day (40 mcg/puff: 2-6 puffs/day or 80 mcg/puff: 1-3 puffs/day)
"Medium" dose: >240-480 mcg/day (40 mcg/puff: 6-12 puffs/day or 80 mcg/puff: 3-6 puffs/day)
"High" dose: >480 mcg/day (40 mcg/puff: >12 puffs/day or 80 mcg/puff: 6 puffs/day)

Conversion from oral systemic corticosteroid to orally inhaled corticosteroid: Initiation of oral inhalation therapy should begin in patients whose asthma is reasonably stabilized on oral corticosteroids (OCS). A gradual dose reduction of OCS should begin ~7 days after starting inhaled therapy. U.S. labeling recommends reducing prednisone dose no more rapidly than ≤2.5 mg/day (or equivalent of other OCS) every 1-2 weeks in adolescents or adults. If adrenal insufficiency occurs, temporarily increase the OCS dose and follow with a more gradual withdrawal. **Note:** When transitioning from systemic to inhaled corticosteroids, supplemental systemic corticosteroid therapy may be necessary during periods of stress or during severe asthma attacks.

Adult: **Asthma**: Inhalation, oral (doses should be titrated to the lowest effective dose once asthma is controlled):
Patients previously on bronchodilators only: Initial dose 40-80 mcg twice daily; maximum dose: 320 mcg twice day
Patients previously on inhaled corticosteroids: Initial dose 40-160 mcg twice daily; maximum dose: 320 mcg twice daily
NIH Asthma Guidelines (NIH, 2007):
"Low" dose: 80-240 mcg/day
"Medium" dose: >240-480 mcg/day
"High" dose: >480 mcg/day

Conversion from oral systemic corticosteroid to orally inhaled corticosteroid: Initiation of oral inhalation therapy should begin in patients whose asthma is reasonably stabilized on oral corticosteroids (OCS). A gradual dose reduction of OCS should begin ~7 days after starting inhaled therapy. U.S. labeling recommends reducing prednisone dose no more rapidly than ≤2.5 mg/day (or equivalent of other OCS) every 1-2 weeks. If adrenal insufficiency occurs, temporarily increase the OCS dose and follow with a more gradual withdrawal. **Note:** When transitioning from systemic to inhaled corticosteroids, supplemental systemic corticosteroid therapy may be necessary during periods of stress or during severe asthma attacks.

Administration Qvar, metered dose inhaler: Canister does not need to be shaken prior to use. Prime canister by spraying twice into the air prior to initial use or if not in use for >10 days. Avoid spraying in face or eyes. Exhale fully prior to bringing inhaler to mouth. Place inhaler in mouth, close lips around mouthpiece, and inhale slowly and deeply while pressing down on the canister with your finger. Remove inhaler and hold breath for approximately 5-10 seconds. Rinse mouth and throat after use to prevent *Candida* infection. Do not wash or put inhaler in water; mouth piece may be cleaned with a dry tissue or cloth. Discard after the "discard by" date or after labeled number of doses has been used, even if container is not completely empty. Patients using a spacer should inhale immediately due to decreased amount of medication that is delivered with a delayed inspiration. **Note:** Use of Qvar with a spacer device is not recommended in children <5 years of age due to the decreased amount of medication that is delivered with increasing wait times; patients should be instructed to inhale immediately if using a spacer device.

Monitoring Parameters Check mucous membranes for signs of fungal infection; monitor growth in pediatric patients; monitor IOP with therapy >6 weeks. Monitor for symptoms of asthma, FEV_1, peak flow, and/or other pulmonary function tests

Additional Information Qvar: Does not contain chlorofluorocarbons (CFCs), uses hydrofluoroalkane (HFA) as the propellant; is a solution formulation; uses smaller-size particles which results in a higher percent of drug delivered to the respiratory tract and lower recommended doses than other products. An open-label, randomized, multicenter, 12-month study in 300 asthmatic children 5-11 years of age indicated that QVAR provided long-term control of asthma at approximately half the dose compared with a CFC propelled beclomethasone MDI and spacer (Pedersen, 2002).

Dosage Forms Considerations
QVAR 8.7 g canisters contain 120 inhalations.

Dosage Forms Excipient information presented when available (limited, particularly for generics); consult specific product labeling.
Aerosol Solution, Inhalation, as dipropionate:
Qvar: 40 mcg/actuation (8.7 g); 80 mcg/actuation (8.7 g)

◆ **Beclomethasone Dipropionate** *see* Beclomethasone (Nasal) *on page 260*

◆ **Beconase AQ** *see* Beclomethasone (Nasal) *on page 260*

◆ **Belladonna Alkaloids With Phenobarbital** *see* Hyoscyamine, Atropine, Scopolamine, and Phenobarbital *on page 1062*

Belladonna and Opium (bel a DON a & OH pee um)

Medication Safety Issues
Sound-alike/look-alike issues:
B&O may be confused with beano
High alert medication:
The Institute for Safe Medication Practices (ISMP) includes this medication among its list of drug classes which have a heightened risk of causing significant patient harm when used in error.
BEERS Criteria medication:
This drug may be potentially inappropriate for use in geriatric patients (Quality of evidence - moderate; Strength of recommendation - strong).

Therapeutic Category Analgesic, Narcotic; Antispasmodic Agent, Urinary

Generic Availability (US) Yes

Use Relief of moderate to severe pain associated with rectal or bladder tenesmus that may occur in postoperative states and neoplastic situations; relief of pain associated with ureteral spasms not responsive to nonopioid analgesics and to space intervals between injections of opioids

Pregnancy Risk Factor C

Pregnancy Considerations Animal reproduction studies have not been conducted with this combination. See individual agents.

Breast-Feeding Considerations It is not known if morphine or atropine is excreted in breast milk following rectal administration of this combination. The manufacturer recommends that caution be exercised when administering to breast-feeding women. See individual agents.

Contraindications Glaucoma; severe renal or hepatic disease; bronchial asthma; narcotic idiosyncrasies; respiratory depression; convulsive disorders; acute alcoholism; delirium tremens; premature labor

Warnings/Precautions May cause CNS depression, which may impair physical or mental abilities; patients must be cautioned about performing tasks which require mental alertness (eg, operating machinery or driving). Usual precautions of opioid agonist therapy should be observed. Use caution with known idiosyncrasy to atropine or atropine-like compounds; hypersensitivity reactions to other phenanthrene-derivative opioid agonists (codeine, hydrocodone, hydromorphone, levorphanol, oxycodone, oxymorphone); debilitated patients; persons dependent upon opioids; biliary tract impairment; adrenal insufficiency; pancreatitis; cardiac disease; prostatic hyperplasia; increased intracranial pressure; toxic psychosis; myxedema. Avoid long-term use in the elderly due to potent anticholinergic effects and uncertain effectiveness (Beers Criteria). Potentially significant interactions may exist, requiring dose or frequency adjustment, additional monitoring, and/or selection of alternative therapy.

Adverse Reactions

Cardiovascular: Palpitations

Central nervous system: Dizziness, drowsiness

Dermatologic: Pruritus, urticaria

Gastrointestinal: Constipation, nausea, vomiting, xerostomia

Genitourinary: Urinary retention

Ophthalmic: Blurred vision, photophobia

Rare but important or life-threatening: Hypogonadism (Brennan, 2013; Debono, 2011)

Drug Interactions

Metabolism/Transport Effects None known.

Avoid Concomitant Use

Avoid concomitant use of Belladonna and Opium with any of the following: Aclidinium; Azelastine (Nasal); Eluxadoline; Glucagon; Ipratropium (Oral Inhalation); Mixed Agonist / Antagonist Opioids; Orphenadrine; Paraldehyde; Potassium Chloride; Thalidomide; Tiotropium; Umeclidinium

Increased Effect/Toxicity

Belladonna and Opium may increase the levels/effects of: AbobotulinumtoxinA; Alcohol (Ethyl); Alvimopan; Analgesics (Opioid); Anticholinergic Agents; Azelastine (Nasal); CNS Depressants; Desmopressin; Diuretics; Eluxadoline; Glucagon; Hydrocodone; Methotrimeprazine; Metyrosine; Mirabegron; Mirtazapine; OnabotulinumtoxinA; Orphenadrine; Paraldehyde; Potassium Chloride; Pramipexole; RimabotulinumtoxinB; ROPINIRole; Rotigotine; Selective Serotonin Reuptake Inhibitors; Suvorexant; Thalidomide; Thiazide Diuretics; Tiotropium; Topiramate; Zolpidem

The levels/effects of Belladonna and Opium may be increased by: Aclidinium; Amphetamines; Anticholinergic Agents; Antipsychotic Agents (Phenothiazines); Brimonidine (Topical); Cannabis; Doxylamine; Dronabinol; Droperidol; HydrOXYzine; Ipratropium (Oral Inhalation); Kava Kava; Magnesium Sulfate; MAO Inhibitors; Methotrimeprazine; Mianserin; Nabilone; Perampanel; Pramlintide; Rufinamide; Sodium Oxybate; Succinylcholine; Tapentadol; Tetrahydrocannabinol; Umeclidinium

Decreased Effect

Belladonna and Opium may decrease the levels/effects of: Acetylcholinesterase Inhibitors; Itopride; Metoclopramide; Pegvisomant; Secretin

The levels/effects of Belladonna and Opium may be decreased by: Acetylcholinesterase Inhibitors; Ammonium Chloride; Mixed Agonist / Antagonist Opioids; Naltrexone

Storage/Stability Store at room temperature. Do not refrigerate.

Mechanism of Action The pharmacologically active agents present in the belladonna component are atropine and scopolamine. Atropine blocks the action of acetylcholine at parasympathetic sites in smooth muscle, secretory glands, and the CNS causing a relaxation of smooth muscle and drying of secretions. The principle agent in opium is morphine. Morphine binds to opiate receptors in the CNS, causing inhibition of ascending pain pathways, altering the perception of and response to pain.

Pharmacodynamics Opium: Onset of action: Within 30 minutes

Pharmacokinetics (Adult data unless noted) Metabolism: Hepatic

Dosing: Usual Rectal: Adults: 1 suppository 1-2 times/day, up to 4 doses/day

Administration Rectal: Remove from foil; moisten finger and suppository; insert rectally

Controlled Substance C-II

Dosage Forms Excipient information presented when available (limited, particularly for generics); consult specific product labeling.

Suppository: Belladonna extract 16.2 mg and opium 30 mg; belladonna extract 16.2 mg and opium 60 mg

- ◆ **Benadryl [OTC]** *see* DiphenhydrAMINE (Systemic) *on page 668*
- ◆ **Benadryl (Can)** *see* DiphenhydrAMINE (Systemic) *on page 668*
- ◆ **Benadryl Allergy [OTC]** *see* DiphenhydrAMINE (Systemic) *on page 668*
- ◆ **Benadryl Allergy Childrens [OTC]** *see* DiphenhydrAMINE (Systemic) *on page 668*
- ◆ **Benadryl® Cream (Can)** *see* DiphenhydrAMINE (Topical) *on page 672*
- ◆ **Benadryl Dye-Free Allergy [OTC]** *see* DiphenhydrAMINE (Systemic) *on page 668*
- ◆ **Benadryl Itch Relief [OTC]** *see* DiphenhydrAMINE (Topical) *on page 672*
- ◆ **Benadryl® Itch Relief Stick (Can)** *see* DiphenhydrAMINE (Topical) *on page 672*
- ◆ **Benadryl Itch Stopping [OTC]** *see* DiphenhydrAMINE (Topical) *on page 672*
- ◆ **Benadryl Maximum Strength [OTC]** *see* DiphenhydrAMINE (Topical) *on page 672*
- ◆ **Benadryl® Spray (Can)** *see* DiphenhydrAMINE (Topical) *on page 672*

Benazepril (ben AY ze pril)

Medication Safety Issues

Sound-alike/look-alike issues:

Benazepril may be confused with Benadryl

Lotensin may be confused with Lioresal, lorcaserin, lovastatin

Brand Names: US Lotensin

Brand Names: Canada Lotensin

Therapeutic Category Angiotensin-Converting Enzyme (ACE) Inhibitor; Antihypertensive Agent

Generic Availability (US) Yes

Use Treatment of hypertension, either alone or in combination with a thiazide diuretic (FDA approved in ages ≥6 years and adults)

Pregnancy Risk Factor D

Pregnancy Considerations **[U.S. Boxed Warning]: Drugs that act on the renin-angiotensin system can cause injury and death to the developing fetus. Discontinue as soon as possible once pregnancy is detected.** Benazepril crosses the placenta. Drugs that act on the renin-angiotensin system are associated with oligohydramnios. Oligohydramnios, due to decreased fetal renal function, may lead to fetal lung hypoplasia and skeletal malformations. Their use in pregnancy is also associated with anuria, hypotension, renal failure, skull hypoplasia, and death in the fetus/neonate. Teratogenic effects may occur following maternal use of an ACE inhibitor during the first trimester, although this finding may be confounded by maternal disease. Because adverse fetal events are well documented with exposure later in pregnancy, ACE inhibitor use in pregnant women is not recommended (Seely 2014; Weber 2014). Infants exposed to an ACE inhibitor in utero should be monitored for hyperkalemia, hypotension, and oliguria. Oligohydramnios may not appear until after irreversible fetal injury has occurred. Exchange transfusions or dialysis may be required to reverse hypotension or improve renal function, although data related to the effectiveness in neonates is limited.

Chronic maternal hypertension itself is also associated with adverse events in the fetus/infant and mother. ACE inhibitors are not recommended for the treatment of uncomplicated hypertension in pregnancy (ACOG 2013) and they are specifically contraindicated for the treatment of hypertension and chronic heart failure during pregnancy by some guidelines (Regitz-Zagrosek 2011). In addition, ACE inhibitors should generally be avoided in women of reproductive age (ACOG 2013). If treatment for hypertension or chronic heart failure in pregnancy is needed, other agents should be used (ACOG 2013; Regitz-Zagrosek 2011).

Breast-Feeding Considerations Small amounts of benazepril and benazeprilat are found in breast milk. Some guidelines consider benazepril to be acceptable for use in breast-feeding women. Monitoring of the nursing child's weight for the first 4 weeks is recommended (Regitz-Zagrosek 2011).

Contraindications Hypersensitivity to benazepril or any component of the formulation; patients with a history of angioedema (with or without prior ACE inhibitor therapy); concomitant use with aliskiren in patients with diabetes mellitus

Canadian labeling: Additional contraindications (not in U.S. labeling): Concomitant use with aliskiren in patients with moderate to severe renal impairment (GFR <60 mL/minute/1.73 m^2); pregnancy; breast-feeding; rare hereditary problems of galactose intolerance (eg, galactosemia, Lapp Lactase deficiency or glucose-galactose malabsorption)

Warnings/Precautions Anaphylactic reactions may occur rarely with ACE inhibitors. At any time during treatment (especially following first dose) angioedema may occur rarely with ACE inhibitors. It may involve the head and neck (potentially compromising airway) or the intestine (presenting with abdominal pain). African-Americans and patients with idiopathic or hereditary angioedema may be at an increased risk. Prolonged frequent monitoring may be required especially if tongue, glottis, or larynx are involved as they are associated with airway obstruction. Patients with a history of airway surgery may have a higher risk of airway obstruction. Aggressive early and appropriate management is critical. Contraindicated in patients with history of angioedema with or without prior ACE inhibitor therapy. Hypersensitivity reactions may be seen during hemodialysis (eg, CVVHD) with high-flux dialysis membranes (eg, AN69), and rarely, during low density lipoprotein apheresis with dextran sulfate cellulose. Rare cases of anaphylactoid reactions have been reported in patients undergoing sensitization treatment with hymenoptera (bee, wasp) venom while receiving ACE inhibitors.

Symptomatic hypotension with or without syncope can occur with ACE inhibitors (usually with the first several doses); effects are most often observed in volume depleted patients; close monitoring of patient is required especially with initial dosing and dosing increases; blood pressure must be lowered at a rate appropriate for the patient's clinical condition. Initiation of therapy in patients with ischemic heart disease or cerebrovascular disease warrants close observation due to the potential consequences posed by falling blood pressure (eg, MI, stroke). Use with caution in hypertrophic cardiomyopathy with outflow tract obstruction and severe aortic stenosis. In patients on chronic ACE inhibitor therapy, intraoperative hypotension may occur with induction and maintenance of general anesthesia; use with caution before, during, or immediately after major surgery. Cardiopulmonary bypass, intraoperative blood loss, or vasodilating anesthesia increases endogenous renin release. Use of ACE inhibitors perioperatively will blunt angiotensin II formation and may result in hypotension. However, discontinuation of therapy prior to surgery is controversial. If continued preoperatively, avoidance of hypotensive agents during surgery is prudent (Hillis, 2011). **[U.S. Boxed Warning]: Drugs that act on the renin-angiotensin system can cause injury and death to the developing fetus. Discontinue as soon as possible once pregnancy is detected.**

Hyperkalemia may occur with ACE inhibitors; risk factors include renal dysfunction, diabetes mellitus, concomitant use of potassium-sparing diuretics, potassium supplements and/or potassium-containing salts. Use cautiously, if at all, with these agents and monitor potassium periodically. Cough may occur with ACE inhibitors. Other causes of cough should be considered (eg, pulmonary congestion in patients with heart failure) and excluded prior to discontinuation. Use with caution in patients with diabetes receiving insulin or oral antidiabetic agents; may be at increased risk for episodes of hypoglycemia.

May be associated with deterioration of renal function and/or increases in serum creatinine, particularly in patients with low renal blood flow (eg, renal artery stenosis, heart failure) whose glomerular filtration rate (GFR) is dependent on efferent arteriolar vasoconstriction by angiotensin II; deterioration may result in oliguria, acute renal failure, and progressive azotemia. Small increases in serum creatinine may occur following initiation; consider discontinuation only in patients with progressive and/or significant deterioration in renal function. Use with caution in patients with unstented unilateral/bilateral renal artery stenosis. When unstented bilateral renal artery stenosis is present, use is generally avoided due to the elevated risk of deterioration in renal function unless possible benefits outweigh risks. Potentially significant drug-drug interactions may exist, requiring dose or frequency adjustment, additional monitoring, and/or selection of alternative therapy.

Rare toxicities associated with ACE inhibitors include cholestatic jaundice (which may progress to fulminant hepatic necrosis), agranulocytosis, neutropenia, or leukopenia with myeloid hypoplasia. Patients with collagen vascular diseases (especially with concomitant renal impairment) or renal impairment alone may be at increased risk for hematologic toxicity; periodically monitor CBC with differential in these patients.

Warnings: Additional Pediatric Considerations In pediatric patients, an isolated dry hacking cough lasting >3 weeks was reported in seven of 42 pediatric patients (17%) receiving ACE inhibitors (von Vigier, 2000); a review of pediatric randomized, controlled ACE inhibitor trials reported a lower incidence of 3.2%; a higher incidence of cough has been reported in pediatric patients receiving benazepril (15.2%); however, this may have resulted from differences in study methodology (Baker-Smith, 2010).

Adverse Reactions

Central nervous system: Dizziness, drowsiness, headache, orthostatic dizziness

Renal: Increased serum creatinine, renal insufficiency (may occur in patients with bilateral renal artery stenosis or hypovolemia)

Respiratory: Cough

Rare but important or life-threatening: Agranulocytosis, alopecia, anaphylactoid reaction, angina pectoris, angioedema (includes head, neck, and intestinal angioedema), arthralgia, arthritis, asthma, dermatitis, dyspnea, ECG changes, eosinophilia, flushing, gastritis, hemolytic anemia, hyperbilirubinemia, hyperglycemia, hyperkalemia, hypersensitivity, hypertonia, hyponatremia, hypotension, impotence, increased blood urea nitrogen (transient), increased serum transaminases, increased uric acid, insomnia, leukopenia, myalgia, neutropenia, orthostatic hypotension, palpitations, pancreatitis, paresthesia, pemphigus, peripheral edema, proteinuria, pruritus, shock, skin photosensitivity, skin rash, Stevens-Johnson syndrome, syncope, thrombocytopenia, vomiting

Anaphylaxis, eosinophilic pneumonitis, neutropenia, agranulocytosis, renal failure, and renal insufficiency have been reported with other ACE inhibitors. In addition, a syndrome including arthralgia, elevated ESR, eosinophilia, fever, interstitial nephritis, myalgia, rash, and vasculitis has been reported to be associated with ACE inhibitors.

Drug Interactions

Metabolism/Transport Effects None known.

Avoid Concomitant Use There are no known interactions where it is recommended to avoid concomitant use.

Increased Effect/Toxicity

Benazepril may increase the levels/effects of: Allopurinol; Amifostine; Antihypertensives; AzaTHIOprine; Ciprofloxacin (Systemic); Drospirenone; DULoxetine; Ferric Gluconate; Gold Sodium Thiomalate; Grass Pollen Allergen Extract (5 Grass Extract); Hypotensive Agents; Iron Dextran Complex; Levodopa; Lithium; Nonsteroidal Anti-Inflammatory Agents; Obinutuzumab; Pregabalin; RisperiDONE; RiTUXimab; Sodium Phosphates

The levels/effects of Benazepril may be increased by: Alfuzosin; Aliskiren; Angiotensin II Receptor Blockers; Barbiturates; Brimonidine (Topical); Canagliflozin; Dapoxetine; Diazoxide; DPP-IV Inhibitors; Eplerenone; Everolimus; Heparin; Heparin (Low Molecular Weight); Herbs (Hypotensive Properties); Hydrochlorothiazide; Loop Diuretics; MAO Inhibitors; Nicorandil; Pentoxifylline; Phosphodiesterase 5 Inhibitors; Potassium Salts; Potassium-Sparing Diuretics; Prostacyclin Analogues; Sirolimus; Temsirolimus; Thiazide Diuretics; TiZANidine; Tolvaptan; Trimethoprim

Decreased Effect

Benazepril may decrease the levels/effects of: Hydrochlorothiazide

The levels/effects of Benazepril may be decreased by: Aprotinin; Herbs (Hypertensive Properties); Icatibant; Lanthanum; Methylphenidate; Nonsteroidal Anti-Inflammatory Agents; Salicylates; Yohimbine

Storage/Stability Store at ≤30°C (86°F). Protect from moisture.

Mechanism of Action Competitive inhibition of angiotensin I being converted to angiotensin II, a potent vasoconstrictor, through the angiotensin I-converting enzyme (ACE) activity, with resultant lower levels of angiotensin II which causes an increase in plasma renin activity and a reduction in aldosterone secretion

Pharmacodynamics Adults:

Maximum effect:

Reduction in plasma angiotensin-converting enzyme (ACE) activity: 1-2 hours after 2-20 mg dose

Reduction in blood pressure: Single dose: 2-4 hours; Continuous therapy: 2 weeks

Duration: Reduction in plasma angiotensin-converting enzyme (ACE) activity: >90% inhibition for 24 hours after 5-20 mg dose

Pharmacokinetics (Adult data unless noted)

Absorption: Oral: 37%; rapidly absorbed; **Note:** Metabolite (benazeprilat) is unsuitable for oral administration due to poor absorption

Distribution: V_d: ~8.7 L

Protein binding: Benazepril: 97%; benazeprilat: 95%

Metabolism: Rapidly and extensively metabolized (primarily in the liver) to benazeprilat (active metabolite), via cleavage of ester group; extensive first-pass effect. Benazeprilat is about 200 times more potent than benazepril. Parent and active metabolite undergo glucuronide conjugation

Half-life: Benazeprilat: Terminal:

Children and Adolescents 6-16 years: 5 hours

Adults: 22 hours

Time to peak serum concentration: Oral:

Parent drug: 0.5-1 hour

Active metabolite (benazeprilat):

Fasting: 1-2 hours

Nonfasting: 2-4 hours

Elimination: Hepatic clearance is the main elimination route of unchanged benazepril. Only trace amounts of unchanged benazepril appear in the urine; 20% of dose is excreted in urine as benazeprilat, 8% as benazeprilat glucuronide, and 4% as benazepril glucuronide

Clearance: Nonrenal excretion (ie, biliary) appears to contribute to the elimination of benazeprilat (11% to 12% in healthy adults); biliary clearance may be increased in patients with severe renal impairment

Dialysis: ~6% of metabolite removed within 4 hours of dialysis following 10 mg of benazepril administered 2 hours prior to procedure; parent compound not found in dialysate

Dosing: Usual Hypertension: Note: Dosage must be titrated according to patient's response; use lowest effective dose

Children ≥6 years and Adolescents: Oral: Initial: 0.2 mg/kg/dose once daily as monotherapy; maximum initial dose: 10 mg/**day**; maintenance: 0.1-0.6 mg/kg/dose once daily; maximum daily dose: 40 mg/**day**

Adults: Oral: Initial: 10 mg once daily in patients not receiving a diuretic; maintenance: 20-80 mg/day as a single dose or 2 divided doses; the need for twice daily dosing should be assessed by monitoring peak (2-6 hours after dosing) and trough blood pressure responses

Note: To decrease the risk of hypotension, patients taking diuretics should have diuretics discontinued 2-3 days prior to starting benazepril; diuretic may be resumed if blood pressure is not controlled with benazepril monotherapy. If diuretics cannot be discontinued prior to starting benazepril, then an initial dose of benazepril of 5 mg once daily should be used.

Dosing adjustment in renal impairment:

Children and Adolescents: CrCl <30 mL/minute/1.73 m^2: Use is not recommended (insufficient data exists; dose not established)

Adults: CrCl <30 mL/minute/1.73 m^2: Initial: 5 mg once daily, then increase as required to a maximum of 40 mg/day

Administration Oral: May be administered without regard to food.

Monitoring Parameters Blood pressure (supervise for at least 2 hours after the initial dose or any dosage increase for significant orthostasis); renal function, WBC, serum potassium; monitor for angioedema and anaphylactoid reactions

Dosage Forms Excipient information presented when available (limited, particularly for generics); consult specific product labeling.

Tablet, Oral, as hydrochloride:

Lotensin: 10 mg, 20 mg, 40 mg

Generic: 5 mg, 10 mg, 20 mg, 40 mg

Extemporaneous Preparations A 2 mg/mL oral suspension may be made with tablets. Mix fifteen benazepril 20 mg tablets in an amber polyethylene terephthalate bottle with Ora-Plus® 75 mL. Shake for 2 minutes, allow suspension to stand for ≥1 hour, then shake again for at least 1 additional minute. Add Ora-Sweet® 75 mL to suspension and shake to disperse. Will make 150 mL of a 2 mg/mL suspension. Label "shake well" and "refrigerate". Stable for 30 days.

Lotensin® prescribing information, Novartis Pharmaceuticals Corporation, Suffern, NY, 2015.

- **Benazepril Hydrochloride** *see* Benazepril *on page 265*
- **BeneFIX** *see* Factor IX (Recombinant) *on page 842*
- **BeneFix (Can)** *see* Factor IX (Recombinant) *on page 842*
- **Benemid [DSC]** *see* Probenecid *on page 1767*
- **Benflumetol and Artemether** *see* Artemether and Lumefantrine *on page 200*
- **Benicar** *see* Olmesartan *on page 1551*
- **Benoxyl® (Can)** *see* Benzoyl Peroxide *on page 270*
- **Bensal HP** *see* Salicylic Acid *on page 1894*
- **Bentyl** *see* Dicyclomine *on page 645*
- **Bentylol (Can)** *see* Dicyclomine *on page 645*
- **Benuryl (Can)** *see* Probenecid *on page 1767*
- **Benylin® D for Infants (Can)** *see* Pseudoephedrine *on page 1801*
- **Benylin DM-E (Can)** *see* Guaifenesin and Dextromethorphan *on page 992*
- **Benylin® E Extra Strength (Can)** *see* GuaiFENesin *on page 988*
- **Benzac AC® (Can)** *see* Benzoyl Peroxide *on page 270*
- **Benzac AC Wash** *see* Benzoyl Peroxide *on page 270*
- **BenzaClin** *see* Clindamycin and Benzoyl Peroxide *on page 493*
- **Benzac W® Gel (Can)** *see* Benzoyl Peroxide *on page 270*
- **Benzac W Wash** *see* Benzoyl Peroxide *on page 270*
- **Benzac W® Wash (Can)** *see* Benzoyl Peroxide *on page 270*
- **Benzathine Benzylpenicillin** *see* Penicillin G Benzathine *on page 1654*
- **Benzathine Penicillin G** *see* Penicillin G Benzathine *on page 1654*
- **Benzatropine** *see* Benztropine *on page 272*
- **BenzEFoam** *see* Benzoyl Peroxide *on page 270*
- **BenzEFoamUltra** *see* Benzoyl Peroxide *on page 270*
- **Benzene Hexachloride** *see* Lindane *on page 1267*
- **BenzePrO** *see* Benzoyl Peroxide *on page 270*
- **BenzePrO Creamy Wash** *see* Benzoyl Peroxide *on page 270*
- **BenzePrO Foaming Cloths** *see* Benzoyl Peroxide *on page 270*
- **BenzePrO Short Contact** *see* Benzoyl Peroxide *on page 270*
- **Benzhexol Hydrochloride** *see* Trihexyphenidyl *on page 2124*
- **Benziq** *see* Benzoyl Peroxide *on page 270*
- **Benziq LS** *see* Benzoyl Peroxide *on page 270*
- **Benziq Wash** *see* Benzoyl Peroxide *on page 270*
- **Benzmethyzin** *see* Procarbazine *on page 1772*

Benzocaine (BEN zoe kane)

Medication Safety Issues

Sound-alike/look-alike issues:

Orabase® may be confused with Orinase

Brand Names: US Anacaine; Anbesol Cold Sore Therapy [OTC]; Anbesol JR [OTC]; Anbesol Maximum Strength [OTC]; Anbesol [OTC]; Baby Anbesol [OTC]; Benz-O-Sthetic [OTC]; Benzocaine Oral Anesthetic [OTC]; Bi-Zets/Benzotroches [OTC]; Blistex Medicated [OTC]; Cepacol Dual Relief [OTC]; Cepacol Sensations Hydra [OTC]; Cepacol Sensations Warming [OTC]; Chiggerex [OTC]; Chiggertox [OTC]; Dent-O-Kain/20 [OTC]; Dentapaine [OTC]; Dermoplast [OTC]; Foille [OTC]; HurriCaine One [OTC]; Hurricaine [OTC]; Ivy-Rid [OTC]; Kank-A Mouth Pain [OTC]; Ora-film [OTC]; Oral Pain Relief Max St [OTC] [DSC]; Pinnacaine Otic; Sore Throat Relief [OTC]; Topex Topical Anesthetic; Trocaine Throat [OTC]; Zilactin Baby [OTC]

Brand Names: Canada Anbesol® Baby; Zilactin Baby®; Zilactin-B®

Therapeutic Category Analgesic, Topical; Local Anesthetic, Oral; Local Anesthetic, Topical

Generic Availability (US) May be product dependent

Use Temporary relief of pain associated with pruritic dermatosis, pruritus, minor burns, toothache, minor sore throat pain, canker sores, hemorrhoids, rectal fissures; anesthetic lubricant for passage of catheters and endoscopic tubes

Pregnancy Risk Factor C

Pregnancy Considerations Reproduction studies have not been conducted.

Breast-Feeding Considerations It is not known if benzocaine is excreted in breast milk. The manufacturer recommends that caution be exercised when administering benzocaine to nursing women.

Contraindications Hypersensitivity to benzocaine, other ester-type local anesthetics, or any component of the formulation; secondary bacterial infection of area; ophthalmic use

Warnings/Precautions Methemoglobinemia has been reported following topical use, particularly with higher concentration (14% to 20%) spray formulations applied to the mouth or mucous membranes. When applied as a spray to the mouth or throat, multiple sprays (or sprays of longer than indicated duration) are not recommended. Use caution with breathing problems (asthma, bronchitis, emphysema, in smokers), inflamed/damaged mucosa, heart disease, and hemoglobin or enzyme abnormalities (glucose-6-phosphate dehydrogenase deficiency, hemoglobin-M disease, NADH-methemoglobin reductase deficiency, pyruvate-kinase deficiency). Alternatives to benzocaine sprays, such as topical lidocaine preparations, should be considered for patients at higher risk of this reaction. Due to the heightened risk of methemoglobinemia, not recommended for use in patients <2 years of age unless under the advice and supervision by a healthcare professional.

The classical clinical finding of methemoglobinemia is chocolate brown-colored arterial blood. However, suspected cases should be confirmed by co-oximetry, which yields a direct and accurate measure of methemoglobin levels. Standard pulse oximetry readings or arterial blood gas values are not reliable. Clinically significant methemoglobinemia requires immediate treatment.

When topical anesthetics are used prior to cosmetic or medical procedures, the lowest amount of anesthetic necessary for pain relief should be applied. High systemic levels and toxic effects (eg, methemoglobinemia, irregular heart beats, respiratory depression, seizures, death) have been reported in patients who (without supervision of a trained professional) have applied topical anesthetics in large amounts (or to large areas of the skin), left these products on for prolonged periods of time, or have used wraps/dressings to cover the skin following application.

Benzyl alcohol and derivatives: Some dosage forms may contain benzyl alcohol; large amounts of benzyl alcohol (≥99 mg/kg/day) have been associated with a potentially fatal toxicity ("gasping syndrome") in neonates; the "gasping syndrome" consists of metabolic acidosis, respiratory distress, gasping respirations, CNS dysfunction (including convulsions, intracranial hemorrhage), hypotension and cardiovascular collapse (AAP, 1997; CDC, 1982); some data suggests that benzoate displaces bilirubin from protein binding sites (Ahlfors, 2001); avoid or use dosage forms containing benzyl alcohol with caution in neonates. See manufacturer's labeling.

When used for self-medication (OTC), notify healthcare provider if condition worsens or does not improve within the timeframe noted on the product labeling or if accompanied by additional symptoms (eg, swelling, rash, headache, nausea, vomiting, or fever). Do not use topical products on open wounds; avoid contact with the eyes.

Warnings: Additional Pediatric Considerations The majority of cases of methemoglobinemia associated with benzocaine use have been in infants and children <2 years of age for treatment of teething pain; also at greater risk for development are patients with asthma, bronchitis, emphysema, mucosal damage, or inflammation at the application site, heart disease, and malnutrition. The FDA recommends against using topical OTC medications for teething pain as some products may cause harm; the use of OTC topical anesthetics (eg, benzocaine) for teething pain is also discouraged by AAP, and The American Academy of Pediatric Dentistry (AAP, 2011; AAPD, 2012). The AAP recommends managing teething pain with a chilled (not frozen) teething ring or gently rubbing/massaging with the caregiver's finger.

Some dosage forms may contain propylene glycol; in neonates large amounts of propylene glycol delivered orally, intravenously (eg, >3,000 mg/day), or topically have been associated with potentially fatal toxicities which can include metabolic acidosis, seizures, renal failure, and CNS depression; toxicities have also been reported in children and adults including hyperosmolality, lactic acidosis, seizures and respiratory depression; use caution (AAP, 1997; Shehab, 2009).

Adverse Reactions

Central nervous system: Localized burning, stinging sensation

Dermatologic: Contact dermatitis, localized erythema, localized rash, urticaria

Hematologic & oncologic: Methemoglobinemia

Hypersensitivity: Hypersensitivity

Local: Local pruritus, localized edema, localized tenderness

Drug Interactions

Metabolism/Transport Effects None known.

Avoid Concomitant Use There are no known interactions where it is recommended to avoid concomitant use.

Increased Effect/Toxicity

Benzocaine may increase the levels/effects of: Prilocaine; Sodium Nitrite

The levels/effects of Benzocaine may be increased by: Nitric Oxide

Decreased Effect There are no known significant interactions involving a decrease in effect.

Storage/Stability Store at room temperature.

Mechanism of Action Ester local anesthetic blocks both the initiation and conduction of nerve impulses by decreasing the neuronal membrane's permeability to sodium ions, which results in inhibition of depolarization with resultant blockade of conduction

Pharmacokinetics (Adult data unless noted)

Absorption: Poor after topical administration to intact skin, but well absorbed from mucous membranes and traumatized skin

Metabolism: Hydrolyzed in plasma and to a lesser extent in the liver by cholinesterase

Elimination: Excretion of the metabolites in urine

Dosing: Usual Children and Adults:

Mucous membranes: Dosage varies depending on area to be anesthetized and vascularity of tissues

Oral mouth/throat preparations: Do not administer for >2 days or in children <2 years of age, unless directed by a physician; refer to specific package labeling

Otic: 4-5 drops into ear canal; may repeat every 1-2 hours as needed

Topical: Apply to affected area as needed

Administration

Mucous membranes: Apply to mucous membrane; do not eat for 1 hour after application to oral mucosa

Otic: After instilling into external ear canal, insert cotton pledget into ear canal

Topical: Apply evenly; do not apply to deep or puncture wounds or to serious burns

Monitoring Parameters Monitor patients for signs and symptoms of methemoglobinemia such as pallor, cyanosis, nausea, muscle weakness, dizziness, confusion, agitation, dyspnea, and tachycardia; co-oximetry

Dosage Forms Excipient information presented when available (limited, particularly for generics); consult specific product labeling. [DSC] = Discontinued product

Aerosol, External:

- Dermoplast: Benzocaine 20% and menthol 0.5% (56 g) [contains methylparaben]
- Ivy-Rid: 2% (82.5 mL)

Gel, Mouth/Throat:

- Anbesol: 10% (9 g) [contains benzyl alcohol, brilliant blue fcf (fd&c blue #1), fd&c yellow #10 (quinoline yellow), fd&c yellow #6 (sunset yellow), methylparaben, propylene glycol, saccharin; cool mint flavor]
- Anbesol JR: 10% (9 g) [contains methylparaben]
- Anbesol Maximum Strength: 20% (9 g) [contains brilliant blue fcf (fd&c blue #1), fd&c red #40, fd&c yellow #10 (quinoline yellow), methylparaben, saccharin]
- Baby Anbesol: 7.5% (9 g)
- Benz-O-Sthetic: 20% (15 g) [contains benzyl alcohol, saccharin sodium]
- Benz-O-Sthetic: 20% (29 g) [contains benzyl alcohol, saccharin sodium; bubble-gum flavor]
- Benz-O-Sthetic: 20% (29 g) [contains benzyl alcohol, saccharin sodium; cherry flavor]
- Dentapaine: 20% (11 g)
- Hurricaine: 20% (5.25 g) [contains polyethylene glycol, saccharin sodium]
- Hurricaine: 20% (28.4 g) [contains polyethylene glycol, saccharin sodium; mint flavor]

Hurricaine: 20% (30 g) [contains polyethylene glycol, saccharin sodium; pina colada flavor]
Hurricaine: 20% (30 g) [contains polyethylene glycol, saccharin sodium; watermelon flavor]
Hurricaine: 20% (5.25 g, 30 g) [contains polyethylene glycol, saccharin sodium; wild cherry flavor]
Oral Pain Relief Max St: 20% (14.2 g [DSC]) [contains saccharin sodium]
Zilactin Baby: 10% (9.4 g) [alcohol free, dye free, saccharin free]

Liquid, External:
Chiggertox: 2.1% (30 mL)

Liquid, Mouth/Throat:
Anbesol: 10% (12 mL) [contains brilliant blue fcf (fd&c blue #1), fd&c yellow #10 (quinoline yellow), fd&c yellow #6 (sunset yellow), methylparaben, saccharin; cool mint flavor]
Anbesol Maximum Strength: 20% (12 mL) [contains benzyl alcohol, brilliant blue fcf (fd&c blue #1), fd&c red #40, fd&c yellow #10 (quinoline yellow), methylparaben, polyethylene glycol, propylene glycol, saccharin]
Benz-O-Sthetic: 20% (56 g) [contains benzyl alcohol, brilliant blue fcf (fd&c blue #1), fd&c red #40, fd&c yellow #10 (quinoline yellow), polyethylene glycol, propylene glycol, saccharin]
Cepacol Dual Relief: 5% (22.2 mL) [sugar free; cherry flavor]
Dent-O-Kain/20: 20% (9 mL) [contains benzyl alcohol, brilliant blue fcf (fd&c blue #1), d&c yellow #11 (quinoline yellow ss), fd&c red #40, propylene glycol, saccharin]
Oral Pain Relief Max St: 20% (15 mL [DSC]) [contains benzyl alcohol, brilliant blue fcf (fd&c blue #1), fd&c red #40, fd&c yellow #10 (quinoline yellow), methylparaben, polyethylene glycol, propylene glycol, saccharin]

Lozenge, Mouth/Throat:
Bi-Zets/Benzotroches: 15 mg (10 ea) [orange flavor]
Cepacol Sensations Hydra: 3 mg (20 ea) [contains brilliant blue fcf (fd&c blue #1), fd&c yellow #10 (quinoline yellow)]
Cepacol Sensations Warming: 4 mg (20 ea) [contains fd&c red #40, fd&c yellow #10 (quinoline yellow)]
Sore Throat Relief: 10 mg (2 ea) [wild cherry flavor]
Trocaine Throat: 10 mg (1 ea)

Ointment, External:
Anacaine: 10% (30 g)
Anbesol Cold Sore Therapy: 20 % (9 g) [contains aloe, vitamin e]
Blistex Medicated: (6.3 g) [contains cetyl alcohol, edetate calcium disodium, saccharin sodium, sd alcohol]
Chiggerex: 2% (52.5 g)
Foille: 5% (28 g)

Solution, Mouth/Throat:
Benz-O-Sthetic: 20% (30 mL) [contains polyethylene glycol, saccharin]
Benzocaine Oral Anesthetic: 20% (59.7 g) [contains alcohol, usp, polyethylene glycol, saccharin sodium]
Hurricaine: 20% (57 g) [contains polyethylene glycol, saccharin sodium]
Hurricaine: 20% (30 mL) [contains polyethylene glycol, saccharin sodium; pina colada flavor]
Hurricaine: 20% (57 g, 30 mL) [contains polyethylene glycol, saccharin sodium; wild cherry flavor]
HurriCaine One: 20% (2 ea, 25 ea) [contains polyethylene glycol, saccharin sodium]
Kank-A Mouth Pain: 20% (9.75 mL) [contains benzyl alcohol, propylene glycol, saccharin sodium]
Topex Topical Anesthetic: 20% (57 g) [cherry flavor]

Solution, Otic:
Pinnacaine Otic: 20% (15 mL)

Strip, Mouth/Throat:
Ora-film: 6% (12 ea) [contains brilliant blue fcf (fd&c blue #1), menthol, methylparaben, propylparaben, tartrazine (fd&c yellow #5)]

Swab, Mouth/Throat:
Benz-O-Sthetic: 20% (2 ea [DSC]) [contains benzyl alcohol, polyethylene glycol, saccharin sodium]
Benz-O-Sthetic: 20% (2 ea) [contains benzyl alcohol, polyethylene glycol, saccharin sodium; cherry flavor]
Hurricaine: 20% (72 ea) [contains polyethylene glycol, saccharin sodium; wild cherry flavor]

- **Benzocaine and Antipyrine** *see* Antipyrine and Benzocaine *on page 177*
- **Benzocaine Oral Anesthetic [OTC]** *see* Benzocaine *on page 268*
- **Benz-O-Sthetic [OTC]** *see* Benzocaine *on page 268*

Benzoyl Peroxide (BEN zoe il peer OKS ide)

Medication Safety Issues

Sound-alike/look-alike issues:
Benzoyl peroxide may be confused with benzyl alcohol
Benoxyl may be confused with Brevoxyl, Peroxyl
Benzac may be confused with Benza
Brevoxyl may be confused with Benoxyl
Fostex may be confused with pHisoHex

Brand Names: US Acne Medication 10 [OTC]; Acne Medication 5 [OTC]; Acne Medication [OTC] [DSC]; Acne-Clear [OTC]; AcneFree Severe Clearing Syst [OTC]; Benzac AC Wash; Benzac W Wash; BenzEFoam; BenzEFoamUltra; BenzePrO; BenzePrO Creamy Wash; BenzePrO Foaming Cloths; BenzePrO Short Contact; Benziq; Benziq LS; Benziq Wash; Benzoyl Peroxide Cleanser [OTC]; Benzoyl Peroxide Wash [OTC]; BP Cleansing [OTC]; BP Foam; BP Foaming Wash; BP Gel [OTC]; BP Wash; BP Wash [OTC]; BPO; BPO Creamy Wash [OTC]; BPO Foaming Cloths; BPO-10 Wash [OTC]; BPO-5 Wash [OTC]; Clearplex V [OTC]; Clearplex X; Clearskin [OTC]; Desquam-X Wash [OTC]; Inova; Lavoclen-4 Acne Wash; Lavoclen-4 Creamy Wash; Lavoclen-8 Acne Wash; Lavoclen-8 Creamy Wash; Neutrogena Clear Pore [OTC]; OC8 [OTC]; Oscion Cleanser; PanOxyl Wash [OTC]; PanOxyl [OTC]; PanOxyl-4 Creamy Wash [OTC]; PanOxyl-8 Creamy Wash [OTC]; PR Benzoyl Peroxide Wash; Riax; SE BPO Wash [DSC]; Zaclir Cleansing

Brand Names: Canada Acetoxyl®; Benoxyl®; Benzac AC®; Benzac W® Gel; Benzac W® Wash; Desquam-X®; Oxyderm™; PanOxyl®; Solugel®

Therapeutic Category Acne Products; Topical Skin Product

Generic Availability (US) May be product dependent

Use Treatment of mild to moderate acne vulgaris (FDA approved in ages ≥12 years and adults)

Pregnancy Risk Factor C

Pregnancy Considerations Animal reproduction studies have not been conducted; ~2% of the applied dose is expected to be absorbed systemically (Akhavan, 2003).

Breast-Feeding Considerations It is not known if benzoyl peroxide is excreted in breast milk. The manufacturer recommends that caution be exercised when administering benzoyl peroxide to nursing women.

Contraindications Hypersensitivity to benzoyl peroxide or any other component of the formulation.

Warnings/Precautions For external use only; avoid contact with eye, eyelids, lips, and mucous membranes. Inform patients to use skin protection and minimize prolonged exposure to sun or tanning beds. May bleach hair, colored fabric, or carpet. Discontinue use if severe skin irritation or redness occurs. Concomitant use of benzoyl peroxide with sulfone products (eg, dapsone, sulfacetamide) may cause temporary discoloration (yellow/orange) of facial hair and skin. Application of products at separate times during the day or washing off benzoyl peroxide prior to application of other products may avoid skin discoloration (Dubina 2009).

Rare but serious and potentially life-threatening allergic reactions or severe irritation have been reported with use of topical OTC benzoyl peroxide or salicylic acid containing products; it has not been determined if the reactions are due to the active ingredients (benzoyl peroxide or salicylic acid), the inactive ingredients, or a combination of both. Hypersensitivity reactions may occur within minutes to a day or longer after product use and differ from local skin irritation (redness, burning, dryness, itching, peeling or slight swelling) that may occur at the site of product application. Treatment should be discontinued if hives or itching develop; patients should seek emergency medical attention if reactions such as throat tightness, difficulty breathing, feeling faint, or swelling of the eyes, face, lips, or tongue develop. Before using a topical OTC acne product for the first time, consumers should apply a small amount to 1 or 2 small affected areas for 3 days to make sure hypersensitivity symptoms do not develop (FDA Drug Safety Communication, 2014).

Benzyl alcohol and derivatives: Some dosage forms may contain benzyl alcohol; large amounts of benzyl alcohol (≥99 mg/kg/day) have been associated with a potentially fatal toxicity ("gasping syndrome") in neonates; the "gasping syndrome" consists of metabolic acidosis, respiratory distress, gasping respirations, CNS dysfunction (including convulsions, intracranial hemorrhage), hypotension and cardiovascular collapse (AAP, 1997; CDC, 1982); some data suggests that benzoate displaces bilirubin from protein binding sites (Ahlfors, 2001); avoid or use dosage forms containing benzyl alcohol with caution in neonates. See manufacturer's labeling.

Warnings: Additional Pediatric Considerations Some dosage forms may contain propylene glycol; in neonates large amounts of propylene glycol delivered orally, intravenously (eg, >3,000 mg/day), or topically have been associated with potentially fatal toxicities which can include metabolic acidosis, seizures, renal failure, and CNS depression; toxicities have also been reported in children and adults including hyperosmolality, lactic acidosis, seizures and respiratory depression; use caution (AAP, 1997; Shehab, 2009).

Adverse Reactions Dermatologic: Contact dermatitis, dryness, erythema, irritation, peeling, stinging

Drug Interactions

Metabolism/Transport Effects None known.

Avoid Concomitant Use There are no known interactions where it is recommended to avoid concomitant use.

Increased Effect/Toxicity

Benzoyl Peroxide may increase the levels/effects of: Dapsone (Topical)

Decreased Effect There are no known significant interactions involving a decrease in effect.

Mechanism of Action Releases free-radical oxygen which oxidizes bacterial proteins in the sebaceous follicles decreasing the number of anaerobic bacteria and decreasing irritating-type free fatty acids

Pharmacokinetics (Adult data unless noted)

Absorption: ~5% through the skin

Metabolism: Major metabolite is benzoic acid

Elimination: In the urine as benzoate

Dosing: Usual Children ≥12 years, Adolescents, and Adults: Topical:

Topical formulations: Apply sparingly once daily; gradually increase to 2-3 times/day if needed. If excessive dryness or peeling occurs, reduce dose frequency or concentration. If excessive stinging or burning occurs, remove with mild soap and water; resume use the next day

Topical cleansers: Wash once or twice daily; control amount of drying or peeling by modifying dose frequency or concentration

Administration Topical: Shake lotion before using; cleanse skin before applying; for external use only. Avoid contact with eyes, eyelids, lips, and mucous membranes; rinse with water if accidental contact occurs

Additional Information Granulation may indicate effectiveness; gels are more penetrating than creams and last longer than creams or lotions

Dosage Forms Excipient information presented when available (limited, particularly for generics); consult specific product labeling. [DSC] = Discontinued product

Bar, External:

PanOxyl: 10% (1 ea)

Cream, External:

Clearskin: 10% (30 g)

Foam, External:

BenzEFoam: 5.3% (60 g, 100 g) [contains cetearyl alcohol, disodium edta, methylparaben, propylene glycol, propylparaben]

BenzEFoamUltra: 9.8% (100 g) [contains cetearyl alcohol, disodium edta, methylparaben, propylene glycol, propylparaben]

BenzePrO: 5.3% (60 g, 100 g) [contains cetearyl alcohol, disodium edta, methylparaben, propylene glycol, propylparaben, trolamine (triethanolamine)]

BenzePrO Short Contact: 9.8% (100 g) [contains cetearyl alcohol, disodium edta, methylparaben, propylene glycol, propylparaben]

BP Foam: 5.3% (60 g, 100 g); 9.8% (100 g) [contains methylparaben, propylparaben]

Riax: 5.5% (100 g); 9.5% (100 g) [contains methylparaben, propylparaben]

Generic: 5.3% (60 g, 100 g); 9.8% (100 g)

Gel, External:

Acne Medication 5: 5% (42.5 g) [contains edetate disodium]

Acne Medication 10: 10% (42.5 g) [contains edetate disodium]

Acne-Clear: 10% (42.5 g)

Benziq: 5.25% (50 g) [contains benzyl alcohol, disodium edta, trolamine (triethanolamine)]

Benziq LS: 2.75% (50 g) [contains trolamine (triethanolamine)]

BP Gel: 5% (60 g) [contains benzyl alcohol, edetate disodium, trolamine (triethanolamine)]

BP Gel: 10% (60 g) [contains benzyl alcohol, disodium edta, trolamine (triethanolamine)]

BPO: 4% (42.5 g); 8% (42.5 g) [contains benzyl alcohol, cetyl alcohol]

Clearplex V: 5% (45 g)

Clearplex X: 10% (45 g)

OC8: 7% (45 g) [contains disodium edta, propylene glycol]

PanOxyl: 3% (10 g) [contains disodium edta]

Generic: 2.5% (60 g); 5% (60 g, 90 g); 10% (56 g, 60 g, 90 g)

Kit, External:

AcneFree Severe Clearing Syst: Wash 2.5% and lotion 10% [contains benzalkonium chloride, butylparaben, cetyl alcohol, disodium edta, edetate sodium (tetrasodium), ethylparaben, isobutylparaben, methylisothiazolinone, methylparaben, propylene glycol, propylparaben, soybeans (glycine max)]

Benzoyl Peroxide Wash: Wash 8% (170.1 g) and bar soap 5% (2 x 21 g), Liquid wash 4% (170.1 g) and bar soap 5% (2 x 21 g) [contains cetearyl alcohol, methylparaben]

BPO Creamy Wash: Wash 4% (170.1 g) and bar soap 5% (2 x 21 g), Wash 8% (170.1 g) and bar soap 5% (2 x 21 g) [contains disodium edta, methylparaben]

Inova: Pad 4% (30s) and tocopherol 5% (28s), Pad 8% (30s) and tocopherol 5% (28s) [contains disodium edta, methylparaben]
Lavoclen-4 Acne Wash: 4% [soap free; contains butylparaben, cetearyl alcohol, methylparaben, propylparaben]
Lavoclen-4 Acne Wash: 4% [soap free; contains butylparaben, methylparaben, propylparaben]
Lavoclen-8 Acne Wash: 8% [soap free; contains butylparaben, cetearyl alcohol, methylparaben, propylparaben]
Lavoclen-8 Acne Wash: 8% [soap free; contains butylparaben, methylparaben, propylparaben]

Liquid, External:
Benzac AC Wash: 5% (226 g)
Benzac W Wash: 5% (226 g)
BenzePrO Creamy Wash: 7% (180 g) [contains cetyl alcohol, edetate disodium, propylene glycol]
Benziq Wash: 5.25% (175 g) [contains benzyl alcohol, cetyl alcohol, disodium edta, propylene glycol]
Benzoyl Peroxide Wash: 5% (148 g, 237 g) [contains cetyl alcohol, edetate disodium, propylene glycol]
Benzoyl Peroxide Wash: 5% (142 g, 227 g) [contains edetate disodium]
Benzoyl Peroxide Wash: 10% (148 g, 237 g) [contains cetyl alcohol, edetate disodium, propylene glycol]
Benzoyl Peroxide Wash: 10% (142 g, 227 g) [contains edetate disodium]
BP Foaming Wash: 10% (227 g) [contains cetearyl alcohol, methylparaben]
BP Wash: 2.5% (227 g); 5% (113 g, 142 g, 227 g) [contains cetearyl alcohol, methylparaben]
BP Wash: 5.25% (175 g); 7% (473 mL) [contains benzyl alcohol, cetyl alcohol, propylene glycol, trolamine (triethanolamine)]
BP Wash: 10% (142 g, 227 g) [contains cetearyl alcohol, methylparaben]
BPO-10 Wash: 10% (227 g) [contains methylparaben, propylene glycol, propylparaben]
BPO-5 Wash: 5% (227 g) [contains methylparaben, propylene glycol, propylparaben]
Desquam-X Wash: 5% (140 g); 10% (140 g) [contains edetate disodium]
Lavoclen-4 Creamy Wash: 4% (170.1 g) [contains cetearyl alcohol, methylparaben]
Lavoclen-8 Creamy Wash: 8% (170.1 g) [contains cetearyl alcohol, methylparaben]
Neutrogena Clear Pore: 3.5% (125 mL) [contains disodium edta, menthol]
PanOxyl: 2.5% (156 g) [soap free; contains cetearyl alcohol]
PanOxyl Wash: 10% (156 g) [contains alcohol, usp, methylparaben]
PanOxyl-4 Creamy Wash: 4% (170.1 g) [contains cetearyl alcohol, methylparaben]
PanOxyl-8 Creamy Wash: 8% (170.1 g) [contains cetearyl alcohol, methylparaben]
PR Benzoyl Peroxide Wash: 7% (180 g, 473 mL) [contains cetyl alcohol, edetate disodium, propylene glycol]
SE BPO Wash: 7% (180 g [DSC]) [contains edetate disodium, methylparaben]

Lotion, External:
Acne Medication 5: 5% (29.5 mL, 30 mL) [odorless; contains disodium edta]
Acne Medication: 10% (30 mL [DSC]) [odorless; contains edetate disodium]
Acne Medication 10: 10% (29.5 mL) [odorless; contains edetate disodium]
Benzoyl Peroxide Cleanser: 6% (170.3 g, 340.2 g) [contains cetyl alcohol, edetate disodium, propylene glycol]
BP Cleansing: 4% (297 g) [contains cetyl alcohol, propylene glycol]
Oscion Cleanser: 6% (170.3 g, 340.2 g)
Zaclir Cleansing: 8% (297 g)

Miscellaneous, External:
BenzePrO Foaming Cloths: 6% (60 ea) [contains cetyl alcohol]
BPO Foaming Cloths: 3% (60 ea); 6% (60 ea); 9% (60 ea) [contains methylparaben]

- **Benzoyl Peroxide and Adapalene** *see* Adapalene and Benzoyl Peroxide *on page 71*
- **Benzoyl Peroxide and Clindamycin** *see* Clindamycin and Benzoyl Peroxide *on page 493*
- **Benzoyl Peroxide Cleanser [OTC]** *see* Benzoyl Peroxide *on page 270*
- **Benzoyl Peroxide Wash [OTC]** *see* Benzoyl Peroxide *on page 270*

Benztropine (BENZ troe peen)

Medication Safety Issues

Sound-alike/look-alike issues:

Benztropine may be confused with bromocriptine

BEERS Criteria medication:

This drug may be potentially inappropriate for use in geriatric patients (Parkinson's disease: Quality of evidence - moderate; Strength of recommendation - strong).

Brand Names: US Cogentin

Brand Names: Canada Benztropine Omega; Kynesia; PMS-Benztropine

Therapeutic Category Anti-Parkinson's Agent; Anticholinergic Agent; Antidote, Drug-induced Dystonic Reactions

Generic Availability (US) Yes

Use Adjunctive treatment of parkinsonism (FDA approved in adults); treatment of drug-induced extrapyramidal effects (except tardive dyskinesia) (FDA approved in adults)

Pregnancy Considerations Animal reproduction studies have not been conducted. Paralytic ileus (which resolved rapidly) was reported in two newborns exposed to a combination of benztropine and chlorpromazine during the second and third trimesters and the last 6 weeks of pregnancy, respectively (Falterman, 1980).

Breast-Feeding Considerations It is not known if benztropine is excreted in breast milk. Anticholinergic agents may suppress lactation.

Contraindications Hypersensitivity to benztropine or any component of the formulation; children <3 years of age (due to atropine-like adverse effects)

Warnings/Precautions May cause anticholinergic effects (constipation, xerostomia, blurred vision, urinary retention). Use with caution in children >3 years of age due to its anticholinergic effects (dose has not been established). Use is contraindicated in children <3 years of age. Use with caution in hot weather or during exercise. May cause anhydrosis and hyperthermia, which may be severe. The risk is increased in hot environments, particularly in the elderly, alcoholics, patients with CNS disease, and those with prolonged outdoor exposure. If there is evidence of anhidrosis, consider decreasing dose so the ability to maintain body heat equilibrium by perspiration is not impaired.

Use with caution in patients >65 years of age; response in elderly may be altered. Initiate at low doses in the elderly and increase as needed while monitoring for adverse events. Avoid use of oral benztropine in older adults for prevention of extrapyramidal symptoms with antipsychotics and alternative agents preferred in the treatment of Parkinson's disease. May be inappropriate in older adults depending on comorbidities (eg, dementia, delirium) due to its potent anticholinergic effects (Beers Criteria). Avoid use in angle-closure glaucoma.

Use with caution in patients with tachycardia, glaucoma, prostatic hyperplasia (especially in the elderly), any tendency toward urinary retention, and obstructive disease of the GI or GU tracts. When given in large doses or to susceptible patients, may cause weakness and inability to move particular muscle groups.

May be associated with confusion, visual hallucinations, or excitement (generally at higher dosages). Intensification of symptoms or toxic psychosis may occur in patients with mental disorders. May cause CNS depression, which may impair physical or mental abilities; patients must be cautioned about performing tasks which require mental alertness (eg, operating machinery or driving). Benztropine does not relieve symptoms of tardive dyskinesia and may potentially exacerbate symptoms.

Potentially significant drug-drug interactions may exist, requiring dose or frequency adjustment, additional monitoring, and/or selection of alternative therapy.

Adverse Reactions

Cardiovascular: Tachycardia

Central nervous system: Confusion, depression, disorientation, heatstroke, hyperthermia, lethargy, memory impairment, nervousness, numbness of fingers, psychotic symptoms (exacerbation of pre-existing symptoms), toxic psychosis, visual hallucination

Dermatologic: Skin rash

Gastrointestinal: Constipation, nausea, paralytic ileus, vomiting, xerostomia

Genitourinary: Dysuria, urinary retention

Ophthalmic: Blurred vision, mydriasis

Drug Interactions

Metabolism/Transport Effects **Substrate** of CYP2D6 (minor); **Note:** Assignment of Major/Minor substrate status based on clinically relevant drug interaction potential

Avoid Concomitant Use

Avoid concomitant use of Benztropine with any of the following: Aclidinium; Eluxadoline; Glucagon; Ipratropium (Oral Inhalation); Potassium Chloride; Tiotropium; Umeclidinium

Increased Effect/Toxicity

Benztropine may increase the levels/effects of: AbobotulinumtoxinA; Analgesics (Opioid); Anticholinergic Agents; Cannabinoid-Containing Products; Eluxadoline; Glucagon; Mirabegron; OnabotulinumtoxinA; Potassium Chloride; RimabotulinumtoxinB; Thiazide Diuretics; Tiotropium; Topiramate

The levels/effects of Benztropine may be increased by: Aclidinium; Ipratropium (Oral Inhalation); Mianserin; Pramlintide; Umeclidinium

Decreased Effect

Benztropine may decrease the levels/effects of: Acetylcholinesterase Inhibitors; Ioflupane I 123; Itopride; Metoclopramide; Secretin

The levels/effects of Benztropine may be decreased by: Acetylcholinesterase Inhibitors

Storage/Stability Store at 20°C to 25°C (68°F to 77°F).

Mechanism of Action Possesses both anticholinergic and antihistaminic effects. *In vitro* anticholinergic activity approximates that of atropine; *in vivo* it is only about half as active as atropine. Animal data suggest its antihistaminic activity and duration of action approach that of pyrilamine maleate.

Pharmacodynamics

Onset of action:

Oral: Within 1 hour

Parenteral: Within 15 minutes

Duration: 6-48 hours

Dosing: Usual Note: IV route should be reserved for situations when oral or IM are not appropriate.

Children and Adolescents: **Drug-induced extrapyramidal reaction:** Oral, IM, IV:

Children ≥3 years: 0.02-0.05 mg/kg/dose 1-2 times daily; use in children <3 years should be reserved for life-threatening emergencies (Bellman, 1974; Habre, 1999; Joseph, 1995; Teoh, 2002)

Adolescents: 1-4 mg every 12-24 hours (Nelson, 1996)

Adults:

Acute dystonia: IM, IV: 1-2 mg as a single dose

Drug-induced extrapyramidal symptom: Oral, IM, IV: 1-4 mg 1-2 times daily or 1-2 mg 2-3 times daily for reactions developing soon after initiation of antipsychotic medication; usually provides relief within 1-2 days, but may continue for up to 1-2 weeks; withdraw after 1-2 weeks to reassess continued need for therapy. May reinitiate benztropine if symptoms recur.

Parkinsonism, idiopathic or postencephalitic: Oral, IM, IV: Usual dose: 1-2 mg daily; range: 0.5-6 mg/day in a single dose at bedtime or divided in 2-4 doses; titrate dose in 0.5 mg increments at 5- to 6-day intervals to achieve the desired effect; maximum daily dose: 6 mg/**day**

Note: Dosing should be individualized based on patient age, weight, and type of parkinsonism being treated. Lower initial doses may be appropriate for older and thinner patients. Low initial doses (0.5-1 mg) may also be appropriate for idiopathic parkinsonism and may be adequate for maintenance. Higher initial doses (2 mg daily) may be required for postencephalitic parkinsonism. Dosing schedule should also be individualized; patients may respond more favorably to either once-daily bedtime dosing or 2-4 divided doses throughout the day; however, once-daily bedtime dosing is often effective.

Dosing adjustment in renal impairment: There are no dosage adjustments provided in the manufacturer's labeling.

Dosing adjustment in hepatic impairment: There are no dosage adjustments provided in the manufacturer's labeling.

Administration

Oral: May be given with or without food; administration with food may decrease GI upset.

Parenteral: IV route should be reserved for situations when oral or IM are not appropriate. Manufacturer's labeling states there is no difference in onset of effect after IV or IM injection and therefore there is usually no need to use the IV route. No specific instructions on administering benztropine IV are provided in the labeling. The IV route has been reported in the literature in adults (slow IV push when reported), although specific instructions are lacking (Sachdev, 1993; Schramm, 2002).

Dosage Forms Excipient information presented when available (limited, particularly for generics); consult specific product labeling.

Solution, Injection, as mesylate:

Cogentin: 1 mg/mL (2 mL)

Generic: 1 mg/mL (2 mL)

Tablet, Oral, as mesylate:

Generic: 0.5 mg, 1 mg, 2 mg

◆ **Benztropine Mesylate** *see* Benztropine *on page* 272

◆ **Benztropine Omega (Can)** *see* Benztropine *on page* 272

Benzyl Alcohol (BEN zill AL koe hol)

Medication Safety Issues

Sound-alike/look-alike issues:

Benzyl alcohol may be confused with benzoyl peroxide

Brand Names: US Ulesfia; Zilactin [OTC]

Therapeutic Category Analgesic, Topical; Antiparasitic Agent, Topical; Pediculocide; Topical Skin Product

Generic Availability (US) No

Use

Lotion: Treatment of head lice infestation (FDA approved in ages ≥6 months and adults)

Liquid (topical): Temporary relief of pain caused by cold sores/fever blisters (FDA approved in ages ≥2 years and adults)

Pregnancy Risk Factor B

Pregnancy Considerations Adverse events have not been observed in animal reproduction studies.

Breast-Feeding Considerations It is unknown if benzyl alcohol is excreted in breast milk. The manufacturer recommends that caution be exercised when administering benzyl alcohol to nursing women.

Contraindications There are no contraindications listed in the manufacturer's labeling.

Warnings/Precautions Benzyl alcohol exposure to the eye should be avoided. If exposure occurs, flush immediately. Keep out of the reach of children and only use under direct adult supervision. Lotion for the treatment of head lice is not recommended for infants <6 months due to the potential for increased absorption. Do not use gel for oral pain in infants or children younger than 2 years.

Benzyl alcohol and derivatives: Patients <1 month of age or premature neonates with a corrected gestational age <44 weeks could be at risk if treated with topical benzyl alcohol. Large amounts of benzyl alcohol (≥99 mg/kg/day) have been associated with a potentially fatal toxicity ("gasping syndrome") in neonates; the "gasping syndrome" consists of metabolic acidosis, respiratory distress, gasping respirations, CNS dysfunction (including convulsions, intracranial hemorrhage), hypotension, and cardiovascular collapse (AAP, 1997; CDC, 1982); some data suggests that benzoate displaces bilirubin from protein binding sites (Ahlfors, 2001); avoid or use dosage forms containing benzyl alcohol with caution in neonates. See manufacturer's labeling.

Self-medication (OTC use): Discontinue use and notify health care provider if condition worsens or does not improve within 7 days, or if swelling, rash, or fever develops. Do not use for >7 days unless instructed by health care professional.

Warnings: Additional Pediatric Considerations Some dosage forms may contain propylene glycol; in neonates large amounts of propylene glycol delivered orally, intravenously (eg, >3,000 mg/day), or topically have been associated with potentially fatal toxicities which can include metabolic acidosis, seizures, renal failure, and CNS depression; toxicities have also been reported in children and adults including hyperosmolality, lactic acidosis, seizures and respiratory depression; use caution (AAP, 1997; Shehab, 2009).

Adverse Reactions

Dermatologic: Erythema, pruritus

Local: Anesthesia, hypoesthesia, irritation, pain

Ocular: Ocular irritation

Rare but important or life-threatening: Dandruff, dermatitis, dryness, excoriation, exfoliation, paresthesia, rash, thermal burn

Drug Interactions

Metabolism/Transport Effects None known.

Avoid Concomitant Use There are no known interactions where it is recommended to avoid concomitant use.

Increased Effect/Toxicity There are no known significant interactions involving an increase in effect.

Decreased Effect There are no known significant interactions involving a decrease in effect.

Storage/Stability

Gel: Store at 15°C to 30°C (59°F to 68°F). Keep away from fire or flame.

Lotion: Store at 20°C to 25°C (68°F to 77°F); excursions are permitted between 15°C and 30°C (59°F and 86°F); do not freeze.

Mechanism of Action Inhibits respiration of lice by obstructing respiratory spiracles causing lice asphyxiation. No ovicidal activity.

Pharmacokinetics (Adult data unless noted) Absorption: Quantifiable serum plasma concentrations reported following prolonged exposure (30 minutes) in patients 6 months to 11 years of age

Dosing: Usual

Lotion (Ulesfia™): Treatment of head lice infestation: Children ≥6 months of age and adults: Apply appropriate volume for hair length to dry hair, saturate the scalp completely, leave on for 10 minutes, rinse thoroughly with water; repeat in 7 days.

- Hair length 0-2 inches: 4-6 ounces
- Hair length 2-4 inches: 6-8 ounces
- Hair length 4-8 inches: 8-12 ounces
- Hair length 8-16 inches: 12-24 ounces
- Hair length 16-22 inches: 24-32 ounces
- Hair length >22 inches: 32-48 ounces

Liquid (topical) [Zilactin®-L (OTC)]: Cold sores/fever blisters: Children ≥2 years of age and adults: Moisten cotton swab with several drops of liquid; apply to affected area up to 4 times/day; do not use for more than 7 days

Administration For topical use only. Do not swallow liquid or lotion.

Lotion (Ulesfia™): Apply under adult supervision to dry hair, until entire scalp and hair are saturated. Leave on for 10 minutes then rinse thoroughly. Avoid contact with eyes. Wash hands after application. A lice comb may be used to remove dead lice after both treatments.

Liquid (topical) [Zilactin®-L (OTC)]: Apply to affected area only with moistened cotton swab. Allow to dry for 15 seconds. Avoid contact with eyes.

Dosage Forms Excipient information presented when available (limited, particularly for generics); consult specific product labeling.

Gel, Mouth/Throat:

Zilactin: 10% (7.1 g) [contains propylene glycol, sd alcohol]

Lotion, External:

Ulesfia: 5% (227 g) [contains polysorbate 80, trolamine (triethanolamine)]

◆ **Benzylpenicillin Benzathine** *see* Penicillin G Benzathine *on page 1654*

◆ **Benzylpenicillin Potassium** *see* Penicillin G (Parenteral/Aqueous) *on page 1656*

◆ **Benzylpenicillin Sodium** *see* Penicillin G (Parenteral/Aqueous) *on page 1656*

Benzylpenicilloyl Polylysine

(BEN zil pen i SIL oyl pol i LIE seen)

Brand Names: US Pre-Pen

Therapeutic Category Diagnostic Agent

Generic Availability (US) No

Use Adjunct in assessing the risk of administering penicillin (penicillin G or benzylpenicillin) in patients suspected of a clinical penicillin hypersensitivity [FDA approved in pediatric patients (age not specified) and adults]. Has also been used as an adjunct in assessment of hypersensitivity to other beta-lactam antibiotics (penicillins and cephalosporins) to determine the safety of penicillin administration in patients with a history of reaction to cephalosporins

Pregnancy Risk Factor C

Pregnancy Considerations Animal reproduction studies have not been conducted with benzylpenicilloyl polylysine. The Centers for Disease Control and Prevention (CDC) states that penicillin skin testing may be useful in assessing suspected penicillin hypersensitivity in pregnant women diagnosed with syphilis (of any stage) due to a lack of proven alternatives to the use of penicillin in this population (CDC, 2006).

Contraindications Systemic or marked local reaction to a previous administration of benzylpenicilloyl polylysine skin test; patients with a known severe hypersensitivity to penicillin should not be tested

Warnings/Precautions Rare systemic allergic reactions, including anaphylaxis, have been associated with penicillin skin testing. Penicillin skin testing should only be performed by skilled medical personnel under direct supervision of a physician, and testing should be performed only in an appropriate healthcare setting prepared for the immediate treatment with epinephrine. To decrease the risk of a systemic allergic reaction, the manufacturer recommends puncture skin testing prior to intradermal testing. Patients with a reliable history of a severe life-threatening penicillin allergy, including Stevens-Johnson syndrome or TEN, should **NOT** receive penicillin skin testing. Responses to skin testing may be attenuated by concurrent administration of antihistamines. Consider delaying testing until antihistamines can be withheld to allow time for their effects to dissipate.

According to the manufacturer, a negative skin test is associated with an incidence of immediate allergic reactions of <5% after penicillin administration and a positive skin test may indicate >50% incidence of allergic reaction occurring after penicillin administration.

Adequate penicillin skin testing should ideally involve reagents of both the major antigenic determinant (penicilloyl-polylysine) and minor determinants (penicilloate or penilloate). Benzylpenicilloyl polylysine alone does not identify those patients who react to a minor antigenic determinant. The minor determinant mixture (MDM) is not commercially available in the U.S.; however, diluted penicillin G (concentration: 10,000 units/mL) has been used as a minor determinant for skin testing purposes (Bernstein, 2008). Penicillin skin testing does not predict the occurrence of late reactions (eg, type II, III, IV or idiopathic reactions).

Adverse Reactions

Cardiovascular: Hypotension

Dermatologic: Angioneurotic edema, pruritus, erythema, urticaria

Local: Inflammation (intense; at skin test site), wheal (locally)

Respiratory: Dyspnea

Miscellaneous: Systemic allergic reactions (including anaphylaxis; rare)

Drug Interactions

Metabolism/Transport Effects None known.

Avoid Concomitant Use There are no known interactions where it is recommended to avoid concomitant use.

Increased Effect/Toxicity There are no known significant interactions involving an increase in effect.

Decreased Effect

The levels/effects of Benzylpenicilloyl Polylysine may be decreased by: Alpha-/Beta-Agonists; Alpha1-Agonists; Antihistamines

Storage/Stability Refrigerate at 2°C to 8°C (36°F to 46°F); discard if left at room temperature for longer than 1 day.

Mechanism of Action Benzylpenicilloyl polylysine, a conjugate of the benzylpenicilloyl structural group (hapten) and the poly-l-lysine carrier (protein), is an antigen which reacts with benzylpenicilloyl IgE antibodies to elicit the release of chemical mediators, thereby producing type I (immediate or accelerated) urticarial reactions in patients hypersensitive to penicillins.

Dosing: Usual Children and Adults: **Note:** Benzylpenicilloyl polylysine should always be applied first via the puncture technique. **Do not administer intradermally to patients who have positive reactions to a puncture test.**

Puncture scratch test: Apply a small drop of the skin test solution using a 22-28 gauge needle and to make a single shallow puncture of the epidermis through the drop of solution. A positive reaction consists of a pale wheal surrounding the puncture site which develops within 10 minutes and ranges from 5-15 mm or more in diameter (wheal may be surrounded by erythema and variable degrees of itching). If a positive response is evident, the solution should be wiped off immediately. If the puncture test is negative or equivocal (<5 mm wheal, with little or no erythema and no itching) 15 minutes following the puncture test, an intradermal test may be performed.

Intradermal test: Using a 0.5 to 1 mL tuberculin syringe with a 3/8 to 5/8 inch, 26- to 30-gauge short bevel needle; inject a volume of skin test solution sufficient to raise a small intradermal bleb ~3 mm in diameter intradermally and duplicate at least 2 cm apart. A control of 0.9% sodium chloride or allergen-diluting solution should be injected at least 5 cm from the antigen test site. Most skin responses to the intradermal test will develop within 5-15 minutes. A response to the skin test is read at 20 minutes.

Interpretation of intradermal test:

- (-) Negative: No increase in size of original bleb or no greater reaction compared to the control site.
- (±) Ambiguous: Wheal only slightly larger than original bleb with or without erythematous flare and slightly larger than control site; **or** discordance between duplicate test sites.
- (+) Positive: Itching and marked increase in size of original bleb to ≥5 mm. Wheal may exhibit pseudopods and be >20 mm in diameter.

Control site should be reactionless. If wheal >2-3 mm develops at control site, repeat the test. If same reaction occurs, consultation is necessary.

Administration

Puncture test: Administer initially by puncture technique on the inner volvar aspect of the forearm; observe 15 minutes for reaction. If negative reaction, follow with an intradermal injection.

Intradermal test: Do **not** administer intradermally to patients with a positive reaction to a puncture test (wheal of 5-15 mm or more in diameter). Administer the intradermal test on the upper, outer arm, below the deltoid muscle in the event a severe hypersensitivity reaction occurs and a tourniquet needs to be applied. During the skin test, immediate treatment with epinephrine should also be available. Observe 20 minutes for reaction.

Monitoring Parameters Observe 15 minutes (puncture) or 20 minutes (intradermal) for reaction.

Additional Information Penicillin skin testing is the preferred method of evaluating patients with possible penicillin specific IgE-mediated (Type I) immediate hypersensitivity reactions, when performed using the appropriate major and minor determinant reagents. Testing detects the presence or absence of penicillin-specific IgE antibodies; therefore, it is not useful to detect non-IgE mediated reactions. Patients testing positive to benzylpenicilloyl polylysine possess IgE antibodies against the benzylpenicilloyl structural group (B-lactam ring). The possibility exists for patients to have selective IgE antibodies directed against the R-group side chain structure of certain penicillins, rather than the core beta-lactam structure. Therefore, these patients may test negative to the penicillin major and minor determinants, but be allergic to semisynthetic penicillins (eg, amoxicillin, ampicillin) only and tolerate other penicillin compounds (Bernstein, 2008). Skin testing has also been used in some centers to determine safety of penicillin administration in patients with prior reactions to cephalosporins.

Dosage Forms Excipient information presented when available (limited, particularly for generics); consult specific product labeling.

Injection, solution:

Pre-Pen®: 6 x 10^{-5} M (0.25 mL)

◆ **Benzylpenicilloyl-polylysine** *see* Benzylpenicilloyl Polylysine *on page 274*

Beractant (ber AKT ant)

Medication Safety Issues

Sound-alike/look-alike issues:

Survanta® may be confused with Sufenta®

Brand Names: US Survanta

Brand Names: Canada Survanta®

Therapeutic Category Lung Surfactant

Generic Availability (US) No

Use Prevention and treatment of respiratory distress syndrome (RDS) in premature infants

Prophylactic therapy: Infants with body weight <1250 g who are at risk for developing or with evidence of surfactant deficiency

Rescue therapy: Treatment of infants with RDS confirmed by x-ray and requiring mechanical ventilation

Pregnancy Considerations Beractant is only indicated for use in premature infants.

Contraindications There are no contraindications listed within the FDA-approved labeling

Warnings/Precautions For endotracheal administration only. Rapidly affects oxygenation and lung compliance; restrict use to a highly-supervised clinical setting with immediate availability of clinicians experienced in intubation and ventilatory management of premature infants. Transient episodes of bradycardia and decreased oxygen saturation occur. Discontinue dosing procedure and initiate measures to alleviate the condition; may reinstitute after the patient is stable. Produces rapid improvements in lung oxygenation and compliance that may require frequent adjustments to oxygen delivery and ventilator settings.

Warnings: Additional Pediatric Considerations Use of beractant in neonates <600 g birth weight or >1750 g birth weight has not been evaluated.

Adverse Reactions During the dosing procedure:

Cardiovascular: Transient bradycardia

Respiratory: Oxygen desaturation

Rare but important or life-threatening: Apnea, endotracheal tube blockage, hypercarbia, hyper-/hypotension, post-treatment nosocomial sepsis probability increased, pulmonary air leaks, pulmonary interstitial emphysema, vasoconstriction

Drug Interactions

Metabolism/Transport Effects None known.

Avoid Concomitant Use

Avoid concomitant use of Beractant with any of the following: Ceritinib

Increased Effect/Toxicity

Beractant may increase the levels/effects of: Bradycardia-Causing Agents; Ceritinib; Ivabradine; Lacosamide

The levels/effects of Beractant may be increased by: Bretylium; Ruxolitinib; Tofacitinib

Decreased Effect There are no known significant interactions involving a decrease in effect.

Storage/Stability **Refrigerate**; protect from light. Prior to administration, warm by standing at room temperature for 20 minutes or held in hand for 8 minutes. **Artificial warming methods should not be used.** Unused, unopened vials warmed to room temperature may be returned to the refrigerator within 24 hours of warming only once.

Mechanism of Action Replaces deficient or ineffective endogenous lung surfactant in neonates with respiratory distress syndrome (RDS) or in neonates at risk of developing RDS. Surfactant prevents the alveoli from collapsing during expiration by lowering surface tension between air and alveolar surfaces.

Dosing: Neonatal Endotracheal:

Prophylactic treatment: 4 mL/kg (100 mg phospholipids/kg) as soon as possible; as many as 4 doses may be administered during the first 48 hours of life, no more frequently than 6 hours apart. The need for additional doses is determined by evidence of continuing respiratory distress or if the infant is still intubated and requiring at least 30% inspired oxygen to maintain a PaO_2 ≤80 torr.

Rescue treatment: 4 mL/kg (100 mg phospholipids/kg) as soon as the diagnosis of RDS is made; may repeat if needed, no more frequently than every 6 hours to a maximum of 4 doses

Administration Endotracheal: For endotracheal administration only. Do not shake; if settling occurs during storage, gently swirl. Suction infant prior to administration; inspect solution to verify complete mixing of the suspension. Administer endotracheally by instillation through a 5-French end-hole catheter inserted into the infant's endotracheal tube. Administer the dose in four 1 mL/kg aliquots. Each quarter-dose is instilled over 2-3 seconds; each quarter-dose is administered with the infant in a different position; slightly downward inclination with head turned to the right, then repeat with head turned to the left; then slightly upward inclination with head turned to the right, then repeat with head turned to the left.

Monitoring Parameters Continuous heart rate and transcutaneous O_2 saturation should be monitored during administration; frequent ABG sampling is necessary to prevent postdosing hyperoxia and hypocarbia.

Dosage Forms Excipient information presented when available (limited, particularly for generics); consult specific product labeling.

Suspension, Inhalation:

Survanta: Phospholipids 25 mg/mL (4 mL, 8 mL)

◆ **Berinert** *see* C1 Inhibitor (Human) *on page 333*

Besifloxacin (be si FLOX a sin)

Brand Names: US Besivance

Brand Names: Canada Besivance™

Therapeutic Category Antibiotic, Fluoroquinolone; Antibiotic, Ophthalmic; Ophthalmic Agent

Generic Availability (US) No

Use Treatment of bacterial conjunctivitis (FDA approved in ages ≥1 year and adults)

Pregnancy Risk Factor C

Pregnancy Considerations Adverse events were observed in some animal reproduction studies. Systemic concentrations of besifloxacin following ophthalmic administration are low. If ophthalmic agents are needed during pregnancy, the minimum effective dose should be used in combination with punctual occlusion for 3 to 5 minutes after application to decrease potential exposure to the fetus (Samples 1988).

Breast-Feeding Considerations It is not known if besifloxacin is excreted into breast milk. The manufacturer recommends that caution be exercised when administering besifloxacin to nursing women.

Contraindications There are no contraindications listed in the manufacturer's labeling.

Warnings/Precautions Severe hypersensitivity reactions, including anaphylaxis, have occurred with systemic quinolone therapy. Prompt discontinuation of drug should occur if skin rash or other symptoms arise. Prolonged use may result in fungal or bacterial superinfection; discontinue use and initiate alternative therapy if superinfection occurs. Do not inject ophthalmic solution subconjunctivally or introduce directly into the anterior chamber of the eye. Contact lenses should not be worn during treatment of ophthalmic infections.

Adverse Reactions

Central nervous system: Headache

Ocular: Blurred vision, conjunctival redness, irritation, pain, pruritus

Drug Interactions

Metabolism/Transport Effects None known.

Avoid Concomitant Use There are no known interactions where it is recommended to avoid concomitant use.

Increased Effect/Toxicity There are no known significant interactions involving an increase in effect.

Decreased Effect There are no known significant interactions involving a decrease in effect.

Storage/Stability Store between 15°C to 25°C (59°F to 77°F). Protect from light.

Mechanism of Action Inhibits both DNA gyrase and topoisomerase IV. DNA gyrase is an essential bacterial enzyme required for DNA replication, transcription, and repair. Topoisomerase IV is an essential bacterial enzyme required for decatenation during cell division. Inhibition effect is bactericidal.

Pharmacokinetics (Adult data unless noted) Half-life elimination: ~7 hours

Dosing: Usual Ophthalmic: Children ≥1 year and Adults: Bacterial conjunctivitis: Instill 1 drop into affected eye(s) 3 times/day (4-12 hours apart) for 7 days

Administration Ophthalmic: Wash hands before and after instillation. Shake bottle once prior to each administration. Avoid contaminating the applicator tip with affected eye(s).

Monitoring Parameters Signs and symptoms of infection or hypersensitivity reaction

Dosage Forms Excipient information presented when available (limited, particularly for generics); consult specific product labeling.

Suspension, Ophthalmic:

Besivance: 0.6% (5 mL) [contains benzalkonium chloride, edetate disodium dihydrate]

◆ **Besifloxacin Hydrochloride** *see* Besifloxacin *on page 276*

◆ **Besivance** *see* Besifloxacin *on page 276*

◆ **Besivance™ (Can)** *see* Besifloxacin *on page 276*

◆ **9-Beta-D-Ribofuranosyladenine** *see* Adenosine *on page 73*

◆ **Betacaine (Can)** *see* Lidocaine (Topical) *on page 1258*

◆ **Beta Care Betatar Gel [OTC]** *see* Coal Tar *on page 523*

◆ **Betaderm (Can)** *see* Betamethasone (Topical) *on page 280*

◆ **Betagan** *see* Levobunolol *on page 1238*

◆ **Betagan® (Can)** *see* Levobunolol *on page 1238*

◆ **Beta HC [OTC]** *see* Hydrocortisone (Topical) *on page 1041*

Betaine (BAY ta een)

Medication Safety Issues

Sound-alike/look-alike issues:

Betaine may be confused with Betadine

Cystadane may be confused with cysteamine, cysteine

Brand Names: US Cystadane

Brand Names: Canada Cystadane

Therapeutic Category Homocystinuria, Treatment Agent

Generic Availability (US) May be product dependent

Use Treatment of homocystinuria to reduce elevated homocysteine blood concentrations (FDA approved in ages 24 days to 17 years and adults); homocystinuria includes deficiencies or defects in cystathionine beta-synthase (CBS), 5,10-methylenetetrahydrofolate reductase (MTHFR), and cobalamin cofactor metabolism (cbl)

Prescribing and Access Restrictions Cystadane may be obtained by contacting AnovoRx at wholesale@anovorx.com.

Pregnancy Risk Factor C

Pregnancy Considerations Animal reproduction studies have not been conducted.

Breast-Feeding Considerations It is not known if betaine is excreted in breast milk. According to the manufacturer, use in nursing women only if clearly needed.

Contraindications There are no contraindications listed in the manufacturer's labeling.

Warnings/Precautions Use caution in patients with cystathionine beta-synthase (CBS) deficiency; treatment with betaine may cause large increases of plasma methionine concentrations. Cerebral edema may be associated with hypermethioninemia.

Adverse Reactions

Gastrointestinal: Diarrhea, dysgeusia, GI distress, nausea

Rare but important or life-threatening: Alopecia, anorexia, agitation, cerebral edema (associated with hypermethioninemia), dental disorders, depression, hives, glossitis, irritability, personality disorder, sleep disturbances, skin odor abnormalities, urinary incontinence, vomiting

Drug Interactions

Metabolism/Transport Effects None known.

Avoid Concomitant Use There are no known interactions where it is recommended to avoid concomitant use.

Increased Effect/Toxicity There are no known significant interactions involving an increase in effect.

Decreased Effect There are no known significant interactions involving a decrease in effect.

Storage/Stability Store at 15°C to 30°C (59°F to 86°F). Protect from moisture

Mechanism of Action Betaine is an endogenous metabolite of choline. Betaine acts as a methyl group donor in the remethylation of homocysteine to methionine. Homocystinuria is an inborn error of metabolism in which elevated plasma homocysteine levels can lead to mental retardation, ocular abnormalities, osteoporosis, premature atherosclerosis and thromboembolic disease. Remethylation is one of the two divergent pathways in the metabolism of homocysteine. The second pathway involves transulfuration of homocysteine to produce cysteine. A number of enzymes and cofactors are also involved in these pathways.

Dosing: Neonatal Oral: PNA ≥24 days (PMA not specified): 100 mg/kg/day divided into 2 doses; increase at weekly intervals in 50 mg/kg/day increments; minimal benefit has been shown in patients treated with >150 mg/kg/day or exceeding a twice daily dosing schedule

Dosing: Usual Oral: **Note:** Minimal benefit has been seen with dosages >150 mg/kg/day or >20 g/day or exceeding a twice daily dosing schedule.

Infants and Children <3 years: 100 mg/kg/day divided into 2 doses; increase at weekly intervals in 50 mg/kg/day increments

Children ≥3 years, Adolescents, and Adults: 3 g twice daily; doses up to 20 g/day have been needed to control homocysteine plasma concentrations in some patients

Preparation for Administration Oral: Shake lightly before removing cap from bottle. Measure prescribed amount with provided measuring scoop and dissolve in 120 to 180 mL of water, juice, milk, or formula, or mix with food for immediate ingestion.

Administration Oral: Administer without regard to food immediately after reconstitution; do not use if powder does not completely dissolve or gives a colored solution.

Monitoring Parameters Plasma homocysteine concentration (should be low or undetectable); plasma methionine (CBS patients)

Additional Information Vitamin B_6, vitamin B_{12}, and folate have been helpful in the management of homocystinuria and are often used in conjunction.

Dosage Forms Excipient information presented when available (limited, particularly for generics); consult specific product labeling.

Powder, Oral, as anhydrous:

Cystadane: 1 g/scoop (180 g)

Tablet, Oral, as anhydrous:

Generic: 300 mg

◆ **Betaine Anhydrous** *see* Betaine *on page 277*

◆ **Betaject (Can)** *see* Betamethasone (Systemic) *on page 278*

◆ **Betaloc (Can)** *see* Metoprolol *on page 1418*

Betamethasone (Systemic) (bay ta METH a sone)

Related Information

Corticosteroids Systemic Equivalencies *on page 2260*

Brand Names: US Celestone Soluspan; Celestone [DSC]

Brand Names: Canada Betaject; Celestone Soluspan

Therapeutic Category Corticosteroid, Systemic

Generic Availability (US) May be product dependent

Use

IM: Anti-inflammatory or immunosuppressant agent in the treatment of a variety of diseases when oral therapy not feasible including those of allergic, hematologic, dermatologic, endocrine, gastrointestinal, ophthalmic, neoplastic, rheumatic, autoimmune, nervous system, renal, and respiratory origin (FDA approved in pediatric patients [age not specified] and adults)

Intra-articular or soft tissue administration: Adjunctive therapy for short-term administration (to tide the patient over an acute episode or exacerbation) in acute gouty arthritis, acute and subacute bursitis, acute nonspecific tenosynovitis, epicondylitis, rheumatoid arthritis, synovitis of osteoarthritis (FDA approved in pediatric patients [age not specified] and adults)

Intralesional: Treatment of alopecia areata; discoid lupus erythematosus; keloids; localized hypertrophic, infiltrated, inflammatory lesions of granuloma annulare, lichen planus, lichen simplex chronicus (neurodermatitis), and psoriatic plaques; necrobiosis lipoidica diabeticorum (FDA approved in pediatric patients [age not specified] and adults); has also been used for treatment of infantile hemangioma.

Pregnancy Risk Factor C

Pregnancy Considerations Adverse events have been observed with corticosteroids in animal reproduction studies. Betamethasone crosses the placenta (Brownfoot, 2013); and is partially metabolized by placental enzymes to an inactive metabolite (Murphy, 2007). Some studies have shown an association between first trimester systemic corticosteroid use and oral clefts (Park-Wyllie, 2000; Pradat, 2003). Systemic corticosteroids may have an effect on fetal growth (decreased birth weight); however, information is conflicting (Lunghi, 2010). Hypoadrenalism may occur in newborns following maternal use of corticosteroids during pregnancy; monitor.

Because antenatal corticosteroid administration may reduce the incidence of intraventricular hemorrhage, necrotizing enterocolitis, neonatal mortality, and respiratory distress syndrome, the injection is often used in patients with preterm premature rupture of membranes (membrane rupture between 24 0/7 weeks and 34 0/7 weeks of gestation) who are at risk of preterm delivery (ACOG, 2013). When systemic corticosteroids are needed in pregnancy, it is generally recommended to use the lowest effective dose for the shortest duration of time, avoiding high doses during the first trimester (Leachman, 2006; Lunghi, 2010; Makol, 2011; Østensen, 2009).

Women exposed to betamethasone during pregnancy for the treatment of an autoimmune disease may contact the OTIS Autoimmune Diseases Study at 877-311-8972.

Breast-Feeding Considerations Corticosteroids are excreted in human milk. The onset of milk secretion after birth may be delayed and the volume of milk produced may be decreased by antenatal betamethasone therapy; this affect was seen when delivery occurred 3-9 days after the betamethasone dose in women between 28 and 34 weeks gestation. Antenatal betamethasone therapy did not affect milk production when birth occurred <3 days or >10 days of treatment (Henderson, 2008).

The manufacturer notes that when used systemically, maternal use of corticosteroids have the potential to cause adverse events in a nursing infant (eg, growth suppression, interfere with endogenous corticosteroid production) and therefore recommends that caution be exercised when administering betamethasone to nursing women. If there is concern about exposure to the infant, some guidelines recommend waiting 4 hours after the maternal dose of an oral systemic corticosteroid before breast-feeding in order to decrease potential exposure to the infant (based on a study using prednisolone) (Bae, 2011; Leachman, 2006; Makol, 2011; Ost, 1985).

Contraindications

Hypersensitivity to any component of the formulation; IM administration contraindicated in idiopathic thrombocytopenic purpura.

Documentation of allergenic cross-reactivity for glucocorticoids is limited. However, because of similarities in chemical structure and/or pharmacologic actions, the possibility of cross-sensitivity cannot be ruled out with certainty.

Warnings/Precautions Avoid concurrent use of other corticosteroids.

May cause hypercorticism or suppression of hypothalamic-pituitary-adrenal (HPA) axis, particularly in younger children or in patients receiving high doses for prolonged periods. HPA axis suppression may lead to adrenal crisis. Withdrawal and discontinuation of a corticosteroid should be done slowly and carefully. Particular care is required when patients are transferred from systemic corticosteroids to inhaled products due to possible adrenal insufficiency or withdrawal from steroids, including an increase in allergic symptoms. Patients receiving >20 mg per day of prednisone (or equivalent) may be most susceptible. Fatalities have occurred due to adrenal insufficiency in asthmatic patients during and after transfer from systemic corticosteroids to aerosol steroids; aerosol steroids do not provide the systemic steroid needed to treat patients having trauma, surgery, or infections. In stressful situations, HPA axis-suppressed patients should receive adequate supplementation with natural glucocorticoids (hydrocortisone or cortisone) rather than betamethasone (due to lack of mineralocorticoid activity).

Acute myopathy has been reported with high-dose corticosteroids, usually in patients with neuromuscular transmission disorders; may involve ocular and/or respiratory muscles; monitor creatine kinase; recovery may be delayed. Corticosteroid use may cause psychiatric disturbances, including depression, euphoria, insomnia, mood swings, and personality changes. Preexisting psychiatric conditions may be exacerbated by corticosteroid use. Prolonged use of corticosteroids may also increase the incidence of secondary infection, mask acute infection (including fungal infections), prolong or exacerbate viral infections, or limit response to killed or inactivated vaccines. Special pathogens (*Amoeba*, *Candida*, *Cryptococcus*, *Mycobacterium*, *Nocardia*, *Pneumocystis*, *Strongyloides*, or *Toxoplasma*) may be activated or an infection exacerbation may occur (may be fatal). Amebiasis or *Strongyloides* infections should be particularly ruled out. Exposure to varicella zoster (chickenpox) should be avoided; corticosteroids should not be used to treat ocular herpes simplex. Corticosteroids should not be used for cerebral malaria or viral hepatitis. Close observation is required in patients with latent tuberculosis and/or TB reactivity; restrict use in active TB (only in conjunction with antituberculosis treatment). Prolonged treatment with corticosteroids has been associated with the development of Kaposi sarcoma (case reports); if noted, discontinuation of therapy should be considered. High-dose corticosteroids should not be used to manage acute head injury. Rare cases of anaphylactoid reactions have been observed in patients receiving corticosteroids.

Use with caution in patients with thyroid disease, hepatic impairment, renal impairment, cardiovascular disease, diabetes, glaucoma, cataracts, myasthenia gravis, patients at risk for osteoporosis, patients at risk for seizures, or GI diseases (diverticulitis, fresh intestinal anastomoses, peptic ulcer, ulcerative colitis) due to perforation risk. Use caution following acute MI (corticosteroids have been associated with myocardial rupture). Use with caution in patients with HF and/or hypertension; long-term use has been associated with fluid retention and electrolyte disturbances. Dietary modifications may be necessary. Use with caution in patients with a recent history of myocardial infarction (MI); left ventricular free wall rupture has been reported after the use of corticosteroids. Use with caution in patients with renal impairment; fluid and sodium retention and increased potassium and calcium excretion may occur. Dietary modifications may be necessary. Not recommended for the treatment of optic neuritis; may increase frequency of new episodes. Intra-articular injection may result in joint tissue damage. Injection into an infected site should be avoided. Injection into a previously infected join is usually not recommended. If infection is suspected, joint fluid examination is recommended. If septic arthritis occurs after injection, institute appropriate antimicrobial therapy. Suspension for injection is for intramuscular, intra-articular or intralesional use only, do not administer intravenously. Corticosteroids are not approved for epidural injection. Serious neurologic events (eg, spinal cord infarction, paraplegia, quadriplegia, cortical blindness, stroke), some resulting in death, have been reported with epidural injection of corticosteroids, with and without use of fluoroscopy. Intra-articular injected corticosteroids may be systemically absorbed. May produce systemic as well as local effects. Appropriate examination of any joint fluid present is necessary to exclude a septic process. Avoid injection into an infected site. Do not inject into unstable joints. Intra-articular injection may result in damage to joint tissues. Potentially significant drug-drug interactions may exist, requiring dose or frequency adjustment, additional monitoring, and/or selection of alternative therapy. Because of the risk of adverse effects, systemic corticosteroids should be used cautiously in the elderly in the smallest possible effective dose for the shortest duration. Withdraw therapy with gradual tapering of dose.

Prolonged use in children may affect growth velocity; growth should be routinely monitored in pediatric patients.

Warnings: Additional Pediatric Considerations Adrenal suppression with failure to thrive has been reported in infants after receiving intralesional corticosteroid injections for treatment of hemangioma (Goyal, 2004). May cause osteoporosis (at any age) or inhibition of bone growth in pediatric patients. Use with caution in patients with osteoporosis. In a population-based study of children, risk of fracture was shown to be increased with >4 courses of corticosteroids; underlying clinical condition may also impact bone health and osteoporotic effect of corticosteroids (Leonard, 2007).

Adverse Reactions

Cardiovascular: Congestive heart failure, edema, hyper-/hypotension

Central nervous system: Dizziness, headache, insomnia, intracranial pressure increased, lightheadedness, nervousness, pseudotumor cerebri, seizure, vertigo

Dermatologic: Ecchymoses, facial erythema, fragile skin, hirsutism, hyper-/hypopigmentation, perioral dermatitis (oral), petechiae, striae, wound healing impaired

Endocrine & metabolic: Amenorrhea, Cushing's syndrome, diabetes mellitus, growth suppression, hyperglycemia, hypokalemia, menstrual irregularities, pituitary-adrenal axis suppression, protein catabolism, sodium retention, water retention

Local: Injection site reactions (intra-articular use), sterile abscess

Neuromuscular & skeletal: Arthralgia, muscle atrophy, fractures, muscle weakness, myopathy, osteoporosis, necrosis (femoral and humeral heads)

Ocular: Cataracts, glaucoma, intraocular pressure increased

Miscellaneous: Anaphylactoid reaction, diaphoresis, hypersensitivity, secondary infection

Drug Interactions

Metabolism/Transport Effects None known.

Avoid Concomitant Use

Avoid concomitant use of Betamethasone (Systemic) with any of the following: Aldesleukin; BCG; BCG (Intravesical); Indium 111 Capromab Pendetide; Mifepristone; Natalizumab; Pimecrolimus; Tacrolimus (Topical); Tofacitinib

Increased Effect/Toxicity

Betamethasone (Systemic) may increase the levels/effects of: Acetylcholinesterase Inhibitors; Amphotericin B; Androgens; Ceritinib; Deferasirox; Leflunomide; Loop Diuretics; Natalizumab; Nicorandil; NSAID (COX-2 Inhibitor); NSAID (Nonselective); Quinolone Antibiotics; Thiazide Diuretics; Tofacitinib; Vaccines (Live); Warfarin

The levels/effects of Betamethasone (Systemic) may be increased by: Aprepitant; CYP3A4 Inhibitors (Strong); Denosumab; Estrogen Derivatives; Fosaprepitant; Indacaterol; Mifepristone; Neuromuscular-Blocking Agents (Nondepolarizing); Pimecrolimus; Roflumilast; Salicylates; Tacrolimus (Topical); Telaprevir; Trastuzumab

Decreased Effect

Betamethasone (Systemic) may decrease the levels/effects of: Aldesleukin; Antidiabetic Agents; BCG; BCG (Intravesical); Calcitriol (Systemic); Coccidioides immitis Skin Test; Corticorelin; Hyaluronidase; Indium 111 Capromab Pendetide; Isoniazid; Salicylates; Sipuleucel-T; Telaprevir; Urea Cycle Disorder Agents; Vaccines (Inactivated); Vaccines (Live)

The levels/effects of Betamethasone (Systemic) may be decreased by: CYP3A4 Inducers (Strong); Echinacea; Mifepristone; Mitotane

Storage/Stability Store at 25°C (77°F); excursions are permitted between 15°C and 30°C (59°F and 86°F). Protect from light.

Mechanism of Action Controls the rate of protein synthesis; depresses the migration of polymorphonuclear leukocytes, fibroblasts; reverses capillary permeability and lysosomal stabilization at the cellular level to prevent or control inflammation

Dosing: Usual Note: Dosages expressed as combined amount of betamethasone sodium phosphate and betamethasone acetate; 1 mg is equivalent to betamethasone sodium phosphate 0.5 mg and betamethasone acetate 0.5 mg. Dosage should be based on severity of disease and patient response; use lowest effective dose for shortest period of time to avoid HPA axis suppression

Pediatric:

General dosing, treatment of inflammatory and allergic conditions: Infants, Children, and Adolescents: IM: Initial: 0.02 to 0.3 mg/kg/day (0.6 to 9 mg/m^2/day) in 3 or 4 divided doses

Infantile hemangioma, severe: Limited data available: Infants and Children: Intralesional: Dosage dependent upon size of lesion: Commonly reported: 6 mg administered as a 6 mg/mL (in combination with triamcinolone injection) divided into multiple injections along the lesion perimeter; reported range: 1.5 to 18 mg/dose; doses usually administered every 8 to 14 weeks; reported range: 6 to 25 weeks (Buckmiller, 2008; Chowdri, 1994; Kushner, 1985; Praseyono, 2011). Dosing based on small trials and case-series, mostly reported in infants and children ≤4 years of age. The largest experience (n=70, age range: 2 months to 12 years) prospectively used a betamethasone/triamcinolone combination injection (1.5 to 18 mg betamethasone acetate) and showed that 89.23% of lesions with an initial volume <20 cc^3 regressed by more than 50%, but only 22.2% of lesions with an initial volume >20 cc^3 displayed a good or excellent response (Chowdri, 1994). Another trial (n=25, age range: 7 weeks to 2 years) used lower doses of 3 to 12 mg (in combination with triamcinolone); 16 patients experienced a marked response (Kushner, 1985).

Adult: **Note:** Dosages expressed as combined amount of betamethasone sodium phosphate and betamethasone acetate; 1 mg is equivalent to betamethasone sodium phosphate 0.5 mg and betamethasone acetate 0.5 mg. Base dosage on severity of disease and patient response

General dosing: IM: Initial: 0.25 to 9 mg/day

Antenatal fetal maturation: IM: In women with preterm premature rupture of membranes (membrane rupture between 24 0/7 weeks and 34 0/7 weeks of gestation), a single course of corticosteroids is recommended if there is a risk of preterm delivery (ACOG, 2013). Although the optimal corticosteroid and dose have not been determined, betamethasone 12 mg every 24 hours for a total of 2 doses has been used in most studies (Brownfoot, 2013).

Bursitis (other than of the foot), tenosynovitis, peritendinitis: Intrabursal: 3 to 6 mg (0.5 to1 mL) for 1 dose; several injections may be required for acute exacerbations or chronic conditions; reduced doses may be warranted for repeat injections

Dermatologic: Intralesional: 1.2 mg/cm^2 (0.2 mL/cm^2) for 1 dose (maximum: 6 mg [1 mL] weekly)

Foot disorders: Intra-articular: 1.5 mg to 6 mg (0.25 to1 mL) per dose at 3- to 7-day intervals. Dose is based upon condition:

Bursitis: 1.5 mg to 3 mg (0.25 to 0.5 mL)

Tenosynovitis: 3 mg (0.5 mL)

Acute gouty arthritis: 3 mg to 6 mg (0.5 to1 mL)

Multiple sclerosis: IM: 30 mg daily for 1 week, followed by 12 mg every other day for 4 weeks

Rheumatoid and osteoarthritis: Intra-articular: 3 mg to 12 mg (0.5 to 2 mL) for 1 dose. Dose is based upon the joint size:

Very large (eg, hip): 6 to 12 mg (1 to 2 mL)

Large (eg, knee, ankle, shoulder): 6 mg (1 mL)

Medium (eg, elbow, wrist): 3 to 6 mg (0.5 to 1 mL)

Small (eg, inter- or metacarpophalangeal, sternoclavicular): 1.5 mg to 3 mg (0.25 to 0.5 mL)

Dosing adjustment in renal impairment: There are no dosage adjustments provided in the manufacturer's labeling.

Dosing adjustment in hepatic impairment: There are no dosage adjustments provided in the manufacturer's labeling.

Preparation for Administration If suspension is coadministered with a local anesthetic, it may be mixed in syringe with 1% or 2% lidocaine HCl (without parabens). Withdraw the dose of betamethasone suspension from the vial into the syringe, then draw up the local anesthetic into the syringe, and shake the syringe briefly. Do not inject the local anesthetic directly into the suspension vial.

Administration Note: May be coadministered with a local anesthetic.

IM: Do **not** give injectable suspension IV

Intrabursal: Tendinitis, tenosynovitis: Inject into affected tendon sheaths (not directly into tendons)

Intralesional: Using a 25-gauge tuberculin syringe with 1/2-inch needle inject a uniform depot; for infantile hemangioma, 26- and 27-gauge needles have been used for administration. Should be injected directly into the lesion area. Do **not** inject subcutaneously.

Monitoring Parameters Intraocular pressure (if therapy >6 weeks); weight, height, and linear growth (with chronic use); assess HPA suppression. Monitor blood pressure, serum glucose, potassium, calcium, hemoglobin, occult blood loss, and clinical presence of adverse effects.

Test Interactions May suppress the wheal and flare reactions to skin test antigens

Dosage Forms Excipient information presented when available (limited, particularly for generics); consult specific product labeling. [DSC] = Discontinued product

Solution, Oral, as base:

Celestone: 0.6 mg/5 mL (118 mL [DSC]) [cherry-orange flavor]

Suspension, Injection:

Celestone Soluspan: Betamethasone sodium phosphate 3 mg and betamethasone acetate 3 mg per 1 mL (5 mL) [contains benzalkonium chloride, edetate disodium]

Generic: Betamethasone sodium phosphate 3 mg and betamethasone acetate 3 mg per 1 mL (5 mL)

Betamethasone (Topical) (bay ta METH a sone)

Medication Safety Issues

Sound-alike/look-alike issues:

Luxiq may be confused with Lasix

Related Information

Corticosteroids Systemic Equivalencies *on page 2260*

Topical Corticosteroids *on page 2262*

Brand Names: US AlphaTrex; Diprolene; Diprolene AF; Luxiq

Brand Names: Canada Betaderm; Betnesol; Celestoderm V; Celestoderm V/2; Diprolene; Diprosone; Luxiq; Prevex B; ratio-Ectosone; Ratio-Topilene; Ratio-Topisone; Rivasone; Rolene; Rosone; Taro-Sone; Valisone Scalp Lotion

Therapeutic Category Corticosteroid, Topical

Generic Availability (US) Yes

Use

Betamethasone dipropionate (augmented): Treatment of inflammation and pruritus associated with corticosteroid-responsive dermatoses of the skin (Cream, lotion, and ointment: FDA approved in ages ≥13 years and adults; Gel: FDA approved in ages ≥12 years and adults)

Betamethasone valerate:

Cream, lotion, and ointment: Treatment of inflammation and pruritus associated with corticosteroid-responsive dermatoses of the skin (FDA approved in pediatric patients [age not specified] and adults)

Foam: Treatment of inflammation and pruritus associated with corticosteroid-responsive dermatoses of the scalp including psoriasis (FDA approved in adults)

Pregnancy Risk Factor C

Pregnancy Considerations Adverse events have been observed with corticosteroids in animal reproduction studies. Topical corticosteroids are preferred over systemic for treating conditions, such as psoriasis or atopic dermatitis in pregnant women; high potency corticosteroids are not recommended during the first trimester. Topical products are not recommended for extensive use, in large quantities, or for long periods of time in pregnant women (Bae, 2011; Koutroulis, 2011; Leachman, 2006). Refer to the Betamethasone (Systemic) monograph for additional information.

Breast-Feeding Considerations Corticosteroids are excreted in human milk. It is not known if systemic absorption following topical administration results in detectable quantities in human milk. Do not apply topical corticosteroids to nipples; hypertension was noted in a nursing infant exposed to a topical corticosteroid while nursing (Leachman, 2006).

The manufacturer notes that when used systemically, maternal use of corticosteroids have the potential to cause adverse events in a nursing infant (eg, growth suppression, interfere with endogenous corticosteroid production) and therefore recommends that caution be exercised when administering betamethasone to nursing women.

Contraindications Hypersensitivity to betamethasone, other corticosteroids, or any component of the formulation

Warnings/Precautions Very high potency topical products are not for treatment of rosacea, perioral dermatitis; not for use on face, groin, or axillae; not for use in a diapered area. Avoid concurrent use of other corticosteroids.

May cause hypercorticism or suppression of hypothalamic-pituitary-adrenal (HPA) axis, particularly in younger children or in patients receiving high doses for prolonged periods. HPA axis suppression may lead to adrenal crisis. Patients receiving large doses of potent topical steroids, steroids to large surface areas, using occlusive dressings, or with liver failure should be periodically evaluated for HPA axis suppression using ACTH stimulation test. Withdrawal and discontinuation of a corticosteroid should be done slowly and carefully by reducing the frequency of application or substitution of a less potent steroid. Recovery is usually prompt and complete upon drug discontinuation, but may require supplemental systemic corticosteroids if signs and symptoms of steroid withdrawal occur. In stressful situations, HPA axis-suppressed patients should receive adequate supplementation with glucocorticoids (hydrocortisone or cortisone) rather than betamethasone (due to lack of mineralocorticoid activity).

Topical corticosteroids may be absorbed percutaneously. Absorption of topical corticosteroids may cause manifestations of Cushing syndrome (rare), hyperglycemia, or glycosuria. Absorption is increased by the use of occlusive dressings, application to denuded skin, application to large surface areas, or prolonged use. Potentially significant interactions may exist, requiring dose or frequency adjustment, additional monitoring, and/or selection of alternative therapy.

Discontinue if skin irritation or contact dermatitis should occur; do not use in patients with decreased skin circulation. Withdraw therapy with gradual tapering of dose by reducing the frequency of application or substitution of a less potent steroid.

Augmented (eg very high potency) product use in patients <13 years of age is not recommended. Not for treatment of rosacea, perioral dermatitis, or if skin atrophy is present at treatment site; not for facial, groin, axillary, oral, ophthalmic, or intravaginal use. Children may absorb proportionally larger amounts after topical application and may be more prone to systemic effects. HPA axis suppression, intracranial hypertension, and Cushing syndrome have been reported in children receiving topical corticosteroids. Prolonged use may affect growth velocity; growth should be routinely monitored in pediatric patients. Use lowest dose possible for shortest period of time to avoid HPA axis suppression. Foam contains flammable propellants. Avoid fire, flame, and smoking during and immediately following administration.

Warnings: Additional Pediatric Considerations The extent of percutaneous absorption is dependent on several factors, including epidermal integrity (intact vs abraded skin), formulation, age of the patient, prolonged duration of use, and the use of occlusive dressings. Percutaneous absorption of topical steroids is increased in neonates (especially preterm neonates), infants, and young children. Infants and small children may be more susceptible to HPA axis suppression, intracranial hypertension, Cushing syndrome, or other systemic toxicities due to larger skin surface area to body mass ratio. HPA axis suppression was observed in 32% of infants and children (age range: 3 months to 12 years) being treated with betamethasone dipropionate cream (0.05%) for atopic dermatitis in an open-label trial (n=60); the incidence was greater younger patients vs older children (mean reported incidence for age ranges: ≤1 year: 50%; 2 to 8 years: 32% to 38%; 9 to 12 years: 17%).

Some dosage forms may contain propylene glycol; in neonates large amounts of propylene glycol delivered orally, intravenously (eg, >3,000 mg/day), or topically have been associated with potentially fatal toxicities which can include metabolic acidosis, seizures, renal failure, and CNS depression; toxicities have also been reported in children and adults including hyperosmolality, lactic acidosis, seizures and respiratory depression; use caution (AAP 1997; Shehab 2009).

Adverse Reactions

Dermatologic: Acneiform eruptions, allergic dermatitis, burning, dry skin, erythema, folliculitis, hypertrichosis, irritation, miliaria, pruritus, skin atrophy, striae, vesiculation

Endocrine and metabolic effects have occasionally been reported with topical use.

Drug Interactions

Metabolism/Transport Effects None known.

Avoid Concomitant Use

Avoid concomitant use of Betamethasone (Topical) with any of the following: Aldesleukin

Increased Effect/Toxicity

Betamethasone (Topical) may increase the levels/effects of: Ceritinib; Deferasirox

The levels/effects of Betamethasone (Topical) may be increased by: Telaprevir

Decreased Effect

Betamethasone (Topical) may decrease the levels/effects of: Aldesleukin; Corticorelin; Hyaluronidase; Telaprevir

Storage/Stability

Cream, lotion, ointment: Store at 15°C to 30°C (59°F to 86°F).

Foam: Store at 20°C to 25°C (68°F to 77°F). Avoid fire, flame, or smoking during use. Do not puncture or incinerate container. Do not expose to heat or store at temperatures above 49°C (120°F).

Mechanism of Action Topical corticosteroids have anti-inflammatory, antipruritic, and vasoconstrictive properties. May depress the formation, release, and activity of endogenous chemical mediators of inflammation (kinins, histamine, liposomal enzymes, prostaglandins) through the induction of phospholipase A_2 inhibitory proteins (lipocortins) and sequential inhibition of the release of arachidonic acid. Betamethasone has intermediate to very high range potency (dosage-form dependent).

Pharmacokinetics (Adult data unless noted)

Absorption: Topical corticosteroids are absorbed percutaneously. The extent of absorption is dependent on several factors, including epidermal integrity (intact vs abraded skin), formulation, age of the patient, prolonged duration of use, and the use of occlusive dressings. Percutaneous absorption of topical steroids is increased in neonates (especially preterm neonates), infants, and young children.

Metabolism: Hepatic

Elimination: Urine and bile

Dosing: Usual Dosage should be based on severity of disease and patient response; use smallest amount for shortest period of time to avoid HPA axis suppression. **Note:** Therapy should be discontinued when control is achieved.

Pediatric: **Dermatoses (corticosteroid-responsive):** Topical:

Betamethasone valerate:

Cream/ointment: Children and Adolescents: Apply a thin film to the affected area once to 3 times daily; usually once or twice daily application is effective.

Lotion: Children and Adolescents: Apply a few drops to the affected area twice daily; in some cases, more frequent application may be necessary; following improvement reduce to once daily application

Betamethasone dipropionate (augmented formulation):

Cream/ointment: Adolescents: Apply a thin film to affected area once or twice daily; maximum dose: 50 g/week; evaluate continuation of therapy if no improvement within 2 weeks of treatment.

Gel: Children and Adolescents ≥12 years: Apply a thin layer to the affected area once or twice daily; rub in gently; maximum dose: 50 g/week; not recommended for use longer than 2 weeks

Lotion: Adolescents: Apply a few drops to the affected area once or twice daily; rub in gently; maximum dose: 50 **mL**/week; not recommended for use for longer than 2 weeks.

Adult: **Note:** Base dosage on severity of disease and patient response.

Corticosteroid-responsive dermatoses: Topical: **Note:** Therapy should be discontinued when control is achieved.

Cream, augmented formulation: Betamethasone dipropionate 0.05%: Apply once or twice daily. Maximum dose: 50 g/week

Cream, unaugmented formulation:

Betamethasone dipropionate 0.05%: Apply once daily; may increase to twice daily if needed

Betamethasone valerate 0.1%: Apply 1 to 3 times daily. **Note:** Once- or twice-daily applications are usually effective.

Foam: Apply to the scalp twice daily, once in the morning and once at night. **Note:** Reassess if no improvement after 2 weeks of treatment.

Gel, augmented formulation: Apply once or twice daily; rub in gently. Maximum: 50 g/week. **Note:** Reassess if no improvement after 2 weeks of treatment.

Lotion, augmented formulation: Betamethasone dipropionate 0.05%: Apply a few drops once or twice daily. Maximum dose: 50 mL/week. **Note:** Reassess if no improvement after 2 weeks of treatment.

Lotion, unaugmented formulation:

Betamethasone dipropionate 0.05%: Apply a few drops twice daily

Betamethasone valerate 0.1%: Apply a few drops twice daily; may consider increasing dose for resistant cases. Following improvement, may apply once daily.

Ointment, augmented formulation: Betamethasone dipropionate 0.05%: Apply once or twice daily. Maximum dose: 50 g/week. **Note:** Reassess if no improvement after 2 weeks of treatment.

Ointment, unaugmented formulation:

Betamethasone dipropionate 0.05%: Apply once daily; may increase to twice daily if needed

Betamethasone valerate 0.1%: Apply 1 to 3 times daily. **Note:** Once- or twice-daily applications are usually effective.

Psoriasis: Topical: Foam: Apply to the scalp twice daily, once in the morning and once at night. **Note:** Therapy should be discontinued when control is achieved; reassess if no improvement after 2 weeks of treatment.

Dosing adjustment in renal impairment: There are no dosage adjustments provided in the manufacturer's labeling.

Dosing adjustment in hepatic impairment: There are no dosage adjustments provided in the manufacturer's labeling.

Administration Topical: For external use only. Apply sparingly to affected areas. Not for use on broken skin or in areas of infection. Do not apply to wet skin unless directed; do not cover with occlusive dressing. Do not apply very high potency agents to face, groin, axillae, or diaper area.

Betamethasone valerate:

Foam: Invert can and dispense a small amount onto a saucer or other cool surface. Do not dispense directly into hands as foam will begin to melt immediately upon contact with warm skin. Pick up small amounts of foam and gently massage into affected areas until foam disappears. Repeat until entire affected scalp area is treated. Avoid fire, flame, and/or smoking during and immediately following application.

Lotion: Shake well prior to use.

Monitoring Parameters Growth in pediatric patients; assess HPA axis suppression (eg, ACTH stimulation test, morning plasma cortisol test, urinary free cortisol test)

Test Interactions May suppress the wheal and flare reactions to skin test antigens

Additional Information

Very high potency (super high potency): Augmented betamethasone dipropionate ointment, lotion, gel

High potency: Augmented betamethasone dipropionate cream, betamethasone dipropionate cream and ointment

Intermediate potency: Betamethasone dipropionate lotion, betamethasone valerate cream

Dosage Forms Excipient information presented when available (limited, particularly for generics); consult specific product labeling.

Cream, External, as dipropionate [strength expressed as base]:

Generic: 0.05% (15 g, 45 g)

Cream, External, as dipropionate augmented [strength expressed as base]:

Diprolene AF: 0.05% (15 g, 50 g)

Generic: 0.05% (15 g, 50 g)

Cream, External, as valerate [strength expressed as base]:

Generic: 0.1% (15 g, 45 g)

Foam, External, as valerate:
Luxiq: 0.12% (50 g, 100 g) [contains alcohol, usp, cetyl alcohol, propylene glycol]
Generic: 0.12% (50 g, 100 g)
Gel, External, as dipropionate augmented [strength expressed as base]:
AlphaTrex: 0.05% (15 g, 50 g)
Generic: 0.05% (15 g, 50 g)
Lotion, External, as dipropionate [strength expressed as base]:
Generic: 0.05% (60 mL)
Lotion, External, as dipropionate augmented [strength expressed as base]:
Diprolene: 0.05% (30 mL, 60 mL) [contains isopropyl alcohol, propylene glycol]
Generic: 0.05% (30 mL, 60 mL)
Lotion, External, as valerate [strength expressed as base]:
Generic: 0.1% (60 mL)
Ointment, External, as dipropionate [strength expressed as base]:
Generic: 0.05% (15 g, 45 g)
Ointment, External, as dipropionate augmented [strength expressed as base]:
Diprolene: 0.05% (15 g, 50 g)
Generic: 0.05% (15 g, 45 g, 50 g)
Ointment, External, as valerate [strength expressed as base]:
Generic: 0.1% (15 g, 45 g)

- **Betamethasone Acetate** *see* Betamethasone (Systemic) *on page 278*
- **Betamethasone Dipropionate** *see* Betamethasone (Topical) *on page 280*
- **Betamethasone Dipropionate, Augmented** *see* Betamethasone (Topical) *on page 280*
- **Betamethasone Sodium Phosphate** *see* Betamethasone (Systemic) *on page 278*
- **Betamethasone Valerate** *see* Betamethasone (Topical) *on page 280*
- **Betapace** *see* Sotalol *on page 1963*
- **Betapace AF** *see* Sotalol *on page 1963*
- **Betaquik [OTC]** *see* Medium Chain Triglycerides *on page 1338*
- **Betasal [OTC]** *see* Salicylic Acid *on page 1894*
- **Betasept Surgical Scrub [OTC]** *see* Chlorhexidine Gluconate *on page 434*
- **Betaxin (Can)** *see* Thiamine *on page 2048*

Betaxolol (Ophthalmic) (be TAKS oh lol)

Medication Safety Issues
Sound-alike/look-alike issues:
Betoptic S may be confused with Betagan, Timoptic
Brand Names: US Betoptic-S
Brand Names: Canada Betoptic S; Sandoz-Betaxolol
Therapeutic Category Beta-Adrenergic Blocker; Beta-Adrenergic Blocker, Ophthalmic
Generic Availability (US) May be product dependent
Use Treatment of elevated intraocular pressure in patients with chronic open-angle glaucoma or ocular hypertension (ophthalmic solution: FDA approved in adults; ophthalmic suspension [Betoptic S]: FDA approved in pediatric patients [age not specified] and adults)
Pregnancy Risk Factor C
Pregnancy Considerations Animal reproduction studies have not been conducted; therefore, the manufacturer classifies Betaxolol (Ophthalmic) as pregnancy category C. When administered orally, betaxolol crosses the placenta, and can be detected in the amniotic fluid and umbilical cord blood. Refer to the Betaxolol (Systemic) monograph for details. The amount of betaxolol available systemically following topical application of the ophthalmic drops is significantly less in comparison to oral doses; however, a minor effect on maternal heart rate and blood pressure may be observed.
Breast-Feeding Considerations When administered orally, betaxolol is excreted into breast milk. Refer to the Betaxolol (Systemic) monograph for details. The amount of betaxolol available systemically following topical application of the ophthalmic drops is significantly less in comparison to oral doses.
Contraindications Hypersensitivity to betaxolol or any component of the formulation; sinus bradycardia; heart block greater than first-degree (except in patients with a functioning artificial pacemaker); cardiogenic shock; uncompensated cardiac failure
Warnings/Precautions Systemic absorption of betaxolol and adverse effects may occur with ophthalmic use, including severe respiratory and cardiac reactions. Use with caution in patients with compensated heart failure and monitor for a worsening of the condition. Discontinue at first signs of cardiac failure. In general, patients with bronchospastic disease should not receive beta-blockers; if used at all, should be used cautiously with close monitoring; asthma exacerbation and pulmonary distress has been reported during betaxolol use. Use with caution in patients with cardiovascular insufficiency; if signs of decreased cerebral blood flow occur, consider alternative therapy. Use with caution in patients with diabetes mellitus; may potentiate hypoglycemia and/or mask signs and symptoms. May mask signs of hyperthyroidism (eg, tachycardia); if hyperthyroidism is suspected, carefully manage and monitor; abrupt withdrawal may exacerbate symptoms of hyperthyroidism or precipitate thyroid storm. Use with caution in patients with myasthenia gravis; may worsen disease. Use caution with history of severe anaphylaxis to allergens; patients taking beta-blockers may become more sensitive to repeated challenges. Treatment of anaphylaxis (eg, epinephrine) in patients taking beta-blockers may be ineffective or promote undesirable effects.

Should not be used alone in angle-closure glaucoma (has no effect on pupillary constriction). Ophthalmic solutipon/suspension contains benzalkonium chloride which may be absorbed by contact lenses; remove contact lens prior to administration and wait 15 minutes before reinserting. Inadvertent contamination of multiple-dose ophthalmic solutions has caused bacterial keratitis. Choroidal detachment has been reported with aqueous suppressant therapy after filtration procedures.
Adverse Reactions
Ocular: Allergic reaction, anisocoria, blurred vision, choroidal detachment, corneal punctate keratitis, corneal punctate staining (with or without dendritic formations), corneal sensitivity decreased, corneal staining, crusty lashes, discharge, dry eyes, edema, erythema, foreign body sensation, inflammation, keratitis, ocular pain, photophobia, sensation of itching, tearing, visual acuity decreased
Rare but important or life-threatening: Alopecia, asthma, bradycardia, bronchial secretions thickened, bronchospasm, depression, dizziness, dyspnea, glossitis, heart block, heart failure, headache, hives, insomnia, lethargy, myasthenia gravis exacerbation, respiratory failure, smell/taste perversion, toxic epidermal necrolysis, vertigo
Drug Interactions
Metabolism/Transport Effects Substrate of CYP1A2 (major), CYP2D6 (minor); **Note:** Assignment of Major/Minor substrate status based on clinically relevant drug interaction potential; **Inhibits** CYP2D6 (weak)

Avoid Concomitant Use

Avoid concomitant use of Betaxolol (Ophthalmic) with any of the following: Floctafenine; Methacholine; Rivastigmine

Increased Effect/Toxicity

Betaxolol (Ophthalmic) may increase the levels/effects of: Alpha-/Beta-Agonists (Direct-Acting); Alpha1-Blockers; Alpha2-Agonists; Antipsychotic Agents (Phenothiazines); ARIPiprazole; Bupivacaine; Cardiac Glycosides; Cholinergic Agonists; Disopyramide; DULoxetine; Ergot Derivatives; Fingolimod; Grass Pollen Allergen Extract (5 Grass Extract); Hypotensive Agents; Insulin; Levodopa; Lidocaine (Systemic); Lidocaine (Topical); Mepivacaine; Methacholine; Midodrine; RisperiDONE; Sulfonylureas

The levels/effects of Betaxolol (Ophthalmic) may be increased by: Abiraterone Acetate; Acetylcholinesterase Inhibitors; Alpha2-Agonists; Aminoquinolines (Antimalarial); Amiodarone; Anilidopiperidine Opioids; Antipsychotic Agents (Phenothiazines); Barbiturates; Calcium Channel Blockers (Nondihydropyridine); CYP1A2 Inhibitors (Moderate); CYP1A2 Inhibitors (Strong); Deferasirox; Dipyridamole; Disopyramide; Dronedarone; Floctafenine; MAO Inhibitors; Nicorandil; NIFEdipine; Peginterferon Alfa-2b; Propafenone; Regorafenib; Reserpine; Rivastigmine; Vemurafenib

Decreased Effect

Betaxolol (Ophthalmic) may decrease the levels/effects of: Beta2-Agonists; Theophylline Derivatives

The levels/effects of Betaxolol (Ophthalmic) may be decreased by: Barbiturates; Nonsteroidal Anti-Inflammatory Agents; Rifamycin Derivatives

Storage/Stability Store ophthalmic suspension upright at 2°C to 25°C (36°F to 77°F). Store ophthalmic solution at 20°C to 25°C (68°F to 77°F).

Mechanism of Action Competitively blocks $beta_1$-receptors, with little or no effect on $beta_2$-receptors; with ophthalmic use, reduces intraocular pressure by reducing the production of aqueous humor

Pharmacodynamics

Onset of action: Within 30 minutes

Peak effect: Intraocular pressure reduction: ~2 hours

Duration: ≥12 hours

Pharmacokinetics (Adult data unless noted)

Absorption: Rapidly absorbed into the systemic circulation (concentrations ~1/10 to 1/20 of oral dosing) (Vainio-Jylhä, 2001)

Excretion: Urine (>80%, as unchanged drug [15%] and inactive metabolites)

Dosing: Neonatal Elevated intraocular pressure: Neonates ≥1 week PNA: Ophthalmic suspension (Betopic S): Instill 1 drop into affected eye(s) twice daily (Plager, 2009)

Dosing: Usual

Pediatric: **Elevated intraocular pressure:** Infants, Children, and Adolescents: Ophthalmic suspension (Betoptic S): Instill 1 drop into affected eye(s) twice daily

Adult: **Glaucoma:** Ophthalmic:

Solution: Instill 1 to 2 drops into affected eye(s) twice daily

Suspension (Betoptic S): Instill 1 drop into affected eye(s) twice daily

Dosing adjustment in renal impairment: Infants, Children, Adolescents, and Adults: There are no dosage adjustments provided in manufacturer's labeling (has not been studied).

Dosing adjustment in hepatic impairment: Infants, Children, Adolescents, and Adults: There are no dosage adjustments provided in manufacturer's labeling (has not been studied).

Administration Ophthalmic: Administer other topically applied ophthalmic medications at least 10 minutes before Betopic S; wash hands before use; invert closed bottle and shake bottle; remove cap carefully so that tip does not touch anything; hold bottle between thumb and index finger; use index finger of other hand to pull down the lower eyelid to form a pocket for the eye drop, tilt head back and instill in eye(s); **do not allow the dispenser tip to touch the eye**. Apply gentle pressure to lacrimal sac during and immediately following instillation (1 minute) or instruct patient to gently close eyelid after administration to decrease systemic absorption of ophthalmic drops (Urrti, 1993; Zimmerman, 1982). Some solutions contain benzalkonium chloride; wait at least 15 minutes after instilling solution before inserting soft contact lenses.

Monitoring Parameters Intraocular pressure

Dosage Forms Excipient information presented when available (limited, particularly for generics); consult specific product labeling.

Solution, Ophthalmic:

Generic: 0.5% (5 mL, 10 mL, 15 mL)

Suspension, Ophthalmic:

Betoptic-S: 0.25% (10 mL, 15 mL)

◆ **Betaxolol Hydrochloride** *see* Betaxolol (Ophthalmic) *on page 283*

Bethanechol (be THAN e kole)

Medication Safety Issues

Sound-alike/look-alike issues:

Bethanechol may be confused with betaxolol

Brand Names: US Urecholine

Brand Names: Canada Duvoid; PHL-Bethanechol; PMS-Bethanechol

Therapeutic Category Cholinergic Agent

Generic Availability (US) Yes

Use Treatment of nonobstructive urinary retention and retention due to neurogenic bladder; gastroesophageal reflux

Pregnancy Risk Factor C

Pregnancy Considerations Animal reproduction studies have not been conducted.

Breast-Feeding Considerations It is not known if bethanechol is excreted in breast milk. Due to the potential for serious adverse reactions in the nursing infant, a decision should be made whether to discontinue nursing or to discontinue the drug, taking into account the importance of treatment to the mother.

Contraindications Hypersensitivity to bethanechol or any component of the formulation; hyperthyroidism, peptic ulcer disease, epilepsy, asthma, pronounced bradycardia or hypotension, vasomotor instability, coronary artery disease, or parkinsonism; mechanical obstruction of the GI or GU tract or when the strength or integrity of the GI or bladder wall is in question; when increased muscular activity of the GI tract or bladder might prove harmful (eg, following urinary bladder surgery, GI resection and anastomosis, possible GI obstruction), bladder neck obstruction, spastic GI disturbances, acute inflammatory lesions of the GI tract, peritonitis, marked vagotonia.

Warnings/Precautions Potential for reflux infection in bacteriuric patients if the sphincter fails to relax as bethanechol contracts the bladder.

Adverse Reactions

Cardiovascular: Flushing, hypotension, tachycardia

Central nervous system: Colic, headache, malaise, seizure

Dermatologic: Diaphoresis

Gastrointestinal: Abdominal cramps, borborygmi, diarrhea, eructation, nausea, salivation, vomiting

Genitourinary: Urinary urgency

Ophthalmic: Lacrimation, miosis

Respiratory: Asthma, bronchoconstriction

Drug Interactions

Metabolism/Transport Effects None known.

Avoid Concomitant Use There are no known interactions where it is recommended to avoid concomitant use.

Increased Effect/Toxicity

The levels/effects of Bethanechol may be increased by: Acetylcholinesterase Inhibitors; Beta-Blockers

Decreased Effect There are no known significant interactions involving a decrease in effect.

Storage/Stability Store at 20°C to 25°C (68°F to 77°F).

Mechanism of Action Due to stimulation of the parasympathetic nervous system, bethanechol increases bladder muscle tone causing contractions which initiate urination. Bethanechol also stimulates gastric motility, increases gastric tone and may restore peristalsis.

Pharmacodynamics

Onset of action: Oral: 30-90 minutes

Duration: Oral: Up to 6 hours

Pharmacokinetics (Adult data unless noted)

Absorption: Oral: Variable

Metabolic fate and excretion have not been determined

Dosing: Usual Oral:

Children:

Abdominal distention or urinary retention: 0.6 mg/kg/day divided 3-4 times/day

Gastroesophageal reflux: 0.1-0.2 mg/kg/dose or 3 mg/m^2/dose given 30 minutes to 1 hour before each meal to a maximum of 4 times/day

Adults: 10-50 mg 2-4 times/day

Administration Oral: Administer on an empty stomach to reduce nausea and vomiting

Dosage Forms Excipient information presented when available (limited, particularly for generics); consult specific product labeling.

Tablet, Oral, as chloride:

Urecholine: 5 mg, 10 mg [scored]

Urecholine: 25 mg, 50 mg [scored; contains fd&c yellow #10 (quinoline yellow), fd&c yellow #6 (sunset yellow)]

Generic: 5 mg, 10 mg, 25 mg, 50 mg

Extemporaneous Preparations A 1 mg/mL solution may be made with tablets. Crush twelve 10 mg tablets in a mortar and reduce to a fine powder. Add small portions of sterile water and mix to a uniform paste; mix while adding sterile water in incremental proportions to **almost** 120 mL; transfer to a calibrated bottle, rinse mortar with sterile water, and add quantity of sterile water sufficient to make 120 mL. Label "shake well" and "refrigerate". Stable for 30 days (Schlatter, 1997).

A 5 mg/mL suspension may be made with tablets and either a 1:1 mixture of Ora-Plus® and Ora-Sweet® or Ora-Plus® and Ora-Sweet® SF or 1:4 concentrated cherry syrup and simple syrup, NF mixture. Crush twelve 50 mg tablets in a mortar and reduce to a fine powder. Add small portions of chosen vehicle and mix to a uniform paste; mix while adding the vehicle in incremental proportions to **almost** 120 mL; transfer to a calibrated bottle, rinse mortar with vehicle, and add quantity of vehicle sufficient to make 120 mL. Label "shake well" and "refrigerate". Stable for 60 days refrigerated (preferred) or at room temperature (Allen, 1998; Nahata, 2004).

Allen LV Jr and Erickson MA, "Stability of Bethanechol Chloride, Pyrazinamide, Quinidine Sulfate, Rifampin, and Tetracycline Hydrochloride in Extemporaneously Compounded Oral Liquids," *Am J Health Syst Pharm*, 1998, 55(17):1804-9.

Nahata MC, Pai VB, and Hipple TF, *Pediatric Drug Formulations*, 5th ed, Cincinnati, OH: Harvey Whitney Books Co, 2004.

Schlatter JL and Saulnier JL, "Bethanechol Chloride Oral Solutions: Stability and Use in Infants," *Ann Pharmacother*, 1997, 31(3):294-6.

◆ **Bethanechol Chloride** *see* Bethanechol *on page 284*

◆ **Bethkis** *see* Tobramycin (Systemic, Oral Inhalation) *on page 2073*

◆ **Betimol** *see* Timolol (Ophthalmic) *on page 2067*

◆ **Betnesol (Can)** *see* Betamethasone (Topical) *on page 280*

◆ **Betoptic-S** *see* Betaxolol (Ophthalmic) *on page 283*

◆ **Betoptic S (Can)** *see* Betaxolol (Ophthalmic) *on page 283*

Bevacizumab (be vuh SIZ uh mab)

Medication Safety Issues

Sound-alike/look-alike issues:

Avastin may be confused with Astelin

Bevacizumab may be confused with brentuximab, cetuximab, ranibizumab, riTUXimab

High alert medication:

This medication is in a class the Institute for Safe Medication Practices (ISMP) includes among its list of drug classes which have a heightened risk of causing significant patient harm when used in error.

International issues:

Avastin [U.S., Canada, and multiple international markets] may be confused with Avaxim, a brand name for hepatitis A vaccine [Canada and multiple international markets]

Related Information

Prevention of Chemotherapy-Induced Nausea and Vomiting in Children *on page 2368*

Brand Names: US Avastin

Brand Names: Canada Avastin

Therapeutic Category Antineoplastic Agent, Monoclonal Antibody; Antineoplastic Agent, Vascular Endothelial Growth Factor (VEGF) Inhibitor; Vascular Endothelial Growth Factor (VEGF) Inhibitor

Generic Availability (US) No

Use Treatment of metastatic colorectal cancer (FDA approved in adults); treatment of unresectable, locally advanced recurrent or metastatic nonsquamous, non-small cell lung cancer (FDA approved in adults); glioblastoma with progressive disease following prior therapy as single agent (FDA approved in adults); and metastatic renal cell cancer (FDA approved in adults). Has also been used in the treatment of pediatric refractory solid tumors and primary CNS tumors; has been used intravitreally for retinopathy of prematurity (Stage 3+).

Pregnancy Considerations Based on its mechanism of action, bevacizumab would be expected to cause fetal harm if administered to a pregnant woman. Information from postmarketing reports following exposure in pregnancy is limited. Adequate contraception during therapy and for ≥6 months following the last dose is recommended due to the long half-life of bevacizumab. Bevacizumab treatment may also increase the risk of ovarian failure and impair fertility; long term effects on fertility are not known.

Breast-Feeding Considerations It is not known if bevacizumab is excreted in breast milk. Immunoglobulins are excreted in breast milk, and it is assumed that bevacizumab may appear in breast milk. Because of the potential for serious adverse reactions in the nursing infant, breast-feeding is not recommended. The half-life of bevacizumab is up to 50 days (average 20 days), and this should be considered when decisions are made concerning breast-feeding resumption.

Note: Canadian labeling recommends to discontinue breast-feeding during treatment and to avoid breast-feeding a minimum of 6 months following discontinuation of treatment.

Contraindications

There are no contraindications listed in the manufacturer's labeling.

Canadian labeling: Hypersensitivity to bevacizumab, any component of the formulation, Chinese hamster ovary cell products or other recombinant human or humanized antibodies; untreated CNS metastases

Warnings/Precautions [US Boxed Warning]: Gastrointestinal (GI) perforation (sometimes fatal) has occurred in 0.3 to 3.2% of clinical study patients receiving bevacizumab; discontinue (permanently) if GI perforation occurs. All cervical cancer patients with GI perforation had a history of prior pelvic radiation. GI perforation was observed in patients with platinum-resistant ovarian cancer, although patients with evidence of recto-sigmoid involvement (by pelvic exam), bowel involvement (on CT scan), or clinical symptoms of bowel obstruction were excluded from the study; avoid bevacizumab use in these ovarian cancer patient populations. Most cases occur within 50 days of treatment initiation; monitor patients for signs/symptoms (eg, fever, abdominal pain with constipation and/or nausea/vomiting). GI fistula (including enterocutaneous, esophageal, duodenal, and rectal fistulas), and intra-abdominal abscess have been reported in patients receiving bevacizumab for colorectal cancer, ovarian cancer, and other cancers (not related to treatment duration). Non-GI fistula formation (including tracheoesophageal, bronchopleural, biliary, vaginal, vesical, renal, bladder, and female tract fistulas) has been observed (rarely fatal), most commonly within the first 6 months of treatment. Gastrointestinal-vaginal fistulas have been reported in cervical cancer patients, all of whom had received prior pelvic radiation; patients may also have bowel obstructions requiring surgical intervention and diverting ostomies. Permanently discontinue in patients who develop internal organ fistulas, tracheoesophageal (TE) fistula, or any grade 4 fistula. **[US Boxed Warning]: The incidence of wound healing and surgical complications, including serious and fatal events, is increased in patients who have received bevacizumab; discontinue with wound dehiscence. Although the appropriate interval between withholding bevacizumab and elective surgery has not been defined, bevacizumab should be discontinued at least 28 days prior to surgery and should not be reinitiated for at least 28 days after surgery and until wound is fully healed.** In a retrospective review of central venous access device placements, a greater risk of wound dehiscence was observed when port placement and bevacizumab administration were separated by <14 days (Erinjeri, 2011).

[US Boxed Warning]: Severe or fatal hemorrhage, including hemoptysis, gastrointestinal bleeding, central nervous system hemorrhage, epistaxis, and vaginal bleeding have been reported (up to 5 times more frequently if receiving bevacizumab). Avoid use in patients with serious hemorrhage or recent hemoptysis (≥2.5 mL blood). Serious or fatal pulmonary hemorrhage has been reported in patients receiving bevacizumab (primarily in patients with non–small cell lung cancer with squamous cell histology [not an FDA-approved indication]). Intracranial hemorrhage, including cases of grade 3 or 4 hemorrhage, has occurred in patients with previously treated glioblastoma. Treatment discontinuation is recommended in all patients with intracranial or other serious hemorrhage. Use with caution in patients with CNS metastases; once case of CNS hemorrhage was observed in an ongoing study of NSCLC patients with CNS metastases. Use in patients with untreated CNS metastases is contraindicated in the Canadian labeling. Use with caution in patients at risk for thrombocytopenia.

Bevacizumab is associated with an increased risk for arterial thromboembolic events (ATE), including cerebral infarction, stroke, MI, TIA, angina, and other ATEs, when used in combination with chemotherapy. History of ATE, diabetes, or ≥65 years of age may present an even greater risk. Although patients with cancer are already at risk for venous thromboembolism (VTE), a meta-analysis of 15 controlled trials has demonstrated an increased risk for VTE in patients who received bevacizumab (Nalluri, 2008). Cervical cancer patients receiving bevacizumab plus chemotherapy may be at increased risk of grade 3 or higher VTE compared to those patients who received chemotherapy alone. Permanently discontinue therapy in patients with severe ATE or life-threatening (grade 4) VTE, including pulmonary embolism; the safety of treatment reinitiation after ATE has not been studied.

Use with caution in patients with cardiovascular disease. Among approved and nonapproved uses evaluated thus far, the incidence of heart failure (HF) and/or left ventricular dysfunction (including LVEF decline), is higher in patients receiving bevacizumab plus chemotherapy when compared to chemotherapy alone. Bevacizumab may potentiate the cardiotoxic effects of anthracyclines. HF is more common with prior anthracycline exposure and/or left chest wall irradiation. The safety of therapy resumption or continuation in patients with cardiac dysfunction has not been studied. In studies of patients with metastatic breast cancer (an off-label use), the incidence of grades 3 or 4 HF was increased in patients receiving bevacizumab plus paclitaxel, compared to the control arm. Patients with metastatic breast cancer who had received prior anthracycline therapy had a higher rate of HF compared to those receiving paclitaxel alone (3.8% vs 0.6% respectively). A meta-analysis of 5 studies which enrolled patients with metastatic breast cancer who received bevacizumab suggested an association with an increased risk of heart failure; all trials included in the analysis enrolled patients who either received prior or were receiving concurrent anthracycline therapy (Choueiri, 2011).

Bevacizumab may cause and/or worsen hypertension; the incidence of severe hypertension in increased with bevacizumab. Use caution in patients with preexisting hypertension and monitor BP closely (every 2 to 3 weeks during treatment; regularly after discontinuation if bevacizumab induced hypertension occurs or worsens). Permanent discontinuation is recommended in patients who experience a hypertensive crisis or hypertensive encephalopathy. Temporarily discontinue in patients who develop uncontrolled hypertension. An increase in diastolic and systolic blood pressures were noted in a retrospective review of patients with renal insufficiency (CrCl ≤60 mL/minute) who received bevacizumab for renal cell cancer (Gupta, 2011). Cases of posterior reversible encephalopathy syndrome (PRES) have been reported. Symptoms (which include headache, seizure, confusion, lethargy, blindness and/or other vision or neurologic disturbances) may occur from 16 hours to 1 year after treatment initiation. Resolution of symptoms usually occurs within days after discontinuation; however neurologic sequelae may remain. PRES may be associated with hypertension; discontinue bevacizumab and begin management of hypertension, if present. The safety of treatment reinitiation after PRES is not known.

Infusion reactions (eg, hypertension, hypertensive crisis, wheezing, oxygen desaturation, hypersensitivity [including anaphylactic/anaphylactoid reactions], chest pain, rigors, headache, diaphoresis) may occur with the first infusion (uncommon); interrupt therapy in patients experiencing severe infusion reactions and administer appropriate therapy; there are no data to address routine premedication use or reinstitution of therapy in patients who experience severe infusion reactions. Cases of necrotizing fasciitis, including fatalities, have been reported (rarely); usually secondary to wound healing complications, GI perforation or fistula formation. Discontinue in patients who develop necrotizing fasciitis. Proteinuria and/or nephrotic syndrome have been associated with bevacizumab; risk may be increased in patients with a history of hypertension; thrombotic microangiopathy has been associated with bevacizumab-induced proteinuria. Withhold treatment for ≥2 g proteinuria/24 hours and resume when proteinuria is <2 g/24 hours; discontinue in patients with nephrotic syndrome. Elderly patients (≥65 years of age) are at higher risk for adverse events, including thromboembolic events and proteinuria; serious adverse events occurring more frequently in the elderly also include weakness, deep thrombophlebitis, sepsis, hyper-/hypotension, MI, CHF, diarrhea, constipation, anorexia, leukopenia, anemia, dehydration, hypokalemia, and hyponatremia. Potentially significant drug-drug interactions may exist, requiring dose or frequency adjustment, additional monitoring, and/or selection of alternative therapy. Microangiopathic hemolytic anemia (MAHA) has been reported when bevacizumab has been used in combination with sunitinib. Concurrent therapy with sunitinib and bevacizumab is also associated with dose-limiting hypertension in patients with metastatic renal cell cancer. The incidence of hand-foot syndrome is increased in patients treated with bevacizumab plus sorafenib in comparison to those treated with sorafenib monotherapy. When used in combination with myelosuppressive chemotherapy, increased rates of severe or febrile neutropenia and neutropenic infection were reported. Bevacizumab, in combination with chemotherapy (or biologic therapy), is associated with an increased risk of treatment-related mortality; a higher risk of fatal adverse events was identified in a meta-analysis of 16 trials in which bevacizumab was used for the treatment of various cancers (breast cancer, colorectal cancer, non–small cell lung cancer, pancreatic cancer, prostate cancer, and renal cell cancer) and compared to chemotherapy alone (Ranpura, 2011). When bevacizumab is used in combination with myelosuppressive chemotherapy, increased rates of severe or febrile neutropenia and neutropenic infection have been reported. In premenopausal women receiving bevacizumab in combination with mFOLFOX (fluorouracil/oxaliplatin based chemotherapy) the incidence of ovarian failure (amenorrhea ≥3 months) was higher (34%) compared to women who received mFOLFOX alone (2%); ovarian function recovered in some patients after treatment was discontinued; premenopausal women should be informed of the potential risk of ovarian failure. Serious eye infections and vision loss due to endophthalmitis have been reported from intravitreal administration (off-label use/route).

Warnings: Additional Pediatric Considerations Some experts recommend caution regarding use in premature neonates for retinopathy of prematurity (ROP) outside of controlled, clinical trials (Quinn, 2011); systemic absorption after intravitreal administration with decreases in VEGF serum concentration (as low as 9% of baseline systemic concentration) have been reported in a case series of 11 neonates (Sato, 2012); short- and long-term implications of systemic exposure are unknown; monitoring is recommended. Osteonecrosis of the jaw has been associated with bevacizumab use alone or in combination with other chemotherapies, steroids, and bisphosphonates. A report of three pediatric patients (ages: 10 years, 13 years, and 17 years) has also described cases of osteonecrosis of the wrist and knee (Fangusaro, 2013).

Adverse Reactions Reported monotherapy and as part of combination chemotherapy regimens.

Cardiovascular: Arterial thrombosis, deep vein thrombosis, hypertension, hypotension, intra-abdominal thrombosis (venous), left ventricular dysfunction, peripheral edema, pulmonary embolism, syncope, thrombosis, venous thromboembolism, venous thromboembolism (secondary; with oral anticoagulants)

Central nervous system: Anxiety, dizziness, fatigue, headache, pain, peripheral sensory neuropathy, taste disorder, voice disorder

Dermatologic: Acne vulgaris, alopecia, cellulitis, dermal ulcer, exfoliative dermatitis, palmar-plantar erythrodysesthesia, xeroderma

Endocrine & metabolic: Dehydration, hyperglycemia, hypoalbuminemia, hypokalemia, hypomagnesemia, hyponatremia, ovarian failure, weight loss

Gastrointestinal: Abdominal pain, anorexia, colitis, constipation, decreased appetite, diarrhea, dyspepsia, gastritis, gastrointestinal fistula, gastrointestinal hemorrhage, gastrointestinal perforation, gastroesophageal reflux disease, gingival hemorrhage (minor), gingival pain, gingivitis, intestinal obstruction, nausea, oral mucosa ulcer, rectal pain, stomatitis, vomiting, xerostomia

Genitourinary: Pelvic pain, proteinuria (median onset: 5.6 months; median time to resolution: 6.1 months), urinary tract infection, vaginal hemorrhage

Hematologic & oncologic: Febrile neutropenia, hemorrhage (CNS), leukopenia, lymphocytopenia, neutropenia, neutropenic infection, pulmonary hemorrhage, thrombocytopenia

Infection: Abscess (tooth), infection (serious; pneumonia, catheter infection, or wound infection)

Neuromuscular & skeletal: Back pain, dysarthria, myalgia, weakness

Ophthalmic: Blurred vision

Otic: Deafness, tinnitus

Renal: Increased serum creatinine

Respiratory: Dyspnea, epistaxis, pneumonitis, rhinitis, upper respiratory tract infection

Miscellaneous: Fistula (anal, gastrointestinal-vaginal), infusion related reaction, postoperative wound complication (including dehiscence)

Rare but important or life-threatening: Angina pectoris, antibody development (anti-bevacizumab and neutralizing), bladder fistula, bronchopleural fistula, cerebral infarction, conjunctival hemorrhage, endophthalmitis (infectious and sterile), fistula of bile duct, fulminant necrotizing fasciitis, gallbladder perforation, gastrointestinal ulcer, hemolytic anemia (microangiopathic; when used in combination with sunitinib), hemoptysis, hemorrhagic stroke, hypersensitivity, hypertensive crisis, hypertensive encephalopathy, increased intraocular pressure, intestinal necrosis, intraocular inflammation (iritis, vitritis), mesenteric thrombosis, myocardial infarction, nasal septum perforation, ocular hyperemia, osteonecrosis of the jaw, ovarian failure, pancytopenia, polyserositis, pulmonary hypertension, rectal fistula, renal failure, renal fistula, renal thrombotic microangiopathy, retinal detachment, retinal hemorrhage, reversible posterior leukoencephalopathy syndrome, sepsis, tracheoesophageal fistula, vaginal fistula, vitreous hemorrhage, vitreous opacity

Drug Interactions

Metabolism/Transport Effects None known.

Avoid Concomitant Use

Avoid concomitant use of Bevacizumab with any of the following: BCG (Intravesical); Belimumab; CloZAPine; Dipyrone; SUNItinib

Increased Effect/Toxicity

Bevacizumab may increase the levels/effects of: Antineoplastic Agents (Anthracycline, Systemic); Belimumab; Bisphosphonate Derivatives; CloZAPine; Irinotecan; SORAfenib; SUNItinib

The levels/effects of Bevacizumab may be increased by: Dipyrone; SUNItinib

Decreased Effect

Bevacizumab may decrease the levels/effects of: BCG (Intravesical)

Storage/Stability Store intact vials at 2°C to 8°C (36°F to 46°F) in original carton; do not freeze. Protect from light; do not shake. Diluted solutions are stable for up to 8 hours under refrigeration. Discard unused portion of vial.

Mechanism of Action Bevacizumab is a recombinant, humanized monoclonal antibody which binds to, and neutralizes, vascular endothelial growth factor (VEGF), preventing its association with endothelial receptors, Flt-1 and KDR. VEGF binding initiates angiogenesis (endothelial proliferation and the formation of new blood vessels). The inhibition of microvascular growth is believed to retard the growth of all tissues (including metastatic tissue).

Pharmacokinetics (Adult data unless noted)

Half-life:

IV:

Pediatric patients (age: 1-21 years): Median: 11.8 days (range: 4.4-14.6 days) (Glade-Bender, 2008)

Adults: 20 days (range: 11-50 days)

Intravitreal: ~5-10 days (Bakri, 2007; Krohne, 2008)

Dosing: Neonatal Retinopathy of prematurity (ROP): Limited data available; dosing regimens variable; dose not established: PMA ≥31 weeks and PNA ≥28 days: Intravitreal injection: Usual dosing: 0.625 mg (0.025 mL) as a single dose in the affected eye; dosing was used in 70 premature neonates (140 eyes) with Stage 3+ ROP in a prospective, randomized comparative trial with laser therapy; the primary outcome studied was recurrence of ROP, which was lower in the treatment group (6%) compared to conventional laser therapy (26%) (Mintz-Hittner, 2011). This same dose was used in a larger retrospective trial of 85 preterm neonates (162 eyes) with Stage 3 ROP as either primary therapy or salvage therapy after laser treatment; ROP regression occurred in 83% of treated eyes (Wu, 2013). Other doses reported range from 0.37-1.25 mg in the affected eye (Harder, 2013, Micieli, 2009; Spandau, 2013). Some experts recommend caution regarding use outside of a clinical trial (Quinn, 2011); systemic absorption with decreases in VEGF serum concentration have been reported in a case series of 11 neonates after intravitreal administration of doses consistent with those in reported in the literature (Sato, 2012).

Dosing: Usual Refer to individual protocols; details concerning dosing in combination regimens should also be consulted.

Children and Adolescents:

Refractory solid tumor: Limited data available: IV: 5-15 mg/kg/dose every 2 weeks in a 28-day course (Glade-Bender, 2008) **or** 5-10 mg/kg every 2-3 weeks (Benesch, 2008)

Primary CNS tumor; recurrent/refractory (high/low grade gliomas, medulloblastoma): Limited data available; efficacy results variable: IV: 10 mg/kg/dose every 2 weeks (Aguilera, 2011; Aguilera, 2013; Packer, 2009; Parekh, 2011; Reismüller, 2010) or days 1 and 15 of each 28 day cycle (Kang, 2008); mostly used in combination with irinotecan with/without temozolmide **or** 15 mg/kg/dose every 3 weeks has also been used (Parekh, 2011; Reismüller, 2010). In general, when treating high-grade glioma, patients with contrast-enhancing disease showed greater response or remained stable, while patients with noncontrast-enhancing disease had disease progression (Parekh, 2011); others have observed only minimal efficacy in patients with high grade glioma (Narayana, 2010)

Adults:

Colorectal cancer, metastatic, in combination with fluorouracil-based chemotherapy: IV: 5 mg/kg every 2 weeks in combination with bolus IFL **or** 10 mg/kg every 2 weeks in combination with FOLFOX4

Colorectal cancer, metastatic, following first-line therapy containing bevacizumab: IV: 5 mg/kg every 2 weeks **or** 7.5 mg/kg every 3 weeks in combination with fluoropyrimidine-irinotecan or fluoropyrimidine-oxaliplatin based regimen

Non-small cell lung cancer (nonsquamous): IV: 15 mg/kg every 3 weeks in combination with carboplatin and paclitaxel

Glioblastoma: IV: 10 mg/kg every 2 weeks as monotherapy

Renal cell cancer, metastatic: IV: 10 mg/kg every 2 weeks in combination with interferon alfa

Dosing adjustment for renal impairment: There are no dosage adjustments provided in manufacturer's labeling.

Dosing adjustment for hepatic impairment: There are no dosage adjustments provided in manufacturer's labeling.

Preparation for Administration IV infusion: Dilute in 100 mL NS prior to infusion (the manufacturer recommends a total volume of 100 mL). Do not mix with dextrose-containing solutions (concentration-dependent degradation may occur).

Administration

Parenteral: IV infusion: Infuse the initial dose over 90 minutes; second infusion may be shortened to 60 minutes if the initial infusion is well-tolerated. Third and subsequent infusions may be shortened to 30 minutes if the 60-minute infusion is well-tolerated. Do **not** administer via IV push.

Intravitreal injection: Inject undiluted bevacizumab solution. The major clinical trial for ROP used an insulin syringe (0.3 mL syringe with a 31 gauge, 5/16 inch needle) to accurately deliver the dose; each 1 unit on an insulin syringe is equivalent to 0.01 mL; typical bevacizumab dose of 0.625 mg would equate to 2.5 units on an insulin syringe using a 25 mg/mL solution. In this ROP trial, the injection site was anesthetized with a drop of tetracaine hydrochloride 0.5% ophthalmic solution or proparacaine hydrochloride 0.5% ophthalmic solution prior to bevacizumab administration and sterilized before and after administration with a drop of povidone-iodine 5% ophthalmic solution. Following the procedure, a topical ophthalmic antibiotic drop was also administered every 6 hours for 7 days (Mintz-Hittner 2011).

Monitoring Parameters

IV administration: Monitor for signs of an infusion reaction during infusion; blood pressure (continue to monitor blood pressure during and after bevacizumab has been discontinued). Monitor CBC with differential; signs/symptoms of GI perforation or abscess (abdominal pain, constipation, vomiting, fever); signs/symptoms of bleeding including hemoptysis, GI bleeding, CNS bleeding, epistaxis. Signs of wound dehiscence or healing complications. Urinalysis for proteinuria, nephrotic syndrome

Intravitreal administration: Monitor blood pressure, heart rate, respiratory rate, and oxygen saturation prior to, during, and after the procedure; monitor for signs and symptoms of infection or ocular inflammation; consider short- and long-term monitoring for sequelae of systemic absorption when used in neonates (Sato, 2012)

Dosage Forms Excipient information presented when available (limited, particularly for generics); consult specific product labeling.

Solution, Intravenous [preservative free]:

Avastin: 100 mg/4 mL (4 mL); 400 mg/16 mL (16 mL)

◆ **Bexsero** *see* Meningococcal Group B Vaccine *on page 1351*

◆ **Biaxin** *see* Clarithromycin *on page 482*

◆ **Biaxin XL** *see* Clarithromycin *on page 482*

◆ **Biaxin XL Pac** *see* Clarithromycin *on page 482*

◆ **Biaxin BID (Can)** *see* Clarithromycin *on page 482*

◆ **Bicillin L-A** *see* Penicillin G Benzathine *on page 1654*

◆ **Bicitra** *see* Sodium Citrate and Citric Acid *on page 1942*

- ◆ **BiCNU** *see* Carmustine *on page 377*
- ◆ **Bidex [OTC]** *see* GuaiFENesin *on page 988*
- ◆ **BIG-IV** *see* Botulism Immune Globulin (Intravenous-Human) *on page 299*
- ◆ **Biltricide** *see* Praziquantel *on page 1751*
- ◆ **Bio-D-Mulsion [OTC]** *see* Cholecalciferol *on page 448*
- ◆ **Bio-D-Mulsion Forte [OTC]** *see* Cholecalciferol *on page 448*
- ◆ **Bio-Amitriptyline (Can)** *see* Amitriptyline *on page 131*
- ◆ **Bio-Amlodipine (Can)** *see* AmLODIPine *on page 133*
- ◆ **Biobase (Can)** *see* Alcohol (Ethyl) *on page 86*
- ◆ **Biobase-G (Can)** *see* Alcohol (Ethyl) *on page 86*
- ◆ **Bio-Celecoxib (Can)** *see* Celecoxib *on page 418*
- ◆ **Bio-Diazepam (Can)** *see* Diazepam *on page 635*
- ◆ **Bio-Ezetimibe (Can)** *see* Ezetimibe *on page 832*
- ◆ **Bio-Flurazepam (Can)** *see* Flurazepam *on page 913*
- ◆ **Bio-Furosemide (Can)** *see* Furosemide *on page 951*
- ◆ **Bio-Hydrochlorothiazide (Can)** *see* Hydrochlorothiazide *on page 1028*
- ◆ **Bio-K+ (Can)** *see Lactobacillus on page 1203*
- ◆ **Bio-Letrozole (Can)** *see* Letrozole *on page 1224*
- ◆ **Bioniche Promethazine (Can)** *see* Promethazine *on page 1777*
- ◆ **Bion® Tears [OTC]** *see* Artificial Tears *on page 201*
- ◆ **BioQuin Durules (Can)** *see* QuiNIDine *on page 1822*
- ◆ **Bio-Statin** *see* Nystatin (Oral) *on page 1537*

Biotin (BYE oh tin)

Therapeutic Category Biotinidase Deficiency, Treatment Agent; Nutritional Supplement; Vitamin, Water Soluble

Use Treatment of primary biotinidase deficiency; nutritional biotin deficiency; component of the vitamin B complex

Mechanism of Action Functions as a coenzyme; involved in carboxylation, transcarboxylation, and decarboxylation reactions of gluconeogenesis, lipogenesis, fatty acid synthesis, propionate metabolism, and the catabolism of leucine

Dosing: Neonatal Oral:

Adequate intake (AI): 5 mcg/day (~0.7 mcg/kg/day)

Biotinidase deficiency: 5-10 mg once daily

Dosing: Usual Oral:

Adequate intake (AI): Infants, Children, and Adults: There is no official RDA.

- Infants:
  - 1 to <6 months: 5 mcg/day (~0.7 mcg/kg/day)
  - 6-12 months: 6 mcg/day (~0.7 mcg/kg/day)
- Children:
  - 1-3 years: 8 mcg/day
  - 4-8 years: 12 mcg/day
  - 9-13 years: 20 mcg/day
  - 14-18 years: 25 mcg/day
- Adults: 30 mcg/day

Biotinidase deficiency: Infants, Children, and Adults: 5-10 mg once daily

Biotin deficiency: Children and Adults: 5-20 mg once daily

Administration Oral: May be administered without regard to meals

Reference Range Serum biotinidase activity

Dosage Forms Capsule: 1 mg

- ◆ **Biphentin (Can)** *see* Methylphenidate *on page 1402*
- ◆ **Bisac-Evac [OTC]** *see* Bisacodyl *on page 289*

Bisacodyl (bis a KOE dil)

Medication Safety Issues

Sound-alike/look-alike issues:

Doxidan may be confused with doxepin

Dulcolax (bisacodyl) may be confused with Dulcolax (docusate)

Related Information

Oral Medications That Should Not Be Crushed or Altered *on page 2476*

Brand Names: US Bisac-Evac [OTC]; Bisacodyl EC [OTC]; Bisacodyl Laxative [OTC]; Biscolax [OTC]; Correct [OTC]; Ducodyl [OTC]; Dulcolax [OTC]; Ex-Lax Ultra [OTC]; Fleet Bisacodyl [OTC]; Fleet Laxative [OTC]; Gentle Laxative [OTC]; Laxative [OTC]; Stimulant Laxative [OTC]; The Magic Bullet [OTC]; Womens Laxative [OTC]

Brand Names: Canada Apo-Bisacodyl [OTC]; Bisacodyl-Odan [OTC]; Bisacolax [OTC]; Carter's Little Pills [OTC]; Codulax [OTC]; Dulcolax For Women [OTC]; Dulcolax [OTC]; PMS-Bisacodyl [OTC]; ratio-Bisacodyl [OTC]; Silver Bullet Suppository [OTC]; Soflax EX [OTC]; The Magic Bullett [OTC]; Woman's Laxative [OTC]

Therapeutic Category Laxative, Stimulant

Generic Availability (US) May be product dependent

Use Treatment of constipation (OTC products; FDA approved in ages ≥6 years and adults); bowel cleansing prior to procedures or examination (FDA approved in children ≥12 years and adults; consult specific product formulations for appropriate age groups)

Pregnancy Considerations Plasma concentrations of BHPM (the active metabolite of bisacodyl) are low (median: 61 ng/mL; range: 21-194 ng/mL) following doses of 10 mg/day for 7 days (Friedrich, 2011). Although not first choice for the treatment of constipation in pregnant women, short-term use of stimulant laxatives is generally considered safe in pregnancy; long-term use should be avoided (Cullen, 2007; Prather, 2004; Wald, 2003).

Breast-Feeding Considerations Neither bisacodyl nor its active metabolite (BHPM) were detectable in breast milk following administration of bisacodyl 10 mg once daily for 7 days to eight lactating women (limit of detection: 1 ng/mL) (Friedrich, 2011).

Contraindications Hypersensitivity to bisacodyl or any component of the formulation; abdominal pain or obstruction, nausea, or vomiting

Adverse Reactions Rare but important or life-threatening: Abdominal cramps (mild), electrolyte disturbance (metabolic acidosis or alkalosis, hypocalcemia), nausea, rectal irritation (burning), vertigo, vomiting

Drug Interactions

Metabolism/Transport Effects None known.

Avoid Concomitant Use There are no known interactions where it is recommended to avoid concomitant use.

Increased Effect/Toxicity There are no known significant interactions involving an increase in effect.

Decreased Effect

The levels/effects of Bisacodyl may be decreased by: Antacids

Storage/Stability Store enteric-coated tablets and rectal suppositories at <30°C.

Mechanism of Action Stimulates peristalsis by directly irritating the smooth muscle of the intestine, possibly the colonic intramural plexus; alters water and electrolyte secretion producing net intestinal fluid accumulation and laxation

Pharmacodynamics Onset of action:

Oral: Within 6 to 10 hours

Rectal: 15 to 60 minutes

Pharmacokinetics (Adult data unless noted)

Absorption: Oral, rectal: <5% absorbed systemically

Metabolism: In the liver

Elimination: Conjugated metabolites excreted in breast milk, bile, and urine

Dosing: Usual

Pediatric: **Constipation:**

Oral:

Manufacturer's labeling:

Children 6 to 12 years: 5 mg once daily

Children ≥12 years and Adolescents: 5 to 15 mg once daily

Alternate dosing: Limited data available (Tabbers [NASPGHAN/ESPGHAN], 2014):

Children ≥3 years to <10 years: 5 mg once daily

Children ≥10 years and Adolescents: 5 to 10 mg once daily

Rectal:

Manufacturer's labeling:

Suppository:

Children 6 to ≤12 years: 5 mg (1/2 suppository) once daily

Children ≥12 years and Adolescents: 10 mg once daily

Enema: Children ≥12 years and Adolescents: 10 mg once daily

Alternate dosing: Limited data available (Tabbers [NASPGHAN/ESPGHAN] 2014): Suppository/enema:

Children ≥2 to <10 years: 5 mg (1/2 suppository) once daily

Children ≥10 years and Adolescents: 5 to 10 mg once daily

Adult: **Constipation:**

Oral: 5 to 15 mg as single dose (up to 30 mg when complete evacuation of bowel is required)

Rectal: Suppository: 10 mg as single dose

Enema: 10 mg as single dose

Dosing adjustment in renal impairment: There are no dosage adjustment provided in manufacturer's labeling.

Dosing adjustment in hepatic impairment: There are no dosage adjustment provided in manufacturer's labeling.

Administration

Oral: Administer on an empty stomach with water; patient should swallow tablet whole; do not break or chew enteric-coated tablet; do not administer within 1 hour of ingesting antacids, alkaline material, milk, or dairy products

Rectal:

Suppository: Remove foil, insert into rectum with pointed end first. Retain in rectum for 15 to 20 minutes.

Enema: Shake well; remove protective shield, insert tip into rectum with slight side to side movement; squeeze the bottle until nearly all liquid expelled (some liquid will remain in unit after use). Gently remove the unit, a small amount of liquid will remain in unit after use.

Dosage Forms Excipient information presented when available (limited, particularly for generics); consult specific product labeling. [DSC] = Discontinued product

Enema, Rectal:

Fleet Bisacodyl: 10 mg/30 mL (37 mL)

Suppository, Rectal:

Bisac-Evac: 10 mg (1 ea, 8 ea, 12 ea, 50 ea, 100 ea, 500 ea, 1000 ea)

Bisacodyl Laxative: 10 mg (12 ea)

Biscolax: 10 mg (12 ea, 100 ea)

Dulcolax: 10 mg (4 ea, 8 ea, 16 ea, 28 ea, 50 ea)

Gentle Laxative: 10 mg (4 ea, 8 ea, 12 ea)

Laxative: 10 mg (12 ea, 100 ea)

The Magic Bullet: 10 mg (10 ea, 12 ea [DSC], 100 ea)

Generic: 10 mg (12 ea, 50 ea, 100 ea)

Tablet Delayed Release, Oral:

Bisacodyl EC: 5 mg

Bisacodyl EC: 5 mg [contains fd&c yellow #10 (quinoline yellow), fd&c yellow #6 (sunset yellow)]

Bisacodyl EC: 5 mg [contains fd&c yellow #10 aluminum lake, fd&c yellow #6 aluminum lake]

Bisacodyl EC: 5 mg [contains fd&c yellow #10 aluminum lake, fd&c yellow #6 aluminum lake, methylparaben, propylparaben, sodium benzoate]

Correct: 5 mg

Ducodyl: 5 mg

Dulcolax: 5 mg [contains fd&c yellow #10 (quinoline yellow), methylparaben, propylparaben, sodium benzoate]

Ex-Lax Ultra: 5 mg [contains fd&c yellow #6 (sunset yellow), methylparaben]

Fleet Laxative: 5 mg

Gentle Laxative: 5 mg

Stimulant Laxative: 5 mg

Stimulant Laxative: 5 mg [contains fd&c yellow #10 aluminum lake, fd&c yellow #6 aluminum lake]

Womens Laxative: 5 mg

Womens Laxative: 5 mg [contains fd&c blue #1 aluminum lake, sodium benzoate, tartrazine (fd&c yellow #5)]

- **Bisacodyl EC [OTC]** *see* Bisacodyl *on page 289*
- **Bisacodyl Laxative [OTC]** *see* Bisacodyl *on page 289*
- **Bisacodyl-Odan [OTC] (Can)** *see* Bisacodyl *on page 289*
- **Bisacolax [OTC] (Can)** *see* Bisacodyl *on page 289*
- **bis(chloroethyl) nitrosourea** *see* Carmustine *on page 377*
- **bis-chloronitrosourea** *see* Carmustine *on page 377*
- **Biscolax [OTC]** *see* Bisacodyl *on page 289*
- **Bismatrol** *see* Bismuth Subsalicylate *on page 290*
- **Bismatrol [OTC]** *see* Bismuth Subsalicylate *on page 290*
- **Bismatrol Maximum Strength [OTC]** *see* Bismuth Subsalicylate *on page 290*

Bismuth Subsalicylate (BIZ muth sub sa LIS i late)

Medication Safety Issues

Sound-alike/look-alike issues:

Kaopectate may be confused with Kayexalate

Other safety concerns:

Maalox Total Relief is a different formulation than other Maalox liquid antacid products which contain aluminum hydroxide, magnesium hydroxide, and simethicone.

Canadian formulation of Kaopectate does not contain bismuth; the active ingredient in the Canadian formulation is attapulgite.

Related Information

H. pylori Treatment in Pediatric Patients *on page 2358*

Brand Names: US Bismatrol Maximum Strength [OTC]; Bismatrol [OTC]; Diotame [OTC]; Geri-Pectate [OTC]; Kao-Tin [OTC]; Peptic Relief [OTC]; Pepto-Bismol To-Go [OTC]; Pepto-Bismol [OTC]; Pink Bismuth [OTC]; Stomach Relief Max St [OTC]; Stomach Relief Plus [OTC]; Stomach Relief [OTC]

Therapeutic Category Gastrointestinal Agent, Miscellaneous

Generic Availability (US) Yes

Use

Subsalicylate formulation: Symptomatic treatment of mild, nonspecific diarrhea including traveler's diarrhea; chronic infantile diarrhea; adjunctive treatment of *Helicobacter pylori*-associated antral gastritis

Subgallate formulation: An aid to reduce fecal odors from a colostomy or ileostomy

Pregnancy Considerations Following oral administration, bismuth and salicylates cross the placenta. The use of salicylates in pregnancy may adversely affect the newborn (Lione, 1988). Use during pregnancy is not recommended (Mahadevan, 2007).

Breast-Feeding Considerations Low amounts of salicylates enter breast milk; refer to the Aspirin monograph for additional information (Bar-Oz, 2004). A case report describes bowel obstruction in a breast-fed infant whose mother applied a bismuth-containing ointment to her nipples prior to breast-feeding (Anonymous, 1974).

Contraindications OTC labeling: When used for self-medication, do not use if you have an ulcer, bleeding problem or bloody/black stool

Warnings/Precautions Bismuth subsalicylate should be used with caution if patient is taking aspirin. Bismuth products may be neurotoxic with very large doses.

When used for self-medication (OTC labeling): Children and teenagers who have or are recovering from chickenpox or flu-like symptoms should not use subsalicylate. Changes in behavior (along with nausea and vomiting) may be an early sign of Reye's syndrome; patients should be instructed to contact their healthcare provider if these occur. Patients should be instructed to contact healthcare provider for diarrhea lasting >2 days, hearing loss, or ringing in the ears. Not labeled for OTC use in children <12 years of age.

Adverse Reactions Subsalicylate formulation:

Central nervous system: Anxiety, confusion, depression, headache, slurred speech

Gastrointestinal: Fecal discoloration (grayish black; impaction may occur in infants and debilitated patients), tongue discoloration (darkening)

Neuromuscular & skeletal: Muscle spasm, weakness

Otic: Hearing loss, tinnitus

Drug Interactions

Metabolism/Transport Effects None known.

Avoid Concomitant Use

Avoid concomitant use of Bismuth Subsalicylate with any of the following: Bismuth Subcitrate; Dexketoprofen; Influenza Virus Vaccine (Live/Attenuated)

Increased Effect/Toxicity

Bismuth Subsalicylate may increase the levels/effects of: Anticoagulants; Bismuth Subcitrate; Blood Glucose Lowering Agents; Carbonic Anhydrase Inhibitors; Corticosteroids (Systemic); Dexketoprofen; Methotrexate; PRALAtrexate; Salicylates; Thrombolytic Agents; Valproic Acid and Derivatives; Varicella Virus-Containing Vaccines; Vitamin K Antagonists

The levels/effects of Bismuth Subsalicylate may be increased by: Agents with Antiplatelet Properties; Ammonium Chloride; Calcium Channel Blockers (Nondihydropyridine); Ginkgo Biloba; Herbs (Anticoagulant/Antiplatelet Properties); Influenza Virus Vaccine (Live/Attenuated); Loop Diuretics; NSAID (Nonselective); Potassium Acid Phosphate; Treprostinil

Decreased Effect

Bismuth Subsalicylate may decrease the levels/effects of: ACE Inhibitors; Dexketoprofen; Hyaluronidase; Loop Diuretics; NSAID (Nonselective); Probenecid; Tetracycline Derivatives

The levels/effects of Bismuth Subsalicylate may be decreased by: Corticosteroids (Systemic); Dexketoprofen; NSAID (Nonselective)

Mechanism of Action Bismuth subsalicylate exhibits both antisecretory and antimicrobial action. This agent may provide some anti-inflammatory action as well. The salicylate moiety provides antisecretory effect and the bismuth exhibits antimicrobial directly against bacterial and viral gastrointestinal pathogens.

Pharmacokinetics (Adult data unless noted)

Absorption: Bismuth is minimally absorbed (<1%) across the GI tract while salicylate salt is readily absorbed (80%)

Distribution: Salicylate: V_d: 170 mL/kg

Protein binding, plasma: Bismuth and salicylate: >90%

Metabolism: Bismuth salts undergo chemical dissociation after oral administration; salicylate is extensively metabolized in the liver

Half-life:

Bismuth: Terminal: 21-72 days

Salicylate: Terminal: 2-5 hours

Elimination:

Bismuth: Renal, biliary

Salicylate: Only 10% excreted unchanged in urine

Dosing: Usual Oral: Bismuth subsalicylate: **(bismuth subsalicylate liquid dosages expressed in mL of 262 mg/15 mL concentration):**

Nonspecific diarrhea: Children: 100 mg/kg/day divided into 5 equal doses for 5 days (maximum: 4.19 g/day) **or**

Children: Up to 8 doses/24 hours:

3-6 years: 1/3 tablet or 5 mL (87 mg) every 30 minutes to 1 hour as needed

6-9 years: 2/3 tablet or 10 mL (175 mg) every 30 minutes to 1 hour as needed

9-12 years: 1 tablet or 15 mL (262 mg) every 30 minutes to 1 hour as needed

Adults: 2 tablets or 30 mL (524 mg) every 30 minutes to 1 hour as needed up to 8 doses/24 hours

Chronic infantile diarrhea:

2-24 months: 2.5 mL (44 mg) every 4 hours

24-48 months: 5 mL (87 mg) every 4 hours

48-70 months: 10 mL (175 mg) every 4 hours

Prevention of traveler's diarrhea: Adults: 2.1 g/day or 2 tablets 4 times/day before meals and at bedtime

Helicobacter pylori-associated antral gastritis: Dosage in children is not well established, the following dosages have been used [in conjunction with ampicillin and metronidazole or (in adults) tetracycline and metronidazole]:

Children ≤10 years: 15 mL (262 mg) 4 times/day for 6 weeks

Children >10 years and Adults: 30 mL (524 mg) solution or two 262 mg tablets 4 times/day for 6 weeks

Dosing adjustment in renal impairment: Avoid use in patients with renal failure

Administration Oral: Shake liquid well before using; chew tablets or allow to dissolve in mouth before swallowing

Test Interactions Increased uric acid, increased AST; bismuth absorbs x-rays and may interfere with diagnostic procedures of GI tract

Additional Information Bismuth subsalicylate: 262 mg = 130 mg nonaspirin salicylate; 525 mg = 236 mg nonaspirin salicylate

Dosage Forms Excipient information presented when available (limited, particularly for generics); consult specific product labeling. [DSC] = Discontinued product

Suspension, Oral, as subsalicylate:

Bismatrol: 262 mg/15 mL (236 mL) [contains benzoic acid, d&c red #22 (eosine), saccharin sodium; wintergreen flavor]

Bismatrol Maximum Strength: 525 mg/15 mL (236 mL) [contains benzoic acid, d&c red #22 (eosine), saccharin sodium; wintergreen flavor]

Geri-Pectate: 262 mg/15 mL (355 mL)

Kao-Tin: 262 mg/15 mL (236 mL, 473 mL) [contains fd&c red #40, saccharin sodium, sodium benzoate]

Peptic Relief: 262 mg/15 mL (237 mL) [sugar free; contains benzoic acid, d&c red #22 (eosine), saccharin sodium; mint flavor]

Pepto-Bismol: 262 mg/15 mL (473 mL) [contains benzoic acid, d&c red #22 (eosine), saccharin sodium]

Pink Bismuth: 262 mg/15 mL (236 mL)

Pink Bismuth: 262 mg/15 mL (237 mL) [contains benzoic acid, d&c red #22 (eosine), saccharin sodium]

Stomach Relief: 262 mg/15 mL (237 mL, 355 mL) [contains d&c red #22 (eosine), saccharin sodium]

Stomach Relief: 527 mg/30 mL (240 mL, 480 mL)

Stomach Relief Max St: 525 mg/15 mL (237 mL) [contains d&c red #22 (eosine), saccharin sodium]

Stomach Relief Plus: 525 mg/15 mL (240 mL, 480 mL)

Tablet Chewable, Oral, as subsalicylate:

Bismatrol: 262 mg [contains aspartame]

Diotame: 262 mg
Peptic Relief: 262 mg [DSC]
Peptic Relief: 262 mg [contains saccharin sodium]
Pepto-Bismol To-Go: 262 mg [sugar free; contains fd&c red #40 aluminum lake, saccharin sodium; cherry flavor]
Pink Bismuth: 262 mg
Pink Bismuth: 262 mg [contains saccharin sodium]
Generic: 262 mg

- **Bis-POM PMEA** *see* Adefovir *on page 72*
- **Bistropamide** *see* Tropicamide *on page 2132*
- **Bivalent Human Papillomavirus Vaccine** *see* Papillomavirus (Types 16, 18) Vaccine (Human, Recombinant) *on page 1628*
- **Bivigam** *see* Immune Globulin *on page 1089*
- **Bi-Zets/Benzotroches [OTC]** *see* Benzocaine *on page 268*
- **BL4162A** *see* Anagrelide *on page 163*
- **Black Widow Spider Species Antivenin** *see* Antivenin (*Latrodectus mactans*) *on page 181*
- **Black Widow Spider Species Antivenom** *see* Antivenin (*Latrodectus mactans*) *on page 181*
- **Blenoxane** *see* Bleomycin *on page 292*
- **Bleo** *see* Bleomycin *on page 292*

Bleomycin (blee oh MYE sin)

Medication Safety Issues

Sound-alike/look-alike issues:

Bleomycin may be confused with Cleocin

High alert medication:

This medication is in a class the Institute for Safe Medication Practices (ISMP) includes among its list of drugs which have a heightened risk of causing significant patient harm when used in error.

International issues:

Some products available internationally may have vial strength and dosing expressed as international units or milligrams (instead of units or USP units). Refer to prescribing information for specific strength and dosing information.

Related Information

Management of Drug Extravasations *on page 2298*
Prevention of Chemotherapy-Induced Nausea and Vomiting in Children *on page 2368*
Safe Handling of Hazardous Drugs *on page 2455*

Brand Names: Canada Blenoxane; Bleomycin Injection, USP

Therapeutic Category Antineoplastic Agent, Antibiotic

Generic Availability (US) Yes

Use Palliative treatment of squamous cell carcinoma (of the head and neck, penis, cervix, or vulva), testicular carcinoma, Hodgkin's lymphoma, and non-Hodgkin's lymphoma; sclerosing agent to control malignant effusions (FDA approved in adults); has also been used in the treatment of germ cell tumors and pediatric Hodgkin's lymphoma

Pregnancy Risk Factor D

Pregnancy Considerations Adverse effects were observed in animal reproduction studies. Women of childbearing potential should avoid becoming pregnant during treatment.

Breast-Feeding Considerations It is not known if bleomycin is excreted in breast milk. Due to the potential for serious adverse reactions in the nursing infant, the manufacturer recommends against breast-feeding during treatment.

Contraindications Hypersensitivity to bleomycin or any component of the formulation

Warnings/Precautions Hazardous agent - use appropriate precautions for handling and disposal (NIOSH 2014 [group 1]). **[U.S. Boxed Warning]: Occurrence of pulmonary fibrosis (commonly presenting as pneumonitis; occasionally progressing to pulmonary fibrosis) is the most severe toxicity. Risk is higher in elderly patients or patients receiving >400 units total lifetime dose;** other possible risk factors include smoking and patients with prior radiation therapy or receiving concurrent oxygen (especially high inspired oxygen doses). A review of patients receiving bleomycin for the treatment of germ cell tumors suggests risk for pulmonary toxicity is increased in patients >40 years of age, with glomerular filtration rate <80 mL/minute, advanced disease, and cumulative doses >300 units (O'Sullivan, 2003). Pulmonary toxicity may include bronchiolitis obliterans and organizing pneumonia (BOOP), eosinophilic hypersensitivity, and interstitial pneumonitis, progressing to pulmonary fibrosis (Sleijfer, 2001); pulmonary toxicity may be due to a lack of the enzyme which inactivates bleomycin (bleomycin hydrolase) in the lungs (Morgan, 2011; Sleijfer, 2001). If pulmonary changes occur, withhold treatment and investigate if drug-related. In children, a younger age at treatment, cumulative dose ≥400 units/m^2 (combined with chest irradiation), and renal impairment are associated with a higher incidence of pulmonary toxicity (Huang, 2011).

A severe idiosyncratic reaction consisting of hypotension, mental confusion, fever, chills, and wheezing (similar to anaphylaxis) has been reported in 1% of lymphoma patients treated with bleomycin. Since these reactions usually occur after the first or second dose, careful monitoring is essential after these doses. Use caution when administering O_2 during surgery to patients who have received bleomycin; the risk of bleomycin-related pulmonary toxicity is increased. Use caution with renal impairment (CrCl <50 mL/minute), may require dose adjustment. May cause renal or hepatic toxicity. **[U.S. Boxed Warning]: Should be administered under the supervision of an experienced cancer chemotherapy physician.** Potentially significant drug-drug interactions may exist, requiring dose or frequency adjustment, additional monitoring, and/or selection of alternative therapy. Some products available internationally may have vial strength and dosing expressed as international units or milligrams (instead of units or USP units); refer to prescribing information for specific dosing information.

Adverse Reactions

Dermatologic: Diffuse scleroderma, erythema, hyperkeratosis, induration, onycholysis, pain at the tumor site, phlebitis, pruritus, rash, skin thickening, striae, vesiculation; peeling of the skin (particularly on the palmar and plantar surfaces of the hands and feet); hyperpigmentation, alopecia, nailbed changes may also occur (appear dose related and reversible with discontinuation)

Gastrointestinal: Anorexia, stomatitis and mucositis, weight loss

Respiratory: Death, hypoxia, Interstitial pneumonitis (acute or chronic), pulmonary fibrosis, rales, tachypnea; symptoms include cough, dyspnea, and bilateral pulmonary infiltrates. The pathogenesis is not certain, but may be due to damage of pulmonary, vascular, or connective tissue. Response to steroid therapy is variable and somewhat controversial.

Miscellaneous: Acute febrile reactions; anaphylactoid-like reactions (characterized by hypotension, confusion, fever, chills, and wheezing; onset may be immediate or delayed for several hours); idiosyncratic reactions

Rare but important or life-threatening: Angioedema, cerebrovascular accident, cerebral arteritis, chest pain, coronary artery disease, flagellate hyperpigmentation, hepatotoxicity, malaise, MI, myelosuppression (rare), myocardial ischemia, nausea, pericarditis, Raynaud's phenomenon, renal toxicity, scleroderma-like skin changes, Stevens-Johnson syndrome, thrombotic microangiopathy, toxic epidermal necrolysis, vomiting

Drug Interactions

Metabolism/Transport Effects None known.

Avoid Concomitant Use

Avoid concomitant use of Bleomycin with any of the following: BCG; BCG (Intravesical); Brentuximab Vedotin; Natalizumab; Pimecrolimus; Tacrolimus (Topical); Tofacitinib; Vaccines (Live)

Increased Effect/Toxicity

Bleomycin may increase the levels/effects of: Leflunomide; Natalizumab; Tofacitinib; Vaccines (Live)

The levels/effects of Bleomycin may be increased by: Brentuximab Vedotin; Denosumab; Filgrastim; Gemcitabine; Pimecrolimus; Roflumilast; Sargramostim; Tacrolimus (Topical); Trastuzumab

Decreased Effect

Bleomycin may decrease the levels/effects of: BCG; BCG (Intravesical); Coccidioides immitis Skin Test; Phenytoin; Sipuleucel-T; Vaccines (Inactivated); Vaccines (Live)

The levels/effects of Bleomycin may be decreased by: Echinacea

Storage/Stability Refrigerate intact vials of powder. Intact vials are stable for up to 4 weeks at room temperature. Solutions reconstituted in NS are stable for up to 28 days refrigerated and 14 days at room temperature; however, the manufacturer recommends stability of 24 hours in NS at room temperature.

Mechanism of Action Inhibits synthesis of DNA; binds to DNA leading to single- and double-strand breaks; also inhibits (to a lesser degree) RNA and protein synthesis

Pharmacokinetics (Adult data unless noted)

Absorption: IM and intrapleural administration: 30% to 50% of IV serum concentrations; intraperitoneal and SubQ routes produce serum concentrations equal to those of IV

Distribution: V_d: 22 L/m^2; highest concentrations in skin, kidney, lung, and heart tissues; lowest in testes and GI tract; does not cross blood-brain

Protein binding: 1%

Metabolism: Via several tissues, including hepatic, GI tract, skin, pulmonary, renal, and serum

Half-life elimination: Biphasic (renal function dependent):

Children: 2.1 to 3.5 hours

Adults:

Normal renal function: Initial: 1.3 hours; Terminal: 9 hours

End-stage renal disease: Initial: 2 hours; Terminal: 30 hours

Time to peak serum concentration: IM: Within 30 minutes

Elimination: Urine (50% to 70% as active drug)

Dosing: Usual Note: An international consideration with use is that dosages below are expressed as USP units; 1 USP unit = 1 mg (by potency) = 1000 international units (Stefanou, 2001). The risk for pulmonary toxicity increases with cumulative lifetime dose >400 units. Refer to individual protocols for specific dosage and interval information.

Pediatric:

Test dose for lymphoma patients: Children and Adolescents: IM, IV, SubQ: Because of the possibility of an anaphylactoid reaction, the manufacturer recommends administering 1 to 2 units of bleomycin before the first 1 to 2 doses; monitor vital signs every 15 minutes; wait a minimum of 1 hour before administering remainder of dose; if no acute reaction occurs, then the regular dosage schedule may be followed. **Note:** Test doses may not be predictive of a reaction (Lam, 2005) and/or may produce false-negative results.

Hodgkin lymphoma (combination regimen):

ABVD regimen: Children and Adolescents: IV: 10 units/m^2 on days 1 and 15 of a 28-day treatment cycle in combination with doxorubicin, vinblastine, dacarbazine (Hutchinson, 1998)

BEACOPP regimen: Children and Adolescents: IV 10 units/m^2 on day 7 of a 21-day treatment cycle in combination with etoposide, doxorubicin, cyclophosphamide, vincristine, procarbazine, and prednisone (Kelly, 2002)

Stanford V: Adolescent ≥16 years: 5 units/m^2/dose in weeks 2, 4, 6, 8, 10, and 12 in combination with mechlorethamine, vinblastine, vincristine, doxorubicin, etoposide, and prednisone (Horning, 2000; Horning, 2002)

Malignant germ cell cancer (combination therapy) (Cushing, 2004): IV:

Infants: 0.5 **mg**/kg/dose day 1 of a 21-day treatment cycle for 4 cycles

Children and Adolescents: 15 units/m^2 day 1 of a 21-day treatment cycle for 4 cycles

Adults:

Test dose for lymphoma patients: IM, IV, SubQ: Because of the possibility of an anaphylactoid reaction, the manufacturer recommends administering 1 to 2 units of bleomycin before the first 1 to 2 doses; monitor vital signs every 15 minutes; wait a minimum of 1 hour before administering remainder of dose; if no acute reaction occurs, then the regular dosage schedule may be followed. **Note:** Test doses may not be predictive of a reaction (Lam, 2005) and/or may produce false-negative results.

Hodgkin's lymphoma (combination regimens): IV:

ABVD: 10 units/m^2 days 1 and 15 of a 28-day treatment cycle (Straus, 2004)

BEACOPP: 10 units/m^2 day 8 of a 21-day treatment cycle (Dann, 2007; Diehl, 2003)

Stanford V: 5 units/m^2/dose in weeks 2, 4, 6, 8, 10, and 12 (Horning, 2000; Horning, 2002)

Malignant pleural effusion: Intrapleural: 60 units as a single instillation; mix in 50-100 mL of NS and instill into the pleural cavity via a thoracostomy tube

Dosing adjustment in obesity: Adults: Fixed doses (dosing which is independent of body weight or BSA) are used in some protocols (eg, testicular cancer); due to toxicity concerns, the same fixed dose should also be considered for obese patients (Griggs, 2012).

Dosing adjustment in renal impairment: Adults:

Manufacturer's labeling: **Note:** Creatinine clearance should be estimated using the Cockcroft-Gault formula:

CrCl >50 mL/minute: No dosage adjustment necessary

CrCl 40 to 50 mL/minute: Administer 70% of normal dose

CrCl 30 to 40 mL/minute: Administer 60% of normal dose

CrCl 20 to 30 mL/minute: Administer 55% of normal dose

CrCl 10 to 20 mL/minute: Administer 45% of normal dose

CrCl 5 to 10 mL/minute: Administer 40% of normal dose

The following guidelines have been used by some clinicians:

Aronoff, 2007: Continuous renal replacement therapy (CRRT): Administer 75% of dose

Kintzel, 1995:

CrCl 46 to 60 mL/minute: Administer 70% of dose

CrCl 31 to 45 mL/minute: Administer 60% of dose

CrCl <30 mL/minute: Consider use of alternative drug

Dosing adjustment in hepatic impairment: There are no dosage adjustments provided in the manufacturer's labeling (has not been studied); however, adjustment for hepatic impairment is not necessary (King, 2001).

Dosing adjustment for toxicity:

Pulmonary changes: Discontinue until determined not to be drug-related.

Pulmonary diffusion capacity for carbon monoxide (DL_{CO}) <30% to 35% of baseline: Discontinue treatment.

Preparation for Administration Hazardous agent; use appropriate precautions for handling and disposal (NIOSH 2014 [group 1]).

Parenteral:

IV: Reconstitute 15-unit vial with 5 mL with NS and the 30-unit vial with 10 mL NS; may be further diluted in NS for continuous IV infusion.

IM or SubQ: Reconstitute 15-unit vial with 1 to 5 mL of SWFI, bacteriostatic water for injection, or NS and the 30-unit vial with 2 to 10 mL of SWFI, bacteriostatic water for injection, or NS.

Intrapleural: Adults: Mix in 50 to 100 mL of NS

Administration Hazardous agent; use appropriate precautions for handling and disposal (NIOSH 2014 [group 1]).

Parenteral:

IM, SubQ: May cause pain at injection site

IV: Administer IV slowly over at least 10 minutes; may be further diluted for administration by continuous IV infusion; administration by continuous infusion may produce less severe pulmonary toxicity.

Intrapleural: Adults: Use of topical anesthetics or opioid analgesia is usually not necessary.

Vesicant/Extravasation Risk May be an irritant

Monitoring Parameters Pulmonary function tests, including total lung volume, forced vital capacity, diffusion capacity for carbon monoxide; vital capacity, total lung capacity, and pulmonary capillary blood volume may be better indicators of changes induced by bleomycin (Sleijfer, 2001), chest x-ray; renal function, hepatic function, vital signs, and temperature initially; CBC with differential and platelet count; check body weight at regular intervals

Dosage Forms Excipient information presented when available (limited, particularly for generics); consult specific product labeling.

Solution Reconstituted, Injection:

Generic: 15 units (1 ea); 30 units (1 ea)

Solution Reconstituted, Injection [preservative free]:

Generic: 15 units (1 ea); 30 units (1 ea)

- ◆ **Bleomycin Injection, USP (Can)** *see* Bleomycin *on page 292*
- ◆ **Bleomycin Sulfate** *see* Bleomycin *on page 292*
- ◆ **Bleph-10** *see* Sulfacetamide (Ophthalmic) *on page 1981*
- ◆ **Bleph 10 DPS (Can)** *see* Sulfacetamide (Ophthalmic) *on page 1981*
- ◆ **Blistex Medicated [OTC]** *see* Benzocaine *on page 268*
- ◆ **BLM** *see* Bleomycin *on page 292*
- ◆ **Bloxiverz** *see* Neostigmine *on page 1505*
- ◆ **BMS-188667** *see* Abatacept *on page 41*
- ◆ **BMS-232632** *see* Atazanavir *on page 210*
- ◆ **BMS 337039** *see* ARIPiprazole *on page 193*
- ◆ **B&O** *see* Belladonna and Opium *on page 264*
- ◆ **BOL-303224-A** *see* Besifloxacin *on page 276*
- ◆ **Boostrix** *see* Diphtheria and Tetanus Toxoids, and Acellular Pertussis Vaccine *on page 681*

Bosentan (boe SEN tan)

Medication Safety Issues

Sound-alike/look-alike issues:

Tracleer may be confused with TriCor

Related Information

Management of Drug Extravasations *on page 2298*

Oral Medications That Should Not Be Crushed or Altered *on page 2476*

Safe Handling of Hazardous Drugs *on page 2455*

Brand Names: US Tracleer

Brand Names: Canada ACT Bosentan; Mylan-Bosentan; PMS-Bosentan; Sandoz-Bosentan; Teva-Bosentan; Tracleer

Therapeutic Category Endothelin Receptor Antagonist

Generic Availability (US) No

Use Treatment of pulmonary arterial hypertension (PAH) [WHO Group I] in patients with NYHA Class II, III, or IV symptoms to improve exercise capacity and decrease the rate of clinical deterioration (FDA approved in ages >12 years and adults); **Note:** Clinical trials establishing effectiveness included primarily patients with NYHA Functional Class II-IV symptoms.

Prescribing and Access Restrictions As a requirement of the REMS program, access to this medication is restricted. Bosentan (Tracleer®) is only available through Tracleer® Access Program (T.A.P.). Only prescribers and pharmacies registered with T.A.P. may prescribe and dispense bosentan. Further information may be obtained from the manufacturer, Actelion Pharmaceuticals (1-866-228-3546 or http://www.tracleer.com/hcp/prescribing-tracleer.asp).

Medication Guide Available Yes

Pregnancy Risk Factor X

Pregnancy Considerations [U.S. Boxed Warning]: May cause birth defects; use in pregnancy is contraindicated. Exclude pregnancy prior to initiation of therapy and obtain pregnancy tests monthly during treatment. Reliable contraception must be used during therapy and for 1 month after stopping treatment. Hormonal contraceptives (oral, injectable, transdermal, or implantable) may not be effective and a second method of contraception (nonhormonal) is required. Patients with tubal ligation or an implanted IUD (Copper T 380A or LNg 20) do not need additional contraceptive measures. When a hormonal or barrier contraceptive is used, one additional method of contraception is still needed if a male partner has had a vasectomy. When initiating treatment for women of reproductive potential, a negative pregnancy test should be documented within the first 5 days of a normal menstrual period and ≥11 days after the last unprotected intercourse. A missed menses or suspected pregnancy should be reported to a healthcare provider and prompt immediate pregnancy testing. Sperm counts may be reduced in men during treatment. Women of childbearing potential should avoid splitting, crushing, or handling broken tablets and exposure to the generated dust (tablet splitting is currently outside of product labeling).

Breast-Feeding Considerations Due to the potential risk of adverse events in a nursing infant, a decision should be made to discontinue nursing or discontinue therapy.

Contraindications Hypersensitivity to bosentan or any component of the formulation; concurrent use of cyclosporine or glyburide; pregnancy

Canadian labeling: Additional contraindications (not in U.S. labeling): Moderate-to-severe hepatic impairment and/or baseline ALT or AST >3 times the upper limit of normal (ULN), particularly when total bilirubin >2 times ULN

Warnings/Precautions Hazardous agent - use appropriate precautions for handling and disposal (NIOSH 2014 [group 3]). **[U.S. Boxed Warning]: May cause hepatotoxicity; has been associated with a high incidence (~11%) of significant transaminase elevations (ALT or AST ≥3 times ULN) with or without elevations in bilirubin and rare cases of unexplained hepatic cirrhosis (after >12 months of therapy) or hepatic failure.**

Monitor transaminases at baseline then monthly thereafter. Adjust dosage if elevations in liver enzymes occur without symptoms of hepatic injury or elevated bilirubin. Treatment should be stopped in patients who develop elevated transaminases either in combination with symptoms of hepatic injury (unusual fatigue, jaundice, nausea, vomiting, abdominal pain, and/or fever) or elevated bilirubin (≥2 times ULN); safety of reintroduction is unknown. Avoid use in patients with baseline serum transaminases >3 times ULN or moderate-to-severe hepatic impairment. Transaminase elevations are dose dependent, generally asymptomatic, occur both early and late in therapy, progress slowly, and are usually reversible after treatment interruption or discontinuation. Consider the benefits of treatment versus the risk of hepatotoxicity when initiating therapy in patients with WHO Class II symptoms.

[U.S. Boxed Warning]: May cause birth defects; use in pregnancy is contraindicated. Exclude pregnancy prior to initiation of therapy and obtain pregnancy tests monthly during treatment. Reliable contraception must be used during therapy and for 1 month after stopping treatment. Hormonal contraceptives (oral, injectable, transdermal, or implantable) may not be effective and a second method of contraception (nonhormonal) is required. Patients with tubal ligation or an implanted IUD (Copper T 380A or LNg 20) do not need additional contraceptive measures. (See Pregnancy Considerations.)

[U.S. Boxed Warning]: Because of the risks of hepatic impairment and the high likelihood of teratogenic effects, bosentan is only available through the T.A.P. restricted distribution program. Patients, prescribers, and pharmacies must be registered with and meet conditions of T.A.P. Call 1-866-228-3546 or visit http://www.tracleer.com/hcp/prescribing-tracleer.asp for more information.

A reduction in hematocrit/hemoglobin may be observed within the first few weeks of therapy with subsequent stabilization of levels. Hemoglobin reductions >15% have been observed in some patients. Measure hemoglobin prior to initiating therapy, at 1 and 3 months, and every 3 months thereafter. Significant decreases in hemoglobin in the absence of other causes may warrant the discontinuation of therapy.

Development of peripheral edema due to treatment and/or disease state (pulmonary arterial hypertension) may occur. There have also been postmarketing reports of fluid retention requiring treatment (eg, diuretics, fluid management, hospitalization). Further evaluation may be necessary to determine cause and appropriate treatment or discontinuation of therapy. Bosentan should be discontinued in any patient with pulmonary edema suggestive of pulmonary veno-occlusive disease (PVOD). Bosentan may interact with many medications, resulting in potentially serious and/or life-threatening adverse events (see Drug Interactions).

Adverse Reactions

Cardiovascular: Chest pain, edema, flushing, hypotension, palpitations, syncope
Central nervous system: Headache
Dermatologic: Pruritus
Genitourinary: Spermatogenesis inhibition
Hematologic & oncologic: Anemia, decreased hemoglobin (typically in first 6 weeks of therapy)
Hepatic: Hepatic insufficiency, increased serum transaminases (≥3 times ULN; dose-related)
Neuromuscular & skeletal: Arthralgia
Respiratory: Respiratory tract infection, sinusitis
Rare but important or life-threatening: Anaphylaxis, angioedema, hepatic cirrhosis (prolonged therapy), hepatic failure (rare), hyperbilirubinemia, hypersensitivity, hypersensitivity angiitis, jaundice, leukopenia, neutropenia, peripheral edema, skin rash, thrombocytopenia, weight gain, worsening of heart failure

Drug Interactions

Metabolism/Transport Effects Substrate of CYP2C9 (minor), CYP3A4 (minor), SLCO1B1; **Note:** Assignment of Major/Minor substrate status based on clinically relevant drug interaction potential; **Induces** CYP2C9 (weak/moderate), CYP3A4 (moderate)

Avoid Concomitant Use

Avoid concomitant use of Bosentan with any of the following: Axitinib; Bedaquiline; Bosutinib; CycloSPORINE (Systemic); Enzalutamide; GlyBURIDE; Nisoldipine; Olaparib; Palbociclib; Simeprevir; Ulipristal

Increased Effect/Toxicity

Bosentan may increase the levels/effects of: Clarithromycin; Ifosfamide

The levels/effects of Bosentan may be increased by: Atazanavir; Boceprevir; Clarithromycin; Cobicistat; CycloSPORINE (Systemic); CYP2C9 Inhibitors (Moderate); CYP2C9 Inhibitors (Strong); CYP3A4 Inhibitors (Moderate); CYP3A4 Inhibitors (Strong); Darunavir; Eltrombopag; Fosamprenavir; GlyBURIDE; Indinavir; Lopinavir; Nelfinavir; Phosphodiesterase 5 Inhibitors; Rifampin; Ritonavir; Saquinavir; Telaprevir; Teriflunomide; Tipranavir

Decreased Effect

Bosentan may decrease the levels/effects of: ARIPiprazole; Atazanavir; Axitinib; Bedaquiline; Boceprevir; Bosutinib; Clarithromycin; Contraceptives (Estrogens); Contraceptives (Progestins); CycloSPORINE (Systemic); CYP3A4 Substrates; Darunavir; Dasabuvir; Enzalutamide; FentaNYL; Fosamprenavir; GlyBURIDE; HMG-CoA Reductase Inhibitors; Hydrocodone; Ibrutinib; Ifosfamide; Indinavir; Lopinavir; Nelfinavir; NiMODipine; Nisoldipine; Olaparib; Ombitasvir; Palbociclib; Paritaprevir; Phosphodiesterase 5 Inhibitors; Saquinavir; Saxagliptin; Simeprevir; Telaprevir; Tipranavir; Ulipristal; Vitamin K Antagonists

The levels/effects of Bosentan may be decreased by: GlyBURIDE; Rifampin

Food Interactions Bioavailability of bosentan is not affected by food. Bosentan serum concentrations may be increased by grapefruit juice. Management: Avoid grapefruit/grapefruit juice.

Storage/Stability Store at 20°C to 25°C (68°F to 77°F); excursions permitted to 15°C to 30°C (59°F to 86°F).

Mechanism of Action Blocks endothelin receptors on vascular endothelium and smooth muscle. Stimulation of these receptors is associated with vasoconstriction. Although bosentan blocks both ET_A and ET_B receptors, the affinity is higher for the A subtype.

Pharmacokinetics (Adult data unless noted)

Distribution: Does not distribute into RBCs; V_d: ~18 L
Protein binding: >98% to plasma proteins (primarily albumin)
Metabolism: Extensive in the liver via cytochrome P450 isoenzymes CYP2C9 and CYP3A4 to three metabolites (one has pharmacologic activity and may account for 10% to 20% of drug effect); steady-state plasma concentrations are 50% to 65% of those attained after single dose (most likely due to autoinduction of liver enzymes); steady-state is attained within 3-5 days
Bioavailability: ~50%
Half-life: Healthy subjects: 5 hours; half-life may be prolonged in PAH, as AUC is 2-fold greater in adults with PAH versus healthy subjects
Time to peak serum concentration: Oral: Within 3-5 hours
Elimination: Biliary excretion; urine (<3% as unchanged drug)

Dialysis: Not likely to be removed (due to extensive protein binding and high molecular weight)

Dosing: Neonatal Persistant pulmonary hypertension (PPHN): Very limited data available: Full-term neonate: Oral: 1 mg/kg/dose twice daily short-term use (2 to 16 days) in three full-term neonates has been reported. In the initial report, two full-term neonates (8 days and 14 days old) with persistent pulmonary hypertension of the newborn (PPHN) and transposition of the great arteries received bosentan prior to cardiac surgery; patients also received other therapies (Goissen 2008). A case report describes the use of bosentan monotherapy for PPHN in a full-term neonate as primary course of treatment initiated at 29 hours of life; therapy was weaned after 72 hours through the following dose reductions: 0.5 mg/kg/dose twice daily followed by 0.5 mg/kg once daily and subsequent discontinuation at 96 hours of treatment (Nakwan 2009).

Dosing: Usual

Pediatric:

Pulmonary arterial hypertension:

Infants ≥7 months and Children: Limited data available (Barst 2003; Ivy 2004; Maiya 2006; Rosenzweig 2005):

Fixed dosing:

5 to <10 kg: Initial: 15.6 mg daily for 4 weeks; increase to maintenance dose of 15.6 mg twice daily

10 to 20 kg: Initial: 31.25 mg daily for 4 weeks; increase to maintenance dose of 31.25 mg twice daily

>20 to 40 kg: Initial: 31.25 mg twice daily for 4 weeks; increase to maintenance dose of 62.5 mg twice daily

>40 kg: Initial: 62.5 mg twice daily for 4 weeks; increase to maintenance dose of 125 mg twice daily

Weight-based dosing: Children ≥2 years: Initial: 0.75 to 1 mg/kg/dose twice daily for 4 weeks (maximum dose: 62.5 mg); then increase to maintenance dose of 2 mg/kg/dose twice daily (maximum dose: ≤40 kg: 62.5 mg; maximum dose: >40 kg: 125 mg); a higher daily dose of 4 mg/kg/dose twice daily has been studied but has not been shown to produce higher serum concentrations than 2 mg/kg/dose and is not recommended by authors of the trial (Beghetti 2009; Beghetti 2009a, Villanueva 2006)

Adolescents <40 kg: Initial and maintenance: 62.5 mg twice daily

Adolescents ≥40 kg: Initial: 62.5 mg twice daily for 4 weeks; increase to maintenance dose of 125 mg twice daily; **Note:** Doses >125 mg twice daily do not provide additional benefit sufficient to offset the increased risk of hepatic injury. When discontinuing treatment, consider a reduction in dosage to 62.5 mg twice daily for 3 to 7 days to avoid clinical deterioration.

Adult:

Pulmonary arterial hypertension: Initial: 62.5 mg twice daily for 4 weeks; increase to maintenance dose of 125 mg twice daily; adults <40 kg should be maintained at 62.5 mg twice daily.

Note: Doses >125 mg twice daily do not provide additional benefit sufficient to offset the increased risk of hepatic injury. When discontinuing treatment, consider a reduction in dosage to 62.5 mg twice daily for 3 to 7 days (to avoid clinical deterioration).

Coadministration with protease inhibitor regimen:

Adults:

Dosage adjustment for concurrent use with atazanavir/ritonavir, darunavir/ritonavir, fosamprenavir, lopinavir/ritonavir, ritonavir, saquinavir/ritonavir, tipranavir/ritonavir:

Coadministration of bosentan in patients currently receiving one of these protease inhibitor regimens for at least 10 days: Begin with bosentan 62.5 mg once daily or every other day based on tolerability

Coadministration of one of these protease inhibitor regimens in patients currently receiving bosentan: Discontinue bosentan at least 36 hours prior to the initiation of an above protease inhibitor regimen. After at least 10 days of the protease inhibitor regimen, resume bosentan 62.5 mg once daily or every other day based on tolerability

Dosage adjustment for concurrent use with indinavir or nelfinavir:

Coadministration of bosentan in patients currently receiving indinavir or nelfinavir: Begin with bosentan 62.5 mg once daily or every other day based on tolerability

Coadministration of indinavir or nelfinavir in patients currently receiving bosentan: Adjust bosentan to 62.5 mg once daily or every other day based on tolerability

Dosing adjustment in renal impairment: No dosage adjustment required.

Dosing adjustment in hepatic impairment: Adolescents and Adults:

Mild impairment (Child-Pugh class A): No dosage adjustment necessary.

Moderate to severe impairment (Child-Pugh class B and C) and/or baseline transaminase >3 times ULN: Use not recommended; systemic exposure significantly increased in patients with moderate impairment (not studied in patients with severe impairment).

Dosing adjustment based on serum transaminase elevation: Adults: If any elevation, regardless of degree, is accompanied by clinical symptoms of hepatic injury (unusual fatigue, nausea, vomiting, abdominal pain, fever, or jaundice) or a serum bilirubin ≥2 times ULN, treatment should be stopped.

AST/ALT >3 times but ≤5 times ULN: Confirm elevation with additional test; if confirmed, reduce dose to 62.5 mg or interrupt treatment. Monitor transaminase levels at least every 2 weeks. May continue or reintroduce treatment, as appropriate, following return to pretreatment aminotransferase values. When reintroducing treatment, begin with starting dose and recheck transaminases within 3 days and at least every 2 weeks thereafter.

AST/ALT >5 times but ≤8 times upper limit of normal: Confirm elevation with additional test; if confirmed, stop treatment. Monitor transaminase levels at least every 2 weeks. May reintroduce treatment, as appropriate, following return to pretreatment aminotransferase values. When reintroducing treatment, begin with starting dose and recheck transaminases within 3 days and at least every 2 weeks thereafter.

AST/ALT >8 times upper limit of normal: Stop treatment and do not reintroduce.

Administration Hazardous agent; use appropriate precautions for handling and disposal (NIOSH 2014 [group 3]).

Oral: May be administered without regard to meals. Avoid grapefruit and grapefruit juice. Women of childbearing potential should avoid splitting, crushing, or handling broken tablets and exposure to the generated dust (tablets should be dissolved in water if necessary).

Monitoring Parameters Serum transaminase (AST and ALT) and bilirubin should be determined prior to the initiation of therapy and at monthly intervals thereafter.

Monitor for clinical signs and symptoms of liver injury (eg, abdominal pain, fatigue, fever, jaundice, nausea, vomiting). Hemoglobin and hematocrit should be measured at baseline, after 1 and 3 months of treatment, and every 3 months thereafter.

A woman of childbearing potential must have a negative pregnancy test prior to the initiation of therapy, monthly thereafter, and 1 month after stopping therapy.

Additional Information The addition of bosentan to epoprostenol therapy in 8 children (8-18 years of age) with idiopathic PAH allowed for a reduction in the epoprostenol dose (and its associated side effects) in 7 of the 8 children. Epoprostenol was able to be discontinued in 3 of the 8 children (Ivy, 2004). The results from the European post-marketing surveillance program in children 2-11 years of age confirm the need for monthly measurement of liver aminotransferases in pediatric patients for the duration of bosentan treatment (Beghetti, 2008).

Clinical studies in adults have shown that bosentan was **not** effective in the treatment of CHF in patients with left ventricular dysfunction; hospitalizations for CHF were more common during the first 1-2 months after initiation of the drug.

Dosage Forms Excipient information presented when available (limited, particularly for generics); consult specific product labeling.

Tablet, Oral:

Tracleer: 62.5 mg, 125 mg

Extemporaneous Preparations Hazardous agent; use appropriate precautions for handling and disposal (NIOSH 2014 [group 3]).

Note: Tablets are not scored; a commercial pill cutter should be used to prepare a 31.25 mg dose from the 62.5 mg tablet; the half-cut 62.5 mg tablets are stable for up to 4 weeks when stored at room temperature in the high-density polyethylene plastic bottle provided by the manufacturer. Since bosentan is classified as a teratogen (Pregnancy Risk Factor X), individuals should avoid exposure to bosentan powder (dust) by taking appropriate measures (eg, using gloves and mask); women of childbearing potential should avoid exposure to dust generated from broken or split tablets.

Crushing of the tablets is not recommended; bosentan tablets will disintegrate rapidly (within 5 minutes) in 5-25 mL of water to create a suspension. An appropriate aliquot of the suspension can be used to deliver the prescribed dose. Any remaining suspension should be discarded. Bosentan should not be mixed or dissolved in liquids with a low (acidic) pH (eg, fruit juices) due to poor solubility; the drug is most soluble in solutions with a pH >8.5.

◆ **Botox** *see* OnabotulinumtoxinA *on page 1561*

◆ **Botox Cosmetic** *see* OnabotulinumtoxinA *on page 1561*

◆ **Botulinum Antitoxin** *see* Botulism Antitoxin, Heptavalent *on page 297*

◆ **Botulinum Toxin Type A** *see* OnabotulinumtoxinA *on page 1561*

◆ **Botulinum Toxin Type B** *see* RimabotulinumtoxinB *on page 1863*

◆ **Botulism Antitoxin** *see* Botulism Antitoxin, Heptavalent *on page 297*

Botulism Antitoxin, Heptavalent

(BOT yoo lism an tee TOKS in hep ta VAY lent)

Therapeutic Category Antitoxin

Generic Availability (US) Yes

Use Treatment of symptomatic botulism following documented or suspected exposure to any of the seven serotypes of botulinum neurotoxin serotypes (serotypes A, B, C, D, E, F, or G) (FDA approved in pediatric patients [age not specified] and adults)

Prescribing and Access Restrictions Heptavalent botulism antitoxin is not available for general public use. All supplies are currently owned by the federal government for inclusion in the Strategic National Stockpile and are distributed by the Centers for Disease Control and Prevention (CDC). Clinicians who suspect botulism in a patient are instructed to call their state health department's emergency 24-hour telephone number; the state health department will contact the CDC to request release of botulism antitoxin, if indicated. State health departments can contact the CDC at their 24-hour telephone number at (770) 488-7100.

Pregnancy Risk Factor C

Pregnancy Considerations Animal reproduction studies have not been conducted. Based on limited information with the use of the previous equine products (BAT-AB; BAT-E), there is no indication that treatment of pregnant patients with botulism should differ from standard therapy (Arnon, 2001). In general, medications used as antidotes should take into consideration the health and prognosis of the mother; antidotes should be administered to pregnant women if there is a clear indication for use and should not be withheld because of fears of teratogenicity (Bailey, 2003).

Breast-Feeding Considerations It is not known if botulism antitoxin is excreted in breast milk. The manufacturer recommends that caution be exercised when administering botulism antitoxin to nursing women.

Contraindications There are no contraindications listed in the manufacturer's labeling.

Warnings/Precautions Severe hypersensitivity reactions, including anaphylaxis and anaphylactoid reactions, may occur. The risk is greatest in patients with a history of hypersensitivity to horses or equine blood products, asthma, or hay fever; pretreatment skin sensitivity testing may be considered in these patient populations and initiation at the lowest achievable infusion rate (<0.01 mL/minute) is recommended. Monitor all patients for acute allergic reactions during and following the infusion; discontinue antitoxin administration in patients who develop a hypersensitivity reaction. Immediate treatment (including epinephrine 1:1000) should be available. Delayed allergic reaction or serum sickness (eg, arthralgia, fever, lymphadenopathy, myalgia, urticarial or maculopapular rash) may occur 10-21 days after administration. Monitor all patients for delayed allergic reactions and administer appropriate medical care as needed.

Infusion reactions (eg, arthralgia, chills, fatigue, fever, headache, myalgia, nausea, vasovagal reactions, vomiting) may occur; monitor all patients for infusion reactions during and following the infusion. In patients who develop an infusion reaction, decrease the infusion rate and treat symptomatically; if symptoms worsen, discontinue the infusion. Product of equine (horse) plasma; may potentially contain infectious agents (eg, viruses) which could transmit disease. Infections thought to be transmitted by this product should be reported to the manufacturer at 1-800-768-2304.

Antitoxin is most effective if administered as early as possible (ideally within 12-48 hours) after the onset of neurologic symptoms (Fagan, 2011a). Antitoxin does not reverse existing paralysis, but it arrests its progression.

Each vial contains a minimum antitoxin potency. The total volume contained in one vial (regardless of vial size) will differ by lot number (~10-22 mL per vial); therefore, withdrawal of the entire vial contents will be required to calculate the dose. May contain maltose which may falsely elevate glucose readings. Some dosage forms may contain polysorbate 80 (also known as Tweens). Hypersensitivity reactions, usually a delayed reaction, have been reported following exposure to pharmaceutical products containing polysorbate 80 in certain individuals (Isaksson, 2002; Lucente 2000; Shelley, 1995). Thrombocytopenia, ascites, pulmonary deterioration, and renal and hepatic failure have been reported in premature neonates after receiving parenteral products containing polysorbate 80 (Alade, 1986; CDC, 1984). See manufacturer's labeling.

Warnings: Additional Pediatric Considerations The safety and efficacy information in pediatric patients is derived from animal model studies. Dosing in pediatric patients is based on the Salisbury Rule. Limited pediatric data safety data available; a CDC expanded access clinical study including 15 pediatric subjects (age range: 10 days to 17 years) reported adverse reactions in two patients; one subject experienced tachycardia, bradycardia, and asystole during infusion; pyrexia was reported in the other patient.

Adverse Reactions

Cardiovascular: Edema

Central nervous system: Chills, fever, headache

Dermatologic: Pruritus, skin rash, urticaria

Gastrointestinal: Nausea, sore throat

Rare but important or life-threatening: Anaphylactoid reaction, anaphylaxis, hypersensitivity, infusion reaction, serum sickness

Drug Interactions

Metabolism/Transport Effects None known.

Avoid Concomitant Use There are no known interactions where it is recommended to avoid concomitant use.

Increased Effect/Toxicity There are no known significant interactions involving an increase in effect.

Decreased Effect There are no known significant interactions involving a decrease in effect.

Storage/Stability Store intact vials frozen at ≤-15°C (≤5°F) until use; once thawed, may be stored at 2°C to 8°C (36°F to 48°F) for up to 36 months or until 48 months from date of manufacture (whichever comes first). Prior to dilution, vials should be brought to room temperature; frozen vials may be thawed by either placing in the refrigerator for ~14 hours or at room temperature for 1 hour followed by a water bath at 98.6°F (37°C) until thawed. Do not use a microwave to thaw; do not refreeze.

Mechanism of Action Contains toxin-specific $F(ab')_2$ and $F(ab')_2$-related antibody fragments which bind and neutralize free botulinum neurotoxin A, B, C, D, E, F, and G. As a result, the neurotoxins are prevented from interacting with the cholinergic nerve ending and internalizing into target cells, thereby minimizing nerve damage and severity of the disease. Clinicians should note that botulism antitoxin does not reverse preexisting toxic manifestations.

Pharmacokinetics (Adult data unless noted)

Distribution: V_d:

- Antitoxin serotype A: 3.6 L
- Antitoxin serotype B: 9.6 L
- Antitoxin serotype C: 6.1 L
- Antitoxin serotype D: 1.5 L
- Antitoxin serotype E: 14.2 L
- Antitoxin serotype F: 3.4 L
- Antitoxin serotype G: 2.4 L

Half-life elimination:

- Antitoxin serotype A: 8.6 hours
- Antitoxin serotype B: 34.2 hours
- Antitoxin serotype C: 29.6 hours
- Antitoxin serotype D: 7.5 hours
- Antitoxin serotype E: 7.8 hours
- Antitoxin serotype F: 14.1 hours
- Antitoxin serotype G: 11.7 hours

Dosing: Neonatal Note: Consider a pretreatment skin sensitivity test in patients at risk for severe hypersensitivity reaction. The total volume contained in one vial (regardless of vial size) will differ by lot number (~10 to 22 mL per vial). In order to calculate partial vial doses (eg, neonatal dosing), withdrawal of the entire contents of the vial to determine the total volume in the vial is required.

Skin sensitivity test: Intradermal: 0.02 mL of a 1:1000 dilution in NS administered intradermally on the volar surface of the forearm; if the test is negative, repeat the test using a 1:100 dilution. Perform concurrent positive (histamine) and negative (saline) control tests. A positive reaction is a wheal with surrounding erythema ≥3 mm larger than the negative control test (saline) when read at 15 to 20 minutes. The histamine control test must be positive for valid interpretation. A negative reaction does not rule out the possibility of an immediate or delayed reaction with treatment.

Botulism, treatment: IV: 10% of the adult dose (one vial), regardless of body weight

Dosing: Usual Note: Consider a pretreatment skin sensitivity test in patients at risk for severe hypersensitivity reactions. The total volume contained in one vial (regardless of vial size) will differ by lot number (~10 to 22 mL per vial). In order to calculate partial vial doses (eg, pediatric dosing), withdrawal of the entire contents of the vial to determine the total volume in the vial is required.

Pediatric:

Skin sensitivity test: Infants, Children, and Adolescents: Intradermal: 0.02 mL of a 1:1000 dilution in NS administered intradermally on the volar surface of the forearm; if the test is negative, repeat the test using a 1:100 dilution. Perform concurrent positive (histamine) and negative (saline) control tests. A positive reaction is a wheal with surrounding erythema ≥3 mm larger than the negative control test (saline) when read at 15 to 20 minutes. The histamine control test must be positive for valid interpretation. A negative reaction does not rule out the possibility of an immediate or delayed reaction with treatment.

Botulism, treatment: IV:

Infants <1 year: 10% of the adult dose (one vial), regardless of body weight

Children ≥1 year and Adolescents <17 years: 20% to 100% of the adult dose dependent upon patient weight; minimum dose: 20% of one vial; maximum dose: One vial

The percentage of the adult dose to be administered is based on patient weight according to the following Salisbury Rule equations:

- ≤30 kg: Percentage (%) of Adult Dose to be Administered = Weight (kg) x 2
- >30 kg: Percentage (%) of Adult Dose to be Administered = Weight (kg) + 30

The following doses are recommended using the above equations:

- 10 to 14 kg: 20% of one vial
- 15 to 19 kg: 30% of one vial
- 20 to 24 kg: 40% of one vial
- 25 to 29 kg: 50% of one vial
- 30 to 34 kg: 60% of one vial
- 35 to 39 kg: 65% of one vial
- 40 to 44 kg: 70% of one vial
- 45 to 49 kg: 75% of one vial
- 50 to 54 kg: 80% of one vial
- ≥55 kg: One vial

Adolescents ≥17 years: One vial

Adult:

Skin sensitivity test: Intradermal: 0.02 mL of a 1:1000 dilution given intradermally on the volar surface of the forearm; if the test is negative, repeat the test using a 1:100 dilution. Perform concurrent positive (histamine) and negative (saline) control tests. A positive reaction is a wheal with surrounding erythema ≥3 mm larger than the negative control test (saline) when read at 15 to 20 minutes. The histamine control test must be positive for valid interpretation. A negative reaction does not rule out the possibility of an immediate or delayed reaction with treatment.

Botulism, treatment: IV: One vial

Dosing adjustment in renal impairment: There are no dosage adjustment provided in manufacturer's labeling (has not been studied).

Dosing adjustment in hepatic impairment: There are no dosage adjustment provided in manufacturer's labeling (has not been studied).

Preparation for Administration Bring vial to room temperature prior to preparation. Do not shake vial during preparation to avoid foaming.

Intradermal: Skin sensitivity testing: Dilute in NS to a 1:1,000 dilution (first step) or 1:100 dilution (second step)

IV: Botulism treatment: Dilute to a 1:10 dilution in NS. The total volume contained in one vial (regardless of vial size) will differ by lot number (~10 to 22 mL per vial); therefore, in patients receiving a dose equal to 1 vial, 90 to 200 mL of NS will be required to prepare a 1:10 dilution. In order to calculate partial vial doses (eg, neonatal/pediatric dosing), withdraw the entire contents of the vial to determine the total volume in the vial since varies with lot number and then calculate percentage partial dose and diluent volume to prepare 1:10 dilution. Do not use if the solution is turbid, cloudy, or contains particles. Discard any unused portion.

Administration

Intradermal: Skin sensitivity testing: Administer enough diluted antitoxin intradermally on the volar surface of the forearm to raise a small wheal; perform concurrent positive (histamine) and negative (saline) control tests.

IV: Botulism treatment: Consider a pretreatment skin sensitivity test in patients at risk for severe hypersensitivity reactions. Treatment doses should be diluted to a 1:10 dilution prior to administration. Use of an in-line filter is optional. A slower infusion rate should be used during the first 30 minutes of treatment; if tolerated, may increase rate every 30 minutes up to the maximum infusion rate for the remainder of the infusion. Monitor vital signs throughout the infusion. Initiate and increase the infusion rate as follows:

Pediatric:

Infants <1 year: Initial: 0.01 mL/kg/minute; may increase the rate by 0.01 mL/kg/minute every 30 minutes to a maximum infusion rate of 0.03 mL/kg/minute

Children ≥1 year and Adolescents <17 years: Initial: 0.01 mL/kg/minute (maximum initial rate: 0.5 mL/minute); may increase the rate by 0.01 mL/kg/minute every 30 minutes to a maximum infusion rate of 0.03 mL/kg/minute (maximum rate: 2 mL/minute)

Adolescents ≥17 years: Initial: 0.5 mL/minutes; may double the infusion rate, if tolerated, every 30 minutes to a maximum infusion rate of 2 mL/minute

Adult: Initial: 0.5 mL/minutes; may double the infusion rate, if tolerated, every 30 minutes to a maximum infusion rate of 2 mL/minute

Monitoring Parameters Monitor vital signs and for the presence of infusion-related reactions and acute hypersensitivity reactions during and immediately following infusion; monitor for delayed allergic reactions for 10 to 21 days after administration.

Test Interactions Blood glucose: Administration may result in falsely elevated blood glucose concentrations due to the presence of maltose in the botulism antitoxin, specifically when blood glucose is measured using glucose dehydrogenase pyrroloquinoline-quinone (GDH-PQQ) method.

Dosage Forms Excipient information presented when available (limited, particularly for generics); consult specific product labeling.

Injection, solution [preservative free]: Each vial contains no less than serotype A antitoxin 4500 units, serotype B antitoxin 3300 units, serotype C antitoxin 3000 units, serotype D antitoxin 600 units, serotype E antitoxin 5100 units, serotype F antitoxin 3000 units, and serotype G antitoxin 600 units (20 mL, 50 mL)

Botulism Immune Globulin (Intravenous-Human)

(BOT yoo lism i MYUN GLOB you lin, in tra VEE nus, YU man)

Medication Safety Issues

Sound-alike/look-alike issues:

BabyBIG may be confused with HBIG

Brand Names: US BabyBIG®

Therapeutic Category Immune Globulin

Generic Availability (US) No

Use Treatment of infant botulism caused by toxin type A or B (FDA approved in ages <1 year)

Prescribing and Access Restrictions Access to botulism immune globulin is restricted through the Infant Botulism Treatment and Prevention Program (IBTPP). Healthcare providers must contact the IBTPP on-call physician at (510) 231-7600 to review treatment indications and to obtain the medication. For more information, refer to http://www.infantbotulism.org or contact IBTPP@infantbotulism.org.

Pregnancy Considerations Botulism immune globulin is only indicated for use in neonates.

Contraindications Hypersensitivity to human immune globulin preparations or any component of the formulation; selective immunoglobulin A deficiency

Warnings/Precautions Hypersensitivity and anaphylactic reactions can occur; immediate treatment (including epinephrine 1:1000) should be available. Aseptic meningitis syndrome (AMS) has been reported with intravenous immune globulin administration (rare); may occur with high doses (≥2 g/kg). Immune globulin intravenous (IGIV) has been associated with antiglobulin hemolysis; monitor for signs of hemolytic anemia. Hyperproteinemia, increased serum viscosity, and hyponatremia may occur following administration of IGIV products; distinguish hyponatremia from pseudohyponatremia to prevent volume depletion, a further increase in serum viscosity, and a higher risk of thrombotic events. These adverse events have not reported with botulism immune globulin. Thrombotic events have been reported with administration of IGIV; use with caution in patients with a history of atherosclerosis or cardiovascular and/or thrombotic risk factors or patients with known/suspected hyperviscosity. Consider a baseline assessment of blood viscosity in patients at risk for hyperviscosity. Infuse at lowest practical rate in patients at risk for thrombotic events. Monitor for transfusion-related acute lung injury (TRALI); noncardiogenic pulmonary edema has been reported with IGIV use. TRALI is characterized by severe respiratory distress, pulmonary edema, hypoxemia, and fever in the presence of normal left ventricular function. Usually occurs within 1-6 hours after infusion.

Acute renal dysfunction (increased serum creatinine, oliguria, acute renal failure) can rarely occur; usually within 7 days of use (more likely with products stabilized with sucrose). Use with caution in patients with renal disease, diabetes mellitus, volume depletion, sepsis, paraproteinemia, and nephrotoxic medications due to risk of renal dysfunction. In patients at risk of renal dysfunction, the rate of infusion and concentration of solution should be minimized. Patients should not be volume depleted prior to therapy. Product of human plasma; may potentially contain infectious agents which could transmit disease. Screening of donors, as well as testing and/or inactivation or removal of certain viruses, reduces the risk. Infections thought to be transmitted by this product should be reported to the manufacturer. For IV infusion only; do not exceed recommended rate of administration. Not indicated for use in adults. Safety and efficacy established for infants <1 year of age; not indicated for children ≥1 year of age.

Adverse Reactions

Cardiovascular: Blood pressure increased/decreased, cardiac murmur, edema, pallor, peripheral coldness, tachycardia

Central nervous system: Agitation, body temperature decreased, irritability, pyrexia

Dermatologic: Contact dermatitis, erythematous rash

Endocrine & metabolic: Dehydration, hyponatremia, metabolic acidosis

Gastrointestinal: Abdominal distension, dysphagia, loose stools, vomiting

Hematologic: Anemia, hemoglobin decreased

Local: Injection site erythema, injection site reaction

Otic: Otitis media

Renal: Neurogenic bladder

Respiratory: Atelectasis, breath sounds decreased cough, dyspnea, lower respiratory tract infection, nasal congestion, oxygen saturation decreased, rales, rhonchi, stridor, tachypnea

Miscellaneous: Infusion rate reactions (includes back pain, chills, fever, muscle cramps, nausea, vomiting, wheezing), oral candidiasis, intubation

Drug Interactions

Metabolism/Transport Effects None known.

Avoid Concomitant Use There are no known interactions where it is recommended to avoid concomitant use.

Increased Effect/Toxicity There are no known significant interactions involving an increase in effect.

Decreased Effect

Botulism Immune Globulin (Intravenous-Human) may decrease the levels/effects of: Vaccines (Live)

Storage/Stability Prior to reconstitution, store between 2°C to 8°C (36°F to 46°F). Infusion should begin within 2 hours of reconstitution and be completed within 4 hours of reconstitution.

Mechanism of Action BIG-IV is purified immunoglobulin derived from the plasma of adults immunized with botulinum toxoid types A and B. BIG-IV provides antibodies to neutralize circulating toxins.

Pharmacodynamics Duration: ~6 months with a single infusion

Pharmacokinetics (Adult data unless noted) Half-life: Infants: ~28 days

Dosing: Neonatal **Infant botulism:** Dosage is specific to the manufactured lot. As of November 2013: IV: Total dose is 50 mg/kg as a single IV infusion. Start as soon as diagnosis of infant botulism is made; refer to product specific information.

Dosing: Usual Pediatric: **Infant botulism:** Infants: Dosage is specific to the manufactured lot. As of November 2013: IV: Total dose is 50 mg/kg as a single IV infusion. Start as soon as diagnosis of infant botulism is made; refer to product specific information.

Dosing adjustment for toxicity: Infusion reactions: Slow the infusion rate or temporarily interrupt infusion for minor reaction (ie, flushing). Discontinue infusion and administer epinephrine for anaphylactic reaction or significant hypotension.

Dosing adjustment in renal impairment: Infants: There are no dosage adjustments provided in the manufacturer's labeling. Use with caution; the rate of infusion and concentration of solution should be minimized in patients with renal impairment or those at risk for renal dysfunction.

Dosing adjustment in hepatic impairment: There are no dosage adjustments provided in the manufacturer's labeling.

Preparation for Administration IV infusion: Reconstitute 100 mg vial with 2 mL SWFI; swirl gently to wet powder; do not shake. Allow ~30 minutes for powder to dissolve; resulting concentration 50 mg/mL.

Administration IV infusion: Infusion should be started within 2 hours of reconstitution and be completed within 4 hours of reconstitution. **Do not administer IM or SubQ.**

Initial: Begin at 25 mg/kg/hour for the first 15 minutes; if well tolerated may increase to a maximum rate of 50 mg/kg/hour; infusion should take 67.5 minutes to complete at the recommended rates and should be concluded within 4 hours of reconstitution (unless infusion rate is decreased or temporarily interrupted due to an adverse reaction). Use low volume tubing for administration via a separate line. If this is not possible, piggyback BabyBIG into a preexisting line containing either NS or a dextrose solution ($D_{2.5}W$, D_5W, $D_{10}W$, or $D_{20}W$) with or without added NaCl. Do not dilute more than 1:2 with any of the above solutions. Drug concentration should be no less than 25 mg/mL. Administer via an in-line or syringe-tip filter (18 micron). Do not administer if solution is turbid. Infusion should be slowed or temporarily interrupted for minor side effects; discontinue in case of hypotension or anaphylaxis. Epinephrine should be available for the treatment of acute allergic reaction.

Monitoring Parameters Vital signs and blood pressure monitored continuously during the infusion. BUN and serum creatinine should be monitored prior to initial infusion. Periodic monitoring of renal function tests and urine output in patients at risk for developing renal failure. Aseptic meningitis syndrome (may occur hours to days following IGIV therapy). Signs of relapse (may occur up to 1 month following recovery).

Additional Information Prior to November 2013, dosing recommendations were for **Lot 4** for a total dose of 75 mg/kg/dose.

Dosage Forms Excipient information presented when available (limited, particularly for generics); consult specific product labeling.

Injection, powder for reconstitution [preservative free]:

BabyBIG®: ~100 mg [contains albumin (human), sucrose; supplied with diluent]

- **Boudreaux's® Butt Paste [OTC]** *see* Zinc Oxide *on page* 2214
- **Bovine Lung Surfactant** *see* Beractant *on page* 276
- **Bovine Lung Surfactant** *see* Calfactant *on page* 355
- **BP Cleansing [OTC]** *see* Benzoyl Peroxide *on page* 270
- **BP Foam** *see* Benzoyl Peroxide *on page* 270
- **BP Foaming Wash** *see* Benzoyl Peroxide *on page* 270
- **BP Gel [OTC]** *see* Benzoyl Peroxide *on page* 270
- **BPO** *see* Benzoyl Peroxide *on page* 270
- **BPO-5 Wash [OTC]** *see* Benzoyl Peroxide *on page* 270
- **BPO-10 Wash [OTC]** *see* Benzoyl Peroxide *on page* 270
- **BPO Creamy Wash [OTC]** *see* Benzoyl Peroxide *on page* 270
- **BPO Foaming Cloths** *see* Benzoyl Peroxide *on page* 270
- **BProtected Pedia D-Vite [OTC]** *see* Cholecalciferol *on page* 448
- **BProtected Pedia Iron [OTC]** *see* Ferrous Sulfate *on page* 871
- **BProtected Vitamin C [OTC]** *see* Ascorbic Acid *on page* 202

- **BP Wash** *see* Benzoyl Peroxide *on page 270*
- **Brethaire** *see* Terbutaline *on page 2024*
- **Brethine** *see* Terbutaline *on page 2024*
- **Brevibloc** *see* Esmolol *on page 789*
- **Brevibloc in NaCl** *see* Esmolol *on page 789*
- **Brevibloc Premixed (Can)** *see* Esmolol *on page 789*
- **Brevital (Can)** *see* Methohexital *on page 1389*
- **Brevital Sodium** *see* Methohexital *on page 1389*
- **Bricanyl** *see* Terbutaline *on page 2024*
- **Bricanyl® Turbuhaler® (Can)** *see* Terbutaline *on page 2024*

Brimonidine (Ophthalmic) (bri MOE ni deen)

Medication Safety Issues

Sound-alike/look-alike issues:

Brimonidine may be confused with bromocriptine

Brand Names: US Alphagan P

Brand Names: Canada Alphagan; Apo-Brimonidine; Apo-Brimonidine P; PMS-Brimonidine Tartrate; ratio-Brimonidine; Sandoz-Brimonidine

Therapeutic Category Alpha-Adrenergic Agonist, Ophthalmic; Glaucoma, Treatment Agent

Generic Availability (US) Yes

Use Lowering of IOP in patients with open-angle glaucoma or ocular hypertension (FDA approved in ages ≥2 years and adults)

Pregnancy Risk Factor B

Pregnancy Considerations Teratogenic effects were not observed in animal reproduction studies.

Breast-Feeding Considerations It is not known if brimonidine is excreted in breast milk. Due to the potential for serious adverse reactions in the nursing infant, a decision should be made whether to discontinue nursing or to discontinue the drug, taking into account the importance of treatment to the mother.

Contraindications Hypersensitivity to brimonidine tartrate or any component of the formulation; children <2 years of age

Canadian labeling: Additional contraindications (not in U.S. labeling): Patients receiving MAO inhibitor therapy

Warnings/Precautions Exercise caution in treating patients with severe cardiovascular disease. Use with caution in patients with depression, cerebral or coronary insufficiency, Raynaud's phenomenon, orthostatic hypotension, or thromboangiitis obliterans. Use with caution in patients with hepatic or renal impairment. Systemic absorption has been reported; children are at higher risk of systemic adverse events (Levy, 2004); use contraindicated in children <2 years of age. May cause CNS depression, which may impair physical or mental abilities; patients must be cautioned about performing tasks which require mental alertness (eg, operating machinery or driving).

Some formulations may contain benzalkonium chloride which may be absorbed by soft contact lenses; remove contacts prior to administration and wait 15 minutes before reinserting. The IOP-lowering efficacy observed with brimonidine tartrate during the first of month of therapy may not always reflect the long-term level of IOP reduction. Routinely monitor IOP.

Warnings: Additional Pediatric Considerations

May cause CNS depression, particularly in young children; the most common adverse effect reported in a study of pediatric glaucoma patients was somnolence and decreased alertness (50% to 83% in children 2 to 6 years of age); these effects resulted in a 16% discontinuation of treatment rate; children >7 years (>20 kg) had a much lower rate of somnolence (25%); apnea, bradycardia, hypotension, hypothermia, hypotonia, and somnolence have been reported in infants receiving brimonidine.

Adverse Reactions Adverse reactions may be formulation dependent; reactions reported with Alphagan P:

Cardiovascular: Hypertension, hypotension

Central nervous system: Dizziness, drowsiness (more common in children), fatigue, foreign body sensation of eye, headache, impaired consciousness (children), insomnia

Dermatologic: Erythema of eyelid, skin rash

Endocrine & metabolic: Hypercholesterolemia

Gastrointestinal: Dyspepsia, xerostomia

Hypersensitivity: Local ocular hypersensitivity reaction (5% to 9%), hypersensitivity reaction

Infection: Infection

Neuromuscular & skeletal: Weakness

Ophthalmic: Allergic conjunctivitis, blepharitis, blepharoconjunctivitis, blurred vision, burning sensation of eyes, cataract, conjunctival edema, conjunctival hemorrhage, conjunctival hyperemia, conjunctivitis, decreased visual acuity, dry eye syndrome, epiphora, eye discharge, eye irritation, eyelid disease, eyelid edema, eye pain, eye pruritus, follicular conjunctivitis, keratitis, photophobia, stinging of eyes, superficial punctate keratitis, visual disturbance, visual field defect, vitreous detachment, vitreous opacity, watery eyes

Respiratory: Bronchitis, cough, dyspnea, flu-like symptoms, pharyngitis, rhinitis, sinus infection, sinusitis

Rare but important or life-threatening: Anterior uveitis, apnea (infants), bradycardia, corneal erosion, depression, dermatological reaction (erythema, eyelid pruritus, vasodilatation), dry nose, dysgeusia, hordeolum, hypothermia (infants), hypotonia (infants), iritis, keratoconjunctivitis sicca, miosis, nausea, tachycardia

Drug Interactions

Metabolism/Transport Effects None known.

Avoid Concomitant Use

Avoid concomitant use of Brimonidine (Ophthalmic) with any of the following: Azelastine (Nasal); Iobenguane I 123; Mianserin; Orphenadrine; Paraldehyde; Thalidomide

Increased Effect/Toxicity

Brimonidine (Ophthalmic) may increase the levels/effects of: Alcohol (Ethyl); Azelastine (Nasal); Beta-Blockers; Buprenorphine; CNS Depressants; DULoxetine; Hydrocodone; Hypotensive Agents; Levodopa; Methotrimeprazine; Metyrosine; Orphenadrine; Paraldehyde; Pramipexole; RisperiDONE; ROPINIRole; Rotigotine; Selective Serotonin Reuptake Inhibitors; Suvorexant; Thalidomide; Zolpidem

The levels/effects of Brimonidine (Ophthalmic) may be increased by: Barbiturates; Beta-Blockers; Brimonidine (Topical); Cannabis; Doxylamine; Dronabinol; Droperidol; HydrOXYzine; Kava Kava; Magnesium Sulfate; MAO Inhibitors; Methotrimeprazine; Nabilone; Nicorandil; Perampanel; Rufinamide; Sodium Oxybate; Tapentadol; Tetrahydrocannabinol

Decreased Effect

Brimonidine (Ophthalmic) may decrease the levels/effects of: Iobenguane I 123

The levels/effects of Brimonidine (Ophthalmic) may be decreased by: Mianserin; Mirtazapine; Serotonin/Norepinephrine Reuptake Inhibitors; Tricyclic Antidepressants

Storage/Stability Store between 15°C to 25°C (59°F to 77°F).

Mechanism of Action Selective agonism for alpha$_2$-receptors; causes reduction of aqueous humor formation and increased uveoscleral outflow

Pharmacodynamics Maximum effect: 2 hours

Pharmacokinetics (Adult data unless noted)
Metabolism: Extensive in liver
Half-life: 2 hours
Time to peak serum concentration: Ophthalmic: Within 0.5-2.5 hours

Dosing: Usual Glaucoma, ocular hypertension: Children ≥2 years, Adolescents, and Adults: Ophthalmic: Instill 1 drop into lower conjunctival sac of affected eye(s) 3 times daily (approximately every 8 hours)

Administration Ophthalmic: Instill into conjunctival sac avoiding contact of bottle tip with skin or eye; apply finger pressure to lacrimal sac during and for 1-2 minutes after instillation to decrease risk of absorption and systemic effects. Administer other topical ophthalmic medications at least 5 minutes apart; generic formulation contains benzalkonium chloride which may be absorbed by soft contact lenses; wait at least 15 minutes after administration to insert soft contact lenses.

Monitoring Parameters IOP

Dosage Forms Excipient information presented when available (limited, particularly for generics); consult specific product labeling.
Solution, Ophthalmic, as tartrate:
Alphagan P: 0.1% (5 mL, 10 mL, 15 mL); 0.15% (5 mL, 10 mL, 15 mL) [contains carboxymethylcellulose sodium]
Generic: 0.15% (5 mL, 10 mL, 15 mL); 0.2% (5 mL, 10 mL, 15 mL)

◆ **Brimonidine and Brinzolamide** *see* Brinzolamide and Brimonidine *on page* 302

◆ **Brimonidine Tartrate** *see* Brimonidine (Ophthalmic) *on page* 301

Brinzolamide and Brimonidine

(brin ZOH la mide & bri MOE ni deen)

Brand Names: US Simbrinza
Brand Names: Canada Simbrinza
Therapeutic Category $Alpha_2$ Agonist, Ophthalmic; Carbonic Anhydrase Inhibitor (Ophthalmic); Ophthalmic Agent, Antiglaucoma

Use Reduction of elevated intraocular pressure (IOP) in patients with ocular hypertension or open-angle glaucoma (FDA approved in ages ≥2 years and adults)

Pregnancy Risk Factor C

Pregnancy Considerations Animal reproduction studies have not been conducted with this combination product; refer to individual monographs.

Breast-Feeding Considerations It is not known if brinzolamide or brimonidine are excreted into breast milk following ophthalmic application. Due to the potential for serious adverse reactions in the nursing infant, the manufacturer recommends a decision be made whether to discontinue nursing or to discontinue the drug, taking into account the importance of treatment to the mother.

Contraindications Hypersensitivity to brinzolamide, brimonidine, or any component of the formulation; children <2 years of age

Warnings/Precautions See individual agents.

Adverse Reactions Also see individual agents.
Gastrointestinal: Dysgeusia, xerostomia
Hypersensitivity: Local ocular hypersensitivity reaction
Ophthalmic: Blurred vision, eye irritation

Drug Interactions

Metabolism/Transport Effects Refer to individual components.

Avoid Concomitant Use
Avoid concomitant use of Brinzolamide and Brimonidine with any of the following: Azelastine (Nasal); Carbonic Anhydrase Inhibitors; Iobenguane I 123; Mianserin; Orphenadrine; Paraldehyde; Thalidomide

Increased Effect/Toxicity
Brinzolamide and Brimonidine may increase the levels/effects of: Alcohol (Ethyl); Alpha-/Beta-Agonists (Indirect-Acting); Azelastine (Nasal); Beta-Blockers; Buprenorphine; Carbonic Anhydrase Inhibitors; CNS Depressants; DULoxetine; Hydrocodone; Hypotensive Agents; Levodopa; Methotrimeprazine; Metyrosine; Orphenadrine; Paraldehyde; Pramipexole; RisperiDONE; ROPINIRole; Rotigotine; Selective Serotonin Reuptake Inhibitors; Suvorexant; Thalidomide; Zolpidem

The levels/effects of Brinzolamide and Brimonidine may be increased by: Barbiturates; Beta-Blockers; Brimonidine (Topical); Cannabis; CYP3A4 Inhibitors (Strong); Doxylamine; Dronabinol; Droperidol; HydrOXYzine; Kava Kava; Magnesium Sulfate; MAO Inhibitors; Methotrimeprazine; Nabilone; Nicorandil; Perampanel; Rufinamide; Sodium Oxybate; Tapentadol; Tetrahydrocannabinol

Decreased Effect
Brinzolamide and Brimonidine may decrease the levels/effects of: Iobenguane I 123

The levels/effects of Brinzolamide and Brimonidine may be decreased by: Mianserin; Mirtazapine; Serotonin/Norepinephrine Reuptake Inhibitors; Tricyclic Antidepressants

Storage/Stability Store at 2°C to 25°C (36°F to 77°F).

Mechanism of Action
Brinzolamide inhibits carbonic anhydrase, leading to decreased aqueous humor secretion. This results in a reduction of intraocular pressure (IOP).
Brimonidine has selective agonism for $alpha_2$-receptors and causes reduction of aqueous humor formation and increased uveoscleral outflow

Pharmacodynamics
Maximum effect: Ocular hypotensive effect:
Brimonidine: 2 hours
Brinzolamide: 2 to 3 hours

Pharmacokinetics (Adult data unless noted)
Absorption: Brinzolamide: Topical: Into systemic circulation
Distribution: Brinzolamide: Accumulates extensively in red blood cells, binding to carbonic anhydrase (brinzolamide and metabolite)
Protein binding: Brinzolamide: ~60%
Metabolism:
Brimonidine: Extensively, hepatic
Brinzolamide: To N-desethyl brinzolamide
Half life:
Brimonidine: 2 to 3 hours
Brinzolamide: 111 days
Time to peak serum concentration: Brimonidine: Within 0.5 to 4 hours
Elimination:
Brimonidine: Urine (74%)
Brinzolamide: Urine (predominantly as unchanged drug)

Dosing: Usual
Pediatric: **Elevated intraocular pressure:** Ophthalmic: Children ≥2 years and Adolescents: Instill 1 drop in affected eye(s) 3 times daily
Adult: **Elevated intraocular pressure:** Ophthalmic: Instill 1 drop in affected eye(s) 3 times daily

Dosing adjustment in renal impairment:
Mild to moderate renal impairment (CrCl ≥30 ml/minute): There are no dosage adjustment provided in the manufacturer's labeling; brinzolamide and metabolite are excreted predominately by the kidney; use with caution.
Severe renal impairment (CrCl <30 mL/minute): Use is not recommended (has not been studied); brinzolamide and metabolite are excreted predominately by the kidney.

Dosing adjustment in hepatic impairment: There are no dosage adjustments provided in manufacturer's labeling (has not been studied); use with caution.

Administration Shake bottle well prior to administration. If using additional topical ophthalmic preparations, separate administration by at least 5 minutes. Remove contact lenses prior to administration and wait 15 minutes after administration before reinserting. Apply gentle pressure to lacrimal sac immediately following instillation (1 minute) or instruct patient to gently close eyelid after administration to decrease systemic absorption of ophthalmic drops (Urtti, 1993; Zimmerman, 1982). Instruct patients to avoid allowing the tip of the dispensing container to contact the eye or surrounding structures. Ocular solutions can become contaminated by common bacteria known to cause ocular infections. Serious damage to the eye and subsequent loss of vision may occur from using contaminated solutions.

Monitoring Parameters Ophthalmic exams and IOP periodically

Dosage Forms Excipient information presented when available (limited, particularly for generics); consult specific product labeling.

Suspension, ophthalmic:

Simbrinza: Brinzolamide 1% and brimonidine tartrate 0.2% (8 mL) [contains benzalkonium chloride]

- **Brinzolamide and Brimonidine Tartrate** *see* Brinzolamide and Brimonidine *on page 302*
- **Brisdelle** *see* PARoxetine *on page 1634*
- **British Anti-Lewisite** *see* Dimercaprol *on page 665*
- **BRL 43694** *see* Granisetron *on page 981*

Bromocriptine (broe moe KRIP teen)

Medication Safety Issues

Sound-alike/look-alike issues:

Bromocriptine may be confused with benztropine, brimonidine

Cycloset may be confused with Glyset

Parlodel may be confused with pindolol, Provera

Related Information

Serotonin Syndrome *on page 2447*

Brand Names: US Cycloset; Parlodel

Brand Names: Canada Dom-Bromocriptine; PMS-Bromocriptine

Therapeutic Category Anti-Parkinson's Agent, Dopamine Agonist; Antidiabetic Agent, Dopamine Agonist; Antidiabetic Agent, Oral; Ergot Derivative

Generic Availability (US) Yes

Use Treatment of dysfunctions associated with hyperprolactinemia, including amenorrhea with or without galactorrhea, infertility, or hypogonadism (FDA approved in adults); treatment of prolactin-secreting adenomas (FDA approved in ages ≥11 years and adults); treatment of acromegaly (FDA approved in adults); treatment of Parkinson's disease (FDA approved in adults); treatment of type 2 diabetes mellitus as an adjunct to diet and exercise (Cycloset®: FDA approved in adults); has also been used for neuroleptic malignant syndrome

Pregnancy Risk Factor B

Pregnancy Considerations No evidence of teratogenicity or fetal toxicity in animal studies. Bromocriptine is used for ovulation induction in women with hyperprolactinemia. In general, therapy should be discontinued if pregnancy is confirmed unless needed for treatment of macroprolactinoma. Data collected from women taking bromocriptine during pregnancy suggest the incidence of birth defects is not increased with use. However, the majority of women discontinued use within 8 weeks of pregnancy. Women not seeking pregnancy should be advised to use appropriate contraception.

Breast-Feeding Considerations A previous indication for prevention of postpartum lactation was withdrawn voluntarily by the manufacturer following reports of serious adverse reactions, including stroke, MI, seizures, and severe hypertension. Use during breast-feeding is specifically contraindicated in the product labeling for Cycloset®. Use in postpartum women with a history of coronary artery disease or other severe cardiovascular conditions is specifically contraindicated in the product labeling for Parlodel® (unless withdrawal of medication is medically contraindicated). Based on the risk/benefit assessment, other treatments should be considered for lactation suppression.

Contraindications

Hypersensitivity to bromocriptine, ergot alkaloids, or any component of the formulation

Additional product-specific contraindications:

Cycloset: Syncopal migraine; breast-feeding

Parlodel: Uncontrolled hypertension; pregnancy (risk to benefit evaluation must be performed in women who become pregnant during treatment for acromegaly, prolactinoma, or Parkinson disease - hypertension during treatment should generally result in efforts to withdraw); postpartum women with a history of coronary artery disease or other severe cardiovascular conditions (unless withdrawal of medication is medically contraindicated)

Warnings/Precautions Complete evaluation of pituitary function should be completed prior to initiation of treatment of any hyperprolactinemia-associated dysfunction. Use caution in patients with a history of peptic ulcer disease, dementia, or cardiovascular disease (myocardial infarction, arrhythmia). Use with extreme caution or avoid in patients with psychosis. Symptomatic hypotension may occur in a significant number of patients. In addition, hypertension, seizures, MI, and stroke have been rarely associated with bromocriptine therapy. Severe headache or visual changes may precede events. The onset of reactions may be immediate or delayed (often may occur in the second week of therapy). Sudden sleep onset and somnolence have been reported with use, primarily in patients with Parkinson's disease. Patients must be cautioned about performing tasks which require mental alertness.

Potentially significant drug-drug interactions may exist, requiring dose or frequency adjustment, additional monitoring, and/or selection of alternative therapy. Instruct patients to limit or avoid concomitant ethanol use; may potentiate the side effects.

Dopamine agonists have been associated with compulsive behaviors and/or loss of impulse control, which has manifested as new or increased gambling urges, sexual urges, uncontrolled spending, or other urges. Dose reduction or discontinuation of therapy reverses these behaviors in some, but not all cases. Visual or auditory hallucinations may occur when administered alone or concomitantly with levodopa; dose reductions or discontinuation may be necessary. Symptoms may persist for several weeks following discontinuation. Risk for melanoma development is increased in Parkinson disease patients; drug causation or factors contributing to risk have not been established. Patients should be monitored closely and periodic skin examinations should be performed. Avoid use of Parlodel in patients with rare hereditary problems of galactose intolerance, severe lactase deficiency, or glucose-galactose malabsorption.

In the treatment of acromegaly, discontinuation is recommended if tumor expansion occurs during therapy. Digital vasospasm (cold sensitive) may occur in some patients with acromegaly; may require dosage reduction. Patients who receive bromocriptine during and immediately following pregnancy as a continuation of previous therapy (eg, acromegaly) should be closely monitored for cardiovascular effects. Should not be used postpartum in women with coronary artery disease or other cardiovascular disease. Use of bromocriptine to control or prevent lactation or in patients with uncontrolled hypertension is not recommended.

Monitoring and careful evaluation of visual changes during the treatment of hyperprolactinemia is recommended to differentiate between tumor shrinkage and traction on the optic chiasm; rapidly progressing visual field loss requires neurosurgical consultation. Discontinuation of bromocriptine in patients with macroadenomas has been associated with rapid regrowth of tumor and increased prolactin serum levels. Cases of pleural and pericardial effusions, as well as pleural, pulmonary and/or retroperitoneal fibrosis and constrictive pericarditis have been reported with prolonged and high-dose daily use. Cardiac valvular fibrosis has also been associated with ergot alkaloids.

In the management of type 2 diabetes mellitus, Cycloset ("quick-release" tablet) should not be interchanged with any other bromocriptine product due to formulation differences and resulting pharmacokinetics. Therapy is not appropriate in patients with diabetic ketoacidosis (DKA) or type 1 diabetes mellitus due to lack of efficacy in these patient populations. There is limited efficacy of use in combination with thiazolidinediones or in combination with insulin. Combination therapy with other hypoglycemic agents may increase risk for hypoglycemic events; dose reduction of concomitant hypoglycemics may be warranted.

Cerebrospinal fluid rhinorrhea has been observed in some prolactin-secreting adenoma patients. Dopaminergic agents have been associated with a syndrome resembling neuroleptic malignant syndrome on abrupt withdrawal or significant dosage reduction after long-term use; gradual dosage reduction is recommended when discontinuing therapy.

Adverse Reactions

Cardiovascular: Hypotension (including postural/orthostatic), Raynaud's phenomenon, syncope, vasospasm (digital)

Central nervous system: Dizziness, drowsiness, fatigue, headache, lightheadedness

Endocrine & metabolic: Hypoglycemia

Gastrointestinal: Abdominal cramps, anorexia, constipation, diarrhea, dyspepsia, gastrointestinal hemorrhage, nausea, vomiting, xerostomia

Infection: Increased susceptibility to infection

Neuromuscular & skeletal: Weakness

Ophthalmic: Amblyopia

Respiratory: Flu-like symptoms, nasal congestion, rhinitis. sinusitis

Rare but important or life-threatening: Acquired valvular heart disease, alopecia, bradycardia, cardiac arrhythmia, cerebrovascular accident (postpartum), confusion, constrictive pericarditis, depression, dysphagia, epileptiform seizures, ergot alkaloids toxicity, erythromelalgia, gastrointestinal ulcer, hallucination, hypertension (postpartum), increased cerebrospinal fluid pressure, insomnia, myocardial infarction (postpartum), narcolepsy, paresthesia, pericardial effusion, peripheral edema, pleural effusion, pleurisy, psychomotor agitation, pulmonary fibrosis, retroperitoneal fibrosis, seizure (postpartum), status epilepticus (postpartum), tachycardia, transient blindness, urinary incontinence, urinary retention, vasodepressor syncope, ventricular tachycardia

Drug Interactions

Metabolism/Transport Effects Substrate of CYP3A4 (major); **Note:** Assignment of Major/Minor substrate status based on clinically relevant drug interaction potential; **Inhibits** CYP1A2 (weak)

Avoid Concomitant Use

Avoid concomitant use of Bromocriptine with any of the following: Alpha-/Beta-Agonists; Alpha1-Agonists; Amisulpride; Conivaptan; Dapoxetine; Fusidic Acid (Systemic); Idelalisib; Lorcaserin; Nitroglycerin; Protease Inhibitors; Serotonin 5-HT1D Receptor Agonists

Increased Effect/Toxicity

Bromocriptine may increase the levels/effects of: Alcohol (Ethyl); Alpha-/Beta-Agonists; Alpha1-Agonists; BuPROPion; CycloSPORINE (Systemic); Hypoglycemia-Associated Agents; Metoclopramide; Serotonin 5-HT1D Receptor Agonists; Serotonin Modulators; TiZANidine

The levels/effects of Bromocriptine may be increased by: Alcohol (Ethyl); Alpha-Lipoic Acid; Androgens; Antiemetics (5HT3 Antagonists); Aprepitant; Beta-Blockers; Conivaptan; CYP3A4 Inhibitors (Moderate); CYP3A4 Inhibitors (Strong); Dapoxetine; Dasatinib; Fosaprepitant; Fusidic Acid (Systemic); Idelalisib; Ivacaftor; Lorcaserin; Luliconazole; Macrolide Antibiotics; MAO Inhibitors; Methylphenidate; Mifepristone; Netupitant; Nitroglycerin; Palbociclib; Pegvisomant; Protease Inhibitors; Quinolone Antibiotics; Salicylates; Serotonin 5-HT1D Receptor Agonists; Simeprevir; Somatostatin Analogs; Stiripentol; Tedizolid

Decreased Effect

Bromocriptine may decrease the levels/effects of: Amisulpride; Antipsychotic Agents (First Generation [Typical]); Nitroglycerin

The levels/effects of Bromocriptine may be decreased by: Amisulpride; Antipsychotic Agents (First Generation [Typical]); Antipsychotic Agents (Second Generation [Atypical]); Hyperglycemia-Associated Agents; Metoclopramide; Quinolone Antibiotics; Thiazide Diuretics

Storage/Stability Store below 25°C (77°F); protect from light.

Mechanism of Action Semisynthetic ergot alkaloid derivative and a dopamine receptor agonist which activates postsynaptic dopamine receptors in the tuberoinfundibular (inhibiting pituitary prolactin secretion) and nigrostriatal pathways (enhancing coordinated motor control).

In the treatment of type 2 diabetes mellitus, the mechanism of action is unknown; however, bromocriptine is believed to affect circadian rhythms which are mediated, in part, by dopaminergic activity, and are believed to play a role in obesity and insulin resistance. It is postulated that bromocriptine (when administered during the morning and released into the systemic circulation in a rapid, 'pulse-like' dose) may reset hypothalamic circadian activities which have been altered by obesity, thereby resulting in the reversal of insulin resistance and decreases in glucose production, without increasing serum insulin concentrations.

Pharmacodynamics Reduction of prolactin concentrations (Parlodel®):

Onset of action: 1-2 hours

Maximum effect: 5-10 hours

Duration: 8-12 hours

Pharmacokinetics (Adult data unless noted)

Bioavailability: Parlodel®: 28%; Cycloset®: 65% to 95%

Distribution: V_d: ~61L

Protein binding: 90% to 96%

Metabolism: Primarily hepatic via CYP3A4; extensive first-pass biotransformation (93%)

Half-life: Parlodel®: ~5 hours; Cycloset®: 6 hours

Time to peak serum concentration:

Parlodel®: 2.5 ± 2 hours

Cycloset®: 53 minutes (fasted); 90-120 minutes (high-fat meal)

Elimination: Feces (82%); urine (2% to 6% as unchanged drug)

Dosing: Usual

Children and Adolescents: **Hyperprolactinemia:**

Children and Adolescents 11-15 years (based on limited information): Oral: Initial: 1.25-2.5 mg daily; dosage may be increased as tolerated to achieve a therapeutic response; usual dosage range: 2.5-10 mg daily

Adolescents ≥16 years: Oral: Initial: 1.25-2.5 mg daily; may be increased by 2.5 mg/day as tolerated every 2-7 days until optimal response; usual dosage range: 2.5-15 mg daily

Adults:

Acromegaly: Oral: Initial: 1.25-2.5 mg daily increasing by 1.25-2.5 mg daily as necessary every 3-7 days; usual dose: 20-30 mg/day (maximum: 100 mg/day)

Hyperprolactinemia: Oral: Initial: 1.25-2.5 mg daily; may be increased by 2.5 mg daily as tolerated every 2-7 days until optimal response; usual dosage range: 2.5-15 mg daily

Neuroleptic malignant syndrome (NMS): Oral: 2.5 mg (orally or via gastric tube) every 8-12 hours, increased to a maximum of 45 mg daily, if needed; continue therapy until NMS is controlled, then taper slowly (Gortney, 2009; Strawn, 2007)

Parkinsonism: Oral: 1.25 mg twice daily, increased by 2.5 mg/day in 2- to 4-week intervals as needed (maximum daily dose: 100 mg/day)

Type 2 diabetes mellitus (Cycloset®): Oral: Initial: 0.8 mg once daily; may increase at weekly intervals in 0.8 mg increments as tolerated; usual dose: 1.6-4.8 mg daily (maximum: 4.8 mg daily)

Dosing adjustment in hepatic impairment: No guidelines are available; however, may be necessary due to extensive metabolism

Administration Oral: May be taken with food to decrease GI distress

Cycloset®: Administer within 2 hours of waking in the morning

Monitoring Parameters Monitor blood pressure closely as well as hepatic, hematopoietic, and cardiovascular function; visual field monitoring is recommended (prolactinoma); pregnancy testing during amenorrheic period; growth hormone and prolactin levels; Hb A_{1c} and serum glucose (type 2 diabetes mellitus)

Additional Information Usually used with levodopa or levodopa/carbidopa to treat Parkinson's disease. When adding bromocriptine, the dose of levodopa/carbidopa can usually be decreased.

Dosage Forms Excipient information presented when available (limited, particularly for generics); consult specific product labeling. [DSC] = Discontinued product

Capsule, Oral:

Parlodel: 5 mg

Generic: 5 mg

Tablet, Oral:

Cycloset: 0.8 mg

Parlodel: 2.5 mg [DSC] [scored]

Generic: 2.5 mg

◆ **Bromocriptine Mesylate** *see* Bromocriptine *on page 303*

Brompheniramine and Pseudoephedrine

(brome fen IR a meen & soo doe e FED rin)

Brand Names: US Brotapp [OTC]; BroveX PSB [OTC]; J-Tan D PD [OTC]; Lodrane D [OTC]; LoHist PSB [OTC] [DSC]; Q-Tapp Cold & Allergy [OTC]; Rynex PSE [OTC]

Therapeutic Category Antihistamine/Decongestant Combination

Generic Availability (US) Yes

Use Temporary relief of symptoms associated with allergic rhinitis; **Note:** Approved ages and uses for generic products may vary; consult labeling for specific information.

Oral:

Capsules (Lodrane-D): FDA approved in ages >12 years and adults

Drops (J-Tan D PD): FDA approved in ages 2-12 years

Elixir (Q-Tapp): FDA approved in ages ≥6 years and adults

Liquid:

Brotapp: FDA approved in ages ≥6 years and adults

Rynex PSE: FDA approved in ages ≥2 years and adults

Contraindications Hypersensitivity to brompheniramine, pseudoephedrine, or any component of the formulation; concomitant MAO inhibitor therapy (or 2 weeks following MAO inhibitor use)

Warnings/Precautions May cause CNS depression, which may impair physical or mental abilities; patients must be cautioned about performing tasks which require mental alertness (eg, operating machinery or driving). Effects may be potentiated when used with other sedative drugs or ethanol. Use caution with hypertension, ischemic heart disease, hyperthyroidism, asthma, increased intraocular pressure, diabetes mellitus, and BPH. Use with caution in the elderly; may be more sensitive to adverse effects.

Benzyl alcohol and derivatives: Some dosage forms may contain sodium benzoate/benzoic acid; benzoic acid (benzoate) is a metabolite of benzyl alcohol; large amounts of benzyl alcohol (≥99 mg/kg/day) have been associated with a potentially fatal toxicity ("gasping syndrome") in neonates; the "gasping syndrome" consists of metabolic acidosis, respiratory distress, gasping respirations, CNS dysfunction (including convulsions, intracranial hemorrhage), hypotension, and cardiovascular collapse (AAP, 1997; CDC, 1982); some data suggests that benzoate displaces bilirubin from protein binding sites (Ahlfors, 2001); avoid or use dosage forms containing benzyl alcohol derivative with caution in neonates. See manufacturer's labeling.

When used for self-medication (OTC), notify healthcare provider if symptoms do not improve within 7 days or are accompanied by fever. Discontinue and contact healthcare provider if nervousness, dizziness, or sleeplessness occur. Antihistamines may cause excitation in young children.

Warnings: Additional Pediatric Considerations Safety and efficacy for the use of cough and cold products in pediatric patients <4 years of age is limited; the AAP warns against the use of these products for respiratory illnesses in this age group. Serious adverse effects including death have been reported (in some cases, high blood concentrations of pseudoephedrine were found). Many of these products contain multiple active ingredients, increasing the risk of accidental overdose when used with other products. The FDA notes that there are no approved OTC uses for these products in pediatric patients <2 years of age. Health care providers are reminded to ask caregivers about the use of OTC cough and cold products in order to avoid exposure to multiple medications containing the same ingredient. Multiple concentrations of oral liquid formulations (drops, elixir, and liquid) exist; close attention must be paid to the concentration when ordering or administering. Antihistamines should not be used to make an infant or child sleepy (AAP 2012; FDA 2008).

Some dosage forms may contain propylene glycol; in neonates large amounts of propylene glycol delivered orally, intravenously (eg, >3,000 mg/day), or topically have been associated with potentially fatal toxicities which can include metabolic acidosis, seizures, renal failure, and CNS depression; toxicities have also been reported in children and adults including hyperosmolality, lactic

acidosis, seizures and respiratory depression; use caution (AAP, 1997; Shehab, 2009).

Adverse Reactions

Cardiovascular: Arrhythmias, flushing, hypertension, pallor, palpitation, tachycardia

Central nervous system: Convulsions, CNS stimulation, dizziness, excitability (children; rare), giddiness, hallucinations, headache, insomnia, irritability, lassitude, nervousness, sedation

Gastrointestinal: Anorexia, diarrhea, dyspepsia, nausea, vomiting, xerostomia

Genitourinary: Dysuria, urinary retention (with BPH)

Neuromuscular skeletal: Tremors, weakness

Ocular: Diplopia

Renal: Polyuria

Respiratory: Respiratory difficulty

Drug Interactions

Metabolism/Transport Effects None known.

Avoid Concomitant Use

Avoid concomitant use of Brompheniramine and Pseudoephedrine with any of the following: Aclidinium; Azelastine (Nasal); Eluxadoline; Ergot Derivatives; Glucagon; Iobenguane I 123; Ipratropium (Oral Inhalation); MAO Inhibitors; Orphenadrine; Paraldehyde; Potassium Chloride; Thalidomide; Tiotropium; Umeclidinium

Increased Effect/Toxicity

Brompheniramine and Pseudoephedrine may increase the levels/effects of: AbobotulinumtoxinA; Alcohol (Ethyl); Analgesics (Opioid); Anticholinergic Agents; Azelastine (Nasal); Buprenorphine; CNS Depressants; Eluxadoline; Glucagon; Hydrocodone; Methotrimeprazine; Metyrosine; Mirabegron; Mirtazapine; OnabotulinumtoxinA; Orphenadrine; Paraldehyde; Potassium Chloride; Pramipexole; RimabotulinumtoxinB; ROPINIRole; Rotigotine; Selective Serotonin Reuptake Inhibitors; Suvorexant; Sympathomimetics; Thalidomide; Thiazide Diuretics; Tiotropium; Topiramate; Zolpidem

The levels/effects of Brompheniramine and Pseudoephedrine may be increased by: Aclidinium; Alkalinizing Agents; AtoMOXetine; Brimonidine (Topical); Cannabis; Carbonic Anhydrase Inhibitors; Doxylamine; Dronabinol; Droperidol; Ergot Derivatives; HydrOXYzine; Ipratropium (Oral Inhalation); Kava Kava; Linezolid; Magnesium Sulfate; MAO Inhibitors; Methotrimeprazine; Mianserin; Nabilone; Perampanel; Pramlintide; Rufinamide; Serotonin/Norepinephrine Reuptake Inhibitors; Sodium Oxybate; Tapentadol; Tedizolid; Tetrahydrocannabinol; Umeclidinium

Decreased Effect

Brompheniramine and Pseudoephedrine may decrease the levels/effects of: Acetylcholinesterase Inhibitors; Benzylpenicilloyl Polylysine; Betahistine; FentaNYL; Hyaluronidase; Iobenguane I 123; Itopride; Metoclopramide; Secretin

The levels/effects of Brompheniramine and Pseudoephedrine may be decreased by: Acetylcholinesterase Inhibitors; Alpha1-Blockers; Amphetamines; Spironolactone; Urinary Acidifying Agents

Storage/Stability Store at room temperature.

Mechanism of Action Brompheniramine maleate is an antihistamine with H_1-receptor activity; pseudoephedrine, a sympathomimetic amine and isomer of ephedrine, acts as a decongestant in respiratory tract mucous membranes with less vasoconstrictor action than ephedrine in normotensive individuals.

Pharmacodynamics See individual monograph for Pseudoephedrine.

Brompheniramine component only:

Maximum effect: Within 3 to 9 hours

Duration: 4 to 6 hours

Pharmacokinetics (Adult data unless noted) See individual monograph for Pseudoephedrine.

Brompheniramine component only:

Distribution: V_d: Children 6 to 12 years: ~20 L/kg (Simons 1999), Adults: ~12 L/kg (Simons 1982)

Metabolism: Hepatic, extensive (Simons 2004)

Half-life: Children 6 to 12 years: 12.4 hours (Simons 1999), Adults: ~25 hours (Simons 1982)

Time to peak serum concentration: Oral: ~3 hours; similar data reported in children 6 to 12 years (Simons 1982; Simons 1999)

Elimination: Urine (50%, as inactive metabolites) (Bruce 1968)

Dosing: Usual Note: Multiple concentrations of oral liquid formulations (drops, elixir, and liquid) exist; close attention must be paid to the concentration when ordering or administering

Pediatric: **Allergic rhinitis and nasal congestion:**

Capsules (Brompheniramine 4 mg and pseudoephedrine 60 mg): Oral: Adolescents: 1 capsule every 4 to 6 hours as needed; maximum daily dose: 4 capsules/**24 hours**

Concentrated Drops (Brompheniramine 1mg and pseudoephedrine 7.5 mg per 1 mL): Oral:

Children 2 to <6 years: 1 mL (1 dropperful) every 4 to 6 hours as needed; maximum daily dose 6 mL/**24 hours**

Children 6 to 12 years: 2 mL (2 dropperfuls) every 4 to 6 hours as needed; maximum daily dose: 12 mL/**24 hours**

Liquid and elixir (Brompheniramine 1 mg and 15 mg pseudoephedrine per 5 mL): Oral:

Children 2 to <6 years: 5 mL every 4 to 6 hours as needed; maximum daily dose: 20 mL/**24 hours**

Children 6 to <12 years: 10 mL every 4 to 6 hours as needed; maximum daily dose: 40 mL/**24 hours**

Children ≥12 and Adolescents: 20 mL every 4 to 6 hours as needed; maximum daily dose: 80 mL/**24 hours**

Adult: **Rhinitis and nasal congestion:** Oral:

Capsules (brompheniramine 4 mg and pseudoephedrine 60 mg): 1 capsule every 4 to 6 hours; maximum daily dose: 4 capsules/**24 hours**

Elixir (Brompheniramine 1 mg and pseudoephedrine 15 mg per 5 mL): 20 mL every 4 to 6 hours as needed; maximum daily dose: 80 mL/**24 hours**

Liquid (Brompheniramine 1mg and pseudoephedrine 15 mg per 5 mL): 20 mL every 4 to 6 hours as needed; maximum daily dose: 80 mL/**24 hours**

Dosing adjustment in renal impairment: \There are no dosage adjustments provided in manufacturer's labeling.

Dosing adjustment in hepatic impairment: There are no dosage adjustments provided in manufacturer's labeling.

Test Interactions See individual agents.

Dosage Forms Excipient information presented when available (limited, particularly for generics); consult specific product labeling. [DSC] = Discontinued product

Capsule, oral:

Lodrane D: Brompheniramine maleate 4 mg and pseudoephedrine hydrochloride 60 mg

Liquid, oral:

Brotapp: Brompheniramine maleate 1 mg and pseudoephedrine hydrochloride 15 mg per 5 mL (120 mL, 240 mL, 480 mL) [ethanol free, sugar free; contains propylene glycol, sodium benzoate; grape flavor]

BroveX PSB: Brompheniramine maleate 4 mg and pseudoephedrine hydrochloride 20 mg per 5 mL (473 mL) [dye free, ethanol free, sugar free; contains propylene glycol; cotton candy flavor]

LoHist PSB: Brompheniramine maleate 4 mg and pseudoephedrine hydrochloride 20 mg per 5 mL (473 mL) [dye free, ethanol free, sugar free; cherry flavor] [DSC]

Q-Tapp Cold & Allergy: Brompheniramine maleate 1 mg and pseudoephedrine hydrochloride 15 mg per 5 mL (118 mL, 237 mL) [ethanol free; contains propylene glycol, sodium 2 mg/5 mL, sodium benzoate; grape flavor]

Rynex PSE: Brompheniramine maleate 1 mg and pseudoephedrine hydrochloride 15 mg per 5 mL (473 mL) (ethanol free, sugar free; contains propylene glycol; orange flavor)

Liquid, oral [drops]:

J-Tan D PD: Brompheniramine maleate 1 mg and pseudoephedrine hydrochloride 7.5 mg per 1 mL (30 mL) [dye free, ethanol free, sugar free; contains propylene glycol; cotton candy flavor]

- ◆ **Brompheniramine Maleate and Pseudoephedrine Hydrochloride** *see* Brompheniramine and Pseudoephedrine *on page 305*
- ◆ **Brompheniramine Maleate and Pseudoephedrine Sulfate** *see* Brompheniramine and Pseudoephedrine *on page 305*
- ◆ **Broncho Saline [OTC]** *see* Sodium Chloride *on page 1938*
- ◆ **Brotapp [OTC]** *see* Brompheniramine and Pseudoephedrine *on page 305*
- ◆ **BroveX PSB [OTC]** *see* Brompheniramine and Pseudoephedrine *on page 305*
- ◆ **BSS** *see* Bismuth Subsalicylate *on page 290*
- ◆ **BTX-A** *see* OnabotulinumtoxinA *on page 1561*
- ◆ **Buckleys Chest Congestion [OTC]** *see* GuaiFENesin *on page 988*
- ◆ **Budeprion SR [DSC]** *see* BuPROPion *on page 324*

Budesonide (Systemic, Oral Inhalation)

(byoo DES oh nide)

Related Information

Inhaled Corticosteroids *on page 2261*

Oral Medications That Should Not Be Crushed or Altered *on page 2476*

Brand Names: US Entocort EC; Pulmicort; Pulmicort Flexhaler; Uceris

Brand Names: Canada Entocort; Pulmicort Turbuhaler

Therapeutic Category Adrenal Corticosteroid; Anti-inflammatory Agent; Antiasthmatic; Corticosteroid, Inhalant (Oral); Glucocorticoid

Generic Availability (US) May be product dependent

Use

Inhalation:

Nebulization: Maintenance therapy and prophylaxis of bronchial asthma (FDA approved in ages 1-8 years); **not** indicated for the relief of acute bronchospasm

Oral inhalation: Maintenance therapy and prophylaxis of bronchial asthma with or without oral corticosteroids (FDA approved in ages ≥6 years and adults); **not** indicated for the relief of acute bronchospasm

Oral:

Entocort® EC: Treatment of mild to moderate active Crohn's disease of the ileum and/or ascending colon and maintenance of remission for up to 3 months (FDA approved in adults); has also been used for treatment of protein-losing enteropathy in patients after Fontan procedure

Uceris™ ER: Induction of remission from active, mild to moderate ulcerative colitis (FDA approved in adults)

Pregnancy Risk Factor C (capsule, tablet)/B (inhalation)

Pregnancy Considerations Adverse events have been observed with corticosteroids in animal reproduction studies. Some studies have shown an association between first trimester systemic corticosteroid use and oral clefts (Park-Wyllie 2000; Pradat 2003). Systemic corticosteroids may also influence fetal growth (decreased birth weight); however, information is conflicting (Lunghi 2010). Hypoadrenalism may occur in newborns following maternal use of corticosteroids in pregnancy; monitor. When systemic corticosteroids are needed in pregnancy, it is generally recommended to use the lowest effective dose for the shortest duration of time, avoiding high doses during the first trimester (Leachman 2006; Lunghi 2010). Budesonide may be used for the induction of remission in pregnant women with inflammatory bowel disease (Habal 2012).

Based on available data, an overall increased risk of congenital malformations or a decrease in fetal growth has not been associated with maternal use of inhaled corticosteroids during pregnancy (Bakhireva 2005; NAEPP 2005; Namazy 2004). In addition, studies of pregnant women specifically using inhaled budesonide have not demonstrated an increased risk of congenital abnormalities. Uncontrolled asthma is associated with adverse events on pregnancy (increased risk of perinatal mortality, pre-eclampsia, preterm birth, low birth weight infants). Inhaled corticosteroids are recommended for the treatment of asthma during pregnancy; budesonide is preferred (ACOG 2008; NAEPP 2005).

Breast-Feeding Considerations Following use of the powder for oral inhalation, ~0.3% to 1% of the maternal dose was found in breast milk. The maximum concentration appeared within 45 minutes of dosing. Plasma budesonide levels obtained from infants ~90 minutes after breast-feeding (~140 minutes after maternal dose) were below the limit of quantification. Concentrations of budesonide in breast milk are expected to be higher following administration of oral capsules/tablets than after an inhaled dose.

Due to the potential for serious adverse reactions in the nursing infant, the manufacturers of the oral tablets and capsules recommend a decision be made whether to discontinue nursing or to discontinue the drug, taking into account the importance of treatment to the mother. If there is concern about exposure to the infant, some guidelines recommend waiting 4 hours after the maternal dose of an oral systemic corticosteroid before breast-feeding in order to decrease potential exposure to the nursing infant (based on a study using prednisolone) (Habal 2012; Ost, 1985).

According to the manufacturer of the product for inhalation, the decision to continue or discontinue breast-feeding during therapy should take into account the risk of minimal exposure to the infant and the benefits of breast-feeding to the mother. The use of inhaled corticosteroids is not considered a contraindication to breast-feeding (NAEPP 2005).

Contraindications

Hypersensitivity to budesonide or any component of the formulation; primary treatment of status asthmaticus, acute episodes of asthma; not for relief of acute bronchospasm

Canadian labeling: Additional contraindications (not in US labeling): Moderate-to-severe bronchiectasis, pulmonary tuberculosis (active or quiescent), untreated respiratory infection (bacterial, fungal, or viral)

Warnings/Precautions May cause hypercorticism or suppression of hypothalamic-pituitary-adrenal (HPA) axis, particularly in younger children, in patients receiving high doses for prolonged periods, or with concomitant CYP3A4 inhibitor use. HPA axis suppression may lead to adrenal crisis. Withdrawal and discontinuation of a corticosteroid should be done slowly and carefully. Particular care is required when patients are transferred from systemic corticosteroids to inhaled products or corticosteroids with lower systemic effect due to possible adrenal insufficiency or withdrawal from steroids, including an increase in allergic symptoms. Adult patients receiving >20 mg per day of prednisone (or equivalent) may be most susceptible. Fatalities have occurred due to adrenal insufficiency in asthmatic patients during and after transfer from systemic corticosteroids to aerosol steroids; aerosol steroids do not provide the systemic steroid needed to treat patients having trauma, surgery, or infections. Do not use this product to transfer patients directly from oral corticosteroid therapy. Select surgical patients on long-term, high-dose, inhaled corticosteroid (ICS), should be given stress doses of hydrocortisone intravenously during the surgical period and the dose reduced rapidly within 24 hours after surgery (NAEPP 2007).

Bronchospasm may occur with wheezing after inhalation; if this occurs stop steroid and treat with a fast-acting bronchodilator (eg, albuterol). Supplemental steroids (oral or parenteral) may be needed during stress or severe asthma attacks. Not to be used in status asthmaticus or for the relief of acute bronchospasm. Acute myopathy has been reported with high-dose corticosteroids, usually in patients with neuromuscular transmission disorders; may involve ocular and/or respiratory muscles; monitor creatine kinase; recovery may be delayed. Corticosteroid use may cause psychiatric disturbances, including depression, euphoria, insomnia, mood swings, and personality changes. Preexisting psychiatric conditions may be exacerbated by corticosteroid use. Prolonged use of corticosteroids may also increase the incidence of secondary infection, mask acute infection (including fungal infections), prolong or exacerbate viral infections, or limit response to vaccines. Exposure to chickenpox should be avoided; corticosteroids should not be used to treat ocular herpes simplex. Corticosteroids should not be used for viral hepatitis. Close observation is required in patients with latent tuberculosis and/or TB reactivity; restrict use in active TB (only in conjunction with antituberculosis treatment). *Candida albicans* infections may occur in the mouth and pharynx; rinsing (and spitting) with water after inhaler use may decrease risk. Prolonged treatment with corticosteroids has been associated with the development of Kaposi's sarcoma (case reports); if noted, discontinuation of therapy should be considered.

Use with caution in patients with thyroid disease, hepatic impairment, renal impairment, cardiovascular disease, diabetes, glaucoma, cataracts, myasthenia gravis, patients at risk for osteoporosis, patients at risk for seizures, or GI diseases (diverticulitis, peptic ulcer, ulcerative colitis) due to perforation risk. Use caution following acute MI (corticosteroids have been associated with myocardial rupture). Because of the risk of adverse effects, systemic corticosteroids should be used cautiously in the elderly in the smallest possible effective dose for the shortest duration.

Potentially significant interactions may exist, requiring dose or frequency adjustment, additional monitoring, and/or selection of alternative therapy.

Orally-inhaled corticosteroids may cause a reduction in growth velocity in pediatric patients (~1 centimeter per year [range: 0.3-1.8 cm per year] and related to dose and duration of exposure). To minimize the systemic effects of orally-inhaled corticosteroids, each patient should be titrated to the lowest effective dose. Growth should be routinely monitored in pediatric patients. Withdraw systemic therapy with gradual tapering of dose. There have been reports of systemic corticosteroid withdrawal symptoms (eg, joint/muscle pain, lassitude, depression) when withdrawing oral inhalation therapy. Pulmicort Flexhaler contains lactose; very rare anaphylactic reactions have been reported in patients with severe milk protein allergy. Some dosage forms may contain polysorbate 80 (also known as Tweens). Hypersensitivity reactions, usually a delayed reaction, have been reported following exposure to pharmaceutical products containing polysorbate 80 in certain individuals (Isaksson 2002; Lucente 2000; Shelley, 1995). Thrombocytopenia, ascites, pulmonary deterioration, and renal and hepatic failure have been reported in premature neonates after receiving parenteral products containing polysorbate 80 (Alade, 1986; CDC, 1984). See manufacturer's labeling.

Warnings: Additional Pediatric Considerations A 12-week study in infants (n=141; 6 to 12 months of age) receiving budesonide nebulizations (0.5 mg or 1 mg once daily) vs placebo demonstrated a budesonide dose dependent suppression of linear growth; in addition, although mean changes from baseline did not indicate budesonide-induced adrenal suppression, six infants who received budesonide had subnormal stimulated cortisol levels at week 12. Children and adolescents (n=18; 6 to 15 years) receiving budesonide nebulizations of 1 and 2 mg twice daily showed a significant reduction in urinary cortisol excretion; this reduction was not seen when patients were dosed at 1 mg/day (maximum recommended dose). Long-term effects of chronic use of budesonide nebulization on immunological or developmental processes of upper airways, mouth, and lung are unknown.

Adverse Reactions

Oral capsules:

Cardiovascular: Chest pain, edema, facial edema, flushing, hypertension, palpitations, tachycardia

Central nervous system: Agitation, amnesia, confusion, dizziness, drowsiness, headache, insomnia, malaise, nervousness, paresthesia, sleep disorder, vertigo

Dermatologic: Acne vulgaris, alopecia, atrophic striae, dermatitis, dermatological disease, eczema

Endocrine & metabolic: Adrenocortical insufficiency, hirsutism, hypokalemia, intermenstrual bleeding, menstrual disease, redistribution of body fat (moon face, buffalo hump), weight gain

Gastrointestinal: Anus disease, dental disease, diarrhea, dyspepsia, enteritis, epigastric pain, exacerbation of Crohn's disease, gastrointestinal fistula, glossitis, hemorrhoids, increased appetite, intestinal obstruction, nausea, oral candidiasis

Genitourinary: Dysuria, hematuria, nocturia, pyuria, urinary frequency, urinary tract infection

Hematologic & oncologic: Abnormal neutrophils, anemia, bruise, C-reactive protein increased, increased erythrocyte sedimentation rate, leukocytosis, purpura

Hepatic: Increased serum alkaline phosphatase

Hypersensitivity: Tongue edema

Infection: Abscess, viral infection

Neuromuscular & skeletal: Arthralgia, arthritis, hyperkinesia, muscle cramps, myalgia, tremor, weakness

Ophthalmic: Eye disease, visual disturbance

Otic: Otic infection

Respiratory: Bronchitis, dyspnea, flu-like symptoms, pharyngeal disease, respiratory tract infection, rhinitis, sinusitis

Miscellaneous: Abscess, C-reactive protein increased, diaphoresis, fat redistribution (moon face, buffalo hump), flu-like syndrome, erythrocyte sedimentation rate increased, viral infection

Rare but important or life-threatening: Anaphylaxis, intracranial hypertension (benign)

Oral inhaler (Pulmicort Flexhaler):

Cardiovascular: Syncope

Central nervous system: Headache, hypertonia, insomnia, pain, voice disorder

Endocrine & metabolic: Weight gain

Gastrointestinal: Abdominal pain, dysgeusia, dyspepsia, nausea, oral candidiasis, viral gastroenteritis, vomiting, xerostomia

Hematologic & oncologic: Bruise

Infection: Infection

Neuromuscular & skeletal: Arthralgia, back pain, bone fracture, myalgia, neck pain, weakness
Otic: Otitis media
Respiratory: Allergic rhinitis, cough, nasal congestion, nasopharyngitis, pharyngitis, respiratory tract infection, rhinitis, sinusitis, viral upper respiratory tract infection
Miscellaneous: Fever
Rare but important or life-threatening: Adrenocortical insufficiency, aggressive behavior, cataract, depression, glaucoma, hypercorticoidism, hypersensitivity (immediate and delayed [includes rash, contact dermatitis, angioedema, bronchospasm, urticaria]), increased intraocular pressure, psychosis, wheezing (patients with severe milk allergy)

Oral tablets:
Central nervous system: Emotional lability, fatigue, headache
Dermatologic: Acne vulgaris
Endocrine & metabolic: Decreased cortisol, hirsutism
Gastrointestinal: Abdominal distension, constipation, flatulence, nausea, upper abdominal pain
Genitourinary: Urinary tract infection
Neuromuscular & skeletal: Arthralgia
Rare but important or life-threatening: Anaphylaxis, intracranial hypertension (benign)

Suspension for nebulization:
Cardiovascular: Chest pain
Central nervous system: Emotional lability, fatigue, voice disorder
Dermatologic: Contact dermatitis, eczema, pruritus, pustular rash, skin rash
Gastrointestinal: Abdominal pain, anorexia, diarrhea, gastroenteritis, vomiting
Hematologic & oncologic: Cervical lymphadenopathy, purpura
Hypersensitivity: Hypersensitivity reaction
Infection: Candidiasis, herpes simplex infection, infection, viral infection
Neuromuscular & skeletal: Bone fracture, hyperkinesia, myalgia
Ophthalmic: Conjunctivitis, eye infection
Otic: Otalgia, otic infection, otitis externa, otitis media
Respiratory: Cough, epistaxis, flu-like symptoms, respiratory tract infection, rhinitis, stridor
Rare but important or life-threatening: Adrenocortical insufficiency, aggressive behavior, avascular necrosis of femoral head, bronchitis, cataract, depression, glaucoma, growth suppression, hypercorticoidism, hypersensitivity (immediate and delayed [includes angioedema, bronchospasm, urticaria]), increased intraocular pressure, osteoporosis, psychosis

Drug Interactions

Metabolism/Transport Effects **Substrate** of CYP3A4 (major); **Note:** Assignment of Major/Minor substrate status based on clinically relevant drug interaction potential

Avoid Concomitant Use

Avoid concomitant use of Budesonide (Systemic, Oral Inhalation) with any of the following: Aldesleukin; BCG; BCG (Intravesical); Conivaptan; Fusidic Acid (Systemic); Grapefruit Juice; Idelalisib; Loxapine; Natalizumab; Pimecrolimus; Tacrolimus (Topical); Tofacitinib

Increased Effect/Toxicity

Budesonide (Systemic, Oral Inhalation) may increase the levels/effects of: Amphotericin B; Deferasirox; Leflunomide; Loop Diuretics; Loxapine; Natalizumab; Thiazide Diuretics; Tofacitinib

The levels/effects of Budesonide (Systemic, Oral Inhalation) may be increased by: Conivaptan; CYP3A4 Inhibitors (Moderate); CYP3A4 Inhibitors (Strong); Dasatinib; Denosumab; Fusidic Acid (Systemic); Grapefruit Juice; Idelalisib; Ivacaftor; Luliconazole; Mifepristone; Palbociclib; Pimecrolimus; Simeprevir; Stiripentol; Tacrolimus (Topical); Telaprevir; Trastuzumab

Decreased Effect

Budesonide (Systemic, Oral Inhalation) may decrease the levels/effects of: Aldesleukin; BCG; BCG (Intravesical); Coccidioides immitis Skin Test; Corticorelin; Hyaluronidase; Sipuleucel-T; Vaccines (Inactivated)

The levels/effects of Budesonide (Systemic, Oral Inhalation) may be decreased by: Antacids; Bile Acid Sequestrants; Echinacea

Food Interactions Grapefruit juice may double systemic exposure of orally administered budesonide. Administration of capsules with a high-fat meal delays peak concentration, but does not alter the extent of absorption; administration of tablets with a high-fat meal decreases peak concentration (~27%). Management: Avoid grapefruit juice when using oral capsules or tablets.

Storage/Stability
Oral capsules and tablets: Store at 25°C (77°F); excursions permitted to 15°C to 30°C (59°F to 86°F); keep container tightly closed.
Oral inhaler (Pulmicort Flexhaler): Store at controlled room temperature of 20°C to 25°C (68°F to 77°F). Protect from moisture.
Suspension for nebulization: Store upright at 20°C to 25°C (68°F to 77°F). Protect from light. Do not refrigerate or freeze. Once aluminum package is opened, solution should be used within 2 weeks. Continue to protect from light.

Mechanism of Action Controls the rate of protein synthesis; depresses the migration of polymorphonuclear leukocytes, fibroblasts; reverses capillary permeability and lysosomal stabilization at the cellular level to prevent or control inflammation. Has potent glucocorticoid activity and weak mineralocorticoid activity.

Pharmacodynamics Clinical effects are due to direct local effect, rather than systemic absorption.
Onset of action:
Nebulization (control of asthma symptoms): Within 2-8 days
Oral inhalation: Within 24 hours
Maximum effect:
Nebulization: 4-6 weeks
Oral inhalation: ≥1-2 weeks

Pharmacokinetics (Adult data unless noted)
Distribution: V_d:
Children 4-6 years: 3 L/kg
Adults: 2.2-3.9 L/kg
Protein binding: 85% to 90%
Metabolism: Extensive hepatic metabolism via cytochrome P450 CYP3A isoenzyme to 2 major metabolites: 16α-hydroxyprednisolone and 6β-hydroxybudesonide; both are <1% as active as parent
Bioavailability:
Nebulization: Children 4-6 years: 6%
Oral inhalation: 39% of an inhaled metered dose is available systemically
Oral: 9% in healthy volunteers and 21% in patients with Crohn's disease (large first pass effect); **Note:** Oral bioavailability is 2.5-fold higher in patients with hepatic cirrhosis
Half-life:
Children 4-6 years: 2.3 hours (after nebulization)
Children 10-14 years: 1.5 hours
Adults: 2-3.6 hours
Time to peak serum concentration:
Nebulization: 20 minutes
Oral inhalation (Pulmicort Flexhaler®): 10 minutes
Oral capsules (Entocort® EC): 0.5-10 hours
Oral tablets, extended release (Uceris™): ~13 hours
Elimination: Urine (60% as metabolites; no unchanged drug) and feces (metabolites)

Clearance:
Children 4-6 years: 0.5 L/minute (~50% greater than healthy adults after weight adjustment)
Adults: 0.9-1.8 L/minute

Dosing: Usual

Pediatric:

Asthma: Note: Doses should be titrated to the lowest effective dose once asthma is controlled:

Nebulization: Pulmicort Respules:

Infants: Limited data available: Initial: 0.25 mg twice daily or 0.5 mg once daily; maximum daily dose: 1 mg/day (Baker 1999; GINA 2009)

Children and Adolescents:

Manufacturer's labeling: Children ≤8 years or Children >8 years and Adolescents unable to effectively use metered-dose inhalers:

Previously treated with bronchodilators alone: Initial: 0.25 mg twice daily or 0.5 mg once daily; maximum daily dose: 0.5 mg/**day**

Previously treated with inhaled corticosteroids: Initial: 0.25 mg twice daily or 0.5 mg once daily; maximum daily dose: 1 mg/**day**

Previously treated with oral corticosteroids: Initial: 0.5 mg twice daily or 1 mg once daily; maximum daily dose: 1 mg/**day**

Symptomatic children not responding to nonsteroidal asthma medications: Initial: 0.25 mg once daily may be considered

NIH Asthma Guidelines (NAEPP 2007): Administer once daily or in divided doses twice daily

Children ≤4 years:
"Low" dose: 0.25 to 0.5 mg/**day**
"Medium" dose: >0.5 to 1 mg/**day**
"High" dose: >1 mg/**day**

Children 5 to 11 years:
"Low" dose: 0.5 mg/**day**
"Medium" dose: 1 mg/**day**
"High" dose: 2 mg/**day**

Oral inhalation: Pulmicort Flexhaler:

Manufacturer's labeling:

Children and Adolescents age 6 to 17 years: Initial: 180 mcg twice daily (some patients may be initiated at 360 mcg twice daily); maximum single dose: 360 mcg

Adolescents ≥18 years: Initial: 360 mcg twice daily (some patients may be initiated at 180 mcg twice daily); maximum single dose: 720 mcg

Alternate dosing: NIH Asthma Guidelines (NAEPP 2007): Administer in divided doses twice daily

Children 5 to 11 years:
"Low" dose: 180 to 400 mcg/**day** (90 mcg/inhalation, 2 to 4 inhalations per day or 180 mcg/inhalation, 1 to 2 inhalations per day)
"Medium" dose: >400 to 800 mcg/**day** (180 mcg/inhalation, 2 to 4 inhalations per day)
"High" dose: >800 mcg/**day** (180 mcg/inhalation, >4 inhalations per day)

Children ≥12 years and Adolescents:
"Low" dose: 180 to 600 mcg/**day** (90 mcg/inhalation, 2 to 6 inhalations per day or 180 mcg/inhalation, 1 to 3 inhalations per day)
"Medium" dose: >600 to 1200 mcg/**day** (180 mcg/inhalation, 3 to 6 inhalations per day)
"High" dose: >1200 mcg/**day** (180 mcg/inhalation, >6 inhalations per day)

Conversion from oral systemic corticosteroid to orally inhaled corticosteroid: Initiation of oral inhalation therapy should begin in patients whose asthma is reasonably stabilized on oral corticosteroids (OCS). A gradual dose reduction of OCS should begin ~7 to 10 days after starting inhaled therapy. Manufacturer's labeling recommends reducing prednisone dose by 2.5 mg/day (or equivalent of other OCS) on a weekly basis (patients using oral inhaler) or by ≤25% every 1 to 2 weeks (patients using respules). When transitioning from systemic to inhaled corticosteroids, supplemental systemic corticosteroid therapy may be necessary during periods of stress or during severe asthma attacks.

Crohn disease; treatment, mild to moderate: Children ≥6 years and Adolescents: Limited data available: Oral capsule (Entocort EC): Induction: 9 mg once daily or in divided doses every 8 hours for 7 to 8 weeks, followed by a maintenance dose of 6 mg daily for 3 to 4 weeks; therapy was discontinued after a total duration of 10 to 12 weeks (Escher 2004; Levine 2003; Levine 2009). In another study of patients 10 to 19 years of age, a trend for higher remission rates using an initial dose of 12 mg daily for 4 weeks, followed by 9 mg daily for 3 weeks, followed by 6 mg daily for 3 weeks was observed (Levine 2009). A retrospective study used doses of 0.45 mg/kg/day up to a maximum daily dose of 9 mg/day (n= 62; age range: 9.5 to 18 years; final dose in all patients: 9 mg/day) (Levine 2002)

Protein-losing enteropathy (PLE) following Fontan: Limited data available: Children ≥7 years and Adolescents: Oral capsule (Entocort EC): Initial: 9 mg once daily or in divided doses every 8 hours; after clinical improvement and albumin >3 g/dL may then wean dose over several weeks to 3 mg once daily or every other day; if during the weaning process the serum albumin decreases to <2.5 g/dL, do not further reduce dose, consider dosage increase. Dosing based on several case series describing institutional experiences, the majority of pediatric patients described were ≥7 years of age (n=17) (John 2011; Schumacher 2011; Thacker 2010; Turner 2012). Reported experience in children <7 years is very limited (n=1); in one report, an initial dose of 6 mg once daily was recommended for children <4 years (Thacker 2010).

Adult:

Asthma: Oral inhalation:

Manufacturer's labeling: Pulmicort Flexhaler: Initial: 360 mcg twice daily (selected patients may be initiated at 180 mcg twice daily); may increase dose after 1 to 2 weeks of therapy in patients who are not adequately controlled; maximum: 720 mcg twice daily; **Note:** Doses should be titrated to the lowest effective dose once asthma is controlled.

NIH Asthma Guidelines (NAEPP 2007):
"Low" dose: 180 to 600 mcg/**day** (180 mcg/inhalation, 1 to 3 inhalations per day)
"Medium" dose: >600 to 1200 mcg/**day** (180 mcg/inhalation, 3 to 6 inhalations per day)
"High" dose: >1200 mcg/**day** (180 mcg/inhalation, >6 inhalations per day)

Conversion from oral systemic corticosteroid to orally inhaled corticosteroid: Initiation of oral inhalation therapy should begin in patients whose asthma is reasonably stabilized on oral corticosteroids (OCS). A gradual dose reduction of OCS should begin ~7 to 10 days after starting inhaled therapy. Manufacturer's labeling recommends reducing prednisone dose by 2.5 mg/day (or equivalent of other OCS) on a weekly basis (patients using oral inhaler) or by ≤25% every 1 to 2 weeks (patients using respules). When transitioning from systemic to inhaled corticosteroids, supplemental systemic corticosteroid therapy may be necessary during periods of stress or during severe asthma attacks.

Crohn's Disease, active: Oral: Capsule (Entocort EC):

Treatment: 9 mg once daily in the morning for ≤8 weeks; may repeat the 8-week course for recurring episodes of active Crohn disease; **Note:** When switching patients from oral prednisolone to oral budesonide, do not stop prednisolone abruptly; prednisolone taper should begin at the same time that budesonide is started.

Maintenance of remission: Following treatment of active disease and control of symptoms (Crohn Disease Activity Index <150), use 6 mg once daily for up to 3 months; if symptoms are still controlled at 3 months, taper the dose to complete cessation; continuing remission dose >3 months has not been demonstrated to result in substantial benefit

Ulcerative colitis, active: Oral: Tablet (Ulceris): 9 mg once daily in the morning for ≤8 weeks

Dosing adjustment in renal impairment: Inhalation, Nebulization, Oral: There are no dosage adjustments provided in the manufacturer's labeling (has not been studied).

Dosing adjustment in hepatic impairment:

Inhalation, Nebulization, Oral: There are no dosage adjustments provided in the manufacturer's labeling (has not been studied). However, budesonide undergoes hepatic metabolism; drug may accumulate with hepatic impairment; use with caution; monitor closely.

Oral: There are no specific dosage adjustments provided in the manufacturer's labeling. Budesonide undergoes hepatic metabolism; bioavailability is increased in cirrhosis; monitor closely for signs and symptoms of hypercorticism.

Moderate to severe liver disease:

Capsule (Entocort EC): Manufacturer's labeling: Consider dosage reduction

Tablet (Uceris): Manufacturer's labeling: Consider discontinuing use

Administration

Inhalation:

Nebulization: Shake gently with a circular motion before use. Administer only with a compressed air driven jet nebulizer; do not use an ultrasonic nebulizer; do not mix with other medications; use adequate flow rates and administer via appropriate size face mask or mouthpiece. Avoid exposure of nebulized medication to eyes. Rinse mouth following treatments to decrease risk of oral candidiasis (wash face if using face mask).

Oral inhaler: Pulmicort Flexhaler®: Hold inhaler in upright position (mouthpiece up) to load dose. Do not shake prior to use. Unit should be primed prior to first use. It will not need to be primed again, even if not used for a long time. Place mouthpiece between lips and inhale forcefully and deeply. Do not exhale through inhaler; do not use a spacer. Dose indicator does not move with every dose, usually only after 5 doses. Discard when dose indicator reads "0". Rinse mouth with water after use to reduce incidence of candidiasis.

Oral: May be administered without regard to meals.

Capsule: Manufacturer's labeling: Swallow whole; do not break, chew, or crush. Opening the capsule and sprinkling over applesauce has been evaluated *in vitro* and no change in the release properties of budesonide was found (Espmarker, 2002); this method of administration has also been used in patients unable to swallow the capsules in a study evaluating budesonide use in Crohn's disease (Thacker, 2010).

Tablet: Swallow whole; do not break, chew, or crush.

Monitoring Parameters Monitor growth in pediatric patients; inhalation: Check mucous membranes for signs of fungal infection; Asthma: FEV_1, peak flow, and/or other pulmonary function tests; Long-term use: Regular eye examinations and IOP, blood pressure, glucose, signs and symptoms of hypercorticism, or adrenal suppression.

Additional Information Budesonide capsules (Entocort™ EC) contain granules in a methylcellulose matrix; the granules are coated with a methacrylic acid polymer to protect from dissolution in the stomach; the coating dissolves at a pH >5.5 (duodenal pH); the methylcellulose matrix controls the release of drug in a time-dependent manner (until the drug reaches the ileum and ascending colon).

Dosage Forms Considerations

Pulmicort Flexhaler 180 mcg/actuation canisters contain 120 actuations and the 90 mcg/actuation canisters contain 60 inhalations.

Dosage Forms Excipient information presented when available (limited, particularly for generics); consult specific product labeling.

Aerosol Powder Breath Activated, Inhalation:

Pulmicort Flexhaler: 90 mcg/actuation (1 ea); 180 mcg/actuation (1 ea) [contains milk protein]

Capsule Extended Release 24 Hour, Oral:

Entocort EC: 3 mg

Generic: 3 mg

Suspension, Inhalation:

Pulmicort: 0.25 mg/2 mL (2 mL); 0.5 mg/2 mL (2 mL); 1 mg/2 mL (2 mL) [contains disodium edta, polysorbate 80]

Generic: 0.25 mg/2 mL (2 mL); 0.5 mg/2 mL (2 mL)

Tablet Extended Release 24 Hour, Oral:

Uceris: 9 mg

Budesonide (Nasal) (byoo DES oh nide)

Brand Names: US Rhinocort Aqua

Brand Names: Canada Mylan-Budesonide AQ; Rhinocort Aqua; Rhinocort Turbuhaler

Therapeutic Category Adrenal Corticosteroid; Anti-inflammatory Agent; Corticosteroid, Intranasal; Glucocorticoid

Generic Availability (US) Yes

Use Management of nasal symptoms associated with seasonal or perennial allergic rhinitis (FDA approved in ages ≥6 years and adults)

Intranasal corticosteroids have also been used as an adjunct to antibiotics in empiric treatment of acute bacterial rhinosinusitis primarily in patients with history of allergic rhinitis (Chow, 2012) and in pediatric patients with mild obstructive sleep apnea syndrome who cannot undergo adenotonsillectomy or who still have symptoms after surgery (Marcus, 2012).

Pregnancy Risk Factor B

Pregnancy Considerations Adverse events have been observed with corticosteroids in animal reproduction studies. Hypoadrenalism may occur in newborns following maternal use of corticosteroids in pregnancy; monitor. Studies of pregnant women using intranasal budesonide have not demonstrated an increased risk of abnormalities. Intranasal corticosteroids are recommended for the treatment of rhinitis during pregnancy; the lowest effective dose should be used (NAEPP, 2005; Wallace, 2008); budesonide is preferred (Wallace, 2008).

Breast-Feeding Considerations Following use of budesonide powder for oral inhalation, ~0.3% to 1% of the maternal dose was found in breast milk. The maximum concentration appeared within 45 minutes of dosing. Plasma budesonide levels obtained from infants ~90 minutes after breast-feeding (~140 minutes after maternal dose) were below the limit of quantification. Milk concentrations following the use of the nasal inhaler are expected to be similar. The use of inhaled corticosteroids is not considered a contraindication to breast-feeding (NAEPP, 2005). The manufacturer recommends using only when clinically appropriate, at the lowest effective dose, and administering the dose following a feeding in order to minimize potential exposure to the nursing infant.

Contraindications Hypersensitivity to budesonide or any component of the formulation

Canadian labeling: Additional contraindications (not in U.S. labeling): Pulmonary tuberculosis (active or quiescent), untreated respiratory infection (bacterial, fungal, or viral); use in patients <6 years of age

Warnings/Precautions May delay wound healing; avoid nasal corticosteroid use in patients with recent nasal septal ulcers, nasal surgery or nasal trauma until healing has occurred. Localized *Candida albicans* infections of the nose and/or pharynx may occur (rarely). Prolonged use of corticosteroids may also increase the incidence of secondary infection, mask acute infection (including fungal infections), prolong or exacerbate viral infections, or limit response to vaccines. Exposure to chickenpox should be avoided. Close observation is required in patients with latent tuberculosis and/or TB reactivity restrict use in active TB (only in conjunction with antituberculosis treatment).

Avoid using higher than recommended dosages; suppression of linear growth (ie, reduction of growth velocity), reduced bone mineral density, or hypercorticism (Cushing syndrome) may occur; titrate to lowest effective dose. Reduction in growth velocity may occur when corticosteroids are administered to pediatric patients, even at recommended doses via intranasal route (monitor growth).

Adverse Reactions Reaction severity varies by dose and duration; not all adverse reactions have been reported with each dosage form.

Respiratory: Bronchospasm, cough, epistaxis, nasal congestion, nasal irritation, pharyngitis, throat irritation

Rare but important or life-threatening: Anosmia, growth suppression, hypersensitivity reactions (immediate and delayed [includes rash, contact dermatitis, angioedema, bronchospasm]), nasal septum perforation, pharyngeal disorders (irritation, throat pain, itchy throat)

Drug Interactions

Metabolism/Transport Effects Substrate of CYP3A4 (minor); **Note:** Assignment of Major/Minor substrate status based on clinically relevant drug interaction potential

Avoid Concomitant Use There are no known interactions where it is recommended to avoid concomitant use.

Increased Effect/Toxicity

Budesonide (Nasal) may increase the levels/effects of: Ceritinib

The levels/effects of Budesonide (Nasal) may be increased by: Cobicistat; CYP3A4 Inhibitors (Strong); Telaprevir

Decreased Effect There are no known significant interactions involving a decrease in effect.

Storage/Stability

Nasal inhaler: Store with valve up at 15°C to 30°C (59°F to 86°F). Protect from high humidity.

Nasal spray: Store with valve up at 20°C to 25°C (68°F to 77°F); do not freeze. Protect from light.

Mechanism of Action Controls the rate of protein synthesis; depresses the migration of polymorphonuclear leukocytes, fibroblasts; reverses capillary permeability and lysosomal stabilization at the cellular level to prevent or control inflammation. Has potent glucocorticoid activity and weak mineralocorticoid activity.

Pharmacodynamics Clinical effects are due to direct local effect, rather than systemic absorption.

Onset of action: Within 10 hours

Maximum effect: 2 weeks

Duration after discontinuation: Several days

Pharmacokinetics (Adult data unless noted)

Distribution: V_d: 2-3 L/kg

Protein binding: 85% to 90%

Metabolism: Extensively metabolized by the liver via cytochrome P450 CYP3A isoenzyme to 2 major metabolites: 16α-hydroxyprednisolone and 6β-hydroxybudesonide; both are <1% as active as parent

Bioavailability: Intranasal 34%, Oral ~10%

Half-life: 2-3 hours

Time to peak serum concentration: 30 minutes

Elimination: 60% to 66% of dose renally excreted as metabolites; no unchanged drug found in urine; remainder via feces as metabolites

Dosing: Usual

Children ≥6 years and Adolescents: **Seasonal or perennial rhinitis:** Intranasal (Rhinocort® Aqua®): Initial: 64 mcg once daily delivered as 32 mcg (1 spray) **per nostril** once daily; dose may be increased if needed

Maximum daily dose:

Children <12 years: 128 mcg once daily delivered as 64 mcg (2 sprays) **per nostril** once daily

Children and Adolescents ≥12 years: 256 mcg once daily delivered as 128 mcg (4 sprays) **per nostril** once daily

Adults: **Seasonal or perennial rhinitis:** Intranasal (Rhinocort® Aqua®): Initial: 64 mcg once daily delivered as 32 mcg (1 spray) **per nostril** once daily; dose may be increased if needed; maximum daily dose: 256 mcg once daily delivered as 128 mcg (4 sprays) **per nostril** once daily

Dosing adjustment in renal impairment: There are no dosage adjustments provided in the manufacturer's labeling (not studied).

Dosing adjustment in hepatic impairment: There are no dosage adjustments provided in the manufacturer's labeling. Systemic availability of budesonide may be increased in patients with hepatic impairment; monitor closely for signs and symptoms of hypercorticism; dosage reduction may be required.

Administration Shake gently prior to each use. Before first use, prime by pressing pump 8 times or until a fine spray appears. If ≥2 days between use, repeat priming with 1 spray or until a fine spray appears. If >14 days between use, rinse applicator and repeat priming with 2 sprays or until a fine spray appears. Blow nose to clear nostrils before each use. Insert applicator into nostril, keeping bottle upright, and close off the other nostril. Breathe in through nose. While inhaling, press pump to release spray. After administration lean head backward for a few seconds; avoid blowing nose for 15 minutes after use. Do not spray into eyes or mouth. Discard after labeled number of doses has been used, even if bottle is not completely empty.

Monitoring Parameters Mucous membranes for signs of fungal infection, growth (pediatric patients), signs/symptoms of HPA axis suppression/adrenal insufficiency; ocular changes

Additional Information When used short term as adjunctive therapy in acute bacterial rhinosinusitis (ABRS), intranasal steroids show modest symptomatic improvement and few adverse effects; improvement is primarily due to increased sinus drainage. Use should be considered optional in ABRS; however, intranasal corticosteroids should be routinely prescribed to ABRS patients who have a history of or concurrent allergic rhinitis (Chow, 2012).

Product Availability Rhinocort Allergy OTC: FDA approved March 2015; anticipated availability is currently unknown.

Dosage Forms Considerations

Rhinocort Aqua 8.6 g bottles contain 120 sprays.

Dosage Forms Excipient information presented when available (limited, particularly for generics); consult specific product labeling.

Suspension, Nasal:

Rhinocort Aqua: 32 mcg/actuation (8.6 g) [contains disodium edta, polysorbate 80]

Generic: 32 mcg/actuation (8.6 g)

◆ **Budesonide and Eformoterol** *see* Budesonide and Formoterol *on page* 313

Budesonide and Formoterol
(byoo DES oh nide & for MOH te rol)

Brand Names: US Symbicort

Brand Names: Canada Symbicort

Therapeutic Category Adrenal Corticosteroid; Adrenergic Agonist Agent; Anti-inflammatory Agent; Antiasthmatic; Beta$_2$-Adrenergic Agonist; Bronchodilator; Corticosteroid, Inhalant (Oral); Glucocorticoid

Use Maintenance treatment of asthma (FDA approved in ages ≥12 years and adults); maintenance treatment of airflow obstruction associated with chronic obstructive pulmonary disease (COPD), including chronic bronchitis and emphysema (FDA approved in adults); **NOT** indicated for the relief of acute bronchospasm

Medication Guide Available Yes

Pregnancy Risk Factor C

Pregnancy Considerations Adverse events were observed in animal reproduction studies using this combination. Refer to individual agents.

Breast-Feeding Considerations It is not known if formoterol is excreted into breast milk; budesonide is excreted in small amounts. The manufacturer does not recommend use of this combination product in breast-feeding women. Refer to individual agents.

Contraindications Hypersensitivity to budesonide, formoterol, or any component of the formulation; need for acute bronchodilation in COPD or asthma (including status asthmaticus)

Canadian labeling: Additional contraindications (not in U.S. labeling): Hypersensitivity to inhaled lactose

Warnings/Precautions [U.S. Boxed Warning]: Long-acting beta$_2$-agonists (LABAs), such as formoterol, increase the risk of asthma-related deaths; budesonide and formoterol should only be used in patients not adequately controlled on a long-term asthma control medication (ie, inhaled corticosteroid) or whose disease severity requires initiation of two maintenance therapies. In a large, randomized, placebo-controlled U.S. clinical trial (SMART, 2006), salmeterol was associated with an increase in asthma-related deaths (when added to usual asthma therapy); risk is considered a class effect among all LABAs. Data are not available to determine if the addition of an inhaled corticosteroid lessens this increased risk of death associated with LABA use. Assess patients at regular intervals once asthma control is maintained on combination therapy to determine if step-down therapy is appropriate (without loss of asthma control), and the patient can be maintained on an inhaled corticosteroid only. LABAs are not appropriate in patients whose asthma is adequately controlled on low- or medium-dose inhaled corticosteroids. **[U.S. Boxed Warning]: LABAs may increase the risk of asthma-related hospitalization in pediatric and adolescent patients.**

Do **not** use for acute bronchospasm or acute symptomatic COPD. Short-acting beta$_2$-agonist (eg, albuterol) should be used for acute symptoms and symptoms occurring between treatments. Do **not** initiate in patients with significantly worsening or acutely deteriorating asthma or COPD. Increased use and/or ineffectiveness of short-acting beta$_2$-agonists may indicate rapidly deteriorating disease and should prompt re-evaluation of the patient's condition. Patients must be instructed to seek medical attention in cases where acute symptoms are not relieved by short-acting beta-agonist (not formoterol) or a previous level of response is diminished. Medical evaluation must not be delayed. Patients using inhaled, short acting beta$_2$-agonists should be instructed to discontinue routine use of these medications prior to beginning treatment with Symbicort®; short acting agents should be reserved for symptomatic relief of acute symptoms. Data are not available to determine if LABA use increases the risk of death in patients with COPD.

Immediate hypersensitivity reactions (urticaria, angioedema, rash, bronchospasm) have been reported. Do not exceed recommended dose; serious adverse events, including fatalities, have been associated with excessive use of inhaled sympathomimetics. Rarely, paradoxical bronchospasm may occur with use of inhaled bronchodilating agents; this should be distinguished from inadequate response. Pneumonia and other lower respiratory tract infections have been reported in patients with COPD following the use of inhaled corticosteroids; monitor COPD patients closely since pneumonia symptoms may overlap symptoms of exacerbations.

Use caution in patients with cardiovascular disease (arrhythmia or hypertension or HF), seizure disorders, diabetes, hepatic impairment, ocular disease, osteoporosis, thyroid disease, or hypokalemia. Beta agonists may cause elevation in blood pressure, heart rate, and result in CNS stimulation/excitation. Beta$_2$-agonists may increase risk of arrhythmia, increase serum glucose, or decrease serum potassium. Long-term use may affect bone mineral density in adults. Infections with *Candida albicans* in the mouth and throat (thrush) have been reported with use. Use with caution in patients taking strong CYP3A4 inhibitors (see Drug Interactions); consider alternative agents that avoid or lessen the potential for CYP-mediated interactions.

Budesonide may cause hypercorticism and/or suppression of hypothalamic-pituitary-adrenal (HPA) axis, particularly in younger children or in patients receiving high doses for prolonged periods. Caution is required when patients are transferred from systemic corticosteroids to products with lower systemic bioavailability (ie, inhalation). May lead to possible adrenal insufficiency or withdrawal symptoms, including an increase in allergic symptoms. Patients receiving prolonged therapy ≥20 mg per day of prednisone (or equivalent) may be most susceptible. Aerosol steroids do **not** provide the systemic steroid needed to treat patients having trauma, surgery, or infections.

Orally-inhaled and intranasal corticosteroids may cause a reduction in growth velocity in pediatric patients (~1 centimeter per year [range 0.3-1.8 cm per year] and related to dose and duration of exposure). To minimize the systemic effects of orally-inhaled and intranasal corticosteroids, each patient should be titrated to the lowest effective dose. Growth should be routinely monitored in pediatric patients.

Prolonged use of corticosteroids may also increase the incidence of secondary infection, mask acute infection (including fungal infections), prolong or exacerbate viral infections, or limit response to vaccines. Exposure to chickenpox should be avoided; corticosteroids should not be used to treat ocular herpes simplex. Corticosteroids should not be used for cerebral malaria. Close observation is required in patients with latent tuberculosis and/or TB reactivity restrict use in active TB (only in conjunction with antituberculosis treatment).

Some products available in Canada contain lactose; very rare anaphylactic reactions have been reported in patients with severe milk protein allergy. Withdraw systemic therapy with gradual tapering of dose. There have been reports of systemic corticosteroid withdrawal symptoms (eg, joint/muscle pain, lassitude, depression) when withdrawing oral inhalation therapy.

Adverse Reactions Note: Adverse events may be dose related; causation not established. Also see individual agents.

Central nervous system: Dizziness, headache

Gastrointestinal: Abdominal distress, oral candidiasis, vomiting

Infection: Influenza
Neuromuscular & skeletal: Back pain
Respiratory: Bronchitis, lower respiratory tract infection, nasal congestion, nasopharyngitis, pharyngolaryngeal pain, sinusitis, upper respiratory tract infection
Miscellaneous: Influenza
Rare but important or life-threatening: Agitation, anaphylaxis, angina pectoris, angioedema, anxiety, atrial arrhythmia, behavioral changes, bronchospasm, bruise, cataract, cough, decreased linear skeletal growth rate (pediatric patients), depression, dermatitis, extrasystoles, glaucoma, hypercorticoidism signs and symptoms, hyperglycemia, hypersensitivity reaction, hypertension, hypokalemia, hypotension, immunosuppression, increased intraocular pressure, insomnia, muscle cramps, nausea, nervousness, palpitations, pruritus, restlessness, skin rash, tachycardia, throat irritation, tremor, urticaria, ventricular arrhythmia, voice disorder

Drug Interactions

Metabolism/Transport Effects Refer to individual components.

Avoid Concomitant Use

Avoid concomitant use of Budesonide and Formoterol with any of the following: Aldesleukin; BCG; BCG (Intravesical); Beta-Blockers (Nonselective); Conivaptan; Fusidic Acid (Systemic); Grapefruit Juice; Idelalisib; Iobenguane I 123; Long-Acting Beta2-Agonists; Loxapine; Natalizumab; Pimecrolimus; Tacrolimus (Topical); Tofacitinib

Increased Effect/Toxicity

Budesonide and Formoterol may increase the levels/effects of: Amphotericin B; Atosiban; Deferasirox; Highest Risk QTc-Prolonging Agents; Leflunomide; Long-Acting Beta2-Agonists; Loop Diuretics; Loxapine; Moderate Risk QTc-Prolonging Agents; Natalizumab; Sympathomimetics; Thiazide Diuretics; Tofacitinib

The levels/effects of Budesonide and Formoterol may be increased by: AtoMOXetine; Caffeine and Caffeine Containing Products; Cannabinoid-Containing Products; Conivaptan; CYP3A4 Inhibitors (Moderate); CYP3A4 Inhibitors (Strong); Dasatinib; Denosumab; Fusidic Acid (Systemic); Grapefruit Juice; Idelalisib; Inhalational Anesthetics; Ivacaftor; Linezolid; Luliconazole; MAO Inhibitors; Mifepristone; Palbociclib; Pimecrolimus; Simeprevir; Stiripentol; Tacrolimus (Topical); Tedizolid; Telaprevir; Theophylline Derivatives; Trastuzumab; Tricyclic Antidepressants

Decreased Effect

Budesonide and Formoterol may decrease the levels/effects of: Aldesleukin; BCG; BCG (Intravesical); Coccidioides immitis Skin Test; Corticorelin; Hyaluronidase; Iobenguane I 123; Sipuleucel-T; Vaccines (Inactivated)

The levels/effects of Budesonide and Formoterol may be decreased by: Antacids; Beta-Blockers (Beta1 Selective); Beta-Blockers (Nonselective); Betahistine; Bile Acid Sequestrants; Echinacea

Storage/Stability

Symbicort 80/4.5, Symbicort 160/4.5: Store at room temperature of 20°C to 25°C (68°F to 77°F) with mouthpiece down. Do not puncture, incinerate, or store near heat or open flame. Discard inhaler after the labeled number of inhalations have been used or within 3 months after removal from foil pouch.

Symbicort Turbuhaler: Store at room temperature of 15°C to 30°C. Protect from heat and moisture.

Mechanism of Action Formoterol relaxes bronchial smooth muscle by selective action on beta$_2$ receptors with little effect on heart rate. Formoterol has a long-acting effect. Budesonide is a corticosteroid which controls the rate of protein synthesis, depresses the migration of polymorphonuclear leukocytes/fibroblasts, and reverses capillary permeability and lysosomal stabilization at the cellular level to prevent or control inflammation.

Pharmacodynamics See individual agents.

Pharmacokinetics (Adult data unless noted) See individual agents.

Dosing: Usual

Pediatric: **Asthma; maintenance treatment:** Oral inhalation:

Children 5 to 11 years: Budesonide 80 mcg/formoterol 4.5 mcg (Symbicort 80/4.5): 2 inhalations twice daily. Do not exceed 4 inhalations/day (Morice, 2008; NAEPP, 2007)

Children and Adolescents ≥12 years not controlled on low-medium dose inhaled corticosteroids: Budesonide 80 mcg/formoterol 4.5 mcg (Symbicort 80/4.5): 2 inhalations twice daily. Do not exceed 4 inhalations/day. In patients not adequately controlled following 2 weeks of therapy, consider the higher dose combination.

Children and Adolescents ≥12 years not controlled on medium-high dose inhaled corticosteroids: Budesonide 160 mcg/formoterol 4.5 mcg (Symbicort 160/4.5): 2 inhalations twice daily. Do not exceed 4 inhalations/day.

Adult:

Asthma: Oral inhalation: Symbicort 80/4.5, Symbicort 160/4.5: 2 inhalations twice daily. Do not exceed 4 inhalations/day. Recommended starting dose combination is determined according to asthma severity. In patients not adequately controlled on the lower combination dose following 1 to 2 weeks of therapy, consider the higher dose combination.

COPD: Oral inhalation: Symbicort 160/4.5: 2 inhalations twice daily. Do not exceed 4 inhalations/day.

Administration Prior to first use, inhaler must be primed by releasing 2 test sprays into the air (away from the face); shake well for 5 seconds before each use. Inhaler must be reprimed if inhaler has not been used for >7 days or has been dropped. Discard after labeled number of inhalations has been used or within 3 months after foil wrap has been removed; do not use immerse in water or use "float test" to determine number of inhalations left.

Monitoring Parameters Pulmonary function tests, vital signs, CNS stimulation, serum glucose, serum potassium; check mucous membranes for signs of fungal infection; monitor growth in pediatric patients

Dosage Forms Excipient information presented when available (limited, particularly for generics); consult specific product labeling.

Aerosol for oral inhalation:

Symbicort 80/4.5: Budesonide 80 mcg and formoterol fumarate dihydrate 4.5 mcg per actuation (6.9 g) [60 metered inhalations]; budesonide 80 mcg and formoterol fumarate dihydrate 4.5 mcg per actuation (10.2 g) [120 metered inhalations]

Symbicort 160/4.5: Budesonide 160 mcg and formoterol fumarate dihydrate 4.5 mcg per actuation (6 g) [60 metered inhalations]; budesonide 160 mcg and formoterol fumarate dihydrate 4.5 mcg per actuation (10.2 g) [120 metered inhalations]

◆ **Buffasal [OTC]** *see* Aspirin *on page* 206

◆ **Bufferin [OTC]** *see* Aspirin *on page* 206

◆ **Bufferin Extra Strength [OTC]** *see* Aspirin *on page* 206

◆ **Buffinol [OTC]** *see* Aspirin *on page* 206

Bumetanide (byoo MET a nide)

Medication Safety Issues

Sound-alike/look-alike issues:

Bumetanide may be confused with Buminate

Bumex may be confused with Brevibloc, Buprenex

International issues:

Bumex [U.S.] may be confused with Permax brand name for pergolide [multiple international markets]

Brand Names: Canada Burinex

Therapeutic Category Antihypertensive Agent; Diuretic, Loop

Generic Availability (US) Yes

Use Management of edema secondary to heart failure or hepatic or renal disease, including nephrotic syndrome (FDA approved in adults); has also been used to reverse oliguria in preterm neonates and for the treatment of hypertension alone or in combination with other antihypertensive agents

Pregnancy Risk Factor C

Pregnancy Considerations Adverse events have been observed in some animal reproduction studies.

Breast-Feeding Considerations It is not known if bumetanide is excreted in breast milk. Breast-feeding is not recommended by the manufacturer. Diuretics have the potential to decrease milk volume and suppress lactation.

Contraindications Hypersensitivity to bumetanide or any component of the formulation; anuria; patients with hepatic coma or in states of severe electrolyte depletion until the condition improves or is corrected

Warnings/Precautions [U.S. Boxed Warning]: Excessive amounts can lead to profound diuresis with fluid and electrolyte loss; close medical supervision and dose evaluation are required. Potassium supplementation and/or use of potassium-sparing diuretics may be necessary to prevent hypokalemia. In contrast to thiazide diuretics, a loop diuretic can also lower serum calcium concentrations. Electrolyte disturbances can predispose a patient to serious cardiac arrhythmias. In cirrhosis, initiate bumetanide therapy with conservative dosing and close monitoring of electrolytes; avoid sudden changes in fluid and electrolyte balance and acid/base status which may lead to hepatic encephalopathy. *In vitro* studies using pooled sera from critically-ill neonates have shown bumetanide to be a potent displacer of bilirubin; avoid use in neonates at risk for kernicterus. Coadministration of antihypertensives may increase the risk of hypotension.

Monitor fluid status and renal function in an attempt to prevent oliguria, azotemia, and reversible increases in BUN and creatinine; close medical supervision of aggressive diuresis required. Larger doses may be necessary in patients with impaired renal function to obtain the same therapeutic response (Brater, 1998). Diuretic resistance may occur in some patients, despite higher doses of loop diuretic treatment, and can usually be overcome by intravenous administration, the use of two diuretics together (eg, furosemide and chlorothiazide), or the use of a diuretic with a positive inotropic agent. When such combinations are used, serum electrolytes need to be monitored even more closely (ACC/AHA [Yancy, 2013]; Cody, 1994; HFSA, 2010). Bumetanide-induced ototoxicity (usually transient) may occur with rapid IV administration, renal impairment, excessive doses, and concurrent use of other ototoxins (eg, aminoglycosides). Asymptomatic hyperuricemia has been reported with use. If given the morning of surgery, bumetanide may render the patient volume depleted and blood pressure may be labile during general anesthesia.

Benzyl alcohol and derivatives: Some dosage forms may contain benzyl alcohol; large amounts of benzyl alcohol (≥99 mg/kg/day) have been associated with a potentially fatal toxicity ("gasping syndrome") in neonates; the "gasping syndrome" consists of metabolic acidosis, respiratory distress, gasping respirations, CNS dysfunction (including convulsions, intracranial hemorrhage), hypotension and cardiovascular collapse (AAP, 1997; CDC, 1982); some data suggests that benzoate displaces bilirubin from protein binding sites (Ahlfors, 2001); avoid or use dosage forms containing benzyl alcohol with caution in neonates. See manufacturer's labeling.

Sulfonamide ("sulfa") allergy: The FDA-approved product labeling for many medications containing a sulfonamide chemical group includes a broad contraindication in patients with a prior allergic reaction to sulfonamides. There is a potential for cross-reactivity between members of a specific class (eg, two antibiotic sulfonamides). However, concerns for cross-reactivity have previously extended to all compounds containing the sulfonamide structure (SO_2NH_2). An expanded understanding of allergic mechanisms indicates cross-reactivity between antibiotic sulfonamides and nonantibiotic sulfonamides may not occur or at the very least this potential is extremely low (Brackett 2004; Johnson 2005; Slatore 2004; Tornero 2004). In particular, mechanisms of cross-reaction due to antibody production (anaphylaxis) are unlikely to occur with nonantibiotic sulfonamides. T-cell-mediated (type IV) reactions (eg, maculopapular rash) are less well understood and it is not possible to completely exclude this potential based on current insights. In cases where prior reactions were severe (Stevens-Johnson syndrome/TEN), some clinicians choose to avoid exposure to these classes.

Adverse Reactions

Central nervous system: Dizziness

Endocrine & metabolic: abnormal serum calcium, abnormal lactate dehydrogenase, hyponatremia, hyperglycemia, phosphorus change, variations in bicarbonate

Genitourinary: Azotemia

Neuromuscular & skeletal: Muscle cramps

Renal: Increased serum creatinine

Respiratory: Variations in CO_2 content

Rare but important or life-threatening: Abdominal pain, abnormal alkaline phosphatase, abnormal bilirubin levels, abnormal hematocrit, abnormal hemoglobin level, abnormal transaminase, arthritic pain, asterixis, auditory impairment, blood cholesterol abnormal, brain disease (in patients with preexisting liver disease), change in creatinine clearance, change in prothrombin time, change in WBC count, chest pain, dehydration, diaphoresis, diarrhea, dyspepsia, ECG changes, erectile dysfunction, fatigue, glycosuria, headache, hyperventilation, hypotension, musculoskeletal pain, nausea, nipple tenderness, orthostatic hypotension, otalgia, ototoxicity, premature ejaculation, proteinuria, pruritus, renal failure, skin rash, Stevens-Johnson syndrome, thrombocytopenia, toxic epidermal necrolysis, urticaria, vertigo, vomiting, weakness, xerostomia

Drug Interactions

Metabolism/Transport Effects None known.

Avoid Concomitant Use

Avoid concomitant use of Bumetanide with any of the following: Mecamylamine

Increased Effect/Toxicity

Bumetanide may increase the levels/effects of: ACE Inhibitors; Allopurinol; Amifostine; Aminoglycosides; Antihypertensives; Cardiac Glycosides; CISplatin; Dofetilide; DULoxetine; Foscarnet; Hypotensive Agents; Ivabradine; Levodopa; Lithium; Mecamylamine; Methotrexate; Neuromuscular-Blocking Agents; Obinutuzumab; RisperiDONE; RiTUXimab; Salicylates; Sodium Phosphates; Topiramate

The levels/effects of Bumetanide may be increased by: Alfuzosin; Analgesics (Opioid); Barbiturates; Beta2-Agonists; Brimonidine (Topical); Canagliflozin; Corticosteroids (Orally Inhaled); Corticosteroids (Systemic); CycloSPORINE (Systemic); Diazoxide; Herbs (Hypotensive Properties); Licorice; MAO Inhibitors; Methotrexate; Nicorandil; Pentoxifylline; Phosphodiesterase 5 Inhibitors; Probenecid; Prostacyclin Analogues

Decreased Effect

Bumetanide may decrease the levels/effects of: Antidiabetic Agents; Lithium; Neuromuscular-Blocking Agents

The levels/effects of Bumetanide may be decreased by: Bile Acid Sequestrants; Fosphenytoin; Herbs (Hypertensive Properties); Methotrexate; Methylphenidate; Nonsteroidal Anti-Inflammatory Agents; Phenytoin; Probenecid; Salicylates; Yohimbine

Food Interactions Bumetanide serum levels may be decreased if taken with food. Management: It has been recommended that bumetanide be administered without food (Bard, 2004).

Storage/Stability

IV: Store vials at 15°C to 30°C (59°F to 86°F). Infusion solutions should be used within 24 hours after preparation. Light sensitive; discoloration may occur when exposed to light.

Tablet: Store at 15°C to 30°C (59°F to 86°F); protect from light.

Mechanism of Action Inhibits reabsorption of sodium and chloride in the ascending loop of Henle and proximal renal tubule, interfering with the chloride-binding cotransport system, thus causing increased excretion of water, sodium, chloride, magnesium, phosphate, and calcium; it does not appear to act on the distal tubule

Pharmacodynamics

Onset of action:
- Oral, IM: Within 30-60 minutes
- IV: Within a few minutes

Maximum effect:
- Oral, IM: 1-2 hours
- IV: 15-30 minutes

Duration:
- Oral: 4-6 hours
- IV: 2-3 hours

Pharmacokinetics (Adult data unless noted)

Distribution: V_d: Neonates and infants: 0.26-0.39 L/kg

Protein binding: 95%
- Neonates: 97%

Metabolism: Partial metabolism occurs in the liver

Bioavailability: 59% to 89% (median: 80%)

Half-life:
- Premature and full term neonates: 6 hours (range up to 15 hours)
- Infants <2 months: 2.5 hours
- Infants 2-6 months: 1.5 hours
- Adults: 1-1.5 hours

Time to peak serum concentration: 0.5-2 hours

Elimination: Unchanged drug excreted in urine (45%); biliary/fecal (2%)

Clearance:
- Preterm and full term neonates: 0.2-1.1 mL/minute/kg
- Infants <2 months: 2.17 mL/minute/kg
- Infants 2-6 months: 3.8 mL/minute/kg
- Adults: 2.9 ± 0.2 mL/minute/kg

Dosing: Neonatal Oral, IM, IV: **Note:** Doses in the higher end of the range may be required for patients with heart failure:

Preterm neonates: 0.01-0.05 mg/kg/dose every 24-48 hours (Lopez-Samplas, 1997; Shankaran, 1995); a retrospective trial reported a mean dose of 0.03 mg/kg/dose every 12-24 hours for oliguric acute renal failure (n=35; PMA: 24-36 weeks) (maximum reported dose: 0.06 mg/kg/dose) (Oliveros, 2011)

Term neonates: 0.01-0.05 mg/kg/dose every 12-24 hours (Sullivan, 1996; Ward, 1977)

Dosing: Usual Note: Dose equivalency for adult patients with normal renal function (approximate): Bumetanide 1 mg = furosemide 40 mg = torsemide 20 mg = ethacrynic acid 50 mg

Infants and Children: Oral, IM, IV: 0.015-0.1 mg/kg/dose every 6-24 hours (maximum dose: 10 mg/day) (Kliegman, 2007); a prospective, open-label dose-range study in infants (mean age: 2 months; range: 0-6 months) reported a maximal diuretic response at doses 0.035-0.04 mg/kg/dose every 6-8 hours, and no additional clinical benefit (ie, urine output) at doses >0.05 mg/kg/dose (Sullivan, 1996)

Adults:

Edema:
- Oral: 0.5-2 mg/dose 1-2 times/day; if diuretic response to initial dose is not adequate, may repeat in 4-5 hours for up to 2 doses (maximum daily dose: 10 mg/**day**)
- IM, IV: 0.5-1 mg/dose; may repeat in 2-3 hours for up to 2 doses if needed (maximum daily dose: 10 mg/**day**)

Hypertension: Oral: 0.5 mg daily (maximum daily dose: 5 mg/**day**); usual dosage range (JNC 7): 0.5-2 mg divided twice daily (Chobanian, 2003)

Preparation for Administration Parenteral: Intermittent IV infusion: May be diluted in D_5W, LR, or NS (Rudy 1991)

Administration

Oral: Administer with food to decrease GI irritation

Parenteral:
- IV: Administer undiluted by direct IV injection over 1 to 2 minutes
- Intermittent IV infusion: Further dilute and administer over 5 minutes (Rudy 1991)

Monitoring Parameters Blood pressure, serum electrolytes, renal function, urine output

Additional Information Patients with impaired hepatic function must be monitored carefully, often requiring reduced doses; larger doses may be necessary in patients with impaired renal function to obtain the same therapeutic response

Dosage Forms Excipient information presented when available (limited, particularly for generics); consult specific product labeling.

Solution, Injection:
- Generic: 0.25 mg/mL (2 mL, 4 mL, 10 mL)

Tablet, Oral:
- Generic: 0.5 mg, 1 mg, 2 mg

◆ **Bumex** *see* Bumetanide *on page 314*

◆ **Buminate** *see* Albumin *on page 79*

◆ **Buminate-5% (Can)** *see* Albumin *on page 79*

◆ **Buminate-25% (Can)** *see* Albumin *on page 79*

◆ **Bunavail** *see* Buprenorphine and Naloxone *on page 322*

◆ **Buphenyl** *see* Sodium Phenylbutyrate *on page 1948*

Bupivacaine (byoo PIV a kane)

Medication Safety Issues

Sound-alike/look-alike issues:

Bupivacaine may be confused with mepivacaine, ropivacaine

Marcaine® may be confused with Narcan®

High alert medication:

The Institute for Safe Medication Practices (ISMP) includes this medication (epidural administration) among its list of drug classes which have a heightened risk of causing significant patient harm when used in error.

Brand Names: US Bupivacaine Spinal; Marcaine; Marcaine Preservative Free; Marcaine Spinal; Sensorcaine; Sensorcaine-MPF; Sensorcaine-MPF Spinal

Brand Names: Canada Marcaine®; Sensorcaine®

Therapeutic Category Local Anesthetic, Injectable

Generic Availability (US) Yes

Use Local anesthetic (injectable) for peripheral nerve block, infiltration, sympathetic block, caudal or epidural block, retrobulbar block

Pregnancy Risk Factor C

Pregnancy Considerations Adverse events were observed in animal reproduction studies. Bupivacaine crosses the placenta. Bupivacaine is approved for use at term in obstetrical anesthesia or analgesia. **[U.S. Boxed Warning]: The 0.75% is not recommended for obstetrical anesthesia.** Bupivacaine 0.75% solutions have been associated with cardiac arrest following epidural anesthesia in obstetrical patients and use of this concentration is not recommended for this purpose. Use in obstetrical paracervical block anesthesia is contraindicated.

Breast-Feeding Considerations Bupivacaine is excreted in breast milk. Due to the potential for serious adverse reactions in the nursing infant, a decision should be made whether to discontinue nursing or to discontinue the drug, taking into account the importance of treatment to the mother.

Contraindications Hypersensitivity to bupivacaine hydrochloride, amide-type local anesthetics, or any component of the formulation; obstetrical paracervical block anesthesia

Note: Use as intravenous regional anesthesia (Bier block) is considered contraindicated per accepted clinical practice.

Warnings/Precautions Do not use solutions containing preservatives for caudal or epidural block. Use with caution in patients with hepatic impairment. Local anesthetics have been associated with rare occurrences of sudden respiratory arrest; convulsions due to systemic toxicity leading to cardiac arrest have also been reported, presumably following unintentional intravascular injection. Intravenous regional anesthesia (Bier block) is **not** recommended; cardiac arrest and death have occurred with this method of administration. **[U.S. Boxed Warning]: The 0.75% concentration is not recommended for obstetrical epidural anesthesia; cardiac arrest with difficult resuscitation or death has occurred.** A test dose is recommended prior to epidural administration (prior to initial dose) and all reinforcing doses with continuous catheter technique. Use caution with cardiovascular dysfunction including patients with hypotension or heart block. Bupivacaine-containing products have been associated with rare occurrences of arrhythmias, cardiac arrest, and death. Use caution in debilitated, elderly, or acutely ill patients; dose reduction may be required. Resuscitative equipment, oxygen, and other resuscitative drugs should be available for immediate use. Continuous intra-articular infusion of local anesthetics after arthroscopic or other surgical procedures is **not** an approved use; chondrolysis (primarily shoulder joint) has occurred following infusion, with some requiring arthroplasty or shoulder replacement.

Warnings: Additional Pediatric Considerations Infants may be at greater risk for bupivacaine toxicity because α_1-acid-glycoprotein, the major serum protein to which bupivacaine is bound, is lower in infants compared with older children; use epidural infusions with caution in infants and monitor closely; increased toxicity may be minimized by limiting the duration of infusion to ≤48 hours (McCloskey, 1992).

Adverse Reactions Note: Most effects are dose related, and are often due to accelerated absorption from the injection site, unintentional intravascular injection, or slow metabolic degradation. The development of any central nervous system symptoms may be an early indication of more significant toxicity (seizure).

Cardiovascular: Bradycardia, cardiac arrest, heart block, hypotension, palpitations, ventricular arrhythmia
Central nervous system: Anxiety, dizziness, restlessness
Gastrointestinal: Nausea, vomiting
Hypersensitivity: Anaphylactoid reaction, hypersensitivity reaction (urticaria, pruritus, angioedema)
Neuromuscular & skeletal: Chondrolysis (continuous intra-articular administration), weakness
Ophthalmic: Blurred vision, miosis
Otic: Tinnitus
Respiratory: Apnea, hypoventilation (usually associated with unintentional subarachnoid injection during high spinal anesthesia)
Rare but important or life-threatening: Seizure; usually associated with unintentional subarachnoid injection during high spinal anesthesia: cranial nerve palsy, fecal incontinence, headache, loss of anal sphincter control, loss of perineal sensation, paralysis, paresthesia, persistent anesthesia, septic meningitis, sexual disorder (loss of function), urinary incontinence

Drug Interactions

Metabolism/Transport Effects Substrate of CYP1A2 (minor), CYP2C19 (minor), CYP2D6 (minor), CYP3A4 (minor); **Note:** Assignment of Major/Minor substrate status based on clinically relevant drug interaction potential

Avoid Concomitant Use There are no known interactions where it is recommended to avoid concomitant use.

Increased Effect/Toxicity

The levels/effects of Bupivacaine may be increased by: Beta-Blockers; Hyaluronidase

Decreased Effect

Bupivacaine may decrease the levels/effects of: Technetium Tc 99m Tilmanocept

Storage/Stability Store at controlled room temperature of 20°C to 25°C (68°F to 77°F).

Mechanism of Action Blocks both the initiation and conduction of nerve impulses by decreasing the neuronal membrane's permeability to sodium ions, which results in inhibition of depolarization with resultant blockade of conduction

Pharmacodynamics

Onset of anesthetic action: Dependent on total dose, concentration, and route administered, but generally occurs within 4-10 minutes
Duration: 1.5-8.5 hours (depending upon route of administration)

Pharmacokinetics (Adult data unless noted)

Distribution: V_d:
- Infants: 3.9 ± 2 L/kg
- Children: 2.7 ± 0.2 L/kg

Protein binding: 84% to 95%
Metabolism: In the liver
Half-life (age-dependent):
- Neonates: 8.1 hours
- Adults: 2.7 hours

Time to peak serum concentration: Caudal, epidural, or peripheral nerve block: 30-45 minutes
Elimination: Small amounts (~6%) excreted in urine unchanged
- Clearance:
  - Infants: 7.1 ± 3.2 mL/kg/minute
  - Children: 10 ± 0.7 mL/kg/minute

Dosing: Neonatal Dose varies with procedure, depth of anesthesia, vascularity of tissues, duration of anesthesia, and condition of patient. Continuous epidural (caudal or lumbar) infusion: Limited data available (Berde, 1992):
Loading dose: 2-2.5 mg/kg (0.8-1 mL/kg of 0.25% bupivacaine)
Infusion dose:
- Dose: 0.2-0.25 mg/kg/**hour**
- Dose (using 0.25% solution): 0.08-0.1 mL/kg/**hour**
- Dose (using 0.125% solution): 0.16-0.2 mL/kg/**hour**
- Dose (using 0.05% solution): 0.4-0.5 mL/kg/**hour**

Dosing: Usual Dose varies with procedure, depth of anesthesia, vascularity of tissues, duration of anesthesia, and condition of patient.

Caudal block (with or without epinephrine, **preservative free**):
- Children: 1-3.7 mg/kg
- Adults: 15-30 mL of 0.25% or 0.5%

Epidural block, **preservative free** (other than caudal block):
Children: 1.25 mg/kg/dose
Adults: 10-20 mL of 0.25%, 0.5%, or 0.75%
Peripheral nerve block: 5 mL dose of 0.25% or 0.5% (12.5-25 mg); maximum dose: 400 mg/day
Sympathetic nerve block: 20-50 mL of 0.25% (no epinephrine) solution
Continuous epidural (caudal or lumbar) infusion: Limited information in infants and children:
Loading dose: 2-2.5 mg/kg (0.8-1 mL/kg of 0.25% bupivacaine)
Infusion dose: See table

Bupivacaine Infusion Dose

Age	Dose	Dose (using 0.25% solution)	Dose (using 0.125% solution)	Dose (using 0.05% solution)
Infants ≤4 mo	0.2-0.25 mg/kg/h	0.08-0.1 mL/kg/h	0.16-0.2 mL/kg/h	0.4-0.5 mL/kg/h
Infants >4 mo and children	0.4-0.5 mg/kg/h	0.16-0.2 mL/kg/h	0.32-0.4 mL/kg/h	0.8-1 mL/kg/h
Adults	5-20 mg/h	2-8 mL/h	4-16 mL/h	10-40 mL/h

Administration Solutions containing preservatives should not be used for epidural or caudal blocks; for epidural infusion, may use undiluted or diluted with preservative free NS

Reference Range Toxicity: 2-4 mcg/mL (however, some experts have suggested that the rate of rise of the serum level is more predictive of toxicity than the actual value; Scott, 1975)

Additional Information For epidural infusion, lower dosages of bupivacaine may be effective when used in combination with opioid analgesics

Dosage Forms Excipient information presented when available (limited, particularly for generics); consult specific product labeling.
Solution, Injection, as hydrochloride:
Marcaine: 0.25% (50 mL); 0.5% (50 mL) [contains methylparaben]
Sensorcaine: 0.25% (50 mL); 0.5% (50 mL) [contains methylparaben]
Sensorcaine-MPF: 0.25% (10 mL, 30 mL); 0.5% (10 mL, 30 mL); 0.75% (10 mL, 30 mL) [methylparaben free]
Generic: 0.25% (10 mL, 30 mL, 50 mL); 0.5% (10 mL, 30 mL, 50 mL); 0.75% (10 mL, 30 mL)
Solution, Injection, as hydrochloride [preservative free]:
Marcaine: 0.75% (10 mL, 30 mL)
Marcaine Preservative Free: 0.25% (10 mL, 30 mL); 0.5% (10 mL, 30 mL)
Generic: 0.25% (10 mL, 20 mL, 30 mL); 0.5% (10 mL, 20 mL, 30 mL); 0.75% (10 mL, 20 mL, 30 mL)
Solution, Intrathecal, as hydrochloride [preservative free]:
Bupivacaine Spinal: 0.75% [7.5 mg/mL] (2 mL)
Marcaine Spinal: 0.75% [7.5 mg/mL] (2 mL)
Sensorcaine-MPF Spinal: 0.75% [7.5 mg/mL] (2 mL)

◆ **Bupivacaine Hydrochloride** *see* Bupivacaine *on page 316*

◆ **Bupivacaine Spinal** *see* Bupivacaine *on page 316*

◆ **Buprenex** *see* Buprenorphine *on page 318*

Buprenorphine (byoo pre NOR feen)

Medication Safety Issues
Sound-alike/look-alike issues:
Buprenex may be confused with Brevibloc, Bumex
High alert medication:
The Institute for Safe Medication Practices (ISMP) includes this medication among its list of drug classes which have a heightened risk of causing significant patient harm when used in error.

Related Information
Patient Information for Disposal of Unused Medications *on page 2453*

Brand Names: US Buprenex; Butrans

Brand Names: Canada Butrans

Therapeutic Category Analgesic, Narcotic; Opioid Partial Agonist

Generic Availability (US) May be product dependent

Use
Oral: Sublingual tablet: Treatment of opioid dependence (FDA approved in ages ≥16 years and adults)
Parenteral: Management of moderate to severe pain (FDA approved in ages ≥2 years and adults)
Transdermal: Management of moderate to severe chronic pain in patients requiring an around-the-clock opioid analgesic for an extended period of time (FDA approved in adults)

Prescribing and Access Restrictions Prescribing of tablets for opioid dependence is limited to physicians who have met the qualification criteria and have received a DEA number specific to prescribing this product. Tablets will be available through pharmacies and wholesalers which normally provide controlled substances.

Medication Guide Available Yes

Pregnancy Risk Factor C

Pregnancy Considerations Adverse effects have been observed in some animal reproduction studies. Buprenorphine crosses the placenta; buprenorphine and norbuprenorphine can be detected in newborn serum, urine, and meconium following in utero exposure (CSAT, 2004). **[U.S. Boxed Warning]: Prolonged use can result in neonatal opioid withdrawal syndrome. If not recognized and treated, this may be life-threatening and require management according to protocols developed by neonatology experts.** Following chronic opioid therapy in pregnancy, adverse events in the newborn (including withdrawal) may occur; monitoring of the neonate is recommended. The minimum effective dose should be used if opioids are needed (Chou, 2009). The onset of withdrawal in infants of women receiving buprenorphine during pregnancy ranged from day 1 to day 8 of life, most occurring on day 1. Symptoms of withdrawal may include agitation, apnea, bradycardia, convulsions, hypertonia, myoclonus, respiratory depression, and tremor.

Buprenorphine is currently considered an alternate treatment for pregnant women who need therapy for opioid addiction (CSAT, 2004; Dow, 2012); however, use in pregnancy for this purpose is increasing (ACOG, 2012; Soyka, 2013). Buprenorphine should not be used to treat pain during labor. Women receiving buprenorphine for the treatment of addiction should be maintained on their daily dose of buprenorphine in addition to receiving the same pain management options during labor and delivery as opioid-naive women; maintenance doses of buprenorphine will not provide adequate pain relief. Narcotic agonist-antagonists should be avoided for the treatment of labor pain in women maintained on buprenorphine due to the risk of precipitating acute withdrawal. In addition, buprenorphine should not be given to women in labor taking methadone (ACOG, 2012).

Amenorrhea may develop secondary to substance abuse; pregnancy may occur following the initiation of buprenorphine maintenance treatment. Contraception counseling is recommended to prevent unplanned pregnancies (Dow, 2012). Long-term opioid use may cause secondary hypogonadism, which may lead to sexual dysfunction or infertility (Brennan, 2013).

Breast-Feeding Considerations Buprenorphine is excreted in breast milk. Breast-feeding is not recommended by the manufacturer. Nursing infants exposed to large doses of opioids should be monitored for apnea and sedation (Montgomery, 2012).

When buprenorphine is used to treat opioid addiction in nursing women, most guidelines do not contraindicate breast-feeding as long as the infant is tolerant to the dose and other contraindications do not exist; caution should be used when nursing infants not previously exposed (ACOG, 2012; CSAT, 2004; Montgomery, 2012). If additional illicit substances are being abused, women treated with buprenorphine should pump and discard breast milk until sobriety is established (ACOG, 2012; Dow, 2012).

Contraindications Hypersensitivity to buprenorphine or any component of the formulation

Transdermal patch: Additional contraindications: Significant respiratory depression; acute or severe asthma; known or suspected paralytic ileus

Documentation of allergenic cross-reactivity for morphine and related drugs in this class is limited. However, because of similarities in chemical structure and/or pharmacologic actions, the possibility of cross-sensitivity cannot be ruled out with certainty.

Warnings/Precautions An opioid-containing analgesic regimen should be tailored to each patient's needs and based upon the type of pain being treated (acute versus chronic), the route of administration, degree of tolerance for opioids (naive versus chronic user), age, weight, and medical condition. The optimal analgesic dose varies widely among patients. Doses should be titrated to pain relief/prevention.

May cause CNS depression, which may impair physical or mental abilities; patients must be cautioned about performing tasks which require mental alertness (eg, operating machinery or driving). Elderly may be more sensitive to CNS depressant and constipating effects. May cause respiratory depression - use caution in patients with respiratory disease or preexisting respiratory depression. Hypersensitivity reactions, including bronchospasm, angioneurotic edema, and anaphylactic shock, have also been reported. Potential for drug dependency exists, abrupt cessation may precipitate withdrawal. Use caution in elderly, debilitated, cachectic, pediatric patients, depression or suicidal tendencies. Tolerance, psychological and physical dependence may occur with prolonged use. Partial antagonist activity may precipitate acute opioid withdrawal in opioid-dependent individuals.

Hepatitis has been reported with buprenorphine use; hepatic events ranged from transient, asymptomatic transaminase elevations to hepatic failure; in many cases, patients had preexisting hepatic dysfunction. Monitor liver function tests in patients at increased risk for hepatotoxicity (eg, history of alcohol abuse, preexisting hepatic dysfunction, IV drug abusers) prior to and during therapy. Use with caution in patients with moderate hepatic impairment; dosage adjustment recommended in severe hepatic impairment.

Use with caution in patients with pulmonary or renal function impairment. Also use caution in patients with head injury or increased ICP, biliary tract dysfunction, pancreatitis, patients with history of hyperthyroidism, morbid obesity, adrenal insufficiency, prostatic hyperplasia, urinary stricture, toxic psychosis, pancreatitis, alcoholism, delirium tremens, or kyphoscoliosis. Avoid use in patients with CNS depression or coma as these patients are susceptible to intracranial effects of CO_2 retention. May cause severe hypotension, including orthostatic hypotension and syncope; use with caution in patients with hypovolemia, cardiovascular disease (including acute MI), or drugs which may exaggerate hypotensive effects (including phenothiazines or general anesthetics). May obscure diagnosis or clinical course of patients with acute abdominal conditions. Use with caution in patients with a history of ileus or bowel obstruction; use of transdermal patch is contraindicated in patients with known or suspected paralytic ileus. Opioid therapy may lower seizure threshold; use caution in patients with a history of seizure disorders. Potentially significant drug-drug interactions may exist, requiring dose or frequency adjustment, additional monitoring, and/or selection of alternative therapy.

Transdermal patch: Indicated for the management of pain severe enough to require daily, around the clock, long-term opioid treatment; should not be used for as-needed pain relief. **[U.S. Boxed Warning]: May cause potentially life-threatening respiratory depression; monitor for respiratory depression, especially during initiation or dose escalation. Misuse or abuse by chewing, swallowing, snorting, or injecting buprenorphine extracted from the transdermal system will result in the uncontrolled delivery of buprenorphine and pose a significant risk of overdose and death. Accidental exposure to even one dose, especially in children, can result in a fatal overdose.** Do not exceed one 20 **mcg**/hour transdermal patch due to the risk of QTc-interval prolongation. Avoid using in patients with a personal or family history of long QT syndrome or in patients with predisposing factors increasing the risk of QT abnormalities (eg, concurrent medications such as antiarrhythmics, hypokalemia, unstable heart failure, unstable atrial fibrillation). **[U.S. Boxed Warning]: Abuse, misuse, and addiction, which can lead to overdose and death, may occur.** Risk of opioid abuse is increased in patients with a history or family history of alcohol or drug abuse or mental illness (eg, major depression). Assess each patient's risk before prescribing, and monitor all patients for the development of these behaviors or conditions. The misuse of transdermal buprenorphine by placing it in the mouth, chewing it, swallowing it, or using it in ways other than indicated may cause choking, overdose, and death. To properly dispose of Butrans patch, fold it over on itself and flush down the toilet; alternatively, seal the used patch in the provided Patch-Disposal Unit and dispose of in the trash. Avoid exposure of application site and surrounding area to direct external heat sources (eg, heating pads, electric blankets, heating lamps, saunas, hot water, or direct sunlight). Buprenorphine release from the patch is temperature-dependent and may result in overdose. Patients who experience fever or increase in core temperature should be monitored closely and adjust dose if signs or respiratory depression or central nervous system depression occur. Application site reactions, including rare cases of severe reactions (eg, vesicles, discharge, "burns"), have been observed with use; onset varies from days to months after initiation; patients should be instructed to report severe reactions promptly. Therapy with the transdermal patch is not appropriate for use in the management of addictions. **[U.S. Boxed Warning]: Prolonged use during pregnancy may result in neonatal abstinence syndrome (NAS) in neonates and infants. If not recognized and treated, this may be life-threatening and require management according to protocols developed by neonatology experts.** Monitor neonate closely. Signs and symptoms include irritability, hyperactivity and abnormal sleep pattern, high pitched cry, tremor, vomiting, diarrhea and failure to gain weight. Onset, duration and severity depend on the drug used, duration of use, maternal dose, and rate of drug elimination by the newborn.

Reversal of partial opioid agonists or mixed opioid agonist/antagonists (eg, buprenorphine, pentazocine) may be incomplete and large doses of naloxone may be required. Concurrent use of agonist/antagonist analgesics may precipitate withdrawal symptoms and/or reduced analgesic efficacy in patients following prolonged therapy with mu opioid agonists. Abrupt discontinuation following prolonged use may also lead to withdrawal symptoms and is not recommended; taper dose gradually when discontinuing.

Sublingual tablets, which are used for induction treatment of opioid dependence, should not be started until effects of withdrawal are evident.

Adverse Reactions

Injection:

Cardiovascular: Hypotension

Central nervous system: Dizziness, headache, sedation

Dermatologic: Diaphoresis

Gastrointestinal: Nausea, vomiting

Ophthalmic: Miosis

Respiratory: Respiratory depression

Rare but important or life-threatening: Amblyopia, anaphylactic shock, apnea, bradycardia, conjunctivitis, coma, cyanosis, depersonalization, depression, diplopia, euphoria, hallucination, hypersensitivity, hypertension, hypogonadism (Brennan, 2013; Debono, 2011), injection site reaction, psychosis, seizure, slurred speech, tachycardia, urinary retention, Wenckebach period on ECG

Tablet:

Central nervous system: Anxiety, chills, depression, dizziness, drowsiness, headache, insomnia, nervousness, pain, withdrawal syndrome

Dermatologic: Diaphoresis

Gastrointestinal: Abdominal pain, constipation, diarrhea, dyspepsia, nausea, vomiting

Infection: Abscess, infection

Neuromuscular & skeletal: Back pain, weakness

Ophthalmic: Lacrimation

Respiratory: Cough, flu-like symptoms, pharyngitis, rhinitis

Miscellaneous: Fever

Rare but important or life-threatening: Anaphylactic shock, angioedema, hepatic encephalopathy, hepatic failure, hepatic necrosis, hepatitis (including cytolytic), hepatorenal syndrome, hypersensitivity, hypogonadism (Brennan, 2013; Debono, 2011), increased serum transaminases

Transdermal patch:

Cardiovascular: Chest pain, hypertension, peripheral edema

Central nervous system: Anxiety, depression, dizziness, drowsiness, fatigue, headache, hypoesthesia, insomnia, migraine, paresthesia

Dermatologic: Diaphoresis, pruritus, rash

Gastrointestinal: Abdominal distress, anorexia, constipation, diarrhea, dyspepsia, nausea, upper abdominal pain, vomiting, xerostomia

Genitourinary: Urinary tract infection

Local: Application site erythema, application site irritation, application site rash, local pruritus

Neuromuscular & skeletal: Arthralgia, back pain, joint swelling, limb pain, muscle spasm, musculoskeletal pain, myalgia, neck pain, tremor, weakness

Respiratory: Bronchitis, cough, dyspnea, flu-like symptoms, nasopharyngitis, pharyngolaryngeal pain, sinusitis, upper respiratory tract infection

Miscellaneous: Fever

Rare but important or life-threatening: Angina pectoris, angioedema, application site dermatitis, bradycardia, contact dermatitis, diverticulitis, exacerbation of asthma, hallucination, hyperventilation, hypersensitivity reaction, hypogonadism (Brennan, 2013; Debono, 2011), hypotension, hypoventilation, increased serum ALT, intestinal obstruction, loss of consciousness, memory impairment, mental deficiency, mental status changes, miosis (dose-related), orthostatic hypotension, psychosis, respiratory depression, respiratory distress, respiratory failure, syncope, tachycardia, urinary incontinence, urinary retention, vasodilatation, visual disturbance, withdrawal syndrome

Drug Interactions

Metabolism/Transport Effects **Substrate** of CYP3A4 (major); **Note:** Assignment of Major/Minor substrate status based on clinically relevant drug interaction potential; **Inhibits** CYP1A2 (weak), CYP2A6 (weak), CYP2C19 (weak), CYP2D6 (weak)

Avoid Concomitant Use

Avoid concomitant use of Buprenorphine with any of the following: Analgesics (Opioid); Atazanavir; Azelastine (Nasal); Conivaptan; Eluxadoline; Fusidic Acid (Systemic); Idelalisib; MAO Inhibitors; Mixed Agonist / Antagonist Opioids; Orphenadrine; Paraldehyde; Thalidomide

Increased Effect/Toxicity

Buprenorphine may increase the levels/effects of: Alvimopan; Azelastine (Nasal); Desmopressin; Diuretics; Eluxadoline; MAO Inhibitors; Methotrimeprazine; Metyrosine; Orphenadrine; Paraldehyde; Pramipexole; ROPINIRole; Rotigotine; Selective Serotonin Reuptake Inhibitors; Suvorexant; Thalidomide; TiZANidine; Zolpidem

The levels/effects of Buprenorphine may be increased by: Alcohol (Ethyl); Amphetamines; Anticholinergic Agents; Aprepitant; Atazanavir; Boceprevir; Brimonidine (Topical); Cannabis; CNS Depressants; Cobicistat; Conivaptan; CYP3A4 Inhibitors (Moderate); CYP3A4 Inhibitors (Strong); Dasatinib; Dronabinol; Droperidol; Fosaprepitant; Fusidic Acid (Systemic); Idelalisib; Ivacaftor; Kava Kava; Luliconazole; Magnesium Sulfate; Methotrimeprazine; Mifepristone; Nabilone; Netupitant; Palbociclib; Perampanel; Rufinamide; Simeprevir; Sodium Oxybate; Stiripentol; Succinylcholine; Tetrahydrocannabinol

Decreased Effect

Buprenorphine may decrease the levels/effects of: Analgesics (Opioid); Atazanavir; Pegvisomant

The levels/effects of Buprenorphine may be decreased by: Ammonium Chloride; Boceprevir; Bosentan; CYP3A4 Inducers (Moderate); CYP3A4 Inducers (Strong); Dabrafenib; Deferasirox; Efavirenz; Etravirine; Mitotane; Mixed Agonist / Antagonist Opioids; Naltrexone; Siltuximab; St Johns Wort; Tocilizumab

Storage/Stability

Injection: Protect from excessive heat >40°C (>104°F). Protect from light.

Patch, tablet: Store at room temperature of 25°C (77°F); excursions permitted between 15°C to 30°C (59°F to 86°F).

Mechanism of Action Buprenorphine exerts its analgesic effect via high affinity binding to μ opiate receptors in the CNS; displays partial mu agonist and weak kappa antagonist activity. Due to it being a partial mu agonist, its analgesic effects plateau at higher doses and it then behaves like an antagonist.

Pharmacodynamics IM:

Onset of action: 15 minutes

Maximum effect: 1 hour

Duration: ≥6 hours

Pharmacokinetics (Adult data unless noted)

Absorption: IM, SubQ: 30% to 40%

Distribution: CSF concentrations are ~15% to 25% of plasma concentrations

V_d:

- Premature neonates (GA: 27-32 weeks): 6.2 ± 2.1 L/kg (Barrett, 1993)
- Children 4-7 years: 3.2 ± 2 L/kg (Olkkola, 1989)
- Adults: 430 L

Protein binding: 96%, primarily to alpha and beta globulin

Metabolism: Hepatic, via both N-dealkylation (to an active metabolite, norbuprenorphine) and glucuronidation; norbuprenorphine also undergoes glucuronidation; extensive first-pass effect

Bioavailability: Relative to IV administration:
- IM: 70%
- Sublingual tablet: 29%
- Transdermal patch: 15%

Half-life:
- IV:
  - Premature neonates (GA: 27-32 weeks): 20 ± 8 hours (Barrett, 1993)
  - Children 4-7 years: ~1 hour (Olkkola, 1989)
  - Adults: 2.2 hours
- Sublingual: 37 hours
- Transdermal patch (apparent half-life): ~26 hours

Time to peak serum concentration:
- Sublingual: 30 minutes to 1 hour (Kuhlman, 1996)
- Transdermal patch: Steady state achieved by day 3

Elimination: 30% of the dose is excreted in the urine (1% as unchanged drug; 9.4% as conjugated drug; 2.7% as norbuprenorphine; and 11% as conjugated norbuprenorphine) and 69% in feces (33% as unchanged drug; 5% as conjugated drug; 21% as norbuprenorphine; and 2% as conjugated norbuprenorphine)
- Clearance: Related to hepatic blood flow
  - Premature neonates (GA: 27-32 weeks): 0.23 ± 0.07 L/hour/kg (Barrett, 1993)
  - Children 4-7 years: 3.6 ± 1.1 L/hour/kg (Olkkola, 1989)
  - Adults: 0.78-1.32 L/hour/kg

Dosing: Neonatal Neonatal abstinence syndrome (NAS): Very limited data available: Full-term neonates: Sublingual solution (0.075 mg/mL): Initial: 5.3 mcg/kg/dose every 8 hours; dosing based on birth weight; may increase dose in 25% increments based on targeted NAS scores; a rescue dose of 50% of the previous dose may be used for inadequate control between scheduled doses; once a maximum daily dose of 60 mcg/kg/day reached, phenobarbital therapy may be added. After 3 days of dose stabilization, buprenorphine may be weaned based on NAS scores using 10% daily dose reductions. Dosing based on an open-label comparative trial with morphine (each treatment group, n= 12); in the clinical trial, doses were increased if a single NAS score was ≥12 or NAS scale scores ≥24 total on three measures; neonates with maternal concomitant benzodiazepine or chronic alcohol abuse were excluded from the trial; results showed a significant decrease in length of NAS treatment and hospital stay compared to morphine treatment arm (Kraft, 2011). In the pilot trial, a lower initial dose of sublingual buprenorphine (4.4 mcg/kg/dose every 8 hours) was used; clinically the majority of patients had NAS symptoms controlled; no differences in outcome variables (length of treatment and hospital) were detected and pharmacokinetic analysis showed >98% of serum concentrations were less than the target concentration needed to control abstinence symptoms in adults (Kraft, 2008).

Dosing: Usual Note: Dose should be titrated to appropriate effect. Use 1/2 of the dose listed in patients with preexisting respiratory depression, decreased respiratory reserve, hypoxia, hypercapnia, significant COPD, or cor pulmonale, and in those receiving medications with CNS or respiratory depressant effects.

Children and Adolescents:

Moderate to severe pain:

Children 2-12 years: IM, slow IV injection: 2-6 **mcg**/kg every 4-6 hours; **Note:** 3 mcg/kg/dose has been most commonly studied; not all children have faster clearance rates than adults; some children may require dosing intervals of every 6-8 hours; observe clinical effects to establish the proper dosing interval

Adolescents: IM, slow IV injection: Initial: Opioid-naive: 0.3 mg every 6-8 hours as needed; initial dose may be repeated once in 30-60 minutes if clinically needed

Opioid dependence: Note: Do not start induction with buprenorphine until objective and clear signs of withdrawal are apparent (otherwise withdrawal may be precipitated). Adolescents ≥16 years: Sublingual:

Induction: Target range: 12-16 mg/day (doses during one induction study used 8 mg on day 1, followed by 16 mg on day 2; other studies accomplished induction over 3-4 days). Treatment should begin at least 4 hours after last use of heroin or short-acting opioid, preferably when first signs of withdrawal appear. Titrating dose to clinical effect should be done as rapidly as possible to prevent undue withdrawal symptoms and patient drop-out during the induction period. There is little controlled experience with induction in patients on methadone or other long-acting opioids; consult expert physician experienced with this procedure.

Maintenance: **Note:** Patients should be switched to the buprenorphine/naloxone combination product for maintenance and for unsupervised therapy; initial target dose: 12-16 mg/day; then adjust dose in 2-4 mg increments/decrements to a dose that adequately suppresses opioid withdrawal; usual range: 4-24 mg/day

Adults:

Moderate to severe pain: IM, slow IV injection: Initial: Opioid-naive: 0.3 mg every 6-8 hours as needed; initial dose may be repeated once in 30-60 minutes if clinically needed; **Note:** In adults, single doses of up to 0.6 mg administered IM may occasionally be required; usual dosage range: 0.15-0.6 mg every 4-8 hours as needed

Opioid dependence: Note: Do not start induction with buprenorphine until objective and clear signs of withdrawal are apparent (otherwise withdrawal may be precipitated). Sublingual:

Induction: Target range: 12-16 mg/day (doses during one induction study used 8 mg on day 1, followed by 16 mg on day 2; other studies accomplished induction over 3-4 days). Treatment should begin at least 4 hours after last use of heroin or short-acting opioid, preferably when first signs of withdrawal appear. Titrating dose to clinical effect should be done as rapidly as possible to prevent undue withdrawal symptoms and patient drop-out during the induction period. There is little controlled experience with induction in patients on methadone or other long-acting opioids; consult expert physician experienced with this procedure.

Maintenance: **Note:** Patients should be switched to the buprenorphine/naloxone combination product for maintenance and for unsupervised therapy; initial target dose: 12-16 mg/day; then adjust dose in 2-4 mg increments/decrements to a dose that adequately suppresses opioid withdrawal; usual range: 4-24 mg/day

Chronic pain (moderate to severe):

Transdermal patch:

Opioid-naive patients: Initial: 5 **mcg**/hour applied once every 7 days

Opioid-experienced patients (conversion from other opioids to buprenorphine): Taper the current around-the-clock opioid for up to 7 days to ≤30 mg/day of oral morphine or equivalent before initiating therapy. Short-acting analgesics as needed may be continued until analgesia with transdermal buprenorphine is attained. There is a potential for buprenorphine to precipitate withdrawal in patients already receiving opioids.

Patients who were receiving daily dose of <30 mg of oral morphine equivalents: Initial: 5 **mcg**/hour applied once every 7 days

Patients who were receiving daily dose of 30-80 mg of oral morphine equivalents: Initial: 10 **mcg**/hour applied once every 7 days

Patient who were receiving daily dose of >80 mg of oral morphine equivalents: Buprenorphine transdermal patch, even at the maximum dose of 20 **mcg**/hour applied once every 7 days, may **not** provide adequate analgesia; **consider the use of an alternate analgesic.**

Dose titration (opioid-naive or opioid-experienced patients): May increase dose, based on patient's supplemental short-acting analgesic requirements, with a minimum titration interval of 72 hours. Maximum dose: 20 **mcg**/hour applied once every 7 days; risk for QTc prolongation increases with doses ≥20 **mcg**/hour patch

Discontinuation of therapy: Taper dose gradually every 7 days to prevent withdrawal; consider initiating immediate-release opioids, if needed.

Dosing adjustment in renal impairment: There are no dosage adjustments provided in manufacturer's labeling (has not been studied).

Dosing adjustment in hepatic impairment:

Injection, sublingual tablet: Children, Adolescents, and Adults: Use caution due to extensive hepatic metabolism; dosage adjustments recommended although no specific recommendations are provided by the manufacturer.

Transdermal patch: Adults:

Mild to moderate impairment: Initial: No dosage adjustment needed; peak plasma levels (C_{max}) and exposure (AUC) were not increased in patients with mild to moderate hepatic impairment following intravenous administration.

Severe impairment: Not studied; consider alternative therapy with more flexibility for dosing adjustments.

Administration

Oral:

Sublingual solution: In neonates, place dose under tongue; insert pacifier to help reduce swallowing of dose (Kraft, 2008; Kraft, 2011)

Sublingual tablet: Place tablet under the tongue until dissolved; do not swallow. If 2 or more tablets are needed per dose, all tablets may be placed under the tongue at once, or 2 tablets may be placed under the tongue at a time; to ensure consistent bioavailability, subsequent doses should always be taken the same way.

Parenteral:

IM: Administer via deep IM injection

IV: Administer slowly, over at least 2 minutes

Topical: Transdermal patch: Apply patch to intact, non-irritated skin only. Apply to a hairless or nearly hairless skin site. If hairless site is not available, do not shave skin (as absorption from patch can be increased); hair at application site should be clipped. Prior to application, if the site must be cleaned, clean with clear water and allow to dry completely; do not use soaps, alcohol, lotions, or abrasives due to potential for increased skin absorption. Do not use any patch that has been damaged, cut, or manipulated in any way. Remove patch from protective pouch immediately before application. Remove the protective backing, and apply the sticky side of the patch to one of eight possible application sites (upper outer arm, upper chest, upper back, or the side of the chest [each site on either side of the body]). Firmly press patch in place and hold for ~15 seconds. Change patch every 7 days. Rotate patch application sites; wait ≥21 days before reapplying another patch to the same skin site. Avoid exposing application site to external heat sources (eg, heating pad, electric blanket, heat lamp, hot tub). If there is difficulty with patch adhesion, the edges of the system may be taped in place with first-aid tape. If the patch falls off during the 7-day dosing interval, dispose of the patch and apply a new patch to a different skin site. To properly dispose of Butrans® patch, fold it over on itself and flush down the toilet; alternatively, seal the used patch in the provided Patch-Disposal Unit and dispose of in the trash.

Monitoring Parameters Pain relief, respiratory rate, mental status, blood pressure; liver enzymes (baseline and periodic), symptoms of withdrawal, CNS depression, application site reactions (transdermal patch)

Additional Information Equianalgesic doses (parenteral): Buprenorphine 0.3 mg = morphine 10 mg; buprenorphine has a longer duration of action than morphine

Symptoms of overdose include CNS and respiratory depression, pinpoint pupils, hypotension, and bradycardia; treatment is supportive; naloxone may have limited effects in reversing respiratory depression; doxapram has also been used as a respiratory stimulant.

Controlled Substance C-III

Dosage Forms Excipient information presented when available (limited, particularly for generics); consult specific product labeling.

Patch Weekly, Transdermal:

Butrans: 5 mcg/hr (4 ea); 7.5 mcg/hr (4 ea); 10 mcg/hr (4 ea); 15 mcg/hr (4 ea); 20 mcg/hr (4 ea)

Solution, Injection:

Buprenex: 0.3 mg/mL (1 mL)

Generic: 0.3 mg/mL (1 mL)

Tablet Sublingual, Sublingual:

Generic: 2 mg, 8 mg

Extemporaneous Preparations A 0.075 mg/mL solution can be made using the 0.3 mg/mL injection, 95% ethanol, and simple syrup. Add 1.26 mL of 95% ethanol to 0.3 mg buprenorphine obtained from an 0.3 mg/1 mL ampule, mix well, and add quantity of simple syrup sufficient to obtain 4 mL (final volume). Solution is stable under refrigeration and at room temperature for 30 days when stored in amber glass bottles and for 7 days when stored in oral syringes (Anagnostis, 2011; Anagnostis, 2013).

Anagnostis EA, Sadaka RE, Sailor LA, et al, "Formulation of Buprenorphine for Sublingual Use in Neonates," *J Pediatr Pharmacol Ther*, 2011, 16(4):281-4.

Anagnostis EA, personal communication, March 2013.

Buprenorphine and Naloxone

(byoo pre NOR feen & nal OKS one)

Medication Safety Issues

High alert medication:

The Institute for Safe Medication Practices (ISMP) includes this medication among its list of drug classes which have a heightened risk of causing significant patient harm when used in error.

Other safety concerns:

Potential for over- or underdosing when switching among various formulations and between strengths of the sublingual films: **Not all strengths of sublingual tablets and films are bioequivalent to one another.** In addition, systemic exposure between the various strengths of sublingual films may be different; pharmacists should not substitute one or more film strengths for another (eg, dispense three 4 mg films for one 12 mg film, or vice-versa) without physician approval. Any patient switching between sublingual tablet and sublingual film formulation or between one or more strengths of the sublingual films should be monitored for over- or underdosing.

Related Information

Patient Information for Disposal of Unused Medications *on page 2453*

Brand Names: US Bunavail; Suboxone; Zubsolv

Brand Names: Canada Mylan-Buprenorphine/Naloxone; Suboxone; Teva-Buprenorphine/Naloxone

Therapeutic Category Analgesic, Narcotic; Opioid Partial Agonist

Generic Availability (US) Yes: Sublingual tablet

Use Maintenance treatment of opioid dependence as part of a complete plan that includes counseling and psychosocial support (Sublingual tablet: FDA approved in ages ≥16 years and adults; Sublingual film: FDA approved in adults)

Prescribing and Access Restrictions In the US prescribing of tablets for opioid dependence is limited to physicians who have met the qualification criteria and have received a DEA number specific to prescribing this product. Tablets will be available through pharmacies and wholesalers which normally provide controlled substances.

In Canada, buprenorphine/naloxone sublingual tablets may be prescribed only by physicians experienced in substitution treatment in opioid dependence and who have completed a recognized buprenorphine/naloxone education program. Components of the program include: Training of physicians in the use of buprenorphine/naloxone; maintenance of a list of physicians who have completed training; daily dosing supervision by a healthcare professional for at least 2 months; take-home doses should only be considered after 2 months based upon clinical stability, length of time in treatment and ability to safely store buprenorphine/naloxone. Take-home doses should be assessed and reviewed regularly. Physicians should not prescribe buprenorphine/naloxone unless supervision of daily dosing by a health care professional for at least 2 months (excluding weekends and holidays) can be ensured. Further information about the program may be obtained by contacting the manufacturer.

Medication Guide Available Yes

Pregnancy Risk Factor C

Pregnancy Considerations Animal reproduction studies have not been conducted with this combination.

Breast-Feeding Considerations Buprenorphine and its active metabolite, norbuprenorphine, are excreted in breast milk. It is not known if naloxone is excreted into breast milk, however, systemic absorption following oral administration is low (Smith, 2012) and any exposure of naloxone to a nursing infant would therefore be limited.

The US labeling recommends that caution be exercised when administering this specific combination product to nursing women. The Canadian labeling contraindicates use in nursing women.

Contraindications

Hypersensitivity to buprenorphine, naloxone, or any component of the formulation

Documentation of allergenic cross-reactivity for opioids is limited. However, because of similarities in chemical structure and/or pharmacologic actions, the possibility of cross-sensitivity cannot be ruled out with certainty.

Canadian labeling (sublingual tablets): Additional contraindications (not in US labeling): Opioid naïve patients; severe respiratory insufficiency; severe hepatic impairment; acute alcoholism; delirium tremens; breastfeeding

Warnings/Precautions See individual agents.

Adverse Reactions Also see individual agents.

Cardiovascular: Vasodilatation

Dermatologic: Diaphoresis

Central nervous system: Headache, pain, withdrawal syndrome

Gastrointestinal: Glossodynia (film), oral hypoesthesia (film), oral mucosa erythema (film), vomiting

Drug Interactions

Metabolism/Transport Effects Refer to individual components.

Avoid Concomitant Use

Avoid concomitant use of Buprenorphine and Naloxone with any of the following: Analgesics (Opioid); Atazanavir; Azelastine (Nasal); Conivaptan; Eluxadoline; Fusidic Acid (Systemic); Idelalisib; MAO Inhibitors; Methylnaltrexone; Mixed Agonist / Antagonist Opioids; Naloxegol; Orphenadrine; Paraldehyde; Thalidomide

Increased Effect/Toxicity

Buprenorphine and Naloxone may increase the levels/effects of: Alvimopan; Azelastine (Nasal); Desmopressin; Diuretics; Eluxadoline; MAO Inhibitors; Methotrimeprazine; Metyrosine; Naloxegol; Orphenadrine; Paraldehyde; Pramipexole; ROPINIRole; Rotigotine; Selective Serotonin Reuptake Inhibitors; Suvorexant; Thalidomide; TiZANidine; Zolpidem

The levels/effects of Buprenorphine and Naloxone may be increased by: Alcohol (Ethyl); Amphetamines; Anticholinergic Agents; Aprepitant; Atazanavir; Boceprevir; Brimonidine (Topical); Cannabis; CNS Depressants; Cobicistat; Conivaptan; CYP3A4 Inhibitors (Moderate); CYP3A4 Inhibitors (Strong); Dasatinib; Dronabinol; Droperidol; Fosaprepitant; Fusidic Acid (Systemic); Idelalisib; Ivacaftor; Kava Kava; Luliconazole; Magnesium Sulfate; Methotrimeprazine; Methylnaltrexone; Mifepristone; Nabilone; Netupitant; Palbociclib; Perampanel; Rufinamide; Simeprevir; Sodium Oxybate; Stiripentol; Succinylcholine; Tetrahydrocannabinol

Decreased Effect

Buprenorphine and Naloxone may decrease the levels/effects of: Analgesics (Opioid); Atazanavir; Pegvisomant

The levels/effects of Buprenorphine and Naloxone may be decreased by: Ammonium Chloride; Boceprevir; Bosentan; CYP3A4 Inducers (Moderate); CYP3A4 Inducers (Strong); Dabrafenib; Deferasirox; Efavirenz; Etravirine; Mitotane; Mixed Agonist / Antagonist Opioids; Naltrexone; Siltuximab; St Johns Wort; Tocilizumab

Storage/Stability Store at 25°C (77°F); excursions are permitted between 15°C and 30°C (59°F and 86°F). Protect from freezing and moisture.

Mechanism of Action

Buprenorphine: Buprenorphine exerts its analgesic effect via high affinity binding to mu opiate receptors in the CNS; displays partial mu agonist and weak kappa antagonist activity

Naloxone: Pure opioid antagonist that competes and displaces opioids at opioid receptor sites

Pharmacodynamics Maximum effect: Buprenorphine: 100 minutes; Naloxone: No clinically significant effect when administered sublingually

Pharmacokinetics (Adult data unless noted) Also see individual agents.

Absorption: High variability among patients, but low variability within each individual patient.

Protein binding: Buprenorphine: ~96%; Naloxone: ~45%

Bioavailability: Potential for greater bioavailability with certain strengths of the sublingual film compared to the same strength of the sublingual tablet exists. Although pharmacokinetics were similar between the sublingual formulations, bioequivalence is variable. In addition, the sizes and compositions between the sublingual film strengths are different which may result in different systemic exposures.

Half-life: Film: Buprenorphine: 24-42 hours; Naloxone: 2-12 hours

Dosing: Usual Note: Sublingual tablets and film contain a free-base ratio of buprenorphine:naloxone of 4:1. Doses based on buprenorphine content; titrate to appropriate effect.

Opioid dependence, maintenance treatment: Sublingual: Adolescents ≥16 years (sublingual tablets) and Adults (sublingual film or sublingual tablets):

Manufacturer's labeling:

Induction: Not recommended; initial treatment should begin using buprenorphine sublingual tablets (see Buprenorphine monograph)

Maintenance: Target dose: 16 mg/day as a single daily dose; dosage should be adjusted in increments of 2 mg or 4 mg to a dose that adequately suppresses opioid withdrawal; usual range: 4-24 mg/day; **Note:** Combination product for maintenance and for unsupervised therapy (if patient's clinical stability permits)

Alternate dosing [Center for Substance Abuse Treatment Guidelines (CSAT), 2004]:

Induction (for patients dependent on **short-acting** opioids and whose last dose of opioids was >12-24 hours prior to induction):

Day 1: Initial: 4 mg; may repeat dose after >2 hours if withdrawal symptoms not relieved; Day 1 maximum daily dose: 8 mg/**day**

Day 2:
- If no withdrawal symptoms, repeat total daily dose from Day 1
- If withdrawal symptoms are present, increase Day 1 dose by 4 mg; if withdrawal symptoms not relieved after >2 hours, may administer an additional 4 mg; Day 2 maximum daily dose: 16 mg/**day**

Subsequent induction days:
- If withdrawal symptoms are not present, daily dose is established (stabilization dose).
- If withdrawal symptoms are present, increase dose in increments of 2 mg or 4 mg each day as needed for symptom relief. Target daily dose by the end of the first week: 12 mg or 16 mg/day; maximum daily dose: 32 mg/**day**

Stabilization: Usual dose: 16-24 mg/day; maximum dose: 32 mg/**day**

Switching between sublingual tablets and sublingual film: Same dosage should be used as the previous administered product. **Note:** Potential for greater bioavailability with the sublingual film compared to the sublingual tablet exists; monitor closely for either over- or underdosing when switching patients from one formulation to another.

Switching between different strengths of sublingual films: Systemic exposure may be different with various combinations of sublingual film strengths; pharmacists should not substitute one or more film strengths for another (eg, switching from three 4 mg films to a single 12 mg film, or vice-versa) without physician approval and patients should be monitored closely for either over- or underdosing when switching between film strengths.

Dosing adjustment in renal impairment: There are no dosage adjustments are provided in manufacturer's labeling.

Dosing adjustment in hepatic impairment: Moderate to severe impairment: Dosage adjustments recommended; however, no specific dosage adjustment recommendations provided by manufacturer; monitor patients closely.

Administration

Sublingual film: Film should be placed under the tongue. Keep under the tongue until film dissolves completely; film should not be chewed, swallowed, or moved after placement. If more than 1 film is needed, the additional film should be placed under the tongue on the opposite side from the first film to minimize overlapping as much as possible.

Sublingual tablets: Place tablet under the tongue until dissolved; do not swallow. If 2 or more tablets are needed per dose, all tablets may be placed under the tongue at once, or 2 tablets may be placed under the tongue at a time; to ensure consistent bioavailability, subsequent doses should always be taken the same way.

Monitoring Parameters Symptoms of withdrawal, respiratory rate, mental status, blood pressure; liver function tests (baseline and periodically during therapy)

Additional Information Naloxone has been added to the formulation to decrease the abuse potential of dissolving tablets or film in water and using as an injection (precipitation of severe withdrawal would occur in opioid dependent patients if the tablets or film were misused in this manner).

Product Availability

Zubsolv new SL tablet strength (11.4 mg/2.9 mg): FDA approved December 2014; availability is anticipated later in 2015.

Zubsolv new SL strength (2.9 mg/0.71 mg): FDA approved June 2015; availability anticipated in the second half of 2015.

Controlled Substance C-III

Dosage Forms Excipient information presented when available (limited, particularly for generics); consult specific product labeling.

Film, buccal:

Bunavail: Buprenorphine 2.1 mg and naloxone 0.3 mg (30s); buprenorphine 4.2 mg and naloxone 0.7 mg (30s); buprenorphine 6.3 mg and naloxone 1 mg (30s) [citrus flavor]

Film, sublingual:

Suboxone: Buprenorphine 2 mg and naloxone 0.5 mg (30s); buprenorphine 4 mg and naloxone 1 mg (30s); buprenorphine 8 mg and naloxone 2 mg (30s); buprenorphine 12 mg and naloxone 3 mg (30s) [lime flavor]

Tablet, sublingual: Buprenorphine 2 mg and naloxone 0.5 mg; buprenorphine 8 mg and naloxone 2 mg

Zubsolv: Buprenorphine 1.4 mg and naloxone 0.36 mg; buprenorphine 5.7 mg and naloxone 1.4 mg; buprenorphine 8.6 mg and naloxone 2.1 mg [menthol flavor]

◆ **Buprenorphine Hydrochloride** *see* Buprenorphine *on page 318*

◆ **Buprenorphine Hydrochloride and Naloxone Hydrochloride Dihydrate** *see* Buprenorphine and Naloxone *on page 322*

◆ **Buproban** *see* BuPROPion *on page 324*

BuPROPion (byoo PROE pee on)

Medication Safety Issues

Sound-alike/look-alike issues:

Aplenzin may be confused with Albenza, Relenza
BuPROPion may be confused with busPIRone
Forfivo XL may be confused with Forteo
Wellbutrin XL may be confused with Wellbutrin SR
Zyban may be confused with Diovan

Related Information

Antidepressant Agents *on page 2257*

Oral Medications That Should Not Be Crushed or Altered *on page 2476*

Brand Names: US Aplenzin; Budeprion SR [DSC]; Buproban; Forfivo XL; Wellbutrin; Wellbutrin SR; Wellbutrin XL; Zyban

Brand Names: Canada Bupropion SR; Mylan-Bupropion XL; Novo-Bupropion SR; PMS-Bupropion SR; ratio-Bupropion SR; Sandoz-Bupropion SR; Wellbutrin SR; Wellbutrin XL; Zyban

Therapeutic Category Antidepressant, Dopamine-Reuptake Inhibitor; Smoking Cessation Aid

Generic Availability (US) Yes

Use Treatment of major depressive disorder (Aplenzin™, Forfivo™ XL, Wellbutrin®, Wellbutrin SR®, Wellbutrin XL®: FDA approved in adults), seasonal affective disorder (SAD) (Aplenzin™, Wellbutrin XL®: FDA approved in adults); adjunct in smoking cessation (Buproban®, Zyban®: FDA approved in adults); has also been used to treat ADHD

Medication Guide Available Yes

Pregnancy Risk Factor C

Pregnancy Considerations Adverse events have been observed in some animal reproduction studies. Bupropion and its metabolites were found to cross the placenta in *in vitro* studies (Earhart, 2012). An increased risk of congenital malformations has not been observed following maternal use of bupropion during pregnancy; however, data specific to cardiovascular malformations is inconsistent. The long-term effects on development and behavior have not been studied. The ACOG recommends that antidepressant therapy during pregnancy be individualized; treatment of depression during pregnancy should incorporate the clinical expertise of the mental health clinician, obstetrician, primary healthcare provider, and pediatrician. According to the American Psychiatric Association (APA), the risks of medication treatment should be weighed against other treatment options and untreated depression. For women who discontinue antidepressant medications during pregnancy and who may be at high risk for postpartum depression, the medications can be restarted following delivery. Treatment algorithms have been developed by the ACOG and the APA for the management of depression in women prior to conception and during pregnancy (ACOG, 2008; APA, 2010; Yonkers, 2009). There is insufficient information related to the use of bupropion to recommend use in pregnancy (ACOG, 2010).

Breast-Feeding Considerations Bupropion and its metabolites are excreted into breast milk. The estimated dose to a nursing infant varies by study and has been reported as ~2% of the weight-adjusted maternal dose (range: 1.4% to 10.6%) (Davis, 2009; Haas, 2004). Adverse events have been reported with some antidepressants and a seizure was noted in one 6-month old nursing infant exposed to bupropion (a causal effect could not be confirmed) (Chaudron, 2004; Hale, 2010). Recommendations for use in nursing women vary by manufacturer labeling.

Contraindications Hypersensitivity to bupropion or any component of the formulation; seizure disorder; history of anorexia/bulimia; patients undergoing abrupt discontinuation of ethanol or sedatives, including benzodiazepines, barbiturates, or antiepileptic drugs; use of MAO inhibitors or MAO inhibitors intended to treat psychiatric disorders (concurrently or within 14 days of discontinuing either bupropion or the MAO inhibitor); initiation of bupropion in a patient receiving linezolid or intravenous methylene blue; patients receiving other dosage forms of bupropion

Aplenzin, Wellbutrin XL: Additional contraindications: Other conditions that increase seizure risk, including arteriovenous malformation, severe head injury, severe stroke, CNS tumor, CNS infection

Warnings/Precautions **[U.S. Boxed Warning]: Use in treating psychiatric disorders: Antidepressants increase the risk of suicidal thinking and behavior in children, adolescents, and young adults (18 to 24 years of age) with major depressive disorder (MDD) and other psychiatric disorders;** consider risk prior to prescribing. Short-term studies did not show an increased risk in patients >24 years of age and showed a decreased risk in patients ≥65 years. All patients must be closely monitored for clinical worsening, suicidality, or unusual changes in behavior, especially during the initiation of therapy (generally first 1 to 2 months) or following an increase or decrease in dosage. The patient's family or caregiver should be instructed to closely observe the patient and communicate condition with healthcare provider. A medication guide should be dispensed with each prescription.

[U.S. Boxed Warning]: Use in smoking cessation: Serious neuropsychiatric events have occurred in patients taking bupropion for smoking cessation, including changes in mood (eg, depression, mania), psychosis, hallucinations, paranoia, delusions, homicidal ideation, hostility, agitation, aggression, anxiety, panic, suicidal ideation, suicide attempt and completed suicide. **The majority occurred during bupropion treatment; some occurred during treatment discontinuation. A causal relationship is uncertain as depressed mood may be a symptom of nicotine withdrawal. Some cases also occurred in patients taking bupropion who continued to smoke. Observe all patients taking bupropion for neuropsychiatric reactions. Instruct patients to contact a health care provider if neuropsychiatric reactions occur.**

The possibility of a suicide attempt is inherent in major depression and may persist until remission occurs. Worsening depression and severe abrupt suicidality that are not part of the presenting symptoms may require discontinuation or modification of drug therapy. Use caution in high-risk patients during initiation of therapy. Prescriptions should be written for the smallest quantity consistent with good patient care. The patient's family or caregiver should be alerted to monitor patients for the emergence of suicidality and associated behaviors such as anxiety, agitation, panic attacks, insomnia, irritability, hostility, impulsivity, akathisia, hypomania, and mania; patients should be instructed to notify their healthcare provider if any of these symptoms or worsening depression or psychosis occur.

May cause delusions, hallucinations, psychosis, concentration disturbance, paranoia, and confusion; most common in depressed patients and patients with a diagnosis of bipolar disorder. Symptoms may abate with dose reduction and/or withdrawal of treatment. May precipitate a manic, mixed, or hypomanic episode; risk is increased in patients with bipolar disorder or who have risk factors for bipolar disorder. Screen patients for a history of bipolar disorder and the presence of risk factors including a family history of bipolar disorder, suicide, or depression. **Bupropion is not FDA approved for bipolar depression.**

May cause a dose-related risk of seizures. Use is contraindicated in patients with a history of seizures or certain conditions with high seizure risk (eg, arteriovenous malformation, severe head injury, severe stroke, CNS tumor, or CNS infection, history of anorexia/bulimia, or patients undergoing abrupt discontinuation of ethanol, benzodiazepines, barbiturates, or antiepileptic drugs). Use caution with concurrent use of antipsychotics, antidepressants, theophylline, systemic corticosteroids, stimulants (including cocaine), anorectants, or hypoglycemic agents, or with excessive use of ethanol, benzodiazepines, sedative/hypnotics, or opioids. Use with caution in seizure-potentiating metabolic disorders (hypoglycemia, hyponatremia, severe hepatic impairment, and hypoxia). The dose-dependent risk of seizures may be reduced by gradual dose increases and by not exceeding the maximum daily dose. Use of multiple bupropion formulations is contraindicated. Permanently discontinue if seizure occurs during therapy. Chewing, crushing, or dividing long-acting products may increase seizure risk.

May cause CNS stimulation (restlessness, anxiety, insomnia) or anorexia. May increase the risks associated with electroconvulsive therapy (ECT). Consider discontinuing, when possible, prior to ECT. May cause weight loss; use caution in patients where weight loss is not desirable. The incidence of sexual dysfunction with bupropion is generally lower than with SSRIs.

May elevate blood pressure and cause hypertension. Events have been observed in patients with or without ▶

evidence of preexisting hypertension. The risk is increased when used concomitantly with monoamine oxidase inhibitors, nicotine replacement, or other drugs that increase dopaminergic or noradrenergic activity. Assess blood pressure before treatment and monitor periodically. Use caution in patients with cardiovascular disease. All children diagnosed with ADHD who may be candidates for stimulant medications should have a thorough cardiovascular assessment to identify risk factors for sudden cardiac death prior to initiation of drug therapy. Use with caution in patients with hepatic or renal dysfunction and in elderly patients; reduced dose and/or frequency may be recommended; Forfivo XL is not recommended in patients with hepatic or renal impairment. Elderly patients may be at greater risk of accumulation during chronic dosing. May cause motor or cognitive impairment in some patients; use with caution if tasks requiring alertness such as operating machinery or driving are undertaken. May cause mild pupillary dilation, which in susceptible individuals can lead to an episode of narrow-angle glaucoma. Consider evaluating patients who have not had an iridectomy for narrow-angle glaucoma risk factors. Anaphylactoid/anaphylactic reactions have occurred, with symptoms of pruritus, urticaria, angioedema, and dyspnea. Serious reactions have been (rarely) reported, including erythema multiforme, Stevens-Johnson syndrome and anaphylactic shock. Arthralgia, myalgia, and fever with rash and other symptoms suggestive of delayed hypersensitivity resembling serum sickness have been reported. Potentially significant drug-drug interactions may exist, requiring dose or frequency adjustment, additional monitoring, and/or selection of alternative therapy.

Extended release tablet: Insoluble tablet shell may remain intact and be visible in the stool.

Warnings: Additional Pediatric Considerations The American Heart Association recommends that all children diagnosed with ADHD who may be candidates for medication, such as bupropion, should have a thorough cardiovascular assessment prior to initiation of therapy. These recommendations are based upon reports of serious cardiovascular adverse events (including sudden death) in patients (both children and adults) taking usual doses of stimulant medications. Most of these patients were found to have underlying structural heart disease (eg, hypertrophic obstructive cardiomyopathy). This assessment should include a combination of thorough medical history, family history, and physical examination. An ECG is not mandatory but should be considered.

Adverse Reactions

Cardiovascular: Cardiac arrhythmia, chest pain, flushing, hypertension, hypotension, palpitations, tachycardia

Central nervous system: Abnormal dreams, agitation, akathisia, anxiety, central nervous system stimulation, confusion, depression, dizziness, drowsiness, headache, hostility, insomnia, irritability, memory impairment, migraine, nervousness, pain, paresthesia, sensory disturbance, sleep disorder, twitching

Dermatologic: Diaphoresis, pruritus, skin rash, urticaria

Endocrine & metabolic: Decreased libido, hot flash, menstrual disease, weight gain, weight loss

Gastrointestinal: Abdominal pain, anorexia, increased appetite, constipation, diarrhea, dysgeusia, dyspepsia, dysphagia, flatulence, nausea, vomiting, xerostomia

Genitourinary: Urinary tract infection, urinary urgency, vaginal hemorrhage

Hypersensitivity: Hypersensitivity reaction (including anaphylaxis, pruritus, urticaria)

Infection: Infection

Neuromuscular & skeletal: Arthralgia, arthritis, myalgia, neck pain, tremor, weakness

Ophthalmic: Blurred vision

Otic: Auditory disturbance, tinnitus

Renal: Polyuria

Respiratory: Cough, pharyngitis, sinusitis, upper respiratory infection

Miscellaneous: Fever

Rare but important or life-threatening: Abnormal accommodation, akinesia, alopecia, amnesia, anaphylactic shock, anaphylactoid reaction, anemia, angioedema, angle-closure glaucoma, aphasia, ataxia, atrioventricular block, cerebrovascular accident, colitis, coma, cystitis, deafness, delayed hypersensitivity, delirium, delusions, depersonalization, derealization, diplopia, dysarthria, dyskinesia, dyspareunia, dysphoria, dystonia, dysuria, edema, EEG pattern changes, erythema multiforme, esophagitis, euphoria, exfoliative dermatitis, extrapyramidal reaction, extrasystoles, facial edema, gastric ulcer, gastroesophageal reflux disease, gastrointestinal hemorrhage, gingival hemorrhage, glossitis, glycosuria, gynecomastia, hallucination, hepatic injury, hepatic insufficiency, hepatitis, hirsutism, hyperglycemia, hyperkinesia, hypertonia, hypoglycemia, hypokinesia, hypomania, impotence, increased intraocular pressure, increased libido, intestinal perforation, jaundice, leukocytosis, leukopenia, lymphadenopathy, manic behavior, myasthenia, mydriasis, myocardial infarction, myoclonus, neuralgia, neuropathy, orthostatic hypotension, painful erection, pancreatitis, pancytopenia, paranoia, pneumonia, psychiatric signs and symptoms, pulmonary embolism, rhabdomyolysis, salpingitis, sciatica, seizure (dose-related), SIADH, skin photosensitivity, Stevens-Johnson syndrome, stomatitis, suicidal ideation, syncope, tardive dyskinesia, thrombocytopenia, tongue edema, urinary incontinence, urinary retention, vasodilatation

Drug Interactions

Metabolism/Transport Effects Substrate of CYP1A2 (minor), CYP2A6 (minor), CYP2B6 (major), CYP2C9 (minor), CYP2D6 (minor), CYP2E1 (minor), CYP3A4 (minor); **Note:** Assignment of Major/Minor substrate status based on clinically relevant drug interaction potential; **Inhibits** CYP2D6 (strong), OCT2

Avoid Concomitant Use

Avoid concomitant use of BuPROPion with any of the following: MAO Inhibitors; Mequitazine; Pimozide; Tamoxifen; Thioridazine

Increased Effect/Toxicity

BuPROPion may increase the levels/effects of: Alcohol (Ethyl); ARIPiprazole; AtoMOXetine; Citalopram; CYP2D6 Substrates; DOXOrubicin (Conventional); Eliglustat; Fesoterodine; FLUoxetine; FluvoxaMINE; Iloperidone; Lorcaserin; Mequitazine; Metoprolol; Nebivolol; OCT2 Substrates; PARoxetine; Pimozide; Propafenone; Tamsulosin; Tetrabenazine; Thioridazine; TraMADol; Tricyclic Antidepressants; Vortioxetine

The levels/effects of BuPROPion may be increased by: Alcohol (Ethyl); Anti-Parkinson's Agents (Dopamine Agonist); CYP2B6 Inhibitors (Moderate); MAO Inhibitors; Mifepristone; Quazepam

Decreased Effect

BuPROPion may decrease the levels/effects of: Codeine; Hydrocodone; Iloperidone; Ioflupane I 123; Tamoxifen; TraMADol

The levels/effects of BuPROPion may be decreased by: CYP2B6 Inducers (Strong); Dabrafenib; Efavirenz; Isavuconazonium Sulfate; Lopinavir; Ritonavir

Storage/Stability Store at 15°C to 30°C (59°F to 86°F).

Wellbutrin, Wellbutrin XL, Zyban: Protect from light and moisture.

Mechanism of Action Aminoketone antidepressant structurally different from all other marketed antidepressants; like other antidepressants the mechanism of bupropion's activity is not fully understood. Bupropion is a relatively weak inhibitor of the neuronal uptake of norepinephrine and dopamine, and does not inhibit monoamine oxidase or the reuptake of serotonin. Metabolite inhibits the reuptake of norepinephrine. The primary mechanism of action is thought to be dopaminergic and/or noradrenergic.

Pharmacodynamics

Onset of action: 1 to 2 weeks

Maximum effect: 8 to 12 weeks

Duration: 1 to 2 days

Pharmacokinetics (Adult data unless noted)

Absorption: Rapid

Distribution: V_d: ~20 to 47 L/kg (Laizure, 1985)

Protein binding: 84%

Metabolism: Extensively hepatic via CYP2B6 to hydroxybupropion; non-CYP-mediated metabolism to erythrohydrobupropion and threohydrobupropion; these three metabolites are active. Preliminary studies suggest hydroxybupropion is 50% and erythrohydrobupropion and threohydrobupropion are 20% as active as parent drug. Bupropion also undergoes oxidation to form the glycine conjugate of meta-chlorobenzoic acid, the major urinary metabolite.

Half-life:

Children and Adolescents:

Extended release: Bupropion hydrochloride (Wellbutrin XL): Children 11 to 16 years: 16.5 ± 3.9 hours (Daviss, 2006)

Sustained release: (Wellbutrin SR): Children and Adolescents ≥11 years (n=19); 12.1 ± 3.3 hours; Metabolites: Hydroxybupropion: 21.8 ± 6.6 hours; Erythrohydrobupropion: 32.7 ± 16 hours; Threohydrobupropion: 26.9 ± 11.9 hours (Daviss, 2005)

Adults: 20 ± 5 hours; Metabolites: Hydroxybupropion: 20 ± 5 hours; Erythrohydrobupropion: 33 ± 10 hours; Threohydrobupropion: 37 ± 13 hours

Extended release: Bupropion hydrobromide: (Aplenzin): 21 ± 7 hours; Metabolites: Hydroxybupropion: 24 ± 5 hours; Erythrohydrobupropion: 31 ± 8 hours; Threohydrobupropion: 51 ± 9 hours

Time to peak serum concentration: Bupropion: Immediate release: ~2 hours; sustained release: ~3 hours; extended release: ~5 hours [Forfivo XL: 5 hours (fasting); 12 hours (fed)]

Metabolites: Hydroxybupropion, erythrohydrobupropion, threohydrobupropion: ~7 hours

Elimination: Urine (87%); feces (10%); only 0.5% of the dose is excreted as unchanged drug

Dosing: Usual Note: Bupropion is available as either hydrochloride or hydrobromide (Aplenzin™) salt formulations which are not interchangeable on a mg per mg basis; dosage expressed in terms of the salt formulation.

Pediatric:

Attention-deficit/hyperactivity disorder: Limited data available: Children and Adolescents: Oral:

Immediate release, hydrochloride salts: Initial: 3 mg/kg/**day** in 2 to 3 divided doses; maximum initial dose: 150 mg/**day**; titrate dose as needed to a maximum daily dose of 6 mg/kg/**day** or 300 mg/**day** with no single dose >150 mg (Dopheide 2009; Pliszka 2007).

Sustained release (Wellbutrin SR) and extended release (Wellbutrin XL), hydrochloride salts: May be used in place of regular tablets, once the daily dose is titrated using the immediate release product and the titrated 12-hour dosage corresponds to a sustained release tablet (Wellbutrin SR) or the 24-hour dosage range corresponds to an extended release tablet size (Wellbutrin XL)

Depression, refractory to SSRIs: Limited data available; **Note:** May be most beneficial in patients with comorbid ADHD, conduct disorder, substance abuse problems or who want to quit smoking (Dopheide 2006). Treatment should be periodically evaluated at appropriate intervals to ensure lowest effective dose is used.

Immediate release, hydrochloride salt: Children ≤11 years: Oral: Initial: 37.5 mg twice daily; titrate to response; usual dosage range: 100 to 400 mg/**day** (Dopheide 2006)

Sustained release, hydrochloride salt (Wellbutrin SR): Children ≥11 years and Adolescents: Oral: Initial: 2 mg/kg up to 100 mg administered as a morning dose; may titrate as needed every 2 to 3 weeks using the following titration schedule: Step 2: Increase up to 3 mg/kg every morning; Step 3: Increase up to 3 mg/kg every morning and 2 mg/kg at 5 pm; Step 4: Increase up to 3 mg/kg/dose twice daily; maximum dose: 150 mg; reported mean effective dose: Morning: 2.2 mg/kg and afternoon: 1.7 mg/kg (Daviss 2001)

Extended release, hydrochloride salt (Wellbutrin XL): Children ≥12 years and Adolescents: Oral: Initial: 150 mg once daily; may titrate after 2 weeks to 300 mg once daily if adequate response not achieved; dosing based on a pharmacokinetic study in eight patients with depression (Daviss 2006); doses as high as 400 mg/**day** have been reported (Dopheide 2006); may also be used once the daily dose is titrated using the immediate release product and the 24-hour dosage range corresponds to an extended release tablet size (Wellbutrin XL).

Smoking cessation: Limited data available: Adolescents ≥14 years and ≥40.5 kg: Sustained release, hydrochloride salt (Buproban, Zyban): Oral: Initial: 150 mg once daily for 3 days; increase to 150 mg twice daily; treatment should start while the patient is still smoking in order to allow drug to reach steady-state levels prior to smoking cessation; generally, patients should stop smoking during the second week of treatment; maximum daily dose: 300 mg/**day**; short-term efficacy was demonstrated in 104 adolescents who received therapy for 7 weeks with cessation counseling (Muramoto 2007).

Adult:

Depression: Note: Treatment should be periodically evaluated at appropriate intervals to ensure lowest effective dose is used.

Immediate release, hydrochloride salt: Initial: 100 mg twice daily; after 3 days may increase to the usual dose of 100 mg 3 times daily; if no clinical improvement after several weeks, may increase to a maximum dose of 150 mg 3 times daily

Sustained release, hydrochloride salt: Initial: 150 mg daily in the morning; if tolerated, as early as day 4, may increase to a target dose of 150 mg twice daily; if no clinical improvement after several weeks, may increase to a maximum dose of 200 mg twice daily; **Note:** Interval between successive doses should be at least 8 hours.

Extended release:

Hydrochloride salt: Initial: 150 mg once daily in the morning; if tolerated, as early as day 4, may increase to 300 mg once daily; if no clinical improvement after several weeks, may increase to maximum dose of 450 mg once daily; **Note:** Forfivo XL may only be used after initial dose titration with other bupropion products.

Hydrochloride salt (Forfivo XL): Switching from Wellbutrin immediate release, SR, or XL to Forfivo XL: Patients receiving 300 mg daily of bupropion hydrochloride for at least 2 weeks and requiring a dose increase or patients already taking 450 mg daily of bupropion hydrochloride may switch to Forfivo XL 450 mg once daily.

Hydrobromide salt (Aplenzin): Initial: 174 mg once daily in the morning; may increase as early as day 4 of dosing to 348 mg once daily (target); maximum dose: 522 mg daily (if no improvement seen after several weeks on 348 mg); **Note:** In patients receiving 348 mg once daily, taper dose down to 174 mg once daily prior to discontinuing.

Switching from hydrochloride salt formulation (eg, Wellbutrin immediate release, SR, XL, or Forfivo XL) to hydrobromide salt formulation (Aplenzin):

Bupropion hydrochloride 150 mg daily is equivalent to bupropion hydrobromide 174 mg once daily

Bupropion hydrochloride 300 mg daily is equivalent to bupropion hydrobromide 348 mg once daily

Bupropion hydrochloride 450 mg daily is equivalent to bupropion hydrobromide 522 mg once daily

Seasonal affective disorder (SAD): Initial: 150 mg once daily (Wellbutrin XL) or 174 mg once daily (Aplenzin) in the morning; if tolerated, may increase after 1 week to 300 mg once daily (Wellbutrin XL) or 348 mg once daily (Aplenzin) in the morning.

Note: Prophylactic treatment should be reserved for those patients with frequent depressive episodes and/or significant impairment. Initiate treatment in the autumn prior to symptom onset, and discontinue in early spring with dose tapering to 150 mg once daily for 2 weeks (Wellbutrin XL) or 174 mg once daily (Aplenzin), then discontinue. Doses >300 mg daily (Wellbutrin XL) or >348 mg daily (Aplenzin) have not been studied in SAD.

Smoking cessation (Zyban, Buproban): Initial: 150 mg once daily for 3 days; increase to 150 mg twice daily; treatment should continue for 7 to 12 weeks

Note: Therapy should begin at least 1 week before target quit date. Target quit dates are generally in the second week of treatment. If patient successfully quits smoking after 7 to 12 weeks, may consider ongoing maintenance therapy based on individual patient risk:benefit. Efficacy of maintenance therapy (300 mg daily) has been demonstrated for up to 6 months. Conversely, if significant progress has not been made by the seventh week of therapy, success is unlikely and treatment discontinuation should be considered.

Dosing conversion between hydrochloride salt immediate (Wellbutrin), sustained (Wellbutrin SR), and extended release (Wellbutrin XL, Forfivo XL) products: Convert using same total daily dose (up to the maximum recommended dose for a given dosage form), but adjust frequency as indicated for sustained (twice daily) or extended (once daily) release products.

Dosing adjustment in renal impairment: Adults: Immediate release, sustained release, and extended release formulations: There are no dosage adjustments provided in the manufacturer's labeling; however, limited pharmacokinetic information suggests elimination of bupropion and/or the active metabolites may be reduced. Use with caution and consider a reduction in dose and/or dosing frequency; closely monitor for adverse effects.

Forfivo XL: Use is not recommended.

Dosage adjustment in hepatic impairment: Adults:

Mild to moderate hepatic impairment: Immediate release, sustained release, and extended release formulations: Use with caution; consider reduced dosage and/or frequency.

Forfivo XL: Use is not recommended.

Severe hepatic cirrhosis: Use with extreme caution; maximum dose:

Aplenzin: 174 mg every other day

Forfivo XL: Use is not recommended.

Wellbutrin: 75 mg once daily

Wellbutrin SR: 100 mg once daily or 150 mg every other day

Wellbutrin XL: 150 mg every other day

Zyban: 150 mg every other day

Administration Oral: May be taken without regard to meals. Do not crush, chew, or divide sustained or extended release tablets (hydrochloride and hydrobromide salt formulations); swallow whole. The insoluble shell of the extended-release tablet may remain intact during GI transit and is eliminated in the feces.

Monitoring Parameters Heart rate, blood pressure, mental status, weight. Monitor patient periodically for symptom resolution; monitor for worsening depression, suicidality, and associated behaviors (especially at the beginning of therapy or when doses are increased or decreased), anxiety, social functioning, mania, panic attacks, tics.

ADHD: Evaluate patients for cardiac disease prior to initiation of therapy for ADHD with thorough medical history, family history, and physical exam; consider ECG; perform ECG and echocardiogram if findings suggest cardiac disease; promptly conduct cardiac evaluation in patients who develop chest pain, unexplained syncope, or any other symptom of cardiac disease during treatment.

Reference Range Therapeutic levels (trough, 12 hours after last dose): 50 to 100 ng/mL

Test Interactions May interfere with urine detection of amphetamine/methamphetamine (false-positive). Decreased prolactin levels.

Dosage Forms Excipient information presented when available (limited, particularly for generics); consult specific product labeling. [DSC] = Discontinued product

Tablet, Oral, as hydrochloride:

Wellbutrin: 75 mg, 100 mg

Generic: 75 mg, 100 mg

Tablet Extended Release 12 Hour, Oral:

Generic: 100 mg, 150 mg

Tablet Extended Release 12 Hour, Oral, as hydrochloride:

Budeprion SR: 100 mg [DSC] [contains tartrazine (fd&c yellow #5)]

Budeprion SR: 150 mg [DSC]

Buproban: 150 mg

Wellbutrin SR: 100 mg, 150 mg, 200 mg

Zyban: 150 mg

Generic: 100 mg, 150 mg, 200 mg

Tablet Extended Release 24 Hour, Oral, as hydrobromide:

Aplenzin: 174 mg, 348 mg, 522 mg

Tablet Extended Release 24 Hour, Oral, as hydrochloride:

Forfivo XL: 450 mg

Wellbutrin XL: 150 mg, 300 mg

Generic: 150 mg, 300 mg

◆ **Bupropion Hydrobromide** *see* BuPROPion *on page 324*

◆ **Bupropion Hydrochloride** *see* BuPROPion *on page 324*

◆ **Bupropion SR (Can)** *see* BuPROPion *on page 324*

◆ **Burinex (Can)** *see* Bumetanide *on page 314*

◆ **Burow's Solution** *see* Aluminum Acetate *on page 110*

◆ **Buscopan (Can)** *see* Scopolamine (Systemic) *on page 1907*

◆ **BuSpar** *see* BusPIRone *on page 328*

BusPIRone (byoo SPYE rone)

Medication Safety Issues

Sound-alike/look-alike issues:

BusPIRone may be confused with buPROPion

Brand Names: Canada Apo-Buspirone; Dom-Buspirone; PMS-Buspirone; Riva-Buspirone; Teva-Buspirone

Therapeutic Category Antianxiety Agent

Generic Availability (US) Yes

Use Management of anxiety disorders

Pregnancy Risk Factor B

Pregnancy Considerations Adverse events have not been observed in animal reproduction studies.

Breast-Feeding Considerations It is not known if buspirone is excreted in breast milk. Breast-feeding is not recommended by the manufacturer.

Contraindications Hypersensitivity to buspirone or any component of the formulation

Warnings/Precautions Use in severe hepatic or renal impairment is not recommended. Low potential for cognitive or motor impairment; until effects on patient known, patients should be warned to use caution when performing tasks which require mental alertness (eg, operating machinery or driving). Effects may be potentiated when used with other sedative drugs or ethanol. Use with MAO inhibitors may result in hypertensive reactions; concurrent use is not recommended. Restlessness syndrome has been reported in small number of patients; may be attributable to buspirone's antagonism of central dopamine receptors. Monitor for signs of any dopamine-related movement disorders (eg, dystonia, akathisia, pseudo-parkinsonism). Buspirone does not exhibit cross-tolerance with benzodiazepines or other sedative/hypnotic agents. If substituting buspirone for any of these agents, gradually withdraw the drug(s) prior to initiating buspirone.

Warnings: Additional Pediatric Considerations Buspirone does not possess antipsychotic activity and should not be used in place of appropriate antipsychotic treatment; two pediatric cases of possible psychotic deterioration have been reported (Soni, 1992).

Adverse Reactions

Cardiovascular: Chest pain

Central nervous system: Abnormal dreams, ataxia, confusion, dizziness, drowsiness, excitement, headache, nervousness, numbness, outbursts of anger, paresthesia

Dermatologic: Diaphoresis, skin rash

Gastrointestinal: Diarrhea, nausea, sore throat

Neuromuscular & skeletal: Musculoskeletal pain, tremor, weakness

Ophthalmic: Blurred vision

Otic: Tinnitus

Respiratory: Nasal congestion

Rare but important or life-threatening: Alcohol abuse, alopecia, amenorrhea, angioedema, anorexia, bradycardia, bruise, cardiac failure, cardiomyopathy, cerebrovascular accident, claustrophobia, cogwheel rigidity, conjunctivitis, dyskinesia, dystonia, edema, eosinophilia, epistaxis, extrapyramidal reaction, galactorrhea, hallucination, hemorrhagic diathesis, hypersensitivity reaction, hypertension, hyperventilation, hypotension, increased intraocular pressure, increased serum ALT, increased serum AST, increased serum transaminases, irritable bowel syndrome, leukopenia, memory impairment, menstrual disease, myocardial infarction, parkinsonian-like syndrome, pelvic inflammatory disease, personality disorder, photophobia, psychosis, rectal hemorrhage, restless leg syndrome, seizure, serotonin syndrome, slowed reaction time, slurred speech, suicidal ideation, syncope, thrombocytopenia, thyroid disease, urinary incontinence, visual disturbance (tunnel vision)

Drug Interactions

Metabolism/Transport Effects **Substrate** of CYP2D6 (minor), CYP3A4 (major); **Note:** Assignment of Major/Minor substrate status based on clinically relevant drug interaction potential

Avoid Concomitant Use

Avoid concomitant use of BusPIRone with any of the following: Azelastine (Nasal); Conivaptan; Dapoxetine; Fusidic Acid (Systemic); Idelalisib; MAO Inhibitors; Methylene Blue; Orphenadrine; Paraldehyde; Thalidomide

Increased Effect/Toxicity

BusPIRone may increase the levels/effects of: Alcohol (Ethyl); Antidepressants (Serotonin Reuptake Inhibitor/Antagonist); Antipsychotic Agents; Azelastine (Nasal); Buprenorphine; CNS Depressants; Hydrocodone; MAO Inhibitors; Methotrimeprazine; Methylene Blue; Metoclopramide; Metyrosine; Orphenadrine; Paraldehyde; Pramipexole; ROPINIRole; Rotigotine; Selective Serotonin Reuptake Inhibitors; Serotonin Modulators; Suvorexant; Thalidomide; Zolpidem

The levels/effects of BusPIRone may be increased by: Antiemetics (5HT3 Antagonists); Antifungal Agents (Azole Derivatives, Systemic); Antipsychotic Agents; Aprepitant; Brimonidine (Topical); Calcium Channel Blockers (Nondihydropyridine); Cannabis; Conivaptan; CYP3A4 Inhibitors (Moderate); CYP3A4 Inhibitors (Strong); Dapoxetine; Dasatinib; Doxylamine; Dronabinol; Droperidol; Fosaprepitant; Fusidic Acid (Systemic); Grapefruit Juice; HydrOXYzine; Idelalisib; Ivacaftor; Kava Kava; Luliconazole; Macrolide Antibiotics; Magnesium Sulfate; Methotrimeprazine; Mifepristone; Nabilone; Netupitant; Palbociclib; Perampanel; Rufinamide; Selective Serotonin Reuptake Inhibitors; Simeprevir; Sodium Oxybate; Stiripentol; Tapentadol; Tetrahydrocannabinol

Decreased Effect

BusPIRone may decrease the levels/effects of: Ioflupane I 123

The levels/effects of BusPIRone may be decreased by: Bosentan; CYP3A4 Inducers (Moderate); CYP3A4 Inducers (Strong); Dabrafenib; Deferasirox; Mitotane; Rifamycin Derivatives; Siltuximab; St Johns Wort; Tocilizumab; Yohimbine

Food Interactions Food may decrease the absorption of buspirone, but it may also decrease the first-pass metabolism, thereby increasing the bioavailability of buspirone. Grapefruit juice may cause increased buspirone concentrations. Management: Administer with or without food, but must be consistent. Avoid intake of large quantities of grapefruit juice.

Storage/Stability Store at 25°C (77°F); excursions permitted between 15°C to 30°C (59°F to 86°F). Protect from light.

Mechanism of Action The mechanism of action of buspirone is unknown. Buspirone has a high affinity for serotonin 5-HT_{1A} and 5-HT_2 receptors, without affecting benzodiazepine-GABA receptors. Buspirone has moderate affinity for dopamine D_2 receptors.

Pharmacodynamics

Onset of action: Within 2 weeks

Maximum effect: 3-4 weeks, up to 4-6 weeks

Pharmacokinetics (Adult data unless noted)

Absorption: Rapid and complete, but bioavailability is limited by extensive first-pass effect; only 1.5% to 13% (mean 4%) of the oral dose reaches the systemic circulation unchanged

Protein binding: 86%

Distribution: V_d: Adults: 5.3 L/kg

Metabolism: In the liver by oxidation (by cytochrome P450 isoenzyme CYP3A4) to several metabolites including 1-pyrimidinyl piperazine (about 1/4 as active as buspirone)

Half-life: Adults: Mean: 2-3 hours; increased with renal or liver dysfunction

Time to peak serum concentration: 40-90 minutes

Elimination: 29% to 63% excreted in urine (primarily as metabolites)

Dosing: Usual

Pediatric: **Anxiety disorders:** Children and Adolescents: Oral: Limited information is available; dose is not well established. One pilot study of 15 children, 6-14 years of age (mean 10 years), with mixed anxiety disorders, used initial doses of 5 mg daily; doses were individualized with increases in increments of 5 mg/day every week as needed to a maximum dose of 20 mg/day divided into 2 doses; the mean dose required: 18.6 mg/day (Simeon, 1994). Some authors (Carrey, 1996 and Kutcher, 1992), based on their clinical experience, recommend higher doses (eg, 15-30 mg/day in 2 divided doses). An open-label study in 25 prepubertal inpatients (mean age: 8 ± 1.8 years; range: 5-11 years) with anxiety symptoms and moderately aggressive behavior used initial doses of 5 mg daily; doses were titrated upwards (over 3 weeks) by 5-10 mg every 3 days to a maximum dose of 50 mg/day; doses >5 mg/day were administered in 2 divided doses/day; buspirone was discontinued in 25% of the children due to increased aggression and agitation or euphoric mania; mean optimal dose (n=19): 28 mg/day; range: 10-50 mg/day; median: 30 mg/day (Pfeffer, 1997). Two placebo-controlled 6-week trials in children and adolescents (n=559; age: 6-17 years) with generalized anxiety disorder studied doses of 7.5-30 mg twice daily (15-60 mg/day); no significant differences between buspirone and placebo with respect to generalized anxiety disorder symptoms were observed (see package insert).

Adult: **Generalized anxiety disorders:** Oral: Initial: 7.5 mg twice daily; may increase every 2-3 days in increments of 2.5 mg twice daily to a maximum of 30 mg twice daily; a dose of 10-15 mg twice daily was most often used in clinical trials that allowed for dose titration

Dosing adjustment in renal impairment: Patients with impaired renal function demonstrated increased plasma levels and a prolonged half-life of buspirone. Use in patients with severe renal impairment not recommended.

Dosing adjustment in hepatic impairment: Patients with impaired hepatic function demonstrated increased plasma levels and a prolonged half-life of buspirone. Use in patients with severe hepatic impairment not recommended.

Administration Oral: Administer in a consistent manner in relation to food (ie, either always with food or always without food); may administer with food to decrease GI upset

Monitoring Parameters Mental status, signs and symptoms of anxiety, liver and renal function; signs of dopamine-related movement disorders (eg, dystonia, akathisia, pseudo-parkinsonism).

Test Interactions The presence of buspirone may result in a false positive on a urinary assay for metanephrine/catecholamine; discontinue buspirone ≥48 hours prior to collection of urine sample for catecholamines

Additional Information Not appropriate for "as needed" (prn) use or for brief, situational anxiety; buspirone is equipotent to diazepam on a milligram to milligram basis in the treatment of anxiety; however, unlike diazepam, the onset of buspirone is delayed

Dosage Forms Excipient information presented when available (limited, particularly for generics); consult specific product labeling.

Tablet, Oral, as hydrochloride:

Generic: 5 mg, 7.5 mg, 10 mg, 15 mg, 30 mg

◆ **Buspirone Hydrochloride** *see* BusPIRone *on page 328*

◆ **Bussulfam** *see* Busulfan *on page 330*

Busulfan (byoo SUL fan)

Medication Safety Issues

Sound-alike/look-alike issues:

Myleran may be confused with Alkeran, Leukeran, melphalan, Mylicon

High alert medication:

This medication is in a class the Institute for Safe Medication Practices (ISMP) includes among its list of drug classes which have a heightened risk of causing significant patient harm when used in error.

Other safety concerns:

A solvent in IV busulfan, N, N-dimethylacetamide, is incompatible with many closed system transfer devices (CSTDs) used for preparing injectable antineoplastics. The plastic components of CSTDs may dissolve and result in subsequent leakage and potential infusion of dissolved plastic into the patient (ISMP [Smetzer 2015]).

Related Information

Management of Drug Extravasations *on page 2298*

Prevention of Chemotherapy-Induced Nausea and Vomiting in Children *on page 2368*

Safe Handling of Hazardous Drugs *on page 2455*

Brand Names: US Busulfex; Myleran

Brand Names: Canada Busulfex; Myleran

Therapeutic Category Antineoplastic Agent, Alkylating Agent

Generic Availability (US) No

Use

Oral: Palliative treatment of chronic myelogenous leukemia (CML) [FDA approved in pediatric patients (age not specified) and adults]; has also been used as a conditioning regimen prior to hemapoietic stem cell transplant

Parenteral: Conditioning regimen prior to allogeneic hematopoietic progenitor cell transplantation for CML in combination with cyclophosphamide [FDA approved in adults]

Pregnancy Risk Factor D

Pregnancy Considerations Adverse events were observed in animal reproduction studies. May cause fetal harm if administered during pregnancy. The solvent in IV busulfan, DMA, is also associated with teratogenic effects and may impair fertility. Women and men of childbearing potential should use effective contraception to avoid pregnancy during and after busulfan treatment.

Breast-Feeding Considerations It is not known if busulfan is excreted in breast milk. According to the manufacturer, the decision to discontinue breast-feeding during therapy or to discontinue busulfan should take into account the benefits of treatment to the mother; breast-feeding should be discontinued during IV busulfan treatment.

Contraindications Hypersensitivity to busulfan or any component of the formulation; oral busulfan is contraindicated in patients without a definitive diagnosis of CML

Warnings/Precautions Hazardous agent - use appropriate precautions for handling and disposal (NIOSH 2014 [group 1]). **[US Boxed Warning]: Severe and prolonged bone marrow suppression commonly occurs; reduce dose or discontinue oral busulfan for unusual suppression; may require bone marrow biopsy. Hematopoietic progenitor cell transplantation is required to prevent potentially fatal complications from prolonged myelosuppression due to IV busulfan.** May result in severe neutropenia, thrombocytopenia, anemia, bone marrow failure, and/or severe pancytopenia; pancytopenia may be prolonged (1 month up to 2 years) and may be reversible. When used for transplantation, monitor CBC with differential daily during treatment and until engraftment. The onset of neutropenia is a median of 4 days post-transplant; recovery is within a median of 13 days following allogeneic transplant (with prophylactic G-CSF use in most patients). Thrombocytopenia occurred at a median of 5 to 6 days. Use with caution in patients with compromised bone marrow reserve (due to prior treatment or radiation therapy). Monitor closely for signs of infection (due to neutropenia) or bleeding (due to thrombocytopenia). May require antibiotic therapy and platelet and red blood cell support.

Seizures have been reported with IV busulfan and with high-dose oral busulfan. When using as a conditioning regimen for transplant, initiate prophylactic anticonvulsant therapy (eg, phenytoin, levetiracetam, benzodiazepines, or valproic acid) prior to treatment. Use with caution in patients predisposed to seizures, with a history of seizures, head trauma, or with other medications associated with inducing seizures. Phenytoin increases busulfan clearance by ≥15%; busulfan kinetics and dosing recommendations for high-dose HSCT conditioning were studied with concomitant phenytoin. If alternate anticonvulsants are used, busulfan clearance may be decreased and dosing should be monitored accordingly.

Bronchopulmonary dysplasia with pulmonary fibrosis ("busulfan lung") is associated with chronic busulfan use; onset is delayed with symptoms occurring at an average of 4 years (range: 4 months to 10 years) after treatment; may be fatal. Symptoms generally include a slow onset of cough, dyspnea, and fever (low-grade), although acute symptomatic onset may also occur. Diminished diffusion capacity and decreased pulmonary compliance have been noted with pulmonary function testing. Differential diagnosis should rule out opportunistic pulmonary infection or leukemic pulmonary infiltrates; may require lung biopsy. Discontinue busulfan if toxicity develops. Pulmonary toxicity may be additive if administered with other cytotoxic agents also associated with pulmonary toxicity. Cardiac tamponade as been reported in children with thalassemia treated with high-dose oral busulfan in combination with cyclophosphamide. Abdominal pain and vomiting preceded tamponade in most children. Monitor for signs/symptoms and evaluate/treat promptly if cardiac tamponade is suspected. Busulfan has been causally related to the development of secondary malignancies (tumors and acute leukemias); chromosomal alterations may also occur. Chronic low-dose busulfan has been associated with ovarian failure (including failure to achieve puberty). Busulfan is associated with a moderate emetic potential (depending on dose and/or administration route); antiemetics may be recommended to prevent nausea and vomiting (Dupuis 2011).

High busulfan area under the concentration versus time curve (AUC) values (>1500 micromolar•minute) are associated with increased risk of hepatic sinusoidal obstruction syndrome (SOS; formerly called veno-occlusive disease [VOD]) due to conditioning for allogenic HSCT; patients with a history of radiation therapy, prior chemotherapy (≥3 cycles), or prior stem cell transplantation are at increased risk; monitor liver function tests (serum transaminases, alkaline phosphatase, and bilirubin) daily until 28 days post-transplant to detect hepatotoxicity (which may preclude hepatic SOS). Oral busulfan doses above 16 mg/kg (based on IBW) and concurrent use with alkylating agents may also increase the risk for hepatic SOS. The solvent in IV busulfan, dimethylacetamide (DMA), may impair fertility. N,N-dimethylacetamide is incompatible with many closed-system transfer devices (CSTDs) used for preparing injectable antineoplastics (ISMP [Smetzer 2015]). DMA may also be associated with hepatotoxicity, hallucinations, somnolence, lethargy, and confusion. **[US Boxed Warning]: According to the manufacturer, oral busulfan should not be used until CML diagnosis has been established. The responsible health care provider should be experienced in assessing response to chemotherapy.** Cellular dysplasia in many organs has been observed (in addition to lung dysplasia); giant hyperchromatic nuclei have been noted in adrenal glands, liver, lymph nodes, pancreas, thyroid, and bone marrow. May obscure routine diagnostic cytologic exams (eg, cervical smear). Potentially significant drug-drug interactions may exist, requiring dose or frequency adjustment, additional monitoring, and/or selection of alternative therapy.

Adverse Reactions

IV:

Cardiovascular: Arrhythmia, atrial fibrillation, cardiomegaly, chest pain, ECG abnormal, edema, heart block, heart failure, hyper-/hypotension, hypervolemia, pericardial effusion, tachycardia, tamponade, thrombosis, vasodilation, ventricular extrasystoles

Central nervous system: Agitation, anxiety, cerebral hemorrhage, chills, confusion, delirium, depression, dizziness, encephalopathy, fever, hallucination, headache, insomnia, lethargy, pain, seizure, somnolence

Dermatologic: Acne, alopecia, erythema nodosum, exfoliative dermatitis, maculopapular rash, pruritus, rash, skin discoloration, vesicular rash, vesiculobullous rash

Endocrine & metabolic: Hyperglycemia, hypocalcemia, hypokalemia, hypomagnesemia, hyponatremia, hypophosphatemia

Gastrointestinal: Abdominal fullness, abdominal pain, anorexia, constipation, diarrhea, dyspepsia, esophagitis, hematemesis, ileus, mucositis/stomatitis, nausea, pancreatitis, rectal disorder, vomiting, weight gain, xerostomia,

Hematologic: Anemia, lymphopenia, myelosuppression, neutropenia (median recovery: 13 days), prothrombin time increased, thrombocytopenia (median onset: 5-6 days)

Hepatic: Alkaline phosphatase increased, ALT increased, hepatic sinusoidal obstruction syndrome (SOS; veno-occlusive disease), hepatomegaly, hyperbilirubinemia, jaundice

Local: Injection site inflammation/pain

Neuromuscular & skeletal: Arthralgia, back pain, myalgia, weakness

Renal: BUN/creatinine increased, dysuria, hematuria, hemorrhagic cystitis, oliguria

Respiratory: Alveolar hemorrhage, asthma, atelectasis, cough, dyspnea, epistaxis, hemoptysis, hiccup, hyperventilation, hypoxia, lung disorder, pharyngitis, pleural effusion, pneumonia, rhinitis, sinusitis

Miscellaneous: Allergic reaction, infection (includes severe bacterial, viral [CMV], and fungal infections)

Oral:

Dermatologic: Hyperpigmentation of skin, rash

Endocrine & metabolic: Amenorrhea, ovarian suppression

Gastrointestinal: Xerostomia

Hematologic: Myelosuppression (anemia, leukopenia, thrombocytopenia)

IV and/or Oral: Rare but important or life-threatening: Acute leukemias, adrenal insufficiency, alopecia (permanent), aplastic anemia (may be irreversible), azoospermia, bronchopulmonary dysplasia, capillary leak syndrome, cataracts (rare), cheilosis, cholestatic jaundice, corneal thinning, dry skin, endocardial fibrosis, erythema multiforme, esophageal varices, gynecomastia, hepatic dysfunction, hepatocellular atrophy, hyperuricemia, hyperuricosuria, interstitial pulmonary fibrosis, malignant tumors, myasthenia gravis, neutropenic fever, ocular (lens) changes, ovarian failure, pancytopenia, porphyria cutanea tarda, pulmonary fibrosis, radiation myelopathy, radiation recall (skin rash), sepsis, sterility, testicular atrophy, thrombotic microangiopathy (TMA), tumor lysis syndrome, urticaria

Drug Interactions

Metabolism/Transport Effects None known.

Avoid Concomitant Use

Avoid concomitant use of Busulfan with any of the following: BCG; BCG (Intravesical); CloZAPine; Dipyrone; Natalizumab; Pimecrolimus; Tacrolimus (Topical); Tofacitinib; Vaccines (Live)

Increased Effect/Toxicity

Busulfan may increase the levels/effects of: CloZAPine; Ifosfamide; Leflunomide; Natalizumab; Tofacitinib; Vaccines (Live)

The levels/effects of Busulfan may be increased by: Acetaminophen; Antifungal Agents (Azole Derivatives, Systemic); Denosumab; Dipyrone; MetroNIDAZOLE (Systemic); Pimecrolimus; Roflumilast; Tacrolimus (Topical); Trastuzumab

Decreased Effect

Busulfan may decrease the levels/effects of: BCG; BCG (Intravesical); Coccidioides immitis Skin Test; Sipuleucel-T; Vaccines (Inactivated); Vaccines (Live)

The levels/effects of Busulfan may be decreased by: Echinacea; Fosphenytoin; Phenytoin

Storage/Stability

Injection: Store intact vials under refrigeration at 2°C to 8°C (36°F to 46°F). Solutions diluted in sodium chloride (NS) injection or dextrose 5% in water (D_5W) for infusion are stable for up to 8 hours at room temperature (25°C [77°F]); the infusion must also be completed within that 8-hour timeframe. Dilution of busulfan injection in NS is stable for up to 12 hours refrigerated (2°C to 8°C); the infusion must be completed within that 12-hour timeframe.

Tablet: Store at 25°C (77°F); excursions permitted to 15°C to 30°C (59°F to 86°F).

Mechanism of Action Busulfan is an alkylating agent which reacts with the N-7 position of guanosine and interferes with DNA replication and transcription of RNA. Busulfan has a more marked effect on myeloid cells than on lymphoid cells and is also very toxic to hematopoietic stem cells. Busulfan exhibits little immunosuppressive activity. Interferes with the normal function of DNA by alkylation and cross-linking the strands of DNA.

Pharmacokinetics (Adult data unless noted)

Absorption: Oral: Rapid and complete

Distribution: V_d: ~1 L/kg; distributes into CSF with levels equal to plasma

Protein binding: 32% plasma proteins; 47% to red blood cells

Metabolism: Extensively hepatic (may increase with multiple doses); glutathione conjugation followed by oxidation

Bioavailability: Oral: Highly variable: Children 1.5-6 years: 68% (range: 22% to 120%); adolescents and adults: 80% (range: 47% to 103%)

Half-life: Mean: 2.69 hours (± 0.49)

Time to peak serum concentration: Oral: Within 1-2 hours; IV: Within 5 minutes

Elimination: Urine (25% to 60% predominantly as metabolites; <2% as unchanged drug)

Clearance:

Children: 3.37 mL/minute/kg

Adults: 2.52 mL/minute/kg (range: 1.49-4.31 mL/minute/kg)

Dosing: Usual Dose, frequency, number of doses, and/or start date may vary by protocol and treatment phase. Refer to individual protocols. **Note:** Premedicate with prophylactic anticonvulsant therapy (eg, phenytoin) prior to high-dose busulfan treatment. Prophylactic antiemetics may be necessary for high-dose (HSCT) regimens.

Pediatric:

Chronic myelogenous leukemia (CML), palliation:

Infants, Children, and Adolescents: Oral:

Remission induction: 0.06 mg/kg/dose once daily **or** 1.8 mg/m²/day once daily; titrate dose (or withhold) to maintain a leukocyte count >15,000/mm³; doses >4 mg/day should be reserved for patients with the most compelling symptoms

Maintenance: When leukocyte count ≥50,000/mm³: Resume induction dose **or** (if remission <3 months) 1-3 mg/day (to control hematologic status and prevent relapse)

Hematopoietic stem cell transplant (HSCT) conditioning regimen: Limited data available:

IV: Infants, Children, and Adolescents: **Note:** Dosing based on actual body weight:

≤12 kg: 1.1 mg/kg/dose every 6 hours for 16 doses

>12 kg: 0.8 mg/kg/dose every 6 hours for 16 doses

Adjust dose to desired AUC (1125 micromolar•minute) using the following formula:

Adjusted dose (mg) = Actual dose (mg) x [target AUC (micromolar•minute) / actual AUC (micromolar•minute)]

Reduced intensity conditioning regimen: Infants, Children, and Adolescents: 0.8 mg/kg/dose for one dose on either day -7 (related donor) or day -10 (unrelated donor or cord recipient) prior to transplant, followed by 7 additional doses of ~0.8 mg/kg/dose every 6 hours (actual dose based on pharmacokinetic analysis after initial dose) beginning days -3 and -2 (related donor) or days -6 and -5 (unrelated donor or cord recipient) prior to transplant; used in combination with fludarabine and antithymocyte globulin (rabbit). In clinical trials, there was no minimum age for inclusion; the youngest patient treated was 2 years (Pulsipher, 2009).

Oral:

Infants and Children <3 years:

Ewing sarcoma: 1 mg/kg/dose every 6 hours for 16 doses on days -6 to -3 prior to transplant in combination with melphalan (Drabo, 2012)

Thalessemia major: 1.25 mg/kg every 6 hours for 16 doses on day -9 to day -6 prior to transplant in combination with cyclophosphamide and antithymocyte globulin (horse); data is from patients who were considered Class 1 or Class 2 (ie, low risk for GVHD or transplant mortality (Hussein, 2013)

Children ≥3 years and Adolescents: 1 mg/kg/dose every 6 hours for 16 doses prior to transplant; days of administration and combination therapy varied by disease: In Ewing sarcoma, on days -6 to -3 prior to transplant in combination with melphalan (Drabco, 2012); in thalassemia major, on days -9 to -6 in combination with cyclophosphamide and antithymocyte globulin (horse) (in this trial, patients were considered Class 1 or Class 2; ie, low risk for GVHD or transplant mortality) (Hussein, 2013) and in acute myeloid leukemia (AML), on days -9 to -6 in combination with cyclophosphamide (in this trial, patients were ≥16 years) (Cassileth, 1998).

Reduced intensity conditioning regimen: Children ≥10 years and Adolescents: 2 mg/kg/dose every 12 hours for 4 doses on days -8 and -7 in combination with fludarabine and antithymocyte globulin (horse); data is from patients with thalessmia major who were considered Class 3 (all risk factors with extensive liver damage and iron overload) (Hussein, 2013)

Adults:

Chronic myelogenous leukemia (CML), palliation:

Oral:

Remission induction: 0.06 mg/kg/dose once daily or 1.8 mg/m²/dose once daily; usual range: 4-8 mg/day; titrate dose (or withhold) to maintain leukocyte counts ≥15,000/mm³; doses >4 mg/day should be reserved for patients with the most compelling symptoms

Maintenance: When leukocyte count ≥50,000/mm³: Resume induction dose **or** (if remission <3 months) 1-3 mg/day (to control hematologic status and prevent relapse)

Hematopoietic stem cell (HSCT) conditioning regimen: IV: 0.8 mg/kg/dose every 6 hours for 4 days (a total of 16 doses); **Note:** Use ideal body weight or actual body weight, (whichever is lower) for dosing.

Obesity: For obese or severely-obese patients, use of an adjusted body weight [IBW + 0.25 x (actual – IBW)] is recommended.

Reduced intensity conditioning regimen: 0.8 mg/kg/day for 4 days starting 5 days prior to transplant (in combinations with fludarabine) (Ho, 2009)

Dosing adjustment in renal impairment:

IV: There are no dosage adjustment provided in the manufacturer's labeling (has not been studied).

Oral: There are no dosage adjustments are provided in the manufacturer's labeling; elimination appears to be independent of renal function; some clinicians suggest adjustment is not necessary (Aronoff, 2007).

Dosing adjustment in hepatic impairment:

IV: There are no dosage adjustments provided in the manufacturer's labeling (has not been studied).

Oral: There are no dosage adjustments provided in the manufacturer's labeling.

Preparation for Administration Hazardous agent; use appropriate precautions for handling and disposal (NIOSH 2014 [group 1]).

Parenteral: Dilute with NS or D_5W. The dilution volume should be 10 times the volume of busulfan injection, ensuring that the final concentration of busulfan is 0.5 mg/mL. Always add busulfan to the diluent, and not the diluent to the busulfan. Mix with several inversions. Do not use polycarbonate syringes or filter needles for preparation or administration.

Administration Hazardous agent; use appropriate precautions for handling and disposal (NIOSH 2014 [group 1]).

Oral: May be administered without regard to meals. To facilitate ingestion of high doses (for HSCT), may insert multiple tablets into clear gelatin capsules for administration.

Parenteral: Infuse over 2 hours through a central venous catheter; flush line before and after each infusion with D_5W or NS. Do **not** use polycarbonate syringes or filter needles for preparation or administration.

Vesicant/Extravasation Risk May be an irritant

Monitoring Parameters CBC with differential and platelet count (weekly for palliative treatment; daily until engraftment for HSCT); liver function tests, bilirubin, and alkaline phosphatase daily thru BMT day +28.

If conducting therapeutic drug monitoring for AUC calculations in HSCT, monitor busulfan plasma concentrations at appropriate collection times (record collection times); for IV infusion: For calculating AUC:

After first dose, collect at 2 hours (end of infusion), 4 hours, and 6 hours (immediately prior to the next dose).

Any other dose, collect a pre-infusion concentration, then at 2 hours (end of infusion), 4 hours, and 6 hours (immediately prior to the next dose).

Dosage Forms Excipient information presented when available (limited, particularly for generics); consult specific product labeling.

Solution, Intravenous:

Busulfex: 6 mg/mL (10 mL)

Tablet, Oral:

Myleran: 2 mg

Extemporaneous Preparations Hazardous agent: Use appropriate precautions for handling and disposal (NIOSH 2014 [group 1]). When manipulating tablets, NIOSH recommends double gloving, a protective gown, and preparation in a controlled device; if not prepared in a controlled device, respiratory and eye protection as well as ventilated engineering controls are recommended (NIOSH 2014).

A 2 mg/mL oral suspension can be prepared in a vertical flow hood with tablets and simple syrup. Crush one-hundred-twenty 2 mg tablets in a mortar and reduce to a fine powder. Add small portions of simple syrup and mix to a uniform paste; mix while adding the simple syrup in incremental proportions to **almost** 120 mL; transfer to a graduated cylinder, rinse mortar and pestle with simple syrup, and add quantity of vehicle sufficient to make 120 mL. Transfer contents of the graduated cylinder into an amber prescription bottle. Label "shake well", "refrigerate", and "caution chemotherapy". Stable for 30 days.

Allen LV, "Busulfan Oral Suspension," *US Pharm*, 1990, 15:94-5.

- ◆ **Busulfanum** *see* Busulfan *on page 330*
- ◆ **Busulfex** *see* Busulfan *on page 330*
- ◆ **Busulphan** *see* Busulfan *on page 330*
- ◆ **Butrans** *see* Buprenorphine *on page 318*
- ◆ **BW-430C** *see* LamoTRIgine *on page 1211*
- ◆ **BW524W91** *see* Emtricitabine *on page 739*
- ◆ **C1 Esterase Inhibitor** *see* C1 Inhibitor (Human) *on page 333*
- ◆ **C1-INH** *see* C1 Inhibitor (Human) *on page 333*
- ◆ **C1-Inhibitor** *see* C1 Inhibitor (Human) *on page 333*
- ◆ **C1INHRP** *see* C1 Inhibitor (Human) *on page 333*
- ◆ **C2B8 Monoclonal Antibody** *see* RiTUXimab *on page 1875*
- ◆ **C-500 [OTC]** *see* Ascorbic Acid *on page 202*

C1 Inhibitor (Human) (cee won in HIB i ter HYU man)

Brand Names: US Berinert; Cinryze

Brand Names: Canada Berinert

Therapeutic Category Blood Product Derivative

Generic Availability (US) No

Use

Berinert: Treatment of acute abdominal, facial, or laryngeal attacks of hereditary angioedema (HAE) (FDA approved in adolescents and adults)

Cinryze: Routine prophylaxis against angioedema attacks in patients with HAE (FDA approved in adolescents and adults); has also been used for treatment of acute abdominal, facial, and laryngeal attacks of HAE

Prescribing and Access Restrictions Assistance with procurement and reimbursement of Cinryze is available for healthcare providers and patients through the CINRYZE-*Solutions* program (telephone: 1-877-945-1000) or at http://www.cinryze.com/Cinryze_Solutions/Default.aspx

Pregnancy Risk Factor C

Pregnancy Considerations Animal reproduction studies have not been conducted. Although information related to use during pregnancy is limited, plasma-derived human C1 inhibitor concentrate is the preferred treatment for HAE during pregnancy (Baker, 2013; Caballero, 2012). Women with HAE should be monitored closely during pregnancy and for at least 72 hours after delivery (Caballero, 2012).

Breast-Feeding Considerations It is not known if these products are excreted into breast milk. The manufacturers recommend caution be used if needed in a nursing woman. Lactation may increase the frequency of attacks and women should be monitored closely. Plasma-derived human C1 inhibitor concentrate is the preferred treatment for HAE during lactation (Caballero, 2012).

Contraindications History of anaphylactic or life-threatening hypersensitivity reactions to human C1 inhibitor or any component of the formulation

Warnings/Precautions Severe hypersensitivity reactions (eg, urticaria, hives, tightness of the chest, wheezing, hypotension, anaphylaxis) may occur during or after administration. Signs/symptoms of hypersensitivity reactions may be similar to the attacks associated with hereditary angioedema, therefore, consideration should be given to treatment methods. In the event of acute hypersensitivity reactions to C1 inhibitor therapy, treatment should be discontinued and epinephrine should be available. Serious arterial and venous thromboembolic events have been reported at recommended doses and when used off-label at doses higher than recommended. Risk factors may include the presence of an indwelling venous catheter/access device, prior history of thrombosis, underlying atherosclerosis, use of oral contraceptives or certain androgens, morbid obesity, and immobility. Consider potential risk of thrombosis with use, and closely monitor patients with preexisting risks for thrombotic events. Product of human plasma; may potentially contain infectious agents (eg, viruses and, theoretically, the Creutzfeldt-Jakob disease [CJD] agent) that could transmit disease. Screening of donors, as well as testing and/or inactivation or removal of certain viruses, reduces the risk. Infections thought to be transmitted by this product should be reported to the manufacturer. Due to the potential for airway obstruction, patients suffering from an acute laryngeal HAE attack and self-administering should be informed to immediately seek medical attention following treatment.

Adverse Reactions

Central nervous system: Dizziness, fever, headache

Dermatologic: Erythema, pruritus, rash

Gastrointestinal: Abdominal pain/discomfort, abnormal taste, nausea, vomiting, xerostomia

Genitourinary: Vulvovaginal fungal infection

Local: Infusion-related reactions

Respiratory: Nasopharyngitis,upper respiratory tract infection

Miscellaneous: Flu-like syndrome, hereditary angioedema attack symptoms exacerbated, viral infection

Rare but important or life-threatening: Anaphylactic reaction, chills, hypersensitivity reaction, injection site erythema, injection site pain, shock, stroke, thrombotic events, transient ischemic attack

Drug Interactions

Metabolism/Transport Effects None known.

Avoid Concomitant Use There are no known interactions where it is recommended to avoid concomitant use.

Increased Effect/Toxicity

The levels/effects of C1 Inhibitor (Human) may be increased by: Androgens; Estrogen Derivatives; Progestins

Decreased Effect There are no known significant interactions involving a decrease in effect.

Storage/Stability Store intact vials at 2°C to 25°C (36°F to 77°F); do not freeze. Store in original carton; protect from light. Use within 3 hours (Cinryze) or 8 hours (Berinert) of reconstitution (Canadian labeling recommends immediate use after reconstitution); do not refrigerate or freeze reconstituted solution. Discard any unused product.

Mechanism of Action C1 inhibitor, one of the serine proteinase inhibitors found in human blood, plays a role in regulating the complement and intrinsic coagulation (contact system) pathway, and is also involved in the fibrinolytic and kinin pathways. C1 inhibitor therapy in patients with C1 inhibitor deficiency, such as HAE, is believed to suppress contact system activation via inactivation of plasma kallikrein and factor XIIa, thus preventing bradykinin production. Unregulated bradykinin production is thought to contribute to the increased vascular permeability and angioedema observed in HAE.

Pharmacodynamics Onset of action:

C1-INH plasma concentration increase: Cinryze: 1 hour or less

Symptom relief; laryngeal:

Berinert: Median: 15 minutes per attack

Cinryze: Pediatric patients 6-17 years: Median: 30 minutes per attack; for the majority of patient unequivocal symptom relief reported within 1 hour (range: 15-135 minutes) (Lumry, 2013)

Duration of Action: Time to complete resolution of HAE symptoms: Berinert: Median: 8.4 hours

Pharmacokinetics (Adult data unless noted)

Distribution: V_{ss}: Berinert:

Children and Adolescents: (6-13 years, n=5): 0.02 L/kg (range: 0.017-0.026 L/kg)

Adults: 0.018 L/kg (range: 0.011-0.028 L/kg)

Half-life elimination:

Berinert:

Children 3 to <12 years: 16.7 hours

Adults: 22 hours (range: 17-24 hours)

Cinryze: 56 hours (range: 11-108 hours)

Time to peak serum concentration: Cinryze: ~4 hours

Dosing: Usual Note: Products are not interchangeable; one unit of Cinryze is **NOT** equivalent to 1 unit of Berinert.

Pediatric:

Hereditary angioedema (HAE) attacks; routine prophylaxis: Cinryze: Children ≥6 years (Limited data available) and Adolescents: IV: 1000 units every 3-4 days (ie, twice weekly) (Lumry, 2013)

Hereditary angioedema (HAE) attacks (abdominal, facial or laryngeal); treatment:

Berinert: Children ≥6 years (Limited data available) and Adolescents: IV: 20 units/kg (Farkas, 2013; Wahn, 2012)

Cinryze: Limited data available: Children ≥6 years and Adolescents: IV: 1000 units; may repeat dose in 1 hour if needed (Lumry, 2013)

Adult:

Hereditary angioedema (HAE) attacks; routine prophylaxis: Cinryze: IV: 1000 units every 3-4 days

Hereditary angioedema (HAE) attacks (abdominal, facial, or laryngeal); treatment: Berinert: IV: 20 units/kg

Preparation for Administration Parenteral: IV: Product should come to room temperature before combining with diluent (SWFI). The provided filter needle or transfer set should be used to withdraw the reconstituted product. Remove filter needle and attach reconstituted solution to infusion set or appropriate needle for infusion.

Berinert: Reconstitute each vial with 10 mL of SWFI using the provided transfer set; final concentration: 50 units/mL. After combining with diluent, gently swirl (do not shake) vial to completely dissolve powder. Do not use if turbid, discolored, or contains particles.

Cinryze: Do not use product if there is no vacuum in the vial. Reconstitute each vial with 5 mL of SWFI using the provided transfer set; final concentration 100 units/mL. After combining with diluent, gently swirl (do not shake) vial to completely dissolve powder. Reconstituted product should be clear and colorless or slightly blue; do not use if turbid, discolored, or contains particles. A silicone-free syringe is recommended for reconstitution and administration.

Administration Parenteral: IV:

Berinert: Administer IV at recommended infusion rate: 4 mL/minute (200 units/minute); use within 8 hours of reconstitution; discard any unused product.

Cinryze: A silicone-free syringe is recommended for administration. Administer IV at recommended infusion rate: 1 mL/minute (over 10 minutes; 100 units/minute); use within 3 hours of reconstitution; discard any unused product.

Self-administration: Following patient or caregiver training and instructions on self-administration, patient or caregiver may self-administer treatment (Berinert) or prophylaxis (Cinryze) therapy. Epinephrine should be available during self-administration in the event of an acute, severe hypersensitivity reaction. Patient suffering from an acute laryngeal HAE attack and self-administering should be informed to seek immediate medical attention following treatment (potential for airway obstruction to occur).

Monitoring Parameters Monitor patient closely for hypersensitivity reaction and thrombotic events during or after administration.

Additional Information

Cinryze: 1 unit corresponds to C1 inhibitor present in 1 mL of normal fresh plasma

Berinert: A single 500 unit vial contains 400-625 units of C1 inhibitor

Dosage Forms Excipient information presented when available (limited, particularly for generics); consult specific product labeling.

Kit, Intravenous:

Berinert: 500 units

Solution Reconstituted, Intravenous [preservative free]:

Cinryze: 500 units (1 ea)

◆ **CaEDTA** *see* Edetate CALCIUM Disodium *on page* 728

◆ **Cafcit** *see* Caffeine *on page* 335

◆ **CAFdA** *see* Clofarabine *on page* 500

◆ **Cafergor (Can)** *see* Ergotamine and Caffeine *on page* 776

◆ **Cafergot** *see* Ergotamine and Caffeine *on page* 776

Caffeine (KAF een)

Brand Names: US Cafcit; Keep Alert [OTC]; No Doz Maximum Strength [OTC]; Stay Awake Maximum Strength [OTC]; Stay Awake [OTC]; Vivarin [OTC]

Therapeutic Category Central Nervous System Stimulant; Diuretic; Respiratory Stimulant

Generic Availability (US) Yes: Tablet, caffeine and sodium benzoate injection, injection, oral solution

Use

Treatment of idiopathic apnea of prematurity **(caffeine citrate)**

Emergency stimulant in acute circulatory failure; diuretic; treatment of spinal puncture headaches **(caffeine sodium benzoate)**

Pregnancy Risk Factor C

Pregnancy Considerations Adverse events were observed in animal reproduction studies. Caffeine crosses the placenta; serum concentrations in the fetus are similar to those in the mother (Grosso, 2005). Based on current studies, usual dietary exposure to caffeine is unlikely to cause congenital malformations (Brent, 2011). However, available data shows conflicting results related to maternal caffeine use and the risk of other adverse events, such as spontaneous abortion or growth retardation (Brent, 2011; Jahanfar, 2013). The half-life of caffeine is prolonged during the second and third trimesters of pregnancy and maternal and fetal exposure is also influenced by maternal smoking or drinking (Brent, 2011; Koren, 2000). Current guidelines recommend limiting caffeine intake from all sources to ≤200 mg/day (ACOG, 2010).

Breast-Feeding Considerations Caffeine is detected in breast milk (Berlin, 1981; Hildebrant, 1983; Ryu, 1985a); concentrations may be dependent upon maternal consumption and her ability to metabolize (eg, smoker versus nonsmoker) (Brent, 2011). The ability of the breast-feeding child to metabolize caffeine is age-dependent (Hildebrant, 1983). Irritability and jitteriness have been reported in the nursing infant exposed to high concentrations of caffeine in breast milk (Martin, 2007). Infant heart rates and sleep patterns were not found to be affected in normal, full-term infants exposed to lesser amounts of caffeine (Ryu, 1985b).

Contraindications Hypersensitivity to caffeine or any component of the formulation; sodium benzoate is not for use in neonates

Warnings/Precautions Use with caution in patients with a history of peptic ulcer, gastroesophageal reflux, impaired renal or hepatic function, seizure disorders, or cardiovascular disease. Avoid use in patients with symptomatic cardiac arrhythmias, agitation, anxiety, or tremor. Over-the-counter [OTC] products contain an amount of caffeine similar to one cup of coffee; limit the use of other caffeine-containing beverages or foods.

Caffeine citrate should not be interchanged with caffeine and sodium benzoate. Avoid use of products containing sodium benzoate in neonates; has been associated with a potentially fatal toxicity ("gasping syndrome"). Neonates receiving caffeine citrate should be closely monitored for the development of necrotizing enterocolitis. Caffeine serum levels should be closely monitored to optimize therapy and prevent serious toxicity. Concomitant use with transcutaneous electrical nerve stimulation may lessen analgesia (Marchand, 1995).

Warnings: Additional Pediatric Considerations During a Cafcit double-blind, placebo-controlled study, six of 85 patients developed necrotizing enterocolitis (NEC); five of these six patients had received caffeine citrate; although no causal relationship has been established, neonates who receive caffeine citrate should be closely monitored for the development of NEC. Caffeine serum levels should be closely monitored to optimize therapy and prevent serious toxicity.

Adverse Reactions Primarily serum-concentration related.

Cardiovascular: Angina pectoris, chest pain, flushing, palpitations, sinus tachycardia, supraventricular tachycardia, vasodilatation, ventricular arrhythmia

Central nervous system: Agitation, delirium, dizziness, hallucination, headache, insomnia, irritability, psychosis, restlessness

Dermatologic: Urticaria

Gastrointestinal: Esophageal motility disorder (sphincter tone decreased), gastritis

Genitourinary: Diuresis

Neuromuscular & skeletal: Fasciculations

Ophthalmic: Increased intraocular pressure (>180 mg caffeine), miosis

Drug Interactions

Metabolism/Transport Effects Substrate of CYP1A2 (major), CYP2C9 (minor), CYP2D6 (minor), CYP2E1 (minor), CYP3A4 (minor); **Note:** Assignment of Major/Minor substrate status based on clinically relevant drug interaction potential; **Inhibits** CYP1A2 (weak)

Avoid Concomitant Use

Avoid concomitant use of Caffeine with any of the following: Iobenguane I 123; Stiripentol

Increased Effect/Toxicity

Caffeine may increase the levels/effects of: Formoterol; Indacaterol; Olodaterol; Sympathomimetics; TiZANidine

The levels/effects of Caffeine may be increased by: Abiraterone Acetate; AtoMOXetine; Cannabinoid-Containing Products; CYP1A2 Inhibitors (Moderate); CYP1A2 Inhibitors (Strong); Deferasirox; Linezolid; Norfloxacin; Peginterferon Alfa-2b; Stiripentol; Tedizolid; Vemurafenib

Decreased Effect

Caffeine may decrease the levels/effects of: Adenosine; Iobenguane I 123; Lithium; Regadenoson

The levels/effects of Caffeine may be decreased by: Teriflunomide

Storage/Stability Store at 20°C to 25°C (68°F to 77°F).

Caffeine citrate: Injection and oral solution contain no preservatives; injection is chemically stable for at least 24 hours at room temperature when diluted to 10 mg/mL (as caffeine citrate) with D_5W, $D_{50}W$, Intralipid® 20%, and Aminosyn® 8.5%; also compatible with dopamine (600 mcg/mL), calcium gluconate 10%, heparin (1 unit/mL), and fentanyl (10 mcg/mL) at room temperature for 24 hours.

Mechanism of Action Increases levels of 3'5' cyclic AMP by inhibiting phosphodiesterase; CNS stimulant which increases medullary respiratory center sensitivity to carbon dioxide, stimulates central inspiratory drive, and improves skeletal muscle contraction (diaphragmatic contractility); prevention of apnea may occur by competitive inhibition of adenosine

Pharmacokinetics (Adult data unless noted)

Distribution: V_d:

Neonates: 0.8-0.9 L/kg

Children >9 months to Adults: 0.6 L/kg

Protein binding: 17%

Metabolism: Interconversion between caffeine and theophylline has been reported in preterm neonates (caffeine levels are ~25% of measured theophylline after theophylline administration and ~3% to 8% of caffeine would be expected to be converted to theophylline)

Half-life:

Neonates: 72-96 hours (range: 40-230 hours)

Infants >9 months, Children, and Adults: 5 hours

Time to peak serum concentration: Oral: Within 30 minutes to 2 hours

Elimination:

Neonates ≤1 month: 86% excreted unchanged in urine

Infants >1 month and Adults: Extensively liver metabolized to a series of partially demethylated xanthines and methyluric acids

Clearance:

Neonates: 8.9 mL/hour/kg (range: 2.5-17)

Adults: 94 mL/hour/kg

Dosing: Neonatal Oral, IV: Apnea of prematurity: **Caffeine citrate: Note:** Dose expressed as caffeine citrate; caffeine base is 1/2 the dose of the caffeine citrate:

Loading dose: Minimum dose: 20 mg/kg caffeine citrate; loading doses as high as 80 mg/kg of caffeine citrate have been reported (Steer, 2004); some centers repeat a load of 20 mg/kg as caffeine citrate to a maximum cumulative dose load of 80 mg/kg as caffeine citrate in refractory patients (Schmidt, 2006; Schmidt, 2007; Steer, 2004)

Maintenance dose: 5-10 mg/kg/day caffeine citrate once daily starting 24 hours after the loading dose; some centers increase maintenance dose in 5 mg/kg/day increments of caffeine citrate to a maximum of 20 mg/kg/day in refractory patients based on clinical response ± serum caffeine concentrations (Schmidt, 2006; Schmidt, 2007; Steer, 2004)

Dosing: Usual

Stimulant/diuretic: **Caffeine sodium benzoate:** Adults: IM, IV: 500 mg as a single dose

Treatment of spinal puncture headache: **Caffeine sodium benzoate:** Adults: IV: 500 mg as a single dose; may repeat in 4 hours if headache unrelieved

Preparation for Administration Parenteral:

Caffeine citrate: May further dilute with D_5W to 10 mg caffeine citrate/mL.

Caffeine sodium benzoate: For spinal headaches, dilute in 1,000 mL NS.

Administration

Oral: May be administered without regard to feedings or meals; may administer injectable formulation (caffeine citrate) orally

Parenteral:

Caffeine citrate: May administer undiluted or further diluted with D_5W. Infuse loading dose over at least 30 minutes; maintenance dose may be infused over at least 10 minutes.

Caffeine sodium benzoate: IV as slow direct injection; for spinal headaches, further dilute and infuse over 1 hour; follow with 1,000 mL NS, infuse over 1 hour; administer IM undiluted

Monitoring Parameters Heart rate, number and severity of apnea spells, serum caffeine levels

Reference Range

Therapeutic: Apnea of prematurity: 8-20 mcg/mL

Potentially toxic: >20 mcg/mL

Toxic: >50 mcg/mL

Dosage Forms Excipient information presented when available (limited, particularly for generics); consult specific product labeling. [DSC] = Discontinued product

Injection, solution, as citrate [preservative free]:

Cafcit: 60 mg/3 mL (3 mL) [equivalent to 10 mg/mL caffeine base]

Generic: 60 mg/3 mL (3 mL) [equivalent to 10 mg/mL caffeine base]

Injection, solution [with sodium benzoate]:

Generic: Caffeine 125 mg/mL and sodium benzoate 125 mg/mL (2 mL) [DSC]

Solution, oral, as citrate [preservative free]:

Cafcit: 60 mg/3 mL (3 mL) [equivalent to 10 mg/mL caffeine base] [DSC]

Generic: 60 mg/3 mL (3 mL) [equivalent to 10 mg/mL caffeine base]

Tablet, oral:

Keep Alert: 200 mg

NoDoz Maximum Strength: 200 mg

Stay Awake: 200 mg

Stay Awake Maximum Strength: 200 mg

Vivarin: 200 mg

Generic: 200 mg

Extemporaneous Preparations A 10 mg/mL oral solution of caffeine (as citrate) may be prepared from 10 g citrated caffeine powder combined with 10 g citric acid USP and dissolved in 1000 mL sterile water. Label "shake well". Stable for 3 months at room temperature (Nahata, 2004).

A 20 mg/mL oral solution of caffeine (as citrate) may be made from 10 g citrated caffeine powder and dissolved in 250 mL sterile water for irrigation. Stir solution until completely clear, then add a 2:1 mixture of simple syrup and cherry syrup in sufficient quantity to make 500 mL. Label "shake well" and "refrigerate". Stable for 90 days (Eisenberg, 1984).

Eisenberg MG and Kang N, "Stability of Citrated Caffeine Solutions for Injectable and Enteral Use," *Am J Hosp Pharm*, 1984, 41(11):2405-6.

Nahata MC, Pai VB, and Hipple TF, *Pediatric Drug Formulations*, 5th ed, Cincinnati, OH: Harvey Whitney Books Co, 2004.

◆ **Caffeine and Ergotamine** *see* Ergotamine and Caffeine *on page* 776

◆ **Caffeine and Sodium Benzoate** *see* Caffeine *on page* 335

◆ **Caffeine Citrate** *see* Caffeine *on page* 335

◆ **Caffeine Sodium Benzoate** *see* Caffeine *on page* 335

Calamine (KAL a meen)

Therapeutic Category Topical Skin Product

Generic Availability (US) Yes

Use Employed primarily as an astringent, protectant, and soothing agent to relieve itching, pain, and discomfort for conditions such as poison ivy, poison oak, poison sumac, sunburn, insect bites, or minor skin irritations (FDA approved in ages ≥6 months and adults)

Contraindications Hypersensitivity to any component of the formulation

Warnings/Precautions For external use only; avoid contact with eyes and mucous membranes. When using for self-medication (OTC use), discontinue use and contact healthcare provider if needed for >7 days or if condition worsens.

Drug Interactions

Metabolism/Transport Effects None known.

Avoid Concomitant Use There are no known interactions where it is recommended to avoid concomitant use.

Increased Effect/Toxicity There are no known significant interactions involving an increase in effect.

Decreased Effect There are no known significant interactions involving a decrease in effect.

Storage/Stability Store at room temperature of 15°C to 30°C (59°F to 86°F).

Dosing: Usual Skin protectant: Infants, Children, Adolescents, and Adults: Topical: Apply to affected area as often as needed; **Note:** For patients <6 months, consult a physician prior to use.

Administration Topical: Shake well before using. Apply to clean, dry skin; may apply using cotton or a soft cloth. Avoid contact with the eyes and mucous membranes; do not use on open wounds or burns.

Additional Information Active ingredients: Calamine, zinc oxide

Dosage Forms Excipient information presented when available (limited, particularly for generics); consult specific product labeling.

Lotion, External:

Generic: 8% (120 mL, 180 mL, 240 mL)

- ◆ **Calamine Lotion** *see* Calamine *on page* 336
- ◆ **Calan** *see* Verapamil *on page* 2170
- ◆ **Calan SR** *see* Verapamil *on page* 2170
- ◆ **Calax [OTC] (Can)** *see* Docusate *on page* 697
- ◆ **Calcarb 600 [OTC]** *see* Calcium Carbonate *on page* 343
- ◆ **Cal-Carb Forte [OTC]** *see* Calcium Carbonate *on page* 343
- ◆ **Calci-Chew [OTC]** *see* Calcium Carbonate *on page* 343
- ◆ **Calcidol [OTC]** *see* Ergocalciferol *on page* 772
- ◆ **Calciferol [OTC]** *see* Ergocalciferol *on page* 772
- ◆ **Calcijex (Can)** *see* Calcitriol *on page* 338
- ◆ **Calcimar (Can)** *see* Calcitonin *on page* 337
- ◆ **Calci-Mix [OTC] [DSC]** *see* Calcium Carbonate *on page* 343
- ◆ **Calcionate [OTC]** *see* Calcium Glubionate *on page* 349
- ◆ **Calcite-500 (Can)** *see* Calcium Carbonate *on page* 343

Calcitonin (kal si TOE nin)

Medication Safety Issues

Sound-alike/look-alike issues:

Calcitonin may be confused with calcitriol

Fortical may be confused with Foradil

Miacalcin may be confused with Micatin

Administration issues:

Calcitonin nasal spray is administered as a single spray into **one** nostril daily, using alternate nostrils each day.

Brand Names: US Fortical; Miacalcin

Brand Names: Canada Calcimar

Therapeutic Category Antidote, Hypercalcemia

Generic Availability (US) Yes

Use

Parenteral: Treatment of Paget's disease of bone; adjunctive therapy for hypercalcemia; postmenopausal osteoporosis (FDA approved in adults); has also been used for osteogenesis imperfecta

Intranasal: Postmenopausal osteoporosis in women >5 years postmenopause with low bone mass (FDA approved in adults)

Pregnancy Risk Factor C

Pregnancy Considerations Adverse events have been observed in animal reproduction studies. Calcitonin does not cross the placenta.

Breast-Feeding Considerations It is not known if calcitonin is excreted in human breast milk. Calcitonin has been shown to decrease milk production in animals. The manufacturer recommends that caution be exercised when administering calcitonin to nursing women.

Contraindications Hypersensitivity to calcitonin salmon or any component of the formulation

Warnings/Precautions A skin test should be performed prior to initiating therapy of calcitonin salmon in patients with suspected sensitivity; anaphylactic shock, anaphylaxis, bronchospasm, and swelling of the tongue or throat have been reported; have epinephrine immediately available for a possible hypersensitivity reaction. A detailed skin testing protocol is available from the manufacturers. Rhinitis and epistaxis have been reported; mucosal alterations may occur. Perform nasal examinations with visualization of the nasal mucosa, turbinates, septum and mucosal blood vessels prior to initiation of therapy, periodically during therapy, and at any time nasal symptoms occur. Temporarily withdraw use if ulceration of nasal mucosa occurs. Discontinue for severe ulcerations >1.5 mm, those that penetrate below the mucosa, or those associated with heavy bleeding. Patients >65 years of age may experience a higher incidence of nasal adverse events with calcitonin nasal spray.

Hypocalcemia with tetany and seizure activity has been reported. Hypocalcemia and other disorders affecting mineral metabolism (eg, vitamin D deficiency) should be corrected before initiating therapy; monitor serum calcium and symptoms of hypocalcemia during therapy. Administer in conjunction with calcium and vitamin D. Fracture reduction efficacy has not been demonstrated; use has not been shown to increase spinal bone mineral density in early postmenopausal women. Use should be reserved for patients for whom alternative treatments are not suitable (eg, patients for whom other therapies are contraindicated or for patients who are intolerant or unwilling to use other therapies). Analyses of randomized controlled trials (in osteoporosis and osteoarthritis) using the nasal spray and oral formulations have demonstrated a statistically significant increase in the risk of the development of cancer in calcitonin-treated patients (compared to placebo). The risk for malignancies is associated with long-term use of calcitonin (trials ranged from 6 months to 5 years in duration). Periodically reassess continued use of calcitonin therapy, carefully considering the risks versus benefits. Similar risk for other routes (subcutaneous, IM, IV) cannot be ruled out. Definitive efficacy of calcitonin-salmon in decreasing fractures is lacking compared to other agents approved for osteoporosis treatment; consider potential benefits of therapy against risks in osteoporosis treatment, including the potential risk for malignancy with long-term use.

Adverse Reactions

Cardiovascular: Flushing

Central nervous system: Depression, dizziness, paresthesia

Dermatologic: Erythematous rash

Gastrointestinal: Abdominal pain, nausea

Hematologic & oncologic: Lymphadenopathy, malignant neoplasm

Infection: Infection

Local: Injection site reaction (injection)

Neuromuscular & skeletal: Back pain, myalgia, osteoarthritis
Ophthalmic: Abnormal lacrimation, conjunctivitis
Respiratory: Bronchospasm, flu-like symptoms, rhinitis (including ulcerative), sinusitis, upper respiratory tract infection
Rare but important or life-threatening; all routes): Alopecia, altered sense of smell, anorexia, antibody development (drug efficacy can be affected), edema, excoriation (nasal mucosa), hearing loss, hypersensitivity reaction, nocturia, polyuria, tachycardia

Drug Interactions

Metabolism/Transport Effects None known.

Avoid Concomitant Use There are no known interactions where it is recommended to avoid concomitant use.

Increased Effect/Toxicity

Calcitonin may increase the levels/effects of: Zoledronic Acid

Decreased Effect

Calcitonin may decrease the levels/effects of: Lithium

Storage/Stability

Injection: Store under refrigeration at 2°C to 8°C (36°F to 46°F); protect from freezing. The following stability information has also been reported: May be stored at room temperature for up to 14 days (Cohen, 2007).
Nasal: Store unopened bottle under refrigeration at 2°C to 8°C (36°F to 46°F); do not freeze.
Fortical: After opening, store for up to 30 days at 20°C to 25°C (68°F to 77°F); excursions permitted to 15°C to 30°C (59°F to 86°F). Store in upright position.
Miacalcin: After opening, store for up to 35 days at room temperature of 15°C to 30°C (59°F to 86°F). Store in upright position.

Mechanism of Action Peptide sequence similar to human calcitonin; functionally antagonizes the effects of parathyroid hormone. Directly inhibits osteoclastic bone resorption; promotes the renal excretion of calcium, phosphate, sodium, magnesium, and potassium by decreasing tubular reabsorption; increases the jejunal secretion of water, sodium, potassium, and chloride

Pharmacodynamics

Onset of action:
Hypercalcemia: IM, SubQ: ~2 hours
Paget's disease: Within a few months; may take up to 1 year for neurologic symptom improvement
Duration: Hypercalcemia: IM, SubQ: 6-8 hours

Pharmacokinetics (Adult data unless noted)

Absorption: Intranasal: Rapidly but highly variable and lower than IM administration
Metabolism: Rapidly in the kidneys, blood, and peripheral tissues
Bioavailability: IM 66%; SubQ: 71%
Half-life, elimination (terminal): IM: 58 minutes; SubQ: 59-64 minutes
Time to peak serum concentration: SubQ ~23 minutes
Elimination: As inactive metabolites in urine
Clearance: Salmon calcitonin: 3.1 mL/kg/minute

Dosing: Usual

Pediatric: **Osteogenesis imperfecta:** Infants >6 months, Children, and Adolescents: IM, SubQ: 2 units/kg/dose 3 times/week (Castells, 1979)
Adult:
Paget's disease: Miacalcin: IM, SubQ: Initial: 100 units/day; maintenance dose: 50 units/day or 50-100 units every 1-2 days; may be preferable to maintain doses of 100 units daily for serious deformity or neurologic involvement
Hypercalcemia: Miacalcin: Initial: IM, SubQ: 4 units/kg every 12 hours for 1-2 days; may increase up to 8 units/kg every 12 hours; if the response remains unsatisfactory after 2 additional days, a further increase up to a maximum of 8 units/kg every 6 hours may be considered
Postmenopausal osteoporosis:
Miacalcin: IM, SubQ: 100 units every other day
Fortical, Miacalcin: Intranasal: 200 units (1 spray) into **one** nostril daily

Administration

Intranasal: Before first use, allow bottle to reach room temperature, then prime pump by releasing at least 5 sprays until full spray is produced. To administer, place nozzle into nostril with head in upright position. Spray into **one** nostril daily; alternate nostrils to reduce irritation. Do not prime pump before each daily use. Discard after 30 doses.
Parenteral: May be administered SubQ or IM; do not exceed 2 mL volume per injection site; SubQ is preferred for outpatient self administration unless the injection volume is >2 mL; IM is preferred if the injection volume is >2 mL (use multiple injection sites if dose volume is >2 mL).

Monitoring Parameters Serum electrolytes and calcium, alkaline phosphatase and 24-hour urine collection for hydroxyproline excretion (Paget's disease); urinalysis (urine sediment); serum calcium; periodic nasal exams (intranasal use only)

Dosage Forms Excipient information presented when available (limited, particularly for generics); consult specific product labeling.
Solution, Injection:
Miacalcin: 200 units/mL (2 mL)
Solution, Nasal:
Fortical: 200 units/actuation (3.7 mL)
Miacalcin: 200 units/actuation (3.7 mL)
Generic: 200 units/actuation (3.7 mL)

◆ **Calcitonin (Salmon)** *see* Calcitonin *on page 337*
◆ **Cal-Citrate [OTC]** *see* Calcium Citrate *on page 348*

Calcitriol (kal si TRYE ole)

Medication Safety Issues

Sound-alike/look-alike issues:
Calcitriol may be confused with alfacalcidol, Calciferol, calcitonin, calcium carbonate, captopril, colestipol, paricalcitol, ropinirole
Administration issues:
Dosage is expressed in mcg (micrograms), **not** mg (milligrams); rare cases of acute overdose have been reported

Brand Names: US Rocaltrol; Vectical

Brand Names: Canada Calcijex; Calcitriol Injection; Calcitriol-Odan; Rocaltrol; Silkis

Therapeutic Category Rickets, Treatment Agent; Vitamin D Analog; Vitamin, Fat Soluble

Generic Availability (US) Yes

Use

Oral/Injection: Management of secondary hyperparathyroidism and resultant metabolic bone disease in patients with moderate-to-severe chronic renal failure not yet on dialysis (FDA approved in ages ≥3 years and adults); management of hypocalcemia and resultant metabolic bone disease in patients on chronic renal dialysis (FDA approved in ages ≥18 years); management of hypocalcemia in patients with hypoparathyroidism (FDA approved in ages ≥1 year and adults) and pseudohypoparathyroidism (FDA approved in ages ≥6 years and adults)
Topical: Management of mild-to-moderate plaque psoriasis (FDA approved in ages ≥18 years)

Pregnancy Risk Factor C

Pregnancy Considerations Teratogenic effects have been observed in some animal reproduction studies. Mild hypercalcemia has been reported in a newborn following maternal use of calcitriol during pregnancy. Adverse effects on fetal development were not observed with use of calcitriol during pregnancy in women (N=9) with pseudovitamin D-dependent rickets. Doses were adjusted every 4 weeks to keep calcium concentrations within normal limits (Edouard, 2011). If calcitriol is used for the management of hypoparathyroidism in pregnancy, dose adjustments may be needed as pregnancy progresses and again following delivery. Vitamin D and calcium levels should be monitored closely and kept in the lower normal range.

Breast-Feeding Considerations Low levels are found in breast milk (~2 pg/mL)

Contraindications

U.S. labeling:

Oral, injection: Hypersensitivity to calcitriol or any component of the formulation; hypercalcemia, vitamin D toxicity

Topical: There are no contraindications listed in the manufacturer's labeling.

Canadian labeling:

Oral, injection: Hypersensitivity to calcitriol, vitamin D or its analogues or derivatives, or any component of the formulation or container; hypercalcemia, vitamin D toxicity

Topical: Ophthalmic or internal use; hypercalcemia or a history of abnormal calcium metabolism; concurrent systemic treatment of calcium homeostasis; severe renal impairment or end-stage renal disease (ESRD)

Warnings/Precautions Oral, injection: Adequate dietary (supplemental) calcium is necessary for clinical response to vitamin D. Excessive vitamin D may cause severe hypercalcemia, hypercalciuria, and hyperphosphatemia. Discontinue use immediately in adult patients with a calcium-phosphate product (serum calcium times phosphorus) >70 mg^2/dL^2, may resume therapy at decreased doses when levels are appropriate. Other forms of vitamin D should be withheld during therapy to avoid the potential for hypercalcemia to develop. In addition, several months may be required for ergocalciferol levels to return to baseline in patients switching from ergocalciferol therapy to calcitriol. Monitor calcium levels closely with initiation of therapy and with dose adjustments; discontinue use promptly in patients who develop hypercalcemia. Avoid abrupt dietary modifications (eg, increased intake of dairy products) which may lead to hypercalcemia; adjust calcium intake if indicated and maintain adequate hydration. Chronic hypercalcemia can result in generalized vascular and soft tissue calcification. Immobilized patients may be at a higher risk for hypercalcemia.

Use oral calcitriol with caution in patients with malabsorption syndromes (efficacy may be limited and/or response may be unpredictable). Use of calcitriol for the treatment of secondary hyperparathyroidism associated with CKD is not recommended in patients with rapidly worsening kidney function or in noncompliant patients. Increased serum phosphate levels in patients with renal failure may lead to calcification; the use of an aluminum-containing phosphate binder is recommended along with a low phosphate diet in these patients. Use with caution in patients taking cardiac glycosides; digitalis toxicity is potentiated by hypocalcemia. Concomitant use with magnesium-containing products such as antacids may lead to hypermagnesemia in patients receiving chronic renal dialysis.

Aluminum: The parenteral product may contain aluminum; toxic aluminum concentrations may be seen with high doses, prolonged use, or renal dysfunction. Premature neonates are at higher risk due to immature renal function and aluminum intake from other parenteral sources. Parenteral aluminum exposure of >4 to 5 mcg/kg/day is associated with CNS and bone toxicity; tissue loading may occur at lower doses (Federal Register, 2002). See manufacturer's labeling. Products may contain coconut (capsule) or palm seed oil (oral solution). Some products may contain tartrazine.

Topical: May cause hypercalcemia; if alterations in calcium occur, discontinue treatment until levels return to normal. For external use only; not for ophthalmic, oral, or intravaginal use. Do not apply to facial skin, eyes, or lips. Absorption may be increased with occlusive dressings. Avoid or limit excessive exposure to natural or artificial sunlight, or phototherapy. The safety and effectiveness has not been evaluated in patients with erythrodermic, exfoliative, or pustular psoriasis. Canadian labeling does not recommend use in patients with hepatic or renal impairment.

Warnings: Additional Pediatric Considerations Monitor serum calcium levels closely; the calcitriol dosage should be adjusted accordingly; serum calcium times phosphorus product (Ca x P) should not exceed 65 mg^2/dL^2 for infants and children <12 years of age and 55 mg^2/dL^2 for adolescents.

Adverse Reactions

Oral, IV:

Cardiovascular: Cardiac arrhythmia, hypertension

Central nervous system: Apathy, drowsiness, headache, hyperthermia, metallic taste, psychosis, sensory disturbance

Dermatologic: Erythema, erythema multiforme, pruritus, skin rash, urticaria

Endocrine & metabolic: Albuminuria, calcinosis, decreased libido, dehydration, growth suppression, hypercalcemia, hypercholesterolemia, polydipsia, weight loss

Gastrointestinal: Abdominal pain, anorexia, constipation, nausea, pancreatitis, stomach pain, vomiting, xerostomia

Genitourinary: Hypercalciuria, nocturia, urinary tract infection

Hepatic: Increased serum ALT, increased serum AST

Hypersensitivity: Hypersensitivity reaction

Local: Pain at injection site (mild)

Neuromuscular & skeletal: Dystrophy, myalgia, ostealgia, weakness

Ophthalmic: Conjunctivitis, photophobia

Renal: Calcium nephrolithiasis, increased blood urea nitrogen, increased serum creatinine, polyuria

Respiratory: Rhinorrhea

Rare but important or life-threatening: Anaphylaxis

Topical:

Dermatologic: Pruritus, psoriasis, skin discomfort

Endocrine & metabolic: Hypercalcemia

Genitourinary: Urine abnormality, hypercalciuria

Rare but important or life-threatening: Kidney stones

Drug Interactions

Metabolism/Transport Effects Substrate of CYP3A4 (major); **Note:** Assignment of Major/Minor substrate status based on clinically relevant drug interaction potential; **Induces** CYP3A4 (weak)

Avoid Concomitant Use

Avoid concomitant use of Calcitriol with any of the following: Aluminum Hydroxide; Conivaptan; Fusidic Acid (Systemic); Idelalisib; Multivitamins/Fluoride (with ADE); Multivitamins/Minerals (with ADEK, Folate, Iron); Sucralfate; Vitamin D Analogs

Increased Effect/Toxicity

Calcitriol may increase the levels/effects of: Aluminum Hydroxide; Cardiac Glycosides; Magnesium Salts; Sucralfate; Vitamin D Analogs

The levels/effects of Calcitriol may be increased by: Aprepitant; Calcium Salts; Ceritinib; Conivaptan; CYP3A4 Inhibitors (Moderate); CYP3A4 Inhibitors

(Strong); Danazol; Dasatinib; Fosaprepitant; Fusidic Acid (Systemic); Idelalisib; Ivacaftor; Luliconazole; Mifepristone; Multivitamins/Fluoride (with ADE); Multivitamins/Minerals (with ADEK, Folate, Iron); Netupitant; Palbociclib; Simeprevir; Stiripentol; Thiazide Diuretics

Decreased Effect

Calcitriol may decrease the levels/effects of: ARIPiprazole; Hydrocodone; Saxagliptin

The levels/effects of Calcitriol may be decreased by: Bile Acid Sequestrants; Bosentan; Corticosteroids (Systemic); CYP3A4 Inducers (Moderate); CYP3A4 Inducers (Strong); Dabrafenib; Deferasirox; Mineral Oil; Mitotane; Orlistat; Sevelamer; Siltuximab; St Johns Wort; Tocilizumab

Storage/Stability

Oral capsule, injection, solution: Store at room temperature of 15°C to 30°C (59°F to 86°F). Protect from light.

Topical: Store at room temperature of 25°C (77°F); excursions permitted to 15°C to 30°C (59°F to 86°F); do not refrigerate; do not freeze.

Mechanism of Action Calcitriol, the active form of vitamin D (1,25 hydroxyvitamin D_3), binds to and activates the vitamin D receptor in kidney, parathyroid gland, intestine, and bone, stimulating intestinal calcium transport and absorption. It reduces PTH levels and improves calcium and phosphate homeostasis by stimulating bone resorption of calcium and increasing renal tubular reabsorption of calcium. Decreased renal conversion of vitamin D to its primary active metabolite (1,25 hydroxyvitamin D) in chronic renal failure leads to reduced activation of vitamin D receptor, which subsequently removes inhibitory suppression of parathyroid hormone (PTH) release; increased serum PTH (secondary hyperparathyroidism) reduces calcium excretion and enhances bone resorption.

The mechanism by which calcitriol is beneficial in the treatment of psoriasis has not been established.

Pharmacodynamics Oral:

Onset of action: 2 hours

Maximum effect: 10 hours

Duration: 3-5 days

Pharmacokinetics (Adult data unless noted)

Distribution: Breast milk: Very low (levels 2.2 ± 0.1 pg/mL)

Protein binding: 99.9%

Metabolism: Primarily to 1,24,25-trihydroxycholecalciferol and 1,24,25-trihydroxy ergocalciferol

Half-life:

- Children 1.8-16 years undergoing peritoneal dialysis: 27.4 hours
- Adults without renal dysfunction: 5-8 hours
- Adults with CRF: 16.2-21.9 hours

Time to peak serum concentration: Oral: 3-6 hours

Elimination: Feces 27% and urine 7% excreted unchanged in 24 hours

- Clearance: Children 1.8-16 years undergoing peritoneal dialysis: 15.3 mL/hour/kg

Dosing: Neonatal

Hypocalcemia secondary to hypoparathyroidism: Oral: 1 mcg once daily for the first 5 days of life

- Alternate regimen: Oral: 0.02-0.06 mcg/kg/day; similar dosage has also been described in neonates with DiGeorge syndrome (Miller, 1983)

Hypocalcemic tetany:

- IV: 0.05 mcg/kg once daily for 5-12 days
- Oral: Initial: 0.25 mcg/dose once daily, followed by 0.01-0.10 mcg/kg/day divided in 2 doses (maximum daily dose: 2 mcg)

Dosing: Usual

Management of hypocalcemia in patients with chronic kidney disease (CKD): Indicated for therapy when serum levels of 25(OH)D are >30 ng/mL (75 nmol/L) and serum levels of intact parathyroid hormone (iPTH) are above the target range for the stage of CKD; serum levels of corrected total calcium are <9.5-10 mg/dL (2.37 mmol/L) and serum levels of phosphorus in children are less than age-appropriate upper limits of normal or in adults <4.6 mg/dL (1.49 mmol/L) (K/DOQI Guidelines, 2005):

Children and Adolescents: CKD Stages 2-4: Oral:

- <10 kg: 0.05 mcg every other day
- 10-20 kg: 0.1-0.15 mcg daily
- >20 kg: 0.25 mcg daily
- Dosage adjustment:
  - If iPTH decrease is <30% after 3 months of therapy and serum levels of calcium and phosphorus are within the target ranges based upon the CKD Stage, increase dosage by 50%
  - If iPTH decrease < target range for CKD stage hold calcitriol therapy until iPTH increases to above target range; resume therapy at half the previous dosage (if dosage <0.25 mcg capsule or 0.05 mcg liquid, use every other day therapy)
  - If serum levels of total corrected calcium exceed 10.2 mg/dL (2.37 mmol/L) hold calcitriol therapy until serum calcium decreased to <9.8 mg/dL (2.37 mmol/L); resume therapy at half the previous dosage (if dosage <0.25 mcg capsule or 0.05 mcg liquid, use every other day therapy)
  - If serum levels of phosphorus increase to > age-appropriate upper limits, hold calcitriol therapy (initiate or increase phosphate binders until the levels of serum phosphorus decrease to age-appropriate limits); resume therapy at half the previous dosage

Children and Adolescents: CKD Stage 5: Oral, IV: Serum calcium times phosphorus product (Ca x P) should not exceed 65 mg^2/dL^2 for infants and children <12 years of age and 55 mg^2/dL^2 for adolescents, serum phosphorus should be within target, serum calcium <10 mg/dL (2.37 mmol/L):

- iPTH 300-500 pg/mL: 0.0075 mcg/kg per dialysis session (3 times/week); not to exceed 0.25 mcg daily
- iPTH >500-1000 pg/mL: 0.015 mcg/kg per dialysis session (3 times/week); not to exceed 0.5 mcg daily
- iPTH >1000 pg/mL: 0.025 mcg/kg per dialysis session (3 times/week); not to exceed 1 mcg daily
- Dosage adjustment: If iPTH decrease is <30% after 3 months of therapy and serum levels of calcium and phosphorus are within the target ranges based upon the CKD Stage 5, increase dosage by 50%

Adult CKD Stages 3 or 4: Serum calcium <9.5 mg/dL (2.37 mmol/L), serum phosphorus <5.5 mg/dL (1.77 mmol/L), serum calcium times phosphorus product (Ca x P) <55 mg^2/dL^2:

- iPTH 300-600 pg/mL: Oral, IV: 0.5-1.5 mcg per dialysis session (3 times/week)
- iPTH 600-1000 pg/mL: IV: 1-3 mcg per dialysis session (3 times/week); Oral: 1-4 mcg per dialysis session (3 times/week)
- iPTH >1000 pg/mL: IV 3-5 mcg per dialysis session (3 times/week); Oral: 3-7 mcg per dialysis session (3 times/week)
- Dosage adjustment:
  - If iPTH decrease < target range for CKD stage 5 hold calcitriol therapy until iPTH increases to above target range; resume therapy at half the previous dosage (if dosage <0.25 mcg capsule or 0.05 mcg liquid, use every other day therapy)

If serum levels of total corrected calcium exceed 9.5 mg/dL (2.37 mmol/L) hold calcitriol therapy until serum calcium decreased to <9.5 mg/dL (2.37 mmol/L); resume therapy at half the previous dosage (if dosage <0.25 mcg capsule or 0.05 mcg liquid, use every other day therapy)

If serum levels of phosphorus increase to >4.6 mg/dL (1.49 mmol/L), hold calcitriol therapy (initiate or increase phosphate binders until the levels of serum phosphorus decrease to 4.6 mg/dL (1.49 mmol/L); resume therapy at prior dosage

Note: Intermittent administration of calcitriol by IV or oral routes is more effective than daily oral calcitriol in lowering iPTH levels.

Hypoparathyroidism/pseudohypoparathyroidism: Oral (evaluate dosage at 2- to 4-week intervals):
- Infants <1 year: 0.04-0.08 mcg/kg once daily
- Children 1-5 years: 0.25-0.75 mcg once daily
- Children >6 years and Adults: 0.5-2 mcg once daily

Vitamin D-dependent rickets: Children and Adults: Oral: 1 mcg once daily

Vitamin D-resistant rickets (familial hypophosphatemia): Children and Adults: Oral: Initial: 0.015-0.02 mcg/kg once daily; maintenance: 0.03-0.06 mcg/kg once daily; maximum dose: 2 mcg once daily

Psoriasis: Adults: Topical: Apply twice daily to affected areas (maximum: 200 g/week)

Administration

Oral: May be administered with or without meals; when administering small doses from the liquid-filled capsules, consider the following concentration for Rocaltrol®:
- 0.25 mcg capsule = 0.25 mcg per 0.17 mL
- 0.5 mcg capsule = 0.5 mcg per 0.17 mL

Parenteral: May be administered undiluted as a bolus dose IV through the catheter at the end of hemodialysis

Topical: Apply externally; not for ophthalmic, oral, or intravaginal use

Monitoring Parameters Signs and symptoms of vitamin D intoxication

Serum calcium and phosphorus:
- IV: Twice weekly during initial phase, then at least monthly once dose established
- Oral: At least every 2 weeks for 3 months or following dose adjustment, then monthly for 3 months, then every 3 months

Serum or plasma intact parathyroid hormone (iPTH): At least every 2 weeks for 3 months or following dose adjustment, then monthly for 3 months, then as per K/DOQI Guidelines below.

Per Kidney Disease Outcome Quality Initiative Practice Guidelines: Children (K/DOQI, 2005):
- Stage 3 CKD: iPTH every 6 months
- Stage 4 CKD: iPTH every 3 months
- Stage 5 CKD: iPTH every 3 months

Per Kidney Disease Outcome Quality Initiative Practice Guidelines: Adults (K/DOQI, 2003):
- Stage 3 CKD: iPTH every 12 months
- Stage 4 CKD: iPTH every 3 months
- Stage 5 CKD: iPTH every 3 months

Reference Range

Chronic kidney disease (CKD) is defined either as kidney damage or GFR <60 mL/minute/1.73 m^2 for ≥3 months); stages of CKD are described below:
- CKD Stage 1: Kidney damage with normal or increased GFR; GFR >90 mL/minute/1.73m^2
- CKD Stage 2: Kidney damage with mild decrease in GFR; GFR 60-89 mL/minute/1.73 m^2
- CKD Stage 3: Moderate decrease in GFR; GFR 30-59 mL/minute/1.73 m^2
- CKD Stage 4: Severe decrease in GFR; GFR 15-29 mL/minute/1.73 m^2
- CKD Stage 5: Kidney failure; GFR <15 mL/minute/1.73 m^2 or dialysis

Target range for iPTH:
- Stage 2 CKD: Children: 35-70 pg/mL (3.85-7.7 pmol/L)
- Stage 3 CKD: Children and Adults: 35-70 pg/mL (3.85-7.7 pmol/L)
- Stage 4 CKD: Children and Adults: 70-110 pg/mL (7.7-12.1 pmol/L)
- Stage 5 CKD:
  - Children: 200-300 pg/mL (22-33 pmol/L)
  - Adults: 150-300 pg/mL (16.5-33 pmol/L)

Serum phosphorous:
- Stages 1-4 CKD: Children: At or above the age-appropriate lower limits and no higher than age-appropriate upper limits
- Stage 3 and 4 CKD: Adults: ≥2.7 to <4.6 mg/dL (≥0.87 to <1.49 mmol/L)
- Stage 5 CKD:
  - Children 1-12 years: 4-6 mg/dL (1.29-1.94 mmol/L)
  - Children >12 years and Adults: 3.5-5.5 mg/dL (1.13-1.78 mmol/L)

Dosage Forms Excipient information presented when available (limited, particularly for generics); consult specific product labeling.

Capsule, Oral:
- Rocaltrol: 0.25 mcg, 0.5 mcg [contains fd&c yellow #6 (sunset yellow), methylparaben, propylparaben]
- Generic: 0.25 mcg, 0.5 mcg

Ointment, External:
- Vectical: 3 mcg/g (100 g)
- Generic: 3 mcg/g (100 g)

Solution, Intravenous:
- Generic: 1 mcg/mL (1 mL)

Solution, Oral:
- Rocaltrol: 1 mcg/mL (15 mL)
- Generic: 1 mcg/mL (15 mL)

◆ **Calcitriol Injection (Can)** *see* Calcitriol *on page 338*

◆ **Calcitriol-Odan (Can)** *see* Calcitriol *on page 338*

◆ **Calcium 600 [OTC]** *see* Calcium Carbonate *on page 343*

Calcium Acetate (KAL see um AS e tate)

Medication Safety Issues

Sound-alike/look-alike issues:

PhosLo® may be confused with Phos-Flur®, ProSom

Brand Names: US Calphron [OTC]; Eliphos; PhosLo; Phoslyra

Brand Names: Canada PhosLo®

Therapeutic Category Calcium Salt; Electrolyte Supplement, Parenteral

Generic Availability (US) May be product dependent

Use Treatment of hyperphosphatemia in end-stage renal failure (FDA approved in adults)

Pregnancy Risk Factor C

Pregnancy Considerations Animal reproduction studies have not been conducted. Calcium crosses the placenta. The amount of calcium reaching the fetus is determined by maternal physiological changes. Intestinal absorption of calcium increases during pregnancy. If use is required in pregnant patients with end stage renal disease, fetal harm is not expected if maternal calcium concentrations are monitored and maintained within normal limits as recommended (IOM, 2011).

Breast-Feeding Considerations Calcium is excreted in breast milk. The amount of calcium in breast milk is homeostatically regulated and not altered by maternal calcium intake (IOM, 2011).

Contraindications Hypersensitivity to any component of the formulation; hypercalcemia, renal calculi

Warnings/Precautions Constipation, bloating, and gas are common with calcium supplements. Hypercalcemia and hypercalciuria are most likely to occur in hypoparathyroid patients receiving high doses of vitamin D. Use with caution in patients who may be at risk of cardiac arrhythmias. Use with caution in digitalized patients; hypercalcemia may precipitate cardiac arrhythmias. Calcium administration interferes with absorption of some minerals and drugs; use with caution. Oral solution may contain maltitol (a sugar substitute) which may cause a laxative effect. Multiple salt forms of calcium exist; close attention must be paid to the salt form when ordering and administering calcium; incorrect selection or substitution of one salt for another without proper dosage adjustment may result in serious over or under dosing.

Warnings: Additional Pediatric Considerations Some dosage forms may contain propylene glycol; in neonates large amounts of propylene glycol delivered orally, intravenously (eg, >3,000 mg/day), or topically have been associated with potentially fatal toxicities which can include metabolic acidosis, seizures, renal failure, and CNS depression; toxicities have also been reported in children and adults including hyperosmolality, lactic acidosis, seizures and respiratory depression; use caution (AAP, 1997; Shehab, 2009).

Adverse Reactions

Endocrine & metabolic: Hypercalcemia

Gastrointestinal: Diarrhea (oral solution), nausea, vomiting

Rare but important or life-threatening: Dizziness, edema, pruritus, weakness

Drug Interactions

Metabolism/Transport Effects None known.

Avoid Concomitant Use

Avoid concomitant use of Calcium Acetate with any of the following: Calcium Salts

Increased Effect/Toxicity

Calcium Acetate may increase the levels/effects of: Cardiac Glycosides; CefTRIAXone; Vitamin D Analogs

The levels/effects of Calcium Acetate may be increased by: Calcium Salts; Multivitamins/Fluoride (with ADE); Multivitamins/Minerals (with ADEK, Folate, Iron); Thiazide Diuretics

Decreased Effect

Calcium Acetate may decrease the levels/effects of: Alpha-Lipoic Acid; Bisphosphonate Derivatives; Calcium Channel Blockers; Deferiprone; DOBUTamine; Dolutegravir; Eltrombopag; Estramustine; Multivitamins/Fluoride (with ADE); Phosphate Supplements; Quinolone Antibiotics; Strontium Ranelate; Tetracycline Derivatives; Thyroid Products; Trientine

The levels/effects of Calcium Acetate may be decreased by: Alpha-Lipoic Acid; Trientine

Food Interactions Foods that contain maltitol may have an additive laxative effect with the oral solution formulation (contains maltitol).

Mechanism of Action Combines with dietary phosphate to form insoluble calcium phosphate which is excreted in feces

Pharmacokinetics (Adult data unless noted)

Absorption: 30% to 40%

Elimination: Primarily in the feces as unabsorbed calcium

Dosing: Usual Note: Dose expressed in mg of **calcium acetate**. Phosphate binding capacity: Calcium acetate 1 g binds 45 mg of phosphorus (KDOQI 2005)

Pediatric: **Control of hyperphosphatemia in end-stage renal failure:** Limited data available; dose should be individualized: Children and Adolescents: Oral: Reported initial dose: 667 to 1,000 mg with each meal; titrate (every 2 to 4 weeks) to response and as serum calcium levels allow (Gulati 2010; Wallot 1996). **Note:** KDOQI guidelines recommend limiting the calcium provided from phosphate binders to 1,500 mg elemental calcium per day and total intake to 2,000 mg elemental calcium from all sources (KDOQI 2010)

Adult: **Control of hyperphosphatemia (ESRD, on dialysis):** Oral: Initial: 1,334 mg with each meal; may increase gradually (ie, every 2 to 3 weeks) to bring the serum phosphate value <6 mg/dL as long as hypercalcemia does not develop. Usual dose: 2,001 to 2,668 mg calcium acetate with each meal; do not give additional calcium supplements

Dosing adjustment in renal impairment: No dosage adjustment necessary.

Dosing adjustment in hepatic impairment: There are no dosage adjustments provided in the manufacturer's labeling.

Administration Oral: Administer with plenty of fluids with meals to optimize effectiveness

Monitoring Parameters Serum calcium (twice weekly during initial dose adjustments), serum phosphorus; serum calcium-phosphorus product; intact parathyroid hormone (iPTH)

Reference Range

Corrected total serum calcium: Children, Adolescents, and Adults: CKD stages 2 to 5D: Maintain normal ranges; preferably on the lower end for stage 5 (KDIGO 2009; KDOQI 2005)

Phosphorus (KDIGO 2009):

CKD stages 3 to 5: Maintain normal ranges

CKD stage 5D: Lower elevated phosphorus levels toward the normal range

Additional Information Due to a poor correlation between the serum ionized calcium (free) and total serum calcium, particularly in states of low albumin or acid/base imbalances, direct measurement of ionized calcium is recommended. If ionized calcium is unavailable, in low albumin states, the corrected **total** serum calcium may be estimated by this equation (assuming a normal albumin of 4 g/dL); [(4 – patient's albumin) x 0.8] + patient's measured total calcium

Elemental Calcium Content of Calcium Salts

Calcium Salt	Elemental Calcium (mg/1 g of salt form)	Calcium (mEq/g)
Calcium acetate	253	12.7
Calcium carbonate	400	20
Calcium chloride	273	13.6
Calcium citrate	211	10.5
Calcium glubionate	63.8	3.2
Calcium gluconate	93	4.65
Calcium lactate	130	6.5
Calcium phosphate (tribasic)	390	19.3

Chronic kidney disease (CKD) (KDIGO 2013; KDOQI 2002): Children ≥2 years, Adolescents, and Adults: GFR <60 mL/minute/1.73 m^2 or kidney damage for >3 months; stages of CKD are described below:

CKD Stage 1: Kidney damage with normal or increased GFR; GFR >90 mL/minute/1.73 m^2

CKD Stage 2: Kidney damage with mild decrease in GFR; GFR 60 to 89 mL/minute/1.73 m^2

CKD Stage 3: Moderate decrease in GFR; GFR 30 to 59 mL/minute/1.73 m^2

CKD Stage 4: Severe decrease in GFR; GFR 15 to 29 mL/minute/1.73 m^2

CKD Stage 5: Kidney failure; GFR <15 mL/minute/1.73 m^2 or dialysis

Dosage Forms Considerations

Calcium acetate is approximately 25% elemental calcium

Calcium acetate 667 mg = elemental calcium 169 mg = calcium 8.45 mEq = calcium 4.23 mmol

Dosage Forms Excipient information presented when available (limited, particularly for generics); consult specific product labeling.

Capsule, Oral:

PhosLo: 667 mg

Generic: 667 mg

Solution, Oral:

Phoslyra: 667 mg/5 mL (473 mL) [contains methylparaben, propylene glycol]

Tablet, Oral:

Calphron: 667 mg

Eliphos: 667 mg

Generic: 667 mg, 668 mg

- ◆ **Calcium Acetate and Aluminum Sulfate** *see* Aluminum Acetate *on page 110*
- ◆ **Calcium Antacid [OTC]** *see* Calcium Carbonate *on page 343*
- ◆ **Calcium Antacid Extra Strength [OTC]** *see* Calcium Carbonate *on page 343*
- ◆ **Calcium Antacid Ultra Max St [OTC]** *see* Calcium Carbonate *on page 343*

Calcium Carbonate (KAL see um KAR bun ate)

Medication Safety Issues

Sound-alike/look-alike issues:

Calcium carbonate may be confused with calcitriol

Children's Pepto may be confused with Pepto-Bismol products

Maalox and Children's Maalox may be confused with other Maalox products

Mylanta may be confused with Mynatal

Os-Cal [DSC] may be confused with Asacol

International issues:

Remegel [Hungary, Great Britain, and Ireland] may be confused with Renagel brand name for sevelamer [U.S., Canada, and multiple international markets]

Remegel: Brand name for calcium carbonate [Hungary, Great Britain, and Ireland], but also the brand name for aluminum hydroxide and magnesium carbonate [Netherlands]

Brand Names: US Alcalak [OTC]; Antacid Calcium Extra Strength [OTC]; Antacid Calcium [OTC]; Antacid Extra Strength [OTC]; Antacid [OTC]; Cal-Carb Forte [OTC]; Cal-Gest Antacid [OTC]; Cal-Mint [OTC]; Calcarb 600 [OTC]; Calci-Chew [OTC]; Calci-Mix [OTC] [DSC]; Calcium 600 [OTC]; Calcium Antacid Extra Strength [OTC]; Calcium Antacid Ultra Max St [OTC]; Calcium Antacid [OTC]; Calcium High Potency [OTC]; Caltrate 600 [OTC]; Florical [OTC]; Maalox Childrens [OTC]; Maalox [OTC]; Os-Cal [OTC] [DSC]; Oysco 500 [OTC]; Titralac [OTC]; Tums Chewy Delights [OTC]; Tums E-X 750 [OTC]; Tums Freshers [OTC]; Tums Kids [OTC]; Tums Lasting Effects [OTC]; Tums Smoothies [OTC]; Tums Ultra 1000 [OTC]; Tums [OTC]

Brand Names: Canada Apo-Cal; Calcite-500; Caltrate; Caltrate Select; Os-Cal; Tums Chews Extra Strength; Tums Extra Strength; Tums Regular Strength; Tums Smoothies; Tums Ultra Strength

Therapeutic Category Antacid; Calcium Salt; Electrolyte Supplement, Oral

Generic Availability (US) May be product dependent

Use Symptomatic relief of hyperacidity associated with peptic ulcer, gastritis, esophagitis, and hiatal hernia; treatment of hyperphosphatemia in end-stage renal failure; dietary supplement; prevention and treatment of calcium deficiency; topical treatment of hydrofluoric acid burns; adjunctive prevention and treatment of osteoporosis

Pregnancy Considerations Calcium crosses the placenta. Intestinal absorption of calcium increases during pregnancy. The amount of calcium reaching the fetus is determined by maternal physiological changes. Calcium requirements are the same in pregnant and nonpregnant females (IOM, 2011). Calcium-based antacids are considered low risk during pregnancy; excessive use should be avoided (Mahadevan, 2006).

Breast-Feeding Considerations Calcium is excreted in breast milk. The amount of calcium in breast milk is homeostatically regulated and not altered by maternal calcium intake. Calcium requirements are the same in lactating and nonlactating females (IOM 2011). Calcium-based antacids are probably compatible with breast-feeding (Mahadevan, 2006).

Contraindications Hypersensitivity to any component of the formulation

Warnings/Precautions Constipation, bloating, and gas are common with calcium supplements. Calcium absorption is impaired in achlorhydria; administration is followed by increased gastric acid secretion within 2 hours of administration especially with high doses. Common in the elderly; use an alternate salt (eg, citrate) and administer with food. Hypercalcemia and hypercalciuria are most likely to occur in hypoparathyroid patients receiving high doses of vitamin D. Use caution when administering calcium supplements to patients with a history of kidney stones. Patients with renal insufficiency are more sensitive or susceptible to the effects of excess calcium; use with caution. It is recommended to concomitantly administer vitamin D for optimal calcium absorption when used for the treatment or prevention of conditions related to bone health (eg, osteoporosis). Multiple salt forms of calcium exist; close attention must be paid to the salt form when ordering and administering calcium; incorrect selection or substitution of one salt for another without proper dosage adjustment may result in serious over or under dosing.

Adverse Reactions Well tolerated

Central nervous system: Headache, laxative effect

Endocrine & metabolic: Hypercalcemia, hypophosphatemia, milk-alkali syndrome (with very high, chronic dosing and/or renal failure [headache, nausea, irritability, and weakness or alkalosis, hypercalcemia, renal impairment])

Gastrointestinal: Abdominal pain, anorexia, constipation, flatulence, hyperacidity (acid rebound), nausea, vomiting, xerostomia

Drug Interactions

Metabolism/Transport Effects None known.

Avoid Concomitant Use

Avoid concomitant use of Calcium Carbonate with any of the following: Calcium Acetate

Increased Effect/Toxicity

Calcium Carbonate may increase the levels/effects of: Amphetamines; Calcium Acetate; Calcium Polystyrene Sulfonate; Cardiac Glycosides; Dexmethylphenidate; Methylphenidate; QuiNIDine; Sodium Polystyrene Sulfonate; Vitamin D Analogs

The levels/effects of Calcium Carbonate may be increased by: Multivitamins/Fluoride (with ADE); Thiazide Diuretics

Decreased Effect

Calcium Carbonate may decrease the levels/effects of: Allopurinol; Alpha-Lipoic Acid; Antipsychotic Agents (Phenothiazines); Atazanavir; Bisacodyl; Bismuth Subcitrate; Bisphosphonate Derivatives; Bosutinib; Calcium Channel Blockers; Captopril; Cefditoren; Cefpodoxime; Cefuroxime; Chloroquine; Corticosteroids (Oral); Dabigatran Etexilate; Dabrafenib; Dasatinib; Deferiprone; Delavirdine; DOBUTamine; Dolutegravir; Eltrombopag; Elvitegravir; Erlotinib; Estramustine; Fosinopril; Gabapentin; HMG-CoA Reductase Inhibitors; Hyoscyamine; Iron Salts; Isoniazid; Itraconazole; Ketoconazole (Systemic); Ledipasvir; Mesalamine; Methenamine; Multivitamins/Fluoride (with ADE); Multivitamins/Minerals (with ADEK, Folate, Iron); Mycophenolate; Nilotinib;

PAZOPanib; PenicillAMINE; Phosphate Supplements; Potassium Acid Phosphate; Quinolone Antibiotics; Rilpivirine; Riociguat; Sotalol; Strontium Ranelate; Sulpiride; Tetracycline Derivatives; Thyroid Products; Trientine

The levels/effects of Calcium Carbonate may be decreased by: Alpha-Lipoic Acid; Trientine

Food Interactions Food may increase calcium absorption. Calcium may decrease iron absorption. Bran, foods high in oxalates, or whole grain cereals may decrease calcium absorption. Management: Administer with food.

Storage/Stability Store between 15°C to 30°C (59°F to 86°F). Protect oral suspension from freezing.

Mechanism of Action As dietary supplement, used to prevent or treat negative calcium balance; in osteoporosis, it helps to prevent or decrease the rate of bone loss. Calcium is an integral component of the skeleton and also moderates nerve and muscle performance and allows normal cardiac function. Also used to treat hyperphosphatemia in patients with chronic kidney disease by combining with dietary phosphate to form insoluble calcium phosphate, which is excreted in feces. Calcium salts as antacids neutralize gastric acidity resulting in increased gastric and duodenal bulb pH; they additionally inhibit proteolytic activity of pepsin if the pH is increased >4 and increase lower esophageal sphincter tone (IOM, 2011).

Pharmacodynamics Acid neutralizing capacity: Tums® 500 mg: 10 mEq, Tums® E-X 750 mg: 15mEq; Tums® Ultra 1000 mg: 20 mEq

Pharmacokinetics (Adult data unless noted)

Absorption: 25% to 35%; varies with age (infants 60%, prepubertal children 28%, pubertal children 34%, young adults 25%); decreased absorption occurs in patients with achlorhydria, renal osteodystrophy, steatorrhea, or uremia

Protein binding: 45%

Elimination: Primarily in the feces as unabsorbed calcium

Dosing: Neonatal Oral:

Adequate intake (AI): 200 mg/day of **elemental calcium**; requirements may vary on prematurity, postnatal age, and other clinical factors; serum calcium concentrations should be monitored closely to determine patient-specific needs

Hypocalcemia: Dose depends on clinical condition and serum calcium concentration: Dose expressed in mg of **elemental calcium**: 50-150 mg/kg/day in 4-6 divided doses; not to exceed 1000 mg/day (Avery, 1994; Riga, 2007; Thomas, 2012)

Dosing: Usual Oral:

Adequate intake (AI): Dosage expressed in terms of **elemental calcium:**

1-6 months: 200 mg/day

7-12 months: 260 mg/day

Recommended daily allowance (RDA): Dosage expressed in terms of **elemental calcium;** during pregnancy and lactation, requirements may change:

1-3 years: 700 mg/day

4-8 years: 1000 mg/day

9-18 years: 1300 mg/day

Females 19-50 years, males 19-70 years: 1000 mg/day

Females ≥51 years, males ≥71 years: 1200 mg/day

Antacid:

Children 2-5 years: Children's Pepto: 1 tablet (400 mg calcium carbonate) as symptoms occur; not to exceed 3 tablets/day

Children >5-11 years: Children's Pepto: 2 tablets (800 mg calcium carbonate) as symptoms occur; not to exceed 6 tablets/day

Children >11 years and Adults:

Tums®, Tums® E-X: Chew 2-4 tablets as symptoms occur; not to exceed 15 tablets (Tums®) or 10 tablets (Tums® E-X) per day

Tums® Ultra: Chew 2-3 tablets as symptoms occur; not to exceed 7 tablets per day

Hypocalcemia: Dose depends on clinical condition and serum calcium concentration: Dose expressed as **elemental calcium**:

Infants and Children: 45-65 mg/kg/day in 4 divided doses (Nelson, 1996)

Adults: 1-2 g or more per day in 3-4 divided doses

Treatment of hyperphosphatemia in end-stage renal failure: Children and Adults: Dose expressed as **calcium carbonate**: 1 g with each meal; increase as needed; range: 4-7 g/day

Adjunctive prevention and treatment of osteoporosis: Adults: 500 mg **elemental calcium** 2-3 times/day; recommended dosage includes dietary intake and should be adjusted depending upon the patient's diet; to improve absorption do not administer more than 500 mg **elemental calcium**/dose

Hydrofluoric acid (HF) burns (HF concentration <20%): Topical: Various topical calcium preparations have been used anecdotally for treatment of dermal exposure to HF solutions; calcium carbonate at concentrations ranging from 2.5% to 33% has been used; a topical calcium carbonate preparation must be compounded; apply topically as needed

Dosage adjustment in renal impairment: CrCl <25 mL/minute may require dosage adjustment depending upon serum calcium level

Administration

Oral: Administer with plenty of fluids with or immediately following meals; if using for phosphate-binding, administer with meals

Suspension: Shake well before administration

Chewable tablets: Thoroughly chew tablets before swallowing

Topical: Massage calcium carbonate slurry into exposed area for 15 minutes

Monitoring Parameters Serum calcium (ionized calcium preferred if available), phosphate, magnesium, heart rate, ECG

Reference Range

Calcium: Newborns: 7-12 mg/dL; 0-2 years: 8.8-11.2 mg/dL; 2 years to adults: 9-11 mg/dL

Calcium, ionized, whole blood: 4.4-5.4 mg/dL

Additional Information Due to a poor correlation between the serum ionized calcium (free) and total serum calcium, particularly in states of low albumin or acid/base imbalances, direct measurement of ionized calcium is recommended. If ionized calcium is unavailable, in low albumin states, the corrected **total** serum calcium may be estimated by this equation (assuming a normal albumin of 4 g/dL); [(4 – patient's albumin) x 0.8] + patient's measured total calcium

Elemental Calcium Content of Calcium Salts

Calcium Salt	Elemental Calcium (mg/1 g of salt form)	Calcium (mEq/g)
Calcium acetate	253	12.7
Calcium carbonate	400	20
Calcium chloride	273	13.6
Calcium citrate	211	10.5
Calcium glubionate	63.8	3.2
Calcium gluconate	93	4.65
Calcium lactate	130	6.5
Calcium phosphate (tribasic)	390	19.3

Dosage Forms Considerations 1 g calcium carbonate = elemental calcium 400 mg = calcium 20 mEq = calcium 10 mmol

Dosage Forms Excipient information presented when available (limited, particularly for generics); consult specific product labeling. [DSC] = Discontinued product

Capsule, Oral:
- Calci-Mix: 1250 mg [DSC]
- Florical: 364 mg

Powder, Oral:
- Generic: 800 mg/2 g (480 g)

Suspension, Oral:
- Generic: 1250 mg/5 mL (5 mL, 473 mL, 500 mL)

Tablet, Oral:
- Cal-Carb Forte: 1250 mg
- Calcarb 600: 1500 mg [scored]
- Calcium 600: 600 mg [scored]
- Calcium 600: 600 mg [contains fd&c yellow #6 aluminum lake, soy polysaccarides]
- Calcium High Potency: 600 mg
- Caltrate 600: 1500 mg [scored]
- Florical: 364 mg
- Oysco 500: 500 mg [contains brilliant blue fcf (fd&c blue #1), tartrazine (fd&c yellow #5)]
- Generic: 500 mg, 600 mg, 648 mg, 1250 mg

Tablet, Oral [preservative free]:
- Calcium 600: 600 mg [lactose free, salt free, sugar free]
- Generic: 500 mg, 600 mg, 1250 mg

Tablet Chewable, Oral:
- Alcalak: 420 mg [mint flavor]
- Antacid: 420 mg [mint flavor]
- Antacid: 500 mg
- Antacid: 500 mg [assorted fruit flavor]
- Antacid: 500 mg [peppermint flavor]
- Antacid: 500 mg [contains brilliant blue fcf (fd&c blue #1), fd&c yellow #10 (quinoline yellow), fd&c yellow #6 (sunset yellow)]
- Antacid: 500 mg [contains fd&c blue #1 aluminum lake, fd&c red #40 aluminum lake, fd&c yellow #5 aluminum lake, fd&c yellow #6 aluminum lake]
- Antacid Calcium: 500 mg [gluten free; peppermint flavor]
- Antacid Calcium Extra Strength: 750 mg [gluten free; contains fd&c blue #1 aluminum lake, fd&c red #40 aluminum lake; assorted fruit flavor]
- Antacid Extra Strength: 750 mg [contains brilliant blue fcf (fd&c blue #1), fd&c red #40]
- Antacid Extra Strength: 750 mg [contains fd&c red #40, fd&c yellow #6 (sunset yellow), tartrazine (fd&c yellow #5)]
- Cal-Gest Antacid: 500 mg [DSC] [contains fd&c blue #1 aluminum lake, fd&c yellow #10 aluminum lake, fd&c yellow #6 aluminum lake]
- Cal-Gest Antacid: 500 mg [contains fd&c blue #1 aluminum lake, fd&c yellow #10 aluminum lake, fd&c yellow #6 aluminum lake; assorted fruit flavor]
- Cal-Mint: 260 mg [animal products free, gelatin free, gluten free, lactose free, no artificial color(s), no artificial flavor(s), starch free, sugar free, yeast free]
- Calci-Chew: 1250 mg [cherry flavor]
- Calcium Antacid: 500 mg [DSC] [assorted fruit flavor]
- Calcium Antacid: 500 mg [DSC] [peppermint flavor]
- Calcium Antacid: 500 mg [contains brilliant blue fcf (fd&c blue #1), fd&c red #40, fd&c yellow #6 (sunset yellow), soybeans (glycine max), tartrazine (fd&c yellow #5); assorted flavor]
- Calcium Antacid: 500 mg [contains fd&c blue #1 aluminum lake]
- Calcium Antacid: 500 mg [contains fd&c blue #1 aluminum lake, fd&c yellow #10 aluminum lake, fd&c yellow #6 aluminum lake; assorted fruit flavor]
- Calcium Antacid Extra Strength: 750 mg [assorted fruit flavor]
- Calcium Antacid Extra Strength: 750 mg [contains brilliant blue fcf (fd&c blue #1), fd&c red #40, fd&c yellow #6 (sunset yellow), tartrazine (fd&c yellow #5); assorted flavor]
- Calcium Antacid Extra Strength: 750 mg [contains fd&c blue #1 aluminum lake, fd&c red #40 aluminum lake]
- Calcium Antacid Extra Strength: 750 mg [gluten free; contains brilliant blue fcf (fd&c blue #1), fd&c yellow #10 (quinoline yellow), fd&c yellow #6 (sunset yellow)]
- Calcium Antacid Ultra Max St: 1000 mg [contains brilliant blue fcf (fd&c blue #1), fd&c red #40, fd&c yellow #6 (sunset yellow), soybeans (glycine max), tartrazine (fd&c yellow #5)]
- Maalox: 600 mg [contains aspartame; wild berry flavor]
- Maalox Childrens: 400 mg [contains aspartame; wild berry flavor]
- Os-Cal: 1250 mg [DSC]
- Titralac: 420 mg [low sodium, sugar free; contains saccharin]
- Tums: 500 mg [gluten free]
- Tums: 500 mg [gluten free; contains fd&c blue #1 aluminum lake, fd&c red #40 aluminum lake, fd&c yellow #6 aluminum lake, tartrazine (fd&c yellow #5)]
- Tums Chewy Delights: 1177 mg [contains fd&c red #40 aluminum lake, soybean lecithin; cherry flavor]
- Tums E-X 750: 750 mg
- Tums E-X 750: 750 mg [assorted flavor]
- Tums E-X 750: 750 mg [gluten free; contains fd&c blue #1 aluminum lake, fd&c red #40 aluminum lake; assorted berries flavor]
- Tums E-X 750: 750 mg [gluten free; contains fd&c blue #1 aluminum lake, fd&c red #40 aluminum lake, fd&c yellow #5 aluminum lake, fd&c yellow #6 aluminum lake; assorted fruit flavor]
- Tums E-X 750: 750 mg [sugar free]
- Tums Freshers: 500 mg [gluten free; contains brilliant blue fcf (fd&c blue #1); mint flavor]
- Tums Kids: 750 mg [scored; contains fd&c blue #1 aluminum lake, fd&c red #40 aluminum lake; cherry flavor]
- Tums Lasting Effects: 500 mg [contains fd&c red #40 aluminum lake, fd&c yellow #6 aluminum lake, tartrazine (fd&c yellow #5)]
- Tums Smoothies: 750 mg [peppermint flavor]
- Tums Smoothies: 750 mg [contains fd&c blue #1 aluminum lake, fd&c red #40 aluminum lake, fd&c yellow #6 aluminum lake, soybeans (glycine max); assorted tropical fruit flavor]
- Tums Smoothies: 750 mg [contains fd&c blue #1 aluminum lake, fd&c red #40 aluminum lake, soybeans (glycine max); berry flavor]
- Tums Smoothies: 750 mg [gluten free; contains fd&c blue #1 aluminum lake, fd&c red #40 aluminum lake, fd&c yellow #5 aluminum lake, fd&c yellow #6 aluminum lake, milk (cow)]
- Tums Ultra 1000: 1000 mg [peppermint flavor]
- Tums Ultra 1000: 1000 mg [contains fd&c blue #1 aluminum lake, fd&c red #40 aluminum lake, fd&c yellow #5 aluminum lake, fd&c yellow #6 aluminum lake; assorted berries flavor]
- Tums Ultra 1000: 1000 mg [contains fd&c red #40 aluminum lake, fd&c yellow #6 aluminum lake, tartrazine (fd&c yellow #5); assorted tropical fruit flavor]
- Tums Ultra 1000: 1000 mg [DSC] [gluten free]
- Tums Ultra 1000: 1000 mg [gluten free; contains fd&c blue #1 aluminum lake, fd&c red #40 aluminum lake, fd&c yellow #6 aluminum lake, tartrazine (fd&c yellow #5)]
- Generic: 260 mg, 500 mg, 750 mg

Tablet Chewable, Oral [preservative free]:
- Generic: 500 mg

Calcium Chloride (KAL see um KLOR ide)

Medication Safety Issues

Sound-alike/look-alike issues:

Calcium chloride may be confused with calcium gluconate

Administration issues:

Calcium chloride may be confused with calcium gluconate.

Confusion with the different intravenous salt forms of calcium has occurred. There is a threefold difference in the primary cation concentration between calcium chloride (in which 1 g = 14 mEq [270 mg] of elemental Ca++) and calcium gluconate (in which 1 g = 4.65 mEq [90 mg] of elemental Ca++).

Prescribers should specify which salt form is desired. Dosages should be expressed either as mEq, mg, or grams of the salt form.

Related Information

Management of Drug Extravasations *on page 2298*

Therapeutic Category Calcium Salt; Electrolyte Supplement, Parenteral

Generic Availability (US) Yes

Use Treatment of hypocalcemia and conditions secondary to hypocalcemia (eg, tetany, seizures, arrhythmias); treatment of cardiac disturbances secondary to hyperkalemia; adjunctive treatment of magnesium sulfate overdose [All indications: FDA approved in pediatric patients (age not specified) and adults]; has also been used for calcium channel blocker toxicity, or beta-blocker toxicity refractory to glucagon and vasopressors

Pregnancy Risk Factor C

Pregnancy Considerations Animal reproduction studies have not been conducted. Calcium crosses the placenta. The amount of calcium reaching the fetus is determined by maternal physiological changes. Calcium requirements are the same in pregnant and nonpregnant females (IOM, 2011). Information related to use as an antidote in pregnancy is limited. In general, medications used as antidotes should take into consideration the health and prognosis of the mother; antidotes should be administered to pregnant women if there is a clear indication for use and should not be withheld because of fears of teratogenicity (Bailey, 2003).

Breast-Feeding Considerations Calcium is excreted in breast milk. The amount of calcium in breast milk is homeostatically regulated and not altered by maternal calcium intake. Calcium requirements are the same in lactating and nonlactating females (IOM, 2011).

Contraindications Known or suspected digoxin toxicity; not recommended as routine treatment in cardiac arrest (includes asystole, ventricular fibrillation, pulseless ventricular tachycardia, or pulseless electrical activity)

Warnings/Precautions For IV use only; do not inject SubQ or IM; avoid rapid IV administration (do not exceed 100 mg/minute except in emergency situations). Vesicant; ensure proper catheter or needle position prior to and during infusion; avoid extravasation; extravasation may result in severe necrosis and sloughing. Monitor the IV site closely. Use with caution in patients with hyperphosphatemia, respiratory acidosis, renal impairment, or respiratory failure; acidifying effect of calcium chloride may potentiate acidosis. Use with caution in patients with chronic renal failure to avoid hypercalcemia; frequent monitoring of serum calcium and phosphorus is necessary. Use with caution in hypokalemic or digitalized patients since acute rises in serum calcium levels may precipitate cardiac arrhythmias; use is contraindicated with known or suspected digoxin toxicity. Hypomagnesemia is a common cause of hypocalcemia; therefore, correction of hypocalcemia may be difficult in patients with concomitant hypomagnesemia. Evaluate serum magnesium and correct hypomagnesemia (if necessary), particularly if initial treatment of hypocalcemia is refractory. The parenteral product may contain aluminum; toxic aluminum concentrations may be seen with high doses, prolonged use, or renal dysfunction. Premature neonates are at higher risk due to immature renal function and aluminum intake from other parenteral sources. Parenteral aluminum exposure of >4 to 5 mcg/kg/day is associated with CNS and bone toxicity; tissue loading may occur at lower doses (Federal Register 2002). See manufacturer's labeling. Avoid metabolic acidosis (ie, administer only up to 2 to 3 days then change to another calcium salt).

Ceftriaxone may complex with calcium causing precipitation. Fatal lung and kidney damage associated with calcium-ceftriaxone precipitates has been observed in premature and term neonates. Due to reports of precipitation reaction in neonates, do not coadminister ceftriaxone with calcium-containing solutions, even via separate infusion lines/sites or at different times in any neonate. Ceftriaxone should not be administered simultaneously with any calcium-containing solution via a Y-site in any patient. However, ceftriaxone and calcium-containing solutions may be administered sequentially of one another for use in patients **other than neonates** if infusion lines are thoroughly flushed (with a compatible fluid) between infusions. Multiple salt forms of calcium exist; close attention must be paid to the salt form when ordering and administering calcium; incorrect selection or substitution of one salt for another without proper dosage adjustment may result in serious over or under dosing.

Adverse Reactions IV:

Cardiovascular (following rapid IV injection): Bradycardia, cardiac arrest, cardiac arrhythmia, hypotension, syncope, vasodilatation

Central nervous system: Feeling abnormal (sense of oppression; with rapid IV injection), tingling sensation (with rapid IV injection)

Endocrine & metabolic: Hot flash (with rapid IV injection), hypercalcemia

Gastrointestinal: Dysgeusia (chalky taste), gastrointestinal irritation, increased serum amylase

Local: Local tissue necrosis (following extravasation)

Renal: Nephrolithiasis

Rare but important or life-threatening: Cutaneous calcification

Drug Interactions

Metabolism/Transport Effects None known.

Avoid Concomitant Use

Avoid concomitant use of Calcium Chloride with any of the following: Calcium Acetate

Increased Effect/Toxicity

Calcium Chloride may increase the levels/effects of: Calcium Acetate; Cardiac Glycosides; CefTRIAXone; Vitamin D Analogs

The levels/effects of Calcium Chloride may be increased by: Multivitamins/Fluoride (with ADE); Multivitamins/Minerals (with ADEK, Folate, Iron); Thiazide Diuretics

Decreased Effect

Calcium Chloride may decrease the levels/effects of: Bisphosphonate Derivatives; Calcium Channel Blockers; Deferiprone; DOBUTamine; Dolutegravir; Eltrombopag; Multivitamins/Fluoride (with ADE); Phosphate Supplements; Tetracycline Derivatives; Thyroid Products; Trientine

The levels/effects of Calcium Chloride may be decreased by: Trientine

Storage/Stability Store intact vials at 20°C to 25°C (68°F to 77°F); excursions permitted to 15°C to 30°C (59°F to 86°F). Do not refrigerate solutions; IV infusion solutions are stable for 24 hours at room temperature.

Although calcium chloride is not routinely used in the preparation of parenteral nutrition, it is important to note that phosphate salts may precipitate when mixed with calcium salts. Solubility is improved in amino acid parenteral nutrition solutions. Check with a pharmacist to determine compatibility.

Mechanism of Action Moderates nerve and muscle performance via action potential excitation threshold regulation

Pharmacokinetics (Adult data unless noted)

Protein binding: 40%, primarily to albumin (Wills, 1971)

Elimination: Primarily feces (80% as insoluble calcium salts); urine (20%)

Dosing: Neonatal

Daily maintenance calcium: IV: Dosage expressed in terms of **elemental calcium**: 3-4 **mEq**/kg/**day**

Parenteral nutrition, maintenance requirement (Mirtallo, 2004): IV: Dosage expressed in terms of **elemental calcium**: 2-4 **mEq**/kg/**day**

Hypocalcemia: IV: Dosage expressed in mg of **calcium chloride**: 10-20 mg/kg/dose, repeat every 4-6 hours if needed

Cardiac arrest in the presence of hyperkalemia or hypocalcemia, hypermagnesemia, or calcium channel blocker toxicity: IV, I.O.: Dosage expressed in mg of **calcium chloride**: 20 mg/kg; may repeat in 10 minutes if necessary; if effective, consider IV infusion of 20-50 mg/kg/**hour**

Tetany: IV: Dosage expressed in mg of **calcium chloride**: 10 mg/kg over 5-10 minutes; may repeat after 6 hours or follow with an infusion with a maximum dose of 200 mg/kg/**day**

Dosing: Usual Infants, Children, and Adolescents: **Note:** One gram of calcium chloride salt is equal to 270 mg of elemental calcium.

Daily maintenance calcium: IV: Dosage expressed in terms of **elemental calcium**

Infants and Children <25 kg: 1-2 **mEq**/kg/**day**

Children 25-45 kg: 0.5-1.5 **mEq**/kg/**day**

Children >45 kg and Adolescents: 0.2-0.3 **mEq**/kg/**day** or 10-20 **mEq**/**day**

Parenteral nutrition, maintenance requirement (Mirtallo, 2004): IV: **Note:** Dosage expressed in terms of **elemental calcium**

Infants and Children ≤50 kg: 0.5-4 **mEq**/kg/**day**

Children >50 kg and Adolescents: 10-20 **mEq**/**day**

Hypocalcemia: Note: In general, IV calcium gluconate is preferred over IV calcium chloride in nonemergency settings due to the potential for extravasation with calcium chloride. Dosage expressed in mg of **calcium chloride**

Manufacturer's recommendations: IV: 2.7-5 mg/kg/dose every 4-6 hours; maximum dose: 1000 mg

Alternative dosing: IV: 10-20 mg/kg/dose; maximum dose: 1000 mg; repeat every 4-6 hours if needed

Cardiac arrest in the presence of hyperkalemia or hypocalcemia, hypermagnesemia, or calcium channel antagonist toxicity (PALS recommendations): IV, I.O.: Dosage expressed in mg of **calcium chloride:** 20 mg/kg/dose (maximum dose: 2000 mg); may repeat in 10 minutes if necessary; if effective, consider IV infusion of 20-50 mg/kg/**hour**; **Note:** Routine use in cardiac arrest is not recommended due to the lack of improved survival (Hegenbarth, 2008; Kleinman, 2010)

Calcium channel blocker toxicity: IV: Dosage expressed in mg of **calcium chloride**: 20 mg/kg/dose infused over 5-10 minutes; if effective, consider IV infusion of 20-50 mg/kg/**hour** (Kleinman, 2010)

Hypocalcemia secondary to citrated blood infusion: IV: 0.45 mEq **elemental** calcium for each 100 mL citrated blood infused

Tetany:

IV: Dosage expressed in mg of **calcium chloride**: 10 mg/kg over 5-10 minutes; may repeat after 6 hours or follow with an infusion with a maximum dose of 200 mg/kg/**day**

Adults: **Dosages are expressed in terms of the calcium chloride salt based on a solution concentration of 100 mg/mL (10%) containing 1.4 mEq (27 mg)/mL elemental calcium.**

Hypocalcemia: IV:

Acute, symptomatic: Manufacturer's recommendations: 200-1000 mg every 1-3 days

Severe, symptomatic (eg, seizure, tetany): 1000 mg over 10 minutes; may repeat every 60 minutes until symptoms resolve (French, 2012)

Cardiac arrest or cardiotoxicity in the presence of hyperkalemia, hypocalcemia, or hypermagnesemia (ACLS recommendations): IV: 500-1000 mg over 2-5 minutes; may repeat as necessary (Vanden Hoek, 2010). **Note:** Routine use in cardiac arrest is not recommended due to the lack of improved survival (Neumar, 2010).

Dosing adjustment in renal impairment: No initial dosage adjustment necessary; however, accumulation may occur with renal impairment and subsequent doses may require adjustment based on serum calcium concentrations

Dosing adjustment in hepatic impairment: No initial dosage adjustment necessary; subsequent doses should be guided by serum calcium concentrations.

Preparation for Administration Parenteral: IV infusion: Dilute to a maximum concentration of 20 mg/mL.

Administration Parenteral: Do not use scalp vein or small hand or foot veins for IV administration; central-line administration is the preferred route. Not for endotracheal administration. Do not inject calcium salts IM or administer SubQ since severe necrosis and sloughing may occur; extravasation of calcium can result in severe necrosis and tissue sloughing. Stop the infusion if the patient complains of pain or discomfort. Warm solution to body temperature prior to administration. Do not infuse calcium chloride in the same IV line as phosphate-containing solutions.

IV: For direct IV injection infuse slow IVP over 3 to 5 minutes or at a maximum rate of 50 to 100 mg calcium chloride/minute; in situations of cardiac arrest, calcium chloride may be administered over 10 to 20 seconds.

IV infusion: Further dilute and administer 45 to 90 mg calcium chloride/kg over 1 hour; 0.6 to 1.2 mEq calcium/kg over 1 hour

Parenteral nutrition solution: Although calcium chloride is not routinely used in the preparation of parenteral nutrition, it is important to note that calcium-phosphate stability in parenteral nutrition solutions is dependent upon the pH of the solution, temperature, and relative concentration of each ion. The pH of the solution is primarily dependent upon the amino acid concentration. The higher the percentage amino acids, the lower the pH and the more soluble the calcium and phosphate. Individual commercially available amino acid solutions vary significantly with respect to pH lowering potential and consequent calcium phosphate compatibility; consult product specific labeling for additional information.

Vesicant; ensure proper needle or catheter placement prior to and during IV infusion. Avoid extravasation. If extravasation occurs, stop infusion immediately and disconnect (leave needle/cannula in place); gently aspirate extravasated solution (do **NOT** flush the line); initiate hyaluronidase antidote (see Management of Drug Extravasations for more details); remove needle/cannula; apply dry cold compresses (Hurst 2004); elevate extremity.

Vesicant/Extravasation Risk Vesicant

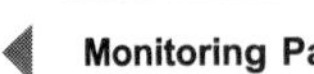

Monitoring Parameters Serum calcium (ionized calcium preferred if available), phosphate, magnesium, heart rate, ECG

Reference Range

	Age	Normal Values Serum Concentration
Calcium, total	Cord blood	9-11.5 mg/dL
	Newborn 3-24 hours	9-10.6 mg/dL
	Newborn 24-48 hours	7-12 mg/dL
	4-7 days	9-10.9 mg/dL
	Child	8.8-10.8 mg/dL
	Adolescent to Adult	8.4-10.2 mg/dL
Calcium, ionized, whole blood	Cord blood	5-6 mg/dL
	Newborn 3-24 hours	4.3-5.1 mg/dL
	Newborn 24-48 hours	4-4.7 mg/dL
	≥2 days	4.8-4.92 mg/dL (2.24-2.46 mEq/L)

Additional Information Due to a poor correlation between the serum ionized calcium (free) and total serum calcium, particularly in states of low albumin or acid/base imbalances, direct measurement of ionized calcium is recommended. If ionized calcium is unavailable, in low albumin states, the corrected **total** serum calcium may be estimated by this equation (assuming a normal albumin of 4 g/dL); [(4 – patient's albumin) x 0.8] + patient's measured total calcium

Elemental Calcium Content of Calcium Salts

Calcium Salt	Elemental Calcium (mg/1 g of salt form)	Calcium (mEq/g)
Calcium acetate	253	12.7
Calcium carbonate	400	20
Calcium chloride	273	13.6
Calcium citrate	211	10.5
Calcium glubionate	63.8	3.2
Calcium gluconate	93	4.65
Calcium lactate	130	6.5
Calcium phosphate (tribasic)	390	19.3

Dosage Forms Considerations 1 g calcium chloride = elemental calcium 273 mg = calcium 13.6 mEq = calcium 6.8 mmol

Dosage Forms Excipient information presented when available (limited, particularly for generics); consult specific product labeling.

Solution, Intravenous:

Generic: 10% (10 mL)

Solution, Intravenous [preservative free]:

Generic: 10% (10 mL)

Calcium Citrate (KAL see um SIT rate)

Medication Safety Issues

Sound-alike/look-alike issues:

Citracal® may be confused with Citrucel®

Brand Names: US Cal-Citrate [OTC]; Calcitrate [OTC]

Brand Names: Canada Osteocit®

Therapeutic Category Calcium Salt; Electrolyte Supplement, Oral

Generic Availability (US) Yes

Use Treatment of hyperphosphatemia in end-stage renal failure; dietary supplement; prevention and treatment of calcium deficiency; adjunctive prevention and treatment of osteoporosis

Pregnancy Considerations Calcium crosses the placenta. Intestinal absorption of calcium increases during pregnancy. The amount of calcium reaching the fetus is determined by maternal physiological changes. Calcium requirements are the same in pregnant and nonpregnant females (IOM, 2011).

Breast-Feeding Considerations Calcium is excreted in breast milk. The amount of calcium in breast milk is homeostatically regulated and not altered by maternal calcium intake. Calcium requirements are the same in lactating and nonlactating females (IOM, 2011).

Contraindications Hypersensitivity to any component of the formulation

Warnings/Precautions Constipation, bloating, and gas are common with calcium supplements. Use with caution in patients with renal failure to avoid hypercalcemia; frequent monitoring of serum calcium and phosphorus is necessary. Use caution when administering calcium supplements to patients with a history of kidney stones. Hypercalcemia and hypercalciuria are most likely to occur in hypoparathyroid patients receiving high doses of vitamin D. Calcium absorption is impaired in achlorhydria; common in elderly. Citrate may be preferred because better absorbed. Calcium administration interferes with absorption of some minerals and drugs; use with caution. It is recommended to concomitantly administer vitamin D for optimal calcium absorption. Taking calcium (≤500 mg) with food improves absorption. Multiple salt forms of calcium exist; close attention must be paid to the salt form when ordering and administering calcium; incorrect selection or substitution of one salt for another without proper dosage adjustment may result in serious over or under dosing.

Adverse Reactions

Central nervous system: Headache

Endocrine & metabolic: Hypercalcemia, hypophosphatemia

Gastrointestinal: Abdominal pain, anorexia, constipation, nausea, vomiting

Mild hypercalcemia (calcium: >10.5 mg/dL) may be asymptomatic or manifest itself as anorexia, constipation, nausea, and vomiting

More severe hypercalcemia (calcium: >12 mg/dL) is associated with coma confusion, delirium, and stupor

Miscellaneous: Thirst

Drug Interactions

Metabolism/Transport Effects None known.

Avoid Concomitant Use

Avoid concomitant use of Calcium Citrate with any of the following: Calcium Acetate

Increased Effect/Toxicity

Calcium Citrate may increase the levels/effects of: Aluminum Hydroxide; Calcium Acetate; Cardiac Glycosides; Vitamin D Analogs

The levels/effects of Calcium Citrate may be increased by: Multivitamins/Fluoride (with ADE); Multivitamins/Minerals (with ADEK, Folate, Iron); Thiazide Diuretics

Decreased Effect

Calcium Citrate may decrease the levels/effects of: Alpha-Lipoic Acid; Bisphosphonate Derivatives; Calcium Channel Blockers; Deferiprone; DOBUTamine; Dolutegravir; Eltrombopag; Estramustine; Multivitamins/Fluoride (with ADE); Phosphate Supplements; Quinolone Antibiotics; Strontium Ranelate; Tetracycline Derivatives; Thyroid Products; Trientine

The levels/effects of Calcium Citrate may be decreased by: Alpha-Lipoic Acid; Trientine

Storage/Stability Store at room temperature.

Mechanism of Action Moderates nerve and muscle performance via action potential excitation threshold regulation

Pharmacokinetics (Adult data unless noted)

Absorption: 25% to 35%; varies with age (infants 60%, prepubertal children 28%, pubertal children 34%, young adults 25%); decreased absorption occurs in patients with achlorhydria, renal osteodystrophy, steatorrhea, or uremia

Protein binding: 45%

Elimination: Primarily in the feces as unabsorbed calcium

Dosing: Neonatal Oral:

Adequate intake (AI): 200 mg/day of **elemental calcium**; requirements may vary on prematurity, postnatal age, and other clinical factors; serum calcium concentrations should be monitored closely to determine patient-specific needs

Hypocalcemia: Dose depends on clinical condition and serum calcium concentration: Dose expressed in mg of **elemental calcium:** 50-150 mg/kg/day in 4-6 divided doses; not to exceed 1000 mg/day

Dosing: Usual Oral:

Adequate intake (AI): Dosage expressed in terms of **elemental calcium:**

1-6 months: 200 mg/day

7-12 months: 260 mg/day

Recommended daily allowance (RDA): Dosage expressed in terms of **elemental calcium;** during pregnancy and lactation, requirements may change:

1-3 years: 700 mg/day

4-8 years: 1000 mg/day

9-18 years: 1300 mg/day

Females 19-50 years, males 19-70 years: 1000 mg/day

Females ≥51 years, males ≥71 years: 1200 mg/day

Hypocalcemia: Dose depends on clinical condition and serum calcium concentration: Dose expressed as **elemental calcium:**

Children: 45-65 mg/kg/day in 4 divided doses

Adults: 1-2 g or more per day in 3-4 divided doses

Dietary supplement: Adults: 500 mg to 2 g divided 2-4 times/day

Adjunctive prevention and treatment of osteoporosis: Adults: 500 mg **elemental calcium** 2-3 times/day; recommended dosage includes dietary intake and should be adjusted depending upon the patient's diet; to improve absorption do not administer more than 500 mg **elemental calcium**/dose

Dosage adjustment in renal impairment: CrCl <25 mL/minute may require dosage adjustment depending upon serum calcium level

Administration Oral: Administer with plenty of fluids; may administer without regard to food when using to treat/prevent deficiency conditions; administer with food when treating hyperphosphatemia or when administering granule formulation

Monitoring Parameters Serum calcium (ionized calcium preferred if available), phosphate, magnesium, heart rate, ECG

Reference Range

Calcium: Newborns: 7-12 mg/dL; 0-2 years: 8.8-11.2 mg/dL; 2 years to adults: 9-11 mg/dL

Calcium, ionized, whole blood: 4.4-5.4 mg/dL

Additional Information Due to a poor correlation between the serum ionized calcium (free) and total serum calcium, particularly in states of low albumin or acid/base imbalances, direct measurement of ionized calcium is recommended. If ionized calcium is unavailable, in low albumin states, the corrected **total** serum calcium may be estimated by this equation (assuming a normal albumin of 4 g/dL); [(4 – patient's albumin) x 0.8] + patient's measured total calcium

Elemental Calcium Content of Calcium Salts

Calcium Salt	Elemental Calcium (mg/1 g of salt form)	Calcium (mEq/g)
Calcium acetate	253	12.7
Calcium carbonate	400	20
Calcium chloride	273	13.6
Calcium citrate	211	10.5
Calcium glubionate	63.8	3.2
Calcium gluconate	93	4.65
Calcium lactate	130	6.5
Calcium phosphate (tribasic)	390	19.3

Dosage Forms Considerations 1 g calcium citrate = elemental calcium 211 mg = calcium 10.5 mEq = calcium 5.25 mmol

Dosage Forms Excipient information presented when available (limited, particularly for generics); consult specific product labeling.

Capsule, Oral [preservative free]:

Cal-Citrate: 150 mg [dye free]

Granules, Oral:

Generic: 760 mg/3.5 g (480 g)

Tablet, Oral:

Generic: 250 mg, 950 mg, 1040 mg

Tablet, Oral [preservative free]:

Calcitrate: 950 mg [lactose free, milk derivatives/products, no artificial color(s), no artificial flavor(s), sodium free, soy free, sugar free, wheat free, yeast free]

◆ **Calcium Disodium Edetate** *see* Edetate CALCIUM Disodium *on page 728*

◆ **Calcium Disodiumethylenediaminetetraacetic Acid** *see* Edetate CALCIUM Disodium *on page 728*

◆ **Calcium Folinate** *see* Leucovorin Calcium *on page 1226*

Calcium Glubionate (KAL see um gloo BYE oh nate)

Medication Safety Issues

Sound-alike/look-alike issues:

Calcium glubionate may be confused with calcium gluconate

Brand Names: US Calcionate [OTC]

Therapeutic Category Calcium Salt; Electrolyte Supplement, Oral

Generic Availability (US) Yes

Use Treatment and replacement of calcium deficiency; dietary supplement; adjunctive prevention and treatment of osteoporosis

Pregnancy Considerations Calcium crosses the placenta. Intestinal absorption of calcium increases during pregnancy. The amount of calcium reaching the fetus is determined by maternal physiological changes. Calcium requirements are the same in pregnant and nonpregnant females (IOM, 2011).

Breast-Feeding Considerations Calcium is excreted in breast milk. The amount of calcium in breast milk is homeostatically regulated and not altered by maternal calcium intake. Calcium requirements are the same in lactating and nonlactating females (IOM, 2011).

Warnings/Precautions Constipation, bloating, and gas are common with calcium supplements. Calcium absorption is impaired in achlorhydria; administration is followed by increased gastric acid secretion within 2 hours of administration especially with high doses. Common in the elderly, use an alternate salt (eg, citrate) and administer with food. Hypercalcemia and hypercalciuria are most likely to occur in hypoparathyroid patients receiving high doses of vitamin D. Use caution when administering calcium supplements to patients with a history of kidney stones. Calcium administration interferes with absorption of some minerals and drugs; use with caution. It is recommended to concomitantly administer vitamin D for optimal calcium absorption. Taking calcium (≤500 mg) with food improves absorption. Multiple salt forms of calcium exist; close attention must be paid to the salt form when ordering and administering calcium; incorrect selection or substitution of one salt for another without proper dosage adjustment may result in serious over or under dosing.

Adverse Reactions Symptoms reported with hypercalcemia:

Gastrointestinal: Abdominal pain, anorexia, constipation, nausea, thirst, vomiting, xerostomia

Genitourinary: Polyuria

Drug Interactions

Metabolism/Transport Effects None known.

Avoid Concomitant Use

Avoid concomitant use of Calcium Glubionate with any of the following: Calcium Acetate

Increased Effect/Toxicity

Calcium Glubionate may increase the levels/effects of: Calcium Acetate; Cardiac Glycosides; Vitamin D Analogs

The levels/effects of Calcium Glubionate may be increased by: Multivitamins/Fluoride (with ADE); Multivitamins/Minerals (with ADEK, Folate, Iron); Thiazide Diuretics

Decreased Effect

Calcium Glubionate may decrease the levels/effects of: Alpha-Lipoic Acid; Bisphosphonate Derivatives; Calcium Channel Blockers; Deferiprone; DOBUTamine; Dolutegravir; Eltrombopag; Estramustine; Multivitamins/Fluoride (with ADE); Phosphate Supplements; Quinolone Antibiotics; Strontium Ranelate; Tetracycline Derivatives; Thyroid Products; Trientine

The levels/effects of Calcium Glubionate may be decreased by: Alpha-Lipoic Acid; Trientine

Food Interactions Food may increase calcium absorption. Calcium may decrease iron absorption. Bran, foods high in oxalates, or whole grain cereals may decrease calcium absorption. Management: Administer preferably with food.

Storage/Stability

Store at room temperature.

Mechanism of Action As dietary supplement, used to prevent or treat negative calcium balance. The calcium in calcium salts moderates nerve and muscle performance and allows normal cardiac function.

Pharmacokinetics (Adult data unless noted)

Absorption: 25% to 35%; varies with age (infants 60%, prepubertal children 28%, pubertal children 34%, young adults 25%); decreased absorption occurs in patients with achlorhydria, renal osteodystrophy, steatorrhea, or uremia

Protein binding: 45%

Elimination: Primarily in the feces as unabsorbed calcium

Dosing: Neonatal Oral:

Adequate intake (AI): 200 mg/day of **elemental calcium**; requirements may vary on prematurity, postnatal age, and other clinical factors; serum calcium concentrations should be monitored closely to determine patient-specific needs

Hypocalcemia: Dose depends on clinical condition and serum calcium concentration:

Dose expressed in mg of **elemental calcium**: 50-150 mg/kg/day in 4-6 divided doses; not to exceed 1000 mg/day

Dose expressed in mg of **calcium glubionate**: 1200 mg/kg/day in 4-6 divided doses

Dosing: Usual Oral:

Adequate intake (AI): Dosage expressed in terms of **elemental calcium:**

1-6 months: 200 mg/day

7-12 months: 260 mg/day

Recommended daily allowance (RDA): Dosage expressed in terms of **elemental calcium;** during pregnancy and lactation, requirements may change:

1-3 years: 700 mg/day

4-8 years: 1000 mg/day

9-18 years: 1300 mg/day

Females 19-50 years, males 19-70 years: 1000 mg/day

Females ≥51 years, males ≥71 years: 1200 mg/day

Dietary supplement: Dosage below based on product containing: 1.8 g calcium glubionate/5 mL (115 mg **elemental calcium**/5 mL)

Infants <12 months: 5 mL/dose 5 times a day; may mix with juice or formula

Children <4 years: 10 mL/dose 3 times a day

Children ≥4 years and Adolescents: 15 mL/dose 3 times a day

Adults: 15 mL/dose 3 times a day

Pregnant or lactating women: 15 mL/dose 4 times a day

Hypocalcemia: Dose depends on clinical condition and serum calcium concentration:

Dose expressed as **elemental calcium**:

Children: 45-65 mg/kg/day in 4 divided doses

Adults: 1-2 g or more per day in 3-4 divided doses

Dose expressed as **calcium glubionate**:

Infants and Children: 600-2000 mg/kg/day in 4 divided doses up to a maximum of 9 g/day

Adults: 6-18 g/day in divided doses

Adjunctive prevention and treatment of osteoporosis: Adults: 500 mg **elemental calcium** 2-3 times/day; recommended dosage includes dietary intake and should be adjusted depending upon the patient's diet; to improve absorption do not administer more than 500 mg **elemental calcium**/dose

Dosage adjustment in renal impairment: CrCl <25 mL/minute may require dosage adjustment depending upon serum calcium level

Administration Oral: Administer with plenty of fluids with or following meals; for phosphate binding, administer on an empty stomach before meals to optimize effectiveness

Monitoring Parameters Serum calcium (ionized calcium preferred if available), phosphate, magnesium, heart rate, ECG

Reference Range

Calcium: Newborns: 7-12 mg/dL; 0-2 years: 8.8-11.2 mg/dL; 2 years to adults: 9-11 mg/dL

Calcium, ionized, whole blood: 4.4-5.4 mg/dL

Test Interactions Decreased magnesium

Additional Information Due to a poor correlation between the serum ionized calcium (free) and total serum calcium, particularly in states of low albumin or acid/base imbalances, direct measurement of ionized calcium is recommended. If ionized calcium is unavailable, in low albumin states, the corrected **total** serum calcium may be estimated by this equation (assuming a normal albumin of 4 g/dL); [(4 – patient's albumin) x 0.8] + patient's measured total calcium

Elemental Calcium Content of Calcium Salts

Calcium Salt	Elemental Calcium (mg/1 g of salt form)	Calcium (mEq/g)
Calcium acetate	253	12.7
Calcium carbonate	400	20
Calcium chloride	273	13.6
Calcium citrate	211	10.5
Calcium glubionate	63.8	3.2
Calcium gluconate	93	4.65
Calcium lactate	130	6.5
Calcium phosphate (tribasic)	390	19.3

Dosage Forms Considerations
1 g calcium glubionate = elemental calcium 63.8 mg = calcium 3.2 mEq = calcium 1.6 mmol

Dosage Forms Excipient information presented when available (limited, particularly for generics); consult specific product labeling.

Syrup, Oral:
Calcionate: 1.8 g/5 mL (473 mL) [fruit flavor]

Calcium Gluconate (KAL see um GLOO koe nate)

Medication Safety Issues

Sound-alike/look-alike issues:

Calcium gluconate may be confused with calcium glubionate, cupric sulfate

Administration issues:

Calcium gluconate may be confused with calcium chloride.

Confusion with the different intravenous salt forms of calcium has occurred. There is a threefold difference in the primary cation concentration between calcium gluconate (in which 1 g = 4.65 mEq [90 mg] of elemental Ca++) and calcium chloride (in which 1 g = 14 mEq [270 mg] of elemental Ca++).

Prescribers should specify which salt form is desired. Dosages should be expressed either as mEq, mg, or grams of the salt form.

Related Information

Management of Drug Extravasations *on page 2298*

Brand Names: US Cal-Glu [OTC]

Therapeutic Category Antidote, Hydrofluoric Acid; Calcium Salt; Electrolyte Supplement, Oral; Electrolyte Supplement, Parenteral

Generic Availability (US) Yes

Use

Parenteral: Treatment of hypocalcemia and conditions secondary to hypocalcemia (eg, tetany, seizures, arrhythmias); treatment of cardiac disturbances secondary to hyperkalemia; adjunctive treatment of rickets, osteomalacia, and magnesium sulfate overdose; decrease capillary permeability in allergic conditions, nonthrombocytopenic purpura, and exudative dermatoses (eg, dermatitis herpetiformis, pruritus secondary to certain drugs) (All indications: FDA approved in all ages); has also been used for calcium channel blocker toxicity and as a supplement in total parenteral nutrition admixtures

Oral: Dietary supplementation of calcium (OTC: FDA approved in adults)

Pregnancy Risk Factor C

Pregnancy Considerations Animal reproduction studies have not been conducted. Calcium crosses the placenta. The amount of calcium reaching the fetus is determined by maternal physiological changes. Calcium requirements are the same in pregnant and nonpregnant females (IOM, 2011). Information related to use as an antidote in pregnancy is limited. In general, medications used as antidotes should take into consideration the health and prognosis of the mother; antidotes should be administered to pregnant women if there is a clear indication for use and should not be withheld because of fears of teratogenicity (Bailey, 2003).

Breast-Feeding Considerations Calcium is excreted in breast milk. The amount of calcium in breast milk is homeostatically regulated and not altered by maternal calcium intake. Calcium requirements are the same in lactating and nonlactating females (IOM, 2011).

Contraindications Ventricular fibrillation; hypercalcemia; concomitant use of IV calcium gluconate and ceftriaxone in neonates

Warnings/Precautions Multiple salt forms of calcium exist; close attention must be paid to the salt form when ordering and administering calcium; incorrect selection or substitution of one salt for another without proper dosage adjustment may result in serious over or under dosing. Avoid too rapid IV administration (do not exceed 200 mg/minute except in emergency situations);may result in vasodilation, hypotension, bradycardia, arrhythmias, and cardiac arrest. Parenteral calcium is a vesicant; ensure proper catheter or needle position prior to and during infusion. Avoid extravasation; may result in necrosis. Monitor the IV site closely. Use with caution in severe hyperphosphatemia or severe hypokalemia. Hypercalcemia may occur in patients with renal failure; frequent determination of serum calcium is necessary. Use caution with chronic renal disease. Use caution when administering calcium supplements to patients with a history of kidney stones. Hypomagnesemia is a common cause of hypocalcemia; therefore, correction of hypocalcemia may be difficult in patients with concomitant hypomagnesemia. Evaluate serum magnesium and correct hypomagnesemia (if necessary), particularly if initial treatment of hypocalcemia is refractory.

The parenteral product may contain aluminum; toxic aluminum concentrations may be seen with high doses, prolonged use, or renal dysfunction. Premature neonates are at higher risk due to immature renal function and aluminum intake from other parenteral sources. Parenteral aluminum exposure of >4 to 5 mcg/kg/day is associated with CNS and bone toxicity; tissue loading may occur at lower doses (Federal Register, 2002). See manufacturer's labeling.

Constipation, bloating, and gas are common with oral calcium supplements (especially carbonate salt). Administering oral calcium with food and vitamin D will optimize calcium absorption. Some products may contain tartrazine, which may cause allergic reactions in susceptible individuals.

Potentially significant drug-drug interactions may exist, requiring dose or frequency adjustment, additional monitoring, and/or selection of alternative therapy.

Adverse Reactions

IV:

Cardiovascular (with rapid IV injection): Arrhythmia, bradycardia, cardiac arrest, hypotension, syncope, vasodilation

Central nervous system: Sense of oppression (with rapid IV injection)

Endocrine & metabolic: Hypercalcemia

Gastrointestinal: Chalky taste

Neuromuscular & skeletal: Tingling sensation (with rapid IV injection)

Miscellaneous: Heat waves (with rapid IV injection)

Postmarketing and/or case reports: Calcinosis cutis

Oral: Gastrointestinal: Constipation

Drug Interactions

Metabolism/Transport Effects None known.

Avoid Concomitant Use

Avoid concomitant use of Calcium Gluconate with any of the following: Calcium Acetate

Increased Effect/Toxicity

Calcium Gluconate may increase the levels/effects of: Calcium Acetate; Cardiac Glycosides; CefTRIAXone; Vitamin D Analogs

The levels/effects of Calcium Gluconate may be increased by: Multivitamins/Fluoride (with ADE); Multivitamins/Minerals (with ADEK, Folate, Iron); Thiazide Diuretics

Decreased Effect

Calcium Gluconate may decrease the levels/effects of: Alpha-Lipoic Acid; Bisphosphonate Derivatives; Calcium Channel Blockers; Deferiprone; DOBUTamine; Dolutegravir; Eltrombopag; Estramustine; Multivitamins/Fluoride (with ADE); Phosphate Supplements; Quinolone Antibiotics; Strontium Ranelate; Tetracycline Derivatives; Thyroid Products; Trientine

The levels/effects of Calcium Gluconate may be decreased by: Alpha-Lipoic Acid; Trientine

Storage/Stability

IV: Store intact vials at 20°C to 25°C (68°F to 77°F); excursions are permitted between 15°C and 30°C (59°F and 86°F). Do not freeze. Calcium-phosphate stability in parenteral nutrition solutions is dependent upon the pH of the solution, temperature, and relative concentration of each ion. The pH of the solution is primarily dependent upon the amino acid concentration. The higher the percentage amino acids the lower the pH, the more soluble the calcium and phosphate. Individual commercially available amino acid solutions vary significantly with respect to pH lowering potential and consequent calcium phosphate compatibility.

Oral: Store at room temperature; consult product labeling for specific requirements.

Mechanism of Action Moderates nerve and muscle performance via action potential threshold regulation.

In hydrogen fluoride exposures, calcium gluconate provides a source of calcium ions to complex free fluoride ions and prevent or reduce toxicity; administration also helps to correct fluoride-induced hypocalcemia.

Pharmacokinetics (Adult data unless noted)

Absorption: Requires vitamin D; varies with age: Infants 60%, prepubertal children 28%, pubertal children 34%, young adults 25%; calcium is absorbed in soluble, ionized form; absorption increased in an acidic environment; decreased absorption occurs in patients with achlorhydria, renal osteodystrophy, steatorrhea, or uremia

Protein binding: ~40%, primarily to albumin (Wills, 1971)

Elimination: Primarily feces (as unabsorbed calcium salts); urine (20%)

Dosing: Neonatal

Adequate intake (AI): Oral: 200 mg/day of **elemental calcium**; requirements may vary on prematurity, postnatal age, and other clinical factors; serum calcium concentrations should be monitored closely to determine patient-specific needs (IOM, 2011)

Enteral nutrition, maintenance requirement (dietary intake; formula, breastmilk): Preterm neonates, birth weight <2000 g: Oral: 150 to 220 mg/kg/day of **elemental calcium** (Abrams, 2013)

Cardiac arrest in the presence of hyperkalemia or hypocalcemia, hypermagnesemia, or calcium channel blocker toxicity: Dose expressed as calcium gluconate: IV, I.O.: 60 to 100 mg/kg/**dose**; may repeat in 10 minutes if necessary; if effective, consider IV infusion (Avery, 1994; Hegenbarth, 2008)

Hypocalcemia: Dose depends on clinical condition and serum calcium concentration; monitor closely:

General dosing:

Dose expressed as **calcium gluconate**: IV: 200 mg/kg every 6 to 12 hours or 400 mg/kg/day as a continuous infusion (Avery, 1994; Scott, 1984)

Dose expressed as **elemental calcium**:

IV: Usual range: 40 to 50 mg/kg/day as a continuous infusion; for asymptomatic hypocalcemia tapering regimen has been suggested: Initial: 80 mg/kg/day as a continuous infusion for 48 hours then reduce to 40 mg/kg/day continuous infusion typically for 24 hours (once normal serum calcium concentration documented) (Cloherty, 2012; Jain, 2010)

Oral: 50 to 150 mg/kg/day in 4 to 6 divided doses; not to exceed 1000 mg/**day** (Avery, 1994; Rigo, 2007). **Note:** In general, other calcium salts may be more preferable oral dosage forms in neonatal patients; however, the 10% calcium gluconate injection may be given orally (Mimouni, 1994).

Symptomatic (ie, seizures, tetany): Dose expressed as **calcium gluconate**: IV: 100 to 200 mg/kg/**dose** over 5 to 10 minutes; followed by a continuous infusion 500 to 800 mg/kg/day (Cloherty, 2012; Jain, 2010; Mimouni, 1994; Nelson, 1996; Root, 1976; Zhou, 2009)

Parenteral nutrition, maintenance requirement: Dose expressed as **elemental calcium**: IV: 2 to 4 **mEq**/kg/day (Mirtallo, 2004)

Rickets (radiographic evidence), treatment: Dose expressed as **elemental calcium**: Oral: Initial: 20 mg/kg/day in 2 to 4 divided doses, increased as tolerated to usual range of 60 to 70 mg/kg/day in 2 to 4 divided doses; maximum daily dose of 80 mg/kg/day (Abrams, 2013; Avery, 1994)

Dosing: Usual

Pediatric:

Adequate intake (AI) (IOM, 2011): Dose expressed as **elemental calcium:** Oral:

1 to 6 months: 200 mg/day

7 to 12 months: 260 mg/day

Recommended daily allowance (RDA) (IOM, 2011): Dose expressed as **elemental calcium;** during pregnancy and lactation, requirements may change: Oral:

1 to 3 years: 700 mg/day

4 to 8 years: 1000 mg/day

9 to 18 years: 1300 mg/day

Parenteral nutrition, maintenance requirement (Mirtallo, 2004): **Note:** Dose expressed as **elemental calcium:** IV:

Infants and Children ≤50 kg: 0.5 to 4 **mEq**/kg/day

Children >50 kg and Adolescents: 10 to 20 **mEq**/day

Hypocalcemia: Dose depends on clinical condition and serum calcium concentration:

General dosing: Infants, Children, and Adolescents: Dose expressed as **calcium gluconate**: IV: 200 to 500 mg/kg/day as a continuous infusion or in 4 divided doses; maximum dose: Infants and Children: 1000 mg/dose; Adolescents: 2000 to 3000 mg/dose (Edmondson, 1990; Zhou, 2009)

Symptomatic (ie, seizures, tetany): Infants, Children, and Adolescents: Dose expressed as **calcium gluconate**: IV: 100 to 200 mg/kg/dose over 5 to 10 minutes; usual adult dose: 1000 to 2000 mg/dose; may repeat after 6 hours or follow with a continuous infusion of 200 to 800 mg/kg/day (Edmondson, 1990; Kelly, 2013; Misra, 2008; Nelson, 1996; Zhou, 2009)

Chronic therapy in asymptomatic patient: Infants and Children: Dose expressed as **calcium gluconate**: Oral: 500 mg/kg/day in divided doses every 4 to 8 hours (Nelson, 1996); **Note:** In general, other oral calcium salts (eg, carbonate, glubionate) are a more preferable oral dosage form option in young pediatric patients; however, the 10% calcium gluconate injection may be given orally (Mimouni, 1994).

Rickets (due to vitamin D deficiency); treatment: Infants and Children: Dose expressed as **elemental calcium**: Oral: 30 to 75 mg/kg/day in 3 divided doses; begin at higher end of range and titrate downward over 2 to 4 weeks (Misra, 2008). **Note:** In general, other oral calcium salts (eg, carbonate, glubionate) are a more preferable oral dosage formulation option in young pediatric patients; however, the 10% calcium gluconate injection may be given orally (Mimouni, 1994).

Cardiac arrest in the presence of hyperkalemia or hypocalcemia, hypermagnesemia, or calcium channel blocker toxicity: Infants, Children, and Adolescents: Dose expressed as **calcium gluconate**: IV, I.O.: 60 to 100 mg/kg/**dose** (maximum dose: 3000 mg); may repeat in 10 minutes if necessary; if effective, consider IV infusion (Hegenbarth, 2008). **Note:** Routine use in cardiac arrest is not recommended due to the lack of improved survival (PALS [Kleinman], 2010).

Calcium channel blocker toxicity; hypotension/conduction disturbances: Infants, Children, and Adolescents: Dose expressed in mg of **calcium gluconate**: IV, I.O.: 60 mg/kg/**dose** administered over 30 to 60 minutes (Hegenbarth, 2008). **Note:** Calcium chloride may provide a more rapid increase of ionized calcium in critically ill children. Calcium gluconate may be substituted if calcium chloride is not available.

Adult: **Note:** Dose expressed in terms of the **calcium gluconate salt** (unless otherwise specified as elemental calcium). Doses expressed in terms of the **calcium gluconate salt** are based on a solution concentration of 100 mg/mL (10%) containing 0.465 mEq (9.3 mg)/mL elemental calcium, except where noted.

Recommended daily allowance (RDA) (IOM, 2011): **Note:** Expressed in terms of elemental calcium: Oral: Females/Males:
- 19 to 50 years: 1000 mg elemental calcium daily
- ≥51 years, females: 1200 mg elemental calcium daily
- 51 to 70 years, males: 1000 mg elemental calcium daily
- Females, pregnant/lactating: Requirements are the same as in nonpregnant or nonlactating females

Hypocalcemia:

Intermittent IV:
- Mild [ionized calcium: 4 to 5 mg/dL (1 to 1.2 mmol/L)]: 1000-2000 mg over 2 hours; asymptomatic patients may be given oral calcium (Ariyan, 2004; French, 2012)
- Moderate to severe [without seizure or tetany; ionized calcium: <4 mg/dL (<1 mmol/L)]: 4000 mg over 4 hours (French, 2012)
- Severe symptomatic (eg, seizure, tetany): 1000 to 2000 mg over 10 minutes; repeat every 60 minutes until symptoms resolve (French, 2012)
- **Note:** Repeat ionized calcium measurement 6 to 10 hours after completion of administration. Check for hypomagnesemia and correct if present. Consider continuous infusion if hypocalcemia is likely to recur due to ongoing losses (French, 2012).
- Continuous IV infusion: 5 to 20 mg/kg/hour (Pai, 2011)

Cardiac arrest or cardiotoxicity in the presence of hyperkalemia, hypocalcemia, or hypermagnesemia: IV: 1500 to 3000 mg over 2 to 5 minutes (Vanden Hoek, 2010); **Note:** Routine use in cardiac arrest is not recommended due to the lack of improved survival (Neumar, 2010).

Maintenance electrolyte requirements for parenteral nutrition: IV (Mirtallo, 2004): **Note:** Expressed in terms of elemental calcium: 10-20 mEq daily

Dosing adjustment in renal impairment: Infants, Children, Adolescents, and Adults: No initial dosage adjustment necessary; however, accumulation may occur with renal impairment and subsequent doses may require adjustment based on serum calcium concentrations.

Dosing adjustment in hepatic impairment: Infants, Children, Adolescents, and Adults: No initial dosage adjustment necessary; subsequent doses should be guided by serum calcium concentrations. In adult patients in the anhepatic stage of liver transplantation, equal rapid increases in ionized concentrations occur suggesting that calcium gluconate does not require hepatic metabolism for release of ionized calcium (Martin, 1990).

Preparation for Administration Parenteral: Observe the vial for the presence of particulates. If particulates are observed, place vial in a 60°C to 80°C water bath for 15 to 30 minutes (or until solution is clear); occasionally shake to dissolve; cool to body/room temperature before use. Do not use vial if particulates do not dissolve. **Note:** Due to the potential presence of particulates, American Regent, Inc recommends the use of a 5 micron filter when preparing calcium gluconate-containing IV solutions (Important Drug Administration Information, American Regent 2013); a similar recommendation has not been noted by other manufacturers.

IV infusion: Further dilute in D_5W or NS; a maximum concentration of 50 mg/mL has been used by some centers. Usual adult concentrations: 1,000 mg/100 mL D_5W or NS; 2,000 mg/100 mL D_5W or NS. Maximum concentration in parenteral nutrition solutions is variable depending upon concentration and solubility (consult detailed reference).

Administration

Oral: Administer with plenty of fluids with or following meals. The 10% calcium gluconate injection may be administered orally in young pediatric patients (Mimouni 1994)

Parenteral: Do not inject calcium salts IM or administer SubQ since severe necrosis and sloughing may occur; extravasation of calcium can result in severe necrosis and tissue sloughing. Do not use scalp vein or small hand or foot veins for IV administration. Not for endotracheal administration.

IV: Administer undiluted slowly (~1.5 mL calcium gluconate 10% per minute; not to exceed 200 mg/minute except in emergency situations; consider cardiac monitoring) through a small needle into a large vein in order to avoid too rapid increases in the serum calcium and extravasation. In acute situations of symptomatic hypocalcemia, infusions over 5 to 10 minutes have been described in pediatric patients (Kelly 2013; Misra 2008)

IV infusion: Administer at a rate not to exceed 200 mg/minute. **Note:** Due to the potential presence of particulates, American Regent, Inc recommends the use of a 0.22 micron in-line filter for IV administration of admixture (1.2 micron filter if admixture contains lipids) (Important Drug Administration Information, American Regent 2013); a similar recommendation has not been noted by other manufacturers.

Parenteral nutrition solution: Calcium-phosphate stability in parenteral nutrition solutions is dependent upon the pH of the solution, temperature, and relative concentration of each ion. The pH of the solution is primarily dependent upon the amino acid concentration. The higher the percentage amino acids the lower the pH, the more soluble the calcium and phosphate. Individual commercially available amino acid solutions vary significantly with respect to pH lowering potential and consequent calcium phosphate compatibility; consult product specific labeling for additional information.

Vesicant; ensure proper needle or catheter placement prior to and during IV infusion. Avoid extravasation. If extravasation occurs, stop infusion immediately and disconnect (leave needle/cannula in place); gently aspirate extravasated solution (do NOT flush the line); initiate hyaluronidase antidote (See Management of Drug Extravasations for more details); remove needle/cannula; apply dry cold compresses (Hurst 2004); elevate extremity.

Vesicant/Extravasation Risk Vesicant

Monitoring Parameters Serum calcium (ionized calcium preferred if available), phosphate, magnesium, heart rate, ECG

Reference Range

	Age	Normal Values Serum Concentration
Calcium, total	Cord blood	9 to 11.5 mg/dL
	Newborn 3 to 24 hours	9 to 10.6 mg/dL
	Newborn 24 to 48 hours	7 to 12 mg/dL
	4 to 7 days	9 to 10.9 mg/dL
	Child	8.8 to 10.8 mg/dL
	Adolescent to Adult	8.4 to 10.2 mg/dL
Calcium, ionized, whole blood	Cord blood	5 to 6 mg/dL
	Newborn 3 to 24 hours	4.3 to 5.1 mg/dL
	Newborn 24 to 48 hours	4 to 4.7 mg/dL
	≥2 days	4.8 to 4.92 mg/dL (2.24 to 2.46 mEq/L)

Test Interactions IV administration may produce falsely decreased serum and urine magnesium concentrations

Additional Information Due to a poor correlation between the serum ionized calcium (free) and total serum calcium, particularly in states of low albumin or acid/base imbalances, direct measurement of ionized calcium is recommended. If ionized calcium is unavailable, in low albumin states, the corrected **total** serum calcium may be estimated by this equation (assuming a normal albumin of 4 g/dL); [(4 – patient's albumin) x 0.8] + patient's measured total calcium

Elemental Calcium Content of Calcium Salts

Calcium Salt	Elemental Calcium (mg/1 g of salt form)	Calcium (mEq/g)
Calcium acetate	253	12.7
Calcium carbonate	400	20
Calcium chloride	273	13.6
Calcium citrate	211	10.5
Calcium glubionate	63.8	3.2
Calcium gluconate	93	4.65
Calcium lactate	130	6.5
Calcium phosphate (tribasic)	390	19.3

Dosage Forms Considerations 1 g calcium gluconate = elemental calcium 93 mg = calcium 4.65 mEq = calcium 2.33 mmol

Dosage Forms Excipient information presented when available (limited, particularly for generics); consult specific product labeling. [DSC] = Discontinued product

Capsule, Oral [preservative free]:
  Cal-Glu: 500 mg [dye free]

Solution, Intravenous:
  Generic: 10% (10 mL, 50 mL, 100 mL)

Solution, Intravenous [preservative free]:
  Generic: 10% (100 mL)

Tablet, Oral:
  Generic: 50 mg, 500 mg, 648 mg [DSC]

◆ **Calcium High Potency [OTC]** *see* Calcium Carbonate *on page 343*

Calcium Lactate (KAL see um LAK tate)

Brand Names: US Cal-Lac [OTC]

Therapeutic Category Calcium Salt; Electrolyte Supplement, Oral

Generic Availability (US) Yes

Use Prevention and treatment of calcium deficiency; dietary supplement; adjunctive prevention and treatment of osteoporosis

Pregnancy Considerations Calcium crosses the placenta. Intestinal absorption of calcium increases during pregnancy. The amount of calcium reaching the fetus is determined by maternal physiological changes. Calcium requirements are the same in pregnant and nonpregnant females (IOM, 2011).

Breast-Feeding Considerations Calcium is excreted in breast milk. The amount of calcium in breast milk is homeostatically regulated and not altered by maternal calcium intake. Calcium requirements are the same in lactating and nonlactating females (IOM, 2011).

Warnings/Precautions Constipation, bloating, and gas are common with calcium supplements. Use with caution in patients with renal failure to avoid hypercalcemia; frequent monitoring of serum calcium and phosphorus is necessary. Use caution when administering calcium supplements to patients with a history of kidney stones. Hypercalcemia and hypercalciuria are most likely to occur in hypoparathyroid patients receiving high doses of vitamin D. Calcium absorption is impaired in achlorhydria; common in elderly, use an alternate salt (eg, citrate) and administer with food. Calcium administration interferes with absorption of some minerals and drugs; use with caution. It is recommended to concomitantly administer vitamin D for optimal calcium absorption. Taking calcium (≤500 mg) with food improves absorption. Multiple salt forms of calcium exist; close attention must be paid to the salt form when ordering and administering calcium; incorrect selection or substitution of one salt for another without proper dosage adjustment may result in serious over or under dosing.

Adverse Reactions Rare but important or life-threatening: Constipation, dizziness, dry mouth, headache, hypercalcemia, hypercalciuria, hypomagnesemia, hypophosphatemia, mental confusion, milk-alkali syndrome, nausea, vomiting

Drug Interactions

Metabolism/Transport Effects None known.

Avoid Concomitant Use

Avoid concomitant use of Calcium Lactate with any of the following: Calcium Acetate

Increased Effect/Toxicity

Calcium Lactate may increase the levels/effects of: Calcium Acetate; Cardiac Glycosides; Vitamin D Analogs

The levels/effects of Calcium Lactate may be increased by: Multivitamins/Fluoride (with ADE); Multivitamins/Minerals (with ADEK, Folate, Iron); Thiazide Diuretics

Decreased Effect

Calcium Lactate may decrease the levels/effects of: Alpha-Lipoic Acid; Bisphosphonate Derivatives; Calcium Channel Blockers; Deferiprone; DOBUTamine; Dolutegravir; Eltrombopag; Estramustine; Multivitamins/Fluoride (with ADE); Phosphate Supplements; Quinolone Antibiotics; Strontium Ranelate; Tetracycline Derivatives; Thyroid Products; Trientine

The levels/effects of Calcium Lactate may be decreased by: Alpha-Lipoic Acid; Trientine

Storage/Stability Store at room temperature.

Mechanism of Action As dietary supplement, used to prevent or treat negative calcium balance; in osteoporosis, it helps to prevent or decrease the rate of bone loss. The calcium in calcium salts moderates nerve and muscle performance and allows normal cardiac function.

Pharmacokinetics (Adult data unless noted)

Absorption: 25% to 35%; varies with age (infants 60%, prepubertal children 28%, pubertal children 34%, young adults 25%); decreased absorption occurs in patients with achlorhydria, renal osteodystrophy, steatorrhea, or uremia

Protein binding: 45%

Elimination: Primarily in the feces as unabsorbed calcium

Dosing: Neonatal Oral:

Adequate intake (AI): 200 mg/day of **elemental calcium**; requirements may vary on prematurity, postnatal age, and other clinical factors; serum calcium concentrations should be monitored closely to determine patient-specific needs

Hypocalcemia: Dose depends on clinical condition and serum calcium concentration:

Dose expressed in mg of **elemental calcium**: 50-150 mg/kg/day in 4-6 divided doses; not to exceed 1000 mg/day

Dose expressed in mg of **calcium lactate**: 400-500 mg/kg/day divided every 4-6 hours

Dosing: Usual Oral:

Adequate intake (AI): Dosage expressed in terms of **elemental calcium:**

1-6 months: 200 mg/day

7-12 months: 260 mg/day

Recommended daily allowance (RDA): Dosage expressed in terms of **elemental calcium;** during pregnancy and lactation, requirements may change:

1-3 years: 700 mg/day

4-8 years: 1000 mg/day

9-18 years: 1300 mg/day

Females 19-50 years, males 19-70 years: 1000 mg/day

Females ≥51 years, males ≥71 years: 1200 mg/day

Hypocalcemia: Dose depends on clinical condition and serum calcium concentration:

Dose expressed as **elemental calcium**:

Children: 45-65 mg/kg/day in 4 divided doses

Adults: 1-2 g or more per day in 3-4 divided doses

Dose expressed as **calcium lactate**:

Infants: 400-500 mg/kg/day divided every 4-6 hours

Children: 500 mg/kg/day divided every 6-8 hours; maximum daily dose: 9 g

Adults: 1.5-3 g/day divided every 8 hours; maximum daily dose: 9 g

Adjunctive prevention and treatment of osteoporosis: Adults: 500 mg **elemental calcium** 2-3 times/day; recommended dosage includes dietary intake and should be adjusted depending upon the patient's diet; to improve absorption do not administer more than 500 mg **elemental calcium**/dose

Dosage adjustment in renal impairment: CrCl <25 mL/minute may require dosage adjustment depending upon serum calcium level

Administration Oral: Administer with plenty of fluids with or following meals

Monitoring Parameters Serum calcium (ionized calcium preferred if available), phosphate, magnesium, heart rate, ECG

Reference Range

Calcium: Newborns: 7-12 mg/dL; 0-2 years: 8.8-11.2 mg/dL; 2 years to adults: 9-11 mg/dL

Calcium, ionized, whole blood: 4.4-5.4 mg/dL

Additional Information Due to a poor correlation between the serum ionized calcium (free) and total serum calcium, particularly in states of low albumin or acid/base imbalances, direct measurement of ionized calcium is recommended. If ionized calcium is unavailable, in low albumin states, the corrected **total** serum calcium may be estimated by this equation (assuming a normal albumin of 4 g/dL); [(4 – patient's albumin) x 0.8] + patient's measured total calcium

Elemental Calcium Content of Calcium Salts

Calcium Salt	Elemental Calcium (mg/1 g of salt form)	Calcium (mEq/g)
Calcium acetate	253	12.7
Calcium carbonate	400	20
Calcium chloride	273	13.6
Calcium citrate	211	10.5
Calcium glubionate	63.8	3.2
Calcium gluconate	93	4.65
Calcium lactate	130	6.5
Calcium phosphate (tribasic)	390	19.3

Dosage Forms Considerations 648 mg calcium lactate = elemental calcium 84 mg = calcium 4.2 mEq = calcium 2.1 mmol

Dosage Forms Excipient information presented when available (limited, particularly for generics); consult specific product labeling.

Capsule, Oral [preservative free]:

Cal-Lac: 500 mg [dye free]

Tablet, Oral:

Generic: 100 mg

Tablet, Oral [preservative free]:

Generic: 648 mg

◆ **Calcium Leucovorin** *see* Leucovorin Calcium *on page 1226*

◆ **Calcium Levoleucovorin** *see* LEVOleucovorin *on page 1248*

◆ **Caldolor** *see* Ibuprofen *on page 1064*

Calfactant (kaf AKT ant)

Brand Names: US Infasurf

Therapeutic Category Lung Surfactant

Generic Availability (US) No

Use Prevention and treatment of respiratory distress syndrome (RDS) in premature infants

Prophylactic therapy: Infants <29 weeks at significant risk for RDS

Treatment: Infants ≤72 hours of age with RDS (confirmed by clinical and radiologic findings and requiring endotracheal intubation)

Contraindications

There are no contraindications listed in the manufacturer's labeling.

Warnings/Precautions For intratracheal administration only. Rapidly affects oxygenation and lung compliance; restrict use to a highly-supervised clinical setting with immediate availability of clinicians experienced in intubation and ventilatory management of premature infants. Transient episodes of bradycardia, decreased oxygen saturation, endotracheal tube blockage or reflux of calfactant into endotracheal tube may occur. Discontinue dosing procedure and initiate measures to alleviate the condition; may reinstitute after the patient is stable. Produces rapid improvements in lung oxygenation and compliance that may require frequent adjustments to oxygen delivery and ventilator settings.

Adverse Reactions

Cardiovascular: Bradycardia, cyanosis

Respiratory: Airway obstruction, reflux, reintubation, requirement for manual ventilation

Drug Interactions

Metabolism/Transport Effects None known.

Avoid Concomitant Use

Avoid concomitant use of Calfactant with any of the following: Ceritinib

Increased Effect/Toxicity

Calfactant may increase the levels/effects of: Bradycardia-Causing Agents; Ceritinib; Ivabradine; Lacosamide

The levels/effects of Calfactant may be increased by: Bretylium; Ruxolitinib; Tofacitinib

Decreased Effect There are no known significant interactions involving a decrease in effect.

Storage/Stability Gentle swirling or agitation of the vial of suspension is often necessary for redispersion. **Do not shake.** Visible flecks of the suspension and foaming under the surface are normal. Calfactant should be stored upright (3 mL vial) and under refrigeration at 2°C to 8°C (36°F to 46°F); protect from light; document date and time removed from refrigeration. Warming before administration is not necessary. Unopened and unused vials of calfactant that have been warmed to room temperature can be returned to refrigeration storage within 24 hours for future use. Repeated warming to room temperature should be avoided. Each single-use vial should be entered only once and the vial with any unused material should be discarded after the initial entry.

Mechanism of Action Endogenous lung surfactant is essential for effective ventilation because it modifies alveolar surface tension, thereby stabilizing the alveoli. Lung surfactant deficiency is the cause of respiratory distress syndrome (RDS) in premature infants and lung surfactant restores surface activity to the lungs of these infants.

Dosing: Neonatal Endotracheal: 3 mL/kg every 12 hours up to a total of 3 doses in the first 96 hours of life; repeat doses have been administered as frequently as every 6 hours for a total of up to 4 doses (if the neonate was still intubated and required at least 30% inspired oxygen to maintain arterial oxygen saturations >90% or with a PaO_2 ≤80 torr on >30% inspired oxygen) (Bloom, 2005; Kattwinkel, 2000)

Administration Intratracheal: Gently swirl to redisperse suspension; do not shake; administer dosage divided into two aliquots of 1.5 mL/kg each into the endotracheal tube; after each instillation, reposition the infant with either the right or left side dependent; administration is made while ventilation is continued over 20-30 breaths for each aliquot, with small bursts timed only during the inspiratory cycles; a pause followed by evaluation of the respiratory status and repositioning should separate the two aliquots; calfactant dosage has also been divided into four equal aliquots and administered with repositioning in four different positions (prone, supine, right and left lateral)

Monitoring Parameters Continuous heart rate and transcutaneous O_2 saturation should be monitored during administration; frequent ABG sampling is necessary to prevent postdosing hyperoxia and hypocarbia

Dosage Forms Excipient information presented when available (limited, particularly for generics); consult specific product labeling.

Suspension, Inhalation:

Infasurf: 35 mg phospholipids and 0.7 mg protein per mL (3 mL, 6 mL)

◆ **Cal-Gest Antacid [OTC]** *see* Calcium Carbonate *on page 343*

◆ **Cal-Glu [OTC]** *see* Calcium Gluconate *on page 351*

◆ **Calicylic [OTC]** *see* Salicylic Acid *on page 1894*

◆ **Cal-Lac [OTC]** *see* Calcium Lactate *on page 354*

◆ **Cal-Mint [OTC]** *see* Calcium Carbonate *on page 343*

◆ **Calphron [OTC]** *see* Calcium Acetate *on page 341*

◆ **Caltrate (Can)** *see* Calcium Carbonate *on page 343*

◆ **Caltrate 600 [OTC]** *see* Calcium Carbonate *on page 343*

◆ **Caltrate Select (Can)** *see* Calcium Carbonate *on page 343*

◆ **Cambia** *see* Diclofenac (Systemic) *on page 641*

◆ **Camila** *see* Norethindrone *on page 1530*

◆ **Camphorated Tincture of Opium (error-prone synonym)** *see* Paregoric *on page 1630*

◆ **Camptosar** *see* Irinotecan *on page 1159*

◆ **Camptothecin-11** *see* Irinotecan *on page 1159*

Canakinumab (can a KIN ue mab)

Brand Names: US Ilaris

Brand Names: Canada Ilaris

Therapeutic Category Interleukin-1 Receptor Antagonist; Monoclonal Antibody

Generic Availability (US) No

Use Treatment of cryopyrin-associated periodic syndromes (CAPS), including familial cold autoinflammatory syndrome (FCAS) and Muckle-Wells syndrome (MWS) (FDA approved in ages ≥4 years and adults); treatment of active systemic for juvenile idiopathic arthritis (SJIA) (FDA approved in ages ≥2 years weighing at least 7.5 kg)

Medication Guide Available Yes

Pregnancy Risk Factor C

Pregnancy Considerations Adverse events were observed in animal reproduction studies. The Canadian product labeling recommends women of reproductive potential use effective contraception during treatment and for 3 months after the last dose.

Breast-Feeding Considerations It is not known if canakinumab is excreted into breast milk. The U.S. manufacturer labeling recommends caution be used if administered to nursing women. The Canadian labeling recommends avoiding use in nursing women.

Contraindications Confirmed hypersensitivity to canakinumab or any component of the formulation

Canadian labeling: Additional contraindications (not in U.S. labeling): Active, severe infections

Warnings/Precautions Hypersensitivity reactions (excluding anaphylactic reactions) have been reported with use; symptoms may be similar to those that are disease-related. Use is contraindicated in patients with known hypersensitivity to canakinumab. Caution should be exercised when considering use in patients with a history of new/recurrent infections, with conditions that predispose them to infections, or with latent or localized infections. Therapy should not be initiated in patients with active or chronic infections. Patients should be evaluated for latent tuberculosis infection with a tuberculin skin test prior to starting therapy. Treat latent TB infections prior to initiating canakinumab therapy. During and following treatment, monitor for signs/symptoms of active TB. Macrophage activation syndrome (MAS may develop in patients with SJIA and should be treated aggressively. Infection or worsening SJIA may be triggers for MAS

Use may impair defenses against malignancies; impact on the development and course of malignancies is not fully defined. Neutropenia (ANC <1500/mm^3) has been reported with use. The Canadian labeling recommends assessing neutrophil counts prior to initiating canakinumab, after 1 to 2 months of therapy, and periodically thereafter. Patients with neutropenia prior to initiation are not recommended for therapy. If a patient becomes neutropenic, close monitoring of the ANC and consideration of treatment discontinuation is also recommended (Ilaris Canadian product monograph, 2013).

Potentially significant drug-drug interactions may exist, requiring dose or frequency adjustment, additional monitoring, and/or selection of alternative therapy. Immunizations should be up to date including pneumococcal and influenza vaccines before initiating therapy. Live vaccines should not be given concurrently. Administration of inactivated (killed) vaccines while on therapy may not be effective.

Some dosage forms may contain polysorbate 80 (also known as Tweens). Hypersensitivity reactions, usually a delayed reaction, have been reported following exposure to pharmaceutical products containing polysorbate 80 in certain individuals (Isaksson, 2002; Lucente 2000; Shelley, 1995). Thrombocytopenia, ascites, pulmonary deterioration, and renal and hepatic failure have been reported in premature neonates after receiving parenteral products containing polysorbate 80 (Alade, 1986; CDC, 1984). See manufacturer's labeling.

Warnings: Additional Pediatric Considerations Influenza reported in 17% of patients during clinical trials. Vertigo has been reported exclusively in patients with MWS (9% to 14%); events appear self-resolving with continued therapy. Infection reported more frequently in children than adults (Kuemmerle-Deschner 2011) for both CAPS and JIA. Treatment for CAPS has been associated with higher incidence of reported adverse reactions including diarrhea (20%), nasopharyngitis (34%), and rhinitis (17%).

Adverse Reactions

Adverse events reported in treatment of CAPS unless otherwise noted.

Central nervous system: Headache, vertigo

Endocrine & metabolic: Decreased serum calcium (Lachmann, 2009), weight gain

Gastrointestinal: Diarrhea, gastroenteritis, nausea, upper abdominal pain (SJIA)

Genitourinary: Proteinuria (Lachmann, 2009)

Hematologic & oncologic: Decreased neutrophils (transient; SJIA), decreased white blood cell count (SJIA), eosinophilia (Lachmann, 2009), thrombocytopenia (mild, transient, SJIA)

Hepatic: Increased serum alkaline phosphatase (Lachmann, 2009), Increased serum ALT (Lachmann, 2009), increased serum AST (Lachmann, 2009), increased serum bilirubin (Lachmann, 2009), increased serum transaminases (SJIA)

Immunologic: Antibody development (non-neutralizing; more common in SJIA)

Infection: Infection (SJIA), influenza

Local: Injection site reaction (more common in SJIA)

Neuromuscular and skeletal: Musculoskeletal pain

Renal: Decreased creatinine clearance (Lachmann, 2009)

Respiratory: Bronchitis, nasopharyngitis, pharyngitis, rhinitis

Rare but important or life-threatening: Hypersensitivity reaction, increased blood pressure, neutropenia (SJIA)

Drug Interactions

Metabolism/Transport Effects None known.

Avoid Concomitant Use

Avoid concomitant use of Canakinumab with any of the following: Anti-TNF Agents; BCG; BCG (Intravesical); Belimumab; Interleukin-1 Inhibitors; Interleukin-1 Receptor Antagonist; Natalizumab; Pimecrolimus; Tacrolimus (Topical); Tofacitinib; Vaccines (Live)

Increased Effect/Toxicity

Canakinumab may increase the levels/effects of: Belimumab; Leflunomide; Natalizumab; Tofacitinib; Vaccines (Live)

The levels/effects of Canakinumab may be increased by: Anti-TNF Agents; Denosumab; Interleukin-1 Inhibitors; Interleukin-1 Receptor Antagonist; Pimecrolimus; Roflumilast; Tacrolimus (Topical); Trastuzumab

Decreased Effect

Canakinumab may decrease the levels/effects of: BCG; BCG (Intravesical); Coccidioides immitis Skin Test; Sipuleucel-T; Vaccines (Inactivated); Vaccines (Live)

The levels/effects of Canakinumab may be decreased by: Echinacea

Storage/Stability Store powder in refrigerator at 2°C to 8°C (36°F to 46°F); do not freeze. Protect from light. After reconstitution, vials may be stored at controlled room temperature for up to 1 hour or in a refrigerator for up to 4 hours.

Mechanism of Action Canakinumab reduces inflammation by binding to interleukin-1 beta (IL-1β) (no binding to IL-1 alpha or IL-1 receptor antagonist) and preventing interaction with cell surface receptors. Cryopyrin-associated periodic syndromes (CAPS) refers to rare genetic syndromes caused by mutations in the nucleotide-binding domain, leucine rich family (NLR), pyrin domain containing 3 (NLRP-3) gene or the cold-induced autoinflammatory syndrome-1 (CIAS1) gene. Cryopyrin, a protein encoded by this gene, regulates IL-1β activation. Deficiency of cryopyrin results in excessive inflammation.

Pharmacodynamics Maximum effect: Within 8 days CRP and serum amyloid normalization

Pharmacokinetics (Adult data unless noted)

Distribution: Varies according to body weight: V_{dss}: Children: 0.097 L/kg (3.2 L in 33 kg); Adults: 0.086 L/kg (6 L in 70 kg)

Protein binding: Binds to serum IL-1β

Bioavailability: SubQ: 66%

Half-life elimination: Pediatric patients ≥4 years: 23 to 26 days; Adults: 26 days

Time to peak serum concentration: Pediatric patients ≥4 years: 2 to 7 days; Adults: ~7 days

Elimination: Clearance: Varies according to body weight (NCT 00685373, 2011):

- Pediatric patients ≤40 kg: 0.083 L/day (0.11 L/day in 33 kg)
- Pediatric patients >40 kg and Adults: 0.18 L/day (0.17 L/day in 70 kg)

Dosing: Usual

Pediatric:

Cryopyrin-associated periodic syndromes (CAPS): Patient syndromes included in trials were: Familial cold autoinflammatory syndrome (FCAS), Muckle-Wells syndrome (MWS), chronic infantile neurological cutaneous articular syndrome/neonatal onset multisystemic inflammatory disease (CINCA/NOMID), and familial cold urticaria (FCU); data has shown that pediatric patients require higher doses than adults (Kuemmerle-Deschner 2011).

Manufacturer's labeling: Children ≥4 years and Adolescents:

- 15 to ≤40 kg: SubQ: Initial: 2 mg/kg/dose every 8 weeks; may increase to 3 mg/kg/dose if response inadequate
- >40 kg: SubQ: 150 mg/dose every 8 weeks

Alternate dosing: Limited data available:

- Children 2 to <4 years and weighing ≥7.5 kg: SubQ: 4 mg/kg/dose every 8 weeks; if no response after 7 days, may repeat 4 mg/kg dose, if response achieved then may continue patient on intensified maintenance of 8 mg/kg/dose every 8 weeks (European Medicines Agency [Ilaris prescribing information 2014])

Children ≥4 years and Adolescents:

≥7.5 kg to <15 kg: SubQ: 4 mg/kg/dose every 8 weeks. If no response after 7 days, may administered a second 4 mg/kg/dose, if full treatment response achieved then may continue patient on intensified maintenance of 8 mg/kg/dose every 8 weeks (European Medicines Agency [Ilaris prescribing information] 2014)

15 kg to ≤40 kg: SubQ: 2 mg/kg/dose every 8 weeks. If response not satisfactory after 7 days, may repeat 2 mg/kg dose, if full treatment response achieved then may continue patient on intensified maintenance of 4 mg/kg/dose every 8 weeks. If after 7 days (ie, day 14) a satisfactory response still not achieved, may administer another 4 mg/kg dose, if full treatment response achieved then may continue patient on intensified maintenance of 8 mg/kg/dose every 8 weeks (European Medicines Agency [Ilaris prescribing information] 2014; Kuemmerle-Deschner 2011). Another dose-escalation regimen describes titration in 2 mg/kg/dose increments every 7 days up to a maximum dose of 8 mg/kg/dose (Ilaris Canadian product monograph, 2013)

>40 kg: SubQ: 150 mg every 8 weeks. If response not satisfactory after 7 days, may repeat 150 mg/dose, if full treatment response achieved then may continue patient on intensified maintenance of 300 mg every 8 weeks. If after 7 days (ie, day 14) a satisfactory response still not achieved, may administer another 300 mg/dose, if full treatment response achieved then may continue patient on intensified maintenance of 600 mg every 8 weeks (European Medicines Agency [Ilaris prescribing information] 2014; Kuemmerle-Deschner 2011). Another dose-escalation regimen describes titration in 150 mg increments every 7 days up to a maximum dose of 600 mg (Ilaris prescribing information [Canada] 2013).

Juvenile idiopathic arthritis; systemic: Children ≥2 years weighing at least 7.5 kg and Adolescents: SubQ: 4 mg/kg/dose every 4 weeks; maximum dose: 300 mg

Adult: **Cryopyrin-associated periodic syndromes (CAPS):**

Manufacturer's labeling: Patient weight >40 kg: SubQ: 150 mg/dose every 8 weeks

Alternate dosing: 150 mg every 8 weeks; if inadequate response after 7 days may consider further titration by 150 mg every 7 days up to a maximum dose of 600 mg. The dose at which a satisfactory response is achieved should be maintained and administered every 8 weeks (Ilaris prescribing information [Canada] 2013).

Dosing adjustment in renal impairment: Children ≥2 years, Adolescents, and Adults: There are no dosage adjustments provided in the manufacturer's labeling; has not been studied.

Dosing adjustment in hepatic impairment: Children ≥2 years, Adolescents, and Adults: There are no dosage adjustments provided in the manufacturer's labeling; has not been studied.

Preparation for Administration SubQ: Reconstitute vial with 1 mL SWFI (preservative free). Swirl the vial at a 45-degree angle for ~1 minute (do not shake), then allow solution to sit for 5 minutes. Continue product dissolution by gently turning vial (without touching rubber stopper) upside down and back 10 times; do not shake. Allow to sit at room temperature for ~15 minutes until solution is clear. Do not shake. Solution may have a slight brownish-yellow tint; do not use if distinctly brown in color or if particulate matter is present in the solution. Each reconstituted vial results in a final concentration of 150 mg/mL.

Administration SubQ: Administer subcutaneously by a health care provider; avoid sites with scar tissue.

Monitoring Parameters CBC with differential, C-reactive protein (CRP), serum amyloid A; signs or symptoms of infection; latent TB screening (prior to initiating therapy), body weight. Eye examinations for patients with CAPS (Caorsi 2013) and symptoms of disease for patients with CAPS or SJIA (Caorsi 2013; Lachmann 2009; Ruperto 2012) were also monitored in clinical trials.

Dosage Forms Excipient information presented when available (limited, particularly for generics); consult specific product labeling.

Solution Reconstituted, Subcutaneous [preservative free]:

Ilaris: 180 mg (1 ea) [contains polysorbate 80]

◆ **Canasa** *see* Mesalamine *on page 1368*

◆ **Cancidas** *see* Caspofungin *on page 383*

◆ **Cancidas® (Can)** *see* Caspofungin *on page 383*

Candesartan (kan de SAR tan)

Medication Safety Issues

Sound-alike/look-alike issues:

Atacand may be confused with antacid

Brand Names: US Atacand

Brand Names: Canada ACH Candesartan; Apo-Candesartan; Atacand; CO Candesartan; DOM-Candesartan; JAMP-Candesartan; Mylan-Candesartan; PMS-Candesartan; Ran-Candesartan; Sandoz-Candesartan; Teva-Candesartan

Therapeutic Category Angiotensin II Receptor Blocker; Antihypertensive Agent

Generic Availability (US) Yes

Use Treatment of hypertension alone or in combination with other antihypertensive agents (FDA approved in ages ≥1 year and adults); treatment of heart failure (NYHA class II-IV) (FDA approved in adults)

Pregnancy Risk Factor D

Pregnancy Considerations [U.S. Boxed Warning]: Drugs that act on the renin-angiotensin system can cause injury and death to the developing fetus. Discontinue as soon as possible once pregnancy is detected. The use of drugs which act on the renin-angiotensin system are associated with oligohydramnios. Oligohydramnios, due to decreased fetal renal function, may lead to fetal lung hypoplasia and skeletal malformations. Use is also associated with anuria, hypotension, renal failure, skull hypoplasia, and death in the fetus/neonate. The exposed fetus should be monitored for fetal growth, amniotic fluid volume, and organ formation. Infants exposed *in utero* should be monitored for hyperkalemia, hypotension, and oliguria (exchange transfusions or dialysis may be needed). These adverse events are generally associated with maternal use in the second and third trimesters.

Untreated chronic maternal hypertension is also associated with adverse events in the fetus, infant, and mother. The use of angiotensin II receptor blockers is not recommended to treat chronic uncomplicated hypertension in pregnant women and should generally be avoided in women of reproductive potential (ACOG, 2013).

Breast-Feeding Considerations It is not known if candesartan is excreted into breast milk. Due to the potential for serious adverse reactions in the nursing infant, the manufacturer recommends a decision be made whether to discontinue nursing or to discontinue the drug, taking into account the importance of treatment to the mother. The Canadian labeling contraindicates use in breast-feeding women.

Contraindications

Hypersensitivity to candesartan or any component of the formulation; concomitant use with aliskiren in patients with diabetes mellitus

Canadian labeling: Additional contraindications (not in U.S. labeling): Concomitant use with aliskiren in patients with moderate-to-severe renal impairment (GFR <60 mL/minute/1.73 m^2); pregnancy; breast-feeding; children <1 year of age; rare hereditary problems of galactose intolerance, Lapp lactase deficiency or glucose-galactose malabsorption

Warnings/Precautions [U.S. Boxed Warning]: Drugs that act on the renin-angiotensin system can cause injury and death to the developing fetus. Discontinue as soon as possible once pregnancy is detected. May cause hyperkalemia; avoid potassium supplementation unless specifically required by healthcare provider. Avoid use or use a smaller dose in patients who are volume depleted; correct depletion first. May be associated with deterioration of renal function and/or increases in serum creatinine, particularly in patients with low renal blood flow (eg, renal artery stenosis, heart failure) whose glomerular filtration rate (GFR) is dependent on efferent arteriolar vasoconstriction by angiotensin II; deterioration may result in oliguria, acute renal failure, and progressive azotemia. Small increases in serum creatinine may occur following initiation; consider discontinuation only in patients with progressive and/or significant deterioration in renal function. Use with caution in unstented unilateral/bilateral renal artery stenosis, preexisting renal insufficiency, or significant aortic/mitral stenosis. Systemic exposure increases in hepatic impairment. U.S. manufacturer labeling recommends a dosage adjustment in patients with moderate hepatic impairment; pharmacokinetics have not been studied in severe hepatic impairment. Use caution when initiating in heart failure; may need to adjust dose, and/or concurrent diuretic therapy, because of candesartan-induced hypotension. In surgical patients on chronic angiotensin receptor blocker (ARB) therapy, intraoperative hypotension may occur with induction and maintenance of general anesthesia Potentially significant drug-drug interactions may exist, requiring dose or frequency adjustment, additional monitoring, and/or selection of alternative therapy. Pediatric patients with a GFR <30 mL/minute/1.73 m^2 should not receive candesartan; has not been evaluated. Avoid use in infants <1 year of age due to potential effects on the development of immature kidneys.

Angioedema has been reported rarely with some angiotensin II receptor antagonists (ARBs) and may occur at any time during treatment (especially following first dose). It may involve the head and neck (potentially compromising airway) or the intestine (presenting with abdominal pain). Patients with idiopathic or hereditary angioedema or previous angioedema associated with ACE-inhibitor therapy may be at an increased risk. Prolonged frequent monitoring may be required, especially if tongue, glottis, or larynx are involved, as they are associated with airway obstruction. Patients with a history of airway surgery may have a higher risk of airway obstruction. Discontinue therapy immediately if angioedema occurs. Aggressive early management is critical. Intramuscular (IM) administration of epinephrine may be necessary. Do not readminister to patients who have had angioedema with ARBs.

Adverse Reactions

Cardiovascular: Angina pectoris, hypotension, myocardial infarction, palpitations, tachycardia

Central nervous system: Anxiety, depression, dizziness, drowsiness, headache, paresthesia, vertigo

Dermatologic: Diaphoresis, skin rash

Endocrine & metabolic: Hyperglycemia, hyperkalemia, hypertriglyceridemia, hyperuricemia

Gastrointestinal: Dyspepsia, gastroenteritis

Genitourinary: Hematuria

Neuromuscular & skeletal: Back pain, increased creatine phosphokinase, myalgia, weakness

Renal: Increased serum creatinine

Respiratory: Dyspnea, epistaxis, pharyngitis, rhinitis, upper respiratory tract infection

Miscellaneous: Fever

Rare but important or life-threatening: Atrial fibrillation, bradycardia, cardiac failure, cerebrovascular accident, confusion, hepatic insufficiency, hepatitis, hypersensitivity, leukopenia, loss of consciousness, pancreatitis, pneumonia, presyncope, pulmonary edema, renal failure, rhabdomyolysis, thrombocytopenia

Drug Interactions

Metabolism/Transport Effects Substrate of CYP2C9 (minor); **Note:** Assignment of Major/Minor substrate status based on clinically relevant drug interaction potential; **Inhibits** CYP2C8 (weak), CYP2C9 (weak)

Avoid Concomitant Use

Avoid concomitant use of Candesartan with any of the following: Amodiaquine

Increased Effect/Toxicity

Candesartan may increase the levels/effects of: ACE Inhibitors; Amifostine; Amodiaquine; Antihypertensives; Ciprofloxacin (Systemic); CycloSPORINE (Systemic); Drospirenone; DULoxetine; Hypotensive Agents; Levodopa; Lithium; Nonsteroidal Anti-Inflammatory Agents; Obinutuzumab; Potassium-Sparing Diuretics; RisperiDONE; RiTUXimab; Sodium Phosphates

The levels/effects of Candesartan may be increased by: Alfuzosin; Aliskiren; Barbiturates; Brimonidine (Topical); Canagliflozin; Dapoxetine; Diazoxide; Eplerenone; Heparin; Heparin (Low Molecular Weight); Herbs (Hypotensive Properties); MAO Inhibitors; Nicorandil; Pentoxifylline; Phosphodiesterase 5 Inhibitors; Potassium Salts; Prostacyclin Analogues; Tolvaptan; Trimethoprim

Decreased Effect

The levels/effects of Candesartan may be decreased by: Herbs (Hypertensive Properties); Methylphenidate; Nonsteroidal Anti-Inflammatory Agents; Yohimbine

Storage/Stability Store at 25°C (77°F); excursions permitted to 15°C to 30°C (59°F to 86°F).

Mechanism of Action Candesartan is an angiotensin receptor antagonist. Angiotensin II acts as a vasoconstrictor. In addition to causing direct vasoconstriction, angiotensin II also stimulates the release of aldosterone. Once aldosterone is released, sodium as well as water are reabsorbed. The end result is an elevation in blood pressure. Candesartan binds to the AT1 angiotensin II receptor. This binding prevents angiotensin II from binding to the receptor thereby blocking the vasoconstriction and the aldosterone secreting effects of angiotensin II.

Pharmacodynamics

Antihypertensive effect:

Onset of action: Within 2 weeks

Maximum effect: 4-6 weeks

Pharmacokinetics (Adult data unless noted)

Absorption: Candesartan: Rapid and complete following conversion from candesartan cilexetil by GI esterases

Distribution: V_d: 0.13 L/kg

Protein binding: >99%

Metabolism: Converted to active candesartan, via ester hydrolysis during absorption from GI tract; hepatic (minor) via O-deethylation to inactive metabolite

Bioavailability, absolute: Candesartan: 15%

Half-life elimination: 9 hours; dose-dependent

Time to peak serum concentration: Pediatric patients (1-17 years), adults: 3-4 hours

Elimination: Excreted via biliary and renal routes; feces: 67%; urine: 33% (26% as unchanged drug). The AUC and C_{max} increased 30% and 56% in mild hepatic impairment and 145% and 73% in moderate hepatic impairment, respectively. The pharmacokinetics after candesartan administration have not been investigated in patients with severe hepatic impairment.

Clearance: Total body: 0.37 mL/minute/kg; Renal: 0.19 mL/minute/kg; decreased with severe renal impairment. In hypertensive patients with CrCl <30 mL/min/1.73 m^2, the AUC and C_{max} are approximately doubled. In heart failure patients with renal impairment, AUC is 36% and 65% higher and C_{max} is 15% and 55% higher in patients with mild and moderate renal impairment, respectively.

Dosing: Usual Note: Use of a lower initial dose is recommended in volume- and salt-depleted patients; dosage must be individualized

Children and Adolescents:

Hypertension:

Children 1 to <6 years: Oral: Initial: 0.2 mg/kg/**day** divided once or twice daily; titrate to response (within 2 weeks, antihypertensive effect usually observed); usual range: 0.05-0.4 mg/kg/**day** divided once or twice daily; maximum daily dose: 0.4 mg/kg/**day**; higher doses have not been studied.

Children and Adolescents 6 to <17 years: Oral:

<50 kg: Initial: 4-8 mg/**day** divided once or twice daily; titrate to response (within 2 weeks, antihypertensive effect usually observed); usual range: 2-16 mg/**day** divided once or twice daily; maximum daily dose: 32 mg/**day**; higher doses have not been studied.

>50 kg: Initial: 8-16 mg/**day** divided once or twice daily; titrate to response (within 2 weeks, antihypertensive effect usually observed); usual range: 4-32 mg/**day** divided once or twice daily; maximum daily dose: 32 mg/**day**; higher doses have not been studied.

Adolescents ≥17 years: Oral: Initial: 16 mg once daily (monotherapy); usual range: 8-32 mg/day divided once or twice daily; blood pressure response is dose-related over the range of 2-32 mg; larger doses do not appear to have a greater effect and there is relatively little experience with such doses

Adults:

Hypertension: Oral: Initial: 16 mg once daily (monotherapy); usual range: 8-32 mg/day divided once or twice daily; blood pressure response is dose-related over the range of 2-32 mg; larger doses do not appear to have a greater effect and there is relatively little experience with such doses

Congestive heart failure: Oral: Initial: 4 mg once daily; double the dose at 2-week intervals, as tolerated; target dose: 32 mg/**day**; **Note:** In selected cases, concurrent therapy with an ACE inhibitor may provide additional benefit.

Dosing adjustment in renal impairment:

Children and Adolescents 1 to <17 years:

CrCl ≥30 mL/minute/1.73 m^2: There are no dosage adjustments provided in the manufacturer's labeling; has not been studied in pediatric patients with renal impairment.

CrCl <30 mL/minute/1.73 m^2: Use is not recommended.

Adults: No initial dosage adjustment necessary; however, in patients with severe renal impairment (CrCl <30 mL/minute/1.73m^2) AUC and C_{max} were approximately doubled after repeated dosing.

Not removed by dialysis.

Dosing adjustment in hepatic impairment:

Mild hepatic impairment (Child-Pugh Class A): No initial dosage adjustment required

Moderate hepatic impairment (Child-Pugh Class B): Adults: Initial: 8 mg daily: AUC increased by 145%

Severe hepatic impairment (Child-Pugh Class C): There are no dosage adjustments provided in manufacturer's labeling (has not been studied); however, systemic exposure increases significantly in moderate impairment.

Administration Oral: May be administered without regard to meals.

Monitoring Parameters Blood pressure, serum creatinine, BUN, baseline and periodic electrolytes

Dosage Forms Excipient information presented when available (limited, particularly for generics); consult specific product labeling.

Tablet, Oral, as cilexetil:

Atacand: 4 mg, 8 mg, 16 mg, 32 mg [scored]

Generic: 4 mg, 8 mg, 16 mg, 32 mg

Extemporaneous Preparations Oral suspension may be made in concentrations ranging from 0.1 to 2 mg/mL; typically 1 mg/mL oral suspension suitable for majority of prescribed doses; any strength tablet may be used. A 1 mg/mL (total volume: 160 mL) oral suspension may be made with tablets and a 1:1 mixture of Ora-Plus® and Ora-Sweet SF®. Prepare the vehicle by adding 80 mL of Ora-Plus® and 80 mL of Ora-Sweet SF® or, alternatively, use 160 mL of Ora-Blend SF®. Add a small amount of vehicle to five 32 mg tablets and grind into a smooth paste using a mortar and pestle. Transfer the paste to a calibrated amber PET bottle, rinse the mortar and pestle clean using the vehicle, add this to the bottle, and then add a quantity of vehicle sufficient to make 160 mL. The suspension is stable at room temperature for 100 days unopened or 30 days after the first opening; do not freeze; label "shake well before use." (Atacand prescribing information, 2013).

- ◆ **Candesartan Cilexetil** *see* Candesartan *on page 358*
- ◆ **CanesOral (Can)** *see* Fluconazole *on page 881*
- ◆ **Canesten® Topical (Can)** *see* Clotrimazole (Topical) *on page 518*
- ◆ **Canesten® Vaginal (Can)** *see* Clotrimazole (Topical) *on page 518*
- ◆ **Capastat Sulfate** *see* Capreomycin *on page 360*
- ◆ **Capex** *see* Fluocinolone (Topical) *on page 897*
- ◆ **Capex® (Can)** *see* Fluocinolone (Topical) *on page 897*
- ◆ **Capital/Codeine** *see* Acetaminophen and Codeine *on page 50*
- ◆ **Capoten** *see* Captopril *on page 364*

Capreomycin (kap ree oh MYE sin)

Medication Safety Issues

Sound-alike/look-alike issues:

Capastat® may be confused with Cepastat®

Brand Names: US Capastat Sulfate

Therapeutic Category Antibiotic, Miscellaneous; Antitubercular Agent

Generic Availability (US) No

Use Treatment of pulmonary tuberculosis (TB) in conjunction with at least one other antituberculosis agent when primary anti-TB agents are ineffective (drug-resistant) or patient does not tolerate or resistant tubercle bacilli present (FDA approved in adults)

Pregnancy Risk Factor C

Pregnancy Considerations Capreomycin has been shown to be teratogenic in animal studies. **[U.S. Boxed Warning]: Safety has not been established in pregnant women**; use during pregnancy only if the potential benefit to the mother outweighs the possible risk to the fetus.

Breast-Feeding Considerations It is not known if capreomycin is excreted in breast milk. The manufacturer recommends that caution be exercised when administering capreomycin to nursing women.

Contraindications Hypersensitivity to capreomycin or any component of the formulation

Warnings/Precautions [U.S. Boxed Warnings]: Use in patients with renal insufficiency or preexisting auditory impairment must be undertaken with great caution, and the risk of additional eighth nerve impairment or renal injury should be weighed against the benefits to be derived from therapy. Since other parenteral antituberculous agents (eg, streptomycin) also have similar and sometimes irreversible toxic effects, particularly on eighth cranial nerve and renal function, simultaneous administration of these agents with capreomycin is not recommended. Use with nonantituberculous drugs (ie, aminoglycoside antibiotics) having ototoxic or nephrotoxic potential should be undertaken only with great caution. Use caution with renal dysfunction and in the elderly; dosage reductions are recommended for known or suspected renal impairment. Electrolyte imbalances (hypocalcemia, hypokalemia, and hypomagnesemia) have been reported with use. Prolonged use may result in fungal or bacterial superinfection, including *C. difficile*-associated diarrhea (CDAD) and pseudomembranous colitis; CDAD has been observed >2 months postantibiotic treatment. **[U.S. Boxed Warning]: Safety in pregnant women or pediatric patients not established.**

Warnings: Additional Pediatric Considerations May cause renal injury including tubular necrosis, elevated BUN or serum creatinine, and abnormal urinary sediment; BUN elevation and abnormal urinary sediment are associated with prolonged therapy and the clinical significance of these findings is not fully established. Proteinuria frequently reported; electrolyte disturbances (hypokalemia, hypomagnesemia, and hypocalcemia) may result from renal injury (CDC, 2003). Discontinuation of therapy due to renal toxicity has been reported in 20% to 25% of patients (CDC, 2003). Monitor renal function; urinalysis and electrolytes at baseline and periodically (monthly) throughout therapy (CDC, 2003; Seddon, 2012). May cause hearing loss; some cases may be irreversible. Tinnitus and vertigo have also been reported; more common in elderly patients and patients with preexisting renal impairment. In pediatric patients treated for multidrug-resistant TB, the reported incidence of hearing loss is variable (7% to 24%) with regimens that included either capreomycin or an aminoglycoside; the majority of children received amikacin compared to capreomycin; specific incidence with capreomycin not determined (Drobac, 2006; Seddon, 2013).

Adverse Reactions

Hematologic: Eosinophilia (dose related, mild)

Otic: Ototoxicity

Renal: Nephrotoxicity (increased BUN)

Rare but important or life-threatening: Acute tubular necrosis, Bartter's syndrome, creatinine increased, hypersensitivity (maculopapular rash, urticaria and/or fever), hypocalcemia, hypokalemia, hypomagnesemia, injection site reactions (abscess, bleeding, induration and pain), leukocytosis, leukopenia, liver function decreased (BSP excretion decreased), renal injury, thrombocytopenia (rare), tinnitus, toxic nephritis, urinary sediment abnormal, vertigo

Drug Interactions

Metabolism/Transport Effects None known.

Avoid Concomitant Use

Avoid concomitant use of Capreomycin with any of the following: BCG; BCG (Intravesical); Mecamylamine

Increased Effect/Toxicity

Capreomycin may increase the levels/effects of: Aminoglycosides; Colistimethate; Mecamylamine; Neuromuscular-Blocking Agents; Polymyxin B

Decreased Effect

Capreomycin may decrease the levels/effects of: BCG; BCG (Intravesical); BCG Vaccine (Immunization); Sodium Picosulfate

Storage/Stability Powder for injection should be stored at room temperature of 15°C to 30°C (59°F to 86°F). Following reconstitution, may store under refrigeration for up to 24 hours.

Mechanism of Action Capreomycin is a cyclic polypeptide antimicrobial. It is administered as a mixture of capreomycin IA and capreomycin IB. The mechanism of action of capreomycin is not well understood. Mycobacterial species that have become resistant to other agents are usually still sensitive to the action of capreomycin. However, significant cross-resistance with viomycin, kanamycin, and neomycin occurs.

Pharmacokinetics (Adult data unless noted)

Absorption: Oral: Not absorbed

Half-life elimination:

- Normal renal function: 4-6 hours
- Renal impairment:
  - CrCl 50-80 mL/minute: 7-10 hours
  - CrCl 20-40 mL/minute: 12-20 hours
  - CrCl 10 mL/minute: 29 hours
  - CrCl 0 mL/minute: 55 hours

Time to peak serum concentration: IM: 1-2 hours

Elimination: Urine (within 12 hours: 52% as unchanged drug)

Dosing: Usual

Infants, Children, Adolescents: **Tuberculosis; multidrug resistant (MDR):** Limited data available: **Note:** Usual duration of therapy is 4-6 months although older children may require up to 8 months of therapy; use in combination with at least 2-3 additional anti-TB agents (overall multidrug regimen dependent upon susceptibility profile/patterns); regimens with less frequent dosing (ie, twice or three times weekly) have less clinical experience supporting efficacy (CDC, 2003; Seddon, 2012): IM, IV:

- Infants and Children weighing ≤40 kg: 15-30 mg/kg once daily; maximum daily dose: 1000 mg/**day** (CDC, 2003; DHHS [pediatric], 2013; Seddon, 2012)
- Children weighing >40 kg and Adolescents: 15 mg/kg once daily; maximum daily dose: 1000 mg/**day** (CDC, 2003; DHHS [adult], 2013; Seddon, 2012)

Adults: **Tuberculosis:** IM, IV: 1000 mg once daily (maximum dose: 20 mg/kg/dose) for 60-120 days, followed by 1000 mg 2-3 times/week **or** 15 mg/kg/day (maximum: 1000 mg/dose) for 2-4 months, followed by 15 mg/kg (maximum: 1000 mg/dose) 2-3 times/week (CDC, 2003)

Dosing interval in renal impairment: Adults: IM, IV:

Manufacturer's labeling: Maximum single dose: 1000 mg

- CrCl 110 mL/minute: Administer 13.9 mg/kg every 24 hours
- CrCl 100 mL/minute: Administer 12.7 mg/kg every 24 hours
- CrCl 80 mL/minute: Administer 10.4 mg/kg every 24 hours
- CrCl 60 mL/minute: Administer 8.2 mg/kg every 24 hours
- CrCl 50 mL/minute: Administer 7 mg/kg every 24 hours **or** 14 mg/kg every 48 hours
- CrCl 40 mL/minute: Administer 5.9 mg/kg every 24 hours **or** 11.7 mg/kg every 48 hours
- CrCl 30 mL/minute: Administer 4.7 mg/kg every 24 hours **or** 9.5 mg/kg every 48 hours **or** 14.2 mg/kg every 72 hours
- CrCl 20 mL/minute: Administer 3.6 mg/kg every 24 hours **or** 7.2 mg/kg every 48 hours **or** 10.7 mg/kg every 72 hours
- CrCl 10 mL/minute: Administer 2.4 mg/kg every 24 hours **or** 4.9 mg/kg every 48 hours **or** 7.3 mg/kg every 72 hours
- CrCl 0 mL/minute: Administer 1.3 mg/kg every 24 hours **or** 2.6 mg/kg every 48 hours **or** 3.9 mg/kg every 72 hours

The following guidelines may also be used:

CDC, 2003:

CrCl ≥30 mL/minute: No adjustment required

CrCl <30 mL/minute and/or hemodialysis: 12-15 mg/kg (maximum dose: 1000 mg/dose) 2-3 days per week (**NOT** daily)

Aronoff, 2007:

CrCl ≥10 mL/minute: No adjustment required

CrCl <10 mL/minute: 1000 mg every 48 hours

Hemodialysis: Administer dose after hemodialysis only

Continuous renal replacement therapy (CRRT): 5 mg/kg every 24 hours

Dosing adjustment in hepatic impairment: There are no dosage adjustments provided in the manufacturer's labeling; some suggest that no extra precautions are needed (CDC, 2003).

Preparation for Administration Parenteral: Reconstitute powder for injection with 2 mL of NS or SWFI; allow 2 to 3 minutes for dissolution.

IV: Further dilute in NS 100 mL.

IM: Concentration for administration dependent upon dose

1,000 mg dose: Administer contents of reconstituted vial

Doses <1,000 mg dose: See table:

Capreomycin Dilution for Doses <1,000 mg

Diluent Volume (mL)	Capreomycin Solution Volume (mL)	Final Concentration (approximate)
2.15	2.85	370 mg/mL
2.63	3.33	315 mg/mL
3.3	4	260 mg/mL
4.3	5	210 mg/mL

Administration Parenteral:

IV: Administer over 60 minutes.

IM: Administer by deep IM injection into large muscle mass

Monitoring Parameters

Pediatric patients: Audiometric measurements and vestibular function (baseline, monthly while on therapy, and at 6 months following discontinuation of therapy); renal function (baseline, weekly during therapy or monthly for first 6 months of therapy, then every 3 months and at 6 months following discontinuation of therapy); baseline and frequent assessment of serum electrolytes (including calcium, magnesium, and potassium), liver function tests, growth parameters (CDC, 2003; Seddon, 2012).

Adults: Audiometric measurements and vestibular function at baseline and during therapy; renal function at baseline and weekly during therapy; frequent assessment of serum electrolytes (including calcium, magnesium, and potassium), liver function tests

Additional Information Recommended dosages are designed to achieve a mean serum concentration of 10 mcg/mL which corresponds to the recommended concentration for susceptibility testing (CDC, 2003).

Dosage Forms Excipient information presented when available (limited, particularly for generics); consult specific product labeling.

Solution Reconstituted, Injection, as sulfate:

Capastat Sulfate: 1 g (1 ea)

◆ **Capreomycin Sulfate** *see* Capreomycin *on page 360*

Capsaicin (kap SAY sin)

Medication Safety Issues

Sound-alike/look-alike issues:

Zostrix may be confused with Zestril, Zovirax

Brand Names: US Aflexeryl-MC [OTC]; Aleveer [OTC] [DSC]; Captracin; Capzasin-HP [OTC]; Capzasin-P [OTC]; DiabetAid Pain and Tingling Relief [OTC]; Flexin; Levatio; MaC Patch; Neuvaxin; Qroxin; Qutenza; Releevia; Releevia MC; RelyyT; Renovo; Salonpas Gel-Patch Hot [OTC]; Salonpas Hot [OTC] [DSC]; Sinelee; Solaice; Trixaicin HP [OTC]; Trixaicin [OTC]; Zostrix Diabetic Foot Pain [OTC]; Zostrix [OTC]; Zostrix-HP [OTC]

Brand Names: Canada Zostrix; Zostrix H.P.

Therapeutic Category Analgesic, Topical; Topical Skin Product; Transient Receptor Potential Vanilloid 1 (TRPV1) Agonist

Generic Availability (US) Yes: Cream

Use Topical treatment of pain associated with postherpetic neuralgia (FDA approved in adults); temporary treatment of minor pain associated with muscles and joints due to backache, strains, sprains, bruises, cramps, or arthritis; temporary relief of pain associated with diabetic neuropathy (FDA approved in adults; DiabetAid Pain and Tingling Relief: FDA approved in ages ≥2 years and adults; Salonpas® Hot: FDA approved in ages ≥12 years and adults); has also been used for postsurgical pain, pain associated with psoriasis, chronic neuralgias unresponsive to other forms of therapy, and intractable pruritus

Pregnancy Risk Factor B

Pregnancy Considerations Adverse events have not been observed in animal reproduction studies with capsaicin patch or liquid. Systemic absorption is limited following topical administration of the patch; plasma concentrations are below the limit of detection 3-6 hours after the patch is removed.

Breast-Feeding Considerations Systemic absorption is limited following topical administration of the patch. When using the topical high concentration (capsaicin 8%) patch, Qutenza™, the manufacturer recommends not breastfeeding on the day of treatment after the patch has been applied to reduce any potential infant exposure.

Contraindications There are no contraindications listed in the manufacturer's labeling.

Warnings/Precautions May cause serious burns (eg, first- to third-degree chemical burns) at the application site. In some cases, hospitalization has been required. Discontinue use and seek medical attention if signs of skin injury (eg, pain, swelling, or blistering) occur following application (FDA Drug Safety Communication, 2012).

Topical high-concentration capsaicin patch (Qutenza): Do not apply to face, scalp, or allow contact with eyes or mucous membranes. If an unintended area of skin is inadvertently exposed, the cleansing gel should be used. Post-application pain should be treated with local cooling methods and/or analgesics (opioids may be necessary). Avoid rapid removal of patches to decrease risk of aerosolization of capsaicin; inhalation of airborne capsaicin may result in coughing or sneezing; if shortness of breath occurs, medical care is required; remove patches gently and slowly to decrease risk of aerosolization. Use with caution in patients with uncontrolled hypertension, or a history of cardiovascular or cerebrovascular events; transient increases in blood pressure due to treatment-related pain have occurred during and after application of patch.

Benzyl alcohol and derivatives: Some dosage forms may contain benzyl alcohol; large amounts of benzyl alcohol (≥99 mg/kg/day) have been associated with a potentially fatal toxicity ("gasping syndrome") in neonates; the "gasping syndrome" consists of metabolic acidosis, respiratory distress, gasping respirations, CNS dysfunction (including convulsions, intracranial hemorrhage), hypotension and cardiovascular collapse (AAP, 1997; CDC, 1982); some data suggests that benzoate displaces bilirubin from protein binding sites (Ahlfors, 2001); avoid or use dosage forms containing benzyl alcohol with caution in neonates. See manufacturer's labeling.

Topical OTC products: Apply externally; avoid contact with eyes or mucous membranes. Should not be applied to broken or irritated skin. Treated area should not be exposed to heat or direct sunlight. Affected area should not be bandaged. Transient burning may occur and generally disappears after several days; discontinue use if severe burning develops. Stop use and consult a health care provider if redness or irritation develops, symptoms get worse, or symptoms resolve and then recur.

Adverse Reactions Topical patch (Qutenza™, capsaicin 8%):

Local: Erythema, pain

Cardiovascular: Hypertension (transient)

Dermatologic: Pruritus

Gastrointestinal: Nausea, vomiting

Local: Dryness, edema, erythema, papules, pruritus, swelling

Respiratory: Bronchitis, nasopharyngitis, sinusitis

Rare but important or life-threatening): Application site reactions (bruising, dermatitis, excoriation, exfoliation, hyperesthesia, inflammation, paresthesia, urticaria), burning sensation, cough, dizziness, dysgeusia, headache, hypoesthesia, peripheral edema, peripheral sensory neuropathy, skin odor (abnormal), throat irritation

Drug Interactions

Metabolism/Transport Effects Substrate of CYP2E1 (minor); **Note:** Assignment of Major/Minor substrate status based on clinically relevant drug interaction potential

Avoid Concomitant Use There are no known interactions where it is recommended to avoid concomitant use.

Increased Effect/Toxicity There are no known significant interactions involving an increase in effect.

Decreased Effect There are no known significant interactions involving a decrease in effect.

Storage/Stability

DiabetAid Pain and Tingling Relief, Zostrix®, Zostrix®-HP: Store at 15°C to 30°C (59°F to 86°F).

Qutenza™: Store at room temperature between 20°C to 25°C (68°F to 77°F).

Mechanism of Action Capsaicin, a transient receptor potential vanilloid 1 receptor (TRPV1) agonist, activates TRPV1 ligand-gated cation channels on nociceptive nerve fibers, resulting in depolarization, initiation of action potential, and pain signal transmission to the spinal cord; capsaicin exposure results in subsequent desensitization of the sensory axons and inhibition of pain transmission initiation. In arthritis, capsaicin induces release of substance P, the principal chemomediator of pain impulses from the periphery to the CNS, from peripheral sensory neurons; after repeated application, capsaicin depletes the neuron of substance P and prevents reaccumulation. The functional link between substance P and the capsaicin receptor, TRPV1, is not well understood.

Pharmacodynamics Onset of action:

OTC products (capsaicin 0.025% to 0.1%): 2-4 weeks of continuous therapy

Qutenza™ patch: 1 week after application

Pharmacokinetics (Adult data unless noted)

Absorption: Topical patch (capsaicin 8%): Systemic absorption is transient and low (<5 ng/mL) in approximately one-third of patients when measured following 60-minute application. In patients with quantifiable concentrations, most fell below the limit of quantitation at 3-6 hours postapplication.

Half-life: Topical patch (capsaicin 8%): 1.64 hours (Babbar, 2009)

Dosing: Usual Topical:

Pain relief:

Lotion: Children >2 years, Adolescents, and Adults: OTC labeling (DiabetAid Tingling and Pain Relief): Apply to affected area 3-4 times/day

Patch: Adolescents ≥12 years and Adults: OTC labeling (Salonpas®-Hot): Apply patch to affected area up to 3-4 times/day for 7 days. Patch may remain in place for up to 8 hours

Cream, gel, liquid: Adults: Apply to affected area 3-4 times/day; efficacy may be decreased if used less than 3 times/day; best results seen after 2-4 weeks of continuous use

Postherpetic neuralgia: Patch [Qutenza™ (capsaicin 8%)]: Adults: Apply patch to most painful area for 60 minutes. Up to 4 patches may be applied in a single application. Treatment may be repeated ≥3 months as needed for return of pain (do not apply more frequently than every 3 months). Area should be pretreated with a topical anesthetic prior to patch application.

Administration

Topical products (cream, gel, liquid, lotion): Wear gloves to apply; apply thin film to the affected areas and gently rub in until absorbed; wash hands with soap and water after applying to avoid spreading to eyes or other sensitive areas of the body.

Topical patch (Salonpas®-Hot): Apply patch externally to clean and dry affected area. Backing film should be removed prior to application. Do not use within 1 hour prior to a bath or immediately after bathing. Do not use with a heating pad.

Topical patch [Qutenza™ (capsaicin 8%)]: Patch should only be applied by physician or by a healthcare professional under the close supervision of a physician. The treatment area must be identified and marked by a physician. The patch can be cut to match size/shape of treatment area. If necessary, excessive hair present on and surrounding the treatment area may be clipped (not shaved) to promote adherence. Prior to application, the treatment area should be cleansed with mild soap and water and dried thoroughly. The treatment area should be anesthetized with a topical anesthetic prior to patch application. Anesthetic should be removed with a dry wipe and area should be cleansed again with soap/water, and dried. Patch may then be applied to dry, intact skin within 2 hours of opening the sealed patch; apply patch using nitrile gloves (latex gloves should **NOT** be used). During application, slowly peel back the release liner under the patch. Patch should remain in place for 60 minutes. Do not touch the patch while it is on the skin. Remove patches gently and slowly. Following patch removal, apply cleansing gel to the treatment area and leave in place for at least 1 minute. All treatment materials should be disposed of according to biomedical waste procedures.

Monitoring Parameters Qutenza™: Blood pressure

Additional Information In patients with severe and persistent local discomfort, pretreatment with topical lidocaine 5% ointment or concurrent oral analgesics for the first 2 weeks of therapy have been effective in alleviating the initial burning sensation and enabling continuation of topical capsaicin

Dosage Forms Excipient information presented when available (limited, particularly for generics); consult specific product labeling. [DSC] = Discontinued product

Cream, topical: 0.025% (60 g)

Capzasin-HP: 0.1% (42.5 g) [contains benzyl alcohol]

Capzasin-P: 0.035% (42.5 g) [contains benzyl alcohol]

Trixaicin: 0.025% (60 g) [contains benzyl alcohol]

Trixaicin HP: 0.075% (60 g) [contains benzyl alcohol]

Zostrix: 0.025% (60 g) [contains benzyl alcohol]

Zostrix Diabetic Foot Pain: 0.075% (60 g) [contains benzyl alcohol]

Zostrix-HP: 0.075% (60 g) [contains benzyl alcohol]
Gel, topical:
Capzasin-P: 0.025% (42.5 g) [contains menthol]
Liquid, topical:
Capzasin-P: 0.15% (29.5 mL)
Lotion, topical:
DiabetAid Pain and Tingling Relief: 0.025% (120 mL)
Patch, topical:
Aflexeril MC: 0.0375% (15s) [contains menthol 5%]
Aleveer: 0.0375% (15s) [contains menthol 5%, and aloe] [DSC]
Captracin: 0.0375% (15s) [contains menthol 5%]
Flexin: 0.0375% (15s) [contains menthol 5%]
Levatio: 0.03% (15s) [contains menthol 5%]
MaC Patch: 0.0375% (15s) [contains menthol 5%]
Neuvaxin: 0.0375% (15s) [contains menthol 5%]
Qroxin: 0.0375% (15s) [contains menthol 5%]
Qutenza: 8% (1s, 2s) [contains metal; supplied with cleansing gel]
Releevia: 0.0375% (15s) [contains menthol 5%]
Releevia MC: 0.0375% (15s) [contains menthol 5%]
RelyyT: 0.025% (15s) [contains menthol 5%]
Renovo: 0.0375% (15s) [contains menthol 5%]
Sinelee: 0.0375%, 0.05% (15s) [contains menthol 5%]
Solaice: 0.05% (15s) [contains menthol 5%]
Salonpas Gel-Patch Hot: 0.025% (3s, 6s) [contains menthol]
Salonpas Hot: 0.025% (1s [DSC]) [contains natural rubber/natural latex in packaging]

Captopril (KAP toe pril)

Medication Safety Issues

Sound-alike/look-alike issues:

Captopril may be confused with calcitriol, Capitrol, carvedilol

International issues:

Acepril [Great Britain] may be confused with Accupril which is a brand name for quinapril in the U.S.

Acepril: Brand name for captopril [Great Britain], but also the brand name for enalapril [Hungary, Switzerland]; lisinopril [Malaysia]

Brand Names: Canada Apo-Capto; Dom-Captopril; Mylan-Captopril; PMS-Captopril

Therapeutic Category Angiotensin-Converting Enzyme (ACE) Inhibitor; Antihypertensive Agent

Generic Availability (US) Yes

Use Treatment of hypertension, heart failure, left ventricular dysfunction after myocardial infarction, and diabetic nephropathy (FDA approved in adults)

Pregnancy Risk Factor D

Pregnancy Considerations **[U.S. Boxed Warning]: Drugs that act on the renin-angiotensin system can cause injury and death to the developing fetus. Discontinue as soon as possible once pregnancy is detected.** Captopril crosses the placenta (Hurault de Lingy 1987). Drugs that act on the renin-angiotensin system are associated with oligohydramnios. Oligohydramnios, due to decreased fetal renal function, may lead to fetal lung hypoplasia and skeletal malformations. Their use in pregnancy is also associated with anuria, hypotension, renal failure, skull hypoplasia, and death in the fetus/neonate. Teratogenic effects may occur following maternal use of an ACE inhibitor during the first trimester, although this finding may be confounded by maternal disease. Because adverse fetal events are well documented with exposure later in pregnancy, ACE inhibitor use in pregnant women is not recommended (Seely 2014; Weber 2014). Infants exposed to an ACE inhibitor in utero should be monitored for hyperkalemia, hypotension, and oliguria. Oligohydramnios may not appear until after irreversible fetal injury has occurred. Exchange transfusions or dialysis may be required to reverse hypotension or improve renal function, although data related to the effectiveness in neonates is limited.

Chronic maternal hypertension itself is also associated with adverse events in the fetus/infant and mother. ACE inhibitors are not recommended for the treatment of uncomplicated hypertension in pregnancy (ACOG 2013) and they are specifically contraindicated for the treatment of hypertension and chronic heart failure during pregnancy by some guidelines (Regitz-Zagrosek 2011). In addition, ACE inhibitors should generally be avoided in women of reproductive age (ACOG 2013). If treatment for hypertension or chronic heart failure in pregnancy is needed, other agents should be used (ACOG 2013; Regitz-Zagrosek 2011).

Breast-Feeding Considerations Captopril is excreted in breast milk. According to the manufacturer, the decision to continue or discontinue breast-feeding during therapy should take into account the risk of exposure to the infant and the benefits of treatment to the mother. Some guidelines consider captopril to be acceptable for use in breast-feeding women. Monitoring of the nursing child's weight for the first 4 weeks is recommended (Regitz-Zagrosek 2011).

Contraindications Hypersensitivity to captopril, any other ACE inhibitor, or any component of the formulation; angioedema related to previous treatment with an ACE inhibitor; concomitant use with aliskiren in patients with diabetes mellitus

Warnings/Precautions Anaphylactic reactions may occur rarely with ACE inhibitors. At any time during treatment (especially following first dose) angioedema may occur rarely with ACE inhibitors; may involve the head and neck (potentially compromising airway) or the intestine (presenting with abdominal pain). African-Americans and patients with idiopathic or hereditary angioedema may be at an increased risk. Prolonged frequent monitoring may be required especially if tongue, glottis, or larynx are involved as they are associated with airway obstruction. Patients with a history of airway surgery may have a higher risk of airway obstruction. Aggressive early and appropriate management is critical. Use in patients with previous angioedema associated with ACE inhibitor therapy is contraindicated. Severe anaphylactoid reactions may be seen during hemodialysis (eg, CVVHD) with high-flux dialysis membranes (eg, AN69), and rarely, during low density lipoprotein apheresis with dextran sulfate cellulose. Rare cases of anaphylactoid reactions have been reported in patients undergoing sensitization treatment with hymenoptera (bee, wasp) venom while receiving ACE inhibitors.

Symptomatic hypotension with or without syncope can occur with ACE inhibitors (usually with the first several doses); effects are most often observed in volume depleted patients; close monitoring of patient is required especially with initial dosing and dosing increases; blood pressure must be lowered at a rate appropriate for the patient's clinical condition. Initiation of therapy in patients with ischemic heart disease or cerebrovascular disease warrants close observation due to the potential consequences posed by falling blood pressure (eg, MI, stroke). Use with caution in hypertrophic cardiomyopathy with outflow tract obstruction and severe aortic stenosis. In patients on chronic ACE inhibitor therapy, intraoperative hypotension may occur with induction and maintenance of general anesthesia; use with caution before, during, or immediately after major surgery. Cardiopulmonary bypass, intraoperative blood loss, or vasodilating anesthesia increases endogenous renin release. Use of ACE inhibitors perioperatively will blunt angiotensin II formation and may result in hypotension. However, discontinuation of therapy prior to surgery is controversial. If continued preoperatively, avoidance of hypotensive agents during surgery is prudent (Hillis, 2011). Extemporaneous preparations of liquid formulations may vary; this may affect the rate and extent of absorption causing intrapatient variability regarding dosing and safety profile for the patient; use with caution and monitor closely if dosage formulations are changed (Bhatt, 2011; Mulla, 2007). **[U.S. Boxed Warning]: Drugs that act on the renin-angiotensin system can cause injury and death to the developing fetus. Discontinue as soon as possible once pregnancy is detected.**

Hyperkalemia may occur with ACE inhibitors; risk factors include renal dysfunction, diabetes mellitus, concomitant use of potassium-sparing diuretics, potassium supplements and/or potassium containing salts. Use cautiously, if at all, with these agents and monitor potassium closely. Cough may occur with ACE inhibitors. Other causes of cough should be considered (eg, pulmonary congestion in patients with heart failure) and excluded prior to discontinuation.

May be associated with deterioration of renal function and/or increases in BUN and serum creatinine, particularly in patients with low renal blood flow (eg, renal artery stenosis, heart failure) whose glomerular filtration rate (GFR) is dependent on efferent arteriolar vasoconstriction by angiotensin II; deterioration may result in oliguria, acute renal failure, and progressive azotemia. Small benign increases in serum creatinine may occur following initiation; consider discontinuation only in patients with progressive and/or significant deterioration in renal function (Bakris, 2000). Use with caution in patients with unstented unilateral/bilateral renal artery stenosis. When unstented bilateral renal artery stenosis is present, use is generally avoided due to the elevated risk of deterioration in renal function unless possible benefits outweigh risks. ACE inhibitors effectiveness is less in black patients than in non-blacks. In addition, ACE inhibitors cause a higher rate of angioedema in black than in non-black patients. Potentially significant drug-drug interactions may exist, requiring dose or frequency adjustment, additional monitoring, and/or selection of alternative therapy.

Rare toxicities associated with ACE inhibitors include cholestatic jaundice (which may progress to fulminant hepatic necrosis, some fatal), agranulocytosis, neutropenia with myeloid hypoplasia; anemia and thrombocytopenia have also occurred. If neutropenia develops (neutrophil count <1,000/mm^3), discontinue therapy. Patients with collagen vascular diseases (especially with concomitant renal impairment) or renal impairment alone may be at increased risk for hematologic toxicity; closely monitor CBC with differential for the first 3 months of therapy and periodically thereafter in these patients. Total urinary proteins greater than 1 g per day have been reported (<1%); nephrotic syndrome occurred in about one-fifth of proteinuric patients. In most cases, proteinuria subsided or cleared within six months (whether or not captopril was continued).

Warnings: Additional Pediatric Considerations An observational study of 66 pediatric patients with heart failure reported hypotension in 15% of patients during therapy initiation at typical starting doses; close monitoring in an inpatient setting and low starting doses has been suggested in these patients (Momma, 2006; Orchard, 2010).

An ACE inhibitor cough is a dry, hacking, nonproductive one that usually occurs within the first few months of treatment and should generally resolve within 1 to 4 weeks after discontinuation of the ACE inhibitor; in pediatric patients, an isolated dry hacking cough lasting >3 weeks was reported in seven of 42 pediatric patients (17%) receiving ACE inhibitors (von Vigier, 2000); a review of pediatric randomized-controlled ACE inhibitor trials reported a lower incidence of 3.2% (Baker-Smith, 2010). Other causes of cough should be considered (eg, pulmonary congestion in patients with heart failure) and excluded prior to discontinuation.

Adverse Reactions

Cardiovascular: Angina pectoris, cardiac arrest, cardiac arrhythmia, cardiac failure, chest pain, flushing, hypotension, myocardial infarction, orthostatic hypotension, palpitations, Raynaud's phenomenon, syncope, tachycardia

Central nervous system: Ataxia, cerebrovascular insufficiency, confusion, depression, drowsiness, myasthenia, nervousness

Dermatologic: Bullous pemphigoid, erythema multiforme, exfoliative dermatitis, pallor, pruritus, skin rash (maculopapular or urticarial; in patients with rash, a positive ANA and/or eosinophilia has been noted), Stevens-Johnson syndrome

Endocrine & metabolic: Gynecomastia, hyperkalemia, hyponatremia (symptomatic)

Gastrointestinal: Cholestasis, dysgeusia (loss of taste or diminished perception), dyspepsia, glossitis, pancreatitis

Genitourinary: Impotence, nephrotic syndrome, oliguria, proteinuria, urinary frequency

Hematologic: Agranulocytosis, anemia, neutropenia (in patients with renal insufficiency or collagen-vascular disease), pancytopenia, thrombocytopenia

Hepatic: Hepatic necrosis (rare), hepatitis, increased serum alkaline phosphatase, increased serum bilirubin, increased serum transaminases, jaundice

Hypersensitivity: Anaphylactoid reaction, angioedema, hypersensitivity reaction (rash, pruritus, fever, arthralgia, and eosinophilia; depending on dose and renal function)

Neuromuscular & skeletal: Myalgia, weakness

Ophthalmic: Blurred vision

Renal: Increased serum creatinine, polyuria, renal failure, renal insufficiency, renal insufficiency (worsening; may occur in patients with bilateral renal artery stenosis or hypovolemia)

Respiratory: Bronchospasm, cough, eosinophilic pneumonitis, rhinitis

Rare but important or life-threatening: Alopecia, angina pectoris, anorexia, aphthous stomatitis, aplastic anemia, cholestatic jaundice, eosinophilia, glomerulonephritis, Guillain-Barre syndrome, hemolytic anemia, Huntington's chorea (exacerbation), hyperthermia, increased erythrocyte sedimentation rate, insomnia, interstitial nephritis, Kaposi's sarcoma, peptic ulcer, pericarditis, psoriasis, seizure (in premature infants), systemic lupus erythematosus, vasculitis, visual hallucination (Doane, 2013)

Drug Interactions

Metabolism/Transport Effects Substrate of CYP2D6 (major); **Note:** Assignment of Major/Minor substrate status based on clinically relevant drug interaction potential

Avoid Concomitant Use There are no known interactions where it is recommended to avoid concomitant use.

Increased Effect/Toxicity

Captopril may increase the levels/effects of: Allopurinol; Amifostine; Antihypertensives; AzaTHIOprine; Ciprofloxacin (Systemic); Drospirenone; DULoxetine; Ferric Gluconate; Gold Sodium Thiomalate; Grass Pollen Allergen Extract (5 Grass Extract); Hypotensive Agents; Iron Dextran Complex; Levodopa; Lithium; Nonsteroidal Anti-Inflammatory Agents; Obinutuzumab; Pregabalin; RisperiDONE; RiTUXimab; Sodium Phosphates

The levels/effects of Captopril may be increased by: Abiraterone Acetate; Alfuzosin; Aliskiren; Angiotensin II Receptor Blockers; Barbiturates; Brimonidine (Topical); Canagliflozin; Cobicistat; CYP2D6 Inhibitors (Moderate); CYP2D6 Inhibitors (Strong); Dapoxetine; Darunavir; Diazoxide; DPP-IV Inhibitors; Eplerenone; Everolimus; Heparin; Heparin (Low Molecular Weight); Herbs (Hypotensive Properties); Loop Diuretics; MAO Inhibitors; Nicorandil; Panobinostat; Peginterferon Alfa-2b;

Pentoxifylline; Phosphodiesterase 5 Inhibitors; Potassium Salts; Potassium-Sparing Diuretics; Prostacyclin Analogues; Sirolimus; Temsirolimus; Thiazide Diuretics; TiZANidine; Tolvaptan; Trimethoprim

Decreased Effect

The levels/effects of Captopril may be decreased by: Antacids; Aprotinin; Herbs (Hypertensive Properties); Icatibant; Lanthanum; Methylphenidate; Nonsteroidal Anti-Inflammatory Agents; Peginterferon Alfa-2b; Salicylates; Yohimbine

Food Interactions Captopril serum concentrations may be decreased if taken with food. Long-term use of captopril may lead to a zinc deficiency which can result in altered taste perception. Management: Take on an empty stomach 1 hour before or 2 hours after meals.

Storage/Stability Store at 20°C to 25°C (68°F to 77°F); protect from moisture.

Mechanism of Action Competitive inhibitor of angiotensin-converting enzyme (ACE); prevents conversion of angiotensin I to angiotensin II, a potent vasoconstrictor; results in lower levels of angiotensin II which causes an increase in plasma renin activity and a reduction in aldosterone secretion

Pharmacodynamics

Onset of action: Antihypertensive: Within 15 minutes

Maximum effect: Antihypertensive: 60-90 minutes; may require several weeks of therapy before full hypotensive effect is seen

Duration: Dose-related

Pharmacokinetics (Adult data unless noted)

Absorption: 60% to 75%

Distribution: 7 L/kg

Bioavailability: 75%

Protein binding: 25% to 30%

Metabolism: 50% metabolized

Half-life:

Infants with CHF: 3.3 hours; range: 1.2-12.4 hours (Pereira, 1991)

Children: 1.5 hours; range: 0.98-2.3 hours (Levy, 1991)

Normal adults (dependent upon renal and cardiac function): 1.9 hours

Adults with CHF: 2.1 hours

Anuria: 20-40 hours

Time to peak serum concentration: Within 1-2 hours

Elimination: 95% excreted in urine in 24 hours

Dosing: Neonatal Heart failure (afterload reduction); hypertension: Limited data available: **Note:** Dosage must be titrated according to patient's response; use lowest effective dose; lower doses (~1/2 of those listed) should be used in patients who are sodium and water depleted due to diuretic therapy

Premature neonates: Oral: Initial: 0.01 mg/kg/dose every 8-12 hours; titrate dose

Term neonates, PNA ≤7 days: Oral: Initial: 0.01 mg/kg/dose every 8-12 hours; titrate dose

Term neonates, PNA >7 days: Oral: Initial: 0.05-0.1 mg/kg/dose every 8-24 hours; titrate dose upward to maximum of 0.5 mg/kg/dose given every 6-24 hours

Dosing: Usual

Infants, Children and Adolescents:

Heart failure (afterload reduction): Limited data available: **Note:** Initiate therapy at lower end of range and titrate upward to prevent symptomatic hypotension (Momma, 2006):

Infants: Oral: 0.3-2.5 mg/kg/day divided every 8-12 hours; one study of infants (age: 1-7 months) with left-right shunt reported a mean dose of 1.3 mg/kg/day

Children and Adolescents: Oral: 0.3-6 mg/kg/day divided every 8-12 hours; maximum daily dose: 150 mg/**day**; in clinical trials, usual reported dosage range was 0.9-3.9 mg/kg/day

Hypertension: Limited data available: **Note:** Dosage must be titrated according to patient's response; use lowest effective dose; lower doses (~1/2 of those listed) should be used in patients who are sodium- and water-depleted due to diuretic therapy

Weight-based dosing:

Infants: Oral: Initial: 0.15-0.3 mg/kg/dose; titrate dose upward to maximum of 6 mg/kg/day in 1-4 divided doses; usual required dose: 2.5-6 mg/kg/day

Children and Adolescents: Oral: Initial: 0.3-0.5 mg/kg/dose every 8 hours; may titrate as needed up to maximum daily dose: 6 mg/kg/**day** in 3 divided doses (NHBPEP, 2004; NHLBI, 2011); maximum daily dose: 450 mg/**day**

Fixed dosing:

Older Children: Oral: Initial: 6.25-12.5 mg/dose every 12-24 hours; titrate as needed; maximum daily dose: 6 mg/kg/**day** in 2-4 divided doses; maximum daily dose: 450 mg/**day**

Adolescents: Oral: Initial: 12.5-25 mg/dose given every 8-12 hours; increase by 25 mg/dose at 1-2 week intervals based on patient response; maximum daily dose: 450 mg/**day**; usual dosage range for hypertension (JNC 7): Adolescents ≥18 years: 25-100 mg/day in 2 divided doses

Adults: **Note:** Titrate dose according to patient's response; use lowest effective dose.

Acute hypertension (urgency/emergency): Oral: 12.5-25 mg, may repeat as needed (may be given sublingually, but no therapeutic advantage demonstrated)

Heart failure: Oral:

Initial dose: 6.25-12.5 mg 3 times daily in conjunction with cardiac glycoside and diuretic therapy; initial dose depends upon patient's fluid/electrolyte status

Target dose: 50 mg 3 times daily

Hypertension: Oral: Initial dose: 25 mg 2-3 times daily [a lower initial dose of 12.5 mg 3 times daily may also be considered (VA Cooperative Study Group, 1984)]; may increase by 12.5-25 mg/dose at 1- to 2-week intervals up to 50 mg 3 times daily; add thiazide diuretic, unless severe renal impairment coexists then consider loop diuretic before further dosage increases or consider other treatment options; maximum dose: 150 mg 3 times daily

Usual dose range (JNC 7): 25-100 mg/day in 2 divided doses

LV dysfunction following MI: Oral: Initial: 6.25 mg; if tolerated, follow with 12.5 mg 3 times daily; then increase to 25 mg 3 times daily during next several days and then gradually increase over next several weeks to target dose of 50 mg 3 times daily (some dose schedules are more aggressive to achieve an increased goal dose within the first few days of initiation)

Diabetic nephropathy: Oral: Initial: 25 mg 3 times daily; may be taken with other antihypertensive therapy if required to further lower blood pressure

Dosing adjustment in renal impairment:

Infants, Children and Adolescents: The following adjustments have been recommended (Aronoff, 2007). **Note:** Renally adjusted dose recommendations are based on doses of 0.1-0.5 mg/kg/dose every 6-8 hours; maximum daily dose: 6 mg/kg/**day**.

GFR 10-50 mL/minute/1.73 m^2: Administer 75% of dose

GFR <10 mL/minute/1.73 m^2: Administer 50% of dose

Intermittent hemodialysis: Administer 50% of dose

Peritoneal dialysis (PD): Administer 50% of dose

Continuous renal replacement therapy (CRRT): Administer 75% of dose

Adults:

Manufacturer's labeling: Reduce initial daily dose and titrate slowly (1- to 2-week intervals) with smaller increments. Slowly back titrate to determine the minimum effective dose once the desired therapeutic effect has been reached.

The following adjustments have been recommended (Aronoff, 2007):

CrCl >50 mL/minute: Administer 100% of normal dose every 8-12 hours

CrCl 10-50 mL/minute: Administer 75% of normal dose every 12-18 hours

CrCl <10 mL/minute: Administer 50% of normal dose every 24 hours

Intermittent hemodialysis (IHD): Administer after hemodialysis on dialysis days

Peritoneal dialysis: Administer 75% of normal dose every 12-18 hours; supplemental dose is not necessary

Administration Oral: Administer on an empty stomach 1 hour before meals or 2 hours after meals; if crushing tablet and dissolving in water, allow adequate time for complete dissolution (>10 minutes) (Bhatt, 2011)

Monitoring Parameters Blood pressure, BUN, serum creatinine, renal function, urine dipstick for protein, serum potassium, WBC with differential, especially during first 3 months of therapy for patients with renal impairment and/or collagen vascular disease; monitor for angioedema and anaphylactoid reactions; hypovolemia and postural hypotension when beginning therapy, adjusting dosage, and on a regular basis throughout

Test Interactions Positive Coombs' [direct]; may cause false-positive results in urine acetone determinations using sodium nitroprusside reagent

Dosage Forms Excipient information presented when available (limited, particularly for generics); consult specific product labeling.

Tablet, Oral:

Generic: 12.5 mg, 25 mg, 50 mg, 100 mg

Extemporaneous Preparations A 1 mg/mL oral solution may be made by allowing two 50 mg tablets to dissolve in 50 mL of distilled water. Add the contents of one 500 mg sodium ascorbate injection ampul or one 500 mg ascorbic acid tablet and allow to dissolve. Add quantity of distilled water sufficient to make 100 mL. Label "shake well" and "refrigerate". Stable for 56 days refrigerated.

Nahata MC, Pai VB, and Hipple TF, *Pediatric Drug Formulations*, 5th ed, Cincinnati, OH: Harvey Whitney Books Co, 2004.

- **Captracin** *see* Capsaicin *on page 362*
- **Capzasin-HP [OTC]** *see* Capsaicin *on page 362*
- **Capzasin-P [OTC]** *see* Capsaicin *on page 362*
- **Carafate** *see* Sucralfate *on page 1978*
- **Carbaglu** *see* Carglumic Acid *on page 376*

CarBAMazepine (kar ba MAZ e peen)

Medication Safety Issues

Sound-alike/look-alike issues:

CarBAMazepine may be confused with OXcarbazepine

Epitol may be confused with Epinal

TEGretol, TEGretol-XR may be confused with Mebaral, Toprol-XL, Toradol, TRENtal

High alert medication:

The Institute for Safe Medication Practices (ISMP) includes this medication among its list of drugs that have a heightened risk of causing significant patient harm when used in error.

BEERS Criteria medication:

This drug may be potentially inappropriate for use in geriatric patients (Quality of evidence - moderate; Strength of recommendation - strong).

Related Information

Oral Medications That Should Not Be Crushed or Altered *on page 2476*

Safe Handling of Hazardous Drugs *on page 2455*

Brand Names: US Carbatrol; Epitol; Equetro; TEGretol; TEGretol-XR

Brand Names: Canada Apo-Carbamazepine; Dom-Carbamazepine; Mapezine; Mylan-Carbamazepine CR; Nu-Carbamazepine; PMS-Carbamazepine; Sandoz-Carbamazepine; Taro-Carbamazepine Chewable; Tegretol; Teva-Carbamazepine

Therapeutic Category Anticonvulsant, Miscellaneous

Generic Availability (US) Yes

Use

Carbatrol, Epitol, Tegretol, Tegretol-XR: Treatment of generalized tonic-clonic, partial (especially complex partial), and mixed partial or generalized seizure disorder (Carbatrol,Tegretol: FDA approved in pediatric patients [age not specified] and adults; Tegretol-XR: FDA approved in ages ≥6 years and adults); relief of pain in trigeminal neuralgia or glossopharyngeal neuralgia (Carbatrol, Epitol, Tegretol, Tegretol XR: FDA approved in adults)

Equetro: Treatment of acute manic and mixed episodes associated with bipolar I disorders (FDA approved in adults)

Medication Guide Available Yes

Pregnancy Risk Factor D

Pregnancy Considerations Studies in pregnant women have demonstrated a risk to the fetus. Carbamazepine and its metabolites can be found in the fetus and may be associated with teratogenic effects, including spina bifida, craniofacial defects, cardiovascular malformations, and hypospadias. The risk of teratogenic effects is higher with anticonvulsant polytherapy than monotherapy.

Developmental delays have also been observed following *in utero* exposure to carbamazepine (per manufacturer); however, socioeconomic factors, maternal and paternal IQ, and polytherapy may contribute to these findings. Pregnancy may cause small decreases of carbamazepine plasma concentrations in the second and third trimesters; monitoring should be considered. When used for the treatment of bipolar disorder, use of carbamazepine should be avoided during the first trimester of pregnancy if possible. The use of a single medication for the treatment of bipolar disorder or epilepsy in pregnancy is preferred. Carbamazepine may decrease plasma concentrations of hormonal contraceptives; breakthrough bleeding or unintended pregnancy may occur and alternate or back-up methods of contraception should be considered.

Patients exposed to carbamazepine during pregnancy are encouraged to enroll themselves into the AED Pregnancy Registry by calling 1-888-233-2334. Additional information is available at www.aedpregnancyregistry.org.

Breast-Feeding Considerations Carbamazepine and its active epoxide metabolite are found in breast milk. Carbamazepine can also be detected in the serum of nursing infants. Transient hepatic dysfunction has been observed in some case reports. Nursing should be discontinued if adverse events are observed. According to the manufacturer, the decision to continue or discontinue breast-feeding during therapy should take into account the risk of exposure to the infant and the benefits of treatment to the mother. Respiratory depression, seizures, nausea, vomiting, diarrhea, and/or decreased feeding have been observed in neonates exposed to carbamazepine *in utero* and may represent a neonatal withdrawal syndrome.

Contraindications Hypersensitivity to carbamazepine, tricyclic antidepressants, or any component of the formulation; bone marrow depression; with or within 14 days of MAO inhibitor use; concurrent use of nefazodone;

concomitant use of delavirdine or other non-nucleoside reverse transcriptase inhibitors

Warnings/Precautions Hazardous agent - use appropriate precautions for handling and disposal (NIOSH 2014 [group 2]).

[U.S. Boxed Warning]: The risk of developing aplastic anemia or agranulocytosis is increased during treatment. Monitor CBC, platelets, and differential prior to and during therapy; discontinue if significant bone marrow suppression occurs. A spectrum of hematologic effects has been reported with use (eg, agranulocytosis, aplastic anemia, neutropenia, leukopenia, thrombocytopenia, pancytopenia, and anemias); patients with a previous history of adverse hematologic reaction to any drug may be at increased risk. Early detection of hematologic change is important; advise patients of early signs and symptoms including fever, sore throat, mouth ulcers, infections, easy bruising, and petechial or purpuric hemorrhage.

[U.S. Boxed Warning]: Severe and sometimes fatal dermatologic reactions, including toxic epidermal necrolysis (TENS) and Stevens-Johnson syndrome (SJS), may occur during therapy. The risk is increased in patients with the variant *HLA-B*1502* allele, found almost exclusively in patients of Asian ancestry. Patients of Asian descent should be screened prior to initiating therapy. Avoid use in patients testing positive for the allele; discontinue therapy in patients who have a serious dermatologic reaction. The risk of SJS or TENS may also be increased if carbamazepine is used in combination with other antiepileptic drugs associated with these reactions. Presence of the *HLA-B*1502* allele has not been found to predict the risk of less serious dermatologic reactions such as anticonvulsant hypersensitivity syndrome or nonserious rash. The risk of developing a hypersensitivity reaction may be increased in patients with the variant *HLA-A*3101* allele. These hypersensitivity reactions include SJS/TEN, maculopapular eruptions, and drug reaction with eosinophilia and systemic symptoms (DRESS/multiorgan hypersensitivity). The *HLA-A*3101* allele may occur more frequently patients of African-American, Arabic, Asian, European, Indian, Latin American, and Native American ancestry. Hypersensitivity has also been reported in patients experiencing reactions to other anticonvulsants; the history of hypersensitivity reactions in the patient or their immediate family members should be reviewed. Approximately 25% to 30% of patients allergic to carbamazepine will also have reactions with oxcarbazepine. Potentially serious, sometimes fatal multiorgan hypersensitivity reactions (also known as drug reaction with eosinophilia and systemic symptoms [DRESS]) have been reported with some antiepileptic drugs including carbamazepine; monitor for signs and symptoms of possible disparate manifestations associated with lymphatic, hepatic, renal, and/or hematologic organ systems; gradual discontinuation and conversion to alternate therapy may be required.

Antiepileptics are associated with an increased risk of suicidal behavior/thoughts with use (regardless of indication); patients should be monitored for signs/symptoms of depression, suicidal tendencies, and other unusual behavior changes during therapy and instructed to inform their healthcare provider immediately if symptoms occur.

Administer carbamazepine with caution to patients with history of cardiac damage, ECG abnormalities (or at risk for ECG abnormalities), hepatic or renal disease. Rare cases of a hepatic failure and vanishing bile duct syndrome involving destruction and disappearance of the intrahepatic bile ducts have been reported. Clinical courses of vanishing bile duct syndrome have been variable ranging from fulminant to indolent. Some cases have also had features associated with other immunoallergenic syndromes such as multiorgan hypersensitivity (DRESS syndrome) and serious dermatologic reactions including Stevens-Johnson syndrome. May activate latent psychosis and/or cause confusion or agitation; elderly patients may be at an increased risk for psychiatric effects.

Carbamazepine is not effective in absence, myoclonic, or akinetic seizures; exacerbation of certain seizure types have been seen after initiation of carbamazepine therapy in children with mixed seizure disorders. Abrupt discontinuation is not recommended in patients being treated for seizures. Dizziness or drowsiness may occur; caution should be used when performing tasks which require alertness until the effects are known. Potentially significant interactions may exist, requiring dose or frequency adjustment, additional monitoring, and/or selection of alternative therapy. Carbamazepine has mild anticholinergic activity; use with caution in patients with increased intraocular pressure, or sensitivity to anticholinergic effects. Hyponatremia caused by the syndrome of inappropriate antidiuretic hormone secretion (SIADH) may occur during therapy. Risk may be increased in the elderly or in patients also taking diuretics and may be dose-dependent. Use caution in elderly patients; may cause or exacerbate syndrome of inappropriate antidiuretic hormone secretion or hyponatremia; monitor sodium closely with initiation or dosage adjustments in older adults (Beers Criteria).

Administration of the suspension will yield higher peak and lower trough serum levels than an equal dose of the tablet form; consider a lower starting dose given more frequently (same total daily dose) when using the suspension. The suspension may contain sorbitol; avoid use in patents with hereditary fructose intolerance.

Warnings: Additional Pediatric Considerations Substitution of Tegretol with generic carbamazepine has resulted in decreased carbamazepine levels and increased seizure activity, as well as increased carbamazepine levels and toxicity. Monitoring of carbamazepine serum concentrations is mandatory when patients are switched from any product to another.

Some dosage forms may contain propylene glycol; in neonates large amounts of propylene glycol delivered orally, intravenously (eg, >3,000 mg/day), or topically have been associated with potentially fatal toxicities which can include metabolic acidosis, seizures, renal failure, and CNS depression; toxicities have also been reported in children and adults including hyperosmolality, lactic acidosis, seizures and respiratory depression; use caution (AAP, 1997; Shehab, 2009).

Adverse Reactions

Cardiovascular: Aggravation of coronary artery disease, atrioventricular block, cardiac arrhythmia, cardiac failure, edema, hypertension, hypotension, syncope, thromboembolism, thrombophlebitis

Central nervous system: Abnormality in thinking, agitation, amnesia, ataxia, chills, confusion, depression, dizziness, drowsiness, fatigue, hallucinations, headache, hyperacusis, neuroleptic malignant syndrome (NMS), paresthesia, peripheral neuritis, slurred speech, speech disturbance, talkativeness, twitching, vertigo

Dermatologic: Acute generalized exanthematous pustulosis, alopecia, diaphoresis, dyschromia, erythema multiforme, erythema nodosum, exfoliative dermatitis, onychomadesis, pruritus, skin photosensitivity, skin rash, Stevens-Johnson syndrome, toxic epidermal necrolysis, urticaria

Endocrine & metabolic: Abnormal thyroid function test, albuminuria, glycosuria, hypocalcemia, hyponatremia, porphyria, SIADH

Gastrointestinal: Abdominal pain, anorexia, constipation, diarrhea, gastric distress, glossitis, nausea, pancreatitis, stomatitis, vanishing bile duct syndrome, vomiting, xerostomia

Genitourinary: Azotemia, impotence, oliguria, urinary frequency, urinary retention

Hematologic & oncologic: Agranulocytosis, anemia, aplastic anemia, bone marrow depression, eosinophilia, leukocytosis, leukopenia, lymphadenopathy, pancytopenia, purpura, thrombocytopenia

Hepatic: Abnormal hepatic function tests, hepatic failure, hepatitis, jaundice

Hypersensitivity: Hypersensitivity reaction, multi-organ hypersensitivity

Neuromuscular & skeletal: Arthralgia, exacerbation of systemic lupus erythematosus, leg cramps, myalgia, osteoporosis, tremor, weakness

Ophthalmic: Blurred vision, cataract, conjunctivitis, diplopia, increased intraocular pressure, nystagmus, oculomotor disturbances

Otic: Tinnitus

Renal: Increased blood urea nitrogen, renal failure

Respiratory: Dry throat, pneumonia

Miscellaneous: Fever

Rare but important or life-threatening: Aseptic meningitis, defective spermatogenesis, hepatotoxicity (idiosyncratic) (Chalasani, 2014), hirsutism, lupus-like syndrome, maculopapular rash, paralysis, reduced fertility (male), suicidal ideation

Drug Interactions

Metabolism/Transport Effects **Substrate** of CYP2C8 (minor), CYP3A4 (major); **Note:** Assignment of Major/Minor substrate status based on clinically relevant drug interaction potential; **Induces** CYP1A2 (strong), CYP2B6 (strong), CYP2C19 (strong), CYP2C8 (strong), CYP2C9 (strong), CYP3A4 (strong), P-glycoprotein

Avoid Concomitant Use

Avoid concomitant use of CarBAMazepine with any of the following: Abiraterone Acetate; Apixaban; Apremilast; Artemether; Axitinib; Azelastine (Nasal); BCG (Intravesical); Bedaquiline; Boceprevir; Bortezomib; Bosutinib; Cabozantinib; Ceritinib; CloZAPine; Conivaptan; Crizotinib; Dabigatran Etexilate; Dasabuvir; Dienogest; Dipyrone; Dolutegravir; Dronedarone; Eliglustat; Enzalutamide; Everolimus; Fusidic Acid (Systemic); Ibrutinib; Idelalisib; Irinotecan; Isavuconazonium Sulfate; Itraconazole; Ivabradine; Ivacaftor; Lapatinib; Ledipasvir; Lumefantrine; Lurasidone; Macitentan; MAO Inhibitors; Mifepristone; Naloxegol; Nefazodone; Netupitant; NIFEdipine; Nilotinib; NiMODipine; Nintedanib; Nisoldipine; Olaparib; Ombitasvir; Orphenadrine; Palbociclib; Panobinostat; Paraldehyde; Paritaprevir; PAZOPanib; Pirfenidone; PONATinib; Praziquantel; Ranolazine; Regorafenib; Reverse Transcriptase Inhibitors (Non-Nucleoside); Rivaroxaban; Roflumilast; RomiDEPsin; Simeprevir; Sofosbuvir; SORAfenib; Stiripentol; Suvorexant; Tasimelteon; Telaprevir; Thalidomide; Ticagrelor; Tofacitinib; Tolvaptan; Toremifene; Trabectedin; TraMADol; Ulipristal; Vandetanib; Vemurafenib; VinCRIStine (Liposomal); Vorapaxar; Voriconazole

Increased Effect/Toxicity

CarBAMazepine may increase the levels/effects of: Adenosine; Alcohol (Ethyl); Azelastine (Nasal); Buprenorphine; Clarithromycin; ClomiPRAMINE; CloZAPine; CNS Depressants; Desmopressin; Eslicarbazepine; Fosphenytoin; Hydrocodone; Lacosamide; Lithium; MAO Inhibitors; Methotrimeprazine; Metyrosine; Orphenadrine; Paraldehyde; Phenytoin; Pramipexole; Rotigotine; Thalidomide

The levels/effects of CarBAMazepine may be increased by: Allopurinol; Brimonidine (Topical); Calcium Channel Blockers (Nondihydropyridine); Cannabis; Carbonic Anhydrase Inhibitors; Cimetidine; Ciprofloxacin (Systemic); Clarithromycin; Conivaptan; CYP3A4 Inhibitors (Moderate); CYP3A4 Inhibitors (Strong); Danazol; Darunavir; Dipyrone; Doxylamine; Dronabinol; Droperidol; Fluconazole; Fusidic Acid (Systemic); Grapefruit Juice; HydrOXYzine; Idelalisib; Isoniazid; Kava Kava; LamoTRIgine; Loxapine; Luliconazole; Macrolide Antibiotics; Magnesium Sulfate; Methotrimeprazine; Nabilone; Nefazodone; Protease Inhibitors; QUEtiapine; QuiNINE; Selective Serotonin Reuptake Inhibitors; Sodium Oxybate; Stiripentol; Tapentadol; Telaprevir; Tetrahydrocannabinol; Thiazide Diuretics; TraMADol; Valproic Acid and Derivatives; Zolpidem

Decreased Effect

CarBAMazepine may decrease the levels/effects of: Abiraterone Acetate; Acetaminophen; Afatinib; Albendazole; Apixaban; Apremilast; ARIPiprazole; Artemether; Axitinib; Bazedoxifene; BCG (Intravesical); Bedaquiline; Bendamustine; Boceprevir; Bortezomib; Bosutinib; Brentuximab Vedotin; Cabozantinib; Calcium Channel Blockers (Dihydropyridine); Calcium Channel Blockers (Nondihydropyridine); Canagliflozin; Cannabidiol; Cannabis; Caspofungin; Ceritinib; Clarithromycin; CloZAPine; Cobicistat; Contraceptives (Estrogens); Contraceptives (Progestins); Corticosteroids (Systemic); Crizotinib; CycloSPORINE (Systemic); CYP1A2 Substrates; CYP2B6 Substrates; CYP2C19 Substrates; CYP2C8 Substrates; CYP2C9 Substrates; CYP3A4 Substrates; Dabigatran Etexilate; Dasabuvir; Dasatinib; Dexamethasone (Systemic); Diclofenac (Systemic); Dienogest; Dolutegravir; DOXOrubicin (Conventional); Doxycycline; Dronabinol; Dronedarone; Eliglustat; Elvitegravir; Enzalutamide; Erlotinib; Eslicarbazepine; Everolimus; Exemestane; Ezogabine; Felbamate; FentaNYL; Fingolimod; Flunarizine; Fosphenytoin; Gefitinib; GuanFACINE; Haloperidol; Hydrocortisone (Systemic); Ibrutinib; Idelalisib; Imatinib; Irinotecan; Isavuconazonium Sulfate; Itraconazole; Ivabradine; Ivacaftor; Ixabepilone; Lacosamide; LamoTRIgine; Lapatinib; Ledipasvir; Linagliptin; Lopinavir; Lumefantrine; Lurasidone; Macitentan; Maraviroc; Mebendazole; Methadone; MethylPREDNISolone; Mianserin; Mifepristone; Naloxegol; Nefazodone; Netupitant; NIFEdipine; Nilotinib; NiMODipine; Nintedanib; Nisoldipine; Olaparib; Ombitasvir; OXcarbazepine; Palbociclib; Paliperidone; Panobinostat; Paritaprevir; PAZOPanib; Perampanel; P-glycoprotein/ABCB1 Substrates; Phenytoin; Pirfenidone; PONATinib; Praziquantel; PrednisoLONE (Systemic); PredniSONE; Propafenone; Protease Inhibitors; QUEtiapine; QuiNINE; Ranolazine; Regorafenib; Reverse Transcriptase Inhibitors (Non-Nucleoside); RisperiDONE; Rivaroxaban; Roflumilast; RomiDEPsin; Rufinamide; Saxagliptin; Selective Serotonin Reuptake Inhibitors; Simeprevir; Sofosbuvir; SORAfenib; SUNItinib; Suvorexant; Tadalafil; Tasimelteon; Telaprevir; Temsirolimus; Tetrahydrocannabinol; Theophylline Derivatives; Thyroid Products; Ticagrelor; Tofacitinib; Tolvaptan; Topiramate; Toremifene; Trabectedin; TraMADol; Treprostinil; Tricyclic Antidepressants; Ulipristal; Valproic Acid and Derivatives; Vandetanib; Vecuronium; Vemurafenib; Vilazodone; VinCRIStine (Liposomal); Vitamin K Antagonists; Vorapaxar; Voriconazole; Vortioxetine; Zaleplon; Ziprasidone; Zolpidem; Zuclopenthixol

The levels/effects of CarBAMazepine may be decreased by: Bosentan; CYP3A4 Inducers (Moderate); CYP3A4 Inducers (Strong); Dabrafenib; Deferasirox; Felbamate; Fosphenytoin; Mefloquine; Methylfolate; Mianserin; Mitotane; Orlistat; Phenytoin; Reverse Transcriptase Inhibitors (Non-Nucleoside); Rufinamide; Siltuximab; St Johns Wort; Theophylline Derivatives; Tocilizumab; TraMADol

Food Interactions Carbamazepine serum levels may be increased if taken with food and/or grapefruit juice. Management: Avoid concurrent ingestion of grapefruit juice.

Maintain adequate hydration, unless instructed to restrict fluid intake.

Storage/Stability

Carbatrol®, Equetro®: Store at controlled room temperature (25°C [77°F]); excursions permitted to 15°C to 30°C (59°F to 86°F); protect from light and moisture.

Tegretol®-XR: Store at controlled room temperature, 15°C to 30°C (59°F to 86°F); protect from moisture.

Tegretol® tablets and chewable tablets: Store at ≤30°C (86°F); protect from light and moisture.

Tegretol® suspension: Store at ≤30°C (86°F); shake well before using.

Mechanism of Action In addition to anticonvulsant effects, carbamazepine has anticholinergic, antineuralgic, antidiuretic, muscle relaxant, antimanic, antidepressive, and antiarrhythmic properties; may depress activity in the nucleus ventralis of the thalamus or decrease synaptic transmission or decrease summation of temporal stimulation leading to neural discharge by limiting influx of sodium ions across cell membrane or other unknown mechanisms; stimulates the release of ADH and potentiates its action in promoting reabsorption of water; chemically related to tricyclic antidepressants

Pharmacokinetics (Adult data unless noted)

Absorption: Slowly from the GI tract

Distribution: Carbamazepine and its active epoxide metabolite distribute into breast milk

V_d:

Neonates: 1.5 L/kg

Children: 1.9 L/kg

Adults: 0.59 to 2 L/kg

Protein binding: Carbamazepine: 75% to 90%, bound to alpha$_1$-acid glycoprotein and nonspecific binding sites on albumin; protein binding may be decreased in newborns

Epoxide metabolite: 50% protein bound

Metabolism: Induces liver enzymes to increase metabolism and shorten half-life over time; metabolized in the liver by cytochrome P450 3A4 to active epoxide metabolite; epoxide metabolite is metabolized by epoxide hydrolase to the trans-diol metabolite; ratio of serum epoxide to carbamazepine concentrations may be higher in patients receiving polytherapy (vs monotherapy) and in infants (vs older children); boys may have faster carbamazepine clearances and may, therefore, require higher mg/kg/day doses of carbamazepine compared to girls of similar age and weight

Bioavailability, oral: 75% to 85%; relative bioavailability of extended release tablet to suspension: 89%

Half-life:

Carbamazepine:

Initial: 25 to 65 hours

Multiple dosing:

Children: 8 to 14 hours

Adults: 12 to 17 hours

Epoxide metabolite: 34 ± 9 hours

Time to peak serum concentration: Unpredictable

Immediate release: Multiple doses: Suspension: 1.5 hours; Tablet: 4 to 5 hours

Extended release: Carbatrol, Equetro: 19 hours (single dose), ~6 hours (multiple doses); Tegretol-XR: 3 to 12 hours

Elimination: Urine 72% (1% to 3% as unchanged drug); feces 28%

Dosing: Usual Dosage must be adjusted according to patient's response and serum concentrations.

Pediatric: **Epilepsy:** Oral: To convert from tablets (immediate release or extended release) or capsules to oral suspension, use the same total mg daily dose and divided into 4 daily doses; monitor serum concentrations. **Note:** Carbamazepine suspension may be administered rectally as maintenance doses, if oral therapy is not possible; when using carbamazepine suspension rectally, administer the same total daily dose, but give in small, diluted, multiple doses; dilute the oral suspension with an equal volume of water; if defecation occurs within the first 2 hours, repeat the dose (Graves, 1987).

Infants and Children:

<6 years: Initial: 10 to 20 mg/kg/day divided twice or 3 times daily as immediate release tablets or 4 times daily as suspension; increase dose every week until optimal response and therapeutic levels are achieved; maintenance dose: Divide into 3-4 doses daily (immediate release tablets or suspension); maximum recommended daily dose: 35 mg/kg/**day**

6 to 12 years: Initial: 100 mg twice daily [immediate release tablets or extended release tablets (Tegretol-XR)] or 50 mg of suspension 4 times daily (200 mg/day); increase by up to 100 mg/day at weekly intervals using a twice daily regimen of extended release tablets or 3 to 4 times daily regimen of other formulations until optimal response and therapeutic levels are achieved; usual maintenance: 400 to 800 mg/day; maximum recommended daily dose: 1000 mg/**day**

Adolescents: Initial: 200 mg twice daily (immediate release tablets, extended release tablets [Tegretol-XR], or extended release capsules [Carbatrol]) or 100 mg of suspension 4 times daily (400 mg daily); increase by up to 200 mg/day at weekly intervals using a twice daily regimen of extended release tablets or capsules, or a 3 to 4 times/day regimen of other formulations until optimal response and therapeutic levels are achieved; usual dose: 800 to 1200 mg/day

Maximum recommended daily doses:

Adolescents ≤15 years: 1000 mg/**day**

Adolescents >15 years: 1200 mg/**day**

Adult:

Epilepsy: Oral: Initial: 400 mg/day in 2 divided doses (tablets or extended release tablets or extended release capsules) or 4 divided doses (oral suspension); increase by up to 200 mg/day at weekly intervals using a twice daily regimen of extended release tablets or capsules, or a 3 to 4 times daily regimen of other formulations until optimal response and therapeutic levels are achieved; usual dose: 800 to 1200 mg/day

Maximum recommended daily dose: 1600 mg/**day**; however, some patients have required up to 2400 mg/**day**

Trigeminal or glossopharyngeal neuralgia: Oral:

Initial: 200 mg/day in 2 divided doses (tablets, extended release tablets, or extended release capsules) or 4 divided doses (oral suspension) with food, gradually increasing in increments of 200 mg/day as needed

Maintenance: Usual: 400 to 800 mg daily in 2 divided doses (tablets, extended release tablets, or extended release capsules) or 4 divided doses (oral suspension); maximum daily dose: 1200 mg/**day**

Bipolar disorder: Oral: Initial: 400 mg/day in 2 divided doses (tablets, extended release tablets, or extended release capsules) or 4 divided doses (oral suspension); may adjust by 200 mg/day increments; maximum daily dose: 1600 mg/**day**. **Note:** Equetro is the only formulation specifically approved by the FDA for the management of bipolar disorder.

Dosing adjustment in renal impairment: Dosage adjustments are not required nor recommended in the manufacturer's labeling; however, the following guidelines have been used by some clinicians (Aronoff, 2007):

Infants, Children, and Adolescents: **Note:** Renally adjusted dose recommendations are based on doses of 10 to 20 mg/kg/**day** divided every 8 to 12 hours.

GFR ≥10 mL/minute/1.73 m^2: No dosage adjustment required

GFR <10 mL/minute/1.73 m^2: Administer 75% of normal dose

Intermittent hemodialysis: Administer 75% of normal dose; on dialysis days give dose **after** hemodialysis
Peritoneal dialysis (PD): Administer 75% of normal dose
Continuous renal replacement therapy (CRRT): Administer 75% of normal dose; monitor serum concentrations
Adults:
GFR ≥10 mL/minute: No dosage adjustment required
GFR <10 mL/minute: Administer 75% of dose
Intermittent hemodialysis: Administer 75% of normal dose; on dialysis days give dose **after** hemodialysis
Peritoneal dialysis (PD): Administer 75% of normal dose
Continuous renal replacement therapy (CRRT): No dosage adjustment recommended

Dosing adjustment in hepatic impairment: Infants, Children, Adolescents, and Adults: Use with caution in hepatic impairment; metabolized primarily in the liver.

Administration Hazardous agent; use appropriate precautions for handling and disposal (NIOSH 2014 [group 2]).
Oral: Administer with food to decrease GI upset
Immediate release:
Chewable and conventional tablets: Administer with meals; may be given 2 to 3 times daily.
Oral suspension: Shake well before use; administer with meals; must be given on a 3 to 4 times daily schedule. When carbamazepine suspension has been combined with chlorpromazine or thioridazine solutions, a precipitate forms which may result in loss of effect. Therefore, it is recommended that the carbamazepine suspension dosage form not be administered at the same time with other liquid medicinal agents or diluents.
Extended release:
Capsules (Carbatrol, Equetro): Consists of three different types of beads: Immediate release, extended release, and enteric release. The bead types are combined in a ratio to allow twice daily dosing. Capsules may be opened and contents sprinkled over food such as a teaspoon of applesauce; do not store medication/food mixture for later use; drink fluids after dose to make sure mixture is completely swallowed; may be administered with or without food; do not crush or chew.
Tablet (Tegretol-XR): Administer with meals; should be dosed twice daily; examine XR tablets for cracks or chips or other damage; do not use damaged extended release tablets without release portal. Swallow tablet whole; do not crush or chew.

Monitoring Parameters ***HLA-B*1502*** genotype screening prior to therapy initiation in patients of Asian descent; CBC with platelet count, reticulocytes, serum iron, liver function tests, ophthalmic examinations (including slit-lamp, fundoscopy, and tonometry), urinalysis, BUN, lipid panel, serum drug concentrations, thyroid function tests, serum sodium; pregnancy test; observe patient for excessive sedation especially when instituting or increasing therapy; signs of edema, skin rash, and hypersensitivity reactions; signs and symptoms of suicidality (eg, anxiety, depression, behavior changes).

Reference Range Timing of serum samples: Absorption is slow; peak levels occur 8 to 65 hours after ingestion of the first dose; the half-life ranges from 8 to 60 hours; therefore, steady-state is achieved in 2 to 5 days
Epilepsy: Therapeutic concentrations: 4 to 12 mcg/mL (SI: 17 to 51 micromoles/L). Patients who require higher levels (8 to 12 mcg/mL [SI: 34 to 51 micromoles/L]) should be carefully monitored. Side effects (especially CNS) occur commonly at higher levels. If other anticonvulsants (enzyme inducers) are given, therapeutic range is 4 to 8 mcg/mL (SI: 17 to 34 micromoles/L) due to increase in unmeasured active epoxide metabolite.

Test Interactions May cause false-positive serum TCA screen; may interact with some pregnancy tests

Additional Information Carbamazepine is not effective in absence, myoclonic, akinetic, or febrile seizures; exacerbation of certain seizure types have been seen after initiation of carbamazepine therapy in children with mixed seizure disorders. Rectally administered carbamazepine is not useful in status epilepticus due to its slow absorption.

Investigationally, loading doses of the suspension (10 mg/kg for children <12 years of age and 8 mg/kg for children >12 years) were given (via NG or ND tubes followed by 5 to 10 mL of water to flush through tube) to PICU patients with frequent seizures/status; 5 of 6 patients attained mean plasma concentrations of 4.3 mcg/mL and 7.3 mcg/mL at 1 and 2 hours postload; concurrent enteral feeding or ileus may delay absorption of loading dose (Miles, 1990).

A recent study (Relling, 2000) demonstrated that enzyme-inducing antiepileptic drugs (AEDs) (carbamazepine, phenobarbital, and phenytoin) increased systemic clearance of antileukemic drugs (teniposide and methotrexate) and were associated with a worse event-free survival, CNS relapse, and hematologic relapse, (ie, lower efficacy), in B-lineage ALL children receiving chemotherapy; the authors recommend using nonenzyme-inducing AEDs in patients receiving chemotherapy for ALL.

Dosage Forms Excipient information presented when available (limited, particularly for generics); consult specific product labeling.
Capsule Extended Release 12 Hour, Oral:
Carbatrol: 100 mg [contains fd&c blue #2 (indigotine)]
Carbatrol: 200 mg, 300 mg
Equetro: 100 mg, 200 mg, 300 mg [contains fd&c blue #2 (indigotine)]
Generic: 100 mg, 200 mg, 300 mg
Suspension, Oral:
TEGretol: 100 mg/5 mL (450 mL) [contains fd&c yellow #6 (sunset yellow), propylene glycol; citrus-vanilla flavor]
Generic: 100 mg/5 mL (450 mL)
Tablet, Oral:
Epitol: 200 mg [scored]
TEGretol: 200 mg [scored; contains fd&c red #40]
Generic: 200 mg
Tablet Chewable, Oral:
Generic: 100 mg
Tablet Extended Release 12 Hour, Oral:
TEGretol-XR: 100 mg, 200 mg, 400 mg
Generic: 200 mg, 400 mg

Extemporaneous Preparations Hazardous agent: Use appropriate precautions for handling and disposal (NIOSH 2014 [group 2]).

Note: Commercial oral suspension is available (20 mg/mL)

A 40 mg/mL oral suspension may be made with tablets. Crush twenty 200 mg tablets in a mortar and reduce to a fine powder. Add small portions of Simple Syrup, NF and mix to a uniform paste; mix while adding the vehicle in incremental proportions to **almost** 100 mL; transfer to a calibrated bottle, rinse mortar with vehicle, and add sufficient quantity of vehicle to make 100 mL. Label "shake well" and "refrigerate". Stable for 90 days.

Nahata MC, Pai VB, and Hipple TF, *Pediatric Drug Formulations*, 5th ed, Cincinnati, OH: Harvey Whitney Books Co, 2004.

Carbamide Peroxide (KAR ba mide per OKS ide)

Brand Names: US Auraphene-B [OTC]; Debrox [OTC]; E-R-O Ear Drops [OTC]; E-R-O Ear Wax Removal System [OTC]; Ear Drops Earwax Aid [OTC]; Ear Wax Remover

[OTC] [DSC]; Earwax Treatment Drops [OTC]; Gly-Oxide [OTC]; Thera-Ear [OTC]

Therapeutic Category Otic Agent, Cerumenolytic

Generic Availability (US) Yes

Use

Oral: Relief of minor inflammation of gums, oral mucosal surfaces and lips including canker sores and dental irritation; adjunct in oral hygiene

Otic: Emulsify and disperse ear wax

Warnings/Precautions

Oral: Self-medication (OTC) use: Instruct patient to discontinue use and consult health care provider if swelling, rash, or fever develops or if irritation, pain, or redness persists or worsens. Patients should consult health care provider for use longer than 7 days.

Otic: Self-medication (OTC use): Instruct patient to consult health care provider prior to use if ear drainage or discharge, ear pain, irritation, rash in ear, dizziness, or eardrum perforation is present or if they had recent ear surgery. Patients should consult health care provider for use longer than 4 days or if condition persists.

Warnings: Additional Pediatric Considerations Some dosage forms may contain propylene glycol; in neonates large amounts of propylene glycol delivered orally, intravenously (eg, >3,000 mg/day), or topically have been associated with potentially fatal toxicities which can include metabolic acidosis, seizures, renal failure, and CNS depression; toxicities have also been reported in children and adults including hyperosmolality, lactic acidosis, seizures and respiratory depression; use caution (AAP, 1997, 2009).

Adverse Reactions

Dermatologic: Rash

Local: Irritation, redness

Miscellaneous: Superinfection

Drug Interactions

Metabolism/Transport Effects None known.

Avoid Concomitant Use There are no known interactions where it is recommended to avoid concomitant use.

Increased Effect/Toxicity There are no known significant interactions involving an increase in effect.

Decreased Effect There are no known significant interactions involving a decrease in effect.

Storage/Stability Store at <25°C (77°F). Keep tip on bottle when not in use.

Mechanism of Action Carbamide peroxide releases hydrogen peroxide which serves as a source of nascent oxygen upon contact with catalase; deodorant action is probably due to inhibition of odor-causing bacteria; softens impacted cerumen due to its foaming action

Pharmacodynamics Onset of action: Otic: Slight disintegration of hard ear wax in 24 hours

Dosing: Usual

Oral: Children and Adults: Solution: Apply several drops undiluted to affected area of the mouth 4 times/day after meals and at bedtime for up to 7 days, expectorate after 2-3 minutes; as an adjunct to oral hygiene after brushing, swish 10 drops for 2-3 minutes, then expectorate

Otic: Solution:

Children <12 years: Individualize the dose according to patient size; 3 drops (range: 1-5 drops) twice daily for up to 4 days

Children ≥12 years and Adults: Instill 5-10 drops twice daily for up to 4 days

Administration

Oral: Apply undiluted solution with an applicator or cotton swab to the affected area after meals and at bedtime; or place drops on the tongue, mix with saliva, swish in the mouth for several minutes, then expectorate. Patient should not rinse mouth or drink fluids for 5 minutes after oral administration.

Otic: Instill drops into the external ear canal; keep drops in ear for several minutes by keeping head tilted or placing cotton in ear. Gently irrigate ear canal with warm water to remove loosened cerumen.

Dosage Forms Excipient information presented when available (limited, particularly for generics); consult specific product labeling. [DSC] = Discontinued product

Solution, Mouth/Throat:

Gly-Oxide: 10% (15 mL, 60 mL) [contains propylene glycol]

Solution, Otic:

Auraphene-B: 6.5% (15 mL)

Debrox: 6.5% (15 mL) [contains propylene glycol]

E-R-O Ear Drops: 6.5% (15 mL) [contains glycerin]

E-R-O Ear Wax Removal System: 6.5% (15 mL)

Ear Drops Earwax Aid: 6.5% (15 mL) [contains propylene glycol, trolamine (triethanolamine)]

Ear Wax Remover: 6.5% (15 mL [DSC]) [contains propylene glycol]

Earwax Treatment Drops: 6.5% (15 mL [DSC])

Earwax Treatment Drops: 6.5% (15 mL) [contains propylene glycol, trolamine (triethanolamine)]

Thera-Ear: 6.5% (15 mL)

◆ **Carbatrol** *see* CarBAMazepine *on page* 367

Carbinoxamine (kar bi NOKS a meen)

Medication Safety Issues

BEERS Criteria medication:

This drug may be potentially inappropriate for use in geriatric patients (Quality of evidence - moderate; Strength of recommendation - strong).

Brand Names: US Arbinoxa; Karbinal ER; Palgic [DSC]

Therapeutic Category Antihistamine

Generic Availability (US) May be product dependent

Use Symptomatic treatment of seasonal and perennial allergic rhinitis; vasomotor rhinitis; allergic conjunctivitis; mild manifestations of urticaria and angioedema; dermatographism; adjunct therapy for anaphylactic reactions (after acute manifestations controlled); amelioration of blood and plasma allergic reactions (All indications: FDA approved in ages ≥2 years and adults). **Note:** Approved ages and uses for generic products may vary; consult labeling for specific information.

Pregnancy Risk Factor C

Pregnancy Considerations Animal reproduction studies have not been conducted. Maternal antihistamine use has generally not resulted in an increased risk of birth defects; however, information specific for the use of carbinoxamine during pregnancy has not been located. Although antihistamines are recommended for some indications in pregnant women, the use of other agents with specific pregnancy data may be preferred.

Breast-Feeding Considerations It is not known if carbinoxamine is excreted in breast milk. Premature infants and newborns have a higher risk of intolerance to antihistamines. Use while breast-feeding is contraindicated by the manufacturer. Antihistamines may decrease maternal serum prolactin concentrations when administered prior to the establishment of nursing.

Contraindications Hypersensitivity to carbinoxamine or any component of the formulation; coadministration with monoamine oxidase inhibitors (MAOIs); children <2 years of age; breast-feeding women

Warnings/Precautions Use caution with asthma, increased intraocular pressure, narrow angle glaucoma, hyperthyroidism, cardiovascular disease, hypertension, pyloroduodenal obstruction, stenosing peptic ulcer, symptomatic prostatic hyperplasia, or urinary retention. Causes sedation; caution must be used in performing tasks which require mental alertness (eg, operating machinery or driving). Avoid use of this potent anticholinergic agent in the elderly due to increased risk of confusion, dry mouth, constipation, and other anticholinergic effects; clearance decreases and tolerance develops in patients of advanced age (Beers Criteria). Use is contraindicated in children age <2 years; deaths have been reported in children age <2 years who were taking carbinoxamine-containing products. Use may diminish mental alertness in children; in young children particularly, carbinoxamine-containing products may produce excitation. Some of these products may contain sodium metabisulfite, a sulfite that may cause allergic-type reactions including anaphylaxis and life-threatening or less severe asthmatic episodes, in susceptible patients. Potentially significant interactions may exist, requiring dose or frequency adjustment, additional monitoring, and/or selection of alternative therapy. Consult drug interactions database for more detailed information.

Warnings: Additional Pediatric Considerations Safety and efficacy for the use of cough and cold products in pediatric patients <4 years of age is limited; the AAP warns against the use of these products for respiratory illnesses in this age group. Serious adverse effects including death have been reported. Many of these products contain multiple active ingredients, increasing the risk of accidental overdose when used with other products. Health care providers are reminded to ask caregivers about the use of OTC cough and cold products in order to avoid exposure to multiple medications containing the same ingredient (AAP 2012; FDA 2008).

Some dosage forms may contain propylene glycol; in neonates large amounts of propylene glycol delivered orally, intravenously (eg, >3,000 mg/day), or topically have been associated with potentially fatal toxicities which can include metabolic acidosis, seizures, renal failure, and CNS depression; toxicities have also been reported in children and adults including hyperosmolality, lactic acidosis, seizures and respiratory depression; use caution (AAP, 1997; Shehab, 2009).

Adverse Reactions Frequency not defined.

Cardiovascular: Chest tightness, extrasystoles, hypotension, palpitations, tachycardia

Central nervous system: Ataxia (most frequent), chills, confusion, dizziness (most frequent), drowsiness (most frequent), euphoria, excitability, fatigue, headache, hysteria, insomnia, irritability, nervousness, neuritis, paresthesia, restlessness, sedation (most frequent), seizure, vertigo

Dermatologic: Diaphoresis, skin photosensitivity, skin rash, urticaria

Endocrine & metabolic: Increased uric acid

Gastrointestinal: Anorexia, constipation, diarrhea, epigastric distress (most frequent), nausea, vomiting, xerostomia

Genitourinary: Difficulty in micturition, early menses, urinary frequency, urinary retention

Hematologic & oncologic: Agranulocytosis, hemolytic anemia, thrombocytopenia

Hypersensitivity: Anaphylactic shock, hypersensitivity reaction

Neuromuscular & skeletal: Tremor

Ophthalmic: Blurred vision, diplopia

Otic: Labyrinthitis, tinnitus

Respiratory: Dry nose, dry throat, nasal congestion, thickening of bronchial secretions (most frequent), wheezing

Drug Interactions

Metabolism/Transport Effects None known.

Avoid Concomitant Use

Avoid concomitant use of Carbinoxamine with any of the following: Aclidinium; Azelastine (Nasal); Eluxadoline; Glucagon; Ipratropium (Oral Inhalation); Orphenadrine; Paraldehyde; Potassium Chloride; Thalidomide; Tiotropium; Umeclidinium

Increased Effect/Toxicity

Carbinoxamine may increase the levels/effects of: AbobotulinumtoxinA; Alcohol (Ethyl); Analgesics (Opioid); Anticholinergic Agents; Azelastine (Nasal); Buprenorphine; CNS Depressants; Eluxadoline; Glucagon; Hydrocodone; Methotrimeprazine; Metyrosine; Mirabegron; Mirtazapine; OnabotulinumtoxinA; Orphenadrine; Paraldehyde; Potassium Chloride; Pramipexole; RimabotulinumtoxinB; ROPINIRole; Rotigotine; Selective Serotonin Reuptake Inhibitors; Suvorexant; Thalidomide; Thiazide Diuretics; Tiotropium; Topiramate; Zolpidem

The levels/effects of Carbinoxamine may be increased by: Aclidinium; Brimonidine (Topical); Cannabis; Doxylamine; Dronabinol; Droperidol; HydrOXYzine; Ipratropium (Oral Inhalation); Kava Kava; Magnesium Sulfate; Methotrimeprazine; Mianserin; Nabilone; Perampanel; Pramlintide; Rufinamide; Sodium Oxybate; Tapentadol; Tetrahydrocannabinol; Umeclidinium

Decreased Effect

Carbinoxamine may decrease the levels/effects of: Acetylcholinesterase Inhibitors; Benzylpenicilloyl Polylysine; Betahistine; Hyaluronidase; Itopride; Metoclopramide; Secretin

The levels/effects of Carbinoxamine may be decreased by: Acetylcholinesterase Inhibitors; Amphetamines

Storage/Stability

Arbinoxa™: Store at 20°C to 25°C (68°F to 77°F); protect from light.

Palgic®: Store at 15°C to 30°C (59°F to 86°F); protect from light.

Mechanism of Action Carbinoxamine competes with histamine for H_1-receptor sites on effector cells in the gastrointestinal tract, blood vessels, and respiratory tract.

Pharmacodynamics Duration: 4 hours

Pharmacokinetics (Adult data unless noted)

Absorption: Well absorbed from the GI tract

Metabolism: Extensively hepatic

Half-life: 10 to 20 hours

Time to peak serum concentration: 1.5 to 5 hours

Elimination: Urine (as metabolites)

Dosing: Usual

Pediatric: **Allergic rhinitis/urticaria/allergic reactions:** Oral:

Immediate release:

- Children 2 to 5 years: Oral solution:
  - Weight-directed: 0.2 to 0.4 mg/kg/day in divided doses 3 to 4 times daily
  - Fixed dose: 1 to 2 mg/dose 3 to 4 times daily; maximum daily dose: 0.4 mg/kg/**day**
- Children 6 to 11 years: Oral solution or tablet: 2 to 4 mg/dose 3 to 4 times daily
- Children ≥12 years and Adolescents: Oral solution or tablet: 4 to 8 mg/dose 3 to 4 times daily

Extended release suspension: **Note:** Fixed dose presented in children 2 to 11 years equates to approximately 0.2 to 0.4 mg/kg/day

- Children 2 to 3 years: 3 to 4 mg/dose every 12 hours
- Children 4 to 5 years: 3 to 8 mg/dose every 12 hours
- Children 6 to 11 years: 6 to 12 mg/dose every 12 hours
- Children ≥12 years and Adolescents: 6 to 16 mg/dose every 12 hours

Adult: **Allergic rhinitis/urticaria:** Oral:

Oral extended release suspension: 6 to 16 mg/dose every 12 hours

Oral solution or tablet: 4 to 8 mg/dose 3 to 4 times daily

Dosing adjustment in renal impairment: There are no dosage adjustments provided in manufacturer's labeling.

Dosing adjustment in hepatic impairment: There are no dosage adjustments provided in manufacturer's labeling.

Administration Oral: Administer on an empty stomach with water.

Product Availability Karbinal ER (extended release) oral suspension: FDA approved March 2013; availability anticipated is January 2015. Consult the prescribing information for additional information.

Dosage Forms Excipient information presented when available (limited, particularly for generics); consult specific product labeling. [DSC] = Discontinued product

Liquid Extended Release, Oral, as maleate:

Karbinal ER: 4 mg/5 mL (480 mL) [contains methylparaben, polysorbate 80, propylparaben, sodium metabisulfite; strawberry-banana flavor]

Solution, Oral, as maleate:

Arbinoxa: 4 mg/5 mL (473 mL) [contains methylparaben, propylene glycol, propylparaben; bubble-gum flavor]

Palgic: 4 mg/5 mL (480 mL [DSC]) [contains methylparaben, propylene glycol, propylparaben; bubble-gum flavor]

Generic: 4 mg/5 mL (118 mL, 473 mL)

Tablet, Oral, as maleate:

Arbinoxa: 4 mg [scored]

Palgic: 4 mg [DSC] [scored]

Generic: 4 mg

◆ **Carbinoxamine Maleate** *see* Carbinoxamine *on page 372*

◆ **Carbocaine** *see* Mepivacaine *on page 1362*

◆ **Carbocaine® (Can)** *see* Mepivacaine *on page 1362*

◆ **Carbocaine Preservative-Free** *see* Mepivacaine *on page 1362*

◆ **Carbolith (Can)** *see* Lithium *on page 1284*

CARBOplatin (KAR boe pla tin)

Medication Safety Issues

Sound-alike/look-alike issues:

CARBOplatin may be confused with CISplatin, oxaliplatin

Paraplatin may be confused with Platinol

High alert medication:

This medication is in a class the Institute for Safe Medication Practices (ISMP) includes among its list of drug classes which have a heightened risk of causing significant patient harm when used in error.

BEERS Criteria medication:

This drug may be potentially inappropriate for use in geriatric patients (Quality of evidence - moderate; Strength of recommendation - strong).

Related Information

Management of Drug Extravasations *on page 2298*

Prevention of Chemotherapy-Induced Nausea and Vomiting in Children *on page 2368*

Safe Handling of Hazardous Drugs *on page 2455*

Brand Names: Canada Carboplatin Injection; Carboplatin Injection BP

Therapeutic Category Antineoplastic Agent, Alkylating Agent; Antineoplastic Agent, Platinum Analog

Generic Availability (US) Yes

Use Treatment of advanced ovarian carcinoma (FDA approved in adults); has also been used in the treatment of bladder cancer, breast cancer (metastatic), central nervous system tumors, cervical cancer (recurrent or metastatic), endometrial cancer, esophageal cancer, head and neck cancer, Hodgkin lymphoma (relapsed or refractory), malignant pleural mesothelioma, melanoma (advanced or metastatic), Merkel cell carcinoma, neuroendocrine tumors (adrenal gland and carcinoid tumors), non-Hodgkin lymphomas (relapsed or refractory), non-small cell lung cancer, prostate cancer, sarcomas (Ewing's sarcoma, osteosarcoma), small cell lung cancer, testicular cancer, thymic malignancies, unknown primary adenocarcinoma, Wilm's tumor, and as a conditioning regimen prior to hematopoietic stem cell transplantation

Pregnancy Risk Factor D

Pregnancy Considerations Embryotoxicity and teratogenicity have been observed in animal reproduction studies. May cause fetal harm if administered during pregnancy. Women of childbearing potential should avoid becoming pregnant during treatment.

Breast-Feeding Considerations It is not known if carboplatin is excreted in breast milk. Due to the potential for toxicity in nursing infants, breast-feeding is not recommended.

Contraindications History of severe allergic reaction to carboplatin, cisplatin, other platinum-containing formulations, mannitol, or any component of the formulation; should not be used in patients with severe bone marrow depression or significant bleeding

Warnings/Precautions Hazardous agent - use appropriate precautions for handling and disposal (NIOSH 2014 [group 1]). High doses have resulted in severe abnormalities of liver function tests. **[U.S. Boxed Warning]: Bone marrow suppression, which may be severe, is dose related; may result in infection (due to neutropenia) or bleeding (due to thrombocytopenia); anemia may require blood transfusion;** reduce dosage in patients with bone marrow suppression; cycles should be delayed until WBC and platelet counts have recovered. Patients who have received prior myelosuppressive therapy and patients with renal dysfunction are at increased risk for bone marrow suppression. Anemia is cumulative.

When calculating the carboplatin dose using the Calvert formula and an estimated glomerular filtration rate (GFR), the laboratory method used to measure serum creatinine may impact dosing. Compared to other methods, standardized isotope dilution mass spectrometry (IDMS) may underestimate serum creatinine values in patients with low creatinine values (eg, ≤0.7 mg/dL) and may overestimate GFR in patients with normal renal function. This may result in higher calculated carboplatin doses and increased toxicities. If using IDMS, the Food and Drug Administration (FDA) recommends that clinicians consider capping estimated GFR at a maximum of 125 mL/minute to avoid potential toxicity.

[U.S. Boxed Warning]: Anaphylactic-like reactions have been reported with carboplatin; may occur within minutes of administration. Epinephrine, corticosteroids and antihistamines have been used to treat symptoms. The risk of allergic reactions (including anaphylaxis) is increased in patients previously exposed to platinum therapy. Skin testing and desensitization protocols have been reported (Confina-Cohen, 2005; Lee, 2004; Markman, 2003). When administered as sequential infusions, taxane derivatives (docetaxel, paclitaxel) should be administered before the platinum derivatives (carboplatin, cisplatin) to limit myelosuppression and to enhance efficacy. Ototoxicity may occur when administered concomitantly with aminoglycosides. Clinically significant hearing loss has been reported to occur in pediatric patients when carboplatin was administered at higher than recommended doses in combination with other ototoxic agents (eg, aminoglycosides). In a study of children receiving carboplatin for the treatment of retinoblastoma, those <6 months of age at treatment initiation were more likely to experience ototoxicity; long-term audiology monitoring is recommended (Qaddoumi, 2012). Loss of vision (usually reversible within weeks of discontinuing) has been reported with higher than recommended doses.

Use caution in elderly patients; may cause or exacerbate syndrome of inappropriate antidiuretic hormone secretion or hyponatremia; monitor sodium closely with initiation or dosage adjustments in older adults (Beers Criteria). Peripheral neuropathy occurs infrequently, the incidence of peripheral neuropathy is increased in patients >65 years of age and those who have previously received cisplatin treatment. Patients >65 years of age are more likely to develop severe thrombocytopenia.

Limited potential for nephrotoxicity unless administered concomitantly with aminoglycosides. **[U.S. Boxed Warning]: Vomiting may occur.** Carboplatin is associated with a moderate emetic potential in adult patients and a high emetic potential in pediatric patients; antiemetics are recommended to prevent nausea and vomiting (Basch, 2011; Dupuis, 2011; Roila, 2010). May be severe in patients who have received prior emetogenic therapy. **[U.S. Boxed Warning]: Should be administered under the supervision of an experienced cancer chemotherapy physician.**

Adverse Reactions

Central nervous system: Neurotoxicity, pain, peripheral neuropathy

Dermatologic: Alopecia

Endocrine & metabolic: Hypocalcemia, hypokalemia, hypomagnesemia, hyponatremia

Gastrointestinal: Abdominal pain, constipation, diarrhea, dysgeusia, mucositis, nausea (without vomiting), stomatitis, vomiting

Hematologic & oncologic: Anemia, bleeding complications, bone marrow depression (dose related and dose limiting; nadir at ~21 days with single-agent therapy), hemorrhage, leukopenia, neutropenia, thrombocytopenia

Hepatic: Increased serum alkaline phosphatase, increased serum AST, increased serum bilirubin

Hypersensitivity: Hypersensitivity

Infection: Infection

Neuromuscular & skeletal: Weakness

Ophthalmic: Visual disturbance

Otic: Ototoxicity

Renal: Decreased creatinine clearance, increased blood urea nitrogen, increased serum creatinine

Rare but important or life-threatening: Anaphylaxis, anorexia, bronchospasm, cardiac failure, cerebrovascular accident, dehydration, embolism, erythema, febrile neutropenia, hemolytic anemia (acute), hemolytic-uremic syndrome, hypertension, hypotension, injection site reaction (pain, redness, swelling), limb ischemia (acute), malaise, metastases, pruritus, skin rash, tissue necrosis (associated with extravasation), urticaria, vision loss

Drug Interactions

Metabolism/Transport Effects None known.

Avoid Concomitant Use

Avoid concomitant use of CARBOplatin with any of the following: BCG; BCG (Intravesical); CloZAPine; Dipyrone; Natalizumab; Pimecrolimus; SORAfenib; Tacrolimus (Topical); Tofacitinib; Vaccines (Live)

Increased Effect/Toxicity

CARBOplatin may increase the levels/effects of: Bexarotene (Systemic); CloZAPine; Leflunomide; Natalizumab; Taxane Derivatives; Tofacitinib; Topotecan; Vaccines (Live)

The levels/effects of CARBOplatin may be increased by: Aminoglycosides; Denosumab; Dipyrone; Pimecrolimus; Roflumilast; SORAfenib; Tacrolimus (Topical); Trastuzumab

Decreased Effect

CARBOplatin may decrease the levels/effects of: BCG; BCG (Intravesical); Coccidioides immitis Skin Test; Fosphenytoin-Phenytoin; Sipuleucel-T; Vaccines (Inactivated); Vaccines (Live)

The levels/effects of CARBOplatin may be decreased by: Echinacea

Storage/Stability Store intact vials at room temperature at 25°C (77°F); excursions permitted to 15°C to 30°C (59°F to 86°F). Protect from light. Further dilution to a concentration as low as 0.5 mg/mL is stable at room temperature (25°C) for 8 hours in NS or D_5W. Stability has also been demonstrated for dilutions in D_5W in PVC bags at room temperature for 9 days (Benaji, 1994); however, the manufacturer recommends use within 8 hours due to lack of preservative. Multidose vials are stable for up to 14 days after opening when stored at 25°C (77°F) following multiple needle entries.

Mechanism of Action Carboplatin is a platinum compound alkylating agent which covalently binds to DNA; interferes with the function of DNA by producing interstrand DNA cross-links

Pharmacokinetics (Adult data unless noted)

Distribution: V_d: 16 L (based on a dose of 300-500 mg/m^2)

Protein binding: 0%; however, platinum (from carboplatin) is 30% protein bound

Half-life: Terminal: CrCl >60 mL/minute: Carboplatin: 2.5-5.9 hours (based on a dose of 300-500 mg/m^2); platinum (from carboplatin): ≥5 days

Elimination: Urine (~70% as carboplatin within 24 hours; 3% to 5% as platinum within 1-4 days)

Dosing: Usual IV (refer to individual protocols):

Infants, Children, and Adolescents: **Note:** Some protocols calculate dose on the basis of body weight rather than body surface area in infants and young children (<3 years or ≤12 kg):

BSA-directed dosing:

Bone marrow transplant preparative regimen: Children: 500 mg/m^2/day for 3 days (Gilheeney, 2010)

Glioma (Packer, 1997): Infants ≥3 months, Children, and Adolescents:

Induction: 175 mg/m^2 once weekly for 4 weeks every 6 weeks (2-week recovery period between courses) in combination with vincristine for 2 cycles

Maintenance: 175 mg/m^2 weekly for 4 weeks, with a 3-week recovery period between courses in combination with vincristine for ≤12 cycles

Sarcomas: Ewing's sarcoma, osteosarcoma: Children and Adolescents: 400 mg/m^2/day for 2 days every 21 days (in combination with ifosfamide and etoposide) (Van Winkle, 2005)

Alternative carboplatin dosing: Some investigators calculate pediatric carboplatin doses using a modified Calvert formula: Dosing based on target AUC (modified Calvert formula for use in children): Total dose (mg) = [Target AUC (mg/mL/minute)] x [GFR (mL/minute) + (0.36 x body weight in kilograms)]; **Note:** GFR in this equation is an exact measured value (eg, "raw" in mL/minute) **not** corrected for BSA (ie, **not** mL/minute/1.73 m^2).

Note: Calvert formula was based on using chromic edetate (^{51}Cr-EDTA) plasma clearance to establish GFR. Some clinicians have recommended that methods for estimating CrCl not be substituted for GFR since carboplatin dosing based on such estimates may not be predictive.

Note: The dose of carboplatin calculated is TOTAL mg DOSE not mg/m^2.

Adults:

Note: Doses for adults are commonly calculated by the target AUC using the Calvert formula, where **Total dose (mg) = Target AUC x (GFR + 25)**. If estimating glomerular filtration rate (GFR) instead of measuring GFR, the Food and Drug Administration (FDA) recommends considering capping estimated GFR at a maximum of 125 mL/minute to avoid potential toxicity.

Ovarian cancer, advanced: IV: 360 mg/m^2 every 4 weeks (as a single agent) **or** 300 mg/m^2 every 4 weeks (in combination with cyclophosphamide) **or** target AUC 4-6 (in previously treated patients)

Dosage adjustment for toxicity: Platelets <50,000 cells/mm^3 or ANC <500 cells/mm^3: Administer 75% of dose

Dosage adjustment in renal impairment: Adults: **Note:** Dose determination with Calvert formula uses GFR and, therefore, inherently adjusts for renal dysfunction.

The manufacturer's labeling recommends the following dosage adjustment guidelines for single-agent therapy:

Baseline CrCl 41-59 mL/minute: Initiate at 250 mg/m^2 and adjust subsequent doses based on bone marrow toxicity

Baseline CrCl 16-40 mL/minute: Initiate at 200 mg/m^2 and adjust subsequent doses based on bone marrow toxicity

Baseline CrCl ≤15 mL/minute: No guidelines are available.

The following dosage adjustments have been used by some clinicians (for dosing based on mg/m^2) (Aronoff, 2007):

Hemodialysis: Administer 50% of dose

Continuous ambulatory peritoneal dialysis (CAPD): Administer 25% of dose

Continuous renal replacement therapy (CRRT): 200 mg/m^2

Dosage adjustment in hepatic impairment: Dosage adjustments are not provided in manufacturer's labeling.

Preparation for Administration Hazardous agent; use appropriate precautions for handling and disposal (NIOSH 2014 [group 1]). **Note:** Needles or IV administration sets that contain aluminum should not be used in the preparation or administration of carboplatin; aluminum can react with carboplatin resulting in precipitate formation and loss of potency.

Parenteral: IV: Solution for injection: Manufacturer's labeling states solution can be further diluted to concentrations as low as 0.5 mg/mL in NS or D_5W; in adults, doses are generally diluted in either 100 mL or 250 mL of NS or D_5W.

Concentrations used for desensitization vary based on protocol.

Administration Hazardous agent; use appropriate precautions for handling and disposal (NIOSH 2014 [group 1]). Carboplatin is associated with a moderate emetic potential in adult patients and a high emetic potential in pediatric patients; antiemetics are recommended to prevent nausea and vomiting (Basch 2011; Dupuis 2011; Roila 2010).

Parenteral: **Note:** Needles or IV administration sets that contain aluminum should not be used in the preparation or administration of carboplatin; aluminum can react with carboplatin resulting in precipitate formation and loss of potency.

IV: Administer over 15 to 60 minutes although some protocols may require infusions up to 24 hours. When administered as a part of a combination chemotherapy regimen, sequence of administration may vary by regimen; refer to specific protocol for sequence recommendation.

Vesicant/Extravasation Risk May be an irritant

Monitoring Parameters CBC with differential and platelet count, serum electrolytes, urinalysis, serum creatinine and BUN, creatinine clearance, liver function tests

Dosage Forms Excipient information presented when available (limited, particularly for generics); consult specific product labeling.

Solution, Intravenous:

Generic: 50 mg/5 mL (5 mL); 150 mg/15 mL (15 mL); 450 mg/45 mL (45 mL); 600 mg/60 mL (60 mL)

Solution, Intravenous [preservative free]:

Generic: 50 mg/5 mL (5 mL); 150 mg/15 mL (15 mL); 450 mg/45 mL (45 mL); 600 mg/60 mL (60 mL)

Solution Reconstituted, Intravenous:

Generic: 150 mg (1 ea)

- ◆ **Carboplatin Injection (Can)** *see* CARBOplatin *on page 374*
- ◆ **Carboplatin Injection BP (Can)** *see* CARBOplatin *on page 374*
- ◆ **Carboxypeptidase-G2** *see* Glucarpidase *on page 974*
- ◆ **Cardene IV** *see* NiCARdipine *on page 1513*
- ◆ **Cardene SR [DSC]** *see* NiCARdipine *on page 1513*
- ◆ **Cardizem** *see* Diltiazem *on page 661*
- ◆ **Cardizem CD** *see* Diltiazem *on page 661*
- ◆ **Cardizem LA** *see* Diltiazem *on page 661*
- ◆ **Cardura** *see* Doxazosin *on page 709*
- ◆ **Cardura-1 (Can)** *see* Doxazosin *on page 709*
- ◆ **Cardura-2 (Can)** *see* Doxazosin *on page 709*
- ◆ **Cardura-4 (Can)** *see* Doxazosin *on page 709*
- ◆ **Cardura XL** *see* Doxazosin *on page 709*

Carglumic Acid (kar GLU mik AS id)

Brand Names: US Carbaglu

Therapeutic Category Antidote; Metabolic Alkalosis Agent; Urea Cycle Disorder (UCD) Treatment Agent

Generic Availability (US) No

Use Adjunctive therapy for treatment of acute hyperammonemia due to N-acetylglutamate synthase (NAGS) deficiency (FDA approved in all ages); maintenance therapy for chronic hyperammonemia due to NAGS deficiency (FDA approved in all ages)

Prescribing and Access Restrictions Carbaglu is not available through pharmaceutical wholesalers or retail pharmacies, but only through direct shipping from the Accredo specialty pharmacy. Prescribers must contact Accredo Health Group at 888-454-8860 or refer to www.-accredo.com to initiate patients on this product.

Pregnancy Risk Factor C

Pregnancy Considerations Adverse events have been observed in animal reproduction studies. There are no adequate and well-controlled studies in pregnant women. However, due to the potential for irreversible fetal neurologic damage for untreated NAGS deficiency, women with this condition must remain on treatment throughout pregnancy.

Breast-Feeding Considerations It is not known if carglumic acid is excreted in breast milk. Breast-feeding is not recommended by the manufacturer.

Contraindications There are no contraindications listed in the manufacturer's labeling.

Warnings/Precautions Acute symptomatic hyperammonemia is a life-threatening emergency; management of hyperammonemia due to N-acetylglutamate synthase (NAGS) deficiency should be done in coordination with those experienced in the management of metabolic disorders. With hyperammonemia, complete protein restriction should be maintained for 24-48 hours and caloric supplementation should be maximized to reverse catabolism and nitrogen turnover.

Adverse Reactions

Central nervous system: Fever, headache, somnolence

Dermatologic: Hyperhidrosis, rash

Gastrointestinal: Abdominal pain, anorexia, diarrhea, dysgeusia, vomiting, weight loss

Hematologic: Anemia

Neuromuscular & skeletal: Weakness

Otic: Ear infection

Respiratory: Nasopharyngitis, pneumonia, tonsillitis

Miscellaneous: Infections, influenza

Drug Interactions

Metabolism/Transport Effects None known.

Avoid Concomitant Use There are no known interactions where it is recommended to avoid concomitant use.

Increased Effect/Toxicity There are no known significant interactions involving an increase in effect.

Decreased Effect There are no known significant interactions involving a decrease in effect.

Storage/Stability Before opening, store refrigerated at 2°C to 8°C (36°F to 46°F). After opening, do not refrigerate or store above 30°C (86°F). Protect from moisture. Discard 1 month after opening.

Mechanism of Action N-acetylglutamate synthase (NAGS) is a mitochondrial enzyme which produces N-acetylglutamate (NAG). NAG is a required allosteric activator of the hepatic mitochondrial enzyme, carbamoyl phosphate synthetase 1 (CPS 1), which converts ammonia into urea in the first step of the urea cycle. In NAGS-deficient patients, carglumic acid serves as a replacement for NAG.

Pharmacodynamics Onset of action: Within 24 hours

Pharmacokinetics (Adult data unless noted)

Distribution: V_d: ~2657 L

Metabolism: Via intestinal flora to carbon dioxide

Half-life, elimination: Median: 5.6 hours (range: 4.3-9.5 hours)

Time to peak serum concentration: Median: 3 hours

Elimination: Feces (60% as unchanged drug); urine (9% as unchanged drug)

Dosing: Neonatal

Acute hyperammonemia; adjunct therapy: Oral: 100-250 mg/kg/day given in 2 or 4 divided doses; titrate to age-appropriate plasma ammonia concentrations; concomitant ammonia-lowering therapy recommended.

Chronic hyperammonemia: Oral: Usual dose: <100 mg/kg/day given in 2 or 4 divided doses; titrate to age-appropriate plasma ammonia concentrations

Dosing: Usual

Pediatric:

Acute hyperammonemia: Infants, Children, and Adolescents: Oral: 100 to 250 mg/kg/day given in 2 or 4 divided doses; titrate to age-appropriate plasma ammonia concentrations; concomitant ammonia-lowering therapy recommended

Chronic hyperammonemia: Infants, Children, and Adolescents: Oral: Usual dose: <100 mg/kg/day given in 2 or 4 divided doses; titrate to age-appropriate plasma ammonia concentrations

Adult: **Note:** Dose should be rounded to the nearest 100 mg (1/2 tablet).

Acute hyperammonemia; adjunct therapy: Oral: 100 to 250 mg/kg/day given in 2 or 4 divided doses; titrate to age-appropriate plasma ammonia concentrations; concomitant ammonia-lowering therapy recommended

Chronic hyperammonemia: Oral: Usual dose: <100 mg/kg/day given in 2 or 4 divided doses; titrate to age-appropriate plasma ammonia concentrations

Preparation for Administration

Oral: Each 200 mg tablet should be dispersed in at least 2.5 mL of water (no other foods/liquids) and administered immediately.

Oral syringe: Disperse each 200 mg tablet in 2.5 mL of water to yield a concentration of 80 mg/mL (shake gently in container). Appropriate volume of dispersion should be drawn up in an oral syringe and administered immediately (discard unused dispersion).

Nasogastric tube: Disperse each 200 mg tablet in water (2.5 mL per tablet for pediatric patients; ≥2.5 mL per tablet for adults) and shake gently; administer immediately.

Administration

Oral: Administer immediately before meals.

Tablets should not be crushed or swallowed whole. After dispersion in water, administer immediately. Tablets do not dissolve completely, and some particles may remain; rinse container with water and administer rinse immediately.

Oral syringe: After dispersion of tablets in water, draw up appropriate volume and administer immediately (discard unused dispersion). After initial administration, refill oral syringe with a minimum of 1 to 2 mL of water and administer immediately.

Nasogastric tube: After dispersion of tablets in water, immediately administer through a nasogastric tube, followed by flush with additional water to clear the tube (tablets do not dissolve completely; some particles may remain). Carglumic acid tablets should not be mixed with any other foods or liquids other than water.

Monitoring Parameters Plasma ammonia concentrations; physical signs/symptoms of hyperammonemia (eg, lethargy, ataxia, confusion, vomiting, seizures, memory impairment)

Dosage Forms Excipient information presented when available (limited, particularly for generics); consult specific product labeling.

Tablet, Oral:

Carbaglu: 200 mg [scored]

◆ **Carimune NF** *see* Immune Globulin *on page* 1089

◆ **Caripul (Can)** *see* Epoprostenol *on page* 769

Carmustine (kar MUS teen)

Medication Safety Issues

Sound-alike/look-alike issues:

Carmustine may be confused with bendamustine, lomustine

High alert medication:

This medication is in a class the Institute for Safe Medication Practices (ISMP) includes among its list of drug classes which have a heightened risk of causing significant patient harm when used in error.

Related Information

Management of Drug Extravasations *on page* 2298

Prevention of Chemotherapy-Induced Nausea and Vomiting in Children *on page* 2368

Safe Handling of Hazardous Drugs *on page* 2455

Brand Names: US BiCNU; Gliadel Wafer

Brand Names: Canada BiCNU; Gliadel Wafer

Therapeutic Category Antineoplastic Agent, Alkylating Agent; Antineoplastic Agent, Alkylating Agent (Nitrosourea)

Generic Availability (US) No

Use

Injection: Treatment of brain tumors (glioblastoma, brainstem glioma, medulloblastoma, astrocytoma, ependymoma, and metastatic brain tumor); multiple myeloma, Hodgkin's lymphoma, and non-Hodgkin's lymphomas (relapsed or refractory) (FDA approved in adults)

Wafer (implant): Adjunct to surgery in patients with recurrent glioblastoma multiforme; adjunct to surgery and radiation in patients with newly diagnosed high grade malignant glioma (FDA approved in adults)

Pregnancy Risk Factor D

Pregnancy Considerations Adverse events have been observed in animal reproduction studies. Carmustine may cause fetal harm if administered to a pregnant woman. Women of childbearing potential should use effective contraception to avoid becoming pregnant while on treatment. May impair fertility. Advise males of potential risk of infertility and to seek fertility/family planning counseling prior to receiving carmustine wafer implants.

Breast-Feeding Considerations It is not known if carmustine is excreted in breast milk. Due to the potential for serious adverse reactions in the nursing infant, the manufacturer recommends breast-feeding be discontinued during treatment.

Contraindications

IV: Hypersensitivity to carmustine or any component of the formulation

Implant: There are no contraindications listed in the manufacturer's labeling.

Warnings/Precautions Hazardous agent - use appropriate precautions for handling and disposal (NIOSH 2014 [group 1]).

Injection:

[US Boxed Warning]: Bone marrow suppression, primarily thrombocytopenia (which may lead to bleeding) and leukopenia (which may lead to infection), is the most common and severe toxicity. Hematologic toxicity is generally delayed; monitor blood counts for at least 6 weeks following treatment. The manufacturer suggests not administering more frequently than every 6 weeks for approved doses/uses. Myelosuppression is cumulative; consider nadir blood counts from prior dose for dosage adjustment. Patients must have platelet counts >100,000/mm^3 and leukocytes >4,000/mm^3 for a repeat dose. Myelosuppression generally occurs 4 to 6 weeks after administration; thrombocytopenia occurs at ~4 weeks and persists for 1 to 2 weeks; leukopenia occurs at 5 to 6 weeks and persists for 1 to 2 weeks. Anemia may occur (less common and less severe than leukopenia or thrombocytopenia). Long-term use is associated with the development of secondary malignancies (acute leukemias and bone marrow dysplasias).

[US Boxed Warnings]: Dose-related pulmonary toxicity may occur; patients receiving cumulative doses >1,400 mg/m^2 are at higher risk. Delayed onset of pulmonary fibrosis may occur years after treatment (may be fatal), particularly in children. Pulmonary toxicity has occurred in children up to 17 years after treatment; this occurred in ages 1 to 16 for the treatment of intracranial tumors; cumulative doses ranged from 770 to 1,800 mg/m^2 (in combination with cranial radiotherapy). Pulmonary toxicity is characterized by pulmonary infiltrates and/or fibrosis and has been reported from 9 days to 43 months after nitrosourea treatment (including carmustine). Although pulmonary toxicity generally occurs in patients who have received prolonged treatment, pulmonary fibrosis has been reported with cumulative doses <1,400 mg/m^2. In addition to high cumulative doses, other risk factors for pulmonary toxicity include history of lung disease and baseline predicted forced vital capacity (FVC) or carbon monoxide diffusing capacity (DL_{CO}) <70%. Baseline and periodic pulmonary function tests are recommended. For high-dose treatment (transplant; off-label dose), acute lung injury may occur ~1 to 3 months post transplant; advise patients to contact their transplant physician for dyspnea, cough, or fever; interstitial pneumonia may be managed with a course of corticosteroids. Children are at higher risk of delayed pulmonary toxicity with IV carmustine.

Reversible increases in transaminases, bilirubin, and alkaline phosphatase have been reported (rare). Monitor liver function tests periodically during treatment. Renal failure, progressive azotemia, and decreased kidney size have been reported in patients who have received large cumulative doses or prolonged treatment. Renal toxicity has also been reported in patients who have received lower cumulative doses. Monitor renal function tests periodically during treatment.

Carmustine is associated with a moderate to high emetic potential (dose-related); antiemetics are recommended to prevent nausea and vomiting (Basch, 2011; Dupuis, 2011). Injection site burning and local tissue reactions, including swelling, pain, erythema, and necrosis have been reported. Monitor infusion site closely for infiltration or injection site reactions. Off-label administration (intra-arterial intracarotid route) has been associated with ocular toxicity. Consider initiating IV treatment at the lower end of the dose range in elderly patients. The diluent for IV carmustine contains ethanol.

Wafer implant:

Seizures occurred in patients who received carmustine wafer implants, including new or worsening seizures and treatment-emergent seizures. Just over half of treatment-emergent seizures occurred within 5 days of surgery; the median onset of first new or worsened post-operative seizure was 4 days. Optimal anti-seizure therapy should be initiated prior to surgery. Monitor for seizures. Brain edema has been reported in patients with newly diagnosed glioma, including one report of intracranial mass effect unresponsive to corticosteroids which led to brain herniation. Monitor closely for intracranial hypertension related to brain edema, inflammation, or necrosis of brain tissue surrounding resection. Re-operation to remove wafers (or remnants) may be necessary for refractory cases. Cases of meningitis have occurred in patients with recurrent glioma receiving wafer implants. Two cases were bacterial (one patient required removal of implants 4 days after implantation and the other developed meningitis following reoperation for recurrent tumor). Another case was determined to be chemical meningitis and resolved with corticosteroids. Monitor postoperatively for signs/symptoms of meningitis and CNS infection.

Monitor closely for known craniotomy-related complications (seizure, intracranial infection, abnormal wound healing, brain edema). Wafer migration may occur; avoid communication between the resection cavity and the ventricular system to prevent wafer migration; communications larger than the wafer should be closed prior to implantation; wafer migration into the ventricular system may cause obstructive hydrocephalus. Monitor for signs/symptoms of obstructive hydrocephalus.

Impaired neurosurgical wound healing, including would dehiscence, delayed healing, and subdural, subgleal or wound effusions may occur with carmustine wafer implant treatment; cerebrospinal fluid leaks have also been reported. Monitor post-operatively for impaired neurosurgical wound healing.

[US Boxed Warning]: Should be administered under the supervision of an experienced cancer chemotherapy physician. Potentially significant drug-drug interactions may exist, requiring dose or frequency adjustment, additional monitoring, and/or selection of alternative therapy.

Adverse Reactions

IV:

Cardiovascular: Arrhythmia (with high doses), chest pain, flushing (with rapid infusion), hypotension, tachycardia

Central nervous system: Ataxia, dizziness

Central nervous system: Ethanol intoxication (with high doses), headache

Dermatologic: Hyperpigmentation/skin burning (after skin contact)

Gastrointestinal: Nausea (common; dose related), vomiting (common; dose related), mucositis (with high doses), toxic enterocolitis (with high doses)

Hematologic: Leukopenia (common; onset: 5 to 6 weeks; recovery: After 1 to 2 weeks), thrombocytopenia (common: onset: ~4 weeks; recovery: After 1 to 2 weeks), anemia, neutropenic fever, secondary malignancies (acute leukemia, bone marrow dysplasias)

Hepatic: Alkaline phosphatase increased, bilirubin increased, hepatic sinusoidal obstruction syndrome (SOS; veno-occlusive disease; with high doses), transaminases increased

Local: Injection site reactions (burning, erythema, necrosis, pain, swelling)
Ocular: Conjunctival suffusion (with rapid infusion), neuroretinitis
Renal: Kidney size decreased, progressive azotemia, renal failure
Respiratory: Interstitial pneumonitis (with high doses), pulmonary fibrosis, pulmonary hypoplasia, pulmonary infiltrates
Miscellaneous: Allergic reaction, infection (with high doses)

Wafer:
Cardiovascular: Chest pain
Central nervous system: Cerebral edema, cerebral hemorrhage, depression, intracranial hypertension, meningitis, seizure
Dermatologic: Skin rash
Gastrointestinal: Abdominal pain, constipation, nausea, vomiting
Genitourinary: Urinary tract infection
Infection: Abscess (local)
Neuromuscular & skeletal: Back pain, weakness
Miscellaneous: Fever, wound healing impairment
Rare but important or life-threatening: Sepsis

Drug Interactions

Metabolism/Transport Effects None known.

Avoid Concomitant Use

Avoid concomitant use of Carmustine with any of the following: BCG; BCG (Intravesical); CloZAPine; Dipyrone; Natalizumab; Pimecrolimus; Tacrolimus (Topical); Tofacitinib; Vaccines (Live)

Increased Effect/Toxicity

Carmustine may increase the levels/effects of: CloZAPine; Leflunomide; Natalizumab; Tofacitinib; Vaccines (Live)

The levels/effects of Carmustine may be increased by: Cimetidine; Denosumab; Dipyrone; Melphalan; Pimecrolimus; Roflumilast; Tacrolimus (Topical); Trastuzumab

Decreased Effect

Carmustine may decrease the levels/effects of: BCG; BCG (Intravesical); Coccidioides immitis Skin Test; Sipuleucel-T; Vaccines (Inactivated); Vaccines (Live)

The levels/effects of Carmustine may be decreased by: Echinacea

Storage/Stability

Injection: Store intact vials and provided diluent under refrigeration at 2°C to 8°C (36°F to 46°F). Carmustine has a low melting point (30.5°C to 32°C [86.9°F to 89.6°F]); exposure to temperature at or above the melting point will cause the drug to liquefy and appear as an oil film on the vials. If drug liquefies, discard the vials as this is a sign of decomposition.

Reconstituted solutions are stable for 24 hours refrigerated (2°C to 8°C) and protected from light. Examine reconstituted vials for crystal formation prior to use. If crystals are observed, they may be redissolved by warming the vial to room temperature with agitation.

Solutions diluted to a concentration of 0.2 mg/mL in D_5W are stable for 8 hours at room temperature (25°C) in glass and protected from light. Although the manufacturer recommends only glass containers be used, stability of a 1 mg/mL solution in D_5W has also been demonstrated for up to 6 hours (with a 6% to 7% loss of potency) in polyolefin containers (Trissel, 2006).

Wafer: Store at or below -20°C (-4°F). Unopened outer foil pouches may be kept at room temperature for up to 6 hours at a time for up to 3 cycles within a 30-day period.

Mechanism of Action Interferes with the normal function of DNA and RNA by alkylation and cross-linking the strands of DNA and RNA, and by possible protein modification; may also inhibit enzyme processes by carbamylation of amino acids in protein

Pharmacokinetics (Adult data unless noted)

Distribution: 3.3 L/kg; readily crosses the blood-brain barrier since it is highly lipid soluble; CSF:plasma ratio >50%
Metabolism: Hepatic; rapid; forms active metabolites
Half-life: Biphasic: Initial: 1.4 minutes; Secondary: 20 minutes (active metabolites: plasma half-life of 67 hours)
Elimination: ~60% to 70% excreted as metabolites in the urine within 96 hours and 6% to 10% excreted as CO_2 by the lungs

Dosing: Usual

Pediatric: **Note:** Children are at increased risk for pulmonary toxicity due to carmustine, weigh risk vs benefit before use. Refer to individual protocols; dosing and frequency may vary.

Brain tumors, Myeloablative therapy prior to autologous stem cell rescue: Very limited data available; Infants, Children, and Adolescents: IV: 100 mg/m^2/dose twice daily for 3 days (total: 600 mg/m^2) as part of a high dose combination chemotherapy regimen is most commonly reported in trials with mixed results (Dunkel,1998, Finlay 2008); however, a phase I trial identified a lower dose of 100 mg/m^2 once daily for 3 days (total: 300 mg/m^2) in combination with thiotepa as the maximum tolerated regimen with a high degree of pulmonary toxicity observed (Gilman 2011).

Adult: **Note:** Utilize patient's actual body weight (full weight) for calculation of body surface area- or weight-based dosing, particularly when the intent of therapy is curative; manage regimen-related toxicities in the same manner as for nonobese patients; if a dose reduction is utilized due to toxicity, consider resumption of full weight-based dosing with subsequent cycles, especially if cause of toxicity (eg, hepatic or renal impairment) is resolved (Griggs, 2012).

Brain tumors, Hodgkin lymphoma, multiple myeloma, non-Hodgkin lymphoma:IV: 150 to 200 mg/m^2 every 6 weeks or 75 to 100 mg/m^2/day for 2 days every 6 weeks

Glioblastoma multiforme (recurrent), newly-diagnosed high-grade malignant glioma: Implantation (wafer): 8 wafers placed in the resection cavity (total dose: 61.6 mg); should the size and shape not accommodate 8 wafers, the maximum number of wafers allowed (up to 8) should be placed

Dosing adjustment in renal impairment: Adults: IV: The FDA-approved labeling does not contain renal dosing adjustment guidelines. The following dosage adjustments have been used by some clinicians (Kintzel, 1995):
CrCl 46 to 60 mL/minute: Administer 80% of dose
CrCl 31 to 45 mL/minute: Administer 75% of dose
CrCl ≤30 mL/minute: Consider use of alternative drug

Dosing adjustment in hepatic impairment: Dosage adjustment may be necessary; however, no specific guidelines are available.

Preparation for Administration Hazardous agent; use appropriate precautions for handling and disposal (NIOSH 2014 [group 1]).

Parenteral: Reconstitute initially with 3 mL of supplied diluent (dehydrated alcohol injection, USP); then further dilute with 27 mL SWFI, this provides a concentration of 3.3 mg/mL in ethanol 10%; protect from light. Carmustine should be prepared in either glass or polyolefin containers due to significant absorption to PVC containers.

Administration Hazardous agent; use appropriate precautions for handling and disposal (NIOSH 2014 [group 1]).

Parenteral: Infuse over 2 hours (infusions <2 hours may lead to injection site pain or burning); infuse through a free-flowing saline or dextrose infusion, or administer through a central catheter to alleviate venous pain/irritation. Significant absorption to PVC containers; should be prepared in either glass or polyolefin containers.

High-dose carmustine (transplant dose): Infuse over a least 2 hours to avoid excessive flushing, agitation, and hypotension; was infused over 1 hour in some trials (Chopra 1993). High-dose carmustine may be fatal if not followed by stem cell rescue. Monitor vital signs frequently during infusion; patients should be supine during infusion and may require the Trendelenburg position, fluid support, and vasopressor support.

Wafer: Double glove before handling; outer gloves should be discarded as chemotherapy waste after handling wafers. Any wafer or remnant that is removed upon repeat surgery should be discarded as chemotherapy waste. The outer surface of the external foil pouch is not sterile. Open pouch gently; avoid pressure on the wafers to prevent breakage. Wafer that are broken in half may be used, however, wafers broken into more than 2 pieces should be discarded in a biohazard container. Oxidized regenerated cellulose (Surgicel) may be placed over the wafer to secure; irrigate cavity prior to closure.

Vesicant/Extravasation Risk Irritant; infiltration may result in local pain, erythema, swelling, burning and skin necrosis; the alcohol-based diluent may be an irritant, especially with high doses.

Monitoring Parameters CBC with differential and platelet count (weekly for at least 6 weeks after a dose), pulmonary function tests (FVC, DLCO; at baseline and frequently during treatment), liver function (periodically), renal function tests (periodically); monitor blood pressure and vital signs during administration, monitor infusion site for possible infiltration

Wafer: Complications of craniotomy (seizures, intracranial infection, brain edema)

Dosage Forms Excipient information presented when available (limited, particularly for generics); consult specific product labeling.

Solution Reconstituted, Intravenous:

BiCNU: 100 mg (1 ea) [contains alcohol, usp]

Wafer, Implant:

Gliadel Wafer: 7.7 mg (8 ea) [contains polifeprosan 20]

- **Carmustine Polymer Wafer** *see* Carmustine *on page 377*
- **Carmustine Sustained-Release Implant Wafer** *see* Carmustine *on page 377*
- **Carmustinum** *see* Carmustine *on page 377*
- **Carnitine** *see* LevOCARNitine *on page 1239*
- **Carnitor** *see* LevOCARNitine *on page 1239*
- **Carnitor SF** *see* LevOCARNitine *on page 1239*
- **Carrington Antifungal [OTC]** *see* Miconazole (Topical) *on page 1431*
- **Carter's Little Pills [OTC] (Can)** *see* Bisacodyl *on page 289*
- **Cartia XT** *see* Diltiazem *on page 661*

Carvedilol (KAR ve dil ole)

Medication Safety Issues

Sound-alike/look-alike issues:

Carvedilol may be confused with atenolol, captopril, carbidopa, carteolol

Coreg may be confused with Corgard, Cortef, Cozaar

Related Information

Oral Medications That Should Not Be Crushed or Altered *on page 2476*

Brand Names: US Coreg; Coreg CR

Brand Names: Canada Apo-Carvedilol; Auro-Carvedilol; Dom-Carvedilol; JAMP-Carvedilol; Mylan-Carvedilol; Novo-Carvedilol; PMS-Carvedilol; RAN-Carvedilol; ratio-Carvedilol

Therapeutic Category Antihypertensive Agent; Beta-Adrenergic Blocker, Nonselective With Alpha-Blocking Activity

Generic Availability (US) May be product dependent

Use Treatment of mild to severe chronic heart failure of cardiomyopathic or ischemic origin (usually in addition to standard therapy) (FDA approved in ages ≥18 years and adults); management of hypertension, alone or in combination with other agents (FDA approved in ages ≥18 years and adults); reduction of cardiovascular mortality in patients with left ventricular dysfunction following MI (FDA approved in ages ≥18 years and adults)

Pregnancy Risk Factor C

Pregnancy Considerations Adverse events have been observed in animal reproduction studies. In a cohort study, an increased risk of cardiovascular defects was observed following maternal use of beta-blockers during pregnancy (Lennestål, 2009). Intrauterine growth restriction (IUGR), small placentas, as well as fetal/neonatal bradycardia, hypoglycemia, and/or respiratory depression have been observed following *in utero* exposure to beta-blockers as a class. Adequate facilities for monitoring infants at birth should be available. Untreated chronic maternal hypertension and pre-eclampsia are also associated with adverse events in the fetus, infant, and mother. Carvedilol is not currently recommended for the initial treatment of maternal hypertension during pregnancy (ACOG, 2001; ACOG, 2002).

Breast-Feeding Considerations It is not known if carvedilol is excreted in breast milk. Due to the potential for serious adverse reactions in the nursing infant, the manufacturer recommends a decision be made whether to discontinue nursing or to discontinue the drug, taking into account the importance of treatment to the mother.

Contraindications

Serious hypersensitivity to carvedilol or any component of the formulation; decompensated cardiac failure requiring intravenous inotropic therapy; bronchial asthma or related bronchospastic conditions; second- or third-degree AV block, sick sinus syndrome, and severe bradycardia (except in patients with a functioning artificial pacemaker); cardiogenic shock; severe hepatic impairment

Documentation of allergenic cross-reactivity for drugs alpha/beta adrenergic blocking agents is limited. However, because of similarities in chemical structure and/or pharmacologic actions, the possibility of cross-sensitivity cannot be ruled out with certainty.

Warnings/Precautions Heart failure patients may experience a worsening of renal function (rare); risk factors include ischemic heart disease, diffuse vascular disease, underlying renal dysfunction, and/or systolic BP <100 mm Hg. Initiate cautiously and monitor for possible deterioration in patient status (eg, symptoms of HF). Worsening heart failure or fluid retention may occur during upward titration; dose reduction or temporary discontinuation may be necessary. Adjustment of other medications (ACE inhibitors and/or diuretics) may also be required. Bradycardia may occur; reduce dosage if heart rate drops to <55 beats/minute. Bradycardia may be observed more frequently in elderly patients (>65 years of age); dosage reductions may be necessary.

Symptomatic hypotension with or without syncope may occur with carvedilol (usually within the first 30 days of therapy); close monitoring of patient is required especially with initial dosing and dosing increases; blood pressure must be lowered at a rate appropriate for the patient's clinical condition. Initiation with a low dose, gradual up-titration, and administration with food may help to decrease the occurrence of hypotension or syncope. Advise patients to avoid driving or other hazardous tasks during initiation of therapy due to the risk of syncope. Beta-blocker therapy should not be withdrawn abruptly (particularly in patients with CAD), but gradually tapered to avoid acute tachycardia, hypertension, and/or ischemia. Chronic beta-blocker therapy should not be routinely withdrawn prior to major surgery.

In general, patients with bronchospastic disease should not receive beta-blockers; if used at all, should be used cautiously with close monitoring. May precipitate or aggravate symptoms of arterial insufficiency in patients with PVD; use with caution and monitor for progression of arterial obstruction. Use with caution in patients with diabetes; may potentiate hypoglycemia and/or mask signs and symptoms (eg, sweating, anxiety, tachycardia). In patients with heart failure and diabetes, use of carvedilol may worsen hyperglycemia; may require adjustment of antidiabetic agents. May mask signs of hyperthyroidism (eg, tachycardia); if hyperthyroidism is suspected, carefully manage and monitor; abrupt withdrawal may exacerbate symptoms of hyperthyroidism or precipitate thyroid storm. May induce or exacerbate psoriasis. Use with caution in patients suspected of having Prinzmetal variant angina. Use with caution in patients with myasthenia gravis. Use with caution in patients with mild to moderate hepatic impairment; use is contraindicated in patients with severe impairment. Use with caution in patients with pheochromocytoma; adequate alpha-blockade is required prior to use. Use caution with history of severe anaphylaxis to allergens; patients taking beta-blockers may become more sensitive to repeated challenges. Treatment of anaphylaxis (eg, epinephrine) in patients taking beta-blockers may be ineffective or promote undesirable effects.

Intraoperative floppy iris syndrome has been observed in cataract surgery patients who were on or were previously treated with alpha$_1$-blockers; there appears to be no benefit in discontinuing alpha-blocker therapy prior to surgery. Instruct patients to inform ophthalmologist of carvedilol use when considering eye surgery. Potentially significant interactions may exist, requiring dose or frequency adjustment, additional monitoring, and/or selection of alternative therapy.

Some dosage forms may contain polysorbate 80 (also known as Tweens). Hypersensitivity reactions, usually a delayed reaction, have been reported following exposure to pharmaceutical products containing polysorbate 80 in certain individuals (Isaksson, 2002; Lucente 2000; Shelley, 1995). Thrombocytopenia, ascites, pulmonary deterioration, and renal and hepatic failure have been reported in premature neonates after receiving parenteral products containing polysorbate 80 (Alade, 1986; CDC, 1984). See manufacturer's labeling.

Adverse Reactions

Cardiovascular: Angina, AV block, bradycardia, cerebrovascular accident, edema (including generalized, dependent, and peripheral), hyper-/hypotension, hyper-/hypovolemia, orthostatic hypotension, palpitation, syncope

Central nervous system: Depression, dizziness, fatigue, fever, headache, hypoesthesia, hypotonia, insomnia, malaise, somnolence, vertigo, weakness

Endocrine & metabolic: Diabetes mellitus, gout, hypercholesterolemia, hyper-/hypoglycemia, hyponatremia, hyperkalemia, hypertriglyceridemia, hyperuricemia

Gastrointestinal: Abdominal pain, diarrhea, melena, nausea, periodontitis, vomiting, weight gain/loss

Genitourinary: Impotence

Hematologic: Anemia, prothrombin decreased, purpura, thrombocytopenia

Hepatic: Alkaline phosphatase increased, GGT increased, transaminases increased

Neuromuscular & skeletal: Arthralgia, arthritis, back pain, muscle cramps, paresthesia

Ocular: Blurred vision

Renal: Albuminuria, BUN increased, creatinine increased, glycosuria, hematuria, nonprotein nitrogen increased, renal insufficiency

Respiratory: Cough, dyspnea, nasopharyngitis, dyspnea, nasal congestion, pulmonary edema, rales, rhinitis, sinus congestion

Miscellaneous: Allergy, flu-like syndrome, injury, sudden death

Rare but important or life-threatening: Anaphylactoid reaction, alopecia, angioedema, aplastic anemia, amnesia, asthma, bronchospasm, bundle branch block, cholestatic jaundice, concentration decreased, diaphoresis, erythema multiforme, exfoliative dermatitis, GI hemorrhage, HDL decreased, hearing decreased, hyperbilirubinemia, hypersensitivity reaction, hypokalemia, hypokinesia, interstitial pneumonitis, leukopenia, libido decreased, migraine, myocardial ischemia, nervousness, neuralgia, nightmares, pancytopenia, paresis, peripheral ischemia, photosensitivity, pruritus, rash (erythematous, maculopapular, and psoriaform), respiratory alkalosis, seizure, Stevens-Johnson syndrome, tachycardia, tinnitus, toxic epidermal necrolysis, urinary incontinence, urticaria, xerostomia

Drug Interactions

Metabolism/Transport Effects Substrate of CYP1A2 (minor), CYP2C9 (minor), CYP2D6 (major), CYP2E1 (minor), CYP3A4 (minor), P-glycoprotein; **Note:** Assignment of Major/Minor substrate status based on clinically relevant drug interaction potential; **Inhibits** P-glycoprotein

Avoid Concomitant Use

Avoid concomitant use of Carvedilol with any of the following: Beta2-Agonists; Bosutinib; Ceritinib; Floctafenine; Methacholine; PAZOPanib; Rivastigmine; Silodosin; Topotecan; VinCRIStine (Liposomal)

Increased Effect/Toxicity

Carvedilol may increase the levels/effects of: Afatinib; Alpha-/Beta-Agonists (Direct-Acting); Alpha1-Blockers; Alpha2-Agonists; Amifostine; Antihypertensives; Antipsychotic Agents (Phenothiazines); Bosutinib; Bradycardia-Causing Agents; Brentuximab Vedotin; Bupivacaine; Cardiac Glycosides; Ceritinib; Cholinergic Agonists; Colchicine; CycloSPORINE (Systemic); Dabigatran Etexilate; Digoxin; Disopyramide; DOXOrubicin (Conventional); DULoxetine; Edoxaban; Ergot Derivatives; Everolimus; Fingolimod; Grass Pollen Allergen Extract (5 Grass Extract); Hypotensive Agents; Insulin; Ivabradine; Lacosamide; Ledipasvir; Levodopa; Lidocaine (Systemic); Lidocaine (Topical); Mepivacaine; Methacholine; Midodrine; Naloxegol; Obinutuzumab; PAZOPanib; P-glycoprotein/ABCB1 Substrates; Prucalopride; Rifaximin; RisperiDONE; RiTUXimab; Rivaroxaban; Silodosin; Sulfonylureas; Topotecan; VinCRIStine (Liposomal)

The levels/effects of Carvedilol may be increased by: Abiraterone Acetate; Acetylcholinesterase Inhibitors; Alpha2-Agonists; Aminoquinolines (Antimalarial); Amiodarone; Anilidopiperidine Opioids; Antipsychotic Agents (Phenothiazines); Barbiturates; Bretylium; Brimonidine (Topical); Calcium Channel Blockers (Nondihydropyridine); Cimetidine; Cobicistat; CYP2C9 Inhibitors (Moderate); CYP2C9 Inhibitors (Strong); CYP2D6 Inhibitors (Moderate); CYP2D6 Inhibitors (Strong); Darunavir;

Diazoxide; Digoxin; Dipyridamole; Disopyramide; Dronedarone; Floctafenine; Herbs (Hypotensive Properties); MAO Inhibitors; NiCARdipine; Nicorandil; NIFEdipine; Panobinostat; Peginterferon Alfa-2b; Pentoxifylline; P-glycoprotein/ABCB1 Inhibitors; Phosphodiesterase 5 Inhibitors; Propafenone; Prostacyclin Analogues; Regorafenib; Reserpine; Rivastigmine; Ruxolitinib; Selective Serotonin Reuptake Inhibitors; Tofacitinib

Decreased Effect

Carvedilol may decrease the levels/effects of: Beta2-Agonists; Theophylline Derivatives

The levels/effects of Carvedilol may be decreased by: Barbiturates; Herbs (Hypertensive Properties); Methylphenidate; Nonsteroidal Anti-Inflammatory Agents; Peginterferon Alfa-2b; P-glycoprotein/ABCB1 Inducers; Rifamycin Derivatives; Yohimbine

Food Interactions Food decreases rate but not extent of absorption. Management: Administration with food minimizes risks of orthostatic hypotension.

Storage/Stability

Coreg: Store at <30°C (<86°F). Protect from moisture.

Coreg CR: Store at 25°C (77°F); excursions permitted to 15°C to 30°C (59°F to 86°F). Protect from light.

Mechanism of Action As a racemic mixture, carvedilol has nonselective beta-adrenoreceptor and alpha-adrenergic blocking activity. No intrinsic sympathomimetic activity has been documented. Associated effects in hypertensive patients include reduction of cardiac output, exercise- or beta-agonist-induced tachycardia, reduction of reflex orthostatic tachycardia, vasodilation, decreased peripheral vascular resistance (especially in standing position), decreased renal vascular resistance, reduced plasma renin activity, and increased levels of atrial natriuretic peptide. In CHF, associated effects include decreased pulmonary capillary wedge pressure, decreased pulmonary artery pressure, decreased heart rate, decreased systemic vascular resistance, increased stroke volume index, and decreased right arterial pressure (RAP).

Pharmacodynamics Oral:

Onset of action:

Alpha-blockade: Within 30 minutes

Beta-blockade: Within 1 hour

Maximum effect: Antihypertensive effect: ~1-2 hours

Pharmacokinetics (Adult data unless noted)

Absorption: Oral: Rapid and extensive, but with large first pass effect; first pass effect is stereoselective with R(+) enantiomer achieving plasma concentrations 2-3 times higher than S(-) enantiomer

Distribution: V_d: 115 L; distributes into extravascular tissues

Protein binding: >98%, primarily to albumin

Metabolism: Extensively (98%) hepatic primarily via CYP2D6 and 2C9 and to a lesser extent CYP3A4, 2C19, and 2E1; metabolized predominantly by aromatic ring oxidation and glucuronidation; oxidative metabolites undergo conjugation via glucuronidation and sulfation; three active metabolites (4′-hydroxyphenyl metabolite is 13 times more potent than parent drug for beta-blockade; however, active metabolites achieve plasma concentrations of only 1/10 of those for carvedilol). Metabolism is subject to genetic polymorphism; CYP2D6 poor metabolizers have a 2-3 fold higher plasma concentration of the R(+) enantiomer and a 20% to 25% increase in the S(-) enantiomer compared to extensive metabolizers.

Bioavailability: Immediate release tablets: 25% to 35%; extended release capsules: 85% of immediate release; bioavailability is increased in patients with CHF

Half-life:

Infants and Children 6 weeks to 3.5 years (n=8): 2.2 hours (Laer, 2002)

Children and Adolescents 5.5-19 years (n=7): 3.6 hours (Laer, 2002)

Adults 7-10 hours; some have reported lower values:

Adults 24-37 years (n=9): 5.2 hours (Laer, 2002)

R(+)-carvedilol: 5-9 hours

S(-)-carvedilol: 7-11 hours

Time to peak serum concentration: Extended release capsules: 5 hours

Elimination: <2% excreted unchanged in urine; metabolites are excreted via bile, into the feces

Dialysis: Hemodialysis does not significantly clear carvedilol

Dosing: Usual Note: Immediate release and extended release products are not interchangeable on a mg:mg basis due to pharmacokinetic differences. Individualize dosage for each patient; monitor patients closely during initiation and upwards titration of dose; reduce dosage if bradycardia or hypotension occurs

Infants, Children, and Adolescents: **Note:** Pharmacokinetic data suggests a faster carvedilol elimination in young pediatric patients (< 3.5 years) which may require more frequent dosing (3 times daily) and a higher target dose per kg (Laer, 2002; Shaddy, 2007).

Heart Failure: Limited data available, efficacy results variable; optimal dose not established: Oral: Immediate release tablets: Initial: Reported mean: 0.075-0.08 mg/kg/dose twice daily; titrate as tolerated; may increase dose by typically 50% every 2 weeks; usual reported maintenance (target) dose range: 0.3-0.75 mg/kg/dose twice daily; the usual titration time to reach target dose was 11-14 weeks (Bruns, 2001; Rusconi, 2004); maximum daily dose: 50 mg/**day**. Dosing based on two retrospective analyses of a total 70 pediatric patients (age range: 3 months to 19 years) which showed improvement in left ventricular function and heart failure symptoms (67% to 68% of patients showed improvement in NYHA class). However, in a large, a multicenter, double-blind, placebo-controlled, dose-finding trial in 161 pediatric patients (treatment group: n=103, median age range: 33-43 months), a lower target dose range of 0.2-0.4 mg/kg/dose twice daily did not result in a statistical difference in composite clinical end point scores compared to placebo; the authors suggested multiple factors for negative efficacy findings including that the study may have been underpowered due to unexpected, high improvement of the placebo-arm; a subset analysis suggests ventricular morphology may play a role in efficacy (Shaddy, 2007).

Adolescents ≥18 years and Adults: **Note:** Reduce dosage if heart rate drops to <55 beats/minute.

Heart Failure: Note: Prior to initiating therapy, other CHF medications should be stabilized and fluid retention minimized.

Immediate release tablets: Oral: Initial: 3.125 mg twice daily for 2 weeks; if tolerated, may increase to 6.25 mg twice daily. May double the dose every 2 weeks to the highest dose tolerated by patient.

Maximum recommended dose:

Mild to moderate heart failure:

<85 kg: 25 mg twice daily

>85 kg: 50 mg twice daily

Severe heart failure: 25 mg twice daily

Extended release capsules: Oral: Initial: 10 mg once daily for 2 weeks; if tolerated, may double the dose (eg, 20 mg, 40 mg) every 2 weeks up to 80 mg once daily; maintain on lower dose if higher dose is not tolerated

Hypertension:

Immediate release tablets: Oral: Initial: 6.25 mg twice daily; if tolerated, dose should be maintained for 1-2 weeks, then increased to 12.5 mg twice daily; maximum daily dose: 50 mg/**day**

Extended release capsules: Oral: Initial: 20 mg once daily; if tolerated, dose should be maintained for 1-2 weeks, then increased to 40 mg once daily if necessary; maximum daily dose: 80 mg/**day**

Left ventricular dysfunction following MI: Note: Initiate only after patient is hemodynamically stable and fluid retention has been minimized.

Immediate release tablets: Oral: Initial: 3.125-6.25 mg twice daily; increase dosage incrementally (eg, from 6.25 to 12.5 mg twice daily) at intervals of 3-10 days, as tolerated, to a target dose of 25 mg twice daily

Extended release capsules: Oral: Initial: 10-20 mg once daily; increase dosage incrementally at intervals of 3-10 days, as tolerated, to a target dose of 80 mg once daily

Conversion from immediate release to extended release (Coreg CR®):

Current dose immediate release tablets 3.125 mg twice daily: Convert to extended release capsules 10 mg once daily

Current dose immediate release tablets 6.25 mg twice daily: Convert to extended release capsules 20 mg once daily

Current dose immediate release tablets 12.5 mg twice daily: Convert to extended release capsules 40 mg once daily

Current dose immediate release tablets 25 mg twice daily: Convert to extended release capsules 80 mg once daily

Dosing adjustment in renal impairment: No adjustment required. **Note:** Mean AUCs were 40% to 50% higher in patients with moderate to severe renal dysfunction who received immediate release carvedilol, but the ranges of AUCs were similar to patients with normal renal function

Dosing adjustment in hepatic impairment:

Mild to moderate impairment (Child-Pugh class A or B): There are no dosage adjustments provided in manufacturer's labeling; use with caution; monitor for symptoms of drug-induced toxicity.

Severe impairment (Child-Pugh class C): Use is contraindicated as drug is extensively metabolized by the liver. **Note:** Patients with severe cirrhotic liver disease achieved carvedilol serum concentrations four- to sevenfold higher than normal patients following a single dose of immediate release carvedilol

Administration

Immediate release tablets: Administer with food to decrease the risk of orthostatic hypotension.

Extended release capsules: Administer with food, preferably in the morning; do not crush or chew capsule; swallow whole; do not take in divided doses. Capsule may be opened and contents sprinkled on a spoonful of applesauce; swallow applesauce/medication mixture immediately; do not chew; do not store for later use; do not use warm applesauce; do not sprinkle capsule contents on food other than applesauce; drink fluids after dose to make sure mixture is completely swallowed.

Monitoring Parameters Heart rate, blood pressure (determine need for dosage increase based on trough blood pressure measurements and tolerance on standing systolic pressure 1 hour after dosing), weight; S_{Cr}, BUN, liver function; in patient with increased risk for developing renal dysfunction, monitor renal function during dosage titration

Additional Information CHF: Carvedilol is a nonselective beta blocker with alpha-blocking and antioxidant properties. It is the only beta blocker approved in adults for the treatment of heart failure. Beta blocker therapy, without intrinsic sympathomimetic activity, should be initiated in adult patients with **stable** CHF (NYHA Class II-IV). To date, carvedilol, sustained release metoprolol, and bisoprolol have demonstrated a beneficial effect on morbidity and mortality. It is important that beta blocker therapy be instituted initially at very low doses with gradual and very careful titration. Because carvedilol has alpha-adrenergic blocking effects, it may lower blood pressure to a greater extent. The definitive clinical benefits of the antioxidant property are not known at this time.

Coreg CR® extended release capsules are hard gelatin capsules filled with immediate-release and controlled-release microparticles containing carvedilol phosphate; the microparticles are drug-layered and coated with methacrylic acid copolymers.

Dosage Forms Excipient information presented when available (limited, particularly for generics); consult specific product labeling.

Capsule Extended Release 24 Hour, Oral, as phosphate:
Coreg CR: 10 mg, 20 mg, 40 mg, 80 mg

Tablet, Oral:
Coreg: 3.125 mg, 6.25 mg, 12.5 mg, 25 mg
Generic: 3.125 mg, 6.25 mg, 12.5 mg, 25 mg

Extemporaneous Preparations A 1.25 mg/mL carvedilol oral suspension may be made with tablets and one of two different vehicles (Ora-Blend or 1:1 mixture of Ora-Sweet and Ora-Plus). Crush five 25 mg tablets in a mortar and reduce to a fine powder; add 15 mL of purified water and mix to a uniform paste. Mix while adding chosen vehicle in incremental proportions to almost 100 mL; transfer to a calibrated amber bottle, rinse mortar with vehicle, and add quantity of vehicle sufficient to make 100 mL. Label "shake well". Stable for 84 days when stored in amber prescription bottles at room temperature (Loyd, 2006).

Carvedilol oral liquid suspensions (0.1 mg/mL and 1.67 mg/mL) made from tablets, water, Ora-Plus, and Ora-Sweet were stable for 12 weeks when stored in glass amber bottles at room temperature (25°C). Use one 3.125 mg tablet for the 0.1 mg/mL suspension or two 25 mg tablets for the 1.67 mg/mL suspension; grind the tablet(s) and compound a mixture with 5 mL of water, 15 mL Ora-Plus, and 10 mL Ora-Sweet. Final volume of each suspension: 30 mL; label "shake well" (data on file, GlaxoSmithKline, Philadelphia, PA: DOF #132 [**Note:** Manufacturer no longer disseminates this document]).

Loyd A Jr, "Carvedilol 1.25 mg/mL Oral Suspension," *Int J Pharm Compounding*, 2006, 10(3):220.

Caspofungin (kas poe FUN jin)

Brand Names: US Cancidas

Brand Names: Canada Cancidas®

Therapeutic Category Antifungal Agent, Echinocandin; Antifungal Agent, Systemic

Generic Availability (US) No

Use Treatment of invasive aspergillosis in patients who are refractory to or intolerant of other therapies (ie, amphotericin B, lipid formulations of amphotericin B, and/or itraconazole); candidemia, intra-abdominal abscess, peritonitis, and pleural space infection caused by susceptible *Candida* species; esophageal candidiasis; empiric therapy of presumed fungal infection in febrile neutropenic patients (FDA approved in ages ≥3 months and adults)

Pregnancy Risk Factor C

Pregnancy Considerations Adverse events have been observed in animal reproduction studies. When treatment of invasive *Aspergillus* or *Candida* infections is needed during pregnancy, other agents are preferred (DHHS [adult] 2014; Pappas 2009). Use may be considered in HIV-infected pregnant women with invasive *Aspergillus* or *Candida* infections when refractory to other agents (DHHS [adult] 2014)

Breast-Feeding Considerations It is not known if caspofungin is excreted in breast milk. The manufacturer recommends that caution be exercised when administering caspofungin to nursing women.

Contraindications Hypersensitivity to caspofungin or any component of the formulation

Warnings/Precautions Anaphylaxis and histamine-related reactions (eg, angioedema, facial swelling, bronchospasm, rash, sensation of warmth) have been reported. Discontinue if anaphylaxis occurs; consider discontinuation if histamine-related reactions occur. Administer supportive treatment if needed. Concurrent use of cyclosporine should be limited to patients for whom benefit outweighs risk, due to a high frequency of hepatic transaminase elevations observed during concurrent use. Potentially significant drug-drug interactions may exist, requiring dose or frequency adjustment, additional monitoring, and/or selection of alternative therapy. Use caution in hepatic impairment; increased transaminases and rare cases of liver impairment (including failure and hepatitis) have been reported in pediatric and adult patients. Monitor liver function tests during therapy; if tests become abnormal or worsen, consider discontinuation. Dosage reduction required in adults with moderate hepatic impairment; safety and efficacy have not been established in children with any degree of hepatic impairment and adults with severe hepatic impairment.

Adverse Reactions

Cardiovascular: Hypertension, hypotension, peripheral edema, tachycardia

Central nervous system: Chills, headache

Dermatologic: Erythema, pruritus, skin rash

Endocrine & metabolic: Hyperglycemia, hypokalemia, hypomagnesemia

Gastrointestinal: Abdominal pain, diarrhea, gastric irritation, nausea, vomiting

Hematologic & oncologic: Anemia, decreased hematocrit, decreased hemoglobin, decreased white blood cell count

Hepatic: Decreased serum albumin, increased serum alkaline phosphatase increased, increased serum ALT, increased serum AST, increased serum bilirubin

Immunologic: Graft versus host disease (infants, children, and adolescents

Infection: Sepsis

Local: Catheter infection, localized phlebitis

Renal: Hematuria, increased blood urea nitrogen, increased serum creatinine

Respiratory: Cough, dyspnea, pleural effusion, pneumonia, rales, respiratory distress, respiratory failure

Miscellaneous: Fever, infusion related reaction, septic shock

Rare but important or life-threatening: Abdominal distention, adult respiratory distress syndrome, anaphylaxis, anorexia, anxiety, arthralgia, atrial fibrillation, back pain, bacteremia, blood coagulation disorder, cardiac arrest, confusion, constipation, decreased appetite, decubitus ulcer, depression, dizziness, drowsiness, dyspepsia, dystonia, edema, epistaxis, erythema multiforme, fatigue, febrile neutropenia, flushing, hepatic failure, hepatitis, hepatomegaly, hepatotoxicity, histamine release (including facial swelling, bronchospasm, sensation of warmth), hypercalcemia, hyperkalemia, hypervolemia, hypoxia, increased gamma-glutamyl transferase, infusion site reaction (pain/pruritus/swelling), insomnia, limb pain, myocardial infarction, nephrotoxicity (serum creatinine ≥2 x baseline value or ≥1 mg/dL in patients with serum creatinine above ULN range), pancreatitis, pulmonary edema, pulmonary infiltrates, renal failure, seizure, Stevens-Johnson syndrome, tachypnea, thrombocytopenia, tremor, urinary tract infection, urticaria, weakness

Drug Interactions

Metabolism/Transport Effects None known.

Avoid Concomitant Use

Avoid concomitant use of Caspofungin with any of the following: Saccharomyces boulardii

Increased Effect/Toxicity

The levels/effects of Caspofungin may be increased by: CycloSPORINE (Systemic)

Decreased Effect

Caspofungin may decrease the levels/effects of: Saccharomyces boulardii; Tacrolimus (Systemic)

The levels/effects of Caspofungin may be decreased by: Inducers of Drug Clearance; Rifampin

Storage/Stability Store intact vials at 2°C to 8°C (36°F to 46°F). Reconstituted solution may be stored at ≤25°C (≤77°F) for 1 hour prior to preparation of infusion solution. Solutions diluted for infusion should be used within 24 hours when stored at ≤25°C (≤77°F) or within 48 hours when stored at 2°C to 8°C (36°F to 46°F).

Mechanism of Action Inhibits synthesis of β(1,3)-D-glucan, an essential component of the cell wall of susceptible fungi. Highest activity is in regions of active cell growth. Mammalian cells do not require β(1,3)-D-glucan, limiting potential toxicity.

Pharmacokinetics (Adult data unless noted)

Distribution: CSF concentrations: Nondetectable [<10 ng/mL (n=1)] (Sáez-Llorens, 2009)

Protein binding: 97% to albumin

Metabolism: Via hydrolysis and N-acetylation in the liver; undergoes spontaneous chemical degradation to an open-ring peptide and hydrolysis to amino acids

Half-life: Beta (distribution): 9-11 hours (~8 hours in children <12 years); terminal: 40-50 hours; beta phase half-life is 32% to 43% lower in pediatric patients than in adult patients

Elimination: 35% of dose excreted in feces primarily as metabolites; 41% of dose excreted in urine primarily as metabolites; 1.4% of dose excreted unchanged in urine

Dialysis: Not dialyzable

Dosing: Neonatal Note: Caspofungin treatment duration should be based on patient status and clinical response. Empiric therapy should be given until neutropenia resolves. In neutropenic patients, continue treatment for at least 7 days after both signs and symptoms of infection and neutropenia resolve. In patients with positive cultures, continue treatment for at least 14 days after the last positive culture.

IV: 25 mg/m²/dose once daily; dosing based on a pharmacokinetic study of 18 neonates including preterm neonates that showed similar serum concentrations to standard adult doses. Reported trough concentrations were slightly elevated and not correlated with increased adverse events (Sáez-Llorens 2009). Limited data available.

Dosing: Usual IV: **Note:** Caspofungin treatment duration should be based on patient status and clinical response. Empiric therapy should be given until neutropenia resolves. In neutropenic patients, continue treatment for at least 7 days after both signs and symptoms of infection and neutropenia resolve. In patients with positive cultures, continue treatment for at least 14 days after the last positive culture.

Infants 1 to <3 months: 25 mg/m²/dose once daily; dosing based on a pharmacokinetic study of 18 infants that showed similar serum concentrations to standard adult doses (50 mg/day). Reported trough concentrations were slightly elevated and not correlated with increased adverse events (Sáez-Llorens 2009)

Infants and Children 3 months to 17 years: Initial dose: 70 mg/m²/dose on day 1, subsequent dosing: 50 mg/m²/dose once daily; may increase to 70 mg/m²/dose once daily if clinical response inadequate (maximum dose: 70 mg). Patients receiving carbamazepine, dexamethasone, efavirenz, nevirapine, phenytoin, or rifampin (and possibly other enzyme inducers): Consider 70 mg/m²/dose once daily (maximum: 70 mg/day).

Adults: Loading dose: 70 mg on day 1, followed by 50 mg once daily thereafter; 70 mg daily dose has been administered and well tolerated in patients not clinically responding to the daily 50 mg dose; may need to adjust dose in patients receiving a concomitant enzyme inducer. Doses greater than the standard adult dosing regimen (ie, 150 mg once daily) have not demonstrated increased benefit or toxicity in patients with invasive candidiasis (Betts 2009).

Esophageal candidiasis: 50 mg once daily with no loading dose

Patients receiving concomitant enzyme inducer:

Patients receiving rifampin: 70 mg caspofungin once daily

Patients receiving carbamazepine, dexamethasone, phenytoin, nevirapine, or efavirenz: May require an increase in caspofungin dose to 70 mg once daily

Dosing adjustment in renal impairment: No adjustment needed

Dosing adjustment in hepatic impairment (based on adult data):

Mild hepatic impairment (Child-Pugh score 5 to 6): No dosage adjustment necessary

Moderate hepatic impairment (Child-Pugh score 7 to 9): Decrease daily dose by 30%

Preparation for Administration Bring refrigerated vial to room temperature. Reconstitute vials using 10.8 mL NS, SWFI, or bacteriostatic water for injection, resulting in a concentration of 5 mg/mL for the 50 mg vial, and 7 mg/mL for the 70 mg vial (vials contain overfill). Mix gently to dissolve until clear solution is formed; do not use if cloudy or contains particles. Solution should be further diluted with NS, 1/2 NS, 1/4 NS, or LR to a final concentration not to exceed 0.5 mg/mL.

Administration Administer by slow IV infusion over 1 hour (manufacturer); higher doses (eg, 150 mg) have been infused over ~2 hours (Betts 2009). Monitor during infusion; isolated cases of possible histamine-related reactions have occurred during clinical trials (rash, flushing, pruritus, facial edema).

Monitoring Parameters Periodic liver function tests, serum potassium, CBC, hemoglobin

Dosage Forms Excipient information presented when available (limited, particularly for generics); consult specific product labeling.

Solution Reconstituted, Intravenous, as acetate:

Cancidas: 50 mg (1 ea); 70 mg (1 ea)

◆ **Caspofungin Acetate** *see* Caspofungin *on page* *383*

Castor Oil (KAS tor oyl)

Therapeutic Category Laxative, Stimulant

Generic Availability (US) Yes

Use Preparation for rectal or bowel examination or surgery; rarely used to relieve constipation; also applied to skin as emollient and protectant

Pregnancy Considerations Ingestion of castor oil may be associated with induction of labor. Use of castor oil as a laxative during pregnancy should be avoided (Cullen, 2007; Hall, 2011; Wald, 2003).

Warnings/Precautions Do not use for longer than 1 week or when abdominal pain, nausea, vomiting, or rectal bleeding are present unless directed by health care provider.

Adverse Reactions

Cardiovascular: Hypotension

Central nervous system: Dizziness

Endocrine & metabolic: Electrolyte disturbance

Gastrointestinal: Abdominal cramps, diarrhea, nausea

Genitourinary: Pelvic congestion

Drug Interactions

Metabolism/Transport Effects None known.

Avoid Concomitant Use There are no known interactions where it is recommended to avoid concomitant use.

Increased Effect/Toxicity There are no known significant interactions involving an increase in effect.

Decreased Effect There are no known significant interactions involving a decrease in effect.

Storage/Stability Protect from heat.

Mechanism of Action Acts primarily in the small intestine; hydrolyzed to ricinoleic acid which reduces net absorption of fluid and electrolytes and stimulates peristalsis

Pharmacodynamics Onset of action: Oral: Within 2-6 hours

Dosing: Usual Oral:

Castor oil:

Infants <2 years: 1-5 mL or 15 mL/m^2/dose as a single dose

Children 2-11 years: 5-15 mL as a single dose

Children ≥12 years and Adults: 15-60 mL as a single dose

Emulsified castor oil:

Infants: 2.5-7.5 mL/dose

Children:

<2 years: 5-15 mL/dose

2-11 years: 7.5-30 mL/dose

Children ≥12 years and Adults: 30-60 mL/dose

Administration Oral: Do not administer at bedtime because of rapid onset of action; chill or administer with milk, juice, or carbonated beverage to improve palatability; administer on an empty stomach; castor oil emulsions should be shaken well before use

Monitoring Parameters I & O, serum electrolytes, stool frequency

Dosage Forms Excipient information presented when available (limited, particularly for generics); consult specific product labeling. [DSC] = Discontinued product

Oil, Oral:

Generic: 95% (59 mL [DSC])

◆ **Cataflam [DSC]** *see* Diclofenac (Systemic) *on page* *641*

◆ **Catapres** *see* CloNIDine *on page* *508*

◆ **Catapres® (Can)** *see* CloNIDine *on page* *508*

◆ **Catapres-TTS-1** *see* CloNIDine *on page* *508*

◆ **Catapres-TTS-2** *see* CloNIDine *on page* *508*

◆ **Catapres-TTS-3** *see* CloNIDine *on page* *508*

◆ **Cathflo Activase** *see* Alteplase *on page* *105*

◆ **Caverject** *see* Alprostadil *on page* *103*

◆ **Caverject Impulse** *see* Alprostadil *on page* *103*

◆ **CaviRinse** *see* Fluoride *on page* *899*

◆ **Cayston** *see* Aztreonam *on page* *248*

◆ **CB-1348** *see* Chlorambucil *on page* *430*

◆ **CBDCA** *see* CARBOplatin *on page* *374*

◆ **CBZ** *see* CarBAMazepine *on page* *367*

◆ **ccIIV3 [Flucelvax]** *see* Influenza Virus Vaccine (Inactivated) *on page* *1108*

◆ **CCNU** *see* Lomustine *on page* *1286*

◆ **2-CdA** *see* Cladribine *on page* *480*

◆ **CDCA** *see* Chenodiol *on page* *427*

◆ **CDDP** *see* CISplatin *on page* *473*

◆ **CE** *see* Estrogens (Conjugated/Equine, Systemic) *on page* *801*

◆ **CE** *see* Estrogens (Conjugated/Equine, Topical) *on page* *803*

◆ **Ceclor (Can)** *see* Cefaclor *on page* *386*

◆ **Cedax** *see* Ceftibuten *on page* *409*

◆ **CEE** *see* Estrogens (Conjugated/Equine, Systemic) *on page* *801*

◆ **CEE** *see* Estrogens (Conjugated/Equine, Topical) *on page 803*

◆ **CeeNU** *see* Lomustine *on page 1286*

Cefaclor (SEF a klor)

Medication Safety Issues

Sound-alike/look-alike issues:

Cefaclor may be confused with cephalexin

Related Information

Oral Medications That Should Not Be Crushed or Altered *on page 2476*

Brand Names: Canada Apo-Cefaclor; Ceclor; Novo-Cefaclor; Nu-Cefaclor; PMS-Cefaclor

Therapeutic Category Antibiotic, Cephalosporin (Second Generation)

Generic Availability (US) Yes

Use Infections caused by susceptible bacteria including *Staph aureus*, *S. pneumoniae*, *S. pyogenes*, and *H. influenzae* (excluding β-lactamase negative, ampicillin-resistant strains); treatment of otitis media, sinusitis, and infections involving the respiratory tract, skin and skin structure, bone and joint; treatment of urinary tract infections caused by *E. coli*, *Klebsiella*, and *Proteus mirabilis*

Pregnancy Considerations Adverse events were not observed in animal reproduction studies. An increased risk of teratogenic effects has not been observed following maternal use of cefaclor.

Breast-Feeding Considerations Small amounts of cefaclor are excreted in breast milk. The manufacturer recommends that caution be exercised when administering cefaclor to nursing women. Nondose-related effects could include modification of bowel flora.

Contraindications Hypersensitivity to cefaclor, any component of the formulation, or other cephalosporins

Warnings/Precautions Anaphylactic reactions have occurred. If a serious hypersensitivity reaction occurs, discontinue and institute emergency supportive measures, including airway management and treatment (eg, epinephrine, antihistamines and/or corticosteroids). Use with caution in patients with a history of gastrointestinal disease, particularly colitis. Use with caution in patients with renal impairment. Prolonged use may result in fungal or bacterial superinfection, including *C. difficile*-associated diarrhea (CDAD) and pseudomembranous colitis; CDAD has been observed >2 months postantibiotic treatment. Use with caution in patients with a history of penicillin allergy. An extended-release tablet dose of 500 mg twice daily is clinically equivalent to an immediate-release capsule dose of 250 mg 3 times daily; an extended-release tablet dose of 500 mg twice daily is **NOT** clinically equivalent to 500 mg 3 times daily of other cefaclor formulations. Potentially significant interactions may exist, requiring dose or frequency adjustment, additional monitoring, and/or selection of alternative therapy.

Benzyl alcohol and derivatives: Some dosage forms may contain sodium benzoate/benzoic acid; benzoic acid (benzoate) is a metabolite of benzyl alcohol; large amounts of benzyl alcohol (≥99 mg/kg/day) have been associated with a potentially fatal toxicity ("gasping syndrome") in neonates; the "gasping syndrome" consists of metabolic acidosis, respiratory distress, gasping respirations, CNS dysfunction (including convulsions, intracranial hemorrhage), hypotension, and cardiovascular collapse (AAP, 1997; CDC, 1982); some data suggests that benzoate displaces bilirubin from protein binding sites (Ahlfors, 2001); avoid or use dosage forms containing benzyl alcohol derivative with caution in neonates. See manufacturer's labeling.

Warnings: Additional Pediatric Considerations May cause serum sickness-like reaction (estimated incidence ranges from 0.024% to 0.2% per drug course); majority of reactions have occurred in children <5 years of age with symptoms of fever, rash, erythema multiforme, and arthralgia, often occurring during the second or third exposure.

Adverse Reactions

Dermatologic: Rash (maculopapular, erythematous, or morbilliform)

Gastrointestinal: Diarrhea

Genitourinary: Vaginitis

Hematologic: Eosinophilia

Hepatic: Increased transaminases

Miscellaneous: Moniliasis

Rare but important or life-threatening: Agitation, agranulocytosis, anaphylaxis, angioedema, aplastic anemia, arthralgia, cholestatic jaundice, CNS irritability, confusion, dizziness, hallucinations, hemolytic anemia, hepatitis, hyperactivity, insomnia, interstitial nephritis, nausea, nervousness, neutropenia, paresthesia, PT prolonged, pruritus, pseudomembranous colitis, seizure, serum-sickness, somnolence, Stevens-Johnson syndrome, thrombocytopenia, toxic epidermal necrolysis, urticaria, vomiting

Reactions reported with other cephalosporins: Abdominal pain, cholestasis, fever, hemorrhage, renal dysfunction, superinfection, toxic nephropathy

Drug Interactions

Metabolism/Transport Effects Substrate of OAT3

Avoid Concomitant Use

Avoid concomitant use of Cefaclor with any of the following: BCG; BCG (Intravesical)

Increased Effect/Toxicity

Cefaclor may increase the levels/effects of: Aminoglycosides; Vitamin K Antagonists

The levels/effects of Cefaclor may be increased by: Probenecid; Teriflunomide

Decreased Effect

Cefaclor may decrease the levels/effects of: BCG; BCG (Intravesical); BCG Vaccine (Immunization); Sodium Picosulfate; Typhoid Vaccine

Food Interactions The bioavailability of cefaclor extended-release tablets is decreased 23% and the maximum concentration is decreased 67% when taken on an empty stomach. Management: Administer with food.

Storage/Stability Store at 20°C to 25°C (68°F to 77°F). Refrigerate suspension after reconstitution and discard after 14 days.

Mechanism of Action Inhibits bacterial cell wall synthesis by binding to one or more of the penicillin-binding proteins (PBPs) which in turn inhibits the final transpeptidation step of peptidoglycan synthesis in bacterial cell walls, thus inhibiting cell wall biosynthesis. Bacteria eventually lyse due to ongoing activity of cell wall autolytic enzymes (autolysins and murein hydrolases) while cell wall assembly is arrested.

Pharmacokinetics (Adult data unless noted)

Absorption: Oral: Well absorbed; acid stable

Distribution: Distributes into tissues and fluids including bone, pleural and synovial fluid; crosses the placenta; appears in breast milk

Protein binding: 25%

Half-life: 30-60 minutes (prolonged with renal impairment)

Time to peak serum concentration:

Capsule: 60 minutes

Suspension: 45-60 minutes

Elimination: Most of dose (80%) excreted unchanged in urine by glomerular filtration and tubular secretion

Dialysis: Moderately dialyzable (20% to 50%)

Dosing: Usual Oral:

Infants >1 month and Children: 20-40 mg/kg/day divided every 8-12 hours; maximum dose: 2 g/day (twice daily option is for treatment of otitis media or pharyngitis)

Otitis media: 40 mg/kg/day divided every 12 hours

Pharyngitis: 20 mg/kg/day divided every 12 hours

Adults: 250-500 mg every 8 hours

Dosing adjustment in renal impairment: CrCl <10 mL/minute: Administer 50% of dose

Administration Oral: Capsule, suspension: Administer 1 hour before or 2 hours after a meal; shake suspension well before use

Monitoring Parameters With prolonged therapy, monitor CBC and stool frequency periodically

Test Interactions Positive direct Coombs', false-positive urinary glucose test using cupric sulfate (Benedict's solution, Clinitest, Fehling's solution).

Dosage Forms Excipient information presented when available (limited, particularly for generics); consult specific product labeling.

Capsule, Oral:

Generic: 250 mg, 500 mg

Suspension Reconstituted, Oral:

Generic: 125 mg/5 mL (150 mL); 250 mg/5 mL (150 mL); 375 mg/5 mL (100 mL)

Tablet Extended Release 12 Hour, Oral:

Generic: 500 mg

Cefadroxil (sef a DROKS il)

Medication Safety Issues

Sound-alike/look-alike issues:

Duricef may be confused with Ultracet

Brand Names: Canada Apo-Cefadroxil; PRO-Cefadroxil; Teva-Cefadroxil

Therapeutic Category Antibiotic, Cephalosporin (First Generation)

Generic Availability (US) Yes

Use Treatment of susceptible bacterial infections including group A beta-hemolytic streptococcal pharyngitis or tonsillitis; skin and soft tissue infections caused by streptococci or staphylococci; urinary tract infections caused by *Klebsiella*, *E. coli*, and *Proteus mirabilis*

Pregnancy Risk Factor B

Pregnancy Considerations Adverse events have not been observed in animal reproduction studies. Cefadroxil crosses the placenta. Limited data is available concerning the use of cefadroxil in pregnancy; however, adverse fetal effects were not noted in a small clinical trial.

Breast-Feeding Considerations Very small amounts of cefadroxil are excreted in breast milk. The manufacturer recommends that caution be exercised when administering cefadroxil to nursing women. Nondose-related effects could include modification of bowel flora.

Contraindications Hypersensitivity to cefadroxil, any component of the formulation, or other cephalosporins

Warnings/Precautions Modify dosage in patients with renal impairment (CrCl <50 mL/minute/1.73 m^2). Use with caution in patients with a history of penicillin allergy, especially IgE-mediated reactions (eg, anaphylaxis, angioedema, urticaria). Use with caution in patients with a history of gastrointestinal disease, particularly colitis. Prolonged use may result in fungal or bacterial superinfection, including *C. difficile*-associated diarrhea (CDAD) and pseudomembranous colitis; CDAD has been observed >2 months postantibiotic treatment. Only IM penicillin has been shown to be effective in the prophylaxis of rheumatic fever. Cefadroxil is generally effective in the eradication of streptococci from the oropharynx; efficacy data for cefadroxil in the prophylaxis of subsequent rheumatic fever episodes are not available.

Suspension may contain sulfur dioxide (sulfite); hypersensitivity reactions, including anaphylaxis and/or asthmatic exacerbations, may occur (may be life threatening).

Benzyl alcohol and derivatives: Some dosage forms may contain sodium benzoate/benzoic acid; benzoic acid (benzoate) is a metabolite of benzyl alcohol; large amounts of benzyl alcohol (≥99 mg/kg/day) have been associated with a potentially fatal toxicity ("gasping syndrome") in neonates; the "gasping syndrome" consists of metabolic acidosis, respiratory distress, gasping respirations, CNS dysfunction (including convulsions, intracranial hemorrhage), hypotension, and cardiovascular collapse (AAP, 1997; CDC, 1982); some data suggests that benzoate displaces bilirubin from protein binding sites (Ahlfors, 2001); avoid or use dosage forms containing benzyl alcohol derivative with caution in neonates. See manufacturer's labeling.

Adverse Reactions

Gastrointestinal: Diarrhea

Rare but important or life-threatening: Agranulocytosis, anaphylaxis, angioedema, cholestasis, *Clostridium difficile* associated diarrhea, dyspepsia, erythema multiforme, erythematous rash, genital candidiasis, hepatic failure, increased serum transaminases, maculopapular rash, neutropenia, pseudomembranous colitis, serum sickness, Stevens-Johnson syndrome, thrombocytopenia, vaginitis

Drug Interactions

Metabolism/Transport Effects None known.

Avoid Concomitant Use

Avoid concomitant use of Cefadroxil with any of the following: BCG; BCG (Intravesical)

Increased Effect/Toxicity

Cefadroxil may increase the levels/effects of: Vitamin K Antagonists

The levels/effects of Cefadroxil may be increased by: Probenecid

Decreased Effect

Cefadroxil may decrease the levels/effects of: BCG; BCG (Intravesical); BCG Vaccine (Immunization); Sodium Picosulfate; Typhoid Vaccine

Food Interactions Concomitant administration with food, infant formula, or cow's milk does **not** significantly affect absorption.

Storage/Stability Store capsules, tablets and un-reconstituted oral suspension at 20°C to 25°C (68°F to 77F); excursions are permitted to 15°C to 30°C (59°F to 86°F). After reconstitution, oral suspension may be stored for 14 days under refrigeration (4°C).

Mechanism of Action Inhibits bacterial cell wall synthesis by binding to one or more of the penicillin-binding proteins (PBPs) which in turn inhibits the final transpeptidation step of peptidoglycan synthesis in bacterial cell walls, thus inhibiting cell wall biosynthesis. Bacteria eventually lyse due to ongoing activity of cell wall autolytic enzymes (autolysins and murein hydrolases) while cell wall assembly is arrested.

Pharmacokinetics (Adult data unless noted)

Absorption: Oral: Rapid; well absorbed from GI tract

Distribution: V_d: 0.31 L/kg; crosses the placenta; appears in breast milk

Protein binding: 20%

Half-life: 1-2 hours; 20-24 hours in renal failure

Time to peak serum concentration: Within 70-90 minutes

Elimination: >90% of dose excreted unchanged in urine within 24 hours

Dosing: Usual Oral:

Infants and Children: 30 mg/kg/day divided twice daily up to a maximum of 2 g/day

Adolescents and Adults: 1-2 g/day in 1-2 divided doses; maximum dose for adults: 4 g/day

Dosing interval in renal impairment:

CrCl 10-25 mL/minute: Administer every 24 hours

CrCl <10 mL/minute: Administer every 36 hours

Preparation for Administration Oral: Reconstitute powder for oral suspension with appropriate amount of water as specified on the bottle. Shake vigorously until suspended.

Administration Oral: May be administered without regard to food; administration with food may decrease nausea or vomiting; shake suspension well before use.

Monitoring Parameters Stool frequency, resolution of infection

Test Interactions Positive direct Coombs', false-positive urinary glucose test using cupric sulfate (Benedict's solution, Clinitest®, Fehling's solution), false-positive serum or urine creatinine with Jaffé reaction

Dosage Forms Excipient information presented when available (limited, particularly for generics); consult specific product labeling.

Capsule, Oral:
 Generic: 500 mg

Suspension Reconstituted, Oral:
 Generic: 250 mg/5 mL (100 mL); 500 mg/5 mL (75 mL, 100 mL)

Tablet, Oral:
 Generic: 1 g

◆ **Cefadroxil Monohydrate** *see* Cefadroxil *on page* 387

CeFAZolin (sef A zoe lin)

Medication Safety Issues

Sound-alike/look-alike issues:

CeFAZolin may be confused with cefoTEtan, cefOXitin, cefprozil, cefTAZidime, cefTRIAXone, cephalexin

Related Information

Prevention of Infective Endocarditis *on page* 2378

Brand Names: Canada Cefazolin For Injection; Cefazolin For Injection, USP

Therapeutic Category Antibiotic, Cephalosporin (First Generation)

Generic Availability (US) Yes

Use Treatment of susceptible infections involving the respiratory tract, skin and skin structure, urinary tract, biliary tract, bone and joint, genitals, and septicemia (FDA approved in ages ≥1 month and adults); perioperative prophylaxis (FDA approved in adults); treatment of bacterial endocarditis (FDA approved in adults); has also been used for bacterial endocarditis prophylaxis for dental and upper respiratory procedures

Pregnancy Risk Factor B

Pregnancy Considerations Adverse effects were not observed in animal reproduction studies. Cefazolin crosses the placenta. Adverse events have not been reported in the fetus following administration of cefazolin prior to cesarean section. Cefazolin is recommended for group B streptococcus prophylaxis in pregnant patients with a nonanaphylactic penicillin allergy. It is also one of the antibiotics recommended for prophylactic use prior to cesarean delivery and may be used in certain situations prior to vaginal delivery in women at high risk for endocarditis.

Due to pregnancy-induced physiologic changes, the pharmacokinetics of cefazolin are altered. The half-life is shorter, the AUC is smaller, and the clearance and volume of distribution are increased.

Breast-Feeding Considerations Small amounts of cefazolin are excreted in breast milk. The manufacturer recommends that caution be exercised when administering cefazolin to nursing women. Nondose-related effects could include modification of bowel flora.

Contraindications Known allergy to the cephalosporin group of antibiotics

Warnings/Precautions Modify dosage in patients with severe renal impairment. Use with caution in patients with a history of penicillin allergy, especially IgE-mediated reactions (eg, anaphylaxis, angioedema, urticaria). Prolonged use may result in fungal or bacterial superinfection, including *C. difficile*-associated diarrhea (CDAD) and pseudomembranous colitis; CDAD has been observed >2 months postantibiotic treatment. May be associated with increased INR, especially in nutritionally-deficient patients, prolonged treatment, hepatic or renal disease. Use with caution in patients with a history of seizure disorder; high levels, particularly in the presence of renal impairment, may increase risk of seizures. Potentially significant drug-drug interactions may exist, requiring dose or frequency adjustment, additional monitoring, and/or selection of alternative therapy.

Adverse Reactions

Cardiovascular: Localized phlebitis

Central nervous system: Seizure

Dermatologic: Pruritus, skin rash, Stevens-Johnson syndrome

Gastrointestinal: Abdominal cramps, anorexia, diarrhea, nausea, oral candidiasis, pseudomembranous colitis, vomiting

Genitourinary: Vaginitis

Hepatic: Hepatitis, increased serum transaminases

Hematologic: Eosinophilia, leukopenia, neutropenia, thrombocythemia, thrombocytopenia

Hypersensitivity: Anaphylaxis

Local: Pain at injection site

Renal: Increased blood urea nitrogen, increased serum creatinine, renal failure

Miscellaneous: Fever

Drug Interactions

Metabolism/Transport Effects None known.

Avoid Concomitant Use

Avoid concomitant use of CeFAZolin with any of the following: BCG; BCG (Intravesical)

Increased Effect/Toxicity

CeFAZolin may increase the levels/effects of: Fosphenytoin; Phenytoin; Vitamin K Antagonists

The levels/effects of CeFAZolin may be increased by: Probenecid

Decreased Effect

CeFAZolin may decrease the levels/effects of: BCG; BCG (Intravesical); BCG Vaccine (Immunization); Sodium Picosulfate; Typhoid Vaccine

Storage/Stability Store intact vials at room temperature and protect from temperatures exceeding 40°C. Reconstituted solutions of cefazolin are light yellow to yellow. Protection from light is recommended for the powder and for the reconstituted solutions. Reconstituted solutions are stable for 24 hours at room temperature and for 10 days under refrigeration. Stability of parenteral admixture at room temperature (25°C) is 48 hours. Stability of parenteral admixture at refrigeration temperature (4°C) is 14 days.

DUPLEX: Store at 20°C to 25°C (68°F to 77°F); excursions permitted to 15°C to 30°C (59°F to 86°F) prior to activation. Following activation, stable for 24 hours at room temperature and for 7 days under refrigeration.

Mechanism of Action Inhibits bacterial cell wall synthesis by binding to one or more of the penicillin-binding proteins (PBPs) which in turn inhibits the final transpeptidation step of peptidoglycan synthesis in bacterial cell walls, thus inhibiting cell wall biosynthesis. Bacteria eventually lyse due to ongoing activity of cell wall autolytic enzymes (autolysins and murein hydrolases) while cell wall assembly is arrested.

Pharmacokinetics (Adult data unless noted)

Distribution: CSF penetration is poor; penetrates bone and synovial fluid well; distributes into bile

Protein binding: 74% to 86%

Metabolism: Minimally hepatic

Half-life:
  Neonates: 3-5 hours
  Adults: 90-150 minutes (prolonged with renal impairment)
Time to peak serum concentration:
  IM: Within 0.5-2 hours
  IV: Within 5 minutes
Elimination: 80% to 100% excreted unchanged in urine

Dosing: Neonatal General dosing, susceptible infection (*Red Book*, 2012): IM, IV:
Body weight <2 kg: 25 mg/kg/dose every 12 hours
Body weight >2 kg:
  PNA ≤7 days: 25 mg/kg/dose every 12 hours
  PNA 8-28 days: 25 mg/kg/dose every 8 hours

Dosing: Usual
Infants, Children, and Adolescents:
  General dosing, susceptible infection (*Red Book*, 2012): IM, IV:
    Mild to moderate infections: 25-50 mg/kg/day divided every 8 hours; maximum dose: 1000 mg
    Severe infections: 100-150 mg/kg/day divided every 8 hours; maximum dose: 2000 mg
  Endocarditis, bacterial:
    Prophylaxis for dental and upper respiratory procedures: IM, IV: 50 mg/kg 30-60 minutes before procedure; maximum dose: 1000 mg (Wilson, 2007)
    Treatment: IV: 100 mg/kg/day in divided doses every 8 hours for at least 6 weeks; with or without gentamicin; if prosthetic valve, also use in combination with rifampin; maximum dose: 2000 mg (Baddour, 2005)
  Peritonitis (CAPD) (Warady, 2012):
    Prophylaxis:
      Touch contamination of PD line: Intraperitoneal: 125 mg per liter
      Invasive dental procedures: IV: 25 mg/kg administered 30-60 minutes before procedure; maximum dose: 1000 mg
      Gastrointestinal or genitourinary procedures: IV: 25 mg/kg administered 60 minutes before procedure; maximum dose: 2000 mg
    Treatment: Intraperitoneal:
      Intermittent: 20 mg/kg every 24 hours in the long dwell
      Continuous: Loading dose: 500 mg per liter of dialysate; maintenance: 125 mg per liter of dialysate
  Pneumonia, community-acquired pneumonia (CAP), *S. aureus*, methicillin susceptible: Infants ≥3 months, Children, and Adolescents: IV: 50 mg/kg/dose every 8 hours; maximum dose: 2000 mg (Bradley, 2011)
  Skin and soft tissue infections, *S. aureus*, methicillin susceptible (mild to moderate): IV: 50 mg/kg/day in divided doses 3 times daily; maximum dose: 1000 mg (Stevens, 2005); higher doses may be required in severe cases
  Surgical prophylaxis: Children and Adolescents: IV: 25-30 mg/kg 30-60 minutes before procedure, may repeat in 4 hours; maximum dose dependent upon patient weight: Weight <120 kg: 2000 mg; weight ≥120 kg: 3000 mg (Bratzler, 2013; *Red Book*, 2012)
Adults:
  General dosing, susceptible infection:
    Mild infection with gram-positive cocci: IV: 250-500 mg every 8 hours
    Moderate to severe infections: IV: 500-1000 mg every 6-8 hours
  Group B streptococcus (neonatal prophylaxis): IV: 2000 mg once, then 1000 mg every 8 hours until delivery (CDC, 2010)
  Perioperative prophylaxis: IM, IV: 1000 mg 30-60 minutes prior to surgery (may repeat in 2-5 hours intraoperatively); followed by 500-1000 mg every 6-8 hours for 24 hours postoperatively
  Pneumonia, pneumococcal: IV: 500 mg every 12 hours
  Urinary tract infection; uncomplicated: IM, IV: 1000 mg every 12 hours

Dosing interval in renal impairment: IM, IV:
  Infants >1 month, Children, and Adolescents: After initial loading dose is administered, modify dose based on the degree of renal impairment:
    CrCl >70 mL/minute: No dosage adjustment required
    CrCl 40-70 mL/minute: Administer 60% of the usual daily dose divided every 12 hours
    CrCl 20-40 mL/minute: Administer 25% of the usual daily dose divided every 12 hours
    CrCl 5-20 mL/minute: Administer 10% of the usual daily dose given every 24 hours
    Hemodialysis: 25 mg/kg/dose every 24 hours (Aronoff, 2007)
    Peritoneal dialysis: 25 mg/kg/dose every 24 hours (Aronoff, 2007)
    Continuous renal replacement therapy: 25 mg/kg/dose every 8 hours (Aronoff, 2007)
  Adults: After initial loading dose is administered, modify dose based on the degree of renal impairment:
    CrCl ≥55 mL/minute: No dosage adjustment required
    CrCl 35-54 mL/minute: Administer full dose ≥every 8 hours
    CrCl 11-34 mL/minute: Administer 50% of usual dose every 12 hours
    CrCl ≤10 mL/minute: Administer 50% of usual dose every 18-24 hours
    Intermittent hemodialysis (IHD) (administer after hemodialysis on dialysis days): Dialyzable (20% to 50%): 500-1000 mg every 24 hours **or** use 1000-2000 mg every 48-72 hours (Heintz, 2009); **Note:** Dosing dependent on the assumption of 3 times/week, complete IHD sessions. Alternatively, may administer 15-20 mg/kg (maximum dose: 2000 mg) after dialysis without regularly scheduled dosing (Ahern, 2003; Sowinski, 2001).
    Peritoneal dialysis (PD): 500 mg every 12 hours
    Continuous renal replacement therapy (CRRT) (Heintz, 2009; Trotman, 2005): Drug clearance is highly dependent on the method of renal replacement, filter type, and flow rate. Appropriate dosing requires close monitoring of pharmacologic response, signs of adverse reactions due to drug accumulation, as well as drug concentrations in relation to target trough (if appropriate). The following are general recommendations only (based on dialysate flow/ultrafiltration rates of 1-2 L/hour and minimal residual renal function) and should not supersede clinical judgment:
      CVVH: Loading dose of 2000 mg, followed by 1000-2000 mg every 12 hours
      CVVHD/CVVHDF: Loading dose of 2000 mg, followed by either 1000 mg every 8 hours **or** 2000 mg every 12 hours. **Note:** Dosage of 1000 mg every 8 hours results in similar steady-state concentrations as 2000 mg every 12 hours and is more cost effective (Heintz, 2009).
Dosing adjustment in hepatic impairment: There are no dosage adjustments provided in the manufacturer's labeling.

Preparation for Administration Parenteral:
IM: Dilute 500 mg vial with 2 mL SWFI and 1 g vial with 2.5 mL SWFI resulting in a concentration of 225 mg/mL and 330 mg/mL, respectively.
IVP: Reconstitute appropriate vial size and further dilute to a maximum concentration: 100 mg/mL (Klaus 1989); in fluid-restricted patients, a concentration of 138 mg/mL using SWFI results in a maximum recommended osmolality for peripheral infusion (Robinson 1987).
Intermittent IV infusion: Further dilute to a maximum final concentration of 20 mg/mL

Administration Parenteral:
IM: Deep IM injection into a large muscle mass.
IV: May be administered IVP over 3 to 5 minutes or IV intermittent infusion over 10 to 60 minutes.

Monitoring Parameters Renal function periodically when used in combination with other nephrotoxic drugs, hepatic function tests, and CBC; prothrombin time in patients at risk; number and type of stools/day for diarrhea; monitor for signs of anaphylaxis during first dose

Test Interactions Positive direct Coombs', false-positive urinary glucose test using cupric sulfate (Benedict's solution, Clinitest, Fehling's solution), false-positive serum or urine creatinine with Jaffé reaction.

Some penicillin derivatives may accelerate the degradation of aminoglycosides *in vitro*, leading to a potential underestimation of aminoglycoside serum concentration.

Dosage Forms Excipient information presented when available (limited, particularly for generics); consult specific product labeling.

Solution, Intravenous:
Generic: 1 g (50 mL)

Solution Reconstituted, Injection:
Generic: 500 mg (1 ea); 1 g (1 ea); 10 g (1 ea); 20 g (1 ea); 100 g (1 ea); 300 g (1 ea)

Solution Reconstituted, Injection [preservative free]:
Generic: 500 mg (1 ea); 1 g (1 ea); 10 g (1 ea); 20 g (1 ea)

Solution Reconstituted, Intravenous:
Generic: 1 g (1 ea); 2 g (1 ea)

- **Cefazolin For Injection (Can)** *see* CeFAZolin *on page 388*
- **Cefazolin For Injection, USP (Can)** *see* CeFAZolin *on page 388*
- **Cefazolin Sodium** *see* CeFAZolin *on page 388*

Cefdinir (SEF di ner)

Therapeutic Category Antibiotic, Cephalosporin (Third Generation)

Generic Availability (US) Yes

Use Treatment of susceptible acute bacterial otitis media (FDA approved in ages 6 months to 12 years); treatment of susceptible acute maxillary sinusitis, pharyngitis/tonsillitis, and uncomplicated skin and skin structure infections (FDA approved in ages ≥6 months and adults); treatment of susceptible acute exacerbations of chronic bronchitis and community-acquired pneumonia (FDA approved in adolescents and adults)

Pregnancy Risk Factor B

Pregnancy Considerations Teratogenic events have not been observed in animal reproduction studies. An increase in most types of birth defects was not found following first trimester exposure to cephalosporins.

Breast-Feeding Considerations Cefdinir is not detectable in breast milk following a single cefdinir 600 mg dose. If present in breast milk, nondose-related effects could include modification of bowel flora.

Contraindications Hypersensitivity to cefdinir, any component of the formulation, or other cephalosporins.

Warnings/Precautions Administer cautiously to penicillin-sensitive patients, especially IgE-mediated reactions (eg, anaphylaxis, urticaria). Prolonged use may result in fungal or bacterial superinfection, including *C. difficile*-associated diarrhea (CDAD) and pseudomembranous colitis; CDAD has been observed >2 months postantibiotic treatment. Use with caution in patients with a history of colitis. Use caution with renal dysfunction (CrCl <30 mL/minute); dose adjustment may be required. Potentially significant drug-drug interactions may exist, requiring dose or frequency adjustment, additional monitoring, and/or selection of alternative therapy.

Adverse Reactions

Central nervous system: Headache

Dermatologic: Skin rash

Endocrine & metabolic: Decreased serum bicarbonate, glycosuria, hyperglycemia, hyperphosphatemia, increased gamma-glutamyl transferase, increased lactate dehydrogenase

Gastrointestinal: Abdominal pain, diarrhea, nausea, vomiting

Genitourinary: Proteinuria, occult blood in urine, urine alkalinization, vaginitis, vulvovaginal candidiasis

Hematologic: Change in WBC count, elevated urine leukocytes, eosinophilia, functional disorder of polymorphonuclear neutrophils, lymphocytopenia, lymphocytosis, thrombocythemia

Hepatic: Increased serum alkaline phosphatase, increased serum ALT

Renal: Increased urine specific gravity

Rare but important or life-threatening: Abnormal stools, anaphylaxis, anorexia, asthma, blood coagulation disorder, bloody diarrhea, candidiasis, cardiac failure, chest pain, cholestasis, conjunctivitis, constipation, cutaneous candidiasis, decreased hemoglobin, decreased urine specific gravity, disseminated intravascular coagulation, dizziness, drowsiness, dyspepsia, enterocolitis (acute), eosinophilic pneumonitis, erythema multiforme, erythema nodosum, exfoliative dermatitis, facial edema, fever, flatulence, fulminant hepatitis, granulocytopenia, hemolytic anemia, hemorrhagic colitis, hemorrhagic diathesis, hepatic failure, hepatitis (acute), hyperkalemia, hyperkinesia, hypersensitivity angiitis, hypertension, hypocalcemia, hypophosphatemia, immune thrombocytopenia, increased amylase, increased blood urea nitrogen, increased monocytes, increased serum AST, increased serum bilirubin, insomnia, interstitial pneumonitis (idiopathic), intestinal obstruction, involuntary body movements, jaundice, laryngeal edema, leukopenia, leukorrhea, loss of consciousness, maculopapular rash, melena, myocardial infarction, pancytopenia, peptic ulcer, pneumonia (drug-induced), pruritus, pseudomembranous colitis, renal disease, renal failure (acute), respiratory failure (acute), rhabdomyolysis, serum sickness, shock, Stevens-Johnson syndrome, stomatitis, thrombocytopenia, toxic epidermal necrolysis, upper gastrointestinal hemorrhage, weakness, xerostomia

Drug Interactions

Metabolism/Transport Effects None known.

Avoid Concomitant Use

Avoid concomitant use of Cefdinir with any of the following: BCG; BCG (Intravesical)

Increased Effect/Toxicity

Cefdinir may increase the levels/effects of: Aminoglycosides; Vitamin K Antagonists

The levels/effects of Cefdinir may be increased by: Probenecid

Decreased Effect

Cefdinir may decrease the levels/effects of: BCG; BCG (Intravesical); BCG Vaccine (Immunization); Sodium Picosulfate; Typhoid Vaccine

The levels/effects of Cefdinir may be decreased by: Iron Salts; Multivitamins/Minerals (with ADEK, Folate, Iron)

Storage/Stability Store at 20°C to 25°C (68°F to 77°F). Store reconstituted suspension at room temperature 20°C to 25°C (68°F to 77°F) for 10 days.

Mechanism of Action Inhibits bacterial cell wall synthesis by binding to one or more of the penicillin-binding proteins (PBPs) which in turn inhibits the final transpeptidation step of peptidoglycan synthesis in bacterial cell walls, thus inhibiting cell wall biosynthesis. Bacteria eventually lyse due to ongoing activity of cell wall autolytic enzymes (autolysins and murein hydrolases) while cell wall assembly is arrested.

Pharmacokinetics (Adult data unless noted)
Distribution: Penetrates into blister fluid, middle ear fluid, tonsils, sinus, and lung tissues
V_d:
Children 6 months to 12 years: 0.67 ± 0.38 L/kg
Adults: 0.35 ± 0.29 L/kg
Protein binding: 60% to 70%
Metabolism: Minimal
Bioavailability:
Capsules: 16% to 21%
Suspension: 25%
Half-life, elimination: 1.7 (± 0.6) hours with normal renal function
Time to peak serum concentration: 2 to 4 hours
Elimination: 11.6% to 18.4% of a dose is excreted unchanged in urine
Dialysis: ~63% is removed by hemodialysis (4 hours duration)

Dosing: Usual
Pediatric:
General dosing, susceptible infection (*Red Book* 2012): Mild to moderate infections: Infants, Children, and Adolescents: Oral: 14 mg/kg/day in divided doses 1 to 2 times daily; maximum daily dose: 600 mg/**day**
Bronchitis, acute exacerbation: Oral: Adolescents: 300 mg every 12 hours for 5 to 10 days **or** 600 mg every 24 hours for 10 days
Otitis media, acute: Infants ≥6 months and Children: Oral: 14 mg/kg/day in divided doses every 12 to 24 hours for 5 to 10 days; maximum daily dose: 600 mg/**day**. Variable duration of therapy: If <2 years of age or severe symptoms (any age): 10-day course; if 2 to 5 years of age with mild to moderate symptoms: 7-day course; if ≥6 years of age with mild to moderate symptoms: 5- to 7-day course (AAP [Lieberthal 2013]). **Note:** Recommended by the AAP as an alternative agent for initial treatment in penicillin allergic patients (AAP, [Lieberthal 2013]).
Pharyngitis/Tonsillitis: Note: Although FDA approved at twice daily dosing, duration <10 days is not recommended (Shulman 2012).
Infants ≥6 months and Children: Oral: 7 mg/kg/dose every 12 hours for 5 to 10 days **or** 14 mg/kg/dose every 24 hours for 10 days; maximum daily dose: 600 mg/**day**
Adolescents: Oral: 300 mg every 12 hours for 5 to 10 days **or** 600 mg every 24 hours for 10 days
Pneumonia, community-acquired: Adolescents: Oral: 300 mg every 12 hours for 10 days
Skin and skin structure infection, uncomplicated:
Infants ≥6 months and Children: Oral: 14 mg/kg/day in divided doses twice daily for 10 days; maximum daily dose: 600 mg/**day**
Adolescents: Oral: 300 mg every 12 hours for 10 days
Sinusitis, acute maxillary: Note: Due to decreased *S. pneumonia* sensitivity, cefdinir is no longer recommended as monotherapy for the initial empiric treatment of sinusitis (Chow 2012)
Infants ≥6 months and Children: Oral: 14 mg/kg/day in divided doses every 12 to 24 hours for 10 days; maximum daily dose: 600 mg/**day**
Adolescents: Oral: 300 mg every 12 hours **or** 600 mg every 24 hours for 10 days
Adult:
Bronchitis, acute exacerbation: Oral: 300 mg every 12 hours for 5 to 10 days **or** 600 mg once daily for 10 days
Pharyngitis/tonsillitis: Oral: 300 mg every 12 hours for 5 to 10 days **or** 600 mg once daily for 10 days. **Note:** Although FDA approved at twice daily dosing, duration <10 days is not recommended (Shulman 2012).
Pneumonia, community-acquired: Oral: 300 mg every 12 hours for 10 days
Sinusitis, acute maxillary: Oral: 300 mg every 12 hours **or** 600 mg once daily for 10 days. **Note:** Due to decreased *S. pneumonia* sensitivity, cefdinir is no longer recommended as monotherapy for the initial empiric treatment of sinusitis (Chow 2012).
Skin and skin structure infection (uncomplicated): Oral: 300 mg every 12 hours for 10 days
Dosing adjustment in renal impairment:
Infants, Children, Adolescents, and Adults: CrCl ≥30 mL/minute: No adjustment required
Infants and Children ≥6 months to 12 years: CrCl <30 mL/minute/1.73 m^2: 7 mg/kg/dose once daily; maximum daily dose: 300 mg/**day**
Adolescents and Adults: CrCl <30 mL/minute: 300 mg once daily
Hemodialysis: Infants, Children, Adolescents, and Adults: Initial dose: 7 mg/kg/dose (maximum dose: 300 mg) every other day. At the conclusion of each hemodialysis session, an additional dose (7 mg/kg/dose up to 300 mg) should be given. Subsequent doses should be administered every other day.
Dosing adjustment in hepatic impairment: No dosage adjustments are recommended.

Preparation for Administration Oral: Reconstitute powder for oral suspension with appropriate amount of water as specified on the bottle. Shake vigorously until suspended.

Administration Oral: May administer with or without food; administer with food if stomach upset occurs; administer cefdinir at least 2 hours before or after antacids or iron supplements; shake suspension well before use.

Monitoring Parameters Evaluate renal function before and during therapy; with prolonged therapy, monitor coagulation tests, CBC, liver function test periodically, and number and type of stools/day for diarrhea. Observe for signs and symptoms of anaphylaxis during first dose.

Test Interactions False-positive reaction for urinary ketones may occur with nitroprusside- but not nitroferricyanide-based tests. False-positive urine glucose results may occur when using Clinitest®, Benedict's solution, or Fehling's solution; glucose-oxidase-based reaction systems (eg, Clinistix®, Tes-Tape®) are recommended. May cause positive direct Coombs' test.

Additional Information Oral suspension contains 2.82-2.94 g of sucrose per 5 mL.

Dosage Forms Excipient information presented when available (limited, particularly for generics); consult specific product labeling.
Capsule, Oral:
Generic: 300 mg
Suspension Reconstituted, Oral:
Generic: 125 mg/5 mL (60 mL, 100 mL); 250 mg/5 mL (60 mL, 100 mL)

Cefditoren (sef de TOR en)

Medication Safety Issues
International issues:
Spectracef [US, Great Britain, Mexico, Portugal, Spain] may be confused with Spectrocef brand name for cefotaxime [Italy]

Brand Names: US Spectracef

Therapeutic Category Antibiotic, Cephalosporin

Generic Availability (US) Yes

Use Treatment of mild to moderate infections caused by susceptible bacteria including acute bacterial exacerbation of chronic bronchitis, community-acquired pneumonia, pharyngitis or tonsillitis, and uncomplicated skin and skin-structure infections (FDA approved in ages ≥12 years and adults)

Pregnancy Risk Factor B

Pregnancy Considerations Adverse events have not been observed in animal reproduction studies. An increase in most types of birth defects was not found following first trimester exposure to cephalosporins.

Breast-Feeding Considerations It is not known whether cefditoren is excreted in human milk. The manufacturer recommends caution when using cefditoren during breast-feeding. If cefditoren reaches the breast milk, the limited oral absorption may minimize the effect on the nursing infant. Nondose-related effects could include modification of bowel flora.

Contraindications Hypersensitivity to cefditoren, any component of the formulation, other cephalosporins, or milk protein; carnitine deficiency or inborn errors of metabolism that may result in clinically significant carnitine deficiency.

Warnings/Precautions Use with caution in patients with a history of penicillin allergy, especially IgE-mediated reactions (eg, anaphylaxis, urticaria). Prolonged use may result in fungal or bacterial superinfection, including *C. difficile*-associated diarrhea (CDAD) and pseudomembranous colitis; CDAD has been observed >2 months postantibiotic treatment. Caution in individuals with seizure disorders; high levels, particularly in the presence of renal impairment, may increase risk of seizures. Use caution in patients with renal or hepatic impairment; modify dosage in patients with severe renal impairment. Cefditoren causes renal excretion of carnitine; do not use in patients with carnitine deficiency; not for long-term therapy due to the possible development of carnitine deficiency over time. May prolong prothrombin time; use with caution in patients with a history of bleeding disorder. Cefditoren tablets contain sodium caseinate, which may cause hypersensitivity reactions in patients with milk protein hypersensitivity; this does not affect patients with lactose intolerance.

Warnings: Additional Pediatric Considerations Carnitine deficiency may result from prolonged use; cefditoren causes renal excretion of carnitine; plasma carnitine concentrations usually return to normal range within 7 to 10 days after discontinuation of therapy. Therapy with cefditoren is contraindicated in patients with carnitine deficiency or inborn errors of metabolism that may result in clinically significant carnitine deficiency.

Adverse Reactions

Central nervous system: Headache

Endocrine & metabolic: Glucose increased

Gastrointestinal: Abdominal pain, diarrhea, dyspepsia, nausea, vomiting

Genitourinary: Vaginal moniliasis

Hematologic: Hematocrit decreased

Renal: Hematuria, urinary white blood cells increased

Rare but important or life-threatening): Acute renal failure, albumin decreased, allergic reaction, arthralgia, asthma, BUN increased, calcium decreased, coagulation time increased, eosinophilic pneumonia, erythema multiforme, fungal infection, hyperglycemia, interstitial pneumonia, leukopenia, leukorrhea, positive direct Coombs' test, potassium increased, pseudomembranous colitis, rash, sodium decreased, Stevens-Johnson syndrome, thrombocythemia, thrombocytopenia, toxic epidermal necrolysis, white blood cells increased/decreased

Reactions reported with other cephalosporins: Anaphylaxis, aplastic anemia, cholestasis, hemorrhage, hemolytic anemia, renal dysfunction, reversible hyperactivity, serum sickness-like reaction, toxic nephropathy

Drug Interactions

Metabolism/Transport Effects None known.

Avoid Concomitant Use There are no known interactions where it is recommended to avoid concomitant use.

Increased Effect/Toxicity

Cefditoren may increase the levels/effects of: Vitamin K Antagonists

The levels/effects of Cefditoren may be increased by: Probenecid

Decreased Effect

The levels/effects of Cefditoren may be decreased by: Antacids; H2-Antagonists; Proton Pump Inhibitors

Food Interactions Moderate- to high-fat meals increase bioavailability and maximum plasma concentration. Management: Take with meals. Maintain adequate hydration, unless instructed to restrict fluid intake.

Storage/Stability Store at 25°C (77°F); excursions permitted between 15°C and 30°C (59°F and 86°F). Protect from light and moisture.

Mechanism of Action Inhibits bacterial cell wall synthesis by binding to one or more of the penicillin-binding proteins (PBPs) which in turn inhibits the final transpeptidation step of peptidoglycan synthesis in bacterial cell walls, thus inhibiting cell wall biosynthesis. Bacteria eventually lyse due to ongoing activity of cell wall autolytic enzymes (autolysins and murein hydrolases) while cell wall assembly is arrested.

Pharmacokinetics (Adult data unless noted)

Distribution: V_d: 9.3 ± 1.6 L

Protein binding: 88% *(in vitro)*, primarily to albumin

Metabolism: Cefditoren pivoxil is hydrolyzed by esterases to cefditoren (active) and pivalate; cefditoren is not appreciable metabolized

Bioavailability: ~14% to 16%, increased by moderate to high-fat meal (mean AUC by 70%; maximum plasma concentration by 50%)

Half-life elimination: 1.6 ± 0.4 hours; increased with moderate (2.7 hours) and severe (4.7 hours) renal impairment

Time to peak serum concentration: 1.5 to 3 hours

Elimination: Urine (as cefditoren and pivaloylcarnitine)

Dosing: Usual

Pediatric:

General dosing, susceptible infection; mild to moderate infections: Children ≥12 years and Adolescents: Oral: 200 to 400 mg twice daily (*Red Book* [AAP, 2012])

Bronchitis, chronic; acute bacterial exacerbation: Children ≥12 years and Adolescents: Oral: 400 mg twice daily for 10 days

Pneumonia, community-acquired: Children ≥12 years and Adolescents: Oral: 400 mg twice daily for 14 days

Pharyngitis, tonsillitis:

Manufacturer's labeling: Children ≥12 years and Adolescents: Oral: 200 mg twice daily for 10 days

Alternate dosing: Infants ≥8 months and Children: Limited data available: Oral: 3 mg/kg/dose 3 times daily for 5 days; dosing based on a prospective study comparing 5 days of cefditoren (n=103, age range: 0.7 to 12.4 years) to 10 days of amoxicillin (n=155); efficacy and tolerability were similar for both groups; cefditoren was administered as a granule formulation that is not available in the U.S. (Ozaki, 2008)

Skin and skin structure infections, uncomplicated: Children ≥12 years and Adolescents: Oral: 200 mg twice daily for 10 days

Adult:

Bronchitis, chronic; acute bacterial exacerbation: Oral: 400 mg twice daily for 10 days

Pneumonia, community-acquired: Oral: 400 mg twice daily for 14 days

Pharyngitis, tonsillitis: Oral: 200 mg twice daily for 10 days

Skin and skin structure infections, uncomplicated: Oral: 200 mg twice daily for 10 days

Dosing adjustment in renal impairment: Children ≥12 years, Adolescents, and Adults:

CrCl ≥50 mL/minute/1.73 m²: No dosage adjustment necessary

CrCl 30-49 mL/minute/1.73 m²: Maximum dose: 200 mg twice daily

CrCl <30 mL/minute/1.73 m²: Maximum dose: 200 mg once daily

End stage renal disease: Appropriate dose has not been determined

Dosing adjustment in hepatic impairment: Children ≥12 years, Adolescents, and Adults:

Mild to moderate impairment (Child-Pugh Class A or B): No dosage adjustment necessary.

Severe impairment (Child-Pugh Class C): There are no dosage adjustment guidelines provided in the manufacturer's labeling (not studied).

Administration Oral: Administer with meals.

Monitoring Parameters Assess patient at beginning and throughout therapy for infection; observe for changes in bowel frequency, monitor for signs of anaphylaxis during first dose

Test Interactions May induce a positive direct Coomb's test. May cause a false-negative ferricyanide test. Glucose oxidase or hexokinase methods recommended for blood/plasma glucose determinations. False-positive urine glucose test when using copper reduction based assays (eg, Clinitest®).

Dosage Forms Excipient information presented when available (limited, particularly for generics); consult specific product labeling.

Tablet, Oral:

Spectracef: 200 mg, 400 mg [contains sodium caseinate]

Generic: 200 mg, 400 mg

◆ **Cefditoren Pivoxil** *see* Cefditoren *on page 391*

Cefepime (SEF e pim)

Medication Safety Issues

Sound-alike/look-alike issues:

Cefepime may be confused with cefixime, cefTAZidime

Brand Names: US Maxipime

Brand Names: Canada Maxipime

Therapeutic Category Antibiotic, Cephalosporin (Fourth Generation)

Generic Availability (US) Yes

Use Treatment of pneumonia, uncomplicated skin and soft tissue infections, and complicated and uncomplicated urinary tract infections (including pyelonephritis) caused by susceptible organisms, and as empiric therapy for febrile neutropenic patients (FDA approved in ages ≥2 months and adults); used in combination with metronidazole for complicated intra-abdominal infections (FDA approved in adults). Cefepime is a fourth generation cephalosporin with activity against gram-negative bacteria, including *Pseudomonas aeruginosa*, *E. coli*, *H. influenzae*, *M. catarrhalis*, *M morganii*, *P. mirabilis*, and strains of Acinetobacter, Citrobacter, Enterobacter, Klebsiella, Providencia, and Serratia; active against gram-positive bacteria, such as *Staphylococcus aureus*, *S. pyogenes*, and *S. pneumoniae*

Pregnancy Risk Factor B

Pregnancy Considerations Adverse events were not observed in animal reproduction studies. Cefepime crosses the placenta.

Breast-Feeding Considerations Small amounts of cefepime are excreted in breast milk. The manufacturer recommends that caution be exercised when administering cefepime to nursing women. Nondose-related effects could include modification of bowel flora.

Contraindications Hypersensitivity to cefepime, other cephalosporins, penicillins, other beta-lactam antibiotics, or any component of the formulation

Warnings/Precautions Severe neurological reactions (some fatal) have been reported, including encephalopathy, myoclonus, seizures, and nonconvulsive status epilepticus; risk may be increased in the presence of renal impairment (CrCl ≤60 mL/minute); ensure dose adjusted for renal function or discontinue therapy if patient develops neurotoxicity; effects are often reversible upon discontinuation of cefepime. Serious adverse reactions have occurred in elderly patients with renal insufficiency given unadjusted doses of cefepime, including life-threatening or fatal occurrences of the following: encephalopathy, myoclonus, and seizures. Use with caution in patients with a history of penicillin or cephalosporin allergy, especially IgE-mediated reactions (eg, anaphylaxis, urticaria). Prolonged use may result in fungal or bacterial superinfection, including *C. difficile*-associated diarrhea (CDAD) and pseudomembranous colitis; CDAD has been observed >2 months postantibiotic treatment. Use with caution in patients with a history of gastrointestinal disease, especially colitis. May be associated with increased INR, especially in nutritionally-deficient patients, prolonged treatment, hepatic or renal disease. Use with caution in patients with a history of seizure disorder; high levels, particularly in the presence of renal impairment, may increase risk of seizures.

Warnings: Additional Pediatric Considerations The manufacturer does not recommend the use of cefepime in pediatric patients for the treatment of serious infections due to *Haemophilus influenzae* type b, for suspected meningitis, or for meningeal seeding from a distant infection site. However, limited data suggest that cefepime may be a valuable alternative for treating bacterial meningitis in children in conjunction with other agents like vancomycin in areas with a high incidence of cephalosporin nonsusceptible pneumococci (Haase, 2004).

Adverse Reactions

Cardiovascular: Localized phlebitis

Central nervous system: Headache

Dermatologic: Pruritus, skin rash

Endocrine & metabolic: Hypophosphatemia

Gastrointestinal: Diarrhea, nausea, vomiting

Hematologic & oncologic: Eosinophilia, positive direct Coombs test (without hemolysis)

Hepatic: Abnormal partial thromboplastin time, abnormal prothrombin time, increased serum ALT, increased serum AST

Local: Local pain

Miscellaneous: Fever

Rare but important or life-threatening: Agranulocytosis, anaphylactic shock, anaphylaxis, brain disease, colitis, coma, confusion, decreased hematocrit, hallucination, hypercalcemia, hyperkalemia, hyperphosphatemia, hypocalcemia, increased blood urea nitrogen, increased serum alkaline phosphatase, increased serum bilirubin, increased serum creatinine, leukopenia, neutropenia, oral candidiasis, pseudomembranous colitis, seizure, status epilepticus (nonconvulsive), stupor, thrombocytopenia, urticaria, vaginitis

Drug Interactions

Metabolism/Transport Effects None known.

Avoid Concomitant Use

Avoid concomitant use of Cefepime with any of the following: BCG; BCG (Intravesical)

Increased Effect/Toxicity

Cefepime may increase the levels/effects of: Aminoglycosides; Vitamin K Antagonists

The levels/effects of Cefepime may be increased by: Probenecid

Decreased Effect
Cefepime may decrease the levels/effects of: BCG; BCG (Intravesical); BCG Vaccine (Immunization); Sodium Picosulfate; Typhoid Vaccine

Storage/Stability
Vials: Store intact vials at 20°C to 25°C (68°F to 77°F). Protect from light. After reconstitution, stable in NS and D_5W for 24 hours at room temperature and 7 days refrigerated. Refer to the manufacturer's product labeling for other acceptable reconstitution solutions.
Dual chamber containers: Store unactivated containers at 20°C to 25°C (68°F to 77°F); excursions permitted to 15°C to 30°C (59°F to 85°F). Do not freeze. Following reconstitution, use within 12 hours if stored at room temperature or within 5 days if stored under refrigeration.
Premixed solution: Store frozen at -20°C (-4°F). Thawed solution is stable for 24 hours at room temperature or 7 days under refrigeration; do not refreeze.

Mechanism of Action Inhibits bacterial cell wall synthesis by binding to one or more of the penicillin-binding proteins (PBPs) which in turn inhibits the final transpeptidation step of peptidoglycan synthesis in bacterial cell walls, thus inhibiting cell wall biosynthesis. Bacteria eventually lyse due to ongoing activity of cell wall autolytic enzymes (autolysis and murein hydrolases) while cell wall assembly is arrested.

Pharmacokinetics (Adult data unless noted)
Absorption: IM: Rapid and complete
Distribution: V_d:
- Neonates (Capparelli, 2005):
  - PMA <30 weeks: 0.51 L/kg
  - PMA >30 weeks: 0.39 L/kg
- Infants and Children 2 months to 11 years: 0.3 L/kg
- Adults: 18 L, 0.26 L/kg; penetrates into inflammatory fluid at concentrations ~80% of serum concentrations and into bronchial mucosa at concentrations ~60% of plasma concentrations; crosses the blood-brain barrier

Protein binding: ~20%
Metabolism: Very little
Half-life:
- Neonates: 4-5 hours (Lima-Rogel, 2008)
- Children 2 months to 6 years: 1.77-1.96 hours
- Adults: 2 hours
- Hemodialysis: 13.5 hours
- Continuous peritoneal dialysis: 19 hours

Elimination: At least 85% eliminated as unchanged drug in urine

Dosing: Neonatal
General dosing, susceptible infection (*Red Book*, 2012): IM, IV: 30 mg/kg/dose every 12 hours
Meningitis: IV:
- Body weight <1 kg:
  - PNA 0-14 days: 50 mg/kg/dose every 12 hours
  - PNA ≥14 days: 50 mg/kg/dose every 8 hours
- Body weight 1-2 kg:
  - PNA 0-7 days: 50 mg/kg/dose every 12 hours
  - PNA ≥8 days: 50 mg/kg/dose every 8 hours
- Body weight >2 kg: 50 mg/kg/dose every 8 hours

Pseudomonal infection: IM, IV:
- Body weight <1 kg:
  - PNA 0-14 days: 50 mg/kg/dose every 12 hours
  - PNA ≥14 days: 50 mg/kg/dose every 8 hours
- Body weight 1-2 kg:
  - PNA 0-7 days: 50 mg/kg/dose every 12 hours
  - PNA ≥8 days: 50 mg/kg/dose every 8 hours
- Body weight >2 kg: 50 mg/kg/dose every 8 hours

Dosing: Usual
Infants, Children, and Adolescents:
General dosing, susceptible infection (*Red Book*, 2012): IM, IV:
- Mild to moderate infection: 50 mg/kg/dose every 12 hours; maximum single dose: 2000 mg
- Severe infection: 50 mg/kg/dose every 8-12 hours; maximum single dose: 2000 mg

Cystic fibrosis, acute pulmonary exacerbation: I.V: 50 mg/kg/dose every 8 hours; maximum dose: 2000 mg; patients with more resistant pseudomonal isolates (MIC ≥16 mg/L) may require 50 mg/kg/dose every 6 hours (Zobell, 2013)

Endocarditis, prosthetic valve, treatment within 1 year of replacement: IV: 50 mg/kg/dose every 8 hours in combination with vancomycin and rifampin for 6 weeks plus gentamicin for the first 2 weeks; maximum single dose: 2000 mg (Baddour, 2005)

Febrile neutropenia, empiric therapy: IV: 50 mg/kg/dose every 8 hours; maximum single dose: 2000 mg (*Red Book*, 2012); duration of therapy dependent upon febrile neutropenia risk-status; in high-risk patients, may discontinue empiric antibiotics if all of the following criteria met: Negative blood cultures at 48 hours; afebrile for at least 24 hours, and evidence of marrow recovery. In low-risk patients, may discontinue empiric antibiotics after 72 hours duration in patients with a negative blood culture and who have been afebrile for 24 hours regardless of marrow recovery status; follow-up closely (Lehrnbecher, 2012).

Intra-abdominal infection, complicated: IV: 50 mg/kg/dose every 12 hours in combination with metronidazole; maximum single dose: 2000 mg (Solomkin, 2010)

Meningitis: IV: 50 mg/kg/dose every 8 hours; maximum single dose: 2000 mg (Tunkel, 2004)

Pneumonia, moderate to severe: Infants ≥2 months, Children, and Adolescents: IV: 50 mg/kg/dose every 12 hours for 10 days; maximum single dose: 2000 mg

Skin and skin structure infections, uncomplicated: Infants ≥2 months, Children, and Adolescents: IV: 50 mg/kg/dose every 12 hours for 10 days; maximum single dose: 2000 mg

Urinary tract infection, complicated and uncomplicated: Infants ≥2 months, Children, and Adolescents: IM, IV: 50 mg/kg/dose every 12 hours for 7-10 days; maximum single dose: 2000 mg; duration based on severity of infection: Mild to moderate: 7-10 days; severe/pyelonephritis: 10 days; **Note:** IM may be considered for mild to moderate infection only.

Adults:
Febrile neutropenia, monotherapy: I.V: 2000 mg every 8 hours for 7 days or until the neutropenia resolves

Intra-abdominal infections, complicated, severe (in combination with metronidazole): IV: 2000 mg every 12 hours for 7-10 days. **Note:** 2010 IDSA guidelines recommend 2000 mg every 8-12 hours for 4-7 days (provided source controlled). Not recommended for hospital-acquired intra-abdominal infections (IAI) associated with multidrug-resistant gram-negative organisms or in mild to moderate community-acquired IAIs due to risk of toxicity and the development of resistant organisms (Solomkin [IDSA], 2010).

Pneumonia: IV:
- Nosocomial (HAP/VAP): 1000-2000 mg every 8-12 hours; **Note:** Duration of therapy may vary considerably (7-21 days); usually longer courses are required if *Pseudomonas*. In absence of *Pseudomonas*, and if appropriate empiric treatment used and patient responsive, it may be clinically appropriate to reduce duration of therapy to 7-10 days (American Thoracic Society Guidelines, 2005).
- Community-acquired (including pseudomonal): 1000-2000 mg every 12 hours for 10 days

Skin and skin structure infections, uncomplicated: IV: 2000 mg every 12 hours for 10 days

Urinary tract infections, complicated and uncomplicated:
- Mild to moderate: IM, IV: 500-1000 mg every 12 hours for 7-10 days

Severe: IV: 2000 mg every 12 hours for 10 days

Dosing adjustment in renal impairment:

Infants, Children, and Adolescents:

Manufacturer's labeling: Infants ≥2 months, Children, and Adolescents: There are no dosage adjustments provided in the manufacturer's labeling; however, similar dosage adjustments to adults would be anticipated based on comparable pharmacokinetics between children and adults.

Alternative dosing recommendations (Aronoff, 2007):

Note: Renally adjusted dose recommendations are based on doses of 50 mg/kg/dose every 8-12 hours.

GFR >50 mL/minute/1.73 m^2: No adjustment needed

GFR 10-50 mL/minute/1.73 m^2: 50 mg/kg/dose every 24 hours

GFR <10 mL/minute/1.73 m^2: 50 mg/kg/dose every 48 hours

Intermittent hemodialysis: 50 mg/kg/dose every 24 hours

Peritoneal dialysis (PD): 50 mg/kg/dose every 24 hours

Continuous renal replacement therapy (CRRT): 50 mg/kg/dose every 12 hours

Adults: Recommended maintenance schedule based on creatinine clearance (may be estimated using the Cockcroft-Gault formula), compared to normal dosing schedule: See table.

Cefepime Hydrochloride

Creatinine Clearance (mL/minute)	Recommended Maintenance Schedule			
>60 (normal recommended dosing schedule)	500 mg every 12 hours	1000 mg every 12 hours	2000 mg every 12 hours	2000 mg every 8 hours
30-60	500 mg every 24 hours	1000 mg every 24 hours	2000 mg every 24 hours	2000 mg every 12 hours
11-29	500 mg every 24 hours	500 mg every 24 hours	1000 mg every 24 hours	2000 mg every 24 hours
<11	250 mg every 24 hours	250 mg every 24 hours	500 mg every 24 hours	1000 mg every 24 hours

Continuous ambulatory peritoneal dialysis (CAPD): Removed to a lesser extent than hemodialysis; administer normal recommended dose every 48 hours

Hemodialysis: 68% removed by hemodialysis: Initial: 1000 mg (single dose) on day 1. Maintenance: 500 mg once daily (1000 mg once daily in febrile neutropenic patients)

Continuous renal replacement therapy (CRRT) (Heintz, 2009; Trotman, 2005): Drug clearance is highly dependent on the method of renal replacement, filter type, and flow rate. Appropriate dosing requires close monitoring of pharmacologic response, signs of adverse reactions due to drug accumulation, as well as drug concentrations in relation to target trough (if appropriate). The following are general recommendations only (based on dialysate flow/ultrafiltration rates of 1-2 L/hour and minimal residual renal function) and should not supersede clinical judgment:

CVVH: Loading dose of 2000 mg followed by 1000-2000 mg every 12 hours

CVVHD/CVVHDF: Loading dose of 2000 mg followed by either 1000 mg every 8 hours **or** 2000 g every 12 hours. **Note:** Dosage of 1000 mg every 8 hours results in similar steady-state concentrations as 2000 mg every 12 hours and is more cost-effective (Heintz, 2009).

Note: Consider higher dosage of 4000 mg/day if treating *Pseudomonas* or life-threatening infections in order to maximize time above MIC (Trotman, 2005). Dosage of 2000 mg every 8 hours may be needed for gram-negative rods with MIC ≥4 mg/L (Heintz, 2009).

Dosing adjustment in hepatic impairment: No dosage adjustments are recommended.

Preparation for Administration Parenteral:

IV: Reconstitute vial with a compatible diluent (resulting concentration of 100 mg/mL for 1 g vial and 160 mg/mL for 2 g vial); further dilute in D_5W, NS, $D_{10}W$, D_5NS, or D_5LR; final concentration should not exceed 40 mg/mL.

IM: Reconstitute with SWFI, NS, D_5W, lidocaine 0.5% or 1%, or bacteriostatic water for injection to a final concentration of 280 mg/mL.

Administration Parenteral:

IV: Administer as an intermittent IV infusion over 30 minutes; in adult clinical trials, cefepime has been administered by direct IV injection over 3 to 5 minutes at final concentrations of 40 mg/mL (Garrelts 1999) and 100 mg/mL (Jaruratanasirikul 2002; Lipman 1999) for severe infections

IM: Administer by deep IM injection into large muscle mass

Monitoring Parameters With prolonged therapy, monitor renal and hepatic function periodically; number and type of stools/day for diarrhea; CBC with differential. Observe for signs and symptoms of anaphylaxis during first dose.

Test Interactions Positive direct Coombs', false-positive urinary glucose test using cupric sulfate (Benedict's solution, Clinitest®, Fehling's solution), false-positive serum or urine creatinine with Jaffé reaction, false-positive urinary proteins and steroids

Dosage Forms Excipient information presented when available (limited, particularly for generics); consult specific product labeling.

Solution, Intravenous, as hydrochloride:

Generic: 1 g/50 mL (50 mL); 2% (100 mL)

Solution Reconstituted, Injection, as hydrochloride:

Maxipime: 1 g (1 ea); 2 g (1 ea)

Generic: 1 g (1 ea); 2 g (1 ea)

Solution Reconstituted, Intravenous, as hydrochloride:

Maxipime: 1 g (1 ea); 2 g (1 ea)

Generic: 1 g/50 mL (1 ea); 2 g/50 mL (1 ea)

◆ **Cefepime Hydrochloride** *see* Cefepime *on page* 393

Cefixime (sef IKS eem)

Medication Safety Issues

Sound-alike/look-alike issues:

Cefixime may be confused with cefepime

Suprax® may be confused with Sporanox®

International issues:

Cefiton: Brand name for cefixime [Portugal] may be confused with Ceftim brand name for ceftazidime [Portugal]; Ceftime brand name for ceftazidime [Thailand]; Ceftin brand name for cefuroxime [U.S., Canada]

Brand Names: US Suprax

Brand Names: Canada Auro-Cefixime; Suprax

Therapeutic Category Antibiotic, Cephalosporin (Third Generation)

Generic Availability (US) May be product dependent

Use Treatment of urinary tract infections, otitis media, acute exacerbations of chronic bronchitis due to susceptible organisms which may include *S. pneumoniae* and *pyogenes*, *H. influenzae*, *M. catarrhalis*, *E. coli*, and *P mirabilis*; treatment of pharyngitis and tonsillitis due to *S. pyogenes*; treatment of uncomplicated cervical/urethral gonorrhea due to *N. gonorrhoeae* (All indications: FDA approved in ages ≥6 months and adults); has also been used for management of irinotecan-associated diarrhea,

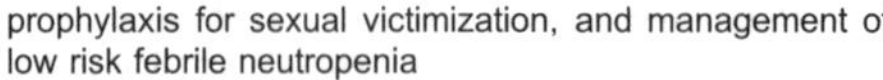

prophylaxis for sexual victimization, and management of low risk febrile neutropenia

Pregnancy Risk Factor B

Pregnancy Considerations Teratogenic effects were not observed in animal reproduction studies. Cefixime crosses the placenta and can be detected in the amniotic fluid (Ozyüncü 2010).

Breast-Feeding Considerations It is not known if cefixime is excreted in breast milk. The manufacturer recommends that consideration be given to discontinuing nursing temporarily during treatment. If present in breast milk, nondose-related effects could include modification of bowel flora.

Contraindications Hypersensitivity to cefixime, any component of the formulation, or other cephalosporins

Warnings/Precautions Prolonged use may result in fungal or bacterial superinfection, including *C. difficile*-associated diarrhea (CDAD) and pseudomembranous colitis; CDAD has been observed >2 months postantibiotic treatment. Modify dosage in patients with renal impairment. Use with caution in patients with a history of penicillin allergy, especially IgE-mediated reactions (eg, anaphylaxis, urticaria).

Chewable tablets contain phenylalanine.

Benzyl alcohol and derivatives: Some dosage forms may contain sodium benzoate/benzoic acid; benzoic acid (benzoate) is a metabolite of benzyl alcohol; large amounts of benzyl alcohol (≥99 mg/kg/day) have been associated with a potentially fatal toxicity ("gasping syndrome") in neonates; the "gasping syndrome" consists of metabolic acidosis, respiratory distress, gasping respirations, CNS dysfunction (including convulsions, intracranial hemorrhage), hypotension, and cardiovascular collapse (AAP, 1997; CDC, 1982); some data suggests that benzoate displaces bilirubin from protein binding sites (Ahlfors, 2001); avoid or use dosage forms containing benzyl alcohol derivative with caution in neonates. See manufacturer's labeling.

Warnings: Additional Pediatric Considerations May cause diarrhea; reported incidence (~16%) similar in children receiving oral suspension and adults receiving tablet dosage form. Use caution when interchanging product formulations; oral suspension and chewable tablets are bioequivalent but oral immediate release tablets are not bioequivalent; for some infections (eg, otitis media), dosing recommendations are product specific.

Adverse Reactions

Gastrointestinal: Abdominal pain, diarrhea, dyspepsia, flatulence, loose stools, nausea

Rare but important or life-threatening: Acute renal failure, anaphylactoid reaction, anaphylaxis, angioedema, candidiasis, dizziness, drug fever, eosinophilia, erythema multiforme, facial edema, fever, headache, hepatitis, hyperbilirubinemia, increased blood urea nitrogen, increased serum creatinine, increased serum transaminases, jaundice, leukopenia, neutropenia, prolonged prothrombin time, pruritus, pseudomembranous colitis, seizure, serum sickness-like reaction, skin rash, Stevens-Johnson syndrome, thrombocytopenia, toxic epidermal necrolysis, urticaria, vaginitis, vomiting

Drug Interactions

Metabolism/Transport Effects None known.

Avoid Concomitant Use

Avoid concomitant use of Cefixime with any of the following: BCG; BCG (Intravesical)

Increased Effect/Toxicity

Cefixime may increase the levels/effects of: Aminoglycosides; Vitamin K Antagonists

The levels/effects of Cefixime may be increased by: Probenecid

Decreased Effect

Cefixime may decrease the levels/effects of: BCG; BCG (Intravesical); BCG Vaccine (Immunization); Sodium Picosulfate; Typhoid Vaccine

Food Interactions Food delays cefixime absorption. Management: May administer with or without food.

Storage/Stability

Capsule, chewable tablet, tablet: Store at 20°C to 25°C (68°F to 77°F).

Powder for suspension: Prior to reconstitution, store at 20°C to 25°C (68°F to 77°F). After reconstitution, suspension may be stored for 14 days at room temperature or under refrigeration.

Mechanism of Action Inhibits bacterial cell wall synthesis by binding to one or more of the penicillin-binding proteins (PBPs); which in turn inhibits the final transpeptidation step of peptidoglycan synthesis in bacterial cell walls, thus inhibiting cell wall biosynthesis. Bacteria eventually lyse due to ongoing activity of cell wall autolytic enzymes (autolysins and murein hydrolases) while cell wall assembly is arrested.

Pharmacokinetics (Adult data unless noted) Note: Chewable tablets and oral suspension are bioequivalent. However, oral suspension and tablet (nonchewable)/capsule formulations are **not** considered bioequivalent (in normal adult volunteers, oral suspension AUC ~10% to 25% greater compared with tablet after doses of 100-400 mg).

Absorption: Oral: 40% to 50%; capsule AUC reduced by ~15% and C_{max} by ~25% when taken with food

Distribution: Widely distributed throughout the body and reaches therapeutic concentration in most tissues and body fluids, including synovial, pericardial, pleural, peritoneal; bile, sputum, and urine; bone, myocardium, gallbladder, and skin and soft tissue

Protein binding: 65%

Half-life:

Normal renal function: 3-4 hours

Renal impairment: Up to 11.5 hours

Time to peak serum concentration: Tablet/suspension: 2-6 hours; capsules: 3-8 hours (delayed with food)

Elimination: Urine (50% of absorbed dose as active drug); feces (10%)

Dosing: Usual

Infants, Children, and Adolescents: **Note:** Unless otherwise specified, any dosage form may be used.

General dosing; susceptible infection (mild-moderate): Oral:

Weight-based:

Infants and Children weighing ≤45 kg: 8 mg/kg/day divided every 12-24 hours; maximum daily dose: 400 mg/**day** (*Red Book*, 2012)

Children weighing >45 kg and Adolescents: 400 mg daily

Fixed dosing: Infants ≥6 months and Children weighing ≤45 kg:

5 to <7.6 kg: 50 mg daily
7.6 to <10.1 kg: 80 mg daily
10.1 to <12.6 kg: 100 mg daily
12.6 to <20.6 kg: 150 mg daily
20.6 to <28.1 kg: 200 mg daily
28.1 to <33.1 kg: 250 mg daily
33.1 to <40.1 kg: 300 mg daily
40.1 to ≤45 kg: 350 mg daily

Febrile neutropenia (low-risk): Limited data available: Oral: Oral suspension: 8 mg/kg/day in divided doses every 12-24 hours; in most trials, cefixime therapy was initiated as step-down therapy after 48-72 hours of empiric parenteral antibiotic therapy with first cefixime dose administered at the end of the last IV infusion (Klassen, 2000; Lehrnbecher, 2012; Paganini, 2000; Shenep, 2001). **Note:** In clinical trials, doses were repeated if patient vomited within 2 hours.

Gonococcal infection, uncomplicated: Children ≥45 kg and Adolescents: 400 mg as a single dose in combination with oral azithromycin (preferred) or oral doxycycline (CDC, 2010). **Note:** CDC no longer recommends cefixime as a first-line agent, only use as an alternative agent with test-of-cure follow up in 7 days (CDC, 2012). In Canada, due to increased antimicrobial resistance, the recommended dose is 800 mg as a single dose for treatment of uncomplicated gonococcal infections in pediatric patients ≥9 years of age (Public Health Agency of Canada, 2012).

Irinotecan-associated diarrhea, prophylaxis: Limited data available: Oral: 8 mg/kg once daily; begin 5 days before oral irinotecan therapy and continue throughout course (Wagner, 2008)

Otitis media, acute: Oral: Oral suspension or chewable tablets:

- Infants and Children weighing ≤45 kg: 8 mg/kg/day divided every 12-24 hours; maximum daily dose: 400 mg/**day**
- Children >45 kg or Adolescents: 400 mg daily in divided doses every 12-24 hours

Pharyngitis or tonsillitis; *S. pyogenes*: Oral: **Note:** Not preferred for treatment in IDSA Guidelines due to unnecessary broad spectrum, and lack of selectivity for antibiotic resistant flora (Schulman, 2012)

- Infants and Children weighing ≤45 kg: 8 mg/kg/day in divided doses every 12-24 hours for ≥10 days; maximum daily dose: 400 mg/day
- Children weighing >45 kg and Adolescents: 400 mg daily in divided doses every 12-24 hours

Pneumonia, community-acquired (CAP); *haemophilus influenza* types A-F or nontypeable; mild infection or step-down therapy: Infants ≥3 months, Children, and Adolescents: Oral: 8 mg/kg/day in divided doses every 12-24 hours; maximum daily dose: 400 mg/**day**(IDSA/PIDS [Bradley, 2011]) *Red Book*, 2012)

Rhinosinusitis, acute bacterial: Oral: 4 mg/kg/dose every 12 hours with concomitant clindamycin for 10-14 days; maximum daily dose: 400 mg/**day**. **Note:** Recommended in patients with non-type I penicillin allergy, after failure of initial therapy or in patients at risk for antibiotic resistance (eg, daycare attendance, age <2 years, recent hospitalization, antibiotic use within the past month) (Chow, 2012).

Sexual victimization, prophylaxis: Children weighing ≥ 45 kg and Adolescents: Oral: 400 mg **plus** azithromycin or doxycycline and completion of hepatitis B virus immunization and consider prophylaxis for trichomoniasis and bacterial vaginosis (*Red Book*, 2012)

Typhoid fever (*Salmonella typhi*): Limited data available; efficacy results variable: Oral: 7.5-10 mg/kg/dose every 12 hours for 7-14 days (Girgis, 1995; Cao, 1999; Stephens, 2002)

Urinary tract infection; acute: Oral:

- Manufacturer 's labeling:
  - Infants ≥6 months and Children weighing ≤45 kg: 8 mg/kg/day in divided doses every 12-24 hours
  - Children weighing >45 kg and Adolescents: 400 mg daily in divided doses every 12-24 hours
- Alternate dosing: Infants and Children ≤2 years: Initial: 8 mg/kg/day every 24 hours for 7-14 days; in patients <24 months, shorter courses (1-3 days) have been shown to be inferior to longer durations of therapy (AAP, 2011)

Adults:

General dosing; susceptible infections: Oral: 400 mg daily in divided doses every 12-24 hours

Gonococcal infection, uncomplicated cervical/urethral/rectal gonorrhea due to *N. gonorrhoeae*: Oral: 400 mg as a single dose in combination with oral azithromycin (preferred) or oral doxycycline (CDC, 2010). **Note:** CDC no longer recommends cefixime as a first-line agent (ceftriaxone is the preferred cephalosporin), if cefixime is used as an alternative agent, test-of-cure follow up in 7 days is recommended; in addition, cefixime is **not** an option for the treatment of uncomplicated gonorrhea of the pharynx (CDC, 2012). In Canada, due to increased antimicrobial resistance, the Public Health Agency of Canada recommends 800 mg as a single dose for treatment of uncomplicated gonococcal infections.

Gonococcal infection, expedited partner therapy: Oral: 400 mg as a single dose in combination with oral azithromycin (CDC, 2012). **Note:** Only used if a heterosexual partner cannot be linked to evaluation and treatment in a timely manner; dose delivered to partner by patient, collaborating pharmacy, or disease investigation specialist.

***S. pyogenes* infections:** Oral: 400 mg daily in divided doses every 12-24 hours for 10 days

Dosing adjustment in renal impairment:

- Infants ≥6 months, Children, and Adolescents: Very limited data available; some clinicians have suggested the following (Daschner, 2005; Dhib, 1991; Guay, 1986):
  - Mild to moderate impairment: No adjustment recommended
  - Severe impairment (GFR ≤10-20 mL/minute/1.73 m^2): Reduce dose by 50%
  - Anuric: Reduce dose by 50%
  - Hemodialysis, peritoneal dialysis: Not significantly removed
- Adults: Manufacturer's labeling:
  - CrCl ≥60 mL/minute: No adjustment required
  - CrCl 21-59 mL/minute: 260 mg once daily
  - CrCl <20 mL/minute:
    - Chewable tablet, tablet: 200 mg once daily
    - 100 mg/5 mL suspension: 172 mg once daily
    - 200 mg/5 mL suspension: 176 mg once daily
    - 500 mg/5 mL suspension: 180 mg once daily
  - Intermittent hemodialysis: Not significantly removed: 260 mg once daily
  - CAPD: Not significantly removed by peritoneal dialysis
    - Chewable tablet, tablet: 200 mg once daily
    - 100 mg/5 mL suspension: 172 mg once daily
    - 200 mg/5 mL suspension: 176 mg once daily
    - 500 mg/5 mL suspension: 180 mg once daily

Dosing adjustment in hepatic impairment: There are no dosage adjustments provided in the manufacturer's labeling.

Preparation for Administration Oral: Powder for suspension: Reconstitute powder for oral suspension with appropriate amount of water as specified on the bottle. Shake vigorously until suspended.

Administration Oral: May be administered with or without food; administer with food to decrease GI distress; shake suspension well before use; chewable tablets must be chewed or crushed before swallowing.

Monitoring Parameters With prolonged therapy, monitor renal and hepatic function periodically; number and type of stools/day for diarrhea. Observe for signs and symptoms of anaphylaxis during first dose. When used as part of alternative treatment for gonococcal infection, test-of-cure 7 days after dose (CDC, 2012).

Test Interactions Positive direct Coombs', false-positive urinary glucose test using cupric sulfate (Benedict's solution, Clinitest®, Fehling's solution), may cause false-positive serum or urine creatinine with the alkaline picrate-based Jaffé reaction for measuring creatinine; false-positive urine ketones using tests with nitroprusside (but not those using nitroferricyanide).

Product Availability Suprax 400 mg tablets have been discontinued in the US for more than 1 year.

Dosage Forms Excipient information presented when available (limited, particularly for generics); consult specific product labeling. [DSC] = Discontinued product

Capsule, Oral:
- Suprax: 400 mg

Suspension Reconstituted, Oral:
- Suprax: 100 mg/5 mL (50 mL) [strawberry flavor]
- Suprax: 200 mg/5 mL (50 mL, 75 mL); 500 mg/5 mL (10 mL, 20 mL) [contains sodium benzoate; strawberry flavor]
- Generic: 100 mg/5 mL (50 mL); 200 mg/5 mL (50 mL, 75 mL)

Tablet, Oral:
- Suprax: 400 mg [DSC] [scored]

Tablet Chewable, Oral:
- Suprax: 100 mg, 200 mg [contains aspartame, fd&c red #40 aluminum lake; tutti-frutti flavor]

◆ **Cefixime Trihydrate** *see* Cefixime *on page* 395

◆ **Cefotan** *see* CefoTEtan *on page* 400

Cefotaxime (sef oh TAKS eem)

Medication Safety Issues

Sound-alike/look-alike issues:

Cefotaxime may be confused with cefOXitin, cefuroxime

International issues:

Spectrocef [Italy] may be confused with Spectracef brand name for cefditoren [U.S., Great Britain, Mexico, Portugal, Spain]

Brand Names: US Claforan; Claforan in D5W

Brand Names: Canada Cefotaxime Sodium For Injection; Claforan

Therapeutic Category Antibiotic, Cephalosporin (Third Generation)

Generic Availability (US) May be product dependent

Use Treatment of susceptible lower respiratory tract, skin and skin structure, bone and joint, intra-abdominal, genitourinary tract, and gynecologic infections, bactermia/septicemia and documented or suspected central nervous system infections (eg, meningitis, ventriculitis) (FDA approved in all ages); prevention of postoperative surgical site infection in contaminated or potentially contaminated surgical procedures [eg, gastrointestinal and genitourinary tract surgeries and hysterectomy (abdominal or vaginal)] and caesarian section (FDA approved in all ages)

Pregnancy Risk Factor B

Pregnancy Considerations Adverse events have not been observed in animal reproduction studies. Cefotaxime crosses the human placenta and can be found in fetal tissue. An increase in most types of birth defects was not found following first trimester exposure to cephalosporins. During pregnancy, peak cefotaxime serum concentrations are decreased and the serum half-life is shorter. Cefotaxime is approved for use in women undergoing cesarean section (consult current guidelines for appropriate use).

Breast-Feeding Considerations Low concentrations of cefotaxime are found in breast milk. The manufacturer recommends that caution be exercised when administering cefotaxime to nursing women. Nondose-related effects could include modification of bowel flora. The pregnancy-related changes in cefotaxime pharmacokinetics continue into the early postpartum period.

Contraindications Hypersensitivity to cefotaxime, any component of the formulation, or other cephalosporins

Warnings/Precautions A potentially life-threatening arrhythmia has been reported in patients who received a rapid (<1 minute) bolus injection via central venous catheter. Granulocytopenia and more rarely agranulocytosis may develop during prolonged treatment (>10 days). Minimize tissue inflammation by changing infusion sites when needed. Use with caution in patients with a history of penicillin allergy, especially IgE-mediated reactions (eg, anaphylaxis, urticaria). Prolonged use may result in fungal or bacterial superinfection, including *C. difficile*-associated diarrhea (CDAD) and pseudomembranous colitis; CDAD has been observed >2 months postantibiotic treatment. Use with caution in patients with renal impairment; dosage adjustment may be required. Use with caution in patients with a history of colitis. Potentially significant drug-drug interactions may exist, requiring dose or frequency adjustment, additional monitoring, and/or selection of alternative therapy.

Adverse Reactions

Dermatologic: Pruritus, skin rash

Gastrointestinal: Colitis, diarrhea, nausea, vomiting

Hematologic & oncologic: Eosinophilia

Local: Induration at injection site (IM), inflammation at injection site (IV), pain at injection site (IM), tenderness at injection site (IM)

Miscellaneous: Fever

Rare but important or life-threatening: Acute generalized exanthematous pustulosis, acute renal failure, agranulocytosis, anaphylaxis, bone marrow failure, brain disease, candidiasis, cardiac arrhythmia (after rapid IV injection via central catheter), cholestasis, *Clostridium difficile* associated diarrhea, erythema multiforme, granulocytopenia, hemolytic anemia, hepatitis, increased blood urea nitrogen, increased gamma-glutamyl transferase, increased lactate dehydrogenase, increased serum alkaline phosphatase, increased serum ALT, increased serum AST, increased serum bilirubin, increased serum creatinine, injection site phlebitis, interstitial nephritis, jaundice, leukopenia, neutropenia, pancytopenia, positive direct Coombs test, pseudomembranous colitis, Stevens-Johnson syndrome, thrombocytopenia, toxic epidermal necrolysis, vaginitis

Drug Interactions

Metabolism/Transport Effects None known.

Avoid Concomitant Use

Avoid concomitant use of Cefotaxime with any of the following: BCG; BCG (Intravesical)

Increased Effect/Toxicity

Cefotaxime may increase the levels/effects of: Aminoglycosides; Vitamin K Antagonists

The levels/effects of Cefotaxime may be increased by: Probenecid

Decreased Effect

Cefotaxime may decrease the levels/effects of: BCG; BCG (Intravesical); BCG Vaccine (Immunization); Sodium Picosulfate; Typhoid Vaccine

Storage/Stability Store intact vials below 30°C (86°F). Protect from light. Reconstituted solution is stable for 12 to 24 hours at room temperature, 7 to 10 days when refrigerated, for 13 weeks when frozen. For IV infusion in NS or D_5W, solution is stable for 24 hours at room temperature, 5 days when refrigerated, or 13 weeks when frozen in Viaflex plastic containers. Thawed solutions of frozen premixed bags are stable for 24 hours at room temperature or 10 days when refrigerated.

Mechanism of Action Inhibits bacterial cell wall synthesis by binding to one or more of the penicillin-binding proteins (PBPs) which in turn inhibits the final transpeptidation step of peptidoglycan synthesis in bacterial cell walls, thus inhibiting cell wall biosynthesis. Bacteria eventually lyse due to ongoing activity of cell wall autolytic enzymes (autolysins and murein hydrolases) while cell wall assembly is arrested. Cefotaxime has activity in the presence of some beta-lactamases, both penicillinases and cephaolsporinases, of gram-negative and gram-positive bacteria. *Enterococcus* species may be intrinsically resistant to cefotaxime. Most extended-spectrum beta-lactamase (ESBL)-producing and carbapenemase-producing isolates are resistant to cefotaxime.

Pharmacokinetics (Adult data unless noted)

Distribution: Into bronchial secretions, middle ear effusions, bone, bile; penetration into CSF when meninges are inflamed

Protein binding: 31% to 50%

Metabolism: Partially metabolized in the liver to active metabolite, desacetylcefotaxime

Half-life:

- Cefotaxime:
  - Neonates, birth weight ≤1500 g: 4.6 hours
  - Neonates, birth weight >1500 g: 3.4 hours
  - Children: 1.5 hours
  - Adults: 1-1.5 hours (prolonged with renal and/or hepatic impairment)
- Desacetylcefotaxime: 1.5-1.9 hours (prolonged with renal impairment)

Time to peak serum concentration: IM: Within 30 minutes

Elimination: Urine (~60% as unchanged drug and metabolites in urine)

Dialysis: Moderately dialyzable (20% to 50%)

Dosing: Neonatal

General dosing, susceptible infection: IM, IV (*Red Book*, 2012):

- Body weight <1 kg:
  - PNA ≤14 days: 50 mg/kg/dose every 12 hours
  - PNA 15-28 days: 50 mg/kg/dose every 8-12 hours
- Body weight 1-2 kg:
  - PNA ≤7 days: 50 mg/kg/dose every 12 hours
  - PNA 8-28 days: 50 mg/kg/dose every 8-12 hours
- Body weight >2 kg:
  - PNA ≤7 days: 50 mg/kg/dose every 12 hours
  - PNA 8-28 days: 50 mg/kg/dose every 8 hours; in some cases, every 6 hours dosing has been used

Gonococcal infection:

- Disseminated or scalp abscess: IM, IV: 25 mg/kg/dose every 12 hours for 7 days; therapy should be extended to 10-14 days if meningitis is documented (CDC, 2010)
- Ophthalmia neonatorum: IM, IV: 100 mg/kg as a single dose (*Red Book*, 2012)

Meningitis (Tunkel, 2004): IV: **Note:** Treat for a minimum of 21 days; use smaller doses and longer intervals for neonates <2 kg.

- PNA ≤7 days and ≥2 kg: 100-150 mg/kg/**day** divided every 8-12 hours
- PNA >7days and ≥2 kg: 150-200 mg/kg/**day** divided every 6-8 hours

Dosing: Usual

Infants, Children, and Adolescents:

General dosing, susceptible infection: Infants, Children and Adolescents: IM, IV:

- AAP recommendations (*Red Book*, 2012):
  - Mild to moderate infection: 50-180 mg/kg/**day** in divided doses every 6-8 hours; maximum daily dose: 6 **g/day**
  - Severe infection: 200-225 mg/kg/day in divided doses every 4-6 hours; up to 300 mg/kg/**day** has been used for meningitis; maximum daily dose: 12 **g/day**
- Manufacturer labeling:
  - <50 kg: 50-180 mg/kg/**day** divided every 4-6 hours
  - ≥50 kg:
    - Uncomplicated infections: IM, IV: 1000 mg every 12 hours
    - Moderate to severe infections: IM, IV: 1000-2000 mg every 8 hours
    - Life-threatening infections: IV: 2000 mg every 4 hours, maximum daily dose: 12 **g/day**

Acute bacterial rhinosinusitis, severe infection requiring hospitalization: Children and Adolescents: IV: 100-200 mg/kg/**day** divided every 6 hours for 10-14 days; maximum dose: 2000 mg (Chow, 2012)

Enteric bacterial infections, empiric treatment (HIV-exposed/-positive): Adolescents: IV: 1000 mg every 8 hours (DHHS [adult], 2013)

Gonorrhea (as an alternative to ceftriaxone) (CDC, 2010; CDC, 2012): Children weighing ≥45 kg and Adolescents:

- Uncomplicated gonorrhea of the cervix, urethra, or rectum: IM: 500 mg as a single dose in combination with oral azithromycin or oral doxycycline
- Disseminated: IV: 1 g every 8 hours for a total duration of at least 7 days

Intra-abdominal infection, complicated: Infants, Children, and Adolescents: IV: 150-200 mg/kg/**day** divided every 6-8 hours; maximum dose: 2000 mg; use in combination with metronidazole (Solomkin, 2010)

Lyme disease, cardiac or CNS manifestations or recurrent arthritis: Infants, Children, and Adolescents: IV: 150-200 mg/kg/**day** in divided doses every 6-8 hours for 14-28 days; maximum daily dose: 6 **g/day** (Halperin, 2007; *Red Book*, 2012; Wormser, 2006)

Meningitis: Infants, Children, and Adolescents: IV: 225-300 mg/kg/**day** divided every 6-8 hours; maximum dose: 2000 mg; use in combination with vancomycin for empiric coverage (*Red Book*, 2012; Tunkel, 2004)

Peritonitis (CAPD) (Warady, 2012): Infants, Children, and Adolescents: Intraperitoneal:

- Intermittent: 30 mg/kg/dose every 24 hours
- Continuous: Loading dose: 500 mg per liter of dialysate; maintenance dose: 250 mg per liter; **Note:** 125 mg/liter has also been recommended as a maintenance dose (Aronoff, 2007)

Pneumonia:

- *Bacterial pneumonia (HIV-exposed/-positive):* IV: 150-200 mg/kg/**day** divided every 6-8 hours; maximum single dose: 2000 mg (DHHS, 2013; DHHS [adult and pediatric], 2013); consider more frequent dosing for severe or life-threatening infections (every 4-6 hours) (*Red Book*, 2012)
- *Community-acquired pneumonia (CAP):* Infants >3 months, Children, and Adolescents: IV: 50 mg/kg/dose every 8 hours; maximum dose: 2000 mg; **Note:** May consider addition of vancomycin or clindamycin to empiric therapy if community-acquired MRSA suspected. In children ≥5 years, a macrolide antibiotic should be added if atypical pneumonia cannot be ruled out (Bradley, 2011).

Salmonellosis (HIV-exposed/-positive): Adolescents: IV: 1000 mg every 8 hours (DHHS [adult], 2013)

Surgical prophylaxis: Children and Adolescents: IV: 50 mg/kg 30-60 minutes prior to the procedure; may repeat in 3 hours; maximum dose: 1000 mg (Bratzler, 2013)

Urinary tract infection: Infants and Children 2-24 months: IM, IV: 150 mg/kg/day divided every 6-8 hours (AAP, 2011)

Adults:

Usual dosage range: IM, IV: 1000-2000 mg every 4-12 hours

- Uncomplicated infections: IM, IV: 1000 mg every 12 hours
- Moderate to severe infections: IM, IV: 1000-2000 mg every 8 hours
- Life-threatening infections: IV: 2000 mg every 4 hours

Caesarean section: IM, IV: 1000 mg as soon as the umbilical cord is clamped, then 1000 mg at 6- and 12-hour intervals

Gonorrhea (CDC, 2010):

- Uncomplicated gonorrhea of the cervix, urethra, or rectum: IM: 500 mg as a single dose in combination with oral azithromycin or oral doxycycline; may also administer 1000 mg as a single dose for rectal gonorrhea in males (per manufacturer labeling)
- Disseminated: IV: 1000 mg every 8 hours for a total duration of at least 7 days

Sepsis: IV: 2000 mg every 6-8 hours

Dosing adjustment in renal impairment:

Infants, Children, and Adolescents: The following adjustments have been recommended (Aronoff, 2007). **Note:** Renally adjusted dose recommendations are based on doses of 100-200 mg/kg/**day** divided every 8 hours.

GFR 30-50 mL/minute/1.73 m^2: 35-70 mg/kg/dose every 8-12 hours

GFR 10-29 mL/minute/1.73 m^2: 35-70 mg/kg/dose every 12 hours

GFR <10 mL/minute/1.73 m^2: 35-70 mg/kg/dose every 24 hours

Intermittent hemodialysis: 35-70 mg/kg/dose every 24 hours

Peritoneal dialysis (PD): 35-70 mg/kg/dose every 24 hours

Continuous renal replacement therapy (CRRT): 35-70 mg/kg/dose every 12 hours

Adults:

Manufacturer's labeling: **Note:** Renal function may be estimated using Cockcroft-Gault formula for dosage adjustment purposes.

CrCl <20 mL/minute/1.73 m^2: Dose should be decreased by 50%.

Alternate Dosing: The following dosage adjustments have been recommended:

GFR >50 mL/minute: Administer every 6 hours (Aronoff, 2007)

GFR 10-50 mL/minute: Administer every 6-12 hours (Aronoff, 2007)

GFR <10 mL/minute: Administer every 24 hours **or** decrease the dose by 50% (and administer at usual intervals) (Aronoff, 2007)

Intermittent hemodialysis (IHD): 1-2 g every 24 hours (on dialysis days, administer after hemodialysis). **Note:** Dosing dependent on the assumption of 3 times/week, complete IHD sessions (Heintz, 2009).

Peritoneal dialysis (PD): 1 g every 24 hours (Aronoff, 2007)

Continuous renal replacement therapy (CRRT) (Heintz, 2009; Trotman, 2005): Drug clearance is highly dependent on the method of renal replacement, filter type, and flow rate. Appropriate dosing requires close monitoring of pharmacologic response, signs of adverse reactions due to drug accumulation, as well as drug concentrations in relation to target trough (if appropriate). The following are general recommendations only (based on dialysate flow/ultrafiltration rates of 1-2 L/hour and minimal residual renal function) and should not supersede clinical judgment:

CVVH: 1-2 g every 8-12 hours

CVVHD: 1-2 g every 8 hours

CVVHDF: 1-2 g every 6-8 hours

Preparation for Administration Parenteral:

IM: Reconstitute powder for injection with SWFI to a final concentration between 230 to 330 mg/mL (see manufacturer labeling for specific details). Shake to dissolve.

IV:

IVP: Reconstitute vials with at least 10 mL SWFI to a maximum concentration of 200 mg/mL.

Intermittent infusion: Reconstitute powder for injection with SWFI, resultant concentration dependent upon product (single dose vials or Pharmacy Bulk vial; see manufacturer labeling for specific details). Dilute dose to a final concentration of 10 to 40 mg/mL with NS, D_5W, $D_{10}W$, D_5NS, $D_5{}^{1/2}NS$, $D_5{}^{1/4}NS$, or LR; some centers have used concentrations up to 60 mg/mL.

Administration Parenteral:

IM: Administer by deep IM injection into a large muscle mass such as the upper outer quadrant of the gluteus maximus. Doses of 2,000 mg should be divided and administered at two different sites.

IV:

IVP: May be administered over 3 to 5 minutes; avoid rapid injection (<1 minute) due to association with arrhythmias

Intermittent infusion: Infuse over 15 to 30 minutes.

Monitoring Parameters Observe for signs and symptoms of anaphylaxis during first dose; monitor infusion site for extravasation; with prolonged therapy, monitor renal, hepatic, and hematologic function periodically; number and type of stools/day for diarrhea

Test Interactions Positive direct Coombs', false-positive urinary glucose test using cupric sulfate (Benedict's solution, Clinitest®, Fehling's solution), false-positive serum or urine creatinine with Jaffé reaction

Dosage Forms Excipient information presented when available (limited, particularly for generics); consult specific product labeling.

Solution, Intravenous:

Claforan in D5W: 1 g/50 mL (50 mL); 2 g/50 mL (50 mL)

Solution Reconstituted, Injection:

Claforan: 500 mg (1 ea); 1 g (1 ea); 2 g (1 ea); 10 g (1 ea)

Generic: 500 mg (1 ea); 1 g (1 ea); 2 g (1 ea); 10 g (1 ea)

Solution Reconstituted, Intravenous:

Claforan: 1 g (1 ea); 2 g (1 ea)

◆ **Cefotaxime Sodium** *see* Cefotaxime *on page 398*

◆ **Cefotaxime Sodium For Injection (Can)** *see* Cefotaxime *on page 398*

CefoTEtan (SEF oh tee tan)

Medication Safety Issues

Sound-alike/look-alike issues:

CefoTEtan may be confused with ceFAZolin, cefOXitin, cefTAZidime, Ceftin®, cefTRIAXone

Therapeutic Category Antibiotic, Cephalosporin (Second Generation)

Generic Availability (US) Yes

Use Treatment of susceptible lower respiratory tract, skin and skin structure, bone and joint, urinary tract, gynecologic, and intra-abdominal infections (FDA approved in adults); surgical prophylaxis (FDA approved in adults)

Pregnancy Risk Factor B

Pregnancy Considerations Adverse events have not been observed in animal reproduction studies. Cefotetan crosses the placenta and produces therapeutic concentrations in the amniotic fluid and cord serum. Cefotetan is one of the antibiotics recommended for prophylactic use prior to cesarean delivery.

Breast-Feeding Considerations Very small amounts of cefotetan are excreted in human milk. The manufacturer recommends caution when giving cefotetan to a breast-feeding mother. Nondose-related effects could include modification of bowel flora.

Contraindications Hypersensitivity to cefotetan, any component of the formulation, or other cephalosporins; previous cephalosporin-associated hemolytic anemia

Warnings/Precautions Modify dosage in patients with severe renal impairment. Although cefotetan contains the methyltetrazolethiol side chain, bleeding has not been a significant problem. Use with caution in patients with a history of penicillin allergy, especially IgE-mediated reactions (eg, anaphylaxis, urticaria). Cefotetan has been associated with a higher risk of hemolytic anemia relative to other cephalosporins (approximately threefold); monitor carefully during use and consider cephalosporin-associated immune anemia in patients who have received cefotetan within 2-3 weeks (either as treatment or prophylaxis). Prolonged use may result in fungal or bacterial superinfection, including *C. difficile*-associated diarrhea (CDAD) and pseudomembranous colitis; CDAD has been observed >2 months postantibiotic treatment. May be associated with increased INR, especially in nutritionally-deficient patients, prolonged treatment, hepatic or renal disease.

Adverse Reactions

Gastrointestinal: Diarrhea

Hepatic: Transaminases increased

Miscellaneous: Hypersensitivity reactions

Rare but important or life-threatening: Agranulocytosis, anaphylaxis, bleeding, BUN increased, creatinine increased, eosinophilia, fever, hemolytic anemia, leukopenia, nausea, nephrotoxicity, phlebitis, prolonged PT, pruritus, pseudomembranous colitis, rash, thrombocytopenia, thrombocytosis, urticaria, vomiting

Reactions reported with other cephalosporins: Agranulocytosis, aplastic anemia, cholestasis, colitis, hemolytic anemia, hemorrhage, pancytopenia, renal dysfunction, seizure, Stevens-Johnson syndrome, superinfection, toxic epidermal necrolysis, toxic nephropathy

Drug Interactions

Metabolism/Transport Effects None known.

Avoid Concomitant Use

Avoid concomitant use of CefoTEtan with any of the following: BCG; BCG (Intravesical)

Increased Effect/Toxicity

CefoTEtan may increase the levels/effects of: Alcohol (Ethyl); Aminoglycosides; Carbocisteine; Vitamin K Antagonists

The levels/effects of CefoTEtan may be increased by: Probenecid

Decreased Effect

CefoTEtan may decrease the levels/effects of: BCG; BCG (Intravesical); BCG Vaccine (Immunization); Sodium Picosulfate; Typhoid Vaccine

Food Interactions Concurrent use with ethanol may cause a disulfiram-like reaction. Management: Monitor patients.

Storage/Stability Reconstituted solution is stable for 24 hours at room temperature and 96 hours when refrigerated. For IV infusion in NS or D_5W solution and after freezing, thawed solution is stable for 24 hours at room temperature or 96 hours when refrigerated. Frozen solution is stable for 12 weeks. Thawed solutions of the commercially available frozen cefotetan injections are stable for 48 hours at room temperature or 21 days when refrigerated.

Mechanism of Action Inhibits bacterial cell wall synthesis by binding to one or more of the penicillin-binding proteins (PBPs) which in turn inhibits the final transpeptidation step of peptidoglycan synthesis in bacterial cell walls, thus inhibiting cell wall biosynthesis. Bacteria eventually lyse due to ongoing activity of cell wall autolytic enzymes (autolysins and murein hydrolases) while cell wall assembly is arrested.

Pharmacokinetics (Adult data unless noted)

Absorption: IM: Completely absorbed

Distribution: Distributes into tissues and fluids including gallbladder, kidney, skin, tonsils, uterus, sputum, prostatic and peritoneal fluids; poor penetration into CSF

Protein binding: 88%

Half-life: 3-4.6 hours, prolonged in patients with moderately impaired renal function (up to 10 hours)

Time to peak serum concentration: IM: Within 1.5-3 hours

Elimination: 51% to 81% excreted as unchanged drug in urine, 20% of dose is excreted in bile

Dosing: Usual

Infants, Children, and Adolescents:

General dosing, susceptible infection (*Red Book*, 2012): IM, IV:

Mild to moderate infection: 30 mg/kg/dose every 12 hours, maximum single dose: 2000 mg

Severe infection: 50 mg/kg/dose every 12 hours; usual maximum single dose: 2000 mg; for life-threatening infections doses as high as 3000 mg every 12 hours have been used

Intra-abdominal infection, complicated: IV: 20-40 mg/kg/dose every 12 hours. **Note:** Due to high rates of *B. fragilis* group resistance, not recommended for the treatment of community-acquired intra-abdominal infections (Solomkin, 2010).

Pelvic inflammatory disease: Adolescents: IV: 2000 mg every 12 hours; used in combination with doxycycline (CDC, 2010)

Surgical prophylaxis: Children and Adolescents: IV: 40 mg/kg 60 minutes prior to procedure; may redose in 6 hours; maximum dose: 2000 mg (Bratzler, 2013)

Adults:

General dosing, susceptible infection: IM, IV: Usual dose: 1000-2000 mg every 12 hours for 5-10 days; 1000-2000 mg may be given every 24 hours for urinary tract infection; maximum single dose: 3000 mg. **Note:** Due to high rates of *B. fragilis* group resistance, not recommended for the treatment of community-acquired intra-abdominal infections (Solomkin, 2010).

Pelvic inflammatory disease: IV: 2000 mg every 12 hours; used in combination with doxycycline (CDC, 2010)

Surgical (perioperative) prophylaxis: IV: 1000-2000 mg 30-60 minutes prior to surgery; when used for cesarean section, dose should be given as soon as umbilical cord is clamped

Urinary tract infection: IM, IV: 500 mg every 12 hours or 1000-2000 mg every 12-24 hours

Dosage adjustment in renal impairment:

Infants, Children, and Adolescents: Dosage adjustments are not provided in the manufacturer's labeling; however, the following guidelines have been used by some clinicians (Aronoff, 2007); **Note:** Renally adjusted dose recommendations are based on doses of 20-40 mg/kg/dose every 12 hours:

GFR ≥30 mL/minute/1.73 m^2: No adjustment required.

GFR 10-29 mL/minute/1.73 m^2: 20-40 mg/kg/dose every 24 hours

GFR <10 mL/minute/1.73 m^2: 20-40 mg/kg/dose every 48 hours

Intermittent hemodialysis: 20-40 mg/kg/dose every 48 hours; give after dialysis on dialysis days

Peritoneal dialysis (PD): 20-40 mg/kg/dose every 48 hours

Continuous renal replacement therapy (CRRT): 20-40 mg/kg/dose every 12 hours

Adults:

CrCl >30 mL/minute: No adjustment required

CrCl 10-30 mL/minute: Administer every 24 hours

CrCl <10 mL/minute: Administer every 48 hours

Hemodialysis: Dialyzable (5% to 20%); administer 1/4 the usual dose every 24 hours on days between dialysis; administer 1/2 the usual dose on the day of dialysis

Dosage adjustment for hepatic impairment: There are no dosage adjustments provided in the manufacturer's labeling.

Preparation for Administration Parenteral:

IM: Reconstitute vial with SWFI, NS, lidocaine 0.5% or 1%, or bacteriostatic water for injection to a final concentration ≤500 mg/mL

IV intermittent: Further dilute reconstituted solution to a concentration of 10 to 40 mg/mL

IV push: Reconstitute with SWFI to a concentration ≤182 mg/mL

Administration

Parenteral:

IM: Inject deep IM into large muscle mass

IV intermittent: Infuse over 20 to 60 minutes

IV push: Inject direct IV over 3 to 5 minutes

Monitoring Parameters CBC, prothrombin time, renal function tests; number and type of stools/day for diarrhea; signs and symptoms of hemolytic anemia; monitor for signs of anaphylaxis during first dose

Test Interactions Positive direct Coombs', false-positive urinary glucose test using cupric sulfate (Benedict's solution, Clinitest®, Fehling's solution), false-positive serum or urine creatinine with Jaffé reaction

Additional Information Sodium content of 1000 mg: 3.5 mEq. Chemical structure contains a methyltetrazolethiol side chain which may be responsible for the disulfiram-like reaction with alcohol and increased risk of bleeding

Dosage Forms Excipient information presented when available (limited, particularly for generics); consult specific product labeling.

Solution Reconstituted, Injection:
Generic: 1 g (1 ea); 2 g (1 ea); 10 g (1 ea)

Solution Reconstituted, Intravenous:
Generic: 1 g (1 ea); 2 g (1 ea)

◆ **Cefotetan Disodium** *see* CefoTEtan *on page 400*

CefOXitin (se FOKS i tin)

Medication Safety Issues

Sound-alike/look-alike issues:

CefOXitin may be confused with ceFAZolin, cefotaxime, cefoTEtan, cefTAZidime, cefTRIAXone, Cytoxan

Mefoxin may be confused with Lanoxin

Brand Names: US Mefoxin

Brand Names: Canada Cefoxitin For Injection

Therapeutic Category Antibiotic, Cephalosporin (Second Generation)

Generic Availability (US) May be product dependent

Use Treatment of susceptible lower respiratory tract, skin and skin structure, bone and joint, genitourinary tract, sepsis, gynecologic, and intra-abdominal infections and surgical prophylaxis (FDA approved in ages ≥3 months and adults)

Pregnancy Risk Factor B

Pregnancy Considerations Adverse events have not been observed in animal reproduction studies. Cefoxitin crosses the placenta and reaches the cord serum and amniotic fluid.

Peak serum concentrations of cefoxitin during pregnancy may be similar to or decreased compared to nonpregnant values. Maternal half-life may be shorter at term. Pregnancy-induced hypertension increases trough concentrations in the immediate postpartum period. Cefoxitin is one of the antibiotics recommended for prophylactic use prior to cesarean delivery.

Breast-Feeding Considerations Very small amounts of cefoxitin are excreted in breast milk. The manufacturer recommends that caution be exercised when administering cefoxitin to nursing women. Nondose-related effects could include modification of bowel flora. Cefoxitin pharmacokinetics may be altered immediately postpartum.

Contraindications Hypersensitivity to cefoxitin, any component of the formulation, or other cephalosporins

Warnings/Precautions Modify dosage in patients with severe renal impairment. Prolonged use may result in superinfection. Use with caution in patients with a history of penicillin allergy, especially IgE-mediated hypersensitivity reactions (eg, anaphylaxis, urticaria). If a hypersensitivity reaction occurs, discontinue immediately. Use with caution in patients with a history of seizures or gastrointestinal disease (particularly colitis). Prolonged use may result in fungal or bacterial superinfection, including *C. difficile*-associated diarrhea (CDAD) and pseudomembranous colitis; CDAD has been observed >2 months post-antibiotic treatment. For group A beta-hemolytic streptococcal infections, antimicrobial therapy should be given for at least 10 days to guard against the risk of rheumatic fever or glomerulonephritis. In pediatric patients ≥3 months of age, higher doses have been associated with an increased incidence of eosinophilia and elevated AST. Elderly patients are more likely to have decreased renal function; use care in dose selection and monitor renal function.

Adverse Reactions

Gastrointestinal: Diarrhea

Rare but important or life-threatening: Anaphylaxis, angioedema, bone marrow depression, dyspnea, eosinophilia, exacerbation of myasthenia gravis, exfoliative dermatitis, fever, hemolytic anemia, hypotension, increased blood urea nitrogen, increased serum creatinine, increased serum transaminases, interstitial nephritis, jaundice, leukopenia, nausea, nephrotoxicity (increased; with aminoglycosides), phlebitis, prolonged prothrombin time, pruritus, pseudomembranous colitis, skin rash, thrombocytopenia, thrombophlebitis, toxic epidermal necrolysis, urticaria, vomiting

Drug Interactions

Metabolism/Transport Effects None known.

Avoid Concomitant Use

Avoid concomitant use of CefOXitin with any of the following: BCG; BCG (Intravesical)

Increased Effect/Toxicity

CefOXitin may increase the levels/effects of: Aminoglycosides; Vitamin K Antagonists

The levels/effects of CefOXitin may be increased by: Probenecid

Decreased Effect

CefOXitin may decrease the levels/effects of: BCG; BCG (Intravesical); BCG Vaccine (Immunization); Sodium Picosulfate; Typhoid Vaccine

Storage/Stability Prior to reconstitution store between 2°C and 25°C (36°F and 77°F). Avoid exposure to temperatures >50°C (122°F). Cefoxitin tends to darken depending on storage conditions; however, product potency is not adversely affected.

Reconstituted solutions of 1 g per 10 mL in sterile water for injection, bacteriostatic water for injection, sodium chloride 0.9% injection, or dextrose 5% injection are stable for 6 hours at room temperature or for 7 days under refrigeration (<5°C [43°F]).

DUPLEX container: Store unactivated container at 20°C to 25°C (68°F to 77°F); excursions permitted to 15°C to 30°C (59°F to 86°F); do not freeze. Following activation, solution is stable for 12 hours at room temperature and 7 days refrigerated.

Mechanism of Action Inhibits bacterial cell wall synthesis by binding to one or more of the penicillin-binding proteins (PBPs) which in turn inhibits the final transpeptidation step of peptidoglycan synthesis in bacterial cell walls, thus inhibiting cell wall biosynthesis. Bacteria eventually lyse due to ongoing activity of cell wall autolytic enzymes (autolysins and murein hydrolases) while cell wall assembly is arrested.

Pharmacokinetics (Adult data unless noted)

Distribution: Distributes into tissues and fluids including ascitic, pleural, bile, and synovial fluids; poor penetration into CSF even with inflamed meninges

Protein binding: 65% to 79%

Half-life:

Neonates and Infants (PNA: 10-53 days): 1.4 hours (Regazzi, 1983)

Adults: 45-60 minutes, increases significantly with renal insufficiency

Time to peak serum concentration: IM: Within 20-30 minutes

Elimination: Urine (85% as unchanged drug)

Dosing: Neonatal General dosing; susceptible infection: Limited data available: IV: 90-100 mg/kg/day divided every 8 hours (Regazzi, 1983; Roos, 1980)

Dosing: Usual

Infants, Children, and Adolescents: Limited data available for infants <3 months:

General dosing, susceptible infection (*Red Book*, 2012): IM, IV:

Mild-moderate infection: 80 mg/kg/day divided every 6-8 hours; maximum daily dose: 4000 mg/**day**

Severe infection: 160 mg/kg/day divided every 6 hours; maximum daily dose: 12 **g/day**

Manufacturer's labeling: Infants ≥3 months, Children, and Adolescents: 80-160 mg/kg/day divided every 4-6 hours; maximum daily dose: 12 **g/day**

Intra-abdominal infections, complicated: IV: 160 mg/kg/day divided every 4-6 hours; maximum daily dose: 8 **g/day** (Solomkin, 2010)

Surgical prophylaxis: IV:

Manufacturer's labeling: Infants ≥3 months, Children, and Adolescents: 30-40 mg/kg 30-60 minutes prior to initial incision, followed by 30-40 mg/kg every 6 hours for up to 24 hours; maximum single dose: 2000 mg

Alternate dosing (ASHP guidelines, endorsed by IDSA): Children and Adolescents: 40 mg/kg 30-60 minutes prior to surgery; may repeat in 2 hours; maximum single dose: 2000 mg [Bratzler, 2013; *Red Book* (AAP, 2012)]

Adults:

General dosing, susceptible infection: IM, IV: 1000-2000 mg every 6-8 hours; maximum daily dose: 12 **g/day**; **Note:** IM injection is painful.

Uncomplicated infections: 1000 mg every 6-8 hours

Moderately severe to severe infections: 1000 mg every 4 hours **or** 2000 mg every 6-8 hours

Infection needing higher dosages (eg, gas gangrene): 2000 mg every 4 hours or 3000 mg every 6 hours

Pelvic inflammatory disease (Workowski, 2010; *Red Book*, 2012):

Inpatients: IV: 2000 mg every 6 hours **plus** doxycycline 100 mg orally every 12 hours until improved, followed by doxycycline to complete 14 days

Outpatients: IM: 2000 mg **plus** probenecid as a single dose, followed by doxycycline for 14 days

Surgical prophylaxis: IM, IV: 2000 mg 30-60 minutes prior to surgery; may repeat in 2 hours intraoperatively (Bratzler, 2013), followed by 2000 mg every 6 hours for no more than 24 hours after surgery depending on the procedure.

Cesarean section: 2000 mg as a single dose administered as soon as the umbilical cord is clamped; may give an additional two doses at 4 and 8 hours after the initial dose.

Dosing adjustment in renal impairment:

Infants, Children, and Adolescents: The manufacturer's labeling suggests dosing modification consistent with the adult recommendations. Some clinicians have used the following guidelines (Aronoff, 2007): **Note:** Renally adjusted dose recommendations are based on doses of 20-40 mg/kg/dose every 6 hours.

GFR >50 mL/minute/1.73 m^2: No adjustment required.

GFR 30-50 mL/minute/1.73 m^2: 20-40 mg/kg/dose every 8 hours

GFR 10-29 mL/minute/1.73 m^2: 20-40 mg/kg/dose every 12 hours

GFR <10 mL/minute/1.73 m^2: 20-40 mg/kg/dose every 24 hours

Intermittent hemodialysis: Moderately dialyzable (20% to 50%): 20-40 mg/kg/dose every 24 hours

Peritoneal dialysis (PD): 20-40 mg/kg/dose every 24 hours

Continuous renal replacement therapy (CRRT): 20-40 mg/kg/dose every 8 hours

Adults: Initial loading dose of 1000-2000 mg, then:

CrCl >50 mL/minute: No adjustment required

CrCl 30-50 mL/minute: 1000-2000 mg every 8-12 hours

CrCl 10-29 mL/minute: 1000-2000 mg every 12-24 hours

CrCl 5-9 mL/minute: 500-1000 mg every 12-24 hours

CrCl <5 mL/minute: 500-1000 mg every 24-48 hours

Hemodialysis: Moderately dialyzable (20% to 50%): Loading dose of 1000-2000 mg after each hemodialysis; maintenance dose as noted above based on CrCl

Continuous arteriovenous or venovenous hemodiafiltration effects: 1000-2000 mg every 8-24 hours

Dosing adjustment in hepatic impairment: There are no dosage adjustments provided in the manufacturer's labeling.

Preparation for Administration Parenteral:

IVP: Reconstitute vials with SWFI, bacteriostatic water for injection, NS, or D_5W to a final concentration of 95 to180 mg/mL; see manufacturer's labeling for specific details.

Intermittent IV infusion: Reconstitute vials with SWFI, bacteriostatic water for injection, NS, or D_5W; see manufacturer's labeling for specific details. Further dilute to a final concentration not to exceed 40 mg/mL in NS, $D_5{}^1/_4$NS, $D_5{}^1/_2$NS, D_5NS, D_5W, $D_{10}W$, LR, D_5LR, mannitol 5% or 10%, or sodium bicarbonate 5%. In fluid restricted patients, a concentration of 125 mg/mL using SWFI results in a maximum recommended osmolality for peripheral infusion (Robinson 1987)

IM: Reconstitute vial with 1 to 2 mL of 0.5% or 1% lidocaine (McCloskey 1979; Sonneville 1977)

Administration Parenteral:

IVP: Administer over 3 to 5 minutes

Intermittent IV infusion: Administer over 10 to 60 minutes

IM: Deep IM injection into a large muscle mass such as the upper outer quadrant of the gluteus maximus. **Note:** IM injection is painful and this route of administration is not described in the prescribing information.

Monitoring Parameters Renal function periodically when used in combination with other nephrotoxic drugs; liver function and hematologic function tests; number and type of stools/day for diarrhea. Observe for signs and symptoms of anaphylaxis during first dose.

Test Interactions Positive direct Coombs', false-positive urinary glucose test using cupric sulfate (Benedict's solution, Clinitest®, Fehling's solution), false-positive serum or urine creatinine with Jaffé reaction

Dosage Forms Excipient information presented when available (limited, particularly for generics); consult specific product labeling.

Solution, Intravenous:

Mefoxin: 1 g (50 mL); 2 g (50 mL)

Solution Reconstituted, Injection:

Generic: 10 g (1 ea)

Solution Reconstituted, Injection [preservative free]:

Generic: 10 g (1 ea)

Solution Reconstituted, Intravenous:

Generic: 1 g (1 ea); 2 g (1 ea)

Solution Reconstituted, Intravenous [preservative free]:

Generic: 1 g (1 ea); 2 g (1 ea)

◆ **Cefoxitin For Injection (Can)** *see* CefOXitin *on page 402*

◆ **Cefoxitin Sodium** *see* CefOXitin *on page 402*

Cefpodoxime (sef pode OKS eem)

Medication Safety Issues

Sound-alike/look-alike issues:

Vantin may be confused with Ventolin

Therapeutic Category Antibiotic, Cephalosporin (Third Generation)

Generic Availability (US) Yes

Use Treatment of the following mild to moderate infections caused by susceptible organisms: Acute otitis media (FDA approved in 2 months to 12 years); pharyngitis or tonsillitis (FDA approved in ages ≥2 months and adults); acute maxillary sinusitis (FDA approved in ages ≥2 months and adults); community acquired pneumonia (FDA approved in ages ≥12 years and adults); acute, bacterial exacerbation of chronic bronchitis (FDA approved in ages ≥12 years and adults); acute uncomplicated urethral and cervical gonorrhea (FDA approved in ages ≥12 years and adults); anorectal gonorrhea (FDA approved in female patients ages ≥12 years and adult); uncomplicated skin and skin structure infections (FDA approved in ages ≥12 years and adults); and uncomplicated urinary tract infections (FDA approved in ages ≥12 years and adults)

Note: CDC no longer recommends oral cephalosporins as a first-line agent for treatment of gonorrhea and cefpodoxime is no longer listed as a recommended option for treatment (CDC 2012).

Pregnancy Risk Factor B

Pregnancy Considerations Teratogenic events were not observed in animal reproduction studies. An increase in most types of birth defects was not found following first trimester exposure to cephalosporins.

Breast-Feeding Considerations Cefpodoxime is excreted in breast milk. The manufacturer recommends discontinuing nursing or discontinuing the medication in breast-feeding women. Nondose-related effects could include modification of bowel flora.

Contraindications Hypersensitivity to cefpodoxime, any component of the formulation, or other cephalosporins

Warnings/Precautions Modify dosage in patients with severe renal impairment. Prolonged use may result in fungal or bacterial superinfection, including *C. difficile*-associated diarrhea (CDAD) and pseudomembranous colitis; CDAD has been observed >2 months postantibiotic treatment. Use with caution in patients with a history of beta-lactam allergy, especially IgE-mediated reactions (eg, anaphylaxis, urticaria).

Potentially significant drug-drug interactions may exist, requiring dose or frequency adjustment, additional monitoring, and/or selection of alternative therapy.

Benzyl alcohol and derivatives: Some dosage forms may contain sodium benzoate/benzoic acid; benzoic acid (benzoate) is a metabolite of benzyl alcohol; large amounts of benzyl alcohol (≥99 mg/kg/day) have been associated with a potentially fatal toxicity ("gasping syndrome") in neonates; the "gasping syndrome" consists of metabolic acidosis, respiratory distress, gasping respirations, CNS dysfunction (including convulsions, intracranial hemorrhage), hypotension, and cardiovascular collapse (AAP 1997; CDC 1982); some data suggests that benzoate displaces bilirubin from protein binding sites (Ahlfors 2001); avoid or use dosage forms containing benzyl alcohol derivative with caution in neonates. See manufacturer's labeling.

Adverse Reactions

Central nervous system: Headache

Dermatologic: Diaper rash, skin rash

Gastrointestinal: Abdominal pain, diarrhea, nausea, vomiting

Genitourinary: Vaginal infection

Rare but important or life-threatening: Anaphylaxis, anxiety, chest pain, cough, decreased appetite, dizziness dysgeusia, epistaxis, eye pruritus, fatigue, fever, flatulence, flushing, fungal skin infection, hypotension insomnia, malaise, nightmares, pruritus, pseudomembranous colitis, purpuric nephritis, tinnitus, vulvovaginal candidiasis, weakness, xerostomia

Drug Interactions

Metabolism/Transport Effects None known.

Avoid Concomitant Use

Avoid concomitant use of Cefpodoxime with any of the following: BCG; BCG (Intravesical)

Increased Effect/Toxicity

Cefpodoxime may increase the levels/effects of: Aminoglycosides; Vitamin K Antagonists

The levels/effects of Cefpodoxime may be increased by: Probenecid

Decreased Effect

Cefpodoxime may decrease the levels/effects of: BCG BCG (Intravesical); BCG Vaccine (Immunization) Sodium Picosulfate; Typhoid Vaccine

The levels/effects of Cefpodoxime may be decreased by: Antacids; H2-Antagonists

Food Interactions Food increases extent of absorption and peak concentration of tablets. Management: Take tablets with food.

Storage/Stability

Suspension: Store at 20°C to 25°C (68°F to 77°F); after reconstitution, suspension may be stored in refrigerator for 14 days.

Tablet: Store at 20°C to 25°C (68°F to 77°F); protect from light.

Mechanism of Action Inhibits bacterial cell wall synthesis by binding to one or more of the penicillin-binding proteins (PBPs) which in turn inhibits the final transpeptidation step of peptidoglycan synthesis in bacterial cell walls, thus inhibiting cell wall biosynthesis. Bacteria eventually lyse due to ongoing activity of cell wall autolytic enzymes (autolysins and murein hydrolases) while cell wall assembly is arrested.

Pharmacokinetics (Adult data unless noted)

Absorption: Tablet: Enhanced in the presence of food or low gastric pH; Oral suspension: Unaffected by food

Distribution: Good tissue penetration, including lung and tonsils; penetrates into pleural fluid

Protein binding: 22% to 33% (in serum); 21% to 29% (in plasma)

Metabolism: De-esterified in the GI tract to the active metabolite, cefpodoxime

Bioavailability: Oral: 50%

Half-life: 2.2 hours (prolonged with renal impairment)

Time to peak serum concentration: Tablets: Within 2 to 3 hours; Oral suspension: Slower in presence of food, 48% increase in T_{max}

Elimination: Urine (29% to 33% of administered dose as unchanged drug)

Dosing: Usual

Pediatric:

General dosing, susceptible infection: Mild to moderate infections: Infants, Children, and Adolescents: Oral: 5 mg/kg/dose every 12 hours; usual maximum dose: 200 mg/dose; however, in patients ≥12 years, higher doses (ie, 400 mg/dose) may be required for some types of infection (*Red Book* [AAP 2015]; Bradley 2015)

Bronchitis, bacterial exacerbation of chronic: Children ≥12 years and Adolescents: Oral: 200 mg every 12 hours for 10 days

Otitis media, acute: Infants and Children 2 months to 12 years: Oral: 5 mg/kg/dose every 12 hours; maximum dose: 200 mg/dose. Variable duration of therapy; the manufacturer suggests 5-day course in all patients, however, AAP guidelines recommend duration based on patient age: If <2 years of age or severe symptoms (any age): 10-day course; if 2 to 5 years of age with mild to moderate symptoms: 7-day course; if ≥6 years of age with mild to moderate symptoms: 5- to 7-day course (AAP [Lieberthal 2013]).

Pharyngitis/tonsillitis:

Infants ≥2 months and Children <12 years: Oral: 5 mg/kg/dose every 12 hours for 5 to 10 days; maximum dose: 100 mg/dose

Children ≥12 years and Adolescents: 100 mg every 12 hours for 5 to 10 days

Pneumonia, acute community-acquired:

Infants ≥3 months and Children <12 years: Limited data available: Oral: 5 mg/kg/dose every 12 hours; maximum dose: 200 mg/dose (Bradley 2015; IDSA [Bradley 2011])

Children ≥12 years and Adolescents: Oral: 200 mg every 12 hours for 14 days

Rhinosinusitis, acute maxillary:

Infants ≥2 months and Children <12 years: Oral: 5 mg/kg/dose every 12 hours for 10 days; maximum dose: 200 mg/dose; **Note:** IDSA recommends use in combination with clindamycin for 10 to 14 days in patients with nontype 1 penicillin allergy, after failure of initial therapy or in patients at risk for antibiotic resistance (eg, daycare attendance, age <2 years, recent hospitalization, antibiotic use within the past month) (Chow 2012).

Children ≥12 years and Adolescents: Oral: 200 mg every 12 hours for 10 days

Skin and skin structure: Children ≥12 years and Adolescents: Oral: 400 mg every 12 hours for 7 to 14 days

Urinary tract infection, uncomplicated: Children ≥12 years and Adolescents: Oral: 100 mg every 12 hours for 7 days

Adult:

Bronchitis, bacterial exacerbation of chronic: Oral: 200 mg every 12 hours for 10 days

Pharyngitis/tonsillitis: Oral: 100 mg every 12 hours for 5 to 10 days

Pneumonia, acute community-acquired: Oral: 200 mg every 12 hours for 14 days

Rhinosinusitis, acute maxillary: Oral: 200 mg every 12 hours for 10 days

Skin and skin structure: Oral: 400 mg every 12 hours for 7 to 14 days

Urinary tract infection, uncomplicated: Oral: 100 mg every 12 hours for 7 days

Dosing adjustment in renal impairment: Infants ≥2 months, Children, Adolescents, and Adults:

CrCl ≥30 mL/minute: No dosage adjustment necessary.

CrCl <30 mL/minute: Administer every 24 hours.

Hemodialysis: Approximately 23% removed during a 3-hour dialysis session. Administer dose 3 times weekly after hemodialysis.

Dosing adjustment in hepatic impairment: Infants ≥ 2 months, Children, Adolescents, and Adults: No dosage adjustment necessary in patient with cirrhosis.

Preparation for Administration Oral suspension: Reconstitute powder for oral suspension with appropriate amount of water as specified on the bottle. Shake vigorously until suspended.

Administration Oral:

Tablet: Administer with food

Suspension: May administer with or without food; shake suspension well before use

Monitoring Parameters Observe patient for diarrhea; with prolonged therapy, monitor renal function periodically. Observe for signs and symptoms of anaphylaxis during first dose.

Test Interactions Positive direct Coombs', false-positive urinary glucose test using cupric sulfate (Benedict's solution, Clinitest®, Fehling's solution), false-positive serum or urine creatinine with Jaffé reaction

Dosage Forms Excipient information presented when available (limited, particularly for generics); consult specific product labeling.

Suspension Reconstituted, Oral:

Generic: 50 mg/5 mL (50 mL, 100 mL); 100 mg/5 mL (50 mL, 100 mL)

Tablet, Oral:

Generic: 100 mg, 200 mg

◆ **Cefpodoxime Proxetil** *see* Cefpodoxime *on page 404*

Cefprozil (sef PROE zil)

Medication Safety Issues

Sound-alike/look-alike issues:

Cefprozil may be confused with ceFAZolin, cefuroxime

Cefzil may be confused with Ceftin

Brand Names: Canada Apo-Cefprozil; Auro-Cefprozil; Ava-Cefprozil; Cefzil; RAN-Cefprozil; Sandoz-Cefprozil

Therapeutic Category Antibiotic, Cephalosporin (Second Generation)

Generic Availability (US) Yes

Use Treatment of mild to moderate infections caused by susceptible organisms involving the upper respiratory tract and skin and skin structure (FDA approved in ages ≥2 years and adults); treatment of mild to moderate acute sinusitis and otitis media (FDA approved in ages ≥6 months and adults)

Pregnancy Risk Factor B

Pregnancy Considerations Adverse events were not observed in animal reproduction studies.

Breast-Feeding Considerations Small amounts of cefprozil are excreted in breast milk. The manufacturer recommends that caution be exercised when administering cefprozil to nursing women. Nondose-related effects could include modification of bowel flora.

Contraindications Hypersensitivity to cefprozil, any component of the formulation, or other cephalosporins

Warnings/Precautions Modify dosage in patients with severe renal impairment. Hypersensitivity reactions have been reported; if hypersensitivity, occurs, discontinue and institute emergency supportive measures, including airway management and treatment (eg, epinephrine, antihistamines and/or corticosteroids). Use with caution in patients with a history of penicillin allergy. Use with caution in patients with a history of gastrointestinal disease, particularly colitis. Prolonged use may result in fungal or bacterial superinfection, including *C. difficile*-associated diarrhea (CDAD) and pseudomembranous colitis; CDAD has been observed >2 months postantibiotic treatment. Potentially significant interactions may exist, requiring dose or frequency adjustment, additional monitoring, and/or selection of alternative therapy. Some products may contain phenylalanine.

Benzyl alcohol and derivatives: Some dosage forms may contain sodium benzoate/benzoic acid; benzoic acid (benzoate) is a metabolite of benzyl alcohol; large amounts of benzyl alcohol (≥99 mg/kg/day) have been associated with a potentially fatal toxicity ("gasping syndrome") in neonates; the "gasping syndrome" consists of metabolic acidosis, respiratory distress, gasping respirations, CNS dysfunction (including convulsions, intracranial hemorrhage), hypotension, and cardiovascular collapse (AAP, 1997; CDC, 1982). Some data suggest that benzoate displaces bilirubin from protein-binding sites (Ahlfors, 2001); avoid or use dosage forms containing benzyl alcohol derivative with caution in neonates. See manufacturer's labeling.

Some dosage forms may contain polysorbate 80 (also known as Tweens). Hypersensitivity reactions, usually a delayed reaction, have been reported following exposure to pharmaceutical products containing polysorbate 80 in certain individuals (Isaksson, 2002; Lucente 2000; Shelley, 1995). Thrombocytopenia, ascites, pulmonary deterioration, and renal and hepatic failure have been reported in premature neonates after receiving parenteral products containing polysorbate 80 (Alade, 1986; CDC, 1984). See manufacturer's labeling.

Adverse Reactions

Central nervous system: Dizziness

Dermatologic: Diaper rash

Gastrointestinal: Abdominal pain, diarrhea, nausea, vomiting

Genitourinary: Genital pruritus, vaginitis

Hepatic: Transaminases increased

Miscellaneous: Superinfection

Rare but important or life-threatening: Anaphylaxis, angioedema, arthralgia, BUN increased, cholestatic jaundice, confusion, creatinine increased, eosinophilia, erythema multiforme, fever, headache, hyperactivity, insomnia, leukopenia, pseudomembranous colitis, rash, serum sickness, somnolence, Stevens-Johnson syndrome, thrombocytopenia, urticaria

Reactions reported with other cephalosporins: Agranulocytosis, aplastic anemia, colitis, hemolytic anemia, hemorrhage, interstitial nephritis, pancytopenia, renal dysfunction, seizure, superinfection, toxic epidermal necrolysis, toxic nephropathy, vaginitis

Drug Interactions

Metabolism/Transport Effects None known.

Avoid Concomitant Use

Avoid concomitant use of Cefprozil with any of the following: BCG; BCG (Intravesical)

Increased Effect/Toxicity

Cefprozil may increase the levels/effects of: Aminoglycosides; Vitamin K Antagonists

The levels/effects of Cefprozil may be increased by: Probenecid

Decreased Effect

Cefprozil may decrease the levels/effects of: BCG; BCG (Intravesical); BCG Vaccine (Immunization); Sodium Picosulfate; Typhoid Vaccine

Food Interactions Food delays cefprozil absorption. Management: May administer with food.

Storage/Stability Store at 20°C to 25°C (68°F to 77°F); excursions permitted to 15°C to 30°C (59°F to 86°F). Refrigerate suspension after reconstitution; discard after 14 days.

Mechanism of Action Inhibits bacterial cell wall synthesis by binding to one or more of the penicillin-binding proteins (PBPs) which in turn inhibits the final transpeptidation step of peptidoglycan synthesis in bacterial cell walls, thus inhibiting cell wall biosynthesis. Bacteria eventually lyse due to ongoing activity of cell wall autolytic enzymes (autolysins and murein hydrolases) while cell wall assembly is arrested.

Pharmacokinetics (Adult data unless noted)

Absorption: Oral: Well absorbed

Distribution: 0.23 L/kg

Protein binding: 36%

Bioavailability: 95%

Half-life, elimination:

Infants and Children (6 months to 12 years): 1.5 hours

Adults:

Normal renal and hepatic function: 1.3 hours

Renal impairment: 5.2 hours

Renal failure: 5.9 hours

Hepatic impairment: 2 hours

Time to peak serum concentration: 1.5 hours (fasting state)

Elimination: 61% excreted unchanged in urine

Dosing: Usual

Infants, Children, and Adolescents:

General dosing, susceptible infection (*Red Book* 2012): Oral: Mild to moderate infection: 7.5-15 mg/kg/dose twice daily; maximum single dose: 500 mg

Bronchitis, acute bacterial exacerbation or secondary bacterial infection: Adolescents: Oral: 500 mg every 12 hours for 10 days

Otitis media, acute: Infants ≥6 months and Children: Oral: 15 mg/kg/dose every 12 hours for 10 days; maximum single dose: 500 mg. **Note:** Cefprozil is not routinely recommended as a treatment option (AAP [Lieberthal, 2013]).

Pharyngitis/tonsillitis: Oral:

Children ≥2 years: 7.5 mg/kg/dose every 12 hours for 10 days; maximum single dose: 500 mg

Adolescents: 500 mg every 24 hours for 10 days

Rhinosinusitis: Oral:

Infants ≥6 months and Children: 7.5-15 mg/kg/dose every 12 hours for 10 days; maximum single dose: 500 mg

Adolescents: 250-500 mg every 12 hours for 10 days

Skin and skin structure infection: Oral:

Children ≥2 years: 20 mg/kg/dose once daily for 10 days; maximum single dose: 500 mg

Adolescents: 250 mg every 12 hours **or** 500 mg every 12-24 hours for 10 days

Urinary tract infection: Oral: Infants and Children 2-24 months: 15 mg/kg/dose twice daily for 7-14 days (AAP, 2011)

Adults:

Bronchitis, acute bacterial exacerbation or secondary bacterial infection: Oral: 500 mg every 12 hours for 10 days

Pharyngitis/tonsillitis: Oral: 500 mg every 24 hours for 10 days

Rhinosinusitis: Oral: 250-500 mg every 12 hours for 10 days

Skin and skin structure infection, uncomplicated: Oral: 250 mg every 12 hours **or** 500 mg every 12-24 hours for 10 days

Dosing adjustment in renal impairment: All patients:

CrCl ≥30 mL/minute: No adjustment required.

CrCl <30 mL/minute: Reduce dose by 50%.

Intermittent hemodialysis: Administer after dialysis; ~55% is removed by hemodialysis. The following guidelines have been used by some clinicians (Aronoff, 2007):

Pediatric patients: Reduce dose by 50%

Adult patients: 250 mg after dialysis

Peritoneal dialysis (Aronoff, 2007): Reduce dose by 50%

Preparation for Administration Oral suspension: Reconstitute powder for oral suspension with appropriate amount of water as specified on the bottle. Shake vigorously until suspended.

Administration Oral: May administer with or without food; administer with food if stomach upset occurs; chilling improves flavor of suspension (do not freeze); shake suspension well before use

Monitoring Parameters Evaluate renal function before and during therapy; with prolonged therapy, monitor coagulation tests, CBC, and liver function tests periodically; monitor for signs of anaphylaxis during first dose.

Test Interactions Positive direct Coombs, false-positive urinary glucose test using cupric sulfate (Benedict's solution, Clinitest, Fehling's solution), but not with enzyme-based tests for glycosuria (eg, Clinistix). A false-negative reaction may occur in the ferricyanide test for blood glucose.

Dosage Forms Excipient information presented when available (limited, particularly for generics); consult specific product labeling.

Suspension Reconstituted, Oral:
Generic: 125 mg/5 mL (50 mL, 75 mL, 100 mL); 250 mg/5 mL (50 mL, 75 mL, 100 mL)
Tablet, Oral:
Generic: 250 mg, 500 mg

CefTAZidime (SEF tay zi deem)

Medication Safety Issues

Sound-alike/look-alike issues:

CefTAZidime may be confused with ceFAZolin, cefepime, cefoTEtan, cefOXitin, cefTRIAXone

Ceptaz may be confused with Septra

Tazicef may be confused with Tazidime

International issues:

Ceftim [Portugal] and Ceftime [Thailand] brand names for ceftazidime may be confused with Ceftin brand name for cefuroxime [U.S., Canada]; Cefiton brand name for cefixime [Portugal]

Brand Names: US Fortaz; Fortaz in D5W; Tazicef

Brand Names: Canada Ceftazidime For Injection; Fortaz

Therapeutic Category Antibiotic, Cephalosporin (Third Generation)

Generic Availability (US) May be product dependent

Use Treatment of susceptible infections of the respiratory tract, urinary tract, gynecologic, skin and skin structure, intra-abdominal, osteomyelitis, sepsis, and meningitis (FDA approved in all ages); has also been used in management of febrile neutropenia and empiric therapy for febrile, granulocytopenic patients

Pregnancy Risk Factor B

Pregnancy Considerations Adverse events have not been observed in animal reproduction studies. Ceftazidime crosses the placenta and reaches the cord serum and amniotic fluid. An increase in most types of birth defects was not found following first trimester exposure to cephalosporins. Maternal peak serum concentration is unchanged in the first trimester. After the first trimester, serum concentrations decrease by approximately 50% of those in nonpregnant patients. Renal clearance is increased during pregnancy.

Breast-Feeding Considerations Very small amounts of ceftazidime are excreted in breast milk. The manufacturer recommends that caution be exercised when administering ceftazidime to nursing women. Ceftazidime in not absorbed when given orally; therefore, any medication that is distributed to human milk should not result in systemic concentrations in the nursing infant. Nondose-related effects could include modification of bowel flora.

Contraindications Clinically significant hypersensitivity to ceftazidime, other cephalosporins, or any component of the formulation

Warnings/Precautions Modify dosage in patients with severe renal impairment. Use with caution in patients with a history of penicillin allergy, especially IgE-mediated reactions (eg, anaphylaxis, urticaria). High ceftazidime levels in patients with renal insufficiency can lead to seizures, encephalopathy, coma, asterixis, myoclonia, and neuromuscular excitability. Reduce total daily dosage. Prolonged use may result in fungal or bacterial superinfection, including *C. difficile*-associated diarrhea (CDAD) and pseudomembranous colitis; CDAD has been observed >2 months postantibiotic treatment. May be associated with increased INR, especially in nutritionally-deficient patients, prolonged treatment, hepatic or renal disease. Use with caution in patients with a history of seizure disorder; high levels may increase risk of seizures.

Adverse Reactions

Cardiovascular: Phlebitis

Endocrine & metabolic: Increased gamma-glutamyl transferase, increased lactate dehydrogenase

Gastrointestinal: Diarrhea

Hematologic & oncologic: Eosinophilia, positive direct Coombs test (without hemolysis), thrombocythemia

Hepatic: Increased serum alkaline phosphatase, increased serum ALT, increased serum AST

Hypersensitivity: Hypersensitivity reactions

Local: Inflammation at injection site, pain at injection site

Rare but important or life-threatening: Agranulocytosis, anaphylaxis, angioedema, asterixis, brain disease, candidiasis, *Clostridium difficile* associated diarrhea, erythema multiforme, hemolytic anemia, hyperbilirubinemia, increased lactate dehydrogenase, leukopenia, lymphocytosis, myoclonus, nausea, neuromuscular excitability, neutropenia, paresthesia, pseudomembranous colitis, renal disease (may be severe, including renal failure), renal insufficiency, seizure, skin rash, Stevens-Johnson syndrome, thrombocytopenia, toxic epidermal necrolysis, vaginitis

Drug Interactions

Metabolism/Transport Effects None known.

Avoid Concomitant Use

Avoid concomitant use of CefTAZidime with any of the following: BCG; BCG (Intravesical)

Increased Effect/Toxicity

CefTAZidime may increase the levels/effects of: Aminoglycosides; Vitamin K Antagonists

The levels/effects of CefTAZidime may be increased by: Probenecid

Decreased Effect

CefTAZidime may decrease the levels/effects of: BCG; BCG (Intravesical); BCG Vaccine (Immunization); Sodium Picosulfate; Typhoid Vaccine

The levels/effects of CefTAZidime may be decreased by: Chloramphenicol

Storage/Stability

Store intact vials at 20°C to 25°C (68°F to 77°F). Protect from light. Reconstituted solution and solution further diluted for IV infusion are stable for 24 weeks when immediately frozen at -20°C (-4°F). After freezing, thawed solution in NS in a Viaflex small volume container for IV administration is stable for 24 hours at room temperature or for 7 days when refrigerated. Do not refreeze the thawed solution. Ceftazidime solutions (concentrations 1 to 40 mg/mL) in NS, D_5W, D_5NS, LR, $D_{10}W$, Ringer's injection, or SWFI are stable for 24 hours at room temperature (20°C to 25°C [68°F to 77°F]) and for 7 days if refrigerated (4°C [39°F]). Consult detailed reference regarding stability of ceftazidime in other solutions.

Premixed frozen solution: Store frozen at -20°C (-4°F). Thawed solution is stable for 8 hours at room temperature or for 3 days under refrigeration; do not refreeze.

Mechanism of Action Inhibits bacterial cell wall synthesis by binding to one or more of the penicillin-binding proteins (PBPs) which in turn inhibits the final transpeptidation step of peptidoglycan synthesis in bacterial cell walls, thus inhibiting cell wall biosynthesis. Bacteria eventually lyse due to ongoing activity of cell wall autolytic enzymes (autolysins and murein hydrolases) while cell wall assembly is arrested.

Pharmacokinetics (Adult data unless noted)

Distribution: Widely distributed throughout the body including bone, bile, skin, CSF (diffuses into CSF at higher concentrations when the meninges are inflamed), endometrium, heart, pleural and lymphatic fluids

Protein binding: <10%

Half-life:

Neonates <23 days: 2.2-4.7 hours

Adults: 1.9 hours (prolonged with renal impairment)

Time to peak serum concentration: IM: Within 60 minutes

Elimination: By glomerular filtration with 80% to 90% of the dose excreted as unchanged drug in urine within 24 hours

Dosing: Neonatal

General dosing, susceptible infection:

Manufacturer's labeling: IV: 30 mg/kg/dose every 12 hours

Alternate dosing (*Red Book*, 2012): IM, IV:

Body weight <1 kg:

PNA ≤14 days: 50 mg/kg/dose every 12 hours; some reports use 25 mg/kg/dose every 24 hours with adequate serum concentrations in premature neonates (Low, 1985; Mulhall, 1985; van den Anker, 1995a; van den Anker, 1995)

PNA 15-28 days: 50 mg/kg/dose every 8-12 hours

Body weight 1-2 kg:

PNA ≤7 days: 50 mg/kg/dose every 12 hours

PNA 8-28 days: 50 mg/kg/dose every 8-12 hours

Body weight >2 kg:

PNA ≤7 days: 50 mg/kg/dose every 12 hours

PNA 8-28 days: 50 mg/kg/dose every 8 hours

Meningitis (Tunkel, 2004): IV:

PNA ≤7 days: 100-150 mg/kg/day divided every 8-12 hours

PNA >7 days: 150 mg/kg/day divided every 8 hours

Dosing: Usual

Infants, Children, and Adolescents:

General dosing, susceptible infection: IM, IV:

Manufacturer's labeling: Infants and Children 1 month to 12 years: 30-50 mg/kg/dose every 8 hours; maximum daily dose: 6 g/**day**

Alternate dosing (*Red Book*, 2012):

Mild to moderate infections: 90-150 mg/kg/day divided every 8 hours; maximum daily dose: 3000 mg/**day**

Severe infections: 200-300 mg/kg/day divided every 8 hours; maximum daily dose: 6 g/**day**

Cystic fibrosis, lung infection caused by *Pseudomonas* spp: IV: 150-200 mg/kg/day divided every 6-8 hours, maximum daily dose: 6 g/**day**; higher doses have been used: 200-400 mg/kg/day divided every 6-8 hours; maximum daily dose: 12 g/**day** (Zobell, 2012)

Febrile neutropenia; empiric: IV: 50-100 mg/kg/dose every 8 hours; maximum daily dose: 6 g/**day** (Hughes, 2002); **Note:** Due to emerging resistance patterns, some centers have found empiric monotherapy is no longer reliable (Freifeld, 2011; Lehrnbecher, 2012).

Intra-abdominal infections, complicated: IV: 50 mg/kg/dose every 8 hours; maximum daily dose: 6 g/**day** (Solomkin, 2010)

Meningitis: IV: 150 mg/kg/day divided every 8 hours; maximum daily dose: 6 g/**day** (Tunkel, 2004)

Peritonitis (CAPD) (Warady, 2012): Intraperitoneal:

Intermittent: 20 mg/kg/dose every 24 hours in the long dwell

Continuous: Loading dose: 500 mg per liter of dialysate; maintenance dose: 125 mg per liter

Urinary tract infection: Infants and Children 2-24 months: IV: 100-150 mg/kg/day divided every 8 hours (AAP, 2011)

Adults:

Bacterial arthritis (gram-negative bacilli): IV: 1000-2000 mg every 8 hours

Bone and joint infections: IV: 2000 mg every 12 hours

Intra-abdominal infection, severe (in combination with metronidazole): IV: 2000 mg every 8 hours for 4-7 days (provided source controlled). Not recommended for hospital-acquired intra-abdominal infections (IAI) associated with multidrug-resistant gram-negative organisms or in mild to moderate community-acquired IAIs due to risk of toxicity and the development of resistant organisms (Solomkin, 2010).

Melioidosis: IV: 40 mg/kg/dose every 8 hours for 10 days, followed by oral therapy with doxycycline or TMP/SMX

Otitis externa: IV: 2000 mg every 8 hours

Peritonitis (CAPD):

Anuric, intermittent: 1000-1500 mg daily

Anuric, continuous (per liter exchange): Loading dose: 250 mg; maintenance dose: 125 mg

Pneumonia: IV:

Uncomplicated: 500-1000 mg every 8 hours

Complicated or severe: 2000 mg every 8 hours

Prosthetic joint infection, *Pseudomonas aeruginosa* (alternative to cefepime or meropenem): IV: 2000 mg every 8 hours for 4-6 weeks (consider addition of an aminoglycoside) (Osmon, 2013)

Skin and soft tissue infections: IV, IM: 500-1000 mg every 8 hours

Severe infections, including meningitis, complicated pneumonia, endophthalmitis, CNS infection, osteomyelitis, gynecological, skin and soft tissue: IV: 2000 mg every 8 hours

Urinary tract infections: IV, IM:

Uncomplicated: 250 mg every 12 hours

Complicated: 500 mg every 8-12 hours

Dosing adjustment in renal impairment:

Infants, Children, and Adolescents: The manufacturer recommends decreasing dosing frequency based on the calculated BSA adjusted creatinine clearance. The following guidelines have been used by some clinicians (Aronoff, 2007): **Note:** Renally adjusted dose recommendations are based on a usual dose of 25-50 mg/kg/dose every 8 hours:

GFR >50 mL/minute: No adjustment required

GFR 30-50 mL/minute: 50 mg/kg/dose every 12 hours

GFR 10-29 mL/minute: 50 mg/kg/dose every 24 hours

GFR ≤10 mL/minute: 50 mg/kg/dose every 48 hours

Hemodialysis: Dialyzable (50% to 100%): 50 mg/kg/dose every 48 hours, give after dialysis on dialysis days

Peritoneal dialysis: 50 mg/kg/dose every 48 hours

Continuous renal replacement therapy (CRRT): 50 mg/kg/dose every 12 hours

Adults:

CrCl >50 mL/minute: No adjustment required

CrCl 31-50 mL/minute: Administer 1000 mg every 12 hours

CrCl 16-30 mL/minute: Administer 1000 mg every 24 hours

CrCl 6-15 mL/minute: Loading dose 1000 mg, then 500 mg every 24 hours

CrCl ≤5 mL/minute: Loading dose 1000 mg, then 500 mg every 48 hours

Hemodialysis: Dialyzable (50% to 100%): Loading dose 1000 mg, then an additional 1000 mg after each dialysis period

Alternate dosing: 500-1000 mg every 24 hours **or** 1000-2000 mg every 48-72 hours (Heintz, 2009). **Note:** Dosing dependent on the assumption of 3 times per week, complete IHD sessions. Administer after hemodialysis on dialysis days.

Peritoneal dialysis: Loading dose 1000 mg, then 500 mg every 24 hours

Continuous renal replacement therapy (CRRT) (Heintz, 2009; Trotman, 2005): Drug clearance is highly dependent on the method of renal replacement, filter type, and flow rate. Appropriate dosing requires close monitoring of pharmacologic response, signs of adverse reactions due to drug accumulation, as well as drug concentrations in relation to target trough (if appropriate). The following are general recommendations only (based on dialysate flow/ultrafiltration rates of 1-2 L/hour and minimal residual renal function) and should not supersede clinical judgment:

CVVH: Loading dose of 2000 mg followed by 1000-2000 mg every 12 hours

CVVHD/CVVHDF: Loading dose of 2000 mg followed by either 1000 mg every 8 hours **or** 2000 mg every

12 hours. **Note:** Dosage of 1000 mg every 8 hours results in similar steady-state concentrations as 2000 mg every 12 hours and is more cost effective. Dosage of 2000 mg every 8 hours may be needed for gram-negative rods with MIC ≥4 mg/L (Heintz, 2009).

Note: For patients receiving CVVHDF, some recommend giving a loading dose of 2000 mg followed by 3000 mg over 24 hours as a continuous IV infusion to maintain concentrations ≥4 times the MIC for susceptible pathogens (Heintz, 2009).

Dosing adjustment in hepatic impairment: No adjustment required.

Preparation for Administration Note: Any carbon dioxide bubbles that may be present in the withdrawn solution should be expelled prior to injection.

IM: Reconstitute the 500 mg vials with 1.5 mL or the 1,000 mg vials with 3 mL of either SWFI, bacteriostatic water, or lidocaine (0.5% or 1%) to a final concentration of 280 mg/mL

IV:

IVP: Reconstitute vial using SWFI to a concentration of 100 to 170 mg/mL; see manufacturer's labeling for specific details.

Intermittent IV infusion: Further dilute to a final concentration ≤40 mg/mL. In fluid restricted patients, a concentration of 125 mg/mL using SWFI results in a maximum recommended osmolality for peripheral infusion (Robinson 1987).

Administration Parenteral: Inadvertent intra-arterial administration may result in distal necrosis.

IM: Deep IM injection into a large muscle mass such as the upper outer quadrant of the gluteus maximus or lateral part of the thigh.

IV:

IVP: Administer over 3 to 5 minutes

Intermittent IV infusion: Administer over 15 to 30 minutes

Monitoring Parameters Renal function periodically when used in combination with aminoglycosides; with prolonged therapy also monitor hepatic and hematologic function periodically; number and type of stools/day for diarrhea. Observe for signs and symptoms of anaphylaxis during first dose. Monitor prothrombin time in patients at risk for increased INR (nutritionally deficient patients, prolonged treatment, hepatic or renal disease)

Test Interactions Positive direct Coombs', false-positive urinary glucose test using cupric sulfate (Benedict's solution, Clinitest®, Fehling's solution), false-positive serum or urine creatinine with Jaffé reaction

Dosage Forms Excipient information presented when available (limited, particularly for generics); consult specific product labeling.

Solution, Intravenous, as sodium [strength expressed as base]:

Fortaz in D5W: 1 g (50 mL); 2 g (50 mL)

Tazicef: 1 g/50 mL (50 mL)

Solution Reconstituted, Injection:

Fortaz: 500 mg (1 ea); 1 g (1 ea); 2 g (1 ea); 6 g (1 ea)

Tazicef: 1 g (1 ea); 2 g (1 ea); 6 g (1 ea)

Generic: 1 g (1 ea); 2 g (1 ea); 6 g (1 ea); 100 g (1 ea)

Solution Reconstituted, Injection [preservative free]:

Generic: 1 g (1 ea); 2 g (1 ea); 6 g (1 ea)

Solution Reconstituted, Intravenous:

Fortaz: 1 g (1 ea); 2 g (1 ea)

Tazicef: 1 g (1 ea); 2 g (1 ea)

Generic: 1 g/50 mL (1 ea); 2 g/50 mL (1 ea)

◆ **Ceftazidime For Injection (Can)** *see* CefTAZidime *on page 407*

Ceftibuten (sef TYE byoo ten)

Medication Safety Issues

Sound-alike/look-alike issues:

Cedax® may be confused with Cidex®

International issues:

Cedax [U.S. and multiple international markets] may be confused with Codex brand name for acetaminophen/codeine [Brazil] and *Saccharomyces boulardii* [Italy]

Brand Names: US Cedax

Therapeutic Category Antibiotic, Cephalosporin (Third Generation)

Generic Availability (US) Yes

Use Treatment of acute exacerbations of chronic bronchitis, acute bacterial otitis media, pharyngitis/tonsillitis due to *H. influenzae* and *M. catarrhalis* (both beta-lactamase-producing and nonproducing strains), *S. pneumoniae* (penicillin-susceptible strains only), and *S. pyogenes*

Pregnancy Risk Factor B

Pregnancy Considerations Teratogenic effects were not observed in animal reproduction studies. An increase in most types of birth defects was not found following first trimester exposure to cephalosporins.

Breast-Feeding Considerations Ceftibuten was not detectable in milk after a single 200 mg dose (limit of detection: 1 mcg/mL). It is not known if it would be detectable after a 400 mg dose or multiple doses. The manufacturer recommends that caution be exercised when administering ceftibuten to nursing women. If ceftibuten does reach the human milk, nondose-related effects could include modification of bowel flora.

Contraindications Hypersensitivity to ceftibuten, any component of the formulation, or other cephalosporins

Warnings/Precautions Modify dosage in patients with moderate-to-severe renal impairment. Prolonged use may result in fungal or bacterial superinfection, including *C. difficile*-associated diarrhea (CDAD) and pseudomembranous colitis; CDAD has been observed >2 months postantibiotic treatment. Use with caution in patients with a history of colitis and other gastrointestinal diseases. Use with caution in patients with a history of penicillin allergy, especially IgE-mediated reactions (eg, anaphylaxis, urticaria).

Oral suspension formulation contains sucrose.

Benzyl alcohol and derivatives: Some dosage forms may contain sodium benzoate/benzoic acid; benzoic acid (benzoate) is a metabolite of benzyl alcohol; large amounts of benzyl alcohol (≥99 mg/kg/day) have been associated with a potentially fatal toxicity ("gasping syndrome") in neonates; the "gasping syndrome" consists of metabolic acidosis, respiratory distress, gasping respirations, CNS dysfunction (including convulsions, intracranial hemorrhage), hypotension, and cardiovascular collapse (AAP, 1997; CDC, 1982); some data suggests that benzoate displaces bilirubin from protein binding sites (Ahlfors, 2001); avoid or use dosage forms containing benzyl alcohol derivative with caution in neonates. See manufacturer's labeling.

Warnings: Additional Pediatric Considerations May cause diarrhea; incidence is higher in younger pediatric patients (8% in patients ≤2 years; 2% in patients >2 years).

Adverse Reactions

Central nervous system: Dizziness, headache

Gastrointestinal: Abdominal pain, diarrhea, dyspepsia, loose stools, nausea, vomiting

Hematologic: Eosinophils increased, hemoglobin decreased, platelets increased

Hepatic: ALT increased, bilirubin increased

Renal: BUN increased

Rare but important or life-threatening: Agitation, alkaline phosphatase increased, anorexia, aphasia, AST increased, constipation, creatinine increased, dehydration, diaper rash, dyspnea, dysuria, eructation, fatigue, fever, flatulence, hematuria, hyperkinesia, insomnia, irritability, jaundice, leukopenia, melena, moniliasis, nasal congestion, paresthesia, platelets increased, pruritus, pseudomembranous colitis, psychosis, rash, rigors, serum-sickness reactions, somnolence, Stevens-Johnson syndrome, stridor, taste perversion, thrombocytopenia, toxic epidermal necrolysis, urticaria, vaginitis, xerostomia

Additional reactions reported with other cephalosporins: Allergic reaction, agranulocytosis, angioedema, aplastic anemia, anaphylaxis, asterixis, cholestasis, drug fever, encephalopathy, erythema multiforme, hemolytic anemia, hemorrhage, interstitial nephritis, neuromuscular excitability, neutropenia, pancytopenia, prolonged PT, renal dysfunction, seizure, superinfection, toxic nephropathy

Drug Interactions

Metabolism/Transport Effects None known.

Avoid Concomitant Use

Avoid concomitant use of Ceftibuten with any of the following: BCG; BCG (Intravesical)

Increased Effect/Toxicity

Ceftibuten may increase the levels/effects of: Aminoglycosides; Vitamin K Antagonists

The levels/effects of Ceftibuten may be increased by: Probenecid

Decreased Effect

Ceftibuten may decrease the levels/effects of: BCG; BCG (Intravesical); BCG Vaccine (Immunization); Sodium Picosulfate; Typhoid Vaccine

The levels/effects of Ceftibuten may be decreased by: Multivitamins/Minerals (with ADEK, Folate, Iron); Multivitamins/Minerals (with AE, No Iron); Zinc Salts

Storage/Stability Store capsules and powder for suspension at 2°C to 25°C (36°F to 77°F). Reconstituted suspension is stable for 14 days when refrigerated at 2°C to 8°C (36°F to 46°F).

Mechanism of Action Inhibits bacterial cell wall synthesis by binding to one or more of the penicillin-binding proteins (PBPs) which in turn inhibits the final transpeptidation step of peptidoglycan synthesis in bacterial cell walls, thus inhibiting cell wall biosynthesis. Bacteria eventually lyse due to ongoing activity of cell wall autolytic enzymes (autolysins and murein hydrolases) while cell wall assembly is arrested.

Pharmacokinetics (Adult data unless noted)

Absorption: Rapid; food decreases peak concentration and lowers AUC

Distribution: Distributes into middle ear fluid, bronchial secretions, sputum, tonsillar tissue, and blister fluid:

V_d:

Children: 0.5 L/kg

Adults: 0.21 L/kg

Protein binding: 65%

Bioavailability: 75% to 90%

Half-life:

Children: 1.9-2.5 hours

Adults: 2-3 hours; CrCl 30-49 mL/minute: 7 hours; CrCl 5-29 mL/minute: 13 hours; CrCl <5 mL/minute: 22 hours

Time to peak serum concentration: 2-3 hours

Elimination: 60% to 70% excreted unchanged in urine

Dialysis: 39% to 65% removed by a 2-4 hour hemodialysis

Dosing: Usual Oral:

Children <12 years: 9 mg/kg/day once daily for 10 days (maximum dose: 400 mg)

Children ≥12 years, Adolescents, and Adults: 400 mg once daily for 10 days

Dosing adjustment in renal impairment:

CrCl ≥50 mL/minute: No adjustment needed

CrCl 30-49 mL/minute: 4.5 mg/kg or 200 mg every 24 hours

CrCl 5-29 mL/minute: 2.25 mg/kg or 100 mg every 24 hours

Hemodialysis: Administer 9 mg/kg (maximum dose: 400 mg) after hemodialysis

Preparation for Administration Oral suspension: Reconstitute powder for oral suspension with appropriate amount of water as specified on the bottle. Shake vigorously until suspended.

Administration

Capsule: Administer without regard to food

Suspension: Shake suspension well before use. Administer 2 hours before or 1 hour after meals.

Monitoring Parameters Observe for signs and symptoms of anaphylaxis during first dose; with prolonged therapy, monitor renal, hepatic, and hematologic function periodically; number and type of stools/day for diarrhea

Test Interactions Positive direct Coombs', false-positive urinary glucose test using cupric sulfate (Benedict's solution, Clinitest®, Fehling's solution), false-positive serum or urine creatinine with Jaffé reaction

Dosage Forms Excipient information presented when available (limited, particularly for generics); consult specific product labeling.

Capsule, Oral:

Cedax: 400 mg [contains butylparaben, edetate calcium disodium, methylparaben, propylparaben]

Generic: 400 mg

Suspension Reconstituted, Oral:

Cedax: 90 mg/5 mL (60 mL, 90 mL, 120 mL) [contains polysorbate 80, sodium benzoate; cherry flavor]

Cedax: 180 mg/5 mL (30 mL, 60 mL) [contains sodium benzoate; cherry flavor]

Generic: 180 mg/5 mL (60 mL)

◆ **Ceftin** *see* Cefuroxime *on page 414*

CefTRIAXone (sef trye AKS one)

Medication Safety Issues

Sound-alike/look-alike issues:

CefTRIAXone may be confused with ceFAZolin, cefoTEtan, cefOXitin, cefTAZidime, Cetraxal

Rocephin may be confused with Roferon

Related Information

Prevention of Infective Endocarditis *on page 2378*

Brand Names: US Rocephin

Brand Names: Canada Ceftriaxone for Injection; Ceftriaxone for Injection USP; Ceftriaxone Sodium for Injection; Ceftriaxone Sodium for Injection BP

Therapeutic Category Antibiotic, Cephalosporin (Third Generation)

Generic Availability (US) Yes

Use Treatment of sepsis, meningitis, infections of the lower respiratory tract, acute bacterial otitis media, skin and skin structure, bone and joint, intra-abdominal and urinary tract due to susceptible organisms (FDA approved in infants, children, adolescents, and adults); surgical prophylaxis (FDA approved in adults); documented or suspected uncomplicated gonococcal infection or pelvic inflammatory disease (FDA approved for adults)

Pregnancy Risk Factor B

Pregnancy Considerations Teratogenic effects have not been observed in animal reproduction studies. Ceftriaxone crosses the placenta and distributes to amniotic fluid. An increase in most types of birth defects was not found following first trimester exposure to cephalosporins. Pregnancy was found to influence the single dose pharmacokinetics of ceftriaxone when administered prior to delivery. The pharmacokinetics of ceftriaxone following multiple doses in the third trimester are similar to those of nonpregnant patients. Ceftriaxone is recommended for use in pregnant women for the treatment of gonococcal infections, Lyme disease, and may be used in certain situations prior to vaginal delivery in women at high risk for endocarditis (consult current guidelines).

Breast-Feeding Considerations Low concentrations of ceftriaxone are excreted in breast milk. The manufacturer recommends that caution be exercised when administering ceftriaxone to nursing women. Nondose-related effects could include modification of bowel flora.

Contraindications Hypersensitivity to ceftriaxone, any component of the formulation, or other cephalosporins; **do not use in hyperbilirubinemic neonates**, particularly those who are premature since ceftriaxone is reported to displace bilirubin from albumin binding sites; concomitant use with intravenous calcium-containing solutions/products in neonates (≤28 days)

Warnings/Precautions Use with caution in patients with a history of penicillin allergy, especially IgE-mediated reactions (eg, anaphylaxis, urticaria). Abnormal gallbladder sonograms have been reported, possibly due to cetriaxone-calcium precipitates; discontinue in patients who develop signs and symptoms of gallbladder disease. Secondary to biliary obstruction, pancreatitis has been reported rarely. Use with caution in patients with a history of GI disease, especially colitis. Severe cases (including some fatalities) of immune-related hemolytic anemia have been reported in patients receiving cephalosporins, including ceftriaxone. Prolonged use may result in fungal or bacterial superinfection, including *C. difficile*-associated diarrhea (CDAD) and pseudomembranous colitis; CDAD has been observed >2 months postantibiotic treatment.

Potentially significant interactions may exist, requiring dose or frequency adjustment, additional monitoring, and/or selection of alternative therapy. May be associated with increased INR (rarely), especially in nutritionally-deficient patients, prolonged treatment, hepatic or renal disease. No adjustment is generally necessary in patients with renal impairment; use with caution in patients with concurrent hepatic dysfunction and significant renal disease, dosage should not exceed 2 g/day. Ceftriaxone may complex with calcium causing precipitation. Fatal lung and kidney damage associated with calcium-ceftriaxone precipitates has been observed in premature and term neonates. Do not reconstitute, admix, or coadminister with calcium-containing solutions, even via separate infusion lines/sites or at different times in any neonatal patient. Ceftriaxone should not be diluted or administered simultaneously with any calcium-containing solution via a Y-site in any patient. However, ceftriaxone and calcium-containing solution may be administered sequentially of one another for use in patients **other than neonates** if infusion lines are thoroughly flushed, with a compatible fluid, between infusions

Adverse Reactions

Dermatologic: Local skin tightening (IM), skin rash

Gastrointestinal: Diarrhea

Hematologic & oncologic: Eosinophilia, leukopenia, thrombocythemia

Hepatic: Increased serum transaminases

Local: Induration at injection site (IM), pain at injection site, tenderness at injection site (IV), warm sensation at injection site (IM)

Renal: Increased blood urea nitrogen

Rare but important or life-threatening: Abdominal pain, agranulocytosis, allergic dermatitis, anaphylaxis, anemia, basophilia, bronchospasm, candidiasis, casts in urine, chills, choledocholithiasis, cholelithiasis, colitis, decreased prothrombin time, diaphoresis, dizziness, dysgeusia, dyspepsia, edema, epistaxis, erythema multiforme, fever, flatulence, flushing, gallbladder sludge, glossitis, glycosuria, headache, hematuria, hemolytic anemia, hypersensitivity pneumonitis, increased monocytes, increased serum alkaline phosphatase, increased serum bilirubin, increased serum creatinine, jaundice, leukocytosis, lymphocytopenia, lymphocytosis, nausea, nephrolithiasis, neutropenia, oliguria, palpitations, pancreatitis, phlebitis, prolonged prothrombin time, pruritus, pseudomembranous colitis, seizure, serum sickness, Stevens-Johnson syndrome, stomatitis, thrombocytopenia, toxic epidermal necrolysis, urticaria, vaginitis, vomiting

Drug Interactions

Metabolism/Transport Effects None known.

Avoid Concomitant Use

Avoid concomitant use of CefTRIAXone with any of the following: BCG; BCG (Intravesical)

Increased Effect/Toxicity

CefTRIAXone may increase the levels/effects of: Aminoglycosides; Vitamin K Antagonists

The levels/effects of CefTRIAXone may be increased by: Calcium Salts (Intravenous); Probenecid; Ringer's Injection (Lactated)

Decreased Effect

CefTRIAXone may decrease the levels/effects of: BCG; BCG (Intravesical); BCG Vaccine (Immunization); Sodium Picosulfate; Typhoid Vaccine

Storage/Stability

Powder for injection: Prior to reconstitution, store at room temperature ≤25°C (≤77°F). Protect from light.

Premixed solution (manufacturer premixed): Store at -20°C; once thawed, solutions are stable for 3 days at room temperature of 25°C (77°F) or for 21 days refrigerated at 5°C (41°F). Do not refreeze.

Stability of reconstituted solutions:

10 to 40 mg/mL: Reconstituted in D_5W, $D_{10}W$, NS, or SWFI: Stable for 2 days at room temperature of 25°C (77°F) or for 10 days when refrigerated at 4°C (39°F). Stable for 26 weeks when frozen at -20°C when reconstituted with D_5W or NS. Once thawed (at room temperature), solutions are stable for 2 days at room temperature of 25°C (77°F) or for 10 days when refrigerated at 4°C (39°F); does not apply to manufacturer's premixed bags. Do not refreeze.

100 mg/mL:

Reconstituted in D_5W, SWFI, or NS: Stable for 2 days at room temperature of 25°C (77°F) or for 10 days when refrigerated at 4°C (39°F).

Reconstituted in lidocaine 1% solution or bacteriostatic water: Stable for 24 hours at room temperature of 25°C (77°F) or for 10 days when refrigerated at 4°C (39°F).

250 to 350 mg/mL: Reconstituted in D_5W, NS, lidocaine 1% solution, bacteriostatic water, or SWFI: Stable for 24 hours at room temperature of 25°C (77°F) or for 3 days when refrigerated at 4°C (39°F).

Mechanism of Action Inhibits bacterial cell wall synthesis by binding to one or more of the penicillin-binding proteins (PBPs) which in turn inhibits the final transpeptidation step of peptidoglycan synthesis in bacterial cell walls, thus inhibiting cell wall biosynthesis. Bacteria eventually lyse due to ongoing activity of cell wall autolytic enzymes (autolysins and murein hydrolases) while cell wall assembly is arrested.

Pharmacokinetics (Adult data unless noted)

Absorption: IM: Complete

Distribution: Widely distributed throughout the body including gallbladder, lungs, bone, bile, CSF (diffuses into the CSF at higher concentrations when the meninges are inflamed)

V_d:

Neonates: 0.34-0.55 L/kg (Richards, 1984)

Infants and Children: 0.3-0.4 L/kg (Richards, 1984)

Adults: 6-14 L

Protein binding: 85% to 95%
Half-life:
Neonates (Martin, 1984):
1-4 days: 16 hours
9-30 days: 9 hours
Pediatric patients (age not specified): 4.1-6.6 hours (Richards, 1984)
Adults: Normal renal and hepatic function: 5-9 hours; renal impairment (mild to severe): 12-16 hours
Time to peak serum concentration: IM: 2-3 hours
Elimination: Unchanged in the urine (33% to 67%) by glomerular filtration and in feces via bile

Dosing: Neonatal Note: Use cefotaxime in place of ceftriaxone if hyperbilirubinemia is present or if patient is receiving calcium-containing intravenous solutions

General dosing, susceptible infection (*Red Book*, 2012): IM, IV: 50 mg/kg/dose every 24 hours

Gonococcal infections (including CNS) (CDC, 2010): IM, IV:
Prophylaxis: 25-50 mg/kg as a single dose; maximum single dose: 125 mg
Treatment: 25-50 mg/kg every 24 hours for 7 days, up to 10-14 days if meningitis is documented; maximum single dose: 125 mg

Meningitis, non-gonococcal: Limited data available, dose not established: **Note:** In neonates, current IDSA guidelines suggest cefotaxime as the preferred nonpseudomonal third-generation cephalosporin; no ceftriaxone dosing is provided in the guidelines (Tunkel, 2004). Dosing based on an open-label prospective trial of 71 patients (age range: PNA 14 days to 15 years) which included 26 patients diagnosed with meningitis and a pharmacokinetic analysis of 20 neonates and infants (n=12 neonates; including six with PNA <14 days) with sepsis or meningitis; both trials reported adequate CSF penetration and favorable response (Martin, 1984; Yogev, 1986). IV:
PNA <14 days: 50 mg/kg/dose once daily
PNA ≥14 days: 100 mg/kg for one dose, followed by 80-100 mg/kg/dose once daily

Ophthalmia neonatorum, treatment: IM, IV: 25-50 mg/kg as a single dose; maximum single dose: 125 mg (CDC, 2010; *Red Book*, 2012)

Dosing: Usual

Infants, Children, and Adolescents:

General dosing, susceptible infection: IM, IV:
Mild to moderate infection: 50-75 mg/kg/dose once daily; maximum single dose: 1000 mg (*Red Book*, 2012)
Severe infection:
AAP recommendation (*Red Book*, 2012): 100 mg/kg/day divided every 12-24 hours
Manufacturer labeling (non-CNS): 50-75 mg/kg/day divided every 12 hours; maximum daily dose: 2000 mg/**day**

Chancroid: IM: 50 mg/kg as a single dose; maximum single dose: 250 mg (*Red Book*, 2012)

Endocarditis, bacterial: IM, IV:
Prophylaxis: 50 mg/kg as a single dose; maximum single dose: 1000 mg (*Red Book*, 2012; Wilson, 2007)
Treatment (Baddour, 2005):
Enterococcal endocarditis (native or prosthetic valve): 100 mg/kg/day divided every 12 hours plus ampicillin for at least 8 weeks
HACEK microorganisms: 100 mg/kg once daily for 4 weeks
Viridans group streptococci and *Streptococcus bovis* (highly penicillin susceptible):
Native valve: 100 mg/kg once daily for 4 weeks or 2 weeks if given with gentamicin
Prosthetic valve: 100 mg/kg once daily for 6 weeks with 2 weeks of gentamicin
Viridans group streptococci and *Streptococcus bovis* (relatively resistant): Native valve: 100 mg/kg once daily for 4 weeks with 2 weeks of gentamicin
Note: American Heart Association (AHA) guidelines now recommend prophylaxis only in patients undergoing invasive procedures and in whom underlying cardiac conditions may predispose to a higher risk of adverse outcomes should infection occur. As of April 2007, routine prophylaxis for GI/GU procedures is no longer recommended by the AHA.

Enteric infection, bacteria, empiric therapy pending diagnostic studies (HIV-exposed/-positive): Adolescents: IV: 1000 mg every 24 hours (DHHS [adult], 2013)

Gonococcal infections: Note: Due to increasing resistance, coadminister with azithromycin, erythromycin, or doxycycline (if ≥8 years) (*Red Book*, 2012):
Epididymitis, acute: IM: 250 mg in a single dose
Uncomplicated cervicitis, pharyngitis, proctitis, urethritis, and vulvovaginitis: Treatment and prophylaxis: IM:
<45 kg: 125 mg as a single dose (CDC, 2010)
≥45 kg: 250 mg as a single dose (CDC, 2010; CDC, 2012)
Complicated: IM, IV:
<45 kg (*Red Book*, 2012):
Disseminated infection: 50 mg/kg once daily for 7 days; maximum single dose: 1000 mg
Conjunctivitis: 50 mg/kg as a single dose; maximum single dose: 1000 mg
Meningitis or endocarditis: 50 mg/kg/day divided every 12 hours for 10-14 days (meningitis) or for 28 days (endocarditis); maximum daily dose: 2000 mg/**day**
≥45 kg (CDC, 2010):
Disseminated infection: 1000 mg once daily for 7 days
Meningitis: 1000-2000 mg every 12 hours for 10-14 days
Endocarditis: 1000-2000 mg every 12 hours for 28 days
Conjunctivitis: IM: 1000 mg in a single dose

Intra-abdominal infection, complicated: IM, IV: 50-75 mg/kg/day divided every 12-24 hours; maximum daily dose: 2000 mg/**day** (Solomkin, 2010)

Lyme disease, neurologic involvement, persistent/recurrent arthritis, heart block, or carditis: IM, IV: 50-75 mg/kg once daily; maximum single dose: 2000 mg; duration dependent on symptoms and response (Halperin, 2007; *Red Book*, 2012; Wormser, 2006)

Meningitis: IM, IV: Loading dose of 100 mg/kg may be administered at the start of therapy
Manufacturer labeling: 100 mg/kg/day divided every 12-24 hours for 7-14 days; maximum daily dose: 4000 mg/**day**
IDSA guidelines (Tunkel, 2004): 80-100 mg/kg/day divided every 12-24 hours; maximum daily dose: 4000 mg/**day**

Meningococcal infection, chemoprophylaxis for high-risk contacts (close exposure to patients with invasive meningococcal disease) (*Red Book*, 2012):
<15 years: IM: 125 mg in a single dose
≥15 years: IM: 250 mg in a single dose

Otitis media, acute (AAP, 2014; AAP [Lieberthal, 2013]):
Acute bacterial: IM, IV: 50 mg/kg in a single dose; maximum single dose: 1000 mg
Persistent or relapsing: IM, IV: 50 mg/kg once daily for 3 days; maximum single dose: 1000 mg

Peritonitis, prophylaxis for patients receiving peritoneal dialysis who require dental procedures: IM, IV: 50 mg/kg administered 30-60 minutes before dental procedure; maximum dose: 1000 mg (Warady, 2012)

Pneumonia:

Bacterial pneumonia (HIV-exposed/-positive): IV: 50-100 mg/kg/day divided every 12-24 hours; maximum daily dose: 4000 mg/**day** (DHHS [adult and pediatric], 2013)

Community-acquired (CAP): (IDSA/PIDS [Bradley, 2011]): Infants >3 months, Children, and Adolescents: IV: 50-100 mg/kg/day divided every 12-24 hours; maximum daily dose 2000 mg/**day**. **Note:** May consider addition of vancomycin or clindamycin to empiric therapy if community-acquired MRSA suspected. Use the higher end of the range for penicillin-resistant *S. pneumoniae*; in children ≥5 years, a macrolide antibiotic should be added if atypical pneumonia cannot be ruled out; preferred in patients not fully immunized for *H. influenzae* type b and S. pneumoniae, or significant local resistance to penicillin in invasive pneumococcal strains

Prophylaxis against sexually transmitted diseases following sexual assault (CDC, 2010):

≤45 kg: IM: 125 mg in a single dose (in combination with azithromycin and metronidazole)

>45 kg: IM, IV: 250 mg in a single dose (in combination with azithromycin and metronidazole)

Rhinosinusitis, acute bacterial:

Ambulatory patients: Children and Adolescents: IM, IV: 50 mg/kg as a single dose; maximum dose: 1000 mg; use for patients who are unable to tolerate oral medication, or unlikely to be adherent to the initial doses of antibiotic (Wald, 2013)

Severe infection requiring hospitalization: IM, IV: 50 mg/kg/day divided every 12 hours for 10-14 days; maximum daily dose: 2000 mg/**day** (Chow, 2012)

Salmonellosis: Note: Salmonella in healthy patients typically does not require antibiotic treatment as it generally resolves in 5-7 days (CDC, 2013)

Infants <6 months of age or who have severe infection, prostheses, valvular heart disease, severe atherosclerosis, malignancy, or uremia: Non-*typhi* species diarrhea: IM, IV: 100 mg/kg/day divided every 12-24 hours for 14 days; or longer if relapsing. **Note:** Not recommended for routine use (Guerrant, 2001).

HIV-exposed/-positive: Adolescents: IV: 1000 mg every 24 hours; duration dependent upon CD4 counts and presence of bactermia (DHHS [adult], 2013)

If CD4 count ≥200 cells/mm^3: 7-14 days; if bacteremia present: At least 14 days or longer for complicated cases

If CD4 count <200 cells/mm^3: 2-6 weeks

Shigellosis: IM, IV: 50-100 mg/kg once daily; usual duration 5 days; may shorten duration to 2 days if clinical response good and no extraintestinal involvement (*Red Book*, 2012; WHO, 2005)

Skin/skin structure infections: IM, IV: 50-75 mg/kg/day in 1-2 divided doses; maximum daily dose: 2000 mg/**day**

***S. pneumoniae* infection, invasive** (*Red Book*, 2012): IV:

CNS infection: 100 mg/kg/day divided every 12-24 hours

Non-CNS infection: 50-75 mg/kg/day divided every 12-24 hours

Surgical prophylaxis: Children and Adolescents: IV: 50-75 mg/kg as a single dose; maximum single dose: 2000 mg (Bratzler, 2013)

Syphilis: Note: Not considered first-line therapy and use should be reserved for special circumstances with close monitoring and follow-up: IM, IV:

Congenital syphilis; treatment: Infants >30 days: 75-100 mg/kg once daily for 10-14 days (CDC, 2010); **Note:** There is insufficient data regarding the use of ceftriaxone for treatment of congenital syphilis (penicillin is recommended); use should be reserved for situations of penicillin shortage

Postexposure prophylaxis (HIV-exposed/-positive): Adolescents: 1000 mg once daily for 8-10 days (DHHS [adult], 2013)

Treatment:

Early syphilis (independent of HIV status): Adolescents: 1000 mg once daily for 10-14 days; optimal dose and duration have not been defined (CDC, 2010)

Neurosyphillis, otic, ocular disease (HIV-exposed/-positive; penicillin-allergic): Adolescents: 2000 mg once daily for 10-14 days. **Note:** Penicillin desensitization is the preferred approach; use should be reserved when desensitization is not feasible (DHHS [adult], 2013).

Typhoid fever: IV: 80 mg/kg once daily for 14 days (Stephens, 2002)

Urinary tract infections: IM, IV:

Infants and Children 2-24 months: 50-75 mg/kg once daily (AAP, 2011; Bradley, 2012)

Children >24 months and Adolescents: 50 mg/kg once daily; maximum single dose: 2000 mg (Bradley, 2012)

Adults:

General dosage, susceptible infection: IM, IV: 1000-2000 mg every 12-24 hours, depending on the type and severity of infection; maximum daily dose: 4000 mg/**day**

Chancroid: IM: 250 mg as single dose (CDC, 2010)

Cholecystitis, mild to moderate: IM, IV: 1000-2000 mg every 12-24 hours for 4-7 days (provided source controlled)

Gonococcal infections (CDC, 2010; CDC, 2012):

Conjunctivitis, complicated: IM, IV: 1000 mg in a single dose

Disseminated: IM, IV: 1000 mg once daily for 24-48 hours; may switch to cefixime (after improvement noted) to complete a total of 7 days of therapy

Endocarditis: IM, IV: 1000-2000 mg every 12 hours for at least 28 days

Epididymitis, acute: IM: 250 mg in a single dose with doxycycline

Meningitis: IM, IV: 1000-2000 mg every 12 hours for 10-14 days

Uncomplicated cervicitis, pharyngitis, urethritis: IM: 250 mg in a single dose with azithromycin (preferred) or doxycycline

Infective endocarditis: IM, IV:

Native valve: 2000 mg once daily for 2-4 weeks; **Note:** If using 2-week regimen, concurrent gentamicin is recommended

Prosthetic valve: 2000 mg once daily for 6 weeks [with or without 2 weeks of gentamicin (dependent on penicillin MIC)]; **Note:** For HACEK organisms, duration of therapy is 4 weeks

Enterococcus faecalis (resistant to penicillin, aminoglycoside, and vancomycin), native or prosthetic valve: 2000 mg twice daily for ≥8 weeks administered concurrently with ampicillin

Prophylaxis: 1000 mg 30-60 minutes before procedure. Intramuscular injections should be avoided in patients who are receiving anticoagulant therapy. In these circumstances, orally administered regimens should be given whenever possible. Intravenously administered antibiotics should be used for patients who are unable to tolerate or absorb oral medications.

Note: American Heart Association (AHA) guidelines now recommend prophylaxis only in patients undergoing invasive procedures and in whom underlying cardiac conditions may predispose to a higher risk of adverse outcomes should infection occur. As of April

2007, routine prophylaxis for GI/GU procedures is no longer recommended by the AHA.

Intra-abdominal infection, complicated, community-acquired, mild to moderate (in combination with metronidazole): IM, IV: 1000-2000 mg every 12-24 hours for 4-7 days (provided source controlled)

Lyme disease: IV: 2000 mg once daily for 14-28 days

Meningitis: IV: 2000 mg every 12 hours for 7-14 days (longer courses may be necessary for selected organisms)

Meningococcal infection, chemoprophylaxis for high-risk contacts (close exposure to patients with invasive meningococcal disease): IM: 250 mg in a single dose

Pelvic inflammatory disease: IM: 250 mg in a single dose plus doxycycline (with or without metronidazole) (CDC, 2010)

Pneumonia, community-acquired: IV: 1000 mg once daily, usually in combination with a macrolide; consider 2000 mg/day for patients at risk for more severe infection and/or resistant organisms (ICU status, age >65 years, disseminated infection)

Prophylaxis against sexually transmitted diseases following sexual assault: IM: 250 mg as a single dose (in combination with azithromycin and metronidazole) (CDC, 2010)

Pyelonephritis (acute, uncomplicated): Females: IV: 1000-2000 mg once daily (Stamm, 1993). Many physicians administer a single parenteral dose before initiating oral therapy (Warren, 1999).

Rhinosinusitis, acute bacterial, severe infection requiring hospitalization: IV: 1000-2000 mg every 12-24 hours for 5-7 days (Chow, 2012)

Surgical prophylaxis: IV: 1000 mg 30 minutes to 2 hours before surgery

Cholecystectomy: 1000-2000 mg every 12-24 hours, discontinue within 24 hours unless infection outside gallbladder suspected

Syphilis: IM, IV: 1000 mg once daily for 10-14 days; **Note:** Alternative treatment for early syphilis, optimal dose, and duration have not been defined (CDC, 2010)

Dosage adjustment in renal impairment: No dosage adjustment is generally necessary in renal impairment; **Note:** Concurrent renal and hepatic dysfunction: Adult maximum daily dose: ≤2000 mg/**day**

Poorly dialyzed; no supplemental dose or dosage adjustment necessary, including patients on intermittent hemodialysis, peritoneal dialysis, or continuous renal replacement therapy (eg, CVVHD).

Dosage adjustment in hepatic impairment: No adjustment is generally necessary in hepatic impairment; **Note:** Concurrent renal and hepatic dysfunction: Adult maximum daily dose: ≤2000 mg/**day**

Preparation for Administration Parenteral: Do not reconstitute with calcium-containing solutions.

IM: Vials should be reconstituted with appropriate volume of diluent (including D_5W, NS, SWFI, bacteriostatic water, or 1% lidocaine) to make a final concentration of 250 mg/mL or 350 mg/mL; more dilute concentrations (100 mg/mL) can be used if needed; see manufacturer's labeling for specific detail.

IV: Reconstitute powder for injection to a concentration of ~100 mg/mL with an appropriate IV diluent (including SWFI, D_5W, $D_{10}W$, NS); see manufacturer's labeling for specific details. Further dilute dose in compatible solution (eg, D_5W or NS) to a final concentration not to exceed 40 mg/mL.

Administration Parenteral: Do not coadminister with calcium-containing solutions.

IM: Administer IM injections deep into a large muscle mass

Intermittent IV infusion: Administer over 30 minutes; shorter infusion times (15 minutes) have been reported (Yogev 1986)

IVP: Administration over 2 to 4 minutes has been reported in pediatric patients >11 years and adults primarily in the outpatient setting (Baumgartner 1983; Garrelts 1988; Poole 1999) and over 5 minutes in pediatric patients ages newborn to 15 years with meningitis (Grubbauer 1990; Martin 1984). Rapid IVP injection over 5 minutes of a 2,000 mg dose resulted in tachycardia, restlessness, diaphoresis, and palpitations in an adult patient (Lossos 1994). IV push administration in young infants may also have been a contributing factor in risk of cardiopulmonary events occurring from interactions between ceftriaxone and calcium (Bradley 2009).

Monitoring Parameters CBC with differential, platelet count, PT, renal and hepatic function tests periodically; number and type of stools/day for diarrhea; observe for signs and symptoms of anaphylaxis

Test Interactions Positive direct Coombs', false-positive urinary glucose test using cupric sulfate (Benedict's solution, Clinitest®, Fehling's solution), false-positive serum or urine creatinine with Jaffé reaction

Additional Information Rocephin® contains 3.6 mEq sodium per gram of ceftriaxone.

Dosage Forms Excipient information presented when available (limited, particularly for generics); consult specific product labeling.

Solution, Intravenous:

Generic: 20 mg/mL (50 mL); 40 mg/mL (50 mL)

Solution Reconstituted, Injection:

Rocephin: 500 mg (1 ea); 1 g (1 ea)

Generic: 250 mg (1 ea); 500 mg (1 ea); 1 g (1 ea); 2 g (1 ea); 100 g (1 ea)

Solution Reconstituted, Intravenous:

Generic: 1 g (1 ea); 2 g (1 ea); 10 g (1 ea)

- ◆ **Ceftriaxone for Injection (Can)** *see* CefTRIAXone *on page 410*
- ◆ **Ceftriaxone for Injection USP (Can)** *see* CefTRIAXone *on page 410*
- ◆ **Ceftriaxone Sodium** *see* CefTRIAXone *on page 410*
- ◆ **Ceftriaxone Sodium for Injection (Can)** *see* CefTRIAXone *on page 410*
- ◆ **Ceftriaxone Sodium for Injection BP (Can)** *see* CefTRIAXone *on page 410*

Cefuroxime (se fyoor OKS eem)

Medication Safety Issues

Sound-alike/look-alike issues:

Cefuroxime may be confused with cefotaxime, cefprozil, deferoxamine

Ceftin may be confused with Cefzil, Cipro

Zinacef may be confused with Zithromax

International issues:

Ceftin [U.S., Canada] may be confused with Cefiton brand name for cefixime [Portugal]; Ceftim brand name for ceftazidime [Portugal]; Ceftime brand name for ceftazidime [Thailand]

Related Information

Oral Medications That Should Not Be Crushed or Altered *on page 2476*

Brand Names: US Ceftin; Zinacef; Zinacef in Sterile Water

Brand Names: Canada Apo-Cefuroxime; Auro-Cefuroxime; Ceftin; Cefuroxime For Injection; Cefuroxime For Injection, USP; PRO-Cefuroxime; ratio-Cefuroxime

Therapeutic Category Antibiotic, Cephalosporin (Second Generation)

Generic Availability (US) May be product dependent

Use

Oral suspension: Treatment of mild to moderate susceptible infections including pharyngitis/tonsillitis, acute bacterial maxillary sinusitis, acute bacterial otitis media, and impetigo (FDA approved in ages 3 months to 12 years)

Oral tablet: Treatment of mild to moderate susceptible infections involving the upper and lower respiratory tract, otitis media, acute bacterial maxillary sinusitis, urinary tract (uncomplicated), skin and soft tissue (uncomplicated), urethral and endocervical gonorrhea (uncomplicated), and early Lyme disease [FDA approved in pediatric patients (age not specified) and adults]

Parenteral: Treatment susceptible infections involving the upper and lower respiratory tract, urinary tract, skin and skin structure, sepsis, uncomplicated and disseminated gonorrhea, and bone and joints (FDA approved in ages ≥3 months and adults); surgical prophylaxis (FDA approved in adults)

Pregnancy Risk Factor B

Pregnancy Considerations Adverse events were not observed in animal reproduction studies. Cefuroxime crosses the placenta and reaches the cord serum and amniotic fluid. Placental transfer is decreased in the presence of oligohydramnios. Several studies have failed to identify an increased teratogenic risk to the fetus following maternal cefuroxime use.

During pregnancy, mean plasma concentrations of cefuroxime are 50% lower, the AUC is 25% lower, and the plasma half-life is shorter than nonpregnant values. At term, plasma half-life is similar to nonpregnant values and peak maternal concentrations after IM administration are slightly decreased. Pregnancy does not alter the volume of distribution. Cefuroxime is one of the antibiotics recommended for prophylactic use prior to cesarean delivery.

Breast-Feeding Considerations Cefuroxime is excreted in breast milk. Manufacturer recommendations vary; caution is recommended if cefuroxime IV is given to a nursing woman and it is recommended to consider discontinuing nursing temporarily during treatment following oral cefuroxime. Nondose-related effects could include modification of bowel flora.

Contraindications Hypersensitivity to cefuroxime, any component of the formulation, or other cephalosporins

Warnings/Precautions Modify dosage in patients with severe renal impairment. Use with caution in patients with a history of penicillin allergy, especially IgE-mediated reactions (eg, anaphylaxis, urticaria). Prolonged use may result in fungal or bacterial superinfection, including *C. difficile*-associated diarrhea (CDAD) and pseudomembranous colitis; CDAD has been observed >2 months postantibiotic treatment. Use with caution in patients with a history of colitis. Use with caution in patients with a history of seizure disorder; cephalosporins have been associated with seizure activity, particularly in patients with renal impairment not receiving dose adjustments. Discontinue if seizures occur. May be associated with increased INR, especially in nutritionally deficient patients, prolonged treatment, hepatic or renal disease. Tablets and oral suspension are not bioequivalent (do not substitute on a mg-per-mg basis). Tablets should not be crushed or chewed due to a strong, persistent bitter taste. Patients unable to swallow whole tablets should be prescribed the oral suspension. Potentially significant drug-drug interactions may exist, requiring dose or frequency adjustment, additional monitoring, and/or selection of alternative therapy.

Benzyl alcohol and derivatives: Some dosage forms may contain sodium benzoate/benzoic acid; benzoic acid (benzoate) is a metabolite of benzyl alcohol; large amounts of benzyl alcohol (≥99 mg/kg/day) have been associated with a potentially fatal toxicity ("gasping syndrome") in neonates; the "gasping syndrome" consists of metabolic acidosis, respiratory distress, gasping respirations, CNS dysfunction (including convulsions, intracranial hemorrhage), hypotension, and cardiovascular collapse (AAP, 1997; CDC, 1982); some data suggests that benzoate displaces bilirubin from protein binding sites (Ahlfors, 2001); avoid or use dosage forms containing benzyl alcohol derivative with caution in neonates. See manufacturer's labeling.

Phenylalanine: Some products may contain phenylalanine.

Adverse Reactions

Cardiovascular: Local thrombophlebitis

Dermatologic: Diaper rash (children)

Endocrine & metabolic: Increased lactate dehydrogenase

Gastrointestinal: Diarrhea (duration-dependent), nausea and vomiting, unpleasant taste

Genitourinary: Vaginitis

Hematologic: Decreased hematocrit, decreased hemoglobin, eosinophilia

Hepatic: Increased serum alkaline phosphatase, increased serum transaminases

Immunologic: Jarisch-Herxheimer reaction

Rare but important or life-threatening: Anaphylaxis, angioedema, anorexia, brain disease, candidiasis, chest tightness, cholestasis, *Clostridium difficile* associated diarrhea, colitis, decreased creatinine clearance, drug fever, dyspepsia, dysuria, erythema, erythema multiforme, gastrointestinal hemorrhage, gastrointestinal infection, glossitis, headache, hearing loss, hemolytic anemia, hepatitis, hyperactivity, hyperbilirubinemia, hypersensitivity, hypersensitivity angiitis, increased blood urea nitrogen, increased liver enzymes, increased serum creatinine, increased thirst, interstitial nephritis, irritability, joint swelling, leukopenia, muscle cramps, muscle rigidity, muscle spasm (neck), neutropenia, oral mucosa ulcer, pancytopenia, positive direct Coombs test, prolonged prothrombin time, pseudomembranous colitis, renal insufficiency, renal pain, seizure, serum sickness-like reaction, sialorrhea, sinusitis, Stevens-Johnson syndrome, swollen tongue, tachycardia, thrombocytopenia (rare), toxic epidermal necrolysis, trismus, upper respiratory tract infection, urethral bleeding, urethral pain, urinary tract infection, vaginal discharge, vaginal irritation, viral infection, vulvovaginal candidiasis, vulvovaginal pruritus

Drug Interactions

Metabolism/Transport Effects

None known.

Avoid Concomitant Use

Avoid concomitant use of Cefuroxime with any of the following: BCG; BCG (Intravesical)

Increased Effect/Toxicity

Cefuroxime may increase the levels/effects of: Aminoglycosides; Vitamin K Antagonists

The levels/effects of Cefuroxime may be increased by: Probenecid

Decreased Effect

Cefuroxime may decrease the levels/effects of: BCG; BCG (Intravesical); BCG Vaccine (Immunization); Sodium Picosulfate; Typhoid Vaccine

The levels/effects of Cefuroxime may be decreased by: Antacids; H2-Antagonists

Food Interactions Bioavailability is increased with food; cefuroxime serum levels may be increased if taken with food or dairy products. Management: Administer tablet without regard to meals; suspension must be administered with food.

Storage/Stability

Injection: Store intact vials at 15°C to 30°C (59°F to 86°F); protect from light. Reconstituted solution is stable for 24 hours at room temperature and 48 hours when refrigerated. IV infusion in NS or D_5W solution is stable for 24 hours at room temperature, 7 days when refrigerated, or 26 weeks when frozen. After freezing, thawed solution is stable for 24 hours at room temperature or 21 days when refrigerated.

Duplex container: Store unactivated units at 20°C to 25°C (68°F to 77°F). Unactivated units with foil strip removed from the drug chamber must be protected from light and used within 7 days. Once activated, may be stored for up to 24 hours at room temperature or for 7 days under refrigeration. Do not freeze.

ADD-Vantage vials: Joined, but not activated, vials are stable for 14 days. Once activated, stable for 24 hours at room temperature and 7 days refrigerated. Do not freeze.

Premix Galaxy plastic containers: Store frozen at -20°C. Thaw container at room temperature or under refrigeration; do not force thaw. Thawed solution is stable for 24 hours at room temperature and 28 days refrigerated; do not refreeze.

Oral suspension: Prior to reconstitution, store at 2°C to 30°C (36°F to 86°F). Reconstituted suspension is stable for 10 days at 2°C to 8°C (36°F to 46°F).

Tablet: Store at 15°C to 30°C (59°F to 86°F).

Mechanism of Action Inhibits bacterial cell wall synthesis by binding to one or more of the penicillin-binding proteins (PBPs) which in turn inhibits the final transpeptidation step of peptidoglycan synthesis in bacterial cell walls, thus inhibiting cell wall biosynthesis. Bacteria eventually lyse due to ongoing activity of cell wall autolytic enzymes (autolysins and murein hydrolases) while cell wall assembly is arrested.

Pharmacokinetics (Adult data unless noted)

Distribution: Into bronchial secretions, synovial and pericardial fluid, kidneys, heart, liver, bone and bile; penetrates into CSF with inflamed meninges

Protein binding: 33% to 50%

Metabolism: Cefuroxime axetil (oral) is hydrolyzed in the intestinal mucosa and blood to cefuroxime

Bioavailability: Oral tablet: Fasting: 37%; following food: 52%; cefuroxime axetil suspension is less bioavailable than the tablet (91% of the AUC for tablets)

Half-life:

Premature neonates:

PNA ≤3 days: Median: 5.8 hours (de Louvois, 1982)

PNA ≥8 days: Median: 1.6-3.8 hours (de Louvois, 1982)

Children and Adolescents: 1.4-1.9 hours

Adults: 1-2 hours (prolonged in renal impairment)

Time to peak serum concentration:

Oral: Children: 3-4 hours; Adults: 2-3 hours

IM: Within 15-60 minutes

Elimination: Primarily 66% to 100% as unchanged drug in urine by both glomerular filtration and tubular secretion

Dosing: Neonatal

General dosing, susceptible infection: IM, IV (*Red Book* [AAP], 2012):

Body weight <1 kg:

PNA ≤14 days: 50 mg/kg/dose every 12 hours

PNA 15 to 28 days: 50 mg/kg/dose every 8 to 12 hours

Body weight 1 to 2 kg:

PNA ≤7 days: 50 mg/kg/dose every 12 hours

PNA 8 to 28 days: 50 mg/kg/dose every 8 to 12 hours

Body weight >2 kg:

PNA ≤7 days: 50 mg/kg/dose every 12 hours

PNA 8 to 28 days: 50 mg/kg/dose every 8 hours

Dosing: Usual Note: Cefuroxime axetil film-coated tablets and oral suspension are not bioequivalent and are not substitutable on a mg/mg basis.

Pediatric:

General dosing, susceptible infection (*Red Book* [AAP], 2012): Infants, Children, and Adolescents:

Mild to moderate infection:

Oral: 20 to 30 mg/kg/day divided twice daily; maximum single dose: 500 mg

IM, IV: 75 to 100 mg/kg/day divided in 3 doses; maximum single dose: 1500 mg

Severe infection: IM, IV: 100 to 200 mg/kg/day divided in 3 to 4 doses; maximum single dose: 1500 mg

Bone and joint infection: Infants ≥3 months, Children, and Adolescents: IM, IV: 50 mg/kg/dose every 8 hours; maximum single dose: 1500 mg

Bronchitis, acute (and exacerbations of chronic bronchitis): Adolescents: Oral tablets: 250 to 500 mg every 12 hours for 10 days

Gonorrhea, uncomplicated: Note: Due to increasing antimicrobial resistance, oral cephalosporins are no longer recommended for treatment of gonococcal infections (CDC, 2012). Adolescents: Oral tablet: 1000 mg as a single dose

Intra-abdominal infection complicated, community-acquired: Infants, Children, and Adolescents: IM, IV: 150 mg/kg/day in divided doses every 6 to 8 hours; maximum single dose: 1500 mg (Solomkin, 2010)

Lyme disease: Infants, Children, and Adolescents:

Acrodermatitis chronica atrophicans: Oral: 15 mg/kg/dose every 12 hours for 21 days; maximum single dose: 500 mg (Wormser, 2006)

Early localized disease: Oral: 15 mg/kg/dose every 12 hours for 14 to 21 days; maximum single dose: 500 mg (*Red Book* [AAP], 2012; Wormser, 2006)

Late disease (arthritis): Oral: 15 mg/kg/dose every 12 hours for 28 days; maximum single dose: 500 mg (Wormser, 2006)

Nervous system disease: **Note:** Use only when doxycycline is contraindicated; doxycycline is the preferred treatment; Oral: 15 mg/kg/dose every 12 hours for 14 days; maximum single dose: 500 mg (Halperin, 2007)

Otitis media, acute:

Manufacturer's labeling: Infants ≥3 months and Children:

Oral suspension: 15 mg/kg/dose twice daily for 10 days; maximum single dose: 500 mg

Oral tablet (patients able to swallow tablet whole): 250 mg twice daily for 10 days

Alternate dosing: AAP recommendations: Infants ≥6 months and Children: Oral suspension: 15 mg/kg/dose twice daily. Variable duration of therapy: If <2 years of age or severe symptoms (any age): 10-day course; if 2 to 5 years of age with mild to moderate symptoms: 7-day course; if ≥6 years of age with mild to moderate symptoms: 5- to 7-day course (AAP [Lieberthal, 2013])

Pharyngitis/tonsillitis:

Infants ≥3 months and Children: Oral suspension: 10 mg/kg/dose twice daily for 10 days; maximum single dose: 250 mg

Adolescents: Oral tablets: 250 mg twice daily for 10 days

Pneumonia, bacterial (HIV-exposed/-positive): Infants and Children: IV: 35 to 50 mg/kg/dose 3 times daily; maximum single dose: 2000 mg (DHHS [pediatric], 2013)

Sinusitis:

Infants ≥3 months and Children:

Oral suspension: 15 mg/kg/dose twice daily for 10 days; maximum single dose: 500 mg

Oral tablet (for patients able to swallow tablet whole): 250 mg twice daily for 10 days

Adolescents: Oral tablet: 250 mg twice daily for 10 days

Skin and skin structure infection:

Animal or human bites (Stevens, 2005): Adolescents:

Oral tablet: 500 mg twice daily

Parenteral: IM, IV: 1000 mg once daily

Impetigo: Infants ≥3 months and Children: Oral suspension: 15 mg/kg/dose twice daily for 10 days; maximum single dose: 500 mg

Uncomplicated skin and skin structure infections: Adolescents: Oral tablet: 250 to 500 mg twice daily for 10 days

Surgical prophylaxis: Children and Adolescents: IV: 50 mg/kg 30 to 60 minutes prior to procedure; may repeat dose in 4 hours; maximum single dose: 1500 mg (Bratzler, 2013)

Urinary tract infection, uncomplicated:

Infants and Children 2 to 24 months: Oral suspension: 10 to 15 mg/kg/dose twice daily (AAP, 2011)

Children >24 months: Moderate to severe disease (possible pyelonephritis): Oral suspension: 20 to 30 mg/kg/day divided twice daily; maximum single dose: 500 mg (Bradley, 2012)

Adolescents: Oral tablet: 250 mg twice daily for 7 to 10 days

Adult:

Bronchitis, acute (and exacerbations of chronic bronchitis):

Oral: 250 to 500 mg every 12 hours for 10 days

IV: 500 to 750 mg every 8 hours (complete therapy with oral dosing)

Cellulitis, orbital: IV: 1500 mg every 8 hours

Cholecystitis, mild to moderate: IV: 1500 mg every 8 hours for 4 to 7 days (provided source controlled)

Gonorrhea:

Disseminated: IM, IV: 750 mg every 8 hours

Uncomplicated:

Oral: 1000 mg as a single dose

IM: 1500 mg as single dose (administer in two different sites with oral probenecid)

Intra-abdominal infection, complicated, community-acquired, mild to moderate (in combination with metronidazole): IV: 1500 mg every 8 hours for 4 to 7 days (provided source controlled) (Solomkin, 2010)

Lyme disease (early): Oral: 500 mg twice daily for 20 days

Pharyngitis/tonsillitis and sinusitis: Oral: 250 mg twice daily for 10 days

Pneumonia, uncomplicated: IM, IV: 750 mg every 8 hours

Severe or complicated infections: IM, IV: 1500 mg every 8 hours (up to 1500 mg every 6 hours in life-threatening infections)

Skin/skin structure infection, uncomplicated:

Oral: 250 to 500 mg every 12 hours for 10 days

IM, IV: 750 mg every 8 hours

Surgical prophylaxis:

Manufacturer's recommendation: IV: 1500 mg 30 minutes to 1 hour prior to procedure (if procedure is prolonged can give 750 mg every 8 hours IV or IM)

Open heart: IV: 1500 mg every 12 hours for a total of 4 doses starting at anesthesia induction

Alternative recommendation: IV: 1500 mg within 60 minutes prior to surgical incision. Doses may be repeated in 4 hours if procedure is lengthy or if there is excessive blood loss (Bratzler, 2013).

Urinary tract infection, uncomplicated:

Oral: 125 to 250 mg twice daily for 7 to 10 days

IV, IM: 750 mg every 8 hours

Dosing interval in renal impairment:

Infants, Children, and Adolescents: The manufacturer's labeling recommends decreasing the frequency similar to adult recommendations. The following guidelines have been used by some clinicians (Aronoff, 2007). **Note:** Renally adjusted dose recommendations are based on doses of 30 mg/kg/day divided every 12 hours (oral) or 75 to 150 mg/kg/day divided every 8 hours (IM, IV). Oral, Parenteral:

GFR ≥30 mL/minute/1.73 m^2: No adjustment required

GFR 10 to 29 mL/minute/1.73 m^2: Administer every 12 hours

GFR <10 mL/minute/1.73 m^2: Administer every 24 hours

Intermittent hemodialysis: Administer every 24 hours

Peritoneal dialysis: Administer every 24 hours

Adults:

Oral: No dosage adjustment required. Dose after dialysis on dialysis days (Aronoff, 2007).

Parenteral:

CrCl >20 mL/minute: No adjustment required

CrCl 10 to 20 mL/minute: 750 mg every 12 hours

CrCl <10 mL/minute: 750 mg every 24 hours

Peritoneal dialysis: Administer every 24 hours

Continuous renal replacement therapy (CRRT): 1000 mg every 12 hours

Dosing adjustment in hepatic impairment: There are no dosage adjustments provided in the manufacturer's labeling.

Preparation for Administration

Oral suspension: Reconstitute powder for oral suspension with appropriate amount of water as specified on the bottle. Shake vigorously until suspended.

Parenteral:

IM: Dilute 750 mg vial with 3 mL SWFI; resultant suspension with a concentration of 225 mg/mL

Intermittent IV infusion: Further dilute reconstituted solution to a final concentration ≤30 mg/mL; in fluid restricted patients, dilution with SWFI to a concentration of 137 mg/mL results in a maximum recommended osmolality for peripheral infusion (Robinson 1987)

IVP: Reconstitute vial to a final concentration of 90 or 95 mg/mL (per manufacturer), some centers have used a final concentration of 100 mg/mL.

Administration

Oral: Cefuroxime axetil suspension must be administered with food; shake suspension well before use; tablets may be administered with or without food; administer with food to decrease GI upset; avoid crushing the tablet due to its bitter taste

Parenteral:

IM: Inject deep IM into large muscle mass; less painful when administered as an injectable suspension rather than a solution, and is less painful when administered into the buttock rather than the thigh

Intermittent IV infusion: Administer over 15 to 30 minutes

IVP: Administer over 3 to 5 minutes

Monitoring Parameters With prolonged therapy, monitor renal, hepatic, and hematologic function periodically; number and type of stools/day for diarrhea; and prothrombin time. Observe for signs and symptoms of anaphylaxis during first dose.

Test Interactions Positive direct Coombs', false-positive urinary glucose test using cupric sulfate (Benedict's solution, Clinitest®, Fehling's solution); false-negative may occur with ferricyanide test. Glucose oxidase or hexokinase-based methods should be used.

Dosage Forms Excipient information presented when available (limited, particularly for generics); consult specific product labeling.

Solution, Intravenous, as sodium [strength expressed as base]:

Zinacef in Sterile Water: 1.5 g (50 mL)

Solution Reconstituted, Injection, as sodium [strength expressed as base]:

Zinacef: 750 mg (1 ea); 1.5 g (1 ea); 7.5 g (1 ea)

Generic: 750 mg (1 ea); 1.5 g (1 ea); 7.5 g (1 ea); 75 g (1 ea); 225 g (1 ea)

Solution Reconstituted, Intravenous, as sodium [strength expressed as base]:

Zinacef: 750 mg (1 ea); 1.5 g (1 ea)

Generic: 750 mg (1 ea); 1.5 g (1 ea); 7.5 g (1 ea)

Suspension Reconstituted, Oral, as axetil [strength expressed as base]:

Ceftin: 125 mg/5 mL (100 mL); 250 mg/5 mL (50 mL, 100 mL) [contains aspartame; tutti-frutti flavor]

Generic: 125 mg/5 mL (100 mL)

Tablet, Oral, as axetil [strength expressed as base]:
Ceftin: 250 mg, 500 mg
Generic: 250 mg, 500 mg

- **Cefuroxime Axetil** *see* Cefuroxime *on page 414*
- **Cefuroxime For Injection (Can)** *see* Cefuroxime *on page 414*
- **Cefuroxime For Injection, USP (Can)** *see* Cefuroxime *on page 414*
- **Cefuroxime Sodium** *see* Cefuroxime *on page 414*
- **Cefzil** *see* Cefprozil *on page 405*
- **CeleBREX** *see* Celecoxib *on page 418*
- **Celebrex (Can)** *see* Celecoxib *on page 418*

Celecoxib (se le KOKS ib)

Medication Safety Issues

Sound-alike/look-alike issues:

CeleBREX may be confused with CeleXA, Cerebyx, Cervarix, Clarinex

Brand Names: US CeleBREX

Brand Names: Canada ACCEL-Celecoxib; ACT Celecoxib; Apo-Celecoxib; Bio-Celecoxib; Celebrex; GD-Celecoxib; JAMP-Celecoxib; Mar-Celecoxib; Mint-Celecoxib; Mylan-Celecoxib; PMS-Celecoxib; Priva-Celecoxib; RAN-Celecoxib; Riva-Celecoxib; Sandoz-Celecoxib; Teva-Celecoxib

Therapeutic Category Nonsteroidal Anti-inflammatory Drug (NSAID), COX-2 Selective

Generic Availability (US) Yes

Use Relief of signs and symptoms of juvenile idiopathic arthritis (JIA) (FDA approved in ages ≥2 years weighing ≥10 kg); relief of sign and symptoms of osteoarthritis, adult rheumatoid arthritis, and ankylosing spondylitis (FDA approved in adults); management of acute pain (FDA approved in adults); treatment of primary dysmenorrhea (FDA approved in adults)

Medication Guide Available Yes

Pregnancy Risk Factor C (prior to 30 weeks gestation)/D (≥30 weeks gestation)

Pregnancy Considerations Teratogenic effects have been observed in some animal studies; therefore, celecoxib is classified as pregnancy category C. Celecoxib is a NSAID that primarily inhibits COX-2 whereas other currently available NSAIDs are nonselective for COX-1 and COX-2. The effects of this selective inhibition to the fetus have not been well studied and limited information is available specific to celecoxib. NSAID exposure during the first trimester is not strongly associated with congenital malformations; however, cardiovascular anomalies and cleft palate have been observed following NSAID exposure in some studies. The use of a NSAID close to conception may be associated with an increased risk of miscarriage. Nonteratogenic effects have been observed following NSAID administration during the third trimester including: Myocardial degenerative changes, prenatal constriction of the ductus arteriosus, fetal tricuspid regurgitation, failure of the ductus arteriosus to close postnatally; renal dysfunction or failure, oligohydramnios; gastrointestinal bleeding or perforation, increased risk of necrotizing enterocolitis; intracranial bleeding (including intraventricular hemorrhage), platelet dysfunction with resultant bleeding; pulmonary hypertension. Because it may cause premature closure of the ductus arteriosus, the use of celecoxib is not recommended ≥30 weeks gestation. The chronic use of NSAIDs in women of reproductive age may be associated with infertility that is reversible upon discontinuation of the medication. A registry is available for pregnant women exposed to autoimmune medications including celecoxib. For additional information contact the Organization of Teratology Information Specialists, OTIS Autoimmune Diseases Study, at 877-311-8972.

Breast-Feeding Considerations Small amounts of celecoxib are found in breast milk. The manufacturer recommends that caution be exercised when administering celecoxib to nursing women.

Contraindications

Hypersensitivity to celecoxib, sulfonamides, aspirin, other NSAIDs, or any component of the formulation; patients who have demonstrated allergic-type reactions to sulfonamides; patients who have experienced asthma, urticaria, or allergic-type reactions after taking aspirin or other NSAIDs; treatment of perioperative pain in the setting of CABG surgery; active gastrointestinal bleeding.

Canadian labeling: Additional contraindications (not in US labeling): Pregnancy (third trimester); women who are breast-feeding; severe, uncontrolled heart failure; active gastrointestinal ulcer (gastric, duodenal, peptic); inflammatory bowel disease; cerebrovascular bleeding; severe liver impairment or active hepatic disease; severe renal impairment (CrCl <30 mL/minute) or deteriorating renal disease; known hyperkalemia; use in patients <18 years of age

Warnings/Precautions [US Boxed Warning]: NSAIDs are associated with an increased risk of serious (and potentially fatal) adverse cardiovascular thrombotic events, including MI and stroke. Risk may be increased with duration of use or preexisting cardiovascular risk factors or disease. Carefully evaluate individual cardiovascular risk profiles prior to prescribing. New-onset or exacerbation of hypertension may occur (NSAIDS may impair response to thiazide or loop diuretics); may contribute to cardiovascular events; monitor blood pressure; use with caution in patients with hypertension. May cause sodium and fluid retention; use with caution in patients with edema, cerebrovascular disease, or ischemic heart disease. Avoid use in patients with heart failure (ACCF/AHA [Yancy, 2013]). Long-term cardiovascular risk in children has not been evaluated.

[US Boxed Warning]: Celecoxib is contraindicated for treatment of perioperative pain in the setting of coronary artery bypass graft (CABG) surgery. Risk of MI and stroke may be increased with use following CABG surgery.

[US Boxed Warning]: NSAIDs may increase risk of serious gastrointestinal ulceration, bleeding, and perforation (may be fatal). These events may occur at any time during therapy and without warning. Use is contraindicated with active GI bleeding. Use caution with a history of GI ulcers, concurrent therapy with aspirin, anticoagulants and/or corticosteroids, smoking, use of alcohol, the elderly or debilitated patients. When used concomitantly with aspirin, a substantial increase in the risk of gastrointestinal complications (eg, ulcer) occurs; concomitant gastroprotective therapy (eg, proton pump inhibitors) is recommended (Bhatt, 2008).

Use the lowest effective dose for the shortest duration of time, consistent with individual patient goals, to reduce risk of cardiovascular or GI adverse events. Alternate therapies should be considered for patients at high risk.

NSAIDs may cause serious skin adverse events including exfoliative dermatitis, Stevens-Johnson syndrome (SJS), and toxic epidermal necrolysis (TEN); may occur without warning and in patients without prior known sulfa allergy. Anaphylactoid reactions may occur, even without prior exposure; patients with "aspirin triad" (bronchial asthma, aspirin intolerance, rhinitis) may be at increased risk. Do not use in patients who have experienced an anaphylactic reaction with NSAID or aspirin therapy. The manufacturer's labeling states to not administer to patients with aspirin-sensitive asthma due to severe and potentially fatal bronchospasm that has been reported in such patients having received aspirin and the potential for cross reactivity with other NSAIDs. The manufacturer also states to use with caution in patients with other forms of asthma. However, in patients with known aspirin-exacerbated respiratory disease (AERD), the use of celecoxib initiated at a low dose with gradual titration in patients with stable, mild-to-moderate persistent asthma has been used without incident (Morales, 2013).

Use with caution in patients with decreased hepatic (dosage adjustments are recommended for moderate hepatic impairment; not recommended for patients with severe hepatic impairment) or renal function. Transaminase elevations have been reported with use; closely monitor patients with any abnormal LFT. Severe hepatic reactions (eg, fulminant hepatitis, liver failure) have occurred with NSAID use, rarely; discontinue if signs or symptoms of liver disease develop, if systemic manifestations occur, or with persistent or worsening abnormal hepatic function tests. NSAID use may compromise existing renal function; dose-dependent decreases in prostaglandin synthesis may result from NSAID use, causing a reduction in renal blood flow which may cause renal decompensation (usually reversible). Patients with impaired renal function, dehydration, heart failure, liver dysfunction, those taking diuretics, ACE inhibitors, angiotensin II receptor blockers, and the elderly are at greater risk for renal toxicity. Rehydrate patient before starting therapy; monitor renal function closely. Not recommended for use in patients with advanced renal disease or severe renal insufficiency; discontinue use with persistent or worsening abnormal renal function tests. Long-term NSAID use may result in renal papillary necrosis. Should not be considered a treatment or replacement of corticosteroid-dependent diseases.

Anaphylactoid reactions may occur, even with no prior exposure to celecoxib. Use with caution in patients with known or suspected deficiency of cytochrome P450 isoenzyme 2C9; poor metabolizers may have higher plasma levels due to reduced metabolism; consider reduced initial doses. Alternate therapies should be considered in patients with JIA who are poor metabolizers of CYP2C9.

Anemia may occur with use; monitor hemoglobin or hematocrit in patients on long-term treatment. Celecoxib does not affect PT, PTT or platelet counts; does not inhibit platelet aggregation at approved doses. Potentially significant drug-drug interactions may exist, requiring dose or frequency adjustment, additional monitoring, and/or selection of alternative therapy.

Use with caution in pediatric patients with systemic-onset juvenile idiopathic arthritis (JIA); serious adverse reactions, including disseminated intravascular coagulation, may occur. The Canadian labeling contraindicates use in patients <18 years of age.

Warnings: Additional Pediatric Considerations Consider alternate therapy in JIA patients who are identified to be CYP2C9 poor metabolizers. In a small pediatric study (n=4), the AUC of celecoxib was ~10 times higher in a child who was homozygous for CYP2C9*3, compared to children who were homozygous for the *1 allele (n=2) or who had the CYP2C9*1/*2 genotype; further studies are needed to determine if carriers of the CYP2C9*3 allele are at increased risk for cardiovascular toxicity or dose related adverse effects of celecoxib, especially with long-term, high-dose use of the drug (Stempak, 2005). Long-term (>6 months) cardiovascular toxicity in children and adolescents has not been studied.

Adverse Reactions

Cardiovascular: Angina pectoris, aortic insufficiency, chest pain, coronary artery disease, edema, facial edema, hypertension (aggravated), myocardial infarction, palpitations, peripheral edema, sinus bradycardia, tachycardia, ventricular hypertrophy

Central nervous system: Anxiety, depression, dizziness, drowsiness, fatigue, headache, hypertonia, hypoesthesia, insomnia, migraine, nervousness, pain, paresthesia, vertigo

Dermatologic: Alopecia, cellulitis, dermatitis, diaphoresis, erythematous rash, maculopapular rash, pruritus, skin photosensitivity, skin rash, urticaria, xeroderma

Endocrine & metabolic: Albuminuria, decreased plasma testosterone, hot flash, hypercholesterolemia, hyperglycemia, hypokalemia, increased nonprotein nitrogen, ovarian cyst, weight gain

Gastrointestinal: Abdominal pain, anorexia, constipation, diarrhea, diverticulitis, dyspepsia, dysphagia, eructation, esophagitis, flatulence, gastritis, gastroenteritis, gastroesophageal reflux disease, gastrointestinal ulcer, hemorrhoids, hiatal hernia, increased appetite, melena, nausea, stomatitis, tenesmus, vomiting, xerostomia

Genitourinary: Cystitis, dysuria, hematuria, urinary frequency

Hematologic & oncologic: Anemia, bruise, thrombocythemia

Hepatic: Increased serum alkaline phosphatase, increased serum transaminases

Hypersensitivity: Hypersensitivity exacerbation, hypersensitivity reaction

Neuromuscular & skeletal: Arthralgia, back pain, increased creatine phosphokinase, leg cramps, myalgia, osteoarthritis, synovitis, tendonitis

Ophthalmic: Conjunctival hemorrhage, vitreous opacity

Otic: Deafness, labyrinthitis, tinnitus

Renal: Increased blood urea nitrogen, increased serum creatinine, nephrolithiasis

Respiratory: Bronchitis, bronchospasm, cough, dyspnea, epistaxis, flu-like symptoms, laryngitis, nasopharyngitis, pharyngitis, pneumonia, rhinitis, sinusitis, upper respiratory tract infection

Miscellaneous: Cyst, fever

Rare but important or life-threatening: Acute renal failure, agranulocytosis, anaphylactoid reaction, angioedema, anosmia, aplastic anemia, aseptic meningitis, cardiac failure, cerebrovascular accident, cholelithiasis, colitis, deep vein thrombosis, dysgeusia, erythema multiforme, esophageal perforation, exfoliative dermatitis, gangrene of skin or other tissue, gastrointestinal hemorrhage, hepatic failure, hepatic necrosis, hepatitis (including fulminant), hypoglycemia, hyponatremia, interstitial nephritis, intestinal obstruction, intestinal perforation, intracranial hemorrhage, jaundice, leukopenia, pancreatitis, pancytopenia, pulmonary embolism, renal papillary necrosis, sepsis, Stevens-Johnson syndrome, syncope, thrombocytopenia, thrombophlebitis, toxic epidermal necrolysis, vasculitis, ventricular fibrillation

Drug Interactions

Metabolism/Transport Effects **Substrate** of CYP2C9 (major), CYP3A4 (minor); **Note:** Assignment of Major/Minor substrate status based on clinically relevant drug interaction potential; **Inhibits** CYP2C8 (moderate), CYP2D6 (moderate)

Avoid Concomitant Use

Avoid concomitant use of Celecoxib with any of the following: Amodiaquine; Dexketoprofen; Floctafenine; Ketorolac (Nasal); Ketorolac (Systemic); Mecamylamine; Morniflumate; Nonsteroidal Anti-Inflammatory Agents; NSAID (COX-2 Inhibitor); Omacetaxine; Thioridazine

Increased Effect/Toxicity

Celecoxib may increase the levels/effects of: 5-ASA Derivatives; Aliskiren; Aminoglycosides; Amodiaquine; Anticoagulants; ARIPiprazole; Bisphosphonate Derivatives; CycloSPORINE (Systemic); CYP2C8 Substrates; CYP2D6 Substrates; Deferasirox; Desmopressin; Digoxin; DOXOrubicin (Conventional); Drospirenone;

Eliglustat; Eplerenone; Estrogen Derivatives; Fesoterodine; Haloperidol; Lithium; Mecamylamine; Methotrexate; Metoprolol; Nebivolol; NSAID (COX-2 Inhibitor); Omacetaxine; Porfimer; Potassium-Sparing Diuretics; PRALAtrexate; Prilocaine; Quinolone Antibiotics; Sodium Nitrite; Tacrolimus (Systemic); Tenofovir; Thioridazine; Vancomycin; Verteporfin; Vitamin K Antagonists

The levels/effects of Celecoxib may be increased by: ACE Inhibitors; Angiotensin II Receptor Blockers; Antidepressants (Tricyclic, Tertiary Amine); Aspirin; Ceritinib; Corticosteroids (Systemic); CycloSPORINE (Systemic); CYP2C9 Inhibitors (Moderate); CYP2C9 Inhibitors (Strong); Dexketoprofen; Floctafenine; Herbs (Anticoagulant/Antiplatelet Properties); Ketorolac (Nasal); Ketorolac (Systemic); Mifepristone; Morniflumate; Nitric Oxide; Nonsteroidal Anti-Inflammatory Agents; Probenecid; Propafenone; Selective Serotonin Reuptake Inhibitors; Sodium Phosphates; Treprostinil

Decreased Effect

Celecoxib may decrease the levels/effects of: ACE Inhibitors; Aliskiren; Angiotensin II Receptor Blockers; Beta-Blockers; Codeine; Eplerenone; HydrALAZINE; Loop Diuretics; Potassium-Sparing Diuretics; Prostaglandins (Ophthalmic); Selective Serotonin Reuptake Inhibitors; Tamoxifen; Thiazide Diuretics; TraMADol

The levels/effects of Celecoxib may be decreased by: Bile Acid Sequestrants; CYP2C9 Inducers (Strong); Dabrafenib

Food Interactions Peak concentrations are delayed and AUC is increased by 10% to 20% when taken with a high-fat meal. Management: Administer without regard to meals.

Storage/Stability Store at 25°C (77°F); excursions permitted to 15°C to 30°C (59°F to 86°F).

Mechanism of Action Inhibits prostaglandin synthesis by decreasing the activity of the enzyme, cyclooxygenase-2 (COX-2), which results in decreased formation of prostaglandin precursors; has antipyretic, analgesic, and anti-inflammatory properties. Celecoxib does not inhibit cyclooxygenase-1 (COX-1) at therapeutic concentrations.

Pharmacokinetics (Adult data unless noted)

Absorption: Prolonged due to low solubility

Distribution: V_d (apparent):

Children and Adolescents ~7-16 years (steady-state): 8.3 ± 5.8 L/kg (Stempak, 2002)

Adults: ~400 L

Protein binding: ~97%; primarily to albumin; binds to alpha 1-acid glycoprotein to a lesser extent

Metabolism: Hepatic via CYP2C9; forms 3 inactive metabolites (a primary alcohol, corresponding carboxylic acid, and its glucuronide conjugate)

Bioavailability: Absolute: Unknown. AUC was increased by 40% and 180% with mild and moderate hepatic impairment, respectively. **Note:** Meta-analysis suggests the AUC is 40% higher in Blacks compared to Caucasians (clinical significance unknown).

Half-life elimination:

Children and Adolescents ~7-16 years (steady-state): 6 ± 2.7 hours (range: 3-10 hours) (Stempak, 2002)

Adults: ~11 hours (fasted)

Time to peak serum concentration:

Children: Median: 3 hours (range: 1-5.8 hours) (Stempak, 2002)

Adults: ~3 hours

Elimination: Feces (57% as metabolites, <3% as unchanged drug); urine (27% as metabolites, <3% as unchanged drug); primary metabolites in feces and urine: Carboxylic acid metabolite (73% of dose); low amounts of glucuronide metabolite appear in urine

Dosing: Usual Note: Use the lowest effective dose for the shortest duration of time, consistent with individual patient goals.

Children ≥2 years and Adolescents: **Juvenile idiopathic arthritis (JIA):** Oral:

≥10 kg to ≤25 kg: 50 mg twice daily

>25 kg: 100 mg twice daily

Adults:

Acute pain or primary dysmenorrhea: Oral: Initial dose: 400 mg, followed by an additional 200 mg if needed on day 1; maintenance dose: 200 mg twice daily as needed

Ankylosing spondylitis: Oral: 200 mg/day as a single dose or in divided doses twice daily; if no effect after 6 weeks, may increase to 400 mg/day. If no response following 6 weeks of treatment with 400 mg/day, consider discontinuation and alternative treatment.

Osteoarthritis: Oral: 200 mg/day as a single dose or in divided doses twice daily

Rheumatoid arthritis: Oral: 100-200 mg twice daily

Dosing adjustment in poor metabolizers of CYP2C9 substrates: Use with caution in patients who are known or suspected poor metabolizers of cytochrome P450 isoenzyme 2C9 substrates.

Children ≥2 years and Adolescents: Consider alternate therapy in JIA patients who are poor metabolizers.

Adults: Consider initiation at 50% of the lowest recommended dose.

Dosing adjustment in renal impairment: Children ≥2 years, Adolescents, and Adults: Use is not recommended in patients with severe renal dysfunction.

Dosing adjustment in hepatic impairment: Children ≥2 years, Adolescents, and Adults:

Moderate hepatic impatient (Child-Pugh Class B): Reduce dose by 50%; monitor closely

Severe hepatic impairment (Child-Pugh Class C): Use is not recommended; has not been studied

Administration Lower doses (up to 200 mg twice daily) may be administered without regard to meals (may administer with food to reduce GI upset); larger doses should be administered with food to improve absorption. Do not administer with antacids. Capsules may be swallowed whole or the entire contents emptied onto a teaspoon of cool or room temperature applesauce; the contents of the capsule sprinkled onto applesauce may be stored under refrigeration for up to 6 hours.

Monitoring Parameters CBC; blood chemistry profile; occult blood loss; periodic liver function tests; renal function (urine output, serum BUN and creatinine); monitor efficacy (eg, in arthritic conditions: Pain, range of motion, grip strength, mobility), inflammation; observe for weight gain, edema; observe for bleeding, bruising; evaluate GI effects (abdominal pain, bleeding, dyspepsia); blood pressure (baseline and throughout therapy)

JIA: Monitor for development of abnormal coagulation tests in patients with systemic-onset JIA

Dosage Forms Excipient information presented when available (limited, particularly for generics); consult specific product labeling.

Capsule, Oral:

CeleBREX: 50 mg, 100 mg, 200 mg, 400 mg

Generic: 50 mg, 100 mg, 200 mg, 400 mg

◆ **Celestoderm V (Can)** *see* Betamethasone (Topical) *on page* 280

◆ **Celestoderm V/2 (Can)** *see* Betamethasone (Topical) *on page* 280

◆ **Celestone [DSC]** *see* Betamethasone (Systemic) *on page* 278

◆ **Celestone Soluspan** *see* Betamethasone (Systemic) *on page* 278

◆ **CeleXA** *see* Citalopram *on page* 476

◆ **Celexa (Can)** *see* Citalopram *on page* 476

◆ **CellCept** *see* Mycophenolate *on page* 1473

- **CellCept Intravenous** *see* Mycophenolate *on page 1473*
- **CellCept I.V. (Can)** *see* Mycophenolate *on page 1473*
- **Cell Culture Inactivated Influenza Vaccine, Trivalent [Flucelvax]** *see* Influenza Virus Vaccine (Inactivated) *on page 1108*
- **Celontin** *see* Methsuximide *on page 1398*
- **Celontin® (Can)** *see* Methsuximide *on page 1398*
- **Celsentri (Can)** *see* Maraviroc *on page 1324*
- **Cemill [OTC]** *see* Ascorbic Acid *on page 202*
- **Cemill SR [OTC]** *see* Ascorbic Acid *on page 202*
- **Centany** *see* Mupirocin *on page 1471*
- **Centany AT** *see* Mupirocin *on page 1471*
- ***Centruroides* Immune FAB2 (Equine)** *see Centruroides* Immune F(ab')$_2$ (Equine) *on page 421*

Centruroides Immune F(ab')$_2$ (Equine)

(sen tra ROY dez i MYUN fab too E kwine)

Brand Names: US Anascorp

Therapeutic Category Antivenin

Generic Availability (US) No

Use Treatment of scorpion envenomation in patients with clinical signs of envenomation including, but not limited to, loss of muscle control, roving or abnormal eye movements, slurred speech, respiratory distress, excessive salivation, frothing at mouth, and vomiting (FDA approved in ages of neonates through adults)

Pregnancy Risk Factor C

Pregnancy Considerations Animal reproduction studies have not been conducted. In general, medications used as antidotes should take into consideration the health and prognosis of the mother; antidotes should be administered to pregnant women if there is a clear indication for use and should not be withheld because of fears of teratogenicity (Bailey 2003). Pregnant women experiencing symptoms refractory to reasonable doses of opioids or other systemic effects which pose a danger to the patient or fetus should be considered for antivenom therapy (Brown 2013).

Breast-Feeding Considerations It is not known if this product is excreted into breast milk. The manufacturer recommends caution be used if administered to a nursing woman.

Contraindications There are no contraindications listed within the manufacturer's labeling.

Warnings/Precautions Derived from equine (horse) immune globulin F(ab')$_2$ fragments; anaphylaxis and anaphylactoid reactions are possible, especially in patients with known allergies to horse protein. Patients who have had previous treatment with *Centruroides* immune F(ab')$_2$ or other equine-derived antivenom/antitoxin may be at a higher risk for acute hypersensitivity reactions. In patients who develop an anaphylactic reaction, discontinue the infusion and administer emergency care. Immediate treatment (eg, epinephrine 1:1000, corticosteroids, diphenhydramine) should be available. In addition, delayed serum sickness may occur, usually within 2 weeks; monitor patients with follow-up visits for signs and symptoms (eg, arthralgia, fever, myalgia, rash).

Product of equine (horse) plasma; may potentially contain infectious agents (eg, viruses) which could transmit disease. May contain small amounts of cresol resulting from the manufacturing process; local reactions and myalgias may occur.

Adverse Reactions

Central nervous system: Fatigue, fever, headache, lethargy

Dermatologic: Pruritus, rash

Gastrointestinal: Diarrhea, nausea, vomiting

Neuromuscular & skeletal: Myalgia

Respiratory: Cough, rhinorrhea

Rare but important or life-threatening: Aspiration, ataxia, chest tightness, eye edema, hypersensitivity, hypoxia, palpitation, pneumonia, respiratory distress, serum sickness (delayed)

Drug Interactions

Metabolism/Transport Effects None known.

Avoid Concomitant Use There are no known interactions where it is recommended to avoid concomitant use.

Increased Effect/Toxicity There are no known significant interactions involving an increase in effect.

Decreased Effect There are no known significant interactions involving a decrease in effect.

Storage/Stability Store unused vials at room temperature of 25°C (77°F); excursions permitted up to 40°C (104°F); do not freeze. Discard partially used vials.

Mechanism of Action Contains venom-specific F(ab')$_2$ fragments of IgG which bind and neutralize venom toxins; thereby helping to remove the toxin from the target tissue and eliminate it from the body.

Pharmacodynamics

Onset: Time to resolution of symptoms: Children: 1.28 ± 0.8 hours; Adults: 1.91 ± 1.4 hours; >95% of all patients will experience resolution of symptoms within 4 hours

Pharmacokinetics (Adult data unless noted)

Distribution: V_{dss}: 13.6 L ± 5.4 L

Half-life: 159 ± 57 hours

Dosing: Neonatal Scorpion envenomation: IV: Initial: 3 vials (~≤360 mg total protein and ≥450 LD50 [mouse] neutralizing units) initiated as soon as possible after scorpion sting; may administer additional vials in 1-vial increments every 30-60 minutes as needed

Dosing: Usual Scorpion envenomation: Infants, Children, Adolescents, and Adults: IV: Initial: 3 vials (~≤360 mg total protein and ≥450 LD50 [mouse] neutralizing units) initiated as soon as possible after scorpion sting; may administer additional vials in 1-vial increments every 30-60 minutes as needed.

Dosing adjustment in renal impairment: There are no dosage adjustments provided in manufacturer's labeling.

Dosing adjustment in hepatic impairment: There are no dosage adjustments provided in manufacturer's labeling.

Preparation for Administration IV: Reconstitute each vial with 5 mL NS; gently swirl to mix. Dilute dose (eg, 1 to 3 vials) with NS to a total volume of 50 mL. Inspect diluted solution; do not use if it contains particulate matter or is discolored or turbid.

Administration IV: Administer over 10 minutes; others have reported beginning infusion slower at 25 to 50 mL/hour and then double the rate every 5 minutes as tolerated (Turri 2011); monitor for return of symptoms of envenomation and repeat as needed. Medications (eg, epinephrine, corticosteroids, diphenhydramine) and equipment for resuscitation should be readily available in case of hypersensitivity reactions. IM administration should generally be avoided since the time to peak blood concentration may be prolonged with this route of administration (Turri 2011; Vasquez 2010). If unable to obtain intravenous access, intraosseous (full dose) and intramuscular (single vial dose) administration have been reported in a neonate and a 16 month old child (Hiller 2010).

Monitoring Parameters Signs and symptoms of envenomation (eg, opsoclonus, involuntary muscle movement, slurred speech, paresthesias, respiratory distress, salivation, frothy sputum, vomiting); signs and symptoms of hypersensitivity reactions; follow-up visits for signs and symptoms of serum sickness (eg, arthralgia, fever, myalgia, rash)

Additional Information Each vial of *Centruroides* immune F(ab')$_2$ (equine) contains ≤120 mg total protein and ≥150 LD50 (mouse) neutralizing units.

Dosage Forms Excipient information presented when available (limited, particularly for generics); consult specific product labeling.

Solution Reconstituted, Intravenous [preservative free]:
Anascorp: (1 ea)

◆ **Cepacol Dual Relief [OTC]** *see* Benzocaine *on page 268*

◆ **Cepacol Sensations Hydra [OTC]** *see* Benzocaine *on page 268*

◆ **Cepacol Sensations Warming [OTC]** *see* Benzocaine *on page 268*

Cephalexin (sef a LEKS in)

Medication Safety Issues

Sound-alike/look-alike issues:

Cephalexin may be confused with cefaclor, ceFAZolin, ciprofloxacin

Keflex may be confused with Keppra, Valtrex

Related Information

Prevention of Infective Endocarditis *on page 2378*

Brand Names: US Keflex

Brand Names: Canada Apo-Cephalex; Dom-Cephalexin; Keflex; PMS-Cephalexin; Teva-Cephalexin

Therapeutic Category Antibiotic, Cephalosporin (First Generation)

Generic Availability (US) Yes

Use Treatment of susceptible bacterial infections, including those caused by group A beta-hemolytic *Streptococcus*, *Staphylococcus*, *Klebsiella pneumoniae*, *E. coli*, and *Proteus mirabilis*; not active against enterococci or methicillin-resistant staphylococci; used to treat susceptible infections of the respiratory tract, skin and skin structure, bone, genitourinary tract, and otitis media; alternative therapy for endocarditis prophylaxis

Pregnancy Risk Factor B

Pregnancy Considerations Adverse events were not observed in animal reproduction studies. Cephalexin crosses the placenta and produces therapeutic concentrations in the fetal circulation and amniotic fluid. An increased risk of teratogenic effects has not been observed following maternal use of cephalexin. Peak concentrations in pregnant patients are similar to those in nonpregnant patients. Prolonged labor may decrease oral absorption.

Breast-Feeding Considerations Small amounts of cephalexin are excreted in breast milk. The manufacturer recommends that caution be exercised when administering cephalexin to nursing women. Maximum milk concentration occurs ~4 hours after a single oral dose and gradually disappears by 8 hours after administration. Non-dose-related effects could include modification of bowel flora.

Contraindications Hypersensitivity to cephalexin, any component of the formulation, or other cephalosporins

Warnings/Precautions Modify dosage in patients with severe renal impairment. Use with caution in patients with a history of penicillin allergy, especially IgE-mediated reactions (eg, anaphylaxis, urticaria). Prolonged use may result in fungal or bacterial superinfection, including *C. difficile*-associated diarrhea (CDAD) and pseudomembranous colitis; CDAD has been observed >2 months post-antibiotic treatment. May be associated with increased INR, especially in nutritionally-deficient patients, prolonged treatment, hepatic or renal disease.

Adverse Reactions

Central nervous system: Agitation, confusion, dizziness, fatigue, hallucination, headache

Dermatologic: Erythema multiforme (rare), genital pruritus, skin rash, Stevens-Johnson syndrome (rare), toxic epidermal necrolysis (rare), urticaria

Gastrointestinal: Abdominal pain, diarrhea, dyspepsia, gastritis, nausea (rare), pseudomembranous colitis, vomiting (rare)

Genitourinary: Genital candidiasis, vaginal discharge, vaginitis

Hematologic & oncologic: Eosinophilia, hemolytic anemia, neutropenia, thrombocytopenia

Hepatic: Cholestatic jaundice (rare), hepatitis (transient, rare), increased serum ALT, increased serum AST

Hypersensitivity: Anaphylaxis, angioedema, hypersensitivity reaction

Neuromuscular & skeletal: Arthralgia, arthritis, arthropathy

Renal: Interstitial nephritis (rare)

Drug Interactions

Metabolism/Transport Effects None known.

Avoid Concomitant Use

Avoid concomitant use of Cephalexin with any of the following: BCG; BCG (Intravesical)

Increased Effect/Toxicity

Cephalexin may increase the levels/effects of: MetFORMIN; Vitamin K Antagonists

The levels/effects of Cephalexin may be increased by: Probenecid

Decreased Effect

Cephalexin may decrease the levels/effects of: BCG; BCG (Intravesical); BCG Vaccine (Immunization); Sodium Picosulfate; Typhoid Vaccine

The levels/effects of Cephalexin may be decreased by: Multivitamins/Minerals (with ADEK, Folate, Iron); Multivitamins/Minerals (with AE, No Iron); Zinc Salts

Food Interactions Peak antibiotic serum concentration is lowered and delayed, but total drug absorbed is not affected. Cephalexin serum levels may be decreased if taken with food. Management: Administer without regard to food.

Storage/Stability

Capsule: Store at 15°C to 30°C (59°F to 86°F).

Powder for oral suspension: Refrigerate suspension after reconstitution; discard after 14 days.

Tablet: Store at 20°C to 25°C (68°F to 77°F).

Mechanism of Action Inhibits bacterial cell wall synthesis by binding to one or more of the penicillin-binding proteins (PBPs) which in turn inhibits the final transpeptidation step of peptidoglycan synthesis in bacterial cell walls, thus inhibiting cell wall biosynthesis. Bacteria eventually lyse due to ongoing activity of cell wall autolytic enzymes (autolysins and murein hydrolases) while cell wall assembly is arrested.

Pharmacokinetics (Adult data unless noted)

Absorption: Rapid (90%); delayed in young children and may be decreased up to 50% in neonates

Distribution: Into tissues and fluids including bone, pleural and synovial fluid; crosses the placenta; appears in breast milk

Protein binding: 6% to 15%

Half-life:

Neonates: 5 hours

Children 3-12 months: 2.5 hours

Adults: 0.5-1.2 hours (prolonged with renal impairment)

Time to peak serum concentration: Oral: Within 60 minutes

Elimination: 80% to 100% of dose excreted as unchanged drug in urine within 8 hours

Dialysis: Moderately dialyzable (20% to 50%)

Dosing: Usual Oral:

Children: 25-50 mg/kg/day divided every 6-8 hours; severe infections: 50-100 mg/kg/day divided every 6-8 hours; maximum dose: 4 g/day

Otitis media: 75-100 mg/kg/day divided every 6 hours

Streptococcal pharyngitis, skin and skin structure infections: 25-50 mg/kg/day divided every 12 hours

Endocarditis prophylaxis: 50 mg/kg 1 hour prior to procedure (maximum: 2 g)
Uncomplicated cystitis: Children >15 years: 500 mg every 12 hours for 7-14 days
Adults: 250-500 mg every 6 hours; maximum dose: 4 g/day
Streptococcal pharyngitis, skin and skin structure infections: 500 mg every 12 hours
Endocarditis prophylaxis: 2 g 1 hour prior to procedure
Uncomplicated cystitis: 500 mg every 12 hours for 7-14 days
Dosing interval in renal impairment:
CrCl 10-40 mL/minute: Administer every 8-12 hours
CrCl <10 mL/minute: Administer every 12-24 hours

Preparation for Administration Oral: Powder for oral suspension: Reconstitute powder for oral suspension with appropriate amount of water as specified on the bottle. Shake vigorously until suspended.

Administration Oral: Administer on an empty stomach (ie, 1 hour prior to, or 2 hours after meals); administer with food if GI upset occurs; shake suspension well before use

Monitoring Parameters With prolonged therapy, monitor renal, hepatic, and hematologic function periodically; number and type of stools/day for diarrhea

Test Interactions Positive direct Coombs', false-positive urinary glucose test using cupric sulfate (Benedict's solution, Clinitest®, Fehling's solution), false-positive serum or urine creatinine with Jaffé reaction, false-positive urinary proteins and steroids

Dosage Forms Excipient information presented when available (limited, particularly for generics); consult specific product labeling.
Capsule, Oral:
Keflex: 250 mg, 500 mg, 750 mg [contains brilliant blue fcf (fd&c blue #1), fd&c yellow #10 (quinoline yellow), fd&c yellow #6 (sunset yellow)]
Generic: 250 mg, 500 mg, 750 mg
Suspension Reconstituted, Oral:
Generic: 125 mg/5 mL (100 mL, 200 mL); 250 mg/5 mL (100 mL, 200 mL)
Tablet, Oral:
Generic: 250 mg, 500 mg

- ◆ **Cephalexin Monohydrate** *see* Cephalexin *on page 422*
- ◆ **Ceprotin** *see* Protein C Concentrate (Human) *on page 1797*
- ◆ **Cerebyx** *see* Fosphenytoin *on page 945*
- ◆ **Cerezyme** *see* Imiglucerase *on page 1082*
- ◆ **Cerubidine** *see* DAUNOrubicin (Conventional) *on page 592*
- ◆ **Cervarix** *see* Papillomavirus (Types 16, 18) Vaccine (Human, Recombinant) *on page 1628*
- ◆ **C.E.S.** *see* Estrogens (Conjugated/Equine, Systemic) *on page 801*
- ◆ **C.E.S.** *see* Estrogens (Conjugated/Equine, Topical) *on page 803*
- ◆ **C.E.S.® (Can)** *see* Estrogens (Conjugated/Equine, Systemic) *on page 801*
- ◆ **Cesamet** *see* Nabilone *on page 1478*
- ◆ **Cetafen [OTC]** *see* Acetaminophen *on page 44*
- ◆ **Cetafen Extra [OTC]** *see* Acetaminophen *on page 44*

Cetirizine (se TI ra zeen)

Medication Safety Issues
Sound-alike/look-alike issues:
Cetirizine may be confused with sertraline, stavudine
ZyrTEC may be confused with Lipitor, Serax, Xanax, Zantac, Zerit, Zocor, ZyPREXA, ZyrTEC-D
ZyrTEC (cetirizine) may be confused with ZyrTEC Itchy Eye (ketotifen)
International issues:
Benadryl international brand name for cetirizine [Great Britain, Phillipines], but also the brand name for acrivastine and pseudoephedrine [Great Britain] and several products containing diphenhydramine [U.S., Canada]

Brand Names: US All Day Allergy Childrens [OTC]; All Day Allergy [OTC]; Cetirizine HCl Allergy Child [OTC]; Cetirizine HCl Childrens Alrgy [OTC]; Cetirizine HCl Childrens [OTC]; Cetirizine HCl Hives Relief [OTC]; ZyrTEC Allergy Childrens [OTC]; ZyrTEC Allergy [OTC]; ZyrTEC Childrens Allergy [OTC]; ZyrTEC Childrens Hives Relief [OTC]; ZyrTEC Hives Relief [OTC]

Brand Names: Canada Aller-Relief [OTC]; Apo-Cetirizine [OTC]; Extra Strength Allergy Relief [OTC]; PMS-Cetirizine; Reactine; Reactine [OTC]

Therapeutic Category Antihistamine

Generic Availability (US) May be product dependent

Use
Prescription products: Oral syrup: Relief of symptoms associated with perennial allergic rhinitis (FDA approved in ages 6 to 23 months); treatment of the uncomplicated skin manifestations of chronic idiopathic urticaria (FDA approved in ages 6 months to 5 years)
OTC products: Relief of symptoms of hay fever or other respiratory allergies, relief of symptoms of common cold (OTC products: oral syrup: FDA approved in ages ≥2 years and adults; tablets: FDA approved in ages ≥6 years and adults). **Note:** Approved ages and uses for generic products may vary; consult labeling for specific information.

Pregnancy Considerations Maternal use of cetirizine has not been associated with an increased risk of major malformations. The use of antihistamines for the treatment of rhinitis during pregnancy is generally considered to be safe at recommended doses. Although safety data is limited, cetirizine may be a preferred second generation antihistamine for the treatment of rhinitis during pregnancy.

Breast-Feeding Considerations Cetirizine is excreted into breast milk.

Contraindications Hypersensitivity to cetirizine, hydroxyzine, or any component of the formulation

Warnings/Precautions Cetirizine should be used cautiously in patients with hepatic or renal impairment; consider dosage adjustment in patients with renal impairment. Use with caution in elderly patients; may be more sensitive to adverse effects. May cause drowsiness; use caution performing tasks which require alertness (eg, operating machinery or driving). Potentially significant drug-drug interactions may exist, requiring dose or frequency adjustment, additional monitoring, and/or selection of alternative therapy. Effects may be potentiated when used with other sedative drugs or ethanol.

Warnings: Additional Pediatric Considerations Safety and efficacy for the use of cough and cold products in pediatric patients <4 years of age is limited; the AAP warns against the use of these products for respiratory illnesses in this age group. Serious adverse effects including death have been reported. Many of these products contain multiple active ingredients, increasing the risk of accidental overdose when used with other products. The FDA notes that there are no approved OTC uses for these products in pediatric patients <2 years of age. Health care providers are reminded to ask caregivers about the use of OTC cough and cold products in order to avoid exposure to multiple medications containing the same ingredient (AAP 2012; FDA 2008).

Some dosage forms may contain propylene glycol; in neonates large amounts of propylene glycol delivered orally, intravenously (eg, >3,000 mg/day), or topically have been associated with potentially fatal toxicities which can include metabolic acidosis, seizures, renal failure, and CNS depression; toxicities have also been reported in children and adults including hyperosmolality, lactic acidosis, seizures and respiratory depression; use caution (AAP 1997; Shehab 2009).

Adverse Reactions

Central nervous system: Dizziness (adults), drowsiness (more common in adults), headache (children), fatigue (adults), insomnia (more common in children), malaise

Gastrointestinal: Abdominal pain (children), diarrhea, nausea, vomiting, xerostomia (adults)

Respiratory: Bronchospasm (children), epistaxis (epistaxis), pharyngitis (children)

Rare but important or life-threatening (as reported in adults and/or children): Aggressive behavior, anaphylaxis, angioedema, ataxia, chest pain, confusion, convulsions, depersonalization, depression, dysgeusia, edema, fussiness, hallucination, hemolytic anemia, hepatic insufficiency, hepatitis, hypertension, hypotension (severe), irritability, nervousness, ototoxicity, palpitations, paralysis, paresthesia, skin photosensitivity, skin rash, suicidal ideation, tongue discoloration, tongue edema, tremor, visual field defect, weakness

Drug Interactions

Metabolism/Transport Effects Substrate of CYP3A4 (minor), P-glycoprotein; **Note:** Assignment of Major/Minor substrate status based on clinically relevant drug interaction potential

Avoid Concomitant Use

Avoid concomitant use of Cetirizine with any of the following: Aclidinium; Azelastine (Nasal); Eluxadoline; Glucagon; Ipratropium (Oral Inhalation); Orphenadrine; Paraldehyde; Potassium Chloride; Thalidomide; Tiotropium; Umeclidinium

Increased Effect/Toxicity

Cetirizine may increase the levels/effects of: AbobotulinumtoxinA; Alcohol (Ethyl); Analgesics (Opioid); Anticholinergic Agents; Azelastine (Nasal); Buprenorphine; CNS Depressants; Eluxadoline; Glucagon; Hydrocodone; Methotrimeprazine; Metyrosine; Mirabegron; Mirtazapine; OnabotulinumtoxinA; Orphenadrine; Paraldehyde; Potassium Chloride; Pramipexole; RimabotulinumtoxinB; ROPINIRole; Rotigotine; Selective Serotonin Reuptake Inhibitors; Suvorexant; Thalidomide; Thiazide Diuretics; Tiotropium; Topiramate; Zolpidem

The levels/effects of Cetirizine may be increased by: Aclidinium; Brimonidine (Topical); Cannabis; Doxylamine; Dronabinol; Droperidol; HydrOXYzine; Ipratropium (Oral Inhalation); Kava Kava; Magnesium Sulfate; Methotrimeprazine; Mianserin; Nabilone; Perampanel; P-glycoprotein/ABCB1 Inhibitors; Pramlintide; Rufinamide; Sodium Oxybate; Tapentadol; Tetrahydrocannabinol; Umeclidinium

Decreased Effect

Cetirizine may decrease the levels/effects of: Acetylcholinesterase Inhibitors; Benzylpenicilloyl Polylysine; Betahistine; Hyaluronidase; Itopride; Metoclopramide; Secretin

The levels/effects of Cetirizine may be decreased by: Acetylcholinesterase Inhibitors; Amphetamines; P-glycoprotein/ABCB1 Inducers

Food Interactions Cetirizine's absorption and maximal concentration are reduced when taken with food. Management: May be taken without regard to meals.

Storage/Stability Store at 20°C to 25°C (68°F to 77°F); excursions are permitted between 15°C and 30°C (59°F and 86°F).

Mechanism of Action Competes with histamine for H_1-receptor sites on effector cells in the gastrointestinal tract, blood vessels, and respiratory tract

Pharmacodynamics

Onset of action: Suppression of skin wheal and flare: 0.7 hours (Simons 1999)

Duration: 24 hours

Pharmacokinetics (Adult data unless noted)

Absorption: Rapid

Distribution: V_d:
- Children: 0.7 L/kg
- Adults: 0.56 L/kg (Simons 1999)

Protein binding: 93%

Metabolism: Limited hepatic metabolism

Half-life:
- Children: 6.2 hours
- Adults: 8 hours

Time to peak serum concentration: 1 hour

Elimination: Urine (70%; 50% as unchanged drug), feces (10%)

Dosing: Usual

Pediatric:

Chronic urticaria: Oral:
- Infants 6 to <12 months: 2.5 mg once daily
- Children 12 to 23 months: Initial: 2.5 mg once daily; dosage may be increased to 2.5 mg twice daily
- Children 2 to 5 years: Initial: 2.5 mg once daily; dosage may be increased to 2.5 mg twice daily or 5 mg once daily; maximum daily dose: 5 mg/**day**

Allergic rhinitis; perennial: Oral:
- Infants 6 to <12 months: 2.5 mg once daily
- Children 12 to 23 months: Initial: 2.5 mg once daily; dosage may be increased to 2.5 mg twice daily

Allergic symptoms, hay fever:
- Children 2 to 5 years: Initial: 2.5 mg once daily; dosage may be increased to 2.5 mg twice daily or 5 mg once daily; maximum daily dose: 5 mg/day
- Children ≥6 years and Adolescents: 5 to 10 mg once daily

Adult: **Upper respiratory allergies/urticaria:** Oral: 5 to 10 mg once daily, depending upon symptom severity; maximum daily dose: 10 mg/day

Dosing adjustment in renal impairment: There are no dosage adjustments provided in the manufacturer's labeling; however, the following adjustments have been recommended (Aronoff 2007):

Infants, Children, and Adolescents:
- GFR ≥30 mL/minute/1.73 m^2: No dosage adjustment necessary.
- GFR 10 to 29 mL/minute/1.73 m^2: Decrease dose by 50%.
- GFR <10 mL/minute/1.73 m^2: Not recommended.
- Intermittent hemodialysis or peritoneal dialysis: Decrease dose by 50%.

Adults:
- GFR >50 mL/minute: No dosage adjustment necessary.
- GFR ≤50 mL/minute: 5 mg once daily
- Intermittent hemodialysis: 5 mg once daily; 5 mg 3 times per week may also be effective.
- Peritoneal dialysis: 5 mg once daily

Dosing adjustment in hepatic impairment: There are no dosage adjustments provided in manufacturer's labeling.

Administration Oral: Administer without regard to food

Chewable tablet: Chew tablet before swallowing; may be taken with or without water.

Dissolving tablet: Allow tablet to melt in mouth; may be taken with our without water.

Test Interactions May cause false-positive serum TCA screen. May suppress the wheal and flare reactions to skin test antigens.

Dosage Forms Excipient information presented when available (limited, particularly for generics); consult specific product labeling. [DSC] = Discontinued product

Capsule, Oral, as hydrochloride:
ZyrTEC Allergy: 10 mg
Solution, Oral, as hydrochloride:
All Day Allergy Childrens: 5 mg/5 mL (118 mL) [contains methylparaben, propylene glycol, propylparaben]
All Day Allergy Childrens: 5 mg/5 mL (118 mL) [dye free, gluten free; contains methylparaben, propylene glycol, propylparaben; grape flavor]
All Day Allergy Childrens: 1 mg/mL (118 mL [DSC]) [dye free, gluten free, sugar free; contains propylene glycol, sodium benzoate; grape flavor]
Cetirizine HCl Allergy Child: 5 mg/5 mL (120 mL) [alcohol free, dye free, gluten free, sugar free; contains methylparaben, propylene glycol, propylparaben; grape flavor]
Cetirizine HCl Allergy Child: 5 mg/5 mL (120 mL) [alcohol free, sugar free; contains methylparaben, propylene glycol, propylparaben]
Cetirizine HCl Childrens: 1 mg/mL (118 mL) [contains methylparaben, propylene glycol, propylparaben]
Cetirizine HCl Hives Relief: 5 mg/5 mL (120 mL) [alcohol free, sugar free; contains methylparaben, propylene glycol, propylparaben; grape flavor]
Generic: 1 mg/mL (120 mL, 473 mL)
Syrup, Oral, as hydrochloride:
Cetirizine HCl Childrens Alrgy: 1 mg/mL (118 mL, 120 mL) [contains methylparaben, propylene glycol, propylparaben; grape flavor]
ZyrTEC Childrens Allergy: 1 mg/mL (118 mL) [contains methylparaben, propylene glycol, propylparaben; banana-grape flavor]
ZyrTEC Childrens Allergy: 1 mg/mL (118 mL) [dye free, sugar free; contains propylene glycol, sodium benzoate]
ZyrTEC Childrens Allergy: 1 mg/mL (118 mL) [dye free, sugar free; contains propylene glycol, sodium benzoate; bubble-gum flavor]
ZyrTEC Childrens Allergy: 5 mg/5 mL (5 mL, 118 mL) [dye free, sugar free; contains propylene glycol, sodium benzoate; grape flavor]
ZyrTEC Childrens Hives Relief: 1 mg/mL (118 mL) [grape flavor]
Generic: 1 mg/mL (120 mL, 473 mL [DSC], 480 mL); 5 mg/5 mL (5 mL, 120 mL [DSC])
Tablet, Oral, as hydrochloride:
All Day Allergy: 10 mg
ZyrTEC Allergy: 10 mg
ZyrTEC Hives Relief: 10 mg
Generic: 5 mg, 10 mg
Tablet Chewable, Oral, as hydrochloride:
All Day Allergy Childrens: 5 mg, 10 mg [tutti-frutti flavor]
ZyrTEC Childrens Allergy: 5 mg [grape flavor]
ZyrTEC Childrens Allergy: 10 mg [contains fd&c blue #2 aluminum lake; grape flavor]
Generic: 5 mg, 10 mg
Tablet Dispersible, Oral, as hydrochloride:
ZyrTEC Allergy Childrens: 10 mg
ZyrTEC Allergy Childrens: 10 mg [citrus flavor]

- ◆ **Cetirizine HCl Allergy Child [OTC]** *see* Cetirizine *on page 423*
- ◆ **Cetirizine HCl Childrens [OTC]** *see* Cetirizine *on page 423*
- ◆ **Cetirizine HCl Childrens Alrgy [OTC]** *see* Cetirizine *on page 423*
- ◆ **Cetirizine HCl Hives Relief [OTC]** *see* Cetirizine *on page 423*
- ◆ **Cetirizine Hydrochloride** *see* Cetirizine *on page 423*
- ◆ **Cetraxal** *see* Ciprofloxacin (Otic) *on page 468*
- ◆ **CFDN** *see* Cefdinir *on page 390*
- ◆ **CG** *see* Chorionic Gonadotropin (Human) *on page 453*
- ◆ **CGP 33101** *see* Rufinamide *on page 1891*
- ◆ **CGP-57148B** *see* Imatinib *on page 1078*
- ◆ **CGS-20267** *see* Letrozole *on page 1224*
- ◆ **Charac-25 [OTC] (Can)** *see* Charcoal, Activated *on page 425*
- ◆ **Charac-50 [OTC] (Can)** *see* Charcoal, Activated *on page 425*
- ◆ **Charactol-25 [OTC] (Can)** *see* Charcoal, Activated *on page 425*
- ◆ **Charactol-50 [OTC] (Can)** *see* Charcoal, Activated *on page 425*

Charcoal, Activated (CHAR kole AK tiv ay ted)

Medication Safety Issues
Sound-alike/look-alike issues:
Actidose® may be confused with Actos®

Related Information
Oral Medications That Should Not Be Crushed or Altered *on page 2476*

Brand Names: US Actidose-Aqua [OTC]; Actidose/Sorbitol [OTC]; Char-Flo with Sorbitol [OTC]; EZ Char [OTC]; Kerr Insta-Char in Sorbitol [OTC]; Kerr Insta-Char [OTC]

Brand Names: Canada Charac-25 [OTC]; Charac-50 [OTC]; Charactol-25 [OTC]; Charactol-50 [OTC]; Charcodote Susp [OTC]; Charcodote TFS [OTC]; Charcodote-Aqueous Sus; Premium Activated Charcoal [OTC]

Therapeutic Category Antidiarrheal; Antidote, Adsorbent; Antiflatulent

Generic Availability (US) May be product dependent

Use Emergency treatment in poisoning by drugs and chemicals (FDA approved in all ages); repetitive doses for GI dialysis in drug overdose to enhance the elimination of certain drugs (theophylline, phenobarbital, carbamazepine, dapsone, quinine) (FDA approved in all ages)

Pregnancy Considerations Activated charcoal is not absorbed systemically following oral administration. Systemic absorption would be required in order for activated charcoal to cross the placenta and reach the fetus. In general, medications used as antidotes should take into consideration the health and prognosis of the mother; antidotes should be administered to pregnant women if there is a clear indication for use and should not be withheld because of fears of teratogenicity (Bailey, 2003).

Breast-Feeding Considerations Activated charcoal is not absorbed systemically following oral administration.

Contraindications There are no absolute contraindications listed within the manufacturer's labeling.

Note: The American Academy of Clinical Toxicology (AACT) and European Association of Poisons Centres and Clinical Toxicologists (EAPCCT) consider the following to be contraindications to the use of charcoal (Chyka, 2005; Vale, 1999): Presence of intestinal obstruction or GI tract not anatomically intact; patients at risk of GI hemorrhage or perforation; patients with an unprotected airway (eg, CNS depression without intubation); if use would increase the risk and severity of aspiration

Warnings/Precautions Charcoal may cause vomiting; the risk appears to be greater when charcoal is administered with sorbitol (Chyka, 2005). IV antiemetics may be required to reduce the risk of vomiting or to control vomiting to facilitate administration (Vale, 1999). Due to the risk of vomiting, avoid the use of charcoal in hydrocarbon and caustic ingestions. Use caution with decreased peristalsis. Some products may contain sorbitol. Coadministration of a cathartic is **not** recommended; cathartics (eg, sorbitol, mannitol, magnesium sulfate) have not been demonstrated to change patient outcome and have no role in the management of the poisoned patient. Cathartics subject the patient to the risk of developing significant fluid and electrolyte abnormalities (AACT, 2004a). Do not use products containing sorbitol in persons with a genetic intolerance to fructose or in patients who are dehydrated; may cause excessive diarrhea. Ipecac should not be administered routinely in the management of poisoned patients (AACT, 2004b).

Not effective in the treatment of poisonings due to the ingestion of low molecular weight compounds such as cyanide, iron, ethanol, methanol, or lithium. Most effective when administered within 30-60 minutes of ingestion. Based on experimental and clinical studies, multidose activated charcoal, in most acute poisonings, has not been shown to reduce morbidity or mortality (Vale, 1999). It may be considered if a patient has ingested a life-threatening amount of carbamazepine, dapsone, phenobarbital, quinine, or theophylline, although no controlled studies have demonstrated clinical benefit.

Benzyl alcohol and derivatives: Some dosage forms may contain sodium benzoate/benzoic acid; benzoic acid (benzoate) is a metabolite of benzyl alcohol; large amounts of benzyl alcohol (≥99 mg/kg/day) have been associated with a potentially fatal toxicity ("gasping syndrome") in neonates; the "gasping syndrome" consists of metabolic acidosis, respiratory distress, gasping respirations, CNS dysfunction (including convulsions, intracranial hemorrhage), hypotension, and cardiovascular collapse (AAP, 1997; CDC, 1982); some data suggests that benzoate displaces bilirubin from protein binding sites (Ahlfors, 2001); avoid or use dosage forms containing benzyl alcohol derivative with caution in neonates. See manufacturer's labeling.

Some dosage forms may contain propylene glycol; large amounts are potentially toxic and have been associated hyperosmolality, lactic acidosis, seizures and respiratory depression; use caution (AAP, 1997; Zar, 2007). Capsules and tablets should not be used for the treatment of poisoning.

Warnings: Additional Pediatric Considerations

Excessive amounts of activated charcoal with sorbitol may cause hypernatremic dehydration in pediatric patients (Farley 1986); use is not recommended in infants <1 year of age. Aspiration may cause tracheal obstruction in infants but usually not a major problem in adults. Aspiration pneumonitis, bronchiolitis obliterans, and ARDS have been reported following aspiration of charcoal; however, these problems may be due to the aspiration of gastric contents and not charcoal per se.

Some dosage forms may contain propylene glycol; in neonates large amounts of propylene glycol delivered orally, intravenously (eg, >3,000 mg/day), or topically have been associated with potentially fatal toxicities which can include metabolic acidosis, seizures, renal failure, and CNS depression; toxicities have also been reported in children and adults including hyperosmolality, lactic acidosis, seizures and respiratory depression; use caution (AAP 1997; Shehab 2009).

Some products contain fructose or sorbitol and should not be administered to patients with a rare autosomal recessive genetic intolerance to fructose.

Adverse Reactions

Gastrointestinal: Abdominal distention, appendicitis, bowel obstruction, constipation, vomiting

Ocular: Corneal abrasion (with direct contact)

Respiratory: Aspiration, respiratory failure

Miscellaneous: Fecal discoloration (black)

Drug Interactions

Metabolism/Transport Effects None known.

Avoid Concomitant Use There are no known interactions where it is recommended to avoid concomitant use.

Increased Effect/Toxicity There are no known significant interactions involving an increase in effect.

Decreased Effect

Charcoal, Activated may decrease the levels/effects of: Leflunomide; Teriflunomide

Food Interactions The addition of some flavoring agents (eg, milk, ice cream, sherbet, marmalade) are known to reduce the adsorptive capacity, and therefore the efficacy, of activated charcoal and should be avoided in preference to activated charcoal-water slurries; nevertheless, these flavoring agents do not completely compromise the effectiveness of activated charcoal and may be necessary in some circumstances (eg, administration in pediatric patients) to enhance compliance (Cooney, 1995; Dagnone, 2002).

Storage/Stability Adsorbs gases from air, store in a closed container.

Mechanism of Action Adsorbs toxic substances, thus inhibiting GI absorption and preventing systemic toxicity. Administration of multiple doses of charcoal may interrupt enteroenteric, enterohepatic, and enterogastric circulation of some drugs; may also adsorb any unabsorbed drug which remains in the gut.

Pharmacodynamics In studies using adult human volunteers: Mean **reduction** in drug absorption following a single dose of ≥50 g activated charcoal (AACT [Chyka 2005]):

Given within 30 minutes after ingestion: 47.3% reduction

Given at 60 minutes after ingestion: 40.07% reduction

Given at 120 minutes after ingestion: 16.5% reduction

Given at 180 minutes after ingestion: 21.13% reduction

Given at 240 minutes after ingestion: 32.5% reduction

Pharmacokinetics (Adult data unless noted)

Absorption: Not absorbed from the GI tract

Elimination: Excreted as charcoal in feces

Dosing: Usual

Pediatric: **Acute poisoning:** Oral, NG:

*Single dose: Charcoal **in water**:*

Age-directed dosing: **Note:** Although dosing by body weight in children (0.5 to 1 g/kg) is recommended by several resources, there are no data or scientific rationale to support this recommendation (Chyka 2005).

- Infants <1 year:
  - Manufacturer's labeling (Actidose-Aqua): 1 g/kg
  - AACT recommendation (Chyka 2005): 10 to 25 g
- Children 1 to 12 years:
  - Manufacturer's labeling:
    - Actidose-Aqua: 25 to 50 g
    - Kerr Insta-Char (Aqueous): Weight ≥16 kg: 1 to 2 g/kg **or** 15 to 30 g
  - AACT recommendation (Chyka 2005): 25 to 50g
- Adolescents:
  - Manufacturer's labeling:
    - Actidose-Aqua: 50 to 100 g
    - Kerr Insta-Char (Aqueous): Weight ≥ 32kg: 1 to 2 g/kg **or** 50 to 100 g
  - AACT recommendation (Chyka 2005): 25 to 100 g

*Single dose: Charcoal **with sorbitol**;* **Note:** Use of oral charcoal with sorbitol as part of a multiple dose activated charcoal regimen is not recommended (AACT [Vale 1999]); however, a single dose may be used to produce catharsis (AACT 2004):

- Infants <1 year: Not recommended
- Children 1 to 12 years (Actidose with Sorbitol):
  - Weight 16 to <32 kg: 25 g
  - Weight ≥ 32 kg: 25 to 50 g
- Adolescents:
  - Actidose with Sorbitol: 50 g
  - Kerr Insta-Char in Sorbitol: Weight ≥32 kg: 1 to 2 g/kg **or** 50 to 100 g

*Multiple dose: Charcoal **in water*** (doses are repeated until clinical observations of toxicity subside and serum drug concentrations have returned to a subtherapeutic range or until the development of absent bowel sounds or ileus); **Note:** Reserve for life threatening ingestions of carbamazepine, dapsone, phenobarbital, quinine, or theophylline (AACT 1999).

Manufacturer's labeling (Actidose-Aqua):

Infants <1 year: 1 g/kg every 4 to 6 hours

Children 1 to 12 years: 25 to 50 g every 4 to 6 hours

Adolescents: 50 to 100 g every 4 to 6 hours

Adult: **Acute poisoning:** Oral, NG: **Note:** Some products may contain sorbitol; coadministration of a cathartic, including sorbitol, is not recommended. Some clinicians still recommend dosing activated charcoal in a 10:1 (charcoal:poison) ratio for optimal efficacy (Gude 2009); however, the amount of poison ingested is commonly unknown, which makes this approach challenging and often impractical (Chyka 2005).

Single dose (Chyka 2005): 25 to 100 g

Multidose: Initial dose: 50 to 100 g followed by 25 to 50 g every 4 hours

Administration Oral: Administer as soon as possible after ingestion, preferably within 1 hour for greatest effect. Shake well before use; may be mixed with chocolate syrup or orange juice to increase palatability. Manufacturer's labeling for Actidose Aqua and Actidose with sorbitol recommends avoiding adding chemicals, syrups, or dairy products.

Instruct patient to drink slowly, rapid administration may increase frequency of vomiting; if patient has persistent vomiting, multiple doses may be administered as a continuous enteral infusion

Monitoring Parameters Check for presence of bowel sounds before administration. Fluid status, sorbitol intake, number of stools, electrolytes if increase in stools or diarrhea occurs; continually assess for active bowel sounds in patients receiving multiple dose activated charcoal

Additional Information The Position Paper on single dose activated charcoal by The American Academy of Clinical Toxicology and The European Association of Poisons Centres and Clinical Toxicologists (Chyka 2005) does not advocate **routine** use of single dose activated charcoal in the treatment of poisoned patients. Scientific literature supports the use of activated charcoal within 1 hour of toxin ingestion, when it will be more likely to produce benefit. Studies in volunteers demonstrate that the effectiveness of activated charcoal decreases as the time of administration after toxin ingestion increases. Therefore, this publication states that activated charcoal may be considered up to 1 hour following ingestion of a potentially toxic amount of poison. In addition, the use of activated charcoal may be considered greater than 1 hour following ingestion, since the potential benefit cannot be excluded. Furthermore, based on current literature, the routine administration of a cathartic with activated charcoal is not recommended; when cathartics are used, only a single dose should be administered so as to decrease adverse effects (AACT 2004).

A policy statement by the American Academy of Pediatrics states that it is currently premature to recommend the **routine** administration of activated charcoal as a home treatment strategy for poisonings (AAP 2003).

Dosage Forms Excipient information presented when available (limited, particularly for generics); consult specific product labeling.

Liquid, Oral:

Actidose-Aqua: 15 g/72 mL (72 mL); 25 g/120 mL (120 mL); 50 g/240 mL (240 mL) [sweet flavor]

Actidose/Sorbitol: 25 g/120 mL (120 mL); 50 g/240 mL (240 mL) [sweet flavor]

Kerr Insta-Char: 25 g/120 mL (120 mL); 50 g/240 mL (240 mL) [contains fd&c red #40, methylparaben sodium, propylene glycol, propylparaben sodium, sodium benzoate; cherry flavor]

Kerr Insta-Char: 50 g/240 mL (240 mL) [contains propylene glycol]

Kerr Insta-Char in Sorbitol: 25 g/120 mL (120 mL); 50 g/240 mL (240 mL) [contains fd&c red #40, methylparaben sodium, propylene glycol, propylparaben sodium, sodium benzoate; cherry flavor]

Suspension, Oral:

Char-Flo with Sorbitol: 25 g (120 mL)

Suspension Reconstituted, Oral:

EZ Char: 25 g (1 ea) [contains bentonite]

◆ **Charcodote-Aqueous Sus (Can)** *see* Charcoal, Activated *on page 425*

◆ **Charcodote Susp [OTC] (Can)** *see* Charcoal, Activated *on page 425*

◆ **Charcodote TFS [OTC] (Can)** *see* Charcoal, Activated *on page 425*

◆ **Char-Flo with Sorbitol [OTC]** *see* Charcoal, Activated *on page 425*

◆ **Chemet** *see* Succimer *on page 1975*

◆ **Chenodal** *see* Chenodiol *on page 427*

◆ **Chenodeoxycholic Acid** *see* Chenodiol *on page 427*

Chenodiol (kee noe DYE ole)

Brand Names: US Chenodal

Therapeutic Category Bile Acid

Generic Availability (US) No

Use Oral dissolution of radiolucent cholesterol gallstones in well-opacifying gallbladders in patients who are not candidates for surgery due to systemic disease or age (FDA approved in adults); has also been used for lipid storage diseases, including cerebrotendinous xanthomatosis, Zellweger syndrome, and other susceptible bile acid biosynthesis defects which result in low chenodeoxycholic acid concentrations

Prescribing and Access Restrictions Prescriptions are only dispensed by a specialty pharmacy, Centric Health Resources, which may be contacted at 866-758-7068.

Pregnancy Risk Factor X

Pregnancy Considerations Hepatic, renal, and adrenal lesions were observed in some animal reproduction studies. Use during pregnancy is contraindicated.

Breast-Feeding Considerations It is not known if chenodiol is excreted in breast milk. The manufacturer recommends that caution be exercised when administering chenodiol to nursing women.

Contraindications Presence of known hepatocyte dysfunction or bile ductal abnormalities (eg, intrahepatic cholestasis, primary biliary cirrhosis, sclerosing cholangitis); use in a patient with a gallbladder confirmed as nonvisualizing after two consecutive single doses of dye; radiopaque stones; gallstone complications or compelling reasons for gallbladder surgery (eg, unremitting acute cholecystitis, cholangitis, biliary obstruction, gallstone pancreatitis, biliary gastrointestinal fistula); pregnancy

Warnings/Precautions Drug-induced liver toxicity may occur (dose-related); close monitoring of serum aminotransferase levels recommended during therapy. Aminotransferase elevations >3 times ULN have been reported; prompt discontinuation recommended. Avoid or use with extreme caution in patients with hepatic impairment or elevated liver enzymes; use contraindicated in patients with known hepatocyte dysfunction or bile ductal abnormalities. Dose-related diarrhea commonly occurs (up to 40% of patients) with use. Diarrhea is usually mild and does not interfere with therapy; however, diarrhea may be severe and a temporary dosage reduction or discontinuation may be required. Epidemiologic studies have suggested that bile acids may increase the risk of colon cancer. Evidence is weak and conflicting; however, a potential link between bile acids and colon cancer cannot be ruled out.

Careful selection of appropriate patients is necessary prior to therapy; studies have shown dissolution rates are higher in patients with small (<15 mm in diameter), radiolucent, and/or floatable stones. Radiopaque (calcified or partially calcified) stones and bile pigment stones do not respond to bile acid dissolution therapy. Response to therapy should be monitored with oral cholecystograms or ultrasonograms. Complete dissolution should be confirmed by one repeat test 1-3 months after continued therapy. If partial dissolution is not observed by 9-12 months, complete dissolution is unlikely. If no response is observed by 18 months, therapy should be discontinued; safety beyond 24 months of use has not been established.

Adverse Reactions

Endocrine & metabolic: LDL cholesterol increased, total cholesterol increased

Gastrointestinal: Abdominal cramps, abdominal pain, anorexia, biliary pain, constipation, diarrhea (including severe diarrhea requiring dose reduction), dyspepsia, flatulence, heartburn, nausea, vomiting

Hematologic: Leukopenia

Hepatic: Aminotransferase increased

Drug Interactions

Metabolism/Transport Effects None known.

Avoid Concomitant Use There are no known interactions where it is recommended to avoid concomitant use.

Increased Effect/Toxicity There are no known significant interactions involving an increase in effect.

Decreased Effect

The levels/effects of Chenodiol may be decreased by: Aluminum Hydroxide; Bile Acid Sequestrants; Estrogen Derivatives; Fibric Acid Derivatives

Storage/Stability Store at 20°C to 20°C (68°F to 77°F).

Mechanism of Action Chenodiol (chenodeoxycholic acid) is a naturally occurring human bile acid, normally constituting one-third of the total bile acid pool. Synthesis of chenodiol is regulated by the relative composition and flux of cholesterol and bile acids through the hepatocyte by a negative feedback effect on the rate-limiting enzymes for synthesis of cholesterol (HMG-CoA reductase) and bile acids (cholesterol 7 alpha-hydroxyl). In patients with cholesterol gallstones, chenodiol is believed to suppress hepatic synthesis of cholesterol and cholic acid, and inhibit biliary cholesterol secretion, which leads to increased production of cholesterol unsaturated bile thereby allowing for dissolution of gallstones.

Pharmacokinetics (Adult data unless noted)

Absorption: Rapid, almost completely absorbed in proximal small intestine (Crosignani 1996)

Distribution: V_d: 1600 L (Crosignani 1996)

Metabolism: Converted hepatically to taurine and glycine conjugates and secreted in bile; extensive first-pass hepatic clearance (60% to 80%); undergoes enterohepatic circulation; further metabolized in colon by bacteria to lithocholic acid; small portion of lithocholate is absorbed and converted to sulfolithocholyl conjugates in the liver

Half-life: 45 hours (Crosignani 1996)

Elimination: Feces (80%, as lithocholate)

Dosing: Usual

Pediatric:

Gallstone dissolution: Limited data available: Oral: Children ≥12 years and Adolescents: 15 mg/kg/day divided 3 times daily with meals; dosing based on reported experience in three obese pediatric patients (age range: 12 to 13 years); **Note:** Not first-line therapy due to frequent side effect (increased LFT, diarrhea) and other therapeutic options available (Podda 1982)

Inborn errors of bile acid biosynthesis: Very limited data available: Oral: Infants, Children and Adolescents: **Note:** Due to the rarity of the disease states, data is limited to small case series and case reports. Adjust dose based upon targeted bile acid or biosynthesis intermediate compound concentrations. Combination therapy with ursodeoxycholic acid (urosdiol) dependent on specific deficiency, and phenotypic presentation of syndrome.

Cerebrotendinous xanthomatosis: Initial: 10 to 15 mg/kg/day divided 1 to 3 times daily; in adolescents, a fixed dose of 750 mg/day has also been reported (Beringer 2010; Kaufman 2012; Setchell 2006; van Heijst 1998)

Steroid dehydrogenase or reductase deficiencies (susceptible): Usual initial range: 5 to 10 mg/kg/day divided once or twice daily; higher initial doses of 11 to 18 mg/kg/day have also been reported; a maintenance dose of 5 mg/kg/day was the most frequently reported and initiated once targeted bile acid normalized or stabilized (depending upon the syndrome) (Clayton 1996; Clayton 2011; Ichimiya 1990; Riello 2010)

Peroxisome deficiency, including Zellweger syndrome: Oral: 100 to 250 mg/day or 5 mg/kg/day have been used (Maeda 2002; Setchell 1992)

Adult: **Gallstone dissolution (monotherapy):** Oral: Initial: 250 mg twice daily for the first 2 weeks and increasing by 250 mg/day each week thereafter until the recommended or maximum tolerated dose is achieved; maintenance: 13 to 16 mg/kg/day in 2 divided doses. **Note:** Dosages <10 mg/kg are usually ineffective and may increase the risk of cholecystectomy.

Dosing adjustment in renal impairment: There are no dosage adjustments provided in manufacturer's labeling.

Dosing adjustment in hepatic impairment: Use extreme caution; contraindicated for use in presence of known hepatocyte dysfunction or bile duct abnormalities.

Administration May be taken without regard to meals.

Monitoring Parameters Serum aminotransferase levels (monthly for first 3 months, then every 3 months during therapy); serum cholesterol (every 6 months); for gallstone dissolution: Oral cholecystograms and/or ultrasonograms (6-9 month intervals for response to therapy); dissolutions of stones should be confirmed 1-3 months later; for bile acid biosynthesis defects: Targeted bile acids or intermediate product concentrations from either serum or blood should be measured (as appropriate) (Clatyon 2011; Setchell, 2006)

Dosage Forms Excipient information presented when available (limited, particularly for generics); consult specific product labeling.

Tablet, Oral:

Chenodal: 250 mg

◆ **Cheracol D [OTC]** *see* Guaifenesin and Dextromethorphan *on page 992*

◆ **Cheracol Plus [OTC]** *see* Guaifenesin and Dextromethorphan *on page 992*

◆ **Cheratussin** *see* GuaiFENesin *on page 988*

◆ **Chew-C [OTC]** *see* Ascorbic Acid *on page 202*

◆ **CHG** *see* Chlorhexidine Gluconate *on page 434*

◆ **Chickenpox Vaccine** *see* Varicella Virus Vaccine *on page 2157*

◆ **Chiggerex [OTC]** *see* Benzocaine *on page 268*

◆ **Chiggertox [OTC]** *see* Benzocaine *on page 268*

◆ **Childrens Advil [OTC]** *see* Ibuprofen *on page 1064*

◆ **Children's Advil® Cold (Can)** *see* Pseudoephedrine and Ibuprofen *on page 1803*

◆ **Childrens Ibuprofen [OTC]** *see* Ibuprofen *on page 1064*

- **Childrens Loratadine [OTC]** *see* Loratadine *on page 1296*
- **Childrens Motrin [OTC]** *see* Ibuprofen *on page 1064*
- **Childrens Motrin Jr Strength [OTC]** *see* Ibuprofen *on page 1064*
- **Childrens Silfedrine [OTC]** *see* Pseudoephedrine *on page 1801*
- **Children's Advil (Can)** *see* Ibuprofen *on page 1064*
- **Children's Europrofen (Can)** *see* Ibuprofen *on page 1064*
- **Children's Motion Sickness Liquid [OTC] (Can)** *see* DimenhyDRINATE *on page 664*
- **ChiRhoStim** *see* Secretin *on page 1911*
- **Chloditan** *see* Mitotane *on page 1446*
- **Chlodithane** *see* Mitotane *on page 1446*
- **Chloral** *see* Chloral Hydrate *on page 429*

Chloral Hydrate (KLOR al HYE drate)

Medication Safety Issues

High alert medication:

The Institute for Safe Medication Practices (ISMP) includes this medication among its list of drugs which have a heightened risk of causing significant patient harm when used in error.

Related Information

Oral Medications That Should Not Be Crushed or Altered *on page 2476*

Preprocedure Sedatives in Children *on page 2444*

Safe Handling of Hazardous Drugs *on page 2455*

Brand Names: Canada PMS-Chloral Hydrate

Therapeutic Category Hypnotic; Sedative

Use Short-term sedative and hypnotic (<2 weeks), sedative/hypnotic prior to nonpainful therapeutic or diagnostic procedures (eg, EEG, CT scan, MRI, ophthalmic exam, dental procedure)

Pregnancy Considerations Animal reproduction studies have not been conducted. Chloral hydrate crosses the placenta, and long-term use may lead to withdrawal symptoms in the neonate.

Breast-Feeding Considerations Chloral hydrate is excreted in breast milk; use by breast-feeding women may cause sedation in the infant.

Contraindications Hypersensitivity to chloral hydrate or any component of the formulation; marked hepatic or renal impairment

Warnings/Precautions May cause CNS depression, which may impair physical or mental abilities; patients must be cautioned about performing tasks that require mental alertness (eg, operating machinery or driving). Effects may be potentiated when used with other sedative drugs or ethanol. Use with caution in patients with porphyria, cardiac disease, gastrointestinal disease, or respiratory disorders. Excessive sedation or other adverse effects may be more likely to occur in elderly patients; dose reduction may be necessary. Life-threatening respiratory obstruction and deaths have been reported with use in children; use with extreme caution. Use with caution in neonates; prolonged use in neonates is associated with direct hyperbilirubinemia (active metabolite [TCE] competes with bilirubin for glucuronide conjugation in the liver). Tolerance to hypnotic effect develops; therefore, not recommended for use >2 weeks. Taper dosage to avoid withdrawal with prolonged use. Health care provider should be alert to problems of abuse and misuse. Patients should be assessed for risk of abuse or addiction prior to therapy and all patients should be monitored for signs of abuse or misuse.

Benzyl alcohol and derivatives: Some dosage forms may contain sodium benzoate/benzoic acid; benzoic acid (benzoate) is a metabolite of benzyl alcohol; large amounts of benzyl alcohol (≥99 mg/kg/day) have been associated with a potentially fatal toxicity ("gasping syndrome") in neonates; the "gasping syndrome" consists of metabolic acidosis, respiratory distress, gasping respirations, CNS dysfunction (including convulsions, intracranial hemorrhage), hypotension, and cardiovascular collapse (AAP, 1997; CDC, 1982); some data suggests that benzoate displaces bilirubin from protein binding sites (Ahlfors, 2001); avoid or use dosage forms containing benzyl alcohol derivative with caution in neonates. See manufacturer's labeling.

Warnings: Additional Pediatric Considerations

Deaths and permanent neurologic injury from respiratory compromise have been reported in children sedated with chloral hydrate; respiratory obstruction may occur in children with tonsillar and adenoidal hypertrophy, obstructive sleep apnea, and Leigh's encephalopathy, and in ASA class III children; depressed levels of consciousness may occur; chloral hydrate should not be administered for sedation by nonmedical personnel or in a nonsupervised medical environment; sedation with chloral hydrate requires careful patient monitoring (Cote, 2000). Animal studies suggest that chloral hydrate may depress the genioglossus muscle and other airway-maintaining muscles in patients who are already at risk for life-threatening airway obstruction (eg, obstructive sleep apnea); alternative sedative agents should be considered for these patients (Hershenson, 1984).

Adverse Reactions

Cardiovascular: Atrial arrhythmia, depression of myocardial contractility, hypotension, shortening of refractory periods, torsades de pointes, ventricular arrhythmia

Central nervous system: Abnormal gait, ataxia, confusion, delirium, dizziness, drowsiness, drug dependence (physical and psychological; with prolonged use or large doses), hallucinations, hangover effect, malaise, nightmares, paradoxical excitation, somnambulism, vertigo

Dermatologic: Skin rash (including erythema, eczematoid dermatitis, urticaria, scarlatiniform exanthems)

Endocrine & metabolic: Acute porphyria, ketonuria

Gastrointestinal: Diarrhea, flatulence, gastric irritation, nausea, vomiting

Hematologic & oncologic: Acute porphyria, eosinophilia, leukopenia

Ophthalmic: Allergic conjunctivitis, blepharoptosis, keratoconjunctivitis

Otic: Increased middle ear pressure (infants and children)

Respiratory: Airway obstruction (young children), laryngeal edema (children)

Miscellaneous: Drug tolerance

Drug Interactions

Metabolism/Transport Effects None known.

Avoid Concomitant Use

Avoid concomitant use of Chloral Hydrate with any of the following: Azelastine (Nasal); Furosemide; Orphenadrine; Paraldehyde; Sodium Oxybate; Thalidomide

Increased Effect/Toxicity

Chloral Hydrate may increase the levels/effects of: Alcohol (Ethyl); Azelastine (Nasal); Buprenorphine; CNS Depressants; Highest Risk QTc-Prolonging Agents; Hydrocodone; Methotrimeprazine; Metyrosine; Mirtazapine; Moderate Risk QTc-Prolonging Agents; Orphenadrine; Paraldehyde; Pramipexole; ROPINIRole; Rotigotine; Selective Serotonin Reuptake Inhibitors; Sodium Oxybate; Suvorexant; Thalidomide; Vitamin K Antagonists; Zolpidem

The levels/effects of Chloral Hydrate may be increased by: Brimonidine (Topical); Cannabis; Doxylamine; Dronabinol; Droperidol; Furosemide; HydrOXYzine; Kava

Kava; Magnesium Sulfate; Methotrimeprazine; Mifepristone; Nabilone; Perampanel; Rufinamide; Tapentadol; Tetrahydrocannabinol

Decreased Effect

The levels/effects of Chloral Hydrate may be decreased by: Flumazenil

Storage/Stability Store syrup and capsules at controlled room temperature. Store syrup in a light-resistant, airtight container; protect from freezing.

Mechanism of Action Central nervous system depressant effects are due to its active metabolite trichloroethanol, mechanism unknown

Pharmacodynamics

Onset of action: 10-20 minutes

Maximum effect: Within 30-60 minutes

Duration: 4-8 hours

Pharmacokinetics (Adult data unless noted)

Absorption: Oral, rectal: Well absorbed

Distribution: Crosses the placenta; distributes to breast milk

Protein binding: Trichloroethanol: 35% to 40%; trichloroacetic acid: ~94% (may compete with bilirubin for albumin binding sites)

Metabolism: Rapidly metabolized by alcohol dehydrogenase to trichloroethanol (active metabolite); trichloroethanol undergoes glucuronidation in the liver; variable amounts of chloral hydrate and trichloroethanol are metabolized in liver and kidney to trichloroacetic acid (inactive)

Half-life:

- Chloral hydrate: Infants: 1 hour
- Trichloroethanol (active metabolite):
  - Neonates: Range: 8.5-66 hours
  - Half-life decreases with increasing postmenstrual age (PMA):
    - Preterm infants (PMA 31-37 weeks): Mean half-life: 40 hours
    - Term infants (PMA 38-42 weeks): Mean half-life: 28 hours
    - Older children (PMA 57-708 weeks): Mean half-life: 10 hours
  - Adults: 8-11 hours
- Trichloroacetic acid: Adults: 67.2 hours

Elimination: Metabolites excreted in urine; small amounts excreted in feces via bile

Dialysis: Dialyzable (50% to 100%)

Dosing: Neonatal Oral, rectal: 25 mg/kg/dose for sedation prior to a procedure; **Note:** Repeat doses should be used with great caution as drug and metabolites accumulate with repeated use; toxicity has been reported after 3 days in a preterm neonate and after 7 days in a term neonate receiving chloral hydrate 40-50 mg/kg every 6 hours

Dosing: Usual Oral, rectal:

Infants and Children:

- Sedation, anxiety: 25-50 mg/kg/day divided every 6-8 hours, maximum dose: 500 mg/dose
- Prior to EEG: 25-50 mg/kg/dose 30-60 minutes prior to EEG; may repeat in 30 minutes to a total maximum of 100 mg/kg or 1 g total for infants and 2 g total for children
- Sedation, nonpainful procedure: 50-75 mg/kg/dose 30-60 minutes prior to procedure; may repeat 30 minutes after initial dose if needed, to a total maximum dose of 120 mg/kg or 1 g total for infants and 2 g total for children
- Hypnotic: 50 mg/kg/dose at bedtime; maximum dose: 1 g/dose; total maximum: 1 g/day for infants and 2 g/day for children

Adults:

- Sedation, anxiety: 250 mg 3 times/day
- Hypnotic: 500-1000 mg at bedtime or 30 minutes prior to procedure, not to exceed 2 g/24 hours

Dosing adjustment in renal impairment:

CrCl ≥50 mL/minute: No dosage adjustment needed

CrCl <50 mL/minute: Avoid use

Administration

Oral: Minimize unpleasant taste and gastric irritation by administering with water, infant formula, fruit juice, or ginger ale; do not crush capsule, contains drug in liquid form with unpleasant taste

Rectal administration: May administer chloral hydrate syrup rectally

Monitoring Parameters Level of sedation; vital signs and O_2 saturation with doses used for sedation prior to procedure

Test Interactions May interfere with copper sulfate tests for glycosuria or with fluorometric urine catecholamine and urinary 17-hydroxycorticosteroid tests.

Additional Information Not an analgesic; osmolality of 500 mg/5 mL syrup is approximately 3500 mOsm/kg

Product Availability Not available in the US

Chlorambucil (klor AM byoo sil)

Medication Safety Issues

Sound-alike/look-alike issues:

Chlorambucil may be confused with Chloromycetin®

Leukeran® may be confused with Alkeran®, leucovorin, Leukine®, Myleran®

High alert medication:

This medication is in a class the Institute for Safe Medication Practices (ISMP) includes among its list of drug classes which have a heightened risk of causing significant patient harm when used in error.

Related Information

Oral Medications That Should Not Be Crushed or Altered *on page 2476*

Prevention of Chemotherapy-Induced Nausea and Vomiting in Children *on page 2368*

Safe Handling of Hazardous Drugs *on page 2455*

Brand Names: US Leukeran

Brand Names: Canada Leukeran®

Therapeutic Category Antineoplastic Agent, Alkylating Agent; Antineoplastic Agent, Alkylating Agent (Nitrogen Mustard)

Generic Availability (US) No

Use Treatment of chronic lymphocytic leukemia (CLL), Hodgkin's and non-Hodgkin's lymphoma (FDA approved in adults); has also been used in the treatment of nephrotic syndrome (unresponsive to conventional therapy) and Waldenström's macroglobulinemia

Pregnancy Risk Factor D

Pregnancy Considerations Animal reproduction studies have demonstrated teratogenicity. Chlorambucil crosses the human placenta. Following exposure during the first trimester, case reports have noted adverse renal effects (unilateral agenesis). Women of childbearing potential should avoid becoming pregnant while receiving treatment. **[U.S. Boxed Warning]: Affects human fertility; probably mutagenic and teratogenic as well**; chromosomal damage has been documented. Reversible and irreversible sterility (when administered to prepubertal and pubertal males), azoospermia (in adult males) and amenorrhea (in females) have been observed. Fibrosis, vasculitis and depletion of primordial follicles have been noted on autopsy of the ovaries.

Breast-Feeding Considerations It is not known if chlorambucil is excreted in breast milk. Due to the potential for serious adverse reactions in the nursing infant, the decision to discontinue chlorambucil or to discontinue breast-feeding should take into account the benefits of treatment to the mother.

Contraindications Hypersensitivity to chlorambucil or any component of the formulation; hypersensitivity to other alkylating agents (may have cross-hypersensitivity); prior (demonstrated) resistance to chlorambucil

Canadian labeling: Additional contraindications (not in U.S. labeling): Use within 4 weeks of a full course of radiation or chemotherapy

Warnings/Precautions Hazardous agent - use appropriate precautions for handling and disposal (NIOSH 2014 [group 1]). Seizures have been observed; use with caution in patients with seizure disorder or head trauma; history of nephrotic syndrome and high pulse doses are at higher risk of seizures. **[U.S. Boxed Warning]: May cause severe bone marrow suppression;** neutropenia may be severe. Reduce initial dosage if patient has received myelosuppressive or radiation therapy within the previous 4 weeks, or has a depressed baseline leukocyte or platelet count. Irreversible bone marrow damage may occur with total doses approaching 6.5 mg/kg. Progressive lymphopenia may develop (recovery is generally rapid after discontinuation). Avoid administration of live vaccines to immunocompromised patients. Rare instances of severe skin reactions (eg, erythema multiforme, Stevens-Johnson syndrome, toxic epidermal necrolysis) have been reported; discontinue promptly if skin reaction occurs.

Chlorambucil is primarily metabolized in the liver. Dosage reductions should be considered in patients with hepatic impairment. **[U.S. Boxed Warning]: Affects human fertility; carcinogenic in humans and probably mutagenic and teratogenic as well;** chromosomal damage has been documented. Reversible and irreversible sterility (when administered to prepubertal and pubertal males), azoospermia (in adult males) and amenorrhea (in females) have been observed. **[U.S. Boxed Warning]: Carcinogenic;** acute myelocytic leukemia and secondary malignancies may be associated with chronic therapy. Duration of treatment and higher cumulative doses are associated with a higher risk for development of leukemia. Potentially significant drug-drug interactions may exist, requiring dose or frequency adjustment, additional monitoring, and/or selection of alternative therapy.

Adverse Reactions

Central nervous system: Agitation (rare), ataxia (rare), confusion (rare), drug fever, fever, focal/generalized seizure (rare), hallucinations (rare)

Dermatologic: Angioneurotic edema, erythema multiforme (rare), rash, skin hypersensitivity, Stevens-Johnson syndrome (rare), toxic epidermal necrolysis (rare), urticaria

Endocrine & metabolic: Amenorrhea, infertility, SIADH (rare)

Gastrointestinal: Diarrhea (infrequent), nausea (infrequent), oral ulceration (infrequent), vomiting (infrequent)

Genitourinary: Azoospermia, cystitis (sterile)

Hematologic: Neutropenia (onset: 3 weeks; recovery: 10 days after last dose), bone marrow failure (irreversible), bone marrow suppression, anemia, leukemia (secondary), leukopenia, lymphopenia, pancytopenia, thrombocytopenia

Hepatic: Hepatotoxicity, jaundice

Neuromuscular & skeletal: Flaccid paresis (rare), muscular twitching (rare), myoclonia (rare), peripheral neuropathy, tremor (rare)

Respiratory: Interstitial pneumonia, pulmonary fibrosis

Miscellaneous: Allergic reactions, malignancies (secondary)

Drug Interactions

Metabolism/Transport Effects None known.

Avoid Concomitant Use

Avoid concomitant use of Chlorambucil with any of the following: BCG; BCG (Intravesical); CloZAPine; Dipyrone; Natalizumab; Pimecrolimus; Tacrolimus (Topical); Tofacitinib; Vaccines (Live)

Increased Effect/Toxicity

Chlorambucil may increase the levels/effects of: CloZAPine; Leflunomide; Natalizumab; Tofacitinib; Vaccines (Live)

The levels/effects of Chlorambucil may be increased by: Denosumab; Dipyrone; Pimecrolimus; Roflumilast; Tacrolimus (Topical); Trastuzumab

Decreased Effect

Chlorambucil may decrease the levels/effects of: BCG; BCG (Intravesical); Coccidioides immitis Skin Test; Sipuleucel-T; Vaccines (Inactivated); Vaccines (Live)

The levels/effects of Chlorambucil may be decreased by: Echinacea

Food Interactions Absorption is decreased when administered with food. Management: Administer preferably on an empty stomach.

Storage/Stability Store in refrigerator at 2°C to 8°C (36°F to 46°F).

Mechanism of Action Alkylating agent; interferes with DNA replication and RNA transcription by alkylation and cross-linking the strands of DNA

Pharmacokinetics (Adult data unless noted)

Absorption: Oral: Rapid and almost completely absorbed from GI tract (>70%); reduced with food

Distribution: V_d: ~0.3 L/kg

Protein binding: ~99%; primarily to albumin

Metabolism: Hepatic (extensively); primarily to an active metabolite, phenylacetic acid mustard

Half-life: Chlorambucil: ~1.5 hours; phenylacetic acid mustard: ~1.8 hours

Time to peak plasma concentration: Chlorambucil: Within 1 hour; phenylacetic acid mustard: Within 1.9 ± 0.7 hours

Elimination: Urine (~20% to 60% excreted in urine within 24 hours principally as metabolites; <1% excreted as unchanged drug or phenylacetic acid mustard in urine)

Dosing: Usual Note: For oncologic uses, dosing and frequency may vary by protocol and/or treatment phase; refer to specific protocol.

Pediatric:

Hodgkin lymphoma: Limited data available: Infants ≥7 months, Children, and Adolescents: ChlVPP regimen: Oral: 6 mg/**m²**/day on days 1 to 14 of a 28-day cycle for 6 to 10 cycles in combination with vinblastine, procarbazine, and prednisolone (Atra, 2002, Capra, 2007, Hall, 2007, Stoneham, 2007)

Nephrotic syndrome; frequently relapsing steroid-sensitive: Children and Adolescents: Oral: 0.1 to 0.2 mg/kg/day once daily for 8 weeks (maximum cumulative dose: 11.2 mg/kg) (Baluarte, 1978, Hodson, 2010; KDIGO, 2012); **Note:** Chlorambucil is not a preferred agent due to a higher incidence of adverse effects with no greater efficacy (Gipson, 2009).

Adult: **Note:** Utilize patient's actual body weight (full weight) for calculation of body surface area- or weight-based dosing, particularly when the intent of therapy is curative; manage regimen-related toxicities in the same manner as for nonobese patients; if a dose reduction is utilized due to toxicity, consider resumption of full weight-based dosing with subsequent cycles, especially if cause of toxicity (eg, hepatic or renal impairment) is resolved (Griggs, 2012). With bone marrow lymphocytic infiltration involvement (in CLL, Hodgkin lymphoma, or NHL), the maximum dose is 0.1 mg/kg/day. While short treatment courses are preferred, if maintenance therapy is required, the maximum dose is 0.1 mg/kg/day.

Chronic lymphocytic leukemia (CLL): Oral: 0.1 mg/kg/day for 3 to 6 weeks or 0.4 mg/kg pulsed doses administered intermittently, biweekly, or monthly (increased by 0.1 mg/kg/dose until response/toxicity observed)

Hodgkin lymphoma: Oral: 0.2 mg/kg/day for 3 to 6 weeks

Non-Hodgkin lymphomas (NHL): Oral: 0.1 mg/kg/day for 3 to 6 weeks

Dosing adjustment in renal impairment: There are no dosage adjustments provided in manufacturer's labeling; however, renal elimination of unchanged chlorambucil and active metabolite (phenylacetic acid mustard) is minimal and renal impairment is not likely to affect elimination. The following adjustments have been recommended: Adults:

Aronoff, 2007:

CrCl >50 mL/minute: No adjustment necessary.

CrCl 10 to 50 mL/minute: Administer 75% of dose.

CrCl <10 mL/minute: Administer 50% of dose.

Peritoneal dialysis (PD): Administer 50% of dose.

Kintzel, 1995: Based on the pharmacokinetics, dosage adjustment is not indicated.

Dosing adjustment in hepatic impairment: Adults: There are no dosing adjustments provided in the manufacturer's labeling (data is insufficient); however, chlorambucil undergoes extensive hepatic metabolism and dosage reduction should be considered in patients with hepatic impairment; monitor closely for toxicity.

Administration Hazardous agent; use appropriate precautions for handling and disposal (NIOSH 2014 [group 1]).

Oral: May be administered as a single daily dose; preferably on an empty stomach.

Monitoring Parameters Liver function tests, CBC with differential (weekly, with WBC monitored weekly during the first 3 to 6 weeks of treatment)

Dosage Forms Excipient information presented when available (limited, particularly for generics); consult specific product labeling.

Tablet, Oral:

Leukeran: 2 mg

Extemporaneous Preparations Hazardous agent: Use appropriate precautions for handling and disposal (NIOSH 2014 [group 1]).

A 2 mg/mL oral suspension may be prepared with tablets. Crush sixty 2 mg tablets in a mortar and reduce to a fine powder. Add small portions of methylcellulose 1% and mix to a uniform paste (total methylcellulose: 30 mL); mix while adding simple syrup in incremental proportions to **almost** 60 mL; transfer to a graduated cylinder, rinse mortar and pestle with simple syrup, and add quantity of vehicle sufficient to make 60 mL. Transfer contents of graduated cylinder to an amber prescription bottle. Label "shake well", "refrigerate", and "protect from light". Stable for 7 days refrigerated.

Dressman JB and Poust RI, "Stability of Allopurinol and of Five Antineoplastics in Suspension," *Am J Hosp Pharm*, 1983, 40(4):616-8.

Nahata MC, Pai VB, and Hipple TF, *Pediatric Drug Formulations*, 5th ed, Cincinnati, OH: Harvey Whitney Books Co, 2004.

◆ **Chlorambucilum** *see* Chlorambucil *on page 430*

◆ **Chloraminophene** *see* Chlorambucil *on page 430*

Chloramphenicol (klor am FEN i kole)

Medication Safety Issues

Sound-alike/look-alike issues:

Chloromycetin® may be confused with chlorambucil, Chlor-Trimeton®

Related Information

Safe Handling of Hazardous Drugs *on page 2455*

Brand Names: Canada Chloromycetin®; Chloromycetin® Succinate; Diochloram®; Pentamycetin®

Therapeutic Category Antibiotic, Miscellaneous

Generic Availability (US) Yes

Use Treatment of serious infections caused by susceptible organisms [eg, Salmonella, rickettsia, *H. influenza* (meningitis), or cystic fibrosis pathogens] when less toxic drugs are ineffective (ie, resistance) or contraindicated (FDA approved in all ages)

Pregnancy Considerations Chloramphenicol crosses the placenta producing cord concentrations approaching maternal serum concentrations. An increased risk of teratogenic effects has not been associated with the use of chloramphenicol in pregnancy (Czeizel, 2000; Heinonen, 1977). "Gray Syndrome" has occurred in premature infants and newborns receiving chloramphenicol. The manufacturer recommends caution if used in a pregnant patient near term or during labor. Chloramphenicol may be used for the treatment of Rocky Mountain spotted fever in pregnant women although caution should be used when administration occurs during the third trimester (CDC, 2006).

Breast-Feeding Considerations Chloramphenicol and its inactive metabolites are excreted in breast milk. Chloramphenicol is well absorbed following oral administration; however, metabolism and excretion are highly variable in infants and children. The half-life is also significantly prolonged in low birth weight infants (Powell, 1982). Due to the potential for serious adverse reactions in the nursing infant, the manufacturer recommends that caution be exercised when administering chloramphenicol to nursing women. Other sources recommended avoiding use while breast-feeding, especially infants <34 weeks postconceptual age or when unusually large doses are needed (Atkinson, 1988; Matsuda, 1984; Plomp, 1983). Non-dose-related effects could include modification of bowel flora.

Contraindications Hypersensitivity to chloramphenicol or any component of the formulation; treatment of trivial or viral infections; bacterial prophylaxis

Warnings/Precautions Hazardous agent - use appropriate precautions for handling and disposal (NIOSH 2014 [group 2]).

Use in neonates (including premature) has resulted in "gray-baby syndrome" characterized by circulatory collapse, cyanosis, acidosis, abdominal distention (with or without emesis), myocardial depression, coma, and death; progression of symptoms is rapid; prompt termination of therapy required. Reaction result from drug accumulation possibly caused by the impaired neonatal hepatic or renal function. Reduce dose with impaired liver function. Use with care in patients with glucose 6-phosphate dehydrogenase deficiency. **[U.S. Boxed Warning]: Serious and fatal blood dyscrasias (aplastic anemia, hypoplastic anemia, thrombocytopenia, and granulocytopenia) have occurred after both short-term and prolonged therapy. Monitor CBC frequently in all patients;** discontinue if evidence of myelosuppression. Irreversible bone marrow suppression may occur weeks or months after therapy. Avoid repeated courses of treatment. Should not be used for minor infections or when less potentially toxic agents are effective. Prolonged use may result in fungal or bacterial superinfection, including *C. difficile*-associated diarrhea (CDAD) and pseudomembranous colitis; CDAD has been observed >2 months postantibiotic treatment.

Adverse Reactions

Central nervous system: Confusion, delirium, depression, fever, headache

Dermatologic: Angioedema, rash, urticaria

Gastrointestinal: Diarrhea, enterocolitis, glossitis, nausea, stomatitis, vomiting

Hematologic: Aplastic anemia, bone marrow suppression, granulocytopenia, hypoplastic anemia, pancytopenia, thrombocytopenia

Ocular: Optic neuritis

Miscellaneous: Anaphylaxis, hypersensitivity reactions, Gray syndrome

Drug Interactions

Metabolism/Transport Effects Inhibits CYP2C19 (strong), CYP2C9 (weak)

Avoid Concomitant Use

Avoid concomitant use of Chloramphenicol with any of the following: BCG; BCG (Intravesical); CloZAPine; Dipyrone

Increased Effect/Toxicity

Chloramphenicol may increase the levels/effects of: Alcohol (Ethyl); Barbiturates; Carbocisteine; Cilostazol; Citalopram; CloZAPine; CycloSPORINE (Systemic); CYP2C19 Substrates; Sulfonylureas; Tacrolimus (Systemic); Vitamin K Antagonists; Voriconazole

The levels/effects of Chloramphenicol may be increased by: Dipyrone

Decreased Effect

Chloramphenicol may decrease the levels/effects of: BCG; BCG (Intravesical); BCG Vaccine (Immunization); CefTAZidime; Clopidogrel; Sodium Picosulfate; Typhoid Vaccine; Vitamin B12

The levels/effects of Chloramphenicol may be decreased by: Barbiturates; Rifampin

Storage/Stability Store at room temperature prior to reconstitution. Reconstituted solutions remain stable for 30 days. Use only clear solutions. Frozen solutions remain stable for 6 months.

Mechanism of Action Reversibly binds to 50S ribosomal subunits of susceptible organisms preventing amino acids from being transferred to growing peptide chains thus inhibiting protein synthesis

Pharmacokinetics (Adult data unless noted)

Distribution: Distributes to most tissues and body fluids; good CSF and brain penetration
- CSF concentration with uninflamed meninges: 21% to 50% of plasma concentration
- CSF concentration with inflamed meninges: 45% to 89% of plasma concentration
  - V_d:
    - Chloramphenicol: 0.5-1 L/kg
    - Chloramphenicol succinate: 0.2-3.1 L/kg; decreased with hepatic or renal dysfunction

Protein binding: Chloramphenicol: 60% decreased with hepatic or renal dysfunction and 30% to 40% in newborn infants

Metabolism:
- Chloramphenicol succinate: Hydrolized in the liver, kidney, and lungs to chloramphenicol (active)
- Chloramphenicol: Hepatic to metabolites (inactive)

Bioavailability:
- Chloramphenicol: Oral: ~80%
- Chloramphenicol succinate: IV: ~70%; highly variable, dependant upon rate and extent of metabolism to chloramphenicol

Half-life:
- Neonates:
  - 1-2 days: 24 hours
  - 10-16 days: 10 hours
- Children: 4-6 hours
- Adults:
  - Normal renal function: ~4 hours
  - Chloramphenicol succinate: ~3 hours
  - End-stage renal disease: 3-7 hours
  - Hepatic disease: Prolonged

Elimination: ~30% as unchanged chloramphenicol succinate in urine; in infants and young children, 6% to 80% of the dose may be excreted unchanged in urine; 5% to 15% as chloramphenicol

Dosing: Neonatal Note: Follow serum concentrations closely to monitor for toxicity and efficacy in neonates due to variability in metabolism; use should be restricted to treatment of serious infections caused by susceptible organisms when less toxic drugs are ineffective (ie, resistance) or contraindicated.

Meningitis (Tunkel, 2004): IV: **Note:** Treat for a minimum of 21 days; use smaller doses and longer intervals for neonates <2 kg:
- PNA ≤7 days: 25 mg/kg/dose every 24 hours
- PNA 8-28 days: 25 mg/kg/dose every 12 hours or 50 mg/kg/dose every 24 hours

Severe infection: IV:
- *Weight-based dosing:* Limited data available (Prober, 1990):
  - Patient weight:
    - <1200 g: 22 mg/kg/dose every 24 hours
    - 1200-2000 g: 25 mg/kg/dose every 24 hours
- *Age-based dosing:* Limited data available:
  - Premature neonate or term neonate with PNA ≤7 days: Dosing regimens variable: 25 mg/kg/dose every 24 hours or initiation with a loading dose of 20 mg/kg followed in 12 hours by a maintenance regimen of 12.5 mg/kg/dose every 12 hours (Rajchgot, 1982; Rajchgot, 1983; Weiss, 1960)
  - Term neonate with PNA >7 days: Dosing regimens variable: 25 mg/kg/dose every 12 hours or 12.5 mg/kg/dose every 6 hours (Rajchgot, 1983; Weiss, 1960)
- *Manufacturer's labeling:* **Note:** Frequency recommended by the manufacturer for this age group is higher than other expert recommendations, which generally recommend no more frequent than every 12 hours; monitor serum concentrations closely.
  - Preterm infants: 6.25 mg/kg/dose every 6 hours
  - Term infants:
    - PNA <14 days: 6.25 mg/kg/dose every 6 hours
    - PNA ≥14 days: 12.5 mg/kg/dose every 6 hours

Dosing: Usual

Infants, Children, and Adolescents: **Note:** Follow serum concentrations closely to monitor for toxicity. Use should be restricted to treatment of serious infections when less toxic drugs are ineffective (ie, resistance) or contraindicated.
- **Meningitis:** IV: 18.75-25 mg/kg/dose every 6 hours (Bradley, 2012; Kliegman, 2011; Tunkel, 2004)
- **Severe infections:** IV:
  - Manufacturer's labeling: 12.5 mg/kg/dose every 6 hours; in some cases higher doses up to 25 mg/kg/dose every 6 hours may be required; higher doses should be promptly decreased when able
  - Alternate dosing: 12.5-25 mg/kg/dose every 6 hours; maximum daily dose: 4000 mg/**day** (AAP, 2012)

Adults: **Systemic infections:** IV: 50-100 mg/kg/day in divided doses every 6 hours

Dosing adjustment in renal impairment: Use with caution; monitor serum concentrations.

Dosing adjustment in hepatic impairment: Use with caution; monitor serum concentrations.

Preparation for Administration Hazardous agent; use appropriate precautions for handling and disposal (NIOSH 2014 [group 2]).

Parenteral: Should not be administered IM; has been shown to be ineffective.
- IV push: Reconstitute with 10 mL SWFI or D_5W for a concentration of 100 mg/mL
- Intermittent IV infusion: Further dilute in D_5W to a final concentration not to exceed 20 mg/mL (Klaus 1998); in neonates, a higher maximum concentration of 25 mg/mL has been used (Prober 1990; Rajchgot 1983)

Administration Hazardous agent; use appropriate precautions for handling and disposal (NIOSH 2014 [group 2]).

Parenteral:
- IV push: Administer over at least 1 minute
- Intermittent IV infusion: Infuse over 30 to 60 minutes (Klaus 1998). In neonates, some centers have

administered as an intermittent IV infusion over 15 minutes (Prober 1990)

Monitoring Parameters CBC with differential and platelet counts (baseline and every 2 days during therapy), serum iron level, iron-binding capacity, periodic liver and renal function tests, serum drug concentration

Reference Range

Therapeutic concentrations:

Meningitis:

Peak: 15-25 mcg/mL

Trough: 5-15 mcg/mL

Other infections:

Peak: 10-20 mcg/mL

Trough: 5-10 mcg/mL

Timing of serum samples: Draw peak concentrations 0.5-1.5 hours after completion of IV dose; and trough immediately before next dose

Test Interactions May cause false-positive results in urine glucose tests when using cupric sulfate (Benedict's solution, Clinitest®).

Additional Information Sodium content of 1 g injection: 2.25 mEq

Dosage Forms Excipient information presented when available (limited, particularly for generics); consult specific product labeling.

Solution Reconstituted, Intravenous:

Generic: 1 g (1 ea)

- **ChloraPrep One Step [OTC]** *see* Chlorhexidine Gluconate *on page 434*
- **Chlorbutinum** *see* Chlorambucil *on page 430*
- **Chlorethazine** *see* Mechlorethamine (Systemic) *on page 1335*
- **Chlorethazine Mustard** *see* Mechlorethamine (Systemic) *on page 1335*

Chlorhexidine Gluconate

(klor HEKS i deen GLOO koe nate)

Medication Safety Issues

Sound-alike/look-alike issues:

Peridex may be confused with Precedex

Brand Names: US Betasept Surgical Scrub [OTC]; ChloraPrep One Step [OTC]; Hibiclens [OTC]; Hibistat [OTC]; Paroex; Peridex; Periogard; Tegaderm CHG Dressing [OTC]

Brand Names: Canada Apo-Chlorhexidine Oral Rinse; Denti-Care Chlorhexidine Gluconate Oral Rinse; GUM Paroex; ORO-Clense; Perichlor; Peridex Oral Rinse; Periogard; X-Pur Chlorhexidine

Therapeutic Category Antibacterial, Topical; Antibiotic, Oral Rinse

Generic Availability (US) May be product dependent

Use Skin cleanser for surgical scrub; cleanser for skin wounds; germicidal hand rinse; antibacterial dental rinse to reduce plaque formation and control gingivitis; prophylactic dental rinse to prevent oral infections in immunocompromised patients, particularly bone marrow transplant patients receiving cytotoxic therapy; and short-term substitute for toothbrushing in situations where the patient is unable to tolerate mechanical stimulation of the gums

Pregnancy Risk Factor B/C (manufacturer specific)

Pregnancy Considerations Adverse events have not been observed in animal reproduction studies following use of the oral rinse; use of periodontal chip has not been studied. Chlorhexidine gluconate oral rinse is poorly absorbed from the gastrointestinal tract.

Breast-Feeding Considerations It is not known if chlorhexidine gluconate is excreted in breast milk. The manufacturer recommends that caution be exercised when administering chlorhexidine gluconate oral rinse to nursing women. However, oral rinse is not intended for ingestion; patient should expectorate after rinsing.

Contraindications Hypersensitivity to chlorhexidine gluconate or any component of the formulation

Warnings/Precautions Serious allergic reactions, including anaphylaxis, have been reported with use.

Oral rinse: Staining of oral surfaces (mucosa, teeth, tooth restorations, dorsum of tongue) may occur; may be visible as soon as 1 week after therapy begins and is more pronounced when there is a heavy accumulation of unremoved plaque and when teeth fillings have rough surfaces. Stain does not have a clinically adverse effect, but because removal may not be possible, patient with frontal restoration should be advised of the potential permanency of the stain. An increase in supragingival calculus has been observed with use; it is not known if the incidence of subgingival calculus is increased. Dental prophylaxis to remove calculus deposits should be performed at least every 6 months. May alter taste perception during use; has rarely been associated with permanent taste alteration.

Periodontal chip: Infectious events (eg, abscesses, cellulitis) have been observed rarely with adjunctive chip placement post scaling and root planing; use with caution in patients with periodontal disease and concomitant diseases potentially decreasing immune status (eg, diabetes, cancer). Use in acute periodontal abscess pocket is not recommended.

Topical: For topical use only. Keep out of eyes, ears, and the mouth; if contact occurs, rinse with cold water immediately; permanent eye injury may result if agent enters and remains in the eye. Deafness has been reported following instillation in the middle ear through perforated ear drums. Avoid applying to wounds that involve more than the superficial skin layers. Avoid repeated use as general skin cleansing of large surfaces (unless necessary for condition). Not for preoperative preparation of face or head; avoid contact with meninges (do not use on lumbar puncture sites). Avoid applying to genital areas; generalized allergic reactions, irritation, and sensitivity have been reported. Solutions may be flammable (products may contain alcohol); avoid exposure to open flame and/or ignition source (eg, electrocautery) until completely dry; avoid application to hairy areas which may significantly delay drying time. Avoid use in children <2 months of age due to potential for increased absorption, and risk of irritation or chemical burns. May cause staining of fabrics (brown stain) due to a chemical reaction between chlorhexidine gluconate bound to fabric and chlorine (if sufficient chlorine is present from certain laundry detergents used during laundering process). When used as a topical antiseptic, improper use may lead to product contamination. Although infrequent, product contamination has been associated with reports of localized and systemic infections. To reduce the risk of infection, ensure antiseptic products are used according to the labeled instructions; avoid diluting products after opening; and apply single-use containers only one time to one patient and discard any unused solution (FDA Drug Safety Communication, 2013).

Warnings: Additional Pediatric Considerations A case of bradycardic episodes after breast-feeding in a 2-day-old neonate whose mother used chlorhexidine gluconate topically on her breasts to prevent mastitis has been reported.

Some dosage forms may contain propylene glycol; in neonates large amounts of propylene glycol delivered orally, intravenously (eg, >3,000 mg/day), or topically have been associated with potentially fatal toxicities which can include metabolic acidosis, seizures, renal failure, and CNS depression; toxicities have also been reported in children and adults including hyperosmolality, lactic

acidosis, seizures and respiratory depression; use caution (AAP, 1997; Shehab, 2009).

Adverse Reactions

Oral:

Dysgeusia, increased tartar formation, mouth discoloration (staining of oral surfaces [mucosa, teeth, dorsum of tongue] may be visible as soon as 1 week after therapy begins and is more pronounced when there is a heavy accumulation of unremoved plaque and when teeth fillings have rough surfaces; stain does not have a clinically adverse effect but because removal may not be possible, patient with frontal restoration should be advised of the potential permanency of the stain), mouth irritation, tongue irritation

Rare but important or life-threatening: Dyspnea, facial edema, nasal congestion

Topical: Allergic sensitization, erythema, hypersensitivity reaction, rough skin, xeroderma

Drug Interactions

Metabolism/Transport Effects None known.

Avoid Concomitant Use There are no known interactions where it is recommended to avoid concomitant use.

Increased Effect/Toxicity There are no known significant interactions involving an increase in effect.

Decreased Effect There are no known significant interactions involving a decrease in effect.

Storage/Stability

Oral rinse: Store at room temperature. Keep out of reach of children.

Periodontal chip: Store at 20°C to 25°C (68°F to 77°F); excursions permitted to 15°C to 30°C (59°F to 86°F).

Topical: Store at room temperature. Alcohol-containing topical products are flammable; keep away from flames or fire.

Mechanism of Action Chlorhexidine has activity against gram-positive and gram-negative organisms, facultative anaerobes, aerobes, and yeast; it is both bacteriostatic and bactericidal, depending on its concentration. The bactericidal effect of chlorhexidine is a result of the binding of this cationic molecule to negatively charged bacterial cell walls and extramicrobial complexes. At low concentrations, this causes an alteration of bacterial cell osmotic equilibrium and leakage of potassium and phosphorous resulting in a bacteriostatic effect. At high concentrations of chlorhexidine, the cytoplasmic contents of the bacterial cell precipitate and result in cell death.

Pharmacokinetics (Adult data unless noted)

Absorption: ~30% of chlorhexidine is retained in the oral cavity following rinsing and is slowly released into the oral fluids; chlorhexidine is poorly absorbed from the GI tract and is not absorbed topically through intact skin

Serum concentrations: Detectable levels are not present in the plasma 12 hours after administration

Elimination: Primarily through the feces (~90%); <1% excreted in the urine

Dosing: Usual

Oral rinse (Peridex® or PerioGard®):

Children and Adults: 15 mL twice daily

Immunocompromised patient: 10-15 mL, 2-3 times/day

Cleanser: Children and Adults: Apply 5 mL per scrub or hand wash; apply 25 mL per body wash or hair wash

Administration

Oral rinse: Precede use of solution by flossing and brushing teeth, completely rinse toothpaste from mouth; swish undiluted oral rinse around in mouth for 30 seconds, then expectorate; caution patient not to swallow the medicine; avoid eating for 2-3 hours after treatment.

Topical:

Surgical scrub: Scrub 3 minutes and rinse thoroughly, wash for an additional 3 minutes

Hand wash: Wash for 15 seconds and rinse

Hand rinse: Rub vigorously for 15 seconds

Body wash: Wet body and/or hair, apply, rinse thoroughly, repeat.

Monitoring Parameters Improvement in gingival inflammation and bleeding; development of teeth or denture discoloration; dental prophylaxis to remove stains at regular intervals of no greater than 6 months.

Test Interactions If chlorhexidine is used as a disinfectant before midstream urine collection, a false-positive urine protein may result (when using dipstick method based upon a pH indicator color change).

Dosage Forms Excipient information presented when available (limited, particularly for generics); consult specific product labeling.

Liquid, External:

Betasept Surgical Scrub: 4% (118 mL, 237 mL, 473 mL, 946 mL, 3780 mL)

Hibiclens: 4% (15 mL, 118 mL, 236 mL, 473 mL, 946 mL, 3790 mL) [contains fd&c red #40, isopropyl alcohol]

Generic: 2% (118 mL); 4% (118 mL, 237 mL, 473 mL, 946 mL, 3800 mL)

Miscellaneous, External:

Hibistat: 0.5% (50 ea) [contains isopropyl alcohol]

Tegaderm CHG Dressing: (Dressing) (1 ea)

Pad, External:

Generic: 2% (2 ea, 6 ea)

Solution, External:

ChloraPrep One Step: 2% (3 mL, 10.5 mL) [latex free]

Solution, Mouth/Throat:

Paroex: 0.12% (473 mL) [alcohol free; contains fd&c red #40, propylene glycol]

Peridex: 0.12% (118 mL, 473 mL) [contains alcohol, usp, brilliant blue fcf (fd&c blue #1), saccharin sodium]

Periogard: 0.12% (473 mL) [mint flavor]

Generic: 0.12% (15 mL, 473 mL)

- **Chlormeprazine** *see* Prochlorperazine *on page 1774*
- **2-Chlorodeoxyadenosine** *see* Cladribine *on page 480*
- **Chloromag** *see* Magnesium Chloride *on page 1310*
- **Chloromycetin® (Can)** *see* Chloramphenicol *on page 432*
- **Chloromycetin® Succinate (Can)** *see* Chloramphenicol *on page 432*

Chloroprocaine (klor oh PROE kane)

Medication Safety Issues

Sound-alike/look-alike issues:

Nesacaine® may be confused with Neptazane™

High alert medication:

The Institute for Safe Medication Practices (ISMP) includes this medication (epidural administration) among its list of drug classes which have a heightened risk of causing significant patient harm when used in error.

Brand Names: US Nesacaine; Nesacaine-MPF

Therapeutic Category Local Anesthetic, Injectable

Generic Availability (US) Yes

Use Production of local or regional analgesia and anesthesia by local infiltration and peripheral nerve block techniques

Pregnancy Risk Factor C

Pregnancy Considerations Animal reproduction studies have not been conducted. Local anesthetics rapidly cross the placenta and may cause varying degrees of maternal, fetal, and neonatal toxicity. Close maternal and fetal monitoring (heart rate and electronic fetal monitoring advised) are required during obstetrical use. Maternal hypotension has resulted from regional anesthesia. Positioning the patient on her left side and elevating the legs may help. Epidural, paracervical, or pudendal anesthesia may alter the forces of parturition through changes in uterine contractility or maternal expulsive efforts. The use of some local anesthetic drugs during labor and delivery may diminish muscle strength and tone for the first day or two of life. Administration as a paracervical block is not recommended with toxemia of pregnancy, fetal distress, or prematurity. Administration of a paracervical block early in pregnancy has resulted in maternal seizures and cardiovascular collapse. Fetal bradycardia and acidosis also have been reported. Fetal depression has occurred following unintended fetal intracranial injection while administering a paracervical and/or pudendal block.

Breast-Feeding Considerations It is not known if chloroprocaine is excreted in breast milk. The manufacturer recommends that caution be exercised when administering chloroprocaine to nursing women.

Contraindications Hypersensitivity to chloroprocaine, other ester type anesthetics, or any component of the formulation; do not use for subarachnoid administration

Warnings/Precautions Use with caution in patients with hepatic impairment or cardiovascular disease. Use with caution in the elderly, debilitated, acutely ill and pediatric patients. Use with extreme caution in patients with myasthenia gravis; may cause significant weakness (Haroutiunian, 2009). **Do not use solutions containing preservatives for caudal or epidural block.** Intravascular injections should be avoided. Continuous intra-articular infusion of local anesthetics after arthroscopic or other surgical procedures is **not** an approved use; chondrolysis (primarily in the shoulder joint) has occurred following infusion, with some cases requiring arthroplasty or shoulder replacement. Careful and constant monitoring of the patient's state of consciousness should be done following each local anesthetic injection; at such times, restlessness, anxiety, tinnitus, dizziness, blurred vision, tremors, depression, or drowsiness may be early warning signs of CNS toxicity. Treatment is primarily symptomatic and supportive. Local anesthetics have been associated with rare occurrences of sudden respiratory arrest, seizures, and cardiac arrest. A test dose is recommended prior to epidural administration. Resuscitative equipment, oxygen, and other resuscitative drugs should be available for immediate use.

Adverse Reactions

Cardiovascular: Bradycardia, cardiac arrest, hypotension, ventricular arrhythmia

Central nervous system: Anxiety, dizziness, restlessness, seizure, tinnitus, unconsciousness

Dermatologic: Angioneurotic edema, erythema, pruritus, urticaria

Neuromuscular & skeletal: Chondrolysis (continuous intra-articular administration)

Ocular: Blurred vision

Respiratory: Respiratory arrest

Miscellaneous: Allergic reactions, anaphylactoid reactions

Drug Interactions

Metabolism/Transport Effects None known.

Avoid Concomitant Use There are no known interactions where it is recommended to avoid concomitant use.

Increased Effect/Toxicity

The levels/effects of Chloroprocaine may be increased by: Hyaluronidase

Decreased Effect

Chloroprocaine may decrease the levels/effects of: Technetium Tc 99m Tilmanocept

Storage/Stability Store at 15°C to 30°C (59°F to 86°F); protect from freezing. Protect from light. Discard Nesacaine®-MPF following single use.

Mechanism of Action Chloroprocaine HCl is benzoic acid, 4-amino-2-chloro-2-(diethylamino) ethyl ester monohydrochloride. Chloroprocaine is an ester-type local anesthetic, which stabilizes the neuronal membranes and prevents initiation and transmission of nerve impulses thereby affecting local anesthetic actions. Local anesthetics including chloroprocaine, reversibly prevent generation and conduction of electrical impulses in neurons by decreasing the transient increase in permeability to sodium. The differential sensitivity generally depends on the size of the fiber; small fibers are more sensitive than larger fibers and require a longer period for recovery. Sensory pain fibers are usually blocked first, followed by fibers that transmit sensations of temperature, touch, and deep pressure. High concentrations block sympathetic somatic sensory and somatic motor fibers. The spread of anesthesia depends upon the distribution of the solution. This is primarily dependent on the volume of drug injected.

Pharmacodynamics

Onset of action: 6-12 minutes

Duration (patient, type of block, concentration, and method of anesthesia dependent): Up to 1 hour

Pharmacokinetics (Adult data unless noted)

Metabolism: Rapidly hydrolyzed by plasma enzymes to 2-chloro-4-aminobenzoic acid and 8-diethylaminoethanol (80% conjugated before elimination)

Half-life (*in vitro*):

- Neonates: 43 ± 2 seconds
- Adult males: 21 ± 2 seconds
- Adult females: 25 ± 1 second

Elimination: Very little excreted as unchanged drug in urine; metabolites: Cloro-aminobenzoic acid and diethylaminoethanol primarily excreted unchanged in urine

Dosing: Usual Dose varies with procedure, desired depth, and duration of anesthesia, desired muscle relaxation, vascularity of tissues, physical condition, and age of patient. The smallest dose and concentration required to produce the desired effect should be used.

Pediatric: **Anesthesia, local injectable:** Children >3 years: Maximum dose without epinephrine: 11 mg/kg

Adult:

Anesthesia, local injectable: Maximum dose: 11 mg/kg; not to exceed 800 mg per treatment; with epinephrine (1:200,000): 14 mg/kg; not to exceed 1,000 mg per treatment

Infiltration and peripheral nerve block:

- Mandibular: 2 to 3 mL (40 to 60 mg) using 2%
- Infraorbital: 0.5 to 1 mL (10 to 20 mg) using 2%
- Brachial plexus: 30 to 40 mL (600 to 800 mg) using 2%
- Digital (without epinephrine): 3 to 4 mL (30 to 40 mg) using 1%
- Pudendal: 10 mL (200 mg) into each side (two sites) using 2%
- Paracervical: 3 mL (30 mg) per each of four sites using 1%

Caudal and lumbar epidural block:

- Caudal: 15 to 25 mL using 2% to 3% solution; may repeat dose at 40- to 60-minute intervals
- Lumbar: 2 to 2.5 mL per segment using 2% to 3% solution; usual total volume 15 to 25 mL; repeated doses 2 to 6 mL less than the original dose may be given at 40- to 50-minutes intervals

Preparation for Administration Parenteral: Dilute with NS. To prepare 1:200,000 epinephrine-chloroprocaine HCl injection, add 0.1 mL of a 1:1000 epinephrine injection to 20 mL of preservative-free chloroprocaine.

Administration Parenteral: Administer in small incremental doses; when using continuous intermittent catheter techniques, use frequent aspirations before and during the injection to avoid intravascular injection

Monitoring Parameters Blood pressure, heart rate, respiration, signs of CNS toxicity (lightheadedness, dizziness, tinnitus, restlessness, tremors, twitching, drowsiness, circumoral paresthesia)

Dosage Forms Excipient information presented when available (limited, particularly for generics); consult specific product labeling.

Solution, Injection, as hydrochloride:
Nesacaine: 1% (30 mL); 2% (30 mL) [contains disodium edta, methylparaben]
Solution, Injection, as hydrochloride [preservative free]:
Nesacaine-MPF: 2% (20 mL); 3% (20 mL) [methylparaben free]
Generic: 2% (20 mL); 3% (20 mL)

◆ **Chloroprocaine Hydrochloride** *see* Chloroprocaine *on page 435*

Chloroquine (KLOR oh kwin)

Medication Safety Issues
International issues:
Aralen [U.S., Mexico] may be confused with Paralen brand name for acetaminophen [Czech Republic]

Brand Names: US Aralen
Brand Names: Canada Aralen; Novo-Chloroquine
Therapeutic Category Amebicide; Antimalarial Agent
Generic Availability (US) Yes

Use Suppression or chemoprophylaxis of malaria in chloroquine-sensitive areas [FDA approved in pediatric patients (age not specified) and adults]; treatment of uncomplicated acute attacks of malaria due to susceptible *Plasmodium* species, except chloroquine-resistant *Plasmodium falciparum* [FDA approved in pediatric patients (age not specified) and adults]; extraintestinal amebiasis (FDA approved in adults); has been used for treatment of rheumatoid arthritis, discoid lupus erythematosus, scleroderma, pemphigus

Pregnancy Considerations In animal reproduction studies, drug accumulated in fetal ocular tissues and remained for several months following drug elimination from the rest of the body. Chloroquine and its metabolites cross the placenta and can be detected in the cord blood and urine of the newborn infant (Akintonwa, 1988; Essien, 1982; Law, 2008). In one study, chloroquine and its metabolites were measurable in the cord blood 89 days (mean) after the last maternal dose (Law, 2008).

Malaria infection in pregnant women may be more severe than in nonpregnant women and has a high risk of maternal and perinatal morbidity and mortality. Therefore, pregnant women and women who are likely to become pregnant are advised to avoid travel to malaria-risk areas. Chloroquine is recommended for the treatment of pregnant women for uncomplicated malaria in chloroquine-sensitive regions; when caused by chloroquine-sensitive *P. vivax* or *P. ovale*, pregnant women should be maintained on chloroquine prophylaxis for the duration of their pregnancy (refer to current guidelines) (CDC, 2011; CDC, 2012).

Breast-Feeding Considerations Chloroquine and its metabolite can be detected in breast milk. Per product labeling, 11 lactating women with malaria were given a single oral dose of chloroquine 600 mg. The maximum daily dose to the breast-feeding infant was calculated to be 0.7% of the maternal dose. Additional information has been published and results are variable. In one study, the relative dose to the nursing infant was calculated to be 2.3% (chloroquine) and 1% (metabolite) of the weight-adjusted maternal dose with the samples obtained a median of 17 days after the last dose. Women in this study received chloroquine phosphate 750 mg daily for 3 days. This report also provides data from other studies, listing relative infant doses of chloroquine ranging from 0.9% to 9.5% of the maternal dose (Law, 2008). Due to the potential for serious adverse reactions in the nursing infant, the manufacturer recommends a decision be made whether to discontinue nursing or to discontinue the drug, taking into account the importance of treatment to the mother. Other sources consider the amount of chloroquine exposure to the nursing infant to be safe when normal maternal doses for malaria are used. However, the amount of chloroquine obtained by a nursing infant from breast milk would not provide adequate protection if therapy for malaria in the infant is needed (CDC, 2012).

Contraindications Hypersensitivity to 4-aminoquinoline compounds or any component of the formulation; the presence of retinal or visual field changes either attributable to 4-aminoquinoline compounds or to any other etiology

Warnings/Precautions Use with caution in patients with hepatic impairment, alcoholism or in conjunction with hepatotoxic drugs. May exacerbate psoriasis or porphyria. Use caution in patients with seizure disorders. Use caution in G6PD deficiency; 4-aminoquinolines such as chloroquine has been associated with hemolysis and renal impairment. Use with caution in patients with preexisting auditory damage; discontinue immediately if hearing defects are noted. Retinopathy, maculopathy, and macular degeneration have occurred; irreversible retinal damage has occurred with prolonged or high dose 4-aminoquinoline therapy; risk factors include age, duration of therapy, and/or high doses. Monitoring is required, especially with prolonged therapy. Discontinue immediately if signs/symptoms occur; visual changes may progress even after therapy is discontinued. Use has been associated with ECG changes, AV block, and cardiomyopathy. May cause QT prolongation and subsequent torsade de pointes; avoid use in patients with diagnosed or suspected congenital long QT syndrome. Rare hematologic reactions including agranulocytosis, aplastic anemia, neutropenia, pancytopenia, and thrombocytopenia; monitor CBC during prolonged therapy. Consider discontinuation if severe blood disorders occur that are unrelated to disease. Acute extrapyramidal disorders may occur, usually resolving after discontinuation of therapy and/or symptomatic treatment. Skeletal muscle myopathy or neuromyopathy, leading to progressive weakness and atrophy of proximal muscle groups have been reported; muscle strength (especially proximal muscles) should be assessed periodically during prolonged therapy; discontinue therapy if weakness occurs. Potentially significant drug-drug interactions may exist, requiring dose or frequency adjustment, additional monitoring, and/or selection of alternative therapy.

Certain strains of *P. falciparum* are resistant to 4-aminoquinoline compounds. Prior to initiation of therapy, it should be determined if chloroquine is appropriate for use in the region to be visited; do not use for the treatment of *P. falciparum* acquired in areas of chloroquine resistance or where chloroquine prophylaxis has failed. Patients should be treated with another antimalarial if patient is infected with a resistant strain of plasmodia. Chloroquine does not prevent relapses in patients with vivax or malariae malaria; will not prevent vivax or malariae infection when administered as a prophylactic. Also consult current CDC guidelines for treatment recommendations.

Adverse Reactions
Cardiovascular: Cardiomyopathy, ECG changes (rare; including prolonged QRS and QTc intervals, T wave inversion or depression), hypotension (rare), torsades de pointes (rare)
Central nervous system: Agitation, anxiety, confusion, decreased deep tendon reflex, delirium, depression, extrapyramidal reaction (dystonia, dyskinesia, protrusion of the tongue, torticollis), hallucination, headache, insomnia, personality changes, polyneuropathy, psychosis, seizure
Dermatologic: Alopecia, bleaching of hair, blue gray skin pigmentation, erythema multiforme (rare), exacerbation of psoriasis, exfoliative dermatitis (rare), lichen planus, pleomorphic rash, pruritus, skin photosensitivity, Stevens-Johnson syndrome (rare), toxic epidermal necrolysis (rare), urticaria

Gastrointestinal: Abdominal cramps, anorexia, diarrhea, nausea, vomiting
Hematologic & oncologic: Agranulocytosis (rare; reversible), aplastic anemia, neutropenia, pancytopenia, thrombocytopenia
Hepatic: Hepatitis, increased liver enzymes
Hypersensitivity: Anaphylactoid reaction, anaphylaxis, angioedema
Immunologic: DRESS syndrome
Neuromuscular & skeletal: Myopathy, neuromuscular disease, proximal myopathy
Ophthalmic: Accommodation disturbances, blurred vision, corneal opacity (reversible), macular degeneration (may be irreversible), maculopathy (may be irreversible), nocturnal amblyopia, retinopathy (including irreversible changes in some patients long-term or high-dose therapy), visual field defects
Otic: Deafness (nerve), hearing loss (risk increased in patients with pre-existing auditory damage), tinnitus

Drug Interactions

Metabolism/Transport Effects **Substrate** of CYP2D6 (major), CYP3A4 (major); **Note:** Assignment of Major/Minor substrate status based on clinically relevant drug interaction potential; **Inhibits** CYP2D6 (moderate)

Avoid Concomitant Use

Avoid concomitant use of Chloroquine with any of the following: Agalsidase Alfa; Agalsidase Beta; Artemether; Conivaptan; Fusidic Acid (Systemic); Highest Risk QTc-Prolonging Agents; Idelalisib; Ivabradine; Lumefantrine; Mefloquine; Mifepristone; Thioridazine

Increased Effect/Toxicity

Chloroquine may increase the levels/effects of: Antipsychotic Agents (Phenothiazines); ARIPiprazole; Beta-Blockers; Cardiac Glycosides; CYP2D6 Substrates; Dapsone (Systemic); Dapsone (Topical); DOXOrubicin (Conventional); Fesoterodine; Highest Risk QTc-Prolonging Agents; Lumefantrine; Mefloquine; Metoprolol; Moderate Risk QTc-Prolonging Agents; Nebivolol; Prilocaine; Sodium Nitrite; Thioridazine

The levels/effects of Chloroquine may be increased by: Abiraterone Acetate; Aprepitant; Artemether; Conivaptan; CYP2D6 Inhibitors (Moderate); CYP2D6 Inhibitors (Strong); CYP3A4 Inhibitors (Moderate); CYP3A4 Inhibitors (Strong); Dapsone (Systemic); Dasatinib; Fosaprepitant; Fusidic Acid (Systemic); Idelalisib; Ivabradine; Ivacaftor; Luliconazole; Mefloquine; Mifepristone; Netupitant; Nitric Oxide; Palbociclib; Panobinostat; Peginterferon Alfa-2b; QTc-Prolonging Agents (Indeterminate Risk and Risk Modifying); Simeprevir; Stiripentol

Decreased Effect

Chloroquine may decrease the levels/effects of: Agalsidase Alfa; Agalsidase Beta; Ampicillin; Anthelmintics; Codeine; Rabies Vaccine; Tamoxifen; TraMADol

The levels/effects of Chloroquine may be decreased by: Antacids; Bosentan; CYP3A4 Inducers (Moderate); CYP3A4 Inducers (Strong); Dabrafenib; Deferasirox; Kaolin; Lanthanum; Mitotane; Peginterferon Alfa-2b; Siltuximab; St Johns Wort; Tocilizumab

Storage/Stability Store at 25°C (77°F); excursions are permitted between 15°C and 30°C (59°F and 86°F); protect from light.

Mechanism of Action Binds to and inhibits DNA and RNA polymerase; interferes with metabolism and hemoglobin utilization by parasites; inhibits prostaglandin effects; chloroquine concentrates within parasite acid vesicles and raises internal pH resulting in inhibition of parasite growth; may involve aggregates of ferriprotoporphyrin IX acting as chloroquine receptors causing membrane damage; may also interfere with nucleoprotein synthesis

Pharmacokinetics (Adult data unless noted)

Absorption: Oral: Rapid
Distribution: Widely distributed in body tissues including eyes, heart, kidneys, liver, leukocytes, and lungs where retention is prolonged; crosses the placenta; appears in breast milk
Protein binding: 50% to 65%
Metabolism: Partially hepatic; main metabolite is desethylchloroquine
Half-life: 3-5 days
Time to peak serum concentration: Oral: Within 1-2 hours
Elimination: ~70% of dose excreted in urine (~35% unchanged); acidification of the urine increases elimination of drug; small amounts of drug may be present in urine months following discontinuation of therapy
Dialysis: Minimally removed by hemodialysis

Dosing: Usual Oral: **Note:** Dosage expressed in terms of base (10 mg base = 16.6 mg chloroquine phosphate):
Malaria:
Suppression or prophylaxis:
Infants and Children: Administer 5 mg base/kg/week on the same day each week (not to exceed 300 mg base/dose); begin 1-2 weeks prior to exposure; continue for 4 weeks after leaving endemic area; if suppressive therapy is not begun prior to exposure, double the initial loading dose to 10 mg base/kg and give in 2 divided doses 6 hours apart, followed by the usual dosage regimen
Adults: 300 mg base on the same day each week; begin 1-2 weeks prior to exposure; continue for 4 weeks after leaving endemic area; if suppressive therapy is not begun prior to exposure, double the initial loading dose to 600 mg base and give in 2 divided doses 6 hours apart, followed by the usual dosage regimen
Acute attack:
Infants and Children: 10 mg base/kg immediately (maximum: 600 mg base/dose), followed by 5 mg base/kg (maximum: 300 mg base/dose) administered at 6, 24, and 48 hours after first dose for a total of 4 doses (CDC, 2009)
Adults: 600 mg base/dose immediately, then 300 mg base/dose at 6, 24, and 48 hours after the first dose
Extraintestinal amebiasis:
Children: 10 mg base/kg once daily for 21 days (up to 600 mg base/day) (Seidel, 1984)
Adults: 600 mg base/day for 2 days followed by 300 mg base/day for at least 2-3 weeks
Rheumatoid arthritis, lupus erythematosus: Adults: 150 mg base once daily

Dosing adjustment in renal impairment: CrCl <10 mL/minute: Administer 50% of dose (Arnoff, 2007)

Administration Oral: Administer with meals to decrease GI upset; chloroquine phosphate tablets have also been mixed with chocolate syrup or enclosed in gelatin capsules to mask the bitter taste

Monitoring Parameters Periodic CBC, examination for muscular weakness, and ophthalmologic examination (visual acuity, slit-lamp, fundoscopic, and visual field tests) in patients receiving prolonged therapy

Additional Information *P. vivax* and *P. ovale* infections treated with chloroquine only can relapse due to hypnozoites; add primaquine to eradicate hypnozoites

Dosage Forms Excipient information presented when available (limited, particularly for generics); consult specific product labeling.
Tablet, Oral, as phosphate:
Aralen: 500 mg [equivalent to chloroquine base 300 mg]
Generic: 250 mg [equivalent to chloroquine base 150 mg], 500 mg [equivalent to chloroquine base 300 mg]

Extemporaneous Preparations A 15 mg chloroquine phosphate/mL oral suspension (equivalent to 9 mg chloroquine base/mL) may be made from tablets and a 1:1 mixture of Ora-Sweet® and Ora-Plus®. Crush three 500 mg chloroquine phosphate tablets (equivalent to

300 mg base/tablet) in a mortar and reduce to a fine powder. Add 15 mL of the vehicle and mix to a uniform paste; mix while adding the vehicle in incremental proportions to **almost** 100 mL; transfer to a calibrated bottle, rinse mortar with vehicle, and add quantity of vehicle sufficient to make 100 mL. Label "shake well before using" and "protect from light". Stable for up to 60 days when stored in the dark at room temperature or refrigerated (preferred).

Allen LV Jr and Erickson MA 3rd, "Stability of Alprazolam, Chloroquine Phosphate, Cisapride, Enalapril Maleate, and Hydralazine Hydrochloride in Extemporaneously Compounded Oral Liquids," *Am J Health Syst Pharm*, 1998, 55(18):1915-20.

◆ **Chloroquine Phosphate** *see* Chloroquine *on page 437*

Chlorothiazide (klor oh THYE a zide)

Medication Safety Issues

International issues:

Diuril [U.S.] may be confused with Duorol brand name for acetaminophen [Spain]

Brand Names: US Diuril; Sodium Diuril

Therapeutic Category Antihypertensive Agent; Diuretic, Thiazide

Generic Availability (US) May be product dependent

Use

Oral: Suspension, tablets: Treatment of edema due to heart failure, hepatic cirrhosis, and estrogen or corticosteroid therapy (FDA approved in infants, children, and adults); treatment of various forms of renal dysfunction, including nephrotic syndrome, acute glomerulonephritis, and chronic renal failure (FDA approved in infants, children, and adults); management of hypertension either alone or in combination with other antihypertensive agents (FDA approved in infants, children, and adults); has also been used for bronchopulmonary dysplasia (BPD) and central diabetes insipidus of infancy; **Note:** Use in pregnancy should be reserved for those cases causing extreme discomfort and unrelieved by rest; should not be routinely used during pregnancy

Parenteral: Treatment of edema due to heart failure, hepatic cirrhosis, and estrogen or corticosteroid therapy (FDA approved in adults); treatment of various forms of renal dysfunction including nephrotic syndrome, acute glomerulonephritis, and chronic renal failure (FDA approved in adults); has also been used for bronchopulmonary dysplasia (BPD); **Note:** Use in pregnancy should be reserved for those cases causing extreme discomfort and unrelieved by rest; should not be routinely used during pregnancy

Pregnancy Risk Factor C

Pregnancy Considerations Adverse events were not observed in animal reproduction studies; however, studies were not complete. Chlorothiazide crosses the placenta and is found in cord blood. Maternal use may cause may cause fetal or neonatal jaundice, thrombocytopenia, or other adverse events observed in adults. Use of thiazide diuretics to treat edema during normal pregnancies is not appropriate; use may be considered when edema is due to pathologic causes (as in the nonpregnant patient); monitor. Untreated chronic maternal hypertension is associated with adverse events in the fetus, infant, and mother (ACOG, 2013). Women who required thiazide diuretics for the treatment of hypertension prior to pregnancy may continue their use (ACOG, 2013).

Breast-Feeding Considerations Chlorothiazide is excreted into breast milk. Due to the potential for serious adverse reactions in the nursing infant, the manufacturer recommends a decision be made whether to discontinue nursing or to discontinue the drug, taking into account the importance of treatment to the mother. Diuretics have the potential to decrease milk volume and suppress lactation.

Contraindications

Hypersensitivity to chlorothiazide, any component of the formulation or sulfonamide-derived drugs; anuria

Note: Although the FDA approved product labeling states this medication is contraindicated with other sulfonamide-containing drug classes, the scientific basis of this statement has been challenged. See "Warnings/Precautions" for more detail.

Warnings/Precautions Hypersensitivity reactions may occur. Use with caution in severe renal disease. Electrolyte disturbances (hypercalcemia, hypokalemia, hypochloremic alkalosis, hyponatremia, hypomagnesemia) can occur. Use with caution in severe hepatic dysfunction; hepatic encephalopathy can be caused by electrolyte disturbances. Gout can be precipitate in certain patients with a history of gout, a familial predisposition to gout, or chronic renal failure. Use caution in patients with diabetes; may see a change in glucose control. Can cause SLE exacerbation or activation. Use with caution in patients with moderate or high cholesterol concentrations. Photosensitization may occur. Correct hypokalemia before initiating therapy. Thiazide diuretics may decrease renal calcium excretion; consider avoiding use in patients with hypercalcemia. Concomitant ethanol use may increase the risk of orthostatic hypotension. If given the morning of surgery, chlorothiazide may render the patient volume depleted and blood pressure may be labile during general anesthesia.

Benzyl alcohol and derivatives: Some dosage forms may contain sodium benzoate/benzoic acid; benzoic acid (benzoate) is a metabolite of benzyl alcohol; large amounts of benzyl alcohol (≥99 mg/kg/day) have been associated with a potentially fatal toxicity ("gasping syndrome") in neonates; the "gasping syndrome" consists of metabolic acidosis, respiratory distress, gasping respirations, CNS dysfunction (including convulsions, intracranial hemorrhage), hypotension, and cardiovascular collapse (AAP, 1997; CDC, 1982); some data suggests that benzoate displaces bilirubin from protein binding sites (Ahlfors, 2001); avoid or use dosage forms containing benzyl alcohol derivative with caution in neonates. See manufacturer's labeling.

Sulfonamide ("sulfa") allergy: The FDA-approved product labeling for many medications containing a sulfonamide chemical group includes a broad contraindication in patients with a prior allergic reaction to sulfonamides. There is a potential for cross-reactivity between members of a specific class (eg, two antibiotic sulfonamides). However, concerns for cross-reactivity have previously extended to all compounds containing the sulfonamide structure (SO_2NH_2). An expanded understanding of allergic mechanisms indicates cross-reactivity between antibiotic sulfonamides and nonantibiotic sulfonamides may not occur or at the very least this potential is extremely low (Brackett 2004; Johnson 2005; Slatore 2004; Tornero 2004). In particular, mechanisms of cross-reaction due to antibody production (anaphylaxis) are unlikely to occur with nonantibiotic sulfonamides. T-cell-mediated (type IV) reactions (eg, maculopapular rash) are less well understood and it is not possible to completely exclude this potential based on current insights. In cases where prior reactions were severe (Stevens-Johnson syndrome/TEN), some clinicians choose to avoid exposure to these classes.

Adverse Reactions

Cardiovascular: Hypotension, necrotizing angiitis, orthostatic hypotension

Central nervous system: Dizziness, headache, paresthesia, restlessness, vertigo

Dermatologic: Alopecia, erythema multiforme, exfoliative dermatitis, skin photosensitivity, skin rash, Stevens-Johnson syndrome, toxic epidermal necrolysis, urticaria

Endocrine & metabolic: Glycosuria, hypercalcemia, hyperglycemia, hyperuricemia, hypochloremic alkalosis, hypokalemia, hypomagnesemia, hyponatremia, increased serum cholesterol, increased serum triglycerides
Gastrointestinal: Abdominal cramps, anorexia, constipation, diarrhea, gastric irritation, nausea, pancreatitis, sialadenitis, vomiting
Genitourinary: Hematuria (IV), impotence
Hematologic & oncologic: Agranulocytosis, aplastic anemia, hemolytic anemia, leukopenia, purpura, thrombocytopenia
Hepatic: Jaundice
Hypersensitivity: Anaphylaxis
Neuromuscular & skeletal: Muscle spasm, systemic lupus erythematosus, weakness
Ophthalmic: Blurred vision, xanthopsia
Renal: Interstitial nephritis, renal failure, renal insufficiency
Respiratory: Pneumonitis, pulmonary edema, respiratory distress
Miscellaneous: Fever

Drug Interactions

Metabolism/Transport Effects None known.

Avoid Concomitant Use

Avoid concomitant use of Chlorothiazide with any of the following: Dofetilide; Mecamylamine

Increased Effect/Toxicity

Chlorothiazide may increase the levels/effects of: ACE Inhibitors; Allopurinol; Amifostine; Antihypertensives; Calcium Salts; CarBAMazepine; Cardiac Glycosides; Cyclophosphamide; Diazoxide; Dofetilide; DULoxetine; Hypotensive Agents; Ivabradine; Levodopa; Lithium; Mecamylamine; Multivitamins/Minerals (with ADEK, Folate, Iron); Multivitamins/Minerals (with AE, No Iron); Obinutuzumab; OXcarbazepine; Porfimer; RisperiDONE; RiTUXimab; Sodium Phosphates; Topiramate; Toremifene; Verteporfin; Vitamin D Analogs

The levels/effects of Chlorothiazide may be increased by: Alcohol (Ethyl); Alfuzosin; Analgesics (Opioid); Anticholinergic Agents; Barbiturates; Beta2-Agonists; Brimonidine (Topical); Corticosteroids (Orally Inhaled); Corticosteroids (Systemic); Dexketoprofen; Diazoxide; Herbs (Hypotensive Properties); Licorice; MAO Inhibitors; Multivitamins/Fluoride (with ADE); Nicorandil; Pentoxifylline; Phosphodiesterase 5 Inhibitors; Prostacyclin Analogues; Selective Serotonin Reuptake Inhibitors

Decreased Effect

Chlorothiazide may decrease the levels/effects of: Antidiabetic Agents

The levels/effects of Chlorothiazide may be decreased by: Bile Acid Sequestrants; Herbs (Hypertensive Properties); Methylphenidate; Nonsteroidal Anti-Inflammatory Agents; Yohimbine

Food Interactions Chlorothiazide serum levels may be increased if taken with food. Management: Administer without regard to food.

Storage/Stability

Powder for injection: Prior to reconstitution, store between 2°C to 25°C (36°F to 77°F). The manufacturer's labeling recommends any unused reconstituted solution be discarded. Precipitation will occur in <24 hours in pH <7.4.
Suspension, tablets: Store at room temperature 15°C to 30°C (59°F to 86°F). Protect from freezing.

Mechanism of Action Inhibits sodium and chloride reabsorption in the distal tubules causing increased excretion of sodium, chloride, and water resulting in diuresis. Loss of potassium, hydrogen ions, magnesium, phosphate, and bicarbonate also occurs.

Pharmacodynamics

Onset of action: Diuresis: Oral: Within 2 hours; IV: Within 15 minutes
Maximum effect: Diuresis: Oral: 4 hours; IV: 30 minutes
Duration: Diuresis: Oral: ~6-12 hours; IV: 2 hours

Pharmacokinetics (Adult data unless noted)

Absorption: Oral: Poor
Bioavailability: 9% to 56%; dose-dependent
Half-life: 45-120 minutes
Time to peak serum concentration: Oral: Within 4 hours; IV: 30 minutes
Elimination: Urine (Oral: 10% to 15% excreted unchanged; IV: 96% excreted unchanged)

Dosing: Neonatal

Edema, heart failure, bronchopulmonary dysplasia: Limited data available; **Note:** The manufacturer states that IV and oral dosing are equivalent; however, some clinicians use lower IV doses due to poor oral absorption.
Oral: 20-40 mg/kg/day in 2 divided doses
IV: 5-10 mg/kg/day in 2 divided doses (Costello, 2007); doses up to 20 mg/kg/day have been used

Hyperinsulinemia hypoglycemia, congenital hyperinsulinism (adjunct therapy): Limited data available: Oral: 7-10 mg/kg/day in 2 divided doses in combination with diazoxide (Aynsley-Green, 2000; Hussain, 2004; Kapoor, 2009)

Diabetes insipidus (central): Limited data available: Oral: 10 mg/kg/day in 2 divided doses; may need to titrate dose to target urine osmolality: 100-150 mOsm/L (Rivkees, 2008)

Dosing: Usual

Infants, Children, and Adolescents: **Note:** The manufacturer states that IV and oral dosing are equivalent; however, some clinicians use lower IV doses due to the poor oral absorption.

Edema (diuresis), heart failure, hypertension:
Manufacturer labeling:
Infants <6 months: Oral: 10-30 mg/kg/day in divided doses once or twice daily
Infants ≥6 months, Children, and Adolescents: Oral: 10-20 mg/kg/day in divided doses once or twice daily
Maximum daily doses:
Infants and Children <2 years: 375 mg/**day**
Children 2-12 years: 1000 mg/**day**
Adolescents: 2000 mg/**day**
Alternate dosing:
Oral: 10-40 mg/kg/day in 2 divided doses
Maximum daily doses:
Infants and Children <2 years: 375 mg/**day**
Children ≥2 years and Adolescents: 1000 mg/**day**
IV: Limited data available: 5-10 mg/kg/day in divided doses once or twice daily (Costello, 2007); in some cases, doses up to 20 mg/kg/day have been used; maximum dose: 500 mg

Diabetes insipidus (central): Infants [breast milk-fed or formula (Similac PM 60/40)-fed]: Limited data available: Oral: 10 mg/kg/day in 2 divided doses; may need to titrate dose to target urine osmolality: 100-150 mOsm/L (Rivkees, 2008)

Adults: **Note:** The manufacturer states that IV and oral dosing are equivalent; however, some clinicians use lower IV doses due to the poor oral absorption.

Hypertension: Oral: 500-2000 mg/day divided in 1-2 doses (manufacturer labeling); doses of 125-500 mg/day have also been recommended (JNC 7)

Edema: Oral, IV: 500-1000 mg once or twice daily; intermittent treatment (eg, therapy on alternative days) may be appropriate for some patients
ACC/AHA 2009 Heart Failure Guidelines:
Oral: 250-500 mg once or twice daily (maximum daily dose: 1000 mg)
IV: 500-1000 mg once or twice daily plus a loop diuretic

Dosage adjustment in renal impairment: Infants, Children, Adolescents, and Adults: CrCl <10 mL/minute: Avoid use. Ineffective with CrCl <30 mL/minute unless in combination with a loop diuretic (Aronoff, 2007).

Note: ACC/AHA 2005 Heart Failure guidelines suggest that thiazides lose their efficacy when CrCl <40 mL/minute.

Preparation for Administration Parenteral: Reconstitute with 18 mL SWFI to provide a concentration of 28 mg/mL. May be further diluted with dextrose or sodium chloride solutions.

Administration

Oral: Administer with food; administer early in day to avoid nocturia; if multiple daily dosing, the last dose should not be administered later than 6:00 pm unless instructed otherwise. Shake suspension well before use.

Parenteral: Administer by direct IV infusion over 3 to 5 minutes or further dilute and infuse over 30 minutes. Avoid extravasation of parenteral solution since it is extremely irritating to tissues. Do **not** administer via IM or SubQ route.

Monitoring Parameters Serum electrolytes, BUN, creatinine, blood pressure, fluid balance, body weight

Test Interactions May interfere with tests for parathyroid function

Dosage Forms Excipient information presented when available (limited, particularly for generics); consult specific product labeling.

Solution Reconstituted, Intravenous, as sodium [strength expressed as base]:

Sodium Diuril: 500 mg (1 ea)

Generic: 500 mg (1 ea)

Suspension, Oral:

Diuril: 250 mg/5 mL (237 mL) [contains alcohol, usp, benzoic acid, fd&c yellow #10 (quinoline yellow), methylparaben, propylparaben, saccharin sodium]

Tablet, Oral:

Generic: 250 mg, 500 mg

Extemporaneous Preparations A 50 mg/mL oral suspension may be made with tablets. Crush ten 500 mg chlorothiazide tablets in a mortar and reduce to a fine powder; mix with a small amount of glycerin to form a uniform paste. Add 2 g carboxymethylcellulose gel (mix 2 g carboxymethylcellulose with 5 to 10 mL water to form a paste; add 40 mL water and heat to 60°C with moderate stirring until dissolution occurs; cool and allow to stand for 1 to 2 hours to form a clear gel). Dissolve 500 mg citric acid in 5 mL water and add to chlorothiazide carboxymethylcellulose mixture with 0.1% parabens. Add a quantity of purified water sufficient to make 100 mL (Nahata, 2004). Label "shake well" and "refrigerate". Stable for 30 days.

Nahata MC, Pai VB, and Hipple TF, *Pediatric Drug Formulations*, 5th ed, Cincinnati, OH: Harvey Whitney Books Co, 2004.

◆ **Chlorphen [OTC]** *see* Chlorpheniramine *on page 441*

◆ **Chlorphenamine** *see* Chlorpheniramine *on page 441*

Chlorpheniramine (klor fen IR a meen)

Medication Safety Issues

Sound-alike/look-alike issues:

Chlor-Trimeton® may be confused with Chloromycetin®

BEERS Criteria medication:

This drug may be potentially inappropriate for use in geriatric patients (Quality of evidence - moderate; Strength of recommendation - strong).

Related Information

Oral Medications That Should Not Be Crushed or Altered *on page 2476*

Brand Names: US Aller-Chlor [OTC]; Allergy 4 Hour [OTC] [DSC]; Allergy Relief [OTC]; Allergy [OTC]; Allergy-Time [OTC]; Chlor-Trimeton Allergy [OTC]; Chlor-Trimeton [OTC]; Chlorphen [OTC]; Ed ChlorPed; Ed Chlorped Jr [OTC]; Ed ChlorPed [OTC]; Ed-Chlor-Tan; Ed-Chlortan [OTC]; Pharbechlor [OTC]

Brand Names: Canada Chlor-Tripolon®; Novo-Pheniram

Therapeutic Category Antihistamine

Generic Availability (US) May be product dependent

Use Perennial and seasonal allergic rhinitis and other allergic symptoms including urticaria (OTC products: Liquid: FDA approved in ages ≥2 years and adults); tablets [immediate release]: FDA approved in ages ≥6 years and adults; tablets [extended release: 12 hours]: FDA approved in ages ≥12 years and adults); **Note:** Approved uses for generic products may vary; consult labeling for specific information.

Pregnancy Considerations Maternal chlorpheniramine use has generally not resulted in an increased risk of birth defects (Aselton, 1985; Gilboa, 2009; Heinonen, 1977; Jick, 1981). Antihistamines are recommended for the treatment of rhinitis, urticaria, and pruritus with rash in pregnant women (although second generation antihistamines may be preferred) (Angier, 2010; Wallace, 2008; Zuberbier, 2009). Antihistamines are not recommended for treatment of pruritus associated with intrahepatic cholestasis in pregnancy (Ambros-Rudolph, 2011; Kremer, 2011).

Breast-Feeding Considerations Chlorpheniramine is excreted into breast milk. Antihistamines may decrease maternal serum prolactin concentrations when administered prior to the establishment of nursing (Messinis, 1985).

Contraindications Hypersensitivity to chlorpheniramine maleate or any component of the formulation; narrow-angle glaucoma; bladder neck obstruction; symptomatic prostate hypertrophy; during acute asthmatic attacks; stenosing peptic ulcer; pyloroduodenal obstruction. Avoid use in premature and term newborns due to possible association with SIDS.

OTC labeling: When used for self-medication, do not use to make a child sleep

Warnings/Precautions Causes sedation, caution must be used in performing tasks which require alertness (eg, operating machinery or driving). Sedative effects of CNS depressants or ethanol are potentiated. Use with caution in patients with urinary tract obstruction, symptomatic prostatic hyperplasia, thyroid dysfunction, increased intraocular pressure, and cardiovascular disease (including hypertension and ischemic heart disease). In the elderly, avoid use of this potent anticholinergic agent due to increased risk of confusion, dry mouth, constipation, and other anticholinergic effects; clearance decreases in patients of advanced age (Beers Criteria). Antihistamines may cause excitation in young children. Not for OTC use in children <2 years of age.

Benzyl alcohol and derivatives: Some dosage forms may contain sodium benzoate/benzoic acid; benzoic acid (benzoate) is a metabolite of benzyl alcohol; large amounts of benzyl alcohol (≥99 mg/kg/day) have been associated with a potentially fatal toxicity ("gasping syndrome") in neonates; the "gasping syndrome" consists of metabolic acidosis, respiratory distress, gasping respirations, CNS dysfunction (including convulsions, intracranial hemorrhage), hypotension, and cardiovascular collapse (AAP, 1997; CDC, 1982); some data suggests that benzoate displaces bilirubin from protein binding sites (Ahlfors, 2001); avoid or use dosage forms containing benzyl alcohol derivative with caution in neonates. See manufacturer's labeling.

Warnings: Additional Pediatric Considerations Safety and efficacy for the use of cough and cold products in pediatric patients <4 years of age is limited; the AAP warns against the use of these products for respiratory illnesses in this age group. Serious adverse effects including death have been reported. Many of these products contain multiple active ingredients, increasing the risk of accidental overdose when used with other products. The FDA notes that there are no approved OTC uses for these products in pediatric patients <2 years of age. Health care providers are reminded to ask caregivers about the use of OTC cough and cold products in order to avoid exposure to multiple medications containing the same ingredient (AAP 2012; FDA 2008).

Some dosage forms may contain propylene glycol; in neonates large amounts of propylene glycol delivered orally, intravenously (eg, >3,000 mg/day), or topically have been associated with potentially fatal toxicities which can include metabolic acidosis, seizures, renal failure, and CNS depression; toxicities have also been reported in children and adults including hyperosmolality, lactic acidosis, seizures and respiratory depression; use caution (AAP 1997; Shehab 2009).

Adverse Reactions

Central nervous system: Dizziness, excitability, fatigue, headache, nervousness, slight to moderate drowsiness

Gastrointestinal: Abdominal pain, diarrhea, increased appetite, nausea, weight gain, xerostomia

Genitourinary: Urinary retention

Neuromuscular & skeletal: Arthralgia, weakness

Ocular: Diplopia

Renal: Polyuria

Respiratory: Pharyngitis, thickening of bronchial secretions

Drug Interactions

Metabolism/Transport Effects **Substrate** of CYP2D6 (major), CYP3A4 (minor); **Note:** Assignment of Major/Minor substrate status based on clinically relevant drug interaction potential; **Inhibits** CYP2D6 (weak)

Avoid Concomitant Use

Avoid concomitant use of Chlorpheniramine with any of the following: Aclidinium; Azelastine (Nasal); Eluxadoline; Glucagon; Ipratropium (Oral Inhalation); Orphenadrine; Paraldehyde; Potassium Chloride; Thalidomide; Tiotropium; Umeclidinium

Increased Effect/Toxicity

Chlorpheniramine may increase the levels/effects of: AbobotulinumtoxinA; Alcohol (Ethyl); Analgesics (Opioid); Anticholinergic Agents; ARIPiprazole; Azelastine (Nasal); Buprenorphine; CNS Depressants; Eluxadoline; Fosphenytoin-Phenytoin; Glucagon; Hydrocodone; Methotrimeprazine; Metyrosine; Mirabegron; Mirtazapine; OnabotulinumtoxinA; Orphenadrine; Paraldehyde; Potassium Chloride; Pramipexole; RimabotulinumtoxinB; ROPINIRole; Rotigotine; Selective Serotonin Reuptake Inhibitors; Suvorexant; Thalidomide; Thiazide Diuretics; Thioridazine; Tiotropium; Topiramate; Zolpidem

The levels/effects of Chlorpheniramine may be increased by: Abiraterone Acetate; Aclidinium; Brimonidine (Topical); Cannabis; Cobicistat; CYP2D6 Inhibitors (Moderate); CYP2D6 Inhibitors (Strong); Darunavir; Doxylamine; Dronabinol; Droperidol; HydrOXYzine; Ipratropium (Oral Inhalation); Kava Kava; Magnesium Sulfate; Methotrimeprazine; Mianserin; Nabilone; Panobinostat; Peginterferon Alfa-2b; Perampanel; Pramlintide; Rufinamide; Sodium Oxybate; Tapentadol; Tetrahydrocannabinol; Thioridazine; Umeclidinium

Decreased Effect

Chlorpheniramine may decrease the levels/effects of: Acetylcholinesterase Inhibitors; Benzylpenicilloyl Polylysine; Betahistine; Hyaluronidase; Itopride; Metoclopramide; Secretin

The levels/effects of Chlorpheniramine may be decreased by: Acetylcholinesterase Inhibitors; Amphetamines; Peginterferon Alfa-2b

Storage/Stability Protect from light.

Mechanism of Action Competes with histamine for H_1-receptor sites on effector cells in the gastrointestinal tract, blood vessels, and respiratory tract

Pharmacokinetics (Adult data unless noted) Note: Data from chlorpheniramine maleate:

Distribution: V_d:

Children and Adolescents 6 to 16 years: 7 ± 2.8 L/kg (Simons, 1982)

Adults: 6 to 12 L/kg (Paton, 1985)

Protein binding: 33% (range: 29% to 37%) (Martínez-Gómez, 2007)

Metabolism: Substantial metabolism in GI mucosa and on first pass through liver

Half-life:

Children and Adolescents 6 to 16 years: 13.1 ± 6.6 hours (range: 6.3 to 23.1 hours) (Simons, 1982)

Adults: 14 to 24 hours (Patton, 1985)

Time to peak serum concentration: Children and Adolescents 6 to 16 years: Oral: 2.5 ± 1.5 hours (range: 1 to 6 hours) (Simons, 1982)

Elimination: Urine (Sharma, 2003)

Dosing: Usual

Pediatric: **Allergic symptoms, allergic rhinitis:** Oral: Chlorpheniramine maleate:

Immediate release (oral liquid, tablets):

Children 2 to <6 years: 1 mg every 4 to 6 hours; maximum daily dose: 6 mg/**day**

Children 6 to 11 years: 2 mg every 4 to 6 hours; maximum daily dose: 12 mg/**day**

Children ≥12 years and Adolescents: 4 mg every 4 to 6 hours; maximum daily dose: 24 mg/**day**

Extended Release: Children ≥12 years and Adolescents: 12 mg every 12 hours; maximum dose: 24 mg in 24 hours

Adult: **Allergic symptoms, allergic rhinitis:** Oral: Chlorpheniramine maleate:

Immediate release: 4 mg every 4 to 6 hours; do not exceed 24 mg/24 hours

Extended release: 12 mg every 12 hours; do not exceed 24 mg/24 hours

Dosing adjustment in renal impairment: There are no dosage adjustments provided in manufacturer's labeling.

Dosing adjustment in hepatic impairment: There are no dosage adjustments provided in manufacturer's labeling.

Administration Oral: May be administered with food or water. Timed release oral forms are to be swallowed whole, not crushed or chewed.

Test Interactions May suppress the wheal and flare reactions to skin test antigens.

Dosage Forms Excipient information presented when available (limited, particularly for generics); consult specific product labeling. [DSC] = Discontinued product

Liquid, Oral, as maleate:

Ed ChlorPed: 2 mg/mL (60 mL) [contains fd&c red #40, propylene glycol, saccharin sodium, sodium benzoate; cotton candy flavor]

Suspension, Oral, as tannate:

Ed ChlorPed: 2 mg/mL (60 mL) [contains aspartame, methylparaben, propylene glycol, propylparaben; cotton candy flavor]

Syrup, Oral, as maleate:

Aller-Chlor: 2 mg/5 mL (118 mL [DSC]) [contains alcohol, usp, fd&c yellow #6 (sunset yellow), menthol, methylparaben, propylene glycol, propylparaben; fruit flavor]

Chlor-Trimeton: 2 mg/5 mL (120 mL) [contains alcohol, usp]

Ed Chlorped Jr: 2 mg/5 mL (118 mL, 473 mL) [alcohol free, sugar free; contains fd&c red #40, methylparaben, propylene glycol, propylparaben; cherry flavor]

Tablet, Oral, as maleate:

Aller-Chlor: 4 mg [scored; contains fd&c yellow #10 aluminum lake]

Allergy: 4 mg [contains fd&c yellow #10 (quinoline yellow)]

Allergy: 4 mg [contains fd&c yellow #10 aluminum lake]

Allergy: 4 mg [scored; contains fd&c yellow #10 aluminum lake]
Allergy 4 Hour: 4 mg [DSC] [contains fd&c yellow #10 (quinoline yellow)]
Allergy Relief: 4 mg [contains fd&c yellow #10 aluminum lake]
Allergy-Time: 4 mg [contains fd&c yellow #10 aluminum lake]
Chlor-Trimeton: 4 mg [scored]
Chlorphen: 4 mg [scored; contains fd&c yellow #10 (quinoline yellow)]
Ed-Chlortan: 4 mg [scored; contains fd&c yellow #10 aluminum lake]
Pharbechlor: 4 mg
Generic: 4 mg

Tablet, Oral, as tannate:
Ed-Chlor-Tan: 8 mg [scored]

Tablet Extended Release, Oral, as maleate:
Chlor-Trimeton Allergy: 12 mg [contains fd&c blue #2 aluminum lake, fd&c yellow #10 aluminum lake, fd&c yellow #6 aluminum lake]
Chlor-Trimeton Allergy: 12 mg [contains fd&c yellow #6 (sunset yellow), fd&c yellow #6 aluminum lake]
Generic: 12 mg

◆ **Chlorpheniramine Maleate** *see* Chlorpheniramine *on page 441*

◆ **Chlorpheniramine Maleate and Hydrocodone Bitartrate** *see* Hydrocodone and Chlorpheniramine *on page 1034*

ChlorproMAZINE (klor PROE ma zeen)

Medication Safety Issues

Sound-alike/look-alike issues:

ChlorproMAZINE may be confused with chlordiazePOXIDE, chlorproPAMIDE, clomiPRAMINE, prochlorperazine, promethazine

Thorazine may be confused with thiamine, thioridazine

BEERS Criteria medication:

This drug may be potentially inappropriate for use in geriatric patients (Quality of evidence - moderate; Strength of recommendation - strong).

Related Information

Prochlorperazine *on page 1774*
Serotonin Syndrome *on page 2447*

Brand Names: Canada Chlorpromazine Hydrochloride Inj; Teva-Chlorpromazine

Therapeutic Category Antiemetic; Antipsychotic Agent, Typical, Phenothiazine; First Generation (Typical) Antipsychotic; Phenothiazine Derivative

Generic Availability (US) Yes

Use Treatment of nausea and vomiting (FDA approved in ages 6 months to 12 years and adults), restlessness and apprehension prior to surgery (FDA approved in ages 6 months to 12 years and adults), severe behavioral problems in children displayed by combativeness and/or explosive hyperexcitable behavior and in short-term treatment of hyperactive children (FDA approved in ages 1-12 years); adjunct in the treatment of tetanus (Parenteral only: FDA approved in ages 6 months to 12 years and adults); schizophrenia (FDA approved in adults), psychotic disorders (FDA approved in adults), mania (FDA approved in adults), acute intermittent porphyria (FDA approved in adults), intractable hiccups (FDA approved in adults); has also been used in management of Tourette's syndrome, neonatal abstinence syndrome, and cyclic vomiting syndrome (prevention); management of chemotherapy-induced nausea and vomiting (CINV); treatment of delirium

Pregnancy Considerations Embryotoxicity was observed in animal reproduction studies. Jaundice or hyper- or hyporeflexia have been reported in newborn infants following maternal use of phenothiazines. Antipsychotic use during the third trimester of pregnancy has a risk for abnormal muscle movements (extrapyramidal symptoms [EPS]) and withdrawal symptoms in newborns following delivery. Symptoms in the newborn may include agitation, feeding disorder, hypertonia, hypotonia, respiratory distress, somnolence, and tremor; these effects may be self-limiting or require hospitalization.

Breast-Feeding Considerations Chlorpromazine and its metabolites have been detected in breast milk; concentrations in the milk do not correlate with those in the mother and may be higher than what is in the maternal plasma.

Contraindications Hypersensitivity to phenothiazines (cross-reactivity between phenothiazines may occur); concomitant use with large amounts of CNS depressants (alcohol, barbiturates, narcotics, etc); comatose states

Warnings/Precautions [U.S. Boxed Warning]: Elderly patients with dementia-related psychosis treated with antipsychotics are at an increased risk of death compared to placebo. Most deaths appeared to be either cardiovascular (eg, heart failure, sudden death) or infectious (eg, pneumonia) in nature. Chlorpromazine is not approved for the treatment of dementia-related psychosis. Highly sedating, use with caution in disorders where CNS depression is a feature and in patients with Parkinson's disease. Use with caution in patients with hemodynamic instability, predisposition to seizures, subcortical brain damage, severe cardiac, hepatic, or renal disease. Use caution in respiratory disease (eg, severe asthma, emphysema) due to potential for CNS effects.

Leukopenia, neutropenia, and agranulocytosis (sometimes fatal) have been reported in clinical trials and postmarketing reports with antipsychotic use; presence of risk factors (eg, preexisting low WBC or history of drug-induced leuko/neutropenia) should prompt periodic blood count assessment. Discontinue therapy at first signs of blood dyscrasias or if absolute neutrophil count $<1000/mm^3$.

Esophageal dysmotility and aspiration have been associated with antipsychotic use; use with caution in patients at risk of aspiration pneumonia (ie, Alzheimer's disease). Use associated with increased prolactin levels; clinical significance of hyperprolactinemia in patients with breast cancer or other prolactin-dependent tumors is unknown. May alter temperature regulation or mask toxicity of other drugs due to antiemetic effects. May alter cardiac conduction; life-threatening arrhythmias have occurred with therapeutic doses of neuroleptics.

Use with caution in patients at risk of hypotension (orthostasis is common) or those who would tolerate transient hypotensive episodes (cerebrovascular disease, cardiovascular disease, or other medications which may predispose). Significant hypotension may occur, particularly with parenteral administration. Injection contains sulfites.

Use with caution in patients with decreased gastrointestinal motility, urinary retention, BPH, xerostomia, or visual problems (ie, narrow-angle glaucoma). Relative to other neuroleptics, chlorpromazine has a moderate potency of cholinergic blockade. May cause pigmentary retinopathy, and lenticular and corneal deposits, particularly with prolonged therapy.

May cause extrapyramidal symptoms, including pseudoparkinsonism, acute dystonic reactions, akathisia, and tardive dyskinesia. Risk of dystonia (and possibly other EPS) may be greater with increased doses, use of conventional antipsychotics, males, and younger patients. Risk of tardive dyskinesia and potential for irreversibility may be increased in elderly patients (particularly women), prolonged therapy, and higher total cumulative dose; antipsychotics may also mask signs/symptoms of tardive dyskinesia. Consider therapy discontinuation with signs/ symptoms of tardive dyskinesia. May cause neuroleptic malignant syndrome (NMS).

Use in elderly patients with dementia is associated with an increased risk of mortality and cerebrovascular accidents; avoid antipsychotic use for behavioral problems associated with dementia unless alternative nonpharmacologic therapies have failed and patient may harm self or others. In addition, may cause or exacerbate syndrome of inappropriate antidiuretic hormone secretion or hyponatremia; monitor sodium closely with initiation or dosage adjustments in older adults. May be inappropriate in older adults depending on comorbidities (eg, delirium) due to its potent anticholinergic effects (Beers Criteria). Increased risk for developing tardive dyskinesia, particularly in elderly women.

Benzyl alcohol and derivatives: Some dosage forms may contain sodium benzoate/benzoic acid; benzoic acid (benzoate) is a metabolite of benzyl alcohol; large amounts of benzyl alcohol (≥99 mg/kg/day) have been associated with a potentially fatal toxicity ("gasping syndrome") in neonates; the "gasping syndrome" consists of metabolic acidosis, respiratory distress, gasping respirations, CNS dysfunction (including convulsions, intracranial hemorrhage), hypotension, and cardiovascular collapse (AAP, 1997; CDC, 1982); some data suggests that benzoate displaces bilirubin from protein binding sites (Ahlfors, 2001); avoid or use dosage forms containing benzyl alcohol derivative with caution in neonates. See manufacturer's labeling. Potentially significant drug-drug interactions may exist, requiring dose or frequency adjustment, additional monitoring, and/or selection of alternative therapy.

Warnings: Additional Pediatric Considerations EPS occurring with chlorpromazine should be differentiated from possible CNS syndromes which may also cause vomiting (eg, Reye's syndrome, encephalopathy); avoid use in pediatric patients whose clinical presentation is suggestive of Reye's syndrome.

Adverse Reactions

Cardiovascular: ECG abnormality (nonspecific QT changes), orthostatic hypotension, tachycardia

Central nervous system: Akathisia, dizziness, drowsiness, dystonia, neuroleptic malignant syndrome, parkinsonian-like syndrome, seizure, tardive dyskinesia

Dermatologic: Dermatitis, skin photosensitivity, skin pigmentation (slate gray)

Endocrine & metabolic: Amenorrhea, gynecomastia, hyperglycemia, hypoglycemia

Gastrointestinal: Constipation, nausea, xerostomia

Genitourinary: Breast engorgement, ejaculatory disorder, false positive pregnancy test, impotence, lactation, urinary retention

Hematologic & oncologic: Agranulocytosis, aplastic anemia, eosinophilia, hemolytic anemia, immune thrombocytopenia, leukopenia

Hepatic: Jaundice

Ophthalmic: Blurred vision, corneal changes, epithelial keratopathy, retinitis pigmentosa

Drug Interactions

Metabolism/Transport Effects Substrate of CYP1A2 (minor), CYP2D6 (major), CYP3A4 (minor); **Note:** Assignment of Major/Minor substrate status based on clinically relevant drug interaction potential; **Inhibits** CYP2D6 (moderate), CYP2E1 (weak)

Avoid Concomitant Use

Avoid concomitant use of ChlorproMAZINE with any of the following: Aclidinium; Amisulpride; Azelastine (Nasal); Eluxadoline; Glucagon; Highest Risk QTc-Prolonging Agents; Ipratropium (Oral Inhalation); Ivabradine; Metoclopramide; Mifepristone; Orphenadrine; Paraldehyde; Potassium Chloride; Sulpiride; Thalidomide; Thioridazine; Tiotropium; Umeclidinium

Increased Effect/Toxicity

ChlorproMAZINE may increase the levels/effects of: AbobotulinumtoxinA; Alcohol (Ethyl); Amisulpride; Analgesics (Opioid); Anticholinergic Agents; Antidepressants (Serotonin Reuptake Inhibitor/Antagonist); ARIPiprazole; Azelastine (Nasal); Beta-Blockers; Buprenorphine; CNS Depressants; CYP2D6 Substrates; Desmopressin; DOXOrubicin (Conventional); Eluxadoline; Fesoterodine; Glucagon; Haloperidol; Highest Risk QTc-Prolonging Agents; Hydrocodone; Mequitazine; Methotrimeprazine; Methylphenidate; Metoprolol; Metyrosine; Mirabegron; Mirtazapine; Moderate Risk QTc-Prolonging Agents; Nebivolol; OnabotulinumtoxinA; Orphenadrine; Paraldehyde; Porfimer; Potassium Chloride; RimabotulinumtoxinB; Selective Serotonin Reuptake Inhibitors; Serotonin Modulators; Sulpiride; Suvorexant; Thalidomide; Thiazide Diuretics; Thiopental; Thioridazine; Tiotropium; Topiramate; Valproic Acid and Derivatives; Verteporfin; Zolpidem

The levels/effects of ChlorproMAZINE may be increased by: Abiraterone Acetate; Acetylcholinesterase Inhibitors (Central); Aclidinium; Antidepressants (Serotonin Reuptake Inhibitor/Antagonist); Antimalarial Agents; Beta-Blockers; Brimonidine (Topical); Cannabis; Cobicistat; CYP2D6 Inhibitors (Moderate); CYP2D6 Inhibitors (Strong); Darunavir; Doxylamine; Dronabinol; Droperidol; Haloperidol; HydrOXYzine; Ipratropium (Oral Inhalation); Ivabradine; Kava Kava; Lithium; Magnesium Sulfate; Methotrimeprazine; Methylphenidate; Metoclopramide; Metyrosine; Mianserin; Mifepristone; Nabilone; Panobinostat; Peginterferon Alfa-2b; Perampanel; Pramlintide; QTc-Prolonging Agents (Indeterminate Risk and Risk Modifying); Rufinamide; Serotonin Modulators; Sodium Oxybate; Tapentadol; Tetrahydrocannabinol; Umeclidinium

Decreased Effect

ChlorproMAZINE may decrease the levels/effects of: Acetylcholinesterase Inhibitors; Amphetamines; Anti-Parkinson's Agents (Dopamine Agonist); Codeine; Itopride; Quinagolide; Secretin; Tamoxifen; TraMADol

The levels/effects of ChlorproMAZINE may be decreased by: Acetylcholinesterase Inhibitors; Antacids; Anti-Parkinson's Agents (Dopamine Agonist); Lithium; Peginterferon Alfa-2b

Storage/Stability

Oral: Store at 20°C to 25°C (68°F to 77°F); protect from light and moisture.

Injection solution: Store at 20°C to 25°C (68°F to 77°F); excursions permitted to 15°C to 30°C (59°F to 86°F). Protect from light. A slightly yellowed solution does not indicate potency loss, but a markedly discolored solution should be discarded.

Mechanism of Action Chlorpromazine is an aliphatic phenothiazine antipsychotic which blocks postsynaptic mesolimbic dopaminergic receptors in the brain; exhibits a strong alpha-adrenergic blocking effect and depresses the release of hypothalamic and hypophyseal hormones; believed to depress the reticular activating system, thus affecting basal metabolism, body temperature, wakefulness, vasomotor tone, and emesis

Pharmacodynamics

Onset of action:

Oral: 30 to 60 minutes

Antipsychotic effects: Gradual, may take up to several weeks

Maximum antipsychotic effect: 6 weeks to 6 months

Duration: Oral: 4 to 6 hours

Pharmacokinetics (Adult data unless noted)

Absorption: Oral: Rapid and virtually complete; large first-pass effect due to metabolism during absorption in the GI mucosa

Distribution: Widely distributed into most body tissues and fluids; crosses blood-brain barrier; V_d: 8 to 160 L/kg

Protein binding: 90% to 99%

Metabolism: Extensively in the liver by demethylation (followed by glucuronide conjugation) and amine oxidation

Bioavailability: Oral: ~32%

Half-life, biphasic:

Initial:

Children: 1.1 hours

Adults: ~2 hours

Terminal:

Children: 7.7 hours

Adults: ~30 hours

Elimination: Urine (<1% as unchanged drug) within 24 hours

Dosing: Neonatal Neonatal abstinence syndrome (withdrawal from maternal opioid use; controls CNS and gastrointestinal symptoms): Limited data available: IM: Initial: 0.55 mg/kg/dose given every 6 hours; change to oral after ~4 days, decrease dose gradually over 2 to 3 weeks. **Note:** Chlorpromazine is rarely used for neonatal abstinence syndrome due to adverse effects such as hypothermia, cerebellar dysfunction, decreased seizure threshold, and eosinophilia; other agents are preferred (AAP Committee on Drugs 1998; Hudak 2012).

Dosing: Usual

Pediatric:

Behavior problems; severe: Note: Begin with low doses and gradually titrate as needed to lowest effective dose; route of administration should be determined by severity of symptoms.

Infants ≥6 months, Children, and Adolescents weighing ≤45.5 kg:

Oral: Initial: 0.55 mg/kg/dose every 4 to 6 hours as needed; may titrate as required; in severe cases, higher doses may be required (50 to 100 mg/**day**); in older children, higher daily doses (200 mg/**day** or higher) may be necessary; maximum daily dose: 500 mg/**day**; daily doses >500 mg have not been shown to further improve behavior in pediatric patients with severe mental impairment

IM, IV: Initial: 0.55 mg/kg/dose every 6 to 8 hours as needed; may titrate as required in severe cases (Kliegman 2007)

Maximum recommended daily doses:

Children <5 years or weighing <22.7 kg: 40 mg/**day**

Children ≥5 years and Adolescents or weighing 22.7 to 45.5 kg: 75 mg/**day**

Adolescents weighing >45.5 kg:

Oral: Range: 30 to 800 mg/**day** in 2 to 4 divided doses, initiate at lower doses and titrate as needed; usual dose is 200 mg/**day**

IM, IV: 25 mg initially, may repeat (25 to 50 mg) in 1 to 4 hours, gradually increase to a maximum of 400 mg/dose every 4 to 6 hours until patient controlled; usual dose 200 to 800 mg/**day** (Kliegman 2007)

Nausea and vomiting, treatment (non-CINV):

Infants ≥6 months, Children, and Adolescents weighing ≤45.5 kg: Oral, IM, IV: 0.55 mg/kg/dose every 6 to 8 hours as needed; in severe cases, higher doses may be needed

Usual maximum daily dose: IM, IV:

Children <5 years or weighing <22.7 kg: 40 mg/**day**

Children ≥5 years and Adolescents or weighing 22.7 to 45.5 kg: 75 mg/**day**

Adolescents weighing >45.5 kg:

Oral: 10 to 25 mg every 4 to 6 hours as needed

IM, IV: Initial: 25 mg; if tolerated (no hypotension), then may give 25 to 50 mg every 4 to 6 hours as needed

Chemotherapy-induced nausea and vomiting (CINV); prevention: Infants ≥6 months, Children, and Adolescents: IV: Initial: 0.5 mg/kg/dose every 6 hours; if not controlled, may increase up to 1 mg/kg/dose; monitor for sedation, maximum dose: 50 mg; recommended in situations where corticosteroids are contraindicated (Dupuis 2013)

Cyclic vomiting syndrome; abortive therapy: Infants ≥6 months, Children, and Adolescents: IV: 0.5 to 1 mg/kg/dose every 6 hours; maximum dose: 50 mg; in combination with diphenhydramine (for possible dystonic reactions) (Li 2008)

Delirium, ICU associated: Limited data available (Silver 2010): Infants ≥6 months, Children, and Adolescents:

Oral: 2.5 to 6 mg/kg/**day** divided every 4 to 6 hours

Maximum daily dose:

Children ≤5 years: 50 mg/**day**

Children >5 years and Adolescents: 200 mg/**day**

IM: 2.5 to 4 mg/kg/**day** divided every 6 to 8 hours; maximum daily dose: 40 mg/**day**

Preoperative sedation, anxiety: Infants ≥6 months, Children, and Adolescents:

Oral: 0.55 mg/kg/dose once 2 to 3 hours before surgery; maximum dose: 50 mg

IM: 0.55 mg/kg/dose once 1 to 2 hours before surgery; maximum dose: 25 mg

Tetanus:

Infants ≥6 months, Children, and Adolescents weighing ≤45.5 kg: IM, IV: 0.55 mg/kg/dose every 6 to 8 hours; in severe cases higher doses may be needed

Usual maximum daily dose:

Children <5 years or weighing <22.7 kg: 40 mg/**day**

Children ≥5 years and Adolescents or weighing 22.7 to 45.5 kg: 75 mg/**day**

Adolescents weighing ≥45.5 kg: IM, IV: 25 to 50 mg every 6 to 8 hours; begin with low dose and increase gradually based upon patient response

Adult:

Intractable hiccups:

Oral, IM: 25 to 50 mg 3 to 4 times daily

IV (refractory to oral or IM treatment): 25 to 50 mg via slow IV infusion

Nausea and vomiting:

Oral: 10 to 25 mg every 4 to 6 hours

IM, IV: 25 to 50 mg every 4 to 6 hours

Schizophrenia/psychoses:

Oral: Range: 30 to 800 mg/day in 1 to 4 divided doses, initiate at lower doses and titrate as needed; usual dose is 200 mg/day; some patients may require 1 to 2 g/**day**

IM, IV: 25 mg initially, may repeat (25 to 50 mg) in 1 to 4 hours, gradually increase to a maximum of 400 mg/dose every 4 to 6 hours until patient controlled; usual dose 300 to 800 mg/**day**

Preparation for Administration Parenteral:

Direct IV injection: Dilute with NS to a maximum concentration of 1 mg/mL.

IV: For treatment of intractable hiccups the manufacturer recommends diluting 25 to 50 mg of chlorpromazine in 500 to 1,000 mL NS.

Administration

Oral: Administer with water, food, or milk to decrease GI upset; brown precipitate may occur when chlorpromazine is mixed with caffeine-containing liquids

Parenteral: Do not administer SubQ (tissue damage and irritation may occur); for direct IV injection, administer diluted solution slow IV at a rate not to exceed 0.5 mg/minute in children and 1 mg/minute in adults. For the treatment of intractable hiccups, infuse as a slow IV infusion. To reduce the risk of hypotension, patients receiving IV chlorpromazine must remain lying down during and for 30 minutes after the injection. **Note:** Avoid skin contact with solution; may cause contact dermatitis.

Monitoring Parameters Vital signs (especially with parenteral use); lipid profile, fasting blood glucose/HgbA_{1c}; BMI; mental status; abnormal involuntary movement scale (AIMS); extrapyramidal symptoms (EPS); CBC in patients with risk factors for leukopenia/neutropenia; periodic eye exam with prolonged therapy

Reference Range Relationship of plasma concentration to clinical response is not well established

Therapeutic: 50 to 300 ng/mL (SI: 157 to 942 nmol/L)

Toxic: >750 ng/mL (SI: >2355 nmol/L)

Test Interactions False-positives for phenylketonuria, amylase, uroporphyrins, urobilinogen. May cause false-positive pregnancy test. May interfere with urine detection of amphetamine/methamphetamine and methadone (false-positives).

Additional Information Although chlorpromazine has been used in combination with meperidine and promethazine as a premedication ("lytic cocktail"), this combination may have a higher rate of adverse effects compared to alternative sedatives/analgesics (AAP, 1995). Use decreased doses in elderly or debilitated patients; dystonic reactions may be more common in patients with hypocalcemia; extrapyramidal reactions may be more common in pediatric patients, especially those with dehydration or acute illnesses (viral or CNS infections).

Dosage Forms Excipient information presented when available (limited, particularly for generics); consult specific product labeling.

Solution, Injection, as hydrochloride:

Generic: 25 mg/mL (1 mL, 2 mL)

Tablet, Oral, as hydrochloride:

Generic: 10 mg, 25 mg, 50 mg, 100 mg, 200 mg

◆ **Chlorpromazine Hydrochloride** *see* ChlorproMAZINE *on page 443*

◆ **Chlorpromazine Hydrochloride Inj (Can)** *see* ChlorproMAZINE *on page 443*

Chlorthalidone (klor THAL i done)

Brand Names: Canada Apo-Chlorthalidone

Therapeutic Category Diuretic, Thiazide

Generic Availability (US) Yes

Use Treatment of edema due to heart failure; hepatic cirrhosis; estrogen or corticosteroid therapy; various forms of renal dysfunction, including nephrotic syndrome, acute glomerulonephritis, and chronic renal failure (FDA approved in adults); management of hypertension either alone or in combination with other antihypertensive agents (FDA approved in adults); **Note:** Use in pregnancy should be reserved for those cases causing extreme discomfort and unrelieved by rest; should not be routinely used during pregnancy.

Pregnancy Risk Factor B

Pregnancy Considerations Adverse events were not observed in animal reproduction studies. Chlorthalidone crosses the placenta and can be detected in cord blood. Maternal use may cause fetal or neonatal jaundice, thrombocytopenia, or other adverse events observed in adults. Use of thiazide diuretics to treat edema during normal pregnancies is not appropriate; use may be considered when edema is due to pathologic causes (as in the nonpregnant patient); monitor. Untreated chronic maternal hypertension is associated with adverse events in the fetus, infant, and mother. Women who require thiazide diuretics for the treatment of hypertension prior to pregnancy may continue their use (ACOG, 2013).

Breast-Feeding Considerations Thiazides are excreted into breast milk. Due to the potential for serious adverse reactions in the nursing infant, the manufacturer recommends a decision be made whether to discontinue nursing or to discontinue the drug, taking into account the importance of treatment to the mother. Diuretics have the potential to decrease milk volume and suppress lactation.

Contraindications

Hypersensitivity to chlorthalidone, other sulfonamide-derived drugs, or any component of the formulation; anuria

Note: Although the FDA approved product labeling states this medication is contraindicated with other sulfonamide-containing drug classes, the scientific basis of this statement has been challenged. See "Warnings/Precautions" for more detail.

Warnings/Precautions Use with caution in severe renal disease. Electrolyte disturbances (hypokalemia, hypochloremic alkalosis, hyponatremia) can occur. Use with caution in severe hepatic dysfunction; hepatic encephalopathy can be caused by electrolyte disturbances. Gout can be precipitate in certain patients with a history of gout, a familial predisposition to gout, or chronic renal failure. Use caution in patients with a history of bronchial asthma; hypersensitivity reactions may occur more readily. Cautious use in prediabetics or diabetics; may see a change in glucose control. Can cause SLE exacerbation or activation. Use with caution in patients with moderate or high cholesterol concentrations. Photosensitization may occur. Correct hypokalemia before initiating therapy. Thiazide diuretics may decrease renal calcium excretion; consider avoiding use in patients with hypercalcemia.

Sulfonamide ("sulfa") allergy: The FDA-approved product labeling for many medications containing a sulfonamide chemical group includes a broad contraindication in patients with a prior allergic reaction to sulfonamides. There is a potential for cross-reactivity between members of a specific class (eg, two antibiotic sulfonamides). However, concerns for cross-reactivity have previously extended to all compounds containing the sulfonamide structure (SO_2NH_2). An expanded understanding of allergic mechanisms indicates cross-reactivity between antibiotic sulfonamides and nonantibiotic sulfonamides may not occur or at the very least this potential is extremely low (Brackett 2004; Johnson 2005; Slatore 2004; Tornero 2004). In particular, mechanisms of cross-reaction due to antibody production (anaphylaxis) are unlikely to occur with nonantibiotic sulfonamides. T-cell-mediated (type IV) reactions (eg, maculopapular rash) are less well understood and it is not possible to completely exclude this potential based on current insights. In cases where prior reactions were severe (Stevens-Johnson syndrome/TEN), some clinicians choose to avoid exposure to these classes.

Adverse Reactions

Dermatologic: Skin photosensitivity

Endocrine & metabolic: Hypokalemia

Gastrointestinal: Anorexia, dyspepsia

Rare but important or life-threatening: Agranulocytosis, aplastic anemia, cholecystitis, diabetes mellitus, gout, hypercalcemia, hyperglycemia, hypersensitivity reaction, hypochloremic alkalosis, hyponatremia, leukopenia, necrotizing angiitis, orthostatic hypotension, pancreatitis, renal insufficiency, thrombocytopenia, toxic epidermal necrolysis, vasculitis, xanthopsia

Drug Interactions

Metabolism/Transport Effects None known.

Avoid Concomitant Use

Avoid concomitant use of Chlorthalidone with any of the following: Dofetilide; Mecamylamine

Increased Effect/Toxicity

Chlorthalidone may increase the levels/effects of: ACE Inhibitors; Allopurinol; Amifostine; Antihypertensives; Calcium Salts; CarBAMazepine; Cardiac Glycosides;

Cyclophosphamide; Diazoxide; Dofetilide; DULoxetine; Hypotensive Agents; Ivabradine; Levodopa; Lithium; Mecamylamine; Multivitamins/Minerals (with ADEK, Folate, Iron); Multivitamins/Minerals (with AE, No Iron); Obinutuzumab; OXcarbazepine; Porfimer; RisperiDONE; RiTUXimab; Sodium Phosphates; Topiramate; Toremifene; Verteporfin; Vitamin D Analogs

The levels/effects of Chlorthalidone may be increased by: Alcohol (Ethyl); Alfuzosin; Analgesics (Opioid); Anticholinergic Agents; Barbiturates; Beta2-Agonists; Brimonidine (Topical); Corticosteroids (Orally Inhaled); Corticosteroids (Systemic); Dexketoprofen; Diazoxide; Herbs (Hypotensive Properties); Licorice; MAO Inhibitors; Multivitamins/Fluoride (with ADE); Nicorandil; Pentoxifylline; Phosphodiesterase 5 Inhibitors; Prostacyclin Analogues; Selective Serotonin Reuptake Inhibitors

Decreased Effect

Chlorthalidone may decrease the levels/effects of: Antidiabetic Agents

The levels/effects of Chlorthalidone may be decreased by: Bile Acid Sequestrants; Herbs (Hypertensive Properties); Methylphenidate; Nonsteroidal Anti-Inflammatory Agents; Yohimbine

Storage/Stability Store at 20°C to 25°C (68°F to 77°F). Protect from light.

Mechanism of Action Sulfonamide-derived diuretic that inhibits sodium and chloride reabsorption in the cortical-diluting segment of the ascending loop of Henle

Pharmacodynamics

Onset of action: Diuresis: ~2 hours

Duration: Diuresis: 24-72 hours

Pharmacokinetics (Adult data unless noted)

Distribution: 0.14 L/kg; sequesters in erythrocytes

Protein binding: ~75%

Bioavailability: Chlorthalidone: ~65%; Thalitone®: 104% to 116% relative to an oral solution

Metabolism: Hepatic

Half-life: 40-60 hours; may be prolonged with renal impairment; Anuria: 81 hours

Time to peak serum concentration: 13.8 hours

Elimination: Urine (~50% to 65% as unchanged drug)

Dosing: Usual

Children and Adolescents: **Hypertension:** Oral: Initial: 0.3 mg/kg once daily; may titrate up to a maximum daily dose: 2 mg/kg/**day** or 50 mg/**day** (NHBPEP, 2004; NHLBI, 2011)

Adults:

Hypertension: Oral: 25-100 mg/day or 100 mg 3 times/week; usual dosage range (JNC 7): 12.5-25 mg/day

Edema: Initial: 50-100 mg/day or 100 mg on alternate days; maximum dose: 200 mg/day

Heart failure-associated edema: 12.5-25 mg once daily; maximum daily dose: 100 mg (ACC/AHA 2009 Heart Failure Guidelines)

Dosing adjustments in renal impairment: Adults: CrCl <10 mL/minute: Avoid use. Ineffective with low GFR (Aronoff, 2007)

Note: ACC/AHA 2009 Heart Failure Guidelines suggest that thiazides lose their efficacy when CrCl <40 mL/minute.

Administration Oral: Administer in the morning with food

Monitoring Parameters Serum electrolytes, BUN, creatinine, blood pressure, fluid balance, body weight

Dosage Forms Excipient information presented when available (limited, particularly for generics); consult specific product labeling.

Tablet, Oral:

Generic: 25 mg, 50 mg, 100 mg

◆ **Chlor-Trimeton [OTC]** *see* Chlorpheniramine *on page 441*

◆ **Chlor-Trimeton Allergy [OTC]** *see* Chlorpheniramine *on page 441*

◆ **Chlor-Tripolon® (Can)** *see* Chlorpheniramine *on page 441*

◆ **Chlor-Tripolon ND® (Can)** *see* Loratadine and Pseudoephedrine *on page 1298*

Chlorzoxazone (klor ZOKS a zone)

Medication Safety Issues

BEERS Criteria medication:

This drug may be potentially inappropriate for use in geriatric patients (Quality of evidence - moderate; Strength of recommendation - strong).

Brand Names: US Lorzone; Parafon Forte DSC

Therapeutic Category Skeletal Muscle Relaxant, Non-paralytic

Generic Availability (US) Yes

Use Symptomatic treatment of muscle spasm and pain associated with acute musculoskeletal conditions

Pregnancy Considerations Animal reproduction studies have not been conducted.

Contraindications Hypersensitivity to chlorzoxazone or any component of the formulation

Warnings/Precautions Rare, serious (including fatal) idiosyncratic and unpredictable hepatocellular toxicity has been reported with use. Discontinue immediately if early signs/symptoms of hepatic toxicity arise (eg, fever, rash, anorexia, nausea, vomiting, fatigue, right upper quadrant pain, dark urine or jaundice). Also discontinue if elevated liver enzymes develop. May cause drowsiness, dizziness, or lightheadedness; effects may be potentiated by ethanol or other CNS depressants. Caution patients about performing tasks which require mental alertness (eg, operating machinery or driving). This class of medication is poorly tolerated by the elderly due to anticholinergic effects, sedation, and weakness. Efficacy is questionable at dosages tolerated by elderly patients (Beers Criteria).

Adverse Reactions

Central nervous system: Dizziness, drowsiness, lightheadedness, paradoxical stimulation, malaise

Dermatologic: Rash (rare), petechiae (rare), ecchymoses (rare), angioedema (very rare)

Gastrointestinal: Diarrhea, GI bleeding (rare), nausea, vomiting

Genitourinary: Urine discoloration

Hepatic: Liver dysfunction

Miscellaneous: Anaphylaxis (very rare)

Drug Interactions

Metabolism/Transport Effects Substrate of CYP1A2 (minor), CYP2A6 (minor), CYP2D6 (minor), CYP2E1 (minor), CYP3A4 (minor); **Note:** Assignment of Major/Minor substrate status based on clinically relevant drug interaction potential; **Inhibits** CYP2E1 (weak)

Avoid Concomitant Use

Avoid concomitant use of Chlorzoxazone with any of the following: Azelastine (Nasal); Orphenadrine; Paraldehyde; Thalidomide

Increased Effect/Toxicity

Chlorzoxazone may increase the levels/effects of: Alcohol (Ethyl); Azelastine (Nasal); Buprenorphine; CNS Depressants; Hydrocodone; Methotrimeprazine; Metyrosine; Mirtazapine; Orphenadrine; Paraldehyde; Pramipexole; ROPINIRole; Rotigotine; Selective Serotonin Reuptake Inhibitors; Suvorexant; Thalidomide; Zolpidem

The levels/effects of Chlorzoxazone may be increased by: Brimonidine (Topical); Cannabis; Disulfiram; Doxylamine; Dronabinol; Droperidol; HydrOXYzine; Isoniazid; Kava Kava; Magnesium Sulfate; Methotrimeprazine; Nabilone; Perampanel; Rufinamide; Sodium Oxybate; Tapentadol; Tetrahydrocannabinol

Decreased Effect There are no known significant interactions involving a decrease in effect.

Mechanism of Action Acts on the spinal cord and subcortical areas of the brain to inhibit polysynaptic reflex arcs involved in causing and maintaining skeletal muscle spasms

Pharmacodynamics

Onset of action: Within 60 minutes

Duration: 3-4 hours

Pharmacokinetics (Adult data unless noted)

Absorption: Oral: Readily

Metabolism: Extensive in the liver by glucuronidation

Half-life: ~60 minutes

Time to peak serum concentration: Adults: 1-2 hours

Elimination: In urine as conjugates; <1% excreted unchanged in urine

Dosing: Usual Oral:

Children: 20 mg/kg/day or 600 mg/m^2/day in 3-4 divided doses

Adults: 250-750 mg 3-4 times/day

Administration Oral: Administer with food

Monitoring Parameters Periodic liver function tests

Dosage Forms Excipient information presented when available (limited, particularly for generics); consult specific product labeling.

Tablet, Oral:

Lorzone: 375 mg [contains sodium benzoate]

Lorzone: 750 mg [scored; contains sodium benzoate]

Parafon Forte DSC: 500 mg [scored; contains brilliant blue fcf (fd&c blue #1), fd&c yellow #10 (quinoline yellow), sodium benzoate]

Generic: 500 mg

Cholecalciferol (kole e kal SI fer ole)

Medication Safety Issues

Sound-alike/look-alike issues:

Cholecalciferol may be confused with alfacalcidol, ergocalciferol

Administration issues:

Liquid vitamin D preparations have the potential for dosing errors when administered to infants. Droppers should be clearly marked to easily provide 400 international units. For products intended for infants, the FDA recommends that accompanying droppers deliver no more than 400 international units per dose.

Brand Names: US Aqueous Vitamin D [OTC]; Bio-D-Mulsion Forte [OTC]; Bio-D-Mulsion [OTC]; BProtected Pedia D-Vite [OTC]; D-3-5 [OTC]; D-Vi-Sol [OTC]; D-Vita [OTC]; D3-50 [OTC]; Decara; Delta D3 [OTC]; Dialyvite Vitamin D 5000 [OTC]; Dialyvite Vitamin D3 Max [OTC]; Pronutrients Vitamin D3 [OTC]; Vitamin D3 Super Strength [OTC]

Brand Names: Canada D-Vi-Sol®

Therapeutic Category Nutritional Supplement; Vitamin D Analog; Vitamin, Fat Soluble

Generic Availability (US) Yes

Use Prevention and treatment of vitamin D deficiency and/or rickets; dietary supplement (FDA approved in all ages)

Pregnancy Considerations Adverse events were observed in animals when high maternal doses of vitamin D were administered during pregnancy. Vitamin D crosses the placenta but the transfer to the fetus from the mother is low. Maternal supplementation has not been shown to affect pregnancy outcomes. Vitamin D requirements are the same in pregnant and nonpregnant females (IOM, 2011).

Breast-Feeding Considerations Small quantities of vitamin D are found in breast milk following normal maternal exposure via sunlight and diet. The amount in breast milk does not correlate with serum levels in the infant. Therefore, vitamin D supplementation is recommended in all infants who are partially or exclusively breast fed. Hypercalcemia has been noted in a breast-feeding infant following maternal use of large doses of ergocalciferol; high doses should be avoided in lactating women (IOM, 2011).

Contraindications Hypercalcemia; hypersensitivity to cholecalciferol or any component of the formulation; malabsorption syndrome; evidence of vitamin D toxicity

Warnings: Additional Pediatric Considerations Some dosage forms may contain propylene glycol; in neonates large amounts of propylene glycol delivered orally, intravenously (eg, >3,000 mg/day), or topically have been associated with potentially fatal toxicities which can include metabolic acidosis, seizures, renal failure, and CNS depression; toxicities have also been reported in children and adults including hyperosmolality, lactic acidosis, seizures and respiratory depression; use caution (AAP, 1997; Shehab, 2009).

Adverse Reactions Endocrine & metabolic: Hypervitaminosis D (signs and symptoms include hypercalcemia, resulting in headache, nausea, vomiting, lethargy, confusion, sluggishness, abdominal pain, bone pain, polyuria, polydipsia, weakness, cardiac arrhythmias [eg, QT shortening, sinus tachycardia], soft tissue calcification, calciuria, and nephrocalcinosis)

Drug Interactions

Metabolism/Transport Effects Inhibits CYP2C19 (weak), CYP2C9 (weak), CYP2D6 (weak)

Avoid Concomitant Use

Avoid concomitant use of Cholecalciferol with any of the following: Aluminum Hydroxide; Multivitamins/Fluoride (with ADE); Multivitamins/Minerals (with ADEK, Folate, Iron); Sucralfate; Vitamin D Analogs

Increased Effect/Toxicity

Cholecalciferol may increase the levels/effects of: Aluminum Hydroxide; ARIPiprazole; Cardiac Glycosides; Sucralfate; Vitamin D Analogs

The levels/effects of Cholecalciferol may be increased by: Calcium Salts; Danazol; Multivitamins/Fluoride (with ADE); Multivitamins/Minerals (with ADEK, Folate, Iron); Thiazide Diuretics

Decreased Effect

The levels/effects of Cholecalciferol may be decreased by: Bile Acid Sequestrants; Mineral Oil; Orlistat

Storage/Stability

Store at room temperature; protect from light.

Pharmacokinetics (Adult data unless noted)

Protein binding: Extensively to vitamin D-binding protein

Metabolism: Hydroxylated in liver to calcifidiol (25-OH-D3) then in kidney to the active form, calcitriol (1α,2-[OH]2 vitamin D_3)

Half-life: 19 to 25 hours

Elimination: As metabolites, urine and feces

Dosing: Neonatal

Adequate intake (AI): Oral: 400 units/day (IOM 2011)

Prevention of Vitamin D deficiency (Greer 2000; Wagner 2008): Oral:

Premature neonates: 400 to 800 units/day or 150 to 400 units/**kg**/day

Breast-fed neonates (fully or partially): 400 units/day beginning in the first few days of life. Continue supplementation until infant is weaned to ≥1,000 mL/day or 1 qt/day of vitamin D-fortified formula or whole milk (after 12 months of age)

Formula-fed neonates ingesting <1,000 mL of vitamin D-fortified formula: 400 units/day

Treatment of Vitamin D deficiency: Oral: **Note:** In addition to calcium and phosphorus supplementation: 2,000 units daily or 50,000 units once weekly for 6 weeks to achieve a serum 25(OH)D level >20 ng/mL; followed by a maintenance dose of 400 to 1,000 units daily (Holick 2011; Golden 2014). **Note:** For patients at high risk of fractures a serum 25(OH)D level >30 ng/mL has been suggested (Golden 2014); some organizations suggest a serum 25(OH)D level >30 ng/mL should be used for all patients (Holick 2011).

Dosing: Usual

Pediatric:

Adequate intake (AI): Oral: Infants: 400 units/day (IOM 2011)

Recommended Daily Allowance (RDA): Oral: Children and Adolescents: 600 units/day (IOM 2011)

Prevention of Vitamin D deficiency: (Greer 2000; Wagner 2008): Oral:

Breast-fed infants (fully or partially): 400 units/day beginning in the first few days of life. Continue supplementation until infant is weaned to ≥1,000 mL/day or 1 qt/day of vitamin D-fortified formula or whole milk (after 12 months of age)

Formula-fed infants ingesting <1000 mL of vitamin D-fortified formula: 400 units/day

Children ingesting <1,000 mL of vitamin D-fortified milk: 400 units/day

Children with increased risk of vitamin D deficiency (chronic fat malabsorption, maintained on chronic antiseizure medications): Higher doses may be required; use laboratory testing [25(OH)D, PTH, bone mineral status] to evaluate

Adolescents without adequate intake: 400 units/day

Treatment Vitamin D deficiency: Oral: **Note:** In addition to calcium and phosphorus supplementation (Holick 2011; Golden 2014):

Infants: 2,000 units daily or 50,000 units once weekly for 6 weeks to achieve a serum 25(OH)D level >20 ng/mL; followed by a maintenance dose of 400 to 1,000 units daily. **Note:** For patients at high risk of fractures a serum 25(OH)D level >30 ng/mL has been suggested (Golden 2014); some organizations suggest a serum 25(OH)D level >30 ng/mL should be used for all patients (Holick 2011).

Children and Adolescents: 2,000 units daily or 50,000 units once weekly for 6 to 8 weeks to achieve serum 25(OH)D level > 20 ng/mL; followed by a maintenance dose of 600 to 1,000 units daily. **Note:** For patients at high risk of fractures a serum 25(OH)D level >30 ng/mL has been suggested (Golden 2014); some organizations suggest a serum 25(OH)D level >30 ng/mL should be used for all patients (Holick 2011).

Children with increased risk of vitamin D deficiency (chronic fat malabsorption, maintained on chronic antiseizure medications, glucocorticoids, HIV medications and antifungals such as ketoconazole, obesity): Higher doses (2 to 3 times higher) may be required; doses of at least 6,000 to 10,000 units daily have been suggested (Holick 2011).

Note: If poor compliance, single high-dose administration (100,000 to 600,000 units over 1 to 5 days) followed by maintenance dosing; intermittently repeating (usually every 3 months) may be needed if poor compliance continues with maintenance dosing (Misra 2008)

Treatment of Vitamin D insufficiency or deficiency associated with CKD (stages 2-5, 5D); serum 25 hydroxyvitamin D [25(OH)D] level ≤30 ng/mL (KDOQI Guidelines 2009): Oral:

Serum 25(OH)D level 16 to 30 ng/mL: Infants, Children, and Adolescents: 2,000 units/day for 3 months or 50,000 units every month for 3 months

Serum 25(OH)D level 5 to 15 ng/mL: Infants, Children, and Adolescents: 4,000 units/day for 12 weeks or 50,000 units every other week for 12 weeks

Serum 25(OH)D level <5 ng/mL: Infants, Children, and Adolescents: 8,000 units/day for 4 weeks then 4,000 units/day for 2 months for total therapy of 3 months or 50,000 units/week for 4 weeks followed by 50,000 units 2 times/month for a total therapy of 3 months

Maintenance dose [once repletion accomplished; serum 25(OH)D level >30 ng/mL]: Infants, Children, and Adolescents: 200 to 1,000 units/day

Prevention and treatment of Vitamin D Deficiency in cystic fibrosis: Oral:

CF guidelines (Tangricha [CF Foundation] 2012):

Recommended inital daily intake to maintain serum 25 (OH)D level ≥30 ng/mL:

Infants: 400 to 500 units/day

Children ≤10 years: 800 to 1,000 units/day

Children >10 years and Adolescents: 800 to 2,000 units/day

Dosing adjustment for serum 25(OH)D level between 20 to 30 ng/mL and patient adherence established (Step 1 increase):

Infants: 800 to 1,000 units/day

Children ≤10 years: 1,600 to 3,000 units/day

Children >10 years and Adolescents: 1,600 to 6,000 units/day

Dosing adjustment for serum 25(OH)D level <20 ng/mL or persistently between 20 to 30 ng/mL and patient adherence established (Step 2 increase):

Infants: Increase up to a maximum 2,000 units/day

Children ≤10 years: Increase to a maximum of 4,000 units/day

Children >10 years and Adolescents: Increase to a maximum of 10,000 units/day

Alternate dosing (Hall 2010):

Initial dose: Serum 25(OH)D level ≤30 ng/mL

Infants: 8,000 units/**week**

Children and Adolescents: 800 units/day

Medium-dose regimen: Serum 25(OH)D level remains ≤30 ng/mL and patient compliance established

Infants and Children <5 years: 12,000 units/week for 12 weeks

Children ≥5 years and Adolescents: 50,000 units/week for 12 weeks

High-dose regimen: Repeat 25(OH)D level remains ≤30 ng/mL and patient compliance established

Infants and Children <5 years: 12,000 units twice weekly for 12 weeks

Children ≥5 years and Adolescents: 50,000 units twice weekly for 12 weeks

Adult:

Recommended Daily Allowance (RDA) (IOM 2011): Oral:

Adults 19 to 70 years: 600 units/day

Female: Pregnancy/lactating: 600 units/day

Osteoporosis prevention and treatment: Oral: 800 to 1,000 units/day (NOF guidelines 2014)

Vitamin D deficiency treatment: Oral: 6,000 units daily or 50,000 units once weekly for 8 weeks to achieve serum 25(OH)D level >30 ng/mL,followed by a maintenance dose of 1,500 to 2,000 units daily (Holick 2011)

Administration May be administered without regard to meals; for oral liquid, use accompanying dropper for dosage measurements

Monitoring Parameters Children at increased risk of vitamin D deficiency (chronic fat malabsorption, chronic antiseizure medication use) require serum 25(OH)D, PTH, and bone-mineral status to evaluate. If vitamin D supplement is required, then 25(OH)D levels should be repeated at 3-month intervals until normal. PTH and bone mineral-status should be monitored every 6 months until normal.

Chronic kidney disease: Monitor serum 25(OH)D, corrected total calcium and phosphorus levels 1 month following initiation of therapy, every 3 months during therapy and with any Vitamin D dose change; alkaline phosphatase, BUN

Reference Range Vitamin D status may be determined by serum 25(OH) D levels (Misra, 2008):

Severe deficiency: ≤5 ng/mL (12.5 nmol/L)

Deficiency: 15 ng/mL (37.5 nmol/L)
Insufficiency: 15-20 ng/mL (37.5-50 nmol/L)
Sufficiency: 20-100 ng/mL (50-250 nmol/L)*
Excess: >100 ng/mL (250 nmol/L)**
Intoxication: 150 ng/mL (375 nmol/L)
*Based on adult data a level of >32 ng/mL (80 nmol/L) is desirable
**Arbitrary designation
Target serum 25(OH) D: >30 ng/mL

Additional Information 1 mcg cholecalciferol provides 40 units of vitamin D activity

Biological potency may be greater with cholecalciferol (vitamin D_3) compared to ergocalciferol (vitamin D_2).

Chronic kidney disease (CKD) (KDIGO, 2013; KDOQI, 2002): Children ≥2 years, Adolescents, and Adults: GFR <60 mL/minute/1.73 m^2 or kidney damage for ≥3 months; stages of CKD are described below:
- CKD Stage 1: Kidney damage with normal or increased GFR; GFR >90 mL/minute/1.73 m^2
- CKD Stage 2: Kidney damage with mild decrease in GFR; GFR 60-89 mL/minute/1.73 m^2
- CKD Stage 3: Moderate decrease in GFR; GFR 30-59 mL/minute/1.73 m^2
- CKD Stage 4: Severe decrease in GFR; GFR 15-29 mL/minute/1.73 m^2
- CKD Stage 5: Kidney failure; GFR <15 mL/minute/1.73 m^2 or dialysis

Dosage Forms Excipient information presented when available (limited, particularly for generics); consult specific product labeling. [DSC] = Discontinued product

Capsule, Oral:
- D-3-5: 5000 units
- Decara: 25,000 units [contains soybean oil]
- Decara: 50,000 units [contains fd&c yellow #10 (quinoline yellow), fd&c yellow #6 (sunset yellow), soybean oil]
- Dialyvite Vitamin D 5000: 5000 units
- Pronutrients Vitamin D3: 1000 units [contains soybean oil]
- Generic: 10,000 units, 50,000 units

Capsule, Oral [preservative free]:
- D-3-5: 5000 units [dye free]
- D3-50: 50,000 units [dye free, sugar free, yeast free]
- Generic: 2000 units, 5000 units

Liquid, Oral:
- Aqueous Vitamin D: 400 units/mL (50 mL) [gluten free, lactose free, sugar free; contains methylparaben, polysorbate 80]
- Bio-D-Mulsion: 400 units/0.03 mL (30 mL)
- Bio-D-Mulsion Forte: 2000 units/0.03 mL (30 mL)
- BProtected Pedia D-Vite: 400 units/mL (50 mL) [alcohol free, sugar free; contains polysorbate 80, propylene glycol, sodium benzoate; cherry flavor]
- D-Vi-Sol: 400 units/mL (50 mL) [gluten free, lactose free, sugar free; contains polysorbate 80]
- D-Vita: 400 units/mL (50 mL) [alcohol free, gluten free, lactose free, sugar free; contains polysorbate 80, propylene glycol, sodium benzoate; fruit flavor]
- Generic: 400 units/mL (50 mL, 52.5 mL)

Liquid, Oral [preservative free]:
- Generic: 5000 units/mL (52.5 mL)

Tablet, Oral:
- Delta D3: 400 units [gelatin free, gluten free, lactose free, no artificial color(s), no artificial flavor(s), starch free, sugar free, yeast free]
- Dialyvite Vitamin D3 Max: 50,000 units [scored]
- Vitamin D3 Super Strength: 2000 units [gluten free]
- Generic: 400 units [DSC], 1000 units, 3000 units, 5000 units

Tablet, Oral [preservative free]:
- Generic: 400 units, 1000 units, 2000 units, 5000 units

Tablet Chewable, Oral:
- Generic: 400 units

Cholestyramine Resin (koe LES teer a meen REZ in)

Brand Names: US Prevalite; Questran; Questran Light

Brand Names: Canada Novo-Cholamine; Novo-Cholamine Light; Olestyr; PMS-Cholestyramine; Questran; Questran Light Sugar Free; ZYM-Cholestyramine-Light; ZYM-Cholestyramine-Regular

Therapeutic Category Antilipemic Agent, Bile Acid Sequestrant

Generic Availability (US) Yes

Use Adjunct in the management of primary hypercholesterolemia (FDA approved in adults); pruritus associated with elevated levels of bile acids (FDA approved in adults); has also been used to manage diarrhea associated with excess fecal bile acids; applied topically to treat diaper dermatitis and as a skin-protectant around enterostomy fistula sites.

Pregnancy Risk Factor C

Pregnancy Considerations Cholestyramine is not absorbed systemically, but may interfere with vitamin absorption; therefore, regular prenatal supplementation may not be adequate. There are no studies in pregnant women; use with caution.

Breast-Feeding Considerations Due to lack of systemic absorption cholestyramine is not expected to be excreted into breast milk; however, the tendency of cholestyramine to interfere with vitamin absorption may have an effect on the nursing infant.

Contraindications Hypersensitivity to bile acid sequestering resins or any component of the formulation; complete biliary obstruction

Warnings/Precautions Secondary causes of hyperlipidemia should be ruled out prior to therapy. Bile acid sequestrants should not be used in patients with baseline fasting triglyceride levels ≥300 mg/dL or type III hyperlipoproteinemia since severe triglyceride elevations may occur. Use bile acid sequestrants with caution in patients with triglyceride levels 250-299 mg/dL and evaluate a fasting lipid panel in 4-6 weeks after initiation; discontinue use if triglycerides are >400 mg/dL (Stone, 2013). Use caution in patients with renal impairment. Not to be taken simultaneously with many other medicines (decreased absorption). Treat any diseases contributing to hypercholesterolemia first. Use with caution in patients susceptible to fat-soluble vitamin deficiencies. Absorption of fat soluble vitamins A, D, E, and K and folic acid may be decreased; patients should take vitamins ≥4 hours before cholestyramine. Chronic use may be associated with bleeding problems (especially in high doses); may be prevented with use of oral vitamin K therapy. May produce or exacerbate constipation problems; fecal impaction may occur; initiate therapy at a reduced dose in patients with a history of constipation. Hemorrhoids may be worsened. Some products may contain phenylalanine.

Warnings: Additional Pediatric Considerations With prolonged use, may potentially cause hypochloremic acidosis due to the exchange of organic anions for chloride; risk may be higher in younger and smaller patients; growth failure and malnutrition may occur in these patients (ASPEN Core Curriculum, 2010). Prolonged exposure to tooth enamel may result in discoloration or erosion; patients should be instructed to avoid sipping or slowly swallowing cholestyramine doses and to maintain good dental hygiene practices. May increase serum triglyceride concentrations; in a trial of children and adolescents (>10 years of age); the serum triglycerides increased 6% to 9% from baseline (not statistically significant) (McCrindle, 1997).

Adverse Reactions

Cardiovascular: Edema, syncope

Central nervous system: Anxiety, dizziness, drowsiness, fatigue, headache, neuralgia, paresthesia, vertigo

Dermatologic: Perianal skin irritation, skin irritation, skin rash, urticaria

Endocrine & metabolic: Hyperchloremic metabolic acidosis (children), increased libido, weight gain, weight loss

Gastrointestinal: Abdominal pain, anorexia, biliary colic, constipation, dental bleeding, dental caries, dental discoloration, diarrhea, diverticulitis, duodenal ulcer with hemorrhage, dysgeusia, dysphagia, eructation, flatulence, gallbladder calcification, gastric ulcer, gastrointestinal hemorrhage, hemorrhoidal bleeding, hiccups, intestinal obstruction (rare), melena, nausea, pancreatitis, rectal pain, steatorrhea, tongue irritation, tooth enamel damage (dental erosion), vomiting

Genitourinary: Diuresis, dysuria, hematuria

Hematologic & oncologic: Adenopathy, anemia, bruise, hemorrhage, hypoprothrombinemia, prolonged prothrombin time, rectal hemorrhage

Hepatic: Abnormal hepatic function tests

Neuromuscular & skeletal: Arthralgia, arthritis, back pain, myalgia, osteoporosis

Ophthalmic: Nocturnal amblyopia (rare), uveitis

Otic: Tinnitus

Respiratory: Asthma, dyspnea, wheezing

Drug Interactions

Metabolism/Transport Effects None known.

Avoid Concomitant Use

Avoid concomitant use of Cholestyramine Resin with any of the following: Mycophenolate

Increased Effect/Toxicity

Cholestyramine Resin may increase the levels/effects of: Spironolactone

Decreased Effect

Cholestyramine Resin may decrease the levels/effects of: Acetaminophen; Amiodarone; AtorvaSTATin; Cardiac Glycosides; Chenodiol; Cholic Acid; Contraceptives (Estrogens); Contraceptives (Progestins); Corticosteroids (Oral); Deferasirox; Ezetimibe; Fibric Acid Derivatives; Fluvastatin; Leflunomide; Lomitapide; Loop Diuretics; Methotrexate; Methylfolate; Multivitamins/Fluoride (with ADE); Multivitamins/Minerals (with ADEK, Folate, Iron); Multivitamins/Minerals (with AE, No Iron); Mycophenolate; Niacin; Nonsteroidal Anti-Inflammatory Agents; PHENobarbital; Pravastatin; Propranolol; Raloxifene; Rosiglitazone; Teriflunomide; Tetracycline Derivatives; Thiazide Diuretics; Thyroid Products; Ursodiol; Vancomycin; Vitamin D Analogs; Vitamin K Antagonists

Food Interactions Cholestyramine (especially high doses or long-term therapy) may decrease the absorption of folic acid, calcium, fat-soluble vitamins (vitamins A, D, E, and K), and iron. Management: Supplementation of folic acid, calcium, fat-soluble vitamins (vitamins A, D, E, and K), and iron may be necessary.

Storage/Stability Store at 20°C to 25°C (68°F to 77°F); excursions permitted to 15°C to 30°C (59°F to 86°F).

Mechanism of Action Forms a nonabsorbable complex with bile acids in the intestine, releasing chloride ions in the process; inhibits enterohepatic reuptake of intestinal bile salts and thereby increases the fecal loss of bile salt-bound low density lipoprotein cholesterol

Pharmacodynamics Maximum effect on serum cholesterol levels: Within 4 weeks

Pharmacokinetics (Adult data unless noted)

Absorption: Not absorbed from the GI tract

Elimination: Forms an insoluble complex with bile acids which is excreted in feces

Dosing: Neonatal Diaper dermatitis: Limited data available: Topical: Apply to affected area with each diaper change; **Note:** Product not commercially available; may be prepared as an extemporaneously compounded ointment or paste in Aquaphor; usual concentration: 5% to 10%; although higher concentrations (up to 20%) have been compounded; some centers have also used petrolatum as the base for compounding (White 2003; Williams 2011)

Dosing: Usual

Pediatric:

Diaper dermatitis: Limited data available: Topical: Infants and Children: Apply to affected area with each diaper change; **Note:** Product not commercially available; may be prepared as an extemporaneously compounded ointment or paste in Aquaphor® or polyethylene glycol; usual concentration 5% to 10%; although higher concentrations (up to 20%) have been compounded; some centers have also used petrolatum as the base for compounding (Preckshot 2001; White 2003; Williams 2011)

Dyslipidemia: Limited data available: Oral: **Note:** Dosages are expressed in terms of anhydrous resin:

Age-directed (fixed-dosing): Children ≥6 years and Adolescents: Initial 2 to 4 g/day for 1 week, then increase as tolerated to 8 g/day; children <10 years of age may only tolerate daily dose of 4 g (McCrindle 2007; Sprecher 1996; Tonstad 1996); lipid-lowering effects are better if dose is administered as a single daily dose with the evening meal (single daily morning doses are less effective); if patients cannot tolerate once daily dosing, the total daily dose may be divided into 2 doses and administered with the morning and evening meals; may also be administered in 3 divided doses daily (Daniels 2002); doses >8 g/day may not provide additional significant cholesterol-lowering effects, but may increase adverse effects (Sprecher 1996)

Weight-directed dosing: Children and Adolescents: 240 mg/kg/day in 3 divided doses; titrate to effect, maximum daily dose: 8 g/**day**

Pruritus secondary to cholestasis: Limited data available: Oral: **Note:** Dosages are expressed in terms of anhydrous resin:

Children ≤10 years: 240 mg/kg/day in 2 or 3 divided doses administered in the morning around breakfast and if necessary, the third dose at lunch; may titrate dose to effect. Some experts have suggested a maximum daily dose of 4 g/day; however, higher doses have been reported to treat pruritus in pediatric patients <10 years; in a case report (age: 9 years), the reported effective dose range was 3.3 to 6.6 g/day; in another case series (n=3; ages: 3-9 years), the reported range was 1.7 to 10 g/day; in some patients, higher doses were associated with increased steatorrhea and required dosage reduction (Cies 2007; Sprecher 1996)

Children >10 years and Adolescents: 240 mg/kg/day administered in the morning before breakfast; may titrate dose to effect. Some experts have suggested a maximum daily dose of 8 g/day; in adult patients, the AASLD guidelines recommend an initial dose of 4 g/day; may titrate up to 16 g/day; in some patients, higher doses have been associated with increased steatorrhea requiring dose reduction (Cies 2007; Iman 2012; Lindor 2009; Sprecher 1996).

Diarrhea secondary to intestinal failure, short-bowel syndrome: Limited data available: Children and Adolescents: Oral: 240 mg/kg/day in 3 divided doses; maximum daily dose: 8 g/day has been suggested (Ching 2009); however, trials have not been completed in pediatric patients and others have recommended avoiding use at this time (ASPEN Core Curriculum 2010).

Adult: **Note:** Dosages are expressed in terms of anhydrous resin: **Dyslipidemia:** Oral: Initial: 4 g 1 to 2 times daily; increase gradually over ≥1-month intervals; maintenance: 8-16 g/day divided in 2 doses; maximum: 24 g/day

Dosing adjustment in renal impairment: There are no dosage adjustment provided in manufacturer's labeling;

however, use with caution in renal impairment; may cause hyperchloremic acidosis.

Dosing adjustment in hepatic impairment: No dosage adjustment necessary; not absorbed from the gastrointestinal tract.

Preparation for Administration Oral: Powder for suspension: Prior to administration, add powder to 60 to 180 mL water or other noncarbonated liquid and mix well. May also be mixed with highly fluid soups, applesauce, or crushed pineapple.

Administration Oral: Administer as prepared suspension; not to be taken in dry form orally; suspension should not be sipped or held in mouth for prolonged periods (may cause tooth discoloration or enamel decay). Administration at mealtime is recommended. Administer other drugs including vitamins or mineral supplements at least 1 hour before or at least 4 to 6 hours after cholestyramine.

Dyslipidemia: Administer as a single dose (preferably) with the evening meal; however, some patients may require divided doses; in pediatric patients, may use 2 to 3 divided doses and in adults up to 6 doses daily.

Pruritus; cholestasis: Administer before breakfast (gall bladder has highest concentration of bile acids available for binding); for patients with an intact gall bladder, it has been suggested to administer the first dose 30 minutes before breakfast, the second dose 30 minutes after breakfast, and the final dose with lunch (Cies 2007)

Monitoring Parameters

Pediatric patients: Fasting lipid profile (baseline, 4 to 6 weeks after initiation, and then every 6 to 12 months), growth, maturation, number of stools per day (NHLBI, 2011)

Adults: Fasting lipid profile before initiating treatment, 3 months after initiation (within 4 to 6 weeks if baseline fasting triglycerides of 250 to 299 mg/dL), and every 6 to 12 months thereafter (Stone, 2013).

Test Interactions Increased prothrombin time

Dosage Forms Excipient information presented when available (limited, particularly for generics); consult specific product labeling. [DSC] = Discontinued product

Packet, Oral:

Prevalite: 4 g (1 ea, 42 ea, 60 ea) [contains aspartame; orange flavor]

Questran: 4 g (1 ea, 60 ea) [orange flavor]

Questran Light: 4 g (1 ea [DSC], 60 ea [DSC]) [sugar free; contains aspartame; orange flavor]

Generic: 4 g (1 ea, 60 ea)

Powder, Oral:

Prevalite: 4 g/dose (231 g) [contains aspartame; orange flavor]

Questran: 4 g/dose (378 g) [orange flavor]

Questran Light: 4 g/dose (210 g) [sugar free; contains aspartame; orange flavor]

Generic: 4 g/dose (210 g, 239.4 g, 378 g)

Choline Magnesium Trisalicylate

(KOE leen mag NEE zhum trye sa LIS i late)

Therapeutic Category Analgesic, Non-narcotic; Anti-inflammatory Agent; Antipyretic; Nonsteroidal Anti-inflammatory Drug (NSAID), Oral; Salicylate

Generic Availability (US) Yes

Use Management of osteoarthritis, rheumatoid arthritis, and other arthritides; treatment of acute painful shoulder, mild to moderate pain, and fever

Pregnancy Risk Factor C

Pregnancy Considerations Animal reproduction studies have not been conducted. Due to the known effects of other salicylates on the fetal cardiovascular system (closure of ductus arteriosus), use during late pregnancy should be avoided.

Breast-Feeding Considerations Excreted in breast milk; peak levels occur up to 9 to 12 hours after dose. The manufacturer recommends that caution be exercised when administering choline magnesium salicylate to nursing women.

Contraindications Hypersensitivity to choline magnesium trisalicylate, other nonacetylated salicylates, or any component of the formulation

Warnings/Precautions Nausea, vomiting, gastric upset, indigestion, heartburn, diarrhea, constipation, and/or epigastric pain may occur frequently. Use with caution in patients with acute or chronic hepatic or renal function, gastritis, asthma, or peptic ulcer disease. Avoid ethanol; may enhance GI adverse effects, including GI bleeding. Children and teenagers who have or are recovering from chickenpox, influenza, or flu-like symptoms should not use salicylate products, including choline magnesium trisalicylate. Changes in behavior (along with nausea and vomiting) may be an early sign of Reye's syndrome; patients should be instructed to contact their health care provider if these occur.

Elderly are a high-risk population for adverse effects from salicylates/NSAIDs. Use lowest effective dose for shortest period possible. Tinnitus is a common adverse effect and may indicate toxicity; reduce dose until tinnitus resolves. Tinnitus may be a difficult and unreliable indication of toxicity due to age-related hearing loss or eighth cranial nerve damage. Potentially significant drug-drug interactions may exist, requiring dose or frequency adjustment, additional monitoring, and/or selection of alternative therapy.

Adverse Reactions

Central nervous system: Dizziness, drowsiness, headache, lethargy, lightheadedness

Gastrointestinal: Constipation, diarrhea, dyspepsia, epigastric, heartburn, nausea, pain, vomiting

Otic: Hearing impairment, tinnitus

Rare but important or life-threatening: Anorexia, asthma, bruising, confusion, duodenal ulceration, dysgeusia, edema, epistaxis, erythema multiforme, esophagitis, hallucinations, hearing loss (irreversible), increased BUN, increased creatinine, increased hepatic enzymes, gastric ulceration, occult bleeding, pruritus, rash, weight gain

Drug Interactions

Metabolism/Transport Effects None known.

Avoid Concomitant Use

Avoid concomitant use of Choline Magnesium Trisalicylate with any of the following: Influenza Virus Vaccine (Live/Attenuated)

Increased Effect/Toxicity

Choline Magnesium Trisalicylate may increase the levels/effects of: Anticoagulants; Blood Glucose Lowering Agents; Carbonic Anhydrase Inhibitors; Corticosteroids (Systemic); Methotrexate; PRALAtrexate; Salicylates; Thrombolytic Agents; Valproic Acid and Derivatives; Varicella Virus-Containing Vaccines; Vitamin K Antagonists

The levels/effects of Choline Magnesium Trisalicylate may be increased by: Agents with Antiplatelet Properties; Ammonium Chloride; Calcium Channel Blockers (Nondihydropyridine); Ginkgo Biloba; Herbs (Anticoagulant/Antiplatelet Properties); Influenza Virus Vaccine (Live/Attenuated); Loop Diuretics; Potassium Acid Phosphate; Treprostinil

Decreased Effect

Choline Magnesium Trisalicylate may decrease the levels/effects of: ACE Inhibitors; Hyaluronidase; Loop Diuretics; Probenecid

The levels/effects of Choline Magnesium Trisalicylate may be decreased by: Corticosteroids (Systemic)

Food Interactions Foods and drugs that alter urine pH may affect renal clearance of salicylate and plasma salicylate concentrations. Curry powder, paprika, licorice, Benedictine liqueur, prunes, raisins, tea, and gherkins may cause salicylate accumulation. These foods contain 6 mg salicylate/100 g. Management: Limit curry powder, paprika, licorice, Benedictine liqueur, prunes, raisins, tea, and gherkins.

Storage/Stability Store between 15°C and 30°C (59°F and 86°F).

Mechanism of Action Weakly inhibits cyclooxygenase enzymes, which results in decreased formation of prostaglandin precursors; antipyretic, analgesic, and anti-inflammatory properties.

Other proposed mechanisms not fully elucidated (and possibly contributing to the anti-inflammatory effect to varying degrees) include inhibiting chemotaxis, altering lymphocyte activity, inhibiting neutrophil aggregation/activation, and decreasing proinflammatory cytokine levels.

Pharmacokinetics (Adult data unless noted)

Absorption: From stomach and small intestine

Distribution: Readily distributes into most body fluids and tissues; crosses the placenta; appears in breast milk

Protein binding: 90% to 95%

Metabolism: Hepatic microsomal enzyme system

Half-life: Dose-dependent, ranging from 2-3 hours at low doses to 30 hours at high doses

Time to peak serum concentration: 20-35 minutes

Elimination: 10% excreted as unchanged drug

Dosing: Usual Oral (based on **total salicylate content**):

Children: 30-60 mg/kg/day given in 3-4 divided doses

Adults: 500 mg to 1.5 g 1-3 times/day

Administration Oral: Administer with food or milk to decrease GI upset; may be mixed with fruit juice just before drinking; do not administer with antacids

Monitoring Parameters Serum salicylate levels; serum magnesium with high doses or in patients with decreased renal function

Reference Range

Salicylate blood levels for anti-inflammatory effect: 150-300 mcg/mL

Analgesia and antipyretic effect: 30-50 mcg/mL

Test Interactions False-negative results for glucose oxidase urinary glucose tests (Clinistix®); false-positives using the cupric sulfate method (Clinitest®); also, interferes with Gerhardt test (urinary ketone analysis), VMA determination; 5-HIAA, xylose tolerance test, and T_3 and T_4; increased PBI

Additional Information Salicylate salts do not inhibit platelet aggregation and, therefore, should not be substituted for aspirin in the prophylaxis of thrombosis (ie, for aspirin's antiplatelet effects)

Dosage Forms Excipient information presented when available (limited, particularly for generics); consult specific product labeling.

Liquid, Oral:

Generic: 500 mg/5 mL (240 mL)

Tablet, Oral:

Generic: 1000 mg

◆ **Chorionic Gonadotropin for Injection (Can)** *see* Chorionic Gonadotropin (Human) *on page 453*

Chorionic Gonadotropin (Human)

(kor ee ON ik goe NAD oh troe pin, HYU man)

Related Information

Safe Handling of Hazardous Drugs *on page 2455*

Brand Names: US Novarel; Pregnyl

Brand Names: Canada Chorionic Gonadotropin for Injection; Pregnyl®

Therapeutic Category Gonadotropin; Ovulation Stimulator

Generic Availability (US) Yes

Use Treatment of hypogonadotropic hypogonadism, prepubertal cryptorchidism; induce ovulation and pregnancy in anovulatory, infertile women

Pregnancy Risk Factor X

Pregnancy Considerations Adverse events have been observed in animal studies at doses intended to induce superovulation (used in combination with gonadotropin). Testicular tumors in otherwise healthy men have been reported when treating secondary infertility.

Breast-Feeding Considerations It is not known if chorionic gonadotropin (human) is excreted in breast milk. The manufacturer recommends that caution be exercised when administering chorionic gonadotropin (human) to nursing women.

Contraindications Hypersensitivity to chorionic gonadotropin or any component of the formulation; precocious puberty; prostatic carcinoma or similar neoplasms; pregnancy

Warnings/Precautions Hazardous agent - use appropriate precautions for handling and disposal (NIOSH 2014 [group 3]).

Use with caution in asthma, seizure disorders, migraine, cardiac or renal disease. **Not** effective in the treatment of obesity.

Cryptorchidism: May induce precocious puberty in children being treated for cryptorchidism; discontinue if signs of precocious puberty occur.

Ovulation induction: These medications should only be used by physicians who are thoroughly familiar with infertility problems and their management. May cause ovarian hyperstimulation syndrome (OHSS). OHSS, an exaggerated response to ovulation induction therapy, is characterized by an increase in vascular permeability which causes a fluid shift from intravascular space to third space compartments (eg, peritoneal cavity, thoracic cavity) (ASRM, 2008; SOGC-CFAS, 2011). This syndrome may begin within 24 hours of treatment, but may become most severe 7 to 10 days after therapy (SOGC-CFAS, 2011). OHSS is typically self-limiting with spontaneous resolution, although it may be more severe and protracted if pregnancy occurs (ASRM, 2008). Symptoms of mild/moderate OHSS may include abdominal distention/discomfort, diarrhea, nausea, and/or vomiting. Severe OHSS symptoms may include abdominal pain that is severe, acute respiratory distress syndrome, anuria/oliguria, ascites, dyspnea, hypotension, nausea/vomiting (intractable), pericardial effusions, tachycardia, or thromboembolism. Decreased creatinine clearance, hemoconcentration, hypoproteinemia, elevated liver enzymes, elevated WBC, and electrolyte imbalances may also be present (ASRM, 2008; Fiedler, 2012; SOGC-CFAS, 2011). If severe OHSS occurs, stop treatment and consider hospitalizing the patient. (ASRM, 2008; SOGC-CFAS, 2011). Treatment is primarily symptomatic and includes fluid and electrolyte management, analgesics, and prevention of thromboembolic complications (ASRM, 2008; SOGC-CFAS, 2011). The ascitic, pleural, and pericardial fluids may be removed if needed to relieve symptoms (eg, pulmonary distress or cardiac tamponade) (ASRM, 2008; SOGC-CFAS, 2011). Women with OHSS should avoid pelvic examination and/or intercourse (ASRM, 2008; SOGC-CFAS, 2011) Multiple births may result from the use of these medications; advise patients of the potential risk of multiple births before starting the treatment.

Benzyl alcohol and derivatives: Some dosage forms may contain benzyl alcohol; large amounts of benzyl alcohol (≥99 mg/kg/day) have been associated with a potentially fatal toxicity ("gasping syndrome") in neonates; the "gasping syndrome" consists of metabolic acidosis, respiratory distress, gasping respirations, CNS dysfunction (including convulsions, intracranial hemorrhage), hypotension and cardiovascular collapse (AAP, 1997; CDC, 1982); some data suggests that benzoate displaces bilirubin from protein binding sites (Ahlfors, 2001); avoid or use dosage forms containing benzyl alcohol with caution in neonates. See manufacturer's labeling.

Warnings: Additional Pediatric Considerations May induce precocious puberty in children being treated for cryptorchidism; discontinue if signs of precocious puberty occur.

Adverse Reactions

Cardiovascular: Edema

Central nervous system: Depression, fatigue, headache, irritability, restlessness

Endocrine & metabolic: Gynecomastia, precocious puberty

Local: Injection site reaction, pain at injection site

Miscellaneous: Hypersensitivity reaction (local or systemic)

Rare but important or life-threatening: Arterial thrombus, ovarian cyst rupture, ovarian hyperstimulation syndrome

Drug Interactions

Metabolism/Transport Effects None known.

Avoid Concomitant Use There are no known interactions where it is recommended to avoid concomitant use.

Increased Effect/Toxicity There are no known significant interactions involving an increase in effect.

Decreased Effect There are no known significant interactions involving a decrease in effect.

Storage/Stability Following reconstitution with the provided diluent, solutions are stable for 30-60 days, depending on the specific preparation, when stored at 2°C to 15°C.

Mechanism of Action Luteinizing hormone obtained from the urine of pregnant women. Stimulates production of gonadal steroid hormones by causing production of androgen by the testes; as a substitute for luteinizing hormone (LH) to stimulate ovulation

Pharmacokinetics (Adult data unless noted)

Distribution: Distributes mainly into the testes in males and into the ovaries in females

Half-life, biphasic:

Initial: 11 hours

Terminal: 23 hours

Time to peak serum concentration: 6 hours

Elimination: Approximately 10% to 12% excreted unchanged in urine within 24 hours; detectable amounts may continue to be excreted in the urine for up to 3-4 days

Dosing: Usual

Children: IM (many regimens have been described):

Prepubertal cryptorchidism:

1000-2000 units/m^2/dose 3 times/week for 3 weeks or 4000 units 3 times/week for 3 weeks

or

5000 units every second day for 4 injections

or

500 units 3 times/week for 4-6 weeks

Hypogonadotropic hypogonadism:

500-1000 units 3 times/week for 3 weeks, followed by the same dose twice weekly for 3 weeks

or

1000-2000 units 3 times/week

or

4000 units 3 times/week for 6-9 months; reduce dosage to 2000 units 3 times/week for additional 3 months

Adults:

Induction of ovulation: Females: 5000-10,000 units the day following the last dose of menotropins

Spermatogenesis induction associated with hypogonadotropic hypogonadism: Male: Treatment regimens vary (range: 1000-2000 units 2-3 times a week). Administer hCG until serum testosterone levels are normal (may require 2-3 months of therapy), then may add follitropin alfa or menopausal gonadotropin if needed to induce spermatogenesis; continue hCG at the dose required to maintain testosterone levels.

Preparation for Administration Hazardous agent; use appropriate precautions for handling and disposal (NIOSH 2014 [group 3]).

Parenteral:

Novarel: Reconstitute with 1 mL of bacteriostatic water for injection for a concentration of 10,000 units/mL or 10 mL for a concentration of 1,000 units/mL

Pregnyl: Reconstitute using provided diluent. Withdraw sterile air from lyophilized vial and inject into diluent vial. Remove 1 to 10 mL from diluent and add to lyophilized vial; agitate gently until powder is completely dissolved in solution.

Administration Hazardous agent; use appropriate precautions for handling and disposal (NIOSH 2014 [group 3]).

Parenteral: Administer IM only.

Monitoring Parameters

Male: Serum testosterone levels, semen analysis

Female: Ultrasound and/or estradiol levels to assess follicle development; ultrasound to assess number and size of follicles; ovulation (basal body temperature, serum progestin level, menstruation, sonography)

Reference Range Depends on application and methodology; <3 milli international units/mL (SI: <3 units/L) usually normal (nonpregnant)

Test Interactions Cross-reacts with radioimmunoassay of gonadotropins, especially LH

Dosage Forms Excipient information presented when available (limited, particularly for generics); consult specific product labeling.

Solution Reconstituted, Intramuscular:

Novarel: 10,000 units (1 ea) [contains benzyl alcohol]

Pregnyl: 10,000 units (1 ea) [contains benzyl alcohol, sodium chloride]

Generic: 10,000 units (1 ea)

◆ **Chromium** *see* Trace Elements *on page* 2097

Ciclesonide (Nasal) (sye KLES oh nide)

Brand Names: US Omnaris; Zetonna

Brand Names: Canada Drymira; Omnaris; Omnaris HFA

Therapeutic Category Corticosteroid, Intranasal

Generic Availability (US) No

Use

Omnaris: Management of seasonal allergic rhinitis (FDA approved in ages ≥6 years and adults); management of perennial allergic rhinitis (FDA approved in ages ≥12 years and adults)

Zetonna: Management of seasonal and perennial allergic rhinitis (FDA approved in ages ≥12 years and adults)

Intranasal corticosteroids have also been used as an adjunct to antibiotics in empiric treatment of acute bacterial rhinosinusitis primarily in patients with history of allergy rhinitis (Chow, 2012) and in pediatric patients with mild obstructive sleep apnea syndrome who cannot undergo adenotonsillectomy or who still have symptoms after surgery (Marcus, 2012)

Pregnancy Risk Factor C

Pregnancy Considerations Adverse events were observed in some animal reproduction studies. Hypoadrenalism may occur in newborns following maternal use of corticosteroids in pregnancy; monitor. Intranasal corticosteroids may be used in the treatment of rhinitis during pregnancy; the lowest effective dose should be used (NAEPP, 2005; Wallace, 2008).

Breast-Feeding Considerations Systemic corticosteroids are excreted in human milk. It is not known if sufficient quantities of ciclesonide are absorbed following nasal inhalation to produce detectable amounts in breast milk; however, oral absorption is limited (<1%). The use of inhaled corticosteroids is not considered a contraindication to breast-feeding (NAEPP, 2005). The manufacturer recommends caution be used if administered to a nursing woman.

Contraindications Hypersensitivity to ciclesonide or any component of the formulation

Warnings/Precautions Avoid nasal corticosteroid use in patients with recent nasal septal ulcers, nasal surgery or nasal trauma until healing has occurred. Avoid using higher than recommended dosages; suppression of linear growth (ie, reduction of growth velocity), reduced bone mineral density, or hypercorticism (Cushing syndrome) may occur; titrate to lowest effective dose. Reduction in growth velocity may occur when corticosteroids are administered to pediatric patients, even at recommended doses via intranasal route (monitor growth). Nasal septal perforation, nasal ulceration, epistaxis, and localized *Candida albicans* infections of the nose and/or pharynx may occur. Monitor patients periodically for adverse nasal effects.

Prolonged use of corticosteroids may increase the incidence of secondary infection, mask acute infection (including fungal infections), prolong or exacerbate viral infections, or limit response to vaccines. Exposure to chickenpox should be avoided; corticosteroids should be used with caution, if at all, in patients with ocular herpes simplex, latent tuberculosis, and/or TB reactivity, or in patients with untreated fungal, viral, or bacterial infections. When used at excessive doses, may cause hypercorticism or suppression of hypothalamic-pituitary-adrenal (HPA) axis, particularly in younger children or in patients receiving high doses for prolonged periods. HPA axis suppression may lead to adrenal crisis. Withdrawal and discontinuation of a corticosteroid should be done slowly and carefully. Particular care is required when patients are transferred from systemic corticosteroids to inhaled products due to possible adrenal insufficiency or withdrawal from steroids, including an increase in allergic symptoms.

Adverse Reactions

Central nervous system: Headache

Gastrointestinal: Nausea

Genitourinary: Urinary tract infection

Infection: Influenza

Neuromuscular & skeletal: Back pain, strain

Otic: Otalgia

Respiratory: Bronchitis, cough (may be dose-responsive), epistaxis, nasal discomfort, nasal septum disorder (may be dose-responsive), nasopharyngitis, oropharyngeal pain, pharyngolaryngeal pain, sinusitis, streptococcal pharyngitis, upper respiratory infection, viral upper respiratory tract infection

Rare but important or life-threatening: ALT increased, angioedema (with swelling of lip/pharynx/tongue), bruising, candidiasis (nasal/pharyngeal), cataract, chest discomfort, dizziness, dry throat, dysgeusia, dyspepsia, GGT increased, growth suppression, intraocular pressure increased, nasal ulcer, palpitation, rash, rhinorrhea, throat irritation, WBC increased, weight gain, wound healing impaired, xerostomia

Drug Interactions

Metabolism/Transport Effects Substrate of CYP3A4 (minor); **Note:** Assignment of Major/Minor substrate status based on clinically relevant drug interaction potential

Avoid Concomitant Use There are no known interactions where it is recommended to avoid concomitant use.

Increased Effect/Toxicity

Ciclesonide (Nasal) may increase the levels/effects of: Ceritinib

Decreased Effect There are no known significant interactions involving a decrease in effect.

Storage/Stability Store at 25°C (77°F); excursions permitted to 15°C to 30°C (59°F to 86°F).

Omnaris®: Do not freeze. Use within 4 months after opening aluminum pouch.

Zetonna™: Protect from heat or open flame (>49°C [120°F]). Do not puncture.

Pharmacodynamics Onset of action: 24-48 hours; further improvement observed over 1-2 weeks in seasonal allergic rhinitis or 5 weeks in perennial allergic rhinitis

Pharmacokinetics (Adult data unless noted)

Absorption: Minimal systemic

Metabolism: Ciclesonide hydrolyzed to active metabolite, des-ciclesonide via esterases in nasal mucosa and lungs; further metabolism via hepatic CYP3A4 and 2D6

Bioavailability: Oral: <1%

Dosing: Usual Note: Product formulations are not interchangeable: Omnaris®: One spray delivers 50 mcg; Zetonna: One spray delivers 37 mcg

Children and Adolescents:

Perennial allergic rhinitis: Intranasal:

Omnaris:

Children 2-11 years: Limited data available: 100 or 200 mcg once daily delivered as 50 mcg (1 spray) or 100 mg (2 sprays) **per nostril** (Berger, 2008; Kim, 2007)

Children ≥12 years and Adolescents: 200 mcg once daily delivered as 100 mcg (2 sprays) **per nostril**; maximum daily dose: 200 mcg/**day**

Zetonna: Children ≥12 years and Adolescents: 74 mcg once daily delivered as 37 mcg (1 spray) **per nostril**; maximum daily dose: 74 mcg/**day**

Seasonal allergic rhinitis: Intranasal:

Omnaris: Children ≥6 years and Adolescents: 200 mcg once daily delivered as 100 mcg (2 sprays) **per nostril**; maximum dose: 200 mcg/**day**

Zetonna: Children ≥12 years and Adolescents: 74 mcg once daily delivered as 37 mcg (1 spray) **per nostril**; maximum daily dose: 74 mcg/**day**

Adults: **Perennial allergic rhinitis, seasonal allergic rhinitis:** Intranasal:

Omnaris: 2 sprays (50 mcg/spray) **per nostril** once daily; maximum: 200 mcg/**day**

Zetonna: 74 mcg once daily delivered as 1 spray (37 mcg/spray) **per nostril** once daily; maximum: 74 mcg/**day**

Dosing adjustment in renal impairment: There are no dosage adjustments provided in the manufacturer's labeling; has not been studied.

Dosing adjustment in hepatic impairment: Children, Adolescents, and Adults: No dosage adjustment necessary.

Administration Intranasal: Blow nose to clear nostrils. Insert applicator into nostril, keeping bottle upright, and close off the other nostril. Breathe in through nose. While inhaling, press pump to release spray. Avoid spraying directly onto the nasal septum or into eyes. Discard after the "discard by" date or after labeled number of doses has been used, even if bottle is not completely empty.

Omnaris: Shake bottle gently before using. Prime pump prior to first use (press 8 times until fine mist appears) or if spray has not been used in 4 consecutive days (press 1 time or until a fine mist appears). Nasal applicator may be removed and rinsed with warm water to clean.

Zetonna: Use nasal canister with supplied nasal actuator only. Prime pump prior to first use (press 3 times until fine mist appears) or if spray has not been used in 10 consecutive days (press 3 times or until a fine mist appears). If canister and actuator become separated, spray 1 test spray in air before using. Clean outside of nose piece with a clean, dry tissue or cloth weekly; do not wash or put in water.

Monitoring Parameters Mucous membranes for signs of fungal infection, growth (pediatric patients), signs/symptoms of HPA axis suppression/adrenal insufficiency; ocular changes

Additional Information When used short term as adjunctive therapy in acute bacterial rhinosinusitis (ABRS), intranasal steroids show modest symptomatic improvement and few adverse effects; improvement is primarily due to increased sinus drainage. Use should be considered optional in ABRS; however, intranasal corticosteroids should be routinely prescribed to ABRS patients who have a history of or concurrent allergic rhinitis (Chow, 2012).

Dosage Forms Considerations

Omnaris 12.5 g bottles contain 120 actuations.

Zetonna 6.1 g canisters contain 60 actuations.

Dosage Forms Excipient information presented when available (limited, particularly for generics); consult specific product labeling.

Aerosol Solution, Nasal:

Zetonna: 37 mcg/actuation (6.1 g)

Suspension, Nasal:

Omnaris: 50 mcg/actuation (12.5 g) [contains edetate sodium (tetrasodium)]

Ciclesonide (Oral Inhalation) (sye KLES oh nide)

Brand Names: US Alvesco

Brand Names: Canada Alvesco

Therapeutic Category Adrenal Corticosteroid; Anti-inflammatory Agent; Antiasthmatic; Corticosteroid, Inhalant (Oral); Glucocorticoid

Generic Availability (US) No

Use Maintenance treatment of asthma (prophylactic management) (FDA approved in ages ≥12 years and adults); **NOT** indicated for the relief of acute bronchospasm; has also been used as daily therapy to manage exercise-induced bronchoconstriction in patients who continue to have symptoms despite the use of short-acting $beta_2$-agonist before exercise (Parsons, 2013)

Pregnancy Risk Factor C

Pregnancy Considerations Adverse events were observed in some animal reproduction studies. Hypoadrenalism may occur in infants born to mothers receiving corticosteroids during pregnancy. Based on available data, an overall increased risk of congenital malformations or a decrease in fetal growth has not been associated with maternal use of inhaled corticosteroids during pregnancy (Bakhireva, 2005; NAEPP, 2005; Namazy, 2004). Uncontrolled asthma is associated with adverse events in pregnancy (increased risk of perinatal mortality, pre-eclampsia, preterm birth, low birth weight infants). Inhaled corticosteroids are recommended for the treatment of asthma during pregnancy (most information available using budesonide) (ACOG, 2008; NAEPP, 2005).

Breast-Feeding Considerations Systemic corticosteroids are excreted in human milk. It is not known if sufficient quantities of ciclesonide are absorbed following oral inhalation to produce detectable amounts in breast milk; however, oral absorption is limited (<1%). The manufacturer recommends that caution be exercised when administering ciclesonide to nursing women. The use of inhaled corticosteroids is not considered a contraindication to breast-feeding (NAEPP, 2005).

Contraindications

Hypersensitivity to ciclesonide or any component of the formulation; primary treatment of acute asthma or status asthmaticus

Canadian labeling: Additional contraindications (not in U.S. labeling): Untreated fungal, bacterial, or tuberculosis infections of the respiratory tract; moderate-to-severe bronchiectasis

Warnings/Precautions May cause hypercorticism or suppression of hypothalamic-pituitary-adrenal (HPA) axis, particularly in younger children or in patients receiving high doses for prolonged periods. HPA axis suppression may lead to adrenal crisis. Withdrawal and discontinuation of a corticosteroid should be done slowly and carefully. Particular care is required when patients are transferred from systemic corticosteroids to inhaled products due to possible adrenal insufficiency or withdrawal from steroids, including an increase in allergic symptoms. Adult patients receiving >20 mg per day of prednisone (or equivalent) may be most susceptible. Fatalities have occurred due to adrenal insufficiency in asthmatic patients during and after transfer from systemic corticosteroids to aerosol steroids; aerosol steroids do **not** provide the systemic steroid needed to treat patients having trauma, surgery, or infections. Select surgical patients on long-term, high-dose, inhaled corticosteroid (ICS), should be given stress doses of hydrocortisone intravenously during the surgical period and the dose reduced rapidly within 24 hours after surgery (NAEPP, 2007).

Bronchospasm may occur with wheezing after inhalation; if this occurs stop steroid and treat with a fast-acting bronchodilator. Supplemental steroids (oral or parenteral) may be needed during stress or severe asthma attacks. Not to be used in status asthmaticus or for the relief of acute bronchospasm. Oropharyngeal thrush due to candida albicans infection may occur with use. Prolonged use of corticosteroids may also increase the incidence of secondary infection, mask acute infection (including fungal infections), prolong or exacerbate viral infections, or limit response to vaccines. Exposure to chickenpox and measles should be avoided; corticosteroids should not be used to treat ocular herpes simplex. Close observation is required in patients with latent tuberculosis and/or TB reactivity; restrict use in active TB (only in conjunction with antituberculosis treatment). Use in patients with TB is contraindicated in the Canadian labeling. Prolonged treatment with corticosteroids has been associated with the development of Kaposi's sarcoma (case reports); if noted, discontinuation of therapy should be considered.

Use with caution in patients with cardiovascular disease, diabetes, severe hepatic impairment, thyroid disease, psychiatric disturbances, myasthenia gravis, glaucoma, cataracts, patients at risk for osteoporosis, and patients at risk for seizures. Use in renally-impaired patients has not been studied; however, ≤20% of drug is eliminated renally. Use with caution in elderly patients.

Orally inhaled corticosteroids may cause a reduction in growth velocity in pediatric patients (~1 cm per year [range: 0.3-1.8 cm per year] and related to dose and duration of exposure). To minimize the systemic effects of orally inhaled corticosteroids, each patient should be titrated to the lowest effective dose. Growth should be routinely monitored in pediatric patients.

Warnings: Additional Pediatric Considerations Relative to other inhaled corticosteroids, ciclesonide may exhibit less effect on HPA function due to it being a prodrug which is activated in the lungs; in four pediatric patients, resolution of HPA suppression was reported after switching from fluticasone to ciclesonide therapy (Heller, 2010).

Adverse Reactions

Cardiovascular: Facial edema

Central nervous system: Dizziness, dysphonia, fatigue, headache

Dermatologic: Urticaria

Gastrointestinal: Gastroenteritis, oral candidiasis

Neuromuscular & Skeletal: Arthralgia, back pain, extremity pain, musculoskeletal chest pain

Ocular: Conjunctivitis

Otic: Ear pain

Respiratory: Hoarseness, nasal congestion, nasopharyngitis, paradoxical bronchospasm, pharyngolaryngeal pain, pneumonia, sinusitis, upper respiratory infection

Miscellaneous: Influenza

Rare but important or life-threatening: ALT increased, angioedema (with swelling of lip/pharynx/tongue), candidiasis (pharyngeal), cataract, chest discomfort, GGT increased, intraocular pressure increased, nausea, palpitation, rash, weight gain, xerostomia

Drug Interactions

Metabolism/Transport Effects Substrate of CYP3A4 (minor); **Note:** Assignment of Major/Minor substrate status based on clinically relevant drug interaction potential

Avoid Concomitant Use

Avoid concomitant use of Ciclesonide (Oral Inhalation) with any of the following: Aldesleukin; Loxapine

Increased Effect/Toxicity

Ciclesonide (Oral Inhalation) may increase the levels/effects of: Amphotericin B; Ceritinib; Deferasirox; Loop Diuretics; Loxapine; Thiazide Diuretics

The levels/effects of Ciclesonide (Oral Inhalation) may be increased by: Telaprevir

Decreased Effect

Ciclesonide (Oral Inhalation) may decrease the levels/effects of: Aldesleukin; Corticorelin; Hyaluronidase; Telaprevir

Storage/Stability Store at 25°C (77°F); excursions to 15°C to 30°C (59°F to 86°F) permitted. Do not puncture. Do not use or store near open flame or heat; canister may burst if exposed to temperatures >49°C (120°F); do not throw canister into fire or incinerator.

Mechanism of Action Ciclesonide is a nonhalogenated, glucocorticoid prodrug that is hydrolyzed to the pharmacologically active metabolite des-ciclesonide following administration. Des-ciclesonide has a high affinity for the glucocorticoid receptor and exhibits anti-inflammatory activity. The mechanism of action for corticosteroids is believed to be a combination of three important properties – anti-inflammatory activity, immunosuppressive properties, and antiproliferative actions.

Pharmacodynamics Onset of action: >4 weeks for maximum benefit

Pharmacokinetics (Adult data unless noted)

Absorption: 52% (lung deposition)

Distribution: V_d: Ciclesonide: 2.9 L/kg; des-ciclesonide: 12.1 L/kg

Protein binding: ≥99%

Metabolism: Ciclesonide hydrolyzed to active metabolite, des-ciclesonide via esterases in nasal mucosa and lungs; further metabolism via hepatic CYP3A4 and 2D6

Half-life: Ciclesonide: 0.7 hours; des-ciclesonide: 6-7 hours

Time to peak serum concentration: ~1 hour (des-ciclesonide)

Elimination: Feces (66%)

Dosing: Usual

Children and Adolescents:

Asthma, maintenance therapy: Note: Doses should be titrated to the lowest effective dose once asthma is controlled: Oral inhalation:

Children 2-4 years: Limited data available; efficacy results variable: 40, 80, or 160 mcg once daily with spacer has been studied in 992 children 2-6 years of age clinically diagnosed with asthma; after 12 weeks of therapy, results showed exacerbation rates were lower in the pooled ciclesonide treatment groups versus placebo; and decreased utility of rescue medications compared to baseline for all groups, including placebo (however, a statistically significant difference was not shown between each ciclesonide group and placebo due to an unusually large and unexpected placebo response); in safety analysis, no untoward effects were observed (Brand, 2011)

Children 5-11 years: Limited data available: 40, 80, or 160 mcg once daily has been used in clinical trials; the majority of data showed statistically significant positive efficacy findings (Gelfand, 2006; Pedersen, 2010). Others have suggested the following (Global Strategy for Asthma Management and Prevention, 2011):

"Low" dose: 80-160 mcg/day

"Medium" dose: >160-320 mcg/day

"High" dose: >320 mcg/day; maximum daily dose: 640 mcg/**day**

Children ≥12 years and Adolescents:

Manufacturer's labeling:

Prior therapy with bronchodilators alone: Initial: 80 mcg twice daily, may increase dose after 4 weeks of therapy if response inadequate; maximum daily dose: 320 mcg/**day**

Prior therapy with inhaled corticosteroids: Initial: 80 mcg twice daily, may increase dose after 4 weeks of therapy if response inadequate; maximum daily dose: 640 mcg/**day**

Prior therapy with oral corticosteroids: Initial: 320 mcg twice daily, may increase dose after 4 weeks of therapy if response inadequate; maximum daily dose: 640 mcg/**day**

Alternate dosing (Global Strategy for Asthma Management and Prevention, 2011): **Note:** Other expert guideline recommendations suggest that doses >200 mcg/day may provide minimal additional benefit while increasing risks for adverse events; add-on therapy should be considered prior to dose increases >200 mcg/day (Lougheed, 2010).

"Low" dose: 80-160 mcg/day

"Medium" dose: >160-320 mcg/day

"High" dose: >320 mcg/day; maximum daily dose: 640 mcg/**day**

Adults:

Asthma, maintenance therapy: Note: Doses should be titrated to the lowest effective dose once asthma is controlled: Oral inhalation:

Manufacturer's labeling:

Prior therapy with bronchodilators alone: Initial: 80 mcg twice daily; maximum daily dose: 320 mcg/**day**

Prior therapy with inhaled corticosteroids: Initial: 80 mcg twice daily; maximum dose: 640 mcg/**day**

Prior therapy with oral corticosteroids: Initial: 320 mcg twice daily; maximum dose: 640 mcg/**day**

Alternate dosing (Global Strategy for Asthma Management and Prevention, 2011):

"Low" dose: 80-160 mcg/day

"Medium" dose: >160-320 mcg/day

"High" dose: >320 mcg/day

Administration Oral inhalation: Shaking inhaler before use is not necessary since drug is formulated as a solution aerosol. With initial use or if inhaler not in use for 7-10 days, prime the inhaler by releasing 3 puffs into the air. Do not spray into eyes or face while priming. Remove mouthpiece cover, place inhaler in mouth, close lips around mouthpiece, and inhale slowly and deeply. Press down on top of inhaler after slow inhalation has begun. Remove inhaler while holding breath for approximately 10 seconds. Breathe out slowly and replace mouthpiece on inhaler. Rinse mouth with water (and spit out) after use to reduce incidence of oral candidiasis. Do not wash any part of inhaler in water; clean mouthpiece using a dry cloth or tissue once weekly. Discard after the "discard by" date or after labeled number of doses has been used, even if container is not completely empty. Dose indicator will turn red when 20 puffs remain; if inhaler dropped, dose indicator may be inaccurate; manual tracking of inhaler actuations recommended.

Monitoring Parameters Check mucus membranes for signs of fungal infection; monitor growth in pediatric patients; monitor IOP with therapy >6 weeks. Monitor for symptoms of asthma, FEV_1, peak flow, and/or other pulmonary function tests

Additional Information When using ciclesonide oral inhalation to help reduce or discontinue oral corticosteroid therapy, begin corticosteroid taper after at least 1 week of ciclesonide inhalation therapy; reduce dose of oral corticosteroid gradually, with next decrease after 1-2 weeks depending on patient's response; do not decrease prednisone faster than 2.5 mg/day in adolescents and adults on a weekly basis; monitor patients for signs of asthma instability and adrenal insufficiency; decrease ciclesonide to lowest effective dose after prednisone reduction is complete.

Dosage Forms Considerations Alvesco 6.1 g canisters contain 60 inhalations.

Dosage Forms Excipient information presented when available (limited, particularly for generics); consult specific product labeling.

Aerosol Solution, Inhalation:

Alvesco: 80 mcg/actuation (6.1 g); 160 mcg/actuation (6.1 g)

◆ **Ciclodan** *see* Ciclopirox *on page 458*

◆ **Ciclodan Cream** *see* Ciclopirox *on page 458*

◆ **Ciclodan Solution** *see* Ciclopirox *on page 458*

Ciclopirox (sye kloe PEER oks)

Brand Names: US Ciclodan; Ciclodan Cream; Ciclodan Solution; Ciclopirox Treatment; CNL8 Nail; Loprox; Pedipirox-4 Nail [DSC]; Penlac

Brand Names: Canada Apo-Ciclopirox; Loprox; Penlac; PMS-Ciclopirox; Stieprox; Taro-Ciclopirox

Therapeutic Category Antifungal Agent, Topical

Generic Availability (US) Yes

Use

Cream/lotion: Treatment of tinea pedis, tinea cruris, and tinea corporis caused by *Trichophyton mentagrophytes*, *T. rubrum*, *Epidermophyton floccosum*, or *Microsporum canis*; treatment of pityriasis versicolor caused by *Malassezia* species; treatment of cutaneous candidiasis caused by *Candida albicans*

Gel: Treatment of tinea corporis and interdigital tinea pedis; treatment of seborrheic dermatitis of the scalp

Shampoo: Treatment of seborrheic dermatitis of the scalp

Solution (lacquer): Treatment of mild to moderate onychomycosis of fingernails and toenails (not involving the lunula) and the immediately adjacent skin caused by *T. rubrum*

Pregnancy Risk Factor B

Pregnancy Considerations Teratogenic effects were not observed in animal studies, however, there are no adequate and well-controlled studies in pregnant women. Use during pregnancy only if clearly needed.

Breast-Feeding Considerations It is not known if ciclopirox is excreted in breast milk. The manufacturer recommends that caution be exercised when administering ciclopirox to nursing women.

Contraindications Hypersensitivity to ciclopirox or any component of the formulation

Warnings/Precautions For external use only; avoid contact with eyes or mucous membranes. Use of occlusive dressings or wrappings should be avoided. Nail lacquer is for topical use only and has not been studied in conjunction with systemic therapy or in patients with type 1 diabetes mellitus (insulin dependent, IDDM). Use has not been evaluated in immunosuppressed or immunocompromised patients. Discontinue treatment if signs and/or symptoms of hypersensitivity are noted.

Benzyl alcohol and derivatives: Some dosage forms may contain benzyl alcohol; large amounts of benzyl alcohol (≥99 mg/kg/day) have been associated with a potentially fatal toxicity ("gasping syndrome") in neonates; the "gasping syndrome" consists of metabolic acidosis, respiratory distress, gasping respirations, CNS dysfunction (including convulsions, intracranial hemorrhage), hypotension and cardiovascular collapse (AAP, 1997; CDC, 1982); some data suggests that benzoate displaces bilirubin from protein binding sites (Ahlfors, 2001); avoid or use dosage forms containing benzyl alcohol with caution in neonates. See manufacturer's labeling.

Warnings: Additional Pediatric Considerations Some dosage forms may contain propylene glycol; in neonates large amounts of propylene glycol delivered orally, intravenously (eg, >3,000 mg/day), or topically have been associated with potentially fatal toxicities which can include metabolic acidosis, seizures, renal failure, and CNS depression; toxicities have also been reported in children and adults including hyperosmolality, lactic acidosis, seizures and respiratory depression; use caution (AAP, 1997; Shehab, 2009).

Adverse Reactions

Cardiovascular: Ventricular tachycardia (shampoo)

Central nervous system: Headache

Dermatologic: Acne, alopecia, contact dermatitis, dry skin, erythema, facial edema, hair discoloration (rare; shampoo formulation in light-haired individuals), nail disorder (shape or color change with lacquer), pruritus, rash

Local: Burning sensation, irritation, pain, or redness

Ocular: Eye pain

Drug Interactions

Metabolism/Transport Effects None known.

Avoid Concomitant Use There are no known interactions where it is recommended to avoid concomitant use.

Increased Effect/Toxicity There are no known significant interactions involving an increase in effect.

Decreased Effect There are no known significant interactions involving a decrease in effect.

Storage/Stability

Cream, shampoo, suspension: Store at 20°C to 25°C (68°F to 77°F).

Lacquer (solution): Store at room temperature of 15°C to 30°C (59°F to 86°F). Flammable; keep away from heat and flame.

Gel: Store at 15°C to 30°C (59°F to 86°F).

Mechanism of Action Inhibiting transport of essential elements in the fungal cell disrupting the synthesis of DNA, RNA, and protein

Pharmacokinetics (Adult data unless noted)

Absorption: Topical: Rapid but minimal with intact skin

Distribution: Present in stratum corneum, dermis, sebaceous glands, nails

Protein binding: 94% to 98%

Metabolism: Conjugated with glucuronic acid

Half-life:

Ciclopirox olamine: 1.7 hours

Ciclopirox gel: 5.5 hours

Elimination: Urine

Dosing: Usual Topical:

Children >10 years, Adolescents, and Adults: Tinea pedis, tinea cruris, tinea corporis, tinea versicolor, and cutaneous candidiasis: Cream/suspension: Apply twice daily for 4 weeks (4-6 weeks for tinea cruris; 2 weeks for tinea versicolor if response is adequate). If no improvement after 4 weeks of treatment, re-evaluate diagnosis.

Children ≥12 years, Adolescents, and Adults: Solution (lacquer): Apply daily as part of a comprehensive management program for onychomycosis; remove with alcohol every 7 days; 48 weeks of continuous therapy may be needed to achieve clear nails

Children >16 years, Adolescents, and Adults:
Tinea pedis, tinea corporis: Gel: Apply twice daily. If no improvement after 4 weeks of treatment, re-evaluate diagnosis.
Seborrheic dermatitis of the scalp:
Gel: Apply twice daily. If no improvement after 4 weeks of treatment, re-evaluate diagnosis.
Shampoo: Apply ~5 mL to wet hair; may use up to 10 mL for longer hair; repeat twice weekly for 4 weeks; allow a minimum of 3 days between applications. If no improvement after 4 weeks of treatment, re-evaluate diagnosis.

Administration Topical:
Cream, gel, suspension: Gently massage into affected areas and surrounding skin.
Lotion: Shake lotion vigorously before application.
Shampoo: Apply to wet hair and scalp, lather, and leave in place ~3 minutes; rinse thoroughly.
Solution (lacquer): Apply evenly over the entire nail plate and 5 mm of surrounding skin using the applicator brush; allow to dry for 30 seconds; apply at bedtime (or allow 8 hours before washing). Solution can be reapplied daily over previous applications; remove with alcohol every 7 days. Avoid contact with eyes and mucous membranes; do not administer orally or intravaginally. Do not occlude affected area with dressings or wrappings.

Monitoring Parameters Resolution of skin or nail infection

Dosage Forms Excipient information presented when available (limited, particularly for generics); consult specific product labeling. [DSC] = Discontinued product
Cream, External, as olamine:
Ciclodan: 0.77% (90 g) [contains benzyl alcohol, cetyl alcohol]
Generic: 0.77% (15 g, 30 g, 90 g)
Gel, External:
Loprox: 0.77% (100 g [DSC]) [contains isopropyl alcohol]
Generic: 0.77% (30 g, 45 g, 100 g)
Kit, External:
Ciclodan Cream: 0.77% [contains benzyl alcohol, cetyl alcohol, edetate disodium, propylene glycol]
Ciclodan Solution: 8% [contains edetate disodium, isopropyl alcohol, menthol]
Ciclopirox Treatment: 8% [contains edetate disodium, isopropyl alcohol, menthol]
CNL8 Nail: 8% [contains isopropyl alcohol]
Pedipirox-4 Nail: 8% [DSC] [contains isopropyl alcohol]
Generic: 8 %
Shampoo, External:
Loprox: 1% (120 mL)
Generic: 1% (120 mL)
Solution, External:
Ciclodan: 8% (6.6 mL) [contains isopropyl alcohol]
Penlac: 8% (6.6 mL) [contains ethyl acetate, isopropyl alcohol]
Generic: 8% (6.6 mL)
Suspension, External, as olamine:
Generic: 0.77% (30 mL, 60 mL)

◆ **Ciclopirox Olamine** *see* Ciclopirox *on page 458*
◆ **Ciclopirox Treatment** *see* Ciclopirox *on page 458*
◆ **Ciclosporin** *see* CycloSPORINE (Ophthalmic) *on page 561*
◆ **Ciclosporin** *see* CycloSPORINE (Systemic) *on page 556*
◆ **Cidecin** *see* DAPTOmycin *on page 582*

Cidofovir (si DOF o veer)

Related Information
Safe Handling of Hazardous Drugs *on page 2455*

Brand Names: US Vistide

Therapeutic Category Antiviral Agent, Parenteral

Generic Availability (US) Yes

Use Treatment of cytomegalovirus (CMV) retinitis in patients with acquired immunodeficiency syndrome (AIDS) (FDA approved in adults). Has also been used for treatment of ganciclovir-resistant CMV, foscarnet-resistant CMV, and adenovirus infections in immunocompromised patients; has also been used intralesionally for the treatment of recurrent respiratory papillomatosis

Pregnancy Risk Factor C

Pregnancy Considerations
[US Boxed Warning]: Possibly carcinogenic and teratogenic based on animal data. May cause hypospermia. Women of childbearing potential should use effective contraception during therapy and for 1 month following treatment. Males should use a barrier contraceptive during therapy and for 3 months following treatment.
The indications for treating CMV retinitis during pregnancy are the same as in nonpregnant HIV infected woman; however systemic therapy should be avoided during the first trimester when possible. When therapy is needed to treat maternal infection, agents other than cidofovir are recommended (DHHS [Adult OI 2014]).

Breast-Feeding Considerations It is not known if cidofovir is excreted in breast milk. Due to the potential for serious adverse reactions in the nursing infant, breast-feeding is not recommended. In addition, HIV-infected mothers are discouraged from breast-feeding to decrease the potential transmission of HIV.

Contraindications Hypersensitivity to cidofovir or any component of the formulation; history of clinically-severe hypersensitivity to probenecid or other sulfa-containing medications; serum creatinine >1.5 mg/dL; CrCl ≤55 mL/minute; urine protein ≥100 mg/dL (≥2+ proteinuria); use with or within 7 days of nephrotoxic agents; direct intraocular injection

Warnings/Precautions Hazardous agent - use appropriate precautions for handling and disposal (NIOSH 2014 [group 2]).

[US Boxed Warning]: Acute renal failure resulting in dialysis and/or contributing to death has occurred with as few as 1 or 2 doses of cidofovir. Renal function (serum creatinine and urine protein) must be monitored within 48 hours prior to each dose of cidofovir and the dose of cidofovir modified as appropriate. Administration must be accompanied by oral probenecid and intravenous saline prehydration. Contraindicated in patients with a baseline serum creatinine >1.5 mg/dL, CrCl ≤55 mL/minute, or urine protein ≥100 mg/dL (≥2+ proteinuria); dosage adjustment or discontinuation of therapy may be required for changes in renal function during treatment. **[US Boxed Warning]: Neutropenia has been reported; monitor neutrophil counts during therapy.** Monitor for signs of metabolic acidosis; decreased sodium bicarbonate with proximal tubule injury and renal wasting syndrome (including Fanconi syndrome), as well as metabolic acidosis with hepatic impairment and pancreatitis (including some fatal cases) have been reported. **[US Boxed Warning]: Possibly carcinogenic and teratogenic based on animal data. May cause hypospermia. [US Boxed Warning]: Indicated only for CMV retinitis treatment in patients with AIDS.** For intravenous use only, **not** for direct intraocular injection; iritis, ocular hypotony, and permanent impairment of vision may occur. Decreased intraocular pressure, sometimes associated with decreased visual acuity, uveitis, or iritis may occur; monitor intraocular pressure for and signs of iritis/uveitis during therapy. If uveitis or iritis occurs, consider treatment with topical corticosteroids with or without topical cycloplegic agents.

Warnings: Additional Pediatric Considerations Administration in children warrants extreme caution due to risk of long-term carcinogenicity and reproductive toxicity. A case of invasive squamous cell cancer has been reported in a pediatric patient receiving intralesional cidofovir for severe, recurrent respiratory papillomatosis; causality not established (Lott, 2009).

Adverse Reactions

Cardiovascular: Cardiomyopathy, cardiovascular disorder, CHF, edema, orthostatic hypotension, shock, syncope, tachycardia

Central nervous system: Agitation, amnesia, anxiety, chills, confusion, convulsion, dizziness, fever, hallucinations, headache, insomnia, malaise, pain, vertigo

Dermatologic: Alopecia, photosensitivity reaction, skin discoloration, urticaria

Endocrine & metabolic: Adrenal cortex insufficiency

Gastrointestinal: Abdominal pain, anorexia, aphthous stomatitis, colitis, constipation, diarrhea, dysphagia, fecal incontinence, gastritis, GI hemorrhage, gingivitis, melena, nausea, proctitis, splenomegaly, stomatitis, tongue discoloration, vomiting

Genitourinary: Urinary incontinence

Hematologic: Anemia, hypochromic anemia, leukocytosis, leukopenia, lymphadenopathy, lymphoma-like reaction, neutropenia, pancytopenia, thrombocytopenia, thrombocytopenic purpura

Local: Injection site reaction

Neuromuscular & skeletal: Tremor, weakness

Ocular: Amblyopia, blindness, cataract, conjunctivitis, corneal lesion, diplopia, intraocular pressure decreased, iritis, ocular hypotony, uveitis, vision abnormal

Otic: Hearing loss

Renal: Creatinine increased, Fanconi syndrome, proteinuria, renal toxicity

Respiratory: Cough, dyspnea, pneumonia

Rare but important or life-threatening: Hepatic failure, metabolic acidosis, pancreatitis

Miscellaneous: Allergic reaction, infection, oral moniliasis, sepsis, serum bicarbonate decreased

Drug Interactions

Metabolism/Transport Effects None known.

Avoid Concomitant Use There are no known interactions where it is recommended to avoid concomitant use.

Increased Effect/Toxicity

Cidofovir may increase the levels/effects of: Tenofovir

Decreased Effect There are no known significant interactions involving a decrease in effect.

Storage/Stability Store intact vials at 20°C to 25°C (68°F to 77°F). Admixtures may be stored for ≤24 hours under refrigeration; however, admixtures must be administered within 24 hours of preparation.

Mechanism of Action Cidofovir is converted to cidofovir diphosphate (the active intracellular metabolite); cidofovir diphosphate suppresses CMV replication by selective inhibition of viral DNA synthesis. Incorporation of cidofovir diphosphate into growing viral DNA chain results in viral DNA synthesis rate reduction.

Pharmacokinetics (Adult data unless noted) Note: Pharmcokinetic data is based on a combination of cidofovir administered with probenecid.

Distribution: V_d: 0.54 L/kg; does not cross significantly into the CSF

Protein binding: <6%

Metabolism: Minimal; Phosphorylated intracellularly to the active metabolite cidofovir diphosphate

Half-life: ~2.6 hours (cidofovir); 17 hours (cidofovir diphosphate)

Elimination: Renal tubular secretion and glomerular filtration

Renal clearance without probenecid: 150 ± 26.9 mL/minute/1.73 m^2

Renal clearance with probenecid: 98.6 ± 27.9 mL/minute/1.73 m^2

Dosing: Usual

Pediatric: **Note:** Administration of cidofovir should be accompanied by concomitant oral probenecid and intravenous normal saline hydration; various regimens have been reported (Anderson, 2008; Bhadri, 2009; Cesaro, 2005; Doan, 2007; Williams, 2009)

Hydration: IV: 20 mL/kg of 0.9% sodium chloride (maximum: 1000 mL) administered for 1 hour before cidofovir infusion and 20 mL/kg of 0.9% sodium chloride (maximum: 1000 mL) over 1 hour during cidofovir infusion, followed by 2 hours of maintenance fluids **or** increase the maintenance fluid infusion rate to 3 times the maintenance rate for 1 hour before cidofovir infusion and continuing until 1 hour after, then decrease to 2 times the maintenance fluid rate for the subsequent 2 hours

Probenecid: Oral: 25-40 mg/kg/dose (maximum dose: 2000 mg) administered 3 hours before cidofovir infusion and 10-20 mg/kg/dose (maximum dose: 1000 mg) at 2-3 hours and 8-9 hours after cidofovir infusion **or** 1-2 g/m^2/dose administered 3 hours prior to cidofovir, followed by 0.5-1.25 g/m^2/dose 1-2 hours and 8 hours after completion

Adenovirus infection, posthematopoietic stem cell transplant; treatment: IV: Limited data available; specific regimens may vary (Legrand, 2001; Ljungman, 2003; Yusuf, 2006): Infants, Children, and Adolescents:

Induction: 5 mg/kg/dose once weekly for 2 consecutive weeks (with hydration and probenecid)

Maintenance: 5 mg/kg/dose once every 2 weeks (with hydration and probenecid) until consecutive negative adenovirus samples. **Note:** Patients requiring longer treatment courses have been switched to 1 mg/kg/dose given 3 times/week (Bhadri, 2009)

Adenovirus infection, postlung transplant; treatment: Very limited data available: Infants ≥6 months and Children <3 years: IV: 1 mg/kg/dose every other day or 3 times weekly for 4 consecutive weeks (with hydration and probenecid); dosing from a case series (n=4, age range: 0.5-2.6 years) (Doan, 2007)

BK virus allograft nephropathy: Limited data available: Children and Adolescents: IV: Initial dose: 0.25 mg/kg/dose every 2-3 weeks; dose may be increased if BK virus PCR counts do not decrease 1 log fold to a maximum dose of 1 mg/kg/dose. Dosing based on reported experience from two case series of 11 renal transplant patients (ages 4-20 years). The reported hydration was $D_5$1/2NS or $D_5$1/4NS for 2 hours before cidofovir and for 2 hours following the infusion; cidofovir was infused over 2 hours and no probenecid was used (Araya, 2008; Araya, 2010).

BK virus hemorrhagic cystitis after stem cell or bone marrow transplant: Limited data available; optimal dose not established: Children and Adolescents: IV: 5 mg/kg/dose once weekly for 2-4 weeks, followed by 5 mg/kg/dose every other week given with probenecid and adequate hydration until cystitis resolved is the most commonly reported dose (Cesaro, 2009, Gaziev, 2010, Megged, 2011). Others have described lower doses of 0.5-1 mg/kg/dose given once weekly with or without probenecid (Faraci, 2009; Cesaro, 2009; Cesaro, 2013).

Cytomegalovirus (CMV) infection: Limited data available. IV:

Allogeneic stem cell transplantation recipients: Treatment: Children and Adolescents: Dosing based on reported experience in 30 pediatric patients (2-14 years) as second-line therapy following allogeneic stem cell transplantation (Cesaro, 2005).

Induction: 5 mg/kg/dose once weekly for 2 consecutive weeks (with hydration, probenecid and antiemetic)
Maintenance: 3-5 mg/kg/dose once every 2 weeks for 2-4 doses (with hydration, probenecid and antiemetic)
HIV-exposed/-positive patients:
CMV retinitis:
Treatment: Adolescents [DHHS (adult), 2013]:
Induction: 5 mg/kg/dose once weekly for 2 consecutive weeks (with hydration and probenecid)
Maintenance: 5 mg/kg/dose every other week (with hydration and probenecid)
Secondary prophylaxis: 5 mg/kg/dose every other week (with hydration and probenecid) [DHHS (adult/pediatric), 2013]
Respiratory papillomatosis, recurrent: Intralesional: 7.5 mg/mL every 2 weeks until complete remission (Naiman, 2006)
Adults:
Cytomegalovirus (CMV) retinitis: Note: Administration of cidofovir should be accompanied by concomitant oral probenecid and intravenous normal saline hydration; administer 2000 mg probenecid orally 3 hours prior to each cidofovir dose and 1000 mg at 2 and 8 hours after completion of the cidofovir infusion (total probenecid dose: 4000 mg); infuse one liter NS over 1-2 hours prior to the cidofovir infusion; may administer second liter of NS over 1-3 hours with or immediately after the cidofovir infusion if tolerated
Induction: IV: 5 mg/kg/dose once weekly for 2 consecutive weeks
Maintenance: IV: 5 mg/kg/dose once every other week
Dosing adjustment in renal impairment: High flux hemodialysis removes ~75%
Infants ≥6 months, Children, and Adolescents If the S_{cr} >1.5 mg/dL, CrCl <90 mL/minute/1.73 m^2, and >2+ proteinuria, the following dosing has been used for treatment of adenovirus post-transplant (Yusuf, 2006):
IV:
Induction: 1 mg/kg/dose 3 times weekly on alternate days for 2 consecutive weeks
Maintenance: 1 mg/kg/dose every other week
Adults:
Preexisting renal impairment: Initiation of cidofovir is contraindicated for Cr >1.5 mg/dL, CrCl ≤55 mL/minute or a urine protein ≥100 mg/dL (≥2+ proteinuria)
During therapy: If the serum creatinine increases by 0.3-0.4 mg/dL above baseline, reduce the cidofovir dose to 3 mg/kg; discontinue cidofovir therapy for increases ≥0.5 mg/dL above baseline or development of ≥3+ proteinuria.
Dosing adjustment in hepatic impairment: There are no dosage adjustments provided in the manufacturer's labeling.

Preparation for Administration Hazardous agent; use appropriate precautions for handling and disposal (NIOSH 2014 [group 2]).
Parenteral: Intermittent infusion: Dilute in 100 mL NS (per manufacturer) or to a final concentration not to exceed 8 mg/mL (Ennis 1997); stability also reported in D_5W
Intralesional: In pediatric trials, has been administered as solution with final concentration of 5 to 10 mg/mL (Bielecki 2009; Naiman 2006).

Administration Hazardous agent; use appropriate precautions for handling and disposal (NIOSH 2014 [group 2]). Do **not** administer by direct intraocular injection due to risk of iritis, ocular hypotony, and permanent visual impairment.
Parenteral: Administer by IV infusion over 1 hour.

Monitoring Parameters Monitor renal function (BUN, serum creatinine) within 48 hours prior to each dose, urinalysis (urine glucose and protein), CBC with differential (neutrophil count) prior to each dose, electrolytes (calcium, magnesium, phosphorus, uric acid), liver function tests (SGOT/SGPT), intraocular pressure and visual acuity

Dosage Forms Excipient information presented when available (limited, particularly for generics); consult specific product labeling.
Solution, Intravenous:
Vistide: 75 mg/mL (5 mL)
Solution, Intravenous [preservative free]:
Generic: 75 mg/mL (5 mL)

◆ **Cilastatin and Imipenem** *see* Imipenem and Cilastatin *on page 1083*

◆ **Ciloxan** *see* Ciprofloxacin (Ophthalmic) *on page 467*

Cimetidine (sye MET i deen)

Medication Safety Issues
Sound-alike/look-alike issues:
Cimetidine may be confused with simethicone

Brand Names: US Cimetidine Acid Reducer [OTC]; Tagamet HB [OTC]

Brand Names: Canada Apo-Cimetidine; Dom-Cimetidine; Mylan-Cimetidine; Novo-Cimetidine; Nu-Cimet; PMS-Cimetidine

Therapeutic Category Gastrointestinal Agent, Gastric or Duodenal Ulcer Treatment; Histamine H_2 Antagonist

Generic Availability (US) Yes

Use Short-term treatment of active duodenal ulcers and benign gastric ulcers; long-term prophylaxis of duodenal ulcer; gastric hypersecretory states; gastroesophageal reflux (GERD); over-the-counter (OTC) formulation for relief of acid indigestion, heartburn, or sour stomach

Pregnancy Risk Factor B

Pregnancy Considerations Teratogenic effects were not observed in animal reproduction studies; therefore, cimetidine is classified as pregnancy category B. Cimetidine crosses the placenta. An increased risk of congenital malformations or adverse events in the newborn has generally not been observed following maternal use of cimetidine during pregnancy. Histamine H_2 antagonists have been evaluated for the treatment of gastroesophageal reflux disease (GERD), as well as gastric and duodenal ulcers during pregnancy. Although if needed, cimetidine is not the agent of choice. Histamine H_2 antagonists may be used for aspiration prophylaxis prior to cesarean delivery.

Breast-Feeding Considerations Cimetidine is excreted into breast milk. The concentration of cimetidine in maternal serum in comparison to breast milk is highly variable. Breast-feeding is not recommended by the manufacturer. Consider the renal function of the breast-feeding infant.

Contraindications Hypersensitivity to cimetidine, any component of the formulation, or other H_2 antagonists

Warnings/Precautions Reversible confusional states, usually clearing within 3-4 days after discontinuation, have been linked to use. Increased age (>50 years) and renal or hepatic impairment are thought to be associated. Use caution in the elderly due to risk of confusion and other CNS effects. Dosage should be adjusted in renal/hepatic impairment or in patients receiving drugs metabolized through the P450 system.

Prolonged treatment (≥2 years) may lead to vitamin B_{12} malabsorption and subsequent vitamin B_{12} deficiency. The magnitude of the deficiency is dose-related and the association is stronger in females and those younger in age (<30 years); prevalence is decreased after discontinuation of therapy (Lam, 2013).

Over the counter (OTC) cimetidine should not be taken by individuals experiencing painful swallowing, vomiting with blood, or bloody or black stools; medical attention should be sought. A physician should be consulted prior to use when pain in the stomach, shoulder, arms or neck is present; if heartburn has occurred for >3 months; or if unexplained weight loss, or nausea and vomiting occur. Frequent wheezing, shortness of breath, lightheadedness, or sweating, especially with chest pain or heartburn, should also be reported. Consultation of a healthcare provider should occur by patients if also taking theophylline, phenytoin, or warfarin; if heartburn or stomach pain continues or worsens; or if use is required for >14 days. Symptoms of GI distress may be associated with a variety of conditions; symptomatic response to H_2 antagonists does not rule out the potential for significant pathology (eg, malignancy). OTC cimetidine is not approved for use in patients <12 years of age.

Warnings: Additional Pediatric Considerations Use of gastric acid inhibitors, including proton pump inhibitors and H_2 blockers, has been associated with an increased risk for development of acute gastroenteritis and community-acquired pneumonia in pediatric patients (Canani, 2006). A large epidemiological study has suggested an increased risk for developing pneumonia in patients receiving H_2 receptor antagonists; however, a causal relationship with ranitidine has not been demonstrated. A cohort analysis including over 11,000 neonates reported an association of H_2 blocker use and an increased incidence of NEC in VLBW neonates (Guillet, 2006). An approximate sixfold increase in mortality, NEC, and infection (ie, sepsis, pneumonia, UTI) was reported in patients receiving ranitidine in a cohort analysis of 274 VLBW neonates (Terrin, 2011).

Adverse Reactions

Cardiovascular: Atrioventricular block, bradycardia, hypotension, tachycardia, vasculitis

Central nervous system: Agitation, confusion, decreased sexual activity, dizziness, drowsiness, headache

Dermatologic: Alopecia, erythema multiforme, exfoliative dermatitis, skin rash, Stevens-Johnson syndrome, toxic epidermal necrolysis

Endocrine & metabolic: Gynecomastia

Gastrointestinal: Diarrhea, nausea, pancreatitis, vomiting

Genitourinary: Breast swelling

Hematologic & oncologic: Agranulocytosis, aplastic anemia, hemolytic anemia (immune-based), neutropenia, pancytopenia, thrombocytopenia

Hepatic: Hepatic fibrosis (case report), increased serum ALT, increased serum AST

Neuromuscular & skeletal: Arthralgia, myalgia, polymyositis

Renal: Increased serum creatinine, interstitial nephritis

Respiratory: Pneumonia (causal relationship not established)

Miscellaneous: Fever

Drug Interactions

Metabolism/Transport Effects Substrate of OAT3, OCT2, P-glycoprotein; **Inhibits** CYP1A2 (weak), CYP2C19 (moderate), CYP2C9 (weak), CYP2D6 (moderate), CYP2E1 (weak), CYP3A4 (weak)

Avoid Concomitant Use

Avoid concomitant use of Cimetidine with any of the following: Dasatinib; Delavirdine; Dofetilide; EPIrubicin; PAZOPanib; Pimozide; Risedronate; Thioridazine

Increased Effect/Toxicity

Cimetidine may increase the levels/effects of: Alfentanil; Amiodarone; ARIPiprazole; Bromazepam; Calcium Channel Blockers; Capecitabine; CarBAMazepine; Carmustine; Carvedilol; Cilostazol; Cisapride; Citalopram; CloZAPine; CYP2C19 Substrates; CYP2D6 Substrates; Dalfampridine; Dexmethylphenidate; Dofetilide; DOXOrubicin (Conventional); Eliglustat; EPIrubicin; Escitalopram; Fesoterodine; Floxuridine; Fluorouracil (Systemic); Fosphenytoin-Phenytoin; Hydrocodone; Lomitapide; Mebendazole; MetFORMIN; Methylphenidate; Metoprolol; Moclobemide; Nebivolol; Nicotine; Pentoxifylline; Pimozide; Pramipexole; Praziquantel; Procainamide; Propafenone; QuiNIDine; QuiNINE; Risedronate; Roflumilast; Saquinavir; Selective Serotonin Reuptake Inhibitors; Sulfonylureas; Tamsulosin; Tegafur; Theophylline Derivatives; Thioridazine; TiZANidine; Tricyclic Antidepressants; Varenicline; Vitamin K Antagonists; Zaleplon; ZOLMitriptan

The levels/effects of Cimetidine may be increased by: AtorvaSTATin; BuPROPion; P-glycoprotein/ABCB1 Inhibitors; Teriflunomide

Decreased Effect

Cimetidine may decrease the levels/effects of: Atazanavir; Bosutinib; Cefditoren; Cefpodoxime; Cefuroxime; Clopidogrel; Codeine; Dabrafenib; Dasatinib; Delavirdine; Erlotinib; Fosamprenavir; Gefitinib; Indinavir; Iron Salts; Itraconazole; Ketoconazole (Systemic); Ledipasvir; Mesalamine; Multivitamins/Minerals (with ADEK, Folate, Iron); Nelfinavir; Nilotinib; PAZOPanib; Posaconazole; Rilpivirine; Tamoxifen; TraMADol

The levels/effects of Cimetidine may be decreased by: P-glycoprotein/ABCB1 Inducers

Food Interactions Prolonged treatment (≥2 years) may lead to malabsorption of dietary vitamin B_{12} and subsequent vitamin B_{12} deficiency (Lam, 2013).

Storage/Stability Tablet: Store between 15°C and 30°C (59°F to 86°F). Protect from light.

Mechanism of Action Competitive inhibition of histamine at H_2 receptors of the gastric parietal cells resulting in reduced gastric acid secretion, gastric volume and hydrogen ion concentration reduced

Pharmacokinetics (Adult data unless noted)

Distribution: Crosses the placenta; breast milk to plasma ratio: 4.6-11.76

Protein binding: 13% to 25%

Metabolism: Hepatic with a sulfoxide as the major metabolite

Bioavailability: 60% to 70%

Half-life:

- Neonates: 3.6 hours
- Children: 1.4 hours
- Adults with normal renal function: 2 hours

Time to peak serum concentration: Oral: 45-90 minutes

Elimination: Primarily in urine (48% unchanged drug); some excretion in bile and feces

Dosing: Neonatal Oral: 5-10 mg/kg/day in divided doses every 8-12 hours

Dosing: Usual Oral:

Infants: 10-20 mg/kg/day divided every 6-12 hours

Children: 20-40 mg/kg/day in divided doses every 6 hours

Adults:

- Short-term treatment of active ulcers: 300 mg 4 times/day or 800 mg at bedtime or 400 mg twice daily for up to 8 weeks
- Duodenal ulcer prophylaxis: 400-800 mg at bedtime
- Gastric hypersecretory conditions: 300-600 mg every 6 hours; dosage not to exceed 2.4 g/day
- GERD: 800 mg twice daily or 400 mg 4 times/day for 12 weeks
- Acid indigestion, heartburn, sour stomach relief (OTC use): 100 mg right before or up to 30 minutes before a meal; no more than 2 tablets per day

Dosing interval in renal impairment using 5-10 mg/kg/dose in children or 300 mg in adults (titrate dose to gastric pH and CrCl):

- CrCl >40 mL/minute: Administer every 6 hours
- CrCl 20-40 mL/minute: Administer every 8 hours or reduce dose by 25%
- CrCl <20 mL/minute: Administer every 12 hours or reduce dose by 50%

Hemodialysis: Administer after dialysis and every 12 hours during the interdialysis period

Dosing adjustment in hepatic impairment: Reduce dosage in severe liver disease

Administration Administer with food; do not administer with antacids

Monitoring Parameters CBC, gastric pH, occult blood with GI bleeding; monitor renal function to correct dose

Dosage Forms Excipient information presented when available (limited, particularly for generics); consult specific product labeling.

Solution, Oral, as hydrochloride [strength expressed as base]:
Generic: 300 mg/5 mL (237 mL, 240 mL)

Tablet, Oral:
Cimetidine Acid Reducer: 200 mg
Tagamet HB: 200 mg
Generic: 200 mg, 300 mg, 400 mg, 800 mg

Extemporaneous Preparations Note: Commercial oral solution is available (strength expressed as base: 60 mg/mL)

A 60 mg/mL oral suspension may be made with tablets. Place twenty-four 300 mg tablets in 5 mL of sterile water for ~3-5 minutes to dissolve film coating. Crush tablets in a mortar and reduce to a fine powder. Add 10 mL of glycerin and mix to a uniform paste; mix while adding Simple Syrup, NF in incremental proportions to **almost** 120 mL; transfer to a calibrated bottle, rinse mortar with vehicle, and add quantity of vehicle sufficient to make 120 mL. Label "shake well" and "refrigerate". Stable for 17 days.

Nahata MC, Pai VB, and Hipple TF, *Pediatric Drug Formulations*, 5th ed, Cincinnati, OH: Harvey Whitney Books Co, 2004.

◆ **Cimetidine Acid Reducer [OTC]** *see* Cimetidine *on page 461*

◆ **Cinryze** *see* C1 Inhibitor (Human) *on page 333*

◆ **Cipralex (Can)** *see* Escitalopram *on page 786*

◆ **Cipralex MELTZ (Can)** *see* Escitalopram *on page 786*

◆ **Cipro** *see* Ciprofloxacin (Systemic) *on page 463*

◆ **Cipro XL (Can)** *see* Ciprofloxacin (Systemic) *on page 463*

◆ **Ciprodex** *see* Ciprofloxacin and Dexamethasone *on page 469*

Ciprofloxacin (Systemic) (sip roe FLOKS a sin)

Medication Safety Issues

Sound-alike/look-alike issues:
Ciprofloxacin may be confused with cephalexin
Cipro may be confused with Ceftin

Brand Names: US Cipro; Cipro in D5W; Cipro XR

Brand Names: Canada ACT Ciprofloxacin; Apo-Ciproflox; Auro-Ciprofloxacin; Cipro; Cipro XL; Ciprofloxacin Injection; Ciprofloxacin Injection USP; Ciprofloxacin Intravenous Infusion; Ciprofloxacin Intravenous Infusion BP; Dom-Ciprofloxacin; JAMP-Ciprofloxacin; Mar-Ciprofloxacin; Mint-Ciproflox; Mint-Ciprofloxacin; Mylan-Ciprofloxacin; PHL-Ciprofloxacin; PMS-Ciprofloxacin; PMS-Ciprofloxacin XL; PRO-Ciprofloxacin; RAN-Ciproflox; ratio-Ciprofloxacin; Riva-Ciprofloxacin; Sandoz-Ciprofloxacin; Septa-Ciprofloxacin; Taro-Ciprofloxacin; Teva-Ciprofloxacin

Therapeutic Category Antibiotic, Quinolone

Generic Availability (US) Yes

Use Treatment of documented or suspected pseudomonal infection of the respiratory or urinary tract, skin and soft tissue, and bone and joint; treatment of complicated UTIs and pyelonephritis in children 1-17 years of age due to *E. coli*; documented multidrug-resistant, aerobic gram-negative bacilli, some gram-positive staphylococci, and *Mycobacterium tuberculosis*; documented infectious diarrhea due to *Campylobacter jejuni*, *Shigella*, or *E. coli*; typhoid fever caused by *Salmonella typhi*; osteomyelitis caused by susceptible organisms in which parenteral therapy is not feasible; uncomplicated cervical and urethral gonorrhea due to *N. gonorrhoeae*; chronic bacterial prostatitis caused by *E. coli* or *Proteus mirabilis*; pulmonary exacerbation of cystic fibrosis; empiric therapy for febrile neutropenia in combination with piperacillin; initial therapy or postexposure prophylaxis for inhalational anthrax; extended release tablet is used for the treatment of UTI and acute uncomplicated pyelonephritis caused by susceptible *E. coli* and *Klebsiella pneumoniae*

Medication Guide Available Yes

Pregnancy Risk Factor C

Pregnancy Considerations Adverse events have been observed in some animal reproduction studies. Ciprofloxacin crosses the placenta and produces measurable concentrations in the amniotic fluid and cord serum (Ludlam 1997). Based on available data, an increased risk of teratogenic effects has not been observed following ciprofloxacin use during pregnancy (Bar-Oz 2009; Padberg 2014). Ciprofloxacin is recommended for prophylaxis and treatment of pregnant women exposed to anthrax (Meaney-Delman 2014). Serum concentrations of ciprofloxacin may be lower during pregnancy than in nonpregnant patients (Giamarellou 1989).

Breast-Feeding Considerations Ciprofloxacin is excreted in breast milk. Due to the potential for serious adverse reactions in the nursing infant, the manufacturer recommends a decision be made whether to discontinue nursing or to discontinue the drug, taking into account the importance of treatment to the mother. However infant serum levels were undetectable (<0.03 mcg/mL) in one report (Gardner 1992). There has been a single case report of perforated pseudomembranous colitis in a breast-feeding infant whose mother was taking ciprofloxacin (Harmon 1992). Ciprofloxacin is recommended for the prophylaxis and treatment of *Bacillus anthracis* in lactating women (Meaney-Delman 2014).

Contraindications Hypersensitivity to ciprofloxacin, any component of the formulation, or other quinolones; concurrent administration of tizanidine

Warnings/Precautions [US Boxed Warning]: There have been reports of tendon inflammation and/or rupture with quinolone antibiotics in all ages; risk may be increased with concurrent corticosteroids, solid organ transplant recipients, and in patients >60 years of age. Rupture of the Achilles tendon sometimes requiring surgical repair has been reported most frequently; but other tendon sites (eg, rotator cuff, biceps) have also been reported. Strenuous physical activity, rheumatoid arthritis, and renal impairment may be an independent risk factor for tendonitis. Inflammation and rupture may occur bilaterally. Cases have been reported within the first 48 hours, during, and up to several months after discontinuation of therapy. Discontinue at first sign of tendon inflammation or pain. Use with caution in patients with rheumatoid arthritis; may increase risk of tendon rupture. Use with caution in patients with a history of tendon disorders.

CNS effects may occur (tremor, restlessness, confusion, and hallucinations, increased intracranial pressure [including pseudotumor cerebri] or seizures). Reactions may occur following the first dose. Use with caution in patients with known or suspected CNS disorder or consider discontinuation if CNS effects develop. Potential for seizures, although very rare, may be increased with concomitant NSAID therapy. Use with caution in individuals at risk of seizures (CNS disorders or concurrent therapy with medications which may lower seizure threshold; status epilepticus has occurred) or if clinically appropriate, consider alternative antimicrobial therapy. Discontinue if seizures occur.

Fluoroquinolones may prolong QTc interval; avoid use in patients with a history of or at risk for QTc prolongation, torsade de pointes, uncorrected hypokalemia, hypomagnesemia, cardiac disease (heart failure, myocardial infarction, bradycardia) or concurrent administration of other medications known to prolong the QT interval (including Class Ia and Class III antiarrhythmics, cisapride, erythromycin, antipsychotics, and tricyclic antidepressants). Hepatocellular, cholestatic, or mixed liver injury has been reported, including hepatic necrosis, life-threatening hepatic events, and fatalities. Acute liver injury can be rapid onset (range: 1-39 days), often associated with hypersensitivity. Most fatalities occurred in patients >55 years of age. Discontinue immediately if signs/symptoms of hepatitis (abdominal tenderness, dark urine, jaundice, pruritus) occur. Additionally, temporary increases in transaminases or alkaline phosphatase or cholestatic jaundice may occur (highest risk in patients with previous liver damage).

Prolonged use may result in fungal or bacterial superinfection, including *C. difficile*-associated diarrhea (CDAD) and pseudomembranous colitis; CDAD has been observed >2 months postantibiotic treatment. Rarely crystalluria has occurred; urine alkalinity may increase the risk. Ensure adequate hydration during therapy. Adverse effects, including those related to joints and/or surrounding tissues, are increased in pediatric patients and therefore, ciprofloxacin should not be considered as drug of choice in children (exception is anthrax treatment). Peripheral neuropathy has been reported (rare); may occur soon after initiation of therapy and may be irreversible; discontinue if symptoms of sensory or sensorimotor neuropathy occur.

Fluoroquinolones have been associated with the development of serious, and sometimes fatal, hypoglycemia, most often in elderly diabetics but also in patients without diabetes. This occurred most frequently with gatifloxacin (no longer available systemically), but may occur at a lower frequency with other quinolones.

Severe hypersensitivity reactions, including anaphylaxis, have occurred with quinolone therapy. Reactions may present as typical allergic symptoms after a single dose, or may manifest as severe idiosyncratic dermatologic, vascular, pulmonary, renal, hepatic, and/or hematologic events, usually after multiple doses. Prompt discontinuation of drug should occur if skin rash or other symptoms arise. **[US Boxed Warning]: Quinolones may exacerbate myasthenia gravis; avoid use (rare, potentially life-threatening weakness of respiratory muscles may occur).** Use caution in renal impairment. Avoid excessive sunlight and take precautions to limit exposure (eg, loose fitting clothing, sunscreen); may cause moderate-to-severe photosensitivity/phototoxicity reactions. Discontinue use if photosensitivity occurs. Since ciprofloxacin is ineffective in the treatment of syphilis and may mask symptoms, all patients should be tested for syphilis at the time of gonorrheal diagnosis and 3 months later. Hemolytic reactions may (rarely) occur with quinolone use in patients with latent or actual glucose-6-phosphate dehydrogenase (G6PD) deficiency.

Potentially significant interactions may exist, requiring dose or frequency adjustment, additional monitoring, and/or selection of alternative therapy. Serious and fatal reactions including seizures, status epilepticus, cardiac arrest and respiratory failure have been reported with concomitant administration of theophylline. If concurrent use is unavoidable, monitor serum theophylline levels and adjust theophylline dose as warranted.

Warnings: Additional Pediatric Considerations

Increased osteochondrosis in immature rats and dogs was observed with ciprofloxacin and fluoroquinolones have caused arthropathy with erosions of the cartilage in weight-bearing joints of immature animals. In an international safety data analysis of ciprofloxacin in approximately 700 pediatric patients (1 to 17 years), the follow-up arthropathy rate at 6 weeks and cumulative arthropathy rate at 1 year were higher in ciprofloxacin treatment group than comparative controls (6 weeks: 9.3% vs 6%; one year: 13.7% to 9.5%). In pediatric patients, fluoroquinolones are not routinely first-line therapy, but after assessment of risks and benefits, can be considered a reasonable alternative for situations where no safe and effective substitute is available [eg, resistance (anthrax, common CF pathogens, multidrug resistant tuberculosis)] or in situations where the only alternative is parenteral therapy and ciprofloxacin offers an oral therapy option (Bradley, 2011). Safety of use in pediatric patients for >14 days of therapy has not been reported; in available pediatric safety data, the typical duration of therapy was approximately 10 days (CAP, AOM) (Bradley, 2011).

Adverse Reactions

Central nervous system: Headache (IV administration), neurological signs and symptoms (children; includes dizziness, insomnia, nervousness, somnolence), restlessness (IV administration)

Dermatologic: Skin rash (more common in children)

Gastrointestinal: Abdominal pain (more common in children), diarrhea (more common in children), dyspepsia (more common in children), nausea, vomiting (more common in children)

Hepatic: Increased serum ALT, increased serum AST (adults)

Local: Injection site reaction (IV administration)

Respiratory: Rhinitis (children)

Miscellaneous: Fever (more common in children)

Rare but important or life-threatening: Abnormal gait, acute generalized exanthematous pustulosis, acute gout attack, acute renal failure, ageusia, agitation, agranulocytosis, albuminuria, anaphylactic shock, anaphylaxis, anemia, angina pectoris, angioedema, anorexia, anosmia, anxiety, arthralgia, ataxia, atrial flutter, bone marrow depression (life-threatening), bronchospasm, candidiasis, candiduria, cardiorespiratory arrest, casts in urine, cerebral thrombosis, chills, cholestatic jaundice, chromatopsia, *Clostridium difficile*-associated diarrhea, confusion, constipation, crystalluria (particularly in alkaline urine), decreased hematocrit, decreased hemoglobin, decreased prothrombin time, delirium, depersonalization, depression (including self-injurious behavior), dizziness, drowsiness, dyspepsia (adults), dysphagia, dysphasia, dyspnea, edema, eosinophilia, erythema multiforme, erythema nodosum, exacerbation of myasthenia gravis, exfoliative dermatitis, fixed drug eruption, flatulence, gastrointestinal hemorrhage, hallucination, headache (oral), hematuria, hemolytic anemia, hepatic failure, hepatic necrosis, hepatotoxicity (idiosyncratic) (Chalasani, 2014), hyperesthesia, hyperglycemia, hyperpigmentation, hypersensitivity reaction, hypertension, hypertonia, hypoglycemia, hypotension, increased blood urea nitrogen, increased creatine phosphokinase, increased INR (in patients treated with vitamin K antagonists), increased intracranial pressure, increased lactate dehydrogenase, increased serum alkaline phosphatase, increased serum bilirubin, increased serum cholesterol, increased serum creatinine, increased serum glucose, increased serum lipase, increased serum triglycerides, increased uric acid, insomnia, interstitial nephritis, intestinal perforation, irritability, jaundice, laryngeal edema, lethargy, lymphadenopathy, malaise, manic behavior, mastalgia, methemoglobinemia, migraine, myalgia, myocardial infarction, myoclonus, nephritis, nephrolithiasis, nightmares, nystagmus, orthostatic hypotension, palpitations, pancreatitis, pancytopenia (life-threatening), paranoia, paresthesia, peripheral neuropathy, petechia, phobia, phototoxicity, pneumonitis, polyneuropathy, prolonged prothrombin time (in patients treated with vitamin K antagonists), pseudotumor cerebri, pulmonary edema, rupture of tendon, seizure (including grand mal), serum sickness-like reaction, skin photosensitivity, status epilepticus, Stevens-Johnson syndrome, suicidal ideation, suicidal tendencies, syncope, tachycardia, tendonitis, thrombocythemia, thrombocytopenia, thrombophlebitis, tinnitus, torsades de pointes, toxic epidermal necrolysis, toxic psychosis, tremor, twitching, unresponsive to stimuli, urethral bleeding, vaginitis, vasculitis, ventricular arrhythmia, ventricular ectopy, visual disturbance, vulvovaginal candidiasis, weakness

Drug Interactions

Metabolism/Transport Effects **Substrate** of OAT3, P-glycoprotein; **Inhibits** CYP1A2 (strong), CYP3A4 (weak)

Avoid Concomitant Use

Avoid concomitant use of Ciprofloxacin (Systemic) with any of the following: Agomelatine; BCG; BCG (Intravesical); CloZAPine; DULoxetine; Highest Risk QTc-Prolonging Agents; Ivabradine; Mifepristone; Pimozide; Pomalidomide; Strontium Ranelate; Tasimelteon; TiZANidine

Increased Effect/Toxicity

Ciprofloxacin (Systemic) may increase the levels/effects of: Agomelatine; ARIPiprazole; Bendamustine; Blood Glucose Lowering Agents; CarBAMazepine; CloZAPine; CYP1A2 Substrates; DULoxetine; Erlotinib; Highest Risk QTc-Prolonging Agents; Hydrocodone; Lomitapide; Methotrexate; Moderate Risk QTc-Prolonging Agents; NiMODipine; Pentoxifylline; Pimozide; Pirfenidone; Pomalidomide; Porfimer; Rasagiline; Roflumilast; ROPINIRole; Ropivacaine; Tasimelteon; Theophylline Derivatives; TiZANidine; Varenicline; Verteporfin; Vitamin K Antagonists

The levels/effects of Ciprofloxacin (Systemic) may be increased by: ACE Inhibitors; Angiotensin II Receptor Blockers; Corticosteroids (Systemic); Fosphenytoin; Ivabradine; Mifepristone; Nonsteroidal Anti-Inflammatory Agents; P-glycoprotein/ABCB1 Inhibitors; Probenecid; QTc-Prolonging Agents (Indeterminate Risk and Risk Modifying); Spironolactone; Teriflunomide

Decreased Effect

Ciprofloxacin (Systemic) may decrease the levels/effects of: BCG; BCG (Intravesical); BCG Vaccine (Immunization); Blood Glucose Lowering Agents; Didanosine; Fosphenytoin; Mycophenolate; Phenytoin; Sodium Picosulfate; Thyroid Products; Typhoid Vaccine

The levels/effects of Ciprofloxacin (Systemic) may be decreased by: Antacids; Calcium Salts; Didanosine; Iron Salts; Lanthanum; Magnesium Salts; Multivitamins/Minerals (with ADEK, Folate, Iron); Multivitamins/Minerals (with AE, No Iron); P-glycoprotein/ABCB1 Inducers; Quinapril; Sevelamer; Strontium Ranelate; Sucralfate; Zinc Salts

Food Interactions Food decreases rate, but not extent, of absorption. Ciprofloxacin serum levels may be decreased if taken with divalent or trivalent cations. Rarely, crystalluria may occur. Enteral feedings may decrease plasma concentrations of ciprofloxacin probably by >30% inhibition of absorption. Management: May administer with food to minimize GI upset. Avoid or take ciprofloxacin 2 hours before or 6 hours after antacids, dairy products, or calcium-fortified juices alone or in a meal containing >800 mg calcium, oral multivitamins, or mineral supplements containing divalent and/or trivalent cations. Ensure adequate hydration during therapy. Ciprofloxacin should not be administered with enteral feedings. The feeding would need to be discontinued for 1-2 hours prior to and after ciprofloxacin administration. Nasogastric administration produces a greater loss of ciprofloxacin bioavailability than does nasoduodenal administration.

Storage/Stability

Injection:

Premixed infusion: Store between 5°C to 25°C (41°F to 77°F); avoid freezing. Protect from light.

Vial: Store between 5°C to 30°C (41°F to 86°F); avoid freezing. Protect from light. Diluted solutions of 0.5-2 mg/mL are stable for up to 14 days refrigerated or at room temperature.

Microcapsules for oral suspension: Prior to reconstitution, store below 25°C (77°F). Protect from freezing. Following reconstitution, store below 30°C (86°F) for up to 14 days. Protect from freezing.

Tablet:

Immediate release: Store between 20°C to 25°C (68°F to 77°F); excursions are permitted between 15°C and 30°C (59°F and 86°F).

Extended release: Store at 25°C (77°F); excursions are permitted between 15°C and 30°C (59°F and 86°F).

Mechanism of Action Inhibits DNA-gyrase in susceptible organisms; inhibits relaxation of supercoiled DNA and promotes breakage of double-stranded DNA

Pharmacokinetics (Adult data unless noted)

Absorption: Oral: Well-absorbed; 500 mg orally every 12 hours produces an equivalent AUC to that produced by 400 mg IV over 60 minutes every 12 hours.

Distribution: Widely distributed into body tissues and fluids with high concentration in bile, saliva, urine, sputum, stool, lungs, liver, skin, muscle, prostate, genital tissue, and bone; low concentration in CSF; crosses the placenta

Protein binding: 16% to 43%

Metabolism: Partially in the liver to four active metabolites

Bioavailability: Oral: 50% to 85%; younger CF patients have a lower bioavailability of 68% vs CF patients >13 years of age with bioavailability of 95%

Half-life:

Children: 4 to 5 hours

Adults with normal renal function: 3 to 5 hours

Time to peak serum concentration: Oral: Immediate release tablet: Within 0.5-2 hours; Extended release tablet: 1 to 4 hours

Elimination: 30% to 50% excreted as unchanged drug in urine via glomerular filtration and active tubular secretion; 20% to 40% excreted in feces primarily from biliary excretion; <1% excreted in bile as unchanged drug

Clearance: After IV:

CF child: 0.84 L/hour/kg

Adult: 0.5 to 0.6 L/hour/kg

Dosing: Neonatal Note: In pediatric patients, ciprofloxacin is not routinely first-line therapy, but after assessment of risks and benefits, can be considered a reasonable alternative for some situations (Bradley, 2011).

Severe infection (eg, sepsis); usually multidrug resistant: Limited data available: IV: 10 mg/kg/dose every 12 hours (Kaguelidou, 2011). A study of 20 neonates (28-36 weeks) showed this dose produced serum concentrations sufficient to treat common gram-negative pathogens. A higher daily dose divided into shorter intervals may be required to achieve serum concentrations sufficient to treat *Staphylococcus aureus* or *Pseudomonas aeruginosa* (Aggarwal, 2004). Reported range: 10 to 60 mg/kg/day (Krcméry, 1999; Schaad, 1995; van den Oever, 1998).

Dosing: Usual

Note: In pediatric patients, ciprofloxacin is not routinely first-line therapy, but after assessment of risks and benefits, can be considered a reasonable alternative for some situations [eg, anthrax, resistance (cystic fibrosis)] or in situations where the only alternative is parenteral therapy and ciprofloxacin offers an oral therapy option (Bradley, 2011).

Note: Extended release tablets and immediate release formulations are not interchangeable. Unless otherwise specified, oral dosing reflects the use of **immediate release** formulation.

Infants, Children, and Adolescents:

General dosing, susceptible infection:

Oral: 20 to 30 mg/kg/day in 2 divided doses; maximum dose: 1.5 g/day

IV: 20 to 30 mg/kg/day divided every 12 hours; maximum dose: 800 mg/day

Inhalational anthrax (postexposure): Initial treatment:

IV: 20 mg/kg/day divided every 12 hours for 60 days; maximum dose: 800 mg/day (substitute oral antibiotics for IV antibiotics as soon as clinical condition improves)

Oral: 30 mg/kg/day divided every 12 hours for 60 days; maximum dose: 1000 mg/day

Complicated UTI or pyelonephritis:

IV: 18 to 30 mg/kg/day divided every 8 hours for 10 to 21 days; maximum dose: 1200 mg/day

Oral: 20 to 40 mg/kg/day divided every 12 hours for 10 to 21 days; maximum dose: 1500 mg/day

Cystic fibrosis:

Oral: 40 mg/kg/day divided every 12 hours; maximum dose: 2 g/day

IV: 30 mg/kg/day divided every 8 to 12 hours; maximum dose: 1.2 g/day

Adults:

Oral: 250 to 750 mg every 12 hours, depending on severity of infection and susceptibility

Acute sinusitis: Mild/moderate: 500 mg every 12 hours for 10 days

Uncomplicated UTI/acute cystitis:

Extended release tablet: 500 mg every 24 hours for 3 days

Immediate release formulation: Acute uncomplicated: 250 mg every 12 hours for 3 days; 250 mg every 12 hours for 7 to 14 days for mild to moderate UTI

Complicated UTI or acute uncomplicated pyelonephritis:

Extended release tablet: 1000 mg every 24 hours for 7 to 14 days

Immediate release formulation: 500 mg every 12 hours for 7 to 14 days

Bone and joint infections:

Mild/moderate: 500 mg every 12 hours for ≥4 to 6 weeks

Severe/complicated: 750 mg every 12 hours for ≥4 to 6 weeks

Chemoprophylaxis regimen for high-risk contacts of invasive meningococcal disease: 500 mg as a single dose

Chronic bacterial prostatitis: 500 mg every 12 hours for 28 days

Infectious diarrhea: 500 mg every 12 hours for 5 to 7 days

Skin and skin structure infections:

Mild/moderate: 500 mg every 12 hours for 7 to 14 days

Severe/complicated: 750 mg every 12 hours for 7 to 14 days

Uncomplicated gonorrhea: 500 mg as a single dose

Chancroid: 500 mg twice daily for 3 days

Lower respiratory tract infection:

Mild/moderate: 500 mg every 12 hours for 7 to 14 days

Severe/complicated: 750 mg every 12 hours for 7 to 14 days

Typhoid fever: 500 mg every 12 hours for 10 days

Inhalational anthrax (postexposure prophylaxis): 500 mg every 12 hours for 60 days

IV: 200-400 mg every 8-12 hours depending on severity of infection

Lower respiratory tract, skin and skin structure infection:

Mild/moderate: 400 mg every 12 hours for 7 to 14 days

Severe/complicated: 400 mg every 8 hours for 7 to 14 days

Treatment of anthrax infection: 400 mg every 12 hours for 60 days (substitute oral antibiotics for IV antibiotics as soon as clinical condition improves)

Empiric therapy in febrile neutropenic patients: 400 mg every 8 hours in combination with piperacillin for 7 to 14 days

Dosing adjustment in renal impairment:

Infants, Children, and Adolescents: Dosage adjustments are not provided in the manufacturer's labeling; however, the following guidelines have been used by some clinicians (Aronoff, 2007): IV, Oral:

GFR ≥30 mL/minute/1.73 m^2: No dosage adjustment necessary

GFR 10 to 29 mL/minute/1.73m^2: 10 to 15 mg/kg/dose every 18 hours

GFR <10 mL/minute/1.73m^2: 10 to 15 mg/kg/dose every 24 hours

Hemodialysis/peritoneal dialysis (PD) (after dialysis on dialysis days): 10 to 15 mg/kg/dose every 24 hours

CRRT: 10 to 15 mg/kg/dose every 12 hours

Adults:

Manufacturer's recommendations:

Oral, immediate release:

CrCl >50 mL/minute: No dosage adjustment necessary

CrCl 30 to 50 mL/minute: Oral: 250 to 500 mg every 12 hours

CrCl 5 to 29 mL/minute: 250 to 500 mg every 18 hours

Hemodialysis/peritoneal dialysis (PD) (administer after dialysis on dialysis days): 250 to 500 mg every 24 hours

Oral, extended release:

CrCl ≥30 mL/minute: No dosage adjustment necessary

CrCl <30 mL/minute: 500 mg every 24 hours

IV:

CrCl ≥30 mL/minute: No dosage adjustment necessary

CrCl 5 to 29 mL/minute: 200 to 400 mg every 18 to 24 hours

Alternate recommendations: Oral (immediate release), IV:

CrCl >50 mL/minute: No dosage adjustment necessary (Aronoff, 2007)

CrCl 10 to 50 mL/minute: Administer 50% to 75% of usual dose every 12 hours (Aronoff, 2007)

CrCl <10 mL/minute: Administer 50% of usual dose every 12 hours (Aronoff, 2007)

Intermittent hemodialysis (IHD) (administer after hemodialysis on dialysis days): Minimally dialyzable (<10%): Oral: 250 to 500 mg every 24 hours or IV: 200 to 400 mg every 24 hours (Heintz, 2009). **Note:** Dosing dependent on the assumption of 3 times/week, complete IHD sessions.

Continuous renal replacement therapy (CRRT) (Heintz, 2009; Trotman, 2005): Drug clearance is highly dependent on the method of renal replacement, filter type, and flow rate. Appropriate dosing requires close monitoring of pharmacologic response, signs of adverse reactions due to drug accumulation, as well as drug concentrations in relation to target trough (if appropriate). The following are general recommendations only (based on dialysate flow/ultrafiltration rates of 1-2 L/hour and minimal residual renal function) and should not supersede clinical judgment:

CVVH/CVVHD/CVVHDF: IV: 200 to 400 mg every 12 to 24 hours

Preparation for Administration

Oral: Reconstitute powder for oral suspension with appropriate amount of water as specified on the bottle. Shake vigorously until suspended.

Parenteral: May be diluted with NS, D_5W, SWFI, $D_{10}W$, $D_5$1/4NS, $D_5$1/2NS, LR to a final concentration not to exceed 2 mg/mL

Administration

Oral: May administer with food to minimize GI upset; divalent and trivalent cations [dairy foods (milk, yogurt) and mineral supplements (eg, iron, zinc, calcium) or calcium-fortified juices] decrease ciprofloxacin absorption; usual dietary calcium intake (including meals which include dairy products) has not been shown to interfere with ciprofloxacin absorption (per manufacturer). Administer immediate release ciprofloxacin and Cipro XR at least 2 hours before or 6 hours after any of these products.

Oral suspension: Should not be administered through feeding tubes (suspension is oil-based and adheres to the feeding tube). Patients should avoid chewing on the microcapsules.

Tablets:

Immediate release: Administering 2 hours after meals is preferable.

Extended release: Do not crush, split, or chew. May be administered with meals containing dairy products (calcium content <800 mg), but not with dairy products alone.

Nasogastric/orogastric tube: Crush immediate release tablet and mix with water. Flush feeding tube before and after administration. Hold tube feedings at least 1 hour before and 2 hours after administration.

Parenteral: Administer by slow IV infusion over 60 minutes to reduce the risk of venous irritation (burning, pain, erythema, and swelling)

Monitoring Parameters Monitor renal, hepatic, and hematopoietic function periodically; monitor number and type of stools/day for diarrhea. Patients receiving concurrent ciprofloxacin and theophylline should have serum levels of theophylline monitored; monitor INR in patients receiving warfarin; patients receiving concurrent ciprofloxacin and cyclosporine should have cyclosporine levels monitored.

Reference Range Therapeutic: 2.6 to 3 mcg/mL

Test Interactions Some quinolones may produce a false-positive urine screening result for opioids using commercially-available immunoassay kits. This has been demonstrated most consistently for levofloxacin and ofloxacin, but other quinolones have shown cross-reactivity in certain assay kits. Confirmation of positive opioid screens by more specific methods should be considered.

Additional Information Although fluoroquinolones are only FDA approved for use in children for complicated UTI, pyelonephritis, and postexposure treatment for inhalational anthrax, the AAP (Bradley, 2011) has identified other appropriate uses for fluoroquinolones once risks and benefits have been assessed to justify its use:

- UTI caused by *Pseudomonas aeruginosa* or other multidrug-resistant, gram-negative bacteria susceptible to fluoroquinolones
- Chronic suppurative otitis media or otitis externa caused by *P. aeruginosa*
- Chronic or acute osteomyelitis or osteochondritis caused by *P. aeruginosa*
- Mycobacterial infections caused by isolates sensitive to fluoroquinolones
- Gram-negative bacterial infections in immunocompromised hosts in which oral therapy is desired or resistance to alternative agents is present

Dosage Forms Excipient information presented when available (limited, particularly for generics); consult specific product labeling.

Solution, Intravenous:

Cipro in D5W: 200 mg/100 mL (100 mL) [latex free]

Generic: 200 mg/100 mL (100 mL); 400 mg/200 mL (200 mL); 200 mg/20 mL (20 mL); 400 mg/40 mL (40 mL)

Solution, Intravenous [preservative free]:

Cipro in D5W: 200 mg/100 mL (100 mL); 400 mg/200 mL (200 mL) [latex free]

Generic: 200 mg/100 mL (100 mL); 400 mg/200 mL (200 mL); 200 mg/20 mL (20 mL); 400 mg/40 mL (40 mL)

Suspension Reconstituted, Oral:

Cipro: 250 mg/5 mL (100 mL); 500 mg/5 mL (100 mL) [strawberry flavor]

Generic: 250 mg/5 mL (100 mL); 500 mg/5 mL (100 mL)

Tablet, Oral, as hydrochloride [strength expressed as base]:

Cipro: 250 mg, 500 mg

Generic: 100 mg, 250 mg, 500 mg, 750 mg

Tablet Extended Release 24 Hour, Oral, as base and hydrochloride [strength expressed as base]:

Cipro XR: 500 mg, 1000 mg

Generic: 500 mg, 1000 mg

Extemporaneous Preparations A 50 mg/mL oral suspension may be made using 2 different vehicles (a 1:1 mixture of Ora-Sweet and Ora-Plus or a 1:1 mixture of Methylcellulose 1% and Simple Syrup, NF). Crush twenty 500 mg tablets and reduce to a fine powder. Add a small amount of vehicle and mix to a uniform paste; mix while adding the vehicle in geometric proportions to **almost** 200 mL; transfer to a calibrated bottle, rinse mortar with vehicle, and add quantity of vehicle sufficient to make 200 mL. Label "shake well" and "refrigerate". Stable 91 days refrigerated and 70 days at room temperature. **Note:** Microcapsules for oral suspension available (50 mg/mL; 100 mg/mL); not for use in feeding tubes.

Nahata MC, Pai VB, and Hipple TF, *Pediatric Drug Formulations*, 5th ed, Cincinnati, OH: Harvey Whitney Books Co, 2004.

Ciprofloxacin (Ophthalmic) (sip roe FLOKS a sin)

Medication Safety Issues

Sound-alike/look-alike issues:

Ciprofloxacin may be confused with cephalexin

Ciloxan may be confused with Cytoxan

Brand Names: US Ciloxan

Brand Names: Canada Ciloxan

Therapeutic Category Antibiotic, Ophthalmic

Generic Availability (US) May be product dependent

Use Treatment of bacterial conjunctivitis due to susceptible organisms (Ointment: FDA approved in ages ≥2 years and adults; Solution: FDA approved in ages ≥1 year and adults); treatment of corneal ulcers (Solution: FDA approved in ages ≥1 year and adults)

Pregnancy Risk Factor C

Pregnancy Considerations Adverse events have been observed in some animal reproduction studies. When administered orally or IV, ciprofloxacin crosses the placenta (Giamarellou 1989; Ludlam 1997). The amount of ciprofloxacin available systemically following topical application of the ophthalmic drops is significantly less in comparison to oral or IV doses. If ophthalmic agents are needed during pregnancy, the minimum effective dose should be used in combination with punctual occlusion for 3 to 5 minutes after application to decrease potential exposure to the fetus (Samples 1988).

Breast-Feeding Considerations It is not known if ciprofloxacin can be detected in breast milk following ophthalmic administration. When administered orally, ciprofloxacin enters breast milk. The manufacturer recommends that caution be exercised when administering ciprofloxacin ophthalmic to nursing women.

Contraindications Hypersensitivity to ciprofloxacin, any component of the formulation, or other quinolones

Warnings/Precautions For ophthalmic use only; not for subconjunctival injection or for introduction into the anterior chamber of the eye. Severe hypersensitivity reactions, including anaphylaxis, have occurred with quinolone therapy (primarily with systemic use). Prompt discontinuation of drug should occur if skin rash or other symptoms arise. Prolonged use may result in fungal or bacterial superinfection. If superinfection is suspected, institute appropriate alternative therapy. Corneal healing may be delayed (ointment). Some products contain benzalkonium chloride which may be absorbed by soft contact lenses; contact lenses should not be worn during treatment of ophthalmologic infections. To avoid contamination, do not touch tip of container to any surface.

Adverse Reactions

Gastrointestinal: Unpleasant taste (immediately after instillation)

Ocular: Conjunctival hyperemia, crystal formation, burning, discomfort, foreign body sensation, itching, keratopathy (ointment), lid margin crusting, white crystalline precipitate (solution; in superficial portion of corneal defect; reversible after completion of therapy)

Rare but important or life-threatening: Corneal infiltrates, corneal staining, hypersensitivity reactions, keratitis, lid edema, nausea, photophobia, tearing, vision decreased

Drug Interactions

Metabolism/Transport Effects None known.

Avoid Concomitant Use There are no known interactions where it is recommended to avoid concomitant use.

Increased Effect/Toxicity There are no known significant interactions involving an increase in effect.

Decreased Effect There are no known significant interactions involving a decrease in effect.

Storage/Stability Store at 2°C to 25°C (36°F to 77°F). Protect from light.

Mechanism of Action Inhibits DNA-gyrase in susceptible organisms; inhibits relaxation of supercoiled DNA and promotes breakage of double-stranded DNA

Dosing: Usual

Children and Adolescents:

Bacterial conjunctivitis; treatment:

Ointment: Children ≥2 years and Adolescents: Apply 1/2" ointment ribbon into the conjunctival sac 3 times daily for 2 days, then twice daily for the next 5 days

Solution: Children ≥1 year and Adolescents: Instill 1-2 drops into the conjunctival sac of the affected eye(s) every 2 hours while awake for 2 days, then 1-2 drops every 4 hours while awake for the next 5 days

Corneal ulcers; treatment: Solution: Children ≥1 year and Adolescents: Instill 2 drops into the conjunctival sac every 15 minutes for the first 6 hours, then 2 drops every 30 minutes for the remainder of the first day; on the second day, 2 drops every hour; on the third day and for the duration of therapy, 2 drops every 4 hours thereafter. Treatment may continue after day 14 if re-epithelialization has not occurred.

Adults:

Bacterial conjunctivitis; treatment:

Ointment: Apply 1/2" ointment ribbon into the conjunctival sac 3 times daily for 2 days, then twice daily for the next 5 days

Solution: Instill 1-2 drops into the conjunctival sac of the affected eye(s) every 2 hours while awake for 2 days, then 1-2 drops every 4 hours while awake for the next 5 days

Corneal ulcers; treatment: Solution: Instill 2 drops into the conjunctival sac every 15 minutes for the first 6 hours, then 2 drops every 30 minutes for the remainder of the first day; on the second day, 2 drops every hour; on the third day and for the duration of therapy, 2 drops every 4 hours thereafter. Treatment may continue after day 14 if re-epithelialization has not occurred.

Administration Ophthalmic: For topical use only. Avoid contacting tip with skin or eye.

Ointment: Instill ointment in the lower conjunctival sac.

Solution: Apply finger pressure to lacrimal sac during and for 1-2 minutes after instillation to decrease risk of absorption and systemic effects.

Dosage Forms Excipient information presented when available (limited, particularly for generics); consult specific product labeling.

Ointment, Ophthalmic, as hydrochloride:

Ciloxan: 0.3% (3.5 g)

Solution, Ophthalmic, as hydrochloride:

Ciloxan: 0.3% (5 mL) [contains benzalkonium chloride, edetate disodium]

Generic: 0.3% (2.5 mL, 5 mL, 10 mL)

Ciprofloxacin (Otic) (sip roe FLOKS a sin)

Medication Safety Issues

Sound-alike/look-alike issues:

Cetraxal® may be confused with cefTRIAXone

Ciprofloxacin may be confused with cephalexin

Brand Names: US Cetraxal

Therapeutic Category Antibiotic, Otic; Antibiotic, Quinolone

Generic Availability (US) Yes

Use Treatment of acute otitis externa (FDA approved in ages ≥1 year and adults)

Pregnancy Risk Factor C

Pregnancy Considerations Animal reproduction studies have not been conducted with ciprofloxacin otic solution. When administered orally or IV, ciprofloxacin crosses the placenta (Giamarellou,1989; Ludlam 1997). The amount of ciprofloxacin available systemically following topical application of the otic drops is expected to be significantly less in comparison to oral or IV doses.

Breast-Feeding Considerations When administered systemically, ciprofloxacin enters breast milk. The amount of ciprofloxacin available systemically following topical application of the otic drops is expected to be significantly less in comparison to oral or IV doses. Due to the potential for serious adverse reactions in the nursing infant, the manufacturer recommends a decision be made whether to discontinue nursing or to discontinue the drug, taking into account the importance of treatment to the mother.

Contraindications Hypersensitivity to ciprofloxacin, any component of the formulation, or other quinolones

Warnings/Precautions For otic use only. If infection is not improved after 1 week, consider culture to identify organism. Severe hypersensitivity reactions have occurred with quinolone therapy. Prompt discontinuation of drug should occur if skin rash or other symptoms of hypersensitivity arise. Prolonged use may result in fungal or bacterial superinfection. If superinfection occurs, discontinue use and institute appropriate alternative therapy. There have been reports of tendon inflammation and/or rupture with systemic quinolone antibiotics. Exposure following otic administration is substantially lower than with systemic therapy. Discontinue at first sign of tendon inflammation or pain.

Adverse Reactions

Central nervous system: Headache

Local: Application site pain, fungal superinfection, pruritus

Drug Interactions

Metabolism/Transport Effects None known.

Avoid Concomitant Use There are no known interactions where it is recommended to avoid concomitant use.

Increased Effect/Toxicity There are no known significant interactions involving an increase in effect.

Decreased Effect There are no known significant interactions involving a decrease in effect.

Storage/Stability Store at 15°C to 25°C (59°F to 77°F). Protect from light. Store unused single-dose containers in foil overwrap pouch until immediately prior to use.

Mechanism of Action Inhibits DNA-gyrase in susceptible organisms; inhibits relaxation of supercoiled DNA and promotes breakage of double-stranded DNA

Dosing: Usual

Pediatric: **Otitis externa, acute:** Children and Adolescents: Otic: Instill 0.25 mL (contents of 1 single-dose container) into affected ear(s) twice daily for 7 days

Adult: **Otitis externa, acute:** Otic: Instill 0.25 mL (contents of 1 single-dose container) into affected ear(s) twice daily for 7 days

Dosing adjustment in renal impairment: Children and Adolescents: There are no dosing adjustments provided in the manufacturer's labeling.

Dosing adjustment in hepatic impairment: Children and Adolescents: There are no dosing adjustments provided in the manufacturer's labeling.

Administration Otic: For otic use only. Prior to use, warm solution by holding container in hands for at least 1 minute. Patient should lie down with affected ear upward. Patients should remain in the position for at least 1 minute to allow penetration of solution.

Dosage Forms Excipient information presented when available (limited, particularly for generics); consult specific product labeling.

Solution, Otic, as hydrochloride [preservative free]:
Cetraxal: 0.2% (1 ea)
Generic: 0.2% (1 ea)

Ciprofloxacin and Dexamethasone

(sip roe FLOKS a sin & deks a METH a sone)

Brand Names: US Ciprodex

Brand Names: Canada Ciprodex

Therapeutic Category Antibiotic/Corticosteroid, Otic

Generic Availability (US) No

Use Treatment of acute otitis media in patients with tympanostomy tubes (FDA approved in ages ≥6 months to 18 years); treatment of acute otitis externa (FDA approved in ages ≥6 months and adults)

Pregnancy Risk Factor C

Pregnancy Considerations Animal reproduction studies have not been conducted with this combination.

Breast-Feeding Considerations Ciprofloxacin and corticosteroids can be detected in breast milk following oral administration. It is not known if serum levels of ciprofloxacin or dexamethasone are high enough following otic administration to produce detectable quantities in breast milk. Due to the potential for serious adverse reactions in the nursing infant, the manufacturer recommends a decision be made whether to discontinue nursing or to discontinue the drug, taking into account the importance of treatment to the mother.

Contraindications Hypersensitivity to ciprofloxacin, other fluoroquinolones, dexamethasone, or any component of the formulation; viral infection of the external canal, including herpes simplex infections

Warnings/Precautions For otic use only; not intended for injection or ophthalmic use. Safety and efficacy have been established in pediatric patients ≥6 months of age, however, the manufacturer states that there are no safety concerns which would preclude the use of this product in younger children. Severe and occasionally fatal hypersensitivity reactions, including anaphylaxis, have occurred with systemic fluoroquinolone therapy. Prompt discontinuation of drug should occur if skin rash or other symptoms of hypersensitivity arise. No clinically relevant changes in hearing function were observed in pediatric patients 4 to 12 years of age treated with ciprofloxacin and dexamethasone and tested for audiometric parameters. Prior to instillation, suspension should be warmed in hands to prevent dizziness which may occur following use of a cold solution. Prolonged use may result in fungal or bacterial superinfection, including *C. difficile*-associated diarrhea (CDAD) and pseudomembranous colitis; if superinfection occurs, discontinue use and institute appropriate therapy. CDAD has been observed >2 months postantibiotic treatment.

Adverse Reactions Also see individual agents.

Dermatologic: Pruritus of ear

Otic: Otalgia

Rare but important or life-threatening: Auditory impairment, oral candidiasis, superinfection

Drug Interactions

Metabolism/Transport Effects None known.

Avoid Concomitant Use There are no known interactions where it is recommended to avoid concomitant use.

Increased Effect/Toxicity There are no known significant interactions involving an increase in effect.

Decreased Effect There are no known significant interactions involving a decrease in effect.

Storage/Stability Store at 20°C to 25°C (68°F to 77°F); excursions are permitted between 15°C and 30°C (59°F and 86°F); avoid freezing. Protect from light.

Mechanism of Action Ciprofloxacin is a fluoroquinolone antibiotic; dexamethasone is a corticosteroid used to decrease inflammation accompanying bacterial infections

Pharmacokinetics (Adult data unless noted)

Absorption: Otic:

Ciprofloxacin: Peak: 0.1% of oral administration peak concentrations

Dexamethasone: Peak: 14% of oral administration peak concentrations

Time to peak serum concentration: 15 minutes to 2 hours post dose application

Dosing: Usual

Pediatric:

Otitis media, acute (with typmanostomy tubes): Infants ≥6 months, Children, and Adolescents: Otic: Instill 4 drops into affected ear(s) twice daily for 7 days

Otitis externa, acute: Infants ≥6 months, Children, and Adolescents: Otic: Instill 4 drops into affected ear(s) twice daily for 7 days

Adult: **Otitis externa, acute:** Otic: Instill 4 drops into affected ear(s) twice daily for 7 days

Dosing adjustment in renal impairment: Infants ≥6 months, Children, and Adolescents: There are no dosing adjustments provided in the manufacturer's labeling.

Dosing adjustment in hepatic impairment: Infants ≥6 months, Children, and Adolescents: There are no dosing adjustments provided in the manufacturer's labeling.

Administration To avoid dizziness which may result from the instillation of a cold solution, warm bottle in hand for 1 to 2 minutes prior to use. Shake suspension well before using; avoid contamination of the tip of the bottle to fingers, ear, or any surfaces. Patient should lie with affected ear upward and maintain position for 60 seconds after suspension is instilled.

Acute otitis media with tympanostomy tubes: Instill drops then gently press the tragus 5 times in a pumping motion to allow the drops to pass through the tube into the middle ear.

Acute otitis externa: Gently pull the outer ear lobe upward and backward to allow the drops to flow down into the ear canal.

Monitoring Parameters Resolution of infection; if infection persists after 1 week of treatment, obtain cultures to guide further treatment. If otorrhea persists after a full course of therapy, or if ≥2 episodes occur within 6 months, evaluate to exclude an underlying condition (eg, cholesteatoma, foreign body, tumor)

Test Interactions See individual agents.

Dosage Forms Excipient information presented when available (limited, particularly for generics); consult specific product labeling.
Suspension, otic:
Ciprodex: Ciprofloxacin 0.3% and dexamethasone 0.1% (7.5 mL) [contains benzalkonium chloride]

Ciprofloxacin and Hydrocortisone

(sip roe FLOKS a sin & hye droe KOR ti sone)

Related Information
Ciprofloxacin (Otic) *on page 468*
Hydrocortisone (Topical) *on page 1041*
Brand Names: US Cipro® HC
Brand Names: Canada Cipro® HC
Therapeutic Category Antibiotic/Corticosteroid, Otic
Generic Availability (US) No
Use Treatment of acute bacterial otitis externa (FDA approved in ages ≥1 year and adults)
Pregnancy Risk Factor C
Pregnancy Considerations Animal reproduction studies have not been conducted with this combination.
Breast-Feeding Considerations Ciprofloxacin can be detected in breast milk following systemic administration. It is not known if serum levels of ciprofloxacin or hydrocortisone are high enough following otic administration to produce detectable quantities in breast milk. Due to the potential for serious adverse reactions in the nursing infant, the manufacturer recommends a decision be made whether to discontinue nursing or to discontinue the drug, taking into account the importance of treatment to the mother.
Contraindications Viral infections of the external canal, including varicella and herpes simplex infections; perforated tympanic membrane; hypersensitivity to hydrocortisone, ciprofloxacin, or any member of the quinolone class of antimicrobial agents.
Warnings/Precautions Severe and occasionally fatal hypersensitivity reactions, including anaphylaxis, have occurred with systemic fluoroquinolone therapy. Prompt discontinuation of drug should occur if skin rash or other symptoms of hypersensitivity arise. Prolonged use may result in fungal or bacterial superinfection, including *C. difficile*-associated diarrhea (CDAD) and pseudomembranous colitis; CDAD has been observed >2 months post-antibiotic treatment. If superinfection occurs, discontinue use and institute appropriate therapy. There have been reports of tendon inflammation and/or rupture with systemic fluoroquinolones. Exposure following otic administration is substantially lower than with systemic therapy. Discontinue at first sign of tendon inflammation or pain.

Benzyl alcohol and derivatives: Some dosage forms may contain benzyl alcohol; large amounts of benzyl alcohol (≥99 mg/kg/day) have been associated with a potentially fatal toxicity ("gasping syndrome") in neonates; the "gasping syndrome" consists of metabolic acidosis, respiratory distress, gasping respirations, CNS dysfunction (including convulsions, intracranial hemorrhage), hypotension and cardiovascular collapse (AAP, 1997; CDC, 1982); some data suggests that benzoate displaces bilirubin from protein binding sites (Ahlfors, 2001); avoid or use dosage forms containing benzyl alcohol with caution in neonates. See manufacturer's labeling.

For otic use only; not intended for injection or ophthalmic use. Prior to instillation, suspension should be warmed in hands to prevent dizziness which may occur following use of a cold solution.
Adverse Reactions Central nervous system: Headache
Rare but important or life-threatening: Alopecia, fungal dermatitis, hypersensitivity reactions, migraine, paresthesia
Drug Interactions
Metabolism/Transport Effects None known.
Avoid Concomitant Use There are no known interactions where it is recommended to avoid concomitant use.
Increased Effect/Toxicity There are no known significant interactions involving an increase in effect.
Decreased Effect There are no known significant interactions involving a decrease in effect.
Storage/Stability Store below 25°C (77°F); avoid freezing. Protect from light.
Dosing: Usual
Pediatric: **Otitis externa, acute:** Children and Adolescents: Otic: Instill 3 drops into the affected ear(s) twice daily for 7 days
Adult: **Otitis externa, acute:** Otic: Instill 3 drops in the affected ear(s) twice daily for 7 days
Dosing adjustment in renal impairment: Children, Adolescents, and Adults: There are no dosing adjustments provided in the manufacturer's labeling.
Dosing adjustment in hepatic impairment: Children, Adolescents, and Adults: There are no dosing adjustments provided in the manufacturer's labeling.
Administration Otic: Prior to use, warm suspension by holding bottle in hands for 1 to 2 minutes; shake suspension well before using; avoid contamination of the tip of the bottle to fingers, ear, or any surfaces; patient should lie with affected ear upward and maintain position for 30 to 60 seconds after suspension is instilled into the ear canal
Test Interactions See individual agents.
Dosage Forms Excipient information presented when available (limited, particularly for generics); consult specific product labeling.
Suspension, otic:
Cipro® HC: Ciprofloxacin hydrochloride 0.2% and hydrocortisone 1% (10 mL) [contains benzyl alcohol]

◆ **Ciprofloxacin Hydrochloride** *see* Ciprofloxacin (Ophthalmic) *on page 467*
◆ **Ciprofloxacin Hydrochloride** *see* Ciprofloxacin (Otic) *on page 468*
◆ **Ciprofloxacin Hydrochloride** *see* Ciprofloxacin (Systemic) *on page 463*
◆ **Ciprofloxacin Hydrochloride and Dexamethasone** *see* Ciprofloxacin and Dexamethasone *on page 469*
◆ **Ciprofloxacin Hydrochloride and Hydrocortisone** *see* Ciprofloxacin and Hydrocortisone *on page 470*
◆ **Ciprofloxacin Injection (Can)** *see* Ciprofloxacin (Systemic) *on page 463*
◆ **Ciprofloxacin Injection USP (Can)** *see* Ciprofloxacin (Systemic) *on page 463*
◆ **Ciprofloxacin Intravenous Infusion (Can)** *see* Ciprofloxacin (Systemic) *on page 463*
◆ **Ciprofloxacin Intravenous Infusion BP (Can)** *see* Ciprofloxacin (Systemic) *on page 463*
◆ **Cipro® HC** *see* Ciprofloxacin and Hydrocortisone *on page 470*
◆ **Cipro in D5W** *see* Ciprofloxacin (Systemic) *on page 463*
◆ **Cipro XR** *see* Ciprofloxacin (Systemic) *on page 463*

Cisapride (SIS a pride)

Medication Safety Issues
Sound-alike/look-alike issues:
Propulsid® may be confused with propranolol
Brand Names: US Propulsid®
Therapeutic Category Gastrointestinal Agent, Prokinetic
Generic Availability (US) No
Use Treatment of nocturnal symptoms of gastroesophageal reflux disease (GERD), also demonstrated effectiveness

for gastroparesis, refractory constipation, and nonulcer dyspepsia in patients failing other therapies

Prescribing and Access Restrictions In U.S., available via limited-access protocol only. Call 877-795-4247 for more information.

Medication Guide Available Yes

Pregnancy Risk Factor C

Pregnancy Considerations Adverse events were observed in animal reproduction studies.

Breast-Feeding Considerations Cisapride is excreted into breast milk. The manufacturer recommends caution be used if administered to a nursing woman.

Contraindications

Hypersensitivity to cisapride or any component of the formulations; GI hemorrhage, mechanical obstruction, GI perforation, or other situations when GI motility stimulation is dangerous

Serious cardiac arrhythmias including ventricular tachycardia, ventricular fibrillation, torsade de pointes, and QT prolongation have been reported in patients taking cisapride with other drugs that inhibit CYP3A4. Some of these events have been fatal. Concomitant oral or intravenous administration of the following drugs with cisapride may lead to elevated cisapride blood levels and is contraindicated:

Antibiotics: Oral or IV erythromycin, clarithromycin, troleandomycin

Antidepressants: Nefazodone

Antifungals: Oral or IV fluconazole, itraconazole, miconazole, oral ketoconazole

Protease inhibitors: Indinavir, ritonavir, amprenavir, atazanavir

Cisapride is also contraindicated for patients with a prolonged electrocardiographic QT intervals (QTc >450 msec), a history of QTc prolongation, or known family history of congenital long QT syndrome; clinically significant bradycardia, renal failure, history of ventricular arrhythmias, ischemic heart disease, and congestive heart failure; uncorrected electrolyte disorders (hypokalemia, hypomagnesemia); respiratory failure; and concomitant medications known to prolong the QT interval and increase the risk of arrhythmia, such as certain antiarrhythmics, certain antipsychotics, certain antidepressants, bepridil, sparfloxacin, and terodiline. The preceding lists of drugs are not comprehensive. Cisapride should not be used in patients with uncorrected hypokalemia or hypomagnesemia or who might experience rapid reduction of plasma potassium such as those administered potassium-wasting diuretics and/or insulin in acute settings.

Warnings/Precautions

[U.S. Boxed Warning]: Serious cardiac arrhythmias including ventricular tachycardia, ventricular fibrillation, torsade de pointes, and QT prolongation have been reported in patients taking this drug. Many of these patients also took drugs expected to increase cisapride blood levels by inhibiting the cytochrome P450 3A4 enzymes that metabolize cisapride. These drugs include clarithromycin, erythromycin, troleandomycin, nefazodone, fluconazole, itraconazole, ketoconazole, indinavir and ritonavir. Some of these events have been fatal. Cisapride is contraindicated in patients taking any of these drugs. **QT prolongation, torsade de pointes (sometimes with syncope), cardiac arrest and sudden death have been reported in patients taking cisapride without the above-mentioned contraindicated drugs.** Recommended doses of cisapride should not be exceeded.

Patients should have a baseline ECG and an electrolyte panel (magnesium, calcium, potassium) prior to initiating cisapride (see Contraindications). Potential benefits should be weighed against risks prior administration of cisapride to patients who have or may develop prolongation of cardiac conduction intervals, particularly QTc. These include patients with conditions that could predispose them to the development of serious arrhythmias, such as multiple organ failure, COPD, apnea and advanced cancer. Cisapride should not be used in patients with uncorrected hypokalemia or hypomagnesemia, such as those with severe dehydration, vomiting or malnutrition, or those taking potassium-wasting diuretics. Cisapride should not be used in patients who might experience rapid reduction of plasma potassium, such as those administered potassium-wasting diuretics and/or insulin in acute settings.

Adverse Reactions

Cardiovascular: Tachycardia

Central nervous system: Anxiety, extrapyramidal effects, fatigue, headache, insomnia, somnolence,

Dermatologic: Rash

Gastrointestinal: Abdominal cramping, constipation, diarrhea (dose dependent), nausea

Respiratory: Coughing, increased incidence of viral infection, rhinitis, sinusitis, upper respiratory tract infection

Rare but important or life-threatening: Apnea, bronchospasm, gynecomastia, hyperprolactinemia, methemoglobinemia, photosensitivity, psychiatric disturbances, seizure (have been reported only in patients with a history of seizure)

Drug Interactions

Metabolism/Transport Effects Substrate of CYP1A2 (minor), CYP2A6 (minor), CYP2B6 (minor), CYP2C19 (minor), CYP2C9 (minor), CYP3A4 (major); **Note:** Assignment of Major/Minor substrate status based on clinically relevant drug interaction potential; **Inhibits** CYP2D6 (weak)

Avoid Concomitant Use

Avoid concomitant use of Cisapride with any of the following: Amitriptyline; Antifungal Agents (Azole Derivatives, Systemic); Aprepitant; Bepridil; Bicalutamide; Boceprevir; Cobicistat; Conivaptan; Fosaprepitant; Fusidic Acid (Systemic); Highest Risk QTc-Prolonging Agents; Idelalisib; Ivabradine; Macrolide Antibiotics; Mifepristone; Moderate Risk QTc-Prolonging Agents; Nefazodone; Protease Inhibitors; Protriptyline; Simeprevir; Telaprevir

Increased Effect/Toxicity

Cisapride may increase the levels/effects of: Alcohol (Ethyl); Bepridil; Highest Risk QTc-Prolonging Agents; NIFEdipine

The levels/effects of Cisapride may be increased by: Amitriptyline; Antifungal Agents (Azole Derivatives, Systemic); Aprepitant; Bicalutamide; Boceprevir; Cimetidine; Cobicistat; Conivaptan; CYP3A4 Inhibitors (Moderate); Fosaprepitant; Fusidic Acid (Systemic); Grapefruit Juice; Idelalisib; Ivabradine; Ivacaftor; Luliconazole; Macrolide Antibiotics; Mifepristone; Moderate Risk QTc-Prolonging Agents; Nefazodone; Netupitant; Palbociclib; Protease Inhibitors; Protriptyline; QTc-Prolonging Agents (Indeterminate Risk and Risk Modifying); Simeprevir; Stiripentol; Telaprevir

Decreased Effect There are no known significant interactions involving a decrease in effect.

Food Interactions Coadministration of grapefruit juice with cisapride increases the bioavailability of cisapride. Management: Avoid consumption of grapefruit/grapefruit juice during cisapride therapy.

Mechanism of Action Enhances the release of acetylcholine at the myenteric plexus. *In vitro* studies have shown cisapride to have serotonin-4 receptor agonistic properties which may increase gastrointestinal motility and cardiac rate; increases lower esophageal sphincter pressure and lower esophageal peristalsis; accelerates gastric emptying of both liquids and solids.

Pharmacodynamics Onset of action: 0.5-1 hour

Pharmacokinetics (Adult data unless noted)
Distribution: Breast milk to plasma ratio: 0.045
Protein binding: 98%
Metabolism: Extensive in liver via cytochrome P450 isoenzyme CYP 3A3/4 to norcisapride, which is eliminated in urine and feces
Bioavailability: 40% to 50%
Half-life: 7-10 hours
Elimination: <10% of dose excreted into feces and urine

Dosing: Neonatal Oral: 0.15-0.2 mg/kg/dose 3-4 times/day; maximum dose: 0.8 mg/kg/day

Dosing: Usual Oral:
Infants and Children: 0.15-0.3 mg/kg/dose 3-4 times/day; maximum dose: 10 mg/dose
Adults: Initial: 10 mg 4 times/day at least 15 minutes before meals and at bedtime; in some patients the dosage will need to be increased to 20 mg to obtain a satisfactory result
Dosage adjustment in liver dysfunction: Reduce daily dosage by 50%

Administration Oral: Administer 15 minutes before meals or feeding

Monitoring Parameters ECG (prior to beginning therapy), serum electrolytes in patients on diuretic therapy (prior to beginning therapy and periodically thereafter)

Cisatracurium (sis a tra KYOO ree um)

Medication Safety Issues
Sound-alike/look-alike issues:
Nimbex may be confused with NovoLOG
High alert medication:
The Institute for Safe Medication Practices (ISMP) includes this medication among its list of drugs which have a heightened risk of causing significant patient harm when used in error.
Other safety concerns:
United States Pharmacopeia (USP) 2006: The Interdisciplinary Safe Medication Use Expert Committee of the USP has recommended the following:
- Hospitals, clinics, and other practice sites should institute special safeguards in the storage, labeling, and use of these agents and should include these safeguards in staff orientation and competency training.
- Healthcare professionals should be on high alert (especially vigilant) whenever a neuromuscular-blocking agent (NMBA) is stocked, ordered, prepared, or administered.

Brand Names: US Nimbex

Brand Names: Canada Nimbex

Therapeutic Category Neuromuscular Blocker Agent, Nondepolarizing; Skeletal Muscle Relaxant, Paralytic

Generic Availability (US) Yes

Use Adjunct to general anesthesia, to facilitate endotracheal intubation, and provide skeletal muscle relaxation during surgery or mechanical ventilation (FDA approved in ages 1 month to 12 years and adults)

Pregnancy Risk Factor B

Pregnancy Considerations Adverse events have not been observed in animal reproduction studies.

Breast-Feeding Considerations It is not known if cisatracurium is excreted in breast milk. The manufacturer recommends that caution be exercised when administering cisatracurium to nursing women.

Contraindications Hypersensitivity to cisatracurium besylate or any component of the formulation; use of the 10 mL multiple-dose vials in premature infants (formulation contains benzyl alcohol)

Warnings/Precautions Maintenance of an adequate airway and respiratory support is critical; certain clinical conditions may result in potentiation or antagonism of neuromuscular blockade:
Antagonism: Respiratory alkalosis, hypercalcemia, demyelinating lesions, peripheral neuropathies, denervation, and muscle trauma
Potentiation: Electrolyte abnormalities (eg, severe hypocalcemia, severe hypokalemia, hypermagnesemia), neuromuscular diseases, metabolic acidosis, metabolic alkalosis, respiratory acidosis, Eaton-Lambert syndrome and myasthenia gravis

Hypothermia may slow Hoffmann elimination thereby prolonging the duration of activity (Greenberg, 2013). Resistance may occur in burn patients (≥20% of total body surface area), usually several days after the injury, and may persist for several months after wound healing. Resistance may occur in patients who are immobilized. Cross-sensitivity with other neuromuscular-blocking agents may occur; use extreme caution in patients with previous anaphylactic reactions to other neuromuscular-blocking agents. Bradycardia may be more common with cisatracurium than with other neuromuscular blocking agents since it has no clinically significant effects on heart rate to counteract the bradycardia produced by anesthetics. Use caution in the elderly. Should be administered by adequately trained individuals familiar with its use.

Benzyl alcohol and derivatives: Some dosage forms may contain benzyl alcohol; large amounts of benzyl alcohol (≥99 mg/kg/day) have been associated with a potentially fatal toxicity ("gasping syndrome") in neonates; the "gasping syndrome" consists of metabolic acidosis, respiratory distress, gasping respirations, CNS dysfunction (including convulsions, intracranial hemorrhage), hypotension and cardiovascular collapse (AAP, 1997; CDC, 1982); some data suggests that benzoate displaces bilirubin from protein binding sites (Ahlfors, 2001); avoid or use dosage forms containing benzyl alcohol with caution in neonates. See manufacturer's labeling.

Adverse Reactions
Effects are minimal and transient.
Rare but important or life-threatening: Bradycardia, bronchospasm, flushing, hypotension, muscle calcification (prolonged use), myopathy (acute quadriplegic syndrome; prolonged use), pruritus, skin rash

Drug Interactions
Metabolism/Transport Effects None known.
Avoid Concomitant Use
Avoid concomitant use of Cisatracurium with any of the following: QuiNINE
Increased Effect/Toxicity
Cisatracurium may increase the levels/effects of: Cardiac Glycosides; Corticosteroids (Systemic); OnabotulinumtoxinA; RimabotulinumtoxinB

The levels/effects of Cisatracurium may be increased by: AbobotulinumtoxinA; Aminoglycosides; Calcium Channel Blockers; Capreomycin; Clindamycin (Topical); Colistimethate; CycloSPORINE (Systemic); Fosphenytoin-Phenytoin; Inhalational Anesthetics; Ketorolac (Nasal); Ketorolac (Systemic); Lincosamide Antibiotics; Lithium; Loop Diuretics; Magnesium Salts; Polymyxin B; Procainamide; QuiNIDine; QuiNINE; Spironolactone; Tetracycline Derivatives; Vancomycin
Decreased Effect
The levels/effects of Cisatracurium may be decreased by: Acetylcholinesterase Inhibitors; Fosphenytoin-Phenytoin; Loop Diuretics

Storage/Stability Refrigerate intact vials at 2°C to 8°C (36°F to 46°F). Use vials within 21 days upon removal from the refrigerator to room temperature of 25°C (77°F). Per the manufacturer, dilutions of 0.1 mg/mL in 0.9% sodium chloride (NS), dextrose 5% in water (D_5W), or D_5NS are stable for up to 24 hours at room temperature or under refrigeration; dilutions of 0.1-0.2 mg/mL in D_5LR are stable for up to 24 hours in the refrigerator. *Additional stability data:* Dilutions of 0.1, 2, and 5 mg/mL in D_5W or NS are stable in the refrigerator for up to 30 days; at room temperature (23°C), dilutions of 0.1 and 2 mg/mL began exhibiting substantial drug loss between 7-14 days; dilutions of 5 mg/mL in D_5W or NS are stable for up to 30 days at room temperature (23°C) (Xu, 1998). Usual concentration: 0.1-0.4 mg/mL.

Mechanism of Action Blocks neural transmission at the myoneural junction by binding with cholinergic receptor sites

Pharmacodynamics

Onset of action: IV: Within 2-3 minutes

Maximum effect: Within 3-5 minutes

Duration: Dose dependent, 35-45 minutes after a single 0.1 mg/kg dose; recovery begins in 20-35 minutes when anesthesia is balanced; recovery is attained in 90% of patients in 25-93 minutes

Pharmacokinetics (Adult data unless noted)

Distribution: V_d: Adults: 0.16 L/kg

Metabolism: Some metabolites are active; 80% of drug clearance is via a rapid nonenzymatic degradation (Hofmann elimination) in the bloodstream; additional metabolism occurs via ester hydrolysis

Half-life: 22-31 minutes

Elimination: <10% of dose excreted as unchanged drug in urine

Clearance:

Children: 5.9 mL/kg/minute

Adults: 5.1 mL/kg/minute

Dosing: Usual Paralysis/skeletal muscle relaxation:

IV:

Infants and Children 1-23 months: 0.15 mg/kg over 5-10 seconds

Children ≥2 years and Adolescents: 0.1-0.15 mg/kg over 5-10 seconds (Martin, 1999; Playfor, 2007)

Adults: Initial: 0.15-0.2 mg/kg followed by maintenance dose of 0.03 mg/kg 40-65 minutes later or as needed to maintain neuromuscular blockade

Continuous IV infusion:

Infants, Children, and Adolescents: 1-4 **mcg**/kg/minute (0.06-0.24 mg/kg/**hour**); 3.9 ± 1.3 **mcg**/kg/minute (0.23 ± 0.08 mg/kg/**hour**) was the mean infusion rate needed to maintain neuromuscular blockade in 19 children (ages 3 months to 16 years) (Burnmester, 2005; Martin, 1999; Playfor, 2007)

Adults: 1-3 **mcg**/kg/minute (0.06-0.18 mg/kg/**hour**); **Note:** There may be wide interpatient variability in dosage (range: 0.5-10 **mcg**/kg/minute in adults) which may increase and decrease over time; optimize patient dosage by utilizing a peripheral nerve stimulator

Preparation for Administration Parenteral: Continuous IV infusion: Further dilute in D_5W or NS to a final concentration of 0.1 to 0.4 mg/mL

Administration

Parenteral: Not for IM injection due to tissue irritation

Rapid IV injection: Administer undiluted over 5 to 10 seconds

Continuous IV infusion: Further dilute in D_5W or NS and administer via infusion pump

Monitoring Parameters Muscle twitch response to peripheral nerve stimulation, heart rate, blood pressure, assisted ventilation status

Additional Information Neuromuscular blocking potency is 3 times that of atracurium; maximum block is up to 2 minutes longer than for equipotent doses of atracurium; laudanosine, a metabolite without neuromuscular blocking activity has been associated with hypotension and seizure activity in animal studies.

Dosage Forms Excipient information presented when available (limited, particularly for generics); consult specific product labeling.

Solution, Intravenous:

Nimbex: 10 mg/5 mL (5 mL)

Nimbex: 20 mg/10 mL (10 mL) [contains benzyl alcohol]

Nimbex: 10 mg/mL (20 mL)

Generic: 20 mg/10 mL (10 mL)

Solution, Intravenous [preservative free]:

Generic: 10 mg/5 mL (5 mL); 10 mg/mL (20 mL)

◆ **Cisatracurium Besylate** *see* Cisatracurium *on page 472*

◆ **cis-DDP** *see* CISplatin *on page 473*

◆ **cis-Diamminedichloroplatinum** *see* CISplatin *on page 473*

CISplatin (SIS pla tin)

Medication Safety Issues

Sound-alike/look-alike issues:

CISplatin may be confused with CARBOplatin, oxaliplatin

Platinol may be confused with Patanol

High alert medication:

This medication is in a class the Institute for Safe Medication Practices (ISMP) includes among its list of drug classes which have a heightened risk of causing significant patient harm when used in error.

BEERS Criteria medication:

This drug may be potentially inappropriate for use in geriatric patients (Quality of evidence - moderate; Strength of recommendation - strong).

Administration issues:

Cisplatin doses >100 mg/m^2 once every 3 to 4 weeks are rarely used and should be verified with the prescriber.

Related Information

Management of Drug Extravasations *on page 2298*

Prevention of Chemotherapy-Induced Nausea and Vomiting in Children *on page 2368*

Safe Handling of Hazardous Drugs *on page 2455*

Brand Names: Canada Cisplatin Injection; Cisplatin Injection BP; Cisplatin Injection, Mylan STD

Therapeutic Category Antineoplastic Agent, Alkylating Agent; Antineoplastic Agent, Platinum Analog

Generic Availability (US) Yes

Use Treatment of metastatic testicular cancer, advanced bladder cancer, and metastatic ovarian cancers (FDA approved in adults); has also been used in the treatment of central nervous system tumors, germ cell tumors, gestational trophoblastic disease (refractory), head and neck cancer, hepatobiliary cancer, hepatoblastoma, Hodgkin lymphoma, medulloblastoma, neuroblastoma, neuroendocrine tumors, non-Hodgkin lymphoma (NHL), osteosarcoma, soft tissue sarcomas, and unknown primary cancers

Pregnancy Risk Factor D

Pregnancy Considerations Adverse effects have been observed in animal reproduction studies. Women of childbearing potential should be advised to avoid pregnancy during treatment. May case fetal harm if administered during pregnancy.

Breast-Feeding Considerations Cisplatin is excreted in breast milk. Breast-feeding is not recommended by the manufacturer.

Contraindications History of allergic reactions to cisplatin, other platinum-containing compounds, or any component of the formulation; preexisting renal impairment; myelosuppressed patients; hearing impairment

Warnings/Precautions Hazardous agent - use appropriate precautions for handling and disposal (NIOSH 2014 [group 1]). **[US Boxed Warning]: Doses >100 mg/m²/cycle (once every 3 to 4 weeks) are rare; verify with the prescriber. Exercise caution to avoid inadvertent overdose due to potential sound-alike/look-alike confusion between CISplatin and CARBOplatin or prescribing practices that fail to differentiate daily doses from the total dose per cycle.** At the approved dose, cisplatin should not be administered more frequently than once every 3 to 4 weeks. Patients should receive adequate hydration, with or without diuretics, prior to and for 24 hours after cisplatin administration. **[US Boxed Warning]: Cumulative renal toxicity associated with cisplatin is severe.** Monitor serum creatinine, blood urea nitrogen, creatinine clearance, and serum electrolytes (calcium, magnesium, potassium, and sodium) closely. According to the manufacturer's labeling, use is contraindicated in patients with preexisting renal impairment and renal function must return to normal prior to administering subsequent cycles; some literature recommends reduced doses with renal impairment. Nephrotoxicity may be potentiated by aminoglycosides.

Use caution in the elderly; may cause or exacerbate syndrome of inappropriate antidiuretic hormone secretion or hyponatremia; monitor sodium closely with initiation or dosage adjustments in older adults (Beers Criteria). Elderly patients may be more susceptible to nephrotoxicity and peripheral neuropathy; select dose cautiously and monitor closely.

[US Boxed Warning]: Dose-related toxicities include myelosuppression, nausea, and vomiting. Cisplatin is associated with a high emetic potential; antiemetics are recommended to prevent nausea and vomiting (Basch, 2011; Dupuis, 2011; Roila, 2010). Nausea and vomiting are dose-related and may be immediate and/or delayed. Diarrhea may also occur. **[US Boxed Warning]: Ototoxicity, which may be more pronounced in children, is manifested by tinnitus and/or loss of high frequency hearing and occasionally, deafness; may be significant.** Ototoxicity is cumulative and may be severe. Audiometric testing should be performed at baseline and prior to each dose. Certain genetic variations in the thiopurine S-methyltransferase (TPMT) gene may be associated with an increased risk of ototoxicity in children administered conventional cisplatin doses (Pussegoda, 2013). Controversy may exist regarding the role of TPMT variants in cisplatin ototoxicity (Ratain, 2013; Yang, 2013); the association has not been consistent across populations and studies. Children without the TPMT gene variants may still be at risk for ototoxicity. Cumulative dose, prior or concurrent exposure to other ototoxic agents (eg, aminoglycosides, carboplatin), prior cranial radiation, younger age, and type of cancer may also increase the risk for ototoxicity in children (Knight, 2005; Landier, 2014). Pediatric patients should receive audiometric testing at baseline, prior to each dose, and for several years after discontinuing therapy. An international grading scale (SIOP Boston scale) has been developed to assess ototoxicity in children (Brock, 2012). Severe (and possibly irreversible) neuropathies (including stocking-glove paresthesias, areflexia, and loss of proprioception/vibratory sensation) may occur with higher than recommended doses or more frequent administration; may require therapy discontinuation. Seizures, loss of motor function, loss of taste, leukoencephalopathy, and posterior reversible leukoencephalopathy syndrome (PRES [formerly RPLS]) have also been described. Serum electrolytes, particularly magnesium and potassium, should be monitored and replaced as needed during and after cisplatin therapy.

[US Boxed Warning]: Anaphylactic-like reactions have been reported; may include facial edema, bronchoconstriction, tachycardia, and hypotension and may occur within minutes of administration; symptoms may be managed with epinephrine, corticosteroids, and/or antihistamines. Hyperuricemia has been reported with cisplatin use, and is more pronounced with doses >50 mg/m²; consider antihyperuricemic therapy to reduce uric acid levels. Local infusion site reactions may occur; monitor infusion site during administration; avoid extravasation. Secondary malignancies have been reported with cisplatin in combination with other chemotherapy agents. Potentially significant drug-drug interactions may exist requiring dose or frequency adjustment, additional monitoring, and/or selection of alternative therapy. **[US Boxed Warning]: Should be administered under the supervision of an experienced cancer chemotherapy physician. Adequate diagnostic and treatment facilities and appropriate management of potential complications should be readily available.** Cisplatin is a vesicant at higher concentrations, and an irritant at lower concentrations; ensure proper needle or catheter placement prior to and during infusion; avoid extravasation. Local infusion site reactions may occur; monitor infusion site during administration.

Adverse Reactions

Central nervous system: Neurotoxicity (peripheral neuropathy is dose and duration dependent)

Gastrointestinal: Nausea and vomiting

Genitourinary: Nephrotoxicity (acute renal failure and chronic renal insufficiency)

Hematologic & oncologic: Anemia, leukopenia (nadir: day 18 to 23; recovery: by day 39; dose related), thrombocytopenia (nadir: day 18 to 23; recovery: by day 39; dose related)

Hepatic: Increased liver enzymes

Local: Local irritation

Otic: Ototoxicity (as tinnitus, high frequency hearing loss; more common in children)

Rare but important or life-threatening: Alopecia (mild), ageusia, anaphylaxis, aortic thrombosis (Fernandes, 2011), autonomic neuropathy, bradycardia (Schlumbrecht, 2015), cardiac arrhythmia, cardiac failure, cerebrovascular accident, extravasation, hemolytic anemia (acute), hemolytic-uremic syndrome, hiccups, hypercholesterolemia, hyperuricemia, hypocalcemia, hypokalemia, hypomagnesemia, hyponatremia, hypophosphatemia, increased serum amylase, leukoencephalopathy, myocardial infarction, neutropenic enterocolitis (Furonaka, 2005), optic neuritis, pancreatitis (Trivedi, 2005), papilledema, peripheral ischemia (acute), phlebitis (Tokuda, 2014), SIADH, tachycardia, thrombotic thrombocytopenic purpura

Drug Interactions

Metabolism/Transport Effects None known.

Avoid Concomitant Use

Avoid concomitant use of CISplatin with any of the following: BCG; BCG (Intravesical); CloZAPine; Dipyrone; Natalizumab; Pimecrolimus; Tacrolimus (Topical); Tofacitinib; Vaccines (Live)

Increased Effect/Toxicity

CISplatin may increase the levels/effects of: Aminoglycosides; CloZAPine; Leflunomide; Natalizumab; Taxane Derivatives; Tofacitinib; Topotecan; Vaccines (Live); Vinorelbine

The levels/effects of CISplatin may be increased by: Denosumab; Dipyrone; Loop Diuretics; Pimecrolimus; Roflumilast; Tacrolimus (Topical); Trastuzumab

Decreased Effect

CISplatin may decrease the levels/effects of: BCG; BCG (Intravesical); Coccidioides immitis Skin Test;

Fosphenytoin-Phenytoin; Sipuleucel-T; Vaccines (Inactivated); Vaccines (Live)

The levels/effects of CISplatin may be decreased by: Alpha-Lipoic Acid; Echinacea

Storage/Stability Store intact vials at 15°C to 25°C (59°F to 77°F). Protect from light. Do not refrigerate solution (precipitate may form). Further dilution **stability is dependent on the chloride ion concentration** and should be mixed in solutions of NS (at least 0.3% NaCl). According to the manufacturer, after initial entry into the vial, solution is stable for 28 days protected from light or for at least 7 days under fluorescent room light at room temperature.

Further dilutions in NS, D_5/0.45% NaCl or D_5/NS to a concentration of 0.05 to 2 mg/mL are stable for 72 hours at 4°C to 25°C.

Mechanism of Action Inhibits DNA synthesis by the formation of DNA cross-links; denatures the double helix; covalently binds to DNA bases and disrupts DNA function; may also bind to proteins; the *cis*-isomer is 14 times more cytotoxic than the *trans*-isomer; both forms cross-link DNA but cis-platinum is less easily recognized by cell enzymes and, therefore, not repaired. Cisplatin can also bind two adjacent guanines on the same strand of DNA producing intrastrand cross-linking and breakage.

Pharmacokinetics (Adult data unless noted)

Distribution: IV: Rapid tissue distribution; high concentrations in kidneys, liver, uterus, and lungs

Protein binding: >90% (O'Dwyer, 2000)

Metabolism: Undergoes nonenzymatic metabolism; inactivated (in both cell and bloodstream) by sulfhydryl groups; covalently binds to glutathione and thiosulfate

Half-life, terminal:

Children:

Free drug: 1.3 hours

Total platinum: 44 hours

Adults: Initial: 14-49 minutes; Beta: 0.7-4.6 hours; Gamma: 24-127 hours (O'Dwyer, 2000)

Elimination: Urine and feces (minimal)

Dosing: Usual Note: Dosing and frequency may vary by protocol and/or treatment phase; refer to specific protocol.

Pediatric: **TO PREVENT POSSIBLE OVERDOSE, VERIFY ANY CISPLATIN DOSE EXCEEDING 100 mg/m^2 PER COURSE. Pretreatment hydration is recommended.**

Germ cell tumors: IV:

Infants: 0.7 mg/**kg**/dose every 3 weeks on days 1-5 in combination with bleomycin and etoposide (Cushing, 2004)

Children and Adolescents: 20 mg/m^2/dose every 3 weeks on days 1-5 in combination with bleomycin and etoposide (Cushing, 2004) **or** 100 mg/m^2 every 3 weeks on day 1 in combination with bleomycin and vinblastine or etoposide (Pinkerton, 1986)

Hepatoblastoma: IV:

Continuous IV infusion:

Infants and Children <10 kg: 2.7 mg/kg continuous infusion over 24 hours every 3 weeks on day 1 in combination with doxorubicin for 4-6 cycles (Pritchard, 2000)

Children ≥10 kg and Adolescents:

Monotherapy: **Note:** For use in standard-risk patients only: 80 mg/m^2 continuous infusion over 24 hours every 2 weeks on day 1

Combination therapy: 80 mg/m^2 continuous infusion over 24 hours every 3 weeks on day 1 in combination with doxorubicin (Perilongo, 2004; Perilongo, 2009; Pritchard, 2000).

Intermittent infusion (over 6 hours):

Infants and Children <10 kg: 3 mg/**kg**/dose given every 3 weeks on day 1 for 4-8 cycles in combination with vincristine and fluorouracil or continuous infusion doxorubicin (Douglass, 1993; Malogolowkin, 2008; Ortega, 2000)

Children ≥10 kg and Adolescents: 90 mg/m^2/dose given every 3 weeks on day 1 for 4-8 cycles in combination with vincristine and fluorouracil or continuous infusion doxorubicin (Douglass, 1993; Malogolowkin, 2008; Ortega, 2000)

Medulloblastoma: Children ≥3 years and Adolescents: IV: 75 mg/m^2/dose every 6 weeks on either day 0 in combination with vincristine and cyclophosphamide or day 1 in combination with lomustine and vincristine of each chemotherapy cycle for 8 cycles (Packer, 2006; Packer, 2013)

Neuroblastoma, high-risk: Infants, Children, and Adolescents: IV: 50 mg/m^2/**day** on days 0-3 every 3 weeks in combination with etoposide (cycles 3 and 5) (Kreissman, 2013; Naranjo, 2011) or 50 mg/m^2/**day** on days 1-4 in combination with etoposide (cycles 3, 5, and 7) (Kushner, 1994)

Osteosarcoma: Children and Adolescents: IV: 60 mg/m^2/**day** for 2 days at weeks 2, 7, 25, and 28 (neoadjuvant) or weeks 5, 10, 25, and 28 (adjuvant) in combination with doxorubicin (Goorin, 2003) or 120 mg/m^2/**day** at weeks 0, 5, 12, and 17 in combination with doxorubicin (Meyers, 2005)

Adult: **TO PREVENT POSSIBLE OVERDOSE, VERIFY ANY CISPLATIN DOSE EXCEEDING 100 mg/m^2 PER COURSE. Pretreatment hydration is recommended.**

Note: Utilize patient's actual body weight (full weight) for calculation of body surface area- or weight-based dosing, particularly when the intent of therapy is curative; manage regimen-related toxicities in the same manner as for nonobese patients; if a dose reduction is utilized due to toxicity, consider resumption of full weight-based dosing with subsequent cycles, especially if cause of toxicity (eg, hepatic or renal impairment) is resolved (Griggs, 2012).

Bladder cancer, advanced: IV: 50-70 mg/m^2 every 3-4 weeks; heavily pretreated patients: 50 mg/m^2 every 4 weeks

Ovarian cancer, metastatic: IV:

Single agent: 100 mg/m^2 every 4 weeks

Combination therapy: 75-100 mg/m^2 every 4 weeks or 75 mg/m^2 every 3 weeks (Ozols, 2003)

Testicular cancer, metastatic: IV: 20 mg/m2/day for 5 days repeated every 3 weeks (Cushing, 2004; Saxman, 1998)

Dosing adjustment in renal impairment: Note: The manufacturer(s) recommend that repeat courses of cisplatin should not be given until serum creatinine is <1.5 mg/dL and/or BUN is <25 mg/dL and use is contraindicated in pre-existing renal impairment. The following adjustments have been recommended:

Aronoff, 2007: All patients:

GFR >50 mL/minute/1.73 m^2: No dosage adjustment necessary

GFR 10-50 mL/minute/1.73 m^2: Administer 75% of dose

GFR <10 mL/minute/1.73 m^2: Administer 50% of dose

Hemodialysis: Partially cleared by hemodialysis: Administer 50% of dose posthemodialysis

Peritoneal dialysis: Administer 50% of dose

Continuous renal replacement therapy (CRRT): Administer 75% of dose

Kintzel, 1995: Adult:

CrCl 46-60 mL/minute: Administer 75% of dose

CrCl 31-45 mL/minute: Administer 50% of dose

CrCl ≤30 mL/minute: Consider use of alternative drug

Dosing adjustment in hepatic impairment: There are no dosage adjustments provided in the manufacturer's labeling; however, cisplatin undergoes nonenzymatic metabolism and predominantly renal elimination; therefore, dosage adjustment is likely not necessary.

Preparation for Administration Hazardous agent; use appropriate precautions for handling and disposal (NIOSH 2014 [group 1]).

Parenteral: The infusion solution should have a final sodium chloride concentration ≥0.2% (Hincal 1979). Needles or IV administration sets that contain aluminum should not be used in the preparation or administration; aluminum can react with cisplatin resulting in precipitate formation and loss of potency.

Administration Hazardous agent; use appropriate precautions for handling and disposal (NIOSH 2014 [group 1]). Cisplatin is associated with a high emetic potential; antiemetics are recommended to prevent nausea and vomiting (Basch 2011; Dupuis 2011; Roila 2010).

Pretreatment hydration is recommended prior to cisplatin administration; adequate posthydration and urinary output (>100 mL/hour in adults) should be maintained for 24 hours after administration.

IV: Infuse over 6 to 8 hours; has also been infused over 30 minutes to 3 hours, at a rate of 1 mg/minute, or as a continuous infusion; infusion rate varies by protocol (refer to specific protocol for infusion details)

Needles or IV administration sets that contain aluminum should not be used for administration; aluminum may react with cisplatin resulting in precipitate formation and loss of potency.

Vesicant (at higher concentrations); ensure proper needle or catheter placement prior to and during infusion; avoid extravasation. If extravasation occurs, stop infusion immediately and disconnect (leave cannula/needle in place); gently aspirate extravasated solution (do **NOT** flush the line); initiate sodium thiosulfate antidote; elevate extremity. Dimethyl sulfoxide (DMSO) may also be considered an option (See Management of Drug Extravasations for more details).

Vesicant/Extravasation Risk Vesicant (>0.4 mg/mL); Irritant (≤0.4 mg/mL)

Monitoring Parameters Renal function tests (serum creatinine, BUN, CrCl), electrolytes (particularly magnesium, calcium, potassium), audiography (baseline and prior to each subsequent dose and following treatment), neurologic exam (with high dose), liver function tests periodically, CBC with differential and platelet count (weekly), urine output, urinalysis

Dosage Forms Excipient information presented when available (limited, particularly for generics); consult specific product labeling.

Solution, Intravenous:

Generic: 50 mg/50 mL (50 mL); 100 mg/100 mL (100 mL)

Solution, Intravenous [preservative free]:

Generic: 50 mg/50 mL (50 mL); 100 mg/100 mL (100 mL); 200 mg/200 mL (200 mL)

- ◆ **Cisplatin Injection (Can)** *see* CISplatin *on page 473*
- ◆ **Cisplatin Injection BP (Can)** *see* CISplatin *on page 473*
- ◆ **Cisplatin Injection, Mylan STD (Can)** *see* CISplatin *on page 473*
- ◆ **cis-platinum** *see* CISplatin *on page 473*
- ◆ ***Cis*-Retinoic Acid** *see* ISOtretinoin *on page 1171*
- ◆ **13-*cis*-Retinoic Acid** *see* ISOtretinoin *on page 1171*
- ◆ **13-*cis*-Vitamin A Acid** *see* ISOtretinoin *on page 1171*

Citalopram (sye TAL oh pram)

Medication Safety Issues

Sound-alike/look-alike issues:

CeleXA may be confused with CeleBREX, Cerebyx, Ranexa, ZyPREXA

BEERS Criteria medication:

This drug may be potentially inappropriate for use in geriatric patients with a history of falls or fractures (Quality of evidence - moderate; Strength of recommendation - strong).

Related Information

Antidepressant Agents *on page 2257*

Brand Names: US CeleXA

Brand Names: Canada Abbott-Citalopram; Accell-Citalopram; ACT Citalopram; AG-Citalopram; Apo-Citalopram; Auro-Citalopram; Celexa; Citalopram-Odan; CTP 30; Dom-Citalopram; ECL-Citalopram; JAMP-Citalopram; Mar-Citalopram; Mint-Citalopram; Mylan-Citalopram; Nat-Citalopram; PHL-Citalopram; PMS-Citalopram; Q-Citalopram; RAN-Citalo; Riva-Citalopram; Sandoz-Citalopram; Septa-Citalopram; Teva-Citalopram

Therapeutic Category Antidepressant, Selective Serotonin Reuptake Inhibitor (SSRI)

Generic Availability (US) Yes

Use Treatment of depression (FDA approved in adults); has also been used to treat obsessive-compulsive disorder (OCD)

Medication Guide Available Yes

Pregnancy Risk Factor C

Pregnancy Considerations Adverse events have been observed in animal reproduction studies. Citalopram and its metabolites cross the human placenta. An increased risk of teratogenic effects, including cardiovascular defects, may be associated with maternal use of citalopram or other SSRIs; however, available information is conflicting. Nonteratogenic effects in the newborn following SSRI/SNRI exposure late in the third trimester include respiratory distress, cyanosis, apnea, seizures, temperature instability, feeding difficulty, vomiting, hypoglycemia, hypo- or hypertonia, hyper-reflexia, jitteriness, irritability, constant crying, and tremor. Symptoms may be due to the toxicity of the SSRIs/SNRIs or a discontinuation syndrome and may be consistent with serotonin syndrome associated with SSRI treatment. Persistent pulmonary hypertension of the newborn (PPHN) has also been reported with SSRI exposure. The long-term effects of *in utero* SSRI exposure on infant development and behavior are not known.

Due to pregnancy-induced physiologic changes, women who are pregnant may require adjusted doses of citalopram to achieve euthymia. The ACOG recommends that therapy with SSRIs or SNRIs during pregnancy be individualized; treatment of depression during pregnancy should incorporate the clinical expertise of the mental health clinician, obstetrician, primary healthcare provider, and pediatrician. According to the American Psychiatric Association (APA), the risks of medication treatment should be weighed against other treatment options and untreated depression. For women who discontinue antidepressant medications during pregnancy and who may be at high risk for postpartum depression, the medications can be restarted following delivery. Treatment algorithms have been developed by the ACOG and the APA for the management of depression in women prior to conception and during pregnancy.

Breast-Feeding Considerations Citalopram and its metabolites are excreted in breast milk. According to the manufacturer, the decision to continue or discontinue breast-feeding during therapy should take into account the risk of exposure to the infant and the benefits of treatment to the mother. Excessive somnolence, decreased feeding, colic, irritability, restlessness, and weight loss have been reported in breast-fed infants. The long-term effects on development and behavior have not been studied; therefore, citalopram should be prescribed to a mother who is breast-feeding only when the benefits outweigh the potential risks. Maternal use of an SSRI during pregnancy may cause delayed milk secretion.

Contraindications

Hypersensitivity to citalopram or any component of the formulation; use of MAO inhibitors intended to treat psychiatric disorders (concurrently or within 14 days of discontinuing either citalopram or the MAO inhibitor); initiation of citalopram in a patient receiving linezolid or intravenous methylene blue; concomitant use with pimozide

Canadian labeling: Additional contraindications (not in US labeling): Known QT interval prolongation or congenital long QT syndrome

Warnings/Precautions [U.S. Boxed Warning]: Antidepressants increase the risk of suicidal thinking and behavior in children, adolescents, and young adults (18-24 years of age) with major depressive disorder (MDD) and other psychiatric disorders; consider risk prior to prescribing. Short-term studies did not show an increased risk in patients >24 years of age and showed a decreased risk in patients ≥65 years. Closely monitor patients for clinical worsening, suicidality, or unusual changes in behavior, particularly during the initial 1-2 months of therapy or during periods of dosage adjustments (increases or decreases); the patient's family or caregiver should be instructed to closely observe the patient and communicate condition with healthcare provider. A medication guide concerning the use of antidepressants should be dispensed with each prescription. **Citalopram is not FDA approved for use in children.**

The possibility of a suicide attempt is inherent in major depression and may persist until remission occurs. Use caution in high-risk patients. Worsening depression and severe abrupt suicidality that are not part of the presenting symptoms may require discontinuation or modification of drug therapy. The patient's family or caregiver should be alerted to monitor patients for the emergence of suicidality and associated behaviors (such as agitation, irritability, hostility, impulsivity, and hypomania) and call healthcare provider.

May worsen psychosis in some patients or precipitate a shift to mania or hypomania in patients with bipolar disorder. Patients presenting with depressive symptoms should be screened for bipolar disorder. Monotherapy in patients with bipolar disorder should be avoided. **Citalopram is not FDA approved for the treatment of bipolar depression.**

Potentially life-threatening serotonin syndrome (SS) has occurred with serotonergic agents (eg, SSRIs, SNRIs), particularly when used in combination with other serotonergic agents (eg, triptans, TCAs, fentanyl, lithium, tramadol, buspirone, St. John's wort, tryptophan) or agents that impair metabolism of serotonin (eg, MAO inhibitors intended to treat psychiatric disorders, other MAO inhibitors [ie, linezolid and intravenous methylene blue]). Discontinue treatment (and any concomitant serotonergic agent) immediately if signs/symptoms arise. May increase the risks associated with electroconvulsive therapy. Has a low potential to impair cognitive or motor performance; caution operating hazardous machinery or driving. Bone fractures have been associated with antidepressant treatment. Consider the possibility of a fragility fracture if an antidepressant-treated patient presents with unexplained bone pain, point tenderness, swelling, or bruising (Rabenda, 2013; Rizzoli, 2012).

Citalopram causes dose-dependent QTc prolongation; torsade de pointes, ventricular tachycardia, and sudden death have been reported. Use is not recommended in patients with congenital long QT syndrome, bradycardia, recent MI, uncompensated heart failure, hypokalemia, and/or hypomagnesemia, or patients receiving concomitant medications which prolong the QT interval; if use is essential and cannot be avoided in these patients, ECG monitoring is recommended. Discontinue therapy in any patient with persistent QTc measurements >500 msec. Serum electrolytes, particularly potassium and magnesium, should be monitored prior to initiation and periodically during therapy in any patient at increased risk for significant electrolyte disturbances; hypokalemia and/or hypomagnesemia should be corrected prior to use. Due to the QT prolongation risk, doses >40 mg/day are not recommended. Additionally, the maximum daily dose should not exceed 20 mg/day in certain populations (eg, CYP2C19 poor metabolizers, patients with hepatic impairment, elderly patients). Potentially significant interactions may exist, requiring dose or frequency adjustment, additional monitoring, and/or selection of alternative therapy. Consult drug interactions database for more detailed information.

Use with caution in patients with a previous seizure disorder or condition predisposing to seizures such as brain damage or alcoholism. May cause or exacerbate sexual dysfunction. Use caution in elderly patients; may be potentially inappropriate in patients with a history of falls or fractures, and may cause hyponatremia/SIADH (elderly at increased risk); volume depletion and diuretics may increase risk. Monitor sodium closely with initiation or dosage adjustments in older adults (Beers Criteria). May cause mild pupillary dilation which in susceptible individuals can lead to an episode of narrow-angle glaucoma. Consider evaluating patients who have not had an iridectomy for narrow-angle glaucoma risk factors. Citalopram is not FDA-approved for use in children; however, if used, monitor weight and growth regularly during therapy due to the potential for decreased appetite and weight loss with SSRI use.

Abrupt discontinuation or interruption of antidepressant therapy has been associated with a discontinuation syndrome. Symptoms arising may vary with antidepressant however commonly include nausea, vomiting, diarrhea, headaches, light-headedness, dizziness, diminished appetite, sweating, chills, tremors, paresthesias, fatigue, somnolence, and sleep disturbances (eg, vivid dreams, insomnia). Greater risks for developing a discontinuation syndrome have been associated with antidepressants with shorter half-lives, longer durations of treatment, and abrupt discontinuation. For antidepressants of short or intermediate half-lives, symptoms may emerge within 2-5 days after treatment discontinuation and last 7-14 days (APA, 2010; Fava, 2006; Haddad, 2001; Shelton, 2001; Warner, 2006).

Warnings: Additional Pediatric Considerations

Selective serotonin reuptake inhibitor (SSRI)-associated behavioral activation (ie, restlessness, hyperkinesis, hyperactivity, agitation) is two- to threefold more prevalent in children compared to adolescents; it is more prevalent in adolescents compared to adults. Somnolence (including sedation and drowsiness) is more common in adults compared to children and adolescents (Safer, 2006). SSRI-associated vomiting is two- to threefold more prevalent in children compared to adolescents and is more prevalent in adolescents compared to adults (Safer, 2006).

Adverse Reactions

Cardiovascular: Bradycardia, hypotension, orthostatic hypotension, prolonged Q-T interval on ECG, tachycardia

Central nervous system: Agitation, amnesia, anxiety, apathy, confusion, depression, drowsiness (dose related), fatigue (dose related), insomnia (dose related), lack of concentration, migraine, paresthesia, yawning (dose related)

Dermatologic: Diaphoresis (dose related), pruritus, skin rash

Endocrine & metabolic: Amenorrhea, decreased libido, weight gain, weight loss

Gastrointestinal: Abdominal pain, anorexia, diarrhea, dysgeusia, dyspepsia, flatulence, increased appetite, nausea, sialorrhea, vomiting, xerostomia
Genitourinary: Dysmenorrhea, ejaculatory disorder, impotence (dose related)
Neuromuscular & skeletal: Arthralgia, myalgia, tremor
Ophthalmic: Accommodation disturbance
Renal: Polyuria
Respiratory: Cough, rhinitis, sinusitis, upper respiratory tract infection
Miscellaneous: Fever
Rare but important or life-threatening: Abnormal serum prolactin levels, acute renal failure, alopecia, anaphylaxis, anemia, angina pectoris, angioedema, angle-closure glaucoma, arthritis, asthma, atrial fibrillation, bronchitis, bundle branch block, bursitis, cardiac arrest, cardiac failure, cataract, catatonia, cerebrovascular accident, cholelithiasis, delirium, delusions, depersonalization, diplopia, diverticulitis, drug dependence, duodenal ulcer, eczema, erythema multiforme, extrapyramidal reaction, extrasystoles, galactorrhea, gastric ulcer, gastrointestinal hemorrhage, granulocytopenia, gynecomastia, hallucination, heavy eyelids, hemolytic anemia, hepatic necrosis, hepatitis, hypersensitivity reaction, hypertension, hypertrichosis, hypoglycemia, hypokalemia, hyponatremia, hypoprothrombinemia, hypothyroidism, ischemic heart disease, leukocytosis, leukopenia, lymphadenopathy, lymphocytopenia, lymphocytosis, melanosis, myasthenia, myocardial infarction, nephrolithiasis, neuroleptic malignant syndrome (Stevens, 2008), obesity, osteoporosis, pancreatitis, phlebitis, pneumonia, priapism, psoriasis, psychosis, pulmonary embolism, rhabdomyolysis, seizure, serotonin syndrome, skin photosensitivity, syncope, thrombocytopenia, thrombosis, tonic-clonic seizures, torsades de pointes, toxic epidermal necrolysis, transient ischemic attacks, urinary incontinence, urinary retention, vaginal hemorrhage, ventricular arrhythmia, withdrawal syndrome

Drug Interactions

Metabolism/Transport Effects Substrate of CYP2C19 (major), CYP2D6 (minor), CYP3A4 (major); **Note:** Assignment of Major/Minor substrate status based on clinically relevant drug interaction potential; **Inhibits** CYP1A2 (weak), CYP2B6 (weak), CYP2C19 (weak), CYP2D6 (weak)

Avoid Concomitant Use

Avoid concomitant use of Citalopram with any of the following: Conivaptan; Dapoxetine; Dosulepin; Fluconazole; Fusidic Acid (Systemic); Highest Risk QTc-Prolonging Agents; Idelalisib; Iobenguane I 123; Ivabradine; Linezolid; MAO Inhibitors; Methylene Blue; Mifepristone; Moderate Risk QTc-Prolonging Agents; Pimozide; Tryptophan; Urokinase

Increased Effect/Toxicity

Citalopram may increase the levels/effects of: Agents with Antiplatelet Properties; Anticoagulants; Antidepressants (Serotonin Reuptake Inhibitor/Antagonist); Antipsychotic Agents; Apixaban; Aspirin; Blood Glucose Lowering Agents; BusPIRone; CarBAMazepine; Collagenase (Systemic); Dabigatran Etexilate; Deoxycholic Acid; Desmopressin; Dextromethorphan; Dosulepin; Highest Risk QTc-Prolonging Agents; Ibritumomab; Methylene Blue; Mexiletine; NSAID (COX-2 Inhibitor); NSAID (Nonselective); Obinutuzumab; Pimozide; Rivaroxaban; Salicylates; Serotonin Modulators; Thiazide Diuretics; Thrombolytic Agents; TiZANidine; Tositumomab and Iodine I 131 Tositumomab; TraMADol; Tricyclic Antidepressants; Urokinase; Vitamin K Antagonists

The levels/effects of Citalopram may be increased by: Alcohol (Ethyl); Analgesics (Opioid); Antiemetics (5HT3 Antagonists); Antipsychotic Agents; Aprepitant; BuPROPion; BusPIRone; Cimetidine; CNS Depressants; Conivaptan; CYP2C19 Inhibitors (Moderate); CYP2C19 Inhibitors (Strong); CYP3A4 Inhibitors (Moderate); CYP3A4 Inhibitors (Strong); Dapoxetine; Fluconazole; Fosaprepitant; Fusidic Acid (Systemic); Glucosamine; Herbs (Anticoagulant/Antiplatelet Properties); Ibrutinib; Idelalisib; Ivabradine; Ivacaftor; Limaprost; Linezolid; Lithium; Luliconazole; MAO Inhibitors; Metoclopramide; Metyrosine; Mifepristone; Moderate Risk QTc-Prolonging Agents; Multivitamins/Fluoride (with ADE); Multivitamins/Minerals (with ADEK, Folate, Iron); Multivitamins/Minerals (with AE, No Iron); Netupitant; Omega-3 Fatty Acids; Palbociclib; Pentosan Polysulfate Sodium; Pentoxifylline; Prostacyclin Analogues; QTc-Prolonging Agents (Indeterminate Risk and Risk Modifying); Simeprevir; Stiripentol; Tedizolid; Tipranavir; TraMADol; Tricyclic Antidepressants; Tryptophan; Vitamin E

Decreased Effect

Citalopram may decrease the levels/effects of: Iobenguane I 123; Ioflupane I 123; Thyroid Products

The levels/effects of Citalopram may be decreased by: Bosentan; CarBAMazepine; CYP2C19 Inducers (Strong); CYP3A4 Inducers (Moderate); CYP3A4 Inducers (Strong); Cyproheptadine; Dabrafenib; Deferasirox; Mitotane; NSAID (COX-2 Inhibitor); NSAID (Nonselective); Rifampin; Siltuximab; St Johns Wort; Tocilizumab

Storage/Stability Store at 25°C (77°F); excursions permitted to 15°C to 30°C (59°F to 86°F). Protect from moisture.

Mechanism of Action A racemic bicyclic phthalane derivative, citalopram selectively inhibits serotonin reuptake in the presynaptic neurons and has minimal effects on norepinephrine or dopamine. Uptake inhibition of serotonin is primarily due to the *S*-enantiomer of citalopram. Displays little to no affinity for serotonin, dopamine, adrenergic, histamine, GABA, or muscarinic receptor subtypes.

Pharmacodynamics

Onset of action: 1-2 weeks
Maximum effect: 8-12 weeks
Duration: 1-2 days

Pharmacokinetics (Adult data unless noted)

Distribution: V_d: Adults: 12 L/kg
Protein binding, plasma: ~80%
Metabolism: Extensively hepatic, primarily via CYP3A4 and CYP2C19; metabolized to N-demethylated, N-oxide, and deaminated metabolites
Bioavailability: 80%; tablets and oral solution are bioequivalent
Half-life elimination: Adults: Range: 24-48 hours; mean: 35 hours (doubled with hepatic impairment)
Time to peak serum concentration: 1 to 6 hours, average within 4 hours
Elimination: Urine (10% as unchanged drug)
Clearance: Hepatic impairment: Decreased by 37%; Mild to moderate renal impairment: Decreased by 17%; Severe renal impairment (CrCl <20 mL/minute): No information available

Dosing: Usual

Children and Adolescents: **Note:** Slower titration of dose every 2-4 weeks may minimize risk of SSRI associated behavioral activation, which has been shown to increase risk of suicidal behavior. Doses >40 mg are not recommended due to risk of QTc prolongation.

Depression: Note: Not FDA approved. Limited information is available; only one randomized, placebo controlled trial has shown citalopram to be effective for the treatment of depression in pediatric patients (Wagner, 2004); other controlled pediatric trials have **not** shown benefit (Sharp, 2006; von Knorring, 2006; Wagner, 2005). Some experts recommend the following doses (Dopheide, 2006):

Children ≤11 years: Initial: 10 mg/day given once daily; increase dose slowly by 5 mg/day every 2 weeks as clinically needed; dosage range: 20-40 mg/day

Children and Adolescents ≥12 years: Initial: 20 mg/day given once daily; increase dose slowly by 10 mg/day every 2 weeks as clinically needed; dosage range: 20-40 mg/day

Obsessive-compulsive disorder: Note: Not FDA approved. Limited information is available; several open label trials have been published (Mukaddes, 2003; Thomsen, 1997; Thomsen, 2001). Some experts recommend the following doses:

Children ≤11 years: Initial: 5-10 mg/day given once daily; increase dose slowly by 5 mg/day every 2 weeks as clinically needed; dosage range: 10-40 mg/day.

Children and Adolescents ≥12 years: Initial: 10-20 mg/day given once daily; increase dose slowly by 10 mg/day every 2 weeks as clinically needed; dosage range: 10-40 mg/day.

Note: Higher mg/kg doses are needed in children compared to adolescents.

Adults: **Depression:**

Patients <60 years: Initial: 20 mg once daily; may increase dose in 20 mg increments at intervals of ≥1 week up to a maximum daily dose: 40 mg/day

Patients ≥60 years, poor metabolizers of CYP2C19 **or** concurrent use of moderate to strong CYP2C19 inhibitors (eg, cimetidine): 20 mg/day

Dosage adjustment in renal impairment: Adults:

Mild or moderate renal impairment: No dosage adjustment needed

Severe renal impairment (CrCl <20 mL/minute): Use with caution

Dosage adjustment in hepatic impairment: Adults: 20 mg once daily due to increased serum concentrations and the risk of QT prolongation

Administration May be administered without regard to meals

Monitoring Parameters ECG; electrolytes (potassium and magnesium concentrations); liver function tests and CBC with continued therapy; monitor patient periodically for symptom resolution; monitor for worsening depression, suicidality, and associated behaviors (especially at the beginning of therapy or when doses are increased or decreased). Monitor for anxiety, social functioning, mania, panic attacks; akathisia

Additional Information If used for an extended period of time, long-term usefulness of citalopram should be periodically re-evaluated for the individual patient. A recent report describes 5 children (age: 8-15 years) who developed epistaxis (n=4) or bruising (n=1) while receiving SSRI therapy (sertraline) (Lake, 2000).

Neonates born to women receiving SSRIs later during the third trimester may experience respiratory distress, apnea, cyanosis, temperature instability, vomiting, feeding difficulty, hypoglycemia, constant crying, irritability, hypotonia, hypertonia, hyper-reflexia, tremor, jitteriness, and seizures; these symptoms may be due to a direct toxic effect, withdrawal syndrome, or (in some cases) serotonin syndrome. Withdrawal symptoms occur in 30% of neonates exposed to SSRIs *in utero*; monitor newborns for at least 48 hours after birth; long-term effects of *in utero* exposure to SSRIs are unknown (Levinson-Castiel, 2006).

Dosage Forms Excipient information presented when available (limited, particularly for generics); consult specific product labeling.

Solution, Oral:
 Generic: 10 mg/5 mL (240 mL)

Tablet, Oral:
 CeleXA: 10 mg
 CeleXA: 20 mg, 40 mg [scored]
 Generic: 10 mg, 20 mg, 40 mg

- ◆ **Citalopram Hydrobromide** *see* Citalopram *on page 476*
- ◆ **Citalopram-Odan (Can)** *see* Citalopram *on page 476*
- ◆ **Citrate of Magnesia** *see* Magnesium Citrate *on page 1311*
- ◆ **Citric Acid and Potassium Citrate** *see* Potassium Citrate and Citric Acid *on page 1738*
- ◆ **Citric Acid and Sodium Citrate** *see* Sodium Citrate and Citric Acid *on page 1942*

Citric Acid, Sodium Citrate, and Potassium Citrate

(SIT rik AS id, SOW dee um SIT rate, & poe TASS ee um SIT rate)

Medication Safety Issues

Sound-alike/look-alike issues:

Polycitra may be confused with Bicitra

Brand Names: US Cytra-3; Virtrate-3

Therapeutic Category Alkalinizing Agent, Oral

Generic Availability (US) May be product dependent

Use As long-term therapy to alkalinize the urine for control and/or dissolution of uric acid and cystine calculi of the urinary tract [FDA approved in pediatric patients (age not specified) and adults]; treatment of chronic metabolic acidosis secondary to renal tubule disorders [FDA approved in pediatric patients (age not specified) and adults]; treatment of gout as adjuvant therapy with uricosuric drugs [FDA approved in pediatric patients (age not specified) and adults]. Has also been used for treatment of chronic metabolic acidosis due chronic diarrhea and some inborn errors of metabolism.

Pregnancy Risk Factor Not established

Pregnancy Considerations Use caution with toxemia of pregnancy.

Contraindications Severe renal impairment with oliguria or azotemia; untreated Addison's disease; severe myocardial damage.

Warnings/Precautions Use with caution in patients with heart failure, peripheral or pulmonary edema, and renal impairment; contains sodium. Conversion to bicarbonate may be impaired in patients who are severely ill, in shock, or with hepatic failure. Use with caution in digitalized patients or those who are receiving concomitant medications that increase potassium. Some dosage forms may contain propylene glycol; large amounts are potentially toxic and have been associated hyperosmolality, lactic acidosis, seizures, and respiratory depression; use caution (AAP, 1997; Zar, 2007).

Benzyl alcohol and derivatives: Some dosage forms may contain sodium benzoate/benzoic acid; benzoic acid (benzoate) is a metabolite of benzyl alcohol; large amounts of benzyl alcohol (≥99 mg/kg/day) have been associated with a potentially fatal toxicity ("gasping syndrome") in neonates; the "gasping syndrome" consists of metabolic acidosis, respiratory distress, gasping respirations, CNS dysfunction (including convulsions, intracranial hemorrhage), hypotension, and cardiovascular collapse (AAP, 1997; CDC, 1982); some data suggests that benzoate displaces bilirubin from protein binding sites (Ahlfors, 2001); avoid or use dosage forms containing benzyl alcohol derivative with caution in neonates. See manufacturer's labeling.

Warnings: Additional Pediatric Considerations Some dosage forms may contain propylene glycol; in neonates large amounts of propylene glycol delivered orally, intravenously (eg, >3,000 mg/day), or topically have been associated with potentially fatal toxicities which can include metabolic acidosis, seizures, renal failure, and CNS depression; toxicities have also been reported in children and adults including hyperosmolality, lactic acidosis, seizures and respiratory depression; use caution (AAP, 1997; Shehab, 2009).

Adverse Reactions

Cardiovascular: Cardiac abnormalities

Endocrine & metabolic: Calcium levels, hyperkalemia, hypernatremia, metabolic alkalosis

Gastrointestinal: Diarrhea

Neuromuscular & skeletal: Tetany

Drug Interactions

Metabolism/Transport Effects None known.

Avoid Concomitant Use There are no known interactions where it is recommended to avoid concomitant use.

Increased Effect/Toxicity

Citric Acid, Sodium Citrate, and Potassium Citrate may increase the levels/effects of: ACE Inhibitors; Aliskiren; Aluminum Hydroxide; Angiotensin II Receptor Blockers; Potassium-Sparing Diuretics

The levels/effects of Citric Acid, Sodium Citrate, and Potassium Citrate may be increased by: Eplerenone; Heparin; Heparin (Low Molecular Weight); Nicorandil

Decreased Effect There are no known significant interactions involving a decrease in effect.

Storage/Stability Store at controlled room temperature of 20°C to 25°C (68°F to 77°F); do not freeze. Protect from excessive heat.

Pharmacokinetics (Adult data unless noted)

Metabolism: ≥95% via hepatic oxidation to bicarbonate

Elimination: <5% unchanged in the urine

Dosing: Neonatal Oral: **Note:** 1 mL of oral solution contains 2 mEq of bicarbonate

Dosing per mEq of bicarbonate: 2-3 mEq bicarbonate/kg/**day** (1-1.5 mL/kg/day) in 3-4 divided doses

Dosing: Usual Oral: **Note:** 1 mL of oral solution contains 2 mEq of bicarbonate

Manufacturer's recommendation: Children: 5-15 mL (10-30 mEq bicarbonate) per dose after meals and at bedtime

Alternative recommendation: Dosing per mEq of bicarbonate:

Infants and Children: 2–3 mEq bicarbonate/kg/**day** (1-1.5 mL/kg/**day**) in 3-4 divided doses

Adults: 15-30 mL (30-60 mEq bicarbonate) per dose after meals and at bedtime

Note: When using to alkalinize the urine, 10-15 mL doses given 4 times daily typically maintain urinary pH 6.5-7.4; doses 15-20 mL4 times daily usually maintain urinary pH at 7.0-7.6

Administration Dose should be diluted in water; may follow dose with additional water if necessary. Administer after meals and at bedtime to prevent osmotic saline laxative effect; shake well before use.

Monitoring Parameters Periodic serum (sodium, potassium, calcium, bicarbonate); urine pH

Additional Information Prior to absorption, citrate ions effects are similar to chloride and therefore, does not affect gastrointestinal pH or disturb digestion.

Oral solution: 1 mL contains 1 mEq potassium, 1 mEq sodium, and 2 mEq of bicarbonate

Dosage Forms Excipient information presented when available (limited, particularly for generics); consult specific product labeling.

Solution, Oral:

Virtrate-3: Citric acid 334 mg, sodium citrate 500 mg, and potassium citrate 550 mg per 5 mL (473 mL) [sugar free; contains fd&c yellow #6 (sunset yellow), polyethylene glycol, propylene glycol, saccharin sodium, sodium benzoate; raspberry flavor]

Generic: Citric acid 334 mg, sodium citrate 500 mg, and potassium citrate 550 mg per 5 mL (473 mL)

Syrup, Oral:

Cytra-3: Citric acid 334 mg, sodium citrate 500 mg, and potassium citrate 550 mg per 5 mL (473 mL) [alcohol free, sugar free; contains fd&c yellow #6 (sunset yellow), polyethylene glycol, propylene glycol, saccharin sodium, sodium benzoate; vanilla flavor]

- ◆ **Citroma [OTC]** *see* Magnesium Citrate *on page 1311*
- ◆ **Citro-Mag (Can)** *see* Magnesium Citrate *on page 1311*
- ◆ **Citrovorum Factor** *see* Leucovorin Calcium *on page 1226*
- ◆ **CL-232315** *see* MitoXANtrone *on page 1448*

Cladribine (KLA dri been)

Medication Safety Issues

Sound-alike/look-alike issues:

Cladribine may be confused with clevidipine, clofarabine, cytarabine, fludarabine

Leustatin may be confused with lovastatin

High alert medication:

This medication is in a class the Institute for Safe Medication Practices (ISMP) includes among its list of drug classes which have a heightened risk of causing significant patient harm when used in error.

Related Information

Management of Drug Extravasations *on page 2298*

Prevention of Chemotherapy-Induced Nausea and Vomiting in Children *on page 2368*

Safe Handling of Hazardous Drugs *on page 2455*

Brand Names: Canada Cladribine Injection

Therapeutic Category Antineoplastic Agent, Antimetabolite (Purine Analog)

Generic Availability (US) Yes

Use Treatment of active hairy cell leukemia (FDA approved in adults); has also been used for acute myeloid leukemia and refractory Langerhans cell histiocytosis (LCH)

Pregnancy Risk Factor D

Pregnancy Considerations Teratogenic effects and fetal mortality were observed in animal reproduction studies. May cause fetal harm if administered during pregnancy. Women of reproductive potential should use highly effective contraception during treatment.

Breast-Feeding Considerations Due to the potential for serious adverse reactions in the nursing infant, the decision to discontinue cladribine or to discontinue breastfeeding should take into account the importance of treatment to the mother.

Contraindications Hypersensitivity to cladribine or any component of the formulation

Warnings/Precautions Hazardous agent - use appropriate precautions for handling and disposal (NIOSH 2014 [group 1]). **[U.S. Boxed Warning]: Dose-dependent, reversible myelosuppression (neutropenia, anemia, and thrombocytopenia) is common and generally reversible;** use with caution in patients with preexisting hematologic or immunologic abnormalities; monitor blood counts, especially during the first 4-8 weeks after treatment. **[U.S. Boxed Warning]: Serious, dose-related neurologic toxicity (including irreversible paraparesis and quadriparesis) has been reported with continuous infusions of higher doses (4-9 times the FDA-approved dose); may also occur at approved doses (rare).** Neurotoxicity may be delayed and may present as progressive, irreversible weakness; diagnostics with electromyography and nerve conduction studies were consistent with demyelinating disease. **[U.S. Boxed Warning]: Acute**

nephrotoxicity (eg, acidosis, anuria, increased serum creatinine), possibly requiring dialysis, has been reported with high doses (4-9 times the FDA-approved dose), particularly when administered with other nephrotoxic agents. Use with caution in patients with renal or hepatic impairment. Fever (>100°F) may occur, with or without neutropenia, observed more commonly in the first month of treatment. Infections (bacterial, viral, and fungal) were reported more commonly in the first month after treatment (generally mild or moderate in severity, although serious infections including sepsis have been reported); the incidence is reduced in the second month; due to neutropenia and T-cell depletion, risk versus benefit of treatment should be evaluated in patients with active infections. Administration of live vaccines is not recommended during treatment with cladribine (may increase the risk of infection due to immunosuppression). Use caution in patients with high tumor burden; tumor lysis syndrome may occur (rare). **[U.S. Boxed Warning]: Should be administered under the supervision of an experienced cancer chemotherapy physician.**

Benzyl alcohol and derivatives: Weekly (7-day) infusion preparation recommends further dilution with bacteriostatic normal saline which contains benzyl alcohol; large amounts of benzyl alcohol (≥99 mg/kg/day) have been associated with a potentially fatal toxicity ("gasping syndrome") in neonates; the "gasping syndrome" consists of metabolic acidosis, respiratory distress, gasping respirations, CNS dysfunction (including convulsions, intracranial hemorrhage), hypotension, and cardiovascular collapse (AAP, 1997; CDC, 1982); some data suggests that benzoate displaces bilirubin from protein binding sites (Ahlfors, 2001); avoid or use dosage forms containing benzyl alcohol with caution in neonates. See manufacturer's labeling.

Adverse Reactions

Cardiovascular: Edema, tachycardia, thrombosis

Central nervous system: Anxiety, chills, dizziness, fatigue, fever, headache, insomnia, malaise, pain

Dermatologic: Bruising, erythema, hyperhidrosis, petechiae, pruritus, purpura, rash

Gastrointestinal: Abdominal pain, appetite decreased, constipation, diarrhea, flatulence, nausea, vomiting

Hematologic: Anemia, myelosuppression, neutropenia, neutropenic fever, thrombocytopenia

Local: Injection site reactions, phlebitis

Neuromuscular & skeletal: Arthralgia, muscle weakness, myalgia, weakness

Respiratory: Abnormal breath sounds, abnormal chest sounds, cough, dyspnea, epistaxis, rales

Miscellaneous: Diaphoresis, infection

Rare but important or life-threatening: Aplastic anemia, bacteremia, CD4 lymphocytopenia (nadir: 4-6 months), cellulitis, consciousness decreased, conjunctivitis, hemolytic anemia, hypereosinophilia, hypersensitivity, myelodysplastic syndrome, opportunistic infections (cytomegalovirus, fungal infections, herpes virus infections, listeriosis, *Pneumocystis jirovecii*), pancytopenia (prolonged), paraparesis, pneumonia, polyneuropathy (with high doses), progressive multifocal leukoencephalopathy (PML), pulmonary interstitial infiltrates, quadriparesis (reported at high doses), renal dysfunction (with high doses), renal failure, septic shock, Stevens-Johnson syndrome, stroke, toxic epidermal necrolysis, tuberculosis reactivation, tumor lysis syndrome

Drug Interactions

Metabolism/Transport Effects

None known.

Avoid Concomitant Use

Avoid concomitant use of Cladribine with any of the following: BCG; BCG (Intravesical); CloZAPine; Dipyrone; Natalizumab; Pimecrolimus; Tacrolimus (Topical); Tofacitinib; Vaccines (Live)

Increased Effect/Toxicity

Cladribine may increase the levels/effects of: CloZAPine; Leflunomide; Natalizumab; Tofacitinib; Vaccines (Live)

The levels/effects of Cladribine may be increased by: Denosumab; Dipyrone; Pimecrolimus; Roflumilast; Tacrolimus (Topical); Trastuzumab

Decreased Effect

Cladribine may decrease the levels/effects of: BCG; BCG (Intravesical); Coccidioides immitis Skin Test; Sipuleucel-T; Vaccines (Inactivated); Vaccines (Live)

The levels/effects of Cladribine may be decreased by: Echinacea

Storage/Stability

Store intact vials refrigerated at 2°C to 8°C (36°F to 46°F). Protect from light. A precipitate may develop at low temperatures and may be resolubilized at room temperature or by shaking the solution vigorously. Inadvertent freezing does not affect the solution; if freezing occurs prior to dilution, allow to thaw naturally prior to reconstitution; do not heat or microwave; do not refreeze.

24-hour continuous infusion: Dilutions for infusion should be used promptly; if not used promptly, the 24-hour infusion may be stored refrigerated for up to 8 hours prior to administration.

7-day continuous infusion: Dilutions for infusion should be used promptly; if not used promptly, the 7-day infusion may be stored refrigerated for up to 8 hours prior to administration. Reconstituted solution is stable for 7 days (when diluted in bacteriostatic NS) in a CADD® medication cassette reservoir. For patients weighing >85 kg, the effectiveness of the preservative in the bacteriostatic diluent may be reduced (due to dilution).

Mechanism of Action

A purine nucleoside analogue; prodrug which is activated via phosphorylation by deoxycytidine kinase to a 5'-triphosphate derivative (2-CaAMP). This active form incorporates into DNA to result in the breakage of DNA strand and shutdown of DNA synthesis and repair. This also results in a depletion of nicotinamide adenine dinucleotide and adenosine triphosphate (ATP). Cladribine is cell-cycle nonspecific.

Pharmacokinetics (Adult data unless noted)

Distribution: V_d:

- Pediatric patients (8 months to 18 years): 12.7 ± 8.5 L/kg; penetrates CSF (CSF concentrations are ~18% of plasma concentration) (Kearns, 1994)
- Adults: ~9 L/kg; penetrates CSF (CSF concentrations are ~25% of plasma concentration)

Protein binding: ~20%

Half-life:

- Pediatric patients (8 months to 18 years): 19.7 ± 3.4 hours (Kearns, 1994)
- Adults: After a 2-hour infusion (with normal renal function): 5.4 hours

Elimination: Urine (18%)

Dosing: Usual

Infants, Children, and Adolescents (details concerning dosing in combination regimens and protocols should be consulted):

Acute myeloid leukemia: Limited data available: IV: 8.9 mg/m²/day continuous infusion for 5 days for 1 or 2 courses (Krance, 2001) or 9 mg/m²/day over 30 minutes for 5 days for 1 course (in combination with cytarabine) (Crews, 2002; Rubnitz, 2009)

Langerhans cell histiocytosis, refractory: Limited data available: IV: 5 mg/m²/day over 2 hours for 5 days every 21 days for up to 6 cycles (Weitzman, 2009)

Adults: Details concerning dosing in combination regimens should also be consulted. **Hairy cell leukemia:** IV: 0.09 mg/kg/day continuous infusion for 7 days for 1 cycle

Dosing adjustment in renal impairment: There are no dosage adjustments provided in the manufacturer's labeling (due to inadequate data); use with caution. The following guidelines have been used by some clinicians (Aronoff, 2007):

Infants, Children, and Adolescents:

GFR >50 mL/minute/1.73 m^2: No adjustment required

GFR 10-50 mL/minute/1.73 m^2: Administer 50% of dose

GFR <10 mL/minute/1.73 m^2: Administer 30% of dose

Hemodialysis: Administer 30% of dose

Continuous renal replacement therapy (CRRT): Administer 50% of dose

Adults:

CrCl 10-50 mL/minute: Administer 75% of dose

CrCl <10 mL/minute: Administer 50% of dose

Continuous ambulatory peritoneal dialysis (CAPD): Administer 50% of dose

Dosing adjustment in hepatic impairment: Adults: There are no dosage adjustments provided in the manufacturer's labeling (due to inadequate data); use with caution.

Preparation for Administration Hazardous agent; use appropriate precautions for handling and disposal (NIOSH 2014 [group 1]).

Parenteral: A precipitate may develop at low temperatures and may be resolubilized at room temperature or by shaking the solution vigorously. Inadvertent freezing does not affect the solution; if freezing occurs prior to dilution, allow to thaw naturally prior to reconstitution; do not heat or microwave; do not refreeze.

To prepare a 24-hour continuous infusion: Further dilute in NS (adults: 500mL). The manufacturer recommends filtering with a 0.22 micron hydrophilic syringe filter prior to adding to infusion bag.

To prepare a 7-day continuous infusion: Further dilute in bacteriostatic NS (Adults: 100 mL); add to CADD medication cassette reservoir. Filter diluent and cladribine with a 0.22 micron hydrophilic filter prior to adding to cassette/reservoir.

Administration Hazardous agent; use appropriate precautions for handling and disposal (NIOSH 2014 [group 1]).

Parenteral: IV: Further dilute prior to use, may be administered over 24 hours as a continuous infusion, or as an intermittent infusion over 30 minutes or 2 hours; dependent upon indication and/or protocol.

Vesicant/Extravasation Risk May be an irritant.

Monitoring Parameters CBC with differential (particularly during the first 4-8 weeks post-treatment); baseline and periodic renal and hepatic function tests; body temperature (fever); bone marrow biopsy (after CBC has normalized; to confirm treatment response); signs and symptoms of neurotoxicity

Dosage Forms Excipient information presented when available (limited, particularly for generics); consult specific product labeling.

Solution, Intravenous [preservative free]:

Generic: 1 mg/mL (10 mL)

- **Cladribine Injection (Can)** *see* Cladribine *on page 480*
- **Claforan** *see* Cefotaxime *on page 398*
- **Claforan in D5W** *see* Cefotaxime *on page 398*
- **Claravis** *see* ISOtretinoin *on page 1171*
- **Clarinex** *see* Desloratadine *on page 605*
- **Clarinex Reditabs** *see* Desloratadine *on page 605*

Clarithromycin (kla RITH roe mye sin)

Medication Safety Issues

Sound-alike/look-alike issues:

Clarithromycin may be confused with Claritin, clindamycin, erythromycin

Related Information

H. pylori Treatment in Pediatric Patients *on page 2358*

Oral Medications That Should Not Be Crushed or Altered *on page 2476*

Prevention of Infective Endocarditis *on page 2378*

Brand Names: US Biaxin; Biaxin XL; Biaxin XL Pac

Brand Names: Canada Accel-Clarithromycin; Apo-Clarithromycin; Apo-Clarithromycin XL; Biaxin; Biaxin BID; Biaxin XL; Dom-Clarithromycin; Mylan-Clarithromycin; PMS-Clarithromycin; RAN-Clarithromycin; Riva-Clarithromycin; Sandoz-Clarithromycin; Teva-Clarithromycin

Therapeutic Category Antibiotic, Macrolide

Generic Availability (US) Yes

Use

Immediate release formulations: Treatment of upper and lower respiratory tract infections, community-acquired pneumonia, acute otitis media, and infections of the skin and skin structure due to susceptible organisms (FDA approved in ages ≥6 months and adults); prophylaxis and treatment of *Mycobacterium avium* complex (MAC) disease in patients with advanced HIV infection (FDA approved in ages ≥20 months and adults); treatment of *Helicobacter pylori* infection (FDA approved in adults); has also been used for infective endocarditis prophylaxis for dental procedures in penicillin-allergic patients; treatment of lyme disease, peritonitis prophylaxis, and post-exposure prophylaxis and treatment of pertussis

Extended release tablets: Treatment of acute maxillary sinusitis, acute bacterial exacerbation of chronic bronchitis, and community acquired pneumonia due to susceptible organisms (FDA approved in adults)

Pregnancy Risk Factor C

Pregnancy Considerations Adverse events have been documented in some animal reproduction studies. Clarithromycin crosses the placenta (Witt, 2003). The manufacturer recommends that clarithromycin not be used in a pregnant woman unless there are no alternative therapies. Clarithromycin is generally not recommended for the treatment or prophylaxis of *Mycobacterium avium* complex (MAC) or bacterial respiratory disease in HIV-infected pregnant patients (DHHS, 2013).

Breast-Feeding Considerations Clarithromycin and its active metabolite (14-hydroxy clarithromycin) are excreted into breast milk. The manufacturer recommends that caution be used if administered to nursing women. Decreased appetite, diarrhea, rash, and somnolence have been noted in nursing infants exposed to macrolide antibiotics (Goldstein, 2009).

Contraindications Hypersensitivity to clarithromycin, erythromycin, any of the macrolide antibiotics, or any component of the formulation; history of cholestatic jaundice/hepatic dysfunction associated with prior use of clarithromycin; history of QT prolongation or ventricular cardiac arrhythmia, including torsade de pointes; concomitant use with cisapride, pimozide, ergotamine, dihydroergotamine, HMG-CoA reductase inhibitors extensively metabolized by CYP3A4 (eg, lovastatin, simvastatin), astemizole or terfenadine (not available in the U.S.); concomitant use with colchicine in patients with renal or hepatic impairment

Warnings/Precautions Use has been associated with QT prolongation and infrequent cases of arrhythmias, including torsade de pointes; use is contraindicated in patients with a history of QT prolongation and ventricular arrhythmias, including torsade de pointes. Systemic exposure is increased in the elderly; may be at increased risk of torsade de pointes, particularly if concurrent severe renal impairment. Use with caution in patients at risk of prolonged cardiac repolarization. Avoid use in patients with uncorrected hypokalemia or hypomagnesemia, clinically significant bradycardia, and patients receiving Class IA (eg, quinidine, procainamide) or Class III (eg, amiodarone, dofetilide, sotalol) antiarrhythmic agents. Use caution in patients with coronary artery disease.

Elevated liver function tests and hepatitis (hepatocellular and/or cholestatic with or without jaundice) have been reported; usually reversible after discontinuation of clarithromycin. May lead to hepatic failure or death (rarely), especially in the presence of preexisting diseases and/or concomitant use of medications. Discontinue immediately if symptoms of hepatitis occur. Dosage adjustment needed in severe renal impairment. Use with caution in patients with myasthenia gravis.

Potentially significant drug-drug interactions may exist, requiring dose or frequency adjustment, additional monitoring, and/or selection of alternative therapy. Colchicine toxicity (including fatalities) has been reported with concomitant use; concomitant use is contraindicated in patients with renal or hepatic impairment. Clarithromycin in combination with ranitidine bismuth citrate should not be used in patients with a history of acute porphyria. Prolonged use may result in fungal or bacterial superinfection, including *C. difficile*-associated diarrhea (CDAD) and pseudomembranous colitis; CDAD has been observed >2 months postantibiotic treatment. Decreased *H. pylori* eradication rates have been observed with short-term (≤7 days) combination therapy. Current guidelines recommend 10 to 14 days of therapy (triple or quadruple) for eradication of *H. pylori* in pediatric and adult patients (Chey, 2007; NASPHGAN [Koletzko 2011]).

Severe acute reactions have (rarely) been reported, including anaphylaxis, Stevens-Johnson syndrome (SJS), toxic epidermal necrolysis (TEN), drug rash with eosinophilia and systemic symptoms (DRESS), and Henoch-Schönlein purpura (IgA vasculitis); discontinue therapy and initiate treatment immediately for severe acute hypersensitivity reactions. The presence of extended release tablets in the stool has been reported, particularly in patients with anatomic (eg, ileostomy, colostomy) or functional GI disorders with decreased transit times. Consider alternative dosage forms (eg, suspension) or an alternative antimicrobial for patients with tablet residue in the stool and no signs of clinical improvement. Some dosage forms may contain propylene glycol; large amounts are potentially toxic and have been associated hyperosmolality, lactic acidosis, seizures, and respiratory depression; use caution (AAP, 1997; Zar, 2007).

Adverse Reactions

Central nervous system: Headache, insomnia
Dermatologic: Skin rash (children)
Gastrointestinal: Abdominal pain, diarrhea, dysgeusia (adults), dyspepsia (adults), nausea (adults), vomiting (children)
Hematologic & oncologic: Prolonged prothrombin time (adults)
Hepatic: Abnormal hepatic function tests
Hypersensitivity: Anaphylactoid reaction
Infection: Candidiasis (including oral)
Renal: Increased blood urea nitrogen
Rare but important or life-threatening: Acne vulgaris, ageusia, altered sense of smell, anxiety, asthma, atrial fibrillation, behavioral changes, cardiac arrest, cellulitis, cholestatic hepatitis, *Clostridium difficile* associated diarrhea, *Clostridium difficile* (colitis), dental discoloration (reversible with dental cleaning), depression, disorientation, DRESS syndrome, drowsiness, dyskinesia, epistaxis, esophagitis, extrasystoles, gastritis, gastroesophageal reflux disease, glossitis, hallucination, hearing loss (reversible), hemorrhage, hepatic failure, hepatotoxicity (idiosyncratic) (Chalasani, 2014), hyperhidrosis, hypersensitivity, hypoglycemia, IgA vasculitis, increased gamma-glutamyl transferase, increased INR, increased lactate dehydrogenase, interstitial nephritis, leukopenia, loss of consciousness, malaise, manic behavior, neck stiffness, neutropenia, pancreatitis, parasominas, paresthesia, prolonged QT interval on ECG, pruritus, pseudomembranous colitis, pulmonary embolism, renal failure, rhabdomyolysis, seizure, Stevens-Johnson syndrome, stomatitis, thrombocytopenia, tinnitus, tongue discoloration, torsades de pointes, vaginal infection, ventricular arrhythmia, ventricular tachycardia

Drug Interactions

Metabolism/Transport Effects Substrate of CYP3A4 (major); **Note:** Assignment of Major/Minor substrate status based on clinically relevant drug interaction potential; **Inhibits** CYP1A2 (weak), CYP3A4 (strong), P-glycoprotein

Avoid Concomitant Use

Avoid concomitant use of Clarithromycin with any of the following: Ado-Trastuzumab Emtansine; Alfuzosin; Apixaban; Astemizole; Avanafil; Axitinib; Barnidipine; BCG; BCG (Intravesical); Bosutinib; Cabozantinib; Ceritinib; Cisapride; Conivaptan; Crizotinib; Dapoxetine; Dihydroergotamine; Disopyramide; Domperidone; Dronedarone; Eplerenone; Ergotamine; Everolimus; Fusidic Acid (Systemic); Halofantrine; Highest Risk QTc-Prolonging Agents; Ibrutinib; Idelalisib; Irinotecan; Isavuconazonium Sulfate; Ivabradine; Lapatinib; Lercanidipine; Lomitapide; Lopinavir; Lovastatin; Lurasidone; Macitentan; Mifepristone; Naloxegol; Nilotinib; NiMODipine; Nisoldipine; Olaparib; Palbociclib; PAZOPanib; Pimozide; QuiNIDine; QuiNINE; Ranolazine; Red Yeast Rice; Regorafenib; Salmeterol; Silodosin; Simeprevir; Simvastatin; Suvorexant; Tamsulosin; Terfenadine; Ticagrelor; Tolvaptan; Topotecan; Toremifene; Trabectedin; Ulipristal; Vemurafenib; VinCRIStine (Liposomal); Vorapaxar

Increased Effect/Toxicity

Clarithromycin may increase the levels/effects of: Ado-Trastuzumab Emtansine; Afatinib; Alfentanil; Alfuzosin; Almotriptan; Alosetron; ALPRAZolam; Antineoplastic Agents (Vinca Alkaloids); Apixaban; ARIPiprazole; Astemizole; AtorvaSTATin; Avanafil; Axitinib; Barnidipine; Bedaquiline; Boceprevir; Bortezomib; Bosentan; Bosutinib; Brentuximab Vedotin; Brinzolamide; Budesonide (Nasal); Budesonide (Systemic, Oral Inhalation); Budesonide (Topical); BusPIRone; Cabazitaxel; Cabergoline; Cabozantinib; Calcium Channel Blockers; Cannabis; CarBAMazepine; Cardiac Glycosides; Ceritinib; Cilostazol; Cisapride; CloZAPine; Cobicistat; Colchicine; Conivaptan; Corticosteroids (Orally Inhaled); Corticosteroids (Systemic); Crizotinib; CYP3A4 Inducers (Strong); CYP3A4 Substrates; Dabigatran Etexilate; Dapoxetine; Dasatinib; Dienogest; Dihydroergotamine; Disopyramide; Domperidone; DOXOrubicin (Conventional); Dronabinol; Dronedarone; Drospirenone; Dutasteride; Edoxaban; Eletriptan; Eplerenone; Ergot Derivatives; Ergotamine; Erlotinib; Estazolam; Etizolam; Everolimus; FentaNYL; Fesoterodine; Fluticasone (Nasal); Fluticasone (Oral Inhalation); GlipiZIDE; GlyBURIDE; GuanFACINE; Halofantrine; Highest Risk QTc-Prolonging Agents; Hydrocodone; Ibrutinib; Imatinib; Imidafenacin; Irinotecan; Isavuconazonium Sulfate; Ivabradine; Ivacaftor; Ixabepilone; Lacosamide; Lapatinib; Ledipasvir; Lercanidipine; Levobupivacaine; Levomilnacipran; Lomitapide; Lopinavir; Lovastatin; Lurasidone; Macitentan; Maraviroc; MedroxyPROGESTERone; MethylPREDNISolone; Midazolam; Moderate Risk QTc-Prolonging Agents; Naloxegol; Nilotinib; NiMODipine; Nintedanib; Nisoldipine; Olaparib; Ospemifene; Oxybutynin; OxyCODONE; Palbociclib; Panobinostat; Parecoxib; Paricalcitol; PAZOPanib; P-glycoprotein/ABCB1 Substrates; Pimecrolimus; Pimozide; Pitavastatin; PONATinib; Pranlukast; Pravastatin; PrednisoLONE (Systemic); PredniSONE; Protease Inhibitors; Prucalopride; QuiNIDine; QuiNINE; Ramelteon; Ranolazine; Red Yeast Rice; Regorafenib; Repaglinide; Retapamulin; Rifaximin; Rilpivirine; Rivaroxaban;

RomiDEPsin; Ruxolitinib; Salmeterol; Saxagliptin; Selective Serotonin Reuptake Inhibitors; Sildenafil; Silodosin; Simeprevir; Simvastatin; Sirolimus; SORAfenib; Suvorexant; Tacrolimus (Topical); Tadalafil; Tamsulosin; Tasimelteon; Telaprevir; Temsirolimus; Terfenadine; Tetrahydrocannabinol; Theophylline Derivatives; Ticagrelor; TiZANidine; Tofacitinib; Tolterodine; Tolvaptan; Topotecan; Toremifene; Trabectedin; TraMADol; Triazolam; Ulipristal; Vardenafil; Vemurafenib; Vilazodone; VinCRIStine (Liposomal); Vitamin K Antagonists; Vorapaxar; Zidovudine; Zopiclone

The levels/effects of Clarithromycin may be increased by: Boceprevir; Bosentan; Cobicistat; Conivaptan; CYP3A4 Inducers (Moderate); CYP3A4 Inducers (Strong); CYP3A4 Inhibitors (Moderate); CYP3A4 Inhibitors (Strong); Fusidic Acid (Systemic); Idelalisib; Ivabradine; Lopinavir; Luliconazole; Mifepristone; Netupitant; Protease Inhibitors; QTc-Prolonging Agents (Indeterminate Risk and Risk Modifying); Stiripentol; Telaprevir

Decreased Effect

Clarithromycin may decrease the levels/effects of: BCG; BCG (Intravesical); BCG Vaccine (Immunization); Clopidogrel; Ifosfamide; Prasugrel; Sodium Picosulfate; Ticagrelor; Typhoid Vaccine; Zidovudine

The levels/effects of Clarithromycin may be decreased by: Bosentan; CYP3A4 Inducers (Moderate); CYP3A4 Inducers (Strong); Dabrafenib; Deferasirox; Efavirenz; Etravirine; Lopinavir; Mitotane; Protease Inhibitors; Siltuximab; St Johns Wort; Tocilizumab

Food Interactions Immediate release: Food delays rate, but not extent of absorption; Extended release: Food increases clarithromycin AUC by ~30% relative to fasting conditions. Management: Administer immediate release products without regard to meals. Administer extended release products with food.

Storage/Stability

Extended release tablets: Store at 20°C to 25°C (68°F to 77°F); excursions are permitted between 15°C and 30°C (59°F and 86°F).

Immediate release tablets:

250 mg: Store at 15°C to 30°C (59°F to 86°F). Protect from light.

500 mg: Store at 20°C to 25°C (68°F to 77°F).

Granules for suspension: Store at 15°C to 30°C (59°F to 86°F) prior to and following reconstitution. Do not refrigerate. Use within 14 days of reconstitution.

Mechanism of Action Exerts its antibacterial action by binding to 50S ribosomal subunit resulting in inhibition of protein synthesis. The 14-OH metabolite of clarithromycin is twice as active as the parent compound against certain organisms.

Pharmacokinetics (Adult data unless noted)

Absorption:

Immediate release: Rapid; food delays rate, but not extent of absorption

Extended release: Fasting is associated with ~30% lower AUC relative to administration with food

Distribution: Widely distributed throughout the body with tissue concentrations higher than serum concentrations; manufacturer reports no data in regards to CNS penetration

Protein binding: 42% to 70% (Peters, 1992)

Metabolism: Partially hepatic via CYP3A4; converted to 14-OH clarithromycin (active metabolite); undergoes extensive first-pass metabolism

Bioavailability: ~50%

Half-life: Dose-dependent, prolonged with renal dysfunction

Clarithromycin:

250 mg dose: 3 to 4 hours

500 mg dose: 5 to 7 hours

14-hydroxy metabolite:

250 mg dose: 5 to 6 hours

500 mg dose: 7 to 9 hours

Time to peak serum concentration: Immediate release formulations: 2 to 3 hours; Extended release: 5 to 8 hours

Elimination: After a 250 mg or 500 mg tablet dose, 20% or 30% is excreted unchanged in urine, respectively; 10% to 15% is excreted as active metabolite 14-OH clarithromycin; feces (29% to 40% mostly as metabolites) (Ferrero, 1990)

Dosing: Usual

Pediatric: **Note:** All pediatric dosing recommendations based on immediate release product formulations (tablet and oral suspension):

General dosing, susceptible infection: Infants, Children, and Adolescents: Oral: 15 mg/kg/day divided every 12 hours; maximum single dose: 500 mg; duration dependent on infection site and severity; usually 7 to 14 days (*Red Book* [AAP], 2012)

Bartonellosis, treatment and secondary prophylaxis in HIV-exposed/-positive patients (excluding CNS infections and endocarditis): Limited data available: Oral:

Infants and Children: 15 mg/kg/day divided every 12 hours for at least 3 months; maximum single dose: 500 mg (CDC, 2009)

Adolescents: 500 mg twice daily administered for at least 3 months (DHHS [adult], 2013)

Endocarditis, prophylaxis; dental procedures in patients allergic to penicillins: Limited data available: Children and Adolescents: Oral: 15 mg/kg; maximum single dose: 500 mg; administer 30 to 60 minutes before procedure. **Note:** As of April 2007, the American Heart Association guidelines now recommend prophylaxis only in patients undergoing invasive procedures and in whom underlying cardiac conditions may predispose to a higher risk of adverse outcomes should infection occur (Wilson, 2007).

Group A streptococcal infection; rheumatic fever, primary prevention and treatment of streptococcal tonsillopharyngitis: Infants, Children, and Adolescents: Oral: 15 mg/kg/day divided every 12 hours for 10 days; maximum single dose: 250 mg (Gerber, 2009; Shulman, 2012)

***Helicobacter pylori* eradication:** Children and Adolescents: Oral: 20 mg/kg/day divided every 12 hours; maximum single dose: 500 mg; initial duration of treatment: 7 to 14 days; as part of triple or quadruple combination regimens with amoxicillin and proton pump inhibitor with or without metronidazole (Koletzko, 2011)

Lyme disease: Limited data available: Children and Adolescents: Oral: 7.5 mg/kg twice daily for 14 to 21 days; maximum single dose: 500 mg (Wormser, 2006)

Mycobacterium avium complex infection (MAC) (HIV-exposed/-positive):

Infants and Children (DHHS [pediatric], 2013)

Prophylaxis: Oral: 15 mg/kg/day divided every 12 hours; maximum single dose: 500 mg; to prevent first episode begin therapy at the following $CD4^+$ T-lymphocyte counts (see below):

Infants <12 months: <750 cells/mm^3

Children 1 to 2 years: <500 cells/mm^3

Children 2 to 5 years: <75 cells/mm^3

Children ≥6 years: <50 cells/mm^3

Recurrence: Oral: 15 mg/kg/day divided every 12 hours; maximum single dose: 500 mg; use in combination with ethambutol with or without rifabutin

Treatment: Oral: 15 to 30 mg/kg/day divided every 12 hours; maximum single dose: 500 mg; use in combination with ethambutol and if severe infection, rifabutin; follow with chronic suppressive therapy

Adolescents (DHHS [adult], 2013):

Prophylaxis:

Primary prophylaxis: Oral: 500 mg twice daily

Secondary prophylaxis: Oral: 500 mg twice daily plus ethambutol; consider additional agents (eg, rifabutin, aminoglycoside, fluoroquinolone) for CD4 <50 cells/mm^3, high mycobacterial load, or ineffective antiretroviral therapy.

Treatment: Oral: 500 mg twice daily in combination with ethambutol: Consider additional agents (eg, rifabutin, aminoglycoside, fluoroquinolone) for CD4 <50 cells/mm^3, high mycobacterial load, or ineffective antiretroviral therapy.

Otitis media, acute (AOM): Infants ≥6 months and Children: Oral: 15 mg/kg/day divided every 12 hours for 10 days; maximum single dose: 500 mg; **Note:** Due to increased *S. pneumoniae* and *H. influenzae* resistance, clarithromycin is not routinely recommended as a treatment option (AAP, [Lieberthal, 2013])

Peritonitis, prophylaxis for patients receiving peritoneal dialysis who require dental procedures: Limited data available: Infants, Children, and Adolescents: Oral: 15 mg/kg 30 to 60 minutes before dental procedure; maximum single dose: 500 mg (Warady, 2012)

Pertussis: Infants, Children, and Adolescents: Oral: 15 mg/kg/day divided every 12 hours for 7 days; maximum single dose: 500 mg (CDC [Tiwari, 2005])

Pneumonia, community-acquired (CAP); presumed atypical pneumonia (*M. pneumoniae, C. pneumoniae, C. trachomatis*); mild infection or step-down therapy: Infants >3 months, Children, and Adolescents: Oral: 15 mg/kg/day every 12 hours for 10 days; shorter courses may be appropriate for mild disease; maximum single dose: 500 mg; **Note:** A beta-lactam antibiotic should be added if typical bacterial pneumonia cannot be ruled out (Bradley, 2011).

Adult:

General dosing, susceptible infection: Oral: 250 to 500 mg every 12 hours **or** 1000 mg (two 500 mg extended release tablets) once daily for 7 to 14 days

Acute exacerbation of chronic bronchitis: Oral:

M. catarrhalis and *S. pneumoniae*: 250 mg every 12 hours for 7 to 14 days **or** 1000 mg (two 500 mg extended release tablets) once daily for 7 days

H. influenzae: 500 mg every 12 hours for 7 to 14 days **or** 1000 mg (two 500 mg extended release tablets) once daily for 7 days

H. parainfluenzae: 500 mg every 12 hours for 7 days **or** 1000 mg (two 500 mg extended release tablets) once daily for 7 days

Acute maxillary sinusitis: Oral: 500 mg every 12 hours **or** 1000 mg (two 500 mg extended release tablets) once daily for 14 days

Mycobacterial infection (prevention and treatment): Oral: 500 mg twice daily (use with other antimycobacterial drugs (eg, ethambutol or rifampin). Continue therapy if clinical response is observed; may discontinue when patient is considered at low risk for disseminated infection.

Peptic ulcer disease: Eradication of *Helicobacter pylori*: Dual or triple combination regimens with bismuth subsalicylate, amoxicillin, an H_2-receptor antagonist, or proton pump inhibitor: Oral: 500 mg every 8 to 12 hours for 10-14 days

Pharyngitis, tonsillitis: Oral: 250 mg every 12 hours for 10 days

Pneumonia: Oral:

C. pneumoniae, *M. pneumoniae*, and *S. pneumoniae*: 250 mg every 12 hours for 7 to 14 days **or** 1000 mg (two 500 mg extended release tablets) once daily for 7 days

H. influenzae: 250 mg every 12 hours for 7 days **or** 1000 mg (two 500 mg extended release tablets) once daily for 7 days

H. parainfluenzae and *M. catarrhalis*: 1000 mg (two 500 mg extended release tablets) once daily for 7 days

Skin and skin structure infection, uncomplicated: Oral: 250 mg every 12 hours for 7 to 14 days

Dosing adjustment in renal impairment:

Infants, Children, and Adolescents: The following adjustments have been recommended (Aronoff, 2007). **Note:** Renally adjusted dose recommendations are based on a dose 15 mg/kg/day divided twice daily.

GFR ≥30 mL/minute/1.73 m^2: No dosage adjustment necessary

GFR 10 to 29 mL/minute/1.73 m^2: 8 mg/kg/day divided every 12 hours

GFR < 10 mL/minute/1.73 m^2: 4 mg/kg once daily

Hemodialysis: Administer after HD session is completed: 4 mg/kg once daily

Peritoneal dialysis: 4 mg/kg once daily

Adult:

CrCl <30 mL/minute: Decrease clarithromycin dose by 50%

Hemodialysis: Administer after HD session is completed (Aronoff, 2007)

In combination with atazanavir or ritonavir:

CrCl 30 to 60 mL/minute: Decrease clarithromycin dose by 50%

CrCl <30 mL/minute: Decrease clarithromycin dose by 75%

Dosing adjustment in hepatic impairment: Adjustment not needed as long as renal function is normal

Preparation for Administration Oral: Powder for oral suspension: Reconstitute powder for oral suspension with appropriate amount of water as specified on the bottle. Shake vigorously until suspended.

Administration

Immediate release tablets and oral suspension: May be administered with or without meals; give every 12 hours rather than twice daily to avoid peak and trough variation. Shake suspension well before each use.

Extended release tablets: Should be given with food. Do not crush or chew extended release tablet.

Monitoring Parameters CBC with differential, serum BUN and creatinine, liver function tests; serum concentration of drugs whose concentrations may be affected in patients receiving concomitant clarithromycin (ie, theophylline, carbamazepine, quinidine, digoxin, anticoagulants, triazolam); hearing (in patients receiving long-term treatment with clarithromycin); observe for changes in bowel frequency

Dosage Forms Excipient information presented when available (limited, particularly for generics); consult specific product labeling.

Suspension Reconstituted, Oral:

Biaxin: 250 mg/5 mL (50 mL, 100 mL) [fruit punch flavor]

Generic: 125 mg/5 mL (50 mL, 100 mL); 250 mg/5 mL (50 mL, 100 mL)

Tablet, Oral:

Biaxin: 250 mg [contains brilliant blue fcf (fd&c blue #1), fd&c yellow #10 (quinoline yellow)]

Biaxin: 500 mg [contains fd&c yellow #10 (quinoline yellow)]

Generic: 250 mg, 500 mg

Tablet Extended Release 24 Hour, Oral:

Biaxin XL: 500 mg [contains fd&c yellow #10 (quinoline yellow)]

Biaxin XL Pac: 500 mg [contains fd&c yellow #10 (quinoline yellow)]

Generic: 500 mg

◆ **Claritin [OTC]** *see* Loratadine *on page 1296*

- **Claritin® (Can)** *see* Loratadine *on page 1296*
- **Claritin-D® 12 Hour Allergy & Congestion [OTC]** *see* Loratadine and Pseudoephedrine *on page 1298*
- **Claritin-D® 24 Hour Allergy & Congestion [OTC]** *see* Loratadine and Pseudoephedrine *on page 1298*
- **Claritin Allergic Decongestant (Can)** *see* Oxymetazoline (Nasal) *on page 1599*
- **Claritin® Extra (Can)** *see* Loratadine and Pseudoephedrine *on page 1298*
- **Claritin Eye [OTC]** *see* Ketotifen (Ophthalmic) *on page 1196*
- **Claritin® Kids (Can)** *see* Loratadine *on page 1296*
- **Claritin® Liberator (Can)** *see* Loratadine and Pseudoephedrine *on page 1298*
- **Claritin Reditabs [OTC]** *see* Loratadine *on page 1296*
- **Clarus (Can)** *see* ISOtretinoin *on page 1171*
- **Clavulanic Acid and Amoxicillin** *see* Amoxicillin and Clavulanate *on page 141*
- **Clavulin (Can)** *see* Amoxicillin and Clavulanate *on page 141*
- **Clear Away 1-Step Wart Remover [OTC]** *see* Salicylic Acid *on page 1894*
- **Clear Eyes Redness Relief [OTC]** *see* Naphazoline (Ophthalmic) *on page 1488*
- **Clearplex V [OTC]** *see* Benzoyl Peroxide *on page 270*
- **Clearplex X** *see* Benzoyl Peroxide *on page 270*
- **Clearskin [OTC]** *see* Benzoyl Peroxide *on page 270*

Clemastine (KLEM as teen)

Medication Safety Issues

BEERS Criteria medication:

This drug may be potentially inappropriate for use in geriatric patients (Quality of evidence - moderate; Strength of recommendation - strong).

Brand Names: US Dayhist Allergy 12 Hour Relief [OTC]; Tavist Allergy [OTC]

Therapeutic Category Antihistamine

Generic Availability (US) Yes

Use Perennial and seasonal allergic rhinitis and other allergic symptoms including urticaria (Oral liquid: FDA approved in ages ≥6 years and adults); relief of symptoms of hay fever or other respiratory allergies (OTC product: FDA approved in ages ≥12 years and adults). **Note:** Approved ages and uses for generic products may vary; consult labeling for specific information.

Pregnancy Risk Factor B

Pregnancy Considerations Maternal clemastine use has generally not resulted in an increased risk of birth defects. Antihistamines are recommended for the treatment of rhinitis, urticaria, and pruritus with rash in pregnant women (although second generation antihistamines may be preferred). Antihistamines are not recommended for treatment of pruritus associated with intrahepatic cholestasis in pregnancy.

Breast-Feeding Considerations Small amounts of clemastine may be excreted in breast milk. Premature infants and newborns have a higher risk of intolerance to antihistamines. Adverse events were observed in single case report of a nursing infant. Use while breast-feeding is contraindicated by the manufacturer. Antihistamines may decrease maternal serum prolactin concentrations when administered prior to the establishment of nursing.

Contraindications Hypersensitivity to clemastine or any component of the formulation; narrow-angle glaucoma

Warnings/Precautions Use caution with bladder neck obstruction, symptomatic prostate hypertrophy, asthmatic attacks, stenosing peptic ulcer, increased intraocular pressure, hyperthyroidism, cardiovascular disease, hypertension, and in the elderly. May cause drowsiness; use caution in performing tasks which require alertness. Effects may be potentiated when used with other sedative drugs or ethanol. In the eldelry, avoid use of this potent anticholinergic agent due to increased risk of confusion, dry mouth, constipation, and other anticholinergic effects; clearance decreases in patients of advanced age (Beers Criteria).

Warnings: Additional Pediatric Considerations Safety and efficacy for the use of cough and cold products in pediatric patients <4 years of age is limited; the AAP warns against the use of these products for respiratory illnesses in this age group. Serious adverse effects including death have been reported. Many of these products contain multiple active ingredients, increasing the risk of accidental overdose when used with other products. The FDA notes that there are no approved OTC uses for these products in pediatric patients <2 years of age. Health care providers are reminded to ask caregivers about the use of OTC cough and cold products in order to avoid exposure to multiple medications containing the same ingredient (AAP 2012; FDA 2008).

The syrup contains 5.5% alcohol.

Adverse Reactions

Cardiovascular: Hypotension, palpitation, tachycardia

Central nervous system: Confusion, dizziness increased, dyscoordination, fatigue, headache, insomnia, irritability, nervousness, restlessness, sedation, sleepiness, somnolence slight to moderate

Dermatologic: Photosensitivity, rash

Gastrointestinal: Constipation, diarrhea, epigastric distress, nausea, vomiting, xerostomia

Genitourinary: Difficult urination, urinary frequency, urinary retention

Hematologic: Agranulocytosis, hemolytic anemia, thrombocytopenia

Ocular: Blurred vision

Otic: Tinnitus

Respiratory: Thickening of bronchial secretions

Miscellaneous: Anaphylaxis

Drug Interactions

Metabolism/Transport Effects Inhibits CYP2D6 (weak)

Avoid Concomitant Use

Avoid concomitant use of Clemastine with any of the following: Aclidinium; Azelastine (Nasal); Eluxadoline; Glucagon; Ipratropium (Oral Inhalation); Orphenadrine; Paraldehyde; Potassium Chloride; Thalidomide; Tiotropium; Umeclidinium

Increased Effect/Toxicity

Clemastine may increase the levels/effects of: AbobotulinumtoxinA; Alcohol (Ethyl); Analgesics (Opioid); Anticholinergic Agents; ARIPiprazole; Azelastine (Nasal); Buprenorphine; CNS Depressants; Eluxadoline; Glucagon; Hydrocodone; Methotrimeprazine; Metyrosine; Mirabegron; Mirtazapine; OnabotulinumtoxinA; Orphenadrine; Paraldehyde; Potassium Chloride; Pramipexole; RimabotulinumtoxinB; ROPINIRole; Rotigotine; Selective Serotonin Reuptake Inhibitors; Suvorexant; Thalidomide; Thiazide Diuretics; Tiotropium; Topiramate; Zolpidem

The levels/effects of Clemastine may be increased by: Aclidinium; Brimonidine (Topical); Cannabis; Doxylamine; Dronabinol; Droperidol; HydrOXYzine; Ipratropium (Oral Inhalation); Kava Kava; Magnesium Sulfate; Methotrimeprazine; Mianserin; Nabilone; Perampanel; Pramlintide; Rufinamide; Sodium Oxybate; Tapentadol; Tetrahydrocannabinol; Umeclidinium

Decreased Effect

Clemastine may decrease the levels/effects of: Acetylcholinesterase Inhibitors; Benzylpenicilloyl Polylysine; Betahistine; Hyaluronidase; Itopride; Metoclopramide; Secretin

The levels/effects of Clemastine may be decreased by: Acetylcholinesterase Inhibitors; Amphetamines

Mechanism of Action Competes with histamine for H_1-receptor sites on effector cells in the gastrointestinal tract, blood vessels, and respiratory tract

Pharmacodynamics

Onset of action: 2 hours after administration
Maximum effect: 5 to 7 hours
Duration: 10 to 12 hours

Pharmacokinetics (Adult data unless noted)

Absorption: Oral: Well absorbed
Distribution: V_d: ~800 L (range: 500 to 1,000 L) (Sharma 2003)
Metabolism: Hepatic; metabolized via unidentified enzymes by O-dealkylation followed by alcohol dehydration, aliphatic oxidation, aromatic oxidation, and direct oxidation; significant first-pass effect (Sharma 2003)
Half-life: ~21 hours (range: 10 to 33 hours) (Sharma 2003)
Time to peak serum concentration: 2 to 5 hours
Elimination: Urine (~42% as metabolites) (Sharma 2003)

Dosing: Usual

Pediatric:

Perennial and seasonal allergic rhinitis: Oral: Syrup:
Children 6 to <12 years: 0.67 mg clemastine fumarate (0.5 mg base) twice daily; dosage may be increased as required; single doses up to 3mg clemastine fumarate (2.25 mg base) have been tolerated; maximum daily dose: 4.02 mg/**day** clemastine fumarate (3 mg/**day** base)
Children ≥12 years and Adolescents: 1.34 mg clemastine fumarate (1 mg base) twice daily; dosage may be increased as required; maximum daily dose 8.04 mg/**day** clemastine fumarate (6 mg/ **day** base)

Allergic symptoms, hayfever: Oral: Tablets: Children ≥12 years and Adolescents: 1.34 mg clemastine fumarate (1 mg base) twice daily; maximum daily dose 2.68 mg/day (2 mg base/**day**)

Urticaria; angioedema: Oral: Syrup:
Children 6 to <12 years: 1.34 mg clemastine fumarate (1 mg base) twice daily; maximum daily dose 4.02 mg/**day** clemastine fumarate 3 mg/**day** base)
Children ≥12 years and Adolescents: 2.68 mg clemastine fumarate (2 mg base) twice daily; maximum daily dose 8.04 mg/**day** clemastine fumarate (6 mg/**day** base)

Adult: **Rhinitis or allergic symptoms (including urticaria):** Oral:
1.34 mg clemastine fumarate (1 mg base) twice daily to 2.68 mg (2 mg base) 3 times/day; do not exceed 8.04 mg/day (6 mg base)
OTC labeling: 1.34 mg clemastine fumarate (1 mg base) twice daily; do not exceed 2 mg base/24 hours

Dosing adjustment in renal impairment: There are no dosage adjustments provided in manufacturer's labeling.

Dosing adjustment in hepatic impairment: There are no dosage adjustments provided in manufacturer's labeling.

Administration Oral: Administer with food

Monitoring Parameters Reduction of rhinitis, urticaria, eczema, pruritus, or other allergic symptoms

Dosage Forms Excipient information presented when available (limited, particularly for generics); consult specific product labeling.

Syrup, Oral, as fumarate:
Generic: 0.67 mg/5 mL (120 mL)
Tablet, Oral, as fumarate:
Dayhist Allergy 12 Hour Relief: 1.34 mg [scored; sodium free]
Tavist Allergy: 1.34 mg [scored; sodium free]
Generic: 1.34 mg, 2.68 mg

- ◆ **Clemastine Fumarate** *see* Clemastine *on page 486*
- ◆ **Cleocin** *see* Clindamycin (Systemic) *on page 487*
- ◆ **Cleocin** *see* Clindamycin (Topical) *on page 491*
- ◆ **Cleocin in D5W** *see* Clindamycin (Systemic) *on page 487*
- ◆ **Cleocin Phosphate** *see* Clindamycin (Systemic) *on page 487*
- ◆ **Cleocin-T** *see* Clindamycin (Topical) *on page 491*
- ◆ **Climara** *see* Estradiol (Systemic) *on page 795*
- ◆ **Clindacin ETZ** *see* Clindamycin (Topical) *on page 491*
- ◆ **Clindacin-P** *see* Clindamycin (Topical) *on page 491*
- ◆ **Clindacin Pac** *see* Clindamycin (Topical) *on page 491*
- ◆ **Clindagel** *see* Clindamycin (Topical) *on page 491*
- ◆ **ClindaMax** *see* Clindamycin (Topical) *on page 491*
- ◆ **Clindamycin IV Infusion (Can)** *see* Clindamycin (Systemic) *on page 487*

Clindamycin (Systemic) (klin da MYE sin)

Medication Safety Issues

Sound-alike/look-alike issues:
Cleocin may be confused with bleomycin, Clinoril, Cubicin, Lincocin
Clindamycin may be confused with clarithromycin, Claritin, vancomycin, lincomycin

Related Information

Prevention of Infective Endocarditis *on page 2378*

Brand Names: US Cleocin; Cleocin in D5W; Cleocin Phosphate

Brand Names: Canada Apo-Clindamycin; Auro-Clindamycin; Ava-Clindamycin; Clindamycin Injection; Clindamycin Injection SDZ; Clindamycin Injection, USP; Clindamycin IV Infusion; Clindamycine; Dalacin C; Mylan-Clindamycin; PMS-Clindamycin; Riva-Clindamycin; Teva-Clindamycin

Therapeutic Category Antibiotic, Anaerobic; Antibiotic, Miscellaneous

Generic Availability (US) Yes

Use Treatment of infections involving the respiratory tract, skin and soft tissue, and female pelvis and genital tract; sepsis and intra-abdominal infections due to susceptible organisms (FDA approved in all ages); has also been used for endocarditis prophylaxis, preoperative prophylaxis, and treatment of babesiosis and malaria

Pregnancy Risk Factor B

Pregnancy Considerations Adverse events were not observed in animal reproduction studies. Clindamycin crosses the placenta and can be detected in the cord blood and fetal tissue (Philipson, 1973; Weinstein, 1976). Clindamycin pharmacokinetics are not affected by pregnancy (Philipson, 1976; Weinstein, 1976). Clindamycin therapy is recommended as an alternative treatment in certain pregnant patients for prophylaxis of group B streptococcal disease in newborns (ACOG 485, 2011); prophylaxis and treatment of *Toxoplasma gondii* encephalitis, or for the treatment of *Pneumocystis* pneumonia (PCP) (DHHS, 2013); bacterial vaginosis (CDC RR12, 2010); or malaria (CDC, 2013). Clindamycin is also one of the antibiotics recommended for prophylactic use prior to cesarean delivery and may be used in certain situations prior to vaginal delivery in women at high risk for endocarditis (ACOG 120, 2011).

Breast-Feeding Considerations Clindamycin can be detected in breast milk; reported concentrations range from 0.7 to 3.8 mcg/mL following maternal doses of 150 mg orally to 600 mg IV. Due to the potential for serious adverse reactions in neonates, breast-feeding is not recommended by the manufacturer. Nondose-related effects could include modification of bowel flora. One case of bloody stools in an infant occurred after a mother received clindamycin while breast-feeding; however, a causal relationship was not confirmed (Mann, 1980).

Contraindications Hypersensitivity to preparations containing clindamycin, lincomycin, or any component of the formulation.

Warnings/Precautions Dosage adjustment may be necessary in patients with severe hepatic dysfunction. **[U.S. Boxed Warning]: Can cause severe and possibly fatal colitis.** Should be reserved for serious infections where less toxic antimicrobial agents are inappropriate. It should not be used in patients with nonbacterial infections such as most upper respiratory tract infections. Hypertoxin producing strains of *C. difficile* cause increased morbidity and mortality, as these infections can be refractory to antimicrobial therapy and may require colectomy. *C. difficile*-associated diarrhea (CDAD) must be considered in all patients who present with diarrhea following antibiotic use. CDAD has been observed >2 months postantibiotic treatment. Use with caution in patients with a history of gastrointestinal disease, particularly colitis. Discontinue drug if significant diarrhea, abdominal cramps, or passage of blood and mucus occurs. Use may result in overgrowth of nonsusceptible organisms, particularly yeast. Should superinfection occur, appropriate measures should be taken as indicated by the clinical situation. May cause hypersensitivity. Serious anaphylactoid reactions require immediate emergency treatment with epinephrine. Oxygen and IV corticosteroids should also be administered as indicated. Severe or fatal reactions such as toxic epidermal necrolysis (TEN) have been reported. Discontinue if severe skin reaction occurs. Premature and low birth weight infants may be more likely to develop toxicity. Some products may contain tartrazine (FD&C yellow no. 5), which may cause allergic reactions in certain individuals. Allergy is frequently seen in patients who also have an aspirin hypersensitivity. Use caution in atopic patients. A subgroup of older patients with associated severe illness may tolerate diarrhea less well. Monitor carefully for changes in bowel frequency. Not appropriate for use in the treatment of meningitis due to inadequate penetration into the CSF. Do not inject IV undiluted as a bolus. Product should be diluted in compatible fluid and infused over 10 to 60 minutes. Potentially significant interactions may exist, requiring dose or frequency adjustment, additional monitoring, and/or selection of alternative therapy.

Benzyl alcohol and derivatives: Some dosage forms may contain benzyl alcohol; large amounts of benzyl alcohol (≥99 mg/kg/day) have been associated with a potentially fatal toxicity ("gasping syndrome") in neonates; the "gasping syndrome" consists of metabolic acidosis, respiratory distress, gasping respirations, CNS dysfunction (including convulsions, intracranial hemorrhage), hypotension and cardiovascular collapse (AAP, 1997; CDC, 1982); some data suggests that benzoate displaces bilirubin from protein binding sites (Ahlfors, 2001); avoid or use dosage forms containing benzyl alcohol with caution in neonates. See manufacturer's labeling.

Adverse Reactions

Cardiovascular: Cardiac arrest (rare; IV administration), hypotension (rare; IV administration), thrombophlebitis (IV)

Central nervous system: Metallic taste (IV)

Dermatologic: Acute generalized exanthematous pustulosis, erythema multiforme (rare), exfoliative dermatitis (rare), maculopapular rash, pruritus, skin rash, Stevens-Johnson syndrome (rare), toxic epidermal necrolysis, urticaria, vesiculobullous dermatitis

Gastrointestinal: Abdominal pain, antibiotic-associated colitis, *Clostridium difficile* associated diarrhea, diarrhea, esophageal ulcer, esophagitis, nausea, pseudomembranous colitis, unpleasant taste (IV), vomiting

Genitourinary: Azotemia, oliguria, proteinuria, vaginitis

Hematologic & oncologic: Agranulocytosis, eosinophilia (transient), neutropenia (transient), thrombocytopenia

Hepatic: Abnormal hepatic function tests, jaundice

Hypersensitivity: Anaphylactoid reaction (rare)

Immunologic: DRESS syndrome

Local: Abscess at injection site (IM), induration at injection site (IM), irritation at injection site (IM), pain at injection site (IM)

Neuromuscular & skeletal: Polyarthritis (rare)

Renal: Renal insufficiency (rare)

Drug Interactions

Metabolism/Transport Effects Substrate of CYP3A4 (minor); **Note:** Assignment of Major/Minor substrate status based on clinically relevant drug interaction potential

Avoid Concomitant Use

Avoid concomitant use of Clindamycin (Systemic) with any of the following: BCG; BCG (Intravesical); Erythromycin (Systemic); Mecamylamine

Increased Effect/Toxicity

Clindamycin (Systemic) may increase the levels/effects of: Mecamylamine; Neuromuscular-Blocking Agents

Decreased Effect

Clindamycin (Systemic) may decrease the levels/effects of: BCG; BCG (Intravesical); BCG Vaccine (Immunization); Erythromycin (Systemic); Sodium Picosulfate; Typhoid Vaccine

The levels/effects of Clindamycin (Systemic) may be decreased by: Kaolin

Food Interactions Peak concentrations may be delayed with food. Management: May administer with food.

Storage/Stability

Capsule: Store at room temperature of 20°C to 25°C (68°F to 77°F).

IV: Infusion solution in NS or D_5W solution is stable for 16 days at room temperature, 32 days refrigerated, or 8 weeks frozen. Prior to use, store vials and premixed bags at controlled room temperature 20°C to 25°C (68°F to 77°F). After initial use, discard any unused portion of vial after 24 hours.

Oral solution: Do not refrigerate reconstituted oral solution (it will thicken). Following reconstitution, oral solution is stable for 2 weeks at room temperature of 20°C to 25°C (68°F to 77°F).

Mechanism of Action Reversibly binds to 50S ribosomal subunits preventing peptide bond formation thus inhibiting bacterial protein synthesis; bacteriostatic or bactericidal depending on drug concentration, infection site, and organism

Pharmacokinetics (Adult data unless noted)

Absorption: Oral: 90% of clindamycin hydrochloride is rapidly absorbed; clindamycin palmitate must be hydrolyzed in the GI tract before it is active

Distribution: No significant levels are seen in CSF, even with inflamed meninges; distributes into saliva, ascites fluid, pleural fluid, bone, and bile

Protein binding: 94%

Bioavailability: Oral: ~90%

Half-life:

- Neonates:
  - Premature: 8.7 hours
  - Full-term: 3.6 hours
- Infants 1 month to 1 year: 3 hours
- Children and Adults with normal renal function: 2-3 hours

Time to peak serum concentration:

- Oral: Within 60 minutes
- IM: Within 1-3 hours

Elimination: Most of the drug is eliminated by hepatic metabolism; 10% of an oral dose excreted in urine and 3.6% excreted in feces as active drug and metabolites

Dosing: Neonatal

General dosing, susceptible infection (*Red Book* [AAP], 2012): IM, IV, Oral:

Body weight <1 kg:

PNA ≤14 days: 5 mg/kg/dose every 12 hours

PNA 15-28 days: 5 mg/kg/dose every 8 hours

Body weight 1-2 kg:

PNA ≤7 days: 5 mg/kg/dose every 12 hours

PNA 8-28 days: 5 mg/kg/dose every 8 hours

Body weight >2 kg:

PNA ≤7 days: 5 mg/kg/dose every 8 hours

PNA 8-28 days: 5 mg/kg/dose every 6 hours

Manufacturer's labeling: Term infant: IM, IV: 15 to 20 mg/kg/day divided every 6 to 8 hours

Dosing: Usual

Infants, Children, and Adolescents:

General dosing, susceptible infection:

IM, IV:

Manufacturer's labeling: Infants, Children, and Adolescents 1 month to 16 years:

Weight-directed dosing: 20 to 40 mg/kg/day divided every 6 to 8 hours

BSA-directed dosing: 350 to 450 mg/m^2/day divided every 6 to 8 hours

Alternate dosing (*Red Book* [AAP], 2012): Infants, Children, and Adolescents:

Mild to moderate infections: 20 mg/kg/day divided every 8 hours; maximum daily dose: 1800 mg/**day**

Severe infections: 40 mg/kg/day divided every 6 to 8 hours; maximum daily dose: 2700 mg/**day**

Oral:

Manufacturer's labeling: Infants, Children, and Adolescents:

Hydrochloride salt (capsule): 8 to 20 mg/kg/day divided every 6 to 8 hours

Palmitate salt (solution): 8 to 25 mg/kg/day divided every 6 to 8 hours; minimum dose: 37.5 mg 3 times daily

Alternate dosing (*Red Book* [AAP]; 2012): Infants, Children, and Adolescents:

Mild to moderate infections: 10 to 25 mg/kg/day divided every 8 hours; maximum daily dose: 1800 mg/**day**

Severe infections: 30 to 40 mg/kg/day divided every 6 to 8 hours; maximum daily dose: 1800 mg/**day**

Babesiosis: Oral: 20 to 40 mg/kg/day divided every 8 hours for 7 to 10 days plus quinine; maximum single dose: 600 mg (*Red Book* [AAP], 2012)

Bacterial endocarditis prophylaxis for dental and upper respiratory procedures in penicillin-allergic patients (*Red Book* [AAP], 2012; Wilson, 2007):

IM, IV: 20 mg/kg 30 minutes before procedure; maximum single dose: 600 mg

Oral: 20 mg/kg 1 hour before procedure; maximum single dose: 600 mg

Note: American Heart Association (AHA) guidelines now recommend prophylaxis only in patients undergoing invasive procedures and in whom underlying cardiac conditions may predispose to a higher risk of adverse outcomes should infection occur. As of April 2007, routine prophylaxis for GI/GU procedures is no longer recommended by the AHA.

Intra-abdominal infection, complicated: IV: **Note:** Not recommended for community-acquired infections due to increasing *Bacteroides fragilis* resistance: 20 to 40 mg/kg/day divided every 6 to 8 hours in combination with gentamicin or tobramycin (Solomkin, 2010)

Malaria, treatment:

Uncomplicated: Oral: 20 mg/kg/day divided every 8 hours for 7 days plus quinine (CDC, 2011; *Red Book* [AAP], 2012)

Severe: IV: Loading dose: 10 mg/kg once followed by 15 mg/kg/day divided every 8 hours plus IV quinidine gluconate; switch to oral therapy (clindamycin and quinine, see above) when able for total treatment duration of 7 days. **Note:** Quinine duration is region specific; consult CDC for current recommendations (CDC, 2011).

Osteomyelitis, septic arthritis, due to MRSA: IV, Oral: 40 mg/kg/day divided every 6 to 8 hours for at least 4 to 6 weeks (osteomyelitis) or 3 to 4 weeks (septic arthritis) (Liu, 2011)

Otitis media, acute: Oral: 30 to 40 mg/kg/day divided every 8 hours; administer with or without a third generation cephalosporin (AAP [Lieberthal, 2013])

Peritonitis (CAPD):

Prophylaxis (Warady, 2012):

Invasive dental procedures: Oral: 20 mg/kg administered 30 to 60 minutes before procedure; maximum dose: 600 mg

Gastrointestinal or genitourinary procedures: IV: 10 mg/kg administered 30 to 60 minutes before procedure; maximum dose: 600 mg

Treatment:

Exit-site and tunnel infection: Oral: 10 mg/kg/dose 3 times daily; maximum single dose: 600 mg (Warady, 2012)

Intraperitoneal, continuous: Loading dose: 300 mg per liter of dialysate; maintenance dose: 150 mg per liter; **Note**: 125 mg/liter has also been recommended as a maintenance dose (Aronoff, 2007; Warady, 2012)

Pharyngitis:

AHA guidelines (Gerber, 2009): Children and Adolescents: Oral: 20 mg/kg/day in divided doses 3 times daily for 10 days; maximum single dose: 600 mg

IDSA guidelines (Shulman, 2012): Children and Adolescents: Oral:

Treatment and primary prevention of rheumatic fever: 21 mg/kg/day in divided doses 3 times daily for 10 days; maximum single dose: 300 mg

Treatment of chronic carriers: 20 to 30 mg/kg/day in divided doses 3 times daily for 10 days; maximum single dose: 300 mg

Pneumococcal disease, invasive: IV: 25 to 40 mg/kg/day divided every 6 to 8 hours (*Red Book* [AAP], 2012)

***Pneumocystis jirovecii* (formerly *carnii*) pneumonia (PCP):**

Non HIV-exposed/-positive (*Red Book* [AAP], 2012):

Mild to moderate disease: Oral: 10 mg/kg 3 to 4 times daily for 21 days; in combination with other agents; maximum single dose: 450 mg

Moderate to severe disease: IV: 15 to 25 mg/kg 3 to 4 times daily for 21 days; give with pentamidine or primaquine; maximum single dose: 600 mg. May switch to oral dose after clinical improvement.

HIV-exposed/-positive: Adolescents (DHHS [adult], 2013):

Mild to moderate disease: Oral: 300 mg every 6 hours **or** 450 mg every 8 hours with primaquine for 21 days

Moderate to severe disease:

Oral: 300 mg every 6 hours **or** 450 mg every 8 hours with primaquine for 21 days

IV: 600 mg every 6 hours **or** 900 mg every 8 hours with primaquine for 21 days

Pneumonia:

Community-acquired pneumonia (CAP) (IDSA/PIDS, Bradley, 2011): Infants ≥3 months, Children, and Adolescents: **Note:** In children ≥5 years, a macrolide antibiotic should be added if atypical pneumonia cannot be ruled out.

Moderate to severe infection: IV: 40 mg/kg/day divided every 6 to 8 hours

Mild infection, step-down therapy: Oral: 30 to 40 mg/kg/day divided every 6 to 8 hours

MRSA pneumonia: IV: 40 mg/kg/day divided every 6 to 8 hours for 7 to 21 days (Liu, 2011)

Rhinosinusitis, acute bacterial: Oral: 30 to 40 mg/kg/day divided every 8 hours with concomitant cefixime or cefpodoxime for 10 to 14 days. **Note:** Recommended in patients with nontype I penicillin allergy, after failure to initial therapy, or in patients at risk for antibiotic resistance (eg, daycare attendance, age <2 years, recent hospitalization, antibiotic use within the past month) (Chow, 2012).

Skin and soft tissue infection:

Impetigo: Oral: 10 to 20 mg/kg/day in divided doses 3 times daily; treatment duration: 7 days; maximum single dose: 400 mg (Stevens, 2005)

MRSA infection (Liu, 2011):

Cellulitis, nonpurulent or purulent: Oral: 40 mg/kg/day divided every 6 to 8 hours; maximum single dose: 450 mg; treatment duration based on clinical response, usually 7 to 14 days

Complicated SSTI infection: IV, Oral: 40 mg/kg/day divided every 6 to 8 hours for 7 to 14 days; maximum single dose range: 450 to 600 mg

MSSA infection (Stevens, 2005): Duration of treatment dependent upon site and severity of infection; cellulitis and abscesses typically require 5 to 10 days of therapy

IV: 25 to 40 mg/kg/day in divided doses 3 times daily; maximum single dose: 600 mg

Oral: 10 to 20 mg/kg/day in divided doses 3 times daily; maximum single dose: 450 mg

Surgical prophylaxis: Children and Adolescents: IV: 10 mg/kg 30 to 60 minutes prior to the procedure; may repeat in 6 hours; maximum single dose: 900 mg (Bratzler, 2013)

Toxoplasmosis (HIV-exposed/positive or hematopoietic cell transplantation recipients):

Infants and Children (CDC, 2009; *Red Book* [AAP], 2012; Tomblyn, 2009):

Treatment, HIV-exposed/-positive: IV, Oral: 5 to 7.5 mg/kg/dose 4 times daily with pyrimethamine and leucovorin; maximum single dose: 600 mg

Secondary prevention:

HIV-exposed/-positive: Oral: 7 to 10 mg/kg/dose every 8 hours and pyrimethamine plus leucovorin; maximum single dose: 600 mg (DHHS [pediatric], 2013)

Hematopoietic cell transplantation recipients: Oral: 5 to 7.5 mg/kg/dose every 6 hours and pyrimethamine plus leucovorin; maximum single dose: 450 mg

Adolescents (DHHS [adult], 2013; *Red Book* [AAP], 2012; Tomblyn, 2009):

Treatment: Oral, IV: 600 mg every 6 hours with pyrimethamine and leucovorin for at least 6 weeks; longer if clinical or radiologic disease is extensive or response is incomplete

Secondary prevention:

HIV-exposed/-positive: Oral: 600 mg every 8 hours with pyrimethamine and leucovorin

Hematopoietic cell transplantation recipients: Oral: 300 to 450 mg every 6 to 8 hours with pyrimethamine and leucovorin

Adults:

General dosing, susceptible infection:

Oral: 150 to 450 mg every 6 to 8 hours

IM, IV: 600 to 2,700 mg/day in 2 to 4 divided doses; up to 4,800 mg IV daily may be used in life-threatening infections

Amnionitis: IV: 450 to 900 mg every 8 hours

Bacterial vaginosis: Oral: 300 mg twice daily for 7 days (CDC, 2010)

Cellulitis due to MRSA: Oral: 300 to 450 mg 3 times daily for 5 to 10 days (Liu, 2011)

Complicated skin/soft tissue infection due to MRSA: IV, Oral: 600 mg 3 times daily for 7 to 14 days (Liu, 2011)

Endocarditis prophylaxis (Wilson, 2007):

Oral: 600 mg 30 to 60 minutes before procedure with no follow-up dose needed

IM, IV: 600 mg 30 to 60 minutes before procedure. Intramuscular injections should be avoided in patients who are receiving anticoagulant therapy. In these circumstances, orally administered regimens should be given whenever possible. Intravenously administered antibiotics should be used for patients who are unable to tolerate or absorb oral medications.

Note: American Heart Association (AHA) guidelines now recommend prophylaxis only in patients undergoing invasive procedures and in whom underlying cardiac conditions may predispose to a higher risk of adverse outcomes should infection occur. As of April 2007, routine prophylaxis for GI/GU procedures is no longer recommended by the AHA.

Gangrenous pyomyositis: IV: 900 mg every 8 hours with penicillin G

Group B Streptococcus (neonatal prophylaxis): IV: 900 mg every 8 hours until delivery (CDC, 2010)

Malaria, severe: IV: Load: 10 mg/kg followed by 15 mg/kg/day divided every 8 hours plus IV quinidine gluconate; switch to oral therapy (clindamycin plus quinine) when able for total clindamycin treatment duration of 7 days (**Note:** Quinine duration is region-specific, consult CDC for current recommendations) (CDC, 2011)

Malaria, uncomplicated treatment: Oral: 20 mg/kg/day divided every 8 hours for 7 days plus quinine (CDC, 2011)

Orofacial/peripharyngeal space infections:

Oral: 150 to 450 mg every 6 hours for at least 7 days; maximum daily dose: 1800 mg/**day**

IV: 600 to 900 mg every 8 hours

Osteomyelitis due to MRSA: IV, Oral: 600 mg 3 times daily for a minimum of 8 weeks (some experts combine with rifampin) (Liu, 2011)

Pelvic inflammatory disease: IV: 900 mg every 8 hours with gentamicin (conventional or single daily dosing); 24 hours after clinical improvement may convert to oral clindamycin 450 mg 4 times daily or oral doxycycline to complete 14 days of total therapy. Avoid doxycycline if tubo-ovarian abscess is present (CDC, 2010).

Pharyngitis, group A streptococci (IDSA, Shulman, 2012): Oral:

Acute treatment in penicillin-allergic patients: 21 mg/kg/day divided every 8 hours for 10 days; maximum single dose: 300 mg

Chronic carrier treatment: 20 to 30 mg/kg/day divided every 8 hours for 10 days; maximum single dose: 300 mg

***Pneumocystis jirovecii* pneumonia:**

IV: 600 mg every 6 hours **or** 900 mg every 8 hours with primaquine for 21 days (DHHS [adult], 2013)

Oral: 300 mg every 6 hours **or** 450 mg every 8 hours with primaquine for 21 days (DHHS [adult], 2013)

Pneumonia due to MRSA: IV, Oral: 600 mg 3 times daily for 7 to 21 days (Liu, 2011)

Prophylaxis in total joint replacement patients undergoing dental procedures which produce bacteremia:

Oral: 600 mg 1 hour prior to procedure (ADA, 2003)

IV: 600 mg 1 hour prior to procedure (for patients unable to take oral medication) (ADA, 2003)

Prosthetic joint infection (Osmon, 2013):
Chronic antimicrobial suppression, staphylococci (oxacillin-susceptible): Oral: 300 mg every 6 hours
Propionibacterium acnes, treatment:
Oral: 300 to 450 mg every 6 hours for 4 to 6 weeks
IV: 600 to 900 mg every 8 hours for 4 to 6 weeks
Septic arthritis due to MRSA: IV, Oral: 600 mg 3 times daily for 3 to 4 weeks (Liu, 2011)
Toxic shock syndrome: IV: 900 mg every 8 hours with penicillin G or ceftriaxone
Toxoplasmosis encephalitis, HIV-exposed/-positive (DHHS [adult], 2013):
Treatment: Oral, IV: 600 mg every 6 hours with pyrimethamine and leucovorin for at least 6 weeks; longer if clinical or radiologic disease is extensive or response is incomplete
Secondary prevention: Oral: 600 mg every 8 hours with pyrimethamine and leucovorin calcium
Dosing adjustment in renal impairment: No adjustment required. Not dialyzable (0% to 5%).
Dosing adjustment in hepatic impairment: No adjustment required. Use caution with severe hepatic impairment.

Preparation for Administration
Oral: Reconstitute powder for oral solution with appropriate amount of water as specified on the bottle. Shake vigorously until suspended.
Parenteral: IV: Dilute to a final concentration not to exceed 18 mg/mL

Administration
Oral: Capsule should be taken with a full glass of water to avoid esophageal irritation; shake oral solution well before use; may administer with or without meals
Parenteral:
IM: Administer undiluted deep IM; rotate sites. Do not exceed 600 mg in a single injection.
IV: Infuse over at least 10 to 60 minutes, at a rate not to exceed 30 mg/minute; hypotension and cardiopulmonary arrest have been reported following rapid IV administration

Monitoring Parameters Observe for changes in bowel frequency; during prolonged therapy, monitor CBC with differential, platelet count, and hepatic and renal function tests periodically.

Dosage Forms Excipient information presented when available (limited, particularly for generics); consult specific product labeling.
Capsule, Oral, as hydrochloride [strength expressed as base]:
Cleocin: 75 mg, 150 mg [contains brilliant blue fcf (fd&c blue #1), tartrazine (fd&c yellow #5)]
Cleocin: 300 mg [contains brilliant blue fcf (fd&c blue #1)]
Generic: 75 mg, 150 mg, 300 mg
Solution, Injection, as phosphate [strength expressed as base]:
Cleocin Phosphate: 300 mg/2 mL (2 mL) [contains benzyl alcohol]
Cleocin Phosphate: 300 mg/2 mL (2 mL); 600 mg/4 mL (4 mL) [contains benzyl alcohol, edetate disodium]
Cleocin Phosphate: 900 mg/6 mL (6 mL) [contains benzyl alcohol]
Cleocin Phosphate: 900 mg/6 mL (6 mL); 9 g/60 mL (60 mL) [contains benzyl alcohol, edetate disodium]
Generic: 300 mg/2 mL (2 mL); 600 mg/4 mL (4 mL); 900 mg/6 mL (6 mL); 9000 mg/60 mL (60 mL); 9 g/60 mL (60 mL)
Solution, Intravenous, as phosphate [strength expressed as base]:
Cleocin in D5W: 300 mg/50 mL (50 mL); 600 mg/50 mL (50 mL); 900 mg/50 mL (50 mL) [contains edetate disodium]
Cleocin Phosphate: 600 mg/4 mL (4 mL) [contains benzyl alcohol, edetate disodium]
Cleocin Phosphate: 900 mg/6 mL (6 mL) [contains benzyl alcohol]
Generic: 300 mg/50 mL (50 mL); 600 mg/50 mL (50 mL); 900 mg/50 mL (50 mL); 300 mg/2 mL (2 mL); 600 mg/4 mL (4 mL); 900 mg/6 mL (6 mL)
Solution Reconstituted, Oral, as palmitate hydrochloride [strength expressed as base]:
Cleocin: 75 mg/5 mL (100 mL) [contains ethylparaben]
Generic: 75 mg/5 mL (100 mL)

Clindamycin (Topical) (klin da MYE sin)

Medication Safety Issues
Sound-alike/look-alike issues:
Cleocin® may be confused with bleomycin, Clinoril®, Cubicin®, Lincocin®
Clindamycin may be confused with clarithromycin, Claritin®, vancomycin
Clindesse may be confused with Clindets [Canada]

Brand Names: US Cleocin; Cleocin-T; Clindacin ETZ; Clindacin Pac; Clindacin-P; Clindagel; ClindaMax; Clindesse; Evoclin

Brand Names: Canada Clinda-T; Clindasol; Clindets; Dalacin T; Dalacin Vaginal; Taro-Clindamycin

Therapeutic Category Acne Products; Antibiotic, Anaerobic; Antibiotic, Miscellaneous

Generic Availability (US) May be product dependent

Use
Topical: Treatment of acne vulgaris (FDA approved in ages ≥12 years and adults)
Vaginal:
Cleocin Vaginal Cream: Treatment of bacterial vaginosis (FDA approved in adults)
Cleocin Ovules, Clindesse cream: Treatment of bacterial vaginosis (FDA approved in nonpregnant, postmenarchal females)

Pregnancy Risk Factor B

Pregnancy Considerations Adverse effects were not observed in animal reproduction studies. Clindamycin has been shown to cross the placenta following oral and parenteral dosing. Refer to the Clindamycin (Systemic) monograph for details. The amount of clindamycin available systemically is less following topical and vaginal application than with IV or oral administration. Oral clindamycin is recommended in certain pregnant patients for the treatment of bacterial vaginosis; however, vaginal therapy is not recommended for use in the second half of pregnancy.

Various clindamycin vaginal products are available for the treatment of bacterial vaginosis. Recommendations for use in pregnant woman vary by product labeling. Current guidelines prefer the use of oral therapy for the treatment of bacterial vaginosis in pregnant women. The CDC notes that vaginal therapy with clindamycin may be associated with adverse outcomes if used in the latter half of pregnancy (CDC, 2010).

If treatment for acne is needed during pregnancy, topical clindamycin may be considered if an antibiotic is needed. To decrease systemic exposure, pregnant women should avoid application to inflamed skin for long periods of time, or to large body surface areas (Kong, 2013).

Breast-Feeding Considerations It is not known if clindamycin is excreted into breast milk following vaginal or topical administration. Due to the potential for serious adverse reactions in the nursing infant, most manufacturers recommend a decision be made whether to discontinue nursing or to discontinue the drug, taking into account the importance of treatment to the mother. If clindamycin is used topically to the chest for the treatment of acne in women who are nursing, care should be taken to avoid accidental ingestion by the infant. To decrease systemic exposure, breast-feeding women should avoid application to inflamed skin for long periods of time, or to large body surface areas (Kong, 2013).

Small amounts of clindamycin transfer to human milk following oral and IV dosing. Refer to the Clindamycin (Systemic) monograph for details. Systemic clindamycin concentrations are less following topical and vaginal application. This minimal absorption should minimize potential exposure to a nursing infant. Nondose-related effects could include modification of bowel flora.

Contraindications Hypersensitivity to clindamycin, lincomycin, or any component of the formulation; previous CDAD (*C. difficile*-associated diarrhea), regional enteritis, ulcerative colitis

Warnings/Precautions Prolonged use may result in fungal or bacterial superinfection, including *C. difficile*-associated diarrhea (CDAD); CDAD has been observed >2 months postantibiotic treatment. Use with caution in patients with a history of gastrointestinal disease. Discontinue drug if significant diarrhea, abdominal cramps, or passage of blood and mucus occurs. Vaginal products may weaken condoms, or contraceptive diaphragms. Barrier contraceptives are not recommended concurrently or for 3-5 days (depending on the product) following treatment. Use caution in atopic patients. Clindamycin foam may cause irritation especially when used with abrasive, desquamating or peeling agents; avoid contact with eyes, mouth, lips, mucous membranes, or broken skin. Topical solution (including pledgets) contains an alcohol base and may cause eye irritation or burning. Rinse with cool tap water if product comes in contact with mucous membranes, abraded skin, or eyes. Use caution when applying near mouth (unpleasant taste).

Benzyl alcohol and derivatives: Some dosage forms may contain benzyl alcohol; large amounts of benzyl alcohol (≥99 mg/kg/day) have been associated with a potentially fatal toxicity ("gasping syndrome") in neonates; the "gasping syndrome" consists of metabolic acidosis, respiratory distress, gasping respirations, CNS dysfunction (including convulsions, intracranial hemorrhage), hypotension and cardiovascular collapse (AAP, 1997; CDC, 1982); some data suggests that benzoate displaces bilirubin from protein binding sites (Ahlfors, 2001); avoid or use dosage forms containing benzyl alcohol with caution in neonates. See manufacturer's labeling.

Warnings: Additional Pediatric Considerations Some dosage forms may contain propylene glycol; in neonates large amounts of propylene glycol delivered orally, intravenously (eg, >3,000 mg/day), or topically have been associated with potentially fatal toxicities which can include metabolic acidosis, seizures, renal failure, and CNS depression; toxicities have also been reported in children and adults including hyperosmolality, lactic acidosis, seizures and respiratory depression; use caution (AAP, 1997; Shehab, 2009).

Adverse Reactions

Topical:

Dermatologic: Burning sensation of skin (gel, lotion, solution), erythema (gel, lotion, solution), exfoliation of skin (lotion, solution), oily skin (gel, lotion, solution), pruritus (gel, lotion, solution), xeroderma (gel, lotion, solution)

Gastrointestinal: Bloody diarrhea, colitis, severe colitis

Rare but important or life-threatening: Abdominal pain, diarrhea (hemorrhagic or severe), folliculitis (gram negative infection), gastrointestinal distress, pseudomembranous colitis

Vaginal:

Dermatologic: Pruritus (non-application site)

Gastrointestinal: Bloody diarrhea, colitis, pseudomembranous colitis, severe colitis

Genitourinary: Trichomonal vaginitis, vaginal moniliasis, vaginal pain, vulvovaginal disease, vulvovaginal pruritus, vulvovaginitis

Infection: Fungal infection

Rare but important or life-threatening: Abdominal pain, application site pain, bacterial infection, diarrhea, dysgeusia, dysuria, edema, endometriosis, epistaxis, fever, flank pain, hypersensitivity reaction, hyperthyroidism, menstrual disease, nausea, pain, pyelonephritis, skin rash, urinary tract infection, vertigo, vomiting

Drug Interactions

Metabolism/Transport Effects None known.

Avoid Concomitant Use

Avoid concomitant use of Clindamycin (Topical) with any of the following: BCG; BCG (Intravesical); Erythromycin (Systemic); Erythromycin (Topical)

Increased Effect/Toxicity

Clindamycin (Topical) may increase the levels/effects of: Neuromuscular-Blocking Agents

Decreased Effect

Clindamycin (Topical) may decrease the levels/effects of: BCG; BCG (Intravesical); BCG Vaccine (Immunization); Sodium Picosulfate

The levels/effects of Clindamycin (Topical) may be decreased by: Erythromycin (Systemic); Erythromycin (Topical)

Storage/Stability

Cream: Store at room temperature.

Foam: Store at room temperature of 20°C to 25°C (68°F to 77°F). Avoid fire, flame, or smoking during or immediately following application.

Gel: Store at room temperature.

Clindagel®: Do not store in direct sunlight.

Lotion: Store at room temperature of 20°C to 25°C (68°F to 77°F).

Ovule: Store at room temperature of 25°C (77°F); avoid heat >30°C (86°F) and high humidity.

Pledget: Store at room temperature.

Topical solution: Store at room temperature of 20°C to 25°C (68°F to 77°F).

Mechanism of Action Reversibly binds to 50S ribosomal subunits preventing peptide bond formation thus inhibiting bacterial protein synthesis; bacteriostatic or bactericidal depending on drug concentration, infection site, and organism

Pharmacokinetics (Adult data unless noted)

Absorption: Topical solution or foam, phosphate: Minimal; Vaginal cream, phosphate: ~5%; Vaginal suppository, phosphate: ~30%

Metabolism: Hepatic; forms metabolites (variable activity); Clindamycin phosphate is converted to clindamycin HCl (active)

Half-life elimination: Vaginal cream: 1.5-2.6 hours following repeated dosing; Vaginal suppository: 11 hours (range: 4-35 hours, limited by absorption rate)

Time to peak, serum: Vaginal cream: ~10-14 hours (range: 4-24 hours); Vaginal suppository: ~5 hours (range: 1-10 hours)

Excretion: Urine (<0.2% with topical foam and solution)

Dosing: Usual Children, Adolescents, and Adults:

Acne vulgaris: Children ≥12 years, Adolescents, and Adults: Topical:

Gel (Clindagel), Foam (Evoclin): Apply to affected area once daily

Gel (Cleocin T), pledget, lotion, solution: Apply a thin film twice daily

Bacterial vaginosis: Adolescents and Adults: Intravaginal:

Cream:

Adolescents: One full applicator inserted intravaginally at bedtime for 7 days (*Red Book*, 2012)

Adults:
Cleocin: One full applicator (100 mg clindamycin) inserted intravaginally once daily before bedtime for 3 or 7 consecutive days in nonpregnant patients and 7 consecutive days in pregnant patients
Clindesse: One full applicator inserted intravaginally as a single dose at anytime during the day in nonpregnant patients
Suppository: Insert one ovule (100 mg clindamycin) intravaginally once daily at bedtime for 3 days

Dosing adjustment in renal impairment: There are no dosage adjustments provided in the manufacturer's labeling; however, no dosage adjustments are required with systemic clindamycin use.

Dosing adjustment in hepatic impairment: There are no dosage adjustments provided in the manufacturer's labeling; however, no dosage adjustments are required with systemic clindamycin use; use caution with severe hepatic impairment.

Administration

Intravaginal: Do not use for topical therapy, instillation in the eye, or oral administration. Wash hands; insert applicator into vagina and expel suppository or cream. Remain lying down for 30 minutes following administration. Wash applicator with soap and water following suppository use; if administering the cream, use each disposable applicator only once.

Topical foam: Do not use intravaginally. Before applying foam, wash affected area with mild soap, then dry. Do not dispense foam directly onto hands or face. Remove cap, hold can at an upright angle, and dispense foam directly into the cap or onto a cool surface. If can is warm or foam is runny, run can under cold water. Use fingertips to pick up small amounts of foam and gently massage into affected area until foam disappears. Avoid fire, flame, or smoking during or immediately following application. Avoid contact with eyes, mouth, lips, mucous membranes, or broken skin.

Topical gel, pledget, solution: Do not use intravaginally, instill in the eye, or administer orally. Solution/pledget contains an alcohol base and if inadvertent contact with mucous membranes occurs, rinse with liberal amounts of water. Remove pledget from foil immediately before use; discard after single use. May use more than one pledget for each application to cover area.

Topical lotion: Shake well immediately before use; apply topically. Do not use intravaginally, instill in the eye, or administer orally.

Monitoring Parameters Observe for changes in bowel frequency.

Dosage Forms Excipient information presented when available (limited, particularly for generics); consult specific product labeling. [DSC] = Discontinued product

Cream, Vaginal, as phosphate [strength expressed as base]:
Cleocin: 2% (40 g) [contains benzyl alcohol]
Clindesse: 2% (5.8 g) [contains disodium edta, methylparaben, propylparaben]
Generic: 2% (40 g)

Foam, External, as phosphate [strength expressed as base]:
Evoclin: 1% (50 g, 100 g) [contains cetyl alcohol, propylene glycol]
Generic: 1% (50 g, 100 g)

Gel, External, as phosphate [strength expressed as base]:
Cleocin-T: 1% (30 g, 60 g) [contains methylparaben, propylene glycol]
Clindagel: 1% (40 mL [DSC], 75 mL) [contains methylparaben, polyethylene glycol, propylene glycol]
ClindaMax: 1% (30 g, 60 g)
Generic: 1% (30 g, 60 g)

Kit, External, as phosphate [strength expressed as base]:
Clindacin ETZ: 1% [contains cetyl alcohol, isopropyl alcohol, propylene glycol]
Clindacin Pac: 1% [contains cetyl alcohol, isopropyl alcohol, propylene glycol]

Lotion, External, as phosphate [strength expressed as base]:
Cleocin-T: 1% (60 mL) [contains cetostearyl alcohol, methylparaben]
ClindaMax: 1% (60 mL)
Generic: 1% (60 mL)

Solution, External, as phosphate [strength expressed as base]:
Cleocin-T: 1% (30 mL, 60 mL) [contains isopropyl alcohol, propylene glycol]
Generic: 1% (30 mL, 60 mL)

Suppository, Vaginal, as phosphate [strength expressed as base]:
Cleocin: 100 mg (3 ea)

Swab, External, as phosphate [strength expressed as base]:
Cleocin-T: 1% (60 ea) [contains isopropyl alcohol, propylene glycol]
Clindacin ETZ: 1% (60 ea) [contains isopropyl alcohol, propylene glycol]
Clindacin-P: 1% (69 ea) [contains isopropyl alcohol, propylene glycol]
Generic: 1% (60 ea)

Clindamycin and Benzoyl Peroxide

(klin da MYE sin & BEN zoe il peer OKS ide)

Brand Names: US Acanya; BenzaClin; Duac; Neuac; Onexton

Brand Names: Canada BenzaClin; Clindoxyl

Therapeutic Category Acne Products; Topical Skin Product

Generic Availability (US) Yes

Use Topical treatment of acne vulgaris (FDA approved in ages ≥12 years and adults)

Pregnancy Risk Factor C

Pregnancy Considerations Animal reproduction studies have not been conducted with this combination. Refer to individual monographs.

Breast-Feeding Considerations It is not known if clindamycin or benzoyl peroxide are excreted into breast milk following topical administration. Due to the potential for serious adverse reactions in the nursing infant, the manufacturers recommend a decision be made whether to discontinue nursing or to discontinue the drug, taking into account the importance of treatment to the mother. Also refer to individual monographs.

Contraindications Hypersensitivity to benzoyl peroxide, clindamycin, lincomycin, or any component of the formulation; history of regional enteritis, ulcerative colitis, pseudomembranous colitis or antibiotic-associated colitis

Warnings/Precautions Systemic absorption may occur after topical use of clindamycin. Anaphylaxis and allergic reactions have been reported. *C. difficile*-associated diarrhea (CDAD) and pseudomembranous colitis have been reported and have been observed >2 months postantibiotic treatment. Use of parenteral and systemic clindamycin has resulted in severe colitis (including fatalities). Discontinue drug if significant diarrhea, abdominal cramps, or passage of blood and mucus occurs. Potentially significant interactions may exist, requiring dose or frequency adjustment, additional monitoring, and/or selection of alternative therapy. Use concomitant topical acne therapy with caution. Concomitant use with erythromycin-containing products is not recommended. Avoid contact with mucous membranes. Inform patients to use skin protection and minimize prolonged exposure to sun and avoid tanning beds and sun lamps. Benzoyl peroxide may bleach hair, colored fabric, or carpeting. Concomitant use of benzoyl peroxide with sulfone products (eg, dapsone, sulfacetamide) may cause temporary discoloration (yellow/orange) of facial hair and skin. Application of products at separate times during the day or washing off benzoyl peroxide prior to application of other products may avoid skin discoloration (Dubina 2009).

Adverse Reactions Also see individual agents.

Dermatologic: Application site scaling, local dryness, sunburn (local)

Local: Application site burning, application site erythema, application site itching, application site reaction, application site stinging, local desquamation

Rare but important or life-threatening: Application site pain, contact dermatitis, hypersensitivity reaction, local skin exfoliation

Drug Interactions

Metabolism/Transport Effects None known.

Avoid Concomitant Use

Avoid concomitant use of Clindamycin and Benzoyl Peroxide with any of the following: BCG; BCG (Intravesical); Erythromycin (Systemic); Erythromycin (Topical)

Increased Effect/Toxicity

Clindamycin and Benzoyl Peroxide may increase the levels/effects of: Dapsone (Topical); Neuromuscular-Blocking Agents

Decreased Effect

Clindamycin and Benzoyl Peroxide may decrease the levels/effects of: BCG; BCG (Intravesical); BCG Vaccine (Immunization); Sodium Picosulfate

The levels/effects of Clindamycin and Benzoyl Peroxide may be decreased by: Erythromycin (Systemic); Erythromycin (Topical)

Storage/Stability

Acanya: Prior to dispensing, store in refrigerator, between 2°C to 8°C (36°F to 46°F); do not freeze. Once dispensed, store at room temperature of ≤25°C (≤77°F), protect from freezing, and use within 10 weeks.

BenzaClin: Store unreconstituted product at room temperature of ≤25°C (≤77°F); do not freeze. Once reconstituted and dispensed, store at room temperature of ≤25°C (≤77°F) and use within 3 months.

Duac: Prior to dispensing, store in refrigerator, between 2°C to 8°C (36°F to 46°F); do not freeze. Once dispensed, store at room temperature of ≤25°C (≤77°F), protect from freezing, and use within 60 days.

Onexton: Prior to dispensing, store in a refrigerator at 2°C to 8°C (36°F to 46°F). Once dispensed, store at or below 25°C (77°F). Protect from freezing.

Mechanism of Action Clindamycin and benzoyl peroxide have activity against *Propionibacterium acnes in vitro*. This organism has been associated with acne vulgaris. Benzoyl peroxide releases free-radical oxygen which oxidizes bacterial proteins in the sebaceous follicles decreasing the number of anaerobic bacteria and decreasing irritating-type free fatty acids. Clindamycin reversibly binds to 50S ribosomal subunits preventing peptide bond formation thus inhibiting bacterial protein synthesis; it is bacteriostatic or bactericidal depending on drug concentration, infection site, and organism.

Pharmacodynamics See individual agents.

Pharmacokinetics (Adult data unless noted) See individual agents.

Dosing: Usual Acne vulgaris: Topical: Children ≥12 years and Adults:

Acanya: Apply pea-sized amount of gel once daily; use >12 weeks has not been studied.

BenzaClin: Apply twice daily (morning and evening)

Duac: Apply once daily in the evening

Preparation for Administration Topical: BenzaClin: Prior to dispensing, tap the vial until powder flows freely. Reconstitute clindamycin with purified water; shake well. Add clindamycin solution to benzoyl peroxide gel and stir until homogenous (60 to 90 seconds).

Administration FOR EXTERNAL USE ONLY. Not for oral, ophthalmic, or intravaginal use.

Topical: Skin should be clean and dry before applying. Apply thin layer to affected areas avoiding contact with eyes, lips, inside of nose, mouth, and all mucous membranes.

Dosage Forms Excipient information presented when available (limited, particularly for generics); consult specific product labeling.

Gel, topical: Clindamycin 1% and benzoyl peroxide 5% (50 g); Clindamycin phosphate 1.2% and benzoyl peroxide 5% (45 g)

Acanya: Clindamycin phosphate 1.2% and benzoyl peroxide 2.5% (50 g)

BenzaClin: Clindamycin 1% and benzoyl peroxide 5% (25 g, 35 g, 50 g)

Duac: Clindamycin phosphate 1.2% and benzoyl peroxide 5% (45 g)

Neuac: Clindamycin phosphate 1.2% and benzoyl peroxide 5% (45 g)

Onexton: Clindamycin phosphate 1.2% and benzoyl peroxide 3.75% (50 g) [contains propylene glycol]

Clindamycin and Tretinoin

(klin da MYE sin & TRET i noyn)

Brand Names: US Veltin; Ziana

Therapeutic Category Acne Products; Antibiotic, Miscellaneous; Retinoic Acid Derivative

Generic Availability (US) No

Use Treatment of acne vulgaris (FDA approved in ages ≥12 years and adults)

Pregnancy Risk Factor C

Pregnancy Considerations Adverse events were observed in animal reproduction studies using this combination topically. See individual agents.

Breast-Feeding Considerations It is not known if clindamycin or tretinoin is excreted into breast milk following topical administration. Due to the potential for serious adverse reactions in nursing infants, the manufacturer recommends a decision be made whether to discontinue nursing or the drug, taking into account the importance of treatment to the mother. See individual agents.

Contraindications Regional enteritis, ulcerative colitis, history of antibiotic-associated colitis

Warnings/Precautions Prolonged use may result in fungal or bacterial superinfection, including *Clostridium difficile*–associated diarrhea (CDAD) and pseudomembranous colitis; CDAD has been observed >2 months postantibiotic treatment. Discontinue drug if significant diarrhea, abdominal cramps, or passage of blood and mucus occurs. Tretinoin use is associated with increased susceptibility/sensitivity to ultraviolet (UV) light; avoid sunlamp or excessive sunlight exposure. Daily sunscreen use and other protective measures recommended. Use is not recommended in patients with sunburn. Treatment can increase skin sensitivity to weather extremes of wind or cold. Also, concomitant topical medications (eg, medicated or abrasive soaps, cleansers, or cosmetics with a strong drying effect) should be used with caution due to increased skin irritation. For external use only; not for ophthalmic, oral, or intravaginal use; avoid mucous membranes, eyes, mouth, and angles of nose. Potentially significant interactions may exist, requiring dose or frequency adjustment, additional monitoring, and/or selection of alternative therapy.

Some dosage forms may contain polysorbate 80 (also known as Tweens). Hypersensitivity reactions, usually a delayed reaction, have been reported following exposure to pharmaceutical products containing polysorbate 80 in certain individuals (Isaksson, 2002; Lucente 2000; Shelley, 1995). Thrombocytopenia, ascites, pulmonary deterioration, and renal and hepatic failure have been reported in premature neonates after receiving parenteral products containing polysorbate 80 (Alade, 1986; CDC, 1984). See manufacturer's labeling.

Adverse Reactions

Dermatologic: Burning, dermatitis, dryness, erythema, exfoliation, irritation, pruritus, scaling, stinging, sunburn

Gastrointestinal: GI symptoms (unspecified)

Respiratory: Nasopharyngitis

Drug Interactions

Metabolism/Transport Effects None known.

Avoid Concomitant Use

Avoid concomitant use of Clindamycin and Tretinoin with any of the following: BCG; BCG (Intravesical); Erythromycin (Systemic); Erythromycin (Topical); Multivitamins/Fluoride (with ADE); Multivitamins/Minerals (with ADEK, Folate, Iron); Multivitamins/Minerals (with AE, No Iron)

Increased Effect/Toxicity

Clindamycin and Tretinoin may increase the levels/effects of: Neuromuscular-Blocking Agents; Porfimer; Verteporfin

The levels/effects of Clindamycin and Tretinoin may be increased by: Multivitamins/Fluoride (with ADE); Multivitamins/Minerals (with ADEK, Folate, Iron); Multivitamins/Minerals (with AE, No Iron)

Decreased Effect

Clindamycin and Tretinoin may decrease the levels/effects of: BCG; BCG (Intravesical); BCG Vaccine (Immunization); Sodium Picosulfate

The levels/effects of Clindamycin and Tretinoin may be decreased by: Erythromycin (Systemic); Erythromycin (Topical)

Storage/Stability Store at 25°C (77°F); excursions permitted to 15°C to 30°C (59°F to 86°F); do not freeze. Protect from heat and light.

Mechanism of Action Clindamycin reversibly binds to 50S ribosomal subunits preventing peptide chain elongation thus inhibiting bacterial protein synthesis. Clindamycin exhibits *in vitro* activity against *Propionibacterium acnes*, an organism associated with acne vulgaris. Topical tretinoin is believed to decrease follicular epithelial cells cohesiveness and increase follicular epithelial cell turnover resulting in decreased microcomedo formation and increased expulsion of comedones.

Pharmacokinetics (Adult data unless noted) Absorption: Tretinoin: Minimal systemic absorption; Clindamycin: Low and variable systemic absorption

Dosing: Usual Acne vulgaris: Children ≥12 years and Adults: Topical: Apply pea-size amount to entire face once daily at bedtime; **Note:** Higher dosages (larger amount or more frequent use) have not been shown to improve efficacy and are associated with increased adverse effects (eg, skin irritation)

Administration Prior to application, clean face with a mild soap and pat dry; place pea-size amount on one fingertip and then dot on chin, cheeks, nose, and forehead. Gently rub over entire face or entire affected area while avoiding eyes, lips, mouth, angles of nose, and mucous membranes. Wash hands after use.

Monitoring Parameters Observe for changes in bowel frequency.

Dosage Forms Excipient information presented when available (limited, particularly for generics); consult specific product labeling.

Gel, topical:

Veltin™: Clindamycin phosphate 1.2% and tretinoin 0.025% (30 g, 60 g)

Ziana®: Clindamycin phosphate 1.2% and tretinoin 0.025% (30 g, 60 g)

- ◆ **Clindamycine (Can)** *see* Clindamycin (Systemic) *on page 487*
- ◆ **Clindamycin Hydrochloride** *see* Clindamycin (Systemic) *on page 487*
- ◆ **Clindamycin Injection (Can)** *see* Clindamycin (Systemic) *on page 487*
- ◆ **Clindamycin Injection SDZ (Can)** *see* Clindamycin (Systemic) *on page 487*
- ◆ **Clindamycin Injection, USP (Can)** *see* Clindamycin (Systemic) *on page 487*
- ◆ **Clindamycin Palmitate** *see* Clindamycin (Systemic) *on page 487*
- ◆ **Clindamycin Phosphate** *see* Clindamycin (Topical) *on page 491*
- ◆ **Clindamycin Phosphate and Benzoyl Peroxide** *see* Clindamycin and Benzoyl Peroxide *on page 493*
- ◆ **Clindamycin Phosphate and Tretinoin** *see* Clindamycin and Tretinoin *on page 494*
- ◆ **Clindasol (Can)** *see* Clindamycin (Topical) *on page 491*
- ◆ **Clinda-T (Can)** *see* Clindamycin (Topical) *on page 491*
- ◆ **Clindesse** *see* Clindamycin (Topical) *on page 491*
- ◆ **Clindets (Can)** *see* Clindamycin (Topical) *on page 491*
- ◆ **Clindoxyl (Can)** *see* Clindamycin and Benzoyl Peroxide *on page 493*
- ◆ **Clinolipid** *see* Fat Emulsion (Plant Based) *on page 850*
- ◆ **Clinoril** *see* Sulindac *on page 1994*
- ◆ **Clinpro 5000** *see* Fluoride *on page 899*

CloBAZam (KLOE ba zam)

Medication Safety Issues

Sound-alike/look-alike issues:

CloBAZam may be confused with clonazePAM

Brand Names: US Onfi

Brand Names: Canada Apo-Clobazam; Clobazam-10; Dom-Clobazam; Frisium; Novo-Clobazam; PMS-Clobazam

Therapeutic Category Anticonvulsant, Benzodiazepine

Generic Availability (US) No

Use Adjunctive treatment of seizures associated with Lennox-Gastaut syndrome (FDA approved in ages ≥2 years and adults); has also been used as monotherapy and adjunctive treatment for other forms of epilepsy

Medication Guide Available Yes

Pregnancy Risk Factor C

Pregnancy Considerations Adverse events were observed in animal reproduction studies. Clobazam crosses the placenta. An increased risk of fetal malformations may be associated with first trimester exposure. The Canadian labeling contraindicates use in the first trimester. Exposure to benzodiazepines immediately prior to or during birth may result in hypothermia, hypotonia, respiratory depression, and difficulty feeding in the neonate; neonates exposed to benzodiazepines late in pregnancy may develop dependence and withdrawal. The incidence of premature birth and low birth weights may be increased following maternal use of benzodiazepines; hypoglycemia and respiratory problems in the neonate may occur following exposure late in pregnancy. Neonatal withdrawal symptoms may occur within days to weeks after birth and "floppy infant syndrome" (which also includes withdrawal symptoms) has been reported with some benzodiazepines (Bergman, 1992; Iqbal, 2002; Wikner, 2007). A combination of factors influences the potential teratogenicity of anticonvulsant therapy. When treating women with epilepsy, monotherapy with the lowest effective dose and avoidance medications known to have a high incidence of teratogenic effects is recommended (Harden, 2009; Wlodarczyk, 2012).

Patients exposed to clobazam during pregnancy are encouraged to enroll themselves into the North American Antiepileptic Drug (NAAED) Pregnancy Registry by calling 1-888-233-2334. Additional information is available at www.aedpregnancyregistry.org.

Breast-Feeding Considerations Clobazam is excreted into breast milk. Due to the potential for serious adverse reactions in the nursing infant, the U.S. manufacturer recommends a decision be made whether to discontinue nursing or to discontinue the drug, taking into account the importance of treatment to the mother. Use in nursing women is contraindicated in the Canadian labeling. Drowsiness, lethargy, or weight loss in nursing infants have been observed in case reports following maternal use of some benzodiazepines (Iqbal, 2002).

Contraindications Hypersensitivity to clobazam or any component of the formulation.

Canadian labeling (not in U.S. labeling): Hypersensitivity to clobazam or any component of the formulation (cross sensitivity with other benzodiazepines may exist); myasthenia gravis; narrow-angle glaucoma; severe hepatic or respiratory disease; sleep apnea; history of substance abuse; use in the first trimester of pregnancy; breast-feeding

Warnings/Precautions Serious reactions, including Stevens-Johnson syndrome (SJS) and toxic epidermal necrolysis (TEN), have been reported. Monitor patients closely for signs and symptoms especially during the first 8 weeks or when reintroducing therapy. Permanently discontinue if SJS/TEN suspected.

Rebound or withdrawal symptoms may occur following abrupt discontinuation or large decreases in dose (more common with prolonged treatment). Cautiously taper dose if drug discontinuation is required. Use with caution in elderly or debilitated patients, patients with mild-to-moderate hepatic impairment or with preexisting muscle weakness or ataxia (may cause muscle weakness). Concentrations of the active metabolite are 3 to 5 times higher in patients who are known CYP2C19 poor metabolizers compared to CYP2C19 extensive metabolizers; dose adjustment is needed in patients who are poor CYP2C19 metabolizers.

Causes CNS depression (dose related) resulting in sedation, dizziness, confusion, or ataxia which may impair physical and mental capabilities. Patients must be cautioned about performing tasks which require mental alertness (eg, operating machinery or driving). Use with caution in patients receiving other CNS depressants or psychoactive agents. Effects with other sedative drugs or ethanol may be potentiated. Use with caution in patients with an impaired gag reflex or respiratory disease.

Tolerance, psychological and physical dependence may occur with prolonged use. Where possible, avoid use in patients with drug abuse, alcoholism, or psychiatric disease (eg, depression, psychosis). May increase risk of suicidal thoughts/behavior.

Acute withdrawal, including seizures, may be precipitated in patients after administration of flumazenil to patients receiving long-term benzodiazepine therapy. Potentially significant interactions may exist, requiring dose or frequency adjustment, additional monitoring, and/or selection of alternative therapy.

Benzodiazepines have been associated with anterograde amnesia. Paradoxical reactions, including hyperactive or aggressive behavior, have been reported with benzodiazepines, particularly in adolescent/pediatric or psychiatric patients. Does not have analgesic, antidepressant, or antipsychotic properties.

Warnings: Additional Pediatric Considerations May cause CNS depression and dose related somnolence and sedation (incidence: 32% with high doses); onset of somnolence and sedation occurs within first month of therapy and may lessen with continued treatment. Paradoxical reactions, including hyperactive or aggressive behavior, have been reported with benzodiazepines, particularly in adolescent/pediatric or psychiatric patients. Decreased bone density and bone length and alterations in behavior have been reported in juvenile animal studies at levels of exposure greater than therapeutic doses; adverse bone effects were reversible upon discontinuation. Administration of high doses to rats for 2 years was associated with an increase in thyroid follicular cell adenomas; implications for human use are uncertain.

Some dosage forms may contain propylene glycol; in neonates large amounts of propylene glycol delivered orally, intravenously (eg, >3,000 mg/day), or topically have been associated with potentially fatal toxicities which can include metabolic acidosis, seizures, renal failure, and CNS depression; toxicities have also been reported in children and adults including hyperosmolality, lactic acidosis, seizures and respiratory depression; use caution (AAP, 1997; Shehab, 2009).

Adverse Reactions

Central nervous system: Aggressive behavior, ataxia, drowsiness, dysarthria, fatigue, insomnia, irritability, lethargy, psychomotor agitation, sedation

Gastrointestinal: Constipation, decreased appetite, dysphagia, increased appetite, sialorrhea, vomiting

Genitourinary: Urinary tract infection

Neuromuscular & skeletal: Dysarthria

Respiratory: Bronchitis, cough, pneumonia, upper respiratory tract infection

Miscellaneous: Fever

Postmarketing and/or case reports (Limited to important or life-threatening): Angioedema, aspiration, behavioral changes, blurred vision, confusion, delirium, delusions, depression, diplopia, eosinophilia, hallucination, hypothermia, leukopenia, lip edema, mood changes, respiratory depression, Stevens-Johnson syndrome, suicidal ideation, suicidal tendencies, thrombocytopenia, toxic epidermal necrolysis, urinary retention, withdrawal syndrome

Drug Interactions

Metabolism/Transport Effects Substrate of CYP2B6 (minor), CYP2C19 (major), CYP3A4 (minor), P-glycoprotein; **Note:** Assignment of Major/Minor substrate status based on clinically relevant drug interaction potential; **Inhibits** CYP2C9 (weak), CYP2D6 (moderate), UGT1A4, UGT1A6, UGT2B4; **Induces** CYP3A4 (weak)

Avoid Concomitant Use

Avoid concomitant use of CloBAZam with any of the following: Azelastine (Nasal); Methadone; OLANZapine; Orphenadrine; Paraldehyde; Sodium Oxybate; Thalidomide; Thioridazine

Increased Effect/Toxicity

CloBAZam may increase the levels/effects of: Azelastine (Nasal); Buprenorphine; CloZAPine; CNS Depressants; CYP2D6 Substrates; Deferiprone; DOXOrubicin (Conventional); Eliglustat; Fesoterodine; Hydrocodone; Methadone; Methotrimeprazine; Metoprolol; Metyrosine; Mirtazapine; Nebivolol; Orphenadrine; Paraldehyde; Pramipexole; ROPINIRole; Rotigotine; Selective Serotonin Reuptake Inhibitors; Sodium Oxybate; Stiripentol; Suvorexant; Thalidomide; Thioridazine; Zolpidem

The levels/effects of CloBAZam may be increased by: Alcohol (Ethyl); Brimonidine (Topical); Cannabis; CYP2C19 Inhibitors (Moderate); CYP2C19 Inhibitors (Strong); Doxylamine; Dronabinol; Droperidol; HydrOXYzine; Kava Kava; Luliconazole; Magnesium Sulfate; Methotrimeprazine; Nabilone; OLANZapine;

Perampanel; Propafenone; Rufinamide; Stiripentol; Tapentadol; Teduglutide; Tetrahydrocannabinol

Decreased Effect

CloBAZam may decrease the levels/effects of: ARIPiprazole; Codeine; Contraceptives (Estrogens); Contraceptives (Progestins); NiMODipine; Saxagliptin; Tamoxifen; TraMADol

The levels/effects of CloBAZam may be decreased by: CYP2C19 Inducers (Strong); Dabrafenib; Theophylline Derivatives; Yohimbine

Food Interactions

Ethanol: Concomitant administration may increase bioavailability of clobazam by 50%. Management: Monitor for increased effects with coadministration.

Food: Serum concentrations may be increased by grapefruit juice. Management: Keep grapefruit consumption consistent.

Storage/Stability Tablets and suspension: Store at 20°C to 25°C (68°F to 77°F). Dispose of unused suspension 90 days after opening bottle.

Mechanism of Action Clobazam is a 1,5 benzodiazepine which binds to stereospecific benzodiazepine receptors on the postsynaptic GABA neuron at several sites within the central nervous system, including the limbic system, reticular formation. Enhancement of the inhibitory effect of GABA on neuronal excitability results by increased neuronal membrane permeability to chloride ions. This shift in chloride ions results in hyperpolarization (a less excitable state) and stabilization. Benzodiazepine receptors and effects appear to be linked to the GABA-A receptors. Benzodiazepines do not bind to GABA-B receptors.

Pharmacodynamics Maximum effect: 5-9 days

Pharmacokinetics (Adult data unless noted)

Absorption: Rapid and extensive; not affected by food or crushing tablet

Distribution: V_{dss}: 100 L; Protein binding: Clobazam: 80% to 90%; N-desmethylclobazam (NCLB): 70%

Metabolism: Hepatic via CYP3A4 and to a lesser extent via CYP2C19 and 2B6; N-demethylation to active metabolite (N-desmethyl) with ~20% activity of clobazam. CYP2C19 primarily mediates subsequent hydroxylation of the N-desmethyl metabolite; metabolic rate increased in children (53% to 69%) (Ng, 2007). Plasma concentrations of NCLB are 5 times higher in CYP2C19 poor metabolizers versus extensive metabolizers.

Bioavailability: 87% (Ng, 2007)

Half-life:

Children: Clobazam: 16 hours (Ng, 2007)

Adults: Clobazam: 36-42 hours

NCLB: 71-82 hours

Time to peak serum concentration: Tablet: 0.5 to 4 hours; Oral suspension: 0.5 to 2 hours

Elimination: Urine: 82% of dose; unchanged drug: 2%, NCLB and other metabolites: ~94%. Feces: 11% of dose; unchanged drug: 1%

Dosing: Usual Note: Dosage should be titrated according to patient tolerability and response.

Pediatric:

Lennox-Gastaut syndrome: Children ≥2 years and Adolescents: Oral:

≤30 kg: Initial: 5 mg once daily for ≥1 week, may then increase to 5 mg twice daily for ≥1 week, then increase to 10 mg twice daily thereafter (maximum daily dose: 20 mg/**day**)

>30 kg: Initial: 5 mg twice daily for ≥1 week, may then increase to 10 mg twice daily for ≥1 week, then increase to 20 mg twice daily thereafter (maximum daily dose: 40 mg/**day**)

Seizures, generalized or partial, monotherapy or adjunctive therapy: Oral: Limited data available [Frisium® prescribing information (U.K.; Canada), 2011; Canadian Study Group, 1998; Ng, 2007]:

Infants and Children <2 years: Initial: 0.5-1 mg/kg/**day** usually in divided doses twice daily; maximum initial daily dose: 5 mg/**day**; may increase dosage slowly (not more often than every 5-7 days); maximum daily dose: 10 mg/**day**

Children 2-16 years: Initial: 5 mg once daily; may increase dosage slowly (not more often than every 5 days), usual range: 10-20 mg/**day** or 0.3-1 mg/kg/**day** in divided doses twice daily; maximum daily dose: 40 mg/**day**

Adults:

Lennox-Gastaut, adjunctive: Oral:

≤30 kg: Initial: 5 mg once daily for ≥1 week, then increase to 5 mg twice daily for ≥1 week, then increase to 10 mg twice daily thereafter

>30 kg: Initial: 5 mg twice daily for ≥1 week, then increase to 10 mg twice daily for ≥1 week, then increase to 20 mg twice daily thereafter

Dosage adjustment in renal impairment: Children, Adolescents, and Adults:

CrCl ≥30 mL/minute: No dosage adjustment required

CrCl <30 mL/minute: Use with caution, has not been studied

Dosage adjustment in hepatic impairment: Children, Adolescents, and Adults:

Mild to moderate impairment (Child-Pugh Score 5-9):

≤30 kg: Initial: 5 mg once daily for ≥2 weeks, then increase to 5 mg twice daily for ≥1 week, may then increase to 10 mg twice daily based on patient tolerability and response

>30 kg: Initial: 5 mg once daily for ≥1 week, then increase to 5 mg twice daily for ≥1 week, then increase to 10 mg twice daily for ≥1 week, may then increase to 20 mg twice daily based on patient tolerability and response

Severe impairment: Use with extreme caution; has not been studied; undergoes extensive hepatic metabolism.

Dosage adjustment for CYP2C19 poor metabolizers: Children, Adolescents, and Adults:

≤30 kg: Initial: 5 mg once daily for ≥2 weeks, then increase to 5 mg twice daily for ≥1 week, may then increase to 10 mg twice daily based on patient tolerability and response

>30 kg: Initial: 5 mg once daily for ≥1 week, then increase to 5 mg twice daily for ≥1 week, then increase to 10 mg twice daily for ≥1 week, may then increase to 20 mg twice daily based on patient tolerability and response

Administration May be administered with or without food.

Tablets: May be administered whole, broken in half along score, or crushed and mixed in applesauce.

Oral suspension: Shake well before use. Measure dosage with manufacturer-provided oral dosing syringe and bottle adapter.

Monitoring Parameters Respiratory and mental status/suicidality (eg, suicidal thoughts, depression, behavioral changes); CBC, liver function, and renal function; some recommend periodic thyroid function tests

Controlled Substance C-IV

Dosage Forms Excipient information presented when available (limited, particularly for generics); consult specific product labeling. [DSC] = Discontinued product

Suspension, Oral:

Onfi: 2.5 mg/mL (120 mL) [contains methylparaben, polysorbate 80, propylene glycol, propylparaben; berry flavor]

Tablet, Oral:
Onfi: 5 mg [DSC]
Onfi: 10 mg, 20 mg [scored]

◆ **Clobazam-10 (Can)** *see* CloBAZam *on page* 495

Clobetasol (kloe BAY ta sol)

Medication Safety Issues

International issues:

Clobex [U.S., Canada, and multiple international markets] may be confused with Codex brand name for *Saccharomyces boulardii* [Italy]

Cloderm: Brand name for clobetasol [China, India, Malaysia, Singapore, Thailand], but also brand name for alclometasone [Indonesia]; clocortolone [U.S., Canada]; clotrimazole [Germany]

Related Information

Topical Corticosteroids *on page* 2262

Brand Names: US Clobetasol Propionate E; Clobex; Clobex Spray; Clodan; Cormax Scalp Application; Olux; Olux-E; Temovate; Temovate E

Brand Names: Canada Clobex; Dermovate; Mylan-Clobetasol; Novo-Clobetasol; Olux-E; PMS-Clobetasol; ratio-Clobetasol; Taro-Clobetasol

Therapeutic Category Adrenal Corticosteroid; Anti-inflammatory Agent; Corticosteroid, Topical; Glucocorticoid

Generic Availability (US) May be product dependent

Use Short-term relief of inflammation and pruritus associated with corticosteroid-responsive dermatoses (cream, emollient cream, gel, ointment, and solution: FDA approved in ages ≥12 and adults; lotion: FDA approved in adults); short-term treatment of mild to moderate plaque psoriasis of nonscalp regions (foam: FDA approved in ages ≥12 years and adults); short-term treatment of moderate- to severe-type plaque psoriasis (emollient cream: FDA approved in ages ≥16 years and adults; lotion, spray: FDA approved in ages ≥18 years and adults); short-term treatment of moderate to severe forms of scalp psoriasis (foam: FDA approved in ages ≥12 years and adults; shampoo: FDA approved in adults)

Pregnancy Risk Factor C

Pregnancy Considerations Adverse events have been observed in animal reproduction studies. Extensive use in pregnant women is not recommended.

Breast-Feeding Considerations It is not known if topical application will result in detectable quantities in breast milk. The manufacturer recommends that caution be exercised when administering clobetasol to nursing women.

Contraindications Hypersensitivity to clobetasol, other corticosteroids, or any component of the formulation; primary infections of the scalp (scalp solution only)

Warnings/Precautions Systemic absorption of topical corticosteroids may cause hypothalamic-pituitary-adrenal (HPA) axis suppression particularly in younger children. HPA axis suppression may lead to adrenal crisis. Allergic contact dermatitis may occur; it is usually diagnosed by failure to heal rather than clinical exacerbation. Prolonged treatment with corticosteroids has been associated with the development of Kaposi sarcoma (case reports); if noted, discontinuation of therapy should be considered. Local effects may occur, including folliculitis, acneiform eruptions, hypopigmentation, perioral dermatitis, allergic contact dermatitis, secondary infection, striae, miliaria, skin atrophy and telangiectasia; may be irreversible. Adverse systemic effects including Cushing syndrome, hyperglycemia, glycosuria, and HPA suppression may occur when used on large surface areas, denuded skin, or with an occlusive dressing. Use in children <12 years of age is not recommended. Children may absorb proportionally larger amounts after topical application and may be more prone to systemic effects. Prolonged use may affect growth velocity; growth should be routinely monitored in pediatric patients. Clobex lotion, Clobex shampoo, Clobex spray, and Clodan shampoo are not recommended for use in pediatric patients ≤17 years.

Do not use on the face, axillae, or groin or for the treatment of rosacea or perioral dermatitis. Emollient cream contains imidurea; may cause allergic sensitization or irritation upon skin contact with the skin. Foam and spray are flammable; do not use near open flame.

Warnings: Additional Pediatric Considerations The extent of percutaneous absorption is dependent on several factors, including epidermal integrity (intact vs abraded skin), formulation, age of the patient, prolonged duration of use, and the use of occlusive dressings. Percutaneous absorption of topical steroids is increased in neonates (especially preterm neonates), infants, and young children. Infants and small children may be more susceptible to HPA axis suppression, intracranial hypertension, Cushing syndrome, or other systemic toxicities due to larger skin surface area to body mass ratio. Due to the high incidence of adrenal suppression noted in clinical studies, clobetasol lotion, shampoo, and spray are not recommended for use in patients <18 years of age. In a study of patients with moderate to severe atopic dermatitis (involving ≥20% BSA) receiving Clobex 0.05% lotion twice daily for 2 weeks, 9 of the14 pediatric patients (12 to 17 years of age) included developed adrenal suppression, compared to 2 of the 10 pediatric patients receiving the cream. In a study of patients receiving Clobex 0.05% shampoo, 5 of 12 pediatric patients (12 to 17 years of age) developed HPA axis suppression.

Some dosage forms may contain propylene glycol; in neonates large amounts of propylene glycol delivered orally, intravenously (eg, >3,000 mg/day), or topically have been associated with potentially fatal toxicities which can include metabolic acidosis, seizures, renal failure, and CNS depression; toxicities have also been reported in children and adults including hyperosmolality, lactic acidosis, seizures and respiratory depression; use caution (AAP, 1997; Shehab, 2009).

Adverse Reactions May depend upon formulation used, length of application, surface area covered, and the use of occlusive dressings.

Central nervous system: Intracranial hypertension (systemic effect reported in children treated with topical corticosteroids), local pain, localized burning, numbness of fingers, stinging sensation

Dermatologic: Atrophic striae (children), eczema asteatotic, erythema, folliculitis, pruritus, skin atrophy, telangiectasia, xeroderma

Endocrine & metabolic: Adrenal suppression, Cushing's syndrome, glucosuria, growth suppression, HPA-axis suppression, hyperglycemia

Local: Local irritation, skin fissure

Respiratory: Nasopharyngitis, streptococcal pharyngitis, upper respiratory tract infection

Rare but important or life-threatening: Alopecia, exfoliation of skin, skin rash, urticaria

Drug Interactions

Metabolism/Transport Effects None known.

Avoid Concomitant Use

Avoid concomitant use of Clobetasol with any of the following: Aldesleukin

Increased Effect/Toxicity

Clobetasol may increase the levels/effects of: Ceritinib; Deferasirox

The levels/effects of Clobetasol may be increased by: Telaprevir

Decreased Effect
Clobetasol may decrease the levels/effects of: Aldesleukin; Corticorelin; Hyaluronidase; Telaprevir

Storage/Stability

Cream, emollient cream, lotion, ointment: Store between 15°C to 30°C (59°F to 86°F); do not refrigerate or freeze.

Foam: Store between 20ºC and 25ºC (68ºF and 77ºF); do not expose to temperatures >49°C (120°F). Avoid fire, flame, or smoking during and immediately following application.

Gel: Store between 2°C and 30°C (36°F and 86°F).

Shampoo: Store between 20°C and 25°C (68°F and 77°F).

Solution: Do not use near an open flame.

Cormax: Store between 15°C to 30°C (59°F to 86°F).

Temovate: Store between 4°C to 25°C (39°F to 77°F).

Spray: Store at room temperature; do not expose to temperatures >30°C (86°F). Do not freeze or refrigerate. Spray is flammable; do not use near open flame.

Mechanism of Action Topical corticosteroids have anti-inflammatory, antipruritic, and vasoconstrictive properties. May depress the formation, release, and activity of endogenous chemical mediators of inflammation (kinins, histamine, liposomal enzymes, prostaglandins) through the induction of phospholipase A_2 inhibitory proteins (lipocortins) and sequential inhibition of the release of arachidonic acid. Clobetasol has very high range potency.

Pharmacokinetics (Adult data unless noted)

Absorption: Percutaneous absorption varies and depends on many factors including vehicle used, integrity of epidermis, dose, and use of occlusive dressing; absorption is increased by occlusive dressings or with decreased integrity of skin (eg, inflammation or skin disease); gel has greater absorption than cream

Metabolism: Hepatic

Elimination: Drug and metabolites are excreted in urine and bile

Dosing: Usual Note: Dosage should be based on severity of disease and patient response; use the smallest amount for the shortest period of time to avoid HPA suppression; discontinue therapy when control is achieved; reassess diagnosis if no improvement is seen within 2 weeks.

Pediatric: **Note:** Due to the high incidence of adrenal suppression noted in clinical studies, clobetasol lotion, shampoo, and spray are not recommended for use in patients <18 years of age.

Dermatoses (steroid-responsive): Children ≥12 years and Adolescents: Topical:

Cream, emollient cream, gel, ointment: Apply sparingly twice daily for up to 2 weeks; maximum weekly dose: 50 g/**week**

Solution: Apply sparingly to affected area of scalp twice daily for up to 2 weeks; maximum weekly dose: 50 mL/**week**

Plaque-type psoriasis of nonscalp areas; mild to moderate: Children ≥12 years and Adolescents: Topical: Foam: Apply sparingly to affected area twice daily for up to 2 weeks; maximum weekly dose: 50 g/**week** or 21 capfuls/**week**

Plaque-type psoriasis; moderate to severe:

Emollient cream: Adolescents ≥16 years: Topical: Apply sparingly twice daily for up to 2 weeks; if response is not adequate, may be used for up to 2 more weeks if application is <10% of body surface area; use with caution; maximum weekly dose: 50 g/**week**

Lotion: Adolescents ≥18 years: Topical: Apply twice daily for up to 2 weeks; maximum weekly dose: 50 g/**week** or 50 mL/**week**)

Spray: Adolescents ≥18 years: Apply by spraying directly onto affected area twice daily and gently rub into skin. Limit treatment to 4 consecutive weeks; treatment beyond 2 weeks should be limited to localized lesions which have not improved sufficiently. Maximum weekly dose: 50 g/**week** or 59 mL/**week**. Do not use more than 26 sprays per application or 52 sprays per day.

Scalp psoriasis, moderate to severe:

Foam: Children ≥12 years and Adolescents: Topical: Apply twice daily for up to 2 weeks; maximum weekly dose: 50 g/**week** or 21 capfuls/**week**)

Shampoo: Adolescents ≥18 years: Topical: Apply thin film to dry scalp once daily; leave in place for 15 minutes, then add water, lather, and rinse thoroughly; maximum weekly dose: 50 g/**week** or 50 mL/**week**. Limit treatment to 4 consecutive weeks.

Adult:

Steroid-responsive dermatoses: Topical: Cream, emollient cream, gel, lotion, ointment, solution: Apply twice daily for up to 2 weeks (maximum weekly dose: 50 g/**week** or 50 mL/**week**)

Mild to moderate plaque-type psoriasis of nonscalp areas: Topical: Foam: Apply twice daily for up to 2 weeks (maximum weekly dose: 50 g/**week** or 21 capfuls/**week**)

Moderate to severe plaque-type psoriasis: Topical:

Emollient cream, lotion: Apply twice daily for up to 2 weeks; can be used for up to 4 weeks when application is <10% of body surface area (maximum weekly dose: 50 g/**week** or 50 mL/**week**). Treatment with lotion beyond 2 weeks should be limited to localized lesions (<10% body surface area) which have not improved sufficiently.

Spray: Apply by spraying directly onto affected area twice daily and gently rub into skin. Limit treatment to 4 consecutive weeks; treatment beyond 2 weeks should be limited to localized lesions which have not improved sufficiently. Maximum weekly dose: 50 g/**week** or 59 mL/**week**. Do not use more than 26 sprays per application or 52 sprays per day.

Scalp psoriasis, moderate to severe: Topical:

Foam: Apply twice daily for up to 2 weeks (maximum weekly dose: 50 g/**week** or 21 capfuls/**week**)

Shampoo: Apply thin film to dry scalp once daily (maximum weekly dose: 50 g/**week** or 50 mL/**week**); leave in place for 15 minutes, then add water, lather, and rinse thoroughly. Limit treatment to 4 consecutive weeks.

Dosing adjustment in renal impairment: There are no dosage adjustments provided in manufacturer's labeling.

Dosing adjustment in hepatic impairment: There are no dosage adjustments provided in manufacturer's labeling.

Administration Topical: Apply the smallest amount that will cover affected area. For topical use only; avoid contact with eyes and mucous membranes. Do not apply to face or intertriginous areas. Do not use if there is atrophy at the treatment site. Minimize contact to nonaffected areas of the body; wash hands after applying. Occlusive dressings not recommended; do not occlude affected area unless directed by a physician; wash hands after applying.

Cream, emollient cream, gel, lotion, ointment, solution: Rub in gently and completely.

Foam: Turn can upside down and spray a small amount (maximum: 1½ capful or about the size of a golf ball) of foam into the cap, other cool surface, or to affected area. If the can is warm or foam is runny, place can under cold, running water. If fingers are warm, rinse with cool water and dry prior to handling (foam will melt on contact with warm skin). Massage foam into affected area. Do not use for diaper dermatitis.

Shampoo: Limit treatment to 4 consecutive weeks. Use on dry scalp; do not wet hair prior to use. Do not use a shower cap or bathing cap while shampoo is on the scalp. Leave in place for 15 minutes, then wet hair, lather, and rinse hair and scalp completely. Although no additional shampoo is necessary to cleanse the hair, a non-medicated shampoo may be used after application if desired.

Spray: Spray directly onto affected area of skin. Gently and completely rub into skin after spraying. Do not use more than 26 sprays per application or 52 sprays per day.

Monitoring Parameters Assess HPA axis suppression in patients using potent topical steroids applied to a large surface area or to areas under occlusion (eg, ACTH stimulation test, morning plasma cortisol test, urinary free cortisol test)

Additional Information Considered to be a super high potency topical corticosteroid; clobetasol is a prednisolone analog with a high level of glucocorticoid activity and slight degree of mineralocorticoid activity.

Dosage Forms Excipient information presented when available (limited, particularly for generics); consult specific product labeling.

Cream, External, as propionate:
- Clobetasol Propionate E: 0.05% (15 g, 30 g, 60 g) [contains cetostearyl alcohol, propylene glycol]
- Clobetasol Propionate E: 0.05% (15 g, 30 g, 60 g) [contains propylene glycol]
- Temovate: 0.05% (30 g, 60 g) [contains cetostearyl alcohol, chlorocresol (chloro-m-cresol), propylene glycol]
- Temovate E: 0.05% (60 g)
- Generic: 0.05% (15 g, 30 g, 45 g, 60 g)

Foam, External, as propionate:
- Olux: 0.05% (50 g, 100 g) [contains cetyl alcohol, propylene glycol]
- Olux-E: 0.05% (50 g, 100 g) [contains cetyl alcohol, propylene glycol]
- Generic: 0.05% (50 g, 100 g)

Gel, External, as propionate:
- Temovate: 0.05% (60 g) [contains propylene glycol]
- Generic: 0.05% (15 g, 30 g, 60 g)

Kit, External, as propionate:
- Clodan: 0.05% [contains alcohol, usp, cetyl alcohol, edetate disodium, propylene glycol]

Liquid, External, as propionate:
- Clobex Spray: 0.05% (59 mL, 125 mL) [contains alcohol, usp]
- Generic: 0.05% (59 mL, 125 mL)

Lotion, External, as propionate:
- Clobex: 0.05% (59 mL, 118 mL)
- Generic: 0.05% (59 mL, 118 mL)

Ointment, External, as propionate:
- Temovate: 0.05% (15 g, 30 g) [contains propylene glycol]
- Generic: 0.05% (15 g, 30 g, 45 g, 60 g)

Shampoo, External, as propionate:
- Clobex: 0.05% (118 mL) [contains alcohol, usp]
- Clodan: 0.05% (118 mL) [contains alcohol, usp]
- Generic: 0.05% (118 mL)

Solution, External, as propionate:
- Cormax Scalp Application: 0.05% (50 mL) [contains isopropyl alcohol]
- Temovate: 0.05% (50 mL)
- Generic: 0.05% (25 mL, 50 mL)

◆ **Clobetasol Propionate** *see* Clobetasol *on page 498*

◆ **Clobetasol Propionate E** *see* Clobetasol *on page 498*

◆ **Clobex** *see* Clobetasol *on page 498*

◆ **Clobex Spray** *see* Clobetasol *on page 498*

◆ **Clodan** *see* Clobetasol *on page 498*

Clofarabine (klo FARE a been)

Medication Safety Issues

Sound-alike/look-alike issues:

Clofarabine may be confused with cladribine, clevidipine, cytarabine, nelarabine

High alert medication:

This medication is in a class the Institute for Safe Medication Practices (ISMP) includes among its list of drug classes which have a heightened risk of causing significant patient harm when used in error.

Related Information

Prevention of Chemotherapy-Induced Nausea and Vomiting in Children *on page 2368*

Safe Handling of Hazardous Drugs *on page 2455*

Brand Names: US Clolar

Brand Names: Canada Clolar

Therapeutic Category Antineoplastic Agent, Antimetabolite; Antineoplastic Agent, Antimetabolite (Purine Antagonist)

Generic Availability (US) No

Use Treatment of relapsed or refractory acute lymphoblastic leukemia (ALL) after at least two prior treatment regimens (FDA approved in ages 1-21 years); has also been used for the treatment of acute myelogenous leukemia (AML)

Pregnancy Risk Factor D

Pregnancy Considerations Adverse events were observed in animal reproduction studies. May cause fetal harm if administered to a pregnant woman. Women of childbearing potential should be advised to use effective contraception and avoid becoming pregnant during therapy.

Breast-Feeding Considerations It is not known if clofarabine is excreted in breast milk. Due to the potential for serious adverse reactions in the nursing infant, breast-feeding should be avoided during clofarabine treatment.

Contraindications

There are no contraindications listed in the manufacturer's U.S. labeling.

Canadian labeling: Hypersensitivity to clofarabine or any component of the formulation; symptomatic CNS involvement; history of serious heart, liver, kidney, or pancreas disease; severe hepatic impairment (AST and/or ALT >5 x ULN, and/or bilirubin >3 x ULN); severe renal impairment (CrCl < 30 mL/minute)

Warnings/Precautions Hazardous agent - use appropriate precautions for handling and disposal (NIOSH 2014 [group 1]). Cytokine release syndrome (eg, tachypnea, tachycardia, hypotension, pulmonary edema) may develop into capillary leak syndrome, systemic inflammatory response syndrome (SIRS), and organ dysfunction; discontinue with signs/symptoms of SIRS or capillary leak syndrome (rapid onset respiratory distress, hypotension, pleural/pericardial effusion, and multiorgan failure) and consider supportive treatment with diuretics, corticosteroids, and/or albumin. Prophylactic corticosteroids may prevent or diminish the signs/symptoms of cytokine release. May require dosage reduction. Monitor blood pressure during 5 days of treatment; discontinue if hypotension develops. Monitor if on concurrent medications known to affect blood pressure. Dose-dependent, reversible myelosuppression (neutropenia, thrombocytopenia, and anemia) is common; may be severe and prolonged. Monitor blood counts and platelets. May be at increased risk for infection due to neutropenia; opportunistic infection or sepsis (may be severe or fatal), is increased due to prolonged neutropenia and immunocompromised state; monitor for signs and symptoms of infection and treat promptly if infection develops. May require therapy discontinuation. Serious and fatal hemorrhages (including cerebral, gastrointestinal, and pulmonary hemorrhage) have occurred, usually associated with thrombocytopenia. Monitor and manage coagulation parameters.

Serious and fatal cases of Stevens-Johnson syndrome (SJS) and toxic epidermal necrolysis (TEN) have been reported. Discontinue clofarabine for exfoliative or bullous rash, or if SJS or TEN are suspected. Clofarabine is associated with a moderate emetic potential; antiemetics are recommended to prevent nausea and vomiting (Basch, 2011; Dupuis, 2011; Roila, 2010). Serious and fatal enterocolitis (including neutropenic colitis, cecitis, and *C. difficile* colitis) has been reported, usually occurring within 30 days of treatment, and when used in combination with other chemotherapy. May lead to complication including necrosis, perforation, hemorrhage or sepsis. Monitor for signs/symptoms of enterocolitis and manage promptly.

Has not been studied in patients with hepatic impairment; use with caution (per manufacturer's labeling). Canadian labeling contraindicates use in severe impairment or in patients with a history of serious hepatic disease. Transaminases and bilirubin may be increased during treatment; transaminase elevations generally occur within 10 days of administration and persist for ≤15 days. In some cases, hepatotoxicity was severe and fatal. The risk for hepatotoxicity, including hepatic sinusoidal obstruction syndrome (SOS; formerly called veno-occlusive disease), is increased in patients who have previously undergone a hematopoietic stem cell transplant. Monitor liver function closely; may require therapy interruption or discontinuation; discontinue if SOS is suspected. Elevated creatinine, acute renal failure, and hematuria were observed in clinical studies. Monitor renal function closely; may require dosage reduction or therapy discontinuation. A pharmacokinetic study demonstrated that systemic exposure increases as creatinine clearance decreases (CrCl <60 mL/minute) (Bonate, 2011). Dosage reduction required for moderate renal impairment (CrCl 30-60 mL/minute); use with caution in patients with CrCl <30 mL/minute (has not been studied). Canadian labeling contraindicates use in severe impairment or in patients with a history of serious kidney disease. Minimize the use of drugs known to cause renal toxicity during the 5-day treatment period; avoid concomitant hepatotoxic medications. Tumor lysis syndrome/hyperuricemia may occur as a consequence of leukemia treatment, including treatment with clofarabine, usually occurring in the first treatment cycle. May lead to life-threatening acute renal failure; adequate hydration and prophylactic antihyperuricemic therapy throughout treatment will reduce the risk/effects of tumor lysis syndrome; monitor closely. Potentially significant drug-drug interactions may exist, requiring dose or frequency adjustment, additional monitoring, and/or selection of alternative therapy.

Adverse Reactions

Cardiovascular: Edema, flushing, hyper-/hypotension, pericardial effusion, tachycardia

Central nervous system: Agitation, anxiety, chills, drowsiness, fatigue, headache, irritability, lethargy, mental status changes, pain

Dermatologic: Cellulitis, erythema, palmar-plantar erythrodysesthesia, pruritic rash, pruritus, skin rash

Gastrointestinal: Abdominal pain, anorexia, diarrhea, gingival bleeding, mouth hemorrhage, mucosal inflammation, nausea, oral candidiasis, pancreatitis, pseudomembranous colitis, rectal pain, stomatitis, typhlitis, vomiting

Genitourinary: Hematuria

Hematologic & oncologic: Anemia, febrile neutropenia, leukopenia, lymphocytopenia, neutropenia, oral mucosal petechiae, petechia, thrombocytopenia, tumor lysis syndrome

Hepatic: Hyperbilirubinemia, increased bilirubin, increased serum ALT, increased serum AST, jaundice

Hypersensitivity: Hypersensitivity

Infection: Bacteremia, candidiasis, herpes simplex infection, herpes zoster, infection (includes bacterial, fungal, and viral), sepsis (including septic shock), sepsis syndrome, staphylococcal bacteremia, staphylococcal sepsis

Local: Catheter infection

Neuromuscular & skeletal: Arthralgia, back pain, limb pain, myalgia, ostealgia, weakness

Renal: Creatinine increased

Respiratory: Dyspnea, epistaxis, pleural effusion, pneumonia, pulmonary edema, respiratory distress, respiratory tract infection, tachypnea

Miscellaneous: Fever

Rare but important or life-threatening: Bone marrow failure, enterocolitis (occurs more frequently within 30 days of treatment and with combination chemotherapy), exfoliative dermatitis, gastrointestinal hemorrhage, hallucination (Jeha, 2006), hepatomegaly (Jeha, 2006), hypokalemia (Jeha, 2006), hyponatremia, hypophosphatemia, increased right ventricular pressure (Jeha, 2006), left ventricular systolic dysfunction (Jeha, 2006), major hemorrhage (including cerebral and pulmonary; majority of cases associated with thrombocytopenia), pancytopenia, Stevens-Johnson syndrome, syncope, toxic epidermal necrolysis

Drug Interactions

Metabolism/Transport Effects None known.

Avoid Concomitant Use

Avoid concomitant use of Clofarabine with any of the following: BCG; BCG (Intravesical); CloZAPine; Dipyrone; Natalizumab; Pimecrolimus; Tacrolimus (Topical); Tofacitinib; Vaccines (Live)

Increased Effect/Toxicity

Clofarabine may increase the levels/effects of: CloZAPine; Leflunomide; Natalizumab; Tofacitinib; Vaccines (Live)

The levels/effects of Clofarabine may be increased by: Denosumab; Dipyrone; Pimecrolimus; Roflumilast; Tacrolimus (Topical); Trastuzumab

Decreased Effect

Clofarabine may decrease the levels/effects of: BCG; BCG (Intravesical); Coccidioides immitis Skin Test; Sipuleucel-T; Vaccines (Inactivated); Vaccines (Live)

The levels/effects of Clofarabine may be decreased by: Echinacea

Storage/Stability Store intact vials at room temperature of 25°C (77°F); excursions permitted to 15°C to 30°C (59°F to 86°F). Solutions diluted for infusion in D_5W or NS may be stored for 24 hours at room temperature.

Mechanism of Action Clofarabine, a purine (deoxyadenosine) nucleoside analog, is metabolized to clofarabine 5'-triphosphate. Clofarabine 5'-triphosphate decreases cell replication and repair as well as causing cell death. To decrease cell replication and repair, clofarabine 5'-triphosphate competes with deoxyadenosine triphosphate for the enzymes ribonucleotide reductase and DNA polymerase. Cell replication is decreased when clofarabine 5'-triphosphate inhibits ribonucleotide reductase from reacting with deoxyadenosine triphosphate to produce deoxynucleotide triphosphate which is needed for DNA synthesis. Cell replication is also decreased when clofarabine 5'-triphosphate competes with DNA polymerase for incorporation into the DNA chain; when done during the repair process, cell repair is affected. To cause cell death, clofarabine 5'-triphosphate alters the mitochondrial membrane by releasing proteins, an inducing factor and cytochrome C.

Pharmacokinetics (Adult data unless noted)

Distribution: V_d: Decreased with increasing age, based on pharmacokinetic simulations: 5.8 L/kg (3 years old); 3.1 L/kg (30 years old); 2.7 L/kg (82 years old) (Bonate, 2011); Children and Adolescents 2-19 years: 172 L/m^2

Protein binding: Children and Adolescents 2-19 years: 47%, primarily to albumin

Metabolism: Intracellularly by deoxycytidine kinase and mono- and di-phosphokinases to active metabolite clofarabine 5'-triphosphate; limited hepatic metabolism (0.2%)

Children and Adolescents 2-19 years: 5.2 hours

Adults: 7 hours; half-life may be increased in patients with renal impairment (Bonate, 2011)

Elimination: Children and Adolescents 2-19 years: 49% to 60% excreted in urine as unchanged drug

Dosing: Usual Dosing and frequency may vary by protocol and/or treatment phase; refer to specific protocol.

Note: Consider prophylactic corticosteroids (hydrocortisone 100 mg/m^2 on days 1-3) to prevent signs/symptoms of capillary leak syndrome or systemic inflammatory response syndrome (SIRS); provide IV hydration, antihyperuricemic agent, and alkalinize urine (to reduce the risk of tumor lysis syndrome/hyperuricemia); consider prophylactic antiemetics.

Pediatric:

Acute lymphocytic leukemia (ALL), relapsed or refractory:

Monotherapy: Children and Adolescents: IV infusion: 52 mg/m^2/day once daily for days 1-5 of each cycle; repeat cycle every 2-6 weeks following recovery or return to baseline organ function; subsequent cycles should begin no sooner than 14 days from the start of the previous cycle and when ANC ≥750/mm^3

Combination therapy: Limited data available: IV Infusion:

Infants: Dosing regimens variable with very limited data available:

Weight-directed dosing: 1.33 mg/kg/day for 5 days in combination with cyclophosphamide and etoposide (O'Connor, 2011)

BSA-directed dosing: 40 mg/m^2/day for 5 days in combination with cyclophosphamide and etoposide (Inaba, 2012); and with topotecan, vinorelbine, thiotepa (TVTC regimen), and dexamethasone in a Phase I trial (Steinherz, 2010)

Children and Adolescents: Usual dose: 40 mg/m^2/day for 5 days in combination with cyclophosphamide and etoposide has been most frequently studied (Hijiya, 2011; Hijiya, 2012; Inaba, 2012; Locatelli, 2009; O'Connor, 2011); and with topotecan, vinorelbine, thiotepa (TVTC regimen), and dexamethasone in a Phase I trial (Steinherz, 2010). In one trial, the protocol included 5 days of clofarabine therapy during induction and 4 days of therapy for consolidation; this study was also amended to exclude patients with prior hematopoietic stem cell transplantation due to a high incidence of veno-occlusive disease (Hijiya, 2011).

Acute myeloid leukemia (AML), relapsed or refractory: Limited data available: Children and Adolescents: IV infusion:

Monotherapy: 52 mg/m^2/day once daily for days 1-5 of each cycle; repeat cycle every 2-6 weeks for up to 12 cycles following recovery or return to baseline organ function; subsequent cycles should begin no sooner than 14 days from the start of the previous cycle and when ANC ≥750/mm^3; the trial did not have minimum exclusion age (patient age ≤21 years at time of diagnosis); the youngest patient was 2 years of age (Jeha, 2009)

Combination therapy: 40 mg/m^2/day once daily for days 1-5 of each cycle in combination with cyclophosphamide and etoposide (Inaba, 2012)

Adults ≤21 years: **Acute lymphocytic leukemia (ALL), relapsed or refractory:** IV infusion: 52 mg/m^2/day once daily for days 1-5 of each cycle; repeat cycle every 2-6 weeks following recovery or return to baseline organ function; subsequent cycles should begin no sooner than 14 days from the start of the previous cycle and when ANC ≥750/mm^3

Dosing adjustment for toxicity: Children, Adolescents, and Adults ≤21 years:

Hematologic toxicity: ANC <500/mm^3 lasting ≥4 weeks: Reduce clofarabine dose by 25% for next cycle

Nonhematologic toxicity:

Clinically significant infection: Withhold treatment until infection is under control, then restart clofarabine at full dose

Grade 3 toxicity, excluding infection, nausea, and vomiting, and transient elevations in transaminases and bilirubin: Withhold treatment; may reinitiate clofarabine with a 25% dose reduction with resolution or return to baseline

Grade ≥3 increase in creatinine or bilirubin: Discontinue clofarabine; may reinitiate with 25% dosage reduction when creatinine or bilirubin return to baseline and patient is stable; administer allopurinol for hyperuricemia

Grade 4 toxicity (noninfectious): Discontinue clofarabine treatment

Capillary leak or systemic inflammatory response syndrome (SIRS) early signs/symptoms (eg, hypotension, tachycardia, tachypnea, pulmonary edema): Discontinue clofarabine; institute supportive measures. May consider reinitiating with a 25% dose-reduction after patient is stable and after organ function recovers to baseline.

Dosing adjustment for renal impairment: Children, Adolescents, and Adults ≤21 years:

CrCl >60 mL/minute: No dosage adjustment recommended

CrCl 30-60 mL/minute: Reduce dose by 50%

CrCl <30 mL/minute: There are no dosage adjustments provided in the manufacturer's labeling; use with caution (has not been studied).

Dosing adjustment for hepatic impairment: There are no dosage adjustments provided in the manufacturer's labeling.

Preparation for Administration Hazardous agent; use appropriate precautions for handling and disposal (NIOSH 2014 [group 1]).

Parenteral: IV infusion: Filter clofarabine through a 0.2 micron syringe filter prior to dilution, and further dilute dose with D_5W or NS to a final concentration of 0.15 to 0.4 mg/mL

Administration Hazardous agent; use appropriate precautions for handling and disposal (NIOSH 2014 [group 1]).

Parenteral: IV infusion: Administer by IV infusion over 2 hours per the manufacturer's labeling and in most trials; a few trials have infused over 1 hour (Federl 2005; Jeha 2004; Kantarian 2003). An inline filter is not needed for administration. Do not administer with any other medications through the same intravenous line.

Monitoring Parameters CBC with differential and platelets (daily during treatment, then 1-2 times weekly or as necessary); liver and kidney function (during 5 days of clofarabine administration); blood pressure, cardiac function, and respiratory status during infusion; signs and symptoms of tumor lysis syndrome, infection, and cytokine release syndrome (tachypnea, tachycardia, hypotension, pulmonary edema); hydration status

Dosage Forms Excipient information presented when available (limited, particularly for generics); consult specific product labeling.

Solution, Intravenous [preservative free]:

Clolar: 1 mg/mL (20 mL)

◆ **Clofarex** *see* Clofarabine *on page 500*

◆ **Clolar** *see* Clofarabine *on page 500*

ClomiPRAMINE (kloe MI pra meen)

Medication Safety Issues

Sound-alike/look-alike issues:

ClomiPRAMINE may be confused with chlorproMAZINE, clevidipine, clomiPHENE, desipramine, Norpramin®

Anafranil may be confused with alfentanil, enalapril, nafarelin

BEERS Criteria medication:

This drug may be potentially inappropriate for use in geriatric patients (Quality of evidence - high [moderate for SIADH]; Strength of recommendation - strong).

Related Information

Antidepressant Agents *on page* 2257

Brand Names: US Anafranil

Brand Names: Canada Anafranil®; Apo-Clomipramine®; CO Clomipramine; Dom-Clomipramine; Novo-Clomipramine

Therapeutic Category Antidepressant, Tricyclic (Tertiary Amine)

Generic Availability (US) Yes

Use Treatment of obsessive-compulsive disorder (OCD) (FDA approved in ages ≥10 years and adults)

Medication Guide Available Yes

Pregnancy Risk Factor C

Pregnancy Considerations Adverse events were observed in some animal reproduction studies. Clomipramine and its metabolite desmethylclomipramine cross the placenta and can be detected in cord blood and neonatal serum at birth (Loughhead, 2006; ter Horst, 2011). Data from five newborns found the half-life for clomipramine in the neonate to be 42 ± 16 hours following *in utero* exposure. Serum concentrations were not found to correlate to withdrawal symptoms (ter Horst, 2011). Withdrawal symptoms (including jitteriness, tremor, and seizures) have been observed in neonates whose mothers took clomipramine up to delivery.

The ACOG recommends that therapy for depression during pregnancy be individualized; treatment should incorporate the clinical expertise of the mental health clinician, obstetrician, primary healthcare provider, and pediatrician (ACOG, 2008). According to the American Psychiatric Association (APA), the risks of medication treatment should be weighed against other treatment options and untreated depression. For women who discontinue antidepressant medications during pregnancy and who may be at high risk for postpartum depression, the medications can be restarted following delivery (APA, 2010). Treatment algorithms have been developed by the ACOG and the APA for the management of depression in women prior to conception and during pregnancy (Yonkers, 2009).

Breast-Feeding Considerations Clomipramine is excreted in breast milk. Based on information from three mother-infant pairs, following maternal use of clomipramine 75-150 mg/day, the estimated exposure to the breast-feeding infant would be 0.4% to 4% of the weight-adjusted maternal dose. Adverse events have not been reported in nursing infants (information from seven cases). Infants should be monitored for signs of adverse events; routine monitoring of infant serum concentrations is not recommended (Fortinguerra, 2009). Due to the potential for serious adverse reactions in the nursing infant, the decision to continue or discontinue breast-feeding during therapy should take into account the risk of exposure to the infant and the benefits of treatment to the mother.

Contraindications Hypersensitivity to clomipramine, other tricyclic agents, or any component of the formulation; use of MAO inhibitors intended to treat psychiatric disorders (concurrently or within 14 days of discontinuing either clomipramine or the MAO inhibitor); initiation of clomipramine in a patient receiving linezolid or intravenous methylene blue; use in a patient during the acute recovery phase of MI

Warnings/Precautions **[U.S. Boxed Warning]: Antidepressants increase the risk of suicidal thinking and behavior in children, adolescents, and young adults (18 to 24 years of age) with major depressive disorder (MDD) and other psychiatric disorders;** consider risk prior to prescribing. Short-term studies did not show an increased risk in patients >24 years of age and showed a decreased risk in patients ≥65 years. Closely monitor patients for clinical worsening, suicidality, or unusual changes in behavior, particularly during the initial 1 to 2 months of therapy or during periods of dosage adjustments (increases or decreases); the patient's family or caregiver should be instructed to closely observe the patient and communicate condition with health care provider. A medication guide should be dispensed with each prescription. **Clomipramine is FDA approved for the treatment of OCD in children ≥10 years of age.**

The possibility of a suicide attempt is inherent in major depression and may persist until remission occurs. Use caution in high-risk patients. Worsening depression and severe abrupt suicidality that are not part of the presenting symptoms may require discontinuation or modification of drug therapy. The patient's family or caregiver should be alerted to monitor patients for the emergence of suicidality and associated behaviors (such as agitation, irritability, hostility, impulsivity, and hypomania) and notify the healthcare provider.

May worsen psychosis in some patients or precipitate a shift to mania or hypomania in patients with bipolar disorder. Patients presenting with depressive symptoms should be screened for bipolar disorder. Monotherapy in patients with bipolar disorder should be avoided. **Clomipramine is not FDA approved for bipolar depression.**

Potentially life-threatening serotonin syndrome (SS) has occurred with serotonergic agents (eg, SSRIs, SNRIs), particularly when used in combination with other serotonergic agents (eg, triptans, TCAs, fentanyl, lithium, tramadol, buspirone, St John's wort, tryptophan) or agents that impair metabolism of serotonin (eg, MAO inhibitors intended to treat psychiatric disorders, other MAO inhibitors [ie, linezolid and intravenous methylene blue]). Discontinue treatment (and any concomitant serotonergic agent) immediately if signs/symptoms arise. TCAs may rarely cause bone marrow suppression; monitor for any signs of infection and obtain CBC if symptoms (eg, fever, sore throat) evident. May cause seizures (relationship to dose and/or duration of therapy) - do not exceed maximum doses. Use caution in patients with a previous seizure disorder or condition predisposing to seizures such as brain damage, alcoholism, or concurrent therapy with other drugs which lower the seizure threshold. May increase the risks associated with electroconvulsive therapy. Bone fractures have been associated with antidepressant treatment. Consider the possibility of a fragility fracture if an antidepressant-treated patient presents with unexplained bone pain, point tenderness, swelling, or bruising (Rabenda, 2013; Rizzoli, 2012). Use with caution in patients with tumors of the adrenal medulla (eg, pheochromocytoma, neuroblastoma); may cause hypertensive crises. Has been associated with a high incidence of sexual dysfunction. Weight gain may occur.

May cause CNS depression, which may impair physical or mental abilities; patients must be cautioned about performing tasks that require mental alertness (eg, operating machinery or driving). The degree of sedation, anticholinergic effects, and conduction abnormalities are high relative to other antidepressants. The risk of orthostasis is moderate to high relative to other antidepressants. Use with caution in patients with a history of cardiovascular disease (including previous MI, stroke, tachycardia, or conduction abnormalities). Use with caution in patients with urinary retention, benign prostatic hyperplasia, narrow-angle glaucoma, xerostomia, visual problems, constipation, or a history of bowel obstruction. Potentially significant drug-drug interactions may exist, requiring dose or frequency adjustment, additional monitoring, and/or selection of alternative therapy.

Recommended by the manufacturer to discontinue prior to elective surgery; risks exist for drug interactions with anesthesia and for cardiac arrhythmias. However, definitive drug interactions have not been widely reported in the literature and continuation of tricyclic antidepressants is generally recommended as long as precautions are taken to reduce the significance of any adverse events that may occur (Pass, 2004). Use with caution in patients with hepatic impairment; increases in ALT/AST have occurred, including rare reports of severe hepatic injury (some fatal); monitor hepatic transaminases periodically in patients with hepatic impairment. Use with caution in patients with renal dysfunction. Avoid use in the elderly due to its potent anticholinergic and sedative properties, and potential to cause orthostatic hypotension. In addition, may also cause or exacerbate syndrome of inappropriate antidiuretic hormone secretion or hyponatremia; monitor sodium closely with initiation or dosage adjustments in older adults (Beers Criteria). May cause mild pupillary dilation which in susceptible individuals can lead to an episode of narrow-angle glaucoma. Consider evaluating patients who have not had an iridectomy for narrow-angle glaucoma risk factors.

Abrupt discontinuation or interruption of antidepressant therapy has been associated with a discontinuation syndrome. Symptoms arising may vary with antidepressant however commonly include nausea, vomiting, diarrhea, headaches, light-headedness, dizziness, diminished appetite, sweating, chills, tremors, paresthesias, fatigue, somnolence, and sleep disturbances (eg, vivid dreams, insomnia). Greater risks for developing a discontinuation syndrome have been associated with antidepressants with shorter half-lives, longer durations of treatment, and abrupt discontinuation. For antidepressants of short or intermediate half-lives, symptoms may emerge within 2-5 days after treatment discontinuation and last 7-14 days (APA, 2010; Fava, 2006; Haddad, 2001; Shelton, 2001; Warner, 2006).

Warnings: Additional Pediatric Considerations Vomiting is two- to threefold more prevalent in children compared to adolescents and is more prevalent in adolescents compared to adults; to help minimize, divide the dose and give with food initially. Once titrated to maintenance therapy, can consolidate to once daily dosing at bedtime.

Adverse Reactions

Cardiovascular: Chest pain (children & adolescents), ECG abnormality, flushing, orthostatic hypotension, palpitations, syncope (children & adolescents), tachycardia

Central nervous system: Abnormal dreams (adults), abnormality in thinking, aggressive behavior (children & adolescents), agitation (adults), anxiety (more common in adults), chills (adults), confusion (more common in adults), depersonalization, depression (adults), dizziness (more common in adults), drowsiness, emotional lability (adults), fatigue, headache (adults), hypertonia, insomnia (more common in adults), irritability (children & adolescents), lack of concentration (adults), memory impairment, migraine (adults), myasthenia, myoclonus (more common in adults), nervousness (more common in adults), pain, panic attack, paresis (children & adolescents), paresthesia (adults), psychosomatic disorder (adults), sleep disorder, speech disturbance (adults), twitching (adults), vertigo, yawning (adults)

Dermatologic: Body odor (children & adolescents), dermatitis (adults), diaphoresis (more common in adults), pruritus (adults), skin rash, urticaria (adults), xeroderma (adults)

Endocrine & metabolic: Amenorrhea (adults), change in libido (adults), hot flash, menstrual disease (adults), weight gain (more common in adults), weight loss (children & adolescents)

Gastrointestinal: Abdominal pain (adults), anorexia, aphthous stomatitis (children & adolescents), constipation (more common in adults), diarrhea, dysgeusia, dyspepsia, dysphagia (adults), esophagitis (adults), flatulence (adults), gastrointestinal disease (adults), halitosis (children & adolescents), increased appetite (adults), nausea (adults), vomiting, xerostomia (more common in adults)

Genitourinary: Breast hypertrophy (adults), cystitis (adults), difficulty in micturition (more common in adults), ejaculation failure (more common in adults), impotence (adults), lactation (nonpuerperal; adults), leukorrhea (adults), mastalgia (adults), urinary frequency (adults), urinary retention (more common in children & adolescents), urinary tract infection (adults), vaginitis (adults)

Hematologic & oncologic: Purpura (adults)

Hepatic: Increased serum ALT (>3 x ULN), increased serum AST (>3 x ULN)

Hypersensitivity: Hypersensitivity reaction (children & adolescents)

Neuromuscular & skeletal: Myalgia (adults), tremor (more common in adults), weakness (more common in children & adolescents)

Ophthalmic: Abnormal lacrimation (adults), anisocoria (children & adolescents), blepharospasm (children & adolescents), conjunctivitis (adults), mydriasis (adults), ocular allergy (children & adolescents), visual disturbance (more common in adults)

Otic: Tinnitus

Respiratory: Bronchospasm (more common in children & adolescents), dyspnea (children & adolescents), epistaxis (adults), laryngitis (children & adolescents), pharyngitis (adults), rhinitis (adults), sinusitis (adults)

Miscellaneous: Fever (adults)

Rare but important or life-threatening: Abnormal electroencephalogram, accommodation disturbance, agranulocytosis, albuminuria, alopecia, anemia, aneurysm, angle-closure glaucoma, anticholinergic syndrome, aphasia, apraxia, ataxia, atrial flutter, blepharitis, bloody stools, bone marrow depression, bradycardia, brain disease, breast fibroadenosis, bronchitis, bundle branch block, cardiac arrest, cardiac arrhythmia, cardiac failure, catalepsy, cellulitis, cerebral hemorrhage, cervical dysplasia, cheilitis, chloasma, cholinergic syndrome, choreoathetosis, chromatopsia, chronic enteritis, colitis, coma, conjunctival hemorrhage, cyanosis, deafness, dehydration, delirium, delusions, dental caries, dermal ulcer, diabetes mellitus, diplopia, duodenitis, dyskinesia, dystonia, edema, edema (oral), endometrial hyperplasia, endometriosis, enlargement of salivary glands, epididymitis, erythematous rash, exophthalmos, exostosis, extrapyramidal reaction, extrasystoles, gastric dilation, gastric ulcer, gastroesophageal reflux disease, glycosuria, goiter, gout, gynecomastia, hallucination, heart block, hematuria, hemiparesis, hemoptysis, hepatic injury (severe), hepatitis, hostility, hyperacusis, hypercholesterolemia, hyperesthesia, hyperglycemia, hyperkinesia, hyperreflexia, hyperthermia, hyperthyroidism, hyperuricemia, hyperventilation, hypnogenic hallucinations, hypoesthesia, hypokalemia, hypokinesia, hypothyroidism, hypoventilation, intestinal obstruction, irritable bowel syndrome, ischemic heart disease, keratitis, laryngismus, leukemoid reaction, leukopenia, lupus erythematous-like rash, lymphadenopathy, maculopapular rash, manic reaction, muscle spasm, mutism, myocardial infarction, myopathy, myositis, nephrolithiasis, neuralgia, neuropathy, nocturnal amblyopia, oculogyric crisis, oculomotor nerve paralysis, ovarian cyst, pancytopenia, paralytic ileus, paranoia, peptic ulcer, periarteritis nodosa, peripheral ischemia, pharyngeal edema, phobia, photophobia, pneumonia, premature ejaculation, pseudolymphoma, psoriasis, psychosis, pyelonephritis, pyuria, rectal hemorrhage, renal cyst, schizophrenic reaction, scleritis, seizure, sensory disturbance, serotonin syndrome, skin hypertrophy, skin photosensitivity, somnambulism, strabismus, stupor, suicidal ideation, thrombocytopenia, thrombophlebitis, tongue ulcer, torticollis, urinary incontinence, uterine hemorrhage, uterine inflammation, vaginal hemorrhage, vasospasm, ventricular tachycardia, visual field defect, voice disorder, withdrawal syndrome

Drug Interactions

Metabolism/Transport Effects Substrate of CYP1A2 (major), CYP2C19 (major), CYP2D6 (major), CYP3A4 (minor); **Note:** Assignment of Major/Minor substrate status based on clinically relevant drug interaction potential; **Inhibits** CYP2D6 (moderate)

Avoid Concomitant Use

Avoid concomitant use of ClomiPRAMINE with any of the following: Aclidinium; Azelastine (Nasal); Dapoxetine; Eluxadoline; Glucagon; Iobenguane I 123; Ipratropium (Oral Inhalation); Linezolid; MAO Inhibitors; Methylene Blue; Moxonidine; Orphenadrine; Paraldehyde; Potassium Chloride; Thalidomide; Thioridazine; Tiotropium; Umeclidinium

Increased Effect/Toxicity

ClomiPRAMINE may increase the levels/effects of: AbobotulinumtoxinA; Alcohol (Ethyl); Alpha-/Beta-Agonists (Direct-Acting); Alpha1-Agonists; Amphetamines; Analgesics (Opioid); Anticholinergic Agents; Antipsychotic Agents; ARIPiprazole; Aspirin; Azelastine (Nasal); Beta2-Agonists; Buprenorphine; Citalopram; CNS Depressants; CYP2D6 Substrates; Desmopressin; DOXOrubicin (Conventional); Eliglustat; Eluxadoline; Escitalopram; Fesoterodine; Glucagon; Highest Risk QTc-Prolonging Agents; Hydrocodone; Methotrimeprazine; Methylene Blue; Metoprolol; Metyrosine; Milnacipran; Mirabegron; Moderate Risk QTc-Prolonging Agents; Nebivolol; Nicorandil; NSAID (COX-2 Inhibitor); NSAID (Nonselective); OnabotulinumtoxinA; Orphenadrine; Paraldehyde; Potassium Chloride; Pramipexole; QuiNIDine; RimabotulinumtoxinB; ROPINIRole; Rotigotine; Serotonin Modulators; Sodium Phosphates; Sulfonylureas; Suvorexant; Thalidomide; Thiazide Diuretics; Thioridazine; Tiotropium; Topiramate; TraMADol; Vitamin K Antagonists; Yohimbine; Zolpidem

The levels/effects of ClomiPRAMINE may be increased by: Abiraterone Acetate; Aclidinium; Altretamine; Antiemetics (5HT3 Antagonists); Antipsychotic Agents; Brimonidine (Topical); BuPROPion; Cannabis; CarBAMazepine; Cimetidine; Cinacalcet; Citalopram; Cobicistat; CYP1A2 Inhibitors (Moderate); CYP1A2 Inhibitors (Strong); CYP2C19 Inhibitors (Moderate); CYP2C19 Inhibitors (Strong); CYP2D6 Inhibitors (Moderate); CYP2D6 Inhibitors (Strong); Dapoxetine; Darunavir; Deferasirox; Dexmethylphenidate; Doxylamine; Dronabinol; Droperidol; DULoxetine; Escitalopram; FLUoxetine; FluvoxaMINE; Grapefruit Juice; HydrOXYzine; Ipratropium (Oral Inhalation); Kava Kava; Linezolid; Lithium; Luliconazole; Magnesium Sulfate; MAO Inhibitors; Methotrimeprazine; Methylphenidate; Metoclopramide; Metyrosine; Mianserin; Mifepristone; Nabilone; Panobinostat; PARoxetine; Peginterferon Alfa-2b; Perampanel; Pramlintide; Propafenone; Protease Inhibitors; QuiNIDine; Rufinamide; Sertraline; Sodium Oxybate; Tapentadol; Tedizolid; Terbinafine (Systemic); Tetrahydrocannabinol; Thyroid Products; TraMADol; Umeclidinium; Valproic Acid and Derivatives; Vemurafenib

Decreased Effect

ClomiPRAMINE may decrease the levels/effects of: Acetylcholinesterase Inhibitors; Alpha1-Agonists; Alpha2-Agonists; Alpha2-Agonists (Ophthalmic); Codeine; Iobenguane I 123; Itopride; Moxonidine; Secretin; Tamoxifen

The levels/effects of ClomiPRAMINE may be decreased by: Acetylcholinesterase Inhibitors; Barbiturates; Cannabis; CYP1A2 Inducers (Strong); CYP2C19 Inducers (Strong); Cyproterone; Dabrafenib; Peginterferon Alfa-2b; St Johns Wort; Teriflunomide

Food Interactions Serum concentrations/toxicity may be increased by grapefruit juice. Management: Avoid grapefruit juice.

Storage/Stability Store at controlled room temperature at 20°C to 25°C (68°F to 77°F).

Mechanism of Action Clomipramine appears to affect serotonin uptake while its active metabolite, desmethylclomipramine, affects norepinephrine uptake

Pharmacodynamics

Onset of action: 1-2 weeks

Maximum effect: 8-12 weeks

Duration: 1-2 days

Pharmacokinetics (Adult data unless noted)

Absorption: Rapid

Distribution: Distributes into CSF, brain, and breast milk; active metabolite (desmethylclomipramine) also distributes into CSF with average CSF to plasma ratio: 2.6

Protein binding: 97%; primarily to albumin

Metabolism: Hepatic to desmethylclomipramine (DMI; active) and other metabolites; extensive first-pass effect; metabolites undergo glucuronide conjugation; metabolism of clomipramine and DMI may be capacity limited (ie, may display nonlinear pharmacokinetics); with multiple dosing, plasma concentrations of DMI are greater than clomipramine

Half-life: Adults (following a 150 mg dose): Clomipramine 19-37 hours (mean: 32 hours); DMI: 54-77 hours (mean: 69 hours)

Elimination: 50% to 60% of dose is excreted in the urine and 24% to 32% in feces; only 0.8% to 1.3% is excreted in urine as parent drug and active metabolite (combined amount)

Dosing: Usual Note: During initial dose titration, divide the dose and give with meals to minimize nausea and vomiting. During maintenance therapy, may administer total daily dose once daily at bedtime to minimize daytime sedation.

Children: **Note:** Controlled clinical trials have not shown tricyclic antidepressants to be superior to placebo for the treatment of depression in children and adolescents (Dopheide, 2006; Wagner, 2005).

<10 years: Safety and efficacy have not been established; specific recommendations cannot be made for use in this age group

≥10 years: OCD: Initial: 25 mg/day; gradually increase, as tolerated, to a maximum of 3 mg/kg/day or 100 mg/day (whichever is smaller) during the first 2 weeks; may then gradually increase, if needed, over the next several weeks to a maximum of 3 mg/kg/day or 200 mg/day (whichever is smaller)

Adults: OCD: Initial: 25 mg/day; gradually increase, as tolerated, to 100 mg/day during the first 2 weeks; may then gradually increase, if needed, over the next several weeks to a total of 250 mg/day maximum

Administration Oral: May administer with food to decrease GI upset.

Monitoring Parameters Monitor patient periodically for symptom resolution; monitor for worsening depression, suicidality, and associated behaviors (especially at the beginning of therapy or when doses are increased or decreased).

Monitor weight, pulse rate and blood pressure prior to and during therapy; ECG and cardiac status in patients with cardiac disease; periodic liver enzymes in patients with liver disease; CBC with differential in patients who develop fever and sore throat during treatment.

Test Interactions Increased glucose; may interfere with urine detection of methadone (false-positive)

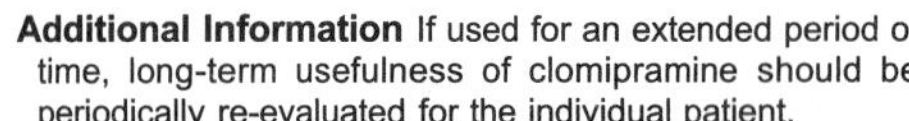

Additional Information If used for an extended period of time, long-term usefulness of clomipramine should be periodically re-evaluated for the individual patient.

Dosage Forms Excipient information presented when available (limited, particularly for generics); consult specific product labeling.

Capsule, Oral, as hydrochloride:
- Anafranil: 25 mg, 50 mg, 75 mg
- Generic: 25 mg, 50 mg, 75 mg

◆ **Clomipramine Hydrochloride** *see* ClomiPRAMINE *on page 502*

◆ **Clonapam (Can)** *see* ClonazePAM *on page 506*

ClonazePAM (kloe NA ze pam)

Medication Safety Issues

Sound-alike/look-alike issues:

ClonazePAM may be confused with cloBAZam, cloNIDine, clorazepate, cloZAPine, LORazepam

KlonoPIN may be confused with cloNIDine, clorazepate, cloZAPine, LORazepam

BEERS Criteria medication:

This drug may be potentially inappropriate for use in geriatric patients (Quality of evidence - high; Strength of recommendation - strong).

Related Information

Safe Handling of Hazardous Drugs *on page 2455*

Brand Names: US KlonoPIN

Brand Names: Canada Apo-Clonazepam; Clonapam; Clonazepam-R; CO Clonazepam; Dom-Clonazepam; Dom-Clonazepam-R; Mylan-Clonazepam; PHL-Clonazepam; PHL-Clonazepam-R; PMS-Clonazepam; PMS-Clonazepam-R; PRO-Clonazepam; ratio-Clonazepam; Riva-Clonazepam; Rivotril; Sandoz-Clonazepam; Teva-Clonazepam; ZYM-Clonazepam

Therapeutic Category Anticonvulsant, Benzodiazepine; Benzodiazepine

Generic Availability (US) Yes

Use Alone or as an adjunct in the treatment of absence (petit mal), petit mal variant (Lennox-Gastaut), infantile spasms, akinetic, and myoclonic seizures; panic disorder with or without agoraphobia

Medication Guide Available Yes

Pregnancy Risk Factor D

Pregnancy Considerations Adverse events have been observed in some animal reproduction studies. Clonazepam crosses the placenta. Teratogenic effects have been observed with some benzodiazepines; however, additional studies are needed. The incidence of premature birth and low birth weights may be increased following maternal use of benzodiazepines; hypoglycemia and respiratory problems in the neonate may occur following exposure late in pregnancy. Neonatal withdrawal symptoms may occur within days to weeks after birth and "floppy infant syndrome" (which also includes withdrawal symptoms) has been reported with some benzodiazepines, including clonazepam (Bergman 1992; Iqbal 2002; Wikner 2007). A combination of factors influences the potential teratogenicity of anticonvulsant therapy. When treating women with epilepsy, monotherapy with the lowest effective dose and avoidance medications known to have a high incidence of teratogenic effects is recommended (Harden 2009; Wlodarczyk 2012).

Patients exposed to clonazepam during pregnancy are encouraged to enroll themselves into the AED Pregnancy Registry by calling 1-888-233-2334. Additional information is available at www.aedpregnancyregistry.org.

Breast-Feeding Considerations Clonazepam is excreted in breast milk. Drowsiness, lethargy, or weight loss in nursing infants have been observed in case reports following maternal use of some benzodiazepines (Iqbal 2002). Breast-feeding is not recommended by the manufacturer.

Contraindications Hypersensitivity to clonazepam, other benzodiazepines, or any component of the formulation; significant liver disease; acute narrow-angle glaucoma

Warnings/Precautions Pooled analysis of trials involving various antiepileptics (regardless of indication) showed an increased risk of suicidal thoughts/behavior (incidence rate: 0.43% treated patients compared to 0.24% of patients receiving placebo); risk observed as early as 1 week after initiation and continued through duration of trials (most trials ≤24 weeks). Monitor all patients for notable changes in behavior that might indicate suicidal thoughts or depression; notify healthcare provider immediately if symptoms occur. Use caution in patients with depression, particularly if suicidal risk may be present.

Benzodiazepines have been associated with anterograde amnesia (Nelson 1999). May cause CNS depression, which may impair physical or mental abilities; patients must be cautioned about performing tasks which require mental alertness (eg, operating machinery or driving Paradoxical reactions, including hyperactive or aggressive behavior, have been reported with benzodiazepines, particularly in adolescent/pediatric or psychiatric patients (Mancuso 2004). Clonazepam may cause respiratory depression and may produce an increase in salivation; use with caution in patients with respiratory disease and in patients who have difficulty handling secretions. May be used in patients with open angle glaucoma who are receiving appropriate therapy; contraindicated in acute narrow angle glaucoma. Use with caution in patients with a history of drug abuse or acute alcoholism; potential for drug dependency exists. Tolerance, psychological and physical dependence may occur with prolonged use. Use with caution in patients with hepatic impairment; accumulation likely to occur. Contraindicated in patients with significant hepatic impairment. Use with caution in patients with renal impairment; clonazepam metabolites are renally eliminated. Use with caution in debilitated patients. Use with extreme caution in patients who are at risk of falls; benzodiazepines have been associated with falls and traumatic injury. In older adults, benzodiazepines increase the risk of impaired cognition, delirium, falls, fractures, and motor vehicle accidents. Due to increased sensitivity in this age group and slower metabolism of long-acting agents (such as clonazepam), avoid use for treatment of insomnia, agitation, or delirium (Beers Criteria).

Does not have analgesic, antidepressant, or antipsychotic properties. Worsening of seizures may occur when added to patients with multiple seizure types. Periodically reevaluate the long-term usefulness of clonazepam for the individual patient. Clonazepam is a long half-life benzodiazepine. Duration of action after a single dose is determined by redistribution rather than metabolism. Tolerance develops to the anticonvulsant effects. It does not develop to the anxiolytic effects (Vinkers 2012). Chronic use of this agent may increase the perioperative benzodiazepine dose needed to achieve desired effect. Rebound or withdrawal symptoms may occur following abrupt discontinuation or large decreases in dose. Use caution when reducing dose or withdrawing therapy; decrease slowly and monitor for withdrawal symptoms. Flumazenil may cause withdrawal in patients receiving long-term benzodiazepine therapy (Brogden 1988). Potentially significant drug-drug interactions may exist, requiring dose or frequency adjustment, additional monitoring, and/or selection of alternative therapy. Use appropriate precautions for handling and disposal (NIOSH 2014 [group 3]).

Adverse Reactions Reactions reported in patients with seizure and/or panic disorder.

Cardiovascular: Edema (ankle or facial), palpitation

Central nervous system: Amnesia, ataxia, behavior problems, coma, confusion, coordination impaired, depression, dizziness, drowsiness, emotional lability, fatigue, fever, hallucinations, headache, hysteria, insomnia, intellectual ability reduced, memory disturbance, nervousness; paradoxical reactions (including aggressive behavior, agitation, anxiety, excitability, hostility, irritability, nervousness, nightmares, sleep disturbance, vivid dreams); psychosis, slurred speech, somnolence, vertigo

Dermatologic: Hair loss, hirsutism, skin rash

Endocrine & metabolic: Dysmenorrhea, libido increased/decreased

Gastrointestinal: Abdominal pain, anorexia, appetite increased/decreased, coated tongue, constipation, dehydration, diarrhea, encopresis, gastritis, gum soreness, nausea, weight changes (loss/gain), xerostomia

Genitourinary: Colpitis, dysuria, ejaculation delayed, enuresis, impotence, micturition frequency, nocturia, urinary retention, urinary tract infection

Hematologic: Anemia, eosinophilia, leukopenia, thrombocytopenia

Hepatic: Alkaline phosphatase increased (transient), hepatomegaly, transaminases increased (transient)

Neuromuscular & skeletal: Choreiform movements, coordination abnormal, dysarthria, hypotonia, muscle pain, muscle weakness, myalgia, tremor

Ocular: Blurred vision, eye movements abnormal, diplopia, nystagmus

Respiratory: Bronchitis, chest congestion, cough, hypersecretions, pharyngitis, respiratory depression, respiratory tract infection, rhinitis, rhinorrhea, shortness of breath, sinusitis

Miscellaneous: Allergic reaction, aphonia, dysdiadochokinesis, "glassy-eyed" appearance, hemiparesis, flu-like syndrome, lymphadenopathy

Rare but important or life-threatening: Apathy, burning skin, chest pain, depersonalization, dyspnea, excessive dreaming, hyperactivity, hypoesthesia, hypotension postural, infection, migraine, organic disinhibition, pain, paresthesia, paresis, periorbital edema, polyuria, suicidal attempt, suicide ideation, thick tongue, twitching, visual disturbance, xerophthalmia

Drug Interactions

Metabolism/Transport Effects Substrate of CYP3A4 (major); **Note:** Assignment of Major/Minor substrate status based on clinically relevant drug interaction potential

Avoid Concomitant Use

Avoid concomitant use of ClonazePAM with any of the following: Azelastine (Nasal); Conivaptan; Fusidic Acid (Systemic); Idelalisib; Methadone; OLANZapine; Orphenadrine; Paraldehyde; Sodium Oxybate; Thalidomide

Increased Effect/Toxicity

ClonazePAM may increase the levels/effects of: Alcohol (Ethyl); Azelastine (Nasal); Buprenorphine; CloZAPine; CNS Depressants; Hydrocodone; Methadone; Methotrimeprazine; Metyrosine; Mirtazapine; Orphenadrine; Paraldehyde; Pramipexole; ROPINIRole; Rotigotine; Selective Serotonin Reuptake Inhibitors; Sodium Oxybate; Suvorexant; Thalidomide; Zolpidem

The levels/effects of ClonazePAM may be increased by: Aprepitant; Brimonidine (Topical); Cannabis; Cobicistat; Conivaptan; Cosyntropin; CYP3A4 Inhibitors (Moderate); CYP3A4 Inhibitors (Strong); Dasatinib; Doxylamine; Dronabinol; Droperidol; Fosaprepitant; Fusidic Acid (Systemic); HydrOXYzine; Idelalisib; Ivacaftor; Kava Kava; Luliconazole; Magnesium Sulfate; Methotrimeprazine; Mifepristone; Nabilone; Netupitant; OLANZapine; Palbociclib; Perampanel; Rufinamide; Simeprevir; Stiripentol; Tapentadol; Teduglutide; Tetrahydrocannabinol; Vigabatrin

Decreased Effect

The levels/effects of ClonazePAM may be decreased by: Bosentan; CYP3A4 Inducers (Moderate); CYP3A4 Inducers (Strong); Dabrafenib; Deferasirox; Mitotane; Siltuximab; St Johns Wort; Theophylline Derivatives; Tocilizumab; Yohimbine

Storage/Stability

Tablets: Store at 20°C to 25°C (68°F to 77°F).

Orally disintegrating tablets: Store at 25°C (77°F); excursions permitted between 15°C and 30°C (59°F and 80°F)

Mechanism of Action The exact mechanism is unknown, but believed to be related to its ability to enhance the activity of GABA; suppresses the spike-and-wave discharge in absence seizures by depressing nerve transmission in the motor cortex.

Pharmacodynamics

Onset of action: 20-60 minutes

Duration:

Infants and young children: Up to 6-8 hours

Adults: Up to 12 hours

Pharmacokinetics (Adult data unless noted)

Absorption: Oral: Well absorbed

Distribution: V_d: Adults: 1.5-4.4 L/kg

Protein binding: 85%

Metabolism: Extensively metabolized in the liver; undergoes nitroreduction to 7-aminoclonazepam, followed by acetylation to 7-acetamidoclonazepam; nitroreduction and acetylation are via cytochrome P450 enzyme system; metabolites undergo glucuronide and sulfate conjugation

Bioavailability: 90%

Half-life:

Children: 22-33 hours

Adults: Usual: 30-40 hours; range: 19-50 hours

Elimination: Metabolites excreted as glucuronide or sulfate conjugates; <2% excreted unchanged in urine

Dosing: Usual Oral:

Seizure disorders:

Infants and Children <10 years or 30 kg:

Initial daily dose: 0.01-0.03 mg/kg/day (maximum initial dose: 0.05 mg/kg/day) given in 2-3 divided doses; increase by no more than 0.5 mg every third day until seizures are controlled or adverse effects seen

Maintenance dose: 0.1-0.2 mg/kg/day divided 3 times/day; not to exceed 0.2 mg/kg/day

Children ≥10 years (>30 kg) and Adults:

Initial daily dose not to exceed 1.5 mg given in 3 divided doses; may increase by 0.5-1 mg every third day until seizures are controlled or adverse effects seen

Maintenance dose: 0.05-0.2 mg/kg/day; do not exceed 20 mg/day

Panic disorder: Adolescents ≥18 years and Adults: Initial: 0.25 mg twice daily; increase in increments of 0.125-0.25 mg twice daily every 3 days; target dose: 1 mg/day; maximum dose: 4 mg/day

Administration Hazardous agent; use appropriate precautions for handling and disposal (NIOSH 2014 [group 3]).

Oral: May administer with food or water to decrease GI distress

Orally-disintegrating tablet: Open pouch and peel back foil on the blister; do not push tablet through foil. Use dry hands to remove tablet and place in mouth. May be swallowed with or without water. Use immediately after removing from package.

Monitoring Parameters Signs and symptoms of suicidality (eg, anxiety, depression, behavior changes). Long-term use: CBC with differential, platelets, liver enzymes

Reference Range Relationship between serum concentration and seizure control is not well established; measurement at random times postdose may contribute to this problem; predose concentrations are recommended

Proposed therapeutic levels: 20-80 ng/mL

Potentially toxic concentration: >80 ng/mL

Additional Information Ethosuximide or valproic acid may be preferred for treatment of absence (petit mal) seizures. Clonazepam-induced behavioral disturbances may be more frequent in mentally handicapped patients. When discontinuing therapy in children, the clonazepam dose may be safely reduced by ≤0.04 mg/kg/week and discontinued when the daily dose is ≤0.04 mg/kg/day. When discontinuing therapy in adults treated for panic disorder, the clonazepam dose may be decreased by 0.125 mg twice daily every 3 days, until the drug is completely withdrawn. Treatment of panic disorder for >9 weeks has not been studied; long-term usefulness of clonazepam for the treatment of panic disorder should be re-evaluated periodically.

Controlled Substance C-IV

Dosage Forms Excipient information presented when available (limited, particularly for generics); consult specific product labeling.

Tablet, Oral:

- KlonoPIN: 0.5 mg [scored]
- KlonoPIN: 1 mg [contains fd&c blue #1 aluminum lake, fd&c blue #2 aluminum lake]
- KlonoPIN: 2 mg
- Generic: 0.5 mg, 1 mg, 2 mg

Tablet Dispersible, Oral:

- Generic: 0.125 mg, 0.25 mg, 0.5 mg, 1 mg, 2 mg

Extemporaneous Preparations Hazardous agent: Use appropriate precautions for handling and disposal (NIOSH 2014 [group 3]).

A 0.1 mg/mL oral suspension may be made with tablets and one of three different vehicles (cherry syrup; a 1:1 mixture of Ora-Sweet® and Ora-Plus®; or a 1:1 mixture of Ora-Sweet® SF and Ora-Plus®). Crush six 2 mg tablets in a mortar and reduce to a fine powder. Add 10 mL of the chosen vehicle and mix to a uniform paste; mix while adding the vehicle in incremental proportions to **almost** 120 mL; transfer to a calibrated bottle, rinse mortar with vehicle, and add quantity of vehicle sufficient to make 120 mL. Label "shake well" and "protect from light". Stable for 60 days when stored in amber prescription bottles in the dark at room temperature or refrigerated.

Allen LV Jr and Erickson MA 3rd, "Stability of Acetazolamide, Allopurinol, Azathioprine, Clonazepam, and Flucytosine in Extemporaneously Compounded Oral Liquids," Am *J Health Syst Pharm* 1996, 53(16):1944-9.

◆ **Clonazepam-R (Can)** *see* ClonazePAM *on page 506*

CloNIDine (KLON i deen)

Medication Safety Issues

Sound-alike/look-alike issues:

CloNIDine may be confused with Clomid, clomiPHENE, clonazePAM, cloZAPine, KlonoPIN, quiNIDine

Catapres may be confused with Cataflam, Combipres

High alert medication:

The Institute for Safe Medication Practices (ISMP) includes this medication (epidural administration) among its list of drug classes which have a heightened risk of causing significant patient harm when used in error.

BEERS Criteria medication:

This drug may be potentially inappropriate for use in geriatric patients (Quality of evidence - low; Strength of recommendation - strong).

Administration issues:

Use caution when interpreting dosing information. Pediatric dose for epidural infusion expressed as mcg/kg/**hour**.

Other safety concerns:

Transdermal patch may contain conducting metal (eg, aluminum); remove patch prior to MRI. Errors have occurred when the inactive, optional adhesive cover has been applied instead of the active clonidine-containing patch.

Related Information

Oral Medications That Should Not Be Crushed or Altered *on page 2476*

Brand Names: US Catapres; Catapres-TTS-1; Catapres-TTS-2; Catapres-TTS-3; Duraclon; Kapvay

Brand Names: Canada Apo-Clonidine®; Catapres®; Dixarit®; Dom-Clonidine; Novo-Clonidine

Therapeutic Category Adrenergic Agonist Agent; Alpha-Adrenergic Agonist; Analgesic, Non-narcotic (Epidural); Antihypertensive Agent

Generic Availability (US) May be product dependent

Use

Oral:

Immediate release: Management of hypertension (monotherapy or as adjunctive therapy) (FDA approved in adults); has also been used for the treatment of attention-deficit/hyperactivity disorder, Tourette syndrome and tic disorders, neonatal abstinence syndrome (opioid withdrawal), and as an aid in the diagnosis of pheochromocytoma and growth hormone deficiency

Extended release: Kapvay™: Treatment of attention deficit hyperactivity disorder (ADHD) (monotherapy or as adjunctive therapy) (FDA approved in ages 6-17 years)

Parenteral: Epidural (Duraclon®): For continuous epidural administration as adjunctive therapy with opioids for treatment of severe cancer pain in patients tolerant to or unresponsive to opioids alone; epidural clonidine is generally more effective for neuropathic pain and less effective (or possibly ineffective) for somatic or visceral pain [FDA approved in pediatric patients (age not specified) and adults]

Transdermal patch: Management of hypertension (monotherapy or as adjunctive therapy) (FDA approved in adults)

Pregnancy Risk Factor C

Pregnancy Considerations Adverse events have been observed in some animal reproduction studies. Clonidine crosses the placenta; concentrations in the umbilical cord plasma are similar to those in the maternal serum and concentrations in the amniotic fluid may be 4 times those in the maternal serum. The pharmacokinetics of clonidine may be altered during pregnancy (Buchanan, 2009). Untreated chronic maternal hypertension is associated with adverse events in the fetus, infant, and mother. If treatment for hypertension during pregnancy is needed, other agents are preferred (ACOG, 2012). **[U.S. Boxed Warning]: Epidural clonidine is not recommended for obstetrical or postpartum pain** due to risk of hemodynamic instability.

Breast-Feeding Considerations Clonidine is excreted in breast milk. Concentrations have been noted as ~7% to 8% of those in the maternal plasma following oral dosing (Atkinson, 1988; Bunjes, 1993) and twice those in the maternal serum following epidural administration. The manufacturer recommends caution be used if administered to nursing women. Another source recommends avoiding use when nursing infants born <34 weeks gestation or when large maternal doses are needed (Atkinson, 1988).

Contraindications Hypersensitivity to clonidine hydrochloride or any component of the formulation

Epidural administration: Injection site infection; concurrent anticoagulant therapy; bleeding diathesis; administration above the C4 dermatome

Warnings/Precautions May cause CNS depression, which may impair physical or mental abilities; patients must be cautioned about performing tasks which require mental alertness (eg, operating machinery or driving). Sedating effects may be potentiated when used with other CNS-depressant drugs or ethanol. Use with caution in patients with severe coronary insufficiency; conduction disturbances; recent MI, CVA, or chronic renal insufficiency. The hemodynamic effects may be prolonged in those with renal impairment; elimination half-life significantly prolonged (up to 41 hours) in patients with severe renal impairment. May cause dose dependent reductions in heart rate; use with caution in patients with preexisting bradycardia or those predisposed to developing bradycardia. Caution in sinus node dysfunction. Use with caution in patients concurrently receiving agents known to reduce SA node function and/or AV nodal conduction (eg, digoxin, diltiazem, metoprolol, verapamil). May cause significant xerostomia. Clonidine may cause eye dryness in patients who wear contact lenses.

[U.S. Boxed Warning]: Must dilute concentrated epidural injectable (500 mcg/mL) solution prior to use. Epidural clonidine is not recommended for perioperative, obstetrical, or postpartum pain due to risk of hemodynamic instability. Clonidine injection should be administered via a continuous epidural infusion device. Monitor closely for catheter-related infection such as meningitis or epidural abscess. Epidural clonidine is not recommended for use in patients with severe cardiovascular disease or hemodynamic instability; may lead to cardiovascular instability (hypotension, bradycardia). Symptomatic hypotension may occur with use; in all patients, use epidural clonidine with caution due to the potential for severe hypotension especially in women and those of low body weight. Most hypotensive episodes occur within the first 4 days of initiation; however, episodes may occur throughout the duration of therapy.

Gradual withdrawal is needed (taper oral immediate release or epidural dose gradually over 2-4 days to avoid rebound hypertension) if drug needs to be stopped. Patients should be instructed about abrupt discontinuation (causes rapid increase in BP and symptoms of sympathetic overactivity). In patients on both a beta-blocker and clonidine where withdrawal of clonidine is necessary, withdraw the beta-blocker first and several days before clonidine withdrawal, then slowly decrease clonidine. In children and adolescents, extended release formulation (Kapvay™) should be tapered in decrements of no more than 0.1 mg every 3-7 days. Discontinue oral immediate release formulations within 4 hours of surgery then restart as soon as possible afterwards. Discontinue oral extended release formulations up to 28 hours prior to surgery, then restart the following day.

Oral formulations of clonidine (immediate release versus extended release) are not interchangeable on a mg:mg basis due to different pharmacokinetic profiles.

Transdermal patch may contain conducting metal (eg, aluminum); remove patch prior to MRI. Due to the potential for altered electrical conductivity, remove transdermal patch before cardioversion or defibrillation. Localized contact sensitization to the transdermal system has been reported; in these patients, allergic reactions (eg, generalized rash, urticaria, angioedema) have also occurred following subsequent substitution of oral therapy.

In the elderly, avoid use as first-line antihypertensive due to high risk of CNS adverse effects; may also cause orthostatic hypotension and bradycardia (Beers Criteria). In pediatric patients, epidural clonidine should be reserved for cancer patients with severe intractable pain, unresponsive to other analgesics or epidural or spinal opioids. Use oral formulations with caution in pediatric patients since children commonly have gastrointestinal illnesses with vomiting and are susceptible to hypertensive episodes due to abrupt inability to take oral medication.

Warnings: Additional Pediatric Considerations The American Heart Association recommends that all children diagnosed with ADHD who may be candidates for medication, such as clonidine, should have a thorough cardiovascular assessment prior to initiation of therapy. These recommendations are based upon reports of serious cardiovascular adverse events (including sudden death) in patients (both children and adults) taking usual doses of stimulant medications. Most of these patients were found to have underlying structural heart disease (eg, hypertrophic obstructive cardiomyopathy). This assessment should include a combination of thorough medical history, family history, and physical examination. An ECG is not mandatory but should be considered. **Note:** ECG abnormalities and four cases of sudden cardiac death have been reported in children receiving clonidine with methylphenidate; reduce dose of methylphenidate by 40% when used concurrently with clonidine; consider ECG monitoring. In patients with ADHD, clonidine may cause hypotension and bradycardia; use with caution in patients with history of hypotension, heart block, bradycardia, cardiovascular disease, syncope, conditions predisposing to syncope (including orthostatic hypotension, dehydration), or receiving concomitant antihypertensive therapy. Patients should be advised to avoid becoming dehydrated or overheated. Heart rate and blood pressure should be monitored at initiation of therapy, with any dose increase, and periodically during therapy.

Adverse Reactions

Oral, Transdermal: Incidence of adverse events may be less with transdermal compared to oral due to the lower peak/trough ratio.

Cardiovascular: Atrioventricular block, bradycardia, cardiac arrhythmia, cardiac failure, cerebrovascular accident, chest pain, ECG abnormality, edema, flushing, localized blanching (transdermal), orthostatic hypotension, palpitations, prolonged Q-T Interval on ECG, Raynaud's phenomenon, syncope, tachycardia

Central Nervous System: Aggressive behavior, agitation, anxiety, behavioral changes, delirium, delusions, depression, dizziness, drowsiness, emotional disturbance, fatigue, hallucination (visual and auditory), headache, insomnia, irritability, lethargy, malaise, nervousness, nightmares, numbness (localized; transdermal), paresthesia, parotid pain (oral), restlessness, sedation, throbbing (transdermal), vivid dream, withdrawal syndrome

Dermatologic: Allergic contact sensitivity (transdermal), alopecia, burning sensation of skin (transdermal), contact dermatitis (transdermal), excoriation (transdermal), hyperpigmentation (transdermal), hypopigmentation (localized; transdermal), localized vesiculation (transdermal), macular eruption, pallor, papule (transdermal), skin rash, transient skin rash (localized; characterized by pruritus and erythema; transdermal), urticaria

Endocrine & metabolic: Decreased libido, gynecomastia, hyperglycemia (transient; oral), increased thirst, weight gain

Gastrointestinal: Abdominal pain (oral), anorexia, constipation, diarrhea, gastrointestinal pseudo-obstruction (oral), nausea, parotitis (oral), sore throat, upper abdominal pain, viral gastrointestinal infection, vomiting, xerostomia

Genitourinary: Erectile dysfunction, nocturia, pollakiuria, sexual disorder, urinary incontinence, urinary retention

Hematologic & oncologic: Thrombocytopenia (oral)

Hepatic: Abnormal hepatic function tests (mild transient abnormalities), hepatitis

Hypersensitivity: Angioedema

Neuromuscular & skeletal: Arthralgia, increased creatine phosphokinase (transient; oral), leg cramps, limb pain, myalgia, tremor, weakness

Ophthalmic: Accommodation disturbance, blurred vision, burning sensation of eyes, decreased lacrimation, dry eye syndrome, increased lacrimation

Otic: Otalgia, otitis media

Respiratory: Asthma, dry nose, epistaxis, flu-like symptoms, nasal congestion, nasopharyngitis, respiratory tract infection, rhinorrhea

Miscellaneous: Crying, fever

Epidural: Note: The following adverse events occurred more often than placebo in cancer patients with intractable pain being treated with concurrent epidural morphine.

Cardiovascular: Chest pain, hypotension, orthostatic hypotension

Central nervous system: Confusion, dizziness, hallucination

Dermatologic: Diaphoresis

Gastrointestinal: Nausea and vomiting, xerostomia

Otic: Tinnitus

Drug Interactions

Metabolism/Transport Effects None known.

Avoid Concomitant Use

Avoid concomitant use of CloNIDine with any of the following: Azelastine (Nasal); Ceritinib; Iobenguane I 123; Orphenadrine; Paraldehyde; Thalidomide

Increased Effect/Toxicity

CloNIDine may increase the levels/effects of: Alcohol (Ethyl); Amifostine; Antihypertensives; Azelastine (Nasal); Beta-Blockers; Bradycardia-Causing Agents; Buprenorphine; Calcium Channel Blockers (Nondihydropyridine); Cardiac Glycosides; Ceritinib; CNS Depressants; DULoxetine; Hydrocodone; Hypotensive Agents; Ivabradine; Lacosamide; Levodopa; Methotrimeprazine; Metyrosine; Obinutuzumab; Orphenadrine; Paraldehyde; Pramipexole; RisperiDONE; RiTUXimab; ROPINIRole; Rotigotine; Selective Serotonin Reuptake Inhibitors; Suvorexant; Thalidomide; Zolpidem

The levels/effects of CloNIDine may be increased by: Alfuzosin; Barbiturates; Beta-Blockers; Bretylium; Brimonidine (Topical); Cannabis; Diazoxide; Doxylamine; Dronabinol; Droperidol; Herbs (Hypotensive Properties); HydrOXYzine; Kava Kava; Magnesium Sulfate; MAO Inhibitors; Methotrimeprazine; Methylphenidate; Nabilone; Nicorandil; Pentoxifylline; Perampanel; Phosphodiesterase 5 Inhibitors; Prostacyclin Analogues; Rufinamide; Ruxolitinib; Sodium Oxybate; Tapentadol; Tetrahydrocannabinol; Tofacitinib

Decreased Effect

CloNIDine may decrease the levels/effects of: Iobenguane I 123

The levels/effects of CloNIDine may be decreased by: Herbs (Hypertensive Properties); Mirtazapine; Serotonin/Norepinephrine Reuptake Inhibitors; Tricyclic Antidepressants; Yohimbine

Storage/Stability

Epidural formulation: Store at 25°C (77°F); excursions permitted to 15°C to 30°C (59°F to 86°F). **Preservative free;** discard unused portion.

Tablets: Store at 25°C (77°F); excursions permitted to 15°C to 30°C (59°F to 86°F). Protect from light.

Extended release tablets: Store at 20°C to 25°C (68°F to 77°F). Protect from light.

Transdermal patches: Store below 30°C (86°F).

Mechanism of Action Stimulates $alpha_2$-adrenoceptors in the brain stem, thus activating an inhibitory neuron, resulting in reduced sympathetic outflow from the CNS, producing a decrease in peripheral resistance, renal vascular resistance, heart rate, and blood pressure; epidural clonidine may produce pain relief at spinal presynaptic and postjunctional $alpha_2$-adrenoceptors by preventing pain signal transmission; pain relief occurs only for the body regions innervated by the spinal segments where analgesic concentrations of clonidine exist. For the treatment of ADHD, the mechanism of action is unknown; it has been proposed that postsynaptic $alpha_2$-agonist stimulation regulates subcortical activity in the prefrontal cortex, the area of the brain responsible for emotions, attentions, and behaviors and causes reduced hyperactivity, impulsiveness, and distractibility.

Pharmacodynamics

Antihypertensive effects:

Onset of action: Oral: Immediate release: 30-60 minutes; Transdermal: Initial application: 2-3 days

Maximum effect: Oral: Immediate release: Within 2-4 hours

Duration: Oral: Immediate release: 6-10 hours

Attention-deficit/hyperactivity disorder: Oral: Extended release: Onset of action: 1-2 weeks (AAP, 2011)

Pharmacokinetics (Adult data unless noted)

Absorption: Oral: Extended release tablets (Kapvay™) are not bioequivalent with immediate release formulations; peak plasma concentrations are 50% lower compared to immediate release formulations

Distribution: V_d: 2 L/kg; highly lipid soluble; distributes readily into extravascular sites; **Note:** Epidurally administered clonidine readily distributes into plasma via the epidural veins and attains clinically significant systemic concentrations.

Protein binding: 20% to 40%

Metabolism: Hepatic to inactive metabolites; undergoes enterohepatic recirculation

Bioavailability: Oral: Immediate release: 75% to 85%; extended release (Kapvay™): 89% (compared to immediate release formulation) (Cunningham, 1994)

Time to peak serum concentration: Oral: Immediate release: 3-5 hours; extended release: 7-8 hours

Half-life:

Oral: Serum half-life:

Neonates: 44-72 hours

Children: 8-12 hours

Adults:

Normal renal function: 12-16 hours

Renal impairment: ≤41 hours

Epidural administration: CSF half-life: 1.3 ± 0.5 hours

Elimination: Urine (40% to 60% as unchanged drug)

Dialysis: Not dialyzable (0% to 5%)

Dosing: Neonatal Note: Compounded oral suspensions may be available in multiple concentrations (up to 10-times more concentrated); precautions should be taken to verify and avoid confusion between the different concentrations; dose should be clearly presented as mcg or mg as appropriate.

Neonatal abstinence syndrome (opioid withdrawal): Limited data available. Oral: 0.5 to 1 **mcg**/kg/dose every 4 to 6 hours (Agthe 2009; Hudak 2012); for premature neonates, a dosing interval of every 6 hours was reported (median GA: 26 weeks and 2 days) and upon stabilization, clonidine doses were stopped or tapered by 0.25 **mcg**/kg every 6 hours if necessary (Leikin 2009)

Dosing: Usual Note: Formulations of clonidine (immediate release vs extended release) are not interchangeable on a mg per mg basis due to different pharmacokinetic profiles. Compounded oral suspensions may be available in multiple concentrations (up to a 10-times more concentrated); precautions should be taken to verify and avoid confusion between the different concentrations; dose should be clearly presented as mcg or mg as appropriate.

Pediatric:

Hypertension: Limited data available:

Oral: Immediate release:

Weight-directed dosing: Children and Adolescents 1 to 17 years: Initial: 5 to 10 **mcg**/kg/day in divided doses every 8 to 12 hours; increase gradually as needed; usual range: 5 to 25 **mcg**/kg/day in divided doses every 6 hours; maximum dose: 0.9 mg/day (Kavey 2010; Rocchini 1984)

Alternate dosing: Fixed dosing: Children and Adolescents ≥12 years: Initial: 0.1 mg twice daily; increase gradually, if needed, by 0.1 mg/day at weekly intervals; usual maintenance dose: 0.2 to 0.6 mg/day in divided doses; maximum recommended dose: 2.4 mg/day (rarely required) (NHBPEP 2004)

Transdermal: Limited data available: Children and Adolescents: May be switched to the transdermal delivery system after oral therapy is titrated to an optimal and stable dose; a transdermal dose approximately equivalent to the total oral daily dose may be used (Hunt 1990).

Hypertension, urgency and emergency: Limited data available: Children and Adolescents 1 to 17 years: Oral: Immediate release: 0.05 to 0.1 mg/dose; may repeat dose(s) up to a maximum total dose of 0.8 mg (NHBPEP 2004)

ADHD: Children ≥6 years and Adolescents:

Oral:

Immediate release: Limited data available (Pliszka 2007):

≤45 kg: Initial: 0.05 mg at bedtime; sequentially increase every 3 to 7 days in 0.05 mg/day increments given as 0.05 mg twice daily, then 3 times daily, then 4 times daily; maximum daily dose weight-dependent: Patient weight: 27 to 40.5 kg: 0.2 mg/day; patient weight: 40.5 to 45 kg; 0.3 mg/day

>45 kg: Initial: 0.1 mg at bedtime; sequentially increase every 3 to 7 days in 0.1 mg/day increments given as 0.1 mg twice daily, then 3 times daily, then 4 times daily; maximum daily dose: 0.4 mg/day

Extended release (Kapvay): Initial: 0.1 mg at bedtime; increase in 0.1 mg/day increments every 7 days until desired response; doses should be administered twice daily (either split equally or with the higher split dosage given at bedtime); maximum: 0.4 mg/day. **Note:** Maintenance treatment for >5 weeks has not been evaluated. When discontinuing therapy, taper daily dose by ≤0.1 mg every 3 to 7 days.

Transdermal: Limited data available: Children and adolescents may be switched to the transdermal delivery system after oral therapy is titrated to an optimal and stable dose; a transdermal dose approximately equivalent to the total oral daily dose may be used (Hunt 1990).

Clonidine tolerance test (test of growth hormone release from the pituitary): Limited data available: Children and Adolescents: Oral: Immediate release: 0.15 mg/m^2 or 5 **mcg**/kg as a single dose; maximum dose: 0.25 mg (250 mcg) (Lanes 1982; Richmond 2008)

Analgesia: Children and Adolescents: Epidural: Continuous infusion: Initial: 0.5 **mcg**/kg/**hour**; adjust with caution, based on clinical effect; usual range: 0.5 to 2 **mcg**/kg/**hour**; do not exceed adult doses. Do not discontinue clonidine abruptly; if needed, gradually reduce dose over 2 to 4 days to avoid withdrawal symptoms. Manufacturer suggests use reserved for cancer patients with severe intractable pain, unresponsive to other opioid analgesics, or epidural or spinal opioids; has also been used for pediatric chronic pain syndromes.

Neuropathic pain: Limited data available: Children and Adolescents:

Oral: Immediate release: Some centers use the following doses (Galloway 2000): Initial: 2 **mcg**/kg/dose every 4 to 6 hours; increase incrementally over several days; range: 2 to 4 **mcg**/kg/dose every 4 to 6 hours

Transdermal: May be switched to the transdermal delivery system after oral therapy is titrated to an optimal and stable dose; a transdermal dose approximately equivalent to the total oral daily dose may be used (Galloway 2000; Hunt 1990).

Tic disorders and Tourette's syndrome: Limited data available: Children ≥7 years and and Adolescents: Oral: Initial: 0.025 to 0.05 mg/day; gradual titration to 3 to 4 times daily schedule using small increments (0.025 mg); target daily dose: 0.2 to 0.3 mg/day; doses up to 0.4 mg/day have been reported (Swain 2007; The Tourette's Syndrome Study Group 2002)

Adult:

Hypertension:

Oral:

Immediate release: Initial dose: 0.1 mg twice daily, usual maintenance dose: 0.2 to 1.2 mg/day in 2 to 4 divided doses; maximum recommended dose: 2.4 mg/day; usual dosage range (JNC 7): 0.1 to 0.8 mg/day in 2 divided doses

Conversion from transdermal to oral: After transdermal patch removal, therapeutic clonidine levels persist for ~8 hours and then slowly decrease over several days. Consider starting oral clonidine no sooner than 8 hours after patch removal.

Transdermal: Applied once weekly as transdermal delivery system; begin therapy with 0.1 mg/day patch applied once every 7 days; increase by 0.1 mg/day at 1 to 2 week intervals based on response; hypotensive action may not begin until 2 to 3 days after initial application; doses >0.6 mg/day do not improve efficacy; usual dosage range (JNC 7): 0.1 to 0.3 mg/day patch applied once weekly. **Note:** If transitioning from oral to transdermal therapy, overlap oral regimen for 1 to 2 days; transdermal route takes 2 to 3 days to achieve therapeutic effects.

Conversion from oral to transdermal:

Day 1: Place Catapres-TTS 1; administer 100% of oral dose.

Day 2: Administer 50% of oral dose.

Day 3: Administer 25% of oral dose.

Day 4: Patch remains; no further oral supplement necessary

Analgesia: Epidural (continuous infusion): Reserved for cancer patients with severe intractable pain, unresponsive to other opioid analgesics: Initial: 30 **mcg/hour**; titrate as required for relief of pain or presence of side effects; minimal experience with doses >40 **mcg/hour**; should be considered an adjunct to intraspinal opioid therapy

Dosing adjustment in renal impairment:

Children and Adolescents: Oral [extended release (Kapvay)], epidural: The manufacturer recommends dosage adjustment according to degree of renal impairment; however, there are no specific dosage adjustment provided in the labeling (has not been studied).

Bradycardia, sedation, and hypotension may be more likely to occur in patients with renal failure; drug is primarily eliminated unchanged in the urine; consider using doses at the lower end of the dosage range; monitor patients closely.

Adults: Oral (immediate release), transdermal, epidural: The manufacturer recommends dosage adjustment according to degree of renal impairment; however, no specific dosage adjustment provided. Bradycardia, sedation, and hypotension may be more likely to occur in patients with renal failure; half-life significantly prolonged in patients with severe renal failure; consider use of lower initial doses and monitor closely.

Hemodialysis: Not dialyzable (0% to 5%); supplemental dose is not necessary. Oral antihypertensive drugs given preferentially at night may reduce the nocturnal surge of blood pressure and minimize the intradialytic hypotension that may occur when taken the morning before a dialysis session (K/DOQI 2005).

Dosing adjustment in hepatic impairment: There are no dosage adjustments provided in the manufacturer labeling.

Preparation for Administration Epidural formulation: Prior to administration, the 500 mcg/mL concentration must be diluted in preservative-free NS to a final concentration of 100 mcg/mL; visually inspect for particulate matter and discoloration

Administration

Epidural: Not for IV use. Visually inspect for particulate matter and discoloration prior to administration (whenever permitted by container and solution). Specialized techniques are required for continuous epidural administration; administration via this route should only be performed by qualified individuals familiar with the techniques of epidural administration and patient management problems associated with this route. Familiarization of the epidural infusion device is essential. Do not discontinue clonidine abruptly; if needed, gradually reduce dose over 2 to 4 days to avoid withdrawal symptoms.

Oral: May be administered without regard to meals. Swallow extended release formulations whole; do not crush or chew. Kapvay should not be split. Do not discontinue clonidine abruptly; if needed, gradually reduce immediate release dose over 2 to 4 days to avoid rebound hypertension; extended release formulation (Kapvay) should be tapered in decrements of ≤0.1 mg every 3 to 7 days.

Transdermal: Patches should be applied at bedtime to a clean, hairless area of the upper arm or chest; rotate patch sites weekly in adults; in children, the patch may need to be changed more frequently (eg, every 3 to 5 days); in adults, redness under patch may be reduced if a topical corticosteroid spray is applied to the area before placement of the patch (Tom 1994); **Note:** Transdermal patch is a membrane-controlled system; do **not** cut the patch to deliver partial doses; rate of drug delivery, reservoir contents, and adhesion may be affected if cut; if partial dose is needed, surface area of patch can be blocked proportionally using adhesive bandage (Lee 1997).

Monitoring Parameters Blood pressure, heart rate; consider ECG monitoring in patients with history of heart disease or concurrent use of medications affecting cardiac conduction. With epidural administration: Blood pressure, heart rate; pulse oximetry with large bolus doses; monitor infusion pump and catheter tubing for obstruction or dislodgment throughout the course of therapy to decrease risk of inadvertent abrupt discontinuation; monitor closely for catheter-related infection, such as meningitis or epidural abscess.

ADHD: Evaluate patients for cardiac disease prior to initiation of therapy for ADHD with thorough medical history, family history, and physical exam; consider ECG; perform ECG and echocardiogram if findings suggest cardiac disease; promptly conduct cardiac evaluation in patients who develop chest pain, unexplained syncope, or any other symptom of cardiac disease during treatment.

Clonidine tolerance test: In addition to growth hormone concentrations, monitor blood pressure and blood glucose (Huang, 2001)

Test Interactions Positive Coombs' test

Additional Information Clonidine-induced symptomatic bradycardia may be treated with atropine. Clonidine hydrochloride 0.1 mg is equal to 0.087 mg of the free base. Medications used to treat ADHD should be part of a total treatment program that may include other components, such as psychological, educational, and social measures. Long-term usefulness of clonidine for the treatment of ADHD should be periodically re-evaluated in patients receiving the drug for extended periods of time.

Dosage Forms Excipient information presented when available (limited, particularly for generics); consult specific product labeling. [DSC] = Discontinued product

Miscellaneous, Oral, as hydrochloride:
- Kapvay: 0.1 mg AM dose, 0.2 mg PM dose (60 ea [DSC])

Patch Weekly, Transdermal:
- Catapres-TTS-1: 0.1 mg/24 hr (4 ea)
- Catapres-TTS-2: 0.2 mg/24 hr (4 ea)
- Catapres-TTS-3: 0.3 mg/24 hr (4 ea)
- Generic: 0.1 mg/24 hr (1 ea, 4 ea); 0.2 mg/24 hr (1 ea, 4 ea); 0.3 mg/24 hr (1 ea, 4 ea)

Solution, Epidural, as hydrochloride:
- Duraclon: 100 mcg/mL (10 mL)
- Generic: 100 mcg/mL (10 mL); 500 mcg/mL (10 mL)

Solution, Epidural, as hydrochloride [preservative free]:
- Duraclon: 100 mcg/mL (10 mL)
- Duraclon: 500 mcg/mL (10 mL) [pyrogen free]
- Generic: 100 mcg/mL (10 mL); 500 mcg/mL (10 mL)

Tablet, Oral, as hydrochloride:
- Catapres: 0.1 mg [scored; contains brilliant blue fcf (fd&c blue #1), fd&c yellow #6 (sunset yellow)]
- Catapres: 0.2 mg, 0.3 mg [scored; contains fd&c yellow #6 (sunset yellow)]
- Generic: 0.1 mg, 0.2 mg, 0.3 mg

Tablet Extended Release 12 Hour, Oral, as hydrochloride:
- Kapvay: 0.1 mg
- Generic: 0.1 mg

Extemporaneous Preparations

0.01 mg/mL concentration

A **0.01** mg/mL oral suspension may be made from tablets. Crush twenty 0.1 mg tablets in a glass mortar and reduce to a fine powder. Slowly add Ora-Blend in ~15 mL increments while mixing to form a uniform paste until approximately half of the total volume (~100 mL) is added. Transfer the suspension to a graduated cylinder. Rinse the mortar and pestle with the remaining vehicle and add quantity to fill the volume within the graduated cylinder to 200 mL. Transfer this amount to a calibrated bottle. Label "shake well". When stored in clear plastic syringes, the suspension is stable for at least 91 days at room temperature (25°C) or refrigerated (4°C).

Ma C, Decarie D, Ensom MHH. Stability of clonidine oral suspension in oral plastic syringes. *Am J Health-Syst Pharm.* 2014;71:657-661.

0.1 mg/mL concentration

A **0.1** mg/mL oral suspension may be made from tablets. Crush thirty 0.2 mg tablets in a glass mortar and reduce to a fine powder. Slowly add 2 mL Purified Water USP and mix to a uniform paste. Slowly add Simple Syrup, NF in 15 mL increments; transfer to a calibrated bottle, rinse mortar with vehicle, and add quantity of vehicle sufficient to make 60 mL. Label "shake well" and "refrigerate". Stable for 28 days when stored in amber glass bottles and refrigerated.

Levinson ML and Johnson CE. Stability of an extemporaneously compounded clonidine hydrochloride oral liquid. *Am J Hosp Pharm.* 1992;49(1):122-125.

◆ **Clonidine Hydrochloride** *see* CloNIDine *on page 508*

Clopidogrel (kloh PID oh grel)

Medication Safety Issues

Sound-alike/look-alike issues:

Plavix may be confused with Elavil, Paxil, Pradax (Canada), Pradaxa

Brand Names: US Plavix

Brand Names: Canada Apo-Clopidogrel; CO Clopidogrel; Dom-Clopidogrel; JAMP-Clopidogrel; Mylan-Clopidogrel; Plavix; PMS-Clopidogrel; RAN-Clopidogrel; Sandoz-Clopidogrel; Teva-Clopidogrel

Therapeutic Category Antiplatelet Agent

Generic Availability (US) Yes

Use Reduction of atherothrombotic events (MI, stroke, and vascular deaths) in patients with recent MI, stroke, or established peripheral arterial disease (FDA approved in adults); reduction of atherothrombotic events in patients with non-ST-segment elevation acute coronary syndrome (unstable angina and non-Q-wave MI) managed medically and through percutaneous coronary intervention (with or without stent) or CABG (FDA approved in adults); reduction of death rate and atherothrombotic events in patients with ST-segment elevation acute MI (STEMI) managed medically (FDA approved in adults).

Medication Guide Available Yes

Pregnancy Risk Factor B

Pregnancy Considerations Adverse events were not observed in animal reproduction studies. Information related to use during pregnancy is limited (Bauer, 2012; DeSantis, 2011; Myers, 2011).

Breast-Feeding Considerations It is not known if clopidogrel is excreted into breast milk. Due to the potential for serious adverse reactions in the nursing infant, the manufacturer recommends a decision be made whether to discontinue nursing or to discontinue the drug, taking into account the importance of treatment to the mother.

Contraindications Hypersensitivity to clopidogrel or any component of the formulation; active pathological bleeding such as peptic ulcer or intracranial hemorrhage

Canadian labeling: Additional contraindications (not in U.S. labeling): Significant liver impairment or cholestatic jaundice

Warnings/Precautions [U.S. Boxed Warning]: Patients with one or more copies of the variant *CYP2C19*2* and/or *CYP2C19*3* alleles (and potentially other reduced-function variants) may have reduced conversion of clopidogrel to its active thiol metabolite. Lower active metabolite exposure may result in reduced platelet inhibition and, thus, a higher rate of cardiovascular events following MI or stent thrombosis following PCI. Although evidence is insufficient to recommend routine genetic testing, tests are available to determine CYP2C19 genotype and may be used to determine therapeutic strategy; alternative treatment or treatment strategies may be considered if patient is identified as a CYP2C19 poor metabolizer. Genetic testing may be considered prior to initiating clopidogrel in patients at moderate or high risk for poor outcomes (eg, PCI in patients with extensive and/or very complex disease). The optimal dose for CYP2C19 poor metabolizers has yet to be determined. After initiation of clopidogrel, functional testing (eg, VerifyNow® P2Y12 assay) may also be done to determine clopidogrel responsiveness (Holmes, 2010).

Use with caution in patients who may be at risk of increased bleeding, including patients with PUD, trauma, or surgery. In patients with coronary stents, premature interruption of therapy may result in stent thrombosis with subsequent fatal and nonfatal MI. Duration of therapy, in general, is determined by the type of stent placed (bare metal or drug eluting) and whether an ACS event was ongoing at the time of placement. Consider discontinuing 5 days before elective surgery (except in patients with cardiac stents that have not completed their full course of dual antiplatelet therapy; patient-specific situations need to be discussed with cardiologist; AHA/ACC/SCAI/ACS/ADA Science Advisory provides recommendations). Discontinue at least 5 days before elective CABG; when urgent CABG is necessary, the ACCF/AHA CABG guidelines recommend discontinuation for at least 24 hours prior to surgery (ACCF/AHA [Hillis, 2011]). The ACCF/AHA STEMI guidelines recommend discontinuation for at least 24 hours prior to *on-pump* CABG if possible; *off-pump* CABG may be performed within 24 hours of clopidogrel administration if the benefits of prompt revascularization outweigh the risks of bleeding (ACCF/AHA [O'Gara, 2013]).

Because of structural similarities, cross-reactivity has been reported among the thienopyridines (clopidogrel, prasugrel, and ticlopidine); use with caution or avoid in patients with hypersensitivity or hematologic reactions to previous thienopyridine use. Use of clopidogrel is contraindicated in patients with hypersensitivity to clopidogrel, although desensitization may be considered for mild-to-moderate hypersensitivity.

Use caution in concurrent treatment with anticoagulants (eg, heparin, warfarin) or other antiplatelet drugs; bleeding risk is increased. Concurrent use with drugs known to inhibit CYP2C19 (eg, proton pump inhibitors) may reduce levels of active metabolite and subsequently reduce clinical efficacy and increase the risk of cardiovascular events; if possible, avoid concurrent use of moderate-to-strong CYP2C19 inhibitors. In patients requiring antacid therapy, consider use of an acid-reducing agent lacking (eg, ranitidine/famotidine) or with less CYP2C19 inhibition. According to the manufacturer, avoid concurrent use of omeprazole (even when scheduled 12 hours apart) or esomeprazole; if a PPI is necessary, the use of an agent with comparatively less effect on the antiplatelet activity of clopidogrel is recommended. Of the PPIs, pantoprazole has the lowest degree of CYP2C19 inhibition *in vitro* (Li, 2004) and has been shown to have has less effect on conversion of clopidogrel to its active metabolite compared to omeprazole (Angiolillo, 2011). Although lansoprazole exhibits the most potent CYP2C19 inhibition *in vitro* (Li, 2004; Ogilvie, 2012), an *in vivo* study of extensive CYP2C19 metabolizers showed less reduction of the active metabolite of clopidogrel by lansoprazole/dexlansoprazole compared to esomeprazole/omeprazole (Frelinger, 2012). Avoidance of rabeprazole appears prudent due to potent *in vitro* CYP2C19 inhibition and lack of sufficient comparative *in vivo* studies with other PPIs. In contrast to these warnings, others have recommended the continued use of PPIs, regardless of the degree of inhibition, in patients with multiple risk factors for GI bleeding who are also receiving clopidogrel since no evidence has established clinically meaningful differences in outcome; however, a clinically-significant interaction cannot be excluded in those who are poor metabolizers of clopidogrel. Staggering PPIs with clopidogrel is not recommended until further evidence is available (Abraham, 2010). Concurrent use of aspirin and clopidogrel is not recommended for secondary prevention of ischemic stroke or TIA in patients unable to take oral anticoagulants due to hemorrhagic risk (Furie, 2011).

Use with caution in patients with severe liver or renal disease (experience is limited). Cases of TTP (usually occurring within the first 2 weeks of therapy), resulting in some fatalities, have been reported; urgent plasmapheresis is required. Use in patients with severe hepatic impairment or cholestatic jaundice is contraindicated in the

Canadian labeling. Cases of TTP (usually occurring within the first 2 weeks of therapy), resulting in some fatalities, have been reported; urgent plasmapheresis is required. In patients with recent lacunar stroke (within 180 days), the use of clopidogrel in addition to aspirin did not significantly reduce the incidence of the primary outcome of stroke recurrence (any ischemic stroke or intracranial hemorrhage) compared to aspirin alone; the use of clopidogrel in addition to aspirin did however increase the risk of major hemorrhage and the rate of all-cause mortality (SPS3 Investigators, 2012).

Assess bleeding risk carefully prior to initiating therapy in patients with atrial fibrillation (Canadian labeling; not an approved use in U.S. labeling); in clinical trials, a significant increase in major bleeding events (including intracranial hemorrhage and fatal bleeding events) were observed in patients receiving clopidogrel plus aspirin versus aspirin alone. Vitamin K antagonist (VKA) therapy (in suitable patients) has demonstrated a greater benefit in stroke reduction than aspirin (with or without clopidogrel).

Adverse Reactions As with all drugs which may affect hemostasis, bleeding is associated with clopidogrel. Hemorrhage may occur at virtually any site. Risk is dependent on multiple variables, including the concurrent use of multiple agents which alter hemostasis and patient susceptibility.

Dermatologic: Pruritus, skin rash

Gastrointestinal: Gastrointestinal hemorrhage

Hematologic & oncologic: Hematoma, minor hemorrhage, major hemorrhage, purpura

Respiratory: Epistaxis

Rare but important or life-threatening: Abnormal hepatic function tests, acute hepatic failure, agranulocytosis, anaphylactoid reaction, angioedema, aplastic anemia, arthralgia, arthritis, bronchospasm, bullous rash, colitis (including ulcerative or lymphocytic), confusion, diarrhea, DRESS syndrome, duodenal ulcer, eczema, eosinophilic pneumonia, erythema multiforme, erythematous rash, exfoliative rash, fever, gastric ulcer, glomerulopathy, hallucination, headache, hemophilia A (acquired), hemophthalmos (including conjunctival and retinal), hemorrhagic stroke, hepatitis, hypersensitivity reaction, hypotension, increased serum creatinine, interstitial pneumonitis, intracranial hemorrhage, lichen planus, maculopapular rash, musculoskeletal bleeding, myalgia, pancreatitis, pancytopenia, pulmonary hemorrhage, respiratory tract hemorrhage, retroperitoneal hemorrhage, serum sickness, Stevens-Johnson syndrome, stomatitis, taste disorder, thrombotic thrombocytopenic purpura, toxic epidermal necrolysis, urticaria, vasculitis, wound hemorrhage

Drug Interactions

Metabolism/Transport Effects Substrate of CYP2C19 (major), CYP3A4 (minor); **Note:** Assignment of Major/Minor substrate status based on clinically relevant drug interaction potential; **Inhibits** CYP2B6 (moderate), CYP2C8 (strong), CYP2C9 (weak), SLCO1B1

Avoid Concomitant Use

Avoid concomitant use of Clopidogrel with any of the following: Amodiaquine; Dasabuvir; Enzalutamide; Esomeprazole; Omeprazole; Urokinase

Increased Effect/Toxicity

Clopidogrel may increase the levels/effects of: Agents with Antiplatelet Properties; Amodiaquine; Anticoagulants; Apixaban; BuPROPion; Collagenase (Systemic); CYP2B6 Substrates; CYP2C8 Substrates; Dabigatran Etexilate; Dasabuvir; Deoxycholic Acid; Enzalutamide; Ibritumomab; Obinutuzumab; Pioglitazone; Rivaroxaban; Rosuvastatin; Salicylates; Thrombolytic Agents; Tositumomab and Iodine I 131 Tositumomab; Treprostinil; Urokinase; Warfarin

The levels/effects of Clopidogrel may be increased by: Dasatinib; FluvoxaMINE; Glucosamine; Herbs (Anticoagulant/Antiplatelet Properties); Ibrutinib; Limaprost; Luliconazole; Multivitamins/Fluoride (with ADE); Multivitamins/Minerals (with ADEK, Folate, Iron); Multivitamins/Minerals (with AE, No Iron); Omega-3 Fatty Acids; Pentosan Polysulfate Sodium; Pentoxifylline; Prostacyclin Analogues; Rifamycin Derivatives; Tipranavir; Vitamin E

Decreased Effect

The levels/effects of Clopidogrel may be decreased by: Amiodarone; Calcium Channel Blockers; Cangrelor; CYP2C19 Inhibitors (Moderate); CYP2C19 Inhibitors (Strong); Dexlansoprazole; Esomeprazole; FluvoxaMINE; Grapefruit Juice; Lansoprazole; Macrolide Antibiotics; Morphine (Liposomal); Morphine (Systemic); Omeprazole; Pantoprazole; RABEprazole

Food Interactions Consumption of three 200 mL glasses of grapefruit juice a day may substantially reduce clopidogrel antiplatelet effects. Management: Avoid or minimize the consumption of grapefruit or grapefruit juice (Holmberg, 2013).

Storage/Stability Store at 25°C (77°F); excursions permitted to 15°C to 30°C (59°F to 86°F).

Mechanism of Action Clopidogrel requires *in vivo* biotransformation to an active thiol metabolite. The active metabolite irreversibly blocks the $P2Y_{12}$ component of ADP receptors on the platelet surface, which prevents activation of the GPIIb/IIIa receptor complex, thereby reducing platelet aggregation. Platelets blocked by clopidogrel are affected for the remainder of their lifespan (~7-10 days).

Pharmacodynamics

Onset of action: Inhibition of platelet aggregation: Detected 2 hours after single oral dose

Maximum effect: Inhibition of platelet aggregation: 3-7 days; average inhibition level at steady-state in adults after receiving 75 mg/day: 40% to 60%.

Duration: Platelet aggregation and bleeding time gradually return to baseline after ~5 days after discontinuation.

Pharmacokinetics (Adult data unless noted)

Absorption: Rapid

Protein binding: Clopidogrel: 98%; main circulating metabolite (carboxylic acid derivative; inactive): 94%

Metabolism: Extensively hepatic via esterase-mediated hydrolysis to a carboxylic acid derivative (inactive) and via CYP450-mediated (CYP2C19 primarily) oxidation with a subsequent metabolism to a thiol metabolite (active).

Half-life: Parent drug: ~6 hours; thiol derivative (active metabolite): ~30 minutes; carboxylic acid derivative (inactive; main circulating metabolite): ~8 hours; **Note:** A clopidogrel radiolabeled study has shown that covalent binding to platelets accounts for 2% of radiolabel and has a half-life of 11 days

Time to peak serum concentration: ~0.75 hours

Elimination: Urine (50%) and feces (46%)

Dosing: Neonatal Antiplatelet effect: Limited data available: Oral: 0.2 mg/kg/dose once daily. A double-blind, placebo-controlled trial of 906 patients (n=461 neonates; n=445 infants ≤3 months) with cyanotic congenital heart disease surgically treated with a systemic-to-pulmonary artery shunt did not demonstrate a clinical benefit compared to placebo. Concomitant aspirin was used in 88% of patients (NCT00396877, 2011). In another trial, 0.2 mg/kg/dose once daily was found to achieve a mean inhibition of platelet aggregation similar to a standard adult dose; **Note:** This study (PICOLO Trial) included 73 evaluable patients [n=34 neonates (with exclusion of patients with weight <2 kg and GA <35 weeks); n=39 infants ≤24 months] with a systemic-to-pulmonary artery shunt, intracardiac or intravascular stent, Kawasaki disease, or arterial graft; 79% of patients received concomitant aspirin (Li 2008).

Dosing: Usual

Pediatric: **Antiplatelet effect:** Limited data available:

Infants and Children ≤24 months: In the PICOLO trial, a dose of 0.2 mg/kg/dose once daily was found to achieve a mean inhibition of platelet aggregation similar to adults receiving the recommended dose; **Note:** This study included pediatric patients with a systemic-to-pulmonary artery shunt, intracardiac or intravascular stent, Kawasaki disease, or arterial graft; 79% of patients received concomitant aspirin (Li 2008).

Children >2 years and Adolescents: Initial dose: 1 mg/kg once daily; titrate to response; in general, do not exceed adult dose (Finkelstein 2005; Soman 2006).

Adult:

Recent MI, recent stroke, or established peripheral arterial disease: 75 mg once daily

Acute coronary syndrome:

Unstable angina, non-ST-segment elevation myocardial infarction (UA/NSTEMI): Initial: 300 mg loading dose, followed by 75 mg once daily for at least 1 month and ideally up to 12 months (in combination with aspirin 75 to 162 mg once daily indefinitely) (Wright 2011)

ST-segment elevation acute myocardial infarction (STEMI): 75 mg once daily (in combination with aspirin 162 t 325 mg initially, followed by 81 to 162 mg/day); **Note:** The CLARITY-TIMI 28 study used a 300 mg loading dose of clopidogrel (with thrombolysis) demonstrating an improvement in the patency rate of the infarct-related artery and reduction in ischemic complications. The duration of therapy was <28 days (usually until hospital discharge) unless nonprimary percutaneous coronary intervention (PCI) was performed (Sabatine 2005).

The American College of Chest Physicians recommends (Goodman 2008):

Patients ≤75 years: Initial: 300 mg loading dose, followed by 75 mg once daily for up to 28 days (in combination with aspirin)

Patients >75 years: 75 mg once daily for up to 28 days (with or without thrombolysis)

Percutaneous coronary intervention (PCI) for UA/NSTEMI or STEMI: Loading dose: 300 to 600 mg (600 mg may be preferred for early invasive strategy with UA/NSTEMI) given as early as possible before or at the time of PCI followed by 75 mg once daily. **Note:** If an initial loading dose of 300 mg was given prior to PCI, a supplemental loading dose of 300 mg (total loading dose: 600 mg) may be administered (Kushner 2009). For patients with UA/NSTEMI, it has been recommended that the loading dose be given at least 2 hours (or 24 hours in patients unable to take aspirin) prior to PCI (*Chest* 2008).

Higher vs standard maintenance dosing: May consider a maintenance dose of 150 mg once daily for 6 days, then 75 mg once daily thereafter in patients not at high risk for bleeding (CURRENT-OASIS 7 Investigators 2010; Wright 2011); however, in another study, in patients with high on-treatment platelet reactivity, the use of 150 mg once daily for 6 months did not demonstrate a difference in 6-month incidence of death from cardiovascular causes, nonfatal MI, or stent thrombosis compared to standard dose therapy (Price 2011).

Duration of clopidogrel (in combination with aspirin) after stent placement: **Premature interruption of therapy may result in stent thrombosis with subsequent fatal and nonfatal MI.** With STEMI, clopidogrel for at least 12 months regardless of stent type (ie, either bare metal or drug eluting stent) is recommended (Kushner, 2009). With UA/NSTEMI, at least 12 months of clopidogrel is recommended in patients receiving a drug eluting stent (DES) unless the risk of bleeding outweighs the benefits. For bare metal stent (BMS) placement, at least 1 month and ideally up to 12 months duration is recommended unless the risk of bleeding outweighs the benefits; then, a minimum of 2 weeks is recommended (Wright, 2011). In either setting, a duration >15 months may be considered in patients with DES placement (Kushner 2009; Wright 2011). For patients without ongoing ACS, clopidogrel should be continued for at least 1 month (for BMS) or at least 12 months (for DES) (Becker 2008).

CYP2C19 poor metabolizers (ie, CYP2C19*2 or *3 carriers): Although routine genetic testing is not recommended in patients treated with clopidogrel undergoing PCI, testing may be considered to identify poor metabolizers who would be at risk for poor outcomes while receiving clopidogrel; if identified, these patients may be considered for an alternative P2Y12 inhibitor (Levine 2011). An appropriate regimen for this patient population has not been established in clinical outcome trials. Although the manufacturer suggests a 600 mg loading dose, followed by 150 mg once daily, it does not appear that this dosing strategy improves outcomes for this patient population (Price 2011).

Dosing adjustment in renal impairment: No dosage adjustment is required; use with caution; experience is limited; **Note:** Plasma concentrations of the main circulating metabolite were lower in adult patients with CrCl 5 to 15 mL/minute versus patients with CrCl 30 to 60 mL/minute or healthy adults. Inhibition of ADP-induced platelet aggregation was 25% lower compared to healthy adults; however, prolongation of bleeding time was similar.

Dosing adjustment in hepatic impairment: Use with caution; experience is limited; **Note:** Inhibition of ADP-induced platelet aggregation and mean bleeding time prolongation were similar in adult patients with severe hepatic impairment compared to healthy subjects after repeated doses of 75 mg once daily for 10 days.

Administration May be administered without regard to food.

Monitoring Parameters Signs of bleeding; hemoglobin and hematocrit periodically. Monitor mean inhibition of platelet aggregation: Goal of 30% to 50% inhibition (similar to adults receiving 75 mg/day). For unstable angina/non-ST-elevation MI in adults, platelet function testing has been used to determine platelet inhibitory response if results of testing may alter management (Wright, 2011).

Additional Information Overdose may lead to prolonged bleeding time with resultant bleeding complications; platelet transfusions may be an appropriate treatment when attempting to rapidly reverse the effects of clopidogrel

Dosage Forms Excipient information presented when available (limited, particularly for generics); consult specific product labeling.

Tablet, Oral:

Plavix: 75 mg, 300 mg

Generic: 75 mg, 300 mg

Extemporaneous Preparations A 5 mg/mL oral suspension may be made using tablets. Crush four 75 mg tablets and reduce to a fine powder. Add a small amount of a 1:1 mixture of Ora-Sweet® and Ora-Plus® and mix to a uniform paste; mix while adding the vehicle in geometric proportions to **almost** 60 mL; transfer to a calibrated bottle, rinse mortar with vehicle, and add quantity of vehicle sufficient to make 60 mL. Label "shake well". Stable 60 days at room temperature or under refrigeration.

Skillman KL, Caruthers RL, and Johnson CE, "Stability of an Extemporaneously Prepared Clopidogrel Oral Suspension," *Am J Health Syst Pharm*, 2010, 67(7):559-61.

◆ **Clopidogrel Bisulfate** *see* Clopidogrel *on page* 513

Clorazepate (klor AZ e pate)

Medication Safety Issues

Sound-alike/look-alike issues:

Clorazepate may be confused with clofibrate, clonazepam, KlonoPIN®

BEERS Criteria medication:

This drug may be potentially inappropriate for use in geriatric patients (Quality of evidence - high; Strength of recommendation - strong).

Brand Names: US Tranxene-T

Brand Names: Canada Apo-Clorazepate®; Novo-Clopate

Therapeutic Category Anticonvulsant, Benzodiazepine; Benzodiazepine; Sedative

Generic Availability (US) Yes

Use Adjunct anticonvulsant in the management of partial seizures (FDA approved in ages ≥9 years and adults); treatment of anxiety disorders (FDA approved in adults); management of alcohol withdrawal (FDA approved in adults)

Medication Guide Available Yes

Pregnancy Considerations Nordiazepam, the active metabolite of clorazepate, crosses the placenta and is measurable in cord blood and amniotic fluid. Teratogenic effects have been observed with some benzodiazepines (including clorazepate); however, additional studies are needed. The incidence of premature birth and low birth weights may be increased following maternal use of benzodiazepines; hypoglycemia and respiratory problems in the neonate may occur following exposure late in pregnancy. Neonatal withdrawal symptoms may occur within days to weeks after birth and "floppy infant syndrome" (which also includes withdrawal symptoms) has been reported with some benzodiazepines (Bergman, 1992; Iqbal, 2002; Patel,1980; Rey, 1979; Wikner, 2007). A combination of factors influences the potential teratogenicity of anticonvulsant therapy. When treating women with epilepsy, monotherapy with the lowest effective dose and avoidance medications known to have a high incidence of teratogenic effects is recommended (Harden, 2009; Wlodarczyk, 2012).

Patients exposed to clorazepate during pregnancy are encouraged to enroll themselves into the AED Pregnancy Registry by calling 1-888-233-2334. Additional information is available at www.aedpregnancyregistry.org.

Breast-Feeding Considerations Nordiazepam, the active metabolite of clorazepate, is found in breast milk and is measurable in the serum of breast-feeding infants. Drowsiness, lethargy, or weight loss in nursing infants have been observed in case reports following maternal use of some benzodiazepines (Iqbal, 2002; Rey, 1979). The manufacturer states that women taking clorazepate should not breast-feed their infants.

Contraindications Hypersensitivity to clorazepate or any component of the formulation (cross-sensitivity with other benzodiazepines may exist); narrow-angle glaucoma

Warnings/Precautions Antiepileptics are associated with an increased risk of suicidal behavior/thoughts with use (regardless of indication); patients should be monitored for signs/symptoms of depression, suicidal tendencies, and other unusual behavior changes during therapy and instructed to inform their healthcare provider immediately if symptoms occur.

Not recommended for use in patients <9 years of age or patients with depressive or psychotic disorders. Use with caution in elderly or debilitated patients, patients with hepatic disease (including alcoholics), or renal impairment. Active metabolites with extended half-lives may lead to delayed accumulation and adverse effects. Use with caution in patients with respiratory disease or impaired gag reflex. Avoid use in patients with sleep apnea.

Causes CNS depression (dose related) resulting in sedation, dizziness, confusion, or ataxia which may impair physical and mental capabilities. Patients must be cautioned about performing tasks which require mental alertness (eg, operating machinery or driving). Use with caution in patients receiving other CNS depressants or psychoactive agents. Effects with other sedative drugs or ethanol may be potentiated. Benzodiazepines have been associated with falls and traumatic injury and should be used with extreme caution in patients who are at risk of these events. In older adults, benzodiazepines increase the risk of impaired cognition, delirium, falls, fractures, and motor vehicle accidents. Due to increased sensitivity in this age group and slower metabolism of long-acting agents (such as clorazepate), avoid use for treatment of insomnia, agitation, or delirium (Beers Criteria).

Use caution in patients with depression, particularly if suicidal risk may be present. Use with caution in patients with a history of drug dependence. Benzodiazepines have been associated with dependence and acute withdrawal symptoms on discontinuation or reduction in dose. Acute withdrawal, including seizures, may be precipitated in patients after administration of flumazenil to patients receiving long-term benzodiazepine therapy. Clorazepate is a long half-life benzodiazepine. Tolerance develops to the anticonvulsant effects. It does not develop to the anxiolytic effects (Vinkers, 2012). Chronic use of this agent may increase the perioperative benzodiazepine dose needed to achieve desired effect.

Benzodiazepines have been associated with anterograde amnesia. Paradoxical reactions, including hyperactive or aggressive behavior, have been reported with benzodiazepines, particularly in adolescent/pediatric or psychiatric patients. Does not have analgesic, antidepressant, or antipsychotic properties.

Adverse Reactions

Cardiovascular: Hypotension

Central nervous system: Anxiety, ataxia, confusion, depression, dizziness, drowsiness, fatigue, headache, insomnia, irritability, lightheadedness, memory impairment, nervousness, slurred speech

Dermatologic: Rash

Endocrine & metabolic: Libido decreased

Gastrointestinal: Appetite increased/decreased, constipation, diarrhea, nausea, salivation decreased, vomiting, xerostomia

Hepatic: Jaundice, transaminase increased

Neuromuscular & skeletal: Dysarthria, tremor

Ocular: Blurred vision, diplopia

Drug Interactions

Metabolism/Transport Effects Substrate of CYP3A4 (major); **Note:** Assignment of Major/Minor substrate status based on clinically relevant drug interaction potential

Avoid Concomitant Use

Avoid concomitant use of Clorazepate with any of the following: Azelastine (Nasal); Conivaptan; Fusidic Acid (Systemic); Idelalisib; Methadone; OLANZapine; Orphenadrine; Paraldehyde; Sodium Oxybate; Thalidomide

Increased Effect/Toxicity

Clorazepate may increase the levels/effects of: Alcohol (Ethyl); Azelastine (Nasal); Buprenorphine; CloZAPine; CNS Depressants; Hydrocodone; Methadone; Methotrimeprazine; Metyrosine; Mirtazapine; Orphenadrine; Paraldehyde; Pramipexole; ROPINIRole; Rotigotine; Selective Serotonin Reuptake Inhibitors; Sodium Oxybate; Suvorexant; Thalidomide; Zolpidem

The levels/effects of Clorazepate may be increased by: Aprepitant; Brimonidine (Topical); Cannabis; Conivaptan; CYP3A4 Inhibitors (Moderate); CYP3A4 Inhibitors

(Strong); Dasatinib; Doxylamine; Dronabinol; Droperidol; Fosamprenavir; Fosaprepitant; Fusidic Acid (Systemic); HydrOXYzine; Idelalisib; Ivacaftor; Kava Kava; Luliconazole; Magnesium Sulfate; MAO Inhibitors; Methotrimeprazine; Mifepristone; Nabilone; Netupitant; OLANZapine; Palbociclib; Perampanel; Ritonavir; Rufinamide; Saquinavir; Simeprevir; Stiripentol; Tapentadol; Teduglutide; Tetrahydrocannabinol

Decreased Effect

The levels/effects of Clorazepate may be decreased by: Bosentan; CYP3A4 Inducers (Moderate); CYP3A4 Inducers (Strong); Dabrafenib; Deferasirox; Mitotane; Siltuximab; St Johns Wort; Theophylline Derivatives; Tocilizumab; Yohimbine

Food Interactions Serum concentrations/toxicity may be increased by grapefruit juice. Management: Keep grapefruit consumption consistent.

Storage/Stability Store at controlled room temperature at 20°C to 25°C (68°F to 77°F). Protect from moisture; keep bottle tightly closed; dispense in tightly closed, light-resistant container.

Mechanism of Action Binds to stereospecific benzodiazepine receptors on the postsynaptic GABA neuron at several sites within the central nervous system, including the limbic system, reticular formation. Enhancement of the inhibitory effect of GABA on neuronal excitability results by increased neuronal membrane permeability to chloride ions. This shift in chloride ions results in hyperpolarization (a less excitable state) and stabilization. Benzodiazepine receptors and effects appear to be linked to the GABA-A receptors. Benzodiazepines do not bind to GABA-B receptors.

Pharmacokinetics (Adult data unless noted)

Distribution: Crosses the placenta

Protein binding: Nordiazepam: 97% to 98%

Metabolism: Rapidly decarboxylated to desmethyldiazepam (nordiazepam; primary metabolite; active) in acidic stomach prior to absorption; hepatically to oxazepam (active)

Half-life:

Nordiazepam: 40-50 hours

Oxazepam: 6-8 hours

Time to peak serum concentration: Oral: Within 1 hour

Elimination: Primarily in urine (62% to 67% of dose); feces (15% to 19%); found in urine as conjugated oxazepam (3-hydroxynordiazepam) (major urinary metabolite) and conjugated p-hydroxynordiazepam and nordiazepam (smaller amounts)

Dosing: Usual Oral:

Anticonvulsant:

Children: Initial dose: 0.3 mg/kg/day; maintenance dose: 0.5-3 mg/kg/day divided 2-4 times/day

or

Children 9-12 years: Initial: 3.75-7.5 mg/dose twice daily; increase dose by 3.75 mg at weekly intervals, not to exceed 60 mg/day in 2-3 divided doses

Children >12 years and Adults: Initial: Up to 7.5 mg/dose 2-3 times/day; increase dose by 7.5 mg at weekly intervals; usual dose: 0.5-1 mg/kg/day; not to exceed 90 mg/day

Anxiety: Adults: 7.5-15 mg 2-4 times/day; usual daily dose: 30 mg/day in divided doses; range: 15-60 mg/day; may be given as single dose of 15 mg at bedtime, with subsequent dosage adjustments based on patient response

Alcohol withdrawal: Adults: Initial: 30 mg, then 15 mg 2-4 times/day on first day; maximum daily dose: 90 mg; gradually decrease dose over subsequent days

Administration Oral: May administer with food or water to decrease GI upset

Monitoring Parameters Excessive CNS depression, respiratory rate, and cardiovascular status; with prolonged use: CBC, liver enzymes, renal function; signs and symptoms of suicidality (eg, anxiety, depression, behavior changes)

Reference Range Therapeutic: 0.12-1 mcg/mL (SI: 0.36-3.01 micromoles/L)

Test Interactions Decreased hematocrit; abnormal liver and renal function tests

Controlled Substance C-IV

Dosage Forms Excipient information presented when available (limited, particularly for generics); consult specific product labeling.

Tablet, Oral, as dipotassium:

Tranxene-T: 3.75 mg [scored; contains fd&c blue #2 (indigotine)]

Tranxene-T: 7.5 mg [scored; contains fd&c yellow #6 (sunset yellow)]

Tranxene-T: 15 mg [scored]

Generic: 3.75 mg, 7.5 mg, 15 mg

◆ **Clorazepate Dipotassium** *see* Clorazepate *on page 516*

◆ **Clotrimaderm (Can)** *see* Clotrimazole (Topical) *on page 518*

◆ **Clotrimazole 3 Day [OTC]** *see* Clotrimazole (Topical) *on page 518*

Clotrimazole (Oral) (kloe TRIM a zole)

Medication Safety Issues

Sound-alike/look-alike issues:

Clotrimazole may be confused with co-trimoxazole

Mycelex may be confused with Myoflex

International issues:

Cloderm: Brand name for clotrimazole [Germany], but also brand name for alclomethasone [Indonesia]; clobetasol [China, India, Malaysia, Singapore, Thailand]; clocortolone [U.S., Canada]

Canesten [multiple international markets] may be confused with Canesten Bifonazol Comp brand name for bifonazole/urea [Austria]; Canesten Extra brand name for bifonazole [China, Germany]; Canesten Extra Nagelset brand name for bifonazole/urea [Denmark]; Canesten Fluconazole brand name for fluconazole [New Zealand]; Canesten Oasis brand name for sodium citrate [Great Britain]; Canesten Once Daily brand name for bifonazole [Australia]; Canesten Oral brand name for fluconazole [United Kingdom]; Cenestin brand name for estrogens (conjugated A/synthetic) [U.S., Canada]

Mycelex: Brand name for clotrimazole [U.S.] may be confused with Mucolex brand name for bromhexine [Malaysia]; carbocisteine [Thailand]

Therapeutic Category Antifungal Agent, Oral Nonabsorbed

Generic Availability (US) Yes

Use Treatment of susceptible fungal infections, including oropharyngeal candidiasis; limited data suggests that the use of clotrimazole troches may be effective for prophylaxis against oropharyngeal candidiasis in neutropenic patients

Pregnancy Risk Factor C

Pregnancy Considerations Adverse events have been observed in animal reproduction studies.

Breast-Feeding Considerations

It is not known if clotrimazole is excreted in breast milk following oral (troche) administration (data not located); however, systemic absorption is low (Sawyer 1975).

Contraindications

Hypersensitivity to clotrimazole or any component of the formulation

Documentation of allergenic cross-reactivity for antifungals is limited. However, because of similarities in chemical structure and/or pharmacologic actions, the possibility of cross-sensitivity can not be ruled out with certainty.

Warnings/Precautions Clotrimazole should not be used for treatment of systemic fungal infection. Abnormal LFTs have been reported, including abnormal aspartate aminotransferase (AST). Elevations are usually minimal. Monitor LFTs periodically, especially in patients with preexisting hepatic impairment. Clotrimazole must be slowly dissolved in the mouth for maximum efficacy. Potentially significant drug-drug interactions may exist, requiring dose or frequency adjustment, additional monitoring, and/or selection of alternative therapy.

Adverse Reactions

Dermatologic: Pruritus

Gastrointestinal: Nausea, vomiting

Hepatic: Abnormal liver function tests

Drug Interactions

Metabolism/Transport Effects **Inhibits** CYP1A2 (weak), CYP2A6 (weak), CYP2B6 (weak), CYP2C19 (weak), CYP2C8 (weak), CYP2C9 (weak), CYP2D6 (weak), CYP2E1 (weak), CYP3A4 (weak)

Avoid Concomitant Use

Avoid concomitant use of Clotrimazole (Oral) with any of the following: Amodiaquine; Pimozide

Increased Effect/Toxicity

Clotrimazole (Oral) may increase the levels/effects of: Amodiaquine; ARIPiprazole; Dofetilide; Hydrocodone; Lomitapide; NiMODipine; Pimozide; Tacrolimus (Systemic); TiZANidine

Decreased Effect There are no known significant interactions involving a decrease in effect.

Storage/Stability Store at 20°C to 25°C (68°F to 77°F). Avoid freezing.

Mechanism of Action Binds to phospholipids in the fungal cell membrane altering cell wall permeability resulting in loss of essential intracellular elements

Pharmacokinetics (Adult data unless noted) Distribution: Following oral administration, clotrimazole is present in saliva for up to 3 hours following 30 minutes of dissolution time in the mouth

Dosing: Usual Children >3 years and Adults: Oral: 10 mg troche dissolved slowly 5 times/day

Administration Dissolve lozenge (troche) in mouth over 15-30 minutes

Monitoring Parameters Periodic liver function tests

Dosage Forms Excipient information presented when available (limited, particularly for generics); consult specific product labeling.

Lozenge, Mouth/Throat:

Generic: 10 mg (70 ea, 140 ea)

Troche, Mouth/Throat:

Generic: 10 mg

Clotrimazole (Topical) (kloe TRIM a zole)

Medication Safety Issues

Sound-alike/look-alike issues:

Clotrimazole may be confused with co-trimoxazole

Lotrimin® may be confused with Lotrisone®

International issues:

Cloderm: Brand name for clotrimazole [Germany], but also brand name for alclomethasone [Indonesia]; clobetasol [China, India, Malaysia, Singapore, Thailand]; clocortolone [U.S., Canada]

Canesten: Brand name for clotrimazole [multiple international markets] may be confused with Canesten Bifonazol Comp brand name for bifonazole/urea [Austria]; Canesten Extra brand name for bifonazole [China, Germany]; Canesten Extra Nagelset brand name for bifonazole/urea [Denmark]; Canesten Fluconazole brand name for fluconazole [New Zealand]; Canesten Oasis brand name for sodium citrate [Great Britain]; Canesten Once Daily brand name for bifonazole [Australia]; Canesten Oral brand name for fluconazole [United Kingdom]; Cenestin® brand name for estrogens (conjugated A/synthetic) [U.S., Canada]

Brand Names: US Alevazol [OTC]; Clotrimazole 3 Day [OTC]; Clotrimazole Anti-Fungal [OTC]; Clotrimazole GRx [OTC]; Desenex [OTC]; Gyne-Lotrimin 3 [OTC]; Gyne-Lotrimin [OTC]; Lotrimin AF For Her [OTC]; Lotrimin AF [OTC]; Shopko Athletes Foot [OTC]

Brand Names: Canada Canesten® Topical; Canesten® Vaginal; Clotrimaderm; Trivagizole-3®

Therapeutic Category Antifungal Agent, Topical; Antifungal Agent, Vaginal

Generic Availability (US) Yes

Use Treatment of susceptible fungal infections, including dermatophytoses, superficial mycoses, cutaneous candidiasis, as well as vulvovaginal candidiasis

Pregnancy Considerations Following topical and vaginal administration, small amounts of imidazoles are absorbed systemically (Duhm, 1974). Vaginal products (7-day therapies) may be considered for the treatment of vulvovaginal candidiasis in pregnant women. This product may weaken latex condoms and diaphragms (CDC, 2010).

Contraindications Hypersensitivity to clotrimazole or any component of the formulation

Warnings/Precautions Avoid contact with eyes.

Benzyl alcohol and derivatives: Some dosage forms may contain benzyl alcohol; large amounts of benzyl alcohol (≥99 mg/kg/day) have been associated with a potentially fatal toxicity ("gasping syndrome") in neonates; the "gasping syndrome" consists of metabolic acidosis, respiratory distress, gasping respirations, CNS dysfunction (including convulsions, intracranial hemorrhage), hypotension and cardiovascular collapse (AAP, 1997; CDC, 1982); some data suggests that benzoate displaces bilirubin from protein binding sites (Ahlfors, 2001); avoid or use dosage forms containing benzyl alcohol with caution in neonates. See manufacturer's labeling.

Adverse Reactions

Vaginal: Genitourinary: Vulvovaginal burning

Rare but important or life-threatening: Burning sensation of the penis (of sexual partner), polyuria, pruritus vulvae, vaginal discharge, vulvar pain, vulvar swelling

Drug Interactions

Metabolism/Transport Effects None known.

Avoid Concomitant Use

Avoid concomitant use of Clotrimazole (Topical) with any of the following: Progesterone

Increased Effect/Toxicity

Clotrimazole (Topical) may increase the levels/effects of: Sirolimus; Tacrolimus (Systemic)

Decreased Effect

Clotrimazole (Topical) may decrease the levels/effects of: Progesterone

Mechanism of Action Binds to phospholipids in the fungal cell membrane altering cell wall permeability resulting in loss of essential intracellular elements

Pharmacokinetics (Adult data unless noted) Absorption: Negligible through intact skin when administered topically; 3% to 10% of an intravaginal dose is absorbed

Dosing: Usual

Children >3 years and Adults: Topical: Apply twice daily

Children >12 years and Adults: Vaginal: 5 g (=1 applicatorful) of vaginal cream daily at bedtime for 3 days (2% vaginal cream) or 7 days (1% vaginal cream)

Administration

Topical: Apply sparingly and rub gently into the cleansed, affected area and surrounding skin; do not apply to the eye.

Vaginal: Wash hands before using. Insert full applicator into vagina gently and expel cream into vagina. Wash applicator with soap and water following use. Remain lying down for 30 minutes following administration.

Dosage Forms Excipient information presented when available (limited, particularly for generics); consult specific product labeling.

Cream, External:

Clotrimazole Anti-Fungal: 1% (14.17 g, 28.35 g) [contains benzyl alcohol, cetyl alcohol]

Clotrimazole GRx: 1% (14 g) [contains benzyl alcohol, cetyl alcohol, polysorbate 80]

Desenex: 1% (15 g, 30 g)

Lotrimin AF: 1% (12 g, 24 g)

Lotrimin AF For Her: 1% (24 g)

Shopko Athletes Foot: 1% (28.4 g) [contains benzyl alcohol, cetostearyl alcohol]

Generic: 1% (15 g, 30 g, 45 g)

Cream, Vaginal:

Clotrimazole 3 Day: 2% (22.2 g)

Gyne-Lotrimin: 1% (45 g) [contains benzyl alcohol]

Gyne-Lotrimin 3: 2% (21 g) [contains benzyl alcohol, cetyl alcohol]

Generic: 1% (45 g)

Ointment, External:

Alevazol: 1% (56.7 g)

Solution, External:

Generic: 1% (10 mL, 30 mL)

◆ **Clotrimazole Anti-Fungal [OTC]** *see* Clotrimazole (Topical) *on page 518*

◆ **Clotrimazole GRx [OTC]** *see* Clotrimazole (Topical) *on page 518*

CloZAPine (KLOE za peen)

Medication Safety Issues

Sound-alike/look-alike issues:

CloZAPine may be confused with clonazePAM, cloNIDine, KlonoPIN

Clozaril may be confused with Clinoril, Colazal

BEERS Criteria medication:

This drug may be potentially inappropriate for use in geriatric patients (Quality of evidence - moderate; Strength of recommendation - strong).

Brand Names: US Clozaril; FazaClo; Versacloz

Brand Names: Canada Apo-Clozapine; Clozaril; Gen-Clozapine

Therapeutic Category Antipsychotic Agent; Second Generation (Atypical) Antipsychotic

Generic Availability (US) May be product dependent

Use Treatment of refractory schizophrenia (FDA approved in adults); to reduce the risk of recurrent suicidal behavior in schizophrenia or schizoaffective disorder (FDA approved in adults)

Prescribing and Access Restrictions

U.S.: Versacloz has a REMS program; Clozaril is deemed to have a REMS program (approval pending from FDA). As a requirement of the REMS program, access to this medication is restricted. Patient-specific registration is required to dispense clozapine. Information specific to each monitoring program is available from the individual manufacturers. If a patient is switched from one brand/manufacturer of clozapine to another, the patient must be entered into a new registry (must be completed by the prescriber and delivered to the dispensing pharmacy). Healthcare providers, including pharmacists dispensing clozapine, should verify the patient's hematological status and qualification to receive clozapine with all existing registries. The manufacturers of clozapine request that health care providers submit all WBC/ANC values following discontinuation of therapy to the registry for all nonrechallengable patients until WBC is ≥3,500/mm^3 and ANC is ≥2,000/mm^3. Further information is available at 1-888-669-6682 (Novartis Pharmaceuticals), 1-877-329-2256 (Jazz Pharmaceuticals), or at the following websites:

Clozaril: http://www.clozarilregistry.com

Fazaclo: https://www.fazacloregistry.com

Versacloz: http://www.versaclozregistry.com

Canada: Currently, there are multiple manufacturers that distribute clozapine and each manufacturer has its own registry and distribution system. Patients must be registered in a database that includes their location, prescribing physician, testing laboratory, and dispensing pharmacist before using clozapine. Information specific to each monitoring program is available from the individual manufacturers.

Pregnancy Risk Factor B

Pregnancy Considerations Adverse events were not observed in animal reproduction studies. Clozapine crosses the placenta and can be detected in the fetal blood and amniotic fluid (Barnas, 1994). Antipsychotic use during the third trimester of pregnancy has a risk for abnormal muscle movements (extrapyramidal symptoms [EPS]) and/or withdrawal symptoms in newborns following delivery. Symptoms in the newborn may include agitation, feeding disorder, hypertonia, hypotonia, respiratory distress, somnolence, and tremor; these effects may be self-limiting or require hospitalization.

Clozapine may theoretically cause agranulocytosis in the fetus and should not routinely be used in pregnancy (NICE, 2007). The American College of Obstetricians and Gynecologists recommends that therapy during pregnancy be individualized; treatment with psychiatric medications during pregnancy should incorporate the clinical expertise of the mental health clinician, obstetrician, primary healthcare provider, and pediatrician. Safety data related to atypical antipsychotics during pregnancy is limited and routine use is not recommended. However, if a woman is inadvertently exposed to an atypical antipsychotic while pregnant, continuing therapy may be preferable to switching to a typical antipsychotic that the fetus has not yet been exposed to; consider risk:benefit (ACOG, 2008). An increased risk of exacerbation of psychosis should be considered when discontinuing or changing treatment during pregnancy and postpartum.

Healthcare providers are encouraged to enroll women 18 to 45 years of age exposed to clozapine during pregnancy in the Atypical Antipsychotics Pregnancy Registry (1-866-961-2388 or http://www.womensmentalhealth.org/pregnancyregistry).

Women with amenorrhea associated with use of other antipsychotic agents may return to normal menstruation when switching to clozapine therapy. Reliable ▶

contraceptive measures should be employed by women of childbearing potential switching to clozapine therapy.

Breast-Feeding Considerations Clozapine was found to accumulate in breast milk in concentrations higher than the maternal plasma (Barnas, 1994). Breast-feeding is not recommended by the manufacturer. Clozapine may theoretically cause agranulocytosis in the nursing infant and should not routinely be used in women who are breast-feeding (NICE, 2007).

Contraindications

Hypersensitivity to clozapine or any component of the formulation (eg, photosensitivity, vasculitis, erythema multiforme, or Stevens-Johnson syndrome [SJS]); history of clozapine-induced agranulocytosis or severe granulocytopenia

Canadian labeling: Additional contraindications (not in U.S. labeling): Myeloproliferative disorders; history of toxic or idiosyncratic agranulocytosis or severe granulocytopenia (unless due to previous chemotherapy); concomitant use with other agents that suppress bone marrow function; active hepatic disease associated with nausea, anorexia, or jaundice; progressive hepatic disease or hepatic failure; paralytic ileus; uncontrolled epilepsy; severe CNS depression or comatose states; severe renal impairment; severe cardiac disease (eg, myocarditis); patients unable to undergo blood testing

Warnings/Precautions **[U.S. Boxed Warning]: Significant risk of potentially life-threatening agranulocytosis, defined as an ANC <500/mm^3. Monitor ANC and WBC prior to and during treatment. ANC must be ≥2,000/mm^3 and WBC must be ≥3,500/mm^3 to begin treatment. Discontinue clozapine and do not rechallenge if ANC <1,000/mm^3 or WBC is <2,000/mm^3. Monitor for symptoms of agranulocytosis and infection (eg, fever, weakness, lethargy, or sore throat). Clozapine is only available through a restricted program requiring enrollment of prescribers, patients, and pharmacies to the Registry.** Do not initiate in patients with a history of clozapine-induced agranulocytosis or granulocytopenia. Reported cases occurred most often in the first 2 to 3 months of therapy. Patients who have developed agranulocytosis or leukopenia are at an increased risk of subsequent episodes. Concurrent use with bone marrow suppressive agents or treatments also leads to an increased risk. The restricted distribution system ensures appropriate WBC and ANC monitoring. Eosinophilia, defined as a blood eosinophil count of >700/mm^3, has been reported to occur with clozapine and usually occurs within the first month of treatment. If eosinophilia develops, evaluate for signs or symptoms of systemic reactions (eg, rash or other allergic symptoms), myocarditis, or organ-specific disease. If systemic disease is suspected, discontinue clozapine immediately. If an eosinophilia cause unrelated to clozapine is identified treat the underlying cause and continue clozapine. In the absence of organ involvement continue clozapine under careful monitoring. If the total eosinophil count continues to increase over several weeks in the absence of systemic disease, base interruption of treatment and rechallenge (after eosinophil count decreases) on overall clinical assessment and consultation with internist or hematologist (**Note:** The Canadian labeling recommends discontinuing therapy for eosinophil count >3,000/mm^3; may resume therapy when eosinophil count <1,000/mm^3).

[U.S. Boxed Warning]: Elderly patients with dementia-related psychosis treated with antipsychotics are at an increased risk of death compared to placebo. Most deaths appeared to be either cardiovascular (eg, heart failure, sudden death) or infectious (eg, pneumonia) in nature. Clozapine is not approved for the treatment of dementia-related psychosis. Avoid antipsychotic use for behavioral problems associated with dementia unless alternative nonpharmacologic therapies have failed and patient may harm self or others. May also be inappropriate in older adults depending on comorbidities (eg, dementia, delirium) due to its potent anticholinergic effects (Beers Criteria). The elderly are more susceptible to adverse effects (including agranulocytosis, cardiovascular, anticholinergic, and tardive dyskinesia). An increased incidence of cerebrovascular effects (eg, transient ischemic attack, stroke), including fatalities, has been reported in placebo-controlled trials of atypical antipsychotics in elderly patients with dementia-related psychosis.

May cause CNS depression, which may impair physical or mental abilities; patients must be cautioned about performing tasks that require mental alertness (eg, operating machinery or driving); use caution in patients receiving general anesthesia. **[U.S. Boxed Warning]: Seizures have been associated with clozapine use in a dose-dependent manner. Initiate treatment with no more than 12.5 mg, titrate gradually using divided dosing. Use with caution in patients at risk of seizures, including those with a history of seizures, head trauma, brain damage, alcoholism, or concurrent therapy with medications which may lower seizure threshold. Patients should be warned that a sudden loss of consciousness may occur with seizures.** Benign transient temperature elevation (>100.4°F) may occur; peaking within the first 3 weeks of treatment. May be associated with an increase or decrease in WBC count. Rule out infection, agranulocytosis, and neuroleptic malignant syndrome (NMS) in patients presenting with fever. However, clozapine may also be associated with severe febrile reactions, including neuroleptic malignant syndrome (NMS). Impaired core body temperature regulation may occur; caution with strenuous exercise, heat exposure, dehydration, and concomitant medication possessing anticholinergic effects (Kerwin, 2004; Safferman, 1991). Clozapine's potential for extrapyramidal symptoms (including tardive dyskinesia) appears to be extremely low. Risk of dystonia (and probably other EPS) may be greater with increased doses, use of conventional antipsychotics, males, and younger patients.

[U.S. Boxed Warning]: Fatalities due to myocarditis and cardiomyopathy have been reported. Upon suspicion of these reactions discontinue clozapine and obtain a cardiac evaluation. Symptoms may include chest pain, tachycardia, palpitations, dyspnea, fever, flu-like symptoms, hypotension, or ECG changes. Patients with Clozaril-related myocarditis or cardiomyopathy should generally not be rechallenged with clozapine. Myocarditis and cardiomyopathy may occur at any period during clozapine treatment, however, typically myocarditis presents within the first 2 months and cardiomyopathy after 8 weeks of treatment. Cases of thromboembolism, including pulmonary embolism and stroke resulting in fatalities, have been associated with clozapine. Clozapine is associated with QT prolongation and ventricular arrhythmias including torsade de pointes; cardiac arrest and sudden death may occur. Use caution in patients with conditions that may increase the risk of QT prolongation, including history of QT prolongation, long QT syndrome, family history of long QT syndrome or sudden cardiac death, significant cardiac arrhythmia, recent myocardial infarction, uncompensated heart failure, treatment with other medications that cause QT prolongation, treatment with medications that inhibit the metabolism of clozapine, hypokalemia, and hypomagnesemia. Consider obtaining a baseline ECG and serum chemistry panel. Correct electrolyte abnormalities prior to initiating therapy. Discontinue clozapine if QTc interval >500 msec. Undesirable changes in lipids have been observed with antipsychotic therapy; incidence varies with product. Periodically monitor total serum cholesterol, triglycerides, LDL, and HDL concentrations.

Potentially significant drug-drug interactions may exist, requiring dose or frequency adjustment, additional monitoring, and/or selection of alternative therapy. Use caution when converting from brand to generic formulation; poor tolerability, including relapse, has been reported usually soon after product switch (1 to 3 months); monitor closely during this time (Bobo, 2010).

May cause anticholinergic effects; use with caution in patients with urinary retention, benign prostatic hyperplasia, narrow-angle glaucoma, xerostomia, visual problems, constipation, or history of bowel obstruction. Because of its potential to significantly decreased GI motility, use is associated with increased risk of paralytic ileus, bowel obstruction, fecal impaction, bowel perforation, and in rare cases death. Bowel regimens and monitoring are recommended. Sialorrhea and drooling may occur with clozapine use; symptoms may be more profound during sleep and may be dose-related. As a result of excessive saliva, patients may initially experience choking sensations that cause nighttime awakening, hoarseness or dysphonia of the voice, and a chronic cough. Skin irritation and infections, aspiration pneumonia, chronic sleep disturbances with daytime fatigue and somnolence, painful swelling of the salivary glands, and symptomatic aerophagia with resultant gas bloating, pain, and flatus may also develop. May cause hyperglycemia; in some cases may be extreme and associated with ketoacidosis, hyperosmolar coma, or death. In some cases, hyperglycemia resolved after discontinuation of the antipsychotic; however, some patients have required continuation of antidiabetic treatment. Monitor for symptoms of hyperglycemia including polydipsia, polyuria, polyphagia, and weakness. Use with caution in patients with diabetes or other disorders of glucose regulation; monitor for worsening of glucose control. Antipsychotic use has been associated with esophageal dysmotility and aspiration; use with caution in patients at risk of aspiration pneumonia (eg, Alzheimer disease). Use with caution in patients with hepatic disease or impairment; monitor hepatic function regularly. Hepatitis has been reported as a consequence of therapy. Use with caution in patients with renal disease.

Use caution with cardiovascular or pulmonary disease; gradually increase dose. **[U.S. Boxed Warning]: Orthostatic hypotension, bradycardia, syncope, and cardiac arrest have been reported with clozapine treatment. Risk is highest during the initial titration period and with rapid dose increases. Symptoms can develop with the first dose and with doses as low as 12.5 mg per day. Initiate treatment with no more than 12.5 mg once daily or twice daily, titrate slowly, and use divided doses. Use with caution in patients at risk for these effects (eg, cerebrovascular disease, cardiovascular disease) or with predisposing conditions for hypotensive episodes (eg, hypovolemia, concurrent antihypertensive medication);** reactions can be fatal. Consider dose reduction if hypotension occurs. May cause tachycardia; tachycardia is not limited to a reflex response to orthostatic hypotension.

The possibility of a suicide attempt is inherent in psychotic illness or bipolar disorder; use caution in high-risk patients during initiation of therapy. Prescriptions should be written for the smallest quantity consistent with good patient care. Medication should not be stopped abruptly; taper off over 1 to 2 weeks. If conditions warrant abrupt discontinuation (eg, leukopenia, myocarditis, cardiomyopathy), monitor patient for psychosis and cholinergic rebound (eg, headache, nausea, vomiting, diarrhea, profuse diaphoresis). Significant weight gain has been observed with antipsychotic therapy; incidence varies with product. Monitor waist circumference and BMI. Clozapine levels may be lower in patients who smoke. Smokers may require twice the daily dose as nonsmokers in order to obtain an equivalent clozapine concentration (Tsuda, 2014). Smoking cessation may cause toxicity in a patient stabilized on clozapine. Monitor change in smoking. Consider baseline serum clozapine levels and/or empiric dosage adjustments (30% to 40% reduction) in patients expected to have a prolonged hospital stay with forced smoking cessation. Case reports suggest symptoms from increasing clozapine concentrations may develop 2 to 4 weeks after smoking cessation (Lowe 2010). Clozapine concentrations may be increased in CYP2D6 poor metabolizers; dose reduction may be necessary. FazaClo oral disintegrating tablets contain phenylalanine.

Warnings: Additional Pediatric Considerations All of the serious adverse effects have also been reported in children and adolescents. Children and adolescents may be more sensitive to neutropenia compared to adults (Sporn, 2007); patients should be carefully monitored and counseled to report mouth sores, flu-like symptoms, or weakness. Incidence of extrapyramidal symptoms, including pseudoparkinsonism, acute dystonic reactions, akathisia may be as high as 15% in children and adolescents (Sporn, 2007).

Adverse Reactions

Cardiovascular: Angina pectoris, ECG changes, hyper-/hypotension, syncope, tachycardia

Central nervous system: Agitation, akathisia, akinesia, anxiety, ataxia, confusion, depression, dizziness, drowsiness, fatigue, headache, insomnia, lethargy, myoclonic seizures, nightmares, pain, restlessness, seizure, slurred speech

Dermatologic: Skin rash

Gastrointestinal: Abdominal discomfort, anorexia, constipation, diarrhea, heartburn, nausea, sialorrhea, sore throat, vomiting, weight gain, xerostomia

Genitourinary: Genitourinary complaint (abnormal ejaculation, retention, urgency, incontinence)

Hematologic: Leukopenia

Hepatic: Abnormal hepatic function tests

Neuromuscular & skeletal: Hyper-/hypokinesia, muscle rigidity, muscle spasm, tremor, weakness

Ocular: Visual disturbances

Respiratory: Dyspnea, nasal congestion

Miscellaneous: Diaphoresis, numbness of tongue

Rare but important or life-threatening: Abnormal electrocephalogram, agranulocytosis, amnesia, anemia, aspiration, bronchitis, cardiac failure, cataplexy, cerebrovascular accident, cholestasis, colitis, deep vein thrombosis, delirium, dermatitis, difficult micturition, dyschromia, edema, eosinophilia, erythema multiforme, fecal impaction, gastric ulcer, gastroenteritis, granulocytopenia, hallucinations, hematemesis, hepatotoxicity, hyperglycemia, hyperosmolar coma, hypersensitivity reaction, hyperuricemia, hypothermia, impotence, increased erythrocyte sedimentation rate, liver steatosis, lower respiratory tract infection, mental retardation, mitral valve insufficiency, myasthenia syndrome, mydriasis, myocarditis, myoclonus, neuroleptic malignant syndrome, obsessive compulsive disorder, orthostatic hypotension, pancreatitis (acute), paralytic ileus, parkinsonian like-syndrome, pheochromocytoma (pseudo), pericardial effusion, pericarditis, periorbital edema, phlebitis, pleural effusion, priapism, prolonged QT interval on ECG, psychosis exacerbated, pulmonary embolism, rectal hemorrhage, renal failure, respiratory arrest, rhabdomyolysis, sialadentitis, sepsis, skin photosensitivity, speech disturbance, status epilepticus, Stevens-Johnson syndrome, syncope, systemic lupus erythematosus, tardive dyskinesia, thrombocytopenia, thrombocytosis, thrombophlebitis, torsade de pointes, weight loss

Drug Interactions

Metabolism/Transport Effects Substrate of CYP1A2 (major), CYP2A6 (minor), CYP2C19 (minor), CYP2C9 (minor), CYP2D6 (minor), CYP3A4 (minor); **Note:** Assignment of Major/Minor substrate status based on clinically relevant drug interaction potential; **Inhibits** CYP1A2 (weak), CYP2C19 (weak), CYP2C9 (weak), CYP2D6 (moderate), CYP2E1 (weak)

Avoid Concomitant Use

Avoid concomitant use of CloZAPine with any of the following: Aclidinium; Amisulpride; Azelastine (Nasal); CarBAMazepine; Ciprofloxacin (Systemic); CYP3A4 Inducers (Strong); Eluxadoline; Glucagon; Highest Risk QTc-Prolonging Agents; Ipratropium (Oral Inhalation); Ivabradine; Metoclopramide; Mifepristone; Myelosuppressive Agents; Orphenadrine; Paraldehyde; Potassium Chloride; St Johns Wort; Sulpiride; Thalidomide; Thioridazine; Tiotropium; Umeclidinium

Increased Effect/Toxicity

CloZAPine may increase the levels/effects of: AbobotulinumtoxinA; Alcohol (Ethyl); Amisulpride; Analgesics (Opioid); Anticholinergic Agents; ARIPiprazole; Azelastine (Nasal); Buprenorphine; CNS Depressants; CYP2D6 Substrates; Eluxadoline; Fesoterodine; Glucagon; Highest Risk QTc-Prolonging Agents; Hydrocodone; Mequitazine; Methotrimeprazine; Methylphenidate; Metoprolol; Metyrosine; Mirabegron; Mirtazapine; Moderate Risk QTc-Prolonging Agents; Nebivolol; OnabotulinumtoxinA; Orphenadrine; Paraldehyde; Potassium Chloride; RimabotulinumtoxinB; Serotonin Modulators; Sulpiride; Suvorexant; Thalidomide; Thiazide Diuretics; Thioridazine; Tiotropium; TiZANidine; Topiramate; Zolpidem

The levels/effects of CloZAPine may be increased by: Abiraterone Acetate; Acetylcholinesterase Inhibitors (Central); Aclidinium; Benzodiazepines; Brimonidine (Topical); Cannabis; CarBAMazepine; Cimetidine; Ciprofloxacin (Systemic); CYP1A2 Inhibitors (Moderate); CYP1A2 Inhibitors (Strong); Deferasirox; Doxylamine; Dronabinol; Droperidol; HydrOXYzine; Ipratropium (Oral Inhalation); Ivabradine; Kava Kava; Lithium; Macrolide Antibiotics; Magnesium Sulfate; MAO Inhibitors; Methotrimeprazine; Methylphenidate; Metoclopramide; Metyrosine; Mianserin; Mifepristone; Myelosuppressive Agents; Nabilone; Nefazodone; Omeprazole; Perampanel; Pramlintide; QTc-Prolonging Agents (Indeterminate Risk and Risk Modifying); Rufinamide; Selective Serotonin Reuptake Inhibitors; Serotonin Modulators; Sodium Oxybate; Tapentadol; Tetrahydrocannabinol; Umeclidinium

Decreased Effect

CloZAPine may decrease the levels/effects of: Acetylcholinesterase Inhibitors; Amphetamines; Antidiabetic Agents; Anti-Parkinson's Agents (Dopamine Agonist); Codeine; Itopride; Quinagolide; Secretin; Tamoxifen; TraMADol

The levels/effects of CloZAPine may be decreased by: Acetylcholinesterase Inhibitors; Cannabis; CarBAMazepine; CYP3A4 Inducers (Strong); Cyproterone; Lithium; Omeprazole; St Johns Wort; Teriflunomide

Storage/Stability

Suspension: Store at ≤25°C (77°F). Protect from light. Do not refrigerate or freeze. Suspension is stable for 100 days after initial bottle opening.

Tablet: Store at ≤30°C (86°F).

Tablet, dispersible: Store at 20°C to 25°C (68°F to 77°F); excursions permitted to 15°C to 30°C (59°F to 86°F). Protect from moisture; do not remove from package until ready to use.

Mechanism of Action The therapeutic efficacy of clozapine (dibenzodiazepine antipsychotic) is proposed to be mediated through antagonism of the dopamine type 2 (D_2) and serotonin type 2A ($5\text{-}HT_{2A}$) receptors. In addition, it acts as an antagonist at alpha-adrenergic, histamine H_1, cholinergic, and other dopaminergic and serotonergic receptors.

Pharmacodynamics

Onset of action: Within 1 week for sedation, improvement in sleep; 6-12 weeks for antipsychotic effects

Adequate trial: 6-12 weeks at a therapeutic dose and blood level

Maximum effect: 6-12 months; improvement may continue 6-12 months after clozapine initiation (Meltzer, 2003)

Duration: Variable

Pharmacokinetics (Adult data unless noted)

Protein binding: 97% to serum proteins

Metabolism: Extensively hepatic; forms metabolites with limited (desmethyl metabolite) or no activity (hydroxylated and N-oxide derivative derivatives). **Note:** A pediatric pharmacokinetic study (n=6; age: 9-16 years) found higher concentrations of the desmethyl metabolite in comparison to clozapine (especially in females) when compared to data from adult studies; the authors suggest that both the parent drug and desmethyl metabolite contribute to the efficacy and adverse effect profile in children and adolescents (Frazier, 2003).

Bioavailability: 12% to 81% (not affected by food); orally disintegrating tablets are bioequivalent to the regular tablets

Half-life: Steady state: 12 hours (range: 4-66 hours)

Time to peak serum concentration: Tablets: 2.5 hours (range: 1-6 hours); orally disintegrating tablets: 2.3 hours (range: 1-6 hours)

Elimination: Urine (~50% of dose) and feces (30%); trace amounts of unchanged drug excreted in urine and feces

Dosing: Usual

Children and Adolescents: **Treatment of refractory childhood-onset schizophrenia or schizoaffective disorder:** Limited data available: Oral: Initial: 12.5 mg once or twice daily; increase daily dose as tolerated every 3-5 days (usually by 25 mg increments) to a target dose of 125-475 mg/day in divided doses (based on patient's age, size, and tolerability). Mean dose in most pediatric studies: 175-200 mg/day (Findling, 2007)

Adults:

Refractory schizophrenia or schizoaffective disorder: Oral: Initial: 12.5 mg once or twice daily; increase as tolerated, in increments of 25-50 mg/day to a target dose of 300-450 mg/day after 2-4 weeks; may increase further if needed, but no more than once or twice weekly, in increments ≤100 mg/day; some patients may require doses as high as 600-900 mg/day in divided doses. Do not exceed 900 mg/day. In some efficacy studies, total daily dosage was administered in three divided doses. **Note:** Due to significant adverse effects, patients who fail to adequately respond clinically, should not be normally continued on therapy for an extended period of time; responding patients should be maintained on the lowest effective dose; patients should be periodically assessed to determine if maintenance treatment is still required.

Reduction of the risk of suicidal behavior in schizophrenia or schizoaffective disorder: Oral: Initial: 12.5 mg once or twice daily; increased, as tolerated, in increments of 25-50 mg/day to a target dose of 300-450 mg/day after 2-4-weeks; may increase further if needed, but no more than once or twice weekly, in increments ≤100 mg/day; mean effective dose is ~300 mg/day (range: 12.5-900 mg). **Note:** A treatment course of at least 2 years is recommended to maintain the decreased risk for suicidal behavior; patients should be reassessed after 2 years for risk of suicidal behavior and periodically thereafter.

Termination of therapy: If dosing is interrupted for ≥48 hours, therapy must be reinitiated at 12.5-25 mg/day; if tolerated, the dose may be increased more rapidly than with initial titration, unless cardiopulmonary arrest occurred during initial titration.

In the event of planned termination of clozapine, gradual reduction in dose over a 1- to 2-week period is recommended. If conditions warrant abrupt discontinuation (eg, leukopenia, eosinophilia), monitor patient for psychosis and cholinergic rebound (headache, nausea, vomiting, diarrhea).

Dosing adjustment for toxicity: Adults: Oral:

Eosinophilia: Interrupt therapy for eosinophil count >4000/mm^3; may resume therapy when eosinophil count <3000/mm^3

Moderate leukopenia or granulocytopenia (WBC 2000-3000/mm^3 and/or ANC 1000-1500/mm^3): Discontinue therapy; may rechallenge patient when WBC is >3500/mm^3 and ANC is >2000/mm^3. **Note:** Patient is at greater risk for developing agranulocytosis.

Severe leukopenia or granulocytopenia (WBC <2000/mm^3 and/or ANC <1000/mm^3): Discontinue therapy and do not rechallenge patient.

Dosing adjustment in renal impairment: There are no dosage adjustments provided in manufacturer's labeling (has not been studied); use with caution.

Dosing adjustment in hepatic impairment: There are no dosage adjustments provided in manufacturer's labeling (has not been studied); use with caution.

Administration May be administered without regard to food.

Orally-disintegrating tablet: Should be removed from foil blister by peeling apart (do not push tablet through the foil). Remove immediately prior to use. Place tablet in mouth and allow to dissolve; swallow with saliva (no water is needed to take the dose). If dosing requires splitting tablet, throw unused portion away.

Monitoring Parameters Mental status, ECG, CBC (see below), liver function tests, vital signs, fasting lipid profile, and fasting blood glucose/Hgb A_{1c} (prior to treatment, at 3 months, then annually, or as symptoms warrant); height, weight, BMI, personal/family history of obesity, waist circumference (weight should be assessed prior to treatment, at 4 weeks, 8 weeks, 12 weeks, and then at quarterly intervals; consider titrating to a different antipsychotic agent for a weight gain ≥5% of the initial weight); blood pressure, pulse, abnormal involuntary movement scale (AIMS).

WBC and ANC should be obtained at baseline and at least weekly for the first 6 months of continuous treatment. If counts remain acceptable (WBC ≥3500/mm^3, ANC ≥2000/mm^3) during this time period, then they may be monitored every other week for the next 6 months. If WBC/ANC continue to remain within these acceptable limits after the second 6 months of therapy, monitoring can be decreased to every 4 weeks. If clozapine is discontinued, a weekly WBC should be conducted for an additional 4 weeks or until WBC is ≥3500/mm^3 and ANC is ≥2000/mm^3. If clozapine therapy is interrupted due to moderate leukopenia, weekly WBC/ANC monitoring is required for 12 months in patients restarted on clozapine treatment. If therapy is interrupted for reasons other than leukopenia/granulocytopenia, the 6-month time period for initiation of biweekly WBCs may need to be reset. This determination depends upon the treatment duration, the length of the break in therapy, and whether or not an abnormal blood event occurred. Consult manufacturer prescribing information for determination of appropriate WBC/ANC monitoring interval.

Interrupt therapy for eosinophil count >4000/mm^3; may resume therapy when eosinophil count <3000/mm^3.

Additional Information Clozapine produces little or no prolactin elevation; this is in contrast to other more typical antipsychotic drugs

Dosage Forms Excipient information presented when available (limited, particularly for generics); consult specific product labeling.

Suspension, Oral:

Versacloz: 50 mg/mL (100 mL) [contains methylparaben sodium, propylparaben sodium]

Tablet, Oral:

Clozaril: 25 mg, 100 mg [scored]

Generic: 25 mg, 50 mg, 100 mg, 200 mg

Tablet Dispersible, Oral:

FazaClo: 12.5 mg, 25 mg, 100 mg, 150 mg, 200 mg [contains aspartame]

◆ **Clozaril** *see* CloZAPine *on page 519*

◆ **4CMenB** *see* Meningococcal Group B Vaccine *on page 1351*

◆ **CMV Hyperimmune Globulin** *see* Cytomegalovirus Immune Globulin (Intravenous-Human) *on page 570*

◆ **CMV-IGIV** *see* Cytomegalovirus Immune Globulin (Intravenous-Human) *on page 570*

◆ **CNL8 Nail** *see* Ciclopirox *on page 458*

◆ **Coagulant Complex Inhibitor** *see* Anti-inhibitor Coagulant Complex (Human) *on page 176*

◆ **Coagulation Factor VIIa** *see* Factor VIIa (Recombinant) *on page 835*

Coal Tar (KOLE tar)

Medication Safety Issues

International issues:

Pentrax [U.S., Canada, Great Britain, Ireland] may be confused with Permax brand name for pergolide [multiple international markets]

Brand Names: US Balnetar [OTC]; Beta Care Betatar Gel [OTC]; Cutar [OTC]; DHS Tar Gel [OTC]; DHS Tar [OTC]; Elta Lite Tar [OTC]; Elta Tar [OTC]; Ionil-T [OTC]; Neutrogena T/Gel Conditioner [OTC]; Neutrogena T/Gel Ex St [OTC]; PC-Tar [OTC]; Pentrax Gold [OTC]; Polytar [OTC]; Psoriasin [OTC]; Scytera [OTC]; Tera-Gel Tar [OTC]; Therapeutic [OTC]; Theraplex T [OTC]; X-Seb T Pearl [OTC]; X-Seb T Plus [OTC]

Brand Names: Canada Doak Oil Forte [OTC]; Doak Oil [OTC]; Emorex Gel [OTC]; Neuotrogena T/Gel Therapeutic Shampoo [OTC]; Odans Liquor Carbonis Detergens [OTC]; Pentrax Gold Shampoo [OTC]; Pentrax Tar Shampoo [OTC]; Psoriasin [OTC]; T/Gel Therapeutic Shampoo Extra Strength [OTC]; Targel® [OTC]; Tersa Tar Shp [OTC]

Therapeutic Category Antipsoriatic Agent, Topical; Antiseborrheic Agent, Topical

Generic Availability (US) May be product dependent

Use Topically for controlling dandruff, seborrheic dermatitis, or psoriasis

Pregnancy Considerations Limited application of coal tar during pregnancy for the treatment of psoriasis appears to be safe in pregnant women (Gelmetti, 2009; Landau, 2011).

Breast-Feeding Considerations A case report describes the absorption of the components of a coal tar containing ointment by a nursing infant. The components were not detected in breast milk, but were assumed to be absorbed by the infant following skin-to-skin contact with the mother while nursing. If coal tar is used in a nursing mother, direct contact by the infant should be avoided (Scheepers, 2009).

Contraindications Hypersensitivity to coal tar or any component of the formulation

Warnings/Precautions For external use only; avoid contact with eyes, genital/rectal areas. May increase photosensitivity; avoid exposure to direct sunlight for 24 hours following application.

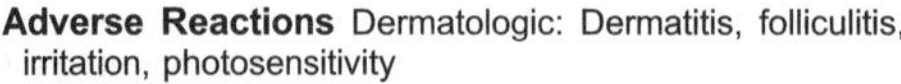

Adverse Reactions Dermatologic: Dermatitis, folliculitis, irritation, photosensitivity

Drug Interactions

Metabolism/Transport Effects None known.

Avoid Concomitant Use There are no known interactions where it is recommended to avoid concomitant use.

Increased Effect/Toxicity There are no known significant interactions involving an increase in effect.

Decreased Effect There are no known significant interactions involving a decrease in effect.

Dosing: Usual Children and Adults: Topical:

Bath: 60-90 mL of a 5% to 20% solution or 15-25 mL of 30% lotion is added to bath water; soak 5-20 minutes, then pat dry; use once daily to once every 3 days

Shampoo: Apply twice weekly for the first 2 weeks then once weekly or more often if needed

Skin: Apply to the affected area 1-4 times/day; decrease frequency to 2-3 times/week once condition has been controlled

Atopic dermatitis: 2% to 5% coal tar cream may be applied once daily or every other day to reduce inflammation

Scalp psoriasis: Tar oil bath or coal tar solution may be painted sparingly to the lesions 3-12 hours before each shampoo

Psoriasis of the body, arms, legs: Apply at bedtime; if thick scales are present, use product with salicylic acid and apply several times during the day

Administration Topical:

Bath: Add appropriate amount of coal tar to lukewarm bath water and mix thoroughly

Shampoo: Rub shampoo onto wet hair and scalp, rinse thoroughly; repeat; leave on 5 minutes; rinse thoroughly

Dosage Forms Excipient information presented when available (limited, particularly for generics); consult specific product labeling.

Bar, External:
- Polytar: Coal tar 0.5% (1 ea)

Cream, External:
- Elta Tar: 2% (107 g)

Emulsion, External:
- Balnetar: 2.5% (221 mL)

Foam, External:
- Scytera: 2% (100 g) [contains disodium edta]

Liquid, External:
- Neutrogena T/Gel Conditioner: 0.5% (130 mL)

Lotion, External:
- Elta Lite Tar: 10% (236 mL)

Oil, External:
- Cutar: 7.5% (177 mL, 3785 mL) [contains methylparaben, polysorbate 80, propylparaben]

Ointment, External:
- Psoriasin: 2% (113 g) [contains alcohol, usp, polysorbate 80]

Shampoo, External:
- Beta Care Betatar Gel: 2.5% (480 mL) [contains trolamine (triethanolamine)]
- DHS Tar: 0.5% (120 mL, 240 mL)
- DHS Tar: 0.5% (120 mL, 240 mL) [fragrance free]
- DHS Tar Gel: 0.5% (240 mL)
- Ionil-T: 1% (473 mL) [contains alcohol, usp, benzalkonium chloride, edetate sodium (tetrasodium), isopropyl alcohol]
- Neutrogena T/Gel Ex St: 1% (177 mL) [contains methylparaben, propylparaben]
- PC-Tar: 1% (177 mL)
- Pentrax Gold: 4% (168 mL)
- Polytar: Coal tar 0.5% (177 mL) [contains alcohol, usp, polysorbate 80, trolamine (triethanolamine)]
- Tera-Gel Tar: 0.5% (118 mL, 235 mL) [contains edetate sodium (tetrasodium), methylparaben, polysorbate 80, propylparaben]
- Therapeutic: 0.5% (251 mL)
- Theraplex T: 1% (240 mL)
- X-Seb T Pearl: 10% (236 mL) [contains brilliant blue fcf (fd&c blue #1), edetate disodium]
- X-Seb T Plus: 10% (236 mL) [contains brilliant blue fcf (fd&c blue #1), edetate disodium]

Solution, External:
- Generic: 20% (100 mL, 500 mL, 4000 mL)

- ◆ **Co-Amoxiclav** *see* Amoxicillin and Clavulanate *on page 141*
- ◆ **Coartem** *see* Artemether and Lumefantrine *on page 200*
- ◆ **CO Atenolol (Can)** *see* Atenolol *on page 215*

Cocaine (koe KANE)

Therapeutic Category Analgesic, Topical; Local Anesthetic, Topical

Generic Availability (US) Yes

Use Topical anesthesia for mucous membranes of the oral, laryngeal, and nasal cavities (FDA approved in children and adults); has also been used for its vasoconstrictive properties in nasal surgery

Pregnancy Risk Factor C

Pregnancy Considerations Animal reproduction studies have not been conducted with this product. Cocaine rapidly crosses the placenta in concentrations equal to those in the mother. Adverse events occur in the fetus (eg, congenital malformations, growth restriction), infant (neonatal abstinence syndrome), and mother (eg, preterm labor, placental abruption) following maternal abuse (Fajemirokun-Odudeyi, 2004).

Breast-Feeding Considerations Cocaine rapidly enters breast milk. Irritability, hypertension, tachypnea, tachycardia, and tremors have been reported in nursing infants (Chasnoff, 1987).

Contraindications Hypersensitivity to cocaine or any component of the formulation

Warnings/Precautions For topical use only. Limit to office and surgical procedures only. Not for ophthalmic use; causes sloughing of the corneal epithelium. Resuscitative equipment and drugs should be immediately available when any local anesthetic is used. Debilitated, elderly patients, acutely ill patients, and children should be given reduced doses consistent with their age and physical status. Use caution in patients with severely traumatized mucosa and sepsis in the region of the proposed application. Use with caution in patients with cardiovascular disease or a history of cocaine abuse. In patients being treated for cardiovascular complication of cocaine abuse, avoid beta-blockers for treatment. Consider anesthesia safe in a cocaine-abusing patient requiring surgery when obvious signs of intoxication are not exhibited (Hill 2006).

Adverse Reactions

Cardiovascular: Arrhythmias (ventricular), cardiac arrhythmia, cardiomyopathy, cerebral vasculitis, CHF, decreased heart rate (low doses), fibrillation (atrial), flutter (atrial), hypertension, myocarditis, pulmonary hypertension, QRS prolongation, Raynaud's phenomenon, sinus bradycardia, sinus tachycardia, tachycardia (moderate doses) tachycardia (supraventricular), thrombosis, vasoconstriction

Central nervous system: Agitation, cerebral vascular accident, clonic-tonic reactions, CNS stimulation, dystonic reactions, euphoria, excitation, fever, hallucinations, headache, hyperthermia, nervousness, paranoia, psychosis, restlessness, seizure, slurred speech, sympathetic storm, vasculitis

Dermatologic: Madarosis, pruritus, skin infarction

Gastrointestinal: Anorexia, colonic ischemia, loss of taste perception, nausea, spontaneous bowel perforation

Genitourinary: Priapism, uterine rupture

Hematologic: Thrombocytopenia

Neuromuscular & skeletal: Chorea (extrapyramidal), fasciculations, paresthesia, tremor
Ocular: Chemosis, iritis, Mydriasis (peak effect at 45 minutes; may last up to 12 hours), sloughing of the corneal epithelium, ulceration of the cornea
Renal: Myoglobinuria, necrotizing vasculitis
Respiratory: Bronchiolitis obliterans organizing pneumonia, hyposmia, nasal congestion, nasal mucosa damage (when snorting), rhinitis, tachypnea
Miscellaneous: Loss of smell, "washed-out" syndrome

Drug Interactions

Metabolism/Transport Effects **Substrate** of CYP3A4 (major); **Note:** Assignment of Major/Minor substrate status based on clinically relevant drug interaction potential; **Inhibits** CYP2D6 (strong)

Avoid Concomitant Use

Avoid concomitant use of Cocaine with any of the following: Conivaptan; Fusidic Acid (Systemic); Idelalisib; Iobenguane I 123; Mequitazine; Pimozide; Tamoxifen; Thioridazine

Increased Effect/Toxicity

Cocaine may increase the levels/effects of: ARIPiprazole; AtoMOXetine; Cannabinoid-Containing Products; CYP2D6 Substrates; DOXOrubicin (Conventional); Eliglustat; Fesoterodine; Iloperidone; Mequitazine; Metoprolol; Nebivolol; Pimozide; Propafenone; Sympathomimetics; Tamsulosin; Tetrabenazine; Thioridazine; TraMADol; Vortioxetine

The levels/effects of Cocaine may be increased by: Aprepitant; Conivaptan; CYP3A4 Inhibitors (Moderate); CYP3A4 Inhibitors (Strong); Dasatinib; Fosaprepitant; Fusidic Acid (Systemic); Idelalisib; Ivacaftor; Linezolid; Luliconazole; Mifepristone; Netupitant; Palbociclib; Simeprevir; Stiripentol; Tedizolid

Decreased Effect

Cocaine may decrease the levels/effects of: Codeine; Hydrocodone; Iloperidone; Iobenguane I 123; Tamoxifen; TraMADol

Storage/Stability Store at 20°C to 25°C (68°F to 77°F); do not freeze.

Mechanism of Action Ester local anesthetic blocks both the initiation and conduction of nerve impulses by decreasing the neuronal membrane's permeability to sodium ions, which results in inhibition of depolarization with resultant blockade of conduction; interferes with the uptake of norepinephrine by adrenergic nerve terminals producing vasoconstriction

Pharmacodynamics Following topical administration to mucosa:
Onset of action: Within 1 minute
Maximum effect: Within 5 minutes
Duration: ≥30 minutes, depending upon route and dosage administered.

Pharmacokinetics (Adult data unless noted)
Absorption: Well absorbed through mucous membranes; ~35% absorbed when applied intranasally with cottonoid pledget (Liao, 1999); absorption is limited by drug-induced vasoconstriction and enhanced by inflammation
Distribution: V_d: ~2 L/kg
Metabolism: Hepatic; major metabolites are ecgonine methyl ester and benzoyl ecgonine
Half-life: 75 minutes
Elimination: Primarily in urine as metabolites and unchanged drug (<10%); cocaine metabolites may appear in the urine of neonates for up to 5 days after birth due to maternal cocaine use shortly before birth

Dosing: Usual Children, Adolescents, and Adults: Topical:
Topical anesthetic: Concentrations of 1% to 4% are used; use lowest effective dose; consider reduced dosages in children, elderly and debilitated patients; dose depends on patient tolerance, anesthetic technique, vascularity of tissue, and area to be anesthetized. Solutions >4% are not recommended due to increased risk and severity of systemic toxicities; maximum total dose: Children: 1-2 mg/kg/dose; Adolescents and Adults: 2-3 mg/kg **or** 200 mg, whichever is lower (Liao, 1999: McGee, 2010).

Administration Topical: Use only on mucous membranes of the oral, laryngeal, and nasal cavities; do not use on extensive areas of broken skin; do not apply commercially available products to the eye

Monitoring Parameters Heart rate, blood pressure, respiratory rate, temperature

Controlled Substance C-II

Dosage Forms Excipient information presented when available (limited, particularly for generics); consult specific product labeling.
Solution, External, as hydrochloride:
Generic: 4% (4 mL, 10 mL); 10% (4 mL)

- ◆ **Cocaine Hydrochloride** *see* Cocaine *on page* 524
- ◆ **CO Candesartan (Can)** *see* Candesartan *on page* 358
- ◆ **CO Clomipramine (Can)** *see* ClomiPRAMINE *on page* 502
- ◆ **CO Clonazepam (Can)** *see* ClonazePAM *on page* 506
- ◆ **CO Clopidogrel (Can)** *see* Clopidogrel *on page* 513
- ◆ **Codar GF** *see* Guaifenesin and Codeine *on page* 990

Codeine (KOE deen)

Medication Safety Issues

Sound-alike/look-alike issues:
Codeine may be confused with Cardene, Cordran, iodine, Lodine

High alert medication:
The Institute for Safe Medication Practices (ISMP) includes this medication among its list of drug classes which have a heightened risk of causing significant patient harm when used in error.

Related Information
Opioid Conversion Table *on page* 2285

Brand Names: Canada Codeine Contin; PMS-Codeine; ratio-Codeine

Therapeutic Category Analgesic, Narcotic; Antitussive; Cough Preparation

Generic Availability (US) Yes

Use Treatment of mild to moderate pain where the use of an opioid is appropriate (FDA approved in adults)

Medication Guide Available Yes

Pregnancy Risk Factor C

Pregnancy Considerations Adverse events have been observed in animal reproduction studies. Opioid analgesics cross the placenta. In humans, birth defects (including some heart defects) have been associated with maternal use of codeine during the first trimester of pregnancy (Broussard 2011). If chronic opioid exposure occurs in pregnancy, adverse events in the newborn (including withdrawal) may occur; monitoring of the neonate is recommended. The minimum effective dose should be used if opioids are needed (Chou 2009). Neonatal abstinence syndrome following opioid exposure may present with autonomic (eg, fever, temperature instability), gastrointestinal (eg, diarrhea, vomiting, poor feeding/weight gain), or neurologic (eg, high pitched crying, increased muscle tone, irritability, seizure, tremor) symptoms (Dow 2012; Hudak 2012).

Breast-Feeding Considerations Codeine and its metabolite (morphine) are found in breast milk and can be detected in the serum of nursing infants. The relative dose to a nursing infant has been calculated to be ~1% of the weight-adjusted maternal dose (Spigset 2000). Higher levels of morphine may be found in the breast milk of lactating mothers who are "ultrarapid metabolizers" of codeine; patients with two or more copies of the variant

CYP2D6*2 allele may have extensive conversion to morphine and thus increased opioid-mediated effects. In one case, excessively high serum concentrations of morphine were reported in a breast-fed infant following maternal use of acetaminophen with codeine. The mother was later found to be an "ultrarapid metabolizer" of codeine; symptoms in the infant included feeding difficulty and lethargy, followed by death. Caution should be used since most persons are not aware if they have the genotype resulting in "ultra-rapid metabolizer" status. When codeine is used in breast-feeding women, it is recommended to use the lowest dose for the shortest duration of time and observe the infant for increased sleepiness, difficulty in feeding or breathing, or limpness (FDA 2007; Koren 2006). The US labeling recommends that caution be used if administered to a nursing woman. Codeine Contin [Canadian product] is contraindicated in nursing women. According to other guidelines, when treatment is needed for pain in nursing women, other agents should be used; if codeine cannot be avoided it should not be used for >4 days (Kahan 2011; Wong 2011).

Contraindications

Hypersensitivity to codeine or any component of the formulation; respiratory depression in the absence of resuscitative equipment; acute or severe bronchial asthma or hypercarbia; presence or suspicion of paralytic ileus; postoperative pain management in children who have undergone tonsillectomy and/or adenoidectomy

Canadian labeling: Additional contraindications (not in US labeling): Hypersensitivity to other opioid analgesics; cor pulmonale; acute alcoholism; delirium tremens; severe CNS depression; convulsive disorders; increased cerebrospinal or intracranial pressure; head injury; obstructive airway disease (in addition to asthma); known or suspected mechanical GI obstruction or any disease that affects bowel transit; suspected surgical abdomen (eg, acute appendicitis or pancreatitis); use with or within 14 days of MAO inhibitors; pregnancy and during labor and delivery; children <12 years of age; Additional product specific contraindications: Codeine Contin: acute pain; intermittent or short duration pain that can be managed with alternative pain medication; breast-feeding

Warnings/Precautions Note: Recommendations between US and Canadian labeling may vary (eg, use of codeine in certain patients/conditions may be contraindicated in the Canadian labeling only; refer to contraindications).

[US Boxed Warning]: Respiratory depression and death have occurred in children who received codeine following tonsillectomy and/or adenoidectomy and were found to have evidence of being ultra-rapid metabolizers of codeine due to a CYP2D6 polymorphism. Deaths have also occurred in nursing infants after being exposed to high concentrations of morphine because the mothers were ultra-rapid metabolizers. Use is contraindicated in the postoperative pain management of children who have undergone tonsillectomy and/or adenoidectomy. The Canadian labeling contraindicates use in children <12 years of age. Use caution in patients with two or more copies of the variant CYP2D6*2 allele; may have extensive conversion to morphine and thus increased opioid-mediated effects. Avoid the use of codeine in these patients; consider alternative analgesics such as morphine or a nonopioid agent (Crews 2012). The occurrence of this phenotype is seen in 0.5% to 1% of Chinese and Japanese, 0.5% to 1% of Hispanics, 1% to 10% of Caucasians, 3% of African-Americans, and 16% to 28% of North Africans, Ethiopians, and Arabs.

May cause dose-related respiratory depression. The risk is increased in elderly patients, debilitated patients, and patients with conditions associated with hypoxia, hypercapnia, or upper airway obstruction. Use with caution in patients with preexisting respiratory compromise (hypoxia), COPD or other obstructive pulmonary disease, and kyphoscoliosis or other skeletal disorder which may alter respiratory function; critical respiratory depression may occur, even at therapeutic dosages.

After chronic maternal exposure to opioids, neonatal withdrawal syndrome may occur in the newborn; monitor neonate closely. Signs and symptoms include irritability, hyperactivity and abnormal sleep pattern, high pitched cry, tremor, vomiting, diarrhea and failure to gain weight. Onset, duration and severity depend on the drug used, duration of use, maternal dose, and rate of drug elimination by the newborn. Opioid withdrawal syndrome in the neonate, unlike in adults, may be life-threatening and should be treated according to protocols developed by neonatology experts.

Use may cause or aggravate constipation; chronic use may result in obstructive bowel disease, particularly in those with underlying intestinal motility disorders. Constipation may also be problematic in patients with unstable angina or those patients post-myocardial infarction. Avoid use in patients with gastrointestinal obstruction, particularly paralytic ileus. May cause hypotension; use with caution in patients with hypovolemia, cardiovascular disease (including acute MI), or drugs which may exaggerate hypotensive effects (including phenothiazines or general anesthetics). May cause CNS depression, which may impair physical or mental abilities; patients must be cautioned about performing tasks which require mental alertness (eg, operating machinery or driving).

Use with extreme caution in patients with head injury, intracranial lesions, or elevated intracranial pressure; exaggerated elevation of ICP may occur. Use with caution in patients with hypersensitivity reactions to other phenanthrene-derivative opioid agonists (hydrocodone, hydromorphone, levorphanol, oxycodone, oxymorphone), adrenal insufficiency (including Addison's disease), biliary tract dysfunction, pancreatitis, thyroid dysfunction, morbid obesity, prostatic hyperplasia and/or urinary stricture, or severe hepatic or renal impairment. Use may obscure diagnosis or clinical course of patients with acute abdominal conditions. May induce or aggravate seizures; use with caution in patients with seizure disorders. Avoid use in patients with CNS depression or coma as these patients are susceptible to intracranial effects of CO_2 retention.

Use with caution in patients with a history of drug abuse or acute alcoholism; potential for drug dependency exists. Tolerance, psychological and physical dependence may occur with prolonged use. Potentially significant drug interactions may exist, requiring dose or frequency adjustment, additional monitoring, and/or selection of alternative therapy. Effects may be potentiated when used with other sedative drugs or ethanol. Concurrent use of agonist/antagonist analgesics may precipitate withdrawal symptoms and/or reduced analgesic efficacy in patients following prolonged therapy with mu opioid agonists. Abrupt discontinuation following prolonged use may also lead to withdrawal symptoms.

Some preparations contain sulfites which may cause allergic reactions. Healthcare provider should be alert to the potential for abuse, misuse, and diversion.

Warnings: Additional Pediatric Considerations In July 2015, the FDA announced that it would be further evaluating the risk of serious adverse effects of codeine-containing products to treat cough and colds in pediatric patients <18 years including slowed or difficulty breathing. In April 2015, the European Medicines Agency (EMA) stated that codeine-containing medicines should not be used in children <12 years, and use is not recommended in pediatric patients 12 to 18 years who have breathing problems including asthma or other chronic breathing problems (FDA 2015).

Adverse Reactions

Cardiovascular: Bradycardia, cardiac arrest, circulatory depression, flushing, hypertension, hypotension, palpitations, shock, syncope, tachycardia

Central nervous system: Abnormal dreams, agitation, anxiety, apprehension, ataxia, chills, depression, disorientation, dizziness, drowsiness, dysphoria, euphoria, fatigue, hallucination, headache, increased intracranial pressure, insomnia, nervousness, paresthesia, sedation, shakiness, taste disorder, vertigo

Dermatologic: Diaphoresis, pruritus, skin rash, urticaria

Gastrointestinal: Abdominal cramps, abdominal pain, anorexia, biliary tract spasm, constipation, diarrhea, nausea, pancreatitis, vomiting, xerostomia

Genitourinary: Urinary hesitancy, urinary retention

Hypersensitivity: Hypersensitivity reaction

Neuromuscular & skeletal: Laryngospasm, muscle rigidity, tremor, weakness

Ophthalmic: Blurred vision, diplopia, miosis, nystagmus, visual disturbance

Respiratory: Bronchospasm, dyspnea, respiratory arrest, respiratory depression

Rare, but important or life-threatening): Hypogonadism (Brennan, 2013; Debono, 2011)

Drug Interactions

Metabolism/Transport Effects **Substrate** of CYP2D6 (major); **Note:** Assignment of Major/Minor substrate status based on clinically relevant drug interaction potential

Avoid Concomitant Use

Avoid concomitant use of Codeine with any of the following: Azelastine (Nasal); Eluxadoline; Mixed Agonist / Antagonist Opioids; Orphenadrine; Paraldehyde; Thalidomide

Increased Effect/Toxicity

Codeine may increase the levels/effects of: Alcohol (Ethyl); Alvimopan; Azelastine (Nasal); CNS Depressants; Desmopressin; Diuretics; Eluxadoline; Hydrocodone; Methotrimeprazine; Metyrosine; Mirtazapine; Orphenadrine; Paraldehyde; Pramipexole; ROPINIRole; Rotigotine; Selective Serotonin Reuptake Inhibitors; Suvorexant; Thalidomide; Zolpidem

The levels/effects of Codeine may be increased by: Amphetamines; Anticholinergic Agents; Antipsychotic Agents (Phenothiazines); Brimonidine (Topical); Cannabis; Doxylamine; Dronabinol; Droperidol; HydrOXYzine; Kava Kava; Magnesium Sulfate; Methotrimeprazine; Nabilone; Perampanel; Rufinamide; Sodium Oxybate; Somatostatin Analogs; Succinylcholine; Tapentadol; Tetrahydrocannabinol

Decreased Effect

Codeine may decrease the levels/effects of: Pegvisomant

The levels/effects of Codeine may be decreased by: Ammonium Chloride; CYP2D6 Inhibitors (Moderate); CYP2D6 Inhibitors (Strong); Mixed Agonist / Antagonist Opioids; Naltrexone

Storage/Stability

Immediate release tablet, oral solution: Store at 15°C to 30°C (59°F to 86°F). Protect from moisture and light.

Controlled release tablet [Canadian product]: Store at 15°C to 30°C (59°F to 86°F).

Mechanism of Action Binds to opioid receptors in the CNS, causing inhibition of ascending pain pathways, altering the perception of and response to pain; causes cough suppression by direct central action in the medulla; produces generalized CNS depression

Pharmacodynamics

Onset of action: Oral: 30-60 minutes

Maximum effect: Oral: 60-90 minutes

Duration: 4-6 hours

Pharmacokinetics (Adult data unless noted)

Absorption: Oral: Adequate

Distribution: 3-6 L/kg

Protein binding: 7% to 25%

Metabolism: Hepatic via UGT2B7 and UGT2B4 to codeine-6-glucuronide, via CYP2D6 to morphine (active), and via CYP3A4 to norcodeine. Morphine is further metabolized via glucuronidation to morphine-3-glucuronide and morphine-6-glucuronide (active).

Bioavailability: 53%

Time to peak serum concentration: 1 hour

Half-life: 2.5-3.5 hours

Elimination: Urine (~90%, ~10% of the total dose as unchanged drug); feces

Dosing: Usual Doses should be titrated to appropriate analgesic effect; use the lowest effective dose for the shortest period of time:

Children and Adolescents: **Pain management; analgesia:** Limited data available: Oral: 0.5-1 mg/kg/dose every 4-6 hours as needed; maximum single dose: 60 mg (APS, 2008); **Note:** Do not use for postoperative tonsillectomy and/or adenoidectomy pain management.

Adults: **Pain management (analgesic):** Oral: Initial: 15-60 mg every 4 hours as needed; maximum total daily dose: 360 mg/**day**; patients with prior opioid exposure may require higher initial doses. **Note:** The American Pain Society recommends an initial dose of 30-60 mg for adults with moderate pain (American Pain Society, 2008).

Dosing adjustment in renal impairment:

Manufacturer's recommendations: Adults: There are no specific dosage adjustments provided in the manufacturer's labeling; however, clearance may be reduced; active metabolites may accumulate. Use with caution; initiate at lower doses or longer dosing intervals followed by careful titration.

Alternate recommendations: The following guidelines have been used by some clinicians (Aronoff, 2007):

Children and Adolescents:

GFR >50 mL/minute/1.73 m^2: No adjustment needed

GFR 10-50 mL/minute/1.73 m^2: Administer 75% of normal dose

GFR <10 mL/minute/1.73 m^2: Administer 50% of normal dose

Hemodialysis: Administer 50% of normal dose

Peritoneal dialysis (PD): Administer 50% of normal dose

CRRT: Administer 75% of normal dose

Adults:

CrCl >50 mL/minute: No adjustment needed

CrCl 10-50 mL/minute: Administer 75% of dose

CrCl <10 mL/minute: Administer 50% of dose

Dosing adjustment in hepatic impairment: Adults: There are no dosage adjustments provided in manufacturer's labeling (has not been studied); however, initial lower doses or longer dosing intervals followed by careful titration are recommended.

Administration Oral: Administer with food or water to decrease nausea and GI upset

Monitoring Parameters Respiratory rate, heart rate, blood pressure, pain relief, CNS status

Test Interactions Some quinolones may produce a false-positive urine screening result for opioids using commercially-available immunoassay kits. This has been demonstrated most consistently for levofloxacin and ofloxacin, but other quinolones have shown cross-reactivity in certain assay kits. Confirmation of positive opioid screens by more specific methods should be considered.

Controlled Substance C-II

Dosage Forms Excipient information presented when available (limited, particularly for generics); consult specific product labeling. [DSC] = Discontinued product

Solution, Oral, as sulfate:
Generic: 30 mg/5 mL (500 mL [DSC])
Tablet, Oral, as sulfate:
Generic: 15 mg, 30 mg, 60 mg

Extemporaneous Preparations A 3 mg/mL oral suspension may be made with codeine phosphate powder, USP. Add 600 mg of powder to a 400 mL beaker. Add 2.5 mL of Sterile Water for Irrigation, USP, and stir to dissolve the powder. Mix for 10 minutes while adding Ora-Sweet to make 200 mL; transfer to a calibrated bottle. Stable 98 days at room temperature.

Dentinger PJ and Swenson CF, "Stability of Codeine Phosphate in an Extemporaneously Compounded Syrup," *Am J Health Syst Pharm*, 2007, 64(24):2569-73.

- ◆ **Codeine and Acetaminophen** *see* Acetaminophen and Codeine *on page 50*
- ◆ **Codeine and Guaifenesin** *see* Guaifenesin and Codeine *on page 990*
- ◆ **Codeine and Promethazine** *see* Promethazine and Codeine *on page 1780*
- ◆ **Codeine Contin (Can)** *see* Codeine *on page 525*
- ◆ **Codeine, Phenylephrine, and Promethazine** *see* Promethazine, Phenylephrine, and Codeine *on page 1782*
- ◆ **Codeine Phosphate** *see* Codeine *on page 525*
- ◆ **Codeine Sulfate** *see* Codeine *on page 525*
- ◆ **Codulax [OTC] (Can)** *see* Bisacodyl *on page 289*
- ◆ **Coenzyme R** *see* Biotin *on page 289*
- ◆ **CO Famciclovir (Can)** *see* Famciclovir *on page 846*
- ◆ **Co-Fentanyl (Can)** *see* FentaNYL *on page 857*
- ◆ **CO Fluconazole (Can)** *see* Fluconazole *on page 881*
- ◆ **CO Fluoxetine (Can)** *see* FLUoxetine *on page 906*
- ◆ **CO Gabapentin (Can)** *see* Gabapentin *on page 954*
- ◆ **Cogentin** *see* Benztropine *on page 272*
- ◆ **Colace [OTC]** *see* Docusate *on page 697*
- ◆ **Colace Clear [OTC]** *see* Docusate *on page 697*
- ◆ **Colazal** *see* Balsalazide *on page 257*

Colchicine (KOL chi seen)

Medication Safety Issues

Sound-alike/look-alike issues:

Colchicine may be confused with Cortrosyn

Related Information

Safe Handling of Hazardous Drugs *on page 2455*

Brand Names: US Colcrys; Mitigare

Brand Names: Canada Jamp-Colchicine; PMS-Colchicine

Therapeutic Category Anti-inflammatory Agent; Antigout Agent

Generic Availability (US) Yes

Use Treatment of familial Mediterranean fever (FMF) (FDA approved in ages ≥4 years and adults); prevention and treatment of acute gout flares (FDA approved in ages >16 years and adults); has also been used for prophylaxis of pseudogout, management of Behçet's disease

Medication Guide Available Yes

Pregnancy Risk Factor C

Pregnancy Considerations Adverse events were observed in animal reproduction studies. Colchicine crosses the human placenta. Use during pregnancy in the treatment of familial Mediterranean fever has not shown an increase in miscarriage, stillbirth, or teratogenic effects (limited data).

Breast-Feeding Considerations Colchicine enters breast milk; exclusively breast-fed infants are expected to receive <10% of the weight-adjusted maternal dose (limited data). The manufacturer recommends that caution be used if administered to a nursing woman.

Contraindications Concomitant use of a P-glycoprotein (P-gp) or strong CYP3A4 inhibitor in presence of renal or hepatic impairment

Mitigare: Patients with both renal and hepatic impairment.

Canadian labeling: Additional contraindications (not in U.S. labeling): Hypersensitivity to colchicine; serious gastrointestinal, hepatic, renal, and cardiac disease

Warnings/Precautions Hazardous agent - use appropriate precautions for handling and disposal (NIOSH 2014 [group 3]). Myelosuppression (eg, thrombocytopenia, leukopenia, granulocytopenia, pancytopenia) and aplastic anemia have been reported in patients receiving therapeutic doses. Neuromuscular toxicity (including rhabdomyolysis) has been reported in patients receiving therapeutic doses; patients with renal dysfunction and elderly patients are at increased risk. Concomitant use of cyclosporine, diltiazem, verapamil, fibrates, and statins may increase the risk of myopathy. Clearance is decreased in renal or hepatic impairment; monitor closely for adverse effects/toxicity. Dosage adjustments may be required depending on degree of impairment or indication, and may be affected by the use of concurrent medication (CYP3A4 or P-gp inhibitors). Concurrent use of P-gp or strong CYP3A4 inhibitors is contraindicated in renal impairment; fatal toxicity has been reported. Colchicine is not an analgesic and should not be used to treat pain from other causes. Potentially significant interactions may exist, requiring dose or frequency adjustment, additional monitoring, and/or selection of alternative therapy.

Adverse Reactions

Central nervous system: Fatigue, headache

Endocrine & metabolic: Gout

Gastrointestinal: Abdominal cramps, abdominal pain, diarrhea, gastrointestinal disease, nausea, vomiting

Respiratory: Pharyngolaryngeal pain

Rare but important or life-threatening: Alopecia, bone marrow depression, dermatitis, disseminated intravascular coagulation, hepatotoxicity, hypersensitivity reaction, increased creatine phosphokinase, lactose intolerance, myalgia, myasthenia, oligospermia, purpura, rhabdomyolysis, toxic neuromuscular disease

Drug Interactions

Metabolism/Transport Effects Substrate of CYP3A4 (major), P-glycoprotein; **Note:** Assignment of Major/Minor substrate status based on clinically relevant drug interaction potential

Avoid Concomitant Use

Avoid concomitant use of Colchicine with any of the following: Conivaptan; Fusidic Acid (Systemic); Idelalisib

Increased Effect/Toxicity

Colchicine may increase the levels/effects of: HMG-CoA Reductase Inhibitors

The levels/effects of Colchicine may be increased by: Conivaptan; CYP3A4 Inhibitors (Moderate); CYP3A4 Inhibitors (Strong); Dasatinib; Digoxin; Fibric Acid Derivatives; Fosamprenavir; Fusidic Acid (Systemic); Idelalisib; Luliconazole; Mifepristone; Palbociclib; P-glycoprotein/ABCB1 Inhibitors; Stiripentol; Telaprevir; Tipranavir

Decreased Effect

Colchicine may decrease the levels/effects of: Choline C 11; Cyanocobalamin; Multivitamins/Fluoride (with ADE); Multivitamins/Minerals (with ADEK, Folate, Iron); Multivitamins/Minerals (with AE, No Iron)

The levels/effects of Colchicine may be decreased by: P-glycoprotein/ABCB1 Inducers

Food Interactions Grapefruit juice may increase colchicine serum concentrations. Management: Administer orally with water and maintain adequate fluid intake. Dose adjustment may be required based on indication if ingesting grapefruit juice. Avoid grapefruit juice with hepatic or renal impairment.

Storage/Stability Store at 20°C to 25°C (68°F to 77°F). Protect from light and moisture.

Mechanism of Action Disrupts cytoskeletal functions by inhibiting β-tubulin polymerization into microtubules, preventing activation, degranulation, and migration of neutrophils associated with mediating some gout symptoms. In familial Mediterranean fever, may interfere with intracellular assembly of the inflammasome complex present in neutrophils and monocytes that mediate activation of interleukin-1β.

Pharmacodynamics Onset of action: Oral: Relief of pain and inflammation occurs after 18-24 hours

Pharmacokinetics (Adult data unless noted)

Bioavailability: <50%

Distribution: Concentrates in leukocytes, kidney, spleen, and liver; distributes into breast milk; crosses the placenta; does not distribute in heart, skeletal muscle, and brain; V_d: 5-8 L/kg

Protein binding: 39%

Metabolism: Hepatic via CYP3A4; three metabolites (2 primary, 1 minor); partially deacetylated and demethylated

Half-life, elimination: 27-31 hours

Time to peak serum concentration: Oral: 1-2 hours (range: 0.5-3 hours)

Excretion: Urine (40% to 65% as unchanged drug), enterohepatic recirculation and biliary excretion also possible

Dialysis: Not dialyzable (0% to 5%)

Dosing: Usual Oral:

Prophylaxis of familial Mediterranean fever (FMF):

Children:

4-6 years: 0.3-1.8 mg/day in 1-2 divided doses

6-12 years: 0.9-1.8 mg/day in 1-2 divided doses

Adolescents >12 years and Adults: 1.2-2.4 mg/day in 1-2 divided doses; titration: Increase or decrease dose in 0.3 mg/day increments based on efficacy or adverse effects; maximum dose: 2.4 mg/day

Gout: Children >16 years and Adults:

Flare treatment: Initial: 1.2 mg at the first sign of flare, followed in 1 hour with a single dose of 0.6 mg (maximum dose: 1.8 mg over 1 hour); **Note:** Current FDA approved dose for gout flare is substantially lower than what has been used historically. Doses larger than the currently recommended dosage for gout flare have not been proven to be more effective. **Note:** Patients receiving prophylaxis treatment may receive treatment dosing; wait 12 hours before resuming prophylactic dose

Prophylaxis: 0.6 mg once or twice daily; maximum dose: 1.2 mg/day

Dosage adjustment for concomitant therapy with CYP3A4 or P-gp inhibitors: Dosage adjustment also required in patients receiving CYP3A4 or P-gp inhibitors up to 14 days prior to initiation of colchicine. **Note:** Treatment of gout flare with colchicine is not recommended in patients receiving prophylactic colchicine and CYP3A4 inhibitors. **Note:** Dosage adjustments may also apply to patients 12-18 years of age with FMF.

Coadministration of **strong** CYP3A4 inhibitor (eg, atazanavir, clarithromycin, indinavir, itraconazole, ketoconazole, nefazodone, nelfinavir, ritonavir, saquinavir, telithromycin):

FMF: Maximum dose: 0.6 mg/day **or** 0.3 mg twice daily

Gout prophylaxis:

If original dose is 0.6 mg twice daily, adjust dose to 0.3 mg once daily

If original dose is 0.6 mg once daily, adjust dose to 0.3 mg every other day

Gout flare treatment: Initial: 0.6 mg, followed in 1 hour by a single dose of 0.3 mg; wait at least 3 days to repeat

Coadministration of **moderate** CYP3A4 inhibitor (eg, amprenavir, aprepitant, diltiazem, erythromycin, fluconazole, fosamprenavir, grapefruit juice, verapamil):

FMF: Maximum dose: 1.2 mg/day **or** 0.6 mg twice daily

Gout prophylaxis:

If original dose is 0.6 mg twice daily, adjust dose to 0.3 mg twice daily **or** 0.6 mg once daily

If original dose is 0.6 mg once daily, adjust dose to 0.3 mg once daily

Gout flare treatment: 1.2 mg as a single dose; wait at least 3 days to repeat days

Coadministration of P-gp inhibitor (eg, cyclosporine, ranolazine):

FMF: Maximum dose: 0.6 mg/day **or** 0.3 mg twice daily

Gout prophylaxis:

If original dose is 0.6 mg twice daily, adjust dose to 0.3 mg once daily

If original dose is 0.6 mg once daily, adjust dose to 0.3 mg every other day

Gout flare treatment: Initial: 0.6 mg as a single dose; wait at least 3 days to repeat

Dosing adjustment in renal impairment: Concurrent use of colchicine and P-gp or strong CYP3A4 inhibitors is **contraindicated** in renal impairment. Use of colchicine to treat gout flares is not recommended in patients with renal impairment receiving prophylatic colchicine.

Children (Kallinich, 2007):

Moderate impairment (CrCl 10-50 mL/minute): Consider dose reduction

Severe impairment (CrCl <10 mL/minute): Reduce dose by 50% or consider discontinuation of therapy; maximum dose: 1 mg/day

Adults:

FMF:

CrCl 30-80 mL/minute: Monitor closely for adverse effects; dose adjustment may be necessary

CrCl <30 mL/minute: Initial dose: 0.3 mg/day; use caution if dose titrated; monitor for adverse effects

Dialysis: Initial dose: 0.3 mg/day; dosing can be increased with close monitoring; monitor for adverse effects. Not removed by dialysis.

Gout prophylaxis:

CrCl 30-80 mL/minute: Dosage adjustment not required; monitor closely for adverse effects

CrCl <30 mL/minute: Initial dose: 0.3 mg/day; use caution if dose titrated; monitor for adverse effects

Dialysis: 0.3 mg twice weekly; monitor closely for adverse effects

Gout flare treatment:

CrCl 30-80 mL/minute: Dosage adjustment not required; monitor closely for adverse effects

CrCl <30 mL/minute: Dosage adjustment may be considered; treatment course should not be repeated more frequently than every 14 days

Dialysis: 0.6 mg as a single dose; wait at least 14 days to repeat

Administration Hazardous agent; use appropriate precautions for handling and disposal (NIOSH 2014 [group 3]).

Oral: Administer without regard to meals and maintain adequate fluid intake

Monitoring Parameters CBC with differential, urinalysis, and renal and hepatic function tests

Test Interactions May cause false-positive results in urine tests for erythrocytes or hemoglobin

Dosage Forms Excipient information presented when available (limited, particularly for generics); consult specific product labeling.

Capsule, Oral:
Mitigare: 0.6 mg [contains brilliant blue fcf (fd&c blue #1), fd&c yellow #10 (quinoline yellow)]
Generic: 0.6 mg
Tablet, Oral:
Colcrys: 0.6 mg [scored; contains fd&c blue #2 (indigotine), fd&c red #40]
Generic: 0.6 mg

◆ **Colcrys** *see* Colchicine *on page* 528

Colesevelam (koh le SEV a lam)

Brand Names: US Welchol
Brand Names: Canada Lodalis
Therapeutic Category Antilipemic Agent, Bile Acid Sequestrant
Generic Availability (US) No
Use Management of heterozygous familial hypercholesterolemia if LDL-C remains ≥190 mg/dL, or ≥160 mg/dL with family history of premature cardiovascular disease, or presence of ≥2 cardiovascular risk factors (FDA approved in ages 10 to 17 years [females ≥1 year postmenarche]); management of elevated LDL in primary hypercholesterolemia (Fredrickson type IIa) when used alone or in combination with an HMG-CoA reductase inhibitor in conjunction with diet and exercise (FDA approved in adults); improve glycemic control in type 2 diabetes mellitus (noninsulin dependent, NIDDM) in conjunction with diet and exercise (FDA approved in adults)
Pregnancy Risk Factor B
Pregnancy Considerations Adverse effects have not been observed in animal reproduction studies. Colesevelam is not absorbed systemically, but may interfere with vitamin absorption; therefore, regular supplementation may not be adequate.
Breast-Feeding Considerations Due to lack of systemic absorption, colesevelam is not expected to be excreted in breast milk; however, the tendency of colesevelam to interfere with the vitamin absorption may have an effect on the nursing infant.
Contraindications
History of bowel obstruction; serum TG concentrations of more than 500 mg/dL; history of hypertriglyceridemia-induced pancreatitis.
Canadian labeling: Hypersensitivity to colesevelam or any component of the formulation; bowel or biliary obstruction
Warnings/Precautions Use with caution in treating patients with serum triglyceride concentrations >300 mg/dL and in patients using insulin, thiazolidinediones, or sulfonylureas (may cause increased concentrations) or in patients susceptible to fat-soluble vitamin deficiencies. Discontinue if triglyceride concentrations exceed 500 mg/dL or hypertriglyceridemia-induced pancreatitis occurs. The American College of Cardiology/American Heart Association recommends to avoid use in patients with baseline fasting triglyceride levels ≥300 mg/dL or type III hyperlipoproteinemia since severe triglyceride elevations may occur. Use bile acid sequestrants with caution in patients with triglyceride levels 250-299 mg/dL and evaluate a fasting lipid panel in 4-6 weeks after initiation; discontinue use if triglycerides are >400 mg/dL (Stone, 2013). Use is not recommended in patients with gastroparesis, other severe GI motility disorders, or a history of major GI tract surgery or patients at risk for bowel obstruction. Use tablets with caution in patients with dysphagia or swallowing disorders; use the oral suspension form of colesevelam due to large tablet size and risk for esophageal obstruction.

Minimal effects are seen on HDL-C and triglyceride levels. Secondary causes of hypercholesterolemia should be excluded before initiation. Colesevelam has not been studied in Fredrickson Type I, III, IV, or V dyslipidemias. Colesevelam is not indicated for the management of type 1 diabetes, particularly in the acute management (eg, DKA). It is also not indicated in type 2 diabetes mellitus as monotherapy and must be used as an adjunct to diet, exercise, and glycemic control with insulin or oral antidiabetic agents. The use of colesevelam in pediatric patients with type 2 diabetes has not been evaluated. Combination with dipeptidyl peptidase 4 inhibitors or thiazolidinediones has not been studied extensively. There is no evidence of macrovascular disease risk reduction with colesevelam.

Use with caution in patients susceptible to fat-soluble vitamin deficiencies. Absorption of fat soluble vitamins A, D, E, and K may be decreased; patients should take vitamins ≥4 hours before colesevelam. Potentially significant drug-drug interactions may exist, requiring dose or frequency adjustment, additional monitoring, and/or selection of alternative therapy. Some products may contain phenylalanine.
Adverse Reactions Unless otherwise noted, adverse effects are reported for adult patients.
Cardiovascular: Cardiovascular toxicity (including myocardial infarction, aortic stenosis, bradycardia), hypertension
Central nervous system: Fatigue (children), headache (children and adults)
Endocrine & metabolic: Hyperglycemia, hypertriglyceridemia, hypoglycemia
Gastrointestinal: Constipation, diarrhea, dyspepsia, gastroesophageal reflux disease, nausea (children and adults), periodontal abscess, vomiting (children)
Hematologic & oncologic: C-reactive protein increased
Neuromuscular & skeletal: Back pain, increased creatine phosphokinase (children and adults), myalgia, weakness
Respiratory: Flu-like symptoms (children), nasopharyngitis (children), pharyngitis, rhinitis (children), upper respiratory tract infection (children and adults)
Rare but important or life-threatening: Dysphagia, esophageal obstruction, fecal impaction, worsening of hemorrhoids, increased serum transaminases, infection, intestinal obstruction, pancreatitis, unstable angina pectoris
Drug Interactions
Metabolism/Transport Effects None known.
Avoid Concomitant Use
Avoid concomitant use of Colesevelam with any of the following: Mycophenolate
Increased Effect/Toxicity There are no known significant interactions involving an increase in effect.
Decreased Effect
Colesevelam may decrease the levels/effects of: Amiodarone; AtorvaSTATin; Chenodiol; Cholic Acid; Contraceptives (Estrogens); Contraceptives (Progestins); Corticosteroids (Oral); CycloSPORINE (Systemic); Deferasirox; Ethinyl Estradiol; Ezetimibe; Glimepiride; GlipiZIDE; GlyBURIDE; Leflunomide; Lomitapide; Loop Diuretics; Methotrexate; Multivitamins/Fluoride (with ADE); Multivitamins/Minerals (with ADEK, Folate, Iron); Multivitamins/Minerals (with AE, No Iron); Mycophenolate; Niacin; Nonsteroidal Anti-Inflammatory Agents; Norethindrone; Olmesartan; Phenytoin; Pravastatin; Propranolol; Raloxifene; Teriflunomide; Tetracycline Derivatives; Thiazide Diuretics; Thyroid Products; Ursodiol; Vancomycin; Vitamin D Analogs; Vitamin K Antagonists
Storage/Stability Store at 25°C (77°F); excursions permitted to 15°C to 30°C (59°F to 86°F). Protect from moisture.
Mechanism of Action Cholesterol is the major precursor of bile acid. Colesevelam binds with bile acids in the intestine to form an insoluble complex that is eliminated in feces. This increased excretion of bile acids results in an increased oxidation of cholesterol to bile acid and a lowering of the serum cholesterol.

Pharmacodynamics

Onset of action:

Lipid-lowering: Within 2 weeks (maximum effect)

Reduction HgA1C (Type II diabetes): 4-6 weeks initial onset, 12-18 weeks maximal effect

Pharmacokinetics (Adult data unless noted)

Absorption: Insignificant

Elimination: Urine (0.05%)

Dosing: Usual

Pediatric: **Note:** Due to large tablet size, the manufacturer recommends packets of oral suspension for some pediatric patients:

Heterozygous familial hypercholesterolemia: Children ≥10 years and Adolescents: Oral:

Once-daily dosing: 3.75 g (oral suspension or 6 tablets) once daily (Stein, 2010)

Twice-daily dosing: 1.875 g (3 tablets) twice daily (Stein, 2010)

Primary hyperlipidemia: Limited data available (NHLBI, 2011): Children ≥10 years and Adolescents: Oral:

Once-daily dosing: 3.75 g (oral suspension or 6 tablets) once daily

Twice-daily dosing: 1.875 g (3 tablets) twice daily

Adult: **Hyperlipidemia, type 2 diabetes mellitus:** Oral:

Once-daily dosing: 3.75 g (oral suspension or 6 tablets) once daily

Twice-daily dosing: 1.875 g (3 tablets) twice daily

Dosing adjustment in renal impairment: There are no dosage adjustments provided in the manufacturer's labeling; however, dosage adjustment unlikely necessary due to low systemic absorption.

Dosing adjustment in hepatic impairment: No dosage adjustment necessary.

Preparation for Administration Granules for oral suspension: Empty 1 packet into a glass; add 4 to 8 ounces of water, fruit juice, or a diet soft drink and mix well.

Administration Educate the patient on dietary guidelines.

Granules for oral suspension: Administer with meals. Do not take in dry form (to avoid GI distress).

Tablets: Due to tablet size, it is recommended that any patient who has trouble swallowing tablets including pediatric patients should avoid use of tablets and use the oral suspension form. Administer with meal(s) and a liquid.

Monitoring Parameters

Pediatric patients: Fasting lipid profile (baseline, 4 to 6 weeks after initiation, and then every 6 to 12 months), growth, maturation, number of stools per day (NHLBI, 2011)

Adults: Fasting lipid profile before initiating treatment, 3 months after initiation (within 4 to 6 weeks if baseline fasting triglycerides of 250 to 299 mg/dL), and every 6 to 12 months thereafter (ACC/AHA [Stone, 2013])

Test Interactions Increased prothrombin time

Dosage Forms Considerations Welchol contains phenylalanine 27 mg per 3.75 gram packet

Dosage Forms Excipient information presented when available (limited, particularly for generics); consult specific product labeling.

Packet, Oral, as hydrochloride:

Welchol: 3.75 g (30 ea) [sugar free; contains aspartame]

Tablet, Oral, as hydrochloride:

Welchol: 625 mg

◆ **Colestid** *see* Colestipol *on page 531*

◆ **Colestid Flavored** *see* Colestipol *on page 531*

Colestipol (koe LES ti pole)

Medication Safety Issues

Sound-alike/look-alike issues:

Colestipol may be confused with calcitriol

Related Information

Oral Medications That Should Not Be Crushed or Altered *on page 2476*

Brand Names: US Colestid; Colestid Flavored; Micronized Colestipol HCl

Brand Names: Canada Colestid

Therapeutic Category Antilipemic Agent, Bile Acid Sequestrant

Generic Availability (US) Yes

Use Adjunct to dietary therapy to decrease elevated serum total and low density lipoprotein cholesterol (LDL-C) in primary hypercholesterolemia (FDA approved in adults)

Pregnancy Considerations Colestipol is not absorbed systemically (<0.17%), but may interfere with vitamin absorption; therefore, regular prenatal supplementation may not be adequate. There are no studies in pregnant women; use with caution.

Breast-Feeding Considerations Due to lack of systemic absorption (<0.17%), colestipol is not expected to be excreted into breast milk; however, the tendency of colestipol to interfere with vitamin absorption may have an effect on the nursing infant.

Contraindications

Hypersensitivity to colestipol or any component of the formulation

Canadian labeling: Additional contraindications (not in U.S. labeling): Complete biliary obstruction; phenylketonurics (Colestid Orange Granules only)

Warnings/Precautions Secondary causes of hyperlipidemia should be ruled out prior to therapy initiation. Bile acid sequestrants should not be used in patients with baseline fasting triglyceride levels ≥300 mg/dL or type III hyperlipoproteinemia because severe triglyceride elevations may occur. Use bile acid sequestrants with caution in patients with triglyceride levels 250 to 299 mg/dL; evaluate a fasting lipid panel in 4 to 6 weeks after initiation and discontinue use if triglycerides are >400 mg/dL (ACC/AHA [Stone, 2013]). Use with caution in patients susceptible to fat-soluble vitamin deficiencies. Absorption of fat-soluble vitamins A, D, E, and K and folic acid may be decreased; patients should take vitamins ≥4 hours before colestipol. Chronic use may be associated with bleeding problems due to hypoprothrombinemia from vitamin K deficiency; may be prevented with use of vitamin K therapy. May produce or exacerbate constipation; fecal impaction may occur, initiate therapy at a reduced dose and increase gradually in patients with a history of constipation. Encourage increased fluid and fiber intake; a stool softener may also be indicated. Hemorrhoids may be worsened. Chronic use may lead to development of hyperchloremic acidosis. There is a theoretical risk of developing hypothyroidism, particularly in patients with limited thyroid reserve; use with caution.

Potentially significant drug-drug interactions may exist, requiring dose or frequency adjustment, additional monitoring, and/or selection of alternative therapy. Not to be taken simultaneously with many other medicines, including vitamin supplements (decreased absorption). Some products may contain phenylalanine. Colestipol granules should never be taken in dry form; may cause esophageal spasm and/or respiratory distress.

Warnings: Additional Pediatric Considerations May raise serum triglyceride concentrations; in a trial of combination therapy of colestipol and pravastatin in children and adolescents (>8 years of age); the serum triglycerides increased by 12% from baseline (McCrindle, 2002).

Adverse Reactions

Cardiovascular: Angina, chest pain, peripheral edema, tachycardia

Central nervous system: Dizziness, fatigue, headache (including migraine and sinus headache), insomnia

Dermatologic: Dermatitis, skin rash, urticaria

Gastrointestinal: Abdominal cramps, abdominal pain, anorexia, bloating, constipation, cholecystitis, cholelithiasis, diarrhea, dyspepsia, dysphagia, esophageal obstruction, flatulence, heartburn, hemorrhoidal bleeding, nausea, peptic ulcer, vomiting
Hepatic: Increased serum alkaline phosphatase, increased serum ALT, increased serum AST
Neuromuscular & skeletal: Arthralgia, arthritis, back pain, myalgia, weakness
Respiratory: Dyspnea

Drug Interactions

Metabolism/Transport Effects None known.

Avoid Concomitant Use

Avoid concomitant use of Colestipol with any of the following: Mycophenolate

Increased Effect/Toxicity There are no known significant interactions involving an increase in effect.

Decreased Effect

Colestipol may decrease the levels/effects of: Amiodarone; AtorvaSTATin; Cardiac Glycosides; Chenodiol; Cholic Acid; Contraceptives (Estrogens); Contraceptives (Progestins); Corticosteroids (Oral); Deferasirox; Diltiazem; Ezetimibe; Fibric Acid Derivatives; Leflunomide; Lomitapide; Loop Diuretics; Methotrexate; Methylfolate; Multivitamins/Fluoride (with ADE); Multivitamins/Minerals (with ADEK, Folate, Iron); Multivitamins/Minerals (with AE, No Iron); Mycophenolate; Niacin; Nonsteroidal Anti-Inflammatory Agents; Pravastatin; Propranolol; Raloxifene; Teriflunomide; Tetracycline Derivatives; Thiazide Diuretics; Thyroid Products; Ursodiol; Vancomycin; Vitamin D Analogs; Vitamin K Antagonists

Storage/Stability Store at 20°C to 25°C (68°F to 77°F).

Mechanism of Action Binds with bile acids to form an insoluble complex that is eliminated in feces; it thereby increases the fecal loss of bile acid-bound low density lipoprotein cholesterol

Pharmacodynamics

Lowering of serum cholesterol: ~1 month
LDL-C reduction: ~19%

Pharmacokinetics (Adult data unless noted)

Absorption: None
Elimination: Feces

Dosing: Usual

Children and Adolescents: **Dyslipidemia:** Limited data available: Oral: Children >8 years and Adolescents: 2-12 g/day; the most recent study produced significant lowering of serum cholesterol utilizing either 10 g once daily or 5 g twice daily (McCrindle, 2002; Tonstad, 1996)

Adults: **Dyslipidemia:** Oral:

Granules: Initial: 5 g 1-2 times/day; maintenance: 5-30 g/day given once or in divided doses; increase by 5 g/day at 1- to 2-month intervals

Tablets: Initial: 2 g 1-2 times/day; maintenance: 2-16 g/day given once or in divided doses; increase by 2 g once or twice daily at 1- to 2-month intervals

Preparation for Administration Oral: Granules: Add granules to at least 90 mL of liquid and stir until completely mixed; may be mixed with any beverage or added to soups, cereal, or pulpy fruits fruits (eg, fruit cocktail, crushed pineapple, peaches, or pears).

Administration Oral: Other drugs should be administered at least 1 hour before or 4 hours after colestipol.

Granules: Do not administer in dry form (to avoid GI distress). Dry granules should be added to at least 90 mL of liquid and stirred until completely mixed; may be mixed with any beverage or added to soups, cereal, or pulpy fruits (eg, fruit cocktail, crushed pineapple, peaches, or pears). After administration, rinse glass with a small amount of liquid to ensure all medication is taken.

Tablets: Administer tablets one at a time, swallowed whole, with plenty of liquid. Do not cut, crush, or chew tablets.

Monitoring Parameters

Pediatric patients: Fasting lipid profile (baseline and every 6 to 12 months), growth, maturation, number of stools per day (NHLBI, 2011)

Adults: Fasting lipid profile before initiating treatment, 3 months after initiation, and every 6 to 12 months thereafter (Stone, 2013).

Dosage Forms Considerations

Colestid tablets contain micronized colestipol. Generic tablets are available in micronized and non-micronized formulations.

Dosage Forms Excipient information presented when available (limited, particularly for generics); consult specific product labeling.

Granules, Oral, as hydrochloride:
Colestid: 5 g (300 g, 500 g) [unflavored flavor]
Colestid Flavored: 5 g (450 g) [contains aspartame; orange flavor]
Generic: 5 g (500 g)

Packet, Oral, as hydrochloride:
Colestid: 5 g (30 ea, 90 ea) [unflavored flavor]
Colestid Flavored: 5 g (60 ea) [contains aspartame; orange flavor]
Generic: 5 g (30 ea, 90 ea)

Tablet, Oral, as hydrochloride:
Colestid: 1 g
Micronized Colestipol HCl: 1 g
Generic: 1 g

◆ **Colestipol Hydrochloride** *see* Colestipol *on page 531*

◆ **CO Lisinopril (Can)** *see* Lisinopril *on page 1280*

Colistimethate (koe lis ti METH ate)

Medication Safety Issues

Other safety concerns:

Due to the potential for dosing errors, it is recommended that prescriptions for colistimethate be expressed as colistin base activity only.

Brand Names: US Coly-Mycin M

Brand Names: Canada Coly-Mycin M

Therapeutic Category Antibiotic, Miscellaneous

Generic Availability (US) Yes

Use Treatment of acute or chronic infections due to sensitive strains of certain gram-negative bacilli (particularly *Pseudomonas aeruginosa*) which are resistant to other antibacterials (FDA approved in all ages); has also been used as inhalation therapy to treat multidrug-resistant gram-negative pneumonia and in cystic fibrosis; intrathecal/intraventricular therapy to treat multidrug resistant gram-negative meningitis.

Pregnancy Risk Factor C

Pregnancy Considerations Adverse events have been observed in animal reproduction studies. Colistimethate crosses the placenta in humans.

Breast-Feeding Considerations Colistin (the active form of colistimethate sodium) and colistin sulphate (another form of colistin) are excreted in human milk. The manufacturer recommends caution if giving colistimethate sodium to a breast-feeding woman. Nondose-related effects could include modification of bowel flora.

Contraindications Hypersensitivity to colistimethate, colistin, or any component of the formulation

Warnings/Precautions Use only to prevent or treat infections strongly suspected or proven to be caused by susceptible bacteria to minimize development of bacterial drug resistance. Nephrotoxicity has been reported; use with caution in patients with preexisting renal disease; dosage adjustments may be required. Withhold treatment if signs of renal impairment occur during treatment. Respiratory arrest has been reported with use; impaired renal function may increase the risk for neuromuscular blockade and apnea. Transient, reversible neurological disturbances (eg, dizziness, numbness, paresthesia, generalized pruritus, slurred speech, tingling, vertigo) may occur. Patients must be cautioned about performing tasks which require mental alertness (eg, operating machinery or driving). Dose reduction may reduce neurologic symptoms; monitor closely. Use of inhaled colistimethate cause bronchoconstriction. Use with caution in patients with hyperactive airways; consider administration of a bronchodilator 15 minutes prior to administration. Colistimethate solutions change to bioactive colistin, a component of which may result in severe pulmonary toxicity. Solutions for inhalation must be mixed immediately prior to administration and used within 24 hours.

Prolonged use may result in fungal or bacterial superinfection, including *C. difficile*-associated diarrhea (CDAD) and pseudomembranous colitis; CDAD has been observed >2 months postantibiotic treatment.

Potentially significant drug-drug interactions may exist, requiring dose or frequency adjustment, additional monitoring, and/or selection of alternative therapy. Use caution when prescribing or dispensing; potential for dosing errors due to lack of standardization in literature when referring to product and dose; colistimethate (inactive prodrug) and colistin base strengths are not interchangeable; verify prescribed dose is expressed in terms of colistin base activity prior to dispensing.

Warnings: Additional Pediatric Considerations Nephrotoxicity is dose dependent and reversible upon discontinuation and has been observed to occur within the first 4 days of therapy in patients with cystic fibrosis (Bosso, 1991). The Cystic Fibrosis Foundation recommends that patients not use colistimethate for inhalation premixed by pharmacies; patients should prepare their colistimethate nebulizer inhalation solutions immediately prior to use. Colistin is comprised of two components: Colistin A (polymyxin E1) and colistin B (polymyxin E2). Polymyxin E1 has been shown to cause localized airway inflammation in animal studies and may result in lung toxicity in humans. Clinicians who continue to prescribe colistimethate for inhalation should be aware of this potentially life-threatening effect and should administer solutions for inhalation promptly following preparation of solution.

Adverse Reactions

Central nervous system: Dizziness, headache, neurotoxicity (Boss 1991; Koch-Weser 1970), oral paresthesia, peripheral paresthesia, slurred speech, vertigo

Dermatologic: Pruritus, skin rash, urticaria

Gastrointestinal: Gastric distress

Genitourinary: Decreased urine output, nephrotoxicity (Dalfino 2012; Oliveira 2009), proteinuria

Neuromuscular & skeletal: Lower extremity weakness

Renal: Acute renal failure (Akajagbor 2013; Deryke 2010), increased blood urea nitrogen, increased serum creatinine

Respiratory: Apnea, respiratory distress

Miscellaneous: Fever

Rare but important or life-threatening: Pulmonary toxicity (acute respiratory tract failure following inhalation, bronchoconstriction, bronchospasm, chest tightness, respiratory distress)

Drug Interactions

Metabolism/Transport Effects None known.

Avoid Concomitant Use

Avoid concomitant use of Colistimethate with any of the following: Bacitracin (Systemic); BCG; BCG (Intravesical); Mecamylamine

Increased Effect/Toxicity

Colistimethate may increase the levels/effects of: Bacitracin (Systemic); Mecamylamine; Neuromuscular-Blocking Agents

The levels/effects of Colistimethate may be increased by: Aminoglycosides; Amphotericin B; Capreomycin; Polymyxin B; Vancomycin

Decreased Effect

Colistimethate may decrease the levels/effects of: BCG; BCG (Intravesical); BCG Vaccine (Immunization); Sodium Picosulfate; Typhoid Vaccine

Storage/Stability Store intact vials (prior to reconstitution) at 20°C to 25°C (68°F to 77°F); excursions permitted to 15°C to 30°C (59°F to 86°F). Reconstituted vials may be refrigerated at 2°C to 8°C (36°F to 46°F) or stored at 20°C to 25°C (68°F to 77°F) for up to 7 days. Solutions for infusion should be freshly prepared; do not use beyond 24 hours.

Mechanism of Action Colistimethate (or the sodium salt [colistimethate sodium]) is the inactive prodrug which is hydrolyzed to colistin, which acts as a cationic detergent and damages the bacterial cytoplasmic membrane causing leaking of intracellular substances and cell death

Pharmacokinetics (Adult data unless noted)

Absorption: Not absorbed from the GI tract, mucous membranes, or intact skin (**Note:** GI absorption has been observed in infants.)

Distribution: Widely distributed to body tissues, such as liver, kidney, heart, and lungs; does not penetrate into CSF, synovial, pleural, or pericardial fluids

V_d: Adolescents and Adults with cystic fibrosis: 0.09 ± 0.03 L/kg (Reed, 2001)

Protein binding: 50%

Half-life:

Infants (including premature infants), Children, Adolescents, and Adults: 2-3 hours

Adolescents and Adults with cystic fibrosis: 3.5 ± 1 hour (Reed, 2001)

Time to peak serum concentration: IM: ~2 hours

Elimination: Primarily by the kidney through glomerular filtration and urinary excretion as unchanged drug

Dosing: Neonatal Note: Dosage expressed in terms of colistin **base**.

General dosing, susceptible infection: IM, IV: 2.5-5 mg/kg/**day** divided every 6-12 hours

Pulmonary infection: Limited data available: Inhalation: 4 mg/kg/dose every 12 hours has been used to treat ventilator-associated pneumonia in neonates [n=8, gestational age: 28-41 weeks; median treatment duration: 9 days (range: 4-14 days)] (Nakwan, 2011)

Dosing: Usual Note: Doses should be based on ideal body weight in obese patients; **Dosage expressed in terms of colistin base:**

Infants, Children, and Adolescents:

General dosing, susceptible infection: Infants, Children, and Adolescents: IM, IV: 2.5-5 mg/kg/**day** divided every 6-12 hours

Cystic fibrosis, pulmonary infection: Limited data available: Children ≥5 years and Adolescents: IV: Usual reported range: 3-5 mg/kg/**day** divided every 8 hours; maximum dose: 100 mg/dose (Bosso, 1991; Reed, 2001; Young, 2013); doses >5 mg/kg/day (up to 8 mg/kg/day) may be required in some situations; however, higher doses are associated with more severe toxicity (Bosso, 1991; Reed, 2001).

Pulmonary infection: Limited data available: Infants, Children, and Adolescents: Inhalation: Usual dose: 75-150 mg in 3 mL of NS (4 mL total volume) via nebulizer twice daily is most frequently reported in clinical practice; reported range: 30-150 mg/dose (Le, 2010; Tramper, 2010)

Adults: **Susceptible infections**: IM, IV: 2.5-5 mg/kg/**day** in 2-4 divided doses

Dosing interval in renal impairment: Adults: IM, IV:

CrCl >80 mL/minute: No dosage adjustment necessary

CrCl 50-79 mL/minute: 2.5-3.8 mg/kg/day in 2 divided doses

CrCl 30-49 mL/minute: 2.5 mg/kg/day in 1-2 divided doses
CrCl 10-29 mL/minute: 1.5 mg/kg every 36 hours
Intermittent hemodialysis (IHD) (administer after hemodialysis on dialysis days): 1.5 mg/kg every 24-48 hours (Heintz, 2009). **Note:** Dosing dependent on the assumption of 3 times/week, complete IHD sessions.
Continuous renal replacement therapy (CRRT) (Heintz, 2009; Trotman, 2005): Drug clearance is highly dependent on the method of renal replacement, filter type, and flow rate. Appropriate dosing requires close monitoring of pharmacologic response, signs of adverse reactions due to drug accumulation, as well as drug concentrations in relation to target trough (if appropriate). The following are general recommendations only (based on dialysate flow/ultrafiltration rates of 1-2 L/hour and minimal residual renal function) and should not supersede clinical judgment:
CVVH/CVVHD/CVVHDF: 2.5 mg/kg every 24-48 hours (frequency dependent upon site or severity of infection or susceptibility of pathogen)
Note: A single case report has demonstrated that the use of 2.5 mg/kg every 48 hours with a dialysate flow rate of 1 L/hour may be inadequate and that dosing every 24 hours was well-tolerated. Based on pharmacokinetic analysis, the authors recommend dosing as frequent as every 12 hours in patients receiving CVVHDF (Li, 2005).

Dosing adjustment in hepatic impairment: There are no dosage adjustments provided in manufacturer's labeling.

Dosing adjustment for toxicity:
CNS toxicity: Dose reduction may reduce neurologic symptoms.
Nephrotoxicity: Withhold treatment if signs of renal impairment occur during treatment.

Preparation for Administration Parenteral:
IV or IM use: Reconstitute vial containing 150 mg of colistin base activity with 2 mL of SWFI resulting in a concentration of 75 mg colistin base/mL; swirl gently to avoid frothing. May further dilute in D_5W or NS for IV infusion.
Continuous IV infusion: The final concentration for continuous infusion should be based on the patient's fluid needs; infusion should be completed within 24 hours of preparation.
Nebulized inhalation: Pediatric patients: Reconstitute vial containing 150 mg of colistin base activity with 2 mL SWFI, resulting in a concentration of 75 mg colistin base activity/mL; further dilute dose to a total volume of 4 mL in NS (Le 2010; Tramper 2010). Storing for >24 hours may increase the risk for potential lung toxicity; preparation immediately prior to administration is recommended (FDA 2007; Le 2010, Wallace 2008).

Administration
Parenteral:
IM: Administer deep into a large muscle mass (eg, gluteal muscle or lateral part of the thigh).
IV push: Administer over 3 to 5 minutes.
Intermittent IV infusion: Administer over 30 minutes.
Continuous IV infusion: Initially, one-half of the total daily dose is administered by direct IV injection over 3 to 5 minutes followed 1 to 2 hours later by the remaining one-half of the total daily dose diluted in a compatible IV solution infused over 22 to 23 hours. Infusion should be completed within 24 hours of preparation.
Inhalation: Administer solution via nebulizer promptly following preparation of solution to decrease possibility of high concentrations of colistin from forming which may lead to potentially life-threatening lung toxicity. Consider use of a bronchodilator (eg, albuterol) within 15 minutes prior to administration (Le 2010).
Note: A case report of fatal lung toxicity implicated in vitro colistin formation from an inhalation solution as a potential etiology, but data regarding the concentration formulation and storage of the inhaled colistin administered to the patient were not reported (FDA 2007 McCoy 2007; Wallace 2008). An acceptable limit of in vitro colistin formation to prevent potential toxicity is unknown. Limited stability data are available regarding the storage of colistin solution for inhaled administration (Healan 2012; Wallace 2008). Storing for >24 hours may increase the risk for potential lung toxicity; preparation immediately prior to administration is recommended (FDA 2007; Le 2010, Wallace 2008).

Monitoring Parameters CBC with differential, renal function tests, urine output; number and type of stools/day for diarrhea; for inhalation therapy: Pre- and post-treatment spirometry; signs of bronchospasm

Additional Information Colistimethate dosing differs between the U.S. and European countries. In the U.S. doses should be expressed as **colistin base**. In European countries, the dose is often expressed as colistimethate sodium and is expressed in terms of units rather than mg:
1 mg colistin base = 2.67 mg colistimethate sodium
1 mg colistimethate sodium = 12,500 units of colistimethate sodium

Dosage Forms Excipient information presented when available (limited, particularly for generics); consult specific product labeling.
Solution Reconstituted, Injection [strength expressed as base]:
Coly-Mycin M: 150 mg (1 ea)
Generic: 150 mg (1 ea)
Solution Reconstituted, Injection [strength expressed as base, preservative free]:
Generic: 150 mg (1 ea)

- ◆ **Colistimethate Sodium** *see* Colistimethate *on page* *532*
- ◆ **Colistin Methanesulfonate** *see* Colistimethate *on page* *532*
- ◆ **Colistin Methanesulphonate** *see* Colistimethate *on page* *532*
- ◆ **Colistin Sulfomethate** *see* Colistimethate *on page* *532*
- ◆ **Colocort** *see* Hydrocortisone (Topical) *on page* *1041*
- ◆ **CO Lovastatin (Can)** *see* Lovastatin *on page* *1305*
- ◆ **Coly-Mycin M** *see* Colistimethate *on page* *532*
- ◆ **Colyte** *see* Polyethylene Glycol-Electrolyte Solution *on page* *1724*
- ◆ **Combantrin (Can)** *see* Pyrantel Pamoate *on page* *1806*
- ◆ **Combivir** *see* Lamivudine and Zidovudine *on page* *1209*
- ◆ **CO Meloxicam (Can)** *see* Meloxicam *on page* *1346*
- ◆ **Compazine** *see* Prochlorperazine *on page* *1774*
- ◆ **Complete Allergy Medication [OTC]** *see* DiphenhydrAMINE (Systemic) *on page* *668*
- ◆ **Complete Allergy Relief [OTC]** *see* DiphenhydrAMINE (Systemic) *on page* *668*
- ◆ **Compound E** *see* Cortisone *on page* *538*
- ◆ **Compound F** *see* Hydrocortisone (Systemic) *on page* *1038*
- ◆ **Compound F** *see* Hydrocortisone (Topical) *on page* *1041*
- ◆ **Compound S** *see* Zidovudine *on page* *2207*
- ◆ **Compound S, Abacavir, and Lamivudine** *see* Abacavir, Lamivudine, and Zidovudine *on page* *38*
- ◆ **Compro** *see* Prochlorperazine *on page* *1774*
- ◆ **Comvax** *see* *Haemophilus* b Conjugate and Hepatitis B Vaccine *on page* *997*
- ◆ **CO Mycophenolate (Can)** *see* Mycophenolate *on page* *1473*
- ◆ **Concerta** *see* Methylphenidate *on page* *1402*

- **Congest (Can)** *see* Estrogens (Conjugated/Equine, Systemic) *on page 801*
- **Conjugated Estrogen** *see* Estrogens (Conjugated/Equine, Systemic) *on page 801*
- **Conjugated Estrogen** *see* Estrogens (Conjugated/Equine, Topical) *on page 803*
- **Constulose** *see* Lactulose *on page 1204*
- **Contac® Cold 12 Hour Relief Non Drowsy (Can)** *see* Pseudoephedrine *on page 1801*
- **ControlRx** *see* Fluoride *on page 899*
- **ControlRx Multi** *see* Fluoride *on page 899*
- **Conventional Amphotericin B** *see* Amphotericin B (Conventional) *on page 147*
- **Conventional Cytarabine** *see* Cytarabine (Conventional) *on page 566*
- **Conventional Daunomycin** *see* DAUNOrubicin (Conventional) *on page 592*
- **Conventional Doxorubicin** *see* DOXOrubicin (Conventional) *on page 713*
- **Conventional Paclitaxel** *see* PACLitaxel (Conventional) *on page 1602*
- **Conventional Vincristine** *see* VinCRIStine *on page 2179*
- **ConZip** *see* TraMADol *on page 2098*
- **CO Ondansetron (Can)** *see* Ondansetron *on page 1564*
- **CO Paroxetine (Can)** *see* PARoxetine *on page 1634*
- **Copegus** *see* Ribavirin *on page 1851*

Copper (KOP er)

Medication Safety Issues

Sound-alike/look-alike issues:

Cupric sulfate may be confused with calcium gluconate

Brand Names: US Coppermin [OTC]; Cu-5 [OTC]

Therapeutic Category Trace Element, Parenteral

Generic Availability (US) May be product dependent

Use Supplement to total parenteral nutrition (TPN) to maintain copper serum concentrations and to prevent depletion of endogenous stores and subsequent deficiency [FDA approved in pediatric patients (age not specified) and adults]

Pregnancy Risk Factor C

Pregnancy Considerations Animal reproduction studies have not been conducted. It is not known whether administration to a pregnant woman can cause fetal harm or can affect reproductive capacity.

Breast-Feeding Considerations It is unknown whether this drug is excreted in human milk. Because many drugs are excreted in human milk, caution should be exercised.

Contraindications There are no contraindications listed in the manufacturer's labeling.

Warnings/Precautions Patients with high output intestinal fistulae may require a larger dose. Use with caution in patients with hepatic impairment. Administration in Wilson's disease is not recommended. The parenteral product may contain aluminum; toxic aluminum concentrations may be seen with high doses, prolonged use, or renal dysfunction. Premature neonates are at higher risk due to immature renal function and aluminum intake from other parenteral sources. Parenteral aluminum exposure of >4 to 5 mcg/kg/day is associated with CNS and bone toxicity; tissue loading may occur at lower doses (Federal Register, 2002). See manufacturer's labeling.

Adverse Reactions Note: Generally well tolerated; excessive copper levels may result in the following adverse effects:

Hepatic: Hepatic dysfunction (including hepatic necrosis)

Drug Interactions

Metabolism/Transport Effects None known.

Avoid Concomitant Use There are no known interactions where it is recommended to avoid concomitant use.

Increased Effect/Toxicity There are no known significant interactions involving an increase in effect.

Decreased Effect

Copper may decrease the levels/effects of: Ascorbic Acid

Storage/Stability Store at controlled room temperature of 20°C to 25°C (68°F to 77°F).

Mechanism of Action Copper is an essential nutrient which serves as a cofactor for serum ceruloplasmin, an oxidase necessary for proper formation of the iron carrier protein, transferrin. It also helps maintain normal rates of red and white blood cell formation and helps prevent development of deficiency symptoms: Leukopenia, neutropenia, anemia, depressed ceruloplasmin levels, impaired transferring formation, secondary iron deficiency and osteoporosis.

Pharmacokinetics (Adult data unless noted) Elimination: Bile (primarily, 80%); intestinal wall (16%); urine (4%)

Dosing: Neonatal

Adequate intake (AI): 200 mcg/day

IV: **Note:** Incorporated into parenteral nutrition solution.

Parenteral nutrition supplementation:

ASPEN Guidelines (Mirtallo, 2004): Preterm and term: 20 mcg/kg/day

Manufacturer recommendation: 20 mcg/kg/day; **Note:** Premature neonates weighing <1.5 kg may have higher daily requirements due to low body reserves and accelerated growth rate.

Dosing: Usual

Infants, Children, and Adolescents:

Adequate intake (AI):

1-6 months: 200 mcg/day

6-12 months: 220 mcg/day

Recommended daily allowances (RDA):

1-3 years: 340 mcg/day

4-8 years: 440 mcg/day

9-13 years: 700 mcg/day

14-18 years: 890 mcg/day

≥19 years: 900 mcg/day

IV: **Note:** Incorporated into parenteral nutrition solution.

Parenteral nutrition supplementation:

ASPEN Guidelines (Mirtallo, 2004):

Infants <10 kg: 20 mcg/kg/day

Infants ≥10 kg and Children ≤40 kg or <12 years: 5-20 mcg/kg/day (maximum dose: 500 mcg/day)

Children ≥12 years or >40 kg and Adolescents: 200-500 mcg/day

Manufacturer recommendation: 20 mcg/kg/day

Adults: **Parenteral nutrition supplementation:** ASPEN Guidelines (Mirtallo, 2004): 0.3-0.5 **mg**/day; manufacturer recommendation: 0.5-1.5 **mg**/day; high output intestinal fistula: Some clinicians may use twice the recommended daily allowance (ASPEN, 2002)

Dosing adjustment in renal impairment: Use caution; contains aluminum

Dosing adjustment in hepatic impairment: Use caution; dosage reduction may be required

Preparation for Administration Parenteral: Must dilute in a volume ≥100 mL.

Administration Parenteral: Not for direct IV or IM injection; must be diluted prior to administration; direct administration of 0.4 mg/mL solution causes tissue irritation

Dosage Forms Excipient information presented when available (limited, particularly for generics); consult specific product labeling.

Capsule, Oral [preservative free]:

Cu-5: 5 mg [dye free]

Solution, Intravenous:

Generic: 0.4 mg/mL (10 mL)

Tablet, Oral:
Coppermin: 5 mg [corn free, rye free, wheat free]

◆ **Copper** *see* Trace Elements *on page 2097*
◆ **Coppermin [OTC]** *see* Copper *on page 535*
◆ **Cordarone** *see* Amiodarone *on page 125*
◆ **Cordran** *see* Flurandrenolide *on page 911*
◆ **Coreg** *see* Carvedilol *on page 380*
◆ **Coreg CR** *see* Carvedilol *on page 380*
◆ **Corgard** *see* Nadolol *on page 1480*
◆ **Coricidin HBP Chest Congestion and Cough [OTC]** *see* Guaifenesin and Dextromethorphan *on page 992*
◆ **Corlopam** *see* Fenoldopam *on page 856*
◆ **Cormax Scalp Application** *see* Clobetasol *on page 498*
◆ **Corn Remover One Step [OTC]** *see* Salicylic Acid *on page 1894*
◆ **Corn Remover Ultra Thin [OTC]** *see* Salicylic Acid *on page 1894*
◆ **CO Rosuvastatin (Can)** *see* Rosuvastatin *on page 1886*
◆ **Correct [OTC]** *see* Bisacodyl *on page 289*
◆ **Correctol Stool Softener [OTC] (Can)** *see* Docusate *on page 697*
◆ **Cortaid Maximum Strength [OTC]** *see* Hydrocortisone (Topical) *on page 1041*
◆ **CortAlo** *see* Hydrocortisone (Topical) *on page 1041*
◆ **Cortamed® (Can)** *see* Hydrocortisone (Topical) *on page 1041*
◆ **Cortef** *see* Hydrocortisone (Systemic) *on page 1038*
◆ **Cortenema** *see* Hydrocortisone (Topical) *on page 1041*
◆ **Cortenema® (Can)** *see* Hydrocortisone (Topical) *on page 1041*
◆ **Corticool [OTC]** *see* Hydrocortisone (Topical) *on page 1041*

Corticotropin (kor ti koe TROE pin)

Medication Safety Issues

Sound-alike/look-alike issues:

Corticotropin may be confused with corticorelin, cosyntropin

Brand Names: US HP Acthar

Therapeutic Category Adrenal Corticosteroid; Infantile Spasms, Treatment

Generic Availability (US) No

Use Treatment of infantile spasms as monotherapy (FDA approved in ages <2 years); treatment of acute exacerbations of multiple sclerosis (FDA approved in adults); adjunctive therapy for exacerbations/acute episodes of rheumatic disorders (eg, psoriatic arthritis, rheumatoid arthritis, juvenile idiopathic arthritis, ankylosing spondylitis) (FDA approved in ages >2 years and adults); exacerbations or maintenance therapy for collagen diseases (eg, systemic lupus erythematosus, systemic dermatomyositis) (FDA approved in ages >2 years and adults); treatment of dermatologic (severe erythema multiforme, Stevens-Johnson syndrome) and allergic (serum sickness) states (FDA approved in ages >2 years and adults); treatment of severe acute/chronic allergic and inflammatory ophthalmic disease (eg, keratitis, iritis, iridocyclitis, diffuse posterior uveitis and choroiditis, optic neuritis, chorioretinitis, anterior segment inflammation) and symptomatic sarcoidosis (FDA approved in ages >2 years and adults); to induce diuresis or remission of proteinuria in patients with nephrotic syndrome without idiopathic uremia or due to lupus erythematosus (FDA approved in ages >2 years and adults)

Prescribing and Access Restrictions H.P. Acthar® Gel is only available through specialty pharmacy distribution and not through traditional distribution sources (eg, wholesalers, retail pharmacies). Hospitals wishing to acquire H.P. Acthar® Gel should contact CuraScript Specialty Distribution (1-877-599-7748).

After treatment is initiated, discharge or outpatient prescriptions should be submitted to the Acthar Support and Access Program (A.S.A.P.) in order to ensure an uninterrupted supply of the medication. The Acthar Referral/Prescription form is available online at http://www.acthar.com/files/Acthar-Prescription-Referral-Form.pdf.

Additional information is available for the A.S.A.P. at http://www.acthar.com/healthcare-professionals/physician-patient-referrals or by calling 1-888-435-2284.

Medication Guide Available Yes

Pregnancy Risk Factor C

Pregnancy Considerations Adverse events were observed in animal reproduction studies. Endogenous corticotropin concentrations are increased near delivery (Smith, 2007).

Some studies have shown an association between first trimester systemic corticosteroid use and oral clefts (Park-Wyllie, 2000; Pradat, 2003). Systemic corticosteroids may also influence fetal growth (decreased birth weight); however, information is conflicting (Lunghi, 2010). When systemic corticosteroids are needed in pregnancy, it is generally recommended to use the lowest effective dose for the shortest duration of time, avoiding high doses during the first trimester (Leachman, 2006; Lunghi, 2010; Makol, 2011; Østensen, 2009).

Breast-Feeding Considerations Corticosteroids are excreted in human milk; information specific to corticotropin has not been located. Due to the potential for serious adverse reactions in the nursing infant, the manufacturer recommends a decision be made whether to discontinue nursing or to discontinue the drug, taking into account the importance of treatment to the mother.

Contraindications Hypersensitivity to proteins of porcine origin, scleroderma, osteoporosis, systemic fungal infections, ocular herpes simplex, peptic ulcer, recent surgery, congestive heart failure (CHF), uncontrolled hypertension, primary adrenocortical insufficiency, adrenocortical hyperfunction, infants with suspected congenital infections, coadministration of live or live attenuated vaccines, IV administration

Warnings/Precautions May cause hypercorticism or suppression of hypothalamic-pituitary-adrenal (HPA) axis, particularly in younger children or in patients receiving high doses for prolonged periods. HPA axis suppression may lead to adrenal crisis. Symptoms of adrenal insufficiency may be difficult to detect in infants treated for infantile spasms. Withdrawal and discontinuation of a corticosteroid should be done slowly and carefully. May affect growth velocity; growth should be routinely monitored in pediatric patients. May increase retention of sodium and wasting of calcium and potassium; sodium restriction and/or potassium supplementation may be required. Changes in thyroid status may necessitate dosage adjustments; metabolic clearance of corticosteroids increases in hyperthyroid patients and decreases in hypothyroid ones.

Prolonged use of corticosteroids may increase the incidence of secondary infection, mask acute infection (including fungal infections), prolong or exacerbate viral infections, or limit response to vaccines. Concomitant use of live or live attenuated vaccines is contraindicated; use caution with inactivated vaccines (response may be variable). Close observation is required in patients with latent tuberculosis (TB) and/or TB reactivity; if therapy is prolonged, prophylaxis should be started. Antibodies may develop following prolonged use and increase the risk of hypersensitivity reactions.

Use with caution in patients with hypertension; use has been associated with fluid retention and hypertension; use is contraindicated with uncontrolled hypertension or congestive heart failure (CHF). Use with caution in patients with diabetes mellitus; may alter glucose production/regulation leading to hyperglycemia. Use with caution in patients with GI disease (diverticulitis, ulcerative colitis, risk of impending perforation, fresh intestinal anastomoses) or abscess/pyogenic infections due to risk of gastric ulcer, GI perforation, and GI bleeding; use is contraindicated with peptic ulcer disease. Use with caution in patients with hepatic impairment, including cirrhosis; long-term use has been associated with fluid retention. Use with caution in patients with myasthenia gravis; exacerbation of symptoms has occurred, especially during initial treatment with corticosteroids. Use with caution in patients with cataracts and/or glaucoma; increased intraocular pressure, open-angle glaucoma, and cataracts have occurred with prolonged corticosteroid use. Consider routine eye exams in chronic users. Contraindicated in patients with ocular herpes simplex. Use with caution in patients of any age at risk for osteoporosis; high doses and/or long-term use of corticosteroids have been associated with increased bone loss and osteoporotic fractures. Use is contraindicated in patients with osteoporosis. Use with caution in patients with renal impairment; fluid retention may occur. May cause psychiatric disturbances, including depression, euphoria, insomnia, irritability (especially in infants), mood swings, personality changes, and psychotic manifestations. Preexisting psychiatric conditions (eg, emotional instability, psychotic tendencies) may be exacerbated by corticosteroid use.

Potentially significant drug-drug interactions may exist, requiring dose or frequency adjustment, additional monitoring, and/or selection of alternative therapy.

Warnings: Additional Pediatric Considerations Use with caution in patients with osteoporosis; underlying clinical condition may also impact bone health and osteoporotic effect of corticosteroids and corticotropin in pediatric patients (Leonard, 2006). Corticosteroid use may cause psychiatric disturbances, including depression, euphoria, insomnia, mood swings, personality changes, and irritability (especially in infants).

Adverse Reactions

Adverse events associated with cortisol elevation; frequency not defined:

- Cardiovascular: Blood pressure increased
- Central nervous system: Behavioral changes, mood changes
- Endocrine & metabolic: Fluid retention, glucose intolerance
- Gastrointestinal: Appetite increased, weight gain

Adverse events associated with infantile spasm treatment:

- Cardiovascular: Cardiac hypertrophy, hypertension
- Central nervous system: Irritability, pyrexia, seizure
- Endocrine & metabolic: Cushingoid syndrome
- Gastrointestinal: Appetite decreased, diarrhea, vomiting, weight gain
- Respiratory: Nasal congestion
- Miscellaneous: Infection

Postmarketing and/or case reports (other adverse events associated with corticosteroids may also occur): Abdominal distension, allergic reactions, carbohydrate intolerance (infants), congestive heart failure, diaphoresis (adults), facial erythema, headache (adults), hirsutism, hypokalemic alkalosis (infants), intracranial hemorrhage (adults), muscle weakness, necrotizing angiitis (adults), pancreatitis (adults), reversible brain shrinkage (secondary to hypertension; infants), skin thinning (adults), subdural hematoma, ulcerative esophagitis, vertebral compression fractures (infants), vertigo (adults)

Drug Interactions

Metabolism/Transport Effects None known.

Avoid Concomitant Use

Avoid concomitant use of Corticotropin with any of the following: Aldesleukin; BCG; BCG (Intravesical); Indium 111 Capromab Pendetide; Mifepristone; Natalizumab; Pimecrolimus; Tacrolimus (Topical); Tofacitinib

Increased Effect/Toxicity

Corticotropin may increase the levels/effects of: Acetylcholinesterase Inhibitors; Amphotericin B; Androgens; Ceritinib; Deferasirox; Leflunomide; Loop Diuretics; Natalizumab; Nicorandil; NSAID (COX-2 Inhibitor); NSAID (Nonselective); Quinolone Antibiotics; Thiazide Diuretics; Tofacitinib; Vaccines (Live); Warfarin

The levels/effects of Corticotropin may be increased by: Aprepitant; CYP3A4 Inhibitors (Strong); Denosumab; Estrogen Derivatives; Fosaprepitant; Indacaterol; Mifepristone; Neuromuscular-Blocking Agents (Nondepolarizing); Pimecrolimus; Roflumilast; Salicylates; Tacrolimus (Topical); Telaprevir; Trastuzumab

Decreased Effect

Corticotropin may decrease the levels/effects of: Aldesleukin; Antidiabetic Agents; BCG; BCG (Intravesical); Calcitriol (Systemic); Coccidioides immitis Skin Test; Corticorelin; Hyaluronidase; Indium 111 Capromab Pendetide; Isoniazid; Salicylates; Sipuleucel-T; Telaprevir; Urea Cycle Disorder Agents; Vaccines (Inactivated); Vaccines (Live)

The levels/effects of Corticotropin may be decreased by: CYP3A4 Inducers (Strong); Echinacea; Mifepristone; Mitotane

Storage/Stability Store in the refrigerator at 2°C to 8°C (36°F to 46°F).

Mechanism of Action Stimulates the adrenal cortex to secrete adrenal steroids (including cortisol), weakly androgenic substances, and aldosterone

Pharmacodynamics

Maximum effect: Cortisol serum concentration: IM, SubQ: 3-12 hours

Duration: Repository: 10-25 hours, up to 3 days

Pharmacokinetics (Adult data unless noted)

Absorption: IM: Over 8-16 hours

Half-life: ACTH: 15 minutes

Elimination: In urine

Dosing: Usual Note: Sudden withdrawal may lead to adrenal insufficiency or recurrent symptoms; tapering the dose prior to discontinuation of therapy may be necessary following prolonged administration.

Pediatric:

Infantile spasms: Infants and Children <2 years: Various regimens have been used (Go 2012; Mackey 2004; Pellock 2010). Some neurologists recommend low-dose ACTH (5 to 40 units/day) for short periods (1-6 weeks), while others recommend larger doses of ACTH (40 to 160 units/day) for long periods of treatment (3 to 12 months); current guidelines recommend consideration to a low-dose ACTH regimen (as an alternative to high-dose); however, literature suggests that the two dosing regimens are probably equally effective for short-term treatment (Go 2012); a recent U.S. consensus report recommends short duration (~2 weeks), followed by a taper (Pellock 2010)

Manufacturer labeling: IM: 75 units/m^2/dose twice daily for 2 weeks, followed by a 2-week taper: 30 units/m^2/dose once daily in the morning for 3 days, followed by 15 units/m^2/dose once daily in the morning for 3 days, followed by 10 units/m^2/dose once daily in the morning for 3 days and 10 units/m^2/dose every other morning for 6 days

Alternative dosing: IM: A prospective, single-blind study (Hrachovy 1994) found no major difference in effectiveness between high-dose long-duration versus low-dose short-duration ACTH therapy. Hypertension, however, occurred more frequently in the high-dose group. Low-dose regimen used in this study: Initial: 20 units/day for 2 weeks, if patient responds, taper and discontinue over a 1-week period; if patient does not respond, increase dose to 30 units/day for 4 weeks then taper and discontinue over a 1-week period.

Anti-inflammatory/immunosuppression: Children >2 years and Adolescents:

Manufacturer labeling: IM, SubQ: 40 to 80 units/dose every 2 to 72 hours

Alternative dosing: IM: 0.8 units/kg/**day or** 25 units/m²/**day** divided every 12 to 24 hours

Adult:

Acute exacerbation of multiple sclerosis: IM, SubQ: 80 to 120 units/**day** for 2 to 3 weeks

All other indications: IM, SubQ: 40 to 80 units/dose every 24 to 72 hours

Administration Parenteral: Warm gel before administration; do not over-pressurize vial when withdrawing product. May be administered IM or SubQ; IM route is recommended for the treatment of infantile spasms; do not administer IV

Monitoring Parameters Blood pressure, serum glucose, potassium, and calcium and clinical presence of adverse effects. Monitor intraocular pressure (if therapy >6 weeks) for signs of secondary ocular infections; linear growth of pediatric patients (with chronic use), assess HPA suppression; for infantile spasms, monitor seizure frequency, type, and duration

Test Interactions May suppress the wheal and flare reactions to skin test antigens

Additional Information Cosyntropin is preferred over corticotropin for diagnostic test of adrenocortical insufficiency (cosyntropin is less allergenic and test is shorter in duration).

Dosage Forms Excipient information presented when available (limited, particularly for generics); consult specific product labeling.

Gel, Injection:

HP Acthar: 80 units/mL (5 mL) [contains phenol]

◆ **Corticotropin, Repository** *see* Corticotropin *on page 536*

◆ **Cortifoam** *see* Hydrocortisone (Topical) *on page 1041*

◆ **Cortifoam™ (Can)** *see* Hydrocortisone (Topical) *on page 1041*

◆ **Cortimyxin (Can)** *see* Neomycin, Polymyxin B, and Hydrocortisone *on page 1503*

◆ **Cortisol** *see* Hydrocortisone (Systemic) *on page 1038*

◆ **Cortisol** *see* Hydrocortisone (Topical) *on page 1041*

Cortisone (KOR ti sone)

Medication Safety Issues

Sound-alike/look-alike issues:

Cortisone may be confused with Cardizem, Cortizone

Related Information

Corticosteroids Systemic Equivalencies *on page 2260*

Therapeutic Category Adrenal Corticosteroid; Anti-inflammatory Agent; Corticosteroid, Systemic; Glucocorticoid

Generic Availability (US) Yes

Use Management of adrenocortical insufficiency

Pregnancy Considerations Adequate reproduction studies have not been conducted. Cortisone crosses the placenta (Migeon, 1957). Some studies have shown an association between first trimester systemic corticosteroid use and oral clefts (Park-Wyllie, 2000; Pradat, 2003). Systemic corticosteroids may also influence fetal growth (decreased birth weight); however, information is conflicting (Lunghi, 2010). Hypoadrenalism may occur in newborns following maternal use of corticosteroids in pregnancy; monitor. When systemic corticosteroids are needed in pregnancy, it is generally recommended to use the lowest effective dose for the shortest duration of time, avoiding high doses during the first trimester (Leachman, 2006; Lunghi, 2010; Makol, 2011; Østensen, 2009).

Women exposed to cortisone during pregnancy for the treatment of an autoimmune disease may contact the OTIS Autoimmune Diseases Study at 877-311-8972.

Breast-Feeding Considerations Corticosteroids are excreted in human milk. The manufacturer notes that when used systemically, maternal use of corticosteroids have the potential to cause adverse events in a nursing infant (eg, growth suppression, interfere with endogenous corticosteroid production). Breast-feeding is not recommended by the manufacturer in women taking pharmacologic doses. If there is concern about exposure to the infant, some guidelines recommend waiting 4 hours after the maternal dose of an oral systemic corticosteroid before breast-feeding in order to decrease potential exposure to the nursing infant (based on a study using prednisolone) (Bae, 2011; Leachman, 2006; Makol, 2011; Ost, 1985).

Contraindications Hypersensitivity to cortisone acetate or any component of the formulation; serious infections except septic shock or tuberculous meningitis; administration of live virus vaccines

Warnings/Precautions Use with caution in patients with thyroid disease, hepatic impairment, renal impairment, cardiovascular disease, diabetes, glaucoma, cataracts, myasthenia gravis, patients at risk for osteoporosis, patients at risk for seizures, or GI diseases (diverticulitis, peptic ulcer, ulcerative colitis) due to perforation risk. Use caution following acute MI (corticosteroids have been associated with myocardial rupture). Because of the risk of adverse effects, systemic corticosteroids should be used cautiously in the elderly in the smallest possible effective dose for the shortest duration. May affect growth velocity; growth should be routinely monitored in pediatric patients. Withdraw therapy with gradual tapering of dose.

May cause hypercorticism or suppression of hypothalamic-pituitary-adrenal (HPA) axis, particularly in younger children or in patients receiving high doses for prolonged periods. HPA axis suppression may lead to adrenal crisis. Withdrawal and discontinuation of a corticosteroid should be done slowly and carefully. Particular care is required when patients are transferred from systemic corticosteroids to inhaled products due to possible adrenal insufficiency or withdrawal from steroids, including an increase in allergic symptoms. Adult patients receiving >20 mg per day of prednisone (or equivalent) may be most susceptible. Fatalities have occurred due to adrenal insufficiency in asthmatic patients during and after transfer from systemic corticosteroids to aerosol steroids; aerosol steroids do not provide the systemic steroid needed to treat patients having trauma, surgery, or infections.

Acute myopathy has been reported with high dose corticosteroids, usually in patients with neuromuscular transmission disorders; may involve ocular and/or respiratory muscles; monitor creatine kinase; recovery may be delayed. Corticosteroid use may cause psychiatric disturbances, including depression, euphoria, insomnia, mood swings, and personality changes. Preexisting psychiatric conditions may be exacerbated by corticosteroid use. Prolonged use of corticosteroids may also increase the incidence of secondary infection, mask acute infection (including fungal infections), prolong or exacerbate viral infections, or limit response to vaccines. Exposure to chickenpox should be avoided; corticosteroids should not be used to treat ocular herpes simplex. Corticosteroids should not be used for cerebral malaria or viral hepatitis. Close observation is required in patients with latent tuberculosis and/or TB reactivity; restrict use in active TB (only in conjunction with antituberculosis treatment). Prolonged treatment with corticosteroids has been associated with the development of Kaposi's sarcoma (case reports); if noted, discontinuation of therapy should be considered.

Warnings: Additional Pediatric Considerations May cause osteoporosis (at any age) or inhibition of bone growth in pediatric patients. Use with caution in patients with osteoporosis. In a population-based study of children, risk of fracture was shown to be increased with >4 courses of corticosteroids; underlying clinical condition may also impact bone health and osteoporotic effect of corticosteroids (Leonard, 2007). Increased IOP may occur, especially with prolonged use; in children, increased IOP has been shown to be dose dependent and produce a greater IOP in children <6 years than older children treated with ophthalmic dexamethasone (Lam, 2005).

Adverse Reactions

Central nervous system: Insomnia, nervousness

Dermatologic: Hirsutism

Endocrine & metabolic: Diabetes mellitus

Gastrointestinal: Increased appetite, indigestion

Neuromuscular & skeletal: Arthralgia

Ocular: Cataracts, glaucoma

Respiratory: Epistaxis

Rare but important or life-threatening: Alkalosis, Cushing's syndrome, delirium, edema, euphoria, fractures, hallucinations, hypersensitivity reactions, hypertension, hypokalemia, muscle wasting, myalgia, osteoporosis, pancreatitis, peptic ulcer, pituitary-adrenal axis suppression, pseudotumor cerebri, psychoses, seizure, skin atrophy, ulcerative esophagitis

Drug Interactions

Metabolism/Transport Effects None known.

Avoid Concomitant Use

Avoid concomitant use of Cortisone with any of the following: Aldesleukin; BCG; BCG (Intravesical); Indium 111 Capromab Pendetide; Mifepristone; Natalizumab; Pimecrolimus; Tacrolimus (Topical); Tofacitinib

Increased Effect/Toxicity

Cortisone may increase the levels/effects of: Acetylcholinesterase Inhibitors; Amphotericin B; Androgens; Ceritinib; Deferasirox; Leflunomide; Loop Diuretics; Natalizumab; Nicorandil; NSAID (COX-2 Inhibitor); NSAID (Nonselective); Quinolone Antibiotics; Thiazide Diuretics; Tofacitinib; Vaccines (Live); Warfarin

The levels/effects of Cortisone may be increased by: Aprepitant; CYP3A4 Inhibitors (Strong); Denosumab; Estrogen Derivatives; Fosaprepitant; Indacaterol; Mifepristone; Neuromuscular-Blocking Agents (Nondepolarizing); Pimecrolimus; Roflumilast; Salicylates; Tacrolimus (Topical); Telaprevir; Trastuzumab

Decreased Effect

Cortisone may decrease the levels/effects of: Aldesleukin; Antidiabetic Agents; BCG; BCG (Intravesical); Calcitriol (Systemic); Coccidioides immitis Skin Test; Corticorelin; Hyaluronidase; Indium 111 Capromab Pendetide; Isoniazid; Salicylates; Sipuleucel-T; Telaprevir; Urea Cycle Disorder Agents; Vaccines (Inactivated); Vaccines (Live)

The levels/effects of Cortisone may be decreased by: Antacids; Bile Acid Sequestrants; CYP3A4 Inducers (Strong); Echinacea; Mifepristone; Mitotane; Somatropin; Tesamorelin

Mechanism of Action Decreases inflammation by suppression of migration of polymorphonuclear leukocytes and reversal of increased capillary permeability

Pharmacodynamics

Maximum effect: Oral: Within 2 hours

Duration: 30-36 hours

Pharmacokinetics (Adult data unless noted)

Distribution: Crosses the placenta; appears in breast milk; distributes to muscles, liver, skin, intestines, and kidneys

Metabolism: In the liver to inactive metabolites

Half-life: 30 minutes

Elimination: In bile and urine

Dosing: Usual Depends upon the condition being treated and the response of the patient. Supplemental doses may be warranted during times of stress in the course of withdrawing therapy. Oral:

Children:

Anti-inflammatory or immunosuppressive: 2.5-10 mg/kg/day or 20-300 mg/m^2/day in divided doses every 6-8 hours

Physiologic replacement: 0.5-0.75 mg/kg/day or 20-25 mg/m^2/day in divided doses every 8 hours

Adults: 20-300 mg/day divided every 12-24 hours

Administration Oral: Administer with meals, food, or milk to decrease GI effects

Monitoring Parameters Long-term use: Electrolytes, glucose, blood pressure, height, weight

Test Interactions May suppress the wheal and flare reactions to skin test antigens

Additional Information Insoluble in water

Dosage Forms Excipient information presented when available (limited, particularly for generics); consult specific product labeling.

Tablet, Oral, as acetate:

Generic: 25 mg

- ◆ **Cortisone Acetate** *see* Cortisone *on page 538*
- ◆ **Cortisporin** *see* Neomycin, Polymyxin B, and Hydrocortisone *on page 1503*
- ◆ **Cortisporin Ointment** *see* Bacitracin, Neomycin, Polymyxin B, and Hydrocortisone *on page 253*
- ◆ **Cortisporin Otic (Can)** *see* Neomycin, Polymyxin B, and Hydrocortisone *on page 1503*
- ◆ **Cortisporin Topical Ointment (Can)** *see* Bacitracin, Neomycin, Polymyxin B, and Hydrocortisone *on page 253*
- ◆ **Cortomycin** *see* Neomycin, Polymyxin B, and Hydrocortisone *on page 1503*
- ◆ **Cortrosyn** *see* Cosyntropin *on page 539*
- ◆ **Cosmegen** *see* DACTINomycin *on page 573*
- ◆ **CO Sotalol (Can)** *see* Sotalol *on page 1963*

Cosyntropin (koe sin TROE pin)

Medication Safety Issues

Sound-alike/look-alike issues:

Cortrosyn may be confused with colchicine, corticorelin, corticotropin, Cotazym

Cosyntropin may be confused with corticorelin, corticotropin

Brand Names: US Cortrosyn

Brand Names: Canada Cortrosyn; Synacthen Depot

Therapeutic Category Adrenal Corticosteroid; Diagnostic Agent, Adrenocortical Insufficiency

Generic Availability (US) Yes

Use Diagnostic test to differentiate primary adrenal from secondary (pituitary) adrenocortical insufficiency [FDA approved in pediatric patients (age not specified) and adults]; has also been used in the diagnosis of congenital adrenal hyperplasia

Pregnancy Risk Factor C

Pregnancy Considerations Animal reproduction studies have not been conducted with cosyntropin; adverse events have been observed with corticosteroids in animal reproduction studies. Some studies have shown an association between first trimester systemic corticosteroid use and oral clefts (Park-Wyllie, 2000; Pradat, 2003). Systemic corticosteroids may also influence fetal growth (decreased birth weight); however, information is conflicting (Lunghi, 2010). When systemic corticosteroids are needed in pregnancy, it is generally recommended to use the lowest effective dose for the shortest duration of time, avoiding high doses during the first trimester (Leachman, 2006; Lunghi, 2010; Makol, 2011; Østensen, 2009).

Breast-Feeding Considerations It is not known if cosyntropin is excreted into breast milk. The manufacturer recommends that caution be exercised when administering cosyntropin to nursing women.

Contraindications Hypersensitivity to cosyntropin or any component of the formulation

Synacthen Depot [Canadian product]: Additional contraindications: Treatment of asthma or other allergic conditions (increased risk of anaphylactic reactions); use in premature babies and neonates <1 month; acute psychosis; untreated bacterial, fungal, and viral infections; active or latent peptic ulcer; refractory heart failure; Cushing's syndrome; treatment of primary adrenocortical insufficiency; adrenogenital syndrome

Warnings/Precautions

Cortrosyn: Use with caution in patients with preexisting allergic disease or a history of allergic reactions to corticotropin.

Synacthen Depot [Canadian product]: Use is contraindicated in patients with allergic conditions. Hypersensitivity reactions (including severe reactions) may occur particularly in patients with asthma or other allergies and often within 30 minutes of administration; monitor for hypersensitivity for ~1 hour after administration. Prolonged use may increase the risk of allergic reactions; contains benzyl alcohol; avoid use in infants and children <3 years of age; contraindicated in neonates. Use caution in patients with hypertension or thromboembolic disease, nonspecific ulcerative colitis, diverticulitis, or recent intestinal anastomosis, hepatic disease, renal disease, myasthenia gravis, osteoporosis, psychiatric disturbances, thyroid disease, and/or ocular disease (cataracts, glaucoma). Avoid use in optic neuritis. Consider routine eye exams in chronic users. Use caution in patients with acute or chronic infections (especially varicella or vaccinia) or exanthematous and fungal diseases. Use with caution in patients with latent tuberculosis; treatment may reactivate latent tuberculosis. Rule out amebiasis prior to initiating therapy; may activate latent amebiasis. Live vaccines should not be given concurrently. Augmentation or resumption of therapy may be necessary in patients undergoing surgery or subjected to trauma during or within 1 year of therapy discontinuation; adjunctive rapid acting corticosteroids may be necessary during periods of stress.

Adverse Reactions Note: Adverse events associated with other corticosteroids may be observed when Synacthen Depot [Canadian product] is used for therapeutic purposes. Refer to corticosteroid monographs for comprehensive lists.

Cardiovascular: Bradycardia, hypertension, peripheral edema, tachycardia

Dermatologic: Skin rash, urticaria at injection site (with erythema)

Hypersensitivity: Anaphylaxis, hypersensitivity reaction

Rare but important or life-threatening: Synacthen Depot (Canadian product): Adrenal hemorrhage

Drug Interactions

Metabolism/Transport Effects None known.

Avoid Concomitant Use

Avoid concomitant use of Cosyntropin with any of the following: Valproic Acid and Derivatives

Increased Effect/Toxicity

Cosyntropin may increase the levels/effects of: ClonazePAM; Diazepam; Nitrazepam; PHENobarbital; Phenytoin; Primidone; Valproic Acid and Derivatives

Decreased Effect There are no known significant interactions involving a decrease in effect.

Storage/Stability

Powder for injection: Store at controlled room temperature of 15°C to 30°C (59°F to 86°F).

IV infusion: Stable for 12 hours at room temperature.

Solution for injection: Store refrigerated between 2°C to 8°C (36°F to 46°F). Protect from light and freezing.

IV infusion: Stable for 12 hours at room temperature.

Suspension for injection: Synacthen Depot [Canadian product]: Store refrigerated between 2°C to 8°C (36°F to 46°F). Protect from light.

Mechanism of Action Stimulates the adrenal cortex to secrete adrenal steroids (including hydrocortisone, cortisone), androgenic substances, and a small amount of aldosterone

Pharmacodynamics

Onset of action: IM, IV: Within 5 minutes increases in plasma cortisol concentrations are observed in healthy individuals

Maximum effect: IM, IV: 45-60 minutes peak plasma cortisol concentration

Dosing: Neonatal Adrenocortical insufficiency, diagnostic test: Note: Cosyntropin injection solution formulation is not recommended for IM administration; use powder for injection formulation.

Preterm neonates: Limited data available; reported range: IM, IV: 0.1-3.5 **mcg**/kg/dose. In 276 ELBW neonates, a dose of 1 **mcg**/kg was found to be superior to 0.1 **mcg**/kg in assessing adrenal function; in addition, the 0.1 **mcg**/kg/dose given IM produced a significantly lower response than when given IV (mean GA: 25.5 weeks; mean birth weight: 743 g) (Watterberg, 2005). Physiologic doses of 0.1 **mcg**/kg were used to test adrenal function in VLBW neonates [mean birth weight 900 g; mean GA: 27 weeks (range: 23-32 weeks)]; only 36% of neonates responded; increasing the dose to 0.2 **mcg**/kg resulted in 67% of the neonates responding, but sensitivity of the test was decreased (Korte, 1996). Doses of 3.5 **mcg**/kg were administered to test adrenal function in 44 preterm neonates (mean birth weight: 823 g; mean GA: 26.2 weeks; mean PMA: 30.1 weeks) during inhaled beclomethasone therapy (Cole, 1999).

Full-term neonates: IM, IV: 15 **mcg**/kg/dose

Dosing: Usual

Infants, Children, and Adolescents:

Adrenocortical insufficiency, diagnostic test: Note: Cosyntropin injection solution formulation is not recommended for IM administration; use powder for injection formulation.

Infants and Children ≤2 years: IM, IV:

Manufacturer's labeling: 0.125 mg

Alternate dosing: 15 **mcg**/kg

Children >2 years and Adolescents:

Manufacturer's labeling:

IM, IV: 0.25 mg; **Note:** Doses in the range of 0.25-0.75 mg have been used in clinical studies; however, maximal response is seen with 0.25 mg dose

IV infusion: 0.25 mg administered over 6 hours (rate: 0.04 mg/hour); may be useful when greater cortisol stimulation required

Alternate dosing (low-dose): Children ≥5 years and Adolescents: IV: 1 **mcg** (Cemeroglu, 2011; Kazlauskaite, 2008)

Congenital adrenal hyperplasia, evaluation: Infants and Children: IM, IV: 0.125-0.25 mg (Speiser, 2010)

Adults: **Adrenocortical insufficiency, diagnostic test:** **Note:** Cosyntropin injection solution formulation is not recommended for IM administration; use powder for injection formulation.

Conventional dose: IM, IV: 0.25 mg; **Note:** Doses in the range of 0.25-0.75 mg have been used in clinical studies; however, maximal response is seen with 0.25 mg dose

IV infusion: 0.25 mg administered over 6 hours (rate: 0.04 mg/hour); may be useful when greater cortisol stimulation required

Low-dose protocol: IM, IV: 1 **mcg** (Abdu, 1999); **Note:** The use of the low-dose protocol has been advocated by some clinicians, particularly in mild or secondary adrenal insufficiency. The low-dose protocol is not recommended in critically ill patients (Marik, 2008).

Preparation for Administration

Parenteral: Following reconstitution, visually inspect solution for discoloration and particulate matter prior to injection. Contains no preservatives; discard unused portion of vial after use.

IM: Reconstituted powder for injection only: Reconstitute 0.25 mg with 1 mL NS; **Note:** Solution for injection not recommended for IM administration per manufacturer.

IV push:

Standard doses: Reconstitute 0.25 mg with 2 to 5 mL NS

Low doses: Concentrations of 1 **mcg**/mL (final volume: 1 mL) and 0.5 **mcg**/mL (final volume: 2 mL) have been reported (Abdu 1999; Cemeroglu 2011)

IV infusion: Mix in NS or D_5W.

Administration Parenteral:

IM:

Powder for injection: Administer as 0.25 mg/mL concentration

Injection solution: Not recommended for IM administration per manufacturer

IV:

IV push: Administer over 2 minutes

IV infusion: Infuse over 4 to 8 hours (~0.04 mg/hour over 6 hours)

Reference Range Plasma cortisol concentrations should be measured immediately before and exactly 30 minutes after the dose; dose should be given in the early morning; normal morning baseline cortisol >5 mcg/dL (SI: >138 nmol/L); normal response 30 minutes after cosyntropin injection: an increase in serum cortisol concentration of ≥7 mcg/dL (SI: ≥193 nmol/L) or peak response >18 mcg/dL (SI: >497 nmol/L). If increase in plasma cortisol levels at 30 minutes is equivocal, consider repeat cortisol sampling at 60 and/or 90 minutes.

Test Interactions Concurrent or recent use of spironolactone, hydrocortisone, cortisone, etomidate, estrogens

Additional Information Each 0.25 mg of cosyntropin is equivalent to 25 units of corticotropin.

Dosage Forms Excipient information presented when available (limited, particularly for generics); consult specific product labeling.

Solution, Intravenous:

Generic: 0.25 mg/mL (1 mL)

Solution Reconstituted, Injection:

Cortrosyn: 0.25 mg (1 ea)

Generic: 0.25 mg (1 ea)

Solution Reconstituted, Injection [preservative free]:

Generic: 0.25 mg (1 ea)

- ◆ **Cotazym (Can)** *see* Pancrelipase *on page 1614*
- ◆ **CO Terbinafine (Can)** *see* Terbinafine (Systemic) *on page 2021*
- ◆ **Co-Trimoxazole** *see* Sulfamethoxazole and Trimethoprim *on page 1986*
- ◆ **Cough DM [OTC]** *see* Dextromethorphan *on page 631*
- ◆ **Cough Syrup [OTC]** *see* GuaiFENesin *on page 988*
- ◆ **Coumadin** *see* Warfarin *on page 2195*
- ◆ **CO Valacyclovir (Can)** *see* ValACYclovir *on page 2138*
- ◆ **Co-Vidarabine** *see* Pentostatin *on page 1668*
- ◆ **Coviracil** *see* Emtricitabine *on page 739*
- ◆ **Cozaar** *see* Losartan *on page 1302*
- ◆ **CPDG2** *see* Glucarpidase *on page 974*
- ◆ **CPG2** *see* Glucarpidase *on page 974*
- ◆ **CPM** *see* Cyclophosphamide *on page 551*
- ◆ **CPT-11** *see* Irinotecan *on page 1159*
- ◆ **CPZ** *see* ChlorproMAZINE *on page 443*
- ◆ **13-CRA** *see* ISOtretinoin *on page 1171*
- ◆ **Creomulsion Adult [OTC]** *see* Dextromethorphan *on page 631*
- ◆ **Creomulsion for Children [OTC]** *see* Dextromethorphan *on page 631*
- ◆ **Creon** *see* Pancrelipase *on page 1614*
- ◆ **Crestor** *see* Rosuvastatin *on page 1886*
- ◆ **Critic-Aid Clear AF [OTC]** *see* Miconazole (Topical) *on page 1431*
- ◆ **Critic-Aid Skin Care® [OTC]** *see* Zinc Oxide *on page 2214*
- ◆ **Crixivan** *see* Indinavir *on page 1098*
- ◆ **CroFab** *see Crotalidae* Polyvalent Immune Fab (Ovine) *on page 543*
- ◆ **Crolom** *see* Cromolyn (Ophthalmic) *on page 543*
- ◆ **Cromoglicate** *see* Cromolyn (Nasal) *on page 542*
- ◆ **Cromoglicate** *see* Cromolyn (Ophthalmic) *on page 543*
- ◆ **Cromoglicate** *see* Cromolyn (Systemic, Oral Inhalation) *on page 541*
- ◆ **Cromoglycic Acid** *see* Cromolyn (Nasal) *on page 542*
- ◆ **Cromoglycic Acid** *see* Cromolyn (Ophthalmic) *on page 543*
- ◆ **Cromoglycic Acid** *see* Cromolyn (Systemic, Oral Inhalation) *on page 541*

Cromolyn (Systemic, Oral Inhalation)

(KROE moe lin)

Brand Names: US Gastrocrom

Brand Names: Canada Nalcrom; Nu-Cromolyn; PMS-Sodium Cromoglycate

Therapeutic Category Antiasthmatic; Inhalation, Miscellaneous

Generic Availability (US) Yes

Use

Nebulization: Prophylactic agent used for long-term (chronic) control of persistent asthma; **NOT** indicated for the relief of acute bronchospasm; also used for the prevention of allergen- or exercise-induced bronchospasm (**Note:** Cromolyn is not as effective as inhaled short-acting beta_2-agonists for exercise-induced bronchospasm; NAEPP, 2007)

Systemic: Mastocytosis, food allergy, and treatment of inflammatory bowel disease

Pregnancy Risk Factor B

Pregnancy Considerations Adverse events were not observed in animal reproduction studies. No data available on whether cromolyn crosses the placenta or clinical effects on the fetus. Available evidence suggests safe use during pregnancy.

Breast-Feeding Considerations No data available on whether cromolyn enters into breast milk or clinical effects on the infant. Use of cromolyn is not considered a contraindication to breast-feeding.

Contraindications Hypersensitivity to cromolyn or any component of the formulation; acute asthma attacks

Warnings/Precautions Severe anaphylactic reactions may occur rarely; cromolyn is a prophylactic drug with no benefit for acute situations; caution should be used when withdrawing the drug or tapering the dose as symptoms may reoccur; use with caution in patients with a history of cardiac arrhythmias. Dosage of oral product should be decreased with hepatic or renal dysfunction.

Warnings: Additional Pediatric Considerations Oral cromolyn increased mortality in neonatal rats when administered at ~9 times the maximum recommended daily dose for infants, but not at ~3 times the maximum recommended daily dose; use of oral cromolyn in infants and children <2 years is not recommended and should be reserved for patients with severe mastocytosis in whom potential benefits clearly outweigh the risks.

Adverse Reactions

Cardiovascular: Angioedema, chest pain, edema, flushing, palpitation, premature ventricular contractions, tachycardia

Central nervous system: Anxiety, behavior changes, convulsions, depression, dizziness, fatigue, hallucinations, headache, irritability, insomnia, lethargy, migraine, nervousness, hypoesthesia, postprandial lightheadedness, psychosis

Dermatologic: Erythema, photosensitivity, pruritus, purpura, rash, urticaria

Gastrointestinal: Abdominal pain, constipation, diarrhea, dyspepsia, dysphagia, esophagospasm, flatulence, glossitis, nausea, stomatitis, vomiting

Genitourinary: Dysuria, urinary frequency

Hematologic: Neutropenia, pancytopenia, polycythemia

Hepatic: Liver function test abnormal

Local: Burning

Neuromuscular & skeletal: Arthralgia, leg weakness, leg stiffness, myalgia, paresthesia

Otic: Tinnitus

Respiratory: Dyspnea, pharyngitis

Miscellaneous: Lupus erythematosus

Drug Interactions

Metabolism/Transport Effects None known.

Avoid Concomitant Use There are no known interactions where it is recommended to avoid concomitant use.

Increased Effect/Toxicity There are no known significant interactions involving an increase in effect.

Decreased Effect There are no known significant interactions involving a decrease in effect.

Storage/Stability Store at room temperature of 15°C to 30°C (59°F to 86°F). Protect from light. Do not use oral solution if solution becomes discolored or forms a precipitate.

Mechanism of Action Prevents the mast cell release of histamine, leukotrienes, and slow-reacting substance of anaphylaxis by inhibiting degranulation after contact with antigens

Pharmacodynamics Not effective for immediate relief of symptoms in acute asthmatic attacks; must be used at regular intervals for 2-4 weeks to be effective; **Note:** Therapeutic response may occur within 2 weeks; however, a trial of 4-6 weeks may be needed to determine maximum benefits.

Pharmacokinetics (Adult data unless noted)

Absorption:

Oral: 0.5% to 2%

Inhalation: ~8% reaches lungs upon inhalation; well absorbed

Half-life: 80-90 minutes

Time to peak serum concentration: Within 15 minutes after inhalation

Elimination: Equally excreted unchanged in urine and feces (via bile); small amounts after inhalation are exhaled

Dosing: Usual

Inhalation, nebulization solution:

Chronic control of asthma: Children ≥2 years and Adults Initial: 20 mg 4 times/day; usual dose: 20 mg 3-4 times/day; **Note:** Once control is achieved, taper frequency to the lowest effective dose (ie, 4 times/day to 3 times/day to twice daily)

Prevention of allergen- or exercise-induced bronchospasm: Children ≥2 years and Adults: Single dose of 20 mg; **Note:** Administer 10-15 minutes prior to exercise or allergen exposure but no longer than 1 hour before

NIH Asthma Guidelines (NAEPP, 2007): Children ≥2 years and Adults: 20 mg 4 times/day

Oral:

Systemic mastocytosis:

Neonates and Preterm Infants: Not recommended

Infants and Children <2 years: Not recommended; reserve use for patients with severe disease in whom potential benefits outweigh risks; 20 mg/kg/day in 4 divided doses; may increase in patients 6 months to 2 years of age if benefits not seen after 2-3 weeks; do not exceed 30 mg/kg/day

Children 2-12 years: 100 mg 4 times/day; not to exceed 40 mg/kg/day

Children >12 years and Adults: 200 mg 4 times/day

Food allergy and inflammatory bowel disease:

Infants and Children <2 years: Not recommended

Children 2-12 years: Initial dose: 100 mg 4 times/day; may double the dose if effect is not satisfactory within 2-3 weeks; not to exceed 40 mg/kg/day

Children >12 years and Adults: Initial dose: 200 mg 4 times/day; may double the dose if effect is not satisfactory within 2-3 weeks; up to 400 mg 4 times/day

Once desired effect is achieved, dose may be tapered to lowest effective dose

Administration Oral concentrate: Open ampul and squeeze contents into glass of water; stir well; administer at least 30 minutes before meals and at bedtime; do not mix with juice, milk, or food

Monitoring Parameters Asthma: Periodic pulmonary function tests; signs and symptoms of disease state when tapering dose

Additional Information The 2007 Expert Panel Report of the National Asthma Education and Prevention Program (NAEPP, 2007) does not recommend cromolyn for initial treatment of persistent asthma in children; inhaled corticosteroids are the preferred agents; cromolyn is considered an alternative medication for the treatment of mild persistent asthma in children. Reserve systemic use in children <2 years of age for severe disease; avoid systemic use in premature infants.

Dosage Forms Excipient information presented when available (limited, particularly for generics); consult specific product labeling.

Concentrate, Oral, as sodium:

Gastrocrom: 100 mg/5 mL (5 mL)

Generic: 100 mg/5 mL (5 mL)

Concentrate, Oral, as sodium [preservative free]:

Generic: 100 mg/5 mL (5 mL)

Nebulization Solution, Inhalation, as sodium:

Generic: 20 mg/2 mL (2 mL)

Cromolyn (Nasal) (KROE moe lin)

Medication Safety Issues

Sound-alike/look-alike issues:

NasalCrom® may be confused with Nasacort®, Nasalide®

Brand Names: US NasalCrom [OTC]

Brand Names: Canada Apo-Cromolyn Nasal Spray [OTC]; Rhinaris-CS Anti-Allergic Nasal Mist

Therapeutic Category Inhalation, Miscellaneous

Generic Availability (US) Yes

Use Management of seasonal or perennial allergic rhinitis

Pregnancy Considerations Animal reproduction studies have not been conducted; however, studies in pregnant women have not shown signs of adverse effects or increased teratogenicity with use during pregnancy (Gilbert, 2005; Mazzotta, 1999).

Breast-Feeding Considerations Use of cromolyn is not considered a contraindication to breast-feeding (NAEPP, 2005).

Contraindications Hypersensitivity to cromolyn or any component of the formulation; acute asthma attacks

Warnings/Precautions Cromolyn is a prophylactic drug with no benefit for acute situations; caution should be used when withdrawing the drug or tapering the dose as symptoms may reoccur.

Adverse Reactions

Central nervous system: Headache

Gastrointestinal: Unpleasant taste

Respiratory: Coughing; hoarseness; increase in burning, irritation, sneezing, or stinging inside of nose; postnasal drip

Rare but important or life-threatening: Epistaxis

Drug Interactions

Metabolism/Transport Effects None known.

Avoid Concomitant Use There are no known interactions where it is recommended to avoid concomitant use.

Increased Effect/Toxicity There are no known significant interactions involving an increase in effect.

Decreased Effect There are no known significant interactions involving a decrease in effect.

Storage/Stability Store at room temperature of 15°C to 30°C (59°F to 86°F). Protect from light.

Dosing: Usual Intranasal: Children ≥2 years and Adults: 1 spray in each nostril 3-4 times/day; maximum dose: 1 spray in each nostril 6 times/day

Administration Clear nasal passages by blowing nose prior to use.

Dosage Forms Excipient information presented when available (limited, particularly for generics); consult specific product labeling.

Aerosol Solution, Nasal, as sodium:

NasalCrom: 5.2 mg/actuation (13 mL, 26 mL) [contains benzalkonium chloride, edetate disodium]

Generic: 5.2 mg/actuation (26 mL)

Cromolyn (Ophthalmic) (KROE moe lin)

Brand Names: Canada Opticrom®

Generic Availability (US) Yes

Use Vernal conjunctivitis, vernal keratoconjunctivitis, and vernal keratitis

Pregnancy Risk Factor B

Pregnancy Considerations Adverse events were not observed in animal reproduction studies.

Breast-Feeding Considerations Use of cromolyn is not considered a contraindication to breast-feeding.

Contraindications Hypersensitivity to cromolyn or any component of the formulation

Warnings/Precautions Severe anaphylactic reactions may occur rarely; cromolyn is a prophylactic drug with no benefit for acute situations; caution should be used when withdrawing the drug or tapering the dose as symptoms may reoccur. Transient burning or stinging may occur.

Adverse Reactions

Ocular: Conjunctival injection, dryness around the eye, edema, eye irritation, immediate hypersensitivity reactions, itchy eyes, puffy eyes, rash, styes, watery eyes

Respiratory: Dyspnea

Drug Interactions

Metabolism/Transport Effects None known.

Avoid Concomitant Use There are no known interactions where it is recommended to avoid concomitant use.

Increased Effect/Toxicity There are no known significant interactions involving an increase in effect.

Decreased Effect There are no known significant interactions involving a decrease in effect.

Storage/Stability Store at room temperature of 15°C to 30°C (59°F to 86°F). Protect from light.

Pharmacokinetics (Adult data unless noted)

Half-life: 80-90 minutes

Elimination: Equally excreted unchanged in urine and feces (via bile)

Dosing: Usual Ophthalmic: Children >4 years and Adults: Instill 1-2 drops 4-6 times/day

Dosage Forms Excipient information presented when available (limited, particularly for generics); consult specific product labeling.

Solution, Ophthalmic, as sodium:

Generic: 4% (10 mL)

- ◆ **Cromolyn Sodium** *see* Cromolyn (Nasal) *on page 542*
- ◆ **Cromolyn Sodium** *see* Cromolyn (Ophthalmic) *on page 543*
- ◆ **Cromolyn Sodium** *see* Cromolyn (Systemic, Oral Inhalation) *on page 541*

Crotalidae Polyvalent Immune Fab (Ovine) (kroe TAL ih die pol i VAY lent i MYUN fab (oh vine))

Brand Names: US CroFab

Therapeutic Category Antivenin

Generic Availability (US) No

Use Management of patients with North American crotalid envenomations [eg, rattlesnakes (*Crotalus, Sistrurus*), copperheads, and cottonmouth/water moccasins (*Agkistrodon*)] [FDA approved in pediatric patients (age not specified) and adults]

Pregnancy Risk Factor C

Pregnancy Considerations Animal reproduction studies have not been conducted. Products contain thimerosal which may be associated with mercury-related toxicities, including neurological and renal toxicities in the fetus and very young children. In general, the health and prognosis of the mother should be taken into consideration when using medications as antidotes; they should be administered to pregnant women if there is a clear indication for use and should not be withheld because of fears of teratogenicity (Bailey, 2003). Experience with the use of antivenom in pregnancy is limited; however, treatment with antivenom should be considered in snake envenomations in which it is usually required as definitive management or in envenomations refractory to supportive care (Brown, 2013).

Breast-Feeding Considerations It is not known if this product is excreted into breast milk. The manufacturer recommends caution be used if administered to a nursing woman.

Contraindications Hypersensitivity to any component of the formulation (including papaya or papain), unless the benefits outweigh the risks and appropriate management for anaphylaxis is readily available

Warnings/Precautions Should be used within 4-6 hours of the envenomation to prevent clinical deterioration and the development of coagulation abnormalities. Coagulation ▶

abnormalities are due directly to snake venom interference with the coagulation cascade. Recurrent coagulopathy occurs in approximately 50% of patients and may persist for 1 to 2 weeks or more; patients who have evidence of coagulopathy during the first 12 hours post antivenom treatment have an ~66% chance of recurrence, which typically occurs 2 to 14 days after completion of antivenom administration (Boyer, 2001). Repeat dosing may be indicated (Miller, 2010; Ruha, 2011). Patients should be monitored for at least 1 week and evaluated for other preexisting conditions associated with bleeding disorders. In severe In severe envenomations, a decrease in platelets may occur, lasting hours to several days, and whole blood transfusions may not be an effective treatment. Anaphylaxis and anaphylactoid reactions are possible due to sheep proteins in the antivenom. Processed with papain and may cause hypersensitivity reactions in patients allergic to papaya, other papaya extracts, papain, chymopapain, or the pineapple-enzyme bromelain. There may also be cross allergy with dust mite and latex allergens. Also contains thimerosal which is a source of mercury.

Warnings: Additional Pediatric Considerations Accumulation of thimerosal has been associated with neurological and renal toxicity; developing fetuses and young infants and children are most susceptible; the presence of thimerosal should not deter use as the risks of untreated crotalid envenomations far outweigh the risk of thimerosal exposure.

Adverse Reactions

Cardiovascular: Hypotension

Central nervous system: Chills, fever

Dermatologic: Pruritus, rash, urticaria

Gastrointestinal: Anorexia, nausea

Respiratory: Asthma, cough, dyspnea, wheezing

Miscellaneous: Anaphylaxis, anaphylactoid reaction, hypersensitivity reactions, serum sickness

Rare but important or life-threatening: Angioedema, chest discomfort, dizziness, erythema, headache, hyperhidrosis, lip swelling, musculoskeletal chest pain, tachycardia, tachypnea, tongue swelling, tracheal edema

Drug Interactions

Avoid Concomitant Use There are no known interactions for which it is recommended to avoid concomitant use.

Increased Effect/Toxicity There are no known significant interactions involving an increase in effect.

Decreased Effect There are no known significant interactions involving a decrease in effect.

Storage/Stability Store at 2°C to 8°C (36°F to 46°F). Do not freeze. Use within 4 hours after reconstitution and dilution.

Mechanism of Action A venom-specific fragment of IgG, which binds and neutralizes venom toxin, helping to remove the toxin from the target tissue and eliminate it from the body.

Pharmacodynamics Onset of action: Stability of patient or reduction in symptoms may be seen within 1 hour of administration

Pharmacokinetics (Adult data unless noted)

Distribution: V_d: Unbound Fab: 110 mL/kg (Seifert, 2001)

Half-life: 12-23 hours (based on limited data)

Elimination: Speculated to occur via reticuloendothelial system (Dart, 1997)

Clearance: Unbound Fab: 5.9 mL/h/kg (Seifert, 2001)

Dosing: Usual IV: Children, Adolescents, and Adults: **Note:** Antivenom dosage is based on venom load and severity of symptoms and not on patient size; therefore, a reduced, weight-based antivenom dose in pediatric patients is **not** recommended (Behm, 2003; Lavonas, 2011a; Offerman, 2002). Clinicians are encouraged to contact their local poison control center or clinical toxicologist for consultation when treating any envenomed patient.

Crotalid envenomation:

Initial dose: 4-6 vials as soon as possible and ideally within 6 hours of snakebite; monitor for 1 hour following infusion to determine if control of envenomation is achieved (arrest of local manifestations and normalization of coagulation studies and other systemic signs). If control is not achieved, repeat with additional dose of 4-6 vials until initial control is achieved. Some experts recommend doubling the initial dose in patients presenting with life-threatening symptoms such as respiratory distress, cardiovascular collapse, significant hemorrhage, or severe neurologic toxicity (Goto, 2009; Lavonas, 2011a).

Maintenance dose (begin once control of envenomation achieved): 2 vials every 6 hours for up to 18 hours. Optimal dosing beyond 18 hours has not been established; however, treatment may be continued if deemed necessary based on patient condition.

Preparation for Administration IV infusion: Reconstitute each vial with 18 mL NS and mix by continuous manual inversion until no solid material is visible. Do not shake. A faster dissolution has been shown using 25 mL SWFI for reconstitution and hand rolling/inverting which may allow for more rapid administration (Quan 2010). Further dilute **total** dose (4 to 6 vials) in 250 mL NS. Due to fluid overload concerns in children who weigh <10 kg, it has been proposed that approximately half of the normal fluid volume for dilution (ie, 125 mL NS) should be used in this patient population (Johnson 2008); lower infusion volumes may also be considered for fluid sensitive patients, such as those with congestive heart failure, chronic lung disease, or renal insufficiency (Goto 2009; Johnson 2008; Offerman 2002; Pizon 2007).

Administration IV infusion: Administer at an initial rate of 25 to 50 mL/hour for the first 10 minutes; if tolerated and no allergic reaction observed, then increase rate so that total dose infuses over 60 minutes, usually to 250 mL/hour. Continue to monitor closely. Epinephrine and diphenhydramine should be available during the infusion. Decreasing the rate of infusion may help control some adverse effects, such as fever, nausea, low back pain, and wheezing.

Monitoring Parameters Vital signs; CBC, platelet count, prothrombin time, aPTT, fibrinogen levels, fibrin split products, clot retraction, bleeding and coagulation times, BUN, electrolytes, bilirubin; size of bite area (repeat every 15-30 minutes); intake and output; signs and symptoms of anaphylaxis/allergy. CBC, platelet counts, and clotting studies should be evaluated at 6-hour intervals until patient is stable.

Additional Information Envenomation Category:

Minimal: Swelling, pain, and bruising are limited to immediate bite site; no systemic signs and symptoms; normal coagulation parameters; no clinical evidence of bleeding

Moderate: Swelling, pain, and bruising are limited to less than a full extremity (or <50 cm if bite was on head or trunk); systemic signs and symptoms are not life-threatening (nausea, vomiting, oral paresthesia, unusual taste, mild hypotension, mild tachycardia, tachypnea); coagulation parameters may be abnormal; no bleeding other than minor hematuria, gum bleeding, or nosebleeds, if not severe

Severe: Swelling, pain, and bruising involve more than the entire extremity or threaten the airway; systemic signs and symptoms are markedly abnormal (severe alteration of mental status, severe hypotension, severe tachycardia, tachypnea, respiratory insufficiency); coagulation parameters are abnormal; serious bleeding or severe threat of bleeding

Dosage Forms Excipient information presented when available (limited, particularly for generics); consult specific product labeling.

Solution Reconstituted, Intravenous:
CroFab: (1 ea) [contains thimerosal]

- ◆ **Crotaline Antivenin, Polyvalent, FAB (Ovine)** *see Crotalidae* Polyvalent Immune Fab (Ovine) *on page 543*
- ◆ **Crotaline Antivenom, Polyvalent, FAB (Ovine)** *see Crotalidae* Polyvalent Immune Fab (Ovine) *on page 543*

Crotamiton (kroe TAM i tonn)

Medication Safety Issues

Sound-alike/look-alike issues:

Eurax may be confused with Efudex, Eulexin, Evoxac, Serax, Urex

International issues:

Eurax [U.S., Canada, and multiple international markets] may be confused with Urex brand name for furosemide [Australia, China,Turkey] and methenamine [U.S., Canada]

Brand Names: US Eurax

Brand Names: Canada Eurax Cream

Therapeutic Category Scabicidal Agent

Generic Availability (US) No

Use Treatment of scabies (*Sarcoptes scabiei*) in infants and children; symptomatic treatment of pruritic skin

Pregnancy Risk Factor C

Pregnancy Considerations Animal reproduction studies have not been conducted; use during pregnancy only if clearly needed.

Breast-Feeding Considerations It is not known if crotamiton is excreted in breast milk.

Contraindications Hypersensitivity to crotamiton or any component of the formulation; patients who manifest a primary irritation response to topical medications

Warnings/Precautions Avoid contact with face, eyes, mucous membranes, and urethral meatus. Do not apply to acutely inflamed, raw, or weeping skin. Discontinue use if severe irritation or sensitization occurs. For external use only.

Adverse Reactions

Dermatologic: Contact dermatitis, pruritus, rash
Local: Local irritation
Miscellaneous: Allergic sensitivity reactions, warm sensation

Drug Interactions

Metabolism/Transport Effects None known.

Avoid Concomitant Use There are no known interactions where it is recommended to avoid concomitant use.

Increased Effect/Toxicity There are no known significant interactions involving an increase in effect.

Decreased Effect There are no known significant interactions involving a decrease in effect.

Storage/Stability Store at room temperature.

Mechanism of Action Crotamiton has scabicidal activity against *Sarcoptes scabiei*; mechanism of action unknown. Antipruritic effects mediated by inhibition of histamine, serotonin, and PAR-2 (Sekine 2012).

Pharmacokinetics (Adult data unless noted) Absorption: Amount of systemic absorption following topical use has not been determined

Dosing: Usual Topical: Infants, Children, and Adults:

Scabicide: Apply over entire body below the head; apply once daily for 2 days followed by a cleansing bath 48 hours after the last application; treatment may be repeated after 7-10 days if mites appear

Pruritus: Massage into affected areas until medication is completely absorbed; may repeat as necessary

Administration Topical: Wash thoroughly and scrub away loose scales, then towel dry; apply a thin layer and gently massage drug onto skin of the entire body from the neck to the toes (with special attention to skin folds, creases, and interdigital spaces); also apply cream or lotion under fingernails after trimming nails short; since scabies can affect the head, scalp, and neck in infants and young children, apply to scalp, neck, and body of this age group; do not apply to the face, eyes, mouth, mucous membranes, or urethral meatus; shake lotion well before use

Additional Information Treatment may be repeated after 7-10 days if live mites are still present

Dosage Forms Excipient information presented when available (limited, particularly for generics); consult specific product labeling.

Cream, External:
Eurax: 10% (60 g)
Lotion, External:
Eurax: 10% (60 g, 454 g)

- ◆ **Crude Coal Tar** *see* Coal Tar *on page 523*
- ◆ **Cruex Prescription Strength [OTC]** *see* Miconazole (Topical) *on page 1431*
- ◆ **Crystalline Penicillin** *see* Penicillin G (Parenteral/Aqueous) *on page 1656*
- ◆ **Crystal Violet** *see* Gentian Violet *on page 970*
- ◆ **Crystapen (Can)** *see* Penicillin G (Parenteral/Aqueous) *on page 1656*
- ◆ **CsA** *see* CycloSPORINE (Ophthalmic) *on page 561*
- ◆ **CsA** *see* CycloSPORINE (Systemic) *on page 556*
- ◆ **C-Time [OTC]** *see* Ascorbic Acid *on page 202*
- ◆ **CTLA-4Ig** *see* Abatacept *on page 41*
- ◆ **CTM** *see* Chlorpheniramine *on page 441*
- ◆ **CTP 30 (Can)** *see* Citalopram *on page 476*
- ◆ **CTX** *see* Cyclophosphamide *on page 551*
- ◆ **Cu-5 [OTC]** *see* Copper *on page 535*
- ◆ **Cubicin** *see* DAPTOmycin *on page 582*
- ◆ **Culturelle® [OTC]** *see Lactobacillus on page 1203*
- ◆ **Cupric Chloride** *see* Copper *on page 535*
- ◆ **Cupric Chloride Dihydrate** *see* Copper *on page 535*
- ◆ **Cuprimine** *see* PenicillAMINE *on page 1652*
- ◆ **Cuprimine® (Can)** *see* PenicillAMINE *on page 1652*
- ◆ **Curosurf** *see* Poractant Alfa *on page 1730*
- ◆ **Cutar [OTC]** *see* Coal Tar *on page 523*
- ◆ **Cutivate** *see* Fluticasone (Topical) *on page 922*
- ◆ **Cuvposa** *see* Glycopyrrolate *on page 979*
- ◆ **CyA** *see* CycloSPORINE (Ophthalmic) *on page 561*
- ◆ **CyA** *see* CycloSPORINE (Systemic) *on page 556*

Cyanocobalamin (sye an oh koe BAL a min)

Brand Names: US Nascobal; Physicians EZ Use B-12

Therapeutic Category Nutritional Supplement; Vitamin, Water Soluble

Generic Availability (US) Yes

Use Treatment of pernicious anemia; vitamin B_{12} deficiency due to dietary deficiencies or malabsorption diseases; inadequate secretion of intrinsic factor, inadequate utilization of B_{12} (eg, during neoplastic treatment); increased B_{12} requirements due to pregnancy, thyrotoxicosis, hemorrhage, malignancy, liver or kidney disease; nutritional supplement

Pregnancy Considerations Animal reproduction studies have not been conducted. Water soluble vitamins cross the placenta. Absorption of vitamin B_{12} may increase during pregnancy. Vitamin B_{12} requirements may be increased in pregnant women compared to nonpregnant women. Serum concentrations of vitamin B_{12} are higher in the neonate at birth than the mother (IOM, 1998).

Breast-Feeding Considerations Vitamin B_{12} is found in breast milk. Milk concentrations are similar to maternal serum concentrations and concentrations may be decreased in women who are vegetarians. Vitamin B_{12} requirements may be increased in nursing women compared to non-nursing women (IOM, 1998).

Contraindications Hypersensitivity to cyanocobalamin, cobalt, or any component of the formulation

Warnings/Precautions IM/SubQ routes are used to treat pernicious anemia; oral and intranasal administration are not indicated until hematologic remission and no signs of nervous system involvement. Treatment of severe vitamin B_{12} megaloblastic anemia may result in thrombocytosis and severe hypokalemia, sometimes fatal, due to intracellular potassium shift upon anemia resolution. Vitamin B_{12} deficiency masks signs of polycythemia vera; use caution in other conditions where folic acid or vitamin B_{12} administration alone might mask true diagnosis, despite hematologic response. Vitamin B_{12} deficiency for >3 months results in irreversible degenerative CNS lesions; neurologic manifestations will not be prevented with folic acid unless vitamin B_{12} is also given. Spinal cord degeneration might also occur when folic acid used as a substitute for vitamin B_{12} in anemia prevention. Use caution in Leber's disease patients; B_{12} treatment may result in rapid optic atrophy. Avoid intravenous route; anaphylactic shock has occurred. Intradermal test dose of vitamin B_{12} is recommended for any patient suspected of cyanocobalamin sensitivity prior to intranasal or injectable administration. Efficacy of intranasal products in patients with nasal pathology or with other concomitant intranasal therapy has not been determined.

Aluminum: The parenteral product may contain aluminum; toxic aluminum concentrations may be seen with high doses, prolonged use, or renal dysfunction. Premature neonates are at higher risk due to immature renal function and aluminum intake from other parenteral sources. Parenteral aluminum exposure of >4 to 5 mcg/kg/day is associated with CNS and bone toxicity; tissue loading may occur at lower doses (Federal Register, 2002). See manufacturer's labeling.

Benzyl alcohol and derivatives: Some dosage forms may contain benzyl alcohol; large amounts of benzyl alcohol (≥99 mg/kg/day) have been associated with a potentially fatal toxicity ("gasping syndrome") in neonates; the "gasping syndrome" consists of metabolic acidosis, respiratory distress, gasping respirations, CNS dysfunction (including convulsions, intracranial hemorrhage), hypotension and cardiovascular collapse (AAP, 1997; CDC, 1982); some data suggests that benzoate displaces bilirubin from protein binding sites (Ahlfors, 2001); avoid or use dosage forms containing benzyl alcohol with caution in neonates. See manufacturer's labeling.

Adverse Reactions

Cardiovascular: Congestive heart failure, peripheral vascular disease, thrombosis (peripheral)

Central nervous system: Abnormal gait, anxiety, ataxia, dizziness, headache, hypoesthesia, nervousness, pain, paresthesia

Dermatologic: Pruritus, skin rash (transient), urticaria

Gastrointestinal: Diarrhea, dyspepsia, glossitis, nausea, sore throat, vomiting

Hematologic & Oncologic: Polycythemia vera

Hypersensitivity: Anaphylaxis (parenteral)

Infection: Infection

Neuromuscular & skeletal: Arthritis, back pain, myalgia, weakness

Respiratory: Dyspnea, pulmonary edema, rhinitis

Drug Interactions

Metabolism/Transport Effects None known.

Avoid Concomitant Use There are no known interactions where it is recommended to avoid concomitant use.

Increased Effect/Toxicity There are no known significant interactions involving an increase in effect.

Decreased Effect

The levels/effects of Cyanocobalamin may be decreased by: Chloramphenicol; Colchicine

Food Interactions Heavy ethanol consumption >2 weeks may impair vitamin B_{12} absorption.

Storage/Stability

Injection: Clear pink to red solutions are stable at room temperature. Protect from light.

Intranasal spray: Store at 15°C to 30°C (59°F to 86°F); do not freeze. Protect from light.

Mechanism of Action Coenzyme for various metabolic functions, including fat and carbohydrate metabolism and protein synthesis, used in cell replication and hematopoiesis

Pharmacodynamics Onset of action:

Megaloblastic anemia: IM:

- Conversion of megaloblastic to normoblastic erythroid hyperplasia within bone marrow: 8 hours
- Increased reticulocytes: 2 to 5 days

Complicated vitamin B_{12} deficiency: IM, SubQ: Resolution of:

- Psychiatric sequelae: 24 hours
- Thrombocytopenia: 10 days
- Granulocytopenia: 2 weeks

Pharmacokinetics (Adult data unless noted)

Absorption: Oral: Drug is absorbed from the terminal ileum in the presence of calcium; for absorption to occur, gastric "intrinsic factor" must be present to transfer the compound across the intestinal mucosa

Distribution: Principally stored in the liver, also stored in the kidneys and adrenals

Protein binding: Bound to transcobalamin II

Metabolism: Converted in the tissues to active coenzymes methylcobalamin and deoxyadenosylcobalamin

Bioavailability:

- Oral: Pernicious anemia: 1.2%
- Intranasal gel: 8.9% (relative to IM formulation)
- Intranasal spray: Nascobal: 6.1% (relative to IM formulation)

Time to peak serum concentration:

- IM, SubQ: 30 minutes to 2 hours
- Intranasal: 1.6 hours

Elimination: 50% to 98% unchanged in the urine

Dosing: Neonatal

Adequate intake (AI): Oral, sublingual: 0.4 mcg/day (~0.05 mcg/kg/day); **Note:** Neonates born to vegan mothers should be supplemented with the AI for vitamin B_{12} from birth; they may have low vitamin B_{12} stores at birth and, if breast-feeding, may only receive a small amount of the vitamin from the mother's milk (Mangels 2001).

Anemia of prematurity: IM: Limited data available; 100 mcg once monthly for 4 months with concomitant folic acid administration produced higher hemoglobin in 34 preterm neonates (GA <36 weeks; birth weight <1,800 g) when compared to placebo or folate monotherapy; all patients received vitamin E and iron supplementation (Worthington-White 1994).

Pernicious anemia; treatment of deficiency: Limited data available: IM, SubQ: Initial: 1,000 mcg/day for 2 to 7 days based upon clinical response; maintenance: 100 mcg/month; **Note:** For severe anemia, a lower initial dose of 0.2 mcg/kg/dose for 2 days followed by the above regimen has been recommended due to potential hypokalemia observed during initial treatment of adults with severe anemia; additional potassium supplementation may also be required (Rasmussen 2001).

Dosing: Usual

Pediatric:

Adequate intake (AI): Oral, sublingual: **Note:** Neonates born to vegan mothers should be supplemented with the AI for vitamin B_{12} from birth; they may have low vitamin B_{12} stores at birth and, if breast-feeding, may only receive a small amount of the vitamin from the mother's milk (Mangels 2001).

Infants 1 to 6 months: 0.4 mcg/day (0.05 mcg/kg/day)

Infants 7 to 12 months: 0.5 mcg/day (0.05 mcg/kg/day)

Recommended daily allowance (RDA): Oral, Sublingual:

Children and Adolescents:

1 to 3 years: 0.9 mcg/day

4 to 8 years: 1.2 mcg/day

9 to 13 years: 1.8 mcg/day

Adolescents ≥14 years: 2.4 mcg/day

Pernicious anemia: Limited data available: Infants, Children, and Adolescents: IM, SubQ: Initial: 1,000 mcg/day for 2 to 7 days based upon clinical response; maintenance: 100 mcg/month; for severe anemia, a lower initial dose of 0.2 mcg/kg/dose for 2 days followed by the above regimen has been recommended; initial low dosage recommended due to potential hypokalemia observed during initial treatment of adults with severe anemia (Rasmussen 2001). Concurrent folic acid supplementation may also be needed.

Vitamin B_{12} deficiency: Infants, Children, and Adolescents: Dosing regimens variable: IM, SubQ: 1000 mcg/day for 2 to 7 days based upon clinical response followed by 100 mcg/week for a month; for severe deficiency, a lower initial dose of 0.2 mcg/kg/dose for 2 days followed by the above regimen has been recommended due to potential hypokalemia observed during initial treatment of adults with severe anemia; additional potassium supplementation may also be required (Rasmussen 2001); for malabsorptive causes of B_{12} deficiency, monthly maintenance doses of 100 mcg have been recommended or as an alternative 100 mcg/day for 10 to 15 days (total dose of 1 to 1.5 mg), then once or twice weekly for several months; may taper to 60 mcg every month

Adult:

Recommended intake: 2.4 mcg/day

Pregnancy: 2.6 mcg/day

Lactation: 2.8 mcg/day

Pernicious anemia: IM, deep SubQ (administer concomitantly with folic acid if needed): 100 mcg daily for 6 to 7 days; if improvement, administer same dose on alternate days for 7 doses; then every 3 to 4 days for 2 to 3 weeks; once hematologic values have returned to normal, maintenance dosage: 100 mcg monthly

Note: Given the lack of toxicity associated with cyanocobalamin, higher doses may be preferred, especially in cases of severe deficiency. Alternate dosing regimens exist with initial doses ranging from 100 to 1,000 mcg every day or every other day for 1 to 2 weeks and maintenance doses of 100 to 1,000 mcg every 1 to 3 months (Oh 2003).

Hematologic remission (without evidence of nervous system involvement):

Intranasal (Nascobal): 500 mcg (1 spray) in one nostril once weekly

Oral: 1,000 to 2,000 mcg daily

IM, SubQ: 100 to 1,000 mcg/month

Vitamin B_{12} deficiency:

Intranasal (Nascobal): 500 mcg (1 spray) in one nostril once weekly

Oral: 1,000 to 2,000 mcg daily for 1 to 2 weeks; maintenance: 1,000 mcg daily (Langan 2011; Oh 2003)

IM, deep SubQ: May use initial treatment similar to that for pernicious anemia depending on severity of deficiency: 100 mcg daily for 6 to 7 days; if improvement, administer same dose on alternate days for 7 doses, then every 3 to 4 days for 2 to 3 weeks; once hematologic values have returned to normal, maintenance dosage: 100 mcg monthly

Note: Given the lack of toxicity associated with cyanocobalamin, higher doses may be preferred, especially in cases of severe deficiency. Alternate dosing regimens exist with initial doses ranging from 100 to 1,000 mcg every day or every other day for 1 to 2 weeks and maintenance doses of 100 to 1,000 mcg every 1 to 3 months (Oh 2003).

Dosing adjustment in renal impairment: There are no dosage adjustments provided in the manufacturer's labeling. Use with caution; some formulations may also contain aluminum, which may accumulate in renal impairment.

Dosing adjustment in hepatic impairment: There are no dosage adjustments provided in the manufacturer's labeling.

Administration

Intranasal: Nascobal nasal spray: Prior to initial dose, activate (prime) spray nozzle by pumping unit quickly and firmly until first appearance of spray, then prime twice more. The unit must be reprimed once immediately before each use. Administer at least one hour before or after ingestion of hot foods or liquids; hot foods can cause nasal secretions and a resulting loss of medication

Oral: Not generally recommended for treatment of severe vitamin B_{12} deficiency due to poor oral absorption (lack of intrinsic factor); oral administration may be used in less severe deficiencies and maintenance therapy; may be administered without regard to food

Parenteral: IM or deep SubQ: Avoid IV administration due to a more rapid system elimination with resulting decreased utilization

Sublingual: Place under the tongue and allow to dissolve; do not swallow whole, chew, or crush

Monitoring Parameters Serum potassium (particularly during initial treatment of deficiency), erythrocyte and reticulocyte count, hemoglobin, hematocrit, platelets, serum cyanocobalamin and folate concentrations; methylmalonate (MMA) and total homocysteine (elevated in Vitamin B_{12} deficiency)

Reference Range Serum vitamin B_{12} levels: Normal: >300 pg/mL; vitamin B_{12} deficiency: <200 pg/mL (200-300 pg/mL borderline result, possible deficiency); megaloblastic anemia: <100 pg/mL

Test Interactions Methotrexate, pyrimethamine, and most antibiotics invalidate folic acid and vitamin B_{12} diagnostic blood assays

Dosage Forms Excipient information presented when available (limited, particularly for generics); consult specific product labeling. [DSC] = Discontinued product

Kit, Injection:

Physicians EZ Use B-12: 1000 mcg/mL [contains benzyl alcohol]

Liquid, Sublingual:

Generic: 3000 mcg/mL (52 mL)

Lozenge, Oral:

Generic: 50 mcg (100 ea); 100 mcg (100 ea); 250 mcg (100 ea, 250 ea); 500 mcg (100 ea, 250 ea)

Solution, Injection:

Generic: 1000 mcg/mL (1 mL, 10 mL, 30 mL)

Solution, Nasal:

Nascobal: 500 mcg/0.1 mL (1 ea, 1.3 mL [DSC]) [contains benzalkonium chloride]

Tablet, Oral:

Generic: 100 mcg, 250 mcg, 500 mcg, 1000 mcg

Tablet, Oral [preservative free]:

Generic: 100 mcg, 500 mcg, 1000 mcg

Tablet Extended Release, Oral:

Generic: 1000 mcg

Tablet Sublingual, Sublingual:
Generic: 2500 mcg
Tablet Sublingual, Sublingual [preservative free]:
Generic: 2500 mcg

◆ **Cyanokit** *see* Hydroxocobalamin *on page 1050*

Cyclobenzaprine (sye kloe BEN za preen)

Medication Safety Issues

Sound-alike/look-alike issues:

Cyclobenzaprine may be confused with cycloSERINE, cyproheptadine

Flexeril may be confused with Floxin

BEERS Criteria medication:

This drug may be potentially inappropriate for use in geriatric patients (Quality of evidence - moderate; Strength of recommendation - strong).

International issues:

Flexin: Brand name for cyclobenzaprine [Chile], but also the brand name for diclofenac [Argentina] and orphenadrine [Israel]

Flexin [Chile] may be confused with Floxin brand name for flunarizine [Thailand], norfloxacin [South Africa], ofloxacin [U.S., Canada], and perfloxacin [Philippines]; Fluoxine brand name for fluoxetine [Thailand]; Flexinol brand name for methocarbamol and paracetamol [India]

Related Information

Oral Medications That Should Not Be Crushed or Altered *on page 2476*

Brand Names: US Active-Cyclobenzaprine; Amrix; EnovaRX-Cyclobenzaprine HCl; Fexmid

Brand Names: Canada Apo-Cyclobenzaprine; Auro-Cyclobenzaprine; Ava-Cyclobenzaprine; Dom-Cyclobenzaprine; JAMP-Cyclobenzaprine; Mylan-Cyclobenzaprine; Novo-Cycloprine; PHL-Cyclobenzaprine; PMS-Cyclobenzaprine; Q-Cyclobenzaprine; ratio-Cyclobenzaprine; Riva-Cycloprine; ZYM-Cyclobenzaprine

Therapeutic Category Skeletal Muscle Relaxant, Nonparalytic

Generic Availability (US) May be product dependent

Use Treatment of muscle spasm associated with acute painful musculoskeletal conditions (immediate release tablets: FDA approved in ages ≥15 years and adults; extended release capsules: FDA approved in adults); has also been used for treatment of muscle spasm associated with acute temporomandibular joint pain (TMJ)

Pregnancy Risk Factor B

Pregnancy Considerations Adverse events have not been observed in animal reproduction studies. The manufacturer recommends avoiding use during pregnancy unless clearly needed.

Breast-Feeding Considerations It is not known if cyclobenzaprine is excreted in breast milk. The manufacturer recommends that caution be exercised when administering cyclobenzaprine to nursing women.

Contraindications Hypersensitivity to cyclobenzaprine or any component of the formulation; during or within 14 days of MAO inhibitors; hyperthyroidism; congestive heart failure; arrhythmias; heart block or conduction disturbances; acute recovery phase of MI

Warnings/Precautions May cause CNS depression, which may impair physical or mental abilities; ethanol and/or other CNS depressants may enhance these effects. Patients must be cautioned about performing tasks which require mental alertness (eg, operating machinery or driving). Cyclobenzaprine shares the toxic potentials of the tricyclic antidepressants (including arrhythmias, tachycardia, and conduction time prolongation) and the usual precautions of tricyclic antidepressant therapy should be observed; use with caution in patients with urinary hesitancy or retention, angle-closure glaucoma or increased intraocular pressure, hepatic impairment, or in the elderly.

Potentially life-threatening serotonin syndrome has occurred with cyclobenzaprine when used in combination with other serotonergic agents (eg, SSRIs, SNRIs, TCAs, meperidine, tramadol, buspirone, MAO inhibitors), bupropion, and verapamil. Monitor patients closely especially during initiation/dose titration for signs/symptoms of serotonin syndrome such as mental status changes (eg, agitation, hallucinations); autonomic instability (eg, tachycardia, labile blood pressure, diaphoresis); neuromuscular changes (eg, tremor, rigidity, myoclonus); GI symptoms (eg, nausea, vomiting, diarrhea); and/or seizures. Discontinue cyclobenzaprine and any concomitant serotonergic agent immediately if signs/symptoms arise. Concomitant use or use within 14 days of discontinuing an MAO inhibitor is contraindicated.

Muscle relaxants are poorly tolerated by the elderly due to potent anticholinergic effects, sedation, and risk of fracture. Efficacy is questionable at dosages tolerated by elderly patients; avoid use (Beers Criteria). Extended release capsules not recommended for use in mild-to-severe hepatic impairment or in the elderly. Potentially significant drug-drug interactions may exist, requiring dose or frequency adjustment, additional monitoring, and/or selection of alternative therapy. Effects may be potentiated when used with other CNS depressants or ethanol.

Warnings: Additional Pediatric Considerations Not effective in the treatment of spasticity due to cerebral or spinal cord disease or in children with cerebral palsy.

Adverse Reactions

Central nervous system: Confusion, decreased mental acuity, dizziness, drowsiness, fatigue, headache, irritability, nervousness

Gastrointestinal: Abdominal pain, acid regurgitation, constipation, diarrhea, dyspepsia, nausea, unpleasant taste, xerostomia

Neuromuscular & skeletal: Weakness

Ophthalmic: Blurred vision

Respiratory: Pharyngitis, upper respiratory tract infection

Rare but important or life-threatening: Anaphylaxis, angioedema, cardiac arrhythmia, convulsions, hepatitis (rare), hypertonia, hypotension, paresthesia, psychosis, seizure, serotonin syndrome, skin rash, syncope, tachycardia

Drug Interactions

Metabolism/Transport Effects Substrate of CYP1A2 (major), CYP2D6 (minor), CYP3A4 (minor); **Note:** Assignment of Major/Minor substrate status based on clinically relevant drug interaction potential

Avoid Concomitant Use

Avoid concomitant use of Cyclobenzaprine with any of the following: Aclidinium; Azelastine (Nasal); Dapoxetine; Eluxadoline; Glucagon; Ipratropium (Oral Inhalation); MAO Inhibitors; Orphenadrine; Paraldehyde; Potassium Chloride; Thalidomide; Tiotropium; Umeclidinium

Increased Effect/Toxicity

Cyclobenzaprine may increase the levels/effects of: AbobotulinumtoxinA; Alcohol (Ethyl); Analgesics (Opioid); Anticholinergic Agents; Antipsychotic Agents; Azelastine (Nasal); Buprenorphine; CNS Depressants; Eluxadoline; Glucagon; Hydrocodone; MAO Inhibitors; Methotrimeprazine; Metoclopramide; Metyrosine; Mirabegron; OnabotulinumtoxinA; Orphenadrine; Paraldehyde; Potassium Chloride; Pramipexole; RimabotulinumtoxinB; ROPINIRole; Rotigotine; Serotonin Modulators; Suvorexant; Thalidomide; Thiazide Diuretics; Tiotropium; Topiramate; TraMADol; Zolpidem

The levels/effects of Cyclobenzaprine may be increased by: Abiraterone Acetate; Aclidinium; Antiemetics (5HT3 Antagonists); Antipsychotic Agents; Brimonidine (Topical); Cannabis; CYP1A2 Inhibitors (Moderate); CYP1A2 Inhibitors (Strong); Dapoxetine; Deferasirox; Doxylamine; Dronabinol; Droperidol; HydrOXYzine; Ipratropium (Oral Inhalation); Kava Kava; Magnesium Sulfate; Methotrimeprazine; Mianserin; Nabilone; Peginterferon Alfa-2b; Perampanel; Pramlintide; Rufinamide; Sodium Oxybate; Tapentadol; Tetrahydrocannabinol; Umeclidinium; Vemurafenib

Decreased Effect

Cyclobenzaprine may decrease the levels/effects of: Acetylcholinesterase Inhibitors; Itopride; Metoclopramide; Secretin

The levels/effects of Cyclobenzaprine may be decreased by: Acetylcholinesterase Inhibitors

Food Interactions Food increases bioavailability (peak plasma concentrations increased by 35% and area under the curve by 20%) of the extended release capsule. Management: Monitor for increased effects if taken with food.

Storage/Stability

Amrix, Flexeril: Store at 25°C (77°F); excursions permitted to 15°C to 30°C (59°F to 86°F). Protect from light.

Fexmid: Store at 20°C to 25°C (68°F to 77°F).

Mechanism of Action Centrally-acting skeletal muscle relaxant pharmacologically related to tricyclic antidepressants; reduces tonic somatic motor activity influencing both alpha and gamma motor neurons

Pharmacodynamics

Onset of action: Immediate release tablet: Within 1 hour

Duration: Immediate release tablet: 12-24 hours

Pharmacokinetics (Adult data unless noted)

Metabolism: Hepatic via CYP3A4, 1A2, and 2D6; may undergo enterohepatic recirculation

Bioavailability: 33% to 55%

Half-life: Normal hepatic function: Range: 8-37 hours; immediate release tablet: 18 hours; extended release capsule: 32 hours; impaired hepatic function: 46.2 hours (range: 22.4-188 hours) (Winchell, 2002)

Time to peak serum concentration: Immediate release tablet: ~4 hours (Winchell, 2002); extended release capsule: 7-8 hours

Elimination: Primarily renal as inactive metabolites and in the feces (via bile) as unchanged drug

Clearance: 0.7 L/minute

Dosing: Usual Oral: **Note:** Do not use longer than 2-3 weeks

Muscle spasm, treatment:

Adolescents ≥15 years: Immediate release tablet: 5 mg 3 times daily; may increase to 7.5-10 mg 3 times daily

Adults:

Immediate release tablet: 5 mg 3 times daily; may increase to 7.5-10 mg 3 times daily

Extended release capsule: 15 mg once daily; may increase to 30 mg once daily

Dosage adjustment in hepatic impairment:

Immediate release tablet:

Mild: 5 mg 3 times daily

Moderate to severe: Use not recommended

Extended release capsule: Mild to severe impairment: Use not recommended

Administration Oral:

Immediate release tablet: May be administered without regard to meals

Extended release capsule: Administer at the same time daily; do not crush or chew

Monitoring Parameters Relief of muscle spasms and pain; improvement in physical activities

Test Interactions May cause false-positive serum TCA screen (Wong, 1995)

Dosage Forms Considerations EnovaRX-Cyclobenzaprine and Active-Cyclobenzaprine creams are compounded from kits. Refer to manufacturer's labeling for compounding instructions.

Dosage Forms Excipient information presented when available (limited, particularly for generics); consult specific product labeling.

Capsule Extended Release 24 Hour, Oral, as hydrochloride:

Amrix: 15 mg

Amrix: 30 mg [contains brilliant blue fcf (fd&c blue #1), fd&c blue #2 (indigotine), fd&c red #40, fd&c yellow #6 (sunset yellow)]

Cream, Transdermal, as hydrochloride:

Active-Cyclobenzaprine: 5% (120 g) [contains chlorocresol (chloro-m-cresol)]

EnovaRX-Cyclobenzaprine HCl: 20 mg/g (120 g) [contains cetearyl alcohol]

Tablet, Oral, as hydrochloride:

Fexmid: 7.5 mg

Generic: 5 mg, 7.5 mg, 10 mg

◆ **Cyclobenzaprine Hydrochloride** *see* Cyclobenzaprine *on page 548*

◆ **Cyclogyl** *see* Cyclopentolate *on page 549*

◆ **Cyclomen® (Can)** *see* Danazol *on page 575*

◆ **Cyclomydril®** *see* Cyclopentolate and Phenylephrine *on page 550*

Cyclopentolate (sye kloe PEN toe late)

Brand Names: US Cyclogyl

Brand Names: Canada AK Pentolate Oph Soln; Cyclogyl; Diopentolate; Minims Cyclopentolate; PMS-Cyclopentolate

Therapeutic Category Anticholinergic Agent, Ophthalmic; Ophthalmic Agent, Mydriatic

Generic Availability (US) Yes

Use Diagnostic procedures requiring mydriasis and cycloplegia

Pregnancy Risk Factor C

Pregnancy Considerations Animal reproduction studies have not been conducted.

Breast-Feeding Considerations It is not known if cyclopentolate is excreted in breast milk. The manufacturer recommends that caution be exercised when administering cyclopentolate to nursing women.

Contraindications Hypersensitivity to cyclopentolate or any component of the formulation; untreated narrow-angle glaucoma; presence of untreated anatomically narrow angles

Warnings/Precautions May result in psychotic reactions and behavioral disturbances in pediatric patients, especially with the 2% solution; increased susceptibility to these effects has been reported in young infants, young children, and in children with spastic paralysis or brain damage; effects usually occur ~30 to 45 minutes after instillation; observe infants for at least 30 minutes following instillation. Feeding intolerance may occur in infants; withhold feeding for 4 hours after examination. May cause a transient elevation in intraocular pressure. Use with caution in the elderly; may be predisposed to increased intraocular pressure. Patients with Down syndrome are predisposed to angle-closure glaucoma; use with caution. To minimize absorption, apply pressure over the nasolacrimal sac for 2 to 3 minutes after instillation. For topical ophthalmic use only. Contains benzalkonium chloride which may be adsorbed by contact lenses; remove contacts prior to administration and wait 15 minutes before reinserting. Potentially significant interactions may exist, requiring dose or frequency adjustment, additional monitoring, and/or selection of alternative therapy.

Adverse Reactions
Cardiovascular: Tachycardia
Central nervous system: Ataxia, hallucinations, hyperactivity, incoherent speech, psychosis, restlessness, seizure
Dermatologic: Burning sensation
Ocular: Intraocular pressure increased, loss of visual accommodation
Miscellaneous: Allergic reaction

Drug Interactions

Metabolism/Transport Effects None known.

Avoid Concomitant Use

Avoid concomitant use of Cyclopentolate with any of the following: Aclidinium; Eluxadoline; Glucagon; Ipratropium (Oral Inhalation); Potassium Chloride; Tiotropium; Umeclidinium

Increased Effect/Toxicity

Cyclopentolate may increase the levels/effects of: AbobotulinumtoxinA; Analgesics (Opioid); Anticholinergic Agents; Cannabinoid-Containing Products; Eluxadoline; Glucagon; Mirabegron; OnabotulinumtoxinA; Potassium Chloride; RimabotulinumtoxinB; Thiazide Diuretics; Tiotropium; Topiramate

The levels/effects of Cyclopentolate may be increased by: Aclidinium; Ipratropium (Oral Inhalation); Mianserin; Pramlintide; Umeclidinium

Decreased Effect

Cyclopentolate may decrease the levels/effects of: Acetylcholinesterase Inhibitors; Itopride; Metoclopramide; Secretin

The levels/effects of Cyclopentolate may be decreased by: Acetylcholinesterase Inhibitors

Storage/Stability Store at 8°C to 27°C (46°F to 80°F).

Mechanism of Action Prevents the muscle of the ciliary body and the sphincter muscle of the iris from responding to cholinergic stimulation, causing mydriasis and cycloplegia

Pharmacodynamics
Maximum effect:
Cycloplegia: 15-60 minutes
Mydriasis: Within 15-60 minutes, with recovery taking up to 24 hours

Dosing: Neonatal Ophthalmic: See Cyclopentolate and Phenylephrine monograph (preferred agent for use in neonates and infants due to lower cyclopentolate concentration and reduced risk for systemic reactions)

Dosing: Usual Ophthalmic:
Infants: See Cyclopentolate and Phenylephrine monograph (preferred agent for use in neonates and infants due to lower cyclopentolate concentration and reduced risk for systemic reactions)
Children: 1 drop of 0.5% or 1% in eye followed by 1 drop of 0.5% or 1% in 5 minutes, if necessary, approximately 40-50 minutes before procedure
Adults: 1 drop of 1% followed by another drop in 5 minutes; approximately 40-50 minutes prior to the procedure, may use 2% solution in heavily pigmented iris

Administration Ophthalmic: Instill drops into conjunctival sac of affected eye(s); avoid contact of bottle tip with skin or eye; to avoid excessive systemic absorption, finger pressure should be applied on the lacrimal sac during and for 1-2 minutes following application

Additional Information Pilocarpine ophthalmic drops applied after the examination may reduce recovery time to 3-6 hours

Dosage Forms Excipient information presented when available (limited, particularly for generics); consult specific product labeling.
Solution, Ophthalmic, as hydrochloride:
Cyclogyl: 0.5% (15 mL); 1% (2 mL, 5 mL, 15 mL); 2% (2 mL, 5 mL, 15 mL)
Generic: 1% (2 mL, 15 mL); 2% (2 mL, 5 mL, 15 mL)

Cyclopentolate and Phenylephrine
(sye kloe PEN toe late & fen il EF rin)

Brand Names: US Cyclomydril®

Therapeutic Category Adrenergic Agonist Agent, Ophthalmic; Anticholinergic Agent, Ophthalmic; Ophthalmic Agent, Mydriatic

Generic Availability (US) No

Use Diagnostic procedures requiring mydriasis and cycloplegia; preferred agent for use in neonates and infants

Pregnancy Risk Factor C

Pregnancy Considerations Animal reproduction studies have not been conducted with this combination.

Breast-Feeding Considerations
It is not known if cyclopentolate or phenylephrine is excreted into breast milk. The manufacturer recommends that caution be exercised when administering to breast-feeding women.

Contraindications
Untreated narrow-angle glaucoma; untreated anatomically narrow angles; hypersensitivity to any component of the formulation

Warnings/Precautions Use caution in patients with cardiovascular disease, hypertension, or hyperthyroidism. May cause a transient elevation in intraocular pressure. Use caution in patients with Down syndrome and in patients predisposed to angle-closure glaucoma.

May cause CNS disturbances. Patients must be cautioned about performing hazardous activities (eg, operating machinery or driving) while pupils are dilated. Psychotic reactions and behavioral disturbances have been reported in children; risk may be increased with brain damage or spastic paralysis. Observe infants for at least 30 minutes following instillation. Feeding intolerance may occur in infants; withhold feeding for 4 hours after examination.

Contains benzalkonium chloride which may be adsorbed by contact lenses; remove contacts prior to administration and wait 15 minutes before reinserting. For topical ophthalmic use and short term administration only. To minimize systemic absorption, apply pressure over the lacrimal sac for 2 to 3 minutes after application.

Warnings: Additional Pediatric Considerations Use of cyclopentolate has been associated with psychotic reactions and behavioral disturbances in pediatric patients; increased susceptibility to these effects has been reported in young infants, young children, and in children with spastic paralysis or brain damage, particularly with concentrations >1%; observe neonates and infants closely for at least 30 minutes after administration; may cause transient elevation of intraocular pressure. The preservative, benzalkonium chloride, may be absorbed by soft contact lenses. Wait at least 10 minutes after instillation before reinserting lenses. Use with caution in patients with Down syndrome, cardiovascular disease, hypertension, and hyperthyroidism; feeding intolerance may follow ophthalmic use of this product in neonates and infants; withhold feedings for 4 hours after examination.

Adverse Reactions See individual agents.

Drug Interactions

Metabolism/Transport Effects None known.

Avoid Concomitant Use

Avoid concomitant use of Cyclopentolate and Phenylephrine with any of the following: Ergot Derivatives; Iobenguane I 123; MAO Inhibitors

Increased Effect/Toxicity

Cyclopentolate and Phenylephrine may increase the levels/effects of: Sympathomimetics

The levels/effects of Cyclopentolate and Phenylephrine may be increased by: AtoMOXetine; Cannabinoid-Containing Products; Ergot Derivatives; Linezolid; MAO Inhibitors; Tedizolid; Tricyclic Antidepressants

Decreased Effect

Cyclopentolate and Phenylephrine may decrease the levels/effects of: Iobenguane I 123

The levels/effects of Cyclopentolate and Phenylephrine may be decreased by: Alpha1-Blockers; Tricyclic Antidepressants

Storage/Stability Store at 8°C to 25°C (46°F to 77°F).

Mechanism of Action The anticholinergic effects of cyclopentolate and the adrenergic effects of phenylephrine cause a greater mydriasis than produced by either agent alone, and cause little cycloplegia.

Pharmacodynamics Onset of action and duration of effect are partially dependent upon eye pigment; dark eyes have a prolonged onset of action and shorter duration than blue eyes

Onset of action: 15-60 minutes

Duration: 4-12 hours

Dosing: Neonatal Ophthalmic: Instill 1 drop into the eye every 5-10 minutes, for up to 3 doses, ~45 minutes before the examination

Dosing: Usual Ophthalmic: Infants, Children, and Adults: Instill 1 drop into the eye every 5-10 minutes, for up to 3 doses, ~40-50 minutes before the examination

Administration Ophthalmic: Instill drops into conjunctival sac of affected eye(s); avoid contact of bottle tip with skin or eye; to avoid excessive systemic absorption, finger pressure should be applied on the lacrimal sac during and for 1-2 minutes following application; preservative absorbed by soft contact lenses; wait at least 10 minutes before reinserting

Additional Information Cyclomydril® is the preferred agent for use in neonates and infants because lower concentrations of both cyclopentolate and phenylephrine provide optimal dilation while minimizing the systemic side effects noted with a higher concentration of each agent used alone

Dosage Forms Excipient information presented when available (limited, particularly for generics); consult specific product labeling.

Solution, ophthalmic:

Cyclomydril: Cyclopentolate hydrochloride 0.2% and phenylephrine hydrochloride 1% (2 mL, 5 mL) [contains benzalkonium chloride]

◆ **Cyclopentolate Hydrochloride** *see* Cyclopentolate *on page 549*

Cyclophosphamide (sye kloe FOS fa mide)

Medication Safety Issues

Sound-alike/look-alike issues:

Cyclophosphamide may be confused with cycloSPORINE, ifosfamide

Cytoxan may be confused with cefOXitin, Ciloxan, cytarabine, CytoGam, Cytosar, Cytosar-U, Cytotec

High alert medication:

This medication is in a class the Institute for Safe Medication Practices (ISMP) includes among its list of drug classes which have a heightened risk of causing significant patient harm when used in error.

Related Information

Management of Drug Extravasations *on page 2298*

Oral Medications That Should Not Be Crushed or Altered *on page 2476*

Prevention of Chemotherapy-Induced Nausea and Vomiting in Children *on page 2368*

Safe Handling of Hazardous Drugs *on page 2455*

Brand Names: Canada Procytox

Therapeutic Category Antineoplastic Agent, Alkylating Agent; Antineoplastic Agent, Alkylating Agent (Nitrogen Mustard); Antirheumatic Miscellaneous; Immunosuppressant Agent

Generic Availability (US) Yes

Use

Oncologic uses: Treatment of Hodgkin lymphoma, non-Hodgkin's lymphomas (including Burkitt's lymphoma), chronic lymphocytic leukemia (CLL), chronic myelocytic leukemia (CML), acute myelocytic leukemia (AML), acute lymphocytic leukemia (ALL), mycosis fungoides, multiple myeloma, neuroblastoma, retinoblastoma, breast cancer, ovarian adenocarcinoma [Oral, parenteral: All indications: FDA approved in pediatric patients (age not specified) and adults]; has also been used for Ewing's sarcoma, rhabdomyosarcoma, Wilms tumor, ovarian germ cell tumors, small cell lung cancer, testicular cancer, pheochromocytoma, hematopoietic stem cell transplant (HSCT) conditioning regimen

Nononcologic uses: Treatment of minimal change nephrotic syndrome [Oral: FDA approved in pediatric patients (age not specified)]; has also been used for aplastic anemia, lupus nephritis, uveitis, and vasculitis (ANCA positive, eg, granulomatosis with polyangiitis [GPA]; Wegener's granulomatosis)

Pregnancy Risk Factor D

Pregnancy Considerations Cyclophosphamide crosses the placenta and can be detected in amniotic fluid (D'Incalci, 1982). Based on the mechanism of action, cyclophosphamide may cause fetal harm if administered during pregnancy. Adverse events (including ectrodactylia) were observed in human studies following exposure to cyclophosphamide. Women of childbearing potential should avoid pregnancy while receiving cyclophosphamide and for up to 1 year after completion of treatment. Males with female partners who are or may become pregnant should use a condom during and for at least 4 months after cyclophosphamide treatment. Cyclophosphamide may cause sterility in males and females (may be irreversible) and amenorrhea in females. When treatment is needed for lupus nephritis, cyclophosphamide should be avoided in women who are pregnant or those who wish to preserve their fertility (Hahn, 2012). Chemotherapy, if indicated, may be administered to pregnant women with breast cancer as part of a combination chemotherapy regimen (common regimens administered during pregnancy include doxorubicin (or epirubicin), cyclophosphamide, and fluorouracil); chemotherapy should not be administered during the first trimester, after 35 weeks gestation, or within 3 weeks of planned delivery (Amant, 2010; Loibl, 2006).

Breast-Feeding Considerations Cyclophosphamide is excreted into breast milk. Leukopenia and thrombocytopenia were noted in an infant exposed to cyclophosphamide while nursing. The mother was treated with one course of cyclophosphamide 6 weeks prior to delivery then cyclophosphamide IV 6 mg/kg (300 mg) once daily for 3 days beginning 20 days postpartum. Complete blood counts were obtained in the breast-feeding infant on each day of therapy; WBC and platelets decreased by day 3 (Durodola, 1979). Due to the potential for serious adverse effects in the nursing infant, a decision should be made to discontinue cyclophosphamide or to discontinue breast-feeding, taking into account the importance of treatment to the mother.

Contraindications

U.S. labeling: Hypersensitivity to cyclophosphamide or any component of the formulation; urinary outflow obstruction

Canadian labeling: Hypersensitivity to cyclophosphamide or its metabolites, urinary outflow obstructions, severe myelosuppression, severe renal or hepatic impairment, active infection (especially varicella zoster), severe immunosuppression

Warnings/Precautions Hazardous agent - use appropriate precautions for handling and disposal (NIOSH 2014 [group 1]).

Cyclophosphamide is associated with the development of hemorrhagic cystitis, pyelitis, ureteritis, and hematuria. Hemorrhagic cystitis may rarely be severe or fatal. Bladder fibrosis may also occur, either with or without cystitis. Urotoxicity is due to excretion of cyclophosphamide metabolites in the urine and appears to be dose- and treatment duration-dependent, although may occur with short-term use. Increased hydration and frequent voiding is recommended to help prevent cystitis; some protocols utilize mesna to protect against hemorrhagic cystitis. Monitor urinalysis for hematuria or other signs of urotoxicity. Severe or prolonged hemorrhagic cystitis may require medical or surgical treatment. While hematuria generally resolves within a few days after treatment is withheld, it may persist in some cases. Discontinue cyclophosphamide with severe hemorrhagic cystitis. Exclude or correct any urinary tract obstructions prior to treatment initiation (use is contraindicated with bladder outlet obstruction). Use with caution (if at all) in patients with active urinary tract infection. Use with caution in patients with renal impairment; dosage adjustment may be needed. Decreased renal excretion and increased serum levels (cyclophosphamide and metabolites) may occur in patients with severe renal impairment (CrCl 10 to 24 mL/minute); monitor for signs/symptoms of toxicity. Use is contraindicated in severe impairment in the Canadian labeling. Cyclophosphamide and metabolites are dialyzable; differences in amount dialyzed may occur due to dialysis system used. If dialysis is required, maintain a consistent interval between administration and dialysis.

Leukopenia, neutropenia, thrombocytopenia, and anemia may commonly occur; may be dose related. Bone marrow failure has been reported. Bone marrow failure and severe immunosuppression may lead to serious (and fatal) infections, including sepsis and septic shock, or may reactive latent infections. Antimicrobial prophylaxis may be considered in appropriate patients. Initiate antibiotics for neutropenic fever; antifungal and antiviral medications may also be necessary. Monitor blood counts during treatment. Avoid use if neutrophils are ≤1500/mm^3 and platelets are <50,000/mm^3. Consider growth factors (primary or secondary prophylaxis) in patients at increased risk for complications due to neutropenia. Platelet and neutrophil nadirs are usually at weeks 1 and 2 of treatment and recovery is expected after ~20 days. Severe myelosuppression may be more prevalent in heavily pretreated patients or in patients receiving concomitant chemotherapy and/or radiation therapy. Monitor for infections; immunosuppression and serious infections may occur; serious infections may require dose reduction, or interruption or discontinuation of treatment.

Cardiotoxicity has been reported (some fatal), usually with high doses associated with transplant conditioning regimens, although may rarely occur with lower doses. Cardiac abnormalities do not appear to persist. Cardiotoxicities reported have included arrhythmias (supraventricular and ventricular), congestive heart failure, heart block, hemorrhagic myocarditis, hemopericardium (secondary to hemorrhagic myocarditis and myocardial necrosis), pericarditis, pericardial effusion including cardiac tamponade, and tachyarrhythmias. Cardiotoxicity is related to endothelial capillary damage; symptoms may be managed with diuretics, ACE inhibitors, beta-blockers, or inotropics (Floyd, 2005). The risk for cardiotoxicity may be increased with higher doses, advanced age, and in patients with prior radiation to the cardiac region, and in patients who have received prior or concurrent cardiotoxic medication. Use with caution in patients with preexisting cardiovascular disease or those at risk for cardiotoxicity. For patients with multiple cardiac risk factors, considering monitoring during treatment (Floyd, 2005).

Pulmonary toxicities, including pneumonitis, pulmonary fibrosis, pulmonary veno-occlusive disease, and acute respiratory distress syndrome, have been reported. Monitor for signs/symptoms of pulmonary toxicity. Consider pulmonary function testing to assess the severity of pneumonitis (Morgan, 2011). Cyclophosphamide-induced pneumonitis is rare and may present as early (within 1 to 6 months) or late onset (several months to years). Early onset may be reversible with discontinuation; late onset is associated with pleural thickening and may persist chronically (Malik, 1996). In addition, late onset pneumonitis (>6 months after therapy initiation) may be associated with increased mortality.

Hepatic sinusoidal obstruction syndrome (SOS), formerly called veno-occlusive liver disease (VOD), has been reported in patients receiving chemotherapy regimens containing cyclophosphamide. A major risk factor for SOS is cytoreductive conditioning transplantation regimens with cyclophosphamide used in combination with total body irradiation or busulfan (or other agents). Other risk factors include preexisting hepatic dysfunction, prior radiation to the abdominal area, and low performance status. Children <3 years of age are reported to be at increased risk for hepatic SOS; monitor for signs or symptoms of hepatic SOS, including bilirubin >1.4 mg/dL, unexplained weight gain, ascites, hepatomegaly, or unexplained right upper quadrant pain (Arndt, 2004). SOS has also been reported in patients receiving long-term lower doses for immunosuppressive indications. Use with caution in patients with hepatic impairment; dosage adjustment may be needed. Use is contraindicated in severe impairment in the Canadian labeling. The conversion between cyclophosphamide to the active metabolite may be reduced in patients with severe hepatic impairment, potentially reducing efficacy.

Nausea and vomiting commonly occur. Cyclophosphamide is associated with a moderate to high emetic potential (depending on dose, regimen, or administration route); antiemetics are recommended to prevent nausea and vomiting (Basch, 2011; Dupuis, 2011; Roila, 2010). Stomatitis/mucositis may also occur. Anaphylactic reactions have been reported; cross-sensitivity with other alkylating agents may occur. Hyponatremia associated with increased total body water, acute water intoxication, and a syndrome resembling SIADH (syndrome of inappropriate secretion of antidiuretic hormone) has been reported; some have been fatal. May interfere with wound healing. May impair fertility; interferes with oogenesis and spermatogenesis. Effect on fertility is generally dependent on dose and duration of treatment and may be irreversible. The age at treatment initiation and cumulative dose were determined to be risk factors for ovarian failure in cyclophosphamide use for the treatment of systemic lupus erythematosus (SLE) (Mok, 1998). Potentially significant drug-drug interactions may exist, requiring dose or frequency adjustment, additional monitoring, and/or selection of alternative therapy. Secondary malignancies (bladder cancer, myelodysplasia, acute leukemias, lymphomas, thyroid cancer, and sarcomas) have been reported with both single-agent and with combination chemotherapy regimens; onset may be delayed (up to several years after treatment). Bladder cancer usually occurs in patients previously experiencing hemorrhagic cystitis; risk may be reduced by preventing hemorrhagic cystitis.

Adverse Reactions

Dermatologic: Alopecia (reversible; onset: 3-6 weeks after start of treatment)

Endocrine & metabolic: Amenorrhea, azoospermia, gonadal suppression, oligospermia, oogenesis impaired, sterility

Gastrointestinal: Abdominal pain, anorexia, diarrhea, mucositis, nausea/vomiting (dose-related), stomatitis

Genitourinary: Hemorrhagic cystitis

Hematologic: Anemia, leukopenia (dose-related; recovery: 7-10 days after cessation), myelosuppression, neutropenia, neutropenic fever, thrombocytopenia

Miscellaneous: Infection

Rare but important or life-threatening: Acute respiratory distress syndrome, anaphylactic reactions, anaphylaxis, arrhythmias (with high-dose [HSCT] therapy), bladder/urinary fibrosis, blurred vision, cardiac tamponade (with high-dose [HSCT] therapy), cardiotoxicity, confusion, dyspnea, ejection fraction decreased, erythema multiforme, gastrointestinal hemorrhage, hearing disorders, heart block, heart failure (with high-dose [HSCT] therapy), hematuria, hemopericardium, hemorrhagic colitis, hemorrhagic myocarditis (with high-dose [HSCT] therapy), hemorrhagic ureteritis, hepatic sinusoidal obstruction syndrome (SOS; formerly called veno-occlusive liver disease), hepatitis, hepatotoxicity, hypersensitivity reactions, hyperuricemia, hypokalemia, hyponatremia, interstitial pneumonitis, interstitial pulmonary fibrosis (with high doses), jaundice, latent infection reactivation, mesenteric ischemia (acute), methemoglobinemia (with high-dose [HSCT] therapy), multiorgan failure, myocardial necrosis (with high-dose [HSCT] therapy), neurotoxicity, neutrophilic eccrine hidradenitis, ovarian fibrosis, pancreatitis, pericarditis, pigmentation changes (skin/fingernails), pneumonia, pulmonary hypertension, pulmonary infiltrates, pulmonary veno-occlusive disease, pyelonephritis, radiation recall, renal tubular necrosis, reversible posterior leukoencephalopathy syndrome (RPLS), rhabdomyolysis, secondary malignancy, septic shock, sepsis, SIADH, Stevens-Johnson syndrome, testicular atrophy, thrombocytopenia (immune mediated), thrombotic disorders (arterial and venous), toxic epidermal necrolysis, toxic megacolon, tumor lysis syndrome, wound healing impaired

Drug Interactions

Metabolism/Transport Effects Substrate of CYP2A6 (minor), CYP2B6 (major), CYP2C19 (minor), CYP2C9 (minor), CYP3A4 (minor); **Note:** Assignment of Major/Minor substrate status based on clinically relevant drug interaction potential; **Induces** CYP2B6 (weak/moderate), CYP2C9 (weak/moderate)

Avoid Concomitant Use

Avoid concomitant use of Cyclophosphamide with any of the following: BCG; BCG (Intravesical); Belimumab; CloZAPine; Dipyrone; Etanercept; Natalizumab; Pimecrolimus; Tacrolimus (Topical); Tofacitinib; Vaccines (Live)

Increased Effect/Toxicity

Cyclophosphamide may increase the levels/effects of: Amiodarone; Antineoplastic Agents (Anthracycline, Systemic); CloZAPine; CycloSPORINE (Systemic); Leflunomide; Natalizumab; Sargramostim; Succinylcholine; Tofacitinib; Vaccines (Live)

The levels/effects of Cyclophosphamide may be increased by: Allopurinol; AzaTHIOprine; Belimumab; CYP2B6 Inhibitors (Moderate); Denosumab; Dipyrone; Etanercept; Filgrastim; Pentostatin; Pimecrolimus; Protease Inhibitors; Quazepam; Roflumilast; Tacrolimus (Topical); Thiazide Diuretics; Trastuzumab

Decreased Effect

Cyclophosphamide may decrease the levels/effects of: BCG; BCG (Intravesical); Coccidioides immitis Skin Test; CycloSPORINE (Systemic); Sipuleucel-T; Vaccines (Inactivated); Vaccines (Live)

The levels/effects of Cyclophosphamide may be decreased by: CYP2B6 Inducers (Strong); Dabrafenib; Echinacea

Storage/Stability

Injection powder for reconstitution: Store intact vials of powder at ≤25°C (77°F). Exposure to excessive temperatures during transport or storage may cause active ingredient to melt (vials with melting may have a clear to yellow viscous liquid which may appear as droplets); do not use vials with signs of melting. Reconstituted solutions in normal saline (NS) are stable for 24 hours at room temperature and for 6 days refrigerated at 2°C to 8°C (36°F to 46°F). Solutions diluted for infusion in ½NS are stable for 24 hours at room temperature and for 6 days refrigerated; solutions diluted in D_5W or D_5NS are stable for 24 hours at room temperature and for 36 hours refrigerated.

Capsules: Store at 20°C to 25°C (68°F to 77°F); excursions are permitted between 15°C and 30°C (59°F and 86°F).

Tablets: Store tablets at ≤25°C (77°F); brief excursions are permitted up to 30°C (86°F); protect from temperatures >30°C (86°F).

Mechanism of Action Cyclophosphamide is an alkylating agent that prevents cell division by cross-linking DNA strands and decreasing DNA synthesis. It is a cell cycle phase nonspecific agent. Cyclophosphamide also possesses potent immunosuppressive activity. Cyclophosphamide is a prodrug that must be metabolized to active metabolites in the liver.

Pharmacokinetics (Adult data unless noted)

Absorption: Oral: Well absorbed

Distribution: V_d: 30 to 50 L (approximates total body water); distributes throughout the body including the brain and CSF, but not in concentrations high enough to treat meningeal leukemia

Protein binding: ~20%; some metabolites: >60%

Metabolism: Hepatic to active metabolites acrolein, 4-aldophosphamide, 4-hydroperoxycyclophosphamide, and nor-nitrogen mustard

Bioavailability: >75%

Half-life: IV: 3 to 12 hours

Children: 4 hours

Adults: 6 to 8 hours

Time to peak serum concentration: Oral: Within 1 hour; IV: Metabolites: 2 to 3 hours

Elimination: Urine (10% to 20% as unchanged drug); feces (4%)

Dosing: Neonatal

Note: For oncology uses, details concerning dosing in combination regimens should also be consulted; antiemetics may be recommended (emetogenic potential varies by dose and combination therapy).

Neuroblastoma

INES 99.1 regimen courses 1 and 2: IV: Newborns or neonates weighing <10 kg: 3.5 mg/kg on days 1 to 5 administered at 2 week intervals for 2 cycles initially, in combination with vincristine (Rubie, 2011)

CE-CAdO regimen courses 3 and 4 (Rubie, 2001): IV:

Newborns: 7 mg/kg on days 1 to 5 every 21 days for 2 cycles

Older neonates: 10 mg/kg on days 1 to 5 every 21 days for 2 cycles

Dosing: Usual Note: For oncology use, details concerning dosing in combination regimens should also be consulted; cyclophosphamide is associated with a moderate to high emetic potential (depending on dose, regimen, or administration route); antiemetics are recommended to prevent nausea and vomiting (Basch, 2011; Dupuis, 2011; Roila, 2010)

Pediatric: **Note:** In pediatric patients, dosing may be based on either BSA (mg/m^2) or weight (mg/kg); use extra precaution to verify dosing parameters during calculations.

Malignancy; general dosing: Infants, Children, and Adolescents:

IV: Initial: 40 to 50 mg/kg in divided doses over 2 to 5 days **or** 10 to 15 mg/kg every 7 to 10 days or 3 to 5 mg/kg twice weekly

Oral: 1 to 5 mg/kg/day (initial and maintenance dosing)

Nephrotic syndrome, minimal change (frequently relapsing): Infants, Children, and Adolescents: Oral: 2 mg/kg/day for 8 to 12 weeks; reported range: 2 to 3 mg/kg/day; maximum cumulative dose: 168 mg/kg; dosing based on ideal bodyweight. (Gipson, 2009; KDIGO, 2012; KDOQI, 2013). Treatment beyond 90 days may increase the potential for sterility in males.

Ewing's sarcoma: *VAC/IE regimen:* Children and Adolescents: IV: 1200 mg/**m²** (plus mesna) on day 1 of a 21-day treatment cycle in combination with vincristine and doxorubicin (then dactinomycin when maximum doxorubicin dose reached), alternate with IE (ifosfamide and etoposide) for a total of 17 cycles (Grier, 2003)

Hodgkin lymphoma: *BEACOPP escalated regimen:* Children and Adolescents: IV: 1200 mg/**m²** on day 0 of a 21-day treatment cycle for 4 cycles in combination with bleomycin, etoposide, doxorubicin, vincristine, prednisone, and procarbazine (Kelly, 2011)

Aplastic anemia, severe; refractory: Limited data available: Children and Adolescents ≥2 years: High-dose therapy: IV: 45 to 50 mg/kg/day for 4 days has been used in several small trials; concurrent prophylactic antimicrobial therapy should be considered (Audino, 2010; Brodsky, 1996; Brodsky, 2010; DeZern, 2011; Jaime-Perez, 2013)

Lupus nephritis; proliferative: Limited data available: Children and Adolescents:

Initial phase; pulse therapy:

IV:

6-month course: Usual range: 500 to 1000 mg/**m²**/dose once monthly (KDIGO, 2012); the following regimen has been used for dosage escalation: Initial: 500 mg/**m²** then titrate as tolerated every 4 weeks in 250 mg/**m²** increments up to 750 or 1000 mg/**m²** every month; maximum monthly dose: 1500 mg/month (Bertsias, 2012; Mina, 2012)

3-month course: 500 mg every 2 weeks for 3 months (Bertsias, 2012; KDIGO, 2012)

Oral: 1 to 1.5 mg/kg/day for 2 to 4 months; maximum daily dose: 150 mg/**day** (KDIGO, 2012); higher doses (2 to 2.5 mg/kg/day for 3 months) may be required in patients with worsening prognostic factors (eg, acute renal function deterioration) (Bertsias, 2012)

Maintenance phase: IV: 500 to 1000 mg/**m²** every 3 months for a total of 1.5 to 3 years has been used; however, current guidelines recommend other oral immunosuppressive agents for maintenance therapy (KDIGO, 2012; Kliegman, 2011; Lehman, 2000)

Neuroblastoma:

INES 99.1 regimen courses 1 and 2: IV: Infants:

<10 kg: 3.5 mg/kg on days 1 to 5 administered at 2-week intervals for 2 cycles initially, in combination with vincristine (Rubie, 2011)

≥10 kg: 5 mg/kg on days 1 to 5 administered at 2-week intervals for 2 cycles initially, in combination with vincristine (Rubie, 2011)

CE-CAdO regimen (courses 3 and 4): IV:

Infants:

Weight-directed: 10 mg/kg on days 1 to 5 every 21 days for 2 cycles (Rubie, 2001)

Body surface area-directed: 150 to 210 mg/**m²** on days 1 to 5 every 21 days for 2 cycles (Rubie, 1998)

Children and Adolescent: Body surface area-directed: Patient weight:

<10 kg: 150 to 210 mg/**m²** on days 1 to 5 every 21 days for 2 cycles (Rubie, 1998)

≥10 kg: 300 mg/**m²** on days 1 to 5 every 21 days for 2 cycles (Rubie, 1998)

HSCT conditioning; myeloablative transplant: Limited data available: Infants, Children, and Adolescents: IV: 50 mg/kg/day for 4 days beginning 5 days before transplant (Champlin, 2007); other regimens have used 60 mg/kg/day for 2 days following busulfan (Locatelli, 2005; Mårtensson, 2013)

Uveitis, severe; recalcitrant, high-risk vision loss: Limited data available: Children and Adolescents: Oral: Initial: 2 mg/kg/day once daily; usual reported range: 1 to 3 mg/kg/day in combination with corticosteroids (which may be decreased while on cyclophosphamide) (Jabs, 2000; Pujari, 2010; Simoni, 2010); dosing based on large, multicenter report of 215 patients with ocular inflammatory disease which included 44 patients with uveitis (age range: 11.5 to 76.4 years); after 12 months of therapy ~89% of patients had no inflammatory disease activity or only slightly active disease. (Pujari, 2010). **Note:** Some data suggests that pulse intravenous therapy may be less effective than oral cyclophosphamide (Pujari, 2010).

Vasculitis, ANCA-associated (eg, granulomatosis with polyangiitis [GPA], Wegener's granulomatosis): Limited data available: Children and Adolescents:

IV: Initial: 15 mg/kg every 2 weeks for 3 doses, then 15 mg/kg every 3 weeks until remission; dosing based on experience from a pediatric case series (n=5) and a larger adult trial (n=76); in the pediatric case series, the median cumulative dose was 90 mg/kg (range: 63 to 115 mg/kg), most patients received 6 to 7 pulses of therapy; in the adult trial, therapy was continue for 3 months after remission (DeGroot, 2009; Krmar, 2013)

Oral: 2 mg/kg/day in combination with corticosteroids until remission; a subsequent decrease in dose to 1.5 mg/kg/day for another 3 months has been reported (DeGroot, 2009; Kliegman, 2011)

Adult: **Malignancy:** For non-HSCT dosing: Utilize patient's actual body weight (full weight) for calculation of body surface area- or weight-based dosing, particularly when the intent of therapy is curative; manage regimen-related toxicities in the same manner as for nonobese patients; if a dose reduction is utilized due to toxicity, consider resumption of full weight-based dosing with subsequent cycles, especially if cause of toxicity (eg, hepatic or renal impairment) is resolved (Griggs, 2012).

IV: 40 to 50 mg/kg in divided doses over 2 to 5 days **or** 10 to 15 mg/kg every 7 to 10 days **or** 3 to 5 mg/kg twice weekly

Oral: 1 to 5 mg/kg/day (initial and maintenance dosing)

Dosing adjustment in renal impairment: There are no dosage adjustments provided in the manufacturer's labeling; decreased renal excretion of cyclophosphamide and its metabolites may occur; monitor patients with severe impairment (CrCl 10 to 24 mL/min) for signs and symptoms of toxicity. The following guidelines have been used by some clinicians:

Pediatric:

Aronoff, 2007: Infants, Children, and Adolescents:

CrCl ≥10 mL/minute: No dosage adjustment required.

CrCl <10 mL/minute: Administer 75% of normal dose.

Hemodialysis: Moderately dialyzable (20% to 50%); administer 50% of normal dose; administer after hemodialysis.

Continuous ambulatory peritoneal dialysis (CAPD): Administer 75% of normal dose.

Continuous renal replacement therapy (CRRT): Administer 100% of normal dose.

KDIGO, 2012: **Lupus nephritis:** Children and Adolescents:

CrCl 25 to 50 mL/minute: Administer 80% of normal dose.

CrCl 10 to <25 mL/minute: Administer 70% of normal dose.

Adult:

Aronoff, 2007:

CrCl ≥10 mL/minute: No dosage adjustment required.

CrCl <10 mL/minute: Administer 75% of normal dose.

Hemodialysis: Moderately dialyzable (20% to 50%); administer 50% of normal dose; administer after hemodialysis.

Continuous ambulatory peritoneal dialysis (CAPD): Administer 75% of normal dose.

Continuous renal replacement therapy (CRRT): Administer 100% of normal dose.

Janus, 2010: Hemodialysis: Administer 75% of normal dose; administer after hemodialysis.

Dosing adjustment in hepatic impairment: There are no dosage adjustment provided in the manufacturer's labeling; in severe hepatic impairment, conversion to an active metabolite may be reduced potentially affecting efficacy. The following adjustments have been recommended (Floyd, 2006): All patients:

Serum bilirubin 3.1 to 5 mg/dL or transaminases >3 times ULN: Administer 75% of dose.

Serum bilirubin >5 mg/mL: Avoid use.

Preparation for Administration Hazardous agent; use appropriate precautions for handling and disposal (NIOSH 2014 [group 1]). Parenteral:

IV push: Reconstitute with NS to a concentration of 20 mg/mL.

IV infusion (intermittent or continuous): Reconstitute with NS or SWFI to a concentration of 20 mg/mL; if reconstituted with NS, may administer undiluted or may further dilute in D_5W, $^1/_2$NS or D_5NS to a concentration no less than 2 mg/mL; if reconstituted with SWFI, must further dilute in D_5W, $^1/_2$NS or D_5NS to a concentration no less than 2 mg/mL.

Administration Hazardous agent; use appropriate precautions for handling and disposal (NIOSH 2014 [group 1]). Cyclophosphamide is associated with a moderate to high emetic potential (depending on dose or regimen); antiemetics are recommended to prevent nausea and vomiting (Basch 2011; Dupuis 2011; Roila 2010).

Oral: Capsules and tablets should be swallowed whole. Tablets are not scored and should not be cut, crushed or chewed. Capsules should not be opened, crushed, or chewed. Wear gloves when handling capsules/tablets and container; avoid exposure to broken capsules. If exposure to capsule contents or crushed/cut tablets, wash hands immediately and thoroughly. Morning administration may be preferred to ensure adequate hydration throughout the day; do not administer tablets/capsules at bedtime.

Parenteral:

IV push: May administer reconstituted solution without further dilution (20 mg/mL); rate may vary based on protocols (refer to specific protocols)

IV infusion (intermittent or continuous): Infusion rate may vary based on protocol (refer to specific protocol for infusion rate); usually over 15 to 60 minutes; larger doses (>1,800 mg/m^2) should be infused over 4 to 6 hours (Phelps 2013)

Bladder toxicity: To minimize bladder toxicity, increase normal fluid intake during and for 1 to 2 days after cyclophosphamide dose. Most adult patients will require a fluid intake of at least 2 L/day. High-dose regimens should be accompanied by vigorous hydration with or without mesna therapy. Morning administration may be preferred to ensure adequate hydration throughout the day.

Hematopoietic stem cell transplant: Adults: Approaches to reduction of hemorrhagic cystitis include infusion of NS 3 L/m^2/24 hours, infusion of NS 3 L/m^2/24 hours with continuous NS bladder irrigation 300 to 1,000 mL/hour, and infusion of NS 1.5 to 3 L/m^2/24 hours with intravenous mesna. Hydration should begin at least 4 hours before cyclophosphamide and continue at least 24 hours after completion of cyclophosphamide. The dose of daily mesna used may be 67% to 100% of the daily dose of cyclophosphamide. Mesna can be administered as a continuous 24-hour intravenous infusion or be given in divided doses every 4 hours. Mesna should begin at the start of treatment, and continue at least 24 hours following the last dose of cyclophosphamide.

Vesicant/Extravasation Risk May be an irritant

Monitoring Parameters CBC with differential and platelet count, BUN, urinalysis, urine specific gravity, serum electrolytes, serum creatinine, monitor for signs/symptoms of hemorrhagic cystitis or other urinary/renal toxicity, pulmonary, cardiac, and/or hepatic toxicity

Dosage Forms Excipient information presented when available (limited, particularly for generics); consult specific product labeling.

Capsule, Oral:

Generic: 25 mg, 50 mg

Solution Reconstituted, Injection:

Generic: 500 mg (1 ea); 1 g (1 ea); 2 g (1 ea)

Tablet, Oral:

Generic: 25 mg, 50 mg

Extemporaneous Preparations Hazardous agent: Use appropriate precautions for handling and disposal (NIOSH 2014 [group 1]).

Liquid solutions for oral administration may be prepared by dissolving cyclophosphamide injection in Aromatic Elixir, N.F. Store refrigerated (in glass container) for up to 14 days.

Cyclophosphamide Prescribing Information, Baxter Healthcare Corporation, Deerfield, Il, May, 2013.

A 10 mg/mL oral suspension may be prepared by reconstituting one 2 g vial for injection with 100 mL of NaCl 0.9%, providing an initial concentration of 20 mg/mL. Mix this solution in a 1:1 ratio with either Simple Syrup, NF or Ora-Plus® to obtain a final concentration of 10 mg/mL. Label "shake well" and "refrigerate". Stable for 56 days refrigerated.

Kennedy R, Groepper D, Tagen M, et al, "Stability of Cyclophosphamide in Extemporaneous Oral Suspensions," *Ann Pharmacother*, 2010, 44(2):295-301.

CycloSERINE (sye kloe SER een)

Medication Safety Issues

Sound-alike/look-alike issues:

CycloSERINE may be confused with cyclobenzaprine, cycloSPORINE

Brand Names: US Seromycin [DSC]

Therapeutic Category Antibiotic, Miscellaneous; Antitubercular Agent

Generic Availability (US) Yes

Use Adjunctive treatment in pulmonary or extrapulmonary tuberculosis; treatment of acute urinary tract infections caused by *E. coli* or *Enterobacter* species when less toxic conventional therapy has failed or is contraindicated

Pregnancy Risk Factor C

Pregnancy Considerations Teratogenic effects have not been observed in animal reproduction studies. Cycloserine crosses the placenta and can be detected in the fetal blood and amniotic fluid. The American Thoracic Society recommends use in pregnant women only if there are no alternatives (CDC, 2003).

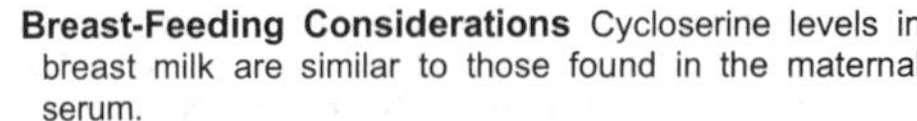

Breast-Feeding Considerations Cycloserine levels in breast milk are similar to those found in the maternal serum.

Contraindications Hypersensitivity to cycloserine or any component of the formulation; epilepsy; depression, severe anxiety, or psychosis; severe renal insufficiency; excessive concurrent use of alcohol

Warnings/Precautions Has been associated with CNS toxicity, including seizures, psychosis, depression, and confusion; decrease dosage or discontinue use if occurs. Use with caution in patients with epilepsy, depression, severe anxiety, psychosis, severe renal insufficiency, chronic alcoholism and patients with potential folate deficiency (malnourished, chronic anticonvulsant therapy, or elderly). Effects may be potentiated when used with other sedative drugs or ethanol. Prolonged use may result in fungal or bacterial superinfection, including *C. difficile*-associated diarrhea (CDAD) and pseudomembranous colitis; CDAD has been observed >2 months postantibiotic treatment.

Adverse Reactions Frequency not defined.

Cardiovascular: Cardiac arrhythmia, heart failure

Central nervous system: Coma, confusion, dizziness, drowsiness, headache, paresis, psychosis, restlessness, seizures, vertigo

Dermatologic: Rash

Endocrine & metabolic: Vitamin B_{12} deficiency

Hematologic: Folate deficiency

Hepatic: Liver enzymes increased

Neuromuscular & skeletal: Dysarthria, hyperreflexia, paresthesia, tremor

Miscellaneous: Allergic manifestations

Drug Interactions

Metabolism/Transport Effects None known.

Avoid Concomitant Use

Avoid concomitant use of CycloSERINE with any of the following: Alcohol (Ethyl); BCG; BCG (Intravesical)

Increased Effect/Toxicity

The levels/effects of CycloSERINE may be increased by: Alcohol (Ethyl); Ethionamide; Isoniazid

Decreased Effect

CycloSERINE may decrease the levels/effects of: BCG; BCG (Intravesical); BCG Vaccine (Immunization); Sodium Picosulfate; Typhoid Vaccine

Food Interactions May increase vitamin B_{12} and folic acid dietary requirements. Management: Vitamin B_{12} and folic acid supplementation may be needed.

Mechanism of Action Inhibits bacterial cell wall synthesis by competing with amino acid (D-alanine) for incorporation into the bacterial cell wall; bacteriostatic or bactericidal

Pharmacokinetics (Adult data unless noted)

Absorption: ~70% to 90% from the GI tract

Distribution: Crosses the placenta; appears in breast milk, bile, sputum, synovial fluid and CSF

Protein binding: Not plasma protein bound

Half-life: Patients with normal renal function: 10 hours

Time to peak serum concentration: Within 3-4 hours

Elimination: 60% to 70% of an oral dose excreted unchanged in urine by glomerular filtration within 72 hours, small amounts excreted in feces, remainder is metabolized

Dosing: Usual Oral:

Tuberculosis:

Children: 10-20 mg/kg/day divided every 12 hours up to 1000 mg/day

Adults: Initial: 250 mg every 12 hours for 14 days, then give 500 mg to 1 g/day in 2 divided doses

Urinary tract infection: Adults: 250 mg every 12 hours for 14 days

Dosing adjustment in renal impairment:

CrCl 10-50 mL/minute: Administer every 24 hours

CrCl <10 mL/minute: Administer every 36-48 hours

Administration Oral: May administer without regard to meals

Monitoring Parameters Periodic renal, hepatic, hematological tests, and plasma cycloserine concentrations

Reference Range Adjust dosage to maintain blood cycloserine concentrations <30 mcg/mL

Dosage Forms Excipient information presented when available (limited, particularly for generics); consult specific product labeling. [DSC] = Discontinued product

Capsule, Oral:

Seromycin: 250 mg [DSC] [contains brilliant blue fcf (fd&c blue #1), fd&c yellow #10 (quinoline yellow), fd&c yellow #6 (sunset yellow)]

Generic: 250 mg

◆ **Cycloset** *see* Bromocriptine *on page 303*

◆ **Cyclosporin A** *see* CycloSPORINE (Ophthalmic) *on page 561*

◆ **Cyclosporin A** *see* CycloSPORINE (Systemic) *on page 556*

CycloSPORINE (Systemic) (SYE kloe spor een)

Medication Safety Issues

Sound-alike/look-alike issues:

CycloSPORINE may be confused with cyclophosphamide, Cyklokapron, cycloSERINE

CycloSPORINE modified (Neoral, Gengraf) may be confused with cycloSPORINE non-modified (SandIMMUNE)

Gengraf may be confused with Prograf

Neoral may be confused with Neurontin, Nizoral

SandIMMUNE may be confused with SandoSTATIN

High alert medication:

This medication is in a class the Institute for Safe Medication Practices (ISMP) includes among its list of drug classes that have a heightened risk of causing significant patient harm when used in error.

Related Information

Oral Medications That Should Not Be Crushed or Altered *on page 2476*

Safe Handling of Hazardous Drugs *on page 2455*

Brand Names: US Gengraf; Neoral; SandIMMUNE

Brand Names: Canada Apo-Cyclosporine; Neoral; Sandimmune I.V.; Sandoz-Cyclosporine

Therapeutic Category Immunosuppressant Agent

Generic Availability (US) Yes

Use Immunosuppressant used with corticosteroids to prevent organ rejection in patients with kidney, liver, lung, heart, and bone marrow transplants; treatment of nephrotic syndrome in patients with documented focal glomerulosclerosis when corticosteroids and cyclophosphamide are unsuccessful; severe psoriasis; severe rheumatoid arthritis not responsive to methotrexate alone; severe autoimmune disease that is resistant to corticosteroids and other therapy; prevention and treatment of graft-versus-host disease in bone marrow transplant patients

Pregnancy Risk Factor C

Pregnancy Considerations Adverse events were not observed following the use of oral cyclosporine in animal reproduction studies (using doses that were not maternally toxic). In humans, cyclosporine crosses the placenta; maternal concentrations do not correlate with those found in the umbilical cord. Cyclosporine may be detected in the serum of newborns for several days after birth (Claris 1993). Based on clinical use, premature births and low birth weight were consistently observed in pregnant transplant patients (additional pregnancy complications also present). Formulations may contain alcohol; the alcohol content should be taken into consideration in pregnant women.

The pharmacokinetics of cyclosporine may be influenced by pregnancy (Grimer 2007). Cyclosporine may be used in pregnant renal, liver, or heart transplant patients (Cowan 2012; EBPG Expert Group on Renal Transplantation 2002; McGuire 2009; Parhar 2012). If therapy is needed for psoriasis, other agents are preferred; however, cyclosporine may be used as an alternative agent along with close clinical monitoring; use should be avoided during the first trimester if possible (Bae 2012). If treatment is needed for lupus nephritis, other agents are recommended to be used in pregnant women (Hahn 2012).

Following transplant, normal menstruation and fertility may be restored within months; however, appropriate contraception is recommended to prevent pregnancy until 1-2 years following the transplant to improve pregnancy outcomes (Cowan 2012; EBPG Expert Group on Renal Transplantation 2002; McGuire 2009; Parhar 2012).

A pregnancy registry has been established for pregnant women taking immunosuppressants following any solid organ transplant (National Transplantation Pregnancy Registry, Temple University, 877-955-6877).

A pregnancy registry has also been established for pregnant women taking Neoral for psoriasis or rheumatoid arthritis (Neoral Pregnancy Registry for Psoriasis and Rheumatoid Arthritis, Thomas Jefferson University, 888-522-5581).

Breast-Feeding Considerations Cyclosporine is excreted in breast milk. Concentrations of cyclosporine in milk vary widely and breast-feeding during therapy is generally not recommended (Bae 2012; Cowan 2012). Due to the potential for serious adverse in the breast-feeding infant, a decision should be made to discontinue cyclosporine or to discontinue breast-feeding, taking into account the importance of treatment to the mother. Formulations may contain alcohol which may be present in breast milk and could be absorbed orally by the breast-feeding infant.

Contraindications

Hypersensitivity to cyclosporine or any component of the formulation. IV cyclosporine is contraindicated in hypersensitivity to polyoxyethylated castor oil (Cremophor EL).

Rheumatoid arthritis and psoriasis patients with abnormal renal function, uncontrolled hypertension, or malignancies. Concomitant treatment with PUVA or UVB therapy, methotrexate, other immunosuppressive agents, coal tar, or radiation therapy are also contraindications for use in patients with psoriasis.

Canadian labeling: Additional contraindications (not in US labeling): Concurrent use with bosentan; rheumatoid arthritis and psoriasis patients with primary or secondary immunodeficiency excluding autoimmune disease, uncontrolled infection, or malignancy (excluding non-melanoma skin cancer).

Warnings/Precautions Hazardous agent - use appropriate precautions for handling and disposal (NIOSH 2014 [group 2]).

[US Boxed Warning]: Increased risk of lymphomas and other malignancies (including fatal outcomes), **particularly skin cancers;** risk is related to intensity/duration of therapy and the use of more than one immunosuppressive agent; all patients should avoid excessive sun/UV light exposure. **[US Boxed Warning]: May cause hypertension; risk is increased with increasing doses/duration.** Use caution when changing dosage forms.

[US Boxed Warning]: Renal impairment, including structural kidney damage has occurred (when used at high doses); risk is increased with increasing doses/duration; monitor renal function closely. Elevations in serum creatinine and BUN generally respond to dosage reductions. Use caution with other potentially nephrotoxic drugs (eg, acyclovir, aminoglycoside antibiotics, amphotericin B, ciprofloxacin); monitor renal function closely with concomitant use. If significant renal impairment occurs, reduce the dose of the coadministered medication or consider alternative treatment. Elevations in serum creatinine and BUN associated with nephrotoxicity generally respond to dosage reductions. In renal transplant patients with rapidly rising BUN and creatinine, carefully evaluate to differentiate between cyclosporine-associated nephrotoxicity and renal rejection episodes. In cases of severe rejection that fail to respond to pulse steroids and monoclonal antibodies, switching to an alternative immunosuppressant agent may be preferred to increasing cyclosporine to excessive blood concentrations.

[US Boxed Warning]: Increased risk of infection with use; serious and fatal infections have been reported. Bacterial, viral, fungal, and protozoal infections (including opportunistic infections) have occurred. Polyoma virus infections, such as the JC virus and BK virus, may result in serious and sometimes fatal outcomes. The JC virus is associated with progressive multifocal leukoencephalopathy (PML), and PML has been reported in patients receiving cyclosporine. PML may be fatal and presents with hemiparesis, apathy, confusion, cognitive deficiencies, and ataxia; consider neurologic consultation as indicated. The BK virus is associated with nephropathy, and polyoma virus-associated nephropathy (PVAN) has been reported in patients receiving cyclosporine. PVAN is associated with serious adverse effects including renal dysfunction and renal graft loss. If PML or PVAN occur in transplant patients, consider reducing immunosuppression therapy as well as the risk that reduced immunosuppression poses to grafts.

Hepatotoxicity (transaminase and bilirubin elevations) and liver injury, including cholestasis, jaundice, hepatitis, and liver failure, has been reported. These events were mainly in patients with confounding factors including infections, coadministration with other potentially hepatotoxic medications, underlying conditions, and significant comorbidities. Fatalities have also been reported rarely, primarily in transplant patients. Increased hepatic enzymes and bilirubin have occurred, usually in the first month and when used at high doses; improvement is usually seen with dosage reduction.

Should be used initially with corticosteroids in transplant patients. Significant hyperkalemia (with or without hyperchloremic metabolic acidosis) and hyperuricemia have occurred with therapy. Syndromes of microangiopathic hemolytic anemia and thrombocytopenia have occurred and may result in graft failure; it is accompanied by platelet consumption within the graft. Syndrome may occur without graft rejection. Although management of the syndrome is unclear, discontinuation or reduction of cyclosporine, in addition to streptokinase and heparin administration or plasmapheresis, has been associated with syndrome resolution. However, resolution seems to be dependent upon early detection of the syndrome via indium 111 labeled platelet scans.

May cause seizures, particularly if used with high-dose corticosteroids. Encephalopathy (including posterior reversible encephalopathy syndrome [PRES]) has also been reported; predisposing factors include hypertension, hypomagnesemia, hypocholesterolemia, high-dose corticosteroids, high cyclosporine serum concentration, and graft-versus-host disease (GVHD). Encephalopathy may be more common in patients with liver transplant compared to kidney transplant. Other neurotoxic events, such as optic disc edema (including papilloedema and potential visual impairment), have been rarely reported primarily in transplant patients.

[US Boxed Warning]: The modified/non-modified formulations are not bioequivalent; cyclosporine (modified) has increased bioavailability as compared to cyclosporine (non-modified) and the products cannot be used interchangeably without close monitoring. Cyclosporine (modified) refers to the oral solution and capsule dosage formulations of cyclosporine in an aqueous dispersion (previously referred to as "microemulsion"). Potentially significant drug-drug/drug-food interactions may exist, requiring dose or frequency adjustment, additional monitoring, and/or selection of alternative therapy. Gingival hyperplasia may occur; avoid concomitant nifedipine in patients who develop gingival hyperplasia (may increase frequency of hyperplasia). Monitor cyclosporine concentrations closely following the addition, modification, or deletion of other medication. Live, attenuated vaccines may be less effective; vaccination should be avoided. Make dose adjustments based on cyclosporine blood concentrations. **[US Boxed Warning]: Cyclosporine non-modified absorption is erratic; monitor blood concentrations closely. [US Boxed Warning]: Prescribing and dosage adjustment should only be under the direct supervision of an experienced physician. Adequate laboratory/medical resources and follow-up are necessary.** Anaphylaxis has been reported with IV use; reserve for patients who cannot take oral form. **[US Boxed Warning]: Risk of skin cancer may be increased in transplant patients.** Due to the increased risk for nephrotoxicity in renal transplantation, avoid using standard doses of cyclosporine in combination with everolimus; reduced cyclosporine doses are recommended; monitor cyclosporine concentrations closely. Cyclosporine and everolimus combination therapy may increase the risk for proteinuria. Cyclosporine combined with either everolimus or sirolimus may increase the risk for thrombotic microangiopathy/thrombotic thrombocytopenic purpura/hemolytic uremic syndrome (TMA/TTP/HUS). Cyclosporine has extensive hepatic metabolism and exposure is increased in patients with severe hepatic impairment; may require dose reduction.

Patients with psoriasis should avoid excessive sun exposure. **[US Boxed Warning]: Risk of skin cancer may be increased with a history of PUVA and possibly methotrexate or other immunosuppressants, UVB, coal tar, or radiation.**

Rheumatoid arthritis: If receiving other immunosuppressive agents, radiation or UV therapy, concurrent use of cyclosporine is not recommended.

Products may contain corn oil, ethanol (consider alcohol content in certain patient populations, including pregnant or breast-feeding women, patients with liver disease, seizure disorders, alcohol dependency, or pediatrics), or propylene glycol; injection also contains the vehicle Cremophor EL (polyoxyethylated castor oil), which has been associated with hypersensitivity (anaphylactic) reactions. Due to the risk for anaphylaxis, IV cyclosporine should be reserved for use in patients unable to take an oral formulation. Some dosage forms may contain propylene glycol; large amounts are potentially toxic and have been associated hyperosmolality, lactic acidosis, seizures, and respiratory depression; use caution (AAP 1997; Zar 2007).

Warnings: Additional Pediatric Considerations Some dosage forms may contain propylene glycol; in neonates large amounts of propylene glycol delivered orally, intravenously (eg, >3,000 mg/day), or topically have been associated with potentially fatal toxicities which can include metabolic acidosis, seizures, renal failure, and CNS depression; toxicities have also been reported in children and adults including hyperosmolality, lactic acidosis, seizures and respiratory depression; use caution (AAP, 1997; Shehab, 2009).

Adverse Reactions Adverse reactions reported with systemic use, including rheumatoid arthritis, psoriasis, and transplantation (kidney, liver, and heart).

Any indication:

- Cardiovascular: Edema, hypertension
- Central nervous system: Headache, paresthesia
- Dermatologic: Hypertrichosis
- Endocrine & metabolic: Female genital tract disease, hirsutism, increased serum triglycerides
- Gastrointestinal: Abdominal distress, diarrhea, dyspepsia, gingival hyperplasia, nausea
- Infection: Increased susceptibility to infection
- Neuromuscular & skeletal: Leg cramps, tremor
- Renal: Increased serum creatinine, renal insufficiency
- Respiratory: Upper respiratory tract infection

Kidney, liver, and heart transplant only:

- Cardiovascular: Chest pain, flushing, glomerular capillary thrombosis, myocardial infarction
- Central nervous system: Anxiety, confusion, convulsions, lethargy, tingling sensation
- Dermatologic: Acne vulgaris, nail disease (brittle fingernails), hair breakage, night sweats, pruritus, skin infection
- Endocrine & metabolic: Gynecomastia, hyperglycemia, hypomagnesemia, weight loss
- Gastrointestinal: Anorexia, aphthous stomatitis, constipation, dysphagia, gastritis, hiccups, pancreatitis, vomiting
- Genitourinary: Hematuria, urinary tract infection (kidney transplant)
- Hematologic & oncologic: Anemia, leukopenia, lymphoma, thrombocytopenia, upper gastrointestinal hemorrhage
- Hepatic: Hepatotoxicity
- Infection: Abscess, cytomegalovirus disease, fungal infection (systemic), localized fungal infection, septicemia, viral infection (kidney transplant)
- Neuromuscular & skeletal: Arthralgia, myalgia, weakness
- Ophthalmic: Conjunctivitis, visual disturbance
- Otic: Hearing loss, tinnitus
- Respiratory: Pneumonia, sinusitis
- Miscellaneous: Fever

Rheumatoid arthritis only:

- Cardiovascular: Abnormal heart sounds, cardiac arrhythmia, cardiac failure, chest pain, myocardial infarction, peripheral ischemia
- Central nervous system: Anxiety, depression, dizziness, drowsiness, emotional lability, hypoesthesia, insomnia, lack of concentration, malaise, migraine, neuropathy, nervousness, pain, paranoia, vertigo
- Dermatologic: Cellulitis, dermatological reaction, dermatitis, diaphoresis, dyschromia, eczema, enanthema, folliculitis, nail disease, pruritus, urticaria, xeroderma
- Endocrine & metabolic: Decreased libido, diabetes mellitus, goiter, hot flash, hyperkalemia, hyperuricemia, hypoglycemia, increased libido, menstrual disease, weight gain, weight loss
- Gastrointestinal: Constipation, dysgeusia, dysphagia, enlargement of salivary glands, eructation, esophagitis, flatulence, gastric ulcer, gastritis, gastroenteritis, gingival hemorrhage, gingivitis, glossitis, peptic ulcer, tongue disease, vomiting, xerostomia
- Genitourinary: Breast fibroadenosis, hematuria, leukorrhea, mastalgia, nocturia, urine abnormality, urinary incontinence, urinary urgency, uterine hemorrhage
- Hematologic & oncologic: Anemia, carcinoma, leukopenia, lymphadenopathy, purpura
- Hepatic: Hyperbilirubinemia

Infection: Abscess (including renal), bacterial infection, candidiasis, fungal infection, herpes simplex infection, herpes zoster, viral infection
Neuromuscular & skeletal: Arthralgia, bone fracture, dislocation, myalgia, stiffness, synovial cyst, tendon disease, weakness
Ophthalmic: Cataract, conjunctivitis, eye pain, visual disturbance
Otic: Tinnitus, deafness, vestibular disturbance
Renal: Abscess (renal), increased blood urea nitrogen, polyuria, pyelonephritis
Respiratory: Abnormal breath sounds, bronchospasm, cough, dyspnea, epistaxis, sinusitis, tonsillitis

Psoriasis only:
Cardiovascular: Chest pain, flushing
Central nervous system: Dizziness, insomnia, nervousness, pain, psychiatric disturbance, vertigo
Dermatologic: Acne vulgaris, folliculitis, hyperkeratosis, pruritus, skin rash, xeroderma
Endocrine & metabolic: Hot flash
Gastrointestinal: Abdominal distention, constipation, gingival hemorrhage, increased appetite
Genitourinary: Urinary frequency
Hematologic & oncologic: Abnormal erythrocytes, altered platelet function, blood coagulation disorder, carcinoma, hemorrhagic diathesis
Hepatic: Hyperbilirubinemia
Neuromuscular & skeletal: Arthralgia
Ophthalmic: Visual disturbance
Respiratory: Bronchospasm, cough, dyspnea, flu-like symptoms, respiratory tract infection, rhinitis
Miscellaneous: Fever

Rare but important or life-threatening; any indication: Anaphylaxis/anaphylactoid reaction (possibly associated with Cremophor EL vehicle in injection formulation), brain disease, central nervous system toxicity, cholestasis, cholesterol increased, exacerbation of psoriasis (transformation to erythrodermic or pustular psoriasis), gout, haemolytic uremic syndrome, hepatic insufficiency, hepatitis, hyperbilirubinemia, hyperkalemia, hyperlipidemia, hypertrichosis, hyperuricemia, hypomagnesemia, impaired consciousness, increased susceptibility to infection (including JC virus and BK virus), jaundice, leg pain (possibly a manifestation of Calcineurin-Inhibitor Induced Pain Syndrome), malignant lymphoma, migraine, myalgia, myopathy, myositis, papilledema, progressive multifocal leukoencephalopathy, pseudotumor cerebri, pulmonary edema (noncardiogenic), renal disease (polyoma virus-associated), reversible posterior leukoencephalopathy syndrome, rhabdomyolysis, thrombotic microangiopathy

Drug Interactions

Metabolism/Transport Effects Substrate of CYP3A4 (major), P-glycoprotein; **Note:** Assignment of Major/Minor substrate status based on clinically relevant drug interaction potential; **Inhibits** BSEP, CYP2C9 (weak), CYP3A4 (weak), P-glycoprotein, SLCO1B1

Avoid Concomitant Use

Avoid concomitant use of CycloSPORINE (Systemic) with any of the following: Aliskiren; AtorvaSTATin; BCG; BCG (Intravesical); Bosentan; Bosutinib; Cholic Acid; Conivaptan; Crizotinib; Dronedarone; Enzalutamide; Eplerenone; Foscarnet; Fusidic Acid (Systemic); Idelalisib; Lercanidipine; Lovastatin; Mifepristone; Natalizumab; PAZOPanib; Pimecrolimus; Pimozide; Pitavastatin; Potassium-Sparing Diuretics; Silodosin; Simeprevir; Simvastatin; Sitaxentan; Tacrolimus (Systemic); Tacrolimus (Topical); Tofacitinib; Topotecan; Vaccines (Live); VinCRIStine (Liposomal)

Increased Effect/Toxicity

CycloSPORINE (Systemic) may increase the levels/effects of: Afatinib; Aliskiren; Ambrisentan; ARIPiprazole; AtorvaSTATin; Boceprevir; Bosentan; Bosutinib; Brentuximab Vedotin; Calcium Channel Blockers (Dihydropyridine); Calcium Channel Blockers (Nondihydropyridine); Caspofungin; Cholic Acid; Colchicine; Dabigatran Etexilate; Dexamethasone (Systemic); Digoxin; Dofetilide; DOXOrubicin (Conventional); Dronedarone; Edoxaban; Eluxadoline; Etoposide; Etoposide Phosphate; Everolimus; Ezetimibe; Fibric Acid Derivatives; Fimasartan; Fluvastatin; Hydrocodone; Imipenem; Ledipasvir; Leflunomide; Lercanidipine; Lomitapide; Loop Diuretics; Lovastatin; Methotrexate; MethylPREDNISolone; Minoxidil (Systemic); Minoxidil (Topical); MitoXANtrone; Naloxegol; Natalizumab; Neuromuscular-Blocking Agents; NiMODipine; Nintedanib; Nonsteroidal Anti-Inflammatory Agents; PAZOPanib; P-glycoprotein/ABCB1 Substrates; Pimozide; Pitavastatin; Pravastatin; PrednisoLONE (Systemic); PredniSONE; Protease Inhibitors; Prucalopride; Repaglinide; Rifaximin; Rivaroxaban; Rosuvastatin; Silodosin; Simeprevir; Simvastatin; Sirolimus; Sitaxentan; Tacrolimus (Systemic); Tacrolimus (Topical); Ticagrelor; Tofacitinib; Topotecan; Vaccines (Live); VinCRIStine (Liposomal)

The levels/effects of CycloSPORINE (Systemic) may be increased by: AcetaZOLAMIDE; Aminoglycosides; Amiodarone; Amphotericin B; Androgens; Angiotensin II Receptor Blockers; Antifungal Agents (Azole Derivatives, Systemic); Aprepitant; Boceprevir; Bromocriptine; Calcium Channel Blockers (Nondihydropyridine); Carvedilol; Chloramphenicol; Conivaptan; Crizotinib; Cyclophosphamide; CYP3A4 Inhibitors (Moderate); CYP3A4 Inhibitors (Strong); Dasatinib; Denosumab; Dexamethasone (Systemic); Eplerenone; Ezetimibe; Fluconazole; Fosaprepitant; Foscarnet; Fusidic Acid (Systemic); GlyBURIDE; Grapefruit Juice; Idelalisib; Imatinib; Imipenem; Ivacaftor; Lercanidipine; Luliconazole; Macrolide Antibiotics; Melphalan; Methotrexate; MethylPREDNISolone; Metoclopramide; Metreleptin; Mifepristone; Netupitant; Nonsteroidal Anti-Inflammatory Agents; Norfloxacin; Omeprazole; Palbociclib; P-glycoprotein/ABCB1 Inhibitors; Pimecrolimus; Potassium-Sparing Diuretics; Pravastatin; PrednisoLONE (Systemic); PredniSONE; Protease Inhibitors; Pyrazinamide; Quinupristin; Ritonavir; Roflumilast; Simeprevir; Sirolimus; Stiripentol; Sulfonamide Derivatives; Tacrolimus (Systemic); Tacrolimus (Topical); Telaprevir; Temsirolimus; Trastuzumab

Decreased Effect

CycloSPORINE (Systemic) may decrease the levels/effects of: BCG; BCG (Intravesical); Coccidioides immitis Skin Test; GlyBURIDE; Mycophenolate; Sipuleucel-T; Vaccines (Inactivated); Vaccines (Live)

The levels/effects of CycloSPORINE (Systemic) may be decreased by: Adalimumab; Armodafinil; Ascorbic Acid; Barbiturates; Bosentan; CarBAMazepine; Colesevelam; Cyclophosphamide; CYP3A4 Inducers (Moderate); CYP3A4 Inducers (Strong); Dabrafenib; Deferasirox; Dexamethasone (Systemic); Echinacea; Efavirenz; Enzalutamide; Fibric Acid Derivatives; Fosphenytoin; Griseofulvin; Imipenem; MethylPREDNISolone; Metreleptin; Mitotane; Modafinil; Multivitamins/Fluoride (with ADE); Multivitamins/Minerals (with ADEK, Folate, Iron); Multivitamins/Minerals (with AE, No Iron); Nafcillin; Orlistat; P-glycoprotein/ABCB1 Inducers; Phenytoin; PrednisoLONE (Systemic); PredniSONE; Rifamycin Derivatives; Sevelamer; Siltuximab; Somatostatin Analogs; St Johns Wort; Sulfinpyrazone; Sulfonamide Derivatives; Tocilizumab; Vitamin E

Food Interactions Grapefruit juice increases cyclosporine serum concentrations. Management: Avoid grapefruit juice.

Storage/Stability

Capsules (modified): Store in the original unit-dose container at 20°C to 25°C (68°F to 77°F).

Capsules (non-modified): Store at 25°C (77°F); excursions are permitted between 15°C and 30°C (59°F and 86°F). An odor may be detected upon opening the unit-dose container, which will dissipate shortly thereafter. This odor does not affect the quality of the product.

Injection: Store below 30°C (86°F) or at controlled room temperature (product dependent). Protect from light. Stability of injection of parenteral admixture at room temperature (25°C) is 6 hours in PVC; 12 to 24 hours in Excel, PAB containers, or glass. The manufacturer recommends discarding diluted infusion solutions after 24 hours.

Oral solution (modified): Store in the original container at 20°C to 25°C (68°F to 77°F). Do not store in the refrigerator. Once opened, use within 2 months. At temperatures below 20°C (68°F), the solution may gel; light flocculation or the formation of a light sediment also may occur. There is no impact on product performance or dosing using the syringe provided. Allow to warm to room temperature (25°C [77°F]) to reverse these changes.

Oral solution (non-modified): Store in the original container at temperatures below 30°C (86°F). Do not store in the refrigerator. Protect from freezing. Once opened, use within 2 months.

Mechanism of Action Inhibition of production and release of interleukin II and inhibits interleukin II-induced activation of resting T-lymphocytes.

Pharmacokinetics (Adult data unless noted)

Absorption: Oral:

Cyclosporine (nonmodified) solution or soft gelatin capsule: Erratically and incompletely absorbed; dependent on the presence of food, bile acids, and GI motility; larger oral doses of cyclosporine are needed in pediatric patients vs adults due to a shorter bowel length resulting in limited intestinal absorption

Cyclosporine (modified) solution in a microemulsion or soft gelatin capsule in a microemulsion: Erratically and incompletely absorbed; increased absorption, up to 30% when compared to cyclosporine (nonmodified); absorption is less dependent on food intake, bile, or GI motility when compared to cyclosporine (nonmodified)

Distribution: Widely distributed in tissues and body fluids including the liver, pancreas, and lungs

V_{dss}: 4-6 L/kg in renal, liver, and marrow transplant recipients (slightly lower values in cardiac transplant patients; children <10 years of age have higher values)

Protein binding: 90% to 98% of dose binds to blood lipoproteins

Metabolism: Undergoes extensive first-pass metabolism following oral administration; extensively metabolized by the cytochrome P450 system in the liver; forms at least 25 metabolites

Bioavailability:

Cyclosporine (nonmodified): Dependent on patient population and transplant type (<10% in adult liver transplant patients and as high as 89% in renal patients). The bioavailability of Sandimmune® capsules and oral solution are equivalent; bioavailability of oral solution is ~30% of the IV solution.

Children: 28% (range: 17% to 42%); with gut dysfunction commonly seen in BMT recipients, oral bioavailability is further reduced

Cyclosporine (modified): Bioavailability of Neoral® capsules and oral solution are equivalent:

Children: 43% (range: 30% to 68%)

Adults: 23% greater than with Sandimmune® in renal transplant patients, 50% greater in liver transplant patients

Half-life: May be prolonged in patients with hepatic impairment and lower in pediatric patients due to a higher metabolic rate

Cyclosporine (nonmodified): Biphasic

Alpha phase: 1.4 hours

Terminal phase: 6-24 hours

Cyclosporine (modified): Biphasic; Terminal: 8.4 hours (range: 5-18 hours)

Time to peak serum concentration:

Cyclosporine (nonmodified): 2-6 hours; some patients have a second peak at 5-6 hours

Cyclosporine (modified): 1.5-2 hours (in renal transplant patients)

Elimination: Primarily biliary with 6% of the dose excreted in urine as unchanged drug (0.1%) and metabolites; clearance is more rapid in pediatric patients than in adults

Dosing: Usual Children and Adults (oral dosage is ~3 times the IV dosage):

Transplantations:

IV: Cyclosporine (non-modified):

Initial: 5-6 mg/kg/dose (1/3 the oral dose) administered 4-12 hours prior to organ transplantation

Maintenance: 2-10 mg/kg/day in divided doses every 8-24 hours; patients should be switched to oral cyclosporine as soon as possible; cyclosporine doses should be adjusted to maintain whole blood HPLC trough concentrations in the reference range

Oral: Cyclosporine (non-modified):

Initial: 14-18 mg/kg/dose administered 4-12 hours prior to organ transplantation; lower initial doses of 10-14 mg/kg/day have been used for renal transplants

Maintenance, postoperative: 5-15 mg/kg/day divided every 12-24 hours; maintenance dose is usually tapered to 3-10 mg/kg/day

When using non-modified formulation, cyclosporine levels may increase in liver transplant patients when the T-tube is closed; may need to decrease dose

Oral: Cyclosporine (modified): Based on the organ transplant population:

Initial: Same as the initial dose for solution or soft gelatin capsule

or

Renal: 9 mg/kg/day (range: 6-12 mg/kg/day) divided every 12 hours

Liver: 8 mg/kg/day (range: 4-12 mg/kg/day) divided every 12 hours

Heart: 7 mg/kg/day (range: 4-10 mg/kg/day) divided every 12 hours

Note: A 1:1 ratio conversion from Sandimmune® to Neoral® has been recommended initially; however, lower doses of Neoral® may be required after conversion to prevent overdose. Total daily doses should be adjusted based on the cyclosporine trough blood concentration and clinical assessment of organ rejection. Cyclosporine blood trough levels should be determined prior to conversion. After conversion to Neoral®, cyclosporine trough levels should be monitored every 4-7 days. **Neoral® and Sandimmune® are not bioequivalent and cannot be used interchangeably.**

Focal segmental glomerulosclerosis: Oral: Initial: 3 mg/kg/day divided every 12 hours

Rheumatoid arthritis: Oral: Cyclosporine (modified): Initial: 2.5 mg/kg/day divided every 12 hours; may increase dose by 0.5-0.75 mg/kg/day if insufficient response is seen after 8 weeks of treatment; maximum dose: 4 mg/kg/day

Psoriasis: Oral: Cyclosporine (modified): Initial: 2.5 mg/kg/day divided every 12 hours; may increase dose by 0.5 mg/kg/day if insufficient response is seen after 4 weeks of treatment; maximum dose: 4 mg/kg/day

Autoimmune diseases: Oral: 1-3 mg/kg/day

Preparation for Administration Hazardous agent; use appropriate precautions for handling and disposal (NIOSH 2014 [group 2])

Parenteral: IV infusion (intermittent or continuous): To minimize leaching of DEHP, non-PVC containers and sets should be used for preparation and administration. Further dilute injection in D_5W or NS to a final concentration not to exceed 2.5 mg/mL.

Administration Hazardous agent; use appropriate precautions for handling and disposal (NIOSH 2014 [group 2]).

Oral: Administer consistently at the same time twice daily; use oral syringe, glass dropper, or glass container (not plastic or styrofoam cup); to improve palatability, oral solution may be mixed with milk, chocolate milk, orange juice, or apple juice that is at room temperature; dilution of Neoral with milk can be unpalatable; stir well and drink at once; do not allow to stand before drinking; rinse with more diluent to ensure that the total dose is taken; after use, dry outside of glass dropper; do not rinse with water or other cleaning agents

Parenteral: To minimize leaching of DEHP, non-PVC containers and sets should be used for administration. May administer by IV intermittent infusion or continuous infusion; for intermittent infusion, administer over 2 to 6 hours. Anaphylaxis has been reported with IV use. Patients should be continuously monitored for at least the first 30 minutes of the infusion and should be monitored frequently thereafter.

Monitoring Parameters Blood/serum drug concentration (trough), blood drug concentration (C_2), renal and hepatic function tests, serum electrolytes, lipid profile, blood pressure, heart rate

Reference Range Reference ranges are method- and specimen-dependent; use the same analytical method consistently; trough levels should be obtained immediately prior to next dose

Therapeutic: Not well-defined; dependent on organ transplanted, time after transplant, organ function, and cyclosporine toxicity. Empiric therapeutic concentration ranges for trough cyclosporine concentrations:
- Kidney: 100-200 ng/mL (serum, RIA)
- BMT: 100-250 ng/mL (serum, RIA)
- Heart: 100-200 ng/mL (serum, RIA)
- Liver: 100-400 ng/mL (blood, HPLC)

Method-dependent (optimum cyclosporine trough concentrations):
- Serum, RIA: 150-300 ng/mL; 50-150 ng/mL (late post-transplant period)
- Whole blood, RIA: 250-800 ng/mL; 150-450 ng/mL (late post-transplant period)
- Whole blood, HPLC: 100-500 ng/mL

C_2 (cyclosporine concentration 2 hours after dose):
- Blood, Fluorescence Polarization Immunoassay (FPIA): 1000-1500 ng/mL (in first 6 months after transplantation)
- Blood, FPIA: 800-900 ng/mL (in second 6 months after transplantation)

Test Interactions Specific whole blood assay for cyclosporine may be falsely elevated if sample is drawn from the same central venous line through which dose was administered (even if flush has been administered and/or dose was given hours before); cyclosporine metabolites cross-react with radioimmunoassay and fluorescence polarization immunoassay

Additional Information Diltiazem has been used to prevent cyclosporine nephrotoxicity, to reduce the frequency of delayed graft function when administered before and after surgery, and to treat the mild hypertension that occurs in most patients after transplantation; diltiazem increases cyclosporine blood concentration by delaying its clearance, resulting in decreased dosage requirements for cyclosporine.

Dosage Forms Considerations

Cyclosporine (modified): Gengraf and Neoral

Cyclosporine (non-modified): SandIMMUNE

Dosage Forms Excipient information presented when available (limited, particularly for generics); consult specific product labeling.

Capsule, Oral:
- Gengraf: 25 mg, 100 mg [contains cremophor el, fd&c blue #2 (indigotine)]
- Neoral: 25 mg, 100 mg [contains alcohol, usp]
- SandIMMUNE: 25 mg [contains alcohol, usp]
- SandIMMUNE: 100 mg
- Generic: 25 mg, 50 mg, 100 mg

Solution, Intravenous:
- SandIMMUNE: 50 mg/mL (5 mL) [contains alcohol, usp, cremophor el]
- Generic: 50 mg/mL (5 mL)

Solution, Oral:
- Gengraf: 100 mg/mL (50 mL) [contains propylene glycol]
- Neoral: 100 mg/mL (50 mL) [contains alcohol, usp]
- SandIMMUNE: 100 mg/mL (50 mL) [contains alcohol, usp]
- Generic: 100 mg/mL (50 mL)

CycloSPORINE (Ophthalmic)

(SYE kloe spor een)

Medication Safety Issues

Sound-alike/look-alike issues:

CycloSPORINE may be confused with cyclophosphamide, Cyklokapron®, cycloSERINE

High alert medication:

This medication is in a class the Institute for Safe Medication Practices (ISMP) includes among its list of drug classes that have a heightened risk of causing significant patient harm when used in error.

Related Information

Safe Handling of Hazardous Drugs *on page 2455*

Brand Names: US Restasis

Brand Names: Canada Restasis®

Therapeutic Category Immunosuppressant Agent

Generic Availability (US) No

Use Increase tear production in patients with moderate to severe keratoconjunctivitis sicca-associated ocular inflammation (FDA approved in ages ≥16 years and adults); has also been used for the treatment and prevention of vernal keratoconjunctivitis

Pregnancy Risk Factor C

Pregnancy Considerations Adverse events were not observed following the use of oral cyclosporine in animal reproduction studies when using doses that were approximately 300,000 times greater than a human ophthalmic dose (assuming complete absorption).

Breast-Feeding Considerations Cyclosporine is found in breast milk following oral administration. Serum concentrations are below the limit of detection (<0.1 ng/mL) following ophthalmic use.

Contraindications Hypersensitivity to cyclosporine or any component of the formulation.

Warnings/Precautions Hazardous agent - use appropriate precautions for handling and disposal (NIOSH 2014 [group 2]).

To avoid contamination, do not touch vial tip to eyelids or other surfaces. Remove contacts prior to administration and wait 15 minutes before reinserting.

Some dosage forms may contain polysorbate 80 (also known as Tweens). Hypersensitivity reactions, usually a delayed reaction, have been reported following exposure to pharmaceutical products containing polysorbate 80 in certain individuals (Isaksson, 2002; Lucente 2000; Shelley, 1995). Thrombocytopenia, ascites, pulmonary deterioration, and renal and hepatic failure have been reported in premature neonates after receiving parenteral products containing polysorbate 80 (Alade, 1986; CDC, 1984). See manufacturer's labeling.

Adverse Reactions Ocular: Blurred vision, burning, conjunctival hyperemia, discharge, epiphora, eye pain, foreign body sensation, pruritus, stinging, visual disturbance

Drug Interactions

Metabolism/Transport Effects None known.

Avoid Concomitant Use There are no known interactions where it is recommended to avoid concomitant use.

Increased Effect/Toxicity There are no known significant interactions involving an increase in effect.

Decreased Effect There are no known significant interactions involving a decrease in effect.

Storage/Stability Store at 15°C to 25°C (59°F to 77°F). Vials are single-use; discard immediately following administration.

Pharmacokinetics (Adult data unless noted) Absorption: Ophthalmic: Serum concentrations were below the quantitation limit of 0.1 ng/mL

Dosing: Usual

Pediatric:

Keratoconjunctivitis sicca: Adolescents ≥16 years: Ophthalmic: Instill 1 drop in each eye every 12 hours

Vernal keratoconjunctivitis (VKC), severe: Limited data available:

Treatment: Children and Adolescents 5 to 14 years: Ophthalmic: Instill 1 drop (0.05%) in affected eye(s) 4 times daily. Dosing based on experience from a prospective trial of 54 pediatric patients (mean age: 9.6 years; range: 5 to 14 years); after 3 months of therapy, improved symptoms were observed, no adverse effects were reported (Keklikci, 2008). A case series in six patients (6 to 14 years) treated with 1 drop twice daily or 4 times daily was also shown to improve symptoms; in four patients cyclosporine was weaned after 6 months (n=1) or 12 months (n=3) of therapy; in three other patients, therapy was still ongoing at the time of publication (Ozcan, 2007). Higher concentrations of cyclosporine have also shown efficacy in clinical trials (1% and 2%); however, those formulations have a different vehicle and are not commercially available in the U.S. (Vichyanond, 2013).

Prevention: Children ≥6 years and Adolescents: Ophthalmic: Instill 1 drop (0.05%) in affected eye(s) twice daily; dosing based on a blinded, comparative (ketotifen) crossover trial in 34 pediatric patients (mean age: 14 ± 7 years) with severe but stable VKC; over a 2-year period, cyclosporine showed a statistically significant reduction in number of recurrences or flare-up compared to ketotifen; both drugs were considered to be well-tolerated (Lambiase, 2011)

Adult: **Keratoconjunctivitis sicca:** Ophthalmic: Instill 1 drop in each eye every 12 hours

Dosing adjustment in renal impairment: There are no dosage adjustments provided in the manufacturer's labeling; however, dosage adjustment unlikely necessary due to low systemic absorption.

Dosing adjustment in hepatic impairment: There are no dosage adjustments provided in the manufacturer's labeling; however, dosage adjustment unlikely necessary due to low systemic absorption.

Administration Hazardous agent; use appropriate precautions for handling and disposal (NIOSH 2014 [group 2]). Invert vial several times prior to use to obtain a uniform emulsion. Avoid contact of vial tip with skin or eye; remove contact lenses prior to administration; lenses may be inserted 15 minutes after instillation. May be used with artificial tears; separate administration by at least 15 minutes.

Dosage Forms Excipient information presented when available (limited, particularly for generics); consult specific product labeling.

Emulsion, Ophthalmic [preservative free]:

Restasis: 0.05% (1 ea) [contains polysorbate 80]

◆ **Cyklokapron** *see* Tranexamic Acid *on page 2100*

Cyproheptadine (si proe HEP ta deen)

Medication Safety Issues

Sound-alike/look-alike issues:

Cyproheptadine may be confused with cyclobenzaprine

Periactin may be confused with Percodan®, Persantine®

BEERS Criteria medication:

This drug may be potentially inappropriate for use in geriatric patients (Quality of evidence - moderate; Strength of recommendation - strong).

International issues:

Periactin brand name for cyproheptadine [U.S., multiple international markets] may be confused with Perative brand name for an enteral nutrition preparation [multiple international markets] and brand name for ketoconazole [Argentina]

Related Information

Serotonin Syndrome *on page 2447*

Brand Names: Canada Euro-Cyproheptadine; PMS-Cyproheptadine

Therapeutic Category Antihistamine

Generic Availability (US) Yes

Use Perennial and seasonal allergic rhinitis and other allergic symptoms including cold urticaria (FDA approved in ages ≥2 years and adults); has also been used to promote weight gain by appetite stimulation in various disease states (eg, cystic fibrosis, cancer-related cachexia); migraine prophylaxis; prevention of episodes of cyclic vomiting; management of dyspeptic symptoms; treatment of spasticity associated with spinal cord damage; and management of serotonin syndrome (eg, following acute SSRI ingestions)

Pregnancy Risk Factor B

Pregnancy Considerations Adverse events have been observed in some animal reproduction studies. Maternal antihistamine use has generally not resulted in an increased risk of birth defects; however, information specific to cyproheptadine is limited. Antihistamines are recommended for the treatment of rhinitis, urticaria, and pruritus with rash in pregnant women (although second generation antihistamines may be preferred). Antihistamines are not recommended for treatment of pruritus associated with intrahepatic cholestasis in pregnancy.

Breast-Feeding Considerations It is not known if cyproheptadine is excreted into breast milk. Premature infants and newborns have a higher risk of intolerance to antihistamines. Use while breast-feeding is contraindicated by the manufacturer. Antihistamines may decrease maternal serum prolactin concentrations when administered prior to the establishment of nursing.

Contraindications Hypersensitivity to cyproheptadine or any component of the formulation; narrow-angle glaucoma; bladder neck obstruction; pyloroduodenal obstruction; symptomatic prostatic hyperplasia; stenosing peptic ulcer; concurrent use of MAO inhibitors; use in debilitated elderly patients; use in premature and term newborns due to potential association with SIDS; breast-feeding

Warnings/Precautions May cause CNS depression, which may impair physical or mental abilities; patients must be cautioned about performing tasks which require mental alertness (eg, operating machinery or driving). Effects may be potentiated when used with other sedative drugs or ethanol. Use with caution in patients with cardiovascular disease; increased intraocular pressure; respiratory disease; or thyroid dysfunction. In the elderly, avoid use of this potent anticholinergic agent due to increased risk of confusion, dry mouth, constipation, and other anticholinergic effects; clearance decreases in patients of advanced age (Beers Criteria). Antihistamines may cause excitation in young children.

Warnings: Additional Pediatric Considerations Excessive dosages of antihistamine in infants and young children may cause hallucinations, CNS depression, seizures, and death. Use with caution and use the lowest effective dose in children ≥2 years of age and avoid concomitant use with other medications having respiratory depressant effects.

Adverse Reactions

Cardiovascular: Extrasystoles, hypotension, palpitations, tachycardia

Central nervous system: Ataxia, chills, confusion, dizziness, drowsiness, euphoria, excitement, fatigue, hallucination, headache, hysteria, insomnia, irritability, nervousness, neuritis, paresthesia, restlessness, sedation, seizure, vertigo

Dermatologic: Diaphoresis, skin photosensitivity, skin rash, urticaria

Gastrointestinal: Abdominal pain, anorexia, cholestasis, constipation, diarrhea, increased appetite, nausea, vomiting, xerostomia

Genitourinary: Difficulty in micturition, urinary frequency, urinary retention

Hematologic & oncologic: Agranulocytosis, hemolytic anemia, leukopenia, thrombocytopenia

Hepatic: Hepatic failure, hepatitis, jaundice

Hypersensitivity: Anaphylactic shock, angioedema, hypersensitivity reaction

Neuromuscular & skeletal: Tremor

Ophthalmic: Blurred vision, diplopia

Otic: Labyrinthitis (acute), tinnitus

Respiratory: Nasal congestion, pharyngitis, thickening of bronchial secretions

Drug Interactions

Metabolism/Transport Effects None known.

Avoid Concomitant Use

Avoid concomitant use of Cyproheptadine with any of the following: Aclidinium; Azelastine (Nasal); Eluxadoline; Glucagon; Ipratropium (Oral Inhalation); MAO Inhibitors; Orphenadrine; Paraldehyde; Potassium Chloride; Thalidomide; Tiotropium; Umeclidinium

Increased Effect/Toxicity

Cyproheptadine may increase the levels/effects of: AbobotulinumtoxinA; Alcohol (Ethyl); Analgesics (Opioid); Anticholinergic Agents; Azelastine (Nasal); Buprenorphine; CNS Depressants; Eluxadoline; Glucagon; Hydrocodone; Methotrimeprazine; Metyrosine; Mirabegron; Mirtazapine; OnabotulinumtoxinA; Orphenadrine; Paraldehyde; Potassium Chloride; Pramipexole; RimabotulinumtoxinB; ROPINIRole; Rotigotine; Suvorexant; Thalidomide; Thiazide Diuretics; Tiotropium; Topiramate; Zolpidem

The levels/effects of Cyproheptadine may be increased by: Aclidinium; Brimonidine (Topical); Cannabis; Doxylamine; Dronabinol; Droperidol; HydrOXYzine; Ipratropium (Oral Inhalation); Kava Kava; Magnesium Sulfate; MAO Inhibitors; Methotrimeprazine; Mianserin; Nabilone; Perampanel; Pramlintide; Rufinamide; Sodium Oxybate; Tapentadol; Tetrahydrocannabinol; Umeclidinium

Decreased Effect

Cyproheptadine may decrease the levels/effects of: Acetylcholinesterase Inhibitors; Benzylpenicilloyl Polylysine; Betahistine; Hyaluronidase; Itopride; MAO Inhibitors; Metoclopramide; Secretin; Selective Serotonin Reuptake Inhibitors

The levels/effects of Cyproheptadine may be decreased by: Acetylcholinesterase Inhibitors; Amphetamines

Storage/Stability

Oral solution: Store at 15°C to 30°C (59°F to 86°F); protect from light.

Oral syrup: Store at 20°C to 25°C (68°F to 77°F); excursions permitted to 15°C to 30°C (59°F to 86°F); protect from light.

Oral tablets: Store at 20°C to 25°C (68°F to 77°F).

Mechanism of Action A potent antihistamine and serotonin antagonist, competes with histamine for H_1-receptor sites on effector cells in the gastrointestinal tract, blood vessels, and respiratory tract

Pharmacokinetics (Adult data unless noted)

Absorption: Well absorbed

Metabolism: Primarily by hepatic glucuronidation via UGT1A (Walker, 1996)

Half-life: 1-4 hours; metabolites: ~16 hours (Paton, 1985)

Time to peak serum concentration: 6-9 hours (Paton, 1985)

Elimination: Urine (~40% primarily as metabolites); feces (2% to 20%, <6% as unchanged drug)

Dosing: Usual

Pediatric:

Allergic conditions: Oral:

Weight-directed or BSA-directed dosing: Children ≥2 years and Adolescents: 0.25 mg/kg/day or 8 mg/m²/day in 2 to 3 divided doses

Fixed-dosing:

2 to 6 years: 2 mg every 8 to 12 hours; maximum daily dose: 12 mg/**day**

7 to 14 years: 4 mg every 8 to 12 hours; maximum daily dose: 16 mg/**day**

≥15 years: Initial: 4 mg every 8 hours; titrate to effect; usual range: 12 to 16 mg/day although some patients may require up to 32 mg; maximum daily dose: 0.5 mg/kg/**day**

Appetite stimulation: Limited data available; dosing regimens variable; Oral:

Weight-directed dosing: Children ≥2 years and Adolescents: 0.25 mg/kg/day divided twice daily; age-dependent maximum daily dose: ≤6 years: 12 mg/**day**; 7 to 14 years: 16 mg/**day**; ≥15 years: 32 mg/**day**. Dosing based on an open-label trial of 66 pediatric cancer patients (median age: 11.7 years; range: 3 to 19 years) which reported 76% response rate (either weight gained or stabilized); mean weight gain: 2.6 kg (range: -0.1 to 10 kg); in a subset analysis, patients >9 years showed a greater response than younger patients as did patients with hematologic malignancies (Couluris 2008).

Fixed dosing: Children ≥5 years and Adolescents: Initial: 2 mg every 6 hours (4 times daily) for 1 week; if tolerated, increase dose to 4 mg every 6 hours; dosing based on a short-term (12-week) double-blind, placebo-controlled trial (n=8 treatment group) and a long-term (1-year) open-label trial (n=12) in cystic fibrosis patients; results showed significant increases in weight gain (3.4 kg vs 1.1 kg in placebo); long-term results showed a generally sustained effect (eg, no further weight loss or some additional weight gain) over study duration (Homnick 2004; Homnick 2005).

Cyclic vomiting syndrome; prevention: Limited data available: Oral: Children 2 to 5 years: 0.25 to 0.5 mg/kg/day in divided doses 2 to 3 times daily; maximum daily dose: 12 mg/**day**; some clinicians have used once daily dose at bedtime to prevent day time sedation (Andersen 1997; Li 2008)

Dyspeptic syndrome; refractory: Limited data available: Oral: Infants ≥9 months and Children <12 years: Reported range: 0.04 to 0.6 mg/kg/day in divided doses 2 to 3 times daily; median effective dose: 0.22 mg/kg/day; dosing based on a retrospective, open-label trial of 80 pediatric patients (median age: 9.8 years; range: 9 months to 20 years) with dyspeptic symptoms (eg, nausea, early satiety, abdominal pain, retching after fundoplication and vomiting) which failed to respond to conventional therapy (eg, diet changes, H_2-blockers, proton pump inhibitors); observed response rate was 55%; a higher response rate (86%) was seen with retching post-Nissen fundoplication (Rodriguez 2013).

Migraine; prophylaxis: Limited data available: Oral: Children ≥3 years and Adolescents: 0.2 to 0.4 mg/kg/day divided twice daily; reported daily dose range: 2 to 8 mg/**day**; maximum daily dose: 0.5 mg/kg/**day**; experience suggests younger patients more tolerant of common cyproheptadine side effects (ie, sedation and increased appetite) (Lewis 2004; Lewis 2004a)

Spasticity associated with spinal cord damage: Limited data available; efficacy results variable: Oral: Children ≥12 years and Adolescents: 4 mg at bedtime; increase by a 4 mg dose every 3 to 4 days; mean daily dose: 16 mg/day in divided doses; maximum daily dose: 36 mg/**day** (Gracie 1997). In the most rigorous evaluation, a double-blind, placebo-controlled, crossover trial of 16 hemiplegic pediatric patients (age range: 4 to 18 years), cyproheptadine (relatively low dose: 1 to 2 mg/day) had no statistical evidence of an effect on gait nor improvement in spasticity parameters (Khodadadeh 1998)

Adult: **Allergic conditions:** Oral: 4 to 20 mg/day divided every 8 hours (not to exceed 0.5 mg/kg/day); some patients may require up to 32 mg/day for adequate control of symptoms

Dosing adjustment in renal impairment: There are no dosage adjustments provided in manufacturer's labeling; however, elimination is diminished in renal insufficiency.

Dosing adjustment in hepatic impairment: There are no dosage adjustments provided in manufacturer's labeling

Administration Oral: Usually administered in 2-4 divided doses (eg, every 6-12 hours); for some uses (eg, cyclic vomiting syndrome), once daily administration at bedtime has been used for some indications to improve tolerability of sedative effects.

Test Interactions Diagnostic antigen skin test results may be suppressed; false positive serum TCA screen

Dosage Forms Excipient information presented when available (limited, particularly for generics); consult specific product labeling.

Syrup, Oral, as hydrochloride:

Generic: 2 mg/5 mL (10 mL, 473 mL)

Tablet, Oral, as hydrochloride:

Generic: 4 mg

◆ **Cyproheptadine Hydrochloride** *see* Cyproheptadine *on page 562*

◆ **Cystadane** *see* Betaine *on page 277*

◆ **Cystagon** *see* Cysteamine (Systemic) *on page 564*

Cysteamine (Systemic) (sis TEE a meen)

Brand Names: US Cystagon; Procysbi

Therapeutic Category Anticystine Agent; Urinary Tract Product

Generic Availability (US) No

Use Management of nephropathic cystinosis

Pregnancy Risk Factor C

Pregnancy Considerations Use only when the potential benefits outweigh the potential hazards to the fetus; in animal studies, cysteamine is teratogenic and fetotoxic. There are no adequate and well-controlled studies in pregnant women.

Breast-Feeding Considerations It is unknown whether cysteamine is excreted in breast milk. Discontinue nursing or discontinue drug during lactation.

Contraindications Hypersensitivity to cysteamine, penicillamine, or any component of the formulation

Warnings/Precautions Initiate therapy as soon as the diagnosis of nephropathic cystinosis has been confirmed. Osteopenia, compression fractures, scoliosis, and genu valgum, accompanied by leg pain and joint hyperextension, have occurred with high doses of the immediate release formulation. Interruption of therapy and subsequent dosage reduction may be required. Depression, lethargy, seizures, somnolence, and encephalopathy have been reported in patients receiving the immediate release formulation; may also occur due to cystinosis not treated with cysteamine. Treatment interruption or dosage reduction may be required in patients with severe or persistent symptoms. Patients should use caution when driving or operating heavy machinery until the effects are known. Skin lesions (eg, molluscoid pseudotumors, skin striae) and skin rashes (including severe rashes such as erythema multiforme bullosa and toxic epidermal necrolysis) have occurred in patients receiving the immediate release formulation. In patients who develop a mild-to-moderate transient rash or skin lesions, interrupt therapy and restart at a lower dose; titrate slowly to therapeutic dose. In patients who develop severe skin rashes, permanently discontinue therapy. Gastrointestinal ulcers and bleeding, nausea, vomiting, anorexia, and abdominal pain have been reported in patients receiving the immediate release formulation. GI symptoms are most commonly seen during the initiation of therapy. If severe symptoms occur, consider a dosage reduction. May cause reversible leukopenia and elevated alkaline phosphatase levels. Intracranial hypertension (pseudotumor cerebri) and/or papilledema have been reported in patients receiving the immediate release formulation; monitor for signs and symptoms of pseudotumor cerebri (eg, headache, tinnitus, dizziness, nausea, diplopia, blurred vision, loss of vision, pain behind the eye or with eye movement). May be managed with diuretics.

Adverse Reactions

Cardiovascular: Hypertension

Central nervous system: Abnormal thinking, ataxia, confusion, depression, dizziness, emotional lability, encephalopathy, fever, hallucinations, headache, impaired cognition, jitteriness, lethargy, nervousness, nightmares, seizure, somnolence

Dermatologic: Rash, urticaria

Endocrine & metabolic: Dehydration

Gastrointestinal: Abdominal pain, constipation, duodenal ulceration, duodenitis, dyspepsia, gastroenteritis, gastrointestinal bleeding, gastrointestinal ulcers, halitosis, nausea

Hematologic: Anemia, leukopenia

Hepatic: Abnormal LFTs

Neuromuscular & skeletal: Hyperkinesia, tremor

Otic: Hearing decreased

Rare but important or life-threatening: Compression fracture, genu valgum, hyperthermia, interstitial nephritis, intracranial hypertension (benign), joint hyperextension, leg pain, molluscoid pseudotumor, osteopenia, papilledema, pseudotumor cerebri, renal failure, scoliosis, skin fragility, skin lesion, skin striae

Drug Interactions

Metabolism/Transport Effects None known.

Avoid Concomitant Use There are no known interactions where it is recommended to avoid concomitant use.

Increased Effect/Toxicity There are no known significant interactions involving an increase in effect.

Decreased Effect There are no known significant interactions involving a decrease in effect.

Food Interactions Concurrent ingestion of food and the delayed release formulation of cysteamine can reduce the systemic exposure of cysteamine. Management: Administer ≥30 minutes before and ≥2 hours after meals; if necessary, patients may eat only a small amount (~4 ounces or 1/2 cup) of food between 1 hour before and 1 hour after administration.

Storage/Stability Store at 20°C to 25°C (68°F to 77°F); excursions permitted to 15°C to 30°C (59°F to 86°F). Protect from light and moisture.

Mechanism of Action Reacts with cystine within the lysosome to convert it to cysteine and to a cysteine-cysteamine mixed disulfide, both of which can then exit the lysosome in patients with cystinosis, an inherited defect of lysosomal transport

Pharmacodynamics
Peak effect: 1.8 hours
Duration: 6 hours

Pharmacokinetics (Adult data unless noted)
Absorption: Rapid
Distribution: V_d: Children: 156 L
Protein binding: Mean: 52%
Half-life: 1 hour
Time to peak serum concentration: 1.4 hours
Elimination: Clearance: Children: 1.2 L/minute

Dosing: Usual Dose-related side effects resulting in withdrawal from research studies occurred more frequently in those patients receiving 1.95 g/m^2/day as compared to 1.3 g/m^2/day; start at the lowest dose and titrate gradually to prevent intolerance.

Oral: Initiate therapy with $^1/_4$ to $^1/_6$ of maintenance dose and titrate slowly over 4-6 weeks:

Children <12 years: Initial: 1.3 g/m^2/day in 4 divided doses; may increase gradually to a maximum of 1.95 g/m^2/day

Children ≥12 years (>110 lbs) and Adults (>110 lbs): 2 g/day in 4 divided doses; dosage may be increased gradually to 1.95 g/m^2/day

Approximate Cysteamine Initial Dose

(to achieve ~1.3 g/m^2/day)

Weight (lbs)	Dose (mg every 6 h)
≤10	100
11-20	150
21-30	200
31-40	250
41-50	300
51-70	350
71-90	400
91-110	450
>110	500

Administration Oral: Contents of capsule may be sprinkled over food; if a dose is missed, take it as soon as possible then return to normal dosing schedule; if identified within 2 hours of next scheduled dose, skip dose; do **not** double the next dose

Monitoring Parameters Blood counts and liver enzymes during therapy; blood pressure; monitor leukocyte cystine measurements to determine adequate dosage and compliance (measure 5-6 hours after administration); monitor skin and bone

Reference Range Leukocyte cystine level goal (measured 5-6 hours after cysteamine dose): <1 nmol of half-cystine/mg protein (some measurable benefits have been seen with levels <2); routine measurements are recommended every 3 months

Dosage Forms Excipient information presented when available (limited, particularly for generics); consult specific product labeling.
Capsule, Oral:
Cystagon: 50 mg, 150 mg
Capsule Delayed Release, Oral:
Procysbi: 25 mg, 75 mg

◆ **Cysteamine Bitartrate** *see* Cysteamine (Systemic) *on page 564*

◆ **Cystech [OTC]** *see* Cysteine *on page 565*

Cysteine (SIS te een)

Brand Names: US Cystech [OTC]

Therapeutic Category Nutritional Supplement

Generic Availability (US) May be product dependent

Use Supplement to crystalline amino acid solutions, in particular the specialized pediatric formulas (eg, Aminosyn® PF, TrophAmine®) to meet the intravenous amino acid nutritional requirements of infants receiving parenteral nutrition (PN)

Pregnancy Considerations Cysteine is generally considered to be a nonessential amino acid in adults because it can be synthesized from methionine (an essential amino acid). The RDA for methionine + cysteine is increased in pregnant women (IOM, 2005).

Breast-Feeding Considerations Cysteine is found in breast milk. The RDA for methionine + cysteine is increased in breast-feeding women (IOM, 2005).

Contraindications Patients with hepatic coma or metabolic disorders involving impaired nitrogen utilization

Warnings/Precautions Metabolic acidosis has occurred in infants related to the "hydrochloride" component of cysteine; each 1 mmol cysteine (175 mg) delivers 1 mEq chloride and 1 mEq hydrogen ion; to balance the extra hydrochloride ions and prevent acidosis addition to the PN solution of a 1 mEq acetate electrolyte salt for each mmol (175 mg) of cysteine may be needed; each 40 mg cysteine (equal to every 1 g amino acid when used in the recommended ratio) adds 0.228 mEq chloride and hydrogen.

Use with caution in patients with diabetes or with risk factors for glucose intolerance; patients with hepatic or renal impairment; or sensitive to volume overload (patients with cardiac insufficiency, pulmonary disease, renal impairment). Patients with hepatic impairment have experienced hyperammonemia, metabolic alkalosis, prerenal azotemia, serum amino acid imbalances, stupor, and coma. Peripheral IV infusion of amino acids in patients with impaired renal or hepatic function could result in an increase in BUN. A slight rise in BUN is to be expected during increased protein intake.

The parenteral product may contain aluminum; toxic aluminum concentrations may be seen with high doses, prolonged use, or renal dysfunction. Premature neonates are at higher risk due to immature renal function and aluminum intake from other parenteral sources. Parenteral aluminum exposure of >4 to 5 mcg/kg/day is associated with CNS and bone toxicity; tissue loading may occur at lower doses (Federal Register, 2002). See manufacturer's labeling.

Use acetate-containing solutions with caution in patients with respiratory or metabolic alkalosis; use potassium-containing solutions with caution in patients with renal impairment, hyperkalemia, or in conditions which potassium retention is present; use sodium-containing solutions with caution in patients with renal impairment, congestive heart failure, and conditions in which edema exists with sodium retention. Concomitant administration with amino acids may reduce the amino acid nitrogen sparing effect.

Adverse Reactions
Cardiovascular: Flushing
Central nervous system: Fever
Endocrine & metabolic: Metabolic acidosis
Gastrointestinal: Nausea
Local: Erythema, phlebitis, thrombosis, warm sensation

Renal: Azotemia, BUN increased

Storage/Stability Store at controlled room temperature 20°C to 25°C (68°F to 77°F); excursions permitted to 15°C to 30°C (59°F to 86°F). Avoid excessive heat; do not freeze. When combined with parenteral amino acid solutions, cysteine is relatively unstable. It is intended to be added immediately prior to administration to the patient. Infusion of the admixture should begin within 1 hour of mixing or may be refrigerated and used within 24 hours. Opened vials must be used within 4 hours of entry.

Mechanism of Action Cysteine is a sulfur-containing amino acid synthesized from methionine via the transsulfuration pathway. It is a precursor of the tripeptide glutathione and also of taurine. Newborn infants have a relative deficiency of the enzyme necessary to affect this conversion. Cysteine may be considered an essential amino acid in infants.

Dosing: Neonatal IV: Added as a fixed ratio to crystalline amino acid solution: 40 mg cysteine per g of amino acids; dosage will vary with the daily amino acid dosage (eg, 0.5-2.5 g/kg/day amino acids would result in 20-100 mg/kg/day cysteine); individual doses of cysteine of 0.8-1 mmol/kg/day have also been added directly to the daily PN solution; the duration of treatment relates to the need for PN

Dosing: Usual IV: Infants: Added as a fixed ratio to crystalline amino acid solution: 40 mg cysteine per g of amino acids; dosage will vary with the daily amino acid dosage (eg, 0.5-2.5 g/kg/day amino acids would result in 20-100 mg/kg/day cysteine); individual doses of cysteine of 0.8-1 mmol/kg/day have also been added directly to the daily PN solution; the duration of treatment relates to the need for PN; patients on chronic PN therapy have received cysteine until 6 months of age and in some cases until 2 years of age

Preparation for Administration Parenteral: IV infusion: Must be diluted into parenteral nutrition solution; dilute with amino acid solution in a ratio of 40 mg cysteine to 1 g amino acid: eg, 500 mg cysteine is added to 12.5 g (250 mL) of 5% amino acid solution

Administration Parenteral: IV infusion: Component of parenteral nutrition solution: Infuse parenteral nutrition solution at rate as directed

Monitoring Parameters BUN, ammonia, electrolytes, pH, acid-base balance, serum creatinine, liver function tests, growth curve

Additional Information Addition of cysteine to PN solutions enhances the solubility of calcium and phosphate by lowering the overall pH of the solution

Dosage Forms Excipient information presented when available (limited, particularly for generics); consult specific product labeling.

Capsule, Oral, as hydrochloride [preservative free]:
 Cystech: 500 mg [dye free]

Solution, Intravenous, as hydrochloride:
 Generic: 50 mg/mL (10 mL, 50 mL)

◆ **Cysteine Hydrochloride** *see* Cysteine *on page 565*

◆ **CYT** *see* Cyclophosphamide *on page 551*

◆ **Cytarabine** *see* Cytarabine (Conventional) *on page 566*

Cytarabine (Conventional)

(sye TARE a been con VEN sha nal)

Medication Safety Issues

Sound-alike/look-alike issues:

Cytarabine may be confused with clofarabine, Cytosar, Cytoxan, vidarabine

Cytarabine (conventional) may be confused with cytarabine liposomal

Cytosar-U may be confused with cytarabine, Cytovene, Cytoxan, Neosar

High alert medication:

This medication is in a class the Institute for Safe Medication Practices (ISMP) includes among its list of drugs classes which have a heightened risk of causing significant patient harm when used in error.

Administration issues:

Intrathecal medication safety: The American Society of Clinical Oncology (ASCO)/Oncology Nursing Society (ONS) chemotherapy administration safety standards (Jacobson, 2009) encourage the following safety measures for intrathecal chemotherapy:

- Intrathecal medication should not be prepared during the preparation of any other agents
- After preparation, store in an isolated location or container clearly marked with a label identifying as "intrathecal" use only
- Delivery to the patient should only be with other medications also intended for administration into the central nervous system

Related Information

Prevention of Chemotherapy-Induced Nausea and Vomiting in Children *on page 2368*

Safe Handling of Hazardous Drugs *on page 2455*

Brand Names: Canada Cytarabine Injection; Cytosar

Therapeutic Category Antineoplastic Agent, Antimetabolite

Generic Availability (US) Yes

Use

IV: Remission induction in acute myeloid leukemia (AML), treatment of acute lymphocytic leukemia (ALL) and chronic myelocytic leukemia (CML; blast phase) (FDA approved in pediatric patients [age not specified] and adults); has also been used in AML consolidation treatment, AML salvage treatment, and treatment of non-Hodgkin lymphomas (NHL)

Intrathecal: Prophylaxis and treatment of meningeal leukemia (FDA approved in pediatric patients [age not specified] and adults)

Pregnancy Risk Factor D

Pregnancy Considerations Adverse effects were demonstrated in animal reproduction studies. Limb and ear defects have been noted in case reports of cytarabine exposure during the first trimester of pregnancy. The following have also been noted in the neonate: Pancytopenia, WBC depression, electrolyte abnormalities, prematurity, low birth weight, decreased hematocrit or platelets. Risk to the fetus is decreased if treatment can be avoided during the first trimester; however, women of childbearing potential should be advised of the potential risks.

Breast-Feeding Considerations It is not known if cytarabine is excreted in breast milk. Due to the potential for serious adverse reactions in the nursing infant, the decision to discontinue cytarabine or to discontinue breastfeeding should take into account the importance of treatment to the mother.

Contraindications Hypersensitivity to cytarabine or any component of the formulation

Warnings/Precautions Hazardous agent - use appropriate precautions for handling and disposal (NIOSH 2014 [group 1]). **[U.S. Boxed Warning]: Myelosuppression (leukopenia, thrombocytopenia and anemia) is the major toxicity of cytarabine.** Use with caution in patients with prior drug-induced bone marrow suppression. Monitor blood counts frequently; once blasts are no longer apparent in the peripheral blood, bone marrow should be monitored frequently. Monitor for signs of infection or neutropenic fever due to neutropenia or bleeding due to thrombocytopenia. **[U.S. Boxed Warning]: Toxicities (less serious) include nausea, vomiting, diarrhea, abdominal pain, oral ulcerations and hepatic**

dysfunction. In adults, doses >1000 mg/m^2 are associated with a moderate emetic potential (Basch, 2011; Roila, 2010). In pediatrics, doses >200 mg/m^2 are associated with a moderate emetic potential and 3000 mg/m^2 is associated with a high emetic potential (Dupuis, 2011); antiemetics are recommended to prevent nausea and vomiting.

High-dose regimens are associated with CNS, gastrointestinal, ocular (reversible corneal toxicity and hemorrhagic conjunctivitis; prophylaxis with ophthalmic corticosteroid drops is recommended), pulmonary toxicities and cardiomyopathy. Neurotoxicity associated with high-dose treatment may present as acute cerebellar toxicity (with or without cerebral impairment), personality changes, or may be severe with seizure and/or coma; may be delayed, occurring up to 3 to 8 days after treatment has begun. Risk factors for neurotoxicity include cumulative cytarabine dose, prior CNS disease and renal impairment; high-dose therapy (>18 g/m^2 per cycle) and age >50 years also increase the risk for cerebellar toxicity (Herzig, 1987). Tumor lysis syndrome and subsequent hyperuricemia may occur; monitor, consider antihyperuricemic therapy and hydrate accordingly. Potentially significant drug-drug interactions may exist, requiring dose or frequency adjustment, additional monitoring, and/or selection of alternative therapy. There have been case reports of fatal cardiomyopathy when high dose cytarabine was used in combination with cyclophosphamide as a preparation regimen for transplantation.

Use with caution in patients with impaired renal and hepatic function; may be at higher risk for CNS toxicities; dosage adjustments may be necessary. Sudden respiratory distress, rapidly progressing to pulmonary edema and cardiomegaly has been reported with high dose cytarabine. May present as severe dyspnea with a rapid onset and refractory hypoxia with diffuse pulmonary infiltrates, leading to respiratory failure; may be fatal (Morgan, 2011). Cytarabine (ARA-C) syndrome is characterized by fever, myalgia, bone pain, chest pain (occasionally), maculopapular rash, conjunctivitis, and malaise; generally occurs 6 to 12 hours following administration; may be managed with corticosteroids. Anaphylaxis resulting in acute cardiopulmonary arrest has been reported (rare). There have been reports of acute pancreatitis in patients receiving continuous infusion cytarabine and in patients receiving cytarabine who were previously treated with L-asparaginase. **[U.S. Boxed Warning]: Should be administered under the supervision of an experienced cancer chemotherapy physician. Due to the potential toxicities, induction treatment with cytarabine should be in a facility with sufficient laboratory and supportive resources.** Some products may contain benzyl alcohol; do not use products containing benzyl alcohol or products reconstituted with bacteriostatic diluent intrathecally or for high-dose cytarabine regimens. Benzyl alcohol is associated with gasping syndrome in premature infants. Delayed progressive ascending paralysis has been reported in two children who received combination chemotherapy with IV and intrathecal cytarabine at conventional doses for the treatment of acute myeloid leukemia (was fatal in one patient). When used for intrathecal administration, should not be prepared during the preparation of any other agents; after preparation, store intrathecal medications in an isolated location or container clearly marked with a label identifying as "intrathecal" use only; delivery of intrathecal medications to the patient should only be with other medications also intended for administration into the central nervous system (Jacobson, 2009).

Adverse Reactions

Cardiovascular: Chest pain, pericarditis

Central nervous system: Dizziness, fever, headache, neural toxicity, neuritis

Dermatologic: Alopecia, pruritus, rash, skin freckling, skin ulceration, urticaria

Gastrointestinal: Abdominal pain, anal inflammation, anal ulceration, anorexia, bowel necrosis, diarrhea, esophageal ulceration, esophagitis, mucositis, nausea, pancreatitis, sore throat, vomiting

Genitourinary: Urinary retention

Hematologic: Myelosuppression, neutropenia (onset: 1 to 7 days; nadir [biphasic]: 7 to 9 days and at 15 to 24 days; recovery [biphasic]: 9 to 12 and at 24 to 34 days), thrombocytopenia (onset: 5 days; nadir: 12 to 15 days; recovery 15 to 25 days), anemia, bleeding, leukopenia, megaloblastosis, reticulocytes decreased

Hepatic: Hepatic dysfunction, jaundice, transaminases increased (acute)

Local: Injection site cellulitis, thrombophlebitis

Ocular: Conjunctivitis

Renal: Renal dysfunction

Respiratory: Dyspnea

Miscellaneous: Allergic edema, anaphylaxis, sepsis

Rare but important or life-threatening: Acute respiratory distress syndrome, amylase increased, angina, aseptic meningitis, cardiopulmonary arrest (acute), cerebral dysfunction, cytarabine syndrome (bone pain, chest pain, conjunctivitis, fever, maculopapular rash, malaise, myalgia); exanthematous pustulosis, hepatic sinusoidal obstruction syndrome (SOS; veno-occlussive disease), hyperuricemia, injection site inflammation (SubQ injection), injection site pain (SubQ injection), interstitial pneumonitis, lipase increased, paralysis (intrathecal and I.V. combination therapy), reversible posterior leukoencephalopathy syndrome (RPLS), rhabdomyolysis, toxic megacolon

Adverse events associated with high-dose cytarabine (CNS, gastrointestinal, ocular, and pulmonary toxicities are more common with high-dose regimens):

Cardiovascular: Cardiomegaly, cardiomyopathy (in combination with cyclophosphamide)

Central nervous system: Cerebellar toxicity, coma, neurotoxicity, personality change, somnolence

Dermatologic: Alopecia (complete), desquamation, rash (severe)

Gastrointestinal: Gastrointestinal ulcer, pancreatitis, peritonitis, pneumatosis cystoides intestinalis

Hepatic: Hyperbilirubinemia, liver abscess, liver damage, necrotizing colitis

Neuromuscular & skeletal: Peripheral neuropathy (motor and sensory)

Ocular: Corneal toxicity, hemorrhagic conjunctivitis

Respiratory: Pulmonary edema, syndrome of sudden respiratory distress

Miscellaneous: Sepsis

Adverse events associated with intrathecal cytarabine administration:

Central nervous system: Accessory nerve paralysis, fever, necrotizing leukoencephalopathy (with concurrent cranial irradiation, intrathecal methotrexate, and intrathecal hydrocortisone), neurotoxicity, paraplegia

Gastrointestinal: Dysphagia, nausea, vomiting

Ocular: Blindness (with concurrent systemic chemotherapy and cranial irradiation), diplopia

Respiratory: Cough, hoarseness

Miscellaneous: Aphonia

Drug Interactions

Metabolism/Transport Effects

None known.

Avoid Concomitant Use

Avoid concomitant use of Cytarabine (Conventional) with any of the following: BCG; BCG (Intravesical); CloZAPine; Dipyrone; Natalizumab; Pimecrolimus; Tacrolimus (Topical); Tofacitinib; Vaccines (Live)

Increased Effect/Toxicity

Cytarabine (Conventional) may increase the levels/effects of: CloZAPine; Leflunomide; Natalizumab; Tofacitinib; Vaccines (Live)

The levels/effects of Cytarabine (Conventional) may be increased by: Denosumab; Dipyrone; Pimecrolimus; Roflumilast; Tacrolimus (Topical); Trastuzumab

Decreased Effect

Cytarabine (Conventional) may decrease the levels/effects of: BCG; BCG (Intravesical); Coccidioides immitis Skin Test; Flucytosine; Sipuleucel-T; Vaccines (Inactivated); Vaccines (Live)

The levels/effects of Cytarabine (Conventional) may be decreased by: Echinacea

Storage/Stability Store intact vials of powder for reconstitution at 20°C to 25°C (68°F to 77°F); store intact vials of solution at 15°C to 30°C (59°F to 86°F).

IV:

Powder for reconstitution: Reconstituted solutions should be stored at room temperature and used within 48 hours.

For IV infusion: Solutions for IV infusion diluted in D_5W or NS are stable for 8 days at room temperature, although the manufacturer recommends administration as soon as possible after preparation.

Intrathecal: Administer as soon as possible after preparation. After preparation, store intrathecal medications in an isolated location or container clearly marked with a label identifying as "intrathecal" use only.

Mechanism of Action Inhibits DNA synthesis. Cytarabine gains entry into cells by a carrier process, and then must be converted to its active compound, aracytidine triphosphate. Cytarabine is a pyrimidine analog and is incorporated into DNA; however, the primary action is inhibition of DNA polymerase resulting in decreased DNA synthesis and repair. The degree of cytotoxicity correlates linearly with incorporation into DNA; therefore, incorporation into the DNA is responsible for drug activity and toxicity. Cytarabine is specific for the S phase of the cell cycle (blocks progression from the G_1 to the S phase).

Pharmacokinetics (Adult data unless noted)

Absorption: Not effective when administered orally; less than 20% absorbed orally

Distribution: V_d: 3 ± 11.9 L/kg; distributed widely and rapidly since it enters the cells readily; crosses blood-brain barrier achieving CSF concentrations 40% to 50% of plasma concentration

Protein binding: 13%

Metabolism: Primarily hepatic; metabolized by deoxycytidine kinase and other nucleotide kinases to aracytidine triphosphate (active); about 86% to 96% of dose is metabolized to inactive uracil arabinoside (ARA-U); intrathecal administration results in little conversion to ARA-U due to the low amount of deaminase in the CSF

Half-life, terminal: 1 to 3 hours; intrathecal: 2 to 6 hours

Time to peak serum concentration: SubQ: 20 to 60 minutes

Elimination: Urine (~80%; 90% as metabolite ARA-U) within 24 hours

Dosing: Usual Note: Dosing and frequency may vary by protocol and/or treatment phase; refer to specific protocol.

Pediatric: **Note:** In pediatric patients, IV dosing may be based on either BSA (mg/m^2) or weight (mg/kg); use extra precaution to verify dosing parameters during calculations. Doses >200 mg/m^2 are associated with a moderate emetic potential and 3000 mg/m^2 is associated with a high emetic potential (Dupuis, 2011); antiemetics are recommended to prevent nausea and vomiting.

Acute lymphocytic leukemia (ALL): POG 8602/PVA regimen, intensification phase: Children and Adolescents: IV: 1000 mg/m^2 continuous infusion over 24 hours day 1 (beginning 12 hours after start of methotrexate) every 3 weeks or every 12 weeks for 6 cycles (Land, 1994)

Acute myeloid leukemia (AML):

Remission induction:

Manufacturer's labeling: Infants, Children, and Adolescents: IV: Standard dose: 100 mg/m^2/day continuous infusion for 7 days or 200 mg/m^2/day continuous infusion (as 100 mg/m^2/dose over 12 hours every 12 hours) for 7 days

Alternate dosing: 7 + 3 regimen (Woods, 1990): Limited data available:

Infants and Children <3 years: IV: 3.3 mg/**kg**/day continuous infusion for 7 days; minimum of 2 courses (in combination with daunorubicin)

Children ≥3 years and Adolescents: IV: 100 mg/m^2/day continuous infusion for 7 days; minimum of 2 courses (in combination with daunorubicin)

Consolidation: Limited data available: 5 + 2 + 5 regimen: Adolescents ≥15 years: IV: 100 mg/m^2/day continuous infusion for 5 days for 2 courses (in combination with daunorubicin and etoposide) (Bishop, 1996)

Salvage treatment for refractory/recurrent disease: Limited data available:

Clofarabine/cytarabine regimen: Children and Adolescents: IV: 1000 mg/m^2/day over 2 hours for 5 days (in combination with clofarabine; administer cytarabine 4 hours after initiation of clofarabine) for up to 2 induction cycles (Cooper, 2014)

FLAG regimen: Children ≥11 years and Adolescents: IV: 2000 mg/m^2/day over 4 hours for 5 days (in combination with fludarabine and G-CSF); may repeat once if needed (Montillo, 1998)

MEC regimen:

Children ≥5 years and Adolescents: IV 1000 mg/m^2/day over 6 hours for 6 days (in combination with etoposide and mitoxantrone) (Amadori, 1991)

Adolescents ≥15 years: IV: 500 mg/m^2/day continuous infusion days 1, 2, and 3 and days 8, 9, and 10 (in combination with mitoxantrone and etoposide); may administer a second course if needed (Archimbaud, 1991; Archimbaud, 1995)

Non-Hodgkin lymphomas:

CODOX-M/IVAC regimen: Children ≥3 years and Adolescents: Cycles 2 and 4 (IVAC): IV: 2000 mg/m^2 every 12 hours days 1 and 2 (total of 4 doses/cycle) (in combination with ifosfamide, mesna, and etoposide; alternate with CODOX-M) (Magrath, 1996)

High-dose cytarabine: Children and Adolescents: IV: 3000 mg/m^2 over 3 hours every 12 hours on days 2 and 3 (secondary phase; total of 4 doses) in combination with methotrexate IV and intrathecal methotrexate/cytarabine (Bowman, 1996)

Meningeal leukemia: Infants, Children, and Adolescent: **Note:** Optimal intrathecal chemotherapy dosing should be based on age (see following information) rather than on body surface area (BSA); CSF volume correlates with age and not to BSA (Bleyer, 1983; Kerr, 2001).

Manufacturer's labeling (based on BSA): Intrathecal: 30 mg/m^2 every 4 days; range: 5 to 75 mg/m^2 once daily for 4 days or once every 4 days until CNS findings normalize, followed by one additional treatment

Alternate dosing: Age-based intrathecal dosing: Intrathecal:

CNS prophylaxis (AML) (Woods, 1990):

<1 years: 20 mg per dose

1 to <2 years: 30 mg per dose

2 to <3 years: 50 mg per dose

≥3 years: 70 mg per dose

CNS prophylaxis (ALL): Dosing regimens variable, age-specific regimens reported from literature:

Gaynon, 1993: Administer on day 0 of induction therapy: Children and Adolescents:
<2 years: 30 mg per dose
2 to <3 years: 50 mg per dose
≥3 years: 70 mg per dose

Matloub, 2006: Administer on day 0 of induction therapy, then as part of triple intrathecal therapy (TIT) on days 7, 14, and 21 during consolidation therapy; as part of TIT on days 0, 28, and 35 for 2 cycles of delayed intensification therapy, and then maintenance treatment as part of TIT on day 0 every 12 weeks for 38 months (boys) or 26 months (girls) from initial induction treatment: Children <10 years:
1 to <2 years: 16 mg per dose
2 to <3 years: 20 mg per dose
3 to 8 years: 24 mg per dose
>8 to <10 years: 30 mg per dose

Pieters, 2007: Administer on day 15 of induction therapy, days 1 and 15 of reinduction phase; and day 1 of cycle 2 of maintenance 1A phase: Infants and young Children (≤12 months at enrollment):
<1 year: 15 mg per dose
≥1 years: 20 mg per dose

Lin, 2007: Administer as part of triple intrathecal therapy (TIT) on days 1 and 15 of induction therapy; days 1, 15, 50, and 64 (standard risk patients) or days 1, 15, 29, and 43 (high-risk patients) during consolidation therapy; day 1 of reinduction therapy, and during maintenance therapy (very high risk patients receive on days 1, 22, 45, and 59 of induction, days 8, 22, 36, and 50 of consolidation therapy, days 8 and 38 of reinduction therapy, and during maintenance): Infants, Children, and Adolescents:
<1 year: 18 mg per dose
1 to <2 years: 24 mg per dose
2 to <3 years: 30 mg per dose
>3 years: 36 mg per dose

Treatment, CNS leukemia (ALL), Very high-risk: Administer as part of triple intrathecal therapy (TIT) weekly until CSF remission, then every 4 weeks throughout continuation treatment (Lin, 2007): Infants, Children, and Adolescents:
<1 year: 18 mg per dose
1 to <2 years: 24 mg per dose
2 to <3 years: 30 mg per dose
≥3 years: 36 mg per dose

Adult: **Note:** Doses >1000 mg/m^2 are associated with a moderate emetic potential in adults (Basch, 2011; Roila, 2010); antiemetics are recommended to prevent nausea and vomiting.

Acute myeloid leukemia (AML) remission induction: IV: 100 mg/m^2/day continuous infusion for 7 days or 200 mg/m^2/day continuous infusion (as 100 mg/m^2 over 12 hours every 12 hours) for 7 days

Meningeal leukemia: Intrathecal: 30 mg/m^2 every 4 days; range: 5 to 75 mg/m^2 once daily for 4 days or once every 4 days until CNS findings normalize, followed by 1 additional treatment. **Note:** Optimal intrathecal chemotherapy dosing should be based on age rather than on body surface area (BSA); CSF volume correlates with age and not to BSA (Bleyer, 1983; Kerr, 2001).

Dosing adjustment in renal impairment: IV: There are no dosage adjustments provided in the manufacturer's labeling; however, the following guidelines have been used by some clinicians:

Infants, Children, and Adolescents: Standard dosing range (100 to 200 mg/m^2): No adjustment necessary (Aronoff, 2007)

Adults:

Aronoff, 2007: Standard dosing range of 100 to 200 mg/m^2: No adjustment necessary

Kintzel, 1995: High-dose cytarabine 1000 to 3000 mg/m^2
CrCl 46 to 60 mL/minute: Administer 60% of dose
CrCl 31 to 45 mL/minute: Administer 50% of dose
CrCl <30 mL/minute: Consider use of alternative drug

Smith, 1997: High-dose cytarabine ≥2000 mg/m^2/dose
Serum creatinine 1.5 to 1.9 mg/dL or increase (from baseline) of 0.5 to 1.2 mg/dL: Reduce dose to 1000 mg/m^2/dose
Serum creatinine ≥2 mg/dL or increase (from baseline) of >1.2 mg/dL: Reduce dose to 100 mg/m^2/day as a continuous infusion

Hemodialysis: In 4-hour dialysis sessions (with high flow polysulfone membrane) 6 hours after cytarabine 1000 mg/m^2 over 2 hours, 63% of the metabolite, ARA-U was extracted from plasma (based in a single adult case report) (Radeski, 2011)

Dosing adjustment in hepatic impairment: IV: Dose may need to be adjusted in patients with liver failure since cytarabine is partially detoxified in the liver. There are no dosage adjustments provided in the manufacturer's labeling; however, the following guidelines have been used by some clinicians: All patients:

Floyd, 2006: Transaminases (any elevation): Administer 50% of dose; may increase subsequent doses in the absence of toxicity

Koren, 1992 (dose not specified): Bilirubin >2 mg/dL: Administer 50% of dose; may increase subsequent doses in the absence of toxicity

Preparation for Administration Hazardous agent; use appropriate precautions for handling and disposal (NIOSH 2014 [group 1]). **Note:** Solutions containing bacteriostatic agents may be used for standard dose (100 to 200 mg/m^2) IV cytarabine preparations, but should not be used for the preparation of either intrathecal doses or high-dose IV therapy preparations

IV:

Powder for reconstitution: Reconstitute with bacteriostatic water for injection (for standard dose) or preservative-free for high-dose preparations.

For IV infusion: Further dilute in 250 to 1,000 mL of NS or D_5W.

Intrathecal: Reconstitute with preservative-free NS; may be further diluted to preferred final volume with Elliott's B solution, preservative-free NS or LR solution; do not use diluents containing benzyl alcohol; the final volume is generally based on institution or practitioner preference; volume range is 3 to 10 mL and may be up to 12 mL and should correspond to an equivalent volume of CSF removed. Intrathecal medications should not be prepared during the preparation of any other agents. After preparation, store intrathecal medications in an isolated location or container clearly marked with a label identifying as "intrathecal" use only.

Intrathecal triple therapy (ITT): Cytarabine 30 to 50 mg with hydrocortisone sodium succinate 15 to 25 mg and methotrexate 12 mg are reported to be compatible together in a syringe (Cheung 1984); other dose-specific combinations: [Cytarabine 18 mg with hydrocortisone 12 mg and methotrexate 6 mg, prepared to a final volume of 6 mL], [cytarabine 24 mg with hydrocortisone 16 mg and methotrexate 8 mg, prepared to a final volume of 8 mL], [cytarabine 30 mg with hydrocortisone 20 mg and methotrexate 10 mg, prepared to a final volume of 10 mL], and [cytarabine 36 mg with hydrocortisone 24 mg and methotrexate 12 mg, prepared to a final volume of 12 mL], have been reported compatible as well (Lin 2008).

Administration Hazardous agent; use appropriate precautions for handling and disposal (NIOSH 2014 [group 1]).

Parenteral: **Note:** In pediatric patients, I.V. doses >200 mg/m^2 are associated with a moderate emetic potential and 3,000 mg/m^2 is associated with a high emetic potential (Dupuis 2011); antiemetics are recommended to prevent nausea and vomiting. In adults, doses >1,000 mg/m^2 are associated with a moderate emetic potential (Basch 2011; Roila 2010).

IV infusion: Infuse as a continuous infusion (standard dose: 100 to 200 mg/m^2/day) or infuse high dose treatments over 1 to 3 hours (infusion rate based on protocol).

IVP: May administer over 15 minutes

Intrathecal administration: Antiemetic therapy should be administered prior to intrathecal doses of cytarabine. Administer as soon as possible after preparation.

Monitoring Parameters Liver function tests, CBC with differential and platelet count, serum creatinine, BUN, serum uric acid; signs of neurotoxicity

Dosage Forms Excipient information presented when available (limited, particularly for generics); consult specific product labeling.

Solution, Injection:

Generic: 20 mg/mL (25 mL); 100 mg/mL (20 mL)

Solution, Injection [preservative free]:

Generic: 20 mg/mL (5 mL, 50 mL); 100 mg/mL (20 mL)

Solution Reconstituted, Injection:

Generic: 100 mg (1 ea); 500 mg (1 ea); 1 g (1 ea)

◆ **Cytarabine Hydrochloride** *see* Cytarabine (Conventional) *on page 566*

◆ **Cytarabine Injection (Can)** *see* Cytarabine (Conventional) *on page 566*

◆ **CytoGam®** *see* Cytomegalovirus Immune Globulin (Intravenous-Human) *on page 570*

Cytomegalovirus Immune Globulin (Intravenous-Human)

(sye toe meg a low VYE rus i MYUN GLOB yoo lin in tra VEE nus HYU man)

Medication Safety Issues

Sound-alike/look-alike issues:

CytoGam® may be confused with Cytoxan, Gamimune® N

Related Information

Centers for Disease Control and Prevention (CDC) and Other Links *on page 2424*

Immunization Administration Recommendations *on page 2411*

Immunization Schedules *on page 2416*

Brand Names: US CytoGam®

Brand Names: Canada CytoGam®

Therapeutic Category Immune Globulin

Generic Availability (US) No

Use Prophylaxis of cytomegalovirus (CMV) disease associated with kidney, lung, liver, pancreas, or heart transplantation [FDA approved in pediatric patients (age not specified) and adults]; concomitant use with ganciclovir should be considered in organ transplants other than kidney from CMV seropositive donors to CMV seronegative recipients; has also been used for CMV treatment in hematopoietic stem cell transplantation

Pregnancy Risk Factor C

Pregnancy Considerations Animal reproduction studies have not been conducted.

Contraindications Hypersensitivity to cytomegalovirus immune globulin (CMV-IGIV), other immunoglobulin preparations, or any component of the formulation; selective immunoglobulin A deficiency

Warnings/Precautions Hypersensitivity and anaphylactic reactions can occur; monitor vital signs during infusion; discontinue immediately for hypotension or anaphylaxis; immediate treatment (including epinephrine 1:1000) should be available. Systemic allergic reactions are rare; may be treated with epinephrine and diphenhydramine. Aseptic meningitis syndrome (AMS) has been reported with intravenous immune globulin administration (rare); may occur with high doses (≥2 g/kg). Symptoms include severe headache, nuchal rigidity, drowsiness, fever, photophobia, painful eye movements and nausea and vomiting. Syndrome usually appears within several hours to 2 days following treatment; usually resolves within several days after discontinuation. Intravenous immune globulin has been associated with antiglobulin hemolysis; monitor for signs of hemolytic anemia. Monitor for adverse pulmonary events including transfusion-related acute lung injury (TRALI); noncardiogenic pulmonary edema has been reported with intravenous immune globulin use. TRALI is characterized by severe respiratory distress, pulmonary edema, hypoxemia, and fever in the presence of normal left ventricular function and usually occurs within 1-6 hours after infusion; may be managed with oxygen and respiratory support.

Acute renal dysfunction (increased serum creatinine, oliguria, osmotic nephrosis, acute renal failure) can rarely occur; usually within 7 days of use (more likely with products stabilized with sucrose). Patients at risk for renal failure include the elderly, patients with preexisting renal disease, diabetes mellitus, volume depletion, sepsis, paraproteinemia, and nephrotoxic medications due to risk of renal dysfunction. In patients at risk of renal dysfunction, the rate of infusion and concentration of solution should be minimized. Discontinue if renal function deteriorates. Patients should not be volume depleted prior to therapy. Thrombotic events have been reported with administration of intravenous immune globulin; patients at risk include those with advanced age or a history of atherosclerosis, cardiovascular and/or thrombotic risk factors, or known/suspected hyperviscosity. Consider a baseline assessment of blood viscosity in patients at risk for hyperviscosity. Use with caution in patients >65 years of age. Product is stabilized with albumin. Product of human plasma; may potentially contain infectious agents which could transmit disease. Screening of donors, as well as testing and/or inactivation or removal of certain viruses, reduces the risk. Infections thought to be transmitted by this product should be reported to the manufacturer. Product is stabilized with sucrose.

Adverse Reactions

Cardiovascular: Flushing

Central nervous system: Chills, fever

Gastrointestinal: Nausea, vomiting

Neuromuscular & skeletal: Arthralgia, back pain, muscle cramps

Respiratory: Wheezing

Rare but important or life-threatening: Abdominal pain, acute renal failure, acute respiratory distress syndrome (ARDS), acute tubular necrosis, allergic reactions (systemic), anaphylactic shock, angioneurotic edema, anuria, apnea, aseptic meningitis syndrome (AMS), blood pressure decreased, bronchospasm, bullous dermatitis, BUN increased, cardiac arrest, coma, Coomb's test positive, cyanosis, dyspnea, epidermolysis, erythema multiforme, hemolysis, hypotension, hypoxemia, leukopenia, liver dysfunction, loss of consciousness, oliguria, osmotic nephrosis, pancytopenia, proximal tubular nephropathy, pulmonary edema, renal dysfunction, rigors, seizure, serum creatinine increased, Stevens-Johnson syndrome, thromboembolism, transfusion-related acute lung injury (TRALI), tremor, vascular collapse

Drug Interactions

Metabolism/Transport Effects None known.

Avoid Concomitant Use There are no known interactions where it is recommended to avoid concomitant use.

Increased Effect/Toxicity There are no known significant interactions involving an increase in effect.

Decreased Effect

Cytomegalovirus Immune Globulin (Intravenous-Human) may decrease the levels/effects of: Vaccines (Live)

Storage/Stability Store refrigerated between 2°C and 8°C (36°F and 46°F). Infusion should begin within 6 hours after entering the vial.

Mechanism of Action CMV-IGIV is a preparation of immunoglobulin G (and trace amounts of IgA and IgM) derived from pooled healthy blood donors and contains a high titer of CMV antibodies; administration provides a passive source of antibodies against cytomegalovirus to attenuate or reduce the incidence of serious CMV disease

Pharmacokinetics (Adult data unless noted) Half-life: 8-24 days

Dosing: Usual

Infants, Children, and Adolescents: **Note:** Refer to individual protocols.

Prophylaxis of CMV disease in kidney transplant: Initial: IV: 150 mg/kg within 72 hours of transplant; 100 mg/kg at weeks 2, 4, 6, and 8 after transplant and 50 mg/kg at weeks 12 and 16 after transplant

Prophylaxis of CMV disease in liver, lung, pancreas, or heart transplant (CMV (+) donor and CMV (-) recipient): IV: 150 mg/kg within 72 hours of transplant, 150 mg/kg at weeks 2, 4, 6, and 8 after transplant; 100 mg/kg at weeks 12 and 16 after transplant

Treatment, CMV disease: Limited data available:

Ganciclovir-resistant infection and disease: IV: 100 mg/kg/dose weekly in combination with other antivirals (eg, ganciclovir, foscarnet, cidofovir); duration of therapy dependent upon CMV antigenemia assay (pp65) or PCR (Bueno, 2002)

Pneumonitis, severe: Children and Adolescents: IV: 400 mg/kg on days 1, 2, and 7 followed by 200 mg/kg on days 14; if still symptomatic, may administer an additional 200 mg/kg on day 21; use in combination with ganciclovir (Reed, 1988)

Adults:

Prophylaxis of CMV disease in kidney transplant: IV:

Initial dose (within 72 hours of transplant): 150 mg/kg/dose

2-, 4-, 6-, and 8 weeks after transplant: 100 mg/kg/dose

12 and 16 weeks after transplant: 50 mg/kg/dose

Prophylaxis of CMV disease in liver, lung, pancreas, or heart transplant: IV:

Initial dose (within 72 hours of transplant): 150 mg/kg/dose

2-, 4-, 6-, and 8 weeks after transplant: 150 mg/kg/dose

12 and 16 weeks after transplant: 100 mg/kg/dose

Dosage adjustment in renal impairment: No dosage adjustment provided in manufacturer's labeling; use with caution. Infuse at minimum rate.

Administration Parenteral: IV infusion: Does not require further dilution; administer as a 50 mg/mL solution through a dedicated IV line containing an in-line 15 micron filter (a 0.2 micron filter is also acceptable) using an infusion pump. Do not mix with other infusions; do not use if turbid. Begin infusion within 6 hours of entering vial, complete infusion within 12 hours of vial entry. Infusion with other products is not recommended; however, if unavoidable, may be piggybacked into an IV line of NS, D_5W, $D_{10}W$, or dextrose 20% in water. Do not dilute more than 1:2.

Initial infusion: Begin at 15 mg/kg/hour; if there are no infusion-related reactions after 30 minutes, increase to 30 mg/kg/hour; if no infusion-related reactions after 30 minutes, increase to 60 mg/kg/hour for the remainder of the infusion; infusion rate should not exceed 75 mL/hour. Monitor closely after each rate change. If patient develops nausea, back pain, or flushing during infusion, slow the rate or temporarily stop the infusion. Discontinue if blood pressure drops or in case of anaphylactic reaction.

Subsequent infusions: Initiate at 15 mg/kg/hour for the first 15 minutes, if no infusion-related reactions, increase to 30 mg/kg/hour for the next 15 minutes; if rate is tolerated, increase to 60 mg/kg/hour and maintain this rate until completion of dose; maximum infusion rate: 60 mg/kg/hour or not to exceed 75 mL/hour.

Monitoring Parameters Renal function (BUN, serum creatinine prior to initial infusion and periodically thereafter); urine output; vital signs, including blood pressure (throughout infusion); signs/symptoms of infusion-related adverse reactions, anaphylaxis; signs and symptoms of hemolytic anemia; blood viscosity (baseline; in patients at risk for hyperviscosity); presence of antineutrophil antibodies (if TRALI is suspected); volume status; weight gain; clinical response

Additional Information

IgA content: Trace

Plasma Source: 2000-5000 donors (5% with top CMV titers)

IgG subclass (%):

IgG_1: 65

IgG_2: 28

IgG_3: 5.2

IgG_4: 1.7

Monomers + dimer (%): ≥95 monomers + dimers

Gamma globulin (%): 99

Albumin: 10 mg/mL

Sodium content: 20-30 mEq/L

Sugar content: 5% sucrose

Osmolality: >200 mOsm/L

Dosage Forms Excipient information presented when available (limited, particularly for generics); consult specific product labeling.

Injection, solution [preservative free]:

CytoGam®: 50 mg (± 10 mg)/mL (50 mL) [contains sodium 20-30 mEq/L, human albumin, and sucrose 50 mg/mL]

- ◆ **Cytomel** *see* Liothyronine *on page 1272*
- ◆ **Cytosar (Can)** *see* Cytarabine (Conventional) *on page 566*
- ◆ **Cytosar-U** *see* Cytarabine (Conventional) *on page 566*
- ◆ **Cytosine Arabinosine Hydrochloride** *see* Cytarabine (Conventional) *on page 566*
- ◆ **Cytotec** *see* Misoprostol *on page 1444*
- ◆ **Cytovene** *see* Ganciclovir (Systemic) *on page 958*
- ◆ **Cytoxan** *see* Cyclophosphamide *on page 551*
- ◆ **Cytra-2** *see* Sodium Citrate and Citric Acid *on page 1942*
- ◆ **Cytra-3** *see* Citric Acid, Sodium Citrate, and Potassium Citrate *on page 479*
- ◆ **Cytra-K** *see* Potassium Citrate and Citric Acid *on page 1738*
- ◆ **D2** *see* Ergocalciferol *on page 772*
- ◆ **D2E7** *see* Adalimumab *on page 67*
- ◆ **D3** *see* Cholecalciferol *on page 448*
- ◆ **D-3-5 [OTC]** *see* Cholecalciferol *on page 448*
- ◆ **D3-50 [OTC]** *see* Cholecalciferol *on page 448*
- ◆ **D-3-Mercaptovaline** *see* PenicillAMINE *on page 1652*
- ◆ **d4T** *see* Stavudine *on page 1970*
- ◆ **D_5W** *see* Dextrose *on page 633*
- ◆ **$D_{10}W$** *see* Dextrose *on page 633*
- ◆ **$D_{25}W$** *see* Dextrose *on page 633*
- ◆ **$D_{30}W$** *see* Dextrose *on page 633*
- ◆ **$D_{40}W$** *see* Dextrose *on page 633*

◆ $D_{50}W$ *see* Dextrose *on page 633*
◆ $D_{60}W$ *see* Dextrose *on page 633*
◆ $D_{70}W$ *see* Dextrose *on page 633*

Dacarbazine (da KAR ba zeen)

Medication Safety Issues

Sound-alike/look-alike issues:

Dacarbazine may be confused with procarbazine

High alert medication:

This medication is in a class the Institute for Safe Medication Practices (ISMP) includes among its list of drugs which have a heightened risk of causing significant patient harm when used in error.

Related Information

Prevention of Chemotherapy-Induced Nausea and Vomiting in Children *on page 2368*

Safe Handling of Hazardous Drugs *on page 2455*

Brand Names: Canada Dacarbazine for Injection

Therapeutic Category Antineoplastic Agent, Miscellaneous

Generic Availability (US) Yes

Use Treatment of malignant melanoma, Hodgkin's disease (FDA approved in adults); has also been used in the treatment of soft tissue sarcomas (fibrosarcomas, rhabdomyosarcoma), islet cell carcinoma, pheochromocytoma, and medullary carcinoma of the thyroid

Pregnancy Risk Factor C

Pregnancy Considerations [U.S. Boxed Warning]: This agent is carcinogenic and/or teratogenic when used in animals; adverse effects have been observed in animal studies. There are no adequate and well-controlled trials in pregnant women; use in pregnancy only if the potential benefit outweighs the potential risk to the fetus.

Breast-Feeding Considerations Due to the potential for serious adverse reactions in the nursing infant, breast-feeding is not recommended.

Contraindications Hypersensitivity to dacarbazine or any component of the formulation

Warnings/Precautions Hazardous agent - use appropriate precautions for handling and disposal (NIOSH 2014 [group 1]). **[U.S. Boxed Warnings]: Bone marrow suppression is a common toxicity;** leukopenia and thrombocytopenia may be severe; may result in treatment delays or discontinuation; monitor closely. **Hepatotoxicity with hepatocellular necrosis and hepatic vein thrombosis has been reported (rare),** usually with combination chemotherapy, but may occur with dacarbazine alone. The half-life is increased in patients with renal and/or hepatic impairment; use caution, monitor for toxicity and consider dosage reduction. Anaphylaxis may occur following dacarbazine administration. Extravasation may result in tissue damage and severe pain. **[U.S. Boxed Warnings]: May be carcinogenic and/or teratogenic. Should be administered under the supervision of an experienced cancer chemotherapy physician.** Carefully evaluate the potential benefits of therapy against the risk for toxicity. Dacarbazine is associated with a high emetic potential; antiemetics are recommended to prevent nausea and vomiting (Basch, 2011; Dupuis, 2011; Roila, 2010).

Adverse Reactions

Dermatologic: Alopecia

Gastrointestinal: Anorexia, nausea and vomiting

Hematologic: Myelosuppression (onset: 5-7 days; nadir: 7-10 days; recovery: 21-28 days), leukopenia, thrombocytopenia

Local: Pain on infusion

Infrequent, postmarketing, and/or case reports: Anaphylactic reactions, anemia, diarrhea, eosinophilia, erythema, facial flushing, facial paresthesia, flu-like syndrome (fever, myalgia, malaise), hepatic necrosis, hepatic vein occlusion, liver enzymes increased (transient), paresthesia, photosensitivity, rash, renal functions test abnormalities, taste alteration, urticaria

Drug Interactions

Metabolism/Transport Effects Substrate of CYP1A2 (major), CYP2E1 (major); **Note:** Assignment of Major/Minor substrate status based on clinically relevant drug interaction potential

Avoid Concomitant Use

Avoid concomitant use of Dacarbazine with any of the following: BCG; BCG (Intravesical); CloZAPine; Dipyrone; Natalizumab; Pimecrolimus; Tacrolimus (Topical); Tofacitinib; Vaccines (Live)

Increased Effect/Toxicity

Dacarbazine may increase the levels/effects of: CloZAPine; Leflunomide; Natalizumab; Tofacitinib; Vaccines (Live)

The levels/effects of Dacarbazine may be increased by: Abiraterone Acetate; CYP1A2 Inhibitors (Moderate); CYP1A2 Inhibitors (Strong); CYP2E1 Inhibitors (Moderate); CYP2E1 Inhibitors (Strong); Deferasirox; Denosumab; Dipyrone; MAO Inhibitors; Peginterferon Alfa-2b; Pimecrolimus; Roflumilast; Tacrolimus (Topical); Trastuzumab; Vemurafenib

Decreased Effect

Dacarbazine may decrease the levels/effects of: BCG; BCG (Intravesical); Coccidioides immitis Skin Test; Sipuleucel-T; Vaccines (Inactivated); Vaccines (Live)

The levels/effects of Dacarbazine may be decreased by: Cannabis; CYP1A2 Inducers (Strong); Cyproterone; Echinacea; SORAfenib; Teriflunomide

Storage/Stability Store intact vials under refrigeration (2°C to 8°C). Protect from light. The following stability information has also been reported: Intact vials are stable for 3 months at room temperature (Cohen, 2007). Reconstituted solution is stable for 24 hours at room temperature (20°C) and 96 hours under refrigeration (4°C) when protected from light, although the manufacturer recommends use within 72 hours if refrigerated and 8 hours at room temperature. Solutions for infusion (in D_5W or NS) are stable for 24 hours at room temperature if protected from light. Decomposed drug turns pink.

Mechanism of Action Alkylating agent which is converted to the active alkylating metabolite MTIC [(methyl-triazene-1-yl)-imidazole-4-carboxamide] via the cytochrome P450 system. The cytotoxic effects of MTIC are manifested through alkylation (methylation) of DNA at the O^6, N^7 guanine positions which lead to DNA double strand breaks and apoptosis. Non-cell cycle specific.

Pharmacokinetics (Adult data unless noted)

Distribution: Distributes to the liver; very little distribution into CSF with CSF concentrations ~14% of plasma concentrations

V_{dss}: Adults: 17 L/m^2

Protein binding: Minimal, 5%

Metabolism: N-demethylated in the liver by microsomal enzymes; metabolites may also have an antineoplastic effect

Half-life, biphasic: Initial: 20-40 minutes; terminal: 5 hours (in patients with normal renal/hepatic function)

Elimination: ~30% to 50% of dose excreted in urine by tubular secretion, 15% to 25% is excreted in urine as unchanged drug

Dosing: Usual IV (refer to individual protocols):

Children:

Pediatric solid tumors: 200-470 mg/m^2/day over 5 days every 21-28 days

Hodgkin's disease: 375 mg/m^2 on days 1 and 15 of treatment course, repeat every 28 days

Adults:

Malignant melanoma: 2-4.5 mg/kg/day for 10 days, repeat in 4 weeks or may use 250 mg/m^2/day for 5 days, repeat in 3 weeks

Hodgkin's disease: 150 mg/m^2/day for 5 days, repeat every 4 weeks **or** 375 mg/m^2 on day 1, repeat in 15 days of each 28-day cycle in combination with other agents

Preparation for Administration Hazardous agent; use appropriate precautions for handling and disposal (NIOSH 2014 [group 1]).

Parenteral: The manufacturer recommends reconstituting 100 mg and 200 mg vials with 9.9 mL and 19.7 mL SWFI, respectively, resulting in a concentration of 10 mg/mL; some institutions use different standard dilutions (eg, 20 mg/mL). May further dilute in D_5W or NS.

Administration Hazardous agent; use appropriate precautions for handling and disposal (NIOSH 2014 [group 1]).

Parenteral: Administer by slow IVP over 2 to 3 minutes or by IV infusion over 15 to 120 minutes

Vesicant/Extravasation Risk May be an irritant

Monitoring Parameters CBC with differential, erythrocytes and platelet count; liver function tests

Dosage Forms Excipient information presented when available (limited, particularly for generics); consult specific product labeling.

Solution Reconstituted, Intravenous:

Generic: 100 mg (1 ea); 200 mg (1 ea)

Solution Reconstituted, Intravenous [preservative free]:

Generic: 200 mg (1 ea)

- **Dacarbazine for Injection (Can)** *see* Dacarbazine *on page 572*
- **DACT** *see* DACTINomycin *on page 573*

DACTINomycin (dak ti noe MYE sin)

Medication Safety Issues

Sound-alike/look-alike issues:

DACTINomycin may be confused with Dacogen, DAPTOmycin, DAUNOrubicin

Actinomycin may be confused with achromycin

High alert medication:

This medication is in a class the Institute for Safe Medication Practices (ISMP) includes among its list of drug classes which have a heightened risk of causing significant patient harm when used in error.

Related Information

Management of Drug Extravasations *on page 2298*

Safe Handling of Hazardous Drugs *on page 2455*

Brand Names: US Cosmegen

Brand Names: Canada Cosmegen

Therapeutic Category Antineoplastic Agent, Antibiotic

Generic Availability (US) No

Use Management (either alone or in combination with other treatment modalities) of Wilms' tumor, childhood rhabdomyosarcoma, Ewing's sarcoma, gestational trophoblastic neoplasms, and metastatic nonseminomatous testicular tumors (FDA approved in ages >6 months and adults); used in regional perfusion (palliative or adjunctive) of locally recurrent or locoregional solid tumors (sarcomas, carcinomas, and adenocarcinomas) (FDA approved in adults). Has also been used for treatment of soft tissue sarcoma (other than rhabdomyosarcoma).

Pregnancy Risk Factor D

Pregnancy Considerations [U.S. Boxed Warning]: Avoid exposure during pregnancy. Adverse effects have been observed in animal reproduction studies. Women of childbearing potential are advised not to become pregnant. When used for gestational trophoblastic neoplasm, unfavorable outcomes have been reported when subsequent pregnancies occur within 6 months of treatment. It is recommended to use effective contraception for 6 months to 1 year after therapy (Matsui 2004; Seckl 2013)

Breast-Feeding Considerations It is not known if dactinomycin is excreted in human breast milk. According to the manufacturer labeling, due to the potential for serious adverse reactions in the nursing infant, the decision to discontinue dactinomycin or to discontinue breast-feeding during therapy should take into account the benefits of treatment to the mother.

Contraindications Hypersensitivity to dactinomycin or any component of the formulation; patients with concurrent or recent chickenpox or herpes zoster

Warnings/Precautions [U.S. Boxed Warning]: Hazardous agent - use appropriate precautions for handling and disposal (NIOSH 2014 [group 1]). If accidental exposure occurs, immediately irrigate copiously for at least 15 minutes with water, saline, or balanced ophthalmic irrigation solution (eye exposure) and at least 15 minutes with water (skin exposure); prompt ophthalmic or medical consultation is also recommended. Contaminated clothing should be destroyed and shoes thoroughly cleaned prior to reuse.

Vesicant; ensure proper needle or catheter placement prior to and during infusion; avoid extravasation. **[U.S. Boxed Warning]: Extremely corrosive to soft tissues; if extravasation occurs during IV use, severe damage to soft tissues will occur; has led to contracture of the arm (rare). Avoid inhalation of vapors or contact with skin, mucous membrane, or eyes; avoid exposure during pregnancy.** Recommended for IV administration only. The manufacturer recommends intermittent ice (15 minutes 4 times/day) for suspected extravasation.

May cause hepatic sinusoidal obstruction syndrome (SOS; formerly called veno-occlusive liver disease); use with caution in hepatobiliary dysfunction. Monitor for signs or symptoms of hepatic SOS, including bilirubin >1.4 mg/dL, unexplained weight gain, ascites, hepatomegaly, or unexplained right upper quadrant pain (Arndt, 2004). The risk of fatal SOS is increased in children <4 years of age.

Dactinomycin potentiates the effects of radiation therapy; use with caution in patients who have received radiation therapy; reduce dosages in patients who are receiving dactinomycin and radiation therapy simultaneously; combination with radiation therapy may result in increased toxicity (eg, GI toxicity, myelosuppression, severe oropharyngeal mucositis). Avoid dactinomycin use within 2 months of radiation treatment for right-sided Wilms' tumor, may increase the risk of hepatotoxicity.

Dactinomycin is associated with a high emetic potential; antiemetics are recommended to prevent nausea and vomiting (Basch, 2011; Dupuis, 2011). Toxic effects may be delayed in onset (2-4 days following a course of treatment) and may require 1-2 weeks to reach maximum severity. Discontinue treatment with severe myelosuppression, diarrhea, or stomatitis. Long-term observation of cancer survivors is recommended due to the increased risk of second primary tumors following treatment with radiation and antineoplastic agents. Regional perfusion therapy may result in local limb edema, soft tissue damage, and possible venous thrombosis; leakage of dactinomycin into systemic circulation may result in hematologic toxicity, infection, impaired wound healing, and mucositis. Dosage is usually expressed in **MICRO**grams and should be calculated on the basis of body surface area (BSA) in obese or edematous adult patients (to relate dose to lean body mass). Avoid administration of live vaccines during dactinomycin treatment. Avoid use in infants <6 months of age (toxic effects may occur more frequently). May be associated with an increased risk of myelosuppression in the elderly; use with caution. **[U.S. Boxed Warning]: Should be administered under the supervision of an experienced cancer chemotherapy physician.** Potentially significant drug-drug interactions may exist, requiring dose or frequency adjustment, additional monitoring, and/or selection of alternative therapy.

Adverse Reactions

Central nervous system: Fatigue, fever, lethargy, malaise

Dermatologic: Acne, alopecia (reversible), cheilitis, erythema multiforme, increased pigmentation, sloughing, or erythema of previously irradiated skin; skin eruptions, Stevens-Johnson syndrome, toxic epidermal necrolysis

Endocrine & metabolic: Growth retardation, hyperuricemia, hypocalcemia

Gastrointestinal: Abdominal pain, anorexia, diarrhea, dysphagia, esophagitis, GI ulceration, mucositis, nausea, pharyngitis, proctitis, stomatitis, vomiting

Hematologic: Agranulocytosis, anemia, aplastic anemia, febrile neutropenia, leukopenia, myelosuppression (onset: 7 days, nadir: 14-21 days, recovery: 21-28 days), neutropenia, pancytopenia, reticulocytopenia, thrombocytopenia, thrombocytopenia (immune mediated)

Hepatic: Ascites, bilirubin increased, hepatic failure, hepatitis, hepatomegaly, hepatopathy thrombocytopenia syndrome, hepatotoxicity, liver function test abnormality, hepatic sinusoidal obstruction syndrome (SOS; veno-occlusive liver disease)

Local: Erythema, edema, epidermolysis, pain, tissue necrosis, and ulceration (following extravasation)

Neuromuscular & skeletal: Myalgia

Renal: Renal function abnormality

Respiratory: Pneumonitis

Miscellaneous: Anaphylactoid reaction, infection, sepsis (including neutropenic sepsis)

Drug Interactions

Metabolism/Transport Effects None known.

Avoid Concomitant Use

Avoid concomitant use of DACTINomycin with any of the following: BCG; BCG (Intravesical); CloZAPine; Dipyrone; Natalizumab; Pimecrolimus; Tacrolimus (Topical); Tofacitinib; Vaccines (Live)

Increased Effect/Toxicity

DACTINomycin may increase the levels/effects of: CloZAPine; Leflunomide; Natalizumab; Tofacitinib; Vaccines (Live)

The levels/effects of DACTINomycin may be increased by: Denosumab; Dipyrone; Pimecrolimus; Roflumilast; Tacrolimus (Topical); Trastuzumab

Decreased Effect

DACTINomycin may decrease the levels/effects of: BCG; BCG (Intravesical); Coccidioides immitis Skin Test; Sipuleucel-T; Vaccines (Inactivated); Vaccines (Live)

The levels/effects of DACTINomycin may be decreased by: Echinacea

Storage/Stability Store at controlled room temperature of 20°C to 25°C (68°F to 77°F). Protect from light and humidity. According to the manufacturer's labeling, recommended final concentrations (≥10 mcg/mL) are stable for 10 hours at room temperature but should be administered within 4 hours due to the lack of preservative.

Mechanism of Action Binds to the guanine portion of DNA intercalating between guanine and cytosine base pairs inhibiting DNA and RNA synthesis and protein synthesis

Pharmacokinetics (Adult data unless noted)

Distribution: Children: Extensive extravascular distribution (59-714 L) (Veal, 2005); does not penetrate blood-brain barrier

Metabolism: Minimal

Half-life, terminal:
- Children: 14-43 hours (Veal, 2005)
- Adults: 36 hours

Elimination: ~30% in urine and feces within 1 week

Dosing: Usual Details concerning dosing in combination regimens should be consulted. **Note: Medication orders for dactinomycin are commonly written in MICROgrams (eg, 150 mcg) although many regimens list the dose in MILLIgrams (eg, mg/kg or mg/m²).** The dose intensity per 2-week cycle for adults and children should not exceed 15 mcg/kg/day for 5 days or 400-600 mcg/m²/day for 5 days. Some practitioners recommend calculation of the dosage for obese or edematous adult patients on the basis of body surface area in an effort to relate dosage to lean body mass.

Infants ≥6 months, Children, and Adolescents:

Ewing's sarcoma: IV: 15 mcg/kg/day for 5 days (in various combination regimens and schedules)

Osteosarcoma: IV: Limited data available: 600 mcg/**m²**/day days 1, 2, and 3 of weeks 15, 31, 34, 39, and 42 (as part of a combination chemotherapy regimen) (Goorin, 2003)

Rhabdomyosarcoma: IV:

Manufacturer's labeling: 15 mcg/kg/day for 5 days (in various combination regimens and schedules)

Alternate dosing: Limited data available: VAC regimen:

Infants ≥6 months: 25 mcg/kg every 3 weeks, weeks 0 to 45 (in combination with vincristine and cyclophosphamide, and mesna); dose omission required following radiation therapy (Raney, 2011)

Children and Adolescents: 45 mcg/kg (maximum dose: 2500 mcg) every 3 weeks, weeks 0 to 45 (in combination with vincristine and cyclophosphamide, and mesna); dose omission required following radiation therapy (Raney, 2011)

Wilms' tumor: IV:

Manufacturer's labeling: 15 mcg/kg/day for 5 days (in various combination regimens and schedules)

Alternate dosing: Limited data available:

DD-4A regimen: Children and Adolescents: 45 mcg/kg on day 1 every 6 weeks for 54 weeks (in combination with doxorubicin and vincristine) (Green, 1998)

EE-4A regimen: Children and Adolescents: 45 mcg/kg on day 1 every 3 weeks for 18 weeks (in combination with vincristine) (Green, 1998)

VAD regimen:

Infants ≥6 months: 750 mcg/**m²** every 6 weeks for 1 year (stage III disease) (in combination with vincristine and doxorubicin) (Pritchard, 1995)

Children and Adolescents: 1500 mcg/**m²** every 6 weeks for 1 year (stage III disease) (in combination with vincristine and doxorubicin) (Pritchard, 1995)

Adults:

Testicular cancer: IV: 1000 mcg/m² on day 1 (as part of a combination chemotherapy regimen)

Gestational trophoblastic neoplasm: IV: 12 mcg/kg/day for 5 days (monotherapy) **or** 500 mcg/dose days 1 and 2 (as part of a combination chemotherapy regimen)

Wilms' tumor, Ewing's sarcoma, rhabdomyosarcoma: IV: 15 mcg/kg/day for 5 days (in various combination regimens and schedules)

Regional perfusion (dosages and techniques may vary by institution; obese patients and patients with prior chemotherapy or radiation therapy may require lower doses): Lower extremity or pelvis: 50 mcg/kg; upper extremity: 35 mcg/kg

Dosing adjustment in renal impairment: There are no dosage adjustments provided in the manufacturer's labeling; however, based on the amount of urinary excretion, dosage adjustments may not be necessary.

Dosing adjustment in hepatic impairment: There are no dosage adjustments provided in the manufacturer's labeling; however, the following adjustments have been recommended: Children, Adolescents and Adults: Any transaminase increase: Reduce dose by 50%; may increase by monitoring toxicities (Floyd, 2006).

Preparation for Administration Hazardous agent; use appropriate precautions for handling and disposal (NIOSH 2014 [group 1]).

Parenteral: Reconstitute initially with 1.1 mL of preservative-free SWFI to yield a concentration of 500 mcg/mL (diluent containing preservatives will cause precipitation). May further dilute in D_5W or NS in glass or polyvinyl chloride (PVC) containers to a recommended concentration of ≥10 mcg/mL; final concentrations <10 mcg/mL are not recommended. Cellulose ester membrane filters may partially remove dactinomycin from solution and should not be used during preparation or administration.

Administration Hazardous agent; use appropriate precautions for handling and disposal (NIOSH 2014 [group 1]).

Parenteral: May administer undiluted into the side-port of a free flowing IV infusion by slow IVP over a few minutes; or may further dilute and administer as IV infusion over 10 to 15 minutes; consider a D_5W or NS flush before and after a dactinomycin dose to ensure venous patency. Cellulose ester membrane filters may partially remove dactinomycin from solution and should not be used during administration. Avoid extravasation; do not give IM or SubQ.

Vesicant; ensure proper needle or catheter placement prior to and during infusion; avoid extravasation. If extravasation occurs, stop infusion immediately and disconnect (leave cannula/needle in place); gently aspirate extravasated solution (do **NOT** flush the line); remove needle/cannula; elevate extremity. Apply dry cold compresses for 20 minutes 4 times a day for 1 to 2 days (Pérez Fidalgo 2012).

Vesicant/Extravasation Risk Vesicant

Monitoring Parameters CBC with differential and platelet count, liver function tests and renal function tests; monitor for signs/symptoms of hepatic SOS, including unexplained weight gain, ascites, hepatomegaly, or unexplained right upper quadrant pain (Arndt, 2004); monitor serum beta-hCG (management of gestational trophoblastic neoplasms)

Test Interactions May interfere with bioassays of antibacterial drug levels

Dosage Forms Excipient information presented when available (limited, particularly for generics); consult specific product labeling.

Solution Reconstituted, Intravenous:

Cosmegen: 0.5 mg (1 ea)

◆ **Dalacin C (Can)** *see* Clindamycin (Systemic) *on page 487*

◆ **Dalacin T (Can)** *see* Clindamycin (Topical) *on page 491*

◆ **Dalacin Vaginal (Can)** *see* Clindamycin (Topical) *on page 491*

◆ **Dalfopristin and Quinupristin** *see* Quinupristin and Dalfopristin *on page 1827*

◆ **Dalmane (Can)** *see* Flurazepam *on page 913*

◆ ***d*-Alpha Tocopherol** *see* Vitamin E *on page 2188*

Danazol (DA na zole)

Medication Safety Issues

Sound-alike/look-alike issues:

Danazol may be confused with Dantrium®

Brand Names: Canada Cyclomen®

Therapeutic Category Androgen

Generic Availability (US) Yes

Use Treatment of endometriosis amenable to hormonal management; fibrocystic breast disease; hereditary angioedema

Pregnancy Risk Factor X

Pregnancy Considerations [U.S. Boxed Warning]: Pregnancy should be ruled out prior to treatment using a sensitive test (beta subunit test, if available). Nonhormonal contraception should be used during therapy. May cause androgenic effects to the female fetus; clitoral hypertrophy, labial fusion, urogenital sinus defect, vaginal atresia, and ambiguous genitalia have been reported. Therapy should be discontinued for 2 months prior to attempting pregnancy (Caballero, 2012).

Breast-Feeding Considerations Use of danazol in nursing women is contraindicated.

Contraindications Hypersensitivity to danazol or any component of the formulation; undiagnosed genital bleeding; pregnancy; breast-feeding; porphyria; markedly impaired hepatic, renal, or cardiac function; androgen-dependent tumor; active or history of thrombosis or thromboembolic disease

Warnings/Precautions [U.S. Boxed Warning]: Peliosis hepatis and benign hepatic adenoma have been reported with long-term use (may be complicated by acute intra-abdominal hemorrhage). Monitor closely for potential hepatotoxicity during therapy. Use with caution in patients with hepatic impairment; use is contraindicated with marked impairment. **[U.S. Boxed Warning]: May cause benign intracranial hypertension (pseudotumor cerebri);** monitor for headache, nausea/vomiting, visual disturbances and/or papilledema. **[U.S. Boxed Warning]: Thromboembolism, thrombotic, and thrombophlebitic events have been reported (including life-threatening or fatal strokes). [U.S. Boxed Warning]: Pregnancy must be ruled out prior to treatment;** a nonhormonal method of contraception should be used during therapy.

Breast cancer should be ruled out prior to treatment for fibrocystic breast disease. Symptoms of pain and tenderness may recur following discontinuation of therapy. Ovulation may not be suppressed at doses used for fibrocystic disease therefore nonhormonal contraception is recommended.

Use with caution in patients with diabetes mellitus; insulin requirements may be increased; monitor carefully. Use with caution in patients with conditions influenced by edema (eg, cardiovascular disease, migraine, seizure disorder, renal impairment); may cause fluid retention. May cause exacerbations of acute intermittent porphyria; use is contraindicated in patients with porphyria. May cause nonreversible androgenic effects. Anabolic steroids may cause blood lipid changes with increased risk of arteriosclerosis.

Adverse Reactions

Cardiovascular: Benign intracranial hypertension (rare), edema, flushing, hypertension, MI, palpitation, tachycardia

Central nervous system: Anxiety (rare), chills (rare), convulsions (rare), depression, dizziness, emotional lability, fainting, fatigue, fever (rare), Guillain-Barré syndrome (rare), headache, nervousness, sleep disorders

Dermatologic: Acne, alopecia, erythema multiforme (rare), mild hirsutism, maculopapular rash, papular rash, petechial rash, pruritus, purpuric rash, seborrhea, Stevens-Johnson syndrome (rare), photosensitivity (rare), urticaria, vesicular rash

Endocrine & metabolic: Amenorrhea (which may continue post therapy), breast size reduction, clitoris hypertrophy (rare), glucose intolerance/glucagon changes, HDL decreased, LDL increased, libido changes, nipple discharge (rare), menstrual disturbances (spotting, altered timing of cycle), semen abnormalities (changes in volume, viscosity, sperm count/motility), sex hormone-binding globulin changes, spermatogenesis reduction, thyroid binding globulin changes

Gastrointestinal: Appetite changes (rare), bleeding gums (rare), constipation, gastroenteritis, nausea, pancreatitis (rare), splenic peliosis (rare), vomiting, weight gain

Genitourinary: Vaginal dryness, vaginal irritation, pelvic pain (rare)

Hematologic: Eosinophilia, erythrocytosis (reversible), leukocytosis, leukopenia, platelet count increased, polycythemia, RBC increased, thrombocytopenia

Hepatic: Cholestatic jaundice, hepatic adenoma, jaundice, liver enzymes increased, malignant tumors (after prolonged use), peliosis hepatis

Neuromuscular & skeletal: Back pain, carpal tunnel syndrome (rare), CPK changes, extremity pain, joint lockup, joint pain, joint swelling, muscle cramps, neck pain, paresthesia, spasms, tremor, weakness

Ocular: Cataracts (rare), visual disturbances

Renal: Hematuria

Respiratory: Interstitial pneumonitis, nasal congestion (rare)

Miscellaneous: Diaphoresis, voice change (hoarseness, sore throat, instability, deepening of pitch)

Rare but important or life-threatening: Hepatotoxicity (idiosyncratic) (Chalasani, 2014)

Drug Interactions

Metabolism/Transport Effects **Inhibits** CYP3A4 (weak)

Avoid Concomitant Use

Avoid concomitant use of Danazol with any of the following: Pimozide; Simvastatin

Increased Effect/Toxicity

Danazol may increase the levels/effects of: ARIPiprazole; C1 inhibitors; CarBAMazepine; CycloSPORINE (Systemic); Dofetilide; HMG-CoA Reductase Inhibitors; Hydrocodone; Lomitapide; NiMODipine; Pimozide; Simvastatin; Tacrolimus (Systemic); Tacrolimus (Topical); Vitamin D Analogs; Vitamin K Antagonists

The levels/effects of Danazol may be increased by: Corticosteroids (Systemic)

Decreased Effect

Danazol may decrease the levels/effects of: Antidiabetic Agents

Food Interactions Food delays time to peak levels. A high-fat meal increases plasma concentration and extent of availability.

Storage/Stability Store at controlled room temperature of 15°C to 30°C (59°F to 86°F).

Mechanism of Action Suppresses pituitary output of follicle-stimulating hormone and luteinizing hormone that causes regression and atrophy of normal and ectopic endometrial tissue; decreases rate of growth of abnormal breast tissue; reduces attacks associated with hereditary angioedema by increasing levels of C4 component of complement

Pharmacodynamics

Endometriosis:

Onset of action: 3 weeks

Fibrocystic breast disease:

Onset of action: 1 month

Maximum effect: 4-6 months

Duration: Symptoms recur in 50% of patients within one year after discontinuation of treatment

Pharmacokinetics (Adult data unless noted)

Absorption: Well absorbed

Metabolism: Extensive hepatic metabolism to inactive metabolites

Half-life: Adults: 4.5 hours

Time to peak serum concentration: 2 hours

Dosing: Usual Adolescents and Adults: Oral: **Note:** Begin treatment during menstruation or obtain appropriate tests to ensure patient is not pregnant:

Endometriosis:

Mild case: 100-200 mg twice daily for 3-6 months; may be continued up to 9 months if necessary

Moderate to severe case: 400 mg twice daily for 3-6 months; may be continued up to 9 months if necessary

Note: A gradual downward titration to a dose sufficient to maintain amenorrhea may be considered depending upon the patient's response

Fibrocystic breast disease: 50-200 mg twice daily

Hereditary angioedema: Initial: 200 mg 2-3 times/day depending upon the patient's response; after a favorable response is obtained, decrease the dosage by 50% or less at intervals of 1-3 months or longer. If an attack occurs, the daily dosage may be increased by up to 200 mg.

Administration Oral: Avoid administration with fatty meals.

Monitoring Parameters Liver function tests, symptomatology and site of disease; serum glucose (if diabetic); HDL and LDL cholesterol; signs and symptoms of pseudotumor cerebri; androgenic effects

Test Interactions Estradiol (Kishino, 2010); testosterone, androstenedione, dehydroepiandrosterone

Additional Information Danazol has seen limited use for treatment of ITP in children refractory to steroids. Ten children, 2.5-17 years of age were treated with 20-30 mg/kg/day in divided doses (maximum: 800 mg/day). Treatment was tapered off after patients responded to therapy (Weinblatt, 1988). Danazol has also been evaluated in hemophilia A in a randomized, double-blind placebo-controlled crossover trial in 19 children. Children <15 years received 150 mg/day and >15 years received 300 mg/day for 3 months. Factor VIII:C levels were increased (Mehta, 1992).

Dosage Forms Excipient information presented when available (limited, particularly for generics); consult specific product labeling.

Capsule, Oral:

Generic: 50 mg, 100 mg, 200 mg

◆ **Dandrex [OTC]** *see* Selenium Sulfide *on page 1913*

◆ **Danocrine** *see* Danazol *on page 575*

◆ **Dantrium** *see* Dantrolene *on page 576*

Dantrolene (DAN troe leen)

Medication Safety Issues

Sound-alike/look-alike issues:

Dantrium may be confused with danazol, Daraprim

Revonto may be confused with Revatio

Related Information

Management of Drug Extravasations *on page 2298*

Serotonin Syndrome *on page 2447*

Brand Names: US Dantrium; Revonto; Ryanodex

Brand Names: Canada Dantrium

Therapeutic Category Antidote, Malignant Hyperthermia; Hyperthermia, Treatment; Skeletal Muscle Relaxant, Nonparalytic

Generic Availability (US) May be product dependent

Use

Parenteral: Management of the fulminant hypermetabolism of skeletal muscle characteristic of malignant hyperthermia (Dantrium, Revonto, Ryanodex: FDA approved in all ages); prevention of malignant hyperthermia in susceptible individuals (preoperative/postoperative administration) (Dantrium, Revonto, Ryanodex: FDA approved in all ages)

Oral: Treatment of spasticity associated with upper motor neuron disorders such as spinal cord injury, stroke, cerebral palsy, or multiple sclerosis (FDA approved in ages ≥5 years and adults); preoperative/postoperative prevention and attenuation of malignant hyperthermia in susceptible individuals (FDA approved in ages ≥5 years and adults)

Note: Dantrolene prophylaxis is not routinely recommended for most malignant hyperthermia susceptible patients, provided there is immediate availability of parenteral dantrolene and adequate perioperative patient management (eg, avoiding known trigger agents [eg, anesthetics] in susceptible patients). Although dantrolene is FDA approved in all ages for malignant hyperthermia, it does not usually occur in patients <12 months of age and has not been reported at <4 months of age (Chamley, 2000; Larach, 2010; Silva, 1999).

Pregnancy Risk Factor C

Pregnancy Considerations Adverse events have been observed in animal reproduction studies. Dantrolene crosses the human placenta. Cord blood concentrations are similar to those in the maternal plasma at term. and dantrolene can be detected in the newborn serum at delivery. Adverse events were not observed in the newborn following maternal doses of 100 mg/day administered orally prior to delivery (Shime, 1988). Uterine atony has been reported following dantrolene injection after delivery; however, this may be due in part to the mannitol contained in the IV preparation (Shin, 1995; Weingarten, 1987). Prophylactic use of dantrolene is not routinely recommended in pregnant women susceptible to MH prior to obstetric surgery, if use is needed, close monitoring of the mother and newborn is recommended (Krause, 2004; Norman, 1995).

Breast-Feeding Considerations Low amounts of dantrolene are excreted into breast milk. Due to the potential for serious adverse reactions in the nursing infant, the manufacturer recommends that a decision be made whether to discontinue nursing or to discontinue the drug, taking into account the importance of treatment to the mother. In a case report, the half-life of dantrolene in breast milk was calculated to be 9 hours; the highest milk concentration was 1.2 mcg/mL following a maternal IV dose; however, the maternal serum concentrations were not reported (Fricker, 1998).

Contraindications

IV: There are no contraindications listed within the manufacturer's labeling.

Oral: Active hepatic disease; should not be used when spasticity is used to maintain posture/balance during locomotion or to obtain/maintain increased function

Warnings/Precautions [U.S. Boxed Warning]: Oral: Has potential for hepatotoxicity. Higher doses (ie, ≥800 mg/day), even sporadic short courses, may increase the risk of severe hepatic injury although hepatic injury may occur at doses <400 mg/day. Overt hepatitis has been most frequently observed between the third and twelfth month of therapy. Hepatic injury appears to be greater in females, in patients >35 years of age, and those taking concurrent medications. A higher incidence of fatal hepatic events have been reported in the elderly, although concurrent disease states and concurrent use of hepatotoxic drugs may have contributed. Idiosyncratic and hypersensitivity reactions (sometimes fatal) of the liver have also occurred. Monitor hepatic function at baseline and as clinically indicated during treatment. Discontinue therapy if abnormal liver function tests occur or benefits are not observed within 45 days when utilized for chronic spasticity.

Loss of grip strength, weakness in the legs, dyspnea, respiratory muscle weakness, dysphagia, and decreased inspiratory capacity has occurred with IV dantrolene. Patients should not ambulate without assistance until they have normal strength and balance. Monitor patients for the adequacy of ventilation and for difficulty swallowing/choking.

Use oral therapy with caution in patients with impaired cardiac, hepatic, or pulmonary function (particularly in obstructive pulmonary disease). Oral therapy may cause photosensitivity. Lightheadedness, dizziness, somnolence, and vertigo may occur and may persist for 48-hours post-dose; patients must be cautioned about performing tasks which require mental alertness (eg, operating machinery or driving).

Injection may contain mannitol. In addition to IV dantrolene, supportive measures must also be utilized for management of malignant hyperthermia; administer diuretics to prevent late kidney injury due to myoglobinuria. Alkaline solution; may cause tissue necrosis if extravasated (vesicant); ensure proper needle or catheter placement prior to and during infusion; avoid extravasation.

Some dosage forms may contain polysorbate 80 (also known as Tweens). Hypersensitivity reactions, usually a delayed reaction, have been reported following exposure to pharmaceutical products containing polysorbate 80 in certain individuals (Isaksson, 2002; Lucente 2000; Shelley, 1995). Thrombocytopenia, ascites, pulmonary deterioration, and renal and hepatic failure have been reported in premature neonates after receiving parenteral products containing polysorbate 80 (Alade, 1986; CDC, 1984). See manufacturer's labeling.

Potentially significant interactions may exist, requiring dose or frequency adjustment, additional monitoring, and/or selection of alternative therapy.

Adverse Reactions

Cardiovascular: Atrioventricular block (intravenous), cardiac failure, flushing (intravenous), phlebitis, tachycardia, variable blood pressure

Central nervous system: chills, choking sensation, confusion, depression, dizziness, drowsiness (may persist for 48 hours post dose), fatigue, feeling abnormal, headache, insomnia, malaise, myasthenia, nervousness, seizure, speech disturbance, voice disorder (intravenous)

Dermatologic: Acneiform eruption (capsules), diaphoresis, eczematous rash, erythema (intravenous), hair disease (abnormal growth), pruritus, urticaria

Gastrointestinal: Abdominal cramps, anorexia, constipation, diarrhea, dysgeusia, dysphagia (use caution at meal time on day of administration as swallowing may be difficult), gastric irritation, gastrointestinal hemorrhage, nausea, sialorrhea, vomiting

Genitourinary: Crystalluria, difficulty in micturition, erectile dysfunction, hematuria, nocturia, urinary frequency, urinary incontinence, urinary retention

Hematologic & oncologic: Anemia, aplastic anemia, leukopenia, lymphocytic lymphoma, thrombocytopenia

Hepatic: Hepatitis

Hypersensitivity: Anaphylaxis

Local: Injection site reaction (intravenous; pain, erythema, swelling), local tissue necrosis (with extravasation due to high product pH)

Neuromuscular & skeletal: Back pain, limb pain (intravenous), myalgia

Ophthalmic: Blurred vision (intravenous), diplopia, epiphora, visual disturbance

Respiratory: Dyspnea (intravenous), pleural effusion (with pericarditis), pulmonary edema (rare), respiratory depression

Miscellaneous: Fever

Rare but important or life-threatening: Decrease in forced vital capacity (intravenous), dyspnea (intravenous), hepatic disease, hepatotoxicity (oral), increased liver enzymes (oral), respiratory muscle failure (intravenous)

Drug Interactions

Metabolism/Transport Effects Substrate of CYP3A4 (major); **Note:** Assignment of Major/Minor substrate status based on clinically relevant drug interaction potential

Avoid Concomitant Use

Avoid concomitant use of Dantrolene with any of the following: Azelastine (Nasal); Calcium Channel Blockers (Nondihydropyridine); Conivaptan; Fusidic Acid (Systemic); Idelalisib; Orphenadrine; Paraldehyde; Thalidomide

Increased Effect/Toxicity

Dantrolene may increase the levels/effects of: Alcohol (Ethyl); Azelastine (Nasal); Buprenorphine; Calcium Channel Blockers (Nondihydropyridine); CNS Depressants; Hydrocodone; Methotrimeprazine; Metyrosine; Mirtazapine; Orphenadrine; Paraldehyde; Pramipexole; ROPINIRole; Rotigotine; Selective Serotonin Reuptake Inhibitors; Suvorexant; Thalidomide; Vecuronium; Zolpidem

The levels/effects of Dantrolene may be increased by: Aprepitant; Brimonidine (Topical); Cannabis; Conivaptan; CYP3A4 Inhibitors (Moderate); CYP3A4 Inhibitors (Strong); Dasatinib; Dexketoprofen; Doxylamine; Dronabinol; Droperidol; Fosaprepitant; Fusidic Acid (Systemic); HydrOXYzine; Idelalisib; Ivacaftor; Kava Kava; Luliconazole; Magnesium Sulfate; Methotrimeprazine; Mifepristone; Nabilone; Netupitant; Palbociclib; Perampanel; Rufinamide; Simeprevir; Sodium Oxybate; Stiripentol; Tapentadol; Tetrahydrocannabinol

Decreased Effect

The levels/effects of Dantrolene may be decreased by: Bosentan; CYP3A4 Inducers (Moderate); CYP3A4 Inducers (Strong); Dabrafenib; Deferasirox; Mitotane; Siltuximab; St Johns Wort; Tocilizumab

Storage/Stability

Capsules: Store at 20°C to 25°C (68°F to 77°F).

Injection, powder for reconstitution: Protect from light. Use reconstituted solution within 6 hours of preparation.

Dantrium: Store unreconstituted vials and reconstituted solutions at 15°C to 30°C (59°F to 86°F).

Revonto: Store unreconstituted vials and reconstituted solutions at 20°C to 25°C (68°F to 77°F).

Ryanodex: Store unreconstituted vials at 20°C to 25°C (68°F to 77°F); excursions are permitted between 15°C and 30°C (59°F and 86°F). Store reconstituted solutions at 20°C to 25°C (68°F to 77°F).

Mechanism of Action Acts directly on skeletal muscle by interfering with release of calcium ion from the sarcoplasmic reticulum; prevents or reduces the increase in myoplasmic calcium ion concentration that activates the acute catabolic processes associated with malignant hyperthermia

Pharmacokinetics (Adult data unless noted)

Absorption: Oral: 70% (Allen, 1988)

Distribution: V_d: 36.4 ± 11.7 L

Metabolism: Extensive; major metabolites are 5-hydroxydantrolene and an acetylamino metabolite of dantrolene

Half-life:

Neonates (at birth): ~20 hours (Shime, 1988)

Children 2 to 7 years: 10 hours (range: 8.1 to 14.8 hours) (Lerman, 1989)

Adults: 4 to 11 hours

Time to peak serum concentration: IV: Dantrolene: 1 minute postdose; 5-hydroxydantrolene: 24 hours postdose

Elimination: Urine (25% as metabolites and unchanged drug); feces (45% to 50%)

Dosing: Usual

Pediatric:

Spasticity: Oral: **Note:** Titrate to desired effect; if no further benefit is observed at a higher dosage, decrease dose to previous lower dose.

Manufacturer's labeling: Children and Adolescents ≥5 years:

Patient weight <50 kg: Initial: 0.5 mg/kg/dose once daily for 7 days, increase to 0.5 mg/kg/dose 3 times daily for 7 days, increase to 1 mg/kg/dose 3 times daily for 7 days, and then increase to 2 mg/kg/dose 3 times daily; some patients may require 2 mg/kg/dose 4 times daily; maximum daily dose: 400 mg/**day**

Patient weight ≥50 kg: Initial: 25 mg once daily for 7 days, then increase to 25 mg 3 times daily for 7 days, then increase to 50 mg 3 times daily for 7 days, and then increase to 100 mg 3 times daily; some patients may require 100 mg 4 times daily; maximum daily dose: 400 mg/**day**

Alternate dosing: Children and Adolescents: Initial: 0.5 mg/kg/dose twice daily (maximum dose: 25 mg); titrate frequency at 4 to 7 days to 3 to 4 times daily; then increase dose by 0.5 mg/kg increments at weekly intervals to effect; maximum daily dose: 12 mg/kg/**day** or 400 mg/**day**, whichever is lower (Krause, 2004)

Malignant hyperthermia: Infants, Children, and Adolescents:

Preoperative prophylaxis: **Note:** Routine use not recommended provided that there is immediate availability of parenteral dantrolene and adequate perioperative patient management (eg, avoiding known trigger agents in susceptible patients):

Oral: 4 to 8 mg/kg/**day** in 3 to 4 divided doses for 1 to 2 days prior to surgery with the last dose administered approximately 3 to 4 hours before scheduled surgery

IV: 2.5 mg/kg/dose administered approximately 1.25 hours prior to surgery; infuse over at least 1 minute (Ryanodex) **or** 1 hour (Dantrium, Revonto) with additional doses as needed and individualized

Crisis: IV:

MHAUS protocol recommendation (available at www.-mhaus.org): 2.5 mg/kg; continuously repeat dose until symptoms subside or a cumulative dose of 10 mg/kg is reached (rarely, some patients may require up to 30 mg/kg for initial treatment).

Manufacturer's labeling: Initial minimum dose: 1 mg/kg; repeat dosing with a minimum of 1 mg/kg until symptoms subside or a cumulative dose of 10 mg/kg is reached

24-hour MH Hotline (for emergencies only):

United States: 1-800-644-9737

Outside the U.S.: 00-1-209-417-3722

Postcrisis follow-up:

MHAUS protocol recommendation: 1 mg/kg every 4 to 6 hours (route not specified) **or** a continuous IV infusion of 0.25 mg/kg/hour for at least 24 hours; further doses may be indicated

Manufacturer's labeling: Oral: 4 to 8 mg/kg/day in 4 divided doses for 1 to 3 days; IV dantrolene may be used to prevent or attenuate recurrence of MH signs when oral therapy is not practical; individualize dosage beginning with 1 mg/kg or more as the clinical situation dictates

Adult:

Spasticity: Note: Dose should be titrated and individualized for maximum effect; use the lowest dose compatible with optimal response. Some patients may not respond until a higher daily dosage is achieved; each dose level should be maintained for 7 days to determine patient response. If no further benefit observed with the higher dose level, then decrease dosage to previous dose level. Because of the potential for hepatotoxicity, stop therapy if benefits are not evident within 45 days.

Initial: Oral: 25 mg once daily for 7 days, increase to 25 mg 3 times daily for 7 days, increase to 50 mg 3 times daily for 7 days, and then increase to 100 mg 3 times daily; some patients may require 100 mg 4 times daily; maximum daily dose: 400 mg/**day**

Malignant hyperthermia:

Preoperative prophylaxis: **Note:** Dantrolene prophylaxis is not recommended for most MH-susceptible patients, provided nontriggering anesthetics are used and an adequate supply of dantrolene is available.

Oral: 4 to 8 mg/kg/**day** in 3 to 4 divided doses for 1 to 2 days prior to surgery with the last dose administered approximately 3 to 4 hours before scheduled surgery

IV: 2.5 mg/kg/dose administered approximately 1.25 hours prior to surgery; infuse over at least 1 minute (Ryanodex) **or** 1 hour (Dantrium, Revonto) with additional doses as needed and individualized

Crisis: IV: 2.5 mg/kg (MHAUS recommendation, available at www.mhaus.org); continuously repeat dose until symptoms subside or a cumulative dose of 10 mg/kg is reached (rarely, some patients may require up to 30 mg/kg for initial treatment). **Note:** Manufacturer's labeling suggests an initial minimum dose of 1 mg/kg.

24-hour MH Hotline (for emergencies only):
United States: 1-800-644-9737
Outside the U.S.: 00-1-209-417-3722

Postcrisis follow-up:

MHAUS protocol suggestion: 1 mg/kg every 4 to 6 hours (route not specified) **or** a continuous IV infusion of 0.25 mg/kg/hour for at least 24 hours; further doses may be indicated

Manufacturer's recommendation: Oral: 4 to 8 mg/kg/day in 4 divided doses for 1 to 3 days; IV dantrolene may be used to prevent or attenuate recurrence of MH signs when oral therapy is not practical; individualize dosage beginning with 1 mg/kg or more as the clinical situation dictates

Dosing adjustment in renal impairment: Infants, Children, Adolescents, and Adults: There are no dosage adjustments provided in the manufacturer's labeling.

Dosing adjustments in hepatic impairment: Infants, Children, Adolescents, and Adults: There are no dosage adjustments provided in the manufacturer's labeling; use of oral dantrolene in patients with active liver disease (hepatitis or cirrhosis) is contraindicated.

Preparation for Administration Parenteral:

Dantrium, Revonto: Reconstitute vial by adding 60 mL of SWFI only **(not bacteriostatic water for injection)**, resultant concentration 0.333 mg/mL; shake vial for ~20 seconds or until solution is clear; no further dilution required; avoid glass bottles for IV infusion due to potential for precipitate formation.

Ryanodex: Reconstitute vial by adding 5 mL of SWFI only **(not bacteriostatic water for injection)**; shake well (suspension is an orange color). Do not dilute or transfer the suspension to another container to infuse the product.

Administration

Oral: Contents of capsule may be mixed with juice or liquid

Parenteral:

Dantrium, Revonto: Administer crisis doses by rapid IV injection; preferably in large-bore IV or central line; for intermittent infusion (prophylaxis doses) over 1 hour or continuous IV infusion.

Ryanodex: Administer crisis doses by rapid IV injection; follow-up doses should be administered over at least 1 minute.

Vesicant; ensure proper needle or catheter placement prior to and during infusion; avoid extravasation. If extravasation occurs, stop infusion immediately and disconnect (leave cannula/needle in place); gently aspirate extravasated solution (do **NOT** flush the line); remove needle/cannula; elevate extremity.

Vesicant/Extravasation Risk Vesicant; because of the high pH (~9.5 to 10.3), may cause tissue necrosis if extravasated.

Monitoring Parameters

Spasticity: Motor performance should be monitored for therapeutic outcomes; nausea, vomiting, and liver function tests (baseline and at appropriate intervals thereafter) should be monitored for potential hepatotoxicity

Malignant hyperthermia: Cardiac, respiratory, and blood pressure monitoring; during and postacute phase: Per MHAUS protocol, patient should be observed in an ICU for at least 24 hours since recrudescence may occur; monitor for arrhythmias; monitor vital signs (including core temperature), electrolytes, ABG, CK, end tidal CO_2 ($EtCO_2$)/capnography, urine output, urine myoglobin

Additional Information MHAUS (www.mhaus.org) provides educational and technical information to patients and healthcare providers. Triggers for the development of malignant hyperthermia in susceptible individuals include: All volatile inhalation anesthetics (desflurane, sevoflurane, isoflurane, halothane, enflurane, ether, methoxyflurane, and cyclopropane) and succinylcholine.

Dosage Forms Excipient information presented when available (limited, particularly for generics); consult specific product labeling. [DSC] = Discontinued product

Capsule, Oral, as sodium:
Dantrium: 25 mg, 50 mg, 100 mg [DSC] [contains fd&c yellow #6 (sunset yellow)]
Generic: 25 mg, 50 mg, 100 mg

Solution Reconstituted, Intravenous, as sodium:
Dantrium: 20 mg (1 ea)
Revonto: 20 mg (1 ea)

Suspension Reconstituted, Intravenous, as sodium:
Ryanodex: 250 mg (1 ea) [contains polysorbate 80]

Extemporaneous Preparations A 5 mg/mL oral suspension may be made with dantrolene capsules, a citric acid solution, and either simple syrup or syrup BP (containing 0.15% w/v methylhydroxybenzoate). Add the contents of five 100 mg dantrolene capsules to a citric acid solution (150 mg citric acid powder in 10 mL water); mix while adding the chosen vehicle in incremental proportions to **almost** 100 mL. Transfer to a calibrated bottle and add quantity of vehicle sufficient to make 100 mL. Label "shake well" and "refrigerate". Simple syrup suspension is stable for 2 days refrigerated; syrup BP suspension is stable for 30 days refrigerated.

Nahata MC, Pai VB, and Hipple TF, *Pediatric Drug Formulations*, 5th ed, Cincinnati, OH: Harvey Whitney Books Co, 2004.

◆ **Dantrolene Sodium** *see* Dantrolene *on page 576*

◆ **Dapcin** *see* DAPTOmycin *on page 582*

Dapsone (Systemic) (DAP sone)

Medication Safety Issues

Sound-alike/look-alike issues:
Dapsone may be confused with Diprosone

Therapeutic Category Antibiotic, Sulfone; Leprostatic Agent

Generic Availability (US) Yes

Use Treatment of leprosy due to susceptible strains [FDA approved in pediatric patients (age not specified) and adults]; treatment of dermatitis herpetiformis [FDA approved in pediatric patients (age not specified) and adults]; has also been used for prophylaxis and treatment of *Pneumocystis jirovecii* pneumonia (PCP); prophylaxis against toxoplasmic encephalitis; treatment of linear IgA bullous dermatosis (LABD) and refractory idiopathic thrombocytopenia purpura (ITP)

Pregnancy Risk Factor C

Pregnancy Considerations Adverse events were observed in some animal reproduction studies. Dapsone crosses the placenta (Brabin, 2004). Per the manufacturer, dapsone has not shown an increased risk of congenital anomalies when given during all trimesters of pregnancy. Several reports have described adverse effects in the newborn after *in utero* exposure to dapsone, including neonatal hemolytic disease, methemoglobinemia, and hyperbilirubinemia (Hocking, 1968; Kabra, 1998; Thornton, 1989). Dapsone may be used in pregnant women requiring maintenance therapy of either leprosy or dermatitis herpetiformis. Dapsone may be used as an alternative agent for prophylaxis of *Pneumocystis jirovecii* pneumonia (PCP) in pregnant, HIV-infected patients (DHHS [OI], 2013).

Breast-Feeding Considerations Dapsone is excreted in breast milk and can be detected in the serum of nursing infants. Hemolytic anemia has been reported in a breastfed infant (Sanders, 1982). Due to the potential for serious adverse reactions in the nursing infant, the manufacturer recommends a decision be made whether to discontinue nursing or to discontinue the drug, taking into account the importance of treatment to the mother.

Contraindications Hypersensitivity to dapsone or any component of the formulation

Warnings/Precautions Use with caution in patients with severe anemia, G6PD, methemoglobin reductase deficiency or hemoglobin M deficiency; hypersensitivity to other sulfonamides; aplastic anemia, agranulocytosis and other severe blood dyscrasias have resulted in death; monitor carefully; serious dermatologic reactions (including toxic epidermal necrolysis) are rare but potential occurrences; sulfone reactions may also occur as potentially fatal hypersensitivity reactions; these, but not leprosy reactional states, require drug discontinuation. Motor loss and muscle weakness have been reported with use. Prolonged use may result in fungal or bacterial superinfection, including *C. difficile*-associated diarrhea and pseudomembranous colitis.

Adverse Reactions

Cardiovascular: Tachycardia

Central nervous system: Fever, headache, insomnia, psychosis (oral/topical), vertigo

Dermatologic: Bullous and exfoliative dermatitis, erythema nodosum, exfoliative dermatitis, morbilliform and scarlatiniform reactions, phototoxicity, Stevens-Johnson syndrome, toxic epidermal necrolysis, urticaria

Endocrine & metabolic: Hypoalbuminemia (without proteinuria), male infertility

Gastrointestinal: Abdominal pain, nausea, pancreatitis, vomiting

Hematologic: Agranulocytosis, anemia, leukopenia, pure red cell aplasia (case report); hemolysis (dose related; seen in patients with and without G6PD deficiency), hemoglobin decrease (1-2 g/dL), reticulocyte increase, methemoglobinemia, red cell life span shortened

Hepatic: Cholestatic jaundice, hepatitis

Neuromuscular & skeletal: Drug-induced lupus erythematosus, lower motor neuron toxicity (prolonged therapy), peripheral neuropathy (rare, nonleprosy patients)

Ocular: Blurred vision

Otic: Tinnitus

Renal: Albuminuria, nephrotic syndrome, renal papillary necrosis

Respiratory: Interstitial pneumonitis, pulmonary eosinophilia

Miscellaneous: Infectious mononucleosis-like syndrome (rash, fever, lymphadenopathy, hepatic dysfunction)

Drug Interactions

Metabolism/Transport Effects Substrate of CYP2C19 (minor), CYP2C8 (minor), CYP2C9 (major), CYP2E1 (minor), CYP3A4 (major); **Note:** Assignment of Major/Minor substrate status based on clinically relevant drug interaction potential

Avoid Concomitant Use

Avoid concomitant use of Dapsone (Systemic) with any of the following: BCG; BCG (Intravesical); Conivaptan; Fusidic Acid (Systemic); Idelalisib

Increased Effect/Toxicity

Dapsone (Systemic) may increase the levels/effects of: Antimalarial Agents; Prilocaine; Sodium Nitrite; Trimethoprim

The levels/effects of Dapsone (Systemic) may be increased by: Antimalarial Agents; Conivaptan; CYP2C9 Inhibitors (Moderate); CYP2C9 Inhibitors (Strong); CYP3A4 Inhibitors (Moderate); CYP3A4 Inhibitors (Strong); Dasatinib; Fosaprepitant; Fusidic Acid (Systemic); Idelalisib; Ivacaftor; Luliconazole; Mifepristone; Netupitant; Nitric Oxide; Palbociclib; Probenecid; Simeprevir; Stiripentol; Trimethoprim

Decreased Effect

Dapsone (Systemic) may decrease the levels/effects of: BCG; BCG (Intravesical); BCG Vaccine (Immunization); Sodium Picosulfate; Typhoid Vaccine

The levels/effects of Dapsone (Systemic) may be decreased by: Bosentan; CYP2C9 Inducers (Strong); CYP3A4 Inducers (Moderate); CYP3A4 Inducers (Strong); Dabrafenib; Deferasirox; Mitotane; Rifamycin Derivatives; Siltuximab; St Johns Wort; Tocilizumab

Storage/Stability Store at 20°C to 25°C (68°F to 76°F). Protect from light.

Mechanism of Action Competitive antagonist of para-aminobenzoic acid (PABA) and prevents normal bacterial utilization of PABA for the synthesis of folic acid

Pharmacokinetics (Adult data unless noted)

Absorption: Rapid and almost complete

Distribution: Distributes into skin, muscle, kidneys, liver, sweat, sputum, saliva, tears, and bile

V_d: 1.5 L/kg

Protein binding: Dapsone: 70% to 90%; Metabolite: ~99%

Metabolism: Hepatic (acetylated and hydroxylated)

Half-life:

Children: 15.1 hours (Mirochnick, 1993)

Adults: 28 hours (range: 10-50 hours)

Time to peak serum concentration: Within 4-8 hours

Elimination: ~85% excreted in urine as metabolites

Dosing: Neonatal Linear IgA bullous dermatosis (LABD): Very limited data available: Term infants: Oral: 0.5 or 1 mg/kg/day; dosing based on experience from two case reports (PNA: 9 days and 20 days) which showed a positive response to dapsone therapy; however, adverse effects hindered treatment course. In the case report involving the youngest patient (PNA: 9 days), the initial dose was 1 mg/kg/day with concurrent prednisolone; the dose was increased to 2 mg/kg/day at which point the neonate developed methemoglobinemia by day 14 of treatment and dapsone was temporarily discontinued; a second course was initiated at 9 months of age for another disease flare at 0.5 mg/kg/day (Gluth, 2004). In the other case report (PNA: 20 days), initial therapy was 0.5 mg/kg/day; the dose was later increased to 1 mg/kg/day; while LABD improved on dapsone therapy, the patient developed pneumonia (highly resistant) which required discontinuation of dapsone (Kishida, 2004).

Dosing: Usual

Pediatric:

Dermatitis herpetiformis: Infants, Children, and Adolescents: Oral: 0.5 to 2 mg/kg/day in 1 to 2 divided doses; maximum initial daily dose in adults: 50 mg/**day**; once lesions controlled, the dose may be decreased as tolerated for chronic therapy; usual range: 0.125 to 0.5 mg/kg/day (Ermacora, 1986; Kliegman, 2011)

Idiopathic thrombocytopenic purpura (ITP), refractory: Limited data available: Children ≥3 years and Adolescents: Oral: 1 to 2 mg/kg/day for at least 2 months. Dosing based on two retrospective reviews. The first was a retrospective cohort analysis of adult and pediatric (age range: 3-61 years, including 35 patients <16 years) with chronic ITP (>6 months with diagnosis) who failed steroid therapy and observed an overall similar response rate for children (65.7%) and adults (Damodar, 2005). Adverse effects occurred in three patients (one with acute hemolysis and two with an erythematous rash). The second was a small retrospective report of seven pediatric patients with acute or chronic refractory, symptomatic ITP (age range: 6-15 years) which also showed a similar response rate (60%); however, a higher incidence [two of seven patients (29%)] of methemoglobinemia was observed (Meeker, 2003).

Leprosy: Infants, Children, and Adolescents: Oral:

Multibacillary leprosy (6 patches or more):

Weight-based: 1 mg/kg/dose once daily; continue for 24 months in combination with other leprosy agents; maximum single dose: 100 mg (*Red Book* [AAP], 2012)

Fixed-dose (WHO, 2010):

Children <10 years: 25 mg once daily; continue treatment for 12 months

Children 10-12 years: 50 mg once daily; continue treatment for 12 months

Paucibacillary leprosy (1-5 patches):

Weight-based: 1 to 2 mg/kg/dose once daily; continue for 12 months in combination with other leprosy agents; maximum single dose: 100 mg (*Red Book* [AAP], 2012)

Fixed-dose (WHO, 2010):

Children <10 years: 25 mg once daily; continue treatment for 6 months

Children 10-12 years: 50 mg once daily; continue treatment for 6 months

Linear IgA bullous dermatosis (LABD): Limited data available: Infants, Children, and Adolescents: Oral: 0.5 to 2 mg/kg/day in 1 to 2 divided doses with or without prednisone; maximum initial daily dose in adults for other indications: 50 to 100 mg/day; may increase if needed at weekly intervals; maximum reported daily dose: 4 mg/kg/**day** (Kenani, 2009; Kliegman, 2011; Thappa, 2003)

***Pneumocystis jirovecii* pneumonia (PCP):** Oral:

Prophylaxis (primary or secondary):

Infants and Children (independent of HIV status including HSCT recipient): 2 mg/kg/dose once daily (maximum single dose: 100 mg) **or** 4 mg/kg/dose once **weekly**; maximum single weekly dose: 200 mg) (CDC/IDSA [Tomblyn], 2009; DHHS [pediatric], 2013; *Red Book* [AAP], 2012)

Adolescents (HIV-exposed/-positive or HSCT recipient): 100 mg/day in 1 or 2 divided doses as monotherapy **or** 50 mg once daily in combination with weekly pyrimethamine and leucovorin **or** 200 mg once **weekly** in combination with weekly pyrimethamine and leucovorin; monotherapy should not be used in patients who are seropositive for *Toxoplasma gondii* (CDC/IDSA [Tomblyn], 2009; DHHS [adult], 2013)

Treatment, mild to moderate disease: Infants, Children, and Adolescents (independent of HIV status): 2 mg/kg/dose once daily in combination with trimethoprim for 21 days; maximum single dose: 100 mg (DHHS [adult], 2013; *Red Book* [AAP], 2012)

***Toxoplasma gondii*, primary prophylaxis:** Oral:

Infants and Children (independent of HIV status): 2 mg/kg/dose **or** 15 mg/m^2/dose once daily in combination with pyrimethamine and leucovorin; maximum single dose: 25 mg; a weekly regimen typically used for PCP prophylaxis but which also covers toxoplasma is 4 mg/kg/dose once **weekly** in combination with weekly pyrimethamine and leucovorin; maximum single weekly dose: 200 mg (DHHS [pediatric], 2013; *Red Book* [AAP], 2012)

Adolescents (HIV-exposed/-positive): 50 mg once daily in combination with weekly pyrimethamine and leucovorin or 200 mg once **weekly** in combination with weekly pyrimethamine and leucovorin (DHHS [adult], 2013)

Adult:

Dermatitis herpetiformis: Oral: Initial: 50 mg once daily; increase to 300 mg daily or higher to achieve full control; reduce dosage to minimal level as soon as possible

Leprosy: Oral: 100 mg once daily in combination with other antileprosy drugs; duration of therapy is variable

Dosing adjustment in renal impairment: There are no dosage adjustments provided in the manufacturer's labeling; however, some clinicians have used the following: Infants, Children, and Adolescents: No adjustment necessary (Aronoff, 2007).

Dosing adjustment in hepatic impairment: There are no dosage adjustments provided in the manufacturer's labeling.

Administration Oral: May administer with meals if GI upset occurs.

Monitoring Parameters CBC with differential (weekly for the first month, monthly for 6 months, then semiannually), reticulocyte count, and liver function tests; check G-6-PD levels prior to initiation of dapsone; monitor for signs of jaundice, hemolysis, or methemoglobinemia.

Additional Information The National Hansen's Disease (Leprosy) Programs (NHDP) may be contacted for further information regarding disease consultation and acquisition of necessary medication (http://www.hrsa.gov/hansensdisease/index.htm)

Dosage Forms Excipient information presented when available (limited, particularly for generics); consult specific product labeling.

Tablet, Oral:

Generic: 25 mg, 100 mg

Extemporaneous Preparations A 2 mg/mL oral suspension may be made with tablets and a 1:1 mixture of Ora-Sweet® and Ora-Plus®. Crush eight 25 mg tablets in a mortar and reduce to a fine powder. Add small portions of vehicle and mix to a uniform paste; mix while adding the vehicle in incremental proportions to **almost** 100 mL; transfer to a calibrated bottle, rinse mortar with vehicle, and add quantity of vehicle sufficient to make 100 mL. Label "shake well". Stable for 90 days at room temperature or refrigerated.

Jacobus Pharmaceutical Company makes a 2 mg/mL proprietary liquid formulation available under an IND for the prophylaxis of *Pneumocystis jirovecii* pneumonia.

Nahata MC, Morosco RS, and Trowbridge JM, "Stability of Dapsone in Two Oral Liquid Dosage Forms," *Ann Pharmacother*, 2000, 34 (7-8):848-50.

Dapsone (Topical) (DAP sone)

Medication Safety Issues

Sound-alike/look-alike issues:

Dapsone may be confused with Diprosone

Brand Names: US Aczone

Brand Names: Canada Aczone

Generic Availability (US) No

Use Topical treatment of acne vulgaris (FDA approved in ages 12-17 years and adults)

Pregnancy Risk Factor C

Pregnancy Considerations Adverse events were observed in some animal reproduction studies. The amount of dapsone available systemically is less following topical application than with oral administration. If treatment for acne is deemed necessary during pregnancy, topical agents other than dapsone are currently recommended (Gollnick, 2003; Meredith, 2013).

Breast-Feeding Considerations Following oral administration, dapsone is excreted into breast milk. Due to the potential for serious adverse reactions in the nursing infant, the manufacturer recommends a decision be made whether to discontinue nursing or to discontinue the drug, taking into account the importance of treatment to the mother

Contraindications

There are no contraindications listed in the manufacturer's labeling.

Canadian labeling: Hypersensitivity to dapsone or any component of the formulation or container.

Warnings/Precautions Changes suggestive of mild hemolysis have been observed in some patients with glucose-6-phosphate dehydrogenase (G6PD) deficiency and using dapsone gel; discontinue use with signs/symptoms of hemolytic anemia. Do not use concomitantly with oral dapsone or other antimalarial agents due to increased risk of hemolytic reactions. Potentially significant drug-drug interactions may exist, requiring dose or frequency adjustment, additional monitoring, and/or selection of alternative therapy. Localized discoloration (yellow or orange) of the skin or facial hair may occur if benzoyl peroxide is used subsequent to dapsone gel; typically resolves in ~1 to 8 weeks. Skin reactions (eg, bullous and exfoliative dermatitis, erythema multiforme, erythema nodosum, morbilliform and scarlatiniform reactions, toxic epidermal necrolysis, urticaria) and peripheral neuropathy have been reported with oral dapsone; similar events were not observed during clinical trials with topical dapsone.

Adverse Reactions

Central nervous system: Suicidal tendencies, tonic-clonic movements

Gastrointestinal: Abdominal pain, pancreatitis, severe vomiting

Respiratory: Pharyngitis, sinusitis

Rare but important or life-threatening: Depression, erythema, facial edema, methemoglobinemia (Swartzentruber 2015), psychosis

Drug Interactions

Metabolism/Transport Effects Substrate of CYP2C19 (minor), CYP2C8 (minor), CYP2C9 (minor), CYP2E1 (minor), CYP3A4 (minor); **Note:** Assignment of Major/Minor substrate status based on clinically relevant drug interaction potential

Avoid Concomitant Use

Avoid concomitant use of Dapsone (Topical) with any of the following: BCG; BCG (Intravesical)

Increased Effect/Toxicity

The levels/effects of Dapsone (Topical) may be increased by: Antimalarial Agents; Benzoyl Peroxide; Trimethoprim

Decreased Effect

Dapsone (Topical) may decrease the levels/effects of: BCG; BCG (Intravesical); BCG Vaccine (Immunization); Sodium Picosulfate

Storage/Stability Store at 20°C to 25°C (68°F to 76°F). Do not freeze.

Dosing: Usual Acne vulgaris: Children ≥12 years, Adolescents, and Adults: Topical: Apply a pea-sized amount of gel to the acne-affected areas twice daily; re-evaluate patient if no improvement after 12 weeks of therapy

Dosage adjustment in renal impairment: No dosage adjustment provided in manufacturer's labeling; has not been studied.

Dosage adjustment in hepatic impairment: No dosage adjustment provided in manufacturer's labeling; has not been studied.

Administration Topical: Wash skin and pat dry then rub in thin layer of gel gently and completely. Wash hands after application.

Dosage Forms Excipient information presented when available (limited, particularly for generics); consult specific product labeling.

Gel, External:

Aczone: 5% (30 g, 60 g, 90 g) [contains methylparaben]

◆ **Daptacel** *see* Diphtheria and Tetanus Toxoids, and Acellular Pertussis Vaccine *on page 681*

DAPTOmycin (DAP toe mye sin)

Medication Safety Issues

Sound-alike/look-alike issues:

Cubicin may be confused with Cleocin

DAPTOmycin may be confused with DACTINomycin

Brand Names: US Cubicin

Brand Names: Canada Cubicin

Therapeutic Category Antibiotic, Cyclic Lipopeptide

Generic Availability (US) No

Use Treatment of complicated skin and skin structure infections caused by susceptible aerobic gram-positive organisms including *S. aureus* [methicillin-susceptible *Staph. aureus* (MSSA) and methicillin-resistant *Staph. aureus* (MRSA)], *S. pyogenes*, *S. agalactiae*, *S. dysgalactiae*, and *E. faecalis* (FDA approved in ages ≥18 years). Treatment of *S. aureus* bacteremia, including right-sided infective endocarditis caused by MSSA or MRSA (FDA approved in ages ≥18 years). Daptomycin is active against bacteria resistant to methicillin, vancomycin, and linezolid.

Pregnancy Risk Factor B

Pregnancy Considerations Adverse events were not observed in animal reproduction studies. Successful use of daptomycin during the second and third trimesters of pregnancy has been described; however, only limited information is available from case reports.

Breast-Feeding Considerations Low concentrations of daptomycin have been detected in breast milk; however, daptomycin is poorly absorbed orally. The manufacturer recommends caution if daptomycin is used during breast-feeding. Per the Canadian product labeling, daptomycin should be discontinued while breast-feeding. Nondose-related effects could include modification of bowel flora.

Contraindications Hypersensitivity to daptomycin

Warnings/Precautions May be associated with an increased incidence of myopathy; discontinue in patients with signs and symptoms of myopathy in conjunction with an increase in CPK (>5 times ULN or 1,000 units/L) or in asymptomatic patients with a CPK ≥10 times ULN. Myopathy may occur more frequently at dose and/or frequency in excess of recommended dosages. Consider temporarily interrupting therapy with other agents associated with an increased risk of myopathy (eg, HMG-CoA reductase inhibitors) during daptomycin therapy. Not indicated for the treatment of pneumonia (inactivation by pulmonary surfactant). Use caution in renal impairment (dosage adjustment required severe renal impairment [CrCl <30 mL/minute]). Limited data (eg, subgroup analysis) from cSSSI and endocarditis trials suggest possibly reduced clinical efficacy (relative to comparators) in patients with baseline moderate renal impairment (<50 mL/minute).

Symptoms suggestive of peripheral neuropathy have been observed with treatment; monitor for new-onset or worsening neuropathy. Prolonged use may result in fungal or bacterial superinfection, including *C. difficile*-associated diarrhea (CDAD) and pseudomembranous colitis; CDAD has been observed >2 months postantibiotic treatment.

Repeat blood cultures in patients with persisting or relapsing *S. aureus* bacteremia/endocarditis or poor clinical response. If culture is positive for *S. aureus*, perform minimum inhibitory concentration (MIC) susceptibility testing of the isolate and diagnostic evaluation of the patient to rule out sequestered foci of infection. Appropriate surgical intervention (eg, debridement, removal of prosthetic devices, valve replacement surgery) and/or consideration of a change in antibacterial therapy may be necessary. Hypersensitivity reactions and anaphylaxis (including angioedema, and drug rash with eosinophilia and systemic symptoms [DRESS]) have been reported with use; discontinue use immediately with signs/symptoms of hypersensitivity and initiate appropriate treatment. Use has been associated with eosinophilic pneumonia; generally develops 2 to 4 weeks after therapy initiation. Monitor for signs/symptoms of eosinophilic pneumonia, including new onset or worsening fever, dyspnea, difficulty breathing, new infiltrates on chest imaging studies, and/or >25% eosinophils present in bronchoalveolar lavage. Discontinue use immediately with signs/symptoms of eosinophilic pneumonia and initiate appropriate treatment (ie, corticosteroids). May reoccur with re-exposure. Although not approved for use in children, the manufacturer recommends to avoid use in pediatric patients <12 months due to risk of potential muscular, neuromuscular, and/or nervous systems effects observed in neonatal canines.

Warnings: Additional Pediatric Considerations Avoid use in neonatal and pediatric patients <12 month (per the manufacturer); neonatal animal models (canine) have shown reversible musculoskeletal, neuromuscular, and nervous system adverse effects including twitching, muscle rigidity of the limbs, and impaired use of the limbs; adverse effects were observed at lower serum concentrations than older canine models (approximately threefold less than juvenile models and ninefold less than adult models) and resolved within 28 days of discontinuation. The neuromuscular/skeletal adverse events occurred with canine doses and drug exposure levels that were higher than the standard adult human dose (6 mg/kg) and corresponding daptomycin exposure levels.

Adverse Reactions

Cardiovascular: Chest pain, hypertension, hypotension, peripheral edema

Central nervous system: Anxiety, dizziness, headache, insomnia

Dermatologic: Diaphoresis, erythema, pruritus, skin rash

Endocrine & metabolic: Hyperkalemia, hyperphosphatemia, hypokalemia

Gastrointestinal: Abdominal pain, constipation, diarrhea, dyspepsia, gastrointestinal hemorrhage, loose stools, nausea, vomiting

Genitourinary: Urinary tract infection

Hematologic & oncologic: Anemia, eosinophilia, increased INR

Hepatic: Increased serum alkaline phosphatase, increased serum transaminases

Infection: Bacteremia, fungal infection, gram-negative organism infection, sepsis

Local: Injection site reaction

Neuromuscular & skeletal: Arthralgia, back pain, increased creatine phosphokinase, limb pain, osteomyelitis, weakness

Renal: Renal failure

Respiratory: Cough, dyspnea, pneumonia, pharyngolaryngeal pain, pleural effusion

Miscellaneous: Fever

Rare but important or life-threatening: Anaphylaxis, atrial fibrillation, atrial flutter, candidiasis, cardiac arrest, *Clostridium difficile* associated diarrhea, coma (post anaesthesia/surgery), eczema, eosinophilic pneumonitis, hallucination, hypomagnesemia, hypersensitivity, jaundice, increased lactate dehydrogenase, lymphadenopathy, mental status changes, neutropenia (Knoll, 2013), oral candidiasis, peripheral neuropathy, proteinuria, prolonged prothrombin time, renal insufficiency, rhabdomyolysis, increased serum bicarbonate, Stevens-Johnson syndrome, stomatitis, supraventricular cardiac arrhythmia, thrombocytopenia, thrombocythemia

Drug Interactions

Metabolism/Transport Effects None known.

Avoid Concomitant Use There are no known interactions where it is recommended to avoid concomitant use.

Increased Effect/Toxicity

The levels/effects of DAPTOmycin may be increased by: HMG-CoA Reductase Inhibitors

Decreased Effect There are no known significant interactions involving a decrease in effect.

Storage/Stability

Store original packages at 2°C to 8°C (36°F to 46°F); avoid excessive heat. Daptomycin vials are for single use only.

U.S. labeling: Reconstituted solution is stable in the vial for 12 hours at room temperature or up to 48 hours if refrigerated at 2°C to 8°C (36°F to 46°F). The diluted solution is stable in the infusion bag for 12 hours at room temperature or 48 hours if refrigerated. The combined time (reconstituted solution in vial and diluted solution in infusion bag) should not exceed 12 hours at room temperature or 48 hours refrigerated.

Canadian labeling: Reconstituted solution is stable in the vial or infusion solution for 12 hours at 25°C (77°F) or up to 10 days if refrigerated at 2°C to 8°C (36°F to 46°F) under normal lighting. The manufacturer recommends using reconstituted solution within 72 hours if stored under refrigeration. The combined time (reconstituted solution in vial and diluted solution in infusion bag) should not exceed 12 hours at up to 25°C (77°F) or 10 days at 2°C to 8°C (36°F to 46°F).

Mechanism of Action Daptomycin binds to components of the cell membrane of susceptible organisms and causes rapid depolarization, inhibiting intracellular synthesis of DNA, RNA, and protein. Daptomycin is bactericidal in a concentration-dependent manner.

Pharmacokinetics (Adult data unless noted)

Distribution: V_d:

- Neonates and Infants <3 months: Median: 0.21 L/kg (range: 0.11-0.34 L/kg) (Cohen-Wolkowiez, 2012)
- Children 2-6 years: 0.14 L/kg (Abdel-Rahman, 2008; Abdel-Rahman, 2011)
- Children 7-17 years: 0.11 ± 0.02 L/kg (Abdel-Rahman, 2008)
- Adults: 0.1 L/kg; Critically ill: V_{ss}: 0.23 ± 0.14 L/kg (Vilay, 2010)

Protein binding: 90% to 93%; patients with renal impairment (CrCl <30 mL/minute): 84% to 88%

Metabolism: Minor amounts of oxidative metabolites have been detected; does not induce or inhibit cytochrome P450 enzymes

Half-life:

- Neonates and Infants <3 months: Median: 6.2 hours (range: 3.7-9 hours) (Cohen-Wolkowiez, 2012)
- Children 2-6 years: Mean range: 5.3-5.7 hours (Abdel-Rahman, 2008; Abdel-Rahman, 2011)
- Children 7-11 years: 5.6 ± 2.2 hours (Abdel-Rahman, 2008)
- Children 12-17 years: 6.7 ± 2.2 hours (Abdel-Rahman, 2008)
- Adults: 8-9 hours; prolonged with renal impairment up to 28 hours

Elimination: 78% of the dose excreted in urine primarily as unchanged drug; feces (6%)

Clearance:

- Neonates and Infants <3 months: Median: 21 mL/hour/kg (range: 16-34 mL/hour/kg) (Cohen-Wolkowiez, 2012)

Children 2-6 years: 19-20 mL/hour/kg (Abdel-Rahman, 2008; Abdel-Rahman, 2011)
Children 7-11 years: 17 mL/hour/kg (Abdel-Rahman, 2008)
Children: 12-17 years: 11 mL/hour/kg (Abdel-Rahman, 2008)
Adults: 8.3-9 mL/hour/kg

Dialysis: 15% removed by 4-hour hemodialysis session; high permeability intermittent hemodialysis removes ~50% during a 4-hour session (Salama, 2010)

Dosing: Neonatal Note: In pediatric patients, daptomycin is not routinely used as first-line therapy. The manufacturer recommends avoiding use in patients <12 months due to musculoskeletal, neuromuscular, and nervous system adverse effects observed in neonatal canine models.

Gram-positive infection, severe: Very limited data available: PMA ≥32 weeks: IV: 6 mg/kg/dose every 12 hours for 10-14 days was used in two neonates [patient age: PMA 32 weeks (PNA: 8 weeks) and PMA: 35 weeks (PNA: 3 weeks)] with normal renal function (Cohen-Wolkowiez, 2008). A pharmacokinetic study of 20 neonates and infants [GA: Median: 32 weeks (range: 23-40 weeks); PNA: Median: 3 days (range: 1-85 days)] evaluated a single 6 mg/kg dose and reported median AUC exposure ~60% of that achieved in adults with standard adult dosing and a faster clearance than adults and adolescents (Cohen-Wolkowiez, 2012).

Dosage adjustment in renal impairment: Data limited to a single case report: A full-term neonate (PNA: 41 days) with decreased renal function (S_{cr}: 0.9 mg/dL), an initial dose of 4 mg/kg/dose every 48 hours was used and increased to 6 mg/kg/dose every 36 hours upon a decrease in serum creatinine (S_{cr}: 0.6 mg/dL) and daptomycin serum concentration evaluation which showed a subtherapeutic peak value (Beneri, 2008).

Dosing: Usual

Pediatric: **Note:** In pediatric patients, daptomycin is not routinely used as first-line therapy. The manufacturer recommends avoiding use in patients <12 months due to musculoskeletal, neuromuscular, and nervous system adverse effects observed in neonatal canine models.

General dosing, susceptible organisms (severe infection): Limited data available:

Children 2-6 years: IV: 8-10 mg/kg/dose once daily (*Red Book*, 2012); in a pharmacokinetic study of 12 children (age: 2-6 years) dosages presented showed similar serum concentrations to standard adult doses (4-6 mg/kg) (Abdel-Rahman, 2011; *Red Book*, 2012)
Children ≥6 years to <12 years: IV: 7 mg/kg/dose once daily (*Red Book*, 2012)
Children ≥12 years and Adolescents: IV: 4-6 mg/kg/dose once daily (*Red Book*, 2012)

MRSA Infection: Limited data available (Lui, 2011):

Bacteremia: Children and Adolescents: IV: 6-10 mg/kg/dose once daily
Endocarditis, infective (prosthetic valve): Children and Adolescents: IV: 6-10 mg/kg/dose once daily
Osteomyeolitis, or septic arthritis: Children and Adolescents: IV: 6-10 mg/kg/dose once daily

Note: IDSA guidelines state ongoing pediatric daptomycin clinical trials focus on an inverse relationship between age and required per kg dose; the following daily doses are under investigation in children and adolescents (Clinicaltrials.gov NCT 00711802)
Children 2-6 years: IV: 9 mg/kg/dose once daily
Children: 7-11 years: IV: 7 mg/kg/dose once daily
Children and Adolescents 12-17 years: IV: 5 mg/kg/dose once daily

Adult:

Skin and/or skin structure infections (complicated): IV: 4 mg/kg/dose once daily for 7-14 days

Bacteremia, right-sided native valve endocarditis caused by MSSA or MRSA: IV: 6 mg/kg/dose once daily for 2-6 weeks [some experts recommend 8-10 mg/kg once daily for complicated bacteremia or infective endocarditis (Liu, 2011)]

Dosage adjustment in renal impairment:

Children ≥2 years and Adolescents: The following dosage adjustments have been recommended (Aronoff, 2007): IV:
GFR >30 mL/minute/1.73 m^2: Administer full dose
GFR 10-29 mL/minute/1.73 m^2: Administer 67% of a full dose every 24 hours
GFR <10 mL/minute/1.73 m^2: Administer 67% of a full dose every 48 hours
Hemodialysis: Administer 67% of a full dose every 48 hours after dialysis
Peritoneal dialysis: Administer 67% of a full dose every 48 hours

Adults: IV:

CrCl <30 mL/minute:
Skin and soft tissue infections: 4 mg/kg/dose every 48 hours
Staphylococcal bacteremia: 6 mg/kg/dose every 48 hours

Intermittent hemodialysis or peritoneal dialysis (PD): Dose as in CrCl <30 mL/minute (administer after hemodialysis on dialysis days) **or** (off-label dosing) may administer 6 mg/kg/dose after hemodialysis 3 times weekly (Salama, 2010)
Note: High permeability intermittent hemodialysis removes ~50% during a 4-hour session (Salama, 2010)

Continuous renal replacement therapy (CRRT) (Heintz, 2009; Trotman, 2005): Drug clearance is highly dependent on the method of renal replacement, filter type, and flow rate. Appropriate dosing requires close monitoring of pharmacologic response, signs of adverse reactions due to drug accumulation, as well as drug concentrations in relation to target trough (if appropriate). The following are general recommendations only (based on dialysate flow/ultrafiltration rates of 1-2 L/hour and minimal residual renal function) and should not supersede clinical judgment:

Continuous veno-venous hemodialysis (CVVHD): 8 mg/kg/dose every 48 hours (Vilay, 2010)
Note: For other forms of CRRT (eg, CVVH or CVVHDF), dosing as with CrCl <30 mL/minute may result in low C_{max}. May consider 4-6 mg/kg/dose every 24 hours (or 8 mg/kg every 48 hours) depending on site or severity of infection or if not responding to standard dosing; therapeutic drug monitoring and/or more frequent serum CPK levels may be necessary (Heintz, 2009).

Slow extended daily dialysis (or extended dialysis): 6 mg/kg/dose every 24 hours (Kielstein, 2010). **Note:** Dialysis should be initiated within 8 hours of administering daptomycin dose to avoid dose accumulation.

Dosage adjustment in hepatic impairment: No adjustment required for mild-to-moderate impairment (Child-Pugh Class A or B); not evaluated in severe hepatic impairment (Child-Pugh Class C)

Preparation for Administration IV: Reconstitute vial with 10 mL NS to a concentration of 50 mg/mL. Add NS to vial and rotate gently to wet powder. Allow vial to stand for 10 minutes, then gently swirl to obtain completely reconstituted solution. Do not shake or agitate vial vigorously.

Neonates: Dilution information has not been reported.
Children 2 to 6 years: Further dilute in 25 mL of NS (Abdel-Rahman 2011)
Children and Adolescents 7 to 17 years: Further dilute in 50 mL of NS (Abdel-Rahman 2008)
Adult: Further dilute in 50 mL NS prior to administration.

Administration IV:

Neonates: Infusion over 60 minutes has been reported in trials (Cohen-Wolkowiez 2012)

Children 2 to 6 years: Infusion over 60 minutes has been reported in trials (Abdel-Rahman 2011)

Children and Adolescents 7 to 17 years: Infusion over 30 minutes has been reported in trials (Abdel-Rahman 2008)

Adults: May administer undiluted IV push over 2 minutes or further dilute and infuse IVPB over 30 minutes

Do not use in conjunction with ReadyMED elastomeric infusion pumps (Cardinal Health, Inc) due to an impurity (2-mercaptobenzothiazole) which leaches from the pump system into the daptomycin solution.

Monitoring Parameters Signs and symptoms of myopathy (muscle pain or weakness, particularly of the distal extremities), weekly CPK levels during therapy (more frequent monitoring if history of current or prior statin therapy and/or renal impairment), signs of peripheral neuropathy; observe for changes in bowel frequency; monitor renal function periodically

Reference Range Adults:

Trough concentrations at steady-state:

4 mg/kg once daily: 5.9 ± 1.6 mcg/mL

6 mg/kg once daily: 6.7 ± 1.6 mcg/mL

Note: Trough concentrations are not predictive of efficacy/toxicity. Daptomycin exhibits concentration-dependent bactericidal activity, so C_{max}:MIC ratios may be a more useful parameter.

Test Interactions Daptomycin may cause false prolongation of the PT and increase of INR with certain recombinant thromboplastin reagents. This appears to be a dose-dependent phenomenon. If PT/INR is elevated, repeat PT/INR immediately prior to next daptomycin dose (eg, trough). If PT/INR remains elevated, repeat PT/INR using alternate reagents (if available) and evaluate for other causes of elevated PT/INR.

Dosage Forms Excipient information presented when available (limited, particularly for generics); consult specific product labeling.

Solution Reconstituted, Intravenous [preservative free]:

Cubicin: 500 mg (1 ea)

◆ **Daraprim** *see* Pyrimethamine *on page 1812*

◆ **Daraprim [DSC] (Can)** *see* Pyrimethamine *on page 1812*

Darbepoetin Alfa (dar be POE e tin AL fa)

Medication Safety Issues

Sound-alike/look-alike issues:

Aranesp may be confused with Aralast, Aricept

Darbepoetin alfa may be confused with dalteparin, epoetin alfa, epoetin beta

Brand Names: US Aranesp (Albumin Free)

Brand Names: Canada Aranesp

Therapeutic Category Colony-Stimulating Factor; Erythropoiesis Stimulating Protein; Hematopoietic Agent

Generic Availability (US) No

Use Treatment of anemia due to chronic kidney disease (FDA approved in ages ≥1 year and adults) or anemia associated with concurrent myelosuppressive chemotherapy for nonmyeloid malignancies receiving chemotherapy (palliative intent) for a planned minimum of 2 additional months of chemotherapy (FDA approved in adults)

Prescribing and Access Restrictions As a requirement of the REMS program, access to this medication is restricted. Healthcare providers and hospitals must be enrolled in the ESA APPRISE (Assisting Providers and Cancer Patients with Risk Information for the Safe use of ESAs) Oncology Program (866-284-8089; http://www.esa-apprise.com) to prescribe or dispense ESAs (ie, darbepoetin alfa, epoetin alfa) to patients with cancer.

Medication Guide Available Yes

Pregnancy Risk Factor C

Pregnancy Considerations Adverse events were observed in animal reproduction studies. Women who become pregnant during treatment with darbepoetin are encouraged to enroll in Amgen's Pregnancy Surveillance Program (800-772-6436).

Breast-Feeding Considerations It is not known if darbepoetin alfa is excreted in breast milk. The manufacturer recommends that caution be exercised when administering darbepoetin alfa to nursing women.

Contraindications Hypersensitivity to darbepoetin or any component of the formulation; uncontrolled hypertension; pure red cell aplasia (due to darbepoetin or other erythropoietin protein drugs)

Warnings/Precautions [U.S. Boxed Warning]: Erythropoiesis-stimulating agents (ESAs) increased the risk of serious cardiovascular events, thromboembolic events, stroke, and/or tumor progression in clinical studies when administered to target hemoglobin levels >11 g/dL (and provide no additional benefit); a rapid rise in hemoglobin (>1 g/dL over 2 weeks) may also contribute to these risks. **[U.S. Boxed Warning]: A shortened overall survival and/or increased risk of tumor progression or recurrence has been reported in studies with breast, cervical, head and neck, lymphoid, and non-small cell lung cancer patients.** It is of note that in these studies, patients received ESAs to a target hemoglobin of ≥12 g/dL; although risk has not been excluded when dosed to achieve a target hemoglobin of <12 g/dL. **[U.S. Boxed Warnings]: To decrease these risks, and risk of cardio- and thrombovascular events, use ESAs in cancer patients only for the treatment of anemia related to concurrent myelosuppressive chemotherapy and use the lowest dose needed to avoid red blood cell transfusions. Discontinue ESA following completion of the chemotherapy course. ESAs are <u>not</u> indicated for patients receiving myelosuppressive therapy when the anticipated outcome is curative.** A dosage modification is appropriate if hemoglobin levels rise >1 g/dL per 2-week time period during treatment (Rizzo, 2010). Use of ESAs has been associated with an increased risk of venous thromboembolism (VTE) without a reduction in transfusions in patients >65 years of age with cancer (Hershman, 2009). Improved anemia symptoms, quality of life, fatigue, or well-being have not been demonstrated in controlled clinical trials. **[U.S. Boxed Warning]: Because of the risks of decreased survival and increased risk of tumor growth or progression, all healthcare providers and hospitals are required to enroll and comply with the ESA APPRISE (Assisting Providers and Cancer Patients with Risk Information for the Safe use of ESAs) Oncology Program prior to prescribing or dispensing ESAs to cancer patients.** Prescribers and patients will have to provide written documentation of discussed risks prior to each course.

[U.S. Boxed Warning]: An increased risk of death, serious cardiovascular events, and stroke was reported in patients with chronic kidney disease (CKD) administered ESAs to target hemoglobin levels ≥11 g/dL; use the lowest dose sufficient to reduce the need for RBC transfusions. An optimal target hemoglobin level, dose or dosing strategy to reduce these risks has not been identified in clinical trials. Hemoglobin rising >1 g/dL in a 2-week period may contribute to the risk (dosage reduction recommended). The American College of Physicians recommends against the use of ESAs in patients with mild to moderate anemia and heart failure or coronary heart disease (ACP [Qaseem, 2013]).

CKD patients who exhibit an inadequate hemoglobin response to ESA therapy may be at a higher risk for cardiovascular events and mortality compared to other patients. ESA therapy may reduce dialysis efficacy (due to increase in red blood cells and decrease in plasma volume); adjustments in dialysis parameters may be needed. Patients treated with epoetin may require increased heparinization during dialysis to prevent clotting of the extracorporeal circuit. CKD patients not requiring dialysis may have a better response to darbepoetin and may require lower doses. An increased risk of DVT has been observed in patients treated with epoetin undergoing surgical orthopedic procedures. Darbepoetin is **not** approved for reduction in allogeneic red blood cell transfusions in patients scheduled for surgical procedures. The risk for seizures is increased with darbepoetin use in patients with CKD; use with caution in patients with a history of seizures. Monitor closely for neurologic symptoms during the first several months of therapy. Use with caution in patients with hypertension; hypertensive encephalopathy has been reported. Use is contraindicated in patients with uncontrolled hypertension. If hypertension is difficult to control, reduce or hold darbepoetin alfa. Due to the delayed onset of erythropoiesis, darbepoetin alfa is **not** recommended for acute correction of severe anemia or as a substitute for emergency transfusion. Consider discontinuing in patients who receive a renal transplant.

Prior to treatment, correct or exclude deficiencies of iron, vitamin B_{12}, and/or folate, as well as other factors which may impair erythropoiesis (inflammatory conditions, infections, bleeding). Prior to and during therapy, iron stores must be evaluated. Supplemental iron is recommended if serum ferritin <100 mcg/L or serum transferrin saturation <20%; most patients with CKD will require iron supplementation. Poor response should prompt evaluation of these potential factors, as well as possible malignant processes and hematologic disease (thalassemia, refractory anemia, myelodysplastic disorder), occult blood loss, hemolysis, osteitis fibrosa cystic, and/or bone marrow fibrosis. Severe anemia and pure red cell aplasia (PRCA) with associated neutralizing antibodies to erythropoietin has been reported, predominantly in patients with CKD receiving SubQ darbepoetin (the IV route is preferred for hemodialysis patients). Cases have also been reported in patients with hepatitis C who were receiving ESAs, interferon, and ribavirin. Patients with a sudden loss of response to darbepoetin (with severe anemia and a low reticulocyte count) should be evaluated for PRCA with associated neutralizing antibodies to erythropoietin; discontinue treatment (permanently) in patients with PRCA secondary to neutralizing antibodies to erythropoietin. Antibodies may cross-react; do not switch to another ESA in patients who develop antibody-mediated anemia.

Potentially serious allergic reactions have been reported (rarely). Discontinue immediately (and permanently) in patients who experience serious allergic/anaphylactic reactions. Some products may contain latex. Some dosage forms may contain polysorbate 80 (also known as Tweens). Hypersensitivity reactions, usually a delayed reaction, have been reported following exposure to pharmaceutical products containing polysorbate 80 in certain individuals (Isaksson, 2002; Lucente 2000; Shelley, 1995). Thrombocytopenia, ascites, pulmonary deterioration, and renal and hepatic failure have been reported in premature neonates after receiving parenteral products containing polysorbate 80 (Alade, 1986; CDC, 1984). See manufacturer's labeling.

Adverse Reactions

Cardiovascular: Angina pectoris, edema, hypotension, myocardial infarction, hypertension, peripheral edema, pulmonary embolism, thromboembolism, thrombosis of vascular graft (arteriovenous), vascular injury (vascular access complications)

Central nervous system: Cerebrovascular disease

Dermatologic: Erythema, skin rash

Endocrine & metabolic: Hypervolemia

Gastrointestinal: Abdominal pain

Respiratory: Cough, dyspnea

Rare but important or life-threatening: Anaphylaxis, anemia (associated with neutralizing antibodies; severe; with or without other cytopenias), angioedema, bronchospasm, cerebrovascular accident, hypersensitivity reaction, hypertensive encephalopathy, pure red cell aplasia, seizure, tumor growth (progression/recurrence; cancer patients), urticaria

Drug Interactions

Metabolism/Transport Effects None known.

Avoid Concomitant Use There are no known interactions where it is recommended to avoid concomitant use.

Increased Effect/Toxicity

Darbepoetin Alfa may increase the levels/effects of: Lenalidomide; Thalidomide

The levels/effects of Darbepoetin Alfa may be increased by: Nandrolone

Decreased Effect There are no known significant interactions involving a decrease in effect.

Storage/Stability Store at 2°C to 8°C (36°F to 46°F); do not freeze. Do not shake. Protect from light. Store in original carton until use. The following stability information has also been reported: May be stored at room temperature for up to 7 days (Cohen, 2007).

Mechanism of Action Induces erythropoiesis by stimulating the division and differentiation of committed erythroid progenitor cells; induces the release of reticulocytes from the bone marrow into the bloodstream, where they mature to erythrocytes. There is a dose response relationship with this effect. This results in an increase in reticulocyte counts followed by a rise in hematocrit and hemoglobin levels. When administered SubQ or IV, darbepoetin's half-life is ~3 times that of epoetin alfa concentrations.

Pharmacodynamics

Onset of action: Several days

Maximum effect: 4-6 weeks

Pharmacokinetics (Adult data unless noted)

Absorption: SubQ: Slow and rate-limiting

Distribution: V_d:
- Children: 51.6 mL/kg (range: 21-73 mL/kg)
- Adults: 52.4 ± 6.6 mL/kg

Bioavailability: SubQ: CKD:
- Children: 54% (range: 32% to 70%)
- Adults: ~37% (range: 30% to 50%)

Half-life:
- Children:
  - IV: Terminal: 22.1 hours (range: 12-30 hours)
  - SubQ: Terminal: 42.8 hours (range: 16-86 hours); Children with cancer: 49.4 hours
- Adults: CKD:
  - IV: Terminal: 21 hours
  - SubQ: Terminal: 49 ± 12.7 hours

Time to peak serum concentration: SubQ:
- CKD patients: 34 hours (range: 24-72 hours)
- Cancer patients:
  - Children: 71.4 hours (median time)
  - Adults: 90 hours (range: 71-123 hours)

Elimination:
- Clearance: IV:
  - Children: 2.29 mL/hour/kg (range: 1.6-3.5 mL/hour/kg)
  - Adults: 1.6 ± 1.0 mL/hour/kg

Dosing: Usual

Children and Adolescents: **Anemia associated with chronic kidney disease (CKD):** Individualize dosing and use the lowest dose necessary to reduce the need for RBC transfusions.

Initial dosing:

Manufacturer labeling:

CKD patients **ON** dialysis (initiate treatment when hemoglobin is <10 g/dL; reduce or interrupt treatment if hemoglobin approaches or exceeds 11 g/dL): Children ≥1 year and Adolescents: Conversion from epoetin alfa: IV (preferred), SubQ: Initial: Epoetin alfa doses of 1500 to ≥90,000 units per week may be converted to doses ranging from 6.25-200 mcg/dose darbepoetin alfa per week (see pediatric column in conversion table).

Alternate dosing: CKD patients darbepoetin alfa-naive (either on dialysis or not on dialysis): Children ≥11 years and Adolescents: IV, SubQ: Initial dose: ~0.45 mcg/kg/dose once weekly; titrate to hemoglobin response (André, 2007)

Dosage adjustment in CKD (either on dialysis or not on dialysis): Children ≥1 year and Adolescents: Do not increase dose more frequently than every 4 weeks (dose decreases may occur more frequently).

If hemoglobin increases >1 g/dL in any 2-week period: Decrease dose by ≥25%

If hemoglobin does not increase by >1 g/dL after 4 weeks: Increase dose by 25%

Inadequate or lack of response: If adequate response is not achieved over 12 weeks, further increases are unlikely to be of benefit and may increase the risk for adverse events; use the minimum effective dose that will maintain a hemoglobin level sufficient to avoid red blood cell transfusions **and** evaluate patient for other causes of anemia; discontinue treatment if responsiveness does not improve

Adults:

Anemia associated with chronic kidney disease (CKD): Individualize dosing and use the lowest dose necessary to reduce the need for RBC transfusions.

CKD patients **ON** dialysis (IV route is preferred for hemodialysis patients; initiate treatment when hemoglobin is <10 g/dL; reduce dose or interrupt treatment if hemoglobin approaches or exceeds 11 g/dL): IV (preferred), SubQ: Initial: 0.45 mcg/kg/dose once weekly or 0.75 mcg/kg/dose once every 2 weeks or epoetin alfa doses of <1500 to ≥90,000 units per week may be converted to doses ranging from 6.25-200 mcg darbepoetin per week (see adult column in conversion table)

CKD patients **NOT** on dialysis (consider initiating treatment when hemoglobin is <10 g/dL; use only if rate of hemoglobin decline would likely result in RBC transfusion and desire is to reduce risk of alloimmunization or other RBC transfusion-related risks; reduce or interrupt dose if hemoglobin exceeds 10 g/dL): IV, SubQ: Initial: 0.45 mcg/kg/dose once every 4 weeks

Dosage adjustment in CKD (either on dialysis or not on dialysis): Do not increase dose more frequently than every 4 weeks (dose decreases may occur more frequently).

If hemoglobin increases >1 g/dL in any 2-week period: Decrease dose by ≥25%

If hemoglobin does not increase by >1 g/dL after 4 weeks: Increase dose by 25%

Inadequate or lack of response: If adequate response is not achieved over 12 weeks, further increases are unlikely to be of benefit and may increase the risk for adverse events; use the minimum effective dose that will maintain a hemoglobin level sufficient to avoid red blood cell transfusions and evaluate patient for other causes of anemia; discontinue treatment if responsiveness does not improve

Anemia due to chemotherapy in cancer patients: Initiate treatment only if hemoglobin <10 g/dL and anticipated duration of myelosuppressive chemotherapy is ≥2 months. Titrate dosage to use the minimum effective dose that will maintain a hemoglobin concentration sufficient to avoid red blood cell transfusions. Discontinue darbepoetin following completion of chemotherapy. SubQ: Initial: 2.25 mcg/kg/dose once weekly **or** 500 mcg once every 3 weeks until completion of chemotherapy

Dosage adjustments:

Increase dose: If hemoglobin does not increase by 1 g/dL **and** remains below 10 g/dL after initial 6 weeks (for patients receiving weekly therapy only), increase dose to 4.5 mcg/kg/dose once weekly (no dosage adjustment if using every-3-week dosing).

Reduce dose by 40% if hemoglobin increases >1 g/dL in any 2-week period **or** hemoglobin reaches a level sufficient to avoid red blood cell transfusion.

Withhold dose if hemoglobin exceeds a level needed to avoid red blood cell transfusion. Resume treatment with a 40% dose reduction when hemoglobin approaches a level where transfusions may be required.

Discontinue: On completion of chemotherapy or if after 8 weeks of therapy there is no hemoglobin response or RBC transfusions still required

Conversion from epoetin alfa to darbepoetin alfa: See table.

Conversion From Epoetin Alfa to Darbepoetin Alfa (IV or SubQ)

(maintain the same route of administration for the conversion)

Previous Weekly Epoetin Alfa Dose (units/wk)	Weekly Darbepoetin Alfa Dosage	
	Pediatric (mcg/wk)	Adults (mcg/wk)
<1500	Not established	6.25
1500-2499	6.25	6.25
2500-4999	10	12.5
5000-10,999	20	25
11,000-17,999	40	40
18,000-33,999	60	60
34,000-89,999	100	100
≥90,000	200	200

Note: Due to the longer serum half-life of darbepoetin alfa, when converting from epoetin alfa, administer darbepoetin alfa once weekly if the patient was receiving epoetin alfa 2-3 times weekly and administer darbepoetin alfa once every two weeks if the patient was receiving epoetin alfa once weekly.

Administration May be administered undiluted IV or SubQ. Do not shake as this may denature the glycoprotein rendering the drug biologically inactive; only use SureClick autoinjectors if administering the full dose. Autoinjectors are for subcutaneous administration only. IV: Infuse over 1 to 3 minutes; IV route preferred for hemodialysis patients.

Monitoring Parameters Hemoglobin (at least once per week until maintenance dose established and after dosage changes; monitor less frequently once hemoglobin is stabilized); CKD patients should be also be monitored at least monthly following hemoglobin stability); iron stores (transferrin saturation and ferritin) prior to and during therapy; serum chemistry (CKD patients)

Cancer patients: Examinations recommended by the ASCO/ASH guidelines (Rizzo, 2010) prior to treatment include peripheral blood smear (in some situations a bone marrow exam may be necessary), assessment for iron, folate, or vitamin B_{12} deficiency, reticulocyte count, renal function status, and occult blood loss; during ESA treatment, assess baseline and periodic iron, total iron-binding capacity, and transferrin saturation or ferritin concentrations.

Additional Information Optimal response is achieved when iron stores are maintained with supplemental iron if necessary; evaluate iron stores prior to and during therapy. Use of ESAs in anemic patients with HIV who have been treated with zidovudine has not been demonstrated in controlled clinical trials to improve the symptoms of anemia, quality of life, fatigue, or well-being.

1 mcg darbepoetin alfa is equivalent to 200 units epoetin alfa.

Dosage Forms Excipient information presented when available (limited, particularly for generics); consult specific product labeling.

Solution, Injection [preservative free]:

Aranesp (Albumin Free): 25 mcg/mL (1 mL); 40 mcg/mL (1 mL); 25 mcg/0.42 mL (0.42 mL); 60 mcg/mL (1 mL); 40 mcg/0.4 mL (0.4 mL); 100 mcg/mL (1 mL); 60 mcg/0.3 mL (0.3 mL); 100 mcg/0.5 mL (0.5 mL); 150 mcg/0.75 mL (0.75 mL); 200 mcg/mL (1 mL); 300 mcg/mL (1 mL); 200 mcg/0.4 mL (0.4 mL); 300 mcg/0.6 mL (0.6 mL) [albumin free; contains polysorbate 80]

Aranesp (Albumin Free): 10 mcg/0.4 mL (0.4 mL) [contains mouse protein (murine) (hamster), polysorbate 80]

Aranesp (Albumin Free): 150 mcg/0.3 mL (0.3 mL); 500 mcg/mL (1 mL) [contains polysorbate 80]

Darunavir (dar OO na veer)

Medication Safety Issues

Sound-alike/look-alike issues:

Prezista may be confused with Prezbicox

High alert medication:

This medication is in a class the Institute for Safe Medication Practices (ISMP) includes among its list of drug classes that have a heightened risk of causing significant patient harm when used in error.

Related Information

Adult and Adolescent HIV *on page 2392*

Pediatric HIV *on page 2380*

Perinatal HIV *on page 2400*

Brand Names: US Prezista

Brand Names: Canada Prezista

Therapeutic Category Antiretroviral Agent; HIV Agents (Anti-HIV Agents); Protease Inhibitor

Generic Availability (US) No

Use Treatment of HIV-1 infection in combination with ritonavir and other antiretroviral agents (FDA approved in ages ≥3 years and adults). **Note:** HIV regimens consisting of **three** antiretroviral agents are strongly recommended.

Pregnancy Risk Factor C

Pregnancy Considerations Teratogenic effects have not been observed in animal reproduction studies. Darunavir has a low level of transfer across the human placenta. Serum concentrations are decreased during pregnancy; therefore, once-daily dosing is not recommended; twice-daily dosing should be used. The DHHS Perinatal HIV Guidelines consider darunavir to be an alternative protease inhibitor (PI) for use in antiretroviral-naive pregnant patients when combined with low-dose ritonavir boosting. A small increased risk of preterm birth has been associated with maternal use of protease inhibitor-based combination antiretroviral (ARV) therapy during pregnancy; however, the benefits of use generally outweigh this risk and PIs should not be withheld if otherwise recommended. Hyperglycemia, new onset of diabetes mellitus, or diabetic ketoacidosis have been reported with PIs; it is not clear if pregnancy increases this risk.

Regardless of CD4 count or HIV RNA copy number, all HIV-infected pregnant women should receive an ARV drug regimen combination of antepartum, intrapartum, and infant ARV prophylaxis. ARV therapy should be started as soon as possible in women with symptomatic infection. Although earlier initiation may be more effective in reducing the perinatal transmission of HIV, initiation may be delayed until after 12 weeks gestation in women who do not require immediate treatment after careful consideration of maternal conditions (eg, nausea and vomiting) and the potential risks of first trimester fetal exposure for specific agents. A scheduled cesarean delivery at 38 weeks gestation is recommended for all women with HIV RNA >1000 copies/mL or unknown concentrations near delivery in order to decrease transmission. If ARV therapy must be interrupted for <24 hours during the peripartum period, stop then restart all medications simultaneously in order to decrease the chance of developing resistance. Long-term follow-up is recommended for all infants exposed to ARV medications. In couples who want to conceive, the HIV-infected partner should attain maximum viral suppression prior to conception.

Healthcare providers are encouraged to enroll pregnant women exposed to antiretroviral medications in the Antiretroviral Pregnancy Registry (1-800-258-4263 or www.APRegistry.com). Healthcare providers caring for HIV-infected women and their infants may contact the National Perinatal HIV Hotline (888-448-8765) for clinical consultation (HHS [perinatal], 2014).

Breast-Feeding Considerations It is not known if darunavir is excreted into breast milk. Maternal or infant antiretroviral therapy does not completely eliminate the risk of postnatal HIV transmission. In addition, multiclass-resistant virus has been detected in breast-feeding infants despite maternal therapy. Therefore, in the United States, where formula is accessible, affordable, safe, and sustainable, and the risk of infant mortality due to diarrhea and respiratory infections is low, complete avoidance of breast-feeding by HIV-infected women is recommended to decrease potential transmission of HIV (HHS [perinatal], 2014).

Contraindications

Coadministration with drugs that are highly dependent on CYP3A for clearance and drugs for which elevated plasma concentrations are associated with serious and/or life-threatening events (narrow therapeutic index) (eg, alfuzosin, dronedarone, colchicine, ranolazine, ergot derivatives [dihydroergotamine, ergonovine, ergotamine, methylergonovine], cisapride, pimozide, midazolam (oral), triazolam, St John's wort, lovastatin, simvastatin, rifampin, sildenafil [for the treatment of pulmonary hypertension]). Must be coadministered with ritonavir; refer to individual monograph for ritonavir for additional contraindication information.

Canadian labeling: Additional contraindications: Hypersensitivity to darunavir or any component of the formulation; coadministration with amiodarone, apixaban, astemizole (not available in Canada), bepridil (not available in Canada), colchicine (in patients with renal and/or hepatic impairment), lidocaine (systemic), quinidine, rivaroxaban, terfenadine (not available in Canada); severe (Child-Pugh class C) hepatic impairment

Warnings/Precautions Darunavir has a high potential for drug interactions requiring dose or frequency adjustment, additional monitoring, and/or selection of alternative therapy.

Use with caution in patients with hepatic impairment, including active chronic hepatitis; consider interruption or discontinuation with worsening hepatic function. Not recommended in severe hepatic impairment (contraindicated in Canadian labeling). Infrequent cases of drug-induced hepatitis (including acute and cytolytic) have been reported. Liver injury has been reported with use (including some fatalities), though generally in patients on multiple medications, with advanced HIV disease, hepatitis B/C coinfection, and/or immune reconstitution syndrome.

Monitor patients closely; consider interrupting or discontinuing therapy if signs/symptoms of liver impairment occur.

May cause fat redistribution (buffalo hump, increased abdominal girth, breast engorgement, facial atrophy). Patients may develop immune reconstitution syndrome resulting in the occurrence of an inflammatory response to an indolent or residual opportunistic infection during initial HIV treatment or activation of autoimmune disorders (eg, Graves disease, polymyositis, Guillain-Barré syndrome) later in therapy; further evaluation and treatment may be required. May increase cholesterol and/or triglycerides. Pancreatitis has been observed with use. Risk for pancreatitis may be increased in patients with elevated triglycerides, advanced HIV disease, or history of pancreatitis. Protease inhibitors have been associated with glucose dysregulation; use caution in patients with diabetes. Initiation or dose adjustments of antidiabetic agents may be required. Use with caution in patients with hemophilia A or B; increased bleeding during protease inhibitor (PI) therapy has been reported. In some patients, additional factor VIII was administered. In more than half the cases, PI therapy was continued or reintroduced if it had been discontinued. Use with caution in patients with sulfonamide allergy (contains sulfa moiety) or hemophilia. Protease inhibitors have been associated with a variety of hypersensitivity events (some severe), including rash, anaphylaxis (rare), angioedema, bronchospasm, erythema multiforme, Stevens-Johnson syndrome (rare), acute generalized exanthematous pustulosis, toxic epidermal necrolysis, and/or drug rash with eosinophilia and systemic symptoms (DRESS). Discontinue treatment if severe skin reactions develop. Severe skin reactions may be accompanied by fever, malaise, fatigue, arthralgias, hepatitis, oral lesion, blisters, conjunctivitis, and/or eosinophilia. Mild-to-moderate rash may occur early in treatment and resolve with continued therapy. Treatment history and resistance data should guide use of darunavir with ritonavir. Do not administer darunavir with ritonavir in pediatric patients younger than 3 years (toxicity and mortality observed in animal studies).

Warnings: Additional Pediatric Considerations Do not use darunavir in children <3 years of age or weighing <10 kg; seizures and death associated with immaturity of the blood-brain barrier and immature hepatic metabolic pathways were observed in juvenile rats (DHHS [pediatric], 2014). Although once daily dosing in treatment-naive pediatric patients or treatment-experienced pediatric patients with no darunavir resistance-associated viral mutations was FDA approved in February 2013, once daily dosing is not recommended in the current DHHS guidelines for: Any patient <12 years, patients 12 to 18 years who are treatment-experienced with prior treatment failure, or patients ≥18 years with darunavir resistance-associated viral mutations (DHHS [pediatric], 2014). Some adverse effects have been reported more frequently in pediatric patients (6 to 18 years) than adults including: Vomiting (13% to 33% vs 2% to 5%); headache (9% vs 3% to 7%); pruritus (8% vs <2%); decreased appetite (8% vs 2%). Darunavir resistance-associated viral mutations include: V11I, V32I, L33F, I47V, I50V, I54L, I54M, T74P, L76V, I84V, and L89V.

Adverse Reactions As a class, protease inhibitors potentially cause dyslipidemias which includes elevated cholesterol and triglycerides and a redistribution of body fat centrally to cause increased abdominal girth, buffalo hump, facial atrophy, and breast enlargement. These agents also cause hyperglycemia. See also Ritonavir monograph.

Central nervous system: Fatigue (more common in children), headache (more common in children)

Dermatologic: Pruritus (more common in children), skin rash (more common in children)

Endocrine & metabolic: Diabetes mellitus, hypercholesterolemia (more common in adults), hyperglycemia, increased amylase (more common in adults), increased LDL cholesterol (more common in adults), increased serum triglycerides

Gastrointestinal: Abdominal distention, abdominal pain (more common in children), anorexia (more common in children), decreased appetite (more common in children), diarrhea (more common in children), dyspepsia, increased serum lipase (more common in adults), nausea (more common in children), vomiting (more common in children)

Hepatic: Increased serum ALT (more common in adults), increased serum AST (more common in adults)

Neuromuscular & skeletal: Weakness

Rare but important or life-threatening: Acute renal failure, alopecia, arthritis, bradycardia, cerebrovascular accident, depression, dermatitis (including dermatitis medicamentosa), DRESS syndrome, facial paralysis, folliculitis, gynecomastia, hematuria, hepatic failure, hepatic neoplasm (malignant), hepatitis (acute and cytolytic), hepatotoxicity, hyperlipidemia, hypersensitivity, hyperthermia, immune reconstitution syndrome, impaired consciousness, infection (including clostridium infection, parasitic infection [cryptosporidiosis], cytomegalovirus disease [encephalitis], hepatitis B, esophageal candidiasis), malignant lymphoma, myocardial infarction, nephrolithiasis, neutropenia, obesity, oropharyngeal ulcer, osteoporosis, pancreatitis, pancytopenia, peripheral neuropathy, pneumothorax, progressive multifocal leukoencephalopathy, pulmonary edema, rectal hemorrhage, redistribution of body fat (eg, buffalo hump, increased abdominal girth, breast engorgement, facial atrophy), respiratory failure, rhabdomyolysis (coadministration with HMG-CoA reductase inhibitors), seizure, sepsis, skin rash (toxic), tachycardia, uveitis

Drug Interactions

Metabolism/Transport Effects Substrate of CYP3A4 (major), P-glycoprotein; **Note:** Assignment of Major/Minor substrate status based on clinically relevant drug interaction potential; **Inhibits** CYP2D6 (weak), CYP3A4 (strong), P-glycoprotein

Avoid Concomitant Use

Avoid concomitant use of Darunavir with any of the following: Ado-Trastuzumab Emtansine; Alfuzosin; Apixaban; Astemizole; Avanafil; Axitinib; Barnidipine; Bosutinib; Cabozantinib; Ceritinib; Cisapride; Conivaptan; Crizotinib; Dapoxetine; Domperidone; Dronedarone; Eplerenone; Ergot Derivatives; Everolimus; Fosphenytoin; Fusidic Acid (Systemic); Halofantrine; Ibrutinib; Idelalisib; Irinotecan; Isavuconazonium Sulfate; Ivabradine; Lapatinib; Lercanidipine; Lomitapide; Lopinavir; Lovastatin; Lurasidone; Macitentan; Midazolam; Naloxegol; Nilotinib; NiMODipine; Nisoldipine; Olaparib; Palbociclib; PAZOPanib; Pimozide; Ranolazine; Red Yeast Rice; Regorafenib; Rifampin; Rifapentine; Rivaroxaban; Salmeterol; Saquinavir; Silodosin; Simeprevir; Simvastatin; St Johns Wort; Suvorexant; Tamsulosin; Telaprevir; Terfenadine; Ticagrelor; Tipranavir; Tolvaptan; Topotecan; Toremifene; Trabectedin; Triazolam; Ulipristal; Vemurafenib; VinCRIStine (Liposomal); Vorapaxar; Voriconazole

Increased Effect/Toxicity

Darunavir may increase the levels/effects of: Ado-Trastuzumab Emtansine; Afatinib; Alfuzosin; Almotriptan; Alosetron; ALPRAZolam; Amiodarone; Apixaban; ARIPiprazole; Astemizole; AtorvaSTATin; Avanafil; Axitinib; Barnidipine; Bedaquiline; Bortezomib; Bosentan; Bosutinib; Brentuximab Vedotin; Brinzolamide; Budesonide (Nasal); Budesonide (Systemic, Oral Inhalation); Budesonide (Topical); Cabazitaxel; Cabozantinib; Calcium Channel Blockers (Dihydropyridine); Calcium Channel Blockers (Nondihydropyridine); Cannabis; CarBAMazepine; Ceritinib; Cilostazol; Cisapride;

Clarithromycin; Colchicine; Conivaptan; Corticosteroids (Orally Inhaled); Corticosteroids (Systemic); Crizotinib; Cyclophosphamide; CycloSPORINE (Systemic); CYP2D6 Substrates; CYP3A4 Substrates; Dabigatran Etexilate; Dapoxetine; Dasatinib; Digoxin; Dofetilide; Domperidone; DOXOrubicin (Conventional); Dronabinol; Dronedarone; Dutasteride; Edoxaban; Efavirenz; Eliglustat; Elvitegravir; Enfuvirtide; Eplerenone; Ergot Derivatives; Erlotinib; Etizolam; Everolimus; FentaNYL; Fesoterodine; Fluticasone (Nasal); Fluticasone (Oral Inhalation); GuanFACINE; Halofantrine; Hydrocodone; Ibrutinib; Iloperidone; Imatinib; Imidafenacin; Irinotecan; Isavuconazonium Sulfate; Itraconazole; Ivabradine; Ivacaftor; Ixabepilone; Ketoconazole (Systemic); Lacosamide; Lapatinib; Ledipasvir; Lercanidipine; Levobupivacaine; Levomilnacipran; Lomitapide; Lovastatin; Lumefantrine; Lurasidone; Macitentan; Maraviroc; Meperidine; MethylPREDNISolone; Midazolam; Mifepristone; Naloxegol; Nefazodone; Nevirapine; Nilotinib; NiMODipine; Nintedanib; Nisoldipine; Olaparib; Ospemifene; Oxybutynin; OxyCODONE; Palbociclib; Panobinostat; Parecoxib; Paricalcitol; PAZOPanib; P-glycoprotein/ABCB1 Substrates; Pimecrolimus; Pimozide; PONATinib; Pranlukast; Pravastatin; PrednisoLONE (Systemic); PredniSONE; Propafenone; Protease Inhibitors; Prucalopride; QUEtiapine; QuiNIDine; Ramelteon; Ranolazine; Red Yeast Rice; Regorafenib; Repaglinide; Retapamulin; Rifabutin; Rifaximin; Rilpivirine; Riociguat; Rivaroxaban; RomiDEPsin; Rosuvastatin; Ruxolitinib; Salmeterol; Saxagliptin; Sildenafil; Silodosin; Simeprevir; Simvastatin; SORAfenib; Suvorexant; Tacrolimus (Systemic); Tacrolimus (Topical); Tadalafil; Tamsulosin; Tasimelteon; Temsirolimus; Tenofovir; Terfenadine; Tetrahydrocannabinol; Ticagrelor; Tofacitinib; Tolterodine; Tolvaptan; Topotecan; Toremifene; Trabectedin; TraMADol; TraZODone; Triazolam; Tricyclic Antidepressants; Ulipristal; Vardenafil; Vemurafenib; Vilazodone; VinCRIStine (Liposomal); Vorapaxar; Zopiclone; Zuclopenthixol

The levels/effects of Darunavir may be increased by: Clarithromycin; Conivaptan; CycloSPORINE (Systemic); CYP3A4 Inhibitors (Moderate); CYP3A4 Inhibitors (Strong); Delavirdine; Enfuvirtide; Fusidic Acid (Systemic); Idelalisib; Itraconazole; Ketoconazole (Systemic); Luliconazole; Mifepristone; Netupitant; Nevirapine; Rifabutin; Simeprevir; Stiripentol; Tenofovir

Decreased Effect

Darunavir may decrease the levels/effects of: Abacavir; Antidiabetic Agents; Boceprevir; Clarithromycin; Contraceptives (Estrogens); Contraceptives (Progestins); Delavirdine; Didanosine; Etravirine; Ifosfamide; Meperidine; Methadone; Norethindrone; PARoxetine; PHENobarbital; Phenytoin; Prasugrel; Sertraline; Telaprevir; Ticagrelor; Valproic Acid and Derivatives; Voriconazole; Warfarin; Zidovudine

The levels/effects of Darunavir may be decreased by: Boceprevir; Bosentan; CYP3A4 Inducers (Moderate); CYP3A4 Inducers (Strong); Dabrafenib; Deferasirox; Efavirenz; Fosphenytoin; Garlic; Lopinavir; Mitotane; Rifampin; Rifapentine; Saquinavir; Siltuximab; St Johns Wort; Telaprevir; Tipranavir; Tocilizumab

Food Interactions Absorption and bioavailability are increased when administered with food. Management: Take with meals.

Storage/Stability

Tablets: Store at 25°C (77°F); excursions are permitted between 15°C and 30°C (59°F and 86°F).

Suspension: Store at 25°C (77°F); excursions are permitted between 15°C and 30°C (59°F and 86°F). Do not refrigerate or freeze.

Mechanism of Action Binds to the site of HIV-1 protease activity and inhibits cleavage of viral Gag-Pol polyprotein precursors into individual functional proteins required for infectious HIV. This results in the formation of immature, noninfectious viral particles.

Pharmacokinetics (Adult data unless noted) Note: All pharmacokinetic parameters derived in the presence of ritonavir coadministration; pharmacokinetic data in pediatric patients (6 to 18 years) reported to be similar to adult data.

Protein binding: ~95%; primarily to alpha$_1$ acid glycoprotein

Metabolism: Hepatic, primarily via CYP3A to minimally active metabolites

Bioavailability: Absolute oral: 82% (darunavir 600 mg single dose with ritonavir twice daily); bioavailability is increased 30% to 40% with food

Half-life elimination: ~15 hours

Time to peak, serum concentration: 2.5 to 4 hours

Elimination: Feces (~80%, 41% as unchanged drug); urine (~14%, 8% as unchanged drug)

Dosing: Usual

Pediatric: **HIV infection, treatment: Note:** Genotypic testing for viral resistance is recommended in therapy experienced patients; coadministration with ritonavir is required; use in combination with other antiretroviral agents.

Note: Darunavir resistance-associated viral mutations include: V11I, V32I, L33F, I47V, I50V, I54L, I54M, T74P, L76V, I84V, and L89V.

Infants and Children <3 years of age or weighing <10 kg: Do not use; seizures and death associated with immaturity of the blood-brain barrier and immature hepatic metabolic pathways were observed in juvenile rats (DHHS [pediatric], 2014)

Treatment-naïve patients or treatment-experienced patients, without darunavir resistance-associated mutation: Children ≥3 years weighing ≥10 kg and Adolescents:

AIDSinfo recommendations (DHHS [pediatric], 2014): Oral:

Weight-directed dosing: Body weight 10 to 15 kg: Darunavir 20 mg/kg (maximum dose: 600 mg) twice daily **plus** ritonavir 3 mg/kg (maximum dose: 100 mg) twice daily

Fixed-dosing:

Twice-daily regimen: Children and Adolescents 3 to <18 years weighing ≥10 kg:

- 10 kg to <11 kg: Darunavir 200 mg **plus** ritonavir 32 mg twice daily
- 11 kg to <12 kg: Darunavir 220 mg **plus** ritonavir 32 mg twice daily
- 12 kg to <13 kg: Darunavir 240 mg **plus** ritonavir 40 mg twice daily
- 13 kg to <14 kg: Darunavir 260 mg **plus** ritonavir 40 mg twice daily
- 14 kg to <15 kg: Darunavir 280 mg **plus** ritonavir 48 mg twice daily
- 15 kg to <30 kg: Darunavir 375 mg **plus** ritonavir 48 twice daily
- 30 kg to <40 kg: Darunavir 450 mg **plus** ritonavir 100 mg twice daily
- ≥40 kg: Darunavir 600 mg **plus** ritonavir 100 mg twice daily

Once-daily regimen: Children and Adolescents ≥12 years

- 30 kg to <40 kg: Darunavir 675 mg **plus** ritonavir 100 mg once daily
- ≥40 kg: Darunavir 800 mg **plus** ritonavir 100 mg once daily

Manufacturer's labeling: Oral: **Note:** Although FDA approved, the Pediatric AIDS*info* guidelines do not recommend once-daily dosing in children <12 years. Alternate weight-directed and fixed-dosing regimens with twice daily dosing are recommended for children >3 year to <12 years of age (see above AIDS*info* recommendations); once-daily dosing is only recommended in patients ≥12 years of age or ≥30 k g without resistant-associated mutations. If once-daily dosing is used in children <12 years of age, therapeutic drug monitoring with measurement of plasma concentrations and inhibitory quotient should be performed (DHHS [pediatric], 2014).

Weight-directed dosing: Body weight 10 to <15 kg: Darunavir 35 mg/kg (maximum dose 800mg) twice daily **plus** ritonavir 7 mg/kg (maximum dose: 100 mg) once daily

Fixed-dosing:

10 kg to <11 kg: Darunavir 350 mg **plus** ritonavir 64 mg once daily

11 kg to <12 kg: Darunavir 385 mg **plus** ritonavir 64 mg once daily

12 kg to <13 kg: Darunavir 420 mg **plus** ritonavir 80 mg once daily

13 kg to <14 kg: Darunavir 455 mg **plus** ritonavir 80 mg once daily

14 kg to <15 kg: Darunavir 490 mg **plus** ritonavir 96 mg once daily

15 kg to <30 kg: Darunavir 600 mg **plus** ritonavir 100 mg once daily

30 kg to <40 kg: Darunavir 675 mg **plus** ritonavir 100 mg once daily

≥40 kg: Darunavir 800 mg **plus** ritonavir 100 mg once daily

Treatment-experienced patients, with at least one darunavir resistance-associated mutation: Children ≥3 years of age weighing ≥10 kg and Adolescents:

Weight-directed dosing: Body weight 10 kg to <15 kg: Darunavir 20 mg/kg (maximum dose: 600 mg) twice daily **plus** ritonavir 3 mg/kg (maximum dose: 100 mg) twice daily

Fixed-dosing:

10 kg to <11 kg: Darunavir 200 mg **plus** ritonavir 32 mg twice daily

11 kg to <12 kg: Darunavir 220 mg **plus** ritonavir 32 mg twice daily

12 kg to <13 kg: Darunavir 240 mg **plus** ritonavir 40 mg twice daily

13 kg to <14 kg: Darunavir 260 mg **plus** ritonavir 40 mg twice daily

14 kg to <15 kg: Darunavir 280 mg **plus** ritonavir 48 mg twice daily

15 kg to <30 kg: Darunavir 375 mg **plus** ritonavir 48 twice daily; **Note:** If weight ≥20 kg, the ritonavir 100 mg tablet may be substituted for liquid formulation to enhance palatability (DHHS [pediatric], 2014).

30 kg to <40 kg: Darunavir 450 mg **plus** ritonavir 60 mg twice daily; **Note:** The ritonavir 100 mg tablet may be substituted for the liquid formulation to enhance palatability (DHHS [pediatric], 2014).

≥40 kg: Darunavir 600 mg **plus** ritonavir 100 mg twice daily

Adult: **HIV infection, treatment:** Oral: **Note:** Genotypic testing for viral resistance is recommended in therapy experienced patients; coadministration with ritonavir is required; use in combination with other antiretroviral agents.

Therapy-naïve: Darunavir 800 mg **plus** ritonavir 100 mg once daily

Therapy-experienced:

With no darunavir resistance-associated substitutions: Darunavir 800 mg **plus** ritonavir 100 mg once daily

With ≥1 darunavir resistance-associated substitution or no genotypic testing: Darunavir 600 mg **plus** ritonavir 100 mg twice daily

Dosing adjustment in renal impairment:

Children ≥3 years of age and Adolescents (DHHS [pediatric], 2014):

CrCl ≥30 mL/minute: No dosage adjustment required

CrCl <30 mL/minute: There are no dosage adjustments provided in manufacturer's labeling (has not been studied).

Adults: No dosage adjustment required (DHHS [adult], 2014).

Dialysis: Darunavir is highly bound to plasma proteins; therefore, removal by hemodialysis or peritoneal dialysis is expected to be minimal.

Dosing adjustment in hepatic impairment:

Mild to moderate impairment (Child-Pugh class A or B): No dosage adjustment necessary

Severe impairment (Child-Pugh class C): Use not recommended

Administration Coadministration with ritonavir and food is required (bioavailability is increased). Shake suspension well prior to each dose; use manufacturer-provided oral dosing syringe to measure dose. In patients taking darunavir once daily, if a dose of darunavir or ritonavir is missed by >12 hours, the next dose should be taken at the regularly scheduled time. If a dose of darunavir or ritonavir is missed by <12 hours, the dose should be taken immediately and then the next dose should be taken at the regularly scheduled time. In patients taking darunavir twice daily, if a dose of darunavir or ritonavir is missed by >6 hours, the next dose should be taken at the regularly scheduled time. If a dose of darunavir or ritonavir is missed by <6 hours, the dose should be taken immediately and then the next dose should be taken at the regularly scheduled time.

Monitoring Parameters Note: Monitor CD4 percentage (if <5 years of age) or CD4 count (if ≥5 years of age) at least every 3 to 4 months (DHHS [pediatric], 2014).

Prior to initiation of therapy: Genotypic resistance testing, CD4 and viral load (every 3 to 4 months), CBC with differential, LFTs, BUN, creatinine, electrolytes, glucose, rinalysis (every 6 to 12 months), and assessment for readiness for adherence with medication regimen. At initiation and with any change in treatment regimen: CBC with differential, electrolytes, calcium, phosphate, glucose, LFTs, bilirubin, urinalysis (at initiation), BUN, creatinine, albumin, total protein, lipid panel (at initiation), CD4, and viral load. After 1 to 2 weeks of therapy: Signs of medication toxicity and adherence. After 2 to 4 weeks of therapy: CBC with differential, viral load, signs of medication toxicity, and adherence; then every 3 to 4 months: CBC with differential, electrolytes, glucose, LFTs, bilirubin, BUN, creatinine, CD4, viral load, signs of medication toxicity, and adherence. Every 6 to 12 months: Lipid panel and urinalysis. CD4 monitoring frequency may be decreased to every 6 to 12 months in children who are adherent to therapy if the value is well above the threshold for opportunistic infections, viral suppression is sustained, and the clinical status is stable for more than 2 to 3 years (DHHS [pediatric], 2014). Monitor for growth and development, signs of HIV-specific physical conditions, HIV disease progression, opportunistic infections, hepatitis, and skin rash.

Reference Range Trough concentration (Limited data available; data is from adult clinical trials that utilized 600 mg twice daily dosing; range utilized in trials): Median: 3300 ng/mL (range: 1255 to 7368 ng/mL) (DHHS [adult, pediatric], 2014)

Dosage Forms Excipient information presented when available (limited, particularly for generics); consult specific product labeling. [DSC] = Discontinued product

Suspension, Oral:

Prezista: 100 mg/mL (200 mL) [contains methylparaben sodium; strawberry cream flavor]

Tablet, Oral:

Prezista: 75 mg, 150 mg

Prezista: 400 mg [DSC], 600 mg [contains fd&c yellow #6 (sunset yellow)]
Prezista: 800 mg

- **Darunavir Ethanolate** *see* Darunavir *on page 588*
- **Daunomycin** *see* DAUNOrubicin (Conventional) *on page 592*

DAUNOrubicin (Conventional)

(daw noe ROO bi sin con VEN sha nal)

Medication Safety Issues

Sound-alike/look-alike issues:

DAUNOrubicin may be confused with DACTINomycin, DAUNOrubicin liposomal, DOXOrubicin, DOXOrubicin liposomal, epirubicin, IDArubicin, valrubicin

High alert medication:

This medication is in a class the Institute for Safe Medication Practices (ISMP) includes among its list of drug classes which have a heightened risk of causing significant patient harm when used in error.

Related Information

Management of Drug Extravasations *on page 2298*

Prevention of Chemotherapy-Induced Nausea and Vomiting in Children *on page 2368*

Safe Handling of Hazardous Drugs *on page 2455*

Brand Names: Canada Cerubidine; Daunorubicin Hydrochloride for Injection

Therapeutic Category Antineoplastic Agent, Anthracycline; Antineoplastic Agent, Antibiotic; Antineoplastic Agent, Topoisomerase II Inhibitor

Generic Availability (US) Yes

Use

Treatment (remission induction) of acute lymphocytic leukemia (ALL) in combination with other chemotherapy (FDA approved in pediatric patients [age not specified] and adults)

Treatment (remission induction) of acute myeloid leukemia (AML) in combination with other chemotherapy (FDA approved in adults)

Pregnancy Risk Factor D

Pregnancy Considerations Adverse events have been observed in animal reproduction studies. Daunorubicin crosses the placenta. Women of reproductive potential should avoid pregnancy.

Breast-Feeding Considerations It is not known if daunorubicin is excreted into breast milk. Due to the potential for serious adverse reactions in the nursing infant, the manufacturer recommends a decision be made whether to discontinue nursing or to discontinue the drug, taking into account the importance of treatment to the mother.

Contraindications Hypersensitivity to daunorubicin or any component of the formulation

Warnings/Precautions Hazardous agent - use appropriate precautions for handling and disposal (NIOSH 2014 [group 1]). **[U.S. Boxed Warning]: Potent vesicant; if extravasation occurs, severe local tissue damage leading to ulceration and necrosis, and pain may occur. For IV administration only. NOT for IM or SubQ administration. Administer through a rapidly flowing IV line.** Ensure proper needle or catheter placement prior to and during infusion. Avoid extravasation. **[U.S. Boxed Warning]: Severe bone marrow suppression may occur when used at therapeutic doses; may lead to infection or hemorrhage.** Use with caution in patients with drug-induced bone marrow suppression (preexisting), unless the therapy benefit outweighs the toxicity risk. Monitor blood counts at baseline and frequently during therapy.

[U.S. Boxed Warning]: May cause cumulative, dose-related myocardial toxicity; may lead to heart failure. May occur either during treatment or may be delayed (months to years after cessations of treatment). The incidence of irreversible myocardial toxicity increases as the total cumulative (lifetime) dosages approach 550 mg/m^2 in adults, 400 mg/m^2 in adults receiving chest radiation, 300 mg/m^2 in children >2 years of age, or 10 mg/kg in children <2 years of age. Total cumulative dose should take into account prior treatment with other anthracyclines or anthracenediones, previous or concomitant treatment with cardiotoxic agents or irradiation of chest. Although the risk increases with cumulative dose, irreversible cardiotoxicity may occur at any dose level. Patients with preexisting heart disease, hypertension, concurrent administration of other antineoplastic agents, prior or concurrent chest irradiation, advanced age; and infants and children are at increased risk. Monitor left ventricular (LV) function (baseline and periodic) with ECHO or MUGA scan; monitor ECG. Cardiotoxicity may occur more frequently in elderly patients. Use with caution in patients with impaired renal function and/or poor marrow reserve due to advanced age; dosage adjustment may be necessary. Infants and children are at increased risk for developing delayed cardiotoxicity; long-term periodic cardiac function monitoring is recommended.

[U.S. Boxed Warning]: Dosage reductions are recommended in patients with renal or hepatic impairment; significant impairment may result in increased toxicities. May cause tumor lysis syndrome and hyperuricemia. Urinary alkalinization and prophylaxis with an antihyperuricemic agent may be necessary. Monitor electrolytes, renal function, and hydration status. Use with caution in patients who have received radiation therapy; reduce dosage in patients who are receiving radiation therapy simultaneously. Secondary leukemias may occur when used with combination chemotherapy or radiation therapy. **[U.S. Boxed Warning]: Should be administered under the supervision of an experienced cancer chemotherapy physician.** Use caution when selecting product for preparation and dispensing; indications, dosages, and adverse event profiles differ between conventional daunorubicin hydrochloride solution and daunorubicin liposomal. Potentially significant drug-drug interactions may exist, requiring dose or frequency adjustment, additional monitoring, and/or selection of alternative therapy.

Warnings: Additional Pediatric Considerations Risk of anthracycline-induced cardiotoxicity (including daunorubicin) is increased in pediatric patients; may occur more frequently and at a lower cumulative dose than adults. Cardiotoxicity in pediatric patients includes impaired left ventricular systolic performance, reduced contractility, congestive heart failure, or death. Cardiotoxicity is dose-dependent and may occur months to years following therapy; may be aggravated by thoracic irradiation. Total dose administered should be taken into account, including all prior anthracycline drugs administered (eg, doxorubicin). Long-term monitoring is recommended for all pediatric patients.

Adverse Reactions

Cardiovascular: Transient ECG abnormalities (supraventricular tachycardia, S-T wave changes, atrial or ventricular extrasystoles); generally asymptomatic and self-limiting. CHF, dose related, may be delayed for 7-8 years after treatment

Dermatologic: Alopecia (reversible); discoloration of saliva, sweat, or tears, radiation recall, skin "flare" at injection site

Endocrine & metabolic: Hyperuricemia

Gastrointestinal: Abdominal pain, diarrhea, GI ulceration, diarrhea, mild nausea or vomiting, stomatitis

Genitourinary: Discoloration of urine (red)

Hematologic: Myelosuppression (onset: 7 days; nadir: 10-14 days; recovery: 21-28 days), primarily leukopenia; thrombocytopenia and anemia

Rare but important or life-threatening: Anaphylactoid reaction, arrhythmia, bilirubin increased, cardiomyopathy, hepatitis, infertility; local (cellulitis, pain, thrombophlebitis at injection site); MI, myocarditis, neutropenic typhlitis, pericarditis, secondary leukemia, skin rash, sterility, systemic hypersensitivity (including urticaria, pruritus, angioedema, dysphagia, dyspnea); transaminases increased

Drug Interactions

Metabolism/Transport Effects **Substrate** of P-glycoprotein

Avoid Concomitant Use

Avoid concomitant use of DAUNOrubicin (Conventional) with any of the following: BCG; BCG (Intravesical); CloZAPine; Dipyrone; Natalizumab; Pimecrolimus; Tacrolimus (Topical); Tofacitinib; Vaccines (Live)

Increased Effect/Toxicity

DAUNOrubicin (Conventional) may increase the levels/effects of: CloZAPine; Leflunomide; Natalizumab; Tofacitinib; Vaccines (Live)

The levels/effects of DAUNOrubicin (Conventional) may be increased by: Bevacizumab; Cyclophosphamide; Denosumab; Dipyrone; P-glycoprotein/ABCB1 Inhibitors; Pimecrolimus; Roflumilast; Tacrolimus (Topical); Taxane Derivatives; Trastuzumab

Decreased Effect

DAUNOrubicin (Conventional) may decrease the levels/effects of: BCG; BCG (Intravesical); Cardiac Glycosides; Coccidioides immitis Skin Test; Sipuleucel-T; Vaccines (Inactivated); Vaccines (Live)

The levels/effects of DAUNOrubicin (Conventional) may be decreased by: Cardiac Glycosides; Echinacea; P-glycoprotein/ABCB1 Inducers

Storage/Stability

Solution: Store intact vials at 2°C to 8°C (36°F to 46°F). Protect from light. Retain in carton until time of use. Solution prepared for infusion may be stored at 20°C to 25°C (68°F to 77°F) for up to 24 hours. Discard unused portion.

Lyophilized powder [Canadian product]: Store intact vials of powder at 15°C to 30°C (59°F to 86°F). Protect from light. Retain in carton until time of use. Reconstituted daunorubicin is stable for 24 hours at room temperature or 48 hours when refrigerated at 2°C to 8°C (36°F to 46°F). Protect reconstituted solution from light.

Mechanism of Action Inhibits DNA and RNA synthesis by intercalation between DNA base pairs and by steric obstruction. Daunomycin intercalates at points of local uncoiling of the double helix. Although the exact mechanism is unclear, it appears that direct binding to DNA (intercalation) and inhibition of DNA repair (topoisomerase II inhibition) result in blockade of DNA and RNA synthesis and fragmentation of DNA.

Pharmacokinetics (Adult data unless noted)

Distribution: Widely distributed in tissues such as spleen, heart, kidneys, liver, and lungs; does not cross the blood-brain barrier

Metabolism: Primarily hepatic to daunorubicinol (active), then to inactive aglycones, conjugated sulfates, and glucuronides

Half-life:

Initial: 45 minutes

Terminal: 18.5 hours

Daunorubicinol, active metabolite: 26.7 hours

Elimination: 40% of dose excreted in bile; 25% excreted in urine as metabolite and unchanged drug

Dosing: Usual **Note:** Dose, frequency, number of doses, and start date may vary by protocol and treatment phase; refer to individual protocols. Daunorubicin is associated with a moderate emetic potential; antiemetics are recommended to prevent nausea and vomiting (Basch 2011; Dupuis 2011; Roila 2010).

Pediatric: **Note:** Dosing presented as both mg/m^2 and mg/kg; use extra precaution and verify dosing units. Cumulative doses above 10 mg/kg in infants and children <2 years of age or above 300 mg/m^2 in children and adolescents >2 years of age are associated with an increased risk of cardiotoxicity.

Acute lymphocytic leukemia (ALL):

Manufacturer's labeling: Remission induction:

Infants and Children <2 years or BSA <0.5 m^2: IV: 1 mg/**kg**/dose on day 1 every week for up to 4 to 6 cycles (in combination with vincristine and prednisone)

Children and Adolescents ≥2 years and BSA ≥0.5 m^2: IV: 25 mg/m2 on day 1 every week for up to 4 to 6 cycles (in combination with vincristine and prednisone)

Alternate dosing:

CCG 1961: Children and Adolescents: IV: Induction: 25 mg/m^2 once weekly for 4 weeks (in combination with vincristine, prednisone, and asparaginase) (Nachman 2009; Siebel 2008)

GRAALL-2003 (Huguet 2009): Adolescents ≥15 years: IV:

Induction: 50 mg/m^2 on days 1, 2, and 3 **and** 30 mg/m^2 on days 15 and 16 (in combination with prednisone, vincristine, asparaginase, cyclophosphamide, and G-CSF support)

Late intensification: 30 mg/m^2 on days 1, 2, and 3 (in combination with prednisone, vincristine, asparaginase, cyclophosphamide, and G-CSF support)

MRC UKALLXII/ECOG E2993: Adolescents ≥15 years: IV: Induction (Phase I): 60 mg/m^2 on days 1, 8, 15, and 22 (in combination with vincristine, asparaginase, and prednisone) (Rowe 2005)

PETHEMA ALL-96 (Ribera 2008): Adolescents ≥15 years: IV:

Induction: 30 mg/m^2 on days 1, 8, 15, and 22 (in combination with vincristine, prednisone, asparaginase, and cyclophosphamide)

Consolidation-2/Reinduction: 30 mg/m^2 on days 1, 2, 8, and 9 (in combination with vincristine, dexamethasone, asparaginase, and cyclophosphamide)

Acute myelogenous leukemia (AML):

Induction:

MRC AML 10/12: Infants and Children ≤16 years: IV: 50 mg/m^2 on days 1, 3, and 5 for 2 cycles (in combination with cytarabine and etoposide) (Gibson 2005)

CCG 2891 (Woods 1996):

Infants and Children <3 years: IV: 0.67 mg/kg/day continuous infusion on days 0 to 4 and 10 to 14 (in combination with dexamethasone, cytarabine, thioguanine, and etoposide)

Children ≥3 years and Adolescents: IV: 20 mg/m^2/day continuous infusion on days 0 to 4 and 10 to 14 (in combination with dexamethasone, cytarabine, thioguanine, and etoposide)

Adult: **Note:** Cumulative doses above 550 mg/m^2 in adults without risk factors for cardiotoxicity and above 400 mg/m^2 in adults receiving chest irradiation are associated with an increased risk of cardiomyopathy.

Acute lymphocytic leukemia (ALL): Manufacturer's labeling: IV: 45 mg/m^2 on days 1, 2, and 3 (in combination with vincristine, prednisone, and asparaginase)

Acute myeloid leukemia (AML): Manufacturer's labeling:

Adults <60 years: Induction: IV: 45 mg/m^2 on days 1, 2, and 3 of the first course of induction therapy; subsequent courses: 45 mg/m^2 on days 1 and 2 (in combination with cytarabine)

Adults ≥60 years: Induction: IV: 30 mg/m^2 on days 1, 2, and 3 of the first course of induction therapy; subsequent courses: 30 mg/m^2 on days 1 and 2 (in combination with cytarabine)

Dosing adjustment in renal impairment:

The manufacturer's labeling recommends the following adjustment: All patients: S_{cr} >3 mg/dL: Administer 50% of normal dose

The following adjustments have also been recommended (Aronof, 2007):

Infants, Children, and Adolescents:

CrCl <30 mL/minute: Administer 50% of dose

Hemodialysis/continuous ambulatory peritoneal dialysis (CAPD): Administer 50% of dose

Adults: No dosage adjustment is necessary

Dosing adjustment in hepatic impairment:

The manufacturer's labeling recommends the following adjustments: All patients:

Serum bilirubin 1.2 to 3 mg/dL: Administer 75% of dose

Serum bilirubin >3 mg/dL: Administer 50% of dose

The following adjustments have also been recommended (Floyd 2006): All patients:

Serum bilirubin 1.2 to 3 mg/dL: Administer 75% of dose

Serum bilirubin 3.1 to 5 mg/dL: Administer 50% of dose

Serum bilirubin >5 mg/dL: Avoid use

Preparation for Administration Hazardous agent; use appropriate precautions for handling and disposal (NIOSH 2014 [group 1]).

Parenteral: IVP: Dilute dose in 10 to 15 mL NS

Administration Hazardous agent; use appropriate precautions for handling and disposal (NIOSH 2014 [group 1]). Daunorubicin is associated with a moderate emetic potential; antiemetics are recommended to prevent nausea and vomiting (Basch 2011; Dupuis 2011; Roila 2010).

Parenteral: Drug is very irritating, do not inject IM or SubQ; further dilute and administer IVP over 1 to 5 minutes into the tubing of a rapidly infusing IV solution of D_5W or NS.

Vesicant; ensure proper needle or catheter placement prior to and during infusion; avoid extravasation. If extravasation occurs, stop infusion immediately and disconnect (leave cannula/needle in place); gently aspirate extravasated solution (do **NOT** flush the line); remove needle/cannula; elevate extremity. Initiate antidote (dimethyl sulfate [DMSO] or dexrazoxane [adult]) (see Management of Drug Extravasations for more details). Apply dry cold compresses for 20 minutes 4 times daily for 1 to 2 days (Pérez Fidalgo 2012); withhold cooling beginning 15 minutes before dexrazoxane infusion; continue withholding cooling until 15 minutes after infusion is completed. Topical DMSO should not be administered in combination with dexrazoxane; may lessen dexrazoxane efficacy.

Vesicant/Extravasation Risk Vesicant

Monitoring Parameters CBC with differential and platelet count, serum bilirubin, serum uric acid, liver function test, ECG, ventricular ejection fraction (echocardiogracphy [ECHO] or multigated radionuclide angiography [MUCA] scan), renal function test; signs/symptoms of extravasation

Dosage Forms Excipient information presented when available (limited, particularly for generics); consult specific product labeling.

Injectable, Intravenous:

Generic: 5 mg/mL (4 mL)

Injectable, Intravenous [preservative free]:

Generic: 5 mg/mL (4 mL, 10 mL)

◆ **DAUNOrubicin Hydrochloride** *see* DAUNOrubicin (Conventional) *on page 592*

◆ **Daunorubicin Hydrochloride for Injection (Can)** *see* DAUNOrubicin (Conventional) *on page 592*

◆ **Dayhist Allergy 12 Hour Relief [OTC]** *see* Clemastine *on page 486*

◆ **Daypro** *see* Oxaprozin *on page 1582*

◆ **Daytrana** *see* Methylphenidate *on page 1402*

◆ **dCF** *see* Pentostatin *on page 1668*

◆ **DDAVP** *see* Desmopressin *on page 607*

◆ **DDAVP Melt (Can)** *see* Desmopressin *on page 607*

◆ **DDAVP Rhinal Tube** *see* Desmopressin *on page 607*

◆ **ddI** *see* Didanosine *on page 646*

◆ **DDP** *see* CISplatin *on page 473*

◆ **1-Deamino-8-D-Arginine Vasopressin** *see* Desmopressin *on page 607*

◆ **Deblitane** *see* Norethindrone *on page 1530*

◆ **Debrox [OTC]** *see* Carbamide Peroxide *on page 371*

◆ **Decadron** *see* Dexamethasone (Systemic) *on page 610*

◆ **Decara** *see* Cholecalciferol *on page 448*

◆ **Declomycin** *see* Demeclocycline *on page 600*

◆ **Decongestant 12Hour Max St [OTC]** *see* Pseudoephedrine *on page 1801*

◆ **Deep Sea Nasal Spray [OTC]** *see* Sodium Chloride *on page 1938*

Deferasirox (de FER a sir ox)

Medication Safety Issues

Sound-alike/look-alike issues:

Deferasirox may be confused with deferiprone, deferoxamine

Brand Names: US Exjade; Jadenu

Brand Names: Canada Exjade

Therapeutic Category Chelating Agent, Oral

Generic Availability (US) No

Use Treatment of chronic iron overload due to blood transfusions (FDA approved in ages ≥2 years and adults); treatment of chronic iron overload due to nontransfusion-dependent thalassemia syndromes with a liver iron concentration (LIC) of at least 5 mg iron per gram of liver dry weight (mg Fe/g dw) and serum ferritin >300 mcg/L (FDA approved in ages ≥10 years and adults)

Prescribing and Access Restrictions Deferasirox (Exjade) is only available through a restricted distribution program called EPASS Complete Care. Prescribers must enroll patients in this program in order to obtain the medication. For patient enrollment, contact 1-888-90-EPASS (1-888-903-7277).

Pregnancy Risk Factor C

Pregnancy Considerations Adverse events were observed in animal reproduction studies. Information related to the use of deferasirox in pregnant women is limited (Vini 2011).

Breast-Feeding Considerations It is not known if deferasirox is excreted in breast milk. Due to the potential for serious adverse reactions in the nursing infant, the manufacturer recommends a decision be made to discontinue breast-feeding or to discontinue the drug, taking into account the importance of treatment to the mother.

Contraindications

Known hypersensitivity to deferasirox or any component of the formulation; CrCl <40 mL/minute or serum creatinine >2 times the age-appropriate ULN; poor performance status; high-risk myelodysplastic syndromes; advanced malignancies; platelet counts <50,000/mm^3

Canadian labeling: Additional contraindications (not in US labeling): MDS patients with <1 year life expectancy; CrCl <60 mL/minute

Warnings/Precautions [US Boxed Warning]: Acute renal failure (including fatalities and cases requiring dialysis) may occur; observed more frequently in patients with comorbid conditions and advanced hematologic malignancies. Obtain serum creatinine and

calculate creatinine clearance in duplicate at baseline prior to initiation, and monitor at least monthly thereafter; in patients with underlying renal dysfunction or at risk for acute renal failure, monitor creatinine weekly during the first month then at least monthly thereafter. Dose reduction, interruption, or discontinuation should be considered for serum creatinine elevations. Monitor serum creatinine and/or creatinine clearance more frequently if creatinine levels are increasing. Use with caution in renal impairment; dosage modification or treatment discontinuation may be required; reductions in initial dose are recommended for patients with CrCl 40 to 60 mL/minute; use is contraindicated in patients with CrCl <40 mL/minute (US labeling) or <60 mL/minute (Canadian labeling) or serum creatinine >2 times age-appropriate ULN. May cause proteinuria; monitor monthly. Renal tubular damage, including Fanconi's syndrome, has also been reported, primarily in pediatric/adolescent patients with beta-thalassemia and serum ferritin levels <1,500 mcg/L.

[US Boxed Warning]: Hepatic injury and failure (including fatalities) may occur. Monitor transaminases and bilirubin at baseline, every 2 weeks for 1 month, then at least monthly thereafter. Hepatitis and elevated transaminases have also been reported. Hepatotoxicity is more common in patients >55 years of age and in patients with significant comorbidities (eg, cirrhosis, multiorgan failure). Reduce dose or temporarily interrupt treatment for severe or persistent increases in transaminases/bilirubin. **[US Boxed Warning]: Avoid use in patients with severe (Child-Pugh class C) hepatic impairment; a dose reduction is required in patients with moderate (Child-Pugh class B) hepatic impairment.** Monitor patients with mild (Child-Pugh class A) or moderate (Child-Pugh class B) impairment closely for efficacy and for adverse reactions requiring dosage reduction.

[US Boxed Warning]: Gastrointestinal (GI) hemorrhage (including fatalities) may occur; observed more frequently in elderly patients with advanced hematologic malignancies and/or low platelet counts; discontinue treatment for suspected GI hemorrhage or ulceration. Other GI effects including irritation and ulceration have been reported. Use caution with concurrent medications that may increase risk of adverse GI effects (eg, NSAIDs, corticosteroids, anticoagulants, oral bisphosphonates). Monitor patients closely for signs/symptoms of GI ulceration/bleeding.

May cause skin rash (dose-related), including erythema multiforme; mild-to-moderate rashes may resolve without treatment interruption; for severe rash, interrupt and consider restarting at a lower dose with dose escalation and oral steroids; discontinue if erythema multiforme is suspected. Severe skin reactions, including Stevens-Johnson syndrome (SJS) and erythema multiforme, have also been reported; discontinue and evaluate if suspected. Hypersensitivity reactions, including severe reactions (anaphylaxis and angioedema) have been reported, onset is usually within the first month of treatment; discontinue if severe. Auditory (decreased hearing and high frequency hearing loss) or ocular disturbances (lens opacities, cataracts, intraocular pressure elevation, and retinal disorders) have been reported (rare); monitor and consider dose reduction or treatment interruption. Bone marrow suppression (including agranulocytosis, neutropenia, thrombocytopenia, and worsening anemia) has been reported, risk may be increased in patients with preexisting hematologic disorders; monitor blood counts regularly; interrupt treatment in patients who develop cytopenias; may reinitiate once cause of cytopenia has been determined; use contraindicated if platelet count <50,000/mm^3. Potentially significant drug-drug interactions may exist, requiring dose or frequency adjustment, additional monitoring, and/or selection of alternative therapy. For transfusion-related iron overload, treatment should be initiated with evidence of chronic iron overload (ie, transfusion of ≥100 mL/kg of packed RBCs [eg, ≥20 units for a 40 kg individual] and serum ferritin consistently >1,000 mcg/L). For non-transfusion-dependent iron overload, initiate with liver iron concentration ≥5 mg Fe/g dry liver weight and serum ferritin >300 mcg/L. Prior to use, consider risk versus anticipated benefit with respect to individual patient's life expectancy and prognosis. Use with caution in the elderly due to the higher incidence of toxicity (eg, hepatotoxicity) and fatal events during use. Overchelation of iron may increase development of toxicity; consider temporary interruption of treatment in transfusional iron overload when serum ferritin <500 mcg/L; in non-transfusion-dependent thalassemia when serum ferritin <300 mcg/L or hepatic iron concentration <3 mg Fe/g dry weight. May contain lactose; Canadian product labeling recommends avoiding use in patients with galactose intolerance, Lapp lactase deficiency, or glucose-galactose malabsorption syndromes. Deferasirox has a low affinity for binding with zinc and copper, may cause variable decreases in the serum concentration of these trace minerals.

Adverse Reactions

Central nervous system: Fatigue, headache (Phatak 2010, Vichinsky 2007)

Dermatologic: Skin rash (dose related)

Gastrointestinal: Abdominal pain (dose related), diarrhea (dose related), nausea (dose related), vomiting (dose related)

Genitourinary: Proteinuria

Hepatic: Increased serum ALT

Infection: Viral infection (Vichinsky 2007)

Neuromuscular & skeletal: Arthralgia (Vichinsky 2007), back pain (Vichinsky 2007)

Renal: Increased serum creatinine (dose related)

Respiratory: Cough (Vichinsky 2007), nasopharyngitis (Vichinsky 2007), pharyngitis (Vichinsky 2007), pharyngolaryngeal pain, respiratory tract infection (Vichinsky 2007)

Rare but important or life-threatening: Abnormal hepatic function tests, acute renal failure, agranulocytosis, alopecia, anaphylaxis, anemia (worsening), angioedema, cataract, cholelithiasis, cytopenia, drug fever, duodenal ulcer, dyschromia, edema, erythema multiforme, Fanconi's syndrome, gastric ulcer, gastritis, gastrointestinal hemorrhage, gastrointestinal perforation, glycosuria, hearing loss (including high frequency), hematuria, fever, hepatic failure, hepatic insufficiency, hepatitis, hyperactivity, hypersensitivity angiitis, hypersensitivity reaction, hypocalcemia, IgA vasculitis, increased intraocular pressure, increased serum bilirubin (Vichinsky 2007), interstitial nephritis, maculopathy, neutropenia, nontuberculous mycobacterial infection, optic neuritis, pancreatitis (associated with gallstones), purpura, renal tubular disease, renal tubular necrosis, retinopathy, sleep disorder, Stevens-Johnson syndrome, thrombocytopenia, visual disturbance

Drug Interactions

Metabolism/Transport Effects Substrate of UGT1A1; **Inhibits** CYP1A2 (moderate), CYP2C8 (moderate); **Induces** CYP3A4 (weak)

Avoid Concomitant Use

Avoid concomitant use of Deferasirox with any of the following: Aluminum Hydroxide; Amodiaquine; Theophylline; TiZANidine

Increased Effect/Toxicity

Deferasirox may increase the levels/effects of: Agomelatine; Amodiaquine; CYP1A2 Substrates; CYP2C8 Substrates; Pirfenidone; Repaglinide; Theophylline; TiZANidine

The levels/effects of Deferasirox may be increased by: Anticoagulants; Bisphosphonate Derivatives; Corticosteroids; Corticosteroids (Systemic); Nonsteroidal Anti-Inflammatory Agents

Decreased Effect

Deferasirox may decrease the levels/effects of: ARIPiprazole; CYP3A4 Substrates; Hydrocodone; NiMODipine; Saxagliptin

The levels/effects of Deferasirox may be decreased by: Aluminum Hydroxide; Bile Acid Sequestrants; Fosphenytoin; PHENobarbital; Phenytoin; Rifampin; Ritonavir

Food Interactions

Tablets for oral suspension: Bioavailability is increased variably when taken with food. Management: Take on an empty stomach at the same time each day at least 30 minutes before food. Maintain adequate hydration, unless instructed to restrict fluid intake.

Tablets: Bioavailability decreased slightly (not clinically meaningful) after a low-fat meal and increased after a high-fat meal. Management: Take on an empty stomach or with a light meal (containing ~250 calories and <7% fat content).

Storage/Stability Store at 25°C (77°F); excursions permitted to 15°C and 30°C (59°F and 86°F). Protect from moisture.

Mechanism of Action Selectively binds iron, forming a complex which is excreted primarily through the feces.

Pharmacokinetics (Adult data unless noted) Note: Systemic exposure has been shown to be less in pediatric patients (2-16 years) compared to adults; in children 2 to 6 years, exposure was reduced by ~50% compared to adults; however, results of safety and efficacy trials using the same dose were similar in pediatric and adult patients. Patients with myelodysplastic syndromes (MDS) and CrCl of 40 to 60 mL/minute had 50% higher mean deferasirox trough concentrations compared to patients with MDS and CrCl >60 mL/minute.

Distribution: 14.4 ± 2.7 L

Protein binding: 99% to serum albumin

Metabolism: Hepatic via glucuronidation by UGT1A1 and UGT1A3; minor oxidation by CYP450; undergoes enterohepatic recirculation

Bioavailability: Tablets for oral suspension: 70%; Tablets: 36% greater than tablet for oral suspension

Half-life: 8 to 16 hours

Time to peak serum concentration: Median range: 1.5 to 4 hours

Elimination: Feces (84%), urine (8%)

Clearance: Females have moderately lower clearance than males (17.5% lower)

Dosing: Usual Note: Calculate dose to the nearest whole tablet size.

Pediatric: Deferasirox is available in two formulations (Exjade: Tablets for oral suspension, Jadenu: Tablets) that are **not** bioequivalent on a mg:mg basis due to bioavailability differences.

Conversion from Exjade to Jadenu: The dose for Jadenu should be ~30% lower than Exjade (doses rounded to the nearest whole tablet).

Blood transfusion; chronic iron overload: Children ≥2 years and Adolescents: Oral: **Note:** Treatment should only be initiated with evidence of chronic iron overload [ie, transfusion of ≥100 mL/kg of packed RBCs (eg, ≥20 units for a 40 kg individual) and serum ferritin consistently >1000 mcg/L].

Exjade (oral tablet for suspension):

Initial: 20 mg/kg once daily

Maintenance: Adjust dose every 3 to 6 months based on serum ferritin levels; increase dose by 5 or 10 mg/kg/day increments; usual range: 20 to 30 mg/kg/day; for serum ferritin levels persistently >2,500 mcg/L without evidence of a decreasing trend, may consider a dose of 40 mg/kg/day; doses >40 mg/kg/day are not recommended. If serum ferritin is <500 mcg/L, interrupt therapy.

Jadenu (oral tablet):

Initial: 14 mg/kg once daily, calculate dose to the nearest whole tablet

Maintenance: Adjust dose every 3 to 6 months based on serum ferritin trends; adjust by 3.5 or 7 mg/kg/day; titrate to individual response and treatment goals. In patients not adequately controlled at a dose of 21 mg/kg/day (eg, serum ferritin levels persistently >2,500 mcg/L and not decreasing over time), then higher doses up to 28 mg/kg/day may be considered; doses >28 mg/kg/day are not recommended). If serum ferritin is <500 mcg/L, interrupt therapy.

Nontransfusion-dependent chronic iron overload; thalassemia syndromes: Children ≥10 years and Adolescents: Oral: **Note:** Treatment should only be initiated with evidence of chronic iron overload (hepatic iron concentration ≥5 mg Fe/g dry weight and serum ferritin >300 mcg/L).

Exjade (oral tablet for suspension):

Initial: 10 mg/kg once daily; after 4 weeks; if baseline hepatic iron concentration was >15 mg Fe/g dry weight, may increase to 20 mg/kg once daily

Maintenance: Dependent upon serum ferritin measurements (monthly) and hepatic iron concentrations (every 6 months)

If serum ferritin is <300 mcg/L: Interrupt therapy and obtain hepatic iron concentration

If hepatic iron concentration:

<3 mg Fe/g dry weight: Interrupt therapy; resume treatment when hepatic iron concentration is >5 mg Fe/g dry weight

3 to 7 mg Fe/g dry weight: Continue treatment at a dose ≤10 mg/kg/day

>7 mg Fe/g dry weight: Consider dose increase to 20 mg/kg/day; repeat measurement and if remains >7 mg Fe/g dry weight, continue current dose; if repeat measurement is 3 to 7 mg Fe/g dry weight, then decrease dose to 10 mg/kg/day

Jadenu (oral tablet):

Initial: 7 mg/kg once daily; after 4 weeks, if hepatic iron concentration was >15 mg Fe/g dry weight, may increase to 14 mg/kg once daily

Maintenance: Dependent upon serum ferritin measurements (monthly) and hepatic iron concentrations (every 6 months)

If serum ferritin is <300 mcg/L: Interrupt therapy and obtain hepatic iron concentration

If hepatic iron concentration:

<3 mg Fe/g dry weight: Interrupt therapy; resume treatment when hepatic iron concentration is >5 mg Fe/g dry weight

3 to 7 mg Fe/g dry weight: Continue treatment at a dose ≤7 mg/kg/day

>7 mg Fe/g dry weight: Consider dose increase to 14 mg/kg/day; repeat measurement and if remains >7 mg Fe/g dry weight, continue current dose; if repeat measurement is 3 to 7 mg Fe/g dry weight, then decrease dose to ≤7 mg/kg/day. Maximum daily dose: 14 mg/kg/day.

Adult:

Conversion from Exjade to Jadenu: The dose for Jadenu should be ~30% lower (rounded to the nearest whole tablet).

Chronic iron overload due to transfusions: Oral: **Note:** Treatment should only be initiated with evidence of chronic iron overload (ie, transfusion of ≥100 mL/kg of packed red blood cells [eg, ≥20 units for a 40 kg individual] and serum ferritin consistently >1,000 mcg/L).

Exjade (oral tablet for suspension):
Initial: 20 mg/kg once daily
Maintenance: **Note**: Consider interrupting therapy for serum ferritin <500 mcg/L (risk of toxicity may be increased). Adjust dose every 3 to 6 months based on serum ferritin trends; adjust by 5 or 10 mg/kg/day; titrate to individual response and treatment goals. In patients not adequately controlled with 30 mg/kg/day, doses up to 40 mg/kg/day may be considered for serum ferritin levels persistently >2,500 mcg/L and not decreasing over time (doses above 40 mg/kg/day are not recommended).
Jadenu (oral tablet):
Initial: 14 mg/kg once daily
Maintenance: **Note:** Consider interrupting therapy for serum ferritin <500 mcg/L (risk of toxicity may be increased). Adjust dose every 3 to 6 months based on serum ferritin trends; adjust by 3.5 or 7 mg/kg/day; titrate to individual response and treatment goals. In patients not adequately controlled with 21 mg/kg/day, doses up to 28 mg/kg/day may be considered for serum ferritin levels persistently >2,500 mcg/L and not decreasing over time (doses above 28 mg/kg/day are not recommended).

Chronic iron overload in nontransfusion-dependent thalassemia syndromes: Oral: **Note:** Treatment should only be initiated with evidence of chronic iron overload (hepatic iron concentration ≥5 mg Fe/g dry weight and serum ferritin >300 mcg/L).
Exjade (oral tablet for suspension):
Initial: 10 mg/kg once daily. Consider increasing to 20 mg/kg once daily after 4 weeks if baseline hepatic iron concentration is >15 mg Fe/g dry weight
Maintenance: Monitor serum ferritin monthly; if serum ferritin is <300 mcg/L, interrupt therapy and obtain hepatic iron concentration. Monitor hepatic iron concentration every 6 months; interrupt therapy if hepatic iron concentration <3 mg Fe/g dry weight. After 6 months of therapy, consider dose adjustment to a maximum of 20 mg/kg/day if hepatic iron concentration >7 mg Fe/g dry weight. Reduce dose to ≤10 mg/kg when hepatic iron concentration is 3 to 7 mg Fe/g dry weight. Do not exceed 20 mg/kg/day. After interruption, resume treatment when hepatic iron concentration >5 mg Fe/g dry weight.
Jadenu (oral tablet):
Initial: 7 mg/kg once daily. Consider increasing to 14 mg/kg once daily after 4 weeks if baseline hepatic iron concentration is >15 mg Fe/g dry weight.
Maintenance: Monitor serum ferritin monthly; if serum ferritin is <300 mcg/L, interrupt therapy and obtain hepatic iron concentration. Monitor hepatic iron concentration every 6 months; interrupt therapy if hepatic iron concentration <3 mg Fe/g dry weight. After 6 months of therapy, consider dose adjustment to a maximum of 14 mg/kg/day if hepatic iron concentration >7 mg Fe/g dry weight. Reduce dose to ≤7 mg/kg when hepatic iron concentration is 3 to7 mg Fe/g dry weight. Do not exceed 14 mg/kg/day. After interruption, resume treatment when hepatic iron concentration >5 mg Fe/g dry weight.

Dosing adjustment with concomitant bile acid sequestrants (eg, cholestyramine, colesevelam, colestipol) or potent UGT inducers (eg, rifampin, phenytoin, phenobarbital, ritonavir): Children ≥2 years, Adolescents, and Adults: Avoid concomitant use; if coadministration necessary, consider increasing the initial deferasirox dose by 50%; monitor serum ferritin and clinical response.

Dosing adjustment in renal impairment:
Baseline: Children ≥2 years, Adolescents, and Adults:
CrCl >60 mL/minute: No dosage adjustment necessary
CrCl 40 to 60 mL/minute: Reduce initial dose by 50%
CrCl <40 mL/minute or serum creatinine >2 x age-appropriate ULN: Use is contraindicated
During therapy: Adjustment dependent upon indication for use.
Transfusional iron overload:
Children ≥2 years and Adolescents <16 years: For increase in serum creatinine ≥33% above the average baseline level and above the age-appropriate ULN: Reduce daily dose **by** 10 mg/kg/day (for Exjade) or 7 mg/kg (for Jadenu)
Adolescents ≥16 years and Adults: If increase in serum creatinine ≥33% above the average baseline: Repeat serum creatinine measurement in 1 week; if still elevated by ≥33%: Reduce daily dose **by** 10 mg/kg/day (for Exjade) or 7 mg/kg (for Jadenu)
All patients: If serum creatinine >2 times age-appropriate ULN or CrCl <40 mL/minute: Discontinue therapy
Nontransfusion-dependent thalassemia syndromes:
Children ≥10 years and Adolescents <16 years: For increase in serum creatinine ≥33% above the average baseline level and above the age-appropriate ULN: Reduce daily dose **by** 5 mg/kg/day (for Exjade) or 3.5 mg/kg (for Jadenu)
Adolescents ≥16 years and Adults: If increase in serum creatinine ≥33% above the average baseline; repeat serum creatinine measurement in 1 week; if still elevated **by** ≥33%:
Exjade: Interrupt therapy if the dose is 5 mg/kg; reduce dose **by** 50% if the dose is 10 or 20 mg/kg
Jadenu: Interrupt therapy if the dose is 3.5 mg/kg; reduce dose **by** 50% if the dose is 7 or 14 mg/kg
All patients: If serum creatinine >2 times age-appropriate ULN or CrCl <40 mL/minute: Discontinue therapy

Dosing adjustment in hepatic impairment: Children ≥2 years, Adolescents, and Adults:
Baseline:
Mild impairment (Child-Pugh class A): No adjustment necessary; monitor closely for efficacy and for adverse reactions requiring dosage reduction
Moderate impairment (Child-Pugh class B): Reduce dose **by** 50%; monitor closely for efficacy and for adverse reactions requiring dosage reduction
Severe impairment (Child-Pugh class C): Avoid use
During therapy: Severe or persistent increases in transaminases/bilirubin: Reduce dose or temporarily interrupt treatment

Dosing adjustment for toxicity:
Bone marrow suppression: Interrupt treatment; may reinitiate once cause of cytopenia has been determined; contraindicated if platelet count <50,000/mm^3
Dermatologic toxicity:
Rash (severe): Interrupt treatment; may reintroduce at a lower dose (with future dose escalation) and short-term oral corticosteroids
Severe skin reaction (Stevens-Johnson syndrome, erythema multiforme): Discontinue and evaluate.
Gastrointestinal: Discontinue treatment for suspected GI ulceration or hemorrhage.
Hearing loss or visual disturbance: Consider dose reduction or treatment interruption

Preparation for Administration Oral tablets for suspension (Exjade): Completely disperse tablets in water, orange juice, or apple juice; use 3.5 ounces for total doses <1,000 mg and 7 ounces for doses ≥1,000 mg; stir to form suspension. Avoid dispersion of tablets in milk (due to slowed dissolution) or carbonated drinks (due to foaming) (Séchaud 2008).

Administration Oral:
Tablets (Jadenu): Administer with water or other liquids at the same time each day. Administer on an empty

stomach or with a light meal (containing less than 7% fat content and ~250 calories). Do not administer simultaneously with aluminum-containing antacids or cholestyramine.

Tablets for oral suspension (Exjade): Administer tablets by making an oral suspension; **do not chew or swallow whole tablets**. Stir to form suspension and drink entire contents. Rinse remaining residue with more fluid; drink. Administer at same time each day on an empty stomach, at least 30 minutes before food. Do not administer simultaneously with aluminum-containing antacids or cholestyramine.

Monitoring Parameters Serum ferritin (baseline, then monthly), iron levels (baseline), CBC with differential, serum creatinine, and/or creatinine clearance [two baseline assessments, then at least monthly; for patients who are at increased risk of complications (eg, pre-existing renal conditions, elderly, comorbid conditions, or receiving other potentially nephrotoxic medications): Two baseline assessments, weekly for the first month then at least monthly thereafter]; urine protein (monthly), serum transaminases (ALT/AST) and bilirubin at baseline, every 2 weeks for 1 month, then monthly; baseline and annual auditory and ophthalmic function (including slit lamp examinations and dilated fundoscopy); performance status (in patients with hematologic malignancies); signs and symptoms of GI ulcers or hemorrhage; cumulative number of RBC units received

Dosage Forms Excipient information presented when available (limited, particularly for generics); consult specific product labeling.

Tablet, Oral:

Jadenu: 90 mg, 180 mg, 360 mg

Tablet Soluble, Oral:

Exjade: 125 mg, 250 mg, 500 mg

Deferoxamine (de fer OKS a meen)

Medication Safety Issues

Sound-alike/look-alike issues:

Deferoxamine may be confused with cefuroxime, deferasirox, deferiprone

Desferal may be confused with desflurane, Desyrel, Dexferrum

International issues:

Desferal [U.S., Canada, and multiple international markets] may be confused with Deseril brand name for methysergide [Australia, Belgium, Great Britain, Netherlands]; Disophrol brand name for dexbrompheniramine and pseudoephedrine [Czech Republic, Poland, Turkey]

Brand Names: US Desferal

Brand Names: Canada Deferoxamine Mesylate for Injection; Desferal; PMS-Deferoxamine

Therapeutic Category Antidote, Aluminum Toxicity; Antidote, Iron Toxicity; Chelating Agent, Parenteral

Generic Availability (US) Yes

Use Adjunct treatment of acute iron intoxication and treatment of chronic iron overload secondary to multiple transfusions (FDA approved in ages ≥3 years and adults); has also been used in the diagnosis and treatment of aluminum accumulation in chronic renal failure

Pregnancy Risk Factor C

Pregnancy Considerations Skeletal anomalies and delayed ossification were observed in some but not all animal reproduction studies. Toxic amounts of iron or deferoxamine have not been noted to cross the placenta. In case of acute iron toxicity, treatment during pregnancy should not be withheld.

Breast-Feeding Considerations It is not known if deferoxamine is excreted in human milk; the manufacturer recommends that caution be used if administered to a breast-feeding woman.

Contraindications Hypersensitivity to deferoxamine or any component of the formulation; patients with severe renal disease or anuria

Note: Canadian labeling does not include severe renal disease or anuria as contraindications.

Warnings/Precautions Flushing of the skin, hypotension urticaria and shock are associated with rapid IV infusion, administer IM, by slow subcutaneous or slow IV infusion only. Auditory disturbances (tinnitus and high frequency hearing loss) have been reported following prolonged administration, at high doses, or in patients with low ferritin levels; generally reversible with early detection and immediate discontinuation. Elderly patients are at increased risk for hearing loss. Audiology exams are recommended with long-term treatment. Ocular disturbances (blurred vision, cataracts, corneal opacities, decreased visual acuity, impaired peripheral, color, and night vision, optic neuritis, retinal pigment abnormalities, scotoma, visual loss/defect) have been reported following prolonged administration, at high doses, or in patients with low ferritin levels; generally reversible with early detection and immediate discontinuation. Elderly patients are at increased risk for ocular disorders. Periodic ophthalmic exams are recommended with long-term treatment.

Deferoxamine has been associated with acute respiratory distress syndrome following excessively high-dose IV treatment of acute iron intoxication or thalassemia (has been reported in children and adults). High deferoxamine doses and concurrent low ferritin levels are also associated with growth retardation. Growth velocity may partially resume to pretreatment velocity rates after deferoxamine dose reduction. Patients with iron overload are at increased susceptibility to infection with *Yersinia enterocolitica* and *Yersinia pseudotuberculosis*; treatment with deferoxamine may enhance this risk; if infection develops, discontinue therapy until resolved. Rare and serious cases of mucormycosis have been reported with use; withhold treatment with signs and symptoms of mucormycosis.

Increases in serum creatinine, acute renal failure and renal tubular disorders have been reported; monitor for changes in renal function. When iron is chelated with deferoxamine, the chelate is excreted renally. Deferoxamine is readily dialyzable. Treatment with deferoxamine in patients with aluminum toxicity may cause hypocalcemia and aggravate hyperparathyroidism. Deferoxamine may cause neurological symptoms (including seizure) in patients with aluminum-related encephalopathy receiving dialysis and may precipitate dialysis dementia onset.

Deferoxamine is **not** indicated for the treatment of primary hemochromatosis (treatment of choice is phlebotomy). Patients should be informed that urine may have a reddish color. Combination treatment with ascorbic acid (>500 mg/day in adults) and deferoxamine may impair cardiac function (rare), reversible upon discontinuation of ascorbic acid. If combination treatment is warranted, initiate ascorbic acid only after one month of regular deferoxamine treatment, do not exceed ascorbic acid dose of 200 mg/day for adults (in divided doses), 100 mg/day for children ≥10 years of age, or 50 mg/day in children <10 years of age; monitor cardiac function. Do not administer deferoxamine in combination with ascorbic acid in patients with preexisting cardiac failure.

Warnings: Additional Pediatric Considerations Growth retardation in pediatric patients especially in patients ≤3 years has been associated with high doses (>60 mg/kg) and concurrent low ferritin levels; a reduction in deferoxamine dosage may partially improve growth velocity; monitor growth in children receiving chronic therapy closely.

Adverse Reactions

Cardiovascular: Flushing, hypotension, shock, tachycardia

Central nervous system: Brain disease (aluminum toxicity/dialysis-related), dizziness, headache, neuropathy (peripheral, sensory, motor, or mixed), paresthesia, seizure

Dermatologic: Skin rash, urticaria

Endocrine & metabolic: Growth suppression (children), hyperparathyroidism (aggravated), hypocalcemia

Gastrointestinal: Abdominal distress, abdominal pain, diarrhea, nausea, vomiting

Genitourinary: Dysuria, urine discoloration (reddish color)

Hematologic & oncologic: Dysplasia (metaphyseal; children <3 years; dose related), leukopenia, thrombocytopenia

Hepatic: Hepatic insufficiency, increased serum transaminases

Hypersensitivity: Anaphylaxis (with or without shock), angioedema, hypersensitivity

Infection: Infection (*Yersinia*, mucormycosis)

Local: Injection site reaction (burning, crust, edema, erythema, eschar, induration, infiltration, irritation, pain, pruritus, swelling, vesicles, wheal formation)

Neuromuscular & skeletal: Arthralgia, muscle spasm, myalgia

Ophthalmic: Blurred vision, cataract, chromatopsia, corneal opacity, decreased peripheral vision, decreased visual acuity, nocturnal amblyopia, optic neuritis, retinal pigment changes, scotoma, vision loss, visual field defect

Otic: Hearing loss, tinnitus

Renal: Acute renal failure, increased serum creatinine, renal tubular disease

Respiratory: Acute respiratory distress (dyspnea, cyanosis, and/or interstitial infiltrates), asthma

Miscellaneous: Fever

Drug Interactions

Metabolism/Transport Effects None known.

Avoid Concomitant Use There are no known interactions where it is recommended to avoid concomitant use.

Increased Effect/Toxicity

Deferoxamine may increase the levels/effects of: Prochlorperazine

The levels/effects of Deferoxamine may be increased by: Ascorbic Acid; Multivitamins/Fluoride (with ADE); Multivitamins/Minerals (with ADEK, Folate, Iron); Multivitamins/Minerals (with AE, No Iron)

Decreased Effect There are no known significant interactions involving a decrease in effect.

Storage/Stability Prior to reconstitution, store at ≤25°C (≤77°F). Following reconstitution, may be stored at room temperature for 24 hours, although the manufacturer recommends use begin within 3 hours of reconstitution. Do not refrigerate reconstituted solution. When stored at 30°C in polypropylene infusion pump syringes, deferoxamine 250 mg/mL in sterile water for injection retained 95% of initial concentration for 14 days (Stiles, 1996).

Mechanism of Action Complexes with trivalent ions (ferric ions) to form ferrioxamine, which is removed by the kidneys, slows accumulation of hepatic iron and retards or eliminates progression of hepatic fibrosis. Also known to inhibit DNA synthesis *in vitro*.

Pharmacokinetics (Adult data unless noted)

Absorption: IM, SubQ: Well absorbed

Distribution: Distributed throughout body fluids

Metabolism: Plasma enzymes; binds with iron to form ferrioxamine (iron complex)

Half-life: 14 hours; plasma: 20-30 minutes (Brittenham, 2011)

Elimination: Primarily urine (as unchanged drug and ferrioxamine); feces (via bile)

Dialysis: Dialyzable

Dosing: Neonatal

Acute iron intoxication: Very limited data available: IV infusion: 5 mg/kg/hour; dosing based on a case report of an oral ferrous sulfate overdose in a former premature neonate (GA: 27 weeks and age at time of treatment PCA: 34 weeks) (Valentine 2009).

Dosing: Usual

Pediatric:

Acute iron intoxication: Limited data available: Children and Adolescents: **Note:** The IV route is used when severe toxicity is evidenced by cardiovascular collapse or systemic symptoms (coma, shock, metabolic acidosis, or gastrointestinal bleeding) or potentially severe intoxications (peak serum iron level >500 mcg/dL) (Perrone 2011). When severe symptoms are not present, the IM may be used.

Continuous IV infusion: Initial: 15 mg/kg/hour and reduce rate as clinically indicated; maximum daily dose: 80 mg/kg/**day** and not to exceed 6 g/**day** [Desferal prescribing information (Canada; UK) 2011]

IV: Initial: 20 mg/kg (maximum dose: 1,000 mg) administered no faster than 15 mg/kg/hour followed by 10 mg/kg (maximum dose: 500 mg) over 4-hour intervals for 2 doses; subsequent doses of 10 mg/kg (maximum dose: 500 mg) over 4 to 12 hours may be repeated depending upon the clinical response; maximum dose: 6 g/**day**; this dosing may also be used IM if symptoms not severe.

IM: 90 mg/kg/dose for one dose, then 45 mg/kg/dose every 4 to 12 hours as needed; maximum single dose: Children: 1,000 mg; Adults: 2,000 mg; maximum daily dose: 6 g/day [Desferal prescribing information (Canada; UK) 2011]; others have used 50 mg/kg/dose every 6 hours with maximum daily dose: 6 **g/day** (Chang 2011); may also use intermittent IV dosing (see above)

Chronic iron overload:

General dosing: Manufacturer's labeling: Children ≥3 years and Adolescents:

IV:

Children and Growing Adolescents: 20 to 40 mg/kg/day over 8 to 12 hours, 5 to 7 days per week, usual maximum daily dose: 40 mg/kg/**day**

Adolescents once growth has ceased: 40 to 50 mg/kg/day over 8 to 12 hours, 5 to 7 days per week, usual maximum daily dose: 60 mg/kg/**day**

SubQ infusion via a portable, controlled infusion device: 20 to 40 mg/kg/day over 8 to 12 hours 3 to 7 days per week; maximum daily dose: 2,000 mg/**day**. Doses >60 mg/kg/day have not been shown to provide additional benefit (Vlachos 2008).

Sickle cell disease, chronic iron overload: Children and Adolescents: SubQ infusion: 25 mg/kg/day over 8 hours; dose and duration may be increased as needed (NHLBI 2005)

Thalassemia, chronic iron overload: **Note:** A lower dose may be required if the ferritin levels are low. In general, the therapeutic index should be kept <0.025 at all times. Therapeutic index = mean daily deferoxamine dose (mg/kg)/ferritin (mcg/L) (Cappellini, 2008):

Children and Growing Adolescents: SubQ infusion: 20 to 40 mg/kg/day over 8 to 12 hours, 6 to 7 nights per week, maximum daily dose: 40 mg/kg/**day**

Adolescents once growth has ceased:

SubQ infusion (preferred): 40 to 60 mg/kg/day over 8 to 12 hours, 6 to 7 nights per week, maximum daily dose: 2,000 mg/**day**

SubQ bolus: 45 mg/kg/dose, 5 times per week.

Aluminum-induced bone disease in chronic renal failure: Limited data available: Children and Adolescents: **Note:** Intended for predialysis serum aluminum concentration of 60-200 mcg/L; do not start chelation therapy if serum aluminum concentration >200 mcg/L; intensive dialysis (6 days per week with a high flux dialysis membrane) should be used until serum aluminum concentration decreases below 200 mcg/L (National Kidney Foundation 2003):

Test (diagnostic) dose: IV: 5 mg/kg as a single dose infused over the last hour of dialysis; measure serum aluminum concentration 2 days later; depending upon the change in serum aluminum concentration, treatment with deferoxamine may be indicated (see Treatment below)

Treatment: IV: Monitor serum aluminum levels closely. See National Kidney Foundation guidelines for additional details on treatment algorithms.

Aluminum rise ≥300 mcg/L or adverse effects with test dose: 5 mg/kg once a week 5 hours before dialysis for 4 months

Aluminum rise <300 mcg/L: 5 mg/kg once a week during the last hour of dialysis for 2 months

Adult:

Acute iron intoxication: Note: The IV route is used when severe toxicity is evidenced by cardiovascular collapse or systemic symptoms (coma, shock, metabolic acidosis, or gastrointestinal bleeding) or potentially severe intoxications (peak serum iron level >500 mcg/dL) (Perrone 2011). When severe symptoms are not present, the IM route may be used.

IM, IV: 1000 mg stat, then 500 mg every 4 hours for 2 doses, additional doses of 500 mg every 4 to 12 hours may be needed depending upon the clinical response; maximum daily dose: 6 **g/day**

Chronic iron overload:

IM: 500 to 1,000 mg/dose; maximum daily dose: 1,000 mg/**day**

IV: 40 to 50 mg/kg/day over 8 to 12 hours for 5 to 7 days per week; maximum daily dose: 6 **g/day**

SubQ via portable, controlled infusion device: 1,000 to 2,000 mg/day or 20 to 40 mg/kg/day over 8 to 24 hours

Dosage adjustment in renal impairment:

Manufacturer's labeling: Severe renal disease or anuria: Use is contraindicated.

Alternate recommendations: The following adjustments have been recommended (Aronoff 2007): Adults:

CrCl >50 mL/minute: No adjustment required

CrCl 10 to 50 mL/minute or CRRT: Administer 25% to 50% of normal dose

CrCl <10 mL/minute, hemodialysis, or peritoneal dialysis: Avoid use

Dosage adjustment in hepatic impairment: There are no dosage adjustments provided in the manufacturer's labeling (not studied).

Preparation for Administration

Parenteral:

IM: Reconstitute with SWFI (500 mg vial with 2 mL SWFI; 2000 mg vial with 8 mL SWFI) to a final concentration of 213 mg/mL

IV: Reconstitute with SWFI (500 mg vial with 5 mL SWFI; 2000 mg vial with 20 mL SWFI) to a final concentration of 95 mg/mL; further dilute for infusion in NS, ½NS, D_5W, or LR.

SubQ: Reconstitute with SWFI (500 mg vial with 5 mL SWFI; 2,000 mg vial with 20 mL SWFI) to a final concentration of 95 mg/mL. Local reactions at the site of SubQ infusion may be minimized by diluting the deferoxamine in 5 to 10 mL SWFI and adding 1 mg hydrocortisone to each mL of deferoxamine solution (Kirking 1991)

Administration

Parenteral:

IM: Preferred route of administration for acute iron ingestion in patients not in shock per the manufacturer's labeling.

IV: Administer as intermittent IV infusion or as continuous IV infusion; maximum rate: 15 mg/kg/hour; may consider reducing infusion rate to <125 mg/hour after the first 1,000 mg have been infused.

SubQ: When administered for chronic iron overload, administration over 8 to 12 hours using a portable infusion pump is generally recommended; however, longer infusion times (24 hours) may also be used. Topical anesthetic or glucocorticoid creams may be used for induration or erythema (Brittenham 2011).

Monitoring Parameters Serum ferritin, iron, total iron binding capacity; CBC with differential, renal function tests, liver function tests, growth velocity (including weight and height) every 3 months, ophthalmologic exam, and audiometry (with chronic use); blood pressure (with IV infusions)

Dialysis patients: Serum aluminum (yearly; every 3 months in patients on aluminum-containing medications)

Aluminum-induced bone disease: Serum aluminum 2 days following test dose; test is considered positive if serum aluminum increases ≥50 mcg/L

Reference Range

Iron, serum: Normal: 50-160 mcg/dL; peak levels >500 mcg/dL associated with toxicity. Consider treatment in symptomatic patients with levels ≥350 mcg/dL; toxicity cannot be excluded with serum iron levels <350 mcg/dL.

Aluminum, serum: <20 mcg/L (National Kidney Foundation, 2003)

Test Interactions TIBC may be falsely elevated with high serum iron concentrations or deferoxamine therapy. Imaging results may be distorted due to rapid urinary excretion of deferoxamine-bound gallium-67; discontinue deferoxamine 48 hours prior to scintigraphy.

Dosage Forms Excipient information presented when available (limited, particularly for generics); consult specific product labeling.

Solution Reconstituted, Injection, as mesylate:

Desferal: 500 mg (1 ea); 2 g (1 ea)

Generic: 500 mg (1 ea); 2 g (1 ea)

- **Deferoxamine Mesylate** *see* Deferoxamine *on page 598*
- **Deferoxamine Mesylate for Injection (Can)** *see* Deferoxamine *on page 598*
- **Dehydral® (Can)** *see* Methenamine *on page 1385*
- **Dehydrobenzperidol** *see* Droperidol *on page 723*
- **Delatestryl (Can)** *see* Testosterone *on page 2025*
- **Delestrogen** *see* Estradiol (Systemic) *on page 795*
- **Delsym [OTC]** *see* Dextromethorphan *on page 631*
- **Delsym Cough Childrens [OTC]** *see* Dextromethorphan *on page 631*
- **Delta-9-tetrahydro-cannabinol** *see* Dronabinol *on page 722*
- **Delta-9 THC** *see* Dronabinol *on page 722*
- **Deltacortisone** *see* PredniSONE *on page 1760*
- **Delta D3 [OTC]** *see* Cholecalciferol *on page 448*
- **Deltadehydrocortisone** *see* PredniSONE *on page 1760*
- **Deltasone** *see* PredniSONE *on page 1760*
- **Delzicol** *see* Mesalamine *on page 1368*
- **Demadex** *see* Torsemide *on page 2095*

Demeclocycline (dem e kloe SYE kleen)

Therapeutic Category Antibiotic, Tetracycline Derivative

Generic Availability (US) Yes

Use Treatment of susceptible bacterial infections (acne, gonorrhea, pertussis, chronic bronchitis, and urinary tract infections) caused by both gram-negative and gram-positive organisms; treatment of chronic syndrome of inappropriate antidiuretic hormone (SIADH) secretion

Pregnancy Risk Factor D

Pregnancy Considerations Tetracyclines, including demeclocycline, cross the placenta and accumulate in developing teeth and long tubular bones. Tetracyclines may discolor fetal teeth following maternal use during pregnancy; the specific teeth involved and the portion of the tooth affected depends on the timing and duration of exposure relative to tooth calcification. As a class, tetracyclines are generally considered second-line antibiotics in pregnant women and their use should be avoided (Gibbons, 1960; Mylonas, 2011).

Breast-Feeding Considerations Tetracyclines are excreted into breast milk. According to the manufacturer, the decision to continue or discontinue breast-feeding during therapy should take into account the risk of exposure to the infant and the benefits of treatment to the mother.

Tetracyclines, including demeclocycline, bind to calcium (Mitrano, 2009). The calcium in maternal milk will significantly decrease the amount of demeclocycline absorbed by the breast-feeding infant. Nondose-related effects could include modification of bowel flora.

Contraindications Hypersensitivity to demeclocycline, tetracyclines, or any component of the formulation

Warnings/Precautions Photosensitivity reactions occur frequently with this drug; avoid prolonged exposure to sunlight and do not use tanning equipment. Use caution in patients with hepatic impairment; dose adjustment and/or adjustment to interval frequency recommended. Hepatotoxicity and hepatic failure have been reported rarely with use. Use with caution in patients with renal impairment; dosage modification required in patients with renal impairment. Nephrotoxicity has also been reported with use, particularly in the setting of cirrhosis. May act as an antianabolic agent and increase BUN. Dose-dependent nephrogenic diabetes insipidus is common with use; however, this adverse event of demeclocycline has been used as a therapeutic advantage in the off-label use of hyponatremia associated with SIADH. Pseudotumor cerebri has been reported with tetracycline use (usually resolves with discontinuation). Prolonged use may result in fungal or bacterial superinfection, including *C. difficile*-associated diarrhea (CDAD) and pseudomembranous colitis; CDAD has been observed >2 months postantibiotic treatment. May cause tissue hyperpigmentation, enamel hypoplasia, or permanent tooth discoloration; use of tetracyclines should be avoided during tooth development (children <8 years of age) unless other drugs are not likely to be effective or are contraindicated. Do not use during pregnancy. In addition to affecting tooth development, tetracycline use has been associated with retardation of skeletal development and reduced bone growth. Concurrent use of tetracyclines and methoxyflurane (not available in the U.S.) is not recommended; fatal renal toxicity has been reported with concurrent use.

Adverse Reactions

Cardiovascular: Pericarditis

Central nervous system: Bulging fontanels (infants), dizziness, headache, pseudotumor cerebri (adults)

Dermatologic: Angioedema, anogenital inflammatory lesions (with monilial overgrowth), erythema multiforme, erythematous rash, exfoliative dermatitis (rare), maculopapular rash, photosensitivity, pigmentation of skin, Stevens-Johnson syndrome (rare), urticaria

Endocrine & metabolic: Microscopic discoloration of thyroid gland (brown/black), nephrogenic diabetes insipidus, thyroid dysfunction (rare)

Gastrointestinal: Anorexia, diarrhea, dysphagia, enterocolitis, esophageal ulcerations, glossitis, nausea, pancreatitis, vomiting

Genitourinary: Balanitis

Hematologic: Eosinophilia, neutropenia, hemolytic anemia, thrombocytopenia

Hepatic: Hepatitis (rare), hepatotoxicity (rare), liver enzymes increased, liver failure (rare)

Neuromuscular & skeletal: Myasthenic syndrome, polyarthralgia, tooth discoloration (children <8 years, rarely in adults)

Ocular: Visual disturbances

Otic: Tinnitus

Renal: Acute renal failure, BUN increased

Respiratory: Pulmonary infiltrates

Miscellaneous: Anaphylaxis, anaphylactoid purpura, fixed drug eruptions (rare), lupus-like syndrome, superinfection, systemic lupus erythematosus exacerbation

Drug Interactions

Metabolism/Transport Effects None known.

Avoid Concomitant Use

Avoid concomitant use of Demeclocycline with any of the following: BCG; BCG (Intravesical); Mecamylamine; Retinoic Acid Derivatives; Strontium Ranelate

Increased Effect/Toxicity

Demeclocycline may increase the levels/effects of: Mecamylamine; Mipomersen; Neuromuscular-Blocking Agents; Porfimer; Retinoic Acid Derivatives; Verteporfin; Vitamin K Antagonists

Decreased Effect

Demeclocycline may decrease the levels/effects of: BCG; BCG (Intravesical); BCG Vaccine (Immunization); Desmopressin; Iron Salts; Penicillins; Sodium Picosulfate; Typhoid Vaccine

The levels/effects of Demeclocycline may be decreased by: Antacids; Bile Acid Sequestrants; Bismuth Subcitrate; Bismuth Subsalicylate; Calcium Salts; Iron Salts; Lanthanum; Magnesium Salts; Multivitamins/Minerals (with ADEK, Folate, Iron); Multivitamins/Minerals (with AE, No Iron); Quinapril; Strontium Ranelate; Sucralfate; Sucroferric Oxyhydroxide; Zinc Salts

Food Interactions Demeclocycline serum levels may be decreased if taken with food, milk, or dairy products. Management: Administer 1 hour before or 2 hours after food, milk, or dairy products.

Storage/Stability Store at controlled room temperature at 20°C to 25°C (68°F to 77°F).

Mechanism of Action Inhibits protein synthesis by binding with the 30S and possibly the 50S ribosomal subunit(s) of susceptible bacteria; may also cause alterations in the cytoplasmic membrane; inhibits the action of ADH in patients with chronic SIADH

Pharmacodynamics Onset of action for diuresis in SIADH: Within 5 days

Pharmacokinetics (Adult data unless noted)

Absorption: ~60% to 80% of dose absorbed from the GI tract; food and dairy products reduce absorption by 50% or more

Distribution: Distributes into pleural fluid, bronchial secretions, sputum, prostatic and seminal fluids, and to body tissues; crosses into breast milk

Protein binding: 36% to 91%

Metabolism: Small amounts metabolized in the liver to inactive metabolites; enterohepatically recycled

Half-life: Adults: 10-17 hours (prolonged with reduced renal function)

Time to peak serum concentration: Oral: Within 3-4 hours

Elimination: Excreted as unchanged drug (42% to 50%) in urine and 31% in feces

Dosing: Usual Oral:

Children >8 years: 8-12 mg/kg/day divided every 6-12 hours

Adults: 150 mg 4 times/day or 300 mg twice daily

Uncomplicated gonorrhea: 600 mg stat, 300 mg every 12 hours for 4 days (3 g total)

SIADH: Initial: 600-1200 mg/day or 13-15 mg/kg/day divided every 6-8 hours; then decrease to 600-900 mg/day

Dosing adjustment in renal impairment: Dose and/or frequency should be modified in response to the degree of renal impairment

Dosing adjustment in hepatic impairment: Not recommended for use

Administration Oral: Administer 1 hour before or 2 hours after food or milk with plenty of fluids; do not administer with food, milk, dairy products, antacids, zinc, or iron supplements

Monitoring Parameters CBC, renal and hepatic function tests, I & O, urine output, serum sodium; observe for changes in bowel frequency

Dosage Forms Excipient information presented when available (limited, particularly for generics); consult specific product labeling.

Tablet, Oral, as hydrochloride:

Generic: 150 mg, 300 mg

- ◆ **Demeclocycline Hydrochloride** *see* Demeclocycline *on page* *600*
- ◆ **Demerol** *see* Meperidine *on page* *1359*
- ◆ **4-Demethoxydaunorubicin** *see* IDArubicin *on page* *1071*
- ◆ **Demethylchlortetracycline** *see* Demeclocycline *on page* *600*
- ◆ **Denavir** *see* Penciclovir *on page* *1651*
- ◆ **Denta 5000 Plus** *see* Fluoride *on page* *899*
- ◆ **DentaGel** *see* Fluoride *on page* *899*
- ◆ **Dentapaine [OTC]** *see* Benzocaine *on page* *268*
- ◆ **Denti-Care Chlorhexidine Gluconate Oral Rinse (Can)** *see* Chlorhexidine Gluconate *on page* *434*
- ◆ **Dent-O-Kain/20 [OTC]** *see* Benzocaine *on page* *268*
- ◆ **Deodorized Tincture of Opium (error-prone synonym)** *see* Opium Tincture *on page* *1569*
- ◆ **2'-Deoxycoformycin** *see* Pentostatin *on page* *1668*
- ◆ **Deoxycoformycin** *see* Pentostatin *on page* *1668*
- ◆ **Depacon** *see* Valproic Acid and Derivatives *on page* *2143*
- ◆ **Depakene** *see* Valproic Acid and Derivatives *on page* *2143*
- ◆ **Depakote** *see* Valproic Acid and Derivatives *on page* *2143*
- ◆ **Depakote ER** *see* Valproic Acid and Derivatives *on page* *2143*
- ◆ **Depakote Sprinkles** *see* Valproic Acid and Derivatives *on page* *2143*
- ◆ **Depen Titratabs** *see* PenicillAMINE *on page* *1652*
- ◆ **Depo-Estradiol** *see* Estradiol (Systemic) *on page* *795*
- ◆ **Depo-Medrol** *see* MethylPREDNISolone *on page* *1409*
- ◆ **Depo-Prevera (Can)** *see* MedroxyPROGESTERone *on page* *1339*
- ◆ **Depo-Provera** *see* MedroxyPROGESTERone *on page* *1339*
- ◆ **Depo-SubQ Provera 104** *see* MedroxyPROGESTERone *on page* *1339*
- ◆ **Depotest 100 (Can)** *see* Testosterone *on page* *2025*
- ◆ **Depo-Testosterone** *see* Testosterone *on page* *2025*
- ◆ **Deprizine FusePaq** *see* Ranitidine *on page* *1836*
- ◆ **DermaFungal [OTC]** *see* Miconazole (Topical) *on page* *1431*
- ◆ **DermaMed [OTC]** *see* Aluminum Hydroxide *on page* *110*
- ◆ **Derma-Smoothe/FS® (Can)** *see* Fluocinolone (Topical) *on page* *897*
- ◆ **Derma-Smoothe/FS Body** *see* Fluocinolone (Topical) *on page* *897*
- ◆ **Derma-Smoothe/FS Scalp** *see* Fluocinolone (Topical) *on page* *897*
- ◆ **Dermasorb HC** *see* Hydrocortisone (Topical) *on page* *1041*
- ◆ **Dermasorb TA** *see* Triamcinolone (Topical) *on page* *2117*
- ◆ **Dermatop** *see* Prednicarbate *on page* *1754*
- ◆ **Dermazole (Can)** *see* Miconazole (Topical) *on page* *1431*
- ◆ **Dermoplast [OTC]** *see* Benzocaine *on page* *268*
- ◆ **DermOtic** *see* Fluocinolone (Otic) *on page* *896*
- ◆ **Dermovate (Can)** *see* Clobetasol *on page* *498*
- ◆ **Desenex [OTC]** *see* Clotrimazole (Topical) *on page* *518*
- ◆ **Desenex [OTC]** *see* Miconazole (Topical) *on page* *1431*
- ◆ **Desenex Jock Itch [OTC]** *see* Miconazole (Topical) *on page* *1431*
- ◆ **Desenex Spray [OTC]** *see* Miconazole (Topical) *on page* *1431*
- ◆ **Desferal** *see* Deferoxamine *on page* *598*
- ◆ **Desferrioxamine** *see* Deferoxamine *on page* *598*
- ◆ **Desiccated Thyroid** *see* Thyroid, Desiccated *on page* *2058*

Desipramine (des IP ra meen)

Medication Safety Issues

Sound-alike/look-alike issues:

Desipramine may be confused with clomiPRAMINE, dalfampridine, diphenhydrAMINE, disopyramide, imipramine, nortriptyline

Norpramin may be confused with clomiPRAMINE, imipramine, Normodyne, Norpace, nortriptyline, Tenormin

BEERS Criteria medication:

This drug may be potentially inappropriate for use in geriatric patients (Quality of evidence - high [moderate for SIADH]; Strength of recommendation - strong).

International issues:

Norpramin: Brand name for desipramine [U.S., Canada], but also the brand name for enalapril/hydrochlorothiazide [Portugal]; omeprazole [Spain]

Related Information

Antidepressant Agents *on page* *2257*

Brand Names: US Norpramin

Brand Names: Canada Dom-Desipramine; Novo-Desipramine; Nu-Desipramine; PMS-Desipramine

Therapeutic Category Antidepressant, Tricyclic (Secondary Amine)

Generic Availability (US) Yes

Use Treatment of depression (FDA approved in adolescents and adults); has also been used in the treatment of attention-deficit/hyperactivity disorder (ADHD)

Medication Guide Available Yes

Pregnancy Considerations Animal reproduction studies are inconclusive. Tricyclic antidepressants may be associated with irritability, jitteriness, and convulsions (rare) in the neonate (Yonkers, 2009).

The ACOG recommends that therapy for depression during pregnancy be individualized; treatment should incorporate the clinical expertise of the mental health clinician, obstetrician, primary healthcare provider, and pediatrician (ACOG, 2008). According to the American Psychiatric Association (APA), the risks of medication treatment should be weighed against other treatment options and untreated depression. For women who discontinue antidepressant medications during pregnancy and who may be at high risk for postpartum depression, the medications can be restarted following delivery (APA, 2010). Treatment algorithms have been developed by the ACOG and the APA for the management of depression in women prior to conception and during pregnancy (Yonkers, 2009).

Breast-Feeding Considerations Desipramine is excreted into breast milk. Based on information from one mother-infant pair, following maternal use of desipramine 300 mg/day, the estimated exposure to the breast-feeding infant would be 2% of the weight-adjusted maternal dose. Adverse events were not reported. Infants should be monitored for signs of adverse events; routine monitoring of infant serum concentrations is not recommended (Fortinguerra, 2009).

Contraindications

Hypersensitivity to desipramine or any component of the formulation; use of MAO inhibitors intended to treat psychiatric disorders (concurrently or within 14 days of stopping desipramine or an MAO inhibitor); initiation of desipramine in a patient receiving linezolid or intravenous methylene blue; use in a patient during the acute recovery phase of MI

Documentation of allergenic cross-reactivity for drugs in this class is limited. However, because of similarities in chemical structure and/or pharmacologic actions, the possibility of cross-sensitivity cannot be ruled out with certainty.

Warnings/Precautions [U.S. Boxed Warning]: Antidepressants increase the risk of suicidal thinking and behavior in children, adolescents, and young adults (18 to 24 years of age) with major depressive disorder (MDD) and other psychiatric disorders; consider risk prior to prescribing. Short-term studies did not show an increased risk in patients >24 years of age and showed a decreased risk in patients ≥65 years. Closely monitor for clinical worsening, suicidality, or unusual changes in behavior, particularly during the initial 1 to 2 months of therapy or during periods of dosage adjustments (increases or decreases); the patient's family or caregiver should be instructed to closely observe the patient and communicate condition with healthcare provider. A medication guide should be dispensed with each prescription. **Desipramine is FDA approved for the treatment of depression in adolescents.**

The possibility of a suicide attempt is inherent in major depression and may persist until remission occurs. Worsening depression and severe abrupt suicidality that are not part of the presenting symptoms may require discontinuation or modification of drug therapy. The patient's family or caregiver should be alerted to monitor patients for the emergence of suicidality and associated behaviors (such as agitation, irritability, hostility, impulsivity, and hypomania) and notify healthcare provider.

May precipitate a shift to mania or hypomania in patients with bipolar disorder. Patients presenting with depressive symptoms should be screened for bipolar disorder including details regarding family history of suicide, bipolar disorder, and depression. Monotherapy in patients with bipolar disorder should be avoided. **Desipramine is not FDA approved for the treatment of bipolar depression.**

Potentially life-threatening serotonin syndrome (SS) has occurred with serotonergic agents (eg, SSRIs, SNRIs), particularly when used in combination with other serotonergic agents (eg, triptans, TCAs, fentanyl, lithium, tramadol, buspirone, St John's wort, tryptophan) or agents that impair metabolism of serotonin (eg, MAO inhibitors intended to treat psychiatric disorders, other MAO inhibitors [ie, linezolid and intravenous methylene blue]). Discontinue treatment (and any concomitant serotonergic agent) immediately if signs/symptoms arise. TCAs may rarely cause bone marrow suppression; monitor for any signs of infection and obtain CBC if symptoms (eg, fever, sore throat) evident. The degree of anticholinergic blockade produced by this agent is low relative to other cyclic antidepressants; however, extreme caution should be used in patients with urinary retention, benign prostatic hyperplasia, narrow-angle glaucoma, xerostomia, visual problems, constipation, or a history of bowel obstruction (APA, 2010). May cause CNS depression, which may impair physical or mental abilities; patients must be cautioned about performing tasks that require mental alertness (eg, operating machinery or driving). May cause orthostatic hypotension (risk is moderate relative to other antidepressants); use with caution in patients at risk of this effect or in those who would not tolerate transient hypotensive episodes (cerebrovascular disease, cardiovascular disease, hypovolemia, or concurrent medication use which may predispose to hypotension/bradycardia) (APA, 2010). Due to risk of conduction abnormalities, use with extreme caution in patients with a history of cardiovascular disease (including previous MI, stroke, tachycardia, or conduction abnormalities) or in patients with a family history of sudden death, dysrhythmias, or conduction abnormalities. Use with caution in patients with diabetes mellitus; may alter glucose regulation (APA, 2010). May cause mild pupillary dilation which in susceptible individuals can lead to an episode of narrow-angle glaucoma. Consider evaluating patients who have not had an iridectomy for narrow-angle glaucoma risk factors.

Recommended by the manufacturer to discontinue prior to elective surgery; risks exist for drug interactions with anesthesia and for cardiac arrhythmias. However, definitive drug interactions have not been widely reported in the literature and continuation of tricyclic antidepressants is generally recommended as long as precautions are taken to reduce the significance of any adverse events that may occur (Pass, 2004). May lower seizure threshold - use extreme caution in patients with a previous seizure disorder or condition predisposing to seizures such as brain damage, alcoholism, or concurrent therapy with other drugs which lower the seizure threshold. In some patients, seizures may precede cardiac dysrhythmias and death. May increase the risks associated with electroconvulsive therapy. Bone fractures have been associated with antidepressant treatment. Consider the possibility of a fragility fracture if an antidepressant-treated patient presents with unexplained bone pain, point tenderness, swelling, or bruising (Rabenda, 2013; Rizzoli, 2012). Use with caution in patients with hepatic or renal dysfunction. Potentially significant interactions may exist, requiring dose or frequency adjustment, additional monitoring, and/or selection of alternative therapy.

Use caution in elderly patients; may cause or exacerbate syndrome of inappropriate antidiuretic hormone secretion or hyponatremia; monitor sodium closely with initiation or dosage adjustments in older adults. May be inappropriate in older adults depending on comorbidities (eg, dementia, delirium) or in patients with a history of falls and fractures due to its potent anticholinergic effects (Beers Criteria). May also increase risk of falling or confusional states.

Abrupt discontinuation or interruption of antidepressant therapy has been associated with a discontinuation syndrome. Symptoms arising may vary with antidepressant however commonly include nausea, vomiting, diarrhea, headaches, lightheadedness, dizziness, diminished appetite, sweating, chills, tremors, paresthesias, fatigue, somnolence, and sleep disturbances (eg, vivid dreams, insomnia). Greater risks for developing a discontinuation syndrome have been associated with antidepressants with shorter half-lives, longer durations of treatment, and abrupt discontinuation. For antidepressants of short or intermediate half-lives, symptoms may emerge within 2 to 5 days after treatment discontinuation and last 7 to 14 days (APA, 2010; Fava, 2006; Haddad, 2001; Shelton, 2001; Warner, 2006).

Warnings: Additional Pediatric Considerations The American Heart Association recommends that all children diagnosed with ADHD who may be candidates for medication, such as desipramine, should have a thorough cardiovascular assessment prior to initiation of therapy. These recommendations are based upon reports of serious cardiovascular adverse events (including sudden death) in patients (both children and adults) taking usual doses of stimulant medications. Most of these patients were found to have underlying structural heart disease (eg, hypertrophic obstructive cardiomyopathy). Asymptomatic ECG changes and minor increases in diastolic blood pressure and heart rate have been noted in children receiving desipramine doses >3.5 mg/kg/day; four cases of sudden death have been reported in children and adolescents 5 to 14 years of age; an association between desipramine and sudden death was not observed in one retrspective study. Pretreatment cardiovascular assessment should include a combination of thorough medical history, family history, and physical examination. An ECG is not mandatory but should be considered.

Adverse Reactions Some reactions listed are based on reports for other agents in this same pharmacologic class, and may not be specifically reported for desipramine.

Cardiovascular: Cardiac arrhythmia, cerebrovascular accident, edema, flushing, heart block, hypertension, hypotension, myocardial infarction, palpitations, premature ventricular contractions, tachycardia, ventricular fibrillation, ventricular tachycardia

Central nervous system: Agitation, anxiety, ataxia, confusion, delusions, disorientation, dizziness, drowsiness, drug fever, EEG pattern changes, extrapyramidal reaction, falling, fatigue, hallucination, headache, hypomania, insomnia, neuroleptic malignant syndrome, nightmares, numbness, peripheral neuropathy, psychosis (exacerbation), restlessness, seizure, tingling of extremities, tingling sensation, withdrawal syndrome

Dermatologic: Alopecia, diaphoresis (excessive), pruritus, skin photosensitivity, skin rash, urticaria

Endocrine & metabolic: Decreased libido, decreased serum glucose, galactorrhea, gynecomastia, increased libido, increased serum glucose, SIADH, weight gain, weight loss

Gastrointestinal: Abdominal cramps, anorexia, constipation, diarrhea, epigastric distress, increased pancreatic enzymes, melanoglossia, nausea, paralytic ileus, parotid gland enlargement, stomatitis, sublingual adenitis, unpleasant taste, vomiting, xerostomia

Genitourinary: Breast hypertrophy, impotence, nocturia, painful ejaculation, testicular swelling, urinary hesitancy, urinary retention, urinary tract dilation

Hematologic & oncologic: Agranulocytosis, eosinophilia, petechia, purpura, thrombocytopenia

Hepatic: Abnormal hepatic function tests, cholestatic jaundice, hepatitis, increased liver enzymes, increased serum alkaline phosphatase

Neuromuscular & skeletal: Tremor, weakness

Ophthalmic: Accommodation disturbance, blurred vision, increased intraocular pressure, mydriasis

Otic: Tinnitus

Renal: Polyuria

Miscellaneous: Fever

Drug Interactions

Metabolism/Transport Effects **Substrate** of CYP1A2 (minor), CYP2D6 (major); **Note:** Assignment of Major/Minor substrate status based on clinically relevant drug interaction potential; **Inhibits** CYP2A6 (moderate), CYP2B6 (moderate), CYP2D6 (moderate), CYP2E1 (weak)

Avoid Concomitant Use

Avoid concomitant use of Desipramine with any of the following: Aclidinium; Artesunate; Azelastine (Nasal); Eluxadoline; Glucagon; Iobenguane I 123; Ipratropium (Oral Inhalation); Linezolid; MAO Inhibitors; Methylene Blue; Moxonidine; Orphenadrine; Paraldehyde; Potassium Chloride; Tegafur; Thalidomide; Thioridazine; Tiotropium; Umeclidinium

Increased Effect/Toxicity

Desipramine may increase the levels/effects of: AbobotulinumtoxinA; Alcohol (Ethyl); Alpha-/Beta-Agonists (Direct-Acting); Alpha1-Agonists; Amphetamines; Analgesics (Opioid); Anticholinergic Agents; Antipsychotic Agents; ARIPiprazole; Artesunate; Azelastine (Nasal); Beta2-Agonists; Buprenorphine; Citalopram; CNS Depressants; CYP2B6 Substrates; CYP2D6 Substrates; Desmopressin; DOXOrubicin (Conventional); Eliglustat; Eluxadoline; Escitalopram; Fesoterodine; Glucagon; Highest Risk QTc-Prolonging Agents; Hydrocodone; Methotrimeprazine; Methylene Blue; Metoprolol; Metyrosine; Moderate Risk QTc-Prolonging Agents; Nebivolol; Nicorandil; OnabotulinumtoxinA; Orphenadrine; Paraldehyde; Potassium Chloride; Pramipexole; QuiNIDine; RimabotulinumtoxinB; ROPINIRole; Rotigotine; Serotonin Modulators; Sodium Phosphates; Sulfonylureas; Suvorexant; Thalidomide; Thiazide Diuretics; Thioridazine; Tiotropium; Topiramate; TraMADol; Vitamin K Antagonists; Yohimbine; Zolpidem

The levels/effects of Desipramine may be increased by: Abiraterone Acetate; Aclidinium; Altretamine; Antiemetics (5HT3 Antagonists); Antipsychotic Agents; Boceprevir; Brimonidine (Topical); BuPROPion; Cannabis; Cimetidine; Cinacalcet; Citalopram; Cobicistat; CYP2D6 Inhibitors (Moderate); CYP2D6 Inhibitors (Strong); Darunavir; Dexmethylphenidate; Doxylamine; Dronabinol; Droperidol; DULoxetine; Escitalopram; FLUoxetine; FluvoxaMINE; HydrOXYzine; Ipratropium (Oral Inhalation); Kava Kava; Linezolid; Lithium; Magnesium Sulfate; MAO Inhibitors; Methotrimeprazine; Methylphenidate; Metoclopramide; Metyrosine; Mianserin; Mifepristone; Mirabegron; Nabilone; Panobinostat; PARoxetine; Peginterferon Alfa-2b; Perampanel; Pramlintide; Propafenone; Protease Inhibitors; QuiNIDine; Rufinamide; Sertraline; Sodium Oxybate; Tapentadol; Tedizolid; Terbinafine (Systemic); Tetrahydrocannabinol; Thyroid Products; TraMADol; Umeclidinium; Valproic Acid and Derivatives

Decreased Effect

Desipramine may decrease the levels/effects of: Acetylcholinesterase Inhibitors; Alpha1-Agonists; Alpha2-Agonists; Alpha2-Agonists (Ophthalmic); Artesunate; Codeine; Iobenguane I 123; Itopride; Moxonidine; Secretin; Tamoxifen; Tegafur

The levels/effects of Desipramine may be decreased by: Acetylcholinesterase Inhibitors; Barbiturates; CarBAMazepine; Peginterferon Alfa-2b; St Johns Wort

Storage/Stability Store at 25°C (77°F); excursions are permitted between 15°C and 30°C (59°F and 86°F). Protect from excessive heat.

Mechanism of Action Traditionally believed to increase the synaptic concentration of norepinephrine (and to a lesser extent, serotonin) in the central nervous system by inhibition of its reuptake by the presynaptic neuronal membrane. However, additional receptor effects have been found including desensitization of adenyl cyclase, down regulation of beta-adrenergic receptors, and down regulation of serotonin receptors.

Pharmacodynamics Antidepressant effects:

Onset of action: Occasionally seen in 2-5 days

Maximum effect: After more than 2 weeks

Pharmacokinetics (Adult data unless noted)

Absorption: Rapidly and well absorbed from the GI tract

Protein binding: 90%

Metabolism: Hepatic

Half-life: Mean range: 18.4 to 21.5 hours (Ciraulo, 1988; Weiner, 1981)

Time to peak serum concentration: ~6 hours (Weiner, 1981)

Elimination: 70% in urine

Dosing: Usual

Pediatric:

Attention-deficit/hyperactivity disorder (ADHD): Limited data available, dosing regimens variable: Titrate dose based on tolerance and response; **Note:** Desipramine should not be used first-line and use reserved for cases where other medications have not been effective or not tolerated (Pliszka, 2007); may be beneficial for patient with comorbid conditions (eg, Tourette's syndrome) (Singer, 1995; Spencer, 1996)

Weight-directed dosing: Children ≥5 years and Adolescents: Oral: Initial: 1.5 mg/kg/day divided twice daily; titrate weekly up to target dose of 3.5 mg/kg/day in 2 divided doses by week 3 (Spencer, 1993; Spencer, 1996; Spencer, 2002). A double-blind, placebo-controlled, parallel trial (n=41, treatment group: n=21) reported a significant reduction in core ADHD symptoms, at mean desipramine dose of 3.4 mg/kg/day; however, a small but statistically significant increase in BP and HR were observed in the treatment group (Spencer, 2002).

Fixed dose: Children ≥7 years and Adolescents ≤13 years: Oral: Initial: 25 mg at bedtime; increase at weekly intervals in 25 mg/day increments up to a maximum dose of 25 mg four times daily (100 mg/day) not to exceed 3 mg/kg/day (Singer, 1995)

Depression: Note: Controlled clinical trials have not shown tricyclic antidepressants to be superior to placebo for the treatment of depression in children and adolescents; not recommended as first-line medication; may be beneficial for patients with comorbid conditions (Birmaher, 2007; Dopheide, 2006; Wagner, 2005).

Children 6 to 12 years: Limited data available: Oral: 1 to 3 mg/kg/day in divided doses; monitor carefully with doses >3 mg/kg/day; maximum daily dose: 5 mg/kg/**day** (Kliegman, 2007)

Adolescents: Oral: Initial dose: Start at the lower range and increase based on tolerance and response; usual maintenance dose: 25 to 100 mg/day; doses up to 150 mg/day may be necessary in severely depressed patients. Maximum daily dose: 150 mg/**day**

Adult: **Depression:** Oral: Initial dose: Start at the lower range and increase based on tolerance and response; usual maintenance dose: 100 to 200 mg/day; doses up to 300 mg/day may be necessary in severely depressed patients

Dosing adjustment for concomitant MAO inhibitor therapy: Adolescents and Adults:

Switching to or from an MAO inhibitor intended to treat psychiatric disorders:

Allow 14 days to elapse between discontinuing an MAO inhibitor intended to treat psychiatric disorders and initiation of desipramine.

Allow 14 days to elapse between discontinuing desipramine and initiation of an MAO inhibitor intended to treat psychiatric disorders.

Use with other MAO inhibitors (linezolid or IV methylene blue):

Do not initiate desipramine in patients receiving linezolid or IV methylene blue; consider other interventions for psychiatric condition.

If urgent treatment with linezolid or IV methylene blue is required in a patient already receiving desipramine and potential benefits outweigh potential risks, discontinue desipramine promptly and administer linezolid or IV methylene blue. Monitor for serotonin syndrome for 2 weeks or until 24 hours after the last dose of linezolid or IV methylene blue, whichever comes first. May resume desipramine 24 hours after the last dose of linezolid or IV methylene blue.

Dosing adjustment in renal impairment: There are no dosage adjustments provided in the manufacturer's labeling; use with caution. Hemodialysis/peritoneal dialysis: Adults: Supplemental dose is not necessary.

Dosing adjustment in hepatic impairment: There are no dosage adjustments provided in the manufacturer's labeling.

Administration Oral: Administer with food to decrease GI upset

Monitoring Parameters Blood pressure, heart rate, ECG, mental status, weight. Monitor patient periodically for symptom resolution; monitor for worsening of depression, suicidality, and associated behaviors (especially at the beginning of therapy or when doses are increased or decreased); signs and symptoms of serotonin syndrome

ADHD: Evaluate patients for cardiac disease prior to initiation of therapy for ADHD with thorough medical history, family history, and physical exam; consider ECG; perform ECG and echocardiogram if findings suggest cardiac disease; promptly conduct cardiac evaluation in patients who develop chest pain, unexplained syncope, or any other symptom of cardiac disease during treatment.

Long-term use: Also monitor CBC with differential, liver enzymes, serum concentrations

Reference Range Plasma concentrations do not always correlate with clinical effectiveness.

Timing of serum samples: Draw trough just before next dose

Therapeutic: 150 to 300 ng/mL (SI: 560 to 1125 nmol/L)

Test Interactions May interfere with urine detection of amphetamines/methamphetamines (false-positive) (Merigan, 1993).

Dosage Forms Excipient information presented when available (limited, particularly for generics); consult specific product labeling.

Tablet, Oral, as hydrochloride:

Norpramin: 10 mg, 25 mg, 50 mg, 75 mg, 100 mg, 150 mg

Generic: 10 mg, 25 mg, 50 mg, 75 mg, 100 mg, 150 mg

- **Desipramine Hydrochloride** *see* Desipramine *on page 602*
- **Desitin® [OTC]** *see* Zinc Oxide *on page 2214*
- **Desitin® Creamy [OTC]** *see* Zinc Oxide *on page 2214*

Desloratadine (des lor AT a deen)

Medication Safety Issues

Sound-alike/look-alike issues:

Clarinex may be confused with Celebrex

Brand Names: US Clarinex; Clarinex Reditabs

Brand Names: Canada Aerius; Aerius Kids; Desloratadine Allergy Control

Therapeutic Category Antihistamine

Generic Availability (US) May be product dependent

Use Symptomatic relief of nasal and non-nasal symptoms of perennial allergic rhinitis (FDA approved in ages ≥6 months and adults); symptomatic relief of nasal and non-nasal symptoms of seasonal allergic rhinitis (FDA approved in ages ≥2 years and adults); symptomatic relief and reduction in number and size of hives in chronic idiopathic urticaria (FDA approved in ages ≥6 months and adults)

Pregnancy Risk Factor C

Pregnancy Considerations Adverse events have been observed in animal reproduction studies; therefore, the manufacturer classifies desloratadine as pregnancy category C. The use of antihistamines for the treatment of rhinitis during pregnancy is generally considered to be safe at recommended doses. Information related to the use of desloratadine during pregnancy is limited; therefore, other agents may be preferred. Desloratadine is the primary metabolite of loratadine; refer to the Loratadine monograph for additional information.

Breast-Feeding Considerations Desloratadine is excreted into breast milk. According to the manufacturer, the decision to continue or discontinue breast-feeding during therapy should take into account the risk of exposure to the infant and the benefits of treatment to the mother.

Contraindications Hypersensitivity to desloratadine, loratadine, or any component of the formulation

Warnings/Precautions Hypersensitivity reactions (including anaphylaxis) have been reported with use; discontinue therapy immediately with signs/symptoms of hypersensitivity. Dose should be adjusted in patients with liver or renal impairment. Use with caution in patients known to be slow metabolizers of desloratadine (incidence of side effects may be increased). Some products may contain phenylalanine.

Benzyl alcohol and derivatives: Some dosage forms may contain sodium benzoate/benzoic acid; benzoic acid (benzoate) is a metabolite of benzyl alcohol; large amounts of benzyl alcohol (≥99 mg/kg/day) have been associated with a potentially fatal toxicity ("gasping syndrome") in neonates; the "gasping syndrome" consists of metabolic acidosis, respiratory distress, gasping respirations, CNS dysfunction (including convulsions, intracranial hemorrhage), hypotension, and cardiovascular collapse (AAP, 1997; CDC, 1982); some data suggests that benzoate displaces bilirubin from protein binding sites (Ahlfors, 2001); avoid or use dosage forms containing benzyl alcohol derivative with caution in neonates. See manufacturer's labeling.

Warnings: Additional Pediatric Considerations Safety and efficacy for the use of cough and cold products in pediatric patients <4 years of age is limited; the AAP warns against the use of these products for respiratory illnesses in this age group. Serious adverse effects including death have been reported. Many of these products contain multiple active ingredients, increasing the risk of accidental overdose when used with other products. Health care providers are reminded to ask caregivers about the use of OTC cough and cold products in order to avoid exposure to multiple medications containing the same ingredient (AAP 2012; FDA 2008).

Some dosage forms may contain propylene glycol; in neonates large amounts of propylene glycol delivered orally, intravenously (eg, >3,000 mg/day), or topically have been associated with potentially fatal toxicities which can include metabolic acidosis, seizures, renal failure, and CNS depression; toxicities have also been reported in children and adults including hyperosmolality, lactic acidosis, seizures and respiratory depression; use caution (AAP 1997; Shehab 2009).

Adverse Reactions Note: Reported in children, unless otherwise noted.

Central nervous system: Dizziness (adults), drowsiness (more common in children), emotional lability, fatigue (adults), headache (adults), irritability, insomnia

Gastrointestinal: Anorexia, appetite increased, diarrhea, dyspepsia (adults), nausea (children and adults), vomiting, xerostomia (adults)

Dermatologic: Erythema, maculopapular rash

Genitourinary: Dysmenorrhea (adults), urinary tract infection

Infection: Parasitic infection, varicella

Neuromuscular & skeletal: Myalgia (adults)

Otic: Otitis media

Respiratory: Bronchitis, cough, epistaxis, pharyngitis (children and adults), rhinorrhea, upper respiratory tract infection

Miscellaneous: Fever

Rare but important or life-threatening: Hepatitis (rare), hypersensitivity reactions (including anaphylaxis, dyspnea, edema, pruritus, rash, urticaria), psychomotor agitation, seizure, tachycardia

Drug Interactions

Metabolism/Transport Effects Substrate of P-glycoprotein

Avoid Concomitant Use

Avoid concomitant use of Desloratadine with any of the following: Aclidinium; Azelastine (Nasal); Eluxadoline; Glucagon; Ipratropium (Oral Inhalation); Orphenadrine; Paraldehyde; Potassium Chloride; Thalidomide; Tiotropium; Umeclidinium

Increased Effect/Toxicity

Desloratadine may increase the levels/effects of: AbobotulinumtoxinA; Alcohol (Ethyl); Analgesics (Opioid); Anticholinergic Agents; Azelastine (Nasal); Buprenorphine; CNS Depressants; Eluxadoline; Glucagon; Hydrocodone; Methotrimeprazine; Metyrosine; Mirabegron; Mirtazapine; OnabotulinumtoxinA; Orphenadrine; Paraldehyde; Potassium Chloride; Pramipexole; RimabotulinumtoxinB; ROPINIRole; Rotigotine; Selective Serotonin Reuptake Inhibitors; Suvorexant; Thalidomide; Thiazide Diuretics; Tiotropium; Topiramate; Zolpidem

The levels/effects of Desloratadine may be increased by: Aclidinium; Brimonidine (Topical); Cannabis; Doxylamine; Dronabinol; Droperidol; HydrOXYzine; Ipratropium (Oral Inhalation); Kava Kava; Magnesium Sulfate; Methotrimeprazine; Mianserin; Nabilone; Perampanel; P-glycoprotein/ABCB1 Inhibitors; Pramlintide; Rufinamide; Sodium Oxybate; Tapentadol; Tetrahydrocannabinol; Umeclidinium

Decreased Effect

Desloratadine may decrease the levels/effects of: Acetylcholinesterase Inhibitors; Benzylpenicilloyl Polylysine; Betahistine; Hyaluronidase; Itopride; Metoclopramide; Secretin

The levels/effects of Desloratadine may be decreased by: Acetylcholinesterase Inhibitors; Amphetamines; P-glycoprotein/ABCB1 Inducers

Food Interactions Food does not affect bioavailability.

Storage/Stability Syrup, tablet, orally-disintegrating tablet: Store at 25°C (77°F); excursions permitted between 15°C to 30°C (59°F to 85°F). Protect from moisture and excessive heat. Use orally-disintegrating tablet immediately after opening blister package. Syrup should be protected from light.

Mechanism of Action Desloratadine, a major active metabolite of loratadine, is a long-acting tricyclic antihistamine with selective peripheral histamine H_1 receptor antagonistic activity.

Pharmacodynamics

Onset of action: 1 hour

Duration: 24 hours

Pharmacokinetics (Adult data unless noted)

Protein binding: 82% to 87% (desloratadine), 85% to 89% (3-hydroxydesloratadine, active metabolite)

Metabolism: Hepatic to an active metabolite (3-hydroxydesloratadine); subsequently undergoes glucuronidation; decreased in slow metabolizers of desloratadine

Half-life: 27 hours

Time to peak serum concentration: 3 hours

Elimination: 87% eliminated via urine and feces as metabolic products

Dosing: Usual

Pediatric:

Perennial allergic rhinitis: Oral:

Infants 6 months to 11 months: 1 mg once daily

Children 1 year to 5 years: 1.25 mg once daily

Children 6 years to 11 years: 2.5 mg once daily

Children ≥12 years and Adolescents: 5 mg once daily

Seasonal allergic rhinitis: Oral:

Children 2 years to 5 years: 1.25 mg once daily

Children 6 years to 11 years: 2.5 mg once daily

Children ≥12 years and Adolescents: 5 mg once daily

Urticaria, chronic idiopathic: Oral:

Infants 6 months to 11 months: 1 mg once daily

Children 1 year to 5 years: 1.25 mg once daily

Children 6 years to 11 years: 2.5 mg once daily

Children ≥12 years and Adolescents: 5 mg once daily

Adult: **Seasonal or perennial allergic rhinitis, chronic idiopathic urticaria:** Oral: 5 mg once daily

Dosing adjustment in renal impairment: Adults: Mild to severe impairment: 5 mg every other day

Dosing adjustment in hepatic impairment: Adults: Mild to severe impairment: 5 mg every other day

Administration Oral: May administer without regard to food.

Orally dissolving tablet: Place orally dissolving tablet directly on the tongue; tablet will disintegrate immediately; may be taken with or without water. Take immediately after removing from blister package.

Syrup: A commercially available measuring dropper or syringe calibrated to deliver 2 mL or 2.5 mL should be used to administer appropriate dose.

Monitoring Parameters Improvement in signs and symptoms of allergic rhinitis or urticaria

Test Interactions May suppress the wheal and flare reactions to skin test antigens

Dosage Forms Excipient information presented when available (limited, particularly for generics); consult specific product labeling.

Syrup, Oral:

Clarinex: 0.5 mg/mL (473 mL) [contains edetate disodium, fd&c yellow #6 (sunset yellow), propylene glycol, sodium benzoate; bubble-gum flavor]

Tablet, Oral:

Clarinex: 5 mg [contains fd&c blue #2 aluminum lake]

Generic: 5 mg

Tablet Dispersible, Oral:

Clarinex Reditabs: 2.5 mg, 5 mg [contains aspartame; tutti-frutti flavor]

Generic: 2.5 mg, 5 mg

◆ **Desloratadine Allergy Control (Can)** *see* Desloratadine *on page 605*

◆ **Desmethylimipramine Hydrochloride** *see* Desipramine *on page 602*

Desmopressin (des moe PRES in)

Medication Safety Issues

Sound-alike/look-alike issues:

Desmopressin may be confused with vasopressin

Brand Names: US DDAVP; DDAVP Rhinal Tube; Stimate

Brand Names: Canada Apo-Desmopressin; DDAVP; DDAVP Melt; Minirin; Nocdurna; Novo-Desmopressin; Octostim; PMS-Desmopressin

Therapeutic Category Antihemophilic Agent; Hemostatic Agent; Hormone, Posterior Pituitary; Vasopressin Analog, Synthetic

Generic Availability (US) Yes

Use Treatment of diabetes insipidus (Tablets: FDA approved in ages ≥4 years and adults; injection: FDA approved in ages ≥12 years and adults; DDAVP nasal spray; DDAVP rhinal tube: FDA approved in ages ≥3 months and adults); control of bleeding in hemophilia A (with factor VIII levels >5%) and mild to moderate type I von Willebrand disease (Injection: FDA approved in ages ≥3 months and adults; Stimate nasal spray: FDA approved in ages ≥11 months and adults); primary nocturnal enuresis (Tablets: FDA approved in ages ≥6 years)

Pregnancy Risk Factor B

Pregnancy Considerations Adverse events were not observed in animal reproduction studies. Anecdotal reports suggest congenital anomalies and low birth weight. However, causal relationship has not been established. Desmopressin has been used safely throughout pregnancy for the treatment of diabetes insipidus (Brewster, 2005; Schrier, 2010). The use of desmopressin is limited for the treatment of von Willebrand disease in pregnant women (NHLBI, 2007).

Breast-Feeding Considerations It is not known if desmopressin is excreted in breast milk. The manufacturer recommends that caution be exercised when administering desmopressin to nursing women.

Contraindications Hypersensitivity to desmopressin or any component of the formulation; hyponatremia or a history of hyponatremia; moderate-to-severe renal impairment (CrCl <50 mL/minute)

Canadian labeling: Additional contraindications (not in U.S. labeling): Type 2B or platelet-type (pseudo) von Willebrand's disease (injection, intranasal, oral, sublingual); known hyponatremia, habitual or psychogenic polydipsia, cardiac insufficiency or other conditions requiring diuretic therapy (intranasal, sublingual); nephrosis, severe hepatic dysfunction (sublingual); primary nocturnal enuresis (intranasal)

Warnings/Precautions Allergic reactions and anaphylaxis have been reported rarely with both the IV and intranasal formulations. Fluid intake should be adjusted downward in the elderly and very young patients to decrease the possibility of water intoxication and hyponatremia. Use may rarely lead to extreme decreases in plasma osmolality, resulting in seizures, coma, and death. Use caution with cystic fibrosis, heart failure, renal dysfunction, polydipsia (habitual or psychogenic [contraindicated in Canadian labeling]), or other conditions associated with fluid and electrolyte imbalance due to potential hyponatremia. Use caution with coronary artery insufficiency or hypertensive cardiovascular disease; may increase or decrease blood pressure leading to changes in heart rate. Consider switching from nasal to intravenous solution if changes in the nasal mucosa (scarring, edema) occur leading to unreliable absorption. Use caution in patients predisposed to thrombus formation; thrombotic events (acute cerebrovascular thrombosis, acute myocardial infarction) have occurred (rare).

Desmopressin (intranasal and IV), when used for hemostasis in hemophilia, is not for use in hemophilia B, type 2B von Willebrand disease, severe classic von Willebrand disease (type 1), or in patients with factor VIII antibodies. In general, desmopressin is also not recommended for use in patients with ≤5% factor VIII activity level, although it may be considered in selected patients with activity levels between 2% and 5%.

Consider switching from nasal to intravenous administration if changes in the nasal mucosa (scarring, edema) occur leading to unreliable absorption. Consider alternative route of administration (IV or intranasal) with inadequate therapeutic response at maximum recommended oral doses. Therapy should be interrupted if patient experiences an acute illness (eg, fever, recurrent vomiting or diarrhea), vigorous exercise, or any condition associated with an increase in water consumption. Some patients may demonstrate a change in response after long-term therapy (>6 months) characterized as decreased response or a shorter duration of response.

Warnings: Additional Pediatric Considerations The FDA has reviewed 61 postmarketing cases of hyponatremia-related seizures associated with the use of desmopressin acetate. Intranasal desmopressin was used in the majority of cases. Many of the patients were children being treated for primary nocturnal enuresis (PNE). An association with at least one concomitant drug or disease that also may cause hyponatremia and/or seizures was noted. As a result, intranasal desmopressin is no longer indicated for the treatment of PNE.

Adverse Reactions

Cardiovascular: Decreased blood pressure (IV), increased blood pressure (IV), flushing (facial)

Central nervous system: Chills (intranasal), dizziness (intranasal), headache, nostril pain (intranasal)

Dermatologic: Skin rash

Endocrine & metabolic: Hyponatremia, water intoxication

Gastrointestinal: Abdominal cramps, abdominal pain (intranasal), gastrointestinal disease (intranasal), nausea (intranasal), sore throat

Hepatic: Increased serum transaminases (transient; associated primarily with tablets)

Local: Burning sensation at injection site, erythema at injection site, swelling at injection site

Neuromuscular & skeletal: Weakness (intranasal)

Ophthalmic: Abnormal lacrimation (intranasal), conjunctivitis (intranasal), ocular edema (intranasal)

Respiratory: Cough, epistaxis (intranasal), nasal congestion, rhinitis (intranasal), upper respiratory infection

Rare but important or life-threatening: Abnormality in thinking, agitation, anaphylaxis (rare), balanitis, cerebral thrombosis (IV; acute), chest pain, coma, diarrhea, drowsiness, dyspepsia, edema, eye pruritus, hypersensitivity reaction (rare), insomnia, localized warm feeling, myocardial infarction (IV), pain, palpitations, photophobia, seizure, tachycardia, vomiting, vulvar pain

Drug Interactions

Metabolism/Transport Effects None known.

Avoid Concomitant Use There are no known interactions where it is recommended to avoid concomitant use.

Increased Effect/Toxicity

Desmopressin may increase the levels/effects of: Lithium

The levels/effects of Desmopressin may be increased by: Analgesics (Opioid); CarBAMazepine; ChlorproMAZINE; LamoTRIgine; Nonsteroidal Anti-Inflammatory Agents; Selective Serotonin Reuptake Inhibitors; Tricyclic Antidepressants

Decreased Effect

The levels/effects of Desmopressin may be decreased by: Demeclocycline; Lithium

Storage/Stability

DDAVP:

Nasal spray: Store at controlled room temperature of 20°C to 25°C (68°F to 77°F). Keep nasal spray in upright position.

Rhinal Tube solution: Store refrigerated at 2°C to 8°C (36°F to 46°F). May store at controlled room temperature of 20°C to 25°C (68°F to 77°F) for up to 3 weeks.

Solution for injection: Store refrigerated at 2°C to 8°C (36°F to 46°F).

Tablet: Store at controlled room temperature of 20°C to 25°C (68°F to 77°F).

DDAVP Melt (CAN; not available in U.S.): Store at 15°C to 25°C (59°F to 77°F) in original container. Protect from moisture.

Stimate nasal spray: Store at room temperature not to exceed 25°C (77°F). Discard 6 months after opening bottle.

Mechanism of Action In a dose dependent manner, desmopressin increases cyclic adenosine monophosphate (cAMP) in renal tubular cells which increases water permeability resulting in decreased urine volume and increased urine osmolality; increases plasma levels of von Willebrand factor, factor VIII, and t-PA contributing to a shortened activated partial thromboplastin time (aPTT) and bleeding time.

Pharmacodynamics

Oral administration:

Onset of ADH action: 1 hour

Maximum effect: 2 to 7 hours

Duration: 6 to 8 hours; **Note:** 0.4 mcg doses have had antidiuretic effects for up to 12 hours

Intranasal administration:

Onset of ADH action: Within 1 hour

Maximum effect: Within 1.5 hours

Duration: 5 to 21 hours

IV infusion:

Onset of increased factor VIII activity: Within 15 to 30 minutes

Maximum effect: 90 minutes to 3 hours

Pharmacokinetics (Adult data unless noted) Note: Due to large differences in bioavailability between product formulations and patient variability in response, dosage conversions between product formulations should be done conservatively titrating to clinical improvement.

Absorption:

Oral tablets: 0.08% to 0.16%; **Note:** Bioavailability of tablet is ~5% of nasal spray.

Nasal solution: 10% to 20%

Nasal spray (1.5 mg/mL concentration): 3.3% to 4.1%

Metabolism: Unknown

Half-life:

Oral: 1.5 to 2.5 hours

IV:

Initial: 7.8 minutes

Terminal: 75.5 minutes (range: 0.4 to 4 hours); severe renal impairment: 9 hours

Intranasal: 3.3 to 3.5 hours

Time to peak serum concentration:

Oral: 0.9 hours

Intranasal: 1.5 hours

Elimination: Primarily in urine

Dosing: Usual Note: Dosing presented is in mcg, mg, and mL (dependent upon product formulation); use extra precaution to verify product formulation and dosing units.

Pediatric:

Diabetes insipidus: Note: Fluid restriction should be observed in these patients; younger patients more susceptible to plasma osmolality shifts and possible hyponatremia. Dosing should be individualized to response.

Oral: Children ≥4 years and Adolescents: Initial: 0.05 **mg** twice daily; titrate to desired response; optimal daily dose range: 0.1 to 0.8 mg/day in 2 to 3 divided doses; reported daily dose range: 0.1 to 1.2 mg/day

Intranasal: DDAVP nasal spray, rhinal tube (100 mcg/mL nasal solution); **Note:** The nasal spray pump can only deliver fixed doses in 10 mcg (0.1 mL) increments; if doses other than this are needed, the rhinal tube delivery system is preferred.

Infants ≥3 months and Children: Initial: 5 mcg/day in 1 to 2 divided doses; usual range: 5 to 30 mcg/day (0.05 to 0.3 mL/day) in divided doses; adjust morning and evening doses separately for an adequate diurnal rhythm of water turnover

Adolescents: 5 to 40 mcg/day in 1 to 3 divided doses; usual adult dose is 20 mcg/day in 2 divided doses;

adjust morning and evening doses separately for an adequate diurnal rhythm of water turnover

IV, SubQ:

Infants and Children <12 years: No definitive dosing available. Adult dosing should not be used in this age group; adverse events such as hyponatremia-induced seizures may occur. Dose should be reduced. Some have suggested an initial dosage range of 0.1 to 1 mcg in 1 or 2 divided doses (Cheetham, 2002). Initiate at low dose and increase as necessary. Closely monitor serum sodium levels and urine output; fluid restriction is recommended.

Children ≥12 years and Adolescents: 2 to 4 mcg/day in 2 divided doses or one-tenth (1/10) of the maintenance intranasal dose; adjust morning and evening doses separately for an adequate diurnal rhythm of water turnover

Hemophilia A and von Willebrand disease (type 1; mild to moderate): Note: Adverse events such as hyponatremia-induced seizures have been reported especially in young children with IV use (Das, 2005; Molnár, 2005; Smith, 1989; Thumfart, 2005; Weinstein, 1989). Fluid restriction and careful monitoring of serum sodium levels and urine output are necessary.

IV: Infants ≥3 months, Children, and Adolescents: 0.3 mcg/kg; if used preoperatively administer 30 minutes before procedure; may repeat dose if needed

Intranasal: Stimate (high concentration spray 1.5 mg/mL): Infants ≥11 months, Children, and Adolescents:

<50 kg: 150 mcg (1 spray)

≥50 kg: 300 mcg (1 spray each nostril)

Repeat use is determined by the patient's clinical condition and laboratory work; if using preoperatively, administer 2 hours before surgery

Nocturnal enuresis: Note: Intranasal formulations are not recommended for nocturnal enuresis treatment.

Oral: Children ≥6 years and Adolescents: Initial: 0.2 mg once before bedtime; titrate as needed to a maximum of 0.6 **mg**; fluid intake should be limited to a minimum from 1 hour before desmopressin administration until the next morning, or at least 8 hours after administration

Adult:

Diabetes insipidus:

IV, SubQ: 2 to 4 mcg/day (0.5 to 1 mL) in 2 divided doses or one-tenth (1/10) of the maintenance intranasal dose. Fluid restriction should be observed.

Intranasal (100 mcg/mL nasal solution): 10 to 40 mcg/day (0.1 to 0.4 mL) divided 1 to 3 times daily; adjust morning and evening doses separately for an adequate diurnal rhythm of water turnover. **Note:** The nasal spray pump can only deliver doses of 10 mcg (0.1 mL) or multiples of 10 mcg (0.1 mL); if doses other than this are needed, the rhinal tube delivery system is preferred. Fluid restriction should be observed.

Oral: Initial: 0.05 mg twice daily; total daily dose should be increased or decreased as needed to obtain adequate antidiuresis (range: 0.1 to 1.2 mg divided 2 to 3 times daily). Fluid restriction should be observed.

Nocturnal enuresis: Oral: 0.2 mg at bedtime; dose may be titrated up to 0.6 mg to achieve desired response

Hemophilia A and mild to moderate von Willebrand disease (type 1):

IV: 0.3 mcg/kg by slow infusion; if used preoperatively, administer 30 minutes before procedure

Intranasal (using high concentration spray 1.5 mg/mL): <50 kg: 150 mcg (1 spray); ≥50 kg: 300 mcg (1 spray each nostril); repeat use is determined by the patient's clinical condition and laboratory work. If using preoperatively, administer 2 hours before surgery.

Dosing adjustment in renal impairment: CrCl <50 mL/minute: Use is contraindicated according to the manufacturer.

Dosing adjustment in hepatic impairment: There are no dosage adjustments provided in manufacturer's labeling.

Preparation for Administration Parenteral: IV infusion: Dilute solution for injection in 10 to 50 mL NS; volume of diluent dependent on patient weight (Infants and children ≤10 kg: 10 mL; Children >10 kg, adolescents and adults: 50 mL)

Administration

Intranasal:

DDAVP (100 mcg/mL): Nasal pump spray: Delivers 0.1 mL (10 mcg); for doses <10 mcg or for other doses which are not multiples, use rhinal tube. DDAVP nasal spray delivers fifty 10 mcg doses in the 5 mL bottle. For 10 mcg dose, administer in one nostril. Any solution remaining after 50 doses should be discarded. Pump must be primed prior to first use.

DDAVP Rhinal tube (100 mcg/mL): Insert top of dropper into tube (arrow marked end) in downward position. Squeeze dropper until solution reaches desired calibration mark. Disconnect dropper. Grasp the tube 3/4-inch from the end and insert tube into nostril until the fingertips reach the nostril. Place opposite end of tube into the mouth (holding breath). Tilt head back and blow with a strong, short puff into the nostril (for very young patients, an adult should blow solution into the child's nose). Reseal dropper after use.

Stimate (1.5 mg/mL): Nasal pump spray: Delivers 0.1 mL (150 mcg); for doses <150 mcg, injection is recommended. Stimate nasal spray delivers twenty-five 150 mcg doses. For 150 mcg dose, administer in one nostril. Any solution remaining after 25 doses should be discarded. Pump must be primed prior to first use or if not used for ≥1 week.

Parenteral:

Central diabetes insipidus: IV push or SubQ: Withdraw dose from ampul into appropriate syringe size (eg, insulin syringe). Further dilution is not required. Administer as direct injection.

Hemophilia A and von Willebrand disease (type 1): IV infusion: Infuse over 15 to 30 minutes.

Monitoring Parameters For all uses, fluid intake, urine volume, and signs and symptoms of hyponatremia should be closely monitored especially in high risk patient subgroups (eg, young children, elderly, patients with heart failure).

Diabetes insipidus: Urine specific gravity, plasma and urine osmolality, serum electrolytes

Nocturnal enuresis: Serum electrolytes if used for >7 days

Hemophilia A: Factor VIII coagulant activity, factor VIII ristocetin cofactor activity, and factor VIII antigen levels, aPTT

von Willebrand disease: Factor VIII coagulant activity, factor VIII ristocetin cofactor activity, and factor VIII von Willebrand antigen levels, bleeding time

Additional Information 1 mcg of desmopressin acetate injection is approximately equal to 4 units of antidiuretic activity; desmopressin acetate injection has an antidiuretic effect about ten times that of an equivalent dose administered intranasally

Dosage Forms Considerations

DDAVP and Minirin 5 mL bottles contain 50 sprays.

Stimate 2.5 mL bottles contain 25 sprays.

Dosage Forms Excipient information presented when available (limited, particularly for generics); consult specific product labeling. [DSC] = Discontinued product

Solution, Injection, as acetate:

DDAVP: 4 mcg/mL (1 mL)

DDAVP: 4 mcg/mL (10 mL) [contains chlorobutanol (chlorobutol)]

Generic: 4 mcg/mL (1 mL, 10 mL)

Solution, Nasal, as acetate:
DDAVP: 0.01% (5 mL) [contains benzalkonium chloride]
DDAVP Rhinal Tube: 0.01% (2.5 mL) [contains chlorobutanol (chlorobutol)]
Stimate: 1.5 mg/mL (2.5 mL) [contains benzalkonium chloride]
Generic: 0.01% (2.5 mL, 5 mL)
Tablet, Oral, as acetate:
DDAVP: 0.1 mg
DDAVP: 0.1 mg [DSC], 0.2 mg [scored]
Generic: 0.1 mg, 0.2 mg

- **Desmopressin Acetate** *see* Desmopressin *on page 607*
- **Desoxyephedrine Hydrochloride** *see* Methamphetamine *on page 1383*
- **Desoxyn** *see* Methamphetamine *on page 1383*
- **Desoxyphenobarbital** *see* Primidone *on page 1766*
- **Desquam-X® (Can)** *see* Benzoyl Peroxide *on page 270*
- **Desquam-X Wash [OTC]** *see* Benzoyl Peroxide *on page 270*
- **Desyrel** *see* TraZODone *on page 2105*
- **Detemir Insulin** *see* Insulin Detemir *on page 1124*
- **Detrol** *see* Tolterodine *on page 2084*
- **Detrol® (Can)** *see* Tolterodine *on page 2084*
- **Detrol LA** *see* Tolterodine *on page 2084*
- **Detrol® LA (Can)** *see* Tolterodine *on page 2084*

Dexamethasone (Systemic)

(deks a METH a sone)

Medication Safety Issues

Sound-alike/look-alike issues:

Dexamethasone may be confused with desoximetasone, dextroamphetamine

Decadron may be confused with Percodan

Related Information

Corticosteroids Systemic Equivalencies *on page 2260*

Brand Names: US Baycadron [DSC]; Dexamethasone Intensol; DexPak 10 Day; DexPak 13 Day; DexPak 6 Day; DoubleDex

Brand Names: Canada Apo-Dexamethasone; Dexasone; Dom-Dexamethasone; PHL-Dexamethasone; PMS-Dexamethasone; PRO-Dexamethasone; ratio-Dexamethasone

Therapeutic Category Adrenal Corticosteroid; Anti-inflammatory Agent; Antiemetic; Corticosteroid, Systemic; Glucocorticoid

Generic Availability (US) May be product dependent

Use Oral, parenteral: Primarily as an anti-inflammatory or immunosuppressant agent in the treatment of a variety of diseases, including those of allergic, hematologic, dermatologic, neoplastic, rheumatic, autoimmune, nervous system, renal, and respiratory origin [FDA approved in pediatric patients (age not specified) and adults]; primary or secondary adrenocorticoid deficiency (not first line) [FDA approved in pediatric patients (age not specified) and adults]; management of cerebral edema, shock, and as a diagnostic agent [FDA approved in pediatric patients (age not specified) and adults]. Has also been used as adjunctive antiemetic agent in the treatment of chemotherapy-induced emesis, treatment of croup (laryngotracheobronchitis), treatment of airway edema prior to extubation, treatment of acute mountain sickness (AMS) and high altitude cerebral edema (HACE), and in neonates with bronchopulmonary dysplasia to facilitate ventilator weaning

Pregnancy Risk Factor C

Pregnancy Considerations Adverse events have been observed with corticosteroids in animal reproduction studies. Betamethasone crosses the placenta (Brownfoot, 2013); and is partially metabolized by placental enzymes to an inactive metabolite (Murphy, 2007). Some studies have shown an association between first trimester systemic corticosteroid use and oral clefts (Park-Wyllie, 2000; Pradat, 2003). Systemic corticosteroids may have an effect on fetal growth (decreased birth weight); however, information is conflicting (Lunghi, 2010). Hypoadrenalism may occur in newborns following maternal use of corticosteroids during pregnancy; monitor.

Because antenatal corticosteroid administration may reduce the incidence of intraventricular hemorrhage, necrotizing enterocolitis, neonatal mortality, and respiratory distress syndrome, the injection is often used in patients with preterm premature rupture of membranes (membrane rupture between 24 0/7 weeks and 34 0/7 weeks of gestation) who are at risk of preterm delivery (ACOG, 2013). When systemic corticosteroids are needed in pregnancy, it is generally recommended to use the lowest effective dose for the shortest duration of time, avoiding high doses during the first trimester (Leachman, 2006; Lunghi, 2010; Makol, 2011; Østensen, 2009).

Women exposed to dexamethasone during pregnancy for the treatment of an autoimmune disease may contact the OTIS Autoimmune Diseases Study at 877-311-8972.

Breast-Feeding Considerations Corticosteroids are excreted in human milk; information specific to dexamethasone has not been located. The manufacturer notes that when used systemically, maternal use of corticosteroids have the potential to cause adverse events in a nursing infant (eg, growth suppression, interfere with endogenous corticosteroid production). Due to the potential for serious adverse reactions in the nursing infant, the manufacturer recommends a decision be made whether to discontinue nursing or to discontinue the drug, taking into account the importance of treatment to the mother. If there is concern about exposure to the infant, some guidelines recommend waiting 4 hours after the maternal dose of an oral systemic corticosteroid before breast-feeding in order to decrease potential exposure to the nursing infant (based on a study using prednisolone) (Bae, 2011; Leachman, 2006; Makol, 2011; Ost, 1985).

Contraindications Hypersensitivity to dexamethasone or any component of the formulation, including sulfites; systemic fungal infections, cerebral malaria

Warnings/Precautions Corticosteroids are not approved for epidural injection. Serious neurologic events (eg, spinal cord infarction, paraplegia, quadriplegia, cortical blindness, stroke), some resulting in death, have been reported with epidural injection of corticosteroids, with and without use of fluoroscopy. Intra-articular injection may produce systemic as well as local effects. Appropriate examination of any joint fluid present is necessary to exclude a septic process. Avoid injection into an infected site. Do not inject into unstable joints. Patients should not overuse joints in which symptomatic benefit has been obtained as long as the inflammatory process remains active. Frequent intra-articular injection may result in damage to joint tissues.

Use with caution in patients with thyroid disease, hepatic impairment, renal impairment, cardiovascular disease, diabetes, glaucoma, cataracts, myasthenia gravis, osteoporosis, seizures, or GI diseases (diverticulitis, intestinal anastomoses, peptic ulcer, ulcerative colitis) due to perforation risk. Avoid ethanol may enhance gastric mucosal irritation. Use caution following acute MI (corticosteroids have been associated with myocardial rupture). Because of the risk of adverse effects, systemic corticosteroids should be used cautiously in the elderly in the smallest possible effective dose for the shortest duration. May affect growth velocity; growth should be routinely monitored in pediatric patients. Withdraw therapy with gradual tapering of dose.

May cause hypercorticism or suppression of hypothalamic-pituitary-adrenal (HPA) axis, particularly in younger children or in patients receiving high doses for prolonged periods. HPA axis suppression may lead to adrenal crisis. Withdrawal and discontinuation of a corticosteroid should be done slowly and carefully. Particular care is required when patients are transferred from systemic corticosteroids to inhaled products due to possible adrenal insufficiency or withdrawal from steroids, including an increase in allergic symptoms. Adult patients receiving >20 mg per day of prednisone (or equivalent) may be most susceptible. Fatalities have occurred due to adrenal insufficiency in asthmatic patients during and after transfer from systemic corticosteroids to aerosol steroids; aerosol steroids do not provide the systemic steroid needed to treat patients having trauma, surgery, or infections. Dexamethasone does not provide adequate mineralocorticoid activity in adrenal insufficiency (may be employed as a single dose while cortisol assays are performed). The lowest possible dose should be used during treatment; discontinuation and/or dose reductions should be gradual. Rare cases of anaphylactoid reactions have been observed in patients receiving corticosteroids. Patients may require higher doses when subject to stress (ie, trauma, surgery, severe infection).

Acute myopathy has been reported with high dose corticosteroids, usually in patients with neuromuscular transmission disorders; may involve ocular and/or respiratory muscles; monitor creatine kinase; recovery may be delayed. Corticosteroid use may cause psychiatric disturbances, including depression, euphoria, insomnia, mood swings, and personality changes. Preexisting psychiatric conditions may be exacerbated by corticosteroid use. Prolonged use of corticosteroids may increase the incidence of secondary infection, mask acute infection (including fungal infections), prolong or exacerbate viral infections, or limit response to vaccines. Exposure to chickenpox or measles should be avoided; corticosteroids should not be used to treat ocular herpes simplex. Corticosteroids should not be used for cerebral malaria, fungal infections, or viral hepatitis. Close observation is required in patients with latent tuberculosis and/or TB reactivity; restrict use in active TB (only fulminating or disseminated TB in conjunction with antituberculosis treatment). Amebiasis should be ruled out in any patient with recent travel to tropic climates or unexplained diarrhea prior to initiation of corticosteroids.

Prolonged treatment with corticosteroids has been associated with the development of Kaposi sarcoma (case reports); if noted, discontinuation of therapy should be considered. High-dose corticosteroids should not be used to manage acute head injury. Some products may contain sodium sulfite, a sulfite that may cause allergic-type reactions including anaphylaxis and life-threatening or less severe asthmatic episodes in susceptible patients. Potentially significant drug-drug interactions may exist, requiring dose or frequency adjustment, additional monitoring, and/or selection of alternative therapy. Some dosage forms may contain propylene glycol; large amounts are potentially toxic and have been associated hyperosmolality, lactic acidosis, seizures, and respiratory depression; use caution (AAP, 1997; Zar, 2007).

Benzyl alcohol and derivatives: Some dosage forms may contain sodium benzoate/benzoic acid; benzoic acid (benzoate) is a metabolite of benzyl alcohol; large amounts of benzyl alcohol (≥99 mg/kg/day) have been associated with a potentially fatal toxicity ("gasping syndrome") in neonates; the "gasping syndrome" consists of metabolic acidosis, respiratory distress, gasping respirations, CNS dysfunction (including convulsions, intracranial hemorrhage), hypotension, and cardiovascular collapse (AAP, 1997; CDC, 1982); some data suggests that benzoate displaces bilirubin from protein binding sites (Ahlfors, 2001); avoid or use dosage forms containing benzyl alcohol derivative with caution in neonates. See manufacturer's labeling.

Warnings: Additional Pediatric Considerations May cause osteoporosis (at any age) or inhibition of bone growth in pediatric patients. Use with caution in patients with osteoporosis. In a population-based study of children, risk of fracture was shown to be increased with >4 courses of corticosteroids; underlying clinical condition may also impact bone health and osteoporotic effect of corticosteroids (Leonard, 2007). In premature neonates, the use of high-dose dexamethasone (approximately >0.5 mg/kg/day) for the prevention or treatment of BPD has been associated with adverse neurodevelopmental outcomes, including higher rates of cerebral palsy without additional clinical benefit over lower doses; current data does not support use of high doses, further studies are needed (Watterberg, 2010). Increased IOP may occur especially with prolonged use; in children, increased IOP has also been shown to be dose-dependent with a greater IOP observed in children <6 years than older children after ophthalmic dexamethasone application; monitor closely (Lam, 2005).

Some dosage forms may contain propylene glycol; in neonates large amounts of propylene glycol delivered orally, intravenously (eg, >3,000 mg/day), or topically have been associated with potentially fatal toxicities which can include metabolic acidosis, seizures, renal failure, and CNS depression; toxicities have also been reported in children and adults including hyperosmolality, lactic acidosis, seizures and respiratory depression; use caution (AAP, 1997; Shehab, 2009).

Adverse Reactions

Cardiovascular: Arrhythmia, bradycardia, cardiac arrest, cardiomyopathy, CHF, circulatory collapse, edema, hypertension, myocardial rupture (post-MI), syncope, thromboembolism, vasculitis

Central nervous system: Depression, emotional instability, euphoria, headache, intracranial pressure increased, insomnia, malaise, mood swings, neuritis, personality changes, pseudotumor cerebri (usually following discontinuation), psychic disorders, seizure, vertigo

Dermatologic: Acne, allergic dermatitis, alopecia, angioedema, bruising, dry skin, erythema, fragile skin, hirsutism, hyper-/hypopigmentation, hypertrichosis, perianal pruritus (following IV injection), petechiae, rash, skin atrophy, skin test reaction impaired, striae, urticaria, wound healing impaired

Endocrine & metabolic: Adrenal suppression, carbohydrate tolerance decreased, Cushing's syndrome, diabetes mellitus, glucose intolerance decreased, growth suppression (children), hyperglycemia, hypokalemic alkalosis, menstrual irregularities, negative nitrogen balance, pituitary-adrenal axis suppression, protein catabolism, sodium retention

Gastrointestinal: Abdominal distention, appetite increased, gastrointestinal hemorrhage, gastrointestinal perforation, nausea, pancreatitis, peptic ulcer, ulcerative esophagitis, weight gain

Genitourinary: Altered (increased or decreased) spermatogenesis

Hepatic: Hepatomegaly, transaminases increased

Local: Postinjection flare (intra-articular use), thrombophlebitis

Neuromuscular & skeletal: Arthropathy, aseptic necrosis (femoral and humoral heads), fractures, muscle mass loss, myopathy (particularly in conjunction with neuromuscular disease or neuromuscular-blocking agents), neuropathy, osteoporosis, parasthesia, tendon rupture, vertebral compression fractures, weakness

Ocular: Cataracts, exophthalmos, glaucoma, intraocular pressure increased
Renal: Glucosuria
Respiratory: Pulmonary edema
Miscellaneous: Abnormal fat deposition, anaphylactoid reaction, anaphylaxis, avascular necrosis, diaphoresis, hiccups, hypersensitivity, impaired wound healing, infections, Kaposi's sarcoma, moon face, secondary malignancy

Drug Interactions

Metabolism/Transport Effects **Substrate** of CYP3A4 (major), P-glycoprotein; **Note:** Assignment of Major/Minor substrate status based on clinically relevant drug interaction potential; **Inhibits** P-glycoprotein; **Induces** CYP2A6 (weak/moderate), CYP2B6 (weak/moderate), CYP2C9 (weak/moderate), CYP3A4 (moderate), P-glycoprotein

Avoid Concomitant Use

Avoid concomitant use of Dexamethasone (Systemic) with any of the following: Aldesleukin; Axitinib; BCG; BCG (Intravesical); Bedaquiline; Bosutinib; Cabozantinib; Conivaptan; Dabigatran Etexilate; Enzalutamide; Fusidic Acid (Systemic); Idelalisib; Indium 111 Capromab Pendetide; Lapatinib; Ledipasvir; Mifepristone; Natalizumab; Nilotinib; Nintedanib; Nisoldipine; Olaparib; Palbociclib; Pimecrolimus; Rilpivirine; RomiDEPsin; Simeprevir; Sofosbuvir; Tacrolimus (Topical); Ticagrelor; Tofacitinib; VinCRIStine (Liposomal)

Increased Effect/Toxicity

Dexamethasone (Systemic) may increase the levels/effects of: Acetylcholinesterase Inhibitors; Amphotericin B; Androgens; Clarithromycin; CycloSPORINE (Systemic); Deferasirox; Fosphenytoin; Ifosfamide; Leflunomide; Lenalidomide; Loop Diuretics; Natalizumab; Nicorandil; NSAID (COX-2 Inhibitor); NSAID (Nonselective); Phenytoin; Quinolone Antibiotics; Thalidomide; Thiazide Diuretics; Tofacitinib; Vaccines (Live); Warfarin

The levels/effects of Dexamethasone (Systemic) may be increased by: Aprepitant; Asparaginase (E. coli); Asparaginase (Erwinia); Conivaptan; CycloSPORINE (Systemic); CYP3A4 Inhibitors (Moderate); CYP3A4 Inhibitors (Strong); Denosumab; Estrogen Derivatives; Fosamprenavir; Fosaprepitant; Fusidic Acid (Systemic); Idelalisib; Indacaterol; Ivacaftor; Luliconazole; Mifepristone; Netupitant; Neuromuscular-Blocking Agents (Nondepolarizing); P-glycoprotein/ABCB1 Inhibitors; Pimecrolimus; Roflumilast; Salicylates; Stiripentol; Tacrolimus (Topical); Telaprevir; Trastuzumab

Decreased Effect

Dexamethasone (Systemic) may decrease the levels/effects of: Afatinib; Aldesleukin; Antidiabetic Agents; ARIPiprazole; Axitinib; BCG; BCG (Intravesical); Bedaquiline; Bosutinib; Brentuximab Vedotin; Cabozantinib; Calcitriol (Systemic); Caspofungin; Clarithromycin; Cobicistat; Coccidioides immitis Skin Test; Corticorelin; CycloSPORINE (Systemic); CYP3A4 Substrates; Dabigatran Etexilate; Dasabuvir; Dasatinib; DOXOrubicin (Conventional); Elvitegravir; Enzalutamide; FentaNYL; Fosamprenavir; Fosphenytoin; Hyaluronidase; Hydrocodone; Ibrutinib; Ifosfamide; Imatinib; Indium 111 Capromab Pendetide; Isoniazid; Ixabepilone; Lapatinib; Ledipasvir; Linagliptin; Nilotinib; NiMODipine; Nintedanib; Nisoldipine; Olaparib; Ombitasvir; Palbociclib; Paliperidone; Paritaprevir; P-glycoprotein/ABCB1 Substrates; Phenytoin; Rilpivirine; RomiDEPsin; Salicylates; Saxagliptin; Simeprevir; Sipuleucel-T; Sofosbuvir; SUNItinib; Telaprevir; Ticagrelor; Triazolam; Urea Cycle Disorder Agents; Vaccines (Inactivated); Vaccines (Live); VinCRIStine (Liposomal)

The levels/effects of Dexamethasone (Systemic) may be decreased by: Antacids; Bile Acid Sequestrants; Bosentan; CYP3A4 Inducers (Moderate); CYP3A4 Inducers (Strong); Dabrafenib; Deferasirox; Echinacea; Fosphenytoin; Mifepristone; Mitotane; P-glycoprotein/ABCB1 Inducers; Phenytoin; Siltuximab; St Johns Wort; Tocilizumab

Storage/Stability

Elixir: Store at 15°C to 30°C (59°F to 86°F); avoid freezing.
Injection: Store intact vials at 20°C to 25°C (68°F to 77°F); excursions permitted to 15°C to 30°C (59°F to 86°F). Protect from light, heat, and freezing. Diluted solutions should be used within 24 hours.
Oral concentrated solution (Intensol): Store at 20°C to 25°C (68°F to 77°F); do not freeze; do not use if precipitate is present; dispense only in original bottle and only with manufacturer-supplied calibrated dropper; discard open bottle after 90 days.
Oral solution: Store at 20°C to 25°C (68°F to 77°F).
Tablets: Store at 20°C to 25°C (68°F to 77°F); protect from moisture.

Mechanism of Action A long acting corticosteroid with minimal sodium-retaining potential. Decreases inflammation by suppression of neutrophil migration, decreased production of inflammatory mediators, and reversal of increased capillary permeability; suppresses normal immune response. Dexamethasone's mechanism of antiemetic activity is unknown.

Pharmacodynamics Duration: Metabolic effects can last for 72 hours

Pharmacokinetics (Adult data unless noted)

Metabolism: In the liver
Half-life: Terminal:
Extremely low birth-weight infants with BPD: 9.3 hours
Children 3 months to 16 years: 4.3 hours
Healthy adults: 3 hours
Time to peak serum concentration:
Oral: Within 1-2 hours
IM: Within 8 hours
Elimination: In urine and bile

Dosing: Neonatal

Airway edema or extubation: Limited data available: IV: 0.25 mg/kg/dose given ~4 hours prior to scheduled extubation then every 8 hours for a total of 3 doses (Couser, 1992); others have used 0.5 mg/kg/dose every 8 hours for 3 doses with last dose administered 1 hour prior to scheduled extubation (Davis, 2001); range: 0.25 to 0.5 mg/kg/dose for 1 to 3 doses; maximum daily dose: 1.5 mg/kg/**day**; limited data available, reported dosing regimens variable. **Note:** A longer duration of therapy may be needed with more severe cases. A recent meta-analysis concluded that future neonatal clinical trials should study a multiple dose strategy with initiation of dexamethasone at least 12 hours before extubation (Khemani, 2009).

Bronchopulmonary dysplasia, facilitation of ventilator wean: Limited data available: PNA ≥7 days: Oral, IV: Initial: 0.15 mg/kg/**day** given in divided doses every 12 hours for 3 days, then tapered every 3 days over 7 days; total dexamethasone dose: 0.89 mg/kg given over 10 days (Doyle, 2006); others have used 0.2 mg/kg/**day** given once daily and tapered every 3 days over 7 days (total dexamethasone dose: 1 mg/kg) (Durand, 2002) or tapered over 14 days (total dexamethasone dose: 1.9 mg/kg) (Whalther, 2003). **Note:** High doses (~0.5 mg/kg/day) do not confer additional benefit over lower doses, are associated with higher incidence of adverse effects (including adverse neurodevelopmental outcomes), and are not recommended for use (Watterberg, 2010). However, a meta-analysis reported total cumulative doses >4 mg/kg reduced the relative risk for the combined outcome, mortality, or bronchopulmonary dysplasia (Onland, 2009).

Dosing: Usual

Pediatric:

Acute mountain sickness (AMS) (moderate)/high altitude cerebral edema (HACE); treatment: Limited data available: Infants, Children, and Adolescents: Oral, IM, IV: 0.15 mg/kg/dose every 6 hours; maximum dose: 4 mg/dose; consider using for high altitude pulmonary edema because of associated HACE with this condition (Luks, 2010; Pollard, 2001)

Airway edema or extubation: Limited data available: Infants, Children, and Adolescents: Oral, IM, IV: 0.5 mg/kg/dose (maximum dose: 10 mg/dose) administered 6 to 12 hours prior to extubation then every 6 hours for 6 doses (total dexamethasone dose: 3 mg/kg) (Anene, 1996; Khemani, 2009; Tellez, 1991)

Anti-inflammatory: Infants, Children, and Adolescents: Oral, IM, IV: Initial dose range: 0.02 to 0.3 mg/kg/**day or** 0.6 to 9 mg/**m²/day** in divided doses every 6 to 12 hours; dose depends upon condition being treated and response of patient; dosage for infants and children should be based on disease severity and patient response; usual adult daily dose range: 0.75 to 9 mg/day

Asthma exacerbation: Limited data available: Infants, Children, and Adolescents: Oral, IM, IV: 0.6 mg/kg once daily as a single dose or once daily for 2 days; maximum dose: 16 mg/dose (Hegenbarth, 2008, Keeney, 2014, Quereshi, 2001); single dose regimens as low as 0.3 mg/kg/dose and as high as 1.7 mg/kg/dose have also been reported (Keeney, 2014; Qureshi, 2001; Shefrin, 2009). **Note:** Duration greater than 2 days is not recommended due to increased risk of metabolic effects (GINA, 2014).

Bacterial meningitis (*H. influenzae* type b): Limited data available: Infants >6 weeks and Children: IV: 0.15 mg/kg/dose every 6 hours for the first 2 to 4 days of antibiotic treatment; start dexamethasone 10 to 20 minutes before or with the first dose of antibiotic; if antibiotics have already been administered, dexamethasone use has not been shown to improve patient outcome and is not recommended (Tunkel, 2004). **Note:** For pneumococcal meningitis, data has not shown clear benefit from dexamethasone administration; risk and benefits should be considered prior to use (*Red Book*, 2012).

Cerebral edema: Infants, Children, and Adolescents: Oral, IM, IV: Loading dose: 1 to 2 mg/kg/dose as a single dose; maintenance: 1 to 1.5 mg/kg/**day** in divided doses every 4 to 6 hours; maximum daily dose: 16 mg/**day** (Kleigman, 2007)

Chemotherapy-induced nausea and vomiting, prevention: Refer to individual protocols and emetogenic potential: Infants, Children, and Adolescents:

POGO recommendations (Dupuis, 2013): **Note:** Reduce dose by 50% if administered concomitantly with aprepitant:

Highly/severely emetogenic chemotherapy: Oral, IV: 6 mg/**m²**/dose every 6 hours

Moderately emetogenic chemotherapy: Oral, IV:

BSA ≤0.6 m²: 2 mg every 12 hours

BSA >0.6 m²: 4 mg every 12 hours

Alternate dosing: *Highly/severely emetogenic chemotherapy:* IV: Usual: 10 mg/**m²**/dose once daily on days of chemotherapy; some patients may require every 12 hour dosing; usual range: 8 to 14 mg/**m²**/dose (Holdsworth, 2006; Jordan, 2010; Phillips, 2010); others have used: Initial: 10 mg/**m²**/dose prior to chemotherapy (maximum dose: 20 mg) then 5 mg/**m²**/dose every 6 hours (Kliegman, 2007)

Congenital adrenal hyperplasia: Adolescents (fully grown): Oral: 0.25 to 0.5 mg once daily; use of a liquid dosage form may be preferable to allow for better dose titration (AAP, 2010; Speiser, 2010). **Note:** For younger patients who are still growing, hydrocortisone or fludrocortisone are preferred.

Croup (laryngotracheobronchitis): Limited data available: Infants and Children: Oral, IM, IV: 0.6 mg/kg once; usual maximum dose: 16 mg (doses as high as 20 mg have been used) (Bjornson, 2004; Hegenbarth, 2008; Rittichier, 2000); **Note:** A single oral dose of 0.15 mg/kg has been shown effective in children with mild to moderate croup (Russell, 2004; Sparrow, 2006).

Physiologic replacement: Infants, Children, and Adolescents: Oral, IM, IV: 0.03 to 0.15 mg/kg/**day** in divided doses every 6 to 12 hours (Kleigman, 2007) **or** Initial: 0.2 to 0.25 mg/**m²/day** administered once daily; some patients may require 0.3 mg/**m²/day** (Gupta, 2008)

Adult:

Acute mountain sickness (AMS)/high altitude cerebral edema (HACE):

Prevention: Oral: 2 mg every 6 hours **or** 4 mg every 12 hours starting on the day of ascent; may be discontinued after staying at the same elevation for 2-3 days or if descent is initiated; do not exceed a 10-day duration (Luks, 2010). **Note:** In situations of rapid ascent to altitudes >3500 meters (such as rescue or military operations), 4 mg every 6 hours may be considered (Luks, 2010).

Treatment: Oral, IM, IV:

AMS: 4 mg every 6 hours (Luks, 2010)

HACE: Initial: 8 mg as a single dose; Maintenance: 4 mg every 6 hours until symptoms resolve (Luks, 2010)

Antiemetic:

Prophylaxis: Oral, IV: 10 to 20 mg 15 to 30 minutes before treatment on each treatment day

Continuous infusion regimen: Oral or IV: 10 mg every 12 hours on each treatment day

Mildly emetogenic therapy: Oral, IM, IV: 4 mg every 4 to 6 hours

Delayed nausea/vomiting: Oral: 4 to 10 mg 1 to 2 times daily for 2 to 4 days **or**

8 mg every 12 hours for 2 days; then

4 mg every 12 hours for 2 days **or**

20 mg 1 hour before chemotherapy; then

10 mg 12 hours after chemotherapy; then

8 mg every 12 hours for 4 doses; then

Anti-inflammatory:

Oral, IM, IV: 0.75 to 9 mg/day in divided doses every 6 to 12 hours

Intra-articular, intralesional, or soft tissue: 0.4 to 6 mg/day

Extubation or airway edema: Oral, IM, IV: 0.5 to 2 mg/kg/day in divided doses every 6 hours beginning 24 hours prior to extubation and continuing for 4 to 6 doses afterwards

4 mg every 12 hours for 4 doses

Multiple myeloma: Oral, IV: 40 mg/day, days 1 to 4, 9 to 12, and 17 to 20, repeated every 4 weeks (alone or as part of a regimen)

Cerebral edema: IV: 10 mg stat, then 4 mg IM/IV (should be given as sodium phosphate) every 6 hours until response is maximized, then switch to oral regimen, then taper off if appropriate; dosage may be reduced after 2 to 4 days and gradually discontinued over 5 to 7 days

Cushing's syndrome, diagnostic: Oral: 1 mg at 11 PM, draw blood at 8 AM; greater accuracy for Cushing syndrome may be achieved by the following:

Dexamethasone: 0.5 mg by mouth every 6 hours for 48 hours (with 24-hour urine collection for 17-hydroxycorticosteroid excretion)

Differentiation of Cushing's syndrome due to ACTH excess from Cushing's due to other causes: Oral: Dexamethasone 2 mg every 6 hours for 48 hours (with

24-hour urine collection for 17-hydroxycorticosteroid excretion)

Multiple sclerosis (acute exacerbation): Oral: 30 mg/day for 1 week, followed by 4 to 12 mg/day for 1 month

Shock, treatment:

Addisonian crisis/shock (eg, adrenal insufficiency/ responsive to steroid therapy): IV: 4 to 10 mg as a single dose, which may be repeated if necessary

Unresponsive shock (eg, unresponsive to steroid therapy): IV: 1 to 6 mg/kg as a single IV dose or up to 40 mg initially followed by repeat doses every 2 to 6 hours while shock persists

Physiological replacement: Oral, IM, IV (should be given as sodium phosphate): 0.03 to 0.15 mg/kg/day **or** 0.6 to 0.75 mg/m^2/day in divided doses every 6 to 12 hours

Dosing adjustment in renal impairment: Infants, Children, Adolescents, and Adults: There are no dosage adjustments provided in the manufacturer's labeling; use with caution. Hemodialysis or peritoneal dialysis: Supplemental dose is not necessary.

Dosage adjustment in hepatic impairment: Infants, Children, Adolescents, and Adults: There are no dosage adjustments provided in the manufacturer's labeling.

Preparation for Administration

Oral: Oral administration of parenteral solution: In some pediatric croup trials, doses were prepared using a parenteral dexamethasone formulation and mixing it with an oral flavored syrup (Bjornson 2004).

IV: May be given undiluted (4 mg/mL or 10 mg/mL). High doses may be further diluted in NS or D_5W (Allan 1986; Bernini 1998). In neonates, use a preservative-free product.

Administration

Oral: May administer with food or milk to decrease GI adverse effects

Parenteral: Use preservative-free dosage forms in neonates.

IM: May administer 4 mg/mL or 10 mg/mL undiluted

IV: May administer as undiluted solution (4 mg/mL or 10 mg/mL) slow IV push, usually over 1 to 4 minutes; rapid administration is associated with perineal discomfort (burning, tingling) (Allan 1986; Neff 2002); may consider further dilution of high doses and administration by IV intermittent infusion over 15 to 30 minutes (Allan 1986; Bernini 1998)

Monitoring Parameters Hemoglobin, occult blood loss, blood pressure, serum potassium and glucose; IOP with systemic use >6 weeks; weight and height in children

Reference Range Dexamethasone suppression test: 8 AM cortisol <6 mcg/100 mL in adults given dexamethasone 1 mg at 11 PM the previous night

Test Interactions May suppress the wheal and flare reactions to skin test antigens

Additional Information Systemic: Due to the long duration of effect (36-54 hours), alternate day dosing does not allow time for adrenal recovery between doses.

Dosage Forms Excipient information presented when available (limited, particularly for generics); consult specific product labeling. [DSC] = Discontinued product

Concentrate, Oral:

Dexamethasone Intensol: 1 mg/mL (30 mL) [contains alcohol, usp; unflavored flavor]

Elixir, Oral:

Baycadron: 0.5 mg/5 mL (237 mL [DSC]) [contains alcohol, usp, benzoic acid, fd&c red #40, propylene glycol; raspberry flavor]

Generic: 0.5 mg/5 mL (237 mL)

Kit, Injection, as sodium phosphate:

DoubleDex: 10 mg/mL

Solution, Oral:

Generic: 0.5 mg/5 mL (240 mL, 500 mL)

Solution, Injection, as sodium phosphate:

Generic: 4 mg/mL (1 mL, 5 mL, 30 mL); 20 mg/5 mL (5 mL); 120 mg/30 mL (30 mL); 10 mg/mL (1 mL, 10 mL [DSC]); 100 mg/10 mL (10 mL)

Solution, Injection, as sodium phosphate [preservative free]:

Generic: 10 mg/mL (1 mL)

Tablet, Oral:

DexPak 10 Day: 1.5 mg [scored; contains fd&c red #40 aluminum lake]

DexPak 13 Day: 1.5 mg [scored; contains fd&c red #40 aluminum lake]

DexPak 6 Day: 1.5 mg [scored; contains fd&c red #40 aluminum lake]

Generic: 0.5 mg, 0.75 mg, 1 mg, 1.5 mg, 2 mg, 4 mg, 6 mg

Dexamethasone (Ophthalmic)

(deks a METH a sone)

Medication Safety Issues

Sound-alike/look-alike issues:

Dexamethasone may be confused with desoximetasone, dextroamphetamine

Maxidex may be confused with Maxzide

Brand Names: US Maxidex; Ozurdex

Brand Names: Canada Diodex; Maxidex; Ozurdex

Therapeutic Category Anti-inflammatory Agent, Ophthalmic; Corticosteroid, Ophthalmic

Generic Availability (US) May be product dependent

Use

Ophthalmic: Management of steroid responsive inflammatory conditions such as allergic conjunctivitis, acne rosacea, superficial punctuate keratitis, herpes zoster keratitis, iritis, cyclitis, or select infective conjunctivitis when benefit of reduced edema and inflammation exceeds steroid use risks (FDA approved in adults); symptomatic treatment of corneal injury from chemical, radiation, or thermal burns, or from penetration of foreign bodies (FDA approved in adults)

Ophthalmic intravitreal implant (Ozurdex®): Treatment of macular edema following branch retinal vein occlusion (BRVO) or central retinal vein occlusion (CRVO) (FDA approved in adults); noninfective uveitis of the posterior segment of the eye (FDA approved in adults)

Otic (using ophthalmic solution): Management of steroid responsive inflammatory conditions such as allergic otitis externa and select infective purulent and nonpurulent otitis externa when benefit of reduced edema and inflammation exceeds steroid use risks (FDA approved in adults)

Pregnancy Risk Factor C

Pregnancy Considerations Adverse events were observed in animal reproduction studies following use of ophthalmic dexamethasone.

Breast-Feeding Considerations Although it is not known if detectable concentrations are found in breast milk following application of ophthalmic dexamethasone, the manufacturer recommends caution be used if administered to a nursing woman.

Contraindications

Hypersensitivity to dexamethasone or any component of the formulation or product

Suspension/solution: Viral disease of the cornea and conjunctiva (including epithelial herpes simplex keratitis, vaccinia, varicella); mycobacterial or fungal infection of the eye; the solution should also not be used for otic indications if perforation of a drum membrane is present

Intravitreal implant: Glaucoma with cup to disc ratios of greater than 0.8; active or suspected ocular or periocular infections including most viral diseases of the cornea and conjunctiva, including active epithelial herpes simplex keratitis (dendritic keratitis), vaccinia, varicella, mycobacterial infections, and fungal diseases; use in patients with a posterior lens capsule that is torn or ruptured

Canadian labeling: Additional contraindications (not in U.S. labeling): Anterior chamber intraocular lens (ACIOL) and rupture of posterior lens capsule; aphakic eyes with rupture of the posterior lens capsule

Warnings/Precautions Avoid prolonged use, which may result in ocular hypertension and/or glaucoma, with damage to the optic nerve, defects in visual acuity and fields of vision, and posterior subcapsular cataract formation. Hypotony of the eyes have also been reported with the implant, some of which were serious [Canadian product]. Monitor intraocular pressure if topical ophthalmic products are used for 10 days or longer. Prolonged use may increase the hazard of secondary ocular infections. Perforations may occur in diseases which cause thinning of the cornea or sclera. May mask infection or enhance existing infection. The possibility of persistent corneal fungal infection should be considered after prolonged use. Corticosteroids should not be used to treat ocular herpes simplex; use caution in patients with a history of ocular herpes simplex; reactivation of viral infection may occur. Ophthalmic solution and suspension contain benzalkonium chloride which may be absorbed by contact lenses; contact lens should not be worn during treatment of ophthalmic infections. Endophthalmitis, ocular inflammation, increased intraocular pressure, and retinal detachments may occur with intravitreal injection. Intraocular pressure elevations peak ~8 weeks following injection; prolonged monitoring of intraocular pressure may be required. A risk of implant migration into the anterior chamber may be present if the posterior capsule of the lens is absent or torn. Temporary blurring may occur following intravitreal injections; patients should not drive until this resolves. Administer adequate anesthesia and a broad-spectrum microbicide prior to procedure.

Intravitreal implant [Canadian product]: For macular edema following CRVO, no more than two consecutive injections should be used, and an interval of ~6 months should be allowed between the two injections. In patients with posterior segment uveitis, the use of a second injection is not recommended. Caution should be exercised if a second injection is considered in cases where the possible benefits are believed to outweigh the risk to the patient; ~6 months should be allowed between the two injections. Patients who experience and retain improved vision and patients who experience a deterioration in vision, which is not slowed by dexamethasone implant, should not be retreated. Repeat doses should only be considered when a patient experiences a response to treatment followed subsequently by a loss in visual acuity and may benefit from re-treatment. Not recommended in patients with macular edema secondary to RVO with significant retinal ischemia. Administration to both eyes is not recommended. Use with caution in aphakic patients.

Warnings: Additional Pediatric Considerations Increased IOP may occur especially with prolonged use; in children, increased IOP has been shown to be dose dependent and produce a greater IOP in children <6 years than older children (Lam, 2005).

Adverse Reactions

Intravitreal implant (Ozurdex):

Cardiovascular: Aneurysm (retinal), hypertension

Central nervous system: Foreign body sensation of eye, headache

Ophthalmic: Anterior chamber inflammation, blepharoptosis, cataract (incidence increases in patients requiring a second injection), conjunctival edema, conjunctival hemorrhage, conjunctival hyperemia, conjunctivitis, corneal erosion, decreased visual acuity, dry eye syndrome, eye pain, increased intraocular pressure, keratitis, retinal hole without detachment, ocular hypertension, vitreous detachment, vitreous opacity

Respiratory: Bronchitis

Rare but important or life-threatening: Corneal edema, decreased intraocular pressure, endophthalmitis, retinal detachment

Ophthalmic solution/suspension: Ophthalmic: Burning sensation of eyes, cataract, decreased visual acuity, eye perforation, filtering blebs, glaucoma (with optic nerve damage), secondary ocular infection, stinging of eyes, visual field defect

Drug Interactions

Metabolism/Transport Effects None known.

Avoid Concomitant Use There are no known interactions where it is recommended to avoid concomitant use.

Increased Effect/Toxicity

Dexamethasone (Ophthalmic) may increase the levels/effects of: Ceritinib

The levels/effects of Dexamethasone (Ophthalmic) may be increased by: NSAID (Ophthalmic)

Decreased Effect There are no known significant interactions involving a decrease in effect.

Storage/Stability

Ocular implant, ophthalmic solution: Store at 15°C to 30°C (59°F to 86°F).

Ophthalmic suspension: Store at 8°C to 27°C (46°F to 80°F).

Mechanism of Action Decreases inflammation by suppression of neutrophil migration, decreased production of inflammatory mediators, and reversal of increased capillary permeability; suppresses normal immune response.

Dosing: Usual

Infants, Children, and Adolescents: **Anti-inflammatory:**

Solution: Limited data available: Ophthalmic: Instill 1-2 drops into conjunctival sac every hour during the day and every other hour during the night; gradually reduce dose to every 3-4 hours, then to 3-4 times/day (Cassidy, 2001)

Suspension: Limited data available: Ophthalmic: Instill 1-2 drops into conjunctival sac up to 4-6 times per day; may use hourly in severe disease in older children; taper prior to discontinuation; others have used 2-4 times/day dosing in children following strabismus surgery; in one study twice daily eye drops controlled inflammation equally well as 4 times daily dosing, but with less increase in IOP (Lam, 2005; Ng, 2000)

Adults:

Ocular inflammation:

Solution: Ophthalmic: Instill 1-2 drops into conjunctival sac every hour during the day and every other hour during the night; gradually reduce dose to every 4 hours, then to 3-4 times/day

Suspension: Ophthalmic: Instill 1-2 drops into conjunctival sac up to 4-6 times per day; may use hourly in severe disease; taper prior to discontinuation

Macular edema (following BRVO or CRVO): Ophthalmic intravitreal implant (Ozurdex®): Intravitreal: 0.7 mg implant injected in affected eye

Noninfective uveitis: Ophthalmic intravitreal implant (Ozurdex®): Intravitreal: 0.7 mg implant injected in affected eye

Otic inflammation: Ophthalmic solution: Initial: Instill 3-4 drops into the aural canal 2-3 times a day; reduce dose gradually once a favorable response is obtained. Alternately, may pack the aural canal with a gauze wick saturated with the solution; remove from the ear after 12-24 hours. Repeat as necessary.

Administration

Ophthalmic: Avoid contact of container tip with skin or eye; remove soft contact lenses prior to using solutions containing benzalkonium chloride. Shake suspension well prior to use.

Intravitreal injection (Ozurdex®): Administer under controlled aseptic conditions (eg, sterile gloves, sterile drape, sterile eyelid speculum). Adequate anesthesia and a broad-spectrum bactericidal agent should be administered prior to injection. In sterile field, open foil pouch, remove applicator, and pull the safety tab straight off of the applicator (do not twist or flex the tab). See package insert for further administration details. If administration is required in the second eye, a new applicator should be used and the sterile field, syringe, gloves, drapes, and eyelid speculum should be changed.

Solution and suspension: Apply finger pressure to lacrimal sac during and for 1-2 minutes after instillation to decrease risk of absorption and systemic effects.

Otic: May use ophthalmic solution otically. Prior to use, clean the aural canal thoroughly and sponge dry.

Monitoring Parameters

Ophthalmic, topical: Intraocular pressure (Lam, 2005)

Ophthalmic intravitreal implant: Following intravitreal injection, monitor for increased IOP and endophthalmitis; check for perfusion of optic nerve head immediately after injection, tonometry within 30 minutes, biomicroscopy between 2-7 days after injection

Dosage Forms Excipient information presented when available (limited, particularly for generics); consult specific product labeling.

Implant, Intraocular [preservative free]:

Ozurdex: 0.7 mg (1 ea)

Solution, Ophthalmic, as phosphate:

Generic: 0.1% (5 mL)

Suspension, Ophthalmic:

Maxidex: 0.1% (5 mL)

◆ **Dexamethasone and Ciprofloxacin** *see* Ciprofloxacin and Dexamethasone *on page 469*

◆ **Dexamethasone Intensol** *see* Dexamethasone (Systemic) *on page 610*

◆ **Dexamethasone, Neomycin, and Polymyxin B** *see* Neomycin, Polymyxin B, and Dexamethasone *on page 1502*

◆ **Dexamethasone Sodium Phosphate** *see* Dexamethasone (Ophthalmic) *on page 614*

◆ **Dexamethasone Sodium Phosphate** *see* Dexamethasone (Systemic) *on page 610*

◆ **Dexasone (Can)** *see* Dexamethasone (Systemic) *on page 610*

Dexchlorpheniramine (deks klor fen EER a meen)

Medication Safety Issues

BEERS Criteria medication:

This drug may be potentially inappropriate for use in geriatric patients (Quality of evidence - moderate; Strength of recommendation - strong).

Therapeutic Category Antihistamine

Generic Availability (US) Yes

Use Perennial and seasonal allergic rhinitis; vasomotor rhinitis; dermographism; mild, uncomplicated allergic skin manifestations of urticaria and angioedema; allergic conjunctivitis due to inhalant allergens and foods; amelioration of allergic reactions to blood or plasma; anaphylactic reactions as adjunctive to epinephrine and other standard measures after the acute manifestations have been controlled (All indications: FDA approved in ages ≥2 years and adults)

Pregnancy Considerations Maternal antihistamine use has generally not resulted in an increased risk of birth defects; however, information specific to dexchlorpheniramine is limited. Dexchlorpheniramine is the *dextro*-isomer of chlorpheniramine. Antihistamines are recommended for the treatment of rhinitis, urticaria, and pruritus with rash in pregnant women (although second generation antihistamines may be preferred). Antihistamines are not recommended for treatment of pruritus associated with intrahepatic cholestasis in pregnancy.

Breast-Feeding Considerations Premature infants and newborns have a higher risk of intolerance to antihistamines. Use while breast-feeding is contraindicated by the manufacturer. Antihistamines may decrease maternal serum prolactin concentrations when administered prior to the establishment of nursing.

Contraindications Hypersensitivity to dexchlorpheniramine maleate, other antihistamines of similar chemical structure, or any component of the formulation; use in newborns or premature infants; breast-feeding mothers; treatment of lower respiratory tract symptoms, including asthma; concomitant MAOI therapy

Warnings/Precautions Causes sedation, caution must be used in performing tasks which require alertness (eg, operating machinery or driving). Effects may be potentiated when used with other sedative drugs or ethanol. Potentially significant interactions may exist, requiring dose or frequency adjustment, additional monitoring, and/or selection of alternative therapy. Use with caution in patients with narrow-angle glaucoma, pyloroduodenal obstruction (including stenotic peptic ulcer), urinary tract obstruction (including bladder neck obstruction and symptomatic prostatic hyperplasia), hyperthyroidism, and cardiovascular disease (including hypertension and ischemic heart disease). In the elderly, avoid use of this potent anticholinergic agent due to increased risk of confusion, dry mouth, constipation, and other anticholinergic effects; clearance decreases in patients of advanced age (Beers Criteria). Antihistamines may cause excitation in young children.

Warnings: Additional Pediatric Considerations Safety and efficacy for the use of cough and cold products in pediatric patients <4 years of age is limited; the AAP warns against the use of these products for respiratory illnesses in this age group. Serious adverse effects including death have been reported. Many of these products contain multiple active ingredients, increasing the risk of accidental overdose when used with other products. Health care providers are reminded to ask caregivers about the use of OTC cough and cold products in order to avoid exposure to multiple medications containing the same ingredient (AAP 2012; FDA 2008).

Some dosage forms may contain propylene glycol; in neonates large amounts of propylene glycol delivered orally, intravenously (eg, >3,000 mg/day), or topically have been associated with potentially fatal toxicities which can include metabolic acidosis, seizures, renal failure, and CNS depression; toxicities have also been reported in children and adults including hyperosmolality, lactic acidosis, seizures and respiratory depression; use caution (AAP 1997; Shehab 2009).

Adverse Reactions

Central nervous system: Dizziness, fatigue, headache, nervousness, slight to moderate drowsiness

Gastrointestinal: Abdominal pain, diarrhea, dry mouth, increased appetite, nausea, weight gain

Neuromuscular & skeletal: Arthralgia

Respiratory: Pharyngitis, thickening of bronchial secretions

Rare but important or life-threatening: Bronchospasm, epistaxis, hepatitis, palpitation

Drug Interactions

Metabolism/Transport Effects None known.

Avoid Concomitant Use

Avoid concomitant use of Dexchlorpheniramine with any of the following: Aclidinium; Azelastine (Nasal);

Eluxadoline; Glucagon; Ipratropium (Oral Inhalation); Orphenadrine; Paraldehyde; Potassium Chloride; Thalidomide; Tiotropium; Umeclidinium

Increased Effect/Toxicity

Dexchlorpheniramine may increase the levels/effects of: AbobotulinumtoxinA; Alcohol (Ethyl); Analgesics (Opioid); Anticholinergic Agents; Azelastine (Nasal); Buprenorphine; CNS Depressants; Eluxadoline; Glucagon; Hydrocodone; Methotrimeprazine; Metyrosine; Mirabegron; Mirtazapine; OnabotulinumtoxinA; Orphenadrine; Paraldehyde; Potassium Chloride; Pramipexole; RimabotulinumtoxinB; ROPINIRole; Rotigotine; Selective Serotonin Reuptake Inhibitors; Suvorexant; Thalidomide; Thiazide Diuretics; Tiotropium; Topiramate; Zolpidem

The levels/effects of Dexchlorpheniramine may be increased by: Aclidinium; Brimonidine (Topical); Cannabis; Doxylamine; Dronabinol; Droperidol; HydrOXYzine; Ipratropium (Oral Inhalation); Kava Kava; Magnesium Sulfate; Methotrimeprazine; Mianserin; Nabilone; Perampanel; Pramlintide; Rufinamide; Sodium Oxybate; Tapentadol; Tetrahydrocannabinol; Umeclidinium

Decreased Effect

Dexchlorpheniramine may decrease the levels/effects of: Acetylcholinesterase Inhibitors; Benzylpenicilloyl Polylysine; Betahistine; Hyaluronidase; Itopride; Metoclopramide; Secretin

The levels/effects of Dexchlorpheniramine may be decreased by: Acetylcholinesterase Inhibitors; Amphetamines

Storage/Stability Store at 20°C to 25°C (68°F to 77°F).

Mechanism of Action Dexchlorpheniramine competes with histamine for H_1-receptor sites on effector cells in the gastrointestinal tract, blood vessels, and respiratory tract. Dexchlorpheniramine is the predominant active isomer of chlorpheniramine and is approximately twice as active as the racemic compound (Moreno 2010).

Pharmacokinetics (Adult data unless noted)

Metabolism: Hepatic (Simons, 2004)

Half-life elimination: 20 to 30 hours (Moreno, 2010)

Time to peak: ~3 hours (Moreno, 2010)

Excretion: Urine

Dosing: Usual

Pediatric: **Perennial and seasonal allergic rhinitis; vasomotor rhinitis; dermographism; mild, uncomplicated allergic skin manifestations of urticaria and angioedema; allergic conjunctivitis due to inhalant allergens and foods; amelioration of allergic reactions to blood or plasma; therapy for anaphylactic reactions as adjunctive to epinephrine and other standard measures after the acute manifestations have been controlled:** Oral:

Children:

2 to 5 years: 0.5 mg every 4 to 6 hours

6 to 11 years: 1 mg every 4 to 6 hours

12 years: 2 mg every 4 to 6 hours

Adolescents: 2 mg every 4 to 6 hours

Adult: **Perennial and seasonal allergic rhinitis and other allergic symptoms including urticaria; vasomotor rhinitis; dermographism; mild, uncomplicated allergic skin manifestations of urticaria and angioedema; allergic conjunctivitis due to inhalant allergens and foods; amelioration of allergic reactions to blood or plasma; therapy for anaphylactic reactions as adjunctive to epinephrine and other standard measures after the acute manifestations have been controlled:** Oral: 2 mg every 4 to 6 hours

Dosing adjustment in renal impairment: There are no dosage adjustments provided in the manufacturer's labeling.

Dosing adjustment in hepatic impairment: There are no dosage adjustments provided in the manufacturer's labeling.

Administration May be administered without regard to meals.

Dosage Forms Excipient information presented when available (limited, particularly for generics); consult specific product labeling. [DSC] = Discontinued product

Syrup, Oral, as maleate:

Generic: 2 mg/5 mL (473 mL [DSC])

- ◆ **Dexchlorpheniramine Maleate** *see* Dexchlorpheniramine *on page 616*
- ◆ **Dexedrine** *see* Dextroamphetamine *on page 625*
- ◆ **Dexferrum [DSC]** *see* Iron Dextran Complex *on page 1164*
- ◆ **Dexiron (Can)** *see* Iron Dextran Complex *on page 1164*

Dexmedetomidine (deks MED e toe mi deen)

Medication Safety Issues

Sound-alike/look-alike issues:

Precedex may be confused with Peridex

High alert medication:

The Institute for Safe Medication Practices (ISMP) includes this medication among its list of drug classes which have a heightened risk of causing significant patient harm when used in error.

Administration issues:

Errors have occurred due to misinterpretation of dosing information; use caution. Maintenance dose expressed as mcg/kg/**hour**.

Brand Names: US Precedex

Brand Names: Canada Precedex

Therapeutic Category Adrenergic Agonist Agent; Alpha-Adrenergic Agonist; Sedative

Generic Availability (US) Yes

Use Sedation of initially intubated and mechanically ventilated patients during treatment in an intensive care setting; sedation prior to and/or during surgical or other procedures of nonintubated patients; duration of infusion should not exceed 24 hours. Other uses include premedication prior to anesthesia induction with thiopental; relief of pain and reduction of opioid dose following laparoscopic tubal ligation; as an adjunct anesthetic in ophthalmic surgery; treatment of shivering; premedication to attenuate the cardiostimulatory and postanesthetic delirium of ketamine. FDA approved in ages ≥18 years.

Pregnancy Risk Factor C

Pregnancy Considerations Adverse effects were observed in some animal reproduction studies. Dexmedetomidine is expected to cross the placenta. Information related to use during pregnancy is limited (El-Tahan, 2012).

Breast-Feeding Considerations It is not known if dexmedetomidine is excreted in breast milk. The manufacturer recommends that caution be exercised when administering dexmedetomidine to nursing women.

Contraindications

There are no contraindications listed in the U.S. manufacturer's labeling.

Canadian labeling: Hypersensitivity to dexmedetomidine or any component of the formulation.

Warnings/Precautions Should be administered only by persons skilled in management of patients in intensive care setting or operating room. Patients should be continuously monitored. Episodes of bradycardia, hypotension, and sinus arrest have been associated with dexmedetomidine. At low concentrations, mean arterial pressure (MAP) may be reduced without changes in other hemodynamic parameters (eg, pulmonary artery occlusion pressure [PAOP]); however, at higher concentrations (>1.9 ng/mL), MAP, CVP, PAOP, PVR, and SVR increase (Ebert, 2000). Use caution in patients with heart block, severe ventricular dysfunction, hypovolemia, diabetes, chronic hypertension, and elderly. Use with caution in patients with hepatic impairment; dosage reductions recommended. Use with caution in patients receiving vasodilators or drugs which decrease heart rate. If medical intervention is required, treatment may include stopping or decreasing the infusion; increasing the rate of IV fluid administration, use of pressor agents, and elevation of the lower extremities. Transient hypertension has been primarily observed during the loading dose administration and is associated with the initial peripheral vasoconstrictive effects of dexmedetomidine. Treatment is generally unnecessary; however, reduction of infusion rate may be required. Patients may be arousable and alert when stimulated. This alone should not be considered as lack of efficacy in the absence of other clinical signs/symptoms. When withdrawn abruptly in patients who have received >24 hours of therapy, withdrawal symptoms similar to clonidine withdrawal may result (eg, hypertension, tachycardia, nervousness, nausea, vomiting, agitation, headaches). Use for >24 hours is not recommended by the manufacturer. Use of infusions >24 hours has been associated with tolerance and tachyphylaxis and dose-related increase in adverse reactions.

Adverse Reactions

Cardiovascular: Atrial fibrillation, bradycardia, edema, hypertension, hypertension (diastolic), hypotension, hypovolemia, peripheral edema, systolic hypertension, tachycardia

Central nervous system: Agitation, anxiety

Endocrine & metabolic: Hyperglycemia, hypocalcemia, hypokalemia, hypoglycemia, hypomagnesemia, increased thirst

Gastrointestinal: Constipation, nausea, xerostomia

Genitourinary: Oliguria

Hematologic & oncologic: Anemia

Renal: Acute renal failure, decreased urine output

Respiratory: Pleural effusion, respiratory depression, wheezing

Miscellaneous: Fever, withdrawal syndrome (ICU sedation)

Rare but important or life-threatening: Acidosis, apnea, atrioventricular block, bronchospasm, cardiac arrest, cardiac disease, chills, confusion, convulsions, decreased visual acuity, delirium, drug tolerance (use >24 hours), extrasystoles, hallucination, heart block, hemorrhage, hepatic insufficiency, hyperbilirubinemia, hypercapnia, hyperkalemia, hyperpyrexia, hypoxia, increased blood urea nitrogen, increased gamma-glutamyl transferase, increased serum alkaline phosphatase, increased serum ALT, increased serum AST, inversion T wave on ECG, myocardial infarction, neuralgia, neuritis, oliguria, photopsia, pulmonary congestion, respiratory acidosis, rigors, seizure, sinoatrial arrest, speech disturbance, supraventricular tachycardia, tachyphylaxis (use >24 hours), variable blood pressure, ventricular arrhythmia, ventricular tachycardia, visual disturbance

Drug Interactions

Metabolism/Transport Effects Substrate of CYP2A6 (major); **Note:** Assignment of Major/Minor substrate status based on clinically relevant drug interaction potential; **Inhibits** CYP1A2 (weak), CYP2C9 (weak)

Avoid Concomitant Use

Avoid concomitant use of Dexmedetomidine with any of the following: Ceritinib; Iobenguane I 123

Increased Effect/Toxicity

Dexmedetomidine may increase the levels/effects of: Beta-Blockers; Bradycardia-Causing Agents; Ceritinib; DULoxetine; Hypotensive Agents; Ivabradine; Lacosamide; Levodopa; RisperiDONE; TiZANidine

The levels/effects of Dexmedetomidine may be increased by: Barbiturates; Beta-Blockers; Bretylium; CYP2A6 Inhibitors (Moderate); CYP2A6 Inhibitors (Strong); MAO Inhibitors; Nicorandil; Ruxolitinib; Tofacitinib

Decreased Effect

Dexmedetomidine may decrease the levels/effects of: Iobenguane I 123

The levels/effects of Dexmedetomidine may be decreased by: Mirtazapine; Serotonin/Norepinephrine Reuptake Inhibitors; Tricyclic Antidepressants

Storage/Stability Store at controlled room temperature of 25°C (77°F); excursions permitted to 15°C to 30°C (59°F to 86°F). The Canadian labeling indicates that following dilution of dexmedetomidine concentrate (100 mcg/mL) in sodium chloride 0.9% to a concentration of 4 mcg/mL, the resultant solution is stable for 25 hours at 15°C to 30°C (59°F to 86°F).

Mechanism of Action Selective alpha$_2$-adrenoceptor agonist with anesthetic and sedative properties thought to be due to activation of G-proteins by alpha$_{2a}$-adrenoceptors in the brainstem resulting in inhibition of norepinephrine release; peripheral alpha$_{2b}$-adrenoceptors are activated at high doses or with rapid IV administration resulting in vasoconstriction.

Pharmacokinetics (Adult data unless noted)

Distribution: V_{dss}: Approximately 118 L

Bioavailability: IM: 73%

Protein binding: 94%

Metabolism: Hepatic via N-glucuronidation, N-methylation, and CYP2A6

Half-life: Distribution: 6 minutes; Terminal: 2 hours

Elimination: Urine (95%); feces (4%)

Clearance: Adults: 39 L/hour; hepatic impairment (Child-Pugh Class A, B, or C): mean clearance values were 74%, 64%, and 53% respectively, of those observed in healthy adults; clearance at birth is approximately 30% of adults, reaching adult values between 6-12 months of age

Dosing: Usual Note: Errors have occurred due to misinterpretation of dosing information. Maintenance dose expressed as mcg/kg/**hour**. **Note:** Individualize and titrate to desired clinical effect: IV:

Children (limited data): Loading dose: 0.5-1 mcg/kg; followed by a maintenance infusion of 0.2-0.7 mcg/kg/**hour**; children <1 year may require higher infusion rates; average infusion range: 0.4 mcg/kg/**hour** vs 0.29 mcg/kg/**hour** in children >1 year; doses as high as 0.75 mcg/kg/**hour** were used (Chrysostomou, 2006). Other studies have used maintenance doses as high as 1 mcg/kg/**hour** (Munro, 2007; Nichols, 2005).

Adults:

ICU sedation: Initial: Loading dose: 1 mcg/kg, followed by a maintenance infusion of 0.2-0.7 mcg/kg/**hour**; adjust rate to desired level of sedation

Procedural sedation: Initial: Loading infusion of 1 mcg/kg [or 0.5 mcg/kg for less invasive procedures (eg, ophthalmic)] over 10 minutes, followed by a maintenance infusion of 0.6 mcg/kg/**hour**, titrate to desired effect; usual range: 0.2-1 mcg/kg/**hour**

Fiberoptic intubation (awake): Initial: Loading infusion of 1 mcg/kg over 10 minutes, followed by a maintenance infusion of 0.7 mcg/kg/**hour** until endotracheal tube is secured

Note: The manufacturer does not recommend that the duration of infusion exceed 24 hours; however, there have been a few studies in adults demonstrating that dexmedetomidine was well tolerated in treatment periods >24 hours; titrate infusion rate so patient awakens slowly; abrupt discontinuation, particularly after prolonged infusions may result in withdrawal symptoms.

Dosage adjustment in hepatic impairment: Dosage reduction may need to be considered. No specific guidelines available.

Usual Infusion Concentrations: Pediatric IV infusion: 4 mcg/mL

Preparation for Administration IV: Must be diluted prior to administration. Dilute 200 mcg (2 mL) in 48 mL NS to achieve a final concentration of 4 mcg/mL. Shake gently to mix.

Administration IV: Administer using a controlled infusion device. Infuse loading dose over 10 minutes; rapid infusions are associated with severe side effects. Dexmedetomidine may adhere to natural rubber; use administration components made with synthetic or coated natural rubber gaskets.

Monitoring Parameters Level of sedation, heart rate, respiration, ECG, blood pressure, pain control

Additional Information As an adjunct to anesthesia, dexmedetomidine has been administered IM 0.5-1.5 mcg/kg/dose, 60 minutes prior to anesthesia.

Dosage Forms Excipient information presented when available (limited, particularly for generics); consult specific product labeling.

Solution, Intravenous [preservative free]:

Precedex: 200 mcg/2 mL (2 mL) [additive free]

Precedex: 200 mcg/50 mL (50 mL); 400 mcg/100 mL (100 mL) [latex free]

Precedex: 80 mcg/20 mL (20 mL)

Generic: 200 mcg/2 mL (2 mL)

◆ **Dexmedetomidine Hydrochloride** *see* Dexmedetomidine *on page 617*

Dexmethylphenidate (dex meth il FEN i date)

Medication Safety Issues

Sound-alike/look-alike issues:

Dexmethylphenidate may be confused with methadone

Focalin may be confused with Focalgin-B, Folotyn

Related Information

Oral Medications That Should Not Be Crushed or Altered *on page 2476*

Brand Names: US Focalin; Focalin XR

Therapeutic Category Central Nervous System Stimulant

Generic Availability (US) Yes

Use Treatment of attention-deficit/hyperactivity disorder (ADHD) (FDA approved in ages ≥6 years and adults)

Medication Guide Available Yes

Pregnancy Risk Factor C

Pregnancy Considerations Teratogenic effects were noted in animal studies. There are no adequate and well-controlled studies in pregnant women. Use only if the potential benefit to the mother outweighs the possible risks to the fetus.

Breast-Feeding Considerations It is not known if dexmethylphenidate is excreted into breast milk. Dexmethylphenidate is the more active *d-threo*-enantiomer of racemic methylphenidate, and methylphenidate is excreted into breast milk. Refer to Methylphenidate monograph for additional information.

Contraindications Marked anxiety, tension, and agitation; hypersensitivity to methylphenidate or any component of the formulation; glaucoma; motor tics; family history or diagnosis of Tourette syndrome; concurrent use with or within 14 days following discontinuation with monoamine oxidase inhibitor (MAOI) therapy.

Warnings/Precautions CNS stimulant use has been associated with serious cardiovascular events including sudden death in patients with preexisting structural cardiac abnormalities or other serious heart problems (sudden death in children and adolescents; sudden death, stroke, and MI in adults). These products should be avoided in patients with known serious structural cardiac abnormalities, cardiomyopathy, serious heart rhythm abnormalities, coronary artery disease (adults), or other serious cardiac problems that could increase the risk of sudden death that these conditions alone carry. Patients should be carefully evaluated for cardiac disease prior to initiation of therapy. Patients who develop exertional chest pain, unexplained syncope, or other symptoms suggestive of cardiac disease should be evaluated promptly. CNS stimulants may increase heart rate (mean increase: 3 to 6 bpm) and blood pressure (mean increase: 2 to 4 mm Hg). Use caution with hypertension, hyperthyroidism, or other cardiovascular conditions (eg, heart failure, recent myocardial infarction, ventricular arrhythmia) that might be exacerbated by increases in blood pressure or heart rate. Stimulants are associated with peripheral vasculopathy, including Raynaud's phenomenon; signs/symptoms are usually mild and intermittent, and generally improve with dose reduction or discontinuation. Digital ulceration and/or soft tissue breakdown have been observed rarely; monitor for digital changes during therapy and seek further evaluation (eg, rheumatology) if necessary.

Use with caution in patients with preexisting psychosis; stimulants may exacerbate symptoms of behavior and thought disorder. Use with caution in patients with bipolar disorder; stimulants may induce mixed/manic episodes. New onset psychosis or mania may occur in children or adolescents with stimulant use. Patients presenting with depressive symptoms should be screened for bipolar disorder, including details regarding family history of suicide, bipolar disorder, and depression. Consider discontinuation if such symptoms (eg, delusional thinking, hallucinations, or mania) occur. May be associated with aggressive behavior or hostility (causal relationship not established); monitor for development or worsening of these behaviors.

Limited information exists regarding amphetamine use in seizure disorder (Cortese, 2013). Use with caution in patients with a history of seizure disorder; may lower seizure threshold leading to new onset or breakthrough seizure activity. Use caution in patients with history of ethanol or drug abuse. May exacerbate symptoms of behavior and thought disorder in psychotic patients. **[US Boxed Warning]: Use with caution in patients with a history of alcohol or drug dependence. Chronic abusive use can lead to marked tolerance and psychological dependence with varying degrees of abnormal behaviors. Frank psychotic episodes can occur, especially with parenteral abuse.** Visual disturbances have been reported (rare). Appetite suppression may occur, particularly in children. Use of stimulants has been associated with weight loss and slowing of growth rate; monitor growth rate and weight during treatment. Treatment interruption may be necessary in patients who are not increasing in height or gaining weight as expected. Prolonged and painful erections (priapism), sometimes requiring surgical intervention, have been reported with stimulant and atomoxetine use in pediatric and adult patients. Priapism has been reported to develop after some time on the drug, often subsequent to an increase in dose and also during a period of drug withdrawal (drug holidays or discontinuation). Patients with certain hematological dyscrasias (eg, sickle cell disease), malignancies, perineal trauma, or concomitant use of alcohol, illicit drugs, or other medications associated with priapism may be at increased risk. Patients who develop abnormally sustained or frequent and painful erections should discontinue therapy and seek immediate medical attention. An emergent urological consultation should be obtained in severe cases. Use has been associated with different dosage forms and products; it is not known if rechallenge with a different formulation will risk recurrence. Avoidance of stimulants and atomoxetine may be preferred in patients with severe cases that were slow to resolve and/or required detumescence (Eiland 2014).

Hypersensitivity reactions including angioedema and anaphylactic reactions have been observed in patients treated with methylphenidate. Use with caution in patients with Tourette syndrome or other tic disorders. Stimulants may exacerbate tics (motor and phonic) and Tourette syndrome; however, evidence demonstrating increased tics is limited. Evaluate for tics and Tourette syndrome prior to therapy initiation (AACAP [Pliszka 2007]). Abrupt discontinuation following high doses or for prolonged periods may result in symptoms of withdrawal including severe depression. Potentially significant drug-drug interactions may exist, requiring dose or frequency adjustment, additional monitoring, and/or selection of alternative therapy.

Warnings: Additional Pediatric Considerations Serious cardiovascular events, including sudden death, may occur in patients with preexisting structural cardiac abnormalities or other serious heart problems. Sudden death has been reported in children and adolescents; sudden death, stroke, and MI have been reported in adults. Avoid the use of CNS stimulants in patients with known serious structural cardiac abnormalities, cardiomyopathy, serious heart rhythm abnormalities, coronary artery disease, or other serious cardiac problems that could place patients at an increased risk to the sympathomimetic effects of a stimulant drug. Patients should be carefully evaluated for cardiac disease prior to initiation of therapy. The American Heart Association recommends that all children diagnosed with ADHD who may be candidates for medication, such as dexmethylphenidate, should have a thorough cardiovascular assessment prior to initiation of therapy. This assessment should include a combination of medical history, family history, and physical examination focusing on cardiovascular disease risk factors. An ECG is not mandatory but should be considered. **Note:** ECG abnormalities and four cases of sudden cardiac death have been reported in children receiving clonidine with methylphenidate; this problem may potentially occur with dexmethylphenidate; consider ECG monitoring and reduction of dexmethylphenidate dose when used concurrently with clonidine.

If a child displays symptoms of cardiovascular disease, including chest pain, dyspnea, or fainting, parents should seek immediate medical care for the child. In a recent retrospective study on the possible association between stimulant medication use and sudden death in children, 564 previously healthy children who died suddenly in motor vehicle accidents were compared to a group of 564 previously healthy children who died suddenly. Two of the 564 (0.4%) children in motor vehicle accidents were taking stimulant medications compared to 10 of 564 (1.8%) children who died suddenly. While the authors of this study conclude there may be an association between stimulant use and sudden death in children, there were a number of limitations to the study and the FDA cannot conclude this information impacts the overall risk:benefit profile of these medications (Gould, 2009). In a large retrospective cohort study involving 1,200,438 children and young adults (aged 2 to 24 years), none of the currently available stimulant medications or atomoxetine were shown to increase the risk of serious cardiovascular events (ie, acute MI, sudden cardiac death, or stroke) in current (adjusted hazard ratio: 0.75; 95% CI: 0.31 to 1.85) or former (adjusted hazard ratio: 1.03; 95% CI: 0.57 to 1.89) users compared to nonusers. It should be noted that due to the upper limit of the 95% CI, the study could not rule out a doubling of the risk, albeit low (Cooper, 2011).

Stimulant medications may increase blood pressure (average increase: 2 to 4 mm Hg) and heart rate (average increase: 3 to 6 bpm); some patients may experience greater increases. Long-term effects in pediatric patients have not been determined. Use of stimulants in children has been associated with growth suppression; monitor growth; treatment interruption may be needed. Appetite suppression may occur; monitor weight during therapy, particularly in children. May exacerbate motor and phonic tics and Tourette syndrome.

Adverse Reactions

Central nervous system: Anxiety, depression (children), dizziness (adults), fever (children), headache, insomnia (children), irritability (children), mood swings (children), restlessness (adults)

Dermatologic: Pruritus (children)

Gastrointestinal: Abdominal pain (children), anorexia (children), appetite decreased (children), dyspepsia, nausea (children), pharyngolaryngeal pain (adults), vomiting (children), xerostomia (adults)

Respiratory: Nasal congestion (children)

Rare but important or life-threatening: Accommodation difficulties, anaphylaxis, hypersensitivity reactions

Also refer to Methylphenidate for adverse effects seen with other methylphenidate products.

Drug Interactions

Metabolism/Transport Effects None known.

Avoid Concomitant Use

Avoid concomitant use of Dexmethylphenidate with any of the following: Iobenguane I 123; MAO Inhibitors

Increased Effect/Toxicity

Dexmethylphenidate may increase the levels/effects of: Fosphenytoin; PHENobarbital; Phenytoin; Primidone; Sympathomimetics; Tricyclic Antidepressants; Vitamin K Antagonists

The levels/effects of Dexmethylphenidate may be increased by: Antacids; AtoMOXetine; Cannabinoid-Containing Products; H2-Antagonists; MAO Inhibitors; Proton Pump Inhibitors; Tedizolid

Decreased Effect

Dexmethylphenidate may decrease the levels/effects of: Iobenguane I 123; Ioflupane I 123

Food Interactions High-fat meal may increase time to peak concentration. Management: Administer without regard to meals.

Storage/Stability Store at 25°C (77°F); excursions permitted to 15°C to 30°C (59°F to 86°F). Protect from light and moisture.

Mechanism of Action Dexmethylphenidate is the more active, *d-threo*-enantiomer, of racemic methylphenidate. It is a CNS stimulant; blocks the reuptake of norepinephrine and dopamine, and increases their release into the extraneuronal space.

Pharmacodynamics

Onset of action: Rapid, within 1-2 hours of an effective dose

Maximum effect: Variable

Duration: Immediate release: 3-5 hours; extended release: 9-12 hours (Dopheide, 2009)

Pharmacokinetics (Adult data unless noted)

Absorption: Immediate release: Rapid; Extended release: Bimodal (with 2 peak concentrations ~4 hours apart)

Distribution: V_d: 2.65 ± 1.11 L/kg

Protein binding: Unknown; racemic methylphenidate: 12% to 15%

Metabolism: Via de-esterification to inactive metabolite, *d*-α-phenyl-piperidine acetic acid (*d*-ritalinic acid)

Bioavailability: 22% to 25%

Half-life:

Children: 2-3 hours

Adults: 2-4.5 hours; **Note:** A few subjects displayed a half-life between 5-7 hours

Time to peak serum concentration:

Immediate release: Fasting: 1-1.5 hours; after a high-fat meal: 2.9 hours

Extended release: First peak: 1.5 hours (range: 1-4 hours); second peak: 6.5 hours (range: 4.5-7 hours)

Elimination: Urine (90%, primarily as inactive metabolite)

Dosing: Usual Note: Reduce dose or discontinue in patients with paradoxical aggravation of symptoms or other adverse events. Discontinue if no improvement is seen after appropriate dosage adjustment over a 1-month period of time.

Children and Adolescents:

Attention-deficit/hyperactivity disorder: Children ≥6 years and Adolescents: Oral:

Patients not currently taking methylphenidate:

Immediate release: Initial: 2.5 mg twice daily; doses should be taken at least 4 hours apart; dosage may be adjusted in increments of 2.5-5 mg at weekly intervals; maximum daily dose: 20 mg/**day** (manufacturer labeling); some experts recommend maximum daily dose: 50 mg/**day** (Dopheide, 2009; Pliszka, 2007)

Extended release: Initial: 5 mg once daily; dosage may be adjusted in increments of 5 mg/day at weekly intervals; maximum daily dose: 30 mg/**day** (manufacturer labeling); some experts recommend maximum daily dose: 50 mg/**day** (Dopheide, 2009; Pliszka, 2007)

Conversion to dexmethylphenidate from methylphenidate:

Immediate release: Initial: Half the total daily dose of racemic methylphenidate; maximum daily dexmethylphenidate dose: 20 mg/**day** (manufacturer labeling); some experts recommend maximum daily dose: 50 mg/**day** (Dopheide, 2009; Pliszka, 2007)

Extended release: Initial: Half the total daily dose of racemic methylphenidate; maximum daily dexmethylphenidate dose: 30 mg/**day** (manufacturer labeling); some experts recommend maximum daily dose: 50 mg/**day** (Dopheide, 2009; Pliszka, 2007)

Conversion from dexmethylphenidate immediate release to dexmethylphenidate extended release: When changing from Focalin® tablets to Focalin® XR capsules, switch to the same daily dose using Focalin® XR; maximum daily dose: 30 mg/**day** (manufacturer labeling); some experts recommend maximum daily dose: 50 mg/**day** (Dopheide, 2009; Pliszka, 2007)

Adults: **Attention-deficit/hyperactivity disorder:** Oral:

Patients not currently taking methylphenidate:

Immediate release: Initial: 2.5 mg twice daily; dosage may be adjusted in increments of 2.5-5 mg at weekly intervals; maximum daily dose: 20 mg/**day**; doses should be taken at least 4 hours apart

Extended release: Initial: 10 mg once daily; dosage may be adjusted in increments of 10 mg/**day** at weekly intervals; maximum daily dose: 40 mg/**day**

Conversion to dexmethylphenidate from methylphenidate:

Immediate release: Initial: Half the total daily dose of racemic methylphenidate; maximum daily dexmethylphenidate dose: 20 mg/**day**

Extended release: Initial: Half the total daily dose of racemic methylphenidate; maximum daily dexmethylphenidate dose: 40 mg/**day**

Conversion from dexmethylphenidate immediate release to dexmethylphenidate extended release: When changing from Focalin® tablets to Focalin® XR capsules, switch to the same daily dose using Focalin® XR; maximum daily dose: 40 mg/**day**

Dosage adjustment in renal impairment: No dosage adjustments provided in the manufacturer's labeling; however, since very little unchanged drug is eliminated in the urine, dosage adjustment in renal impairment is not expected to be required.

Dosage adjustment in hepatic impairment: No dosage adjustments provided in the manufacturer's labeling (not studied); use with caution.

Administration

Immediate release: Twice daily dosing should be administered at least 4 hours apart; may be taken with or without food.

Extended release: Administer once daily in the morning. Do not crush, chew, or divide capsule; swallow whole. Capsule may be opened and contents sprinkled over a spoonful of applesauce; consume immediately and entirely; do not store for future use.

Monitoring Parameters Evaluate patients for cardiac disease prior to initiation of therapy with thorough medical history, family history, and physical exam; consider ECG; perform ECG and echocardiogram if findings suggest cardiac disease; promptly conduct cardiac evaluation in patients who develop chest pain, unexplained syncope, or any other symptom of cardiac disease during treatment. Monitor CNS activity; CBC with differential, platelet count; blood pressure and heart rate (baseline following dose increases and periodically during treatment), sleep, appetite, abnormal movements, height, weight, BMI, growth in children. Patients should be re-evaluated at appropriate intervals to assess continued need of the medication. Observe for signs/symptoms of aggression or hostility, or depression. Monitor for visual disturbances.

Additional Information Treatment with dexmethylphenidate should include "drug holidays" or periodic discontinuation in order to assess the patient's requirements, decrease tolerance, and limit suppression of linear growth and weight. Medications used to treat ADHD should be part of a total treatment program that may include other components such as psychological, educational, and social measures. Long-term use of the immediate release tablets (ie, >6 weeks) and extended release capsules (>7 weeks) has not been studied; long-term usefulness should be periodically re-evaluated for the individual patient.

Focalin® XR capsules use a bimodal release where 1/2 the dose is provided in immediate release beads and 1/2 the dose is in delayed release beads. A single, once-daily dose of a capsule provides the same amount of dexmethylphenidate as two tablets given 4 hours apart. The modified release properties of Focalin® XR capsules are pH dependent; thus, concomitant administration of antacids or acid suppressants might alter the release of dexmethylphenidate.

Controlled Substance C-II

Dosage Forms Excipient information presented when available (limited, particularly for generics); consult specific product labeling.

Capsule Extended Release 24 Hour, Oral, as hydrochloride:

Focalin XR: 5 mg [contains fd&c blue #2 (indigotine)]
Focalin XR: 10 mg
Focalin XR: 15 mg [contains fd&c blue #2 (indigotine)]
Focalin XR: 20 mg
Focalin XR: 25 mg [contains fd&c blue #2 (indigotine)]
Focalin XR: 30 mg
Focalin XR: 35 mg, 40 mg [contains fd&c blue #2 (indigotine)]
Generic: 5 mg, 10 mg, 15 mg, 20 mg, 30 mg, 40 mg

Tablet, Oral, as hydrochloride:

Focalin: 2.5 mg, 5 mg, 10 mg
Generic: 2.5 mg, 5 mg, 10 mg

◆ **Dexmethylphenidate Hydrochloride** *see* Dexmethylphenidate *on page 619*

◆ **DexPak 6 Day** *see* Dexamethasone (Systemic) *on page 610*

◆ **DexPak 10 Day** *see* Dexamethasone (Systemic) *on page 610*

◆ **DexPak 13 Day** *see* Dexamethasone (Systemic) *on page 610*

Dexrazoxane (deks ray ZOKS ane)

Medication Safety Issues

Sound-alike/look-alike issues:

Zinecard may be confused with Gemzar

Related Information

Management of Drug Extravasations *on page 2298*

Prevention of Chemotherapy-Induced Nausea and Vomiting in Children *on page 2368*

Safe Handling of Hazardous Drugs *on page 2455*

Brand Names: US Totect; Zinecard

Brand Names: Canada Zinecard

Therapeutic Category Antidote; Cardioprotective Agent; Chelating Agent; Chemoprotectant Agent

Generic Availability (US) Yes

Use

Zinecard®: Reduction of anthracycline-induced (ie, doxorubicin-induced) cardiotoxicity in women with metastatic breast cancer (FDA approved in adults). Not recommended for use with initial anthracycline therapy; most dexrazoxane studies have been done in women with metastatic breast cancer who had received a cumulative doxorubicin dose of 300 mg/m^2. Has also been used for prevention of doxorubicin cardiomyopathy associated with treatment of acute lymphoblastic leukemia (ALL).

Totect®: Treatment of anthracycline extravasation (FDA approved in adults)

Pregnancy Risk Factor D

Pregnancy Considerations Adverse events were observed in animal reproduction studies using doses less than the equivalent human dose (based on BSA). May cause fetal harm if administered during pregnancy. Women of childbearing potential should use highly effective contraception to prevent pregnancy during treatment.

Breast-Feeding Considerations It is not known if dexrazoxane is excreted in breast milk. Due to the potential for serious adverse reactions in the nursing infant, a decision should be made to discontinue nursing or to discontinue dexrazoxane, taking into account the importance of treatment to the mother.

Contraindications

Zinecard:

US labeling: Use with chemotherapy regimens that do not contain an anthracycline

Canadian labeling: Hypersensitivity to dexrazoxane or any component of the formulation; use with chemotherapy regimens that do not contain an anthracycline;; use as a chemotherapeutic agent

Totect: There are no contraindications listed in the manufacturer's labeling.

Warnings/Precautions Hazardous agent - use appropriate precautions for handling and disposal (NIOSH 2014 [group 2]).

Dexrazoxane may cause mild myelosuppression (leukopenia, neutropenia, and thrombocytopenia); myelosuppression may be additive with concurrently administered chemotherapeutic agents. Does not eliminate the potential for anthracycline-induced cardiac toxicity; carefully monitor cardiac function (LVEF) before and periodically during treatment. Potentially significant drug-drug interactions may exist, requiring dose or frequency adjustment, additional monitoring, and/or selection of alternative therapy. May interfere with the antitumor effect of chemotherapy when given concurrently with fluorouracil, doxorubicin and cyclophosphamide (FAC). Acute myeloid leukemia (AML) and myelodysplastic syndrome (MDS) have been reported in pediatric patients and some adult patients receiving dexrazoxane in combination with chemotherapy. When used for the prevention of cardiomyopathy, doxorubicin should be administered within 30 minutes after the completion of the dexrazoxane infusion (do not administer doxorubicin before dexrazoxane). Dosage adjustment required for moderate or severe renal insufficiency (clearance is reduced). Due to dosage adjustments for doxorubicin in hepatic impairment, a proportional dose reduction in dexrazoxane is recommended to maintain the dosage ratio of 10:1. Do not use DMSO in patients receiving dexrazoxane for anthracycline extravasation; may diminish dexrazoxane efficacy. For IV administration; not for local infiltration into extravasation site.

Warnings: Additional Pediatric Considerations Secondary malignant neoplasms (SMN) have been reported with dexrazoxane and razoxane [racemic mixture of which dexrazoxane is the S(+) enantiomer] use; a multicenter review of pediatric trials reported the incidence of SMN to be very rare; a single case was reported out of 533 pediatric patients evaluated throughout 5-year follow-up (Vrooman, 2011).

Adverse Reactions Note: Most adverse reactions are thought to be attributed to chemotherapy, except for increased myelosuppression, pain at injection site, and phlebitis.

Prevention of doxorubicin cardiomyopathy (reactions listed are those which were greater in the dexrazoxane arm in a comparison of chemotherapy plus dexrazoxane vs chemotherapy alone):

Cardiovascular: Phlebitis

Central nervous system: Fatigue, neurotoxicity

Dermatologic: Erythema

Hematologic & oncologic: Bone marrow depression, granulocytopenia, leukopenia, thrombocytopenia

Infection: Infection, sepsis

Local: Pain at injection site pain

Miscellaneous: Fever

Rare but important or life threatening: Metastases (including acute myeloid leukemia, myelodysplastic syndrome)

Anthracycline extravasation:

Cardiovascular: Localized phlebitis, peripheral edema

Central nervous system: Depression, dizziness, fatigue, headache, insomnia

Dermatologic: Alopecia

Endocrine & metabolic: Hypercalcemia, hyponatremia, increased lactate dehydrogenase

Gastrointestinal: Abdominal pain, anorexia, constipation, diarrhea, nausea, vomiting

Hematologic & oncologic: Anemia, decreased hemoglobin, decreased neutrophils, decreased white blood cell count, febrile neutropenia, leukopenia, neutropenia, thrombocytopenia

Hepatic: Increased serum alkaline phosphatase, increased serum ALT, increased serum AST, increased serum bilirubin

Infection: Postoperative infection

Local: Pain at injection site

Renal: Increased serum creatinine

Respiratory: Cough, dyspnea, pneumonia

Miscellaneous: Fever

Drug Interactions

Metabolism/Transport Effects None known.

Avoid Concomitant Use

Avoid concomitant use of Dexrazoxane with any of the following: BCG (Intravesical); CloZAPine; Dimethyl Sulfoxide; Dipyrone

Increased Effect/Toxicity

Dexrazoxane may increase the levels/effects of: CloZAPine

The levels/effects of Dexrazoxane may be increased by: Dipyrone

Decreased Effect

Dexrazoxane may decrease the levels/effects of: BCG (Intravesical); DOXOrubicin (Conventional)

The levels/effects of Dexrazoxane may be decreased by: Dimethyl Sulfoxide

Storage/Stability Note: Preparation and storage are product specific; refer to individual product labeling for further details. Discard unused solutions.

Totect: Store intact vials at 25°C (77°F); excursions permitted to 15°C to 30°C (59°F to 86°F). Protect from light. When reconstituted with the supplied diluent to a final concentration of 10 mg/mL the reconstituted solution is stable for 2 hours. Solutions for infusion are stable for 4 hours when stored at <25°C (77°F).

Zinecard: Store intact vials at 25°C (77°F); excursions permitted to 15°C to 30°C (59°F to 86°F). When reconstituted with sterile water for injection, the reconstituted solution is stable for 30 minutes at room temperature or 3 hours refrigerated at 2°C to 8°C (36°F to 46°F). Solutions diluted for infusion are stable for 1 hour when stored at room temperature or 4 hours refrigerated.

Dexrazoxane generic formulation (Mylan): Store intact vials at 20°C to 25°C (68°F to 77°F). Reconstituted solutions and solutions diluted for infusion are stable for 6 hours when stored at room temperature or refrigerated at 2°C to 8°C (36°F to 46°F).

Additional stability information: When studied as a 24-hour continuous infusion for the prevention of cardiomyopathy, solutions prepared with sodium lactate diluent and diluted to a final concentration of 0.1 or 0.5 mg/mL in D_5W were found to retain ≥90% of their initial concentration when stored at room temperature (ambient light conditions) for ≤24 hours (Tetef, 2001).

Mechanism of Action Derivative of ethylenediaminetetraacetic acid (EDTA); a potent intracellular chelating agent. As a cardioprotectant, dexrazoxane appears to be converted intracellularly to a ring-opened chelating agent that interferes with iron-mediated oxygen free radical generation thought to be responsible, in part, for anthracycline-induced cardiomyopathy. In the management of anthracycline extravasation, dexrazoxane may act by reversibly inhibiting topoisomerase II, protecting tissue from anthracycline cytotoxicity, thereby decreasing tissue damage.

Pharmacokinetics (Adult data unless noted)

Distribution: Distributes to heart, liver, and kidneys

V_d:

Children: 0.96 L/kg

Adults: 22-25 L/m^2

Protein binding: Insignificant

Metabolism: Hydrolyzed by dihydropyrimidine aminohydrolase and dihydrocrotase

Half-life: Biphasic: Adults:

Distribution half-life: 8-21 minutes

Elimination half-life: 2-3 hours

Elimination: 40% to 60% of dose excreted renally within 24 hours

Dosing: Usual

Infants, Children, and Adolescents: **Prevention of anthracycline cardiomyopathy associated with acute lymphoblastic leukemia (ALL):** IV: A 10:1 dose ratio of dexrazoxane:doxorubicin (example: 300 mg/m^2 dexrazoxane: 30 mg/m^2 doxorubicin) (Lipshultz, 2010; Moghrabi, 2007; Silverman, 2010). **Note:** Cardiac monitoring should continue during dexrazoxane therapy; anthracycline/dexrazoxane should be discontinued in patients who develop a decline in LVEF or clinical CHF.

Adults:

Prevention of doxorubicin cardiomyopathy: IV: A 10:1 ratio of dexrazoxane:doxorubicin (dexrazoxane 500 mg/m^2:doxorubicin 50 mg/m^2). **Note:** Cardiac monitoring should continue during dexrazoxane therapy; doxorubicin/dexrazoxane should be discontinued in patients who develop a decline in LVEF or clinical CHF.

Treatment of extravasation: IV: 1000 mg/m^2 on days 1 and 2 (maximum dose: 2000 mg), followed by 500 mg/m^2 on day 3 (maximum dose: 1000 mg); begin treatment as soon as possible, within 6 hours of extravasation

Dosage adjustment in renal impairment: Adults: **Note:** Renal function may be estimated using the Cockcroft-Gault formula.

Moderate-to-severe (CrCl<40 mL/minute):

Prevention of cardiomyopathy: Reduce dose by 50%, using a 5:1 dexrazoxane:doxorubicin ratio (Example: 250 mg/m^2 dexrazoxane: 50 mg/m^2 doxorubicin)

Anthracycline-induced extravasation: Reduce dose by 50%

Dosage adjustment in hepatic impairment:

Prevention of cardiomyopathy: Since doxorubicin dosage is reduced in hyperbilirubinemia, a proportional reduction in dexrazoxane dosage is recommended (maintain a 10:1 ratio of dexrazoxane:doxorubicin)

Anthracycline-induced extravasation: Use has not been evaluated in patients with hepatic dysfunction

Preparation for Administration Hazardous agent; use appropriate precautions for handling and disposal (NIOSH 2014 [group 2]). **Note:** Preparation and storage are product specific; refer to individual product labeling for further details. Discard unused solutions. I.V.:

Prevention of doxorubicin cardiomyopathy:

Zinecard: Reconstitute vial with SWFI to a concentration of 10 mg/mL. Prior to infusion, further dilute reconstituted dexrazoxane solution in LR to a final concentration of 1.3 to 3 mg/mL.

Dexrazoxane generic formulation (Bedford Laboratories; Mylan, Inc): Reconstitute with the supplied diluent (0.167 molar sodium lactate injection) to a final concentration of 10 mg/mL. Prior to infusion, may further dilute reconstituted dexrazoxane solution with D_5W or NS to a final concentration of 1.3 to 5 mg/mL.

Treatment of anthracycline extravasation: Totect: Reconstitute 500 mg vial with 50 mL of the supplied diluent (0.167 molar sodium lactate injection) to a final concentration of 10 mg/mL. Prior to infusion, further dilute reconstituted dexrazoxane solution in 1,000 mL NS.

Administration Hazardous agent; use appropriate precautions for handling and disposal (NIOSH 2014 [group 2]). **Note:** Preparation and storage are product specific; refer to individual product labeling for further details. Discard unused solutions. Do not mix in the same container with other medications. IV:

Prevention of doxorubicin cardiomyopathy: Administer doxorubicin within 30 minutes after completion of dexrazoxane infusion (do not administer doxorubicin before dexrazoxane).

Zinecard: Administer by rapid drip infusion; do **not** administer by IV push.

Dexrazoxane generic formulation (Mylan): Administer by slow IV push or rapid drip infusion.

Treatment of anthracycline extravasation: Totect: Stop vesicant infusion immediately and disconnect IV line (leave needle/cannula in place); gently aspirate extravasated solution from the IV line (do **NOT** flush the line); remove needle/cannula; elevate extremity. Administer dexrazoxane IV over 1 to 2 hours; begin infusion as soon as possible, within 6 hours of extravasation. Infusion solution should be at room temperature prior to administration. Infuse in a large vein in an area remote from the extravasation. Day 2 and 3 doses should be administered at approximately the same time (±3 hours) as the dose on day 1. For IV administration; not for local infiltration into extravasation.

Apply dry cold compresses for 20 minutes 4 times daily for 1 to 2 days (Pérez Fidalgo 2012); withhold cooling beginning 15 minutes before dexrazoxane infusion; continue withholding cooling until 15 minutes after infusion is completed. Do not use DMSO in combination with dexrazoxane; may lessen efficacy.

Monitoring Parameters CBC with differential (frequent); liver function; serum creatinine; cardiac function (for adults: repeat monitoring at 400 mg/m^2, 500 mg/m^2, and with every 50 mg/m^2 of doxorubicin thereafter); monitor site of extravasation

Dosage Forms Excipient information presented when available (limited, particularly for generics); consult specific product labeling.

Solution Reconstituted, Intravenous:

Totect: 500 mg (1 ea) [pyrogen free]

Zinecard: 250 mg (1 ea); 500 mg (1 ea) [pyrogen free]

Generic: 250 mg (1 ea); 500 mg (1 ea)

Dextran (DEKS tran)

Medication Safety Issues

Sound-alike/look-alike issues:

Dextran may be confused with Dexedrine

Brand Names: US LMD in D5W; LMD in NaCl

Therapeutic Category Plasma Volume Expander

Generic Availability (US) No

Use Adjunctive treatment of shock or impending shock due to trauma (eg, burns, hemorrhage, surgery, surgical complications), a priming fluid in pump oxygenators during extracorporeal circulation, and for venous thrombosis and pulmonary embolism prophylaxis in patients undergoing surgery associated with a high incidence of thromboembolic complications (eg, hip surgery) (All indications: FDA approved in infants, children, adolescents, and adults), **Note:** This is not a substitute for blood or plasma; does not have oxygen-carrying capacity.

Pregnancy Risk Factor C

Pregnancy Considerations Animal reproduction studies have not been conducted.

Breast-Feeding Considerations It is not known if dextran is excreted in breast milk. The manufacturer recommends that caution be exercised when administering dextran to nursing women.

Contraindications Hypersensitivity to dextran or any component of the formulation; marked hemostatic defects (eg, thrombocytopenia, hypofibrinogenemia) of all types including those caused by medications (eg, heparin, warfarin); marked cardiac decompensation; renal disease with severe oliguria or anuria

Warnings/Precautions Hypersensitivity reactions have been reported; discontinue use immediately with signs of hypersensitivity and administer appropriate therapy. Use caution in patients at risk from overexpansion of blood volume (eg, very young, elderly patients, or those with heart failure). Large volumes of dextran (doses >1000 mL) may cause reduction in hemoglobin concentration and excessive dilution of plasma proteins due to hemodilution; transient prolongation of bleeding time or an increase in bleeding tendency may occur with large volumes; use caution to prevent a decrease in hematocrit <30%. Use with caution in patients with thrombocytopenia or active hemorrhage; may increase the risk of more bleeding. Not a substitute for blood or blood components. Renal failure has been reported. Fluid status including urine output should be monitored closely. Use in severe oliguria or anuria is contraindicated.

Adverse Reactions

Cardiovascular: Cardiac arrest, hypotension, tightness of chest

Dermatologic: Urticaria

Gastrointestional: Nausea, vomiting

Hematologic (all dose related): Bleeding time (prolonged), wound bleeding, wound hematoma

Hepatic: Liver function tests (abnormal)

Renal: Acute renal failure

Respiratory: Pulmonary edema (dose related), wheezing

Miscellaneous: Anaphylactoid reaction

Drug Interactions

Metabolism/Transport Effects None known.

Avoid Concomitant Use

Avoid concomitant use of Dextran with any of the following: Abciximab

Increased Effect/Toxicity

Dextran may increase the levels/effects of: Abciximab

Decreased Effect There are no known significant interactions involving a decrease in effect.

Storage/Stability Store at 20°C to 25°C (68°F to 77°F); do not freeze. Do not use if crystalline precipitate forms. Discard partially used containers.

Mechanism of Action Produces plasma volume expansion by virtue of its highly colloidal starch structure.

Pharmacodynamics Duration: Plasma expanding effect lasts 3-4 hours

Pharmacokinetics (Adult data unless noted)

Metabolism: Molecules with molecular weight ≥50,000 are metabolized to glucose

Elimination: Dextran 40: ~75% excreted in urine (unchanged) within 24 hours

Dosing: Usual

Infants, Children, Adolescents: **Note:** Dose and infusion rate are dependent upon the patient's fluid status and must be individualized:

Volume expansion/shock: IV:

Infants: Infuse 5 mL/kg as rapidly as necessary; maximum daily dose: 20 mL/kg/**day** for first 24 hours, 10 mL/kg/**day** thereafter; therapy should not be continued beyond 5 days

Children and Adolescents <50 kg: Infuse 10 mL/kg as rapidly as necessary; maximum daily dose: 20 mL/kg/**day** for first 24 hours, 10 mL/kg/**day** thereafter; therapy should not be continued beyond 5 days

Adolescents ≥50 kg: Infuse 500-1000 mL (~10 mL/kg) as rapidly as necessary; maximum daily dose: 20 mL/kg/**day** for first 24 hours; 10 mL/kg/**day** thereafter; therapy should not be continued beyond 5 days

Pump prime: IV: **Note:** Dose will vary with the volume of the pump oxygenator; doses usually added to the perfusion circuit.

Infants: 5 mL/kg; usual maximum total dose: 20 mL/kg/**day**

Children: 10 mL/kg; usual maximum total dose: 20 mL/kg/**day**

Adolescents: 10-20 mL/kg; usual maximum total dose: 20 mL/kg/**day**

Postoperative prophylaxis of venous thrombosis/pulmonary embolism: IV: **Note:** Current ACCP guidelines for the prevention of venous thromboembolism in surgical patients do not recommend the use of dextran; consider the use of other anticoagulants (Falck-Ytter, 2012; Gould, 2012):

Infants: Begin during surgical procedure and give 5 mL/kg; continue daily for 2-3 days; an additional 5 mL/kg should be administered every 2-3 days during the period of risk (up to 2 weeks postoperatively)

Children and Adolescents (<50 kg): Begin during surgical procedure and give 10 mL/kg; continue daily for 2-3 days; an additional 10 mL/kg should be administered every 2-3 days during the period of risk (up to 2 weeks postoperatively)

Adolescents (≥50 kg): IV: Begin during surgical procedure and give 500-1000 mL (~10 mL/kg); an additional

500 mL should be administered every 2-3 days during the period of risk (up to 2 weeks postoperatively)

Adults:

Volume expansion/shock: IV: Infuse 500-1000 mL (~10 mL/kg) as rapidly as possible; maximum: 20 mL/kg/day for first 24 hours; 10 mL/kg/day thereafter; therapy should not be continued beyond 5 days

Pump prime: IV: Varies with the volume of the pump oxygenator; generally, the solution is added in a dose of 10-20 mL/kg; usual maximum total dose: 20 mL/kg

Postoperative prophylaxis of venous thrombosis/pulmonary embolism: IV: **Note:** Current ACCP guidelines for the prevention of venous thromboembolism in surgical patients do not recommend the use of dextran; consider the use of other anticoagulants (Falck-Ytter, 2012; Gould, 2012): Per the manufacturer, begin during surgical procedure and give 500-1000 mL (~10 mL/kg); continue treatment with 500 mL once daily for 2-3 additional days. Additional 500 mL should be administered every 2-3 days during the period of risk (up to 2 weeks postoperatively).

Administration Parenteral: Do not use if crystalline precipitate forms. For IV infusion only (use an infusion pump or pressure infusion). For volume expansion/shock, may infuse initial volume as rapidly as possible. **Monitor closely for anaphylactic reaction; have epinephrine and resuscitative equipment available.**

Monitoring Parameters Vital signs, signs of allergic/anaphylactoid reaction especially for 30 minutes after starting infusions; coagulation parameters, hemoglobin, hematocrit, acid-base balance, electrolytes, serum protein, signs of circulatory overload (ie, heart rate, blood pressure, central venous pressure, hematocrit), renal function, urine output; urine specific gravity; platelets

Test Interactions Falsely elevated serum glucose when determined by methods that use high concentrations of acid (eg, sulfuric acid, acetic acid); may interfere with bilirubin assays that use alcohol and total protein assays using biuret reagents; dextran 70 may produce erythrocyte aggregation and interfere with blood typing and cross matching of blood

Additional Information Dextran in sodium chloride 0.9% contains sodium chloride 154 mEq/L

Dosage Forms Excipient information presented when available (limited, particularly for generics); consult specific product labeling.

Solution, Intravenous:

LMD in D5W: 10% Dextran 40 (500 mL) [latex free]

LMD in NaCl: 10% Dextran 40 (500 mL) [latex free]

◆ **Dextran 40** *see* Dextran *on page 624*

◆ **Dextran, Low Molecular Weight** *see* Dextran *on page 624*

Dextroamphetamine (deks troe am FET a meen)

Medication Safety Issues

Sound-alike/look-alike issues:

Dexedrine may be confused with dextran, Excedrin

Dextroamphetamine may be confused with dexamethasone

Related Information

Oral Medications That Should Not Be Crushed or Altered *on page 2476*

Brand Names: US Dexedrine; ProCentra; Zenzedi

Brand Names: Canada Dexedrine

Therapeutic Category Amphetamine; Anorexiant; Central Nervous System Stimulant

Generic Availability (US) Yes

Use

Immediate release tablets, oral solution (ProCentra®): Treatment of attention-deficit/hyperactivity disorder (ADHD) (FDA approved in ages 3-16 years); treatment of narcolepsy (FDA approved in ages ≥6 years and adults); has also been used for treatment of obesity secondary to hypothalamic-pituitary dysfunction

Extended/sustained release capsules (Dexedrine® Spansule®): Treatment of attention-deficit/hyperactivity disorder (ADHD) (FDA approved in ages 6-16 years); treatment of narcolepsy (FDA approved in ages ≥6 years and adults)

Medication Guide Available Yes

Pregnancy Risk Factor C

Pregnancy Considerations Adverse effects have been observed in animal reproduction studies. The majority of human data is based on illicit amphetamine/methamphetamine exposure and not from therapeutic maternal use (Golub, 2005). Use of amphetamines during pregnancy may lead to an increased risk of premature birth and low birth weight; newborns may experience symptoms of withdrawal. Behavioral problems may also occur later in childhood (LaGasse, 2012).

Breast-Feeding Considerations The majority of human data is based on illicit amphetamine/methamphetamine exposure and not from therapeutic maternal use (Golub, 2005). Amphetamines are excreted into breast milk and use may decrease milk production. Increased irritability, agitation, and crying have been reported in nursing infants (ACOG, 2011). The manufacturer recommends that mothers taking dextroamphetamine refrain from nursing.

Contraindications

Hypersensitivity or idiosyncrasy to dextroamphetamine, other sympathomimetic amines, or any component of the formulation; advanced arteriosclerosis, symptomatic cardiovascular disease, moderate-to-severe hypertension; hyperthyroidism; glaucoma; agitated states; patients with a history of drug abuse; during or within 14 days following MAO inhibitor therapy.

Documentation of allergenic cross-reactivity for amphetamines is limited. However, because of similarities in chemical structure and/or pharmacologic actions, the possibility of cross-sensitivity cannot be ruled out with certainty.

Warnings/Precautions [U.S. Boxed Warning]: Use has been associated with serious cardiovascular events including sudden death in patients with preexisting structural cardiac abnormalities or other serious heart problems (sudden death in children and adolescents; sudden death, stroke and MI in adults. These products should be avoided in the patients with known serious structural cardiac abnormalities, cardiomyopathy, serious heart rhythm abnormalities, or other serious cardiac problems that could increase the risk of sudden death that these conditions alone carry. Patients should be carefully evaluated for cardiac disease prior to initiation of therapy. Patients who develop symptoms such as exertional chest pain, unexplained syncope, or other symptoms suggestive of cardiac disease during treatment should undergo a prompt cardiac evaluation. Use with caution in patients with hypertension and other cardiovascular conditions that might be exacerbated by increases in blood pressure or heart rate. Amphetamines may impair the ability to engage in potentially hazardous activities. May cause visual disturbances. Stimulants are associated with peripheral vasculopathy, including Raynaud's phenomenon; signs/symptoms are usually mild and intermittent, and generally improve with dose reduction or discontinuation. Digital ulceration and/or soft tissue breakdown have been observed rarely; monitor for digital changes during therapy and seek further evaluation (eg, rheumatology) if necessary.

Limited information exists regarding amphetamine use in seizure disorder (Cortese, 2013). The manufacturer recommends use with caution in patients with a history of seizure disorder; may lower seizure threshold leading to new onset or breakthrough seizure activity. Use with caution in patients with preexisting psychosis or bipolar disorder. May exacerbate symptoms of behavior and thought disorder or induce mixed/manic episode, respectively. New onset psychosis or mania may also occur with stimulant use. Observe for symptoms of aggression and/or hostility. Stimulants may exacerbate tics (motor and phonic) and Tourette syndrome. Evaluate for tics and Tourette syndrome prior to therapy initiation. **[U.S. Boxed Warning]: Potential for drug dependency exists; prolonged use may lead to drug dependency.** Use is contraindicated in patients with history of ethanol or drug abuse. Prescriptions should be written for the smallest quantity consistent with good patient care to minimize possibility of overdose. Abrupt discontinuation following high doses or for prolonged periods may result in symptoms for withdrawal.

Use caution in the elderly due to CNS stimulant adverse effects. Appetite suppression may occur, particularly in children. Use of stimulants has been associated with weight loss and slowing of growth rate; monitor growth rate and weight during treatment. Treatment interruption may be necessary in patients who are not increasing in height or gaining weight as expected.

Benzyl alcohol and derivatives: Some dosage forms may contain sodium benzoate/benzoic acid; benzoic acid (benzoate) is a metabolite of benzyl alcohol; large amounts of benzyl alcohol (≥99 mg/kg/day) have been associated with a potentially fatal toxicity ("gasping syndrome") in neonates; the "gasping syndrome" consists of metabolic acidosis, respiratory distress, gasping respirations, CNS dysfunction (including convulsions, intracranial hemorrhage), hypotension, and cardiovascular collapse (AAP, 1997; CDC, 1982); some data suggests that benzoate displaces bilirubin from protein binding sites (Ahlfors, 2001); avoid or use dosage forms containing benzyl alcohol derivative with caution in neonates. See manufacturer's labeling.

Warnings: Additional Pediatric Considerations Serious cardiovascular events, including sudden death, may occur in patients with preexisting structural cardiac abnormalities or other serious heart problems. Sudden death has been reported in children and adolescents; sudden death, stroke, and MI have been reported in adults. Avoid the use of amphetamines in patients with known serious structural cardiac abnormalities, cardiomyopathy, serious heart rhythm abnormalities, coronary artery disease, or other serious cardiac problems that could place patients at an increased risk to the sympathomimetic effects of amphetamines. Patients should be carefully evaluated for cardiac disease prior to initiation of therapy. The American Heart Association recommends that all children diagnosed with ADHD who may be candidates for medication, such as dextroamphetamine, should have a thorough cardiovascular assessment prior to initiation of therapy. This assessment should include a combination of medical history, family history, and physical examination focusing on cardiovascular disease risk factors. An ECG is not mandatory but should be considered. If a child displays symptoms of cardiovascular disease, including chest pain, dyspnea, or fainting, parents should seek immediate medical care for the child. In a recent retrospective study on the possible association between stimulant medication use and sudden death in children, 564 previously healthy children who died suddenly in motor vehicle accidents were compared to a group of 564 previously healthy children who died suddenly. Two of the 564 (0.4%) children in motor vehicle accidents were taking stimulant medications compared to 10 of 564 (1.8%) children who died suddenly. While the authors of this study conclude there may be an association between stimulant use and sudden death in children, there were a number of limitations to the study and the FDA cannot conclude this information impacts the overall risk:benefit profile of these medications (Gould, 2009). In a large retrospective cohort study involving 1,200,438 children and young adults (aged 2 to 24 years), none of the currently available stimulant medications or atomoxetine were shown to increase the risk of serious cardiovascular events (ie, acute MI, sudden cardiac death, or stroke) in current (adjusted hazard ratio: 0.75; 95% CI: 0.31 to 1.85) or former (adjusted hazard ratio: 1.03; 95% CI: 0.57 to 1.89) users compared to nonusers. It should be noted that due to the upper limit of the 95% CI, the study could not rule out a doubling of the risk, albeit low (Cooper, 2011).

Stimulant medications may increase blood pressure (average increase: 2 to 4 mm Hg) and heart rate (average increase: 3 to 6 bpm); some patients may experience greater increases.

Adverse Reactions Frequency not defined.

Cardiovascular: Cardiomyopathy, hypertension, palpitations, tachycardia

Central nervous system: Aggressive behavior, dizziness, dysphoria, euphoria, exacerbation of tics, Gilles de la Tourette's syndrome, headache, insomnia, mania, overstimulation, psychosis, restlessness

Dermatologic: Urticaria

Endocrine & metabolic: Change in libido, weight loss

Gastrointestinal: Anorexia, constipation, diarrhea, unpleasant taste, xerostomia

Genitourinary: Frequent erections, impotence, prolonged erection

Neuromuscular & skeletal: Dyskinesia, rhabdomyolysis, tremor

Ophthalmic: Accommodation disturbances, blurred vision

Drug Interactions

Metabolism/Transport Effects Substrate of CYP2D6 (minor); **Note:** Assignment of Major/Minor substrate status based on clinically relevant drug interaction potential

Avoid Concomitant Use

Avoid concomitant use of Dextroamphetamine with any of the following: Iobenguane I 123; MAO Inhibitors

Increased Effect/Toxicity

Dextroamphetamine may increase the levels/effects of: Analgesics (Opioid); Sympathomimetics

The levels/effects of Dextroamphetamine may be increased by: Alkalinizing Agents; Antacids; AtoMOXetine; Cannabinoid-Containing Products; Carbonic Anhydrase Inhibitors; Linezolid; MAO Inhibitors; Proton Pump Inhibitors; Tedizolid; Tricyclic Antidepressants

Decreased Effect

Dextroamphetamine may decrease the levels/effects of: Antihistamines; Ethosuximide; Iobenguane I 123; Ioflupane I 123; PHENobarbital; Phenytoin

The levels/effects of Dextroamphetamine may be decreased by: Ammonium Chloride; Antipsychotic Agents; Ascorbic Acid; Gastrointestinal Acidifying Agents; Lithium; Methenamine; Multivitamins/Fluoride (with ADE); Multivitamins/Minerals (with ADEK, Folate, Iron); Multivitamins/Minerals (with AE, No Iron); Urinary Acidifying Agents

Food Interactions Amphetamine serum levels may be reduced if taken with acidic food, juices, or vitamin C. Management: Monitor response when taken concurrently.

Storage/Stability Store at 20°C to 25°C (68°F to 77°F). Protect from light.

Mechanism of Action Amphetamines are noncatecholamine, sympathomimetic amines that promote release of catecholamines (primarily dopamine and norepinephrine) from their storage sites in the presynaptic nerve terminals. A less significant mechanism may include their ability to block the reuptake of catecholamines by competitive inhibition.

Pharmacodynamics

Onset of action: Oral: 60-90 minutes

Duration of action: Immediate release: 4-6 hours; extended release: 8 hours (Dopheide, 2009)

Pharmacokinetics (Adult data unless noted)

Distribution: V_d: 3.5-4.6 L/kg; distributes into CNS; mean CSF concentrations are 80% of plasma

Metabolism: Hepatic via CYP monooxygenase and glucuronidation

Half-life: 12 hours

Time to peak serum concentration: Oral: Immediate release: 3 hours; sustained release: 8 hours

Elimination: In urine as unchanged drug and inactive metabolites; urinary excretion is pH dependent and is increased with acid urine (low pH)

Dosing: Usual Note: Use lowest effective individualized dose.

Pediatric:

Attention-deficit/hyperactivity disorder:

Immediate release tablets; oral solution:

Children 3-5 years: Oral: Initial: 2.5 mg once daily in the morning; increase daily dose by 2.5 mg increments at weekly intervals until optimal response is obtained; maximum daily dose: 40 mg/**day** in 2-3 divided doses; use intervals of 4-6 hours between doses. **Note:** Although FDA approved, current guidelines do not recommend use in children ≤5 years due to insufficient evidence (AAP, 2011).

Children ≥6 years and Adolescents: Oral: Initial: 5 mg once or twice daily with first dose in the morning; increase daily dose by 5 mg increments at weekly intervals until optimal response is obtained, usual range 5-20 mg/**day**; maximum daily dose: 40 mg/**day** in 2-3 divided doses; use intervals of 4-6 hours between doses

Extended/sustained release capsules: Children ≥6 years and Adolescents: Oral: Initial: 5 mg once or twice daily with first dose in the morning; increase daily dose by 5 mg increments at weekly intervals until optimal response is obtained, usual range: 5-20 mg/**day**; maximum daily dose: 40 mg/**day** in 1-2 divided doses; use intervals of 6-8 hours between doses; in patients >50 kg, a maximum daily dose of 60 mg/**day** in divided doses has been used (Dopheide, 2009; Pliszka, 2007)

Narcolepsy:

Immediate release tablets, oral solution:

Children 6-12 years: Oral: Initial: 5 mg daily, may increase at 5 mg increments at weekly intervals until optimal response is obtained; maximum daily dose: 60 mg/**day** in 1-3 divided doses: use intervals of 4-6 hours between doses

Adolescents: Oral: Initial: 10 mg daily, may increase at 10 mg increments at weekly intervals until optimal response is obtained; maximum daily dose: 60 mg/**day** in 1-3 divided doses; use intervals of 4-6 hours between doses

Extended/sustained release capsules:

Children 6-12 years: Oral: Initial: 5 mg daily, may increase at 5 mg increments at weekly intervals until optimal response is obtained; maximum daily dose: 60 mg/**day** in 1-2 divided doses; use intervals of 6-8 hours between doses

Adolescents: Oral: Initial: 10 mg daily, may increase at 10 mg increments at weekly intervals until optimal response is obtained; maximum daily dose: 60 mg/**day** in 1-2 divided doses; use intervals of 6-8 hours between doses

Obesity secondary to hypothalamic-pituitary dysfunction: Limited data available: Immediate release tablet; oral solution: Children ≥6 years and Adolescents: Oral: Initial: 5 mg once daily in the morning; may increase daily dose at 2.5 mg increments at weekly intervals until optimal response is obtained; additional daily doses may be given before lunch and dinner if necessary; dosing based on a small, open-label trial of five children (age: 6-9 years) postsurgical resection for management of craniopharyngioma (Mason, 2002); maximum daily dose: 20 mg/**day** in 3 divided doses.

Adult: **Narcolepsy:** Extended/sustained release capsules; immediate release tablets; oral solution: Oral: Initial: 10 mg daily, may increase at 10 mg increments in weekly intervals until optimal response is obtained; maximum daily dose: 60 mg/**day**

Administration Oral: Administer initial dose upon awakening; do not administer doses late in the evening due to potential for insomnia. Do not crush or chew extended/sustained release preparations.

Monitoring Parameters Evaluate patients for cardiac disease prior to initiation of therapy with thorough medical history, family history, and physical exam; consider ECG; perform ECG and echocardiogram if findings suggest cardiac disease; promptly conduct cardiac evaluation in patients who develop chest pain, unexplained syncope, or any other symptom of cardiac disease during treatment. Monitor CNS activity, blood pressure, heart rate, sleep, appetite, abnormal movements, height, weight, BMI, growth in children. Patients should be re-evaluated at appropriate intervals to assess continued need of the medication. Observe for signs/symptoms of aggression or hostility, or depression. Monitor for visual disturbances.

Test Interactions Amphetamines may elevate plasma corticosteroid levels; may interfere with urinary steroid determinations.

Additional Information Treatment for ADHD should include "drug holiday" or periodic discontinuation in order to assess the patient's requirements, decrease tolerance, and limit suppression of linear growth and weight. Medications used to treat ADHD should be part of a total treatment program that may include other components such as psychological, educational, and social measures. Sustained release capsule (Dexedrine® Spansule®) is formulated to release an initial dose promptly with the remaining medication gradually released over a prolonged time.

Controlled Substance C-II

Dosage Forms Excipient information presented when available (limited, particularly for generics); consult specific product labeling.

Capsule Extended Release 24 Hour, Oral, as sulfate:

Dexedrine: 5 mg, 10 mg, 15 mg [contains brilliant blue fcf (fd&c blue #1), fd&c blue #1 aluminum lake, fd&c red #40, fd&c yellow #10 (quinoline yellow), fd&c yellow #6 (sunset yellow)]

Generic: 5 mg, 10 mg, 15 mg

Solution, Oral, as sulfate:

ProCentra: 5 mg/5 mL (473 mL) [contains benzoic acid, saccharin sodium; bubble-gum flavor]

Generic: 5 mg/5 mL (473 mL)

Tablet, Oral, as sulfate:

Dexedrine: 5 mg, 10 mg [scored]

Zenzedi: 2.5 mg

Zenzedi: 5 mg [scored; contains fd&c yellow #6 (sunset yellow)]

Zenzedi: 7.5 mg [contains brilliant blue fcf (fd&c blue #1), fd&c yellow #10 (quinoline yellow)]

Zenzedi: 10 mg [scored; contains fd&c blue #2 (indigotine), fd&c red #40, fd&c yellow #6 (sunset yellow)]

Zenzedi: 15 mg [contains brilliant blue fcf (fd&c blue #1), fd&c blue #2 (indigotine), fd&c red #40]

Zenzedi: 20 mg [contains brilliant blue fcf (fd&c blue #1)]

Zenzedi: 30 mg [contains fd&c yellow #10 (quinoline yellow)]
Generic: 5 mg, 10 mg

Dextroamphetamine and Amphetamine

(deks troe am FET a meen & am FET a meen)

Medication Safety Issues

Sound-alike/look-alike issues:

Adderall may be confused with Adderall XR, Inderal

Related Information

Dextroamphetamine *on page 625*
Oral Medications That Should Not Be Crushed or Altered *on page 2476*

Brand Names: US Adderall; Adderall XR

Brand Names: Canada Adderall XR

Therapeutic Category Amphetamine; Anorexiant; Central Nervous System Stimulant

Generic Availability (US) Yes

Use

Immediate release tablets (Adderall®): Treatment of attention-deficit/hyperactivity disorder (ADHD) (FDA approved in ages ≥3 years and adults); treatment of narcolepsy (FDA approved in ages ≥6 years and adults)

Extended release capsules (Adderall XR®): Treatment of attention-deficit/hyperactivity disorder (ADHD) (FDA approved in ages ≥6 years and adults)

Medication Guide Available Yes

Pregnancy Risk Factor C

Pregnancy Considerations Adverse effects have been observed in animal reproduction studies. The majority of human data is based on illicit amphetamine/methamphetamine exposure and not from therapeutic maternal use (Golub, 2005). Use of amphetamines during pregnancy may lead to an increased risk of premature birth and low birth weight; newborns may experience symptoms of withdrawal. Behavioral problems may also occur later in childhood (LaGasse, 2012).

Breast-Feeding Considerations The majority of human data is based on illicit amphetamine/methamphetamine exposure and not from therapeutic maternal use (Golub, 2005). Amphetamines are excreted into breast milk and use may decrease milk production. Increased irritability, agitation, and crying have been reported in nursing infants (ACOG, 2011). A case report describes maternal use of amphetamine 20 mg/day throughout pregnancy and while breast-feeding. Milk concentrations were higher in breast milk than the maternal serum. The milk/plasma ratio ranged from 2.8 to 7.5 when measured on days 10 and 42 following delivery (Steiner, 1984). The manufacturer recommends that mothers taking dextroamphetamine/amphetamine refrain from nursing.

Contraindications Hypersensitivity or idiosyncrasy to the sympathomimetic amines; advanced arteriosclerosis; symptomatic cardiovascular disease; moderate-to-severe hypertension; hyperthyroidism; hypersensitivity or idiosyncrasy to the sympathomimetic amines; glaucoma; agitated states; patients with a history of drug abuse; during or within 14 days following MAO inhibitor (hypertensive crisis)

Warnings/Precautions [U.S. Boxed Warning]: Use has been associated with serious cardiovascular events including sudden death in patients with preexisting structural cardiac abnormalities or other serious heart problems (sudden death in children and adolescents; sudden death, stroke and MI in adults. These products should be avoided in the patients with known serious structural cardiac abnormalities, cardiomyopathy, serious heart rhythm abnormalities, or other serious cardiac problems that could increase the risk of sudden death that these conditions alone carry. Patients should be carefully evaluated for cardiac disease prior to initiation of therapy. Patients who develop symptoms such as exertional chest pain, unexplained syncope, or other symptoms suggestive of cardiac disease during treatment should undergo a prompt cardiac evaluation. Use with caution in patients with hypertension and other cardiovascular conditions that might be exacerbated by increases in blood pressure or heart rate. Stimulants are associated with peripheral vasculopathy, including Raynaud phenomenon; signs/symptoms are usually mild and intermittent, and generally improve with dose reduction or discontinuation. Digital ulceration and/or soft tissue breakdown have been observed rarely; monitor for digital changes during therapy and seek further evaluation (eg, rheumatology) if necessary. Amphetamines may impair the ability to engage in potentially hazardous activities. May cause visual disturbances.

Limited information exists regarding amphetamine use in seizure disorder (Cortese, 2013). The manufacturer recommends use with caution in patients with a history of seizure disorder; may lower seizure threshold leading to new onset or breakthrough seizure activity. Use with caution in patients with psychiatric or seizure disorders. May exacerbate symptoms of behavior and thought disorder in psychotic patients; new-onset psychosis or mania may occur with stimulant use; observe for symptoms of aggression and/or hostility. Screen patients with comorbid depressive symptoms prior to initiating treatment to determine if they are at risk for bipolar disorder. Stimulants may unmask tics in individuals with coexisting Tourette syndrome. **[U.S. Boxed Warning]: Potential for drug dependency exists; prolonged use may lead to drug dependency.** Use is contraindicated in patients with history of drug abuse. Prescriptions should be written for the smallest quantity consistent with good patient care to minimize possibility of overdose. Abrupt discontinuation following high doses or for prolonged periods may result in symptoms for withdrawal.

Appetite suppression may occur; monitor weight during therapy, particularly in children. Use of stimulants has been associated with suppression of growth; monitor growth rate during treatment. Not recommended for children younger than 3 years.

Warnings: Additional Pediatric Considerations Serious cardiovascular events, including sudden death, may occur in patients with preexisting structural cardiac abnormalities or other serious heart problems. Sudden death has been reported in children and adolescents; sudden death, stroke, and MI have been reported in adults. Avoid the use of amphetamines in patients with known serious structural cardiac abnormalities, cardiomyopathy, serious heart rhythm abnormalities, coronary artery disease, or other serious cardiac problems that could place patients at an increased risk to the sympathomimetic effects of amphetamines. Patients should be carefully evaluated for cardiac disease prior to initiation of therapy. The American Heart Association recommends that all children diagnosed with ADHD who may be candidates for medication, such as dextroamphetamine and amphetamine, should have a thorough cardiovascular assessment prior to initiation of therapy. This assessment should include a combination of medical history, family history, and physical examination focusing on cardiovascular disease risk factors. An ECG is not mandatory but should be considered. If a child displays symptoms of cardiovascular disease, including chest pain, dyspnea, or fainting, parents should seek immediate medical care for the child. In a recent retrospective study on the possible association between stimulant medication use and sudden death in children, 564 previously healthy children who died suddenly in motor vehicle accidents were compared to a group of 564 previously healthy children who died suddenly. Two of the 564 (0.4%) children in motor vehicle accidents were taking stimulant medications compared to 10 of 564 (1.8%) children who died suddenly. While the authors of this study conclude there may be an association between stimulant use and sudden death in children, there were a number of limitations to the study and the FDA cannot conclude this information impacts the overall risk:benefit profile of these medications (Gould, 2009). In a large retrospective cohort study involving 1,200,438 children and young adults (aged 2 to 24 years), none of the currently available stimulant medications or atomoxetine were shown to increase the risk of serious cardiovascular events (ie, acute MI, sudden cardiac death, or stroke) in current (adjusted hazard ratio: 0.75; 95% CI: 0.31 to 1.85) or former (adjusted hazard ratio: 1.03; 95% CI: 0.57 to 1.89) users compared to nonusers. It should be noted that due to the upper limit of the 95% CI, the study could not rule out a doubling of the risk, albeit low (Cooper, 2011).

Stimulant medications may increase blood pressure (average increase: 2 to 4 mm Hg) and heart rate (average increase: 3 to 6 bpm); some patients may experience greater increases.

Long-term effects in pediatric patients have not been determined. Use of stimulants in children has been associated with growth suppression; monitor growth; treatment interruption may be needed. Appetite suppression may occur; monitor weight during therapy, particularly in children.

Adverse Reactions

As reported with Adderall XR:

Cardiovascular: Palpitations, systolic hypertension (adolescents; dose related; transient), tachycardia (adults)

Central nervous system: Agitation (adults), anxiety (adults), dizziness, drowsiness, emotional lability, headache (adults), insomnia, nervousness, speech disturbance, twitching

Dermatologic: Diaphoresis, skin photosensitivity

Endocrine & metabolic: Decreased libido, dysmenorrhea, weight loss

Gastrointestinal: Abdominal pain, anorexia, constipation, decreased appetite, diarrhea, dyspepsia, nausea, teeth clenching, tooth infection, vomiting, xerostomia

Genitourinary: Impotence, urinary tract infection

Infection: Infection

Respiratory: Dyspnea

Miscellaneous: Fever

Rare but important or life-threatening: Alopecia, cardiomyopathy, cerebrovascular accident, depression, dyskinesia, dysphoria, euphoria, frequent erections, Gilles de la Tourette's syndrome, hypersensitivity, mydriasis, myocardial infarction, prolonged erections, psychosis, Raynaud phenomenon, rhabdomyolysis, seizure, toxic epidermal necrolysis

Drug Interactions

Metabolism/Transport Effects Refer to individual components.

Avoid Concomitant Use

Avoid concomitant use of Dextroamphetamine and Amphetamine with any of the following: Iobenguane I 123; MAO Inhibitors

Increased Effect/Toxicity

Dextroamphetamine and Amphetamine may increase the levels/effects of: Analgesics (Opioid); Sympathomimetics

The levels/effects of Dextroamphetamine and Amphetamine may be increased by: Alkalinizing Agents; Antacids; AtoMOXetine; Cannabinoid-Containing Products; Carbonic Anhydrase Inhibitors; Linezolid; MAO Inhibitors; Proton Pump Inhibitors; Tedizolid; Tricyclic Antidepressants

Decreased Effect

Dextroamphetamine and Amphetamine may decrease the levels/effects of: Antihistamines; Ethosuximide; Iobenguane I 123; Ioflupane I 123; PHENobarbital; Phenytoin

The levels/effects of Dextroamphetamine and Amphetamine may be decreased by: Ammonium Chloride; Antipsychotic Agents; Ascorbic Acid; Gastrointestinal Acidifying Agents; Lithium; Methenamine; Multivitamins/Fluoride (with ADE); Multivitamins/Minerals (with ADEK, Folate, Iron); Multivitamins/Minerals (with AE, No Iron); Urinary Acidifying Agents

Food Interactions Amphetamine serum levels may be reduced if taken with acidic food, juices, or vitamin C. Management: Monitor response when taken concurrently.

Storage/Stability

Immediate release tablets (Adderall®): Store at 20°C to 25°C (68°F to 77°F).

Extended release capsules (Adderall XR®): Store at 25°C (77°F); excursions permitted to 15°C to 30°C (59°F to 86°F).

Mechanism of Action Amphetamines are noncatecholamine, sympathomimetic amines that promote release of catecholamines (primarily dopamine and norepinephrine) from their storage sites in the presynaptic nerve terminals. A less significant mechanism may include their ability to block the reuptake of catecholamines by competitive inhibition.

Pharmacodynamics Oral:

Onset of action: Tablet: 30-60 minutes

Duration: Tablet: 4-6 hours

Pharmacokinetics (Adult data unless noted)

Absorption: Oral: Well-absorbed

Distribution: V_d: 3.5-4.6 L/kg; distributes into CNS, mean CSF concentrations are 80% of plasma

Metabolism: Hepatic via cytochrome P450 mono-oxygenase and glucuronidation; two active metabolites (norephedrine and 4-hydroxyamphetamine) are formed via oxidation

Half-life:

- d-amphetamine:
  - Children 6-12 years: 9 hours
  - Adolescents 13-17 years: 11 hours
  - Adults: 10 hours
- l-amphetamine:
  - Children 6-12 years: 11 hours
  - Adolescents 13-17 years: 13-14 hours
  - Adults: 13 hours

Time to peak serum concentration:

- Tablet (immediate release): 3 hours
- Capsule (extended release): 7 hours

Elimination: 70% of a single dose is eliminated within 24 hours; excreted as unchanged amphetamine (30%), benzoic acid, hydroxyamphetamine, hippuric acid, norephedrine and p-hydroxynorephedrine; **Note:** Urinary recovery of amphetamine is highly dependent on urine flow rates and urinary pH; urinary recovery of amphetamine may range from 1% in alkaline urine to 75% in acidic urine

Clearance: Children have a higher clearance (on a mg/kg basis) than adolescents and adults

Dosing: Usual Note: Use lowest effective individualized dose; administer first dose as soon as awake

Children and Adolescents:

Attention-deficit/hyperactivity disorder:

Immediate release tablets:

Children 3-5 years: Oral: Initial 2.5 mg daily given every morning; increase daily dose by 2.5 mg at weekly intervals until optimal response is obtained; maximum daily dose: 40 mg/**day** given in 1-2 divided doses per day; use intervals of 4-6 hours between doses. **Note:** Select patients may require daily dose to be given in 3 divided doses per day. Although FDA approved, current guidelines do not recommend dextroamphetamine/amphetamine use in children ≤5 years due to insufficient evidence (AAP, 2011).

Children ≥6 years and Adolescents: Oral: Initial: 5 mg once or twice daily; increase daily dose by 5 mg at weekly intervals until optimal response is obtained; usual maximum daily dose: 40 mg/**day** given in 1-2 divided doses per day; use intervals of 4-6 hours between doses; in patients >50 kg a maximum daily dose of 60 mg/**day** in divided doses has been used (Dopheide, 2009; Pliszka, 2007). **Note:** Select patients may require daily dose to be given in 3 divided doses per day.

Extended release capsules: **Note:** Patients taking divided doses of immediate release tablets may be switched to extended release capsule using the same total daily dose (taken once daily); titrate dose at weekly intervals to achieve optimal response.

Children 6-12 years: Oral: Initial: 5-10 mg daily given every morning; increase daily dose by 5 mg or 10 mg at weekly intervals until optimal response is obtained; usual maximum daily dose: 30 mg/**day**; in patients >50 kg a maximum daily dose of 60 mg/**day** has been used (Dopheide, 2009; Pliszka, 2007)

Adolescents 13-17 years: Oral: Initial: 10 mg daily given every morning; may increase to 20 mg daily after 1 week if symptoms are not controlled; usual maximum daily dose: 20 mg/**day**; in patients >50 kg a maximum daily dose of 60 mg/**day** has been used (Dopheide, 2009; Pliszka, 2007)

Narcolepsy:

Children 6-12 years: Immediate release tablets: Oral: Initial: 5 mg daily; increase daily dose by 5 mg at weekly intervals until optimal response is obtained; maximum daily dose: 60 mg/**day** given in 1-3 divided doses per day; use intervals of 4-6 hours between doses

Adolescents: Immediate release tablets: Oral: Initial: 10 mg daily; increase daily dose by 10 mg at weekly intervals until optimal response is obtained; maximum daily dose: 60 mg/**day** given in 1-3 divided doses per day; use intervals of 4-6 hours between doses

Adults:

Attention-deficit/hyperactivity disorder:

Immediate release tablets: Oral: Initial: 5 mg once or twice daily; increase daily dose in 5 mg increments at weekly intervals until optimal response is obtained; usual maximum dose: 40 mg/**day** given in 1-3 divided doses per day; use intervals of 4-6 hours between doses

Extended release capsules: Oral: Initial: 20 mg once daily in the morning; higher doses (up to 60 mg once daily) have been evaluated; however, there is not adequate evidence that higher doses provide additional benefit. **Note:** Patients taking divided doses of immediate release tablets may be switched to extended release capsule using the same total daily dose (taken once daily); titrate dose at weekly intervals to achieve optimal response.

Narcolepsy: Immediate release tablets: Oral: Initial: 10 mg daily; increase daily dose by 10 mg at weekly intervals until optimal response is obtained; maximum daily dose: 60 mg/**day** given in 1-3 divided doses per day; use intervals of 4-6 hours between doses

Dosage adjustment in renal impairment: No dosage adjustments provided in the manufacturer's labeling; use with caution; elimination may be decreased with renal impairment.

Dosage adjustment in hepatic impairment: No dosage adjustments provided in the manufacturer's labeling; use with caution; elimination may be decreased with hepatic impairment.

Administration

Immediate release tablet: To avoid insomnia, last daily dose should be administered no less than 6 hours before retiring

Extended release capsule: Avoid afternoon doses to prevent insomnia. Swallow capsule whole; do not chew or divide. May be administered with or without food. May open capsule and sprinkle contents on applesauce; consume applesauce/medication mixture immediately; do not store; do not chew sprinkled beads from capsule

Monitoring Parameters Evaluate patients for cardiac disease prior to initiation of therapy with thorough medical history, family history, and physical exam; consider ECG; perform ECG and echocardiogram if findings suggest cardiac disease; promptly conduct cardiac evaluation in patients who develop chest pain, unexplained syncope, or any other symptom of cardiac disease during treatment. Monitor CNS activity, blood pressure, heart rate, sleep, appetite, abnormal movements, height, weight, BMI, growth in children. Patients should be re-evaluated at appropriate intervals to assess continued need of the medication. Observe for signs/symptoms of aggression or hostility, or depression. Monitor for visual disturbances.

Test Interactions May interfere with urinary steroid testing

Additional Information Treatment of ADHD should include "drug holidays" or periodic discontinuation of medication in order to assess the patient's requirements, decrease tolerance, and limit suppression of linear growth and weight. Medications used to treat ADHD should be part of a total treatment program that may include other components such as psychological, educational, and social measures. The combination of equal parts of *d, l*-amphetamine aspartate, *d, l*-amphetamine sulfate, dextroamphetamine saccharate and dextroamphetamine sulfate results in a 3:1 ratio of the dextro- and levo-isomers of amphetamine.

The duration of action of Adderall® is longer than methylphenidate; behavioral effects of a single morning dose of Adderall® may last throughout the school day; a single morning dose of Adderall® has been shown in several studies to be as effective as twice daily dosing of methylphenidate for the treatment of ADHD (Manos, 1999; Pelham, 1999; Pliszka, 2000).

Controlled Substance C-II

Dosage Forms Excipient information presented when available (limited, particularly for generics); consult specific product labeling.

Capsule, extended release, oral:

5 mg [dextroamphetamine sulfate 1.25 mg, dextroamphetamine saccharate 1.25 mg, amphetamine aspartate monohydrate 1.25 mg, amphetamine sulfate 1.25 mg (equivalent to amphetamine base 3.1 mg)]

10 mg [dextroamphetamine sulfate 2.5 mg, dextroamphetamine saccharate 2.5 mg, amphetamine aspartate monohydrate 2.5 mg, amphetamine sulfate 2.5 mg (equivalent to amphetamine base 6.3 mg)]

15 mg [dextroamphetamine sulfate 3.75 mg, dextroamphetamine saccharate 3.75 mg, amphetamine aspartate monohydrate 3.75 mg, amphetamine sulfate 3.75 mg (equivalent to amphetamine base 9.4 mg)]

20 mg [dextroamphetamine sulfate 5 mg, dextroamphetamine saccharate 5 mg, amphetamine aspartate monohydrate 5 mg, amphetamine sulfate 5 mg (equivalent to amphetamine base 12.5 mg)]

25 mg [dextroamphetamine sulfate 6.25 mg, dextroamphetamine saccharate 6.25 mg, amphetamine aspartate monohydrate 6.25 mg, amphetamine sulfate 6.25 mg (equivalent to amphetamine base 15.6 mg)]

30 mg [dextroamphetamine sulfate 7.5 mg, dextroamphetamine saccharate 7.5 mg, amphetamine aspartate monohydrate 7.5 mg, amphetamine sulfate 7.5 mg (equivalent to amphetamine base 18.8 mg)]

Adderall XR

5 mg [dextroamphetamine sulfate 1.25 mg, dextroamphetamine saccharate 1.25 mg, amphetamine aspartate monohydrate 1.25 mg, amphetamine sulfate 1.25 mg (equivalent to amphetamine base 3.1 mg)]

10 mg [dextroamphetamine sulfate 2.5 mg, dextroamphetamine saccharate 2.5 mg, amphetamine aspartate monohydrate 2.5 mg, amphetamine sulfate 2.5 mg (equivalent to amphetamine base 6.3 mg)]

15 mg [dextroamphetamine sulfate 3.75 mg, dextroamphetamine saccharate 3.75 mg, amphetamine aspartate monohydrate 3.75 mg, amphetamine sulfate 3.75 mg (equivalent to amphetamine base 9.4 mg)]

20 mg [dextroamphetamine sulfate 5 mg, dextroamphetamine saccharate 5 mg, amphetamine aspartate monohydrate 5 mg, amphetamine sulfate 5 mg (equivalent to amphetamine base 12.5 mg)]

25 mg [dextroamphetamine sulfate 6.25 mg, dextroamphetamine saccharate 6.25 mg, amphetamine aspartate monohydrate 6.25 mg, amphetamine sulfate 6.25 mg (equivalent to amphetamine base 15.6 mg)]

30 mg [dextroamphetamine sulfate 7.5 mg, dextroamphetamine saccharate 7.5 mg, amphetamine aspartate monohydrate 7.5 mg, amphetamine sulfate 7.5 mg (equivalent to amphetamine base 18.8 mg)]

Tablet, oral:

5 mg [dextroamphetamine sulfate 1.25 mg, dextroamphetamine saccharate 1.25 mg, amphetamine aspartate monohydrate 1.25 mg, amphetamine sulfate 1.25 mg (equivalent to amphetamine base 3.13 mg)]

7.5 mg [dextroamphetamine 1.875 mg, dextroamphetamine saccharate 1.875 mg, amphetamine aspartate monohydrate 1.875 mg, amphetamine sulfate 1.875 mg (equivalent to amphetamine base 4.7 mg)]

10 mg [dextroamphetamine sulfate 2.5 mg, dextroamphetamine saccharate 2.5 mg, amphetamine aspartate monohydrate 2.5 mg, amphetamine sulfate 2.5 mg (equivalent to amphetamine base 6.3 mg)]

12.5 mg [dextroamphetamine sulfate 3.125 mg, dextroamphetamine saccharate 3.125 mg, amphetamine aspartate monohydrate 3.125 mg, amphetamine sulfate 3.125 mg (equivalent to amphetamine base 7.8 mg)]

15 mg [dextroamphetamine sulfate 3.75 mg, dextroamphetamine saccharate 3.75 mg, amphetamine aspartate monohydrate 3.75 mg, amphetamine sulfate 3.75 mg (equivalent to amphetamine base 9.4 mg)]

20 mg [dextroamphetamine sulfate 5 mg, dextroamphetamine saccharate 5 mg, amphetamine aspartate monohydrate 5 mg, amphetamine sulfate 5 mg (equivalent to amphetamine base 12.6 mg)]

30 mg [dextroamphetamine sulfate 7.5 mg, dextroamphetamine saccharate 7.5 mg, amphetamine aspartate monohydrate 7.5 mg, amphetamine sulfate 7.5 mg (equivalent to amphetamine base 18.8 mg)]

Adderall:

5 mg [dextroamphetamine sulfate 1.25 mg, dextroamphetamine saccharate 1.25 mg, amphetamine aspartate monohydrate 1.25 mg, amphetamine sulfate 1.25 mg (equivalent to amphetamine base 3.13 mg)]

7.5 mg [dextroamphetamine sulfate 1.875 mg, dextroamphetamine saccharate 1.875 mg, amphetamine aspartate monohydrate 1.875 mg, amphetamine sulfate 1.875 mg (equivalent to amphetamine base 4.7 mg)]

10 mg [dextroamphetamine sulfate 2.5 mg, dextroamphetamine saccharate 2.5 mg, amphetamine aspartate monohydrate 2.5 mg, amphetamine sulfate 2.5 mg (equivalent to amphetamine base 6.3 mg)]

12.5 mg [dextroamphetamine sulfate 3.125 mg, dextroamphetamine saccharate 3.125 mg, amphetamine aspartate monohydrate 3.125 mg, amphetamine sulfate 3.125 mg (equivalent to amphetamine base 7.8 mg)]

15 mg [dextroamphetamine sulfate 3.75 mg, dextroamphetamine saccharate 3.75 mg, amphetamine aspartate monohydrate 3.75 mg, amphetamine sulfate 3.75 mg (equivalent to amphetamine base 9.4 mg)]

20 mg [dextroamphetamine sulfate 5 mg, dextroamphetamine saccharate 5 mg, amphetamine aspartate monohydrate 5 mg, amphetamine sulfate 5 mg (equivalent to amphetamine base 12.6 mg)]

30 mg [dextroamphetamine sulfate 7.5 mg, dextroamphetamine saccharate 7.5 mg, amphetamine aspartate monohydrate 7.5 mg, amphetamine sulfate 7.5 mg (equivalent to amphetamine base 18.8 mg)]

Extemporaneous Preparations A 1 mg/mL oral suspension may be made with tablets. Crush ten 10 mg tablets in a mortar and reduce to a fine powder. Add small portions of Ora-Sweet and mix to a uniform paste; mix while adding the vehicle in equal proportions to **almost** 100 mL; transfer to a calibrated bottle, rinse mortar with vehicle, and add sufficient quantity of vehicle to make 100 mL. Label "shake well". Stable 30 days at room temperature.

Justice J, Kupiec TC, Matthews P, et al, "Stability of Adderall in Extemporaneously Compounded Oral Liquids," *Am J Health Syst Pharm*, 2001, 58(15):1418-21.

◆ **Dextroamphetamine Sulfate** *see* Dextroamphetamine *on page 625*

Dextromethorphan (deks troe meth OR fan)

Medication Safety Issues

Sound-alike/look-alike issues:

Benylin may be confused with Benadryl, Ventolin

Delsym may be confused with Delfen, Desyrel

Brand Names: US Cough DM [OTC]; Creomulsion Adult [OTC]; Creomulsion for Children [OTC]; Delsym Cough Childrens [OTC]; Delsym [OTC]; ElixSure Cough [OTC]; Hold [OTC]; Little Colds Cough Formula [OTC]; Nycoff [OTC]; PediaCare Childrens Long-Act [OTC]; Robafen Cough [OTC]; Robitussin Childrens Cough LA [OTC]; Robitussin CoughGels [OTC]; Robitussin Lingering CoughGels [OTC]; Robitussin Lingering LA Cough [OTC]; Robitussin Maximum Strength [OTC]; Scot-Tussin Diabetes CF [OTC]; Silphen DM Cough [OTC]; Simply Cough [OTC]; Triaminic Long Acting Cough [OTC]; Trocal Cough Suppressant [OTC]; Vicks Nature Fusion Cough [OTC]

Therapeutic Category Antitussive; Cough Preparation

Generic Availability (US) May be product dependent

Use Symptomatic relief of coughs due to minor throat or bronchial irritation caused by the common cold (FDA approved in adults; refer to product specific information regarding FDA approval in pediatric patients). **Note**: Approved ages and uses for generic products may vary; consult labeling for specific information.

Pregnancy Considerations Maternal use of standard OTC doses of dextromethorphan when used as an antitussive during the first trimester of pregnancy has not been found to increase the risk of teratogenic effects. Dextromethorphan is metabolized in the liver via CYP2D6 and CYP3A enzymes. The activity of both enzymes is increased in the mother during pregnancy. In the fetus, CYP2D6 activity is low in the fetal liver and CYP3A4 activity is present by ~17 weeks gestation.

Contraindications Concurrent administration with or within 2 weeks of discontinuing an MAO inhibitor

Warnings/Precautions Symptoms of agitation, confusion, hallucinations, hyper-reflexia, myoclonus, shivering, and tachycardia may occur with concomitant proserotonergic drugs (ie, SSRIs/SNRIs or triptans); especially with higher dextromethorphan doses.

Healthcare providers should be alert to problems of abuse or misuse. Abuse can cause death, brain damage, seizure, loss of consciousness and irregular heartbeat. Use with caution in patients who are sedated, debilitated or confined to a supine position. Use with caution in atopic children. Not for OTC use in children <4 years of age. Some products may contain tartrazine.

Benzyl alcohol and derivatives: Some dosage forms may contain sodium benzoate/benzoic acid; benzoic acid (benzoate) is a metabolite of benzyl alcohol; large amounts of benzyl alcohol (≥99 mg/kg/day) have been associated with a potentially fatal toxicity ("gasping syndrome") in neonates; the "gasping syndrome" consists of metabolic acidosis, respiratory distress, gasping respirations, CNS dysfunction (including convulsions, intracranial hemorrhage), hypotension, and cardiovascular collapse (AAP, 1997; CDC, 1982); some data suggests that benzoate displaces bilirubin from protein binding sites (Ahlfors, 2001); avoid or use dosage forms containing benzyl alcohol derivative with caution in neonates. See manufacturer's labeling.

Self-medication (OTC use): When used for self medication (OTC) notify healthcare provider if symptoms do not improve within 7 days, or are accompanied by fever, rash or persistent headache. Do not use for persistent or chronic cough (as with smoking, asthma, chronic bronchitis, emphysema) or if cough is accompanied by excessive phlegm unless directed to do so by healthcare provider.

Warnings: Additional Pediatric Considerations Safety and efficacy for the use of cough and cold products in pediatric patients <4 years of age is limited; the AAP warns against the use of these products for respiratory illnesses in this age group. Serious adverse effects including death have been reported. Many of these products contain multiple active ingredients, increasing the risk of accidental overdose when used with other products. The FDA notes that there are no approved OTC uses for these products in pediatric patients <2 years of age. Health care providers are reminded to ask caregivers about the use of OTC cough and cold products in order to avoid exposure to multiple medications containing the same ingredient (AAP 2012; FDA 2008).

Anecdotal reports of abuse of dextromethorphan-containing cough/cold products have increased, especially among teenagers.

Some dosage forms may contain propylene glycol; in neonates large amounts of propylene glycol delivered orally, intravenously (eg, >3,000 mg/day), or topically have been associated with potentially fatal toxicities which can include metabolic acidosis, seizures, renal failure, and CNS depression; toxicities have also been reported in children and adults including hyperosmolality, lactic acidosis, seizures and respiratory depression; use caution (AAP, 1997; Shehab, 2009).

Adverse Reactions Central nervous system: Confusion, excitement, irritability, nervousness, serotonin syndrome

Drug Interactions

Metabolism/Transport Effects **Substrate** of CYP2B6 (minor), CYP2C19 (minor), CYP2C9 (minor), CYP2D6 (major), CYP2E1 (minor), CYP3A4 (minor); **Note:** Assignment of Major/Minor substrate status based on clinically relevant drug interaction potential; **Inhibits** CYP2D6 (weak)

Avoid Concomitant Use

Avoid concomitant use of Dextromethorphan with any of the following: Dapoxetine; MAO Inhibitors

Increased Effect/Toxicity

Dextromethorphan may increase the levels/effects of: Antipsychotic Agents; ARIPiprazole; Memantine; Metoclopramide; Serotonin Modulators

The levels/effects of Dextromethorphan may be increased by: Abiraterone Acetate; Antiemetics (5HT3 Antagonists); Antipsychotic Agents; Cobicistat; CYP2D6 Inhibitors (Moderate); CYP2D6 Inhibitors (Strong); Dapoxetine; Darunavir; MAO Inhibitors; Panobinostat; Parecoxib; Peginterferon Alfa-2b; QuiNIDine; Selective Serotonin Reuptake Inhibitors

Decreased Effect

The levels/effects of Dextromethorphan may be decreased by: Peginterferon Alfa-2b

Mechanism of Action Decreases the sensitivity of cough receptors and interrupts cough impulse transmission by depressing the medullary cough center through sigma receptor stimulation; structurally related to codeine

Pharmacodynamics Onset of antitussive action: Within 15 to 30 minutes

Pharmacokinetics (Adult data unless noted)

Metabolism: Hepatic via demethylation via CYP2D6 to dextrorphan (active); CYP3A4 and CYP3A5 form smaller amounts of 3-hydroxy and 3-methoxy derivatives

Half-life: Elimination: Extensive metabolizers: 2 to 4 hours; poor metabolizers: 24 hours

Time to peak serum concentration: 2 to 3 hours

Elimination: Principally in urine as metabolites

Dosing: Usual

Pediatric: **Cough suppressant:** Oral:

- Oral syrup (immediate release):
  - Children: 4 years to <6 years: 5 mg every 4 hours as needed; do not exceed 6 doses in 24 hours
  - Children 6 years to <12 years: 10 mg every 4 hours as needed; do not exceed 6 doses in 24 hours
  - Children ≥12 years and Adolescents: 20 mg every 4 hours as needed; do not exceed 6 doses in 24 hours
- Long-acting liquid:
  - Children 6 years to <12 years: 15 mg every 6 to 8 hours as needed; do not exceed 4 doses in 24 hours
  - Children ≥12 years and Adolescents: 30 mg every 6 to 8 hours as needed; do not exceed 4 doses in 24 hours
- Oral capsule: Children ≥12 years and Adolescents: 30 mg every 6 to 8 hours as needed; do not exceed 4 doses in 24 hours
- Extended release suspension (dextromethorphan polistirex):
  - Children 4 years to <6 years: 15 mg every 12 hours as needed; do not exceed 30 mg in 24 hours
  - Children 6 years to <12 years: 30 mg every 12 hours as needed; do not exceed 60 mg in 24 hours
  - Children ≥12 years and Adolescents: 60 mg every 12 hours as needed; do not exceed 120 mg in 24 hours

Adult: **Cough suppressant:** Oral:

- Oral syrup: 20 mg every 4 hours as needed
- Oral capsule or long-acting liquid: 30 mg every 6 to 8 hours as needed
- Extended release suspension: 60 mg every 12 hours as needed

Administration Oral: May administer without regard to meals

Monitoring Parameters Cough, mental status

Test Interactions False-positive phencyclidine, opioids and heroin urine drug screen

Additional Information Dextromethorphan 15 to 30 mg equals 8 to 15 mg codeine as an antitussive

Dosage Forms Excipient information presented when available (limited, particularly for generics); consult specific product labeling.

Capsule, Oral, as hydrobromide:

- Robafen Cough: 15 mg [contains brilliant blue fcf (fd&c blue #1), fd&c red #40]
- Robitussin CoughGels: 15 mg [contains brilliant blue fcf (fd&c blue #1)]

Robitussin Lingering CoughGels: 15 mg [contains brilliant blue fcf (fd&c blue #1), fd&c red #40, polyethylene glycol, propylene glycol]
Gel, Oral, as hydrobromide:
ElixSure Cough: 7.5 mg/5 mL (120 mL) [alcohol free; contains carbomer 934p, propylene glycol, propylparaben; cherry bubblegum flavor]
Liquid, Oral, as hydrobromide:
Little Colds Cough Formula: 7.5 mg/mL (30 mL) [alcohol free, dye free, saccharin free; contains sodium benzoate; grape flavor]
PediaCare Childrens Long-Act: 7.5 mg/5 mL (118 mL) [contains brilliant blue fcf (fd&c blue #1), saccharin sodium, sodium benzoate]
Robitussin Lingering LA Cough: 15 mg/5 mL (118 mL) [contains alcohol, usp, fd&c red #40, menthol, saccharin sodium, sodium benzoate]
Scot-Tussin Diabetes CF: 10 mg/5 mL (118.3 mL, 480 mL, 3780 mL) [alcohol free, dye free, fructose free, sodium free, sorbitol free, sugar free]
Triaminic Long Acting Cough: 7.5 mg/5 mL (118 mL) [alcohol free, dye free, pseudoephedrine free; contains benzoic acid, propylene glycol]
Vicks Nature Fusion Cough: 15 mg/15 mL (236 mL) [alcohol free, dye free, gluten free; contains polyethylene glycol, propylene glycol; honey flavor]
Liquid Extended Release, Oral:
Cough DM: 30 mg/5 mL (89 mL) [alcohol free; contains fd&c yellow #10 aluminum lake, methylparaben, polysorbate 80, propylparaben, sodium metabisulfite; orange flavor]
Delsym: 30 mg/5 mL (89 mL, 148 mL) [alcohol free; contains brilliant blue fcf (fd&c blue #1), disodium edta, methylparaben, polyethylene glycol, polysorbate 80, propylene glycol, propylparaben; grape flavor]
Delsym: 30 mg/5 mL (89 mL, 148 mL) [alcohol free; contains edetate disodium, fd&c yellow #6 (sunset yellow), methylparaben, polyethylene glycol, polysorbate 80, propylene glycol, propylparaben; orange flavor]
Delsym Cough Childrens: 30 mg/5 mL (89 mL, 148 mL) [alcohol free; contains brilliant blue fcf (fd&c blue #1), edetate disodium, methylparaben, polyethylene glycol, polysorbate 80, propylene glycol, propylparaben, soybean oil; grape flavor]
Delsym Cough Childrens: 30 mg/5 mL (89 mL, 148 mL) [alcohol free; contains edetate disodium, fd&c yellow #6 (sunset yellow), methylparaben, polyethylene glycol, polysorbate 80, propylene glycol, propylparaben, soybean oil; orange flavor]
Generic: 30 mg/5 mL (89 mL)
Lozenge, Mouth/Throat, as hydrobromide:
Hold: 5 mg (10 ea)
Hold: 5 mg (10 ea) [cherry flavor]
Nycoff: 15 mg (500 ea)
Trocal Cough Suppressant: 7.5 mg (1 ea) [cherry flavor]
Strip, Oral, as hydrobromide:
Triaminic Long Acting Cough: 7.5 mg (14 ea, 16 ea) [contains alcohol, usp, fd&c red #40; cherry flavor]
Triaminic Long Acting Cough: 7.5 mg (14 ea) [contains alcohol, usp, fd&c red #40, isopropyl alcohol]
Syrup, Oral, as hydrobromide:
Creomulsion Adult: 20 mg/15 mL (118 mL)
Creomulsion for Children: 5 mg/5 mL (118 mL) [cherry flavor]
Robitussin Childrens Cough LA: 7.5 mg/5 mL (118 mL) [contains fd&c red #40, propylene glycol, saccharin sodium, sodium benzoate]
Robitussin Maximum Strength: 15 mg/5 mL (118 mL) [contains alcohol, usp, fd&c red #40, menthol, saccharin sodium, sodium benzoate; pleasant-tasting flavor]
Silphen DM Cough: 10 mg/5 mL (118 mL) [contains alcohol, usp; strawberry flavor]
Simply Cough: 5 mg/5 mL (120 mL) [alcohol free; cherry-berry flavor]
Triaminic Long Acting Cough: 7.5 mg/5 mL (118 mL) [alcohol free, dye free; contains benzoic acid, edetate disodium, propylene glycol]

◆ **Dextromethorphan and Guaifenesin** *see* Guaifenesin and Dextromethorphan *on page 992*

Dextrose (DEKS trose)

Medication Safety Issues
Sound-alike/look-alike issues:
Glutose™ may be confused with Glutofac®
High alert medication:
The Institute for Safe Medication Practices (ISMP) includes this medication (hypertonic solutions ≥20%) among its list of drugs which have a heightened risk of causing significant patient harm when used in error.
Other safety concerns:
Inappropriate use of low sodium or sodium-free intravenous fluids (eg D_5W, hypotonic saline) in pediatric patients can lead to significant morbidity and mortality due to hyponatremia (ISMP, 2009).

Related Information
Management of Drug Extravasations *on page 2298*
Pediatric Parenteral Nutrition *on page 2359*

Brand Names: US Dextrose Thermoject System; Glucose Nursette [OTC]; Glutol [OTC]; Glutose 15 [OTC]; Glutose 45 [OTC]; Insta-Glucose [OTC]

Therapeutic Category Antidote, Insulin; Antidote, Oral Hypoglycemic; Fluid Replacement, Enteral; Fluid Replacement, Parenteral; Hyperglycemic Agent; Hyperkalemia, Adjunctive Treatment Agent; Intravenous Nutritional Therapy

Generic Availability (US) May be product dependent

Use
IV:
5% and 10% solutions: Peripheral infusion to provide calories and fluid replacement
10% solution: Treatment of hypoglycemia in neonates
25% (hypertonic) solution: Treatment of acute symptomatic episodes of hypoglycemia to restore depressed blood glucose levels; adjunctive treatment of hyperkalemia when combined with insulin (FDA approved in neonates and older infants)
50% (hypertonic) solution: Treatment of insulin-induced hypoglycemia (hyperinsulinemia or insulin shock) and adjunctive treatment of hyperkalemia in adolescents and adults
≥10% solutions: Infusion after admixture with amino acids for nutritional support
Oral: Treatment of hypoglycemia

Pregnancy Risk Factor C (injection, infusion)

Pregnancy Considerations In patients who require parenteral nutrition for treatment of hyperemesis gravidarum, dextrose is part of the parenteral nutrition regimen (ASPEN, 2002).

Contraindications Hypersensitivity to corn or corn products; diabetic coma with hyperglycemia; hypertonic solutions in patients with intracranial or intraspinal hemorrhage; patients with delirium tremens and dehydration; patients with anuria, hepatic coma, or glucose-galactose malabsorption syndrome

Warnings/Precautions Hypertonic solutions (>10%) may cause thrombosis if infused via peripheral veins; administer hypertonic solutions via a central venous catheter. Vesicant (at concentrations ≥10%); ensure proper catheter or needle position prior to and during infusion; avoid extravasation. Rapid administration of hypertonic solutions may produce significant hyperglycemia, glycosuria, and shifts in electrolytes; this may result in dehydration, hyperosmolar syndrome, coma, and death especially in patients with chronic uremia or carbohydrate intolerance. Excessive or rapid dextrose administration in very low birth weight infants has been associated with increased serum osmolality and possible intracerebral hemorrhage.

The parenteral product may contain aluminum; toxic aluminum concentrations may be seen with high doses, prolonged use, or renal dysfunction. Premature neonates are at higher risk due to immature renal function and aluminum intake from other parenteral sources. Parenteral aluminum exposure of >4 to 5 mcg/kg/day is associated with CNS and bone toxicity; tissue loading may occur at lower doses (Federal Register, 2002). See manufacturer's labeling.

Use with caution in patients with diabetes. Hyperglycemia and glycosuria may be functions of the rate of administration of dextrose; to minimize these effects, reduce the rate of infusion; addition of insulin may be necessary. Administration of potassium free IV dextrose solutions may result in significant hypokalemia, particularly if highly concentrated dextrose solutions are used; monitor closely and/or add potassium to dextrose solutions for patients with adequate renal function. Administration of low sodium or sodium-free IV dextrose solutions may result in significant hyponatremia or water intoxication in pediatric patients; monitor serum sodium concentration. Abrupt withdrawal of dextrose solution may be associated with rebound hypoglycemia. An unexpected rise in blood glucose level in an otherwise stable patient may be an early symptom of infection. Do not use oral forms in unconscious patients.

Adverse Reactions Note: Most adverse effects are associated with excessive dosage or rate of infusion.

Cardiovascular: Edema, localized phlebitis, phlebitis, venous thrombosis

Central nervous system: Confusion, loss of consciousness

Endocrine & metabolic: Acidosis, dehydration, glycosuria, hyperglycemia, hyperosmolar syndrome, hypervolemia, hypokalemia, hypomagnesemia, hypophosphatemia, hypovolemia, ketonuria, polydipsia

Gastrointestinal: Diarrhea (oral), nausea

Local: Local pain, local tissue necrosis

Renal: Polyuria

Respiratory: Pulmonary edema, tachypnea

Miscellaneous: Fever

Drug Interactions

Metabolism/Transport Effects None known.

Avoid Concomitant Use There are no known interactions where it is recommended to avoid concomitant use.

Increased Effect/Toxicity There are no known significant interactions involving an increase in effect.

Decreased Effect There are no known significant interactions involving a decrease in effect.

Storage/Stability Stable at room temperature; protect from freezing and extreme heat. Store oral dextrose in airtight containers.

Mechanism of Action Dextrose, a monosaccharide, is a source of calories and fluid for patients unable to obtain an adequate oral intake; may decrease body protein and nitrogen losses; promotes glycogen deposition in the liver. When used in the treatment of hyperkalemia (combined with insulin), dextrose stimulates the uptake of potassium by cells, especially in muscle tissue, lowering serum potassium.

Pharmacodynamics

Onset of action: Treatment of hypoglycemia: Oral: 10 minutes

Maximum effect: Treatment of hyperkalemia: IV: 30 minutes

Pharmacokinetics (Adult data unless noted)

Absorption: Rapidly from the small intestine by an active mechanism

Metabolism: Metabolized to carbon dioxide and water

Time to peak serum concentration: Oral: 40 minutes

Dosing: Neonatal

Hypoglycemia: Note: Doses may be repeated in severe cases:

Age-directed dosing:

GA <34 weeks: IV: 0.1-0.2 g/kg/dose (1-2 mL/kg/dose of $D_{10}W$); followed by continuous IV infusion at a rate of 4-6 **mg**/kg/minute

GA ≥34 weeks: IV: 0.2 g/kg/dose (2 mL/kg/dose of $D_{10}W$) and/or a continuous IV infusion at a rate of 5-8 **mg**/kg/minute to maintain serum glucose concentration to maintain plasma glucose ≥40-50 mg/dL (Adamkin, 2011)

PALS Guidelines (PALS, 2010): IV, I.O.: Newborns: 0.5-1 g/kg/dose (5-10 mL/kg/dose of $D_{10}W$)

Parenteral nutrition: IV: Dextrose component (ASPEN Guidelines, 2002; ASPEN Pediatric Nutrition Support Core Curriculum, 2010):

Preterm neonates: Initial:5-7 **mg**/kg/minute; daily increase: 1-2.5 **mg**/kg/minute or 1% to 2.5% increments; maximum: 18 **mg**/kg/minute

Term neonates: Initial: 6-9 **mg**/kg/minute; daily increase: 1-2 **mg**/kg/minute or 2.5% to 5% increments; maximum: 18 **mg**/kg/minute

Dosing: Usual

Hypoglycemia: Note: Doses may be repeated in severe cases:

Infants and Children:

PALS Guidelines (PALS, 2010): IV, I.O.: Infants and Children: 0.5-1 g/kg/dose (2-4 mL/kg/dose of 25% solution)

Infants 1-6 months: IV: 0.25-0.5 g/kg/dose (1-2 mL/kg/dose of 25% solution; 2.5-5 mL/kg of 10% solution; 0.5-1 mL/kg of 50% solution); maximum: 25 g/dose

Infants >6 months and Children: IV: 0.5-1 g/kg/dose (2-4 mL/kg/dose of 25% solution; 5-10 mL/kg of 10% solution; 1-2 mL/kg of 50% solution); maximum: 25 g/dose

Children >2 years: Oral: 10-20 g as single dose; repeat in 10 minutes if necessary

Adolescents and Adults:

PALS Guidelines (PALS, 2010): IV, I.O.: 0.5-1 g/kg/dose (1-2 mL/kg of 50% solution)

Alternate dosing: IV: 10-25 g (40-100 mL of 25% solution or 20-50 mL of 50% solution)

Oral: 10-20 g as single dose; repeat in 10 minutes if necessary

Hyperkalemia, treatment: IV (in combination with insulin):

Infants and Children: 0.5-1 g/kg (using 25% or 50% solution) combined with regular insulin 1 unit for every 4-5 g dextrose given; infuse over 2 hours (infusions as short as 30 minutes have been recommended); repeat as needed

Adolescents and Adults: 25-50 g dextrose (250-500 mL $D_{10}W$) combined with 10 units regular insulin administered over 30-60 minutes; repeat as needed or as an alternative 25 g dextrose (50 mL $D_{50}W$) combined with 5-10 units regular insulin infused over 5 minutes; repeat as needed

Note: More rapid infusions (<30 minutes) may be associated with hyperglycemia and hyperosmolality and will exacerbate hyperkalemia; avoid use in patients who are already hyperglycemic

Parenteral nutrition: IV: Dextrose component (ASPEN Guidelines, 2002; ASPEN Pediatric Nutrition Support Core Curriculum, 2010):
Infants <1 year: Initial: 6-9 **mg**/kg/minute; daily increase: 1-2.5 **mg**/kg/minute or 1% to 2.5% increments; maximum: 18 **mg**/kg/minute
Children 1-10 years: Initial: 10%; daily increase 1-2 **mg**/kg/minute or 5% increments; maximum: 8-10 **mg**/kg/minute
Children >10 years and Adolescents: Initial: 3.5 **mg**/kg/minute or 10%; daily increase: 1-2 **mg**/kg/minute or 5% increments; maximum: 5-6 **mg**/kg/minute

Preparation for Administration Parenteral: Dilute concentrated dextrose solutions for peripheral venous administration to a maximum concentration of 12.5%; in emergency situations, 25% dextrose has been used peripherally in infants and children and 50% dextrose has been used for adolescents (PALS [Kleinman] 2010).

Administration
Oral: Must be swallowed to be absorbed
Parenteral: For IV administration only, not SubQ or IM. Maximum concentration for peripheral administration is 12.5%; in emergency situations, 25% dextrose has been used peripherally in infants and children and 50% dextrose in adolescents; for direct IV infusion, administer over 1 minute at a rate not to exceed 200 mg/kg; continuous infusion rates vary with tolerance and range from 4.5 to 15 **mg**/kg/minute; hyperinsulinemic neonates may require up to 15 to 25 **mg**/kg/minute infusion rates
Vesicant (at concentrations ≥10%); ensure proper needle or catheter placement prior to and during IV infusion. Avoid extravasation. If extravasation occurs, stop infusion immediately and disconnect (leave needle/cannula in place); gently aspirate extravasated solution (do **NOT** flush the line); initiate hyaluronidase antidote (see Management of Drug Extravasations for more details); remove needle/cannula; apply dry cold compresses (Hurst 2004); elevate extremity.

Vesicant/Extravasation Risk Vesicant (at concentrations >10%)

Monitoring Parameters Serum and urine glucose concentrations; serum electrolytes, I & O, caloric intake

Additional Information
1 g dextrose IV = 3.4 kcal
1 g glucose monohydrate = 1 g anhydrous dextrose
Osmolarity: Dextrose 10%: 505 mOsm/L; Dextrose 25%: 1330 mOsm/L; Normal body fluid: 310 mOsm/L

Dosage Forms Excipient information presented when available (limited, particularly for generics); consult specific product labeling. [DSC] = Discontinued product
Crystals, Oral:
Generic: (120 g [DSC])
Gel, Oral:
Glutose 15: 40% (37.5 g)
Glutose 15: 40% (37.5 g) [lemon flavor]
Glutose 45: 40% (112.5 g) [lemon flavor]
Insta-Glucose: 77.4% (31 g) [contains fd&c red #40, methylparaben, propylparaben, sodium benzoate]
Liquid, Oral:
Glutol: 55% (180 mL) [lemon flavor]
Solution, Injection:
Dextrose Thermoject System: 5% (10 mL)
Solution, Intravenous:
Generic: 250 mg/mL (10 mL); 5% (25 mL, 50 mL, 100 mL, 150 mL, 250 mL, 500 mL, 1000 mL); 10% (250 mL, 500 mL, 1000 mL); 20% (500 mL); 30% (500 mL); 40% (500 mL); 50% (50 mL, 500 mL, 1000 mL, 2000 mL); 70% (500 mL, 1000 mL, 2000 mL)
Solution, Oral:
Glucose Nursette: 5% (59 mL)
Tablet Chewable, Oral:
Generic: 4 g

- ◆ **Dextrose Monohydrate** *see* Dextrose *on page 633*
- ◆ **Dextrose Thermoject System** *see* Dextrose *on page 633*
- ◆ **Dex-Tuss** *see* Guaifenesin and Codeine *on page 990*
- ◆ **dFdC** *see* Gemcitabine *on page 961*
- ◆ **dFdCyd** *see* Gemcitabine *on page 961*
- ◆ **DFM** *see* Deferoxamine *on page 598*
- ◆ **DFMO** *see* Eflornithine *on page 737*
- ◆ **D-Forte (Can)** *see* Ergocalciferol *on page 772*
- ◆ **DHAD** *see* MitoXANtrone *on page 1448*
- ◆ **DHAQ** *see* MitoXANtrone *on page 1448*
- ◆ **DHE** *see* Dihydroergotamine *on page 659*
- ◆ **D.H.E. 45** *see* Dihydroergotamine *on page 659*
- ◆ **DHPG Sodium** *see* Ganciclovir (Systemic) *on page 958*
- ◆ **DHS Sal [OTC]** *see* Salicylic Acid *on page 1894*
- ◆ **DHS Tar [OTC]** *see* Coal Tar *on page 523*
- ◆ **DHS Tar Gel [OTC]** *see* Coal Tar *on page 523*
- ◆ **Diabeta** *see* GlyBURIDE *on page 975*
- ◆ **Diabeta** *see* GlyBURIDE *on page 975*
- ◆ **DiaBeta (Can)** *see* GlyBURIDE *on page 975*
- ◆ **DiabetAid Pain and Tingling Relief [OTC]** *see* Capsaicin *on page 362*
- ◆ **Diabetic Siltussin DAS-Na [OTC]** *see* GuaiFENesin *on page 988*
- ◆ **Diabetic Siltussin-DM DAS-Na [OTC]** *see* Guaifenesin and Dextromethorphan *on page 992*
- ◆ **Diabetic Siltussin-DM DAS-Na Maximum Strength [OTC]** *see* Guaifenesin and Dextromethorphan *on page 992*
- ◆ **Diabetic Tussin [OTC]** *see* GuaiFENesin *on page 988*
- ◆ **Diabetic Tussin DM [OTC]** *see* Guaifenesin and Dextromethorphan *on page 992*
- ◆ **Diabetic Tussin DM Maximum Strength [OTC]** *see* Guaifenesin and Dextromethorphan *on page 992*
- ◆ **Diabetic Tussin Mucus Relief [OTC]** *see* GuaiFENesin *on page 988*
- ◆ **Dialyvite Vitamin D 5000 [OTC]** *see* Cholecalciferol *on page 448*
- ◆ **Dialyvite Vitamin D3 Max [OTC]** *see* Cholecalciferol *on page 448*
- ◆ **Diaminocyclohexane Oxalatoplatinum** *see* Oxaliplatin *on page 1578*
- ◆ **Diaminodiphenylsulfone** *see* Dapsone (Systemic) *on page 579*
- ◆ **Diaminodiphenylsulfone** *see* Dapsone (Topical) *on page 581*
- ◆ **Diamode [OTC]** *see* Loperamide *on page 1288*
- ◆ **Diamox® (Can)** *see* AcetaZOLAMIDE *on page 52*
- ◆ **Diamox Sequels** *see* AcetaZOLAMIDE *on page 52*
- ◆ **Diarr-Eze (Can)** *see* Loperamide *on page 1288*
- ◆ **Diastat (Can)** *see* Diazepam *on page 635*
- ◆ **Diastat AcuDial** *see* Diazepam *on page 635*
- ◆ **Diastat Pediatric** *see* Diazepam *on page 635*
- ◆ **Diazemuls (Can)** *see* Diazepam *on page 635*

Diazepam (dye AZ e pam)

Medication Safety Issues
Sound-alike/look-alike issues:
Diazepam may be confused with diazoxide, diltiazem, Ditropan, LORazepam

Valium® may be confused with Valcyte®

BEERS Criteria medication:

This drug may be potentially inappropriate for use in geriatric patients (Quality of evidence - high; Strength of recommendation - strong).

Related Information

Management of Drug Extravasations *on page 2298*
Patient Information for Disposal of Unused Medications *on page 2453*
Preprocedure Sedatives in Children *on page 2444*
Serotonin Syndrome *on page 2447*

Brand Names: US Diastat AcuDial; Diastat Pediatric; Diazepam Intensol; Valium

Brand Names: Canada Apo-Diazepam; Bio-Diazepam; Diastat; Diazemuls; Diazepam Auto Injector; Diazepam Injection USP; Novo-Dipam; PMS-Diazepam; Valium

Therapeutic Category Antianxiety Agent; Anticonvulsant, Benzodiazepine; Benzodiazepine; Hypnotic; Sedative

Generic Availability (US) Yes

Use

Oral: Management of general anxiety disorders, ethanol withdrawal symptoms, relief of skeletal muscle spasms, muscle spasticity, and tetany; adjunct in the treatment of convulsive disorders (FDA approved in ages ≥6 months and adults)

Parenteral: Management of general anxiety disorders, ethanol withdrawal symptoms, relief of skeletal muscle spasms, muscle spasticity, and tetany; to provide preoperative or preprocedural sedation and amnesia; adjunct treatment of status epilepticus and severe recurrent convulsive disorders (FDA approved in ages >30 days and adults)

Rectal gel: Management of intermittent bouts of increased seizure activity in refractory epilepsy patients on stable AED therapy (FDA approved in ages ≥2 years and adults)

Pregnancy Risk Factor D

Pregnancy Considerations Teratogenic effects have been reported in animal reproduction studies. In humans, diazepam and its metabolites (N-desmethyldiazepam, temazepam, and oxazepam) cross the placenta. Teratogenic effects have been observed with diazepam; however, additional studies are needed. The incidence of premature birth and low birth weights may be increased following maternal use of benzodiazepines; hypoglycemia and respiratory problems in the neonate may occur following exposure late in pregnancy. Neonatal withdrawal symptoms may occur within days to weeks after birth and "floppy infant syndrome" (which also includes withdrawal symptoms) has been reported with some benzodiazepines (including diazepam) (Bergman, 1992; Iqbal, 2002; Wikner, 2007). A combination of factors influences the potential teratogenicity of anticonvulsant therapy. When treating women with epilepsy, monotherapy with the lowest effective dose and avoidance of medications known to have a high incidence of teratogenic effects is recommended (Harden, 2009; Wlodarczyk, 2012).

Breast-Feeding Considerations Diazepam and N-desmethyldiazepam can be found in breast milk; the oxazepam metabolite has also been detected in the urine of a nursing infant. Drowsiness, lethargy, or weight loss in nursing infants have been observed in case reports following maternal use of some benzodiazepines, including diazepam (Iqbal, 2002). Because diazepam and its metabolites may be present in breast milk for prolonged periods following administration, one manufacturer recommends discontinuing breast-feeding for an appropriate period of time.

Contraindications Hypersensitivity to diazepam or any component of the formulation (cross-sensitivity with other benzodiazepines may exist); myasthenia gravis; severe respiratory insufficiency; severe hepatic insufficiency; sleep apnea syndrome; acute narrow-angle glaucoma; not for use in infants <6 months of age (oral)

Warnings/Precautions Withdrawal has also been associated with an increase in the seizure frequency. Use with caution with drugs which may decrease diazepam metabolism. Use with caution in debilitated patients, obese patients, patients with hepatic disease (including alcoholics), or renal impairment. Active metabolites with extended half-lives may lead to delayed accumulation and adverse effects. Use with caution in patients with respiratory disease or impaired gag reflex.

Acute hypotension, muscle weakness, apnea, and cardiac arrest have occurred with parenteral administration. Acute effects may be more prevalent in patients receiving concurrent barbiturates, opioids, or ethanol. Appropriate resuscitative equipment and qualified personnel should be available during administration and monitoring. Avoid use of the injection in patients with shock, coma, or acute ethanol intoxication. Intra-arterial injection or extravasation of the parenteral formulation should be avoided. Some dosage forms may contain propylene glycol; large amounts are potentially toxic and have been associated hyperosmolality, lactic acidosis, seizures, and respiratory depression; use caution (AAP, 1997; Zar, 2007). Administration of rectal gel should only be performed by individuals trained to recognize characteristic seizure activity and monitor response.

IV administration: Vesicant; ensure proper needle or catheter placement prior to and during administration; avoid extravasation.

Benzyl alcohol and derivatives: Some dosage forms may contain benzyl alcohol and/or sodium benzoate/benzoic acid; benzoic acid (benzoate) is a metabolite of benzyl alcohol; large amounts of benzyl alcohol (≥99 mg/kg/day) have been associated with a potentially fatal toxicity ("gasping syndrome") in neonates; the "gasping syndrome" consists of metabolic acidosis, respiratory distress, gasping respirations, CNS dysfunction (including convulsions, intracranial hemorrhage), hypotension, and cardiovascular collapse (AAP, 1997; CDC, 1982); some data suggests that benzoate displaces bilirubin from protein binding sites (Ahlfors, 2001); avoid or use dosage forms containing benzyl alcohol and/or benzyl alcohol derivative with caution in neonates. See manufacturer's labeling.

Causes CNS depression (dose-related) resulting in sedation, dizziness, confusion, or ataxia which may impair physical and mental capabilities. Patients must be cautioned about performing tasks which require mental alertness (eg, operating machinery or driving). Use with caution in patients receiving other CNS depressants or psychoactive agents. Effects with other sedative drugs or ethanol may be potentiated. The dosage of opioids should be reduced by approximately one-third when diazepam is added. Benzodiazepines have been associated with falls and traumatic injury and should be used with extreme caution in patients who are at risk of these events. Benzodiazepines with long half-lives may produce prolonged sedation and increase the risk of falls and fracture. In older adults, benzodiazepines increase the risk of impaired cognition, delirium, falls, fractures, and motor vehicle accidents. Due to increased sensitivity in this age group and slower metabolism of long-acting agents (such as diazepam), avoid use for treatment of insomnia, agitation, or delirium (Beers Criteria).

Use with caution in patients taking strong CYP3A4 inhibitors, moderate or strong CYP3A4 and CYP2C19 inducers and major CYP3A4 substrates.

Use caution in patients with depression or anxiety associated with depression, particularly if suicidal risk may be present. Use with caution in patients with a history of drug dependence. Benzodiazepines have been associated with dependence and acute withdrawal symptoms on discontinuation or reduction in dose. Acute withdrawal, including seizures, may be precipitated in patients after administration of flumazenil to patients receiving long-term benzodiazepine therapy. Diazepam is a long half-life benzodiazepine. Tolerance develops to the sedative, hypnotic, and anticonvulsant effects. It does not develop to the anxiolytic or skeletal muscle relaxing effects (Vinkers, 2012). Chronic use of this agent may increase the perioperative benzodiazepine dose needed to achieve desired effect.

Diazepam has been associated with anterograde amnesia. Psychiatric and paradoxical reactions, including hyperactive or aggressive behavior, have been reported with benzodiazepines, particularly in adolescent/pediatric or elderly patients. Does not have analgesic, antidepressant, or antipsychotic properties.

Warnings: Additional Pediatric Considerations Neonates and young infants have decreased metabolism of diazepam and desmethyldiazepam (active metabolite), both can accumulate with repeated use and cause increased toxicity.

Adverse Reactions Adverse reactions may vary by route of administration.

Cardiovascular: Hypotension, localized phlebitis, vasodilatation

Central nervous system: Amnesia, ataxia, confusion, depression, drowsiness, dysarthria, fatigue, headache, slurred speech, vertigo

Dermatologic: Skin rash

Endocrine & metabolic: Change in libido

Gastrointestinal: Altered salivation (dry mouth or hypersalivation), constipation, diarrhea, nausea

Genitourinary: Urinary incontinence, urinary retention

Hepatic: Jaundice

Local: Pain at injection site

Neuromuscular & skeletal: Tremor, weakness

Ophthalmic: Blurred vision, diplopia

Respiratory: Apnea, asthma, bradypnea

Miscellaneous: Paradoxical reaction (eg, aggressiveness, agitation, anxiety, delusions, hallucinations, inappropriate behavior, increased muscle spasms, insomnia, irritability, psychoses, rage, restlessness, sleep disturbances, stimulation)

Drug Interactions

Metabolism/Transport Effects Substrate of CYP1A2 (minor), CYP2B6 (minor), CYP2C19 (major), CYP2C9 (minor), CYP3A4 (major); **Note:** Assignment of Major/Minor substrate status based on clinically relevant drug interaction potential; **Inhibits** CYP2C19 (weak)

Avoid Concomitant Use

Avoid concomitant use of Diazepam with any of the following: Azelastine (Nasal); Conivaptan; Fusidic Acid (Systemic); Idelalisib; Methadone; OLANZapine; Orphenadrine; Paraldehyde; Sodium Oxybate; Thalidomide

Increased Effect/Toxicity

Diazepam may increase the levels/effects of: Alcohol (Ethyl); Alfentanil; Azelastine (Nasal); Buprenorphine; CloZAPine; CNS Depressants; Hydrocodone; Methadone; Methotrimeprazine; Metyrosine; Mirtazapine; Orphenadrine; Paraldehyde; Pramipexole; ROPINIRole; Rotigotine; Selective Serotonin Reuptake Inhibitors; Sodium Oxybate; Suvorexant; Thalidomide; Zolpidem

The levels/effects of Diazepam may be increased by: Aprepitant; Brimonidine (Topical); Cannabis; Conivaptan; Cosyntropin; CYP2C19 Inhibitors (Moderate); CYP2C19 Inhibitors (Strong); CYP3A4 Inhibitors (Moderate); CYP3A4 Inhibitors (Strong); Dasatinib; Disulfiram; Doxylamine; Dronabinol; Droperidol; Etravirine; Fosamprenavir; Fosaprepitant; Fusidic Acid (Systemic); HydrOXYzine; Idelalisib; Ivacaftor; Kava Kava; Luliconazole; Magnesium Sulfate; Methotrimeprazine; Mifepristone; Nabilone; Netupitant; OLANZapine; Palbociclib; Perampanel; Ritonavir; Rufinamide; Saquinavir; Simeprevir; Stiripentol; Tapentadol; Teduglutide; Tetrahydrocannabinol

Decreased Effect

The levels/effects of Diazepam may be decreased by: Bosentan; CYP2C19 Inducers (Strong); CYP3A4 Inducers (Moderate); CYP3A4 Inducers (Strong); Dabrafenib; Deferasirox; Etravirine; Mitotane; Siltuximab; St Johns Wort; Theophylline Derivatives; Tocilizumab; Yohimbine

Food Interactions Diazepam serum concentrations may be decreased if taken with food. Grapefruit juice may increase diazepam serum concentrations. Management: Avoid concurrent use of grapefruit juice. Maintain adequate hydration, unless instructed to restrict fluid intake.

Storage/Stability

Injection: Store at 20°C to 25°C (68°F to 77°F); excursions permitted to 15°C to 30°C (59°F to 86°F). Protect from light. Potency is retained for up to 3 months when kept at room temperature. Most stable at pH 4-8; hydrolysis occurs at pH <3.

Oral solution: Store at 25°C (77°F); excursions permitted to 15°C to 30°C (59°F to 86°F).

Oral concentrated solution: Store at 25°C (77°F); excursions permitted to 15°C to 30°C (59°F to 86°F); protect from light; discard opened bottle after 90 days.

Rectal gel: Store at 25°C (77°F); excursion permitted to 15°C to 30°C (59°F to 86°F).

Tablet: Store at 15°C to 30°C (59°F to 86°F).

Mechanism of Action Binds to stereospecific benzodiazepine receptors on the postsynaptic GABA neuron at several sites within the central nervous system, including the limbic system, reticular formation. Enhancement of the inhibitory effect of GABA on neuronal excitability results by increased neuronal membrane permeability to chloride ions. This shift in chloride ions results in hyperpolarization (a less excitable state) and stabilization. Benzodiazepine receptors and effects appear to be linked to the GABA-A receptors. Benzodiazepines do not bind to GABA-B receptors.

Pharmacodynamics Status epilepticus:

Onset of action:
- IV: 1-3 minutes
- Rectal: 2-10 minutes

Duration: 15-30 minutes

Pharmacokinetics (Adult data unless noted)

Absorption:
- Oral: 85% to 100%
- IM: Poor
- Rectal (gel): Well absorbed

Distribution: Widely distributed; crosses blood-brain barrier and placenta; distributes into breast milk; V_d: Adults: 0.8-1 L/kg

Protein binding:
- Neonates: 84% to 86%
- Adults: 98%

Metabolism: In the liver to desmethyldiazepam (active metabolite) and N-methyloxazepam (active metabolite); these are metabolized to oxazepam (active) which undergoes glucuronide conjugation before being excreted

Bioavailability: Rectal (gel): 90%

Half-life:
- Diazepam:
  - Neonates: 50-95 hours
  - Infants 1 month to 2 years: 40-50 hours
  - Children 2-12 years: 15-21 hours
  - Children 12-16 years: 18-20 hours
  - Adults: 20-50 hours
  - Increased half-life in those with severe hepatic disorders

Desmethyldiazepam (active metabolite): Adults: 50-100 hours; may be further prolonged in neonates

Time to peak serum concentration:

Oral: Mean: 1-1.5 hours; range: 0.25-2.5 hours

Rectal (gel): 1.5 hours

Elimination: In urine, primarily as conjugated oxazepam (75%), desmethyldiazepam, and N-methyloxazepam

Dialysis: Not dialyzable (0% to 5%)

Dosing: Neonatal Status epilepticus: I.V: (Not recommended as first-line agent; use only after multiple agents have failed; injection contains benzoic acid, sodium benzoate, and benzyl alcohol): 0.1 to 0.3 mg/kg/dose given over 3 to 5 minutes, every 15 to 30 minutes, to a maximum total dose of 2 mg

Rectal gel formulation: Not recommended; product contains benzoic acid, sodium benzoate, benzyl alcohol, ethanol 10%, and propylene glycol; prolonged CNS depression has been reported in neonates receiving diazepam

Dosing: Usual

Anxiety:

Children:

Oral: 0.12 to 0.8 mg/kg/day in divided doses every 6 to 8 hours

IM, IV: 0.04 to 0.3 mg/kg/dose every 2 to 4 hours to a maximum of 0.6 mg/kg within an 8-hour period if needed

Adults:

Oral: 2 to 10 mg 2 to 4 times/day

IM, IV: 2 to 10 mg, may repeat in 3 to 4 hours if needed

Convulsive disorders:

Adjunct: Adults: Oral: 2 to 10 mg 2 to 4 times/day

Acute treatment:

Rectal gel formulation:

Infants 1 to <6 months: Not recommended; product contains benzoic acid, sodium benzoate, benzyl alcohol, ethanol 10%, and propylene glycol

Infants and Children 6 months to 2 years: Dose not established

Children 2 to 5 years: 0.5 mg/kg

Children 6 to 11 years: 0.3 mg/kg

Children ≥12 years and Adults: 0.2 mg/kg

Note: Round dose to the nearest 2.5 mg increment, not exceeding a 20 mg/dose; dose may be repeated in 4 to 12 hours if needed; do not use more than 5 times per month or more than once every 5 days

Rectal: Undiluted 5 mg/mL parenteral formulation (filter if using ampul): 0.5 mg/kg/dose then 0.25 mg/kg/dose in 10 minutes if needed

Febrile seizure prophylaxis: Children: Oral: 1 mg/kg/day divided every 8 hours; initiate therapy at first sign of fever and continue for 24 hours after fever resolves (Rosman, 1993; Steering Committee, 2008)

Status epilepticus:

Infants >30 days and Children: IV: 0.1 to 0.3 mg/kg/dose given over 3 to 5 minutes, every 5 to 10 minutes (maximum: 10 mg/dose) (Hegenbarth, 2008)

Manufacturer's recommendations:

Infants >30 days and Children <5 years: IV: 0.2 to 0.5 mg slow IV every 2 to 5 minutes up to a maximum total dose of 5 mg; repeat in 2-4 hours if needed

Children ≥5 years: IV: 1 mg slow IV every 2 to 5 minutes up to a maximum of 10 mg; repeat in 2 to 4 hours if needed

Adult: IV: Initial: 5 to 10 mg; may repeat every 10 to 15 minutes up to a maximum dose of 30 mg; may repeat in 2 to 4 hours if needed, but residual active metabolites may still be present

Ethanol withdrawal (acute): Adults: Oral: 10 mg 3 to 4 times during first 24 hours, then decrease to 5 mg 3 to 4 times/day as needed

Muscle spasms:

Cerebral palsy-associated spasticity: **Note:** Limited data available. Dose should be individualized and titrated to effect and tolerability. Oral:

Children <12 years and <15 kg (Delgado, 2010; Mathew, 2005):

<8.5 kg: 0.5 to 1 mg at bedtime

8.5 to 15 kg: 1 to 2 mg at bedtime

Children 5 to 16 years and ≥15 kg: Initial: 1.25 mg 3 times daily; may titrate to 5 mg 4 times daily (Engle, 1966)

General muscle spasms: Adults: IV, IM: Initial: 5 to 10 mg; then 5 to 10 mg in 3 to 4 hours, if necessary. Larger doses may be required if associated with tetanus.

Tetanus-associated:

Infants >30 days: IV, IM: 1 to 2 mg/dose every 3 to 4 hours as needed

Children ≥5 years: IV, IM: 5 to 10 mg/dose every 3 to 4 hours as needed

Preoperative medication: Adults: IM: 10 mg before surgery

Sedation or muscle relaxation: Children:

Oral: 0.12 to 0.8 mg/kg/day in divided doses every 6 to 8 hours

IM, IV: 0.04 to 0.3 mg/kg/dose every 2 to 4 hours to a maximum of 0.6 mg/kg within an 8-hour period if needed

Moderate sedation for procedures:

Children:

Oral: 0.2 to 0.3 mg/kg (maximum dose: 10 mg) 45 to 60 minutes prior to procedure

IV: Initial: 0.05 to 0.1 mg/kg over 3 to 5 minutes, titrate slowly to effect (maximum total dose: 0.25 mg/kg) (Krauss, 2006)

Adolescents:

Oral: 10 mg

IV: 5 mg; may repeat with 2.5 mg if needed

Skeletal muscle relaxant (adjunct therapy): Adults: Oral: 2 to 10 mg 3 to 4 times/day

Preparation for Administration Oral: Oral concentrate solution (5 mg/mL): Dilute or mix with water, juice, soda, applesauce, or pudding before use.

Administration

Oral: Administer with food or water.

Oral concentrate solution (5 mg/mL): Dilute or mix product before use. Measure dose only with calibrated dropper provided.

Parenteral: IV: May administer undiluted (5 mg/mL); per manufacturer, do not mix with other medications. Rapid injection may cause respiratory depression or hypotension; infants and children: Do not exceed 1 to 2 mg/minute IV push; adults: Maximum infusion rate: 5 mg/minute; maximum concentration for administration: 5 mg/mL.

Vesicant; ensure proper needle or catheter placement prior to and during infusion; avoid extravasation. If extravasation occurs, stop IV administration immediately and disconnect (leave cannula/needle in place); gently aspirate extravasated solution (do NOT flush the line); remove needle/cannula; elevate extremity. Apply dry cold compresses (Hurst 2004).

Rectal: Diastat AcuDial: Prior to administration, confirm that the syringe is properly set to the correct dose and that the green "ready" band is visible.

Diastat AcuDial and Diastat: Place patient on side (facing person responsible for monitoring), with top leg bent forward. Insert rectal tip (lubricated) gently into rectum until rim fits snug against rectal opening; push plunger gently over 3 seconds. After additional 3 seconds, remove syringe; hold buttocks together while slowly counting to 3 to prevent leakage; keep patient on side, facing towards you and continue to observe patient;

discard any unused medication, syringe, and all used materials safely away from children; do not reuse; see Administration and Disposal Instructions that come with product.

Vesicant/Extravasation Risk Vesicant

Monitoring Parameters Heart rate, respiratory rate, blood pressure, mental status; with long-term therapy: Liver enzymes, CBC

Reference Range Effective therapeutic range not well established

Proposed therapeutic:

Diazepam: 0.2-1.5 mcg/mL (SI: 0.7-5.3 micromoles/L)

N-desmethyldiazepam (nordiazepam): 0.1-0.5 mcg/mL (SI: 0.35-1.8 micromoles/L)

Test Interactions False-negative urinary glucose determinations when using Clinistix® or Diastix®

Additional Information Diazepam does not have any analgesic effects. Diarrhea in a 9 month old infant receiving high-dose oral diazepam was attributed to the diazepam oral solution that contained polyethylene glycol and propylene glycol (both are osmotically active); diarrhea resolved when crushed tablets were substituted for the oral solution (Marshall, 1995).

Diastat® AcuDial™: Prescribed dose must be "dialed in" and locked before dispensing; consult package insert for directions on setting prescribed dose; confirm green "ready" band is visible prior to dispensing product.

Controlled Substance C-IV

Dosage Forms Excipient information presented when available (limited, particularly for generics); consult specific product labeling.

Concentrate, Oral:

Diazepam Intensol: 5 mg/mL (30 mL) [contains alcohol, usp; unflavored flavor]

Generic: 5 mg/mL (30 mL)

Device, Intramuscular:

Generic: 10 mg/2 mL (2 mL)

Gel, Rectal:

Diastat AcuDial: 10 mg (1 ea); 20 mg (1 ea) [contains alcohol, usp, benzoic acid, sodium benzoate]

Diastat Pediatric: 2.5 mg (1 ea) [contains benzoic acid, benzyl alcohol, propylene glycol, sodium benzoate]

Generic: 2.5 mg (1 ea); 10 mg (1 ea); 20 mg (1 ea)

Solution, Injection:

Generic: 5 mg/mL (2 mL, 10 mL)

Solution, Oral:

Generic: 1 mg/mL (5 mL, 500 mL)

Tablet, Oral:

Valium: 2 mg, 5 mg, 10 mg [scored]

Generic: 2 mg, 5 mg, 10 mg

◆ **Diazepam Auto Injector (Can)** *see* Diazepam *on page 635*

◆ **Diazepam Injection USP (Can)** *see* Diazepam *on page 635*

◆ **Diazepam Intensol** *see* Diazepam *on page 635*

Diazoxide (dye az OKS ide)

Medication Safety Issues

Sound-alike/look-alike issues:

Diazoxide may be confused with diazepam, Dyazide®

Brand Names: US Proglycem

Brand Names: Canada Proglycem®

Therapeutic Category Antihypoglycemic Agent; Vasodilator

Generic Availability (US) No

Use

Management of hypoglycemia related to hyperinsulinism secondary to the following conditions: Islet cell adenoma, adenomatosis, or hyperplasia; extrapancreatic malignancy; nesidioblastosis (persistent hyperinsulinemic hypoglycemia of infancy); leucine sensitivity (All indications: FDA approved in neonates, infants, and children)

Management of hypoglycemia related to hyperinsulinism secondary to the following conditions: Inoperable islet cell adenoma or carcinoma; extrapancreatic malignancy (FDA approved in adults)

Pregnancy Risk Factor C

Pregnancy Considerations Adverse events have been observed in animal studies. Diazoxide crosses the human placenta. Altered carbohydrate metabolism, hyperbilirubinemia, or thrombocytopenia have been reported in the fetus or neonate. Alopecia and hypertrichosis lanuginosa have also been reported in infants following maternal use of diazoxide during the last 19-60 days of pregnancy.

Breast-Feeding Considerations It is not known if diazoxide is excreted in breast milk. Due to the potential for serious adverse reactions in the nursing infant, a decision should be made whether to discontinue nursing or to discontinue the drug, taking into account the importance of treatment to the mother.

Contraindications Hypersensitivity to diazoxide or to other thiazides; functional hypoglycemia

Warnings/Precautions Use with caution in patients with heart failure, hepatic impairment, hyperuricemia or a history of gout. Use caution with renal impairment; a reduced dose should be considered. Ketoacidosis or nonketotic hyperosmolar coma may occur during treatment; usually in patients with concomitant illness. Transient cataracts have been reported which subside following correction of hyperosmolarity. May displace bilirubin from albumin; use caution in newborns with hyperbilirubinemia.

Some dosage forms may contain propylene glycol; large amounts are potentially toxic and have been associated hyperosmolality, lactic acidosis, seizures, and respiratory depression; use caution (AAP, 1997; Zar, 2007).

Benzyl alcohol and derivatives: Some dosage forms may contain sodium benzoate/benzoic acid; benzoic acid (benzoate) is a metabolite of benzyl alcohol; large amounts of benzyl alcohol (≥99 mg/kg/day) have been associated with a potentially fatal toxicity ("gasping syndrome") in neonates; the "gasping syndrome" consists of metabolic acidosis, respiratory distress, gasping respirations, CNS dysfunction (including convulsions, intracranial hemorrhage), hypotension, and cardiovascular collapse (AAP, 1997; CDC, 1982); some data suggests that benzoate displaces bilirubin from protein binding sites (Ahlfors, 2001); avoid or use dosage forms containing benzyl alcohol derivative with caution in neonates. See manufacturer's labeling.

Warnings: Additional Pediatric Considerations Transient cataracts have been reported in an infant in association with hyperosmolar coma; cataracts subsided following correction of hyperosmolarity. Abnormal facial features have been reported in four children who received diazoxide for >4 years for the treatment of hypoglycemia hyperinsulinism.

Adverse Reactions

Cardiovascular: Cardiac failure (due to sodium and water retention), chest pain (rare), hyperosmolar coma (nonketotic), hypertension (transient), hypotension, palpitations, tachycardia

Central nervous system: Anxiety, dizziness, extrapyramidal reaction, headache, insomnia, malaise, paresthesia, peripheral neuritis (poly)

Dermatologic: Cutaneous candidiasis, loss of scalp hair, pruritus, purpura, skin rash

Endocrine & metabolic: Albuminuria, diabetic ketoacidosis, fluid retention, galactorrhea, glycosuria, gout, hirsutism, hyperglycemia, sodium retention

Gastrointestinal: Abdominal pain, acute pancreatitis, ageusia (transient), anorexia, diarrhea, intestinal obstruction, nausea, pancreatic necrosis, vomiting

Genitourinary: Azotemia, decreased urine output, hematuria, lump in breast (enlargement), nephrotic syndrome (reversible), uricosuria

Hematologic & oncologic: Decreased hematocrit, decreased hemoglobin, decreased serum immunoglobulins (IgG), eosinophilia, hemorrhage (excessive), lymphadenopathy, neutropenia (transient), thrombocytopenia

Hepatic: Increased serum alkaline phosphatase, increased serum AST

Infection: Herpes virus infection

Neuromuscular & skeletal: Accelerated bone maturation, craniofacial abnormality (children with chronic use), weakness

Ophthalmic: Blurred vision, cataract (transient), diplopia, lacrimation, scotoma (ring), subconjunctival hemorrhage

Renal: Decreased creatinine clearance

Miscellaneous: Fever

Drug Interactions

Metabolism/Transport Effects None known.

Avoid Concomitant Use There are no known interactions where it is recommended to avoid concomitant use.

Increased Effect/Toxicity

Diazoxide may increase the levels/effects of: Antihypertensives

The levels/effects of Diazoxide may be increased by: MAO Inhibitors; Thiazide Diuretics; Thiopental

Decreased Effect

Diazoxide may decrease the levels/effects of: Antidiabetic Agents; Fosphenytoin; Phenytoin

Storage/Stability Store at 25°C (77°F); excursions permitted to 15°C to 30°C (59°F to 86°F). Protect from light. Store in carton until ready to use.

Mechanism of Action Opens ATP-dependent potassium channels on pancreatic beta cells in the presence of ATP and Mg^{2+}, resulting in hyperpolarization of the cell and inhibition of insulin release. Diazoxide binds to a different site on the potassium channel than the sulfonylureas (Doyle, 2003).

Pharmacodynamics

Hyperglycemic effects (oral):

Onset of action: Within 1 hour

Duration (normal renal function): 8 hours

Pharmacokinetics (Adult data unless noted)

Protein binding: >90%

Half-life:

Children: 9-24 hours

Adults: 24-36 hours

Elimination: 50% excreted unchanged in urine

Dosing: Neonatal Hyperinsulinemic hypoglycemia: Oral: Initial: 10 mg/kg/day in divided doses every 8 hours; usual range: 5-15 mg/kg/day in divided doses every 8 hours (Hussain, 2004; Kapoor, 2009); **Note:** Often given in conjunction with chlorothiazide

Dosing: Usual Note: Dose should be individualized based on the severity of the hypoglycemic condition, blood glucose concentration, and clinical response of patient. Use the least amount of drug that achieves the desired clinical and laboratory results.

Infants, Children, and Adolescents: **Hyperinsulinemic hypoglycemia:**

Infants: Oral: Initial: 10 mg/kg/day in divided doses every 8 hours; usual range: 8-15 mg/kg/day in divided doses every 8-12 hours; range of 5-20 mg/kg/day in divided doses every 8 hours has been used (Kapoor, 2009)

Children and Adolescents: Oral: Initial: 3 mg/kg/day in divided doses every 8 hours; usual range: 3-8 mg/kg/day in divided doses every 8-12 hours. **Note:** In certain instances, patients with refractory hypoglycemia may require higher doses.

Adults: **Hyperinsulinemic hypoglycemia:** Oral: Initial: 3 mg/kg/day in divided doses every 8 hours; usual range: 3-8 mg/kg/day in divided doses every 8-12 hours. **Note:** In certain instances, patients with refractory hypoglycemia may require higher doses.

Dosing adjustment in renal impairment: Half-life may be prolonged with renal impairment; a reduced dose should be considered.

Dosing adjustment in hepatic impairment: There are no dosage adjustments provided in the manufacturer's labeling.

Administration Shake suspension well before use; suspension comes with calibrated dropper (to deliver dose of 10-50 mg, in 10 mg increments).

Monitoring Parameters Blood glucose, serum uric acid, electrolytes, BUN; renal function; AST, CBC with differential, platelets; urine glucose and ketones; blood pressure, heart rate

Test Interactions Serum renin concentrations may be increased. Serum cortisol concentrations may be decreased.

Additional Information The injectable form of diazoxide, which was used for the emergency treatment of hypertension, is no longer available.

Dosage Forms Excipient information presented when available (limited, particularly for generics); consult specific product labeling.

Suspension, Oral:

Proglycem: 50 mg/mL (30 mL) [chocolate mint flavor]

◆ **Dibenzyline** *see* Phenoxybenzamine *on page 1683*

Dibucaine (DYE byoo kane)

Brand Names: US Nupercainal [OTC]

Therapeutic Category Analgesic, Topical; Local Anesthetic, Topical

Generic Availability (US) Yes

Use Fast, temporary relief of pain and itching due to hemorrhoids, minor burns, other minor skin conditions

Pregnancy Considerations Dibucaine is not absorbed systemically following topical administration on intact skin. Systemic absorption would be required in order for dibucaine to cross the placenta and reach the fetus.

Breast-Feeding Considerations No data reported; however, topical administration is probably compatible.

Contraindications Hypersensitivity to amide-type anesthetics, ophthalmic use

Warnings/Precautions When topical anesthetics are used prior to cosmetic or medical procedures, the lowest amount of anesthetic necessary for pain relief should be applied. High systemic levels and toxic effects (eg, methemoglobinemia, irregular heart beats, respiratory depression, seizures, death) have been reported in patients who (without supervision of a trained professional) have applied topical anesthetics in large amounts (or to large areas of the skin), left these products on for prolonged periods of time, or have used wraps/dressings to cover the skin following application.

Adverse Reactions

Dermatologic: Angioedema, contact dermatitis

Local: Burning

Drug Interactions

Metabolism/Transport Effects None known.

Avoid Concomitant Use There are no known interactions where it is recommended to avoid concomitant use.

Increased Effect/Toxicity There are no known significant interactions involving an increase in effect.

Decreased Effect There are no known significant interactions involving a decrease in effect.

Storage/Stability Darkens on light exposure.

Mechanism of Action Local anesthetics bind selectively to the intracellular surface of sodium channels to block influx of sodium into the axon. As a result, depolarization necessary for action potential propagation and subsequent nerve function is prevented. The block at the sodium channel is reversible. When drug diffuses away from the axon, sodium channel function is restored and nerve propagation returns.

Pharmacodynamics

Onset of action: Within 15 minutes

Duration: 2-4 hours

Pharmacokinetics (Adult data unless noted) Absorption: Poor through intact skin, but well absorbed through mucous membranes and excoriated skin

Dosing: Usual Children and Adults:

Rectal: Hemorrhoids: Administer each morning, evening, and after each bowel movement

Topical: Apply gently to the affected areas; no more than 30 g for adults or 7.5 g for children should be used in any 24-hour period

Administration

Rectal: Insert ointment into rectum using a rectal applicator

Topical: Apply gently to affected areas; do not use near the eyes or over denuded surfaces or blistered areas

Dosage Forms Excipient information presented when available (limited, particularly for generics); consult specific product labeling.

Ointment, External:

Nupercainal: 1% (56.7 g)

Generic: 1% (28 g, 28.35 g)

Ointment, Rectal:

Nupercainal: 1% (28.4 g, 56.7 g, 60 g)

◆ **DIC** *see* Dacarbazine *on page 572*

Diclofenac (Systemic) (dye KLOE fen ak)

Medication Safety Issues

Sound-alike/look-alike issues:

Diclofenac may be confused with Diflucan

Cataflam may be confused with Catapres

Voltaren may be confused with traMADol, Ultram, Verelan

BEERS Criteria medication:

This drug may be potentially inappropriate for use in geriatric patients (Quality of evidence - moderate; Strength of recommendation - strong).

International issues:

Diclofenac may be confused with Duphalac brand name for lactulose [multiple international markets]

Flexin: Brand name for diclofenac [Argentina], but also the brand name for cyclobenzaprine [Chile] and orphenadrine [Israel]

Flexin [Argentina] may be confused with Floxin brand name for flunarizine [Thailand], norfloxacin [South Africa], and ofloxacin [U.S.]

Related Information

Oral Medications That Should Not Be Crushed or Altered *on page 2476*

Brand Names: US Cambia; Cataflam [DSC]; Voltaren-XR [DSC]; Zipsor; Zorvolex

Brand Names: Canada Apo-Diclo; Apo-Diclo Rapide; Apo-Diclo SR; Cambia; Diclofenac EC; Diclofenac ECT; Diclofenac K; Diclofenac SR; Diclofenac-SR; Dom-Diclofenac; Dom-Diclofenac SR; PMS-Diclofenac; PMS-Diclofenac K; PMS-Diclofenac-SR; PRO-Diclo-Rapide; Sandoz-Diclofenac; Sandoz-Diclofenac Rapide; Sandoz-Diclofenac SR; Teva-Diclofenac; Teva-Diclofenac EC; Teva-Diclofenac K; Teva-Diclofenac SR; Voltaren; Voltaren Rapide; Voltaren SR

Therapeutic Category Analgesic, Non-narcotic; Anti-inflammatory Agent; Nonsteroidal Anti-inflammatory Drug (NSAID), Oral

Generic Availability (US) May be product dependent

Use Oral:

Capsule: Relief of mild to moderate acute pain (FDA approved in ages ≥18 years and adults)

Immediate release tablet: Relief of mild to moderate pain; primary dysmenorrhea; acute and chronic treatment of rheumatoid arthritis and osteoarthritis (all indications: FDA approved in adults); has also been used for juvenile idiopathic arthritis

Delayed release tablet: Acute and chronic treatment of rheumatoid arthritis, osteoarthritis, and ankylosing spondylitis (FDA approved in adults)

Extended release tablet: Chronic treatment of osteoarthritis and rheumatoid arthritis (FDA approved in adults)

Oral solution: Treatment of acute migraine with or without aura (FDA approved in ages ≥18 years and adults)

Medication Guide Available Yes

Pregnancy Risk Factor C (oral, injection)/D (≥30 weeks gestation [oral, injection])

Pregnancy Considerations Adverse events were not observed in the initial animal reproduction studies; therefore, manufacturers classify most dosage forms of diclofenac as pregnancy category C (oral, injection: Category D ≥30 weeks gestation). Diclofenac crosses the placenta and can be detected in fetal tissue and amniotic fluid. NSAID exposure during the first trimester is not strongly associated with congenital malformations; however, cardiovascular anomalies and cleft palate have been observed following NSAID exposure in some studies. The use of a NSAID close to conception may be associated with an increased risk of miscarriage. Nonteratogenic effects have been observed following NSAID administration during the third trimester including: Myocardial degenerative changes, prenatal constriction of the ductus arteriosus, fetal tricuspid regurgitation, failure of the ductus arteriosus to close postnatally; renal dysfunction or failure, oligohydramnios; gastrointestinal bleeding or perforation, increased risk of necrotizing enterocolitis; intracranial bleeding (including intraventricular hemorrhage), platelet dysfunction with resultant bleeding; pulmonary hypertension. Because they may cause premature closure of the ductus arteriosus, use of NSAIDs in pregnancy (particularly late pregnancy) should be avoided. Product labeling for Cambia, Zipsor, and Zorvolex specifically notes that use at ≥30 weeks' gestation should be avoided. Use in the third trimester is contraindicated in the Canadian labeling. The chronic use of NSAIDs in women of reproductive age may be associated with infertility that is reversible upon discontinuation of the medication. A registry is available for pregnant women exposed to autoimmune medications including diclofenac. For additional information contact the Organization of Teratology Information Specialists, OTIS Autoimmune Diseases Study, at 877-311-8972

Breast-Feeding Considerations Low concentrations of diclofenac can be found in breast milk. Breast-feeding is not recommended by most manufacturers. The manufacturers of the injection recommend that caution be exercised when administering diclofenac to breast-feeding women. Use while breast-feeding is contraindicated in Canadian labeling.

Contraindications

Hypersensitivity to diclofenac (eg, anaphylactoid reactions, serious skin reactions) or bovine protein (Zipsor only) or any component of the formulation; patients who have experienced asthma, urticaria, or other allergic-type reactions after taking aspirin or other NSAIDs; treatment of perioperative pain in the setting of CABG surgery; patients with moderate to severe renal impairment in the perioperative period and who are at risk for volume depletion (injection only)

Canadian labeling: Additional contraindications (not in U.S. labeling): Severe uncontrolled heart failure, active gastric/duodenal/peptic ulcer; active GI bleed or perforation; regional ulcer, gastritis, or ulcerative colitis; cerebrovascular bleeding or other bleeding disorders; inflammatory bowel disease; severe hepatic impairment; active hepatic disease; severe renal impairment (CrCl <30 mL/minute) or deteriorating renal disease; known hyperkalemia; patients <16 years of age; breast-feeding; pregnancy (third trimester); use of diclofenac suppository if recent history of bleeding or inflammatory lesions of rectum/anus

Warnings/Precautions **[U.S. Boxed Warning]: NSAIDs are associated with an increased risk of adverse cardiovascular thrombotic events, including MI and stroke.** Risk may increase with dose and duration of use or preexisting cardiovascular risk factors or disease. Carefully evaluate individual cardiovascular risk profiles (eg, hypertension, ischemic heart disease, diabetes, smoking) and consider alternative agents if appropriate) prior to prescribing. May cause new-onset hypertension or worsening of existing hypertension. Monitor blood pressure closely. Use caution with fluid retention. Avoid use in heart failure (ACCF/AHA [Yancy, 2013]). Concurrent administration of ibuprofen, and potentially other nonselective NSAIDs, may interfere with aspirin's cardioprotective effect. **[U.S. Boxed Warning]: Use is contraindicated for treatment of perioperative pain in the setting of coronary artery bypass graft (CABG) surgery.** Risk of MI and stroke may be increased with use following CABG surgery.

NSAID use may compromise existing renal function; dose-dependent decreases in prostaglandin synthesis may result from NSAID use, reducing renal blood flow which may cause renal decompensation. NSAID use may increase the risk for hyperkalemia (Canadian labeling contraindicates use with known hyperkalemia). Patients with impaired renal function, dehydration, heart failure, liver dysfunction, those taking diuretics and ACEI, and the elderly are at greater risk of renal toxicity and hyperkalemia. Rehydrate patient before starting therapy; monitor renal function closely. Not recommended for use in patients with advanced renal disease. Injection is not recommended in patients with moderate to severe renal impairment and is contraindicated in patients with moderate to severe renal impairment in the perioperative period and who are at risk for volume depletion. Long-term NSAID use may result in renal papillary necrosis while persistent urinary symptoms (eg, dysuria, bladder pain), cystitis, or hematuria may occur any time after initiating NSAID therapy. Discontinue therapy with symptom onset and evaluate for origin.

[U.S. Boxed Warning]: NSAIDs may increase risk of gastrointestinal irritation, inflammation, ulceration, bleeding, and perforation. These events may occur at any time during therapy and without warning. Use caution with a history of GI disease (bleeding or ulcers), concurrent therapy with aspirin, anticoagulants and/or corticosteroids, smoking, use of alcohol, the elderly or debilitated patients. When used concomitantly with aspirin, a substantial increase in the risk of gastrointestinal complications (eg, ulcer) occurs; concomitant gastroprotective therapy (eg, proton pump inhibitors) is recommended (Bhatt, 2008).

Use the lowest effective dose for the shortest duration of time, consistent with individual patient goals, to reduce risk of cardiovascular or GI adverse events. Alternate therapies should be considered for patients at high risk. Canadian labeling contraindicates use in patients with active gastric/duodenal/peptic ulcer; active GI bleed or perforation; or regional ulcer, gastritis, or ulcerative colitis.

NSAIDs may cause photosensitivity or serious skin adverse events including exfoliative dermatitis, Stevens-Johnson syndrome (SJS), and toxic epidermal necrolysis (TEN); discontinue use at first sign of skin rash or hypersensitivity. Anaphylactoid reactions may occur, even without prior exposure; patients with "aspirin triad" (bronchial asthma, aspirin intolerance, rhinitis) may be at increased risk. Do not use in patients who experience bronchospasm, asthma, rhinitis, or urticaria with NSAID or aspirin therapy. Use caution in other forms of asthma. Platelet adhesion and aggregation may be decreased; may prolong bleeding time; patients with coagulation disorders or who are receiving anticoagulants should be monitored closely. Anemia may occur; patients on long-term NSAID therapy should be monitored for anemia. Rarely, NSAID use may cause severe blood dyscrasias (eg, agranulocytosis, aplastic anemia, thrombocytopenia).

Use with caution in patients with impaired hepatic function (Canadian labeling contraindicates use in severe hepatic impairment or active hepatic disease). Closely monitor patients with any abnormal LFT. Transaminase elevations have been observed with use, generally within the first 2 months of therapy, but may occur at any time. Risk may be higher with diclofenac than other NSAIDS (Laine, 2009; Rostom, 2005). Significant elevations in transaminases (eg, >3 x ULN) occur before patients become symptomatic; initiate monitoring 4 to 8 weeks into therapy. Rarely, severe hepatic reactions (eg, fulminant hepatitis, liver failure) have occurred; discontinue all formulations if signs or symptoms of liver disease develop, or if systemic manifestations occur. Use with caution in hepatic porphyria (may trigger attack; Jose, 2008).

NSAIDS may cause drowsiness, dizziness, blurred vision, and other neurologic effects which may impair physical or mental abilities; patients must be cautioned about performing tasks which require mental alertness (eg, operating machinery or driving). Discontinue use with blurred or diminished vision and perform ophthalmologic exam. Monitor vision with long-term therapy. May increase the risk of aseptic meningitis, especially in patients with systemic lupus erythematosus (SLE) and mixed connective tissue disorders. In the elderly, avoid chronic use (unless alternative agents ineffective and patient can receive concomitant gastroprotective agent); nonselective oral NSAID use is associated with an increased risk of GI bleeding and peptic ulcer disease in older adults in high risk category (eg, >75 years or age or receiving concomitant oral/parenteral corticosteroids, anticoagulants, or antiplatelet agents) (Beers Criteria).

Withhold for at least 4 to 6 half-lives prior to surgical or dental procedures.

Different formulations of oral diclofenac are not bioequivalent, even if the milligram strength is the same; do not interchange products. Zipsor (capsule) contains gelatin; use is contraindicated in patients with history of hypersensitivity to bovine protein. Oral solution is only indicated for the acute treatment of migraine; not indicated for migraine prophylaxis or cluster headache; contains phenylalanine. Injection is not indicated for long-term use.

Adverse Reactions

Injection:

Cardiovascular: Cerebrovascular accident, edema, hypertension, myocardial infarction, significant cardiovascular event

Central nervous system: Dizziness, headache

Dermatologic: Exfoliative dermatitis, pruritus, skin rash, Stevens-Johnson syndrome, toxic epidermal necrolysis

Endocrine & metabolic: Fluid retention

Gastrointestinal: Abdominal pain, constipation, diarrhea, dyspepsia, esophageal perforation, flatulence,

gastrointestinal ulcer (including gastric/duodenal), heartburn, intestinal perforation, nausea, vomiting
Hematologic & oncologic: Anemia, hemorrhage, prolonged bleeding time
Hepatic: Increased liver enzymes, increased serum ALT, increased serum AST, increased serum transaminases
Hypersensitivity: Anaphylactoid reaction
Local: Extravasation, infusion site reaction
Otic: Tinnitus
Renal: Renal insufficiency
Miscellaneous: Gastrointestinal inflammation, wound healing impairment
Rare but important or life-threatening: Abnormal Dreams, agranulocytosis, alopecia, anaphylaxis, angioedema, anxiety, aplastic anemia, asthma, auditory impairment, blurred vision, cardiac arrhythmia, change in appetite, colitis, coma, confusion, congestive heart failure, conjunctivitis, convulsions, cystitis, depression, diaphoresis, drowsiness, dyspnea, dysuria, ecchymoses, eosinophilia, eructation, erythema multiforme, esophagitis, exfoliative dermatitis, fever, fulminant hepatitis, gastritis, gastrointestinal hemorrhage, glossitis, hallucination, hematemesis, hematuria, hemolytic anemia, hepatic failure, hepatic necrosis, hepatitis, hepatotoxicity, hyperglycemia, hypertension, hypotension, infection, insomnia, interstitial nephritis, jaundice, leukopenia, lymphadenopathy, malaise, melena, meningitis, nervousness, oliguria, palpitations, pancreatitis, pancytopenia, paresthesia, pneumonia, polyuria, proteinuria, purpura, rectal hemorrhage, renal failure, respiratory depression, sepsis, skin photosensitivity, stomatitis, syncope, tachycardia, thrombocytopenia, toxic epidermal necrolysis, tremor, urticaria, vasculitis, vertigo, weakness, weight changes

Oral:
Cardiovascular: Edema, hypertension
Central nervous system: Dizziness, falling, headache, procedural pain
Dermatologic: Pruritus, skin rash
Gastrointestinal: Abdominal discomfort, abdominal pain, constipation, diarrhea, duodenal ulcer, dyspepsia, flatulence, GI adverse effects (gastric ulcer, hemorrhage, and perforation; risk increases with therapy duration), heartburn, nausea, vomiting
Genitourinary: Urinary tract infection
Hematologic & oncologic: Anemia, bruise, prolonged bleeding time
Hepatic: Increased serum ALT, increased serum AST, increased serum transaminases
Neuromuscular & skeletal: Arthralgia, back pain, limb pain, osteoarthritis
Otic: Tinnitus
Renal: Renal function abnormality
Respiratory: Bronchitis, cough, nasopharyngitis, sinusitis, upper respiratory tract infection
Rare but important or life-threatening: Agranulocytosis, alopecia, anaphylactoid reaction, aplastic anemia, aseptic meningitis, asthma, cardiac arrhythmia, cardiac failure, cerebrovascular accident, colitis, coma, conjunctivitis, cystitis, decreased hemoglobin, depression, diplopia, eosinophilia, erythema multiforme, esophageal ulcer, esophagitis, gastritis, hearing loss, hemolytic anemia, hepatic failure, hepatitis, hyperglycemia, hypotension, interstitial nephritis, intestinal perforation, lymphadenopathy, memory impairment, meningitis, myocardial infarction, pancreatitis, pancytopenia, peptic ulcer, pneumonia, psychotic reaction, purpura, rectal hemorrhage, renal failure, respiratory depression, seizure, sepsis, skin photosensitivity, Stevens-Johnson syndrome, tachycardia, toxic epidermal necrolysis, vasculitis

Rectal suppository [Canadian product]:
Also refer to adverse reactions associated with oral formulations.
Rare but important or life-threatening: Local hemorrhage, hemorrhoids (exacerbation), proctitis

Drug Interactions

Metabolism/Transport Effects Substrate of CYP1A2 (minor), CYP2B6 (minor), CYP2C19 (minor), CYP2C8 (minor), CYP2C9 (minor), CYP2D6 (minor), CYP3A4 (minor); **Note:** Assignment of Major/Minor substrate status based on clinically relevant drug interaction potential; **Inhibits** CYP1A2 (weak), CYP2C9 (weak), CYP2E1 (weak), UGT1A6

Avoid Concomitant Use

Avoid concomitant use of Diclofenac (Systemic) with any of the following: Dexketoprofen; Floctafenine; Ketorolac (Nasal); Ketorolac (Systemic); Morniflumate; NSAID (COX-2 Inhibitor); Omacetaxine; Urokinase

Increased Effect/Toxicity

Diclofenac (Systemic) may increase the levels/effects of: 5-ASA Derivatives; Agents with Antiplatelet Properties; Aliskiren; Aminoglycosides; Anticoagulants; Apixaban; Bisphosphonate Derivatives; Collagenase (Systemic); CycloSPORINE (Systemic); Dabigatran Etexilate; Deferasirox; Deferiprone; Deoxycholic Acid; Desmopressin; Digoxin; Drospirenone; Eplerenone; Haloperidol; Ibritumomab; Lithium; Methotrexate; Nonsteroidal Anti-Inflammatory Agents; NSAID (COX-2 Inhibitor); Obinutuzumab; Omacetaxine; PEMEtrexed; Porfimer; Potassium-Sparing Diuretics; PRALAtrexate; Quinolone Antibiotics; Rivaroxaban; Salicylates; Tacrolimus (Systemic); Tenofovir; Thrombolytic Agents; TiZANidine; Tositumomab and Iodine I 131 Tositumomab; Urokinase; Vancomycin; Verteporfin; Vitamin K Antagonists

The levels/effects of Diclofenac (Systemic) may be increased by: ACE Inhibitors; Angiotensin II Receptor Blockers; Antidepressants (Tricyclic, Tertiary Amine); Corticosteroids (Systemic); CycloSPORINE (Systemic); CYP2C9 Inhibitors (Strong); Dasatinib; Dexketoprofen; Floctafenine; Glucosamine; Herbs (Anticoagulant/Antiplatelet Properties); Ibrutinib; Ketorolac (Nasal); Ketorolac (Systemic); Limaprost; Morniflumate; Multivitamins/Fluoride (with ADE); Multivitamins/Minerals (with ADEK, Folate, Iron); Multivitamins/Minerals (with AE, No Iron); Omega-3 Fatty Acids; Pentosan Polysulfate Sodium; Pentoxifylline; Probenecid; Prostacyclin Analogues; Selective Serotonin Reuptake Inhibitors; Serotonin/Norepinephrine Reuptake Inhibitors; Sodium Phosphates; Tipranavir; Treprostinil; Vitamin E; Voriconazole

Decreased Effect

Diclofenac (Systemic) may decrease the levels/effects of: ACE Inhibitors; Aliskiren; Angiotensin II Receptor Blockers; Beta-Blockers; Eplerenone; HydrALAZINE; Loop Diuretics; Potassium-Sparing Diuretics; Prostaglandins (Ophthalmic); Salicylates; Selective Serotonin Reuptake Inhibitors; Thiazide Diuretics

The levels/effects of Diclofenac (Systemic) may be decreased by: Bile Acid Sequestrants; CYP2C9 Inducers (Strong); Salicylates

Storage/Stability
Capsule, powder for oral solution: Store at 25°C (77°F); excursions permitted to 15°C to 30°C (59°F to 86°F). Protect from moisture.
Injection: Store at 20°C to 25°C (68°F to 77°F). Do not freeze. Protect from light.
Suppository [Canadian product]: Store at 15°C to 30°C (59°F to 86°F); protect from heat.
Tablet: Store immediate-release and ER tablets below 30°C (86°F); store delayed-release tablets at 20°C to 25°C (68°F to 77°F). Protect from moisture.

Mechanism of Action Reversibly inhibits cyclooxygenase-1 and 2 (COX-1 and 2) enzymes, which results in decreased formation of prostaglandin precursors; has antipyretic, analgesic, and anti-inflammatory properties

Other proposed mechanisms not fully elucidated (and possibly contributing to the anti-inflammatory effect to varying degrees), include inhibiting chemotaxis, altering lymphocyte activity, inhibiting neutrophil aggregation/activation, and decreasing proinflammatory cytokine levels.

Pharmacokinetics (Adult data unless noted)

Distribution: V_d: 1.4 L/kg

Protein binding: >99%

Metabolism: Hepatic; undergoes first-pass metabolism; in the liver, undergoes hydroxylation then glucuronide and sulfate conjugation

Bioavailability: 50%

Half-life: 2.3 hours

Time to peak serum concentration:

Cambia™: 0.25 hours

Cataflam®: 1 hour

Voltaren®: 2.22 hours

Voltaren®-XR: 5.25 hours

Elimination: About 65% of the dose is eliminated in the urine and ~35% in the bile (primarily as conjugated forms); little or no unchanged drug is excreted in urine or bile

Dosing: Usual Note: Different oral formulations are not bioequivalent; do not interchange products.

Children and Adolescents <18 years: **Juvenile idiopathic arthritis:** Limited data available: Oral: Immediate release tablet: 2-3 mg/kg/day divided 2-4 times/day; maximum daily dose: 200 mg/**day** (Haapasaari, 1983; Hashkes, 2005)

Adolescents ≥18 years and Adults:

Analgesia: Oral:

Immediate release capsule: 25 mg 4 times/day

Immediate release tablet: Adults: Initial: 50 mg 3 times/day [maximum dose: 150 mg/day; may administer 100 mg loading dose, followed by 50 mg every 8 hours; initial maximum daily dose (day 1): 200 mg/day; maximum dose day 2 and thereafter: 150 mg/day]

Ankylosing spondylitis: Adults: Oral: Delayed release tablet: 100-125 mg/day in 4-5 divided doses

Migraine: Oral: Oral solution: 50 mg (one packet) as a single dose at the time of migraine onset; safety and efficacy of a second dose have not been established

Osteoarthritis: Adults: Oral:

Immediate release tablet: 150-200 mg/day in 3-4 divided doses

Delayed release tablet: 150-200 mg/day in 2-4 divided doses

Extended release tablet: 100 mg/day; may increase dose to 200 mg/day in 2 divided doses

Primary dysmenorrhea: Adults: Oral: Immediate release tablet: Initial: 50 mg 3 times/day (maximum dose: 150 mg/day); may administer 100 mg loading dose, followed by 50 mg every 8 hours

Rheumatoid arthritis: Adults: Oral:

Immediate release tablet: 150-200 mg/day in 3-4 divided doses

Delayed release tablet: 150-200 mg/day in 2-4 divided doses

Extended release tablet: 100 mg/day; may increase dose to 200 mg/day in 2 divided doses

Dosing adjustment in renal impairment: Not recommended in patients with advanced renal disease or significant renal impairment.

Dosing adjustment in hepatic impairment: May require dosage adjustment; use oral solution only if benefits outweigh risks.

Preparation for Administration Oral solution: Empty contents of packet into 1-2 ounces (30-60 mL) of water (do not use other liquids); mix well and administer immediately.

Administration Administer with milk or food to decrease GI upset; take with full glass of water to enhance absorption.

Delayed or extended release dosage form: Do not chew or crush delayed release or extended release tablets, swallow whole.

Oral solution: Empty contents of packet into 1-2 ounces (30-60 mL) of water (do not use other liquids); mix well and administer right away. Food may reduce effectiveness.

Monitoring Parameters CBC, liver enzymes (periodically during chronic therapy starting 4-8 weeks after initiation); monitor urine output, BUN, serum creatinine in patients receiving diuretics

Additional Information Diclofenac potassium = Cataflam®; potassium content: 5.8 mg (0.15 mEq) per 50 mg tablet

Product Availability

Dyloject injection: FDA approved December 2014; anticipated availability is currently unknown.

Dyloject is indicated as monotherapy for the management of mild to severe pain or in combination with opioid analgesics for the management of moderate to severe pain.

Dosage Forms Excipient information presented when available (limited, particularly for generics); consult specific product labeling. [DSC] = Discontinued product

Capsule, Oral, as base:

Zorvolex: 18 mg, 35 mg [contains brilliant blue fcf (fd&c blue #1), fd&c blue #2 (indigotine)]

Capsule, Oral, as potassium:

Zipsor: 25 mg [contains gelatin (bovine)]

Packet, Oral, as potassium:

Cambia: 50 mg (1 ea, 9 ea) [contains aspartame, saccharin sodium; anise-mint flavor]

Tablet, Oral, as potassium:

Cataflam: 50 mg [DSC]

Generic: 50 mg

Tablet Delayed Release, Oral, as sodium:

Generic: 25 mg, 50 mg, 75 mg

Tablet Extended Release 24 Hour, Oral, as sodium:

Voltaren-XR: 100 mg [DSC]

Generic: 100 mg

- **Diclofenac EC (Can)** *see* Diclofenac (Systemic) *on page 641*
- **Diclofenac ECT (Can)** *see* Diclofenac (Systemic) *on page 641*
- **Diclofenac K (Can)** *see* Diclofenac (Systemic) *on page 641*
- **Diclofenac Potassium** *see* Diclofenac (Systemic) *on page 641*
- **Diclofenac Sodium** *see* Diclofenac (Systemic) *on page 641*
- **Diclofenac SR (Can)** *see* Diclofenac (Systemic) *on page 641*

Dicloxacillin (dye kloks a SIL in)

Therapeutic Category Antibiotic, Penicillin (Antistaphylococcal)

Generic Availability (US) Yes

Use Treatment of skin and soft tissue infections, pneumonia and follow-up therapy of osteomyelitis caused by susceptible penicillinase-producing staphylococci

Pregnancy Risk Factor B

Pregnancy Considerations Adverse events have not been observed in animal reproduction studies. Dicloxacillin crosses the placenta (Depp 1970). Maternal use of penicillins has generally not resulted in an increased risk of birth defects.

Breast-Feeding Considerations Small amounts of dicloxacillin can be detected in breast milk (Matsuda 1984). The manufacturer recommends that caution be exercised when administering dicloxacillin to nursing women. Dicloxacillin has been recommended to treat mastitis in lactating women (Amir 2014).

Contraindications Hypersensitivity to dicloxacillin, penicillin, or any component of the formulation

Warnings/Precautions Monitor PT if patient concurrently on warfarin. Use with caution in neonates; elimination of drug is slow. Serious and occasionally severe or fatal hypersensitivity (anaphylactoid) reactions have been reported in patients on penicillin therapy, especially with a history of beta-lactam hypersensitivity, history of sensitivity to multiple allergens, or previous IgE-mediated reactions (eg, anaphylaxis, angioedema, urticaria). Use with caution in asthmatic patients. Prolonged use may result in fungal or bacterial superinfection, including *C. difficile*-associated diarrhea and pseudomembranous colitis.

Adverse Reactions

Gastrointestinal: Abdominal pain, diarrhea, nausea

Rare but important or life-threatening: Agranulocytosis, eosinophilia, hemolytic anemia, hepatotoxicity, hypersensitivity, interstitial nephritis, leukopenia, neutropenia, prolonged PT, pseudomembranous colitis, rash (maculopapular to exfoliative), seizure with extremely high doses and/or renal failure, serum sickness-like reactions, thrombocytopenia, vaginitis, vomiting

Drug Interactions

Metabolism/Transport Effects **Induces** CYP3A4 (weak)

Avoid Concomitant Use

Avoid concomitant use of Dicloxacillin with any of the following: BCG; BCG (Intravesical); Probenecid

Increased Effect/Toxicity

Dicloxacillin may increase the levels/effects of: Methotrexate

The levels/effects of Dicloxacillin may be increased by: Probenecid

Decreased Effect

Dicloxacillin may decrease the levels/effects of: ARIPiprazole; BCG; BCG (Intravesical); BCG Vaccine (Immunization); Hydrocodone; Mycophenolate; NiMODipine; Saxagliptin; Sodium Picosulfate; Typhoid Vaccine; Vitamin K Antagonists

The levels/effects of Dicloxacillin may be decreased by: Tetracycline Derivatives

Food Interactions Food decreases drug absorption rate and serum concentration. Management: Administer around-the-clock on an empty stomach with a large glass of water 1 hour before or 2 hours after meals.

Mechanism of Action Inhibits bacterial cell wall synthesis by binding to one or more of the penicillin-binding proteins (PBPs) which in turn inhibits the final transpeptidation step of peptidoglycan synthesis in bacterial cell walls, thus inhibiting cell wall biosynthesis. Bacteria eventually lyse due to ongoing activity of cell wall autolytic enzymes (autolysins and murein hydrolases) while cell wall assembly is arrested.

Pharmacokinetics (Adult data unless noted)

Absorption: 35% to 76% absorbed from the GI tract

Distribution: Into bone, bile, pleural fluid, synovial fluid, and amniotic fluid; appears in breast milk

Protein binding: 96% to 98%

Half-life: Adults: 0.6-0.8 hours; slightly prolonged in patients with renal impairment

Time to peak serum concentration: Within 0.5-2 hours

Elimination: Partially eliminated by the liver and excreted in bile; 31% to 65% eliminated in urine as unchanged drug and active metabolite

Neonates: Prolonged

CF patients: More rapid elimination than healthy patients

Dialysis: Not dialyzable (0% to 5%)

Dosing: Usual Oral:

Children <40 kg: 25-50 mg/kg/day divided every 6 hours; doses of 50-100 mg/kg/day in divided doses every 6 hours have been used for follow-up therapy of osteomyelitis; maximum dose: 2 g/day

Children >40 kg and Adults: 125-500 mg every 6 hours; maximum dose: 2 g/day

Administration Oral: Administer with water 1 hour before or 2 hours after meals on an empty stomach

Monitoring Parameters Periodic monitoring of CBC, platelet count, BUN, serum creatinine, urinalysis, and liver enzymes during prolonged therapy

Test Interactions False-positive urine and serum proteins; false-positive in uric acid, urinary steroids; may interfere with urinary glucose tests using cupric sulfate (Benedict's solution, Clinitest®); may inactivate aminoglycosides *in vitro*

Additional Information Sodium content of 250 mg capsule: 0.6 mEq

Dosage Forms Excipient information presented when available (limited, particularly for generics); consult specific product labeling.

Capsule, Oral:

Generic: 250 mg, 500 mg

◆ **Dicloxacillin Sodium** *see* Dicloxacillin *on page 644*

◆ **Dicopanol FusePaq** *see* DiphenhydrAMINE (Systemic) *on page 668*

Dicyclomine (dye SYE kloe meen)

Medication Safety Issues

Sound-alike/look-alike issues:

Dicyclomine may be confused with diphenhydrAMINE, doxycycline, dyclonine

Bentyl may be confused with Aventyl, Benadryl, Bontril, Cantil, Proventil, TRENtal

BEERS Criteria medication:

This drug may be potentially inappropriate for use in geriatric patients (Quality of evidence - moderate; Strength of recommendation - strong).

Brand Names: US Bentyl

Brand Names: Canada Bentylol; Dicyclomine Hydrochloride Injection; Formulex; Jamp-Dicyclomine; Protylol; Riva-Dicyclomine

Therapeutic Category Anticholinergic Agent; Antispasmodic Agent, Gastrointestinal

Generic Availability (US) Yes

Use Treatment of functional bowel/irritable bowel syndrome

Pregnancy Risk Factor B

Pregnancy Considerations Adverse events have not been observed in animal reproduction studies. In epidemiologic studies, birth defects were not observed in pregnant women taking doses up to 40 mg daily throughout the first trimester; information has not been located when used in pregnant women at recommended doses (80-160 mg daily). Use for the treatment of irritable bowel syndrome (IBS) is not recommended during pregnancy (Mahadevan, 2006).

Breast-Feeding Considerations Dicyclomine is excreted in breast milk. Due to the potential for serious adverse reactions in the nursing infant, use in nursing women and infants <6 months of age is contraindicated. In addition, anticholinergics may suppress lactation.

Contraindications Obstructive diseases of the GI tract; severe ulcerative colitis; reflux esophagitis; unstable cardiovascular status in acute hemorrhage; obstructive uropathy; glaucoma; myasthenia gravis; breast-feeding; infants <6 months of age

Canadian labeling: Additional contraindications (not in U.S. labeling): Hypersensitivity to dicyclomine or any component of the formulation

Warnings/Precautions Diarrhea may be a sign of incomplete intestinal obstruction, treatment should be discontinued if this occurs. May cause drowsiness and/or blurred vision, which may impair physical or mental abilities; patients must be cautioned about performing tasks which require mental alertness (eg, operating machinery or driving). Effects may be potentiated when used with other sedative drugs or ethanol. Use with caution in patients with hepatic or renal disease, prostatic hyperplasia (known or suspected), mild-moderate ulcerative colitis (use is contraindicated with severe ulcerative colitis), hyperthyroidism, coronary artery disease, tachyarrhythmias, heart failure, hypertension, or autonomic neuropathy. Evaluate tachycardia prior to administration. Avoid long-term use in the elderly due to potent anticholinergic effects and uncertain effectiveness (Beers Criteria).

Heat prostration may occur in the presence of increased environmental temperature; use caution in hot weather and/or exercise. Psychosis and delirium have been reported in patients with an extreme sensitivity to anticholinergic effects or at excessive dosages, such as the elderly or patients with mental illness. Do not use anticholinergic agents in patients with salmonella dysentery; toxic dilatation of intestine and intestinal perforation may occur. Serious respiratory reactions, central nervous symptoms, and deaths have been reported following administration to infants; use in infants <6 months of age is contraindicated). The injectable formulation is for IM administration only; inadvertent IV administration may cause thrombosis/thrombophlebitis and injection site reactions reactions (eg, pain, edema, skin color change, reflex sympathetic dystrophy).

Warnings: Additional Pediatric Considerations Use with caution in children with Down syndrome, spastic paralysis, or brain damage; increased sensitivity to toxic effects compared to adults has been reported.

Adverse Reactions

Central nervous system: Dizziness, drowsiness, nervousness

Gastrointestinal: Nausea, xerostomia

Neuromuscular & skeletal: Weakness

Ophthalmic: Blurred vision

Rare but important or life-threatening: Abdominal distention, abdominal pain, anaphylactic shock, angioedema, confusion, constipation, cycloplegia, decreased lactation, delirium, dermatitis (allergic), dyspepsia, dyspnea, erythema, facial edema, fatigue, hallucination, headache, hypersensitivity, insomnia, malaise, mydriasis, nasal congestion, palpitations, skin rash, syncope, tachyarrhythmia, vomiting

Drug Interactions

Metabolism/Transport Effects None known.

Avoid Concomitant Use

Avoid concomitant use of Dicyclomine with any of the following: Aclidinium; Eluxadoline; Glucagon; Ipratropium (Oral Inhalation); Potassium Chloride; Tiotropium; Umeclidinium

Increased Effect/Toxicity

Dicyclomine may increase the levels/effects of: AbobotulinumtoxinA; Analgesics (Opioid); Anticholinergic Agents; Cannabinoid-Containing Products; Eluxadoline; Glucagon; Mirabegron; OnabotulinumtoxinA; Potassium Chloride; RimabotulinumtoxinB; Thiazide Diuretics; Tiotropium; Topiramate

The levels/effects of Dicyclomine may be increased by: Aclidinium; Ipratropium (Oral Inhalation); Mianserin; Pramlintide; Umeclidinium

Decreased Effect

Dicyclomine may decrease the levels/effects of: Acetylcholinesterase Inhibitors; Itopride; Metoclopramide; Secretin

The levels/effects of Dicyclomine may be decreased by: Acetylcholinesterase Inhibitors

Storage/Stability

Capsule, tablet: Store at room temperature, preferably below 30°C (86°F). Protect tablet from direct sunlight.

Oral solution: Store at 20°C to 25°C (68°F to 77°F); protect from excessive heat.

Solution for injection: Store at room temperature, preferably below 30°C (86°F); protect from freezing.

Mechanism of Action Blocks the action of acetylcholine at parasympathetic sites in smooth muscle, secretory glands and the CNS

Pharmacodynamics

Onset of action: 1-2 hours

Duration: Up to 4 hours

Pharmacokinetics (Adult data unless noted)

Absorption: Oral: Well absorbed

Distribution: V_d: 3.65 L/kg

Bioavailability: 67%

Half-life:

- Initial phase: 1.8 hours
- Terminal phase: 9-10 hours

Time to peak serum concentration: Oral: 1-1.5 hours

Elimination: 80% in urine; 10% in feces

Dosing: Usual

Infants >6 months: Oral: 5 mg/dose 3-4 times/day

Children: Oral: 10 mg/dose 3-4 times/day

Adults:

- Oral: Initial: 20 mg 4 times/day, then increase up to 40 mg 4 times/day
- IM: 20 mg/dose 4 times/day; oral therapy should replace IM therapy as soon as possible

Administration

Oral: Administer 30 minutes before eating

Parenteral: IM only; not for IV use

Dosage Forms Excipient information presented when available (limited, particularly for generics); consult specific product labeling.

Capsule, Oral, as hydrochloride:

- Bentyl: 10 mg [contains brilliant blue fcf (fd&c blue #1), fd&c red #40]
- Generic: 10 mg

Solution, Intramuscular, as hydrochloride:

- Bentyl: 10 mg/mL (2 mL) [pyrogen free]

Solution, Oral, as hydrochloride:

- Generic: 10 mg/5 mL (473 mL)

Tablet, Oral, as hydrochloride:

- Bentyl: 20 mg
- Generic: 20 mg

◆ **Dicyclomine Hydrochloride** *see* Dicyclomine *on page 645*

◆ **Dicyclomine Hydrochloride Injection (Can)** *see* Dicyclomine *on page 645*

◆ **Dicycloverine Hydrochloride** *see* Dicyclomine *on page 645*

Didanosine (dye DAN oh seen)

Medication Safety Issues

Sound-alike/look-alike issues:

Videx may be confused with Bidex, Lidex

High alert medication:

This medication is in a class the Institute for Safe Medication Practices (ISMP) includes among its list of drug classes that have a heightened risk of causing significant patient harm when used in error.

Related Information

Adult and Adolescent HIV *on page 2392*

Oral Medications That Should Not Be Crushed or Altered *on page 2476*

Pediatric HIV *on page 2380*

Perinatal HIV *on page 2400*

Brand Names: US Videx; Videx EC

Brand Names: Canada Videx; Videx EC

Therapeutic Category Antiretroviral Agent; HIV Agents (Anti-HIV Agents); Nucleoside Reverse Transcriptase Inhibitor (NRTI)

Generic Availability (US) May be product dependent

Use Treatment of HIV infection in combination with other antiretroviral agents (Oral solution: FDA approved in ages ≥2 weeks and adults; Delayed release capsule: FDA approved in ages ≥6 years weighing ≥20 kg and adults); **Note:** HIV regimens consisting of **three** antiretroviral agents are strongly recommended

Medication Guide Available Yes

Pregnancy Risk Factor B

Pregnancy Considerations Adverse events have not been observed in animal reproduction studies. Didanosine has a low to moderate level of transfer across the human placenta. Based on data from the Antiretroviral Pregnancy Registry, an increased rate of birth defects has been observed following maternal use of didanosine during the first trimester and later during pregnancy; no pattern of defects has been observed and clinical relevance is uncertain. Pharmacokinetics are not significantly altered during pregnancy; dose adjustments are not needed. Cases of lactic acidosis/hepatic steatosis syndrome related to mitochondrial toxicity have been reported in pregnant women with prolonged use of nucleoside analogues. It is not known if pregnancy itself potentiates this known side effect; however, women may be at increased risk of lactic acidosis and liver damage. In addition, these adverse events are similar to other rare but life-threatening syndromes which occur during pregnancy (eg, HELLP syndrome). Hepatic enzymes and electrolytes should be monitored in women receiving nucleoside analogues and clinicians should watch for early signs of the syndrome. In addition, mitochondrial dysfunction may develop in infants following in utero exposure. Due to the reports of lactic acidosis, maternal, and neonatal mortality, didanosine and stavudine should not be used in combination during pregnancy. The DHHS Perinatal HIV Guidelines recommend didanosine to be used only in special circumstances during pregnancy; not recommended for initial therapy in antiretroviral-naïve pregnant women due to toxicity (HHS [perinatal], 2014).

Regardless of CD4 count or HIV RNA copy number, all HIV-infected pregnant women should receive a combination antiretroviral (ARV) drug regimen. A combination of antepartum, intrapartum, and infant ARV prophylaxis is recommended. ARV therapy should be started as soon as possible in women with symptomatic infection. Although earlier initiation may be more effective in reducing the perinatal transmission of HIV, initiation may be delayed until after 12 weeks gestation in women who do not require immediate treatment after careful consideration of maternal conditions (eg, nausea and vomiting) and the potential risks of first trimester fetal exposure for specific agents. A scheduled cesarean delivery at 38 weeks gestation is recommended for all women with HIV RNA >1000 copies/mL or unknown concentrations near delivery in order to decrease transmission. If ARV therapy must be interrupted for <24 hours during the peripartum period, stop then restart all medications simultaneously in order to decrease the chance of developing resistance. Long-term follow-up is recommended for all infants exposed to ARV medications. In couples who want to conceive, the HIV-infected partner should attain maximum viral suppression prior to conception.

Healthcare providers are encouraged to enroll pregnant women exposed to antiretroviral medications in the Antiretroviral Pregnancy Registry (1-800-258-4263 or www.APRegistry.com). Health care providers caring for HIV-infected women and their infants may contact the National Perinatal HIV Hotline (888-448-8765) for clinical consultation (HHS [perinatal], 2014).

Breast-Feeding Considerations Maternal or infant antiretroviral therapy does not completely eliminate the risk of postnatal HIV transmission. In addition, multiclass-resistant virus has been detected in breast-feeding infants despite maternal therapy. Therefore, in the United States, where formula is accessible, affordable, safe, and sustainable, and the risk of infant mortality due to diarrhea and respiratory infections is low, complete avoidance of breast-feeding by HIV-infected women is recommended to decrease potential transmission of HIV (HHS [perinatal], 2014).

Contraindications Coadministration with allopurinol or ribavirin

Warnings/Precautions [U.S. Boxed Warning]: Pancreatitis (fatal and nonfatal) has been reported alone or in combination regimens in both treatment-naïve and treatment-experienced patients, regardless of degree of immunosuppression. Suspend use in patients with suspected pancreatitis and discontinue in patients with confirmed pancreatitis; frequency is dose related. In patients with risk factors for pancreatitis, use with extreme caution and only if clearly indicated. Patients with advanced HIV-1 infection, especially the elderly, are at increased risk and should be followed closely. Patients with renal impairment may be at greater risk for pancreatitis if treated without dose adjustment. **[U.S. Boxed Warning]: Lactic acidosis, symptomatic hyperlactatemia, and severe hepatomegaly with steatosis (sometimes fatal) have occurred alone or in combination, including didanosine and other antiretrovirals.** Risk may be increased with female gender, obesity, or prolonged exposure. Fatal lactic acidosis has been reported in pregnant women who received the combination of didanosine and stavudine with other antiretroviral agents. The combination of didanosine and stavudine should be used with caution during pregnancy and is recommended only if the potential benefit clearly outweighs the potential risk. Use caution when administering to patients with known risk factors for liver disease. Hepatotoxicity may occur even in the absence of marked transaminase elevations; suspend therapy in any patient developing clinical/laboratory findings which suggest hepatotoxicity. Hepatotoxicity and hepatic failure (including fatal cases) have been reported in HIV patients receiving combination drug therapy with didanosine and stavudine or hydroxyurea, or didanosine, stavudine, and hydroxyurea; avoid these combinations. Not currently recommended in combination with tenofovir due to failure and resistance. Noncirrhotic portal hypertension may develop within months to years of starting didanosine therapy. Signs may include elevated liver enzymes, esophageal varices, hematemesis, ascites, and splenomegaly. Noncirrhotic portal hypertension may lead to liver failure and/or death. Discontinue use in patients with evidence of this condition. Pregnant women may be at increased risk of lactic acidosis and liver damage. Use with caution in patients with hepatic impairment; safety and efficacy have not been established in patients with significant hepatic disease. Patients on combination antiretroviral therapy with hepatic impairment may be at increased risk of potentially severe and fatal hepatic toxicity; consider interruption or discontinuation of therapy if hepatic impairment worsens.

Peripheral neuropathy (numbness, tingling or pain in the hands or feet) has been reported, more frequently in patients with advanced HIV disease, in patients with a history of neuropathy or in patients being treated with a neurotoxic drug (eg, stavudine). Discontinue therapy if neuropathy occurs. Retinal changes (including retinal depigmentation) and optic neuritis have been reported in adults and children using didanosine. Patients should undergo retinal examination periodically. Potentially significant interactions may exist, requiring dose or frequency adjustment, additional monitoring, and/or selection of alternative therapy. Use caution in renal impairment; dose reduction recommended for CrCl <60 mL/minute. May cause redistribution of fat (eg, buffalo hump, peripheral wasting with increased abdominal girth, cushingoid appearance). Patients may develop immune reconstitution syndrome resulting in the occurrence of an inflammatory response to an indolent or residual opportunistic infection during initial HIV treatment or activation of autoimmune disorders (eg, Graves' disease, polymyositis, Guillain-Barré syndrome) later in therapy; further evaluation and treatment may be required. Dosing recommendations for didanosine powder for oral solution in patients younger than 2 weeks cannot be made because the pharmacokinetics of didanosine in these infants are too variable to determine an appropriate dose. Delayed-release capsules may be used in pediatric patients who weigh at least 20 kg. Didanosine delayed-release capsules are indicated for once-daily use; didanosine powder for oral solution is recommended for use in a twice daily regimen.

Warnings: Additional Pediatric Considerations Fatal and nonfatal pancreatitis is more common in adults than children (1% to 7% vs 3% [normal doses]). Retinal depigmentation in children receiving doses >300 mg/m^2/day may occur; retinal changes and optic neuritis have been reported in pediatric and adult patients; perform periodic retinal examinations. Due to an increased risk of serious toxicities, the combined use of stavudine and didanosine is not recommended for use in adults and adolescents (DHHS [adult], 2014) and is not recommended as part of an initial antiretroviral regimen in pediatric patients; however, it may be considered for use in pediatric regimens if the potential benefit clearly outweighs the risks (DHHS [pediatric], 2014).

Adverse Reactions As reported in monotherapy studies; risk of toxicity may increase when combined with other agent.

Dermatologic: Pruritus, rash

Endocrine & metabolic: Uric acid increased

Gastrointestinal: Abdominal pain, amylase increased, diarrhea, pancreatitis (patients >65 years of age had a higher frequency of pancreatitis than younger patients)

Hepatic: Alkaline phosphatase increased, ALT increased, AST increased

Neuromuscular & skeletal: Peripheral neuropathy

Rare but important or life-threatening: Acute renal impairment, alopecia, anaphylactoid reaction, anemia, anorexia, arthralgia, chills/fever, diabetes mellitus, dry eyes, dyspepsia, flatulence, granulocytopenia, hepatic steatosis, hepatitis, hyper-/hypoglycemia, hyperlactatemia (symptomatic), hypersensitivity, immune reconstitution syndrome, lactic acidosis/hepatomegaly, leukopenia, lipodystrophy, liver failure, myalgia, myopathy, optic neuritis, pain, parotid gland enlargement, portal hypertension (noncirrhotic), retinal depigmentation, rhabdomyolysis, sialoadenitis, Stevens-Johnson syndrome, thrombocytopenia, weakness, xerostomia

Drug Interactions

Metabolism/Transport Effects None known.

Avoid Concomitant Use

Avoid concomitant use of Didanosine with any of the following: Alcohol (Ethyl); Allopurinol; Febuxostat; Hydroxyurea; Ribavirin; Tenofovir

Increased Effect/Toxicity

Didanosine may increase the levels/effects of: Hydroxyurea

The levels/effects of Didanosine may be increased by: Alcohol (Ethyl); Allopurinol; Febuxostat; Ganciclovir-Valganciclovir; Hydroxyurea; Ribavirin; Stavudine; Tenofovir

Decreased Effect

Didanosine may decrease the levels/effects of: Antifungal Agents (Azole Derivatives, Systemic); Atazanavir; Indinavir; Quinolone Antibiotics; Rilpivirine

The levels/effects of Didanosine may be decreased by: Atazanavir; Darunavir; Lopinavir; Methadone; Quinolone Antibiotics; Rilpivirine; Tenofovir; Tipranavir

Food Interactions Food decreases AUC and C_{max}; serum levels may be decreased by 55%. Management: Administer on an empty stomach at least 30 minutes before or 2 hours after eating depending on dosage form.

Storage/Stability Delayed release capsules should be stored in tightly closed bottles at controlled room temperature of 25°C (77°F). Unreconstituted powder should be stored at 15°C to 30°C (59°F to 86°F); reconstituted oral solution is stable for 30 days stored at 2°C to 8°C (36°F to 46°F).

Mechanism of Action Didanosine, a purine nucleoside (adenosine) analog and the deamination product of dideoxyadenosine (ddA), inhibits HIV replication *in vitro* in both T cells and monocytes. Didanosine is converted within the cell to the mono-, di-, and triphosphates of ddA. These ddA triphosphates act as substrate and inhibitor of HIV reverse transcriptase substrate and inhibitor of HIV reverse transcriptase thereby blocking viral DNA synthesis and suppressing HIV replication.

Pharmacokinetics (Adult data unless noted)

Absorption: Subject to degradation by acidic pH of stomach; some formulations are buffered to resist acidic pH. Delayed release capsules contain enteric-coated beadlets which dissolve in the small intestine.

Distribution: Extensive intracellular distribution

- CSF/plasma ratio:
  - Infants 8 months to Adolescents 19 years: 46% (range: 12% to 85%)
  - Adults: 21%
- V_d (apparent):
  - Age-based:
    - Infants 8 months to Adolescents 19 years: 28 ± 15 L/m^2
    - Adults: 43.7 ± 8.9 L/m^2
  - Weight-based:
    - Children 20 kg to <25 kg: 98 ± 30 L
    - Children 25 kg to <60 kg: 155 ± 55 L
    - Children ≥60 kg: 363 ± 138 L
    - Adults ≥60 kg: 308 ± 164 L

Protein binding: <5%

Metabolism: Converted intracellularly to active triphosphate form; presumed to be metabolized via the same metabolic pathway as endogenous purines

Bioavailability: Variable and affected by the presence of food in the GI tract, gastric pH, and the dosage form administered

- Infants 8 months to Adolescents 19 years: 25% ± 20%
- Adults: 42% ± 12%

Half-life:

- Plasma:
  - Newborns (1 day old): 2 ± 0.7 hours
  - Infants 2 weeks to 4 months: 1.2 ± 0.3 hours
  - Infants 8 months to Adolescents 19 years: 0.8 ± 0.3 hours
  - Adults with normal renal function: 1.5 ± 0.4 hours
- Intracellular: Adults: 25 to 40 hours
- Elimination:
  - Children 20 kg to <25 kg: 0.75 ± 0.13 hours
  - Children 25 kg to <60 kg: 0.92 ± 0.09 hours

Children ≥60 kg: 1.26 ± 0.19 hours
Adults ≥60 kg: 1.19 ± 21 hours
Time to peak serum concentration: Delayed release capsules: 2 hours; Oral solution: 0.25 to 1.5 hours
Elimination: Unchanged drug excreted in urine
Infants 8 months to Adolescents 19 years: 18% ± 10%
Adults: 18% ± 8%

Dosing: Neonatal

HIV infection, treatment: Use in combination with other antiretroviral agents:
PNA <14 days: Dose not established; pharmacokinetic parameters are too variable to determine appropriate dosage
PNA ≥14 days: Oral solution:
AIDS*info* recommendation (DHHS [pediatric], 2014): 50 mg/m^2/dose every 12 hours.
Manufacturer's labeling: 100 mg/m^2/dose every 12 hours. **Note:** Not recommended based on pharmacokinetic data; expert panel members suggest toxicity may occur using this dose in this age group (DHHS [pediatric]; 2014).

Dosing adjustment in renal impairment: Insufficient data exists to recommend a specific dosage adjustment; however, a decrease in the dose should be considered in pediatric patients with renal impairment.

Dosing: Usual

Pediatric: **HIV infection, treatment:** Oral: Use in combination with other antiretroviral agents:
Infants 1 to 8 months: Oral solution:
AIDS*info* recommendation (DHHS [pediatric], 2014):
Infants 1 to <3 months: 50 mg/m^2/dose every 12 hours
Infants ≥3 to 8 months: Oral solution: 100 mg/m^2/dose every 12 hours
Manufacturer's labeling: 100 mg/m^2/dose every 12 hours. **Note:** Based on pharmacokinetic data, expert panel members suggest toxicity may occur using manufacturer dosing in infants <3 months (DHHS [pediatric], 2014).
Infants >8 months and Children:
Oral solution:
Manufacturer's labeling: 120 mg/m^2/dose every 12 hours; do not exceed adult dose; once-daily dosing of the oral solution is not FDA approved in children; limited data is available
AIDS*info* recommendation (DHHS [pediatric], 2014): 120 mg/m^2/dose every 12 hours; maximum dose: 200 mg/dose
Alternate once-daily dosing for treatment-naive children ≥3 years: 240 mg/m^2/dose once daily; maximum dose: 400 mg/dose; may also use the delayed release capsule if calculated dose is appropriate and child is able to swallow a capsule whole
Delayed release capsule: Children ≥6 years and ≥20 kg who are able to swallow a capsule whole:
20 kg to <25 kg: 200 mg once daily
25 kg to <60 kg: 250 mg once daily
≥60 kg: 400 mg once daily
Adolescents:
Oral solution: **Note:** Although once-daily dosing is available, it should only be considered for adolescent/adult patients whose management requires once-daily administration (eg, to enhance compliance); the preferred dosing frequency of didanosine oral solution is twice daily because there is more evidence to support the effectiveness of this dosing frequency:
<60 kg: 125 mg every 12 hours **or** 250 mg once daily
≥60 kg: 200 mg every 12 hours or 400 mg once daily using a special Videx solution in double strength antacid which provides 400 mg/20 mL for once-daily dosing
Delayed release capsule:
20 kg to <25 kg: 200 mg once daily
25 kg to <60 kg: 250 mg once daily
≥60 kg: 400 mg once daily

Adult: **HIV infection, treatment:** Oral:
Dosing based on patient weight:
Pediatric powder for oral solution (Videx):
<60 kg: 125 mg twice daily (preferred) or 250 mg once daily
≥60 kg: 200 mg twice daily (preferred) or 400 mg once daily
Delayed release capsule (Videx EC):
25 kg to <60 kg: 250 mg once daily
≥60 kg: 400 mg once daily
When taken with tenofovir: **Note:** Combined use of tenofovir with didanosine is no longer recommended (DHHS [adult], 2014).
<60 kg and CrCl ≥60 mL/minute: 200 mg once daily
≥60 kg and CrCl ≥60 mL/minute: 250 mg once daily
CrCl <60 mL/minute: Dose has not been established

Dosing adjustment in renal impairment:
Infants and Children: Insufficient data exists to recommend a specific dosage adjustment; however, a decrease in the dose should be considered in pediatric patients with renal impairment. The following guidelines have been used by some clinicians (Aronoff, 2007):
GFR >50 mL/minute/1.73 m^2: No adjustment required
GFR 30 to 50 mL/minute/1.73 m^2: 75 mg/m^2/dose every 12 hours
GFR 10 to 29 mL/minute/1.73 m^2: 90 mg/m^2/dose every 24 hours
GFR <10 mL/minute/1.73 m^2: 75 mg/m^2/dose every 24 hours
Hemodialysis: 75 mg/m^2/dose every 24 hours after dialysis
Peritoneal dialysis: 75 mg/m^2/dose every 24 hours
Continuous renal replacement therapy (CRRT): 75 mg/m^2/dose every 12 hours
Adolescents and Adults: Dosing based on patient weight, creatinine clearance, and dosage form:
Dosing for patients <60 kg:
CrCl ≥60 mL/minute: No dosage adjustment required
CrCl 30 to 59 mL/minute:
Oral solution: 75 mg twice daily or 150 mg once daily
Delayed release capsule: 125 mg once daily
CrCl 10 to 29 mL/minute:
Oral solution: 100 mg once daily
Delayed release capsule: 125 mg once daily
CrCl <10 mL/minute:
Oral solution: 75 mg once daily
Delayed release capsule: Use alternate formulation
Dosing for patients ≥60 kg:
CrCl ≥60 mL/minute: No dosage adjustment required
CrCl 30 to 59 mL/minute:
Oral solution: 100 mg twice daily or 200 mg once daily
Delayed release capsule: 200 mg once daily
CrCl 10 to 29 mL/minute:
Oral solution: 150 mg once daily
Delayed release capsule: 125 mg once daily
CrCl <10 mL/minute:
Oral solution: 100 mg once daily
Delayed release capsule: 125 mg once daily

Dosing adjustment in patients requiring continuous ambulatory peritoneal dialysis (CAPD) or hemodialysis: Adults: Use dosing recommendations for patients with CrCl <10 mL/minute; supplemental doses following hemodialysis are not needed

Dosing adjustment in hepatic impairment: No adjustment recommended; Adults: In a single-dose study, mean AUC and peak serum concentrations of didanosine were 13% and 19% higher, respectively, in adults with moderate to severe hepatic impairment (Child-Pugh

Class B or C). However, a similar range and distribution of AUC and peak concentrations were observed. It is important to monitor patients with hepatic impairment closely for didanosine toxicity. Patients with hepatic impairment may be at increased risk for didanosine toxicities.

Preparation for Administration Oral: Pediatric powder for oral solution: Prior to dispensing, add 100 mL or 200 mL purified water, USP to the 2 g or 4 g container, respectively, to achieve a 20 mg/mL solution. Immediately mix the resulting solution with an equal volume of an antacid that contains the active ingredients aluminum hydroxide (400 mg/5 mL), magnesium hydroxide (400 mg/5 mL), and simethicone (40 mg/5 mL) to achieve a final concentration of 10 mg/mL. Dispense in flint glass or plastic (eg, HDPE, PET, or PETG) bottles with child resistant closures.

Administration Oral: Administer oral solution and delayed release capsule on an empty stomach 30 minutes before or at least 2 hours after a meal. Some experts have recommended giving without regard to meals in order to improve compliance (DHHS [pediatric], 2014). Swallow capsule whole; do not break open or chew. If administered with tenofovir, the delayed release capsule may be administered with a light meal or in the fasted state. Administer didanosine at least 1 hour apart from indinavir. Administer didanosine at least 2 hours apart from ritonavir or atazanavir. Didanosine should be given at least 1 hour before or 2 hours after lopinavir/ritonavir. Nelfinavir should be administered 2 hours before or 1 hour after didanosine. Administer buffered formulations of didanosine at least 1 hour apart from fosamprenavir.

Shake oral solution well before use. Undergoes rapid degradation when exposed to an acidic environment; 10% of the drug decomposes to hypoxanthine in <2 minutes at pH <3 at 37°C.

Monitoring Parameters Note: Monitor CD4 percentage (if <5 years of age) or CD4 count (if ≥5 years of age) at least every 3-4 months (DHHS [pediatric], 2014).

Prior to initiation of therapy: Genotypic resistance testing, CD4 and viral load (every 3 to 4 months), CBC with differential, LFTs, BUN, creatinine, electrolytes, glucose, urinalysis (every 6 to 12 months), and assessment of readiness for adherence with medication regimen. At initiation and with any change in treatment regimen: CBC with differential, electrolytes, calcium, phosphate, glucose, LFTs, bilirubin, urinalysis (at initiation), BUN, creatinine, albumin, total protein, lipid panel (at initiation), CD4, and viral load. After 1 to 2 weeks of therapy: Signs of medication toxicity and adherence. After 2 to 4 weeks of therapy: CBC with differential, viral load, signs of medication toxicity, and adherence; then every 3 to 4 months: CBC with differential, electrolytes, glucose, LFTs, bilirubin, BUN, creatinine, CD4, viral load, signs of medication toxicity, and adherence. Lipid panel and urinalysis every 6 to 12 months. CD4 monitoring frequency may be decreased to every 6 to 12 months in children who are adherent to therapy if the value is well above the threshold for opportunistic infections, viral suppression is sustained, and the clinical status is stable for more than 2 to 3 years (DHHS [pediatric], 2014). Monitor for growth and development, signs of HIV-specific physical conditions, HIV disease progression, opportunistic infections, peripheral neuropathy, pancreatitis, or lactic acidosis

To monitor for portal hypertension: CBC with platelet count, splenomegaly on physical exam, liver enzymes, serum bilirubin, albumin, INR, ultrasound

Additional Information Once daily, didanosine delayed-release capsules have been approved for use in children 6 to 18 years of age who are ≥20 kg. This approval was based on pharmacokinetic studies; however, limited published literature exists. In a single-dose pharmacokinetic study in children 4 to 11.5 years of age (n=10; median age: 7.6 years), a dose of 240 mg/m^2 was shown to have a similar plasma AUC as compared to the buffered formulation. However, two patients were excluded from data analysis, one due to extremely low didanosine serum concentrations throughout the dosing interval (King, 2002). Doses of 240 mg/m^2 once daily, with a maximum of 400 mg once daily, are being studied in pediatric clinical trials. **Note:** In PACTG 1021, treatment-naive children (3 to 21 years of age) received 240 mg/m^2/dose once daily (maximum: 400 mg/dose) with good viral suppression (DHHS [pediatric], 2014). Children with a surface area ≥0.45 m^2 who could swallow capsules received the delayed-release capsule; the oral suspension was used for smaller children (McKinney, 2007).

The relative bioavailability of didanosine suspension administered once daily versus twice daily was studied in 24 children, 4.8 ± 2.9 years of age. Didanosine was administered in doses of 90 mg/m^2/dose every 12 hours and 180 mg/m^2/dose once daily. The relative bioavailability of once-daily dosing compared to twice daily dosing was 0.95 ± 0.49 (range: 0.22 to 1.97). The authors suggest these results support the potential clinical use of once-daily dosing in pediatric patients. However, due to the large inter- and intrasubject variability, these 2 regimens would **not** be considered to be bioequivalent based on FDA criteria (Abreu, 2000).

A high rate of early virologic failure in therapy-naive adult HIV patients has been observed with the once-daily three-drug combination therapy of didanosine enteric-coated beadlets (Videx EC), lamivudine, and tenofovir and the once-daily three-drug combination therapy of abacavir, lamivudine, and tenofovir. These combinations should not be used or offered at any time. Any patient currently receiving either of these regimens should be closely monitored for virologic failure and considered for treatment modification. Early virologic failure was also observed in therapy-naive adult HIV patients treated with tenofovir, didanosine enteric-coated beadlets (Videx EC), and either efavirenz or nevirapine; rapid emergence of resistant mutations has also been reported with this combination; the combination of tenofovir, didanosine, and any non-nucleoside reverse transcriptase inhibitor is **not** recommended as initial antiretroviral therapy. **Note:** Didanosine plus tenofovir is **not** recommended as a component of an initial antiretroviral therapy regimen in pediatric patients and is no longer recommended as part of any antiretroviral regimen in adults and adolescents (DHHS [pediatric, adult], 2014).

One major study found an increased risk of MI in patients receiving didanosine; however, other cohort studies did not find an increased cardiovascular risk (DHHS [adult], 2014).

Dosage Forms Excipient information presented when available (limited, particularly for generics); consult specific product labeling.

Capsule Delayed Release, Oral:
  Videx EC: 125 mg, 200 mg, 250 mg, 400 mg
  Generic: 125 mg, 200 mg, 250 mg, 400 mg
Solution Reconstituted, Oral:
  Videx: 2 g (100 mL); 4 g (200 mL)

- ◆ **Dideoxyinosine** *see* Didanosine *on page* 646
- ◆ **Dietary Fiber Laxative [OTC]** *see* Psyllium *on page* 1804
- ◆ **Differin** *see* Adapalene *on page* 70
- ◆ **Differin® (Can)** *see* Adapalene *on page* 70
- ◆ **Differin® XP (Can)** *see* Adapalene *on page* 70
- ◆ **Diflucan** *see* Fluconazole *on page* 881
- ◆ **Diflucan injection (Can)** *see* Fluconazole *on page* 881

- **Diflucan One (Can)** *see* Fluconazole *on page 881*
- **Diflucan PWS (Can)** *see* Fluconazole *on page 881*
- **Difluorodeoxycytidine Hydrochlorothiazide** *see* Gemcitabine *on page 961*

Difluprednate (dye floo PRED nate)

Medication Safety Issues

Sound-alike/look-alike issues:

Durezol may be confused with Durasal

Brand Names: US Durezol

Therapeutic Category Corticosteroid, Ophthalmic

Generic Availability (US) No

Use Treatment of inflammation and pain following ocular surgery (FDA approved in pediatric patients [age not specified] and adults); treatment of endogenous anterior uveitis (FDA approved in adults)

Pregnancy Risk Factor C

Pregnancy Considerations Adverse events have been observed in animal reproduction studies. The amount of difluprednate absorbed systemically following ophthalmic administration is below the limit of quantification (<50 ng/mL).

Breast-Feeding Considerations It is not known if difluprednate is excreted in breast milk; however, systemic corticosteroids are excreted in breast milk. Because systemic absorption may cause adverse effects, the manufacturer recommends that caution be exercised when administering difluprednate to nursing women.

Contraindications Active viral (including herpes simplex keratitis, vaccinia, varicella) infections of the cornea or conjunctiva, fungal infection of ocular structures, or mycobacterial ocular infections

Warnings/Precautions For ophthalmic use only; not for intraocular administration. Steroids may mask infection or enhance existing ocular infection; prolonged use may result in secondary infections due to immunosuppression. The possibility of corneal fungal infections should be considered with persistent corneal ulceration during prolonged therapy; obtain cultures when appropriate. Use caution in patients with a history of ocular herpes simplex. Re-evaluate after 2 days if symptoms have not improved. Use is contraindicated in most viral diseases of the cornea and conjunctiva. Prolonged use may result in posterior subcapsular cataract formation. Use following cataract surgery may delay healing or increase the incidence of bleb formation. Corneal perforation may occur with topical steroids in diseases which cause thinning of the cornea or sclera. Use with caution in presence of glaucoma. Prolonged use of corticosteroids may result in elevated intraocular pressure (IOP); damage to the optic nerve; and defects in visual acuity and fields of vision. Monitor IOP in any patient receiving treatment for ≥10 days. Initial prescription and renewal of medication for >28 days should be made by healthcare provider only after examination with the aid of magnification such as slit lamp biomicroscopy or fluorescein staining (if appropriate). To avoid contamination, do not touch tip of container to any surface. Contains sorbic acid which may be absorbed by contact lenses; remove contacts prior to administration and wait 10 minutes before reinserting.

Warnings: Additional Pediatric Considerations Pediatric patients may be at increased risk for elevations in intraocular pressure (IOP) when using diflurprednate for uveitis (Birnbaum, 2011; Slabaugh, 2012). In one retrospective review (n=27, age range: 6 to 63 years), four of the five children (80%) treated with diflurprednate had an increase in IOP of ≥5 mm Hg (two had increase ≥20 mm Hg) compared to seven out of 22 adults (32%) (three had increase ≥20 mm Hg). Elevation of IOP responded to discontinuation of difluprednate or the addition of glaucoma medications (Birnbaum, 2011). Another retrospective review of pediatric uveitis patients (n=14, age range: 7 to 18 years) described a higher incidence of cataracts in addition to increased IOP in this patient population (Slabaugh, 2012).

Adverse Reactions

Adverse reactions following ocular surgery:

Ophthalmic: Anterior chamber inflammation, blepharitis, cataract (secondary), conjunctival edema, corneal edema, decreased visual acuity, eye pain, hyperemia (ciliary and conjunctival), iritis, photophobia, postoperative ophthalmic inflammation, punctate keratitis

Rare but important or life-threatening: Abnormal healing, corneal changes (pigmentation and striae), crusting of eyelid, episcleritis, eye perforation, eye pruritus, foreign body sensation of eye, increased intraocular pressure, increased lacrimation, injected sclera, local irritation, macular edema, optic nerve damage, secondary infection, uveitis, viral infection

Adverse reactions associated with treatment of endogenous anterior uveitis:

Central nervous system: Headache

Ophthalmic: Anterior chamber inflammation, blurred vision, corneal edema, decreased visual acuity, dry eye syndrome, eye irritation, eye pain, hyperemia (conjunctival and limbal), increased intraocular pressure, iridocyclitis, iritis, photophobia, punctate keratitis, uveitis

Drug Interactions

Metabolism/Transport Effects None known.

Avoid Concomitant Use There are no known interactions where it is recommended to avoid concomitant use.

Increased Effect/Toxicity

Difluprednate may increase the levels/effects of: Ceritinib

The levels/effects of Difluprednate may be increased by: NSAID (Ophthalmic)

Decreased Effect There are no known significant interactions involving a decrease in effect.

Storage/Stability Store at 15°C to 25°C (59°F to 77°F); do not freeze. Protect from light.

Mechanism of Action Corticosteroids inhibit the inflammatory response including edema, capillary dilation, leukocyte migration, and scar formation. Difluprednate penetrates cells readily to induce the production of lipocortins. These proteins modulate the activity of prostaglandins and leukotrienes.

Pharmacokinetics (Adult data unless noted)

Absorption: Systemic: Exposure to active metabolite is negligible with ocular administration

Metabolism: Undergoes deacetylation to an active metabolite (DFB)

Dosing: Usual

Pediatric:

Endogenous anterior uveitis: Children ≥2 years and Adolescents: Ophthalmic: Limited data available: Instill 1 drop into conjunctival sac of the affected eye(s) 4 times daily for 14 days, then taper as clinically indicated (Sheppard, 2014; Slabaugh, 2012)

Inflammation associated with ocular surgery: Infants, Children, and Adolescents: Ophthalmic: Instill 1 drop in conjunctival sac of the affected eye(s) 4 times daily beginning 24 hours after surgery, continue for 2 weeks, then decrease to 2 times daily for 1 week, then taper based on response

Adult:

Endogenous anterior uveitis: Ophthalmic: Instill 1 drop into conjunctival sac of the affected eye(s) 4 times daily for 14 days, then taper as clinically indicated

Inflammation associated with ocular surgery: Ophthalmic: Instill 1 drop in conjunctival sac of the affected eye(s) 4 times daily beginning 24 hours after surgery, continue for 2 weeks, then decrease to 2 times daily for 1 week, then taper based on response

Dosing adjustment in renal impairment: Infants, Children, Adolescents, and Adults: There are no dosage adjustments provided in manufacturer's labeling; however, dosage adjustment unlikely due to low systemic absorption.

Dosing adjustment in hepatic impairment: Infants, Children, Adolescents, and Adults: There are no dosage adjustments provided in manufacture"s labeling; however, dosage adjustment unlikely due to low systemic absorption.

Administration Wash hands prior to use. Avoid contact of bottle tip with skin or eye; ocular solutions can become contaminated by common bacteria known to cause ocular infections. Serious damage to the eye and subsequent loss of vision may occur from using contaminated solutions. Remove contact lenses prior to administration and wait at least 10 minutes before reinserting soft contact lenses. The use of the same bottle for both eyes is not recommended in surgical patients.

Monitoring Parameters Intraocular pressure in any patient receiving treatment for ≥10 days; periodic examination of lens with prolonged use (>28 days)

Dosage Forms Excipient information presented when available (limited, particularly for generics); consult specific product labeling.

Emulsion, Ophthalmic:

Durezol: 0.05% (5 mL) [contains edetate sodium (tetrasodium), polysorbate 80]

- **Digestive Enzyme** *see* Pancrelipase *on page* *1614*
- **Digibind** *see* Digoxin Immune Fab *on page* *657*
- **DigiFab** *see* Digoxin Immune Fab *on page* *657*
- **Digitalis** *see* Digoxin *on page* *652*
- **Digitek** *see* Digoxin *on page* *652*
- **Digox** *see* Digoxin *on page* *652*

Digoxin (di JOKS in)

Medication Safety Issues

Sound-alike/look-alike issues:

Digoxin may be confused with Desoxyn, doxepin

Lanoxin may be confused with Lasix, levothyroxine, Levoxyl, Levsinex, Lomotil, Mefoxin, naloxone, Xanax

High alert medication:

The Institute for Safe Medication Practices (ISMP) includes this medication among its list of drugs which have a heightened risk of causing significant patient harm when used in error.

BEERS Criteria medication:

This drug may be potentially inappropriate for use in geriatric patients (Quality of evidence - moderate; Strength of recommendation - strong).

International issues:

Lanoxin [U.S., Canada, and multiple international markets] may be confused with Limoxin brand name for ambroxol [Indonesia] and amoxicillin [Mexico]

Related Information

Management of Drug Extravasations *on page* *2298*

Brand Names: US Digitek; Digox; Lanoxin; Lanoxin Pediatric

Brand Names: Canada Apo-Digoxin; Digoxin Injection CSD; Lanoxin; Pediatric Digoxin CSD; PMS-Digoxin; Toloxin

Therapeutic Category Antiarrhythmic Agent, Miscellaneous; Cardiac Glycoside

Generic Availability (US) Yes

Use Treatment of mild to moderate heart failure (HF) (Injection, oral solution: FDA approved in all ages; Tablets: FDA approved in ages ≥5 years and adults); chronic atrial fibrillation (rate-control) (all dosage forms: FDA approved in adults). Has also been used for fetal tachycardia with or without hydrops; to slow ventricular rate in supraventricular tachyarrhythmias such as supraventricular tachycardias (SVT), excluding atrioventricular reciprocating tachycardia (AVRT)

Pregnancy Risk Factor C

Pregnancy Considerations Animal reproduction studies have not been conducted. Digoxin crosses the placenta and serum concentrations are similar in the mother and fetus at delivery. Digoxin is recommended as first-line in the treatment of fetal tachycardia determined to be SVT. In pregnant women with SVT, use of digoxin is recommended (Blomström-Lundqvist, 2003).

Breast-Feeding Considerations Digoxin is excreted into breast milk and similar concentrations are found within mother's serum and milk. The manufacturer recommends that caution be used when administered to nursing women.

Contraindications Hypersensitivity to digoxin (rare) or other forms of digitalis, or any component of the formulation; ventricular fibrillation

Warnings/Precautions Watch for proarrhythmic effects (especially with digoxin toxicity). Withdrawal in clinically stable patients with HF may lead to recurrence of HF symptoms. During an episode of atrial fibrillation or flutter in patients with an accessory bypass tract (eg, Wolff-Parkinson-White syndrome) or pre-excitation syndrome, use has been associated with increased anterograde conduction down the accessory pathway leading to ventricular fibrillation; avoid use in such patients (ACLS [Neumar, 2010]; AHA/ACC/HRS [January, 2014]). Because digoxin slows sinoatrial and AV conduction, the drug commonly prolongs the PR interval. Digoxin may cause severe sinus bradycardia or sinoatrial block in patients with preexisting sinus node disease. Avoid use in patients with second- or third-degree heart block (except in patients with a functioning artificial pacemaker) (Yancy, 2013); incomplete AV block (eg, Stokes-Adams attack) may progress to complete block with digoxin administration. Digoxin should be considered for use only in heart failure (HF) with reduced ejection fraction (HFrEF) when symptoms remain despite guideline-directed medical therapy. It may also be considered in patients with both HF and atrial fibrillation; however, beta blockers may offer better ventricular rate control than digoxin (ACCF/AHA [Yancy, 2013]). When used for rate control in patients with atrial fibrillation or heart failure, monitor serum concentrations closely; may be associated with an increased risk of mortality especially when serum concentrations are not properly controlled (Vamos 2015). Avoid use in patients with hypertrophic cardiomyopathy (HCM) and outflow tract obstruction unless used to control ventricular response with atrial fibrillation; outflow obstruction may worsen due to the positive inotropic effects of digoxin. Digoxin is potentially harmful in the treatment of dyspnea in patients with HCM in the absence of atrial fibrillation (Gersh, 2011). In a murine model of viral myocarditis, digoxin in high doses was shown to be detrimental (Matsumori, 1999). If used in humans, therefore, digoxin should be used with caution and only at low doses (Frishman, 2007). The manufacturer recommends avoiding the use of digoxin in patients with myocarditis.

Use with caution in patients with hyperthyroidism (increased digoxin clearance) and hypothyroidism (reduced digoxin clearance). Atrial arrhythmias associated with hypermetabolic (eg, hyperthyroidism) or hyperdynamic (hypoxia, arteriovenous shunt) states are very difficult to treat; treat underlying condition first. Use with caution in patients with an acute MI; may increase myocardial oxygen demand. During an acute coronary syndrome, digoxin administered IV may be used to slow a rapid ventricular response and improve left ventricular (LV) function in the acute treatment of atrial fibrillation associated with severe LV function and heart failure or hemodynamic instability (AHA/ACC/HRS [January, 2014]). Reduce dose with renal impairment and when amiodarone, propafenone, quinidine, or verapamil are added to a patient on digoxin; use with caution in patients taking strong inducers or inhibitors of P-glycoprotein (eg, cyclosporine). Avoid rapid IV administration of calcium in digitalized patients; may produce serious arrhythmias.

Atrial arrhythmias associated with hypermetabolic states are very difficult to treat; treat underlying condition first; if digoxin is used, ensure digoxin toxicity does not occur. Patients with beri beri heart disease may fail to adequately respond to digoxin therapy; treat underlying thiamine deficiency concomitantly. Correct electrolyte disturbances, especially hypokalemia or hypomagnesemia, prior to use and throughout therapy; toxicity may occur despite therapeutic digoxin concentrations. Hypercalcemia may increase the risk of digoxin toxicity; maintain normocalcemia. It is not necessary to routinely reduce or hold digoxin therapy prior to elective electrical cardioversion for atrial fibrillation; however, exclusion of digoxin toxicity (eg, clinical and ECG signs) is necessary prior to cardioversion. If signs of digoxin excess exist, withhold digoxin and delay cardioversion until toxicity subsides (AHA/ACC/HRS [January, 2014]). IV administration: Vesicant; ensure proper needle or catheter placement prior to and during administration; avoid extravasation. Some dosage forms may contain propylene glycol; large amounts are potentially toxic and have been associated hyperosmolality, lactic acidosis, seizures, and respiratory depression; use caution (AAP, 1997; Zar, 2007). Use with caution in the elderly; decreases in renal clearance may result in toxic effects; in general, avoid doses >0.125 mg/day; in heart failure, higher doses may increase the risk of potential toxicity and have not been shown to provide additional benefit (Beers Criteria).

Warnings: Additional Pediatric Considerations Children are more likely to experience cardiac arrhythmia as a sign of excessive dosing. The most common are conduction disturbances or tachyarrhythmia (atrial tachycardia with or without block) and junctional tachycardia. Ventricular tachyarrhythmias are less common. In infants, sinus bradycardia may be a sign of digoxin toxicity. Any arrhythmia seen in a child on digoxin should be considered as digoxin toxicity. The gastrointestinal and central nervous system symptoms are not frequently seen in children.

Some dosage forms may contain propylene glycol; in neonates large amounts of propylene glycol delivered orally, intravenously (eg, >3,000 mg/day), or topically have been associated with potentially fatal toxicities which can include metabolic acidosis, seizures, renal failure, and CNS depression; toxicities have also been reported in children and adults including hyperosmolality, lactic acidosis, seizures and respiratory depression; use caution (AAP, 1997; Shehab, 2009).

Adverse Reactions

Cardiovascular: Accelerated junctional rhythm, asystole, atrial tachycardia with or without block, AV dissociation, first-, second- (Wenckebach), or third-degree heart block, facial edema, PR prolongation, PVCs (especially bigeminy or trigeminy), ST segment depression, ventricular tachycardia or ventricular fibrillation

Central nervous system: Apathy, anxiety, confusion, delirium, depression, dizziness, fever, hallucinations, headache, mental disturbances

Dermatologic: Rash (erythematous, maculopapular [most common], papular, scarlatiniform, vesicular or bullous), pruritus, urticaria, angioneurotic edema

Gastrointestinal: Abdominal pain, anorexia, diarrhea, nausea, vomiting

Neuromuscular & skeletal: Weakness

Ocular: Visual disturbances (blurred or yellow vision)

Respiratory: Laryngeal edema

Rare but important or life-threatening: Asymmetric chorea, gynecomastia, thrombocytopenia, palpitation, intestinal ischemia, hemorrhagic necrosis of the intestines, vaginal cornification, eosinophilia, sexual dysfunction, diaphoresis

Drug Interactions

Metabolism/Transport Effects Substrate of CYP3A4 (minor), P-glycoprotein; **Note:** Assignment of Major/Minor substrate status based on clinically relevant drug interaction potential

Avoid Concomitant Use

Avoid concomitant use of Digoxin with any of the following: Ceritinib

Increased Effect/Toxicity

Digoxin may increase the levels/effects of: Adenosine; Bradycardia-Causing Agents; Carvedilol; Ceritinib; Colchicine; Dronedarone; Ivabradine; Lacosamide; Midodrine

The levels/effects of Digoxin may be increased by: Aminoquinolines (Antimalarial); Amiodarone; Amphotericin B; Antithyroid Agents; AtorvaSTATin; Barnidipine; Beta-Blockers; Boceprevir; Bretylium; Brimonidine (Topical); Calcium Channel Blockers (Nondihydropyridine); Calcium Polystyrene Sulfonate; Calcium Salts; Carvedilol; CloNIDine; Conivaptan; CycloSPORINE (Systemic); Dronedarone; Edrophonium; Eliglustat; Epoprostenol; Etravirine; Flecainide; Glycopyrrolate; Isavuconazonium Sulfate; Itraconazole; Lenalidomide; Licorice; Loop Diuretics; Macrolide Antibiotics; Mifepristone; Milnacipran; Mirabegron; Multivitamins/Fluoride (with ADE); Multivitamins/Minerals (with ADEK, Folate, Iron); Multivitamins/Minerals (with AE, No Iron); Nefazodone; Neuromuscular-Blocking Agents; NIFEdipine; Nonsteroidal Anti-Inflammatory Agents; Parathyroid Hormone; Paricalcitol; P-glycoprotein/ABCB1 Inhibitors; Posaconazole; Potassium-Sparing Diuretics; Propafenone; Protease Inhibitors; QuiNIDine; QuiNINE; Ranolazine; Regorafenib; Reserpine; Ruxolitinib; Simeprevir; SitaGLIPtin; Sodium Polystyrene Sulfonate; Spironolactone; Telaprevir; Telmisartan; Thiazide Diuretics; Ticagrelor; Tofacitinib; Tolvaptan; Trimethoprim; Vandetanib; Vilazodone; Vitamin D Analogs

Decreased Effect

Digoxin may decrease the levels/effects of: Antineoplastic Agents (Anthracycline, Systemic)

The levels/effects of Digoxin may be decreased by: 5-ASA Derivatives; Acarbose; Aminoglycosides; Antineoplastic Agents (Anthracycline, Systemic); Bile Acid Sequestrants; Kaolin; PenicillAMINE; P-glycoprotein/ABCB1 Inducers; Polyethylene Glycol 3350; Polyethylene Glycol 4000; Potassium-Sparing Diuretics; St Johns Wort; Sucralfate

Food Interactions Digoxin peak serum concentrations may be decreased if taken with food. Meals containing increased fiber (bran) or foods high in pectin may decrease oral absorption of digoxin.

Storage/Stability Store at 25°C (77°F); excursions permitted to 15°C to 30°C (59°F to 86°F). Protect elixir, injection, and tablets from light.

Mechanism of Action

Heart failure: Inhibition of the sodium/potassium ATPase pump in myocardial cells results in a transient increase of intracellular sodium, which in turn promotes calcium influx via the sodium-calcium exchange pump leading to increased contractility. May improve baroreflex sensitivity (Gheorghiade, 1991).

Supraventricular arrhythmias: Direct suppression of the AV node conduction to increase effective refractory period and decrease conduction velocity - positive inotropic effect, enhanced vagal tone, and decreased ventricular rate to fast atrial arrhythmias. Atrial fibrillation may decrease sensitivity and increase tolerance to higher serum digoxin concentrations.

Pharmacodynamics

Onset of action: Heart rate control:
- Oral: 1 to 2 hours
- IV: 5 to 60 minutes; dependent upon rate of infusion

Maximum effect: Heart rate control:
- Oral: 2 to 8 hours
- IV: 1 to 6 hours; **Note:** In adult patients with atrial fibrillation, median time to ventricular rate control in one study was 6 hours (range: 3 to 15 hours) (Siu, 2009)

Duration: Adults: 3 to 4 days

Pharmacokinetics (Adult data unless noted)

Absorption: By passive nonsaturable diffusion in the upper small intestine; food may delay but does not affect extent of absorption

Distribution: Distribution phase: 6 to 8 hours
- V_d: Extensive to peripheral tissues; concentrates in heart, liver, kidney, skeletal muscle, and intestines. Heart/serum concentration is 70:1. Pharmacologic effects are delayed and do not correlate well with serum concentrations during distribution phase
  - Neonates, full-term: 7.5 to 10 L/kg
  - Children: 16 L/kg
  - Adults: 7 L/kg
  - Disease-related changes:
    - Hyperthyroidism: Increased V_d
    - Hyperkalemia, hyponatremia: Decreased digoxin distribution to heart and muscle
    - Hypokalemia: Increased digoxin distribution to heart and muscles
    - Chronic renal failure: Decreased V_d: 4 to 6 L/kg
    - Decreased sodium/potassium ATPase activity: Decreased tissue binding

Protein binding: ~25%; in uremic patients, digoxin is displaced from plasma protein binding sites

Metabolism: Via sequential sugar hydrolysis in the stomach or by reduction of lactone ring by intestinal bacteria (in ~10% of population, gut bacteria may metabolize up to 40% of digoxin dose); once absorbed, only ~16% is metabolized to 3-beta-digoxigenin, 3-keto-digoxigenin, and glucuronide and sulfate conjugates; metabolites may contribute to therapeutic and toxic effects of digoxin; metabolism is reduced with decompensated heart failure

Bioavailability:
- Oral solution: 70% to 85%
- Tablets: 60% to 80%

Half-life, elimination:
- Premature: 61 to 170 hours
- Neonates, full-term: 35 to 45 hours
- Infants: 18 to 25 hours
- Children: 35 hours
- Adults: 36 to 48 hours
- Anuric adults: 3.5 to 5 days
- Metabolites: Digoxigenin: 4 hours; Monodigitoxoside: 3 to 12 hours

Time to peak serum concentration: Oral tablets: 1 to 3 hours; oral solution: 30 to 90 minutes

Elimination: Urine (50% to 70% as unchanged drug)

Dosing: Neonatal Heart failure, atrial dysrhythmias:

Injection, Oral solution: Dosage must be individualized due to substantial individual variation. For management of heart failure, a lower serum digoxin concentration may be adequate compared to treatment of cardiac arrhythmias; consider doses at the lower end of the recommended range for treatment of heart failure; a digitalizing dose (loading dose) may not be necessary when treating heart failure (Ross, 2001). For management of atrial dysrhythmias, dose should be titrated to the lowest effective dose.

The dosage tables below list dosage recommendations for normal renal function and are based upon average patient response. **Note:** Doses have been adjusted for clinical usefulness. Total digitalizing dose should be decreased by 50% in patients with end-stage renal disease. **Note:** Total digitalizing dose should be divided (see below). If changing from oral solution to IV therapy, dosage should be reduced by 20% to 25%.

Initial Dosage Recommendations for Digoxin[A] (Digitalizing)

Age	Total Digitalizing Dose Administer in three divided doses[B] (mcg/kg)	
	Oral	IV[C]
Preterm neonates	20 to 30	15 to 25
Full-term neonates	25 to 35	20 to 30

[A]Based on lean body weight and normal renal function for age

[B]Do not give full total digitalizing dose (TDD) at once. Give one-half of the TDD for the initial dose, then give one-quarter of the TDD for each of two subsequent doses at 6- to 8-hour intervals; prior to additional doses, clinical response should be fully evaluated (eg, ECG).

[C]May also be administered IM; however, not usually recommended.

Maintenance Dosage Recommendations for Digoxin[A]

Age	Total Daily Maintenance Dose Administer in equal divided doses every 12 hours (mcg/kg/day)	
	Oral	IV[B,C]
Preterm neonates	5 to 7.5	4 to 6
Full-term neonates	8 to 10	5 to 8

[A]Based on lean body weight and normal renal function for age. Decrease maintenance dose in patients with decreased renal function.

[B]Daily maintenance IV dose is typically 20% to 30% of total IV digitalizing dose.

[C]May also be administered IM; however, not usually recommended.

Dosing: Usual

Infants, Children, and Adolescents: Dosage must be individualized due to substantial individual variation; for management of heart failure, a lower serum digoxin concentration may be adequate compared to treatment of cardiac arrhythmias; consider doses at the lower end of the recommended range for treatment of heart failure; a digitalizing dose (loading dose) may not be necessary when treating heart failure (Ross, 2001). For management of atrial dysrhythmias, dose should be titrated to the lowest effective dose.

The dosage tables below list dosage recommendations for normal renal function and are based on average patient response. **Note:** Doses have been adjusted for clinical usefulness. Total digitalizing dose should be decreased by 50% in patients with end-stage renal disease. **Note:** Total digitalizing dose should be divided (see below). If changing from oral solution or tablets to IV therapy, dosage should be reduced by 20% to 25%.

Initial Dosage Recommendations for Digoxin[A] (Digitalizing)

Age	Total Digitalizing Dose Administer in three divided doses[B] (mcg/kg)		
	Oral Solution	Tablets	IV[C]
1 to 24 months	35 to 60	–	30 to 50
2 to 5 years	30 to 45	–	25 to 35
5 to 10 years	20 to 35	20 to 45	15 to 30
>10 years	10 to 15	10 to 15	8 to 12

[A]Based on lean body weight and normal renal function for age

[B]**Do not give full total digitalizing dose (TDD) at once.** Give one-half of the TDD for the initial dose, then give one-quarter of the TDD for each of two subsequent doses at 6- to 8-hour intervals; prior to additional doses, clinical response should be fully evaluated (eg, ECG).

[C]May also be administered by I.M; however, not recommended.

Maintenance Dosage Recommendations for Digoxin[A]

Age	Daily Maintenance Dose If ≤10 years, administer in equal divided doses twice daily If >10 years, administer once daily (mcg/kg/day)		
	Oral Solution	Tablets	IV[B,C]
1 to 24 months	10 to 15	–	7.5 to 12
2 to 5 years	8 to 10	–	6 to 9
5 to 10 years	5 to 10	6 to 11	4 to 8
>10 years	2.5 to 5	2.5 to 5	2 to 3

[A]Based on lean body weight and normal renal function for age. Decrease maintenance dose in patients with decreased renal function.

[B]May also be administered by I.M; however, not recommended.

[C]Daily maintenance IV dose is typically 20% to 30% of total digitalizing IV dose in pediatric patients ≤24 months and 25% to 35% in older pediatric patients.

Adult: **Note:** When changing from oral (tablets or liquid) or IM to IV therapy, dosage should be reduced by 20% to 25%.

Atrial fibrillation (rate control):

Total digitalizing dose (TDD): IV: 8 to 12 **mcg**/kg; administer half of TDD over 5 minutes with the remaining portion as 25% fractions at 4 to 8 hour intervals (ACLS [Neumar, 2010]) **or** may administer 0.25 mg with repeat dosing to a maximum of 1.5 mg over 24 hours followed by an oral maintenance regimen (AHA/ACC/HRS [January, 2014]).

Maintenance: Oral: 0.125 to 0.25 mg once daily (AHA/ACC/HRS [January, 2014])

Heart failure: Note: Loading dose not recommended; Daily maintenance dose: Oral: 0.125 to 0.25 mg once daily; higher daily doses (up to 0.5 mg/day) are rarely necessary. If patient is >70 years old, has impaired renal function, or has a low lean body mass, low doses (eg, 0.125 mg daily or every other day) should be used initially (ACCF/AHA [Yancy, 2013]. **Note:** IV. digoxin may be used to control ventricular response in patients with atrial fibrillation and heart failure with reduced ejection fraction (HFrEF) who do not have an accessory pathway or preexcitation syndrome (AHA/ACC/HRS [January, 2014]). The addition of a beta-blocker to digoxin is usually more effective in controlling ventricular response, particularly during exercise (ACCF/AHA [Yancy, 2013]).

Supraventricular tachyarrhythmias (rate control):

Initial: Total digitalizing dose:

Oral: 0.75 to 1.5 mg

IV, IM: 0.5 to 1 mg (**Note:** IM not preferred due to severe injection site pain.)

Give 1/2 of the total digitalizing dose (TDD) as the initial dose, then give 1/4 of the TDD in each of two subsequent doses at 6- to 8-hour intervals. Obtain ECG 6 hours after each dose to assess potential toxicity.

Daily maintenance dose:

Oral: 0.125 to 0.5 mg once daily

IV, IM: 0.1 to 0.4 mg once daily (**Note:** IM not preferred due to severe injection site pain.)

Dosing adjustment in renal impairment:

Infants, Children, and Adolescents: There are no dosage adjustments provided in the manufacturer's labeling; however, the following adjustments have been recommended:

Loading dose: Reduce by 50% in end-stage renal disease

Maintenance dose:

Manufacturer's labeling: Dosage reductions and close monitoring recommended; see product labeling for CrCl-specific dosage recommendation

Alternate dosing: The following adjustments have been recommended (Aronoff, 2007):

GFR >50 mL/minute/1.73 m^2: No dosage adjustment necessary

GFR: 30 to 50 mL/minute/1.73 m^2: Administer 75% of normal dose at normal intervals

GFR: 10 to 29 mL/minute/1.73 m^2: Administer 50% of normal dose at normal intervals **or** administer normal dose every 36 hours

GFR: <10 mL/minute/1.73 m^2: Administer 25% of normal dose at normal intervals **or** administer normal dose every 48 hours

Intermittent hemodialysis: Nondialyzable (0% to 5%); administer 25% of normal dose at normal intervals **or** administer normal dose every 48 hours

Peritoneal dialysis (PD): Administer 25% of normal dose at normal intervals **or** administer normal dose every 48 hours

Continuous renal replacement therapy (CRRT): Administer 75% of normal dose at normal intervals; titrate to desired effect; monitor serum concentrations

Adults: There are no dosage adjustments provided in the manufacturer's labeling; however, the following adjustments have been recommended:

Loading dose:

ESRD: If loading dose necessary, reduce by 50% (Aronoff, 2007)

Acute renal failure: Based on expert opinion, if patient in acute renal failure requires ventricular rate control (eg, in atrial fibrillation), consider alternative therapy. If loading digoxin becomes necessary, patient volume of distribution may be increased and reduction in loading dose may not be necessary; however, maintenance dosing will require adjustment as long as renal failure persists.

Maintenance dose (Aronoff, 2007):

CrCl >50 mL/minute: No dosage adjustment necessary

CrCl 10 to 50 mL/minute: Administer 25% to 75% of normal daily dose (divided and given at normal intervals) or administer normal dose every 36 hours

CrCl <10 mL/minute: Administer 10% to 25% of normal daily dose (divided and given at normal intervals) or give normal dose every 48 hours

Continuous renal replacement therapy (CRRT): Administer 25% to 75% of the normal daily dose or administer normal dose every 36 hours; monitor serum concentrations.

Hemodialysis: Not dialyzable; no supplemental dose necessary

Heart failure: Initial maintenance dose (Bauman, 2006; Jusko, 1974; Koup, 1975): **Note:** The following suggested dosing recommendations are intended to achieve a target digoxin concentration of 0.7 ng/mL. Renal function estimated using Cockcroft-Gault formula.

CrCl >120 mL/minute: 0.25 mg once daily

CrCl 80 to 120 mL/minute: Alternate between doses of 0.25 mg and 0.125 mg once daily

CrCl 30 to 80 mL/minute: 0.125 mg once daily

CrCl <30 mL/minute: 0.125 mg every 48 hours

Note: A contemporary digoxin dosing nomogram using creatinine clearance and ideal body weight or height has been published for determining the initial maintenance dose in patients with heart failure to achieve a target digoxin concentration of 0.7 ng/mL (Bauman, 2006).

Dosing adjustment in hepatic impairment: There are no dosage adjustments provided in the manufacturer's labeling.

Preparation for Administration Parenteral:

IV: May be administered undiluted or diluted at least fourfold in D_5W, $D_{10}W$, NS, or SWFI; less than fourfold dilution may lead to drug precipitation.

IM: No dilution required.

Administration

Oral: Administer consistently with relationship to meals; avoid concurrent administration (ie, administer digoxin 1 hour before or 2 hours after) with meals high in fiber or pectin and with drugs that decrease oral absorption of digoxin

Oral solution: Only the calibrated manufacturer-provided dropper or a calibrated oral syringe should be used to measure the dose. For doses <0.2 mL the manufacturer-provided dropper is not accurate and should not be used; use a calibrated oral syringe.

Parenteral:

IV: May be slowly administered IV over ≥5 minutes (usually 5 to 10 minutes); avoid rapid IV infusion since this may result in systemic and coronary arteriolar vasoconstriction

Vesicant; ensure proper needle or catheter placement prior to and during administration; avoid extravasation. If extravasation occurs, stop IV administration immediately and disconnect (leave cannula/needle in place); gently aspirate extravasated solution (do **NOT** flush the line); remove needle/cannula; elevate extremity.

IM: Not usually recommended due to local irritation, pain, and tissue damage; if necessary, administer by deep injection followed by massage at the injection site. May cause intense pain.

Vesicant/Extravasation Risk Vesicant

Monitoring Parameters Heart rate and rhythm, periodic ECG; follow serum potassium, magnesium, and calcium closely (especially in patients receiving diuretics or amphotericin or patient with a history of hypokalemia or hypomagnesemia); decreased serum potassium and magnesium, or increased serum magnesium and calcium may increase digoxin toxicity; assess renal function (serum BUN, S_{cr}) in order to adjust dose; obtain serum drug concentrations at least 8 to 12 hours after a dose, preferably prior to next scheduled dose. Observe patients for noncardiac signs of toxicity, confusion, and depression.

Therapeutic drug monitoring: Digoxin serum concentrations are monitored because digoxin possesses a narrow therapeutic serum concentration range; the therapeutic endpoint is difficult to quantify and digoxin toxicity may be life-threatening. Digoxin serum concentrations should be drawn **at least 6 to 8 hours after the previous dose, regardless of route of administration (optimally 12 to 24 hours after a dose)**. **Note:** Serum digoxin concentrations may decrease in response to exercise due to increased skeletal muscle uptake; a period of rest (eg, ~2 hours) after exercise may be necessary prior to drawing serum digoxin concentrations.

Initiation of therapy:

If a loading dose is given: Digoxin serum concentration may be drawn within 12 to 24 hours after the initial loading dose administration. Concentrations drawn this early may confirm the relationship of digoxin plasma concentrations and response but are of little value in determining maintenance doses.

If a loading dose is not given: Digoxin serum concentration should be obtained after 3 to 5 days of therapy.

Maintenance therapy:

Trough concentrations should be followed just prior to the next dose or at a minimum of 6 to 8 hours after last dose.

Digoxin serum concentrations should be obtained within 5 to 7 days (approximate time to steady-state) after any dosage changes. Continue to obtain digoxin serum concentrations 7 to 14 days after any change in maintenance dose. **Note:** Time to steady state will be longer in patients with decreased renal function (eg, premature neonates or patients with renal impairment). In patients with end-stage renal disease, it may take 15 to 20 days to reach steady-state.

Patients who are receiving electrolyte-altering medications such as diuretics, serum potassium, magnesium, and calcium should be monitored closely.

Digoxin serum concentrations should be obtained whenever any of the following conditions occur:

Questionable patient compliance or to evaluate clinical deterioration following an initial good response

Changing renal function

Suspected digoxin toxicity

Initiation or discontinuation of therapy with drugs (eg, amiodarone, quinidine, verapamil) which potentially interact with digoxin.

Any disease changes (eg, thyroid disease)

Reference Range Digoxin therapeutic serum trough concentrations:

Heart failure: 0.5 to 0.9 ng/mL (ACCF/AHA [Yancy, 2013])

Adults: <0.5 ng/mL (SI: <0.6 nmol/L); probably indicates underdigitalization unless there are special circumstances

Toxic: >2 ng/mL; (SI: >2.6 nmol/L). **Note:** Serum concentration must be used in conjunction with clinical symptoms and ECG to confirm diagnosis of digoxin intoxication.

Digoxin-like immunoreactive substance (DLIS) may cross-react with digoxin immunoassay and falsely increase serum concentrations. DLIS has been found in patients with renal and liver disease, heart failure, neonates, and pregnant women (3rd trimester).

Test Interactions Spironolactone may interfere with digoxin radioimmunoassay.

Dosage Forms Excipient information presented when available (limited, particularly for generics); consult specific product labeling.

Solution, Injection:
- Lanoxin: 0.25 mg/mL (2 mL) [contains alcohol, usp, propylene glycol]
- Lanoxin Pediatric: 0.1 mg/mL (1 mL) [contains alcohol, usp, propylene glycol]
- Generic: 0.25 mg/mL (1 mL, 2 mL)

Solution, Oral:
- Generic: 0.05 mg/mL (60 mL)

Tablet, Oral:
- Digitek: 125 mcg [scored; contains fd&c yellow #10 aluminum lake]
- Digitek: 250 mcg [scored]
- Digox: 125 mcg [scored; contains fd&c yellow #10 aluminum lake]
- Digox: 250 mcg [scored]
- Lanoxin: 62.5 mcg [contains fd&c yellow #6 (sunset yellow)]
- Lanoxin: 125 mcg [scored; contains fd&c yellow #10 (quinoline yellow), fd&c yellow #6 (sunset yellow)]
- Lanoxin: 187.5 mcg
- Lanoxin: 250 mcg [scored]
- Generic: 125 mcg, 250 mcg

Digoxin Immune Fab (di JOKS in i MYUN fab)

Brand Names: US DigiFab

Brand Names: Canada DigiFab

Therapeutic Category Antidote, Digoxin

Generic Availability (US) No

Use Treatment of potentially life-threatening digoxin or digitoxin intoxication in carefully selected patients; acute digoxin ingestion (ie, >10 mg in adults; >0.1 mg/kg or >4 mg in children; ingestions resulting in serum concentrations >10 ng/mL), chronic ingestions leading to steady-state digoxin concentrations >6 ng/mL in adults or >4 ng/mL in children; patients experiencing manifestations of digoxin toxicity due to overdose (eg, life-threatening ventricular arrhythmias, progressive bradycardia, second- or third-degree heart block not responsive to atropine, serum potassium >5.5 mEq/L in adults or >6 mEq/L in children) [FDA approved in pediatric patients (age not specified) and adults]

Pregnancy Risk Factor C

Pregnancy Considerations Animal reproduction studies have not been conducted. In general, medications used as antidotes should take into consideration the health and prognosis of the mother; antidotes should be administered to pregnant women if there is a clear indication for use and should not be withheld because of fears of teratogenicity (Bailey, 2003).

Breast-Feeding Considerations It is not known if digoxin immune fab is excreted in breast milk. The manufacturer recommends caution be exercised when administering to nursing women.

Contraindications There are no contraindications listed in the manufacturer's labeling.

Warnings/Precautions Digoxin immune Fab is derived from ovine (sheep) Fab immunoglobulin fragments; hypersensitivity reactions (eg, anaphylactic or anaphylactoid reactions, delayed allergic reactions) are possible. Patients with allergies to sheep proteins and patients with prior exposure to ovine antibodies or ovine Fab may be at a higher risk for anaphylactic reactions. In patients who develop an anaphylactic reaction, discontinue the infusion immediately and administer emergency care; balance the need for epinephrine against its potential risk in the setting of digitalis toxicity. Processed with papain and may cause hypersensitivity reactions in patients allergic to papaya, other papaya extracts, papain, chymopapain, or the pineapple-enzyme bromelain. There may also be cross allergenicity with dust mite and latex allergens.

Patients experiencing acute digitalis toxicity may present with significant hyperkalemia due to shifting of potassium into the extracellular space. Upon treatment with digoxin immune Fab, potassium shifts back into the intracellular space and may result in hypokalemia. Monitor potassium closely, especially during the first few hours after administration; treat hypokalemia cautiously when clinically indicated.

In patients chronically maintained on digoxin for HF, administration of digoxin immune Fab may result in exacerbation of HF symptoms due to a reduction in digoxin serum concentration. If reinitiation is required, consider postponing until Fab fragments have been eliminated completely; elimination may take several days or longer, especially in patients with renal impairment. Use with caution in patients with renal failure (experience limited); the Fab-digoxin complex will be eliminated more slowly. Toxicity may recur; prolonged monitoring for recurrence of symptoms and evaluation of free (unbound) digoxin concentrations (if test available) may be warranted in this patient population.

Adverse Reactions

Cardiovascular: Heart failure exacerbation (due to withdrawal of digoxin), orthostatic hypotension, rapid ventricular response (patients with atrial fibrillation; due to withdrawal of digoxin)

Endocrine & metabolic: Hypokalemia

Local: Phlebitis

Miscellaneous: Allergic reactions, serum sickness

Drug Interactions

Metabolism/Transport Effects None known.

Avoid Concomitant Use There are no known interactions where it is recommended to avoid concomitant use.

Increased Effect/Toxicity There are no known significant interactions involving an increase in effect.

Decreased Effect There are no known significant interactions involving a decrease in effect.

Storage/Stability Store vials at 2°C to 8°C (36°F to 46°F); do not freeze. Reconstituted solutions are stable for 4 hours when stored at 2°C to 8°C (36°F to 46°F). The following stability information has also been reported: May be stored at room temperature for up to 30 days (Cohen, 2007).

Mechanism of Action Digoxin immune antigen-binding fragments (Fab) are specific antibodies for the treatment of digitalis intoxication in carefully selected patients; binds with molecules of digoxin or DIGIToxin and is then excreted by the kidneys and removed from the body

Pharmacodynamics Onset of action: Improvement in signs and symptoms occurs within 2-30 minutes following IV infusion

Pharmacokinetics (Adult data unless noted)

Distribution: V_d: 0.3 L/kg

Half-life: 15 hours; renal impairment prolongs half-life

Elimination: Renal with concentrations declining to undetectable amounts within 5-7 days

Dosing: Neonatal Acute ingestion of known amount: IV:

Based on amount (in mg) of digoxin ingested:

Step 1: Calculate total body load (mg)

Total body load (mg) = 0.8 x [amount (mg) digoxin tablets or elixir ingested]

Step 2: Calculate number of vials needed

Digoxin Immune Fab Dose (vials) = Total body load (mg) / (0.5)

Based on steady-state serum digoxin concentration: Consider dilution of the reconstituted vial with NS and administer the dose via a tuberculin syringe.

Digoxin Immune Fab Dose (mg) = [(serum digoxin concentration [ng/mL] x weight [kg]) / 100] x 40 mg/vial

Dose Estimates of Digoxin Immune Fab (in mg) From Serum Digoxin Concentration

Patient Weight (kg)	Serum Digoxin Concentration (ng/mL)						
	1	2	4	8	12	16	20
1	0.4 mg[A]	1 mg[A]	1.5 mg[A]	3 mg	5 mg	6.5 mg	8 mg
3	1 mg[A]	2.5 mg[A]	5 mg	10 mg	14 mg	19 mg	24 mg
5	2 mg[A]	4 mg	8 mg	16 mg	24 mg	32 mg	40 mg

[A]Dilution of reconstituted vial to 1 mg/mL may be desirable.

Dosing: Usual Infants, Children, Adolescents, and Adults:

Note: Estimation of the dose is based on the body burden of digitalis. This may be calculated if the amount ingested is known or the postdistribution serum drug concentration is known (round the dose up to the nearest whole vial). If the amount ingested is unknown, general dosing guidelines should be used.

Acute ingestion of unknown amount: IV: 20 vials is adequate to treat most life-threatening ingestions. In small children, it is important to monitor for fluid overload. May give as a single dose or give 10 vials, observe the response, and give a second dose of 10 vials if indicated.

Acute ingestion of known amount: IV:

Based on amount of digoxin ingested:

Step 1: Calculate total body load (mg)

Total body load (mg) = 0.8 x [amount (mg) digoxin tablets or elixir ingested]

Step 2: Calculate number of vials needed

Digoxin Immune Fab Dose (vials) = Total body load (mg) / (0.5)

Based on steady-state serum digoxin concentration: IV:

Digoxin Immune Fab Dose (mg) = [(serum digoxin concentration [ng/mL] x weight [kg]) / 100] x 40 mg/vial

Digoxin Immune Fab Dose (vials) = (serum digoxin concentration [ng/mL] x weight [kg]) / 100

Note: Infants and Children ≤20 kg may require smaller doses; calculate the dose in milligrams (mg), consider dilution of the reconstituted vial with NS, and administer the dose via a tuberculin syringe.

Alternatively, the following table gives an estimation of the amount of Digoxin Immune Fab needed based on the steady-state serum digoxin concentration.

Infants and Children Dose Estimates of Digoxin Immune Fab (in mg) From Serum Digoxin Concentration

Patient Weight (kg)	Serum Digoxin Concentration (ng/mL)						
	1	2	4	8	12	16	20
3	1 mg[A]	2.5 mg[A]	5 mg	10 mg	14 mg	19 mg	24 mg
5	2 mg[A]	4 mg	8 mg	16 mg	24 mg	32 mg	40 mg
10	4 mg	8 mg	16 mg	32 mg	48 mg	64 mg	80 mg
20	8 mg	16 mg	32 mg	64 mg	96 mg	128 mg	160 mg

[A]Dilution of reconstituted vial to 1 mg/mL may be desirable.

Adult Dose Estimate of Digoxin Immune Fab (in # of Vials) From Serum Digoxin Concentration

Patient Weight (kg)	Serum Digoxin Concentration (ng/mL)						
	1	2	4	8	12	16	20
40	0.5 vial	1 vial	2 vials	3 vials	5 vials	7 vials	8 vials
60	0.5 vial	1 vial	3 vials	5 vials	7 vials	10 vials	12 vials
70	1 vial	2 vials	3 vials	6 vials	9 vials	11 vials	14 vials
80	1 vial	2 vials	3 vials	7 vials	10 vials	13 vials	16 vials
100	1 vial	2 vials	4 vials	8 vials	12 vials	16 vials	20 vials

Chronic toxicity (serum digoxin concentration unavailable): IV:

Infants and Children ≤20 kg: 1 vial is adequate to reverse most cases of toxicity

Children >20 kg, Adolescents, and Adults: 6 vials is adequate to reverse most cases of toxicity

Dosing adjustment in renal impairment: No dosage adjustment necessary; however, use with caution since digoxin-digoxin immune Fab complex is renally eliminated. Patients should undergo prolonged monitoring for recurrence of toxicity.

Preparation for Administration Parenteral: IV: Reconstitute each vial to a concentration of 10 mg/mL by adding 4 mL SWFI; gently mix. Add reconstituted digoxin immune Fab to an appropriate volume of NS. For very small doses, the reconstituted vial can be further diluted by adding an additional 36 mL NS to achieve a final concentration of 1 mg/mL. Infants and small children who require very small doses may administer reconstituted digoxin immune Fab undiluted using a tuberculin syringe.

Administration Parenteral: IV: IV infusion over at least 30 minutes is preferred. May also be given by bolus injection if cardiac arrest is imminent (infusion-related reaction may occur). Discontinue the infusion and reinitiate at a slower rate if an infusion-related reaction occurs.

Monitoring Parameters Prior to the first dose of digoxin immune Fab evaluate serum potassium, serum digoxin concentration, and serum creatinine; closely monitor serum potassium (eg, hourly for 4-6 hours; at least daily thereafter), temperature, blood pressure, and electrocardiogram after administration. Total serum digoxin concentrations will rise precipitously following administration of digoxin immune Fab due to the presence of the Fab-digoxin complex; because digoxin bound to Fab fragments is not physiologically active this rise has no clinical meaning. Therefore, avoid monitoring total serum digoxin concentrations until the Fab fragments have been eliminated completely; this may be several days to weeks in patients with renal impairment (Ujhelyi, 1995).

Patients with renal failure may experience a recurrence of toxicity; prolonged monitoring for recurrence of symptoms and evaluation of free (unbound) digoxin concentrations (if test available) may be warranted in this patient population.

Test Interactions Digoxin immune fab may interfere with digitalis immunoassay measurements, thereby resulting in clinically misleading total serum digoxin concentrations until all Fab fragments are eliminated from the body (may take several days to >1 week after administration). Digoxin serum samples should be obtained before digoxin immune fab administration, if possible.

Additional Information Each 40 mg vial (DigiFab™) will bind approximately 0.5 mg digoxin or digitoxin; for individuals at increased risk of sensitivity an intradermal or scratch technique skin test using a 1:100 dilution of reconstituted digoxin immune Fab diluted in NS has been used. Skin test volume is 0.1 mL of 1:100 dilution; evaluate after 20 minutes.

Dosage Forms Excipient information presented when available (limited, particularly for generics); consult specific product labeling.

Solution Reconstituted, Intravenous [preservative free]:
DigiFab: 40 mg (1 ea)

◆ **Digoxin Injection CSD (Can)** *see* Digoxin *on page 652*

Dihydroergotamine (dye hye droe er GOT a meen)

Brand Names: US D.H.E. 45; Migranal

Brand Names: Canada Migranal®

Therapeutic Category Alpha-Adrenergic Blocking Agent, Intranasal; Alpha-Adrenergic Blocking Agent, Parenteral; Antimigraine Agent; Ergot Alkaloid and Derivative

Generic Availability (US) Yes

Use

Intranasal: Treatment of migraine headache with or without aura (FDA approved in adults)

Parenteral: Treatment of headache with or without aura and cluster headaches (FDA approved in adults)

Pregnancy Risk Factor X

Pregnancy Considerations Dihydroergotamine is oxytocic and should not be used during pregnancy.

Breast-Feeding Considerations Ergot derivatives inhibit prolactin and it is known that ergotamine is excreted in breast milk (vomiting, diarrhea, weak pulse, and unstable blood pressure have been reported in nursing infants). It is not known if dihydroergotamine would also cause these effects, however, it is likely that it is excreted in human breast milk. Do not use in nursing women.

Contraindications Hypersensitivity to dihydroergotamine or any component of the formulation; uncontrolled hypertension, ischemic heart disease, angina pectoris, history of MI, silent ischemia, or coronary artery vasospasm including Prinzmetal's angina; hemiplegic or basilar migraine; peripheral vascular disease; sepsis; severe hepatic or renal dysfunction; following vascular surgery; avoid use within 24 hours of sumatriptan, zolmitriptan, other serotonin agonists, or ergot-like agents; avoid during or within 2 weeks of discontinuing MAO inhibitors; concurrent use of peripheral and central vasoconstrictors; ergot alkaloids are contraindicated with potent inhibitors of CYP3A4 (includes protease inhibitors, azole antifungals, and some macrolide antibiotics); pregnancy, breast-feeding

Warnings/Precautions [U.S. Boxed Warning]: Ergot alkaloids are contraindicated with potent inhibitors of CYP3A4 (includes protease inhibitors, azole antifungals, and some macrolide antibiotics); concomitant use associated with an increased risk of vasospasm leading to cerebral ischemia and/or ischemia of the extremities. Do not give to patients with risk factors for CAD until a cardiovascular evaluation has been performed; if evaluation is satisfactory, the healthcare provider should administer the first dose and cardiovascular status should be periodically evaluated. May cause vasospastic reactions; persistent vasospasm may lead to gangrene or death in patients with compromised circulation. Discontinue if signs of vasoconstriction develop. Rare reports of increased blood pressure in patients without history of hypertension. Rare reports of adverse cardiac events (acute MI, life-threatening arrhythmias, death) have been reported following use of the injection. Cerebral hemorrhage, subarachnoid hemorrhage, and stroke have also occurred following use of the injection. Not for prolonged use. Pleural and peritoneal fibrosis have been reported with prolonged daily use. Cardiac valvular fibrosis has also been associated with ergot alkaloids. Use with caution in the elderly.

Migranal® Nasal Spray: Local irritation to nose and throat (usually transient and mild-moderate in severity) can occur; long-term consequences on nasal or respiratory mucosa have not been extensively evaluated.

Warnings: Additional Pediatric Considerations May cause nausea; in pediatric patients, antiemetic prophylaxis (prochlorperazine or metoclopramide) 30 minutes prior to initial dihydroergotamine dose has been used (O'Brien, 2011).

Adverse Reactions

Nasal spray:

Central nervous system: Dizziness,drowsiness, taste disorder

Endocrine & metabolic: Hot flash

Gastrointestinal: Diarrhea, nausea, vomiting

Local: Application site reaction

Neuromuscular & skeletal: Stiffness, weakness

Respiratory: Pharyngitis, rhinitis

Rare but important or life-threatening: Injection and nasal spray: Abdominal pain, anxiety, cerebral hemorrhage, cerebrovascular accident, coronary artery vasospasm, diaphoresis, diarrhea, dizziness, dyspnea, edema, fibrothorax (prolonged use), flushing, headache, hyperkinesia, hypertension, ischemic heart disease, muscle cramps, myalgia, myasthenia, myocardial infarction, palpitations, paresthesia, peripheral cyanosis, peripheral ischemia, retroperitoneal fibrosis (prolonged use), skin rash, subarachnoid hemorrhage, tremor, valvular sclerosis (associated with ergot alkaloids), ventricular fibrillation, ventricular tachycardia (transient)

Drug Interactions

Metabolism/Transport Effects Substrate of CYP3A4 (major); **Note:** Assignment of Major/Minor substrate status based on clinically relevant drug interaction potential

Avoid Concomitant Use

Avoid concomitant use of Dihydroergotamine with any of the following: Alpha-/Beta-Agonists; Alpha1-Agonists; Boceprevir; Clarithromycin; Cobicistat; Conivaptan; Crizotinib; Dapoxetine; Enzalutamide; Fusidic Acid (Systemic); Idelalisib; Itraconazole; Ketoconazole (Systemic); Lorcaserin; Mifepristone; Nitroglycerin; Posaconazole; Protease Inhibitors; Serotonin 5-HT1D Receptor Agonists; Telaprevir; Voriconazole

Increased Effect/Toxicity

Dihydroergotamine may increase the levels/effects of: Alpha-/Beta-Agonists; Alpha1-Agonists; Antipsychotic Agents; Metoclopramide; Serotonin 5-HT1D Receptor Agonists; Serotonin Modulators

The levels/effects of Dihydroergotamine may be increased by: Antiemetics (5HT3 Antagonists); Antipsychotic Agents; Aprepitant; Beta-Blockers; Boceprevir; Clarithromycin; Cobicistat; Conivaptan; Crizotinib; CYP3A4 Inhibitors (Moderate); CYP3A4 Inhibitors (Strong); Dapoxetine; Dasatinib; Fosaprepitant; Fusidic Acid (Systemic); Idelalisib; Itraconazole; Ivacaftor; Ketoconazole (Systemic); Lorcaserin; Luliconazole; Macrolide Antibiotics; Mifepristone; Netupitant; Nitroglycerin; Palbociclib; Posaconazole; Protease Inhibitors; Serotonin 5-HT1D Receptor Agonists; Simeprevir; Stiripentol; Tedizolid; Telaprevir; Voriconazole

Decreased Effect

Dihydroergotamine may decrease the levels/effects of: Nitroglycerin

The levels/effects of Dihydroergotamine may be decreased by: Enzalutamide

Storage/Stability

Injection: Store below 25°C (77°F); do not refrigerate or freeze; protect from heat. Protect from light.

Nasal spray: Prior to use, store below 25°C (77°F); do not refrigerate or freeze. Once spray applicator has been prepared, use within 8 hours; discard any unused solution.

Mechanism of Action Ergot alkaloid alpha-adrenergic blocker directly stimulates vascular smooth muscle to vasoconstrict peripheral and cerebral vessels; also has effects on serotonin receptors

Pharmacodynamics

Onset of action:

IM: 15-30 minutes

Intranasal: 30 minutes

IV: Immediate

Duration: IM: 3-4 hours

Pharmacokinetics (Adult data unless noted)

Distribution: V_d: ~800 L

Bioavailability: Intranasal: 32%

Protein binding: 93%

Metabolism: Extensively in the liver; one active metabolite

Half-life: Biphasic: terminal half-life: ~9-10 hours

Time to peak serum concentration: IM: Within 15-30 minutes; intranasal: 0.5-1 hour; IV: 15 minutes; SubQ: 15-45 minutes

Elimination: Predominately into bile and feces and 10% excreted in urine, mostly as metabolites

Clearance: 1.5 L/minute

Dosing: Usual

Children and Adolescents: **Intractable migraine >72 hours (status migrainosus):** Limited data available; optimal dose not established:

IV: Premedicate with antiemetic (metoclopramide or prochlorperazine have been used)

Low dose regimen:

Children 6 to <10 years: 0.1 mg/dose every 6 hours; improvement usually seen after 5 doses; if improvement noted, continue therapy until headache-free up to a maximum of 16 doses; if no improvement after 5 doses, discontinue therapy (O'Brien, 2011)

Children ≥10 to 12 years: 0.15 mg/dose every 6 hours; improvement usually seen after 5 doses; if improvement noted, continue therapy until headache-free up to a maximum of 16 doses; if no improvement after 5 doses, discontinue therapy. One study reported increasing the dose by 0.05 mg increments as tolerated (ie, no abdominal discomfort). Postmenarche female patients should complete pregnancy screening prior to first dose (Linder, 1994; O'Brien, 2011).

Adolescents ≤16 years: 0.2 mg/dose every 6 hours; improvement usually seen after 5 doses; if improvement noted, continue therapy until headache-free up to a maximum of 16 doses; if no improvement after 5 doses, discontinue therapy. Postmenarche female patients should complete pregnancy screening prior to first dose (O'Brien, 2011).

High dose regimen:

Children 6-9 years or Children ≥10 years and <25 kg: 0.5 mg/dose every 8 hours; improvement usually seen after 5 doses; if improvement noted, continue therapy until headache-free up to a maximum of 20 doses; if no improvement after 5 doses, discontinue therapy; an additional dose after headache subsides has also been suggested (Kabbouche, 2009; O'Brien, 2011). **Note:** An initial test dose (half of the appropriate dose for age and weight) has been used; if test dose tolerated, remainder of dose administered 30 minutes later (Kabbouche, 2009).

Children ≥10 years and >25 kg and Adolescents: 1 mg/dose every 8 hours; improvement usually seen after 5 doses; if improvement noted, continue therapy until headache-free up to a maximum of 20 doses; if no improvement after 5 doses, discontinue therapy (Kabbouche, 2009; O'Brien, 2011). **Note:** An initial test dose (half of the appropriate dose for age and weight) has been used; if test dose tolerated, remainder of dose administered 30 minutes later (Kabbouche, 2009).

Intranasal: Adolescents: 1 spray (0.5 mg) into each nostril (total dose: 1 mg); repeat if needed within 15 minutes up to a total of 4 sprays (2 mg); maximum daily dose: 6 sprays (3 mg)/24-hour period; **Note:** Do not exceed 8 sprays (4 mg)/week.

Adults: **Migraine, cluster headache:**

IM, SubQ: 1 mg at first sign of headache; repeat hourly to a maximum dose of 3 mg/day; maximum dose: 6 mg/week

IV: 1 mg at first sign of headache; repeat hourly up to a maximum dose of 2 mg/day; maximum dose: 6 mg/week

Intranasal: 1 spray (0.5 mg) of nasal spray should be administered into each nostril; if needed, repeat after 15 minutes, up to a total of 4 sprays (2 mg). **Note:** Do not exceed 6 sprays (3 mg) in a 24-hour period and no more than 8 sprays (4 mg) in a week.

Dosing adjustment in renal impairment: Contraindicated in severe renal impairment

Dosing adjustment in hepatic impairment: Dosage reductions are probably necessary but specific guidelines are not available; contraindicated in severe hepatic dysfunction

Administration

Intranasal: Prior to administration, the nasal spray applicator must be primed (pumped 4 times); spray once into each nostril; avoid deep inhalation through the nose while spraying or immediately after spraying; do not tilt head back. For further information, consult manufacturer labeling.

IM, SubQ: Administer without dilution

IV: Administer without dilution slowly over 2-3 minutes

Dosage Forms Considerations Migranal nasal solution contains caffeine 10 mg/mL

Dosage Forms Excipient information presented when available (limited, particularly for generics); consult specific product labeling.

Solution, Injection, as mesylate:

D.H.E. 45: 1 mg/mL (1 mL)

Generic: 1 mg/mL (1 mL)

Solution, Nasal, as mesylate:

Migranal: 4 mg/mL (1 mL)

Generic: 4 mg/mL (1 mL)

- **Dihydroergotamine Mesylate** *see* Dihydroergotamine *on page 659*
- **Dihydrohydroxycodeinone** *see* OxyCODONE *on page 1590*
- **Dihydromorphinone** *see* HYDROmorphone *on page 1044*
- **Dihydroxyanthracenedione** *see* MitoXANtrone *on page 1448*
- **Dihydroxyanthracenedione Dihydrochloride** *see* MitoXANtrone *on page 1448*
- **1,25 Dihydroxycholecalciferol** *see* Calcitriol *on page 338*
- **Dihydroxydeoxynorvinkaleukoblastine** *see* Vinorelbine *on page 2183*
- **Diiodohydroxyquin** *see* Iodoquinol *on page 1155*
- **Dilacor XR [DSC]** *see* Diltiazem *on page 661*
- **Dilantin** *see* Phenytoin *on page 1690*
- **Dilantin Infatabs** *see* Phenytoin *on page 1690*
- **Dilaudid** *see* HYDROmorphone *on page 1044*
- **Dilaudid-HP** *see* HYDROmorphone *on page 1044*
- **Dilt-CD [DSC]** *see* Diltiazem *on page 661*

Diltiazem (dil TYE a zem)

Medication Safety Issues

Sound-alike/look-alike issues:

Cardizem may be confused with Cardene, Cardene SR, Cardizem CD, Cardizem SR, cortisone

Cartia XT may be confused with Procardia XL

Diltiazem may be confused with Calan, diazepam, Dilantin

Tiazac may be confused with Tigan, Tiazac XC [CAN], Ziac

High alert medication:

The Institute for Safe Medication Practices (ISMP) includes this medication (IV formulation) among its list of drug classes which have a heightened risk of causing significant patient harm when used in error.

Administration issues:

Significant differences exist between oral and IV dosing. Use caution when converting from one route of administration to another.

International issues:

Cardizem [U.S., Canada, and multiple international markets] may be confused with Cardem brand name for celiprolol [Spain]

Cartia XT [U.S.] may be confused with Cartia brand name for aspirin [multiple international markets]

Dilacor XR [U.S.] may be confused with Dilacor brand name for verapamil [Brazil]

Dipen [Greece] may be confused with Depen brand name for penicillamine [U.S.]; Depin brand name for nifedipine [India]; Depon brand name for acetaminophen [Greece]

Tiazac: Brand name for diltiazem [U.S, Canada], but also the brand name for pioglitazone [Chile]

Related Information

Oral Medications That Should Not Be Crushed or Altered *on page 2476*

Brand Names: US Cardizem; Cardizem CD; Cardizem LA; Cartia XT; Dilacor XR [DSC]; Dilt-CD [DSC]; Dilt-XR; Diltiazem CD; Diltiazem HCl CD [DSC]; Diltzac [DSC]; Matzim LA; Taztia XT; Tiazac

Brand Names: Canada ACT Diltiazem CD; ACT Diltiazem T; Apo-Diltiaz; Apo-Diltiaz CD; Apo-Diltiaz SR; Apo-Diltiaz TZ; Ava-Diltiazem; Cardizem CD; Diltiazem Hydrochloride Injection; Diltiazem TZ; Diltiazem-CD; PMS-Diltiazem CD; ratio-Diltiazem CD; Sandoz-Diltiazem CD; Sandoz-Diltiazem T; Teva-Diltiazem; Teva-Diltiazem CD; Teva-Diltiazem HCL ER Capsules; Tiazac; Tiazac XC

Therapeutic Category Antianginal Agent; Antihypertensive Agent; Calcium Channel Blocker; Calcium Channel Blocker, Nondihydropyridine

Generic Availability (US) Yes

Use

Oral: Treatment of chronic stable angina or angina from coronary artery spasm; hypertension (**Note:** Only extended release products are FDA approved for the treatment of hypertension) (FDA approved in adults)

Injection: Management of atrial fibrillation or atrial flutter; paroxysmal supraventricular tachycardias (PSVT) (FDA approved in adults); has also been used for stable narrow-complex tachycardia uncontrolled or unconverted by adenosine or vagal maneuvers or if SVT is recurrent

Pregnancy Risk Factor C

Pregnancy Considerations Adverse events have been observed in animal reproduction studies. Untreated chronic maternal hypertension is associated with adverse events in the fetus, infant, and mother. If treatment for hypertension during pregnancy is needed, other agents are preferred (ACOG, 2013). The Canadian labeling contraindicates use in pregnant women or women of child-bearing potential. Women with hypertrophic cardiomyopathy who are controlled with diltiazem prior to pregnancy may continue therapy, but increased fetal monitoring is recommended (Gersh, 2011).

Breast-Feeding Considerations Diltiazem is excreted into breastmilk in concentrations similar to those in the maternal plasma (Okada, 1985). Breast-feeding is not recommended by the manufacturer.

Contraindications

Oral: Hypersensitivity to diltiazem or any component of the formulation; sick sinus syndrome (except in patients with a functioning artificial pacemaker); second- or third-degree AV block (except in patients with a functioning artificial pacemaker); severe hypotension (systolic <90 mm Hg); acute MI and pulmonary congestion

Intravenous (IV): Hypersensitivity to diltiazem or any component of the formulation; sick sinus syndrome (except in patients with a functioning artificial pacemaker); second- or third-degree AV block (except in patients with a functioning artificial pacemaker); severe hypotension (systolic <90 mm Hg); cardiogenic shock; administration concomitantly or within a few hours of the administration of IV beta-blockers; atrial fibrillation or flutter associated with accessory bypass tract (eg, Wolff-Parkinson-White syndrome); ventricular tachycardia (with wide-complex tachycardia, must determine whether origin is supraventricular or ventricular)

Canadian labeling: Additional contraindications (not in U.S. labeling): IV and Oral: Pregnancy; use in women of child-bearing potential; concurrent use with intravenous dantrolene

Warnings/Precautions Can cause first-, second-, and third-degree AV block or sinus bradycardia and risk increases with agents known to slow cardiac conduction. The most common side effect is peripheral edema; occurs within 2-3 weeks of starting therapy. Symptomatic hypotension with or without syncope can rarely occur; blood pressure must be lowered at a rate appropriate for the patient's clinical condition. Ethanol may increase risk of hypotension or vasodilation. Advise patients to avoid ethanol. Use caution when using diltiazem together with a beta-blocker; may result in conduction disturbances, hypotension, and worsened LV function. Simultaneous administration of IV diltiazem and an IV beta-blocker or administration within a few hours of each other may result in asystole and is contraindicated. Use with other agents known to either reduce SA node function and/or AV nodal conduction (eg, digoxin) or reduce sympathetic outflow (eg, clonidine) may increase the risk of serious bradycardia. Use caution in left ventricular dysfunction (may exacerbate condition). The ACCF/AHA heart failure guidelines recommend to avoid use in patients with heart failure due to lack of benefit and/or worse outcomes with calcium channel blockers in general (ACCF/AHA [Yancy, 2013]). Use with caution with hypertrophic obstructive cardiomyopathy; routine use is currently not recommended due to insufficient evidence (Maron, 2003). Use with caution in hepatic or renal dysfunction. Transient dermatologic reactions have been observed with use; if reaction persists, discontinue. May (rarely) progress to erythema multiforme or exfoliative dermatitis.

Adverse Reactions

Cardiovascular: Atrioventricular block (first degree), bradycardia, edema (including lower limb), extrasystoles, flushing, hypotension, palpitations, vasodilatation

Central nervous system: Dizziness, headache, nervousness, pain

Dermatologic: Skin rash

Endocrine & metabolic: Gout

Gastrointestinal: Constipation, diarrhea, dyspepsia, vomiting

Local: Injection site reaction (itching, burning)

Neuromuscular & skeletal: Myalgia, weakness

Respiratory: Bronchitis, dyspnea, pharyngitis, rhinitis sinus congestion

Rare but important or life-threatening: amblyopia, amnesia, atrioventricular block (second or third degree), bundle branch block, cardiac arrhythmia, cardiac failure, depression, dysgeusia, extrapyramidal reaction, gingival hyperplasia, hemolytic anemia, hypersensitivity reaction, increased serum alkaline phosphatase, increased serum ALT, increased serum AST, petechiae, skin photosensitivity, Stevens-Johnson syndrome, syncope, tachycardia, thrombocytopenia, tremor, toxic epidermal necrolysis

Drug Interactions

Metabolism/Transport Effects Substrate of CYP2C9 (minor), CYP2D6 (minor), CYP3A4 (major), P-glycoprotein; **Note:** Assignment of Major/Minor substrate status based on clinically relevant drug interaction potential; **Inhibits** CYP2C9 (weak), CYP2D6 (weak), CYP3A4 (moderate)

Avoid Concomitant Use

Avoid concomitant use of Diltiazem with any of the following: Bosutinib; Ceritinib; Conivaptan; Dantrolene; Domperidone; Fusidic Acid (Systemic); Ibrutinib; Idelalisib; Ivabradine; Lomitapide; Naloxegol; Olaparib; Pimozide; Rifampin; Simeprevir; Tolvaptan; Trabectedin; Ulipristal

Increased Effect/Toxicity

Diltiazem may increase the levels/effects of: Alfentanil; Amifostine; Amiodarone; Antihypertensives; Aprepitant; ARIPiprazole; AtorvaSTATin; Atosiban; Avanafil; Beta-Blockers; Bosentan; Bosutinib; Bradycardia-Causing Agents; Budesonide (Systemic, Oral Inhalation); Budesonide (Topical); BusPIRone; Calcium Channel Blockers (Dihydropyridine); Cannabis; CarBAMazepine; Cardiac Glycosides; Ceritinib; Cilostazol; Colchicine; CycloSPORINE (Systemic); CYP3A4 Substrates; Dapoxetine; Dofetilide; Domperidone; DOXOrubicin (Conventional); Dronabinol; Dronedarone; DULoxetine; Eletriptan; Eliglustat; Eplerenone; Everolimus; FentaNYL; Fingolimod; Fosaprepitant; Fosphenytoin; Halofantrine; Hydrocodone; Hypotensive Agents; Ibrutinib; Imatinib; Ivabradine; Ivacaftor; Lacosamide; Levodopa; Lithium; Lomitapide; Lovastatin; Lurasidone; Magnesium Salts; Midodrine; Naloxegol; Neuromuscular-Blocking Agents (Nondepolarizing); NiMODipine; Nitroprusside; Obinutuzumab; Olaparib; OxyCODONE; Phenytoin; Pimecrolimus; Pimozide; Propafenone; QuiNIDine; Ranolazine; Red Yeast Rice; RisperiDONE; RiTUXimab; Rivaroxaban; Salicylates; Salmeterol; Saxagliptin; Simeprevir; Simvastatin; Suvorexant; Tacrolimus (Systemic); Tacrolimus (Topical); Tetrahydrocannabinol; Tolvaptan; Trabectedin; Ulipristal; Vilazodone; Zopiclone; Zuclopenthixol

The levels/effects of Diltiazem may be increased by: Alfuzosin; Alpha1-Blockers; Anilidopiperidine Opioids; Antifungal Agents (Azole Derivatives, Systemic); Aprepitant; AtorvaSTATin; Barbiturates; Bretylium; Brimonidine (Topical); Calcium Channel Blockers (Dihydropyridine); Cimetidine; CloNIDine; Conivaptan; CycloSPORINE (Systemic); CYP3A4 Inhibitors (Moderate); CYP3A4 Inhibitors (Strong); Dantrolene; Dasatinib; Diazoxide; Dronedarone; Fluconazole; Fosaprepitant; Fusidic Acid (Systemic); Grapefruit Juice; Herbs (Hypotensive Properties); Idelalisib; Ivabradine; Lovastatin; Luliconazole; Macrolide Antibiotics; Magnesium Salts; MAO Inhibitors; Mifepristone; Netupitant; Nicorandil; Palbociclib; Pentoxifylline; P-glycoprotein/ABCB1 Inhibitors; Phosphodiesterase 5 Inhibitors; Prostacyclin Analogues; Protease Inhibitors; Regorafenib; Ruxolitinib; Simvastatin; Stiripentol; Tofacitinib

Decreased Effect

Diltiazem may decrease the levels/effects of: Clopidogrel; Ifosfamide

The levels/effects of Diltiazem may be decreased by: Barbiturates; Bosentan; Calcium Salts; CarBAMazepine; Colestipol; CYP3A4 Inducers (Moderate); CYP3A4 Inducers (Strong); Dabrafenib; Deferasirox; Efavirenz; Herbs (Hypertensive Properties); Methylphenidate; Mitotane; Nafcillin; P-glycoprotein/ABCB1 Inducers; Rifampin; Rifamycin Derivatives; Siltuximab; St Johns Wort; Tocilizumab; Yohimbine

Food Interactions Diltiazem serum levels may be elevated if taken with food. Serum concentrations were not altered by grapefruit juice in small clinical trials.

Storage/Stability

Capsule, tablet: Store at room temperature. Protect from light.

Solution for injection: Store in refrigerator at 2°C to 8°C (36°F to 46°F); do not freeze. May be stored at room temperature for up to 1 month. Following dilution to ≤1 mg/mL with $D_5{}^1/_2NS$, D_5W, or NS, solution is stable for 24 hours at room temperature or under refrigeration.

Mechanism of Action Nondihydropyridine calcium channel blocker which inhibits calcium ion from entering the "slow channels" or select voltage-sensitive areas of vascular smooth muscle and myocardium during depolarization, producing a relaxation of coronary vascular smooth muscle and coronary vasodilation; increases myocardial oxygen delivery in patients with vasospastic angina

Pharmacodynamics

Onset of action:

Oral: Tablet: Immediate release: 30 to 60 minutes

Parenteral (IV bolus): Within 3 minutes

Maximum effect:

Antiarrhythmic (IV bolus): 2 to 7 minutes

Antihypertensive (Oral; multiple dosing): Within 2 weeks

Pharmacokinetics (Adult data unless noted)

Absorption: 80%

Distribution: V_d: 1.7 L/kg; appears in breast milk

Protein binding: 70% to 80%

Metabolism: Extensive first-pass effect; metabolized in the liver; desacetyldiltiazem is an active metabolite (25% to 50% as potent as diltiazem based on coronary vasodilation effects); desacetyldiltiazem may accumulate with plasma concentrations 10% to 20% of diltiazem levels

Bioavailability: Oral: ~40%

Half-life: 3 to 4.5 hours, up to 8 hours with chronic high dosing

Time to peak serum concentration:

Tablet: Immediate release: 2 to 4 hours

Cardizem CD: 10 to 14 hours

Cardizem LA, Matzim LA: 11 to 18 hours

Cardizem SR: 6 to 11 hours

Dilacor XR: 4 to 6 hours

Elimination: In urine and bile mostly as metabolites; 2% to 4% excreted as unchanged drug in urine

Dialysis: Not dialyzable

Dosing: Usual

Hypertension: Oral:

Children: Minimal information available; some centers use the following: Initial: 1.5 to 2 mg/kg/day in 3 to 4 divided doses (extended release formulations may be dosed once or twice daily); maximum dose: 3.5 mg/kg/day; some centers use a maximum dose of 6 mg/kg/day up to 360 mg/day (Flynn 2000); **Note:** Doses up to 8 mg/kg/day given in 4 divided doses have been used for investigational therapy of Duchenne muscular dystrophy.

Adolescents ≥18 years and Adults:

Capsule, extended release (once-daily dosing): **Note:** Usual dosage range (JNC 7): 180 to 420 mg once daily

Cardizem CD, Cartia XT: Initial: 180 to 240 mg once daily; may increase dose after 14 days; usual: 240 to 360 mg once daily; maximum: 480 mg once daily

Dilacor XR, Diltia XT, Dilt-XR: Initial: 180 to 240 mg once daily; may increase after 14 days; usual: 180 to 480 mg once daily; maximum: 540 mg once daily

Taztia XT Tiazac: Initial: 120 to 240 mg once daily; may increase dose after 14 days; maximum: 540 mg once daily

Capsule, extended release (twice-daily dosing): Initial: 60 to 120 mg twice daily; may increase dose after 14 days; usual: 240 to 360 mg/day

Note: Diltiazem is available as a generic intended for either once- or twice-daily dosing, depending on the formulation; verify appropriate extended release capsule formulation is administered.

Tablet, extended release: Cardizem LA, Matzim LA: Initial: 180 to 240 mg once daily; may increase dose after 14 days; limited clinical experience with doses >360 mg/day; maximum dose: 540 mg once daily; usual dosage range (JNC 7): 120 to 540 mg once daily

Tablet, immediate release: 30 to 120 mg 3 to 4 times/day; dosage should be increased gradually, at 1- to 2-day intervals until optimum response is obtained; usual maintenance dose: 180 to 360 mg/day

Angina: Adults: Oral:

Capsule, extended release:

Dilacor XR, Dilt-XR, Diltia XT: Initial: 120 mg once daily; titrate over 7 to 14 days; usual dose range: 120 to 320 mg/day: maximum: 480 mg/day

Cardizem CD, Cartia XT: Initial: 120 to 180 mg once daily; titrate over 7 to 14 days; usual dose range: 120 to 320 mg/day; maximum: 480 mg/day

Tiazac, Taztia XT: Initial: 120 to 180 mg once daily; titrate over 7 to 14 days; usual dose range: 120 to 320 mg/day; maximum: 540 mg/day

Tablet, extended release (Cardizem LA, Matzim LA): 180 mg once daily; may increase at 7- to 14-day intervals; usual dose range: 120 to 320 mg/day; maximum: 360 mg/day

Tablet, immediate release (Cardizem): Usual starting dose: 30 mg 4 times/day; titrate dose gradually at 1- to 2-day intervals; usual dose range: 120 to 320 mg/day

Atrial fibrillation, atrial flutter, PSVT: Adults: IV:

Initial bolus dose: 0.25 mg/kg actual body weight over 2 minutes (average adult dose: 20 mg); ACLS guideline recommends 15 to 20 mg

Repeat bolus dose (may be administered after 15 minutes if the response is inadequate): 0.35 mg/kg actual body weight over 2 minutes (average adult dose: 25 mg); ACLS guideline recommends 20 to 25 mg

Continuous infusion (infusions >24 hours or infusion rates >15 mg/hour are not recommended): Initial infusion rate of 10 mg/hour; rate may be increased in 5 mg/hour increments up to 15 mg/hour as needed; some patients may respond to an initial rate of 5 mg/hour

If diltiazem injection is administered by continuous infusion for >24 hours, the possibility of decreased diltiazem clearance, prolonged elimination half-life, and increased diltiazem and/or diltiazem metabolite plasma concentrations should be considered.

Conversion from IV diltiazem to oral diltiazem: Start first oral dose approximately 3 hours after bolus dose

Oral dose (mg/day) is approximately equal to [(rate in mg/hour x 3) + 3] x 10; Note: Dose per day may need to be divided depending on formulation used

3 mg/hour = 120 mg/day

5 mg/hour = 180 mg/day

7 mg/hour = 240 mg/day

11 mg/hour = 360 mg/day (maximum recommended dose)

Usual Infusion Concentrations: Pediatric IV infusion: 1 mg/mL

Preparation for Administration Parenteral: Continuous IV infusion: Further dilute with NS, D_5W, or $D_5{}^1/_2NS$ to a maximum final concentration of 1 mg/mL

Administration

Oral:

Tablet, immediate release (Cardizem): Administer before meals and at bedtime

Extended release preparations (CD, LA, XR, XT, Tiazac): Swallow whole; do not chew, break, or crush. Do not open Dilacor XR capsules.

Dilacor XR, Dilt-XR, Diltia XT: Take in the morning on an empty stomach

Cardizem CD, Cardizem LA, Cartia XT, Matzim LA: May be administered with or without food, but should be administered consistently with relation to meals; administer with a full glass of water

Taztia XT and Tiazac capsules (extended release) may be opened and sprinkled on applesauce; swallow applesauce immediately, do not chew; follow with some cool water (adults: 1 glass) to ensure complete swallowing; do not use hot applesauce; do not divide capsule contents (ie, do not administer partial doses); do not store mixture of applesauce and capsule contents, use immediately

Parenteral:

IV bolus: Adults: Infuse over 2 minutes; response to bolus may require several minutes to reach maximum.

Continuous IV infusion: Continuous infusion should be via infusion pump. Response may persist for several hours after infusion is discontinued.

Monitoring Parameters Blood pressure, heart rate, renal function, liver enzymes; ECG with IV therapy

Ventricular rate control in patients with atrial fibrillation or flutter (adults): Patients who respond, usually have at least a 20% decrease in ventricular response rate or a rate <100 beats/minute.

Additional Information Cartia XT is the generic version of Cardizem CD; Diltia XT and Dilt-XR are the generic versions of Dilacor XR; Taztia XT is the generic version of Tiazac; Matzim LA is the generic version of Cardizem LA.

Dosage Forms Excipient information presented when available (limited, particularly for generics); consult specific product labeling. [DSC] = Discontinued product

Capsule Extended Release 12 Hour, Oral, as hydrochloride:

Generic: 60 mg, 90 mg, 120 mg

Capsule Extended Release 24 Hour, Oral, as hydrochloride:

Cardizem CD: 120 mg, 180 mg, 240 mg, 300 mg, 360 mg [contains brilliant blue fcf (fd&c blue #1)]

Cartia XT: 120 mg, 180 mg, 240 mg, 300 mg

Dilacor XR: 240 mg [DSC]

Dilt-CD: 120 mg [DSC]

Dilt-CD: 180 mg [DSC], 240 mg [DSC] [contains brilliant blue fcf (fd&c blue #1)]

Dilt-CD: 300 mg [DSC]

Dilt-XR: 120 mg, 180 mg, 240 mg [contains brilliant blue fcf (fd&c blue #1), fd&c red #40, fd&c yellow #10 (quinoline yellow)]

Diltiazem CD: 120 mg

Diltiazem CD: 180 mg [contains brilliant blue fcf (fd&c blue #1), fd&c yellow #10 (quinoline yellow)]

Diltiazem CD: 240 mg [contains fd&c yellow #10 (quinoline yellow)]

Diltiazem HCl CD: 360 mg [DSC] [contains brilliant blue fcf (fd&c blue #1)]

Diltzac: 120 mg [DSC] [contains brilliant blue fcf (fd&c blue #1)]

Diltzac: 180 mg [DSC]

Diltzac: 240 mg [DSC], 300 mg [DSC] [contains brilliant blue fcf (fd&c blue #1)]

Diltzac: 360 mg [DSC]
Taztia XT: 120 mg, 180 mg, 240 mg, 300 mg, 360 mg
Tiazac: 120 mg, 180 mg, 240 mg, 300 mg, 360 mg, 420 mg [contains brilliant blue fcf (fd&c blue #1), fd&c red #40]
Generic: 120 mg, 180 mg, 240 mg, 300 mg, 360 mg, 420 mg

Solution, Intravenous, as hydrochloride:
Generic: 25 mg/5 mL (5 mL, 25 mL); 50 mg/10 mL (10 mL); 125 mg/25 mL (25 mL)

Solution, Intravenous, as hydrochloride [preservative free]:
Generic: 50 mg/10 mL (10 mL); 125 mg/25 mL (25 mL)

Solution Reconstituted, Intravenous, as hydrochloride:
Generic: 100 mg (1 ea)

Tablet, Oral, as hydrochloride:
Cardizem: 30 mg
Cardizem: 30 mg [contains fd&c blue #1 aluminum lake, fd&c yellow #10 aluminum lake]
Cardizem: 60 mg [DSC] [scored]
Cardizem: 60 mg [scored; contains fd&c blue #1 aluminum lake, fd&c yellow #10 aluminum lake, fd&c yellow #6 aluminum lake, methylparaben]
Cardizem: 90 mg [DSC] [scored]
Cardizem: 120 mg [scored; contains fd&c yellow #10 aluminum lake, fd&c yellow #6 aluminum lake, methylparaben]
Generic: 30 mg, 60 mg, 90 mg, 120 mg

Tablet Extended Release 24 Hour, Oral, as hydrochloride:
Cardizem LA: 120 mg, 180 mg, 240 mg, 300 mg, 360 mg, 420 mg
Matzim LA: 180 mg, 240 mg, 300 mg, 360 mg, 420 mg
Generic: 180 mg, 240 mg, 300 mg, 360 mg, 420 mg

Extemporaneous Preparations A 12 mg/mL oral suspension may be made from tablets (regular, not extended release) and one of three different vehicles (cherry syrup, a 1:1 mixture of Ora-Sweet® and Ora-Plus®, or a 1:1 mixture of Ora-Sweet® SF and Ora-Plus®). Crush sixteen 90 mg tablets in a mortar and reduce to a fine powder. Add 10 mL of the chosen vehicle and mix to a uniform paste; mix while adding the vehicle in incremental proportions to **almost** 120 mL; transfer to a calibrated bottle, rinse mortar with vehicle, and add quantity of vehicle sufficient to make 120 mL. Label "shake well" and "protect from light". Stable for 60 days when stored in amber plastic prescription bottles in the dark at room temperature or refrigerated.

Allen LV and Erickson MA, "Stability of Baclofen, Captopril, Diltiazem Hydrochloride, Dipyridamole, and Flecainide Acetate in Extemporaneously Compounded Oral Liquids," *Am J Health Syst Pharm*, 1996, 53(18):2179-84.

◆ **Diltiazem CD** *see* Diltiazem *on page 661*

◆ **Diltiazem-CD (Can)** *see* Diltiazem *on page 661*

◆ **Diltiazem HCl CD [DSC]** *see* Diltiazem *on page 661*

◆ **Diltiazem Hydrochloride** *see* Diltiazem *on page 661*

◆ **Diltiazem Hydrochloride Injection (Can)** *see* Diltiazem *on page 661*

◆ **Diltiazem TZ (Can)** *see* Diltiazem *on page 661*

◆ **Dilt-XR** *see* Diltiazem *on page 661*

◆ **Diltzac [DSC]** *see* Diltiazem *on page 661*

DimenhyDRINATE (dye men HYE dri nate)

Medication Safety Issues

Sound-alike/look-alike issues:

DimenhyDRINATE may be confused with diphenhydrAMINE

BEERS Criteria medication:

This drug may be potentially inappropriate for use in geriatric patients (Quality of evidence - varies based on comorbidity; Strength of recommendation - varies based on comorbidity)

Brand Names: US Dramamine [OTC]; Driminate [OTC]; Motion Sickness [OTC]

Brand Names: Canada Apo-Dimenhydrinate [OTC]; Children's Motion Sickness Liquid [OTC]; Dimenhydrinate Injection; Dinate [OTC]; Gravol IM; Gravol [OTC]; Jamp-Dimenhydrinate [OTC]; Nauseatol [OTC]; Novo-Dimenate [OTC]; PMS-Dimenhydrinate [OTC]; Sandoz-Dimenhydrinate [OTC]; Travel Tabs [OTC]

Therapeutic Category Antiemetic; Antihistamine

Generic Availability (US) May be product dependent

Use Treatment and prevention of nausea, vertigo, and vomiting associated with motion sickness (oral tablets: FDA approved in children ≥2 years and adults; IV product: FDA approved in infants, children, and adults)

Pregnancy Risk Factor B

Pregnancy Considerations Adverse events have not been observed in animal reproduction studies. The risk of fetal abnormalities was not increased following maternal use of dimenhydrinate during any trimester of pregnancy. Dimenhydrinate is recommended for the treatment of nausea and vomiting of pregnancy. Dimenhydrinate may have an oxytocic effect if used during labor.

Breast-Feeding Considerations Small amounts of dimenhydrinate are excreted into breast milk. Irritability in a breast-feeding infant was noted in one study. According to the manufacturer, the decision to continue or discontinue breast-feeding during therapy should take into account the risk of exposure to the infant and the benefits of treatment to the mother. Antihistamines may decrease maternal serum prolactin concentrations when administered prior to the establishment of nursing.

Contraindications Hypersensitivity to dimenhydrinate or any component of the formulation; neonates (injection contains benzyl alcohol)

Warnings/Precautions Causes sedation, caution must be used in performing tasks which require alertness (eg, operating machinery or driving). May mask the symptoms of ototoxicity, use caution if used in conjunction with antibiotics that have the potential to cause ototoxicity. Effects may be potentiated when used with other sedative drugs or ethanol. Use with caution in patients with angle-closure glaucoma, asthma, pyloroduodenal obstruction (including stenotic peptic ulcer), urinary tract obstruction (including bladder neck obstruction and symptomatic prostatic hyperplasia), hyperthyroidism, increased intraocular pressure, and cardiovascular disease (including hypertension and tachycardia). May be inappropriate for use in older adults depending on comorbidities (eg, dementia, delirium) due to its potent anticholinergic effects (Beers Criteria). Use with caution in the elderly; may be more sensitive to adverse effects. Antihistamines may cause excitation in young children. Not for OTC use in children <2 years of age. Parenteral formulation should not be injected intra-arterially.

Benzyl alcohol and derivatives: Some dosage forms may contain benzyl alcohol; large amounts of benzyl alcohol (≥99 mg/kg/day) have been associated with a potentially fatal toxicity ("gasping syndrome") in neonates; the "gasping syndrome" consists of metabolic acidosis, respiratory distress, gasping respirations, CNS dysfunction (including convulsions, intracranial hemorrhage), hypotension and cardiovascular collapse (AAP, 1997; CDC, 1982); some data suggests that benzoate displaces bilirubin from protein binding sites (Ahlfors, 2001); avoid or use dosage forms containing benzyl alcohol with caution in neonates. See manufacturer's labeling.

Adverse Reactions

Cardiovascular: Tachycardia

Central nervous system: Dizziness, drowsiness, excitation, headache, insomnia, lassitude, nervousness, restlessness

Dermatologic: Rash

Gastrointestinal: Anorexia, epigastric distress, nausea, xerostomia
Genitourinary: Dysuria
Ocular: Blurred vision
Respiratory: Thickening of bronchial secretions

Drug Interactions

Metabolism/Transport Effects None known.

Avoid Concomitant Use

Avoid concomitant use of DimenhyDRINATE with any of the following: Aclidinium; Azelastine (Nasal); Eluxadoline; Glucagon; Ipratropium (Oral Inhalation); Orphenadrine; Paraldehyde; Potassium Chloride; Thalidomide; Tiotropium; Umeclidinium

Increased Effect/Toxicity

DimenhyDRINATE may increase the levels/effects of: AbobotulinumtoxinA; Alcohol (Ethyl); Analgesics (Opioid); Anticholinergic Agents; Azelastine (Nasal); Buprenorphine; CNS Depressants; Eluxadoline; Glucagon; Hydrocodone; Methotrimeprazine; Metyrosine; Mirabegron; Mirtazapine; OnabotulinumtoxinA; Orphenadrine; Paraldehyde; Potassium Chloride; Pramipexole; RimabotulinumtoxinB; ROPINIRole; Rotigotine; Selective Serotonin Reuptake Inhibitors; Suvorexant; Thalidomide; Thiazide Diuretics; Tiotropium; Topiramate; Zolpidem

The levels/effects of DimenhyDRINATE may be increased by: Aclidinium; Brimonidine (Topical); Cannabis; Doxylamine; Dronabinol; Droperidol; HydrOXYzine; Ipratropium (Oral Inhalation); Kava Kava; Magnesium Sulfate; Methotrimeprazine; Mianserin; Nabilone; Perampanel; Pramlintide; Rufinamide; Sodium Oxybate; Tapentadol; Tetrahydrocannabinol; Umeclidinium

Decreased Effect

DimenhyDRINATE may decrease the levels/effects of: Acetylcholinesterase Inhibitors; Benzylpenicilloyl Polylysine; Betahistine; Hyaluronidase; Itopride; Metoclopramide; Secretin

The levels/effects of DimenhyDRINATE may be decreased by: Acetylcholinesterase Inhibitors; Amphetamines

Storage/Stability
Solution for injection: Store at 20°C to 25°C (68°F to 77°F). Protect from light.
Suppository [Canadian product]: Store at 15°C to 30°C (59°F to 86°F).

Mechanism of Action Competes with histamine for H_1-receptor sites on effector cells in the gastrointestinal tract, blood vessels, and respiratory tract; blocks chemoreceptor trigger zone, diminishes vestibular stimulation, and depresses labyrinthine function through its central anticholinergic activity

Pharmacodynamics
Onset of action: Oral: Within 15-30 minutes
Duration: ~3-6 hours

Pharmacokinetics (Adult data unless noted)
Absorption: Well absorbed from the GI tract
Metabolism: Extensive in the liver

Dosing: Usual
Children 2-5 years:
Oral:
12.5-25 mg every 6-8 hours; maximum dose: 75 mg/day
or
5 mg/kg/day or 150 mg/m²/day in 4 divided doses, not to exceed 75 mg/day
IM:
1.25 mg/kg
or
37.5 mg/m² 4 times/day; maximum: 75 mg/day
Children: 6-12 years:
Oral:
25-50 mg every 6-8 hours; maximum dose: 150 mg/day
or
5 mg/kg/day or 150 mg/m²/day in 4 divided doses, not to exceed 150 mg/day
IM:
1.25 mg /kg
or
37.5 mg/m² 4 times/day; maximum: 150 mg/day
Children ≥12 years and Adults:
Oral: 50-100 mg every 4-6 hours, not to exceed 400 mg/day
IM, IV: 50-100 mg every 4 hours

Preparation for Administration Parenteral:
IM: No dilution required
IV: Dilute each 50 mg in 10 mL NS

Administration
Oral: Administer with food or water
Parenteral:
IM: Administer undiluted
IV:
Pediatric patients: The IV route is not recommended (per manufacturer)
Adults: May further dilute and administer IV over 2 minutes; do not inject intra-arterially

Dosage Forms Excipient information presented when available (limited, particularly for generics); consult specific product labeling.
Solution, Injection:
Generic: 50 mg/mL (1 mL)
Tablet, Oral:
Dramamine: 50 mg
Dramamine: 50 mg [scored]
Driminate: 50 mg [scored]
Motion Sickness: 50 mg [scored]
Generic: 50 mg
Tablet Chewable, Oral:
Dramamine: 50 mg [contains aspartame, fd&c yellow #6 aluminum lake]
Dramamine: 50 mg [scored; contains aspartame, fd&c yellow #6 aluminum lake]

◆ **Dimenhydrinate Injection (Can)** *see* DimenhyDRINATE *on page 664*

Dimercaprol (dye mer KAP role)

Brand Names: US Bal in Oil

Therapeutic Category Antidote, Arsenic Toxicity; Antidote, Gold Toxicity; Antidote, Lead Toxicity; Antidote, Mercury Toxicity; Chelating Agent, Parenteral

Generic Availability (US) Yes

Use Antidote to gold, arsenic (except arsine), or acute mercury poisoning (except nonalkyl mercury); adjunct to edetate CALCIUM disodium in acute lead poisoning [FDA approved in pediatric patients (age not specified) and adults]

Pregnancy Risk Factor C

Pregnancy Considerations Animal reproduction studies have not been conducted. There are no adequate and well-controlled studies in pregnant women.

Lead poisoning: Lead is known to cross the placenta in amounts related to maternal plasma levels. Prenatal lead exposure may be associated with adverse events such as spontaneous abortion, preterm delivery, decreased birth weight, and impaired neurodevelopment. Some adverse outcomes may occur with maternal blood lead levels <10 mcg/dL. In addition, pregnant women exposed to lead may have an increased risk of gestational hypertension. Consider chelation therapy in pregnant women with confirmed blood lead levels ≥45 mcg/dL (pregnant women with blood lead levels ≥70 mcg/dL should be considered for chelation regardless of trimester); consultation with experts in lead poisoning and high-risk pregnancy is recommended. Encephalopathic pregnant women should be chelated regardless of trimester (CDC, 2010).

Breast-Feeding Considerations It is not known if dimercaprol is excreted in breast milk; however, it is not absorbed orally, which would limit the exposure to a nursing infant. When used for the treatment of lead poisoning, the amount of lead in breast milk may range from 0.6% to 3% of the maternal serum concentration. Women with confirmed blood lead levels ≥40 mcg/dL should not initiated breast-feeding; pumping and discarding breast milk is recommended until blood lead levels are <40 mcg/dL, at which point breast-feeding may resume (CDC, 2010). Calcium supplementation may reduce the amount of lead in breast milk.

Contraindications Hepatic insufficiency (unless due to arsenic poisoning)

Warnings/Precautions Potentially a nephrotoxic drug, use with caution in patients with oliguria; keep urine alkaline to protect the kidneys (prevents dimercaprol-metal complex breakdown). Discontinue or use with extreme caution if renal insufficiency develops during treatment. Hemodialysis may be used to remove dimercaprol-metal chelate in patients with renal dysfunction. Use with caution in patients with glucose 6-phosphate dehydrogenase deficiency; may increase the risk of hemolytic anemia. Administer all injections deep IM at different sites; **not** for IV administration. Fevers may occur in ~30% of children and may persistent for the duration of therapy. Product contains peanut oil; use caution in patients with peanut allergy; medication for the treatment of hypersensitivity reactions should be available for immediate use. When used in the treatment of lead poisoning, investigate, identify, and remove sources of lead exposure prior to treatment; do not permit patients to re-enter the contaminated environment until lead abatement has been completed. Primary care providers should consult experts in the chemotherapy of heavy metal toxicity before using chelation drug therapy. Dimercaprol is not indicated for the treatment of iron, cadmium, or selenium poisoning; use in these patients may result in toxic dimercaprol-metal complexes.

Benzyl alcohol and derivatives: Some dosage forms may contain sodium benzoate/benzoic acid; benzoic acid (benzoate) is a metabolite of benzyl alcohol; large amounts of benzyl alcohol (≥99 mg/kg/day) have been associated with a potentially fatal toxicity ("gasping syndrome") in neonates; the "gasping syndrome" consists of metabolic acidosis, respiratory distress, gasping respirations, CNS dysfunction (including convulsions, intracranial hemorrhage), hypotension, and cardiovascular collapse (AAP, 1997; CDC, 1982); some data suggests that benzoate displaces bilirubin from protein binding sites (Ahlfors, 2001); avoid or use dosage forms containing benzyl alcohol derivative with caution in neonates. See manufacturer's labeling.

Adverse Reactions

Cardiovascular: Chest pain, hypertension (dose related), tachycardia (dose related)

Central nervous system: Anxiety, fever, headache, nervousness

Dermatologic: Abscess

Gastrointestinal: Abdominal pain, burning sensation (lips, mouth, throat), nausea, salivation, throat irritation/pain, vomiting

Genitourinary: Burning sensation (penis)

Hematologic: Leukopenia (polymorphonuclear)

Local: Injection site pain

Neuromuscular & skeletal: Paresthesias (hand), weakness

Ocular: Blepharospasm, conjunctivitis, lacrimation

Renal: Acute renal insufficiency

Respiratory: Rhinorrhea, throat constriction

Miscellaneous: Diaphoresis

Drug Interactions

Metabolism/Transport Effects None known.

Avoid Concomitant Use

Avoid concomitant use of Dimercaprol with any of the following: Iron Salts; Multivitamins/Minerals (with ADEK, Folate, Iron)

Increased Effect/Toxicity

Dimercaprol may increase the levels/effects of: Iron Salts; Multivitamins/Minerals (with ADEK, Folate, Iron)

Decreased Effect There are no known significant interactions involving a decrease in effect.

Storage/Stability Store at 20°C to 25°C (68°F to 77°F).

Mechanism of Action Sulfhydryl group combines with ions of various heavy metals to form relatively stable, nontoxic, soluble chelates which are excreted in urine

Pharmacokinetics (Adult data unless noted)

Absorption: IM: Rapid; Oral: Not absorbed

Distribution: To all tissues including the brain

Metabolism: Hepatic; rapid to inactive metabolites

Time to peak serum concentration: 30-60 minutes

Elimination: Urine and feces via bile

Dosing: Usual Infants, Children, Adolescents, and Adults: **Note:** Premedication with a histamine H_1 antagonist (eg, diphenhydramine) is recommended.

Arsenic or gold poisoning (acute, mild): IM: 2.5 mg/kg/dose every 6 hours for 2 days, then every 12 hours on the third day, and once daily thereafter for 10 days

Arsenic or gold poisoning (acute, severe): IM: 3 mg/kg/dose every 4 hours for 2 days then every 6 hours on the third day, then every 12 hours thereafter for 10 days

Mercury poisoning (acute): IM: 5 mg/kg initially followed by 2.5 mg/kg/dose 1-2 times/day for 10 days

Lead poisoning: IM: **Note:** For the treatment of high blood lead levels in children, the CDC recommends chelation treatment when blood lead levels are >45 mcg/dL (CDC, 2002); however, dimercaprol is only recommended for use (in combination with edetate CALCIUM disodium) in children whose blood lead levels are >70 mcg/dL or in children with lead encephalopathy (AAP, 2005; Chandran, 2010). In adults, available guidelines recommend chelation therapy with blood lead levels >50 mcg/dL and significant symptoms; chelation therapy may also be indicated with blood lead levels ≥100 mcg/dL and/or symptoms (Kosnett, 2007).

Blood lead levels ≥70 mcg/dL, symptomatic lead poisoning, or lead encephalopathy (in conjunction with edetate CALCIUM disodium): 4 mg/kg/dose every 4 hours for 2-7 days; duration of therapy of at least 3 days is recommended by some experts (Chandran, 2010). **Note:** Begin treatment with edetate CALCIUM disodium with the second dimercaprol dose.

Dosing adjustment in renal impairment: There are no adjustments provided in manufacturer's labeling. Use with extreme caution or discontinue if acute renal insufficiency develops during therapy.

Dosing adjustment in hepatic impairment: Use is contraindicated in hepatic insufficiency (except in cases of postarsenical jaundice).

Administration Parenteral: Administer undiluted, **deep** IM; rotate injection sites. Keep urine alkaline to protect renal function. When used in the treatment of lead poisoning, administer in a separate site from edetate CALCIUM disodium

Monitoring Parameters Renal function, urine pH, infusion-related reactions

For lead poisoning: Blood lead levels (baseline and 7-21 days after completing chelation therapy); hemoglobin or hematocrit, iron status, free erythrocyte protoporphyrin, or zinc protoporphyrin; neurodevelopmental changes

For arsenic poisoning: Urine arsenic concentration

Test Interactions Iodine I^{131} thyroidal uptake values may be decreased

Dosage Forms Excipient information presented when available (limited, particularly for generics); consult specific product labeling.

Solution, Intramuscular:

Bal in Oil: 100 mg/mL (3 mL) [contains benzyl benzoate, peanut oil]

◆ **2,3-Dimercapto-1-Propanol** *see* Dimercaprol *on page 665*

◆ **2,3-Dimercaptopropan-1-Ol** *see* Dimercaprol *on page 665*

◆ **2,3-Dimercaptopropanol** *see* Dimercaprol *on page 665*

◆ **β,β-Dimethylcysteine** *see* PenicillAMINE *on page 1652*

Dimethyl Sulfoxide (dye meth il sul FOKS ide)

Medication Safety Issues

Sound-alike/look-alike issues:

Dimethyl sulfoxide may be confused with dimethyl fumarate

Related Information

Management of Drug Extravasations *on page 2298*

Brand Names: US Rimso-50

Brand Names: Canada Dimethyl Sulfoxide Irrigation, USP; Kemsol; Rimso-50

Therapeutic Category Urinary Tract Product

Generic Availability (US) No

Use Symptomatic relief of interstitial cystitis (FDA approved in adults); has also been used for management of extravasation of certain chemotherapeutic agents (eg, anthracyclines, mitomycin)

Pregnancy Risk Factor C

Pregnancy Considerations Adverse events have been observed in some animal reproduction studies.

Breast-Feeding Considerations It is not known if dimethyl sulfoxide is excreted in breast milk. The manufacturer recommends that caution be exercised when administering dimethyl sulfoxide to nursing women.

Contraindications There are no contraindications listed in the manufacturer's labeling.

Warnings/Precautions For bladder instillation or topical administration for extravasation management (off-label use) only; not for IV or IM administration. Do not use in patients receiving dexrazoxane for anthracycline extravasation (Mourdisen, 2007); dimethyl sulfoxide (DMSO) may diminish dexrazoxane efficacy. Hypersensitivity reactions with intravesical administration have been reported rarely; hypersensitivity has also occurred with topical administration. If anaphylactoid symptoms occur, manage appropriately. Use with caution in patients with urinary tract malignancy; may be harmful due to vasodilatory effects. Lens changes and opacities have been observed in animal studies; full eye exams (including slit lamp) are recommended prior to use and periodically during treatment. A garlic-like taste may occur, beginning a few minutes after instillation and lasting for several hours. Garlic odor on the breath and skin may also occur and persist for up to 3 days. Bladder discomfort may occur; generally diminishes with repeated administration.

Adverse Reactions

Dermatologic: Body odor (garlic; duration: Up to 72 hours)

Gastrointestinal: Halitosis/unpleasant taste (garlic; onset: Within a few minutes after instillation; duration: Up to 72 hours)

Genitourinary: Bladder pain, cystitis (transient)

Local: Localized erythema (topical application; Perez Fidalgo, 2012)

Hypersensitivity: Hypersensitivity

Postmarketing and/or case reports: Contact dermatitis, cystitis (eosinophilic), pigment deposits on lens

Drug Interactions

Metabolism/Transport Effects Inhibits CYP2C19 (weak), CYP2C9 (weak)

Avoid Concomitant Use

Avoid concomitant use of Dimethyl Sulfoxide with any of the following: Dexrazoxane

Increased Effect/Toxicity

Dimethyl Sulfoxide may increase the levels/effects of: Sulindac

Decreased Effect

Dimethyl Sulfoxide may decrease the levels/effects of: Dexrazoxane

Storage/Stability Store at 20°C to 25°C (68°F to 77°F). Protect from strong light.

Mechanism of Action For management of cystitis, dimethyl sulfoxide (DMSO) has anti-inflammatory, analgesic, mast cell inhibition, and muscle relaxing effects (Chancellor, 2004). DMSO also has free-radical scavenger properties, which increases removal of vesicant drugs from tissues to minimize tissue damage in extravasation management (Perez Fidalgo, 2012).

Pharmacokinetics (Adult data unless noted)

Absorption: Topical: Well absorbed from application site

Distribution: Topical: Rapidly penetrates tissues (Bertelli, 1995)

Metabolism: Oxidation to dimethyl sulfone; reduction to dimethyl sulfide

Elimination: Urine and feces (as unchanged drug and dimethyl sulfone); skin and lungs (dimethyl sulfide)

Dosing: Usual

Pediatric: **Extravasation management, anthracyclines or mitomycin:** Topical DMSO: Apply to a region covering twice the affected area every 8 hours for 7 days; begin within 10 minutes of extravasation; do not cover with a dressing (Pérez Fidalgo, 2012)

Adult:

Extravasation management, anthracyclines or mitomycin: Topical DMSO: Apply to a region covering twice the affected area every 8 hours for 7 days; begin within 10 minutes of extravasation; do not cover with a dressing (Pérez Fidalgo, 2012)

Interstitial cystitis: Bladder instillation: Instill 50 mL directly into bladder and retain for 15 minutes; repeat every 2 weeks until symptoms are relieved, then increase intervals between treatments

Administration Not for IV or IM use

Topical: Extravasation management, anthracyclines or mitomycin: Stop vesicant infusion immediately and disconnect IV line (leave needle/cannula in place); gently aspirate extravasated solution from the IV line (do **NOT** flush the line); remove needle/cannula; elevate extremity. Apply DMSO topically (within 10 minutes of extravasation) to extravasation site, covering an area twice the size of extravasation; allow to air dry; do not cover with a dressing (Pérez Fidalgo, 2012).

Intravesical: Interstitial cystitis: Instill directly into the bladder via catheter or syringe. To reduce bladder spasm, apply an analgesic lubricant (eg, lidocaine jelly) to urethra prior to catheter insertion; belladonna and opium suppositories may be of benefit.

Dosage Forms Excipient information presented when available (limited, particularly for generics); consult specific product labeling.

Solution, Intravesical:

Rimso-50: 50% (50 mL)

◆ **Dimethylsulfoxide** *see* Dimethyl Sulfoxide *on page 667*

◆ **Dimethyl Sulfoxide Irrigation, USP (Can)** *see* Dimethyl Sulfoxide *on page 667*

DiphenhydrAMINE (Systemic)

(dye fen HYE dra meen)

Medication Safety Issues

Sound-alike/look-alike issues:

DiphenhydrAMINE may be confused with desipramine, dicyclomine, dimenhyDRINATE

Benadryl may be confused with benazepril, Bentyl, Benylin, Caladryl

BEERS Criteria medication:

This drug may be potentially inappropriate for use in geriatric patients (Quality of evidence - moderate; Strength of recommendation - strong).

International issues:

Benadryl brand name for diphenhydramine [U.S., Canada], but also the brand name for cetirizine [Great Britain, Phillipines] and acrivastine and pseudoephedrine [Great Britain]

Sominex brand name for diphenhydramine [U.S., Canada], but also the brand name for promethazine [Great Britain]; valerian [Chile]

Brand Names: US Aler-Dryl [OTC]; Allergy Relief Childrens [OTC]; Allergy Relief [OTC]; Altaryl [OTC]; Anti-Hist Allergy [OTC]; Banophen [OTC]; Benadryl Allergy Childrens [OTC]; Benadryl Allergy [OTC]; Benadryl Dye-Free Allergy [OTC]; Benadryl [OTC]; Complete Allergy Medication [OTC]; Complete Allergy Relief [OTC]; Dicopanol FusePaq; Diphen [OTC]; Diphenhist [OTC]; Genahist [OTC]; Geri-Dryl [OTC]; GoodSense Allergy Relief [OTC]; Naramin [OTC]; Nighttime Sleep Aid [OTC]; Nytol Maximum Strength [OTC]; Nytol [OTC]; PediaCare Childrens Allergy [OTC]; Pharbedryl; Pharbedryl [OTC]; Q-Dryl [OTC]; Quenalin [OTC]; Scot-Tussin Allergy Relief [OTC]; Siladryl Allergy [OTC]; Silphen Cough [OTC]; Simply Allergy [OTC]; Simply Sleep [OTC]; Sleep Tabs [OTC]; Sominex Maximum Strength [OTC]; Sominex [OTC]; Tetra-Formula Nighttime Sleep [OTC]; Total Allergy Medicine [OTC]; Total Allergy [OTC]; Triaminic Cough/Runny Nose [OTC]; ZzzQuil [OTC]

Brand Names: Canada Allerdryl; Allernix; Benadryl; Nytol; Nytol Extra Strength; PMS-Diphenhydramine; Simply Sleep; Sominex

Therapeutic Category Antidote, Drug-induced Dystonic Reactions; Antidote, Hypersensitivity Reactions; Antihistamine; Sedative

Generic Availability (US) May be product dependent

Use

Prescription products:

Oral (Liquid: 12.5 mg per 5 mL): Treatment of allergic reactions caused by histamine release, adjunct to epinephrine in anaphylaxis after acute symptoms have been controlled, relief of other uncomplicated acute allergic conditions including urticaria and angioedema, treatment and prophylaxis of motion sickness, management of Parkinsonian syndrome including drug-induced extrapyramidal symptoms (dystonic reactions) alone or in combination with centrally acting anticholinergic agents, treatment of allergic conjunctivitis, and dermatographism (FDA approved in ages ≥28 days and adults); treatment of occasional insomnia (FDA approved in ages ≥12 years and adults)

Parenteral: Treatment of allergic reactions caused by histamine release; adjunct to epinephrine in anaphylaxis after acute symptoms have been controlled; relief of other uncomplicated acute allergic conditions including urticaria and angioedema; treatment of motion sickness; management of Parkinsonian syndrome including drug-induced extrapyramidal symptoms (dystonic reactions) alone or in combination with centrally acting anticholinergic agents (All indications: FDA approved in ages ≥28 days and adults)

OTC products: Relief of symptoms of hay fever or other respiratory allergies [OTC products: Capsules, tablets, liquid (12.5 mg per 5 mL): FDA approved in ages ≥6 years and adults]; relief of symptoms of common cold (OTC products: Capsules and tablets: FDA approved in ages ≥6 years and adults); treatment of occasional insomnia [OTC products: Capsules, liquid (50 mg per 30 mL): FDA approved in ages ≥12 years and adults]. **Note:** Approved uses for generic products may vary; consult labeling for specific information.

Pregnancy Risk Factor B

Pregnancy Considerations Adverse events have not been observed in animal reproduction studies. Diphenhydramine crosses the placenta. Maternal diphenhydramine use has generally not resulted in an increased risk of birth defects; however, adverse events (withdrawal symptoms, respiratory depression) have been reported in newborns exposed to diphenhydramine *in utero*. Antihistamines are recommended for the treatment of rhinitis, urticaria, and pruritus with rash in pregnant women (although second generation antihistamines may be preferred). Antihistamines are not recommended for treatment of pruritus associated with intrahepatic cholestasis in pregnancy.

Breast-Feeding Considerations Diphenhydramine is excreted into breast milk; drowsiness has been reported in a breast-feeding infant. Premature infants and newborns have a higher risk of intolerance to antihistamines. Breast-feeding is contraindicated by the manufacturer. Antihistamines may decrease maternal serum prolactin concentrations when administered prior to the establishment of nursing.

Contraindications Hypersensitivity to diphenhydramine, other structurally related antihistamines, or any component of the formulation; neonates or premature infants; breast-feeding

Additional contraindications: Parenteral: Use as a local anesthetic

OTC labeling: When used for self-medication, do not use in children <6 years, to make a child sleep, or with any other diphenhydramine-containing products (including topical products)

Warnings/Precautions Causes sedation, caution must be used in performing tasks which require alertness (eg, operating machinery or driving). Potentially significant drug-drug interactions may exist, requiring dose or frequency adjustment, additional monitoring, and/or selection of alternative therapy. Sedative effects of CNS depressants or ethanol are potentiated. Antihistamines may cause excitation in young children. Toxicity (overdose) in pediatric patients may result in hallucinations, convulsions, or death; neonates and young children are highly sensitive to depressive effects of diphenhydramine; use is contraindicated in neonates. Use with caution in patients with angle-closure glaucoma, pyloroduodenal obstruction (including stenotic peptic ulcer), urinary tract obstruction (including bladder neck obstruction and symptomatic prostatic hyperplasia), asthma, hyperthyroidism, increased intraocular pressure, and cardiovascular disease (including hypertension and tachycardia).

Some preparations contain soy protein; avoid use in patients with soy protein or peanut allergies. Some products may contain phenylalanine. Some products may contain alcohol. Some dosage forms may contain propylene glycol; large amounts are potentially toxic and have been associated hyperosmolality, lactic acidosis, seizures, and respiratory depression; use caution (AAP, 1997; Zar, 2007).

Benzyl alcohol and derivatives: Some dosage forms may contain sodium benzoate/benzoic acid; benzoic acid (benzoate) is a metabolite of benzyl alcohol; large amounts of benzyl alcohol (≥99 mg/kg/day) have been associated with a potentially fatal toxicity ("gasping syndrome") in neonates; the "gasping syndrome" consists of metabolic acidosis, respiratory distress, gasping respirations, CNS dysfunction (including convulsions, intracranial hemorrhage), hypotension, and cardiovascular collapse (AAP, 1997; CDC, 1982); some data suggests that benzoate displaces bilirubin from protein binding sites (Ahlfors, 2001); avoid or use dosage forms containing benzyl alcohol derivative with caution in neonates. See manufacturer's labeling.

Some dosage forms may contain polysorbate 80 (also known as Tweens). Hypersensitivity reactions, usually a delayed reaction, have been reported following exposure to pharmaceutical products containing polysorbate 80 in certain individuals (Isaksson, 2002; Lucente 2000; Shelley, 1995). Thrombocytopenia, ascites, pulmonary deterioration, and renal and hepatic failure have been reported in premature neonates after receiving parenteral products containing polysorbate 80 (Alade, 1986; CDC, 1984). See manufacturer's labeling.

Oral products: In the elderly, avoid use of this potent anticholinergic agent due to increased risk of confusion, dry mouth, constipation, and other anticholinergic effects; clearance decreases in patients of advanced age; tolerance develops to hypnotic effects; when used for severe allergic reaction, use may be appropriate (Beers Criteria). Oral solutions are available in two concentrations (ie, 12.5 mg/5 mL and 50 mg/30 mL [eg, ZzzQuil]); precautions should be taken to verify and avoid confusion between the different concentrations; dose should be clearly presented as "mg"; the 50 mg/30 mL oral solution is indicated for the occasional treatment of insomnia.

Parenteral products: Subcutaneous or intradermal use has been associated with tissue necrosis; administer IV or IM only.

Warnings: Additional Pediatric Considerations Safety and efficacy for the use of cough and cold products in pediatric patients <4 years of age is limited; the AAP warns against the use of these products for respiratory illnesses in this age group. Serious adverse effects, including death, have been reported. Many of these products contain multiple active ingredients, increasing the risk of accidental overdose when used with other products. The FDA notes that there are no approved OTC uses for these products in pediatric patients <2 years of age. Health care providers are reminded to ask caregivers about the use of OTC cough and cold products in order to avoid exposure to multiple medications containing the same ingredient. Toxicity (overdosage) in pediatric patients can result in hallucinations, convulsions, or death. Neonates and infants are highly sensitive to depressive effects of diphenhydramine; use is contraindicated in neonates (premature and term); use with extreme caution in infants and young children (AAP 2012; FDA 2008).

Some dosage forms may contain propylene glycol; in neonates large amounts of propylene glycol delivered orally, intravenously (eg, >3,000 mg/day), or topically have been associated with potentially fatal toxicities which can include metabolic acidosis, seizures, renal failure, and CNS depression; toxicities have also been reported in children and adults including hyperosmolality, lactic acidosis, seizures and respiratory depression; use caution (AAP 1997; Shehab 2009).

Adverse Reactions

Cardiovascular: Chest tightness, extrasystoles, hypotension, palpitations, tachycardia

Central nervous system: Ataxia, chills, confusion, dizziness, drowsiness, euphoria, excitement, fatigue, headache, insomnia, irritability, nervousness, neuritis, paradoxical excitation, paresthesia, restlessness, sedation, seizure, vertigo

Dermatologic: Diaphoresis

Endocrine & metabolic: Menstrual disease (early menses)

Gastrointestinal: Anorexia, constipation, diarrhea, dry mucous membranes, epigastric distress, nausea, vomiting, xerostomia

Genitourinary: Difficulty in micturition, urinary frequency, urinary retention

Hematologic & oncologic: Agranulocytosis, hemolytic anemia, thrombocytopenia

Hypersensitivity: Anaphylactic shock

Neuromuscular & skeletal: Tremor

Ophthalmic: Blurred vision, diplopia

Otic: Labyrinthitis (acute), tinnitus

Respiratory: Constriction of the pharynx, nasal congestion, thickening of bronchial secretions, wheezing

Drug Interactions

Metabolism/Transport Effects Inhibits CYP2D6 (moderate)

Avoid Concomitant Use

Avoid concomitant use of DiphenhydrAMINE (Systemic) with any of the following: Aclidinium; Azelastine (Nasal); Eluxadoline; Glucagon; Ipratropium (Oral Inhalation); Orphenadrine; Paraldehyde; Potassium Chloride; Thalidomide; Thioridazine; Tiotropium; Umeclidinium

Increased Effect/Toxicity

DiphenhydrAMINE (Systemic) may increase the levels/effects of: AbobotulinumtoxinA; Alcohol (Ethyl); Analgesics (Opioid); Anticholinergic Agents; ARIPiprazole; Azelastine (Nasal); Buprenorphine; CNS Depressants; CYP2D6 Substrates; DOXOrubicin (Conventional); Eliglustat; Eluxadoline; Fesoterodine; Glucagon; Highest Risk QTc-Prolonging Agents; Hydrocodone; Methotrimeprazine; Metoprolol; Metyrosine; Mirabegron; Mirtazapine; Moderate Risk QTc-Prolonging Agents; Nebivolol; OnabotulinumtoxinA; Orphenadrine; Paraldehyde; Potassium Chloride; Pramipexole; RimabotulinumtoxinB; ROPINIRole; Rotigotine; Selective Serotonin Reuptake Inhibitors; Suvorexant; Thalidomide; Thiazide Diuretics; Thioridazine; Tiotropium; Topiramate; Zolpidem

The levels/effects of DiphenhydrAMINE (Systemic) may be increased by: Aclidinium; Brimonidine (Topical); Cannabis; Doxylamine; Dronabinol; Droperidol; HydrOXYzine; Ipratropium (Oral Inhalation); Kava Kava; Magnesium Sulfate; Methotrimeprazine; Mianserin; Mifepristone; Nabilone; Perampanel; Pramlintide; Propafenone; Rufinamide; Sodium Oxybate; Tapentadol; Tetrahydrocannabinol; Umeclidinium

Decreased Effect

DiphenhydrAMINE (Systemic) may decrease the levels/effects of: Acetylcholinesterase Inhibitors; Benzylpenicilloyl Polylysine; Betahistine; Codeine; Hyaluronidase; Itopride; Metoclopramide; Secretin; Tamoxifen; TraMADol

The levels/effects of DiphenhydrAMINE (Systemic) may be decreased by: Acetylcholinesterase Inhibitors; Amphetamines

Storage/Stability

Injection: Store at room temperature of 20°C to 25°C (68°F to 77°F); protect from light and freezing.

Oral: Store at room temperature. Protect capsules and tablets from moisture. Protect oral solution from freezing and light.

Mechanism of Action Competes with histamine for H_1-receptor sites on effector cells in the gastrointestinal tract, blood vessels, and respiratory tract; anticholinergic and sedative effects are also seen

Pharmacodynamics

Maximum sedative effect: 1-3 hours after administration

Duration: 4-7 hours

Pharmacokinetics (Adult data unless noted)

Absorption: Oral: Well-absorbed but 40% to 60% of an oral dose reaches the systemic circulation due to first-pass metabolism

Distribution: V_d: 3-22 L/kg

Protein-binding: 78%

Metabolism: Extensive hepatic n-demethylation via CYP2D6; minor demethylation via CYP1A2, 2C9, and 2C19; significant first-pass effect

Bioavailability: ~40% to 70%

Half-life: 2-8 hours

Time to peak serum concentration: 2-4 hours

Elimination: Urine (as unchanged drug)

Dosing: Usual Note: Oral solutions are available in two concentrations [ie, 12.5 mg/5 mL and 50 mg/30 mL (eg, ZzzQuil)]; precautions should be taken to verify and avoid confusion between the different concentrations; dose should be clearly presented as "mg;" the 50 mg/30 mL oral solution is indicated for the occasional treatment of insomnia.

Pediatric:

Allergies; hay fever: Infants, Children, and Adolescents:

Oral:

Weight-directed dosing: 5 mg/kg/day divided into 3-4 doses; maximum daily dose: 300 mg/day; age-related maximum daily doses may also be considered: <6 years: 37.5 mg/day; 6-11 years: 150 mg/day; ≥12 years: 300 mg/day

Fixed dosing:

Children 2 to <6 years: Limited data available: 6.25 mg every 4-6 hours; maximum daily dose: 37.5 mg/day (Kliegman, 2011)

Children 6 to <12 years: 12.5-25 mg every 4-6 hours; maximum daily dose: 150 mg/day

Children ≥12 years and Adolescents: 25-50 mg every 4-6 hours; maximum daily dose: 300 mg/day

Allergic reaction (severe)/anaphylaxis (adjunct to epinephrine): Infants, Children, and Adolescents:

Manufacturer's labeling: IV, IM, Oral: 1.25 mg/kg/dose given every 6 hours; maximum daily dose: 300 mg/day

Alternate dosing: IV, IM, Oral: 1-2 mg/kg/dose; maximum single dose: 50 mg/**dose** (Hegenbarth, 2008; Kliegman, 2011; Liberman, 2008; Lieberman, 2010; Simons, 2011)

Rhinitis, sneezing due to common cold: Oral:

Children 6 to <12 years: 25 mg every 4-6 hours; maximum daily dose: 150 mg/day

Children ≥12 years and Adolescents: 25-50 mg every 4-6 hours; maximum daily dose: 300 mg/day

Dystonic reactions: Infants, Children, and Adolescents: IV, IM: 1-2 mg/kg/dose; maximum single dose: 50 mg (Hegenbarth, 2008; Kliegman, 2011); may repeat in 20-30 minutes if necessary

Motion sickness: Infants, Children, and Adolescents:

Prophylaxis: Oral:

Manufacturer's labeling: First dose should be administered 30 minutes before travel.

Weight-directed dosing: 5 mg/kg/day divided into 3-4 doses; maximum daily dose: 300 mg/day

Fixed dosing: 12.5-25 mg 3-4 times daily

Alternate dosing: Children 2-12 years: Limited data available: 0.5-1 mg/kg/dose every 6 hours; maximum single dose: 25 mg. First dose should be administered 1 hour before travel (CDC, 2014).

Treatment:

IV, IM: 1.25 mg/kg/dose every 6 hours; maximum daily dose: 300 mg/day

Oral:

Weight-directed dosing: 5 mg/kg/day divided into 3-4 doses; maximum daily dose: 300 mg/day

Fixed dosing: 12.5-25 mg 3-4 times daily

Insomnia; occasional: Oral:

Children 2-12 years, weighing 10-50 kg: Limited data available: 1 mg/kg administered 30 minutes before bedtime; maximum single dose: 50 mg (Russo, 1976)

Children ≥12 years and Adolescents: 50 mg administered 30 minutes before bedtime

Pruritis (opioid-induced): Limited data available: Infants, Children, and Adolescents: IM, IV, Oral: 0.5-1 mg/kg/dose every 6 hours; maximum daily dose: 100/day (Kliegman, 2011)

Urticaria: Infants, Children, and Adolescents: Oral:

Weight-directed dosing: 5 mg/kg/day divided into 3-4 doses; maximum daily dose: 300 mg/day

Fixed dosing: 12.5-25 mg 3-4 times daily

Adult:

Allergic reactions:

Oral: 25-50 mg every 6-8 hours

IM, IV: 10-50 mg per dose; single doses up to 100 mg may be used if needed; not to exceed 400 mg/day

Antitussive: Oral: 25 mg every 4 hours; maximum: 150 mg/24 hours

Motion sickness:
Oral: 25-50 mg every 6-8 hours
IM, IV: 10-50 mg per dose; single doses up to 100 mg may be used if needed; not to exceed 400 mg/day
Insomnia; occasional: Oral: 50 mg at bedtime
Dystonic reactions: IM, IV: 50 mg in a single dose; may repeat in 20-30 minutes if necessary

Preparation for Administration IV: May further dilute in a compatible IV fluid to a concentration <50 mg/mL

Administration
Oral: May administer without regards to meals; when used to prevent motion sickness, first dose should be given 30 to 60 minutes prior to exposure
Parenteral: For IV or IM administration only. Local necrosis may result with SubQ or intradermal use. For IV administration, may administer IVP undiluted at a rate ≤25 mg/minute or further diluted as an intermittent infusion over 10 to 15 minutes. **Note:** Seizures may be precipitated with too rapid IV administration in pediatric patients (Hegenbarth 2008).

Test Interactions May interfere with urine detection of methadone and phencyclidine (false-positives); may cause false-positive serum TCA screen; may suppress the wheal and flare reactions to skin test antigens

Dosage Forms Considerations Dicopanol FusePaq is a compounding kit for the preparation of an oral suspension. Refer to manufacturer's labeling for compounding instructions.

Dosage Forms Excipient information presented when available (limited, particularly for generics); consult specific product labeling. [DSC] = Discontinued product
Capsule, Oral, as hydrochloride:
Allergy Relief: 25 mg [contains brilliant blue fcf (fd&c blue #1), butylparaben, edetate calcium disodium, fd&c blue #2 (indigotine), fd&c red #40, fd&c yellow #10 (quinoline yellow), methylparaben, polysorbate 80, propylparaben]
Banophen: 25 mg [contains brilliant blue fcf (fd&c blue #1), fd&c red #40, fd&c yellow #6 (sunset yellow), methylparaben, propylparaben]
Banophen: 50 mg [contains brilliant blue fcf (fd&c blue #1), fd&c red #40]
Benadryl: 25 mg
Benadryl Allergy: 25 mg [dye free]
Benadryl Dye-Free Allergy: 25 mg [dye free]
Diphenhist: 25 mg [DSC] [contains brilliant blue fcf (fd&c blue #1), butylparaben, fd&c red #40, methylparaben, propylparaben]
Genahist: 25 mg
Geri-Dryl: 25 mg
GoodSense Allergy Relief: 25 mg [dye free]
Pharbedryl: 25 mg, 50 mg [contains brilliant blue fcf (fd&c blue #1), fd&c red #40]
Q-Dryl: 25 mg [contains brilliant blue fcf (fd&c blue #1), butylparaben, fd&c red #40, methylparaben, propylparaben]
ZzzQuil: 25 mg [contains brilliant blue fcf (fd&c blue #1), fd&c red #40]
Generic: 25 mg, 50 mg
Elixir, Oral, as hydrochloride:
Altaryl: 12.5 mg/5 mL (120 mL, 480 mL, 3840 mL) [contains alcohol, usp]
Generic: 12.5 mg/5 mL (5 mL, 10 mL)
Liquid, Oral, as hydrochloride:
Allergy Relief Childrens: 12.5 mg/5 mL (118 mL, 480 mL) [alcohol free; contains fd&c red #40, sodium benzoate]
Banophen: 12.5 mg/5 mL (118 mL) [alcohol free; cherry flavor]
Banophen: 12.5 mg/5 mL (473 mL) [alcohol free, sugar free; cherry flavor]
Benadryl Allergy Childrens: 12.5 mg/5 mL (118 mL, 236 mL) [alcohol free; contains fd&c red #40, sodium benzoate]
Benadryl Allergy Childrens: 12.5 mg/5 mL (5 mL, 236 mL) [alcohol free; contains fd&c red #40, sodium benzoate; cherry flavor]
Benadryl Allergy Childrens: 12.5 mg/5 mL (118 mL) [alcohol free, dye free, sugar free; contains saccharin sodium, sodium benzoate]
Diphenhist: 12.5 mg/5 mL (118 mL, 473 mL) [alcohol free; contains fd&c red #40, saccharin sodium, sodium benzoate; fruit flavor]
Naramin: 12.5 mg/5 mL (5 mL) [alcohol free; contains fd&c red #40, sodium benzoate; cherry flavor]
PediaCare Childrens Allergy: 12.5 mg/5 mL (118 mL) [alcohol free; contains fd&c red #40, sodium benzoate]
Q-Dryl: 12.5 mg/5 mL (118 mL, 237 mL, 473 mL) [alcohol free; contains fd&c red #40, saccharin sodium, sodium benzoate; cherry flavor]
Scot-Tussin Allergy Relief: 12.5 mg/5 mL (118.3 mL, 240 mL, 480 mL, 3780 mL) [alcohol free, dye free, saccharin free, sodium free, sorbitol free, sugar free]
Siladryl Allergy: 12.5 mg/5 mL (118 mL, 237 mL, 473 mL) [alcohol free, sugar free; contains fd&c red #40, methylparaben, propylene glycol, propylparaben, saccharin sodium; cherry flavor]
Total Allergy Medicine: 12.5 mg/5 mL (118 mL) [alcohol free]
ZzzQuil: 50 mg/30 mL (177 mL, 354 mL) [contains alcohol, usp, brilliant blue fcf (fd&c blue #1), fd&c red #40, propylene glycol, saccharin sodium, sodium benzoate; berry flavor]
Solution, Injection, as hydrochloride:
Generic: 50 mg/mL (1 mL, 10 mL)
Solution, Injection, as hydrochloride [preservative free]:
Generic: 50 mg/mL (1 mL)
Strip, Oral, as hydrochloride:
Triaminic Cough/Runny Nose: 12.5 mg (14 ea) [contains alcohol, usp, brilliant blue fcf (fd&c blue #1), fd&c red #40]
Triaminic Cough/Runny Nose: 12.5 mg (16 ea) [contains alcohol, usp, brilliant blue fcf (fd&c blue #1), fd&c red #40; grape flavor]
Suspension Reconstituted, Oral, as hydrochloride:
Dicopanol FusePaq: 5 mg/mL (150 mL) [contains sodium benzoate]
Syrup, Oral, as hydrochloride:
Altaryl: 12.5 mg/5 mL (120 mL, 480 mL, 3785 mL) [alcohol free; cherry flavor]
Quenalin: 12.5 mg/5 mL (120 mL) [fruit flavor]
Silphen Cough: 12.5 mg/5 mL (118 mL, 237 mL, 473 mL) [contains alcohol, usp, fd&c red #40, menthol, methylparaben, propylene glycol, propylparaben; strawberry flavor]
Tablet, Oral, as hydrochloride:
Aler-Dryl: 50 mg
Allergy Relief: 25 mg [contains polysorbate 80]
Anti-Hist Allergy: 25 mg
Banophen: 25 mg
Benadryl: 25 mg
Benadryl Allergy: 25 mg
Benadryl Allergy: 25 mg [contains edetate calcium disodium, fd&c red #40, methylparaben, polysorbate 80, propylparaben]
Complete Allergy Medication: 25 mg
Complete Allergy Relief: 25 mg
Diphen: 25 mg
Diphenhist: 25 mg [DSC]
Geri-Dryl: 25 mg
Nighttime Sleep Aid: 25 mg [contains fd&c blue #1 aluminum lake, fd&c blue #2 aluminum lake, polysorbate 80]
Nighttime Sleep Aid: 50 mg [DSC] [contains fd&c blue #1 aluminum lake]
Nytol: 25 mg
Nytol Maximum Strength: 50 mg

Simply Allergy: 25 mg
Simply Sleep: 25 mg [contains brilliant blue fcf (fd&c blue #1)]
Sleep Tabs: 25 mg [scored; contains fd&c blue #1 aluminum lake]
Sominex: 25 mg [contains fd&c blue #1 aluminum lake]
Sominex Maximum Strength: 50 mg [contains fd&c blue #1 aluminum lake, polysorbate 80]
Tetra-Formula Nighttime Sleep: 50 mg [contains fd&c blue #1 aluminum lake]
Total Allergy: 25 mg
Generic: 25 mg

Tablet Chewable, Oral, as hydrochloride:
Benadryl Allergy Childrens: 12.5 mg [contains aspartame, fd&c blue #1 aluminum lake; cherry flavor]
Benadryl Allergy Childrens: 12.5 mg [contains aspartame, fd&c blue #1 aluminum lake; grape flavor]

DiphenhydrAMINE (Topical)

(dye fen HYE dra meen)

Medication Safety Issues

Sound-alike/look-alike issues:

DiphenhydrAMINE may be confused with desipramine, dicyclomine, dimenhyDRINATE

Benadryl® may be confused with benazepril, Bentyl®, Benylin®, Caladryl®

Administration issues:

Institute for Safe Medication Practices (ISMP) has reported cases of patients mistakenly *swallowing* Benadryl® Itch Stopping [OTC] gel intended for topical application. Unclear labeling and similar packaging of the topical gel in containers resembling an oral liquid are factors believed to be contributing to the administration errors. The topical gel contains camphor which can be toxic if swallowed. ISMP has requested the manufacturer to make the necessary changes to prevent further confusion.

Brand Names: US Anti-Itch Maximum Strength [OTC]; Anti-Itch [OTC]; Banophen [OTC]; Benadryl Itch Relief [OTC]; Benadryl Itch Stopping [OTC]; Benadryl Maximum Strength [OTC]; Itch Relief [OTC]

Brand Names: Canada Benadryl® Cream; Benadryl® Itch Relief Stick; Benadryl® Spray

Therapeutic Category Antihistamine

Generic Availability (US) May be product dependent

Use Relief of pain and itching associated with insect bites, minor cuts and burns, or rashes

Pregnancy Considerations When administered orally, diphenhydramine crosses the placenta. Diphenhydramine can also be measurable in the serum following topical administration to large areas of the body. Refer to the Diphenhydramine (Systemic) monograph.

Breast-Feeding Considerations When administered orally, diphenhydramine can be detected in breast milk. Diphenhydramine can also be measurable in the serum following topical administration to large areas of the body. Refer to the Diphenhydramine (Systemic) monograph.

Contraindications Hypersensitivity to diphenhydramine or any component of the formulation; neonates or premature infants; breast-feeding

Warnings/Precautions Self-medication (OTC use): Topical products should not be used on large areas of the body, or on chicken pox or measles. Healthcare provider should be contacted if topical use is needed for >7 days. Topical products are not for OTC use in children <2 years of age. Do not use with other products containing diphenhydramine.

Warnings: Additional Pediatric Considerations Some dosage forms may contain propylene glycol; in neonates large amounts of propylene glycol delivered orally, intravenously (eg, >3,000 mg/day), or topically have been associated with potentially fatal toxicities which can include metabolic acidosis, seizures, renal failure, and CNS depression; toxicities have also been reported in children and adults including hyperosmolality, lactic acidosis, seizures and respiratory depression; use caution (AAP, 1997; Shehab, 2009).

Adverse Reactions Dermatologic: Photosensitivity, rash, urticaria

Drug Interactions

Metabolism/Transport Effects None known.

Avoid Concomitant Use

Avoid concomitant use of DiphenhydrAMINE (Topical) with any of the following: Aclidinium; Azelastine (Nasal); Eluxadoline; Glucagon; Ipratropium (Oral Inhalation); Orphenadrine; Paraldehyde; Potassium Chloride; Thalidomide; Tiotropium; Umeclidinium

Increased Effect/Toxicity

DiphenhydrAMINE (Topical) may increase the levels/effects of: AbobotulinumtoxinA; Alcohol (Ethyl); Analgesics (Opioid); Anticholinergic Agents; Azelastine (Nasal); Buprenorphine; CNS Depressants; Eluxadoline; Glucagon; Hydrocodone; Methotrimeprazine; Metyrosine; Mirabegron; Mirtazapine; OnabotulinumtoxinA; Orphenadrine; Paraldehyde; Potassium Chloride; Pramipexole; RimabotulinumtoxinB; ROPINIRole; Rotigotine; Selective Serotonin Reuptake Inhibitors; Suvorexant; Thalidomide; Thiazide Diuretics; Tiotropium; Topiramate; Zolpidem

The levels/effects of DiphenhydrAMINE (Topical) may be increased by: Aclidinium; Brimonidine (Topical); Cannabis; Doxylamine; Dronabinol; Droperidol; HydrOXYzine; Ipratropium (Oral Inhalation); Kava Kava; Magnesium Sulfate; Methotrimeprazine; Mianserin; Nabilone; Perampanel; Pramlintide; Rufinamide; Sodium Oxybate; Tapentadol; Tetrahydrocannabinol; Umeclidinium

Decreased Effect

DiphenhydrAMINE (Topical) may decrease the levels/effects of: Acetylcholinesterase Inhibitors; Benzylpenicilloyl Polylysine; Betahistine; Hyaluronidase; Itopride; Metoclopramide; Secretin

The levels/effects of DiphenhydrAMINE (Topical) may be decreased by: Acetylcholinesterase Inhibitors; Amphetamines

Dosing: Usual Topical cream, gel, spray, or stick:

Children ≥2 to 12 years: Apply 1% concentration not more than 3-4 times/day

Children ≥12 years and Adults: Apply 1% or 2% concentration not more than 3-4 times/day

Administration Shake well (gel); apply thin coat to affected area

Test Interactions May suppress the wheal and flare reactions to skin test antigens

Dosage Forms Excipient information presented when available (limited, particularly for generics); consult specific product labeling.

Cream, External, as hydrochloride:
Anti-Itch: 2% (28.4 g) [contains cetyl alcohol, methylparaben, propylene glycol, propylparaben]
Anti-Itch: 2% (28.4 g) [contains methylparaben, propylparaben]
Anti-Itch Maximum Strength: 2% (30 g)
Banophen: 2% (28 g) [contains cetyl alcohol, methylparaben, propylene glycol, propylparaben]
Benadryl Itch Stopping: 1% (28.3 g) [contains cetyl alcohol]
Itch Relief: 2% (15 g, 30 g, 56.8 g)

Gel, External, as hydrochloride:
Benadryl Itch Stopping: 2% (118 mL) [contains alcohol, usp, methylparaben, propylparaben]

Solution, External, as hydrochloride:
Benadryl Maximum Strength: 2% (60 mL) [contains alcohol, usp]
Stick, External, as hydrochloride:
Benadryl Itch Relief: 2% (14 mL) [contains alcohol, usp]

- **Diphenhydramine Citrate** *see* DiphenhydrAMINE (Systemic) *on page 668*
- **Diphenhydramine Hydrochloride** *see* DiphenhydrAMINE (Systemic) *on page 668*
- **Diphenhydramine Hydrochloride** *see* DiphenhydrAMINE (Topical) *on page 672*
- **Diphenhydramine Tannate** *see* DiphenhydrAMINE (Systemic) *on page 668*

Diphenoxylate and Atropine

(dye fen OKS i late & A troe peen)

Medication Safety Issues

Sound-alike/look-alike issues:

Lomotil may be confused with LaMICtal, LamISIL, lamoTRIgine, Lanoxin, Lasix, loperamide

International issues:

Lomotil [U.S., Canada, and multiple international markets] may be confused with Ludiomil brand name for maprotiline [multiple international markets]

Lomotil: Brand name for diphenoxylate [U.S., Canada, and multiple international markets], but also the brand name for loperamide [Mexico, Philippines]

Brand Names: US Lomotil

Brand Names: Canada Lomotil

Therapeutic Category Antidiarrheal

Generic Availability (US) Yes

Use Treatment of diarrhea

Pregnancy Risk Factor C

Pregnancy Considerations Teratogenic effects were not noted in animal studies; decreased maternal weight, fertility and litter sizes were observed. There are no adequate and well-controlled studies in pregnant women.

Breast-Feeding Considerations Atropine is excreted in breast milk (refer to Atropine monograph); the manufacturer states that diphenoxylic acid may be excreted in breast milk.

Contraindications Hypersensitivity to diphenoxylate, atropine, or any component of the formulation; obstructive jaundice; diarrhea associated with pseudomembranous enterocolitis or enterotoxin-producing bacteria; not for use in children <2 years of age

Warnings/Precautions Use in conjunction with fluid and electrolyte therapy when appropriate. In case of severe dehydration or electrolyte imbalance, withhold diphenoxylate/atropine treatment until corrective therapy has been initiated. Inhibiting peristalsis may lead to fluid retention in the intestine aggravating dehydration and electrolyte imbalance. Reduction of intestinal motility may be deleterious in diarrhea resulting from *Shigella, Salmonella*, toxigenic strains of *E. coli*, and pseudomembranous enterocolitis associated with broad-spectrum antibiotics; use is not recommended.

Use with caution in children. Younger children may be predisposed to toxicity; signs of atropinism may occur even at recommended doses, especially in patients with Down syndrome. Overdose in children may result in severe respiratory depression, coma, and possibly permanent brain damage.

Use caution with acute ulcerative colitis, hepatic or renal dysfunction. If there is no response with 48 hours, this medication is unlikely to be effective and should be discontinued; if chronic diarrhea is not improved symptomatically within 10 days at maximum dosage, control is unlikely with further use. Physical and psychological dependence have been reported with higher than recommended dosing.

Adverse Reactions

Cardiovascular: Flushing, tachycardia

Central nervous system: Confusion, depression, dizziness, drowsiness, euphoria, headache, hyperthermia, lethargy, malaise, numbness, restlessness, sedation

Dermatologic: Pruritus, urticaria, xeroderma

Gastrointestinal: Abdominal distress, anorexia, gingival swelling, nausea, pancreatitis, paralytic ileus, toxic megacolon, vomiting, xerostomia

Genitourinary: Urinary retention

Hypersensitivity: Anaphylaxis, angioedema

Drug Interactions

Metabolism/Transport Effects None known.

Avoid Concomitant Use

Avoid concomitant use of Diphenoxylate and Atropine with any of the following: Aclidinium; Azelastine (Nasal); Eluxadoline; Glucagon; Ipratropium (Oral Inhalation); Orphenadrine; Paraldehyde; Potassium Chloride; Thalidomide; Tiotropium; Umeclidinium

Increased Effect/Toxicity

Diphenoxylate and Atropine may increase the levels/effects of: AbobotulinumtoxinA; Alcohol (Ethyl); Analgesics (Opioid); Anticholinergic Agents; Azelastine (Nasal); Buprenorphine; CNS Depressants; Eluxadoline; Glucagon; Hydrocodone; Methotrimeprazine; Metyrosine; Mirabegron; Mirtazapine; OnabotulinumtoxinA; Orphenadrine; Paraldehyde; Potassium Chloride; Pramipexole; RimabotulinumtoxinB; ROPINIRole; Rotigotine; Selective Serotonin Reuptake Inhibitors; Suvorexant; Thalidomide; Thiazide Diuretics; Tiotropium; Topiramate; Zolpidem

The levels/effects of Diphenoxylate and Atropine may be increased by: Aclidinium; Brimonidine (Topical); Cannabis; Doxylamine; Dronabinol; Droperidol; HydrOXYzine; Ipratropium (Oral Inhalation); Kava Kava; Magnesium Sulfate; Methotrimeprazine; Mianserin; Nabilone; Perampanel; Pramlintide; Rufinamide; Sodium Oxybate; Tapentadol; Tetrahydrocannabinol; Umeclidinium

Decreased Effect

Diphenoxylate and Atropine may decrease the levels/effects of: Acetylcholinesterase Inhibitors; Itopride; Metoclopramide; Secretin

The levels/effects of Diphenoxylate and Atropine may be decreased by: Acetylcholinesterase Inhibitors

Storage/Stability

Oral solution: Store at 20°C to 25°C (68°F to 77°F). Discard opened bottle after 90 days.

Tablet: Store at 20°C to 25°C (68°F to 77°F); protect from light.

Mechanism of Action Diphenoxylate inhibits excessive GI motility and GI propulsion; commercial preparations contain a subtherapeutic amount of atropine to discourage abuse

Pharmacodynamics Antidiarrheal effects:

Onset of action: Within 45-60 minutes

Maximum effect: Within 2 hours

Duration: 3-4 hours

Tolerance to antidiarrheal effects may occur with prolonged use

Pharmacokinetics (Adult data unless noted)

Atropine: See Atropine

Diphenoxylate:

Absorption: Oral: Well absorbed

Distribution: Major metabolite (diphenoxylic acid) may be excreted in breast milk

Metabolism: Extensive in the liver via ester hydrolysis to diphenoxylic acid (active)

Half-life:

Diphenoxylate: 2.5 hours

Diphenoxylic acid: 12-24 hours

Time to peak serum concentration: ~2 hours

Elimination: Primarily (49%) in feces (via bile); ~14% is excreted in urine; <1% excreted unchanged in urine

Dosing: Usual Oral (as diphenoxylate):

Children 2-12 years: **Liquid: Note:** Only the liquid product is recommended for children under 13 years of age; do not exceed recommended doses; reduce dose as soon as symptoms are initially controlled; maintenance doses may be as low as 25% of initial dose; if no improvement within 48 hours of therapy, diphenoxylate is not likely to be effective

Initial: 0.3-0.4 mg/kg/day in 4 divided doses (maximum: 10 mg/day) **or**

Manufacturer's recommendations: Initial:

<2 years: Not recommended

2 years (11-14 kg): 1.5-3 mL 4 times/day

3 years (12-16 kg): 2-3 mL 4 times/day

4 years (14-20 kg): 2-4 mL 4 times/day

5 years (16-23 kg): 2.5-4.5 mL 4 times/day

6-8 years (17-32 kg): 2.5-5 mL 4 times/day

9-12 years (23-55 kg): 3.5-5 mL 4 times/day

Alternative pediatric dosing: Initial:

<2 years: Not recommended

2-5 years: 2 mg 3 times/day

5-8 years: 2 mg 4 times/day

8-12 years: 2 mg 5 times/day

Adults: Initial: 5 mg (2 tablets or 10 mL) 4 times/day until control achieved (maximum: 20 mg/day); then reduced dose as needed; maintenance: 5-15 mg/day in 2-3 divided doses; some patients may be controlled on doses as low as 5 mg/day

Note: Do not exceed recommended doses; reduce dose once symptoms are initially controlled; acute diarrhea usually improves within 48 hours; if chronic diarrhea dose not improve within 10 days at maximum daily doses of 20 mg, diphenoxylate is not likely to be effective.

Administration Oral: May be administered with food to decrease GI upset; use plastic dropper provided when measuring liquid; **Note:** Dropper has a 2 mL (1 mg) capacity and is calibrated in increments of 1/2 mL (0.25 mg)

Monitoring Parameters Bowel frequency, signs and symptoms of atropinism, fluid and electrolytes

Additional Information Naloxone reverses toxicity due to diphenoxylate; Lomotil® solution also contains sorbitol

Controlled Substance C-V

Dosage Forms Excipient information presented when available (limited, particularly for generics); consult specific product labeling. [DSC] = Discontinued product

Solution, oral: Diphenoxylate hydrochloride 2.5 mg and atropine sulfate 0.025 mg per 5 mL (5 mL, 10 mL, 60 mL)

Lomotil: Diphenoxylate hydrochloride 2.5 mg and atropine sulfate 0.025 mg per 5 mL (60 mL) [contains alcohol 15%; cherry flavor] [DSC]

Tablet, oral: Diphenoxylate hydrochloride 2.5 mg and atropine sulfate 0.025 mg

Lomotil: Diphenoxylate hydrochloride 2.5 mg and atropine sulfate 0.025 mg

◆ **Diphenylhydantoin** *see* Phenytoin *on page 1689*

Diphtheria and Tetanus Toxoids

(dif THEER ee a & TET a nus TOKS oyds)

Medication Safety Issues

Sound-alike/look-alike issues:

Diphtheria and Tetanus Toxoids (Td) may be confused with tuberculin purified protein derivative (PPD)

Pediatric diphtheria and tetanus (DT) may be confused with adult tetanus and diphtheria (Td)

Related Information

Centers for Disease Control and Prevention (CDC) and Other Links *on page 2424*

Immunization Administration Recommendations *on page 2411*

Immunization Schedules *on page 2416*

Brand Names: US Tenivac

Brand Names: Canada Td Adsorbed

Therapeutic Category Vaccine; Vaccine, Inactivated Bacteria

Generic Availability (US) Yes

Use

Diphtheria and tetanus toxoids adsorbed for pediatric use (DT): Active immunity against diphtheria and tetanus when pertussis vaccine is contraindicated (FDA approved in ages 6 weeks to 6 years); has also been used for tetanus prophylaxis in wound management

Tetanus and diphtheria toxoids adsorbed for adult use (Td) (Tenivac): Active immunity against diphtheria and tetanus; tetanus prophylaxis in wound management (FDA approved in ages ≥7 years and adults)

The Advisory Committee on Immunization Practices (ACIP) recommends routine vaccination for the following:

- Children ≥7 years, Adolescents, and Adults should receive a booster dose of Td every 10 years; may substitute a single Td booster dose with Tdap (CDC/ACIP 60[1] 2011)
- Children 7 to 10 years, Adolescents, Adults, and the Elderly (≥65 years) who are wounded in bombings or similar mass casualty events who have penetrating injuries or nonintact skin exposure and who cannot confirm receipt of a tetanus booster within the previous 5 years, may also receive a single dose of Td; children ≥11 years, adolescents and adults may also receive Td if Tdap is unavailable (CDC [Chapman 2008])

Medication Guide Available Yes

Pregnancy Risk Factor C

Pregnancy Considerations Reproduction studies have not been conducted. DT is not recommended for use in persons ≥7 years of age. Inactivated bacterial vaccines have not been shown to cause increased risks to the fetus (NCIRD/ACIP, 2011). The Advisory Committee on Immunization Practices (ACIP) recommends a single Tdap vaccination during each pregnancy; ideally between 27 and 36 weeks gestation. Pregnant women who are not immunized or are only partially immunized should complete the primary series with Td. Tetanus immune globulin and a tetanus toxoid containing vaccine are recommended by the ACIP as part of the standard wound management to prevent tetanus in pregnant women; the use of a tetanus-toxoid containing vaccine during pregnancy is recommended for wound management if ≥5 years have passed since the last Td vaccination (CDC/ACIP 2013).

Breast-Feeding Considerations It is not known if this vaccine is excreted into breast milk. The manufacturer recommends that caution be used if administered to breast-feeding women. Inactivated vaccines do not affect the safety of breast-feeding for the mother or the infant. Breast-feeding infants should be vaccinated according to the recommended schedules (NCIRD/ACIP, 2011). ACIP recommends that if Tdap was not administered during pregnancy, it should be administered during the immediate postpartum period; women who are not immunized or are only partially immunized should complete the primary series with Td (CDC/ACIP 2013).

Contraindications Hypersensitivity to diphtheria, tetanus toxoid, or any component of the formulation

Warnings/Precautions Do not confuse pediatric diphtheria and tetanus (DT) with adult tetanus and diphtheria (Td). Pediatric dosage form (DT) should only be used in patients 6 weeks to ≤6 years of age. Td should be administered to children ≥7 years of age, adolescents and adults

Immediate treatment including epinephrine 1:1,000) for anaphylactoid and/or hypersensitivity reactions should be available during vaccine use (NCIRD/ACIP 2011). Patients with a history of severe local reaction (Arthus-type) following a previous tetanus toxoid dose should not be given further routine or emergency doses of Td more frequently than every 10 years, even if using for wound management with wounds that are not clean or minor;.these patients generally have high serum antitoxin levels (NCIRD/ACIP 2011). Use with caution if Guillain-Barré syndrome occurred within 6 weeks of prior tetanus toxoid-containing vaccine. Syncope has been reported with use of injectable vaccines and may result in serious secondary injury (eg, skull fracture, cerebral hemorrhage); typically reported in adolescents and young adults and within 15 minutes after vaccination. Procedures should be in place to avoid injuries from falling and to restore cerebral perfusion if syncope occurs (NCIRD/ACIP 2011).

Use with caution in patients with bleeding disorders (including thrombocytopenia) and patients on anticoagulant therapy; bleeding/hematoma may occur from IM administration; if the patient receives antihemophilia or other similar therapy, IM injection can be scheduled shortly after such therapy is administered (NCIRD/ACIP 2011). The decision to administer or delay vaccination because of current or recent febrile illness depends on the severity of symptoms and the etiology of the disease. Consider deferring administration in patients with moderate or severe acute illness (with or without fever); vaccination should not be delayed for patients with mild acute illness (with or without fever). Use with caution in severely immunocompromised patients (eg, patients receiving chemo/radiation therapy or other immunosuppressive therapy [including high-dose corticosteroids]); may have a reduced response to vaccination. In general, household and close contacts of persons with altered immunocompetence may receive all age appropriate (IDSA [Rubin 2014]; NCIRD/ACIP 2011); inactivated vaccines should be administered ≥2 weeks prior to planned immunosuppression when feasible (IDSA [Rubin 2014]). Vaccination may not result in effective immunity in all patients. Response depends upon multiple factors (eg, type of vaccine, age of patient) and may be improved by administering the vaccine at the recommended dose, route, and interval. Vaccines may not be effective if administered during periods of altered immune competence (NCIRD/ACIP 2011). Antipyretics have not been shown to prevent febrile seizures. Antipyretics may be used to treat fever or discomfort following vaccination (NCIRD/ACIP 2011). One study reported that routine prophylactic administration of acetaminophen to prevent fever prior to vaccination decreased the immune response of some vaccines; the clinical significance of this reduction in immune response has not been established (Prymula 2009). Apnea has occurred following intramuscular vaccine administration in premature infants; consider clinical status implications. In general, preterm infants should be vaccinated at the same chronological age as full-term infants (NCIRD/ACIP 2011). Some products may contain natural latex/natural rubber or thimerosal. In order to maximize vaccination rates, the ACIP recommends simultaneous administration (ie, >1 vaccine on the same day at different anatomic sites) of all age-appropriate vaccines (live or inactivated) for which a person is eligible at a single clinic visit, unless contraindications exist. The use of combination vaccines is generally preferred over separate injections, taking into consideration provider assessment, patient preference, and adverse events. When using combination vaccines, the minimum age for administration is the oldest minimum age for any individual component; the minimum interval between dosing is the greatest minimum interval between any individual component. The ACIP prefers each dose of a specific vaccine in a series come from the same manufacturer when possible (NCIRD/ACIP 2011). Use of this vaccine for specific medical and/or other indications (eg, immunocompromising conditions, hepatic or kidney disease, diabetes) is also addressed in the ACIP Recommended Adult Immunization Schedule (CDC/ACIP [Kim 2015]). Specific recommendations for vaccination in immunocompromised patients with asplenia, cancer, HIV infection, cerebrospinal fluid leaks, cochlear implants, hematopoietic stem cell transplant (prior to or after), sickle cell disease, solid organ transplant (prior to or after), or those receiving immunosuppressive therapy for chronic conditions as well as contacts of immunocompromised patients are available from the IDSA (Rubin 2014).

Warnings: Additional Pediatric Considerations Diphtheria and tetanus toxoid is available in two formulations which contain different amounts of the diphtheria toxoid; DT or "pediatric" formulation has twice the diphtheria toxoid as Td or "adult" toxoid; use of DT in children >7 years and adults is associated with more severe adverse reactions to the diphtheria toxoid than in infants and younger children.

Adverse Reactions All serious adverse reactions must be reported to the U.S. Department of Health and Human Services (DHHS) Vaccine Adverse Event Reporting System (VAERS) 1-800-822-7967 or online at https://vaers.hhs.gov/esub/index. In Canada, adverse reactions may be reported to local provincial/territorial health agencies or to the Vaccine Safety Section at Public Health Agency of Canada (1-866-844-0018).

Central nervous system: Chills, fever, headache, tiredness

Endocrine & metabolic: Lymph node swelling

Gastrointestinal: Diarrhea, nausea, vomiting

Local: Injection site: Erythema, pain, swelling

Neuromuscular & skeletal: Body ache/muscle weakness, sore/swollen joints

Dermatologic: Rash

Rare but important or life-threatening: Allergic reactions (angioedema, rash, urticaria), anaphylactic reactions, arthralgia, chills, dizziness, fatigue, injection site reactions (cellulitis, induration, nodules, warmth), lymphadenopathy, musculoskeletal stiffness, myalgia, pain, pain in extremities, paresthesia, peripheral edema, seizure, syncope, weakness

Drug Interactions

Metabolism/Transport Effects None known.

Avoid Concomitant Use There are no known interactions where it is recommended to avoid concomitant use.

Increased Effect/Toxicity There are no known significant interactions involving an increase in effect.

Decreased Effect

The levels/effects of Diphtheria and Tetanus Toxoids may be decreased by: Belimumab; Fingolimod; Immunosuppressants; Meningococcal Polysaccharide (Groups A / C / Y and W-135) Tetanus Toxoid Conjugate Vaccine

Storage/Stability Store at 2°C to 8°C (35°F to 46°F). Do not freeze; discard if product has been frozen.

Mechanism of Action Promotes active immunity to diphtheria and tetanus by inducing production of specific antibodies.

Dosing: Usual

Primary Immunization:

CDC (ACIP) recommendations (Strikas 2015): Infants and Children 6 weeks to 6 years with contraindication to immunization containing pertussis: **Note:** Preterm infants should be vaccinated according to their chronological age from birth; Pediatric formulation (DT): IM: 0.5 mL per dose for a total of 5 doses administered as follows:

Three doses, usually given at 2-, 4-, and 6 months of age; may be given as early as 6 weeks of age and repeated every 4 to 8 weeks

Fourth dose: Given at ~15 to 18 months of age, but at least 6 months after third dose. The fourth dose may be given as early as 12 months of age, but at least 6 months must have elapsed between the third dose and the fourth dose. The fourth dose does not need to be repeated if administered at least 4 months after the third dose.

Fifth dose: Given at 4 to 6 years of age, prior to starting school or kindergarten; if the fourth dose is given at ≥4 years of age, the fifth dose may be omitted

Catch-up immunization:

CDC (ACIP) Recommendations (Strikas 2015): **Note:** Do not restart the series. If doses have been given, begin the below schedule at the applicable dose number.

Infants and Children who start primary immunization series ≥4 months of age through 6 years (prior to seventh birthday): Pediatric formulation (DT): IM: 0.5 mL per dose for a total of 4 to 5 doses administered as follows: 3 doses at least 4 weeks apart followed 6 months later with dose 4; a fifth dose may be given 6 months later (the fifth dose is not necessary if the child received the fourth dose after 4 years of age)

Children ≥7 years and Adolescents not fully, or never vaccinated against diphtheria, or tetanus, or pertussis, or whose vaccination status is not known: IM: 0.5 mL per dose for a total of 3 to 4 doses given as follows:

First dose given on the elected date: Use Td only if contraindication to vaccine containing pertussis, Tdap (Adacel, Boostrix) is preferred for this dose

Second dose (tetanus and diphtheria, Td) given at least 4 weeks after the first dose

Third dose (tetanus and diphtheria, Td) given at least 4 weeks after the second dose (if first DTaP/DT at <12 months of age) **or** given at least 6 months after the second dose (if first dose DTaP/DT at ≥12 months of age)

Fourth dose (tetanus and diphtheria, Td) given at least 6 months after the third dose; fourth dose is not needed if the first DTaP/DT dose was given at ≥12 months of age.

Manufacturer's labeling: Tenivac: Children ≥7 years, Adolescents, and Adults: IM: Patients previously not immunized should receive 2 primary doses of 0.5 mL each, given at an interval of 8 weeks; plus a third (reinforcing) dose of 0.5 mL given 6 to 8 months later. **Note:** For patients who have not received Tdap, a dose should be included as part of primary immunization (in place of one of the Td doses) (CDC/ACIP [Kim 2015]).

Booster immunization: For routine booster in patients who have completed primary immunization series. The ACIP prefers Tdap for use in in some situations if no contraindications exist; refer to Diphtheria and Tetanus Toxoids, and Acellular Pertussis Vaccine monograph for additional information.

Children 11 to 12 years: IM: 0.5 mL as a single dose when at least 5 years have elapsed since last dose of toxoid-containing vaccine. If not contraindicated, Tdap is the preferred agent for this dose. Subsequent routine doses (Td) are not recommended more often than every 10 years. **Note:** If Tdap is given as part of catch-up dosing at 7 to 10 years of age, the 11 to 12 year booster is not needed. Regular Td booster immunizations should begin 10 years after the last dose of the primary series.

Adolescents and Adults: IM 0.5 mL as a single dose every 10 years

Tetanus prophylaxis in wound management (CDC/ACIP [Broder 2006]): Infants, Children, Adolescents, and Adults: Tetanus prophylaxis in patients with wounds should be based on if the wound is clean or contaminated, the immunization status of the patient. Wound management includes proper use of tetanus toxoid and/or tetanus immune globulin (TIG), wound cleaning, and (if required) surgical debridement and the proper use of antibiotics. Patients with an uncertain or incomplete tetanus immunization status should have additional follow-up to ensure a series is completed. Patients with a history of Arthus reaction following a previous dose of a tetanus toxoid-containing vaccine should not receive a tetanus toxoid-containing vaccine until >10 years after the most recent dose even if they have a wound that is neither clean nor minor. See table.

Tetanus Prophylaxis Wound Management

History of Tetanus Immunization (Doses)	Clean, Minor Wounds		All Other Wounds[1]	
	Tetanus toxoid[2]	TIG	Tetanus toxoid[2]	TIG
Uncertain or <3 doses	Yes	No	Yes	Yes
3 or more doses	No[3]	No	No[4]	No

[1]Such as, but not limited to, wounds contaminated with dirt, feces, soil, and saliva; puncture wounds; wounds from crushing, tears, burns, and frostbite.

[2]Tetanus toxoid in this chart refers to a tetanus toxoid containing vaccine. For children ≤6 years old DTaP (DT, if pertussis vaccine contraindicated) is preferred to tetanus toxoid alone. For children ≥7 years of age and Adults, Td preferred to tetanus toxoid alone; Tdap may be preferred if the patient has not previously been vaccinated with Tdap.

[3]Yes, if ≥10 years since last dose.

[4]Yes, if ≥ 5 years since last dose.

Abbreviations: **DT** = Diphtheria and Tetanus Toxoids (formulation for age ≤6 years); **DTaP** = Diphtheria and Tetanus Toxoids, and Acellular Pertussis (formulation for age ≤6 years; Daptacel, Infanrix); **Td** = Diphtheria and Tetanus Toxoids (formulation for age ≥7 years; Tenivac); **TT** = Tetanus toxoid (adsorbed [formulation for age ≥7 years]); **Tdap** = Diphtheria and Tetanus Toxoids, and Acellular Pertussis (Adacel or Boostrix [formulations for age ≥7 years]); **TIG** = Tetanus Immune Globulin

Dosing adjustment in renal impairment: There are no dosage adjustments provided in the manufacturer's labeling.

Dosing adjustment in hepatic impairment: There are no dosage adjustments provided in the manufacturer's labeling.

Administration IM Prior to use, shake suspension well; not for IV or SubQ administration. To prevent syncope related injuries, adolescents and adults should be vaccinated while seated or lying down (NCIRD/ACIP 2011). US law requires that the date of administration, the vaccine manufacturer, lot number of vaccine, and the administering person's name, title, and address be entered into the patient's permanent medical record.

DT (pediatric use): Administer in either the anterolateral aspect of the thigh or the deltoid muscle; do not inject in the gluteal area

Td: Administer in the deltoid muscle; do not inject in the gluteal area.

For patients at risk of hemorrhage following intramuscular injection, the vaccine should be administered intramuscularly if, in the opinion of the physician familiar with the patient's bleeding risk, the vaccine can be administered by this route with reasonable safety. If the patient receives antihemophilia or other similar therapy, intramuscular vaccination can be scheduled shortly after such therapy is administered. A fine needle (23 gauge or smaller) should be used for the vaccination and firm pressure on the site (without rubbing) for at least 2 minutes. The patient should be instructed concerning the risk of hematoma from the injection. Patients on anticoagulant therapy should be considered to have the same bleeding risks and treated as those with clotting factor disorders (NCIRD/ACIP 2011).

Monitoring Parameters Observe for syncope for 15 minutes following administration (NCIRD/ACIP 2011). If seizure-like activity associated with syncope occurs, maintain patient in supine or Trendelenburg position to reestablish adequate cerebral perfusion.

Dosage Forms Excipient information presented when available (limited, particularly for generics); consult specific product labeling. [DSC] = Discontinued product

Injection, suspension [Td, adult; preservative free]: Diphtheria 2 Lf units and tetanus 2 Lf units per 0.5 mL (0.5 mL)

Tenivac: Diphtheria 2 Lf units and tetanus 5 Lf units per 0.5 mL (0.5 mL) [contains aluminum, may contain natural rubber/natural latex in prefilled syringe]

Injection, suspension [DT, pediatric; preservative free]: Diphtheria 6.7 Lf units and tetanus 5 Lf units per 0.5 mL (0.5 mL) [DSC]; Diphtheria 25 Lf units and tetanus 5 Lf units per 0.5 mL (0.5 mL) [contains aluminum]

Diphtheria and Tetanus Toxoids, Acellular Pertussis, and Poliovirus Vaccine

(dif THEER ee a & TET a nus TOKS oyds, ay CEL yoo lar per TUS sis & POE lee oh VYE rus vak SEEN)

Medication Safety Issues

Sound-alike/look-alike issues:

Adacel (trade name for Diphtheria and Tetanus Toxoids, and Acellular Pertussis Vaccine) should not be confused with Adacel-Polio (trade name for Diphtheria and Tetanus Toxoids, Acellular Pertussis, and Poliovirus Vaccine in Canada)

International issues:

Repevax [Multiple International Markets] may be confused with Revaxis brand name for diphtheria, tetanus, and poliomyelitis vaccine [Multiple International Markets]

Related Information

Centers for Disease Control and Prevention (CDC) and Other Links *on page 2424*

Immunization Administration Recommendations *on page 2411*

Immunization Schedules *on page 2416*

Brand Names: US Kinrix; Quadracel

Brand Names: Canada Adacel-Polio; Quadracel

Therapeutic Category Vaccine; Vaccine, Inactivated Bacteria; Vaccine, Inactivated Virus

Generic Availability (US) No

Use

Kinrix: Active immunization against diphtheria, tetanus, pertussis, and poliomyelitis; used as the fifth dose in the DTaP series and the fourth dose in the IPV series in patients whose previous DTaP vaccine doses have been with Infanrix (DTaP) and/or Pediarix (DTaP, hepatitis B, IPV combined) for the first 3 doses and Infanrix (DTaP) for the fourth dose (FDA approved in ages 4 to 6 years)

Quadracel: Active immunization against diphtheria, tetanus, pertussis, and poliomyelitis; used as the fifth dose in the DTaP series and the fourth or fifth dose in the IPV series in children who have received 4 doses of Pentacel (DTaP, IPV, and *Haemophilus b* combined) and/or Daptacel (DTaP) (FDA approved in ages 4 to 6 years)

The Advisory Committee on Immunization Practices (ACIP) recommends this as routine vaccination for use as the fifth dose in the DTaP series and the fourth dose in the IPV series (CDC/ACIP 57[39] 2008).

Pregnancy Risk Factor C

Pregnancy Considerations Reproduction studies have not been conducted; Kinrix and Quadracel are not indicated for women of childbearing age. Adacel-Polio [Canadian product] is not recommended for use in pregnant women unless a definite risk of pertussis exists. Inactivated bacterial vaccines have not been shown to cause increased risks to the fetus (NCIRD/ACIP 2011).

Breast-Feeding Considerations Kinrix and Quadracel are not indicated for use in patients ≥7 years of age. Use of Adacel-Polio [Canadian product] in lactating women has not been studied. Inactivated bacterial vaccines have not been shown to cause increased risks to the fetus (NCIRD/ACIP 2011).

Contraindications Severe allergic reaction (eg, anaphylaxis) after a previous dose of any diphtheria toxoid, tetanus toxoid, pertussis-containing vaccine, or inactivated poliovirus vaccine, or to any component of DTaP/IPV, including neomycin and polymyxin B; encephalopathy (eg, coma, decreased level of consciousness, prolonged seizures) within 7 days of administration of a previous dose of a pertussis-containing vaccine that is not attributable to another identifiable cause; progressive neurologic disorder, including infantile spasms, uncontrolled epilepsy, or progressive encephalopathy.

Warnings/Precautions Immediate treatment (including epinephrine 1:1,000) for anaphylactoid and/or hypersensitivity reactions should be available during vaccine use (NCIRD/ACIP 2011). Patients with a history of severe local reaction (Arthus-type) following a previous tetanus toxoid dose should not be given further routine or emergency doses of Td more frequently than every 10 years, even if using for wound management with wounds that are not clean or minor; these patients generally have high serum antitoxin levels. Carefully consider use in patients with history of any of the following effects from previous administration of any pertussis-containing vaccine: Fever ≥105°F (40.5°C) within 48 hours of unknown cause; seizures with or without fever occurring within 3 days; persistent, inconsolable crying episodes lasting ≥3 hours and occurring within 48 hours; collapse or shock-like state (hypotonic-hyporesponsive episode) within 48 hours. Kinrix and Quadracel are contraindicated in patients who had encephalopathy within 7 days of a previous pertussis-containing vaccine. Use with caution if Guillain-Barré syndrome occurred within 6 weeks of prior tetanus toxoid-containing vaccine (NCIRD/ACIP 2011). The decision to administer or delay vaccination because of current or recent febrile illness depends on the severity of symptoms and the etiology of the disease. Consider deferring administration in patients with moderate or severe acute illness (with or without fever); vaccination should not be delayed for patients with mild acute illness (with or without fever). Syncope has been reported with use of injectable vaccines and may result in serious secondary injury (eg, skull fracture, cerebral hemorrhage); typically reported in adolescents and young adults and within 15 minutes after vaccination. Procedures should be in place to avoid injuries from falling and to restore cerebral perfusion if syncope occurs (NCIRD/ACIP 2011).

Use with caution in patients with history of seizure disorder, progressive neurologic disease, or conditions predisposing to seizures; ACIP guidelines recommend deferring immunization until health status can be assessed and condition stabilized (NCIRD/ACIP 2011). Use with caution in patients with bleeding disorders (including thrombocytopenia) and/or patients on anticoagulant therapy; bleeding/hematoma may occur from IM administration; if the patient receives antihemophilia or other similar therapy, IM injection can be scheduled shortly after such therapy is administered (NCIRD/ACIP 2011).

Use with caution in severely immunocompromised patients (eg, patients receiving chemo/radiation therapy or other immunosuppressive therapy [including high-dose corticosteroids]); may have a reduced response to vaccination. In general, household and close contacts of persons with altered immunocompetence may receive all age appropriate vaccines (IDSA [Rubin 2014]; NCIRD/ACIP 2011); inactivated vaccines should be administered ≥2 weeks prior to planned immunosuppression when feasible (IDSA [Rubin 2014]).

Contains aluminum, neomycin, or polymyxin B; packaging may contain latex. Some dosage forms may contain polysorbate 80 (also known as Tweens). Hypersensitivity reactions, usually a delayed reaction, have been reported following exposure to pharmaceutical products containing polysorbate 80 in certain individuals (Isaksson 2002; Lucente 2000; Shelley 1995). Thrombocytopenia, ascites, pulmonary deterioration, and renal and hepatic failure have been reported in premature neonates after receiving parenteral products containing polysorbate 80 (Alade 1986; CDC 1984). See manufacturer's labeling.

In order to maximize vaccination rates, the ACIP and the NACI, recommend simultaneous administration (ie, >1 vaccine on the same day at different anatomic sites) of all age-appropriate vaccines (live or inactivated) for which a person is eligible at a single clinic visit, unless contraindications exist. The use of combination vaccines is generally preferred over separate injections, taking into consideration provider assessment, patient preference, and adverse events. When using combination vaccines, the minimum age for administration is the oldest minimum age for any individual component; the minimum interval between dosing is the greatest minimum interval between any individual components. The ACIP prefers each dose of a specific vaccine in a series come from the same manufacturer when possible (NCIRD/ACIP 2011). According to the manufacturer, antipyretics may be considered at the time of and for 24 hours following vaccination to patients at high risk for seizures to reduce the possibility of postvaccination fever. However, antipyretics have not been shown to prevent febrile seizures; antipyretics may be used to treat fever or discomfort following vaccination (NCIRD/ACIP 2011). One study reported that routine prophylactic administration of acetaminophen to prevent fever prior to vaccination decreased the immune response of some vaccines; the clinical significance of this reduction in immune response has not been established (Prymula 2009). Vaccination may not result in effective immunity in all patients. Response depends upon multiple factors (eg, type of vaccine, age of patient) and may be improved by administering the vaccine at the recommended dose, route, and interval. Vaccines may not be effective if administered during periods of altered immune competence (NCIRD/ACIP 2011). If Kinrix is inadvertently administered to children for an earlier dose in the series, it may be counted as a valid dose, provided the minimum interval requirements were met. Safety and efficacy of Kinrix and Quadracel have not been established for use in adults.

Adverse Reactions All serious adverse reactions must be reported to the US Department of Health and Human Services (DHHS) Vaccine Adverse Event Reporting System (VAERS) 1-800-822-7967 or online at https://vaers.hhs.gov/esub/index. In Canada, adverse reactions may be reported to local provincial/territorial health agencies or to the Vaccine Safety Section at Public Health Agency of Canada (1-866-844-0018).

Adverse events reported within 4 to 7 days of vaccination:

>10%:

Cardiovascular: Swelling of injected limb (arm circumference increase), swelling of injected limb (extensive)

Central nervous system: Drowsiness, headache, malaise

Gastrointestinal: Decreased appetite

Local: Injection site: Erythema at injection site, pain at injection site, swelling

Neuromuscular & skeletal: Myalgia

Miscellaneous: Fever

Rare but important or life-threatening: Abscess at injection site, cerebrovascular accident, convulsions, cyanosis, febrile seizures, gastroenteritis, hypernatremia, hypersensitivity reaction, hypotonia, hypotonic/hyporesponsive episode, injection site cellulitis, residual mass at injection site, sterile abscess at injection site, syncope

Drug Interactions

Metabolism/Transport Effects None known.

Avoid Concomitant Use There are no known interactions where it is recommended to avoid concomitant use.

Increased Effect/Toxicity There are no known significant interactions involving an increase in effect.

Decreased Effect

The levels/effects of Diphtheria and Tetanus Toxoids, Acellular Pertussis, and Poliovirus Vaccine may be decreased by: Belimumab; Fingolimod; Immunosuppressants; Meningococcal Polysaccharide (Groups A / C / Y and W-135) Tetanus Toxoid Conjugate Vaccine

Storage/Stability

Kinrix, Quadracel: Store under refrigeration of 2°C to 8°C (36°F to 46°F); do not freeze. Discard if frozen.

Adacel-Polio [Canadian product]: Store under refrigeration of 2°C to 8°C (36°F to 46°F); stable for 72 hours at temperatures up to 25°C (77°F); do not freeze. Discard if frozen.

Mechanism of Action Promotes active immunity to diphtheria, tetanus, pertussis, and poliovirus (types 1, 2 and 3) by inducing production of specific antibodies and antitoxins.

Pharmacodynamics Onset of action: Immune response observed to all components ~1 month following vaccination

Dosing: Usual Pediatric: **Immunization:** Children 4 to 6 years: IM: 0.5 mL as a single dose; **Note:** For use as the fifth dose in the DTaP series and the fourth dose in the IPV series

Dosing adjustment in renal impairment: There are no dosage adjustments provided in the manufacturer's labeling.

Dosing adjustment in hepatic impairment: There are no dosage adjustments provided in the manufacturer's labeling.

Administration Shake well; do not use unless a homogeneous, turbid, white suspension forms; administer IM the deltoid muscle of the upper arm; not for IV or SubQ administration. U.S. law requires that the date of administration, name of the vaccine manufacturer, lot number of vaccine, and the administering person's name, title, and address be entered into the patient's permanent medical record.

For patients at risk of hemorrhage following intramuscular injection, the vaccine should be administered intramuscularly if, in the opinion of the physician familiar with the patient's bleeding risk, the vaccine can be administered by this route with reasonable safety. If the patient receives antihemophilia or other similar therapy, intramuscular vaccination can be scheduled shortly after such therapy is administered. A fine needle (23 gauge or smaller) should be used for the vaccination and firm pressure on the site (without rubbing) for at least 2 minutes. The patient should be instructed concerning the risk of hematoma from the injection. Patients on anticoagulant therapy should be considered to have the same bleeding risks and treated as those with clotting factor disorders (NCIRD/ACIP 2011).

Monitoring Parameters Observe for syncope for 15 minutes following administration (NCIRD/ACIP 2011). If seizure-like activity associated with syncope occurs, maintain patient in supine or Trendelenburg position to reestablish adequate cerebral perfusion.

Additional Information Contains the following three pertussis antigens: Inactivated pertussis toxin (PT), filamentous hemagglutinin (FHA), and pertactin. Contains the same diphtheria, tetanus toxoids, and pertussis antigens found in Infanrix and Pediarix. Contains the same poliovirus antigens found in Infanrix.

Product Availability Quadracel: FDA approved March 2015; anticipated availability is currently unknown.

Dosage Forms Excipient information presented when available (limited, particularly for generics); consult specific product labeling.

Injection, suspension [preservative free]:

Kinrix: Diphtheria toxoid 25 Lf, tetanus toxoid 10 Lf, acellular pertussis antigens [inactivated pertussis toxin 25 mcg, filamentous hemagglutinin 25 mcg, pertactin 8 mcg], type 1 poliovirus 40 D-antigen units, type 2 poliovirus 8 D-antigen units, and type 3 poliovirus 32 D-antigen units per 0.5 mL (0.5 mL) [contains aluminum, neomycin sulfate, polymyxin B, polysorbate 80; may contain natural rubber/natural latex in prefilled syringe]

Quadracel: Diphtheria toxoid 15 Lf, tetanus toxoid 5 Lf, acellular pertussis antigens [detoxified pertussis toxin 20 mcg, filamentous hemagglutinin 20 mcg, pertactin 3 mcg, fimbriae (types 2 and 3) 5 mcg], type 1 poliovirus 40 D-antigen units, type 2 poliovirus 8 D-antigen units, and type 3 poliovirus 32 D-antigen units per 0.5 mL (0.5 mL) [contains aluminum, neomycin sulfate, polymyxin B, polysorbate 80]

Diphtheria and Tetanus Toxoids, Acellular Pertussis, Poliovirus and *Haemophilus* b Conjugate Vaccine

(dif THEER ee a & TET a nus TOKS oyds ay CEL yoo lar per TUS sis POE lee oh VYE rus & hem OF fi lus bee KON joo gate vak SEEN)

Medication Safety Issues

Administration issues:

Pentacel® is supplied in two vials, one containing DTaP-IPV liquid and one containing Hib powder, which must be mixed together in order to administer the recommended vaccine components.

Related Information

Centers for Disease Control and Prevention (CDC) and Other Links *on page 2424*

Immunization Administration Recommendations *on page 2411*

Immunization Schedules *on page 2416*

Brand Names: US Pentacel

Brand Names: Canada Infanrix-IPV/HIB; Pediacel; Pentacel

Therapeutic Category Vaccine; Vaccine, Inactivated Bacteria; Vaccine, Inactivated Virus

Generic Availability (US) No

Use Active immunization against diphtheria, tetanus, pertussis, poliomyelitis, and invasive disease caused by *H. influenzae* type b (FDA approved in ages 6 weeks to ≤4 years)

Advisory Committee on Immunization Practices (ACIP) states that Pentacel (DTaP-IPV/Hib) may be used to provide the recommended DTaP, IPV, and Hib immunization in infants and children ≤4 years of age. Whenever feasible, the same manufacturer should be used to provide the pertussis component; however, vaccination should not be deferred if a specific brand is not known or is not available. The Hib component in Pentacel contains a tetanus toxoid conjugate. A Hib vaccine containing the PRP-OMP conjugate (PedvaxHIB) may provide a more rapid seroconversion following the first dose and may be preferable to use in certain populations (eg, American Indian or Alaska Native children) (CDC 57[39] 2008).

Pregnancy Risk Factor C

Pregnancy Considerations Animal reproduction studies have not been conducted for this combination product. This product is not indicated for use in women of child-bearing age.

Contraindications Severe allergic reaction to any vaccine containing diphtheria toxoid, tetanus toxoid, pertussis, poliovirus, or *Haemophilus* b, or any component of this vaccine; encephalopathy occurring within 7 days of a previous pertussis vaccine not (not attributable to another identifiable cause); progressive neurologic disorders (including infantile spasms, uncontrolled epilepsy, or progressive encephalopathy)

Warnings/Precautions Immediate treatment (including epinephrine 1:1,000) for anaphylactoid and/or hypersensitivity reactions should be available during vaccine use (NCIRD/ACIP 2011). Carefully consider use in patients with history of any of the following effects from previous administration of a pertussis-containing vaccine: Fever ≥105°F (40.5°C) within 48 hours of unknown cause; seizures with or without fever occurring within 3 days; persistent, inconsolable crying episodes lasting ≥3 hours and occurring within 48 hours; or collapse or shock-like state (hypotonic-hyporesponsive episode) occurring within 48 hours. Patients with a history of severe local reaction (Arthus-type) following a previous tetanus toxoid dose should not be given further routine or emergency doses of Td more frequently than every 10 years, even if using for wound management with wounds that are not clean or minor; these patients generally have high serum antitoxin levels (NCIRD/ACIP 2011).

The decision to administer or delay vaccination because of current or recent febrile illness depends on the severity of symptoms and the etiology of the disease. Consider deferring administration in patients with moderate or severe acute illness (with or without fever); vaccination should not be delayed for patients with mild acute illness (with or without fever) (NCIRD/ACIP 2011). Syncope has been reported with use of injectable vaccines and may result in serious secondary injury (eg, skull fracture, cerebral hemorrhage); typically reported in adolescents and young adults and within 15 minutes after vaccination. Procedures should be in place to avoid injuries from falling and to restore cerebral perfusion if syncope occurs (NCIRD/ACIP 2011). Apnea has been reported following IM vaccine administration in premature infants; consider clinical status implications. In general, preterm infants should be vaccinated at the same chronological age as full-term infants (NCIRD/ACIP 2011).

Use with caution in patients with bleeding disorders (including thrombocytopenia) and patients on anticoagulant therapy; bleeding/hematoma may occur from IM administration; if the patient receives antihemophilia or other similar therapy, I.M. injection can be scheduled shortly after such therapy is administered (NCIRD/ACIP 2011). Use with caution if Guillain-Barré syndrome occurred within 6 weeks of prior tetanus toxoid-toxoid containing vaccine (NCIRD/ACIP 2011). Use with caution in patients with history of seizure disorder, progressive neurologic disease, or conditions predisposing to seizures; ACIP guidelines recommend deferring immunization until health status can be assessed and condition stabilized (NCIRD/ACIP 2011). Antipyretics have not been shown to prevent febrile seizures; antipyretics may be used to treat fever or discomfort following vaccination (NCIRD/ACIP 2011). One study reported that routine prophylactic administration of acetaminophen to prevent fever prior to vaccination decreased the immune response of some vaccines; the clinical significance of this reduction in immune response has not been established (Prymula 2009). Vaccination may not result in effective immunity in all patients. Response depends upon multiple factors (eg, type of vaccine, age of patient) and may be improved by administering the vaccine at the recommended dose, route, and interval. Vaccines may not be effective if administered during periods of altered immune competence (NCIRD/ACIP 2011). Use with caution in severely immunocompromised patients (eg, patients receiving chemo/radiation therapy or other immunosuppressive therapy [including high-dose corticosteroids]); may have a reduced response to vaccination. In general, household and close contacts of persons with altered immunocompetence may receive all age appropriate vaccines (IDSA [Rubin 2014]; NCIRD/ACIP 2011); inactivated vaccines should be administered ≥2 weeks prior to planned immunosuppression when feasible (IDSA [Rubin 2014]). In order to maximize vaccination rates, the ACIP recommends simultaneous administration (ie, >1 vaccine on the same day at different anatomic sites) of all age-appropriate vaccines (live or inactivated) for which a person is eligible at a single clinic visit, unless contraindications exist. The use of combination vaccines is generally preferred over separate injections, taking into consideration provider assessment, patient preference, and potential adverse events. When using combination vaccines, the minimum age for administration is the oldest minimum age for any individual component; the minimum interval between dosing is the greatest minimum interval between any individual components. The ACIP prefers each dose of a specific vaccine in a series come from the same manufacturer when possible (NCIRD/ACIP 2011). If inadvertently administered to children ≥5 years as a booster dose, it may be counted as a valid dose (CDC 57[39] 2008). Safety and efficacy have not been established in adults.

Product may contain aluminum, neomycin, or polymyxin B. Some dosage forms may contain polysorbate 80 (also known as Tweens). Hypersensitivity reactions, usually a delayed reaction, have been reported following exposure to pharmaceutical products containing polysorbate 80 in certain individuals (Isaksson 2002; Lucente 2000; Shelley 1995). Thrombocytopenia, ascites, pulmonary deterioration, and renal and hepatic failure have been reported in premature neonates after receiving parenteral products containing polysorbate 80 (Alade 1986; CDC 1984). See manufacturer's labeling.

Adverse Reactions All serious adverse reactions must be reported to the U.S. Department of Health and Human Services (DHHS) Vaccine Adverse Event Reporting System (VAERS) 1-800-822-7967 or online at https://vaers.hhs.gov/esub/index. In Canada, adverse reactions may be reported to local provincial/territorial health agencies or to the Vaccine Safety Section at Public Health Agency of Canada (1-866-844-0018).

Central nervous system: Crying (inconsolable), fever ≥38°C, fussiness/irritability, lethargy/decreased activity

Local: Injection site reactions: Arm circumference increase >5 mm, redness >5 mm, swelling >5 mm, tenderness

Rare but important or life-threatening: Anaphylaxis/anaphylactic reaction, apnea, appetite decreased, asthma, bronchiolitis, consciousness decreased, cough, cyanosis, dehydration, diarrhea, encephalopathy, erythema, gastroenteritis, hypersensitivity reactions, hypotonia, hypotonic-hyporesponsive episodes, injection site reactions (abscess, extensive swelling of injected limb, inflammation, mass), pallor, pneumonia, screaming, seizure, skin discoloration, somnolence, vomiting

Drug Interactions

Metabolism/Transport Effects None known.

Avoid Concomitant Use There are no known interactions where it is recommended to avoid concomitant use.

Increased Effect/Toxicity There are no known significant interactions involving an increase in effect.

Decreased Effect

The levels/effects of Diphtheria and Tetanus Toxoids, Acellular Pertussis, Poliovirus and Haemophilus b Conjugate Vaccine may be decreased by: Belimumab; Fingolimod; Immunosuppressants; Meningococcal Polysaccharide (Groups A / C / Y and W-135) Tetanus Toxoid Conjugate Vaccine

Storage/Stability Store at 2°C to 8°C (35°F to 46°F). Do not freeze; discard if product has been frozen. Use immediately after reconstitution.

Dosing: Usual

Pediatric:

Primary immunization:

Infants and Children 6 weeks to ≤4 years: IM: 0.5 mL per dose for a total of 4 doses administered as follows: 2, 4, 6, and 15 to 18 months of age. The first dose may be administered as early as 6 weeks of age. Following completion of the 4-dose series, children should receive a dose of DTaP vaccine at 4 to 6 years of age (Daptacel recommended due to same pertussis antigen used in both products).

Note: Per the ACIP, polio vaccine is given at 2-, 4-, and 6 to 18 months of age. Use of the minimum age and minimum intervals during the first 6 months of life should only be done when the vaccine recipient is at risk for imminent exposure to circulating poliovirus (shorter intervals and earlier start dates may lead to lower seroconversion) (CDC 58[30] 2009). Pentacel is not indicated for the polio booster dose given at 4 to 6 years of age; Kinrix or IPV should be used.

Use in infants and children previously vaccinated with one or more component, and who are also scheduled to receive all vaccine components:

Infants and Children previously vaccinated with ≥1 dose of Daptacel or IPV vaccines: Pentacel may be used to complete the first 4 doses of the DTaP or IPV series in children scheduled to receive the other components in the vaccine.

Infants and Children previously vaccinated with ≥1 dose of *Haemophilus b* Conjugate vaccine: Pentacel may be used to complete the series in children scheduled to receive the other components in the vaccine; however, if different brands of *Haemophilus b* Conjugate vaccine are administered to complete the series, 3 primary immunizing doses are needed, followed by a booster dose.

Note: Completion of 3 doses of Pentacel provides primary immunization against diphtheria, tetanus, *H. influenzae* type B, and poliomyelitis. Completion of the 4-dose series with Pentacel provides primary immunization against pertussis. It also provides a booster vaccination against diphtheria, tetanus, *H. influenzae* type B, and poliomyelitis.

Dosing adjustment in renal impairment: There are no dosage adjustments provided in manufacturer's labeling.

Dosing adjustment in hepatic impairment: There are no dosage adjustments provided in manufacturer's labeling.

Preparation for Administration IM: Pentacel is supplied in two vials, one containing DTaP-IPV liquid and one containing Hib powder, which must be mixed together before administering. Gently shake vial containing DTaP-IPV component. Withdraw liquid contents and inject into vial containing Hib powder; gently swirl until a cloudy, uniform suspension results.

Administration IM: Administer IM in the anterolateral aspect of thigh in infants <1 year of age or deltoid muscle of upper arm in older children. Do not administer to gluteal area or areas near a major nerve trunk; not for IV or SubQ administration. US law requires that the date of administration, name of the vaccine manufacturer, lot number of vaccine, and the administering person's name, title, and address be entered into the patient's permanent medical record. Lot numbers are different for each component of the DTaP-IPV/Hib vaccine; numbers should be recorded separately for the DTaP-IPV and Hib components. The vaccine components should not be administered separately.

For patients at risk of hemorrhage following intramuscular injection, the vaccine should be administered intramuscularly if, in the opinion of the physician familiar with the patient's bleeding risk, the vaccine can be administered by this route with reasonable safety. If the patient receives antihemophilia or other similar therapy, intramuscular vaccination can be scheduled shortly after such therapy is administered. A fine needle (23 gauge or smaller) should be used for the vaccination and firm pressure on the site (without rubbing) for at least 2 minutes. The patient should be instructed concerning the risk of hematoma from the injection. Patients on anticoagulant therapy should be considered to have the same bleeding risks and treated as those with clotting factor disorders (NCIRD/ACIP 2011).

Monitoring Parameters Observe for syncope for 15 minutes following administration (NCIRD/ACIP 2011). If seizure-like activity associated with syncope occurs, maintain patient in supine or Trendelenburg position to reestablish adequate cerebral perfusion.

Additional Information Contains the following three pertussis antigens: Inactivated pertussis toxin (PT), filamentous hemagglutinin (FHA), and pertactin. Contains the same diphtheria, tetanus toxoids, and pertussis antigens found in Daptacel; the same poliovirus antigens found in IPOL; the same Hib-PRP found in ActHIB.

Dosage Forms Excipient information presented when available (limited, particularly for generics); consult specific product labeling.

Injection, suspension:

Pentacel®: Diphtheria toxoid 15 Lf, tetanus toxoid 5 Lf, acellular pertussis antigens [pertussis toxin detoxified 20 mcg, filamentous hemagglutinin 20 mcg, pertactin 3 mcg, fimbriae (types 2 and 3) 5 mcg], type 1poliovirus 40 D-antigen units; type 2 poliovirus 8 D-antigen units; type 3 poliovirus 32 D-antigen units, and *Haemophilus* b capsular polysaccharide 10 mcg [bound to tetanus toxoid 24 mcg] per 0.5 mL (0.5 mL) [contains albumin, aluminum, neomycin, polymyxin B sulfate, and polysorbate 80; supplied in two vials, one containing DTaP-IPV liquid and one containing Hib powder]

◆ **Diphtheria and Tetanus Toxoids and Acellular Pertussis Adsorbed, and Inactivated Poliovirus Vaccine Combined** *see* Diphtheria and Tetanus Toxoids, Acellular Pertussis, and Poliovirus Vaccine *on page 677*

◆ **Diphtheria and Tetanus Toxoids and Acellular Pertussis Adsorbed, Hepatitis B (Recombinant) and Inactivated Poliovirus Vaccine Combined** *see* Diphtheria, Tetanus Toxoids, Acellular Pertussis, Hepatitis B (Recombinant), and Poliovirus (Inactivated) Vaccine *on page 685*

Diphtheria and Tetanus Toxoids, and Acellular Pertussis Vaccine

(dif THEER ee a & TET a nus TOKS oyds & ay CEL yoo lar per TUS sis vak SEEN)

Medication Safety Issues

Sound-alike/look-alike issues:

Adacel (Tdap) may be confused with Daptacel (DTaP)

Tdap (Adacel, Boostrix) may be confused with DTaP (Daptacel, Infanrix, Tripedia)

Administration issues:

Carefully review product labeling to prevent inadvertent administration of Tdap when DTaP is indicated. Tdap contains lower amounts of diphtheria toxoid and some pertussis antigens than DTaP.

DTaP is indicated for use in persons ≤6 years of age

Tdap is indicated for use in children ≥10 years of age. If needed, Tdap can be used for children 7 to 10 years (CDC/ACIP, 60[1] 2011)

Guidelines are available in case of inadvertent administration of these products; refer to ACIP recommendations, February 2006 available at http://www.cdc.gov/mmwr/preview/mmwrhtml/rr55e223a1.htm

Other safety concerns:

DTaP: Diphtheria and tetanus toxoids and acellular pertussis vaccine

DTP: Diphtheria and tetanus toxoids and pertussis vaccine (unspecified pertussis antigens)

DTwP: Diphtheria and tetanus toxoids and whole-cell pertussis vaccine (no longer available on U.S. market)

Tdap: Tetanus toxoid, reduced diphtheria toxoid, and acellular pertussis vaccine

Related Information

Centers for Disease Control and Prevention (CDC) and Other Links *on page 2424*

Immunization Administration Recommendations *on page 2411*

Immunization Schedules *on page 2416*

Brand Names: US Adacel; Boostrix; Daptacel; Infanrix

Brand Names: Canada Adacel; Boostrix

Therapeutic Category Vaccine; Vaccine, Inactivated Bacteria

Generic Availability (US) No

Use

DTaP (Daptacel, Infanrix): Active immunization for prevention of diphtheria, tetanus, and pertussis (FDA approved in ages 6 weeks through 6 years); has also been used for wound management for the prevention of tetanus

Tdap:

Adacel: Active booster immunization for prevention of diphtheria, tetanus, and pertussis (FDA approved in ages 10 to 64 years)

Boostrix: Active booster immunization for prevention of diphtheria, tetanus, and pertussis (FDA approved in ages ≥10 years); has also been used for wound management for the prevention of tetanus

The Advisory Committee on Immunization Practices (ACIP) recommends routine vaccination for the following:

Infants and Children 6 weeks to <7 years (DTaP):

- For primary immunization against diphtheria, tetanus, and pertussis (Use of diphtheria toxoid [ACIP] 2000)
- Pediatric patients wounded in bombings or similar mass casualty events, have penetrating injuries or nonintact skin exposure, and have an uncertain vaccination history should receive a tetanus booster with DTaP if no contraindications exist (CDC [Chapman 2008])

Children 7 to 10 years (Tdap):

- Children not fully vaccinated against pertussis should receive a single dose of Tdap if no contraindications exist (CDC/ACIP 60[1] 2011)
- Children never vaccinated against diphtheria, tetanus, or pertussis, or whose vaccination status is not known should receive a series of three vaccinations containing tetanus and diphtheria toxoids and the first dose should be with Tdap (CDC/ACIP 60[1] 2011)

Children ≥11 years and Adolescents (Tdap):

- A single dose of Tdap as a booster dose in adolescents who have completed the recommended childhood DTaP vaccination series (preferred age of administration is 11 to 12 years) (CDC/ACIP 60 [1] 2011)

Children ≥11 years, Adolescents, and Adults (Tdap):

- Persons wounded in bombings or similar mass casualty events and who cannot confirm receipt of a tetanus booster within the previous 5 years and who have penetrating injuries or nonintact skin exposure should receive a single dose of Tdap (CDC [Chapman 2008])

Adolescent and Adult females: Pregnant females should receive a single dose with each pregnancy, preferably between 27 to 36 weeks gestation (CDC/ACIP 62 [7] 2013)

Adults ≥19 years (including adults ≥65 years) (Tdap): A single dose of Tdap should be given to all patients who have not previously received Tdap or for whom their vaccine status is unknown. Following administration of Tdap, Td vaccine should be used for routine boosters (CDC/ACIP [Kim 2015]). The following patients, who have not yet received Tdap or for whom vaccine status is not known, should receive a single dose of Tdap as soon as feasible:

- Close contacts of children <12 months of age: Tdap should ideally be administered at least 2 weeks prior to beginning close contact (CDC/ACIP 60[41], 2011; CDC/ACIP [Kretsinger 2006])
- Health care providers with direct patient contact (CDC/ACIP [Kretsinger 2006])

Note: Tdap is currently recommended for a single dose only (all age groups) (CDC/ACIP 60[1] 2011; CDC/ACIP 61[25] 2012) except pregnant females (CDC/ACIP 62 [7] 2013)

Medication Guide Available Yes

Pregnancy Risk Factor B/C (manufacturer specific)

Pregnancy Considerations Animal reproduction studies have not been conducted with all products; when conducted, adverse effects to the fetus were not observed in developmental toxicity studies. Inactivated bacterial vaccines have not been shown to cause increased risks to the fetus (NCIRD/ACIP 2011). Daptacel and Infanrix are not recommended for use in a pregnant woman or any patient ≥7 years of age. Using data collected from 2005-2010 VAERS, there were not any patterns of adverse maternal, fetal, or neonatal outcomes identified following maternal use of the Tdap vaccine (Zheteyeva 2012).

All pregnant females should receive a single dose of Tdap during each pregnancy, regardless of previous vaccination status, preferably between 27-36 weeks gestation. Alternately, administration of Tdap can be given immediately postpartum to all women who have not previously been vaccinated with Tdap in order to protect the mother and infant from pertussis (CDC/ACIP 62[7] 2013). In case of an ongoing local pertussis epidemic, pregnant women should be vaccinated with Tdap for their own protection as is recommended for nonpregnant women, regardless of fetal gestational age. In addition, if a tetanus toxoid–containing vaccine is needed as standard care for wound management, Tdap may be given regardless of fetal gestational age if otherwise indicated. However, if Tdap is used prior to 27-36 weeks gestation in these instances, women should not receive more than 1 dose during the same pregnancy (ACOG 2013).

Pregnancy registries have been established for women who may become exposed to Boostrix (888-452-9622) or Adacel (800-822-2463) while pregnant.

Breast-Feeding Considerations It is not known if this vaccine is excreted into breast milk. The manufacturer recommends that caution be used if administered to a nursing woman. Breast-feeding is not a contraindication to vaccine administration. Women who have not previously had a dose of Tdap should receive a dose postpartum to help prevent pertussis in infants <12 months of age (CDC/ACIP 62[7] 2013). Inactivated vaccines do not affect the safety of breast-feeding for the mother or the infant. Breast-feeding infants should be vaccinated according to the recommended schedules (NCIRD/ACIP 2011).

Contraindications Hypersensitivity to diphtheria, tetanus toxoids, pertussis, or any component of the formulation; progressive neurologic disorder, including infantile spasms, uncontrolled epilepsy or progressive epilepsy (postpone until condition stabilized); encephalopathy occurring within 7 days of administration and not attributable to another cause

Warnings/Precautions The decision to administer or delay vaccination because of current or recent febrile illness depends on the severity of symptoms and the etiology of the disease. Consider deferring administration in patients with moderate or severe acute illness (with or without fever); vaccination should not be delayed for patients with mild acute illness (with or without fever) (NCIRD/ACIP 2011). Carefully consider use in patients with history of any of the following effects from previous administration of any pertussis to containing vaccine: Fever ≥105°F (40.5°C) within 48 hours of unknown cause; seizures with or without fever occurring within 3 days; persistent, inconsolable crying episodes lasting ≥3 hours and occurring within 48 hours; collapse or shock-like state (hypotonic-hyporesponsive episode) within 48 hours. Use with caution if Guillain-Barré syndrome occured within 6 weeks of prior tetanus toxoid-containing vaccine. Patients with a history of severe local reaction (Arthus-type) following a previous tetanus toxoid dose should not be given further routine or emergency doses of Td more frequently than every 10 years, even if using for wound management with wounds that are not clean or minor; these patients generally have high serum antitoxin levels. Apnea has been reported following IM vaccine administration in premature infants; consider risk versus benefit in infants born prematurely. In general, preterm infants should be vaccinated at the same chronological age as full-term infants (NCIRD/ACIP 2011). Syncope has been reported with use of injectable vaccines and may result in serious secondary injury (eg, skull fracture, cerebral hemorrhage); typically reported in adolescents and young adults and within 15 minutes after vaccination. Procedures should be in place to avoid injuries from falling and to restore cerebral perfusion if syncope occurs NCIRD/ACIP 2011).

Use with caution in patients with bleeding disorders (including thrombocytopenia) and patients on anticoagulant therapy; bleeding/hematoma may occur from IM administration; if the patient receives antihemophilia or other similar therapy, IM injection can be scheduled shortly after such therapy is administered (NCIRD/ACIP 2011). Use with caution in severely immunocompromised patients (eg, patients receiving chemo/radiation therapy or other immunosuppressive therapy [including high-dose corticosteroids]); may have a reduced response to vaccination. In general, household and close contacts of persons with altered immunocompetence may receive all age appropriate vaccines (IDSA [Rubin 2014]; NCIRD/ACIP 2011); inactivated vaccines should be administered ≥2 weeks prior to planned immunosuppression when feasible (IDSA [Rubin 2014]). Vaccination may not result in effective immunity in all patients. Response depends upon multiple factors (eg, type of vaccine, age of patient) and may be improved by administering the vaccine at the recommended dose, route, and interval. Vaccines may not be effective if administered during periods of altered immune competence (NCIRD/ACIP 2011). Per the manufacturer, antipyretic prophylaxis may be considered for patients at high risk for seizures. However, antipyretics have not been shown to prevent febrile seizures. Antipyretics may be used to treat fever or discomfort following vaccination (NCIRD/ACIP 2011). One study reported that routine prophylactic administration of acetaminophen to prevent fever prior to vaccination decreased the immune response of some vaccines; the clinical significance of this reduction in immune response has not been established (Prymula 2009). Use with caution in patients with history of seizure disorder, progressive neurologic disease, or conditions predisposing to seizures; ACIP guidelines recommend deferring immunization until health status can be assessed and condition stabilized (NCIRD/ACIP 2011). Packaging may contain natural latex rubber. Immediate treatment (including epinephrine 1:1,000) for anaphylactic/anaphylactoid reaction should be available during vaccine use. In order to maximize vaccination rates, the ACIP recommends simultaneous administration (ie, >1 vaccine on the same day at different anatomic sites) of all age-appropriate vaccines (live or inactivated) for which a person is eligible at a single clinic visit, unless contraindications exist. The use of combination vaccines is generally preferred over separate injections, taking into consideration provider assessment, patient preference, and adverse events. When using combination vaccines, the minimum age for administration is the oldest minimum age for any individual component; the minimum interval between dosing is the greatest minimum interval between any individual components. The ACIP prefers each dose of a specific vaccine in a series come from the same manufacturer when possible (NCIRD/ACIP 2011).

Use of this vaccine for specific medical and/or other indications (eg, immunocompromising conditions, hepatic or kidney disease, diabetes) is also addressed in the ACIP Recommended Adult Immunization Schedule (CDC/ACIP [Kim 2015]). Specific recommendations for vaccination in immunocompromised patients with asplenia, cancer, HIV infection, cerebrospinal fluid leaks, cochlear implants, hematopoietic stem cell transplant (prior to or after), sickle cell disease, solid organ transplant (prior to or after), or those receiving immunosuppressive therapy for chronic conditions as well as contacts of immunocompromised patients are available from the IDSA (Rubin 2014).

Adacel is formulated with the same antigens found in Daptacel, but with reduced quantities of tetanus and pertussis. Boostrix is formulated with the same antigens found in Infanrix, but in reduced quantities. Use of Adacel or Boostrix in the primary immunization series or to complete the primary series has not been evaluated.

Some dosage forms may contain polysorbate 80 (also known as Tweens). Hypersensitivity reactions, usually a delayed reaction, have been reported following exposure to pharmaceutical products containing polysorbate 80 in certain individuals (Isaksson 2002; Lucente 2000; Shelley, 1995). Thrombocytopenia, ascites, pulmonary deterioration, and renal and hepatic failure have been reported in premature neonates after receiving parenteral products containing polysorbate 80 (Alade 1986; CDC 1984). See manufacturer's labeling.

Adverse Reactions All serious adverse reactions must be reported to the U.S. Department of Health and Human Services (DHHS) Vaccine Adverse Event Reporting System (VAERS) 1-800-822-7967 or online at https://vaers.hhs.gov/esub/index. In Canada, adverse reactions may be reported to local provincial/territorial health agencies or to the Vaccine Safety Section at Public Health Agency of Canada (1-866-844-0018).

Daptacel, Infanrix (incidence of erythema, swelling, and fever increases with successive doses):

Central nervous system: Apathy (refusal to play), drowsiness, irritability, lethargy

Gastrointestinal: Decreased appetite, vomiting

Local: Erythema at injection site, local pain, localized edema, tenderness at injection site

Miscellaneous: Crying (prolonged or persistent), fever, fussiness

Rare but important or life-threatening: Anaphylaxis, angioedema, apnea, brain disease, bronchitis, cellulitis, cough, cyanosis, diarrhea, erythema, fatigue, headache, hypersensitivity reaction, hypotonia, hypotonic/hyporesponsive episode, immune thrombocytopenia, infantile spasm, injection site reaction (abscess, cellulitis, induration, mass, nodule, rash), intussusception, lymphadenopathy, nausea, otalgia, peripheral edema, pruritus, respiratory tract infection, screaming, seizure, skin rash, sudden infant death syndrome, thrombocytopenia, urticaria

Adacel; Boostrix:

Central nervous system: Chills, fatigue, headache

Dermatologic: Skin rash

Endocrine & metabolic: Increased arm circumference

Gastrointestinal: Gastrointestinal disease (includes abdominal pain, diarrhea, nausea, and/or vomiting)

Hematologic & oncologic: Adenopathy

Local: erythema at injection site, pain at injection site, swelling at injection site

Neuromuscular & skeletal: Arthralgia, myalgia

Miscellaneous: Fever (≥38°C [≥100.4°F])

Rare but important or life-threatening: Anaphylaxis, back pain, diabetes mellitus, encephalitis, facial paralysis, Guillain-Barre syndrome, hypersensitivity reaction, hypoesthesia, hypotonic/hyporesponsive episode, IgA vasculitis, injection site reaction (bruising, induration, inflammation, mass, nodule, pruritus, sterile abscess, warmth), lymphadenitis, lymphadenopathy, myalgia, myocarditis, myositis, nerve compression, paresthesia, peripheral edema (extensive), pruritus, seizure, syncope, urticaria

Drug Interactions

Metabolism/Transport Effects None known.

Avoid Concomitant Use There are no known interactions where it is recommended to avoid concomitant use.

Increased Effect/Toxicity There are no known significant interactions involving an increase in effect.

Decreased Effect

The levels/effects of Diphtheria and Tetanus Toxoids, and Acellular Pertussis Vaccine may be decreased by: Belimumab; Fingolimod; Immunosuppressants; Meningococcal Polysaccharide (Groups A / C / Y and W-135) Tetanus Toxoid Conjugate Vaccine

Storage/Stability Refrigerate at 2°C to 8°C (35°F to 46°F); do not freeze; discard if frozen. The following stability information has also been reported for Infanrix: May be stored at room temperature for up to 72 hours (Cohen 2007).

Mechanism of Action Promotes active immunity to diphtheria, tetanus, and pertussis by inducing production of specific antibodies.

Dosing: Usual

Primary immunization: Infants and Children 6 weeks to <7 years: **Note:** Whenever possible, the same product should be used for all doses. Preterm infants should be vaccinated according to their chronological age from birth. DTaP (Daptacel, Infanrix): IM: 0.5 mL per dose for a total of 5 doses administered as follows:

Three doses, usually given at 2-, 4-, and 6 months of age; may be given as early as 6 weeks of age and repeated every 4 to 8 weeks

Fourth dose: Given at ~15 to 20 months of age but at least 6 months after third dose. The fourth dose may be given as early as 12 months of age.

Fifth dose: Given at 4 to 6 years of age, prior to starting school or kindergarten; if the fourth dose is given at ≥4 years of age, the fifth dose may be omitted

Catch-up immunization: CDC (ACIP) Recommendations (Strikas 2015): **Note:** Do not restart the series. If doses have been given, begin the below schedule at the applicable dose number.

Infants and children who start primary immunization series ≥4 months of age through 6 years (prior to 7th birthday): DTaP (Daptacel, Infanrix): IM: 0.5 mL per dose for a total of 4 to 5 doses administered as follows: 3 doses at least 4 weeks apart, followed 6 months later with dose 4; a 5th dose may be given 6 months later (the 5th dose is not necessary if the child received the 4th dose after 4 years of age)

Children ≥7 years and Adolescents not fully vaccinated against pertussis, or whose vaccination status is not known: IM: 0.5 mL single dose as part of the catch-up series; any additional doses needed would be Td.

Booster immunization (Adacel, Boostrix): Children ≥10 years, Adolescents, and Adults: **Note:** Tdap can be administered regardless of the interval between the last tetanus or diphtheria toxoid-containing vaccine. Tdap is currently recommended for a single dose only (CDC 60 [1] 2011; CDC/ACIP 61[25] 2012), except pregnant females who should receive a Tdap dose during each pregnancy (preferably between 27 and 36 weeks' gestation) (CDC 62[7] 2013). **Note:** If Tdap was received as part of a catch-up series, Tdap should not be administered as the booster dose; use Td instead.

CDC (ACIP) recommendations:

Children and Adolescents 10 to 18 years: Tdap (Adacel, Boostrix): IM: 0.5 mL per dose as a single dose. Tdap should be given as a single booster dose at age 11 or 12 years in children who have completed a childhood vaccination series, followed by booster doses of Td every 10 years. **Note:** If Tdap was given as part of catch-up dosing at 7 to 10 years of age, the 11 to 12 year booster is not needed. Regular Td booster immunizations should begin 10 years after the last dose of the primary series. Children who have not received Tdap at age 11 or 12 should receive a single dose of Tdap in place of a single Td booster dose (CDC/ACIP [Broder 2006]; CDC 60[1] 2011]; CDC/ACIP [Strikas 2015]).

Adults ≥19 years: Tdap (Adacel, Boostrix): IM: 0.5 mL per dose. A single dose of Tdap should be given to replace a single dose of the 10 year Td booster in patients who have not previously received Tdap or for whom vaccine status is not known. A single dose of Tdap is recommended for health care personnel who have not previously received Tdap and who have direct patient contact (CDC/ACIP [Kretsinger 2006]). Tdap should be administered regardless of interval since last tetanus- or diphtheria-containing vaccine (CDC/ACIP 61[25] 2012).

Manufacturer's labeling: Tdap (Adacel, Boostrix): Children ≥10 years, Adolescents, and Adults: IM: 0.5 mL as a single dose, administered 5 years after last dose of tetanus toxoid, diphtheria toxoid, and/or pertussis-containing vaccine

Tetanus prophylaxis in wound management (CDC/ACIP [Broder 2006]): Children ≥7 years, Adolescents, and Adults: Tdap (Adacel, Boostrix): IM: 0.5 mL as a single dose may be used as an alternative to Td vaccine when a tetanus toxoid-containing vaccine is needed for wound management, and in whom the pertussis component is also indicated. Tetanus prophylaxis in patients with wounds should be based on if the wound is clean or contaminated, the immunization status of the patient. Wound management includes proper use of tetanus toxoid and/or tetanus immune globulin (TIG), wound cleaning, and (if required) surgical debridement and the proper use of antibiotics. Patients with an uncertain or incomplete tetanus immunization status should have additional follow-up to ensure a series is completed. Patients with a history of Arthus reaction following a previous dose of a tetanus toxoid-containing vaccine should not receive a tetanus toxoid-containing vaccine until >10 years after the most recent dose even if they have a wound that is neither clean nor minor. See table.

Tetanus Prophylaxis Wound Management

History of Tetanus Immunization (Doses)	Clean, Minor Wounds		All Other Wounds[1]	
	Tetanus toxoid[2]	TIG	Tetanus toxoid[2]	TIG
Uncertain or <3 doses	Yes	No	Yes	Yes
3 or more doses	No[3]	No	No[4]	No

[1]Such as, but not limited to, wounds contaminated with dirt, feces, soil, and saliva; puncture wounds; wounds from crushing, tears, burns, and frostbite.

[2]Tetanus toxoid in this chart refers to a tetanus toxoid containing vaccine. For children ≤6 years old DTaP (DT, if pertussis vaccine contraindicated) is preferred to tetanus toxoid alone. For children ≥7 years of age, Adolescents, and Adults, Td preferred to tetanus toxoid alone; Tdap may be preferred if the patient has not previously been vaccinated with Tdap.

[3]Yes, if ≥10 years since last dose.

[4]Yes, if ≥ 5 years since last dose.

Abbreviations: **DT** = Diphtheria and Tetanus Toxoids (formulation for age ≤6 years); **DTaP** = Diphtheria and Tetanus Toxoids, and Acellular Pertussis (formulation for age ≤6 years; Daptacel, Infanrix); **Td** = Diphtheria and Tetanus Toxoids (formulation for age ≥7 years; Tenivac™); **TT** = Tetanus toxoid (adsorbed [formulation for age ≥7 years]); **Tdap** = Diphtheria and Tetanus Toxoids, and Acellular Pertussis (Adacel or Boostrix [formulations for age ≥7 years]); **TIG** = Tetanus Immune Globulin

Dosing adjustment in renal impairment: There are no dosage adjustments provided in the manufacturer's labeling.

Dosing adjustment in hepatic impairment: There are no dosage adjustments provided in the manufacturer's labeling.

Administration Shake vial well before withdrawing the dose; administer IM into midlateral aspect of the thigh in infants and small children; administer in the deltoid area to older children and adults; not for IV, intradermal, or SubQ administration. To prevent syncope related injuries, adolescents and adults should be vaccinated while seated or lying down (NCIRD/ACIP 2011). US law requires that the date of administration, the vaccine manufacturer, lot number of vaccine, and the administering person's name, title, and address be entered into the patient's permanent medical record.

For patients at risk of hemorrhage following intramuscular injection, the vaccine should be administered intramuscularly if, in the opinion of the physician familiar with the patient's bleeding risk, the vaccine can be administered by this route with reasonable safety. If the patient receives antihemophilia or other similar therapy, intramuscular vaccination can be scheduled shortly after such therapy is administered. A fine needle (23 gauge or smaller) should be used for the vaccination and firm pressure on the site (without rubbing) for at least 2 minutes. The patient should be instructed concerning the risk of hematoma from the injection. Patients on anticoagulant therapy should be considered to have the same bleeding risks and treated as those with clotting factor disorders (NCIRD/ACIP 2011).

Monitoring Parameters Observe for syncope for 15 minutes following administration (NCIRD/ACIP 2011). If seizure-like activity associated with syncope occurs, maintain patient in supine or Trendelenburg position to reestablish adequate cerebral perfusion.

Additional Information Adacel is formulated with the same antigens found in Daptacel but with reduced quantities of tetanus and pertussis; Boostrix is formulated with the same antigens found in Infanrix but in reduced quantities. Use of Adacel or Boostrix in the primary immunization series or to complete the primary series has not been evaluated.

The following guidance has been given for when the pediatric formulation is inadvertently given to a patient 7 to 18 years of age (CDC/ACIP [Strikas 2015]):

- For patients 7 to 10 years of age, the dose may count as part of the catch-up series. It may also count as the adolescent Tdap booster, or another Tdap booster can be given at age 11 to 12 years.
- For patients 11 to 18 years, the dose should be counted as the adolescent Tdap booster.

Dosage Forms Excipient information presented when available (limited, particularly for generics); consult specific product labeling.

Injection, suspension [Tdap, booster formulation]:

Adacel: Diphtheria 2 Lf units, tetanus 5 Lf units, and acellular pertussis antigens [detoxified pertussis toxin 2.5 mcg, filamentous hemagglutinin 5 mcg, pertactin 3 mcg, fimbriae (types 2 and 3) 5 mcg] per 0.5 mL (0.5 mL) [contains aluminum; may contain natural rubber/natural latex in prefilled syringe]

Boostrix: Diphtheria 2.5 Lf units, tetanus 5 Lf units, and acellular pertussis antigens [inactivated pertussis toxin 8 mcg, filamentous hemagglutinin 8 mcg, pertactin 2.5 mcg] per 0.5 mL (0.5 mL) [contains aluminum and polysorbate 80; may contain natural rubber/natural latex in prefilled syringe]

Injection, suspension [DTaP, active immunization formulation]:

Daptacel: Diphtheria 15 Lf units, tetanus 5 Lf units, and acellular pertussis antigens [detoxified pertussis toxin 10 mcg, filamentous hemagglutinin 5 mcg, pertactin 3 mcg, fimbriae (types 2 and 3) 5 mcg] per 0.5 mL (0.5 mL) [preservative free; contains aluminum]

Infanrix: Diphtheria 25 Lf units, tetanus 10 Lf units, and acellular pertussis antigens [inactivated pertussis toxin 25 mcg, filamentous hemagglutinin 25 mcg, pertactin 8 mcg] per 0.5 mL (0.5 mL) [preservative free; contains aluminum and polysorbate 80]

Infanrix: Diphtheria 25 Lf units, tetanus 10 Lf units, and acellular pertussis antigens [inactivated pertussis toxin 25 mcg, filamentous hemagglutinin 25 mcg, pertactin 8 mcg] per 0.5 mL (0.5 mL) [preservative free; contains aluminum and polysorbate 80; prefilled syringes contain natural rubber/natural latex] [DSC]

◆ **Diphtheria, Tetanus Toxoids, Acellular Pertussis (DTaP)** *see* Diphtheria and Tetanus Toxoids, Acellular Pertussis, and Poliovirus Vaccine *on page 677*

◆ **Diphtheria, Tetanus Toxoids, Acellular Pertussis (DTaP)** *see* Diphtheria and Tetanus Toxoids, Acellular Pertussis, Poliovirus and *Haemophilus* b Conjugate Vaccine *on page 679*

Diphtheria, Tetanus Toxoids, Acellular Pertussis, Hepatitis B (Recombinant), and Poliovirus (Inactivated) Vaccine

(dif THEER ee a, TET a nus TOKS oyds, ay CEL yoo lar per TUS sis, hep a TYE tis bee ree KOM be nant, & POE lee oh VYE rus in ak ti VAY ted vak SEEN)

Related Information

Centers for Disease Control and Prevention (CDC) and Other Links *on page 2424*

Immunization Administration Recommendations *on page 2411*

Immunization Schedules *on page 2416*

Brand Names: US Pediarix

Brand Names: Canada Pediarix

Therapeutic Category Vaccine; Vaccine, Inactivated Bacteria; Vaccine, Inactivated Virus

Generic Availability (US) No

Use Combination vaccine for the active immunization against diphtheria, tetanus, pertussis, hepatitis B virus (all known subtypes), and poliomyelitis (caused by poliovirus types 1, 2, and 3) (FDA approved in ages 6 weeks through 6 years)

The Advisory Committee on Immunization Practices (ACIP) recommends Pediarix for the following (CDC 52 [10] 2003):

- Primary vaccination for DTaP, Hep B, and IPV in children at 2, 4, and 6 months of age.
- To complete the primary vaccination series in children who have received DTaP (Infanrix) or a birth-dose of hepatitis B and who are scheduled to receive the other components of the vaccine. Whenever feasible, the same manufacturer should be used to provide the pertussis component; however, vaccination should not be deferred if a specific brand is not known or is not available. HepB and IPV from different manufacturers are interchangeable.

Pregnancy Risk Factor C

Pregnancy Considerations Reproduction studies have not been conducted; not indicated for women of childbearing age.

Breast-Feeding Considerations Not indicated for women of childbearing age.

Contraindications Hypersensitivity to diphtheria and tetanus toxoids, pertussis, hepatitis B, poliovirus vaccine, or any component of the vaccine; encephalopathy occurring within 7 days of a previous pertussis vaccine not (not attributable to another identifiable cause); progressive neurologic disorders (including infantile spasms, uncontrolled epilepsy, or progressive encephalopathy)

Warnings/Precautions Immediate treatment (including epinephrine 1:1,000) for anaphylactoid and/or hypersensitivity reactions should be available during vaccine use. Infants born of HBsAg-positive mothers should receive monovalent hepatitis B vaccine and hepatitis B immune globulin; infants born of HBsAg-unknown mothers should receive monovalent hepatitis B vaccine; use of combination product in these patients to complete the hepatitis B vaccination series is limited but is considered acceptable by the ACIP. Carefully consider use in patients with history of any of the following effects from previous administration of any pertussis-containing vaccine: Fever ≥105°F (40.5°C) within 48 hours of unknown cause; seizures with or without fever occurring within 3 days; persistent, inconsolable crying episodes lasting ≥3 hours and occurring within 48 hours; collapse or shock-like state (hypotonic-hyporesponsive episode) within 48 hours. Patients with a history of severe local reaction (Arthus-type) following a previous tetanus toxoid dose should not be given further routine or emergency doses of Td more frequently than every 10 years, even if using for wound management with wounds that are not clean or minor; these patients generally have high serum antitoxin levels (NCIRD/ACIP 2011).

Apnea has occurred following IM vaccine administration in premature infants; consider clinical status implications. In general, preterm infants should be vaccinated at the same chronological age as full-term infants (NCIRD/ACIP 2011). Syncope has been reported with use of injectable vaccines and may result in serious secondary injury (eg, skull fracture, cerebral hemorrhage); typically reported in adolescents and young adults and within 15 minutes after vaccination. Procedures should be in place to avoid injuries from falling and to restore cerebral perfusion if syncope occurs (NCIRD/ACIP 2011).

Use with caution if Guillain-Barré syndrome occurred within 6 weeks of prior tetanus toxoid-containing vaccine (NCIRD/ACIP 2011). Use with caution in patients with history of seizure disorder, progressive neurologic disease, or conditions predisposing to seizures; ACIP guidelines recommend deferring immunization until health status can be assessed and condition stabilized (NCIRD/ACIP 2011). The use of Pediarix combination vaccine is associated with higher rates of fever in comparison to the separate administration of individual components. Per the manufacturer, antipyretic prophylaxis may be considered for patients at high risk for seizures. However, antipyretics have not been shown to prevent febrile seizures; antipyretics may be used to treat fever or discomfort following vaccination (NCIRD/ACIP 2011). One study reported that routine prophylactic administration of acetaminophen to prevent fever prior to vaccination decreased the immune response of some vaccines; the clinical significance of this reduction in immune response has not been established (Prymula 2009).

Vaccination may not result in effective immunity in all patients. Response depends upon multiple factors (eg, type of vaccine, age of patient) and may be improved by administering the vaccine at the recommended dose, route, and interval. Vaccines may not be effective if administered during periods of altered immune competence (NCIRD/ACIP 2011). Use with caution in severely immunocompromised patients (eg, patients receiving chemo/radiation therapy or other immunosuppressive therapy [including high-dose corticosteroids]); may have a reduced response to vaccination. In general, household and close contacts of persons with altered immunocompetence may receive all age appropriate vaccines (IDSA [Rubin 2014]; NCIRD/ACIP 2011); inactivated vaccines should be administered ≥2 weeks prior to planned immunosuppression when feasible (IDSA [Rubin 2014]). The decision to administer or delay vaccination because of current or recent febrile illness depends on the severity of symptoms and the etiology of the disease. Consider deferring administration in patients with moderate or severe acute illness (with or without fever); vaccination should not be delayed for patients with mild acute illness (with or without fever) (NCIRD/ACIP 2011).

Use caution in patients with bleeding disorders (including thrombocytopenia) and patients on anticoagulant therapy; bleeding/hematoma may occur from IM administration; if the patient receives antihemophilia or other similar therapy, IM injection can be scheduled shortly after such therapy is administered (NCIRD/ACIP 2011). Not approved for the fourth dose of the IPV series or the fourth and fifth doses of the DTaP series. Product may contain aluminum, neomycin, polymyxin B, and yeast protein; packaging may contain latex. Some dosage forms may contain polysorbate 80 (also known as Tweens). Hypersensitivity reactions, usually a delayed reaction, have been reported following exposure to pharmaceutical products containing polysorbate 80 in certain individuals (Isaksson 2002; Lucente 2000; Shelley 1995). Thrombocytopenia, ascites, pulmonary deterioration, and renal and hepatic failure have been reported in premature neonates after receiving parenteral products containing polysorbate 80 (Alade 1986; CDC 1984). See manufacturer's labeling.

In order to maximize vaccination rates, the ACIP recommends simultaneous administration (ie, >1 vaccine on the same day at different anatomic sites) of all age-appropriate vaccines (live or inactivated) for which a person is eligible at a single clinic visit, unless contraindications exist. The use of combination vaccines is generally preferred over separate injections, taking into consideration provider assessment, patient preference, and adverse events. When using combination vaccines, the minimum age for administration is the oldest minimum age for any individual component; the minimum interval between dosing is the greatest minimum interval between any individual component. The ACIP prefers each dose of a specific vaccine in a series come from the same manufacturer when possible (NCIRD/ACIP 2011).

Adverse Reactions All serious adverse reactions must be reported to the U.S. Department of Health and Human Services (DHHS) Vaccine Adverse Event Reporting System (VAERS) 1-800-822-7967 or online at https://vaers.hhs.gov/esub/index. In Canada, adverse reactions may be reported to local provincial/territorial health agencies or to the Vaccine Safety Section at Public Health Agency of Canada (1-866-844-0018).

Adverse events reported within 4 days of vaccination at 2-, 4-, and 6 months of age in patients given Pediarix® concomitantly with Hib conjugate vaccine and PCV7 vaccine.

Central nervous system: Drowsiness, fever, irritability/fussiness

Gastrointestinal: Loss of appetite

Local: Injection site: Pain, redness, swelling

Additional and postmarketing events: Anaphylactic/anaphylactoid reaction, angioedema, anorexia, apnea, arthus-type hypersensitivity reactions, brachial neuritis, bulging fontanelle, consciousness depressed, cough, cranial mononeuropathy, crying, cyanosis, demyelinating disease, diarrhea, dyspnea, encephalitis, erythema, fatigue, febrile convulsion, Guillain-Barré syndrome, hypersensitivity reaction, hypotonia, hypotonic-hyporesposnive episode, injection site reactions (cellulitis, induration, itching, nodule, warmth, vesicles), insomnia, lethargy, limb pain, limb swelling, liver function test abnormalities, nervousness, pallor, peripheral mononeuropathy, petechiae, rash, restlessness, screaming, seizure, SIDS, somnolence, upper respiratory tract infection, urticaria, vomiting

Drug Interactions

Metabolism/Transport Effects None known.

Avoid Concomitant Use There are no known interactions where it is recommended to avoid concomitant use.

Increased Effect/Toxicity There are no known significant interactions involving an increase in effect.

Decreased Effect

The levels/effects of Diphtheria, Tetanus Toxoids, Acellular Pertussis, Hepatitis B (Recombinant), and Poliovirus (Inactivated) Vaccine may be decreased by: Belimumab; Fingolimod; Immunosuppressants; Meningococcal Polysaccharide (Groups A / C / Y and W-135) Tetanus Toxoid Conjugate Vaccine

Storage/Stability Store under refrigeration at 2°C to 8°C (36°F to 46°F); do not freeze. Discard if frozen. The following stability information has also been reported for Pediarix: May be stored at room temperature for up to 24 hours (Cohen 2007).

Mechanism of Action Promotes active immunity to diphtheria, tetanus, pertussis, hepatitis B and poliovirus (types 1, 2, and 3) by inducing production of specific antibodies and antitoxins.

Dosing: Usual

Pediatric:

Primary immunization: Infants ≥6 weeks and Children <7 years: IM: 0.5 mL per dose for a total of three doses administered as follows: 2, 4, and 6 months of age in 6- to 8-week intervals (preferably 8-week intervals). Vaccination usually begins at 2 months, but may be started as early as 6 weeks of age. Preterm infants should be vaccinated according to their chronological age from birth.

Note: Pediarix is approved for the first 3 doses of polio vaccine. Per the ACIP, polio vaccine is given at 2, 4, and 6 to 18 months of age. Use of the minimum age and minimum intervals during the first 6 months of life should only be done when the vaccine recipient is at risk for imminent exposure to circulating poliovirus (shorter intervals and earlier start dates may lead to lower seroconversion) (CDC 58[30] 2009).

Use in infants and children previously vaccinated with one or more component, and who are also scheduled to receive all vaccine components:

Hepatitis B vaccine: Infants previously vaccinated with 1 or 2 doses of another hepatitis B vaccine may use Pediarix to complete the 3-dose series. Not for use as birth dose of hepatitis B vaccine; infants who received a birth dose of hepatitis B vaccine may receive a 3-dose series of Pediarix (total of 4 hepatitis B vaccine doses). Infants born to HBsAg-positive women should begin dosing with DTaP-HepB-IPV by age 6 to 8 weeks after receiving the single antigen hepatitis B vaccine at birth (CDC/ACIP [Strikas 2015]).

Diphtheria, tetanus toxoids, and acellular pertussis vaccine (DTaP): Infants previously vaccinated with 1 or 2 doses of Infanrix may use Pediarix to complete the first 3 doses of the series; use of Pediarix to complete DTaP vaccination started with products other than Infanrix has not been studied.

Inactivated polio vaccine (IPV): Infants previously vaccinated with 1 or 2 doses of IPV may use Pediarix to complete the first 3 doses of the series.

Dosing adjustment in renal impairment: There are no dosage adjustments provided in the manufacturer's labeling.

Dosing adjustment in hepatic impairment: There are no dosage adjustments provided in the manufacturer's labeling

Administration Shake well; administer IM in either the anterolateral aspect of the thigh or in the deltoid muscle of the upper arm; not for IV or SubQ administration.

U.S. law requires that the date of administration, name of the vaccine manufacturer, lot number of vaccine, and the administering person's name, title, and address be entered into the patient's permanent medical record.

For patients at risk of hemorrhage following intramuscular injection, the vaccine should be administered intramuscularly if, in the opinion of the physician familiar with the patient's bleeding risk, the vaccine can be administered by this route with reasonable safety. If the patient receives antihemophilia or other similar therapy, intramuscular vaccination can be scheduled shortly after such therapy is administered. A fine needle (23 gauge or smaller) should be used for the vaccination and firm pressure on the site (without rubbing) for at least 2 minutes. The patient should be instructed concerning the risk of hematoma from the injection. Patients on anticoagulant therapy should be considered to have the same bleeding risks and treated as those with clotting factor disorders (NCIRD/ACIP 2011).

Monitoring Parameters Observe for syncope for 15 minutes following administration (NCIRD/ACIP 2011). If seizure-like activity associated with syncope occurs, maintain patient in supine or Trendelenburg position to reestablish adequate cerebral perfusion.

Additional Information Contains the following three pertussis antigens: Inactivated pertussis toxin (PT), filamentous hemagglutinin (FHA), and pertactin. Contains the same diphtheria and tetanus toxoids and pertussis antigens found in Infanrix and Kinrix. Contains the same hepatitis B surface antigen (HB_sAg) found in Engerix-B (recombinant vaccine). Thimerosal is used during manufacturing, but removed to less than detectable levels in the final suspension.

Dosage Forms Excipient information presented when available (limited, particularly for generics); consult specific product labeling.

Injection, suspension [preservative free]:

Pediarix: Diphtheria toxoid 25 Lf, tetanus toxoid 10 Lf, acellular pertussis antigens [inactivated pertussis toxin 25 mcg, filamentous hemagglutin 25 mcg, pertactin 8 mcg, HBsAg 10 mcg, type 1 poliovirus 40 D antigen units, type 2 poliovirus 8 D antigen units and type 3 poliovirus 32 D antigen units] per 0.5 mL (0.5 mL) [contains aluminum, neomycin sulfate (trace amounts), polymyxin B (trace amounts), polysorbate 80, and yeast protein ≤5%; may contain natural rubber/natural latex in prefilled syringe]

- **Diphtheria, Tetanus Toxoids, Acellular Pertussis, Hepatitis B (Recombinant), and Poliovirus (Inactivated) Vaccine** *see* Diphtheria, Tetanus Toxoids, Acellular Pertussis, Hepatitis B (Recombinant), and Poliovirus (Inactivated) Vaccine *on page 685*
- **Diphtheria, Tetanus Toxoids, Acellular Pertussis, Hepatitis B (Recombinant), and Poliovirus Vaccine** *see* Diphtheria, Tetanus Toxoids, Acellular Pertussis, Hepatitis B (Recombinant), and Poliovirus (Inactivated) Vaccine *on page 685*
- **Diphtheria Toxoid** *see* Diphtheria and Tetanus Toxoids, Acellular Pertussis, Poliovirus and *Haemophilus* b Conjugate Vaccine *on page 679*
- **Dipivalyl Epinephrine** *see* Dipivefrin *on page 687*

Dipivefrin (dye PI ve frin)

Brand Names: Canada Ophtho-Dipivefrin™; PMS-Dipivefrin; Propine®

Therapeutic Category Adrenergic Agonist Agent, Ophthalmic; Ophthalmic Agent, Vasoconstrictor

Generic Availability (US) No

Use Reduces elevated IOP in chronic open-angle glaucoma; treatment of ocular hypertension

Pregnancy Risk Factor B

Pregnancy Considerations Adverse events have not been observed in animal reproduction studies when administered orally. Systemic adverse events (eg, arrhythmias, hypertension) have been reported following ophthalmic application; use is not recommended in pregnancy (Razeghinejad, 2011).

Breast-Feeding Considerations Systemic adverse events (eg, arrhythmias, hypertension) have been reported following ophthalmic application; use is not recommended in breast-feeding women (Razeghinejad, 2011).

Contraindications Hypersensitivity to dipivefrin, any component of the formulation, or epinephrine; angle-closure glaucoma

Warnings/Precautions Use with caution in patients with hypertension or cardiac disorders and in aphakic patients. Contains sodium metabisulfite.

Adverse Reactions

Central nervous system: Headache

Local: Burning, stinging

Ocular: Blepharoconjunctivitis, blurred vision, bulbar conjunctival follicles, cystoid macular edema, ocular congestion, ocular pain, mydriasis, photophobia

Rare but important or life-threatening: Arrhythmias, hypertension

Drug Interactions

Metabolism/Transport Effects None known.

Avoid Concomitant Use

Avoid concomitant use of Dipivefrin with any of the following: Ergot Derivatives; Iobenguane I 123

Increased Effect/Toxicity

Dipivefrin may increase the levels/effects of: Sympathomimetics

The levels/effects of Dipivefrin may be increased by: AtoMOXetine; Cannabinoid-Containing Products; Ergot

Derivatives; Linezolid; Serotonin/Norepinephrine Reuptake Inhibitors; Tedizolid

Decreased Effect

Dipivefrin may decrease the levels/effects of: Iobenguane I 123

The levels/effects of Dipivefrin may be decreased by: Alpha1-Blockers; Spironolactone

Storage/Stability Avoid exposure to light and air. Discolored or darkened solutions indicate loss of potency.

Mechanism of Action Dipivefrin is a prodrug of epinephrine which is the active agent that stimulates alpha- and/or beta-adrenergic receptors increasing aqueous humor outflow

Pharmacodynamics

Onset of action:

Ocular pressure effects: Within 30 minutes

Mydriasis: Within 30 minutes

Maximum effect: Ocular pressure effects: Within 1 hour

Duration:

Ocular pressure effects: 12 hours or longer

Mydriasis: Several hours

Pharmacokinetics (Adult data unless noted) Absorption: Rapid into the aqueous humor; converted to epinephrine

Dosing: Usual Children and Adults: Ophthalmic: Initial: Instill 1 drop every 12 hours

Administration Ophthalmic: Instill drop into eye; apply finger pressure to lacrimal sac during and for 1-2 minutes after instillation to decrease risk of absorption and systemic effects; avoid contacting bottle tip with skin or eye

Monitoring Parameters IOP

Dosage Forms Excipient information presented when available (limited, particularly for generics); consult specific product labeling. [DSC] = Discontinued product

Solution, ophthalmic, as hydrochloride [drops]:

Propine®: 0.1% (10 mL [DSC]) [contains benzalkonium chloride]

◆ **Dipivefrin Hydrochloride** *see* Dipivefrin *on page 687*

◆ **Diprivan** *see* Propofol *on page 1786*

◆ **Diprolene** *see* Betamethasone (Topical) *on page 280*

◆ **Diprolene AF** *see* Betamethasone (Topical) *on page 280*

◆ **Dipropylacetic Acid** *see* Valproic Acid and Derivatives *on page 2143*

◆ **Diprosone (Can)** *see* Betamethasone (Topical) *on page 280*

Dipyridamole (dye peer ID a mole)

Medication Safety Issues

Sound-alike/look-alike issues:

Dipyridamole may be confused with disopyramide

Persantine® may be confused with Periactin

BEERS Criteria medication:

This drug may be potentially inappropriate for use in geriatric patients (Quality of evidence - moderate; Strength of recommendation - strong).

International issues:

Persantine [U.S., Canada, Belgium, Denmark, France] may be confused with Permitil brand name for sildenafil [Argentina]

Brand Names: US Persantine

Brand Names: Canada Apo-Dipyridamole FC®; Dipyridamole For Injection; Persantine®

Therapeutic Category Antiplatelet Agent; Vasodilator, Coronary

Generic Availability (US) Yes

Use Maintain patency after surgical grafting procedures including coronary artery bypass; with warfarin to decrease thrombosis in patients after artificial heart valve replacement; for chronic management of angina pectoris; with aspirin to prevent coronary artery thrombosis; in combination with aspirin or warfarin to prevent other thromboembolic disorders; dipyridamole may also be given 2 days prior to open heart surgery to prevent platelet activation by extracorporeal bypass pump; diagnostic agent IV (dipyridamole stress test) for coronary artery disease

Pregnancy Risk Factor B

Pregnancy Considerations Adverse events have not been observed in animal reproduction studies.

Breast-Feeding Considerations Dipyridamole is excreted in breast milk. The manufacturer recommends that caution be exercised when administering dipyridamole to nursing women.

Contraindications Hypersensitivity to dipyridamole or any component of the formulation

Warnings/Precautions Use with caution in patients with hypotension, unstable angina, and/or recent MI. Use with caution in hepatic impairment. Avoid use of oral dipyridamole in this age group due to risk of orthostatic hypotension and availability of more efficacious alternative agents (Beers Criteria). Use caution in patients on other antiplatelet agents or anticoagulation. Severe adverse reactions have occurred with IV administration (rarely); use the IV form with caution in patients with bronchospastic disease or unstable angina. Aminophylline should be available in case of urgency or emergency with IV use.

Adverse Reactions

Oral:

Cardiovascular: Angina pectoris, flushing

Central nervous system: Dizziness, headache

Dermatologic: Pruritus, skin rash

Gastrointestinal: Abdominal distress, diarrhea, vomiting

Hepatic: Hepatic insufficiency

Rare but important or life-threatening: Alopecia, arthritis, cholelithiasis, dyspepsia, fatigue, hepatitis, hypersensitivity reaction, hypotension, laryngeal edema, malaise, myalgia, nausea, palpitations, paresthesia, tachycardia, thrombocytopenia

IV:

Cardiovascular: Altered blood pressure, ECG abnormality (ST-T changes, extrasystoles), exacerbation of angina pectoris, flushing, hypertension, hypotension, tachycardia

Central nervous system: Dizziness, fatigue, headache, pain, paresthesia

Gastrointestinal: Nausea

Respiratory: Dyspnea

Rare but important or life-threatening: Abdominal pain, arthralgia, ataxia, back pain, bronchospasm, cardiac arrhythmia (ventricular tachycardia, bradycardia, AV block, SVT, atrial fibrillation, asystole), cardiomyopathy, cough, depersonalization, diaphoresis, dysgeusia, dyspepsia, dysphagia, ECG abnormality (unspecified), edema, eructation, flatulence, hypersensitivity reaction, hypertonia, hyperventilation, increased appetite, increased thirst, injection site reaction, leg cramps (intermittent claudication), malaise, mastalgia, muscle rigidity, myalgia, myocardial infarction, orthostatic hypotension, otalgia, palpitations, perineal pain, pharyngitis, pleuritic chest pain, pruritus, renal pain, rhinitis, skin rash, syncope, tenesmus, tinnitus, tremor, urticaria, vertigo, visual disturbance, vomiting, weakness, xerostomia

Drug Interactions

Metabolism/Transport Effects Inhibits BCRP, P-glycoprotein

Avoid Concomitant Use

Avoid concomitant use of Dipyridamole with any of the following: Bosutinib; PAZOPanib; Riociguat; Silodosin; Topotecan; Urokinase; VinCRIStine (Liposomal)

Increased Effect/Toxicity

Dipyridamole may increase the levels/effects of: Adenosine; Afatinib; Agents with Antiplatelet Properties; Anticoagulants; Apixaban; Beta-Blockers; Bosutinib; Brentuximab Vedotin; Colchicine; Collagenase (Systemic); Dabigatran Etexilate; Deoxycholic Acid; DOXOrubicin (Conventional); DULoxetine; Edoxaban; Everolimus; Hypotensive Agents; Ibritumomab; Ledipasvir; Levodopa; Naloxegol; Obinutuzumab; PAZOPanib; P-glycoprotein/ABCB1 Substrates; Prucalopride; Regadenoson; Rifaximin; Riociguat; RisperiDONE; Rivaroxaban; Salicylates; Silodosin; Thrombolytic Agents; Topotecan; Tositumomab and Iodine I 131 Tositumomab; Urokinase; VinCRIStine (Liposomal)

The levels/effects of Dipyridamole may be increased by: Barbiturates; Dasatinib; Glucosamine; Herbs (Anticoagulant/Antiplatelet Properties); Ibrutinib; Limaprost; Multivitamins/Fluoride (with ADE); Multivitamins/Minerals (with ADEK, Folate, Iron); Multivitamins/Minerals (with AE, No Iron); Nicorandil; Omega-3 Fatty Acids; Pentosan Polysulfate Sodium; Pentoxifylline; Prostacyclin Analogues; Tipranavir; Vitamin E

Decreased Effect

Dipyridamole may decrease the levels/effects of: Acetylcholinesterase Inhibitors

Storage/Stability IV: Store between 15°C to 25°C (59°F to 77°F); do not freeze. Protect from light.

Mechanism of Action Inhibits the activity of adenosine deaminase and phosphodiesterase, which causes an accumulation of adenosine, adenine nucleotides, and cyclic AMP; these mediators then inhibit platelet aggregation and may cause vasodilation; may also stimulate release of prostacyclin or PGD_2; causes coronary vasodilation

Pharmacokinetics (Adult data unless noted) Oral:

Absorption: Slow and variable

Distribution: Distributes to breast milk

V_d: Adults: 2-3 L/kg

Protein binding: 91% to 99%

Metabolism: In the liver to glucuronide conjugate

Bioavailability: 27% to 66%

Half-life, terminal: 10-12 hours

Time to peak serum concentration: Oral: 75 minutes

Elimination: In feces via bile as glucuronide conjugates and unchanged drug

Dosing: Usual

Children:

Oral: 3-6 mg/kg/day in 3 divided doses

Doses of 4-10 mg/kg/day have been used investigationally to treat proteinuria in pediatric renal disease

Mechanical prosthetic heart valves: 2-5 mg/kg/day [used in combination with an oral anticoagulant in children who have systemic embolism despite adequate oral anticoagulant therapy (INR 2.5-3.5), and used in combination with low-dose oral anticoagulation (INR 2-3) plus aspirin in children in whom full-dose oral anticoagulation is contraindicated] (Monagle, 2001). **Note:** The *Chest* guidelines (Monagle, 2004) do not mention the use of dipyridamole for prophylaxis for mechanical prosthetic heart valves in children; an oral anticoagulant plus aspirin is recommended for the patient groups mentioned above.

Adults:

Prophylaxis of thromboembolism after cardiac valve replacement (adjunctive use): Oral: 75-100 mg 4 times/day

Dipyridamole stress test (for evaluation of myocardial perfusion): IV: 0.142 mg/kg/minute for a total of 4 minutes (0.57 mg/kg total); maximum dose: 60 mg; inject thallium 201 within 5 minutes after end of injection of dipyridamole

Preparation for Administration Parenteral: IV: Prior to administration, dilute solution for injection to a ≥1:2 ratio in NS, ½NS, or D_5W. Total volume should be ~20 to 50 mL.

Administration

Oral: Administer with water on an empty stomach 1 hour before or 2 hours after meals; may take with milk or food to decrease GI upset

Parenteral: IV: Infuse diluted solution over 4 minutes

Monitoring Parameters Blood pressure, heart rate

Test Interactions Concurrent caffeine or theophylline use may demonstrate a false-negative result with dipyridamole-thallium myocardial imaging.

Dosage Forms Excipient information presented when available (limited, particularly for generics); consult specific product labeling.

Solution, Intravenous:

Generic: 5 mg/mL (2 mL, 10 mL)

Tablet, Oral:

Persantine: 25 mg, 50 mg, 75 mg [contains fd&c yellow #10 aluminum lake, methylparaben, propylparaben, sodium benzoate]

Generic: 25 mg, 50 mg, 75 mg

Extemporaneous Preparations A 10 mg/mL oral suspension may be made with tablets and one of three different vehicles (cherry syrup, a 1:1 mixture of Ora-Sweet® and Ora-Plus®, or a 1:1 mixture of Ora-Sweet® SF and Ora-Plus®). Crush twenty-four 50 mg tablets in a mortar and reduce to a fine powder. Add 20 mL of the chosen vehicle and mix to a uniform paste; mix while adding the vehicle in incremental proportions to **almost** 120 mL; transfer to a calibrated bottle, rinse mortar with vehicle, and add quantity of vehicle sufficient to make 120 mL. Label "shake well" and "protect from light". Stable for 60 days when stored in amber plastic prescription bottles in the dark at room temperature or refrigerated.

Allen LV and Erickson III MA, "Stability of Baclofen, Captopril, Diltiazem, Hydrochloride, Dipyridamole, and Flecainide Acetate in Extemporaneously Compounded Oral Liquids," *Am J Health Syst Pharm*, 1996, 53:2179-84.

◆ **Dipyridamole For Injection (Can)** *see* Dipyridamole *on page 688*

◆ **Disodium Cromoglycate** *see* Cromolyn (Nasal) *on page 542*

◆ **Disodium Cromoglycate** *see* Cromolyn (Ophthalmic) *on page 543*

◆ **Disodium Cromoglycate** *see* Cromolyn (Systemic, Oral Inhalation) *on page 541*

◆ **Disodium Thiosulfate Pentahydrate** *see* Sodium Thiosulfate *on page 1955*

◆ ***d*-Isoephedrine Hydrochloride** *see* Pseudoephedrine *on page 1801*

Disopyramide (dye soe PEER a mide)

Medication Safety Issues

Sound-alike/look-alike issues:

Disopyramide may be confused with desipramine, dipyridamole

Norpace may be confused with Norpramin

BEERS Criteria medication:

This drug may be potentially inappropriate for use in geriatric patients (Quality of evidence - low; Strength of recommendation - strong).

Related Information

Oral Medications That Should Not Be Crushed or Altered *on page 2476*

Brand Names: US Norpace; Norpace CR

Brand Names: Canada Norpace; Rythmodan; Rythmodan-LA

Therapeutic Category Antiarrhythmic Agent, Class I-A

Generic Availability (US) May be product dependent

Use Treatment of life-threatening ventricular arrhythmias; suppression and prevention of unifocal and multifocal ventricular premature complexes, coupled ventricular premature complexes, and/or paroxysmal ventricular tachycardia; also effective in the conversion and prevention of recurrence of atrial fibrillation, atrial flutter, and paroxysmal atrial tachycardia

Pregnancy Risk Factor C

Pregnancy Considerations Adverse events have been observed in animal reproduction studies. Disopyramide levels have been reported in human fetal blood. Disopyramide may stimulate contractions in pregnant women. In a case report, disopyramide use in the third trimester resulted in painful uterine contractions after the first dose and hemorrhage after the second dose (Abbi, 1999).

Breast-Feeding Considerations Disopyramide is excreted in breast milk. Due to the potential for serious adverse reactions in nursing infants, the manufacturer recommends a decision be made whether to discontinue nursing or to discontinue the drug, taking into account the importance of the treatment to the mother.

Contraindications Hypersensitivity to disopyramide or any component of the formulation; cardiogenic shock; preexisting second- or third-degree heart block (except in patients with a functioning artificial pacemaker); congenital long QT syndrome; sick sinus syndrome

Warnings/Precautions Watch for proarrhythmic effects; may cause QTc prolongation and subsequent torsade de pointes; avoid use in patients with diagnosed or suspected congenital long QT syndrome. Monitor and adjust dose to prevent QTc prolongation. Increases in QTc >25% over baseline should result in cessation or reduction in disopyramide dosing. Initiate within the hospital with cardiac monitoring. The incidence of proarrhythmic effects and mortality may be increased with Class Ia antiarrhythmic agents in patients with pre-existing disease. Avoid concurrent use with other medications that prolong QT interval or decrease myocardial contractility. Correct hypokalemia before initiating therapy; may worsen toxicity. **[U.S. Boxed Warning]: In the Cardiac Arrhythmia Suppression Trial (CAST), recent (>6 days but <2 years ago) myocardial infarction patients with asymptomatic, non-life-threatening ventricular arrhythmias did not benefit and may have been harmed by attempts to suppress the arrhythmia with flecainide or encainide. An increased mortality or nonfatal cardiac arrest rate (7.7%) was seen in the active treatment group compared with patients in the placebo group (3%). The applicability of the CAST results to other populations is unknown. Antiarrhythmic agents should be reserved for patients with life-threatening ventricular arrhythmias.** Use with caution or avoid in patients with any degree of left ventricular dysfunction or history of heart failure (HF); may precipitate or exacerbate HF. Due to significant anticholinergic effects, do not use in patients with urinary retention, BPH, glaucoma, or myasthenia gravis. Reduce dosage in renal or hepatic impairment. Avoid use in the elderly due to a risk of developing heart failure (potent negative inotrope) and adverse effects associated with potent anticholinergic properties; alternative antiarrhythmic agents preferred (Beers Criteria). Controlled release form is not recommended for CrCl ≤40 mL/minute. In patients with atrial fibrillation or flutter, block the AV node before initiating. Use caution in Wolff-Parkinson-White syndrome or bundle branch block. Monitor closely for hypotension during the initiation of therapy.

Adverse Reactions The most common adverse effects are related to cholinergic blockade. The most serious adverse effects of disopyramide are CHF and hypotension.

Cardiovascular: Cardiac conduction disturbance, chest pain CHF, edema, hypotension, syncope

Central nervous system: Dizziness, fatigue, headache, malaise, nervousness

Dermatologic: Generalized dermatoses, pruritus, rash

Endocrine & metabolic: Cholesterol increased, hypokalemia, triglycerides increased

Gastrointestinal: Abdominal bloating, abdominal distension, anorexia, constipation, diarrhea, dry throat, flatulence, nausea, vomiting, weight gain, xerostomia

Genitourinary: Impotence, urinary frequency, urinary hesitancy, urinary retention, urinary urgency

Neuromuscular & skeletal: Muscular pain, muscle weakness

Ocular: Blurred vision, dry eyes

Respiratory: Dyspnea

Rare but important or life-threatening: Agranulocytosis, AV block, BUN increased, cholestatic jaundice, creatinine increased, depression, dysuria, gynecomastia, hepatotoxicity, hypoglycemia, insomnia, new or worsened arrhythmia (proarrhythmic effect), paresthesia, psychotic reaction, respiratory distress, thrombocytopenia, transaminases increased. Rare cases of lupus have been reported (generally in patients previously receiving procainamide), peripheral neuropathy, psychosis, toxic cutaneous blisters.

Drug Interactions

Metabolism/Transport Effects Substrate of CYP3A4 (major); **Note:** Assignment of Major/Minor substrate status based on clinically relevant drug interaction potential

Avoid Concomitant Use

Avoid concomitant use of Disopyramide with any of the following: Aclidinium; Amiodarone; Conivaptan; Eluxadoline; Fingolimod; Fusidic Acid (Systemic); Glucagon; Highest Risk QTc-Prolonging Agents; Idelalisib; Ipratropium (Oral Inhalation); Itraconazole; Ivabradine; Ketoconazole (Systemic); Macrolide Antibiotics; Mifepristone; Moderate Risk QTc-Prolonging Agents; Potassium Chloride; Propafenone; Tiotropium; Umeclidinium; Verapamil

Increased Effect/Toxicity

Disopyramide may increase the levels/effects of: AbobotulinumtoxinA; Analgesics (Opioid); Anticholinergic Agents; Beta-Blockers; Cannabinoid-Containing Products; Eluxadoline; Fosphenytoin; Glucagon; Highest Risk QTc-Prolonging Agents; Hypoglycemia-Associated Agents; Lidocaine (Systemic); Lidocaine (Topical); OnabotulinumtoxinA; Potassium Chloride; RimabotulinumtoxinB; Thiazide Diuretics; Tiotropium; Topiramate

The levels/effects of Disopyramide may be increased by: Aclidinium; Amiodarone; Androgens; Antidiabetic Agents; Aprepitant; Beta-Blockers; Conivaptan; CYP3A4 Inhibitors (Moderate); CYP3A4 Inhibitors (Strong); Fingolimod; Fosaprepitant; Fusidic Acid (Systemic); Herbs (Hypoglycemic Properties); Idelalisib; Ipratropium (Oral Inhalation); Itraconazole; Ivabradine; Ivacaftor; Ketoconazole (Systemic); Luliconazole; Lurasidone; Macrolide Antibiotics; MAO Inhibitors; Mifepristone; Moderate Risk QTc-Prolonging Agents; Netupitant; Palbociclib; Pegvisomant; Pramlintide; Propafenone; QTc-Prolonging Agents (Indeterminate Risk and Risk Modifying); Quinolone Antibiotics; Salicylates; Selective Serotonin Reuptake Inhibitors; Simeprevir; Stiripentol; Umeclidinium; Verapamil

Decreased Effect

Disopyramide may decrease the levels/effects of: Acetylcholinesterase Inhibitors; Itopride; Secretin

The levels/effects of Disopyramide may be decreased by: Acetylcholinesterase Inhibitors; Bosentan; CYP3A4 Inducers (Moderate); CYP3A4 Inducers (Strong); Dabrafenib; Deferasirox; Etravirine; Fosphenytoin; Mitotane; PHENobarbital; Phenytoin; Quinolone Antibiotics; Rifampin; Siltuximab; St Johns Wort; Tocilizumab

Storage/Stability Store at 25°C (77°F); excursions permitted to 15°C to 30°C (59°F to 86°F).

Mechanism of Action Class Ia antiarrhythmic: Decreases myocardial excitability and conduction velocity; reduces disparity in refractory between normal and infarcted myocardium; possesses anticholinergic, peripheral vasoconstrictive, and negative inotropic effects

Pharmacodynamics

Capsules, regular:

Onset of action: 30-210 minutes

Duration: 1.5-8.5 hours

Pharmacokinetics (Adult data unless noted)

Protein binding: Concentration dependent, stereoselective, and ranges from 20% to 60%

Distribution: V_d: Children: 1 L/kg

Metabolism: In the liver; major metabolite has anticholinergic and antiarrhythmic effects

Bioavailability: 60% to 83%

Half-life:

Children: 3.15 hours

Adults: 4-10 hours (mean: 6.7 hours), increased half-life with hepatic or renal disease

Elimination: 40% to 60% excreted unchanged in urine and 10% to 15% in feces

Clearance is greater and half-life shorter in children vs adults; clearance (children): 3.76 mL/minute/kg

Dosing: Usual Oral:

Children (start with lower dose listed):

<1 year: 10-30 mg/kg/day in 4 divided doses

1-4 years: 10-20 mg/kg/day in 4 divided doses

4-12 years: 10-15 mg/kg/day in 4 divided doses

12-18 years: 6-15 mg/kg/day in 4 divided doses

Adults: **Note:** Some patients may require initial loading dose; see product information for details

<50 kg: 100 mg every 6 hours **or** 200 mg every 12 hours (controlled release)

>50 kg: 150 mg every 6 hours **or** 300 mg every 12 hours (controlled release); if no response, may increase to 200 mg every 6 hours; maximum dose required for patients with severe refractory ventricular tachycardia is 400 mg every 6 hours. **Note:** Use lower doses (100 mg of nonsustained release every 6-8 hours) in adults with cardiomyopathy or cardiac decompensation.

Adult dosing adjustment in renal impairment: 100 mg (nonsustained release) given at the following intervals: See table

Creatinine Clearance (mL/min)	Dosage Interval
30-40	Every 8 h
15-30	Every 12 h
<15	Every 24 h

Administration Oral: Administer on an empty stomach; do not crush, break, or chew controlled release capsules, swallow whole

Monitoring Parameters Blood pressure, ECG, drug level; serum potassium, glucose, cholesterol, triglycerides, and liver enzymes; especially important to monitor ECG in patients with hepatic or renal disease, heart disease, or others with increased risk of adverse effects

Reference Range Therapeutic:

Atrial arrhythmias: 2.8-3.2 mcg/mL (SI: 8.3-9.4 micromoles/L)

Ventricular arrhythmias: 3.3-7.5 mcg/mL (SI: 9.7-22 micromoles/L)

Toxic: >7 mcg/mL (SI: >20.7 micromoles/L)

Dosage Forms Excipient information presented when available (limited, particularly for generics); consult specific product labeling.

Capsule, Oral:

Norpace: 100 mg, 150 mg

Generic: 100 mg, 150 mg

Capsule Extended Release 12 Hour, Oral:

Norpace CR: 100 mg, 150 mg

Extemporaneous Preparations A 1 mg/mL oral suspension may be made with a tablet and Simple Syrup, NF. Crush one 100 mg tablet in a mortar and reduce to a fine powder. Add small portions of the vehicle and mix to a uniform paste; mix while adding the vehicle in incremental proportions to **almost** 100 mL; transfer to a calibrated bottle, rinse mortar with vehicle, and add quantity of vehicle sufficient to make 100 mL. Label "shake well" and "refrigerate". Stable for 28 days.

A 10 mg/mL oral suspension may be made with tablets and Simple Syrup, NF. Crush ten 100 mg tablets in a mortar and reduce to a fine powder. Add small portions of the vehicle and mix to a uniform paste; mix while adding the vehicle in incremental proportions to **almost** 100 mL; transfer to a calibrated bottle, rinse mortar with vehicle, and add quantity of vehicle sufficient to make 100 mL. Label "shake well" and "refrigerate". Stable for 28 days.

Nahata MC, Pai VB, and Hipple TF, *Pediatric Drug Formulations*, 5th ed, Cincinnati, OH: Harvey Whitney Books Co, 2004.

- ◆ **Disopyramide Phosphate** *see* Disopyramide *on page 689*
- ◆ **Dithioglycerol** *see* Dimercaprol *on page 665*
- ◆ **Ditropan** *see* Oxybutynin *on page 1588*
- ◆ **Ditropan XL** *see* Oxybutynin *on page 1588*
- ◆ **Diuril** *see* Chlorothiazide *on page 439*
- ◆ **Divalproex Sodium** *see* Valproic Acid and Derivatives *on page 2143*
- ◆ **Divigel** *see* Estradiol (Systemic) *on page 795*
- ◆ **Dixarit® (Can)** *see* CloNIDine *on page 508*
- ◆ **5071-1DL(6)** *see* Megestrol *on page 1344*
- ◆ ***dl*-Alpha Tocopherol** *see* Vitamin E *on page 2188*
- ◆ ***D*-Mannitol** *see* Mannitol *on page 1321*
- ◆ **4-DMDR** *see* IDArubicin *on page 1071*
- ◆ **DMSA** *see* Succimer *on page 1975*
- ◆ **DMSO** *see* Dimethyl Sulfoxide *on page 667*
- ◆ **Doak Oil [OTC] (Can)** *see* Coal Tar *on page 523*
- ◆ **Doak Oil Forte [OTC] (Can)** *see* Coal Tar *on page 523*

DOBUTamine (doe BYOO ta meen)

Medication Safety Issues

Sound-alike/look-alike issues:

DOBUTamine may be confused with DOPamine

High alert medication:

The Institute for Safe Medication Practices (ISMP) includes this medication among its list of drugs which have a heightened risk of causing significant patient harm when used in error.

Related Information

Emergency Drip Calculations *on page 2229*

Management of Drug Extravasations *on page 2298*

Brand Names: Canada Dobutamine Injection, USP; Dobutrex

Therapeutic Category Adrenergic Agonist Agent; Sympathomimetic

Generic Availability (US) Yes

Use Short-term management of patients with cardiac decompensation

Pregnancy Risk Factor B

Pregnancy Considerations Adverse events have not been observed in animal reproduction studies.

Breast-Feeding Considerations It is not known if dobutamine is excreted in breast milk. The manufacturer recommends that caution be exercised when administering dobutamine to nursing women.

Contraindications Hypersensitivity to dobutamine or sulfites (some contain sodium metabisulfate), or any component of the formulation; hypertrophic cardiomyopathy with outflow tract obstruction (formerly known as idiopathic hypertrophic subaortic stenosis [IHSS])

Warnings/Precautions May cause dose-related increases in heart rate. Patients with atrial fibrillation may experience an increase in ventricular response. An increase in blood pressure is more common due to augmented cardiac output, but occasionally a patient may become hypotensive. May exacerbate ventricular ectopy (dose-related). If needed, correct hypovolemia first to optimize hemodynamics. Ineffective therapeutically in the presence of mechanical obstruction such as severe aortic stenosis. Use caution post-MI (can increase myocardial oxygen demand). Use cautiously in the elderly starting at lower end of the dosage range. Use with extreme caution in patients taking MAO inhibitors. Dobutamine in combination with stress echo may be used diagnostically. The ACCF/AHA 2013 heart failure guidelines do not recommend long-term use of intravenous inotropic therapy except for palliative purposes in end-stage disease (ACCF/AHA [Yancy, 2013]). Product may contain sodium sulfite.

Adverse Reactions

Cardiovascular: Ventricular premature contractions (5%; dose related), angina pectoris (1% to 3%), chest pain (1% to 3%; nonspecific), palpitations (1% to 3%), hypotension, increased blood pressure, increased heart rate, localized phlebitis, ventricular ectopy (increased)

Central nervous system: Headache (1% to 3%), paresthesia

Dermatologic: Skin necrosis (isolated cases)

Endocrine & metabolic: Decreased serum potassium (slight)

Gastrointestinal: Nausea (1% to 3%)

Hematologic & oncologic: Thrombocytopenia (isolated cases)

Local: Local inflammation, local pain (from infiltration)

Neuromuscular & skeletal: Leg cramps (mild)

Respiratory: Dyspnea (1% to 3%)

Miscellaneous: Fever (1% to 3%)

Drug Interactions

Metabolism/Transport Effects Substrate of COMT

Avoid Concomitant Use

Avoid concomitant use of DOBUTamine with any of the following: Iobenguane I 123

Increased Effect/Toxicity

DOBUTamine may increase the levels/effects of: Sympathomimetics

The levels/effects of DOBUTamine may be increased by: AtoMOXetine; Cannabinoid-Containing Products; COMT Inhibitors; Linezolid; Tedizolid

Decreased Effect

DOBUTamine may decrease the levels/effects of: Iobenguane I 123

The levels/effects of DOBUTamine may be decreased by: Calcium Salts

Storage/Stability Store reconstituted solution under refrigeration for 48 hours or 6 hours at room temperature. Stability of parenteral admixture at room temperature (25°C) is 48 hours; at refrigeration (4°C) stability is 7 days. Remix solution every 24 hours. Pink discoloration of solution indicates slight oxidation but no significant loss of potency.

Mechanism of Action Dobutamine, a racemic mixture, stimulates myocardial $beta_1$-adrenergic receptors primarily by the (+) enantiomer and some $alpha_1$ receptor agonism by the (-) enantiomer, resulting in increased contractility and heart rate, and stimulates both $beta_2$- and $alpha_1$-receptors in the vasculature. Although $beta_2$ and $alpha_1$ adrenergic receptors are also activated, the effects of $beta_2$ receptor activation may equally offset or be slightly greater than the effects of $alpha_1$ stimulation, resulting in some vasodilation in addition to the inotropic and chronotropic actions (Leier, 1988; Majerus, 1989; Ruffolo, 1987). Lowers central venous pressure and wedge pressure, but has little effect on pulmonary vascular resistance (Leier, 1977; Leier, 1978).

Pharmacodynamics

Onset of action: IV: 1-10 minutes

Maximum effect: Within 10-20 minutes

Pharmacokinetics (Adult data unless noted)

Metabolism: In tissues and the liver to inactive metabolites

Half-life: 2 minutes

Dosing: Neonatal Continuous IV infusion: 2-20 mcg/kg/minute; titrate to desired response

Dosing: Usual Continuous IV infusion: Infants, Children, and Adults: 2.5-15 mcg/kg/minute, titrate to desired response; maximum dose: 40 mcg/kg/minute

Usual Infusion Concentrations: Neonatal Note: Premixed solutions available.

IV infusion: 1000 **mcg**/mL, 2000 **mcg**/mL, **or** 4000 **mcg**/mL

Usual Infusion Concentrations: Pediatric Note: Premixed solutions available.

IV infusion: 1000 **mcg**/mL, 2000 **mcg**/mL, **or** 4000 **mcg**/mL

Preparation for Administration Parenteral: Dilute in D_5W or NS to a maximum concentration of 5,000 mcg/mL (5 mg/mL); ISMP and Vermont Oxford Network recommends a standard concentration of 2,000 mcg/mL (2 mg/mL) for neonates (ISMP 2011)

Administration Parenteral: Administer as a continuous IV infusion via an infusion device; administer into large vein.

Rate of infusion (mL/hour) = dose (mcg/kg/minute) x weight (kg) x 60 minutes/hour divided by the concentration (mcg/mL)

Monitoring Parameters ECG, heart rate, CVP, MAP, urine output; if pulmonary artery catheter is in place, monitor CI, PCWP, RAP, and SVR. Dobutamine lowers central venous pressure and wedge pressure but has little effect on pulmonary vascular resistance.

Dosage Forms Excipient information presented when available (limited, particularly for generics); consult specific product labeling.

Solution, Intravenous, as hydrochloride:

Generic: 1 mg/mL (250 mL); 2 mg/mL (250 mL); 4 mg/mL (250 mL); 250 mg/20 mL (20 mL); 500 mg/40 mL (40 mL)

◆ **Dobutamine Hydrochloride** *see* DOBUTamine *on page 691*

◆ **Dobutamine Injection, USP (Can)** *see* DOBUTamine *on page 691*

◆ **Dobutrex (Can)** *see* DOBUTamine *on page 691*

◆ **Docefrez** *see* DOCEtaxel *on page 692*

DOCEtaxel (doe se TAKS el)

Medication Safety Issues

Sound-alike/look-alike issues:

DOCEtaxel may be confused with cabazitaxel, PACLitaxel

Taxotere may be confused with Taxol

High alert medication:

This medication is in a class the Institute for Safe Medication Practices (ISMP) includes among its list of

drug classes which have a heightened risk of causing significant patient harm when used in error.

Administration issues:

Multiple concentrations: Docetaxel is available as a one-vial formulation at concentrations of 10 mg/mL (generic formulation) and 20 mg/mL (concentrate; Taxotere), and as a lyophilized powder (Docefrez) which is reconstituted (with provided diluent) to 20 mg/0.8 mL (20 mg vial) or 24 mg/mL (80 mg vial). Docetaxel was previously available as a two-vial formulation (a concentrated docetaxel solution vial and a diluent vial) resulting in a reconstituted concentration of 10 mg/mL. The two-vial formulation has been discontinued by the Taxotere manufacturer (available generically). Admixture errors have occurred due to the availability of various docetaxel concentrations.

Related Information

Management of Drug Extravasations *on page 2298*

Prevention of Chemotherapy-Induced Nausea and Vomiting in Children *on page 2368*

Safe Handling of Hazardous Drugs *on page 2455*

Brand Names: US Docefrez; Taxotere

Brand Names: Canada Docetaxel for Injection; Taxotere

Therapeutic Category Antineoplastic Agent, Antimicrotubular; Antineoplastic Agent, Taxane Derivative

Generic Availability (US) May be product dependent

Use Treatment of breast cancer (locally advanced/metastatic or adjuvant treatment of operable node-positive); locally advanced or metastatic non-small cell lung cancer (NSCLC); and hormone refractory, metastatic prostate cancer (Docefrez, Taxotere: FDA approved in adults); advanced gastric adenocarcinoma; locally advanced squamous cell head and neck cancer (Taxotere: FDA approved in adults); has also been used in the treatment of soft tissue sarcoma; Ewing's sarcoma, osteosarcoma, and unknown primary adenocarcinoma

Pregnancy Risk Factor D

Pregnancy Considerations Adverse events have been observed in animal reproduction studies. An *ex vivo* human placenta perfusion model illustrated that docetaxel crossed the placenta at term. Placental transfer was low and affected by the presence of albumin; higher albumin concentrations resulted in lower docetaxel placental transfer (Berveiller, 2012). Some pharmacokinetic properties of docetaxel may be altered in pregnant women (van Hasselt, 2014). Women of childbearing potential should avoid becoming pregnant during therapy. A pregnancy registry is available for all cancers diagnosed during pregnancy at Cooper Health (877-635-4499).

Breast-Feeding Considerations It is not known if docetaxel is excreted into breast milk. Due to the potential for serious adverse reactions in nursing the infant, the manufacturer recommends a decision be made whether to discontinue breast-feeding or the drug, taking into account the importance of treatment to the mother.

Contraindications

Severe hypersensitivity to docetaxel or any component of the formulation; severe hypersensitivity to other medications containing polysorbate 80; neutrophil count <1500/mm^3

Canadian labeling: Additional contraindications (not in U.S. labeling): Severe hepatic impairment; pregnancy; breast-feeding

Warnings/Precautions Hazardous agent - use appropriate precautions for handling and disposal (NIOSH 2014 [group 1]). **[U.S. Boxed Warning]: Avoid use in patients with bilirubin exceeding upper limit of normal (ULN) or AST and/or ALT >1.5 times ULN in conjunction with alkaline phosphatase >2.5 times ULN; patients with isolated transaminase elevations >1.5 times ULN also had a higher rate of neutropenic fever, although no increased incidence of toxic death.** Patients with abnormal liver function are also at increased risk of other treatment-related adverse events, including grade 4 neutropenia, infections, and severe thrombocytopenia, stomatitis, skin toxicity or toxic death; obtain liver function tests prior to each treatment cycle. Canadian labeling contraindicates use in severe hepatic impairment. Canadian labeling contraindicates use in severe hepatic impairment. **[U.S. Boxed Warnings]: Severe hypersensitivity reactions, characterized by generalized rash/erythema, hypotension, bronchospasms, or anaphylaxis may occur (may be fatal; has occurred in patients receiving corticosteroid premedication); minor reactions including flushing or localized skin reactions may also occur; do not administer to patients with a history of severe hypersensitivity to docetaxel or polysorbate 80 (component of formulation). Severe fluid retention, characterized by pleural effusion (requiring immediate drainage, ascites, peripheral edema (poorly tolerated), dyspnea at rest, cardiac tamponade, generalized edema, and weight gain, has been reported.** Fluid retention may begin as lower extremity peripheral edema and become generalized with a median weight gain of 2 kg. In patients with breast cancer, the median cumulative dose to onset of moderate or severe fluid retention was 819 mg/m^2; fluid retention resolves in a median of 16 weeks after discontinuation. Observe for hypersensitivity, especially with the first two infusions. Discontinue for severe reactions; do not rechallenge if severe. Patients should be premedicated with a corticosteroid (starting one day prior to administration) to reduce the incidence and severity of hypersensitivity reactions and fluid retention; severity is reduced with dexamethasone premedication starting one day prior to docetaxel administration. Premedication with oral corticosteroids is recommended to decrease the incidence and severity of fluid retention and severity of hypersensitivity reactions. The manufacturer recommends dexamethasone 16 mg/day (8 mg twice daily) orally for 3 days, starting the day before docetaxel administration; for prostate cancer, when prednisone is part of the antineoplastic regimen, dexamethasone 8 mg orally is administered at 12 hours, 3 hours, and 1 hour prior to docetaxel.

[U.S. Boxed Warning]: Patients with abnormal liver function, those receiving higher doses, and patients with non–small cell lung cancer and a history of prior treatment with platinum derivatives who receive single-agent docetaxel at a dose of 100 mg/m^2 are at higher risk for treatment-related mortality.

Neutropenia is the dose-limiting toxicity. Patients with increased liver function tests experienced more episodes of neutropenia with a greater number of severe infections. **[U.S. Boxed Warning]: Patients with an absolute neutrophil count <1,500/mm^3 should not receive docetaxel.** Platelets should recover to >100,000/mm^3 prior to treatment. Monitor blood counts and liver function tests frequently; dose reduction or therapy discontinuation may be necessary.

Cutaneous reactions including erythema (with edema) and desquamation have been reported; may require dose reduction. Cystoid macular edema (CME) has been reported; if vision impairment occurs, a prompt comprehensive ophthalmic exam is recommended. If CME is diagnosed, initiate appropriate CME management and discontinue docetaxel (consider non-taxane treatments). In a study of patients receiving docetaxel for the adjuvant treatment of breast cancer, a majority of patients experienced tearing, which occurred in patients with and without lacrimal duct obstruction at baseline; onset was generally after cycle 1, but subsided in most patients within 4 months after therapy completion (Chan, 2013). Dosage adjustment is recommended with severe neurosensory symptoms (paresthesia, dysesthesia, pain); persistent symptoms may require discontinuation; reversal of symptoms may be delayed after discontinuation. Some docetaxel formulations contain alcohol (content varies by formulation), which may affect the central nervous system and cause symptoms of alcohol intoxication. Consider alcohol content and use with caution in patients for whom alcohol intake should be avoided or minimized. Patients should avoid driving or operating machinery immediately after the infusion. Treatment-related acute myeloid leukemia or myelodysplasia occurred in patients receiving docetaxel in combination with anthracyclines and/or cyclophosphamide. Fatigue and weakness (may be severe) have been reported; symptoms may last a few days up to several weeks; in patients with progressive disease, weakness may be associated with a decrease in performance status. Potentially significant drug-drug interactions may exist, requiring dose or frequency adjustment, additional monitoring, and/or selection of alternative therapy. Docetaxel is an irritant with vesicant-like properties; ensure proper needle or catheter placement prior to and during infusion; avoid extravasation.

Some dosage forms may contain polysorbate 80 (also known as Tweens). Hypersensitivity reactions, usually a delayed reaction, have been reported following exposure to pharmaceutical products containing polysorbate 80 in certain individuals (Isaksson, 2002; Lucente 2000; Shelley, 1995). Thrombocytopenia, ascites, pulmonary deterioration, and renal and hepatic failure have been reported in premature neonates after receiving parenteral products containing polysorbate 80 (Alade, 1986; CDC, 1984). See manufacturer's labeling.

Adverse Reactions Frequency of adverse effects may vary depending on diagnosis, dose, liver function, prior treatment, and premedication. The incidence of adverse events was usually higher in patients with elevated liver function tests.

Cardiovascular: Decreased left ventricular ejection fraction, hypotension

Central nervous system: Central nervous system toxicity (including neuropathy), peripheral motor neuropathy (mainly distal extremity weakness)

Dermatologic: Alopecia, dermatological reaction, nail disease

Endocrine & metabolic: Fluid retention (dose dependent)

Gastrointestinal: Diarrhea, dysgeusia, nausea, stomatitis, vomiting

Hematologic & oncologic: Anemia (dose dependent), febrile neutropenia (dose dependent), leukopenia, neutropenia (nadir [median]: 7 days, duration [severe neutropenia]: 7 days; dose dependent), thrombocytopenia (dose dependent)

Hepatic: Increased serum alkaline phosphatase, increased serum bilirubin, increased serum transaminases

Hypersensitivity: Hypersensitivity

Infection: Infection (dose dependent)

Local: Infusion site reactions (including hyperpigmentation, inflammation, redness, dryness, phlebitis, extravasation, swelling of the vein)

Neuromuscular & skeletal: Arthralgia, myalgia, neuromuscular reaction, weakness

Ophthalmic: Epiphora (associated with canalicular stenosis)

Respiratory: Pulmonary reaction

Miscellaneous: Hypersensitivity (including with premedication), infection (dose dependent)

Rare but important or life-threatening: Acute myelocytic leukemia, acute respiratory distress, anaphylactic shock, anorexia, ascites, atrial fibrillation, atrial flutter, atrioventricular block, bradycardia, bronchospasm, cardiac arrhythmia, cardiac failure, cardiac tamponade, chest pain, chest tightness, colitis, confusion, conjunctivitis, constipation, cystoid macular edema, deep vein thrombosis, dehydration, disease of the lacrimal apparatus (duct obstruction), disseminated intravascular coagulation, drug fever, duodenal ulcer, dyspnea, ECG abnormality, erythema multiforme, esophagitis, gastrointestinal hemorrhage, gastrointestinal obstruction, gastrointestinal perforation, hearing loss, hemorrhagic diathesis, hepatitis, hypertension, hyponatremia, intestinal obstruction, interstitial pulmonary disease, ischemic colitis, ischemic heart disease, loss of consciousness (transient), lymphedema (peripheral), multiorgan failure, myelodysplastic syndrome, myocardial infarction, neutropenic enterocolitis, ototoxicity, palmar-plantar erythrodysesthesia, pericardial effusion, pleural effusion, pneumonia, pneumonitis, pruritus, pulmonary edema, pulmonary embolism, pulmonary fibrosis, radiation pneumonitis, radiation recall phenomenon, renal failure, renal insufficiency, respiratory failure, skin changes (scleroderma-like), seizure, sepsis, sinus tachycardia, Stevens-Johnson syndrome, subacute cutaneous lupus erythematosus, syncope, toxic epidermal necrolysis, tachycardia, thrombophlebitis, unstable angina pectoris, visual disturbance (transient)

Drug Interactions

Metabolism/Transport Effects Substrate of CYP3A4 (major), P-glycoprotein; **Note:** Assignment of Major/Minor substrate status based on clinically relevant drug interaction potential

Avoid Concomitant Use

Avoid concomitant use of DOCEtaxel with any of the following: BCG; BCG (Intravesical); CloZAPine; Conivaptan; Dipyrone; Fusidic Acid (Systemic); Idelalisib; Natalizumab; Pimecrolimus; Tacrolimus (Topical); Tofacitinib; Vaccines (Live)

Increased Effect/Toxicity

DOCEtaxel may increase the levels/effects of: Antineoplastic Agents (Anthracycline, Systemic); CloZAPine; Leflunomide; Natalizumab; Tofacitinib; Vaccines (Live)

The levels/effects of DOCEtaxel may be increased by: Antifungal Agents (Azole Derivatives, Systemic); Conivaptan; CYP3A4 Inhibitors (Moderate); CYP3A4 Inhibitors (Strong); Dasatinib; Denosumab; Dipyrone; Dronedarone; Fusidic Acid (Systemic); Idelalisib; Ivacaftor; Luliconazole; Mifepristone; Netupitant; Palbociclib; P-glycoprotein/ABCB1 Inhibitors; Pimecrolimus; Platinum Derivatives; Roflumilast; Simeprevir; SORAfenib; Stiripentol; Tacrolimus (Topical); Trastuzumab

Decreased Effect

DOCEtaxel may decrease the levels/effects of: BCG; BCG (Intravesical); Coccidioides immitis Skin Test; Sipuleucel-T; Vaccines (Inactivated); Vaccines (Live)

The levels/effects of DOCEtaxel may be decreased by: Bosentan; CYP3A4 Inducers (Moderate); CYP3A4 Inducers (Strong); Dabrafenib; Deferasirox; Echinacea; Mitotane; P-glycoprotein/ABCB1 Inducers; Siltuximab; St Johns Wort; Tocilizumab

Storage/Stability Storage and stability may vary by manufacturer, refer to specific prescribing information.

Docetaxel 10 mg/mL: Store intact vials between 2°C to 25°C (36°F to 77°F) (actual recommendations may vary by generic manufacturer; consult manufacturer's labeling). Protect from bright light. Freezing does not adversely affect the product. Multi-use vials (80 mg/8 mL and 160 mg/16 mL) are stable for up to 28 days after first entry when stored between 2°C to 8°C (36°F to 46°F) and protected from light. Solutions diluted for infusion should be used within 4 hours of preparation, including infusion time.

Docetaxel 20 mg/mL concentrate:

Taxotere: Store intact vials between 2°C to 25°C (36°F to 77°F). Protect from bright light. Freezing does not adversely affect the product. Solutions diluted for infusion in non-PVC containers should be used within 6 hours of preparation, including infusion time, when stored between 2°C to 25°C (36°F to 77°F) or within 48 hours when stored between 2°C to 8°C (36°F to 46°F).

Generic formulations: Store intact vials at 25°C (77°F); excursions permitted between 15°C to 30°C (59°F to 86°F). Protect from light. Solutions diluted for infusion should be used within 4 hours of preparation, including infusion time.

Docetaxel lyophilized powder (Docefrez): Store intact vials between 2°C to 8°C (36°F to 46°F). Protect from light. Allow vials (and provided diluent) to stand at room temperature for 5 minutes prior to reconstitution. After reconstitution, may be stored refrigerated or at room temperature for up to 8 hours. Solutions diluted for infusion should be used within 6 hours of preparation, including infusion time. According to the manufacturer, physical and chemical in-use stability of the infusion solution (prepared as recommended) has been demonstrated in non-PVC bags up to 48 hours when stored between 2°C and 8°C (36°F and 46°F).

Two-vial formulation *(generic; concentrate plus diluent formulation)*: Reconstituted solutions of the two-vial formulation are stable in the vial for 8 hours at room temperature or under refrigeration. Solutions diluted for infusion in polyolefin containers should be used within 4 hours of preparation, including infusion time.

Mechanism of Action Docetaxel promotes the assembly of microtubules from tubulin dimers, and inhibits the depolymerization of tubulin which stabilizes microtubules in the cell. This results in inhibition of DNA, RNA, and protein synthesis. Most activity occurs during the M phase of the cell cycle.

Pharmacokinetics (Adult data unless noted) Exhibits linear pharmacokinetics at the recommended dosage range

Distribution: Extensive extravascular distribution and/or tissue binding; V_d: 80-90 L/m^2, V_{dss}: 113 L (mean steady state)

Protein binding: ~94% to 97%, primarily to alpha$_1$-acid glycoprotein, albumin, and lipoproteins

Metabolism: Hepatic; oxidation via CYP3A4 to metabolites

Half-life: Terminal: 11 hours

Elimination: Feces (75%, <8% as unchanged drug); urine (6%)

Dosing: Usual Dose, frequency, number of doses, and start date may vary by protocol and treatment phase. Refer to individual protocols: **Note:** Premedicate with corticosteroids, beginning the day before docetaxel administration (administer corticosteroids for 1-3 days), to reduce the severity of hypersensitivity reactions and pulmonary/peripheral edema.

Pediatric: **Ewing's Sarcoma; osteosarcoma (recurrent or progressive):** Limited data available: Children and Adolescents: IV: 75-125 mg/m^2 every 21 days; administer on day 8 of treatment cycle if given in combination with other chemotherapy (Mora, 2009; Navid, 2008; Zwerdling, 2006)

Adult: **Note:** Utilize patient's actual body weight (full weight) for calculation of body surface area- or weight-based dosing, particularly when the intent of therapy is curative; manage regimen-related toxicities in the same manner as for nonobese patients; if a dose reduction is utilized due to toxicity, consider resumption of full weight-based dosing with subsequent cycles, especially if cause of toxicity (eg, hepatic or renal impairment) is resolved (Griggs, 2012).

Breast cancer: IV:

Locally-advanced or metastatic: 60-100 mg/m^2 every 3 weeks as a single agent

Operable, node-positive (adjuvant treatment): 75 mg/m^2 every 3 weeks for 6 courses (in combination with doxorubicin and cyclophosphamide)

Non-small cell lung cancer: IV: 75 mg/m^2 every 3 weeks (as monotherapy or in combination with cisplatin)

Prostate cancer: IV: 75 mg/m^2 every 3 weeks (in combination with prednisone)

Gastric adenocarcinoma: IV: 75 mg/m^2 every 3 weeks (in combination with cisplatin and fluorouracil)

Head and neck cancer: IV: 75 mg/m^2 every 3 weeks (in combination with cisplatin and fluorouracil) for 3 or 4 cycles, followed by radiation therapy

Dosing adjustment for concomitant CYP3A4 inhibitors: Adults: Avoid the concomitant use of strong CYP3A4 inhibitors with docetaxel. If concomitant use of a strong CYP3A4 inhibitor cannot be avoided, consider reducing the docetaxel dose by 50% (based on limited pharmacokinetic data).

Dosing adjustment for toxicity: Adults: **Note:** Toxicity includes febrile neutropenia, neutrophils ≤500/mm^3 for >1 week, severe or cumulative cutaneous reactions; in non-small cell lung cancer, this may also include platelets <25,000/mm^3 and other grade 3/4 nonhematologic toxicities.

Breast cancer (single agent): Patients dosed initially at 100 mg/m^2; reduce dose to 75 mg/m^2; **Note:** If the patient continues to experience these adverse reactions, the dosage should be reduced to 55 mg/m^2 or therapy should be discontinued; discontinue for peripheral neuropathy ≥ grade 3. Patients initiated at 60 mg/m^2 who do not develop toxicity may tolerate higher doses.

Breast cancer, adjuvant treatment (combination chemotherapy): TAC regimen should be administered when neutrophils are ≥1500/mm^3. Patients experiencing febrile neutropenia should receive G-CSF in all subsequent cycles. Patients with persistent febrile neutropenia (while on G-CSF), patients experiencing severe/cumulative cutaneous reactions, moderate neurosensory effects (signs/symptoms) or grade 3 or 4 stomatitis should receive a reduced dose (60 mg/m^2) of docetaxel. Discontinue therapy with persistent toxicities after dosage reduction.

Non-small cell lung cancer:

Monotherapy: Patients dosed initially at 75 mg/m^2 should have dose held until toxicity is resolved, then resume at 55 mg/m^2; discontinue for peripheral neuropathy ≥ grade 3.

Combination therapy (with cisplatin): Patients dosed initially at 75 mg/m^2 should have the docetaxel dosage reduced to 65 mg/m^2 in subsequent cycles; if further adjustment is required, dosage may be reduced to 50 mg/m^2

Prostate cancer: Reduce dose to 60 mg/m^2; discontinue therapy if toxicities persist at lower dose.

Gastric cancer, head and neck cancer: Note: Cisplatin may require dose reductions/therapy delays for peripheral neuropathy, ototoxicity, and/or nephrotoxicity. Patients experiencing febrile neutropenia, documented infection with neutropenia or neutropenia >7 days should receive G-CSF in all subsequent cycles. For neutropenic complications despite G-CSF use, further reduce dose to 60 mg/m^2. Dosing with neutropenic complications in subsequent cycles should be further reduced to 45 mg/m^2. Patients who experience grade 4 thrombocytopenia should receive a dose reduction from 75 mg/m^2 to 60 mg/m^2. Discontinue therapy for persistent toxicities.

Gastrointestinal toxicity for docetaxel in combination with cisplatin and fluorouracil for treatment of gastric cancer or head and neck cancer:

Diarrhea, grade 3:

First episode: Reduce fluorouracil dose by 20%

Second episode: Reduce docetaxel dose by 20%

Diarrhea, grade 4:

First episode: Reduce fluorouracil and docetaxel doses by 20%

Second episode: Discontinue treatment

Stomatitis, grade 3:

First episode: Reduce fluorouracil dose by 20%

Second episode: Discontinue fluorouracil for all subsequent cycles

Third episode: Reduce docetaxel dose by 20%

Stomatitis, grade 4:

First episode: Discontinue fluorouracil for all subsequent cycles

Second episode: Reduce docetaxel dose by 20%

Dosing adjustment in renal impairment: Adults: Renal excretion is minimal; therefore, the need for dosage adjustments for renal dysfunction is unlikely (Janus, 2010; Li, 2007). Not removed by hemodialysis; may be administered before or after hemodialysis (Janus, 2010).

Dosing adjustment in hepatic impairment: Adults:

Manufacturer's labeling:

Total bilirubin greater than the ULN, or AST/ALT >1.5 times ULN concomitant with alkaline phosphatase >2.5 times ULN: Use is not recommended.

Hepatic impairment dosing adjustment specific for gastric or head and neck cancer:

AST/ALT >2.5 to ≤5 times ULN and alkaline phosphatase ≤2.5 times ULN: Administer 80% of dose

AST/ALT >1.5 to ≤5 times ULN and alkaline phosphatase >2.5 to ≤5 times ULN: Administer 80% of dose

AST/ALT >5 times ULN and /or alkaline phosphatase >5 times ULN: Discontinue docetaxel

The following guidelines have been used by some clinicians (Floyd, 2006):

AST/ALT 1.6-6 times ULN: Administer 75% of dose

AST/ALT >6 times ULN: Use clinical judgment

Preparation for Administration Hazardous agent; use appropriate precautions for handling and disposal (NIOSH 2014 [group 1]). Preparation instructions may vary by manufacturer, refer to specific prescribing information. **Note:** Some formulations contain overfill.

Note: Multiple concentrations: Docetaxel is available as a one-vial formulation at concentrations of 10 mg/mL (generic formulation) and 20 mg/mL (concentrate; Taxotere), and as a lyophilized powder (Docefrez) which is reconstituted (with provided diluent) to 20 mg/0.8 mL (20 mg vial) or 24 mg/mL (80 mg vial). Admixture errors have occurred due to the availability of various concentrations. Docetaxel was previously available as a two-vial formulation which included two vials (a concentrated docetaxel vial and a diluent vial), resulting in a reconstituted concentration of 10 mg/mL; the two-vial formulation has been discontinued by the Taxotere manufacturer (available generically).

One-vial formulations: Further dilute for infusion in 250 to 500 mL of NS or D_5W in a non-DEHP container (eg, glass, polypropylene, polyolefin) to a final concentration of 0.3 to 0.74 mg/mL. Gently rotate and invert manually to mix thoroughly; avoid shaking or vigorous agitation.

Taxotere: Use **only** a 21-gauge needle to withdraw docetaxel from the vial (larger bore needles, such as 18-gauge or 19-gauge needles, may cause stopper coring and rubber precipitates). If intact vials were stored refrigerated, allow to stand at room temperature for 5 minutes prior to dilution. Inspect vials prior to dilution; solution is supersaturated and may crystalize over time; do not use if crystalized.

Lyophilized powder: Allow vials (and provided diluent) to stand at room temperature for 5 minutes prior to reconstitution. Reconstitute with the provided diluent (contains ethanol in polysorbate 80); add 1 mL to each 20 mg vial (resulting concentration is 20 mg/0.8 mL) and 4 mL to each 80 mg vial (resulting concentration is 24 mg/mL). Shake well to dissolve completely. Reconstituted solution is supersaturated and could crystallize over time; if crystals appear, discard the solution (should no longer be used). If air bubbles are present, allow to stand for a few minutes while air bubbles dissipate. Further dilute in 250 mL of NS or D_5W in a non-DEHP container (eg, glass, polypropylene, polyolefin) to a final concentration of 0.3 to 0.74 mg/mL (for doses >200 mg, use a larger volume of NS or D_5W, not to exceed a final concentration of 0.74 mg/mL). Mix thoroughly by manual agitation.

Two-vial formulation *(generic; concentrate plus diluent formulation):* Vials should be diluted with 13% (w/w) polyethylene glycol 400/water (provided with the drug) to a final concentration of 10 mg/mL. Do not shake. Further dilute for infusion in 250 to 500 mL of NS or D_5W in a non-DEHP container (eg, glass, polypropylene, polyolefin) to a final concentration of 0.3 to 0.74 mg/mL. Gently rotate to mix thoroughly. Do not use the two-vial formulation with the one-vial formulation for the same admixture product.

Administration Hazardous agent; use appropriate precautions for handling and disposal (NIOSH 2014 [group 1]).

Administer as an IV infusion over 1 hour through nonsorbing polyethylene lined (non-DEHP) tubing; in-line filter is not necessary (the use of a filter during administration is not recommended by the manufacturer). Infusion should be completed within 4 hours of preparation. **Note:** Premedication with corticosteroids for 3 days, beginning the day before docetaxel administration, is recommended to prevent hypersensitivity reactions and pulmonary/peripheral edema. Some docetaxel formulations contain alcohol (content varies by formulation); use with caution in patients for whom alcohol intake should be avoided or minimized.

Irritant with vesicant-like properties; avoid extravasation. Assure proper needle or catheter position prior to administration. If extravasation occurs, stop infusion immediately and disconnect (leave cannula/needle in place); gently aspirate extravasated solution (do **NOT** flush the line); remove needle/cannula; elevate extremity. Information conflicts regarding the use of warm or cold compresses (Pérez Fidalgo 2012; Polovich 2009).

Vesicant/Extravasation Risk Irritant with vesicant-like properties

Monitoring Parameters CBC with differential, liver function tests, bilirubin, alkaline phosphatase, renal function; monitor for hypersensitivity reactions, neurosensory symptoms, gastrointestinal toxicity (eg, diarrhea, stomatitis), cutaneous reactions, fluid retention, epiphora, and canalicular stenosis

Additional Information Premedication with oral corticosteroids is recommended to decrease the incidence and severity of fluid retention and severity of hypersensitivity reactions. The manufacturer recommends dexamethasone 16 mg (8 mg twice daily) orally for 3 days. In one pediatric clinical trial, dexamethasone 3 mg/m^2 orally or IV every 6 hours for 2 doses, starting 12 hours before docetaxel administration has been described (Zwerdling, 2006).

Dosage Forms Excipient information presented when available (limited, particularly for generics); consult specific product labeling.

Concentrate, Intravenous:

Taxotere: 20 mg/mL (1 mL); 80 mg/4 mL (4 mL) [contains alcohol, usp, polysorbate 80]

Generic: 20 mg/mL (1 mL); 80 mg/4 mL (4 mL); 160 mg/8 mL (8 mL); 20 mg/0.5 mL (0.5 mL); 80 mg/2 mL (2 mL)
Concentrate, Intravenous [preservative free]:
Generic: 20 mg/mL (1 mL); 80 mg/4 mL (4 mL); 140 mg/7 mL (7 mL)
Solution, Intravenous:
Generic: 20 mg/2 mL (2 mL); 80 mg/8 mL (8 mL); 160 mg/16 mL (16 mL); 200 mg/20 mL (20 mL)
Solution Reconstituted, Intravenous:
Docefrez: 20 mg (1 ea); 80 mg (1 ea) [contains alcohol, usp, polysorbate 80]

- ◆ **Docetaxel for Injection (Can)** *see* DOCEtaxel *on page 692*
- ◆ **DocQLace [OTC]** *see* Docusate *on page 697*
- ◆ **Doc-Q-Lax [OTC]** *see* Docusate and Senna *on page 698*
- ◆ **Docu [OTC]** *see* Docusate *on page 697*
- ◆ **Docuprene [OTC]** *see* Docusate *on page 697*

Docusate (DOK yoo sate)

Medication Safety Issues
Sound-alike/look-alike issues:
Colace may be confused with Calan, Cozaar
Dulcolax (docusate) may be confused with Dulcolax (bisacodyl)
International issues:
Docusate may be confused with Doxinate brand name for doxylamine and pyridoxine [India]

Related Information
Oral Medications That Should Not Be Crushed or Altered *on page 2476*

Brand Names: US Colace Clear [OTC]; Colace [OTC]; D.O.S. [OTC]; Diocto [OTC]; DocQLace [OTC]; Docu Soft [OTC]; Docu [OTC]; Docuprene [OTC]; Docusil [OTC]; DocuSol Kids [OTC]; DocuSol Mini [OTC]; DOK [OTC]; Dulcolax Stool Softener [OTC]; Enemeez Mini [OTC]; Healthy Mama Move It Along [OTC]; Kao-Tin [OTC]; KS Stool Softener [OTC]; Laxa Basic [OTC]; Pedia-Lax [OTC]; Promolaxin [OTC]; Silace [OTC]; Sof-Lax [OTC]; Stool Softener Laxative DC [OTC]; Stool Softener [OTC]; Sur-Q-Lax [OTC]; Vacuant Mini-Enema [OTC] [DSC]

Brand Names: Canada Apo-Docusate Calcium [OTC]; Apo-Docusate Sodium [OTC]; Calax [OTC]; Colace [OTC]; Correctol Stool Softener [OTC]; Docusate Sodium Odan [OTC]; Dom-Docusate Sodium [OTC]; Dosolax [OTC]; Euro-Docusate C [OTC]; Jamp-Docusate [OTC]; Novo-Docusate Calcium [OTC]; Novo-Docusate Sodium [OTC]; PHL-Docusate Sodium [OTC]; PMS-Docusate Calcium [OTC]; PMS-Docusate Sodium [OTC]; ratio-Docusate Sodium [OTC]; Selax [OTC]; Silace [OTC]; Sirop Docusate De Sodium [OTC]; Soflax C [OTC]; Soflax Pediatric Drops [OTC]; Soflax [OTC]; Taro-Docusate [OTC]; Teva-Docusate Sodium [OTC]

Therapeutic Category Laxative, Surfactant; Stool Softener

Generic Availability (US) May be product dependent

Use
Docusate sodium: Stool softener in patients who should avoid straining during defecation (OTC products: Oral: FDA approved in ages ≥2 years and adults); relief of occasional constipation (OTC products: Oral, rectal enema: FDA approved in ages ≥2 and adults); has also been used as a ceruminolytic
Docusate calcium: Relief of occasional constipation (OTC products: FDA approved in ages ≥12 years and adults)

Pregnancy Considerations The short-term use of docusate for the treatment of constipation is generally considered safe during pregnancy (Mahadevan, 2006). Hypomagnesemia was reported in a newborn following chronic maternal overuse throughout pregnancy (Schindler, 1984).

Breast-Feeding Considerations Maternal use of docusate is considered to be compatible with breast-feeding (Mahadevan, 2006).

Contraindications Hypersensitivity to docusate or any component of the formulation; concomitant use of mineral oil; intestinal obstruction, acute abdominal pain, nausea, or vomiting

Warnings/Precautions Prolonged, frequent, or excessive use may result in dependence or electrolyte imbalance

Warnings: Additional Pediatric Considerations Some dosage forms may contain propylene glycol; in neonates large amounts of propylene glycol delivered orally, intravenously (eg, >3,000 mg/day), or topically have been associated with potentially fatal toxicities which can include metabolic acidosis, seizures, renal failure, and CNS depression; toxicities have also been reported in children and adults including hyperosmolality, lactic acidosis, seizures and respiratory depression; use caution (AAP 1997; Shehab 2009).

Adverse Reactions
Gastrointestinal: Abdominal cramping, diarrhea, Intestinal obstruction
Miscellaneous: Throat irritation

Drug Interactions
Metabolism/Transport Effects None known.
Avoid Concomitant Use There are no known interactions where it is recommended to avoid concomitant use.
Increased Effect/Toxicity There are no known significant interactions involving an increase in effect.
Decreased Effect There are no known significant interactions involving a decrease in effect.

Mechanism of Action Reduces surface tension of the oil-water interface of the stool resulting in enhanced incorporation of water and fat allowing for stool softening

Pharmacodynamics Onset of action: Oral: 12 to 72 hours; rectal: 2 to 15 minutes

Dosing: Usual
Pediatric: **Constipation (occasional), treatment; stool softener:**
Docusate sodium:
Oral:
Manufacturer's labeling:
Children 2 years to <12 years: 50 to 150 mg/day in single or divided doses
Children ≥12 years and Adolescents: 50 to 360 mg/day in single or divided doses
Alternate dosing:
Weight-directed dosing: Infants and Children: 5 mg/kg/day in 1 to 4 divided doses (Nelson 1996)
Age-directed (fixed) dosing:
Infants ≥6 months and Children <2 years: 12.5 mg 3 times daily (NICE 2010)
Children ≥2 and Adolescents: 40 to 150 mg/day in 1 to 4 divided doses (Kliegman 2011); in children ≥12 years and adolescents, doses up to 500 mg/day divided may be used (NICE 2010)
Rectal:
Children 2 to <12 years:
100 mg/5 mL: 100 mg (1 unit) once daily
283 mg/5 mL: 283 mg (1 unit) once daily
Children ≥12 years and Adolescents: 283 mg/5mL: 283 mg (1 unit) 1 to 3 times daily
Docusate calcium: Children ≥12 years and Adolescents: 240 mg once daily
Adult: **Note:** Docusate salts are interchangeable; the amount of sodium, calcium, or potassium per dosage unit is clinically insignificant. **Stool softener:**
Oral: 50 to 500 mg/day in 1 to 4 divided doses

Rectal: Add 50 to 100 mg of docusate liquid to enema fluid (saline or water); give as retention or flushing enema

Administration

Oral: Docusate liquid products may have bitter taste due to active ingredient, consider mixing with milk, fruit juice, or infant formula to mask taste; ensure adequate fluid intake

Rectal: Empty contents of enema into rectum, discard disposable administration device

Test Interactions Decreased potassium (S), decreased chloride (S)

Additional Information Docusate sodium 5 to 10 mg/mL **liquid** instilled in the ear as a ceruminolytic produces substantial ear wax disintegration within 15 minutes and complete disintegration after 24 hours (Chen 1991)

Dosage Forms Excipient information presented when available (limited, particularly for generics); consult specific product labeling. [DSC] = Discontinued product

Capsule, Oral, as calcium:

- Kao-Tin: 240 mg [sodium free; contains brilliant blue fcf (fd&c blue #1), fd&c red #40, fd&c yellow #6 (sunset yellow)]
- Kao-Tin: 240 mg [sodium free; contains fd&c red #40]
- Stool Softener: 240 mg [contains brilliant blue fcf (fd&c blue #1), fd&c red #40, fd&c yellow #6 (sunset yellow)]
- Stool Softener Laxative DC: 240 mg [contains fd&c red #40]
- Sur-Q-Lax: 240 mg
- Generic: 240 mg

Capsule, Oral, as sodium:

- Colace: 50 mg [DSC]
- Colace: 100 mg [contains fd&c red #40, fd&c yellow #6 (sunset yellow)]
- Colace Clear: 50 mg [dye free]
- D.O.S.: 250 mg
- DocQLace: 100 mg [contains fd&c red #40, fd&c yellow #6 (sunset yellow)]
- Docu Soft: 100 mg
- Docusil: 100 mg
- DOK: 100 mg [contains fd&c red #40, fd&c yellow #6 (sunset yellow)]
- DOK: 250 mg
- DOK: 250 mg [contains fd&c red #40, fd&c yellow #6 (sunset yellow)]
- Dulcolax Stool Softener: 100 mg [contains fd&c red #40, fd&c yellow #6 (sunset yellow)]
- KS Stool Softener: 100 mg [stimulant free; contains brilliant blue fcf (fd&c blue #1), fd&c red #40, methylparaben, propylparaben, tartrazine (fd&c yellow #5)]
- Laxa Basic: 100 mg
- Sof-Lax: 100 mg
- Stool Softener: 100 mg
- Stool Softener: 100 mg, 250 mg [contains fd&c red #40, fd&c yellow #6 (sunset yellow)]
- Stool Softener: 100 mg [stimulant free; contains brilliant blue fcf (fd&c blue #1), fd&c red #40, fd&c yellow #6 (sunset yellow)]
- Stool Softener: 100 mg, 250 mg [stimulant free; contains fd&c red #40, fd&c yellow #6 (sunset yellow)]
- Generic: 100 mg, 250 mg

Enema, Rectal, as sodium:

- DocuSol Kids: 100 mg/5 mL (5 ea) [contains polyethylene glycol]
- DocuSol Mini: 283 mg (5 ea)
- Enemeez Mini: 283 mg (5 mL)
- Vacuant Mini-Enema: 283 mg (5 mL [DSC])

Liquid, Oral, as sodium:

- Diocto: 50 mg/5 mL (473 mL) [contains fd&c red #40, methylparaben, polyethylene glycol, propylene glycol, propylparaben; vanilla flavor]
- Diocto: 50 mg/5 mL (473 mL) [contains parabens, polyethylene glycol]
- Docu: 50 mg/5 mL (10 mL, 473 mL) [contains methylparaben, polyethylene glycol, propylene glycol, propylparaben, sodium benzoate; vanilla flavor]
- Pedia-Lax: 50 mg/15 mL (118 mL) [contains edetate disodium, methylparaben, polyethylene glycol, propylene glycol, propylparaben; fruit punch flavor]
- Silace: 150 mg/15 mL (473 mL) [lemon-vanilla flavor]
- Generic: 50 mg/5 mL (10 mL)

Syrup, Oral, as sodium:

- Diocto: 60 mg/15 mL (473 mL) [contains fd&c red #40, menthol, methylparaben, polyethylene glycol, propylparaben, sodium benzoate; peppermint flavor]
- Diocto: 60 mg/15 mL (473 mL [DSC]) [contains fd&c red #40, methylparaben, propylene glycol, propylparaben, sodium benzoate; peppermint flavor]
- Diocto: 60 mg/15 mL (473 mL) [contains fd&c red #40, propylene glycol, saccharin sodium, sodium benzoate]
- Silace: 60 mg/15 mL (473 mL) [contains alcohol, usp; peppermint flavor]

Tablet, Oral, as sodium:

- Docuprene: 100 mg [contains sodium benzoate]
- DOK: 100 mg [scored]
- Healthy Mama Move It Along: 100 mg [scored; stimulant free; contains sodium benzoate]
- Promolaxin: 100 mg [scored; contains sodium benzoate]
- Stool Softener: 100 mg [contains sodium benzoate]
- Generic: 100 mg

Docusate and Senna (DOK yoo sate & SEN na)

Medication Safety Issues

Sound-alike/look-alike issues:

Senokot may be confused with Depakote

Brand Names: US Doc-Q-Lax [OTC]; Dok Plus [OTC]; Geri-Stool [OTC]; Peri-Colace [OTC]; Senexon-S [OTC]; Senna Plus [OTC]; SennaLax-S [OTC]; Senokot-S [OTC]; SenoSol-SS [OTC]

Therapeutic Category Laxative, Stimulant; Laxative, Surfactant; Stool Softener

Generic Availability (US) Yes

Use Treatment of constipation generally associated with dry, hard stools and decreased intestinal motility; prevention of opiate-induced constipation

Pregnancy Considerations See individual agents.

Breast-Feeding Considerations See individual agents.

Contraindications If abdominal pain, nausea or vomiting are present; concurrent use of mineral oil; duration of >1 week

Warnings/Precautions Not recommended for over-the-counter (OTC) use in patients experiencing stomach pain, nausea, vomiting, or a sudden change in bowel movements which lasts >2 weeks. OTC labeling does not recommend for use longer than 1 week. Not recommended for OTC use in children <2 years of age. Discontinue use and contact healthcare provider if rectal bleeding occurs.

Adverse Reactions

Gastrointestinal: Abdominal cramps, diarrhea, nausea, vomiting

Genitourinary: Urine discoloration (red/brown)

Mechanism of Action Docusate is a stool softener; sennosides are laxatives

Pharmacodynamics Onset of action: Within 6-12 hours

Pharmacokinetics (Adult data unless noted) Senna:

Metabolism: Senna is metabolized in the liver

Elimination: In the feces (via bile) and in urine

Dosing: Usual Oral:

Children 2 to <6 years: 1/2 tablet once daily at bedtime; maximum: 1 tablet twice daily

Children 6 to <12 years: 1 tablet once daily at bedtime; maximum: 2 tablets twice daily

Children ≥12 years, Adolescents, and Adults: 2 tablets once daily at bedtime; maximum: 4 tablets twice daily

Administration Administer with water, preferably in the evening

Monitoring Parameters I & O, frequency of bowel movements, serum electrolytes if severe diarrhea develops

Dosage Forms Excipient information presented when available (limited, particularly for generics); consult specific product labeling.

Tablet, oral: Docusate sodium 50 mg and sennosides 8.6 mg

Doc-Q-Lax: Docusate sodium 50 mg and sennosides 8.6 mg

Dok Plus: Docusate sodium 50 mg and sennosides 8.6 mg [contains sodium benzoate]

Geri-Stool: Docusate sodium 50 mg and sennosides 8.6 mg

Peri-Colace: Docusate sodium 50 mg and sennosides 8.6 mg

Senexon-S: Docusate sodium 50 mg and sennosides 8.6 mg [contains calcium 20 mg/tablet, sodium 6 mg/tablet]

SennaLax-S: Docusate sodium 50 mg and sennosides 8.6 mg [contains sodium benzoate]

Senna Plus: Docusate sodium 50 mg and sennosides 8.6 mg

Senokot-S: Docusate sodium 50 mg and sennosides 8.6 mg [sugar free; contains sodium 4 mg/tablet]

SenoSol-SS: Docusate sodium 50 mg and sennosides 8.6 mg [contains sodium 3 mg/tablet]

- ◆ **Docusate and Sennosides** *see* Docusate and Senna *on page 698*
- ◆ **Docusate Calcium** *see* Docusate *on page 697*
- ◆ **Docusate Potassium** *see* Docusate *on page 697*
- ◆ **Docusate Sodium** *see* Docusate *on page 697*
- ◆ **Docusate Sodium Odan [OTC] (Can)** *see* Docusate *on page 697*
- ◆ **Docusil [OTC]** *see* Docusate *on page 697*
- ◆ **Docu Soft [OTC]** *see* Docusate *on page 697*
- ◆ **DocuSol Kids [OTC]** *see* Docusate *on page 697*
- ◆ **DocuSol Mini [OTC]** *see* Docusate *on page 697*
- ◆ **Dofus [OTC]** *see Lactobacillus on page 1203*
- ◆ **DOK [OTC]** *see* Docusate *on page 697*
- ◆ **Dok Plus [OTC]** *see* Docusate and Senna *on page 698*

Dolasetron (dol A se tron)

Medication Safety Issues

Sound-alike/look-alike issues:

Anzemet may be confused with Aldomet, Antivert, Avandamet

Dolasetron may be confused with granisetron, ondansetron, palonosetron

Brand Names: US Anzemet

Brand Names: Canada Anzemet

Therapeutic Category Antiemetic; Selective 5-HT_3 Receptor Antagonist

Generic Availability (US) No

Use

Parenteral solution: Prevention and treatment of postoperative nausea and vomiting (FDA approved in ages ≥2 years and adults)

Tablets: Prevention of nausea and vomiting associated with moderately emetogenic cancer chemotherapy (initial and repeat courses) (FDA approved in ages ≥2 years and adults)

Pregnancy Risk Factor B

Pregnancy Considerations Adverse events have not been observed in animal reproduction studies.

Breast-Feeding Considerations It is not known if dolasetron is excreted in breast milk. The manufacturer recommends that caution be exercised when administering dolasetron to nursing women.

Contraindications

U.S. labeling:

Injection: Hypersensitivity to dolasetron or any component of the formulation; intravenous administration is contraindicated when used for prevention of chemotherapy-associated nausea and vomiting

Tablet: Hypersensitivity to dolasetron or any component of the formulation

Canadian labeling: Hypersensitivity to dolasetron or any component of the formulation; use in children and adolescents <18 years of age; use for the prevention or treatment of postoperative nausea and vomiting; concomitant use with apomorphine

Warnings/Precautions Dolasetron is associated with a number of dose-dependent increases in ECG intervals (eg, PR, QRS duration, QT/QTc, JT), usually occurring 1-2 hours after IV administration and usually lasting 6-8 hours; however, may last ≥24 hours and rarely lead to heart block or arrhythmia. Clinically relevant QT-interval prolongation may occur resulting in torsade de pointes, when used in conjunction with other agents that prolong the QT interval (eg, Class I and III antiarrhythmics). Avoid use in patients at greater risk for QT prolongation (eg, patients with congenital long QT syndrome, medications known to prolong QT interval, electrolyte abnormalities, and cumulative high-dose anthracycline therapy) and/or ventricular arrhythmia. Correct potassium or magnesium abnormalities prior to initiating therapy. IV formulations of 5-HT_3 antagonists have more association with ECG interval changes, compared to oral formulations. Reduction in heart rate may also occur with the 5-HT_3 antagonists. Use with caution in children and adolescents who have or may develop QTc prolongation; rare cases of supraventricular and ventricular arrhythmias, cardiac arrest, and MI have been reported in this population. ECG monitoring is recommended in patients with renal impairment and in the elderly.

Serotonin syndrome has been reported with 5-HT_3 receptor antagonists, predominantly when used in combination with other serotonergic agents (eg, SSRIs, SNRIs, MAOIs, mirtazapine, fentanyl, lithium, tramadol, and/or methylene blue). Some of the cases have been fatal. The majority of serotonin syndrome reports due to 5-HT_3 receptor antagonist have occurred in a post-anesthesia setting or in an infusion center. Serotonin syndrome has also been reported following overdose of another 5-HT_3 receptor antagonist. Monitor patients for signs of serotonin syndrome, including mental status changes (eg, agitation, hallucinations, delirium, coma); autonomic instability (eg, tachycardia, labile blood pressure, diaphoresis, dizziness, flushing, hyperthermia); neuromuscular changes (eg, tremor, rigidity, myoclonus, hyperreflexia, incoordination); gastrointestinal symptoms (eg, nausea, vomiting, diarrhea); and/or seizures. If serotonin syndrome occurs, discontinue 5-HT_3 receptor antagonist treatment and begin supportive management.

Use with caution in patients allergic to other 5-HT_3 receptor antagonists; cross-reactivity has been reported with other 5-HT_3 receptor antagonists. **For chemotherapy-associated nausea and vomiting, should be used on a scheduled basis, not on an "as needed" (PRN) basis,** since data support the use of this drug only in the prevention of nausea and vomiting (due to antineoplastic therapy) and not in the rescue of nausea and vomiting. Not intended for treatment of nausea and vomiting or for chronic continuous therapy. If the prophylaxis dolasetron dose for postoperative nausea and vomiting has failed, a repeat dose should not be administered as rescue or treatment for postoperative nausea and vomiting. Potentially significant drug-drug interactions may exist, requiring dose or frequency adjustment, additional monitoring, and/or selection of alternative therapy.

Some dosage forms may contain polysorbate 80 (also known as Tweens). Hypersensitivity reactions, usually a delayed reaction, have been reported following exposure to pharmaceutical products containing polysorbate 80 in certain individuals (Isaksson, 2002; Lucente 2000; Shelley, 1995). Thrombocytopenia, ascites, pulmonary deterioration, and renal and hepatic failure have been reported in premature neonates after receiving parenteral products containing polysorbate 80 (Alade, 1986; CDC, 1984). See manufacturer's labeling.

Adverse Reactions Adverse events may vary according to indication and route of administration.

Cardiovascular: Bradycardia (may be severe after IV administration), edema, facial edema, flushing, hypotension (may be severe after IV administration), orthostatic hypotension, peripheral edema, peripheral ischemia, phlebitis, sinus arrhythmia, tachycardia, thrombophlebitis

Central nervous system: Abnormal dreams, agitation, anxiety, ataxia, chills, confusion, depersonalization, dizziness, fatigue (oral), headache (more common in oral), pain, paresthesia, shivering sleep disorder, twitching, vertigo

Dermatologic: Diaphoresis, skin rash, urticaria

Endocrine & metabolic: Increased gamma-glutamyl transferase

Gastrointestinal: Abdominal pain, anorexia, constipation, diarrhea (oral), dysgeusia, dyspepsia, pancreatitis

Genitourinary: Dysuria, hematuria

Hematologic and oncologic: Anemia, hematoma, prolonged prothrombin time, prolonged partial thromboplastin time, purpura, thrombocytopenia

Hepatic: Hyperbilirubinemia, increased serum alkaline phosphatase

Hypersensitivity: Anaphylaxis

Local: Burning sensation at injection site (IV), pain at injection site (IV)

Neuromuscular & skeletal: Arthralgia, myalgia, tremor

Ophthalmic: Photophobia, visual disturbance

Otic: Tinnitus

Renal: Acute renal failure, polyuria

Respiratory: Bronchospasm, dyspnea, epistaxis

Rare but important or life-threatening: Abnormal T waves on ECG, appearance of U waves on ECG, atrial fibrillation, atrioventricular block, bundle branch block (left and right), chest pain, extrasystoles (APCs or VPCs), increased serum ALT (transient), increased serum AST (transient), ischemic heart disease, nodal arrhythmia, prolongation P-R interval on ECG (dose-dependent), prolonged Q-T interval on ECG, serotonin syndrome, slow R wave progression, ST segment changes on ECG, supraventricular cardiac arrhythmia, syncope (may be severe after IV administration), torsades de pointes, ventricular arrhythmia (may be serious), ventricular fibrillation cardiac arrest (intravenous), wide complex tachycardia (intravenous), widened QRS complex on ECG (dose-dependent)

Drug Interactions

Metabolism/Transport Effects **Substrate** of CYP2C9 (minor), CYP3A4 (minor); **Note:** Assignment of Major/Minor substrate status based on clinically relevant drug interaction potential; **Inhibits** CYP2D6 (weak)

Avoid Concomitant Use

Avoid concomitant use of Dolasetron with any of the following: Apomorphine; Highest Risk QTc-Prolonging Agents; Ivabradine; Mequitazine; Mifepristone

Increased Effect/Toxicity

Dolasetron may increase the levels/effects of: Apomorphine; ARIPiprazole; Highest Risk QTc-Prolonging Agents; Mequitazine; Moderate Risk QTc-Prolonging Agents; Panobinostat; Serotonin Modulators

The levels/effects of Dolasetron may be increased by: Ivabradine; Mifepristone; QTc-Prolonging Agents (Indeterminate Risk and Risk Modifying)

Decreased Effect

Dolasetron may decrease the levels/effects of: Tapentadol; TraMADol

Food Interactions Food does not affect the bioavailability of oral doses.

Storage/Stability

Injection: Store intact vials at 20°C to 25°C (68°F to 77°F); excursions are permitted to 15°C to 30°C (59°F to 86°F). Protect from light. Solutions diluted for infusion are stable under normal lighting conditions at room temperature for 24 hours or under refrigeration for 48 hours.

Tablets: Store at 20°C to 25°C (68°F to 77°F). Protect from light.

Mechanism of Action Selective serotonin receptor ($5\text{-}HT_3$) antagonist, blocking serotonin both peripherally (primary site of action) and centrally at the chemoreceptor trigger zone

Pharmacokinetics (Adult data unless noted) Due to the rapid metabolism of dolasetron to hydrodolasetron (primary active metabolite), the majority of the following pharmacokinetic parameters relate to hydrodolasetron:

Absorption: Oral: Rapid and complete

Distribution:

- Children: 5.9 to 7.4 L/kg
- Adults: 5.8 L/kg

Metabolism: Hepatic; rapidly converted by carbonyl reductase to active major metabolite, hydrodolasetron; hydrodolasetron is metabolized by the cytochrome P450 CYP2D6 and CYP3A enzyme systems and flavin mono-oxygenase

Bioavailability: Oral: Children: 59% (formulation not specified), adults: 75% (not affected by food)

Protein binding: 69% to 77% (active metabolite)

Half-life, elimination:

- Dolasetron: IV: <10 minutes
- Hydrodolasetron:
  - Oral: Children: 5.5 hours, adolescents: 6.4 hours, adults: 8.1 hours
  - IV: Children: 4.8 hours, adults: 7.3 hours

Time to peak serum concentration:

- Oral: ~1 hours
- IV: 0.6 hours

Elimination: Urine ~67% (Dolasetron: <1% excreted unchanged in urine; hydrodolasetron: 53% to 61% of total dose); feces ~33%

Dosing: Usual

Pediatric:

Chemotherapy-induced nausea and vomiting (CINV); prevention: Note: Due to increased risk of QTc prolongation, IV administration of dolasetron for CINV is contraindicated; however, the parenteral formulation may be administered orally to patients who cannot swallow tablets or in whom the tablet strength is an inappropriate dose.

Children ≥2 years and Adolescents ≤16 years: Oral (tablet or using the parenteral formulation): 1.8 mg/kg as a single dose within 1 hour before chemotherapy; maximum dose: 100 mg/dose

Adolescents >16 years: Oral: 100 mg as a single dose within 1 hour before chemotherapy

Postoperative nausea and vomiting: Note: If the prophylaxis dolasetron dose has failed, a repeat dose should not be administered as rescue or treatment.

Prevention:
Oral (using parenteral formulation administered orally): Children and Adolescents 2-16 years: 1.2 mg/kg administered within 2 hours before surgery; maximum dose: 100 mg
IV:
Children ≥2 years and Adolescents ≤16 years: 0.35 mg/kg administered ~15 minutes before cessation of anesthesia; maximum dose: 12.5 mg/dose
Adolescents >16 years: 12.5 mg administered ~15 minutes before cessation of anesthesia (do not exceed the recommended dose)
Treatment: IV:
Children ≥2 years and Adolescents ≤16 years: 0.35 mg/kg as soon as nausea or vomiting present; maximum dose: 12.5 mg/dose
Adolescents >16 years: 12.5 mg as soon as nausea or vomiting present (do not exceed the recommended dose)

Adult:
Chemotherapy-induced nausea and vomiting, prevention (including initial and repeat courses): Oral: 100 mg within 1 hour before chemotherapy
Postoperative nausea and vomiting:
Prevention: IV: 12.5 mg ~15 minutes before cessation of anesthesia (do not exceed the recommended dose)
Treatment: IV: 12.5 mg as soon as nausea or vomiting present (do not exceed the recommended dose)

Dosing adjustment in renal impairment: Children ≥2 years, Adolescents, and Adults: No dosage adjustment necessary; however, ECG monitoring is recommended in patients with renal impairment.

Dosing adjustment in hepatic impairment: Children ≥2 years, Adolescents, and Adults: No dosage adjustment necessary.

Preparation for Administration
Oral: Oral administration of parenteral solution: Dilute in apple or apple-grape juice; dilution is stable for 2 hours at room temperature (Anzemet prescribing information 2014).
Parenteral: IV: Solution for IV infusion: May dilute in up to 50 mL of a compatible solution (ie, NS, D_5W, $D_5{}^1/_2NS$, D_5LR, LR, and 10% mannitol injection); usual concentration range: 0.25 to 2 mg/mL (Phelps 2013)

Administration
Oral: May be administered with or without food; parenteral solution may be administered orally
Parenteral: IV:
IV push: May administer undiluted (20 mg/mL) over 30 seconds
IV infusion: Infuse over ≤15 minutes; flush line before and after dolasetron administration

Monitoring Parameters ECG (in patients with cardiovascular disease, elderly, renally impaired, those at risk of developing hypokalemia and/or hypomagnesemia); serum potassium and magnesium

Dosage Forms Excipient information presented when available (limited, particularly for generics); consult specific product labeling.
Solution, Intravenous, as mesylate:
Anzemet: 20 mg/mL (0.625 mL, 5 mL, 25 mL)
Tablet, Oral, as mesylate:
Anzemet: 50 mg, 100 mg

Extemporaneous Preparations Dolasetron injection may be diluted in apple or apple-grape juice and taken orally; this dilution is stable for 2 hours at room temperature (Anzemet prescribing information, 2013).

A 10 mg/mL oral suspension may be prepared with tablets and either a 1:1 mixture of Ora-Plus and Ora-Sweet SF or a 1:1 mixture of strawberry syrup and Ora-Plus. Crush twelve 50 mg tablets in a mortar and reduce to a fine powder. Slowly add chosen vehicle to **almost** 60 mL; transfer to a calibrated bottle, rinse mortar with vehicle, and add quantity of vehicle sufficient to make 60 mL. Label "shake well" and "refrigerate". Stable for 90 days refrigerated.

Anzemet® prescribing information, sanofi-aventis U.S. LLC, Bridgewater, NJ, 2013.
Johnson CE, Wagner DS, and Bussard WE, "Stability of Dolasetron in Two Oral Liquid Vehicles," *Am J Health Syst Pharm*, 2003, 60 (21):2242-4.

◆ **Dolasetron Mesylate** *see* Dolasetron *on page* 699
◆ **Dolophine** *see* Methadone *on page* 1379
◆ **Doloral (Can)** *see* Morphine (Systemic) *on page* 1461

Dolutegravir (doe loo TEG ra vir)

Medication Safety Issues
High alert medication:
This medication is in a class the Institute for Safe Medication Practices (ISMP) includes among its list of drug classes that have a heightened risk of causing significant patient harm when used in error.

Related Information
Adult and Adolescent HIV *on page* 2392
Pediatric HIV *on page* 2380
Perinatal HIV *on page* 2400

Brand Names: US Tivicay
Brand Names: Canada Tivicay
Therapeutic Category Antiretroviral, Integrase Inhibitor (Anti-HIV); Antiviral Agent; HIV Agents (Anti-HIV Agents); Integrase Inhibitor
Generic Availability (US) No
Use Treatment of HIV-1 infection in combination with other antiretroviral agents (FDA approved in ages ≥12 years weighing ≥40 kg and adults). **Note:** HIV regimens consisting of **three** antiretroviral agents are strongly recommended.
Medication Guide Available Yes
Pregnancy Risk Factor B/C (manufacturer specific)
Pregnancy Considerations Adverse events were observed in some animal reproduction studies. It is not known if dolutegravir crosses the placenta. The DHHS Perinatal HIV Guidelines note there are insufficient data to recommend use in pregnancy.

Regardless of CD4 count or HIV RNA copy number, all HIV-infected pregnant women should receive a combination antiretroviral (ARV) drug regimen. A combination of antepartum, intrapartum, and infant ARV prophylaxis is recommended. ARV therapy should be started as soon as possible in women with symptomatic infection. Although earlier initiation may be more effective in reducing the perinatal transmission of HIV, initiation may be delayed until after 12 weeks gestation in women who do not require immediate treatment after careful consideration of maternal conditions (eg, nausea and vomiting) and the potential risks of first trimester fetal exposure for specific agents. A scheduled cesarean delivery at 38 weeks gestation is recommended for all women with HIV RNA >1000 copies/mL or unknown concentrations near delivery in order to decrease transmission. If ARV therapy must be interrupted for <24 hours during the peripartum period, stop then restart all medications simultaneously in order to decrease the chance of developing resistance. Long-term follow-up is recommended for all infants exposed to ARV medications. In couples who want to conceive, the HIV-infected partner should attain maximum viral suppression prior to conception.

Health care providers are encouraged to enroll pregnant women exposed to antiretroviral medications in the Antiretroviral Pregnancy Registry (1-800-258-4263 or www.APRegistry.com). Health care providers caring for HIV-infected women and their infants may contact the National Perinatal HIV Hotline (888-448-8765) for clinical consultation (DHHS [perinatal], 2014).

Breast-Feeding Considerations It is not known if dolutegravir is excreted into breast milk. Maternal or infant antiretroviral therapy does not completely eliminate the risk of postnatal HIV transmission. In addition, multiclass-resistant virus has been detected in breast-feeding infants despite maternal therapy. Therefore, in the United States, where formula is accessible, affordable, safe, and sustainable, and the risk of infant mortality due to diarrhea and respiratory infections is low, complete avoidance of breast-feeding by HIV-infected women is recommended to decrease potential transmission of HIV (DHHS [perinatal], 2014). The manufacturer notes that women should be instructed not to breast-feed their infants while on dolutegravir therapy.

Contraindications Hypersensitivity to dolutegravir or any component of the formulation; concurrent use with dofetilide

Warnings/Precautions Hypersensitivity reactions such as rash, constitutional findings, and organ dysfunction (eg, liver injury) have been reported. Discontinue immediately if signs of hypersensitivity occur. Monitor clinical status and liver function tests, and initiate supportive therapy as appropriate. If hypersensitivity occurs, do not reinitiate therapy with dolutegravir. May cause redistribution of fat (eg, buffalo hump, peripheral wasting with increased abdominal girth, cushingoid appearance). Patients may develop immune reconstitution syndrome resulting in the occurrence of an inflammatory response to an indolent or residual opportunistic infection during initial HIV treatment or activation of autoimmune disorders (eg, Graves' disease, polymyositis, Guillain-Barré syndrome) later in therapy; further evaluation and treatment may be required. Patients with underlying hepatic disease (such as hepatitis B or C coinfection) may be at increased risk of development or worsening of transaminase elevations; use with caution. Elevation in transaminases may be concurrent with development of immune reconstitution syndrome or hepatitis B reactivation (especially if antihepatitis therapy has been discontinued). Monitor transaminases at baseline and during therapy. Potentially significant drug-drug interactions may exist, requiring dose or frequency adjustment, additional monitoring, and/or selection of alternative therapy.

Adverse Reactions Adverse reactions reported with combination therapy.

Central nervous system: Depression, fatigue, headache, insomnia, suicidal ideation, suicidal tendencies

Dermatologic: Pruritus

Endocrine & metabolic: Hyperglycemia

Gastrointestinal: Abdominal distress, abdominal pain, diarrhea, flatulence, increased serum lipase, nausea, upper abdominal pain, vomiting

Hepatic: Hepatitis, hyperbilirubinemia, increased serum ALT (includes patients with hepatitis B and/or C infections), increased serum AST

Hematologic & oncologic: Leukopenia, neutropenia

Hypersensitivity: Hypersensitivity reaction

Neuromuscular & skeletal: Increased creatine phosphokinase, myositis

Renal: Renal insufficiency

Drug Interactions

Metabolism/Transport Effects Substrate of BCRP, CYP3A4 (minor), P-glycoprotein, UGT1A1, UGT1A3, UGT1A9; **Note:** Assignment of Major/Minor substrate status based on clinically relevant drug interaction potential; **Inhibits** OCT2

Avoid Concomitant Use

Avoid concomitant use of Dolutegravir with any of the following: CarBAMazepine; Dofetilide; Fosphenytoin-Phenytoin; Nevirapine; OXcarbazepine; PHENobarbital; Primidone; St Johns Wort

Increased Effect/Toxicity

Dolutegravir may increase the levels/effects of: Dofetilide; MetFORMIN

Decreased Effect

The levels/effects of Dolutegravir may be decreased by: Aluminum Hydroxide; Calcium Salts; CarBAMazepine; Efavirenz; Etravirine; Fosamprenavir; Fosphenytoin-Phenytoin; Iron Salts; Magnesium Salts; Multivitamins/Minerals (with ADEK, Folate, Iron); Multivitamins/Minerals (with AE, No Iron); Nevirapine; OXcarbazepine; PHENobarbital; Primidone; Rifampin; Selenium; St Johns Wort; Sucralfate; Tipranavir; Zinc Salts

Storage/Stability Store at 25°C (77°F); excursions permitted 15°C to 30°C (59°F to 86°F).

Mechanism of Action Binds to the integrase active site and inhibits the strand transfer step of HIV-1 DNA integration necessary for the HIV replication cycle.

Pharmacokinetics (Adult data unless noted) Note: The pharmacokinetics of dolutegravir in HIV-1-infected pediatric patients aged 12 to <18 years were similar to those observed in HIV-1-infected adults.

Absorption: Food increased the extent of absorption and slowed the rate of absorption of dolutegravir. Low-, moderate-, and high-fat meals increased dolutegravir AUC by 33%, 41%, and 66%, respectively; increased C_{max} by 46%, 52%, and 67%, respectively; and prolonged T_{max} to 3, 4, and 5 hours from 2 hours under fasted conditions, respectively.

Distribution: V_d/F = ~17.4 L

Protein binding: ≥98.9%

Metabolism: Primarily metabolized via UGT1A1 with some contribution from CYP3A

Bioavailability: Has not been established

Half-life elimination: ~14 hours

Time to peak serum concentration: 2 to 3 hours

Elimination: Feces (53% as unchanged drug); urine (~31% as metabolites, <1% as unchanged drug)

Dosing: Usual

Pediatric: **HIV infection, treatment:** Children ≥12 years and Adolescents weighing ≥40 kg: Oral: **Note:** Use in combination with other antiretroviral agents.

Treatment-naive or treatment-experienced integrase strand transfer inhibitor (INSTI)-naive: 50 mg once daily

Treatment-naive or treatment-experienced INSTI-naive when coadministered ***with efavirenz, fosamprenavir/ritonavir, tipranavir/ritonavir or rifampin:*** 50 mg twice daily

Adult: **HIV treatment:** Oral: **Note:** Use in combination with other antiretroviral agents.

Treatment-naive or treatment-experienced integrase strand transfer inhibitor (INSTI)-naive: 50 mg once daily

Treatment-naive or treatment-experienced INSTI-naive when coadministered ***with efavirenz, fosamprenavir/ritonavir, tipranavir/ritonavir, or rifampin:*** 50 mg twice daily

INSTI-experienced ***with certain INSTI-associated resistance substitutions or clinically suspected INSTI resistance*** (**Note:** Consult prescribing information for details): 50 mg twice daily

Dosing adjustment in renal impairment:

Treatment-naive or treatment-experienced INSTI-naive: Children ≥12 years, Adolescents, and Adults: Mild, moderate, or severe impairment: No dosage adjustment required.

INSTI-experienced ***with certain INSTI-associated resistance substitutions or clinically suspected INSTI resistance:*** Adults:

CrCl ≥30 mL/minute: No dosage adjustment necessary.

CrCl <30 mL/minute: Use with caution since the reduction in dolutegravir concentrations may result in loss of therapeutic effect and development of resistance to dolutegravir or other coadministered antiretroviral agents.

ESRD including hemodialysis: Has not been studied.

Dosing adjustment in hepatic impairment: Children ≥12 years, Adolescents, and Adults:

Mild to moderate impairment (Child-Pugh class A or B): No dosage adjustment necessary.

Severe impairment (Child-Pugh class C): Not recommended (has not been studied).

Administration Oral: May be administered without regard to meals. Take 2 hours before or 6 hours after cation-containing antacids or laxatives, sucralfate, oral supplements containing iron or calcium, or buffered medications. Alternatively, dolutegravir and supplements containing calcium or iron can be taken together with food.

Monitoring Parameters Note: Monitor CD4 percentage (if <5 years of age) or CD4 count (if ≥5 years of age) at least every 3 to 4 months (DHHS [pediatric], 2014).

Prior to initiation of therapy: Genotypic resistance testing, CD4 and viral load (every 3 to 4 months), CBC with differential, LFTs, BUN, creatinine, electrolytes, glucose, urinalysis (every 6 to 12 months), and assessment of readiness for adherence with mediation regimen. At initiation and with any change in treatment regimen: CBC with differential, electrolytes, calcium, phosphate, glucose, LFTs, bilirubin, urinalysis (at initiation), BUN, creatinine, albumin, total protein, lipid panel (at initiation), CD4, and viral load. After 1 to 2 weeks of therapy: Signs of medication toxicity and adherence. After 2 to 4 weeks of therapy: CBC with differential, viral load, signs of medication toxicity, and adherence; then every 3 to 4 months: CBC with differential, electrolytes, glucose, LFTs, bilirubin, BUN, creatinine, CD4, viral load, signs of medication toxicity, and adherence. Every 6 to 12 months: Lipid panel and urinalysis. CD4 monitoring frequency may be decreased to every 6 to 12 months in children who are adherent to therapy if the value is well above the threshold for opportunistic infections, viral suppression is sustained, and the clinical status is stable for more than 2 to 3 years (DHHS [pediatric], 2014). Monitor for growth and development, signs of HIV-specific physical conditions, HIV disease progression, opportunistic infections and hypersensitivity.

Additional Information In clinical trials, poor virologic response was observed in patients with an INSTI-resistance Q148 substitution (Q148H/R) plus ≥2 additional INSTI-resistance substitutions including L741/M, E138A/D/K/T, G140A/S, Y143H/R, E157Q, G163E/K/Q/R/S, or G193E/R treated with dolutegravir 50 mg twice daily.

Dosage Forms Excipient information presented when available (limited, particularly for generics); consult specific product labeling.

Tablet, Oral:

Tivicay: 50 mg

- ◆ **Dolutegravir Sodium** *see* Dolutegravir *on page 701*
- ◆ **Dom-Amantadine (Can)** *see* Amantadine *on page 112*
- ◆ **Dom-Amiodarone (Can)** *see* Amiodarone *on page 125*
- ◆ **Dom-Amlodipine (Can)** *see* AmLODIPine *on page 133*
- ◆ **Dom-Anagrelide (Can)** *see* Anagrelide *on page 163*
- ◆ **Dom-Atenolol (Can)** *see* Atenolol *on page 215*
- ◆ **DOM-Atomoxetine (Can)** *see* AtoMOXetine *on page 217*
- ◆ **Dom-Atorvastatin (Can)** *see* AtorvaSTATin *on page 220*
- ◆ **Dom-Azithromycin (Can)** *see* Azithromycin (Systemic) *on page 242*
- ◆ **Dom-Baclofen (Can)** *see* Baclofen *on page 254*
- ◆ **Dom-Bromocriptine (Can)** *see* Bromocriptine *on page 303*
- ◆ **Dom-Buspirone (Can)** *see* BusPIRone *on page 328*
- ◆ **DOM-Candesartan (Can)** *see* Candesartan *on page 358*
- ◆ **Dom-Captopril (Can)** *see* Captopril *on page 364*
- ◆ **Dom-Carbamazepine (Can)** *see* CarBAMazepine *on page 367*
- ◆ **Dom-Carvedilol (Can)** *see* Carvedilol *on page 380*
- ◆ **Dom-Cephalexin (Can)** *see* Cephalexin *on page 422*
- ◆ **Dom-Cimetidine (Can)** *see* Cimetidine *on page 461*
- ◆ **Dom-Ciprofloxacin (Can)** *see* Ciprofloxacin (Systemic) *on page 463*
- ◆ **Dom-Citalopram (Can)** *see* Citalopram *on page 476*
- ◆ **Dom-Clarithromycin (Can)** *see* Clarithromycin *on page 482*
- ◆ **Dom-Clobazam (Can)** *see* CloBAZam *on page 495*
- ◆ **Dom-Clomipramine (Can)** *see* ClomiPRAMINE *on page 502*
- ◆ **Dom-Clonazepam (Can)** *see* ClonazePAM *on page 506*
- ◆ **Dom-Clonazepam-R (Can)** *see* ClonazePAM *on page 506*
- ◆ **Dom-Clonidine (Can)** *see* CloNIDine *on page 508*
- ◆ **Dom-Clopidogrel (Can)** *see* Clopidogrel *on page 513*
- ◆ **Dom-Cyclobenzaprine (Can)** *see* Cyclobenzaprine *on page 548*
- ◆ **Dom-Desipramine (Can)** *see* Desipramine *on page 602*
- ◆ **Dom-Dexamethasone (Can)** *see* Dexamethasone (Systemic) *on page 610*
- ◆ **Dom-Diclofenac (Can)** *see* Diclofenac (Systemic) *on page 641*
- ◆ **Dom-Diclofenac SR (Can)** *see* Diclofenac (Systemic) *on page 641*
- ◆ **Dom-Divalproex (Can)** *see* Valproic Acid and Derivatives *on page 2143*
- ◆ **Dom-Docusate Sodium [OTC] (Can)** *see* Docusate *on page 697*
- ◆ **Dom-Doxazosin (Can)** *see* Doxazosin *on page 709*
- ◆ **Dom-Doxycycline (Can)** *see* Doxycycline *on page 717*
- ◆ **Domeboro [OTC]** *see* Aluminum Acetate *on page 110*
- ◆ **Dom-Fluconazole (Can)** *see* Fluconazole *on page 881*
- ◆ **Dom-Fluoxetine (Can)** *see* FLUoxetine *on page 906*
- ◆ **Dom-Fluvoxamine (Can)** *see* FluvoxaMINE *on page 928*
- ◆ **Dom-Furosemide (Can)** *see* Furosemide *on page 951*
- ◆ **Dom-Gabapentin (Can)** *see* Gabapentin *on page 954*
- ◆ **Dom-Glyburide (Can)** *see* GlyBURIDE *on page 975*
- ◆ **Dom-Irbesartan (Can)** *see* Irbesartan *on page 1158*
- ◆ **Dom-Isoniazid (Can)** *see* Isoniazid *on page 1168*
- ◆ **Dom-Levetiracetam (Can)** *see* LevETIRAcetam *on page 1234*
- ◆ **Dom-Lisinopril (Can)** *see* Lisinopril *on page 1280*
- ◆ **Dom-Loperamide (Can)** *see* Loperamide *on page 1288*
- ◆ **Dom-Lorazepam (Can)** *see* LORazepam *on page 1299*
- ◆ **Dom-Lovastatin (Can)** *see* Lovastatin *on page 1305*
- ◆ **Dom-Medroxyprogesterone (Can)** *see* MedroxyPROGESTERone *on page 1339*
- ◆ **Dom-Meloxicam (Can)** *see* Meloxicam *on page 1346*
- ◆ **Dom-Metformin (Can)** *see* MetFORMIN *on page 1375*
- ◆ **Dom-Methimazole (Can)** *see* Methimazole *on page 1386*
- ◆ **Dom-Metoprolol-L (Can)** *see* Metoprolol *on page 1418*

DOPamine (DOE pa meen)

Medication Safety Issues

Sound-alike/look-alike issues:

DOPamine may be confused with DOBUTamine, Dopram

High alert medication:

The Institute for Safe Medication Practices (ISMP) includes this medication among its list of drugs which have a heightened risk of causing significant patient harm when used in error.

Related Information

Adult ACLS Algorithms *on page 2236*

Emergency Drip Calculations *on page 2229*

Management of Drug Extravasations *on page 2298*

Therapeutic Category Adrenergic Agonist Agent; Sympathomimetic

Generic Availability (US) Yes

Use Increase cardiac output, blood pressure, and urine flow as an adjunct in the treatment of shock or hypotension which persists after adequate fluid volume replacement; in low dosage to increase renal perfusion

Pregnancy Risk Factor C

Pregnancy Considerations Adverse events have been observed in some animal reproduction studies. It is not known if dopamine crosses the placenta.

Breast-Feeding Considerations It is not known if dopamine is excreted in breast milk. The manufacturer recommends that caution be exercised when administering dopamine to nursing women.

Contraindications Hypersensitivity to sulfites (commercial preparation contains sodium bisulfite); pheochromocytoma; ventricular fibrillation

Warnings/Precautions Use with caution in patients with cardiovascular disease or cardiac arrhythmias or patients with occlusive vascular disease. Correct hypovolemia and electrolytes when used in hemodynamic support. May cause increases in HR increasing the risk of tachycardia and other tachyarrhythmia. Use with caution in patients with recent myocardial infarction; may increase myocardial oxygen consumption. Use has been associated with a higher incidence of adverse events (eg, tachyarrhythmias) in adult patients with shock compared to norepinephrine. Higher 28-day mortality was also seen in patients with septic shock; the use of norepinephrine in patients with shock may be preferred. The 2012 Surviving Sepsis Campaign (SSC) guidelines suggest dopamine use as an alternative to norepinephrine only in patients with low risk of tachyarrhythmias and absolute or relative bradycardia (SCCM [Dellinger, 2013]). Use with extreme caution in patients taking MAO inhibitors.

Vesicant; ensure proper needle or catheter placement prior to and during infusion. Avoid extravasation; infuse into a large vein if possible. Avoid infusion into leg veins. Watch IV site closely. **[U.S. Boxed Warning]: If extravasation occurs, infiltrate the area with diluted phentolamine (5 to 10 mg in 10 to 15 mL of saline) with a fine hypodermic needle. Phentolamine should be administered as soon as possible after extravasation is noted to prevent sloughing/necrosis.** Product may contain sodium metabisulfite.

Adverse Reactions

Cardiovascular: Angina pectoris, atrial fibrillation, bradycardia, ectopic beats, hypertension, hypotension, palpitations, tachycardia, vasoconstriction, ventricular arrhythmia, ventricular conduction, widened QRS complex on ECG

Central nervous system: Anxiety, headache

Dermatologic: Gangrene (high dose), piloerection

Endocrine & metabolic: Increased serum glucose (usually not above normal limits)

Gastrointestinal: Nausea, vomiting

Genitourinary: Azotemia

Ophthalmic: Increased intraocular pressure, mydriasis

Renal: Polyuria

Respiratory: Dyspnea

Miscellaneous: Tissue necrosis

Drug Interactions

Metabolism/Transport Effects Substrate of COMT, OCT2

Avoid Concomitant Use
Avoid concomitant use of DOPamine with any of the following: Ergot Derivatives; Inhalational Anesthetics; Iobenguane I 123; Lurasidone

Increased Effect/Toxicity
DOPamine may increase the levels/effects of: Lurasidone; Sympathomimetics

The levels/effects of DOPamine may be increased by: AtoMOXetine; Beta-Blockers; BuPROPion; Cannabinoid-Containing Products; COMT Inhibitors; Ergot Derivatives; Hyaluronidase; Inhalational Anesthetics; Linezolid; Serotonin/Norepinephrine Reuptake Inhibitors; Tedizolid; Tricyclic Antidepressants

Decreased Effect
DOPamine may decrease the levels/effects of: Benzylpenicilloyl Polylysine; Iobenguane I 123

The levels/effects of DOPamine may be decreased by: Alpha1-Blockers; Spironolactone

Storage/Stability Protect from light. Solutions that are darker than slightly yellow should not be used.

Mechanism of Action Stimulates both adrenergic and dopaminergic receptors, lower doses are mainly dopaminergic stimulating and produce renal and mesenteric vasodilation, higher doses also are both dopaminergic and beta$_1$-adrenergic stimulating and produce cardiac stimulation and renal vasodilation; large doses stimulate alpha-adrenergic receptors

Pharmacodynamics
Onset of action: Adults: 5 minutes
Duration: Due to its short duration of action (<10 minutes) a continuous infusion must be used

Pharmacokinetics (Adult data unless noted)
Metabolism: In plasma, kidneys, and liver; 75% to inactive metabolites by monoamine oxidase and catechol-o-methyltransferase and 25% to norepinephrine (active)
Half-life: 2 minutes
Clearance: Neonatal clearance varies and appears to be age related. Clearance is more prolonged with combined hepatic and renal dysfunction. Dopamine has exhibited nonlinear kinetics in children; dose changes in children may not achieve steady-state for approximately 1 hour rather than 20 minutes seen in adults.

Dosing: Neonatal Continuous IV infusion: 1-20 mcg/kg/minute; titrate to desired response
The hemodynamic effects of dopamine are dose-dependent:
Low dosage: 1-5 mcg/kg/minute, increased renal blood flow and urine output
Intermediate dosage: 5-15 mcg/kg/minute, increased renal blood flow, heart rate, cardiac contractility, cardiac output, and blood pressure
High dosage: >15 mcg/kg/minute, alpha-adrenergic effects begin to predominate, vasoconstriction, increased blood pressure

Dosing: Usual Continuous IV infusion:
The hemodynamic effects of dopamine are dose-dependent:
Low dosage: 1-5 mcg/kg/minute, increased renal blood flow and urine output
Intermediate dosage: 5-15 mcg/kg/minute, increased renal blood flow, heart rate, cardiac contractility, cardiac output, and blood pressure
High dosage: >15 mcg/kg/minute, alpha-adrenergic effects begin to predominate, vasoconstriction, increased blood pressure
Infants and Children: 1-20 mcg/kg/minute, maximum dose: 50 mcg/kg/minute continuous infusion, titrate to desired response
Adults: 1 mcg/kg/minute up to 50 mcg/kg/minute, titrate to desired response
If dosages >20-30 mcg/kg/minute are needed, a more direct-acting pressor may be beneficial (ie, epinephrine, norepinephrine)

Usual Infusion Concentrations: Neonatal Note: Premixed solutions available.
IV infusion: 1600 **mcg**/mL **or** 3200 **mcg**/mL

Usual Infusion Concentrations: Pediatric Note: Premixed solutions available.
IV infusion: 1600 **mcg**/mL **or** 3200 **mcg**/mL

Preparation for Administration Parenteral: Vials (concentrated solution) must be diluted prior to administration; maximum concentration: 3,200 mcg/mL (3.2 mg/mL); concentrations as high as 6,000 mcg/mL have been infused into large veins, safely and with efficacy, in cases of extreme fluid restriction (Murray 2014). ISMP and Vermont Oxford Network recommend a standard concentration of 1,600 mcg/mL (1.6 mg/mL) for neonates (ISMP 2011).

Administration Parenteral: Administer as a continuous IV infusion with the use of an infusion pump. Administer into large vein to prevent the possibility of extravasation (central-line administration); administration into an umbilical arterial catheter is not recommended. Monitor continuously for free flow; use infusion device to control rate of flow; when discontinuing the infusion, gradually decrease the dose of dopamine (sudden discontinuation may cause hypotension).
Rate of infusion (mL/hour) = dose (mcg/kg/minute) x weight (kg) x 60 minutes/hour divided by concentration (mcg/mL)
Vesicant; ensure proper needle or catheter placement prior to and during infusion; avoid extravasation. If extravasation occurs, stop infusion immediately and disconnect (leave cannula/needle in place); gently aspirate extravasated solution (do **NOT** flush the line); remove needle/cannula; elevate extremity. Initiate phentolamine (or alternative) antidote (see Management of Drug Extravasations for more details). Apply dry warm compresses (Hurst 2004).

Vesicant/Extravasation Risk Vesicant

Monitoring Parameters ECG, heart rate, CVP, MAP, urine output; if pulmonary artery catheter is in place, monitor CI, PWCP, SVR, RAP, and PVR

Dosage Forms Excipient information presented when available (limited, particularly for generics); consult specific product labeling.
Solution, Intravenous, as hydrochloride:
Generic: 0.8 mg/mL (250 mL, 500 mL); 1.6 mg/mL (250 mL, 500 mL); 3.2 mg/mL (250 mL); 40 mg/mL (5 mL, 10 mL); 80 mg/mL (5 mL); 160 mg/mL (5 mL)

◆ **Dopamine Hydrochloride** *see* DOPamine *on page 704*
◆ **Dopram** *see* Doxapram *on page 707*

Dornase Alfa (DOOR nase AL fa)

Brand Names: US Pulmozyme
Brand Names: Canada Pulmozyme
Therapeutic Category Enzyme, Inhalant; Mucolytic Agent
Generic Availability (US) No
Use Management of cystic fibrosis patients to reduce the frequency of respiratory infections that require parenteral antibiotics in patients with FVC ≥40% of predicted; in conjunction with standard therapies to improve pulmonary function (FDA approved in ages ≥5 years and adults)
Pregnancy Considerations Adverse events have not been observed in animal reproduction studies.
Breast-Feeding Considerations Measurable amounts would not be expected in breast milk following inhalation; however, it is not known if dornase alfa is excreted in human milk. According to the manufacturer, the decision to breastfeed during therapy should take into account the

risk of exposure to the infant and the benefits of treatment to the mother.

Contraindications Hypersensitivity to dornase alfa, Chinese hamster ovary cell products, or any component of the formulation

Warnings/Precautions In patients with pulmonary function <40% of normal, dornase alfa does not significantly reduce the risk of respiratory infections that require parenteral antibiotics. Safety studies included children ≥3 months, however experience is limited in children <5 years of age

Warnings: Additional Pediatric Considerations Use with caution in infants and children <5 years of age; safety studies included infants down to 3 months; limit use to those infants and children <5 years to those with potential for benefit in pulmonary function or in risk of respiratory tract infection. Some adverse effects were reported more frequently in infants and children <5 years of age than older children (5 to 10 years of age) including: Cough (45% vs 30%) and rhinitis (35% vs 27%).

Adverse Reactions Adverse events were similar in children using the PARI BABY™ nebulizer (facemask as opposed to mouthpiece) with the addition of cough.

Cardiovascular: Chest pain

Central nervous system: Fever

Dermatologic: Rash

Gastrointestinal: Dyspepsia

Ocular: Conjunctivitis

Respiratory: Dyspnea, FVC decrease ≥10% of predicted, laryngitis, pharyngitis, rhinitis

Miscellaneous: Dornase alfa serum antibodies, voice alteration

Rare but important or life-threatening: Headache, urticaria

Drug Interactions

Metabolism/Transport Effects None known.

Avoid Concomitant Use There are no known interactions where it is recommended to avoid concomitant use.

Increased Effect/Toxicity There are no known significant interactions involving an increase in effect.

Decreased Effect There are no known significant interactions involving a decrease in effect.

Storage/Stability Store at 2°C to 8°C (36°F to 46°F) in protective foil to protect from light. Refrigerate during transport and do not expose to room temperatures for ≥24 hours.

Mechanism of Action The hallmark of cystic fibrosis lung disease is the presence of abundant, purulent airway secretions composed primarily of highly polymerized DNA. The principal source of this DNA is the nuclei of degenerating neutrophils, which is present in large concentrations in infected lung secretions. The presence of this DNA produces a viscous mucous that may contribute to the decreased mucociliary transport and persistent infections that are commonly seen in this population. Dornase alfa is a deoxyribonuclease (DNA) enzyme produced by recombinant gene technology. Dornase selectively cleaves DNA, thus reducing mucous viscosity and as a result, airflow in the lung is improved and the risk of bacterial infection may be decreased.

Pharmacodynamics Onset of improved pulmonary function tests (PFTs): 3-8 days; PFTs will return to baseline 2-3 weeks after discontinuation of therapy

Pharmacokinetics (Adult data unless noted) Following nebulization, enzyme levels are measurable in the sputum within 15 minutes and decline rapidly thereafter

Dosing: Usual

Infants and Children ≤5 years: Not approved for use, however studies using this therapy in small numbers of children as young as 3 months of age have reported efficacy and similar side effects.

Children >5 years and Adults: Inhalation: 2.5 mg/day through selected nebulizers in conjunction with a Pulmo-Aide®, Pari-Proneb®, Mobilaire™, Porta-Neb®, or Pari Baby™ compressor system

Note: While some patients, especially older than 21 years of age or with forced vital capacity (FVC) >85%, may benefit from twice daily administration, another study (Fuchs, 1994) reported no difference between once or twice daily therapy; in a randomized crossover trial involving 48 children, alternate day treatment was as effective as daily treatment over a 12-week period (Suri, 2001).

Administration Nebulization: Should not be diluted or mixed with any other drugs in the nebulizer, this may inactivate the drug

Dosage Forms Excipient information presented when available (limited, particularly for generics); consult specific product labeling.

Solution, Inhalation:

Pulmozyme: 1 mg/mL (2.5 mL)

◆ **Doryx** *see* Doxycycline *on page 717*

Dorzolamide (dor ZOLE a mide)

Brand Names: US Trusopt

Brand Names: Canada Sandoz-Dorzolamide; Trusopt

Therapeutic Category Carbonic Anhydrase Inhibitor, Ophthalmic

Generic Availability (US) Yes

Use Treatment of elevated intraocular pressure in patients with ocular hypertension or open-angle glaucoma [FDA approved in pediatric patients (age not specified) and adults]

Pregnancy Risk Factor C

Pregnancy Considerations Adverse events have been observed in animal reproduction studies following systemic administration. IOP is usually lower during pregnancy. If topical medications for the treatment of glaucoma in pregnant women cannot be discontinued because small increases in IOP cannot be tolerated, the minimum effective dose should be used in combination with punctual occlusion to decrease exposure to the fetus (Johnson, 2001).

Breast-Feeding Considerations It is not known if dorzolamide is excreted in breast milk. Due to the potential for serious adverse reactions in the nursing infant, the manufacturer recommends a decision be made whether to discontinue nursing or to discontinue the drug, taking into account the importance of treatment to the mother.

Contraindications Hypersensitivity to dorzolamide or any component of the formulation

Warnings/Precautions Dorzolamide is a sulfonamide; although administered ocularly, systemic absorption may occur and could result in hypersensitivity. Discontinue use if signs of hypersensitivity or a serious reaction occur. Local ocular adverse effects (primarily conjunctivitis and lid reactions) were reported with chronic administration; many resolved upon discontinuation of drug therapy. Choroidal detachment has been reported after filtration procedures. Systemic absorption and adverse effects (similar to sulfonamides) including, blood dyscrasias, Stevens-Johnson syndrome, toxic epidermal necrolysis, fulminant hepatic necrosis, agranulocytosis, aplastic anemia, and other blood dyscrasias may occur with ophthalmic use. Use with caution in patients with low endothelial cell counts; may be at increased risk of corneal edema. Use with caution in patients with hepatic impairment (has not been studied). Use is not recommended in patients with severe renal impairment (CrCl <30 mL/minute; has not been studied).

Should be used in combination with therapeutic interventions for the treatment of acute angle-closure glaucoma. Some products contain benzalkonium chloride which may be absorbed by soft contact lenses; remove lens prior to administration and wait 15 minutes before reinserting. Inadvertent contamination of multiple-dose ophthalmic solutions has caused bacterial keratitis. Potentially significant drug-drug interactions may exist, requiring dose or frequency adjustment, additional monitoring, and/or selection of alternative therapy.

Adverse Reactions

Gastrointestinal: Bitter taste following administration

Ocular: Blurred vision; burning, stinging, or discomfort immediately following administration; conjunctivitis; dryness; lid reactions; photophobia; signs and symptoms of ocular allergic reaction; superficial punctate keratitis; redness; tearing

Rare but important or life-threatening: Allergic reaction (systemic), angioedema, bronchospasm, choriodal detachment (following filtration procedures), dyspnea, epistaxis, myopia (transient), ocular pain, paresthesia, pharyngitis, Stevens-Johnson syndrome, throat irritation, toxic epidermal necrolysis

Drug Interactions

Metabolism/Transport Effects Substrate of CYP2C9 (minor), CYP3A4 (minor); **Note:** Assignment of Major/Minor substrate status based on clinically relevant drug interaction potential

Avoid Concomitant Use

Avoid concomitant use of Dorzolamide with any of the following: Carbonic Anhydrase Inhibitors

Increased Effect/Toxicity

Dorzolamide may increase the levels/effects of: Alpha-/Beta-Agonists (Indirect-Acting); Carbonic Anhydrase Inhibitors

Decreased Effect There are no known significant interactions involving a decrease in effect.

Storage/Stability Store at 15°C to 30°C (59°F to 86°F). Protect from light.

Mechanism of Action Reversible inhibition of the enzyme carbonic anhydrase resulting in reduction of hydrogen ion secretion at renal tubule and an increased renal excretion of sodium, potassium, bicarbonate, and water to decrease production of aqueous humor; also inhibits carbonic anhydrase in central nervous system to retard abnormal and excessive discharge from CNS neurons

Pharmacodynamics

Maximum effect: 2 hours

Duration: 8-12 hours

Pharmacokinetics (Adult data unless noted)

Absorption: Topical: Reaches systemic circulation

Distribution: Accumulates in RBCs during chronic administration as a result of binding to CA-II

Protein binding: 33%

Metabolism: Hepatic to active but less potent metabolite, N-desethyl dorzolamide

Half-life: Terminal RBC half-life: 147 days; washes out of RBCs nonlinearly, resulting in rapid decline of drug concentration initially, followed by a slower elimination phase with a half-life of ~4 months

Elimination: Primarily unchanged in the urine

Dosing: Neonatal Reduction of intraocular pressure: GA ≥36 weeks and PNA ≥7 days: Ophthalmic: 1 drop to affected eye(s) 3 times daily (Ott, 2005)

Dosing: Usual

Pediatric: **Reduction of intraocular pressure:** Infants, Children, and Adolescents: Ophthalmic: 1 drop to affected eye(s) 3 times/daily

Adult: **Reduction of intraocular pressure:** Ophthalmic: 1 drop to affected eye(s) 3 times/daily

Dosing adjustment in renal impairment:

CrCl ≥30 mL/minute: There are no dosage adjustments provided in the manufacturer's labeling.

CrCl <30 mL/minute: All patients: Use is not recommended (has not been studied).

Dosing adjustment in hepatic impairment: There are no dosage adjustments provided in the manufacturer's labeling (has not been studied); use with caution.

Administration Ophthalmic: Wash hands before use. Unscrew the cap by turning in the direction of the arrows on top of the cap. Pull lower eyelid down slightly to form a pocket for the eye drop and tilt head back; administer 1 drop. Apply gentle pressure to lacrimal sac immediately following instillation (1 minute) or instruct patient to gently close eyelid after administration to decrease systemic absorption of ophthalmic drops (Urtti, 1993; Zimmerman, 1982). Avoid contact of bottle tip with skin or eye; ocular solutions can become contaminated by common bacteria known to cause ocular infections. Serious damage to the eye and subsequent loss of vision may occur from using contaminated solutions. Some solutions contain benzalkonium chloride; remove contact lenses prior to administration and wait at least 15 minutes after instillation before reinserting soft contact lenses. If more than one topical ophthalmic drug is being used, separate administration by at least 5 minutes.

Monitoring Parameters Periodic ophthalmic exams, intraocular pressure

Dosage Forms Excipient information presented when available (limited, particularly for generics); consult specific product labeling.

Solution, Ophthalmic:

Trusopt: 2% (10 mL)

Generic: 2% (10 mL)

◆ **Dorzolamide Hydrochloride** *see* Dorzolamide *on page* *706*

◆ **D.O.S. [OTC]** *see* Docusate *on page* *697*

◆ **Dosolax [OTC] (Can)** *see* Docusate *on page* *697*

◆ **DOSS** *see* Docusate *on page* *697*

◆ **DoubleDex** *see* Dexamethasone (Systemic) *on page* *610*

◆ **Double Tussin DM [OTC]** *see* Guaifenesin and Dextromethorphan *on page* *992*

Doxapram (DOKS a pram)

Medication Safety Issues

Sound-alike/look-alike issues:

Doxapram may be confused with doxazosin, doxepin, DOXOrubicin

Dopram® may be confused with DOPamine

International issues:

Doxapram may be confused with Doxinate brand name for doxylamine and pyridoxine [Italy]

Brand Names: US Dopram

Therapeutic Category Central Nervous System Stimulant; Respiratory Stimulant

Generic Availability (US) Yes

Use Respiratory and CNS stimulant for treatment of respiratory depression secondary to anesthesia, drug-induced CNS depression, and acute hypercapnia secondary to COPD (FDA approved in ages ≥12 years and adults); has also been used for idiopathic apnea of prematurity refractory to xanthines

Pregnancy Risk Factor B

Pregnancy Considerations Adverse events have not been observed in animal reproduction studies.

Breast-Feeding Considerations It is not known if doxapram is excreted in breast milk. The manufacturer recommends that caution be exercised when administering doxapram to nursing women.

Contraindications Hypersensitivity to doxapram or any component of the formulation; significant cardiovascular impairment (eg, uncompensated heart failure, severe coronary artery disease); severe hypertension (including severe hypertension associated with hyperthyroidism or pheochromocytoma); cerebral edema, cerebral vascular accident, epilepsy, head injury; mechanical disorders of ventilation (eg, mechanical obstruction, muscle paresis, neuromuscular blockade, flail chest, pneumothorax, acute asthma, pulmonary fibrosis); pulmonary embolism

Warnings/Precautions Adequate airway required prior to use; consider airway protection in case of vomiting. Resuscitative equipment (in addition to anticonvulsants and oxygen) should be readily available; doxapram alone may not be sufficient to stimulate spontaneous breathing or provide sufficient arousal. Doxapram is neither an antagonist to skeletal muscle relaxants nor an opioid antagonist. Use with caution in patients with hypermetabolic states (eg, hyperthyroidism, pheochromocytoma). May cause dysrhythmias; monitor for disturbances of cardiac rhythm. If sudden hypotension develops during use, discontinue. Increases in blood pressure are generally modest; use is contraindicated in patients with severe hypertension. May cause severe CNS stimulation, including seizures; anticonvulsants (as well as oxygen and resuscitative equipment) should be available to manage potential excessive CNS stimulation.

Do **not** use in patients on mechanical ventilation. Use with caution in treating pulmonary disease; a pressor effect on pulmonary circulation may result in a fall in arterial pO_2. If sudden dyspnea develops during use, discontinue. Doxapram causes patients to increase the work of breathing; therefore, do not increase the rate of infusion in an attempt to lower the pCO_2 in severely-ill COPD patients. Use with caution in patients with cerebrovascular disease; lowered pCO_2 induced by hyperventilation produces cerebral vasoconstriction and decreased circulation. Use with caution in patients with hepatic or renal impairment. If patient has received anesthesia with a volatile agent known to sensitize the myocardium to catecholamines, avoid use of doxapram until anesthetic has been eliminated to decrease the risk of ventricular tachycardia or ventricular fibrillation. Use caution with coadministration of MAO inhibitors of sympathomimetics; additive pressor effect may occur. Avoid extravasation; doxapram may cause thrombophlebitis or local skin irritation. Hemolysis may result from rapid infusion.

Benzyl alcohol and derivatives: Some dosage forms may contain benzyl alcohol; large amounts of benzyl alcohol (≥99 mg/kg/day) have been associated with a potentially fatal toxicity ("gasping syndrome") in neonates; the "gasping syndrome" consists of metabolic acidosis, respiratory distress, gasping respirations, CNS dysfunction (including convulsions, intracranial hemorrhage), hypotension and cardiovascular collapse (AAP, 1997; CDC, 1982); some data suggests that benzoate displaces bilirubin from protein binding sites (Ahlfors, 2001); avoid or use dosage forms containing benzyl alcohol with caution in neonates. See manufacturer's labeling.

Warnings: Additional Pediatric Considerations Recommended doses of doxapram for treatment of neonatal apnea will deliver 5.4 to 27 mg/kg/day of benzyl alcohol; the use of doxapram should be reserved for neonates who are unresponsive to the treatment of apnea with therapeutic serum concentrations of theophylline or caffeine. Use with caution in premature neonates and infants; hypertension (dose related), irritability, seizures, excessive crying, sleep disturbances, abdominal distention, vomiting, NEC, increased gastric residuals, bloody stools, hyperglycemia, and glycosuria have been reported.

Adverse Reactions

Cardiovascular: Arrhythmia, blood pressure increased, chest pain, chest tightness, flushing, heart rate changes, T waves lowered, ventricular tachycardia, ventricular fibrillation

Central nervous system: Apprehension, Babinski turns positive, disorientation, dizziness, hallucinations, headache, hyperactivity, pyrexia, seizure

Dermatologic: Burning sensation, pruritus

Gastrointestinal: Defecation urge, diarrhea, nausea, vomiting

Genitourinary: Spontaneous voiding, urinary retention

Hematologic: Hematocrit decreased, hemoglobin decreased, hemolysis, red blood cell count decreased

Local: Phlebitis

Neuromuscular & skeletal: Clonus, deep tendon reflexes increase, fasciculations, involuntary muscle movement, muscle spasm, paresthesia

Ocular: Pupillary dilatation

Renal: Albuminuria, BUN increased

Respiratory: Bronchospasm, cough, dyspnea, hiccups, hyperventilation, laryngospasm, rebound hypoventilation, tachypnea

Miscellaneous: Diaphoresis

Rare but important or life-threatening: Emergence agitation, second-degree AV block (premature neonates), QT-interval prolonged (premature neonates)

Drug Interactions

Metabolism/Transport Effects None known.

Avoid Concomitant Use

Avoid concomitant use of Doxapram with any of the following: Iobenguane I 123

Increased Effect/Toxicity

Doxapram may increase the levels/effects of: Sympathomimetics

The levels/effects of Doxapram may be increased by: AtoMOXetine; Cannabinoid-Containing Products; Linezolid; MAO Inhibitors; Tedizolid

Decreased Effect

Doxapram may decrease the levels/effects of: Iobenguane I 123

Storage/Stability Store intact vials at 20°C to 25°C (68°F to 77°F).

Mechanism of Action Stimulates respiration through action on peripheral carotid chemoreceptors; respiratory center in medulla is also directly stimulated as dosage is increased

Pharmacodynamics Following a single IV injection:

Onset of respiratory stimulation: Within 20-40 seconds

Maximum effect: Within 1-2 minutes

Duration: 5-12 minutes

Pharmacokinetics (Adult data unless noted)

Metabolism: Extensive in the liver to active metabolite (keto-doxapram)

Distribution: V_d: Neonates: 4-7.3 L/kg

Half-life:

Neonates, premature: 6.6-12 hours

Adults: Mean: 3.4 hours (range: 2.4-4.1 hours)

Clearance: Neonates, premature: 0.44-0.7 L/hour/kg

Dosing: Neonatal IV: Apnea of prematurity: Initial loading dose: 2.5-3 mg/kg followed by a continuous IV infusion of 1 mg/kg/**hour**; titrate to the lowest rate at which apnea is controlled (maximum dose: 2.5 mg/kg/**hour**); **Note:** Typically considered third-line agent.

Dosing: Usual IV:

Respiratory depression following anesthesia: Adults: Titrate to sustain the desired level of respiratory stimulation with a minimum of side effects:

Initial: 0.5-1 mg/kg; may repeat at 5-minute intervals; maximum total dose: 2 mg/kg

Continuous IV infusion: Initial: 5 mg/minute until adequate response or adverse effects seen; decrease to 1-3 mg/minute; usual total infusion dose: 0.5-4 mg/kg or 300 mg

Drug-induced CNS depression: Adults: Mild to moderate depression: Initial: 1-2 mg/kg; may repeat in 5 minutes; may repeat at 1-2 hour intervals (until sustained consciousness); maximum dose: 3 g/day; if depression recurs, may repeat in 24 hours. As an alternative, after the initial doses, a continuous infusion of 1-3 mg/minute may be used. Discontinue if patient begins to waken; do not infuse for more than 2 hours.

Hypercapnia associated with COPD: Adults: Continuous infusion of 1-2 mg/minute for 2 hours; may increase to 3 mg/minute if needed. Do not infuse for more than 2 hours. Monitor arterial blood gases closely (in a minimum of 30-minute intervals)

Preparation for Administration Parenteral: Dilute in NS **or** dextrose (D_5W or $D_{10}W$) to 1 mg/mL; maximum concentration: 2 mg/mL

Indication-specific preparation for IV infusion: Adults:

Drug-induced CNS depression or postanesthesia: Mix doxapram 250 mg in 250 mL of D_5W, $D_{10}W$, or NS.

COPD-associated hypercapnia: Mix doxapram 400 mg in 180 mL of D_5W, $D_{10}W$, or NS.

Administration Parenteral: IV: Administer as an intermittent bolus over 15 to 30 minutes or as an IV infusion. Avoid rapid infusion. Avoid extravasation; irritating to tissues.

Monitoring Parameters Pulse oximetry, blood pressure, heart rate, arterial blood gases, deep tendon reflexes; for apnea: number, duration, and severity of apneic episodes

Reference Range Initial studies suggest a therapeutic serum level of at least 1.5 mg/L; toxicity becomes frequent at serum levels >5 mg/L

Dosage Forms Excipient information presented when available (limited, particularly for generics); consult specific product labeling.

Solution, Intravenous, as hydrochloride:

Dopram: 20 mg/mL (20 mL) [contains benzyl alcohol]

Generic: 20 mg/mL (20 mL)

◆ **Doxapram Hydrochloride** *see* Doxapram *on page 707*

Doxazosin (doks AY zoe sin)

Medication Safety Issues

Sound-alike/look-alike issues:

Doxazosin may be confused with doxapram, doxepin, DOXOrubicin

Cardura may be confused with Cardene, Cordarone, Cordran, Coumadin, K-Dur, Ridaura

BEERS Criteria medication:

This drug may be potentially inappropriate for use in geriatric patients (Quality of evidence - moderate; Strength of recommendation - strong).

Related Information

Oral Medications That Should Not Be Crushed or Altered *on page 2476*

Brand Names: US Cardura; Cardura XL

Brand Names: Canada Apo-Doxazosin; Cardura-1; Cardura-2; Cardura-4; Dom-Doxazosin; Doxazosin-1; Doxazosin-2; Doxazosin-4; Mylan-Doxazosin; PMS-Doxazosin; Teva-Doxazosin

Therapeutic Category Alpha-Adrenergic Blocking Agent, Oral; Antihypertensive Agent; Vasodilator

Generic Availability (US) May be product dependent

Use

Immediate release tablets: Treatment of hypertension alone or in combination with diuretics, beta-blockers, calcium channel blockers, or ACE inhibitors (FDA approved in adults); treatment of urinary outflow obstruction and/or obstructive and irritative symptoms associated with benign prostatic hyperplasia (BPH) (FDA approved in adults); has also been used for treatment of dysfunctional voiding and primary bladder neck dysfunction

Extended release tablets: Treatment of signs and symptoms of benign prostatic hyperplasia (BPH) (FDA approved in adults)

Pregnancy Risk Factor C

Pregnancy Considerations Adverse events were observed in some animal reproduction studies. Untreated chronic maternal hypertension is associated with adverse events in the fetus, infant, and mother. If treatment for hypertension during pregnancy is needed, other agents are generally preferred (ACOG, 2013).

Breast-Feeding Considerations Doxazosin is excreted into breast milk. Information is available from a single case report following a maternal dose of doxazosin 4 mg every 24 hours for 2 doses. Milk samples were obtained at various intervals over 24 hours, beginning ~17 hours after the first dose. Maternal serum samples were obtained at nearly the same times, beginning ~1 hour later. The highest serum and milk concentrations of doxazosin were observed ~1 hour after the dose. Using the highest milk concentration (4.15 mcg/L), the estimated dose to the nursing infant was calculated to be <1% of the weight-adjusted maternal dose (Jensen, 2013). The manufacturer recommends that caution be used if administered to nursing women.

Contraindications Hypersensitivity to quinazolines (prazosin, terazosin), doxazosin, or any component of the formulation

Warnings/Precautions Can cause significant orthostatic hypotension and syncope, especially with first dose; anticipate a similar effect if therapy is interrupted for a few days, if dosage is rapidly increased, or if another antihypertensive drug (particularly vasodilators) or a PDE-5 inhibitor is introduced. Discontinue if symptoms of angina occur or worsen. Patients should be cautioned about performing hazardous tasks when starting new therapy or adjusting dosage upward. Priapism has been associated with use (rarely). Prostate cancer should be ruled out before starting for BPH. Use with caution in mild-to-moderate hepatic impairment; not recommended in severe dysfunction. Intraoperative floppy iris syndrome has been observed in cataract surgery patients who were on or were previously treated with alpha$_1$-blockers. Causality has not been established and there appears to be no benefit in discontinuing alpha-blocker therapy prior to surgery. In the elderly, avoid use as an antihypertensive due to high risk of orthostatic hypotension; alternative agents preferred due to a more favorable risk/benefit profile (Beers Criteria).

The extended release formulation consists of drug within a nondeformable matrix; following drug release/absorption, the matrix/shell is expelled in the stool. The use of nondeformable products in patients with known stricture/narrowing of the GI tract has been associated with symptoms of obstruction. Use caution in patients with increased GI retention (eg, chronic constipation) as doxazosin exposure may be increased. Extended release formulation is not indicated for use in women or for the treatment of hypertension.

Adverse Reactions

Cardiovascular: Arrhythmia, edema, facial edema, flushing, hypotension, orthostatic hypotension

Central nervous system: Anxiety, ataxia, dizziness, fatigue, headache, hypertonia, insomnia, malaise, movement disorder, pain, somnolence, vertigo

Endocrine & metabolic: Sexual dysfunction

Gastrointestinal: Abdominal pain, dyspepsia, nausea, xerostomia

Genitourinary: Impotence, incontinence, polyuria, urinary tract infection

Neuromuscular & skeletal: Arthritis,muscle cramps, muscle weakness, myalgia

Ocular: Abnormal vision

Otic: Tinnitus

Respiratory: Dyspnea, epistaxis, respiratory disorder, rhinitis

Rare but important or life-threatening: Abnormal lacrimation, abnormal thinking, agitation, allergic reaction, alopecia, amnesia, angina, anorexia, appetite increased, arthralgia, back pain, blurred vision, bradycardia, breast pain, bronchospasm, cerebrovascular accident, chest pain, cholestasis, confusion, cough, depersonalization, diaphoresis increased, diarrhea, dry skin, dysuria, earache, eczema, emotional lability, fecal incontinence, fever, gastroenteritis, gout, gynecomastia, hematuria, hepatitis, hot flashes, hypoesthesia, hypokalemia, impaired concentration, impotence, infection, influenza-like syndrome, intraoperative floppy iris syndrome (cataract surgery), jaundice, leukopenia, liver function tests increased, libido decreased, lymphadenopathy, micturition abnormality, migraine, MI, neutropenia, nocturia, pallor, palpitation, paranoia, paresis, parosmia, peripheral ischemia, pharyngitis, photophobia, priapism, pruritus, purpura, renal calculus, rigors, sinusitis, skin rash, syncope, taste perversion, thirst, thrombocytopenia, tremor, twitching, urticaria, vomiting, weight gain/loss

Drug Interactions

Metabolism/Transport Effects Substrate of CYP2C19 (minor), CYP2D6 (minor), CYP3A4 (major); **Note:** Assignment of Major/Minor substrate status based on clinically relevant drug interaction potential

Avoid Concomitant Use

Avoid concomitant use of Doxazosin with any of the following: Alpha1-Blockers; Boceprevir; Conivaptan; Fusidic Acid (Systemic); Idelalisib

Increased Effect/Toxicity

Doxazosin may increase the levels/effects of: Alpha1-Blockers; Amifostine; Antihypertensives; Calcium Channel Blockers; DULoxetine; Hypotensive Agents; Levodopa; Obinutuzumab; RisperiDONE; RiTUXimab

The levels/effects of Doxazosin may be increased by: Aprepitant; Barbiturates; Beta-Blockers; Boceprevir; Brimonidine (Topical); Conivaptan; CYP3A4 Inhibitors (Moderate); CYP3A4 Inhibitors (Strong); Dapoxetine; Dasatinib; Diazoxide; Fosaprepitant; Fusidic Acid (Systemic); Herbs (Hypotensive Properties); Idelalisib; Ivacaftor; Luliconazole; MAO Inhibitors; Mifepristone; Netupitant; Nicorandil; Palbociclib; Pentoxifylline; Phosphodiesterase 5 Inhibitors; Prostacyclin Analogues; Simeprevir; Stiripentol

Decreased Effect

Doxazosin may decrease the levels/effects of: Alpha-/Beta-Agonists; Alpha1-Agonists

The levels/effects of Doxazosin may be decreased by: Bosentan; CYP3A4 Inducers (Moderate); CYP3A4 Inducers (Strong); Dabrafenib; Deferasirox; Herbs (Hypertensive Properties); Methylphenidate; Mitotane; Siltuximab; St Johns Wort; Tocilizumab; Yohimbine

Storage/Stability Store at 25°C (77°F); excursions permitted between 15°C to 30°C (59°F to 86°F).

Mechanism of Action

Hypertension: Competitively inhibits postsynaptic alpha$_1$-adrenergic receptors which results in vasodilation of veins and arterioles and a decrease in total peripheral resistance and blood pressure; ~50% as potent on a weight by weight basis as prazosin.

BPH: Competitively inhibits postsynaptic alpha$_1$-adrenergic receptors in prostatic stromal and bladder neck tissues. This reduces the sympathetic tone-induced urethral stricture causing BPH symptoms.

Pharmacodynamics

Onset of action: Urinary outflow effects (immediate release): 1-2 weeks

Maximum effect: Antihypertensive effect (immediate release): 2-6 hours

Duration: Antihypertensive effect (immediate release): >24 hours

Pharmacokinetics (Adult data unless noted)

Protein binding: ~98%

Metabolism: Extensively hepatic to active metabolites; primarily via CYP3A4; secondary pathways involve CYP2D6 and 2C19; may undergo enterohepatic recycling

Bioavailability: Immediate release: ~65%; Extended release relative to immediate release: 54% to 59%

Half-life: Immediate release: ~22 hours; Extended release: 15-19 hours; prolonged in patients with hepatic impairment

Time to peak serum concentration: Immediate release: 2-3 hours; Extended release: 8-9 hours

Elimination: Feces (63%, primarily as metabolites); urine (9%, primarily as metabolites; trace amounts as unchanged drug)

Dosing: Usual Note: If drug is discontinued for greater than several days, consider beginning with initial dose and retitrate as needed.

Children and Adolescents:

Dysfunctional voiding: Limited data available, efficacy results variable: Children ≥3 years and Adolescents: Oral: Immediate release: Initial: 0.5 mg once daily at bedtime; some trials maintained a fixed dose; others titrated at weekly or biweekly intervals to effect as tolerated (maximum daily dose: 2 mg/**day**) (Austin, 1999; Cain, 2003; El-Hefnawy, 2012; Yucel, 2005). In some trials, a larger initial dose (1 mg/**day**) was used in patients weighing >40-50 kg (Austin, 1999; Yucel, 2005).

Hypertension: Limited data available: Children and Adolescents: Oral: Immediate release: Initial: 1 mg/**day**; maximum daily dose: 4 mg/**day** (NHBPEP, 2004; NHLBI, 2011)

Adults:

Benign prostatic hypertrophy (BPH): Oral:

Immediate release: 1 mg once daily in morning or evening; may be increased to 2 mg once daily. Thereafter titrate upwards, if needed, over several weeks, balancing therapeutic benefit with doxazosin-induced postural hypotension. Usual range: 4-8 mg/day; maximum dose: 8 mg/day

Reinitiation of therapy: If therapy is discontinued for several days, restart at 1 mg dose and titrate as before

Extended release: 4 mg once daily with breakfast; titrate based on response and tolerability every 3-4 weeks to maximum recommended dose of 8 mg/day

Reinitiation of therapy: If therapy is discontinued for several days, restart at 4 mg dose and titrate as before

Note: Conversion to extended release from immediate release: Omit final evening dose of immediate release prior to starting morning dosing with extended release product; initiate extended release product using 4 mg once daily

Hypertension: Oral: Immediate release: 1 mg once daily in morning or evening; may be increased to 2 mg once daily. Thereafter titrate upwards, if needed, over several weeks, balancing therapeutic benefit with doxazosin-induced postural hypotension. Maximum dose: 16 mg/day

Reinitiation of therapy: If therapy is discontinued for several days, restart at 1 mg dose and titrate as before

Dosing adjustment in hepatic impairment: Adults: Use with caution in mild-to-moderate hepatic dysfunction. Do not use with severe impairment.

Dosing adjustment in renal impairment: There are no dosage adjustments provided in manufacturer's labeling; however, limited data suggest renal impairment does not significantly alter pharmacokinetic parameters.

Administration Oral:

Immediate release: Administer without regard to meals at the same time each day

Extended release (Cardura® XL): Tablets should be swallowed whole; do not crush, chew, or divide. Administer with morning meal.

Monitoring Parameters Standing and sitting/supine blood pressure, especially 2-6 hours after the initial dose, then prior to doses (to ensure adequate control throughout the dosing interval); urinary symptoms if used for dysfunctional voiding or BPH treatment.

Dosage Forms Excipient information presented when available (limited, particularly for generics); consult specific product labeling.

Tablet, Oral:

Cardura: 1 mg, 2 mg, 4 mg, 8 mg [scored]

Generic: 1 mg, 2 mg, 4 mg, 8 mg

Tablet Extended Release 24 Hour, Oral:

Cardura XL: 4 mg, 8 mg

◆ **Doxazosin-1 (Can)** *see* Doxazosin *on page 709*

◆ **Doxazosin-2 (Can)** *see* Doxazosin *on page 709*

◆ **Doxazosin-4 (Can)** *see* Doxazosin *on page 709*

◆ **Doxazosin Mesylate** *see* Doxazosin *on page 709*

Doxepin (Systemic) (DOKS e pin)

Medication Safety Issues

Sound-alike/look-alike issues:

Doxepin may be confused with digoxin, doxapram, doxazosin, Doxidan, doxycycline

SINEquan may be confused with saquinavir, SEROquel, Singulair, Zonegran

BEERS Criteria medication:

This drug may be potentially inappropriate for use in geriatric patients (Quality of evidence - high [moderate for SIADH]; Strength of recommendation - strong).

International issues:

Deptran [Australia] may be confused with Deralin brand name for propranolol [Australia, Israel]

Doxal [Finland] may be confused with Doxil brand name for doxorubicin (liposomal) [US, Israel]

Doxal brand name for doxepin [Finland] but also brand name for pyridoxine/thiamine [Brazil]

Related Information

Antidepressant Agents *on page 2257*

Brand Names: US Silenor

Brand Names: Canada Apo-Doxepin; Novo-Doxepin; Silenor; Sinequan; Zonalon

Therapeutic Category Antianxiety Agent; Antidepressant, Tricyclic (Tertiary Amine)

Generic Availability (US) May be product dependent

Use Treatment of various forms of depression and anxiety disorders associated with psychoneurosis, alcoholism, organic disease, and manic-depressive disorders (FDA approved in ages ≥12 years and adults); treatment of insomnia with difficulty of sleep maintenance (Silanor®: FDA approved in adults)

Medication Guide Available Yes

Pregnancy Risk Factor C

Pregnancy Considerations Adverse events were observed in animal reproduction studies. Tricyclic antidepressants may be associated with irritability, jitteriness, and convulsions (rare) in the neonate (Yonkers 2009).

The ACOG recommends that therapy for depression during pregnancy be individualized; treatment should incorporate the clinical expertise of the mental health clinician, obstetrician, primary healthcare provider, and pediatrician (ACOG 2008). According to the American Psychiatric Association (APA), the risks of medication treatment should be weighed against other treatment options and untreated depression. For women who discontinue antidepressant medications during pregnancy and who may be at high risk for postpartum depression, the medications can be restarted following delivery (APA 2010). Treatment algorithms have been developed by the ACOG and the APA for the management of depression in women prior to conception and during pregnancy (Yonkers 2009).

Breast-Feeding Considerations Doxepin and N-desmethyldoxepin are excreted into breast milk (Frey, 1999; Kemp, 1985). Drowsiness, vomiting, poor feeding, and muscle hypotonia were noted in a nursing infant following maternal use of doxepin. Symptoms began to resolve 24 hours after feedings with breast milk were discontinued (Frey, 1999). In addition, product labeling notes that drowsiness and apnea have been reported in a nursing infant following maternal use of doxepin for depression. The manufacturer recommends that caution be used if administered to a nursing woman.

Contraindications

Hypersensitivity to doxepin, dibenzoxepins, or any component of the formulation; glaucoma; urinary retention; use of MAO inhibitors within 14 days

Documentation of allergenic cross-reactivity for tricyclic antidepressants is limited. However, because of similarities in chemical structure and/or pharmacologic actions, the possibility of cross-sensitivity cannot be ruled out with certainty.

Warnings/Precautions [US Boxed Warning]: Antidepressants increase the risk of suicidal thinking and behavior in children, adolescents, and young adults (18-24 years of age) with major depressive disorder (MDD) and other psychiatric disorders; consider risk prior to prescribing. Short-term studies did not show an increased risk in patients >24 years of age and showed a decreased risk in patients ≥65 years. Closely monitor for clinical worsening, suicidality, or unusual changes in behavior, particularly during the initial 1 to 2 months of therapy or during periods of dosage adjustments (increases or decreases); the patient's family or caregiver should be instructed to closely observe the patient and communicate condition with healthcare provider. A medication guide should be dispensed with each prescription. **Doxepin is not approved for use in pediatric patients.**

The possibility of a suicide attempt is inherent in major depression and may persist until remission occurs. Use caution in high-risk patients. Worsening depression and severe abrupt suicidality that are not part of the presenting symptoms may require discontinuation or modification of drug therapy. The patient's family or caregiver should be alerted to monitor patients for the emergence of suicidality and associated behaviors (such as agitation, irritability, hostility, impulsivity, and hypomania) and call healthcare provider.

Risk of suicidal behavior may be increased regardless of doxepin dose; antidepressant doses of doxepin are 10- to 100-fold higher than doses for insomnia.

May precipitate a shift to mania or hypomania in patients with bipolar disorder. Patients presenting with depressive symptoms should be screened for bipolar disorder. Monotherapy in patients with bipolar disorder should be avoided. **Doxepin is not FDA approved for the treatment of bipolar depression.**

Should only be used for insomnia after evaluation of potential causes of sleep disturbance. Failure of sleep disturbance to resolve after 7 to 10 days may indicate psychiatric or medical illness. An increased risk for hazardous sleep-related activities has been noted; discontinue use with any sleep-related episodes. The risks of sedative and anticholinergic effects are high relative to other antidepressant agents. Anxiety, psychosis, and other neuropsychiatric symptoms may occur unpredictably. May cause

CNS depression, which may impair physical or mental abilities; patients must be cautioned about performing tasks that require mental alertness (eg, operating machinery or driving). Also use caution in patients with benign prostatic hyperplasia, xerostomia, visual problems, constipation, or history of bowel obstruction.

May cause orthostatic hypotension or conduction disturbances (risks are moderate relative to other antidepressants). Use with caution in patients with a history of cardiovascular disease (including previous MI, stroke, tachycardia, or conduction abnormalities). Use with caution in patients with respiratory compromise or sleep apnea; use of Silenor is generally not recommended with severe sleep apnea.

Use caution in patients with a previous seizure disorder or condition predisposing to seizures such as brain damage, alcoholism, or concurrent therapy with other drugs which lower the seizure threshold (APA 2010). Bone fractures have been associated with antidepressant treatment. Consider the possibility of a fragility fracture if an antidepressant-treated patient presents with unexplained bone pain, point tenderness, swelling, or bruising (Rabenda 2013; Rizzoli 2012). Use with caution in patients with hepatic dysfunction. May cause mild pupillary dilation which in susceptible individuals can lead to an episode of narrow-angle glaucoma. Consider evaluating patients who have not had an iridectomy for narrow-angle glaucoma risk factors. Potentially significant drug-drug interactions may exist, requiring dose or frequency adjustment, additional monitoring, and/or selection of alternative therapy.

May cause confusion and over sedation in the elderly. In the elderly, avoid doses >6 mg/day in this age group due to its potent anticholinergic and sedative properties, and potential to cause orthostatic hypotension; safety of doses ≤6 mg/day is comparable to placebo. In addition, may also cause or exacerbate syndrome of inappropriate antidiuretic hormone secretion or hyponatremia; monitor sodium closely with initiation or dosage adjustments in older adults (Beers Criteria).

Abrupt discontinuation or interruption of antidepressant therapy has been associated with a discontinuation syndrome. Symptoms arising may vary with antidepressant however commonly include nausea, vomiting, diarrhea, headaches, lightheadedness, dizziness, diminished appetite, sweating, chills, tremors, paresthesias, fatigue, somnolence, and sleep disturbances (eg, vivid dreams, insomnia). Greater risks for developing a discontinuation syndrome have been associated with antidepressants with shorter half-lives, longer durations of treatment, and abrupt discontinuation. For antidepressants of short or intermediate half-lives, symptoms may emerge within 2-5 days after treatment discontinuation and last 7 to 14 days (APA 2010; Fava 2006; Haddad 2001; Shelton 2001; Warner 2006).

Adverse Reactions May be dependent on diagnosis.

Cardiovascular: Edema, flushing, hypertension (chronic insomnia patients), hypotension, tachycardia

Central nervous system: Ataxia, chills, confusion, disorientation, dizziness (chronic insomnia patients), drowsiness, extrapyramidal reaction, fatigue, hallucination, headache, numbness, paresthesia, sedation (chronic insomnia patients), seizure, tardive dyskinesia

Dermatologic: Alopecia, diaphoresis (excessive), pruritus, skin photosensitivity, skin rash

Endocrine & metabolic: Altered serum glucose, change in libido, galactorrhea, gynecomastia, SIADH, weight gain

Gastrointestinal: Anorexia, aphthous stomatitis, constipation, diarrhea, dysgeusia, dyspepsia, gastroenteritis (chronic insomnia patients), nausea (chronic insomnia patients), vomiting, xerostomia

Genitourinary: Breast hypertrophy, testicular swelling, urinary retention

Hematologic & oncologic: Agranulocytosis, eosinophilia, leukopenia, purpura, thrombocytopenia

Hepatic: Jaundice

Neuromuscular & skeletal: Tremor, weakness

Ophthalmic: Blurred vision

Otic: Tinnitus

Respiratory: Exacerbation of asthma, upper respiratory tract infection (chronic insomnia patients)

Rare but important or life-threatening: Adenocarcinoma (lung, stage I), adjustment disorder, anemia, angle-closure glaucoma, atrioventricular block, bone fracture, breast cyst, cerebrovascular accident, chest pain, decreased neutrophils, decreased performance on neuropsychometrics, decreased range of motion (joints), depression, ECG abnormality (ST-T segment, QRS complex, QRS axis), eye infection, fungal infection, gastroesophageal reflux disease, hematochezia, hematoma, hemoglobinuria, hyperbilirubinemia, hyperkalemia, hypermagnesemia, hypersensitivity, hypoacusis, hypokalemia, increased serum ALT, increased serum transaminases, malignant melanoma, migraine, peripheral edema, pneumonia, sleep paralysis, somnambulism (complex sleep-related behavior [sleep-driving, cooking or eating food, making phone calls]), staphylococcal cellulitis, syncope, tenosynovitis, tooth infection, urinary incontinence, urinary tract infection, viral infection

Drug Interactions

Metabolism/Transport Effects **Substrate** of CYP1A2 (minor), CYP2C19 (minor), CYP2D6 (major), CYP3A4 (minor); **Note:** Assignment of Major/Minor substrate status based on clinically relevant drug interaction potential

Avoid Concomitant Use

Avoid concomitant use of Doxepin (Systemic) with any of the following: Aclidinium; Azelastine (Nasal); Dapoxetine; Eluxadoline; Glucagon; Iobenguane I 123; Ipratropium (Oral Inhalation); Linezolid; MAO Inhibitors; Methylene Blue; Moxonidine; Orphenadrine; Paraldehyde; Potassium Chloride; Thalidomide; Tiotropium; Umeclidinium

Increased Effect/Toxicity

Doxepin (Systemic) may increase the levels/effects of: AbobotulinumtoxinA; Alcohol (Ethyl); Alpha-/Beta-Agonists (Direct-Acting); Alpha1-Agonists; Amphetamines; Analgesics (Opioid); Anticholinergic Agents; Antipsychotic Agents; Aspirin; Azelastine (Nasal); Beta2-Agonists; Buprenorphine; Citalopram; CNS Depressants; Desmopressin; Eluxadoline; Escitalopram; Glucagon; Highest Risk QTc-Prolonging Agents; Hydrocodone; Methotrimeprazine; Methylene Blue; Metyrosine; Mirabegron; Moderate Risk QTc-Prolonging Agents; Nicorandil; NSAID (COX-2 Inhibitor); NSAID (Nonselective); OnabotulinumtoxinA; Orphenadrine; Paraldehyde; Potassium Chloride; Pramipexole; QuiNIDine; RimabotulinumtoxinB; ROPINIRole; Rotigotine; Serotonin Modulators; Sodium Phosphates; Sulfonylureas; Suvorexant; Thalidomide; Thiazide Diuretics; Tiotropium; Topiramate; TraMADol; Vitamin K Antagonists; Yohimbine; Zolpidem

The levels/effects of Doxepin (Systemic) may be increased by: Abiraterone Acetate; Aclidinium; Altretamine; Antiemetics (5HT3 Antagonists); Antipsychotic Agents; Brimonidine (Topical); BuPROPion; Cannabis; Cimetidine; Cinacalcet; Citalopram; Cobicistat; CYP2D6 Inhibitors (Moderate); CYP2D6 Inhibitors (Strong); Dapoxetine; Darunavir; Dexmethylphenidate; Doxylamine; Dronabinol; Droperidol; DULoxetine; Escitalopram; FLUoxetine; FluvoxaMINE; HydrOXYzine; Ipratropium (Oral Inhalation); Kava Kava; Linezolid; Lithium; Magnesium Sulfate; MAO Inhibitors; Methotrimeprazine; Methylphenidate; Metoclopramide; Metyrosine; Mianserin; Mifepristone; Nabilone; Panobinostat; PARoxetine; Peginterferon Alfa-2b; Perampanel; Pramlintide; Protease Inhibitors; QuiNIDine; Rufinamide; Sertraline; Sodium Oxybate; Tapentadol; Tedizolid; Terbinafine

(Systemic); Tetrahydrocannabinol; Thyroid Products; TraMADol; Umeclidinium; Valproic Acid and Derivatives

Decreased Effect

Doxepin (Systemic) may decrease the levels/effects of: Acetylcholinesterase Inhibitors; Alpha1-Agonists; Alpha2-Agonists; Alpha2-Agonists (Ophthalmic); Iobenguane I 123; Itopride; Moxonidine; Secretin

The levels/effects of Doxepin (Systemic) may be decreased by: Acetylcholinesterase Inhibitors; Barbiturates; CarBAMazepine; Peginterferon Alfa-2b; St Johns Wort

Food Interactions Administration with a high-fat meal increases the bioavailability of Silenor and delays the peak plasma concentration by ~3 hours. Management: Silenor should not be taken during or within 3 hours of a meal.

Storage/Stability Store at room temperature. Protect from light.

Mechanism of Action

Increases the synaptic concentration of serotonin and norepinephrine in the central nervous system by inhibition of their reuptake by the presynaptic neuronal membrane (Pinder, 1977); antagonizes the histamine (H_1) receptor for sleep maintenance.

Efficacy of doxepin in the off-label use of chronic urticaria is believed to be related to its potent H_1 and H_2 receptor antagonist activity (Kozel 2004).

Pharmacodynamics

Onset: Sedation: ~30 minutes

Maximum effects: Antidepressant: Usually >2 weeks; anxiolytic: May occur sooner

Pharmacokinetics (Adult data unless noted)

Distribution: Widely throughout body tissues; V_d: ~12,000 L

Protein binding: 80% to 85%

Metabolism: Hepatic primarily via CYP2C19 and 2D6 to metabolites, including N-desmethyldoxepin (active); N-desmethyldoxepin undergoes glucuronide conjugation

Half-life: Doxepin: ~15 hours; N-desmethyldoxepin: 31 hours

Time to peak serum concentration: Fasting: Silanor®: 3.5 hours

Elimination: Urine (mainly excreted as glucuronide conjugates; <3% as unchanged drug or N-desmethyldoxepin)

Dosing: Usual

Children and Adolescents: **Depression and/or anxiety:**

Oral:

Children 7-11 years: Limited data available; efficacy results variable; controlled clinical trials have not shown tricyclic antidepressants to be superior to placebo for the treatment of depression in children and have not recommended them for use (Dopheide, 2006; USPTF, 2009; Wagner, 2005); some centers have used the following doses: 1-3 mg/kg/day in single or divided doses

Children ≥12 years and Adolescents: **Note:** Controlled clinical trials have not shown tricyclic antidepressants to be superior to placebo for the treatment of depression in adolescents and have not recommended them for use (Dopheide, 2006; USPTF, 2009; Wagner, 2005); Initial: 25-75 mg/day at bedtime or in 2-3 divided doses; begin at the low end of range and gradually titrate; select patients may respond to 25-50 mg/day; maximum single dose: 150 mg; maximum daily dose: 300 mg/**day**

Adults:

Depression and/or anxiety: Oral: Initial: 25-150 mg/day at bedtime or in 2-3 divided doses; may gradually increase up to 300 mg/day; single dose should not exceed 150 mg; select patients may respond to 25-50 mg/day

Insomnia (Silenor®): Oral: 3-6 mg once daily 30 minutes prior to bedtime; maximum dose: 6 mg/day

Preparation for Administration Oral: Concentrated solution: Must dilute with water, whole or skimmed milk, or orange, grapefruit, tomato, prune, or pineapple juice prior to administration (use ~120 mL for adults). Do not mix with carbonated beverages (physically incompatible).

Administration

Oral:

Depression/anxiety: Administer with food to decrease GI upset.

Insomnia (Silenor): Administer within 30 minutes prior to bedtime; do not take within 3 hours of a meal; **Note:** Not taking Silenor within 3 hours of a meal will give a faster onset and help minimize the risk for next day effects.

Monitoring Parameters Blood pressure, heart rate, mental status, weight, liver enzymes, and CBC with differential. Monitor patient periodically for symptom resolution; monitor for worsening depression, suicidality, and associated behaviors (especially at the beginning of therapy or when doses are increased or decreased).

Reference Range Utility of serum concentration monitoring is controversial

Doxepin plus desmethyldoxepin:

Proposed therapeutic concentration: 110-250 ng/mL (394-895 nmol/L)

Toxic concentration: >500 ng/mL (>1790 nmol/L) (toxicities may be seen at lower concentrations in some patients)

Additional Information For treatment of insomnia, use beyond 3 months has not been evaluated.

Dosage Forms Excipient information presented when available (limited, particularly for generics); consult specific product labeling.

Capsule, Oral:

Generic: 10 mg, 25 mg, 50 mg, 75 mg, 100 mg, 150 mg

Concentrate, Oral:

Generic: 10 mg/mL (118 mL, 120 mL)

Tablet, Oral:

Silenor: 3 mg [contains brilliant blue fcf (fd&c blue #1)]

Silenor: 6 mg [contains brilliant blue fcf (fd&c blue #1), fd&c yellow #10 (quinoline yellow)]

◆ **Doxepin Hydrochloride** *see* Doxepin (Systemic) *on page 711*

DOXOrubicin (Conventional)

(doks oh ROO bi sin con VEN sha nal)

Medication Safety Issues

Sound-alike/look-alike issues:

Conventional formulation (Adriamycin) may be confused with the liposomal formulation (Doxil)

DOXOrubicin may be confused with DACTINomycin, DAUNOrubicin, DAUNOrubicin liposomal, doxapram, doxazosin, DOXOrubicin liposomal, epirubicin, IDArubicin, valrubicin

Adriamycin may be confused with achromycin, Aredia, Idamycin

High alert medication:

This medication is in a class the Institute for Safe Medication Practices (ISMP) includes among its list of drug classes which have a heightened risk of causing significant patient harm when used in error.

Administration issues:

Use caution when selecting product for preparation and dispensing; indications, dosages, rate of administration, and adverse event profiles differ between conventional DOXOrubicin hydrochloride solution and DOXOrubicin liposomal. Both formulations are the same concentration. As a result, serious errors have occurred.

Other safety concerns:

ADR is an error-prone abbreviation

International issues:

Doxil may be confused with Doxal which is a brand name for doxepin in Finland, a brand name for doxycycline in Austria, and a brand name for pyridoxine/thiamine combination in Brazil

Rubex, a discontinued brand name for DOXOrubicin in the U.S, is a brand name for ascorbic acid in Ireland

Related Information

Management of Drug Extravasations *on page 2298*

Prevention of Chemotherapy-Induced Nausea and Vomiting in Children *on page 2368*

Safe Handling of Hazardous Drugs *on page 2455*

Brand Names: US Adriamycin

Brand Names: Canada Adriamycin PFS; Doxorubicin Hydrochloride For Injection, USP; Doxorubicin Hydrochloride Injection

Therapeutic Category Antineoplastic Agent, Anthracycline; Antineoplastic Agent, Antibiotic; Antineoplastic Agent, Topoisomerase II Inhibitor

Generic Availability (US) Yes

Use Treatment of metastatic cancers or disseminated neoplastic conditions including acute lymphocytic leukemia (ALL), acute myeloid leukemia (AML), Hodgkin lymphoma, non-Hodgkin lymphoma, soft tissue and bone sarcomas, breast cancer, thyroid cancer, bronchiogenic carcinoma in which the small cell histologic type is the most responsive compared to other cell types, gastric carcinoma, ovarian cancer, transitional cell bladder carcinoma, neuroblastoma, and Wilms tumor [FDA approved in pediatric patients (age not specified) and adults]; treatment component of adjuvant therapy in women with evidence of axillary lymph node involvement following resection of primary breast cancer (FDA approved in adults), has also been used for the treatment of multiple myeloma, endometrial carcinoma, uterine sarcoma, head and neck cancer, liver cancer, and kidney cancer.

Pregnancy Risk Factor D

Pregnancy Considerations Adverse events have been observed in animal reproduction studies. Based on the mechanism of action, doxorubicin may cause fetal harm if administered during pregnancy (according to the manufacturer's labeling). Advise patients (females of reproductive potential and males with female partners of reproductive potential) to use effective nonhormonal contraception during and for 6 months following therapy. Limited information is available from a retrospective study of women who received doxorubicin (in combination with cyclophosphamide) during the second or third (prior to week 35) trimester for the treatment of pregnancy-associated breast cancer (Ring, 2005). Some pharmacokinetic properties of doxorubicin may be altered in pregnant women (van Hasselt, 2014). The European Society for Medical Oncology (ESMO) has published guidelines for diagnosis, treatment, and follow-up of cancer during pregnancy (Peccatori 2013); the guidelines recommend referral to a facility with expertise in cancer during pregnancy and encourage a multidisciplinary team (obstetrician, neonatologist, oncology team). If chemotherapy is indicated, it should **not** be administered in the first trimester, but may begin in the second trimester. There should be a 3-week time period between the last chemotherapy dose and anticipated delivery, and chemotherapy should not be administered beyond week 33 of gestation.

A pregnancy registry is available for all cancers diagnosed during pregnancy at Cooper Health (877-635-4499).

Breast-Feeding Considerations Doxorubicin and its metabolites are excreted in breast milk. Due to the potential for serious adverse reactions in the nursing infant, the manufacturer recommends a decision be made whether to discontinue nursing or to discontinue the drug, taking into account the importance of treatment to the mother.

Contraindications Hypersensitivity (including anaphylaxis) to doxorubicin, any component of the formulation, or to other anthracyclines or anthracenediones; recent MI (within past 4 to 6 weeks), severe myocardial insufficiency, severe arrhythmia; previous therapy with high cumulative doses of doxorubicin, daunorubicin, idarubicin, or other anthracycline and anthracenediones; severe persistent drug-induced myelosuppression or baseline neutrophil count <1500/mm^3; severe hepatic impairment (Child-Pugh class C or bilirubin >5 mg/dL)

Warnings/Precautions Hazardous agent - use appropriate precautions for handling and disposal (NIOSH 2014 [group 1]). **[U.S. Boxed Warning]: May cause cumulative, dose-related, myocardial toxicity (early or delayed, including acute left ventricular failure and HF). The risk of cardiomyopathy increases with cumulative exposure and with concomitant cardiotoxic therapy; the incidence of irreversible myocardial toxicity increases as the total cumulative (lifetime) dosages approach 300 to 500 mg/m^2. Assess left ventricular ejection fraction (LVEF) with either an echocardiogram or MUGA scan before, during, and after therapy; increase the frequency of assessments as the cumulative dose exceeds 300 mg/m^2.** Cardiotoxicity is dose-limiting. Delayed cardiotoxicity may occur late in treatment or within months to years after completion of therapy, and is typically manifested by LVEF reduction and/or heart failure (may be life threatening). Subacute effects such as pericarditis and myocarditis may also occur. Early toxicity may consist of tachyarrhythmias, including sinus tachycardia, premature ventricular contractions, and ventricular tachycardia, as well as bradycardia. Electrocardiographic changes including ST-T wave changes, atrioventricular and bundle-branch block have also been reported. These effects are not necessarily predictive of subsequent delayed cardiotoxicity. Total cumulative dose should take into account prior treatment with other anthracyclines or anthracenediones, previous or concomitant treatment with other cardiotoxic agents or irradiation of chest. Although the risk increases with cumulative dose, irreversible cardiotoxicity may occur at any dose level. Patients with active or dominant cardiovascular disease, concurrent administration of cardiotoxic drugs, prior therapy with other anthracyclines or anthracenediones, prior or concurrent chest irradiation, advanced age, and infants and children are at increased risk. Alternative administration schedules (weekly or continuous infusions) have are associated with less cardiotoxicity.

[U.S. Boxed Warning]: Vesicant; if extravasation occurs, severe local tissue damage leading to tissue injury, blistering, ulceration, and necrosis may occur. Discontinue infusion immediately and apply ice to the affected area. For IV administration only. Do not administer IM or SubQ. Ensure proper needle or catheter placement prior to and during infusion. Avoid extravasation.

[U.S. Boxed Warning]: May cause severe myelosuppression, which may result in serious infection, septic shock, transfusion requirements, hospitalization, and death. Myelosuppression may be dose-limiting and primarily manifests as leukopenia and neutropenia; anemia and thrombocytopenia may also occur. The nadir typically occurs 10 to 14 days after administration with cell count recovery around day 21. Monitor blood counts at baseline and regularly during therapy.

[U.S. Boxed Warning]: Secondary acute myelogenous leukemia (AML) and myelodysplastic syndrome (MDS) have been reported following treatment. AML and MDS typically occur within one to three years of treatment; risk factors for development of secondary AML or MDS include treatment with anthracyclines in combination with DNA-damaging antineoplastics (eg, alkylating agents) and/or radiation therapy, heavily pretreated patients, and escalated anthracycline doses. May cause tumor lysis syndrome and hyperuricemia (in patients with rapidly growing tumors). Urinary alkalinization and prophylaxis with an antihyperuricemic agent may be necessary. Monitor electrolytes, renal function, and hydration status. **[U.S. Boxed Warning]: Dosage modification is recommended in patients with impaired hepatic function;** toxicities may be increased in patients with hepatic impairment. Use is contraindicated in patients with severe impairment (Child-Pugh class C or bilirubin >5 mg/dL). Monitor hepatic function tests (eg, transaminases, alkaline phosphatase, and bilirubin) closely. Use with caution in patients who have received radiation therapy; radiation recall may occur. May increase radiation-induced toxicity to the myocardium, mucosa, skin, and liver. Doxorubicin is associated with a moderate or high emetic potential (depending on dose or regimen); antiemetics are recommended to prevent nausea and vomiting (Basch, 2011; Dupuis, 2011; Roila, 2010). Potentially significant drug-drug interactions may exist, requiring dose or frequency adjustment, additional monitoring, and/or selection of alternative therapy.

In men, doxorubicin may damage spermatozoa and testicular tissue, resulting in possible genetic fetal abnormalities; may also result in oligospermia, azoospermia, and permanent loss of fertility (sperm counts have been reported to return to normal levels in some men, occurring several years after the end of therapy). In females of reproductive potential, doxorubicin may cause infertility and result in amenorrhea; premature menopause can occur. Children are at increased risk for developing delayed cardiotoxicity; long-term cardiac function monitoring is recommended. Doxorubicin may contribute to prepubertal growth failure in children; may also contribute to gonadal impairment (usually temporary). Radiation recall pneumonitis has been reported in children receiving concomitant dactinomycin and doxorubicin. **[U.S. Boxed Warning]: Should be administered under the supervision of an experienced cancer chemotherapy physician.** Use caution when selecting product for preparation and dispensing; indications, dosages and adverse event profiles differ between conventional doxorubicin hydrochloride solution and doxorubicin liposomal. Both formulations are the same concentration. As a result, serious errors have occurred.

Warnings: Additional Pediatric Considerations

Pediatric patients are at increased risk for developing delayed cardiac toxicity and CHF during early adulthood due to an increasing census of long-term survivors; risk factors include young treatment age (<5 years), cumulative exposure, and concomitant cardiotoxic therapy. Up to 40% of pediatric patients may have subclinical cardiac dysfunction and 5% to 10% may develop heart failure. Long-term monitoring is recommended for all pediatric patients.

Adverse Reactions

Cardiovascular:

Acute cardiotoxicity: Atrioventricular block, bradycardia, bundle branch block, ECG abnormalities, extrasystoles (atrial or ventricular), sinus tachycardia, ST-T wave changes, supraventricular tachycardia, tachyarrhythmia, ventricular tachycardia

Delayed cardiotoxicity: LVEF decreased, CHF (manifestations include ascites, cardiomegaly, dyspnea, edema, gallop rhythm, hepatomegaly, oliguria, pleural effusion, pulmonary edema, tachycardia); myocarditis, pericarditis

Central nervous system: Malaise

Dermatologic: Alopecia, itching, photosensitivity, radiation recall, rash; discoloration of saliva, sweat, or tears

Endocrine & metabolic: Amenorrhea, dehydration, infertility (may be temporary), hyperuricemia

Gastrointestinal: Abdominal pain, anorexia, colon necrosis, diarrhea, GI ulceration, mucositis, nausea, vomiting

Genitourinary: Discoloration of urine

Hematologic: Leukopenia/neutropenia (nadir: 10-14 days; recovery: by day 21); thrombocytopenia and anemia

Local: Skin "flare" at injection site, urticaria

Neuromuscular & skeletal: Weakness

Rare but important or life-threatening: Anaphylaxis, azoospermia, bilirubin increased, coma (when in combination with cisplatin or vincristine), conjunctivitis, fever, gonadal impairment (children), growth failure (prepubertal), hepatitis, hyperpigmentation (nail, skin & oral mucosa), infection, keratitis, lacrimation, myelodysplastic syndrome, neutropenic fever, neutropenic typhlitis, oligospermia, peripheral neurotoxicity (with intra-arterial doxorubicin), phlebosclerosis, radiation recall pneumonitis (children), secondary acute myelogenous leukemia, seizure (when in combination with cisplatin or vincristine), sepsis, shock, Stevens-Johnson syndrome, systemic hypersensitivity (including urticaria, pruritus, angioedema, dysphagia, and dyspnea), toxic epidermal necrolysis, transaminases increased, urticaria

Drug Interactions

Metabolism/Transport Effects Substrate of CYP2D6 (major), CYP3A4 (major), P-glycoprotein; **Note:** Assignment of Major/Minor substrate status based on clinically relevant drug interaction potential; **Inhibits** CYP2B6 (moderate), CYP2D6 (weak); **Induces** P-glycoprotein

Avoid Concomitant Use

Avoid concomitant use of DOXOrubicin (Conventional) with any of the following: BCG; BCG (Intravesical); CloZAPine; Conivaptan; Dabigatran Etexilate; Dipyrone; Fusidic Acid (Systemic); Idelalisib; Ledipasvir; Natalizumab; Pimecrolimus; Sofosbuvir; Tacrolimus (Topical); Tofacitinib; Vaccines (Live); VinCRIStine (Liposomal)

Increased Effect/Toxicity

DOXOrubicin (Conventional) may increase the levels/effects of: ARIPiprazole; CloZAPine; CYP2B6 Substrates; Leflunomide; Mercaptopurine; Natalizumab; Tofacitinib; Vaccines (Live); Zidovudine

The levels/effects of DOXOrubicin (Conventional) may be increased by: Abiraterone Acetate; Bevacizumab; Conivaptan; Cyclophosphamide; CycloSPORINE (Systemic); CYP2D6 Inhibitors (Moderate); CYP2D6 Inhibitors (Strong); CYP3A4 Inhibitors (Moderate); CYP3A4 Inhibitors (Strong); Dasatinib; Denosumab; Dipyrone; Fusidic Acid (Systemic); Idelalisib; Luliconazole; Mifepristone; Palbociclib; Panobinostat; Peginterferon Alfa-2b; P-glycoprotein/ABCB1 Inhibitors; Pimecrolimus; Roflumilast; SORAfenib; Stiripentol; Tacrolimus (Topical); Taxane Derivatives; Trastuzumab

Decreased Effect

DOXOrubicin (Conventional) may decrease the levels/effects of: Afatinib; BCG; BCG (Intravesical); Brentuximab Vedotin; Cardiac Glycosides; Coccidioides immitis Skin Test; Dabigatran Etexilate; Ledipasvir; Linagliptin; P-glycoprotein/ABCB1 Substrates; Sipuleucel-T; Sofosbuvir; Stavudine; Vaccines (Inactivated); Vaccines (Live); VinCRIStine (Liposomal); Zidovudine

The levels/effects of DOXOrubicin (Conventional) may be decreased by: Bosentan; Cardiac Glycosides; CYP3A4 Inducers (Moderate); CYP3A4 Inducers (Strong); Dabrafenib; Deferasirox; Dexrazoxane; Echinacea; Mitotane; Peginterferon Alfa-2b; P-glycoprotein/ABCB1 Inducers; Siltuximab; St Johns Wort; Tocilizumab

Storage/Stability

Lyophilized powder: Store powder at 20°C to 25°C (68°F to 77°F). Protect from light. Retain in carton until time of use. Discard unused portion from single-dose vials. Reconstituted doxorubicin is stable for 7 days at room temperature under normal room lighting and for 15 days when refrigerated at 2°C to 8°C (36°F to 46°F). Protect reconstituted solution from light.

Solution: Store refrigerated at 2°C to 8°C (36°F to 46°F). Protect from light. Retain in carton until time of use. Discard unused portion. Storage of vials of solution under refrigeration may result in formation of a gelled product; if gelling occurs, place vials at room temperature for 2 to 4 hours to return the product to a slightly viscous, mobile solution.

Mechanism of Action Inhibition of DNA and RNA synthesis by intercalation between DNA base pairs by inhibition of topoisomerase II and by steric obstruction. Doxorubicin intercalates at points of local uncoiling of the double helix. Although the exact mechanism is unclear, it appears that direct binding to DNA (intercalation) and inhibition of DNA repair (topoisomerase II inhibition) result in blockade of DNA and RNA synthesis and fragmentation of DNA. Doxorubicin is also a powerful iron chelator; the iron-doxorubicin complex can bind DNA and cell membranes and produce free radicals that immediately cleave the DNA and cell membranes.

Pharmacokinetics (Adult data unless noted)

Distribution: V_d: 809 to 1214 L/m^2 does not penetrate into CSF

Protein binding: ~75%

Metabolism: Primarily hepatic to doxorubicinol (active), then to inactive aglycones, conjugated sulfates, and glucuronides

Half-life, multiphasic:
- Distribution: ~5 minutes
- Terminal: 20 to 48 hours
  - Male: 54 hours
  - Female: 35 hours

Elimination: Feces (40% as unchanged drug); urine (5% to 12% as unchanged drug and metabolites)
- Clearance:
  - Infants and Children <2 years: 813 mL/minute/m^2
  - Children and Adolescents >2 years: 1540 mL/minute/m^2
  - Adults: 324 to 809 mL/minutes/m^2

Dosing: Usual Note: Dose, frequency, number of doses, and start date may vary by protocol and treatment phase; refer to individual protocols.

Lower dosages should be considered for patients with inadequate marrow reserve (due to advanced age, prior treatment, or neoplastic marrow infiltration). Cumulative doses above 550 mg/m^2 are associated with an increased risk of cardiomyopathy.

Doxorubicin is associated with a moderate to high emetic potential (depending on dose or regimen); antiemetics are recommended to prevent nausea and vomiting (Basch, 2011).

Pediatric:

Malignancy (metastatic solid tumors, leukemia, or lymphoma; general dosing): Manufacturer's labeling: IV: Infants, Children, and Adolescents:
- Single-agent therapy: 60 to 75 mg/m^2 every 21 days
- Combination therapy: 40 to 75 mg/m^2 every 21 to 28 days

Acute lymphoblastic leukemia: IV: Children and Adolescents:

DFCI Consortium Protocol 00-01 (Vrooman, 2013):
- Induction: 30 mg/m^2/dose on days 0 and 1 of a 4-week cycle (in combination with vincristine, methotrexate, *E.coli* asparaginase, prednisone, intrathecal cytarabine, and intrathecal methotrexate/cytarabine/hydrocortisone)
- CNS therapy: High-risk patients: 30 mg/m^2 on day 1 of a 3-week cycle (in combination with dexrazoxane, vincristine, 6-mercaptopurine, and intrathecal methotrexate/cytarabine)
- Intensification: High-risk patients: 30 mg/m^2 on day 1 of every 3-week cycle (in combination with dexrazoxane, vincristine, 6-mercaptopurine, *E.coli* asparaginase, prednisone or dexamethasone, and intrathecal methotrexate/cytarabine/hydrocortisone); cumulative doxorubicin dose: 300 mg/m^2

Ewing's sarcoma: IV: Children and Adolescents:
- *VAC/IE regimen:* 75 mg/m^2 on day 1 every 21 days for 5 cycles (in combination with vincristine and cyclophosphamide; after 5 cycles, dactinomycin replaced doxorubicin), alternating cycles with ifosfamide and etoposide for a total of 17 cycles (Grier, 2003)
- *VAIA regimen:* 30 mg/m^2/day on days 1 and 2 every 21 days (doxorubicin alternates with dactinomycin; in combination with vincristine and ifosfamide) for 14 cycles (Paulussen, 2008)
- *VIDE regimen:* 20 mg/m^2/day over 4 hours on days 1 to 3 every 21 days for 6 cycles (in combination with vincristine, ifosfamide, and etoposide) (Juergens, 2006)

Hodgkin lymphoma: IV: Children and Adolescents:
- *BEACOPP regimen*: 35 mg/m^2 administered on day 0 of a 21 day treatment cycle (in combination with bleomycin, etoposide, cyclophosphamide, vincristine, procarbazine, and prednisone) (Kelly, 2002)

Osteosarcoma: IV: Children and Adolescents:
- *Cisplatin/doxorubicin regimen* (Bramwell, 1992): 25 mg/m^2 (bolus infusion) on days 1 to 3 every 21 days (in combination with cisplatin)
- *High-dose methotrexate/cisplatin/doxorubicin/ifosfamide regimen* (Bacci, 2003):
  - Preoperative: 75 mg/m^2 administered as a continuous infusion over 24 hours on day 3 of weeks 1 and 7 (in combination with methotrexate, cisplatin, and ifosfamide; refer to protocol for criteria, frequency, and other specific information)
  - Postoperative: 90 mg/m^2 administered as a continuous infusion over 24 hours on weeks 13, 22, and 31 (alternating methotrexate, cisplatin, and ifosfamide)
- *High-dose methotrexate/cisplatin/doxorubicin regimen* (Bacci, 2000):
  - Preoperative: 60 mg/m^2 over 8 hours on days 9 and 36 (in combination with methotrexate and cisplatin)
  - Postoperative: 45 mg/m^2/day over 4 hours for 2 consecutive days (in alternating cycles of methotrexate, ifosfamide, and cisplatin/etoposide; refer to protocol for criteria, frequency, and other specific information)

Rhabdomyosarcoma: IV: Children and Adolescents:
- *VAC/IE regimen:* 37.5 mg/m^2 on days 1 and 2 (administered over 18 hours each day) every 6 weeks (in combination with vincristine and cyclophosphamide), alternating cycles with ifosfamide and etoposide (Arndt, 1998)

Adult: **Note:** Utilize patient's actual body weight (full weight) for calculation of body surface area- or weight-based dosing, particularly when the intent of therapy is curative; manage regimen-related toxicities in the same manner as for nonobese patients; if a dose reduction is utilized due to toxicity, consider resumption of full weight-based dosing with subsequent cycles, especially if cause of toxicity (eg, hepatic or renal impairment) is resolved (Griggs, 2012).

Breast cancer: IV: 60 mg/m^2 on day 1 of a 21-day cycle (in combination with cyclophosphamide) for 4 cycles

Metastatic solid tumors, leukemia, or lymphoma: IV:
- Single-agent therapy: 60 to 75 mg/m^2 every 21 days
- Combination therapy: 40 to 75 mg/m^2 every 21 to 28 days

Dosing adjustment in renal impairment: All patients: Mild, moderate, or severe impairment: There are no dosage adjustments provided in the manufacturers' labeling (has not been studied); however, adjustments are likely not necessary given limited renal excretion. The following adjustments have also been recommended (Aronoff, 2007):

CrCl <50 mL/minute: No dosage adjustment necessary.

Hemodialysis: Supplemental dose is not necessary.

Dosing adjustment in hepatic impairment: All patients: The manufacturers' labeling recommends the following adjustments:

Serum bilirubin 1.2 to 3 mg/dL: Administer 50% of dose.

Serum bilirubin 3.1 to 5 mg/dL: Administer 25% of dose.

Severe hepatic impairment (Child-Pugh class C or bilirubin >5 mg/dL): Use is contraindicated.

The following adjustments have also been recommended (Floyd, 2006):

Transaminases 2 to 3 times ULN: Administer 75% of dose.

Transaminases >3 times ULN: Administer 50% of dose.

Preparation for Administration Hazardous agent; use appropriate precautions for handling and disposal (NIOSH 2014 [group 1]).

Parenteral: Reconstitute lyophilized powder with NS (using 5 mL for the 10 mg vial, 10 mL for the 20 mg vial, or 25 mL for the 50 mg vial) to a final concentration of 2 mg/mL; gently shake until contents are dissolved. May further dilute doxorubicin solution or reconstituted doxorubicin solution in 50 to 1,000 mL D_5W or NS for infusion. Unstable in solutions with a pH <3 or >7.

Administration Hazardous agent; use appropriate precautions for handling and disposal (NIOSH 2014 [group 1]). Doxorubicin is associated with a moderate to high emetic potential (depending on dose or regimen); antiemetics are recommended to prevent nausea and vomiting (Basch 2011).

Parenteral: Administer IV push over at least 3 to 10 minutes or by continuous IV infusion (infusion via central venous line recommended). Do not administer IM or SubQ. Rate of administration varies by protocol, refer to individual protocol for details. Protect from light until completion of infusion. Avoid contact with alkaline solutions. Monitor for local erythematous streaking along vein and/or facial flushing (may indicate rapid infusion rate); decrease rate if occurs.

Vesicant; ensure proper needle or catheter placement prior to and during infusion; avoid extravasation. If extravasation occurs, stop infusion immediately and disconnect (leave cannula/needle in place); gently aspirate extravasated solution (do **NOT** flush the line); remove needle/cannula; elevate extremity. Initiate antidote (dexrazoxane (adults) or dimethyl sulfate [DMSO]) (see Management of Drug Extravasations for more details). Apply dry cold compresses for 20 minutes 4 times daily for 1 to 2 days (Perez Fidalgo 2012); withhold cooling beginning 15 minutes before dexrazoxane infusion; continue withholding cooling until 15 minutes after infusion is completed. Topical DMSO should not be administered in combination with dexrazoxane; may lessen dexrazoxane efficacy.

Vesicant/Extravasation Risk Vesicant

Monitoring Parameters CBC with differential and platelet count; liver function tests (bilirubin, ALT/AST, alkaline phosphatase); serum uric acid, calcium, potassium, phosphate and creatinine; hydration status; cardiac function (baseline, periodic, and followup): ECG, left ventricular ejection fraction (echocardiography [ECHO] or multigated radionuclide angiography [MUGA]); monitor infusion site

Dosage Forms Excipient information presented when available (limited, particularly for generics); consult specific product labeling. [DSC] = Discontinued product

Solution, Intravenous, as hydrochloride:

Adriamycin: 2 mg/mL (5 mL, 10 mL, 25 mL, 100 mL)

Generic: 2 mg/mL (5 mL, 10 mL, 25 mL, 100 mL)

Solution, Intravenous, as hydrochloride [preservative free]:

Generic: 2 mg/mL (5 mL, 10 mL, 25 mL, 75 mL, 100 mL)

Solution Reconstituted, Intravenous, as hydrochloride:

Adriamycin: 10 mg (1 ea); 20 mg (1 ea); 50 mg (1 ea)

Generic: 50 mg (1 ea)

Solution Reconstituted, Intravenous, as hydrochloride [preservative free]:

Generic: 10 mg (1 ea); 50 mg (1 ea [DSC])

- ◆ **Doxorubicin HCl** *see* DOXOrubicin (Conventional) *on page 713*
- ◆ **Doxorubicin Hydrochloride** *see* DOXOrubicin (Conventional) *on page 713*
- ◆ **Doxorubicin Hydrochloride For Injection, USP (Can)** *see* DOXOrubicin (Conventional) *on page 713*
- ◆ **Doxorubicin Hydrochloride Injection (Can)** *see* DOXOrubicin (Conventional) *on page 713*
- ◆ **Doxy 100** *see* Doxycycline *on page 717*
- ◆ **Doxycin (Can)** *see* Doxycycline *on page 717*

Doxycycline (doks i SYE kleen)

Medication Safety Issues

Sound-alike/look-alike issues:

Doxycycline may be confused with dicyclomine, doxepin, doxylamine

Doxy100 may be confused with Doxil

Monodox may be confused with Maalox

Oracea may be confused with Orencia

Vibramycin may be confused with vancomycin, Vibativ

International issues:

Oracea (U.S brand name) is marketed in Canada under the brand name Apprilon

Related Information

Oral Medications That Should Not Be Crushed or Altered *on page 2476*

Brand Names: US Acticlate; Adoxa; Adoxa Pak 1/100; Adoxa Pak 1/150; Adoxa Pak 2/100; Alodox Convenience [DSC]; Avidoxy; Doryx; Doxy 100; Monodox; Morgidox; NicAzelDoxy 30 [DSC]; NicAzelDoxy 60 [DSC]; Ocudox [DSC]; Oracea; TargaDOX; Vibramycin

Brand Names: Canada Apo-Doxy; Apo-Doxy Tabs; Apprilon; Dom-Doxycycline; Doxycin; Doxytab; Periostat; PHL-Doxycycline; PMS-Doxycycline; Teva-Doxycycline; Vibra-Tabs; Vibramycin

Therapeutic Category Antibiotic, Tetracycline Derivative

Generic Availability (US) May be product dependent

Use Treatment of infections caused by susceptible *Rickettsia*, *Chlamydia*, and *Mycoplasma*; alternative to mefloquine for malaria prophylaxis; treatment for syphilis, uncomplicated *Neisseria gonorrhoeae*, *Listeria*, *Actinomyces israelii*, *Fusobacterium fusiforme*, and *Clostridium* infections in penicillin-allergic patients; used for community-acquired pneumonia and other common infections due to susceptible organisms; anthrax due to *Bacillus anthracis*, including inhalational anthrax (postexposure); treatment of infections caused by uncommon susceptible gram-negative and gram-positive organisms, including *Borrelia recurrentis*, *Ureaplasma urealyticum*, *Haemophilus ducreyi*, *Yersinia pestis*, *Francisella tularensis*, *Vibrio cholerae*, *Campylobacter fetus*, *Brucella* spp, *Bartonella bacilliformis*, and *Calymmatobacterium granulomatis*, Q fever, Lyme disease; treatment of inflammatory lesions associated with rosacea; adjunct to amebicides for intestinal amebiasis; adjunct for treatment of severe acne (FDA approved in ages ≥8 years and adults); treatment of inflammatory lesions (papules and pustules) associated with rosacea (Oracea®: FDA approved in adults). Has also been used for community-acquired MRSA cellulitis, in ehrlichiosis and management of malignant pleural effusions with intrapleural administration.

Pregnancy Risk Factor D

Pregnancy Considerations Tetracyclines cross the placenta and accumulate in developing teeth and long tubular bones. Therapeutic doses of doxycycline during pregnancy are unlikely to produce substantial teratogenic risk, but data are insufficient to say that there is no risk. In general, reports of exposure have been limited to short durations of therapy in the first trimester. Tetracyclines may discolor fetal teeth following maternal use during pregnancy; the specific teeth involved and the portion of the tooth affected depends on the timing and duration of exposure relative to tooth calcification. As a class, tetracyclines are generally considered second-line antibiotics in pregnant women and their use should be avoided. Tetracycline medications should be used during pregnancy only when other medications are contraindicated or ineffective (Mylonas 2011).

Breast-Feeding Considerations Doxycycline is excreted in breast milk (Chung 2002). According to the manufacturer, the decision to continue or discontinue breast-feeding during therapy should take into account the risk of exposure to the infant and the benefits of treatment to the mother. Although nursing is not specifically contraindicated, the effects of long-term exposure via breast milk are not known. Oral absorption of doxycycline is not markedly influenced by simultaneous ingestion of milk; therefore, oral absorption of doxycycline by the breast-feeding infant would not be expected to be diminished by the calcium in the maternal milk. Nondose-related effects could include modification of bowel flora.

Contraindications

US labeling: Hypersensitivity to doxycycline, tetracycline, or any component of the formulation

Canadian labeling: Hypersensitivity to doxycycline, tetracycline, or any component of the formulation; myasthenia gravis

Periostat, Apprilon: Additional contraindications: Use in infants and children <8 years of age or during second or third trimester of pregnancy; breast-feeding

Warnings/Precautions Photosensitivity reaction may occur with this drug; avoid prolonged exposure to sunlight or tanning equipment. Antianabolic effects of tetracyclines can increase BUN (dose-related). Hypersensitivity syndromes have been reported, including drug rash with eosinophilia and systemic symptoms (DRESS), urticaria, angioneurotic edema, anaphylaxis, anaphylactoid purpura, serum sickness, pericarditis, and systemic lupus erythematosus exacerbation. Hepatotoxicity rarely occurs; if symptomatic, conduct LFT and discontinue drug. Intracranial hypertension (headache, blurred vision, diplopia, vision loss, and/or papilledema) has been associated with use. Women of childbearing age who are overweight or have a history of intracranial hypertension are at greater risk. Concomitant use of isotretinoin (known to cause pseudotumor cerebri) and doxycycline should be avoided. Intracranial hypertension typically resolves after discontinuation of treatment; however, permanent visual loss is possible. If visual symptoms develop during treatment, prompt ophthalmologic evaluation is warranted. Intracranial pressure can remain elevated for weeks after drug discontinuation; monitor patients until they stabilize. Prolonged use may result in fungal or bacterial superinfection, including *C. difficile*-associated diarrhea (CDAD) and pseudomembranous colitis; CDAD has been observed >2 months postantibiotic treatment. May cause tissue hyperpigmentation, tooth enamel hypoplasia, or permanent tooth discoloration; use of tetracyclines should be avoided during tooth development (last half or pregnancy, infancy, and children <8 years of age) unless other drugs are not likely to be effective or are contraindicated. However, recommended in treatment of anthrax exposure, tickborne rickettsial diseases, and Q fever. Do not use during pregnancy. In addition to affecting tooth development, tetracycline use has been associated with retardation of skeletal development and reduced bone growth. When used for malaria prophylaxis, does not completely suppress asexual blood stages of *Plasmodium* strains. Doxycycline does not suppress *Plasmodium falciparum*'s sexual blood stage gametocytes. Patients completing a regimen may still transmit the infection to mosquitoes outside endemic areas.

Oracea (US labeling) or Apprilon (Canadian labeling): Additional specific warnings: Should not be used for the treatment or prophylaxis of bacterial infections, since the lower dose of drug per capsule may be subefficacious and promote resistance. Syrup contains sodium metabisulfite. Effectiveness of products intended for use in periodontitis has not been established in patients with coexistent oral candidiasis; use with caution in patients with a history or predisposition to oral candidiasis.

Warnings: Additional Pediatric Considerations

Administration of tetracycline 25 mg/kg/day was associated with decreased fibular growth rate in premature infants (reversible with discontinuation of drug); bulging fontanels have been reported in infants.

Some dosage forms may contain propylene glycol; in neonates large amounts of propylene glycol delivered orally, intravenously (eg, >3,000 mg/day), or topically have been associated with potentially fatal toxicities which can include metabolic acidosis, seizures, renal failure, and CNS depression; toxicities have also been reported in children and adults including hyperosmolality, lactic acidosis, seizures and respiratory depression; use caution (AAP, 1997; Shehab, 2009).

Adverse Reactions

Central nervous system: Bulging fontanel (infants), headache, intracranial hypertension (adults), pericarditis

Dermatologic: Discoloration of thyroid gland (brown/black, no dysfunction reported), erythema multiforme, erythematous rash, exfoliative dermatitis, maculopapular rash, skin hyperpigmentation, skin photosensitivity, Stevens-Johnson syndrome, toxic epidermal necrolysis, urticaria

Endocrine & metabolic: Hypoglycemia

Gastrointestinal: Anorexia, *Clostridium difficile* associated diarrhea, dental discoloration (children), diarrhea, dysphagia, enterocolitis, esophageal ulcer, esophagitis, glossitis, nausea, upper abdominal pain, vomiting

Genitourinary: Vaginitis (bacterial, 3%), vulvovaginal disease (mycotic infection, 2%), inflammatory anogenital lesion

Hematologic & oncologic: Anaphylactoid purpura, eosinophilia, hemolytic anemia, neutropenia, thrombocytopenia

Hepatic: Hepatotoxicity (rare)

Hypersensitivity: Anaphylaxis, angioedema, serum sickness

Neuromuscular & skeletal: Exacerbation of systemic lupus erythematosus

Renal: Increased blood urea nitrogen (dose related)

Note: Additional adverse reactions not listed above that have been reported with Oracea or Periostat (Canadian availability; not available in the U.S.):

Periostat: Arthralgia (6%), dyspepsia (6%), dysmenorrhea (4%), pain (4%), bronchitis (3%)

Oracea: Nasopharyngitis (5%), hypertension (3%), sinusitis (3%), anxiety (2%), fungal infection (2%), increased blood pressure (2%), increased lactate dehydrogenase (2%), increased serum AST (2%), influenza (2%), pain (2%), abdominal pain (1% to 2%), back pain (1%), hyperglycemia (1%), sinus headache (1%), xerostomia (1%)

Drug Interactions

Metabolism/Transport Effects None known.

Avoid Concomitant Use

Avoid concomitant use of Doxycycline with any of the following: BCG; BCG (Intravesical); Mecamylamine; Retinoic Acid Derivatives; Strontium Ranelate

Increased Effect/Toxicity

Doxycycline may increase the levels/effects of: Mecamylamine; Mipomersen; Neuromuscular-Blocking Agents; Porfimer; Retinoic Acid Derivatives; Verteporfin; Vitamin K Antagonists

Decreased Effect

Doxycycline may decrease the levels/effects of: BCG; BCG (Intravesical); BCG Vaccine (Immunization); Iron Salts; Penicillins; Sodium Picosulfate; Typhoid Vaccine

The levels/effects of Doxycycline may be decreased by: Antacids; Barbiturates; Bile Acid Sequestrants; Bismuth Subcitrate; Bismuth Subsalicylate; Calcium Salts; CarBAMazepine; Fosphenytoin; Iron Salts; Lanthanum; Magnesium Salts; Multivitamins/Minerals (with ADEK, Folate, Iron); Multivitamins/Minerals (with AE, No Iron); Phenytoin; Quinapril; Rifampin; Strontium Ranelate; Sucralfate; Sucroferric Oxyhydroxide

Food Interactions

Ethanol: Chronic ethanol ingestion may reduce the serum concentration of doxycycline.

Food: Doxycycline serum levels may be slightly decreased if taken with food or milk. Administration with iron or calcium may decrease doxycycline absorption. May decrease absorption of calcium, iron, magnesium, zinc, and amino acids. Management: Doryx tablets can be administered without regard to meals.

Storage/Stability

Capsule, tablet: Store at 20°C to 25°C (68°F to 77°F); excursions are permitted between 15°C and 30°C (59°F and 86°F). Protect from light and moisture.

Syrup, oral suspension: Store below 30°C (86°F); protect from light.

IV infusion: Protect from light. Stability varies based on solution.

Mechanism of Action Inhibits protein synthesis by binding with the 30S and possibly the 50S ribosomal subunit(s) of susceptible bacteria; may also cause alterations in the cytoplasmic membrane

Periostat capsules (Canadian availability; not available in the US): Proposed mechanism: Has been shown to inhibit collagenase activity *in vitro*. Also has been noted to reduce elevated collagenase activity in the gingival crevicular fluid of patients with periodontal disease. Systemic levels do not reach inhibitory concentrations against bacteria.

Pharmacokinetics (Adult data unless noted)

Absorption: Almost completely from the GI tract; absorption can be reduced by food or milk by 20%

Distribution: Widely distributed into body tissues and fluids including synovial and pleural fluid, bile, bronchial secretions; poor penetration into the CSF; appears in breast milk

Protein binding: 80% to 85%

Metabolism: Not metabolized in the liver; partially inactivated in the GI tract by chelate formation

Bioavailability: Reduced at high pH; may be clinically significant in patients with gastrectomy, gastric bypass surgery, or who are otherwise deemed achlorhydric

Half-life: 12-15 hours (usually increases to 22-24 hours with multiple dosing); Oracea®: 21hours

Time to peak serum concentration: Oral: Within 1.5-4 hours

Elimination: In the urine (23%) and feces (30%)

Dialysis: Not dialyzable (0% to 5%)

Dosing: Usual

Children <8 years:

Anthrax: Note: In the presence of systemic involvement, extensive edema, and/or lesions on head/neck, doxycycline should initially be administered IV Initial treatment should include two or more agents per CDC recommendations. Agents suggested for use in conjunction with doxycycline include rifampin, vancomycin, penicillin, ampicillin, chloramphenicol, imipenem, clindamycin, or clarithromycin. For bioterrorism postexposure, continue combined therapy for 60 days; if natural exposure, 7-10 days of therapy.

Treatment: IV: 2.2 mg/kg/dose every 12 hours (maximum dose: 100 mg/dose); may switch to oral therapy (same dosing) when clinically appropriate (CDC, 2001)

Prophylaxis; postexposure (inhalation or cutaneous): Oral: 2.2 mg/kg/dose every 12 hours for 60 days (maximum dose: 100 mg/dose) (CDC, 2001; *Red Book*, 2009)

Ehrlichiosis: Oral, IV: 2 mg/kg/dose every 12 hours (maximum dose: 100 mg/dose) for 3 days after defervescence and at least 7 days total (*Red Book*, 2009)

Tickborne rickettsial disease: Oral, IV: 2.2 mg/kg/dose every 12 hours (maximum dose: 100 mg/dose) for 5-7 days. Severe or complicated disease may require longer treatment; human granulocytotropic anaplasmosis (HGA) should be treated for 10-14 days (CDC, 2006)

Children ≥8 years:

General dosing: Oral, IV: 2-4 mg/kg/**day** divided every 12-24 hours, maximum daily dose: 200 mg/**day**

Anthrax (if strain is proven susceptible): Note: In the presence of systemic involvement, extensive edema, and/or lesions on head/neck, doxycycline should initially be administered IV Initial treatment should include two or more agents per CDC recommendations. Agents suggested for use in conjunction with doxycycline include rifampin, vancomycin, penicillin, ampicillin, chloramphenicol, imipenem, clindamycin, or clarithromycin. For bioterrorism postexposure, continue combined therapy for 60 days; if natural exposure, administer 7-10 days of therapy.

Treatment: IV: 2.2 mg/kg/dose every 12 hours (maximum dose: 100 mg/dose); may switch to oral therapy (same dosing) when clinically appropriate

Prophylaxis; postexposure (inhalation or cutaneous): Oral: 2.2 mg/kg/dose every 12 hours for 60 days (maximum dose: 100 mg/dose)

Brucellosis: Oral: 1-2 mg/kg/dose twice daily for 6 weeks (maximum dose: 100 mg/dose); use in combination with rifampin

Chlamydial infections, uncomplicated: Oral: 100 mg/dose twice daily for 7 days

Lyme disease, Q fever, or Tularemia: Oral: 100 mg/dose twice daily for 14-21 days

Malaria:

Treatment: Oral, IV: 2.2 mg/kg/dose twice daily for 7 days (maximum dose: 100 mg/dose) (CDC, 2011); for uncomplicated cases, combination therapy with quinine sulfate is recommended; in severe cases, combination therapy with quinidine gluconate should be used; **Note:** Duration of either quinine sulfate or quinidine gluconate is region-specific; consult CDC for current recommendations.

Prophylaxis: Oral: 2.2 mg/kg/dose once daily (maximum dose: 100 mg/day) starting 1-2 days before travel to the area with endemic infection, continuing daily during travel and for 4 weeks after leaving endemic area; maximum duration of prophylaxis: 4 months

MRSA, community-acquired cellulitis (purulent); skin/soft tissue infections: Oral:

≤45 kg: 2 mg/kg/dose every 12 hours for 5-10 days

>45 kg: 100 mg twice daily for 5-10 days (Liu, 2011)

Tickborne rickettsial disease or Ehrlichiosis: >45 kg: Oral, IV: 100 mg every 12 hours. Severe or complicated disease may require longer treatment; HGA should be treated for 10-14 days

Adolescents and Adults:

General dosing: Oral, IV: 100-200 mg/day in 1-2 divided doses

Anthrax (if strain is proven susceptible): Refer to Children's dosing for **"Note"** on route, combined therapy, and duration

Treatment: IV: 100 mg every 12 hours for 60 days (substitute oral antibiotics for IV antibiotics as soon as clinical condition improves)

Prophylaxis; postexposure (inhalation or cutaneous): Oral: 100 mg every 12 hours for 60 days

Chlamydial infections, uncomplicated: Oral: 100 mg/dose twice daily for 7 days

Lyme disease, Q fever, or Tularemia: Oral: 100 mg/dose twice daily for 14-21 days

Malaria:

Treatment: Oral, IV: 100 mg twice daily for 7 days (CDC, 2011); for uncomplicated cases, combination therapy with quinine sulfate is recommended; in severe cases, combination therapy with quinidine gluconate should be used; **Note:** Duration of either quinine sulfate or quinidine gluconate is region-specific; consult CDC for current recommendations.

Prophylaxis: Oral: 100 mg/dose once daily starting 1-2 days before travel to the area with endemic infection, continuing daily during travel, and for 4 weeks after leaving endemic area; maximum duration of prophylaxis: 4 months

MRSA, community-acquired cellulitis (purulent): Oral: 100 mg twice daily for 5-10 days (Liu, 2011)

Nongonococcal urethritis caused by *C. trachomatis* or *U. urealyticum*: Oral: 100 mg/dose twice daily for 7 days

Pelvic inflammatory disease:

Treatment, inpatient: Oral, IV: 100 mg every 12 hours for 14 days administered with cefoxitin or cefotetan; may transition to oral doxycycline (add clindamycin or metronidazole if tubo-ovarian abscess present) to complete the 14 days of therapy (CDC, 2010)

Treatment, outpatient: Oral: 100 mg every 12 hours for 14 days (with or without metronidazole); preceded by a single IM dose of cefoxitin (plus oral probenecid) or ceftriaxone (CDC, 2010)

Periodontitis: Oral (Periostat®): 20 mg twice daily as an adjunct following scaling and root planing; may be administered for up to 9 months

Rosacea: Oral (Oracea®): 40 mg once daily in the morning. **Note:** Oracea® capsules are not bioequivalent to other doxycycline products.

Sclerosing agent for pleural effusion: 500 mg in 25-30 mL of NS instilled into the pleural space to control pleural effusions associated with metastatic tumors; or for recurrent malignant pleural effusions: 500 mg in 250 mL NS

Tickborne rickettsial disease or ehrlichiosis: Oral, IV: 100 mg every 12 hours. Severe or complicated disease may require longer treatment; HGA should be treated for 10-14 days

Dosing adjustment in renal impairment: No adjustment necessary

Preparation for Administration Parenteral: IV: Reconstitute each 100 mg vial with 10 mL SWFI or other compatible solution, resulting in a concentration of 10 mg/mL; following reconstitution, further dilute with a compatible solution to a final concentration of 0.1 to 1 mg/mL.

Administration

Oral: Administer capsules or tablets with adequate amounts of fluid; avoid antacids, infant formula, milk, dairy products, and iron for 1 hour before or 2 hours after administration of doxycycline (unless extemporaneously prepared in the instance of public health emergency when milk or pudding is appropriate); may be administered with food to decrease GI upset; shake suspension well before use

Doryx: May break up the tablet and sprinkle the delayed release pellets on a spoonful of applesauce. Do **not** crush or damage the delayed release pellets; loss or damage of pellets prevents using the dose. Swallow the Doryx/applesauce mixture immediately without chewing. Discard mixture if it cannot be used immediately.

Parenteral: For IV use only; administer over 1 to 4 hours; avoid rapid infusion

Sclerosing agent:

To control pleural effusions associated with metastatic tumors: Instill into the pleural space through a thoracostomy tube following drainage of the accumulated pleural fluid; clamp the tube then remove the fluid

For recurrent malignant pleural effusions: Administer via chest tube lavage, clamp tube for 24 hours then drain

Monitoring Parameters Periodic monitoring of renal, hematologic, and hepatic function tests; observe for changes in bowel frequency

Test Interactions Injectable tetracycline formulations (if they contain large amounts of ascorbic acid) may result in a false-negative urine glucose using glucose oxidase tests (eg, Clinistix, Diastix, Tes-Tape); false elevations of urinary catecholamines with fluorescence

Additional Information Injection contains ascorbic acid. According to the CDC, staining of the teeth is negligible with short courses of doxycycline and is of minimal consequence in children >6 or 7 years of age because visible tooth formation is complete by this age. Benefits outweigh the risks for rickettsial infections, ehrlichiosis, anthrax, and cholera (CDC, 2006; *Red Book*, 2009). Oracea® capsules are not bioequivalent to other doxycycline products.

Dosage Forms Considerations

Alodox Convenience kits contain doxycycline tablets 20 mg, plus eyelid cleanser

Morgidox kits contain doxycycline capsules 100 mg, plus AcuWash moisturizing Daily Cleanser

NizAzel Doxy kits contain doxycycline tablets 100 mg, plus NicAzel FORTE dietary supplement tablets

Ocudox kits contain doxycycline capsules 50 mg, plus eyelid cleanser and Tears Again Advanced eyelid spray

Dosage Forms Excipient information presented when available (limited, particularly for generics); consult specific product labeling. [DSC] = Discontinued product

Capsule, Oral, as hyclate [strength expressed as base]:

Morgidox: 100 mg [contains brilliant blue fcf (fd&c blue #1)]

Vibramycin: 100 mg [contains brilliant blue fcf (fd&c blue #1)]

Generic: 50 mg, 100 mg

Capsule, Oral, as monohydrate [strength expressed as base]:

Adoxa: 150 mg [contains fd&c red #40, fd&c yellow #6 (sunset yellow)]

Monodox: 75 mg, 100 mg

Generic: 50 mg, 75 mg, 100 mg, 150 mg

Capsule Delayed Release, Oral, as monohydrate [strength expressed as base]:

Oracea: 40 mg

Generic: 40 mg

Kit, Combination, as hyclate [strength expressed as base]:

Alodox Convenience: 20 mg [DSC]

Morgidox: 1 x 100 mg, 2 x 100 mg [contains brilliant blue fcf (fd&c blue #1), cetyl alcohol, edetate disodium]

Ocudox: 50 mg [DSC] [contains brilliant blue fcf (fd&c blue #1)]

Kit, Oral, as monohydrate [strength expressed as base]:
NicAzelDoxy 30: 100 mg [DSC] [contains brilliant blue fcf (fd&c blue #1), fd&c yellow #10 aluminum lake, fd&c yellow #6 (sunset yellow), fd&c yellow #6 aluminum lake, tartrazine (fd&c yellow #5)]
NicAzelDoxy 60: 100 mg [DSC] [contains brilliant blue fcf (fd&c blue #1), fd&c yellow #10 aluminum lake, fd&c yellow #6 (sunset yellow), fd&c yellow #6 aluminum lake, tartrazine (fd&c yellow #5)]
Solution Reconstituted, Intravenous, as hyclate [strength expressed as base, preservative free]:
Doxy 100: 100 mg (1 ea)
Generic: 100 mg (1 ea)
Suspension Reconstituted, Oral, as monohydrate:
Generic: 25 mg/5 mL (60 mL)
Suspension Reconstituted, Oral, as monohydrate [strength expressed as base]:
Vibramycin: 25 mg/5 mL (60 mL) [contains brilliant blue fcf (fd&c blue #1), methylparaben, propylparaben; raspberry flavor]
Generic: 25 mg/5 mL (60 mL)
Syrup, Oral, as calcium [strength expressed as base]:
Vibramycin: 50 mg/5 mL (473 mL) [contains butylparaben, propylene glycol, propylparaben, sodium metabisulfite; raspberry-apple flavor]
Tablet, Oral, as hyclate [strength expressed as base]:
Acticlate: 75 mg [contains brilliant blue fcf (fd&c blue #1), fd&c yellow #6 (sunset yellow)]
Acticlate: 150 mg [scored; contains fd&c blue #2 (indigotine)]
TargaDOX: 50 mg [contains fd&c blue #2 (indigotine), fd&c yellow #6 (sunset yellow)]
Generic: 20 mg, 100 mg
Tablet, Oral, as monohydrate [strength expressed as base]:
Adoxa: 50 mg
Adoxa: 75 mg [contains fd&c yellow #10 aluminum lake, fd&c yellow #6 (sunset yellow)]
Adoxa: 100 mg
Adoxa Pak 1/100: 100 mg [contains fd&c yellow #10 aluminum lake, fd&c yellow #6 (sunset yellow)]
Adoxa Pak 2/100: 100 mg [contains fd&c yellow #10 aluminum lake, fd&c yellow #6 (sunset yellow)]
Adoxa Pak 1/150: 150 mg [scored; contains fd&c yellow #6 (sunset yellow)]
Avidoxy: 100 mg [contains fd&c yellow #10 aluminum lake, fd&c yellow #6 aluminum lake]
Generic: 50 mg, 75 mg, 100 mg, 150 mg
Tablet Delayed Release, Oral, as hyclate [strength expressed as base]:
Doryx: 50 mg
Doryx: 150 mg, 200 mg [scored]
Generic: 75 mg, 100 mg, 150 mg

Extemporaneous Preparations If a public health emergency is declared and liquid doxycycline is unavailable for the treatment of anthrax, emergency doses may be prepared for children or adults who cannot swallow tablets.

Add 20 mL of water to one 100 mg tablet. Allow tablet to soak in the water for 5 minutes to soften. Crush into a fine powder and stir until well mixed. Appropriate dose should be taken from this mixture. To increase palatability, mix with food or drink. If mixing with drink, add 15 mL of milk, chocolate milk, chocolate pudding, or apple juice to the appropriate dose of mixture. If using apple juice, also add 4 teaspoons of sugar. Doxycycline and water mixture may be stored at room temperature for up to 24 hours.

US Food and Drug Administration, Center for Drug Evaluation and Research, "Public Health Emergency Home Preparation Instructions for Doxycycline." Available at http://www.fda.gov/Drugs/EmergencyPreparedness/BioterrorismandDrugPreparedness/ucm130996.htm

◆ **Doxycycline Calcium** *see* Doxycycline *on page 717*

◆ **Doxycycline Hyclate** *see* Doxycycline *on page 717*

◆ **Doxycycline Monohydrate** *see* Doxycycline *on page 717*

Doxylamine (dox IL a meen)

Medication Safety Issues

Sound-alike/look-alike issues:

Doxylamine may be confused with doxycycline

BEERS Criteria medication:

This drug may be potentially inappropriate for use in geriatric patients (Quality of evidence - moderate; Strength of recommendation - strong).

Brand Names: US Aldex AN [OTC]; Doxytex; Nitetime Sleep-Aid [OTC]; Sleep Aid [OTC]

Brand Names: Canada Unisom-2

Therapeutic Category Antihistamine

Generic Availability (US) May be product dependent

Use

Oral liquid: Temporary relief of rhinorrhea; sneezing; itchy nose or throat; and itchy, watery eyes due to hay fever or other respiratory allergies (FDA approved in ages 2 to <6 years)

Tablets: Treatment of short-term insomnia (with difficulty of sleep onset) (OTC products: FDA approved in ages ≥12 years and adults)

Pregnancy Risk Factor C

Pregnancy Considerations Animal reproduction studies were not conducted by the manufacturer. Maternal use of doxylamine in combination with pyridoxine during pregnancy has not been shown to increase the baseline risk of major malformations. Doxylamine is recommended for the treatment of nausea and vomiting of pregnancy (ACOG 2004). Antihistamines are recommended for the treatment of rhinitis in pregnant women (although second generation antihistamines may be preferred) (Wallace 2008).

Breast-Feeding Considerations Use of doxylamine is contraindicated in nursing women. Doxylamine succinate is expected to be found in breast milk and adverse events (unusual excitement, irritability, sedation) may be expected in a nursing infant. Infants with apnea or other respiratory conditions may be more vulnerable.

Contraindications Hypersensitivity to doxylamine or any component of the formulation; newborns; breast-feeding women

Documentation of allergenic cross-reactivity for antihistamines is limited. However, because of similarities in chemical structure and/or pharmacologic actions, the possibility of cross-sensitivity cannot be ruled out with certainty.

OTC labeling: Do not use in children <12 years of age.

Canadian labeling: Additional contraindications (not in U.S. labeling): Narrow angle glaucoma; asthmatic attack; prostatic hypertrophy; stenosing peptic ulcer, pyloroduodenal obstruction; bladder-neck obstruction; concurrent use with monoamine oxidase-inhibitors.

Warnings/Precautions May cause drowsiness; patient should avoid tasks requiring alertness (eg, driving, operating machinery) until effects are known. Effects may be potentiated when used with other sedative drugs or ethanol. Antihistamines may cause paradoxical excitation in young children. Use with caution in patients with angle-closure glaucoma, respiratory disease, urinary tract obstruction (including bladder neck obstruction and symptomatic prostatic hyperplasia), pyloroduodenal obstruction (including stenotic peptic ulcer), thyroid dysfunction, increased intraocular pressure, and cardiovascular disease (including hypertension and ischemic heart disease); Canadian labeling contraindicates use in narrow angle (ie, angle-closure) glaucoma, prostatic hypertrophy and bladder-neck obstruction, pyloroduodenal obstruction (including stenotic peptic ulcer), and asthmatic attack. If sleeplessness persists for >2 weeks, consult health care provider. In the elderly, avoid use of this potent anticholinergic agent due to increased risk of confusion, dry mouth, constipation, and other anticholinergic effects; clearance decreases in patients of advanced age; tolerance develops to hypnotic effects (Beers Criteria). Do not use for insomnia in children <12 years of age. Potentially significant interactions may exist, requiring dose or frequency adjustment, additional monitoring, and/or selection of alternative therapy. Consult drug interactions database for more detailed information.

Warnings: Additional Pediatric Considerations Safety and efficacy for the use of cough and cold products in pediatric patients <4 years of age is limited; the AAP warns against the use of these products for respiratory illnesses in this age group. Serious adverse effects including death have been reported. Many of these products contain multiple active ingredients, increasing the risk of accidental overdose when used with other products. The FDA notes that there are no approved OTC uses for these products in pediatric patients <2 years of age. Health care providers are reminded to ask caregivers about the use of OTC cough and cold products in order to avoid exposure to multiple medications containing the same ingredient (AAP 2012; FDA 2008).

Adverse Reactions

Cardiovascular: Palpitation, tachycardia

Central nervous system: Dizziness, disorientation, drowsiness, headache, paradoxical CNS stimulation, vertigo

Gastrointestinal: Anorexia, dry mucous membranes, diarrhea, constipation, epigastric pain, xerostomia

Genitourinary: Dysuria, urinary retention

Ocular: Blurred vision, diplopia

Drug Interactions

Metabolism/Transport Effects None known.

Avoid Concomitant Use

Avoid concomitant use of Doxylamine with any of the following: Aclidinium; Azelastine (Nasal); Eluxadoline; Glucagon; Ipratropium (Oral Inhalation); Orphenadrine; Paraldehyde; Potassium Chloride; Thalidomide; Tiotropium; Umeclidinium

Increased Effect/Toxicity

Doxylamine may increase the levels/effects of: AbobotulinumtoxinA; Anticholinergic Agents; Azelastine (Nasal); Buprenorphine; CNS Depressants; Eluxadoline; Glucagon; Hydrocodone; Methotrimeprazine; Metyrosine; Mirabegron; Mirtazapine; OnabotulinumtoxinA; Orphenadrine; Paraldehyde; Potassium Chloride; Pramipexole; RimabotulinumtoxinB; ROPINIRole; Rotigotine; Selective Serotonin Reuptake Inhibitors; Suvorexant; Thalidomide; Thiazide Diuretics; Tiotropium; Topiramate; Zolpidem

The levels/effects of Doxylamine may be increased by: Aclidinium; Alcohol (Ethyl); Brimonidine (Topical); Cannabis; Dronabinol; Droperidol; HydrOXYzine; Ipratropium (Oral Inhalation); Kava Kava; Magnesium Sulfate; MAO Inhibitors; Methotrimeprazine; Mianserin; Nabilone; Perampanel; Pramlintide; Rufinamide; Sodium Oxybate; Tapentadol; Tetrahydrocannabinol; Umeclidinium

Decreased Effect

Doxylamine may decrease the levels/effects of: Acetylcholinesterase Inhibitors; Benzylpenicilloyl Polylysine; Betahistine; Hyaluronidase; Itopride; Metoclopramide; Secretin

The levels/effects of Doxylamine may be decreased by: Acetylcholinesterase Inhibitors; Amphetamines

Storage/Stability Store at 15°C to 30°C (59°F to 86°F).

Mechanism of Action Doxylamine competes with histamine for H_1-receptor sites on effector cells; blocks chemoreceptor trigger zone, diminishes vestibular stimulation, and depresses labyrinthine function through its central anticholinergic activity.

Pharmacokinetics (Adult data unless noted)

Metabolism: Hepatic by N-dealkylation to metabolites

Half-life: 10 to 12 hours (Friedman, 1985; Paton, 1985)

Time to peak: 2 to 4 hours (Friedman, 1985; Friedman, 1989; Paton, 1985)

Elimination: Urine (primarily as metabolites)

Dosing: Usual

Pediatric:

Allergies; hay fever: Children 2 to <6 years: Liquid: Oral: 2.5 mg every 4 to 6 hours; maximum daily dose: 15 mg in 24 hours or as instructed by health care professional

Insomnia: Children ≥12 years and Adolescents: Tablets: Oral: 25 mg once daily before bedtime or as instructed by health care professional

Adult: **Insomnia:** Oral: 25 mg once daily before bedtime or as instructed by health care professional

Dosing adjustment in renal impairment: Children ≥2 years, Adolescents, and Adults. There are no dosage adjustments provided in manufacturer's labeling.

Dosing adjustment in hepatic impairment: Children ≥2 years, Adolescents, and Adults. There are no dosage adjustments provided in manufacturer's labeling.

Administration Oral: Take 30 minutes prior to bedtime

Test Interactions May interfere with urine detection of methadone (false-positive) (Hausmann, 1983).

Dosage Forms Excipient information presented when available (limited, particularly for generics); consult specific product labeling.

Liquid, Oral, as succinate:

Doxytex: 2.5 mg/2.5 mL (473 mL) [alcohol free, sugar free; apple sauce flavor]

Tablet, Oral, as succinate:

Nitetime Sleep-Aid: 25 mg [scored]

Sleep Aid: 25 mg [scored; contains fd&c blue #1 aluminum lake]

Tablet Chewable, Oral, as succinate:

Aldex AN: 5 mg [contains fd&c red #40, fd&c yellow #10 (quinoline yellow); orange flavor]

- ◆ **Doxylamine Succinate** *see* Doxylamine *on page* 721
- ◆ **Doxytab (Can)** *see* Doxycycline *on page* 717
- ◆ **Doxytex** *see* Doxylamine *on page* 721
- ◆ **DPA** *see* Valproic Acid and Derivatives *on page* 2143
- ◆ **DPE** *see* Dipivefrin *on page* 687
- ◆ **D-Penicillamine** *see* PenicillAMINE *on page* 1652
- ◆ **DPH** *see* Phenytoin *on page* 1690
- ◆ **Dramamine [OTC]** *see* DimenhyDRINATE *on page* 664
- ◆ **Dramamine Less Drowsy [OTC]** *see* Meclizine *on page* 1337
- ◆ **Dr Gs Clear Nail [OTC]** *see* Tolnaftate *on page* 2083
- ◆ **Driminate [OTC]** *see* DimenhyDRINATE *on page* 664
- ◆ **Drisdol** *see* Ergocalciferol *on page* 772
- ◆ **Dristan Long Lasting Nasal (Can)** *see* Oxymetazoline (Nasal) *on page* 1599
- ◆ **Dristan Spray [OTC]** *see* Oxymetazoline (Nasal) *on page* 1599
- ◆ **Drixoral Nasal (Can)** *see* Oxymetazoline (Nasal) *on page* 1599
- ◆ **Drixoral® ND (Can)** *see* Pseudoephedrine *on page* 1801

Dronabinol (droe NAB i nol)

Medication Safety Issues

Sound-alike/look-alike issues:

Dronabinol may be confused with droperidol

Brand Names: US Marinol

Therapeutic Category Antiemetic

Generic Availability (US) Yes

Use Treatment of nausea and vomiting secondary to cancer chemotherapy in patients who have not responded to conventional antiemetics; treatment of anorexia associated with weight loss in AIDS patients

Pregnancy Risk Factor C

Pregnancy Considerations Adverse events have been observed in animal reproduction studies.

Breast-Feeding Considerations Dronabinol is excreted in breast milk. Breast-feeding is not recommended by the manufacturer.

Contraindications Hypersensitivity to dronabinol, cannabinoids, sesame oil, or any component of the formulation.

Warnings/Precautions Use with caution in patients with seizure disorders and in the elderly. May cause occasional hypotension, possible hypertension, syncope, or tachycardia; use with caution in patients with cardiac disorders. May cause CNS depression, which may impair physical or mental abilities; patients must be cautioned about performing tasks that require mental alertness (eg, operating machinery, driving).

Administration with phenothiazines (eg, prochlorperazine) for the management of chemotherapy-induced nausea and vomiting may result in improved efficacy (compared to either drug alone) without additional toxicity. Use with caution in patients with a history of substance abuse, including alcohol abuse or dependence; potential for drug dependency exists. Tolerance, psychological and physical dependence may occur with prolonged use. May cause withdrawal symptoms upon abrupt discontinuation. Use with caution in patients with mania, depression, or schizophrenia; careful psychiatric monitoring is recommended.

Adverse Reactions

Cardiovascular: Palpitations, tachycardia, vasodilation/facial flushing

Central nervous system: Abnormal thinking, amnesia, anxiety, ataxia, depersonalization, dizziness, euphoria, hallucination, paranoia, somnolence

Gastrointestinal: Abdominal pain, nausea, vomiting

Neuromuscular & skeletal: Weakness

Rare but important or life-threatening: Conjunctivitis, depression, diarrhea, fatigue, fecal incontinence, flushing, hypotension, myalgia, nightmares, seizure, speech difficulties, tinnitus, vision difficulties

Drug Interactions

Metabolism/Transport Effects Substrate of CYP2C9 (minor), CYP3A4 (minor); **Note:** Assignment of Major/Minor substrate status based on clinically relevant drug interaction potential

Avoid Concomitant Use There are no known interactions where it is recommended to avoid concomitant use.

Increased Effect/Toxicity

Dronabinol may increase the levels/effects of: Alcohol (Ethyl); CNS Depressants; Sympathomimetics

The levels/effects of Dronabinol may be increased by: Anticholinergic Agents; Cocaine; CYP2C9 Inhibitors (Moderate); CYP2C9 Inhibitors (Strong); CYP3A4 Inhibitors (Moderate); CYP3A4 Inhibitors (Strong); MAO Inhibitors; Ritonavir

Decreased Effect

The levels/effects of Dronabinol may be decreased by: CYP3A4 Inducers (Strong)

Storage/Stability Store in a cool environment between 8°C and 15°C (46°F and 59°F) or refrigerated; protect from freezing.

Mechanism of Action Dronabinol (synthetic delta-9-tetrahydrocannabinol [delta-9-THC]), an active cannabinoid and natural occurring component of *Cannabis sativa L.* (marijuana), activates cannabinoid receptors CB_1 and CB_2. Activation of the CB_1 receptor produces marijuana-like effects on psyche and circulation, whereas activation of the CB_2 receptor does not. Dronabinol has approximately equal affinity for the CB_1 and CB_2 receptors; however, efficacy is less at CB_2 receptors. Activation of the cannabinoid system with dronabinol causes psychological effects that can be divided into 4 groups: affective (euphoria and easy laughter); sensory (increased perception of external stimuli and of the person's own body); somatic (feeling of the body floating or sinking in the bed); and cognitive (distortion of time perception, memory lapses, difficulty in concentration). Most effects (eg, analgesia, appetite enhancement, muscle relaxation, hormonal actions) are mediated by central cannabinoid receptors (CB_1), their distribution reflecting many of the medicinal benefits and adverse effects (Grotenhermen 2003).

Pharmacodynamics

Onset of action: 30 minutes to 1 hour

Maximum effect: 2-4 hours

Duration:

Psychoactive effects: 4-6 hours

Appetite stimulation: 24 hours

Pharmacokinetics (Adult data unless noted)

Absorption: Oral: 90% to 95%; first-pass metabolism results in low systemic bioavailability

Distribution: V_d: ~10L/kg

Protein binding: ~97%

Metabolism: Extensive first-pass; metabolized in the liver to several metabolites some of which are active

Bioavailability: 10% to 20%

Half-life:

Biphasic: Alpha: 4 hours

Terminal: 25-36 hours

Dronabinol metabolites: 44-59 hours

Time to peak serum concentration: Within 0.5-4 hours

Elimination: Biliary excretion is the major route of elimination; 50% excreted in feces within 72 hours; 10% to 15% excreted in urine within 72 hours

Clearance: Adults: Mean 0.2 L/kg/hour (highly variable)

Dosing: Usual Oral:

Antiemetic: Children and Adults: 5 mg/m^2 1-3 hours before chemotherapy, then give 5 mg/m^2/dose every 2-4 hours after chemotherapy for a total of 4-6 doses/day; dose may be increased in 2.5 mg/m^2 increments to a maximum of 15 mg/m^2 per dose if needed

Alternative dosing: Adults: 5 mg 3-4 times/day; dosage may be escalated during a chemotherapy cycle or at subsequent cycles depending upon response

Appetite stimulant: Adults: 2.5 mg twice daily before lunch and dinner; if intolerant, a dosage of 2.5 mg once daily at night may be tried; maximum dosage (escalating): 10 mg twice daily

Administration May be administered without regard to meals; take before meals if used to stimulate appetite

Monitoring Parameters Heart rate, blood pressure

Controlled Substance C-III

Dosage Forms Excipient information presented when available (limited, particularly for generics); consult specific product labeling.

Capsule, Oral:

Marinol: 2.5 mg, 5 mg, 10 mg [contains sesame oil]

Generic: 2.5 mg, 5 mg, 10 mg

Droperidol (droe PER i dole)

Medication Safety Issues

Sound-alike/look-alike issues:

Droperidol may be confused with dronabinol

Brand Names: Canada Droperidol Injection, USP

Therapeutic Category Antiemetic

Generic Availability (US) Yes

Use Reduce the incidence of nausea and vomiting associated with surgical and diagnostic procedures in patients for whom other treatments are ineffective or inappropriate (FDA approved in ages ≥2 years and adults)

Pregnancy Risk Factor C

Pregnancy Considerations Adverse events were observed in some animal reproduction studies. Although use in pregnancy has been reported, due to cases of QT prolongation and torsade de pointes (some fatal), use of other agents in pregnant women is preferred (ACOG, 2004).

Breast-Feeding Considerations It is not known if droperidol is excreted in breast milk. The manufacturer recommends that caution be exercised when administering droperidol to nursing women.

Contraindications Hypersensitivity to droperidol or any component of the formulation; known or suspected QT prolongation, including congenital long QT syndrome (prolonged QTc is defined as >440 msec in males or >450 msec in females)

Canadian labeling: Additional contraindications (not in U.S. labeling): Not for use in children ≤2 years of age

Warnings/Precautions May alter cardiac conduction. **[U.S. Boxed Warning]: Cases of QT prolongation and torsade de pointes, including some fatal cases, have been reported.** Use extreme caution in patients with bradycardia (<50 bpm), cardiac disease, concurrent MAO inhibitor therapy, Class I and Class III antiarrhythmics or other drugs known to prolong QT interval, and electrolyte disturbances (hypokalemia or hypomagnesemia), including concomitant drugs which may alter electrolytes (diuretics).

Use with caution in patients with seizures or severe liver disease. May be sedating, use with caution in disorders where CNS depression is a feature. Caution in patients with hemodynamic instability, predisposition to seizures, subcortical brain damage, pheochromocytoma or renal disease. Esophageal dysmotility and aspiration have been associated with antipsychotic use - use with caution in patients at risk of pneumonia (ie, Alzheimer's disease). Caution in breast cancer or other prolactin-dependent tumors (may elevate prolactin levels). May alter temperature regulation or mask toxicity of other drugs due to antiemetic effects. May cause orthostatic hypotension - use with caution in patients at risk of this effect or those who would tolerate transient hypotensive episodes (cerebrovascular disease, cardiovascular disease, or other medications which may predispose). Significant hypotension may occur.

May cause anticholinergic effects (confusion, agitation, constipation, xerostomia, blurred vision, urinary retention). Therefore, they should be used with caution in patients with decreased gastrointestinal motility, urinary retention, BPH, xerostomia, visual problems, or narrow-angle glaucoma (screening is recommended). Relative to other neuroleptics, droperidol has a low potency of cholinergic blockade.

May cause extrapyramidal symptoms, including pseudoparkinsonism, acute dystonic reactions, akathisia, and tardive dyskinesia. Risk of dystonia (and possibly other EPS) may be greater with increased doses, use of conventional antipsychotics, males, and younger patients. Risk of tardive dyskinesia and potential for irreversibility may be increased in elderly patients (particularly women), prolonged therapy, and higher total cumulative dose. May be associated with neuroleptic malignant syndrome (NMS). May mask toxicity of other drugs or conditions (eg, intestinal obstruction, Reye's syndrome, brain tumor) due to antiemetic effects. Use with caution in the elderly; reduce initial dose.

Warnings: Additional Pediatric Considerations Not recommended for routine use in children for ambulatory operative procedures unless patient is being admitted to the hospital and other antiemetic therapies have failed (Gan, 2007).

Adverse Reactions

Cardiovascular: Cardiac arrest, hypertension, hypotension (especially orthostatic), QTc prolongation (dose dependent), tachycardia, torsade de pointes, ventricular tachycardia

Central nervous system: Anxiety, chills, depression (postoperative, transient), dizziness, drowsiness (postoperative) increased, dysphoria, extrapyramidal symptoms (akathisia, dystonia, oculogyric crisis), hallucinations (postoperative), hyperactivity, neuroleptic malignant syndrome (NMS) (rare), restlessness

Respiratory: Bronchospasm, laryngospasm

Miscellaneous: Anaphylaxis, shivering

Drug Interactions

Metabolism/Transport Effects None known.

Avoid Concomitant Use

Avoid concomitant use of Droperidol with any of the following: Aclidinium; Amisulpride; Azelastine (Nasal); Eluxadoline; Glucagon; Highest Risk QTc-Prolonging Agents; Ipratropium (Oral Inhalation); Ivabradine; Metoclopramide; Mifepristone; Orphenadrine; Paraldehyde; Potassium Chloride; Sulpiride; Thalidomide; Tiotropium; Umeclidinium

Increased Effect/Toxicity

Droperidol may increase the levels/effects of: AbobotulinumtoxinA; Alcohol (Ethyl); Amisulpride; Anticholinergic Agents; Azelastine (Nasal); Buprenorphine; CNS Depressants; Eluxadoline; Glucagon; Highest Risk QTc-Prolonging Agents; Hydrocodone; Mequitazine; Methotrimeprazine; Methylphenidate; Metoclopramide; Mirabegron; Moderate Risk QTc-Prolonging Agents; OnabotulinumtoxinA; Orphenadrine; Paraldehyde; Potassium Chloride; RimabotulinumtoxinB; Selective Serotonin Reuptake Inhibitors; Serotonin Modulators; Sulpiride; Suvorexant; Thalidomide; Thiazide Diuretics; Tiotropium; Zolpidem

The levels/effects of Droperidol may be increased by: Acetylcholinesterase Inhibitors (Central); Aclidinium; Brimonidine (Topical); Cannabis; Dronabinol; Ipratropium (Oral Inhalation); Ivabradine; Kava Kava; Lithium; Magnesium Sulfate; MAO Inhibitors; Methotrimeprazine; Methylphenidate; Metyrosine; Mifepristone; Nabilone; Perampanel; Pramlintide; QTc-Prolonging Agents (Indeterminate Risk and Risk Modifying); Rufinamide; Serotonin Modulators; Sodium Oxybate; Tapentadol; Tetrahydrocannabinol; Umeclidinium

Decreased Effect

Droperidol may decrease the levels/effects of: Acetylcholinesterase Inhibitors; Amphetamines; Anti-Parkinson's Agents (Dopamine Agonist); Itopride; Quinagolide; Secretin

The levels/effects of Droperidol may be decreased by: Acetylcholinesterase Inhibitors; Anti-Parkinson's Agents (Dopamine Agonist); Lithium

Storage/Stability Store at 20°C to 25°C (68°F to 77°F); excursions permitted to 15°C to 30°C (59°F to 86°F). Protect from light. Solutions diluted in NS or D_5W are stable at room temperature for up to 7 days in PVC bags or glass bottles. Solutions diluted in LR are stable at room temperature for 24 hours in PVC bags and up to 7 days in glass bottles.

Mechanism of Action Droperidol is a butyrophenone antipsychotic; antiemetic effect is a result of blockade of dopamine stimulation of the chemoreceptor trigger zone. Other effects include alpha-adrenergic blockade, peripheral vascular dilation, and reduction of the pressor effect of epinephrine resulting in hypotension and decreased peripheral vascular resistance; may also reduce pulmonary artery pressure

Pharmacodynamics

Onset of action: 3-10 minutes

Maximum effect: Within 30 minutes

Duration: 2-4 hours (up to 12 hours)

Pharmacokinetics (Adult data unless noted)

V_d: Children: ~0.6 L/kg; Adults: ~1.5 L/kg (McKeage, 2006)

Absorption: IM: Rapid (Cressman, 1973)

Protein binding: 85% to 90% (McKeage, 2006)

Metabolism: Hepatic, to *p*-fluorophenylacetic acid, benzimidazolone, *p*-hydroxypiperidine

Half-life: Children: 1.7 hours; adults: 1.7 to 2.2 hours (McKeage, 2006)

Elimination: In urine (75%; <1% as unchanged drug) and feces (22%) (Cressman, 1973; McKeage, 2006)

Dosing: Usual Dosage must be individualized, based on age, body weight, underlying medical conditions, physical status, concomitant medications, type of anesthesia, and surgical procedure

Children 2-12 years:

Postoperative nausea and vomiting (PONV):

Prevention, if high risk for PONV: IM, IV: 0.01-0.015 mg/kg/dose given near the end of surgery (Gan, 2007); maximum dose: 1.25 mg; administer additional doses after at least 6 hours with caution and only if potential benefit outweighs risks; **Note:** Previous reports suggested a higher dose of 0.075 mg/kg as effective; however, due to side-effects associated with the higher doses, doses >0.05 mg/kg are considered excessive and no longer recommended (Gan, 2007; Henzi, 2000).

Treatment (not first line): IV:

Manufacturer's labeling: **Maximum** initial dose: 0.1 mg/kg/dose; administer additional doses with extreme caution and only if potential benefit outweighs risks

Alternate dosing: Doses as low as 0.01-0.015 mg/kg/dose (up to 0.03 mg/kg) may be effective for breakthrough nausea and vomiting; maximum initial dose: 0.1 mg/kg; administer additional doses after at least 6 hours with caution and only if potential benefit outweighs risks

Adults:

Prevention of PONV: IM, IV:

Manufacturer labeling: Maximum initial dose: 2.5 mg; additional doses of 1.25 mg may be administered with caution to achieve desired effect

Consensus guideline recommendations: 0.625-1.25 mg IV administered at the end of surgery (Gan, 2007)

Dosage adjustment in renal impairment: Specific dosing recommendations are not provided; use with caution.

Dosage adjustment in hepatic impairment: Specific dosing recommendations are not provided; use with caution.

Administration Parenteral: Administer undiluted IM or by slow IV injection over 2 to 5 minutes

Monitoring Parameters Prior to use: 12-lead ECG to identify patients with QT prolongation (use is contraindicated); continuous ECG during and for 2-3 hours after dosage administration is recommended. Blood pressure, heart rate, respiratory rate; serum potassium and magnesium; observe for dystonias, extrapyramidal side effects; temperature

Dosage Forms Excipient information presented when available (limited, particularly for generics); consult specific product labeling.

Solution, Injection:

Generic: 2.5 mg/mL (2 mL)

◆ **Droperidol Injection, USP (Can)** *see* Droperidol *on page 723*

◆ **Droxia** *see* Hydroxyurea *on page 1055*

◆ **Dr. Smith's Diaper Rash [OTC]** *see* Zinc Oxide *on page 2214*

◆ **DRV** *see* Darunavir *on page 588*

◆ **Drymira (Can)** *see* Ciclesonide (Nasal) *on page 454*

◆ **DSCG** *see* Cromolyn (Nasal) *on page 542*

◆ **DSCG** *see* Cromolyn (Ophthalmic) *on page 543*

◆ **DSCG** *see* Cromolyn (Systemic, Oral Inhalation) *on page 541*

◆ **DSS** *see* Docusate *on page 697*

◆ **DT** *see* Diphtheria and Tetanus Toxoids *on page 674*

◆ **DTaP** *see* Diphtheria and Tetanus Toxoids, and Acellular Pertussis Vaccine *on page 681*

◆ **DTaP-HepB-IPV** *see* Diphtheria, Tetanus Toxoids, Acellular Pertussis, Hepatitis B (Recombinant), and Poliovirus (Inactivated) Vaccine *on page 685*

◆ **DTaP-IPV** *see* Diphtheria and Tetanus Toxoids, Acellular Pertussis, and Poliovirus Vaccine *on page 677*

◆ **DTaP-IPV/Hib** *see* Diphtheria and Tetanus Toxoids, Acellular Pertussis, Poliovirus and *Haemophilus* b Conjugate Vaccine *on page 679*

◆ **DTIC** *see* Dacarbazine *on page 572*

◆ **DTIC-Dome** *see* Dacarbazine *on page 572*

◆ **DTO (error-prone abbreviation)** *see* Opium Tincture *on page 1569*

◆ **Duac** *see* Clindamycin and Benzoyl Peroxide *on page 493*

◆ **Ducodyl [OTC]** *see* Bisacodyl *on page 289*

◆ **Dulcolax [OTC]** *see* Bisacodyl *on page 289*

◆ **Dulcolax For Women [OTC] (Can)** *see* Bisacodyl *on page 289*

◆ **Dulcolax Milk of Magnesia [OTC]** *see* Magnesium Hydroxide *on page 1313*

◆ **Dulcolax Stool Softener [OTC]** *see* Docusate *on page 697*

◆ **Dulera** *see* Mometasone and Formoterol *on page 1457*

◆ **Duofilm (Can)** *see* Salicylic Acid *on page 1894*

◆ **Duoforte 27 (Can)** *see* Salicylic Acid *on page 1894*

◆ **DuP 753** *see* Losartan *on page 1302*

◆ **Duraclon** *see* CloNIDine *on page 508*

◆ **Duragesic** *see* FentaNYL *on page 857*

◆ **Duragesic MAT (Can)** *see* FentaNYL *on page 857*

◆ **Duramorph** *see* Morphine (Systemic) *on page 1461*

◆ **Durela (Can)** *see* TraMADol *on page 2098*

◆ **Durezol** *see* Difluprednate *on page 651*

◆ **Duricef** *see* Cefadroxil *on page 387*

◆ **Duvoid (Can)** *see* Bethanechol *on page 284*

◆ **D-Vi-Sol [OTC]** *see* Cholecalciferol *on page 448*

◆ **D-Vi-Sol® (Can)** *see* Cholecalciferol *on page 448*

◆ **D-Vita [OTC]** *see* Cholecalciferol *on page 448*

◆ **DX-88** *see* Ecallantide *on page 726*

Dyclonine (DYE kloe neen)

Medication Safety Issues

Sound-alike/look-alike issues:

Dyclonine may be confused with dicyclomine

Brand Names: US Sucrets® Children's [OTC]; Sucrets® Maximum Strength [OTC]; Sucrets® Regular Strength [OTC]

Therapeutic Category Local Anesthetic, Oral

Generic Availability (US) No

Use Used topically for temporary relief of pain associated with oral mucosa

Contraindications Hypersensitivity to dyclonine or any component of the formulation

Warnings/Precautions When used for self-medication (OTC) patients should contact healthcare provider if symptoms worsen or last for >7 days. When treating a severe sore throat, patients should contact healthcare provider if symptoms lasts >2 days, occur with fever, headache, rash, nausea, or vomiting. Not for OTC use in children <2 years of age.

Adverse Reactions

Local: Irritation, numbness, pain, stinging

Miscellaneous: Allergic reactions, cold/heat sensation

Drug Interactions

Metabolism/Transport Effects None known.

Avoid Concomitant Use There are no known interactions where it is recommended to avoid concomitant use.

Increased Effect/Toxicity There are no known significant interactions involving an increase in effect.

Decreased Effect There are no known significant interactions involving a decrease in effect.

Dosing: Usual

Children >3 years: Topical: Slowly dissolve 1 lozenge (1.2 mg) in mouth every 2 hours, if necessary

Children >12 years and Adults: Topical: Slowly dissolve 1 lozenge (3 mg) in mouth every 2 hours, if necessary

Administration Topical: Apply to mucous membranes of the mouth or throat area: food should not be ingested for 60 minutes following application in the mouth or throat area

Dosage Forms Excipient information presented when available (limited, particularly for generics); consult specific product labeling. [DSC] = Discontinued product

Lozenge, oral, as hydrochloride:

- Sucrets® Children's: 1.2 mg (18s) [cherry flavor]
- Sucrets® Maximum Strength: 3 mg (18s) [black-cherry flavor]
- Sucrets® Maximum Strength: 3 mg (18s) [wintergreen flavor]
- Sucrets® Regular Strength: 2 mg (18s)
- Sucrets® Regular Strength: 2 mg (18s [DSC]) [wild cherry flavor]

- ◆ **Dyclonine Hydrochloride** *see* Dyclonine *on page* 725
- ◆ **Dyloject** *see* Diclofenac (Systemic) *on page* 641
- ◆ **Dymista** *see* Azelastine and Fluticasone *on page* 241
- ◆ **Dyrenium** *see* Triamterene *on page* 2119
- ◆ **Dyspel [OTC]** *see* Ibuprofen *on page* 1064
- ◆ **E-400 [OTC]** *see* Vitamin E *on page* 2188
- ◆ **E-400-Clear [OTC]** *see* Vitamin E *on page* 2188
- ◆ **E-400-Mixed [OTC]** *see* Vitamin E *on page* 2188
- ◆ **E 2080** *see* Rufinamide *on page* 1891
- ◆ **EACA** *see* Aminocaproic Acid *on page* 121
- ◆ **Ear Drops Earwax Aid [OTC]** *see* Carbamide Peroxide *on page* 371
- ◆ **Ear Wax Remover [OTC] [DSC]** *see* Carbamide Peroxide *on page* 371
- ◆ **Earwax Treatment Drops [OTC]** *see* Carbamide Peroxide *on page* 371

Ecallantide (e KAL lan tide)

Brand Names: US Kalbitor

Therapeutic Category Kallikrein Inhibitor

Generic Availability (US) No

Use Treatment of acute attacks of hereditary angioedema (HAE) (FDA approved in ages ≥12 years and adults)

Medication Guide Available Yes

Pregnancy Risk Factor C

Pregnancy Considerations Adverse effects were observed in animal reproduction studies. If treatment for HAE is needed during pregnancy, other agents are preferred (Caballero, 2012).

Breast-Feeding Considerations It is not known if ecallantide is excreted in breast milk. The manufacturer recommends that caution be exercised when administering ecallantide to nursing women.

Contraindications Hypersensitivity to ecallantide or any component of the formulation

Warnings/Precautions [U.S. Boxed Warning]: Serious hypersensitivity reactions, including anaphylaxis have been reported; administer only by healthcare provider in presence of appropriate medical support to manage anaphylaxis and hereditary angioedema. Do not administer to patients with known hypersensitivity to ecallantide. Reactions usually occur within 1 hour and may include chest discomfort, flushing, hypotension, nasal congestion, pharyngeal edema, pruritus, rash, rhinorrhea, sneezing, throat irritation, urticaria, and wheezing. Signs/symptoms of hypersensitivity reactions may be similar to those associated with hereditary angioedema attacks, therefore, consideration should be given to treatment methods; monitor patients closely. Some patients may develop antibodies to ecallantide during therapy; seroconversion may increase the risk of hypersensitivity reaction.

Adverse Reactions

Central nervous system: Fatigue, headache

Dermatologic: Pruritus, skin rash, urticaria

Gastrointestinal: Diarrhea, nausea, upper abdominal pain, vomiting

Hypersensitivity: Anaphylaxis

Immunologic: Antibody development

Local: Injection site reaction (includes bruising, erythema, irritation, pain, pruritus, urticaria)

Respiratory: Nasopharyngitis, upper respiratory tract infection

Miscellaneous: Fever

Rare but important or life-threatening: Hypersensitivity reaction (chest discomfort, flushing, pharyngeal edema, rhinorrhea, sneezing, nasal congestion, throat irritation, wheezing, hypotension)

Drug Interactions

Metabolism/Transport Effects None known.

Avoid Concomitant Use There are no known interactions where it is recommended to avoid concomitant use.

Increased Effect/Toxicity There are no known significant interactions involving an increase in effect.

Decreased Effect There are no known significant interactions involving a decrease in effect.

Storage/Stability Store at 2°C to 8°C (36°F to 46°F). Protect from light. May be stored for up to 14 days at <30°C (<86°F).

Mechanism of Action Ecallantide is a recombinant protein which inhibits the conversion of high molecular weight kininogen to bradykinin by selectively and reversibly inhibiting plasma kallikrein. Unregulated bradykinin production is thought to contribute to the increased vascular permeability and angioedema observed in HAE.

Pharmacodynamics Onset: <4 hours (median time <30 minutes) (Epstein, 2008)

Pharmacokinetics (Adult data unless noted)

Distribution: V_d: 26.4 ± 7.8 L

Half-life elimination: 2 ± 0.5 hours

Time to peak serum concentration: ~2 to 3 hours

Elimination: Primarily urine

Dosing: Usual

Pediatric: **Hereditary angioedema (HAE), treatment:**

Children 8 to <12 years of age: Limited data available: SubQ: 30 mg (as three 10 mg [1 mL] injections); dosing based on data pooled from four clinical studies (n=29, ages 9 to 17 years including 25 who received at least one dose of ecallantide) (MacGinnitie, 2013) and a single case report in an 8-year old (Dy, 2013); efficacy was observed with no adverse events reported.

Children ≥12 years and Adolescents: SubQ: 30 mg (as three 10 mg [1 mL] injections); if attack persists, may repeat an additional 30 mg within 24 hours

Adult: **Hereditary angioedema (HAE), treatment:** SubQ: 30 mg (as three 10 mg [1 mL] injections); if attack persists, may repeat an additional 30 mg within 24 hours

Dosing adjustment in renal impairment: There are no dosage adjustments provided in the manufacturer's labeling (has not been studied).

Dosing adjustment in hepatic impairment: There are no dosage adjustments provided in the manufacturer's labeling (has not been studied).

Administration Administer as 3 (10 mg/mL each) injections subcutaneously into skin of abdomen, upper arm, or thigh (do not administer at site of attack). Recommended needle size is 27-gauge. Separate injections by 2 inches (5 cm). May inject all doses in same or different location; rotation of sites is not necessary. Monitor/observe for hypersensitivity.

Monitoring Parameters Monitor for hypersensitivity reaction

Dosage Forms Excipient information presented when available (limited, particularly for generics); consult specific product labeling.

Solution, Subcutaneous [preservative free]:

Kalbitor: 10 mg/mL (1 mL)

◆ **ECL-Citalopram (Can)** *see* Citalopram *on page 476*

◆ **ECL-Metformin (Can)** *see* MetFORMIN *on page 1375*

◆ **EC-Naprosyn** *see* Naproxen *on page 1489*

Econazole (e KONE a zole)

Brand Names: US Ecoza

Therapeutic Category Antifungal Agent, Topical

Generic Availability (US) May be product dependent

Use Topical treatment of tinea pedis, tinea cruris, tinea corporis, tinea versicolor, and cutaneous candidiasis

Pregnancy Risk Factor C

Pregnancy Considerations Adverse events were observed in some animal reproduction studies. The manufacturer recommends avoiding use during pregnancy, especially during the first trimester.

Breast-Feeding Considerations It is not known if econazole is excreted in breast milk. The manufacturer recommends that caution be exercised when administering econazole to nursing women.

Contraindications

Cream: Hypersensitivity to econazole or any component of the formulation

Foam: There are no contraindications listed in the manufacturer's labeling. Documentation of allergenic cross-reactivity for imidazole antifungals is limited. However, because of similarities in chemical structure and/or pharmacologic actions, the possibility of cross-sensitivity cannot be ruled out with certainty.

Warnings/Precautions For topical use only; avoid contact with eyes, mouth, nose, or other mucous membranes. Discontinue if sensitivity or irritation occurs. Avoid heat, flame and smoking during and immediately following application; topical foam is flammable.

Warnings: Additional Pediatric Considerations Some dosage forms may contain propylene glycol; in neonates large amounts of propylene glycol delivered orally, intravenously (eg, >3,000 mg/day), or topically have been associated with potentially fatal toxicities which can include metabolic acidosis, seizures, renal failure, and CNS depression; toxicities have also been reported in children and adults including hyperosmolality, lactic acidosis, seizures, and respiratory depression; use caution (AAP, 1997; Shehab, 2009).

Adverse Reactions

Dermatologic: Burning sensation of skin, erythema, pruritus, stinging of the skin

Rare but important or life-threatening: Application site reaction, pruritic rash

Drug Interactions

Metabolism/Transport Effects Inhibits CYP2E1 (weak)

Avoid Concomitant Use There are no known interactions where it is recommended to avoid concomitant use.

Increased Effect/Toxicity

Econazole may increase the levels/effects of: Vitamin K Antagonists

Decreased Effect There are no known significant interactions involving a decrease in effect.

Storage/Stability

Cream: Store below 30°C (86°F).

Foam: Store at 20°C to 25°C (68°F to 77°F); excursions are permitted between 15°C and 30°C (59°F and 86°F). Do not expose to heat and/or store at temperatures >49°C (120°F) even when the container is empty. Do not store in direct sunlight. Do not refrigerate or freeze.

Mechanism of Action Alters fungal cell wall membrane permeability; may interfere with RNA and protein synthesis, and lipid metabolism

Pharmacokinetics (Adult data unless noted)

Absorption: Following topical administration, <10% is percutaneously absorbed

Metabolism: In the liver to >20 metabolites

Elimination: <1% of an applied dose recovered in urine or feces

Dosing: Usual Children and Adults: Topical:

Tinea cruris, corporis, pedis, and tinea versicolor: Apply once daily

Cutaneous candidiasis: Apply twice daily

Administration Topical: Apply a sufficient amount of cream to cover affected areas; do not apply to the eye or intravaginally

Additional Information Candidal infections and tinea cruris, versicolor, and corporis should be treated for 2 weeks and tinea pedis for 1 month; occasionally, longer treatment periods may be required

Product Availability Ecoza topical foam: FDA approved October 2013; anticipated availability currently unknown

Dosage Forms Excipient information presented when available (limited, particularly for generics); consult specific product labeling.

Cream, External, as nitrate:

Generic: 1% (15 g, 30 g, 85 g)

Foam, External, as nitrate:

Ecoza: 1% (70 g) [contains propylene glycol, trolamine (triethanolamine)]

◆ **Econazole Nitrate** *see* Econazole *on page 727*

◆ **Econopred** *see* PrednisoLONE (Ophthalmic) *on page 1758*

◆ **Ecotrin [OTC]** *see* Aspirin *on page 206*

◆ **Ecotrin Arthritis Strength [OTC]** *see* Aspirin *on page 206*

◆ **Ecotrin Low Strength [OTC]** *see* Aspirin *on page 206*

◆ **Ecoza** *see* Econazole *on page 727*

◆ **Ecoza** *see* Econazole *on page 727*

◆ **Ed A-Hist PSE [OTC]** *see* Triprolidine and Pseudoephedrine *on page 2129*

◆ **Ed ChlorPed** *see* Chlorpheniramine *on page 441*

◆ **Ed Chlorped Jr [OTC]** *see* Chlorpheniramine *on page 441*

◆ **Ed-Chlor-Tan** *see* Chlorpheniramine *on page 441*

◆ **Edecrin** *see* Ethacrynic Acid *on page* 809

Edetate CALCIUM Disodium

(ED e tate KAL see um dye SOW dee um)

Medication Safety Issues

Sound-alike look-alike issues:

To avoid potentially serious errors, the abbreviation "EDTA" should **never** be used.

Edetate CALCIUM disodium (CaEDTA) may be confused with edetate disodium (Na_2EDTA) (not commercially available in the U.S. or Canada). CDC recommends that edetate disodium should **never** be used for chelation therapy in children. Fatal hypocalcemia may result if edetate disodium is used for chelation therapy instead of edetate calcium disodium. ISMP recommends confirming the diagnosis to help distinguish between the two drugs prior to dispensing and/or administering either drug.

Edetate CALCIUM disodium may be confused with etomidate

Therapeutic Category Antidote, Lead Toxicity; Chelating Agent, Parenteral

Generic Availability (US) Yes

Use Treatment of symptomatic acute and chronic lead poisoning [FDA approved pediatric patients (age not specified) and adults]

Pregnancy Risk Factor B

Pregnancy Considerations Adverse events were observed in some animal reproduction studies; there are no well controlled studies of edetate CALCIUM disodium in pregnant women. Lead is known to cross the placenta in amounts related to maternal plasma levels. Prenatal lead exposure may be associated with adverse events such as spontaneous abortion, preterm delivery, decreased birth weight, and impaired neurodevelopment. Some adverse outcomes may occur with maternal blood lead levels <10 mcg/dL. In addition, pregnant women exposed to lead may have an increased risk of gestational hypertension. Consider chelation therapy in pregnant women with confirmed blood lead levels ≥45 mcg/dL (pregnant women with blood lead levels ≥70 mcg/dL should be considered for chelation regardless of trimester); consultation with experts in lead poisoning and high-risk pregnancy is recommended. Encephalopathic pregnant women should be chelated regardless of trimester (CDC, 2010).

Breast-Feeding Considerations If present in breast milk, oral absorption of edetate CALCIUM disodium is poor (<5%) which would limit exposure to a nursing infant. However, edetate CALCIUM disodium is not used orally because it may increase lead absorption from the GI tract. The amount of lead in breast milk may range from 0.6% to 3% of the maternal serum concentration. Women with confirmed blood lead levels ≥40 mcg/dL should not initiate breast-feeding; pumping and discarding breast milk is recommended until blood lead levels are <40 mcg/dL, at which point breast-feeding may resume (CDC, 2010). Calcium supplementation may reduce the amount of lead in breast milk.

Contraindications Active renal disease or anuria; hepatitis

Warnings/Precautions [U.S. Boxed Warning]: Use with extreme caution in patients with lead encephalopathy and cerebral edema. In these patients, IV infusion has been associated with lethal increase in intracranial pressure; IM injection is preferred.

Edetate CALCIUM disodium is potentially nephrotoxic. Renal tubular acidosis and fatal nephrosis may occur, especially with high doses; do not exceed the recommended daily dose. If anuria, increasing proteinuria, or hematuria occurs during therapy, discontinue use. Minimize nephrotoxicity by providing adequate hydration, establishment of good urine output, avoidance of excessive doses, and limit continuous administration to ≤5 days. Monitor for arrhythmias and ECG changes during IV therapy.

Exercise caution in the ordering, dispensing, and administration of this drug. Edetate CALCIUM disodium (CaEDTA) may be confused with edetate disodium (Na_2EDTA) (not commercially available in the U.S. or Canada). The CDC and FDA recommend that edetate disodium should never be used for chelation therapy (especially in children) (Mitka, 2008). Death has occurred following the use of edetate disodium for chelation therapy in pediatric patients with autism (Baxter, 2008). Fatal hypocalcemia may result if edetate disodium is used for the treatment of lead poisoning instead of edetate CALCIUM disodium (Baxter, 2008). Investigate, identify, and remove sources of lead exposure prior to treatment. Primary care providers should consult experts in chemotherapy of lead toxicity before using chelation drug therapy. Do not permit patients to re-enter the contaminated environment until lead abatement has been completed.

Adverse Reactions

Cardiovascular: Arrhythmia, ECG changes, hypotension

Central nervous system: Chills, fatigue, fever, headache, malaise

Dermatologic: Cheilosis, dermatitis, rash

Endocrine & metabolic: Hypercalcemia, hypokalemia

Gastrointestinal: Anorexia, GI upset, nausea, thirst (excessive), vomiting

Hematologic: Anemia, bone marrow suppression (transient)

Hepatic: Alkaline phosphatase decreased, liver function test increased (mild)

Local: Pain at injection site (IM injection), thrombophlebitis (IV infusion when concentration >5 mg/mL)

Neuromuscular & skeletal: Arthralgia, myalgia, numbness, paresthesia, tremor

Ocular: Lacrimation

Renal: Glucosuria, microscopic hematuria, nephrosis, nephrotoxicity, proteinuria, renal tubular necrosis, urinary frequency/urgency

Respiratory: Nasal congestion, sneezing

Miscellaneous: Iron, magnesium, and/or zinc deficiency (with chronic therapy)

Drug Interactions

Metabolism/Transport Effects None known.

Avoid Concomitant Use

Avoid concomitant use of Edetate CALCIUM Disodium with any of the following: BCG (Intravesical); CloZAPine; Dipyrone

Increased Effect/Toxicity

Edetate CALCIUM Disodium may increase the levels/effects of: CloZAPine; Insulin

The levels/effects of Edetate CALCIUM Disodium may be increased by: Dipyrone

Decreased Effect

Edetate CALCIUM Disodium may decrease the levels/effects of: BCG (Intravesical)

Storage/Stability Store at 25°C (77°F); excursion permitted to 15°C to 30°C (59°F to 86°F).

Mechanism of Action Calcium is displaced by divalent and trivalent heavy metals, forming a nonionizing soluble complex that is excreted in urine

Pharmacodynamics

Onset of chelation with IV administration: 1 hour

Maximum excretion of chelated lead with IV administration: 24-48 hours

Pharmacokinetics (Adult data unless noted)

Absorption: IM, SubQ: Well absorbed; Oral: <5%

Distribution: Into extracellular fluid; minimal CSF penetration (~5%)
Metabolism: Almost none of the drug is metabolized
Half-life, plasma: 20 to 60 minutes
Elimination: Urine (as metal chelates or unchanged drug); decreased GFR decreases elimination

Dosing: Usual

Pediatric: **Lead poisoning, treatment:** Infants, Children, and Adolescents: **Note:** For the treatment of high blood lead levels in children, the CDC recommends chelation treatment when blood lead levels are >45 mcg/dL (CDC 2002). The AAP recommends succimer as the drug used for initial management in asymptomatic children when blood lead levels are >45 mcg/dL and <70 mcg/dL. Edetate CALCIUM disodium can be used in children allergic to succimer (AAP 2005; Chandran 2010). Combination therapy with edetate CALCIUM disodium and dimercaprol is recommended for use in children whose blood lead levels are ≥70 mcg/dL or in children with lead encephalopathy (AAP 2005; Chandran 2010). Depending upon the blood lead level, additional courses may be necessary; at least 2 to 4 days should elapse before repeat treatment is initiated.

Blood lead levels <70 mcg/dL and asymptomatic: IM, IV: 1,000 mg/m²/day for 5 days **or** 50 mg/kg/day for 5 days with a suggested maximum daily dose of 1,000 mg/day in children or 2,000 mg/day in adults (Chandran 2010; Howland 2011)

Blood lead levels ≥70 mcg/dL or symptomatic lead poisoning (in conjunction with dimercaprol): **Note:** Begin treatment with edetate CALCIUM disodium with the second dimercaprol dose: IM, IV: 1,000 mg/m²/day **or** 25 to 50 mg/kg/day for 5 days with a suggested maximum daily dose of 1,000 mg/day in children or 2,000 to 3,000 mg/day in adults (Chandran 2010; Howland 2011)

Lead encephalopathy (in conjunction with dimercaprol): **Note:** Begin treatment with edetate CALCIUM disodium with the second dimercaprol dose: IM, IV: 1,500 mg/m²/day **or** 50 to 75 mg/kg/day for 5 days with a suggested (maximum daily dose of: 1,000 mg/day in children or 2,000 to 3,000 mg in adults) (Chandran 2010; Howland 2011)

Adult: **Lead poisoning: Note:** Available guidelines recommend chelation therapy with blood lead levels >50 mcg/dL and significant symptoms; chelation therapy may also be indicated with blood lead levels ≥100 mcg/dL and/or symptoms (Kosnett 2007). Depending upon the blood lead level, additional courses may be necessary; at least 2 to 4 days should elapse before repeat treatment is initiated.

Blood lead levels <70 mcg/dL and asymptomatic: IM, IV: 1,000 mg/m²/day for 5 days

Blood lead levels ≥70 mcg/dL or symptomatic lead poisoning (in conjunction with dimercaprol): **Note:** Begin treatment with edetate CALCIUM disodium with the second dimercaprol dose: IM, IV: 1,000 mg/m²/day **or** 25 to 50 mg/kg/day for 5 days; a maximum dose of 3,000 mg has been suggested (Howland 2011)

Lead encephalopathy (in conjunction with dimercaprol): **Note:** Begin treatment with edetate CALCIUM disodium with the second dimercaprol dose: IM, IV: 1,500 mg/m²/day or 50 to 75 mg/kg/day for 5 days; a maximum dose of 3,000 mg has been suggested (Howland 2011)

Lead nephropathy: An alternative dosing regimen reflecting the reduction in renal clearance is based upon the serum creatinine; **Note:** Repeat regimen monthly until lead levels are reduced to an acceptable level: IM, IV:
S_{cr} 2 to 3 mg/dL: 500 mg/m² every 24 hours for 5 days
S_{cr} 3 to 4 mg/dL: 500 mg/m² every 48 hours for 3 doses
S_{cr} >4 mg/dL: 500 mg/m² once weekly

Dosing adjustment in renal impairment: Infants, Children, Adolescents, and Adults: Dose should be reduced with preexisting mild renal disease. Limiting the daily dose to 1,000 mg in children and 2,000 mg in adults may decrease risk of nephrotoxicity, although larger doses may be needed in the treatment of lead encephalopathy (Howland 2011).

Dosing adjustment in hepatic impairment: There are no dosage adjustments provided in the manufacturer's labeling.

Preparation for Administration Parenteral:

IV infusion: Dilute total daily dose in 250 to 500 mL of NS or D_5W. Concentrations >0.5% (5 mg/mL) should be avoided.

IM: Procaine or lidocaine should be added to solutions given by IM injection to minimize pain at the injection site. The final lidocaine or procaine concentration of 5 mg/mL (0.5%) can be obtained by adding 0.25 mL of lidocaine 10% solution per 5 mL edetate CALCIUM disodium or 1 mL of 1% lidocaine or procaine solution per mL of edetate CALCIUM disodium.

Administration Parenteral: For IM or IV use; IV is generally preferred; however, the IM route is preferred when cerebral edema is present.

IV infusion: Administer the daily dose as a diluted solution over 8 to 12 hours or continuously over 24 hours (Howland 2011). Avoid rapid infusion.

IM injection: Daily dose should be divided into 2 to 3 equal doses spaced 8 to 12 hours apart. Procaine hydrochloride or lidocaine may be added to the edetate CALCIUM disodium to minimize pain at injection site. Administer by deep IM injection. When used in conjunction with dimercaprol, inject into a separate site.

Monitoring Parameters Urinary output; urinalysis; renal function, hepatic function, serum electrolytes (baseline and daily [severe lead poisoning] or at days 2 and 5 [less severe lead poisoning]); ECG (with IV therapy); blood lead levels (baseline and 7 to 21 days after completing chelation therapy); hemoglobin or hematocrit; iron status; free erythrocyte protoporphyrin or zinc protoporphyrin; neurodevelopmental changes

Test Interactions If edetate CALCIUM disodium is given as a continuous IV infusion, stop the infusion for at least 1 hour before blood is drawn for lead concentration to avoid a falsely elevated value

Dosage Forms Excipient information presented when available (limited, particularly for generics); consult specific product labeling. [DSC] = Discontinued product

Solution, Injection:

Generic: 500 mg/2.5 mL (2.5 mL [DSC]); 1 g/5 mL (5 mL)

◆ **Edetate Disodium CALCIUM** *see* Edetate CALCIUM Disodium *on page 728*

◆ **Edex** *see* Alprostadil *on page 103*

◆ **Edluar** *see* Zolpidem *on page 2220*

Edrophonium (ed roe FOE nee um)

Brand Names: US Enlon

Brand Names: Canada Enlon®; Tensilon®

Therapeutic Category Antidote, Neuromuscular Blocking Agent; Cholinergic Agent; Diagnostic Agent, Myasthenia Gravis

Generic Availability (US) No

Use Diagnosis of myasthenia gravis; differentiation of cholinergic crises from myasthenia crises; reversal of nondepolarizing neuromuscular blockers; treatment of paroxysmal atrial tachycardia

Pregnancy Considerations Animal reproduction studies have not been conducted.

Breast-Feeding Considerations It is not known if edrophonium is excreted in breast milk. According to the manufacturer, if administration is required, avoid breast-feeding the infant immediately after use due to the potential for adverse events in the nursing infant.

Contraindications Hypersensitivity to edrophonium, sulfites, or any component of the formulation; GI or GU obstruction

Warnings/Precautions Use with caution in patients with bronchial asthma and those receiving a cardiac glycoside; atropine sulfate should always be readily available as an antagonist. Overdosage can cause cholinergic crisis which may be fatal. IV atropine should be readily available for treatment of cholinergic reactions. Use with caution in patients with cardiac arrhythmias (eg, bradyarrhythmias). Avoid use in myasthenia gravis; may exacerbate muscular weakness. Products may contain sodium sulfite.

Adverse Reactions

Cardiovascular: Arrhythmias (especially bradycardia), AV block, carbon monoxide decreased, cardiac arrest, ECG changes (nonspecific), flushing, hypotension, nodal rhythm, syncope, tachycardia

Central nervous system: Convulsions, dizziness, drowsiness, dysarthria, dysphonia, headache, loss of consciousness

Dermatologic: Skin rash, thrombophlebitis (IV), urticaria

Gastrointestinal: Diarrhea, dysphagia, flatulence, hyperperistalsis, nausea, salivation, stomach cramps, vomiting

Genitourinary: Urinary urgency

Neuromuscular & skeletal: Arthralgias, fasciculations, muscle cramps, spasms, weakness

Ocular: Lacrimation, small pupils

Respiratory: Bronchiolar constriction, bronchospasm, dyspnea, bronchial secretions increased, laryngospasm, respiratory arrest, respiratory depression, respiratory muscle paralysis

Miscellaneous: Allergic reactions, anaphylaxis, diaphoresis increased

Drug Interactions

Metabolism/Transport Effects None known.

Avoid Concomitant Use There are no known interactions where it is recommended to avoid concomitant use.

Increased Effect/Toxicity

Edrophonium may increase the levels/effects of: Beta-Blockers; Cardiac Glycosides; Cholinergic Agonists; Succinylcholine

The levels/effects of Edrophonium may be increased by: Corticosteroids (Systemic)

Decreased Effect

Edrophonium may decrease the levels/effects of: Anticholinergic Agents; Neuromuscular-Blocking Agents (Nondepolarizing)

The levels/effects of Edrophonium may be decreased by: Anticholinergic Agents; Dipyridamole

Mechanism of Action Inhibits destruction of acetylcholine by acetylcholinesterase. This facilitates transmission of impulses across myoneural junction and results in increased cholinergic responses such as miosis, increased tonus of intestinal and skeletal muscles, bronchial and ureteral constriction, bradycardia, and increased salivary and sweat gland secretions.

Pharmacodynamics

Onset of action:
- IM: 2-10 minutes
- IV: 30-60 seconds

Duration:
- IM: 5-30 minutes
- IV: 5-10 minutes

Pharmacokinetics (Adult data unless noted)

Distribution: V_d:
- Infants: 1.18 ± 0.2 L/kg
- Children: 1.22 ± 0.74 L/kg
- Adults: 0.9 ± 0.13 L/kg

Half-life:
- Infants: 73 ± 30 minutes
- Children: 99 ± 31 minutes
- Adults: 126 ± 59 minutes

Elimination: Clearance:
- Infants: 17.8 mL/kg/minute
- Children: 14.2 mL/kg/minute
- Adults: 8.3 ± 2.9 mL/kg/minute

Dosing: Usual Usually administered IV, however, if not possible, IM or SubQ may be used

Infants: Diagnosis of myasthenia gravis: Initial:
- IM, SubQ: 0.5-1 mg
- IV: Initial: 0.1 mg, followed by 0.4 mg (if no response); total dose = 0.5 mg

Children:

Diagnosis of myasthenia gravis: Initial:
- IM, SubQ: ≤34 kg: 2 mg; >34 kg: 5 mg
- IV: 0.04 mg/kg given over 1 minute followed by 0.16 mg/kg given within 45 seconds (if no response) (maximum dose: 10 mg total)

  or

  Alternative (manufacturer's recommendations):
  - ≤34 kg: 1 mg; if no response after 45 seconds, it may be repeated in 1 mg increments every 30-45 seconds to a total of 5 mg
  - >34 kg: 2 mg; if no response after 45 seconds, it may be repeated in 1 mg increments every 30-45 seconds to a total of 10 mg

Titration of oral anticholinesterase therapy: IV: 0.04 mg/kg once given 1 hour after oral intake of the drug being used in treatment; if strength improves, an increase in neostigmine or pyridostigmine dose is indicated

Adults:

Diagnosis of myasthenia gravis: Initial:
- IM, SubQ: Initial: 10 mg; if no cholinergic reaction occurs, administer 2 mg 30 minutes later to rule out false-negative reaction
- IV: 2 mg test dose administered over 15-30 seconds; 8 mg given 45 seconds later (if no response is seen); test dose may be repeated after 30 minutes.

Titration of oral anticholinesterase therapy: IV: 1-2 mg given 1 hour after oral dose of anticholinesterase; if strength improves, an increase in neostigmine or pyridostigmine dose is indicated

Differentiation of cholinergic from myasthenic crisis: IV: 1 mg, may repeat after 1 minute (**Note:** Intubation and controlled ventilation may be required if patient has cholinergic crises.)

Reversal of nondepolarizing neuromuscular blocking agents (neostigmine with atropine usually preferred): IV: 10 mg over 30-45 seconds, may repeat every 5-10 minutes up to 40 mg total dose

Termination of paroxysmal atrial tachycardia: IV: 5-10 mg

Dosing adjustment in renal impairment: Dose may need to be reduced in patients with chronic renal failure

Administration Parenteral: Edrophonium is administered by direct IV or IM injection

Monitoring Parameters Pre- and postinjection strength (cranial musculature is most useful); heart rate, respiratory rate, blood pressure, changes in fasciculations

Test Interactions Increased aminotransferase [ALT/AST] (S), amylase (S)

Dosage Forms Excipient information presented when available (limited, particularly for generics); consult specific product labeling.

Solution, Injection, as chloride:
- Enlon: 10 mg/mL (15 mL) [contains phenol]

◆ **Edrophonium Chloride** *see* Edrophonium *on page* 729

Efavirenz (e FAV e renz)

Medication Safety Issues

High alert medication:

This medication is in a class the Institute for Safe Medication Practices (ISMP) includes among its list of drug classes that have a heightened risk of causing significant patient harm when used in error.

Related Information

Adult and Adolescent HIV *on page 2392*

Oral Medications That Should Not Be Crushed or Altered *on page 2476*

Pediatric HIV *on page 2380*

Perinatal HIV *on page 2400*

Brand Names: US Sustiva

Brand Names: Canada Mylan-Efavirenz; Sustiva; Teva-Efavirenz

Therapeutic Category Antiretroviral Agent; HIV Agents (Anti-HIV Agents); Non-nucleoside Reverse Transcriptase Inhibitor (NNRTI)

Generic Availability (US) No

Use Treatment of HIV-1 infection in combination with other antiretroviral agents (FDA approved in ages ≥3 months weighing at least 3.5 kg and adults). **Note:** HIV regimens consisting of **three** antiretroviral agents are strongly recommended.

Prescribing and Access Restrictions Efavirenz oral solution is available only through an expanded access (compassionate use) program. Enrollment information may be obtained by calling 877-372-7097.

Pregnancy Considerations Teratogenic effects have been observed in primates receiving efavirenz. Efavirenz has a moderate level of transfer across the human placenta. Based on data from the Antiretroviral Pregnancy Registry, an increased risk of overall birth defects has not been observed following first trimester exposure to efavirenz; however, neural tube and other CNS defects have been reported. Due to the low number of first trimester exposures and the low incidence of neural tube defects in the general population, available data are insufficient to evaluate risk. Other antiretroviral agents should strongly be considered for use in women of childbearing potential who are planning to become pregnant or who are sexually active and not using effective contraception. Nonpregnant women of reproductive age should undergo pregnancy testing prior to initiation of efavirenz. Barrier contraception should be used in combination with other (hormonal) methods of contraception during therapy and for 12 weeks after efavirenz is discontinued. Neural tube defects would occur following exposure during the first 5 to 6 weeks of gestation (most pregnancies are not detected before 4 to 6 weeks gestation). For women who present in the first trimester already on an efavirenz-containing regimen and who have adequate viral suppression, efavirenz may be continued; changing regimens may lead to loss of viral control and increase the risk of perinatal transmission. Pharmacokinetic data from available studies do not suggest dose alterations are needed during pregnancy. The DHHS Perinatal HIV Guidelines consider efavirenz to be a preferred NNRTI for use in antiretroviral-naive pregnant women after 8 weeks gestation. Hypersensitivity reactions (including hepatic toxicity and rash) are more common in women on NNRTI therapy; it is not known if pregnancy increases this risk.

Regardless of CD4 count or HIV RNA copy number, all HIV-infected pregnant women should receive a combination antiretroviral (ARV) drug regimen. A combination of antepartum, intrapartum, and infant ARV prophylaxis is recommended. ARV therapy should be started as soon as possible in women with symptomatic infection. Although earlier initiation may be more effective in reducing the perinatal transmission of HIV, initiation may be delayed until after 12 weeks gestation in women who do no require immediate treatment after careful consideration of maternal conditions (eg, nausea and vomiting) and the potential risks of first trimester fetal exposure for specific agents. A scheduled cesarean delivery at 38 weeks gestation is recommended for all women with HIV RNA >1000 copies/mL or unknown concentration near delivery in order to decrease transmission. If ARV therapy must be interrupted for <24 hours during the peripartum period, stop then restart all medications simultaneously in order to decrease the chance of developing resistance. Long-term follow-up is recommended for all infants exposed to ARV medications. In couples who want to conceive, the HIV-infected partner should attain maximum viral suppression prior to conception.

Health care providers are encouraged to enroll pregnant women exposed to antiretroviral medications in the Antiretroviral Pregnancy Registry (1-800-258-4263 or www.-APRegistry.com). Health care providers caring for HIV-infected women and their infants may contact the National Perinatal HIV Hotline (888-448-8765) for clinical consultation (HHS [perinatal], 2014).

Breast-Feeding Considerations Efavirenz is excreted into breast milk. Although breast-feeding is not recommended, plasma concentrations of efavirenz in nursing infants have been reported as ~13% of maternal plasma concentrations.

Maternal or infant antiretroviral therapy does not completely eliminate the risk of postnatal HIV transmission. In addition, multiclass-resistant virus has been detected in breast-feeding infants despite maternal therapy. Therefore, in the United States, where formula is accessible, affordable, safe, and sustainable, and the risk of infant mortality due to diarrhea and respiratory infections is low, complete avoidance of breast-feeding by HIV-infected women is recommended to decrease potential transmission of HIV (HHS [perinatal], 2014).

Contraindications Hypersensitivity (eg, Stevens-Johnson syndrome, erythema multiforme, toxic skin eruptions) to efavirenz or any component of the formulation

Warnings/Precautions Do not use as single-agent therapy. Avoid pregnancy; women of childbearing potential should undergo pregnancy testing prior to initiation of therapy. Use caution with other agents metabolized by cytochrome P450 isoenzyme 3A4 (see Contraindications); concomitant use of other efavirenz-containing products should be avoided (unless needed for dosage adjustment with concomitant rifampin treatment). Use caution with history of mental illness/drug abuse (predisposition to psychological reactions); may cause CNS and psychiatric symptoms, which include impaired concentration, dizziness or drowsiness (avoid potentially hazardous tasks such as driving or operating machinery if these effects are noted); CNS effects may be potentiated when used with other psychoactive drugs or ethanol. Serious psychiatric side effects have been associated with efavirenz, including severe depression, suicidal ideation, nonfatal suicide attempts, paranoia, and mania; instruct patients to contact healthcare provider if serious psychiatric effects occur. May cause mild-to-moderate maculopapular rash; usually occurs within 2 weeks of starting therapy;

discontinue if severe rash (involving blistering, desquamation, mucosal involvement, or fever) develops; contraindicated in patients with a history of a severe cutaneous reaction (eg, Stevens-Johnson syndrome). Children are more susceptible.

Caution in patients with known or suspected hepatitis B or C infection or Child-Pugh class A hepatic impairment; not recommended in Child-Pugh class B or C hepatic impairment. Persistent elevations of serum transaminases >5 times the upper limit of normal should prompt evaluation - benefit of continued therapy should be weighed against possible risk of hepatotoxicity. Hepatic failure has been reported, including patients with no preexisting hepatic disease or other identifiable risk factors. Monitor liver function tests in patients with underlying hepatic disease (eg, hepatitis B or C, marked transaminase elevations or taking concomitant medications that may cause hepatotoxicity). Ethanol may increase hepatotoxic potential; instruct patients to limit or avoid alcohol. Increases in total cholesterol and triglycerides have been reported; screening should be done prior to therapy and periodically throughout treatment. May cause redistribution of fat (eg, buffalo hump, peripheral wasting with increased abdominal girth, cushingoid appearance). Patients may develop immune reconstitution syndrome resulting in the occurrence of an inflammatory response to an indolent or residual opportunistic infection during initial HIV treatment or activation of autoimmune disorders (eg, Graves' disease, polymyositis, Guillain-Barré syndrome) later in therapy; further evaluation and treatment may be required. Use with caution in patients with a history of seizure disorder; seizures have been associated with use. Efavirenz administered as monotherapy or added on to a failing regimen may result in rapid viral resistance to efavirenz. Consider cross-resistance when adding antiretroviral agents on to efavirenz therapy.

Warnings: Additional Pediatric Considerations Efavirenz is hepatically metabolized, primarily via highly polymorphic CYP2B6 enzymes; individuals with the CYP2B6 516 T/T genotype have been shown to have reduced metabolism, resulting in greater exposure compared to the G/G or G/T genotypes (extensive metabolizers); this has particularly been demonstrated in infants and children <3 years of age. The T/T genotype has an allele frequency of 20% in African-Americans. Although FDA approved in pediatric patients ≥3 months of age and weighing ≥3.5 kg, current guidelines recommend that efavirenz not be used in infants and children <3 years of age in general; pharmacokinetic data suggest that FDA approved dosing may result in subtherapeutic levels in extensive metabolizers and supratherapeutic in slow metabolizers. In infants and children 3 months to <3 years of age and weighing ≥3 kg, evaluate CYP2B6 genotype prior to efavirenz therapy; in those with T/T genotype (slow metabolizer), dosage reduction and therapeutic drug level monitoring recommended (DHHS [pediatric], 2014).

Efavirenz may cause a rash, which usually presents as pruritic maculopapular skin eruptions; incidence is more common and more severe in children than in adults (incidence: Children 32%; adults 26%, median onset: Children: 28 days [range: 3 to 1642 days]; adults: 11 days). In adults, most rashes appeared within 14 days after starting therapy and the mean duration was 16 days. Rash may be treated with antihistamines and corticosteroids and usually resolves within 1 month while continuing therapy. Discontinue if severe rash (involving blistering, desquamation, mucosal involvement, ulceration, or fever) occurs. Consider prophylaxis with antihistamines in children due to frequency and severity of rash reported in children.

The overall reported incidence of CNS adverse effects was 53% (all patients) vs 25% in controls; nervous system symptoms in children were reported to be 18%. Fever has been reported with use (children: 21%).

May cause diarrhea or loose stools; reported incidence in children is 39%. Cough may occur; reported incidence in children is 16%.

Adverse Reactions

Central nervous system: Abnormal dreams, anxiety, depression, dizziness, fatigue, fever, hallucinations, headache, impaired concentration, insomnia, nervousness, pain, severe depression, somnolence

Dermatologic: Pruritus, rash

Endocrine & metabolic: HDL increased, hyperglycemia, total cholesterol increased, triglycerides increased

Gastrointestinal: Abdominal pain, amylase increased, anorexia, diarrhea, dyspepsia, nausea, vomiting

Hematologic: Neutropenia

Hepatic: ALT increased, AST increased

Respiratory: Cough

Rare but important or life-threatening: Allergic reaction, ataxia, body fat accumulation/redistribution, cerebellar coordination disturbances, delusions, dermatitis (photoallergic), erythema multiforme, gynecomastia, hepatic failure, hepatitis, immune reconstitution syndrome, malabsorption, mania, neuropathy, neurosis, palpitations, pancreatitis, paranoia, psychosis, seizures, Stevens-Johnson syndrome, suicide attempts, suicidal ideation, visual abnormalities

Drug Interactions

Metabolism/Transport Effects Substrate of CYP2B6 (major), CYP3A4 (major); **Note:** Assignment of Major/Minor substrate status based on clinically relevant drug interaction potential; **Inhibits** CYP2C19 (moderate), CYP2C8 (moderate), CYP2C9 (moderate); **Induces** CYP2B6 (weak/moderate), CYP3A4 (moderate)

Avoid Concomitant Use

Avoid concomitant use of Efavirenz with any of the following: Amodiaquine; Atovaquone; Axitinib; Azelastine (Nasal); Bedaquiline; Boceprevir; Bosutinib; CarBAMazepine; Dasabuvir; Elvitegravir; Enzalutamide; Etravirine; Itraconazole; Ketoconazole (Systemic); Nevirapine; Nisoldipine; Olaparib; Orphenadrine; Palbociclib; Paraldehyde; Paritaprevir; Posaconazole; Reverse Transcriptase Inhibitors (Non-Nucleoside); Rilpivirine; Simeprevir; St Johns Wort; Thalidomide; Ulipristal

Increased Effect/Toxicity

Efavirenz may increase the levels/effects of: Alcohol (Ethyl); Amodiaquine; Azelastine (Nasal); Bosentan; Cannabis; Carvedilol; Cilostazol; Citalopram; CNS Depressants; CYP2C19 Substrates; CYP2C8 Substrates; CYP2C9 Substrates; Dasabuvir; Dronabinol; Etravirine; Fosphenytoin; Hydrocodone; Ifosfamide; Methotrimeprazine; Metyrosine; Mirtazapine; Nevirapine; Orphenadrine; Paraldehyde; Paritaprevir; Phenytoin; Pramipexole; Rilpivirine; Ritonavir; ROPINIRole; Rotigotine; Selective Serotonin Reuptake Inhibitors; Suvorexant; Tetrahydrocannabinol; Thalidomide; Vitamin K Antagonists; Zolpidem

The levels/effects of Efavirenz may be increased by: Boceprevir; Brimonidine (Topical); Cannabis; CYP2B6 Inhibitors (Moderate); Darunavir; Doxylamine; Dronabinol; Droperidol; HydrOXYzine; Kava Kava; Magnesium Sulfate; Methotrimeprazine; Mifepristone; Nabilone; Nevirapine; Perampanel; Quazepam; Reverse Transcriptase Inhibitors (Non-Nucleoside); Ritonavir; Rufinamide; Saquinavir; Sodium Oxybate; Tapentadol; Tetrahydrocannabinol; Voriconazole

Decreased Effect

Efavirenz may decrease the levels/effects of: Alcohol (Ethyl); ARIPiprazole; Artemether; Atazanavir; AtorvaSTATin; Atovaquone; Axitinib; Bedaquiline; Boceprevir;

Bosutinib; Buprenorphine; BuPROPion; Calcium Channel Blockers; Canagliflozin; CarBAMazepine; Caspofungin; Clarithromycin; Clopidogrel; Contraceptives (Progestins); CycloSPORINE (Systemic); CYP3A4 Substrates; Darunavir; Dasabuvir; Diltiazem; Dolutegravir; Elvitegravir; Enzalutamide; Etonogestrel; Etravirine; Everolimus; FentaNYL; Fosamprenavir; Ibrutinib; Ifosfamide; Indinavir; Itraconazole; Ketoconazole (Systemic); Lopinavir; Lovastatin; Maraviroc; Methadone; NiMODipine; Nisoldipine; Norgestimate; Olaparib; Ombitasvir; Palbociclib; Paritaprevir; Posaconazole; Pravastatin; Proguanil; Rifabutin; Rilpivirine; Saquinavir; Saxagliptin; Sertraline; Simeprevir; Simvastatin; Sirolimus; Tacrolimus (Systemic); Telaprevir; Ulipristal; Vitamin K Antagonists; Voriconazole

The levels/effects of Efavirenz may be decreased by: Bosentan; CarBAMazepine; CYP2B6 Inducers (Strong); CYP3A4 Inducers (Moderate); CYP3A4 Inducers (Strong); Dabrafenib; Deferasirox; Fosphenytoin; Ginkgo Biloba; Mitotane; Nevirapine; Phenytoin; Reverse Transcriptase Inhibitors (Non-Nucleoside); Rifabutin; Rifampin; Siltuximab; St Johns Wort; Telaprevir; Tocilizumab

Food Interactions High-fat/high-caloric meals increase the absorption of efavirenz. CNS effects are possible. Management: Avoid high-fat/high-caloric meals. Administer at or before bedtime on an empty stomach unless using capsule sprinkle method in patients unable to swallow capsules or tablets. If capsule sprinkle method is used, patient should not consume additional food for 2 hours after administration.

Storage/Stability Store at 25°C (77°F); excursion permitted to 15°C to 30°C (59°F to 86°F).

Mechanism of Action As a non-nucleoside reverse transcriptase inhibitor, efavirenz has activity against HIV-1 by binding to reverse transcriptase. It consequently blocks the RNA-dependent and DNA-dependent DNA polymerase activities including HIV-1 replication. It does not require intracellular phosphorylation for antiviral activity.

Pharmacokinetics (Adult data unless noted)

Absorption: Increased by high-fat/high-caloric meals

Distribution: CSF concentrations are 0.69% of plasma (range: 0.26% to 1.2%); however, CSF:plasma concentration ratio is 3 times higher than free fraction in plasma

Protein binding: 99.5% to 99.8%, primarily to albumin

Metabolism: Hepatic via CYP3A and CYP2B6 to hydroxylated metabolites which then undergo glucuronidation; induces P450 enzymes and its own metabolism

Bioavailability: 42%

Half-life:

Single dose: 52 to 76 hours

Multiple doses: 40 to 55 hours

Time to peak serum concentration: 3 to 5 hours

Elimination: <1% excreted unchanged in the urine; 14% to 34% excreted as metabolites in the urine and 16% to 61% in feces (primarily as unchanged drug)

Dosing: Neonatal Not recommended for use; limited pharmacokinetic data demonstrate that target trough concentrations are difficult to achieve (DHHS [pediatric], 2014); additional studies are needed to determine the appropriate dosage.

Dosing: Usual

Pediatric: **HIV infection, treatment:** Use in combination with other antiretroviral agents; dosage adjustments for concomitant drug administration may be required; see below Dosage adjustment for concomitant drugs:

Infants <3 months or <3 kg: Not recommended for use

Infants ≥3 months weighing ≥3 kg and Children <3 years: Oral:

AIDSinfo recommendation: Very limited data available: **Note:** In general, current guidelines do not recommend efavirenz use in patients <3 years of age unless use is unavoidable due to the clinical situation; CYP2B6 genotype testing should be performed prior to therapy initiation. The following doses are under investigation and have been suggested by the expert panel based on pharmacokinetic data (DHHS [pediatric], 2014)

Extensive metabolizers (CYP2B6 516 G/G or G/T genotypes):

3 kg to <5 kg: 200 mg once daily
5 kg to <7 kg: 300 mg once daily
7 kg to <14 kg: 400 mg once daily
14 kg to <17 kg: 500 mg once daily
≥17 kg: 600 mg once daily

Slow metabolizer (CYP 2B6 516 T/T genotype):

3.3 kg to <7 kg: 50 mg once daily
7 kg to <14 kg: 100 mg once daily
≥14 kg: 150 mg once daily

Manufacturer's labeling: **Note:** Although FDA approved in pediatric patients ≥3 months of age and weighing ≥3.5 kg, pharmacokinetic data suggest that the FDA approved dosing may result in subtherapeutic levels in extensive metabolizers and supratherapeutic in slow metabolizers and use should be avoided.

3.5 kg to <5 kg: 100 mg once daily
5 kg to <7.5 kg: 150 mg once daily
7.5 kg to <15 kg: 200 mg once daily
15 kg to <20 kg: 250 mg once daily

Children ≥3 years and Adolescents:

Weight-directed dosing: Oral:

10 kg to <15 kg: 200 mg once daily
15 kg to <20 kg: 250 mg once daily
20 kg to <25 kg: 300 mg once daily
25 kg to <32.5 kg: 350 mg once daily
32.5 kg to <40 kg: 400 mg once daily
≥40 kg: 600 mg once daily

BSA-directed dosing: Oral: 367 mg/$\mathbf{m^2}$/dose once daily, maximum dose: 600 mg; recommended by some experts due to concern of underdosing at the upper end of each weight range (DHHS [pediatric], 2014)

Adult: **HIV infection, treatment: Note:** Use in combination with other antiretroviral agents: Oral: 600 mg once daily (DHHS [adult], 2014)

Dosage adjustment for concomitant rifampin:

Pediatric patients weighing ≤50 kg and Adults ≤50 kg: There are no dosage adjustments provided in manufacturer's labeling; however, efavirenz dosage increase may be considered.

Pediatric patients weighing >50 kg and Adults >50 kg: Oral: Increase efavirenz dose to 800 mg once daily

Dosage adjustment for concomitant voriconazole:

Infants ≥3 months, Children, and Adolescents: There are no dosage adjustments provided in manufacturer's labeling; however, efavirenz dose reduction and voriconazole dosage increase may be considered.

Adults: Oral: Reduce efavirenz dose to 300 mg once daily (use capsule formulation) and increase voriconazole dose to 400 mg every 12 hours

Dosing adjustment in renal impairment: Infants ≥3 months, Children, Adolescents, and Adults: There are no dosage adjustments provided in manufacturer's labeling; however, drug undergoes minimal renal excretion.

Dosing adjustment in hepatic impairment: Infants ≥3 months, Children, Adolescents, and Adults:

Mild impairment (Child-Pugh class A): No dosage adjustment recommended; use with caution

Moderate to severe impairment (Child-Pugh class B or C): Use not recommended; not studied

Administration Administer dose at bedtime to decrease CNS adverse effects; administer with water on an empty stomach (administration with food may increase efavirenz concentrations and adverse effects). Capsules and tablets should be swallowed intact. For patients who cannot swallow capsules or tablets, the capsules may be opened and added to 1 to 2 teaspoons of age-appropriate soft food (eg, applesauce, grape jelly, or yogurt) or 10 mL of room temperature infant formula. **Note:** Efavirenz tastes peppery (grape jelly may be used to improve taste). After administration, an additional small amount (2 teaspoons) of food or formula must be added to the empty mixing container, stirred to disperse any remaining efavirenz residue, and administered to the patient. Administer the efavirenz food or formula mixture within 30 minutes of mixing; do not save for future use. No additional food should be consumed for 2 hours after administration. Refer to the detailed "Instructions of Use" (found in the product labeling) for preparing a dose of efavirenz using the capsule sprinkle method.

Monitoring Parameters **Note:** Monitor CD4 percentage (if <5 years of age) or CD4 count (if ≥5 years of age) at least every 3 to 4 months (DHHS [pediatric], 2014).

Prior to initiation of therapy: Genotypic resistance testing, CD4 and viral load (every 3 to 4 months), CBC with differential, LFTs, BUN, creatinine, electrolytes, glucose, urinalysis (every 6 to 12 months), and assessment of readiness for adherence with medication regimen. At initiation and with any change in treatment regimen: CBC with differential, electrolytes, calcium, phosphate, glucose, LFTs, bilirubin, urinalysis (at initiation), BUN, creatinine, albumin, total protein, lipid panel (at initiation), CD4, and viral load. After 1 to 2 weeks of therapy: Signs of medication toxicity and adherence. After 2 to 4 weeks of therapy: CBC with differential, viral load, and signs of medication toxicity, and adherence; then every 3 to 4 months: CBC with differential, electrolytes, glucose, LFTs, bilirubin, BUN, creatinine, CD4, viral load, signs of medication toxicity, and adherence. Every 6 to 12 months: Lipid panel and urinalysis. CD4 monitoring frequency may be decreased to every 6 to 12 months in children who are adherent to therapy if the value is well above the threshold for opportunistic infections, viral suppression is sustained, and the clinical status is stable for more than 2 to 3 years (DHHS [pediatric], 2014). Monitor for growth and development, signs of HIV-specific physical conditions, HIV disease progression, opportunistic infections, signs and symptoms of rash, serum amylase, and CNS and psychiatric effects.

Additional monitoring for patients 3 months to <3 years of age weighing ≥3kg: CYP 2B6 genotype prior to therapy; efavirenz serum trough concentrations 2 weeks after initiation and at 3 years of age (DHHS [pediatric], 2014)

Reference Range Trough concentration: >1000 ng/mL (DHHS [adult, pediatric], 2014)

Test Interactions False-positive tests for cannabinoids have been reported when the CEDIA DAU Multilevel THC assay is used. False-positive results with other assays for cannabinoids have not been observed. False-positive tests for benzodiazepines have been reported and are likely due to the 8-hydroxy-efavirenz major metabolite.

Additional Information An oral liquid formulation of efavirenz (strawberry/mint-flavored solution) is available on an investigational basis from Bristol-Myers Squibb Company as part of an expanded access program for HIV-infected children and adolescents 3 to 16 years of age; for further details call 877-372-7097. **Note:** The bioavailability of the investigational liquid was found to be 20% lower than that of the capsules in adult volunteers; a recent pediatric study used initial doses of the liquid formulation that were 20% higher than pediatric capsule doses; these higher doses resulted in AUC values that were similar to AUCs achieved with the capsules (Starr, 2002).

Early virologic failure and rapid emergence of resistant mutations have been observed in therapy-naïve adult HIV patients treated with tenofovir, didanosine enteric-coated beadlets (Videx® EC), and either efavirenz or nevirapine; the combination of tenofovir, didanosine, and any non-nucleoside reverse transcriptase inhibitor is **not** recommended as initial antiretroviral therapy.

Dosage Forms Excipient information presented when available (limited, particularly for generics); consult specific product labeling.

Capsule, Oral:
Sustiva: 50 mg, 200 mg

Tablet, Oral:
Sustiva: 600 mg

Efavirenz, Emtricitabine, and Tenofovir

(e FAV e renz, em trye SYE ta been, & ten OF oh vir)

Medication Safety Issues

High alert medication:

This medication is in a class the Institute for Safe Medication Practices (ISMP) includes among its list of drug classes that have a heightened risk of causing significant patient harm when used in error.

Related Information

Adult and Adolescent HIV *on page 2392*
Pediatric HIV *on page 2380*
Perinatal HIV *on page 2400*

Brand Names: US Atripla

Brand Names: Canada Atripla

Therapeutic Category Antiretroviral Agent; HIV Agents (Anti-HIV Agents); Non-nucleoside Reverse Transcriptase Inhibitor (NNRTI); Nucleoside Reverse Transcriptase Inhibitor (NRTI); Nucleotide Reverse Transcriptase Inhibitor (NRTI)

Generic Availability (US) No

Use Treatment of HIV infection either alone or in combination with other antiretroviral agents (FDA approved in ages ≥12 years weighing at least 40 kg and adults)

Pregnancy Risk Factor D

Pregnancy Considerations Adverse events have been observed in some animal reproduction studies. The manufacturer of this combination recommends pregnancy testing prior to therapy and effective contraception in women of reproductive potential during treatment and for 12 weeks after therapy is discontinued. See individual agents.

Breast-Feeding Considerations Efavirenz, emtricitabine, and tenofovir are excreted into breast milk. See individual agents.

Contraindications

History of clinically-significant hypersensitivity (eg, Stevens-Johnson syndrome, erythema multiforme, or toxic skin reactions) to efavirenz; concurrent use of bepridil, cisapride, midazolam, triazolam, voriconazole, ergot alkaloids (includes dihydroergotamine, ergotamine, ergonovine, methylergonovine), St John's wort, pimozide

Canadian labeling: Additional contraindications (not in US labeling): Hypersensitivity to any component of the formulation; concomitant use with astemizole or terfenadine (not marketed in Canada)

Warnings/Precautions **[U.S. Boxed Warning]: Lactic acidosis and severe hepatomegaly with steatosis have been reported with nucleoside analogues, including fatal cases.** Not recommended in patients with moderate or severe hepatic impairment (Child-Pugh class B, C). Use caution in patients with mild hepatic impairment (Child-Pugh class A), HBV or HCV coinfection, elevated transaminases or use of concomitant hepatotoxic drugs. Use caution in hepatic impairment. Use with caution in patients with risk factors for liver disease (risk may be increased in obese patients or prolonged exposure) and suspend treatment in any patient who develops clinical or laboratory findings suggestive of lactic acidosis or hepatotoxicity (transaminase elevation may/may not accompany hepatomegaly and steatosis). Persistent elevations of serum transaminases >5 times the upper limit of normal should prompt evaluation - benefit of continued therapy should be weighed against possible risk of hepatotoxicity. Ethanol may increase hepatotoxic potential; instruct patients to limit or avoid alcohol. May cause redistribution of fat (eg, buffalo hump, peripheral wasting with increased abdominal girth, cushingoid appearance).

[U.S. Boxed Warning]: Safety and efficacy during coinfection of HIV and HBV have not been established; acute, severe exacerbations of HBV have been reported following discontinuation of antiretroviral therapy. All patients with HIV should be tested for HBV prior to initiation of treatment. Caution in patients with known or suspected hepatitis B or C infection (monitoring of liver function is recommended). In HBV coinfected patients, monitor hepatic function closely for several months following discontinuation.

Potentially significant drug-drug interactions may exist, requiring dose or frequency adjustment, additional monitoring, and/or selection of alternative therapy. Patients may develop immune reconstitution syndrome resulting in the occurrence of an inflammatory response to an indolent or residual opportunistic infection during initial HIV treatment or activation of autoimmune disorders (eg, Graves' disease, polymyositis, Guillain-Barré syndrome) later in therapy; further evaluation and treatment may be required. Discontinue if severe rash (involving blistering, desquamation, mucosal involvement or fever) develops. Consider alternative therapy in the case of life-threatening cutaneous reactions (see Contraindications). Children are more susceptible to development of rash (median time to onset: 28 days); prophylactic antihistamines may be used. To avoid duplicate therapy, do not use concurrently with efavirenz emtricitabine, tenofovir, or any combination of these drugs; however, coadministration with efavirenz may be required for dose-adjustment with concomitant rifampin therapy.

Use caution with history of mental illness/drug abuse (predisposition to psychological reactions); may cause CNS and psychiatric symptoms, which include impaired concentration, dizziness or drowsiness (avoid potentially hazardous tasks such as driving or operating machinery if these effects are noted); serious psychiatric side effects have been associated with efavirenz, including severe depression, suicidal ideation, paranoia, and mania. CNS effects may be potentiated when used with other sedative drugs or ethanol. Seizures have been associated with efavirenz use; use caution in patients with a history of seizure disorder.

May cause osteomalacia with proximal renal tubulopathy. Bone pain, extremity pain, fractures, arthralgias, weakness and muscle pain have been reported. In patients at risk for renal dysfunction, persistent or worsening bone or muscle symptoms should be evaluated for hypophosphatemia and osteomalacia. May cause acute renal failure or Fanconi syndrome; use caution with other nephrotoxic agents (including high dose or multiple NSAID use or those which compete for active tubular secretion). Acute renal failure has occurred in HIV-infected patients with risk factors for renal impairment who were on a stable tenofovir regimen to which a high dose or multiple NSAID therapy was added. Consider alternatives to NSAIDS in patients taking tenofovir and at risk for renal impairment. IDSA guidelines recommend discontinuing tenofovir in HIV infected patients who develop a decline in GFR (a >25% decrease in GFR from baseline and to a level of <60 mL/minute/1.73 m^2) during use, particularly in presence of proximal tubular dysfunction (eg, euglycemic glycosuria, increased urinary phosphorus excretion and hypophosphatemia, proteinuria [new onset or worsening]) (IDSA [Lucas 2014]).

Product is a fixed-dose combination and is not appropriate for use in renal impairment (CrCl <50 mL/minute).

In clinical trials, use has been associated with decreases in bone mineral density in HIV-1 infected adults and increases in bone metabolism markers. Serum parathyroid hormone and 1,25 vitamin D levels were also higher. Decreases in bone mineral density have also been observed in clinical trials of HIV-1 infected pediatric patients. Observations in chronic hepatitis B infected pediatric patients (aged 12-18 years) were similar.

Avoid pregnancy; women of childbearing potential should undergo pregnancy testing prior to initiation of therapy. Two forms of contraception should be used during and for 12 weeks after discontinuation of therapy. Fixed-dose combination product; safety and efficacy have not been established in pediatric patients <12 years of age and <40 kg. In children <40 kg, the dose of efavirenz would be excessive.

Warnings: Additional Pediatric Considerations Efavirenz may cause a rash, which usually presents as pruritic maculopapular skin eruptions; incidence is more common and more severe in children than in adults (incidence: Adults 26%, children 46%; median onset: Adults: 11 days, children: 9 days [range: 6 to 205 days]). Most rashes in children appeared within 14 days after starting therapy [median duration: Adults: 16 days, children: 6 days (range: 2 to 37 days)]. Median duration of rash in children who continued therapy was 9 days; rash may be treated with antihistamines and corticosteroids and usually resolves within 1 month while continuing therapy. Discontinue if severe rash (involving blistering, desquamation, mucosal involvement, ulceration, or fever) occurs. Consider prophylaxis with antihistamines in children due to frequency and severity of rash reported in children.). The overall reported incidence of CNS adverse effects was 53% vs 25% in controls; nervous system symptoms in children were reported to be 18%. Fever has been reported with use (children: 21%).

Emtricitabine-associated hyperpigmentation may occur at a higher frequency in pediatric patients compared to adults (children: 32%; adults: 2% to 6%).

Recent studies suggest that tenofovir-related bone loss may be greater in children who are less mature (eg, Tanner stage 1-2) than in those who are more physically mature (Tanner ≥3). A significant decrease in lumbar spine BMD (>6%) was reported in five of 15 pediatric patients who received a tenofovir-containing regimen for 48 weeks. No orthopedic fractures occurred, but two patients required discontinuation of tenofovir. All five patients with a decrease in BMD were virologic responders and prepubertal (Tanner Stage 1). This study found a moderately strong correlation between decreases in bone mineral density z scores at week 48 and age at baseline. No correlation between decreases in bone mineral density z scores and tenofovir dose or pharmacokinetics was observed; BMD loss may limit the usefulness of tenofovir in prepubertal children (DHHS [pediatric], 2014; Giacomet, 2005; Hazra, 2005; Purdy, 2008). Monitor BMD for potential bone toxicities during therapy; supplementation with calcium and vitamin D may be beneficial but has not been studied.

Adverse Reactions The complete adverse reaction profile of combination therapy has not been established. **See individual agents.** The following adverse effects were noted in clinical trials with combination therapy:

Central nervous system: Abnormal dreams, anxiety, depression, dizziness, fatigue, headache, insomnia, somnolence

Dermatologic: Rash
Endocrine & metabolic: Bone mineral density decreased, hypercholesterolemia, hyperglycemia, triglycerides increased
Gastrointestinal: Diarrhea, nausea, serum amylase increased, vomiting
Hematologic: Neutropenia
Hepatic: Alkaline phosphatase increased, ALT increased, AST increased
Neuromuscular & skeletal: Creatine increased
Renal: Hematuria
Respiratory: Nasopharyngitis, sinusitis, upper respiratory infection
Rare but important or life-threatening: Glycosuria

Drug Interactions

Metabolism/Transport Effects Refer to individual components.

Avoid Concomitant Use

Avoid concomitant use of Efavirenz, Emtricitabine, and Tenofovir with any of the following: Adefovir; Amodiaquine; Atovaquone; Axitinib; Azelastine (Nasal); Bedaquiline; Boceprevir; Bosutinib; CarBAMazepine; Dasabuvir; Didanosine; Elvitegravir; Enzalutamide; Etravirine; Itraconazole; Ketoconazole (Systemic); LamiVUDine; Nevirapine; Nisoldipine; Olaparib; Orphenadrine; Palbociclib; Paraldehyde; Paritaprevir; Posaconazole; Reverse Transcriptase Inhibitors (Non-Nucleoside); Rilpivirine; Simeprevir; St Johns Wort; Thalidomide; Ulipristal

Increased Effect/Toxicity

Efavirenz, Emtricitabine, and Tenofovir may increase the levels/effects of: Adefovir; Alcohol (Ethyl); Aminoglycosides; Amodiaquine; Azelastine (Nasal); Bosentan; Cannabis; Carvedilol; Cilostazol; Citalopram; CNS Depressants; CYP2C19 Substrates; CYP2C8 Substrates; CYP2C9 Substrates; Dasabuvir; Didanosine; Dronabinol; Etravirine; Fosphenytoin; Hydrocodone; Ifosfamide; Methotrimeprazine; Metyrosine; Mirtazapine; Nevirapine; Orphenadrine; Paraldehyde; Paritaprevir; Phenytoin; Pramipexole; Rilpivirine; Ritonavir; ROPINIRole; Rotigotine; Selective Serotonin Reuptake Inhibitors; Suvorexant; Tetrahydrocannabinol; Thalidomide; TiZANidine; Vitamin K Antagonists; Zolpidem

The levels/effects of Efavirenz, Emtricitabine, and Tenofovir may be increased by: Acyclovir-Valacyclovir; Adefovir; Aminoglycosides; Atazanavir; Boceprevir; Brimonidine (Topical); Cannabis; Cidofovir; Cobicistat; CYP2B6 Inhibitors (Moderate); Darunavir; Diclofenac (Systemic); Doxylamine; Dronabinol; Droperidol; Ganciclovir-Valganciclovir; HydrOXYzine; Kava Kava; LamiVUDine; Ledipasvir; Magnesium Sulfate; Methotrimeprazine; Mifepristone; Nabilone; Nevirapine; Nonsteroidal Anti-Inflammatory Agents; Perampanel; Quazepam; Reverse Transcriptase Inhibitors (Non-Nucleoside); Ribavirin; Ritonavir; Rufinamide; Saquinavir; Sodium Oxybate; Tapentadol; Tetrahydrocannabinol; Voriconazole

Decreased Effect

Efavirenz, Emtricitabine, and Tenofovir may decrease the levels/effects of: Alcohol (Ethyl); ARIPiprazole; Artemether; Atazanavir; AtorvaSTATin; Atovaquone; Axitinib; Bedaquiline; Boceprevir; Bosutinib; Buprenorphine; BuPROPion; Calcium Channel Blockers; Canagliflozin; CarBAMazepine; Caspofungin; Clarithromycin; Clopidogrel; Contraceptives (Progestins); CycloSPORINE (Systemic); CYP3A4 Substrates; Darunavir; Dasabuvir; Didanosine; Diltiazem; Dolutegravir; Elvitegravir; Enzalutamide; Etonogestrel; Etravirine; Everolimus; FentaNYL; Fosamprenavir; Ibrutinib; Ifosfamide; Indinavir; Itraconazole; Ketoconazole (Systemic); Lopinavir; Lovastatin; Maraviroc; Methadone; NiMODipine; Nisoldipine; Norgestimate; Olaparib; Ombitasvir; Palbociclib; Paritaprevir; Posaconazole; Pravastatin; Proguanil; Rifabutin; Rilpivirine; Saquinavir; Saxagliptin; Sertraline; Simeprevir; Simvastatin; Sirolimus; Tacrolimus (Systemic); Telaprevir; Tipranavir; Ulipristal; Vitamin K Antagonists; Voriconazole

The levels/effects of Efavirenz, Emtricitabine, and Tenofovir may be decreased by: Adefovir; Bosentan; CarBAMazepine; CYP2B6 Inducers (Strong); CYP3A4 Inducers (Moderate); CYP3A4 Inducers (Strong); Dabrafenib; Deferasirox; Fosphenytoin; Ginkgo Biloba; Mitotane; Nevirapine; Phenytoin; Reverse Transcriptase Inhibitors (Non-Nucleoside); Rifabutin; Rifampin; Siltuximab; St Johns Wort; Telaprevir; Tipranavir; Tocilizumab

Food Interactions See individual agents.

Storage/Stability Store at 25°C (77°F); excursions permitted between 15°C to 30°C (59°F to 86°F). Dispense only in original container; do not use if seal on bottle is broken or missing.

Mechanism of Action See individual agents.

Pharmacokinetics (Adult data unless noted) One Atripla® tablet is bioequivalent to one efavirenz 600 mg tablet plus one emtricitabine 200 mg capsule plus one tenofovir 300 mg tablet (single dose study); see individual agents

Dosing: Usual

Pediatric: **HIV infection, treatment:** May be used alone or in combination with other antiretroviral agents:
- Children <12 years or <40 kg: Product is a fixed-dose combination; safety and efficacy have not been established; use in patients <40 kg would result in an excessive efavirenz dose
- Children ≥12 years and Adolescents; weighing ≥40 kg: Oral: 1 tablet once daily

Adult: **HIV infection, treatment:** Oral: 1 tablet once daily

Dosing adjustment in renal impairment: Children ≥12 years, Adolescents, and Adults: CrCl <50 mL/minute: Use not recommended.

Dosing adjustment in hepatic impairment: Children ≥12 years, Adolescents, and Adults:
- Mild hepatic impairment (Child-Pugh class A): Use with caution; limited clinical experience
- Moderate to severe hepatic impairment (Child-Pugh class B, C): Not recommended

Administration Administer dose at bedtime to decrease CNS adverse effects. Administer with water on an empty stomach; administration with food may increase efavirenz concentrations and adverse effects.

Monitoring Parameters Note: Monitor CD4 percentage (if <5 years of age) or CD4 count (if ≥5 years of age) at least every 3 to 4 months (DHHS [pediatric], 2014).

Patients should be screened for hepatitis B infection before starting therapy. Prior to initiation of therapy: Genotypic resistance testing, CD4 and viral load (every 3 to 4 months), CBC with differential, LFTs, BUN, creatinine, creatinine clearance, electrolytes, glucose, urinalysis (every 6 to 12 months), and assessment of readiness for adherence with medication regimen. At initiation and with any change in treatment regimen: CBC with differential, electrolytes, calcium, phosphorus, glucose, LFTs, bilirubin, urinalysis (at initiation), BUN, creatinine, albumin, total protein, lipid panel (at initiation), CD4, and viral load. After 1 to 2 weeks of therapy: Signs of medication toxicity and adherence. After 2 to 4 weeks of therapy: CBC with differential, viral load, and signs of medication toxicity, and adherence; then every 3 to 4 months: CBC with differential, electrolytes, glucose, LFTs, bilirubin, BUN, creatinine, CD4, viral load, signs of medication toxicity, and adherence. Every 6 to 12 months: Lipid panel and urinalysis. CD4 monitoring frequency may be decreased to every 6 to 12 months in children who are adherent to therapy if the value is well above the threshold for opportunistic infections, viral suppression is sustained, and the clinical status is stable for more than 2 to 3 years (DHHS [pediatric], 2014). Monitor for growth and development, signs of HIV-specific physical conditions, HIV disease progression, opportunistic infections, rash, CNS and psychiatric effects, bone abnormalities, hyperpigmentation, or lactic acidosis. Consider bone mineral density assessment for all patients with a history of pathologic bone fractures or other risk factors for osteoporosis or bone loss. Some experts recommend obtaining a DXA scan prior to therapy and 6 months into therapy, especially for patients in pre- and early puberty (Tanner stages 1 and 2) (DHHS [pediatric], 2014).

Reference Range Efavirenz: Trough concentration: >1000 ng/mL (DHHS [adult, pediatric], 2014)

Test Interactions False-positive test for cannabinoids have been reported with some screening assays used in HIV-infected and uninfected subjects receiving efavirenz. Confirmation of screening tests for cannabinoids by a more specific method is recommended.

Dosage Forms Excipient information presented when available (limited, particularly for generics); consult specific product labeling.

Tablet, oral:

Atripla: Efavirenz 600 mg, emtricitabine 200 mg, and tenofovir disoproxil fumarate 300 mg

◆ **Effexor XR** *see* Venlafaxine *on page 2166*

Eflornithine (ee FLOR ni theen)

Medication Safety Issues

Sound-alike/look-alike issues:

Vaniqa® may be confused with Viagra®

Brand Names: US Vaniqa

Brand Names: Canada Vaniqa®

Therapeutic Category Antiprotozoal; Topical Skin Product

Generic Availability (US) No

Use Reduce unwanted hair from face and adjacent areas under the chin (Cream: FDA approved in females ≥12 years and adults); injectable (available through WHO). Used for treatment of meningoencephalitic stage of *Trypanosoma brucei gambiense* infection (sleeping sickness). **Note:** Eflornithine has specific activity against *T.b. gambiense* in early and late stages (not effective for *T.b. rhodesiense*).

Prescribing and Access Restrictions Injectable eflornithine is donated to World Health Organization (WHO) by the manufacturer. Further information may be found on WHO website at http://www.who.int/trypanosomiasis_african/diagnosis/en/index.html or by contacting the CDC Drug Service (404-639-3670).

Pregnancy Risk Factor C

Pregnancy Considerations When administered topically, teratogenic effects were not observed in animal reproduction studies. Discontinuation or not initiating therapy should be considered since information related to topical use in pregnancy is limited.

Breast-Feeding Considerations It is not known if eflornithine is excreted in breast milk. The manufacturer recommends that caution be exercised when administering eflornithine to nursing women.

Contraindications Hypersensitivity to eflornithine or any component of the formulation

Warnings/Precautions

Cream: For topical use by females only. Discontinue if hypersensitivity occurs.

Injection: For IV use only; not for IM administration. Must be diluted before use; frequent monitoring for myelosuppression should be done; use with caution in patients with a history of seizures and in patients with renal impairment; serial audiograms should be obtained; due to the potential for relapse, patients should be followed up for at least 24 months.

Adverse Reactions

Injection (Priotto, 2009):

Cardiovascular: Arrhythmia, chest pain, edema, hyper-/hypotension, shock

Central nervous system: Amnesia, anxiety, ataxia, coma, confusion, depression, dizziness, fever, hallucination, headache, insomnia, lethargy, seizure

Dermatologic: Pruritus, rash

Endocrine & metabolic: Dehydration

Gastrointestinal: Abdominal pain, anorexia, constipation, diarrhea, dysphagia, nausea, taste disturbance, vomiting, xerostomia

Genitourinary: Urinary frequency/urgency, urinary incontinence

Hematologic: Anemia, leukopenia, neutropenia, thrombocytopenia

Local: Extravasation, injection site reaction

Neuromuscular & skeletal: Arthralgia, myalgia, peripheral neuropathy, tremor, weakness

Otic: Inner ear disturbance

Renal: ALT altered, bilirubin altered, creatinine altered

Respiratory: Cough, dyspnea, epistaxis, respiratory distress

Miscellaneous: Hiccups, infection

Topical:

Central nervous system: Dizziness, headache

Dermatologic: Acne, alopecia, burning skin, dry skin, erythema, folliculitis, ingrown hair, pruritus, pseudofolliculitis barbae, rash, skin irritation, stinging, tingling skin

Gastrointestinal: Anorexia, dyspepsia

Rare but important or life-threatening: Bleeding skin, cheilitis, contact dermatitis, facial edema, herpes simplex, lip swelling, nausea, numbness, rosacea, vertigo, weakness

Drug Interactions

Metabolism/Transport Effects None known.

Avoid Concomitant Use There are no known interactions where it is recommended to avoid concomitant use.

Increased Effect/Toxicity There are no known significant interactions involving an increase in effect.

Decreased Effect There are no known significant interactions involving a decrease in effect.

Storage/Stability

Cream: Store at controlled room temperature 25°C (77°F); excursions permitted to 15°C to 30°C (59 °F to 86°F); do not freeze.

Injection: Use within 24 hours of preparation.

Mechanism of Action

Cream: Eflornithine inhibits the enzyme ornithine decarboxylase (ODC) which inhibits cell division and synthetic functions and thereby affects the rate of hair growth.

Injection: Eflornithine exerts antitumor and antiprotozoal effects through specific, irreversible ("suicide") inhibition of the enzyme ornithine decarboxylase (ODC). ODC is the rate-limiting enzyme in the biosynthesis of putrescine, spermine, and spermidine, the major polyamines in nucleated cells. Polyamines are necessary for the synthesis of DNA, RNA, and proteins and are, therefore, necessary for cell growth and differentiation. Although many microorganisms and higher plants are able to produce polyamines from alternate biochemical pathways, all mammalian cells depend on ornithine decarboxylase to produce polyamines. Eflornithine inhibits ODC and rapidly depletes animal cells of putrescine and spermidine; the concentration of spermine remains the same or may even increase. Rapidly dividing cells appear to be most susceptible to the effects of eflornithine.

Pharmacodynamics Reduced hair growth: Topical:

Onset of action: 4 to 8 weeks

Duration: Continues until ~8 weeks after discontinuing treatment

Pharmacokinetics (Adult data unless noted)

Absorption: Topical: <1%

Half-life elimination: IV: 3 to 3.5 hours; Topical: 8 hours

Elimination: Primarily urine (as unchanged drug)

Dosing: Usual

Pediatric:

Reduction of unwanted facial hair: Topical: Cream: Female Children ≥12 years and Adolescents: Apply thin layer of cream to affected areas of face and adjacent chin twice daily, at least 8 hours apart

Treatment of infections caused by *Trypanosoma brucei gambiense* infection (sleeping sickness): Limited data available (WHO, 2013):

NECT regimen: Children and Adolescents: IV: 200 mg/kg/dose every 12 hours for 7 days in combination with nifurtimox

Monotherapy: IV:

Children <12 years: 150 mg/kg/dose every 6 hours for 14 days

Children ≥12 years and Adolescents: 100 mg/kg/dose every 6 hours for 14 days

Adult: **Reduction unwanted facial hair:** Topical: Apply thin layer of cream to affected areas of face and adjacent chin twice daily, at least 8 hours apart

Dosing adjustment in renal impairment:

Injection: Dose should be adjusted although no specific guidelines are available.

Topical: There are no dosage adjustments provided in manufacturer's labeling; however, dosage adjustment unlikely due to limited systemic absorption.

Dosing adjustment in hepatic impairment: Topical: There are no dosage adjustments provided in manufacturer's labeling; however, dosage adjustment unlikely due to limited systemic absorption.

Preparation for Administration Parenteral: IV: Dilute 100 mL ampul with 400 mL normal saline.

Administration

Parenteral: IV: Administer diluted solution by IV infusion over 45 to 120 minutes; not for IM administration

Topical: For external use only. Rub in thoroughly. Hair removal techniques must still be continued; wait at least 5 minutes after removing hair to apply cream. Do not wash affected area for at least 8 hours following application. Makeup and sunscreen may be used over treated area(s) after cream has dried.

Monitoring Parameters Parenteral: CBC with platelet counts

Dosage Forms Excipient information presented when available (limited, particularly for generics); consult specific product labeling.

Cream, External, as hydrochloride:

Vaniqa: 13.9% (45 g) [contains cetearyl alcohol, methylparaben, propylparaben]

◆ **Eflornithine Hydrochloride** *see* Eflornithine *on page 737*

◆ **Eformoterol** *see* Formoterol *on page 934*

◆ **Eformoterol and Budesonide** *see* Budesonide and Formoterol *on page 313*

◆ **Eformoterol and Mometasone** *see* Mometasone and Formoterol *on page 1457*

◆ **Efraloctocog Alfa** *see* Antihemophilic Factor (Recombinant) *on page 168*

◆ **EHDP** *see* Etidronate *on page 815*

◆ **Elaprase** *see* Idursulfase *on page 1073*

◆ **Elavil** *see* Amitriptyline *on page 131*

◆ **Electrolyte Lavage Solution** *see* Polyethylene Glycol-Electrolyte Solution *on page 1724*

◆ **Elepsia XR** *see* LevETIRAcetam *on page 1234*

◆ **Elestat** *see* Epinastine *on page 759*

◆ **Elestrin** *see* Estradiol (Systemic) *on page 795*

◆ **Elidel** *see* Pimecrolimus *on page 1702*

◆ **Eligard** *see* Leuprolide *on page 1229*

◆ **Elimite** *see* Permethrin *on page 1675*

◆ **Eliphos** *see* Calcium Acetate *on page 341*

◆ **Elitek** *see* Rasburicase *on page 1839*

◆ **Elixophyllin** *see* Theophylline *on page 2044*

◆ **ElixSure Congestion [OTC]** *see* Pseudoephedrine *on page 1801*

◆ **ElixSure Cough [OTC]** *see* Dextromethorphan *on page 631*

◆ **Elocom (Can)** *see* Mometasone (Topical) *on page 1456*

◆ **Elocon** *see* Mometasone (Topical) *on page 1456*

◆ **Eloctate** *see* Antihemophilic Factor (Recombinant) *on page 168*

Elosulfase Alfa (el oh SUL fase AL fa)

Brand Names: US Vimizim

Therapeutic Category Enzyme

Generic Availability (US) No

Use Treatment of mucopolysaccharidosis type IVA (MPS IVA; Morquio A syndrome) (FDA approved in ages ≥5 years and adults)

Pregnancy Risk Factor C

Pregnancy Considerations Adverse events were observed in some animal reproduction studies. Mucopolysaccharidosis type IVA (MPS IVA) has the potential to cause adverse events in both the mother and fetus. A pregnancy registry is available for women who may be exposed to elosulfase alfa for the treatment of MPS IVA during pregnancy (MARS@bmrn.com or 1-800-983-4587).

Breast-Feeding Considerations It is not known if elosulfase alfa is excreted into breast milk. The manufacturer recommends that caution be used if administered to nursing women. The pregnancy registry also collects data from women using elosulfase alfa for the treatment of MPS IVA and who are breast-feeding.

Contraindications There are no contraindications listed in the manufacturer's labeling.

Warnings/Precautions [U.S. Boxed Warning]: Serious hypersensitivity reactions, including life-threatening anaphylactic reactions have occurred, regardless of treatment course duration. Anaphylaxis may present as abdominal pain, chest discomfort, cough, cyanosis, dyspnea, erythema, flushing, hypotension, nausea, rash, retching, throat tightness, urticaria, and vomiting. Monitor closely during and after infusion. Appropriate medical support should be readily available. Patients with acute respiratory disease are at risk of serious acute exacerbation or respiratory compromise due to hypersensitivity; additional monitoring may be required. Discontinue immediately if anaphylactic or acute reaction occurs. Patients experiencing initial severe or refractory reactions may need prolonged monitoring. Use caution with readministration. Infusion-related reactions have been reported; may be sporadic and/or severe. Hypersensitivity reactions may occur as early as 30 minutes from the start of infusion and have also been reported as late as 6 days after infusion; reactions may occur as late as the 47th infusion. Patients should be premedicated with antihistamines with or without antipyretics prior to infusion; evaluate airway prior to therapy (due to possible effects of antihistamine use). In case of reaction, decrease the rate of infusion, temporarily discontinue the infusion, and/or administer additional antipyretics/ antihistamines and possibly corticosteroids. Discontinue treatment immediately if severe reaction occurs; use caution with readministration.

Consider delaying treatment in patients with an acute febrile or respiratory illness; may be increased risk of life-threatening complications from hypersensitivity reactions. Use with caution in patients with sleep apnea; antihistamine pretreatment may increase the risk of apneic episodes. Apnea treatment options (eg, supplemental oxygen or continuous positive airway pressure) should be readily available. Patients with MPA IVA may experience spinal/cervical cord compression (SCC) as a part of their disease. Monitor patients for signs and symptoms of SCC (eg, back pain, limb paralysis, urinary and fecal incontinence). All patients developed anti-drug antibodies and neutralizing antibodies during clinical trials; it is unknown if presence of antibodies is related to a higher risk of infusion reactions or clinical efficacy treatment effect, respectively.

Adverse Reactions

Central nervous system: Chills, fatigue, headache
Gastrointestinal: Abdominal pain, nausea, vomiting
Hypersensitivity: Hypersensitivity reaction
Immunologic: Immunogenicity
Miscellaneous: Fever

Drug Interactions

Metabolism/Transport Effects None known.

Avoid Concomitant Use There are no known interactions where it is recommended to avoid concomitant use.

Increased Effect/Toxicity There are no known significant interactions involving an increase in effect.

Decreased Effect There are no known significant interactions involving a decrease in effect.

Storage/Stability Prior to use, store intact vials under refrigeration at 2°C to 8°C (36°F to 46°F); do not freeze or shake. Protect from light. Following dilution, use immediately. If unable to use immediately, may store for up to 24 hours under refrigeration followed by up to 24 hours at 23°C to 27°C (73°F to 81°F) during administration.

Mechanism of Action Elosulfase alfa is a recombinant form of N-acetylgalactosamine-6-sulfatase, produced in Chinese hamster cells. A deficiency of this enzyme leads to accumulation of the glycosaminoglycan (GAG) substrates (keratan sulfate and chondroitin-6-sulfate) in tissues, causing cellular, tissue and organ dysfunction. Elosulfase alfa provides the exogenous enzyme (N-acetylgalactosamine-6-sulfatase) that is taken into lysosomes and thereby increases the catabolism of the GAG substrates (eg, keratan sulfate and chondroitin-6-sulfate).

Pharmacokinetics (Adult data unless noted)

Distribution: V_d: Week 0: 396 mL/kg; Week 22: 650 mL/kg
Half-life elimination: Week 0: ~8 minutes; Week 22: ~36 minutes
Time to peak serum concentration: Week 0: 172 minutes; Week 22: 202 minutes

Dosing: Usual Note: Premedicate with antihistamines with or without antipyretics 30 to 60 minutes prior to infusion.

Pediatric: **Mucopolysaccharidosis type IVA (MPS IVA; Morquio A syndrome):** Children ≥5 years and Adolescents: IV: 2 mg/kg once weekly

Adult: **Mucopolysaccharidosis type IVA (MPS IVA; Morquio A syndrome):** IV: 2 mg/kg once weekly

Dosing adjustment in renal impairment: There are no dosage adjustments provided in manufacturer's labeling.

Dosing adjustment in hepatic impairment: There are no dosage adjustments provided in manufacturer's labeling.

Preparation for Administration IV: Dilute calculated dose in NS to a final volume of 100 mL (for patients weighing <25 kg) or 250 mL (for patients weighing ≥25 kg). Gently rotate to distribute. Do not shake or agitate. Use immediately. Vials are for single use only; discard any unused product.

Administration IV: Administer using a low protein-binding infusion set with in-line low protein-binding 0.2 micrometer filter. Pretreatment with antihistamines with or without antipyretics is recommended 30 to 60 minutes prior to infusion.

Patients <25 kg: Infuse solution at 3 mL/hour for the first 15 minutes. If well-tolerated, increase to 6 mL/hour for the next 15 minutes. If well-tolerated, increase rate every 15 minutes in 6 mL/hour increments; maximum infusion rate: 36 mL/hour. The total volume of the infusion should be delivered over ≥3.5 hours.

Patients ≥25 kg: Infuse 250 mL solution at 6 ml/hour for the first 15 minutes. If well-tolerated, increase to 12 mL/hour for the next 15 minutes. If well-tolerated, increase rate every 15 minutes in 12 mL/hour increments; maximum infusion rate: 72 mL/hour. The total volume of the infusion should be delivered over ≥4.5 hours.

The infusion can be slowed, temporarily stopped, or discontinued if a hypersensitivity reaction occurs. Discontinue immediately if severe reaction occurs. Do not infuse with other products in the infusion tubing. Administration should be completed within 48 hours from time of dilution.

Monitoring Parameters Monitor for infusion/hypersensitivity reactions; signs/symptoms of spinal or cervical compression.

Dosage Forms

Excipient information presented when available (limited, particularly for generics); consult specific product labeling.

Solution, Intravenous [preservative free]:
Vimizim: 5 mg/5 mL (5 mL) [contains mouse protein (murine) (hamster)]

- ◆ **Elosulfase alfa** *see* Elosulfase Alfa *on page 738*
- ◆ **Eloxatin** *see* Oxaliplatin *on page 1578*
- ◆ **Elta Lite Tar [OTC]** *see* Coal Tar *on page 523*
- ◆ **Elta Seal Moisture Barrier [OTC]** *see* Zinc Oxide *on page 2214*
- ◆ **Elta Tar [OTC]** *see* Coal Tar *on page 523*
- ◆ **Eltor® (Can)** *see* Pseudoephedrine *on page 1801*
- ◆ **Eltroxin (Can)** *see* Levothyroxine *on page 1250*
- ◆ **E-Max-1000 [OTC]** *see* Vitamin E *on page 2188*
- ◆ **Emend** *see* Aprepitant *on page 186*
- ◆ **Emend** *see* Fosaprepitant *on page 939*
- ◆ **Emend® IV (Can)** *see* Fosaprepitant *on page 939*
- ◆ **EMLA** *see* Lidocaine and Prilocaine *on page 1263*
- ◆ **Emo-Cort® (Can)** *see* Hydrocortisone (Topical) *on page 1041*
- ◆ **Emorex Gel [OTC] (Can)** *see* Coal Tar *on page 523*
- ◆ **Emtec** *see* Acetaminophen and Codeine *on page 50*

Emtricitabine (em trye SYE ta been)

Medication Safety Issues

High alert medication:

This medication is in a class the Institute for Safe Medication Practices (ISMP) includes among its list of drug classes that have a heightened risk of causing significant patient harm when used in error.

Related Information

Adult and Adolescent HIV *on page 2392*
Pediatric HIV *on page 2380*
Perinatal HIV *on page 2400*

Brand Names: US Emtriva

Brand Names: Canada Emtriva®

Therapeutic Category Antiretroviral Agent; HIV Agents (Anti-HIV Agents); Nucleoside Reverse Transcriptase Inhibitor (NRTI)

Generic Availability (US) No

Use Treatment of HIV infection in combination with other antiretroviral agents (FDA approved in all ages). **Note:** HIV regimens consisting of **three** antiretroviral agents are strongly recommended.

Pregnancy Risk Factor B

Pregnancy Considerations Adverse events were not observed in animal studies. Emtricitabine has a high level of transfer across the human placenta; no increased risk of overall birth defects has been observed according to data collected by the antiretroviral pregnancy registry. Cases of lactic acidosis/hepatic steatosis syndrome related to mitochondrial toxicity have been reported in pregnant women with prolonged use of nucleoside analogues. It is not known if pregnancy itself potentiates this known side effect; however, women may be at increased risk of lactic acidosis and liver damage. In addition, these adverse events are similar to other rare but life-threatening syndromes which occur during pregnancy (eg, HELLP syndrome). Hepatic enzymes and electrolytes should be monitored in women receiving nucleoside analogues and clinicians should watch for early signs of the syndrome. In addition, mitochondrial dysfunction may develop in infants following in utero exposure. A pharmacokinetic study shows a slight decrease in emtricitabine serum levels during the third trimester and immediately postpartum; however, there is no clear need to adjust the dose. The DHHS Perinatal HIV Guidelines consider emtricitabine with tenofovir to be a preferred NRTI backbone in antiretroviral-naive pregnant women. The DHHS Perinatal HIV Guidelines consider emtricitabine plus tenofovir a recommended dual NRTI/NtRTI backbone for HIV/HBV coinfected pregnant women.

Regardless of CD4 count or HIV RNA copy number, all HIV-infected pregnant women should receive a combination antiretroviral (ARV) drug regimen. A combination of antepartum, intrapartum, and infant ARV prophylaxis is recommended. ARV therapy should be started as soon as possible in women with symptomatic infection. Although earlier initiation may be more effective in reducing the perinatal transmission of HIV, initiation may be delayed until after 12 weeks gestation in women who do not require immediate treatment after careful consideration of maternal conditions (eg, nausea and vomiting) and the potential risks of first trimester fetal exposure for specific agents. A scheduled cesarean delivery at 38 weeks gestation is recommended for all women with HIV RNA >1,000 copies/mL or unknown concentrations near delivery in order to decrease transmission. If ARV therapy must be interrupted for <24 hours during the peripartum period, stop then restart all medications simultaneously in order to decrease the chance of developing resistance. Long-term follow-up is recommended for all infants exposed to ARV medications. In couples who want to conceive, the HIV-infected partner should attain maximum viral suppression prior to conception.

Health care providers are encouraged to enroll pregnant women exposed to antiretroviral medications in the Antiretroviral Pregnancy Registry (1-800-258-4263 or www.APRegistry.com). Healthcare providers caring for HIV-infected women and their infants may contact the National Perinatal HIV Hotline (888-448-8765) for clinical consultation (HHS [perinatal], 2014).

Breast-Feeding Considerations Emtricitabine is excreted into breast milk. Maternal or infant antiretroviral therapy does not completely eliminate the risk of postnatal HIV transmission. In addition, multiclass-resistant virus has been detected in breast-feeding infants despite maternal therapy. Therefore, in the United States, where formula is accessible, affordable, safe, and sustainable, and the risk of infant mortality due to diarrhea and respiratory infections is low, complete avoidance of breast-feeding by HIV-infected women is recommended to decrease potential transmission of HIV (HHS [perinatal], 2014).

Contraindications Hypersensitivity to emtricitabine or any component of the formulation

Warnings/Precautions [U.S. Boxed Warning]: Lactic acidosis, severe hepatomegaly with steatosis, and hepatic failure have occurred rarely with emtricitabine (similar to other nucleoside analogues). Some cases have been fatal; stop treatment if lactic acidosis or hepatotoxicity occur. Prior liver disease, obesity, extended duration of therapy, and female gender may represent risk factors for severe hepatic reactions. Testing for hepatitis B is recommended prior to the initiation of therapy; **[U.S. Boxed Warnings]: Hepatitis B may be exacerbated following discontinuation of emtricitabine; not indicated for treatment of chronic hepatitis B; safety and efficacy in HIV/HBV coinfected patients not established.** May be associated with fat redistribution (buffalo hump, increased abdominal girth, breast engorgement, facial atrophy, and dyslipidemia). Immune reconstitution syndrome may develop resulting in the occurrence of an inflammatory response to an indolent or residual opportunistic infection during initial HIV treatment or activation of autoimmune disorders (eg, Graves' disease, polymyositis, Guillain-Barré syndrome) later in therapy; further evaluation and treatment may be required. Use caution in patients with renal impairment (dosage adjustment required). Concomitant use of other emtricitabine-containing products should be avoided. Concomitant use of lamivudine or lamivudine-containing products should be avoided; cross-resistance may develop.

Warnings: Additional Pediatric Considerations Hyperpigmentation may occur at a higher frequency in pediatric patients compared to adults (children: 32%; adults: 2% to 6%).

Some dosage forms may contain propylene glycol; in neonates large amounts of propylene glycol delivered orally, intravenously (eg, >3,000 mg/day), or topically have been associated with potentially fatal toxicities which can include metabolic acidosis, seizures, renal failure, and CNS depression; toxicities have also been reported in children and adults including hyperosmolality, lactic acidosis, seizures, and respiratory depression; use caution (AAP, 1997; Shehab, 2009).

Adverse Reactions

Central nervous system: Abnormal dreams, depression, dizziness, headache, insomnia, neuropathy/neuritis

Dermatologic: Hyperpigmentation (primarily of palms and/or soles but may include tongue, arms, lip and nails; generally mild and nonprogressive without associated local reactions such as pruritus or rash), rash (includes pruritus, maculopapular rash, vesiculobullous rash, pustular rash, and allergic reaction)

Endocrine & metabolic: Disordered glucose homeostasis, serum amylase increased, serum triglycerides increased

Gastrointestinal: Abdominal pain, diarrhea, dyspepsia, nausea, serum amylase increased, vomiting

Genitourinary: Hematuria

Hematologic: Anemia, neutropenia

Hepatic: Alkaline phosphatase increased, bilirubin increased, transaminases increased

Neuromuscular & skeletal: Arthralgia, CPK increased, creatinine kinase increased, myalgia, paresthesia, weakness

Respiratory: Cough, respiratory tract infection (upper), pharyngitis, rhinitis, sinusitis

Rare but important or life-threatening: Immune reconstitution syndrome

Drug Interactions

Metabolism/Transport Effects None known.

Avoid Concomitant Use

Avoid concomitant use of Emtricitabine with any of the following: LamiVUDine

Increased Effect/Toxicity

The levels/effects of Emtricitabine may be increased by: Ganciclovir-Valganciclovir; LamiVUDine; Ribavirin

Decreased Effect There are no known significant interactions involving a decrease in effect.

Food Interactions Food decreases peak plasma concentrations, but does not alter the extent of absorption or overall systemic exposure. Management: Administer without regard to meals.

Storage/Stability

Capsules: Store at 25°C (77°F); excursions permitted to 15°C to 30°C (59°F to 86°F).

Oral solution: Store at 2°C to 8°C (36°F to 46°F). Use within 3 months if stored at 25°C (77°F) with excursions permitted to 15°C to 30°C (59°F to 86°F).

Mechanism of Action Nucleoside reverse transcriptase inhibitor; emtricitabine is a cytosine analogue which is phosphorylated intracellularly to emtricitabine 5'-triphosphate which interferes with HIV viral RNA dependent DNA polymerase resulting in inhibition of viral replication.

Pharmacokinetics (Adult data unless noted)

Absorption: Rapid, extensive

Protein binding: <4%

Metabolism: Converted intracellularly to the active triphosphate form; undergoes minimal biotransformation via oxidation and glucuronide conjugation

Bioavailability:

Capsules: 93%

Oral solution: 75%

Note: Relative bioavailability of solution to capsule: 80%

Half-life: Normal renal function:

Infants, Children, and Adolescents: Elimination half-life (emtricitabine):

Single dose: 11 hours

Multiple dose: 7.9 to 9.5 hours

Infants 0 to 3 months (n=20; median age: 26 days): 12.1 ± 3.1 hours

Infants 3 to 24 months (n=14): 8.9 ± 3.2 hours

Children 25 months to 6 years (n=19): 11.3 ± 6.4 hours

Children 7 to 12 years (n=17): 8.2 ± 3.2 hours

Adolescents 13 to 17 years (n=27): 8.9 ± 3.3 hours

Adults:

Elimination half-life (emtricitabine): 10 hours

Intracellular half-life (emtricitabine 5'-triphosphate): 39 hours

Time to peak serum concentration: 1 to 2 hours

Elimination: Urine (86% of dose, primarily as unchanged drug; 13% as metabolites; 9% of dose as oxidative metabolite; 4% as glucuronide metabolite); feces (14% of dose)

Clearance: Renal clearance is greater than creatinine clearance; thus, emtricitabine may be eliminated by both glomerular filtration and active tubular secretion

Dosing: Neonatal HIV infection, treatment: Note: Use in combination with other antiretroviral agents. Oral solution: 3 mg/kg/dose once daily

Dosing adjustment in renal impairment: Monitor clinical response and renal function closely. There are no dosage adjustments provided in the manufacturer's labeling (not studied); however, consider a reduction in the dose and/or an increase in the dosing interval similar to dosage adjustments for adults.

Dosing: Usual

Pediatric: **HIV infection, treatment: Note:** Use in combination with other antiretroviral agents. Oral:

Infants 1 to <3 months: Oral solution: 3 mg/kg/dose once daily

Infants ≥3 months, Children, and Adolescents:

Oral solution: 6 mg/kg/dose once daily; maximum daily dose: 240 mg/**day**

Capsules: Patient weight >33 kg and able to swallow capsule whole: 200 mg once daily

Adolescents ≥18 years:

Capsules: 200 mg once daily

Oral solution: 240 mg once daily

Adult: **HIV infection, treatment: Note:** Use in combination with other antiretroviral agents. Oral:

Capsules: 200 mg once daily

Oral solution: 240 mg once daily

Dosing adjustment in renal impairment: Monitor clinical response and renal function closely. Dialysis: 30% of the dose is removed by hemodialysis (over 3 hours)

Infants, Children, and Adolescents <18 years: There are no dosage adjustments provided in the manufacturer's labeling; however, may consider a reduction in the dose and/or an increase in the dosing interval similar to dosage adjustments for adults.

Adolescents ≥18 years and Adults:

CrCl ≥50 mL/minute: No dosage adjustment necessary

CrCl 30 to 49 mL/minute: Capsule: 200 mg every 48 hours; oral solution: 120 mg every 24 hours

CrCl 15 to 29 mL/minute: Capsule: 200 mg every 72 hours; oral solution: 80 mg every 24 hours

CrCl <15 mL/minute (including hemodialysis patients): **Note:** If dose is given on day of dialysis, administer dose after dialysis: Capsule: 200 mg every 96 hours; oral solution: 60 mg every 24 hours

Dosing adjustment in hepatic impairment: There are no dosage adjustments provided in the manufacturer's labeling; however, emtricitabine is not metabolized by liver enzymes so the impact of liver impairment should be minimal; monitor patients closely.

Administration May be administered without regard to food

Monitoring Parameters Note: Monitor CD4 percentage (if <5 years of age) or CD4 count (if ≥5 years of age) at least every 3 to 4 months (DHHS [pediatric], 2014)

Patients should be screened for hepatitis B infection before starting therapy. Prior to initiation of therapy: Genotypic resistance testing, CD4 and viral load (every 3 to 4 months), CBC with differential, LFTs, BUN, creatinine, electrolytes, glucose, urinalysis (every 6 to 12 months), and assessment of readiness for adherence with medication regimen. At initiation and with any change in treatment regimen: CBC with differential, electrolytes, calcium, phosphorus, glucose, LFTs, bilirubin, urinalysis (at initiation), BUN, creatinine, albumin, total protein, lipid panel (at initiation), CD4, and viral load. After 1 to 2 weeks of therapy: Signs of medication toxicity and adherence. After 2 to 4 weeks of therapy: CBC with differential, viral load, signs of medication toxicity, and adherence; then every 3 to 4 months: CBC with differential, electrolytes, glucose, LFTs, bilirubin, BUN, creatinine, CD4, viral load, signs of medication toxicity, and adherence. Every 6 to 12 months: Lipid panel and urinalysis. CD4 monitoring frequency may be decreased to every 6 to 12 months in children who are adherent to therapy if the value is well above the threshold for opportunistic infections, viral suppression is sustained, and the clinical status is stable for more than 2 to 3 years (DHHS [pediatric], 2014). Monitor for growth and development, signs of HIV-specific physical conditions, HIV disease progression, opportunistic infections, skin rash, or hyperpigmentation.

Additional Information Emtricitabine is the (-) enantiomer of 2', 3'-dideoxy-5-fluoro-3'-thiacytidine (FTC), a fluorinated derivative of lamivudine.

Mutation in the HIV reverse transcriptase gene at codon 184, M184V/I (ie, substitution of methionine by valine or isoleucine) is associated with resistance to emtricitabine.

Emtricitabine-resistant isolates (M184V/I) are cross-resistant to lamivudine and zalcitabine. HIV-1 isolates containing the K65R mutation show reduced susceptibility to emtricitabine.

Dosage Forms Excipient information presented when available (limited, particularly for generics); consult specific product labeling.

Capsule, Oral:

Emtriva: 200 mg [contains fd&c blue #2 (indigotine)]

Solution, Oral:

Emtriva: 10 mg/mL (170 mL) [contains edetate disodium, fd&c yellow #6 (sunset yellow), methylparaben, propylene glycol, propylparaben; cotton candy flavor]

Emtricitabine and Tenofovir

(em trye SYE ta been & ten OF oh vir)

Medication Safety Issues

High alert medication:

This medication is in a class the Institute for Safe Medication Practices (ISMP) includes among its list of drug classes that have a heightened risk of causing significant patient harm when used in error.

Related Information

Adult and Adolescent HIV *on page 2392*

Pediatric HIV *on page 2380*

Perinatal HIV *on page 2400*

Brand Names: US Truvada

Brand Names: Canada Truvada

Therapeutic Category Antiretroviral Agent; HIV Agents (Anti-HIV Agents); Nucleoside Reverse Transcriptase Inhibitor (NRTI); Nucleotide Reverse Transcriptase Inhibitor (NRTI)

Generic Availability (US) No

Use Treatment of HIV infection in combination with other antiretroviral agents (FDA approved in ages ≥12 years weighing at least 35 kg and adults); **Note:** HIV regimens consisting of **three** antiretroviral agents are strongly recommended; pre-exposure prophylaxis (PrEP) in combination with safer sex practices for prevention of HIV infection in adults at high risk (FDA approved in adults)

Medication Guide Available Yes

Pregnancy Risk Factor B

Pregnancy Considerations Animal reproduction studies have not been conducted with this combination. Although approved for use in combination with safer sex practices for the prevention of HIV-1 infection in adults who are at high risk for acquiring HIV (preexposure prophylaxis [PrEP]), data on use in heterosexual HIV serodiscordant couples wishing to conceive are under study. Women of reproductive age should have a pregnancy test prior to starting PrEP and at regular intervals during therapy. In addition to pregnancy testing, uninfected women considering PrEP therapy should also undergo screening for HIV and other sexually transmitted diseases. Serodiscordant couples wishing to conceive should seek expert consultation to determine the safest approach for their specific situation. If HIV infection is documented during PrEP therapy, the antiretroviral agents should be discontinued in order to minimize drug resistance. If pregnancy is detected during therapy, the potential risks and benefits of continuing PrEP during pregnancy should be discussed (HHS [perinatal], 2014). Refer to individual monographs for additional information.

The DHHS Perinatal HIV Guidelines consider emtricitabine in combination with tenofovir to be a preferred NRTI backbone for use in antiretroviral-naive pregnant women (HHS [perinatal], 2014).

Healthcare providers are encouraged to enroll pregnant women exposed to antiretroviral medications in the Antiretroviral Pregnancy Registry (1-800-258-4263 or www.APRegistry.com). Healthcare providers caring for HIV-infected women and their infants may contact the National Perinatal HIV Hotline (888-448-8765) for clinical consultation (HHS [perinatal], 2014).

Breast-Feeding Considerations Emtricitabine and tenofovir are excreted into breast milk. Refer to individual monographs. Use in combination with safer sex practices for preexposure prophylaxis (PrEP) in lactating women who are HIV-uninfected is limited (HHS [perinatal], 2014).

Contraindications

U.S. labeling: Do not use for preexposure prophylaxis in patients with unknown or HIV-1 positive status. For HIV-1 treatment, use only in HIV-1-infected patients in combination with other antiretrovirals.

Canadian labeling: Previously demonstrated hypersensitivity to any component of the formulation.

Warnings/Precautions Not recommended as a component of a triple nucleoside regimen.

[U.S. Boxed Warning]: Lactic acidosis and severe hepatomegaly with steatosis have been reported with nucleoside and nucleotide analogues (eg, tenofovir), including fatal cases. Use with caution in patients with risk factors for liver disease (risk may be increased in obese patients or prolonged exposure) and suspend treatment in any patient who develops clinical or laboratory findings suggestive of lactic acidosis (transaminase elevation may/may not accompany hepatomegaly and steatosis). Use caution in hepatic impairment; no dosage adjustment is required; limited studies indicate the pharmacokinetics of tenofovir are not altered in hepatic dysfunction.

HIV-1 treatment: Use caution in moderate renal impairment (CrCl <50 mL/minute); dosage adjustment required. May cause acute renal failure or Fanconi syndrome; use caution with other nephrotoxic agents (including high dose or multiple NSAID use or those which compete for active tubular secretion). Acute renal failure has occurred in HIV-infected patients with risk factors for renal impairment who were on a stable tenofovir regimen to which a high dose or multiple NSAID therapy was added. Consider alternatives to NSAIDS in patients taking tenofovir and at risk for renal impairment. Calculate creatinine clearance prior to initiation in all patients; monitor renal function during therapy (including recalculation of creatinine clearance and serum phosphorus) in patients at risk for renal impairment, including those with previous renal decline on adefovir. In clinical trials, use has been associated with decreases in bone mineral density in HIV-1 infected adults and increases in bone metabolism markers. Serum parathyroid hormone and 1,25 vitamin D levels were also higher. Decreases in bone mineral density have also been observed in clinical trials of HIV-1 infected pediatric patients. Observations in chronic hepatitis B infected pediatric patients (aged 12-18 years) were similar. Consider monitoring of bone density in adult and pediatric patients with a history of pathologic fractures or with other risk factors for bone loss or osteoporosis. Consider calcium and vitamin D supplementation for all patients; effect of supplementation has not been studied but may be beneficial. Long-term bone health and fracture risk unknown. Skeletal growth (height) appears to be unaffected in tenofovir-treated children and adolescents. May cause osteomalacia with proximal renal tubulopathy. Bone pain, extremity pain, fractures, arthralgias, weakness and muscle pain have been reported. In patients at risk for renal dysfunction, persistent or worsening bone or muscle symptoms should be evaluated for hypophosphatemia and osteomalacia. Avoid use in patients with CrCl <30 mL/minute. IDSA guidelines recommend avoiding tenofovir in HIV patients with preexisting kidney disease (CrCl <50 mL/minute and not on hemodialysis or GFR <60 mL/minute/1.73 m^2) when other effective HIV treatment options exist because data suggest risk of chronic kidney disease (CKD) is increased (IDSA [Lucas 2014]). IDSA guidelines also recommend discontinuing tenofovir in HIV infected patients who develop a decline in GFR (a >25% decrease in GFR from baseline and to a level of <60 mL/minute/1.73 m^2) during use, particularly in presence of proximal tubular dysfunction (eg, euglycemic glycosuria, increased urinary phosphorus excretion and hypophosphatemia, proteinuria [new onset or worsening]) (IDSA [Lucas 2014]). Monitor for possible bone abnormalities during therapy. All patients with HIV should be tested for HBV prior to initiation of treatment.

Pre-exposure prophylaxis (PrEP): Routinely monitor patients with mild renal impairment. Calculate creatinine clearance prior to initiation in all patients; monitor renal function during therapy (including recalculation of creatinine clearance and serum phosphorus). Do not use in CrCl <60 mL/minute. PrEP should be accompanied by a comprehensive HIV-1 prevention program (eg, risk reduction counseling, access to condoms), with particular emphasis on medication adherence. In addition, regular monitoring (eg, HIV status of patient and partner(s), risk behavior, adherence, adverse effects, sexually transmitted infections that facilitate HIV-1 transmission) is highly recommended.

[U.S. Boxed Warning]: Safety and efficacy during coinfection of HIV and HBV have not been established; acute, severe exacerbations of HBV have been reported following discontinuation of antiretroviral therapy. In HBV coinfected patients, monitor hepatic function closely for several months following discontinuation. May cause redistribution of fat (eg, buffalo hump, peripheral wasting with increased abdominal girth, cushingoid appearance). Patients may develop immune reconstitution syndrome resulting in the occurrence of an inflammatory response to an indolent or residual opportunistic infection during initial HIV treatment or activation of autoimmune disorders (eg, Graves' disease, polymyositis, Guillain-Barré syndrome) later in therapy; further evaluation and treatment may be required. Do not use concurrently with adefovir, emtricitabine, tenofovir, lamivudine, or lamivudine-combination products.

[U.S. Boxed Warning]: Confirm HIV-1 negative status immediately before and at least every 3 months during therapy. Risk of drug resistant HIV-1 variants with PrEP use if patient had undetected acute HIV-1 infection. Some HIV-1 tests (eg, rapid tests) do not detect acute HIV-1 infection. Screen PrEP candidates for acute viral infections and potential exposure events ≤1 month of starting PrEP. If infections or events exist, wait 1 month to start PrEP and reconfirm HIV-1 negative status. Do not start PrEP if signs or symptoms of acute HIV-1 infection are present unless HIV-1 negative status is confirmed by a test approved by the Food and Drug Administration (FDA) as an aid to detect HIV-1 infection (including acute or primary infection).

Warnings: Additional Pediatric Considerations Emtricitabine-associated hyperpigmentation may occur at a higher frequency in pediatric patients compared to adults (children: 32%; adults: 2% to 6%).

Recent studies suggest that tenofovir-related bone loss may be greater in children who are less mature (eg, Tanner stage 1-2) than in those who are more physically mature (Tanner ≥3). A significant decrease in lumbar spine BMD (>6%) was reported in five of 15 pediatric patients who received a tenofovir-containing regimen for 48 weeks. No orthopedic fractures occurred, but two patients required discontinuation of tenofovir. All five patients with a decrease in BMD were virologic responders and prepubertal (Tanner Stage 1). This study found a moderately strong correlation between decreases in bone mineral density z scores at week 48 and age at baseline. No correlation between decreases in bone mineral density z scores and tenofovir dose or pharmacokinetics was observed; BMD loss may limit the usefulness of tenofovir in prepubertal children ([DHHS [pediatric], 2014; Giacomet, 2005; Hazra, 2005; Purdy, 2008). Monitor BMD for potential bone toxicities during therapy; supplementation with calcium and vitamin D may be beneficial but has not been studied.

Adverse Reactions The adverse reaction profile of combination therapy has not been established. See individual agents.

Drug Interactions

Metabolism/Transport Effects Refer to individual components.

Avoid Concomitant Use

Avoid concomitant use of Emtricitabine and Tenofovir with any of the following: Adefovir; Didanosine; LamiVUDine

Increased Effect/Toxicity

Emtricitabine and Tenofovir may increase the levels/effects of: Adefovir; Aminoglycosides; Darunavir; Didanosine; TiZANidine

The levels/effects of Emtricitabine and Tenofovir may be increased by: Acyclovir-Valacyclovir; Adefovir; Aminoglycosides; Atazanavir; Cidofovir; Cobicistat; Darunavir; Diclofenac (Systemic); Ganciclovir-Valganciclovir; LamiVUDine; Ledipasvir; Lopinavir; Nonsteroidal Anti-Inflammatory Agents; Ribavirin; Simeprevir; Telaprevir

Decreased Effect

Emtricitabine and Tenofovir may decrease the levels/effects of: Atazanavir; Didanosine; Simeprevir; Tipranavir

The levels/effects of Emtricitabine and Tenofovir may be decreased by: Adefovir; Tipranavir

Food Interactions See individual agents.

Storage/Stability Store tablets at 25°C (77°F); excursions permitted to 15°C to 30°C (59°F to 86°F). Dispense only in original container; do not use if seal on bottle is broken or missing.

Mechanism of Action Nucleoside and nucleotide reverse transcriptase inhibitor combination; emtricitabine is a cytosine analogue while tenofovir disoproxil fumarate (TDF) is an analog of adenosine 5'-monophosphate. Each drug interferes with HIV viral RNA dependent DNA polymerase resulting in inhibition of viral replication.

Pharmacokinetics (Adult data unless noted) One Truvada tablet is bioequivalent to one emtricitabine 200 mg capsule and one tenofovir 300 mg tablet (single dose study); see individual agents

Dosing: Usual

Pediatric: **HIV infection, treatment:** Use in combination with other antiretroviral agents.

Children and Adolescents <12 years or <35 kg: Not intended for use; product is a fixed-dose combination; safety and efficacy have not been established in these patients

Children and Adolescents ≥12 years and ≥35 kg: Oral: One tablet once daily

Adult:

HIV infection, treatment: Oral: One tablet once daily

Pre-exposure prophylaxis (PrEP) for prevention of HIV infection in uninfected high-risk individuals: Oral: One tablet once daily

Dosing adjustment in renal impairment: Note: Closely monitor clinical response and renal function in these patients; clinical effectiveness and safety of these guidelines have not been evaluated.

HIV infection, treatment:

Children ≥12 years and Adolescents: CrCl <30 mL/minute or patients requiring hemodialysis: Use not recommended (DHHS [pediatric], 2014).

Adults: Manufacturer's labeling:
CrCl ≥50 mL/minute: No adjustment necessary.
CrCl 30-49 mL/minute: Administer every 48 hours.
CrCl <30 mL/minute or patients requiring hemodialysis: Use not recommended.

Pre-exposure prophylaxis (PrEP): Adults:
CrCl >60 mL/minute: No adjustment necessary.
CrCl <60 mL/minute: Use not recommended.

Dosing adjustment in hepatic impairment: There are no dosage adjustments provided in the manufacturer's labeling; however, no dosing adjustments are necessary for tenofovir in hepatic impairment. No specific data is available on emtricitabine in hepatic impairment, but given its limited hepatic metabolism, the impact of liver impairment should be minimal; need for dose adjustment is unlikely.

Administration May be administered without regard to food

Monitoring Parameters

HIV treatment: Note: Monitor CD4 percentage (if <5 years of age) or CD4 count (if ≥5 years of age) at least every 3 to 4 months (DHHS [pediatric], 2014).

Patients should be screened for hepatitis B infection before starting therapy. Prior to initiation of therapy: HIV genotypic resistance testing, CD4 and viral load (every 3 to 4 months), CBC with differential, LFTs, BUN, creatinine, urine dipstick for protein and glucose, electrolytes, glucose, urinalysis (every 6 to 12 months), and assessment of readiness for adherence with medication regimen. At initiation and with any change in treatment regimen: CBC with differential, electrolytes, calcium, phosphate, glucose, LFTs, bilirubin, urinalysis (at initiation), BUN, creatinine, albumin, total protein, lipid panel (at initiation), CD4, and viral load. After 1 to 2 weeks of therapy: Signs of medication toxicity and adherence. After 2 to 4 weeks of therapy: CBC with differential, viral load, signs of medication toxicity, and adherence; then every 3 to 4 months: CBC with differential, electrolytes, glucose, LFTs, bilirubin, BUN, creatinine, CD4, viral load, signs of medication toxicity, and adherence. Every 6 to 12 months: Lipid panel and urinalysis. CD4 monitoring frequency may be decreased to every 6 to 12 months in children who are adherent to therapy if the value is well above the threshold for opportunistic infections, viral suppression is sustained, and the clinical status is stable for more than 2 to 3 years (DHHS [pediatric], 2014). Monitor for growth and development, signs of HIV-specific physical conditions, HIV disease progression, opportunistic infections, lactic acidosis, hyperpigmentation, or bone abnormalities. Consider bone mineral density assessment for all patients with a history of pathologic bone fractures or other risk factors for osteoporosis or bone loss. Some experts recommend obtaining a DXA scan prior to therapy and 6 months into therapy, especially for patients in pre- and early puberty (Tanner stages 1 and 2) (DHHS [pediatric], 2014). In patients coinfected with HBV, monitor hepatic function closely (clinically and with laboratory tests) for at least several months after discontinuing emtricitabine and tenofovir therapy.

HIV-1 pre-exposure prophylaxis (PrEP): Pregnancy test for women receiving PrEP (every visit); documented negative HIV test (immediately prior to use, every 2 to 3 months, and following discontinuation of PrEP), assess risk behaviors and symptoms of sexually transmitted infections (STIs) or acute HIV-1 infection and provide condoms (immediately prior to use, then every 2 to 3 months during therapy); BUN and serum creatinine (prior to initiation, 3 months after initiation, then every 6 months); testing for HBV (prior to initiation) and STIs (prior to initiation, then at least every 6 months, even if asymptomatic) (CDC, 2011; CDC, 2012)

Additional Information Emtricitabine is the (-) enantiomer of 2', 3'-dideoxy-5-fluoro-3'-thiacytidine (FTC), a fluorinated derivative of lamivudine.

Mutation in the HIV reverse transcriptase gene at codon 184, M184V/I (ie, substitution of methionine by valine or isoleucine) is associated with resistance to emtricitabine. Emtricitabine-resistant isolates (M184V/I) are cross-resistant to lamivudine and zalcitabine. HIV-1 isolates containing the K65R mutation show reduced susceptibility to emtricitabine.

Dosage Forms Excipient information presented when available (limited, particularly for generics); consult specific product labeling.

Tablet:
Truvada: Emtricitabine 200 mg and tenofovir disoproxil fumarate 300 mg

- ◆ **Emtricitabine, Efavirenz, and Tenofovir** *see* Efavirenz, Emtricitabine, and Tenofovir *on page 734*
- ◆ **Emtriva** *see* Emtricitabine *on page 739*
- ◆ **Emtriva® (Can)** *see* Emtricitabine *on page 739*

Enalapril (e NAL a pril)

Medication Safety Issues

Sound-alike/look-alike issues:
Enalapril may be confused with Anafranil, Elavil, Eldepryl, ramipril

Administration issues:
Significant differences exist between oral and IV dosing. Use caution when converting from one route of administration to another.

International issues:
Acepril [Hungary, Switzerland] may be confused with Accupril which is a brand name for quinapril [U.S., Canada, multiple international markets]
Acepril: Brand name for enalapril [Hungary, Switzerland], but also brand name for captopril [Great Britain]; lisinopril [Malaysia]

Brand Names: US Epaned; Vasotec

Brand Names: Canada ACT-Enalapril; Apo-Enalapril; Mylan-Enalapril; PMS-Enalapril; PRO-Enalapril; RAN-Enalapril; Riva-Enalapril; Sandoz-Enalapril; Sig-Enalapril; Taro-Enalapril; Teva-Enalapril; Vasotec

Therapeutic Category Angiotensin-Converting Enzyme (ACE) Inhibitor

Generic Availability (US) May be product dependent

Use Management of mild to severe hypertension (FDA approved in ages 1 month to 16 years and adults), CHF (FDA approved in adults), and asymptomatic left ventricular dysfunction (FDA approved in adults); has also been used to treat proteinuria in steroid-resistant nephrotic syndrome patients

Pregnancy Risk Factor D

Pregnancy Considerations [U.S. Boxed Warning]: Drugs that act on the renin-angiotensin system can cause injury and death to the developing fetus. Discontinue as soon as possible once pregnancy is detected. Enalaprilat, the active metabolite of enalapril, crosses the placenta; teratogenic effects may occur following maternal use during pregnancy. Drugs that act on the renin-angiotensin system are associated with oligohydramnios. Oligohydramnios, due to decreased fetal renal function, may lead to fetal lung hypoplasia and skeletal malformations. The use of these drugs in pregnancy is also associated with anuria, hypotension, renal failure, skull hypoplasia, and death in the fetus/neonate. Chronic maternal hypertension itself is also associated with adverse events in the fetus/infant. ACE inhibitors are not recommended during pregnancy to treat maternal hypertension or heart failure. Use of an ACE inhibitor should also be avoided in any woman of reproductive age. Women who are planning a pregnancy should be considered for other medication options if an ACE inhibitor is currently prescribed or the ACE inhibitor should be discontinued as soon as possible once pregnancy is detected. The exposed fetus should be monitored for fetal growth, amniotic fluid volume, and organ formation. Infants exposed to an ACE inhibitor *in utero* should be monitored for hyperkalemia, hypotension, and oliguria (exchange transfusions or dialysis may be needed). These adverse events are generally associated with maternal use in the second and third trimesters.

Untreated chronic maternal hypertension is also associated with adverse events in the fetus, infant, and mother. The use of ACE inhibitors is not recommended to treat chronic uncomplicated hypertension in pregnant women and should generally be avoided in women of reproductive potential (ACOG, 2013).

Breast-Feeding Considerations Enalapril and enalaprilat are excreted in breast milk. Breast-feeding is not recommended by the manufacturer.

Contraindications

Hypersensitivity to enalapril or any component of the formulation; angioedema related to previous treatment with an ACE inhibitor; patients with idiopathic or hereditary angioedema; concomitant use with aliskiren in patients with diabetes mellitus

Documentation of allergenic cross-reactivity for ACE inhibitors is limited. However, because of similarities in chemical structure and/or pharmacologic actions, the possibility of cross-sensitivity cannot be ruled out with certainty.

Canadian labeling: Additional contraindications (not in U.S. labeling): Concomitant use with aliskiren-containing drugs in patients with moderate-to-severe renal impairment (GFR <60 mL/minute/1.73 m^2)

Warnings/Precautions Anaphylactic reactions may occur rarely with ACE inhibitors. At any time during treatment (especially following first dose) angioedema may occur rarely with ACE inhibitors; it may involve the head and neck (potentially compromising airway) or the intestine (presenting with abdominal pain). African-Americans may be at an increased risk. Prolonged frequent monitoring may be required especially if tongue, glottis, or larynx are involved as they are associated with airway obstruction. Patients with a history of airway surgery may have a higher risk of airway obstruction. Aggressive early and appropriate management is critical. Use in patients with idiopathic or hereditary angioedema or previous angioedema associated with ACE inhibitor therapy is contraindicated. Severe anaphylactoid reactions may be seen during hemodialysis (eg, CVVHD) with high-flux dialysis membranes (eg, AN69), and rarely, during low density lipoprotein apheresis with dextran sulfate cellulose. Rare cases of anaphylactoid reactions have been reported in patients undergoing sensitization treatment with hymenoptera (bee, wasp) venom while receiving ACE inhibitors.

Symptomatic hypotension with or without syncope can occur with ACE inhibitors (usually with the first several doses); effects are most often observed in volume depleted patients; correct volume depletion prior to initiation; close monitoring of patient is required especially with initial dosing and dosing increases; blood pressure must be lowered at a rate appropriate for the patient's clinical condition. Initiation of therapy in patients with ischemic heart disease or cerebrovascular disease warrants close observation due to the potential consequences posed by falling blood pressure (eg, MI, stroke). Use with caution in hypertrophic cardiomyopathy with outflow tract obstruction and severe aortic stenosis. In patients on chronic ACE inhibitor therapy, intraoperative hypotension may occur with induction and maintenance of general anesthesia; use with caution before, during, or immediately after major surgery. Cardiopulmonary bypass, intraoperative blood loss, or vasodilating anesthesia increases endogenous renin release. Use of ACE inhibitors perioperatively will blunt angiotensin II formation and may result in hypotension. However, discontinuation of therapy prior to surgery is controversial. If continued preoperatively, avoidance of hypotensive agents during surgery is prudent (Hillis, 2011). **[U.S. Boxed Warning]: Drugs that act on the renin-angiotensin system can cause injury and death to the developing fetus. Discontinue as soon as possible once pregnancy is detected.**

Hyperkalemia may occur with ACE inhibitors; risk factors include renal dysfunction, diabetes mellitus, concomitant use of potassium-sparing diuretics, potassium supplements, and/or potassium-containing salts. Use cautiously, if at all, with these agents and monitor potassium closely. Cough may occur with ACE inhibitors. Other causes of cough should be considered (eg, pulmonary congestion in patients with heart failure) and excluded prior to discontinuation.

May be associated with deterioration of renal function and/or increases in serum creatinine, particularly in patients with low renal blood flow (eg, renal artery stenosis, heart failure) whose glomerular filtration rate (GFR) is dependent on efferent arteriolar vasoconstriction by angiotensin II; deterioration may result in oliguria, acute renal failure, and progressive azotemia. Small increases in serum creatinine may occur following initiation; consider discontinuation only in patients with progressive and/or significant deterioration in renal function. Use with caution in patients with unstented unilateral/bilateral renal artery stenosis. When unstented bilateral renal artery stenosis is present, use is generally avoided due to the elevated risk of deterioration in renal function unless possible benefits outweigh risks. Potentially significant drug-drug interactions may exist, requiring dose or frequency adjustment, additional monitoring, and/or selection of alternative therapy.

Rare toxicities associated with ACE inhibitors include cholestatic jaundice (which may progress to fulminant hepatic necrosis), agranulocytosis, neutropenia or leukopenia with myeloid hypoplasia. Patients with collagen vascular diseases (especially with concomitant renal impairment) or renal impairment alone may be at increased risk for hematologic toxicity; periodically monitor CBC with differential in these patients.

Warnings: Additional Pediatric Considerations In pediatric patients, an isolated dry hacking cough lasting >3 weeks was reported in seven of 42 pediatric patients (17%) receiving ACE inhibitors (von Vigier, 2000); a review of pediatric randomized-controlled ACE inhibitor trials reported a lower incidence of 3.2% (Baker-Smith, 2010). Other causes of cough should be considered (eg, pulmonary congestion in patients with heart failure) and excluded prior to discontinuation.

Adverse Reactions

Cardiovascular: Chest pain, hypotension, orthostatic effect, orthostatic hypotension, syncope

Central nervous system: Dizziness, fatigue, headache

Dermatologic: Skin rash

Gastrointestinal: Abdominal pain, anorexia, constipation, diarrhea, dysgeusia, nausea, vomiting

Neuromuscular & skeletal: Weakness

Renal: Increased serum creatinine, renal insufficiency (in patients with bilateral renal artery stenosis or hypovolemia)

Respiratory: Bronchitis, cough, dyspnea

Rare but important or life-threatening: Acute generalized exanthematous pustulosis, agranulocytosis, alopecia, anaphylactoid reaction, angina pectoris, angioedema, anosmia, arthritis, asthma, ataxia, atrial fibrillation, atrial tachycardia, bone marrow depression, bradycardia, cardiac arrest, cardiac arrhythmia, cerebrovascular accident, cholestatic jaundice, confusion, conjunctivitis, depression, eosinophilia, eosinophilic pneumonitis, erythema multiforme, exfoliative dermatitis, giant-cell arteritis, gynecomastia, hallucination, hemolysis (with G6PD), herpes zoster, IgA vasculitis, increased erythrocyte sedimentation rate, intestinal obstruction, insomnia, interstitial nephritis, leukocytosis, lichenoid eruption, melena, myocardial infarction, myositis, neutropenia, ototoxicity, pancreatitis, pemphigus, pemphigus foliaceus, peripheral neuropathy, positive ANA titer, psychosis, pulmonary edema, pulmonary embolism, pulmonary infarct, pulmonary infiltrates, Raynaud's phenomenon, serositis, Sjogren's syndrome, skin photosensitivity, Stevens-Johnson syndrome, stomatitis, systemic lupus erythematosus, thrombocytopenia, toxic epidermal necrolysis, upper respiratory tract infection, vasculitis, visual hallucination (Doane, 2013)

Drug Interactions

Metabolism/Transport Effects None known.

Avoid Concomitant Use There are no known interactions where it is recommended to avoid concomitant use.

Increased Effect/Toxicity

Enalapril may increase the levels/effects of: Allopurinol; Amifostine; Antihypertensives; AzaTHIOprine; Ciprofloxacin (Systemic); Drospirenone; DULoxetine; Ferric Gluconate; Gold Sodium Thiomalate; Grass Pollen Allergen Extract (5 Grass Extract); Hypotensive Agents; Iron Dextran Complex; Levodopa; Lithium; Nonsteroidal Anti-Inflammatory Agents; Obinutuzumab; Pregabalin; RisperiDONE; RiTUXimab; Sodium Phosphates

The levels/effects of Enalapril may be increased by: Alfuzosin; Aliskiren; Angiotensin II Receptor Blockers; Barbiturates; Brimonidine (Topical); Canagliflozin; Dapoxetine; Diazoxide; DPP-IV Inhibitors; Eplerenone; Everolimus; Heparin; Heparin (Low Molecular Weight); Herbs (Hypotensive Properties); Loop Diuretics; MAO Inhibitors; Nicorandil; Pentoxifylline; Phosphodiesterase 5 Inhibitors; Potassium Salts; Potassium-Sparing Diuretics; Prostacyclin Analogues; Sirolimus; Temsirolimus; Thiazide Diuretics; TiZANidine; Tolvaptan; Trimethoprim

Decreased Effect

The levels/effects of Enalapril may be decreased by: Aprotinin; Herbs (Hypertensive Properties); Icatibant; Lanthanum; Methylphenidate; Nonsteroidal Anti-Inflammatory Agents; Salicylates; Yohimbine

Storage/Stability

Solution kit: Store at 25°C (77°F); excursions are permitted between 15°C and 30°C (59°F and 86°F). Do not freeze. Protect from moisture. Once reconstituted, the solution should be stored at 15°C to 30°C (59°F to 86°F) and may be stored for up to 60 days.

Tablet: Store at 25°C (77°F); excursions permitted to 15°C to 30°C (59°F to 86°F). Protect from moisture.

Mechanism of Action Competitive inhibitor of angiotensin-converting enzyme (ACE); prevents conversion of angiotensin I to angiotensin II, a potent vasoconstrictor; results in lower levels of angiotensin II which causes an increase in plasma renin activity and a reduction in aldosterone secretion

Pharmacodynamics Antihypertensive effect:

Onset of action: Within 1 hour

Maximum effect: Within 4-8 hours

Duration: 12-24 hours

Pharmacokinetics (Adult data unless noted)

Absorption: 55% to 75%

Protein binding: 50% to 60%

Metabolism: Enalapril is a prodrug (inactive) and undergoes biotransformation to enalaprilat (active) in the liver

Half-life:

Enalapril:

CHF: Neonates (n=3, PNA: 10-19 days): 10.3 hours (range: 4.2-13.4 hours) (Nakamura, 1994)

CHF: Infants and Children ≤6.5 years of age (n=11): 2.7 hours (range: 1.3-6.3 hours) (Nakamura, 1994)

Healthy Adults: 2 hours

CHF: Adults: 3.4-5.8 hours

Enalaprilat (active metabolite):

CHF: Neonates (n=3, PNA: 10-19 days): 11.9 hours (range: 5.9-15.6 hours) (Nakamura, 1994)

CHF: Infants and Children ≤6.5 years of age (n=11): 11.1 hours (range: 5.1-20.8 hours) (Nakamura, 1994)

Infants 6 weeks to 8 months: 6-10 hours

Adults: 35-38 hours

Time to peak serum concentration:

Enalapril: Within 0.5-1.5 hours

Enalaprilat (active): Within 3-4.5 hours

Elimination: Principally in urine (60% to 80%) with some fecal excretion

Dosing: Neonatal Use lower listed initial dose in patients with hyponatremia, hypovolemia, severe CHF, decreased renal function, or in those receiving diuretics

Hypertension: Oral: Initial: 0.04-0.1 mg/kg/day every 24 hours; initiate at the lower end of the range and titrate to effect as required every few days; hypotension and oliguria have been associated with initial doses of 0.1 mg/kg (Dutta, 2003; Schilder, 1995); maximum reported dose: 0.27 mg/kg/day (Leversha, 1994)

Dosing adjustment in renal impairment: Use in neonates with GFR <30 mL/minute/1.73 m^2 is not recommended; no dosing data available

Dosing: Usual Use lower listed initial dose in patients with hyponatremia, hypovolemia, severe CHF, decreased renal function, or in those receiving diuretics.

Pediatric:

Heart Failure: Limited data available: Infants, Children, and Adolescents: Oral: Initial: 0.1 mg/kg/day in 1 to 2 divided doses; increase as required over 2 weeks to maximum of 0.5 mg/kg/day; mean dose required for CHF improvement in 39 children (mean age: 4 years) was 0.36 mg/kg/day; select individuals have been treated with doses up to 0.94 mg/kg/day (Leversha 1994; Momma 2006)

Hypertension: Infants, Children, and Adolescents: Oral: Initial: 0.08 mg/kg once daily (maximum dose: 5 mg); adjust dose according to blood pressure readings; doses >0.58 mg/kg (or >40 mg) have not been studied

Proteinuria, nephrotic syndrome: Limited data available: Oral:

Fixed dosing: Children ≥7 years and Adolescents: 2.5-5 mg/day was reported in a retrospective study in normotensive pediatric patients as either monotherapy (n=17; mean age: 13.7 years; range: 8-17 years) or with prednisone (n=11; mean age: 12.6 years; range: 7-16 years); significant decrease in proteinuria (with or without nephrotic syndrome) occurred; no significant change in blood pressure was observed (Sasinka, 1999); a case series of three adolescents with sickle anemia nephropathy reported an initial dose of 5 mg/day; one patient required an increase to 7.5 mg/day (Fitzhugh, 2005)

Weight-directed dosing: Children and Adolescents: Initial: 0.2 mg/kg/day; titrate to response at 4- to 12-week intervals; range: 0.2-0.6 mg/kg/day; maximum daily dose: 20 mg/**day**; a crossover dose comparison trial showed effects on proteinuria were dose-dependent (Bagga, 2004; Chandar, 2007; Delucchi, 2000; Lama, 2000; White, 2003); if combined with other angiotensin blockade (ARB), lower doses have been reported (0.1-0.16 mg/kg/day) (Chandar, 2007)

Adult:

Asymptomatic left ventricular dysfunction: Oral: Initial: 2.5 mg twice daily; increase as tolerated; usual dose: 20 mg/day in 2 divided doses

Heart failure: Oral: Initial: 2.5 mg once or twice daily (usual range: 5-40 mg/day in 2 divided doses); titrate slowly at 1- to 2-week intervals. Target dose: 10-20 mg twice daily (ACC/AHA 2009 Heart Failure Guidelines)

Hypertension: Oral: 2.5-5 mg/day then increase as required, usually at 1- to 2-week intervals; usual dose range (JNC 7): 2.5-40 mg/day in 1-2 divided doses. **Note:** Initiate with 2.5 mg if patient is taking a diuretic which cannot be discontinued. May add a diuretic if blood pressure cannot be controlled with enalapril alone.

Dosing adjustment in renal impairment:

Infants, Children, and Adolescents:

Manufacturer's labeling: Use in infants, children, and adolescents ≤16 years of age with GFR <30 mL/minute/1.73 m^2 is not recommended; no dosing data available in this population

Alternate recommendations (Aronoff, 2007):

GFR >50 mL/minute/1.73 m^2: No dosage adjustment necessary

GFR 10-50 mL/minute/1.73 m^2: Administer 75% of usual dose

GFR <10 mL/minute/1.73 m^2: Administer 50% of usual dose

Adults:

Manufacturer's labeling:

CrCl >30 mL/minute: No dosage adjustment necessary

CrCl ≤30 mL/minute: Administer 2.5 mg/day; titrate upward until blood pressure is controlled

Alternate recommendations (Aronoff, 2007):

GFR >50 mL/minute: No dosage adjustment necessary

GFR 10-50 mL/minute: Administer 50% to 100% of usual dose

GFR <10 mL/minute: Administer 25% of usual dose

Peritoneal dialysis: Supplemental dose is not necessary, although some removal of drug occurs

Preparation for Administration Oral: Epaned: Solution kit (for 150 mL, enalapril solution 1 mg/mL): Kit contains 1 bottle of enalapril powder and 1 bottle of Ora-Sweet SF dilution to be added to the enalapril powder prior to dispensing. Firmly tap the enalapril powder for oral solution bottle on a hard surface 5 times. Add approximately one-half (75 mL) of the Ora-Sweet SF diluent to the enalapril 150 mL oral solution bottle and shake well for 30 seconds. Add the remainder of the Ora-Sweet SF diluent and shake well for an additional 30 seconds.

Administration May administer without regard to food

Monitoring Parameters Blood pressure, renal function, WBC, serum potassium, serum glucose; monitor for angioedema and anaphylactoid reactions

Test Interactions Positive Coombs' [direct]; may cause false-positive results in urine acetone determinations using sodium nitroprusside reagent

Additional Information Severe hypotension was reported in a **preterm** neonate (birth weight: 835 g, gestational age: 26 weeks, postnatal age: 9 days) who was treated with enalapril 0.1 mg/kg orally; hypotension responded to IV plasma and dopamine; the authors suggest starting enalapril in preterm infants at 0.01 mg/kg and increasing upwards in a stepwise fashion with very close monitoring of blood pressure and urine output. However, in this case report, oral enalapril at doses of 0.01 mg/kg to 0.04 mg/kg did not adequately control blood pressure. Further studies are needed (Schilder, 1995).

Dosage Forms Excipient information presented when available (limited, particularly for generics); consult specific product labeling.

Solution Reconstituted, Oral, as maleate:

Epaned: 1 mg/mL (150 mL) [contains methylparaben, propylparaben, saccharin sodium; berry-citrus flavor]

Tablet, Oral, as maleate:

Vasotec: 2.5 mg, 5 mg, 10 mg, 20 mg [scored]

Generic: 2.5 mg, 5 mg, 10 mg, 20 mg

Extemporaneous Preparations Note: Commercial oral solution kit is available (1 mg/mL).

A 1 mg/mL oral suspension may be made with tablets, Bicitra [discontinued] or equivalent, and Ora-Sweet SF. Place ten 20 mg tablets in a 200 mL polyethylene terephthalate bottle; add 50 mL of Bicitra [discontinued] or equivalent and shake well for at least 2 minutes. Let stand for 1 hour then shake for 1 additional minute; add 150 mL of Ora-Sweet SF and shake well. Label "shake well" and "refrigerate". Stable for 30 days when stored in a polyethylene terephthalate bottle and refrigerated (Vasotec prescribing information, 2011).

A 1 mg/mL oral suspension may be made with tablets and one of three different vehicles (cherry syrup, a 1:1 mixture of Ora-Sweet and Ora-Plus, or a 1:1 mixture of Ora-Sweet SF and Ora-Plus). Crush six 20 mg tablets in a mortar and reduce to a fine powder. Add 15 mL of the chosen vehicle and mix to a uniform paste; mix while adding the vehicle in incremental proportions to **almost** 120 mL; transfer to a calibrated bottle, rinse mortar with vehicle, and add quantity of vehicle sufficient to make 120 mL. Label "shake well" and "protect from light". Stable for 60 days when stored in amber plastic prescription bottles in the dark at room temperature or refrigerated (Allen, 1998).

A 1 mg/mL oral suspension may be made with tablets and one of three different vehicles (deionized water, citrate buffer solution at pH 5.0, or a 1:1 mixture of Ora-Sweet and Ora-Plus). Crush twenty 10 mg tablets in a mortar and reduce to a fine powder. Add small portions of the chosen vehicle and mix to a uniform paste; mix while adding vehicle in incremental proportions to **almost** 200 mL; transfer to a graduated cylinder, rinse mortar with vehicle, and add quantity of vehicle sufficient to make 200 mL. Label "shake well" and "protect from light". Preparations made in citrate buffer solution at pH 5.0 and the 1:1 mixture of Ora-Sweet and Ora-Plus are stable for 91 days when stored in plastic prescription bottles in the dark at room temperature or refrigerated. Preparation made in deionized water is stable for 91 days refrigerated or 56 days at room temperature when stored in plastic prescription bottles in the dark. **Note:** To prepare the isotonic citrate buffer solution (pH 5.0), see reference (Nahata, 1998).

A more dilute, 0.1 mg/mL oral suspension may be made with tablets and an isotonic buffer solution at pH 5.0. Grind one 20 mg tablet in a glass mortar and reduce to a fine powder; mix with isotonic citrate buffer (pH 5.0) and filter; add quantity of buffer solution sufficient to make 200 mL. Label "shake well", "protect from light", and "refrigerate". Stable for 90 days (Boulton, 1994).

Allen LV Jr and Erickson MA 3rd, "Stability of Alprazolam, Chloroquine Phosphate, Cisapride, Enalapril Maleate, and Hydralazine Hydrochloride in Extemporaneously Compounded Oral Liquids," *Am J Health Syst Pharm*, 1998, 55(18):1915-20.

Boulton DW, Woods DJ, Fawcett JP, et al, "The Stability of an Enalapril Maleate Oral Solution Prepared From Tablets," *Aust J Hosp Pharm*, 1994, 24(2):151-6.

Nahata MC, Morosco RS, and Hipple TF, "Stability of Enalapril Maleate in Three Extemporaneously Prepared Oral Liquids," *Am J Health Syst Pharm*, 1998, 55(11):1155-7.

Vasotec® prescribing information, Valeant Pharmaceuticals North America LLC, Bridgewater, NJ; 2011.

Enalaprilat (en AL a pril at)

Medication Safety Issues

Administration issues:

Significant differences exist between oral and IV dosing. Use caution when converting from one route of administration to another.

Brand Names: Canada Vasotec IV

Therapeutic Category Angiotensin-Converting Enzyme (ACE) Inhibitor

Generic Availability (US) Yes

Use Treatment of hypertension when oral therapy is not practical (FDA approved in adults); has also been used for heart failure

Pregnancy Risk Factor C (1st trimester); D (2nd and 3rd trimesters)

Pregnancy Considerations [U.S. Boxed Warning]: Drugs that act on the renin-angiotensin system can cause injury and death to the developing fetus. Discontinue as soon as possible once pregnancy is detected. Enalaprilat, the active metabolite of enalapril, crosses the placenta; teratogenic effects may occur following maternal use during pregnancy. Drugs that act on the renin-angiotensin system are associated with oligohydramnios. Oligohydramnios, due to decreased fetal renal function, may lead to fetal lung hypoplasia and skeletal malformations. The use of these drugs in pregnancy is also associated with anuria, hypotension, renal failure, skull hypoplasia, and death in the fetus/neonate. Chronic maternal hypertension itself is also associated with adverse events in the fetus/infant. ACE inhibitors are not recommended during pregnancy to treat maternal hypertension or heart failure. Use of an ACE inhibitor should also be avoided in any woman of reproductive age. Women who are planning a pregnancy should be considered for other medication options if an ACE inhibitor is currently prescribed or the ACE inhibitor should be discontinued as soon as possible once pregnancy is detected. The exposed fetus should be monitored for fetal growth, amniotic fluid volume, and organ formation. Infants exposed to an ACE inhibitor *in utero* should be monitored for hyperkalemia, hypotension, and oliguria (exchange transfusions or dialysis may be needed). These adverse events are generally associated with maternal use in the second and third trimesters.

Untreated chronic maternal hypertension is also associated with adverse events in the fetus, infant, and mother. The use of ACE inhibitors is not recommended to treat chronic uncomplicated hypertension in pregnant women and should generally be avoided in women of reproductive potential (ACOG, 2013).

Breast-Feeding Considerations Enalapril and enalaprilat are excreted in breast milk. Breast-feeding is not recommended by the manufacturer.

Contraindications Hypersensitivity to enalapril or enalaprilat; angioedema related to previous treatment with an ACE inhibitor; patients with idiopathic or hereditary angioedema; concomitant use with aliskiren in patients with diabetes mellitus

Warnings/Precautions Anaphylactic reactions may occur rarely with ACE inhibitors. At any time during treatment (especially following first dose) angioedema may occur rarely with ACE inhibitors; it may involve the head and neck (potentially compromising airway) or the intestine (presenting with abdominal pain). African-Americans may be at an increased risk. Prolonged frequent monitoring may be required especially if tongue, glottis, or larynx are involved as they are associated with airway obstruction. Patients with a history of airway surgery may have a higher risk of airway obstruction. Aggressive early and appropriate management is critical. Use in patients with idiopathic or hereditary angioedema or previous angioedema associated with ACE inhibitor therapy is contraindicated. Severe anaphylactoid reactions may be seen during hemodialysis (eg, CVVHD) with high-flux dialysis membranes (eg, AN69), and rarely, during low density lipoprotein apheresis with dextran sulfate cellulose. Rare cases of anaphylactoid reactions have been reported in patients undergoing sensitization treatment with hymenoptera (bee, wasp) venom while receiving ACE inhibitors.

Symptomatic hypotension with or without syncope can occur with ACE inhibitors (usually with the first several doses); effects are most often observed in volume-depleted patients; correct volume depletion prior to initiation; close monitoring of patient is required especially with initial dosing and dosing increases; blood pressure must be lowered at a rate appropriate for the patient's clinical condition. Initiation of therapy in patients with ischemic heart disease or cerebrovascular disease warrants close observation due to the potential consequences posed by falling blood pressure (eg, MI, stroke). Use with caution in hypertrophic cardiomyopathy with outflow tract obstruction and severe aortic stenosis. In patients on chronic ACE inhibitor therapy, intraoperative hypotension may occur with induction and maintenance of general anesthesia; use with caution before, during, or immediately after major surgery. Cardiopulmonary bypass, intraoperative blood loss, or vasodilating anesthesia increases endogenous renin release. Use of ACE inhibitors perioperatively will blunt angiotensin II formation and may result in hypotension. However, discontinuation of therapy prior to surgery is controversial. If continued preoperatively, avoidance of hypotensive agents during surgery is prudent (Hillis, 2011). **[U.S. Boxed Warning]: Based on human data, ACEIs can cause injury and death to the developing fetus when used in the second and third trimesters. ACEIs should be discontinued as soon as possible once pregnancy is detected.**

Hyperkalemia may occur with ACE inhibitors; risk factors include renal dysfunction, diabetes mellitus, concomitant use of potassium-sparing diuretics, potassium supplements, and/or potassium-containing salts. Use cautiously, if at all, with these agents and monitor potassium closely. Cough may occur with ACE inhibitors. Other causes of cough should be considered (eg, pulmonary congestion in patients with heart failure) and excluded prior to discontinuation.

May be associated with deterioration of renal function and/or increases in serum creatinine, particularly in patients with low renal blood flow (eg, renal artery stenosis, heart failure) whose glomerular filtration rate (GFR) is dependent on efferent arteriolar vasoconstriction by angiotensin II; deterioration may result in oliguria, acute renal failure, and progressive azotemia. Small increases in serum creatinine may occur following initiation; consider discontinuation only in patients with progressive and/or significant deterioration in renal function. Use with caution in patients with unstented unilateral/bilateral renal artery stenosis. When unstented bilateral renal artery stenosis is present, use is generally avoided due to the elevated risk of deterioration in renal function unless possible benefits outweigh risks. Concomitant use of an angiotensin receptor blocker (ARB) or renin inhibitor (eg, aliskiren) is associated with an increased risk of hypotension, hyperkalemia, and renal dysfunction; concomitant use with aliskiren should be avoided in patients with GFR <60 mL/minute and is contraindicated in patients with diabetes mellitus (regardless of GFR).

Rare toxicities associated with ACE inhibitors include cholestatic jaundice (which may progress to fulminant hepatic necrosis), agranulocytosis, neutropenia, or leukopenia with myeloid hypoplasia. Patients with collagen vascular diseases (especially with concomitant renal impairment) or renal impairment alone may be at increased risk for hematologic toxicity; periodically monitor CBC with differential in these patients.

Benzyl alcohol and derivatives: Some dosage forms may contain benzyl alcohol; large amounts of benzyl alcohol (≥99 mg/kg/day) have been associated with a potentially fatal toxicity ("gasping syndrome") in neonates; the "gasping syndrome" consists of metabolic acidosis, respiratory distress, gasping respirations, CNS dysfunction (including convulsions, intracranial hemorrhage), hypotension and cardiovascular collapse (AAP, 1997; CDC, 1982); some data suggests that benzoate displaces bilirubin from protein binding sites (Ahlfors, 2001); avoid or use dosage forms containing benzyl alcohol with caution in neonates. See manufacturer's labeling.

Adverse Reactions Note: Since enalapril is converted to enalaprilat, adverse reactions associated with enalapril may also occur with enalaprilat (also refer to Enalapril monograph).

Cardiovascular: Hypotension

Central nervous system: Headache

Gastrointestinal: Nausea

Rare but important or life-threatening: Angioedema, constipation, cough, dizziness, fatigue, fever, MI, rash

Drug Interactions

Metabolism/Transport Effects None known.

Avoid Concomitant Use There are no known interactions where it is recommended to avoid concomitant use.

Increased Effect/Toxicity

Enalaprilat may increase the levels/effects of: Allopurinol; Amifostine; Antihypertensives; AzaTHIOprine; Ciprofloxacin (Systemic); Drospirenone; DULoxetine; Ferric Gluconate; Gold Sodium Thiomalate; Grass Pollen Allergen Extract (5 Grass Extract); Hypotensive Agents; Iron Dextran Complex; Levodopa; Lithium; Nonsteroidal Anti-Inflammatory Agents; Obinutuzumab; Pregabalin; RisperiDONE; RiTUXimab; Sodium Phosphates

The levels/effects of Enalaprilat may be increased by: Alfuzosin; Aliskiren; Angiotensin II Receptor Blockers; Barbiturates; Brimonidine (Topical); Canagliflozin; Dapoxetine; Diazoxide; DPP-IV Inhibitors; Eplerenone; Everolimus; Heparin; Heparin (Low Molecular Weight); Herbs (Hypotensive Properties); Loop Diuretics; MAO Inhibitors; Nicorandil; Pentoxifylline; Phosphodiesterase 5 Inhibitors; Potassium Salts; Potassium-Sparing Diuretics; Prostacyclin Analogues; Sirolimus; Temsirolimus; Thiazide Diuretics; TiZANidine; Tolvaptan; Trimethoprim

Decreased Effect

The levels/effects of Enalaprilat may be decreased by: Aprotinin; Herbs (Hypertensive Properties); Icatibant; Methylphenidate; Nonsteroidal Anti-Inflammatory Agents; Salicylates; Yohimbine

Storage/Stability Enalaprilat is a clear, colorless solution which should be stored at <30°C (86°F). IV is stable for 24 hours at room temperature in D_5W, NS, D_5NS, or D_5LR.

Mechanism of Action Competitive inhibitor of angiotensin-converting enzyme (ACE); prevents conversion of angiotensin I to angiotensin II, a potent vasoconstrictor; results in lower levels of angiotensin II which causes an increase in plasma renin activity and a reduction in aldosterone secretion

Pharmacodynamics Antihypertensive effect:

Onset of action: Within 15 minutes

Maximum effect: Within 1-4 hours

Duration: Dose dependent, usually 4-6 hours

Pharmacokinetics (Adult data unless noted)

Protein binding: 50% to 60%

Half-life:

CHF: Neonates (n=3; PNA: 10-19 days): 11.9 hours (range: 5.9-15.6 hours) (Nakamura, 1994)

CHF: Infants and Children ≤6.5 years of age (n=11): 11.1 hours (range: 5.1-20.8 hours) (Nakamura, 1994)

Infants 6 weeks to 8 months: 6-10 hours

Adults: 35-38 hours

Elimination: Principally in urine (60% to 80%) with some fecal excretion

Dosing: Neonatal Use lower listed initial dose in patients with hyponatremia, hypovolemia, severe CHF, decreased renal function, or in those receiving diuretics

Hypertension: IV: 5-10 **mcg**/kg/dose every 8-24 hours as determined by clinical response (eg, blood pressure readings); monitor patients carefully; some patients may require higher doses

Dosing adjustment in renal impairment: Note: Use in neonates with GFR <30 mL/minute/1.73 m^2 is not recommended; no dosing data available

Dosing: Usual Use lower listed initial dose in patients with hyponatremia, hypovolemia, severe CHF, decreased renal function, or in those receiving diuretics

Infants and Children: **Hypertension:** IV: 5-10 **mcg**/kg/dose every 8-24 hours; maximum dose:1.25 mg/dose; frequency determined by clinical response (eg, blood pressure readings); monitor patients carefully; some patients may require higher doses (NHBPEP, 2005)

Adolescents and Adults: **Hypertension:** IV: 0.625-1.25 mg/dose every 6 hours; doses as high as 5 mg/dose every 6 hours have been tolerated for up to 36 hours; little experience with doses >20 mg/day

Dosing adjustment in renal impairment:

Infants, Children, and Adolescents:

Aronoff, 2007:

GFR >50 mL/minute/1.73 m^2: No dosage adjustment necessary

GFR 10-50 mL/minute/1.73 m^2: Administer 75% of usual dose

GFR <10 mL/minute/1.73 m^2: Administer 50% of usual dose

Alternate recommendations: Others suggest avoiding use in infants, children, and adolescents ≤16 years of age with GFR <30 mL/minute/1.73 m^2.

Adults:

Manufacturer's labeling:

CrCl >30 mL/minute: No dosage adjustment necessary

CrCl ≤30 mL/minute: Initiate with 0.625 mg; if after 1 hour clinical response is unsatisfactory, may repeat. May then administer 1.25 mg every 6 hours

Alternate recommendations (Aronoff, 2007):

GFR >50 mL/minute: No dosage adjustment necessary

GFR 10-50 mL/minute: Administer 50% to 100% of usual dose

GFR <10 mL/minute: Administer 25% to 50% of usual dose

Peritoneal dialysis: Supplemental dose is not necessary, although some removal of drug occurs.

Preparation for Administration IV: May be diluted in a compatible solution to a final concentration ≤25 mcg/mL; for example, 0.625 to 1.25 mg in up to 50 mL of a compatible solution

Administration Administer as IV infusion over 5 minutes (undiluted or further diluted)

Monitoring Parameters Blood pressure, renal function, WBC, serum potassium, serum glucose; monitor for angioedema and anaphylactoid reactions

Dosage Forms Excipient information presented when available (limited, particularly for generics); consult specific product labeling.

Injectable, Intravenous:

Generic: 1.25 mg/mL (1 mL, 2 mL)

◆ **Enalapril Maleate** *see* Enalapril *on page 744*

◆ **Enbrel** *see* Etanercept *on page 806*

◆ **Enbrel SureClick** *see* Etanercept *on page 806*

◆ **Endocet** *see* Oxycodone and Acetaminophen *on page 1594*

◆ **Endodan®** *see* Oxycodone and Aspirin *on page 1597*

◆ **Enemeez Mini [OTC]** *see* Docusate *on page 697*

Enfuvirtide (en FYOO vir tide)

Medication Safety Issues

High alert medication:

This medication is in a class the Institute for Safe Medication Practices (ISMP) includes among its list of drug classes that have a heightened risk of causing significant patient harm when used in error.

Related Information

Adult and Adolescent HIV *on page 2392*

Pediatric HIV *on page 2380*

Perinatal HIV *on page 2400*

Brand Names: US Fuzeon

Brand Names: Canada Fuzeon

Therapeutic Category Antiretroviral Agent; Fusion Inhibitor; HIV Agents (Anti-HIV Agents)

Generic Availability (US) No

Use Treatment of HIV-1 infection in combination with other antiretroviral agents in treatment-experienced patients who are failing current antiretroviral therapy (FDA approved in ages ≥6 years and adults). **Note:** HIV regimens consisting of **three** antiretroviral agents are strongly recommended. However, in published studies, enfuvirtide was added onto a new optimized background regimen of 3 to 5 antiretroviral agents, in patients failing their current antiretroviral regimen. Selection of the new optimized regimen was based on medication history, genotyping, and phenotyping. Due to the lack of studies, enfuvirtide cannot be recommended as initial therapy in patients who are antiretroviral naïve.

Pregnancy Risk Factor B

Pregnancy Considerations Teratogenic effects were not observed in animal studies. Enfuvirtide has minimal to low transfer across the human placenta. The DHHS Perinatal HIV Guidelines note that data are insufficient to recommend use during pregnancy.

Regardless of CD4 count or HIV RNA copy number, all HIV-infected pregnant women should receive a combination antiretroviral (ARV) drug regimen. A combination of antepartum, intrapartum, and infant ARV prophylaxis is recommended. ARV therapy should be started as soon as possible in women with symptomatic infection. Although earlier initiation may be more effective in reducing the perinatal transmission of HIV, initiation may be delayed until after 12 weeks gestation in women who do not require immediate treatment after careful consideration of maternal conditions (eg, nausea and vomiting) and the potential risks of first trimester fetal exposure for specific agents. A scheduled cesarean delivery at 38 weeks gestation is recommended for all women with HIV RNA >1000 copies/mL or unknown concentrations near delivery in order to decrease transmission. If ARV therapy must be interrupted for <24 hours during the peripartum period, stop then restart all medications simultaneously in order to decrease the chance of developing resistance. Long-term follow-up is recommended for all infants exposed to ARV medications. In couples who want to conceive, the HIV-infected partner should attain maximum viral suppression prior to conception.

Healthcare providers are encouraged to enroll pregnant women exposed to antiretroviral medications in the Antiretroviral Pregnancy Registry (1-800-258-4263 or www.APRegistry.com). Healthcare providers caring for HIV-infected women and their infants may contact the National Perinatal HIV Hotline (888-448-8765) for clinical consultation (HHS [perinatal], 2014).

Breast-Feeding Considerations It is not known if enfuvirtide is excreted into breast milk. Maternal or infant antiretroviral therapy does not completely eliminate the risk of postnatal HIV transmission. In addition, multiclass-resistant virus has been detected in breast-feeding infants despite maternal therapy. Therefore, in the United States, where formula is accessible, affordable, safe, and sustainable, and the risk of infant mortality due to diarrhea and respiratory infections is low, complete avoidance of breast-feeding by HIV-infected women is recommended to decrease potential transmission of HIV (HHS [perinatal], 2014).

Contraindications Hypersensitivity to enfuvirtide or any component of the formulation

Warnings/Precautions Use is not recommended in antiretroviral therapy-naive patients (HHS [adult], 2014). Monitor closely for signs/symptoms of pneumonia; associated with an increased incidence during clinical trials, particularly in patients with a low CD4 cell count, high initial viral load, IV drug use, smoking, or a history of lung disease. May cause hypersensitivity reactions (symptoms may include rash, fever, nausea, vomiting, chills, rigors, hypotension, and/or elevated transaminases). Discontinue therapy immediately if systemic reactions occur; do not rechallenge patient. In addition, local injection site reactions are common. Patients may develop immune reconstitution syndrome resulting in the occurrence of an inflammatory response to an indolent or residual opportunistic infection during initial HIV treatment or activation of autoimmune disorders (eg, Graves' disease, polymyositis, Guillain-Barré syndrome) later in therapy; further evaluation and treatment may be required. Administration using a needle-free device has been associated with nerve pain (including neuralgia and/or paresthesia lasting up to 6 months), bruising, and hematomas when administered at sites where large nerves are close to the skin; only administer medication in recommended sites and use caution in patients with coagulation disorders (eg, hemophilia) or receiving anticoagulants.

Adverse Reactions

Central nervous system: Fatigue, insomnia

Dermatologic: Folliculitis

Gastrointestinal: Abdominal pain, anorexia, appetite decreased, diarrhea, nausea, pancreatitis, weight loss, xerostomia

Hematologic: Eosinophilia

Hepatic: Transaminases increased

Local: Injection site infection, injection site reactions (may include pain, erythema, induration, pruritus, ecchymosis, nodule or cyst formation)

Neuromuscular & skeletal: CPK increased, limb pain, myalgia

Ocular: Conjunctivitis

Respiratory: Bacterial pneumonia, cough, sinusitis

Miscellaneous: Flu-like syndrome, herpes simplex, infection, lymphadenopathy

Rare but important or life-threatening: Abacavir hypersensitivity worsening, amylase increased, angina, anxiety, constipation, depression, GGT increased, glomerulonephritis, Guillain-Barré syndrome, hepatic steatosis, hyperglycemia; hypersensitivity reactions (symptoms may include rash, fever, nausea, vomiting, hypotension, and transaminase increases); insomnia, lipase increased, lymphadenopathy, neutropenia, peripheral neuropathy, pneumopathy, renal failure, renal insufficiency, respiratory distress, sepsis, sixth nerve palsy, suicide attempt, taste disturbances, thrombocytopenia, toxic hepatitis, triglycerides increased, tubular necrosis, weakness

Drug Interactions

Metabolism/Transport Effects None known.

Avoid Concomitant Use There are no known interactions where it is recommended to avoid concomitant use.

Increased Effect/Toxicity

Enfuvirtide may increase the levels/effects of: Protease Inhibitors

The levels/effects of Enfuvirtide may be increased by: Protease Inhibitors

Decreased Effect There are no known significant interactions involving a decrease in effect.

Storage/Stability Store intact vials at 25°C (77°F); excursions are permitted between 15°C and 30°C (59°F and 86°F). Store reconstituted solution in the original vial at 2°C to 8°C (36°F to 46°F); use within 24 hours. Vials are for single use only; discard unused portion.

Mechanism of Action Binds to the first heptad-repeat (HR1) in the gp41 subunit of the viral envelope glycoprotein. Inhibits the fusion of HIV-1 virus with CD4 cells by blocking the conformational change in gp41 required for membrane fusion and entry into CD4 cells

Pharmacokinetics (Adult data unless noted)

Absorption: SubQ: Absorption is comparable when injected into abdomen, arm, or thigh

Distribution: V_d (mean ± SD): 5.5 ± 1.1 L

CSF concentrations (2 to 18 hours after administration; n=4): Nondetectable (<0.025 mcg/mL)

Protein Binding: 92%; primarily to albumin, but also to alpha-1 acid glycoprotein (to a lesser extent)

Metabolism: Expected to undergo catabolism via peptidases and proteinases in the liver and kidneys to amino acids; amino acids would then be recycled in the body pool. A deaminated metabolite (with 20% activity compared to parent drug) was formed via hydrolysis during *in vitro* human microsomal and hepatocyte studies.

Bioavailability:

Oral: Not bioavailable by this route

SubQ: Absolute: 84.3% ± 15.5%; **Note:** Bioequivalence was found to be similar in a study comparing standard administration using a needle versus a needle-free device.

Half-life: 3.8 ± 0.6 hours

Time to peak serum concentration: SubQ:

Single dose: Median: 8 hours (range: 3 to 12 hours)

Multiple dosing: Median: 4 hours (range: 4 to 8 hours)

Clearance:

Plasma clearance is decreased in adults with lower body weight and in females after adjusting for body weight (clearance in adults females is 20% lower compared to adults males). However, no adjustment in dose is recommended for gender or weight.

Compared to patients with normal renal function, enfuvirtide clearance is decreased by 38% in patients with severe renal impairment (CrCl 11 to 35 mL/minute) and by 14% to 28% in patients with end-stage renal disease who are maintained on dialysis. However, no adjustment in dose is recommended for patients with renal impairment.

Apparent clearance: Multiple dosing:

Children: 40 ± 17 mL/hour/kg

Adults: 30.6 ± 10.6 mL/hour/kg

Dosing: Usual

Pediatric: **HIV infection, treatment:** Treatment-experienced patients only. Use not recommended in antiretroviral therapy naïve patients (DHHS [pediatric, adult], 2014): **Note:** Use in combination with other antiretroviral agents:

Age-directed dosing:

Children and Adolescents 6 to 16 years: SubQ: 2 mg/kg twice daily; maximum dose: 90 mg/dose

Adolescents >16 years: SubQ: 90 mg twice daily (DHHS [pediatric], 2014)

Weight-directed, fixed dosing: Children ≥6 years and Adolescents: SubQ:

11 to 15.5 kg: 27 mg twice daily
15.6 to 20 kg: 36 mg twice daily
20.1 to 24.5 kg: 45 mg twice daily
24.6 to 29 kg: 54 mg twice daily
29.1 to 33.5 kg: 63 mg twice daily
33.6 to 38 kg: 72 mg twice daily
38.1 to 42.5 kg: 81 mg twice daily
≥42.6 kg: 90 mg twice daily

Adult: **HIV infection, treatment:** Treatment-experienced patients only. Use not recommended in antiretroviral therapy naïve patients (DHHS [adult], 2014): **Note:** Use in combination with other antiretroviral agents: SubQ: 90 mg twice daily

Dosing adjustment in renal impairment: Adults:

CrCl >35 mL/minute: Clearance of enfuvirtide is not affected; no dosage adjustment required.

CrCl ≤35 mL/minute: Limited data showed decreased clearance; however, no dosage adjustment recommended.

End-stage renal disease (on dialysis): Limited data showed decreased clearance; however, no dosage adjustment recommended. **Note:** Hemodialysis does not significantly affect clearance of enfuvirtide.

Dosing adjustment in hepatic impairment: No dosage adjustment required.

Preparation for Administration SubQ: Reconstitute with 1 mL SWFI; tap vial for 10 seconds and roll gently between the hands to avoid foaming and to ensure contact with diluent; then allow to stand until complete dissolution; may require up to 45 minutes to form solution; allow more time if solution is foamy or jelled; to reduce reconstitution time, may gently roll vial between hands until drug is completely dissolved. Visually inspect vial to ensure complete dissolution of drug; solution should be clear, colorless, and without particulate matter or bubbles. Use immediately or refrigerate reconstituted solution and use within 24 hours; bring refrigerated solution to room temperature before administration.

Administration SubQ: Bring refrigerated reconstituted vials to room temperature before injection and visually inspect vial again; solution should be clear, colorless, and without particulate matter or bubbles.

Inject SubQ into upper arm, abdomen, or anterior thigh. Do not inject IM (severity of reactions is increased). Do not inject into skin abnormalities including directly over a blood vessel, into moles, bruises, scar tissue, near the navel, surgical scars, burn sites, or tattoos. Do not inject in or near sites where large nerves are close to the skin including near the elbow, knee, groin, and inferior or medial sections of the buttocks. Rotate injection site (ie, give injections at a site different from the preceding injection site); do not inject into any site where an injection site reaction is present. After injection, apply heat or ice to injection site or gently massage area to better disperse the dose, to minimize local injection reactions (DHHS [pediatric] 2014); discard unused portion of the vial (vial is for single use only).

Monitoring Parameters Note: Monitor CD4 percentage (if <5 years of age) or CD4 count (if ≥5 years of age) at least every 3 to 4 months (DHHS [pediatric], 2014).

Prior to initiation of therapy: Genotypic resistance testing, CD4 and viral load (every 3 to 4 months), CBC with differential, LFTs, BUN, creatinine, electrolytes, glucose, and urinalysis (every 6 to 12 months), and assessment of readiness for adherence with medication regimen. At initiation and with any change in treatment regimen: CBC with differential, electrolytes, calcium, phosphate, glucose, LFTs, bilirubin, urinalysis (at initiation), BUN, creatinine, albumin, total protein, lipid panel (at initiation), CD4, and viral load. After 1 to 2 weeks of therapy: Signs of medication toxicity and adherence. After 2 to 4 weeks of therapy: CBC with differential, viral load, signs of medication toxicity, and adherence; then every 3 to 4 months: CBC with differential, electrolytes, glucose, LFTs, bilirubin, BUN, creatinine, CD4, viral load, signs of medication toxicity, and adherence. Every 6 to 12 months: Lipid panel and urinalysis. CD4 monitoring frequency may be decreased to every 6 to 12 months in children who are adherent to therapy if the value is well above the threshold for opportunistic infections, viral suppression is sustained, and the clinical status is stable for more than 2 to 3 years (DHHS [pediatric], 2014). Monitor for growth and development, signs of HIV-specific physical conditions, HIV disease progression, opportunistic infections, local injection site reactions, local infection, cellulitis, and signs and symptoms of pneumonia, especially in patients at risk.

Additional Information Reconstituted injection has a pH ~9.0.

Dosage Forms Excipient information presented when available (limited, particularly for generics); consult specific product labeling.

Solution Reconstituted, Subcutaneous:

Fuzeon: 90 mg (1 ea)

- **Engerix-B** *see* Hepatitis B Vaccine (Recombinant) *on page 1015*
- **Enhanced-Potency Inactivated Poliovirus Vaccine** *see* Poliovirus Vaccine (Inactivated) *on page 1721*
- **Enlon** *see* Edrophonium *on page 729*
- **Enlon® (Can)** *see* Edrophonium *on page 729*
- **EnovaRX-Baclofen** *see* Baclofen *on page 254*
- **EnovaRX-Cyclobenzaprine HCl** *see* Cyclobenzaprine *on page 548*
- **EnovaRX-Ibuprofen** *see* Ibuprofen *on page 1064*
- **EnovaRX-Lidocaine HCl** *see* Lidocaine (Topical) *on page 1258*
- **EnovaRX-Naproxen** *see* Naproxen *on page 1489*
- **EnovaRX-Tramadol** *see* TraMADol *on page 2098*

Enoxaparin (ee noks a PA rin)

Medication Safety Issues

Sound-alike/look-alike issues:

Lovenox may be confused with Lasix, Levaquin, Levemir, Lotronex, Protonix

High alert medication:

The Institute for Safe Medication Practices (ISMP) includes this medication among its list of drugs which have a heightened risk of causing significant patient harm when used in error.

National Patient Safety Goals:

The Joint Commission (TJC) requires healthcare organizations that provide anticoagulant therapy to have a process in place to reduce the risk of anticoagulant-associated patient harm. Patients receiving anticoagulants should receive individualized care through a defined process that includes standardized ordering, dispensing, administration, monitoring and education. This does not apply to routine short-term use of anticoagulants for prevention of venous thromboembolism when the expectation is that the patient's laboratory values will remain within or close to normal values (NPSG.03.05.01).

Brand Names: US Lovenox

Brand Names: Canada Lovenox; Lovenox HP; Lovenox With Preservative

Therapeutic Category Anticoagulant; Low Molecular Weight Heparin (LMWH)

Generic Availability (US) Yes

Use Prophylaxis and treatment of thromboembolic disorders, specifically prevention of DVT following hip or knee replacement surgery, abdominal surgery in patients at thromboembolic risk (ie, >40 years of age, obese, general anesthesia >30 minutes, malignancy, history of DVT, or pulmonary embolism), and in medical patients at thromboembolic risk due to severely restricted mobility during acute illness (FDA approved in adults). Administered with warfarin: For inpatient treatment of acute DVT (with or without pulmonary embolism) and outpatient treatment of acute DVT (without pulmonary embolism) (FDA approved in adults). Administered with aspirin: For prevention of ischemic complications of non-Q-wave MI and unstable angina and for the treatment of acute ST-segment elevation myocardial infarction (STEMI) (FDA approved in adults)

Pregnancy Risk Factor B

Pregnancy Considerations Adverse events were not observed in animal reproduction studies. Low molecular weight heparin (LMWH) does not cross the placenta; increased risks of fetal bleeding or teratogenic effects have not been reported (Bates, 2012).

LMWH is recommended over unfractionated heparin for the treatment of acute venous thromboembolism (VTE) in pregnant women. LMWH is also recommended over unfractionated heparin for VTE prophylaxis in pregnant women with certain risk factors (eg, homozygous factor V Leiden, antiphospholipid antibody syndrome with ≥3 previous pregnancy losses). Prophylaxis is not routinely recommended for women undergoing assisted reproduction therapy; however, LMWH therapy is recommended for women who develop severe ovarian hyperstimulation syndrome. LMWH should be discontinued at least 24 hours prior to induction of labor or a planned cesarean delivery. For women undergoing cesarean section and who have additional risk factors for developing VTE, the prophylactic use of LMWH may be considered (Bates, 2012).

LMWH may also be used in women with mechanical heart valves (consult current guidelines for details) (Bates, 2012; Nishimura, 2014). Women who require long-term anticoagulation with warfarin and who are considering pregnancy, LMWH substitution should be done prior to conception when possible. When choosing therapy, fetal outcomes (ie, pregnancy loss, malformations), maternal outcomes (ie, VTE, hemorrhage), burden of therapy, and maternal preference should be considered (Bates, 2012). Monitoring antifactor Xa levels is recommended (Bates, 2012; Nishimura, 2014).

Multiple-dose vials contain benzyl alcohol (avoid in pregnant women due to association with gasping syndrome in premature infants); use of preservative-free formulations is recommended.

Breast-Feeding Considerations Small amounts of LMWH have been detected in breast milk; however, because it has a low oral bioavailability, it is unlikely to cause adverse events in a nursing infant. Enoxaparin product labeling does not recommend use in nursing women; however, antithrombotic guidelines state that use of LMWH may be continued in breast-feeding women (Guyatt, 2012).

Contraindications

Hypersensitivity to enoxaparin, heparin, pork products, or any component of the formulation (including benzyl alcohol in multiple-dose vials); thrombocytopenia associated with a positive *in vitro* test for antiplatelet antibodies in the presence of enoxaparin; active major bleeding

Canadian labeling: Additional contraindications (not in U.S. labeling): Use of multiple-dose vials in newborns or premature neonates; history of confirmed or suspected immunologically-mediated heparin-induced thrombocytopenia; acute or subacute bacterial endocarditis; major blood clotting disorders; active gastric or duodenal ulcer; hemorrhagic cerebrovascular accident (except if there are systemic emboli); severe uncontrolled hypertension; diabetic or hemorrhagic retinopathy; other conditions or diseases involving an increased risk of hemorrhage; injuries to and operations on the brain, spinal cord, eyes, and ears; spinal/epidural anesthesia when repeated dosing of enoxaparin (1 mg/kg every 12 hours or 1.5 mg/kg daily) is required, due to increased risk of bleeding.

Note: Use of enoxaparin in patients with current heparin-induced thrombocytopenia (HIT) or HIT with thrombosis is **not** recommended and considered contraindicated due to high cross-reactivity to heparin-platelet factor-4 antibody (Guyatt [ACCP], 2012; Warkentin, 1999).

Warnings/Precautions **[U.S. Boxed Warning]: Spinal or epidural hematomas, including subsequent long-term or permanent paralysis, may occur with recent or anticipated neuraxial anesthesia (epidural or spinal anesthesia) or spinal puncture in patients anticoagulated with LMWH or heparinoids. Consider risk versus benefit prior to spinal procedures; risk is increased by the use of concomitant agents which may alter hemostasis, the use of indwelling epidural catheters, a history of spinal deformity or spinal surgery, as well as a history of traumatic or repeated epidural or spinal punctures. Optimal timing between neuraxial procedures and enoxaparin administration is not known.** Delay placement or removal of catheter for at least 12 hours after administration of low-dose enoxaparin (eg, 30 to 60 mg/day) and at least 24 hours after high-dose enoxaparin (eg, 0.75 to 1 mg/kg twice daily or 1.5 mg/kg once daily) and consider doubling these times in patients with creatinine clearance <30 mL/minute; risk of neuraxial hematoma may still exist since antifactor Xa levels are still detectable at these time points. Patients receiving twice daily high-dose enoxaparin should have the second dose withheld to allow a longer time period prior to catheter placement or removal. Upon removal of catheter, consider withholding enoxaparin for at least 4 hours. **Patient should be observed closely for bleeding and signs and symptoms of neurological impairment if therapy is administered during or immediately following diagnostic lumbar puncture, epidural anesthesia, or spinal anesthesia. If neurological compromise is noted, urgent treatment is necessary.** If spinal hematoma is suspected, diagnose and treat immediately; spinal cord decompression may be considered although it may not prevent or reverse neurological sequelae.

Do not administer intramuscularly. Discontinue use 12 to 24 hours prior to CABG and dose with unfractionated heparin per institutional practice (ACCF/AHA [Anderson, 2013]). Not recommended for thromboprophylaxis in patients with prosthetic heart valves (especially pregnant women). Not to be used interchangeably (unit for unit) with heparin or any other low molecular weight heparins. Monitor patient closely for signs or symptoms of bleeding. Certain patients are at increased risk of bleeding. Risk factors include bacterial endocarditis; congenital or acquired bleeding disorders; active ulcerative or angiodysplastic GI diseases; severe uncontrolled hypertension; hemorrhagic stroke; use shortly after brain, spinal, or ophthalmic surgery; patients treated concomitantly with platelet inhibitors; recent GI bleeding or ulceration; renal dysfunction and hemorrhage; thrombocytopenia or platelet defects or history of heparin-induced thrombocytopenia; severe liver disease; hypertensive or diabetic retinopathy; or in patients undergoing invasive procedures. Protamine may be considered as a partial reversal agent in overdose situations (consult Protamine monograph for dosing recommendations). To minimize risk of bleeding following PCI, achieve hemostasis at the puncture site after PCI. If a closure device is used, sheath can be removed immediately. If manual compression is used, remove sheath 6 hours after the last IV/SubQ dose of enoxaparin. Do not administer further doses until 6 to 8 hours after sheath removal; observe for signs of bleeding/hematoma formation. Cases of enoxaparin-induced thrombocytopenia and thrombosis (similar to heparin-induced thrombocytopenia [HIT]), some complicated by organ infarction, limb ischemia, or death, have been observed. Use with extreme caution or avoid in patients with history of HIT, especially if administered within 100 days of HIT episode (Warkentin, 2001); monitor platelet count closely. Use is contraindicated in patients with thrombocytopenia associated with a positive *in vitro* test for antiplatelet antibodies in the presence of enoxaparin. Discontinue therapy and consider alternative treatment if platelets are <100,000/mm^3 and/or thrombosis develops. Use caution in patients with congenital or drug-induced thrombocytopenia or platelet defects. Risk of bleeding may be increased in women <45 kg and in men <57 kg. Use caution in patients with renal failure; dosage adjustment needed if CrCl <30 mL/minute. Use with caution in the elderly (delayed elimination may occur); dosage alteration/adjustment may be required (eg, omission of IV bolus in acute STEMI in patients ≥75 years of age). Monitor for hyperkalemia; can cause hyperkalemia possibly by suppressing aldosterone production.

Benzyl alcohol and derivatives: Some dosage forms may contain benzyl alcohol and should not be used in pregnant women. In neonates, large amounts of benzyl alcohol (≥99 mg/kg/day) have been associated with a potentially fatal toxicity ("gasping syndrome"); the "gasping syndrome" consists of metabolic acidosis, respiratory distress, gasping respirations, CNS dysfunction (including convulsions, intracranial hemorrhage), hypotension, and cardiovascular collapse (AAP, 1997; CDC, 1982); some data suggests that benzoate displaces bilirubin from protein binding sites (Ahlfors, 2001); avoid or use dosage forms containing benzyl alcohol with caution in neonates. See manufacturer's labeling.

Safety and efficacy of prophylactic dosing of enoxaparin has not been established in patients who are obese (>30 kg/m^2) nor is there a consensus regarding dosage adjustments. The American College of Chest Physicians Practice Guidelines suggest consulting with a pharmacist regarding dosing in bariatric surgery patients and other obese patients who may require higher doses of LMWH (ACCP [Gould, 2012]).

Adverse Reactions As with all anticoagulants, bleeding is the major adverse effect of enoxaparin. Hemorrhage may occur at virtually any site. Risk is dependent on multiple variables. At the recommended doses, single injections of enoxaparin do not significantly influence platelet aggregation or affect global clotting time (ie, PT or aPTT).

Central nervous system: Confusion, pain
Gastrointestinal: Diarrhea, nausea
Hematologic & oncologic: Anemia, bruise, major hemorrhage (includes cases of intracranial, retroperitoneal, or intraocular hemorrhage; incidence varies with indication/population), thrombocytopenia
Hepatic: Increased serum ALT, increased serum AST
Local: Bruising at injection site, erythema at injection site, hematoma at injection site, irritation at injection site, pain at injection site
Renal: Hematuria
Miscellaneous: Fever
Rare but important or life-threatening: Alopecia, anaphylaxis, anaphylactoid reaction, eczematous rash (plaques), eosinophilia, epidural hematoma (spinal; after neuroaxial anesthesia or spinal puncture; risk may be increased with indwelling epidural catheter or concomitant use of other drugs affecting hemostasis), headache, hepatic injury (hepatocellular and cholestatic),

hyperkalemia, hyperlipidemia (very rare), hypersensitivity angiitis, hypersensitivity reaction, hypertriglyceridemia, intracranial hemorrhage (up to 0.8%), osteoporosis (following long-term therapy), pruritic erythematous rash (patches), pruritus, purpura, retroperitoneal hemorrhage, severe anemia (hemorrhagic), shock, skin necrosis, thrombocythemia, thrombocytopenia, thrombosis (prosthetic value [in pregnant females] or associated with enoxaparin-induced thrombocytopenia; can cause limb ischemia or organ infarction), urticaria, vesicobullous rash

Drug Interactions

Metabolism/Transport Effects None known.

Avoid Concomitant Use

Avoid concomitant use of Enoxaparin with any of the following: Apixaban; Dabigatran Etexilate; Edoxaban; Omacetaxine; Rivaroxaban; Urokinase; Vorapaxar

Increased Effect/Toxicity

Enoxaparin may increase the levels/effects of: ACE Inhibitors; Aliskiren; Angiotensin II Receptor Blockers; Anticoagulants; Canagliflozin; Collagenase (Systemic); Deferasirox; Deoxycholic Acid; Eplerenone; Ibritumomab; Nintedanib; Obinutuzumab; Omacetaxine; Palifermin; Potassium Salts; Potassium-Sparing Diuretics; Rivaroxaban; Tositumomab and Iodine I 131 Tositumomab

The levels/effects of Enoxaparin may be increased by: 5-ASA Derivatives; Agents with Antiplatelet Properties; Apixaban; Dabigatran Etexilate; Dasatinib; Edoxaban; Herbs (Anticoagulant/Antiplatelet Properties); Ibrutinib; Limaprost; Nonsteroidal Anti-Inflammatory Agents; Omega-3 Fatty Acids; Pentosan Polysulfate Sodium; Pentoxifylline; Prostacyclin Analogues; Salicylates; Sugammadex; Thrombolytic Agents; Tibolone; Tipranavir; Urokinase; Vitamin E; Vorapaxar

Decreased Effect

The levels/effects of Enoxaparin may be decreased by: Estrogen Derivatives; Progestins

Storage/Stability Store at 25°C (77°F); excursions permitted to 15°C to 30°C (59°F to 86°F); do not freeze. Do not store multiple-dose vials for >28 days after first use.

Mechanism of Action Standard heparin consists of components with molecular weights ranging from 4000 to 30,000 daltons with a mean of 16,000 daltons. Heparin acts as an anticoagulant by enhancing the inhibition rate of clotting proteases by antithrombin III impairing normal hemostasis and inhibition of factor Xa. Low molecular weight heparins have a small effect on the activated partial thromboplastin time and strongly inhibit factor Xa. Enoxaparin is derived from porcine heparin that undergoes benzylation followed by alkaline depolymerization. The average molecular weight of enoxaparin is 4500 daltons which is distributed as (≤20%) 2000 daltons (≥68%) 2000 to 8000 daltons, and (≤15%) >8000 daltons. Enoxaparin has a higher ratio of antifactor Xa to antifactor IIa activity than unfractionated heparin.

Pharmacodynamics Antifactor Xa and antithrombin (antifactor IIa) activities:

Maximum effect: SubQ: 3-5 hours

Duration: ~12 hours following a 40 mg daily dose given SubQ

Pharmacokinetics (Adult data unless noted) Based on antifactor Xa activity

Distribution: Does not cross the placental barrier

Mean V_d: Adults: 4.3 L

Protein binding: Does not bind to most heparin binding proteins

Metabolism: Primarily in the liver via desulfation and depolymerization to lower molecular weight molecules with very low biological activity

Bioavailability: Adults: SubQ: ~100%

Half-life: SubQ: Adults: Single dose: 4.5 hours; repeat dosing: 7 hours

Elimination: 40% of IV dose is excreted in urine as active and inactive fragments; 10% of dose is excreted by kidneys as active enoxaparin fragments; 8% to 20% of antifactor Xa activity is recovered within 24 hours in the urine

Clearance: Decreased by 30% in patients with CrCl <30 mL/minute

Dosing: Neonatal SubQ:

Initial therapy:

Chest, 2008 recommendations (Monagle, 2008):

Prophylaxis: 0.75 mg/kg/dose every 12 hours

Treatment: 1.5 mg/kg/dose every 12 hours

Alternate dosing: Treatment: **Note:** Several recent studies suggest that doses higher than those recommended in the *Chest* guidelines are required in neonates (Malowany, 2007; Malowany, 2008; Sanchez de Toledo, 2010). Some centers have used the following:

Premature neonates: 2 mg/kg/dose every 12 hours

Full-term neonates: 1.7 mg/kg/dose every 12 hours

Maintenance therapy: *Chest*, 2008 recommendations (Monagle, 2008): See **Dosage Titration** table: **Note:** In a prospective study of 177 courses of enoxaparin in pediatric patients (146 treatment courses; 31 prophylactic courses) considerable variation in maintenance dosage requirements was observed (Dix, 2000).

Enoxaparin Dosage Titration

Antifactor Xa	Dose Titration	Time to Repeat Antifactor Xa Level
<0.35 units/mL	Increase dose by 25%	4 h after next dose
0.35-0.49 units/mL	Increase dose by 10%	4 h after next dose
0.5-1 unit/mL	Keep same dosage	Next day, then 1 wk later, then monthly (4 h after dose)
1.1-1.5 units/mL	Decrease dose by 20%	Before next dose
1.6-2 units/mL	Hold dose for 3 h and decrease dose by 30%	Before next dose, then 4 h after next dose
>2 units/mL	Hold all doses until antifactor Xa is 0.5 units/mL, then decrease dose by 40%	Before next dose and every 12 h until antifactor Xa <0.5 units/mL

Modified from Monagle P, Michelson AD, Bovill E, et al, "Antithrombotic Therapy in Children," *Chest*, 2001, 119:344S-70S.

Dosing: Usual

Infants and Children: SubQ:

Initial therapy:

Chest, 2008 recommendations (Monagle, 2008):

Infants 1 to <2 months:

Prophylaxis: 0.75 mg/kg/dose every 12 hours

Treatment: 1.5 mg/kg/dose every 12 hours

Infants ≥2 months and Children ≤18 years:

Prophylaxis: 0.5 mg/kg/dose every 12 hours

Treatment: 1 mg/kg/dose every 12 hours

Alternate dosing: Treatment: **Note:** Several recent studies suggest that doses higher than those recommended in the *Chest* guidelines are required in pediatric patients (especially in young infants) (Bauman, 2009; Malowany, 2007; Malowany, 2008). Some centers have used the following:

1 to <3 months: 1.8 mg/kg/dose every 12 hours

3-12 months: 1.5 mg/kg/dose every 12 hours

1-5 years: 1.2 mg/kg/dose every 12 hours

6-18 years: 1.1 mg/kg/dose every 12 hours

Maintenance therapy: *Chest*, 2008 recommendations (Monagle, 2008): See **Dosage Titration** table: **Note:** In a prospective study of 177 courses of enoxaparin in pediatric patients (146 treatment courses; 31 prophylactic courses) considerable variation in maintenance dosage requirements was observed (Dix, 2000).

Enoxaparin Dosage Titration

Antifactor Xa	Dose Titration	Time to Repeat Antifactor Xa Level
<0.35 units/mL	Increase dose by 25%	4 h after next dose
0.35-0.49 units/mL	Increase dose by 10%	4 h after next dose
0.5-1 unit/mL	Keep same dosage	Next day, then 1 wk later, then monthly (4 h after dose)
1.1-1.5 units/mL	Decrease dose by 20%	Before next dose
1.6-2 units/mL	Hold dose for 3 h and decrease dose by 30%	Before next dose, then 4 h after next dose
>2 units/mL	Hold all doses until antifactor Xa is 0.5 units/mL, then decrease dose by 40%	Before next dose and every 12 h until antifactor Xa <0.5 units/mL

Modified from Monagle P, Michelson AD, Bovill E, et al, "Antithrombotic Therapy in Children," *Chest*, 2001, 119:344S-70S.

Adults: **Note:** Consider lower doses for patients <45 kg

Prevention of DVT: SubQ:

Knee replacement surgery: 30 mg every 12 hours; give first dose 12-24 hours after surgery (provided hemostasis has been established); average duration 7-10 days, up to 14 days

Hip replacement surgery: Initial phase: 30 mg every 12 hours with first dose 12-24 hours after surgery (provided hemostasis has been established) or consider 40 mg once daily with first dose given 12 ± 3 hours prior to surgery; average duration of initial phase: 7-10 days, up to 14 days; after initial phase, give 40 mg once daily for 3 weeks

Abdominal surgery in patients at risk: 40 mg once daily; give first dose 2 hours prior to surgery; average duration: 7-10 days, up to 12 days

Medical patients at risk due to severely restricted mobility during acute illness: 40 mg once daily; average duration: 6-11 days, up to 14 days

Treatment of acute DVT and pulmonary embolism: SubQ: **Note:** Initiate warfarin therapy on the same day of starting enoxaparin; continue enoxaparin for a minimum of 5 days (average 7 days) until INR is therapeutic (between 2 and 3) for 24 hours (Kearon, 2008).

Inpatient treatment of acute DVT with or without pulmonary embolism: 1 mg/kg every 12 hours or 1.5 mg/kg once daily

Outpatient treatment of acute DVT without pulmonary embolism: 1 mg/kg every 12 hours

Prevention of ischemic complications of non-Q-wave MI or unstable angina: SubQ: 1 mg/kg every 12 hours in conjunction with oral aspirin (100-325 mg once daily); continue treatment for a minimum of 2 days until patient is clinically stabilized (usually 2-8 days; up to 12.5 days)

Treatment of acute ST-segment elevation myocardial infarction (STEMI): Note: Optimal duration is not defined; in the major clinical trial, therapy was continued for 8 days or until hospital discharge; optimal duration may be >8 days. All patients should receive aspirin (75-325 mg once daily) as soon as they are identified as having STEMI. In patients with STEMI receiving thrombolytics, initiate enoxaparin dosing between 15 minutes before and 30 minutes after fibrinolytic therapy. In patients undergoing percutaneous coronary intervention (PCI), if balloon inflation occurs ≤8 hours after the last SubQ enoxaparin dose, no additional dosing is needed. If balloon inflation occurs 8-12 hours after last SubQ enoxaparin dose, a single IV dose of 0.3 mg/kg should be administered (Hirsh, 2008; King, 2007).

Adults <75 years of age: Initial: 30 mg single IV bolus **plus** 1 mg/kg (maximum: 100 mg/dose for the first 2 doses only) SubQ every 12 hours. The first SubQ dose should be administered with the IV bolus. Maintenance: After first 2 doses, administer 1 mg/kg SubQ every 12 hours.

Adults ≥75 years of age: Dosage adjustment required; see package insert

Dosage adjustment in renal impairment:

CrCl ≥30 mL/minute: No specific adjustment recommended; monitor patients closely for bleeding

CrCl <30 mL/minute: **Note:** Monitor antifactor Xa activity closely. Adults:

DVT prophylaxis in abdominal surgery, hip replacement, knee replacement, or in medical patients during acute illness: SubQ: 30 mg once daily

DVT treatment in conjunction with warfarin (in inpatients with or without pulmonary embolism and in outpatients without pulmonary embolism): SubQ: 1 mg/kg once daily

Prevention of ischemic complications of non-Q-wave MI or unstable angina (with aspirin): SubQ: 1 mg/kg once daily

Treatment of STEMI:

Adults <75 years: Initial: 30 mg single IV bolus **plus** 1 mg/kg SubQ (administered at the same time as the IV bolus); maintenance: SubQ: 1 mg/kg once daily

Adults ≥75 years: See package insert

Dosage adjustment in hepatic impairment: Dosage adjustment not established; use with caution in patients with hepatic impairment

Administration Parenteral: Do not administer IM For SubQ use, administer by deep SubQ injection; do not rub injection site after SubQ administration as bruising may occur. When administering 30 mg or 40 mg SubQ from a commercially prefilled syringe, do not expel the air bubble from the syringe prior to injection (in order to avoid loss of drug). IV administration is indicated as part of treatment of STEMI only; flush IV access with NS or D_5W before and after enoxaparin IV bolus administration (to clear drug from port)

Monitoring Parameters CBC with platelets, stool occult blood tests, serum creatinine and potassium; antifactor Xa activity in select patients (eg, neonates, infants, children, obese patients, and patients with significant renal impairment, active bleeding, or abnormal coagulation parameters); **Note**: Routine monitoring of PT and APTT is not warranted since PT and APTT are relatively insensitive measures of low molecular weight heparin activity; consider monitoring bone density in infants and children with long-term use

Reference Range Antifactor Xa: **Note:** The following are suggested peak values of antifactor Xa. Once daily dosing in pediatric patients is not feasible due to faster enoxaparin clearance and lower drug exposure in pediatric patients compared to adults (O'Brien, 2007).

Therapeutic:

Neonates and Children: 0.5-1.0 units/mL, measured 4-6 hours after SubQ administration **or** 0.5-0.8 units/mL, measured 2-6 hours after SubQ administration (Monagle, 2012)

Adults:

Once-daily dosing: >1 anti-Xa units/mL (Garcia, 2012); the manufacturer recommends a range of 1-2 anti-Xa units/mL

Twice-daily dosing: 0.6-1 anti-Xa units/mL (Garcia, 2012)

Prophylactic:

Children: Prevention of central venous access device related DVT: 0.1-0.3 units/mL (Monagle, 2012)

Adults: 0.2-0.4 units/mL (Nutescu, 2009)

Additional Information Each 10 mg of enoxaparin sodium equals ~1000 units of antifactor Xa activity.

Enoxaparin contains fragments of unfractionated heparin produced by alkaline degradation (depolymerization) of heparin benzyl ester; enoxaparin has mean molecular weights of 3500-5600 daltons, which are much lower than mean molecular weights of unfractionated heparin (12,000-15,000 daltons). Low molecular weight heparins (LMWH) have several advantages over unfractionated heparin: Better SubQ bioavailability, more convenient administration (SubQ versus IV), longer half-life (longer dosing interval), more predictable pharmacokinetics and pharmacodynamic (anticoagulant) effect, less intensive laboratory monitoring, reduced risk of heparin-induced thrombocytopenia, potential for outpatient use, and probable reduced risk of osteoporosis (further studies are needed).

Accidental overdosage of enoxaparin may be treated with protamine sulfate; 1 mg protamine sulfate neutralizes 1 mg enoxaparin; first dose of protamine sulfate should equal the dose of enoxaparin injected, if enoxaparin was given in the previous 8 hours; use 0.5 mg protamine sulfate per 1 mg enoxaparin if enoxaparin was given >8 hours prior to protamine or if a second dose of protamine is needed; a second dose of protamine sulfate (0.5 mg per 1 mg enoxaparin) may be given if APTT remains prolonged 2-4 hours after first dose; protamine may not be required ≥12 hours after enoxaparin administration; avoid overdosage with protamine

Some centers dispense pediatric doses in an insulin syringe for greater delivery accuracy and to avoid errors associated with dilutions. Each 1 unit on a 30, 50, or 100 unit graduated insulin syringe is 0.01 mL; using a **100 mg/mL** enoxaparin injection, each "1 unit" on the insulin syringe would provide 1 mg of enoxaparin (Bauman, 2009a).

Dosage Forms Excipient information presented when available (limited, particularly for generics); consult specific product labeling.

Solution, Injection, as sodium:

Lovenox: 300 mg/3 mL (3 mL) [contains benzyl alcohol, pork (porcine) protein]

Generic: 300 mg/3 mL (3 mL)

Solution, Subcutaneous, as sodium [preservative free]:

Lovenox: 30 mg/0.3 mL (0.3 mL); 40 mg/0.4 mL (0.4 mL); 60 mg/0.6 mL (0.6 mL); 80 mg/0.8 mL (0.8 mL); 100 mg/mL (1 mL); 120 mg/0.8 mL (0.8 mL); 150 mg/mL (1 mL) [contains pork (porcine) protein]

Generic: 30 mg/0.3 mL (0.3 mL); 40 mg/0.4 mL (0.4 mL); 60 mg/0.6 mL (0.6 mL); 80 mg/0.8 mL (0.8 mL); 100 mg/mL (1 mL); 120 mg/0.8 mL (0.8 mL); 150 mg/mL (1 mL)

◆ **Enoxaparin Sodium** *see* Enoxaparin *on page 752*

Entecavir (en TE ka veer)

Related Information

Safe Handling of Hazardous Drugs *on page 2455*

Brand Names: US Baraclude

Brand Names: Canada Apo-Entecavir; Baraclude; PMS-Entecavir

Therapeutic Category Antiviral Agent

Generic Availability (US) May be product dependent

Use Treatment of chronic hepatitis B infection with evidence of active viral replication and either evidence of persistent transaminase elevations or histologically active disease (FDA approved in ages ≥2 years weighing ≥10 kg and adults). **Note:** In children, indication is based on data in patients with compensated liver disease only; in adults, indication is based on data in patients with compensated and decompensated liver disease.

Pregnancy Risk Factor C

Pregnancy Considerations Teratogenic effects have been observed in animal studies. Information related to use in pregnancy is limited; use only if other options are inappropriate (DHHS [OI], 2013). Pregnant women taking entecavir should enroll in the pregnancy registry by calling 1-800-258-4263.

Breast-Feeding Considerations It is not known if entecavir is excreted in breast milk. Due to the potential for serious adverse reactions in the nursing infant, the manufacturer recommends a decision be made whether to discontinue nursing or to discontinue the drug, taking into account the importance of treatment to the mother.

Contraindications There are no contraindications listed in the manufacturer's U.S. labeling.

Canadian labeling: Hypersensitivity to entecavir or any component of the formulation

Warnings/Precautions Hazardous agent - use appropriate precautions for handling and disposal (NIOSH 2014 [group 2]).

[U.S. Boxed Warning]: Lactic acidosis and severe hepatomegaly with steatosis (including fatal cases) have been reported with nucleoside analogue inhibitors; use with caution in patients with risk factors for liver disease (risk may be increased with female gender, decompensated liver disease, obesity, or prolonged nucleoside inhibitor exposure) and suspend treatment in any patient who develops clinical or laboratory findings suggestive of lactic acidosis or hepatotoxicity (transaminase elevation may/may not accompany hepatomegaly and steatosis)

[U.S. Boxed Warning]: Severe, acute exacerbation of hepatitis B may occur upon discontinuation of antihepatitis B therapy, including entecavir. Monitor liver function for at least several months after stopping treatment; reinitiation of antihepatitis B therapy may be required. Use caution in patients with renal impairment or in patients receiving concomitant therapy which may reduce renal function; dose adjustment recommended for CrCl <50 mL/minute. Cross-resistance may develop in patients failing previous therapy with lamivudine. There are limited data available on the use of entecavir in lamivudine-experienced pediatric patients; use in these patients only if the potential benefit justifies the potential risk to the child.

HIV: **[U.S. Boxed Warning]: May cause the development of HIV resistance in chronic hepatitis B patients with unrecognized or untreated HIV infection.** Determine HIV status prior to initiating treatment with entecavir. **Not recommended for HIV/HBV coinfected patients unless also receiving highly active antiretroviral therapy (HAART).** The manufacturer's labeling states that entecavir does not exhibit any clinically-relevant activity against human immunodeficiency virus (HIV type 1). However, a small number of case reports have indicated declines in virus levels during entecavir therapy. HIV resistance to a common HIV drug has been reported in an HIV/HBV-infected patient receiving entecavir as monotherapy for HBV.

Dose adjustment not required in patients with hepatic impairment. Limited data supporting treatment of chronic hepatitis B in patients with decompensated liver disease; observe for increased adverse reactions, including hepatorenal dysfunction.

Some dosage forms may contain polysorbate 80 (also known as Tweens). Hypersensitivity reactions, usually a delayed reaction, have been reported following exposure to pharmaceutical products containing polysorbate 80 in certain individuals (Isaksson, 2002; Lucente 2000; Shelley, 1995). Thrombocytopenia, ascites, pulmonary deterioration, and renal and hepatic failure have been reported in premature neonates after receiving parenteral products containing polysorbate 80 (Alade, 1986; CDC, 1984). See manufacturer's labeling.

Adverse Reactions Adverse reactions are generally similar in adult and pediatric patients.

Cardiovascular: Peripheral edema (with decompensated liver disease)

Central nervous system: Dizziness, fatigue, headache

Dermatologic: Skin rash

Endocrine & metabolic: Decreased serum bicarbonate (with decompensated liver disease), glycosuria, hyperglycemia

Gastrointestinal: Abdominal pain, diarrhea, dyspepsia, increased serum amylase, increased serum lipase, nausea, unpleasant taste, vomiting

Genitourinary: Hematuria

Hepatic: Ascites (with decompensated liver disease), increased serum ALT, increased serum bilirubin, hepatic encephalopathy

Hematologic & oncologic: Hepatic carcinoma (with decompensated liver disease)

Renal: Increased serum creatinine

Respiratory: Upper respiratory tract infection (with decompensated liver disease)

Miscellaneous: Fever (with decompensated liver disease)

Rare but important or life-threatening: Alopecia, anaphylactoid reaction, hepatomegaly, insomnia, lactic acidosis, macular edema (Muqit, 2011), renal failure, thrombocytopenia

Drug Interactions

Metabolism/Transport Effects None known.

Avoid Concomitant Use There are no known interactions where it is recommended to avoid concomitant use.

Increased Effect/Toxicity

The levels/effects of Entecavir may be increased by: Ganciclovir-Valganciclovir; Ribavirin

Decreased Effect There are no known significant interactions involving a decrease in effect.

Food Interactions Food delays absorption and reduces AUC by 18% to 20%. Management: Administer on an empty stomach 2 hours before or after a meal.

Storage/Stability Store at 25°C (77°F); excursions permitted to 15°C to 30°C (59°F to 86°F). Protect from light. After opening, oral solution can be used up to expiration date on the bottle.

Mechanism of Action Entecavir is intracellularly phosphorylated to guanosine triphosphate which competes with natural substrates to effectively inhibit hepatitis B viral polymerase; enzyme inhibition blocks reverse transcriptase activity thereby reducing viral DNA synthesis.

Pharmacokinetics (Adult data unless noted) Note: The pharmacokinetics of pediatric patients ≥2 years are similar to adult values.

Distribution: Extensive to tissues (V_d in excess of total body water)

Protein binding: ~13%

Metabolism: Minor hepatic glucuronide/sulfate conjugation

Bioavailability: Tablet and oral solution are bioequivalent.

Half-life elimination: Terminal: 5 to 6 days; accumulation: 24 hours

Time to peak serum concentration: 0.5 to 1.5 hours

Elimination: Urine (62% to 73% as unchanged drug); undergoes glomerular filtration and tubular secretion

Dosing: Usual Note: Oral tablets and solution may be used interchangeably on a mg:mg basis.

Pediatric:

Hepatitis B infection (HBV), chronic: Oral: **Note:** Optimal duration of treatment not established for nucleoside analogs, a minimum of 12 months and typically longer required; consolidation therapy of at least 6 months after seroconversion and complete viral suppression has been suggested (Jonas 2010).

Children and Adolescents 2 to <16 years with compensated liver diseases:

Treatment naive:

- 10 to 11 kg: 0.15 mg oral solution once daily
- >11 to 14 kg: 0.2 mg oral solution once daily
- >14 to 17 kg: 0.25 mg oral solution once daily
- >17 to 20 kg: 0.3 mg oral solution once daily
- >20 to 23 kg: 0.35 mg oral solution once daily
- >23 to 26 kg: 0.4 mg oral solution once daily
- >26 to 30 kg: 0.45 mg oral solution once daily
- >30 kg: 0.5 mg oral solution or tablet once daily

Lamivudine-experienced:

- 10 to 11 kg: 0.3 mg oral solution once daily
- >11 to 14 kg: 0.4 mg oral solution once daily
- >14 to 17 kg: 0.5 mg oral solution once daily
- >17 to 20 kg: 0.6 mg oral solution once daily
- >20 to 23 kg: 0.7 mg oral solution once daily
- >23 to 26 kg: 0.8 mg oral solution once daily
- >26 to 30 kg: 0.9 mg oral solution once daily
- >30 kg: 1 mg oral solution or tablet once daily

Adolescents ≥16 years:

Nucleoside treatment naïve with compensated liver disease: 0.5 mg once daily

Lamivudine-refractory or known lamivudine or telbivudine-resistant mutations: 1 mg once daily

HIV/Hepatitis B virus coinfection: Limited data available: **Note:** Only recommended in patients who cannot take tenofovir; must be used in addition to a fully suppressive antiretroviral therapy regimen (DHHS [adult/pediatric] 2013): Oral:

Nucleoside treatment naive: Adolescents: 0.5 mg once daily (DHHS [adult] 2013)

Lamivudine-refractory or -resistant with decompensated liver disease:

Children 12 years of age: 0.5 mg once daily (DHHS [pediatric] 2013)

Adolescents: 1 mg once daily (DHHS [adult] 2013)

HBV reinfection prophylaxis, postliver transplant (with or without HBIG): Limited data available: Adolescents ≥16 years: Oral: 1 mg once daily has been reported in an open-label trial of 65 patients (age range: 16 years and older); however, a lower dose of 0.5 mg once daily has also been used in adult patients (age range: 23 to 65 years) (Fung 2011; Perrillo 2012).

Adult: **Hepatitis B virus (HBV) infection, treatment:** Oral:

Nucleoside treatment naive: 0.5 mg once daily

Lamivudine-refractory or -resistant viremia (or known lamivudine- or telbivudine-resistant mutations): 1 mg once daily

Decompensated liver disease: 1 mg once daily

Treatment duration (AASLD Practice Guidelines [Lok], 2009):

Hepatitis Be antigen (HBeAg) positive chronic hepatitis: Treat ≥1 year until HBeAg seroconversion and undetectable serum HBV DNA; continue therapy for ≥6 months after HBeAg seroconversion

HBeAg negative chronic hepatitis: Treat >1 year until hepatitis B surface antigen (HBsAg) clearance

Decompensated liver disease: Lifelong treatment is recommended.

Note: Patients not achieving a primary response (<2 log decrease in serum HBV DNA) after at least 6 months of therapy should either receive additional treatment or be switched to an alternative therapy.

Dosing adjustment in renal impairment:

Children and Adolescents: There are no dosage adjustments provided in the manufacturer's labeling; insufficient data to recommend a specific dose adjustment in pediatric patients with renal impairment; a reduction in the dose or an increase in the dosing interval similar to adjustments for adults should be considered.

Adults: Daily dosage regimen preferred:

CrCl ≥50 mL/minute: No adjustment necessary

CrCl 30 to 49 mL/minute: Administer 50% of usual dose once daily or administer the normal dose every 48 hours

CrCl 10 to 29 mL/minute: Administer 30% of usual dose once daily or administer the normal dose every 72 hours

CrCl <10 mL/minute: Administer 10% of usual dose once daily or administer the normal dose every 7 days

Hemodialysis and peritoneal dialysis (CAPD): Minimally removed by hemodialysis (13% over 4 hours) and CAPD (0.3% over 7 days): Administer 10% of usual dose once daily or administer the normal dose every 7 days; administer after hemodialysis

Dosing adjustment in hepatic impairment: Children ≥ 2 years, Adolescents, and Adults: No adjustment necessary.

Administration Hazardous agent; use appropriate precautions for handling and disposal (NIOSH 2014 [group 2]).

Oral: Administer on an empty stomach (2 hours before or after a meal).

Oral solution: Do not dilute or mix oral solution with water or other beverages; use calibrated oral dosing syringe.

Monitoring Parameters HIV status (prior to initiation of therapy); liver function tests, renal function; in HBV/HIV-coinfected patients, monitor HIV viral load and CD4 count; HBeAg, HBV DNA; in patients with lamivudine-refractory or -resistant viremia (or known lamivudine- or telbivudine-resistance mutations) entecavir resistance can develop rapidly. Monitor HBV DNA every 3 months (DHHS [adults], 2013).

Dosage Forms Excipient information presented when available (limited, particularly for generics); consult specific product labeling.

Solution, Oral:

Baraclude: 0.05 mg/mL (210 mL) [contains methylparaben, propylparaben; orange flavor]

Tablet, Oral:

Baraclude: 0.5 mg, 1 mg

Generic: 0.5 mg, 1 mg

◆ **Entocort (Can)** *see* Budesonide (Systemic, Oral Inhalation) *on page 307*

◆ **Entocort EC** *see* Budesonide (Systemic, Oral Inhalation) *on page 307*

◆ **Entre-Hist PSE** *see* Triprolidine and Pseudoephedrine *on page 2129*

◆ **Entrophen (Can)** *see* Aspirin *on page 206*

◆ **Entsol [OTC]** *see* Sodium Chloride *on page 1938*

◆ **Entsol Nasal [OTC]** *see* Sodium Chloride *on page 1938*

◆ **Entsol Nasal Wash [OTC]** *see* Sodium Chloride *on page 1938*

◆ **Enulose** *see* Lactulose *on page 1204*

◆ **Envarsus XR** *see* Tacrolimus (Systemic) *on page 1999*

◆ **Epaned** *see* Enalapril *on page 744*

◆ **EPEG** *see* Etoposide *on page 819*

EPHEDrine (Systemic) (e FED rin)

Medication Safety Issues

Sound-alike/look-alike issues:

EPHEDrine may be confused with Epifrin, EPINEPHrine

High alert medication:

The Institute for Safe Medication Practices (ISMP) includes this medication among its list of drugs which have a heightened risk of causing significant patient harm when used in error.

Therapeutic Category Adrenergic Agonist Agent; Sympathomimetic

Generic Availability (US) Yes

Use

Oral: Temporary relief of bronchial asthma symptoms (shortness of breath, tightness of chest, and wheezing) (OTC labeling: FDA approved in ages ≥12 years and adults); **Note:** Not recommended for routine management and treatment of asthma (NAEPP, 2007); has also been used for nasal decongestion and congenital myasthenic syndromes

Parenteral: Treatment of anesthesia-induced hypotension; treatment of hypotension following induced sympathectomy or following overdosage of antihypertensive drugs [FDA approved in pediatric patients (age not specified) and adults]; has also been used for idiopathic orthostatic hypotension and bronchodilation; **Note:** Not recommended for routine management and treatment of asthma (NAEPP, 2007) nor septic shock (Brierley, 2009).

Pregnancy Risk Factor C

Pregnancy Considerations Animal reproduction studies have not been conducted. Ephedrine crosses the placenta (Hughes, 1985). Ephedrine injection is used at delivery for the prevention and/or treatment of maternal hypotension associated with spinal anesthesia in women undergoing cesarean section (ASA, 2007).

Contraindications Hypersensitivity to ephedrine or any component of the formulation; angle-closure glaucoma; concurrent use of other sympathomimetic agents

Warnings/Precautions Blood volume depletion should be corrected before injectable ephedrine therapy is instituted; use caution in patients with unstable vasomotor symptoms, diabetes, hyperthyroidism, prostatic hyperplasia or a history of seizures; also use caution in the elderly and those patients with cardiovascular disorders such as coronary artery disease, arrhythmias, and hypertension. Ephedrine may cause hypertension. Long-term use may cause anxiety and symptoms of paranoid schizophrenia. Use with caution in the elderly, since it crosses the blood-brain barrier and may cause confusion. Use with extreme caution in patients taking MAO inhibitors.

Warnings: Additional Pediatric Considerations Safety and efficacy for the use of cough and cold products in children <2 years of age is limited. Serious adverse effects including death have been reported. The FDA notes that there are no approved OTC uses for these products in children <2 years of age. Health care providers are reminded to ask caregivers about the use of OTC cough and cold products in order to avoid exposure to multiple medications containing the same ingredient.

Adverse Reactions

Cardiovascular: Angina pectoris, cardiac arrhythmia, hypertension, palpitations, tachycardia

Central nervous system: Anxiety, confusion, delirium, dizziness, hallucination, headache, insomnia, intracranial hemorrhage, nervousness, precordial pain, restlessness, tension, vertigo

Dermatologic: Diaphoresis, pallor

Gastrointestinal: Anorexia, nausea, vomiting

Genitourinary: Dysuria, urinary retention (males with prostatism)

Neuromuscular & skeletal: Tremor, vesicle sphincter spasm, weakness
Respiratory: Dyspnea

Drug Interactions

Metabolism/Transport Effects None known.

Avoid Concomitant Use

Avoid concomitant use of EPHEDrine (Systemic) with any of the following: Ergot Derivatives; Inhalational Anesthetics; Iobenguane I 123; MAO Inhibitors

Increased Effect/Toxicity

EPHEDrine (Systemic) may increase the levels/effects of: Droxidopa; Inhalational Anesthetics; Sympathomimetics

The levels/effects of EPHEDrine (Systemic) may be increased by: Alkalinizing Agents; AtoMOXetine; Cannabinoid-Containing Products; Carbonic Anhydrase Inhibitors; Ergot Derivatives; Hyaluronidase; Linezolid; MAO Inhibitors; Serotonin/Norepinephrine Reuptake Inhibitors; Tedizolid

Decreased Effect

EPHEDrine (Systemic) may decrease the levels/effects of: Benzylpenicilloyl Polylysine; FentaNYL; Iobenguane I 123

The levels/effects of EPHEDrine (Systemic) may be decreased by: Alpha1-Blockers; Spironolactone; Urinary Acidifying Agents

Storage/Stability Protect all dosage forms from light.
Injection solution: Store at room temperature. **Note:** Storage guidelines vary; check product labeling for exact temperature range.

Mechanism of Action Releases tissue stores of norepinephrine and thereby produces an alpha- and beta-adrenergic stimulation; longer-acting and less potent than epinephrine

Pharmacodynamics Pressor/cardiac effects: Duration:
Oral: 4 hours
SubQ: 1 hour

Pharmacokinetics (Adult data unless noted)
Absorption: Oral: Complete
Metabolism: Minimally hepatic by oxidative deamination, demethylation, aromatic hydroxylation, and conjugation
Bioavailability: Oral: 85%
Half-life: 3-6 hours
Elimination: Dependent upon urinary pH with greatest excretion in acid pH; urine pH 5: 74% to 99% excreted unchanged; urine pH 8: 22% to 25% excreted unchanged

Dosing: Neonatal Myasthenic syndromes, congenital: Limited data available: Oral: Initial: 1 mg/kg/**day** in 3 divided doses, may increase to 3 mg/kg/**day** in 3 divided doses (Kliegman, 2011)

Dosing: Usual
Pediatric:
Asthma, bronchodilation: Children ≥12 years and Adolescents: Oral: 12.5-25 mg every 4 hours; if symptoms do not improve after 1 hour from initial dose, physician should be contacted and continuation of therapy evaluated; maximum daily dose: 150 mg/**day**; **Note:** Not recommended for routine management and treatment of asthma and **NOT** indicated for the relief of acute bronchospasm (NAEPP, 2007)
Hypotension, anesthesia-induced: Use the smallest effective dose for the shortest time; **Note:** Not recommended for use in management of septic shock (Brierley, 2009):
Infants, Children, and Adolescents ≤15 years: Limited data available: Slow IV push: 0.1-0.3 mg/kg/dose every 4-6 hours; maximum dose: 25 mg (Taguchi, 1996)
Adolescents >15 years: IV: 5-25 mg/dose slow IV push repeated after 5-10 minutes as needed, then every 3-4 hours; maximum dose: 150 mg/24 hours
Myasthenic syndromes, congenital: Infants, Children, and Adolescents: Limited data available: Oral: Initial: 1 mg/kg/**day** in 3 divided doses, may increase to 3 mg/kg/**day** in 3 divided doses (Engel, 2007; Kliegman, 2011)
Adult:
Hypotension, anesthesia-induced: IV: 5-25 mg/dose slow IV push repeated after 5-10 minutes as needed, then every 3-4 hours (maximum: 150 mg/24 hours)
Idiopathic orthostatic hypotension: Oral: 25-50 mg 3 times/**day**; maximum daily dose: 150 mg/**day**; **Note:** Not considered first-line for this indication.

Preparation for Administration Parenteral: IV: Dilution to a concentration of 5 or 10 mg/mL has been used for doses of 5 to 25 mg; in a pediatric hypotension trial, ephedrine doses of 0.1 mg/kg and 0.2 mg/kg were diluted to 1 mg/mL and 2 mg/mL, respectively (Taguchi 1996)

Administration
Oral: May be administered without regard to food
Parenteral: IV: Administer by slow IV push

Monitoring Parameters Blood pressure, pulse, respiratory symptoms

Test Interactions Can cause a false-positive amphetamine EMIT assay

Additional Information Because ephedrine and pseudoephedrine have been used to synthesize methamphetamine, the DEA has placed them in the category of "Schedule Listed Products"; restrictions are in place to reduce the potential for misuse (diversion) and abuse (eg, storage requirements, additional documentation of sale); the DEA limit for a single transaction to a single individual for drug products containing ephedrine or pseudoephedrine is 3.6 g/24 hours, 9 g/30 days, or if mail-order transaction 7.5 g/30 days.

Dosage Forms Excipient information presented when available (limited, particularly for generics); consult specific product labeling. [DSC] = Discontinued product
Capsule, Oral, as sulfate:
Generic: 25 mg [DSC]
Solution, Injection, as sulfate:
Generic: 50 mg/mL (1 mL)
Solution, Injection, as sulfate [preservative free]:
Generic: 50 mg/mL (1 mL)

◆ **Ephedrine Sulfate** *see* EPHEDrine (Systemic) *on page 758*

◆ **E-Pherol [OTC]** *see* Vitamin E *on page 2188*

◆ **Epi-Clenz [OTC]** *see* Alcohol (Ethyl) *on page 86*

◆ **Epiduo®** *see* Adapalene and Benzoyl Peroxide *on page 71*

Epinastine (ep i NAS teen)

Brand Names: US Elestat

Therapeutic Category Antiallergic, Ophthalmic

Generic Availability (US) Yes

Use Prevention of itching associated with allergic conjunctivitis (FDA approved in ages ≥2 years and adults)

Pregnancy Risk Factor C

Pregnancy Considerations Teratogenic effects were not observed in animal studies. There are no adequate and well-controlled studies in pregnant women.

Breast-Feeding Considerations It is not known if epinastine is excreted in breast milk. The manufacturer recommends that caution be exercised when administering epinastine to nursing women.

Contraindications There are no contraindications listed in the manufacturer's labeling.

Warnings/Precautions Contains benzalkonium chloride; contact lenses should be removed prior to use, wait 10 minutes before reinserting. Not for the treatment of contact lens irritation; do not wear contact lenses if eye is red. Inadvertent contamination of multiple-dose ophthalmic solutions has caused bacterial keratitis.

Adverse Reactions

Central nervous system: Headache

Ocular: Burning sensation, folliculosis, hyperemia, pruritus

Respiratory: Cough, pharyngitis, rhinitis, sinusitis

Miscellaneous: Infection (defined as cold symptoms and upper respiratory infection)

Rare but important or life-threatening: Lacrimation increased

Drug Interactions

Metabolism/Transport Effects None known.

Avoid Concomitant Use There are no known interactions where it is recommended to avoid concomitant use.

Increased Effect/Toxicity There are no known significant interactions involving an increase in effect.

Decreased Effect There are no known significant interactions involving a decrease in effect.

Storage/Stability Store at controlled room temperature of 15°C to 25°C (59°F to 77°F). Keep tightly closed.

Mechanism of Action Selective H_1-receptor antagonist; inhibits release of histamine from the mast cell; also has affinity for the H_2, $alpha_1$, $alpha_2$, and the 5-HT_2 receptors

Pharmacodynamics

Onset of action: 3-5 minutes

Duration: 8 hours

Pharmacokinetics (Adult data unless noted)

Absorption: Low systemic absorption following topical application

Distribution: Does not cross blood-brain barrier

Protein binding: 64%

Metabolism: <10% metabolized

Half-life: 12 hours

Elimination: IV: Urine (55%); feces (30%)

Dosing: Usual Children ≥2 years, Adolescents, and Adults: **Allergic Conjunctivitis:** Ophthalmic: Instill 1 drop into each eye twice daily; continue throughout period of exposure, even in the absence of symptoms

Dosing adjustment in renal impairment: There are no dosage adjustments provided in the manufacturer's labeling; however, dosage adjustment unlikely necessary due to low systemic absorption.

Dosing adjustment in hepatic impairment: There are no dosage adjustments provided in the manufacturer's labeling; however, dosage adjustment unlikely necessary due to low systemic absorption.

Administration For ophthalmic use only; avoid touching tip of applicator to eye or other surfaces. Contact lenses should be removed prior to application; may be reinserted after 10 minutes. Do not wear contact lenses if eyes are red.

Dosage Forms Excipient information presented when available (limited, particularly for generics); consult specific product labeling.

Solution, Ophthalmic, as hydrochloride:

Elestat: 0.05% (5 mL) [contains benzalkonium chloride]

Generic: 0.05% (5 mL)

◆ **Epinastine Hydrochloride** *see* Epinastine *on page 759*

EPINEPHrine (Systemic, Oral Inhalation)

(ep i NEF rin)

Medication Safety Issues

Sound-alike/look-alike issues:

EPINEPHrine may be confused with ePHEDrine

Epifrin may be confused with ephedrine, EpiPen

High alert medication:

The Institute for Safe Medication Practices (ISMP) includes this medication among its list of drugs which have a heightened risk of causing significant patient harm when used in error.

Administration issues:

Medication errors have occurred due to confusion with epinephrine products expressed as ratio strengths (eg, 1:1000 vs 1:10,000).

Epinephrine 1:1000 = 1 mg/mL and is most commonly used IM

Epinephrine 1:10,000 = 0.1 mg/mL and is used IV

Medication errors have occurred when topical epinephrine 1 mg/mL (1:1000) has been inadvertently injected. Vials of injectable and topical epinephrine look very similar. Epinephrine should always be appropriately labeled with the intended administration.

International issues:

EpiPen [U.S., Canada, and multiple international markets] may be confused with Epigen brand name for glycyrrhizinic acid [Argentina, Mexico, Russia] and Epopen brand name for epoetin alfa [Spain] and Epigent brand name for gentamicin [multiple international markets]

Related Information

Adult ACLS Algorithms *on page 2236*

Emergency Drip Calculations *on page 2229*

Management of Drug Extravasations *on page 2298*

Newborn Resuscitation Algorithm *on page 2231*

Pediatric ALS (PALS) Algorithms *on page 2233*

Safe Handling of Hazardous Drugs *on page 2455*

Serotonin Syndrome *on page 2447*

Brand Names: US Adrenaclick; Adrenalin; Asthmanefrin Refill [OTC]; Asthmanefrin Starter Kit [OTC]; Auvi-Q; EpiPen 2-Pak; EpiPen Jr 2-Pak; Micronefrin [OTC] [DSC]; S2 [OTC]

Brand Names: Canada Adrenalin; Allerject; Anapen; Anapen Junior; EpiPen; EpiPen Jr; S2; Twinject

Therapeutic Category Adrenergic Agonist Agent; Antiasthmatic; Antidote, Hypersensitivity Reactions; Bronchodilator; Sympathomimetic

Generic Availability (US) May be product dependent

Use

Parenteral:

Injection: Treatment of bronchospasms, bronchial asthma, anaphylactic reactions, cardiac arrest, and attacks of transitory atrioventricular (AV) heart block with syncopal seizures (Stokes-Adams Syndrome); added to local anesthetics to decrease systemic absorption of intraspinal and local anesthetics and increase duration of action; induction and maintenance of mydriasis during intraocular surgery [FDA approved in pediatric patients (age not specified) and adults]

Autoinjectors (eg, Auvi-Q™, EpiPen®): Emergency treatment (immediate administration) of severe allergic reactions including anaphylaxis in patient at increased risk or previous history of anaphylactic reactions (FDA approved in patients weighing ≥15 kg)

Oral inhalation (nebulization): Racemic epinephrine: Treatment of bronchial asthma (OTC labeling: FDA approved in ages ≥4 years and adults); has also been used to treat upper airway obstruction and croup

Pregnancy Risk Factor C

Pregnancy Considerations Teratogenic effects have been observed in animal reproduction studies. Epinephrine crosses the placenta and may cause fetal anoxia. Use during pregnancy when the potential benefit to the mother outweighs the possible risk to the fetus.

Breast-Feeding Considerations It is not known if epinephrine is excreted in breast milk. The manufacturer recommends that caution be exercised when administering epinephrine to nursing women.

Contraindications

There are no absolute contraindications to the use of injectable epinephrine (including Adrenaclick, Auvi-Q,

EpiPen, EpiPen Jr, Allerject [Canadian product], and Twinject [Canadian product]) in a life-threatening situation. Some products include the following contraindications: Hypersensitivity to sympathomimetic amines; general anesthesia with halogenated hydrocarbons (eg, halothane) or cyclopropane; narrow angle glaucoma; nonanaphylactic shock; in combination with local anesthesia of certain areas such as fingers, toes, and ears; use in situations where vasopressors may be contraindicated (eg, thyrotoxicosis, diabetes, in obstetrics when maternal blood pressure is in excess of 130/80 mm Hg and in hypertension and other cardiovascular disorders)

Injectable solution (Adrenalin, Epinephrine injection, USP): There are no contraindications listed in the manufacturer's labeling.

Oral inhalation (OTC labeling): Concurrent use or within 2 weeks of MAO inhibitors

Warnings/Precautions Use with caution in elderly patients, patients with diabetes mellitus, cardiovascular diseases (eg, coronary artery disease, hypertension), thyroid disease, cerebrovascular disease, in patients with prostate enlargement or urinary retention, or Parkinson's disease. May induce cardiac arrhythmias; use with caution especially in patients with cardiac disease or those receiving drugs that sensitize the myocardium. Due to peripheral constriction and cardiac stimulation, pulmonary edema may occur. Due to renal blood vessel constriction, decreased urine output may occur. In hypovolemic patients, correct blood volume depletion before administering any vasopressor. Some products contain sulfites as preservatives; the presence of sulfites in some products should not deter administration during a serious allergic or other emergency situation even if the patient is sulfite-sensitive. Potentially significant drug-drug interactions may exist, requiring dose or frequency adjustment, additional monitoring, and/or selection of alternative therapy.

IV administration: Rapid IV administration may cause death from cerebrovascular hemorrhage or cardiac arrhythmias. However, rapid IV administration during pulseless arrest is necessary. Vesicant; ensure proper needle or catheter placement prior to and during infusion; avoid extravasation. Accidental injection into digits, hands, or feet may result in local reactions, including injection site pallor, coldness and hypoesthesia or injury, resulting in bruising, bleeding, discoloration, erythema, or skeletal injury; patient should seek immediate medical attention if this occurs. Rapid IV administration may cause death from cerebrovascular hemorrhage or cardiac arrhythmias; however, rapid IV administration during pulseless arrest is necessary. Prior to intraocular use, must dilute 1:**1000** (1 mg/mL) solution to a concentration of 1:**100,000** to 1:**1,000,000** (10 **mcg**/mL to 1 **mcg**/mL) prior to intraocular use. When used undiluted, has been associated with corneal endothelial damage.

Self medication (OTC use): Oral inhalation: Prior to self-medication, patients should contact healthcare provider. The product should only be used in persons with a diagnosis of asthma. If symptoms are not relieved in 20 minutes or become worse do not continue to use the product - seek immediate medical assistance. The product should not be used more frequently or at higher doses than recommended unless directed by a healthcare provider. This product should not be used in patients who have required hospitalization for asthma or if a patient is taking prescription medication for asthma. Use with caution in patients with prostate enlargement or urinary retention. Do not use if you have taken a MAO inhibitor (certain drugs used for depression, Parkinson's disease, or other conditions) within 2 weeks.

Adverse Reactions

Cardiovascular: Angina, cardiac arrhythmia, chest pain, flushing, hypertension, pallor, palpitation, sudden death, tachycardia (parenteral), vasoconstriction, ventricular ectopy, ventricular fibrillation

Central nervous system: Anxiety (transient), apprehensiveness, cerebral hemorrhage, dizziness, headache, insomnia, lightheadedness, nervousness, restlessness

Gastrointestinal: Dry throat, loss of appetite, nausea, vomiting, xerostomia

Genitourinary: Acute urinary retention in patients with bladder outflow obstruction

Neuromuscular & skeletal: Tremor, weakness

Ocular: Allergic lid reaction, burning, corneal endothelial damage (intraocular use), eye pain, ocular irritation, precipitation of or exacerbation of narrow-angle glaucoma, transient stinging

Respiratory: Dyspnea, pulmonary edema

Miscellaneous: Diaphoresis

Drug Interactions

Metabolism/Transport Effects Substrate of COMT

Avoid Concomitant Use

Avoid concomitant use of EPINEPHrine (Systemic, Oral Inhalation) with any of the following: Ergot Derivatives; Iobenguane I 123; Lurasidone

Increased Effect/Toxicity

EPINEPHrine (Systemic, Oral Inhalation) may increase the levels/effects of: Lurasidone; Sympathomimetics

The levels/effects of EPINEPHrine (Systemic, Oral Inhalation) may be increased by: AtoMOXetine; Beta-Blockers; Cannabinoid-Containing Products; COMT Inhibitors; Ergot Derivatives; Hyaluronidase; Inhalational Anesthetics; Linezolid; MAO Inhibitors; Serotonin/Norepinephrine Reuptake Inhibitors; Tedizolid; Tricyclic Antidepressants

Decreased Effect

EPINEPHrine (Systemic, Oral Inhalation) may decrease the levels/effects of: Antidiabetic Agents; Benzylpenicilloyl Polylysine; Iobenguane I 123

The levels/effects of EPINEPHrine (Systemic, Oral Inhalation) may be decreased by: Alpha1-Blockers; Promethazine; Spironolactone

Storage/Stability Epinephrine is sensitive to light and air. Protection from light is recommended. Oxidation turns drug pink, then a brown color. **Solutions should not be used if they are discolored or contain a precipitate.**

Adrenaclick: Store between 20°C to 25°C (68°F to 77°F); excursions permitted to 15°C to 30°C (59°F to 86°F); do not freeze or refrigerate. Protect from light.

Adrenalin: Store between 20°C to 25°C (68°F to 77°F); do not freeze. Protect from light.

Allerject [Canadian product]: Store between 15°C to 30°C (59°F to 86°F); do not refrigerate. Protect from light.

Asthmanefrin: Store between 20°C to 25°C (68°F to 77°F); protect from light and excessive heat.

Auvi-Q: Store between 20°C to 25°C (68°F to 77°F); excursions permitted to 15°C to 30°C (59°F to 86°F); do not refrigerate. Protect from light by storing in outer case provided.

Epinephrine injection, USP: Store between 20°C to 25°C (68°F to 77°F); do not refrigerate; protect from freezing. Protect from light until ready for use.

EpiPen and EpiPen Jr: Store at 25°C (77°F); excursions permitted to 15°C to 30°C (59°F to 86°F); do not freeze or refrigerate. Protect from light by storing in carrier tube provided.

Twinject [Canadian product]: Store between 20°C to 25°C (68°F to 77°F); excursions permitted to 15°C to 30°C (59°F to 86°F); do not freeze or refrigerate. Protect from light.

S2, Asthmanefrin: Store between 2°C to 20°C (36°F to 68°F). Protect from light.

Stability of injection of parenteral admixture at room temperature (25°C) or refrigeration (4°C) is 24 hours.

Mechanism of Action Stimulates alpha-, beta$_1$-, and beta$_2$-adrenergic receptors resulting in relaxation of smooth muscle of the bronchial tree, cardiac stimulation (increasing myocardial oxygen consumption), and dilation of skeletal muscle vasculature; small doses can cause vasodilation via beta$_2$-vascular receptors; large doses may produce constriction of skeletal and vascular smooth muscle

Pharmacodynamics

Local vasoconstriction:

Onset of action: 5 minutes

Duration: <1 hour

Onset of bronchodilation:

Inhalation: Within 1 minute

SubQ: Within 5-10 minutes

Pharmacokinetics (Adult data unless noted)

Absorption: Orally ingested doses are rapidly metabolized in GI tract and liver; pharmacologically active concentrations are not achieved

Distribution: Does not cross blood-brain barrier

Metabolism: Taken up into the adrenergic neuron and metabolized by monoamine oxidase and catechol-o-methyltransferase; circulating drug hepatically metabolized

Excretion: Urine (as inactive metabolites, metanephrine, and sulfate and hydroxy derivatives of mandelic acid; small amounts as unchanged drug)

Dosing: Neonatal Cardiopulmonary resuscitation (Kattwinkel, 2010):

IV: 0.01-0.03 mg/kg (0.1-0.3 mL/kg of **1:10,000** solution) every 3-5 minutes as needed

Endotracheal: **Note:** IV route preferred: E.T.: 0.05-0.1 mg/kg (0.5-1 mL/kg of **1:10,000** solution) every 3-5 minutes until IV access established or return of spontaneous circulation

Dosing: Usual

Infants, Children, and Adolescents:

Asthma, bronchodilation:

Nebulization: Racemic epinephrine (2.25% solution): Children ≥4 years and Adolescents: Manufacturer labeling: 0.5 mL diluted with 3-5 mL of NS; administer with jet nebulizer over ~15 minutes every 3-4 hours as needed. **Note:** Not recommended for routine management and treatment of asthma (NAEPP, 2007).

Asystole or pulseless arrest (AHA, 2010):

IV, I.O.: 0.01 mg/kg (0.1 mL/kg of **1:10,000** solution) (maximum single dose: 1 mg); every 3-5 minutes until return of spontaneous circulation

Endotracheal: 0.1 mg/kg (0.1 mL/kg of **1:1000** solution) (maximum single dose: 2.5 mg) every 3-5 minutes until return of spontaneous circulation or IV/I.O. access established. **Note:** Recent clinical studies suggest that lower epinephrine concentrations delivered by endotracheal administration may produce transient β-adrenergic effects which may be detrimental (eg, hypotension, lower coronary artery perfusion pressure). IV or I.O. are the preferred methods of administration.

Bradycardia (AHA, 2010):

IV, I.O.: 0.01 mg/kg (0.1 mL/kg of **1:10,000** solution) (maximum dose: 1 mg or 10 mL); may repeat every 3-5 minutes as needed

Endotracheal: 0.1 mg/kg (0.1 mL/kg of **1:1000** solution) (maximum single dose: 2.5 mg); doses as high as 0.2 mg/kg may be effective; may repeat every 3-5 minutes as needed until IV/I.O. access established

Continuous infusion: IV, I.O.: 0.1-1 **mcg**/kg/**minute**; titrate dosage to desired effect

Croup (laryngotracheobronchitis), airway edema:

Nebulization: Infants, Children, and Adolescents: **Note:** Typically relief of symptoms occurs within 10-30 minutes and lasts 2-3 hours; patients should be observed for rapid symptom recurrence and possible repeat treatment.

Racemic epinephrine (2.25% solution): 0.05-0.1 mL/kg (maximum dose: 0.5 mL) diluted in 2 mL NS, may repeat dose every 20 minutes; others have reported use of 0.5 mL as a fixed dose for all patients; use lower end of dosing range for younger infants (Hegenbarth, 2008; Rosekrans, 1998; Rotta, 2003; Wright, 2002)

L-epinephrine: 0.5 mL/kg of **1:1000** solution (maximum dose: 5 mL) diluted in NS, may repeat dose every 20 minutes; **Note:** Racemic epinephrine 10 mg = 5 mg L-epinephrine (Hegenbarth, 2008)

Hypersensitivity/Allergic reactions: Note: SubQ administration results in slower absorption and is less reliable. IM administration in the anterolateral aspect of the middle third of the thigh is preferred in the setting of anaphylaxis (ACLS guidelines, 2010; Kemp, 2008). For self-administration following severe allergic reactions (eg, insect stings, food), the World Health Organization (WHO) and Anaphylaxis Canada recommend the availability of one dose for every 10-20 minutes of travel time to a medical emergency facility.

IM, SubQ: 0.01 mg/kg (0.01 mL/kg/dose of **1:1000** solution) not to exceed 0.3-0.5 mg every 5-15 minutes (Hegenbarth, 2008; Kemp, 2008)

IM: Autoinjector dose:

AAP/World Allergy Organization recommendations (Kemp, 2008; Sicherer, 2007):

10-25 kg: 0.15 mg

>25 kg: 0.3 mg

Manufacturer labeling (Auvi-Q™, EpiPen® Jr, EpiPen®, Twinject®):

15-29 kg: 0.15 mg; if anaphylactic symptoms persist, dose may be repeated in 5-15 minutes

≥30 kg: 0.3 mg; if anaphylactic symptoms persist, dose may be repeated in 5-15 minutes

IV: 0.01 mg/kg (0.1 mL/kg of **1:10,000** solution) not to exceed 0.5 mg every 20 minutes; may use continuous infusion (0.1 mcg/kg/minute) to prevent frequent doses in more severe reactions

Hypotension/shock, fluid-resistant: Continuous IV infusion: 0.1-1 **mcg**/kg/**minute**; doses up to 5 mcg/kg/minute may rarely be necessary, may be combined with inotropic support (Hegenbarth, 2008)

SubQ: 0.01 mg/kg (0.01 mL/kg of **1:1000** solution) (maximum single dose: 0.5 mg) every 20 minutes for 3 doses (Hegenbarth, 2008)

Inotropic support: Continuous IV infusion: 0.1-1 **mcg**/kg/**minute**; titrate dosage to desired effect

Postresuscitation infusion to maintain cardiac output or stabilize: Continuous IV/I.O. infusion rate: 0.1-1 mcg/kg/minute; doses <0.3 mcg/kg/minute generally produce β-adrenergic effects and higher doses (>0.3 mcg/kg/minute) generally produce alpha-adrenergic vasoconstriction; titrate dosage to desired effect

Adults:

Asystole/pulseless arrest, pulseless VT/VF (ACLS, 2010):

IV, I.O.: 1 mg every 3-5 minutes until return of spontaneous circulation; if this approach fails, higher doses of epinephrine (up to 0.2 mg/kg) have been used for treatment of specific problems (eg, beta-blocker or calcium channel blocker overdose)

Endotracheal: 2-2.5 mg every 3-5 minutes until IV/I.O. access established or return of spontaneous circulation; dilute in 5-10 mL NS or sterile water. **Note:** Absorption may be greater with sterile water (Naganobu, 2000).

Bradycardia (symptomatic; unresponsive to atropine or pacing): IV infusion: 2-10 mcg/minute **or** 0.1-0.5 mcg/kg/minute (7-35 mcg/minute in a 70 kg patient); titrate to desired effect (ACLS, 2010)

Bronchodilator:

Nebulization: S2® (racemic epinephrine, OTC labeling): 0.5 mL: Repeat no more frequently than every 3-4 hours as needed.

SubQ: 0.3-0.5 mg (**1:1000** solution) every 20 minutes for 3 doses

Hypersensitivity reactions: Note: SubQ administration results in slower absorption and is less reliable. IM administration in the anterolateral aspect of the middle third of the thigh is preferred in the setting of anaphylaxis (ACLS guidelines, 2010; Kemp, 2008).

IM, SubQ: 0.2-0.5 mg (**1:1000** solution) every 5-15 minutes in the absence of clinical improvement (ACLS, 2010; Kemp, 2008; Lieberman, 2010). If clinician deems appropriate, the 5-minute interval between injections may be shortened to allow for more frequent administration (Lieberman, 2010).

IV: 0.1 mg (**1:10,000** solution) over 5 minutes; may infuse at 1-4 mcg/minute to prevent the need to repeat injections frequently **or** may initiate with an infusion at 5-15 mcg/minute (with crystalloid administration) (ACLS, 2010; Brown, 2004). In general, IV administration should only be done in patients who are profoundly hypotensive or are in cardiopulmonary arrest refractory to volume resuscitation and several epinephrine injections (Lieberman, 2010).

Self-administration following severe allergic reactions (eg, insect stings, food): **Note:** The World Health Organization (WHO) and Anaphylaxis Canada recommend the availability of one dose for every 10-20 minutes of travel time to a medical emergency facility. More than 2 doses should only be administered under direct medical supervision.

Auvi-Q™: IM, SubQ: 0.3 mg; if anaphylactic symptoms persist, dose may be repeated

Twinject®: IM, SubQ: 0.3 mg; if anaphylactic symptoms persist, dose may be repeated in 5-15 minutes using the same device after partial disassembly

EpiPen®: IM, SubQ: 0.3 mg; if anaphylactic symptoms persist, dose may be repeated in 5-15 minutes using an additional EpiPen®

Hypotension/shock, severe and fluid resistant: IV infusion: Initial: 0.1-0.5 mcg/kg/minute (7-35 mcg/minute in a 70 kg patient); titrate to desired response (ACLS, 2010)

Induction and maintenance of mydriasis during intraocular surgery: Intraocular: Must dilute 1:**1000** (1 mg/mL) solution to a concentration of 1:**100,000** to 1:**1,000,000** (10 **mcg**/mL to 1 **mcg**/mL) prior to intraocular use: May use as an irrigation solution as needed during the procedure or may administer intracamerally (ie, directly into the anterior chamber of the eye) with a bolus dose of 0.1 mL of a 1:**100,000** to 1:**400,000** (10 **mcg**/mL to 2.5 **mcg**/mL) dilution.

Dosing adjustment in renal impairment: There are no dosage adjustment provided in manufacturer's labeling.

Dosing adjustment in hepatic impairment: There are no dosage adjustment provided in manufacturer's labeling.

Usual Infusion Concentrations: Neonatal IV infusion: 10 **mcg**/mL, 16 **mcg**/mL, 32 **mcg**/mL, or 64 **mcg**/mL

Usual Infusion Concentrations: Pediatric IV infusion: 16 **mcg**/mL, 32 **mcg**/mL, or 64 **mcg**/mL

Preparation for Administration

Endotracheal: Pediatric patients: May dilute in 1 to 5 mL NS based on patient size (Hegenbarth 2008). Adults: Dilute in NS or sterile water (ACLS [Neumar 2010]). Absorption may be greater with sterile water (Naganobu 2000).

Intraocular: Dilute 1 mL of 1 mg/mL (1:**1,000**) solution in 100 mL to 1,000 mL of an ophthalmic irrigation fluid for a final concentration of 1:**100,000** to 1:**1,000,000** (10 **mcg**/mL to 1 **mcg**/mL); may use this solution as an irrigation as needed during the procedure. May also prepare a dilution of 1:**100,000** to 1:**400,000** (10 **mcg**/mL to 2.5 **mcg**/mL) for intracameral administration.

Nebulization: S2, Asthmanefrin: If using jet nebulizer, must be diluted; manufacturer recommends diluting in 3 to 5 mL NS; some have recommended diluting in as little as 2 to 2.5 mL NS in the treatment of croup (Hegenbarth 2008; Rosenkrans 1998). If using handheld rubber bulb nebulizer, dilution is not required.

Parenteral:

Direct IV or I.O. administration: Dilute to a maximum concentration of 100 mcg/mL; if using **1:10,000** concentration, no dilution is necessary

Continuous IV infusion: Dilute to a maximum concentration of 64 mcg/mL (Phillips 2011). ISMP and Vermont Oxford Network recommend a standard concentration of 10 mcg/mL for neonates (ISMP 2011). **Note:** Although the manufacturer recommends dilution in dextrose containing solutions (provides protection against significant loss of potency by oxidation) and does not recommend dilution in NS alone, dilution in NS has been reported to be physically compatible (Trissel 2014).

Administration

Endotracheal:

Neonates: Use 0.1 mg/mL (**1:10,000**) solution

Infants, Children, and Adolescents: Use 1 mg/mL solution (**1:1000**); administer and flush with a minimum of 5 mL NS, followed by 5 manual ventilations

Nebulization: If using jet nebulizer: Administer over ~15 minutes

Parenteral:

Direct IV or I.O. administration: If using **1:10,000** concentration, no dilution is necessary; **1:1,000** concentration must be further diluted

Continuous IV infusion: When administering as a continuous infusion, central line administration is preferred. IV infusions require an infusion pump. If central line not available, as a temporary measure, may administer through a large vein. Avoid use of ankle veins (due to potential for gangrene), leg veins in elderly patients, or leg veins in those suffering from occlusive vascular diseases (eg, diabetic endarteritis, Buerger's disease, arteriosclerosis, atherosclerosis).

Rate of infusion (mL/hour) = dose (mcg/kg/minute) x weight (kg) x 60 minutes/hour divided by the concentration (mcg/mL)

Vesicant; ensure proper needle or catheter placement prior to and during infusion; avoid extravasation. If extravasation occurs, stop infusion immediately and disconnect (leave cannula/needle in place); gently aspirate extravasated solution (do **NOT** flush the line); remove needle/cannula; elevate extremity. Initiate phentolamine (or alternative antidote) (see Management of Drug Extravasations for more details). Apply dry warm compresses (Hurst, 2004).

IM (Auvi-Q, EpiPen, EpiPen Jr): Intramuscularly into anterolateral aspect of the middle third of the thigh; Auvi-Q and EpiPen products are single-use products and a new device should be used for each dose. **Note:** In overweight or obese children, because skin surface to muscle depth is greater in the upper half of the thigh, administration into the lower half of the thigh may be preferred. In very obese children, injection into the calf will provide an even greater chance of intramuscular administration (Arkwright 2013).

SubQ: Use only **1:1000** solution

Vesicant/Extravasation Risk Vesicant

Monitoring Parameters ECG, heart rate, blood pressure, site of infusion for excessive blanching/extravasation, rebound respiratory symptoms, cardiac monitor and blood pressure monitor required during continuous infusion

Dosage Forms Excipient information presented when available (limited, particularly for generics); consult specific product labeling. [DSC] = Discontinued product

Device, Injection:
- Auvi-Q: 0.15 mg/0.15 mL (2 ea); 0.3 mg/0.3 mL (2 ea) [contains sodium bisulfite]
- EpiPen 2-Pak: 0.3 mg/0.3 mL (2 ea) [latex free; contains sodium metabisulfite]
- EpiPen Jr 2-Pak: 0.15 mg/0.3 mL (2 ea) [contains sodium metabisulfite]

Nebulization Solution, Inhalation:
- Asthmanefrin Refill: 2.25% (1 ea) [contains edetate disodium]
- Asthmanefrin Starter Kit: 2.25% (1 ea) [contains edetate disodium]
- Micronefrin: 2.25% (15 mL [DSC], 30 mL [DSC])

Nebulization Solution, Inhalation [preservative free]:
- S2: 2.25% (1 ea) [sulfite free; contains edetate disodium]

Solution, Injection:
- Adrenalin: 1 mg/mL (1 mL) [contains sodium metabisulfite]
- Adrenalin: 30 mg/30 mL (30 mL) [contains chlorobutanol (chlorobutol), sodium metabisulfite]
- Generic: 0.1 mg/mL (10 mL); 1 mg/mL (1 mL)

Solution, Intravenous [preservative free]:
- Generic: 1 mg/mL (1 mL)

Solution, Injection, as hydrochloride:
- Adrenalin: 1 mg/mL (30 mL [DSC]) [contains chlorobutanol (chlorobutol), sodium bisulfite]
- Adrenalin: 1 mg/mL (1 mL [DSC]) [contains sodium bisulfite]
- Generic: 1 mg/mL (1 mL, 30 mL)

Solution Auto-injector, Injection:
- Adrenaclick: 0.15 mg/0.15 mL (2 ea); 0.3 mg/0.3 mL (2 ea) [latex free; contains chlorobutanol (chlorobutol), sodium bisulfite]
- Generic: 0.15 mg/0.15 mL (1 ea, 2 ea); 0.3 mg/0.3 mL (1 ea, 2 ea)

Solution Prefilled Syringe, Injection:
- Generic: 0.1 mg/mL (10 mL)

EPINEPHrine (Nasal) (ep i NEF rin)

Medication Safety Issues

Sound-alike/look-alike issues:

EPINEPHrine may be confused with ePHEDrine

Related Information

Safe Handling of Hazardous Drugs *on page 2455*

Brand Names: US Adrenalin

Brand Names: Canada Adrenalin®

Therapeutic Category Decongestant, Nasal

Generic Availability (US) No

Use Nasal decongestant, decrease superficial hemorrhage

Pregnancy Considerations Refer to the EPINEPHrine (Systemic) monograph.

Breast-Feeding Considerations Refer to the EPINEPHrine (Systemic) monograph.

Warnings/Precautions Use with caution in elderly patients, patients with diabetes mellitus, cardiovascular diseases (eg, coronary artery disease, hypertension), thyroid disease, cerebrovascular disease, Parkinson's disease, or patients taking tricyclic antidepressants.

Adverse Reactions

Cardiovascular: Angina, cardiac arrhythmia, chest pain, flushing, hypertension, pallor, palpitation, sudden death, tachycardia (parenteral), vasoconstriction, ventricular ectopy

Central nervous system: Anxiety (transient), apprehensiveness, cerebral hemorrhage, dizziness, headache, insomnia, lightheadedness, nervousness, restlessness

Gastrointestinal: Dry throat, loss of appetite, nausea, vomiting, xerostomia

Genitourinary: Acute urinary retention in patients with bladder outflow obstruction

Neuromuscular & skeletal: Tremor, weakness

Ocular: Allergic lid reaction, burning, eye pain, ocular irritation, precipitation of or exacerbation of narrow-angle glaucoma, transient stinging

Respiratory: Dyspnea, pulmonary edema

Miscellaneous: Diaphoresis

Drug Interactions

Metabolism/Transport Effects Substrate of COMT

Avoid Concomitant Use

Avoid concomitant use of EPINEPHrine (Nasal) with any of the following: Ergot Derivatives; Iobenguane I 123

Increased Effect/Toxicity

EPINEPHrine (Nasal) may increase the levels/effects of: Sympathomimetics

The levels/effects of EPINEPHrine (Nasal) may be increased by: AtoMOXetine; Beta-Blockers; Cannabinoid-Containing Products; COMT Inhibitors; Ergot Derivatives; Inhalational Anesthetics; Linezolid; MAO Inhibitors; Serotonin/Norepinephrine Reuptake Inhibitors; Tedizolid; Tricyclic Antidepressants

Decreased Effect

EPINEPHrine (Nasal) may decrease the levels/effects of: Iobenguane I 123

The levels/effects of EPINEPHrine (Nasal) may be decreased by: Alpha1-Blockers; Promethazine; Spironolactone

Storage/Stability Epinephrine is sensitive to light and air. Protection from light is recommended. Oxidation turns drug pink, then a brown color. **Solutions should not be used if they are discolored or contain a precipitate.**

Mechanism of Action Stimulates alpha-, $beta_1$-, and $beta_2$-adrenergic receptors resulting in local vasoconstriction and relief of nasal congestion

Pharmacodynamics Local vasoconstriction (topical):

Onset of action: 5 minutes

Duration: <1 hour

Pharmacokinetics (Adult data unless noted)

Distribution: Crosses placenta but not blood-brain barrier

Metabolism: Extensive in the liver and other tissues by the enzymes catechol-o-methyltransferase and monoamine oxidase

Dosing: Usual Children ≥6 years and Adults: Apply drops locally as needed; do not exceed 1 mL every 15 minutes

Administration Apply as drops or with sterile swab.

Monitoring Parameters Heart rate, blood pressure

Dosage Forms Excipient information presented when available (limited, particularly for generics); consult specific product labeling.

Solution, Nasal, as hydrochloride:
- Adrenalin: 0.1% (30 mL)

- ◆ **Epinephrine and Lidocaine** *see* Lidocaine and Epinephrine *on page 1262*
- ◆ **Epinephrine Bitartrate** *see* EPINEPHrine (Systemic, Oral Inhalation) *on page 760*
- ◆ **Epinephrine Hydrochloride** *see* EPINEPHrine (Nasal) *on page 764*
- ◆ **Epinephrine Hydrochloride** *see* EPINEPHrine (Systemic, Oral Inhalation) *on page 760*
- ◆ **EpiPen (Can)** *see* EPINEPHrine (Systemic, Oral Inhalation) *on page 760*
- ◆ **EpiPen 2-Pak** *see* EPINEPHrine (Systemic, Oral Inhalation) *on page 760*
- ◆ **EpiPen Jr (Can)** *see* EPINEPHrine (Systemic, Oral Inhalation) *on page 760*
- ◆ **EpiPen Jr 2-Pak** *see* EPINEPHrine (Systemic, Oral Inhalation) *on page 760*

- ◆ **Epipodophyllotoxin** *see* Etoposide *on page 819*
- ◆ **Epitol** *see* CarBAMazepine *on page 367*
- ◆ **Epival (Can)** *see* Valproic Acid and Derivatives *on page 2143*
- ◆ **Epival ECT (Can)** *see* Valproic Acid and Derivatives *on page 2143*
- ◆ **Epivir** *see* LamiVUDine *on page 1205*
- ◆ **Epivir HBV** *see* LamiVUDine *on page 1205*
- ◆ **EPO** *see* Epoetin Alfa *on page 765*

Epoetin Alfa (e POE e tin AL fa)

Medication Safety Issues

Sound-alike/look-alike issues:

Epoetin alfa may be confused with darbepoetin alfa, epoetin beta

Epogen may be confused with Neupogen

International issues:

Epopen [Spain] may be confused with EpiPen brand name for epinephrine [U.S., Canada, and multiple international markets]

Brand Names: US Epogen; Procrit

Brand Names: Canada Eprex

Therapeutic Category Colony-Stimulating Factor; Growth Factor; Hematopoietic Agent; Recombinant Human Erythropoietin

Generic Availability (US) No

Use Treatment of anemia associated with chronic kidney disease (CKD) in patients on dialysis (FDA approved in ages 1 month to 16 years and adults); treatment of anemia associated with CKD without dialysis (FDA approved in adults); anemia in cancer patients with nonmyeloid malignancies receiving concurrent myelosuppressive chemotherapy (palliative intent) when chemotherapy is a planned for a minimum of 2 months (FDA approved in ages ≥5 years and adults); anemia related to HIV therapy with zidovudine (FDA approved in adults); reduction of allogeneic RBC transfusion for elective, noncardiac, nonvascular surgery when perioperative hemoglobin is >10 to ≤13 g/dL and with high risk for blood loss (FDA approved in adults); has also been used for anemia of prematurity; treatment of symptomatic anemia in myelodysplastic syndrome

Prescribing and Access Restrictions As a requirement of the REMS program, access to this medication is restricted. Healthcare providers and hospitals must be enrolled in the ESA APPRISE (Assisting Providers and Cancer Patients with Risk Information for the Safe use of ESAs) Oncology Program (866-284-8089; http://www.esa-apprise.com) to prescribe or dispense ESAs (ie, epoetin alfa, darbepoetin alfa) to patients with cancer.

Medication Guide Available Yes

Pregnancy Risk Factor C

Pregnancy Considerations Adverse events were observed in animal reproduction studies. In vitro studies suggest that recombinant erythropoietin does not cross the human placenta (Reisenberger, 1997). Polyhydramnios and intrauterine growth retardation have been reported with use in women with chronic kidney disease (adverse effects also associated with maternal disease). Hypospadias and pectus excavatum have been reported with first trimester exposure (case report).

Recombinant erythropoietin alfa has been evaluated as adjunctive treatment for severe pregnancy associated iron deficiency anemia (Breymann, 2001; Krafft, 2009) and has been used in pregnant women with iron-deficiency anemia associated with chronic kidney disease (CKD) (Furaz-Czerpak 2012; Josephson, 2007).

Amenorrheic premenopausal women should be cautioned that menstruation may resume following treatment with recombinant erythropoietin (Furaz-Czerpak, 2012). Multidose formulations containing benzyl alcohol are contraindicated for use in pregnant women; if treatment during pregnancy is needed, single dose preparations should be used.

Women who become pregnant during treatment with epoetin are encouraged to enroll in Amgen's Pregnancy Surveillance Program (1-800-772-6436).

Breast-Feeding Considerations Endogenous erythropoietin is found in breast milk (Semba, 2002). It is not known if recombinant erythropoietin alfa is excreted into breast milk. The manufacturer recommends caution be used if the single dose vial preparation is administered to nursing women; use of the multiple dose vials containing benzyl alcohol is contraindicated in breast-feeding women. When administered enterally to neonates (mixed with human milk or infant formula), recombinant erythropoietin did not significantly increase serum EPO concentrations. If passage via breast milk does occur, risk to a nursing infant appears low (Juul, 2003).

Contraindications Hypersensitivity to epoetin or any component of the formulation; uncontrolled hypertension; pure red cell aplasia (due to epoetin or other epoetin protein drugs); multidose vials contain benzyl alcohol and are contraindicated in neonates, infants, pregnant women, and nursing women

Warnings/Precautions **[U.S. Boxed Warning]: Erythropoiesis-stimulating agents (ESAs) increased the risk of serious cardiovascular events, thromboembolic events, stroke, mortality, and/or tumor progression in clinical studies when administered to target hemoglobin levels >11 g/dL** (and provide no additional benefit); a rapid rise in hemoglobin (>1 g/dL over 2 weeks) may also contribute to these risks. **[U.S. Boxed Warning]: A shortened overall survival and/or increased risk of tumor progression or recurrence has been reported in studies with breast, cervical, head and neck, lymphoid, and non-small cell lung cancer patients.** It is of note that in these studies, patients received ESAs to a target hemoglobin of ≥12 g/dL; although risk has not been excluded when dosed to achieve a target hemoglobin of <12 g/dL. **[U.S. Boxed Warnings]: To decrease these risks, and risk of cardio- and thrombovascular events, use the lowest dose needed to avoid red blood cell transfusions. Use ESAs in cancer patients only for the treatment of anemia related to concurrent myelosuppressive chemotherapy; discontinue ESA following completion of the chemotherapy course. ESAs are not indicated for patients receiving myelosuppressive therapy when the anticipated outcome is curative.** A dosage modification is appropriate if hemoglobin levels rise >1 g/dL per 2-week time period during treatment (Rizzo, 2010). Use of ESAs has been associated with an increased risk of venous thromboembolism (VTE) without a reduction in transfusions in patients with cancer (Hershman, 2009). Improved anemia symptoms, quality of life, fatigue, or well-being have not been demonstrated in controlled clinical trials. **[U.S. Boxed Warning]: Because of the risks of decreased survival and increased risk of tumor growth or progression, all healthcare providers and hospitals are required to enroll and comply with the ESA APPRISE (Assisting Providers and Cancer Patients with Risk Information for the Safe use of ESAs) Oncology Program prior to prescribing or dispensing ESAs to cancer patients.** Prescribers and patients will have to provide written documentation of discussed risks prior to each new course.

[U.S. Boxed Warning]: An increased risk of death, serious cardiovascular events, and stroke was reported in chronic kidney disease (CKD) patients

administered ESAs to target hemoglobin levels ≥11 g/dL; use the lowest dose sufficient to reduce the need for RBC transfusions. An optimal target hemoglobin level, dose or dosing strategy to reduce these risks has not been identified in clinical trials. Hemoglobin rising >1 g/dL in a 2-week period may contribute to the risk (dosage reduction recommended). The American College of Physicians recommends against the use of ESAs in patients with mild to moderate anemia and heart failure or coronary heart disease (ACP [Qaseem, 2013]). The ACCF/AHA 2013 Heart Failure Guidelines do not provide a clear recommendation on the use of erythropoiesis-stimulating agents (ESA) in anemic heart failure patients.

Chronic kidney disease patients who exhibit an inadequate hemoglobin response to ESA therapy may be at a higher risk for cardiovascular events and mortality compared to other patients. ESA therapy may reduce dialysis efficacy (due to increase in red blood cells and decrease in plasma volume); adjustments in dialysis parameters may be needed. Patients treated with epoetin may require increased heparinization during dialysis to prevent clotting of the extracorporeal circuit. **[U.S. Boxed Warning]: DVT prophylaxis is recommended in perisurgery patients due to the risk of DVT.** Increased mortality was also observed in patients undergoing coronary artery bypass surgery who received epoetin alfa; these deaths were associated with thrombotic events. Epoetin is **not** approved for reduction of red blood cell transfusion in patients undergoing cardiac or vascular surgery and is **not** indicated for surgical patients willing to donate autologous blood.

Use with caution in patients with hypertension (contraindicated in uncontrolled hypertension) or with a history of seizures; hypertensive encephalopathy and seizures have been reported. If hypertension is difficult to control, reduce or hold epoetin alfa. An excessive rate of rise of hemoglobin is associated with hypertension or exacerbation of hypertension; decrease the epoetin dose if the hemoglobin increase exceeds 1 g/dL in any 2-week period. Blood pressure should be controlled prior to start of therapy and monitored closely throughout treatment. The risk for seizures is increased with epoetin use in patients with CKD; monitor closely for neurologic symptoms during the first several months of therapy. Due to the delayed onset of erythropoiesis, epoetin alfa is **not** recommended for acute correction of severe anemia or as a substitute for emergency transfusion.

Prior to treatment, correct or exclude deficiencies of iron, vitamin B_{12}, and/or folate, as well as other factors which may impair erythropoiesis (inflammatory conditions, infections). Prior to and periodically during therapy, iron stores must be evaluated. Supplemental iron is recommended if serum ferritin <100 mcg/L or serum transferrin saturation <20%; most patients with chronic kidney disease will require iron supplementation. Poor response should prompt evaluation of these potential factors, as well as possible malignant processes and hematologic disease (thalassemia, refractory anemia, myelodysplastic disorder), occult blood loss, hemolysis, ostetis fibrosa cystic, and/or bone marrow fibrosis. Severe anemia and pure red cell aplasia (PRCA) with associated neutralizing antibodies to erythropoietin has been reported, predominantly in patients with CKD receiving SubQ epoetin (the IV route is preferred for hemodialysis patients). Cases have also been reported in patients with hepatitis C who were receiving ESAs, interferon, and ribavirin. Patients with a sudden loss of response to epoetin alfa (with severe anemia and a low reticulocyte count) should be evaluated for PRCA with associated neutralizing antibodies to erythropoietin; discontinue treatment (permanently) in patients with PRCA secondary to neutralizing antibodies to epoetin.

Potentially serious allergic reactions have been reported (rarely). Discontinue immediately (and permanently) in patients who experience serious allergic/anaphylactic reactions.

Some dosage forms may contain polysorbate 80 (also known as Tweens). Hypersensitivity reactions, usually a delayed reaction, have been reported following exposure to pharmaceutical products containing polysorbate 80 in certain individuals (Isaksson, 2002; Lucente 2000; Shelley, 1995). Thrombocytopenia, ascites, pulmonary deterioration, and renal and hepatic failure have been reported in premature neonates after receiving parenteral products containing polysorbate 80 (Alade, 1986; CDC, 1984). See manufacturer's labeling.

Some products may contain albumin.

Benzyl alcohol and derivatives: Some dosage forms may contain benzyl alcohol; large amounts of benzyl alcohol (≥99 mg/kg/day) have been associated with a potentially fatal toxicity ("gasping syndrome") in neonates; the "gasping syndrome" consists of metabolic acidosis, respiratory distress, gasping respirations, CNS dysfunction (including convulsions, intracranial hemorrhage), hypotension and cardiovascular collapse (AAP, 1997; CDC, 1982); some data suggests that benzoate displaces bilirubin from protein binding sites (Ahlfors, 2001); avoid or use dosage forms containing benzyl alcohol with caution in neonates. See manufacturer's labeling.

Warnings: Additional Pediatric Considerations May be associated with an increased risk of retinopathy of prematurity (ROP); an increase in ROP has been observed in neonates receiving epoetin alfa for anemia of prematurity, with a reported incidence of 15% to 17%; however, a direct association with the drug has not been established. A meta-analysis of early treatment with epoetin alfa showed that neonates treated within the first week of life did not have a significant increased incidence in stage ≥3 ROP; however, a post-ad hoc data analysis of all neonates (regardless of age at treatment) showed an increased risk (Ohlsson 2014); a meta-analysis of late treatment showed an overall trend toward increased incidence of ROP (all stages) and at stage ≥ 3 (Aher 2014). Risks and benefits should be assessed prior to initiation.

Adverse Reactions

Cardiovascular: Deep vein thrombosis, edema, hypertension, thrombosis

Central nervous system: Chills, depression, dizziness, fever, headache, insomnia

Dermatologic: Pruritus, rash,urticaria

Endocrine & metabolic: Hyperglycemia, hypokalemia

Gastrointestinal: Dysphagia, nausea, stomatitis, vomiting, weight loss

Hematologic: Leukopenia

Local: Clotted vascular access, injection site reaction

Neuromuscular & skeletal: Arthralgia, bone pain, muscle spasm, myalgia

Respiratory: Cough, pulmonary embolism, respiratory congestion, upper respiratory infection

Rare but important or life-threatening: Allergic reaction, anaphylactic reaction, angioedema, bronchospasm, erythema, hypersensitivity reactions, hypertensive encephalopathy, microvascular thrombosis, MI, neutralizing antibodies, porphyria, pure red cell aplasia (PRCA), renal vein thrombosis, retinal artery thrombosis, seizure, stroke, tachycardia, temporal vein thrombosis, thrombophlebitis, TIA, tumor progression

Drug Interactions

Metabolism/Transport Effects None known.

Avoid Concomitant Use There are no known interactions where it is recommended to avoid concomitant use.

Increased Effect/Toxicity

Epoetin Alfa may increase the levels/effects of: Lenalidomide; Thalidomide

The levels/effects of Epoetin Alfa may be increased by: Nandrolone

Decreased Effect There are no known significant interactions involving a decrease in effect.

Storage/Stability Vials should be stored at 2°C to 8°C (36°F to 46°F); **do not freeze or shake**. Protect from light.

Single-dose 1 mL vial contains no preservative: Use one dose per vial. Do not re-enter vial; discard unused portions.

Single-dose vials (except 40,000 units/mL vial) are stable for 2 weeks at room temperature (Cohen, 2007). Single-dose 40,000 units/mL vial is stable for 1 week at room temperature.

Multidose 1 mL or 2 mL vial contains preservative. Store at 2°C to 8°C after initial entry and between doses. Discard 21 days after initial entry.

Multidose vials (with preservative) are stable for 1 week at room temperature (Cohen, 2007).

Prefilled syringes containing the 20,000 units/mL formulation with preservative are stable for 6 weeks refrigerated (2°C to 8°C) (Naughton, 2003).

Dilutions of 1:10 and 1:20 (1 part epoetin:19 parts sodium chloride) are stable for 18 hours at room temperature (Ohls, 1996).

Prior to SubQ administration, preservative free solutions may be mixed with bacteriostatic NS containing benzyl alcohol 0.9% in a 1:1 ratio (Corbo, 1992).

Dilutions of 1:10 in $D_{10}W$ with human albumin 0.05% or 0.1% are stable for 24 hours.

Mechanism of Action Induces erythropoiesis by stimulating the division and differentiation of committed erythroid progenitor cells; induces the release of reticulocytes from the bone marrow into the bloodstream, where they mature to erythrocytes. There is a dose response relationship with this effect. This results in an increase in reticulocyte counts followed by a rise in hematocrit and hemoglobin levels.

Pharmacodynamics

Onset of action: Several days

Maximum effect (hemoglobin level): 2 to 6 weeks

Pharmacokinetics (Adult data unless noted) Note: While a much higher peak plasma concentration is achieved after IV bolus administration, it declines at a more rapid rate than after subcutaneous administration (McMahon, 1990; Salmonson, 1990)

Absorption: SubQ: Slow (McMahon, 1990; Salmonson, 1990)

Distribution: Similar to extracelluar plasma volume in adults (McMahon, 1990; Salmonson, 1990); reported to be higher in premature neonates on body weight basis (Brown, 1993)

Metabolism: Some degradation does occur

Bioavailability: SubQ: Premature neonates: 42% (Brown, 1993); Adults: 36% (Salmonson, 1990)

Half-life:

Neonates: With high doses, nonlinear kinetics have been observed (Wu, 2012)

Anemia of prematurity:

PMA <32 week (weight: 800 ± 206 grams): IV: 8.1 ± 2.7 hours; SubQ: 7.1 ± 4.1 hours (Brown, 1993)

PMA ≥32 weeks (weight range: 1330 to 1740 g): SubQ: Median: 7.9 hours (range: 5.6 to 19.4 hours) (Krishnan, 1996)

Neuroprotective/hypoxic ischemia encephalopathy (HIE) (Wu, 2012): ≥36 weeks GA; IV:

250 units/kg: 7.6 ± 6.9 hours

500 units/kg: 7.2 ± 1.9 hours

1,000 units/kg: 15 ± 4.5 hours

2,500 units/kg: 18.7 ± 4.7 hours

Infants, Children, and Adolescents: Chronic kidney disease: IV: 4 to 13 hours

Adults:

Chronic kidney disease: IV: 4 to 13 hours

Cancer: SubQ: 16 to 67 hours

Time to peak serum concentration: Pediatric patients >1 month and Adults: Chronic kidney disease: SubQ: 5 to 24 hours

Elimination: Feces (majority); urine (small amounts, 10% unchanged in healthy volunteers)

Dosing: Neonatal

Anemia of prematurity: Limited data available; dosing regimens and efficacy results variable: **Note:** Role in therapy not determined; some experts recommend to avoid use due to increased risk of adverse effects (eg, retinopathy of prematurity) (Aher 2014; Ohlsson 2014): IV, SubQ: Reported range: 150 to 1,500 units/kg/**week** divided into 2 to 5 doses (Alarcon 2005); a commonly accepted regimen is 250 units/kg/dose 3 times weekly for 10 doses; supplement with oral iron therapy (Kenner 2007; Maier 1994); a small trial used a weekly dose of 1,200 units/kg once weekly and reported increased reticulocytes and maintained hematocrit similar to 3 times a week dosing in 10 neonates (GA: 27.9 ± 0.6 weeks; birth weight: 922 ± 75 g) (Ohls 2012)

Neuroprotective/hypoxic ischemia encephalopathy (HIE): Limited data available, dosing regimens variable:

Low dose: Initial dose: SubQ: 300 or 500 units/kg/dose; maintenance dose: IV: 300 or 500 units/kg/dose every other day for 2 weeks beginning within first 48 hours of life was used in 73 neonates diagnosed with moderate HIE; improved neurologic outcomes were reported at 18 months of age (Zhu 2009)

High dose: IV, SubQ: 1,000 or 2,500 units/kg/dose once daily for 3 to 5 days beginning within first 24 hours of life; dosing based on a Phase I/II safety and pharmacokinetic, case-control study of 30 ELBW neonates (mean GA: 26.1 weeks, birth weight: 745 g) which showed dosing ≥1,000 units/kg IV provided proposed target serum concentration for neuroprotective effects (>6,000 mIU/mL) and reported a diminished severity of ICH in treatment groups (Juul, 2008). In a prospective, case-controlled pilot efficacy trial, 15 term neonates diagnosed with HIE received SubQ administration of 2,500 units/kg/dose for 5 days beginning within first 24 hours of life; short-term findings (PNA: 2 weeks) included decreased nitric oxide serum concentrations and fewer seizures; long-term finding (PNA: 6 months) included fewer neurologic abnormalities (Elmahdy 2010)

Dosing: Usual Dosing schedules need to be individualized and careful monitoring of patients receiving the drug is recommended. Use has not been demonstrated in controlled clinical trials to improve symptoms of anemia, quality of life, fatigue, or patient well-being.

Pediatric:

Anemia in chronic kidney disease (ON dialysis): Note: IV route is preferred for hemodialysis patients; initiate treatment when hemoglobin is <10 g/dL; reduce dose or interrupt treatment if hemoglobin approaches or exceeds 11 g/dL:

Initial dose:

Infants, Children, and Adolescents ≤16 years: IV, SubQ: 50 units/kg/dose 3 times weekly

Adolescents >16 years: 50 to 100 units/kg 3 times/week

Dosage adjustments:

If hemoglobin does **not** increase by >1 g/dL after 4 weeks: Increase dose by 25%; do not increase the dose more frequently than once every 4 weeks

If hemoglobin increases >1 g/dL in any 2-week period: Reduce dose by ≥25%; dose reductions can occur more frequently than once every 4 weeks; avoid frequent dosage adjustments

Inadequate or lack of response over a 12-week escalation period: Further increases are unlikely to improve response and may increase risks; use the minimum effective dose that will maintain an Hgb level sufficient to avoid RBC transfusions and evaluate patient for other causes of anemia. Discontinue therapy if responsiveness does not improve.

Anemia in chronic kidney disease (NOT on dialysis): Adolescents >16 years: **Note:** Consider initiating treatment when hemoglobin is <10 g/dL; use only if rate of hemoglobin decline would likely result in RBC transfusion and desire is to reduce risk of alloimmunization or other RBC transfusion-related risks; reduce dose or interrupt treatment if hemoglobin exceeds 10 g/dL: IV, SubQ:

Initial dose: 50 to 100 units/kg 3 times/week

Dosage adjustments:

If hemoglobin does **not** increase by >1 g/dL after 4 weeks: Increase dose by 25%; do not increase the dose more frequently than once every 4 weeks

If hemoglobin increases >1 g/dL in any 2-week period: Reduce dose by ≥25%; dose reductions can occur more frequently than once every 4 weeks; avoid frequent dosage adjustments

Inadequate or lack of response over a 12-week escalation period: Further increases are unlikely to improve response and may increase risks; use the minimum effective dose that will maintain a Hgb level sufficient to avoid RBC transfusions and evaluate patient for other causes of anemia. Discontinue therapy if responsiveness does not improve.

Anemia due to myelosuppressive chemotherapy (palliative) in cancer patients: Note: Initiate treatment only if hemoglobin <10 g/dL and anticipated duration of myelosuppressive chemotherapy is ≥2 months. Titrate dosage to use the minimum effective dose that will maintain a hemoglobin level sufficient to avoid red blood cell transfusions. Children ≥5 years and Adolescents: IV:

Initial dose: 600 units/kg/dose once weekly until completion of chemotherapy

Dosage adjustments:

If hemoglobin does not increase by >1 g/dL **and** remains <10 g/dL after initial 4 weeks: Increase to 900 units/kg/dose (maximum dose: 60,000 units/dose); discontinue after 8 weeks of treatment if RBC transfusions are still required or there is no hemoglobin response

If hemoglobin exceeds a level needed to avoid red blood cell transfusion: Withhold dose; resume treatment with a 25% dose reduction when hemoglobin approaches a level where transfusions may be required

If hemoglobin increases >1 g/dL in any 2-week period **or** hemoglobin reaches a level sufficient to avoid red blood cell transfusion: Reduce dose by 25%

Anemia due to zidovudine in HIV-infected patients: Limited data available: **Note:** Titrate dosage to use the minimum effective dose that will maintain a hemoglobin level sufficient to avoid red blood cell transfusions. Infants ≥3 months, Children, and Adolescents ≤17 years: IV, SubQ: Doses ranging from 50 to 400 units/kg/dose 2 to 3 times weekly have been reported; withhold dose if hemoglobin exceeds 12 g/dL, may resume treatment with a 25% dose reduction once hemoglobin <11 g/dL (Ferri, 2002)

Adult:

Anemia associated with chronic kidney disease: Individualize dosing and use the lowest dose necessary to reduce the need for RBC transfusions.

Chronic kidney disease patients **ON dialysis** (IV route is preferred for hemodialysis patients; initiate treatment when hemoglobin is <10 g/dL; reduce dose or interrupt treatment if hemoglobin approaches or exceeds 11 g/dL): IV, SubQ: Initial dose: 50 to 100 units/kg/dose 3 times weekly

Chronic kidney disease patients **NOT on dialysis** (consider initiating treatment when hemoglobin is <10 g/dL; use only if rate of hemoglobin decline would likely result in RBC transfusion and desire is to reduce risk of alloimmunization or other RBC transfusion-related risks; reduce dose or interrupt treatment if hemoglobin exceeds 10 g/dL): IV, SubQ: Initial dose: 50 to 100 units/kg/dose 3 times/week

Dosage adjustments for chronic kidney disease patients (either on dialysis or not on dialysis):

If hemoglobin does not increase by >1 g/dL after 4 weeks: Increase dose by 25%; do not increase the dose more frequently than once every 4 weeks

If hemoglobin increases >1 g/dL in any 2-week period: Reduce dose by ≥25%; dose reductions can occur more frequently than once every 4 weeks; avoid frequent dosage adjustments

Inadequate or lack of response over a 12-week escalation period: Further increases are unlikely to improve response and may increase risks; use the minimum effective dose that will maintain an Hgb level sufficient to avoid RBC transfusions and evaluate patient for other causes of anemia. Discontinue therapy if responsiveness does not improve.

Anemia due to chemotherapy in cancer patients: Initiate treatment only if hemoglobin <10 g/dL and anticipated duration of myelosuppressive chemotherapy is ≥2 months. Titrate dosage to use the minimum effective dose that will maintain a hemoglobin level sufficient to avoid red blood cell transfusions. Discontinue erythropoietin following completion of chemotherapy. SubQ: Initial dose: 150 units/kg/dose 3 times weekly or 40,000 units once weekly until completion of chemotherapy.

Dosage adjustments:

If hemoglobin does not increase by >1 g/dL **and** remains below 10 g/dL after initial 4 weeks: Increase to 300 units/kg/dose 3 times weekly or 60,000 units weekly; discontinue after 8 weeks of treatment if RBC transfusions are still required or there is no hemoglobin response

If hemoglobin exceeds a level needed to avoid red blood cell transfusion: Withhold dose; resume treatment with a 25% dose reduction when hemoglobin approaches a level where transfusions may be required

If hemoglobin increases >1 g/dL in any 2-week period **or** hemoglobin reaches a level sufficient to avoid red blood cell transfusion: Reduce dose by 25%

Anemia due to zidovudine in HIV-infected patients: Titrate dosage to use the minimum effective dose that will maintain a hemoglobin level sufficient to avoid red blood cell transfusions. Hemoglobin levels should not exceed 12 g/dL.

Serum erythropoietin levels ≤500 mUnits/mL and zidovudine doses ≤4200 mg/week): IV, SubQ: Initial: 100 units/kg/dose 3 times weekly; if hemoglobin does not increase after 8 weeks, increase dose by ~50 to 100 units/kg/dose at 4 to 8 week intervals until hemoglobin reaches a level sufficient to avoid RBC transfusion; maximum dose: 300 units/kg/dose. Withhold dose if hemoglobin exceeds 12 g/dL, may resume treatment with a 25% dose reduction once hemoglobin <11 g/dL. Discontinue if hemoglobin increase is not achieved with 300 units/kg/dose for 8 weeks.

Surgery patients (perioperative hemoglobin should be >10 g/dL and ≤13 g/dL; DVT prophylactic anticoagulation is recommended): SubQ: Initial dose:

300 units/kg/day beginning 10 days before surgery, on the day of surgery, and for 4 days after surgery **or**

600 units/kg once weekly for 4 doses, given 21, 14, and 7 days before surgery, and on the day of surgery

Dosing adjustment in renal impairment: Infants, Children, Adolescents, and Adults: No dosage adjustment necessary.

Dosing adjustment in hepatic impairment: Infants, Children, Adolescents, and Adults: There are no dosage adjustments provided in the manufacturer's labeling.

Preparation for Administration Parenteral: Do not shake as this may denature the glycoprotein rendering the drug biologically inactive; do not use if product has been shaken or frozen.

IV: Some institutions may dilute with an equal volume of NS; in some neonatal trials, doses were diluted in dextrose solutions containing at least 0.05% protein as either amino acids or albumin (Ohls 1996; Ohls 1997)

SubQ: Preservative free solutions may be mixed with bacteriostatic NS containing benzyl alcohol 0.9% in a 1:1 ratio; acts as a local anesthetic to reduce pain at the injection site. Do not use in neonates and infants; risk of benzyl alcohol toxicity.

Administration Parenteral: Do not shake as this may denature the glycoprotein rendering the drug biologically inactive; do not use if product has been shaken or frozen.

SubQ: Preferred route of administration except in patients with CKD on hemodialysis; 1:1 dilution with bacteriostatic NS (containing benzyl alcohol) acts as a local anesthetic to reduce pain at the injection site. Multiple-dose vials already contain benzyl alcohol.

IV: Manufacturer recommends administering without dilution; some institutions may further dilute with NS; infuse over 1 to 3 minutes; it may be administered into the venous line at the end of the dialysis procedure. In neonates, may be infused over 4 hours when diluted in parenteral nutrition or dextrose containing IVF with at least 0.05% protein (amino acids or albumin) (Ohls 1996; Ohls 1997)

Monitoring Parameters Transferrin saturation and serum ferritin (prior to and during treatment); hemoglobin (weekly after initiation and following dose adjustments until stable and sufficient to minimize need for RBC transfusion, CKD patients should be also be monitored at least monthly following hemoglobin stability); blood pressure; seizures (CKD patients following initiation for first few months, includes new-onset or change in seizure frequency or premonitory symptoms)

Cancer patients: Examinations recommended by the ASCO/ASH guidelines (Rizzo, 2010) prior to treatment include: Peripheral blood smear (in some situations a bone marrow exam may be necessary), assessment for iron, folate, or vitamin B_{12} deficiency, reticulocyte count, renal function status, and occult blood loss; during ESA treatment, assess baseline and periodic iron, total iron-binding capacity, and transferrin saturation or ferritin levels

Reference Range Adult zidovudine-treated HIV patients: Available evidence indicates patients with endogenous serum erythropoietin concentrations >500 mIU/mL are unlikely to respond

Dosage Forms Excipient information presented when available (limited, particularly for generics); consult specific product labeling.

Solution, Injection:

Epogen: 10,000 units/mL (2 mL); 20,000 units/mL (1 mL) [contains benzyl alcohol]

Procrit: 10,000 units/mL (2 mL); 20,000 units/mL (1 mL) [contains benzyl alcohol]

Solution, Injection [preservative free]:

Epogen: 2000 units/mL (1 mL); 3000 units/mL (1 mL); 4000 units/mL (1 mL); 10,000 units/mL (1 mL)

Procrit: 2000 units/mL (1 mL); 3000 units/mL (1 mL); 4000 units/mL (1 mL); 10,000 units/mL (1 mL); 40,000 units/mL (1 mL)

◆ **Epogen** *see* Epoetin Alfa *on page* 765

Epoprostenol (e poe PROST en ole)

Medication Safety Issues

High alert medication:

The Institute for Safe Medication Practices (ISMP) includes this medication among its list of drugs which have a heightened risk of causing significant patient harm when used in error.

Brand Names: US Flolan; Veletri

Brand Names: Canada Caripul; Flolan

Therapeutic Category Prostaglandin

Generic Availability (US) Yes

Use Treatment of pulmonary arterial hypertension (PAH) (WHO Group I) to improve exercise capacity. **Note:** Efficacy has been established in patients with NYHA Class III or IV symptoms with idiopathic or heritable PAH or PAH associated with connective tissue diseases (FDA approved in adults)

Has also been used diagnostically as a short-term IV infusion in patients with pulmonary hypertension in the cardiac catheterization laboratory to screen for responsiveness to other oral vasodilating agents (eg, calcium channel blockers). **Note:** Responsiveness to short-term (acute) IV infusions of epoprostenol predicts responsiveness to long-term treatment with oral calcium channel blockers; however, it does not predict responsiveness to long-term IV epoprostenol therapy. Patients who do not respond acutely to epoprostenol may respond to the drug when used chronically.

Other potential uses include treatment of secondary pulmonary hypertension associated with ARDS, SLE, congenital heart disease, congenital diaphragmatic hernia, neonatal pulmonary hypertension, cardiopulmonary bypass surgery, hemodialysis, peripheral vascular disorders, portal hypertension, and neonatal purpura fulminans.

Prescribing and Access Restrictions Orders for epoprostenol are distributed by two sources in the United States. Information on orders or reimbursement assistance may be obtained from either Accredo Health, Inc (1-866-344-4874) or CVS Caremark (1-877-242-2738).

Pregnancy Risk Factor B

Pregnancy Considerations Adverse events have not been observed in animal reproduction studies. Women with PAH are encouraged to avoid pregnancy (McLaughlin 2009).

Breast-Feeding Considerations It is not known if epoprostenol is excreted in breast milk. Due to the potential for serious adverse reactions in the nursing infant, the manufacturer of Flolan recommends a decision be made whether to discontinue nursing or to discontinue the drug, taking into account the importance of treatment to the mother. The manufacturer of Veletri recommends that caution be exercised when administering epoprostenol to nursing women.

Contraindications Hypersensitivity to epoprostenol, to structurally-related compounds; or any component of the formulationFlolan: Additional contraindications: Heart failure caused by reduced left ventricular ejection fractionVeletri: Additional contraindications: Chronic use in patients with heart failure due to severe left ventricular systolic dysfunction; chronic use patients who develop pulmonary edema during dose initiation

Warnings/Precautions Epoprostenol is a potent pulmonary and systemic vasodilator and can cause hypotension and other reactions such as flushing, nausea, vomiting, dizziness, and headache. Monitor blood pressure and symptoms regularly during initiation and after dose change. Initiation or transition to epoprostenol requires specialized cardiopulmonary monitoring in a critical care setting where clinicians are experienced in advanced management of pulmonary arterial hypertension. To reduce the risk of thromboembolism during chronic use, anticoagulants should be coadministered unless contraindicated. Avoid abrupt interruptions or large sudden reductions in dosage; may result in rebound pulmonary hypertension (eg, dyspnea, dizziness, asthenia). A fatal case occurred following interruption; immediate access to medication or pump and infusion sets is essential to prevent treatment interruptions. Some patients with PAH have developed pulmonary edema during dosing adjustment and acute vasodilator testing (an off-label use), which may be associated with concomitant heart failure (LV systolic dysfunction with significantly elevated left heart filling pressures) or pulmonary veno-occlusive disease/ pulmonary capillary hemangiomatosis. If pulmonary edema develops during therapy initiation, discontinue and do not readminister. Epoprostenol is a potent inhibitor of platelet aggregation; use with caution in patients with other risk factors for bleeding. Chronic continuous IV infusion of epoprostenol via a chronic indwelling central venous catheter (CVC) has been associated with local infections and serious blood stream infections.

Warnings: Additional Pediatric Considerations Although the use of anticoagulants in adult patients with primary pulmonary hypertension has been shown to improve survival, such efficacy has not been demonstrated in pediatric patients. Some studies have reported the routine use of warfarin in pediatric patients receiving long-term (chronic) infusions of epoprostenol for pulmonary hypertension (Barst, 1999; Rosenzweig, 1999), while other studies have routinely discontinued anticoagulants prior to the initiation of epoprostenol therapy (Higenbottam, 1993). Epoprostenol is a potent inhibitor of platelet aggregation; monitor patients for bleeding, especially those with other risk factors or medications which may increase the risk for hemorrhage. Further studies are needed to assess the risks and benefits of routine anticoagulation in pediatric patients treated with epoprostenol.

Adverse Reactions Note: Adverse events reported during dose initiation and escalation include flushing, headache, nausea/vomiting, hypotension, anxiety/nervousness/ agitation, chest pain; dizziness, abdominal pain, bradycardia, musculoskeletal pain, dyspnea, back pain, diaphoresis, dyspepsia, hypoesthesia/paresthesia, and tachycardia are also reported. Although some adverse reactions may be related to the underlying disease state, abdominal pain, anxiety/nervousness/agitation, arthralgia, bleeding, bradycardia, diarrhea, diaphoresis, flu-like syndrome, flushing, headache, hypotension, jaw pain, nausea, pain, pulmonary edema, rash, tachycardia, thrombocytopenia, and vomiting are clearly contributed to epoprostenol. The following adverse events have been reported during chronic administration for idiopathic or heritable PAH:

Cardiovascular: Flushing, hypotension, tachycardia

Central nervous system: Agitation, anxiety, chills, dizziness, fever, flu-like syndrome, headache, nervousness, sepsis, tremor

Dermatologic: Dermal ulcer, eczema, skin rash, urticaria

Gastrointestinal: Anorexia, diarrhea, nausea, vomiting

Local: Injection site reactions: Infection, pain

Neuromuscular & skeletal: Arthralgia, hyperesthesia, hypoesthesia, jaw pain, musculoskeletal pain, myalgia, neck pain, pain, paresthesia

Rare but important or life-threatening: Abdominal pain, anemia, ascites, dyspnea, fatigue, hemorrhage, hepatic failure, hyperthyroidism, pancytopenia, pulmonary edema, pulmonary embolism, splenomegaly, thrombocytopenia

Drug Interactions

Metabolism/Transport Effects None known.

Avoid Concomitant Use There are no known interactions where it is recommended to avoid concomitant use.

Increased Effect/Toxicity

Epoprostenol may increase the levels/effects of: Agents with Antiplatelet Properties; Anticoagulants; Antihypertensives; Digoxin

The levels/effects of Epoprostenol may be increased by: Thrombolytic Agents

Decreased Effect There are no known significant interactions involving a decrease in effect.

Storage/Stability

Flolan: Prior to use, store intact vials and diluent at 15°C to 25°C (59°F to 77°F); do not freeze. Protect from light. Following reconstitution, solution must be stored at 2°C to 8°C (36°F to 46°F) if not used immediately; do not freeze. Protect from light. Storage and administration limits for reconstituted solution are dependent on type of diluent use during reconstitution:

Sterile diluent for Flolan: When used at 15°C to 25°C (59°F to 77°F), reconstituted solutions are stable for up to 8 hours following reconstitution or removal from refrigerator. May also be stored for up to 40 hours at 2°C to 8°C (36°F to 46°F) before use. When used with a cold pack, reconstituted solutions are stable for up to 24 hours; may also be stored at 2°C to 8°C (36°F to 46°F) before use as long as the total time of refrigerated storage and infusion does not exceed 48 hours. Change cold packs every 12 hours.

pH 12 sterile diluent for Flolan: Freshly prepared reconstituted solutions or reconstituted solutions that have been stored at 2°C to 8°C (36°F to 46°F) for no longer than 8 days can be administered up to 72 hours at up to 25°C (77°F); 48 hours at up to 30°C (86°F); 24 hours at up to 35°C (95°F); 12 hours at up to 40°C (104°F).

Veletri: Prior to use, store intact vials at 20°C to 25°C (68°F to 77°F); do not freeze. Protect from light. Reconstituted vials must be further diluted prior to use.

Caripul [Canadian product]: Prior to use, store intact vials at 15°C to 30°C (59°F to 86°F); do not freeze. Reconstituted vials must be further diluted prior to use.

Reconstituted solutions of Veletri or Caripul immediately diluted to a final concentration within a drug delivery reservoir may be administered immediately or stored at 2°C to 8°C (36°F to 46°F) for up to 8 days; do not freeze. Protect from light.

If administered immediately, the following maximum durations of administration at room temperature (25°C [77°F]) according to solution concentration are recommended:

U.S. labeling (Veletri):

3000 to <15,000 ng/mL: 48 hours

15,000 to <60,000 ng/mL: 48 hours

≥60,000 ng/mL: 72 hours

Canadian labeling (Caripul):

3000 to <15,000 ng/mL: 48 hours

≥15,000: 48 hours

If stored at 2°C to 8°C (36°F to 46°F) for up to 8 days, the following maximum durations of administration at room temperature (25°C [77°F]) according to solution concentration are recommended:

3000 to <15,000 ng/mL: 24 hours

15,000 to <60,000 ng/mL: 48 hours

≥60,000 ng/mL: 48 hours

Short excursions at 40°C (104°F) are permitted as follows:

Solution concentration <15,000 ng/mL: Up to 2 hours

Solution concentration 15,000 to <60,000 ng/mL: Up to 4 hours

Solution concentration ≥60,000 ng/mL: Up to 8 hours

The following maximum durations of administration at temperatures >25°C to 40°C (>77°F up to 104°F) administered either immediately or after up to 8 days storage at 2°C to 8°C (36°F to 46°F) according to solution concentration are recommended:

Use at temperature >25°C to 30°C (>77°F up to 86°F):

U.S. labeling (Veletri):

<60,000 ng/mL: 24 hours

≥60,000 ng/mL: 48 hours

Canadian labeling (Caripul): All concentrations: 24 hours

Use at temperature up to 40°C (104°F):

U.S. labeling (Veletri): ≥60,000 ng/mL: 24 hours (immediately administered after preparation)

Mechanism of Action Epoprostenol is also known as prostacyclin and PGI_2. It is a strong vasodilator of all vascular beds. In addition, it is a potent endogenous inhibitor of platelet aggregation. The reduction in platelet aggregation results from epoprostenol's activation of intracellular adenylate cyclase and the resultant increase in cyclic adenosine monophosphate concentrations within the platelets. Additionally, it is capable of decreasing thrombogenesis and platelet clumping in the lungs by inhibiting platelet aggregation.

Pharmacokinetics (Adult data unless noted)

Metabolism: Rapidly hydrolyzed at a neutral pH in blood; also metabolized by enzymatic degradation; two primary metabolites with pharmacologic activity less than epoprostenol are formed: 6-keto-PGF_{1alpha} (via spontaneous degradation) and 6,15-diketo-13,14-dihydro-PGF_{1alpha} (via enzymatic degradation); 14 minor metabolites have also been isolated in the urine

Half-life: ≤6 minutes

Elimination: Urine (84% of dose); feces (4%)

Dosing: Neonatal Note: Doses are expressed in units of **nanograms** (ng)/kg/minute.

Pulmonary hypertension: Very limited data available; efficacy results variable. **Note:** Avoid abrupt withdrawal or sudden large dose reductions when discontinuing therapy to prevent rebound pulmonary hypertension.

Continuous IV infusion:

Low-dose regimen: Initial: 2 ng/kg/minute slowly titrated to 20 ng/kg/minute over ~3 hours was described in a single case report; epoprostenol was used in a full-term neonate (PNA: 72 hours) for PPHN refractory to inhaled nitric oxide and showed initial improvement in oxygenation index (Golzand 2005)

High-dose regimen: Initial: 20 ng/kg/minute, slowly titrated (according to oxygenation) at 30-minute intervals over 4 to 12 hours to a mean dose of 60 ng/kg/minute (range: 30 to 120 ng/kg/minute) and continued for a mean of 5.3 days (range: 3 to 10.5 days) was used in an open-label trial of eight neonates (GA: 34 to 42 weeks; PNA: 3 to 32 hours) with PPHN (excluding CHD and congenital diaphragmatic hernia) (Eronen 1997)

Dosing: Usual Note: Doses are expressed in units of **nanograms** (ng)/kg/minute.

Pulmonary hypertension: Infants, Children, Adolescents, and Adults: Continuous IV infusion:

Initial: 1 to 2 ng/kg/minute, increase dose in increments of 1 to 2 ng/kg/minute every 15 minutes or longer until dose-limiting side effects are noted or tolerance limit to epoprostenol is observed

Dose adjustment:

Increase dose: 1 to 2 ng/kg/minute increments at intervals of at least 15 minutes if symptoms of pulmonary hypertension persist or recur following improvement. In clinical trials, dosing increases occurred at intervals of 24 to 48 hours or longer.

Decrease dose: 2 ng/kg/minute decrements at intervals of at least 15 minutes in case of dose-limiting pharmacologic (adverse) events. Avoid abrupt withdrawal or sudden large dose reductions.

Chronic dosing: The need for increased doses should be expected with chronic use; incremental increases occur more frequently during the first few months after the drug is initiated. The optimal dose in children is not well defined. The mean chronic dose at 1 year of therapy is 20 to 40 ng/kg/minute in adults, but is 50-80 ng/kg/minute in children (particularly younger children); significant variability in optimal dose occurs in pediatric patients (Barst 1999; Rosenweig 1999; Widlitz 2003).

Preparation for Administration

Flolan: Reconstitute with the manufacturer-supplied sterile diluent only (see Preparation of Epoprostenol Infusion table on next page). The final volume (usually 100 mL) is a 24-hour supply and may be divided into 3 equal parts (ie, three 8-hour infusion aliquots); one portion to be administered at present and the two other portions should be stored in the refrigerator until time of administration.

Veletri: Reconstitute with SWFI or NS (see Preparation of Epoprostenol Infusion table below). Reconstituted solutions immediately diluted to a final concentration within a drug delivery reservoir may be administered immediately or stored at 2°C to 8°C (36°F to 46°F) for up to 8 days; maximum infusion duration is dependent on concentration and time to initiation of therapy (see Storage/Stability).

Preparation of Epoprostenol Infusion

To make solution with concentration:	Flolan Instructions	Veletri Instructions
	Note: Flolan may only be prepared with sterile diluent provided.	**Note:** Veletri may only be prepared with sterile water for injection (SWFI) or NS.
3,000 ng/mL	Dissolve one 0.5 mg vial with 5 mL supplied diluent, withdraw 3 mL, and add to a sufficient volume of supplied diluent to make a total of 100 mL.	Dissolve one 0.5 mg vial with 5 mL of SWFI or NS, withdraw 3 mL, and add to a sufficient volume of the identical diluent to make a total of 100 mL.
5,000 ng/mL	Dissolve one 0.5 mg vial with 5 mL supplied diluent, withdraw entire vial contents, and add to a sufficient volume of supplied diluent to make a total of 100 mL.	Dissolve one 0.5 mg vial with 5 mL of SWFI or NS, withdraw entire vial contents, and add to a sufficient volume of the identical diluent to make a total of 100 mL.
10,000 ng/mL	Dissolve two 0.5 mg vials each with 5 mL supplied diluent, withdraw entire vial contents, and add to a sufficient volume of supplied diluent to make a total of 100 mL.	Dissolve two 0.5 mg vials each with 5 mL of SWFI or NS, withdraw entire vial contents, and add to a sufficient volume of the identical diluent to make a total of 100 mL.
15,000 ng/mL	Dissolve one 1.5 mg vial with 5 mL supplied diluent, withdraw entire vial contents, and add to a sufficient volume of supplied diluent to make a total of 100 mL.	Dissolve one 1.5 mg vial with 5 mL of SWFI or NS, withdraw entire vial contents, and add to a sufficient volume of the identical diluent to make a total of 100 mL.
20,000 ng/mL	Dissolve two 0.5 mg vials each with 5 mL supplied diluent, withdraw entire vial contents, and add to a sufficient volume of supplied diluent to make a total of **50 mL** (DeWet, 2004).	
30,000 ng/mL		Dissolve two 1.5 mg vials each with 5 mL of SWFI or NS, withdraw entire vial contents, and add to a sufficient volume of the identical diluent to make a total of 100 mL.

Administration Continuous IV infusion: Administer through a central venous catheter; peripheral infusion may be used temporarily until central line is established. Epoprostenol should be infused using an infusion pump through a dedicated lumen exclusive of any other drugs; consider a multilumen catheter if other IV medications are routinely administered. Use infusion sets with an in-line 0.22 micron filter for Veletri infusions. Flolan labeling does not specifically recommend filtering; however, the use of an in-line 0.22 micron filter was used during clinical trials. Avoid abrupt withdrawal, interruptions in delivery, or sudden large reductions in dosing. Patients should have access to a backup infusion pump and infusion sets. Patients may be discharged using an ambulatory infusion pump. Appropriate ambulatory infusion pump should be small and lightweight; be able to adjust infusion rates in 2 ng/kg/minute increments; have occlusion, end of infusion, and low battery alarms; have ± 6% accuracy of the programmed rate; and be positive continuous or pulsatile pressure-driven with intervals ≤3 minutes between pulses. The reservoir should be made of polypropylene, polyvinyl chloride, or glass. Immediate access to back up pump, infusion sets and medication is essential to prevent treatment interruptions.

Monitoring Parameters Hemodynamic effects (pulmonary vascular resistance, pulmonary arterial pressure, systemic blood pressure, heart rate). Monitor blood pressure (standing and supine) and heart rate closely for several hours following dosage adjustments. Monitor for improvements in exercise capacity, exertional dyspnea, fatigue, syncope, chest pain, and quality of life. Monitor the infusion pump device and catheters to avoid drug delivery system related failures. Monitor weight; serum potassium.

Additional Information The primary role of epoprostenol is in the treatment of primary pulmonary hypertension in patients unresponsive to other therapy. Response to initial therapy is evaluated in a controlled setting before chronic therapy is administered. The role of epoprostenol in the treatment of heart failure confers a negative impact on cardiovascular morbidity and mortality. Clinical trials in adults showed improvement of heart failure symptoms and exercise tolerance, but an increase in mortality.

Dosage Forms Excipient information presented when available (limited, particularly for generics); consult specific product labeling.

Solution Reconstituted, Intravenous:
- Flolan: 0.5 mg (1 ea); 1.5 mg (1 ea)
- Veletri: 0.5 mg (1 ea); 1.5 mg (1 ea)
- Generic: 0.5 mg (1 ea); 1.5 mg (1 ea)

- ◆ **Epoprostenol Sodium** *see* Epoprostenol *on page 769*
- ◆ **Eprex (Can)** *see* Epoetin Alfa *on page 765*
- ◆ **Epsilon Aminocaproic Acid** *see* Aminocaproic Acid *on page 121*
- ◆ **Epsom Salt [OTC]** *see* Magnesium Sulfate *on page 1317*
- ◆ **Epsom Salts** *see* Magnesium Sulfate *on page 1317*
- ◆ **EPT** *see* Teniposide *on page 2015*
- ◆ **Eptacog Alfa (Activated)** *see* Factor VIIa (Recombinant) *on page 835*
- ◆ **Epuris (Can)** *see* ISOtretinoin *on page 1171*
- ◆ **Epzicom** *see* Abacavir and Lamivudine *on page 36*
- ◆ **Equalizer Gas Relief [OTC]** *see* Simethicone *on page 1927*
- ◆ **Equetro** *see* CarBAMazepine *on page 367*
- ◆ **Equipto-Baclofen** *see* Baclofen *on page 254*
- ◆ **Equipto-Naproxen** *see* Naproxen *on page 1489*
- ◆ **Erdol (Can)** *see* Ergocalciferol *on page 772*

Ergocalciferol (er goe kal SIF e role)

Medication Safety Issues

Sound-alike/look-alike issues:

Calciferol may be confused with calcitriol

Drisdol may be confused with Drysol

Ergocalciferol may be confused with alfacalcidol, cholecalciferol

Administration issues:

Liquid vitamin D preparations have the potential for dosing errors when administered to infants. Droppers should be clearly marked to easily provide 400 international units. For products intended for infants, the FDA recommends that accompanying droppers deliver no more than 400 international units per dose.

Related Information

Oral Medications That Should Not Be Crushed or Altered *on page 2476*

Brand Names: US Calcidol [OTC]; Calciferol [OTC]; Drisdol; Drisdol [OTC]

Brand Names: Canada D-Forte; Erdol

Therapeutic Category Nutritional Supplement; Vitamin D Analog; Vitamin, Fat Soluble

Generic Availability (US) Yes

Use Prevention and treatment of vitamin D deficiency and/or rickets or osteomalacia (FDA approved in all ages); treatment of familial hypophosphatemia; treatment of hypoparathyroidism; prevention and treatment of vitamin D deficiency and insufficiency in patients with chronic kidney disease (CKD); dietary supplement

Pregnancy Risk Factor C

Pregnancy Considerations

Adverse events were observed in some animal reproduction studies. The ergocalciferol (vitamin D_2) metabolite, 25 (OH)D, crosses the placenta; maternal serum concentrations correlate with fetal concentrations at birth (Misra, 2008; Wagner, 2008).

Vitamin D deficiency in a pregnant woman may lead to a vitamin D deficiency in the neonate (Misra, 2008; Wagner, 2008). Serum 25(OH)D concentrations should be measured in pregnant women considered to be at increased risk of deficiency (ACOG, 2011). The amount of vitamin D contained in prenatal vitamins may not be adequate to treat a deficiency during pregnancy; although larger doses may be needed, current guidelines recommend a total of 1000 to 2000 units/day until more safety data is available (ACOG, 2011; Holick, 2011). In women not at risk for deficiency, doses larger than the RDA should be avoided during pregnancy (ACOG, 2011).

Breast-Feeding Considerations

The 25(OH)D metabolite can be detected in breast milk. The manufacturer recommends that caution be used if ergocalciferol is administered to nursing women. Hypercalcemia has been noted in a breast-feeding infant following maternal use of large amounts of vitamin D; calcium serum concentrations should be monitored in nursing infants exposed to large doses.

Small quantities of vitamin D are found in breast milk following normal maternal exposure via sunlight and diet. The amount in breast milk does not correlate with serum levels in the infant and the vitamin D content of human milk is not enough to meet the recommended intake for a nursing infant. Therefore, vitamin D supplementation is recommended in all infants who are partially or exclusively breast fed (Misra, 2008; Wagner, 2008).

Contraindications

Hypercalcemia; malabsorption syndrome; abnormal sensitivity to the toxic effects of vitamin D; hypervitaminosis D

Documentation of allergenic cross-reactivity for drugs in this class is limited. However, because of similarities in chemical structure and/or pharmacologic actions, the possibility of cross-sensitivity can not be ruled out with certainty.

Warnings/Precautions Normal serum phosphorous concentrations must be maintained in patients treated for hyperphosphatemia to prevent metastatic calcification. Concomitant treatment with intravenous calcium, parathyroid hormone, and/or dihydrotachysterol may also be required when treating hypoparathyroidism. Adults with a BMI >30 kg/m^2 are at high risk for vitamin D deficiency due to storage of vitamin D in adipose tissue. Doses higher than the RDA may be required, but must be carefully monitored to avoid toxicity (Holick, 2011). Metabolism of vitamin D may be altered in patients with chronic kidney disease. Supplementation with ergocalciferol may be needed; close monitoring is required (KDOQI, 2003).The range between therapeutic and toxic doses is narrow in vitamin D-resistant rickets; adjust dose based on clinical response to avoid toxicity. Potentially significant drug-drug interactions may exist, requiring dose or frequency adjustment, additional monitoring, and/or selection of alternative therapy.

Oral solutions may contain propylene glycol; toxicities may occur if large doses of vitamin D are required. Alternate dosage forms/products should be used (Misra, 2008). Products may contain tartrazine, which may cause allergic reactions in certain individuals.

Adequate calcium supplementation is required; calcium and phosphorous levels must be monitored during therapy. All sources of vitamin D (eg, dietary supplements, fortified foods, medication) should be evaluated. Effects of vitamin D toxicity can last ≥2 months after therapy is discontinued.

Warnings: Additional Pediatric Considerations Some dosage forms may contain propylene glycol; in neonates large amounts of propylene glycol delivered orally, intravenously (eg, >3,000 mg/day), or topically have been associated with potentially fatal toxicities which can include metabolic acidosis, seizures, renal failure, and CNS depression; toxicities have also been reported in children and adults including hyperosmolality, lactic acidosis, seizures, and respiratory depression; use caution (AAP, 1997; Shehab, 2009).

Adverse Reactions Endocrine & metabolic: Hypervitaminosis D (signs and symptoms include hypercalcemia, resulting in headache, nausea, vomiting, lethargy, confusion, sluggishness, abdominal pain, bone pain, polyuria, polydipsia, weakness, cardiac arrhythmias [eg, QT shortening, sinus tachycardia], soft tissue calcification, calciuria, and nephrocalcinosis)

Drug Interactions

Metabolism/Transport Effects None known.

Avoid Concomitant Use

Avoid concomitant use of Ergocalciferol with any of the following: Aluminum Hydroxide; Multivitamins/Fluoride (with ADE); Multivitamins/Minerals (with ADEK, Folate, Iron); Sucralfate; Vitamin D Analogs

Increased Effect/Toxicity

Ergocalciferol may increase the levels/effects of: Aluminum Hydroxide; Cardiac Glycosides; Sucralfate; Vitamin D Analogs

The levels/effects of Ergocalciferol may be increased by: Calcium Salts; Danazol; Multivitamins/Fluoride (with ADE); Multivitamins/Minerals (with ADEK, Folate, Iron); Thiazide Diuretics

Decreased Effect

The levels/effects of Ergocalciferol may be decreased by: Bile Acid Sequestrants; Mineral Oil; Orlistat

Storage/Stability Store at 15°C to 30°C (59°F to 86°F). Protect from light.

Mechanism of Action Ergocalciferol (vitamin D_2) is a provitamin. The active metabolite, 1,25-dihydroxyvitamin D (calcitriol), stimulates calcium and phosphate absorption from the small intestine, promotes secretion of calcium from bone to blood; promotes renal tubule phosphate resorption.

Pharmacodynamics Maximum effect occurs in ~1 month following daily doses

Pharmacokinetics (Adult data unless noted)

Absorption: Readily absorbed from GI tract; absorption requires intestinal presence of bile

Metabolism: Inactive until hydroxylated in the liver and the kidney to calcifediol and then to calcitriol (most active form)

Dosing: Neonatal Note: 1 mcg = 40 USP units

Adequate Intake (AI): Oral: 10 mcg/day (400 units)

Prevention of Vitamin D deficiency (Greer, 2000; Wagner, 2008): Oral:
Premature neonates: 10-20 mcg/day (400-800 units), up to 750 mcg/day (30,000 units)
Breast-fed neonates (fully or partially): 10 mcg/day (400 units/day) beginning in the first few days of life. Continue supplementation until infant is weaned to ≥1000 mL/day or 1 qt/day of vitamin D-fortified formula (after 12 months of age)
Formula-fed neonates ingesting <1000 mL of vitamin D-fortified formula: 10 mcg/day (400 units/day)

Vitamin D-dependent rickets: In addition to calcium supplementation: Oral: 25 mcg/day (1000 units) for 2-3 months; once radiologic evidence of healing is observed, dose should be decreased to 10 mcg/day (400 units/day)

Dosing: Usual Note: 1 mcg = 40 USP units

Infants, Children, and Adolescents:

Adequate Intake (AI): Oral: Infants: 10 mcg/day (400 units)

Recommended Daily Allowance (RDA): Oral: Children and Adolescents: 15 mcg/day (600 units)

Prevention of Vitamin D Deficiency (Greer, 2000; Wagner, 2008): Oral:
Breast-fed infants (fully or partially): 10 mcg/day (400 units/day) beginning in the first few days of life. Continue supplementation until infant is weaned to ≥1000 mL/day or 1 qt/day of vitamin D-fortified formula or whole milk (after 12 months of age)
Formula-fed infants ingesting <1000 mL of vitamin D-fortified formula or milk: 10 mcg/day (400 units/day)
Children ingesting <1000 mL of vitamin D-fortified milk: 10 mcg/day (400 units/day)
Children with increased risk of vitamin D deficiency (chronic fat malabsorption, maintained on chronic antiseizure medications): Higher doses may be required. Use laboratory testing [25(OH)D, PTH, bone mineral status] to evaluate.
Adolescents without adequate intake: 10 mcg/day (400 units/day)

Vitamin D insufficiency or deficiency associated with CKD (stages 2-5, 5D); serum 25 hydroxyvitamin D (25[OH]D) level <30 ng/mL: (K/DOQI Guidelines, 2009): Oral:
Serum 25(OH)D level 16-30 ng/mL: Children: 2000 units/day for 3 months or 50,000 units every month for 3 months
Serum 25(OH)D level 5-15 ng/mL: Children: 4000 units/day for 12 weeks or 50,000 units every other week for 12 weeks
Serum 25(OH)D level <5 ng/mL: Children: 8000 units/day for 4 weeks then 4000 units/day for 2 months for total therapy of 3 months or 50,000 units/week for 4 weeks followed by 50,000 units 2 times/month for a total therapy of 3 months
Maintenance dose [once repletion accomplished; serum 25(OH)D level >30 ng/mL]: 200-1000 units/day
Dosage adjustment: Monitor 25(OH)D, corrected total calcium and phosphorus levels 1 month following initiation of therapy, every 3 months during therapy and with any Vitamin D dose change.

Hypoparathyroidism: Oral: Children: 1.25-5 mg/day (50,000-200,000 units) with calcium supplements

Vitamin D-dependent rickets: Oral: **Note:** In addition to calcium supplementation:
Infants 1-12 months: 25-125 mcg/day (1000-5000 units) for 2-3 months; once radiologic evidence of healing is observed, dose should be decreased to 10 mcg/day (400 units/day)
Children >12 months: 125-250 mcg/day (5000-10,000 units) for 2-3 months; once radiologic evidence of healing is observed, dose should be decreased to 10 mcg/day (400 units/day)

Prevention and treatment vitamin D Deficiency in cystic fibrosis: Oral: Recommended daily intake (Borowitz 2002):
Infants <1 year: 400 units/day
Children >1 year: 400-800 units/day

Nutritional rickets and osteomalacia: Oral:
Children with normal absorption: 25-125 mcg/day (1000-5000 units) for 6-12 weeks
Children with malabsorption: 250-625 mcg/day (10,000-25,000 units)

Familial hypophosphatemia: Oral: Children: Initial: 1000-2000 mcg/day (40,000-80,000 units) with phosphate supplements; daily dosage is increased at 3- to 4-month intervals in 250-500 mcg (10,000-20,000 units) increments

Adults:

Dietary Reference Intake for Vitamin D: Oral:
Adults 19-70 years: RDA: 600 units/day
Female: Pregnancy/lactating: RDA: 600 units/day

Vitamin D deficiency treatment: Oral: 50,000 units once per week for 8 weeks, followed by 50,000 units every 2-4 weeks thereafter for maintenance of adequate levels (Holick, 2007) **or** 50,000 units twice per week for 5 weeks (Stechschulte, 2009)

Vitamin D deficiency/insufficiency in patients with CKD stages 3-4 (K/DOQI guidelines): Oral: Dose is based on 25-hydroxyvitamin D serum level [25(OH) D]: Treatment duration should be a total of 6 months:
Serum 25(OH)D 16-30 ng/mL: 50,000 units/month
Serum 25(OH)D 5-15 ng/mL: 50,000 units/week for 4 weeks, then 50,000 units/month
Serum 25(OH)D <5 ng/mL: 50,000 units/week for 12 weeks, then 50,000 units/month

Hypoparathyroidism: Oral: 625 mcg to 5 mg/day (25,000-200,000 units) and calcium supplements

Nutritional rickets and osteomalacia: Oral:
Adults with normal absorption: 25-125 mcg/day (1000-5000 units)
Adults with malabsorption: 250-7500 mcg (10,000-300,000 units)

Vitamin D-dependent rickets: Oral: 250 mcg to 1.5 mg/day (10,000-60,000 units)

Vitamin D-resistant rickets: Oral: 12,000-500,000 units/day

Familial hypophosphatemia: Oral: 10,000-60,000 units plus phosphate supplements

Administration Oral: May be administered without regard to meals; for oral liquid, use accompanying dropper for dosage measurements

Monitoring Parameters Children at increased risk of vitamin D deficiency (chronic fat malabsorption, chronic antiseizure medication use) require serum 25(OH)D, PTH, and bone-mineral status to evaluate. If vitamin D supplement is required, then 25(OH)D levels should be repeated at 3-month intervals until normal. PTH and bone mineral-status should be monitored every 6 months until normal.

Chronic kidney disease: Serum calcium and phosphorus levels (in CKD: After 1 month and then at least every 3 months); alkaline phosphatase, BUN; bone x-ray (hypophosphatemia or hypoparathyroidism); 25(OH)D (in CKD: After 3 months of treatment and as needed thereafter)

Reference Range Vitamin D status may be determined by serum 25(OH) D levels (Misra, 2008):
Severe deficiency: ≤5 ng/mL (12.5 nmol/L)
Deficiency: 15 ng/mL (37.5 nmol/L)
Insufficiency: 15-20 ng/mL (37.5-50 nmol/L)
Sufficiency: 20-100 ng/mL (50-250 nmol/L)*
Excess: >100 ng/mL (250 nmol/L)**
Intoxication: 150 ng/mL (375 nmol/L)
*Based on adult data a level of >32 ng/mL (80 nmol/L) is desirable
**Arbitrary designation

Target serum 25(OH) D: >30 ng/mL

Additional Information 1.25 mg ergocalciferol provides 50,000 units of vitamin D activity; 1 drop of 8000 units/mL = 200 units (40 drops = 1 mL)

Chronic kidney disease (CKD) (KDIGO, 2013; KDOQI, 2002): Children ≥2 years, Adolescents, and Adults: GFR <60 mL/minute/1.73 m^2 or kidney damage for ≥3 months; stages of CKD are described below:

CKD Stage 1: Kidney damage with normal or increased GFR; GFR >90 mL/minute/1.73 m^2

CKD Stage 2: Kidney damage with mild decrease in GFR; GFR 60-89 mL/minute/1.73 m^2

CKD Stage 3: Moderate decrease in GFR; GFR 30-59 mL/minute/1.73 m^2

CKD Stage 4: Severe decrease in GFR; GFR 15-29 mL/minute/1.73 m^2

CKD Stage 5: Kidney failure; GFR <15 mL/minute/1.73 m^2 or dialysis

Dosage Forms Excipient information presented when available (limited, particularly for generics); consult specific product labeling.

Capsule, Oral:

Drisdol: 50,000 units [contains brilliant blue fcf (fd&c blue #1), soybean oil, tartrazine (fd&c yellow #5)]

Generic: 50,000 units

Solution, Oral:

Calcidol: 8000 units/mL (60 mL) [contains propylene glycol]

Calciferol: 8000 units/mL (60 mL) [contains propylene glycol]

Drisdol: 8000 units/mL (60 mL) [contains propylene glycol]

Generic: 8000 units/mL (60 mL)

Tablet, Oral:

Generic: 400 units, 2000 units

◆ **Ergomar** *see* Ergotamine *on page 775*

Ergotamine (er GOT a meen)

Related Information

Oral Medications That Should Not Be Crushed or Altered *on page 2476*

Brand Names: US Ergomar

Therapeutic Category Alpha-Adrenergic Blocking Agent, Oral; Antimigraine Agent; Ergot Alkaloid

Generic Availability (US) No

Use Prevent or abort vascular headaches, such as migraine and migraine variants also known as "histaminic cephalalgia"

Pregnancy Risk Factor X

Pregnancy Considerations May cause prolonged constriction of the uterine vessels and/or increased myometrial tone leading to reduced placental blood flow. This has contributed to fetal growth retardation in animals.

Breast-Feeding Considerations Ergotamine is excreted in breast milk and may cause vomiting, diarrhea, weak pulse, and unstable blood pressure in the nursing infant. Consider discontinuing the drug or discontinuing nursing.

Contraindications Hypersensitivity to ergotamine or any component of the formulation; peripheral vascular disease; hepatic or renal impairment; coronary artery disease; hypertension; sepsis; ergot alkaloids are contraindicated with strong inhibitors of CYP3A4 (includes protease inhibitors, azole antifungals, and some macrolide antibiotics); pregnancy

Warnings/Precautions Ergot alkaloids have been associated with fibrotic valve thickening (eg, aortic, mitral, tricuspid); usually associated with long-term, chronic use; vasospasm or vasoconstriction can occur; ergot alkaloid use may result in ergotism (intense vasoconstriction) resulting in peripheral vascular ischemia and possible gangrene; rare cases of pleural and/or retroperitoneal fibrosis have been reported with prolonged daily use. Discontinuation after extended use may result in withdrawal symptoms (eg, rebound headache). Avoid use in the elderly.

[U.S. Boxed Warning]: Ergot alkaloids are contraindicated with potent inhibitors of CYP3A4 (includes protease inhibitors, azole antifungals, and some macrolide antibiotics); concomitant use associated with acute ergot toxicity (ergotism).

Adverse Reactions

Cardiovascular: Absence of pulse, bradycardia, cardiac valvular fibrosis, cyanosis, ECG changes, edema, gangrene, hypertension, ischemia, precordial distress and pain, tachycardia, vasospasm

Central nervous system: Vertigo

Dermatologic: Itching

Gastrointestinal: Nausea, vomiting

Genitourinary: Retroperitoneal fibrosis

Neuromuscular & skeletal: Muscle pain, numbness, paresthesia, weakness

Respiratory: Pleuropulmonary fibrosis

Miscellaneous: Cold extremities

Drug Interactions

Metabolism/Transport Effects Substrate of CYP3A4 (major); **Note:** Assignment of Major/Minor substrate status based on clinically relevant drug interaction potential

Avoid Concomitant Use

Avoid concomitant use of Ergotamine with any of the following: Alpha-/Beta-Agonists; Alpha1-Agonists; Boceprevir; Clarithromycin; Cobicistat; Conivaptan; Crizotinib; Dapoxetine; Enzalutamide; Fusidic Acid (Systemic); Idelalisib; Itraconazole; Ketoconazole (Systemic); Lorcaserin; Mifepristone; Nitroglycerin; Posaconazole; Protease Inhibitors; Serotonin 5-HT1D Receptor Agonists; Telaprevir; Voriconazole

Increased Effect/Toxicity

Ergotamine may increase the levels/effects of: Alpha-/Beta-Agonists; Alpha1-Agonists; Antipsychotic Agents; Metoclopramide; Serotonin 5-HT1D Receptor Agonists; Serotonin Modulators

The levels/effects of Ergotamine may be increased by: Antiemetics (5HT3 Antagonists); Antipsychotic Agents; Aprepitant; Beta-Blockers; Boceprevir; Clarithromycin; Cobicistat; Conivaptan; Crizotinib; CYP3A4 Inhibitors (Moderate); CYP3A4 Inhibitors (Strong); Dapoxetine; Dasatinib; Fosaprepitant; Fusidic Acid (Systemic); Idelalisib; Itraconazole; Ivacaftor; Ketoconazole (Systemic); Lorcaserin; Luliconazole; Macrolide Antibiotics; Mifepristone; Netupitant; Nitroglycerin; Palbociclib; Posaconazole; Protease Inhibitors; Serotonin 5-HT1D Receptor Agonists; Simeprevir; Stiripentol; Tedizolid; Telaprevir; Voriconazole

Decreased Effect

Ergotamine may decrease the levels/effects of: Nitroglycerin

The levels/effects of Ergotamine may be decreased by: Enzalutamide

Food Interactions Grapefruit juice may cause increased blood levels of ergotamine, leading to increased toxicity. Management: Avoid grapefruit juice.

Storage/Stability Store at 20°C to 25°C (68°F to 77°F); excursions permitted to 15°C to 30°C (59°F to 86°F). Protect from heat and light.

Mechanism of Action Has partial agonist and/or antagonist activity against tryptaminergic, dopaminergic and alpha-adrenergic receptors depending upon their site; is a highly active uterine stimulant; it causes constriction of peripheral and cranial blood vessels and produces depression of central vasomotor centers

Pharmacokinetics (Adult data unless noted)
Absorption: Oral, rectal: Erratic
Distribution: V_d: Adults: 1.85 L/kg
Metabolism: Extensive in the liver
Bioavailability: Poor overall (<5%)
Half-life: Adults: 2-2.5 hours
Time to peak serum concentration: Oral: Within 0.5-3 hours
Elimination: In bile as metabolites (90%)

Dosing: Usual Adolescents and Adults: **Note:** Not for chronic daily administration: Sublingual: 1 tablet under tongue at first sign, then 1 tablet every 30 minutes; maximum: 3 tablets/24 hours, 5 tablets/week

Administration Sublingual: Place tablet under the tongue; do not crush; may administer without regard to meals.

Dosage Forms Excipient information presented when available (limited, particularly for generics); consult specific product labeling.
Tablet Sublingual, Sublingual, as tartrate:
Ergomar: 2 mg [contains fd&c blue #1 aluminum lake, fd&c yellow #10 aluminum lake, saccharin sodium]

Ergotamine and Caffeine

(er GOT a meen & KAF een)

Medication Safety Issues
Sound-alike/look-alike issues:
Cafergot may be confused with Carafate

Brand Names: US Cafergot; Migergot

Brand Names: Canada Cafergor

Therapeutic Category Alpha-Adrenergic Blocking Agent, Oral; Antimigraine Agent; Ergot Alkaloid

Generic Availability (US) Yes: Tablet

Use Prevent or abort vascular headaches, such as migraine and migraine variants also known as "histaminic cephalalgia"

Pregnancy Risk Factor X

Pregnancy Considerations Animal reproduction studies have not been conducted with this combination. Ergotamine and caffeine both cross the placenta and may cause prolonged constriction of the uterine vessels and/or increased myometrial tone leading to reduced placental blood flow. Use is contraindicated in pregnant women.

Breast-Feeding Considerations Caffeine is excreted in breast milk and may cause adverse events in a nursing infant (Atkinson, 1988; Berlin, 1984). Ergotamine is excreted in breast milk and may cause vomiting, diarrhea, weak pulse, and unstable blood pressure in the nursing infant. Due to the potential for serious adverse reactions in the nursing infant, the manufacturer recommends a decision be made whether to discontinue nursing or to discontinue the drug, taking into account the importance of treatment to the mother.

Contraindications Hypersensitivity to ergotamine, caffeine, or any component of the formulation; peripheral vascular disease; hepatic or renal impairment; coronary heart disease; hypertension; sepsis; concomitant use of ergot alkaloids with strong inhibitors of CYP3A4 (includes protease inhibitors [indinavir, nelfinavir, ritonavir], azole antifungals [eg, ketoconazole, itraconazole], and some macrolide antibiotics [clarithromycin, erythromycin, troleandomycin]); pregnancy

Warnings/Precautions Ergot alkaloids have been associated (rarely) with fibrotic valve thickening (eg, aortic, mitral, tricuspid); usually associated with long-term, chronic use; vasospasm or vasoconstriction can occur possibly resulting in cyanosis, decreased cerebral blood flow, bradycardia or tachycardia, asystole and hypertension; sustained vasoconstriction may also lead to intermittent claudication, precordial distress and pain. Do not use is any patient at risk or predisposed to vascular effects of ergot alkaloids. Ergot alkaloid use may result in ergotism resulting in peripheral vascular ischemia and possible gangrene; rare cases of pleural and/or retroperitoneal fibrosis have been reported with prolonged daily use. Discontinuation after extended use may result in withdrawal symptoms (eg, rebound headache). Additional potentially significant drug-drug interactions may exist, requiring dose or frequency adjustment, additional monitoring, and/or selection of alternative therapy. Solitary rectal or anal ulcers have occurred rarely when suppositories are used in higher than recommended doses or with continual use of recommended doses for prolonged periods of time. After discontinuation, spontaneous healing occurs within 4 to 8 weeks. Avoid use in the elderly.

[U.S. Boxed Warning]: Ergot alkaloids are contraindicated with potent inhibitors of CYP3A4 (includes protease inhibitors and some macrolide antibiotics). Serum levels of ergotamines may be elevated, leading to increased risk of vasospasm leading to cerebral ischemia and or ischemia of extremities. Serious and/or life-threatening peripheral ischemia has been associated with concomitant use.

Adverse Reactions
Cardiovascular: Absence of pulse, bradycardia, cardiac valvular fibrosis, cyanosis, ECG changes, edema, gangrene, hypertension, ischemia, precordial distress and pain, tachycardia, vasospasm
Central nervous system: Vertigo
Dermatologic: Itching
Gastrointestinal: Anal or rectal ulcer (with overuse of suppository), nausea, vomiting
Genitourinary: Retroperitoneal fibrosis
Neuromuscular & skeletal: Muscle pain, numbness, paresthesia, weakness
Respiratory: Pleuropulmonary fibrosis
Miscellaneous: Cold extremities

Drug Interactions

Metabolism/Transport Effects Refer to individual components.

Avoid Concomitant Use
Avoid concomitant use of Ergotamine and Caffeine with any of the following: Alpha-/Beta-Agonists; Alpha1-Agonists; Boceprevir; Clarithromycin; Cobicistat; Conivaptan; Crizotinib; Dapoxetine; Enzalutamide; Fusidic Acid (Systemic); Idelalisib; Iobenguane I 123; Itraconazole; Ketoconazole (Systemic); Lorcaserin; Mifepristone; Nitroglycerin; Posaconazole; Protease Inhibitors; Serotonin 5-HT1D Receptor Agonists; Stiripentol; Telaprevir; Voriconazole

Increased Effect/Toxicity
Ergotamine and Caffeine may increase the levels/effects of: Alpha-/Beta-Agonists; Alpha1-Agonists; Antipsychotic Agents; Formoterol; Indacaterol; Metoclopramide; Olodaterol; Serotonin 5-HT1D Receptor Agonists; Serotonin Modulators; Sympathomimetics; TiZANidine

The levels/effects of Ergotamine and Caffeine may be increased by: Abiraterone Acetate; Antiemetics (5HT3 Antagonists); Antipsychotic Agents; Aprepitant; AtoMOXetine; Beta-Blockers; Boceprevir; Cannabinoid-Containing Products; Clarithromycin; Cobicistat; Conivaptan; Crizotinib; CYP1A2 Inhibitors (Moderate); CYP1A2 Inhibitors (Strong); CYP3A4 Inhibitors (Moderate); CYP3A4 Inhibitors (Strong); Dapoxetine; Dasatinib; Deferasirox; Fosaprepitant; Fusidic Acid (Systemic); Idelalisib; Itraconazole; Ivacaftor; Ketoconazole (Systemic); Linezolid; Lorcaserin; Luliconazole; Macrolide Antibiotics; Mifepristone; Netupitant; Nitroglycerin; Norfloxacin; Palbociclib; Peginterferon Alfa-2b; Posaconazole; Protease Inhibitors; Serotonin 5-HT1D Receptor Agonists; Simeprevir; Stiripentol; Tedizolid; Telaprevir; Vemurafenib; Voriconazole

Decreased Effect

Ergotamine and Caffeine may decrease the levels/effects of: Adenosine; Iobenguane I 123; Nitroglycerin; Regadenoson

The levels/effects of Ergotamine and Caffeine may be decreased by: Enzalutamide; Teriflunomide

Food Interactions See individual agents.

Storage/Stability

Suppositories: Store refrigerated at 2°C to 8°C (36°F to 46°F) in sealed foil.

Tablet: Store at 20°C to 25°C (68°F to 77°F). Protect from light.

Mechanism of Action Has partial agonist and/or antagonist activity against tryptaminergic, dopaminergic and alpha-adrenergic receptors depending upon their site; is a highly active uterine stimulant; it causes constriction of peripheral and cranial blood vessels and produces depression of central vasomotor centers

Pharmacokinetics (Adult data unless noted)

Absorption: Oral, rectal: Erratic; absorption is enhanced by caffeine coadministration

Metabolism: Extensive in the liver

Bioavailability: Poor overall (<5%)

Half-life: 2-2.5 hours

Time to peak serum concentration: Oral: Within 0.5-3 hours

Elimination: In bile as metabolites (90%)

Dosing: Usual Adolescents and Adults: **Note:** Not for chronic daily administration:

Oral: 2 mg at onset of attack; then 1-2 mg every 30 minutes as needed; maximum dose: 6 mg per attack; do not exceed 10 mg/week

Rectal, suppositories: 1 suppository at first sign of an attack; follow with second dose after 1 hour, if needed; maximum dose: 2 per attack; do not exceed 5/week

Administration Oral: Tablets may be taken without regard to meals.

Dosage Forms Excipient information presented when available (limited, particularly for generics); consult specific product labeling.

Suppository, rectal:

Migergot: Ergotamine tartrate 2 mg and caffeine 100 mg (12s)

Tablet, oral: Ergotamine tartrate 1 mg and caffeine 100 mg

Cafergot: Ergotamine tartrate 1 mg and caffeine 100 mg

◆ **Ergotamine Tartrate** *see* Ergotamine *on page 775*

◆ **Ergotamine Tartrate and Caffeine** *see* Ergotamine and Caffeine *on page 776*

◆ **E-R-O Ear Drops [OTC]** *see* Carbamide Peroxide *on page 371*

◆ **E-R-O Ear Wax Removal System [OTC]** *see* Carbamide Peroxide *on page 371*

◆ **Errin** *see* Norethindrone *on page 1530*

◆ **Ertaczo** *see* Sertaconazole *on page 1915*

Ertapenem (er ta PEN em)

Medication Safety Issues

Sound-alike/look-alike issues:

Ertapenem may be confused with doripenem, imipenem, meropenem

INVanz may be confused with AVINza, IV vancomycin

Brand Names: US INVanz

Brand Names: Canada Invanz

Therapeutic Category Antibiotic, Carbapenem

Generic Availability (US) No

Use Treatment of moderate to severe, complicated intra-abdominal infections, acute pelvic infections, complicated skin and skin structure infections (including diabetic foot infections without osteomyelitis), community-acquired pneumonia, and complicated urinary tract infections (including pyelonephritis) caused by susceptible organisms (FDA approved in ages ≥3 months and adults); prophylaxis of surgical site infection following colorectal surgery (FDA approved in adults)

Pregnancy Risk Factor B

Pregnancy Considerations Teratogenic effects were not observed in animal reproduction studies. Ertapenem is approved for the treatment of postpartum endomyometritis, septic abortion, and postsurgical infections. Information related to use during pregnancy has not been located.

Breast-Feeding Considerations Ertapenem is excreted in breast milk. The low concentrations in milk and low oral bioavailability suggest minimal exposure risk to the infant. The manufacturer recommends that caution be exercised when administering ertapenem to nursing women. Non-dose-related effects could include modification of bowel flora.

Contraindications Known hypersensitivity to any component of this product or to other drugs in the same class or in patients who have demonstrated anaphylactic reactions to beta-lactams; known hypersensitivity to local anesthetics of the amide type due to the use of lidocaine as a diluent (IM use only).

Warnings/Precautions Use caution with renal impairment. Dosage adjustment required in patients with moderate to severe renal dysfunction; elderly patients often require lower doses (based upon renal function). Use may result in fungal or bacterial superinfection, including *C. difficile*-associated diarrhea (CDAD) and pseudomembranous colitis; CDAD has been observed >2 months postantibiotic treatment. Carbapenems have been associated with CNS adverse effects, including confusional states and seizures (myoclonic); use caution with CNS disorders (eg, brain lesions and history of seizures) and adjust dose in renal impairment to avoid drug accumulation, which may increase seizure risk. Serious hypersensitivity reactions, including anaphylaxis, have been reported (some without a history of previous allergic reactions to beta-lactams). Doses for IM administration are mixed with lidocaine; consult Lidocaine (Systemic) information for associated Warnings/Precautions. May decrease divalproex sodium/valproic acid concentrations leading to breakthrough seizures; concomitant use not recommended.

Adverse Reactions

Cardiovascular: Chest pain, edema, hypotension, phlebitis, thrombophlebitis

Central nervous system: Altered mental status (ie, agitation, confusion, disorientation, mental acuity decreased, somnolence, stupor), dizziness, headache, hypothermia (infants, children, and adolescents), insomnia

Dermatologic: Diaper rash (infants and children), genital rash (infants, children, and adolescents), pruritus, skin lesion (infants, children, and adolescents), skin rash

Gastrointestinal: Abdominal pain, constipation, decreased appetite (infants, children, and adolescents), diarrhea, nausea, vomiting

Genitourinary: Erythrocyturia, vaginitis

Hematologic & oncologic: Decreased hematocrit, decreased hemoglobin, decreased neutrophils, eosinophilia, leukocyturia, leukopenia, thrombocythemia

Hepatic: Increased serum alkaline, increased serum ALT, increased serum AST

Infection: Herpes simplex infection (infants, children, and adolescents)

Local: Infused vein complication

Neuromuscular & skeletal: Arthralgia (infants, children, and adolescents)

Otic: Otic infection (infants, children, and adolescents)

Respiratory: Cough, dyspnea, nasopharyngitis (infants, children, and adolescents), rhinitis (infants, children, and adolescents), rhinorrhea (infants, children, and adolescents), upper respiratory tract infection (infants, children, and adolescents), wheezing (infants, children, and adolescents)

Miscellaneous: Fever

Rare but important or life-threatening: Anaphylactoid reaction, anaphylaxis, anuria, asthma, asystole, atrial fibrillation, bradycardia, bronchoconstriction, cardiac arrest, cardiac arrhythmia, cardiac failure, cholelithiasis, *Clostridium difficile* associated diarrhea, delirium, DRESS syndrome, extravasation, gastrointestinal hemorrhage, gout, heart murmur, hemoptysis, hyperglycemia, hyperkalemia, hypertension, hypoxemia, impaired consciousness, intestinal obstruction, jaundice, oral candidiasis, oliguria, pancreatitis, pleural effusion, prolonged prothrombin time, renal insufficiency, seizure, septicemia, septic shock, subdural hematoma, tachycardia, thrombocytopenia, tissue necrosis, ventricular tachycardia

Drug Interactions

Metabolism/Transport Effects None known.

Avoid Concomitant Use

Avoid concomitant use of Ertapenem with any of the following: BCG; BCG (Intravesical)

Increased Effect/Toxicity

Ertapenem may increase the levels/effects of: Tacrolimus (Systemic)

The levels/effects of Ertapenem may be increased by: Probenecid

Decreased Effect

Ertapenem may decrease the levels/effects of: BCG; BCG (Intravesical); BCG Vaccine (Immunization); Sodium Picosulfate; Typhoid Vaccine; Valproic Acid and Derivatives

Storage/Stability Prior to reconstitution, store vials at ≤25°C (77°F). The reconstituted IM solution should be used within 1 hour after preparation. The reconstituted IV solution may be stored at room temperature (25°C [77°F]) and used within 6 hours, or stored for 24 hours under refrigeration (5°C [41°F]) and used within 4 hours after removal from refrigeration. Do not freeze.

Mechanism of Action Inhibits bacterial cell wall synthesis by binding to one or more of the penicillin-binding proteins; which in turn inhibits the final transpeptidation step of peptidoglycan synthesis in bacterial cell walls, thus inhibiting cell wall biosynthesis. Bacteria eventually lyse due to ongoing activity of cell wall autolytic enzymes (autolysins and murein hydrolases) while cell wall assembly is arrested.

Pharmacokinetics (Adult data unless noted)

Absorption: IM: Almost complete

Distribution: V_d:

- Infants ≥3 months and Children: ~0.2 L/kg
- Adolescents: 0.16 L/kg
- Adults: 0.12 L/kg

Protein binding: 85% to 95% (concentration-dependent, primarily to albumin)

Metabolism: Non-CYP-mediated hydrolysis to inactive metabolite

Bioavailability: IM: 90%

Half-life:

- Infants ≥3 months and Children: 2.5 hours
- Adolescents and Adults: 4 hours

Time to peak serum concentration: IM: 2.3 hours

Elimination: Urine [80% (38% as unchanged drug)] and feces (10%)

Dosing: Usual Note: IV therapy may be administered for up to 14 days; IM for up to 7 days.

Infants, Children, and Adolescents:

General dosing, susceptible infection: IM, IV:

Infants and Children (*Red Book* [AAP], 2012): Severe infections: 15 mg/kg/dose twice daily; maximum single dose: 500 mg

Adolescents: 1000 mg once daily

Intra-abdominal infection, complicated: IM, IV: **Note:** IDSA guidelines recommend a treatment duration of 4-7 days (provided source controlled) for community-acquired, mild to moderate infections (Solomkin, 2010)

Infants <3 months: 15 mg/kg/dose twice daily (*Red Book* [AAP], 2012)

Infants ≥3 months and Children: 15 mg/kg/dose twice daily for 5-14 days; maximum single dose: 500 mg

Adolescents: 1000 mg once daily for 5-14 days

Pelvic infections, acute: IM, IV:

Infants <3 months: 15 mg/kg/dose twice daily (*Red Book* [AAP], 2012)

Infants ≥3 months and Children: 15 mg/kg/dose twice daily for 3-10 days; maximum single dose: 500 mg

Adolescents: 1000 mg once daily for 3-10 days

Pneumonia, community acquired: IM, IV: **Note:** Duration includes possible switch to appropriate oral step-down therapy after at least 3 days of parenteral treatment, once clinical improvement demonstrated.

Infants <3 months: 15 mg/kg/dose twice daily (*Red Book* [AAP], 2012)

Infants ≥3 months and Children: 15 mg/kg/dose twice daily for 10-14 days; maximum single dose: 500 mg

Adolescents: 1000 mg once daily for 10-14 days

Skin and skin structure infections, complicated: IM, IV:

Infants <3 months: 15 mg/kg/dose twice daily (*Red Book* [AAP], 2012)

Infants ≥3 months and Children: 15 mg/kg/dose twice daily for 7-14 days; maximum single dose: 500 mg

Adolescents: 1000 mg once daily for 7-14 days

Surgical prophylaxis: IV: Children and Adolescents: 15 mg/kg 60 minutes before procedure; maximum dose: 1000 mg (Bratzler, 2013)

Urinary tract infections (including pyelonephritis): IM, IV: **Note:** Duration includes possible switch to appropriate oral therapy after at least 3 days of parenteral treatment, once clinical improvement demonstrated.

Infants <3 months: 15 mg/kg/dose twice daily (*Red Book* [AAP], 2012)

Infants ≥3 months and Children: 15 mg/kg/dose twice daily for 10-14 days; maximum single dose: 500 mg

Adolescents: 1000 mg once daily for 10-14 days

Adults:

General dosing, susceptible infection: IM, IV:1000 mg once daily

Prophylaxis of surgical site infection following colorectal surgery: IV: Single 1000 mg dose administered 1 hour prior to surgical procedure

Dosing adjustment in renal impairment: Adults:

CrCl >30 mL/minute/1.73 m^2: No dosage adjustment required.

CrCl ≤30 mL/minute/1.73 m^2: 500 mg once daily

Continuous Ambulatory Peritoneal Dialysis (CAPD): 500 mg daily (Cardone, 2011)

Hemodialysis: ~30% removed by hemodialysis (Curran, 2003). If daily dose is given within 6 hours prior to hemodialysis, a supplementary dose of 150 mg should be given following hemodialysis.

Dosing adjustment in hepatic impairment: There are no dosage adjustments provided in the manufacturer's labeling.

Preparation for Administration

Parenteral:

IM: Reconstitute 1,000 mg vial with 3.2 mL of 1% lidocaine HCl injection (without epinephrine); resultant concentration: 312.5 mg/mL. Shake well.

Intermittent IV infusion: Reconstitute 1000 mg vial with 10 mL of SWFI, NS, or bacteriostatic water for injection; resultant concentration: 100 mg/mL. Shake well. Further dilute dose with NS; for adolescents and adults, transfer dose to 50 mL NS; for children, dilute dose to a final concentration ≤20 mg/mL.

Administration Parenteral:

IM: Administer deep into a large muscle mass such as the gluteus maximus or lateral part of the thigh. Avoid injection into a blood vessel.

Intermittent IV infusion: Infuse over 30 minutes. Do not coinfuse with other medications. **Do not infuse with dextrose-containing solutions.**

Monitoring Parameters Periodic renal, hepatic, and hematologic function tests; neurological assessment

Additional Information Sodium content: 1000 mg ertapenem contains 6 mEq

Dosage Forms Excipient information presented when available (limited, particularly for generics); consult specific product labeling.

Solution Reconstituted, Injection:

INVanz: 1 g (1 ea)

Solution Reconstituted, Intravenous:

INVanz: 1 g (1 ea)

- ◆ **Ertapenem Sodium** *see* Ertapenem *on page 777*
- ◆ **Erwinase (Can)** *see* Asparaginase (*Erwinia*) *on page 204*
- ◆ **Erwinaze** *see* Asparaginase (*Erwinia*) *on page 204*
- ◆ ***Erwinia chrysanthemi*** *see* Asparaginase (*Erwinia*) *on page 204*
- ◆ **Ery** *see* Erythromycin (Topical) *on page 783*
- ◆ **Erybid (Can)** *see* Erythromycin (Systemic) *on page 779*
- ◆ **Eryc (Can)** *see* Erythromycin (Systemic) *on page 779*
- ◆ **Erygel** *see* Erythromycin (Topical) *on page 783*
- ◆ **EryPed 200** *see* Erythromycin (Systemic) *on page 779*
- ◆ **EryPed 400** *see* Erythromycin (Systemic) *on page 779*
- ◆ **Erysol (Can)** *see* Erythromycin (Topical) *on page 783*
- ◆ **Ery-Tab** *see* Erythromycin (Systemic) *on page 779*
- ◆ **Erythrocin Lactobionate** *see* Erythromycin (Systemic) *on page 779*
- ◆ **Erythrocin Stearate** *see* Erythromycin (Systemic) *on page 779*

Erythromycin (Systemic) (er ith roe MYE sin)

Medication Safety Issues

Sound-alike/look-alike issues:

Erythromycin may be confused with azithromycin, clarithromycin

Eryc may be confused with Emcyt, Ery-Tab

Related Information

Oral Medications That Should Not Be Crushed or Altered *on page 2476*

Brand Names: US E.E.S. 400; E.E.S. Granules; Ery-Tab; EryPed 200; EryPed 400; Erythrocin Lactobionate; Erythrocin Stearate; PCE

Brand Names: Canada Apo-Erythro Base; Apo-Erythro E-C; Apo-Erythro-ES; Apo-Erythro-S; EES; Erybid; Eryc; Novo-Rythro Estolate; Novo-Rythro Ethylsuccinate; Nu-Erythromycin-S; PCE

Therapeutic Category Antibiotic, Macrolide

Generic Availability (US) May be product dependent

Use Treatment of mild to moderately severe infections of the upper and lower respiratory tract and skin infections due to susceptible *streptococcus* and *staphylococcus* sp. and *Haemophilus influenzae*; other susceptible bacterial infections, including *Mycoplasma pneumoniae*, *Legionella pneumonia*, nongonococcal urethritis, Lyme disease, diphtheria, pertussis, chancroid, *Chlamydia*, *Ureaplasma*, and *Campylobacter* gastroenteritis, syphilis, prophylaxis of recurrent rheumatic fever in penicillin- or sulfa-allergic patients (all indications: FDA approved in all ages); has also been used in conjunction with neomycin for decontaminating the bowel for surgery; prophylaxis of pneumococcal infections in children with sickle cell disease (SCD), and functional or anatomic asplenia who are penicillin allergic

Pregnancy Risk Factor B

Pregnancy Considerations Adverse events were not observed in animal reproduction studies. Erythromycin crosses the placenta and low concentrations are found in the fetal serum. Cardiovascular anomalies following exposure in early pregnancy have been reported in some observational studies. Serum concentrations of erythromycin may be variable in pregnant women (Kiefer 1955; Philipson 1976).

In patients with acute infections during pregnancy, erythromycin may be given if an antibiotic is required and appropriate based on bacterial sensitivity (ACOG No. 120 2011). Erythromycin is the antibiotic of choice for preterm premature rupture of membranes (with membrane rupture between 24 0/7 to 33 6/7 weeks gestation) (ACOG 2013), the treatment of granuloma inguinale, and lymphogranuloma venereum in pregnancy (CDC [RR-12] 2010), and the treatment of or long-term suppression of *Bartonella* infection in HIV-infected pregnant patients [DHHS 2013]. Erythromycin may be appropriate as an alternative agent for the treatment of chlamydial infections in pregnant women (consult current guidelines) (CDC [RR-12] 2010).

Breast-Feeding Considerations Erythromycin is excreted in breast milk; therefore, the manufacturer recommends that caution be exercised when administering erythromycin to breast-feeding women. Decreased appetite, diarrhea, rash, and somnolence have been reported in nursing infants exposed to macrolide antibiotics (Goldstein 2009).

One case report and a cohort study raise the possibility for a connection with pyloric stenosis in neonates exposed to erythromycin via breast milk and an alternative antibiotic may be preferred for breast-feeding mothers of infants in this age group (Sorensen 2003; Stang 1986).

Contraindications Hypersensitivity to erythromycin, any macrolide antibiotics, or any component of the formulation

Concomitant use with pimozide, cisapride, ergotamine or dihydroergotamine, terfenadine, astemizole, lovastatin, or simvastatin

Warnings/Precautions Use caution with hepatic impairment with or without jaundice has occurred, it may be accompanied by malaise, nausea, vomiting, abdominal colic, and fever; discontinue use if these occur. Potentially significant drug-drug interactions may exist, requiring dose or frequency adjustment, additional monitoring, and/or selection of alternative therapy. Use caution with other medication relying on CYP3A4 metabolism; high potential for drug interactions exists. Prolonged use may result in fungal or bacterial superinfection, including *C. difficile*-associated diarrhea (CDAD) and pseudomembranous colitis; CDAD has been observed >2 months postantibiotic treatment. Use in infants has been associated with infantile hypertrophic pyloric stenosis (IHPS). Macrolides have been associated with rare QTc prolongation and ventricular arrhythmias, including torsade de pointes; avoid use in patients with prolonged QT interval, uncorrected hypokalemia or hypomagnesemia, clinically significant bradycardia, or concurrent use of Class IA (eg, quinidine, procainamide) or Class III (eg, amiodarone, dofetilide, sotalol) antiarrhythmic agents. Avoid concurrent use with strong CYP3A inhibitors; may increase the risk of sudden cardiac death (Ray 2004). Use caution in elderly patients, as risk of adverse events may be increased. Use caution in myasthenia gravis patients; erythromycin may aggravate muscular weakness.

Benzyl alcohol and derivatives: Some dosage forms may contain benzyl alcohol; large amounts of benzyl alcohol (≥99 mg/kg/day) have been associated with a potentially fatal toxicity ("gasping syndrome") in neonates; the "gasping syndrome" consists of metabolic acidosis, respiratory distress, gasping respirations, CNS dysfunction (including convulsions, intracranial hemorrhage), hypotension and cardiovascular collapse (AAP 1997; CDC 1982); some data suggests that benzoate displaces bilirubin from protein binding sites (Ahlfors 2001); avoid or use dosage forms containing benzyl alcohol with caution in neonates. See manufacturer's labeling.

Warnings: Additional Pediatric Considerations Hepatic impairment with or without jaundice has occurred primarily in older children and adults; reported incidence in children is ~0.1% and in adults is 0.25%; it may be accompanied by malaise, nausea, vomiting, abdominal colic, and fever; discontinue use if these occur. Infantile hypertrophic pyloric stenosis with symptoms of nonbilious vomiting or irritability with feeding has been reported in 5% of infants who received erythromycin for pertussis prophylaxis.

Adverse Reactions

Cardiovascular: QTc prolongation, torsade de pointes, ventricular arrhythmia, ventricular tachycardia

Central nervous system: Seizure

Dermatologic: Erythema multiforme, pruritus, rash, Stevens-Johnson syndrome, toxic epidermal necrolysis

Gastrointestinal: Abdominal pain, anorexia, diarrhea, infantile hypertrophic pyloric stenosis, nausea, oral candidiasis, pancreatitis, pseudomembranous colitis, vomiting

Hepatic: Cholestatic jaundice (most common with estolate), hepatitis, liver function tests abnormal

Local: Phlebitis at the injection site, thrombophlebitis

Neuromuscular & skeletal: Weakness

Otic: Hearing loss

Miscellaneous: Allergic reactions, anaphylaxis, hypersensitivity reactions, interstitial nephritis, urticaria

Drug Interactions

Metabolism/Transport Effects **Substrate** of CYP2B6 (minor), CYP3A4 (major), P-glycoprotein; **Note:** Assignment of Major/Minor substrate status based on clinically relevant drug interaction potential; **Inhibits** CYP3A4 (moderate), P-glycoprotein

Avoid Concomitant Use

Avoid concomitant use of Erythromycin (Systemic) with any of the following: Barnidipine; BCG; BCG (Intravesical); Bosutinib; Cisapride; Clindamycin (Topical); Conivaptan; Disopyramide; Domperidone; Fluconazole; Fusidic Acid (Systemic); Highest Risk QTc-Prolonging Agents; Ibrutinib; Idelalisib; Ivabradine; Lincosamide Antibiotics; Lomitapide; Lovastatin; Mequitazine; Mifepristone; Naloxegol; Olaparib; PAZOPanib; Pimozide; QuiNIDine; QuiNINE; Silodosin; Simeprevir; Simvastatin; Terfenadine; Tolvaptan; Topotecan; Trabectedin; Ulipristal; VinCRIStine (Liposomal)

Increased Effect/Toxicity

Erythromycin (Systemic) may increase the levels/effects of: Afatinib; Alfentanil; ALPRAZolam; Antineoplastic Agents (Vinca Alkaloids); ARIPiprazole; AtorvaSTATin; Avanafil; Barnidipine; Bosentan; Bosutinib; Brentuximab Vedotin; Budesonide (Systemic, Oral Inhalation); Budesonide (Topical); BusPIRone; Calcium Channel Blockers; Cannabis; CarBAMazepine; Cardiac Glycosides; Cilostazol; Cisapride; CloZAPine; Colchicine; CycloSPORINE (Systemic); CYP3A4 Substrates; Dabigatran Etexilate; Dapoxetine; Disopyramide; Domperidone; DOXOrubicin (Conventional); Dronabinol; Edoxaban; Eletriptan; Eplerenone; Ergot Derivatives; Estazolam; Everolimus; FentaNYL; Fexofenadine; Highest Risk QTc-Prolonging Agents; Hydrocodone; Ibrutinib; Imatinib; Ivabradine; Ivacaftor; Ledipasvir; Lomitapide; Lovastatin; Lurasidone; Mequitazine; Midazolam; Moderate Risk QTc-Prolonging Agents; Naloxegol; Nintedanib; Olaparib; OxyCODONE; PAZOPanib; P-glycoprotein/ABCB1 Substrates; Pimecrolimus; Pimozide; Pitavastatin; Pravastatin; QuiNIDine; QuiNINE; Ranolazine; Repaglinide; Rifamycin Derivatives; Rifaximin; Rilpivirine; Rivaroxaban; Salmeterol; Saxagliptin; Selective Serotonin Reuptake Inhibitors; Sildenafil; Silodosin; Simeprevir; Simvastatin; Sirolimus; Suvorexant; Tacrolimus (Systemic); Tacrolimus (Topical); Telaprevir; Temsirolimus; Terfenadine; Tetrahydrocannabinol; Theophylline Derivatives; Tolvaptan; Topotecan; Trabectedin; Triazolam; Ulipristal; Vardenafil; Vilazodone; VinCRIStine (Liposomal); Vitamin K Antagonists; Zopiclone

The levels/effects of Erythromycin (Systemic) may be increased by: Aprepitant; Conivaptan; CYP3A4 Inhibitors (Moderate); CYP3A4 Inhibitors (Strong); Dasatinib; Fluconazole; Fosaprepitant; Fusidic Acid (Systemic); Idelalisib; Ivabradine; Luliconazole; Mifepristone; Netupitant; Palbociclib; P-glycoprotein/ABCB1 Inhibitors; QTc-Prolonging Agents (Indeterminate Risk and Risk Modifying); Stiripentol; Telaprevir

Decreased Effect

Erythromycin (Systemic) may decrease the levels/effects of: BCG; BCG (Intravesical); BCG Vaccine (Immunization); Clindamycin (Topical); Clopidogrel; Ifosfamide; Sodium Picosulfate; Typhoid Vaccine; Zafirlukast

The levels/effects of Erythromycin (Systemic) may be decreased by: Bosentan; CYP3A4 Inducers (Moderate); CYP3A4 Inducers (Strong); Dabrafenib; Deferasirox; Etravirine; Lincosamide Antibiotics; Mitotane; P-glycoprotein/ABCB1 Inducers; Siltuximab; St Johns Wort; Tocilizumab

Food Interactions

Ethanol: Ethanol may decrease absorption of erythromycin or enhance effects of ethanol. Management: Avoid ethanol.

Food: Erythromycin serum levels may be altered if taken with food (formulation-dependent). GI upset, including diarrhea, is common. Management: May be taken with food to decrease GI upset, otherwise take around-the-clock with a full glass of water. Do not give with milk or acidic beverages (eg, soda, juice).

Storage/Stability

Injection: Store unreconstituted vials at 20°C to 25°C (68°F to 77°F). Reconstituted solution (50 mg/mL) is stable for 2 weeks when refrigerated or for 24 hours at room temperature. Erythromycin IV infusion solution is stable at pH 6 to 8; stability of lactobionate is pH dependent; IV form has longest stability in NS. Parenteral admixture in NS is stable for 24 hours at 4°C. Admixtures in NS (including Add-Vantage containers) should be infused within 8 hours of preparation.

Oral suspension:

Granules: Prior to mixing, store at <30°C (86°F). After mixing, store under refrigeration and use within 10 days.

Powder: Prior to mixing, store at <30°C (86°F). After mixing, store at ≤25°C (77°F) and use within 35 days.

Tablet and capsule formulations: Store at <30°C (86°F).

Mechanism of Action Inhibits RNA-dependent protein synthesis at the chain elongation step; binds to the 50S ribosomal subunit resulting in blockage of transpeptidation

Pharmacokinetics (Adult data unless noted)

Absorption: Variable, but better with salt forms than with base; 18% to 45% absorbed orally; ethylsuccinate may be better absorbed with food

Distribution: Poor penetration into the CSF

V_d: 0.64 L/kg

Protein binding: 73% to 81%

Metabolism: In the liver by demethylation via CYP3A4

Half-life:

Neonates (≤15 days of age): 2.1 hours

Adults: 1.5-2 hours
ESRD: 5-6 hours
Time to peak serum concentration: Oral:
Base: 4 hours
Stearate: 3 hours
Ethylsuccinate: 0.5-2.5 hours
Elimination: 2% to 5% unchanged drug excreted in urine, major excretion in feces (via bile)
Dialysis: Not removed by peritoneal dialysis or hemodialysis

Dosing: Neonatal

General dosing: Oral (ethylsuccinate); IV (lactobionate): (*Red Book*, 2012):
Body weight <1 kg:
PNA ≤14 days: 10 mg/kg/dose every 12 hours
PNA 15-28 days: 10 mg/kg/dose every 8 hours
Body weight 1-2 kg:
PNA ≤7 days: 10 mg/kg/dose every 12 hours
PNA 8-28 days: 10 mg/kg/dose every 8 hours
Bodyweight >2 kg:
PNA ≤7 days: 10 mg/kg/dose every 12 hours
PNA 8-28 days: 10 mg/kg/dose every 8 hours

Chlamydial conjunctivitis or chlamydial pneumonia: Oral: Ethylsuccinate or base: Full-term neonates: 50 mg/kg/**day** divided every 6 hours for 14 days; a repeat course may be necessary (*Red Book*, 2012)

Pertussis; treatment or postexposure prophylaxis: Oral: Ethylsuccinate: 10 mg/kg/dose 4 times daily for 14 days; **Note:** Due to association of erythromycin and infantile hypertrophic pyloric stenosis in neonates, azithromycin is considered first-line agent in infants <1 month of age (*Red Book*, 2012)

Prokinetic (GI motility) agent: Limited data available; efficacy results variable: PNA ≥14 days:
Low-dose regimen: Oral: 1.5-2.5 mg/kg/dose every 6 hours; therapy started after initiation of enteral feeds; has been studied in GA <32 weeks (Chicella, 2005; Oei, 2001)
Intermediate-dose regimen: Oral: 5 mg/kg/dose every 6 hours; therapy started after initiation of enteral feeds; dosing based on a randomized, controlled trial of 45 VLBW neonates (n=19 treatment group; mean GA: 28.4 weeks); treatment was initiated at a mean PNA: 21.9 + 7.7 days and continued for 14 days (Ng, 2012)
High-dose regimens (antimicrobial doses): Oral: 10-12.5 mg/kg/dose every 6-8 hours orally have been used after initiation of enteral feeds; efficacy has not been demonstrated in the majority of trials. Exposure to these doses in neonates with PNA ≤14 days has been associated with a 10-fold increase in the risk of hypertrophic pyloric stenosis (Chicella, 2005)

Dosing: Usual

Infants, Children, and Adolescents:
General dosing, susceptible infection:
Manufacturer's labeling:
Oral: Base, ethylsuccinate, stearate: 30-50 mg/kg/**day** divided every 6-8 hours usually; for severe infection may double dose; maximum daily dose: Mild to moderate infection: 2000 mg/**day**; severe infection: 4000 mg/**day**
IV: Lactobionate: 15-20 mg/kg/**day** divided every 6 hours; maximum daily dose: 4000 mg/**day**
Alternate dosing (*Red Book*, 2012):
Mild to moderate infection: Oral: 50 mg/kg/**day** divided every 6-8 hours; maximum daily dose: 2000 mg/**day**
Severe infection: IV: Lactobionate: 5 mg/kg/dose every 6 hours, maximum daily dose: 4000 mg/**day**

Acne, moderate to severe; treatment: Children and Adolescents: Oral: 250-500 mg 1-2 times daily in conjunction with topical therapy (eg, benzoyl peroxide); maximum daily dose: 50 mg/kg/**day**; duration of 4-8 weeks of therapy usually necessary to evaluate initial clinical response with a longer duration for a maximum effect (3-6 months); resistance problematic with therapy, use typically reserved for patients <8 years who cannot receive tetracycline derivatives (Eichenfield, 2013)

Anthrax, cutaneous, community-acquired (Stevens, 2005):
Oral: 10 mg/kg/dose every 6 hours; treatment duration of 5-9 days usually adequate in most cases
IV: 20-40 mg/kg/**day** divided every 6 hours; maximum daily dose: 4000 mg; treatment duration of 5-9 days usually adequate in most cases

***Bartonella* sp infections [bacillary angiomatosis (BA), peliosis hepatis (PH)]:**
Non-HIV-exposed/-positive; treatment: Oral: Ethylsuccinate: 10 mg/kg/ dose 4 times daily; maximum daily dose: 2000 mg/day; treatment duration: BA: 3 months; PH: 4 months (Rolain, 2004)
HIV-exposed/-positive:
Prophylaxis: Infants and Children (CDC, 2009): Oral: 30-50 mg/kg/day divided into 2-4 doses daily; maximum daily dose: 2000 mg/**day**
Treatment: Duration of therapy: ≥3 months (of sufficient duration to prevent relapse)
Infants and Children (CDC, 2009):
Oral: 30-50 mg/kg/day divided into 2-4 doses daily; maximum daily dose: 2000 mg/**day**
IV: 15-50 mg/kg/day divided into 4 doses daily; maximum daily dose: 2000 mg/**day**
Adolescents: IV, Oral: 500 mg every 6 hours with or without rifampin (DHHS [adult], 2013)

***Chlamydia trachomatis* infection** (CDC, 2010; *Red Book*, 2012):
Conjunctivitis or pneumonia: Oral (base or ethylsuccinate): 50 mg/kg/**day** divided every 6 hours for 14 days; maximum daily dose: 2000 mg/**day**; a repeat course may be necessary; for severe trachoma, longer durations may be necessary (40 days)
Anogenital tract infection:
Children and Adolescents <45 kg: Oral (base or ethylsuccinate): 50 mg/kg/**day** divided every 6 hours for 14 days; maximum daily dose: 2000 mg/**day**
Adolescents ≥45 kg: Oral:
Base: 500 mg 4 times daily for 7 days
Ethylsuccinate: 800 mg 4 times daily for 7 days
Lymphogranuloma venereum (LGV): Adolescents ≥45 kg: Oral (base): 500 mg 4 times daily for 21 days

Impetigo: Oral: 10 mg/kg/dose 4 times daily (Stevens, 2005)

Lyme Disease: Oral: 50 mg/kg/day divided every 6 hours for 14-21 days; maximum dose: 500 mg (Wormser, 2006)

Peritonitis, exit-site and tunnel infection: Oral (base): 30-50 mg/kg/day divided 3-4 times daily; maximum single dose: 500 mg (Warady, 2012)

Pertussis (CDC, 2005; *Red Book*, 2012):
Infants 1-5 months: Oral: 10 mg/kg/dose 4 times daily for 14 days
Infants ≥6 months and Children: Oral: 10 mg/kg/dose 4 times daily for 7-14 days; maximum daily dose: 2000 mg/**day**
Adolescents: Oral: 500 mg 4 times daily for 7-14 days

Pneumonia, community-acquired (CAP) (Bradley, 2011): Infants >3 months, Children, and Adolescents: **Note:** A beta-lactam antibiotic should be added if typical bacterial pneumonia cannot be ruled out.
Presumed atypical (*M. pneumoniae, C. pneumoniae, C. trachomatis*); mild infection or step-down therapy: Oral: 10 mg/kg/dose every 6 hours; maximum daily dose: 2000 mg/**day**
Moderate to severe atypical infection: IV: Lactobionate: 5 mg/kg/dose every 6 hours; maximum daily dose: 4000 mg/**day**

Preoperative bowel preparation: Children and Adolescents: Oral: Base: 20 mg/kg; maximum dose: 1000 mg administered at 1, 2, and 11 PM on the day before surgery combined with mechanical cleansing of the large intestine and oral neomycin (Bratzler, 2013)

Prokinetic (GI motility) agent: Limited data available:

Diagnosis; gastric emptying study (provocative testing): IV: 2.8 mg/kg infused over 20 minutes was reported from one center's experience; maximum dose: 250 mg (Waseem, 2012)

Treatment: Oral: 3 mg/kg/dose 4 times daily; may increase as needed to effect; maximum dose: 10 mg/kg or 250 mg (Rodriguez, 2012)

Pneumococcal, prophylaxis in penicillin-allergic patients with sickle cell disease (SCD) and functional or anatomic asplenia (Knight-Madden, 2001): Oral:

Infants and Children: 4 months to <3 years: 125 mg twice daily; salt not specified

Children 3-4 years: 250 mg twice daily; salt not specified

Adults:

General dosing: Note: Due to differences in absorption, 400 mg erythromycin ethylsuccinate produces the same serum levels as 250 mg erythromycin base or stearate.

IV: Lactobionate: 15-20 mg/kg/day divided every 6 hours or given as a continuous infusion over 24 hours, not to exceed 4 g/day

Oral:

Base, delayed release: 333 mg every 8 hours

Stearate or base: 250-500 mg every 6-12 hours

Ethylsuccinate: 400-800 mg every 6-12 hours

Chancroid: Oral: Base: 500 mg 3 times/day for 7 days

Chlamydia trachomatis: Oral:

Base: 500 mg 4 times/day for 7 days **or**

Ethylsuccinate: 800 mg 4 times/day for 7 days

Pertussis: Oral: 500 mg every 6 hours for 14 days

Preoperative bowel preparation: Oral: 1 g erythromycin base at 1, 2, and 11 PM on the day before surgery combined with mechanical cleansing of the large intestine and oral neomycin

Dosing adjustment in renal impairment: Infants, Children, and Adolescents: The following adjustments have been recommended (Aronoff, 2007). **Note:** Renally adjusted dose recommendations are based on oral doses of 30-50 mg/kg/**day** divided every 6-8 hours.

GFR ≥10 mL/minute/1.73 m^2: No adjustment required

GFR <10 mL/minute/1.73 m^2: Intermittent hemodialysis, peritoneal dialysis: Not removed by peritoneal dialysis or hemodialysis: 10-17 mg/kg/dose every 8 hours

Dosing adjustment in hepatic impairment: There are no dosage adjustments provided in the manufacturer's labeling.

Preparation for Administration Parenteral: Reconstitute with SWFI (preservative free) to a concentration of 50 mg/mL; other diluents for reconstitution may cause precipitation (gel) to occur. Must further dilute reconstituted solution prior to administration to a concentration of ≤1 mg/mL (continuous infusion) or 1 to 5 mg/mL (intermittent infusion) in NS (preferred, longest stability) or LR. Dextrose containing diluents (D_5W, D_5LR, and D_5NS) may be used but require the addition of sodium bicarbonate to the solution so the pH is in the optimal range for erythromycin stability; acidic solutions of erythromycin are unstable and lose their potency rapidly. Manufacturer recommends adding 1 mL of 4% sodium bicarbonate (Neut) per 100 mL of solution or may add 0.5 mL of the 8.4% sodium bicarbonate solution per each 100 mL of D_5W.

Administration

Oral: Avoid milk and acidic beverages 1 hour before or after a dose; administer after food to decrease GI discomfort; ethylsuccinate chewable tablets should not be swallowed whole; do not chew or break delayed release capsule or enteric coated tablets, swallow whole

Parenteral: Administer by intermittent IV infusion over 20 to 60 minutes or as a continuous infusion. Intermittent IV infusion may be very irritating to the vein; per the manufacturer, continuous infusion is preferable due to slower infusion rate and lower concentration. For intermittent IV infusion, prolonging the infusion duration over 60 minutes or longer has been recommended to decrease the cardiotoxic effects of erythromycin (Farrar 1993; Sims 1994).

Monitoring Parameters Assess results of culture and sensitivity tests and patient's previous allergy history prior to therapy; liver function tests, observe for changes in bowel frequency; with IV use: Blood pressure, heart rate

Test Interactions False-positive urinary catecholamines (fluorometric assay), 17-hydroxycorticosteroids and 17-ketosteroids

Additional Information Treatment of erythromycin-associated cardiac toxicity with prolongation of the QT interval and ventricular tachydysrhythmias includes discontinuing erythromycin and administering magnesium.

Dosage Forms Excipient information presented when available (limited, particularly for generics); consult specific product labeling.

Capsule Delayed Release Particles, Oral, as base:

Generic: 250 mg

Solution Reconstituted, Intravenous, as lactobionate:

Erythrocin Lactobionate: 500 mg (1 ea); 1000 mg (1 ea)

Suspension Reconstituted, Oral, as ethylsuccinate:

E.E.S. Granules: 200 mg/5 mL (100 mL, 200 mL) [cherry flavor]

EryPed 200: 200 mg/5 mL (100 mL) [fruit flavor]

EryPed 400: 400 mg/5 mL (100 mL) [banana flavor]

Tablet, Oral, as base:

Generic: 250 mg, 500 mg

Tablet, Oral, as ethylsuccinate:

E.E.S. 400: 400 mg [contains fd&c red #40, fd&c yellow #10 (quinoline yellow)]

Generic: 400 mg

Tablet, Oral, as stearate:

Erythrocin Stearate: 250 mg

Tablet Delayed Release, Oral, as base:

Ery-Tab: 250 mg, 333 mg, 500 mg

PCE: 333 mg

PCE: 500 mg [dye free, no artificial color(s)]

Erythromycin (Ophthalmic) (er ith roe MYE sin)

Medication Safety Issues

Sound-alike/look-alike issues:

Erythromycin may be confused with azithromycin

Brand Names: US Ilotycin; Romycin [DSC]

Brand Names: Canada Diomycin®; PMS-Erythromycin

Therapeutic Category Antibiotic, Macrolide; Antibiotic, Ophthalmic

Generic Availability (US) Yes

Use Treatment of superficial eye infections involving the conjunctiva or cornea; prevention of ophthalmia neonatorum due to *Neisseria gonorrhoeae* or *Chlamydia trachomatis* [FDA approved in pediatric patients (all ages) and adults]; has also been used for the treatment of chlamydial ophthalmic infections

Pregnancy Risk Factor B

Pregnancy Considerations Adverse events were not observed in animal reproduction studies. Erythromycin has been shown to cross the placenta following oral dosing. Refer to the Erythromycin (Systemic) monograph for details. The amount of erythromycin available systemically following ophthalmic application is not known.

Systemic absorption would be required in order for erythromycin to cross the placenta and reach the fetus.

Breast-Feeding Considerations It is not known of erythromycin is excreted into breast milk following ophthalmic application. The manufacturer recommends that caution be exercised when administering erythromycin ophthalmic ointment to nursing women. Erythromycin has been shown to enter breast milk following oral dosing. Refer to the Erythromycin (Systemic) monograph for details. Systemic absorption would be required in order for erythromycin to enter breast milk and reach the nursing infant.

Contraindications Hypersensitivity to erythromycin or any component of the formulation

Warnings/Precautions For ophthalmic use only. Avoid contamination. Do not touch tip of applicator or let tip of applicator touch eye.

Adverse Reactions Ocular: Hypersensitivity, minor ocular irritation, redness

Drug Interactions

Metabolism/Transport Effects None known.

Avoid Concomitant Use There are no known interactions where it is recommended to avoid concomitant use.

Increased Effect/Toxicity

Erythromycin (Ophthalmic) may increase the levels/effects of: Vitamin K Antagonists

Decreased Effect There are no known significant interactions involving a decrease in effect.

Storage/Stability Store at 20°C to 25°C (68°F to 77°F); protect from freezing and excessive heat.

Mechanism of Action Inhibits RNA-dependent protein synthesis at the chain elongation step; binds to the 50S ribosomal subunit resulting in blockage of transpeptidation

Dosing: Neonatal Ophthalmic: Prophylaxis of neonatal gonococcal or chlamydial ophthalmia: Ointment: Instill 1 cm ribbon into each conjunctival sac once

Dosing: Usual Ophthalmic: Conjunctivitis: Infants, Children, and Adults: Ointment: Instill 1 cm ribbon one or more times daily up to 6 times daily depending on the severity of the infection

Administration Ophthalmic ointment for prevention of neonatal ophthalmia: Wipe each eyelid gently with sterile cotton; instill 1 cm ribbon of ointment in each lower conjunctival sac; massage eyelids gently to spread the ointment; after 1 minute, excess ointment can be wiped away with sterile cotton. Avoid contact of applicator tip with skin or eye.

Dosage Forms Excipient information presented when available (limited, particularly for generics); consult specific product labeling. [DSC] = Discontinued product

Ointment, Ophthalmic:

Ilotycin: 5 mg/g (1 g)

Romycin: 5 mg/g (3.5 g [DSC])

Generic: 5 mg/g (1 g, 3.5 g)

Erythromycin (Topical) (er ith roe MYE sin)

Medication Safety Issues

Sound-alike/look-alike issues:

Erythromycin may be confused with azithromycin, clarithromycin

Brand Names: US Akne-Mycin [DSC]; Ery; Erygel

Brand Names: Canada Erysol

Therapeutic Category Antibiotic, Macrolide; Antibiotic, Topical

Generic Availability (US) May be product dependent

Use Treatment of acne vulgaris

Pregnancy Risk Factor B

Pregnancy Considerations Adverse events were not observed in animal reproduction studies. Erythromycin has been shown to cross the placenta following oral dosing. Refer to the Erythromycin (Systemic) monograph for details. The amount of erythromycin available systemically following topical application is considered to be very low (Akhavan, 2003). Systemic absorption would be required in order for erythromycin to cross the placenta and reach the fetus. Topical erythromycin may be used for the treatment of acne in pregnancy (Dréno, 2013; Eichenfield, 2013; Gollnick, 2003).

Breast-Feeding Considerations It is not known if erythromycin is excreted into breast milk following topical application. The manufacturer recommends that caution be exercised when administering to nursing women. Erythromycin has been shown to enter breast milk following oral dosing. Refer to the Erythromycin (Systemic) monograph for details. The amount of erythromycin available systemically following topical application is considered to be very low (Akhavan, 2003). Systemic absorption would be required in order for erythromycin to enter breast milk and reach the nursing infant.

Contraindications

Hypersensitivity to erythromycin or any component of the formulation

Documentation of allergenic cross-reactivity for erythromycin is limited. However, because of similarities in chemical structure and/or pharmacologic actions, the possibility of cross-sensitivity cannot be ruled out with certainty.

Warnings/Precautions For topical use only; not for ophthalmic use. Avoid contact with eyes, nose, mouth, mucous membranes, or broken skin. Lack of improvement or worsening of acne may indicate microbial resistance. Alternative therapy may be required for severe acne (eg, nodular). Consider alternate therapy in patients with poor tolerance to macrolides or clindamycin. Prolonged use may result in fungal or bacterial superinfection, including *C. difficile*-associated diarrhea (CDAD) and pseudomembranous colitis; CDAD has been observed >2 months postantibiotic treatment. Discontinue if significant diarrhea, abdominal cramps, or passage of blood and mucus occurs. Use caution with concurrent use of other agents used to treat acne, especially with peeling, desquamating or abrasive agents; irritation may be cumulative. Discontinue use if irritation or dermatitis occurs. Topical gel may be flammable; keep away from heat and flame.

Warnings: Additional Pediatric Considerations Some dosage forms may contain propylene glycol; in neonates large amounts of propylene glycol delivered orally, intravenously (eg, >3,000 mg/day), or topically have been associated with potentially fatal toxicities which can include metabolic acidosis, seizures, renal failure, and CNS depression; toxicities have also been reported in children and adults including hyperosmolality, lactic acidosis, seizures, and respiratory depression; use caution (AAP, 1997; Shehab, 2009).

Adverse Reactions

Dermatologic: Erythema, dryness, oiliness, peeling, pruritus, tenderness, urticaria

Ocular: Eye irritation

As reported with Erysol [Canadian product]:

Dermatologic: Coriaceousness, desquamation, fissure (around mouth), oiliness, scaling

Local: Application site: Irritation (burning, dryness, erythema, stinging, tenderness)

Rare but important or life-threatening: Abdominal discomfort/pain, allergic reaction, diarrhea, facial edema, pruritus, rash, skin exfoliation, urticaria

Drug Interactions

Metabolism/Transport Effects None known.

Avoid Concomitant Use

Avoid concomitant use of Erythromycin (Topical) with any of the following: BCG; BCG (Intravesical); Clindamycin (Topical)

Increased Effect/Toxicity There are no known significant interactions involving an increase in effect.

Decreased Effect

Erythromycin (Topical) may decrease the levels/effects of: BCG; BCG (Intravesical); BCG Vaccine (Immunization); Clindamycin (Topical); Sodium Picosulfate

Storage/Stability

Akne-Mycin: Store below 27°C (80°F).

Ery: Store at 20°C to 25°C (68°F to 77°F).

Erygel: Store at 20°C to 25°C (68°F to 77°F). Protect from heat and flame.

Erysol [Canadian product]: Store at 15°C to 30°C (59°F to 86°F). Protect from heat and flame.

Mechanism of Action Antibacterial activity is due to inhibition of RNA-dependent protein synthesis at the chain elongation step; binds to the 50S ribosomal subunit resulting in blockage of transpeptidation. Alcohol component induces skin drying and peeling.

Dosing: Usual Children and Adults: Apply 2% solution over the affected area twice daily after the skin has been thoroughly washed and patted dry

Administration Apply thin film to the cleansed, affected area.

Dosage Forms Excipient information presented when available (limited, particularly for generics); consult specific product labeling. [DSC] = Discontinued product

Gel, External:

Erygel: 2% (30 g, 60 g)

Generic: 2% (30 g, 60 g)

Ointment, External:

Akne-Mycin: 2% (25 g [DSC]) [contains cetostearyl alcohol]

Pad, External:

Ery: 2% (60 ea) [contains propylene glycol]

Generic: 2% (60 ea)

Solution, External:

Generic: 2% (60 mL)

Erythromycin and Sulfisoxazole

(er ith roe MYE sin & sul fi SOKS a zole)

Medication Safety Issues

Sound-alike/look-alike issues:

Pediazole® may be confused with Pediapred®

Brand Names: US E.S.P.®

Brand Names: Canada Pediazole®

Therapeutic Category Antibiotic, Macrolide; Antibiotic, Sulfonamide Derivative

Generic Availability (US) Yes

Use Treatment of otitis media caused by susceptible strains of *Haemophilus influenzae* (FDA approved in ages 2 months to 12 years)

Pregnancy Risk Factor C

Pregnancy Considerations Animal reproduction studies have not been conducted with this combination. Erythromycin and sulfisoxazole cross the placenta. Most reports do not identify an increase in risk for congenital abnormalities due to prenatal exposure to erythromycin. Cardiovascular anomalies following exposure in early pregnancy have been reported in some observational studies; see Erythromycin (Systemic) monograph for additional information. Based on available information, an increased risk for congenital malformations has not been observed after use of sulfisoxazole during pregnancy (Aselton, 1985; Heinonen, 1977; Hibbard, 1967; Jick 1981); however, studies with sulfonamides as a class have shown mixed results (ACOG No. 494, 2011).

Individually, erythromycin and sulfonamides may be used to treat infections in pregnant women when clinically appropriate for confirmed infections caused by susceptible organisms. Use of sulfonamides during the first trimester should be limited to situations where no alternative therapies are available (ACOG No. 120, 2011; ACOG No. 494, 2011). Erythromycin/sulfisoxazole is contraindicated in late pregnancy because sulfonamides may cause kernicterus in the newborn. Neonatal healthcare providers should be informed if maternal sulfonamide therapy is used near the time of delivery (DHHS, 2013).

Breast-Feeding Considerations Erythromycin and sulfisoxazole are both excreted into breast milk. Per the manufacturer, this combination is contraindicated in mothers nursing infants <2 months of age because sulfonamides distribute into breast milk and may cause kernicterus in the newborn. Sulfonamides should not be used while nursing an infant with G6PD deficiency or hyperbilirubinemia (Della-Giustina, 2003). See Erythromycin (Systemic) monograph for information specific to the use of erythromycin in nursing women. Nondose-related effects could include modification of bowel flora.

Contraindications

Hypersensitivity to erythromycin, sulfonamides, or any component of the formulation; pregnant women at term; nursing mothers of infants <2 months of age; infants <2 months of age (sulfas compete with bilirubin for binding sites)

Note: Although the FDA approved product labeling states this medication is contraindicated with other sulfonamide-containing drug classes, the scientific basis of this statement has been challenged. See "Warnings/Precautions" for more detail.

Warnings/Precautions Use with caution in patients with impaired renal or hepatic function, myasthenia gravis, G6PD deficiency (hemolysis may occur). Macrolides have been associated with rare QTc prolongation and ventricular arrhythmias, including torsade de pointes; use with caution in patients at risk of prolonged cardiac repolarization.

Fatalities associated with severe reactions including agranulocytosis, aplastic anemia, and other blood dyscrasias; hepatic necrosis, Stevens-Johnson syndrome, and toxic epidermal necrolysis have occurred with sulfonamides; discontinue use at first sign of rash or signs of serious adverse reactions. Use with caution in patients with allergies or asthma.

Prolonged use may result in fungal or bacterial superinfection, including *C. difficile*-associated diarrhea (CDAD) and pseudomembranous colitis; CDAD has been observed >2 months postantibiotic treatment.

Some dosage forms may contain polysorbate 80 (also known as Tweens). Hypersensitivity reactions, usually a delayed reaction, have been reported following exposure to pharmaceutical products containing polysorbate 80 in certain individuals (Isaksson, 2002; Lucente 2000; Shelley, 1995). Thrombocytopenia, ascites, pulmonary deterioration, and renal and hepatic failure have been reported in premature neonates after receiving parenteral products containing polysorbate 80 (Alade, 1986; CDC, 1984). See manufacturer's labeling.

Sulfonamide ("sulfa") allergy: Traditionally, concerns for cross-reactivity have extended to all compounds containing the sulfonamide structure (SO_2NH_2). An expanded understanding of allergic mechanisms indicates cross-reactivity between antibiotic sulfonamides and nonantibiotic sulfonamides may not occur, or at the very least this potential is extremely low (Brackett 2004; Johnson 2005; Slatore 2004; Tornero 2004). In particular, mechanisms of cross-reaction due to antibody production (anaphylaxis) are unlikely to occur with nonantibiotic sulfonamides and antibiotic sulfonamides. A nonantibiotic sulfonamide compound which contains the arylamine structure and therefore may cross-react with antibiotic sulfonamides is sulfasalazine (Zawodniak 2010). T-cell-mediated (type IV) reactions (eg, maculopapular rash) are less understood and it is not possible to completely exclude this potential based on current insights. In cases where prior reactions were severe (Stevens-Johnson syndrome/TEN), some clinicians choose to avoid exposure to these classes.

Adverse Reactions Adverse events specific to this combination have not been identified.

Cardiovascular: Allergic myocarditis, arteritis, cyanosis, edema (including periorbital), flushing, intracranial hypertension, palpitations, periarteritis nodosa, syncope, tachycardia, torsade de pointes, vasculitis, ventricular arrhythmia

Central nervous system: Anxiety, ataxia, depression, disorientation, dizziness, drowsiness, fatigue, fever, hallucinations, headache, insomnia, psychosis, seizure, vertigo

Dermatologic: Angioedema, erythema multiforme, exfoliative dermatitis, photosensitivity, pruritus, purpura, rash, Stevens-Johnson syndrome, toxic epidermal necrolysis, urticaria

Endocrine & metabolic: Goiter (rare), hypoglycemia (rare)

Gastrointestinal: Abdominal pain, anorexia, diarrhea, flatulence, gastrointestinal hemorrhage, glossitis, hypertrophic pyloric stenosis, melena, nausea, oral candidiasis, pancreatitis, pseudomembranous colitis, salivary gland swelling, stomatitis, vomiting

Genitourinary: Urinary retention

Hematologic: Agranulocytosis, anemia, aplastic anemia, clotting disorders (including hypoprothrombinemia, hypofibrinogenemia, sulfhemoglobinemia, methemoglobinemia), eosinophilia, hemolytic anemia, leukopenia, thrombocytopenia

Hepatic: Hepatotoxicity (including hepatitis, hepatic necrosis, and cholestatic jaundice), liver enzymes increased

Neuromuscular & skeletal: Paresthesia, peripheral neuritis, rigors, weakness

Otic: Hearing loss (reversible), tinnitus

Renal: Acute renal failure, blood urea nitrogen increased, crystalluria, diuresis (rare), hematuria, nephritis, serum creatinine increased, toxic nephrosis (with oliguria and anuria)

Respiratory: Cough, dyspnea, pneumonitis, pulmonary infiltrates

Miscellaneous: Anaphylaxis, hypersensitivity reactions, serum sickness, systemic lupus erythematosus (SLE)

Drug Interactions

Metabolism/Transport Effects Refer to individual components.

Avoid Concomitant Use

Avoid concomitant use of Erythromycin and Sulfisoxazole with any of the following: Barnidipine; BCG; BCG (Intravesical); Bosutinib; Cisapride; Clindamycin (Topical); Conivaptan; Disopyramide; Domperidone; Fluconazole; Fusidic Acid (Systemic); Highest Risk QTc-Prolonging Agents; Ibrutinib; Idelalisib; Ivabradine; Lincosamide Antibiotics; Lomitapide; Lovastatin; Mecamylamine; Mequitazine; Methenamine; Mifepristone; Naloxegol; Olaparib; PAZOPanib; Pimozide; Potassium P-Aminobenzoate; Procaine; QuiNIDine; QuiNINE; Silodosin; Simeprevir; Simvastatin; Terfenadine; Tolvaptan; Topotecan; Trabectedin; Ulipristal; VinCRIStine (Liposomal)

Increased Effect/Toxicity

Erythromycin and Sulfisoxazole may increase the levels/effects of: Afatinib; Alfentanil; ALPRAZolam; Antineoplastic Agents (Vinca Alkaloids); ARIPiprazole; AtorvaSTATin; Avanafil; Barnidipine; Bosentan; Bosutinib; Brentuximab Vedotin; Budesonide (Systemic, Oral Inhalation); Budesonide (Topical); BusPIRone; Calcium Channel Blockers; Cannabis; CarBAMazepine; Cardiac Glycosides; Carvedilol; Cilostazol; Cisapride; CloZAPine; Colchicine; CycloSPORINE (Systemic); CYP2C9 Substrates; CYP3A4 Substrates; Dabigatran Etexilate; Dapoxetine; Diclofenac (Systemic); Disopyramide; Domperidone; DOXOrubicin (Conventional); Dronabinol; Edoxaban; Eletriptan; Eplerenone; Ergot Derivatives; Estazolam; Everolimus; FentaNYL; Fexofenadine; Highest Risk QTc-Prolonging Agents; Hydrocodone; Hypoglycemia-Associated Agents; Ibrutinib; Imatinib; Ivabradine; Ivacaftor; Lacosamide; Ledipasvir; Lomitapide; Lovastatin; Lurasidone; Mecamylamine; Mequitazine; Methotrexate; Midazolam; Moderate Risk QTc-Prolonging Agents; Naloxegol; Nintedanib; Olaparib; Ospemifene; OxyCODONE; Parecoxib; PAZOPanib; P-glycoprotein/ABCB1 Substrates; Pimecrolimus; Pimozide; Pitavastatin; Porfimer; Pravastatin; QuiNIDine; QuiNINE; Ramelteon; Ranolazine; Repaglinide; Rifamycin Derivatives; Rifaximin; Rilpivirine; Rivaroxaban; Salmeterol; Saxagliptin; Selective Serotonin Reuptake Inhibitors; Sildenafil; Silodosin; Simeprevir; Simvastatin; Sirolimus; Sulfonylureas; Suvorexant; Tacrolimus (Systemic); Tacrolimus (Topical); Telaprevir; Temsirolimus; Terfenadine; Tetrahydrocannabinol; Theophylline Derivatives; Thiopental; Tolvaptan; Topotecan; Trabectedin; Triazolam; Ulipristal; Vardenafil; Verteporfin; Vilazodone; VinCRIStine (Liposomal); Vitamin K Antagonists; Zopiclone

The levels/effects of Erythromycin and Sulfisoxazole may be increased by: Androgens; Antidiabetic Agents; Cannabis; Conivaptan; CYP2C9 Inhibitors (Moderate); CYP2C9 Inhibitors (Strong); CYP3A4 Inhibitors (Moderate); CYP3A4 Inhibitors (Strong); Dasatinib; Dexketoprofen; Fluconazole; Fosaprepitant; Fusidic Acid (Systemic); Herbs (Hypoglycemic Properties); Idelalisib; Ivabradine; Luliconazole; MAO Inhibitors; Methenamine; Mifepristone; Netupitant; Palbociclib; Pegvisomant; P-glycoprotein/ABCB1 Inhibitors; QTc-Prolonging Agents (Indeterminate Risk and Risk Modifying); Quinolone Antibiotics; Salicylates; Selective Serotonin Reuptake Inhibitors; Stiripentol; Telaprevir

Decreased Effect

Erythromycin and Sulfisoxazole may decrease the levels/effects of: BCG; BCG (Intravesical); BCG Vaccine (Immunization); Clindamycin (Topical); Clopidogrel; CycloSPORINE (Systemic); Ifosfamide; Sodium Picosulfate; Typhoid Vaccine

The levels/effects of Erythromycin and Sulfisoxazole may be decreased by: Bosentan; CYP2C9 Inducers (Strong); CYP3A4 Inducers (Moderate); CYP3A4 Inducers (Strong); Dabrafenib; Deferasirox; Etravirine; Lincosamide Antibiotics; Mitotane; P-glycoprotein/ABCB1 Inducers; Potassium P-Aminobenzoate; Procaine; Quinolone Antibiotics; Siltuximab; St Johns Wort; Tocilizumab

Storage/Stability Prior to reconstitution, store at room temperature. After reconstitution, store in refrigerator for up to 14 days.

Mechanism of Action Erythromycin inhibits bacterial protein synthesis; sulfisoxazole competitively inhibits bacterial synthesis of folic acid from para-aminobenzoic acid

Pharmacokinetics (Adult data unless noted)

Erythromycin ethylsuccinate:

Absorption: Well absorbed from the GI tract; improved in presence of food

Distribution: Widely distributed into most body tissues and fluids; poor penetration into CSF

Protein binding: 75% to 90%

Metabolism: In the liver by demethylation via CYP3A4

Half-life: 1-1.5 hours

Elimination: Unchanged drug is excreted and concentrated in bile; <5% of dose eliminated in urine

Dialysis: Not removed by peritoneal dialysis or hemodialysis

Sulfisoxazole acetyl:

Absorption: Rapid and complete; the small intestine is the major site of absorption

Distribution: Into extracellular space; CSF concentration ranges from 8% to 57% of blood concentration in patients with normal meninges

Protein binding: 85%; primarily to albumin

Metabolism: Undergoes N-acetylation and N-glucuronide conjugation in the liver

Half-life: 4.6-7.8 hours, prolonged in renal impairment

Time to peak serum concentration: 2.5 hours (range: 1-4 hours)

Elimination: Urine (97%; 52% as unchanged drug)

Dialysis: >50% removed by hemodialysis

Dosing: Usual Infants ≥2 months and Children: **Otitis media, acute:** 40 to 50 mg/kg/day of erythromycin in divided doses every 6 to 8 hours; maximum daily dose: 2,000 mg/**day** of erythromycin; if dosing based on sulfisoxazole component: 150 mg/kg/day of sulfisoxazole in divided doses every 6 to 8 hours; maximum daily dose: 6 g/**day** sulfisoxazole. **Note:** Due to resistance of *S. pneumoniae*, should not be used in patients that fail first-line amoxicillin therapy (AAP [Lieberthal, 2013]).

Dosing adjustment in renal impairment: There are no dosage adjustments provided in manufacturer's labeling.

Dosing adjustment in hepatic impairment: There are no dosage adjustments provided in manufacturer's labeling; use with caution.

Preparation for Administration Oral suspension: Reconstitute granules for oral suspension with appropriate amount of water as specified on the bottle. Shake well until suspended.

Administration Oral suspension: Administer without regard to food; shake suspension well before use

Monitoring Parameters CBC with differential and platelet count, urinalysis; periodic liver function and renal function tests; urinalysis, observe patient for diarrhea

Test Interactions False-positive urinary protein; false-positive urinary catecholamines, 17-hydroxycorticosteroids and 17-ketosteroids

Dosage Forms Excipient information presented when available (limited, particularly for generics); consult specific product labeling.

Powder for oral suspension: Erythromycin ethylsuccinate 200 mg and sulfisoxazole acetyl 600 mg per 5 mL (100 mL, 150 mL, 200 mL)

E.S.P.®: Erythromycin ethylsuccinate 200 mg and sulfisoxazole acetyl 600 mg per 5 mL (100 mL, 150 mL, 200 mL) [cheri beri flavor]

◆ **Erythromycin Base** *see* Erythromycin (Ophthalmic) *on page 782*

◆ **Erythromycin Base** *see* Erythromycin (Systemic) *on page 779*

◆ **Erythromycin Ethylsuccinate** *see* Erythromycin (Systemic) *on page 779*

◆ **Erythromycin Lactobionate** *see* Erythromycin (Systemic) *on page 779*

◆ **Erythromycin Stearate** *see* Erythromycin (Systemic) *on page 779*

◆ **Erythropoiesis-Stimulating Agent (ESA)** *see* Darbepoetin Alfa *on page 585*

◆ **Erythropoiesis-Stimulating Agent (ESA)** *see* Epoetin Alfa *on page 765*

◆ **Erythropoiesis-Stimulating Protein** *see* Darbepoetin Alfa *on page 585*

◆ **Erythropoietin** *see* Epoetin Alfa *on page 765*

Escitalopram (es sye TAL oh pram)

Medication Safety Issues

Sound-alike/look-alike issues:

Lexapro may be confused with Loxitane [DSC]

BEERS Criteria medication:

This drug may be potentially inappropriate for use in geriatric patients with a history of falls or fractures (Quality of evidence - high [moderate for SIADH]; Strength of recommendation - strong).

International issues:

Zavesca: Brand name for escitalopram [in multiple international markets; ISMP April 21, 2010], but also brand name for miglustat [Canada, U.S., and multiple international markets]

Related Information

Antidepressant Agents *on page 2257*

Brand Names: US Lexapro

Brand Names: Canada ACT Escitalopram; Apo-Escitalopram; Cipralex; Cipralex MELTZ; JAMP-Escitalopram; Mar-Escitalopram; Mylan-Escitalopram; PMS-Escitalopram; Priva-Escitalopram; RAN-Escitalopram; Riva-Escitalopram; Sandoz Escitalopram; Teva-Escitalopram

Therapeutic Category Antidepressant, Selective Serotonin Reuptake Inhibitor (SSRI)

Generic Availability (US) Yes

Use Treatment of major depressive disorder (FDA approved in ages 12-17 years and adults); treatment of generalized anxiety disorders (GAD) (FDA approved in adults); has also been studied in children and adolescents with social anxiety disorders and pervasive developmental disorders (PDD) including autism

Medication Guide Available Yes

Pregnancy Risk Factor C

Pregnancy Considerations Adverse events have been observed in animal reproduction studies. Escitalopram crosses the placenta and is distributed into the amniotic fluid. An increased risk of teratogenic effects, including cardiovascular defects, may be associated with maternal use of escitalopram or other SSRIs; however, available information is conflicting. Nonteratogenic effects in the newborn following SSRI/SNRI exposure late in the third trimester include respiratory distress, cyanosis, apnea, seizures, temperature instability, feeding difficulty, vomiting, hypoglycemia, hypo- or hypertonia, hyper-reflexia, jitteriness, irritability, constant crying, and tremor. Symptoms may be due to the toxicity of the SSRIs/SNRIs or a discontinuation syndrome and may be consistent with serotonin syndrome associated with SSRI treatment. Persistent pulmonary hypertension of the newborn (PPHN) has also been reported with SSRI exposure. The long-term effects of *in utero* SSRI exposure on infant development and behavior are not known. Escitalopram is the S-enantiomer of the racemic derivative citalopram; also refer to the Citalopram monograph.

Due to pregnancy-induced physiologic changes, some pharmacokinetic parameters of escitalopram may be altered. The ACOG recommends that therapy with SSRIs or SNRIs during pregnancy be individualized; treatment of depression during pregnancy should incorporate the clinical expertise of the mental health clinician, obstetrician, primary healthcare provider, and pediatrician. According to the American Psychiatric Association (APA), the risks of medication treatment should be weighed against other treatment options and untreated depression. For women who discontinue antidepressant medications during pregnancy and who may be at high risk for postpartum depression, the medications can be restarted following delivery. Treatment algorithms have been developed by the ACOG and the APA for the management of depression in women prior to conception and during pregnancy.

Breast-Feeding Considerations Escitalopram and its metabolite are excreted into breast milk. Limited data is available concerning the effects escitalopram may have in the nursing infant and the long-term effects on development and behavior have not been studied. Adverse effects have been reported in nursing infants exposed to some SSRIs. According to the manufacturer, the decision to continue or discontinue breast-feeding during therapy should take into account the risk of exposure to the infant and the benefits of treatment to the mother. Maternal use of an SSRI during pregnancy may cause delayed milk secretion. Escitalopram is the S-enantiomer of the racemic derivative citalopram; also refer to the Citalopram monograph.

Contraindications Hypersensitivity to escitalopram, citalopram, or any component of the formulation; use of MAO inhibitors intended to treat psychiatric disorders (concurrently or within 14 days of discontinuing either escitalopram or the MAO inhibitor); initiation of escitalopram in a patient receiving linezolid or intravenous methylene blue; concurrent use of pimozide

Canadian labeling: Additional contraindications (not in U.S. labeling): Known QT-interval prolongation or congenital long QT syndrome

Warnings/Precautions [U.S. Boxed Warning]: Antidepressants increase the risk of suicidal thinking and behavior in children, adolescents, and young adults (18-24 years of age) with major depressive disorder (MDD) and other psychiatric disorders; consider risk prior to prescribing. Short-term studies did not show an increased risk in patients >24 years of age and showed a decreased risk in patients ≥65 years. Closely monitor patients for clinical worsening, suicidality, or unusual changes in behavior, particularly during the initial 1-2 months of therapy or during periods of dosage adjustments (increases or decreases); the patient's family or caregiver should be instructed to closely observe the patient and communicate condition with healthcare provider. A medication guide concerning the use of antidepressants should be dispensed with each prescription. **Escitalopram is not FDA approved for use in children <12 years of age.**

The possibility of a suicide attempt is inherent in major depression and may persist until remission occurs. Use caution in high-risk patients. Worsening depression and severe abrupt suicidality that are not part of the presenting symptoms may require discontinuation or modification of drug therapy. The patient's family or caregiver should be alerted to monitor patients for the emergence of suicidality and associated behaviors (such as agitation, irritability, hostility, impulsivity, and hypomania) and call healthcare provider.

May precipitate a shift to mania or hypomania in patients with bipolar disorder. Patients presenting with depressive symptoms should be screened for bipolar disorder. Monotherapy in patients with bipolar disorder should be avoided. Escitalopram is not FDA approved for the treatment of bipolar depression.

Potentially life-threatening serotonin syndrome (SS) has occurred with serotonergic agents (eg, SSRIs, SNRIs), particularly when used in combination with other serotonergic agents (eg, triptans, TCAs, fentanyl, lithium, tramadol, buspirone, St John's wort, tryptophan) or agents that impair metabolism of serotonin (eg, MAO inhibitors intended to treat psychiatric disorders, other MAO inhibitors [ie, linezolid and intravenous methylene blue]). Discontinue treatment (and any concomitant serotonergic agent) immediately if signs/symptoms arise. May increase the risks associated with electroconvulsive therapy. Has a low potential to impair cognitive or motor performance; caution operating hazardous machinery or driving. Bone fractures have been associated with antidepressant treatment. Consider the possibility of a fragility fracture if an antidepressant-treated patient presents with unexplained bone pain, point tenderness, swelling, or bruising (Rabenda, 2013; Rizzoli, 2012).

Use with caution in patients with a recent history of MI or unstable heart disease. Use has been associated with dose-dependent QT-interval prolongation with doses of 10 mg and 30 mg/day in healthy subjects (mean change from baseline: 4.3 msec and 10.7 msec, respectively); prolongation of QT interval and ventricular arrhythmia (including torsade de pointes) have been reported, particularly in females with preexisting QT prolongation or other risk factors (eg, hypokalemia, other cardiac disease).

Use caution with a previous seizure disorder or condition predisposing to seizures such as brain damage, alcoholism, or concurrent therapy with other drugs which lower the seizure threshold. May cause hyponatremia/SIADH (elderly at increased risk); volume depletion (diuretics may increase risk) may occur. Use caution in patients with metabolic disease. May cause or exacerbate sexual dysfunction. Use caution in elderly patients; may be potentially inappropriate in patients with a history of falls or fractures, and may cause or exacerbate syndrome of inappropriate antidiuretic hormone secretion or hyponatremia; monitor sodium closely with initiation or dosage adjustments in older adults (Beers Criteria). Bioavailability and half-life are increased by 50% in the elderly. Use caution with severe renal impairment or liver impairment; concomitant CNS depressants. May cause mild pupillary dilation which in susceptible individuals can lead to an episode of narrow-angle glaucoma. Consider evaluating patients who have not had an iridectomy for narrow-angle glaucoma risk factors. Use with caution in patients who are hemodynamically unstable. Potentially significant drug-drug interactions may exist, requiring dose or frequency adjustment, additional monitoring, and/or selection of alternative therapy. Escitalopram systemic exposure may be increased in CYP2C19 poor metabolizers; Canadian labeling recommends a dosage adjustment in this patient population.

Abrupt discontinuation or interruption of antidepressant therapy has been associated with a discontinuation syndrome. Symptoms arising may vary with antidepressant however commonly include nausea, vomiting, diarrhea, headaches, light-headedness, dizziness, diminished appetite, sweating, chills, tremors, paresthesias, fatigue, somnolence, and sleep disturbances (eg, vivid dreams, insomnia). Greater risks for developing a discontinuation syndrome have been associated with antidepressants with shorter half-lives, longer durations of treatment, and abrupt discontinuation. For antidepressants of short or intermediate half-lives, symptoms may emerge within 2-5 days after treatment discontinuation and last 7-14 days (APA, 2010; Fava, 2006; Haddad, 2001; Shelton, 2001; Warner, 2006). Some dosage forms may contain propylene glycol; large amounts are potentially toxic and have been associated hyperosmolality, lactic acidosis, seizures, and respiratory depression; use caution (AAP, 1997; Zar, 2007).

Warnings: Additional Pediatric Considerations SSRI-associated behavioral activation (ie, restlessness, hyperkinesis, hyperactivity, agitation) is two- to threefold more prevalent in children compared to adolescents; it is more prevalent in adolescents compared to adults. Somnolence (including sedation and drowsiness) is more common in adults compared to children and adolescents (Safer, 2006). Escitalopram may impair cognitive or motor performance. SSRI-associated vomiting is two- to threefold more prevalent in children compared to adolescents and is more prevalent in adolescents compared to adults (Safer, 2006).

Some dosage forms may contain propylene glycol; in neonates large amounts of propylene glycol delivered orally, intravenously (eg, >3,000 mg/day), or topically have been associated with potentially fatal toxicities which can include metabolic acidosis, seizures, renal failure, and CNS depression; toxicities have also been reported in children and adults including hyperosmolality, lactic acidosis, seizures, and respiratory depression; use caution (AAP, 1997; Shehab, 2009).

Adverse Reactions

Central nervous system: Abnormal dreams, anorgasmia, dizziness, drowsiness, fatigue, headache, insomnia, lethargy, paresthesia, yawning

Dermatologic: Diaphoresis

Endocrine & metabolic: Decreased libido, menstrual disease

Gastrointestinal: Abdominal pain, constipation, decreased appetite, diarrhea, dyspepsia, flatulence, nausea, toothache, vomiting, xerostomia

Genitourinary: Ejaculatory disorder, impotence, urinary tract infection (children)

Neuromuscular & skeletal: Back pain (children), neck pain, shoulder pain

Respiratory: Flu-like symptoms, nasal congestion (children), rhinitis, sinusitis

Rare but important or life-threatening: Abdominal cramps, abnormal gait, acute renal failure, aggressive behavior, agitated depression, agitation, agranulocytosis, akathisia, alopecia, amnesia, anaphylaxis, anemia, angioedema, angle-closure glaucoma, anxiety, apathy, aplastic anemia, arthralgia, ataxia, atrial fibrillation, blurred vision, bradycardia, bronchitis, cardiac failure, cerebrovascular accident, chest pain, choreoathetosis, deep vein thrombosis, delirium, delusions, depersonalization, dermatitis, diabetes mellitus, diplopia, dyskinesia, dysmenorrhea, dysphagia, dyspnea, dystonia, dysuria, ecchymoses, edema, epistaxis, erythema multiforme, extrapyramidal reaction, fever, flushing, gastroenteritis, gastroesophageal reflux disease, gastrointestinal hemorrhage, hallucination, heartburn, hemolytic anemia, hepatic failure, hepatic necrosis, hepatitis, hot flash, hypercholesterolemia, hyperglycemia, hypermenorrhea, hyperprolactinemia, hypersensitivity reaction, hypertension, hypertensive crisis, hypoesthesia, hypoglycemia, hypokalemia, hyponatremia, hypoprothrombinemia, hypotension, immune thrombocytopenia, increased appetite, increased INR, increased liver enzymes, increased serum bilirubin, irritability, jaw tightness, lack of concentration, leukopenia, limb pain, migraine, myalgia, myasthenia, mydriasis, myocardial infarction, myoclonus, neuroleptic malignant syndrome (Stevens, 2008), nightmares, nystagmus, orthostatic hypotension, palpitations, pancreatitis, panic, paranoia, Parkinsonian-like syndrome, phlebitis, priapism, prolonged Q-T interval on ECG, psychosis, pulmonary embolism, rectal hemorrhage, rhabdomyolysis, seizure, serotonin syndrome, SIADH, sinus congestion, sinus headache, skin photosensitivity, skin rash, spontaneous abortion, Stevens-Johnson syndrome, suicidal ideation, suicidal tendencies, syncope, tachycardia, tardive dyskinesia, thrombocytopenia, thrombosis, tinnitus, torsades de pointes, toxic epidermal necrolysis, tremor, urinary frequency, urinary retention, urticaria, ventricular arrhythmia, ventricular tachycardia, vertigo, visual disturbance, withdrawal syndrome

Drug Interactions

Metabolism/Transport Effects Substrate of CYP2C19 (major), CYP3A4 (major); **Note:** Assignment of Major/Minor substrate status based on clinically relevant drug interaction potential; **Inhibits** CYP2D6 (weak)

Avoid Concomitant Use

Avoid concomitant use of Escitalopram with any of the following: Conivaptan; Dapoxetine; Dosulepin; Fusidic Acid (Systemic); Highest Risk QTc-Prolonging Agents; Idelalisib; Iobenguane I 123; Ivabradine; Linezolid; MAO Inhibitors; Methylene Blue; Mifepristone; Moderate Risk QTc-Prolonging Agents; Pimozide; Tryptophan; Urokinase

Increased Effect/Toxicity

Escitalopram may increase the levels/effects of: Agents with Antiplatelet Properties; Anticoagulants; Antidepressants (Serotonin Reuptake Inhibitor/Antagonist); Antipsychotic Agents; Apixaban; Aspirin; Blood Glucose Lowering Agents; BusPIRone; CarBAMazepine; Collagenase (Systemic); Dabigatran Etexilate; Deoxycholic Acid; Desmopressin; Dextromethorphan; Dosulepin; Highest Risk QTc-Prolonging Agents; Ibritumomab; Methylene Blue; Mexiletine; NSAID (COX-2 Inhibitor); NSAID (Nonselective); Obinutuzumab; Pimozide; Rivaroxaban; Salicylates; Serotonin Modulators; Thiazide Diuretics; Thrombolytic Agents; Tositumomab and Iodine I 131 Tositumomab; TraMADol; Tricyclic Antidepressants; Urokinase; Vitamin K Antagonists

The levels/effects of Escitalopram may be increased by: Alcohol (Ethyl); Analgesics (Opioid); Antiemetics (5HT3 Antagonists); Antipsychotic Agents; Aprepitant; BusPIRone; Cimetidine; CNS Depressants; Conivaptan; CYP2C19 Inhibitors (Moderate); CYP2C19 Inhibitors (Strong); CYP3A4 Inhibitors (Moderate); CYP3A4 Inhibitors (Strong); Dapoxetine; Fosaprepitant; Fusidic Acid (Systemic); Glucosamine; Herbs (Anticoagulant/Antiplatelet Properties); Ibrutinib; Idelalisib; Ivabradine; Ivacaftor; Limaprost; Linezolid; Lithium; Luliconazole; MAO Inhibitors; Metoclopramide; Metyrosine; Mifepristone; Moderate Risk QTc-Prolonging Agents; Multivitamins/Fluoride (with ADE); Multivitamins/Minerals (with ADEK, Folate, Iron); Multivitamins/Minerals (with AE, No Iron); Netupitant; Omega-3 Fatty Acids; Omeprazole; Palbociclib; Pentosan Polysulfate Sodium; Pentoxifylline; Prostacyclin Analogues; QTc-Prolonging Agents (Indeterminate Risk and Risk Modifying); Stiripentol; Tedizolid; Tipranavir; TraMADol; Tricyclic Antidepressants; Tryptophan; Vitamin E

Decreased Effect

Escitalopram may decrease the levels/effects of: Iobenguane I 123; Ioflupane I 123; Simeprevir; Thyroid Products

The levels/effects of Escitalopram may be decreased by: Boceprevir; Bosentan; CarBAMazepine; CYP2C19 Inducers (Strong); CYP3A4 Inducers (Moderate); CYP3A4 Inducers (Strong); Cyproheptadine; Dabrafenib; Deferasirox; Mitotane; NSAID (COX-2 Inhibitor); NSAID (Nonselective); Siltuximab; St Johns Wort; Telaprevir; Tocilizumab

Storage/Stability Store at 25°C (77°F); excursions permitted to 15°C to 30°C (59°F to 86°F). Cipralex MELTZ [Canadian product] should be stored in original package and protected from light.

Mechanism of Action Escitalopram is the S-enantiomer of the racemic derivative citalopram, which selectively inhibits the reuptake of serotonin with little to no effect on norepinephrine or dopamine reuptake. It has no or very low affinity for $5\text{-HT}_{1\text{-}7}$, alpha- and beta-adrenergic, $D_{1\text{-}5}$, $H_{1\text{-}3}$, $M_{1\text{-}5}$, and benzodiazepine receptors. Escitalopram does not bind to or has low affinity for Na^+, K^+, Cl^-, and Ca^{++} ion channels.

Pharmacodynamics

Onset of action: 1-2 weeks

Maximum effect: 8-12 weeks

Pharmacokinetics (Adult data unless noted)

Distribution: V_d: Adults: 12 L/kg

Protein binding, plasma: ~56%

Metabolism: Extensively hepatic via CYP2C19 and 3A4 to S-demethylcitalopram (S-DCT; 1/7 the activity of escitalopram); S-DCT is metabolized to S-didemethylcitalopram (S-DDCT; active; 1/27 the activity of escitalopram) via CYP2D6

Bioavailability: 80%; tablets and oral solution are bioequivalent
Half-life elimination: Mean:
Adults: 27-32 hours
Adolescents: 19 hours
Time to peak serum concentration: Adults: 5 hours; Adolescents: 2.9 hours
Elimination: Urine (8% as unchanged drug)
Clearance (citalopram):
Hepatic impairment: Decreased by 37%
Mild-to-moderate renal impairment: Decreased by 17%
Severe renal impairment (CrCl <20 mL/minute): No information available

Dosing: Usual
Pediatric:
Depression: Oral:
Children <12 years: Limited data available; only one randomized, placebo-controlled trial has been published; efficacy was not demonstrated for children <12 years of age (Wagner 2006)
Children and Adolescents ≥12 years: Initial: 10 mg once daily; may be increased to 20 mg/day after at least 3 weeks
Autism and PDD: Limited data available: Oral: Children and Adolescents 6 to 17 years: Initial: 2.5 mg once daily; may increase if needed to 5 mg/day after 1 week; may then increase at weekly intervals by 5 mg/day if needed and as tolerated; maximum dose: 20 mg/day. Dosing based on a prospective, 10-week, open-labeled, forced dose-titration trial of 28 children and adolescents 6 to 17 years of age (mean age: 10.4 years) (Owley 2005). Mean severity outcome scores showed significant improvement; mean final dose: 11.1 ± 6.5 mg/day (range: 0 to 20 mg/day); no significant correlation between final tolerated dose and weight was shown; 10 of 28 treated subjects could not tolerate a 10 mg/day dose
Social anxiety disorder: Limited data available: Oral: Children and Adolescents 10-17 years: Initial: 5 mg once daily for 7 days, then 10 mg/day for 7 days; may then increase at weekly intervals by 5 mg/day if needed, based on clinical response and tolerability; maximum dose: 20 mg/day. Dosing based on a prospective, 12-week, open-labeled trial of 20 children and adolescents 10-17 years of age (mean age: 15 years) (Isolan 2007). At the end of the 12 weeks, 65% of patients met overall response criteria and all symptomatic and quality of life outcome measures showed significant improvements; mean final dose: 13 ± 4.1 mg/day
Adult: **Depression, generalized anxiety disorder:** Oral: Initial: 10 mg once daily; dose may be increased to 20 mg/day after at least 1 week
Dosage adjustment in renal impairment:
Mild-to-moderate impairment: No dosage adjustment needed
Severe impairment: CrCl <20 mL/minute: Use with caution
Dosage adjustment in hepatic impairment: Adolescents >12 years and Adults: 10 mg/day

Administration Administer once daily (morning or evening); may be administered with or without food.

Monitoring Parameters Monitor patient periodically for symptom resolution; monitor for worsening depression, suicidality, and associated behaviors (especially at the beginning of therapy or when doses are increased or decreased). Monitor for anxiety, social functioning, mania, panic attacks; akathisia. Monitor for signs and symptoms of serotonin syndrome or neuroleptic malignant syndrome-like reactions.

Additional Information If used for an extended period of time, long-term usefulness of escitalopram should be periodically re-evaluated for the individual patient. A recent report describes 5 children (age: 8-15 years) who developed epistaxis (n=4) or bruising (n=1) while receiving SSRI therapy (sertraline) (Lake, 2000).

Neonates born to women receiving SSRIs later during the third trimester may experience respiratory distress, apnea, cyanosis, temperature instability, vomiting, feeding difficulty, hypoglycemia, constant crying, irritability, hypotonia, hypertonia, hyper-reflexia, tremor, jitteriness, and seizures; these symptoms may be due to a direct toxic effect, withdrawal syndrome, or (in some cases) serotonin syndrome. Withdrawal symptoms occur in 30% of neonates exposed to SSRIs *in utero*; monitor newborns for at least 48 hours after birth; long-term effects of *in utero* exposure to SSRIs are unknown (Levinson-Castiel, 2006).

Dosage Forms Excipient information presented when available (limited, particularly for generics); consult specific product labeling.
Solution, Oral:
Lexapro: 5 mg/5 mL (240 mL) [contains methylparaben, propylene glycol, propylparaben; peppermint flavor]
Generic: 5 mg/5 mL (240 mL)
Tablet, Oral:
Lexapro: 5 mg
Lexapro: 10 mg, 20 mg [scored]
Generic: 5 mg, 10 mg, 20 mg

◆ **Escitalopram Oxalate** *see* Escitalopram *on page 786*
◆ **Eserine Salicylate** *see* Physostigmine *on page 1697*
◆ **Eskalith** *see* Lithium *on page 1284*

Esmolol (ES moe lol)

Medication Safety Issues
Sound-alike/look-alike issues:
Esmolol may be confused with Osmitrol
Brevibloc may be confused with Brevital, Bumex, Buprenex
High alert medication:
The Institute for Safe Medication Practices (ISMP) includes this medication among its list of drugs which have a heightened risk of causing significant patient harm when used in error.

Related Information
Management of Drug Extravasations *on page 2298*
Serotonin Syndrome *on page 2447*

Brand Names: US Brevibloc; Brevibloc in NaCl

Brand Names: Canada Brevibloc; Brevibloc Premixed

Therapeutic Category Antiarrhythmic Agent, Class II; Antihypertensive Agent; Beta-Adrenergic Blocker

Generic Availability (US) Yes

Use Treatment of supraventricular tachycardia (primarily to control ventricular rate in patients with atrial fibrillation or flutter) (FDA approved in adults); noncompensatory sinus tachycardia (FDA approved in adults); perioperative tachycardia and hypertension (FDA approved in adults)

Pregnancy Risk Factor C

Pregnancy Considerations Adverse events were observed in some animal reproduction studies. Esmolol has been shown to decrease fetal heart rate. Adverse fetal/neonatal events have also been observed with the chronic use of beta-blockers during pregnancy. Esmolol is a short-acting beta-blocker and not indicated for the chronic treatment of hypertension. Esmolol has been evaluated for use during intubation as an agent to offset the exaggerated pressor response observed in pregnant women with hypertension undergoing surgery (Bansal, 2002).

Breast-Feeding Considerations It is not known if esmolol is excreted into breast milk. Due to the potential for serious adverse reactions in the nursing infant, the manufacturer recommends a decision be made whether to discontinue nursing or to discontinue the drug, taking into account the importance of treatment to the mother. The short half-life and the fact that it is not intended for chronic use should limit any potential exposure to the nursing infant.

Contraindications Hypersensitivity to esmolol or any component of the formulation; severe sinus bradycardia; heart block greater than first degree (except in patients with a functioning artificial ventricular pacemaker); sick sinus syndrome; cardiogenic shock; decompensated heart failure; IV administration of calcium channel blockers (eg, verapamil) in close proximity to esmolol (ie, while effects of other drug are still present); pulmonary hypertension

Canadian labeling: Additional contraindications (not in U.S. labeling): Patients requiring inotropic agents and/or vasopressors to maintain cardiac output and systolic blood pressure; hypotension; right ventricular failure secondary to pulmonary hypertension; untreated pheochromocytoma

Warnings/Precautions Can cause bradycardia including sinus pause, heart block, severe bradycardia, and cardiac arrest. Consider preexisting conditions such as first degree AV block, sick sinus syndrome, or other conduction disorders before initiating; use is contraindicated in patients with sick sinus syndrome or second- or third-degree AV block (except in patients with a functioning artificial ventricular pacemaker). Bradycardia may be observed more frequently in elderly patients (>65 years of age); dosage reductions may be necessary. Hypotension is common; patients need close blood pressure monitoring. If an unacceptable drop in blood pressure occurs, reduction in dose or discontinuation may reverse hypotension (usually within 30 minutes). Avoid use in patients with hypovolemia; treat hypovolemia first, otherwise, use of esmolol may attenuate reflex tachycardia and further increase the risk of hypotension. Administer cautiously in compensated heart failure and monitor for a worsening of the condition; use is contraindicated in patients with decompensated heart failure.

Esmolol has been associated with elevations in serum potassium and development of hyperkalemia especially in patients with risk factors (eg, renal impairment); monitor serum potassium during therapy. Use with caution in patients with myasthenia gravis. Use caution in patients with renal dysfunction (active metabolite retained). Adequate alpha-blockade is required prior to use of any beta-blocker for patients with untreated pheochromocytoma; Canadian labeling contraindicates use in this patient population. Use beta-blockers cautiously in patients with bronchospastic disease; monitor pulmonary status closely. Use cautiously in patients with diabetes because it can mask prominent hypoglycemic symptoms. May mask signs of hyperthyroidism (eg, tachycardia); if hyperthyroidism is suspected, carefully manage and monitor; abrupt withdrawal may exacerbate symptoms of hyperthyroidism or precipitate thyroid storm. Use esmolol with caution in patients with hypertension associated with hypothermia; monitor vital signs closely and titrate esmolol slowly. Use caution with history of severe anaphylaxis to allergens; patients taking beta-blockers may become more sensitive to repeated challenges. Treatment of anaphylaxis (eg, epinephrine) in patients taking beta-blockers may be ineffective or promote undesirable effects. Can precipitate or aggravate symptoms of arterial insufficiency in patients with PVD and Raynaud's disease; use with caution and monitor for progression of arterial obstruction.

Use caution with concurrent use of digoxin, verapamil or diltiazem; bradycardia or heart block can occur (may be fatal). Use is contraindicated when IV calcium channel blockers have been administered in close proximity to esmolol (ie, while effects of other drug are still present). Beta-blocker therapy should not be withdrawn abruptly (particularly in patients with CAD), but gradually tapered to avoid acute tachycardia, hypertension, and/or ischemia. Vesicant; ensure proper needle or catheter placement prior to and during infusion; avoid extravasation. Extravasation can lead to skin necrosis and sloughing; avoid infusions into small veins or through a butterfly catheter.

Adverse Reactions

Cardiovascular: Asymptomatic hypotension, blood pressure decreased, peripheral ischemia, symptomatic hypotension

Central nervous system: Agitation, confusion, dizziness, headache, somnolence

Gastrointestinal: Nausea, vomiting

Local: Infusion site reaction (including irritation, inflammation, and severe reactions associated with extravasation [eg, thrombophlebitis, necrosis, and blistering])

Rare but important or life-threatening: Abdominal discomfort, abnormal thinking, angioedema, anorexia, anxiety, bradycardia, bronchospasm, cardiac arrest, constipation, coronary arteriospasm, decompensated heart failure, depression, dyspepsia, flushing, heart block, hyperkalemia, lightheadedness, pallor, paresthesia, psoriasis, renal tubular acidosis, seizure, severe bradycardia/asystole (rare), syncope, urinary retention, urticaria, xerostomia

Drug Interactions

Metabolism/Transport Effects None known.

Avoid Concomitant Use

Avoid concomitant use of Esmolol with any of the following: Ceritinib; Floctafenine; Methacholine; Rivastigmine

Increased Effect/Toxicity

Esmolol may increase the levels/effects of: Alpha-/Beta-Agonists (Direct-Acting); Alpha1-Blockers; Alpha2-Agonists; Amifostine; Antihypertensives; Antipsychotic Agents (Phenothiazines); Bradycardia-Causing Agents; Bupivacaine; Cardiac Glycosides; Ceritinib; Cholinergic Agonists; Disopyramide; DULoxetine; Ergot Derivatives; Fingolimod; Grass Pollen Allergen Extract (5 Grass Extract); Hypotensive Agents; Insulin; Ivabradine; Lacosamide; Levodopa; Lidocaine (Systemic); Lidocaine (Topical); Mepivacaine; Methacholine; Midodrine; Obinutuzumab; RisperiDONE; RiTUXimab; Sulfonylureas

The levels/effects of Esmolol may be increased by: Acetylcholinesterase Inhibitors; Alpha2-Agonists; Aminoquinolines (Antimalarial); Amiodarone; Anilidopiperidine Opioids; Antipsychotic Agents (Phenothiazines); Barbiturates; Bretylium; Brimonidine (Topical); Calcium Channel Blockers (Nondihydropyridine); Diazoxide; Dipyridamole; Disopyramide; Dronedarone; Floctafenine; Herbs (Hypotensive Properties); MAO Inhibitors; Nicorandil; NIFEdipine; Pentoxifylline; Phosphodiesterase 5 Inhibitors; Propafenone; Prostacyclin Analogues; Regorafenib; Reserpine; Rivastigmine; Ruxolitinib; Tofacitinib

Decreased Effect

Esmolol may decrease the levels/effects of: Beta2-Agonists; Theophylline Derivatives

The levels/effects of Esmolol may be decreased by: Barbiturates; Herbs (Hypertensive Properties); Methylphenidate; Nonsteroidal Anti-Inflammatory Agents; Rifamycin Derivatives; Yohimbine

Storage/Stability Clear, colorless to light yellow solution which should be stored at 25°C (77°F); excursions permitted to 15°C to 30°C (59°F to 86°F); do not freeze. Protect from excessive heat. Stable for at least 24 hours (under refrigeration or at controlled room temperature) at a final concentration of 10 mg/mL.

Mechanism of Action Class II antiarrhythmic: Competitively blocks response to beta$_1$-adrenergic stimulation with little or no effect of beta$_2$-receptors except at high doses, no intrinsic sympathomimetic activity, no membrane stabilizing activity

Pharmacodynamics

Onset of action: IV: Beta blockade occurs within 2 to 10 minutes (onset of effects is quickest when loading doses are administered)

Duration: Short (10 to 30 minutes), prolonged following higher cumulative doses, extended duration of use

Pharmacokinetics (Adult data unless noted)

Protein binding: Esmolol 55%; acid metabolite 10%

Distribution: V_d:

Children ≥2.5 years and Adolescents ≤16 years: 2 ± 1.4 L/kg (range: 0.5 to 3.6 L/kg) (Wiest 1991)

Adults: Esmolol: ~3.4 L/kg; Acid metabolite: ~0.4 L/kg

Metabolism: In blood by red blood cell esterases; forms acid metabolite (negligible activity; produces no clinically important effects) and methanol (does not achieve concentrations associated with methanol toxicity)

Half-life, elimination:

Children ≥18 months and Adolescents ≤16 years: Variable; mean range: 2.7 to 4.8 minutes (reported full range: 0.2 to 9.9 minutes) (Cuneo 1994; Tabbutt 2008b; Wiest 1991; Wiest 1998)

Adults: Esmolol: 9 minutes; Acid metabolite: 3.7 hours; elimination of metabolite decreases with end-stage renal disease

Elimination: Urine (73% to 88% as metabolites and <2% as unchanged drug)

Dosing: Neonatal Note: Dose must be titrated individual response and tolerance.

Postoperative hypertension: Limited data available; further studies are needed. An open-label trial used the following dosing guidelines to treat postoperative hypertension following cardiac surgery; dose was titrated until blood pressure was ≤90th percentile for age; final dose required was significantly higher in patients with aortic coarctation repair than in patients with repair of other congenital heart defects (Wiest 1998):

Term neonates: Continuous IV infusion: PNA 0 to 7 days: Initial: 50 mcg/kg/minute; titrate dose by 25 to 50 mcg/kg/minute every 20 minutes

Term neonates: Continuous IV infusion: PNA 8 to 28 days: Initial: 75 mcg/kg/minute; titrate dose by 50 mcg/kg/minute every 20 minutes

Note: Maximum dose: 1,000 mcg/kg/minute; higher doses have not been evaluated

Dosing: Usual Note: Dose must be titrated to individual response and tolerance.

Pediatric:

Hypertensive emergency/urgency: Infants, Children, and Adolescents: Continuous IV infusion: 100 to 500 mcg/kg/minute infusion (NHBPEP Working Group 2004); another approach is to initiate therapy with a bolus of 100 to 500 mcg/kg over 1 minute, followed by an infusion of 25 to 100 mcg/kg/minute; titrating as needed up to 500 mcg/kg/minute (Chandar 2012; Temple 2000)

Postoperative hypertension: Limited data available; large effective dose range reported: Infants and Children: Initial IV bolus: 100 to 500 mcg/kg, followed by continuous IV infusion: Initial rate: 100 to 500 mcg/kg/minute; titrate to effect; range of effective doses: 125 to 1,000 mcg/kg/minute (Talbutt 2008a; Talbutt 2008b; Wiest 1998). Dosing based on several trials. In the largest trial, patients (n=118, weight ≥2.5 kg, age <6 years, mean age: ~18 months) experiencing hypertension after coarctation of aorta repair received a median maximum dose of 521 mcg/kg/minute (Talbutt 2008b); the need for coadministration of nitroprusside infusion increased with patient age (age ≤30 days: 27%, >30 days to <2 years: 54%; age 2 to 6 years: 69%). In a smaller trial (n=20, age: 1 month to 12 years, median age: 25.6 months), patients experiencing hypertension after heart surgery (including 10 with coarctation of the aorta) a higher mean effective dose of 700 mcg/kg/minute was reported. In this trial, infants were initiated at 100 mcg/kg/minute, then titrated by 50 mcg/kg/minute every 10 minutes; patients with aortic coarctation repair required a significantly higher dose (mean: 830 ± 153 mcg/kg/minute) than patients with repair of other congenital heart defects (mean: 570 ± 230 mcg/kg/minute) (Wiest 1998).

Supraventricular tachycardia (SVT): Limited data available: Children and Adolescents: Initial IV bolus: 100 to 500 mcg/kg over 1 minute followed by a continuous IV infusion: Initial rate: 25 to 100 mcg/kg/minute, titrate in 25 to 50 mcg/kg/minute increments; usual maintenance dose: 50 to 500 mcg/kg/minute (Park 2014); doses up to 1,000 mcg/kg/minute have been reported (Trippel 1991). One electrophysiologic study assessing esmolol-induced beta-blockade (n=20, age range: 2 to 16 years) used an initial dose of 600 mcg/kg over 2 minutes followed by an infusion of 200 mcg/kg/minute; the infusion was titrated upward by 50 to 100 mcg/kg/minute every 5 to 10 minutes until a reduction >10% in heart rate or mean blood pressure occurred. Mean dose required: 550 mcg/kg/minute with a range of 300 to 1,000 mcg/kg/minute (Trippel 1991).

Adult:

Intraoperative and postoperative tachycardia and/or hypertension: IV:

Immediate control: Initial bolus: 1,000 mcg/kg over 30 seconds, followed by a 150 mcg/kg/minute infusion, if necessary. Adjust infusion rate as needed to maintain desired heart rate and/or blood pressure (up to 300 mcg/kg/minute)

Gradual control: Initial bolus: 500 mcg/kg over 1 minute, followed by a 50 mcg/kg/minute infusion for 4 minutes. Infusion may be continued at 50 mcg/kg/minute or, if the response is inadequate, titrated upward in 50 mcg/kg/minute increments (increased no more frequently than every 4 minutes) to a maximum of 300 mcg/kg/minute; may administer an optional loading dose equal to the initial bolus (500 mcg/kg over 1 minute) prior to each increase in infusion rate.

For control of tachycardia, doses >200 mcg/kg/minute provide minimal additional effect. *For control of postoperative hypertension,* as many as one-third of patients may require higher doses (250 to 300 mcg/kg/minute) to control blood pressure; the safety of doses >300 mcg/kg/minute has not been studied.

Supraventricular tachycardia (SVT) or noncompensatory sinus tachycardia: IV: Loading dose (optional): 500 mcg/kg over 1 minute; follow with a 50 mcg/kg/minute infusion for 4 minutes; response to this initial infusion rate may be a rough indication of the responsiveness of the ventricular rate

Infusion may be continued at 50 mcg/kg/minute or, if the response is inadequate, titrated upward in 50 mcg/kg/minute increments (increased no more frequently than every 4 minutes) to a maximum of 200 mcg/kg/minute.

To achieve more rapid response, following the initial loading dose and 50 mcg/kg/minute infusion, administer with a second 500 mcg/kg loading dose over 1 minute, and increase the maintenance infusion to 100 mcg/kg/minute for 4 minutes. If necessary, a third (and final) 500 mcg/kg loading dose may be administered, prior to increasing to an infusion rate of 150 mcg/kg/minute. After 4 minutes of the 150 mcg/kg/minute infusion, the infusion rate may be increased to a maximum rate of 200 mcg/kg/minute (without a bolus dose).

Note: If a loading dose is not administered, a continuous infusion at a fixed dose reaches steady-state in ~30 minutes. In general, the usual effective dose is 50 to 200 mcg/kg/minute; doses as low as 25 mcg/kg/minute may be adequate. Maintenance infusions may be continued for up to 48 hours.

Guidelines for transfer to oral therapy (beta-blocker, calcium channel blocker):

Infusion should be reduced by 50% thirty minutes following the first dose of the alternative agent.

Manufacturer suggests following the second dose of the alternative drug, patient's response should be monitored and if control is adequate for the first hour, esmolol may be discontinued.

Dosing adjustment in renal impairment: Adults: No dosage adjustments are required for maintenance infusion of 150 mcg/kg/minute for 4 hours. There is no information on higher rates or longer duration.

Dosing adjustment in hepatic impairment: Adults: No dosage adjustment required.

Usual Infusion Concentrations: Pediatric Note: Premixed solutions available.

IV infusion: 10,000 **mcg**/mL or 20,000 **mcg**/mL

Administration Parenteral: IV: Commercially available concentrations (10 mg/mL and 20 mg/mL) are iso-osmotic and can be used for direct IV use; loading doses (eg, Adults: 500 **mcg**/kg) may be administered over 30 seconds to 1 minute depending on how urgent the need for effect. Do not introduce additives into the premixed bags. Medication port of premixed bag should be used to withdraw only the initial bolus; do not use medication port to withdraw additional bolus doses (sterility cannot be assured).

Vesicant; ensure proper needle or catheter placement prior to and during infusion; avoid extravasation. If extravasation occurs, stop infusion immediately and disconnect (leave cannula/needle in place); gently aspirate extravasated solution (do **NOT** flush the line); remove needle/cannula; elevate extremity.

Vesicant/Extravasation Risk Vesicant

Monitoring Parameters Blood pressure, ECG, heart rate, respiratory rate, IV site; serum potassium (especially with renal impairment)

Dosage Forms Excipient information presented when available (limited, particularly for generics); consult specific product labeling.

Solution, Intravenous, as hydrochloride:
- Brevibloc: 10 mg/mL (10 mL)
- Brevibloc in NaCl: 2000 mg (100 mL); 2500 mg (250 mL)
- Generic: 10 mg/mL (10 mL)

Solution, Intravenous, as hydrochloride [preservative free]:
- Generic: 10 mg/mL (10 mL); 100 mg/10 mL (10 mL)

◆ **Esmolol Hydrochloride** *see* Esmolol *on page 789*

Esomeprazole (es oh ME pray zol)

Medication Safety Issues

Sound-alike/look-alike issues:

Esomeprazole may be confused with ARIPiprazole, omeprazole

NexIUM may be confused with NexAVAR

Related Information

Oral Medications That Should Not Be Crushed or Altered *on page 2476*

Brand Names: US NexIUM; Nexium 24HR [OTC]; NexIUM I.V.

Brand Names: Canada Apo-Esomeprazole; Mylan-Esomeprazole; Nexium; PMS-Esomeprazole DR

Therapeutic Category Gastric Acid Secretion Inhibitor; Gastrointestinal Agent, Gastric or Duodenal Ulcer Treatment; Proton Pump Inhibitor

Generic Availability (US) May be product dependent

Use

Oral: Short-term treatment (up to 6 weeks) of erosive esophagitis associated with gastroesophageal reflux disease (GERD) (FDA approved in ages 1 month to <1 year); short-term treatment (4-8 weeks) and maintenance of healing of severe erosive esophagitis (FDA approved in ages ≥1 year and adults); short-term treatment (4-8 weeks) of symptomatic gastroesophageal reflux disease (GERD) (FDA approved in children ≥1 year and adults); adjunctive treatment of duodenal ulcers associated with *Helicobacter pylori*; prevention of gastric ulcers associated with continuous NSAID therapy in patients at high risk; long-term treatment of pathological hypersecretory conditions including Zollinger-Ellison syndrome (FDA approved in adults)

IV: Short-term alternative treatment (≤10 days) of GERD with erosive esophagitis when oral therapy is not possible or appropriate (FDA approved in ages ≥1 month and adults)

Medication Guide Available Yes

Pregnancy Risk Factor C

Pregnancy Considerations Adverse events have been observed in some animal reproduction studies. An increased risk of hypospadias was reported following maternal use of proton pump inhibitors (PPIs) during pregnancy (Anderka, 2012), but this was based on a small number of exposures and the same association was not found in another study (Erichsen, 2012). An increased risk of major birth defects following maternal use of PPIs during pregnancy was not observed in an additional study (Pasternak, 2010). Esomeprazole is the s-isomer of omeprazole; refer to the Omeprazole monograph for additional information. When treating GERD in pregnancy, PPIs may be used when clinically indicated (Katz, 2013).

Breast-Feeding Considerations Esomeprazole and strontium (limited data) are excreted in breast milk. The manufacturer of esomeprazole recommends that caution be exercised when administering to nursing women. The manufacturer of esomeprazole strontium recommends a decision be made whether to discontinue nursing or to discontinue the drug, taking into account the importance of treatment to the mother. Esomeprazole is the s-isomer of omeprazole and omeprazole is excreted in breast milk; refer to Omeprazole monograph for additional information.

Contraindications Hypersensitivity (eg, anaphylaxis, anaphylactic shock, angioedema, bronchospasm, acute interstitial nephritis, urticaria) to esomeprazole, other substituted benzimidazole proton pump inhibitors, or any component of the formulation

Warnings/Precautions Use of proton pump inhibitors (PPIs) may increase the risk of gastrointestinal infections (eg, *Salmonella, Campylobacter*). Relief of symptoms does not preclude the presence of a gastric malignancy. Atrophic gastritis (by biopsy) has been noted with long-term omeprazole therapy; this may also occur with esomeprazole. No reports of enterochromaffin-like (ECL) cell carcinoids, dysplasia, or neoplasia have occurred. Use of PPIs may increase risk of CDAD, especially in hospitalized patients; consider CDAD diagnosis in patients with persistent diarrhea that does not improve. Use the lowest dose and shortest duration of PPI therapy appropriate for the condition being treated. Safety and efficacy of IV therapy for GERD >10 days have not been established; transition from IV to oral therapy as soon possible. Bioavailability may be increased in Asian populations, the elderly, and patients with hepatic dysfunction. Decreased *H. pylori* eradication rates have been observed with short-term (≤7 days) combination therapy. The American College of Gastroenterology recommends 10-14 days of therapy (triple or quadruple) for eradication of *H. pylori* (Chey, 2007).

PPIs may diminish the therapeutic effect of clopidogrel, thought to be due to reduced formation of the active metabolite of clopidogrel. The manufacturer of clopidogrel recommends either avoidance of both omeprazole (even when scheduled 12 hours apart) and esomeprazole or use of a PPI with comparatively less effect on the active metabolite of clopidogrel (eg, pantoprazole). In contrast to these warnings, others have recommended the continued use of PPIs, regardless of the degree of inhibition, in patients with a history of GI bleeding or multiple risk factors for GI bleeding who are also receiving clopidogrel since no evidence has established clinically meaningful differences in outcome; however, a clinically-significant interaction cannot be excluded in those who are poor metabolizers of clopidogrel (Abraham, 2010; Levine, 2011). Additionally, potentially significant drug-drug interactions may exist, requiring dose or frequency adjustment, additional monitoring, and/or selection of alternative therapy.

Increased incidence of osteoporosis-related bone fractures of the hip, spine, or wrist may occur with PPI therapy. Patients on high-dose or long-term therapy should be monitored. Use the lowest effective dose for the shortest duration of time, use vitamin D and calcium supplementation, and follow appropriate guidelines to reduce risk of fractures in patients at risk. Acute interstitial nephritis has been observed in patients taking PPIs; may occur at any time during therapy and is generally due to an idiopathic hypersensitivity reaction. Discontinue if acute interstitial nephritis develops.

Hypomagnesemia, reported rarely, usually with prolonged PPI use of >3 months (most cases >1 year of therapy); may be symptomatic or asymptomatic; severe cases may cause tetany, seizures, and cardiac arrhythmias. Consider obtaining serum magnesium concentrations prior to beginning long-term therapy, especially if taking concomitant digoxin, diuretics, or other drugs known to cause hypomagnesemia; and periodically thereafter. Hypomagnesemia may be corrected by magnesium supplementation, although discontinuation of esomeprazole may be necessary; magnesium levels typically return to normal within 1 week of stopping.

Prolonged treatment (≥2 years) may lead to vitamin B_{12} malabsorption and subsequent vitamin B_{12} deficiency. The magnitude of the deficiency is dose-related and the association is stronger in females and those younger in age (<30 years); prevalence is decreased after discontinuation of therapy (Lam, 2013).

Severe liver dysfunction may require dosage reductions. Dosage adjustments are not necessary for any degree of renal impairment when using esomeprazole magnesium or esomeprazole sodium; however, since pharmacokinetics of the strontium may be reduced in mild to moderate renal impairment, esomeprazole strontium is not recommended for use in severe impairment (has not been studied). Esomeprazole strontium competes with calcium for intestinal absorption and is incorporated into bone; use of esomeprazole strontium in pediatric patients is not recommended. When used for self-medication (OTC), do not use for >14 days.

Serum chromogranin A (CgA) levels increase secondary to drug-induced decreases in gastric acid. May cause false positive results in diagnostic investigations for neuroendocrine tumors. Temporarily stop omeprazole treatment ≥14 days before CgA test; if CgA level high, repeat test to confirm. Use same commercial lab for testing to prevent variable results.

Adverse Reactions

Central nervous system: Dizziness, drowsiness, headache

Dermatologic: Pruritus

Gastrointestinal: Abdominal pain, constipation, diarrhea, flatulence, nausea, xerostomia

Local: Injection site reaction (IV)

Rare but important or life-threatening: Aggression, agranulocytosis, alopecia, anaphylaxis, anemia, angioedema, anorexia, benign polyps/nodules, blurred vision, bone fracture, cervical lymphadenopathy, chest pain, *Clostridium difficile*-associated diarrhea (CDAD), conjunctivitis, cyanocobalamin deficiency, cystitis, depression, dermatitis, dysgeusia, dysmenorrhea, epistaxis, erythema multiforme, exacerbation of arthritis, exacerbation of asthma, fibromyalgia syndrome, fungal infection, gastric carcinoid tumor, gastroenteritis, GI dysplasia, GI moniliasis, goiter, gynecomastia, hallucinations, hematuria, hepatic encephalopathy, hepatic failure, hepatitis, hepatotoxicity (idiosyncratic) (Chalasani, 2014), hernia, hyperhidrosis, hyperparathyroidism, hypersensitivity reactions, hypertension, hypertonia, hyperuricemia, hypoesthesia, hypokalemia, hypomagnesemia (with or without hypocalcemia and/or hypokalemia), hyponatremia, impotence, increased gastrin, increased serum alkaline phosphatase, increased serum ALT, increased serum AST, increased serum creatinine, increased thyroid-stimulating hormone, insomnia, interstitial nephritis, jaundice, laryngeal edema, leukocytosis, leukopenia, microscopic colitis, migraine, moniliasis, myasthenia, otitis media, pancreatitis, pancytopenia, parosmia, pathological fracture due to osteoporosis, phlebitis, photosensitivity, pneumonia, polymyalgia rheumatica, proteinuria, pruritus ani, rigors, skin rash (erythematous and maculopapular), Stevens-Johnson syndrome, stomatitis, tachycardia, thrombocytopenia, thrombophlebitis, toxic epidermal necrolysis, vaginitis, visual field defect, weight changes

Drug Interactions

Metabolism/Transport Effects Substrate of CYP2C19 (major), CYP3A4 (minor); **Note:** Assignment of Major/Minor substrate status based on clinically relevant drug interaction potential; **Inhibits** CYP2C19 (moderate)

Avoid Concomitant Use

Avoid concomitant use of Esomeprazole with any of the following: Clopidogrel; Dasatinib; Delavirdine; Erlotinib; Nelfinavir; PAZOPanib; Rifampin; Rilpivirine; Risedronate; St Johns Wort

Increased Effect/Toxicity

Esomeprazole may increase the levels/effects of: Amphetamine; Cilostazol; Citalopram; CYP2C19 Substrates; Dexmethylphenidate; Dextroamphetamine; Methotrexate; Methylphenidate; Raltegravir; Risedronate; Saquinavir; Tacrolimus (Systemic); Vitamin K Antagonists; Voriconazole

The levels/effects of Esomeprazole may be increased by: Fluconazole; Ketoconazole (Systemic); Voriconazole

Decreased Effect

Esomeprazole may decrease the levels/effects of: Atazanavir; Bisphosphonate Derivatives; Bosutinib; Cefditoren; Clopidogrel; Dabigatran Etexilate; Dabrafenib; Dasatinib; Delavirdine; Erlotinib; Gefitinib; Indinavir; Iron Salts; Itraconazole; Ketoconazole (Systemic); Ledipasvir; Mesalamine; Multivitamins/Minerals (with ADEK, Folate, Iron); Mycophenolate; Nelfinavir; Nilotinib; PAZOPanib; Posaconazole; Rilpivirine; Riociguat; Risedronate

The levels/effects of Esomeprazole may be decreased by: CYP2C19 Inducers (Strong); Dabrafenib; Rifampin; St Johns Wort; Tipranavir

Food Interactions Prolonged treatment (≥2 years) may lead to malabsorption of dietary vitamin B_{12} and subsequent vitamin B_{12} deficiency (Lam, 2013).

Storage/Stability

Capsules: Keep container tightly closed.

Esomeprazole magnesium: Store at 25°C (77°F); excursions permitted to 15°C to 30°C (59°F to 86°F).

Esomeprazole strontium: Store at 20°C to 25°C (68°F to 77°F); excursions permitted to 15°C to 30°C (59°F to 86°F).

Granules: Store at 25°C (77°F); excursions permitted to 15°C to 30°C (59°F to 86°F).

Powder for injection: Store at 25°C (77°F); excursions permitted to 15°C to 30°C (59°F to 86°F). Protect from light. Per the manufacturer, following reconstitution, solution for injection prepared in NS, and solution for infusion prepared in NS or LR should be used within 12 hours; solution for infusion prepared in D_5W should be used within 6 hours. Refrigeration is not required following reconstitution.

Additional stability data: Following reconstitution, solutions for infusion prepared in D_5W, NS, or LR in PVC bags are chemically and physically stable for 48 hours at room temperature (25°C) and for at least 120 hours under refrigeration (4°C) (Kupiec, 2008).

Mechanism of Action Proton pump inhibitor suppresses gastric acid secretion by inhibition of the H^+/K^+-ATPase in the gastric parietal cell. Esomeprazole is the S-isomer of omeprazole.

Pharmacokinetics (Adult data unless noted)

Distribution: V_d: 16 L

Protein binding: 97%

Metabolism: Hepatic via CYP2C19 primarily and to a lesser extent via 3A3/4 isoenzymes to hydroxy, desmethyl, and sulfone metabolites (all inactive)

Bioavailability: 64% after a single dose; 90% with repeated administration

Half-life:
- Infants: 0.93 hours
- Children 1-5 years: 0.42-0.74 hours (Zhao, 2006)
- Children 6-11 years: 0.73-0.88 hours (Zhao, 2006)
- Adolescents 12-17 years: 0.82-1.22 hours (Li, 2006)
- Adults: 1-1.5 hours

Time to peak serum concentration: Oral:
- Infants: Median: 3 hours
- Children 1-5 years: 1.33-1.44 hours (Zhao, 2006)
- Children 6-11 years: 1.75-1.79 hours (Zhao, 2006)
- Adolescents 12-17 years: 1.96-2.04 hours (Li, 2006)
- Adults: 1.6 hours

Elimination: Urine (80%, primarily as inactive metabolites; <1% excreted as active drug); feces (20%)

Clearance (with repeated dosing):
- Children 1-5 years: 6-19.44 L/hour (Zhao, 2006)
- Children 6-11 years: 7.84-9.22 L/hour (Zhao, 2006)
- Adolescents 12-17 years: 8.36-15.88 L/hour (Li, 2006)

Dosing: Neonatal GERD: Oral: 0.5 mg/kg/dose given once daily for 7 days; has been shown to reduce esophageal acid exposure and gastric acidity, but did not decrease bolus reflux in 26 preterm and term infants with symptoms of GERD (GA: 23-41 weeks) (Omari, 2009)

Dosing: Usual

Infants, Children, and Adolescents:

Erosive esophagitis associated with GERD:

Oral:

Infants: **Note:** Safety and efficacy of doses >1.33 mg/kg/**day** and/or therapy beyond 6 weeks have not been studied.
- 3-5 kg: 2.5 mg once daily
- >5-7.5 kg: 5 mg once daily
- >7.5 kg: 10 mg once daily

Children 1-11 years: **Note:** Safety and efficacy of doses >1 mg/kg/**day** and/or therapy beyond 8 weeks have not been established.
- <20 kg: 10 mg once daily
- >20 kg: 10 or 20 mg once daily

Children ≥12 years and Adolescents: 20-40 mg once daily for 4 to 8 weeks

IV: **Note:** Indicated only in cases where oral therapy is inappropriate or not possible; safety and efficacy >10 days has not been established.

Infants: 0.5 mg/kg/dose once daily

Children 1-17 years:
- <55 kg: 10 mg once daily
- ≥55 kg: 20 mg once daily

GERD, symptomatic: Oral:

Manufacturer's labeling:

Children 1-11 years: 10 mg once daily for up to 8 weeks. **Note:** Safety and efficacy of doses >1 mg/kg/**day** and/or therapy beyond 8 weeks have not been established.

Children ≥12 years and Adolescents: 20 mg once daily for 4-8 weeks

Alternate dosing (AAP recommendation): Infants, Children, and Adolescents: 0.7-3.3 mg/kg/**day** (Lightdale, 2013)

Adults:

Erosive esophagitis (healing): Oral: Initial: 20-40 mg once daily for 4-8 weeks; if incomplete healing, continue for an additional 4-8 weeks; maintenance: 20 mg once daily (controlled studies did not extend beyond 6 months)

GERD, short-term treatment: IV: 20 mg or 40 mg once daily. **Note:** Indicated only in cases where oral therapy is inappropriate or not possible; safety and efficacy ≥10 days has not been established.

GERD, symptomatic: Oral: 20 mg once daily for 4 weeks; may consider an additional 4 weeks of treatment if symptoms do not resolve

***Helicobacter pylori* eradication:** Oral: 40 mg once daily (in combination with antibiotic therapy) for 10 days

Pathological hypersecretory conditions including Zollinger-Ellison syndrome: Oral: 40 mg twice daily; adjust regimen to individual patient needs; doses up to 240 mg daily have been administered

Prevention of NSAID-induced gastric ulcers: Oral: 20-40 mg once daily for up to 6 months. **Note:** 40 mg daily did not show additional benefit over 20 mg daily in clinical trials.

Dosing adjustment in renal impairment: Infants, Children, Adolescents, and Adults: Oral, IV: No dosage adjustments are recommended.

Dosing adjustment in hepatic impairment: Adults: Oral, IV:

Mild to moderate liver impairment (Child-Pugh Class A or B): No dosage adjustments are recommended.

Severe liver impairment (Child-Pugh Class C): Use with caution; do not exceed 20 mg daily.

Usual Infusion Concentrations: Pediatric IV infusion: 0.4 mg/mL **or** 0.8 mg/mL

Preparation for Administration

Oral: Granules: Mix contents of the 2.5 mg or 5 mg packet with 5 mL of water or the 10 mg, 20 mg, or 40 mg packet with 15 mL of water and stir; leave 2 to 3 minutes to thicken.

IV:

For IV injection (≥3 minutes): Adults: Reconstitute powder with 5 mL NS.

For IV infusion (10 to 30 minutes): Infants, Children, Adolescents, and Adults: Reconstitute powder (20 mg or 40 mg) with 5 mL of NS, LR, or D_5W; further dilute to a final volume of 50 mL to achieve a final concentration of 0.4 mg/mL or 0.8 mg/mL, respectively

For IV infusion (loading dose and continuous infusion): Adults: Prepare the 80 mg loading dose by reconstituting two 40 mg vials with NS (5 mL each); the contents of the two vials should then be further diluted in NS 100 mL. To prepare the continuous infusion, also reconstitute two 40 mg vials with NS (5 mL each); the contents of the two vials should then be further diluted in NS 100 mL.

Administration

Oral: Administer at least 1 hour before food or meals

Capsule: Swallow whole, do not chew or crush. For patients with difficulty swallowing the capsule, capsule may be opened and the enteric coated pellets may be mixed with 1 tablespoon of applesauce (applesauce should not be hot) and swallowed immediately; do not chew or crush granules; do not store mixture for future use.

Nasogastric tube administration: Open capsule and place intact granules into a 60 mL catheter-tipped syringe; mix with 50 mL of water. Replace plunger and shake vigorously for 15 seconds. Ensure that no granules remain in syringe tip. Do not administer if pellets dissolve or disintegrate. Use immediately after preparation. After administration, flush nasogastric tube with additional water.

Granules: Mix contents of the 2.5 mg or 5 mg packet with 5 mL of water or the 10 mg, 20 mg, or 40 mg packet with 15 mL water and stir; leave for 2-3 minutes to thicken; stir and drink within 30 minutes. If any medicine remains after drinking, add more water, stir and drink immediately.

Nasogastric or gastric tube administration: If using a 2.5 mg or 5 mg packet, first add 5 mL of water to a catheter-tipped syringe, then add granules from packet. If using a 10 mg, 20 mg, or 40 mg packet, first add 15 mL of water to a catheter-tipped syringe, then add granules from packet. Shake the syringe, leave 2-3 minutes to thicken. Shake the syringe and administer through nasogastric or gastric tube (French size 6 or greater) within 30 minutes. Refill the syringe with an equal amount (5 mL or 15 mL) of water, shake and flush tube.

IV: Flush line prior to and after administration with NS, LR, or D_5W.

Infants, Children, and Adolescents: Administer desired dose by intermittent infusion over 10 to 30 minutes. The manufacturer recommends that children receive intravenous esomeprazole by intermittent infusion only.

Adults:

Treatment of GERD: May be administered by injection over ≥3 minutes or by intermittent infusion over 10 to 30 minutes

Prevention of recurrent gastric or duodenal ulcer bleeding postendoscopy: Administer the loading dose over 30 minutes, followed by the continuous infusion over 71.5 hours (adjust rate of continuous infusion in patients with hepatic dysfunction)

Test Interactions Esomeprazole may falsely elevate serum chromogranin A (CgA) levels. The increased CgA level may cause false-positive results in the diagnosis of a neuroendocrine tumor. Temporarily stop esomeprazole ≥14 days prior to assessing CgA level; repeat level if initially elevated; use the same laboratory for all testing of CgA levels.

Product Availability Esomeprazole strontium 24.65 mg capsules have been discontinued for more than 1 year.

Dosage Forms Considerations Esomeprazole strontium 49.3 mg is equivalent to 40 mg of esomeprazole base.

Dosage Forms Excipient information presented when available (limited, particularly for generics); consult specific product labeling. [DSC] = Discontinued product

Capsule Delayed Release, Oral, as magnesium [strength expressed as base]:

NexIUM: 20 mg, 40 mg [contains brilliant blue fcf (fd&c blue #1), fd&c red #40, fd&c yellow #10 (quinoline yellow)]

Nexium 24HR: 20 mg [contains brilliant blue fcf (fd&c blue #1), fd&c red #40]

Generic: 20 mg, 40 mg

Capsule Delayed Release, Oral, as strontium:

Generic: 24.65 mg [DSC], 49.3 mg [DSC]

Packet, Oral, as magnesium [strength expressed as base]:

NexIUM: 2.5 mg (30 ea); 5 mg (30 ea); 10 mg (30 ea); 20 mg (30 ea); 40 mg (30 ea)

Solution Reconstituted, Intravenous, as sodium [strength expressed as base]:

NexIUM I.V.: 20 mg (1 ea [DSC]); 40 mg (1 ea)

Generic: 20 mg (1 ea); 40 mg (1 ea)

- ◆ **Esomeprazole Magnesium** *see* Esomeprazole *on page 792*
- ◆ **Esomeprazole Sodium** *see* Esomeprazole *on page 792*
- ◆ **Esomeprazole Strontium** *see* Esomeprazole *on page 792*
- ◆ **E.S.P.®** *see* Erythromycin and Sulfisoxazole *on page 784*
- ◆ **Estrace** *see* Estradiol (Systemic) *on page 795*
- ◆ **Estradiol** *see* Estradiol (Systemic) *on page 795*

Estradiol (Systemic) (es tra DYE ole)

Medication Safety Issues

Sound-alike/look-alike issues:

Alora may be confused with Aldara

Elestrin may be confused with alosetron

BEERS Criteria medication:

This drug may be potentially inappropriate for use in geriatric patients (Quality of evidence - high [oral and transdermal patch]; Strength of recommendation - strong [oral and transdermal patch]).

Other safety issues:

Transdermal patch may contain conducting metal (eg, aluminum); remove patch prior to MRI.

International issues:

Vivelle: Brand name for estradiol [US and multiple international markets, but also the brand name for ethinyl estradiol and norgestimate [Austria]

Related Information

Contraceptive Comparison Table *on page 2309*

Safe Handling of Hazardous Drugs *on page 2455*

Brand Names: US Alora; Climara; Delestrogen; Depo-Estradiol; Divigel; Elestrin; Estrace; Estrasorb [DSC]; Estrogel; Evamist; Femring; Menostar; Minivelle; Vivelle-Dot

Brand Names: Canada Climara; Depo-Estradiol; Divigel; Estradot; EstroGel; Menostar; Oesclim; Sandoz-Estradiol Derm 100; Sandoz-Estradiol Derm 50; Sandoz-Estradiol Derm 75

Therapeutic Category Estrogen Derivative

Generic Availability (US) May be product dependent

Use Treatment of hypoestrogenism due to hypogonadism, castration, or primary ovarian failure; treatment of moderate to severe vasomotor symptoms of menopause, moderate to severe symptoms of vulvar and vaginal atrophy due to menopause, palliative treatment of breast cancer in select patients, palliative treatment of androgen-dependent prostate cancer, and prevention of osteoporosis in postmenopausal women (All indications: FDA approved in adults); has also been used for management of Turner Syndrome and for induction of puberty in patients with delayed puberty

Pregnancy Risk Factor X

Pregnancy Considerations In general, the use of estrogen and progestin as in combination hormonal contraceptives has not been associated with teratogenic effects when inadvertently taken early in pregnancy. These products are contraindicated for use during pregnancy.

Breast-Feeding Considerations Estrogens are excreted in breast milk and have been shown to decrease the quantity and quality of human milk. The manufacturer recommends that caution be used if administered to breast-feeding women. Monitor the growth of the infant closely.

Contraindications

Angioedema, anaphylactic reaction, or hypersensitivity to estradiol or any component of the formulation; undiagnosed abnormal genital bleeding; DVT or PE (current or history of); active or history of arterial thromboembolic disease (eg, stroke, MI); breast cancer (known, suspected or history of), except in appropriately selected patients being treated for metastatic disease; estrogen-dependent tumor (known or suspected); hepatic impairment or disease; known protein C, protein S, antithrombin deficiency or other known thrombophilic disorders; pregnancy.

Documentation of allergenic cross-reactivity for estrogens is limited. However, because of similarities in chemical structure and/or pharmacologic actions, the possibility of cross-sensitivity cannot be ruled out with certainty.

Warnings/Precautions Hazardous agent: Use appropriate precautions for handling and disposal (NIOSH 2014 [group 2]).

Anaphylaxis requiring emergency medical management has been reported and may develop at any time during therapy. Angioedema involving the face, feet, hands, larynx, and tongue has also been reported.

[US Boxed Warning]: Based on data from the Women's Health Initiative (WHI) studies, an increased risk of invasive breast cancer was observed in postmenopausal women using conjugated estrogens (CE) in combination with medroxyprogesterone acetate (MPA). This risk may be associated with duration of use and declines once combined therapy is discontinued (Chlebowski 2009). The risk of invasive breast cancer was decreased in postmenopausal women with a hysterectomy using CE only, regardless of weight. However, the risk was not significantly decreased in women at high risk for breast cancer (family history of breast cancer, personal history of benign breast disease) (Anderson 2012). An increase in abnormal mammogram findings has also been reported with estrogen alone or in combination with progestin therapy. Estrogen use may lead to severe hypercalcemia in patients with breast cancer and bone metastases; discontinue estrogen if hypercalcemia occurs. Postmenopausal estrogens with or without progestins may increase the risk of ovarian cancer; however, the absolute risk to an individual woman is small. Although results from various studies are not consistent, risk does not appear to be significantly associated with the duration, route, or dose of therapy. In one study, the risk decreased after 2 years following discontinuation of therapy (Mørch 2009). Although the risk of ovarian cancer is rare, women who are at an increased risk (eg, family history) should be counseled about the association (NAMS 2012).

[US Boxed Warning]: Estrogens with or without progestin should not be used to prevent cardiovascular disease. Using data from the Women's Health Initiative (WHI) studies, an increased risk of deep vein thrombosis (DVT) and stroke has been reported with CE and an increased risk of DVT, stroke, pulmonary emboli (PE) and myocardial infarction (MI) has been reported with CE with MPA in postmenopausal women 50 to 79 years of age. Additional risk factors include diabetes mellitus, hypercholesterolemia, hypertension, SLE, obesity, tobacco use, and/or history of venous thromboembolism (VTE). Risk factors should be managed appropriately; discontinue use if adverse cardiovascular events occur or are suspected. Use is contraindicated in women with active DVT, PE, active arterial thromboembolic disease or a history of these conditions.

[US Boxed Warning]: Estrogens with or without progestin should not be used to prevent dementia. In the Women's Health Initiative Memory Study (WHIMS), an increased incidence of probable dementia was observed in women ≥65 years of age taking CE alone or in combination with MPA.

[US Boxed Warning]: The use of unopposed estrogen in women with a uterus is associated with an increased risk of endometrial cancer. The addition of a progestin to estrogen therapy may decrease the risk of endometrial hyperplasia, a precursor to endometrial cancer. Adequate diagnostic measures, including endometrial sampling if indicated, should be performed to rule out malignancy in postmenopausal women with undiagnosed abnormal vaginal bleeding. There is no evidence that the use of natural estrogens results in a different endometrial risk profile than synthetic estrogens at equivalent estrogen doses. The risk of endometrial cancer is dose and duration dependent; risk appears to be greatest with use ≥5 years and may persist following discontinuation of therapy. The use of a progestin is not generally required when low doses of estrogen are used locally for vaginal atrophy (NAMS 2012; NAMS 2013). Estrogens may exacerbate endometriosis. Malignant transformation of residual endometrial implants has been reported posthysterectomy with unopposed estrogen therapy. Consider adding a progestin in women with residual endometriosis posthysterectomy.

[US Boxed Warning]: Estrogens with or without progestin should be used for the shortest duration possible at the lowest effective dose consistent with treatment goals and risks for the individual woman. Patients should be reevaluated as clinically appropriate to determine if treatment is still necessary. Available data related to treatment risks are from Women's Health Initiative (WHI) studies, which evaluated oral CE 0.625 mg with or without MPA 2.5 mg relative to placebo in postmenopausal women. Other combinations and dosage forms of estrogens and progestins were not studied. **Outcomes reported from clinical trials using CE with or without MPA should be assumed to be similar for other doses and other dosage forms of estrogens and progestins until comparable data becomes available.** Women who are early in menopause, who are in good cardiovascular health, and who are at low risk for adverse cardiovascular events can be considered candidates for estrogen with or without progestin therapy for the relief of menopausal symptoms (ACOG 565 2013). Use of a transdermal product should be considered over an oral agent in women requiring systemic therapy who have risk factors for venous thromboembolism or coronary heart disease (ACOG 556 2013; Schenck-Gustafsson 2011; Tremollieres 2011).

Topical estradiol may be transferred to another person following skin-to-skin contact with the application site. **[US Boxed Warning]: Breast budding and breast masses in prepubertal females and gynecomastia and breast masses in prepubertal males have been reported following unintentional contact with application sites of women using topical estradiol (Evamist). Patients should strictly adhere to instructions for use in order to prevent secondary exposure. In most cases, conditions resolved with removal of estradiol exposure.** If unexpected changes in sexual development occur in prepubertal children, the possibility of unintentional estradiol exposure should be evaluated by a health care provider. Discontinue if conditions for the safe use of the topical spray cannot be met.

Women with inherited thrombophilias (eg, protein C or S deficiency) may have increased risk of venous thromboembolism (DeSancho 2010; van Vlijmen 2011). Use is contraindicated in women with protein C, protein S, antithrombin deficiency, or other known thrombophilic disorders. Estrogen compounds are generally associated with lipid effects such as increased HDL-cholesterol and decreased

LDL-cholesterol. Triglycerides may also be increased in women with preexisting hypertriglyceridemia; discontinue if pancreatitis occurs. The use of estrogens and/or progestins may change the results of some laboratory tests (eg, coagulation factors, lipids, glucose tolerance, binding proteins). The dose, route, and the specific estrogen/progestin influence these changes. In addition, personal risk factors (eg, cardiovascular disease, smoking, diabetes, age) also contribute to adverse events; use of specific products may be contraindicated in women with certain risk factors. Estrogens may increase thyroid-binding globulin (TBG) levels leading to increased circulating total thyroid hormone levels. Women on thyroid replacement therapy may require higher doses of thyroid hormone while receiving estrogens. Potentially significant interactions may exist, requiring dose or frequency adjustment, additional monitoring, and/or selection of alternative therapy.

Estrogens may cause retinal vascular thrombosis; discontinue if migraine, loss of vision, proptosis, diplopia, or other visual disturbances occur; discontinue permanently if papilledema or retinal vascular lesions are observed on examination. Use caution with asthma, epilepsy, hepatic hemangiomas, migraine, porphyria, SLE; may exacerbate disease. May have adverse effects on glucose tolerance; use caution in women with diabetes. Use caution with diseases which may be exacerbated by fluid retention, including cardiac or renal dysfunction. Use of postmenopausal estrogen may be associated with an increased risk of gallbladder disease requiring surgery. Estrogens are poorly metabolized in patients with hepatic dysfunction. Use caution with a history of cholestatic jaundice associated with prior estrogen use or pregnancy. Discontinue if jaundice develops or if acute or chronic hepatic disturbances occur. Use is contraindicated with hepatic impairment or disease. Exogenous estrogens may exacerbate angioedema symptoms in women with hereditary angioedema. Use caution with hypoparathyroidism; estrogen-induced hypocalcemia may occur.

Whenever possible, estrogens should be discontinued at least 4 to 6 weeks prior to elective surgery associated with an increased risk of thromboembolism or during periods of prolonged immobilization.

Avoid oral and transdermal patch estrogen products (with or without progestins) in the elderly due to potential of increased risk of breast and endometrial cancers, and lack of proven cardioprotection and cognitive protection (Beers Criteria).

Prior to puberty, estrogens may cause premature closure of the epiphyses. Premature breast development, vaginal bleeding and vaginal cornification may be induced in girls. Modification of the normal puberty process may occur in boys.

Osteoporosis use: For use only in women at significant risk of osteoporosis and for who other nonestrogen medications are not considered appropriate.

Vulvar and vaginal atrophy use: Moderate-to-severe symptoms of vulvar and vaginal atrophy include vaginal dryness, dyspareunia, and atrophic vaginitis. When used solely for the treatment of vulvar and vaginal atrophy, topical vaginal products should be considered. Use caution applying topical products to severely atrophic vaginal mucosa. Use of a progestin is normally not required when low-dose estrogen is applied locally and only for this purpose (NAMS 2012; NAMS 2013).

Topical emulsion, gel: Absorption of the topical emulsion (Estrasorb) and topical gel (Elestrin) is increased by application of sunscreen; do not apply sunscreen within close proximity of estradiol. Application of sunscreen or lotion after EstroGel decreases absorption of estradiol; the effect of applying sunscreen or lotion prior to Estrogel has not been studied. Application of Divigel with sunscreen has not been evaluated.

Topical spray: When sunscreen is applied ~1 hour prior to the topical spray (Evamist), no change in absorption was observed (estradiol absorption was decreased when sunscreen is applied 1 hour after Evamist).

Transdermal patch: May contain conducting metal (eg, aluminum); remove patch prior to MRI.

Vaginal ring: Use may not be appropriate in women with narrow vagina, vaginal stenosis, vaginal infections, cervical prolapse, rectoceles, cystoceles, or other conditions which may increase the risk of vaginal irritation, ulceration, or increase the risk of expulsion. Ring should be removed in case of ulceration, erosion, or adherence to vaginal wall; do not reinsert until healing is complete. Ensure proper vaginal placement of the ring to avoid inadvertent urinary bladder insertion.

Some dosage forms may contain benzyl alcohol; large amounts of benzyl alcohol (≥99 mg/kg/day) have been associated with a potentially fatal toxicity ("gasping syndrome") in neonates; the "gasping syndrome" consists of metabolic acidosis, respiratory distress, gasping respirations, CNS dysfunction (including convulsions, intracranial hemorrhage), hypotension and cardiovascular collapse (AAP, 1997; CDC, 1982); some data suggests that benzoate displaces bilirubin from protein binding sites (Ahlfors 2001); avoid or use dosage forms containing benzyl alcohol with caution in neonates. See manufacturer's labeling. Some products may contain chlorobutanol (a chloral derivative) as a preservative, which may be habit forming. Some products may contain tartrazine.

Warnings: Additional Pediatric Considerations Some dosage forms may contain propylene glycol; in neonates large amounts of propylene glycol delivered orally, intravenously (eg, >3,000 mg/day), or topically have been associated with potentially fatal toxicities which can include metabolic acidosis, seizures, renal failure, and CNS depression; toxicities have also been reported in children and adults including hyperosmolality, lactic acidosis, seizures, and respiratory depression; use caution (AAP, 1997; Shehab, 2009).

Adverse Reactions Some adverse reactions observed with estrogen and/or progestin combination therapy.

Cardiovascular: Cerebrovascular accident, deep vein thrombosis, edema, hypertension, local thrombophlebitis, myocardial infarction, pulmonary thromboembolism, retinal thrombosis, thrombophlebitis, venous thromboembolism

Central nervous system: Anxiety, chorea, dementia, depression, dizziness, exacerbation of epilepsy, headache, hypoesthesia, irritability, migraine, mood disorder, nervousness, nipple pain, pain

Dermatologic: Chloasma, erythema multiforme, erythema nodosum, localized erythema (transdermal patch), loss of scalp hair, pruritus, skin discoloration (melasma), skin rash, urticaria

Endocrine & metabolic: Change in libido, change in menstrual flow (alterations in frequency and flow of bleeding patterns), exacerbation of diabetes mellitus, exacerbation of porphyria, fibrocystic breast changes, fluid retention, galactorrhea, hirsutism, hot flash, hypocalcemia, increased serum triglycerides, weight gain, weight loss

Gastrointestinal: Abdominal cramps, abdominal pain, bloating, carbohydrate intolerance, constipation, diarrhea, dyspepsia, flatulence, gallbladder disease, gastroenteritis, nausea, pancreatitis, vomiting

Genitourinary: Abnormal uterine bleeding, breakthrough bleeding, breast hypertrophy, breast tenderness, cervical polyp, change in cervical ectropion, change in cervical secretions, dysmenorrhea, endometrial hyperplasia, endometrium disease, leukorrhea, mastalgia, nipple discharge, spotting, urinary tract infection, uterine fibroids (size increased), uterine pain, vaginal discomfort (vaginal ring; burning, irritation, itching), vaginal hemorrhage, vaginitis, vulvovaginal candidiasis

Hematologic & oncologic: Hemorrhagic eruption, hypercoagulability state, malignant neoplasm of breast, ovarian cancer

Hepatic: Cholestatic jaundice, exacerbation of hepatic hemangioma

Hypersensitivity: Anaphylactoid reaction, anaphylaxis, angioedema, hypersensitivity reaction

Infection: Fungal infection, infection

Local: Application site reaction (gel, spray, transdermal patch)

Neuromuscular & skeletal: Arthralgia, arthropathy, back pain, exacerbation of systemic lupus erythematosus, leg cramps, limb pain, myalgia, neck pain, weakness

Ophthalmic: Change in corneal curvature (steepening), conjunctivitis, contact lens intolerance

Otic: Otitis media

Respiratory: asthma, bronchitis, cough, exacerbation of asthma, flu-like symptoms, nasopharyngitis, pharyngitis, rhinitis, sinus congestion, sinus headache, sinusitis, upper respiratory tract infection

Miscellaneous: Accidental injury, cyst

Rare but important or life-threatening: Bowel obstruction (vaginal ring), genitourinary complaint (inadvertent ring insertion into the bladder should be considered with unexplained urinary complaints), hemorrhage, mechanical complication of genitourinary device (ring adherence to vaginal or bladder wall), portal vein thrombosis, toxic shock syndrome (vaginal ring), unstable angina pectoris

Drug Interactions

Metabolism/Transport Effects **Substrate** of CYP1A2 (major), CYP2A6 (minor), CYP2B6 (minor), CYP2C19 (minor), CYP2C9 (minor), CYP2D6 (minor), CYP2E1 (minor), CYP3A4 (major), P-glycoprotein; **Note:** Assignment of Major/Minor substrate status based on clinically relevant drug interaction potential; **Inhibits** CYP1A2 (weak), CYP2C8 (weak); **Induces** CYP3A4 (weak)

Avoid Concomitant Use

Avoid concomitant use of Estradiol (Systemic) with any of the following: Amodiaquine; Anastrozole; Dehydroepiandrosterone; Exemestane; Indium 111 Capromab Pendetide; Ospemifene

Increased Effect/Toxicity

Estradiol (Systemic) may increase the levels/effects of: Amodiaquine; Anthrax Immune Globulin (Human); C1 inhibitors; Corticosteroids (Systemic); Immune Globulin; Lenalidomide; Ospemifene; ROPINIRole; Thalidomide; Theophylline Derivatives; Tipranavir; TiZANidine

The levels/effects of Estradiol (Systemic) may be increased by: Ascorbic Acid; Dehydroepiandrosterone; Herbs (Estrogenic Properties); NSAID (COX-2 Inhibitor); P-glycoprotein/ABCB1 Inhibitors

Decreased Effect

Estradiol (Systemic) may decrease the levels/effects of: Anastrozole; Anticoagulants; Antidiabetic Agents; ARIPiprazole; Chenodiol; Exemestane; Hyaluronidase; Hydrocodone; Indium 111 Capromab Pendetide; NiMODipine; Ospemifene; Saxagliptin; Somatropin; Thyroid Products; Ursodiol

The levels/effects of Estradiol (Systemic) may be decreased by: Bosentan; Cannabis; CYP1A2 Inducers (Strong); CYP3A4 Inducers (Moderate); CYP3A4 Inducers (Strong); Cyproterone; Dabrafenib; Deferasirox; Mitotane; P-glycoprotein/ABCB1 Inducers; Siltuximab; St Johns Wort; Teriflunomide; Tipranavir; Tocilizumab

Food Interactions Folic acid absorption may be decreased. Routine use of ethanol increases estrogen level and risk of breast cancer; may also increase the risk of osteoporosis. Management: Avoid ethanol.

Storage/Stability

Store all products at controlled room temperature. In addition:

Depo-Estradiol: Protect from light.

Evamist: Do not freeze.

Femring: Store in pouch.

Transdermal patch (all products): Store in protective pouch.

Climara, Menostar: Do not store >30°C (>86°F).

Mechanism of Action Estrogens are responsible for the development and maintenance of the female reproductive system and secondary sexual characteristics. Estradiol is the principle intracellular human estrogen and is more potent than estrone and estriol at the receptor level; it is the primary estrogen secreted prior to menopause. Following menopause, estrone and estrone sulfate are more highly produced. Estrogens modulate the pituitary secretion of gonadotropins, luteinizing hormone, and follicle-stimulating hormone through a negative feedback system; estrogen replacement reduces elevated levels of these hormones in postmenopausal women.

Pharmacokinetics (Adult data unless noted)

Absorption: Well-absorbed from the gastrointestinal tract, mucous membranes, and the skin. Average serum estradiol concentrations (C_{avg}) vary by product and dose

Injection: Estradiol valerate and estradiol cypionate are absorbed over several weeks following IM injection

Transdermal:

Elestrin: Exposure increased by 55% with application of sunscreen 10 minutes prior to dose

Estrasorb: Exposure increased by 35% with application of sunscreen 10 minutes prior to dose

Distribution: Widely distributes throughout the body; sex hormone target organs contain higher concentrations

Protein binding: Primarily bound to sex hormone-binding globulin and albumin

Metabolism: Hepatic; partial metabolism via CYP3A4 enzymes; estradiol is reversibly converted to estrone and estriol; oral estradiol also undergoes enterohepatic recirculation by conjugation in the liver, followed by excretion of sulfate and glucuronide conjugates into the bile, then hydrolysis in the intestine and estrogen reabsorption. Sulfate conjugates are the primary form found in postmenopausal women. With transdermal application, less estradiol is metabolized leading to higher circulating concentrations of estradiol and lower concentrations of estrone and conjugates.

Elimination: Primarily urine (as estradiol, estrone, estriol, and their glucuronide and sulfate conjugates)

Dosing: Usual Note: Use lowest effective dose for shortest duration possible that is consistent with an individual's treatment goals and risks; all dosage needs to be adjusted based upon the patient's response.

Pediatric:

Constitutional delay of growth and puberty (CDGP) (females): Limited data available: Children ≥12 years and Adolescents: **Note:** Begin with the lowest available dose and gradually increase. Obtain bone age every 6 months to avoid premature epiphyseal closure. If treatment continues beyond 1 year or breast growth is significant and has plateaued or breakthrough bleeding occurs, add cyclic progesterone. Continue until menstruation has been established, or longer if clinically indicated (Palmert 2012; Santos 2014; Sperling 2014).

Oral (micronized, Estrace): Initial dose: 5 mcg/kg once daily; after 6 to 12 months of therapy, may increase to 10 mcg/kg once daily (Palmert 2012). Using currently available dosage forms, some have recommended starting at a fixed dose of 0.25 mg once daily (1/2 of the 0.5 mg tablet) and increasing to 0.5 mg once daily after 6 to 12 months.

Transdermal: Initial dose: 3.1 to 6.2 mcg/day patch (eg, 1/8 to 1/4 of a 25 mcg/day patch), apply at night, remove in the morning. Increase by 3.1 to 6.2 mcg/day patch every 6 months (Palmert 2012). **Note:** The practice of cutting patches to achieve low doses is cited frequently in the literature (Ankarberg-Lindgren 2001; Davenport 2010; Hindmarsh 2009; Palmert 2012); however, product specific data may not be available for all transdermal products due to product availability/ manufacturing changes.

Hypogonadism (females): Limited data available: Children ≥12 years and Adolescents: **Note:** Begin with the lowest available dose and gradually increase. Obtain bone age every 6 months to avoid premature epiphyseal closure. Once breast growth is significant and has plateaued or breakthrough bleeding occurs, add cyclic progesterone. Continue until menstruation has been established, or longer if clinically indicated (Palmert 2012; Sperling 2014).

Oral (micronized): Initial dose: 5 mcg/kg once daily for 6 to 12 months; may then increase to 10 mcg/kg/day for 6 to 12 months; dose may be increased at every 6 to 12 month intervals by 5 mcg/kg/day, up to 20 mcg/kg/ day. Do not exceed adult dose of 2 mg daily (Palmert 2012).

Transdermal: Initial dose: 3.1 to 6.2 mcg/day patch (eg, 1/8 to 1/4 of a 25 mcg/day patch), apply at night, remove in the morning. Increase by 3.1 to 6.2 mcg/day patch every 6 months; Do not exceed adult dose of 50 to 100 mcg/24 hours (Palmert 2012). Note: The practice of cutting patches to achieve low doses is cited frequently in the literature (Ankarberg-Lindgren 2001; Davenport 2010; Hindmarsh 2009; Palmert 2012); however, product specific data may not be available for all transdermal products due to product availability/ manufacturing changes.

Turner syndrome (females): Limited data available: Children ≥12 years and Adolescents: Begin at ~12 years of age using a low dose and gradually increase dose over 2 to 4 years to full adult dose. After 2 years of estrogen or when breakthrough bleeding occurs, add cyclic progesterone. **Note:** Full dose estrogen will be needed until at least age 30 years (Bondy 2007).

IM: Cypionate (Depot-Estradiol): Initial: 0.2 to 0.4 mg every 4 weeks, slowly increase dose over about 2 years to the goal adult dose: 3 mg/month; one trial started at 0.2 mg/dose, then increased dose at 6 month intervals in 0.2 mg/dose increments until dose of 1 mg reached and then increased in 0.5 mg/dose increments thereafter to a final dose of 3 mg (Bondy 2007; Rosenfield 2005)

Oral (micronized, Estrace): Initial dose: 5 mcg/kg once daily for the first 2 years, followed by 7.5 mcg/kg for the 3rd year, then 10 mcg/kg thereafter; once final height is attained, increase to adult dose of 1 to 2 mg/day (Bannink 2009). A fixed dose of 0.25 mg once daily; increasing to the adult dose of 2 to 4 mg/day over the course of 2 years has also been suggested (Bondy 2007). **Note:** Due to extensive first-pass metabolism, other routes of administration may be preferable.

Topical gel (Divigel): Initial: 0.1 mg of estradiol once daily for the first year, 0.2 mg of estradiol once daily for the second year, 0.5 mg of estradiol once daily for the third year, 1 mg of estradiol once daily for the fourth year, and 1.5 mg of estradiol once daily for the fifth year. Dosing based on a trial of 23 girls that followed development for 5 years; long-term dose is unknown. Due to lack of commercially available product for lower doses, individual sachets of 0.1 mg estradiol were prepared (Piippo 2004).

Transdermal patch: Initial: 6.25 mcg/day patch; slowly increase over about 2 years to the goal adult dose: 100 to 200 mcg/day patch (Bondy 2007)

Note: The lowest-dose commercially available patches deliver 14 and 25 µg daily; preferred dose fractionation method has not been established (eg, administering a partial patch, limiting to overnight use, or administering whole patches for 7 to 10 days per month). Product specific data may not be available for splitting/cutting some transdermal patches; one center has used the following titration method using Vivelle-Dot product (Davenport 2010):

Treatment month:

- 0 to <6 months of treatment: 3.125 mcg to 4.17 mcg/dose (equals 1/8 to 1/6 of a 25 mcg/day patch), apply at night, remove in the morning (not continuous)
- 6 to <12 months of treatment: 3.125 mcg to 4.17 mcg/dose (equals 1/8 to 1/6 of a 25 mcg/day patch) apply twice weekly (continuous)
- 12 to <18 months of treatment: 6.25 mcg to 8.33 mcg/dose (equals 1/4 to 1/3 of a 25 mcg/day patch), apply twice weekly (continuous)
- 18 to <24 months of treatment: 12.5 mcg/dose (equals 1/2 of a 25 mcg/day patch), apply twice weekly (continuous)
- ≥24 months of treatment: 25 mcg/day patch, apply twice weekly (continuous); then increase by one patch strength every 6 months to a final goal of 100 mcg/day continuously

Adult: **Note:** See package insert for doses related to postmenopausal symptoms, prevention of osteoporosis in postmenopausal women, and palliative treatment of breast cancer or androgen-dependent prostate cancer in adults.

Hypoestrogenism (female) due to hypogonadism, castration, or primary ovarian failure:

Oral (Estrace): Initial: 1 to 2 mg once daily; titrate as necessary to control symptoms using minimal effective dose for maintenance therapy

IM: Valerate (Delestrogen): 10 to 20 mg every 4 weeks

Transdermal:

Alora: Apply 0.05 mg patch twice weekly

Climara: Apply 0.025 mg/day patch once weekly. Adjust dose as necessary to control symptoms.

Vivelle-Dot: Apply 0.0375 mg patch twice weekly

Hypoestrogenism (female) due to hypogonadism: IM: Cypionate (Depo-Estradiol): 1.5 to 2 mg once monthly

Dosing adjustment in renal impairment: For most products, there are no dosage adjustments provided in the manufacturer's labeling (has not been studied).

Dosing adjustment in hepatic impairment: For most products, there are no dosage adjustments provided in the manufacturer's labeling (has not been studied); use is contraindicated with hepatic dysfunction or disease.

Administration Hazardous agent; use appropriate precautions for handling and disposal (NIOSH 2014 [group 2]).

Oral: May administer with food or after a meal to reduce GI upset

Parenteral: Injection for IM use only

Cypionate: Inspect for any particulate (particularly crystals); warming and shaking the vial should redissolve any crystals

Valerate: Should be injected into the upper outer quadrant of the gluteal muscle; administer with a dry needle (solution may become cloudy with wet needle).

Transdermal: **Note:** See package insert for administration related to postmenopausal symptoms, prevention of osteoporosis in postmenopausal women, and palliative treatment of breast cancer or androgen-dependent prostate cancer in adults.

Gel (Divigel): Apply to clean, dry, unbroken skin at the same time each day. Apply entire contents of packet to right or left upper thigh each day (alternate sites). Do not apply to face, breasts, vaginal area, or irritated skin. Apply over an area ~5x7 inches. Do not wash application site for 1 hour. Allow to dry for 5 minutes prior to dressing. Gel is flammable; avoid fire or flame until dry. After application, wash hands with soap and water. Prior to the first use, pump must be primed.

Transdermal patch: Do not apply transdermal system to breasts, but place on trunk of body (preferably abdomen). Rotate application sites allowing a 1-week interval between applications at a particular site. Do not apply to oily, damaged or irritated skin; avoid waistline or other areas where tight clothing may rub the patch off. Apply patch immediately after removing from protective pouch. In general, if patch falls off, the same patch may be reapplied or a new system may be used for the remainder of the dosing interval (not recommended with all products) When replacing patch, reapply to a new site. Swimming, bathing, or showering are not expected to affect use of the patch. Note the following exceptions:

Climara, Menostar, Minivelle: Swimming, bathing, or wearing patch while in a sauna have not been studied; adhesion of patch may be decreased or delivery of estradiol may be affected. Showering is not expected to cause the Minivelle patch to fall off. Remove patch slowly after use to avoid skin irritation. If any adhesive remains on the skin after removal, first allow skin to dry for 15 minutes, then gently rub area with an oil-based cream or lotion. If patch falls off, a new patch should be applied for the remainder of the dosing interval.

Monitoring Parameters Blood pressure, weight, height, serum calcium, glucose, liver enzymes; bone maturation and epiphyseal effects in young patients in whom bone growth is not complete; breast exam, mammogram, Papanicolaou smear, signs for endometrial cancer in female patients with a uterus; bone density measurement if used for prevention of osteoporosis

Turner Syndrome and CDPG (puberty induction): Adolescents: Signs of puberty progression, ovarian tissue growth/changes (pelvic ultrasound), height, weight, growth parameters, breast exam, mammogram, Papanicolaou smear (Sperling 2014)

Reference Range

Pediatric patients (Janfaza 2006):

Tanner stage 1: Females: 5.9 ± 9.7 pmol/L, Males: 1.5 ± 4.1

Tanner stage 2: Females: 25.3 ± 4.0 pmol/L, Males: 2.6 ± 3.0

Tanner stage 3: Females: 84.1 ± 120.5 pmol/L, Males: 8.7 ± 11.0

Tanner stage 4: Females: 97.3 ± 137.7 pmol/L, Males: 13.0 ± 9.4

Tanner stage 5: Females: 174.3 ± 239.5 pmol/L, Males: 15.5 ± 9.4

Adults:

Females:

Premenopausal: 30 to 400 pg/mL (SI: 110 to 1,468 pmol/L) (depending on phase of menstrual cycle)

Postmenopausal: 0 to 30 pg/mL (SI: 0 to 110 pmol/L)

Adult males: 10 to 50 pg/mL (SI: 37 to 184 pmol/L)

Test Interactions Reduced response to metyrapone test.

Dosage Forms Excipient information presented when available (limited, particularly for generics); consult specific product labeling. [DSC] = Discontinued product

Emulsion, Transdermal, as hemihydrate:

Estrasorb: 4.35 mg/1.74 g (1.74 g [DSC]) [contains polysorbate 80, soybean oil]

Gel, Transdermal:

Divigel: 0.25 mg/0.25 g (1 ea); 0.5 mg/0.5 g (1 ea); 1 mg/g (1 g) [contains propylene glycol, trolamine (triethanolamine)]

Elestrin: 0.06% (26 g) [contains edetate disodium, propylene glycol, trolamine (triethanolamine)]

Estrogel: 0.06% (50 g) [contains alcohol, usp, trolamine (triethanolamine)]

Oil, Intramuscular, as cypionate:

Depo-Estradiol: 5 mg/mL (5 mL)

Oil, Intramuscular, as valerate:

Delestrogen: 10 mg/mL (5 mL) [contains chlorobutanol (chlorobutol), sesame oil]

Delestrogen: 20 mg/mL (5 mL); 40 mg/mL (5 mL) [contains benzyl alcohol]

Generic: 10 mg/mL (5 mL [DSC]); 20 mg/mL (5 mL); 40 mg/mL (5 mL)

Patch Twice Weekly, Transdermal:

Alora: 0.025 mg/24 hr (1 ea, 8 ea); 0.05 mg/24 hr (1 ea, 8 ea); 0.075 mg/24 hr (1 ea, 8 ea); 0.1 mg/24 hr (1 ea, 8 ea)

Minivelle: 0.025 mg/24 hr (8 ea); 0.0375 mg/24 hr (8 ea); 0.05 mg/24 hr (8 ea); 0.075 mg/24 hr (8 ea); 0.1 mg/24 hr (8 ea)

Vivelle-Dot: 0.025 mg/24 hr (8 ea); 0.0375 mg/24 hr (1 ea, 8 ea); 0.05 mg/24 hr (1 ea, 8 ea); 0.075 mg/24 hr (1 ea, 8 ea); 0.1 mg/24 hr (1 ea, 8 ea)

Generic: 0.025 mg/24 hr (8 ea); 0.0375 mg/24 hr (8 ea); 0.05 mg/24 hr (8 ea); 0.075 mg/24 hr (8 ea); 0.1 mg/24 hr (8 ea)

Patch Weekly, Transdermal:

Climara: 0.025 mg/24 hr (4 ea); 0.0375 mg/24 hr (4 ea); 0.05 mg/24 hr (1 ea, 4 ea); 0.06 mg/24 hr (4 ea); 0.075 mg/24 hr (4 ea); 0.1 mg/24 hr (1 ea, 4 ea)

Menostar: 14 mcg/24 hr (4 ea)

Generic: 0.025 mg/24 hr (4 ea); 0.0375 mg/24 hr (4 ea); 0.05 mg/24 hr (4 ea); 0.06 mg/24 hr (4 ea); 0.075 mg/24 hr (4 ea); 0.1 mg/24 hr (4 ea)

Ring, Vaginal, as acetate:

Femring: 0.05 mg/24 hr (1 ea); 0.1 mg/24 hr (1 ea)

Solution, Transdermal:

Evamist: 1.53 mg/spray (8.1 mL) [contains alcohol, usp, octyl salicylate]

Tablet, Oral:

Estrace: 0.5 mg, 1 mg, 2 mg [scored]

Generic: 0.5 mg, 1 mg, 2 mg

◆ **Estradiol Acetate** *see* Estradiol (Systemic) *on page 795*

◆ **Estradiol Transdermal** *see* Estradiol (Systemic) *on page 795*

◆ **Estradiol Valerate** *see* Estradiol (Systemic) *on page 795*

◆ **Estradot (Can)** *see* Estradiol (Systemic) *on page 795*

◆ **Estrasorb [DSC]** *see* Estradiol (Systemic) *on page 795*

◆ **Estrogel** *see* Estradiol (Systemic) *on page 795*

◆ **EstroGel (Can)** *see* Estradiol (Systemic) *on page 795*

◆ **Estrogenic Substances, Conjugated** *see* Estrogens (Conjugated/Equine, Systemic) *on page 801*

◆ **Estrogenic Substances, Conjugated** *see* Estrogens (Conjugated/Equine, Topical) *on page 803*

Estrogens (Conjugated/Equine, Systemic) (ES troe jenz KON joo gate ed, EE kwine)

Medication Safety Issues

Sound-alike/look-alike issues:

Premarin® may be confused with Primaxin®, Provera®, Remeron®

BEERS Criteria medication:

This drug may be potentially inappropriate for use in geriatric patients (Quality of evidence - high [oral]; Strength of recommendation - strong [oral]).

Related Information

Contraceptive Comparison Table *on page 2309*

Safe Handling of Hazardous Drugs *on page 2455*

Brand Names: US Premarin

Brand Names: Canada C.E.S.®; Congest; PMS-Conjugated Estrogens C.S.D.; Premarin®

Therapeutic Category Estrogen Derivative

Generic Availability (US) No

Use Treatment of dysfunctional uterine bleeding, hypoestrogenism (due to hypogonadism, castration, or primary ovarian failure), moderate to severe vasomotor symptoms of menopause; moderate to severe symptoms of vulvar and vaginal atrophy due to menopause; palliative treatment of breast cancer in select patients; palliative treatment of androgen-dependent prostate cancer; prevention of osteoporosis in postmenopausal women; **Note:** Intravenous product is indicated for short-term use only

Pregnancy Considerations Estrogens are not indicated for use during pregnancy or immediately postpartum. In general, the use of estrogen and progestin as in combination hormonal contraceptives have not been associated with teratogenic effects when inadvertently taken early in pregnancy. These products are contraindicated for use during pregnancy.

Breast-Feeding Considerations Estrogen has been shown to decrease the quantity and quality of human milk. Use only if clearly needed. Monitor the growth of the infant closely.

Contraindications Angioedema or anaphylactic reaction to estrogens or any component of the formulation; undiagnosed abnormal vaginal bleeding; history of or current thrombophlebitis or venous thromboembolic disorders (including DVT, PE); active or history of arterial thromboembolic disease (eg, stroke, MI); carcinoma of the breast (except in appropriately selected patients being treated for metastatic disease); estrogen-dependent tumor; hepatic dysfunction or disease; known protein C, protein S, antithrombin deficiency or other known thrombophilic disorders; pregnancy

Canadian labeling: Additional contraindications (not in U.S. labeling): Endometrial hyperplasia; partial or complete vision loss due to ophthalmic vascular disease; migraine with aura

Warnings/Precautions Hazardous agent - use appropriate precautions for handling and disposal (NIOSH 2014 [group 2]).

Anaphylaxis requiring emergency medical management has been reported within minutes to hours of taking conjugated estrogen (CE) tablets. Angioedema involving the face, feet, hands, larynx, and tongue has also been reported. Exogenous estrogens may exacerbate symptoms in women with hereditary angioedema.

[U.S. Boxed Warning]: Based on data from the Women's Health Initiative (WHI) studies, an increased risk of invasive breast cancer was observed in postmenopausal women using conjugated estrogens (CE) in combination with medroxyprogesterone acetate (MPA). This risk may be associated with duration of use and declines once combined therapy is discontinued (Chlebowski, 2009). The risk of invasive breast cancer was decreased in postmenopausal women with a hysterectomy using CE only, regardless of weight. However, the risk was not significantly decreased in women at high risk for breast cancer (family history of breast cancer, personal history of benign breast disease) (Anderson, 2012). An increase in abnormal mammogram findings has also been reported with estrogen alone or in combination with progestin therapy. Estrogen use may lead to severe hypercalcemia in patients with breast cancer and bone metastases; discontinue estrogen if hypercalcemia occurs. **[U.S. Boxed Warning]: The use of unopposed estrogen in women with an intact uterus is associated with an increased risk of endometrial cancer. The addition of a progestin to estrogen therapy may decrease the risk of endometrial hyperplasia, a precursor to endometrial cancer. Adequate diagnostic measures, including endometrial sampling if indicated, should be performed to rule out malignancy in postmenopausal women with undiagnosed abnormal vaginal bleeding.** Estrogens may exacerbate endometriosis. Malignant transformation of residual endometrial implants has been reported posthysterectomy with unopposed estrogen therapy. Consider adding a progestin in women with residual endometriosis posthysterectomy. Postmenopausal estrogen therapy and combined estrogen/progesterone therapy may increase the risk of ovarian cancer; however, the absolute risk to an individual woman is small. Although results from various studies are not consistent, risk does not appear to be significantly associated with the duration, route, or dose of therapy. In one study, the risk decreased after 2 years following discontinuation of therapy (Mørch, 2009). Although the risk of ovarian cancer is rare, women who are at an increased risk (eg, family history) should be counseled about the association (NAMS, 2012).

[U.S. Boxed Warning]: Estrogens with or without progestin should not be used to prevent cardiovascular disease. Using data from the Women's Health Initiative (WHI) studies, an increased risk of deep vein thrombosis (DVT) and stroke has been reported with CE and an increased risk of DVT, stroke, pulmonary emboli (PE) and myocardial infarction (MI) has been reported with CE with MPA in postmenopausal women. Additional risk factors include diabetes mellitus, hypercholesterolemia, hypertension, SLE, obesity, tobacco use, and/or history of venous thromboembolism (VTE). Adverse cardiovascular events have also been reported in males taking estrogens for prostate cancer. Risk factors should be managed appropriately; discontinue use if adverse cardiovascular events occur or are suspected. Women with inherited thrombophilias (eg, protein C or S deficiency) may have increased risk of venous thromboembolism (DeSancho, 2010; van Vlijmen, 2011). Use is contraindicated in women with protein C, protein S, antithrombin deficiency, or other known thrombophilic disorders.

[U.S. Boxed Warning]: Estrogens with or without progestin should not be used to prevent dementia. In the Women's Health Initiative Memory Study (WHIMS), an increased incidence of dementia was observed in women ≥65 years of age taking CE alone or in combination with MPA.

Estrogen compounds are generally associated with lipid effects such as increased HDL-cholesterol and decreased LDL-cholesterol. Triglycerides may also be increased; discontinue if pancreatitis occurs. Use with caution in patients with familial defects of lipoprotein metabolism. Estrogens may increase thyroid-binding globulin (TBG) levels leading to increased circulating total thyroid hormone levels. Women on thyroid replacement therapy may require higher doses of thyroid hormone while receiving estrogens. Use caution in patients with hypoparathyroidism; estrogen-induced hypocalcemia may occur. May have adverse effects on glucose tolerance; use caution in women with diabetes. Use caution in patients with asthma, epilepsy, hepatic hemangiomas, porphyria, or SLE; may exacerbate disease. Use with caution in patients with diseases which may be exacerbated by fluid retention, including cardiac or renal dysfunction. Use of postmenopausal estrogen may be associated with an increased risk of gallbladder disease requiring surgery. Use caution with migraine; may exacerbate disease. Canadian labeling contraindicates use in migraine with aura. Estrogens may cause retinal vascular thrombosis; discontinue if migraine, loss of vision, proptosis, diplopia, or other visual disturbances occur; discontinue permanently if papilledema or retinal vascular lesions are observed on examination.

Estrogens are poorly metabolized in patients with hepatic dysfunction. Use caution with a history of cholestatic jaundice associated with prior estrogen use or pregnancy. Discontinue if jaundice develops or if acute or chronic hepatic disturbances occur. Use is contraindicated with hepatic disease.

Whenever possible, estrogens should be discontinued at least 4-6 weeks prior to elective surgery associated with an increased risk of thromboembolism or during periods of prolonged immobilization. Avoid use of oral estrogen (with or without progestins) in the elderly due to potential of increased risk of breast and endometrial cancers, and lack of proven cardioprotection and cognitive protection (Beers Criteria). Prior to puberty, estrogens may cause premature closure of the epiphyses, premature breast development in girls or gynecomastia in boys. Vaginal bleeding and vaginal cornification may also be induced in girls. The use of estrogens and/or progestins may change the results of some laboratory tests (eg, coagulation factors, lipids, glucose tolerance, binding proteins). The dose, route, and the specific estrogen/progestin influences these changes. In addition, personal risk factors (eg, cardiovascular disease, smoking, diabetes, age) also contribute to adverse events; use of specific products may be contraindicated in women with certain risk factors.

[U.S. Boxed Warning]: Estrogens with or without progestin should be used for the shortest duration possible at the lowest effective dose consistent with treatment goals. Before prescribing estrogen therapy to postmenopausal women, the risks and benefits must be weighed for each patient. Women should be informed of these risks and benefits, as well as possible effects of progestin when added to estrogen therapy. Patients should be reevaluated as clinically appropriate to determine if treatment is still necessary. Available data related to treatment risks are from Women's Health Initiative (WHI) studies, which evaluated oral CE 0.625 mg with or without MPA 2.5 mg relative to placebo in postmenopausal women. Other combinations and dosage forms of estrogens and progestins were not studied. **Outcomes reported from clinical trials using CE with or without MPA should be assumed to be similar for other doses and other dosage forms of estrogens and progestins until comparable data becomes available.**

Benzyl alcohol and derivatives: Some dosage forms may contain benzyl alcohol; large amounts of benzyl alcohol (≥99 mg/kg/day) have been associated with a potentially fatal toxicity ("gasping syndrome") in neonates; the "gasping syndrome" consists of metabolic acidosis, respiratory distress, gasping respirations, CNS dysfunction (including convulsions, intracranial hemorrhage), hypotension and cardiovascular collapse (AAP, 1997; CDC, 1982); some data suggests that benzoate displaces bilirubin from protein binding sites (Ahlfors, 2001); avoid or use dosage forms containing benzyl alcohol with caution in neonates. See manufacturer's labeling.

Vulvar and vaginal atrophy use: Moderate-to-severe symptoms of vulvar and vaginal atrophy include vaginal dryness, dyspareunia, and atrophic vaginitis. When used solely for the treatment of vulvar and vaginal atrophy, topical vaginal products should be considered (NAMS, 2007).

Osteoporosis use: For use only in women at significant risk of osteoporosis and for who other nonestrogen medications are not considered appropriate.

Adverse Reactions

Central nervous system: Depression, dizziness, headache, nervousness, pain

Dermatologic: Pruritus

Endocrine & metabolic: Breast pain

Gastrointestinal: Abdominal pain, diarrhea, flatulence

Genitourinary: Leukorrhea, vaginal hemorrhage, vaginal moniliasis, vaginitis

Neuromuscular & skeletal: Arthralgia, back pain, leg cramps, weakness

Respiratory: Cough increased, pharyngitis, sinusitis

Additional adverse reactions reported with injection; frequency not defined: Local: injection site: Edema, pain, phlebitis

Rare but important or life-threatening: Alopecia, anaphylaxis, angioedema, asthma exacerbation, benign meningioma (possible growth), bloating, breast cancer, breast discharge/enlargement/tenderness, cervical secretion changes, chloasma, cholestatic jaundice, contact lens intolerance, dementia, deep vein thrombosis (DVT), dysmenorrhea, edema, endometrial cancer, endometrial hyperplasia, epilepsy exacerbation, erythema multiforme, erythema nodosum, fibrocystic breast changes, galactorrhea, gallbladder disease, glucose intolerance, gynecomastia (males), hepatic hemangiomas (enlargement), hirsutism, hypersensitivity reactions, hypertension, irritability, ischemic colitis, libido changes, melasma, MI, migraine, mood disturbances, nausea, ovarian cancer, pancreatitis, pulmonary emboli (PE), pelvic pain, porphyria exacerbation, rash, retinal vascular thrombosis, stroke, superficial venous thrombosis, thrombophlebitis, triglyceride increase, urticaria, uterine bleeding (abnormal), uterine leiomyomata (increase in size), vaginal candidiasis, vomiting, weight changes

Drug Interactions

Metabolism/Transport Effects Substrate of CYP1A2 (major), CYP2A6 (minor), CYP2B6 (minor), CYP2C19 (minor), CYP2C9 (minor), CYP2D6 (minor), CYP2E1 (minor), CYP3A4 (major); **Note:** Assignment of Major/Minor substrate status based on clinically relevant drug interaction potential; **Inhibits** CYP1A2 (weak); **Induces** CYP3A4 (weak)

Avoid Concomitant Use

Avoid concomitant use of Estrogens (Conjugated/Equine, Systemic) with any of the following: Anastrozole; Dehydroepiandrosterone; Exemestane; Indium 111 Capromab Pendetide; Ospemifene

Increased Effect/Toxicity

Estrogens (Conjugated/Equine, Systemic) may increase the levels/effects of: Anthrax Immune Globulin (Human); C1 inhibitors; Corticosteroids (Systemic); Immune Globulin; Lenalidomide; Ospemifene; ROPINIRole; Thalidomide; Theophylline Derivatives; Tipranavir; TiZANidine

The levels/effects of Estrogens (Conjugated/Equine, Systemic) may be increased by: Ascorbic Acid; Dehydroepiandrosterone; Herbs (Estrogenic Properties); NSAID (COX-2 Inhibitor)

Decreased Effect

Estrogens (Conjugated/Equine, Systemic) may decrease the levels/effects of: Anastrozole; Anticoagulants; Antidiabetic Agents; ARIPiprazole; Chenodiol; Exemestane; Hyaluronidase; Hydrocodone; Indium 111 Capromab

Pendetide; NiMODipine; Ospemifene; Saxagliptin; Somatropin; Thyroid Products; Ursodiol

The levels/effects of Estrogens (Conjugated/Equine, Systemic) may be decreased by: Bosentan; Cannabis; CYP1A2 Inducers (Strong); CYP3A4 Inducers (Moderate); CYP3A4 Inducers (Strong); Cyproterone; Dabrafenib; Deferasirox; Mitotane; Siltuximab; St Johns Wort; Teriflunomide; Tipranavir; Tocilizumab

Food Interactions Folic acid absorption may be decreased. Routine use of ethanol increases estrogen level and risk of breast cancer; may also increase the risk of osteoporosis. Management: Avoid ethanol.

Storage/Stability

Injection: Refrigerate at 2°C to 8°C (36°F to 46°F) prior to reconstitution. Use immediately following reconstitution.

Tablets: Store at room temperature 20°C to 25°C (68°F to 77°F).

Mechanism of Action Conjugated estrogens contain a mixture of estrone sulfate, equilin sulfate, 17 alpha-dihydroequilin, 17 alpha-estradiol and 17 beta-dihydroequilin. Estrogens are responsible for the development and maintenance of the female reproductive system and secondary sexual characteristics. Estradiol is the principle intracellular human estrogen and is more potent than estrone and estriol at the receptor level; it is the primary estrogen secreted prior to menopause. Following menopause, estrone and estrone sulfate are more highly produced. Estrogens modulate the pituitary secretion of gonadotropins, luteinizing hormone, and follicle-stimulating hormone through a negative feedback system; estrogen replacement reduces elevated levels of these hormones in postmenopausal women.

Pharmacokinetics (Adult data unless noted)

Absorption: Oral, transmucosal, transdermal: Well absorbed

Distribution: Widely distributes throughout the body; sex hormone target organs contain higher concentrations; distributes into breast milk

Protein binding: Primarily bound to sex hormone-binding globulin and albumin

Metabolism: Hepatic, via cytochrome P450 isoenzyme CYP3A4; estradiol is converted to estrone and estriol; estrone is also converted to estriol and is converted to estradiol (**Note:** A dynamic equilibrium of metabolic interconversions between estrogens exists in the circulation); estrogens also undergo hepatic sulfate and glucuronide conjugation and enterohepatic recirculation

Elimination: Excreted in the urine as estradiol, estrone, estriol (major urinary metabolite), and glucuronide and sulfate conjugates

Dosing: Usual Adolescents and Adults: **Note:** Use lowest effective dose for the shortest duration possible that is consistent with an individual's treatment goals and risks:

Female castration or primary ovarian failure: Oral: Cyclic regimen: 1.25 mg/day for 3 weeks, then no drug for the 4th week per cycle; repeat; titrate dose to response; use lowest effective dose

Female hypogonadism: Oral:

Manufacturer's recommendation: Cyclic regimen: 0.3-0.625 mg/day for 3 weeks, then no drug for the 4th week per cycle; titrate dose to response; use lowest effective dose

Alternative dosing: 2.5-7.5 mg/day in divided doses for 20 days, off 10 days and repeat until menses occur

Dysfunctional uterine bleeding:

Stable hematocrit: Oral: 1.25 mg twice daily for 21 days; if bleeding persists after 48 hours, increase to 2.5 mg twice daily; if bleeding persists after 48 more hours, increase to 2.5 mg 4 times/day; some recommend starting at 2.5 mg 4 times/day (**Note:** Medroxyprogesterone acetate 10 mg/day is also given on days 17-21; Neistein, 1991)

Alternatively: Oral: 2.5-5 mg/day for 7-10 days; then decrease to 1.25 mg/day for 2 weeks

Unstable hematocrit: Oral, IV: 5 mg 2-4 times/day; if bleeding is profuse, 20-40 mg every 4 hours up to 24 hours may be used; **Note:** A progestational-weighted contraception pill should also be given (eg, Ovral® 2 tablets stat and 1 tablet 4 times/day or medroxyprogesterone acetate 5-10 mg 4 times/day; Neistein, 1991)

Alternatively: IM, IV: 25 mg every 6-12 hours until bleeding stops

Preparation for Administration Hazardous agent; use appropriate precautions for handling and disposal (NIOSH 2014 [group 2]).

Parenteral: Reconstitute with 5 mL SWFI; slowly inject diluent against side wall of the vial. Agitate gently; do not shake violently.

Administration Hazardous agent; use appropriate precautions for handling and disposal (NIOSH 2014 [group 2]).

Oral: Administer with food or after eating to reduce GI upset; administration of dose at bedtime may decrease adverse effects

Parenteral: Administer slow IV to avoid vascular flushing; may be administered IM for dysfunctional uterine bleeding, but IV use is preferred (more rapid response)

Monitoring Parameters Blood pressure, weight, serum calcium, glucose, liver enzymes; dysfunctional uterine bleeding: Hematocrit, hemoglobin, PT; bone maturation and epiphyseal effects in young patients in whom bone growth is not complete; breast exam, mammogram, Papanicolaou smear, signs for endometrial cancer in female patients with a uterus; bone density measurement if used for prevention of osteoporosis

Test Interactions Reduced response to metyrapone test.

Additional Information See package insert for doses related to postmenopausal symptoms, prevention of osteoporosis in postmenopausal women, and palliative treatment of breast cancer or androgen-dependent prostate cancer in adults.

Dosage Forms Excipient information presented when available (limited, particularly for generics); consult specific product labeling.

Solution Reconstituted, Injection:

Premarin: 25 mg (1 ea) [contains benzyl alcohol]

Tablet, Oral:

Premarin: 0.3 mg [contains fd&c blue #2 (indigotine), fd&c yellow #10 (quinoline yellow)]

Premarin: 0.45 mg [contains fd&c blue #2 (indigotine)]

Premarin: 0.625 mg [contains fd&c blue #2 (indigotine), fd&c red #40]

Premarin: 0.9 mg

Premarin: 1.25 mg [contains fd&c yellow #10 (quinoline yellow), fd&c yellow #6 (sunset yellow)]

Estrogens (Conjugated/Equine, Topical)

(ES troe jenz KON joo gate ed, EE kwine)

Medication Safety Issues

Sound-alike/look-alike issues:

Premarin® may be confused with Primaxin®, Provera®, Remeron®

BEERS Criteria medication:

This drug may be potentially inappropriate for use in geriatric patients (Quality of evidence - moderate [topical]; Strength of recommendation - weak [topical]).

Related Information

Contraceptive Comparison Table *on page 2309*

Safe Handling of Hazardous Drugs *on page 2455*

Brand Names: US Premarin

Brand Names: Canada Premarin®

Therapeutic Category Estrogen Derivative; Estrogen Derivative, Vaginal

Generic Availability (US) No

Use Treatment of vulvar and vaginal atrophy; moderate to severe dyspareunia (pain during intercourse) due to vaginal/vulvar atrophy of menopause

Pregnancy Considerations Estrogens are not indicated for use during pregnancy or immediately postpartum. In general, the use of estrogen and progestin as in combination hormonal contraceptives have not been associated with teratogenic effects when inadvertently taken early in pregnancy. These products are contraindicated for use during pregnancy. Use of the vaginal cream may weaken latex found in condoms, diaphragms, or cervical caps.

Breast-Feeding Considerations Estrogen has been shown to decrease the quantity and quality of human milk. Use only if clearly needed. Monitor the growth of the infant closely.

Contraindications Undiagnosed abnormal vaginal bleeding; history of or current thrombophlebitis or venous thromboembolic disorders (including DVT, PE); active or history of arterial thromboembolic disease (eg, stroke, MI); carcinoma of the breast; estrogen-dependent tumor; hepatic dysfunction or disease; known protein C, protein S, antithrombin deficiency or other known thrombophilic disorders; pregnancy

Canadian labeling: Additional contraindications (not in U.S. labeling): Hypersensitivity to estrogens or any component of the formulation; endometrial hyperplasia; partial or complete vision loss due to ophthalmic vascular disease

Warnings/Precautions Hazardous agent - use appropriate precautions for handling and disposal (NIOSH 2014 [group 2]).

[U.S. Boxed Warning]: Based on data from the Women's Health Initiative (WHI) studies, an increased risk of invasive breast cancer was observed in postmenopausal women using conjugated estrogens (CE) in combination with medroxyprogesterone acetate (MPA). This risk may be associated with duration of use and declines once combined therapy is discontinued (Chlebowski, 2009). The risk of invasive breast cancer was decreased in postmenopausal women with a hysterectomy using CE only, regardless of weight. However, the risk was not significantly decreased in women at high risk for breast cancer (family history of breast cancer, personal history of benign breast disease) (Anderson, 2012). An increase in abnormal mammogram findings has also been reported with estrogen alone or in combination with progestin therapy. Estrogen use may lead to severe hypercalcemia in patients with breast cancer and bone metastases; discontinue estrogen if hypercalcemia occurs. Use is contraindicated in patients with known or suspected breast cancer. **[U.S. Boxed Warning]: The use of unopposed estrogen in women with an intact uterus is associated with an increased risk of endometrial cancer. The addition of a progestin to estrogen therapy may decrease the risk of endometrial hyperplasia, a precursor to endometrial cancer. Adequate diagnostic measures, including endometrial sampling if indicated, should be performed to rule out malignancy in postmenopausal women with undiagnosed abnormal vaginal bleeding.** Estrogens may exacerbate endometriosis. Malignant transformation of residual endometrial implants has been reported posthysterectomy with unopposed estrogen therapy. Consider adding a progestin in women with residual endometriosis posthysterectomy. Postmenopausal estrogen therapy and combined estrogen/progesterone therapy may increase the risk of ovarian cancer; however, the absolute risk to an individual woman is small. Although results from various studies are not consistent, risk does not appear to be significantly associated with the duration, route, or dose of therapy. In one study, the risk decreased after 2 years following discontinuation of therapy (Mørch, 2009). Although the risk of ovarian cancer is rare, women who are at an increased risk (eg, family history) should be counseled about the association (NAMS, 2012).

[U.S. Boxed Warning]: Estrogens with or without progestin should not be used to prevent cardiovascular disease. Using data from the Women's Health Initiative (WHI) studies, an increased risk of deep vein thrombosis (DVT) and stroke has been reported with CE and an increased risk of DVT, stroke, pulmonary emboli (PE) and myocardial infarction (MI) has been reported with CE with MPA in postmenopausal women. Additional risk factors include diabetes mellitus, hypercholesterolemia, hypertension, SLE, obesity, tobacco use, and/or history of venous thromboembolism (VTE). Risk factors should be managed appropriately; discontinue use if adverse cardiovascular events occur or are suspected. Women with inherited thrombophilias (eg, protein C or S deficiency) may have increased risk of venous thromboembolism (DeSancho, 2010; van Vlijmen 2011). Use is contraindicated in women with protein C, protein S, antithrombin deficiency, or other known thrombophilic disorders.

[U.S. Boxed Warning]: Estrogens with or without progestin should not be used to prevent dementia. In the Women's Health Initiative Memory Study (WHIMS), an increased incidence of dementia was observed in women ≥65 years of age taking CE alone or in combination with MPA.

Estrogen compounds are generally associated with lipid effects such as increased HDL-cholesterol and decreased LDL-cholesterol. Triglycerides may also be increased; discontinue if pancreatitis occurs. Use with caution in patients with familial defects of lipoprotein metabolism. Estrogens may increase thyroid-binding globulin (TBG) levels leading to increased circulating total thyroid hormone levels. Women on thyroid replacement therapy may require higher doses of thyroid hormone while receiving estrogens. Use caution in patients with hypoparathyroidism; estrogen induced hypocalcemia may occur. May have adverse effects on glucose tolerance; use caution in women with diabetes. Use caution in patients with asthma, epilepsy, hepatic hemangiomas, migraine, porphyria or SLE; may exacerbate disease. Use with caution in patients with diseases which may be exacerbated by fluid retention, including cardiac or renal dysfunction. Use of postmenopausal estrogen may be associated with an increased risk of gallbladder disease requiring surgery. Estrogens may cause retinal vascular thrombosis; discontinue if migraine, loss of vision, proptosis, diplopia, or other visual disturbances occur; discontinue permanently if papilledema or retinal vascular lesions are observed on examination. Exogenous estrogens may exacerbate angioedema symptoms in women with hereditary angioedema. The use of estrogens and/or progestins may change the results of some laboratory tests (eg, coagulation factors, lipids, glucose tolerance, binding proteins). The dose, route, and the specific estrogen/progestin influences these changes. In addition, personal risk factors (eg, cardiovascular disease, smoking, diabetes, age) also contribute to adverse events; use of specific products may be contraindicated in women with certain risk factors.

Estrogens are poorly metabolized in patients with hepatic dysfunction. Use caution with a history of cholestatic jaundice associated with prior estrogen use or pregnancy. Discontinue if jaundice develops or if acute or chronic hepatic disturbances occur. Use is contraindicated with hepatic disease.

In the elderly, low-dose intravaginal estrogen may be appropriate for use in the management of vaginal symptoms, lower urinary tract infections, and dyspareunia; in addition, evidence has shown that vaginal estrogens (particularly at estradiol doses of <25 mcg twice weekly) in the treatment of vaginal dryness is safe and effective in women with breast cancer. (Beers Criteria).

Vulvar and vaginal atrophy use: When used solely for the treatment of vulvar and vaginal atrophy, topical vaginal products should be considered. Use caution applying topical products to severely atrophic vaginal mucosa.

Whenever possible, estrogens should be discontinued at least 4-6 weeks prior to elective surgery associated with an increased risk of thromboembolism or during periods of prolonged immobilization.

[U.S. Boxed Warning]: Estrogens with or without progestin should be used for the shortest duration possible at the lowest effective dose consistent with treatment goals. Before prescribing estrogen therapy to postmenopausal women, the risks and benefits must be weighed for each patient. Women should be informed of these risks and benefits, as well as possible effects of progestin when added to estrogen therapy. Patients should be reevaluated as clinically appropriate to determine if treatment is still necessary. Available data related to treatment risks are from Women's Health Initiative (WHI) studies, which evaluated oral CE 0.625 mg with or without MPA 2.5 mg relative to placebo in postmenopausal women. Other combinations and dosage forms of estrogens and progestins were not studied. **Outcomes reported from clinical trials using CE with or without MPA should be assumed to be similar for other doses and other dosage forms of estrogens and progestins until comparable data becomes available.**

Moderate-to-severe symptoms of vulvar and vaginal atrophy include vaginal dryness, dyspareunia, and atrophic vaginitis. When used solely for the treatment of vulvar and vaginal atrophy, topical vaginal products should be considered. Use caution applying topical products to severely atrophic vaginal mucosa. Use of a progestin is normally not required when low-dose estrogen is applied locally and only for this purpose (NAMS, 2007).

Benzyl alcohol and derivatives: Some dosage forms may contain benzyl alcohol; large amounts of benzyl alcohol (≥99 mg/kg/day) have been associated with a potentially fatal toxicity ("gasping syndrome") in neonates; the "gasping syndrome" consists of metabolic acidosis, respiratory distress, gasping respirations, CNS dysfunction (including convulsions, intracranial hemorrhage), hypotension and cardiovascular collapse (AAP, 1997; CDC, 1982); some data suggests that benzoate displaces bilirubin from protein binding sites (Ahlfors, 2001); avoid or use dosage forms containing benzyl alcohol with caution in neonates. See manufacturer's labeling.

Use of the vaginal cream may weaken latex found in condoms, diaphragms or cervical caps. Systemic absorption occurs following vaginal use; warnings, precautions, and adverse events observed with oral therapy should be considered.

Warnings: Additional Pediatric Considerations Some dosage forms may contain propylene glycol; in neonates large amounts of propylene glycol delivered orally, intravenously (eg, >3,000 mg/day), or topically have been associated with potentially fatal toxicities which can include metabolic acidosis, seizures, renal failure, and CNS depression; toxicities have also been reported in children and adults including hyperosmolality, lactic acidosis, seizures, and respiratory depression; use caution (AAP, 1997; Shehab, 2009).

Adverse Reactions Due to systemic absorption, other adverse effects associated with systemic therapy may also occur. Reported with daily use:

Cardiovascular: Vasodilatation

Central nervous system: Pain

Endocrine & metabolic: Breast pain

Gastrointestinal: Abdominal pain

Genitourinary: Vaginitis

Neuromuscular & skeletal: Back pain, weakness

Rare but important or life-threatening: Anaphylactic reactions, breast cancer, deep vein thrombosis (DVT), dementia, depression, endometrial cancer, gallbladder disease, gynecomastia (males), hypertension, leukorrhea, MI, pulmonary emboli (PE), retinal vascular thrombosis, stroke, uterine leiomyomata (increase in size)

Drug Interactions

Metabolism/Transport Effects Substrate of CYP1A2 (major), CYP2A6 (minor), CYP2B6 (minor), CYP2C19 (minor), CYP2C9 (minor), CYP2D6 (minor), CYP2E1 (minor), CYP3A4 (major); **Note:** Assignment of Major/Minor substrate status based on clinically relevant drug interaction potential; **Inhibits** CYP1A2 (weak); **Induces** CYP3A4 (weak)

Avoid Concomitant Use

Avoid concomitant use of Estrogens (Conjugated/Equine, Topical) with any of the following: Anastrozole; Dehydroepiandrosterone; Exemestane; Indium 111 Capromab Pendetide; Ospemifene

Increased Effect/Toxicity

Estrogens (Conjugated/Equine, Topical) may increase the levels/effects of: Anthrax Immune Globulin (Human); C1 inhibitors; Corticosteroids (Systemic); Immune Globulin; Lenalidomide; Ospemifene; ROPINIRole; Thalidomide; Theophylline Derivatives; Tipranavir; TiZANidine

The levels/effects of Estrogens (Conjugated/Equine, Topical) may be increased by: Ascorbic Acid; Dehydroepiandrosterone; Herbs (Estrogenic Properties); NSAID (COX-2 Inhibitor)

Decreased Effect

Estrogens (Conjugated/Equine, Topical) may decrease the levels/effects of: Anastrozole; Anticoagulants; Antidiabetic Agents; ARIPiprazole; Chenodiol; Exemestane; Hyaluronidase; Hydrocodone; Indium 111 Capromab Pendetide; NiMODipine; Ospemifene; Saxagliptin; Somatropin; Thyroid Products; Ursodiol

The levels/effects of Estrogens (Conjugated/Equine, Topical) may be decreased by: Bosentan; Cannabis; CYP1A2 Inducers (Strong); CYP3A4 Inducers (Moderate); CYP3A4 Inducers (Strong); Cyproterone; Dabrafenib; Deferasirox; Mitotane; Siltuximab; St Johns Wort; Teriflunomide; Tipranavir; Tocilizumab

Storage/Stability Vaginal cream: Store at room temperature of 20°C to 25°C (68°F to 77°F); excursions permitted to 15°C to 30°C (59°F to 86°F).

Mechanism of Action Conjugated estrogens contain a mixture of estrone sulfate, equilin sulfate, 17 alpha-dihydroequilin, 17 alpha-estradiol and 17 beta-dihydroequilin. Estrogens are responsible for the development and maintenance of the female reproductive system and secondary sexual characteristics. Estradiol is the principle intracellular human estrogen and is more potent than estrone and estriol at the receptor level; it is the primary estrogen secreted prior to menopause. Following menopause, estrone and estrone sulfate are more highly produced. Estrogens modulate the pituitary secretion of gonadotropins, luteinizing hormone, and follicle-stimulating hormone through a negative feedback system; estrogen replacement reduces elevated levels of these hormones in postmenopausal women.

Pharmacokinetics (Adult data unless noted) Absorption: Transmucosal, transdermal: Well absorbed

Dosing: Usual Adults: Female:

Moderate to severe dyspareunia: Intravaginal: 0.5 g twice weekly (eg, Monday and Thursday) **or** once daily cyclically*

Vulvar and vaginal atrophy: Intravaginal: 0.5-2 g/day given cyclically*

***Cyclic administration:** Either 3 weeks on, 1 week off **or** 25 days on, 5 days off

Administration Hazardous agent; use appropriate precautions for handling and disposal (NIOSH 2014 [group 2]).

Intravaginal: Use marked stopping points on applicator to measure prescribed dose; to administer, lay down on back and draw knees up; gently insert applicator into vagina and press plunger downward to deliver medication; wash plunger and barrel with mild soap and water after use; do not boil or use hot water.

Monitoring Parameters Blood pressure, weight, serum calcium, glucose, liver enzymes; dysfunctional uterine bleeding; hematocrit, hemoglobin, PT; bone maturation and epiphyseal effects in young patients in whom bone growth is not complete; breast exam, mammogram, Papanicolaou smear, signs for endometrial cancer in female patients with a uterus

Test Interactions Reduced response to metyrapone test.

Dosage Forms Excipient information presented when available (limited, particularly for generics); consult specific product labeling.

Cream, Vaginal:

Premarin: 0.625 mg/g (30 g) [contains benzyl alcohol, cetyl alcohol, propylene glycol monostearate]

Etanercept (et a NER sept)

Medication Safety Issues

Sound-alike/look-alike issues:

Enbrel may be confused with Levbid

Brand Names: US Enbrel; Enbrel SureClick

Brand Names: Canada Enbrel

Therapeutic Category Antirheumatic, Disease Modifying; Tumor Necrosis Factor (TNF) Blocking Agent

Generic Availability (US) No

Use Treatment of moderately- to severely-active polyarticular juvenile idiopathic arthritis (FDA approved in ages ≥2 years);treatment of signs and symptoms of moderately- to severely-active rheumatoid arthritis, psoriatic arthritis, and active ankylosing spondylitis (FDA approved in ages ≥18 years and adults); treatment of chronic (moderate to severe) plaque psoriasis in patients who are candidates for systemic therapy or phototherapy (FDA approved in ages ≥18 years and adults); has also been used as adjunctive therapy Kawasaki disease and for treatment of familial Mediterranean fever (colchicine refractory or colchicine intolerant), scleroderma, and chronic nonbacterial osteomyelitis

Medication Guide Available Yes

Pregnancy Risk Factor B

Pregnancy Considerations Adverse events have not been observed in animal reproduction studies. Etanercept crosses the placenta. Following in utero exposure, concentrations in the newborn at delivery are 3% to 32% of the maternal serum concentration.

A pregnancy registry has been established to monitor outcomes of women exposed to etanercept during pregnancy (800-772-6436).

Breast-Feeding Considerations Etanercept is excreted into breast milk in low concentrations and is minimally absorbed by a nursing infant (limited data). The manufacturer recommends that caution be used if administered to a nursing woman, taking into account the importance of the drug to the mother and potential effects to the nursing infant. A lactation surveillance program has been established to monitor outcomes of breastfed infants exposed to etanercept (800-772-6436).

Contraindications Sepsis

Warnings/Precautions [US Boxed Warning]: Patients receiving etanercept are at increased risk for serious infections which may result in hospitalization and/or fatality; infections usually developed in patients receiving concomitant immunosuppressive agents (eg, methotrexate or corticosteroids) and may present as disseminated (rather than local) disease. Active tuberculosis (or reactivation of latent tuberculosis), invasive fungal (including aspergillosis, blastomycosis, candidiasis, coccidioidomycosis, histoplasmosis, and pneumocystosis) and bacterial, viral or other opportunistic infections (including legionellosis and listeriosis) have been reported in patients receiving TNF-blocking agents, including etanercept. Monitor closely for signs/symptoms of infection. Discontinue for serious infection or sepsis. Consider risks versus benefits prior to use in patients with a history of chronic or recurrent infection. Consider empiric antifungal therapy in patients who are at risk for invasive fungal infection and develop severe systemic illness. Caution should be exercised when considering use in the elderly or in patients with conditions that predispose them to infections (eg, diabetes) or residence/travel from areas of endemic mycoses (blastomycosis, coccidioidomycosis, histoplasmosis), or with latent or localized infections. Do not initiate etanercept therapy with clinically important active infection. Patients who develop a new infection while undergoing treatment should be monitored closely. **[US Boxed Warning]: Tuberculosis (disseminated or extrapulmonary) has been reported in patients receiving etanercept; both reactivation of latent infection and new infections have been reported.** Patients should be evaluated for tuberculosis risk factors and for latent tuberculosis infection with a tuberculin skin test prior to starting therapy. Treatment of latent tuberculosis should be initiated before etanercept therapy; consider antituberculosis treatment if adequate course of treatment cannot be confirmed in patients with a history of latent or active tuberculosis or with risk factors despite negative skin test. Some patients who tested negative prior to therapy have developed active infection; tests for latent tuberculosis infection may be falsely negative while on etanercept therapy. Monitor for signs and symptoms of tuberculosis in all patients. Rare reactivation of hepatitis B virus (HBV) has occurred in chronic virus carriers, usually in patients receiving concomitant immunosuppressants; evaluate for HBV prior to initiation in all patients. Monitor during and for several months following discontinuation of treatment in HBV carriers; interrupt therapy if reactivation occurs and treat appropriately with antiviral therapy; if resumption of therapy is deemed necessary, exercise caution and monitor patient closely. Patients should be brought up to date with all immunizations before initiating therapy. Live vaccines should not be given concurrently with etanercept; there is no data available concerning secondary transmission of live vaccines in patients receiving therapy. Patients with a significant exposure to varicella virus should temporarily discontinue etanercept. Treatment with varicella zoster immune globulin should be considered.

[US Boxed Warning]: Lymphoma and other malignancies have been reported in children and adolescent patients receiving TNF-blocking agents, including etanercept. Half of the malignancies reported in children were lymphomas (Hodgkin and non-Hodgkin) while other cases varied and included malignancies not typically observed in this population. The impact of etanercept on the development and course of malignancy is not fully defined. Compared to the general population, an increased risk of lymphoma has been noted in clinical trials; however, rheumatoid arthritis alone has been previously associated with an increased rate of lymphoma. Lymphomas and other malignancies were also observed (at rates higher than expected for the general population) in adult patients receiving etanercept. Etanercept is not recommended for use in patients with Wegener's granulomatosis who are receiving immunosuppressive therapy due to higher incidence of noncutaneous solid malignancies. Hepatosplenic T-cell lymphoma (HSTCL), a rare T-cell lymphoma, has also been associated with TNF-blocking agents, primarily reported in adolescent and young adult males with Crohn disease or ulcerative colitis. Melanoma, nonmelanoma skin cancer, and Merkel cell carcinoma have been reported in patients receiving TNF-blocking agents, including etanercept. Perform periodic skin examinations in all patients during therapy, particularly those at increased risk of skin cancer. Positive antinuclear antibody titers have been detected in patients (with negative baselines). Rare cases of autoimmune disorder, including lupus-like syndrome or autoimmune hepatitis, have been reported; monitor and discontinue if symptoms develop.

Allergic reactions may occur; if an anaphylactic reaction or other serious allergic reaction occurs, administration should be discontinued immediately and appropriate therapy initiated. Use with caution in patients with preexisting or recent onset CNS demyelinating disorders; rare cases of new-onset or exacerbation of CNS demyelinating disorders have occurred; may present with mental status changes and some may be associated with permanent disability. Optic neuritis, transverse myelitis, multiple sclerosis, Guillain-Barré syndrome, other peripheral demyelinating neuropathies, and new-onset or exacerbation of seizures have been reported. Use with caution in patients with heart failure or decreased left ventricular function; worsening and new-onset heart failure has been reported, including in patients without known preexisting cardiovascular disease. Use caution in patients with a history of significant hematologic abnormalities; has been associated with pancytopenia and aplastic anemia (rare). Patients must be advised to seek medical attention if they develop signs and symptoms suggestive of blood dyscrasias; discontinue if significant hematologic abnormalities are confirmed. Use with caution in patients with moderate to severe alcoholic hepatitis. Compared to placebo, the mortality rate in patients treated with etanercept was similar at one month but significantly higher after 6 months.

Due to a higher incidence of serious infections, concomitant use with anakinra is not recommended. Hypoglycemia has been reported in patients receiving concomitant therapy with etanercept and antidiabetic medications; dose reduction of antidiabetic medication may be necessary. Use with caution in patient with diabetes; monitor blood glucose as clinically necessary. Some dosage forms may contain dry natural rubber (latex).

Benzyl alcohol and derivatives: Diluent for injection may contain benzyl alcohol; large amounts of benzyl alcohol (≥99 mg/kg/day) have been associated with a potentially fatal toxicity ("gasping syndrome") in neonates; the "gasping syndrome" consists of metabolic acidosis, respiratory distress, gasping respirations, CNS dysfunction (including convulsions, intracranial hemorrhage), hypotension and cardiovascular collapse (AAP, 1997; CDC, 1982); some data suggests that benzoate displaces bilirubin from protein binding sites (Ahlfors, 2001); avoid or use dosage forms containing benzyl alcohol with caution in neonates. See manufacturer's labeling.

Warnings: Additional Pediatric Considerations In an analysis of children and adolescents who had received TNF-blockers (etanercept and infliximab), the FDA identified 48 cases of malignancy. Of the 48 cases, ~50% were lymphomas (eg, Hodgkin and non-Hodgkin lymphoma) and other malignancies, such as leukemia, melanoma, and solid organ tumors, were also reported; malignancies rarely seen in children (eg, leiomyosarcoma, hepatic malignancies, and renal cell carcinoma) were also observed. Overall, in pediatric patients, the median onset of malignancy was after 30 months of therapy (range: 1 to 84 months); most of these cases (88%) were receiving other immunosuppressive medications (eg, azathioprine and methotrexate). As compared to the general population, an increased risk of lymphoma has been noted in clinical trials; however, rheumatoid arthritis has been previously associated with an increased rate of lymphoma. The role of TNF-blockers in the development of malignancies in children cannot be excluded. The FDA also reviewed 147 postmarketing reports of leukemia (including acute myeloid leukemia, chronic lymphocytic leukemia, and chronic myeloid leukemia) in patients (children and adults) using TNF-blockers. Average onset time to development of leukemia was within the first 1 to 2 years of TNF blocker initiation. Although most patients were receiving other immunosuppressive agents, the role of TNF blockers in the development of leukemia could not be excluded. The FDA concluded that there is a possible association with the development of leukemia and the use of TNF-blockers. Patients should be monitored closely for signs and symptoms suggestive of malignancy, evidence of which should result in prompt discontinuation of the medication and appropriate diagnostic evaluation.

In JIA patients, rare inflammatory bowel disease has also been reported (van Dijken, 2011); monitor and discontinue therapy if symptoms develop.

Adverse Reactions

Central nervous system: Dizziness, headache

Dermatologic: Pruritus, skin rash

Gastrointestinal: Abdominal pain (more common in children), diarrhea, nausea (children), vomiting

Infection: Infection

Local: Injection site reaction (bleeding, bruising, erythema, itching, pain, or swelling)

Neuromuscular & skeletal: Weakness

Respiratory: Cough, pharyngitis, respiratory distress, respiratory tract infection, rhinitis, sinusitis, upper respiratory tract infection

Miscellaneous: Antibody development (positive antidouble-stranded DNA antibodies), fever, positive ANA titer

Rare but important or life-threatening: Abscess, adenopathy, anemia, angioedema, anorexia, aplastic anemia, appendicitis, aseptic meningitis, aspergillosis, autoimmune hepatitis, blood coagulation disorder, bursitis, cardiac failure, cerebral ischemia, cerebrovascular accident, cholecystitis, cutaneous lupus erythematous, deep vein thrombosis, demyelinating disease of the central nervous system (suggestive of multiple sclerosis, transverse myelitis, or optic neuritis), depression, dermal ulcer, erythema multiforme, gastritis, gastroenteritis, gastrointestinal hemorrhage, glomerulopathy (membranous), hepatotoxicity (idiosyncratic) (Chalasani, 2014), herpes zoster, hydrocephalus (with normal pressure), hypersensitivity, hypersensitivity reaction, hypertension, hypotension, inflammatory bowel disease, interstitial pulmonary disease, intestinal perforation, ischemic heart disease, leukemia, leukopenia, lupus-like syndrome, lymphadenopathy, malignant lymphoma, malignant melanoma, malignant neoplasm, Merkel cell carcinoma, myocardial infarction, multiple sclerosis, nephrolithiasis, neutropenia, optic neuritis, oral mucosa ulcer, pancreatitis, pancytopenia, pneumonia due to *Pneumocystis carinii*, polymyositis, psoriasis (including new onset, palmoplantar, pustular, or exacerbation), pulmonary disease, pulmonary embolism, reactivation of HBV, sarcoidosis, scleritis, seizure, skin carcinoma, Stevens-Johnson syndrome, subcutaneous nodule, thrombocytopenia, thrombophlebitis, toxic epidermal necrolysis, tuberculosis, tuberculous arthritis, urinary tract infection, uveitis, varicella zoster infection, vasculitis (cutaneous and systemic), weight gain

Drug Interactions

Metabolism/Transport Effects None known.

Avoid Concomitant Use

Avoid concomitant use of Etanercept with any of the following: Abatacept; Anakinra; BCG; BCG (Intravesical); Belimumab; Canakinumab; Certolizumab Pegol; Cyclophosphamide; InFLIXimab; Natalizumab; Pimecrolimus; Rilonacept; Tacrolimus (Topical); Tocilizumab; Tofacitinib; Vaccines (Live); Vedolizumab

Increased Effect/Toxicity

Etanercept may increase the levels/effects of: Abatacept; Anakinra; Belimumab; Canakinumab; Certolizumab Pegol; Cyclophosphamide; InFLIXimab; Leflunomide; Natalizumab; Rilonacept; Tofacitinib; Vaccines (Live); Vedolizumab

The levels/effects of Etanercept may be increased by: Denosumab; Pimecrolimus; Roflumilast; Tacrolimus (Topical); Tocilizumab; Trastuzumab

Decreased Effect

Etanercept may decrease the levels/effects of: BCG; BCG (Intravesical); Coccidioides immitis Skin Test; Sipuleucel-T; Vaccines (Inactivated); Vaccines (Live)

The levels/effects of Etanercept may be decreased by: Echinacea

Storage/Stability

Refrigerate at 2°C to 8°C (36°F to 46°F). Do not freeze. Do not store in extreme heat or cold. Store in the original carton to protect from light or physical damage.

Individual autoinjectors, prefilled syringes, or dose trays (containing multi-use vials and diluent syringes) may be stored at room temperature for a maximum single period of 14 days with protection from light and sources of heat, and humidity. Once an autoinjector, prefilled syringe or dose tray has been stored at room temperature, it should not be placed back into the refrigerator; discard after 14 days.

Once the multi-use vial has been reconstituted, use the reconstituted solution immediately or refrigerate at 2°C to 8°C (36°F to 46°F). Reconstituted solution must be used within 14 days; discard after 14 days.

Mechanism of Action Etanercept is a recombinant DNA-derived protein composed of tumor necrosis factor receptor (TNFR) linked to the Fc portion of human IgG1. Etanercept binds tumor necrosis factor (TNF) and blocks its interaction with cell surface receptors. TNF plays an important role in the inflammatory processes and the resulting joint pathology of rheumatoid arthritis (RA), polyarticular-course juvenile idiopathic arthritis (JIA), ankylosing spondylitis (AS), and plaque psoriasis.

Pharmacodynamics

Onset of action: RA: 1-2 weeks

Maximum effect: RA: Full effect is usually seen within 3 months

Pharmacokinetics (Adult data unless noted)

Absorption: Absorbed slowly after SubQ injection

Distribution: V_d: 1.78-3.39 L/m^2

Bioavailability: SubQ: 60%

Half-life:

Children: 70-94.8 hours

Adults: 102 ± 30 hours

Time to peak serum concentration: SubQ: 69 ± 34 hours

Elimination: Clearance:

Children and Adolescents 4-17 years: 46 mL/hour/m^2

Adults: 160 ± 80 mL/hour

Dosing: Usual

Pediatric:

Juvenile idiopathic arthritis: Children ≥2 years and Adolescents: SubQ:

Once-weekly dosing: 0.8 mg/kg/dose once weekly; maximum dose: 50 mg/dose

Twice-weekly dosing: 0.4 mg/kg/dose twice weekly, given 72 to 96 hours apart; maximum dose: 25 mg/dose (Lovell, 2006)

Kawasaki disease; acute, adjunct therapy: Limited data available: Infants ≥6 months and Children <6 years: SubQ: 0.8 mg/kg/dose for 3 doses; administer first dose within 24 hours after completion of IV immunoglobulin (day 0), the second dose at day 7, and third dose at day 14; maximum dose: 50 mg/dose. Dosing based on an open-labeled pilot trial of 15 pediatric patients (mean age: 2.6 years); all patients also received standard aspirin therapy; no patients required retreatment or rescue therapy for signs/symptoms of Kawasaki disease (Choueiter, 2010). A large double-blind, placebo-controlled trial is ongoing [EATAK trial (NCT00841789)] utilizing the same dosage regimen; results pending (Portman, 2011).

Mediterranean fever; familial (FMF) (intolerance or resistance to colchicine): Very limited data available; efficacy results variable: Children ≥11 years and Adolescents: SubQ: 0.8 mg/kg once weekly; maximum dose: 50 mg/dose; dosing based on a case series (n=3); results showed fewer attacks with treatment, median duration of therapy was 3 months and all patients continued colchicine therapy if able; over time, therapy was eventually changed to anakinra due to clinician determined unsatisfactory response (Akgul, 2012; Özen, 2011; Sakallioglu, 2006; Soriano, 2013); a case series in adult patients (n=5, age range: 20-40 years) reported no further attacks (80%) or decrease frequency (20%) with etanercept (25 mg twice weekly) therapy (Bilgen, 2011).

Plaque psoriasis:

Children and Adolescents 4 to 17 years: Limited data available: SubQ: 0.8 mg/kg/dose once weekly; maximum dose: 50 mg/dose; results of a long-term study (96 weeks) showed efficacy maintained and therapy generally well-tolerated (Paller, 2008; Paller, 2010; Siegfried, 2010)

Adolescents ≥18 years: SubQ: Initial: 50 mg twice weekly administered 72 to 96 hours apart for 3 months; **Note:** Initial doses of 25 mg or 50 mg per week were also shown to be efficacious; maintenance dose: 50 mg once weekly

Rheumatoid arthritis, psoriatic arthritis, ankylosing spondylitis: Adolescents ≥18 years: SubQ:

Once-weekly dosing: 50 mg once weekly

Twice-weekly dosing: 25 mg given twice weekly (individual doses should be separated by 72 to 96 hours); maximum amount administered at a single injection site: 25 mg; rheumatoid arthritis: Maximum weekly dose: 50 mg/week

Adult:

Plaque psoriasis: SubQ: Initial: 50 mg twice weekly (administered 72 to 96 hours apart) for 3 months; **Note:** Initial doses of 25 mg or 50 mg per week were also shown to be efficacious; maintenance dose: 50 mg once weekly.

Rheumatoid arthritis, psoriatic arthritis, ankylosing spondylitis: SubQ:

Once-weekly dosing: 50 mg once weekly

Twice-weekly dosing: 25 mg given twice weekly (individual doses should be separated by 72 to 96 hours); maximum amount administered at a single injection site: 25 mg; rheumatoid arthritis: Maximum weekly dose: 50 mg/week

Dosing adjustment in renal impairment: There are no dosage adjustment provided in manufacturer's labeling (has not been studied).

Dosing adjustment in hepatic impairment: There are no dosage adjustment provided in manufacturer's labeling (has not been studied).

Preparation for Administration Multiple-use vial: Reconstitute by adding 1 mL of bacteriostatic water for injection (supplied) slowly to 25 mg vial, gently swirl; do not shake or agitate vigorously; dissolution generally complete in <10 minutes; resulting solution is 25 mg/mL. Do not filter reconstituted solution during preparation or administration.

Administration Administer subcutaneously into front of the thigh (preferred), abdomen (avoiding the area around the navel [2 inches in adults]), or outer area of the upper arm. Rotate injection sites. New injections should be given at least 1 inch from an old site and never into areas where the skin is tender, bruised, red, or hard or into any raised thick, red, or scaly skin patches or lesions. For a more comfortable injection, autoinjectors, prefilled syringes, and dose trays may be allowed to reach room temperature by removing from the refrigerator 15 to 30 minutes prior to injection. **Note:** If the prescriber determines that it is appropriate, patients may self-inject after proper training in injection technique.

Multiple-use vial: Do not administer >25 mg at a single injection site if the multiple-use vial is used to prepare the dose.

Single-use prefilled syringe or autoinjector: Do not remove needle cover or needle shield while allowing to reach room temperature. Visually inspect for particulate matter and discoloration prior to administration; solution may have small white particles of protein, which is normal for a proteinaceous solution; should not be used if cloudy, discolored or if foreign matter is present.

Monitoring Parameters Monitor improvement of symptoms and physical function assessments (eg, joint swelling, pain, and tenderness; ESR or C-reactive protein level). Latent TB screening prior to initiating and during therapy; signs/symptoms of infection (prior to, during, and following therapy); CBC with differential; signs/symptoms/ worsening of heart failure; HBV screening prior to initiating (all patients), HBV carriers (during and for several months following therapy); signs and symptoms of hypersensitivity reaction; symptoms of lupus-like syndrome; signs/symptoms of malignancy (eg, splenomegaly, hepatomegaly, abdominal pain, persistent fever, night sweats, weight loss).

Dosage Forms Excipient information presented when available (limited, particularly for generics); consult specific product labeling.

Kit, Subcutaneous [preservative free]:
 Enbrel: 25 mg [contains benzyl alcohol, tromethamine]

Solution Auto-injector, Subcutaneous [preservative free]:
 Enbrel SureClick: 50 mg/mL (0.98 mL)

Solution Prefilled Syringe, Subcutaneous [preservative free]:
 Enbrel: 25 mg/0.5 mL (0.51 mL); 50 mg/mL (0.98 mL)

◆ **Ethacrynate Sodium** *see* Ethacrynic Acid *on page 809*

Ethacrynic Acid (eth a KRIN ik AS id)

Medication Safety Issues

Sound-alike/look-alike issues:

Edecrin may be confused with Eulexin, Ecotrin

Brand Names: US Edecrin; Sodium Edecrin

Brand Names: Canada Edecrin; Sodium Edecrin

Therapeutic Category Antihypertensive Agent; Diuretic, Loop

Generic Availability (US) No

Use Management of edema secondary to CHF, hepatic or renal disease; hypertension

Pregnancy Risk Factor B

Pregnancy Considerations Adverse events were not observed in animal reproduction studies.

Breast-Feeding Considerations It is not known if ethacrynic acid is excreted in breast milk. Due to the potential for serious adverse reactions in the nursing infant, a decision should be made whether to discontinue nursing or to discontinue the drug, taking into account the importance of treatment to the mother.

Contraindications Hypersensitivity to ethacrynic acid or any component of the formulation; anuria; history of severe watery diarrhea caused by this product; infants

Warnings/Precautions Loop diuretics are potent diuretics; excess amounts can lead to profound diuresis with fluid and electrolyte loss; close medical supervision and dose evaluation are required. Watch for and correct electrolyte disturbances; adjust dose to avoid dehydration. In contrast to thiazide diuretics, a loop diuretic can also lower serum calcium concentrations. Electrolyte disturbances can predispose a patient to serious cardiac arrhythmias. In cirrhosis, avoid electrolyte and acid/base imbalances that might lead to hepatic encephalopathy. Monitor fluid status and renal function in an attempt to prevent oliguria, azotemia, and reversible increases in BUN and creatinine; close medical supervision of aggressive diuresis required. Diuretic resistance may occur in some patients, despite higher doses of loop diuretic treatment. Diuretic resistance can usually be overcome by intravenous administration, the use of two diuretics together (eg, furosemide and chlorothiazide), or the use of a diuretic with a positive inotropic agent. Rapid IV administration, renal impairment, excessive doses, and concurrent use of other ototoxins is associated with ototoxicity; has been associated with a higher incidence of ototoxicity than other loop diuretics. Hypersensitivity reactions can rarely occur, however, ethacrynic acid has no cross-reactivity to sulfonamides or sulfonylureas. Coadministration of antihypertensives may increase the risk of hypotension. If given the morning of surgery, ethacrynic acid may render the patient volume depleted and blood pressure may be labile during general anesthesia.

Adverse Reactions

Central nervous system: Apprehension, chills, confusion, encephalopathy (patients with pre-existing liver disease), fatigue, fever, headache, vertigo

Dermatologic: Henoch-Schönlein purpura (IgA vasculitis) (in patient with rheumatic heart disease), skin rash

Endocrine & metabolic: Gout; hyperglycemia; hypoglycemia (occurred in two uremic patients who received doses above those recommended); hyponatremia; reversible hyperuricemia; variations in phosphorus, CO_2 content, bicarbonate, and calcium

Gastrointestinal: Abdominal discomfort or pain, acute pancreatitis (rare), anorexia, diarrhea, dysphagia, gastrointestinal bleeding, malaise, nausea, vomiting

Genitourinary: Hematuria

Hepatic: Abnormal liver function tests, jaundice

Hematology: Agranulocytosis, severe neutropenia, thrombocytopenia

Local: Local irritation and pain, thrombophlebitis (with intravenous use)

Ocular: Blurred vision

Otic: Temporary or permanent deafness, tinnitus

Renal: Increased serum creatinine

Drug Interactions

Metabolism/Transport Effects None known.

Avoid Concomitant Use

Avoid concomitant use of Ethacrynic Acid with any of the following: Furosemide; Mecamylamine

Increased Effect/Toxicity

Ethacrynic Acid may increase the levels/effects of: ACE Inhibitors; Allopurinol; Amifostine; Aminoglycosides;

Antihypertensives; Cardiac Glycosides; CISplatin; Dofetilide; DULoxetine; Foscarnet; Hypotensive Agents; Ivabradine; Levodopa; Lithium; Mecamylamine; Methotrexate; Neuromuscular-Blocking Agents; Obinutuzumab; RisperiDONE; RiTUXimab; Salicylates; Sodium Phosphates; Topiramate; Vitamin K Antagonists

The levels/effects of Ethacrynic Acid may be increased by: Alfuzosin; Analgesics (Opioid); Barbiturates; Beta2-Agonists; Brimonidine (Topical); Canagliflozin; Corticosteroids (Orally Inhaled); Corticosteroids (Systemic); CycloSPORINE (Systemic); Diazoxide; Furosemide; Herbs (Hypotensive Properties); Licorice; MAO Inhibitors; Methotrexate; Nicorandil; Pentoxifylline; Phosphodiesterase 5 Inhibitors; Probenecid; Prostacyclin Analogues

Decreased Effect

Ethacrynic Acid may decrease the levels/effects of: Antidiabetic Agents; Lithium; Neuromuscular-Blocking Agents

The levels/effects of Ethacrynic Acid may be decreased by: Bile Acid Sequestrants; Fosphenytoin; Herbs (Hypertensive Properties); Methotrexate; Methylphenidate; Nonsteroidal Anti-Inflammatory Agents; Phenytoin; Probenecid; Salicylates; Yohimbine

Storage/Stability Store at 25°C (77°F); excursions permitted to 15°C to 30°C (59°F to 86°F). Discard unused reconstituted solution after 24 hours.

Mechanism of Action Inhibits reabsorption of sodium and chloride in the ascending loop of Henle and distal renal tubule, interfering with the chloride-binding cotransport system, thus causing increased excretion of water, sodium, chloride, magnesium, and calcium

Pharmacodynamics

Onset of action:
- Oral: Within 30 minutes
- IV: 5 minutes

Peak effect:
- Oral: 2 hours
- IV: 15-30 minutes

Duration:
- Oral: 6-8 hours
- IV: 2 hours

Pharmacokinetics (Adult data unless noted)

Absorption: Oral: Rapid

Protein binding: >90%

Metabolism: In the liver to active cysteine conjugate (35% to 40%)

Elimination: In bile, 30% to 60% excreted unchanged in urine

Dosing: Usual Note: Dose equivalency for adult patients with normal renal function (approximate): Bumetanide 1 mg = furosemide 40 mg = torsemide 20 mg = ethacrynic acid 50 mg

Children:
- Oral: 1 mg/kg/dose once daily, increase at intervals of 2-3 days to a maximum of 3 mg/kg/day
- IV: 1 mg/kg/dose; repeat doses are not routinely recommended, however if indicated, repeat doses every 8-12 hours

Adults:
- Oral: 25-400 mg/day in 1-2 divided doses
- IV: 0.5-1 mg/kg/dose (maximum dose: 100 mg/dose); repeat doses not routinely recommended, however if indicated, repeat every 8-12 hours

Preparation for Administration Parenteral: Reconstitute with 50 mL D_5W or NS resulting in 1 mg/mL concentration per the manufacturer; maximum concentration: 2 mg/mL (Sparrow 1968).

Administration

Oral: Administer with food or milk

Parenteral: IV: May be infused without further dilution over a period of several minutes or infused slowly through the tubing of a running infusion; should not to be administered IM or SubQ due to local pain and irritation

Monitoring Parameters Serum electrolytes, blood pressure, renal function, hearing

Additional Information Injection contains thimerosal

Dosage Forms Excipient information presented when available (limited, particularly for generics); consult specific product labeling.

Solution Reconstituted, Intravenous, as ethacrynate sodium:
- Sodium Edecrin: 50 mg (1 ea)

Tablet, Oral:
- Edecrin: 25 mg [scored]

Extemporaneous Preparations A 1 mg/mL oral suspension may be made with ethacrynic acid powder. Dissolve 120 mg ethacrynic acid powder in a small amount of 10% alcohol. Add a small amount of 50% sorbitol solution and stir. Adjust pH to 7 with 0.1N sodium hydroxide solution. Add sufficient quantity of 50% sorbitol solution to make a final volume of 120 mL. Add methylparaben 6 mg and propylparaben 2.4 mg as preservatives. Stable for 220 days at room temperature.

Das Gupta V, Gibbs CW Jr, and Ghanekar AG, "Stability of Pediatric Liquid Dosage Forms of Ethacrynic Acid, Indomethacin, Methyldopate Hydrochloride, Prednisone and Spironolactone," *Am J Hosp Pharm*, 1978, 35(11):1382-5.

Handbook on Extemporaneous Formulations, Bethesda, MD: American Society of Hospital Pharmacists, 1987.

Ethambutol (e THAM byoo tole)

Medication Safety Issues

Sound-alike/look-alike issues:

Myambutol® may be confused with Nembutal

Brand Names: US Myambutol

Brand Names: Canada Etibi

Therapeutic Category Antitubercular Agent

Generic Availability (US) Yes

Use Treatment of pulmonary tuberculosis (FDA approved in ages ≥13 years and adults) and other mycobacterial diseases in conjunction with other antimycobacterial agents

Pregnancy Risk Factor C

Pregnancy Considerations Teratogenic effects have been seen in animals. There are no adequate and well-controlled studies in pregnant women; there have been reports of ophthalmic abnormalities in infants born to women receiving ethambutol as a component of antitubercular therapy. Use only during pregnancy if benefits outweigh risks.

Breast-Feeding Considerations The manufacturer suggests use during breast-feeding only if benefits to the mother outweigh the possible risk to the infant. Some references suggest that exposure to the infant is low and does not produce toxicity, and breast-feeding should not be discouraged. Other references recommend if breast-feeding, monitor the infant for rash, malaise, nausea, or vomiting.

Contraindications Hypersensitivity to ethambutol or any component of the formulation; optic neuritis (risk vs benefit decision); use in young children, unconscious patients, or any other patient who may be unable to discern and report visual changes

Warnings/Precautions May cause optic neuritis (unilateral or bilateral), resulting in decreased visual acuity or other vision changes. Discontinue promptly in patients with changes in vision, color blindness, or visual defects (effects normally reversible, but reversal may require up to a year). Irreversible blindness has been reported. Monitor visual acuity prior to and during therapy. Evaluation of visual acuity changes may be more difficult in patients with cataracts, optic neuritis, diabetic retinopathy, and inflammatory conditions of the eye; consideration should be given to whether or not visual changes are related to disease progression or effects of therapy. Use only in children whose visual acuity can accurately be determined and monitored (not recommended for use in children <13 years of age unless the benefit outweighs the risk). Dosage modification is required in patients with renal insufficiency; monitor renal function prior to and during treatment. Hepatic toxicity has been reported, possibly due to concurrent therapy; monitor liver function prior to and during treatment.

Adverse Reactions

Cardiovascular: Myocarditis, pericarditis

Central nervous system: Confusion, disorientation, dizziness, fever, hallucinations, headache, malaise

Dermatologic: Dermatitis, erythema multiforme, exfoliative dermatitis, pruritus, rash

Endocrine & metabolic: Acute gout or hyperuricemia

Gastrointestinal: Abdominal pain, anorexia, GI upset, nausea, vomiting

Hematologic: Eosinophilia, leukopenia, lymphadenopathy, neutropenia, thrombocytopenia

Hepatic: Hepatitis, hepatotoxicity (possibly related to concurrent therapy), LFTs abnormal

Neuromuscular & skeletal: Arthralgia, peripheral neuritis

Ocular: Optic neuritis; symptoms may include decreased acuity, scotoma, color blindness, or visual defects (usually reversible with discontinuation, irreversible blindness has been described)

Renal: Nephritis

Respiratory: Infiltrates (with or without eosinophilia), pneumonitis

Miscellaneous: Anaphylaxis, anaphylactoid reaction; hypersensitivity syndrome (cutaneous reactions, eosinophilia, and organ-specific inflammation)

Drug Interactions

Metabolism/Transport Effects None known.

Avoid Concomitant Use There are no known interactions where it is recommended to avoid concomitant use.

Increased Effect/Toxicity There are no known significant interactions involving an increase in effect.

Decreased Effect

The levels/effects of Ethambutol may be decreased by: Aluminum Hydroxide

Storage/Stability Store at controlled room temperature of 20°C to 25°C (68°F to 77°F).

Mechanism of Action Inhibits arabinosyl transferase resulting in impaired mycobacterial cell wall synthesis

Pharmacokinetics (Adult data unless noted)

Absorption: Oral: ~80%

Distribution: Well distributed throughout the body with high concentrations in kidneys, lungs, saliva, and red blood cells; concentrations in CSF are low; crosses the placenta; excreted into breast milk

Protein binding: 20% to 30%

Metabolism: 20% by the liver to inactive metabolite

Half-life: 2.5-3.6 hours (up to 7 hours or longer with renal impairment)

Time to peak serum concentration: Within 2-4 hours

Elimination: ~50% in urine and 20% excreted in feces as unchanged drug

Dialysis: Slightly dialyzable (5% to 20%)

Dosing: Usual Oral:

Infants and Children:

Tuberculosis, active: **Note:** Used as part of a multidrug regimen; treatment regimens consist of an initial 2-month phase, followed by a continuation phase of 4 or 7 additional months; frequency of dosing may differ depending on phase of therapy

HIV negative: 15-20 mg/kg/day once daily (maximum: 1 g/day) **or** 50 mg/kg/dose twice weekly (maximum: 2.5 g/dose) (*MMWR*, 2003)

HIV-exposed/-infected: 15-25 mg/kg/day once daily (maximum: 2.5 g/day) (CDC, 2009)

MAC, secondary prophylaxis or treatment in HIV-exposed/-infected: 15-25 mg/kg/day once daily (maximum: 2.5 g/day) with clarithromycin (or azithromycin) with or without rifabutin (CDC, 2009)

Nontuberculous mycobacterial infection: 15-25 mg/kg/day once daily (maximum: 2.5 g/day)

Adolescents and Adults:

Disseminated *Mycobacterium avium* (MAC) treatment in patients with advanced HIV infection: 15 mg/kg ethambutol in combination with clarithromycin or azithromycin with/without rifabutin (Griffith, 2007)

Nontuberculous mycobacterium (*M. kansasii*): Adults: 15 mg/kg/day ethambutol for duration to include 12 months of culture-negative sputum; typically used in combination with rifampin and isoniazid; **Note:** Previous recommendations stated to use 25 mg/kg/day for the initial 2 months of therapy; however, IDSA guidelines state this may be unnecessary given the success of rifampin-based regimens with ethambutol 15 mg/kg/day or omitted altogether (Griffith, 2007)

Tuberculosis, active: **Note:** Used as part of a multidrug regimen; treatment regimens consist of an initial 2-month phase, followed by a continuation phase of 4 or 7 additional months; frequency of dosing may differ depending on phase of therapy.

Initial: 15 mg/kg once daily; Retreatment (previous antituberculosis therapy): 25 mg/kg once daily

Suggested doses by lean body weight (*MMWR*, 2003):

Daily therapy: 15-25 mg/kg
- 40-55 kg: 800 mg
- 56-75 kg: 1200 mg
- 76-90 kg: 1600 mg (maximum dose regardless of weight)

Twice weekly directly observed therapy (DOT): 50 mg/kg
- 40-55 kg: 2000 mg
- 56-75 kg: 2800 mg
- 76-90 kg: 4000 mg (maximum dose regardless of weight)

Three times/week DOT: 25-30 mg/kg (maximum: 2.5 g)
- 40-55 kg: 1200 mg
- 56-75 kg: 2000 mg
- 76-90 kg: 2400 mg (maximum dose regardless of weight)

Dosing interval in renal impairment: Aronoff, 2007:

CrCl 10-50 mL/minute: Administer every 24-36 hours

CrCl <10 mL/minute: Administer every 48 hours

Hemodialysis: Slightly dialyzable (5% to 20%); Administer dose postdialysis

Peritoneal dialysis: Dose for CrCl <10 mL/minute: Administer every 48 hours

Continuous arteriovenous or venovenous hemofiltration: Dose for CrCl 10-50 mL/minute: Administer every 24-36 hours

MMWR, 2003: Adults: CrCl <30 mL/minute and hemodialysis: 15-25 mg/kg/dose 3 times weekly

Administration Oral: Administer with or without food; if GI upset occurs, administer with food. Tablet may be pulverized and mixed with apple juice or apple sauce. Do not mix with other juices or syrups since they do not mask ethambutol's bitter taste or are not stable. Administer ethambutol at least 4 hours before aluminum hydroxide.

Monitoring Parameters Monthly examination of visual acuity and color discrimination in patients receiving >15 mg/kg/day; periodic renal, hepatic, and hematologic function tests

Dosage Forms Excipient information presented when available (limited, particularly for generics); consult specific product labeling.

Tablet, Oral, as hydrochloride:

Myambutol: 100 mg

Myambutol: 400 mg [scored]
Generic: 100 mg, 400 mg

- **Ethambutol Hydrochloride** *see* Ethambutol *on page 810*
- **Ethanoic Acid** *see* Acetic Acid *on page 55*
- **Ethanol** *see* Alcohol (Ethyl) *on page 86*
- **Etherified Starch** *see* Tetrastarch *on page 2037*

Ethiodized Oil (eth EYE oh dyezd oyl)

Therapeutic Category Diagnostic Agent, Radiologic Examination of GI Tract

Use Radio-opaque contrast agent used for: Lymphography (FDA approved in pediatric patients [age not specified] and adults); hysterosalpingography (FDA approved in adults); selective hepatic intra-arterial use for imaging tumors with known hepatocellular carcinoma (FDA approved in adults)

Pregnancy Risk Factor C

Pregnancy Considerations Animal reproduction studies have not been conducted using the indicated routes of administration; however, adverse events have not been observed in animal reproduction studies following oral administration. Ethiodized oil use during pregnancy causes iodine transfer and may interfere with thyroid function of the fetus; brain damage and permanent hypothyroidism may occur.

Breast-Feeding Considerations Ethiodized oil is excreted in breast milk. Breast-feeding is not recommended by the manufacturer; if breast-feeding is continued, thyroid function of the infant should be monitored.

Contraindications Hypersensitivity to ethiodized oil; patients with hyperthyroidism, traumatic injuries, recent hemorrhage or bleeding

Hysterosalpingography: Pregnancy, acute pelvic inflammatory disease, marked cervical erosion, endocervicitis and intrauterine bleeding, in the immediate pre- or postmenstrual phase, or within 30 days of curettage or conization

Lymphography: Right to left cardiac shunt, advanced pulmonary disease, tissue trauma or hemorrhage advanced neoplastic disease with expected lymphatic obstruction, previous surgery interrupting the lymphatic system, radiation therapy to the examined area

Selective hepatic intra-arterial injection: Presence of dilated bile ducts unless external biliary drainage was performed before injection

Warnings/Precautions [U.S. Boxed Warning]: Pulmonary and cerebral embolism may result from inadvertent intravascular injection or intravasation of ethiodized oil; may occur immediately or a few hours to days after administration. Avoid use in patients with severely impaired lung function, cardiorespiratory failure, or right-sided cardiac overload. Radiological monitoring should be performed during injection; do not exceed the maximum recommended dose and rate of injection. To decrease the risk of pulmonary embolism during lymphography, obtain radiographic confirmation of intralymphatic injection and discontinue the procedure when ethiodized oil becomes visible in the thoracic duct or lymphatic obstruction is observed.

Serious and life-threatening anaphylactoid and anaphylactic reactions with cardiovascular, respiratory, or cutaneous manifestations may occur. Avoid use in patients with a history of sensitivity to other iodine-based contrast media, bronchial asthma, or allergic disorders due to increased risk of hypersensitivity to ethiodized oil. Equipment for resuscitation and trained personnel experienced in handling emergencies should be immediately available. Most reactions occur within 30 minutes; delayed reactions may occur up to several days after administration. Monitor for ≥30 minutes following administration. Use with caution in patients receiving hepatic intra-arterial administration; procedural risks include vascular complications and infections. Hepatic intra-arterial use may exacerbate: portal hypertension and cause variceal bleeds; hepatic ischemia and cause liver enzyme elevations, fever, and abdominal pain; and hepatic failure and cause ascites and encephalopathy. Hepatic vein thrombosis, irreversible liver insufficiency, and death have also been reported. Hyperthyroidism or hypothyroidism may occur following administration of iodinated contrast media; use caution in patients at risk (eg, patients with latent hyperthyroidism, Hashimoto thyroiditis, or history of thyroid irradiation). Diagnostic tests may be affected for up to 2 years after lymphography. Prior to use in women for hysterosalpingography, exclude the presence of pregnancy, uterine bleeding, endocervicitis, acute pelvic inflammatory disease, the immediate pre- or postmenstrual phase, or within 30 days of curettage or conization. **[U.S. Boxed Warning]: For intralymphatic, intrauterine, and selective hepatic intra-arterial use only. Administer slowly with radiologic monitoring; do not exceed recommended dose.**

Adverse Reactions

Cardiovascular: Cerebral embolism, ischemia (hepatic; exacerbation), portal hypertension (exacerbation), pulmonary embolism

Hepatic: Hepatic failure (exacerbation), hepatic insufficiency (irreversible), hepatic vein thrombosis

Hypersensitivity: Anaphylactoid reaction, anaphylaxis

Rare but important or life-threatening: Acute respiratory distress, allergic dermatitis, circulatory shock, diarrhea, edema, foreign body reaction, granuloma (including lipogranuloma), hepatic dysfunction (transitory), hypersensitivity, hyperthyroidism, hypothyroidism, iodism (headache, soreness of mouth and pharynx, coryza, and skin rash), liver decompensation, liver enzyme disorder, lymphangitis, lymphedema (exacerbation), nausea, pain, pelvic inflammatory disease (exacerbation), renal insufficiency, retinal vein occlusion, thrombophlebitis, thyroiditis, wound healing impairment

Drug Interactions

Metabolism/Transport Effects None known.

Avoid Concomitant Use There are no known interactions where it is recommended to avoid concomitant use.

Increased Effect/Toxicity

The levels/effects of Ethiodized Oil may be increased by: Aldesleukin

Decreased Effect There are no known significant interactions involving a decrease in effect.

Storage/Stability Store at 15°C to 30°C (59°F to 86°F). Protect from light.

Mechanism of Action Ethiodized oil is used as a radio-paque contrast agent composed of iodine combined with ethyl esters of fatty acids of poppy seed oil, primarily as ethyl monoiodostearate and ethyl diiodostearate.

Pharmacodynamics Duration: Hepatic: ~2 to 4 weeks after intra-arterial administration; retention in liver tumor is prolonged in hepatocellular carcinoma

Dosing: Usual Use the smallest possible dose based on anatomical area to be visualized; dose varies with procedure. Refer to prescribing information for detailed dosing and administration information.

Pediatric: **Lymphography:** Infants, Children, and Adolescents: Injection: 1 to 6 mL according to area to be visualized; maximum dose: 0.25 mL/kg/dose

Note: Inject into lymphatic vessel under radiological monitoring. Interrupt injection if patient experiences pain; discontinue injection if lymphatic blockage is present (to minimize entry into the venous circulation via lymphovenous channels) and/or as soon as ethiodized oil is radiographically evident in the thoracic duct (to minimize entry into the subclavian vein and pulmonary embolization). Obtain immediate postinjection images; reimage at 24 to 48 hours to evaluate nodal architecture.

Adult:

Hysterosalpingography: Injection: Inject in 2 mL increments into the endometrial cavity until tubal patency is determined; discontinue use if excessive discomfort develops. Reimage after 24 hours to determine if ethiodized oil has entered the peritoneal cavity.

Lymphography: Injection: **Note:** Inject into lymphatic vessel under radiological monitoring. Interrupt injection if patient experiences pain; discontinue injection if lymphatic blockage is present (to minimize into the venous circulation via lymphovenous channels) and/or as soon as ethiodized oil is radiographically evident in the thoracic duct (to minimize entry into the subclavian vein and pulmonary embolization). Obtain immediate postinjection images; reimage at 24 to 48 hours to evaluate nodal architecture.

Unilateral lymphography of upper extremities: 2 to 4 mL
Unilateral lymphography of lower extremities: 6 to 8 mL
Penile lymphography: 2 to 3 mL
Cervical lymphography: 1 to 2 mL

Selective hepatic intra-arterial injection: Note: Dose depends on tumor size, local blood flow in liver and tumor: Dosage range: 1.5 to 15 mL administered slowly under continuous radiologic monitoring; discontinue administration when stagnation or reflux is evident. Limit dose to the quantity required for adequate visualization; maximum total dose: 20 mL

Dosing adjustment for renal impairment: There are no dosage adjustments provided in the manufacturer's labeling.

Dosage adjustment for hepatic impairment: There are no dosage adjustments provided in the manufacturer's labeling.

Administration Ethiodized oil is a clear, pale yellow to amber colored oil; do not use if the color has darkened. Draw solution into a glass syringe and use promptly; discard any unused portion of Lipiodol. For intralymphatic, intrauterine, and selective hepatic intra-arterial use only. Route of administration varies by indication.

Hysterosalpingography: Inject into endometrial cavity with fluoroscopic control.

Lymphography: Inject into a lymphatic vessel under radiologic guidance to prevent inadvertent venous administration or intravasation. Upper or lower extremities administration: Start injection into lymphatic channel at a rate not to exceed 0.2 mL/min; inject total dose in no less than 1.25 hours.

Selective hepatic intra-arterial injection: Inject amount slowly under continuous radiologic monitoring.

Monitoring Parameters Renal function prior to administration and after administration in patients with a history of renal impairment; monitor for hypersensitivity reactions for at least 30 minutes following administration

Dosage Forms Excipient information presented when available (limited, particularly for generics); consult specific product labeling.

Injection: Iodine 37% (10 mL)

◆ **Ethiofos** *see* Amifostine *on page 115*

Ethionamide (e thye on AM ide)

Brand Names: US Trecator

Brand Names: Canada Trecator®

Therapeutic Category Antitubercular Agent

Generic Availability (US) No

Use In conjunction with other antituberculosis agents in the treatment of tuberculosis and other mycobacterial diseases

Pregnancy Risk Factor C

Pregnancy Considerations Ethionamide crosses the placenta; teratogenic effects were observed in animal studies. Use during pregnancy is not recommended.

Breast-Feeding Considerations If ethionamide is used while breast-feeding, monitor the infant for adverse effects.

Contraindications Hypersensitivity to ethionamide or any component of the formulation; severe hepatic impairment

Warnings/Precautions Use with caution in patients with diabetes mellitus or thyroid dysfunction; use with caution in patients receiving cycloserine or isoniazid. Cross-resistance to isoniazid has been reported if inhA mutation is present. May cause hepatotoxicity; monitor liver function tests monthly. Use not recommended in patients with porphyria; animal and *in vitro* studies have shown porphyria-inducing effects. Periodic eye exams are recommended. Drug-resistant tuberculosis develops rapidly if ethionamide is used alone; must administer with at least one other antituberculosis agent. Instruct patients to avoid excessive ethanol; psychotic reaction may occur.

Adverse Reactions

Cardiovascular: Orthostatic hypotension

Central nervous system: Depression, dizziness, drowsiness, headache, psychiatric disturbances, restlessness, seizure

Dermatologic: Acne, alopecia, photosensitivity, purpura, rash

Endocrine & metabolic: Gynecomastia, hypoglycemia, hypothyroidism or goiter, menstrual irregularities, pellagra-like syndrome

Gastrointestinal: Abdominal pain, anorexia, diarrhea, excessive salivation, metallic taste, nausea, stomatitis, vomiting, weight loss

Genitourinary: Impotence

Hematologic: Leukopenia, thrombocytopenia

Hepatic: Bilirubin increased, hepatitis, jaundice, liver function tests increased

Neuromuscular & skeletal: Arthralgia, peripheral neuritis

Ocular: Blurred vision, diplopia, optic neuritis

Respiratory: Olfactory disturbances

Miscellaneous: Hypersensitivity reaction

Drug Interactions

Metabolism/Transport Effects None known.

Avoid Concomitant Use There are no known interactions where it is recommended to avoid concomitant use.

Increased Effect/Toxicity

Ethionamide may increase the levels/effects of: CycloSERINE; Isoniazid

The levels/effects of Ethionamide may be increased by: Alcohol (Ethyl)

Decreased Effect There are no known significant interactions involving a decrease in effect.

Storage/Stability Store at 20°C to 25°C (68°F to 77°F). Keep containers tightly closed.

Mechanism of Action Inhibits peptide synthesis; bacteriostatic

Pharmacokinetics (Adult data unless noted)

Absorption: ~80% is rapidly absorbed from the GI tract

Distribution: Crosses the placenta; widely distributed into body tissues and fluids including liver, kidneys, and CSF

Protein binding: 10%

Metabolism: In the liver to active and inactive metabolites

Bioavailability: 80%

Half-life: 2-3 hours

Time to peak serum concentration: Oral: Within 3 hours

Elimination: As metabolites (active and inactive) and parent drug in the urine

Dosing: Usual Oral:

Children: 15-20 mg/kg/day in 2-3 divided doses, not to exceed 1 g/day

Adults: 500-1000 mg/day in 1-3 divided doses

Administration Oral: Administer with meals to decrease GI distress

Monitoring Parameters Initial and periodic serum AST and ALT, blood glucose, thyroid function tests, periodic ophthalmologic exams

Dosage Forms Excipient information presented when available (limited, particularly for generics); consult specific product labeling.

Tablet, Oral:

Trecator: 250 mg [contains fd&c yellow #6 (sunset yellow)]

Ethosuximide (eth oh SUKS i mide)

Medication Safety Issues

Sound-alike/look-alike issues:

Ethosuximide may be confused with methsuximide

Zarontin® may be confused with Neurontin®, Xalatan®, Zantac®, Zaroxolyn®

Brand Names: US Zarontin

Brand Names: Canada Zarontin®

Therapeutic Category Anticonvulsant, Succinimide

Generic Availability (US) Yes

Use Management of absence (petit mal) epilepsy (FDA approved in ages ≥3 years and adults); also used for management of myoclonic seizures and akinetic epilepsy

Medication Guide Available Yes

Pregnancy Considerations Ethosuximide crosses the placenta. Cases of birth defects have been reported in infants. Epilepsy itself, the number of medications, genetic factors, or a combination of these probably influence the teratogenicity of anticonvulsant therapy.

Patients exposed to ethosuximide during pregnancy are encouraged to enroll themselves into the NAAED Pregnancy Registry by calling 1-888-233-2334. Additional information is available at www.aedpregnancyregistry.org.

Breast-Feeding Considerations Ethosuximide is excreted into breast milk. The manufacturer recommends caution be used if administered to a nursing woman.

Contraindications History of hypersensitivity to succinimides

Warnings/Precautions Antiepileptics are associated with an increased risk of suicidal behavior/thoughts with use (regardless of indication); patients should be monitored for signs/symptoms of depression, suicidal tendencies, and other unusual behavior changes during therapy and instructed to inform their healthcare provider immediately if symptoms occur. Severe reactions, including Stevens-Johnson syndrome, have been reported with an onset usually within 28 days, but may be observed later. Drug should be discontinued if there are any signs of rash. If SJS is suspected do not resume ethosuximide and consider alternative therapy.

Use with caution in patients with hepatic or renal disease; abrupt withdrawal of the drug may precipitate absence status; ethosuximide may increase tonic-clonic seizures when used alone in patients with mixed seizure disorders; ethosuximide must be used in combination with other anticonvulsants in patients with both absence and tonic-clonic seizures. Succinimides have been associated with severe blood dyscrasias and cases of systemic lupus erythematosus. Consider evaluation of blood counts in patients with signs/symptoms of infection. May cause CNS depression, which may impair physical or mental abilities; patients must be cautioned about performing tasks which require mental alertness (eg, operating machinery or driving). Effects with other sedative drugs or ethanol may be potentiated.

Benzyl alcohol and derivatives: Some dosage forms may contain sodium benzoate/benzoic acid; benzoic acid (benzoate) is a metabolite of benzyl alcohol; large amounts of benzyl alcohol (≥99 mg/kg/day) have been associated with a potentially fatal toxicity ("gasping syndrome") in neonates; the "gasping syndrome" consists of metabolic acidosis, respiratory distress, gasping respirations, CNS dysfunction (including convulsions, intracranial hemorrhage), hypotension, and cardiovascular collapse (AAP, 1997; CDC, 1982); some data suggests that benzoate displaces bilirubin from protein binding sites (Ahlfors, 2001); avoid or use dosage forms containing benzyl alcohol derivative with caution in neonates. See manufacturer's labeling.

Adverse Reactions

Central nervous system: Aggressiveness, ataxia, concentration impaired, dizziness, drowsiness, euphoria, fatigue, headache, hyperactivity, irritability, lethargy, mental depression (with cases of overt suicidal intentions), night terrors, paranoid psychosis, sleep disturbance

Dermatologic: Hirsutism, pruritus, rash, Stevens-Johnson syndrome, urticaria

Endocrine & metabolic: Libido increased

Gastrointestinal: Abdominal pain, anorexia, cramps, diarrhea, epigastric pain, gastric upset, gum hypertrophy, nausea, tongue swelling, vomiting, weight loss

Genitourinary: Hematuria (microscopic), vaginal bleeding

Hematologic: Agranulocytosis, eosinophilia, leukopenia, pancytopenia

Ocular: Myopia

Miscellaneous: Allergic reaction, drug rash with eosinophilia and systemic symptoms (DRESS), hiccups, systemic lupus erythematosus

Drug Interactions

Metabolism/Transport Effects Substrate of CYP3A4 (major); **Note:** Assignment of Major/Minor substrate status based on clinically relevant drug interaction potential

Avoid Concomitant Use

Avoid concomitant use of Ethosuximide with any of the following: Azelastine (Nasal); Conivaptan; Fusidic Acid (Systemic); Idelalisib; Orphenadrine; Paraldehyde; Thalidomide

Increased Effect/Toxicity

Ethosuximide may increase the levels/effects of: Alcohol (Ethyl); Azelastine (Nasal); Buprenorphine; CNS Depressants; Fosphenytoin; Hydrocodone; Methotrimeprazine; Metyrosine; Mirtazapine; Orphenadrine; Paraldehyde; Phenytoin; Pramipexole; ROPINIRole; Rotigotine; Selective Serotonin Reuptake Inhibitors; Suvorexant; Thalidomide; Zolpidem

The levels/effects of Ethosuximide may be increased by: Aprepitant; Brimonidine (Topical); Cannabis; Cobicistat; Conivaptan; CYP3A4 Inhibitors (Moderate); CYP3A4 Inhibitors (Strong); Dasatinib; Doxylamine; Dronabinol; Droperidol; Fosaprepitant; Fusidic Acid (Systemic); HydrOXYzine; Idelalisib; Ivacaftor; Kava Kava; Luliconazole; Magnesium Sulfate; Methotrimeprazine; Mifepristone; Nabilone; Netupitant; Palbociclib; Perampanel; Rufinamide; Simeprevir; Sodium Oxybate; Stiripentol; Tapentadol; Tetrahydrocannabinol; Valproic Acid and Derivatives

Decreased Effect

Ethosuximide may decrease the levels/effects of: Valproic Acid and Derivatives

The levels/effects of Ethosuximide may be decreased by: Amphetamines; Bosentan; CYP3A4 Inducers (Moderate); CYP3A4 Inducers (Strong); Dabrafenib; Deferasirox; Fosphenytoin; Mefloquine; Mianserin; Mitotane; Orlistat; Phenytoin; Siltuximab; St Johns Wort; Tocilizumab

Storage/Stability

Capsules: Store at 25°C (77°F); excursions permitted to 15°C to 30°C (59°F to 86°F).

Solution: Store below 30°C (86°F); do not freeze. Protect from light.

Mechanism of Action Increases the seizure threshold and suppresses paroxysmal spike-and-wave pattern in absence seizures; depresses nerve transmission in the motor cortex

Pharmacokinetics (Adult data unless noted)

Distribution: V_d: Adults: 0.62-0.72 L/kg; crosses the placenta; excreted in human breast milk

Protein binding: <10%

Metabolism: ~80% metabolized in the liver to three inactive metabolites

Half-life:

Children: 30 hours

Adults: 50-60 hours

Time to peak serum concentration:

Capsule: Within 2-4 hours

Solution: <2-4 hours

Elimination: Slow in urine as metabolites (50%) and as unchanged drug (10% to 20%); small amounts excreted in feces

Dialysis: Removed by hemodialysis and peritoneal dialysis

Dosing: Usual

Children and Adolescents: **Management of absence (petit mal) seizures:** Oral:

Children <6 years (Limited data available in children <3 years): Initial: 15 mg/kg/day in 2 divided doses; maximum single dose: 250 mg; may increase every 4-7 days; usual maintenance dose: 15-40 mg/kg/day in 2 divided doses; maximum daily dose: 1500 mg/**day**

Children ≥6 years and Adolescents: Initial: 250 mg twice daily; may increase every 4-7 days in 250 mg/**day** increments; maximum daily dose: 1500 mg/**day** in 2 divided doses; usual maintenance dose: 20-40 mg/kg/day in 2 divided doses

Adults: **Management of absence (petit mal) seizures:** Oral: Initial: 500 mg/day; increase by 250 mg as needed every 4-7 days up to 1500 mg/day in divided doses

Dosing adjustment in renal impairment: There are no dosage adjustment provided in manufacturer's labeling; use with caution.

Dosing adjustment in hepatic impairment: There are no dosage adjustment provided in manufacturer's labeling; use with caution.

Administration Oral: Administer with food or milk to decrease GI upset

Monitoring Parameters Seizure frequency, trough serum concentrations; CBC with differential, platelets, liver enzymes, urinalysis, renal function; signs and symptoms of suicidality (eg, anxiety, depression, behavior changes)

Reference Range

Therapeutic: 40-100 mcg/mL (SI: 280-710 micromoles/L)

Toxic: >150 mcg/mL (SI: >1062 micromoles/L)

Additional Information Considered to be a drug of choice for simple absence seizures

Dosage Forms Excipient information presented when available (limited, particularly for generics); consult specific product labeling.

Capsule, Oral:

Zarontin: 250 mg [contains fd&c yellow #10 (quinoline yellow)]

Generic: 250 mg

Solution, Oral:

Zarontin: 250 mg/5 mL (474 mL) [raspberry flavor]

Generic: 250 mg/5 mL (473 mL, 474 mL)

◆ **Ethoxynaphthamido Penicillin Sodium** *see* Nafcillin *on page 1481*

◆ **Ethyl Alcohol** *see* Alcohol (Ethyl) *on page 86*

◆ **Ethyl Aminobenzoate** *see* Benzocaine *on page 268*

◆ **Ethyol** *see* Amifostine *on page 115*

◆ **Etibi (Can)** *see* Ethambutol *on page 810*

Etidronate (e ti DROE nate)

Medication Safety Issues

Sound-alike/look-alike issues:

Etidronate may be confused with etomidate

Brand Names: Canada ACT Etidronate; Mylan-Etidronate

Therapeutic Category Antidote, Hypercalcemia; Bisphosphonate Derivative

Generic Availability (US) Yes

Use Symptomatic treatment of Paget's disease of bone and prevention and treatment of heterotopic ossification following spinal cord injury or total hip replacement (FDA approved in adults)

Pregnancy Risk Factor C

Pregnancy Considerations Adverse events were observed in some animal reproduction studies. It is not known if bisphosphonates cross the placenta, but fetal exposure is expected (Djokanovic, 2008; Stathopoulos, 2011). Bisphosphonates are incorporated into the bone matrix and gradually released over time. The amount available in the systemic circulation varies by dose and duration of therapy. Theoretically, there may be a risk of fetal harm when pregnancy follows the completion of therapy; however, available data have not shown that exposure to bisphosphonates during pregnancy significantly increases the risk of adverse fetal events (Djokanovic, 2008; Levy, 2009; Stathopoulos, 2011). Until additional data is available, most sources recommend discontinuing bisphosphonate therapy in women of reproductive potential as early as possible prior to a planned pregnancy; use in premenopausal women should be reserved for special circumstances when rapid bone loss is occurring (Bhalla, 2010; Pereira, 2012; Stathopoulos, 2011). Because hypocalcemia has been described following *in utero* bisphosphonate exposure, exposed infants should be monitored for hypocalcemia after birth (Djokanovic, 2008; Stathopoulos, 2011).

Breast-Feeding Considerations It is not known if etidronate is excreted into breast milk. The manufacturer recommends caution be exercised when administering etidronate to nursing women.

Contraindications Hypersensitivity to bisphosphonates or any component of the formulation; overt osteomalacia; patients with abnormalities of the esophagus (eg, stricture, achalasia) which delay esophageal emptying

Warnings/Precautions Ensure adequate calcium and vitamin D intake. Etidronate may retard mineralization of bone; treatment may need delayed or interrupted until callus is present. Use caution in patients with renal impairment. Use caution with enterocolitis; diarrhea has been reported at high doses and therapy may need to be withheld.

Osteonecrosis of the jaw (ONJ) has been reported in patients receiving bisphosphonates. Risk factors include invasive dental procedures (eg, tooth extraction, dental implants, boney surgery); a diagnosis of cancer, with concomitant chemotherapy or corticosteroids; poor oral hygiene, ill-fitting dentures; and comorbid disorders (anemia, coagulopathy, infection, preexisting dental disease); risk may increase with duration of bisphosphonate use. Most reported cases occurred after IV bisphosphonate therapy; however, cases have been reported following oral therapy. A dental exam and preventative dentistry should be performed prior to placing patients with risk factors on chronic bisphosphonate therapy. The manufacturer's labeling states that discontinuing bisphosphonates in patients requiring invasive dental procedures may reduce the risk of ONJ. However, other experts suggest that there is no evidence that discontinuing therapy reduces the risk of developing ONJ (Assael, 2009). The benefit/risk must be assessed by the treating physician and/or dentist/surgeon prior to any invasive dental procedure. Patients developing ONJ while on bisphosphonates should receive care by an oral surgeon.

Infrequently, severe (and occasionally debilitating) bone, joint, and/or muscle pain have been reported during bisphosphonate treatment. The onset of pain ranged from a single day to several months. Consider discontinuing therapy in patients who experience severe symptoms; symptoms usually resolve upon discontinuation. Some patients experienced recurrence when rechallenged with same drug or another bisphosphonate; avoid use in patients with a history of these symptoms in association with bisphosphonate therapy. Do not exceed recommended dose or use continuously for >6 months in patients with Paget's disease; risk of osteomalacia or fractures may be increased. Long bones with predominantly lytic lesions may be prone to fracture, particularly in patients unresponsive to treatment. Potentially significant drug-drug interactions may exist, requiring dose or frequency adjustment, additional monitoring, and/or selection of alternative therapy.

Adverse Reactions

Gastrointestinal: Diarrhea, nausea

Neuromuscular & skeletal: Ostealgia

Postmarketing and/or case reports: Agranulocytosis, alopecia, amnesia, angioedema, arthralgia, arthritis, asthma exacerbation, bone fracture, confusion, depression, esophageal cancer, esophagitis, follicular eruption, gastritis, glossitis, hallucination, headache, hypersensitivity reactions, leg cramps, leukopenia, macular rash, maculopapular rash, musculoskeletal pain (sometimes severe and/or incapacitating), osteomalacia, pancytopenia, paresthesia, peptic ulcer disease exacerbation, pruritus, Stevens-Johnson syndrome, urticaria

Drug Interactions

Metabolism/Transport Effects None known.

Avoid Concomitant Use There are no known interactions where it is recommended to avoid concomitant use.

Increased Effect/Toxicity

Etidronate may increase the levels/effects of: Deferasirox

The levels/effects of Etidronate may be increased by: Aminoglycosides; Nonsteroidal Anti-Inflammatory Agents; Systemic Angiogenesis Inhibitors

Decreased Effect

The levels/effects of Etidronate may be decreased by: Antacids; Calcium Salts; Iron Salts; Magnesium Salts; Multivitamins/Minerals (with ADEK, Folate, Iron); Multivitamins/Minerals (with AE, No Iron); Proton Pump Inhibitors

Food Interactions Food and/or supplements decrease the absorption and bioavailability of the drug. Management: Administer tablet on an empty stomach with a full glass of plain water or fruit juice (6-8 oz) 2 hours before food. Avoid administering foods/supplements with calcium, iron, or magnesium within 2 hours of drug. Do not take with mineral water or other beverages.

Storage/Stability Store at controlled room temperature of 25°C (77°F).

Mechanism of Action Decreases bone resorption by inhibiting osteocystic osteolysis; decreases mineral release and matrix or collagen breakdown in bone

Pharmacodynamics

Onset of therapeutic effects: Within 1-3 months of therapy

Duration: Persists for 12 months without continuous therapy

Pharmacokinetics (Adult data unless noted)

Absorption: ~3%

Half-life: 1-6 hours

Elimination: Primarily as unchanged drug in urine (50%) with unabsorbed drug eliminated in feces

Dosing: Usual Oral:

Heterotopic ossification: Children and Adults:

Spinal cord injury: 20 mg/kg once daily (or in divided doses if GI discomfort occurs) for 2 weeks, then 10 mg/kg/day for 10 weeks

Total hip replacement: 20 mg/kg/day 1 month before and 3 months after surgery

Note: This dosage when used in children for >1 year has been associated with a rachitic syndrome.

Paget's disease: Adults: Initial: 5-10 mg/kg/day (not to exceed 6 months) or 11-20 mg/kg/day (not to exceed 3 months). Doses >20 mg/kg/day are **not** recommended. Higher doses should be used only when lower doses are ineffective or there is a need to suppress rapid bone turnover (eg, potential for irreversible neurologic damage) or reduce elevated cardiac output. Daily dose may be divided if adverse GI effects occur; courses of therapy should be separated by drug-free periods of at least 3 months.

Dosing adjustment in renal impairment: Adult:

S_{cr} 2.5-4.9 mg/dL: Use with caution

S_{cr} ≥5 mg/dL: **Not recommended**

Administration Oral: Administer on an empty stomach with a full glass of plain water (6-8 oz), 2 hours before meals. Patients should be instructed to stay upright (not to lie down) after taking the medication.

Monitoring Parameters Serum calcium, phosphate, creatinine, BUN, alkaline phosphatase, 25(OH)D, pain

Test Interactions Bisphosphonates may interfere with diagnostic imaging agents such as technetium-99m-diphosphonate in bone scans.

Dosage Forms Excipient information presented when available (limited, particularly for generics); consult specific product labeling.

Tablet, Oral, as disodium:

Generic: 200 mg, 400 mg

◆ **Etidronate Disodium** *see* Etidronate *on page 815*

Etodolac (ee toe DOE lak)

Medication Safety Issues

Sound-alike/look-alike issues:

Lodine may be confused with codeine, iodine, Lopid

BEERS Criteria medication:

This drug may be potentially inappropriate for use in geriatric patients (Quality of evidence - moderate; Strength of recommendation - strong).

Brand Names: Canada Apo-Etodolac; Utradol

Therapeutic Category Analgesic, Non-narcotic; Anti-inflammatory Agent; Nonsteroidal Anti-inflammatory Drug (NSAID), Oral

Generic Availability (US) Yes

Use Oral:

Immediate release: Acute and long-term management of osteoarthritis and rheumatoid arthritis; management of acute pain (All indications: FDA approved in ages ≥18 years and adults)

Extended release: Relief of the signs and symptoms of JIA (FDA approved in ages 6-16 years weighing at least 20 kg); relief of signs and symptoms of osteoarthritis and rheumatoid arthritis (FDA approved in adults)

Medication Guide Available Yes

Pregnancy Risk Factor C

Pregnancy Considerations Adverse events were not observed in the initial animal reproduction studies; therefore, the manufacturer classifies etodolac as pregnancy category C. NSAID exposure during the first trimester is not strongly associated with congenital malformations; however, cardiovascular anomalies and cleft palate have been observed following NSAID exposure in some studies. The use of an NSAID close to conception may be associated with an increased risk of miscarriage. Nonteratogenic effects have been observed following NSAID administration during the third trimester including: Myocardial degenerative changes, prenatal constriction of the ductus arteriosus, fetal tricuspid regurgitation, failure of the ductus arteriosus to close postnatally; renal dysfunction or failure, oligohydramnios; gastrointestinal bleeding or perforation, increased risk of necrotizing enterocolitis; intracranial bleeding (including intraventricular hemorrhage), platelet dysfunction with resultant bleeding; pulmonary hypertension. Because they may cause premature closure of the ductus arteriosus, use of NSAIDs late in pregnancy should be avoided (use after 31 or 32 weeks gestation is not recommended by some clinicians). The chronic use of NSAIDs in women of reproductive age may be associated with infertility that is reversible upon discontinuation of the medication.

Breast-Feeding Considerations It is not known if etodolac is excreted into breast milk. Use of etodolac while breast-feeding is not recommended by the manufacturer.

Contraindications Hypersensitivity to etodolac, aspirin, other NSAIDs, or any component of the formulation; perioperative pain in the setting of coronary artery bypass graft (CABG) surgery

Warnings/Precautions **[U.S. Boxed Warning]: NSAIDs are associated with an increased risk of adverse cardiovascular thrombotic events, including MI and stroke.** Risk may be increased with duration of use or preexisting cardiovascular risk factors or disease. Carefully evaluate individual cardiovascular risk profiles prior to prescribing. May cause new-onset hypertension or worsening of existing hypertension. Use caution with fluid retention. Avoid use in heart failure (ACCF/AHA [Yancy, 2013]). Concurrent administration of ibuprofen, and potentially other nonselective NSAIDs, may interfere with aspirin's cardioprotective effect. **[U.S. Boxed Warning]: Use is contraindicated for treatment of perioperative pain in the setting of coronary artery bypass graft (CABG) surgery**. Risk of MI and stroke may be increased with use following CABG surgery.

[U.S. Boxed Warning]: NSAIDs may increase risk of gastrointestinal irritation, inflammation, ulceration, bleeding, and perforation. These events may occur at any time during therapy and without warning. Use caution with a history of GI disease (bleeding or ulcers), concurrent therapy with aspirin, anticoagulants and/or corticosteroids, smoking, use of alcohol, the elderly or debilitated patients. When used concomitantly with aspirin, a substantial increase in the risk of gastrointestinal complications (eg, ulcer) occurs; concomitant gastroprotective therapy (eg, proton pump inhibitors) is recommended (Bhatt, 2008).

Platelet adhesion and aggregation may be decreased; may prolong bleeding time; patients with coagulation disorders or who are receiving anticoagulants should be monitored closely. Anemia may occur; patients on long-term NSAID therapy should be monitored for anemia. Rarely, NSAID use may cause severe blood dyscrasias (eg, agranulocytosis, aplastic anemia, thrombocytopenia).

NSAID use may compromise existing renal function; dose-dependent decreases in prostaglandin synthesis may result from NSAID use, reducing renal blood flow which may cause renal decompensation. NSAID use may increase the risk for hyperkalemia. Patients with impaired renal function, dehydration, heart failure, liver dysfunction, those taking diuretics and ACE inhibitors, and the elderly are at greater risk for renal toxicity and hyperkalemia. Rehydrate patient before starting therapy; monitor renal function closely. Not recommended for use in patients with advanced renal disease. Long-term NSAID use may result in renal papillary necrosis.

Use the lowest effective dose for the shortest duration of time, consistent with individual patient goals, to reduce risk of cardiovascular or GI adverse events. Alternate therapies should be considered for patients at high risk.

NSAIDs may cause serious skin adverse events including exfoliative dermatitis, Stevens-Johnson syndrome (SJS), and toxic epidermal necrolysis (TEN); discontinue use at first sign of skin rash or hypersensitivity. Anaphylactoid reactions may occur, even without prior exposure; patients with "aspirin triad" (bronchial asthma, aspirin intolerance, rhinitis) may be at increased risk. Do not use in patients who experience bronchospasm, asthma, rhinitis, or urticaria with NSAID or aspirin therapy. Use caution in other forms of asthma.

Use with caution in patients with decreased hepatic function. Closely monitor patients with any abnormal LFT. Severe hepatic reactions (eg, fulminant hepatitis, liver failure) have occurred with NSAID use, rarely; discontinue if signs or symptoms of liver disease develop, or if systemic manifestations occur.

NSAIDS may cause drowsiness, dizziness, blurred vision and other neurologic effects which may impair physical or mental abilities; patients must be cautioned about performing tasks which require mental alertness (eg, operating machinery or driving). Discontinue use with blurred or diminished vision and perform ophthalmologic exam. Monitor vision with long-term therapy. In the elderly, avoid chronic use (unless alternative agents ineffective and patient can receive concomitant gastroprotective agent); nonselective oral NSAID use is associated with an increased risk of GI bleeding and peptic ulcer disease in older adults in high risk category (eg, >75 years or age or receiving concomitant oral/parenteral corticosteroids, anticoagulants, or antiplatelet agents) (Beers Criteria).

Withhold for at least 4-6 half-lives prior to surgical or dental procedures.

Use of extended release product consisting of a nondeformable matrix should be avoided in patients with stricture/narrowing of the GI tract; symptoms of obstruction have been associated with nondeformable products.

Adverse Reactions

Central nervous system: Chills, depression, dizziness, nervousness

Dermatologic: Pruritus, skin rash

Gastrointestinal: Abdominal cramps, constipation, diarrhea, dyspepsia, flatulence, gastritis, melena, nausea, vomiting

Genitourinary: Dysuria

Neuromuscular & skeletal: Weakness

Ophthalmic: Blurred vision

Otic: Tinnitus

Renal: Polyuria

Miscellaneous: Fever

Rare but important or life-threatening: Abnormal uterine bleeding, agranulocytosis, alopecia, anaphylactoid reaction, anaphylaxis, anemia, angioedema, anorexia, aphthous stomatitis, aseptic meningitis, asthma, cardiac arrhythmia, cardiac failure, cerebrovascular accident, confusion, conjunctivitis, cystitis, duodenitis, dyspnea, ecchymosis, edema, erythema multiforme, esophagitis (+/- stricture or cardiospasm), exfoliative dermatitis, gastrointestinal ulceration, hallucination, headache, hearing loss, hematemesis, hematuria, hepatic failure, hepatitis, hepatotoxicity (idiosyncratic) (Chalasani, 2014), hyperglycemia (in controlled patients with diabetes), hyperpigmentation, hypersensitivity angiitis, hypersensitivity reaction, hypertension, increased liver function tests, infection, insomnia, interstitial nephritis, jaundice, leukopenia, myocardial infarction, necrotizing angiitis, nephrolithiasis, palpitations, pancreatitis, pancytopenia, paresthesia, peptic ulcer (+/- bleeding/perforation), peripheral neuropathy, photophobia, prolonged bleeding time, pulmonary infiltrates (eosinophilia), rectal bleeding, renal failure, renal insufficiency, shock, prolonged bleeding time, skin photosensitivity, Stevens-Johnson syndrome, syncope, thrombocytopenia, toxic epidermal necrolysis, urticaria, vesiculobullous dermatitis, renal papillary necrosis, visual disturbance

Drug Interactions

Metabolism/Transport Effects None known.

Avoid Concomitant Use

Avoid concomitant use of Etodolac with any of the following: Dexketoprofen; Floctafenine; Ketorolac (Nasal); Ketorolac (Systemic); Morniflumate; NSAID (COX-2 Inhibitor); Omacetaxine; Urokinase

Increased Effect/Toxicity

Etodolac may increase the levels/effects of: 5-ASA Derivatives; Agents with Antiplatelet Properties; Aliskiren; Aminoglycosides; Anticoagulants; Apixaban; Bisphosphonate Derivatives; Collagenase (Systemic); CycloSPORINE (Systemic); Dabigatran Etexilate; Deferasirox; Deoxycholic Acid; Desmopressin; Digoxin; Drospirenone; Eplerenone; Haloperidol; Ibritumomab; Lithium; Methotrexate; Nonsteroidal Anti-Inflammatory Agents; NSAID (COX-2 Inhibitor); Obinutuzumab; Omacetaxine; PEMEtrexed; Porfimer; Potassium-Sparing Diuretics; PRALAtrexate; Quinolone Antibiotics; Rivaroxaban; Salicylates; Tacrolimus (Systemic); Tenofovir; Thrombolytic Agents; Tositumomab and Iodine I 131 Tositumomab; Urokinase; Vancomycin; Verteporfin; Vitamin K Antagonists

The levels/effects of Etodolac may be increased by: ACE Inhibitors; Angiotensin II Receptor Blockers; Antidepressants (Tricyclic, Tertiary Amine); Corticosteroids (Systemic); CycloSPORINE (Systemic); Dasatinib; Dexketoprofen; Diclofenac (Systemic); Floctafenine; Glucosamine; Herbs (Anticoagulant/Antiplatelet Properties); Ibrutinib; Ketorolac (Nasal); Ketorolac (Systemic); Limaprost; Morniflumate; Multivitamins/Fluoride (with ADE); Multivitamins/Minerals (with ADEK, Folate, Iron); Multivitamins/Minerals (with AE, No Iron); Omega-3 Fatty Acids; Pentosan Polysulfate Sodium; Pentoxifylline; Probenecid; Prostacyclin Analogues; Selective Serotonin Reuptake Inhibitors; Serotonin/Norepinephrine Reuptake Inhibitors; Sodium Phosphates; Tipranavir; Treprostinil; Vitamin E

Decreased Effect

Etodolac may decrease the levels/effects of: ACE Inhibitors; Aliskiren; Angiotensin II Receptor Blockers; Beta-Blockers; Eplerenone; HydrALAZINE; Loop Diuretics; Potassium-Sparing Diuretics; Prostaglandins (Ophthalmic); Salicylates; Selective Serotonin Reuptake Inhibitors; Thiazide Diuretics

The levels/effects of Etodolac may be decreased by: Bile Acid Sequestrants; Salicylates

Food Interactions Etodolac peak serum levels may be decreased if taken with food. Management: Administer with food to decrease GI upset.

Storage/Stability Store at 20°C to 25°C (68°F to 77°F). Protect from moisture.

Mechanism of Action Reversibly inhibits cyclooxygenase-1 and 2 (COX-1 and 2) enzymes, which results in decreased formation of prostaglandin precursors; has antipyretic, analgesic, and anti-inflammatory properties

Other proposed mechanisms not fully elucidated (and possibly contributing to the anti-inflammatory effect to varying degrees), include inhibiting chemotaxis, altering lymphocyte activity, inhibiting neutrophil aggregation/activation, and decreasing proinflammatory cytokine levels.

Pharmacodynamics

Acute pain: Immediate release:

Onset of action: 30 minutes

Maximum effect: 1-2 hours

Duration of action: Mean range: 4-6 hours

Arthritis (chronic management): Onset of action: Typically within 2 weeks

Pharmacokinetics (Adult data unless noted)

Absorption: Immediate release: Rapid

Distribution:

Immediate release: Pediatric patients (6-16 years; n=11): Terminal V_d: 0.49 L/kg (Boni, 1999); Adults: Apparent V_d: 0.49 L/kg

Extended release: Apparent V_d: 0.57 L/kg

Protein binding: ≥99%, primarily albumin

Metabolism: Hepatic to several hydroxylated metabolites and etodolac glucuronide; hydroxylated metabolites undergo further glucuronidation

Bioavailability: ≥80%

Half-life elimination: Terminal:

Immediate release: Pediatric patients (6-16 years, n=11): 6.5 hours (Boni, 1999); Adults: 6.4 hours

Extended release: Pediatric patients (6-16 years, n=72): 12 hours; Adults: 8.4 hours

Time to peak serum concentration:

Immediate release: Pediatric patients (6-16 years, n=11): 1.4 hours (Boni, 1999); Adults: 1-2 hours

Extended release: 6-7 hours

Elimination: Urine 73% (1% unchanged); feces 16%; clearance similar in pediatric patients and adults (~0.05 L/hour/kg) (Boni, 1999)

Dosing: Usual Note: Dosage should be titrated to the lowest effective dose for the shortest duration possible. For chronic conditions, therapeutic response may take 1-2 weeks of treatment.

Children and Adolescents:

Analgesia, acute pain: Limited data available in ages <18 years: Oral: Immediate release capsules or tablets:

Manufacturer's labeling: Adolescents ≥18 years: 200-400 mg every 6-8 hours, as needed; maximum daily dose: 1000 mg/**day**

Alternate dosing (American Pain Society, 2008): Children and Adolescents:

Patient weight <50 kg: 7.5-10 mg/kg/dose every 12 hours; maximum daily dose: 1000 mg/**day**

Patient weight ≥50 kg: 300-400 mg every 8-12 hours; maximum daily dose: 1000 mg/**day**

Juvenile idiopathic arthritis: Children and Adolescents:

Oral: Extended release tablets:

20-30 kg: 400 mg once daily

31-45 kg: 600 mg once daily

46-60 kg: 800 mg once daily

>60 kg: 1000 mg once daily

Rheumatoid arthritis, osteoarthritis: Oral: Adolescents ≥18 years:

Immediate release capsules and tablets: 300-500 mg twice daily or 300 mg 3 times daily; maximum daily dose: 1000 mg/**day**

Extended release tablets: 400-1000 mg once daily

Adults:

Acute pain: Oral: Immediate release capsules or tablets: 200-400 mg every 6-8 hours, as needed; maximum daily dose: 1000 mg/**day**

Rheumatoid arthritis, osteoarthritis: Oral:

Immediate release capsules or tablets: 400 mg 2 times/day **or** 300 mg 2-3 times/day **or** 500 mg 2 times/day; doses >1000 mg/day have not been evaluated

Extended release tablets: 400-1000 mg once daily

Dosing adjustment in renal impairment:

Immediate release: Adolescents ≥18 years and Adults:

Mild to moderate: No adjustment required.

Severe: No dosing adjustment necessary.

Hemodialysis: Not removed; dosing adjustment not necessary.

Extended release: There are no dosing adjustments provided in the manufacturer's labeling; has not been studied.

Dosing adjustment in hepatic impairment: No adjustment required.

Administration May be administered with food to decrease GI upset.

Monitoring Parameters Periodic CBC, liver enzymes, serum BUN and creatinine, signs and symptoms of GI bleeding

Test Interactions False-positive for urinary bilirubin and ketone

Dosage Forms Excipient information presented when available (limited, particularly for generics); consult specific product labeling.

Capsule, Oral:
Generic: 200 mg, 300 mg

Tablet, Oral:
Generic: 400 mg, 500 mg

Tablet Extended Release 24 Hour, Oral:
Generic: 400 mg, 500 mg, 600 mg

◆ **Etodolic Acid** *see* Etodolac *on page* 816

◆ **EtOH** *see* Alcohol (Ethyl) *on page* 86

Etomidate (e TOM i date)

Medication Safety Issues

Sound-alike/look-alike issues:

Etomidate may be confused with etidronate

High alert medication:

The Institute for Safe Medication Practices (ISMP) includes this medication among its list of drugs which have a heightened risk of causing significant patient harm when used in error.

Brand Names: US Amidate

Therapeutic Category General Anesthetic

Generic Availability (US) Yes

Use Induction and maintenance of general anesthesia particularly in patients with diminished cardiovascular function; sedation for short procedures

Pregnancy Risk Factor C

Pregnancy Considerations Adverse events have been observed in animal reproduction studies.

Breast-Feeding Considerations It is not known if etomidate is excreted in breast milk. The manufacturer recommends that caution be exercised when administering etomidate to nursing women.

Contraindications Hypersensitivity to etomidate or any component of the formulation

Warnings/Precautions Etomidate inhibits 11-B-hydroxylase, an enzyme important in adrenal steroid production. A single induction dose blocks the normal stress-induced increase in adrenal cortisol production for 4-8 hours, up to 24 hours in elderly and debilitated patients. Continuous infusion of etomidate for sedation in the ICU may increase mortality because patients may not be able to respond to stress. No increase in mortality has been identified with a single dose for induction of anesthesia. Consider exogenous corticosteroid replacement in patients undergoing severe stress.

Warnings: Additional Pediatric Considerations Some dosage forms may contain propylene glycol; in neonates large amounts of propylene glycol delivered orally, intravenously (eg, >3,000 mg/day), or topically have been associated with potentially fatal toxicities which can include metabolic acidosis, seizures, renal failure, and CNS depression; toxicities have also been reported in children and adults including hyperosmolality, lactic acidosis, seizures, and respiratory depression; use caution (AAP, 1997; Shehab, 2009).

Adverse Reactions

Gastrointestinal: Hiccups, nausea, vomiting on emergence from anesthesia

Local: Pain at injection site

Neuromuscular & skeletal: Myoclonus, transient skeletal movements, uncontrolled eye movements

Rare but important or life-threatening: Apnea, arrhythmia, bradycardia, decreased cortisol synthesis, hyper-/hypotension, hyper-/hypoventilation, laryngospasm, tachycardia

Drug Interactions

Metabolism/Transport Effects None known.

Avoid Concomitant Use There are no known interactions where it is recommended to avoid concomitant use.

Increased Effect/Toxicity There are no known significant interactions involving an increase in effect.

Decreased Effect There are no known significant interactions involving a decrease in effect.

Storage/Stability Store at room temperature.

Mechanism of Action Ultrashort-acting nonbarbiturate hypnotic (benzylimidazole) used for the induction of anesthesia; chemically, it is a carboxylated imidazole which produces a rapid induction of anesthesia with minimal cardiovascular effects; produces EEG burst suppression at high doses

Pharmacodynamics

Onset of action: 30-60 seconds

Maximum effect: 1 minute

Duration: Dose dependent: 2-3 minutes (0.15 mg/kg dose); 4-10 minutes (0.3 mg/kg dose); rapid recovery is due to rapid redistribution

Pharmacokinetics (Adult data unless noted)

Distribution: V_d: 3.6-4.5 L/kg

Protein binding: 76%; decreased protein binding resulting in an increased percentage of "free" etomidate in patients with renal failure or hepatic cirrhosis

Metabolism: Hepatic and plasma esterases

Half-life, elimination: Terminal: 2.6-3.5 hours

Time to peak serum concentration: 7 minutes

Excretion: 75% excreted in urine over 24 hours; 2% excreted unchanged

Dosing: Usual IV:

Induction & maintenance of anesthesia: Children >10 years and Adults: Initial: 0.2-0.6 mg/kg over 30-60 seconds; maintenance: 10-20 mcg/kg/minute; smaller doses may be used to supplement subpotent anesthetic agents

Procedural sedation: Limited data in children; initial doses 0.1-0.3 mg/kg have been used; repeat doses may be needed depending upon the duration of the procedure and the response of the patient

Administration IV: Administer IV push over 30-60 seconds; very irritating; avoid administration into small vessels on the dorsum of the head or hand; preadministration of lidocaine may be beneficial

Monitoring Parameters Cardiac monitoring, blood pressure, respiratory rate, sedation score (procedural sedation)

Dosage Forms Excipient information presented when available (limited, particularly for generics); consult specific product labeling.

Solution, Intravenous:
Amidate: 2 mg/mL (10 mL, 20 mL) [contains propylene glycol]
Generic: 2 mg/mL (10 mL, 20 mL)

Solution, Intravenous [preservative free]:
Generic: 2 mg/mL (10 mL, 20 mL)

Etoposide (e toe POE side)

Medication Safety Issues

Sound-alike/look-alike issues:

Etoposide may be confused with teniposide

Etoposide may be confused with etoposide phosphate (a prodrug of etoposide which is rapidly converted in the plasma to etoposide)

VePesid may be confused with Versed

High alert medication:

This medication is in a class the Institute for Safe Medication Practices (ISMP) includes among its list of drug classes which have a heightened risk of causing significant patient harm when used in error.

Related Information

Management of Drug Extravasations *on page 2298*

Oral Medications That Should Not Be Crushed or Altered *on page 2476*

Prevention of Chemotherapy-Induced Nausea and Vomiting in Children *on page 2368*

Safe Handling of Hazardous Drugs *on page 2455*

Brand Names: US Toposar

Brand Names: Canada Etoposide Injection; Etoposide Injection USP; Vepesid

Therapeutic Category Antineoplastic Agent, Mitotic Inhibitor; Antineoplastic Agent, Topoisomerase Inhibitor

Generic Availability (US) Yes

Use Treatment of refractory testicular tumors (Parenteral: FDA approved in adults) and small cell lung cancer (Oral and parenteral: FDA approved in adults); has also been used for malignant lymphoma, Hodgkin's disease, leukemias (ALL, ANLL, AML), neuroblastoma; treatment of Ewing's sarcoma, rhabdomyosarcoma, osteosarcoma, Wilms' tumor, CNS tumors; conditioning regimen with hematopoietic stem cell transplantation

Pregnancy Risk Factor D

Pregnancy Considerations Adverse events were observed in animal reproduction studies. Etoposide may cause fetal harm if administered during pregnancy. Women of childbearing potential should be advised to avoid pregnancy.

Breast-Feeding Considerations It is not known if etoposide is excreted in breast milk. Due to the potential for serious adverse reactions in the nursing infant, the decision to discontinue etoposide or to discontinue breast-feeding during treatment should take into account the benefits of treatment to the mother.

Contraindications Hypersensitivity to etoposide or any component of the formulation

Canadian labeling: Additional contraindications (not in U.S. labeling): Severe leukopenia or thrombocytopenia; severe hepatic impairment; severe renal impairment

Warnings/Precautions Hazardous agent - use appropriate precautions for handling and disposal (NIOSH 2014 [group 1]). **[U.S. Boxed Warning]: Severe dose-limiting and dose-related myelosuppression with resulting infection or bleeding may occur.** Treatment should be withheld for platelets <50,000/mm^3 or absolute neutrophil count (ANC) <500/mm^3. May cause anaphylactic-like reactions manifested by chills, fever, tachycardia, bronchospasm, dyspnea, and hypotension. In addition, facial/tongue swelling, coughing, chest tightness, cyanosis, laryngospasm, diaphoresis, hypertension, back pain, loss of consciousness, and flushing have also been reported less commonly. Incidence is primarily associated with intravenous administration (up to 2%) compared to oral administration (<1%). Infusion should be interrupted and medications for the treatment of anaphylaxis should be available for immediate use. High drug concentration and rate of infusion, as well as presence of benzyl alcohol in the etoposide intravenous formulation have been suggested as contributing factors to the development of hypersensitivity reactions. Etoposide intravenous formulations may contain benzyl alcohol, while etoposide phosphate (the water soluble prodrug of etoposide) intravenous formulation does not contain benzyl alcohol. Case reports have suggested that etoposide phosphate has been used successfully in patients with previous hypersensitivity reactions to etoposide (Collier, 2008; Siderov, 2002). The use of concentrations higher than recommended were associated with higher rates of anaphylactic-like reactions in children.

Secondary acute leukemias have been reported with etoposide, either as monotherapy or in combination with other chemotherapy agents. Must be diluted; do not give IV push, infuse over at least 30 to 60 minutes; hypotension is associated with rapid infusion. If hypotension occurs, interrupt infusion and administer IV hydration and supportive care; decrease infusion upon reinitiation. Etoposide is an irritant; tissue irritation and inflammation have occurred following extravasation. Do not administer IM or SubQ. Dosage should be adjusted in patients with hepatic or renal impairment (Canadian labeling contraindicates use in severe hepatic and/or renal impairment). Use with caution in patients with low serum albumin; may increase risk for toxicities. Use with caution in elderly patients; may be more likely to develop severe myelosuppression and/or GI effects (eg, nausea/vomiting). **[U.S. Boxed Warning]: Should be administered under the supervision of an experienced cancer chemotherapy physician.**

Oral etoposide is associated with a low (adults) or moderate (children) emetic potential; antiemetics may be recommended to prevent nausea and vomiting (Dupuis, 2011; Roila, 2010). Potentially significant drug-drug interactions may exist, requiring dose or frequency adjustment, additional monitoring, and/or selection of alternative therapy.

Benzyl alcohol and derivatives: Some dosage forms may contain benzyl alcohol; large amounts of benzyl alcohol (≥99 mg/kg/day) have been associated with a potentially fatal toxicity ("gasping syndrome") in neonates; the "gasping syndrome" consists of metabolic acidosis, respiratory distress, gasping respirations, CNS dysfunction (including convulsions, intracranial hemorrhage), hypotension, and cardiovascular collapse (AAP, 1997; CDC, 1982); some data suggests that benzoate displaces bilirubin from protein binding sites (Ahlfors, 2001); avoid or use dosage forms containing benzyl alcohol with caution in neonates. See manufacturer's labeling.

Injectable formulation contains alcohol (~33% v/v); may contribute to adverse reactions, especially with higher etoposide doses.

Polysorbate 80: Some dosage forms may contain polysorbate 80 (also known as Tweens). Hypersensitivity reactions, usually a delayed reaction, have been reported following exposure to pharmaceutical products containing polysorbate 80 in certain individuals (Isaksson, 2002; Lucente 2000; Shelley, 1995). Thrombocytopenia, ascites, pulmonary deterioration, and renal and hepatic failure have been reported in premature neonates after receiving parenteral products containing polysorbate 80 (Alade, 1986; CDC, 1984). See manufacturer's labeling.

Adverse Reactions Note: The following may occur with higher doses used in stem cell transplantation: Alopecia, ethanol intoxication, hepatitis, hypotension (infusion-related), metabolic acidosis, mucositis, nausea and vomiting (severe), secondary malignancy, skin lesions (resembling Stevens-Johnson syndrome).

Cardiovascular: Hypotension (due to rapid infusion)

Dermatologic: Alopecia

Gastrointestinal: Abdominal pain, anorexia, diarrhea, nausea/vomiting, stomatitis

Hematologic: Anemia, leukopenia (nadir: 7-14 days; recovery: By day 20), thrombocytopenia (nadir: 9-16 days; recovery: By day 20)

Hepatic: Hepatic toxicity

Neuromuscular & skeletal: Peripheral neuropathy

Miscellaneous: Anaphylactic-like reaction (including chills, fever, tachycardia, bronchospasm, dyspnea)

Rare but important or life-threatening: Amenorrhea, blindness (transient/cortical), cyanosis, extravasation (induration/necrosis), facial swelling, hypersensitivity, hypersensitivity-associated apnea, interstitial pneumonitis, laryngospasm, maculopapular rash, metabolic acidosis, MI, mucositis, myocardial ischemia, optic neuritis, perivasculitis, pruritus, pulmonary fibrosis, radiation-recall dermatitis, rash, reversible posterior leukoencephalopathy syndrome (RPLS), seizure, Stevens-Johnson syndrome, tongue swelling, toxic epidermal necrolysis, toxic megacolon, vasospasm

Drug Interactions

Metabolism/Transport Effects Substrate of CYP1A2 (minor), CYP2E1 (minor), CYP3A4 (major), P-glycoprotein; **Note:** Assignment of Major/Minor substrate status based on clinically relevant drug interaction potential; **Inhibits** CYP2C9 (weak)

Avoid Concomitant Use

Avoid concomitant use of Etoposide with any of the following: BCG; BCG (Intravesical); CloZAPine; Conivaptan; Dipyrone; Fusidic Acid (Systemic); Idelalisib; Natalizumab; Pimecrolimus; Tacrolimus (Topical); Tofacitinib; Vaccines (Live)

Increased Effect/Toxicity

Etoposide may increase the levels/effects of: CloZAPine; Leflunomide; Natalizumab; Tofacitinib; Vaccines (Live); Vitamin K Antagonists

The levels/effects of Etoposide may be increased by: Aprepitant; Atovaquone; Conivaptan; CycloSPORINE (Systemic); CYP3A4 Inhibitors (Moderate); CYP3A4 Inhibitors (Strong); Dasatinib; Denosumab; Dipyrone; Fosaprepitant; Fusidic Acid (Systemic); Idelalisib; Ivacaftor; Luliconazole; Mifepristone; Netupitant; Palbociclib; P-glycoprotein/ABCB1 Inhibitors; Pimecrolimus; Roflumilast; Simeprevir; Stiripentol; Tacrolimus (Topical); Trastuzumab

Decreased Effect

Etoposide may decrease the levels/effects of: BCG; BCG (Intravesical); Coccidioides immitis Skin Test; Sipuleucel-T; Vaccines (Inactivated); Vaccines (Live)

The levels/effects of Etoposide may be decreased by: Barbiturates; Bosentan; CYP3A4 Inducers (Moderate); CYP3A4 Inducers (Strong); Dabrafenib; Deferasirox; Fosphenytoin; Mitotane; P-glycoprotein/ABCB1 Inducers; Phenytoin; Siltuximab; St Johns Wort; Tocilizumab

Storage/Stability

Capsules: Store oral capsules at 2°C to 8°C (36°F to 46°F); do not freeze. Dispense in a light-resistant container.

Injection: Store intact vials of injection at 20°C to 25°C (68°F to 77°F; do not freeze. According to the manufacturer's labeling, stability for solutions diluted for infusion in D_5W or NS (in glass or plastic containers) varies based on concentration; 0.2 mg/mL solutions are stable for 96 hours at room temperature and 0.4 mg/mL solutions are stable for 24 hours at room temperature (precipitation may occur at concentrations above 0.4 mg/mL).

Etoposide injection contains polysorbate 80 which may cause leaching of diethylhexyl phthalate (DEHP), a plasticizer contained in polyvinyl chloride (PVC) bags and tubing. Higher concentrations and longer storage time after preparation in PVC bags may increase DEHP leaching. Preparation in glass or polyolefin containers will minimize patient exposure to DEHP. When undiluted etoposide injection is stored in acrylic or ABS (acrylonitrile, butadiene and styrene) plastic containers, the containers may crack and leak.

Mechanism of Action Etoposide has been shown to delay transit of cells through the S phase and arrest cells in late S or early G_2 phase. The drug may inhibit mitochondrial transport at the NADH dehydrogenase level or inhibit uptake of nucleosides into HeLa cells. It is a topoisomerase II inhibitor and appears to cause DNA strand breaks. Etoposide does not inhibit microtubular assembly.

Pharmacokinetics (Adult data unless noted)

Absorption: Oral: Large variability

Distribution: CSF concentration is <5% of plasma concentration

Children: V_{dss}: 10 L/m^2

Adults: V_{dss}: 7-17 L/m^2

Protein binding: 94% to 97%

Metabolism: In the liver (with a biphasic decay)

Bioavailability: Averages 50% (range: 25% to 75%)

Half-life, terminal:

Children: 6-8 hours

Adults: 4-15 hours with normal renal and hepatic function

Elimination: Both unchanged drug and metabolites are excreted in urine and a small amount (2% to 16%) in feces; up to 55% of an IV dose is excreted unchanged in urine in children

Dosing: Usual

Pediatric: **Note:** Dose, frequency, number of doses, and start date may vary by protocol and treatment phase; refer to individual protocols; limited data available:

Acute lymphocytic leukemia (ALL), relapsed: Children and Adolescents: IV: *Consolidation:* 100 mg/m^2/dose once daily on days 15-19 (in combination with other chemotherapeutic agents) (Parker, 2010)

Acute myeloid leukemia (AML):

Induction:

Age-directed dosing (Gibson, 2011):

Infants <1 year: IV: 75 mg/m^2/dose once daily on days 1-5 (in combination with cytarabine and daunorubicin or mitoxantrone)

Children ≥1 year and Adolescents: IV: 100 mg/m^2/dose once daily on days 1-5 (in combination with cytarabine and daunorubicin or mitoxantrone)

BSA-directed dosing (Cooper, 2012): Infants, Children, and Adolescents: IV:

BSA <0.6 m^2: 3.3 mg/**kg**/dose once daily on days 1-5 (in combination with other chemotherapeutic agents)

BSA ≥0.6 m^2: 100 mg/m^2/dose once daily on days 1-5 (in combination with other chemotherapeutic agents)

Intensification: BSA-directed dosing (Cooper, 2012): Infants, Children, and Adolescents: IV:

BSA <0.6 m^2: 5 mg/**kg**/dose once daily on days 1-5 (in combination with cytarabine)

BSA ≥0.6 m^2: 150 mg/m^2/dose once daily on days 1-5 (in combination with cytarabine)

Consolidation: Infants, Children, and Adolescents: IV: 100 mg/m^2/dose once daily for 4-5 days, administered over 1 hour (in combination with cytarabine and daunorubicin or amsacrine) (Gibson, 2012; Perel, 2002); 75 mg/m^2/dose once daily on days 1-5 (in combination with cytarabine and amsacrine) was administered to infants <1 year in one study (Gibson, 2012)

CNS tumor:

Infants and Children <3 years: IV: 6.5 mg/**kg**/dose administered on days 3 and 4 (in combination with cisplatin as Cycle B regimen) for 28 day cycle alternating with Cycle A regimen (cyclophosphamide and vincristine); therapy initiated 2-4 weeks after tumor resection (Duffner, 1993)

Children ≥3 years and Adolescents: IV: 100 mg/m^2/dose once daily on days 1, 2, and 3 (in combination with vincristine and carboplatin or cyclophosphamide) every 3 weeks for 4 cycles prior to radiation (Taylor, 2003)

Children ≥6 years and Adolescents: IV: 150 mg/m^2/dose once daily on days 3 and 4 (in combination with cisplatin) every 3 weeks for 4 cycles prior to radiation (Kovnar, 1990)

Hematopoietic stem cell transplantation (HSCT), conditioning regimen: Children ≥1 year and Adolescents: IV: 30 **or** 60 mg/kg/dose administered over 4-8 hours as a single dose 3 or 4 days prior to transplantation (Biagi, 2000; Duerst, 2000; Horning, 1994; Snyder, 1993; Zander, 1997)

Hodgkin's lymphoma, advanced stage (BEACOPP regimen): *Induction:* Children ≥4 years and Adolescents: IV: 200 mg/m^2/dose once daily on days 0-2 (3 doses) every 3 weeks for 4 cycles (in combination with bleomycin, doxorubicin, cyclophosphamide, vincristine, procarbazine, and prednisone); 4 additional cycles may be given to slow early responders (Kelly, 2002; Kelly, 2011)

Neuroblastoma, high-risk: Children ≥1 year and Adolescents:

Induction: IV: 100-200 mg/m^2/dose infused over 1-2 hours once daily for 3-5 consecutive days (in combination with other chemotherapy agents) (Kaneko, 2002; Kushner, 2004; Simon, 2007; Simon, 2007a); other reported regimens include 100 mg/m^2/dose on day 2 and 5 (in combination with cisplatin, doxorubicin, and cyclophosphamide) every 28 days for 5 cycles (Matthay, 1999)

Myeloablative therapy with stem cell rescue:

IV: 100-200 mg/m^2/day for 4-5 days beginning 8-9 days prior to transplantation was used in 301 patients (Kaneko, 2002)

Continuous IV infusion: 640 mg/m^2 infused over 96 hours beginning 8 days prior to transplant (Matthany, 1999; Park, 2009)

Sarcoma: Children ≥1 year and Adolescents: IV: 100 mg/m^2/dose once daily for 5 doses on days 0-4 every 3 weeks [in combination with ifosfamide and carboplatin (ICE regimen)] (Van Winkle, 2005); other reported regimens include: 150 mg/m^2/dose once daily for 3 doses on days 1-3 in combination with vincristine, doxorubicin, cyclophosphamide, and ifosfamide (VACIE regimen) (Navid, 2006)

Wilms tumor (ICE Regimen): Children and Adolescents: IV: 100 mg/m^2/dose once daily for 3-5 doses (in combination with ifosfamide and carboplatin); repeat cycle every 21 days (Abu-Ghosh, 2002; Daw, 2009)

Adult: **Note:** Utilize patient's actual body weight (full weight) for calculation of body surface area- or weight-based dosing, particularly when the intent of therapy is curative (excludes HSCT dosing); manage regimen-related toxicities in the same manner as for nonobese patients; if a dose reduction is utilized due to toxicity, consider resumption of full weight-based dosing with subsequent cycles, especially if cause of toxicity (eg, hepatic or renal impairment) is resolved (Griggs, 2012).

Small cell lung cancer (in combination with other chemotherapy agents):

IV: 35 mg/m^2/day for 4 days, up to 50 mg/m^2/day for 5 days every 3-4 weeks

Oral: Due to poor bioavailability, oral doses should be twice the IV dose (and rounded to the nearest 50 mg)

Testicular cancer (in combination with other chemotherapy agents): IV: 50-100 mg/m^2/day on days 1-5 **or** 100 mg/m^2/day on days 1, 3, and 5 repeated every 3-4 weeks

Dosing adjustment in renal impairment:

Infants, Children, and Adolescents: Dosage adjustments are not provided in the manufacturer's labeling; however, the following adjustments have been recommended (Aronoff, 2007):

GFR >50 mL/minute/1.73 m^2: No dosage adjustment necessary

GFR 10-50 mL/minute/1.73m^2: Administer 75% of dose

GFR <10 mL/minute/1.73m^2: Administer 50% of dose

Hemodialysis/peritoneal dialysis (PD) (after dialysis on dialysis days): Administer 50% of dose

Continuous renal replacement therapy (CRRT): Administer 75% of dose and reduce for hyperbilirubinemia

Adults:

Manufacturer's labeling:

CrCl >50 mL/minute: No adjustment required.

CrCl 15-50 mL/minute: Administer 75% of dose

CrCl <15 mL minute: Data not available; consider further dose reductions

The following guidelines have been used by some clinicians:

Aronoff, 2007:

CrCl >50 mL/minute: No adjustment required.

CrCl 10-50 mL/minute: Administer 75% of normal dose

CrCl <10 mL/minute: Administer 50% of normal dose

Hemodialysis: Administer 50% of dose; supplemental posthemodialysis dose is not necessary

Peritoneal dialysis: Administer 50% of dose; supplemental dose is not necessary

Continuous renal replacement therapy (CRRT): Administer 75% of dose

Janus, 2010: Hemodialysis: Reduce dose by 50%; not removed by hemodialysis so may be administered before or after dialysis

Kintzel, 1995:

CrCl 46-60 mL/minute: Administer 85% of dose

CrCl 31-45 mL/minute: Administer 80% of dose

CrCl ≤30 mL/minute: Administer 75% of dose

Dosing adjustment in hepatic impairment:

Infants, Children, and Adolescents: The following adjustments have been recommended (Floyd, 2006): Bilirubin 1.5-3 mg/dL or AST >3 times ULN: Administer 50% of dose

Adults: There are no dosage adjustments provided in manufacturer's labeling; however, the following adjustments have been recommended.

Donelli, 1998: Liver dysfunction may reduce the metabolism and increase the toxicity of etoposide. Normal doses of IV etoposide should be given to patients with liver dysfunction (dose reductions may result in subtherapeutic concentrations); however, use caution with concomitant liver dysfunction (severe) and renal dysfunction as the decreased metabolic clearance cannot be compensated by increased renal clearance.

Floyd, 2006: Bilirubin 1.5-3 mg/dL or AST >3 times ULN: Administer 50% of dose

King, 2001; Koren, 1992: Bilirubin 1.5-3 mg/dL or AST >180 units/L: Administer 50% of dose

Dosage adjustment for toxicity: Adults:

Infusion (hypersensitivity) reactions: Interrupt infusion

ANC <500/mm^3 or platelets <50,000/mm^3: Withhold treatment until recovery

Severe adverse reactions (nonhematologic): Reduce dose or discontinue treatment

Preparation for Administration Hazardous agent; use appropriate precautions for handling and disposal (NIOSH 2014 [group 1]).

Oral: The injection may be used for oral administration either as an extemporaneous preparation (see Extemporaneous Preparations) or by mixing dose with orange juice, apple juice, or lemonade at a final concentration not to exceed 0.4 mg/mL.

Parenteral: IV: Etoposide should be diluted in D_5W or NS to a final concentration of 0.2 to 0.4 mg/mL; concentrations >0.4 mg/mL are very unstable and may precipitate within a few minutes. However, more concentrated IV solutions (0.6 to 1 mg/mL) may be used cautiously in some protocols. Undiluted etoposide (20 mg/mL) has been used for HSCT conditioning regimens and prepared in a glass syringe (Horning 1994). Higher than recommended concentrations of etoposide infusions may crack hard plastic in chemo venting pins and infusion lines; inspect infusion solution for particulate matter and plastic devices for cracks and leaks. Diluted solutions have concentration-dependent stability: More concentrated solutions have shorter stability times.

Administration Hazardous agent; use appropriate precautions for handling and disposal (NIOSH 2014 [group 1]).

Oral: In adults, doses ≤200 mg/day should be given as a single daily dose; doses >400 mg should be given in 2 to 4 divided doses. If necessary, the injection may be used for oral administration either as an extemporaneous preparation or by mixing dose with orange juice, apple juice, or lemonade at a final concentration not to exceed 0.4 mg/mL.

Parenteral: IV: For IV infusion only; do not administer by rapid IV injection or by intrathecal, intraperitoneal, or intrapleural routes due to possible severe toxicity. Administer by continuous IV infusion or IV intermittent infusion via an in-line 0.22 micron filter over at least 60 minutes at a rate not to exceed 100 mg/m^2/hour (or 3.3 mg/**kg**/hour). HSCT conditioning regimens have infused etoposide through a central venous catheter over 4 to 8 hours (Biagi 2000; Duerst 2000; Horning 1994; Snyder 1993; Zander 1997). Higher than recommended concentrations of etoposide infusions may crack hard plastic in chemo venting pins and infusion lines; inspect infusion solution for particulate matter and plastic devices for cracks and leaks.

Vesicant/Extravasation Risk May be an irritant

Monitoring Parameters CBC with differential and platelet count, hemoglobin, vital signs (blood pressure), albumin, bilirubin, liver and renal function tests

Dosage Forms Excipient information presented when available (limited, particularly for generics); consult specific product labeling.

Capsule, Oral:

Generic: 50 mg

Solution, Intravenous:

Toposar: 100 mg/5 mL (5 mL); 500 mg/25 mL (25 mL); 1 g/50 mL (50 mL) [contains alcohol, usp, polyethylene glycol 300, polysorbate 80]

Generic: 100 mg/5 mL (5 mL); 500 mg/25 mL (25 mL); 1 g/50 mL (50 mL)

Extemporaneous Preparations Hazardous agent: Use appropriate precautions for handling and disposal (NIOSH 2014 [group 1]).

Etoposide 10 mg/mL oral solution: Dilute etoposide for injection 1:1 with normal saline to a concentration of 10 mg/mL. This solution is stable in plastic oral syringes for 22 days at room temperature. Prior to oral administration, further mix with fruit juice (orange, apple, or lemon; **NOT** grapefruit juice) to a concentration of <0.4 mg/mL; once mixed with fruit juice, use within 3 hours.

McLeod HL and Relling MV, "Stability of Etoposide Solution for Oral Use," *Am J Hosp Pharm*, 1992, 49(11):2784-5.

◆ **Etoposide Injection (Can)** *see* Etoposide *on page 819*

◆ **Etoposide Injection USP (Can)** *see* Etoposide *on page 819*

◆ **ETR** *see* Etravirine *on page 823*

Etravirine (et ra VIR een)

Medication Safety Issues

High alert medication:

This medication is in a class the Institute for Safe Medication Practices (ISMP) includes among its list of drug classes that have a heightened risk of causing significant patient harm when used in error.

International issues:

Etravirine [U.S. and multiple international markets] may be confused with ethaverine [multiple international markets]

Related Information

Adult and Adolescent HIV *on page 2392*

Oral Medications That Should Not Be Crushed or Altered *on page 2476*

Pediatric HIV *on page 2380*

Perinatal HIV *on page 2400*

Brand Names: US Intelence

Brand Names: Canada Intelence®

Therapeutic Category Antiretroviral Agent; HIV Agents (Anti-HIV Agents); Non-nucleoside Reverse Transcriptase Inhibitor (NNRTI)

Generic Availability (US) No

Use Treatment of HIV-1 infection in combination with other antiretroviral agents (FDA approved in ages ≥6 years weighing at least 16 kg and adults); **Note:** HIV regimens consisting of **three** antiretroviral agents are strongly recommended.

Pregnancy Risk Factor B

Pregnancy Considerations Adverse events have not been noted in animal reproduction studies. Etravirine crosses the placenta. Based on limited data, dose adjustments are not needed in pregnant women. However, because available data in pregnant women are insufficient, the DHHS Perinatal HIV Guidelines do not recommend use in antiretroviral-naive women unless other alternatives are not available. Hypersensitivity reactions (including hepatic toxicity and rash) are more common in women on NNRTI therapy; it is not known if pregnancy increases this risk.

Regardless of CD4 count or HIV RNA copy number, all HIV-infected pregnant women should receive a combination antiretroviral (ARV) drug regimen. A combination of antepartum, intrapartum, and infant ARV prophylaxis is recommended. ARV therapy should be started as soon as possible in women with symptomatic infection. Although earlier initiation may be more effective in reducing the perinatal transmission of HIV, initiation may be delayed until after 12 weeks gestation in women who do not require immediate treatment after careful consideration of maternal conditions (eg, nausea and vomiting) and the potential risks of first trimester fetal exposure for specific agents. A scheduled cesarean delivery at 38 weeks gestation is recommended for all women with HIV RNA >1000 copies/mL or unknown concentrations near delivery in order to decrease transmission. If ARV therapy must be interrupted for <24 hours during the peripartum period, stop then restart all medications simultaneously in order to decrease the chance of developing resistance. Long-term follow-up is recommended for all infants exposed to ARV medications. In couples who want to conceive, the HIV-infected partner should attain maximum viral suppression prior to conception.

Health care providers are encouraged to enroll pregnant women exposed to antiretroviral medications in the Antiretroviral Pregnancy Registry (1-800-258-4263 or www.APRegistry.com). Health care providers caring for HIV-infected women and their infants may contact the National Perinatal HIV Hotline (888-448-8765) for clinical consultation (HHS [perinatal], 2014).

Breast-Feeding Considerations It is not known if etravirine is excreted into breast milk. Maternal or infant antiretroviral therapy does not completely eliminate the risk of postnatal HIV transmission. In addition, multiclass-resistant virus has been detected in breast-feeding infants despite maternal therapy. Therefore, in the United States, where formula is accessible, affordable, safe, and sustainable, and the risk of infant mortality due to diarrhea and respiratory infections is low, complete avoidance of breastfeeding by HIV-infected women is recommended to decrease potential transmission of HIV (HHS [perinatal], 2014).

Contraindications There are no contraindications listed in the manufacturer's U.S. labeling.

Canadian labeling: Hypersensitivity to etravirine or any component of the formulation.

Warnings/Precautions Severe and possibly life-threatening skin reactions (including Stevens-Johnson syndrome, toxic epidermal necrolysis, and erythema multiforme) and hypersensitivity reactions ranging from rash (including drug rash with eosinophilia and systemic symptoms [DRESS]) and/or constitutional symptoms to occasional organ dysfunction (including hepatic failure) have been reported; discontinue immediately with signs or symptoms of severe skin reaction or hypersensitivity. Self-limiting (with continued therapy) mild-to-moderate rashes (higher incidence in females) were also observed in clinical trials (pediatric and adult), usually during second week of therapy initiation. Not for use in treatment-naive patients, or experienced patients without evidence of viral mutations conferring resistance to NNRTIs and PIs. May cause redistribution of fat (eg, buffalo hump, peripheral wasting with increased abdominal girth, cushingoid appearance). Patients may develop immune reconstitution syndrome resulting in the occurrence of an inflammatory response to an indolent or residual opportunistic infection during initial HIV treatment or activation of autoimmune disorders (eg, Graves' disease, polymyositis, Guillain-Barré syndrome) later in therapy; further evaluation and treatment may be required.

High potential for drug interactions; concomitant use of etravirine with some drugs may require cautious use, may not be recommended, or may require dosage adjustments.

Warnings: Additional Pediatric Considerations Rash is more common and severe in pediatric patients (6 years to <18 years) than in adults; usually described as pruritic, maculopapular skin eruptions (incidence: Pediatric patients: 15%, adults 10%). In pediatric patients, rashes usually appeared within 14 days of starting therapy and generally resolved within a week. Discontinue etravirine if severe rash (involving blistering, desquamation, mucosal involvement, ulceration, or fever) occurs.

Adverse Reactions

Dermatologic: Rash

Endocrine & metabolic: Cholesterol (total) increased, hyperglycemia, LDL increased, triglycerides increased

Gastrointestinal: Amylase increased, diarrhea (children and adolescents), nausea

Hepatic: ALT increased, AST increased

Neuromuscular & skeletal: Peripheral neuropathy

Renal: Creatinine increased

Rare but important or life-threatening: Amnesia, anemia (including hemolytic), angina, angioedema, anorexia, atrial fibrillation, diabetes mellitus, drug rash with eosinophilia and systemic symptoms (DRESS), erythema multiforme, GERD, gynecomastia, hemorrhagic stroke, hematemesis, hepatic failure, hepatic steatosis, hepatitis, hepatomegaly, hypersensitivity reaction, hypersomnia, hypoesthesia, immune reconstitution syndrome, insomnia, lipohypertrophy/dystrophy, MI, pancreatitis, paresthesia, renal failure, rhabdomyolysis, seizure, Stevens-Johnson syndrome, syncope, toxic epidermal necrolysis

Drug Interactions

Metabolism/Transport Effects **Substrate** of CYP2C19 (major), CYP2C9 (major), CYP3A4 (major); **Note:** Assignment of Major/Minor substrate status based on clinically relevant drug interaction potential; **Inhibits** CYP2C19 (moderate), CYP2C9 (moderate); **Induces** CYP3A4 (moderate)

Avoid Concomitant Use

Avoid concomitant use of Etravirine with any of the following: Axitinib; Bedaquiline; Boceprevir; Bosutinib; CarBAMazepine; Efavirenz; Enzalutamide; Fosamprenavir; Fosphenytoin; Nisoldipine; Olaparib; Palbociclib; PHENobarbital; Phenytoin; Primidone; Reverse Transcriptase Inhibitors (Non-Nucleoside); Rifamycin Derivatives; Rilpivirine; Ritonavir; Simeprevir; St Johns Wort; Tipranavir

Increased Effect/Toxicity

Etravirine may increase the levels/effects of: Antifungal Agents (Azole Derivatives, Systemic); Artemether; Bosentan; Cannabis; Carvedilol; Cilostazol; Citalopram; Clarithromycin; CYP2C19 Substrates; CYP2C9 Substrates; Diazepam; Digoxin; Dronabinol; Efavirenz; Fosamprenavir; Ifosfamide; Protease Inhibitors; Rilpivirine; Tetrahydrocannabinol

The levels/effects of Etravirine may be increased by: Antifungal Agents (Azole Derivatives, Systemic); Artemether; Atazanavir; Reverse Transcriptase Inhibitors (Non-Nucleoside)

Decreased Effect

Etravirine may decrease the levels/effects of: Amiodarone; Antifungal Agents (Azole Derivatives, Systemic); ARIPiprazole; Artemether; Atazanavir; Axitinib; Bedaquiline; Bepridil; Bosutinib; Buprenorphine; CarBAMazepine; Clarithromycin; Clopidogrel; CYP3A4 Substrates; Dasabuvir; Diazepam; Disopyramide; Dolutegravir; Efavirenz; Enzalutamide; FentaNYL; Flecainide; HMG-CoA Reductase Inhibitors; Hydrocodone; Ibrutinib; Ifosfamide; Lidocaine (Systemic); Macrolide Antibiotics; Maraviroc; Methadone; Mexiletine; NiMODipine; Nisoldipine; Olaparib; Ombitasvir; Palbociclib; Paritaprevir; Phosphodiesterase 5 Inhibitors; Propafenone; QuiNIDine; Rilpivirine; Saxagliptin; Simeprevir; Telaprevir

The levels/effects of Etravirine may be decreased by: Boceprevir; Bosentan; CarBAMazepine; CYP2C19 Inducers (Strong); CYP2C9 Inducers (Strong); CYP3A4 Inducers (Moderate); Dabrafenib; Darunavir; Deferasirox; Fosphenytoin; Mitotane; PHENobarbital; Phenytoin; Primidone; Protease Inhibitors; Reverse Transcriptase Inhibitors (Non-Nucleoside); Rifabutin; Rifamycin Derivatives; Ritonavir; Siltuximab; St Johns Wort; Tipranavir; Tocilizumab

Food Interactions Food increases absorption of etravirine by ~50%. Management: Take after meals and maintain adequate hydration, unless instructed to restrict fluid intake.

Storage/Stability Store at USP controlled room temperature of 25°C (77°F); excursions permitted to 15°C to 30°C (59°F to 86°F). Protect from moisture.

Mechanism of Action As a non-nucleoside reverse transcriptase inhibitor, etravirine has activity against HIV-1 by binding to reverse transcriptase. It consequently blocks the RNA-dependent and DNA-dependent DNA polymerase activities, including HIV-1 replication. It does not require intracellular phosphorylation for antiviral activity.

Pharmacokinetics (Adult data unless noted) Note: Pharmacokinetic data suggests that with comparable dosing, exposure in pediatric patients ≥6 years is similar to adult patients.

Absorption: Decreased under fasting conditions

Protein binding: ~99.9%; primarily to albumin and alpha$_1$-acid glycoprotein

Metabolism: Hepatic, primarily by CYP3A4, 2C9, and 2C19; major metabolites exhibit ~10% of parent drug activity against wild-type HIV

Half-life elimination: 41 hours ± 20 hours

Time to peak serum concentration: 2.5-4 hours

Elimination: Feces (up to 86% as unchanged drug)

Hemodialysis: Due to extensive protein binding, significant removal by hemodialysis or peritoneal dialysis is unlikely

Dosing: Usual

Pediatric: **HIV infection, treatment:** Use in combination with other antiretroviral agents.

Children <6 years or pediatric patients <16 kg: Not recommended for use; no dosing recommendations available.

Children ≥6 years and Adolescents, antiretroviral-experienced: Oral:

16 kg to <20 kg: 100 mg twice daily
20 kg to <25 kg: 125 mg twice daily
25 kg to <30 kg: 150 mg twice daily
≥30 kg: 200 mg twice daily

Adult: **HIV infection, treatment:** Use in combination with other antiretroviral agents.

Oral: Antiretroviral-experienced: 200 mg twice daily

Dosing adjustment in renal impairment: Children, Adolescents, and Adults: No dosage adjustments required (DHHS [adult, pediatric], 2014).

Dosing adjustment in hepatic impairment:

Mild to moderate impairment (Child-Pugh class A or B): Children, Adolescents, and Adults: No dosage adjustments required (DHHS [adult, pediatric], 2014).

Severe impairment (Child-Pugh class C): Adolescents and Adults: There are no dosage adjustments provided in manufacturer's labeling (has not been studied).

Administration Oral: Administer after meals. Swallow tablet whole with water; do not chew. If unable to swallow tablets, may disperse tablets in 5 mL water (enough to cover tablets), stir well (until milky appearance), add additional water (or may add milk or orange juice), and drink immediately. Rinse glass several times (with water, milk, or orange juice) and swallow entire contents to ensure administration of full dose. Do not use grapefruit juice, carbonated beverages, or warm (>40°C) drinks (including warm water).

Monitoring Parameters Note: Monitor CD4 percentage (if <5 years of age) or CD4 count (if ≥5 years of age) at least every 3 to 4 months (DHHS [pediatric], 2014).

Prior to initiation of therapy: Genotypic resistance testing, CD4 and viral load (every 3 to 4 months), CBC with differential, LFTs, BUN, creatinine, electrolytes, glucose, urinalysis (every 6 to 12 months), and assessment of readiness for adherence with medication regimen. At initiation and with any change in treatment regimen: CBC with differential, electrolytes, calcium, phosphate, glucose, LFTs, bilirubin, urinalysis (at initiation), BUN, creatinine, albumin, total protein, lipid panel, CD4, and viral load. After 1 to 2 weeks of therapy: Signs of medication toxicity and adherence. After 2 to 4 weeks of therapy: CBC with differential, viral load, signs of medication toxicity, and adherence; then every 3 to 4 months: CBC with differential, electrolytes, glucose, LFTs, bilirubin, BUN, creatinine, CD4, viral load, signs of medication toxicity, and adherence. Every 6 to 12 months: Lipid panel and urinalysis. CD4 monitoring frequency may be decreased to every 6 to 12 months in children who are adherent to therapy if the value is well above the threshold for opportunistic infections, viral suppression is sustained, and the clinical status is stable for more than 2 to 3 years (DHHS [pediatric], 2014). Monitor for growth and development, signs of HIV-specific physical conditions, HIV disease progression, opportunistic infections, skin rash, or hypersensitivity.

Reference Range Trough concentration (Limited data available; range utilized in trials): Adolescents and Adults: Median: 275 ng/mL (range: 81 to 2980 ng/mL) (DHHS [adult], 2014)

Dosage Forms Excipient information presented when available (limited, particularly for generics); consult specific product labeling.

Tablet, Oral:

Intelence: 25 mg [scored]
Intelence: 100 mg, 200 mg

◆ **Euglucon (Can)** *see* GlyBURIDE *on page 975*

◆ **Eurax** *see* Crotamiton *on page 545*

◆ **Eurax Cream (Can)** *see* Crotamiton *on page 545*

◆ **Euro-Cyproheptadine (Can)** *see* Cyproheptadine *on page 562*

◆ **Euro-Docusate C [OTC] (Can)** *see* Docusate *on page 697*

◆ **Euro-Lac (Can)** *see* Lactulose *on page 1204*

◆ **Eutectic Mixture of Lidocaine and Tetracaine** *see* Lidocaine and Tetracaine *on page 1266*

◆ **Evac [OTC]** *see* Psyllium *on page 1804*

◆ **Evamist** *see* Estradiol (Systemic) *on page 795*

Everolimus (e ver OH li mus)

Medication Safety Issues

Sound-alike/look-alike issues:

Everolimus may be confused with sirolimus, tacrolimus, temsirolimus

Afinitor may be confused with afatinib

High alert medication:

This medication is in a class the Institute for Safe Medication Practices (ISMP) includes among its list of drug classes which have a heightened risk of causing significant patient harm when used in error.

Administration issues:

Tablets (Afinitor, Zortress) and tablets for oral suspension (Afinitor Disperz) are not interchangeable; do not combine formulations to achieve total desired dose.

Related Information

Oral Medications That Should Not Be Crushed or Altered *on page 2476*

Prevention of Chemotherapy-Induced Nausea and Vomiting in Children *on page 2368*

Safe Handling of Hazardous Drugs *on page 2455*

Brand Names: US Afinitor; Afinitor Disperz; Zortress

Brand Names: Canada Afinitor

Therapeutic Category Antineoplastic Agent, mTOR Kinase Inhibitor; Immunosuppressant Agent

Generic Availability (US) No

Use

Afinitor: Treatment of subependymal giant cell astrocytoma (SEGA) associated with tuberous sclerosis complex (TSC) which requires intervention, but cannot be curatively resected (FDA approved in ages ≥1 year and adults); treatment of advanced hormone receptor-positive, HER2-negative breast cancer in postmenopausal women (in combination with exemestane and after letrozole or anastrozole failure (FDA approved in adults); treatment of advanced renal cell cancer (RCC), after sunitinib or sorafenib failure (FDA approved in adults); treatment of renal angiomyolipoma with TSC not requiring immediate surgery (FDA approved in adults); treatment of advanced, metastatic, or unresectable pancreatic neuroendocrine tumors (PNET) (FDA approved in adults)

Afinitor Disperz: Treatment of SEGA associated with TSC which requires intervention, but cannot be curatively resected (FDA approved in ages ≥1 year and adults)

Zortress: Prophylaxis of organ rejection in patients at low-moderate immunologic risk receiving renal or liver transplants (FDA approved in adults)

Medication Guide Available Yes

Pregnancy Risk Factor D (Afinitor) / C (Zortress)

Pregnancy Considerations Adverse events were observed in animal reproduction studies with exposures lower than expected with human doses. Based on the mechanism of action, may cause fetal harm if administered during pregnancy. Women of reproductive potential should be advised to avoid pregnancy and use highly effective birth control during treatment and for up to 8 weeks after everolimus discontinuation.

The National Transplantation Pregnancy Registry (NTPR) (Temple University) is a registry for pregnant women taking immunosuppressants following any solid organ transplant. The NTPR encourages reporting of all immunosuppressant exposures during pregnancy in transplant recipients at 877-955-6877.

Breast-Feeding Considerations It is not known if everolimus is excreted in breast milk. Due to the potential for serious adverse reactions in the nursing infant, breast-feeding should be avoided.

Contraindications Hypersensitivity to everolimus, sirolimus, other rapamycin derivatives, or any component of the formulation.

Warnings/Precautions Hazardous agent - use appropriate precautions for handling and disposal (NIOSH 2014 [group 1]). To avoid potential contact with everolimus, caregivers should wear gloves when preparing suspension from tablets for oral suspension. Noninfectious pneumonitis, interstitial lung disease (ILD), and/or noninfectious fibrosis have been observed with mTOR inhibitors including everolimus; some cases were fatal. Symptoms include dyspnea, cough, hypoxia and/or pleural effusion; promptly evaluate worsening respiratory symptoms. Consider opportunistic infections such as *Pneumocystis jiroveci* pneumonia (PCP) when evaluating clinical symptoms. May require treatment interruption followed by dose reduction (pneumonitis has developed even with reduced doses) and/or corticosteroid therapy; discontinue for grade 4 pneumonitis. Consider discontinuation for recurrence of grade 3 toxicity after dosage reduction. In patients who require steroid therapy for symptom management, consider PCP prophylaxis. Imaging may overestimate the incidence of clinical pneumonitis. **[U.S. Boxed Warning]: Everolimus has immunosuppressant properties which may result in infection;** the risk of developing bacterial (including mycobacterial), viral, fungal and protozoal infections and for local, opportunistic (including polyomavirus infection), and/or systemic infections is increased; may lead to sepsis, respiratory failure, hepatic failure, or fatality. Polyomavirus infection in transplant patients may be serious and/or fatal. Polyoma virus-associated nephropathy (due to BK virus), which may result in serious cases of deteriorating renal function and renal graft loss, has been observed with use. JC virus-associated progressive multiple leukoencephalopathy (PML) may also be associated with everolimus use in transplantation. Reduced immunosuppression (taking into account the risks of rejection) should be considered with evidence of polyoma virus infection or PML. Reactivation of hepatitis B has been observed in patients receiving everolimus. Resolve preexisting invasive fungal infections prior to treatment initiation. Cases (some fatal) of *Pneumocystis jiroveci* pneumonia (PCP) have been reported with everolimus use. Consider PCP prophylaxis in patients receiving concomitant corticosteroid or other immunosuppressant therapy. In addition, transplant recipient patients should receive prophylactic therapy for PCP and for cytomegalovirus (CMV). Monitor for signs and symptoms of infection during treatment. Discontinue if invasive systemic fungal infection is diagnosed (and manage with appropriate antifungal therapy).

[U.S. Boxed Warning]: Immunosuppressant use may result in the development of malignancy, including lymphoma and skin cancer. The risk is associated with treatment intensity and the duration of therapy. To minimize the risk for skin cancer, limit exposure to sunlight and ultraviolet light; wear protective clothing and use effective sunscreen.

[U.S. Boxed Warning]: Due to the increased risk for nephrotoxicity in renal transplantation, avoid standard doses of cyclosporine in combination with everolimus; reduced cyclosporine doses are recommended when everolimus is used in combination with cyclosporine. Therapeutic monitoring of cyclosporine and everolimus concentrations is recommended. Monitor for proteinuria; the risk of proteinuria is increased when everolimus is used in combination with cyclosporine, and with higher serum everolimus concentrations. Everolimus and cyclosporine combination therapy may increase the risk for thrombotic microangiopathy/thrombotic thrombocytopenic purpura/hemolytic uremic syndrome (TMA/TTP/HUS); monitor blood counts. In liver transplantation, the tacrolimus dose and target range should be reduced to minimize the risk of nephrotoxicity. Eliminating calcineurin inhibitors from the immunosuppressive regimen may result in acute rejection. Elevations in serum creatinine (generally mild), renal failure, and proteinuria have been also observed with everolimus use; monitor renal function (BUN, creatinine, and/or urinary protein). Risk of nephrotoxicity may be increased when administered with calcineurin inhibitors (eg, cyclosporine, tacrolimus); dosage adjustment of calcineurin inhibitor is necessary. An increased incidence of rash, infection and dose interruptions have been reported in patients with renal insufficiency (CrCl ≤60 mL/minute) who received mTOR inhibitors for the treatment of renal cell cancer (Gupta, 2011); serum creatinine elevations and proteinuria have been reported. Monitor renal function (BUN, serum creatinine, urinary protein) at baseline and periodically, especially if risk factors for further impairment exist; pharmacokinetic studies have not been conducted; dosage adjustments are not required based on renal impairment. **[U.S. Boxed Warning]: An increased risk of renal arterial and venous thrombosis has been reported with use in renal transplantation, generally within the first 30 days after transplant; may result in graft loss.** MTOR inhibitors are associated with an increase in hepatic artery thrombosis, most cases have been reported within 30 days after transplant and usually proceeded to graft loss or death; do not use everolimus prior to 30 days post liver transplant.

Potentially significant drug-drug/drug-food interactions may exist, requiring dose or frequency adjustment, additional monitoring, and/or selection of alternative therapy. In transplant patients, avoid the use of certain HMG-CoA reductase inhibitors (eg, simvastatin, lovastatin); may increase the risk for rhabdomyolysis due to the potential interaction with cyclosporine (which may be given in combination with everolimus for transplantation).

Use is associated with mouth ulcers, mucositis and stomatitis; manage with topical therapy; avoid the use of alcohol-, hydrogen peroxide-, iodine-, or thyme-based mouthwashes (due to the high potential for drug interactions, avoid the use of systemic antifungals unless fungal infection has been diagnosed). Everolimus is associated with the development of angioedema; concomitant use with other agents known to cause angioedema (eg, ACE inhibitors) may increase the risk. Everolimus use may delay wound healing and increase the occurrence of wound-related complications (eg, wound dehiscence, infection, incisional hernia, lymphocele, seroma); may require surgical intervention; use with caution in the peri-surgical period. Generalized edema, including peripheral edema and lymphedema, and local fluid accumulation (eg, pericardial effusion, pleural effusion, ascites) may also occur.

Everolimus exposure is increased in patients with hepatic impairment. For patients with breast cancer, PNET, RCC, or renal angiomyolipoma with mild and moderate hepatic impairment, reduced doses are recommended; in patients with severe hepatic impairment, use is recommended (at reduced doses) if the potential benefit outweighs risks. Reduced doses are recommended in transplant patients with hepatic impairment; pharmacokinetic information does not exist for renal transplant patients with severe impairment (Child-Pugh class B or C); monitor whole blood trough levels closely for patients with SEGA, reduced doses may be needed for mild and moderate hepatic impairment (based on therapeutic drug monitoring), and are recommended in severe hepatic impairment; monitor whole blood trough levels. The Canadian labeling recommends against the use of everolimus in patients <18 years of age with SEGA and hepatic impairment.

[U.S. Boxed Warning]: Increased mortality (usually associated with infections) within the first 3 months after transplant was noted in a study of patients with *de novo* heart transplant receiving immunosuppressive regimens containing everolimus (with or without induction therapy). Use in heart transplantation is not recommended. Hyperglycemia, hyperlipidemia, and hypertriglyceridemia have been reported. Higher serum everolimus concentrations are associated with an increased risk for hyperlipidemia. Use has not been studied in patients with baseline cholesterol >350 mg/dL. Monitor fasting glucose and lipid profile prior to treatment initiation and periodically thereafter; monitor more frequently in patients with concomitant medications affecting glucose. Manage with appropriate medical therapy (if possible, optimize glucose control and lipids prior to treatment initiation). Antihyperlipidemic therapy may not normalize levels. May alter insulin and/or oral hypoglycemic therapy requirements in patients with diabetes; the risk for new onset diabetes is increased with everolimus use after transplantation. Decreases in hemoglobin, neutrophils, platelets, and lymphocytes have been reported; monitor blood counts at baseline and periodically. Increases in serum glucose are common; may alter insulin and/or oral hypoglycemic therapy requirements in patients with diabetes; the risk for new-onset diabetes is increased with everolimus use after transplantation. Patients should not be immunized with live viral vaccines during or shortly after treatment and should avoid close contact with recently vaccinated (live vaccine) individuals; consider the timing of routine immunizations prior to the start of therapy in pediatric patients treated for SEGA. In pediatric patients treated for SEGA, complete recommended series of live virus childhood vaccinations prior to treatment (if immediate everolimus treatment is not indicated); an accelerated vaccination schedule may be appropriate. Continue treatment with everolimus for renal cell cancer as long as clinical benefit is demonstrated or until occurrence of unacceptable toxicity. Safety and efficacy have not been established for the use of everolimus in the treatment of carcinoid tumors.

Tablets (Afinitor, Zortress) and tablets for oral suspension (Afinitor Disperz) are not interchangeable; Afinitor Disperz is only indicated in conjunction with therapeutic monitoring for the treatment of SEGA. Do not combine formulations to achieve total desired dose. May cause infertility; in females, menstrual irregularities, secondary amenorrhea, and increases in luteinizing hormone and follicle-stimulating hormone have occurred; azoospermia and oligospermia have been observed in males. Avoid use in patients with hereditary galactose intolerance, Lapp lactase deficiency, or glucose-galactose malabsorption; may result in diarrhea and malabsorption. The safety and efficacy of everolimus in renal transplantation patients with high-immunologic risk or in solid organ transplant other than renal or liver have not been established. **[U.S. Boxed Warning]: In transplantation, everolimus should only be used by physicians experienced in immunosuppressive therapy and management of transplant patients. Adequate laboratory and supportive medical resources must be readily available.** For indications requiring whole blood trough concentrations to determine dosage adjustments, a consistent method should be used; concentration values from different assay methods may not be interchangeable.

Adverse Reactions

Cardiovascular: Angina pectoris, atrial fibrillation, cardiac failure, chest discomfort, chest pain, deep vein thrombosis, edema (generalized), hypertension (including hypertensive crisis), hypotension, palpitations, peripheral edema, pulmonary embolism, renal artery thrombosis, syncope, tachycardia, venous thromboembolism

Central nervous system: Agitation, behavioral changes (anxiety/aggression/behavioral disturbance; SEGA), chills, depression, dizziness, drowsiness, fatigue, hallucination, headache, hemiparesis, hypoesthesia, insomnia, lethargy, malaise, migraine, neuralgia, paresthesia, seizure

Dermatologic: Acneiform eruption, acne vulgaris, alopecia, cellulitis (SEGA), contact dermatitis, eczema, erythema, excoriation, hyperhidrosis, hypertrichosis, nail disease (including onychoclasis), night sweats, palmar-plantar erythrodysesthesia (hand-foot syndrome), papule, pityriasis rosea, pruritus, skin lesion, skin rash, xeroderma

Endocrine & metabolic: Amenorrhea, cushingoid appearance, cyanocobalamin deficiency, decreased serum albumin, decreased serum bicarbonate, dehydration, diabetes mellitus (new onset; more common in liver transplant), exacerbation of diabetes mellitus, gout, hirsutism, hypercalcemia, hypercholesterolemia, hyperglycemia, hyperkalemia (renal transplant), hyperlipidemia (renal, liver transplant), hypermenorrhea, hyperparathyroidism, hyperphosphatemia, hypertriglyceridemia, hyperuricemia, hypocalcemia, hypoglycemia, hypokalemia, hypomagnesemia (renal transplant), hyponatremia, hypophosphatemia, increased follicle-stimulating hormone, increased luteinizing hormone, iron deficiency, irregular menses, lipid metabolism disorder (renal transplant), menstrual disease, ovarian cyst

Gastrointestinal: Abdominal distention, abdominal pain, ageusia, anorexia, constipation, decreased appetite, diarrhea, dysgeusia, dyspepsia, dysphagia, epigastric distress, flatulence, gastritis, gastroenteritis, gastroesophageal reflux disease, gingival hyperplasia, hematemesis, hemorrhoids, intestinal obstruction, mucositis, nausea, oral herpes, peritonitis, stomatitis (more common in oncology uses), vomiting, weight loss, xerostomia

Genitourinary: Bladder spasm, dysmenorrhea, dysuria (renal transplant), erectile dysfunction, hematuria (renal transplant), irregular menses, pollakiuria, proteinuria, pyuria, scrotal edema, urinary retention, urinary tract infection, urinary urgency, vaginal hemorrhage

Hematologic & oncologic: Anemia, hemorrhage, leukocytosis, leukopenia (more common in oncology uses), lymphadenopathy, lymphocytopenia, neoplasm (liver transplant), neutropenia, pancytopenia (renal, liver transplant), prolonged partial thromboplastin time (SEGA), thrombocytopenia (more common in oncology uses)

Hepatic: Abnormal hepatic function tests (liver transplant), ascites (liver transplant), increased serum alkaline phosphatase (more common in oncology uses), increased serum ALT, increased serum AST, increased serum bilirubin, increased serum transaminases

Hypersensitivity: Hypersensitivity (including anaphylaxis, dyspnea, flushing, chest pain, angioedema)

Infection: BK virus, candidiasis, herpes virus infection, infection, sepsis

Neuromuscular & skeletal: Arthralgia, back pain, jaw pain, joint swelling, limb pain, muscle spasm, musculoskeletal pain, myalgia, osteonecrosis, osteopenia, osteoporosis, spondylitis, tremor, weakness

Ophthalmic: Blurred vision, cataract, conjunctivitis, eyelid edema, ocular hyperemia

Otic: Otitis

Renal: Hydronephrosis, increased blood urea nitrogen, increased serum creatinine, interstitial nephritis, polyuria, renal failure, renal insufficiency

Respiratory: Atelectasis, bronchitis, cough, dyspnea, epistaxis, lower respiratory tract infection, nasal congestion, nasopharyngitis, oropharyngeal pain, pharyngolaryngeal pain, pharyngitis, pleural effusion, pneumonia, pneumonitis (including alveolitis, interstitial lung disease, lung infiltrate, pulmonary alveolar hemorrhage, pulmonary toxicity), pulmonary edema, rhinitis, rhinorrhea, sinus congestion, sinusitis, upper respiratory tract infection, wheezing

Miscellaneous: Fever, postoperative wound complication (including incisional hernia), wound healing impairment (more common in renal and liver transplant)

Rare but important or life-threatening: Aspergillosis, azoospermia, cardiac arrest, cholecystitis, cholelithiasis, decreased plasma testosterone, fluid retention, hemolytic uremic syndrome, hepatic artery thrombosis, influenza, intrahepatic cholestasis, malignant lymphoma, oligospermia, pancreatitis, pneumonia due to *pneumocystis jiroveci*, progressive multifocal leukoencephalopathy, reactivation of HBV, respiratory distress, skin neoplasm, synovitis (severe), thrombosis of vascular graft, thrombotic thrombocytopenic purpura

Drug Interactions

Metabolism/Transport Effects Substrate of CYP3A4 (major), P-glycoprotein; **Note:** Assignment of Major/Minor substrate status based on clinically relevant drug interaction potential

Avoid Concomitant Use

Avoid concomitant use of Everolimus with any of the following: BCG; BCG (Intravesical); CloZAPine; Conivaptan; CYP3A4 Inducers (Strong); CYP3A4 Inhibitors (Strong); Dipyrone; Fusidic Acid (Systemic); Grapefruit Juice; Idelalisib; Natalizumab; Pimecrolimus; St Johns Wort; Tacrolimus (Topical); Tofacitinib; Vaccines (Live); Voriconazole

Increased Effect/Toxicity

Everolimus may increase the levels/effects of: ACE Inhibitors; CloZAPine; Leflunomide; Natalizumab; Tofacitinib; Vaccines (Live)

The levels/effects of Everolimus may be increased by: Conivaptan; CycloSPORINE (Systemic); CYP3A4 Inhibitors (Moderate); CYP3A4 Inhibitors (Strong); Dasatinib; Denosumab; Dipyrone; Fusidic Acid (Systemic); Grapefruit Juice; Idelalisib; Luliconazole; Mifepristone; Palbociclib; P-glycoprotein/ABCB1 Inhibitors; Pimecrolimus; Roflumilast; Stiripentol; Tacrolimus (Topical); Trastuzumab; Voriconazole

Decreased Effect

Everolimus may decrease the levels/effects of: Antidiabetic Agents; BCG; BCG (Intravesical); Coccidioides immitis Skin Test; Sipuleucel-T; Vaccines (Inactivated); Vaccines (Live)

The levels/effects of Everolimus may be decreased by: Bosentan; CYP3A4 Inducers (Moderate); CYP3A4 Inducers (Strong); Dabrafenib; Deferasirox; Echinacea; Efavirenz; P-glycoprotein/ABCB1 Inducers; Siltuximab; St Johns Wort; Tocilizumab

Food Interactions Grapefruit juice may increase levels of everolimus. Absorption with food may be variable. Management: Avoid grapefruit juice. Take with or without food, but be consistent with regard to food.

Storage/Stability Tablets and tablets for suspension: Store at room temperature of 25°C (77°F); excursions permitted to 15°C to 30°C (59°F to 86°F). Protect from light; protect from moisture.

Mechanism of Action Everolimus is a macrolide immunosuppressant and a mechanistic target of rapamycin (mTOR) inhibitor which has antiproliferative and antiangiogenic properties, and also reduces lipoma volume in patients with angiomyolipoma. Reduces protein synthesis and cell proliferation by binding to the FK binding protein-12 (FKBP-12), an intracellular protein, to form a complex that inhibits activation of mTOR (mechanistic target of rapamycin) serine-threonine kinase activity. Also reduces angiogenesis by inhibiting vascular endothelial growth factor (VEGF) and hypoxia-inducible factor (HIF-1) expression. Angiomyolipomas may occur due to unregulated mTOR activity in TSC-associated renal angiomyolipoma (Budde, 2012); everolimus reduces lipoma volume (Bissler, 2012).

Pharmacokinetics (Adult data unless noted)

Absorption: Rapid but moderate

Distribution: V_d apparent: 128 to 589 L; volume of distribution in pediatric patients (3 to 16 years) lower than adults (Van-Damme-Lombaerts, 2002)

Protein binding: ~74%

Metabolism: Extensively metabolized via CYP3A4; forms 6 weak metabolites

Bioavailability:

Tablets: ~30%; systemic exposure reduced by 22% with a high-fat meal and by 32% with a light-fat meal

Tablets for suspension: AUC equivalent to tablets although peak concentrations are 20% to 36% lower; steady-state concentrations are similar; systemic exposure reduced by 12% with a high-fat meal and by 30% with a low-fat meal

Half-life elimination: ~30 hours; in pediatric patients (3 to 16 years), half-life similar to adult data (Van-Damme-Lombaerts, 2002)

Time to peak serum concentration: 1 to 2 hours

Elimination: Feces (80%, based on solid organ transplant studies); urine (~5%, based on solid organ transplant studies); clearance in pediatric patients lower than adults possibly due to distributive differences (Van-Damme-Lombaerts, 2002)

Dosing: Usual Note: Tablets (Afinitor, Zortress) and/or tablets for oral suspension (Afinitor Disperz) are not interchangeable. Afinitor Disperz is only indicated for the treatment of subependymal giant cell astrocytoma (SEGA), in conjunction with therapeutic monitoring. Do not combine formulations to achieve total desired dose.

Pediatric:

Subependymal giant cell astrocytoma (SEGA): Children ≥1 year and Adolescents:

Afinitor; Afinitor Disperz: Oral: Initial: 4.5 mg/m^2 once daily; round to nearest tablet (tablet or tablet for oral suspension) size; continue until disease progression or unacceptable toxicity

Therapeutic drug monitoring: Assess trough concentration ~2 weeks after initiation or dosage modification, if dosage form switched (tablets or tablets for oral suspension), hepatic function changes, or concurrent therapy with a CYP3A4 or p-glycoprotein (P-gp) inducer or inhibitor is modified (initiated, dose change, or discontinued). Adjust maintenance dose if needed at 2-week intervals to achieve and maintain trough concentrations between 5 and 15 ng/mL; once stable dose is attained and BSA is stable throughout treatment, monitor trough concentrations every 6 to 12 months; monitor every 3-6 months if BSA is changing.

If trough <5 ng/mL: Increase dose by 2.5 mg/day (tablets) or 2 mg/day (tablets for oral suspension).

If trough >15 ng/mL: Reduce dose by 2.5 mg/day (tablets) or 2 mg/day (tablets for oral suspension). **Note:** If dose reduction necessary in patients receiving the lowest strength available, administer every other day.

Transplantation; renal, rejection prophylaxis: Zortress: Limited data available: Children ≥1 year and Adolescents: Oral: Initial: 0.8 mg/m²/dose twice daily (maximum single dose: 1.5 mg) to maintain concentration: 3 to 6 ng/mL; reported start time of therapy variable: Within 48 hours post-transplantation was used in a multicenter, international trial of 19 pediatric patients; another trial began at 2 weeks after transplantation (single center, n=20 pediatric patients); a trial evaluating use for 3 years in pediatric patients (<16 years), the mean reported dose was 1.53 mg/m²/day and no untoward adverse effects were noted (Ettenger, 2008; Hoyer, 2003; Pape, 2007; Pape, 2010; Pape, 2011; Van-Damme-Lombaerts, 2002; Vester, 2002).

Adult:

Breast cancer, advanced, hormone receptor-positive, HER2-negative: Afinitor: Oral: 10 mg once daily (in combination with exemestane); continue treatment until no longer clinically beneficial or until unacceptable toxicity

Pancreatic neuroendocrine tumors, advanced (PNET): Afinitor: Oral: 10 mg once daily; continue treatment until no longer clinically benefiting or until unacceptable toxicity

Renal cell cancer (RCC), advanced: Afinitor: Oral: 10 mg once daily; continue treatment until no longer clinically benefiting or until unacceptable toxicity

Renal angiomyolipoma: Afinitor: Oral: 10 mg once daily; continue treatment until no longer clinically beneficial or until unacceptable toxicity

Subependymal giant cell astrocytoma (SEGA): Afinitor: Body surface area-based dosing: Oral: Initial dose: 4.5 mg/m² once daily; round to nearest tablet (tablet or tablet for oral suspension) size.

Therapeutic drug monitoring: Assess trough concentration ~2 weeks after initiation or dosage modification, if dosage form switched (tablets or tablets for oral suspension), hepatic function changes, or therapy with a CYP3A4 or p-glycoprotein (P-gp) inducer or inhibitor is modified (initiated, dose change, or discontinued). Adjust maintenance dose if needed at 2-week intervals to achieve and maintain trough concentrations between 5 and 15 ng/mL; once stable dose is attained and BSA is stable throughout treatment, monitor trough concentrations every 6 to 12 months; monitor every 3 to 6 months if BSA is changing.

If trough <5 ng/mL: Increase dose by 2.5 mg/day (tablets) or 2 mg/day (tablets for oral suspension).

If trough >15 ng/mL: Reduce dose by 2.5 mg/day (tablets) or 2 mg/day (tablets for oral suspension). **Note:** If dose reduction necessary in patients receiving the lowest strength available, administer every other day.

Transplantation; liver, rejection prophylaxis (begin at least 30 days post-transplant): Zortress: Oral: Initial: 1 mg twice daily; adjust maintenance dose if needed at a 4- to 5-day interval (from prior dose adjustment) based on concentrations, tolerability, and response; goal concentration is between 3 and 8 ng/mL (based on an LC/MS/MS assay method). If trough is <3 ng/mL, double total daily dose (using available tablet strengths); if trough >8 ng/mL on 2 consecutive measures, decrease dose by 0.25 mg twice daily. Administer in combination with tacrolimus (reduced dose required) and corticosteroids.

Transplantation; renal, rejection prophylaxis: Zortress: Initial: 0.75 mg twice daily; adjust maintenance dose if needed at a 4- to 5-day interval (from prior dose adjustment) based on concentrations, tolerability, and response; goal concentration is between 3 and 8 ng/mL (based on an LCMSMS assay method). If trough is <3 ng/mL, double total daily dose (using available tablet strengths); if trough >8 ng/mL on 2 consecutive measures, decrease dose by 0.25 mg twice daily. **Note:** For use in renal transplantation, administer in combination with basiliximab induction and concurrently with cyclosporine (dose adjustment required) and corticosteroids.

Dosage adjustment for concomitant CYP3A4 inhibitors/inducers and/or P-glycoprotein (P-gp) inhibitors: Breast cancer, PNET, RCC, renal angiomyolipoma: Adults:

CYP3A4/P-gp inducers: Strong inducers: Avoid concomitant administration with strong CYP3A4 inducers (eg, carbamazepine, phenobarbital, phenytoin, rifabutin, rifampin, rifapentine, St John's wort); if concomitant use cannot be avoided, consider doubling the everolimus dose, using increments of 5 mg or less, with careful monitoring. If the strong CYP3A4/P-gp enzyme inducer is discontinued, consider allowing 3 to 5 days to elapse prior to reducing the everolimus to the dose used prior to initiation of the CYP3A4/P-gp inducer.

CYP3A4/P-gp inhibitors:

Strong inhibitors: Avoid concomitant administration with strong CYP3A4 inhibitors (eg, atazanavir, clarithromycin, indinavir, itraconazole, ketoconazole, nefazodone, nelfinavir, ritonavir, saquinavir, telithromycin, voriconazole).

Moderate inhibitors (eg, amprenavir, aprepitant, diltiazem, erythromycin, fluconazole, fosamprenavir, verapamil): Reduce dose to 2.5 mg once daily; may consider increasing from 2.5 mg to 5 mg once daily based on patient tolerance. When the moderate inhibitor is discontinued, allow ~2 to 3 days to elapse prior to adjusting the everolimus upward to the dose used prior to initiation of the moderate inhibitor.

SEGA: Children, Adolescents, and Adults:

CYP3A4/P-gp inducers: Strong inducers: Avoid concomitant administration with strong CYP3A4 inducers (eg, carbamazepine, phenobarbital, phenytoin, rifabutin, rifampin, rifapentine, St John's wort); if concomitant use cannot be avoided, an initial starting everolimus dose of 9 mg/m² once daily is recommended, or double the everolimus dose and assess tolerability; evaluate trough concentration after ~2 weeks; adjust dose as necessary based on therapeutic drug monitoring to maintain target trough concentrations of 5 to 15 ng/mL. If the strong CYP3A4/P-gp enzyme inducer is discontinued, reduce the everolimus by ~50% or to the dose used prior to initiation of the CYP3A4/P-gp inducer; reassess trough concentration after ~2 weeks.

CYP3A4/P-gp inhibitors:

Strong inhibitors: Avoid concomitant administration with strong CYP3A4/P-gp inhibitors (eg, atazanavir, clarithromycin, indinavir, itraconazole, ketoconazole, nefazodone, nelfinavir, ritonavir, saquinavir, telithromycin, voriconazole).

Moderate inhibitors (eg, amprenavir, aprepitant, diltiazem, erythromycin, fluconazole, fosamprenavir, verapamil):

Initiating everolimus therapy with concurrent moderate CYP3A4/P-gp inhibitor: Initial everolimus dose: 2.5 mg/m² once daily

Currently taking everolimus and starting a moderate CYP3A4/P-gp inhibitor: Reduce everolimus dose by ~50%; if dose reduction is required for patients receiving the lowest strength available, consider alternate-day dosing.

Discontinuing a moderate CYP3A4/P-gp inhibitor after concomitant use with everolimus: Discontinue moderate inhibitor and allow 2 to 3 days to elapse prior to resuming the everolimus dose used prior to initiation of the moderate inhibitor.

Therapeutic drug monitoring: Assess trough concentrations ~2 weeks after everolimus initiation or dosage modifications, or initiation or changes to concurrent CYP3A4/P-gp inhibitor therapy; adjust everolimus maintenance dose if needed at 2-week intervals to achieve and maintain trough concentrations between 5 and 15 ng/mL.

Transplantation; renal: Children, Adolescents, and Adults: Dosage adjustments may be necessary based on everolimus whole blood trough concentrations.

Dosing adjustment in renal impairment: No adjustment necessary

Dosing adjustment in hepatic impairment:

Mild hepatic impairment (Child-Pugh class A):

Breast cancer, PNET, RCC, renal angiomyolipoma: Adults: Reduce dose to 7.5 mg once daily; if not tolerated, may further reduce to 5 mg once daily.

SEGA: Children, Adolescents, and Adults: Adjustment to initial dose may not be necessary; subsequent dosing is based on therapeutic drug monitoring (monitor 2 weeks after initiation, dosage modifications, or after any change in hepatic status; target trough concentration: 5-15 ng/mL).

Transplantation, liver or renal: Adults: Reduce initial dose by ~33%; individualize subsequent dosing based on therapeutic drug monitoring (target trough concentration: 3 to 8 ng/mL).

Moderate hepatic impairment (Child-Pugh class B):

Breast cancer, PNET, RCC, renal angiomyolipoma: Adults: Reduce dose to 5 mg once daily if not tolerated, may further reduce to 2.5 mg once daily.

SEGA: Children, Adolescents, and Adults: Adjustment to initial dose may not be necessary; subsequent dosing is based on therapeutic drug monitoring (monitor 2 weeks after initiation, dosage modifications, or after any change in hepatic status; target trough concentration: 5 to 15 ng/mL).

Transplantation, liver or renal: Adults: Reduce initial dose by ~50%; individualize subsequent dosing based on therapeutic drug monitoring (target trough concentration: 3 to 8 ng/mL).

Severe hepatic impairment (Child-Pugh class C):

Breast cancer, PNET, RCC, renal angiomyolipoma: Adults: If potential benefit outweighs risks, a maximum dose of 2.5 mg once daily may be used.

SEGA: Children, Adolescents, and Adults: Reduce initial dose to 2.5 mg/m^2 once daily (or current dose by ~50%); subsequent dosing is based on therapeutic drug monitoring (monitor ~2 weeks after initiation, dosage modifications, or after any change in hepatic status; target trough concentration: 5 to 15 ng/mL).

Transplantation, liver or renal: Adults: Reduce initial dose by ~50%; individualize subsequent dosing based on therapeutic drug monitoring (target trough concentration: 3 to 8 ng/mL).

Dosage adjustment for toxicity: Children, Adolescents, and Adults:

Breast cancer (adjustments apply to everolimus), PNET, RCC, renal angiomyolipoma: Toxicities may require temporary dose interruption (with or without a subsequent dose reduction) or discontinuation: Reduce everolimus dose by ~50% if dosage adjustment is necessary.

Noninfectious pneumonitis:

Grade 1 (asymptomatic radiological changes suggestive of pneumonitis): No dosage adjustment necessary; monitor appropriately.

Grade 2 [symptomatic but not interfering with activities of daily living (ADL)]: Consider interrupting treatment, rule out infection, and consider corticosteroids until symptoms improve to ≤ grade 1; reinitiate at a lower dose. Discontinue if recovery does not occur within 4 weeks.

Grade 3 (symptomatic, interferes with ADL; oxygen indicated): Interrupt treatment until symptoms improve to ≤ grade 1; rule out infection and consider corticosteroid treatment; may reinitiate at a lower dose. If grade 3 toxicity recurs, consider discontinuing.

Grade 4 (life-threatening; ventilatory support indicated): Discontinue treatment; rule out infection; consider corticosteroid treatment.

Stomatitis (avoid the use of products containing alcohol, hydrogen peroxide, iodine, or thyme derivatives):

Grade 1 (minimal symptoms, normal diet): No dosage adjustment necessary; manage with mouth wash (nonalcoholic or salt water) several times a day.

Grade 2 (symptomatic but can eat and swallow modified diet): Interrupt treatment until symptoms improve to ≤ grade 1; reinitiate at same dose; if stomatitis recurs at grade 2, interrupt treatment until symptoms improve to ≤ grade 1 and then reinitiate at a lower dose. Also manage with topical (oral) analgesics (eg, benzocaine, butyl aminobenzoate, tetracaine, menthol, or phenol) ± topical (oral) corticosteroids (eg, triamcinolone oral paste).

Grade 3 (symptomatic and unable to orally aliment or hydrate adequately): Interrupt treatment until symptoms improve to ≤ grade 1; then reinitiate at a lower dose. Also manage with topical (oral) analgesics (eg, benzocaine, butyl aminobenzoate, tetracaine, menthol, or phenol) ± topical (oral) corticosteroids (eg, triamcinolone oral paste).

Grade 4 (life-threatening symptoms): Discontinue treatment; initiate appropriate medical intervention.

Metabolic toxicity (eg, hyperglycemia, dyslipidemia):

Grade 1: No dosage adjustment necessary; initiate appropriate medical intervention and monitor.

Grade 2: No dosage adjustment necessary; manage with appropriate medical intervention and monitor.

Grade 3: Temporarily interrupt treatment; reinitiate at a lower dose; manage with appropriate medical intervention and monitor.

Grade 4: Discontinue treatment; manage with appropriate medical intervention.

Nonhematologic toxicities (excluding pneumonitis, stomatitis, and metabolic toxicity):

Grade 1: If toxicity is tolerable, no dosage adjustment necessary; initiate appropriate medical intervention and monitor.

Grade 2: If toxicity is tolerable, no dosage adjustment necessary; initiate appropriate medical intervention and monitor. If toxicity becomes intolerable, temporarily interrupt treatment until improvement to ≤ grade 1 and reinitiate at the same dose; if toxicity recurs at grade 2, temporarily interrupt treatment until improvement to ≤ grade 1 and then reinitiate at a lower dose.

Grade 3: Temporarily interrupt treatment until improvement to ≤ grade 1; initiate appropriate medical intervention and monitor. May reinitiate at a lower dose; if toxicity recurs at grade 3, consider discontinuing.

Grade 4 (life-threatening symptoms): Discontinue treatment; initiate appropriate medical intervention.

SEGA: *Severe/intolerable adverse reactions:* Temporarily interrupt or permanently discontinue treatment; if dose reduction is required upon reinitiation, reduce dose by ~50%; if dose reduction is required for patients receiving the lowest available strength, consider alternate day dosing.

Transplantation, liver or renal:

Evidence of polyoma virus infection or PML: Consider reduced immunosuppression (taking into account the allograft risks associated with decreased immunosuppression).

Pneumonitis (grade 4 symptoms) or invasive systemic fungal infection: Discontinue.

Preparation for Administration Hazardous agent; use appropriate precautions for handling and disposal (NIOSH 2014 [group 1]). To avoid potential contact with everolimus, caregivers should wear gloves when preparing suspension from tablets for oral suspension.

Oral: Tablets for oral suspension:

Preparation in an oral syringe: Place dose into 10 mL oral syringe (maximum: 10 mg/syringe; use an additional syringe for doses >10 mg). Draw ~5 mL of water and ~4 mL of air into oral syringe; allow to sit (tip up) in a container until tablets are in suspension (3 minutes). Gently invert syringe 5 times immediately prior to administration; administer contents (dose), and then add ~5 mL water and ~4 mL of air to same syringe, swirl to suspend remaining particles, and administer entire contents.

Preparation in a small glass: Place dose into a small glass (≤100 mL) containing ~25 mL water (maximum: 10 mg/glass; use an additional glass for doses >10 mg); allow to sit until tablets are in suspension (3 minutes). Stir gently with spoon immediately prior to administration; administer contents, then add ~25 mL water to same glass, swirl with same spoon to suspend remaining particles and administer entire contents.

Administration Hazardous agent; use appropriate precautions for handling and disposal (NIOSH 2014 [group 1]). To avoid potential contact with everolimus, caregivers should wear gloves when preparing suspension from tablets for oral suspension.

Oral: May be taken with or without food; to reduce variability, take consistently with regard to food; if using for SEGA, breast cancer, PNET, renal angiolipoma, or RCC, administer at the same time each day; if using for liver or renal transplantation, administer consistently ~12 hours apart and at the same time as tacrolimus (liver transplant) or cyclosporine (renal transplant).

Tablets: Swallow tablet whole with a glass of water; do not chew or crush; do not use tablets that are crushed or broken; avoid contact with or exposure to crushed or broken tablets.

Tablets for oral suspension: Administer as a suspension only. Administer immediately after preparation; discard if not administered within 60 minutes after preparation. Prepare suspension in water only. Do not break or crush tablets. May be prepared in an oral syringe or small glass.

Monitoring Parameters CBC with differential (baseline and periodic), liver function, serum creatinine, urinary protein, and BUN (baseline and periodic); fasting serum glucose and lipid profile (baseline and periodic); monitor for signs and symptoms of infection, noninfectious pneumonitis, or malignancy

SEGA: Monitor everolimus whole blood trough concentrations approximately 2 weeks after treatment initiation, 2 weeks after dose modifications, and after initiation or dose modification of concomitant CYP3A4 and/or P-gp inducers or inhibitors.

Transplantation; liver or renal: Monitor whole blood trough concentrations (based on an LCMSMS assay method), especially in patients with hepatic impairment, with concomitant CYP3A4/P-gp inhibitors and inducers, and when cyclosporine formulations or doses are changed; dosage adjustments should be made on trough concentrations obtained 4 to 5 days after previous dosage adjustment; monitor cyclosporine concentrations and proteinuria.

Reference Range Recommended range for everolimus whole blood trough concentrations:

SEGA: 5 to 15 ng/mL (high concentrations may be associated with larger reductions in SEGA volumes; responses have been observed at concentrations as low as 5 ng/mL)

Transplantation; liver or renal: 3 to 8 ng/mL (based on LCMSMS assay method); in pediatric studies, reported target range: 3 to 6 ng/mL

Dosage Forms Excipient information presented when available (limited, particularly for generics); consult specific product labeling.

Tablet, Oral:

Afinitor: 2.5 mg, 5 mg, 7.5 mg, 10 mg

Zortress: 0.25 mg, 0.5 mg, 0.75 mg

Tablet Soluble, Oral:

Afinitor Disperz: 2 mg, 3 mg, 5 mg

Extemporaneous Preparations Hazardous agent: Use appropriate precautions for handling and disposal (NIOSH 2014 [group 1]).

Tablets: An oral liquid may be prepared using tablets. Disperse tablet in ~30 mL (1 oz) of water; gently stir. Administer and rinse container with additional 30 mL (1 oz) water and administer to ensure entire dose is administered. Administer immediately after preparation.

Afinitor (everolimus) [prescribing information]. East Hanover, NJ: Novartis Pharmaceuticals Corporation; July 2012.

Tablets for oral suspension: Administer as a suspension only. Administer immediately after preparation; discard if not administered within 60 minutes after preparation. Prepare suspension in water only. Do not break or crush tablets.

Preparation in an oral syringe: Place dose into 10 mL oral syringe (maximum 10 mg/syringe; use an additional syringe for doses >10 mg). Draw ~5 mL of water and ~4 mL of air into oral syringe; allow to sit (tip up) in a container until tablets are in suspension (3 minutes). Gently invert syringe 5 times immediately prior to administration; administer contents, then add ~5 mL water and ~4 mL of air to same syringe, swirl to suspend remaining particles and administer entire contents.

Preparation in a small glass: Place dose into a small glass (≤100 mL) containing ~25 mL water (maximum 10 mg/glass; use an additional glass for doses >10 mg); allow to sit until tablets are in suspension (3 minutes). Stir gently with spoon immediately prior to administration; administer contents, then add ~25 mL water to same glass, swirl with same spoon to suspend remaining particles and administer entire contents.

Administer immediately after preparation; discard if not administered within 60 minutes after preparation.

Afinitor and Afinitor Disperz (everolimus) [prescribing information]. East Hanover, NJ: Novartis Pharmaceuticals Corporation; August 2012.

- ◆ **Everone 200 (Can)** *see* Testosterone *on page 2025*
- ◆ **Evithrom®** *see* Thrombin (Topical) *on page 2056*
- ◆ **Evoclin** *see* Clindamycin (Topical) *on page 491*
- ◆ **Evzio** *see* Naloxone *on page 1485*
- ◆ **Exalgo** *see* HYDROmorphone *on page 1044*
- ◆ **Exjade** *see* Deferasirox *on page 594*
- ◆ **Ex-Lax [OTC]** *see* Senna *on page 1914*
- ◆ **Ex-Lax Maximum Strength [OTC]** *see* Senna *on page 1914*
- ◆ **Ex-Lax Ultra [OTC]** *see* Bisacodyl *on page 289*
- ◆ **Extina** *see* Ketoconazole (Topical) *on page 1191*
- ◆ **Extra Strength Allergy Relief [OTC] (Can)** *see* Cetirizine *on page 423*
- ◆ **Exuviance Blemish Treatment [OTC]** *see* Salicylic Acid *on page 1894*

◆ **Eye-Sed [OTC]** *see* Zinc Sulfate *on page 2214*

◆ **EZ Char [OTC]** *see* Charcoal, Activated *on page 425*

Ezetimibe (ez ET i mibe)

Medication Safety Issues

Sound-alike/look-alike issues:

Ezetimibe may be confused with ezogabine

Zetia may be confused with Zebeta, Zestril

Brand Names: US Zetia

Brand Names: Canada ACH-Ezetimibe; ACT Ezetimibe; Apo-Ezetimibe; Bio-Ezetimibe; Ezetrol; JAMP-Ezetimibe; Mar-Ezetimibe; Mint-Ezetimibe; Mylan-Ezetimibe; PMS-Ezetimibe; Priva-Ezetimibe; RAN-Ezetimibe; Riva-Ezetimibe; Sandoz Ezetimibe; Teva-Ezetimibe

Therapeutic Category Antilipemic Agent; Cholesterol Absorption Inhibitor

Generic Availability (US) No

Use Adjunct to dietary therapy in combination with simvastatin in patients with heterozygous familial hypercholesterolemia (FDA approved in boys and postmenarchal girls 10-17 years of age); adjunct to dietary therapy (monotherapy or in combination with HMG-CoA reductase inhibitor in patients with primary hypercholesterolemia (heterozygous familial and nonfamilial) (FDA approved in adults); in combination with atorvastatin or simvastatin in the treatment of homozygous familial hypercholesterolemia (FDA approved in adults); in combination with fenofibrate in the treatment of mixed hyperlipidemia (FDA approved in adults); adjunct to dietary therapy for the reduction of elevated sitosterol and campesterol levels in patients with homozygous familial sitosterolemia (FDA approved in adults)

Pregnancy Risk Factor C

Pregnancy Considerations Use is contraindicated in women who are or who may become pregnant.

Breast-Feeding Considerations It is not known if ezetimibe is excreted in breast milk. According to the manufacturer, the decision to continue or discontinue breast-feeding during therapy should take into account the risk of exposure to the infant and the benefits of treatment to the mother. Use is contraindicated in nursing women who require combination therapy with an HMG-CoA reductase inhibitor.

Contraindications Hypersensitivity to ezetimibe or any component of the formulation; concomitant use with an HMG-CoA reductase inhibitor (statin) in patients with active hepatic disease or unexplained persistent elevations in serum transaminases; pregnancy and breast-feeding (when used concomitantly with a statin)

Warnings/Precautions Secondary causes of hyperlipidemia should be ruled out prior to therapy. Use caution with severe renal (CrCl ≤30 mL/minute/1.73 m^2); systemic exposure is increased ~1.5-fold. If using concurrent simvastatin in patients with moderate to severe renal impairment (CrCl <60 mL/minute/1.73m^2), the manufacturer of ezetimibe recommends that simvastatin doses exceeding 20 mg be used with caution and close monitoring for adverse events (eg, myopathy). Myopathy, including rhabdomyolysis, has been reported (rarely) with ezetimibe monotherapy; risk may be increased with concomitant use of a statin or fibrate. Discontinue ezetimibe and statin or fibrate immediately if myopathy is suspected or confirmed (symptomatic patient with CPK >10 x ULN).

A higher incidence of elevated transaminases (≥3 x ULN) has been observed with concomitant use of ezetimibe and statins compared to statin monotherapy; transaminase changes were generally not associated with symptoms or cholestasis and returned to baseline with or without discontinuation of therapy. Consider discontinuation of ezetimibe and/or the statin for persistently elevated transaminases (ALT or AST ≥3 x ULN). Systemic exposure is increased in hepatic impairment. Use caution with mild hepatic impairment (Child-Pugh class A); use is not recommended in patients with moderate or severe hepatic impairment (Child-Pugh classes B and C). Potentially significant drug-drug interactions may exist, requiring dose or frequency adjustment, additional monitoring, and/or selection of alternative therapy.

Adverse Reactions

Central nervous system: Fatigue

Gastrointestinal: Diarrhea

Hepatic: Transaminases increased (with HMG-CoA reductase inhibitors) (≥3 x ULN)

Neuromuscular & skeletal: Arthralgia, pain in extremity

Respiratory: Sinusitis, upper respiratory tract infection

Miscellaneous: Influenza

Rare but important or life-threatening: Abdominal pain, anaphylaxis, angioedema, autoimmune hepatitis (Stolk, 2006), cholecystitis, cholelithiasis, cholestatic hepatitis (Stolk, 2006), CPK increased, depression, dizziness, erythema multiforme, headache, hepatitis, hypersensitivity reactions, myalgia, myopathy, nausea, pancreatitis, paresthesia, rash, rhabdomyolysis, thrombocytopenia, urticaria

Drug Interactions

Metabolism/Transport Effects Substrate of SLCO1B1

Avoid Concomitant Use

Avoid concomitant use of Ezetimibe with any of the following: Bezafibrate; Gemfibrozil

Increased Effect/Toxicity

Ezetimibe may increase the levels/effects of: CycloSPORINE (Systemic)

The levels/effects of Ezetimibe may be increased by: Bezafibrate; CycloSPORINE (Systemic); Eltrombopag; Fenofibrate and Derivatives; Gemfibrozil; Teriflunomide

Decreased Effect

The levels/effects of Ezetimibe may be decreased by: Bile Acid Sequestrants

Storage/Stability Store at 25°C (77°F); excursions are permitted between 15°C and 30°C (59°F and 86°F). Protect from moisture.

Mechanism of Action Inhibits absorption of cholesterol at the brush border of the small intestine via the sterol transporter, Niemann-Pick C1-Like1 (NPC1L1). This leads to a decreased delivery of cholesterol to the liver, reduction of hepatic cholesterol stores and an increased clearance of cholesterol from the blood; decreases total C, LDL-cholesterol (LDL-C), ApoB, and triglycerides (TG) while increasing HDL-cholesterol (HDL-C).

Pharmacodynamics

Onset of action: Within 1 week

Maximum effect: 2-4 weeks

Pharmacokinetics (Adult data unless noted) Note: Pharmacokinetic data in children and adolescents ≥10 years of age are reported to be similar to that in adult patients.

Protein binding: >90%

Metabolism: Extensive glucuronide conjugation in the small intestine and liver to a pharmacologically active metabolite; may undergo enterohepatic recycling

Bioavailability: Variable

Hepatic impairment: Moderate hepatic impairment (Child-Pugh score 7-9): AUC increased 3-4 times; severe hepatic impairment (Child-Pugh 10-15): AUC increased 5-6 times

Renal impairment: Severe renal dysfunction (CrCl <30 mL/minute/1.73 m^2): AUC increased 1.5 times

Half-life: 22 hours (ezetimibe and metabolite)

Time to peak serum concentration: 4-12 hours (ezetimibe); 1-2 hours (active metabolite)

Elimination: Feces (78%, 69% as ezetimibe): urine (11%, 9% as metabolite)

Dosing: Usual

Pediatric: **Hyperlipidemia:**

Children 5 to 9 years: Limited data available: Oral: 10 mg once daily; dosing based on two studies of monotherapy; a prospective trial (n=17 including six patients ≤9 years) and a retrospective review (n=36, age range: 8 to 17 years) showed significant decreases in total cholesterol and LDL-C; patients were followed up to a mean of 13.6 months, no untoward effects were noted (Clauss 2009; Yeste 2009)

Children ≥10 years and Adolescents: Oral: 10 mg once daily in combination with simvastatin. Has also been shown in small pediatric trials to decrease TC and LDL-C when used as monotherapy as adjunct to dietary changes (Clauss 2009; Yeste 2009)

Adult: **Homozygous familial hypercholesterolemia, primary hyperlipidemia, homozygous sitosterolemia:** Oral: 10 mg once daily

Dosing adjustment in renal impairment: No dosage adjustments are recommended.

Dosing adjustment in hepatic impairment:

Mild hepatic impairment (Child-Pugh score 5-6): No dosage adjustments are recommended.

Moderate to severe impairment (Child-Pugh score 7-15): Use is not recommended.

Administration Oral: May be taken without regard to meals or time of day; may be administered with an HMG-CoA reductase inhibitor (eg, atorvastatin, simvastatin) or fenofibrate. Administer ≥2 hours before or ≥4 hours after bile acid sequestrants.

Monitoring Parameters Total cholesterol profile prior to therapy, and when clinically indicated and/or periodically thereafter. When used in combination with fenofibrate, monitor LFTs and signs and symptoms of cholelithiasis.

2013 ACC/AHA Blood Cholesterol Guideline recommendations (Stone, 2013): Baseline LFTs (reasonable); when used in combination with statin therapy, monitor LFTs when clinically indicated; discontinue use of ezetimibe if ALT elevations >3 times upper limit of normal persist.

Dosage Forms Excipient information presented when available (limited, particularly for generics); consult specific product labeling.

Tablet, Oral:

Zetia: 10 mg

Ezetimibe and Simvastatin

(ez ET i mibe & SIM va stat in)

Medication Safety Issues

Sound-alike/look-alike issues:

Vytorin may be confused with Vyvanse

Brand Names: US Vytorin

Therapeutic Category Antilipemic Agent; Cholesterol Absorption Inhibitor; HMG-CoA Reductase Inhibitor

Generic Availability (US) No

Use As an adjunct to diet for the reduction of elevated total cholesterol (total-C) and low-density lipoprotein cholesterol (LDL-C) in patients with homozygous familial hypercholesterolemia, as an adjunct to other lipid-lowering treatments (eg, LDL apheresis), or if such treatments are unavailable. As an adjunct to diet for the reduction of elevated total-C, LDL-C, apolipoprotein B (apo B), triglycerides, and non-high-density lipoprotein cholesterol (HDL-C), and to increase HDL-C in patients with primary (heterozygous familial and nonfamilial) hyperlipidemia or mixed hyperlipidemia (All indications: FDA approved in adults)

Limitations of use: No incremental benefit of ezetimibe/simvastatin on cardiovascular morbidity and mortality over and above that demonstrated for simvastatin has been established. Ezetimibe/simvastatin has not been studied in Fredrickson type I, III, IV, and V dyslipidemias.

Pregnancy Risk Factor X

Pregnancy Considerations Use is contraindicated in pregnant women or women who may become pregnant. See individual agents.

Breast-Feeding Considerations It is not known if ezetimibe or simvastatin are excreted into breast milk. Use is contraindicated in nursing women. See individual agents.

Contraindications Coadministration with strong CYP3A4 inhibitors (eg, itraconazole, ketoconazole, posaconazole, voriconazole, HIV protease inhibitors, boceprevir, telaprevir, erythromycin, clarithromycin, telithromycin, nefazodone, cobicistat-containing products), gemfibrozil, cyclosporine, or danazol; hypersensitivity to ezetimibe, simvastatin, or any component of this medication; active liver disease or unexplained persistent elevations in hepatic transaminases; pregnancy or use in women who may become pregnant; breast-feeding

Warnings/Precautions See individual agents.

Adverse Reactions Also see individual agents.

Central nervous system: Headache

Gastrointestinal: Diarrhea

Hepatic: ALT increased

Neuromuscular & skeletal: Myalgia, myopathy, pain in extremity

Respiratory: Upper respiratory infection

Miscellaneous: Influenza

Drug Interactions

Metabolism/Transport Effects Refer to individual components.

Avoid Concomitant Use

Avoid concomitant use of Ezetimibe and Simvastatin with any of the following: Amodiaquine; Bezafibrate; Boceprevir; Clarithromycin; Conivaptan; CycloSPORINE (Systemic); CYP3A4 Inhibitors (Strong); Danazol; Erythromycin (Systemic); Fusidic Acid (Systemic); Gemfibrozil; Grapefruit Juice; Idelalisib; Mifepristone; Protease Inhibitors; Red Yeast Rice; Telaprevir; Telithromycin

Increased Effect/Toxicity

Ezetimibe and Simvastatin may increase the levels/effects of: Amodiaquine; ARIPiprazole; DAPTOmycin; Diltiazem; PAZOPanib; Trabectedin; Vitamin K Antagonists

The levels/effects of Ezetimibe and Simvastatin may be increased by: Acipimox; Amiodarone; AmLODIPine; Aprepitant; Azithromycin (Systemic); Bezafibrate; Boceprevir; Ciprofibrate; Clarithromycin; Colchicine; Conivaptan; CycloSPORINE (Systemic); CYP3A4 Inhibitors (Moderate); CYP3A4 Inhibitors (Strong); Cyproterone; Danazol; Dasatinib; Diltiazem; Dronedarone; Eltrombopag; Erythromycin (Systemic); Fenofibrate and Derivatives; Fluconazole; Fosaprepitant; Fusidic Acid (Systemic); Gemfibrozil; Grapefruit Juice; Green Tea; Idelalisib; Imatinib; Ivacaftor; Lercanidipine; Lomitapide; Luliconazole; Mifepristone; Netupitant; Niacin; Niacinamide; Palbociclib; Protease Inhibitors; QuiNINE; Raltegravir; Ranolazine; Red Yeast Rice; Sildenafil; Simeprevir; Stiripentol; Telaprevir; Telithromycin; Teriflunomide; Ticagrelor; Verapamil

Decreased Effect

Ezetimibe and Simvastatin may decrease the levels/effects of: Lanthanum

The levels/effects of Ezetimibe and Simvastatin may be decreased by: Antacids; Bile Acid Sequestrants; Bosentan; CYP3A4 Inducers (Moderate); CYP3A4 Inducers (Strong); Dabrafenib; Deferasirox; Efavirenz; Eslicarbazepine; Etravirine; Fosphenytoin; Mitotane; Phenytoin; Rifamycin Derivatives; Siltuximab; St Johns Wort; Tocilizumab

Food Interactions See individual agents.

Storage/Stability Store at 20°C to 25°C (68°F to 77°F).

Mechanism of Action

Ezetimibe: Inhibits absorption of cholesterol at the brush border of the small intestine, leading to a decreased delivery of cholesterol to the liver. Ezetimibe inhibits the enzyme Niemann-Pick C1-Like1 (NPC1L1), a sterol transporter.

Simvastatin: A methylated derivative of lovastatin that acts by competitively inhibiting 3-hydroxy-3-methylglutaryl-coenzyme A (HMG-CoA) reductase, the enzyme that catalyzes the rate-limiting step in cholesterol biosynthesis. In addition to the ability of HMG-CoA reductase inhibitors to decrease levels of high-sensitivity C-reactive protein (hsCRP), they also possess pleiotropic properties including improved endothelial function, reduced inflammation at the site of the coronary plaque, inhibition of platelet aggregation, and anticoagulant effects (de Denus, 2002; Ray, 2005).

Pharmacodynamics

Onset of action (simvastatin): >3 days

Maximum effect (simvastatin): ≥2 weeks

Pharmacokinetics (Adult data unless noted) See individual agents.

Bioavailability: Vytorin is equivalent to coadministered ezetimibe and simvastatin.

Dosing: Usual

Pediatric: **Note:** A lower, conservative dosing regimen may be necessary in patient populations predisposed to myopathy, including patients of Chinese descent or those concurrently receiving other lipid-lowering agents (eg, niacin, fibric acid derivatives), amiodarone, amlodipine, diltiazem, dronedarone, ranolazine, verapamil (see the following conservative, maximum adult doses)

Heterozygous familial hypercholesterolemia: Limited data available: Children ≥10 years and Adolescents (males and postmenarchal females): Oral: Initial: Ezetimibe 10 mg and simvastatin 10 to 20 mg once daily in the evening. Reported final dosing range: Ezetimibe 10 mg and simvastatin 10 to 40 mg once daily (van der Graaf, 2008); maximum dose: Ezetimibe 10 mg and simvastatin 40 mg

Adult: **Note: Dosing limitation: Simvastatin 80 mg is limited to patients that have been taking this dose for >12 consecutive months without evidence of myopathy and are not currently taking or beginning to take a simvastatin dose-limiting or contraindicated interacting medication.** If patient is unable to achieve low-density lipoprotein-cholesterol (LDL-C) goal using the 40 mg dose of simvastatin, increasing to 80 mg dose is not recommended. Instead, switch patient to an alternative LDL-C-lowering treatment providing greater LDL-C reduction. After initiation or titration, monitor lipid response after ≥2 weeks and adjust dose as necessary.

Homozygous familial hypercholesterolemia: Oral: Ezetimibe 10 mg and simvastatin 40 mg once daily in the evening

Primary hyperlipidemias: Oral: Initial: Ezetimibe 10 mg and simvastatin 10 to 20 mg once daily in the evening. Start patients who require >55% reduction in LDL-C at ezetimibe 10 mg and simvastatin 40 mg once daily in the evening. Dosing range: Ezetimibe 10 mg and simvastatin 10 to 40 mg once daily

Dosing adjustment with concomitant medications: Oral: Adults: **Note:** Patients currently tolerating and requiring a dose of simvastatin 80 mg who require initiation of an interacting drug with a dose cap for simvastatin should be switched to an alternative statin with less potential for drug-drug interaction.

Amiodarone, amlodipine, or ranolazine: Simvastatin dose should **not** exceed 20 mg once daily

Diltiazem, dronedarone, or verapamil: Simvastatin dose should **not** exceed 10 mg once daily

Lomitapide: Reduce simvastatin dose by 50% when initiating lomitapide. Simvastatin dose should **not** exceed 20 mg once daily (or 40 mg once daily for those who previously tolerated simvastatin 80 mg daily for ≥1 year without evidence of muscle toxicity).

Dosing adjustment in Chinese patients on niacin doses ≥1 g/day: Adults: Oral: Use caution with simvastatin doses exceeding 20 mg/day; because of an increased risk of myopathy, do not administer simvastatin 80 mg.

Dosing adjustment in renal impairment:

Manufacturer's labeling: Adults:

GFR ≥60 mL/minute/1.73 m^2: No adjustment required.

GFR <60 mL/minute/1.73 m^2: Maximum dose: 10 mg ezetimibe/20 mg simvastatin daily; use with caution and monitor closely if higher doses are needed.

KDIGO recommendations (KDIGO, 2013): Children and Adolescents: Multidrug regimens (including ezetimibe and simvastatin) are not recommended for pediatric patients with chronic kidney disease, regardless of severity of LDL elevation.

Dosing adjustment for hepatic impairment: Adults: Use is contraindicated in patients with active liver disease or with unexplained transaminase elevations.

Administration Oral: May be administered without regard to meals. Administration with the evening meal or at bedtime has been associated with somewhat greater LDL-C reduction. Ezetimibe/simvastatin should be taken ≥2 hours before or ≥4 hours after administration of a bile acid sequestrant.

Monitoring Parameters

Pediatric patients: Baseline: ALT, AST, and creatine phosphokinase levels (CPK); fasting lipid panel (FLP) and repeat ALT and AST should be checked after 4 weeks of therapy; if no myopathy symptoms or laboratory abnormalities, then monitor FLP, ALT, and AST every 3 to 4 months during the first year and then every 6 months thereafter (NHLBI, 2011)

Adults:

2013 ACC/AHA Blood Cholesterol Guideline recommendations (Stone, 2013):

Lipid panel (total cholesterol, HDL, LDL, triglycerides): Baseline lipid panel; fasting lipid profile within 4 to 12 weeks after initiation or dose adjustment and every 3 to 12 months (as clinically indicated) thereafter. If 2 consecutive LDL levels are <40 mg/dL, consider decreasing the dose.

Hepatic transaminase levels: Baseline measurement of hepatic transaminase levels (ie, ALT); measure hepatic function if symptoms suggest hepatotoxicity (eg, unusual fatigue or weakness, loss of appetite, abdominal pain, dark-colored urine or yellowing of skin or sclera) during therapy.

CPK: CPK should not be routinely measured. Baseline CPK measurement is reasonable for some individuals (eg, family history of statin intolerance or muscle disease, clinical presentation, concomitant drug therapy that may increase risk of myopathy). May measure CPK in any patient with symptoms suggestive of myopathy (pain, tenderness, stiffness, cramping, weakness, or generalized fatigue).

Evaluate for new-onset diabetes mellitus during therapy; if diabetes develops, continue statin therapy and encourage adherence to a heart-healthy diet, physical activity, a healthy body weight, and tobacco cessation.

If patient develops a confusional state or memory impairment, may evaluate patient for nonstatin causes (eg, exposure to other drugs), systemic and neuropsychiatric causes, and the possibility of adverse effects associated with statin therapy.

Manufacturer recommendations: Baseline liver function tests and repeat when clinically indicated thereafter.

Upon initiation or titration, lipid panel should be analyzed after ≥2 weeks.

Dosage Forms Excipient information presented when available (limited, particularly for generics); consult specific product labeling.

Tablet:

Vytorin 10/10: Ezetimibe 10 mg and simvastatin 10 mg
Vytorin 10/20: Ezetimibe 10 mg and simvastatin 20 mg
Vytorin 10/40: Ezetimibe 10 mg and simvastatin 40 mg
Vytorin 10/80: Ezetimibe 10 mg and simvastatin 80 mg

- ◆ **Ezetrol (Can)** *see* Ezetimibe *on page 832*
- ◆ **EZFE 200 [OTC]** *see* Polysaccharide-Iron Complex *on page 1728*
- ◆ **F_3T** *see* Trifluridine *on page 2124*
- ◆ **FA-8 [OTC]** *see* Folic Acid *on page 931*
- ◆ **FabAV, FAB (Ovine)** *see Crotalidae* Polyvalent Immune Fab (Ovine) *on page 543*
- ◆ **Fabior** *see* Tazarotene *on page 2010*
- ◆ **Fabrazyme** *see* Agalsidase Beta *on page 76*

Factor VIIa (Recombinant)

(FAK ter SEV en aye ree KOM be nant)

Brand Names: US NovoSeven RT

Brand Names: Canada Niastase; Niastase RT

Therapeutic Category Antihemophilic Agent

Generic Availability (US) No

Use Treatment of bleeding episodes and prevention of bleeding in surgical interventions in patients with either hemophilia A or B when inhibitors to factor VIII or factor IX are present, acquired hemophilia, or congenital factor VII deficiency [FDA approved in pediatrics (age not specified) and adults]

Pregnancy Risk Factor C

Pregnancy Considerations Adverse events have been observed in animal reproduction studies.

Breast-Feeding Considerations It is not known if factor VIIa (recombinant) is excreted in breast milk. Due to the potential for serious adverse reactions in the nursing infant, a decision should be made whether to discontinue nursing or to discontinue the drug, taking into account the importance of treatment to the mother.

Contraindications There are no contraindications listed in the manufacturer's labeling.

Warnings/Precautions [US Boxed Warning]: Serious arterial and venous thrombotic events following administration of Factor VIIa (recombinant) have been reported. Discuss the risks and explain the signs and symptoms of thrombotic and thromboembolic events to patients who will receive factor VIIa (recombinant). Monitor patients for signs and symptoms of activation of the coagulation system and for thrombosis. All patients receiving factor VIIa should be monitored for signs and symptoms of activation of the coagulation system or thrombosis; thrombotic events due to circulating tissue factor or predisposing coagulopathy may be increased in patients with disseminated intravascular coagulation (DIC), advanced atherosclerotic disease, septicemia, crush injury, concomitant treatment with activated or nonactivated prothrombin complex concentrates, or uncontrolled postpartum hemorrhage. Use with caution in patients with an increased risk of thromboembolic complications (eg, coronary heart disease, liver disease, DIC, postoperative immobilization, elderly patients, and neonates). Decreased dosage or discontinuation is warranted with confirmed intravascular coagulation or presence of clinical thrombosis.

Hypersensitivity reactions, including anaphylaxis, have been reported with use. Use with caution in patients with known hypersensitivity to mouse, hamster, or bovine proteins, or factor VIIa, or any components of the product. If hypersensitivity reaction occurs, discontinue use and administer appropriate treatment; carefully consider the benefits versus the risk of continued treatment with factor VIIa. Some dosage forms may contain polysorbate 80 (also known as Tweens). Hypersensitivity reactions, usually a delayed reaction, have been reported following exposure to pharmaceutical products containing polysorbate 80 in certain individuals (Isaksson, 2002; Lucente 2000; Shelley, 1995). Thrombocytopenia, ascites, pulmonary deterioration, and renal and hepatic failure have been reported in premature neonates after receiving parenteral products containing polysorbate 80 (Alade, 1986; CDC, 1984). See manufacturer's labeling. A number of factors influence the efficacy of factor VIIa, including hypothermia, thrombocytopenia, acidosis, and the amount of blood products transfused prior to administration (Dunkley, 2008). In patients with factor VII deficiency, if factor VIIa activity does not reach the expected level, prothrombin time is not corrected, or bleeding is uncontrolled (with recommended doses), suspect antibody formation and perform antibody analysis. Prothrombin time and factor VII coagulant activity should be measured before and after administration in patients with factor VII deficiency.

Adverse Reactions

Cardiovascular: Bradycardia, edema, hypertension, hypotension, thrombosis

Central nervous system: Cerebrovascular disease, headache, pain

Dermatologic: Pruritus, skin rash

Endocrine & metabolic: Decreased serum fibrinogen

Gastrointestinal: Vomiting

Hematologic & oncologic: Decreased prothrombin time, disseminated intravascular coagulation, increased fibrinolysis, purpura

Hepatic: Abnormal hepatic function tests

Hypersensitivity: Hypersensitivity reaction

Local: Injection site reaction

Neuromuscular & skeletal: Osteoarthrosis

Renal: Renal function abnormality

Respiratory: Pneumonia

Miscellaneous: Decreased therapeutic response, fever

Rare but important or life-threatening: Anaphylactic shock, anaphylaxis, angina pectoris, angioedema, antibody development, arterial embolism (retinal), arterial thrombosis, arterial thrombosis (limb, retinal), bowel infarction, cerebral infarction, cerebral ischemia, cerebrovascular accident, deep vein thrombosis, hepatic artery thrombosis, hypersensitivity, immunogenicity, increased fibrin degradation products (including D-dimer elevation), intracardiac thrombus, local phlebitis, myocardial infarction, myocardial ischemia, nausea, occlusion of cerebral arteries, peripheral ischemia, portal vein thrombosis, pulmonary embolism, renal artery thrombosis, thrombophlebitis, venous thrombosis at injection site

Drug Interactions

Metabolism/Transport Effects None known.

Avoid Concomitant Use There are no known interactions where it is recommended to avoid concomitant use.

Increased Effect/Toxicity

The levels/effects of Factor VIIa (Recombinant) may be increased by: Factor XIII A-Subunit (Recombinant)

Decreased Effect There are no known significant interactions involving a decrease in effect.

Storage/Stability NovoSeven RT: Prior to reconstitution, store between 2°C and 25°C (36°F and 77°F); do not freeze. Protect from light. Reconstituted solutions may be stored at room temperature or under refrigeration, but must be infused within 3 hours of reconstitution. Do not freeze reconstituted solutions. Do not store reconstituted solutions in syringes.

Mechanism of Action Recombinant factor VIIa, a vitamin K-dependent glycoprotein, promotes hemostasis by activating the extrinsic pathway of the coagulation cascade. It replaces deficient activated coagulation factor VII, which complexes with tissue factor and may activate coagulation factor X to Xa and factor IX to IXa. When complexed with other factors, coagulation factor Xa converts prothrombin to thrombin, a key step in the formation of a fibrin-platelet hemostatic plug.

Pharmacodynamics

Onset of action: 10-20 minutes

Maximum effect: 6 hours

Pharmacokinetics (Adult data unless noted)

Distribution: V_d: Children: 130 mL/kg; Adults: 103-105 mL/kg (range: 78-139 mL/kg)

Half-life: Elimination: Children: 1.32 hours; Adults: 2.3 hours (range: 1.7-2.7 hours)

Time to peak serum concentration: 15 minutes

Elimination: Clearance: Children: 67 mL/kg/hour; Adults: 30-36 mL/kg/hour (range: 27-49 mL/kg/hour)

Dosing: Usual IV: Children and Adults:

Hemophilia A or B with inhibitors:

Bleeding episodes: 90 mcg/kg every 2 hours until hemostasis is achieved or until the treatment is judged ineffective. The dose and interval may be adjusted based upon the severity of bleeding and the degree of hemostasis achieved. Doses between 35-120 mcg/kg have been used successfully in clinical trials. The dose, interval, and duration of therapy may be adjusted based on severity of bleeding and the degree of hemostasis achieved. For patients treated for joint or muscle bleeds, a decision on the outcome of treatment was reached within 8 doses in the majority of patients, although more doses were required for severe bleeds; adverse effects were reported most commonly in patients treated with 12 or more doses. For patients experiencing severe bleeds to maintain the hemostatic plug, dosing should be continued at 3- to 6-hour intervals; the duration of posthemostatic dosing should be minimized.

Surgical interventions: 90 mcg/kg immediately before surgery; repeat at 2-hour intervals for the duration of surgery. Continue every 2 hours for 48 hours, then every 2-6 hours until healed for minor surgery; continue every 2 hours for 5 days, then every 4 hours until healed for major surgery

Congenital factor VII deficiency: Bleeding episodes and surgical interventions: 15-30 mcg/kg every 4-6 hours until hemostasis is achieved. Doses as low as 10 mcg/kg have been effective; individualized dosing is recommended.

Acquired hemophilia: 70-90 mcg/kg every 2-3 hours until hemostasis is achieved

Preparation for Administration Parenteral: Prior to reconstitution, bring vials to room temperature. Add recommended diluent along wall of vial; do not inject directly onto powder. Gently swirl until dissolved.

NovoSeven RT: Reconstitute each vial to a final concentration of 1 mg/mL using the provided histidine diluent as follows:

1 mg vial: 1.1 mL histidine diluent vial or 1 mL prefilled histidine diluent syringe

2 mg vial: 2.1 mL histidine diluent vial or 2 mL prefilled histidine diluent syringe

5 mg vial: 5.2 mL histidine diluent vial or 5 mL prefilled histidine diluent syringe

8 mg vial: 8.1 mL histidine diluent vial or 8 mL prefilled histidine diluent syringe

Administration Parenteral: IV administration only: Administer as a slow bolus over 2 to 5 minutes (depending on the dose administered). Use NS to flush line (if necessary) before and after administration. Administer within 3 hours after reconstitution.

Monitoring Parameters Monitor for evidence of hemostasis; although the prothrombin time/INR, aPTT, and factor VII clotting activity have no correlation with achieving clinical hemostasis, these parameters may be useful as adjunct tests to evaluate efficacy and guide dose or interval adjustments

Additional Information Each mg factor VIIa contains 0.4 mEq sodium and 0.01 mEq calcium; "off-label" uses in limited patient populations have been reported (primarily adult patients) including reversal of anticoagulant over dose and reduction in bleeding associated with thrombocytopenia, trauma, hepatic dysfunction, and cardiac bypass surgery; further randomized, blinded clinical trials are needed to determine efficacy, dosage, and safety for these indications (Ghorashian, 2004; Tobias, 2004)

Dosage Forms Excipient information presented when available (limited, particularly for generics); consult specific product labeling.

Solution Reconstituted, Intravenous [preservative free]:

NovoSeven RT: 1 mg (1 ea); 2 mg (1 ea); 5 mg (1 ea); 8 mg (1 ea) [contains polysorbate 80]

◆ **Factor VIII Concentrate** *see* Antihemophilic Factor/von Willebrand Factor Complex (Human) *on page 173*

◆ **Factor VIII (Human)** *see* Antihemophilic Factor (Human) *on page 167*

◆ **Factor VIII (Human)/von Willebrand Factor** *see* Antihemophilic Factor/von Willebrand Factor Complex (Human) *on page 173*

◆ **Factor VIII Inhibitor Bypassing Activity** *see* Anti-inhibitor Coagulant Complex (Human) *on page 176*

◆ **Factor VIII (Recombinant)** *see* Antihemophilic Factor (Recombinant) *on page 168*

Factor IX Complex (Human) [(Factors II, IX, X)] (FAK ter nyne KOM pleks HYU man FAKter too nyne ten)

Medication Safety Issues

Sound-alike/look-alike issues:

Factor IX Complex may be confused with Factor IX

Safety concern:

Factor IX Complex may be confused with Factor IX

The term "Prothrombin Complex Concentrate" or "PCC" has been used to describe both Factor IX Complex (Human) [Factors II, IX, X] and Prothrombin Complex Concentrate (Human) [(Factors II, VII, IX, X), Protein C, Protein S]. **Factor IX Complex (Human) [Factors II, IX, X] (Bebulin, Profilnine) contains low or nontherapeutic levels of factor VII component** and should not be confused with Prothrombin Complex Concentrate (Human) [(Factors II, VII, IX, X), Protein C, Protein S] (Kcentra, Octaplex) which contains therapeutic levels of factor VII.

Brand Names: US Bebulin; Bebulin VH; Profilnine SD

Therapeutic Category Antihemophilic Agent; Blood Product Derivative

Generic Availability (US) No

Use Prevention and control of bleeding in patients with factor IX deficiency (hemophilia B or Christmas disease) (Profilnine® SD: FDA approved in ages >16 years and adults; Bebulin® VH: FDA approved in adults)

Pregnancy Risk Factor C

Pregnancy Considerations Animal reproduction studies have not been conducted. Factor IX concentrations do not change significantly in pregnant women with coagulation disorders and women with factor IX deficiency may be at increased risk of postpartum hemorrhage. Pregnant women should have clotting factors monitored, particularly at 28 and 34 weeks gestation and prior to invasive procedures. Prophylaxis may be needed if factor IX concentrations are <50 units/mL at term and treatment should continue for 3-5 days postpartum depending on route of delivery. Because parvovirus infection may cause hydrops fetalis or fetal death, a recombinant product is preferred if prophylaxis or treatment is needed. The neonate may also be at an increased risk of bleeding following delivery and should be tested for the coagulation disorder (Chi, 2012; Kadir, 2009; Lee, 2006).

Contraindications There are no contraindications listed in the manufacturer's labeling.

Warnings/Precautions Factor IX Complex (Human) [Factors II, IX, X] (Bebulin, Profilnine) contains low or nontherapeutic levels of factor VII component and should not be confused with Prothrombin complex concentrate (Human) [(Factors II, VII, IX, X), Protein C, Protein S] (Kcentra, Octaplex) which contains therapeutic levels of factor VII. Factor IX Complex (Human) [Factors II, IX, X] (Bebulin, Profilnine) should not be used for the treatment of factor VII deficiency. When treating warfarin associated hemorrhage (off-label use), administration of additional fresh frozen plasma (FFP) or factor VIIa should be considered. Hypersensitivity and anaphylactic reactions have been reported with use. Delayed reactions (up to 20 days after infusion) in previously untreated patients may also occur. Due to potential for allergic reactions, the initial ~10-20 administrations should be performed under appropriate medical supervision. The development of factor IX antibodies (or inhibitors) has been reported with factor IX therapy (usually occurs within the first 10-20 exposure days); the risk of severe hypersensitivity reactions occurring may be greater in these patients. Patients experiencing allergic reactions should be evaluated for factor IX inhibitors. When clinical response is suboptimal or patient is to undergo surgical procedure, screen for inhibitors. Patients with severe gene defects (eg, gene deletion or inversion) are more likely to develop inhibitors (WFH [Srivastava 2005]).

Observe closely for signs or symptoms of intravascular coagulation or thrombosis. Use with caution when administering to patients with liver disease, postoperatively, neonates, or patients at risk of thromboembolic phenomena, disseminated intravascular coagulation or patients with signs of fibrinolysis due to the potential risk of thromboembolic complications. Use with caution in patients with liver dysfunction; may be at increased risk of developing thrombosis or DIC. Product of human plasma; may potentially contain infectious agents which could transmit disease. Screening of donors, as well as testing and/or inactivation or removal of certain viruses, reduces the risk. Infections thought to be transmitted by this product should be reported to the manufacturer. Some products may contain heparin. Use with caution in patients with a history of heparin-induced thrombocytopenia. Some product packaging may contain natural rubber latex.

Adverse Reactions

Cardiovascular: Flushing, thrombosis (sometimes fatal)

Central nervous system: Chills, fever, headache, lethargy, somnolence

Dermatologic: Rash, urticaria

Gastrointestinal: Nausea, vomiting

Hematologic: DIC

Neuromuscular & skeletal: Paresthesia

Respiratory: Dyspnea

Miscellaneous: Anaphylactic shock, clotting factor antibodies (development of), heparin-induced thrombocytopenia (with products containing heparin)

Drug Interactions

Metabolism/Transport Effects None known.

Avoid Concomitant Use

Avoid concomitant use of Factor IX Complex (Human) [(Factors II, IX, X)] with any of the following: Aminocaproic Acid

Increased Effect/Toxicity

The levels/effects of Factor IX Complex (Human) [(Factors II, IX, X)] may be increased by: Aminocaproic Acid

Decreased Effect There are no known significant interactions involving a decrease in effect.

Storage/Stability

Bebulin® VH: Prior to use, store under refrigeration at 2°C to 8°C (36°F to 46°F); avoid freezing. Following reconstitution, do not refrigerate and use within 3 hours.

Profilnine® SD: Prior to use, store under refrigeration at 2°C to 8°C (36°F to 46°F); avoid freezing; may also stored at room temperature (not to exceed 30°C) for up to 3 months. Following reconstitution, do not refrigerate and use within 3 hours.

Mechanism of Action Replaces deficient clotting factor including factor X; hemophilia B, or Christmas disease, is an X-linked recessively inherited disorder of blood coagulation characterized by insufficient or abnormal synthesis of the clotting protein factor IX. Factor IX is a vitamin K-dependent coagulation factor which is synthesized in the liver. Factor IX is activated by factor XIa in the intrinsic coagulation pathway. Activated factor IX (IXa), in combination with factor VII:C, activates factor X to Xa, resulting ultimately in the conversion of prothrombin to thrombin and the formation of a fibrin clot. The infusion of exogenous factor IX to replace the deficiency present in hemophilia B temporarily restores hemostasis.

Pharmacokinetics (Adult data unless noted) Half-life: Cleared rapidly from the serum in two phases:

First phase: 4-6 hours

Terminal: 22.5 hours

Dosing: Usual

Hemophilia B: Children, Adolescents, and Adults: IV: Dosage is expressed in units of factor IX activity and must be individualized based on severity of factor IX deficiency, extent and location of bleeding, and clinical status of patient (WHF, 2013). When multiple doses are required, administer at 24-hour intervals unless otherwise specified.

Formula for units required to raise blood level %:

Bebulin® VH: In general, 1 unit/kg of factor IX will increase the plasma factor IX level by 0.8%

Number of Factor IX units required = body weight (kg) x desired factor IX increase (as % of normal) x 1.2 units/kg

For example, to increase factor IX level to 25% of normal in a 70 kg patient: Number of factor IX units needed = 70 kg x 25 x 1.2 unit/kg = 2100 units

Profilnine® SD: In general, 1 unit/kg of factor IX will increase the plasma factor IX level by 1%:

Number of factor IX units required = bodyweight (kg) x desired factor IX increase (as % of normal) x 1 unit/kg

For example, to increase factor IX level to 25% of normal in a 70 kg patient: Number of factor IX units needed = 70 kg x 25 x 1 unit/kg = 1750 units

As a general rule, the level of factor IX required for treatment of different conditions is listed below:

Hemorrhage:

Minor bleeding (early hemarthrosis, minor epistaxis, gingival bleeding, mild hematuria):

Bebulin® VH: Raise factor IX level to 20% of normal [typical initial dose: 25-35 units/kg]; generally a single dose is sufficient

Profilnine® SD: Mild to moderate bleeding: Raise factor IX level to 20% to 30% of normal; generally a single dose is sufficient

Moderate bleeding (severe joint bleeding, early hematoma, major open bleeding, minor trauma, minor hemoptysis, hematemesis, melena, major hematuria):

Bebulin® VH: Raise factor IX level to 40% of normal [typical initial dose: 40-55 units/kg]; average duration of treatment is 2 days or until adequate wound healing

Profilnine® SD: Mild to moderate bleeding: Raise factor IX level to 20% to 30% of normal

Major bleeding (severe hematoma, major trauma, severe hemoptysis, hematemesis, melena):

Bebulin® VH: Raise factor IX level to ≥60% of normal [typical initial dose: 60-70 units/kg]; average duration of treatment is 2-3 days or until adequate wound healing. Do not raise >60% in patients who may be predisposed to thrombosis.

Profilnine® SD: Raise factor IX level to 30% to 50% of normal; daily infusions are usually required

Surgical procedures:

Dental surgery:

Bebulin® VH: Raise factor IX level to 40% to 60% of normal on day of surgery [typical dose: 50-60 units/kg]. One infusion, administered 1 hour prior to surgery, is generally sufficient for the extraction of one tooth; for the extraction of multiple teeth, replacement therapy may be required for up to 1 week (see dosing guidelines for Minor Surgery).

Profilnine® SD: Raise factor IX level to 50% of normal immediately prior to procedure; administer additional doses if bleeding recurs

Minor surgery:

Bebulin® VH: Raise factor IX level to 40% to 60% of normal on day of surgery [typical initial dose: 50-60 units/kg]. Decrease factor IX level from 40% of normal to 20% of normal during initial postoperative period (1-2 weeks or until adequate wound healing) [typical dose: 55 units/kg decreasing to 25 units/kg]. The preoperative dose should be given 1 hour prior to surgery. The average dosing interval may be every 12 hours initially, then every 24 hours later in the postoperative period.

Profilnine® SD: Raise factor IX level to 30% to 50% of normal for at least 1 week following surgery

Major surgery:

Bebulin® VH: Raise factor IX level to ≥60% of normal on day of surgery [typical initial dose: 70-95 units/kg]; do not raise >60% in patients who may be predisposed to thrombosis. Decrease factor IX level from 60% of normal to 20% of normal during initial postoperative period (1-2 weeks) [typical dose: 70 units/kg decreasing to 35 units/kg]; further decrease to maintain a factor IX level of 20% of normal during late postoperative period (≥3 weeks) and continuing until adequate wound healing is achieved [typical dose: 35 units/kg decreasing to 25 units/kg]. The preoperative dose should be given 1 hour prior to surgery. The average dosing interval may be every 12 hours initially, then every 24 hours later in the postoperative period.

Profilnine® SD: Raise factor IX level to 30% to 50% of normal for at least 1 week following surgery

Prophylaxis, hemorrhage (long-term management): Bebulin® VH: 20-30 units/kg/dose once or twice a week may reduce frequency of spontaneous hemorrhage; dosing regimen should be individualized.

Preparation for Administration Parenteral: Bring diluent and concentrate to room temperature; gently rotate or agitate to dissolve.

Bebulin VH: Prior to reconstitution, warm both diluent (SWFI) and concentrate vials to room temperature (but not above 37°C [98.6°F]). Using the supplied double ended needle, insert one end into the diluent stopper. Invert diluent vial over concentrate vial and insert remaining needle into concentrate stopper. Diluent will be drawn into the concentrate vial by vacuum. Disconnect the 2 vials by removing the needle from the concentrate vial. Gently agitate or rotate the concentrate vial until dissolved. After reconstitution, attach the enclosed filter needle to a sterile syringe. Inject appropriate amount of air into vial, invert vial, and withdraw concentrate solution. Remove and discard filter needle. Attach appropriate IV needle or infusion set winged adapter.

Profilnine SD:

Prior to reconstitution, allow diluent (SWFI) and concentrate vials to warm to room temperature (but not above 37°C [98.6°F]). Aseptically push the plastic spike at the blue end of the Mix2Vial transfer set through the center of the stopper of the diluent vial. After carefully removing only the clear package from the Mix2Vial transfer set, invert the diluent vial with the transfer set still attached and push the plastic spike through the center of the stopper of concentrate vial; diluent will automatically transfer. While still attached, gently swirl concentrate vial to ensure product is dissolved; do not shake. Disconnect the 2 vials; contents of concentrate vial are now available for removal by screwing a syringe onto the transfer set. Inject appropriate amount of air into vial, invert vial, and withdraw amount needed. Remove syringe from transfer set and attach an administration set to the syringe. **Note:** If more than one vial of concentrate is to be administered to the same patient, then contents of 2 vials may be drawn into the same syringe through a separate unused Mix2Vial set before attaching administration set.

After reconstitution, parenteral drug products should be inspected for particulate matter and discoloration prior to administration, whenever solution and container permit. When reconstitution process is strictly followed, a few small particles may occasionally remain. The Mix2-Vial set will remove particles and the labeled potency will not be reduced.

Administration Parenteral: IV administration only. Visually inspect for particulate matter and discoloration prior to administration whenever permitted by solution or container. Infuse slowly; rate of administration should be individualized for patient's comfort; rapid IV administration may cause vasomotor reactions; maximum rates of administration: Bebulin VH: 2 mL/minute; Profilnine SD: 10 mL/minute; **Note:** Slowing the rate of infusion, changing the lot of medication, or administering antihistamines may relieve some adverse reactions.

Monitoring Parameters Levels of factors II, IX, and X; signs/symptoms of hypersensitivity reactions and bleeding; hemoglobin, hematocrit; screen for factor IX inhibitors by measuring inhibitor titers (children: Every 3-12 months or 10-20 exposure days)

Reference Range Patients with severe hemophilia will have factor IX levels <1%, often undetectable. Moderate forms of the disease have levels of 1% to 5% while some mild cases may have 5% to 49% of normal factor IX. Plasma concentration is about 4 mg/L.

Dosage Forms Considerations

Strengths expressed as an approximate value. Consult individual vial labels for exact potency within each vial.

Bebulin VH packaged contents may contain natural rubber latex.

Dosage Forms Excipient information presented when available (limited, particularly for generics); consult specific product labeling.

Solution Reconstituted, Intravenous:

Bebulin: 200-1200 units (1 ea)

Bebulin VH: 200-1200 units (1 ea)

Profilnine SD: 500 units (1 ea); 1000 units (1 ea); 1500 units (1 ea) [contains polysorbate 80]

◆ **Factor Eight Inhibitor Bypassing Activity** *see* Anti-inhibitor Coagulant Complex (Human) *on page 176*

Factor IX (Human) (FAK ter nyne HYU man)

Medication Safety Issues

Sound-alike/look-alike issues:

Factor IX may be confused with Factor IX Complex

Brand Names: US AlphaNine SD; Mononine

Brand Names: Canada Immunine VH

Therapeutic Category Antihemophilic Agent; Blood Product Derivative

Generic Availability (US) No

Use

AlphaNine SD: Prevention and control of bleeding in factor IX deficiency (hemophilia B or Christmas disease) (FDA approved in ages ≥16 years and adults)

Mononine: Prevention and control of bleeding in factor IX deficiency (hemophilia B or Christmas disease) (FDA approved in all ages)

NOTE: Contains **nondetectable levels of factors II, VII, and X**; therefore, **NOT INDICATED** for replacement therapy of any other clotting factor besides factor IX or for reversal of anticoagulation due to either vitamin K antagonists or other anticoagulants (eg, dabigatran), for hemophilia A patients with factor VIII inhibitors, or for patients in a hemorrhagic state caused by reduced production of liver-dependent coagulation factors (eg, hepatitis, cirrhosis).

Pregnancy Risk Factor C

Pregnancy Considerations Animal reproduction studies have not been conducted. Factor IX concentrations do not change significantly in pregnant women with coagulation disorders and women with factor IX deficiency may be at increased risk of postpartum hemorrhage. Pregnant women should have clotting factors monitored, particularly at 28 and 34 weeks gestation and prior to invasive procedures. Prophylaxis may be needed if factor IX concentrations are <50 units/mL at term and treatment should continue for 3 to 5 days postpartum depending on route of delivery. Because parvovirus infection may cause hydrops fetalis or fetal death, a recombinant product is preferred if prophylaxis or treatment is needed. The neonate may also be at an increased risk of bleeding following delivery and should be tested for the coagulation disorder (Chi, 2012; Kadir, 2009; Lee, 2006).

Contraindications

AlphaNine SD: There are no contraindications listed in the manufacturer's labeling.

Mononine: Hypersensitivity to mouse protein

Warnings/Precautions Hypersensitivity and anaphylactic reactions have been reported with use. Delayed reactions (up to 20 days after infusion) in previously untreated patients may also occur. Due to potential for allergic reactions, the initial ~10 to 20 administrations should be performed under appropriate medical supervision. Hypersensitivity reactions may be associated with factor IX inhibitor development; patients experiencing allergic reactions should be evaluated for factor IX inhibitors (WFH [Srivastava 2013]). The development of factor IX antibodies (or inhibitors) has been reported with factor IX therapy (usually occurs within the first 10 to 20 exposure days); the risk of severe hypersensitivity reactions occurring may be greater in these patients. When clinical response is suboptimal, the patient has reached a specified number of exposure days, or patient is to undergo surgical procedure, screen for inhibitors. Patients with severe hemophilia compared to those with mild or moderate hemophilia are more likely to develop inhibitors (WFH [Srivastava 2013]).

Observe closely for signs or symptoms of intravascular coagulation or thrombosis; risk is generally associated with the use of factor IX complex concentrates (containing therapeutic amounts of additional factors); however, potential risk exists with use of factor IX products (containing only factor IX). Use with caution when administering to patients with liver disease, postoperatively, neonates, or patients at risk of thromboembolic phenomena, disseminated intravascular coagulation or patients with signs of fibrinolysis due to the potential risk of thromboembolic complications.

Some dosage forms may contain polysorbate 80 (also known as Tweens). Hypersensitivity reactions, usually a delayed reaction, have been reported following exposure to pharmaceutical products containing polysorbate 80 in certain individuals (Isaksson, 2002; Lucente 2000; Shelley, 1995). Thrombocytopenia, ascites, pulmonary deterioration, and renal and hepatic failure have been reported in premature neonates after receiving parenteral products containing polysorbate 80 (Alade, 1986; CDC, 1984). See manufacturer's labeling.

Contains **nondetectable levels of factors II, VII, and X**. Therefore, **NOT INDICATED** for replacement therapy of any other clotting factor besides factor IX. In addition, factor IX concentrate is **NOT INDICATED** for reversal of anticoagulation due to either vitamin K antagonists or other anticoagulants (eg, dabigatran), hemophilia A patients with factor VIII inhibitors, or patients in a hemorrhagic state caused by reduced production of liver-dependent coagulation factors (eg, hepatitis, cirrhosis). Product of human plasma; despite purification methods (AlphaNine SD - solvent detergent treated/virus filtered; Mononine - virus filtered); products may potentially contain infectious agents which could transmit disease. Screening of donors, as well as testing and/or inactivation or removal of certain viruses, reduces the risk. Infections thought to be transmitted by this product should be reported to the manufacturer. Safety and efficacy have not been established with factor IX products in immune tolerance induction. Nephrotic syndrome has occurred following immune tolerance induction in patients with factor IX inhibitors and a history of allergic reactions to therapy.

Warnings: Additional Pediatric Considerations Use with caution when administering to neonates; the safety and efficacy of continuous infusion administration has not been established; thrombotic events have been reported in patients receiving continuous infusion of recombinant Factor IX through a central venous catheter, including life-threatening superior vena cava syndrome in neonates.

Adverse Reactions

Cardiovascular: Flushing, thrombosis

Central nervous system: Burning sensation (in jaw/skull), chills, headache, lethargy, paresthesia, rigors

Dermatologic: Skin photosensitivity, urticaria

Gastrointestinal: Diarrhea, nausea, vomiting

Hematologic & oncologic: Disseminated intravascular coagulation

Hepatic: Increased serum alkaline phosphatase, increased serum ALT, increased serum AST

Hypersensitivity: Anaphylaxis, hypersensitivity reaction

Local: Discomfort at injection site (stinging, burning), injection site reaction, pain at injection site

Neuromuscular & skeletal: Neck tightness

Ophthalmic: Visual disturbance

Respiratory: Allergic rhinitis, asthma, laryngeal edema, pulmonary disease

Miscellaneous: Fever (including transient fever following rapid administration)

Rare, but important or life-threatening: Cerebral hemorrhage (intrathalamic [Douvas, 2004]), cyanosis, decreased therapeutic response, factor IX inhibitor development, hypotension, myocardial infarction (high doses), pulmonary embolism (high doses), superior vena cava syndrome (neonates [Douvas, 2004])

Drug Interactions

Metabolism/Transport Effects None known.

Avoid Concomitant Use

Avoid concomitant use of Factor IX (Human) with any of the following: Aminocaproic Acid

Increased Effect/Toxicity
The levels/effects of Factor IX (Human) may be increased by: Aminocaproic Acid

Decreased Effect There are no known significant interactions involving a decrease in effect.

Storage/Stability When stored at refrigerator temperature, 2°C to 8°C (36°F to 46°F), factor IX is stable for the period indicated by the expiration date on its label. Avoid freezing which may damage container for the diluent.

AlphaNine SD: May also be stored at room temperature not to exceed 30°C (86°F) for up to 1 month. Reconstituted solution should be used within 3 hours of preparation.

Mononine: May also be stored at room temperature not to exceed 25°C (77°F) for up to 1 month. Reconstituted solution should be at room temperature and used within 3 hours of preparation.

Mechanism of Action Replaces deficient clotting factor IX. Hemophilia B, or Christmas disease, is an X-linked inherited disorder of blood coagulation characterized by insufficient or abnormal synthesis of the clotting protein factor IX. Factor IX is a vitamin K-dependent coagulation factor which is synthesized in the liver. Factor IX is activated by factor XIa in the intrinsic coagulation pathway. Activated factor IX (IXa), in combination with factor VII:C activates factor X to Xa, resulting ultimately in the conversion of prothrombin to thrombin and the formation of a fibrin clot. The infusion of exogenous factor IX to replace the deficiency present in hemophilia B temporarily restores hemostasis.

Pharmacokinetics (Adult data unless noted) Half-life: Factor IX component: ~21-25 hours

Dosing: Neonatal Note: Contains **nondetectable levels of factors II, VII, and X**; therefore, **NOT INDICATED** for replacement therapy of any other clotting factor besides factor IX or for reversal of anticoagulation due to either vitamin K antagonists or other anticoagulants (eg, dabigatran), for hemophilia A patients with factor VIII inhibitors, or for patients in a hemorrhagic state caused by reduced production of liver-dependent coagulation factors (eg, hepatitis, cirrhosis).

Control or prevention of bleeding in patients with factor IX deficiency (hemophilia B or Christmas disease): IV: Dosage is expressed in units of factor IX activity and must be individualized based on formulation, severity of factor IX deficiency, extent and location of bleed, and clinical situation of patient.

Formula for units required to raise blood level:

Mononine:

Number of Factor IX Units Required = body weight (in kg) x desired Factor IX level increase (% or units/dL) x 1 unit/kg

For example, for a 100% level in a 3 kg patient who has an actual level of 20%: Number of Factor IX Units needed = 3 kg x 80% x 1 unit/kg = 240 units

Intermittent IV: Desired Factor IX level, dosing interval, and duration based on hemorrhage type:

Minor hemorrhage (eg, bruising, cuts/scrapes, uncomplicated joint hemorrhage)/Prophylaxis:
- Desired factor IX levels (% or units/dL): 15 to 25
- Frequency of dosing: Every 24 hours
- Duration of treatment: 1 to 2 days

Major trauma or surgery:
- Desired factor IX levels (% or units/dL): 25 to 50
- Frequency of dosing: Every 18 to 30 hours; interval dependent upon half-life and measured factor IX levels
- Duration of treatment: Up to 10 days depending on nature of insult

Dosing: Usual NOTE: Contains **nondetectable levels of factors II, VII, and X**; therefore, **NOT INDICATED** for replacement therapy of any other clotting factor besides factor IX or for reversal of anticoagulation due to either vitamin K antagonists or other anticoagulants (eg, dabigatran), for hemophilia A patients with factor VIII inhibitors, or for patients in a hemorrhagic state caused by reduced production of liver-dependent coagulation factors (eg, hepatitis, cirrhosis).

Pediatric:

Control or prevention of bleeding in patients with factor IX deficiency (hemophilia B or Christmas disease): Infants, Children, and Adolescents: IV: Dosage is expressed in units of factor IX activity and must be individualized based on formulation, severity of factor IX deficiency, extent and location of bleed, and clinical situation of patient.

Formula for units required to raise blood level:

Number of Factor IX Units Required = body weight (in kg) x desired Factor IX level increase (% or units/dL) x 1 unit/kg

For example, for a 100% level in a 25 kg patient who has an actual level of 20%: Number of Factor IX Units needed = 25 kg x 80% x 1 unit/kg = 2000 units

Manufacturer's labeling: AlphaNine SD, Mononine: Infants, Children, and Adolescents: Intermittent IV:

Desired Factor IX Level, Dosing Interval and Duration based on Hemorrhage Type:

Minor hemorrhage (eg, bruising, cuts/scrapes, uncomplicated joint hemorrhage):
- Desired factor IX levels (% or units/dL): 15 to 30
- Frequency of dosing: Every 12 to 24 hours
- Duration of treatment: 1 to 2 days

Moderate hemorrhage (eg, epistaxis, oropharyngeal bleeds, dental extractions, hematuria):
- Desired factor IX levels (% or units/dL): 25 to 50
- Frequency of dosing: Every 12 to 24 hours
- Duration of treatment: 2 to 7 days

Major hemorrhage [eg, joint and muscle (especially large muscles) hemorrhage, intracranial or intraperitoneal hemorrhage], major trauma, or surgical prophylaxis:
- Desired factor IX levels (% or units/dL): 50 to 100 (depending on the clinical situation, desired Factor IX level may be reduced following active treatment period for hemorrhage or >48 hours postop)
- Frequency of dosing: Every 12 to 24 hours (AlphaNine SD) or 18 to 30 hours (Mononine), interval dependent upon product used, half-life, and measured factor IX levels (after 3 to 5 days, maintain at least 20% activity)
- Duration of treatment: 7 to 10 days, depending upon nature of insult

Alternate dosing: **Note:** The following recommendations reflect general dosing requirements; may vary from those found within prescribing information or practitioner preference:

Prophylaxis, primary: Infants, Children, and Adolescents: IV: 15 to 30 units/kg twice weekly (WFH guidelines [Srivastava 2013] [Utrecht protocol]) **or** 25 to 40 units/kg twice weekly [WFH guidelines (Srivastava 2013) (Malmö protocol)] **or** 40 to 100 units/kg 2 to 3 times weekly (National Hemophilia Foundation, MASAC recommendation 2007); however, the optimum regimen has yet to be defined.

Hemorrhage, treatment (when no significant resource constraints exist) [WFH guidelines (Srivastava 2013)]: **Note:** Factor IX level may either be expressed as units/dL or as %. Dosing frequency most commonly corresponds to the half-life of factor IX but should be determined based on an assessment of factor IX levels before the next dose. Infants, Children, and Adolescents:

Intermittent IV: Desired Factor IX Level to Maintain and Duration Based on Site of Hemorrhage/Clinical Situation:

Joint: 40 to 60 units/dL for 1-2 days, may be longer if response is inadequate

Superficial muscle (no neurovascular compromise): 40 to 60 units/dL for 2-3 days, sometimes longer if response is inadequate

Iliopsoas and deep muscle with neurovascular injury, or substantial blood loss: Initial: 60 to 80 units/dL for 1 to 2 days; Maintenance: 30 to 60 units/dL for 3 to 5 days, sometimes longer as secondary prophylaxis during physiotherapy

CNS/head: Initial: 60 to 80 units/dL for 1 to 7 days; Maintenance: 30 units/dL for 8 to 21 days

Throat and neck: Initial: 60 to 80 units/dL for 1 to 7 days; Maintenance: 30 units/dL for 8 to 14 days

Gastrointestinal: Initial: 60 to 80 units/dL for 7 to 14 days; Maintenance: 30 units/dL (duration not specified)

Renal: 40 units/dL for 3 to 5 days

Deep laceration: 40 units/dL for 5 to 7 days

Surgery (major):

Preop: 60 to 80 units/dL

Postop: 40 to 60 units/dL for 1 to 3 days, then 30 to 50 units/dL for 4 to 6 days, then 20 to 40 units/dL for 7 to 14 days

Surgery (minor):

Preop: 50 to 80 units/dL

Postop: 30 to 80 units/dL for 1 to 5 days depending on procedure type

Continuous IV infusion: Very limited data available; only data with Mononine product available: **Note:** Used for patients who require prolonged periods of treatment (eg, intracranial hemorrhage or surgery) to avoid peaks and troughs associated with intermittent infusions [Batorova 2002; Hoots 2003; Morfini 2008; Poon 2012; WFH guidelines (Srivastava 2013)]:

Following initial bolus to achieve the desired factor IX level: Initial dosing: 4 to 6 units/kg/hour; adjust dose based on frequent factor IX assays and calculation of factor IX clearance at steady-state using the following equations:

Factor IX clearance (mL/kg/hour) = (current infusion rate in units/kg/hour)/(plasma Factor IX level in units/**mL**)

New infusion rate (units/kg/hour) = (factor IX clearance in mL/kg/hour) x (desired plasma level in units/**mL**)

The median reported dose in post-operative patients (7-85 years) was 3.84 units/kg/hour (range: 1.74 to 7.3 units/kg/hour) (Hoots 2003)

Adult: **Control or prevention of bleeding in patients with factor IX deficiency (hemophilia B or Christmas disease):** IV: AlphaNine SD, Mononine: Dosage is expressed in units of factor IX activity; dosing must be individualized based on severity of factor IX deficiency, extent and location of bleeding, and clinical status of patient. Refer to product information for specific manufacturer recommended dosing. Alternatively, the WFH has recommended general dosing for factor IX products.

Formula for units required to raise blood level: **Note**: If patient has severe hemophilia (ie, baseline factor IX level is or presumed to be <1%), then may just use "desired factor IX level" instead of "desired factor IX level increase".

Number of factor IX units required = patient weight (in kg) x desired factor IX level increase (as % or units/dL) x 1 unit/kg

For example, to attain an 80% level in a 70 kg patient who has a baseline level of 20%: Number of factor IX units needed = 70 kg x 60% x 1 unit/kg = 4,200 units

WFH guidelines (Srivastava 2013): **Note:** The following recommendations may vary from those found within prescribing information or practitioner preference.

Prophylaxis: IV: 15 to 30 units/kg twice weekly [WFH guidelines (Srivastava 2013) (Utrecht protocol)] **or** 25 to 40 units/kg twice weekly [WFH guidelines (Srivastava 2013) (Malmö protocol)] **or** 40 to 100 units/kg administered 2 to 3 times weekly (National Hemophilia Foundation, MASAC recommendation 2007); optimum regimen has yet to be defined.

Treatment:

Intermittent IV: 2013 World Federation of Hemophilia Treatment Recommendations (When No Significant Resource Constraint Exists): **Note:** Factor IX level may either be expressed as units/dL or as %. Dosing frequency most commonly corresponds to the half-life of factor IX but should be determined based on an assessment of factor IX levels before the next dose.

Desired Factor IX Level to Maintain and Duration Based on Site of Hemorrhage/Clinical Situation:

Joint: 40 to 60 units/dL for 1 to 2 days, may be longer if response is inadequate

Superficial muscle (no neurovascular compromise): 40 to 60 units/dL for 2 to 3 days, sometimes longer if response is inadequate

Iliopsoas and deep muscle with neurovascular injury, or substantial blood loss: Initial: 60 to 80 units/dL for 1 to 2 days; Maintenance: 30 to 60 units/dL for 3 to 5 days, sometimes longer as secondary prophylaxis during physiotherapy

CNS/head: Initial: 60 to 80 units/dL for 1 to 7 days; Maintenance: 30 units/dL for 8 to 21 days

Throat and neck: Initial: 60 to 80 units/dL for 1 to 7 days; Maintenance: 30 units/dL for 8 to 14 days

Gastrointestinal: Initial: 60 to 80 units/dL for 7 to 14 days; Maintenance: 30 units/dL (duration not specified)

Renal: 40 units/dL for 3 to 5 days

Deep laceration: 40 units/dL for 5 to 7 days

Surgery (major):

Preop: 60 to 80 units/dL

Postop: 40 to 60 units/dL for 1 to 3 days, then 30 to 50 units/dL for 4 to 6 days, then 20 to 40 units/dL for 7 to 14 days

Surgery (minor):

Preop: 50 to 80 units/dL

Postop: 30 to 80 units/dL for 1 to 5 days depending on procedure type

Continuous IV infusion: **Note:** For patients who require prolonged periods of treatment (eg, intracranial hemorrhage or surgery) to avoid peaks and troughs associated with intermittent infusion [Batorova 2002; Poon 2012; Rickard 1995; WFH guidelines (Srivastava 2013)]: Following initial bolus to achieve the desired factor IX level: Initiate 4 to 6 units/kg/hour; adjust dose based on frequent factor assays and calculation of factor IX clearance at steady-state using the following equations:

Factor IX clearance (mL/kg/hour) = (current infusion rate in units/kg/hour) divided by (plasma level in units/**mL**)

New infusion rate (units/kg/hour) = (factor IX clearance in mL/kg/hour) x (desired plasma level in units/**mL**)

Preparation for Administration

IV bolus: Refer to instructions for individual products. Exact potency labeled on each vial. Diluent and factor IX should come to room temperature before combining.

Continuous IV infusion: Mononine: Reconstitute to 100 units/mL; may be further diluted in NS to either 5 units/mL or 10 units/mL. The preparation of solution for infusion is dependent upon prescriber discretion and should be replaced every 12 hours (Hoots 2003).

Administration Solution should be infused at room temperature. With patients who have had allergic reactions during factor IX infusion, administration of hydrocortisone prior to infusion may be necessary [WFH guidelines (Srivastava 2013)].

IV bolus: Should be infused **slowly over several minutes**: Rate of administration should be determined by the response and comfort of the patient.

AlphaNine SD: Administer IV at a rate not exceeding 10 mL/minute

Mononine: Administer IV at a rate of ~2 mL/minute. Administration rates of up to 225 **units**/minute have been regularly tolerated without incident (when reconstituted as directed to ~100 units/mL).

WFH recommendations (Srivastava 2013): Infuse at a rate determined by age: Young children: 100 **units**/minute; Adults: 3 mL/minute

Continuous IV infusion: In an open-label, multicenter trial (age range: 7 to 85 years), Mononine was administered as a continuous infusion either as the reconstituted solution or further diluted. The preparation of solution for infusion is dependent upon prescriber discretion and should be replaced every 12 hours (Hoots 2003).

Monitoring Parameters Factor IX levels [measure 15 minutes after infusion to verify calculated doses [WFH guidelines (Srivastava 2013)], aPTT, BP, HR, signs of hypersensitivity reactions; screen for factor IX inhibitors if the patient experiences hypersensitivity reaction or when patient is to undergo surgery, if suboptimal response to treatment occurs, if patient is being intensively treated for >5 days within 4 weeks of the last infusion, or at the following intervals [WFH guidelines (Srivastava 2013)]:

Children: Screen for inhibitors every 5 exposure days until 20 exposure days, every 10 exposure days between 21-50 exposure days, and at a minimum of twice a year until 150 exposure days is reached.

Adults (with >150 exposure days apart from a 6-12 monthly review): Screen for inhibitors when suboptimal response occurs.

Reference Range Average normal factor IX levels are 50% to 150%; patients with severe hemophilia B will have levels <1%, often undetectable. Moderate forms of the disease have levels of 1% to 5% while some mild cases may have 5% to 49% of normal factor IX.

Additional Information In absence of inhibitors, 1 unit/kg factor IX human administered will increase plasma factor IX level by 1 unit/dL [WFH guidelines (Srivastava, 2013)].

Dosage Forms Considerations Strengths expressed with approximate values. Consult individual vial labels for exact potency within each vial.

Dosage Forms Excipient information presented when available (limited, particularly for generics); consult specific product labeling.

Solution Reconstituted, Intravenous [preservative free]:

AlphaNine SD: 500 units (1 ea); 1000 units (1 ea); 1500 units (1 ea) [contains polysorbate 80]

Mononine: 250 units (1 ea); 500 units (1 ea); 1000 units (1 ea) [contains polysorbate 80]

Factor IX (Recombinant)

(FAK ter nyne ree KOM be nant)

Medication Safety Issues

Sound-alike/look-alike issues:

Factor IX may be confused with Factor IX Complex

Brand Names: US Alprolix; BeneFIX; Ixinity; Rixubis

Brand Names: Canada BeneFix

Therapeutic Category Antihemophilic Agent

Generic Availability (US) Yes

Use

BeneFIX: Prevention and control of bleeding in patients with hemophilia B (congenital factor IX deficiency or Christmas disease); perioperative management in patients with hemophilia B [All indications: FDA approved in pediatric patients (age not specified) and adults]

Rixubis: Prevention and control of bleeding episodes in patients with hemophilia B (congenital factor IX deficiency or Christmas disease); perioperative management in patients with hemophilia B; routine prophylaxis to prevent or reduce the frequency of bleeding episodes in patients with hemophilia B (All indications: FDA approved in adults)

NOTE: Contains **only factor IX**. Therefore, **NOT INDICATED** for replacement therapy of any other clotting factor besides factor IX or for reversal of anticoagulation due to either vitamin K antagonists or other anticoagulants (eg, dabigatran), for hemophilia A patients with factor VIII inhibitors, or for patients in a hemorrhagic state caused by reduced production of liver-dependent coagulation factors (eg, hepatitis, cirrhosis).

Pregnancy Risk Factor C

Pregnancy Considerations Animal reproduction studies have not been conducted. Factor IX concentrations do not change significantly in pregnant women with coagulation disorders and women with factor IX deficiency may be at increased risk of postpartum hemorrhage. Pregnant women should have clotting factors monitored, particularly at 28 and 34 weeks gestation and prior to invasive procedures. Prophylaxis may be needed if factor IX concentrations are <50 units/mL at term and treatment should continue for 3 to 5 days postpartum depending on route of delivery. Because parvovirus infection may cause hydrops fetalis or fetal death, a recombinant product is preferred if prophylaxis or treatment is needed. The neonate may also be at an increased risk of bleeding following delivery and should be tested for the coagulation disorder (Chi, 2012; Kadir, 2009; Lee, 2006).

Breast-Feeding Considerations It is not known if factor IX (recombinant) is excreted in breast milk. The manufacturer recommends that caution be exercised when administering factor IX (recombinant) to nursing women.

Contraindications Life-threatening, immediate hypersensitivity reactions (including anaphylaxis) to factor IX, hamster protein (BeneFix, Ixinity, and Rixubis), or any component of the formulation; disseminated intravascular coagulation (Rixubis); signs of fibrinolysis (Rixubis)

Warnings/Precautions Contains **only factor IX**. Therefore, **NOT INDICATED** for replacement therapy of any other clotting factor besides factor IX or for reversal of anticoagulation due to either vitamin K antagonists or other anticoagulants (eg, dabigatran), for hemophilia A patients with factor VIII inhibitors, or for patients in a hemorrhagic state caused by reduced production of liver-dependent coagulation factors (eg, hepatitis, cirrhosis).

Hypersensitivity and anaphylactic reactions have been reported with use. Risk is highest during the early phases of initial exposure in previously untreated patients, especially those with high-risk gene mutations. Delayed reactions (up to 20 days after infusion) in previously untreated patients may also occur. Due to potential for allergic reactions, the initial ~10 to 20 administrations should be performed under appropriate medical supervision. Hypersensitivity reactions may be associated with factor IX inhibitor development; patients experiencing allergic reactions should be evaluated for factor IX inhibitors (WFH [Srivastava 2013]). If severe hypersensitivity reactions occur, consider the use of alternative hemostatic measures.

The development of factor IX antibodies (or inhibitors) has been reported with factor IX therapy (usually occurs within the first 10 to 20 exposure days); the risk of severe hypersensitivity reactions occurring may be greater in these patients. When clinical response is suboptimal, the patient has reached a specified number of exposure days, or patient is to undergo surgical procedure, screen for inhibitors. Patients with severe hemophilia compared to those with mild or moderate hemophilia are more likely to develop inhibitors (WFH [Srivastava 2013]).

Observe closely for signs or symptoms of intravascular coagulation or thrombosis; risk is generally associated with the use of factor IX complex concentrates (containing therapeutic amounts of additional factors); however, potential risk exists with use of factor IX products (containing only factor IX) especially when administered as a continuous infusion through a central venous catheter. Use with caution when administering to patients with liver disease, postoperatively, neonates, patients at risk of thromboembolic phenomena or disseminated intravascular coagulation, or patients with signs of fibrinolysis due to the potential risk of thromboembolic complications.

Safety and efficacy have not been established with factor IX products in immune tolerance induction. Nephrotic syndrome has occurred following immune tolerance induction in patients with factor IX inhibitors and a history of allergic reactions to therapy.

Warnings: Additional Pediatric Considerations Use with caution when administering to neonates; the safety and efficacy of continuous infusion administration has not been established; thrombotic events have been reported in patients receiving continuous infusion of recombinant Factor IX through a central venous catheter, including life-threatening superior vena cava syndrome in neonates.

Adverse Reactions

Cardiovascular: Chest tightness, flushing, thromboembolic complications, thromboembolism

Central nervous system: Apathy, chills, depression, dizziness, drowsiness, headache, lethargy

Dermatologic: Pruritic rash, skin rash, urticaria

Gastrointestinal: Dysgeusia, nausea, oral paresthesia, vomiting

Hematologic & oncologic: Hemophilia

Hypersensitivity: Hypersensitivity reaction

Immunologic: Antibody development

Infection: Influenza

Local: Cellulitis at injection site, discomfort at injection site, injection site phlebitis, injection site reaction, pain at injection site

Neuromuscular & skeletal: Limb pain, tremor, weakness

Ophthalmic: Blurred vision

Renal: Renal infarction

Respiratory: Cough, dyspnea, hypoxia

Miscellaneous: Fever

Rare but important or life-threatening: Anaphylaxis, hypotension, nephrotic syndrome (associated with immune tolerance induction), obstructive uropathy, palpitations, superior vena cava syndrome (neonates)

Drug Interactions

Metabolism/Transport Effects None known.

Avoid Concomitant Use

Avoid concomitant use of Factor IX (Recombinant) with any of the following: Aminocaproic Acid

Increased Effect/Toxicity

The levels/effects of Factor IX (Recombinant) may be increased by: Aminocaproic Acid

Decreased Effect There are no known significant interactions involving a decrease in effect.

Storage/Stability

Alprolix: Store at 2°C to 8°C (36°F to 46°F); do not freeze. May be stored at room temperature (not to exceed 30°C [86°F]) for up to 6 months. After removal from refrigeration, do not return to refrigerator. Following reconstitution, may be stored at room temperature (not to exceed 30°C [86°F]) for no longer than 3 hours. Protect from direct sunlight.

BeneFIX:

Product labeled for room temperature storage: May either store at 2°C to 30°C (36°F to 86°F) or refrigerated at 2°C to 8°C (36°F to 46°F). Avoid freezing which may damage the diluent syringe. Reconstituted solution should be at room temperature and used within 3 hours of preparation.

Product labeled for refrigerated storage: Store at 2°C to 8°C (36°F to 46°F). May be stored at room temperature (not to exceed 30°C [86°F]) for up to 6 months; do not use after this 6-month period has elapsed even if the expiration date on the carton has not been exceeded. If date of removal from refrigeration is not recorded on the carton, the assigned expiration date (printed on the end flap of the carton) **must be reduced by 12 months**. Avoid freezing which may damage the diluent syringe. Reconstituted solution should be at room temperature and used within 3 hours of preparation.

Ixinity: Store at 2°C to 25°C (36°F to 77°F). Do not freeze. Keep vial in the carton and protect from light. Infuse reconstituted solution immediately or within 3 hours when stored at room temperature. Do not refrigerate after reconstitution.

Rixubis: Store at 2°C to 8°C (36°F to 46°F) for up to 24 months; do not freeze. May store at room temperature not to exceed 30°C (86°F) for up to 12 months within the 24-month time period; do not return to refrigerator.

Mechanism of Action Replaces deficient clotting factor IX. Hemophilia B, or Christmas disease, is an X-linked inherited disorder of blood coagulation characterized by insufficient or abnormal synthesis of the clotting protein factor IX. Factor IX is a vitamin K-dependent coagulation factor which is synthesized in the liver. Factor IX is activated by factor XIa in the intrinsic coagulation pathway. Activated factor IX (IXa) in combination with factor VII:C activates factor X to Xa, resulting ultimately in the conversion of prothrombin to thrombin and the formation of a fibrin clot. The infusion of exogenous factor IX to replace the deficiency present in hemophilia B temporarily restores hemostasis.

Pharmacokinetics (Adult data unless noted)

Half-life elimination:

BeneFIX:

Children ≥2 years and Adolescents ≤15 years: 14 to 28 hours

Adolescents ≥16 years and Adults: 11 to 36 hours

Rixubis: Adolescents ≥15 years and Adults: 16 to 52 hours

Dosing: Neonatal NOTE: Contains **only factor IX**. Therefore, **NOT INDICATED** for replacement therapy of any other clotting factor besides factor IX or for reversal of anticoagulation due to either vitamin K antagonists or other anticoagulants (eg, dabigatran), for hemophilia A patients with factor VIII inhibitors, or for patients in a hemorrhagic state caused by reduced production of liver-dependent coagulation factors (eg, hepatitis, cirrhosis).

Control or prevention of bleeding in patients with factor IX deficiency (hemophilia B or Christmas disease): IV: Dosage is expressed in units of factor IX activity and must be individualized based on formulation, severity of factor IX deficiency, extent and location of bleed, and clinical situation of patient.

Formula for units required to raise blood level:

BeneFIX:

Number of Factor IX Units Required = body weight (in kg) x desired factor IX level increase (% or units/dL) x 1.4 units/kg per units/dL

For example, for a 100% level in a 3 kg patient who has an actual level of 20%: Number of Factor IX Units needed = 3 kg x 80% x 1.4 units/kg per units/dL = 336 units

Intermittent IV: Desired factor IX level, dosing interval and duration based on hemorrhage type:

Minor hemorrhage (uncomplicated joint hemorrhage, superficial muscle, or soft tissue):

Desired factor IX levels (% or units/dL): 20 to 30

Frequency of dosing: Every 12 to 24 hours

Duration of treatment: 1 to 2 days

Moderate hemorrhage (intramuscular or soft tissue with dissection, mucous membrane, dental extractions, or hematuria):

Desired factor IX levels (% or units/dL): 25 to 50

Frequency of dosing: Every 12 to 24 hours

Duration of treatment: Until bleeding stops and healing begins, ~2 to 7 days

Major hemorrhage (pharynx, retorpharnynx, retroperitoneum, CNS, surgery):

Desired factor IX levels (% or units/dL): 50 to 100

Frequency of dosing: Every 12 to 24 hours

Duration of treatment: 7 to 10 days

Dosing: Usual NOTE: Contains **only factor IX**; therefore, **NOT INDICATED** for replacement therapy of any other clotting factor besides factor IX or for reversal of anticoagulation due to either vitamin K antagonists or other anticoagulants (eg, dabigatran), for hemophilia A patients with factor VIII inhibitors, or for patients in a hemorrhagic state caused by reduced production of liver-dependent coagulation factors (eg, hepatitis, cirrhosis).

Pediatric: **Control or prevention of bleeding in patients with factor IX deficiency (hemophilia B or Christmas disease):** IV: Dosage is expressed in units of factor IX activity and must be individualized based on formulation, severity of factor IX deficiency, extent and location of bleeding, and clinical status of patient.

Formula for units required to raise blood level:

Infants, Children, and Adolescents <15 years: BeneFIX: Number of factor IX units required = patient weight (in kg) x desired factor IX level increase (as % or units/dL) x 1.4 units/kg per units/dL

For example, for a 100% level in a 25 kg patient who has an actual level of 20%: Number of factor IX Units needed = 25 kg x 80% x 1.4 units/kg per units/dL = 2,800 units

Adolescents ≥15 years: BeneFIX: Number of factor IX units required = patient weight (in kg) x desired factor IX level increase (as % or units/dL) x 1.3 units/kg per units/dL

For example, for a 100% level in a 70 kg patient who has an actual level of 20%: Number of factor IX Units needed = 70 kg x 80% x 1.3 units/kg per units/dL = 7,280 units

Manufacturer's labeling: BeneFIX: Infants, Children, and Adolescents: Intermittent IV:

Desired factor IX level, dosing interval and duration based on hemorrhage type:

Minor hemorrhage (uncomplicated joint hemorrhage, superficial muscle, or soft tissue):

Desired factor IX levels (% or units/dL): 20 to 30

Frequency of dosing: Every 12 to 24 hours

Duration of treatment: 1 to 2 days

Moderate hemorrhage (intramuscular or soft tissue with dissection, mucous membrane, dental extractions, or hematuria):

Desired factor IX levels (% or units/dL): 25 to 50

Frequency of dosing: Every 12 to 24 hours

Duration of treatment: Until bleeding stops and healing begins, ~2 to 7 days

Major hemorrhage (pharynx, retorpharnynx, retroperitoneum, CNS, surgery):

Desired factor IX levels (% or units/dL): 50 to 100

Frequency of dosing: Every 12 to 24 hours

Duration of treatment: 7 to 10 days

Alternative dosing: **Note:** The following recommendations reflect general dosing requirements; may vary from those found within prescribing information or practitioner preference:

Prophylaxis, primary: Infants, Children, and Adolescents: IV: 15 to 30 units/kg twice weekly [WFH guidelines (Srivastava 2013) (Utrecht protocol)] **or** 25 to 40 units/kg twice weekly [WFH guidelines (Srivastava 2013) (Malmö protocol)] **or** 40 to 100 units/kg administered 2 to 3 times weekly (National Hemophilia Foundation, MASAC recommendation 2007); optimum regimen has yet to be defined.

Hemorrhage, treatment: **Note:** Factor IX level may either be expressed as units/dL or as %. Dosing frequency most commonly corresponds to the half-life of factor IX but should be determined based on an assessment of factor IX levels before the next dose. Infants, Children, and Adolescents: IV:

Desired Factor IX Level to Maintain and Duration Based on Site of Hemorrhage/Clinical Situation (when no significant resource constraints exist) [WFH guidelines (Srivastava 2013)]:

Joint: 40 to 60 units/dL for 1 to 2 days, may be longer if response is inadequate

Superficial muscle (no neurovascular compromise): 40 to 60 units/dL for 2 to 3 days, sometimes longer if response is inadequate

Iliopsoas and deep muscle with neurovascular injury, or substantial blood loss: Initial: 60 to 80 units/dL for 1 to 2 days; Maintenance: 30 to 60 units/dL for 3 to 5 days, sometimes longer as secondary prophylaxis during physiotherapy

CNS/head: Initial: 60 to 80 units/dL for 1 to 7 days; Maintenance: 30 units/dL for 8 to 21 days

Throat and neck: Initial: 60 to 80 units/dL for 1 to 7 days; Maintenance: 30 units/dL for 8 to 14 days

Gastrointestinal: Initial: 60 to 80 units/dL for 7 to 14 days; Maintenance: 30 units/dL (duration not specified)

Renal: 40 units/dL for 3 to 5 days

Deep laceration: 40 units/dL for 5 to 7 days

Surgery (major):

Preop: 60 to 80 units/dL

Postop: 40 to 60 units/dL for 1 to 3 days; then 30 to 50 units/dL for 4 to 6 days; then 20 to 40 units/dL for 7 to 14 days

Surgery (minor):

Preop: 50 to 80 units/dL

Postop: 30 to 80 units/dL for 1 to 5 days depending on procedure type

Adult:

Control or prevention of bleeding in patients with factor IX deficiency (hemophilia B or Christmas disease): IV: Dosage is expressed in units of factor IX activity; dosing must be individualized based on severity of factor IX deficiency, extent and location of bleeding, and clinical status of patient. Refer to product information for specific manufacturer recommended dosing. Alternatively, the World Federation of Hemophilia (WFH) has recommended general dosing for factor IX products.

Formula for units required to raise blood level: **Note:** If patient has severe hemophilia (ie, baseline factor IX level is or presumed to be <1%), then may just use "desired factor IX level" instead of "desired factor IX level increase".

Number of factor IX units required = patient weight (in kg) x desired factor IX level increase (as % or units/dL) x 1.3 units/kg per units/dL

World Federation of Hemophilia (WFH) Guidelines (Srivastava 2013): **Note:** The following recommendations may vary from those found within prescribing information or practitioner preference.

Prophylaxis, primary: IV: 15 to 30 units/kg twice weekly [WFH guidelines (Srivastava 2013) (Utrecht protocol)] **or** 25 to 40 units/kg twice weekly [WFH guidelines (Srivastava 2013) (Malm□ protocol)] **or** 40 to 100 units/kg 2 or 3 times weekly (National Hemophilia Foundation, MASAC recommendation 2007); however, the optimum regimen has yet to be defined.

Treatment: Intermittent IV: 2013 World Federation of Hemophilia Treatment Recommendations (When No Significant Resource Constraint Exists): **Note:** Factor IX level may either be expressed as units/dL or as %. Dosing frequency most commonly corresponds to the half-life of factor IX but should be determined based on an assessment of factor IX levels before the next dose.

Desired Factor IX Level to Maintain and Duration Based on Site of Hemorrhage/Clinical Situation:

Joint: 40 to 60 units/dL for 1 to 2 days, may be longer if response is inadequate

Superficial muscle (no neurovascular compromise): 40 to 60 units/dL for 2 to 3 days, sometimes longer if response is inadequate

Iliopsoas and deep muscle with neurovascular injury, or substantial blood loss: Initial: 60 to 80 units/dL for 1 to 2 days; Maintenance: 30 to 60 units/dL for 3 to 5 days, sometimes longer as secondary prophylaxis during physiotherapy

CNS/head: Initial: 60 to 80 units/dL for 1 to 7 days; Maintenance: 30 units/dL for 8 to 21 days

Throat and neck: Initial: 60 to 80 units/dL for 1 to 7 days; Maintenance: 30 units/dL for 8 to 14 days

Gastrointestinal: Initial: 60 to 80 units/dL for 7 to 14 days; Maintenance: 30 units/dL (duration not specified)

Renal: 40 units/dL for 3 to 5 days

Deep laceration: 40 units/dL for 5 to 7 days

Surgery (major):

Preop: 60 to 80 units/dL

Postop: 40 to 60 units/dL for 1 to 3 days; then 30 to 50 units/dL for 4 to 6 days; then 20 to 40 units/dL for 7 to 14 days

Surgery (minor):

Preop: 50 to 80 units/dL

Postop: 30 to 80 units/dL for 1 to 5 days depending on procedure type

Continuous IV infusion: **Note:** For patients who require prolonged periods of treatment (eg, intracranial hemorrhage or surgery) to avoid peaks and troughs associated with intermittent infusions [Batorova 2002; Poon 2012; Rickard 1995; WFH guidelines (Srivastava 2013)]: Following initial bolus to achieve the desired factor IX level: Initiate 4 to 6 units/kg/hour; adjust dose based on frequent factor assays and calculation of factor IX clearance at steady-state using the following equations:

Factor IX clearance (mL/kg/hour) = (current infusion rate in units/kg/hour)/(plasma level in units/**mL**)

Factor IX clearance (mL/kg/hour) = (current infusion rate in units/kg/hour)/(plasma level in units/mL)

New infusion rate (units/kg/hour) = (factor IX clearance in mL/kg/hour) x (desired plasma level in units/mL)

New infusion rate (units/kg/hour) = (factor IX clearance in mL/kg/hour) x (desired plasma level in units/**mL**)

Routine prophylaxis to prevent bleeding episodes in patients with factor IX deficiency (hemophilia B or Christmas disease): Rixubis: IV: 40 to 60 units/kg twice weekly; may titrate dose depending upon age, bleeding pattern, and physical activity

Preparation for Administration

IV bolus: Refer to instructions provided by the manufacturer. If refrigerated, diluent and factor IX should come to room temperature before combining.

Continuous IV infusion: Limited data available: One study reconstituted with SWFI to a final concentration of 100 units/mL for continuous administration; some patients also had heparin added to the infusion at a final concentration of 4 units/mL; solutions with or without heparin retained 90% clotting activity for 14 days when stored at 4°C; when stored at room temperature nonheparin-containing solutions retained over 90% activity until day 7 and heparin-containing solutions were the least stable and fell below 90% activity after 4 days (Chowdary 2001).

Administration Solution should be infused at room temperature. With patients who have had allergic reactions during factor IX infusion, administration of hydrocortisone prior to infusion may be necessary [WFH guidelines (Srivastava 2013)].

IV bolus:

BeneFIX: Should be infused **slowly over several minutes**. Rate of administration should be determined by the response and comfort of the patient.

Rixubis: Bolus infusion; maximum rate of administration is 10 mL/minute

WFH recommendations (Srivastava 2013): Infuse at a rate determined by age: Young children: 100 **units**/minute; Adults: 3 mL/minute

Continuous IV infusion: Limited data available in select patients: Infuse as directed. Evidence supporting the use of continuous infusion is primarily with BeneFix (Chowdary 2001). The safety and efficacy of Rixubis and Alprolix administration by continuous infusion has not been established.

Monitoring Parameters Factor IX levels [measure 15 minutes after infusion to verify calculated doses [WFH guidelines (Srivastava 2013)], aPTT, BP, HR, signs of hypersensitivity reactions; screen for factor IX inhibitors if the patient experiences hypersensitivity reaction or when patient is to undergo surgery, if suboptimal response to treatment occurs, if patient is being intensively treated for >5 days within 4 weeks of the last infusion, or at the following intervals [WFH guidelines (Srivastava 2013)]:

Children: Screen for inhibitors every 5 exposure days until 20 exposure days, every 10 exposure days between 21 to 50 exposure days, and at a minimum of twice a year until 150 exposure days is reached.

Adults (with >150 exposure days apart from a 6 to 12 monthly review): Screen for inhibitors when suboptimal response occurs.

Reference Range Average normal factor IX levels are 50% to 150%; patients with severe hemophilia will have levels <1%, often undetectable. Moderate forms of the disease have levels of 1% to 5% while some mild cases may have 5% to 49% of normal factor IX.

Additional Information In absence of inhibitors, 1 unit/kg of factor IX ***recombinant*** will increase plasma factor IX level by 0.7 unit/dL in children <15 years and 0.8 units/dL in adults (WFH guidelines [Srivastava, 2013]).

Dosage Forms Considerations Strengths expressed with approximate values. Consult individual vial labels for exact potency within each vial.

Dosage Forms Excipient information presented when available (limited, particularly for generics); consult specific product labeling.

Solution Reconstituted, Intravenous [preservative free]:

Alprolix: 500 units (1 ea); 1000 units (1 ea); 2000 units (1 ea); 3000 units (1 ea)

BeneFIX: 250 units (1 ea); 500 units (1 ea); 1000 units (1 ea); 2000 units (1 ea) [contains polysorbate 80]

Ixinity: 500 units (1 ea); 1000 units (1 ea); 1500 units (1 ea) [contains mouse protein (murine) (hamster), polysorbate 80]

Rixubis: 250 units (1 ea); 500 units (1 ea); 1000 units (1 ea); 2000 units (1 ea); 3000 units (1 ea) [contains polysorbate 80]

◆ **3 Factor PCC** *see* Factor IX Complex (Human) [(Factors II, IX, X)] *on page 836*

Famciclovir (fam SYE kloe veer)

Medication Safety Issues

Sound-alike/look-alike issues:

Famvir® may be confused with Femara®

Brand Names: US Famvir

Brand Names: Canada Apo-Famciclovir®; Ava-Famciclovir; CO Famciclovir; Famvir®; PMS-Famciclovir; Sandoz-Famciclovir

Therapeutic Category Antiviral Agent, Oral

Generic Availability (US) Yes

Use Treatment of acute herpes zoster (shingles); treatment or suppression of recurrent episodes of genital herpes in immunocompetent patients; treatment of recurrent episodes of herpes labialis (cold sores) in immunocompetent patients; treatment of recurrent episodes of mucocutaneous herpes simplex infections in HIV patients (FDA approved in ages ≥18 years)

Pregnancy Risk Factor B

Pregnancy Considerations Teratogenic effects were not observed in animal reproduction studies. Data in pregnant women is limited. A registry has been established for women exposed to famciclovir during pregnancy (888-669-6682).

Breast-Feeding Considerations There is no specific data describing the excretion of famciclovir in breast milk. Breast-feeding is not recommended by the manufacturer unless the potential benefits outweigh any possible risk. If herpes lesions are on breast, breast-feeding should be avoided in order to avoid transmission to infant.

Contraindications Hypersensitivity to famciclovir, penciclovir, or any component of the formulation

Warnings/Precautions Has not been established for use in immunocompromised patients (except HIV-infected patients with orolabial or genital herpes, patients with ophthalmic or disseminated zoster or with initial episode of genital herpes, and in Black and African American patients with recurrent episodes of genital herpes. Acute renal failure has been reported with use of inappropriate high doses in patients with underlying renal disease. Dosage adjustment is required in patients with renal insufficiency. Tablets contain lactose; do not use with galactose intolerance, severe lactase deficiency, or glucose-galactose malabsorption syndromes.

Adverse Reactions

Central nervous system: Fatigue, headache, migraine

Dermatologic: Pruritus, rash

Endocrine & metabolic: Dysmenorrhea

Gastrointestinal: Abdominal pain, diarrhea, flatulence, nausea, vomiting

Hematologic: Neutropenia

Hepatic: Bilirubin increased, transaminases increased

Neuromuscular & skeletal: Paresthesia

Rare but important or life-threatening: Anemia, angioedema (eyelid, face, periorbital, pharyngeal edema), cholestatic jaundice, confusion, delirium, disorientation, dizziness, erythema multiforme, hallucinations, leukocytoclastic vasculitis, palpitations, somnolence, Stevens-Johnson syndrome, thrombocytopenia, toxic epidermal necrolysis, urticaria

Drug Interactions

Metabolism/Transport Effects None known.

Avoid Concomitant Use

Avoid concomitant use of Famciclovir with any of the following: Varicella Virus Vaccine; Zoster Vaccine

Increased Effect/Toxicity There are no known significant interactions involving an increase in effect.

Decreased Effect

Famciclovir may decrease the levels/effects of: Varicella Virus Vaccine; Zoster Vaccine

Food Interactions Rate of absorption and/or conversion to penciclovir and peak concentration are reduced with food, but bioavailability is not affected. Management: Administer without regard to meals.

Storage/Stability Store at 25°C (77°F); excursions permitted to 15°C to 30°C (59°F to 86°F).

Mechanism of Action Famciclovir undergoes rapid biotransformation to the active compound, penciclovir (prodrug), which is phosphorylated by viral thymidine kinase in HSV-1, HSV-2, and VZV-infected cells to a monophosphate form; this is then converted to penciclovir triphosphate and competes with deoxyguanosine triphosphate to inhibit HSV-2 polymerase, therefore, herpes viral DNA synthesis/replication is selectively inhibited.

Pharmacokinetics (Adult data unless noted) Penciclovir:

Absorption: Rapid

Distribution: V_{dss}: Healthy adults: 1.08 ± 0.17 L/kg

Protein binding: <20%

Metabolism: Famciclovir is a prodrug which is metabolized via deacetylation and oxidation in the intestinal wall and liver to penciclovir (active) during extensive first-pass metabolism

Bioavailability: 77% ± 8%

Half-life:

Serum: Mean: 2-3 hours; increased with renal dysfunction

Mean half-life, terminal:

CrCl >80 mL/minute: 2.15 hours

CrCl 60-80 mL/minute: 2.47 hours

CrCl 30-59 mL/minute: 3.87 hours

CrCl <29 mL/minute: 9.85 hours

Intracellular penciclovir triphosphate: HSV 1: 10 hours; HSV 2: 20 hours; VZV: 7 hours

Time to peak serum concentration: ~1 hour

Elimination: Primarily excreted via the kidneys; after oral administration, 73% is excreted in the urine (predominantly as penciclovir) and 27% in feces; penciclovir undergoes tubular secretion; requires dosage adjustment with renal impairment

Dialysis: Hemodialysis: May enhance elimination of penciclovir

Dosing: Usual Oral:

Children and Adolescents: Insufficient clinical data exists to identify an appropriate pediatric dose (AAP, 2006):

Adults:

Herpes zoster: 500 mg every 8 hours for 7 days; initiate as soon as diagnosed; initiation of therapy within 48 hours of rash onset may be more beneficial; no efficacy data available for treatment initiated >72 hours after onset of rash

Genital herpes: Treatment of initial clinical episode: 250 mg 3 times/day for 7-10 days; **Note:** Treatment may be continued if healing is not complete after 10 days of therapy (CDC, 2006)

Recurrent genital herpes in immunocompetent patients:

Treatment: 1000 mg twice daily for 1 day or 125 mg twice daily for 5 days (CDC, 2006); initiate at first sign or symptom; efficacy is not established if treatment is started >6 hours after onset of lesions or symptoms

Suppression: 250 mg twice daily for up to 1 year

Recurrent herpes labialis (cold sores): 1500 mg as a single dose; initiate at first sign or symptom such as tingling, burning, or itching; efficacy established for initiation of treatment within 1 hour of symptom onset

Recurrent orolabial or genital herpes in HIV patients: Treatment: 500 mg twice daily for 7 days

Recurrent genital herpes in HIV patients: Suppression: 500 mg twice daily (CDC, 2006)

Dosing interval in renal impairment: Adults:

Herpes zoster:

CrCl ≥60 mL/minute: Administer 500 mg every 8 hours

CrCl 40-59 mL/minute: Administer 500 mg every 12 hours

CrCl 20-39 mL/minute: Administer 500 mg every 24 hours

CrCl <20 mL/minute: Administer 250 mg every 24 hours

Patients on hemodialysis: Administer 250 mg after each dialysis session

Recurrent genital herpes: Treatment (single day regimen):

CrCl ≥60 mL/minute: Administer 1000 mg every 12 hours for 1 day

CrCl 40-59 mL/minute: Administer 500 mg every 12 hours for 1 day

CrCl 20-39 mL/minute: Administer 500 mg as a single dose

CrCl <20 mL/minute: Administer 250 mg as a single dose

Patients on hemodialysis: Administer 250 mg as a single dose after dialysis session

Recurrent genital herpes: Suppression:

CrCl ≥40 mL/minute: Administer 250 mg every 12 hours

CrCl 20-39 mL/minute: Administer 125 mg every 12 hours

CrCl <20 mL/minute: Administer 125 mg every 24 hours

Patients on hemodialysis: Administer 125 mg after each dialysis session

Recurrent herpes labialis: Treatment (single dose regimen):

CrCl ≥60 mL/minute: Administer 1500 mg as a single dose

CrCl 40-59 mL/minute: Administer 750 mg as a single dose

CrCl 20-39 mL/minute: Administer 500 mg as a single dose

CrCl <20 mL/minute: Administer 250 mg as a single dose

Patients on hemodialysis: Administer 250 mg as a single dose after dialysis session

Recurrent orolabial or genital herpes in HIV infected patients:

CrCl ≥40 mL/minute: Administer 500 mg every 12 hours

CrCl 20-39 mL/minute: Administer 500 mg every 24 hours

CrCl <20 mL/minute: Administer 250 mg every 24 hours

Patients on hemodialysis: Administer 250 mg after each dialysis session

Administration Oral: May be administered without regard to meals; may be administered with food to decrease GI upset

Monitoring Parameters Resolution of rash, renal function, WBC, liver enzymes

Dosage Forms Excipient information presented when available (limited, particularly for generics); consult specific product labeling.

Tablet, Oral:

Famvir: 125 mg, 250 mg, 500 mg

Generic: 125 mg, 250 mg, 500 mg

Famotidine (fa MOE ti deen)

Medication Safety Issues

Sound-alike/look-alike issues:

Famotidine may be confused with FLUoxetine, furosemide

Brand Names: US Acid Reducer Maximum Strength [OTC]; Acid Reducer [OTC]; Heartburn Relief Max St [OTC]; Heartburn Relief [OTC]; Pepcid

Brand Names: Canada Acid Control; Apo-Famotidine; Famotidine Omega; Maximum Strength Pepcid AC; Mylan-Famotidine; Pepcid AC; Pepcid Complete; Peptic guard; Teva-Famotidine; Ulcidine

Therapeutic Category Gastrointestinal Agent, Gastric or Duodenal Ulcer Treatment; Histamine H_2 Antagonist

Generic Availability (US) Yes

Use

Oral: Short-term therapy for gastroesophageal reflux disease (FDA approved in all ages); short-term therapy and treatment of duodenal ulcer and active benign gastric ulcer (FDA approved in ages 1 to 16 years and adults); treatment of pathological hypersecretory conditions (eg, Zollinger-Ellison syndrome, multiple endocrine adenomas) (FDA approved in ages ≥17 years and adults) relief of heartburn, acid indigestion, and sour stomach (OTC products: FDA approved in ages >12 years and adults); has also been used symptomatic relief in gastritis

IV: Short-term therapy and treatment for gastroesophageal reflux disease, duodenal ulcer, and active benign gastric ulcer until oral famotidine therapy can be initiated (FDA approved in ages 1 to 16 years and adults); treatment of pathological hypersecretory conditions (eg, Zollinger-Ellison syndrome, multiple endocrine adenomas) until oral famotidine therapy can be initiated (FDA approved in ages ≥17 years and adults); has also been used for stress ulcer prophylaxis and gastric acid suppression in critically ill patients

Pregnancy Risk Factor B

Pregnancy Considerations Adverse events have not been observed in animal reproduction studies; therefore, famotidine is classified as pregnancy category B. Famotidine crosses the placenta. An increased risk of congenital malformations or adverse events in the newborn has generally not been observed following maternal use of famotidine during pregnancy. Histamine H_2 antagonists have been evaluated for the treatment of gastroesophageal reflux disease (GERD), as well as gastric and duodenal ulcers, during pregnancy. Although if needed, famotidine is not the agent of choice. Histamine H_2 antagonists may be used for aspiration prophylaxis prior to cesarean delivery.

Breast-Feeding Considerations Famotidine is excreted into breast milk with peak concentrations occurring ~6 hours after the maternal dose. According to the manufacturer, the decision to continue or discontinue breast-feeding during therapy should take into account the risk of exposure to the infant and the benefits of treatment to the mother.

Contraindications Hypersensitivity to famotidine, other H_2 antagonists, or any component of the formulation

Warnings/Precautions Modify dose in patients with moderate-to-severe renal impairment. Prolonged QT interval has been reported in patients with renal dysfunction. The FDA has received reports of torsade de pointes occurring with famotidine (Poluzzi, 2009). Relief of symptoms does not preclude the presence of a gastric malignancy. Reversible confusional states, usually clearing within 3-4 days after discontinuation, have been linked to use. Prolonged treatment (≥2 years) may lead to vitamin B_{12} malabsorption and subsequent vitamin B_{12} deficiency. The magnitude of the deficiency is dose-related and the association is stronger in females and those younger in age (<30 years); prevalence is decreased after discontinuation of therapy (Lam, 2013). Increased age (>50 years) and renal or hepatic impairment are thought to be associated.

Benzyl alcohol and derivatives: Some dosage forms may contain benzyl alcohol and/or sodium benzoate/benzoic acid; benzoic acid (benzoate) is a metabolite of benzyl alcohol; large amounts of benzyl alcohol (≥99 mg/kg/day) have been associated with a potentially fatal toxicity ("gasping syndrome") in neonates; the "gasping syndrome" consists of metabolic acidosis, respiratory distress, gasping respirations, CNS dysfunction (including convulsions, intracranial hemorrhage), hypotension, and cardiovascular collapse (AAP, 1997; CDC, 1982); some data suggests that benzoate displaces bilirubin from protein binding sites (Ahlfors, 2001); avoid or use dosage forms containing benzyl alcohol and/or benzyl alcohol derivative with caution in neonates. See manufacturer's labeling.

OTC labeling: When used for self-medication, patients should be instructed not to use if they have difficulty swallowing, are vomiting blood, or have bloody or black stools. Not for use with other acid reducers.

Warnings: Additional Pediatric Considerations Use of gastric acid inhibitors, including proton pump inhibitors and H_2 blockers, has been associated with an increased risk for development of acute gastroenteritis and community-acquired pneumonia in pediatric patients (Canani, 2006). A large epidemiological study has suggested an increased risk for developing pneumonia in patients receiving H_2 receptor antagonists; however, a causal relationship with ranitidine has not been demonstrated. A cohort analysis including over 11,000 neonates reported an association of H_2 blocker use and an increased incidence of NEC in VLBW neonates (Guillet, 2006). An approximate sixfold increase in mortality, NEC, and infection (ie, sepsis, pneumonia, UTI) was reported in patients receiving ranitidine in a cohort analysis of 274 VLBW neonates (Terrin, 2011).

Adverse Reactions

Central nervous system: Dizziness, headache

Gastrointestinal: Constipation, diarrhea, necrotizing enterocolitis (VLBW neonates; Guillet, 2006)

Rare but important or life-threatening: Abdominal discomfort, acne, agitation, agranulocytosis, allergic reaction, alopecia, anaphylaxis, angioedema, anorexia, anxiety, arrhythmia, arthralgia, AV block, bronchospasm, cholestatic jaundice, confusion, conjunctival injection, depression, dry skin, facial edema, fatigue, fever, flushing, hallucinations, hepatitis, injection site reactions, insomnia, interstitial pneumonia, leukopenia, libido decreased, liver function tests increased, muscle cramps, nausea, palpitation, pancytopenia, paresthesia, pruritus, QT-interval prolongation, rash, rhabdomyolysis, seizure, somnolence, Stevens-Johnson syndrome, taste disorder, tinnitus, thrombocytopenia, torsade de pointes, toxic epidermal necrolysis, urticaria, vomiting, weakness, xerostomia

Drug Interactions

Metabolism/Transport Effects **Substrate** of OCT2

Avoid Concomitant Use

Avoid concomitant use of Famotidine with any of the following: Dasatinib; Delavirdine; PAZOPanib; Risedronate

Increased Effect/Toxicity

Famotidine may increase the levels/effects of: Dexmethylphenidate; Highest Risk QTc-Prolonging Agents; Methylphenidate; Moderate Risk QTc-Prolonging Agents; Risedronate; Saquinavir; Varenicline

The levels/effects of Famotidine may be increased by: BuPROPion; Mifepristone

Decreased Effect

Famotidine may decrease the levels/effects of: Atazanavir; Bosutinib; Cefditoren; Cefpodoxime; Cefuroxime; Dabrafenib; Dasatinib; Delavirdine; Erlotinib; Fosamprenavir; Gefitinib; Indinavir; Iron Salts; Itraconazole; Ketoconazole (Systemic); Ledipasvir; Mesalamine; Multivitamins/Minerals (with ADEK, Folate, Iron); Nelfinavir; Nilotinib; PAZOPanib; Posaconazole; Rilpivirine

Food Interactions Prolonged treatment (≥2 years) may lead to malabsorption of dietary vitamin B_{12} and subsequent vitamin B_{12} deficiency (Lam, 2013).

Storage/Stability

Oral:

Powder for oral suspension: Prior to mixing, dry powder should be stored at controlled room temperature of 25°C (77°F). Reconstituted oral suspension is stable for 30 days at room temperature; do not freeze.

Tablet: Store controlled room temperature. Protect from moisture.

IV:

Solution for injection: Prior to use, store at 2°C to 8°C (36°F to 46°F). If solution freezes, allow to solubilize at controlled room temperature. May be stored at room temperature for up to 3 months (data on file [Bedford Laboratories, 2011]).

IV push: Following preparation, solutions for IV push should be used immediately, or may be stored in refrigerator and used within 48 hours.

Infusion: Following preparation, the manufacturer states may be stored for up to 48 hours under refrigeration; however, solutions for infusion have been found to be physically and chemically stable for 7 days at room temperature.

Solution for injection, premixed bags: Store at controlled room temperature of 25°C (77°F); avoid excessive heat.

Mechanism of Action Competitive inhibition of histamine at H_2 receptors of the gastric parietal cells, which inhibits gastric acid secretion

Pharmacodynamics Antisecretory effect:

Onset: IV; Oral: Within 1 hour

Maximum effect:

IV: 30 minutes

Oral: 1 to 4 hours

Duration: 10 to 12 hours

Pharmacokinetics (Adult data unless noted)

Absorption: Oral: Incompletely

Distribution: V_d:

Neonates and infants:

0 to 3 months: 1.4 ± 0.4 L/kg to 1.8 ± 0.3 L/kg

>3 to 12 months: 2.3 ± 0.7 L/kg

Children: 2 ± 1.5 L/kg

Adolescents: 1.5 ± 0.4 L/kg

Adults: 0.94 to 1.33 L/kg

Protein binding: 15% to 20%

Metabolism: 30% to 35%; minimal first-pass metabolism; forms one metabolite (S-oxide)

Bioavailability: Oral: 40% to 45%

Half-life:

Neonates and infants:

0 to 3 months: 8.1 ± 3.5 hours to 10.5 ± 5.4 hours

>3 to 12 months: 4.5 ± 1.1 hours

Children: 3.3 ± 2.5 hours
Adolescents: 2.3 ± 0.4 hours
Adults: 2.5 to 3.5 hours; increases with renal impairment; if CrCl <10 mL/minute, half-life ≥20 hours
Anuria: 24 hours
Time to peak serum concentration: Oral: 1 to 3 hours; orally disintegrating tablet: 2.5 hours
Elimination: 65% to 70% unchanged drug in urine
Clearance:
Neonates and infants:
0 to 3 months: 0.13 to 0.21 ± 0.06 L/hour/kg
>3 to 12 months: 0.49 ± 0.17 L/hour/kg
Children 1 to 11 years: 0.54 ± 0.34 L/hour/kg
Adolescents: 0.48 ± 0.14 L/hour/kg
Adults: 0.39 ± 0.14 L/hour/kg

Dosing: Neonatal

Gastric acid suppression, GERD: Oral:
Manufacturer's labeling: 0.5 mg/kg/dose once daily
Alternate dosing: Limited data available: PMA ≥37 weeks: Initial: 0.5 mg/kg/dose once daily; if not effective, may increase to 1 mg/kg/dose once daily; in the trial, the minimum GA for inclusion was ≥32 weeks and no minimum PNA inclusion criteria; the youngest patient reported to receive the higher 1 mg/kg/dose was 1.3 months PNA (median: 3.7 months; range: 1.3 to 10.5 months) (Orenstein, 2003)
Stress ulcer prophylaxis, gastric acid suppression: Limited data available: IV: 0.25 to 0.5 mg/kg/dose once daily has been used; some data have suggested that the lower dose of 0.25 mg/kg may have a less favorable pharmacodynamics profile (eg, duration of gastric pH >4) than the higher 0.5 mg/kg dosage (Crill, 1999; James, 1998; Wenning, 2005)

Dosing: Usual

Pediatric:
GERD, esophagitis: Oral:
Infants 1 to <3 months:
Manufacturer's labeling: 0.5 mg/kg/dose once daily for up to 8 weeks
Alternate dosing: Limited data available: Initial: 0.5 mg/kg/dose once daily; if not effective, may increase to 1 mg/kg/dose once daily (Orenstein, 2003)
Infants ≥3 months to <1 year:
Manufacturer's labeling: 0.5 mg/kg/dose twice daily for up to 8 weeks
Alternate dosing: Limited data available: Initial: 0.5 mg/kg/dose twice daily; if not effective, may increase to 1 mg/kg/dose twice daily (Orenstein, 2003)
Children and Adolescents 1 to 16 years: 0.5 mg/kg/dose twice daily (maximum dose: 40 mg/dose); doses up to 1 mg/kg/dose twice daily have been reported
Adolescents ≥17 years: 20 mg twice daily for up to 6 weeks; for esophagitis and accompanying symptoms due to GERD, may use 20 to 40 mg twice daily for up to 12 weeks
Patients unable to take oral medication: IV:
Infants: 0.25 to 0.5 mg/kg/dose once daily (Crill, 1999; James, 1998; Wenning, 2005)
Children and Adolescents 1 to 16 years: Initial: 0.25 mg/kg/dose every 12 hours (maximum dose: 20 mg/dose); doses up to 0.5 mg/kg/dose every 12 hours have been reported
Adolescents ≥17 years: 20 mg every 12 hours
Peptic ulcer disease: Oral:
Children and Adolescents 1 to 16 years: 0.5 mg/kg/**day** once daily at bedtime or divided twice daily (maximum daily dose: 40 mg/day); doses up to 1 mg/kg/**day** have been used
Adolescents ≥17 years:
Duodenal ulcer: Acute therapy: 40 mg once daily at bedtime (or 20 mg twice daily) for 4 to 8 weeks; maintenance therapy: 20 mg once daily at bedtime
Gastric ulcer: Acute therapy: 40 mg once daily at bedtime
Stress ulcer prophylaxis, gastric acid suppression: Limited data available: IV: Infants, Children, and Adolescents: 0.5 to 1 mg/kg/dose every 12 hours; maximum dose: 20 mg/dose (Crill, 1999)
Hypersecretory conditions: Oral: Adolescents ≥17 years: Initial: 20 mg every 6 hours, may increase up to 160 mg every 6 hours
Heartburn, acid indigestion, or sour stomach (OTC use): Oral: Children ≥12 years and Adolescents: 10 to 20 mg every 12 hours; dose may be taken 15 to 60 minutes before eating foods known to cause heartburn; maximum daily dose: 2 tablets/day (20 to 40 mg dependent upon OTC product)
Adult:
Duodenal ulcer: Oral: Acute therapy: 40 mg once daily at bedtime (or 20 mg twice daily) for 4 to 8 weeks; maintenance therapy: 20 mg once daily at bedtime
Gastric ulcer: Oral: Acute therapy: 40 mg once daily at bedtime
Hypersecretory conditions: Oral: Initial: 20 mg every 6 hours, may increase in increments up to 160 mg every 6 hours
GERD: Oral: 20 mg twice daily for 6 weeks
Esophagitis and accompanying symptoms due to GERD: Oral: 20 mg or 40 mg twice daily for up to 12 weeks
Patients unable to take oral medication: IV: 20 mg every 12 hours
Heartburn, indigestion, sour stomach OTC labeling: Oral: 10 to 20 mg every 12 hours; dose may be taken 15 to 60 minutes before eating foods known to cause heartburn

Dosing adjustment in renal impairment:
Infants, Children, and Adolescents: There are no specific dosage adjustments provided in the manufacturer's labeling; however, decreased doses or extended dosing intervals are recommended in patients with moderate to severe renal impairment; some have suggested the following (Aronoff, 2007): **Note:** Renally adjusted dose recommendations are based on doses of 0.5 to 1 mg/kg/day divided every 12 hours.
GFR 30 to 50 mL/minute/1.73 m^2: 0.5 mg/kg/dose every 24 hours
GFR 10 to 29 mL/minute/1.73 m^2: 0.25 mg/kg/dose every 24 hours
GFR <10 mL/minute/1.73 m^2: 0.125 mg/kg/dose every 24 hours
Intermittent hemodialysis: 0.125 mg/kg/dose every 24 hour
Peritoneal dialysis (PD): 0.125 mg/kg/dose every 24 hours
Continuous renal replacement therapy (CRRT): 0.5 mg/kg/dose every 24 hours
Adults: CrCl <50 mL/minute: Manufacturer recommendation: Administer 50% of dose or increase the dosing interval to every 36 to 48 hours (to limit potential CNS adverse effects)

Dosing adjustment in hepatic impairment: There are no dosage adjustments provided in the manufacturer's labeling.

Preparation for Administration

Oral: Reconstitute powder for oral suspension with appropriate amount of water as specified on the bottle. Shake vigorously until suspended.

Parenteral:

IV push: Dilute famotidine with NS (or another compatible solution) to a maximum concentration of 4 mg/mL; in adults may also administer undiluted (Lipsy 1995)

IV Infusion: Dilute to 0.2 mg/mL in an appropriate diluent; in adolescents or adults typically prepared with 100 mL D_5W or another compatible solution

Administration

Oral: May administer with food and antacids; shake suspension vigorously for 10 to 15 seconds prior to each use

Parenteral:

IV push: May be administered at a rate of ≤10 mg/minute over at least 2 minutes

IV infusion: Infuse over 15 to 30 minutes

Dosage Forms Excipient information presented when available (limited, particularly for generics); consult specific product labeling. [DSC] = Discontinued product

Solution, Intravenous:

Generic: 20 mg (50 mL); 20 mg/2 mL (2 mL); 40 mg/4 mL (4 mL); 200 mg/20 mL (20 mL); 500 mg/50 mL (50 mL)

Solution, Intravenous [preservative free]:

Generic: 20 mg/2 mL (2 mL); 40 mg/4 mL (4 mL [DSC])

Suspension Reconstituted, Oral:

Pepcid: 40 mg/5 mL (50 mL) [contains methylparaben sodium, propylparaben sodium, sodium benzoate; cherry banana mint flavor]

Generic: 40 mg/5 mL (50 mL)

Tablet, Oral:

Acid Reducer: 10 mg

Acid Reducer Maximum Strength: 20 mg

Heartburn Relief: 10 mg

Heartburn Relief Max St: 20 mg

Pepcid: 20 mg

Pepcid: 20 mg [DSC] [scored]

Pepcid: 40 mg

Pepcid: 40 mg [DSC] [scored]

Generic: 10 mg, 20 mg, 40 mg

Extemporaneous Preparations An 8 mg/mL oral suspension may be made with tablets. Crush seventy 40 mg tablets in a mortar and reduce to a fine powder. Add small portions of sterile water and mix to a uniform paste. Mix while adding a 1:1 mixture of Ora-Plus® and Ora-Sweet® in incremental proportions to **almost** 350 mL; transfer to a calibrated bottle, rinse mortar with vehicle, and add quantity of vehicle sufficient to make 350 mL. Label "shake well". Stable for 95 days at room temperature.

Dentinger PJ, Swenson CF, and Anaizi NH, "Stability of Famotidine in an Extemporaneously Compounded Oral Liquid," *Am J Health Syst Pharm*, 2000, 57(14):1340-2.

- **Famotidine Omega (Can)** *see* Famotidine *on page* *847*
- **Famvir** *see* Famciclovir *on page* *846*
- **Famvir® (Can)** *see* Famciclovir *on page* *846*
- **Fanatrex FusePaq** *see* Gabapentin *on page* *954*
- **2F-ara-AMP** *see* Fludarabine *on page* *888*
- **Faslodex** *see* Fulvestrant *on page* *950*
- **Fasturtec (Can)** *see* Rasburicase *on page* *1839*

Fat Emulsion (Plant Based)

(fat e MUL shun plant baste)

Medication Safety Issues

Sound-alike/look-alike issues:

Intralipid may be confused with ViperSlide (lubricant used during atherectomy procedures)

Related Information

Pediatric Parenteral Nutrition *on page* *2359*

Brand Names: US Intralipid; Liposyn III; Nutrilipid

Brand Names: Canada Intralipid

Therapeutic Category Caloric Agent; Intravenous Nutritional Therapy

Generic Availability (US) Yes

Use

Intralipid, Liposyn III: Source of calories and essential fatty acids for patients requiring parenteral nutrition of extended duration (FDA approved in all ages); prevention and treatment of essential fatty acid deficiency (EFAD) (FDA approved in all ages); has also been used for treatment of local anesthetic-induced cardiac arrest unresponsive to conventional resuscitation

Nutrilipid: Source of calories and essential fatty acids for patients requiring parenteral nutrition for extended periods of time or when oral or enteral nutrition is not possible, insufficient, or contraindicated (FDA approved in all ages)

Clinolipid: Source of calories and essential fatty acids for patients requiring parenteral nutrition of extended duration (FDA approved in adults)

Pregnancy Risk Factor C

Pregnancy Considerations Animal reproductive studies have not been conducted. Indications for fat emulsion therapy in pregnant women are the same as in nonpregnant women. The ASPEN guidelines for parenteral and enteral nutrition state that intravenous fat emulsion may be used safely in pregnant women to provide calories and prevent essential fatty acid deficiency (ASPEN Guidelines, 2002).

Breast-Feeding Considerations The fatty acids found in fat emulsion (eg, linoleic acid, linolenic acid) are endogenous to human milk and concentrations are influenced by maternal diet (IOM, 2005). The manufacturers recommend that caution be exercised when administering fat emulsion therapy to nursing women.

Contraindications

Clinolipid, Nutrilipid: Known hypersensitivity to egg or soybean proteins or to any component of the formulation; severe hyperlipidemia (serum triglyceride concentrations above 1,000 mg/dL) or severe disorders of lipid metabolism characterized by hypertriglyceridemia.

Intralipid 20%, 30%: Disturbances in normal fat metabolism such as pathologic hyperlipemia, lipoid nephrosis, or acute pancreatitis if accompanied by hyperlipidemia; pharmacy bulk package is not intended for direct IV administration.

Liposyn III (10%, 20%, 30%): Disturbances in normal fat metabolism such as pathologic hyperlipemia, lipoid nephrosis, or acute pancreatitis if accompanied by hyperlipidemia; pharmacy bulk package is not intended for direct IV administration; use of product in which there appears to be an oiling out of the emulsion; partly used containers stored for later use.

Additional contraindications (10% and 20% only): Addition of additives to product bottle (except heparin at 1 to 2 units/mL of fat emulsion); use of a filter.

Warnings/Precautions [U.S. Boxed Warning]: Deaths in preterm infants following administration of fat emulsion have been reported; autopsy findings included intravascular fat accumulation in the lungs. Premature infants, low birth weight infants, and small for gestational age infants clear intravenous fat emulsion poorly and have increased free fatty acid plasma levels following fat emulsion infusion. Strict adherence to proper infusion rates, dosing, and monitoring are necessary; infusion rate should be as low as possible; strict monitoring of metabolic tolerance and elimination of infused fat from the circulation must occur. To avoid hyperlipidemia and/or fat deposition, do not exceed recommended daily doses and consider administering less than the maximum recommended doses in preterm and small for gestational age infants. Clinolipid is not indicated for use in pediatric patients. Pediatric clinical studies did not establish that Clinolipid provides sufficient amounts of essential fatty acids (EFA) in pediatric patients, which may predispose them to neurologic complications due to EFA insufficiency. Because free fatty acids displace bilirubin from albumin binding sites, the use of lipid infusions in jaundiced or premature infants should be done with caution.

Allergic reactions to lipid emulsion may occur; discontinue infusion immediately if signs or symptoms of hypersensitivity or allergic reactions occur. The too-rapid administration of fat emulsion can cause fluid and/or fat overloading, resulting in dilution of serum electrolyte concentrations, overhydration, congested states, pulmonary edema, impaired pulmonary diffusion capacity, or metabolic acidosis. All formulations contain soybean oil and egg yolk phospholipids; the manufacturer's labeling of some products contraindicates use in patients with known hypersensitivity to soybean proteins or egg yolk phospholipids. Use caution in patients with renal and/or hepatic impairment. Monitor by appropriate laboratory evaluation (eg, triglycerides). Use caution in patients with pancreatitis without hyperlipidemia; ensure triglyceride levels remain <400 mg/dL. Lipid emulsion in a three-in-one mixture may obscure the presence of a precipitate; follow compounding guidelines, especially for calcium and phosphate additions.

The parenteral product may contain aluminum; toxic aluminum concentrations may be seen with high doses, prolonged use, or renal dysfunction. Premature neonates are at higher risk due to immature renal function and aluminum intake from other parenteral sources. Parenteral aluminum exposure of >4 to 5 mcg/kg/day is associated with CNS and bone toxicity; tissue loading may occur at lower doses (Federal Register, 2002). See manufacturer's labeling.

Successful resuscitation following the administration of fat emulsion has been reported in animal studies and several human case reports in which cardiovascular toxicity was unresponsive to conventional resuscitation and antidotal measures. Successful resuscitation following the administration of fat emulsion in a pediatric patient experiencing local anesthetic cardiovascular toxicity has been reported (Ludot, 2008). Additional information is available at http://www.lipidrescue.org. Consider use when local anesthetic toxicity is likely and conventional methods are unsuccessful. Continue CPR throughout treatment with lipid emulsion.

Parenteral nutrition: Although the exact etiology is unknown and likely multifactorial, parenteral nutrition associated liver disease (PNALD) has been reported in patients receiving parenteral nutrition for extended periods of time, especially preterm infants, and can present as cholestasis or steatohepatitis, fibrosis and cirrhosis, possibly leading to hepatic failure; cholecystitis and cholelithiasis have also been observed. Consider discontinuation or dose reduction in patients who develop abnormal LFTs. Refeeding severely undernourished patients with parenteral nutrition may result in the refeeding syndrome (eg, intracellular shift of potassium, phosphorus, and magnesium as the patient becomes anabolic); thiamine deficiency and fluid retention may also develop. Carefully monitor severely undernourished patients and slowly increase their nutrient intakes, while avoiding overfeeding.

Although rare, a reduced or limited ability to metabolize lipids accompanied by prolonged plasma clearance resulting in a sudden deterioration in the patient's condition accompanied by fever, anemia, leukopenia, thrombocytopenia, coagulation disorders, hyperlipidemia, liver fatty infiltration (hepatomegaly), deteriorating liver function, and CNS (eg, coma) can occur; usually reversible upon discontinuation.

The use of fat emulsion has been associated with anemia likely due to hemodilution (Zellner, 1967). Use with caution in patients with anemia. Use with caution in patients with bleeding disorders. Potentially significant interactions may exist, requiring dose or frequency adjustment, additional monitoring, and/or selection of alternative therapy.

Adverse Reactions

Endocrine & metabolic: Hyperglycemia, hyperlipidemia

Gastrointestinal: Gallbladder disorder, nausea and vomiting

Genitourinary: Urinary tract infection

Hematologic & oncologic: Hypoproteinemia

Hepatic: Abnormal hepatic function tests, hepatic abnormality

Infection: Septicemia

Miscellaneous: Fever

Rare but important or life-threatening: Cholestasis, cyanosis, decreased INR, hepatic effects (brown pigment deposition in the reticuloendothelial system ["intravenous fat pigment"]), hepatomegaly, hypercoagulability state, hypersensitivity reaction, infusion site irritation, jaundice, leukopenia, liver steatosis, overloading syndrome (focal seizures, fever, leukocytosis, hepatomegaly, splenomegaly, shock), pancreatitis, thrombocytopenia, thrombophlebitis

Storage/Stability

Do not freeze. If accidentally frozen, discard. Do not store partly used containers; fat emulsion can support the growth of various organisms. Do not use if the emulsion appears to be oiling out. Once the closure is penetrated, the contents should be used as soon as possible; the transfer of contents to suitable TPN admixture containers must be completed within 4 hours of closure penetration. Admixtures prepared using fat emulsion should be used promptly or stored under refrigeration at 2°C to 8°C (36°F to 46°F) for 24 hours or less and used completely within 24 hours after removal from refrigeration.

Intralipid, Nutrilipid: Store below 25°C (77°F).

Liposyn III: Store at 20°C to 25°C (68°F to 77°F).

Clinolipid: Store at 20°C to 25°C (68°F to 77°F); excursions permitted between 15°C and 30°C (59°F and 86°F). Avoid excessive heat. Store in overpouch until ready to use.

Mechanism of Action Fat emulsion is metabolized and utilized as an energy source; provides the essential fatty acids, linoleic acid, and alpha linolenic acid necessary for normal structure and function of cell membranes; in local anesthetic toxicity, lipid emulsion probably extracts lipophilic local anesthesia from cardiac muscle

In local anesthetic toxicity, exogenous lipids provide an alternative source of binding of lipid-soluble local anesthetics (Rowlingson, 2008), commonly known as the "lipid sink" effect. This is more relevant to bupivacaine, levobupivacaine, and ropivacaine than mepivacaine and prilocaine. High lipid partition constant and large volumes of distribution are good predictors of success when using lipid therapy (French, 2011). Lipid administration may also affect the heart in a metabolically advantageous way by improving fatty acid transport (Weinberg, 2006).

Dosing: Neonatal

Parenteral nutrition: Intralipid, Liposyn III, Nutrilipid: **Note:** Fat emulsion should not exceed 60% of the total daily calories. At the onset of therapy, the patient should be observed for any immediate allergic reactions such as dyspnea, cyanosis, and fever.

Premature neonates: IV: Initial dose: 1 to 2 g/kg/day, increase by 0.5 to 1 g/kg/day to a maximum of 3 to 3.5 g/kg/day depending upon the needs/nutritional goals; daily dose infused over 24 hours; total infusion time may be incrementally increased (ie, cycled) to a maximum daily infusion over 12 hours (ASPEN Guidelines, 2002; ASPEN Pediatric Nutrition Support Core Curriculum, 2010); do not exceed 1 g/kg in 4 hours

Term neonates: IV: Initial dose: 1 to 2 g/kg/day, increase by 0.5 to 1 g/kg/day to a maximum of 3 g/kg/day depending upon the needs/nutritional goals; daily dose infused over 24 hours; total infusion time may be incrementally increased (ie, cycled) to a maximum daily infusion over 12 hours (ASPEN Guidelines, 2002; ASPEN Pediatric Nutrition Support Core Curriculum, 2010)

Localized anesthetic toxicity: Full-term neonate: Very limited data available: 20% fat emulsion: IV: 1 **mL**/kg was reported in a single case report in a 2-day-old neonate undergoing caudal epidural block for a urologic procedure (Lin, 2010)

Dosing: Usual

Pediatric:

Parenteral nutrition: Intralipid, Liposyn III, Nutrilipid: **Note:** Fat emulsion should not exceed 60% of the total daily calories. At the onset of therapy, the patient should be observed for any immediate allergic reactions such as dyspnea, cyanosis, and fever.

Infants: IV: Initial dose: 1 to 2 g/kg/day, increase by 0.5 to 1 g/kg/day to a maximum of 3 g/kg/day depending upon the needs/nutritional goals; daily dose infused over 24 hours; total infusion time may be incrementally increased (ie, cycled) to a maximum daily infusion over 12 hours (ASPEN Guidelines, 2002; ASPEN Pediatric Nutrition Support Core Curriculum, 2010)

Children 1 to 10 years: IV: Initial dose: 1 to 2 g/kg/day, increase by 0.5 to 1 g/kg/day to a maximum of 2 to 3 g/kg/day depending upon the needs/nutritional goals; daily dose infused over 24 hours; total infusion time may be incrementally increased (ie, cycled) to a maximum daily infusion over 12 hours (ASPEN Guidelines, 2002; ASPEN Pediatric Nutrition Support Core Curriculum, 2010)

Children ≥11 years and Adolescents: IV: Initial dose: 1 g/kg/day; not to exceed 500 mL 20% fat emulsion on the first day of therapy, increase by 1 g/kg/day to a maximum of 2.5 g/kg/day; daily dose infused over 24 hours; total infusion time may be incrementally increased (ie, cycled) to a maximum daily infusion over 12 hours (ASPEN Guidelines, 2002; ASPEN Pediatric Nutrition Support Core Curriculum, 2010)

Essential fatty acid deficiency (EFAD), prevention: Intralipid, Liposyn III: Infants, Children, and Adolescents: IV: Administer 8% to 10% of total caloric intake as fat emulsion; infuse 2 to 3 times weekly; may need to increase dose during stress

Local anesthetic toxicity: Infants, Children, and Adolescents: Limited data available: 20% fat emulsion: IV: 0.8 to 3 **mL**/kg bolus has been used successfully in several pediatric case reports (1 month to 13 years) (Fuzaylov, 2010; Ludot, 2008; Shah, 2009; Wong, 2010); a single case report in a 6-year-old described use of a continuous IV infusion at 0.25 **mL**/kg/minute to a total dose of 8 **mL**/kg following the bolus dose (Wong, 2010)

Adult:

Caloric source: IV: **Note:** Fat emulsion should not exceed 60% of the total daily calories. Initial dose: 1 to 1.5 g/kg/day (not to exceed 500 mL Intralipid 10% or 20% or 330 mL Intralipid 30% [over 4 to 6 hours] on the first day of therapy); daily dose may be infused over 12 to 24 hours; maximum daily dose: 2.5 g/kg/day

Essential fatty acid deficiency (EFAD), prevention: IV: Administer at least 2% to 4% of total caloric intake as linoleic acid and 0.25% to 0.5% as alpha linolenic acid (Mirtallo, 2004; Mirtallo, 2010)

Essential fatty acid deficiency (EFAD), treatment: Intralipid, Liposyn III: IV: Administer 8% to 10% of total caloric intake as fat emulsion; may infuse up to once daily (Riella, 1975). If EFAD occurs with stress, the dosage needed to correct EFAD may be increased.

Dosing adjustment in renal impairment: There are no dosage adjustments provided in manufacturer's labeling; use with caution.

Dosing adjustment in hepatic impairment: There are no dosage adjustments provided in manufacturer's labeling; use with caution.

Preparation for Administration Do not add additives directly to the fat emulsion (there may be some instances when heparin may be added for piggy-back administration through a Y-connector). When preparing parenteral nutrition admixture, do not add fat emulsion to the TPN container first; destabilization of the lipid emulsion may occur when other solutions (eg, dextrose) are added. Minimize pH-related problems by ensuring that dextrose solutions, which are typically acidic, are not mixed with lipid emulsions alone. First transfer dextrose solution to the TPN admixture container; then transfer amino acid injection; then transfer lipid emulsion. Amino acid injection, dextrose injection, and lipid emulsions may be simultaneously transferred to the admixture container; use gentle agitation during admixing to minimize localized concentration effects; may shake bags gently after each addition. Do not use administration sets and lines that contain di-2-ehtylhexyl phthalate (DEHP).

Clinolipid: When preparing total parenteral nutrition admixture, do not use the EXACTAMIX Inlet H938173 with an EXACTAMIX compounder to transfer Clinolipid injection; associated with dislodgement of the administration port membrane into the Clinolipid injection bag.

Administration

Note: Preparation and administration dependent upon use.

Parenteral nutrition:

Intralipid: Do not use <1.2 micron filter. Prior to opening the overwrap, the integrity indicator should be inspected. If the indicator is black, the overwrap is damaged; do not use.

Liposyn III: Do not use a filter.

Nutrilipid: Use a 1.2 micron in-line filter. To avoid air embolism, use a nonvented infusion set or close the air vent on a vented set and use a dedicated line without any connections. Prior to opening the overwrap, the oxygen indicator should be inspected; if the indicator is pink or dark pink, do not use. May be infused concurrently into the same vein as carbohydrate-amino acid solutions by means of a Y-connector located near the infusion site; flow rates of each solution should be controlled separately by infusion pumps. Do not use administration sets and lines that contain di-2-ethylhexyl phthalate (DEHP). See prescribing information for detailed administration information.

Clinolipid: Do not use <1.2 micron filter. Prior to opening the overwrap of Clinolipid, check the color of the oxygen indicator and compare to the reference color next to the OK symbol. If the color of the oxygen absorber/indicator does not correspond to the reference color, do not use. After opening the bag, use the contents immediately and do not store for a subsequent infusion. Do not connect flexible bags in series to avoid air embolism due to possible residual gas contained in the primary bag. When preparing total parenteral nutrition admixture, do not use the EXACTAMIX Inlet H938173 with an EXACTAMIX compounder to transfer Clinolipid injection; associated with dislodgement of the administration port membrane into the Clinolipid injection bag.

Administer via peripheral line or by central venous infusion. At the onset of therapy, the patient should be observed for any immediate allergic reactions such as dyspnea, cyanosis, and fever. Change tubing after each infusion. The 10% and 20% fat emulsions may be simultaneously infused with amino acid and dextrose mixtures by means of Y-connector located near infusion site into either central or peripheral line or administered in total nutrient mixtures (3-in-1) with amino acids, dextrose, and other nutrients. Fat emulsions of 30% should only be administered in total nutrient mixtures

(3-in-1) with amino acids, dextrose, and other nutrients; not intended for direct infusion; must be further diluted to a final concentration not to exceed 20%. At the bedside, fat emulsion solution should be elevated higher than other parenteral fluids to prevent it running up into other IV lines due to its low specific gravity.

Neonates, Infants, Children, and Adolescents:

Infusion rate: Premature and/or septic neonates and infants may require reduced infusion rates; manufacturers recommend not exceeding 1 g/kg in 4 hours in this population; however, in general for all pediatric patients, lower rates of ≤0.15 to 0.17 g/kg/hour have been recommended by some groups (ASPEN Pediatric Nutrition Support Core Curriculum 2010); in adults, a maximum rate of 0.125 g/kg/hour has been suggested (Mirtallo 2004).

Product-specific infusion rates (volume):

10% emulsions: **Note:** Avoid use of 10% fat emulsion in preterm infants as a greater accumulation of plasma lipids occurs with the greater phospholipid load of the 10% fat emulsion. Liposyn III: Initiate at 0.1 **mL**/minute for 15 minutes, may increase to ≤100 **mL/hour** if tolerated

20% emulsions:

Intralipid: Initiate at ≤0.05 **mL**/minute for 10-15 minutes; if no untoward effects occur, the infusion rate may be increased to 0.5 **mL**/kg/**hour**

Liposyn III: Initiate at 0.1 **mL**/minute for 15 minutes, may increase to ≤50 **mL/hour** if tolerated

Nutrilipid:

Neonates, Infants, Children, and Adolescents <17 years: Initiate at 0.05 **mL**/minute for 10 to 15 minutes; if no untoward effects the infusion may be gradually increased to required rate; maximum rate of infusion: Neonates, Infants and Children ≤10 years: 0.75 **mL**/kg/**hour**; Children and Adolescents 11 to 16 years: 0.5 **mL**/kg/**hour**

Adolescents ≥ 17 years: Initiate at 0.5 **mL**/minute for 15 to 30 minutes; if no untoward effects the infusion may be gradually increased; maximum rate of infusion: 0.5 **mL**/kg/**hour**

Adults:

Intralipid, Liposyn III:

10% emulsions: Initiate at 1 **mL**/minute for 15 to 30 minutes; if no untoward effects occur, the infusion rate may be increased to 2 **mL**/minute

20% emulsions: Initiate at 0.5 mL/minute for 15 to 30 minutes; if no untoward effects occur, the infusion rate may be increased to 1 **mL**/minute

Nutrilipid: Initiate at 0.5 **mL**/minute for 15 to 30 minutes; if no untoward effects the infusion may be gradually increased; maximum rate of infusion: 0.5 **mL**/kg/**hour**

Clinolipid: Initiate at 0.5 **mL**/minute for 15 to 30 minutes; if no untoward effects the infusion may be gradually increased to the required rate.

Local anesthetic toxicity: 20% emulsion: Administer initial bolus undiluted over 1 minute; may be administered either peripherally or centrally; bolus may be followed by a continuous infusion depending on clinical scenario. Chest compressions should continue during administration if patient is in cardiac arrest. Continue the infusion for at least 10 minutes after hemodynamic stability is restored. The infusion rate may be increased if hemodynamic instability recurs (ACMT 2010; Neal 2012).

Monitoring Parameters Monitor for signs and symptoms of infection (including vascular access device complications); fluid and electrolyte status; serum osmolarity; blood glucose; blood counts (including platelets and coagulation parameters); signs and symptoms of essential fatty acid deficiency, refeeding syndrome, and/or hypersensitivity reactions

Monitor liver and renal function tests periodically. Monitor triglycerides before initiation of lipid therapy and at least weekly during therapy (or until triglycerides are stable and when changes are made in the amount of fat administered) (ASPEN Guidelines, 2002); monitor especially closely in premature infants, septic infants, and patients with pancreatitis or liver disease.

Additional Information

Caloric content: 10% emulsion = 1.1 Kcal/mL; 20% emulsion = 2 Kcal/mL; 30% emulsion = 3 Kcal/mL

Phosphorus: ~1.5 mMol/100 mL of emulsion

10% and 20% emulsions are isotonic and may be administered peripherally

Product Availability Clinolipid: FDA approved October 2013; anticipated availability is currently unknown. Refer to the prescribing information for additional information.

Dosage Forms Considerations Product oil source for Intralipid, Liposyn III, and Nutrilipid: soybean

Dosage Forms Excipient information presented when available (limited, particularly for generics); consult specific product labeling. [DSC] = Discontinued product

Emulsion, Intravenous:

Intralipid: 20% (100 mL, 250 mL, 500 mL, 1000 mL); 30% (500 mL) [contains egg yolk phospholipids, glycerin]

Liposyn III: 10% (200 mL, 250 mL, 500 mL); 20% (200 mL, 250 mL, 500 mL)

Liposyn III: 30% (500 mL [DSC]) [contains egg phosphatides]

Nutrilipid: 20% (250 mL, 500 mL, 1000 mL) [contains egg yolk phospholipids, glycerin]

◆ **FazaClo** *see* CloZAPine *on page 519*

◆ **5-FC** *see* Flucytosine *on page 886*

◆ **FEIBA** *see* Anti-inhibitor Coagulant Complex (Human) *on page 176*

◆ **FEIBA NF** *see* Anti-inhibitor Coagulant Complex (Human) *on page 176*

◆ **FEIBA VH** *see* Anti-inhibitor Coagulant Complex (Human) *on page 176*

Felbamate (FEL ba mate)

Brand Names: US Felbatol

Therapeutic Category Anticonvulsant, Miscellaneous

Generic Availability (US) Yes

Use Not a first-line agent; reserved for patients who do not adequately respond to alternative agents and whose epilepsy is so severe that the benefit outweighs the risk of liver failure or aplastic anemia; used as monotherapy and adjunctive therapy in patients with partial seizures with and without secondary generalization (FDA approved in ages ≥14 years and adults); adjunctive therapy in children who have partial and generalized seizures associated with Lennox-Gastaut syndrome (FDA approved in ages 2–14 years)

Prescribing and Access Restrictions A patient "informed consent" form should be completed and signed by the patient and physician. Copies are available from MEDA Pharmaceuticals by calling 800-526-3840.

Medication Guide Available Yes

Pregnancy Risk Factor C

Pregnancy Considerations Adverse events were not observed in animal reproduction studies. Postmarketing case reports in humans include fetal death, genital malformation, anencephaly, encephalocele, and placental disorder.

Patients exposed to felbamate during pregnancy are encouraged to enroll themselves into the North American Antiepileptic Drug (AED) Pregnancy Registry by calling 1-888-233-2334. Additional information is available at www.aedpregnancyregistry.org.

Breast-Feeding Considerations Felbamate has been detected in human milk.

Contraindications Hypersensitivity to felbamate or any component of the formulation; known sensitivity to other carbamates; history of any blood dyscrasia or hepatic dysfunction

Warnings/Precautions [U.S. Boxed Warning]: Felbamate is associated with an increased risk of aplastic anemia. [U.S. Boxed Warning]: Felbamate has been associated with rare cases of hepatic failure (estimated >6 cases per 75,000 patients per year). Do not initiate treatment in patients with pre-existing hepatic dysfunction. Use caution in patients with renal impairment (dose adjustment recommended); half-life may be increased. Not indicated for use as a first-line antiepileptic treatment; only recommended in those patients who respond inadequately to alternative treatments and whose epilepsy is so severe that a substantial risk of aplastic anemia and/or liver failure is deemed acceptable in light of the benefits conferred by its use. Antiepileptics are associated with an increased risk of suicidal behavior/thoughts with use (regardless of indication); patients should be monitored for signs/symptoms of depression, suicidal tendencies, and other unusual behavior changes during therapy and instructed to inform their healthcare provider immediately if symptoms occur. CNS effects may be potentiated when used with other sedative drugs or ethanol. Antiepileptic drugs should not be suddenly discontinued because of the possibility of increasing seizure frequency.

Adverse Reactions

Cardiovascular: Chest pain, facial edema, palpitation, tachycardia

Central nervous system: Abnormal thinking, agitation, aggressive reaction, ataxia, depression, dizziness, emotional lability, euphoria, fatigue. fever, hallucinations, headache, insomnia, malaise, migraine, nervousness, psychological disturbances, somnolence, stupor, suicide attempt

Dermatologic: Acne, bullous eruption, pruritus, purpura, skin rash, urticaria

Endocrine and metabolic: Hypokalemia, hyponatremia, hypophosphatemia, intramenstrual bleeding

Gastrointestinal: Abdominal pain, anorexia, appetite increased, constipation, diarrhea, dyspepsia, esophagitis, hiccup, nausea, taste perversion, vomiting, weight gain/loss, xerostomia

Genitourinary: Urinary tract infection

Hematologic: Granulocytopenia, leukocytosis, leukopenia, lymphadenopathy, thrombocytopenia

Hepatic: Alkaline phosphatase increased, liver function tests increased

Neuromuscular & skeletal: Abnormal gait, dystonia, myalgia, pain, paresthesia, tremor, weakness

Ocular: Abnormal vision, diplopia, miosis

Otic: Otitis media

Respiratory: Cough, pharyngitis, rhinitis, sinusitis, upper respiratory infection

Miscellaneous: Flu-like syndrome, LDH increased

Rare but important or life-threatening: Acute renal failure, agranulocytosis, allergic reaction, alopecia, anaphylactoid reaction, anemia, aplastic anemia, atrial arrhythmia, atrial fibrillation, bradycardia, cardiac arrest, cardiac failure, cerebrovascular disorder, cerebral edema, choreoathetosis, coagulation disorder, coma, concentration impaired, confusion, CPK increased, delusion, diaphoresis, DIC, dysphagia, dyspnea, dysarthria, dyskinesia, dysuria, embolism, encephalopathy, enteritis, eosinophilia, epistaxis, extrapyramidal disorder, flushing, gastric ulcer, gastritis, gastroesophageal reflux, GI hemorrhage, gingival bleeding, glossitis, hematemesis, hematuria, hemolytic anemia, Henoch-Schönlein vasculitis, hepatic failure, hepatitis, hepatorenal syndrome, hyperammonemia, hyper-/hypoglycemia, hyper-/hypotension, hypernatremia, hypocalcemia, hypomagnesemia, hypoxia, ileus, ischemic necrosis, jaundice, manic reaction, mononeuritis, nephrosis, nystagmus, pancreatitis, pancytopenia, paralysis, paranoid reaction, peripheral ischemia, photosensitivity, platelet disorder, pleural effusion, pneumonitis, psychosis, pulmonary hemorrhage, rectal hemorrhage, renal function abnormal, respiratory depression, rhabdomyolysis, SIADH, status epilepticus, Stevens-Johnson syndrome, sudden death, suicidal behavior/ideation, SVT, thrombophlebitis, torsade de pointes, toxic epidermal necrolysis, ulcerative stomatitis, urinary retention, urticaria

Drug Interactions

Metabolism/Transport Effects Substrate of CYP2E1 (minor), CYP3A4 (major); **Note:** Assignment of Major/Minor substrate status based on clinically relevant drug interaction potential; **Inhibits** CYP2C19 (weak); **Induces** CYP3A4 (weak)

Avoid Concomitant Use

Avoid concomitant use of Felbamate with any of the following: Azelastine (Nasal); Conivaptan; Fusidic Acid (Systemic); Idelalisib; Orphenadrine; Paraldehyde; Thalidomide; Ulipristal

Increased Effect/Toxicity

Felbamate may increase the levels/effects of: Alcohol (Ethyl); Azelastine (Nasal); Barbiturates; Buprenorphine; CNS Depressants; Fosphenytoin; Highest Risk QTc-Prolonging Agents; Hydrocodone; Methotrimeprazine; Metyrosine; Mirtazapine; Moderate Risk QTc-Prolonging Agents; Orphenadrine; Paraldehyde; PHENobarbital; Phenytoin; Pramipexole; Primidone; ROPINIRole; Rotigotine; Selective Serotonin Reuptake Inhibitors; Suvorexant; Thalidomide; Valproic Acid and Derivatives; Zolpidem

The levels/effects of Felbamate may be increased by: Aprepitant; Brimonidine (Topical); Cannabis; Conivaptan; CYP3A4 Inhibitors (Moderate); CYP3A4 Inhibitors (Strong); Dasatinib; Doxylamine; Dronabinol; Droperidol; Fosaprepitant; Fusidic Acid (Systemic); HydrOXYzine; Idelalisib; Ivacaftor; Kava Kava; Luliconazole; Magnesium Sulfate; Methotrimeprazine; Mifepristone; Nabilone; Netupitant; Palbociclib; Perampanel; Rufinamide; Simeprevir; Sodium Oxybate; Stiripentol; Tapentadol; Tetrahydrocannabinol

Decreased Effect

Felbamate may decrease the levels/effects of: ARIPiprazole; CarBAMazepine; Contraceptives (Estrogens); Contraceptives (Progestins); NiMODipine; Saxagliptin; Ulipristal

The levels/effects of Felbamate may be decreased by: Barbiturates; Bosentan; CarBAMazepine; CYP3A4 Inducers (Moderate); CYP3A4 Inducers (Strong); Dabrafenib; Deferasirox; Fosphenytoin; Mefloquine; Mianserin; Mitotane; Orlistat; PHENobarbital; Phenytoin; Primidone; Siltuximab; St Johns Wort; Tocilizumab

Food Interactions Tablet: Food does not affect absorption. Management: Administer without regard to meals.

Storage/Stability Store in tightly closed container at controlled room temperature of 20°C to 25°C (68°F to 77°F).

Mechanism of Action Mechanism of action is unknown but has properties in common with other marketed anticonvulsants; has weak inhibitory effects on GABA-receptor binding, benzodiazepine receptor binding, and is devoid of activity at the MK-801 receptor binding site of the NMDA receptor-ionophore complex.

Pharmacokinetics (Adult data unless noted)

Absorption: Oral: Rapid and almost complete

Distribution: V_d: Adults: Mean: 0.75 L/kg; range: 0.7-1.1 L/kg

Protein binding: 20% to 25%, primarily to albumin

Metabolism: In the liver via hydroxylation and conjugation
Bioavailability: >90%
Half-life: Adults: Mean: 20-30 hours; shorter (ie, 14 hours) with concomitant enzyme-inducing drugs; half-life is prolonged (by 9-15 hours) in patients with renal dysfunction
Time to peak serum concentration: 1-4 hours
Elimination: 40% to 50% excreted as unchanged drug and 40% as inactive metabolites in urine
Clearance, apparent: Clearance is decreased (by 40% to 50%) in patients with renal impairment
Children 2-9 years: 61.3 ± 8.2 mL/kg/hour
Children 10-12 years: 34.3 ± 4.3 mL/kg/hour

Dosing: Usual See Warnings/Precautions regarding concomitant antiepileptic drugs

Children 2-14 years with Lennox-Gastaut: Adjunctive therapy: Initial: 15 mg/kg/day in 3-4 divided doses; increase dose by 15 mg/kg/day increments at weekly intervals; maximum dose: 45 mg/kg/day or 3600 mg/day (whichever is less). Decrease dose of concomitant anticonvulsants (ie, carbamazepine, phenytoin, phenobarbital, valproic acid) by 20% at initiation of felbamate; further dosage reductions of concurrent anticonvulsants may be needed.

Children ≥14 years and Adults:

Adjunctive therapy: Initial: 1200 mg/day in 3-4 divided doses; increase daily dose by 1200 mg increments every week to a maximum dose of 3600 mg/day. Decrease dose of concomitant anticonvulsants (ie, carbamazepine, phenytoin, phenobarbital, valproic acid) by 20% at initiation of felbamate; further dosage reductions of concurrent anticonvulsants may be needed.

Conversion to monotherapy: Initial: 1200 mg/day in 3 or 4 divided doses; at week 2, increase daily dose by 1200 mg increments every week up to a maximum dose of 3600 mg/day. Decrease dose of other anticonvulsants by 1/3 their original dose at initiation of felbamate, and when felbamate dose is increased at week 2; continue to reduce other anticonvulsants as clinically needed.

Monotherapy: Initial: 1200 mg/day in 3 or 4 divided doses; titrate dosage upward according to clinical response and monitor patients closely; increase daily dose in 600 mg increments every 2 weeks to 2400 mg/day; maximum dose: 3600 mg/day

Dosage adjustment in renal impairment: Use with caution; reduce initial and maintenance doses by 50%

Administration Oral: May be administered without regard to meals; shake suspension well before use

Monitoring Parameters Serum concentrations of concomitant anticonvulsant therapy; CBC with differential and platelet count before, during, and for a significant time after discontinuing felbamate therapy; liver enzyme tests and bilirubin before initiation and periodically during therapy; signs and symptoms of suicidality (eg, anxiety, depression, behavior changes)

Reference Range Not necessary to routinely monitor serum drug levels; dose should be titrated to clinical response; therapeutic range not fully determined; proposed 30-100 mcg/mL

Additional Information Monotherapy has not been associated with gingival hyperplasia, impaired concentration, weight gain, or abnormal thinking; felbamate has also been used in a small number of patients with infantile spasms (Pellock, 1999); an open-label study in children with refractory partial seizures (n=30; mean age: 9 years; range: 2-17 years) found that children >10 years of age had a more favorable response; this was thought to be related to the higher felbamate serum concentrations (and lower apparent clearance) in children >10 years of age compared to those <10 years; the faster apparent clearance in children <10 years of age should be considered when using this agent (Carmant, 1994)

Dosage Forms Excipient information presented when available (limited, particularly for generics); consult specific product labeling.
Suspension, Oral:
Felbatol: 600 mg/5 mL (237 mL, 946 mL)
Generic: 600 mg/5 mL (237 mL, 240 mL, 473 mL, 946 mL)
Tablet, Oral:
Felbatol: 400 mg, 600 mg [scored]
Generic: 400 mg, 600 mg

◆ **Felbatol** *see* Felbamate *on page 853*
◆ **Feldene** *see* Piroxicam *on page 1710*

Felodipine (fe LOE di peen)

Medication Safety Issues
Sound-alike/look-alike issues:
Plendil may be confused with Isordil, pindolol, Pletal, PriLOSEC, Prinivil

Related Information
Oral Medications That Should Not Be Crushed or Altered *on page 2476*

Brand Names: Canada Plendil; Sandoz-Felodipine

Therapeutic Category Antihypertensive Agent; Calcium Channel Blocker; Calcium Channel Blocker, Dihydropyridine

Generic Availability (US) Yes

Use Treatment of hypertension alone or in combination with other antihypertensives (FDA approved in adults)

Pregnancy Risk Factor C

Pregnancy Considerations Adverse events were observed in animal reproduction studies. Untreated chronic maternal hypertension is associated with adverse events in the fetus, infant, and mother. If treatment for hypertension during pregnancy is needed, other agents are preferred (ACOG, 2013). The Canadian labeling contraindicates use in women of childbearing potential and during pregnancy.

Breast-Feeding Considerations It is not known if felodipine is excreted in breast milk. Due to the potential for serious adverse reactions in the nursing infant, the U.S. labeling recommends a decision be made whether to discontinue nursing or to discontinue the drug, taking into account the importance of treatment to the mother. The Canadian labeling contraindicates use in nursing women.

Contraindications
Hypersensitivity to felodipine or any component of the formulation.
Canadian labeling: Additional contraindications (not in U.S. labeling): Hypersensitivity to other dihydropyridines; women of childbearing potential, in pregnancy, and during lactation.

Warnings/Precautions Increased angina and/or MI has occurred with initiation or dosage titration of dihydropyridine calcium channel blockers, reflex tachycardia may occur resulting in angina and/or MI in patients with obstructive coronary disease especially in the absence of concurrent beta-blockade. Use with extreme caution in patients with severe aortic stenosis. Use caution in patients with hypertrophic cardiomyopathy with outflow tract obstruction. The ACCF/AHA heart failure guidelines recommend to avoid use in patients with heart failure due to lack of benefit and/or worse outcomes with calcium channel blockers in general (Yancy, 2013). Elderly patients and patients with hepatic impairment should start off with a lower dose. Peripheral edema (dose dependent) is the most common side effect (occurs within 2 to 3 weeks of starting therapy). Symptomatic hypotension with or without syncope can rarely occur; blood pressure must be lowered at a rate appropriate for the patient's clinical condition. Potentially significant drug-drug interactions may exist, requiring dose or frequency adjustment, additional monitoring, and/or selection of alternative therapy. May contain lactose; if necessary, consider alternative agents in patients intolerant of lactose.

Adverse Reactions

Cardiovascular: Flushing, peripheral edema, tachycardia

Central nervous system: Headache

Rare but important or life-threatening: Angina, angioedema, anxiety, arrhythmia, CHF, CVA, decreased libido, depression, dizziness, gingival hyperplasia, dyspnea, dysuria, gynecomastia, hypotension, impotence, insomnia, irritability, leukocytoclastic vasculitis, MI, nervousness, paresthesia, somnolence, syncope, urticaria, vomiting

Drug Interactions

Metabolism/Transport Effects Substrate of CYP3A4 (major); **Note:** Assignment of Major/Minor substrate status based on clinically relevant drug interaction potential; **Inhibits** CYP2C8 (moderate), CYP2C9 (weak), CYP2D6 (weak)

Avoid Concomitant Use

Avoid concomitant use of Felodipine with any of the following: Amodiaquine; Conivaptan; Fusidic Acid (Systemic); Idelalisib; Itraconazole; Ketoconazole (Systemic)

Increased Effect/Toxicity

Felodipine may increase the levels/effects of: Amifostine; Amodiaquine; Antihypertensives; ARIPiprazole; Atosiban; Calcium Channel Blockers (Nondihydropyridine); CYP2C8 Substrates; DULoxetine; Fosphenytoin; Hypotensive Agents; Levodopa; Magnesium Salts; Neuromuscular-Blocking Agents (Nondepolarizing); Nitroprusside; Obinutuzumab; Phenytoin; RisperiDONE; RiTUXimab; Tacrolimus (Systemic)

The levels/effects of Felodipine may be increased by: Alfuzosin; Alpha1-Blockers; Antifungal Agents (Azole Derivatives, Systemic); Aprepitant; Barbiturates; Bitter Orange; Brimonidine (Topical); Calcium Channel Blockers (Nondihydropyridine); Cimetidine; Conivaptan; CycloSPORINE (Systemic); CYP3A4 Inhibitors (Moderate); CYP3A4 Inhibitors (Strong); Dapoxetine; Dasatinib; Diazoxide; Fluconazole; Fosaprepitant; Fusidic Acid (Systemic); Grapefruit Juice; Herbs (Hypotensive Properties); Idelalisib; Itraconazole; Ivacaftor; Ketoconazole (Systemic); Luliconazole; Macrolide Antibiotics; Magnesium Salts; MAO Inhibitors; Mifepristone; Netupitant; Nicorandil; Palbociclib; Pentoxifylline; Phosphodiesterase 5 Inhibitors; Prostacyclin Analogues; Protease Inhibitors; Simeprevir; Stiripentol

Decreased Effect

Felodipine may decrease the levels/effects of: Clopidogrel

The levels/effects of Felodipine may be decreased by: Barbiturates; Bosentan; Calcium Salts; CarBAMazepine; CYP3A4 Inducers (Moderate); CYP3A4 Inducers (Strong); Dabrafenib; Deferasirox; Efavirenz; Herbs (Hypertensive Properties); Melatonin; Methylphenidate; Mitotane; Nafcillin; Rifamycin Derivatives; Siltuximab; St Johns Wort; Tocilizumab; Yohimbine

Food Interactions

Ethanol: Ethanol increases felodipine absorption. Management: Monitor for a greater hypotensive effect if ethanol is consumed.

Food: Compared to a fasted state, felodipine peak plasma concentrations are increased up to twofold when taken after a meal high in fat or carbohydrates. Grapefruit juice similarly increases felodipine C_{max} by twofold. Increased therapeutic and vasodilator side effects, including severe hypotension and myocardial ischemia, may occur. Management: May be taken with a small meal that is low in fat and carbohydrates; avoid grapefruit juice during therapy.

Storage/Stability Store below 30°C (86°F); protect from light.

Mechanism of Action Inhibits calcium ions from entering the "slow channels" or select voltage-sensitive areas of vascular smooth muscle and myocardium during depolarization, producing a relaxation of coronary vascular smooth muscle and coronary vasodilation; increases myocardial oxygen delivery in patients with vasospastic angina

Pharmacodynamics

Onset of action: Antihypertensive: 2-5 hours

Duration: Antihypertensive: 24 hours

Pharmacokinetics (Adult data unless noted)

Absorption: ~100%

Distribution: V_d: 10 L/kg

Protein binding: >99%

Metabolism: Hepatic; CYP3A4 substrate (major); extensive first-pass effect

Bioavailability: 20%; extensive first-pass metabolism

Half-life: 11-16 hours

Time to peak serum concentration: 2.5-5 hours

Elimination: Urine (70% as metabolites); feces 10%

Dosing: Usual

Children ≥6 years and Adolescents: **Hypertension:** Oral: Initial: 2.5 mg once daily; may increase as needed at 2-week intervals to a maximum daily dose: 10 mg/**day** (NHLBI, 2011)

Adults: **Hypertension:** Oral: 2.5-10 mg once daily; increase by 5 mg at 2-week intervals, as needed, to a maximum of 20 mg/day; usual dose range (JNC 7): 2.5-20 mg once daily

Dosing adjustment for renal impairment: Adults: Usually not required

Dosing adjustment for hepatic impairment: Adults: Initial dose: 2.5 mg/day; **Note:** Clearance is reduced to ~60% of normal in patients with hepatic disease; monitor closely

Administration Oral: Must be swallowed whole; do not crush or chew; should be taken either without food or with a light meal.

Monitoring Parameters Blood pressure, peripheral edema, liver enzymes

Dosage Forms Excipient information presented when available (limited, particularly for generics); consult specific product labeling.

Tablet Extended Release 24 Hour, Oral:

Generic: 2.5 mg, 5 mg, 10 mg

- **Femara** *see* Letrozole *on page* 1224
- **Femring** *see* Estradiol (Systemic) *on page* 795
- **Fenesin DM IR [OTC]** *see* Guaifenesin and Dextromethorphan *on page* 992
- **Fenesin IR [OTC]** *see* GuaiFENesin *on page* 988

Fenoldopam (fe NOL doe pam)

Brand Names: US Corlopam

Therapeutic Category Dopamine Agonist

Generic Availability (US) Yes

Use Short-term reduction in blood pressure (up to 4 hours) [FDA approved in ages <1 month (full term or ≥2 kg) to 12 years and adults]; treatment of severe hypertension (up to 48 hours), including in patients with renal compromise (FDA approved in adults); has also been used for augmentation of urine output and prevention of acute renal injury in critically ill patients (for 24 hours)

Pregnancy Risk Factor B

Pregnancy Considerations Fetal harm was not observed in animal studies; however, safety and efficacy have not been established for use during pregnancy. Use during pregnancy only if clearly needed.

Breast-Feeding Considerations It is not known if fenoldopam is excreted in breast milk. The manufacturer recommends that caution be exercised when administering fenoldopam to nursing women.

Contraindications There are no contraindications listed within the manufacturer's approved labeling.

Warnings/Precautions Use with caution in patients with open-angle glaucoma or intraocular hypertension; fenoldopam causes a dose-dependent increase in intraocular pressure. Dose-related tachycardia can occur, especially at infusion rates >0.1 mcg/kg/minute. Use with extreme caution in patients with obstructive coronary disease or ongoing angina pectoris; can increase myocardial oxygen demand due to tachycardia leading to angina pectoris. Serum potassium concentrations <3 mEq/L were observed within 6 hours of fenoldopam initiation; monitor potassium concentrations appropriately. Use with caution in patients with increased intracranial pressure; use has not been studied in this population. For continuous infusion only (no bolus doses). Some dosage forms may contain propylene glycol; large amounts are potentially toxic and have been associated hyperosmolality, lactic acidosis, seizures, and respiratory depression; use caution (AAP, 1997; Zar, 2007). Contains sulfites; may cause allergic reaction in susceptible individuals.

Warnings: Additional Pediatric Considerations A dose related tachycardia can occur, especially at infusion rates >0.1 mcg/kg/minute; in pediatric patients at doses >0.8 mcg/kg/minute, tachycardia has been shown to persist for at least 4 hours. Close monitoring of blood pressure is necessary; hypotension can occur.

Some dosage forms may contain propylene glycol; in neonates large amounts of propylene glycol delivered orally, intravenously (eg, >3,000 mg/day), or topically have been associated with potentially fatal toxicities which can include metabolic acidosis, seizures, renal failure, and CNS depression; toxicities have also been reported in children and adults including hyperosmolality, lactic acidosis, seizures, and respiratory depression; use caution (AAP, 1997; Shehab, 2009).

Adverse Reactions

Cardiovascular: Angina, bradycardia, chest pain, cutaneous flushing, extrasystoles, heart failure, hypotension, MI, orthostatic hypotension, palpitation, ST-T abnormalities, T-wave inversion, tachycardia

Central nervous system: Anxiety, dizziness, fever, headache, insomnia

Endocrine & metabolic: Hyperglycemia, hypokalemia, LDH increased

Gastrointestinal: Abdominal pain/fullness, constipation, diarrhea, nausea, vomiting

Genitourinary: Urinary tract infection

Hematologic: Bleeding, leukocytosis

Hepatic: Transaminases increased

Local: Injection site reactions

Neuromuscular & skeletal: Back pain, limb cramps

Ocular: Intraocular pressure increased

Renal: BUN increased, creatinine increased, oliguria

Respiratory: Dyspnea, nasal congestion

Miscellaneous: Diaphoresis

Drug Interactions

Metabolism/Transport Effects None known.

Avoid Concomitant Use There are no known interactions where it is recommended to avoid concomitant use.

Increased Effect/Toxicity There are no known significant interactions involving an increase in effect.

Decreased Effect There are no known significant interactions involving a decrease in effect.

Storage/Stability Store undiluted product at 2°C to 30°C (35°F to 86°F). Following dilution, store at room temperature and use solution within 24 hours.

Mechanism of Action A selective postsynaptic dopamine agonist (D_1-receptors) which exerts hypotensive effects by decreasing peripheral vasculature resistance with increased renal blood flow, diuresis, and natriuresis; 6 times as potent as dopamine in producing renal vasodilatation; has minimal adrenergic effects

Pharmacodynamics

Onset of action: Children: 5 minutes; Adults: 10 minutes; **Note:** Majority of effect of a given infusion rate is attained within 15 minutes.

Duration of effect (after stopping infusion): 30-60 minutes

Pharmacokinetics (Adult data unless noted)

Distribution: V_d: 0.6 L/kg

Metabolism: Hepatic via methylation, glucuronidation, and sulfation; the 8-sulfate metabolite may have some activity; extensive first-pass effect

Half-life, elimination: Children: 3-5 minutes; Adults: ~5 minutes

Elimination: Urine (90%); feces (10%)

Clearance: Children: 3 L/hour/kg

Dosing: Usual IV:

Children: Initial: 0.2 mcg/kg/minute; may be increased every 20-30 minutes to 0.3-0.5 mcg/kg/minute; maximum dose: 0.8 mcg/kg/minute (higher doses have been shown to worsen tachycardia without any additional blood pressure benefits)

Adults: Initial: 0.1-0.3 mcg/kg/minute (lower initial doses may be associated with less reflex tachycardia); may be increased in increments of 0.05-0.1 mcg/kg/minute every 15 minutes until target blood pressure is reached; the maximal infusion rate reported in clinical studies was 1.6 mcg/kg/minute

Dosage adjustment for renal impairment: No guidelines are available.

Usual Infusion Concentrations: Pediatric IV infusion: 60 **mcg**/mL

Preparation for Administration Continuous IV infusion: Must be diluted prior to infusion; dilute in NS or D_5W to a maximum final concentration of 60 mcg/mL for children and 40 mcg/mL for adults.

Administration Continuous IV infusion: Administer using an infusion pump

Monitoring Parameters Blood pressure, heart rate, ECG, renal/hepatic function tests

Additional Information Fenoldopam infusion can be abruptly discontinued or gradually tapered prior to discontinuation.

Dosage Forms Excipient information presented when available (limited, particularly for generics); consult specific product labeling.

Solution, Intravenous:

Corlopam: 10 mg/mL (1 mL); 20 mg/2 mL (2 mL) [contains propylene glycol, sodium metabisulfite]

Generic: 10 mg/mL (1 mL); 20 mg/2 mL (2 mL)

◆ **Fenoldopam Mesylate** *see* Fenoldopam *on page* 856

FentaNYL (FEN ta nil)

Medication Safety Issues

Sound-alike/look-alike issues:

FentaNYL may be confused with alfentanil, SUFentanil

High alert medication:

The Institute for Safe Medication Practices (ISMP) includes this medication among its list of drug classes which have a heightened risk of causing significant patient harm when used in error.

Administration issues:

Fentanyl transdermal system patches: Leakage of fentanyl gel from the patch has been reported; patch may be less effective; do not use. Thoroughly wash any skin surfaces coming into direct contact with gel with water (do not use soap). May contain conducting metal (eg, aluminum); remove patch prior to MRI.

Other safety concerns:

Fentanyl transdermal system patches:

Dosing of transdermal fentanyl patches may be confusing. Transdermal fentanyl patches should always be prescribed in mcg/hour, not size. Patch dosage form of Duragesic-12 actually delivers 12.5 mcg/hour of fentanyl. Use caution, as orders may be written as "Duragesic 12.5" which can be erroneously interpreted as a 125 mcg dose.

Patches should be stored and disposed of with care to avoid accidental exposure to children. The FDA has issued numerous safety advisories to warn users of the possible consequences (including hospitalization and death) of inappropriate storage or disposal of patches.

Abstral, Actiq, Fentora, Onsolis, and Subsys are not interchangeable; do not substitute doses on a mcg-per-mcg basis.

Related Information

Opioid Conversion Table *on page 2285*

Oral Medications That Should Not Be Crushed or Altered *on page 2476*

Patient Information for Disposal of Unused Medications *on page 2453*

Preprocedure Sedatives in Children *on page 2444*

Brand Names: US Abstral; Actiq; Duragesic; Fentora; Ionsys; Lazanda; Onsolis [DSC]; Subsys

Brand Names: Canada Abstral; Apo-Fentanyl Matrix; Co-Fentanyl; Duragesic MAT; Fentanyl Citrate Injection, USP; Fentora; Mylan-Fentanyl Matrix Patch; PMS-Fentanyl MTX; RAN-Fentanyl Matrix Patch; Sandoz Fentanyl Patch; Teva-Fentanyl

Therapeutic Category Analgesic, Narcotic; General Anesthetic

Generic Availability (US) Yes: Injection, lozenge, patch

Use

Parenteral: Relief of pain; preoperative medication; adjunct to general or regional anesthesia (FDA approved in ages ≥2 years and adults); has also been used for sedation and intranasally for analgesia

Transdermal patch (Duragesic®): Treatment of persistent, moderate-to-severe chronic pain in opioid-tolerant patients who are currently receiving opioids (FDA approved in ages ≥2 years and adults); see **Note**

Transmucosal products:

Buccal film (Onsolis®): Breakthrough cancer pain in opioid-tolerant patients who are currently receiving around-the-clock opioids for persistent cancer pain (FDA approved in ≥18 years and adults); see **Note**

Buccal tablet (Fentora®): Breakthrough cancer pain in opioid-tolerant patients who are currently receiving around-the-clock opioids for persistent cancer pain (FDA approved in ≥18 years and adults); see **Note**

Nasal spray (Lazanda®): Breakthrough cancer pain in opioid-tolerant patients who are currently receiving around-the-clock opioids for persistent cancer pain (FDA approved in ≥18 years and adults); see **Note**

Oral lozenge (Actiq®): Breakthrough cancer pain in opioid-tolerant patients who are currently receiving around-the-clock opioids for persistent cancer pain (FDA approved in ages ≥16 years and adults); see **Note**

Sublingual spray (Subsys®): Breakthrough cancer pain in opioid-tolerant patients who are currently receiving around-the-clock opioids for persistent cancer pain (FDA approved in ≥18 years and adults); see **Note**

Sublingual tablet (Abstral®): Breakthrough cancer pain in opioid-tolerant patients who are currently receiving around-the-clock opioids for persistent cancer pain (FDA approved in ≥18 years and adults); see **Note**

Note: Patients are considered opioid-tolerant if they are receiving around-the-clock opioids at a dose of at least 60 mg/day of morphine, 25 mcg/hour of transdermal fentanyl, 30 mg/day of oral oxycodone, 8 mg/day of oral hydromorphone, or an equivalent dose of another opioid for 1 week or longer.

Prescribing and Access Restrictions As a requirement of the REMS program, access is restricted.

Transmucosal immediate-release fentanyl products (eg, sublingual tablets and spray, oral lozenges, buccal tablets and soluble film, nasal spray) are only available through the Transmucosal Immediate-Release Fentanyl (TIRF) REMS ACCESS program. Enrollment in the program is required for outpatients, prescribers for outpatient use, pharmacies (inpatient and outpatient), and distributors. Enrollment is not required for inpatient administration (eg, hospitals, hospices, long-term care facilities), inpatients, and prescribers who prescribe to inpatients. Further information is available at 1-866-822-1483 or at www.TIRFREMSaccess.com

Note: Effective December, 2011, individual REMs programs for TIRF products were combined into a single access program (TIRF REMS Access). Prescribers and pharmacies that were enrolled in at least one individual REMS program for these products will automatically be transitioned to the single access program.

Medication Guide Available Yes

Pregnancy Risk Factor C

Pregnancy Considerations Adverse events have been observed in some animal reproduction studies. Fentanyl crosses the placenta.

Fentanyl injection may be used for the management of pain during labor (ACOG, 2002). When used for pain relief during labor, opioids may temporarily affect the heart rate of the fetus (ACOG, 2002). Transient muscular rigidity has been observed in the neonate with fentanyl; symptoms of respiratory or neurological depression were not different than those observed in infants of untreated mothers.

[U.S. Boxed Warning]: Prolonged maternal use of opioids during pregnancy can cause neonatal withdrawal syndrome in the newborn which may be life-threatening if not recognized and treated according to protocols developed by neonatology experts. If prolonged opioid therapy is required in a pregnant woman, ensure treatment is available and warn patient of risk to the neonate. If chronic opioid exposure occurs in pregnancy, adverse events in the newborn (including withdrawal) may occur; monitoring of the neonate is recommended. The minimum effective dose should be used if opioids are needed (Chou, 2009). Symptoms characteristic of neonatal abstinence syndrome have been observed following chronic fentanyl use in pregnant women. Neonatal abstinence syndrome following opioid exposure may present with autonomic (eg, fever, temperature instability), gastrointestinal (eg, diarrhea, vomiting, poor feeding/weight gain), or neurologic (eg, high pitched crying, increased muscle tone, irritability, seizure, tremor) symptoms (Dow, 2012; Hudak, 2012).

Long-term opioid use may cause secondary hypogonadism, which may lead to sexual dysfunction or infertility (Brennan, 2013).

Transdermal patch, transmucosal lozenge, nasal spray (Lazanda), sublingual tablet, sublingual spray (Subsys), buccal tablet (Fentora), and buccal film (Onsolis) are not recommended for analgesia during labor and delivery. Transdermal patch Canadian labeling contraindicates use in pregnant women and during labor and delivery.

Breast-Feeding Considerations Fentanyl is excreted in low concentrations in breast milk and breast-feeding is not recommended by the manufacturers.

Parenteral opioids used during labor have the potential to interfere with a newborn's natural reflex to nurse within the first few hours after birth. When needed, a short-acting opioid, such as fentanyl, is preferred for women who will be nursing (Montgomery, 2012)

Breast-feeding is considered acceptable following single doses to the mother; however, limited information is available when used long-term (Spigset, 2000). Nursing infants exposed to large doses of opioids should be monitored for apnea and sedation (Montgomery, 2012).

Note: Transdermal patch, transmucosal lozenge, sublingual tablet, sublingual spray (Subsys), buccal tablet (Fentora), and buccal film (Onsolis) are not recommended in nursing women due to potential for sedation and/or respiratory depression. Transdermal patch Canadian labeling contraindicates use in nursing women. Sublingual tablet Canadian labeling recommends that breast-feeding not be started until 48 hours after the last dose of fentanyl.

Contraindications Hypersensitivity to fentanyl or any component of the formulation

Additional contraindications for transdermal device (eg, Ionsys): Significant respiratory depression; acute or severe bronchial asthma; known or suspected paralytic ileus and GI obstruction; hypersensitivity to cetylpyridinium chloride (eg, Cepacol)

Additional contraindications for transdermal patches (eg, Duragesic): Severe respiratory disease or depression including acute asthma (unless patient is mechanically ventilated); paralytic ileus; patients requiring short-term therapy, management of acute or intermittent pain, postoperative or mild pain, and in patients who are **not** opioid tolerant

Additional contraindications for transmucosal buccal tablets (Fentora), buccal films (Onsolis), lozenges (eg, Actiq), sublingual tablets (Abstral), sublingual spray (Subsys), nasal spray (Lazanda): Contraindicated in the management of acute or postoperative pain (including headache, migraine, or dental pain), and in patients who are **not** opioid tolerant. Abstral and Onsolis also are contraindicated for acute pain management in the emergency room.

Canadian labeling: Additional contraindication (not in US labeling):

Injection: Septicemia; severe hemorrhage or shock; local infection at proposed injection site; disturbances in blood morphology and/or anticoagulant therapy or other concomitant drug therapy or medical conditions which could contraindicate the technique of epidural administration

Sublingual tablets (Abstral): Severe respiratory depression or severe obstructive lung disease.

Transdermal patch: Hypersensitivity to other opioids; suspected surgical abdomen (eg, acute appendicitis, pancreatitis); known or suspected mechanical GI obstruction (eg, bowel obstruction, strictures); acute alcoholism, delirium tremens, and convulsive disorders; severe CNS depression, increased cerebrospinal or intracranial pressure and head injury; concurrent use of monoamine oxidase (MAO) inhibitors or within 14 days of therapy; women who are nursing, pregnant, or during labor and delivery

Warnings/Precautions An opioid-containing analgesic regimen should be tailored to each patient's needs and based upon the type of pain being treated (acute versus chronic), the route of administration, degree of tolerance for opioids (naive versus chronic user), age, weight, and medical condition. The optimal analgesic dose varies widely among patients. Doses should be titrated to pain relief/prevention. May cause CNS depression, which may impair physical or mental abilities; patients must be cautioned about performing tasks which require mental alertness (eg, operating machinery or driving). Effects may be potentiated when used with other sedative drugs or ethanol. Fentanyl shares the toxic potentials of opioid agonists, and precautions of opioid agonist therapy should be observed; use with caution in patients with bradycardia or bradyarrhythmias; rapid IV infusion may result in skeletal muscle and chest wall rigidity leading to respiratory distress and/or apnea, bronchoconstriction, laryngospasm; inject slowly over 3 to 5 minutes. Monitor for respiratory depression in patients with significant chronic obstructive pulmonary disease or cor pulmonale, and patients having a substantially decreased respiratory reserve, hypoxia, hypercarbia, or preexisting respiratory depression, particularly when initiating therapy and titrating with fentanyl; even therapeutic doses may decrease respiratory drive to the point of apnea. Consider the use of alternative nonopioid analgesics in these patients. **[U.S. Boxed Warning]: Users are exposed to the risks of addiction, abuse, and misuse, potentially leading to overdose and death. Assess each patient's risk prior to prescribing; monitor all patients for development of these behaviors or conditions.** The risk for opioid abuse is increased in patients with a personal or family history of substance abuse (including drug or alcohol abuse or addiction) or mental illness (eg, major depression). Tolerance or drug dependence may result from extended use. The elderly may be particularly susceptible to the CNS depressant and constipating effects of opioids. Use extreme caution in patients with COPD or other chronic respiratory conditions (some products may be contraindicated). Use caution with biliary tract impairment, pancreatitis, head injuries (some products may be contraindicated), morbid obesity, renal impairment, or hepatic dysfunction. **[U.S. Boxed Warning]: Use with strong or moderate CYP3A4 inhibitors may result in increased effects and potentially fatal respiratory depression. In addition, discontinuation of a concomitant CYP 3A4 inducer may result in increased fentanyl concentrations. Monitor patients receiving any CYP 3A4 inhibitor or inducer.** Concurrent use of mixed agonist/antagonist analgesics (eg, pentazocine, nalbuphine, butorphanol) or partial agonist (eg, buprenorphine) analgesics may precipitate withdrawal symptoms and/or reduced analgesic efficacy in patients following prolonged therapy with mu opioid agonists. Abrupt discontinuation following prolonged use may also lead to withdrawal symptoms. May aggravate convulsions in patients with convulsive disorders, and may induce or aggravate seizures in some clinical settings. Monitor patients with a history of seizure disorders for worsened seizure control. May cause severe hypotension including orthostatic hypotension and syncope in ambulatory patients; risk is increased in patients whose ability to maintain blood pressure has already been compromised by a reduced blood volume; monitor these patients for signs of hypotension after initiating therapy. Potentially significant interactions may exist, requiring dose or frequency adjustment, additional monitoring, and/or selection of alternative therapy.

Pediatric patients: **[U.S. Boxed Warning]: Buccal film, buccal tablet, nasal spray, sublingual tablet, sublingual spray, and lozenge preparations contain an amount of medication that can be fatal to children. Keep all used and unused products out of the reach of children at all times and discard products properly.** Patients and caregivers should be counseled on the dangers to children including the risk of exposure to partially-consumed products.

[U.S. Boxed Warning] Abstral, Actiq, Duragesic, Fentora, Ionsys, Lazanda, Onsolis, Subsys: May cause serious, life-threatening, or fatal respiratory depression, even when used as recommended. Monitor closely for respiratory depression, especially during initiation or dose escalation. Abstral, Actiq, Duragesic, Fentora, Lazanda, Onsolis, or Subsys should only be prescribed for opioid-tolerant patients. Risk of respiratory depression increased in elderly patients, debilitated patients, and patients with conditions associated with hypoxia or hypercapnia; usually occurs after administration of initial dose in nontolerant patients or when given with other drugs that depress respiratory function.

Transmucosal (buccal film/tablet, sublingual spray/tablet, lozenge) and nasal spray: **[U.S. Boxed Warning]: Transmucosal and nasal fentanyl formulations are contraindicated in the management of acute or postoperative pain and in opioid nontolerant patients.** Should be used only for the care of opioid-tolerant cancer patients with breakthrough pain and is intended for use by specialists who are knowledgeable in treating cancer pain. **[U.S. Boxed Warning]: Substantial differences exist in the pharmacokinetic profile of fentanyl products. Do not convert patients on a mcg-per-mcg basis from one fentanyl product to another fentanyl product; the substitution of one fentanyl product for another fentanyl product may result in a fatal overdose. [U.S. Boxed Warning]: Available only through the TIRF REMS ACCESS program, a restricted distribution program with outpatients, prescribers who prescribe to outpatients, pharmacies (inpatient and outpatient), and distributor-required enrollment.** Avoid use of topical nasal decongestants (eg, oxymetazoline) during episodes of rhinitis when using fentanyl nasal spray; response to fentanyl may be delayed or reduced. Avoid use of sublingual spray in cancer patients with grade 2 or higher mucositis (fentanyl exposure increased); use with caution in patients with grade 1 mucositis, and closely monitor for respiratory and CNS depression.

Transdermal device: **[U.S. Boxed Warning]: Available only through a restricted program under a Risk Evaluation and Mitigation Strategy (REMS) called the Ionsys REMS Program. [U.S. Boxed Warning]: For use only in patients in the hospital. Discontinue treatment before patients leave the hospital. Only the patient should activate Ionsys dosing. Accidental exposure to an intact Ionsys device or to the hydrogel component, especially by children, through contact with skin or contact with mucous membranes, can result in a fatal overdose of fentanyl.** Following accidental contact with the device or its components, immediately rinse the affected area thoroughly with water. Do not use soap, alcohol, or other solvent because they may enhance the drug's ability to penetrate the skin; monitor for signs of respiratory or CNS depression. If the device is not handled correctly using gloves, healthcare professionals are at risk of accidental exposure to a fatal overdose of fentanyl. Ionsys device is considered magnetic resonance unsafe. The device contains metal parts and must be removed and properly disposed of before an MRI procedure to avoid injury to the patient and damage to device. It is unknown if exposure to an MRI procedure increases release of fentanyl from the device. Monitor any patients wearing the device with inadvertent exposure to an MRI for signs of CNS and respiratory depression. Use of Ionsys device during cardioversion, defibrillation, X-ray, CT, or diathermy can damage the device from the strong electromagnetic fields set up by these procedures. The device contains radio-opaque components and may interfere with an X-ray image or CT scan. Remove and properly dispose of the device prior to cardioversion, defibrillation, X-ray, CT, or diathermy. Avoid contact with synthetic materials (such as carpeted flooring) to reduce the possibility of electrostatic discharge and damage to the device. Avoid exposing the device to electronic security systems to reduce the possibility of damage. Use near communications equipment (eg, base stations for radio telephones and land mobile radios, amateur radio, AM and FM radio broadcast and TV broadcast Radio) and Radio Frequency Identification (RFID) transmitters can damage the device. Depending on the rated maximum output power and frequency of the transmitter, the recommended separation distance between the device and communications equipment or the RFID transmitter ranges between 0.12 and 23 meters. The low-level electrical current provided by the device does not result in electromagnetic interference with other electromechanical devices like pacemakers or electrical monitoring equipment. If exposure to the procedures listed above, electronic security systems, electrostatic discharge, communications equipment, or RFID transmitters occurs, and if the device does not appear to function normally, remove and replace with a new device. Topical skin reactions (erythema, sweating, vesicles, papules/pustules) may occur with use and are typically limited to the application site area. If a severe skin reaction is observed, remove device and discontinue further use. Ionsys is not for use in patients who are not alert and able to follow directions; avoid use in patients with impaired consciousness or coma. Avoid use in patients with circulatory shock; may cause vasodilation that can further reduce cardiac output and blood pressure.

Transdermal patch (Duragesic): **[U.S. Boxed Warning]: Transdermal patch is contraindicated for use as an as-needed analgesic, in the management of acute or postoperative pain, or in patients who are opioid non-tolerant. Monitor closely for respiratory depression during use, particularly during initiation of therapy or after dose increases.** Should only be prescribed by health care professionals who are knowledgeable in the use of potent opioids in the management of chronic pain. For patients undergoing cordotomy or other pain-relieving procedures, the Canadian labeling recommends withholding transdermal fentanyl within 72 hours prior to the procedure and in the immediate postoperative period; dose adjustment may be necessary upon resuming therapy. **[U.S. Boxed Warning]: Exposure of application site and surrounding area to direct external heat sources (eg, heating pads, electric blankets, heat or tanning lamps, sunbathing, hot tubs) may increase fentanyl absorption and has resulted in fatalities. Patients who experience fever or increase in core body temperature should be monitored closely.** Serum fentanyl concentrations may increase by approximately one-third for patients with a body temperature of 40°C (104°F) secondary to a temperature-dependent increase in fentanyl release from the patch and increased skin permeability. **[U.S. Boxed Warning]: Accidental exposure to fentanyl transdermal patch has resulted in fatal overdose in children and adults. Strict adherence to recommended handling and disposal instructions is necessary to prevent accidental exposures.** Avoid unclothed/unwashed application site exposure, inadvertent person-to-person patch transfer (eg, while hugging), incidental exposure (eg, sharing same bed, sitting on patch), intentional exposure (eg, chewing), or accidental exposure by caregivers when applying/removing patch. **[U.S. Boxed Warning]: Prolonged maternal use of opioids during pregnancy can cause neonatal withdrawal syndrome in the newborn which may be life-threatening if not recognized and treated according to protocols developed by neonatology experts. If prolonged opioid therapy is required in a pregnant woman, patient should be warned of risk to the neonate and ensure treatment is available.** Should be applied only to intact skin. Use of a patch that has been cut, damaged, or altered in any way may result in overdosage. Patients who experience adverse reactions should be monitored for at least 24 hours after removal of the patch. Drug continues to be absorbed from the skin for 24 hours or more following removal of the patch. May contain conducting metal (eg, aluminum); remove patch prior to MRI.

Warnings: Additional Pediatric Considerations

Opioid withdrawal may occur after conversion of one dosage form to another or after dosage adjustment; with prolonged use, taper dose to prevent withdrawal symptoms. Neonates who receive a total fentanyl dose >1.6 mg/kg or continuous infusion duration >5 days are more likely to develop opioid withdrawal symptoms; for infants and children 1 week to 22 months of age, those who receive a total dose of 1.5 mg/kg or duration >5 days have a 50% chance of developing opioid withdrawal and those receiving a total dose >2.5 mg/kg or duration of infusion >9 days have a 100% chance of developing withdrawal.

Dosage form specific:

Use transdermal patch in pediatric patients only if they are opioid-tolerant, receiving at least 60 mg oral morphine equivalents per day, and ≥2 years of age.

Use of Actiq was evaluated in a clinical trial of 15 opioid-tolerant pediatric patients (age: 5 to 15 years) with breakthrough pain; 12 of the 15 patients received doses of 200 mcg to 600 mcg; no conclusions about safety and efficacy could be drawn due to the small sample size.

Some dosage forms may contain propylene glycol; in neonates large amounts of propylene glycol delivered orally, intravenously (eg, >3,000 mg/day), or topically have been associated with potentially fatal toxicities which can include metabolic acidosis, seizures, renal failure, and CNS depression; toxicities have also been reported in children and adults including hyperosmolality, lactic acidosis, seizures, and respiratory depression; use caution (AAP, 1997; Shehab, 2009).

Adverse Reactions

Cardiovascular: Bradycardia, cardiac arrhythmia, cardiorespiratory arrest, chest pain, chest wall rigidity (high dose IV), deep vein thrombosis, edema, flushing, hypertension, hypotension, orthostatic hypotension, palpitations, peripheral edema, pulmonary embolism (nasal spray), sinus tachycardia, syncope, tachycardia, vasodilatation

Central nervous system: Abnormal dreams, abnormal gait, abnormality in thinking, agitation, altered sense of smell, amnesia, anxiety, ataxia, central nervous system depression, chills, confusion, depression, disorientation, dizziness, drowsiness, dysphoria, euphoria, fatigue, hallucination, headache, hypoesthesia, insomnia, irritability, lack of concentration, lethargy, malaise, mental status changes, migraine, nervousness, neuropathy, paranoia, paresthesia, restlessness, rigors, sedation, speech disturbance, stupor, vertigo, withdrawal syndrome

Dermatologic: Alopecia, cellulitis, decubitus ulcer, diaphoresis, erythema, hyperhidrosis, night sweats, pallor, papule, pruritus, skin rash

Endocrine & metabolic: Dehydration, hot flash, hypercalcemia, hyperglycemia, hypoalbuminemia, hypocalcemia, hypoglycemia, hypokalemia, hypomagnesemia, hyponatremia, weight loss

Gastrointestinal: Abdominal distention, abdominal pain, anorexia, biliary tract spasm, constipation, decreased appetite, diarrhea, dysgeusia, dyspepsia, dysphagia (buccal tablet/film/sublingual spray), flatulence, gastritis, gastroenteritis, gastroesophageal reflux disease, gastrointestinal hemorrhage, gastrointestinal ulcer (gingival, lip, mouth; transmucosal use/nasal spray), gingival pain (buccal tablet), gingivitis (lozenge), glossitis (lozenge), hematemesis, hiccups, intestinal obstruction, nausea, periodontal abscess (lozenge/buccal tablet), rectal pain, stomatitis (lozenge/buccal tablet/sublingual tablet/sublingual spray), tongue disease (sublingual tablet), vomiting, xerostomia

Genitourinary: Dysuria, erectile dysfunction, mastalgia, urinary incontinence, urinary retention, urinary tract infection, vaginal hemorrhage, vaginitis

Hematologic & oncologic: Anemia, bruise, leukopenia, lymphadenopathy, neutropenia, thrombocytopenia

Hepatic: Ascites, increased serum alkaline phosphatase, increased serum AST, jaundice

Hypersensitivity: Hypersensitivity

Local: Application site erythema, application site irritation, application site pain

Neuromuscular & skeletal: Arthralgia, back pain, limb pain, muscle rigidity, myalgia, tremor, weakness

Ophthalmic: Blepharoptosis, blurred vision, diplopia, dry eye syndrome, miosis, strabismus, swelling of eye

Renal: Renal failure

Respiratory: Apnea, asthma, bronchitis, cough, dyspnea, dyspnea (exertional), epistaxis, flu-like symptoms, hemoptysis, hypoventilation, hypoxia, laryngitis, nasal congestion (nasal spray), nasal discomfort (nasal spray), nasopharyngitis, pharyngitis, pharyngolaryngeal pain, pneumonia, postnasal drip (nasal spray), respiratory depression, rhinitis, rhinorrhea (nasal spray), sinusitis, upper respiratory tract infection, wheezing

Miscellaneous: Fever

Rare but important or life-threatening: Amblyopia, anaphylaxis, angina pectoris, aphasia, bladder pain, bronchospasm, central nervous system stimulation, delirium, depersonalization, dizziness (paradoxical), drug dependence (physical and psychological; with prolonged use), dysesthesia, emotional lability, esophageal stenosis, exfoliative dermatitis, fecal impaction, genitourinary tract spasm, gingival hemorrhage (lozenge), gum line erosion (lozenge), hematuria, hostility, hypertonia, hypogonadism (Brennan, 2013; Debono, 2011), hypotonia, laryngospasm, myasthenia, nocturia, oliguria, pancytopenia, pleural effusion, polyuria, pustules, seizure, stertorous breathing, tooth loss (lozenge), urticaria, vertigo

Drug Interactions

Metabolism/Transport Effects Substrate of CYP3A4 (major); **Note:** Assignment of Major/Minor substrate status based on clinically relevant drug interaction potential

Avoid Concomitant Use

Avoid concomitant use of FentaNYL with any of the following: Azelastine (Nasal); Conivaptan; Crizotinib; Dapoxetine; Eluxadoline; Enzalutamide; Fusidic Acid (Systemic); Idelalisib; MAO Inhibitors; Mifepristone; Mixed Agonist / Antagonist Opioids; Orphenadrine; Paraldehyde; Thalidomide

Increased Effect/Toxicity

FentaNYL may increase the levels/effects of: Alcohol (Ethyl); Alvimopan; Antipsychotic Agents; Azelastine (Nasal); Beta-Blockers; Calcium Channel Blockers (Nondihydropyridine); CNS Depressants; Desmopressin; Diuretics; Eluxadoline; Hydrocodone; MAO Inhibitors; Methotrimeprazine; Metoclopramide; Metyrosine; Orphenadrine; Paraldehyde; Pramipexole; ROPINIRole; Rotigotine; Serotonin Modulators; Suvorexant; Thalidomide; Zolpidem

The levels/effects of FentaNYL may be increased by: Amphetamines; Anticholinergic Agents; Antiemetics (5HT3 Antagonists); Antipsychotic Agents; Antipsychotic Agents (Phenothiazines); Brimonidine (Topical); Cannabis; Conivaptan; Crizotinib; CYP3A4 Inhibitors (Moderate); CYP3A4 Inhibitors (Strong); Dapoxetine; Dasatinib; Doxylamine; Dronabinol; Droperidol; Fusidic Acid (Systemic); HydrOXYzine; Idelalisib; Ivacaftor; Kava Kava;

Luliconazole; Magnesium Sulfate; Methotrimeprazine; Mifepristone; Nabilone; Palbociclib; Perampanel; Rufinamide; Simeprevir; Sodium Oxybate; Stiripentol; Succinylcholine; Tapentadol; Tetrahydrocannabinol

Decreased Effect

FentaNYL may decrease the levels/effects of: Ioflupane I 123; Pegvisomant

The levels/effects of FentaNYL may be decreased by: Alpha-/Beta-Agonists (Indirect-Acting); Alpha1-Agonists; Ammonium Chloride; CYP3A4 Inducers (Moderate); CYP3A4 Inducers (Strong); Enzalutamide; Mixed Agonist / Antagonist Opioids; Naltrexone; St Johns Wort

Food Interactions Fentanyl concentrations may be increased by grapefruit juice. Management: Avoid concurrent intake of large quantities (>1 quart/day) of grapefruit juice.

Storage/Stability

Injection formulation: Store intact vials/ampules at controlled room temperature of 20°C to 25°C (68°F to 77°F). Protect from light. Canadian labeling (not in U.S. labeling) recommends that when admixing injection formulation in NS for epidural administration, the resulting solution be used within 24 hours.

Nasal spray: Do not store above 25°C (77°F); do not freeze. Protect from light. Bottle should be stored in the provided child-resistant container when not in use and kept out of the reach of children at all times.

Transdermal device: Store at 25°C (77°F); excursions permitted to 15°C to 30°C (59°F to 86° F).

Transdermal patch: Do not store above 25°C (77°F). Keep out of the reach of children.

Transmucosal (buccal film, buccal tablet, lozenge, sublingual spray, sublingual tablet): Store at controlled room temperature of 20°C to 25°C (68°F to 77°F). Protect from freezing and moisture. Keep out of the reach of children.

Mechanism of Action Binds with stereospecific receptors at many sites within the CNS, increases pain threshold, alters pain reception, inhibits ascending pain pathways

Pharmacodynamics Respiratory depressant effect may last longer than analgesic effect

Onset of action: Analgesia:

- IM: 7-8 minutes
- Intranasal: Children 3-12 years: 5-10 minutes (Borland, 2002)
- IV: Almost immediate
- Transdermal patch (initial placement): 6 hours
- Transmucosal: 5-15 minutes

Maximum effect:

- Transdermal patch (initial placement): 24 hours
- Transmucosal: 15-30 minutes

Duration:

- IM: 1-2 hours
- IV: 0.5-1 hour
- Transdermal patch (removal of patch/no placement): 17 hours
- Transmucosal: Related to blood level; respiratory depressant effect may last longer than analgesic effect

Pharmacokinetics (Adult data unless noted) Note: Fentanyl serum concentrations are ~twofold higher in children 1.5-5 years old who are not opioid-tolerant and are receiving the transdermal patch. Pharmacokinetic parameters in older pediatric patients are similar to adults.

Absorption:

Transdermal: Drug is released at a nearly constant rate from the transdermal matrix system into the skin, where it accumulates; this results in a depot of fentanyl in the outer layer of the skin. Fentanyl is absorbed into the systemic circulation from the depot. This results in a gradual increase in serum concentrations over the first 12-24 hours, followed by a fairly constant concentration for the remainder of the dosing interval. Absorption is decreased in cachectic patients (compared to normal size patients). Pharmacokinetics of transdermal patch with or without Bioclusive™ overlay (polyurethane film dressing) were bioequivalent. Exposure to external heat increases drug absorption from patch.

Transmucosal:

- Buccal film and buccal tablet: Rapid; ~50% from the buccal mucosa; 50% swallowed with saliva and slowly absorbed from GI tract
- Transmucosal lozenge: Rapid; ~25% absorbed from buccal mucosa; 75% swallowed with saliva and slowly absorbed from GI tract

Distribution: Highly lipophilic, redistributes into muscle and fat; crosses placenta; **Note:** IV fentanyl exhibits a 3-compartment distribution model. Changes in blood pH may alter ionization of fentanyl and affect its distribution between plasma and CNS

- V_{dss}: Children: 0.05-14 years of age (after long-term continuous infusion): ~15 L/kg (range: 5-30 L/kg)
- V_{dss}: Adults: 4-6 L/kg

Protein binding: 80% to 85%, primarily to alpha-1-acid glycoprotein; also binds to albumin and erythrocytes; **Note:** Free fraction increases with acidosis

Metabolism: >90% metabolized in the liver via cytochrome P450 isoenzyme CYP3A4 by N-dealkylation (to norfentanyl) and hydroxylation to other inactive metabolites

Bioavailability: **Note:** Comparative studies have found the buccal film to have a 40% greater systemic exposure (ie, AUC) than the transmucosal lozenge, and the buccal tablet to have a 30% to 50% greater exposure than the transmucosal lozenge

- Buccal film: 71% (mucositis did not have a clinically significant effect on peak concentration and AUC; however, bioavailability is expected to decrease if film is inappropriately chewed and swallowed)
- Buccal tablet: 65%
- Oral lozenge: 47%
- Sublingual spray: 76%
- Sublingual tablet: 54%

Half-life:

IV:

- Pediatric patients 5 months to 4.5 years: 2.4 hours
- Pediatric patients 6 months to 14 years (after long-term continuous infusion): ~21 hours (range: 11-36 hours)
- Adults: 2-4 hours; **Note:** Using a 3-compartment model, fentanyl displayed an initial distribution half-life of 6 minutes; second distribution half-life of 1 hour and terminal half-life of 16 hours

Transdermal patch: 17 hours (range: 13-22 hours, apparent half-life is influenced by extended absorption)

Transmucosal products: 3-14 hours (dose-dependent)

- Buccal film: ~14 hours
- Buccal tablet: 100-200 mcg: 3-4 hours; 400-800 mcg: 11-12 hours
- Nasal spray: 15-25 hours (based on a multiple-dose pharmacokinetic study when doses are administered in the same nostril and separated by a 1-, 2-, or 4-hour time lapse)

Time to peak serum concentration:

Transdermal patch: 24-72 hours, after several sequential 72-hour applications, steady state serum concentrations are reached

Transmucosal products:

- Buccal film: Median: 1 hour (range: 0.75-4 hours)
- Buccal tablet: Median: 47 minutes (range: 20-240 minutes)
- Nasal spray: Median: 15-21 minutes
- Oral lozenge: Median: 20-40 minutes (range: 20-480 minutes), measured after the start of dose administration
- Sublingual spray: Median: 90 minutes (range: 10-120 minutes)
- Sublingual tablet: Median: 30-60 minutes (range: 15-240 minutes)

Elimination: Urine 75% (primarily as metabolites, <7% to 10% as unchanged drug); feces ~9%

Clearance: Newborn infants: Clearance may be significantly correlated to gestational age and birth weight (Saarenmaa, 2000)

Dosing: Neonatal Note: Doses should be titrated to appropriate effects; wide range of doses exist, dependent upon desired degree of analgesia/anesthesia, clinical environment, patient's status, and presence of opioid tolerance. Lower initial doses are recommended for nonventilated patients (WHO, 2012).

Analgesia: Limited data available:

International Evidence-Based Group for Neonatal Pain recommendations (Anand, 2001): Opioid-naive:

Intermittent doses: Slow IV push: 0.5-3 mcg/kg/dose

Continuous IV infusion: 0.5-2 mcg/kg/**hour**

WHO Guidelines for Pediatric Pain (WHO, 2012): Opioid-naive:

Intermittent doses: Slow IV push: Initial: 1-2 mcg/kg/dose; may repeat every 2-4 hours, titrate dose to effectiveness

Continuous IV infusion: Initial IV bolus: Slow IV push: 1-2 mcg/kg, then 0.5-1 mcg/kg/**hour**; titrate upward; usual range: 1-3 mcg/kg/**hour**

Alternate dosing: Intermittent doses: Some centers have used the following: Slow IV push: 1-4 mcg/kg/dose; may repeat every 2-4 hours (Nelson, 1996)

Continuous analgesia/sedation; mechanically ventilated patient: Limited data available: Initial IV bolus: 1-2 mcg/kg, then 0.5-1 mcg/kg/**hour**; titrate carefully to effect. Dosing based on a trial of 20 neonates ventilated for respiratory distress syndrome; mean required dose was age-dependent: GA <34 weeks (n=12): 0.64 mcg/kg/**hour** and for GA ≥34 weeks (n=8): 0.75 mcg/kg/**hour** (Roth, 1991).

Continuous analgesia/sedation during ECMO: Limited data available: Initial IV bolus: 5-10 mcg/kg slow IV push over 10 minutes, then 1-5 mcg/kg/**hour**; titrate carefully to effect; tolerance may develop; higher doses (up to 20 mcg/kg/**hour**) may be needed by day 6 of ECMO (Arnold, 1991; Leuschen, 1993).

Endotracheal intubation: Limited data available: IV: 1-4 mcg/kg slow IV push (Cloherty, 2012; Kumar, 2010)

Dosing: Usual Note: Doses should be titrated to appropriate effects; wide range of doses exist, dependent upon desired degree of analgesia/anesthesia, clinical environment, patient's status, and presence of opioid tolerance.

Infants and Children:

Acute pain: IV: Opioid-naive:

Infants: Limited data available: Initial: 1-2 mcg/kg/dose; may repeat at 2-4 hour intervals; in opioid-tolerant or younger infants, titration to higher doses may be required (up to 4 mcg/kg/dose) (Hegenbarth, 2008; Nelson, 1996; WHO, 2012)

Children: Limited data available in children <2 years: Initial: 1-2 mcg/kg/dose; may repeat at 30- to 60-minute intervals; in opioid-tolerant children, titration to higher doses may be required (Hegenbarth, 2008; Nelson, 1996; WHO, 2012)

Analgesia for minor procedures/sedation: Limited data available in children <2 years:

IM, IV: 1-2 mcg/kg/dose; administer 3 minutes before the procedure; maximum dose: 50 mcg; may repeat 1/2 original dose every 3-5 minutes if necessary; titrate to effect (Cramton, 2012; Krauss, 2006; Zeltzer, 1990)

Intranasal (using parenteral preparation): Limited data available: Infants and Children ≥10 kg: 1.5 mcg/kg once (maximum: 100 mcg/dose); reported range: 1-2 mcg/kg; some studies that used an initial dose of 1.5 mcg/kg allowed for additional incremental doses of 0.3-0.5 mcg/kg to be administered every 5 minutes, not to exceed a total dose of 3 mcg/kg depending on pain type and severity (Borland, 2002; Borland, 2005; Borland, 2007; Chung, 2010; Cole, 2009; Crellin, 2010; Herd, 2009; Manjushree, 2002; Saunders, 2010)

Anesthesia, adjunct: IM, IV: Children 2-12 years: 2-3 mcg/kg/dose

Continuous analgesia/sedation: Limited data available in children <2 years: Initial IV bolus: 1-2 mcg/kg then 1 mcg/kg/**hour**; titrate to effect; usual: 1-3 mcg/kg/**hour**; some require 5 mcg/kg/**hour** (WHO, 2012)

Chronic pain, moderate to severe: Transdermal patch: Children ≥2 years who are opioid-tolerant receiving at least 60 mg oral morphine equivalents per day: Initial: 25 mcg/**hour** system or higher, based on conversion to fentanyl equivalents and administration of equianalgesic dosage (see package insert for further information); use short-acting analgesics for first 24 hours with supplemental PRN doses thereafter (for breakthrough pain); dose may be increased after 3 days, based on the daily dose of supplementary PRN opioids required; use the ratio of 45 mg of oral morphine equivalents per day to a 12.5 mcg/**hour** increase in transdermal patch dosage; change patch every 72 hours; **Note:** Dosing intervals less than every 72 hours are **not** recommended for children and adolescents. Initiation of the transdermal patch in children taking <60 mg of oral morphine equivalents per day has not been studied in controlled clinical trials; in open-label trials, children 2-18 years of age who were receiving at least 45 mg of oral morphine equivalents per day were started with an initial transdermal dose of 25 mcg/**hour** (or higher, depending upon equianalgesic dose of opioid received).

Endotracheal intubation, emergent: Limited data available: IV: 1-5 mcg/kg/dose (Hegenbarth, 2008)

Patient-controlled analgesia (PCA): Limited data available: IV: Children ≥5 years; opioid-naïve: **Note:** PCA has been used in children as young as 5 years of age; however, clinicians need to assess children 5-8 years of age to determine if they are able to use the PCA device correctly. All patients should receive an initial loading dose of an analgesic (to attain adequate control of pain) before starting PCA for maintenance. Adjust doses, lockouts, and limits based on required loading dose, age, state of health, and presence of opioid tolerance. Use lower end of dosing range for opioid-naïve. Assess patient and pain control at regular intervals and adjust settings if needed (American Pain Society, 2008):

Patient weight ≤50 kg:

Usual concentration: Determined by weight; some centers use the following:

Children <12 kg: 10 mcg/mL

Children 12-30 kg: 25 mcg/mL

Children >30 kg: 50 mcg/mL

Demand dose: Usual initial: 0.5-1 mcg/kg/dose; usual range: 0.5-1 mcg/kg/dose

Lockout: Usual initial: 5 doses/hour

Lockout interval: Range: 6-8 minutes

Usual basal rate: 0-0.5 mcg/kg/**hour**

Patient weight >50 kg:

Usual concentration: 50 mcg/mL

Demand dose: Usual initial: 20 mcg; usual range: 10-50 mcg

Lockout interval: Usual initial: 6 minutes; usual range: 5-8 minutes

Usual basal rate: ≤50 mcg/**hour**

Adolescents and Adults:

Analgesia for minor procedures/sedation: IV: 0.5-1 mcg/kg/dose; may repeat after 30-60 minutes; or 25-50 mcg, repeat full dose in 5 minutes if needed, may repeat 4-5 times with 25 mcg at 5-minute intervals if needed. **Note:** Higher doses are used for major procedures.

Continuous analgesia/sedation:
<50 kg: Initial IV bolus: 1-2 mcg/kg; continuous infusion rate: 1-2 mcg/kg/**hour**
>50 kg: Initial IV bolus: 1-2 mcg/kg **or** 25-100 mcg/dose; continuous infusion rate: 1-2 mcg/kg/**hour or** 25-200 mcg/**hour**

Patient-controlled analgesia (PCA): IV: **Note:** All patients should receive an initial loading dose of an analgesic (to attain adequate control of pain) before starting PCA for maintenance. Adjust doses, lockouts, and limits based on required loading dose, age, state of health, and presence of opioid tolerance. Use lower end of dosing range for opioid-naïve. Assess patient and pain control at regular intervals and adjust settings if needed (American Pain Society, 2008):
Adolescents ≤50 kg; opioid-naïve:
Usual concentration: 50 mcg/mL
Demand dose: Usual initial: 0.5-1 mcg/kg/dose; usual range: 0.5-1 mcg/kg/dose
Lockout: Usual initial: 5 doses/hour
Lockout interval: Range: 6-8 minutes
Usual basal rate: 0-0.5 mcg/kg/**hour**
Adolescents >50 kg and Adults; opioid-naïve:
Usual concentration: 50 mcg/mL
Demand dose: Usual initial: 20 mcg; usual range: 10-50 mcg
Lockout interval: Usual initial: 6 minutes; usual range: 5-8 minutes
Usual basal rate: ≤50 mcg/**hour**

Preoperative sedation, adjunct to regional anesthesia, postoperative pain: IM, IV: 25-100 mcg/dose

Adjunct to general anesthesia: Slow IV:
Low dose: 0.5-2 mcg/kg/dose depending on the indication
Moderate dose: Initial: 2-20 mcg/kg/dose; Maintenance (bolus or infusion): 1-2 mcg/kg/**hour**. Discontinuing fentanyl infusion 30-60 minutes prior to the end of surgery will usually allow adequate ventilation upon emergence from anesthesia. For "fast-tracking" and early extubation following major surgery, total fentanyl doses are limited to 10-15 mcg/kg.
High dose: 20-50 mcg/kg/dose; **Note:** High dose fentanyl as an adjunct to general anesthesia is rarely used, but is still described in the manufacturer's label.

General anesthesia without additional anesthetic agents: IV: 50-100 mcg/kg/dose with O_2 and skeletal muscle relaxant

Moderate to severe chronic pain: Transdermal patch: Opioid-tolerant patients receiving at least 60 mg oral morphine equivalents per day: Initial: 25 mcg/**hour** system or higher, based on conversion to fentanyl equivalents and administration of equianalgesic dosage (see manufacturer labeling for further information); use short-acting analgesics for first 24 hours with supplemental PRN doses thereafter (for breakthrough pain); dose may be increased after 3 days based on the daily dose of supplementary PRN opioids required; use the ratio of 45 mg of oral morphine equivalents per day to a 12.5 mcg/**hour** increase in transdermal patch dosage; transdermal patch is usually administered every 72 hours but select **adult** patients may require every 48-hour administration; dosage increase administered every 72 hours should be tried before 48-hour schedule is used

Breakthrough cancer pain: Adolescents ≥16 years and Adults: Transmucosal lozenge (Actiq®): Opioid-tolerant patients: Titrate dose to provide adequate analgesia: Initial: 200 mcg; may repeat dose only once, 15 minutes after completion of first dose if needed. Do not exceed a maximum of 2 doses per each breakthrough cancer pain episode; patient must wait at least 4 hours before treating another episode. Titrate dose up to next higher strength if treatment of several consecutive breakthrough episodes requires >1 Actiq® per episode; evaluate each new dose over several breakthrough cancer pain episodes (generally 1-2 days) to determine proper dose of analgesia with acceptable side effects. Once dose has been determined, consumption should be limited to ≤4 units/day. Re-evaluate maintenance (around-the-clock) opioid dose if patient requires >4 units/day. If signs of excessive opioid effects occur before a dose is complete, the unit should be removed from the mouth immediately, and subsequent doses decreased.

Adolescents 18 years of age and Adults:

Severe pain:
IM, IV: 50-100 mcg/dose every 1-2 hours as needed; patients with prior opioid exposure may tolerate higher initial doses
Intrathecal (American Pain Society, 2008): **Note: Must use preservative-free.** Doses must be adjusted for age, injection site, and patient's medical condition and degree of opioid tolerance.
Single dose: 5-25 mcg/dose; may provide adequate relief for up to 6 hours
Continuous infusion: Not recommended in acute pain management due to risk of excessive accumulation. For chronic cancer pain, infusion of very small doses may be practical (American Pain Society, 2008).
Epidural (American Pain Society, 2008): **Note: Must use preservative-free.** Doses must be adjusted for age, injection site, and patient's medical condition and degree of opioid tolerance.
Single dose: 25-100 mcg/dose; may provide adequate relief for up to 8 hours
Continuous infusion: 25-100 mcg/**hour**

Breakthrough cancer pain: Opioid-tolerant patients: For patients who are tolerant to and currently receiving opioid therapy for persistent cancer pain; dosing should be individually titrated to provide adequate analgesia with minimal side effects. Dose titration should be done if patient requires more than 1 dose/breakthrough pain episode for several consecutive episodes. Patients experiencing >4 breakthrough pain episodes/day should have the dose of their long-term opioid re-evaluated.
Buccal film (Onsolis®): Initial dose: 200 mcg for all patients; **Note:** Patients previously using another transmucosal product should be initiated at doses of 200 mcg; do **not** switch patients using any other fentanyl product on a mcg-per-mcg basis.
Dose titration: If titration of dose is required, increase dose in 200 mcg increments once per episode using multiples of the 200 mcg film; do not redose within a single episode of breakthrough pain and separate single doses by ≥2 hours. During titration, do not exceed 4 simultaneous applications of the 200 mcg films (800 mcg). If >800 mcg required, treat next episode with one 1200 mcg film (maximum dose: 1200 mcg). Once maintenance dose is determined, all other unused films should be disposed of and that strength (using a single film) should be used. During any pain episode, if adequate relief is not achieved after 30 minutes following buccal film application, a rescue medication (as determined by healthcare provider) may be used.
Maintenance: Determined dose applied as a single film once per episode and separated by ≥2 hours (dose range: 200-1200 mcg); limit to 4 applications/day. Consider increasing the around-the-clock opioid therapy in patients experiencing >4 breakthrough pain episodes/day.
Buccal tablets (Fentora®): Initial dose: 100 mcg; a second 100 mcg dose, if needed, may be administered 30 minutes after the start of the first dose; **Note:** For patients previously using the transmucosal

lozenge (Actiq®), the initial dose should be selected using the conversions listed below (maximum: 2 doses per breakthrough pain episode every 4 hours).

Dose titration: If required, should be done using multiples of the 100 mcg tablets. Patient can take two 100 mcg tablets (one on each side of mouth). If that dose is not successful, can use four 100 mcg tablets (two on each side of mouth). If titration requires >400 mcg/dose, then use 200 mcg tablets. **Note:** Buccal tablet may be administered sublingually once an effective maintenance dose has been established.

Conversion from transmucosal lozenge to buccal tablet (Fentora®): Initial dose:

Lozenge dose 200-400 mcg, then use buccal tablet 100 mcg

Lozenge dose 600-800 mcg, then use buccal tablet 200 mcg

Lozenge dose 1200-1600 mcg, then use buccal tablet 400 mcg

Note: Four 100 mcg buccal tablets deliver approximately 12% and 13% higher values of C_{max} and AUC, respectively, compared to one 400 mcg buccal tablet. To prevent confusion, patient should only have one strength of tablets available at a time. Using more than four buccal tablets at a time has not been studied.

Nasal spray (Lazanda®):

Initial dose: 100 mcg (one 100 mcg spray in one nostril) for all patients. **Note:** Patients previously using another fentanyl product should be initiated at a dose of 100 mcg; do not convert patients from other fentanyl products to Lazanda® on a mcg-per-mcg basis.

Dose titration: If pain is relieved within 30 minutes, that same dose should be used to treat subsequent episodes. If pain is unrelieved, may increase to a higher dose using the recommended titration steps. **Must wait at least 2 hours before treating another episode with nasal spray.** Dose titration steps: If no relief with 100 mcg dose, increase to 200 mcg dose per episode (one 100 mcg spray in each nostril); if no relief with 200 mcg dose, increase to 400 mcg per episode (one 400 mcg spray in one nostril or two 100 mcg sprays in each nostril); if no relief with 400 mcg dose, increase to 800 mcg dose per episode (one 400 mcg spray in each nostril). **Note:** Single doses >800 mcg have not been evaluated. There are no data supporting the use of a combination of dose strengths.

Maintenance dose: Once maintenance dose for breakthrough pain episode has been determined, use that dose for subsequent episodes. For pain that is not relieved after 30 minutes of Lazanda® administration or if a separate breakthrough pain episode occurs within the 2 hour window before the next Lazanda® dose is permitted, a rescue medication may be used. Limit Lazanda® use to ≤4 episodes of breakthrough pain per day. If response to maintenance dose changes (increase in adverse reactions or alterations in pain relief), dose readjustment may be necessary. If patient is experiencing >4 breakthrough pain episodes/day, consider increasing the around-the-clock, long-acting opioid therapy; if long-acting opioid therapy dose is altered, re-evaluate and retitrate Lazanda® dose as needed.

Sublingual spray (Subsys®):

Initial dose: 100 mcg for all patients. If pain is unrelieved, one additional 100 mcg dose may be given 30 minutes after administration of the first dose. A maximum of two doses can be given per breakthrough pain episode; must wait at least 4 hours before treating another episode. **Note:** Patients must remain on around-the-clock opioids during use. Patients previously using other fentanyl products should be initiated at a dose of 100 mcg; do not convert patients from any other fentanyl product (transmucosal, transdermal, or parenteral) to Subsys® on a mcg-per-mcg basis.

Dose titration: If pain is relieved within 30 minutes, that same dose should be used to treat subsequent episodes and no titration is necessary. If pain is unrelieved, may increase to a higher dose using the recommended titration steps. Goal is to determine the dose that provides adequate analgesia (with tolerable side effects) using a single dose per breakthrough pain episode. For each breakthrough pain episode, if pain unrelieved after 30 minutes only one additional dose using the same strength may be given (maximum: Two doses per breakthrough pain episode). **Must wait at least 4 hours before treating another episode with Subsys®.**

Dose titration steps: If no relief with 100 mcg dose, increase to 200 mcg dose per episode (one 200 mcg unit); if no relief with 200 mcg dose, increase to 400 mcg per episode (one 400 mcg unit); if no relief with 400 mcg dose, increase to 600 mcg dose per episode (one 600 mcg unit); if no relief with 600 mcg dose, increase to 800 mcg dose per episode (one 800 mcg unit); if no relief with 800 mcg dose, increase to 1200 mcg dose per episode (two 600 mcg units); if no relief with 1200 mcg dose, increase to 1600 mcg per episode (two 800 mcg units).

Maintenance dose: Once maintenance dose for breakthrough pain episode has been determined, use that dose for subsequent episodes. If occasional episodes of unrelieved breakthrough pain occur following 30 minutes of Subsys® administration, one additional dose using the same strength may be administered (maximum: Two doses per breakthrough pain episode); patient must wait 4 hours before treating another breakthrough pain episode with Subsys®. Once maintenance dose is determined, limit Susbsys® use to ≤4 episodes of breakthrough pain per day. If response to maintenance dose changes (increase in adverse reactions or alterations in pain relief), dose readjustment may be necessary. If patient is experiencing >4 breakthrough pain episodes/day, consider increasing the around-the-clock, long-acting opioid therapy.

Sublingual tablet (Abstral®):

Initial dose: 100 mcg for all patients; if pain is unrelieved, a second dose may be given 30 minutes after administration of the first dose. A maximum of two doses can be given per breakthrough pain episode; must wait at least 2 hours before treating another episode. **Note:** Patients previously using another fentanyl product should be initiated at a dose of 100 mcg; do not convert patients from other fentanyl products to Abstral® on a mcg-per-mcg basis.

Dose titration: If titration required, increase in 100 mcg increments (up to 400 mcg) over consecutive breakthrough episodes. If titration requires >400 mcg/dose, increase in increments of 200 mcg, starting with 600 mcg dose. During titration, patients may use multiples of 100 mcg and/or 200 mcg tablets for any single dose; do not exceed 4 tablets at one time; safety and efficacy of doses >800 mcg have not been evaluated.

Maintenance dose: Once maintenance dose for breakthrough pain episode has been determined, use only one tablet in the appropriate strength per episode; if pain is unrelieved with maintenance dose. A second dose may be given after 30 minutes; maximum of two doses/episode of breakthrough pain; separate treatment of subsequent episodes by ≥2 hours; limit treatment to ≤4 breakthrough episodes/day. Consider increasing the around-the-clock, long-acting opioid therapy in patients experiencing >4 breakthrough pain episodes/day; if long-acting opioid therapy dose altered, re-evaluate and retitrate Abstral® dose as needed.

Dosing adjustment in renal impairment:

Infants, Children, and Adolescents: There are no dosage adjustments provided in the manufacturer's labeling; however, the following guidelines have been used by some clinicians (Aronoff, 2007): The following assumes dosages of 0.5-2 mcg/kg/dose or 1-5 mcg/kg/**hour** in normal renal function: IV:

GFR >50 mL/minute/1.73 m^2: No adjustment required

GFR 10-50 mL/minute/1.73m^2: Administer 75% of usual dose

GFR <10 mL/minute/1.73m^2: Administer 50% of usual dose

Intermittent hemodialysis: Administer 50% of usual dose

Peritoneal dialysis (PD): Administer 50% of usual dose

Continuous renal replacement therapy (CRRT): Administer 75% of usual dose

Adolescents ≥16 years and Adults: Transdermal (patch): Degree of impairment (ie, CrCl) not defined in manufacturer's labeling.

Mild to moderate impairment: Initial: Reduce dose by 50%; monitor patient closely

Severe impairment: Use not recommended

Adolescents ≥18 years and Adults: Transmucosal (buccal film/tablet, sublingual spray/tablet, lozenge) and nasal spray: Although fentanyl pharmacokinetics may be altered in renal disease, fentanyl can be used successfully in the management of breakthrough cancer pain. Use with caution; reduce initial dose and titrate to reach clinical effect with careful monitoring of patients, especially those with severe renal disease.

Dosing adjustment in hepatic impairment:

Transdermal (patch): Adolescents ≥16 years and Adults:

Mild to moderate impairment: Initial: Reduce dose by 50%

Severe impairment: Use not recommended

Transmucosal (buccal film/tablet, sublingual spray/tablet, lozenge) and nasal spray: Adolescents ≥18 years and Adults: Although fentanyl pharmacokinetics may be altered in hepatic disease, fentanyl can be used successfully in the management of breakthrough cancer pain. Use with caution; reduce initial dose and titrate to reach clinical effect with careful monitoring of patients, especially those with severe hepatic disease.

Usual Infusion Concentrations: Neonatal IV infusion: 10 **mcg**/mL

Usual Infusion Concentrations: Pediatric IV infusion: 10 **mcg**/mL

Preparation for Administration Continuous IV infusion: May further dilute in NS or D_5W. ISMP and Vermont Oxford Network recommend a standard concentration of 10 mcg/mL for neonates (ISMP 2011).

Administration

Parenteral: IV: Administer by slow IV push over 3 to 5 minutes or by continuous infusion. Larger bolus doses (>5 mcg/kg) should be given by slow IV push over 5 to 10 minutes.

Transdermal patch: Apply to nonhairy, clean, dry, nonirritated, intact skin of the flat area of front or back of upper torso, flank area, or upper arm; apply to upper back in young children or in people with cognitive impairment to decrease the potential of the patient removing the patch. Monitor the adhesion of the system closely in children. Clip hair prior to application, do **not** shave area; prior to application, skin may be cleaned with clear water (do not use soaps, lotions, alcohol, oils, or other substances which may irritate the skin); allow skin to dry thoroughly prior to application. Apply patch immediately after removing from package; firmly press in place and hold for at least 30 seconds; change patch every 72 hours; remove old patch before applying new patch; do not apply new patch to same place as old patch; wash hands after applying patch. If there is difficulty with patch adhesion, the edges of the system may be taped in place with first-aid tape; if difficulty with adhesion persists, an adhesive film dressing (eg, Bioclusive, Tegaderm) may be applied over the system. If patch falls off before 72 hours, a new patch may be applied to a different skin site.

Note: Transdermal patch is a membrane-controlled system; do **not** cut the patch to deliver partial doses; do **not** use patches that are cut, damaged, or leaking; do **not** use if seal of package is broken; rate of drug delivery may be significantly increased if patch is cut, damaged, or leaking and result in absorption of a potentially fatal dose; reservoir contents and adhesion may be affected if cut; if partial dose is needed, surface area of patch can be blocked proportionally using adhesive bandage (Lee 1997). Do **not** use soap, alcohol, or other solvents to remove transdermal gel if it accidentally touches skin as they may increase transdermal absorption; use copious amounts of water. Avoid exposing application site to external heat sources (eg, electric blanket, heating pad, heat lamp, tanning lamp, sauna, heated water bed, hot tub, hot baths, sunbathing). Dispose of properly.

Transmucosal products:

Buccal film (Onsolis): Foil overwrap should be removed just prior to administration. Prior to placing film, wet inside of cheek using tongue or by rinsing with water. Place film inside mouth with the pink side of the unit against the inside of the moistened cheek. With finger, press the film against cheek and hold for 5 seconds. The film should stick to the inside of cheek after 5 seconds. The film should be left in place until it dissolves (usually within 15 to 30 minutes after application). Liquids may be consumed after 5 minutes of application. Food can be eaten after film dissolves. If using more than one film simultaneously (during titration period), apply films on either side of mouth (do not apply on top of each other). Do not chew or swallow film. Do not cut or tear the film.

Buccal tablet (Fentora®): Do not use if blister package has been opened or tampered with. Blister package should be opened just prior to administration. Peel back the blister backing to expose the tablet; do not push tablet through the blister (damage to the tablet may occur). Administer tablet immediately after removal from blister. Place entire tablet in the buccal cavity (above a rear molar, between the upper cheek and gum) or under the tongue; should dissolve in about 14 to 25 minutes. If remnants remain after 30 minutes they may be swallowed with a glass of water. Use alternate side of mouth for subsequent doses. Do not break, split, suck, chew, or swallow tablet (this will result in decreased effect). If excessive opioid effects appear before tablet is completely dissolved (eg, dizziness, sedation, nausea), instruct patient to rinse mouth with water and spit remaining pieces of tablet into sink or toilet immediately; rinse the sink or flush toilet to dispose of tablet particles.

Intranasal:

Solution (injectable product): Pediatric patients ≥10 kg: If congested, suction nostrils prior to administration. Using a 50 mcg/mL solution, administer half of the dose to each nostril using an atomizer such as the MAD® Nasal Drug delivery device or drip into the nostril slowly with a syringe; higher concentrations (150 mcg/mL and 300 mcg/mL) have been studied to prevent excess volume administration and decrease leakage, but comparative trials have not been performed.

Nasal spray (Lazanda): Prior to initial use, prime device by spraying 4 sprays into the provided pouch (the counting window will show a green bar when the bottle is ready for use). Insert nozzle a short distance into the nose (~1/2 inch or 1 cm) and point towards the bridge of the nose (while closing off the other nostril using one finger). Press on finger grips until a "click" sound is heard and the number in the counting window advances by one. The "click" sound and dose counter are the only reliable methods for ensuring a dose has been administered (spray is not always felt on the nasal mucosa). Patient should remain seated for at least 1 minute following administration. Do not blow nose for ≥30 minutes after administration. Wash hands before and after use. There are 8 full therapeutic sprays in each bottle; do not continue to use bottle after "8" sprays have been used. Dispose of bottle and contents if ≥5 days have passed since last use or if it has been ≥4 days since bottle was primed. Spray the remaining contents into the provided pouch, seal in the child-resistant container, and dispose of in the trash.

Oral lozenge (Actiq): Oral: Do not use if blister package has been opened. Blister package should be opened with scissors just prior to administration; once removed, patient should place the lozenge in mouth and suck it; do not bite or chew lozenge. Place lozenge in mouth between cheek and lower gum; occasionally move lozenge from one side of the mouth to the other; consume lozenge over 15 minutes; remove lozenge from mouth if signs of excessive opioid effects appear before lozenge is totally consumed. Remove handle after lozenge is consumed or patient achieves adequate response.

Sublingual spray (Subsys): Open sealed blister unit with scissors immediately prior to administration. Contents of unit should be sprayed into mouth under the tongue. Dispose of unit immediately after use, using disposal bottle provided.

Sublingual tablet (Abstral): Remove from the blister unit immediately prior to administration. Place tablet directly under the tongue on the floor of the mouth and allow to completely dissolve; do not chew, suck, or swallow. Do not eat or drink anything until tablet is completely dissolved. In patients with a dry mouth, water may be used to moisten the buccal mucosa just before administration.

Monitoring Parameters Respiratory rate, blood pressure, heart rate, oxygen saturation, bowel sounds, abdominal distention; signs of misuse, abuse, or addiction

Transdermal patch: Monitor patient for at least 24 hours after application of first dose

Additional Information Fentanyl is 50-100 times as potent as morphine; morphine 10 mg IM = fentanyl 0.1-0.2 mg IM Fentanyl has less hypotensive effects than morphine or meperidine due to minimal or no histamine release. IV product has a pH of 4.0-7.5.

Product Availability Ionsys (iontophoretic transdermal system): FDA approved May 2015; availability anticipated in the third quarter of 2015. Information pertaining to this product within the monograph is pending revision. Consult prescribing information for additional information.

Controlled Substance C-II

Dosage Forms Excipient information presented when available (limited, particularly for generics); consult specific product labeling. [DSC] = Discontinued product

Film, for buccal application, as citrate [strength expressed as base]:

Onsolis: 200 mcg (30s); 400 mcg (30s); 600 mcg (30s); 800 mcg (30s); 1200 mcg (30s) [DSC]

Injection, solution, as citrate [strength expressed as base, preservative free]:

Generic: 0.05 mg/mL (2 mL, 5 mL, 10 mL, 20 mL, 50 mL)

Liquid, sublingual, as base [spray]:

Subsys: 100 mcg (30s); 200 mcg (30s); 400 mcg (30s); 600 mcg (30s); 800 mcg (30s) [contains dehydrated ethanol 63.6%, propylene glycol]

Lozenge, oral, as citrate [strength expressed as base, transmucosal]:

Actiq: 200 mcg (30s); 400 mcg (30s); 600 mcg (30s); 800 mcg (30s); 1200 mcg (30s); 1600 mcg (30s) [contains sugar 2 g/lozenge; berry flavor]

Generic: 200 mcg (30s); 400 mcg (30s); 600 mcg (30s); 800 mcg (30s); 1200 mcg (30s); 1600 mcg (30s)

Patch, transdermal, as base:

Duragesic: 12 [delivers 12.5 mcg/hr] (5s) [contains ethanol 0.1 mL/10 cm^2; 5 cm^2]

Duragesic: 25 [delivers 25 mcg/hr] (5s) [contains ethanol 0.1 mL/10 cm^2; 10 cm^2]

Duragesic: 50 [delivers 50 mcg/hr] (5s) [contains ethanol 0.1 mL/10 cm^2; 20 cm^2]

Duragesic: 75 [delivers 75 mcg/hr] (5s) [contains ethanol 0.1 mL/10 cm^2; 30 cm^2]

Duragesic: 100 [delivers 100 mcg/hr] (5s) [contains ethanol 0.1 mL/10 cm^2; 40 cm^2]

Ionsys: 40 mcg/actuation (6s) [iontophoretic transdermal system]

Generic: 12 [delivers 12.5 mcg/hr] (5s); 25 [delivers 25 mcg/hr] (5s); 50 [delivers 50 mcg/hr] (5s); 75 [delivers 75 mcg/hr] (5s); 87.5 [delivers 87.5 mcg/hr] (5s); 100 [delivers 100 mcg/hr] (5s)

Powder, for prescription compounding, as citrate: USP: 100% (1 g)

Solution, intranasal, as citrate [strength expressed as base, spray]:

Lazanda: 100 mcg/spray (5 mL); 400 mcg/spray (5 mL) [delivers 8 metered sprays]

Tablet, for buccal application, as citrate [strength expressed as base]:

Fentora: 100 mcg (28s); 200 mcg (28s); 400 mcg (28s); 600 mcg (28s); 800 mcg (28s)

Tablet, sublingual, as citrate [strength expressed as base]:

Abstral: 100 mcg (12s, 32s); 200 mcg (12s, 32s); 300 mcg (12s, 32s); 400 mcg (12s, 32s); 600 mcg (32s); 800 mcg (32s)

- ◆ **Fentanyl Citrate** *see* FentaNYL *on page 857*
- ◆ **Fentanyl Citrate Injection, USP (Can)** *see* FentaNYL *on page 857*
- ◆ **Fentanyl Hydrochloride** *see* FentaNYL *on page 857*
- ◆ **Fentanyl Patch** *see* FentaNYL *on page 857*
- ◆ **Fentora** *see* FentaNYL *on page 857*
- ◆ **Feosol Original** *see* Ferrous Sulfate *on page 871*
- ◆ **Ferate [OTC]** *see* Ferrous Gluconate *on page 870*
- ◆ **Fergon [OTC]** *see* Ferrous Gluconate *on page 870*
- ◆ **Fer-In-Sol [OTC]** *see* Ferrous Sulfate *on page 871*
- ◆ **Fer-In-Sol (Can)** *see* Ferrous Sulfate *on page 871*
- ◆ **Fer-Iron [OTC]** *see* Ferrous Sulfate *on page 871*
- ◆ **Fermalac (Can)** *see Lactobacillus on page 1203*
- ◆ **Ferodan (Can)** *see* Ferrous Sulfate *on page 871*
- ◆ **FeroSul [OTC]** *see* Ferrous Sulfate *on page 871*
- ◆ **Ferretts [OTC]** *see* Ferrous Fumarate *on page 869*
- ◆ **Ferrex 150 [OTC]** *see* Polysaccharide-Iron Complex *on page 1728*

Ferric Gluconate (FER ik GLOO koe nate)

Medication Safety Issues

Sound-alike/look-alike issues:

Ferric gluconate may be confused with ferric carboxymaltose, ferumoxytol

Brand Names: US Ferrlecit

Brand Names: Canada Ferrlecit

Therapeutic Category Iron Salt, Parenteral; Mineral, Parenteral

Generic Availability (US) Yes

Use Treatment of microcytic, hypochromic anemia resulting from iron deficiency in combination with erythropoietin in hemodialysis patients when iron administration is not feasible or ineffective

Pregnancy Risk Factor B

Pregnancy Considerations Adverse events were not observed in animal reproduction studies. It is recommended that pregnant women meet the dietary requirements of iron with diet and/or supplements in order to prevent adverse events associated with iron deficiency anemia in pregnancy. Treatment of iron deficiency anemia in pregnant women is the same as in nonpregnant women and in most cases, oral iron preparations may be used. Except in severe cases of maternal anemia, the fetus achieves normal iron stores regardless of maternal concentrations.

Breast-Feeding Considerations Iron is normally found in breast milk. Breast milk or iron fortified formulas generally provide enough iron to meet the recommended dietary requirements of infants. The amount of iron in breast milk is generally not influenced by maternal iron status.

Contraindications Known hypersensitivity to ferric gluconate or any component of the formulation

Warnings/Precautions Serious hypersensitivity reactions, including anaphylactic-type reactions, have occurred (may be life-threatening). Monitor during administration and for ≥30 minutes after administration and until clinically stable after infusion. Avoid rapid administration. Equipment for resuscitation and trained personnel experienced in handling medical emergencies should always be immediately available. Clinically significant hypotension may occur; usually resolves within 1-2 hours. May augment hemodialysis-induced hypotension. Use with caution in elderly patients. Use only in patients with documented iron deficiency; caution with hemoglobinopathies or other refractory anemias.

Benzyl alcohol and derivatives: Some dosage forms may contain benzyl alcohol; large amounts of benzyl alcohol (≥99 mg/kg/day) have been associated with a potentially fatal toxicity ("gasping syndrome") in neonates; the "gasping syndrome" consists of metabolic acidosis, respiratory distress, gasping respirations, CNS dysfunction (including convulsions, intracranial hemorrhage), hypotension and cardiovascular collapse (AAP, 1997; CDC, 1982); some data suggests that benzoate displaces bilirubin from protein binding sites (Ahlfors, 2001); avoid or use dosage forms containing benzyl alcohol with caution in neonates. See manufacturer's labeling.

Adverse Reactions

Cardiovascular: Angina pectoris, bradycardia, chest pain, edema, hyper-/hypotension, hypervolemia, MI, peripheral edema, syncope, tachycardia, vasodilation

Central nervous system: Agitation, chills, consciousness decreased, dizziness, fatigue, fever, headache, lightheadedness, malaise, rigors, somnolence

Dermatologic: Pruritus, rash

Endocrine & metabolic: Hyper-/hypokalemia, hypoglycemia

Gastrointestinal: Abdominal pain, anorexia, diarrhea, dyspepsia, eructation, flatulence, GI disorder, melena, nausea, rectal disorder, vomiting

Genitourinary: Menorrhagia, UTI

Hematologic: Anemia, erythrocytes abnormal (changes in morphology/color/number), leukocytosis, lymphadenopathy

Local: Injection site reaction

Neuromuscular & skeletal: Arm pain, arthralgia, back pain, cramps, leg cramps, leg edema, paresthesia, weakness

Ocular: Arcus senilis, conjunctivitis, diplopia, puffy eyelids, redness of eyes, rolling of eyes, watery eyes

Otic: Deafness

Respiratory: Cough, dyspnea, pharyngitis, pneumonia, pulmonary edema, rhinitis, upper respiratory infections

Miscellaneous: Abscess, carcinoma, diaphoresis, flu-like symptoms, infection, sepsis

Rare but important or life-threatening: Allergic reaction, anaphylactic reactions, convulsion, facial flushing, hemorrhage, hypertonia, hypoesthesia, loss of consciousness, shock, skin discoloration

Drug Interactions

Metabolism/Transport Effects None known.

Avoid Concomitant Use

Avoid concomitant use of Ferric Gluconate with any of the following: Dimercaprol

Increased Effect/Toxicity

The levels/effects of Ferric Gluconate may be increased by: ACE Inhibitors; Dimercaprol

Decreased Effect There are no known significant interactions involving a decrease in effect.

Storage/Stability Store at 20°C to 25°C (68°F to 77°F); excursions permitted to 15°C to 30°C (59°F to 86°F). Do not freeze. Use immediately after dilution.

Mechanism of Action Supplies a source to elemental iron necessary to the function of hemoglobin, myoglobin and specific enzyme systems; allows transport of oxygen via hemoglobin

Pharmacodynamics

Onset of action: Hematologic response to either oral or parenteral iron salts is essentially the same; red blood cell form and color changes within 3-10 days

Maximum effect: Peak reticulocytosis occurs in 5-10 days, and hemoglobin values increase within 2-4 weeks

Pharmacokinetics (Adult data unless noted)

Following IV doses, the uptake of iron by the reticuloendothelial system appears to be constant at about 40-60 mg/hour

Half-life: 1.31 hours

Elimination: By the reticuloendothelial system and excreted in urine and feces (via bile)

Dialysis: Not dialyzable

Dosing: Usual Multiple forms for parenteral iron exist; close attention must be paid to the specific product when ordering and administering; incorrect selection or substitution of one form for another without proper dosage adjustment may result in serious over- or under-dosing; test doses are recommended before starting therapy. **Note:** Per National Kidney Foundation DOQI Guidelines, initiation of iron therapy, determination of dose, and duration of therapy should be guided by results of iron status tests combined with the Hb level and the dose of the erythropoietin stimulating agent. There is insufficient evidence to recommend IV iron if ferritin level >500 ng/mL.

Dosage expressed in mg **elemental** iron: IV:

Children ≥6 years: 1.5 mg/kg (0.12 mL/kg Ferrlecit®) repeated at each of 8 sequential dialysis sessions not to exceed 125 mg (10 mL) per dose

Adults: 125 mg (10 mL) during hemodialysis; most patients will require a cumulative dose of 1 g over ~8 sequential dialysis treatments to achieve a favorable response

Note: A test dose (25 mg in adult patients) previously recommended in product literature is no longer listed. No pediatric test dose has been recommended by the manufacturer.

Preparation for Administration Parenteral: IV infusion: Dilute dose in NS: Children: 25 mL; adults: 100 mL. In adults, may also administer undiluted.

Administration Parenteral: IV infusion:
Children and Adolescents: Administer diluted over 1 hour
Adults: Administer diluted over 1 hour or administer undiluted slowly at a rate of up to 12.5 mg/minute

Monitoring Parameters Vital signs and other symptoms of anaphylactoid reactions (during IV infusion); reticulocyte count, serum ferritin, hemoglobin, serum iron concentrations, and transferrin saturation (TSAT). Ferritin and TSAT may be inaccurate if measured within 14 days of receiving a large single dose (1000 mg in adults).

Reference Range
Serum iron:
Newborns: 110-270 mcg/dL
Infants: 30-70 mcg/dL
Children: 55-120 mcg/dL
Adults: Male: 75-175 mcg/dL; female: 65-165 mcg/dL
Total iron binding capacity:
Newborns: 59-175 mcg/dL
Infants: 100-400 mcg/dL
Children and Adults: 230-430 mcg/dL
Transferrin: 204-360 mg/dL
Percent transferrin saturation (TSAT): 20% to 50%
Iron levels >300 mcg/dL may be considered toxic; should be treated as an overdosage
Ferritin: 13-300 ng/mL
Chronic kidney disease (CKD): Targets for iron therapy (KDOQI Guidelines, 2007) to maintain Hgb 11-12 g/dL:
Children: Nondialysis CKD, hemodialysis, or peritoneal dialysis: Ferritin: >100 ng/mL and TSAT >20%
Adults: Nondialysis (CKD) or peritoneal dialysis: Ferritin: >100 ng/mL and TSAT >20%
Hemodialysis: Ferritin >200 ng/mL and TSAT >20% or CHr (content of hemoglobin in reticulocytes) >29 pg/cell

Test Interactions Serum or transferrin bound iron levels may be falsely elevated if assessed within 24 hours of ferric gluconate administration. Serum ferritin levels may be falsely elevated for 5 days after ferric gluconate administration.

Additional Information Iron storage may lag behind the appearance of normal red blood cell morphology; use periodic hematologic determination to assess therapy

Dosage Forms Considerations Strength of ferric gluconate injection is expressed as elemental iron.

Dosage Forms Excipient information presented when available (limited, particularly for generics); consult specific product labeling.
Solution, Intravenous:
Ferrlecit: 12.5 mg/mL (5 mL) [contains benzyl alcohol, sucrose]
Generic: 12.5 mg/mL (5 mL)

◆ **Ferric x-150 [OTC]** *see* Polysaccharide-Iron Complex *on page 1728*

◆ **Ferrimin 150 [OTC]** *see* Ferrous Fumarate *on page 869*

◆ **Ferrlecit** *see* Ferric Gluconate *on page 867*

◆ **Ferro-Bob [OTC]** *see* Ferrous Sulfate *on page 871*

◆ **Ferrocite [OTC]** *see* Ferrous Fumarate *on page 869*

Ferrous Fumarate (FER us FYOO ma rate)

Related Information
Oral Medications That Should Not Be Crushed or Altered *on page 2476*

Brand Names: US Ferretts [OTC]; Ferrimin 150 [OTC]; Ferrocite [OTC]; Hemocyte [OTC]

Brand Names: Canada Palafer®

Therapeutic Category Iron Salt; Mineral, Oral

Generic Availability (US) Yes

Use Prevention and treatment of iron deficiency anemias (OTC: FDA approved in adults; see product specific labeling for pediatric approval ages); has also been used as supplemental therapy for patients receiving epoetin alfa

Pregnancy Considerations It is recommended that pregnant women meet the dietary requirements of iron with diet and/or supplements in order to prevent adverse events associated with iron deficiency anemia in pregnancy. Treatment of iron deficiency anemia in pregnant women is the same as in nonpregnant women and in most cases, oral iron preparations may be used. Except in severe cases of maternal anemia, the fetus achieves normal iron stores regardless of maternal concentrations.

Breast-Feeding Considerations Iron is normally found in breast milk. Breast milk or iron-fortified formulas generally provide enough iron to meet the recommended dietary requirements of infants. The amount of iron in breast milk is generally not influenced by maternal iron status.

Contraindications Hypersensitivity to iron salts or any component of the formulation; hemochromatosis, hemolytic anemia

Warnings/Precautions Avoid in patients with peptic ulcer, enteritis, or ulcerative colitis. Administration of iron for >6 months should be avoided except in patients with continuous bleeding or menorrhagia. Anemia in the elderly is often caused by "anemia of chronic disease" or associated with inflammation rather than blood loss. Iron stores are usually normal or increased, with a serum ferritin >50 ng/mL and a decreased total iron binding capacity. Hence, the "anemia of chronic disease" is not secondary to iron deficiency but the inability of the reticuloendothelial system to reclaim available iron stores. Avoid in patients receiving frequent blood transfusions Avoid use in premature infants until the vitamin E stores, deficient at birth, are replenished. Accidental overdose of iron-containing products is a leading cause of fatal poisoning in children under 6 years of age. Keep this product out of the reach of children. In case of accidental overdose call the poison control center immediately.

Warnings: Additional Pediatric Considerations Consider all iron sources when evaluating the dose of iron, including combination products, infant formulas, and liquid nutritional supplements.

Adverse Reactions
Gastrointestinal: Constipation, dark stools, diarrhea, heartburn, nausea, staining of teeth, stomach cramping, vomiting
Genitourinary: Discoloration of urine
Rare but important or life-threatening: Contact irritation

Drug Interactions

Metabolism/Transport Effects None known.

Avoid Concomitant Use
Avoid concomitant use of Ferrous Fumarate with any of the following: Dimercaprol

Increased Effect/Toxicity
The levels/effects of Ferrous Fumarate may be increased by: Dimercaprol

Decreased Effect
Ferrous Fumarate may decrease the levels/effects of: Alpha-Lipoic Acid; Bisphosphonate Derivatives; Cefdinir; Deferiprone; Dolutegravir; Eltrombopag; Levodopa; Levothyroxine; Methyldopa; PenicillAMINE; Phosphate Supplements; Quinolone Antibiotics; Tetracycline Derivatives; Trientine

The levels/effects of Ferrous Fumarate may be decreased by: Alpha-Lipoic Acid; Antacids; H2-Antagonists; Pancrelipase; Proton Pump Inhibitors; Tetracycline Derivatives; Trientine

Food Interactions Cereals, dietary fiber, tea, coffee, eggs, and milk may decrease absorption.

Storage/Stability Store at 15°C to 30°C (59°F to 86°F). Iron is a leading cause of fatal poisoning in children. Store out of children's reach and in child-resistant containers.

Mechanism of Action Replaces iron found in hemoglobin, myoglobin, and enzymes; allows the transportation of oxygen via hemoglobin

Pharmacodynamics

Onset of action: Hematologic response: Red blood cells form within 3-10 days; similar onset as parenteral iron salts

Maximum effect: Peak reticulocytosis occurs in 5-10 days, and hemoglobin values increase within 2-4 weeks

Pharmacokinetics (Adult data unless noted)

Absorption: Oral: Iron is absorbed in the duodenum and upper jejunum; in persons with normal iron stores 10% of an oral dose is absorbed, this is increased to 20% to 30% in persons with inadequate iron stores; food and achlorhydria will decrease absorption

Protein binding: To transferrin

Elimination: Excreted in the urine, sweat, sloughing of intestinal mucosa, and by menses

Dosing: Usual Note: Doses expressed as **elemental** iron.

Ferrous fumarate contains 33% elemental iron:

Pediatric:

Recommended daily allowance (RDA): Oral:

Children 4 to 8 years: 10 mg /day

Children and Adolescents 9 to 13 years: 8 mg /day

Adolescents 14 to 18 years:

Male: 11 mg /day

Female: 15 mg /day

Iron deficiency, prevention: Oral:

Children ≥5 years in areas where anemia prevalence is >40%: 30 mg/day with folic acid (WHO 2001)

Adolescents in areas where anemia prevalence is >40%: 60 mg/day with folic acid (WHO 2001)

Iron deficiency, treatment of iron deficiency: Oral: Children and Adolescents: 3 to 6 mg/kg/day in 3 divided doses (Carney 2010; Kliegman 2011)

Adult:

Recommended daily allowance (RDA): Oral

19 to 50 years:

Males: 8 mg/day

Females 18 mg/day

>50 years: 8 mg/day

Iron deficiency, prevention: Oral: 60 mg once daily (Stoltzfus 1998; WHO 2001)

Iron deficiency, treatment of iron deficiency: Oral: 100 to 200 mg daily in 2 to 3 divided doses (Liu 2012; Stoltzfus 1998; WHO 2001)

Note: To avoid GI upset, start with a single daily dose and increase by 1 tablet/day each week or as tolerated until desired daily dose is achieved.

Administration Oral: Do not chew or crush sustained release preparations; administer with water or juice between meals for maximum absorption; may administer with food if GI upset occurs; do not administer with milk or milk products

Monitoring Parameters Serum iron, total iron binding capacity, reticulocyte count, hemoglobin, ferritin

Reference Range

Serum iron: 22-184 mcg/dL

Total iron binding capacity:

Infants: 100-400 mcg/dL

Children and Adults: 250-400 mcg/dL

Additional Information When treating iron deficiency anemias, treat for 3-4 months after hemoglobin/hematocrit return to normal in order to replenish total body stores

Elemental Iron Content of Iron Salts

Iron Salt	Elemental Iron Content (% of salt form)	Approximate Equivalent Doses (mg of iron salt)
Ferrous fumarate	33	197
Ferrous gluconate	11.6	560
Ferrous sulfate	20	324
Ferrous sulfate, exsiccated	30	217

Dosage Forms Excipient information presented when available (limited, particularly for generics); consult specific product labeling.

Tablet, Oral:

Ferretts: 325 mg (106 mg elemental iron) [scored]

Ferrimin 150: Elemental iron 150 mg

Ferrocite: 324 mg (106 mg elemental iron) [contains fd&c blue #1 aluminum lake, fd&c yellow #5 aluminum lake]

Hemocyte: 324 mg (106 mg elemental iron)

Generic: 90 mg (29.5 mg elemental iron), 324 mg (106 mg elemental iron), Elemental iron 29 mg

Ferrous Gluconate (FER us GLOO koe nate)

Related Information

Oral Medications That Should Not Be Crushed or Altered *on page 2476*

Brand Names: US Ferate [OTC]; Fergon [OTC]

Brand Names: Canada Apo-Ferrous Gluconate®; Novo-Ferrogluc

Therapeutic Category Iron Salt; Mineral, Oral

Generic Availability (US) Yes

Use Prevention and treatment of iron deficiency anemias (OTC: FDA approved in adults); has also been used as supplemental therapy for patients receiving epoetin alfa

Pregnancy Considerations It is recommended that pregnant women meet the dietary requirements of iron with diet and/or supplements in order to prevent adverse events associated with iron deficiency anemia in pregnancy. Treatment of iron deficiency anemia in pregnant women is the same as in nonpregnant women and in most cases, oral iron preparations may be used. Except in severe cases of maternal anemia, the fetus achieves normal iron stores regardless of maternal concentrations.

Breast-Feeding Considerations Iron is normally found in breast milk. Breast milk or iron fortified formulas generally provide enough iron to meet the recommended dietary requirements of infants. The amount of iron in breast milk is generally not influenced by maternal iron status.

Contraindications Hypersensitivity to iron salts or any component of the formulation; hemochromatosis, hemolytic anemia

Warnings/Precautions Avoid in patients with peptic ulcer, enteritis, or ulcerative colitis. Administration of iron for >6 months should be avoided except in patients with continuous bleeding or menorrhagia. Anemia in the elderly is often caused by "anemia of chronic disease" or associated with inflammation rather than blood loss. Iron stores are usually normal or increased, with a serum ferritin >50 ng/mL and a decreased total iron binding capacity. Hence, the "anemia of chronic disease" is not secondary to iron deficiency but the inability of the reticuloendothelial system to reclaim available iron stores. Avoid in patients receiving frequent blood transfusions Avoid use in premature infants until the vitamin E stores, deficient at birth, are replenished. Accidental overdose of iron-containing products is a leading cause of fatal poisoning in children under 6 years of age. Keep this product out of the reach of children. In case of accidental overdose call the poison control center immediately.

Warnings: Additional Pediatric Considerations Consider all iron sources when evaluating the dose of iron, including combination products, infant formulas, and liquid nutritional supplements.

Adverse Reactions

Gastrointestinal: Constipation, dark stools, diarrhea, heartburn, nausea, staining of teeth, stomach cramping, vomiting

Genitourinary: Discoloration of urine

Rare but important or life-threatening: Contact irritation

Drug Interactions

Metabolism/Transport Effects None known.

Avoid Concomitant Use

Avoid concomitant use of Ferrous Gluconate with any of the following: Dimercaprol

Increased Effect/Toxicity

The levels/effects of Ferrous Gluconate may be increased by: Dimercaprol

Decreased Effect

Ferrous Gluconate may decrease the levels/effects of: Alpha-Lipoic Acid; Bisphosphonate Derivatives; Cefdinir; Deferiprone; Dolutegravir; Eltrombopag; Levodopa; Levothyroxine; Methyldopa; PenicillAMINE; Phosphate Supplements; Quinolone Antibiotics; Tetracycline Derivatives; Trientine

The levels/effects of Ferrous Gluconate may be decreased by: Alpha-Lipoic Acid; Antacids; H2-Antagonists; Pancrelipase; Proton Pump Inhibitors; Tetracycline Derivatives; Trientine

Food Interactions Cereals, dietary fiber, tea, coffee, eggs, and milk may decrease absorption.

Storage/Stability Store at 20°C to 25°C (68°F to 77°F). Iron is a leading cause of fatal poisoning in children. Store out of children's reach and in child-resistant containers.

Mechanism of Action Replaces iron found in hemoglobin, myoglobin, and enzymes; allows the transportation of oxygen via hemoglobin

Pharmacodynamics

Onset of action: Hematologic response: Red blood cells form within 3-10 days; similar onset as parenteral iron salts

Maximum effect: Peak reticulocytosis occurs in 5-10 days, and hemoglobin values increase within 2-4 weeks

Pharmacokinetics (Adult data unless noted)

Absorption: Oral: Iron is absorbed in the duodenum and upper jejunum; in persons with normal iron stores 10% of an oral dose is absorbed, this is increased to 20% to 30% in persons with inadequate iron stores; food and achlorhydria will decrease absorption

Protein binding: To transferrin

Elimination: Excreted in the urine, sweat, sloughing of intestinal mucosa, and by menses

Dosing: Usual Note: Doses expressed as **elemental** iron. Ferrous gluconate contains ~12% elemental iron.

Pediatric:

Recommended daily allowance (RDA): Oral:

Children 4 to 8 years: 10 mg /day

Children and Adolescents 9 to 13 years: 8 mg /day

Adolescents 14 to 18 years:

Male: 11 mg /day

Female: 15 mg /day

Iron deficiency, prevention: Oral:

Note: Tablet dosage form may not be suitable for all pediatric doses. When appropriate, consider rounding to nearest whole tablet size.

Children ≥5 years in areas where anemia prevalence is >40%: 30 mg/day with folic acid (WHO 2001)

Adolescents in areas where anemia prevalence is >40%: 60 mg/day with folic acid (WHO 2001)

Iron deficiency, treatment of iron deficiency: Oral: Children and Adolescents: 3 to 6 mg/kg/day in 3 divided doses (Carney 2010; Kleigman 2011)

Adults:

Recommended daily allowance (RDA): Oral:

19 to 50 years:

Males: 8 mg iron/day

Females: 18 mg iron/day

>50 years: 8 mg iron/day

Iron deficiency anemia, prevention: Oral: 60 mg/day (Stoltzfus 1998; WHO 2001)

Iron deficiency anemia, treatment of iron deficiency: Oral: 100 to 200 mg daily in 2 to 3 divided doses (Liu 2012; Stoltzfus 1998; WHO 2001)

Administration Oral: Do not chew or crush sustained release preparations; administer with water or juice between meals for maximum absorption; may administer with food if GI upset occurs; do not administer with milk or milk products

Monitoring Parameters Serum iron, total iron binding capacity, reticulocyte count, hemoglobin, ferritin

Reference Range

Serum iron: 22 to 184 mcg/dL

Total iron binding capacity:

Infants: 100 to 400 mcg/dL

Children and Adults: 250 to 400 mcg/dL

Test Interactions False-positive for blood in stool by the guaiac test

Additional Information When treating iron deficiency anemias, treat for 3-4 months after hemoglobin/hematocrit return to normal in order to replenish total body stores

Elemental Iron Content of Iron Salts

Iron Salt	Elemental Iron Content (% of salt form)	Approximate Equivalent Doses (mg of iron salt)
Ferrous fumarate	33	197
Ferrous gluconate	11.6	560
Ferrous sulfate	20	324
Ferrous sulfate, exsiccated	30	217

Dosage Forms Excipient information presented when available (limited, particularly for generics); consult specific product labeling. [DSC] = Discontinued product

Tablet, Oral:

Fergon: 240 (27 Fe) mg [contains tartrazine (fd&c yellow #5)]

Generic: 240 (27 Fe) mg, 324 (37.5 Fe) mg, 324 (38 Fe) mg, 325 (36 Fe) mg

Tablet, Oral [preservative free]:

Ferate: 240 (27 Fe) mg [corn free, dairy free, egg free, fragrance free, gluten free, no artificial flavor(s), sodium free, soy free, starch free, sugar free, wheat free, yeast free; contains fd&c blue #1 aluminum lake, fd&c yellow #6 aluminum lake]

Ferate: 256 (28 Fe) mg [DSC] [gluten free, lactose free, milk free, no artificial color(s), no artificial flavor(s), sodium free, soy free, sugar free, wheat free, yeast free]

Ferrous Sulfate (FER us SUL fate)

Medication Safety Issues

Sound-alike/look-alike issues:

Feosol® may be confused with Fer-In-Sol®

Fer-In-Sol® may be confused with Feosol®

Slow FE® may be confused with Slow-K®

Administration issues:

Multiple concentrations of liquid iron preparations exist. Fer-In-Sol® drops (manufactured by Mead Johnson)

and a limited number of generic products are available at a concentration of 15 mg/mL. However, a suspension product, MyKidz Iron 10™ drops, is available at a concentration of 15 mg/1.5 mL. Check concentration closely prior to dispensing. Prescriptions written in milliliters (mL) should be clarified.

Related Information

Oral Medications That Should Not Be Crushed or Altered *on page 2476*

Brand Names: US BProtected Pedia Iron [OTC]; Fer-In-Sol [OTC]; Fer-Iron [OTC]; FeroSul [OTC]; Ferro-Bob [OTC]; FerrouSul [OTC]; Iron Supplement Childrens [OTC]; Slow Fe [OTC]; Slow Iron [OTC]; Slow Release Iron [OTC] [DSC]

Brand Names: Canada Apo-Ferrous Sulfate; Fer-In-Sol; Ferodan

Therapeutic Category Iron Salt; Mineral, Oral

Generic Availability (US) Yes

Use Prevention and treatment of iron deficiency anemias (OTC: FDA approved in all ages); has also been used as supplemental therapy for patients receiving epoetin alfa

Pregnancy Considerations Iron crosses the placenta and fetal stores are obtained from the mother (McArdle 2011). Iron requirements are increased in pregnant women compared to nonpregnant females (IOM 2001). All pregnant women should be tested for iron deficiency anemia and treated with supplemental iron if needed (ACOG 2008; CDC 1998). Untreated iron deficiency anemia during pregnancy may be associated with an increased risk of low birth weight, preterm delivery, and perinatal mortality, as well as postpartum depression in the mother and decreased mental functioning in the offspring (ACOG 2008; CDC 1998; IOM 2001). Treatment improves maternal hematologic status and neonatal birth weight (Haider 2013).

Breast-Feeding Considerations Iron is normally found in breast milk. Breast milk has a higher concentration of bioavailable iron than cows' milk or goats' milk. Breast milk or iron-fortified formulas generally provide enough iron to meet the recommended dietary requirements of infants up to 6 months of age (CDC 1998; IOM 2001). Maternal iron requirements are increased in breast-feeding women (IOM 2001). The amount of iron in breast milk is generally not influenced by maternal iron status (IOM 1991).

Contraindications Hypersensitivity to iron salts or any component of the formulation; hemochromatosis, hemolytic anemia

Warnings/Precautions Avoid in patients with peptic ulcer, enteritis, or ulcerative colitis. Administration of iron for >6 months should be avoided except in patients with continuous bleeding or menorrhagia. Anemia in the elderly is often caused by "anemia of chronic disease" or associated with inflammation rather than blood loss. Iron stores are usually normal or increased, with a serum ferritin >50 ng/mL and a decreased total iron binding capacity. Hence, the "anemia of chronic disease" is not secondary to iron deficiency but the inability of the reticuloendothelial system to reclaim available iron stores. Avoid in patients receiving frequent blood transfusions Avoid use in premature infants until the vitamin E stores, deficient at birth, are replenished. Accidental overdose of iron-containing products is a leading cause of fatal poisoning in children under 6 years of age. Keep this product out of the reach of children. In case of accidental overdose call the poison control center immediately.

Polysorbate 80: Some dosage forms may contain polysorbate 80 (also known as Tweens). Hypersensitivity reactions, usually a delayed reaction, have been reported following exposure to pharmaceutical products containing polysorbate 80 in certain individuals (Isaksson 2002; Lucente 2000; Shelley 1995). Thrombocytopenia, ascites, pulmonary deterioration, and renal and hepatic failure have been reported in premature neonates after receiving parenteral products containing polysorbate 80 (Alade 1986; CDC 1984). See manufacturer's labeling.

Propylene glycol: Some dosage forms may contain propylene glycol; large amounts are potentially toxic and have been associated hyperosmolality, lactic acidosis, seizures, and respiratory depression; use caution (AAP 1997; Zar 2007).

Warnings: Additional Pediatric Considerations Consider all iron sources when evaluating the dose of iron, including combination products, infant formulas, and liquid nutritional supplements. Some liquid preparations may temporarily stain the teeth.

Some dosage forms may contain propylene glycol; in neonates large amounts of propylene glycol delivered orally, intravenously (eg, >3,000 mg/day), or topically have been associated with potentially fatal toxicities which can include metabolic acidosis, seizures, renal failure, and CNS depression; toxicities have also been reported in children and adults including hyperosmolality, lactic acidosis, seizures, and respiratory depression; use caution (AAP, 1997; Shehab, 2009).

Adverse Reactions

Gastrointestinal: Constipation, dark stools, diarrhea, epigastric pain, GI irritation, heartburn, nausea, stomach cramping, vomiting

Genitourinary: Discoloration of urine

Miscellaneous: Liquid preparations may temporarily stain the teeth

Rare but important or life-threatening: Contact irritation

Drug Interactions

Metabolism/Transport Effects None known.

Avoid Concomitant Use

Avoid concomitant use of Ferrous Sulfate with any of the following: Dimercaprol

Increased Effect/Toxicity

The levels/effects of Ferrous Sulfate may be increased by: Dimercaprol

Decreased Effect

Ferrous Sulfate may decrease the levels/effects of: Alpha-Lipoic Acid; Bisphosphonate Derivatives; Cefdinir; Deferiprone; Dolutegravir; Eltrombopag; Levodopa; Levothyroxine; Methyldopa; PenicillAMINE; Phosphate Supplements; Quinolone Antibiotics; Tetracycline Derivatives; Trientine

The levels/effects of Ferrous Sulfate may be decreased by: Alpha-Lipoic Acid; Antacids; H2-Antagonists; Pancrelipase; Proton Pump Inhibitors; Tetracycline Derivatives; Trientine

Food Interactions Cereals, dietary fiber, tea, coffee, eggs, and milk may decrease absorption.

Storage/Stability Iron is a leading cause of fatal poisoning in children. Store out of children's reach and in child-resistant containers.

Mechanism of Action Replaces iron, found in hemoglobin, myoglobin, and other enzymes; allows the transportation of oxygen via hemoglobin

Pharmacodynamics

Onset of action: Hematologic response: Red blood cells form within 3 to 10 days; similar onset as parenteral iron salts

Maximum effect: Peak reticulocytosis occurs in 5 to 10 days, and hemoglobin values increase within 2 to 4 weeks

Pharmacokinetics (Adult data unless noted)

Absorption: Oral: Iron is absorbed in the duodenum and upper jejunum; in persons with normal iron stores 10% of an oral dose is absorbed, this is increased to 20% to 30% in persons with inadequate iron stores; food and achlorhydria will decrease absorption

Protein binding: To transferrin

Elimination: Excreted in the urine, sweat, sloughing of intestinal mucosa, and by menses

Dosing: Neonatal Note: Multiple concentrations of ferrous sulfate oral liquid exist; close attention must be paid to the concentration when ordering and administering ferrous sulfate; incorrect selection or substitution of one ferrous sulfate liquid for another without proper dosage volume adjustment may result in serious over- or underdosing.

Note: Doses expressed in terms of **elemental** iron; ferrous sulfate contains ~20% elemental iron; ferrous sulfate exsiccated (dried) contains ~30% elemental iron

Adequate Intake (AI): Oral: 0.27 mg/day

Iron deficiency; prevention in neonates fed human milk: Oral:

Preterm (<37 weeks gestational age): 2 mg/kg/day divided every 12 to 24 hours; begin at 4 to 8 weeks PNA (maximum dose: 15 mg/day) (Baker 2010; WHO 2001)

Full-term: In healthy, term infants, that are full or partially breast-fed, AAP does not recommend routine additional supplementation of iron be considered until at least 4 to 6 months of age, if at all (Baker 2010; Schanler 2011)

Iron deficiency anemia; treatment: Oral:

Treatment, severe iron deficiency anemia: 4 to 6 mg/kg/day in 3 divided doses (Carney 2010; Rao 2009)

Treatment, mild to moderate iron deficiency anemia: 3 mg/kg/day in 1 to 2 divided doses (CDC 1998; IOM 1993)

Supplementation during epoetin use: Limited data available; dosing regimens variable: Usual dose: 6 mg /kg/day in 2 to 3 divided doses; usual range: 3 to 8 mg/kg/day although higher doses (up to 12 mg/kg/day) have been used in some protocols (Kleinman 2009; Meyer 1996; Rao 2009)

Dosing: Usual Note: Multiple concentrations of ferrous sulfate oral liquid exist; close attention must be paid to the concentration when ordering and administering ferrous sulfate; incorrect selection or substitution of one ferrous sulfate liquid for another without proper dosage volume adjustment may result in serious over- or underdosing.

Note: Doses expressed in terms of **elemental** iron; Ferrous sulfate contains ~20% elemental iron; ferrous sulfate exsiccated (dried) contains ~30% elemental iron

Pediatric: **Note:** Pediatric dosages expressed in terms of **elemental** iron.

Adequate intake (AI): Oral: 1-6 months: 0.27 mg iron/day

Recommended daily allowance (RDA): Oral:

Infants 7-12 months: 11 mg iron/day
Children 1-3 years: 7 mg iron/day
Children 4-8 years: 10 mg iron/day
Children and Adolescents 9-13 years: 8 mg iron/day
Adolescents 14-18 years:
Male: 11 mg iron/day
Female: 15 mg iron/day

Iron deficiency anemia; prevention: Oral:

Infants ≥4 months (receiving human milk as only nutritional source or >50% as source of nutrition without iron fortified food): 1 mg iron/kg/day (Baker, 2010); **Note:** In healthy, term infants, AAP does not recommend routine additional supplementation of iron be considered until at least 4-6 months of age if breastfed (full or partial) (Baker, 2010; Schanler, 2011)

Infants and Children 6 months to <2 years in areas where anemia prevalence is >40% and iron fortified foods not available: 2 mg/kg/day (WHO, 2001)

Children 2 years to < 5 years in areas where anemia prevalence is >40%: 2 mg/kg/day; aximum dose: 30 mg/day (WHO, 2001)

Children ≥5 years in areas where anemia prevalence is >40%: 30 mg/day with folic acid (WHO, 2001)

Adolescent in areas where anemia prevalence is >40%: 60 mg/day with folic acid (WHO, 2001)

Treatment of iron deficiency: Infants, Children, and Adolescents: 3 to 6 mg/kg/day in 3 divided doses (Carney, 2010, Kliegman, 2011)

Adults:

Recommended daily allowance (RDA): Oral:

19-50 years:
Males: 8 mg elemental iron/day
Females 18 mg elemental iron/day
>50 years: 8 mg elemental iron/day
Pregnancy: 27 mg elemental iron/day
Lactation: 9-10 mg elemental iron/day

Note: Dose expressed in terms of elemental iron.

Iron deficiency anemia, prevention: Oral: 60 mg once daily (Stoltzfus, 1998; WHO, 2001)

Iron deficiency anemia, treatment: Oral: 100 to 200 mg daily in 2 to 3 divided doses (Liu, 2012; Stoltzfus, 1998; WHO, 2001). **Note:** Extended release tablets are intended for once daily use

Administration Oral: Do not chew or crush extended release preparations; administer with water or juice between meals for maximum absorption; may administer with food if GI upset occurs; do not administer with milk or milk products

Monitoring Parameters Serum iron, total iron binding capacity, reticulocyte count, hemoglobin, ferritin

Reference Range

Serum iron: 22-184 mcg/dL
Total iron binding capacity:
Infants: 100-400 mcg/dL
Children and Adults: 250-400 mcg/dL

Test Interactions False-positive for blood in stool by the guaiac test

Additional Information When treating iron deficiency anemias, treat for 3-4 months after hemoglobin/hematocrit return to normal in order to replenish total body stores.

Elemental Iron Content of Iron Salts

Iron Salt	Elemental Iron Content (% of salt form)	Approximate Equivalent Doses (mg of iron salt)
Ferrous fumarate	33	197
Ferrous gluconate	11.6	560
Ferrous sulfate	20	324
Ferrous sulfate, exsiccated	30	217

Dosage Forms Excipient information presented when available (limited, particularly for generics); consult specific product labeling. [DSC] = Discontinued product

Elixir, Oral:

FeroSul: 220 (44 Fe) mg/5 mL (473 mL) [contains alcohol, usp, fd&c yellow #6 (sunset yellow), propylene glycol, saccharin sodium, sodium benzoate; lemon flavor]

Generic: 220 (44 Fe) mg/5 mL (5 mL, 473 mL)

Liquid, Oral:

Generic: 220 (44 Fe) mg/5 mL (473 mL)

Solution, Oral:

BProtected Pedia Iron: 75 (15 Fe) mg/mL (50 mL) [alcohol free, gluten free; contains sodium metabisulfite; citrus flavor]

Fer-In-Sol: 75 (15 Fe) mg/mL (50 mL) [contains alcohol, usp, sodium bisulfite]

Fer-Iron: 75 (15 Fe) mg/mL (50 mL) [contains sodium metabisulfite; lemon flavor]

Iron Supplement Childrens: 75 (15 Fe) mg/mL (50 mL) [alcohol free, dye free, gluten free, lactose free; contains sodium bisulfite]

Generic: 75 (15 Fe) mg/mL (50 mL)

Syrup, Oral:
Generic: 300 (60 Fe) mg/5 mL (5 mL)
Tablet, Oral:
Ferro-Bob: 325 (65 Fe) mg
Generic: 325 (65 Fe) mg
Tablet, Oral [preservative free]:
FerrouSul: 325 (65 Fe) mg [sodium free, starch free]
Generic: 325 (65 Fe) mg
Tablet Delayed Release, Oral:
Generic: 324 (65 Fe) mg, 325 (65 Fe) mg
Tablet Extended Release, Oral:
Slow Fe: 160 (50 Fe) mg
Slow Fe: 142 (45 Fe) mg [contains fd&c blue #1 aluminum lake, fd&c red #40 aluminum lake, fd&c yellow #6 aluminum lake]
Slow Release Iron: 140 (45 Fe) mg [DSC] [contains brilliant blue fcf (fd&c blue #1), fd&c red #40 aluminum lake, fd&c yellow #6 aluminum lake]
Tablet Extended Release, Oral [preservative free]:
Slow Iron: 160 (50 Fe) mg [gluten free]
Generic: 140 (45 Fe) mg

- ◆ **FerrouSul [OTC]** *see* Ferrous Sulfate *on page 871*
- ◆ **FerUS [OTC] [DSC]** *see* Polysaccharide-Iron Complex *on page 1728*
- ◆ **$FeSO_4$** *see* Ferrous Sulfate *on page 871*
- ◆ **FeverAll Adult [OTC]** *see* Acetaminophen *on page 44*
- ◆ **FeverAll Childrens [OTC]** *see* Acetaminophen *on page 44*
- ◆ **FeverAll Infants [OTC]** *see* Acetaminophen *on page 44*
- ◆ **FeverAll Junior Strength [OTC]** *see* Acetaminophen *on page 44*
- ◆ **Fexmid** *see* Cyclobenzaprine *on page 548*

Fexofenadine (feks oh FEN a deen)

Medication Safety Issues

Sound-alike/look-alike issues:

Allegra may be confused with Allegra Anti-Itch Cream (diphenhydramine/allantoin), Viagra
Fexofenadine may be confused with fesoterodine
Mucinex Allergy may be confused with Mucinex

International issues:

Allegra [U.S, Canada, and multiple international markets] may be confused with Allegro brand name for fluticasone [Israel] and frovatriptan [Germany]

Brand Names: US Allegra Allergy Childrens [OTC]; Allegra Allergy [OTC]; Fexofenadine HCl Childrens [OTC]; Mucinex Allergy [OTC]

Brand Names: Canada Allegra 12 Hour (OTC); Allegra 24 Hour (OTC)

Therapeutic Category Antihistamine

Generic Availability (US) May be product dependent

Use Relief of symptoms due to hayfever or upper respiratory allergies (OTC products: Oral suspension: FDA approved in ages ≥2 years and adults; Meltable tablets: FDA approved in ages ≥6 years and adults; Tablets [12 or 24 hours]: FDA approved in ages ≥12 years and adults); has also been used to treat uncomplicated skin manifestations of urticaria. **Note:** Approved ages and uses for generic products may vary; consult labeling for specific information.

Pregnancy Risk Factor C

Pregnancy Considerations Adverse events have been observed in animal reproduction studies; therefore, the manufacturer classifies fexofenadine as pregnancy category C. The use of antihistamines for the treatment of rhinitis during pregnancy is generally considered to be safe at recommended doses. Information related to the use of fexofenadine during pregnancy is limited; therefore, other agents are preferred.

Breast-Feeding Considerations Following administration of terfenadine to nursing mothers, fexofenadine (active metabolite of terfenadine) was found to cross into human breast milk (Allegra Canadian product monograph, 2006). The U.S. manufacturer recommends that caution be exercised when administering fexofenadine to nursing women. The Canadian labeling recommends avoiding use in nursing women.

Contraindications Hypersensitivity to fexofenadine or any component of the formulation

Warnings/Precautions Use with caution in patients with renal impairment; dosage adjustment recommended. Orally disintegrating tablet contains phenylalanine. Effects may be potentiated when used with other sedative drugs or ethanol.

Warnings: Additional Pediatric Considerations Safety and efficacy for the use of cough and cold products in pediatric patients <4 years of age is limited; the AAP warns against the use of these products for respiratory illnesses in this age group. Serious adverse effects including death have been reported. Many of these products contain multiple active ingredients, increasing the risk of accidental overdose when used with other products. The FDA notes that there are no approved OTC uses for these products in pediatric patients <2 years of age. Health care providers are reminded to ask caregivers about the use of OTC cough and cold products in order to avoid exposure to multiple medications containing the same ingredient (AAP 2012; FDA 2008).

Some dosage forms may contain propylene glycol; in neonates large amounts of propylene glycol delivered orally, intravenously (eg, >3,000 mg/day), or topically have been associated with potentially fatal toxicities which can include metabolic acidosis, seizures, renal failure, and CNS depression; toxicities have also been reported in children and adults including hyperosmolality, lactic acidosis, seizures, and respiratory depression; use caution (AAP 1997; Shehab 2009).

Adverse Reactions

Central nervous system: Dizziness, drowsiness, fatigue, fever, headache, pain, somnolence
Endocrine & metabolic: Dysmenorrhea
Gastrointestinal: Diarrhea, dyspepsia, nausea, vomiting
Neuromuscular & skeletal: Back pain, myalgia, pain in extremities
Otic: Otitis media
Respiratory: Cough, rhinorrhea, sinusitis, upper respiratory tract infection
Miscellaneous: Viral infection
Rare but important or life-threatening: Hypersensitivity reactions (anaphylaxis, angioedema, chest tightness, dyspnea, flushing, pruritus, rash, urticaria); insomnia, nervousness, sleep disorders, paroniria (terrifying dreams)

Drug Interactions

Metabolism/Transport Effects Substrate of CYP3A4 (minor), P-glycoprotein, SLCO1B1; **Note:** Assignment of Major/Minor substrate status based on clinically relevant drug interaction potential; **Inhibits** CYP2D6 (weak)

Avoid Concomitant Use

Avoid concomitant use of Fexofenadine with any of the following: Aclidinium; Azelastine (Nasal); Eluxadoline; Glucagon; Ipratropium (Oral Inhalation); Orphenadrine; Paraldehyde; Potassium Chloride; Thalidomide; Tiotropium; Umeclidinium

Increased Effect/Toxicity

Fexofenadine may increase the levels/effects of: AbobotulinumtoxinA; Alcohol (Ethyl); Analgesics (Opioid); Anticholinergic Agents; ARIPiprazole; Azelastine (Nasal); Buprenorphine; CNS Depressants; Eluxadoline; Glucagon; Hydrocodone; Methotrimeprazine; Metyrosine; Mirabegron; Mirtazapine; OnabotulinumtoxinA;

Orphenadrine; Paraldehyde; Potassium Chloride; Pramipexole; RimabotulinumtoxinB; ROPINIRole; Rotigotine; Selective Serotonin Reuptake Inhibitors; Suvorexant; Thalidomide; Thiazide Diuretics; Tiotropium; Topiramate; Zolpidem

The levels/effects of Fexofenadine may be increased by: Aclidinium; Brimonidine (Topical); Cannabis; Doxylamine; Dronabinol; Droperidol; Eltrombopag; Erythromycin (Systemic); HydrOXYzine; Ipratropium (Oral Inhalation); Itraconazole; Kava Kava; Ketoconazole (Systemic); Magnesium Sulfate; Methotrimeprazine; Mianserin; Nabilone; Perampanel; P-glycoprotein/ABCB1 Inhibitors; Pramlintide; Rifampin; Rufinamide; Sodium Oxybate; Tapentadol; Teriflunomide; Tetrahydrocannabinol; Umeclidinium; Verapamil

Decreased Effect

Fexofenadine may decrease the levels/effects of: Acetylcholinesterase Inhibitors; Benzylpenicilloyl Polylysine; Betahistine; Hyaluronidase; Itopride; Metoclopramide; Secretin

The levels/effects of Fexofenadine may be decreased by: Acetylcholinesterase Inhibitors; Amphetamines; Antacids; Grapefruit Juice; P-glycoprotein/ABCB1 Inducers; Rifampin

Food Interactions High-fat meals decrease the bioavailability of fexofenadine by ~50%. Fruit juice (apple, grapefruit, orange) may decrease bioavailability of fexofenadine by ~36%. Management: Administer with water only, avoid fruit juice.

Storage/Stability

U.S. labeling: Store at controlled room temperature of 20°C to 25°C (68°F to 77°F). Protect from excessive moisture.

Canadian labeling: Store at 15°C to 30°C (59°F to 86°F). Protect from moisture.

Mechanism of Action Fexofenadine is an active metabolite of terfenadine and like terfenadine it competes with histamine for H_1-receptor sites on effector cells in the gastrointestinal tract, blood vessels and respiratory tract; it appears that fexofenadine does not cross the blood-brain barrier to any appreciable degree, resulting in a reduced potential for sedation

Pharmacodynamics

Onset of action: 2 hours (Simons 2004)

Duration: 24 hours (Simons 2004)

Pharmacokinetics (Adult data unless noted)

Absorption: Rapid

Distribution: V_d: Children: 5.4 to 5.8 L/kg

Protein binding: 60% to 70% (Brunton 2011)

Metabolism: 5% hepatic; 3.5% transformed into methylester metabolite found only in feces (possibly transformed by gut microflora)

Half-life: 14.4 hours (Simons 2004)

Time to peak serum concentration: Tablets: 2.6 hours (Simons 2004); ODT: 2 hours (4 hours with high-fat meal); Suspension: 1 hour (Allegra prescribing information 2007)

Elimination: Urine (12% as unchanged drug); feces (80% as unchanged drug) (Simons 2004)

Dosing: Usual

Pediatric:

Allergic symptoms/rhinitis: Oral:

Infants ≥6 months and <10.5kg: Limited data available: Oral suspension: 15 mg twice daily. Dosing from a safety and tolerability study of infants with allergic rhinitis (n=58; mean age 8.8 ±1.6 months); adverse events were similar compared to placebo. **Note:** Five patients received 30 mg twice daily, which also had similar adverse effects compared to placebo (Hampell 2007)

Children ≤2 years and <10.5 kg: Limited data available: Oral suspension: 15 to 30 mg twice daily. Dosing from a safety and tolerability study of patients with allergic rhinitis receiving fexofenadine 15 mg twice daily (n= 27; mean age: 16.1 months) or fexofenadine 30 mg twice daily (n=103; mean age: 17.9 ± 3.2 months) compared to placebo. Adverse events were similar between patients receiving fexofenadine and patients receiving placebo (Hampell 2007)

Children 2 to 11 years: Oral suspension or orally disintegrating tablet (ODT): 30 mg twice daily

Children ≥12 years and Adolescents:

Tablets, orally disintegrating tablet (ODT): 60 mg twice daily

Extended release tablet: 180 mg once daily

Chronic idiopathic urticaria: Note: Dosing based on previous FDA approved manufacturer labeling (Allegra prescribing information 2007): Oral:

Infants ≥6 months to Children <2 years: Oral suspension: 15 mg twice daily

Children 2 to 11 years: Oral suspension or orally disintegrating tablet (ODT): 30 mg twice daily

Children ≥12 years and Adolescents:

Tablets, orally disintegrating tablet (ODT): 60 mg twice daily

Extended release tablet: 180 mg once daily

Adult: **Allergic symptoms, rhinitis:** Oral: 60 mg twice daily or 180 mg once daily

Dosing adjustment in renal impairment:

There are no dosage adjustments provided in the OTC manufacturer's labeling; previous prescribing information (Allegra prescribing information 2007) suggested the following:

Infants ≥6 months to Children <2 years: Any degree of renal impairment: Initial: 15 mg once daily

Children 2 to 11 years: Any degree of renal impairment: 30 mg once daily

Children ≥12 years and Adolescents: 60 mg once daily

Others have suggested the following: Children ≥12 years, Adolescents, and Adults (Aronoff 2007):

CrCl 10 to 50 mL/minute: 60 mg once daily

CrCl < 10 mL/minute: 30 mg once daily

Hemodialysis: Not effectively removed by hemodialysis: 30 mg once daily

Peritoneal dialysis: 30 mg once daily

Dosing adjustment in hepatic impairment: There are no dosage adjustments provided in manufacturer's labeling.

Administration

Suspension, tablet: May administer without respect to food. Take with water; avoid administration with fruit juices; shake suspension well before use.

Orally disintegrating tablet: Take on an empty stomach. Do not remove from blister pack until ready to administer. Using dry hands, place immediately on tongue. Tablet will dissolve within seconds, and may be swallowed with or without liquid; avoid taking with fruit juices. Do not split or chew.

Monitoring Parameters Improvement in signs and symptoms of allergic rhinitis and chronic idiopathic urticaria

Test Interactions May suppress the wheal and flare reactions to skin test antigens.

Dosage Forms Excipient information presented when available (limited, particularly for generics); consult specific product labeling.

Suspension, Oral, as hydrochloride:

Allegra Allergy Childrens: 30 mg/5 mL (240 mL) [alcohol free, dye free; contains butylparaben, edetate disodium, propylene glycol, propylparaben; berry flavor]

Allegra Allergy Childrens: 30 mg/5 mL (120 mL) [alcohol free, dye free; contains butylparaben, edetate disodium, propylene glycol, propylparaben; raspberry creme flavor]

Fexofenadine HCl Childrens: 30 mg/5 mL (118 mL) [alcohol free, dye free; contains butylparaben, edetate disodium, propylene glycol, propylparaben; berry flavor]

Tablet, Oral:
Allegra Allergy: 60 mg
Allegra Allergy: 180 mg [contains brilliant blue fcf (fd&c blue #1)]
Tablet, Oral, as hydrochloride:
Allegra Allergy: 60 mg, 180 mg
Allegra Allergy Childrens: 30 mg
Mucinex Allergy: 180 mg [contains fd&c red #40]
Generic: 60 mg, 180 mg
Tablet Dispersible, Oral, as hydrochloride:
Allegra Allergy Childrens: 30 mg [contains aspartame; orange cream flavor]

◆ **Fexofenadine HCl Childrens [OTC]** *see* Fexofenadine *on page 874*

◆ **Fexofenadine Hydrochloride** *see* Fexofenadine *on page 874*

◆ **Fiber Therapy [OTC]** *see* Psyllium *on page 1804*

Filgrastim (fil GRA stim)

Medication Safety Issues

Sound-alike/look-alike issues:

Filgrastim may be confused with filgrastim-sndz, tbo-filgrastim

Neupogen may be confused with Epogen, Neulasta, Neumega, Nutramigen

International issues:

Neupogen [U.S., Canada, and multiple international markets] may be confused with Neupro brand name for rotigotine [multiple international markets]

Some products available internationally may have vial strength and dosing expressed as units (instead of as micrograms). Refer to prescribing information for specific strength and dosing information.

Brand Names: US Granix; Neupogen

Brand Names: Canada Neupogen

Therapeutic Category Colony-Stimulating Factor; Hematopoietic Agent

Generic Availability (US) No

Use

Cancer patients (nonmyeloid malignancies) receiving myelosuppressive chemotherapy to decrease the incidence of infection (febrile neutropenia) in regimens associated with a high incidence of neutropenia with fever [FDA approved in pediatric patients (age not specified) and adults]

Acute myelogenous leukemia (AML) following induction or consolidation chemotherapy to shorten time to neutrophil recovery and reduce the duration of fever (FDA approved in adults)

Cancer patients (nonmyeloid malignancies) receiving bone marrow transplant to shorten the duration of neutropenia and neutropenia-related events (eg, neutropenic fever) (FDA approved in adults)

Peripheral stem cell transplantation to mobilize hematopoietic progenitor cells for apheresis collection (FDA approved in adults)

Severe chronic neutropenia (SCN; chronic administration) to reduce the incidence and duration of neutropenic complications (fever, infections, oropharyngeal ulcers) in symptomatic patients with congenital, cyclic, or idiopathic neutropenia (FDA approved in ages ≥1 month and adults)

Has also been used for AIDS patients receiving zidovudine; neonatal neutropenia

Pregnancy Risk Factor C

Pregnancy Considerations Adverse events have been observed in animal reproduction studies. Filgrastim has been shown to cross the placenta in humans.

Women who become pregnant during Neupogen treatment are encouraged to enroll in the manufacturer's Pregnancy Surveillance Program (1-800-772-6436).

Breast-Feeding Considerations It is not known if filgrastim, filgrastim-sndz, or tbo-filgrastim is excreted in breast milk. The manufacturers recommend that caution be exercised when administering filgrastim products to breast-feeding women.

Women who are nursing during Neupogen treatment are encouraged to enroll in the manufacturer's Lactation Surveillance program (1-800-772-6436).

Contraindications

Neupogen, Zarxio: History of serious allergic reactions to human granulocyte colony-stimulating factors, such as filgrastim or pegfilgrastim, or any component of the formulation.

Granix: There are no contraindications listed in the manufacturer's labeling

Warnings/Precautions Serious allergic reactions (*including anaphylaxis) have been reported, usually with the initial exposure; may be managed symptomatically with administration of antihistamines, steroids, bronchodilators, and/or epinephrine. Allergic reactions may recur within days after the initial allergy management has been stopped. Do not administer filgrastim products to patients who experienced serious allergic reaction to filgrastim or pegfilgrastim. Permanently discontinue filgrastim products in patients with serious allergic reactions. Rare cases of splenic rupture have been reported (may be fatal); in patients with upper abdominal pain, left upper quadrant pain, or shoulder tip pain, withhold treatment and evaluate for enlarged spleen or splenic rupture. Moderate or severe cutaneous vasculitis has been reported, generally occurring in patients with severe chronic neutropenia on chronic therapy. Withhold treatment if cutaneous vasculitis occurs; may be restarted with a dose reduction once symptoms resolve and the absolute neutrophil count (ANC) has decreased. Capillary leak syndrome (CLS), characterized by hypotension, hypoalbuminemia, edema, and hemoconcentration, may occur in patients receiving human granulocyte colony-stimulating factors (G-CSF). CLS episode may vary in frequency and severity. If CLS develops, monitor closely and manage symptomatically (may require intensive care). CLS may be life-threatening if treatment is delayed.

White blood cell counts of ≥100,000/mm^3 have been reported with filgrastim doses >5 mcg/kg/day. When filgrastim products are used as an adjunct to myelosuppressive chemotherapy, discontinue when ANC exceeds 10,000/mm^3 after the ANC nadir has occurred (to avoid potential excessive leukocytosis). Doses that increase the ANC beyond 10,000/mm^3 may not result in additional clinical benefit. Monitor complete blood cell count (CBC) twice weekly during therapy. In patients receiving myelosuppressive chemotherapy, filgrastim discontinuation generally resulted in a 50% decrease in circulating neutrophils within 1 to 2 days, and a return to pretreatment levels in 1 to 7 days. When used for peripheral blood progenitor cell collection, discontinue filgrastim products if leukocytes >100,000/mm^3. Thrombocytopenia has also been reported with filgrastim products; monitor platelet counts. Filgrastim products should not be routinely used in the treatment of established neutropenic fever. Colony-stimulating factors may be considered in cancer patients with febrile neutropenia who are at high risk for infection-associated complications or who have prognostic factors indicative of a poor clinical outcome (eg, prolonged and severe neutropenia, age >65 years, hypotension, pneumonia, sepsis syndrome, presence of invasive fungal infection, uncontrolled primary disease, hospitalization at the time of fever development) (Freifeld, 2011; Smith, 2006). Do not use filgrastim products in the period 24 hours before to 24 hours after administration of cytotoxic chemotherapy because of the potential sensitivity of rapidly dividing myeloid cells to cytotoxic chemotherapy. Transient increase in neutrophil count is seen 1 to 2 days after filgrastim initiation; however, for sustained neutrophil response, continue until post-nadir ANC reaches 10,000/mm^3. Avoid simultaneous use of filgrastim products with chemotherapy and radiation therapy. Avoid concurrent radiation therapy with filgrastim; safety and efficacy have not been established with patients receiving radiation therapy. The G-CSF receptor through which filgrastim products act has been found on tumor cell lines. May potentially act as a growth factor for any tumor type (including myeloid malignancies and myelodysplasia). When used for stem cell mobilization, may release tumor cells from marrow, which could be collected in leukapheresis product; potential effect of tumor cell reinfusion is unknown.

May precipitate severe sickle cell crises, sometimes resulting in fatalities, in patients with sickle cell disorders (sickle cell trait or sickle cell disease); carefully evaluate potential risks and benefits. Discontinue in patients undergoing sickle cell crisis. Establish diagnosis of severe chronic neutropenia (SCN) prior to initiation; use prior to appropriate diagnosis of SCN may impair or delay proper evaluation and treatment for neutropenia due to conditions other than SCN. Myelodysplastic syndrome (MDS) and acute myeloid leukemia (AML) have been reported to occur in the natural history of congenital neutropenia (without cytokine therapy). Cytogenetic abnormalities and transformation to MDS and AML have been observed with filgrastim when used to manage SCN, although the risk for MDS and AML appears to be in patients with congenital neutropenia. Abnormal cytogenetics and MDS are associated with the development of AML. The effects of continuing filgrastim products in patients who have developed abnormal cytogenetics or MDS are unknown; consider risk versus benefits of continuing treatment. Acute respiratory distress syndrome (ARDS) has been reported. Evaluate patients who develop fever and lung infiltrates or respiratory distress for ARDS; discontinue in patients with ARDS. Reports of alveolar hemorrhage, manifested as pulmonary infiltrates and hemoptysis (requiring hospitalization), have occurred in healthy donors undergoing PBPC mobilization (off-label for use in healthy donors); hemoptysis resolved upon discontinuation.

The packaging of some dosage forms may contain latex.

Some products available internationally may have vial strength and dosing expressed as units (instead of as micrograms). Refer to prescribing information for specific strength and dosing information.

Some dosage forms may contain polysorbate 80 (also known as Tweens). Hypersensitivity reactions, usually a delayed reaction, have been reported following exposure to pharmaceutical products containing polysorbate 80 in certain individuals (Isaksson, 2002; Lucente 2000; Shelley, 1995). Thrombocytopenia, ascites, pulmonary deterioration, and renal and hepatic failure have been reported in premature neonates after receiving parenteral products containing polysorbate 80 (Alade, 1986; CDC, 1984). See manufacturer's labeling.

Adverse Reactions

Cardiovascular: Cardiac arrhythmia, chest pain, hypertension, myocardial infarction

Central nervous system: Dizziness, fatigue, headache, hypoesthesia, pain

Dermatologic: Alopecia, erythema, maculopapular rash, skin rash

Endocrine & metabolic: Increased lactate dehydrogenase (reversible mild to moderate elevations), increased uric acid (reversible mild to moderate elevations)

Gastrointestinal: Nausea, vomiting

Genitourinary: Urinary tract infection

Hematologic & oncologic: Anemia, leukocytosis, petechia, splenomegaly (more common in severe chronic neutropenia, rare in other patients), thrombocytopenia

Hepatic: Increased serum alkaline phosphatase (reversible mild to moderate elevations)

Hypersensitivity: Transfusion reaction

Immunologic: Antibody development (no evidence of neutralizing response)

Neuromuscular & skeletal: Arthralgia, back pain, limb pain, muscle spasm, musculoskeletal pain, ostealgia (dose and cycle related)

Respiratory: Cough, dyspnea, epistaxis, upper respiratory tract infection

Miscellaneous: Fever

Rare but important or life-threatening: Capillary leak syndrome, cerebral hemorrhage, decreased bone mineral density, decreased hemoglobin, diarrhea, erythema nodosum, exacerbation of psoriasis, hematuria, hemoptysis, hepatomegaly, hypersensitivity angiitis, hypersensitivity reaction, oropharyngeal pain, peripheral edema, proteinuria, pulmonary hemorrhage, pulmonary infiltrates, renal insufficiency, respiratory distress syndrome, severe sickle cell crisis, splenic rupture, Sweet syndrome, tachycardia

Drug Interactions

Metabolism/Transport Effects None known.

Avoid Concomitant Use There are no known interactions where it is recommended to avoid concomitant use.

Increased Effect/Toxicity

Filgrastim may increase the levels/effects of: Bleomycin; Cyclophosphamide; Topotecan

Decreased Effect There are no known significant interactions involving a decrease in effect.

Storage/Stability

Neupogen: Store at 2°C to 8°C (36°F to 46°F). Store in the original carton. Protect from light. Protect from direct sunlight. Avoid freezing; if frozen, thaw in the refrigerator before administration. Discard if frozen more than once. Do not shake. Transport via a pneumatic tube has not been studied. Prior to injection, allow to reach room temperature for up to 30 minutes and a maximum of 24 hours. Discard any vial or prefilled syringe left at room temperature for more than 24 hours. Solutions diluted for infusion may be stored at room temperature for up to 24 hours (infusion must be completed within 24 hours of preparation).

Extended storage information may be available for undiluted filgrastim; contact product manufacturer to obtain current recommendations. Sterility has been assessed and maintained for up to 7 days when prepared under strict aseptic conditions (Jacobson, 1996; Singh, 1994). The manufacturer recommends using within 24 hours due to the potential for bacterial contamination.

Granix: Store prefilled syringes at 2°C to 8°C (36°F to 46°F). Protect from light. Do not shake. May be removed from 2°C to 8°C (36°F to 46°F) storage for a single period of up to 5 days between 23°C to 27°C (73°F to 81°F). If not used within 5 days, the product may be returned to 2°C to 8°C (36°F to 46°F) up to the expiration date. Exposure to -1°C to -5°C (23°F to 30°F) for up to 72 hours and temperatures as low as -15°C to -25°C (5°F to -13°F) for up to 24 hours do not adversely affect stability. Discard unused product.

Zarxio: Store at 2°C to 8°C (36°F to 46°F). Store in the original carton. Protect from light. Avoid freezing; if frozen, thaw in the refrigerator before administration. Discard if frozen more than once. Do not shake. Transport via a pneumatic tube has not been studied. Prior to injection, allow to reach room temperature for up to 30 minutes and a maximum of 24 hours. Discard any prefilled syringe left at room temperature for more than 24 hours. Solutions diluted for infusion may be stored at room temperature for up to 24 hours (infusion must be completed within 24 hours of preparation).

Mechanism of Action Filgrastim and tbo-filgrastim are granulocyte colony stimulating factors (G-CSF) produced by recombinant DNA technology. G-CSFs stimulate the production, maturation, and activation of neutrophils to increase both their migration and cytotoxicity.

Pharmacodynamics

Onset of action: Immediate transient leukopenia with the nadir occurring 5 to 15 minutes after an IV dose or 30 to 60 minutes after a SubQ dose followed by a sustained elevation in neutrophil levels within the first 24 hours reaching a plateau in 3 to 5 days

Duration: Upon discontinuation of G-CSF, ANC decreases by 50% within 2 days and returns to pretreatment levels within 1 week; WBC counts return to normal range in 4 to 7 days

Pharmacokinetics (Adult data unless noted)

Distribution: V_d: 150 mL/kg

Bioavailability: Not bioavailable after oral administration

Half-life: Neonates: 4.4 hours; Adults: 1.8 to 3.5 hours

Time to peak serum concentration: SubQ: Within 2 to 6 hours

Dosing: Neonatal Note: International considerations: Dosages below expressed as micrograms; 1 mcg = 100,000 units (Höglund 1998).

Neutropenia with sepsis: IV, SubQ: 10 mcg/kg/day divided every 12 to 24 hours for 3 to 14 days; most trials have used once daily dosing for 3 days (Carr 2009)

Neutropenia, prophylaxis of infection: IV, SubQ: 5 to 10 mcg/kg/day for 3 to 5 days (Carr 2009)

Neutropenia, congenital: SubQ: Initial: 5 mcg/kg/day, followed by 10 mcg/kg/day; then titrate to response using 10 mcg/kg/day increments every 14 days until target ANC (1,000 to 1,500/mm^3) is reached and maintained; if ANC exceeds 5,000/mm^3, dosage should be reduced to lowest effective dose. Typical dose range for response of patients included in the international CN registry is 3 to 10 mcg/kg/day; maximum dose: 120 mcg/kg/day (Boztug 2008; Welte 2006)

Neutropenia, idiopathic or cyclic: SubQ:1 to 5 mcg/kg/day once daily (Ancliff 2003)

Dosing: Usual Note: International considerations: Dosages below expressed as micrograms; 1 mcg = 100,000 units (Höglund 1998).

Infants, Children, and Adolescents: **Note:** Details concerning dosing in combination regimens and institution protocols should also be consulted. For larger doses (eg, adolescents), rounding doses to the nearest vial size may enhance patient convenience and reduce costs without compromising clinical response.

Bone marrow transplantation, cancer patients: Limited data available: IV, SubQ: 5 mcg/kg/day administered ≥24 hours after cytotoxic chemotherapy and ≥24 hours after bone marrow infusion (Schaison 1998; Wagner 2001)

Chemotherapy-induced neutropenia: IV, SubQ: 5 mcg/kg/day once daily beginning ≥24 hours after chemotherapy; recommendations for duration of therapy vary: Manufacturer labeling is for up to 14 days or until ANC reaches 10,000/mm^3; others have suggested a lower target ANC of 5,000/mm^3 (Schaison 1998; Wagner 2001). For subsequent chemotherapy cycles, dose may be increased by 5 mcg/kg based upon patient's previous response to therapy along with duration and severity of neutropenia; reported range: 4 to 8 mcg/kg/day.

Neutropenia, idiopathic or cyclic: SubQ: 1 to 5 mcg/kg/day once daily (Ancliff 2003)

Neutropenia due to zidovudine for HIV treatment: SubQ: 5 to 10 mcg/kg/day once daily (Working Group 2008)

Peripheral blood progenitor cell (PBPC) mobilization, autologous bone marrow transplant: Limited data available: IV, SubQ: 10 mcg/kg/day given for 4 to 5 days before apheresis procedure (Diaz 2000; Wagner 2001)

Adults: Details concerning dosing in combination regimens and institution protocols should also be consulted. Rounding doses to the nearest vial size may enhance patient convenience and reduce costs without compromising clinical response.

Bone marrow transplantation (in patients with cancer; to shorten the duration of neutropenia and neutropenia-related events): IV, SubQ.: 10 mcg/kg/day (administer ≥24 hours after chemotherapy and ≥24 hours after bone marrow infusion); adjust the dose according to the duration and severity of neutropenia; recommended steps based on neutrophil response:

When ANC >1,000/mm^3 for 3 consecutive days: Reduce filgrastim dose to 5 mcg/kg/day.

If ANC remains >1,000/mm^3 for 3 more consecutive days: Discontinue filgrastim.

If ANC decreases to <1,000/mm^3: Resume at 5 mcg/kg/day.

If ANC decreases to <1,000/mm^3 during the 5 mcg/kg/day dose: Increase filgrastim to 10 mcg/kg/day and follow the above step

Chemotherapy-induced neutropenia: IV, SubQ: 5 mcg/kg/day; doses may be increased by 5 mcg/kg (for each chemotherapy cycle) according to the duration and severity of the neutropenia; continue for up to 14 days or until the ANC reaches 10,000/mm^3

Peripheral blood progenitor cell (PBPC) collection: SubQ: 10 mcg/kg/dose once daily, usually for 6 to 7 days. Begin at least 4 days before the first apheresis and continue until the last apheresis; consider dose adjustment for WBC >100,000/mm^3

Severe chronic neutropenia: SubQ:

Congenital: Initial: 6 mcg/kg/dose twice daily; adjust the dose based on ANC and clinical response

Idiopathic/cyclic: Initial: 5 mcg/kg/day; adjust the dose based on ANC and clinical response

Preparation for Administration Parenteral: Visually inspect prior to use; discard if discolored or if particulates are present.

Neupogen: **Do not dilute with saline at any time; product may precipitate.**

SubQ: For continuous infusion, dilute dose in 10 mL D_5W and infuse at a rate of 10 mL/24 hours

IV: Filgrastim may be diluted with D_5W to a concentration of 5 to 15 mcg/mL for IV infusion administration (minimum concentration: 5 mcg/mL). Concentrations of 5 to 15 mcg/mL require addition of albumin (final albumin concentration of 2 mg/mL) to prevent adsorption to plastics; albumin should be added to the D_5W prior to addition of G-CSF. Dilution to <5 mcg/mL is not recommended. Do not shake. Discard unused portion of vial/prefilled syringe.

Administration Parenteral: **Note:** When used for neutropenia associated with chemotherapy or BMT, do not administer in the 24 hours prior to or earlier than 24 hours after cytotoxic chemotherapy.

SubQ: Administer undiluted solution as a bolus injection (preferred) (Smith 2006; Wagner 2001); manufacturer labeling suggests may also be given as a continuous infusion for the following indications: Chemotherapy-induced neutropenia, bone marrow transplantation, and peripheral blood progenitor cell collection.

IV: May be administered as a short infusion over 15 to 30 minutes; manufacturer labeling suggests may also be given as a continuous IV infusion for chemotherapy-induced neutropenia or as a 4- or 24-hour infusion for bone marrow transplantation.

Monitoring Parameters Temperature, CBC with differential and platelet count, hematocrit, uric acid, urinalysis, liver function tests

Reference Range Blood samples for monitoring the hematologic effects of G-CSF should be drawn just before the next dose

Test Interactions May interfere with bone imaging studies; increased hematopoietic activity of the bone marrow may appear as transient positive bone imaging changes

Product Availability Zarxio (filgrastim-sndz): FDA approved March 2015; anticipated availability is currently unknown. Zarxio is biosimilar to Neupogen. Further information can be found at http://www.fda.gov/NewsEvents/Newsroom/PressAnnouncements/ucm436648.htm?source=govdelivery&utm_medium=email&utm_source=govdelivery.

Dosage Forms Considerations

Prefilled syringes: Granix, Neupogen: 300 mcg/0.5 mL (0.5 mL); 480 mcg/0.8 mL (0.8 mL)

Vials: Neupogen: 300 mcg/mL (1 mL); 480 mcg/1.6 mL (1.6 mL)

Dosage Forms Excipient information presented when available (limited, particularly for generics); consult specific product labeling.

Solution, Injection:

Neupogen: 300 mcg/mL (1 mL); 480 mcg/1.6 mL (1.6 mL) [contains polysorbate 80]

Solution, Injection [preservative free]:

Neupogen: 300 mcg/0.5 mL (0.5 mL); 480 mcg/0.8 mL (0.8 mL) [contains polysorbate 80]

Solution Prefilled Syringe, Subcutaneous [preservative free]:

Granix: 300 mcg/0.5 mL (0.5 mL); 480 mcg/0.8 mL (0.8 mL) [contains polysorbate 80]

- ◆ **Filgrastim-Sndz** *see* Filgrastim *on page 876*
- ◆ **Finacea** *see* Azelaic Acid *on page 238*
- ◆ **First-Hydrocortisone** *see* Hydrocortisone (Topical) *on page 1041*
- ◆ **First-Lansoprazole** *see* Lansoprazole *on page 1219*
- ◆ **First-Omeprazole** *see* Omeprazole *on page 1555*
- ◆ **First-Testosterone** *see* Testosterone *on page 2025*
- ◆ **First-Testosterone MC** *see* Testosterone *on page 2025*
- ◆ **First-Vancomycin 25** *see* Vancomycin *on page 2151*
- ◆ **First-Vancomycin 50** *see* Vancomycin *on page 2151*
- ◆ **Fisalamine** *see* Mesalamine *on page 1368*
- ◆ **FK506** *see* Tacrolimus (Systemic) *on page 1999*
- ◆ **Flagyl** *see* MetroNIDAZOLE (Systemic) *on page 1421*
- ◆ **Flagyl ER** *see* MetroNIDAZOLE (Systemic) *on page 1421*
- ◆ **Flamazine® (Can)** *see* Silver Sulfadiazine *on page 1926*
- ◆ **Flanax Pain Relief [OTC]** *see* Naproxen *on page 1489*
- ◆ **Flarex** *see* Fluorometholone *on page 903*
- ◆ **Flarex® (Can)** *see* Fluorometholone *on page 903*
- ◆ **Flebogamma [DSC]** *see* Immune Globulin *on page 1089*
- ◆ **Flebogamma DIF** *see* Immune Globulin *on page 1089*

Flecainide (fle KAY nide)

Medication Safety Issues

Sound-alike/look-alike issues:

Flecainide may be confused with fluconazole

Tambocor [DSC] may be confused with Pamelor, Temodar, tamoxifen, Tamiflu

BEERS Criteria medication:

This drug may be potentially inappropriate for use in geriatric patients (Quality of evidence - high; Strength of recommendation - strong).

Brand Names: US Tambocor [DSC]

Brand Names: Canada Apo-Flecainide®; Tambocor™

Therapeutic Category Antiarrhythmic Agent, Class I-C

Generic Availability (US) Yes

Use Prevention and suppression of documented life-threatening ventricular arrhythmias (ie, sustained ventricular tachycardia); prevention of symptomatic, disabling supraventricular tachycardias in patients without structural heart disease (FDA approved in pediatric patients [age not specified] and adults)

Pregnancy Risk Factor C

Pregnancy Considerations Adverse events have been observed in some animal reproduction studies.

Breast-Feeding Considerations Flecainide is excreted in human breast milk at concentrations as high as 4 times corresponding plasma levels.

Contraindications Hypersensitivity to flecainide or any component of the formulation; pre-existing second- or third-degree AV block or with right bundle branch block when associated with a left hemiblock (bifascicular block) (except in patients with a functioning artificial pacemaker); cardiogenic shock; coronary artery disease (based on CAST study results); concurrent use of ritonavir or amprenavir

Warnings/Precautions **[U.S. Boxed Warning]: In the Cardiac Arrhythmia Suppression Trial (CAST), recent (>6 days but <2 years ago) myocardial infarction patients with asymptomatic, non-life-threatening ventricular arrhythmias did not benefit and may have been harmed by attempts to suppress the arrhythmia with flecainide or encainide.** An increased mortality or nonfatal cardiac arrest rate (7.7%) was seen in the active treatment group compared with patients in the placebo group (3%). The applicability of the CAST results to other populations is unknown. The risks of class 1C agents and the lack of improved survival make use in patients without life-threatening arrhythmias generally unacceptable. **[U.S. Boxed Warning]: Watch for proarrhythmic effects;** monitor and adjust dose to prevent QTc prolongation. Not recommended for patients with chronic atrial fibrillation. In the treatment of atrial fibrillation in the elderly, avoid antiarrhythmics as first-line treatment. In older adults, data suggests rate control may provide more benefits than risks compared to rhythm control for most patients (Beers Criteria). **[U.S. Boxed Warning]: When treating atrial flutter, 1:1 atrioventricular conduction may occur; pre-emptive negative chronotropic therapy (eg, digoxin, beta-blockers) may lower the risk.** Pre-existing hypokalemia or hyperkalemia should be corrected before initiation (can alter drug's effect). A worsening or new arrhythmia may occur (proarrhythmic effect). Use caution in heart failure (may precipitate or exacerbate HF). Dose-related increases in PR, QRS, and QT intervals occur. Use with caution in sick sinus syndrome or with permanent pacemakers or temporary pacing wires (can increase endocardial pacing thresholds). Cautious use in significant hepatic impairment.

Adverse Reactions

Cardiovascular: Chest pain, edema, palpitation, proarrhythmic, sinus node dysfunction, syncope, tachycardia

Central nervous system: Anxiety, ataxia, depression, dizziness, fatigue, fever, headache, hypoesthesia, insomnia, malaise, nervousness, paresis, somnolence, tinnitus, vertigo

Dermatologic: Rash

Gastrointestinal: Abdominal pain, anorexia, constipation, diarrhea, nausea

Neuromuscular & skeletal: Paresthesias, tremor, weakness

Ocular: Blurred vision, diplopia, visual disturbances

Respiratory: Dyspnea

Rare but important or life-threatening: Alopecia, alters pacing threshold, amnesia, angina, AV block, bradycardia, bronchospasm, CHF, corneal deposits, depersonalization, euphoria, exfoliative dermatitis, granulocytopenia, heart block, increased P-R, leukopenia, metallic taste, neuropathy, paradoxical increase in ventricular rate in atrial fibrillation/flutter, paresthesia, photophobia, pneumonitis, pruritus, QRS duration, swollen lips/tongue/mouth, tardive dyskinesia, thrombocytopenia, urinary retention, urticaria, ventricular arrhythmia

Drug Interactions

Metabolism/Transport Effects Substrate of CYP1A2 (minor), CYP2D6 (major); **Note:** Assignment of Major/Minor substrate status based on clinically relevant drug interaction potential; **Inhibits** CYP2D6 (weak)

Avoid Concomitant Use

Avoid concomitant use of Flecainide with any of the following: Fosamprenavir; Highest Risk QTc-Prolonging Agents; Ivabradine; Mifepristone; Ritonavir; Saquinavir; Tipranavir

Increased Effect/Toxicity

Flecainide may increase the levels/effects of: ARIPiprazole; Digoxin; Highest Risk QTc-Prolonging Agents; Moderate Risk QTc-Prolonging Agents

The levels/effects of Flecainide may be increased by: Abiraterone Acetate; Amiodarone; Boceprevir; Carbonic Anhydrase Inhibitors; Cobicistat; CYP2D6 Inhibitors (Moderate); CYP2D6 Inhibitors (Strong); Darunavir; Fosamprenavir; Ivabradine; Mifepristone; Mirabegron; Panobinostat; Peginterferon Alfa-2b; QTc-Prolonging Agents (Indeterminate Risk and Risk Modifying); Ritonavir; Saquinavir; Sodium Bicarbonate; Sodium Lactate; Telaprevir; Tipranavir; Tromethamine; Verapamil

Decreased Effect

The levels/effects of Flecainide may be decreased by: Etravirine; Peginterferon Alfa-2b; Sodium Bicarbonate

Food Interactions Clearance may be decreased in patients following strict vegetarian diets due to urinary pH ≥8. Dairy products (milk, infant formula, yogurt) may interfere with the absorption of flecainide in infants; there is one case report of a neonate (GA 34 weeks PNA >6 days) who required extremely large doses of oral flecainide when administered every 8 hours with feedings ("milk feeds"); changing the feedings from "milk feeds" to 5% glucose feeds alone resulted in a doubling of the flecainide serum concentration and toxicity.

Mechanism of Action Class Ic antiarrhythmic; slows conduction in cardiac tissue by altering transport of ions across cell membranes; causes slight prolongation of refractory periods; decreases the rate of rise of the action potential without affecting its duration; increases electrical stimulation threshold of ventricle, His-Purkinje system; possesses local anesthetic and moderate negative inotropic effects

Pharmacokinetics (Adult data unless noted)

Absorption: Oral: Rapid and nearly complete

Distribution: V_d: 5 to 13.4 L/kg

Protein binding: 40% to 50% ($alpha_1$ glycoprotein)

Metabolism: Hepatic

Bioavailability: 85% to 90%

Half-life, elimination: Increased half-life with CHF or renal dysfunction

Newborns: ~29 hours

Infants: 11 to 12 hours

Children: 8 hours

Adolescents 12 to 15 years: 11 to 12 hours

Adults: ~20 hours (range: 12 to 27 hours)

Time to peak serum concentration: ~3 hours (range: 1 to 6 hours)

Elimination: Urine (as unchanged drug: ~30%, range: 10% to 50% and metabolites)

Dosing: Neonatal Supraventricular tachycardia: Limited data available; optimal dose not established: Oral: Initial: 2 mg/kg/day divided every 12 hours; titrate to clinical response, monitor serum concentration; mean dose required to suppress SVT: 3.35 ± 1.35 mg/kg/day in 17 neonates (n=20 treated neonates; mean PNA: 11.5 days; mean GA: 36.8 weeks; mean birthweight: 2.8 kg); study did not report resultant serum concentrations; **Note:** Acute SVT was initially controlled with IV flecainide (not available in U.S.) and then converted to preventative oral therapy (Ferlini, 2009). In a retrospective analysis of 39 neonates treated with digoxin and/or flecainide for SVT (median PNA at treatment: 12 days), an initial flecainide dose of 6 to 8 mg/kg/day divided every 12 hours was used and titrated to response and serum concentrations; final dosage range of 3.2 to 13.5 mg/kg/day produced successful suppression of SVT in 24 of 25 patients. The authors noted high variability in serum concentrations with initial dosing (0.23 to 1.14 mcg/mL) (O'Sullivan, 1995).

Dosing: Usual

Pediatric: **Arrhythmias:**

Manufacturer's labeling: BSA-directed dosing: Use caution with dose titration, as small change in dose may result in disproportionate increase in plasma concentrations.

Infants ≤6 months: Oral: Initial: 50 mg/m²/day divided every 8 to 12 hours; may titrate dose at 4 day intervals; maximum daily dose: 200 mg/m²/**day**; higher doses have been associated with an increased risk of proarrhythmic effects

Infants >6 months, Children, and Adolescents: Oral: Initial: 100 mg/m²/day divided every 8 to 12 hours; may titrate dose at 4 day intervals; maximum daily dose: 200 mg/m²/**day**; higher doses have been associated with an increased risk of proarrhythmic effects

Alternate dosing: Weight-based dosing: Limited data available; dosing regimens variable: Infants, Children, and Adolescents: Oral: Initial: 1 to 3 mg/kg/day divided every 8 hours; may titrate dose at 4-day intervals; usual maintenance range: 3 to 6 mg/kg/day (Park, 2014); an average effective dose of 4 mg/kg/day was reported in an expert analysis of literature and clinical experience (Perry 1992); maximum daily dose: 8 mg/kg/day (Perry, 1992); higher doses have been associated with an increased risk of proarrhythmic effects

Adult:

Atrial fibrillation or flutter (pharmacological cardioversion): Outpatient: "Pill-in-the-pocket" dose: Oral: 200 mg (patient weight <70 kg), 300 mg (weight ≥70 kg). May not repeat in ≤24 hours (AHA/ACC/HRS [January, 2014]; Alboni, 2004). **Note:** An initial inpatient conversion trial should have been successful before sending patient home on this approach. Patient must be taking an AV nodal-blocking agent (eg, beta-blocker, nondihydropyridine calcium channel blocker) prior to initiation of antiarrhythmic.

Life-threatening ventricular arrhythmias: Oral: Initial: 100 mg every 12 hours, increase by 50 to 100 mg/day (given in 2 doses/day) every 4 days; usual maximum daily dose: 400 mg/**day**; for patients receiving 400 mg/day who are not controlled and have trough concentrations <0.6 mcg/mL, dosage may be increased to 600 mg/**day**

Paroxysmal supraventricular arrhythmias (eg, PSVT, atrial fibrillation) without structural heart disase (maintenance of sinus rhythm): Oral: Initial: 50 mg every 12 hours; increase by 50 mg twice daily at 4-day intervals; maximum daily dose: 300 mg/**day**. The AHA/ACC/HRS atrial fibrillation guidelines recommend a maximum dose of 400 mg per day (January, 2014).

Dosing adjustment in renal failure: Not dialyzable (~1%)

Manufacturer's labeling: Adults: CrCl ≤35 mL/minute/1.73 m²: Initial: 50 mg every 12 hours or 100 mg once daily;

increase dose slowly at intervals >4 days; monitor plasma levels closely

Alternate recommendations: The following guidelines have been used by some clinicians (Aronoff 2007):

GFR ≤50 mL/minute: Decrease dose by 50%; dose increases should be made cautiously at intervals >4 days and serum levels monitored frequently.

Hemodialysis: No supplemental dose recommended.

Peritoneal dialysis: No supplemental dose recommended.

Dosing adjustment in hepatic impairment: Monitoring of plasma levels is recommended because half-life is significantly increased. When transferring from another antiarrhythmic agent, allow for 2 to 4 half-lives of the agent to pass before initiating flecainide therapy.

Administration Oral: Administer around-the-clock to promote less variation in peak and trough serum levels. May be administered in children and adults without regard to food; in infants receiving milk or milk based formulas, avoid concurrent administration with feedings; monitor serum concentrations and decrease the dose when the diet changes to a decreased consumption of milk

Monitoring Parameters ECG, blood pressure, pulse, periodic serum concentrations after at least 5 doses when doses are started or changed or when dietary changes due to maturation or concurrent illness occur, liver enzymes

Reference Range Therapeutic trough: 0.2 to 1 mcg/mL (SI: 0.4 to 2 micromoles/L). **Note**: Pediatric patients may respond at the lower end of the recommended therapeutic range (0.2 to 0.5 mcg/mL) but up to 0.8 mcg/mL may be required.

Additional Information Single oral dose flecainide for termination of PSVT in children and young adults (n=25) and combination therapy of flecainide with amiodarone for refractory tachyarrhythmias in infancy (n=9) have been reported

Dosage Forms Excipient information presented when available (limited, particularly for generics); consult specific product labeling. [DSC] = Discontinued product

Tablet, Oral, as acetate:

Tambocor: 50 mg [DSC], 100 mg [DSC], 150 mg [DSC]

Generic: 50 mg, 100 mg, 150 mg

Extemporaneous Preparations A 20 mg/mL oral liquid suspension may be made from tablets and one of three different vehicles (cherry syrup, a 1:1 mixture of Ora-Sweet® and Ora-Plus®, or a 1:1 mixture of Ora-Sweet® SF and Ora-Plus®). Crush twenty-four 100 mg tablets in a mortar and reduce to a fine powder. Add 20 mL of the chosen vehicle and mix to a uniform paste; mix while adding the vehicle in incremental proportions to **almost** 120 mL; transfer to a calibrated bottle, rinse mortar with vehicle, and add quantity of vehicle sufficient to make 120 mL. Label "shake well" and "protect from light". Stable for 60 days when stored in amber plastic prescription bottles in the dark at room temperature or refrigerated.

Allen LV and Erickson III MA, "Stability of Baclofen, Captopril, Diltiazem, Hydrochloride, Dipyridamole, and Flecainide Acetate in Extemporaneously Compounded Oral Liquids," *Am J Health Syst Pharm*, 1996, 53:2179-84.

- **Flecainide Acetate** *see* Flecainide *on page 879*
- **Fleet Bisacodyl [OTC]** *see* Bisacodyl *on page 289*
- **Fleet Enema [OTC]** *see* Sodium Phosphates *on page 1949*
- **Fleet Enema (Can)** *see* Sodium Phosphates *on page 1949*
- **Fleet Enema Extra [OTC]** *see* Sodium Phosphates *on page 1949*
- **Fleet Laxative [OTC]** *see* Bisacodyl *on page 289*
- **Fleet Liquid Glycerin Supp [OTC]** *see* Glycerin *on page 978*
- **Fleet Oil [OTC]** *see* Mineral Oil *on page 1439*
- **Fleet Pedia-Lax Enema [OTC]** *see* Sodium Phosphates *on page 1949*
- **Flexbumin** *see* Albumin *on page 79*
- **Flexeril** *see* Cyclobenzaprine *on page 548*
- **Flexin** *see* Capsaicin *on page 362*
- **Flolan** *see* Epoprostenol *on page 769*
- **Flomax** *see* Tamsulosin *on page 2008*
- **Flomax CR (Can)** *see* Tamsulosin *on page 2008*
- **Flonase [DSC]** *see* Fluticasone (Nasal) *on page 917*
- **Flonase (Can)** *see* Fluticasone (Nasal) *on page 917*
- **Flonase Allergy Relief [OTC]** *see* Fluticasone (Nasal) *on page 917*
- **Flo-Pred** *see* PrednisoLONE (Systemic) *on page 1755*
- **Floranex™ [OTC]** *see Lactobacillus on page 1203*
- **Flora-Q™ [OTC]** *see Lactobacillus on page 1203*
- **Florical [OTC]** *see* Calcium Carbonate *on page 343*
- **Florinef** *see* Fludrocortisone *on page 891*
- **Florinef® (Can)** *see* Fludrocortisone *on page 891*
- **Flovent** *see* Fluticasone (Oral Inhalation) *on page 919*
- **Flovent Diskus** *see* Fluticasone (Oral Inhalation) *on page 919*
- **Flovent HFA** *see* Fluticasone (Oral Inhalation) *on page 919*
- **Floxin Otic Singles** *see* Ofloxacin (Otic) *on page 1545*
- **Fluad (Can)** *see* Influenza Virus Vaccine (Inactivated) *on page 1108*
- **Fluarix** *see* Influenza Virus Vaccine (Inactivated) *on page 1108*
- **Fluarix Quadrivalent** *see* Influenza Virus Vaccine (Inactivated) *on page 1108*
- **Flubenisolone** *see* Betamethasone (Systemic) *on page 278*
- **Flublok** *see* Influenza Virus Vaccine (Recombinant) *on page 1116*
- **Flucelvax** *see* Influenza Virus Vaccine (Inactivated) *on page 1108*

Fluconazole (floo KOE na zole)

Medication Safety Issues

Sound-alike/look-alike issues:

Fluconazole may be confused with flecainide, FLUoxetine, furosemide, itraconazole, voriconazole

Diflucan may be confused with diclofenac, Diprivan, disulfiram

International issues:

Canesten (oral capsules) [Great Britain] may be confused with Canesten brand name for clotrimazole (various dosage forms) [multiple international markets]; Cenestin brand name estrogens (conjugated A/synthetic) [U.S., Canada]

Related Information

Safe Handling of Hazardous Drugs *on page 2455*

Brand Names: US Diflucan

Brand Names: Canada ACT Fluconazole; Apo-Fluconazole; CanesOral; CO Fluconazole; Diflucan; Diflucan injection; Diflucan One; Diflucan PWS; Dom-Fluconazole; Fluconazole Injection; Fluconazole Injection SDZ; Fluconazole Omega; Monicure; Mylan-Fluconazole; Novo-Fluconazole; PHL-Fluconazole; PMS-Fluconazole; PRO-Fluconazole; Riva-Fluconazole; Taro-Fluconazole

Therapeutic Category Antifungal Agent, Systemic

Generic Availability (US) Yes

Use Treatment of candidiasis (vaginal, oropharyngeal, esophageal, urinary tract infections, peritonitis, pneumonia, and systemic infections); cryptococcal meningitis; antifungal prophylaxis in allogeneic bone marrow transplant recipients (All indications: FDA approved in all ages); strains of *Candida* with decreased *in vitro* susceptibility to fluconazole are being isolated with increasing frequency; fluconazole is more active against *C. albicans* than other candidal strains like *C. parapsilosis*, *C. glabrata*, and *C. tropicalis*; for some infections, an alternative to amphotericin B in patients with pre-existing renal impairment or when requiring concomitant therapy with other potentially nephrotoxic drugs

Pregnancy Risk Factor C (single dose for vaginal candidiasis)/D (all other indications)

Pregnancy Considerations Adverse events have been observed in some animal reproduction studies. When used in high doses, fluconazole is teratogenic in animal studies. Following exposure during the first trimester, case reports have noted similar malformations in humans when used in higher doses (400 mg/day) over extended periods of time (Aleck, 1997). Abnormalities reported include abnormal facies, abnormal calvarial development, arthrogryposis, brachycephaly, cleft palate, congenital heart disease, femoral bowing, thin ribs and long bones. Use of lower doses (150 mg as a single dose) does not suggest an increase risk to the fetus. Most azole antifungals, including fluconazole, are recommended to be avoided during pregnancy (Pappas, 2009).

Breast-Feeding Considerations Fluconazole is excreted in breast milk. The manufacturer recommends that caution be exercised when administering fluconazole to nursing women. Fluconazole is found in breast milk at concentrations similar to maternal plasma.

Contraindications Hypersensitivity to fluconazole or any component of the formulation (cross-reaction with other azole antifungal agents may occur, but has not been established; use caution); coadministration of terfenadine in adult patients receiving multiple doses of 400 mg or higher or with CYP3A4 substrates which may lead to QTc prolongation (eg, astemizole, cisapride, erythromycin, pimozide, or quinidine)

Warnings/Precautions Hazardous agent; use appropriate precautions for handling and disposal (NIOSH 2014 [group 3]). Serious (and sometimes fatal) hepatic toxicity (eg, hepatitis, cholestasis, fulminant hepatic failure) has been observed. Use with caution in patients with renal and hepatic dysfunction or previous hepatotoxicity from other azole derivatives. Patients who develop abnormal liver function tests during fluconazole therapy should be monitored closely and discontinued if symptoms consistent with liver disease develop. Rare exfoliative skin disorders have been observed; fatal outcomes have been reported in patients with serious concomitant diseases. Monitor patients with deep seated fungal infections closely for rash development and discontinue if lesions progress. In patients with superficial fungal infections who develop a rash attributable to fluconazole, treatment should also be discontinued. Cases of QTc prolongation and torsade de pointes associated with fluconazole use have been reported (usually high dose or in combination with agents known to prolong the QT interval); use caution in patients with concomitant medications or conditions which are arrhythmogenic. Potentially significant drug-drug interactions may exist, requiring dose or frequency adjustment, additional monitoring, and/or selection of alternative therapy. May occasionally cause dizziness or seizures; use caution driving or operating machines.

Powder for oral suspension contains sucrose; use caution with fructose intolerance, sucrose-isomaltase deficiency, or glucose-galactose malabsorption.

Benzyl alcohol and derivatives: Some dosage forms may contain sodium benzoate/benzoic acid; benzoic acid (benzoate) is a metabolite of benzyl alcohol; large amounts of benzyl alcohol (≥99 mg/kg/day) have been associated with a potentially fatal toxicity ("gasping syndrome") in neonates; the "gasping syndrome" consists of metabolic acidosis, respiratory distress, gasping respirations, CNS dysfunction (including convulsions, intracranial hemorrhage), hypotension, and cardiovascular collapse (AAP, 1997; CDC, 1982); some data suggests that benzoate displaces bilirubin from protein binding sites (Ahlfors, 2001); avoid or use dosage forms containing benzyl alcohol derivative with caution in neonates. See manufacturer's labeling.

Adverse Reactions

Cardiovascular: Angioedema (rare)

Central nervous system: Dizziness, headache

Dermatologic: Rash

Gastrointestinal: Abdominal pain, diarrhea, dysgeusia, dyspepsia, nausea, vomiting

Hepatic: Alkaline phosphatase increased, ALT increased, AST increased, hepatic failure (rare), hepatitis, jaundice

Miscellaneous: Anaphylactic reactions (rare)

Rare but important or life-threatening: Agranulocytosis, alopecia, cholestasis, diaphoresis, drug eruption, exanthematous pustulosis, fatigue, fever, hypercholesterolemia, hypertriglyceridemia, hypokalemia, insomnia, leukopenia, malaise, myalgia, neutropenia, paresthesia, QT prolongation, seizure, somnolence, Stevens-Johnson syndrome, thrombocytopenia, torsade de pointes, toxic epidermal necrolysis, tremor, vertigo, weakness, xerostomia

Drug Interactions

Metabolism/Transport Effects Inhibits CYP1A2 (weak), CYP2C19 (strong), CYP2C9 (moderate), CYP3A4 (moderate)

Avoid Concomitant Use

Avoid concomitant use of Fluconazole with any of the following: Bosutinib; Cisapride; Citalopram; Domperidone; Erythromycin (Systemic); Ibrutinib; Ivabradine; Lomitapide; Naloxegol; Olaparib; Ospemifene; Pimozide; QuiNIDine; Saccharomyces boulardii; Simeprevir; Tolvaptan; Trabectedin; Ulipristal; Voriconazole

Increased Effect/Toxicity

Fluconazole may increase the levels/effects of: Alfentanil; Amitriptyline; ARIPiprazole; AtorvaSTATin; Avanafil; Bosentan; Bosutinib; Budesonide (Systemic, Oral Inhalation); Budesonide (Topical); BusPIRone; Busulfan; Calcium Channel Blockers; Cannabis; CarBAMazepine; Carvedilol; Cilostazol; Cisapride; Citalopram; Colchicine; CycloSPORINE (Systemic); CYP2C19 Substrates; CYP2C9 Substrates; CYP3A4 Substrates; Dapoxetine; Domperidone; DOXOrubicin (Conventional); Dronabinol; Eletriptan; Eliglustat; Eplerenone; Erythromycin (Systemic); Etravirine; Everolimus; FentaNYL; Fluvastatin; Fosphenytoin; Halofantrine; Highest Risk QTc-Prolonging Agents; Hydrocodone; Ibrutinib; Imatinib; Ivabradine; Ivacaftor; Lomitapide; Lovastatin; Lurasidone; Methadone; Moderate Risk QTc-Prolonging Agents; Naloxegol; Nevirapine; NiMODipine; Olaparib; Ospemifene; OxyCODONE; Parecoxib; Phenytoin; Pimecrolimus; Pimozide; PredniSONE; Propafenone; Proton Pump Inhibitors; QuiNIDine; Ramelteon; Ranolazine; Red Yeast Rice; Rifamycin Derivatives; Rivaroxaban; Ruxolitinib; Salmeterol; Saxagliptin; Sildenafil; Simeprevir; Simvastatin; Sirolimus; Solifenacin; Sulfonylureas; SUNItinib; Suvorexant; Tacrolimus (Systemic); Tadalafil; Temsirolimus; Tetrahydrocannabinol; Tipranavir; TiZANidine; Tofacitinib; Tolvaptan; Trabectedin; Ulipristal; Vardenafil; Vilazodone; Vitamin K Antagonists; Voriconazole; Zidovudine; Zolpidem; Zopiclone

The levels/effects of Fluconazole may be increased by: Amitriptyline; Etravirine; Mifepristone

Decreased Effect

Fluconazole may decrease the levels/effects of: Amphotericin B; Clopidogrel; Ifosfamide; Losartan; Saccharomyces boulardii

The levels/effects of Fluconazole may be decreased by: Didanosine; Etravirine; Rifamycin Derivatives

Storage/Stability

Tablet: Store at <30°C (86°F).

Powder for oral suspension: Store dry powder at <30°C (86°F). Following reconstitution, store at 5°C to 30°C (41°F to 86°F). Discard unused portion after 2 weeks. Do not freeze.

Injection: Store injection in glass at 5°C to 30°C (41°F to 86°F). Store injection in plastic flexible containers at 5°C to 25°C (41°F to 77°F). Brief exposure of up to 40°C (104°F) does not adversely affect the product. Do not freeze. Do not unwrap unit until ready for use.

Mechanism of Action Interferes with fungal cytochrome P450 activity (lanosterol 14-α-demethylase), decreasing ergosterol synthesis (principal sterol in fungal cell membrane) and inhibiting cell membrane formation

Pharmacokinetics (Adult data unless noted)

Absorption: Oral: Well absorbed; food does not affect extent of absorption

Distribution: ~0.6 L/kg; widely throughout body with good penetration into CSF, eye, peritoneal fluid, sputum, skin, and urine. Relative diffusion blood into CSF: Adequate with or without inflammation; CSF:blood concentration ratio: Independent of degree of meningeal inflammation: 50% to 90%

Protein binding: 11% to 12%

Bioavailability: Oral: >90%

Half-life:

- Premature neonates (GA: 26-29 weeks): 73.6 hours
  - PNA: 6 days: 53 hours
  - PNA: 12 days: 47 hours
- Pediatric patients (9 months to 15 years):
  - 9 months to 13 years: Oral: 19.5-25 hours
  - 5-15 years: IV: 15-18 hours
- Adults: Normal renal function: ~30 hours

Time to peak serum concentration: Oral: 1-2 hours

Elimination: 80% (unchanged in urine); 11% (metabolites in urine)

Dosing: Neonatal Note: Daily dose of fluconazole is the same for oral and IV administration; unless otherwise specified, either dosage form may be used:

Candidiasis: IV, Oral:

Invasive (systemic):

Prophylaxis: Dosing based on IDSA guidelines and a pharmacokinetic simulation. Duration should be guided by presence of risk factors. Optimal criteria and duration of fluconazole prophylaxis need further defined(Healy, 2009).

GA <30 weeks: Consider for neonates with a birth weight <1000 g who are in a nursery with a high rate of invasive candidiasis.

Age at initiation of therapy:

PNA <7 days: IV: 3 mg/kg/dose or 6 mg/kg/dose twice weekly; in ELBW, therapy initiation recommended during first 48-72 hours of life by the IV route and continued for 4-6 weeks or until IV access no longer required for care of the neonate (Pappas, 2009; *Red Book*, 2012). **Note:** Dose selection may be directed by NICU-specific *Candida* sp. susceptibility (ie, use lower dose for an organism with an MIC ≤2 mcg/mL; neither dose has been studied for organisms with an MIC >4 mcg/mL) (Pappas, 2009; Wade, 2009).

PNA ≥7-42 days: 3 mg/kg/dose once daily or 6 mg/kg/dose every 72 hours (Wade, 2009)

PNA >42 days: 6 mg/kg/dose every 48 hours (Wade, 2009)

GA 30-40 weeks: 6 mg/kg/dose every 48 hours (Wade, 2009)

Treatment:

Systemic candidiasis, invasive disease: 12 mg/kg/dose once daily for 21 days; gestational age not specified (Pappas, 2009). Others have recommended a loading dose of 25 mg/kg, followed by 12 mg/kg once daily; an evaluation of this dosing in five neonates (GA: 35-38 weeks; PNA: 16 days) showed all subjects reached target trough concentrations (>8 mcg/mL) within 24 hours (Piper, 2011; Wade, 2008; Wade, 2009). Some experts have suggested 12 mg/kg/dose every 48 hours for PNA <8 days.

Oral (thrush) (Pappas, 2009): Term neonate:

PNA ≤14 days: Initial: 6 mg/kg/dose followed by 3 mg/kg/dose every 24-72 hours for 7-14 days

PNA >14 days: Initial: 6 mg/kg/dose followed by 3 mg/kg/dose once daily for 7-14 days

Esophageal disease (Pappas, 2009): Term neonate:

PNA ≤14 days: Initial: 6 mg/kg/dose followed by 3 mg/kg/dose every 24-72 hours for a minimum of 14-21 days; duration of therapy based upon clinical response; some suggest to continue for 2 weeks after clinical resolution with a minimum of at least 3 weeks of therapy

PNA >14 days: Initial: 6 mg/kg/dose followed by 3 mg/kg/dose once daily for a minimum of 14-21 days; in some cases, doses up to 12 mg/kg may be required; duration of therapy based upon clinical response; continue for 2 weeks after clinical resolution with a minimum of at least 3 weeks of therapy

Cryptococcal, CNS disease (meningitis): IV, Oral: PNA >14 days:

Acute treatment: 12 mg/kg/dose followed by 6-12 mg/kg/day for 10-12 weeks after CSF culture becomes negative

Prevention of relapse: 6 mg/kg/dose once daily

Dosing adjustment in renal impairment: There are no specific neonatal dosage adjustments provided in the manufacturer's labeling; some experts have used the following indication-specific dosing (Wade, 2009): Candidiasis, prophylaxis: IV, Oral:

S_{cr} ≥1.3 mg/dL: 6 mg/kg once weekly

S_{cr} ≤1 mg/dL: Standard dosing

Dosing: Usual

Infants and Children: **Note:** Daily dose of fluconazole is the same for oral and IV administration; unless otherwise specified, either dosage form may be used:

General dosing, susceptible infection: IV, Oral: Initial: 6-12 mg/kg/dose, followed by 3-12 mg/kg/dose once daily; maximum daily dose: 600 mg/**day**; duration and dosage depends on severity of infection

Candidiasis: IV, Oral:

Prophylaxis regimens:

Chemotherapy-induced neutropenia (including stem cell transplantation): 6 mg/kg/dose once daily during induction chemotherapy and period of neutropenia risk; maximum daily dose: 400 mg/**day** (Pappas, 2009)

Postsolid organ transplant: 6 mg/kg/dose once daily for 14 days; maximum daily dose: 400 mg/**day** (Pappas, 2009)

Treatment and suppression regimens:

Esophageal infection:

Non-HIV-exposed/-positive: *Treatment:* 6 mg/kg/dose on Day 1, followed by 3 mg/kg/dose once daily for at least 21 days and at least 2 weeks following symptom resolution. In some cases, higher doses (up to 12 mg/kg/**day**) may be used; maximum daily dose: 400 mg/**day**

HIV-exposed/-positive (CDC, 2009):
Treatment: 6 mg/kg/dose on Day 1, followed by 3-6 mg/kg/dose once daily for 4-21 days; maximum daily dose: 400 mg/**day**
Relapse suppression: 3-6 mg/kg/dose once daily; maximum daily dose: 200 mg/**day**
Oropharyngeal infection:
Non-HIV-exposed/-positive: *Treatment:* 6 mg/kg/dose on Day 1, followed by 3 mg/kg/dose once daily for at least 14 days; maximum daily dose: Day 1: 200 mg/**day**; subsequent days: 100 mg/**day**
HIV-exposed/-positive: *Treatment:* 3-6 mg/kg/dose once daily for 7-14 days; maximum daily dose: 400 mg/**day** (CDC, 2009)
Systemic infection (invasive disease):
Non-HIV-exposed/-positive (neutropenic or non-neutropenic patients; reserve use for stable patients only): *Treatment:* 12 mg/kg/dose on Day 1 (maximum dose: 800 mg), followed by 12 mg/kg/dose once daily or 6 mg/kg/dose twice daily; maximum daily dose: 600 mg/**day**; treatment duration: 2 weeks after clearance from blood and symptom resolution (Filioti, 2007; Pappas, 2009; Zaoutis, 2010)
HIV-exposed/-positive: *Treatment:* 5-6 mg/kg/dose twice daily for minimum of 4 weeks; maximum daily dose: 600 mg/**day**; reserve for documented *C. albicans* or other susceptible species (CDC, 2009)

Coccidioidomycosis, meningeal infection, or in a stable patient with diffuse pulmonary or disseminated disease (HIV-exposed/-positive) (CDC, 2009): IV, Oral:
Treatment: 5-6 mg/kg/dose twice daily; maximum daily dose: 800 mg/**day**, followed by chronic suppressive therapy
Relapse suppression: 6 mg/kg/dose once daily; maximum daily dose: 400 mg/**day**

Cryptococcal infection: IV, Oral:
CNS disease:
Non-HIV-exposed/-positive:
Acute therapy:
Manufacturer's labeling: 12 mg/kg/dose on Day 1, followed by 6 mg/kg/dose once daily; in some cases, doses as high as 12 mg/kg/day once daily may be required dependent upon patient's response to therapy; treatment duration 10-12 weeks after CSF becomes culture negative; maximum daily dose: 800 mg/**day**
Alternate dosing: Consolidation phase: 5-6 mg/kg/dose **twice** daily; treatment duration: 8 weeks followed by maintenance therapy; maximum daily dose: 800 mg/**day** (Perfect, 2010)
Maintenance therapy: 6 mg/kg/dose once daily for 6-12 months; maximum daily dose: 200 mg/**day** (Perfect, 2010)
HIV-exposed/-positive:
Acute therapy, induction: 12 mg/kg /dose on Day 1, followed by 6-12 mg/kg/dose once daily; maximum daily dose: 800 mg/**day**; in combination with flucytosine for at least 2 weeks until significant clinical improvement and negative CSF cultures then begin consolidation therapy; reserve as alternate therapy when amphotericin (including lipid-based products) is not tolerated (CDC, 2009)
Consolidation therapy: 12 mg/kg/dose on Day 1, followed by 6-12 mg/kg/dose once daily for a minimum of 8 weeks; maximum daily dose: 800 mg/**day**; **Note:** CSF cultures should be negative prior to initiating consolidation therapy (CDC, 2009)
Relapse suppression: 6 mg/kg/dose once daily; maximum daily dose: 200 mg/**day**
Localized (non-CNS), disseminated, or pulmonary disease:
Non-HIV-exposed/-positive:
Mild-moderate pulmonary disease or localized infection: *Treatment:* 6 mg/kg once daily; maximum daily dose: 400 mg/**day**; a treatment duration of 6-12 months has been used in organ transplant recipients (Perfect, 2010)
Severe pulmonary disease, or disseminated infection; treatment:
Acute therapy: 12 mg/kg/dose on Day 1, followed by 6 mg/kg/dose once daily; in some cases, doses as high as 12 mg/kg/dose once daily may be used dependent upon patient's response to therapy; treatment duration 10-12 weeks; maximum daily dose: 800 mg/**day** (Perfect, 2010)
Maintenance therapy: 6 mg/kg/dose once daily for 6-12 months; maximum daily dose: 200 mg/**day** (Perfect, 2010)
HIV-exposed/-positive (CDC, 2009):
Treatment: 12 mg/kg/dose on Day 1, followed by 6-12 mg/kg/dose once daily; maximum daily dose: 600 mg/**day**; treatment duration variable and dependent upon infection site, severity, and clinical response; chronic suppressive therapy should be initiated upon treatment completion
Relapse suppression: 6 mg/kg/dose once daily; maximum daily dose: 200 mg/**day**

Histoplasmosis; relapse prevention (HIV-exposed/-positive): IV, Oral: 3-6 mg/kg/dose once daily; maximum daily dose: 200 mg/**day** (CDC, 2009).

Peritonitis (Warady, 2012):
Prophylaxis during antibiotic therapy: IV, Oral: 3-6 mg/kg/dose every 24-48 hours; maximum single dose: 200 mg
Treatment:
Peritonitis: Intraperitoneal, IV, Oral: 6-12 mg/kg/dose every 24-48 hours; maximum single dose: 400 mg
Exit-site and tunnel infections: Oral: 6 mg/kg/dose every 24-48 hours; maximum single dose: 400 mg

Surgical prophylaxis: IV: 6 mg/kg as a single dose 1-2 hours prior to procedure; maximum dose: 400 mg (Bratzler, 2013)

Adolescents:

General dosing, susceptible infection: IV, Oral: Initial: 6-12 mg/kg/dose followed by 3-12 mg/kg/dose once daily; maximum daily dose: 600 mg/**day**; duration and dosage depend on severity of infection

Blastomycosis, CNS disease (independent of HIV status): Oral: *Step-down therapy:* 800 mg once daily; initiate after 4-6 weeks of amphotericin therapy and continue for at least 12 months or until resolution of CNS abnormalities has been recommended in adult patients (Chapman, 2005)

Candidiasis: IV, Oral:
Prophylaxis regimens:
Chemotherapy-induced neutropenia (including stem cell transplantation): 6 mg/kg/dose once daily during induction chemotherapy and period of neutropenia risk; maximum daily dose: 400 mg/**day** (Pappas, 2009)
Postsolid organ transplant: 6 mg/kg/dose once daily for 14 days; maximum daily dose: 400 mg/**day** (Pappas, 2009)
Treatment and suppression regimens:
Esophageal infection:
Non-HIV-exposed/-positive: *Treatment:* 6 mg/kg/dose on Day 1, followed by 3 mg/kg/dose once daily for at least 21 days and at least 2 weeks following symptom resolutions. In some cases, higher doses (up to 12 mg/kg/**day**) may be used; maximum daily dose: 400 mg/**day**

HIV-exposed/-positive (DHHS, 2013):
Treatment: 100 mg once daily for 14-21 days; maximum daily dose: 400 mg/**day**
Relapse suppression: 100-200 mg once daily
Oropharyngeal infection:
Non-HIV-exposed/-positive: *Treatment:* 6 mg/kg/dose on Day 1, followed by 3 mg/kg/dose once daily for at least 14 days; maximum daily dose: Day 1: 200 mg/**day**; subsequent doses: 100 mg/**day**
HIV-exposed/-positive (DHHS, 2013):
Treatment: Oral: 100 mg once daily for 7-14 days
Relapse suppression: Oral: 100 mg once daily or 3 times weekly
Systemic infection (invasive disease): Neutropenic or non-neutropenic patients (non-HIV-exposed/-positive; reserve use for stable patients only): *Treatment:* 12 mg/kg/dose on Day 1 (maximum dose: 800 mg) followed by 12 mg/kg/dose once daily or 6 mg/kg/dose twice daily (maximum daily dose: 600 mg/**day**); treatment duration: 2 weeks after clearance from blood and symptom resolution (Fioliti, 2007; Pappas, 2009; Zaoutis, 2010)
Vulvovaginal infection:
Uncomplicated (independent of HIV status): *Treatment:* Oral: 150 mg single dose (CDC, 2010; CDC, 2013)
Complicated (severe, recurrent) (HIV-exposed/-positive) (DHHS, 2013):
Treatment: 100-200 mg once daily for at least 7 days
Relapse suppression: Oral: 150 mg/dose once weekly

Coccidioidomycosis: IV, Oral:
Non-CNS disease:
Non-HIV-exposed/-positive: *Treatment:* 400-800 mg once daily; for severe disseminated extrapulmonary infection, doses up to 2000 mg/day have been used; total therapy duration (treatment and maintenance) dependent upon site of infection; for pneumonia (diffuse) at least 12 months (if patient immunosuppressed, consider additional suppression therapy); for other disseminated (nonpulmonary infections), treatment duration based upon clinical response and may extend longer than 12 months (Galgiani, 2005)
HIV-exposed/-positive (CDC, 2013):
Prevention, first episode: Oral: 400 mg once daily
Treatment:
Mild infection or focal pneumonia: 400 mg once daily
Severe infection (eg, diffuse pulmonary infection or extrathoracic disseminated disease): 400 mg once daily in combination with amphotericin; continue fluconazole after amphotericin stopped following clinical improvement
Chronic suppressive therapy: Oral: 400 mg once daily
Meningeal infection:
Non-HIV-exposed/-positive: *Treatment:* 400-1000 mg once daily, continue indefinitely (Galgiani, 2005)
HIV-exposed/-positive (DHHS, 2013):
Treatment: 400-800 mg once daily
Suppression: Oral: 400 mg once daily

Cryptococcal infection: IV, Oral:
CNS disease:
Non-HIV-exposed/-positive:
Treatment: Acute therapy: 12 mg/kg/dose on Day 1, followed by 6 mg/kg/dose once daily; in some cases doses as high as 12 mg/kg/dose once daily may be used dependent upon patient's response to therapy; treatment duration 10-12 weeks; maximum daily dose: 800 mg/**day**
Consolidation therapy: Oral: 10-12 mg/kg/dose once daily for 8 weeks; maximum daily dose: 800 mg/**day** (Perfect, 2010)
Maintenance therapy: Oral: 6 mg/kg/dose once daily; maximum daily dose: 200 mg/**day** (Perfect, 2010)
HIV-exposed/-positive (DHHS, 2013):
Induction: Continue therapy for at least 2 weeks
Combination therapy: 800 mg once daily with amphotericin or liposomal amphotericin; if patient unable to tolerate amphotericin (or lipid product formulations) may use 400-800 mg/dose once daily with flucytosine
Monotherapy: 1200 mg once daily
Consolidation therapy: 400 mg once daily for 8 weeks; begin after at least 2 weeks of induction therapy (ie, significant clinical improvement and negative CSF cultures)
Maintenance therapy: Oral: 200 mg once daily for at least 12 months
Localized (non-CNS), disseminated, or pulmonary disease:
Non-HIV-exposed/-positive: Cryptococcal pneumonia: Oral: *Treatment:* 6-12 mg/kg/dose once daily for 6-12 months; maximum daily dose: 800 mg/**day** (Perfect, 2010)
HIV-exposed/-positive (DHHS, 2013):
Diffuse pulmonary disease or extrapulmonary disease:
Induction: Continue therapy for at least 2 weeks
Combination therapy: 800 mg once daily with amphotericin or liposomal amphotericin; if patient unable to tolerate amphotericin (or lipid product formulations) may use 400-800 mg/dose once daily with flucytosine
Monotherapy: 1200 mg once daily
Consolidation therapy: Oral: 400 mg once daily for 8 weeks; begin after at least 2 weeks of induction therapy (ie, significant clinical improvement and negative CSF cultures)
Maintenance therapy: Oral: 200 mg once daily for at least 12 months
Focal pulmonary infiltrates or mild-moderate symptoms: Oral: 400 mg once daily for 12 months

Histoplasmosis: IV, Oral:
Non-HIV-exposed/-positive (Wheat, 2007):
Treatment: 200-800 mg once daily
Maintenance (CNS disease): Following 8 weeks of amphotericin B, fluconazole 200-400 mg once daily for 12 months
HIV-exposed/-positive (DHHS, 2013): Duration of therapy for induction and maintenance at least 12 months
Treatment, less severe disease: Oral: 800 mg once daily
Maintenance (severe disseminated or CNS disease): Oral: 800 mg once daily
Suppression, long-term (severe disseminated or CNS disease): Oral: 400 mg once daily

Penicilliosis; prevention first episode (HIV-exposed/-positive): Oral: 400 mg once weekly (DHHS, 2013)

Peritonitis (Warady, 2012):
Prophylaxis during antibiotic therapy: IV, Oral: 3-6 mg/kg/dose every 24-48 hours; maximum single dose: 200 mg
Treatment:
Peritonitis: Intraperitoneal, IV, Oral: 6-12 mg/kg/dose every 24-48 hours; maximum single dose: 400 mg
Exit-site and tunnel infection: Oral: 6 mg/kg/dose every 24-48 hours; maximum single dose: 400 mg

Surgical prophylaxis: IV: 6 mg/kg as a single dose 1-2 hours prior to procedure; maximum dose: 400 mg (Bratzler, 2013)

Adult: **Usual dosage range:** 150 mg once **or** 200-800 mg/day; duration and dosage depend on severity of infection

Dosing adjustment in renal impairment:
Infants, Children, and Adolescents:
No adjustment for vaginal candidiasis single-dose therapy.
For multiple dosing, administer usual load then adjust daily doses as follows; based upon Schwartz calculations:
CrCl >50 mL/minute/1.73 m^2: No adjustment necessary.
CrCl 10-50 mL/minute/1.73 m^2 (no dialysis): Administer 50% of recommended dose at the normal interval.
CrCl ≤10 mL/minute/1.73 m^2: Administer 50% of recommended dose every 48 hours (Aronoff, 2007).
Intermittent hemodialysis: Dialyzable (50%): May administer 100% of daily dose (according to indication) after each dialysis session; others have suggested the following: Administer 50% of dose every 48 hours; on dialysis days administer dose after dialysis session (Aronoff, 2007)
Peritoneal dialysis: Administer 50% of recommended dose every 48 hours (Aronoff, 2007)
Continuous renal replacement (CRRT): 6 mg/kg/dose every 24 hours (Aronoff, 2007)
Adults:
No adjustment for vaginal candidiasis single-dose therapy.
For multiple dosing, administer usual load then adjust daily doses as follows: Administer loading dose of 50-400 mg, then adjust daily doses as follows:
CrCl ≤50 mL/minute (no dialysis): Administer 50% of recommended dose daily
Intermittent hemodialysis (IHD): Dialyzable (50%): May administer 100% of daily dose (according to indication) after each dialysis session. Alternatively, doses of 200-400 mg every 48-72 hours or 100-200 mg every 24 hours have been recommended (Heintz, 2009). **Note:** Dosing dependent on the assumption of 3 times/week, complete IHD sessions.
Continuous renal replacement therapy (CRRT) (Heintz, 2009; Trotman, 2005): Drug clearance is highly dependent on the method of renal replacement, filter type, and flow rate. Appropriate dosing requires close monitoring of pharmacologic response, signs of adverse reactions due to drug accumulation, as well as drug concentrations in relation to target trough (if appropriate). The following are general recommendations only (based on dialysate flow/ultrafiltration rates of 1-2 L/hour and minimal residual renal function) and should not supersede clinical judgment:
CVVH: Loading dose of 400-800 mg followed by 200-400 mg every 24 hours
CVVHD/CVVHDF: Loading dose of 400-800 mg followed by 400-800 mg every 24 hours (CVVHD or CVVHDF) or 800 mg every 24 hours (CVVHDF)
Note: Higher maintenance doses of 400 mg every 24 hours (CVVH), 800 mg every 24 hours (CVVHD), and 500-600 mg every 12 hours (CVVHDF) may be considered when treating resistant organisms and/or when employing combined ultrafiltration and dialysis flow rates of ≥2 L/hour for CVVHD/CVVHDF (Heintz, 2009; Trotman, 2005).

Dosing adjustment in hepatic impairment: There are no dosage adjustments provided in manufacturer's labeling; use with caution.

Preparation for Administration Hazardous agent; use appropriate precautions for handling and disposal (NIOSH 2014 [group 3]).
Oral: Reconstitute powder for oral suspension with appropriate amount of water as specified on the bottle. Shake vigorously until suspended.

Administration Hazardous agent; use appropriate precautions for handling and disposal (NIOSH 2014 [group 3]).
Oral: Administer without regard to meals; shake suspension well before use
Parenteral: Do not use if cloudy or precipitated. Administered by IV infusion over approximately 1 to 2 hours at a rate not to exceed 200 mg/hour; for pediatric patients receiving doses ≥6 mg/kg, administer IV infusion over 2 hours

Monitoring Parameters Periodic liver function (AST, ALT, alkaline phosphatase), renal function tests, serum potassium, CBC with differential, and platelet count

Additional Information
Dosing equivalency suggested by the manufacturer's labeling:
Pediatric patients 3 mg/kg = Adults 100 mg
Pediatric patients 6 mg/kg = Adults 200 mg
Pediatric patients 12 mg/kg = Adults 400 mg

Dosage Forms Excipient information presented when available (limited, particularly for generics); consult specific product labeling.
Solution, Intravenous:
Generic: 100 mg (50 mL); 200 mg (100 mL); 400 mg (200 mL)
Solution, Intravenous [preservative free]:
Generic: 200 mg (100 mL); 400 mg (200 mL)
Suspension Reconstituted, Oral:
Diflucan: 10 mg/mL (35 mL); 40 mg/mL (35 mL) [orange flavor]
Generic: 10 mg/mL (35 mL); 40 mg/mL (35 mL)
Tablet, Oral:
Diflucan: 50 mg, 100 mg, 150 mg, 200 mg
Generic: 50 mg, 100 mg, 150 mg, 200 mg

◆ **Fluconazole Injection (Can)** *see* Fluconazole *on page 881*

◆ **Fluconazole Injection SDZ (Can)** *see* Fluconazole *on page 881*

◆ **Fluconazole Omega (Can)** *see* Fluconazole *on page 881*

Flucytosine (floo SYE toe seen)

Medication Safety Issues
Sound-alike/look-alike issues:
Flucytosine may be confused with fluorouracil
Ancobon® may be confused with Oncovin
High alert medication:
The Institute for Safe Medication Practices (ISMP) includes this medication among its list of drugs which have a heightened risk of causing significant patient harm when used in error.

Brand Names: US Ancobon

Therapeutic Category Antifungal Agent, Systemic

Generic Availability (US) Yes

Use Treatment of serious infections caused by susceptible strains of Candida (septicemia, endocarditis, pulmonary, urinary tract infections) and/or Cryptococcus (meningitis, pulmonary, septicemia, urinary tract infections) in combination with amphotericin B (FDA approved in adults)

Pregnancy Risk Factor C

Pregnancy Considerations Adverse events have been observed in some animal reproduction studies. Flucytosine is metabolized to fluorouracil which may cause adverse events if administered during pregnancy; refer to the Fluorouracil (Systemic) monograph for additional information.

Breast-Feeding Considerations It is not known if flucytosine is excreted in breast milk. Due to the potential for serious adverse reactions in the nursing infant, a decision should be made whether to discontinue nursing or to discontinue the drug, taking into account the importance of treatment to the mother.

Contraindications Hypersensitivity to flucytosine or any component of the formulation

Warnings/Precautions [U.S. Boxed Warning]: Use with extreme caution in patients with renal dysfunction; dosage adjustment required. Avoid use as monotherapy; resistance rapidly develops. Use with caution in patients with bone marrow depression; patients with hematologic disease or who have been treated with radiation or drugs that suppress the bone marrow may be at greatest risk. Bone marrow toxicity may be irreversible. **[U.S. Boxed Warning]: Closely monitor hematologic, renal, and hepatic status.** Hepatotoxicity and bone marrow toxicity appear to be dose related; monitor levels closely and adjust dose accordingly.

Warnings: Additional Pediatric Considerations Serum flucytosine concentrations are highly variable in neonates; monitor closely (Pasqualotte, 2007); serum concentrations tended to be higher in children <12 years of age; monitor closely (Soltani, 2006).

Adverse Reactions

Cardiovascular: Cardiac arrest, myocardial toxicity, ventricular dysfunction, chest pain

Central nervous system: Ataxia, confusion, fatigue, hallucinations, headache, parkinsonism, psychosis, pyrexia, sedation, seizure, vertigo

Dermatologic: Rash, photosensitivity, pruritus, toxic epidermal necrolysis, urticaria

Endocrine & metabolic: Hypoglycemia, hypokalemia

Gastrointestinal: Abdominal pain, anorexia, diarrhea, duodenal ulcer, enterocolitis, hemorrhage, nausea, ulcerative colitis, vomiting, xerostomia

Hematologic: Agranulocytosis, anemia, aplastic anemia, bone marrow aplasia, eosinophilia, leukopenia, pancytopenia, thrombocytopenia

Hepatic: Acute hepatic injury, bilirubin increased, hepatic dysfunction, jaundice, liver enzymes increased

Neuromuscular & skeletal: Paresthesia, peripheral neuropathy, weakness

Otic: Hearing loss

Renal: Azotemia, BUN increased, crystalluria, renal failure, serum creatinine increased

Respiratory: Dyspnea, respiratory arrest

Miscellaneous: Allergic reaction

Drug Interactions

Metabolism/Transport Effects None known.

Avoid Concomitant Use

Avoid concomitant use of Flucytosine with any of the following: BCG (Intravesical); CloZAPine; Dipyrone; Gimeracil; Saccharomyces boulardii

Increased Effect/Toxicity

Flucytosine may increase the levels/effects of: CloZAPine

The levels/effects of Flucytosine may be increased by: Amphotericin B; Dipyrone; Gimeracil

Decreased Effect

Flucytosine may decrease the levels/effects of: BCG (Intravesical); Saccharomyces boulardii

The levels/effects of Flucytosine may be decreased by: Cytarabine (Conventional)

Food Interactions Food decreases the rate, but not the extent of absorption.

Storage/Stability Store at room temperature of 25°C (77°F); excursions permitted to 15°C to 30°C (59°F to 86°F).

Mechanism of Action Penetrates fungal cells and is converted to fluorouracil which competes with uracil interfering with fungal RNA and protein synthesis

Pharmacokinetics (Adult data unless noted)

Absorption: Oral: Rapid; rate of absorption is delayed in patients with renal impairment; serum concentrations are highly variable in neonates; monitor closely (Pasqualotte, 2007); serum concentrations tended to be higher in children <12 years of age; monitor closely (Soltani, 2006)

Distribution: Widely distributed into body tissues and fluids including CSF, aqueous humor, peritoneal fluid, bronchial secretions, liver, spleen, kidney, heart, and joints

V_d: Adults: 0.68 L/kg

Protein binding: 2.9% to 4%

Metabolism: Minimal hepatic metabolism; deaminated to 5-fluorouracil (probably by gut bacteria)

Bioavailability: 78% to 89%; decreased in neonates

Half-life:

- Neonates: 4-34 hours (Baley, 1990)
- Infants: 7.4 hours
- Adults: 2.5-5 hours
- Anuria: 85 hours (range: 30-250 hours)

Time to peak serum concentration: Oral:

- Infants: 2.5 ± 1.3 hours
- Adults: Within 2 hours

Elimination: 90% excreted unchanged in urine by glomerular filtration; small portion is excreted in the feces

Dialysis: Dialyzable (50% to 100%)

Dosing: Neonatal Note: Administer in combination with amphotericin B or another susceptible antifungal to prevent development of resistance:

General dosing, susceptible infection: Limited data available: Oral: Initial:

Body weight ≤2 kg

- PNA ≤7 days: 75 mg/kg/day divided every 8 hours
- PNA 8-28 days: 75 mg/kg/day divided every 6 hours

Body weight >2 kg: 75 mg/kg/day divided every 6 hours

Note: Monitoring of serum concentrations recommended; reported dosing range: 25-100 mg/kg/day in divided doses every 6-24 hours (Baley, 1990; Fernandez, 2000; Marr, 1994)

Candidal meningitis: Limited data available: Oral: 100 mg/kg/**day** in divided doses every 6-8 hours in combination with amphotericin B; monitoring of serum concentrations should be considered; reported range: 75-100 mg/kg/day; dosing based on a retrospective study and case reports (n=9) including premature neonates (GA: 24-28 weeks; PMA at treatment: 26-29 weeks); treatment duration in some cases was up to 6 weeks (Fernandez, 2000; Marr, 1994; Pahud, 2009)

Dosing: Usual Note: In general, administer in combination with amphotericin B or another susceptible antifungal due to development of resistance.

Infants, Children, and Adolescents:

General dosing, susceptible infections: Oral: 50-150 mg/kg/day in divided doses every 6 hours (*Red Book*, 2012)

Candidiasis (Pappas, 2009): Oral:

Endocarditis or implanted cardiovascular device: 25 mg/kg/dose every 6 hours in combination with amphotericin B; valve replacement or removal of hardware is strongly recommended

Endophthalmitis: 25 mg/kg/dose every 6 hours in combination with amphotericin B

Invasive (including CNS disease), treatment: 25 mg/kg/dose every 6 hours

Urinary tract infection:

- Cystitis, symptomatic: 25 mg/kg/dose every 6 hours for 7-10 days
- Pyelonephritis: 25 mg/kg/dose every 6 hours for 2 weeks; with or without amphotericin B; if fungal balls present, use in combination with amphotericin B and treatment duration should be until symptom resolution and clear urine culture

Cryptococcal disease; disseminated (including CNS disease); treatment (independent of HIV status): Oral: 25 mg/kg/dose every 6 hours in combination with amphotericin B or fluconazole; minimum treatment duration: ≥2 weeks; full treatment duration dependent upon: HIV status, source of infection and concomitant antifungal therapy (DHHS [adult and pediatric], 2013; Perfect, 2010; Tunkel, 2009)

Adults:

General dosing, susceptible infection: Oral: 12.5-37.5 mg/kg/dose every 6 hours

Endocarditis: Oral: 100 mg/kg/day in 3 or 4 divided doses (with amphotericin B) for at least 4-6 weeks after valve replacement (Gould, 2012; Pappas, 2009)

Meningoencephalitis, cryptococcal: Oral: Induction: 25 mg/kg/dose (with amphotericin B) every 6 hours for at least 4 weeks, or if HIV-infected at least 2 weeks; if clinical improvement, may discontinue both amphotericin and flucytosine and follow with an extended course of fluconazole (DHHS [adult], 2013; Perfect, 2010)

Dosing adjustment in renal impairment: Monitor serum concentrations.

Infants, Children, and Adolescents: There are no dosage adjustments provided in the manufacturer labeling; however, the following guidelines have been used by some clinicians:

Aronoff, 2007: Infants, Children, and non-HIV-exposed/-positive Adolescents: Based on a usual dose of 100-150 mg/kg/day divided every 6 hours

GFR 30-50 mL/minute/1.73 m^2: 25-37.5 mg/kg/dose every 8 hours

GFR 10-29 mL/minute/1.73 m^2: 25-37.5 mg/kg/dose every 12 hours

GFR <10 mL/minute/1.73 m^2: 25-37.5 mg/kg/dose every 24 hours

Hemodialysis or peritoneal dialysis: 25-37.5 mg/kg/dose every 24 hours

Continuous renal replacement therapy: 25-37.5 mg/kg/dose every 8 hours; monitor serum concentrations

DHHS [adult], 2013: HIV-exposed/-positive: Adolescents: Based on a usual dose of 25 mg/kg every 6 hours:

CrCl >40 mL/minute: No adjustment recommended

CrCl 20-40 mL/minute: 25 mg/kg every 12 hours

CrCl 10 to <20 mL/minute: 25 mg/kg every 24 hours

CrCl <10 mL/minute: 25 mg/kg every 48 hours

Hemodialysis: Administer dose after hemodialysis: 25-50 mg/kg every 48-72 hours

Adults: The manufacturer's labeling suggests using lower initial dose; the following guidelines have been used by some clinicians

Aronoff, 2007: Based on a usual dose of 37.5 mg/kg every 6 hours:

CrCl >80 mL/minute: No adjustment recommended

CrCl 50-80 mL/minute: 37.5 mg/kg every 12 hours

CrCl 10-50 mL/minute: 37.5 mg/kg every 12-24 hours

CrCl <10 mL/minute: 37.5 mg/kg every 24-48 hours, but monitor drug concentrations frequently

Hemodialysis: Administer dose after hemodialysis

Peritoneal dialysis: 500-1000 mg every 24 hours

Continuous renal replacement therapy: 37.5 mg/kg every 12-24 hours; monitor serum concentrations

DHHS [adult], 2013: Based on a usual dose of 25 mg/kg every 6 hours:

CrCl >40 mL/minute: No adjustment recommended

CrCl 20-40 mL/minute: 25 mg/kg every 12 hours

CrCl 10 to ≤20 mL/minute: 25 mg/kg every 24 hours

CrCl <10 mL/minute: 25 mg/kg every 48 hours

Hemodialysis: Administer dose after hemodialysis: 25-50 mg/kg every 48-72 hours

Dosing adjustment in hepatic impairment: There are no dosage adjustments provided in the manufacturer's labeling, but flucytosine has minimal hepatic metabolism; use caution.

Administration Oral: Administer around-the-clock to promote less variation in peak and trough serum levels; to avoid nausea and vomiting, administer a few capsules at a time over 15 minutes until full dose is taken.

Monitoring Parameters Prior to therapy: Serum electrolytes (especially potassium), CBC with differential, BUN, and creatinine. During therapy: Serum electrolytes, creatinine, BUN, alkaline phosphatase, AST, ALT, CBC, platelet count; serum flucytosine concentrations; *in vitro* susceptibility tests to flucytosine

Reference Range

Therapeutic: Trough: 25-50 mcg/mL; peak: 50-100 mcg/mL; peak concentrations should not exceed 100 mcg/mL to avoid bone marrow toxicity and hepatotoxicity; for patients who are HIV-exposed/-positive a peak concentration of 40-60 mcg/mL is recommended (DHHS [pediatric], 2013)

Trough: Draw just prior to dose administration

Peak: Draw 2 hours after an oral dose administration

Test Interactions Flucytosine causes markedly false elevations in serum creatinine values when the Ektachem® analyzer is used. The Jaffé reaction is recommended for determining serum creatinine.

Dosage Forms Excipient information presented when available (limited, particularly for generics); consult specific product labeling.

Capsule, Oral:

Ancobon: 250 mg, 500 mg

Generic: 250 mg, 500 mg

Extemporaneous Preparations A 10 mg/mL oral suspension may be made with capsules and distilled water. Empty the contents of ten 500 mg capsules in a mortar; add small portions of distilled water and mix to a uniform paste. Mix while adding distilled water in incremental proportions to **almost** 500 mL; transfer to a 500 mL volumetric flask, rinse mortar several times with distilled water, and add sufficient quantity of distilled water to make 500 mL. Store in glass or plastic prescription bottles and label "shake well". Stable for 70 days refrigerated and 14 days at room temperature.

Wintermeyer SM and Nahata MC, "Stability of Flucytosine in an Extemporaneously Compounded Oral Liquid," *Am J Health Syst Pharm*, 1996, 53(4):407-9.

◆ **Fludara** *see* Fludarabine *on page 888*

Fludarabine (floo DARE a been)

Medication Safety Issues

Sound-alike/look-alike issues:

Fludarabine may be confused with cladribine, floxuridine, Flumadine

Fludara may be confused with FUDR

High alert medication:

This medication is in a class the Institute for Safe Medication Practices (ISMP) includes among its list of drug classes which have a heightened risk of causing significant patient harm when used in error.

Related Information

Prevention of Chemotherapy-Induced Nausea and Vomiting in Children *on page 2368*

Safe Handling of Hazardous Drugs *on page 2455*

Brand Names: US Fludara

Brand Names: Canada Fludara; Fludarabine Phosphate for Injection; Fludarabine Phosphate for Injection, USP; Fludarabine Phosphate Injection, PPC STD.

Therapeutic Category Antineoplastic Agent, Antimetabolite; Antineoplastic Agent, Antimetabolite (Purine Analog); Antineoplastic Agent, Antimetabolite (Purine Antagonist)

Generic Availability (US) Yes

Use Treatment of B-cell chronic lymphocytic leukemia (CLL) unresponsive to previous therapy with an alkylating agent-containing regimen (FDA approved in ages ≥18 years); has also been used in the treatment of relapsed acute lymphocytic leukemia (ALL) or acute myeloid leukemia (AML), reduced-intensity conditioning regimens prior to allogeneic hematopoietic stem cell transplantation, non-Hodgkin's lymphomas (NHL), and AML in either refractory or in poor risk patients

Pregnancy Risk Factor D

Pregnancy Considerations Adverse events were observed in animal reproduction studies. Based on the mechanism of action, fludarabine may cause fetal harm if administered during pregnancy. Effective contraception is recommended during and for 6 months after treatment for women and men with female partners of reproductive potential.

Breast-Feeding Considerations It is not known if fludarabine is excreted in breast milk. Due to the potential for serious adverse reactions in the nursing infant, a decision should be made to discontinue breast-feeding or to discontinue fludarabine, taking into account the importance of treatment to the mother.

Contraindications Hypersensitivity of fludarabine or any component of the formulation

Canadian labeling: Additional contraindications (not in U.S. labeling): Severe renal impairment (CrCl <30 mL/minute); decompensated hemolytic anemia; concurrent use with pentostatin

Warnings/Precautions Hazardous agent - use appropriate precautions for handling and disposal (NIOSH 2014 [group 1]). Use with caution in patients with renal insufficiency (clearance of the primary metabolite 2-fluoro-ara-A is reduced); dosage reductions are recommended (monitor closely for excessive toxicity); use of the IV formulation is not recommended if CrCl <30 mL/minute. Canadian labeling contraindicates use of oral and IV formulations if CrCl <30 mL/minute. Use with caution in patients with preexisting hematological disorders (particularly granulocytopenia) or preexisting central nervous system disorder (epilepsy), spasticity, or peripheral neuropathy. **[U.S. Boxed Warning]: Higher than recommended doses are associated with severe neurologic toxicity (delayed blindness, coma, death); similar neurotoxicity (agitation, coma, confusion and seizure) has been reported with standard CLL doses.** Neurotoxicity symptoms due to high doses appear from 21 to 60 days following the last fludarabine dose, although neurotoxicity has been reported as early as 7 days and up to 225 days. Possible neurotoxic effects of chronic administration are unknown. Caution patients about performing tasks which require mental alertness (eg, operating machinery or driving).

[U.S. Boxed Warning]: Life-threatening (and sometimes fatal) autoimmune effects, including hemolytic anemia, autoimmune thrombocytopenia/thrombocytopenic purpura (ITP), Evans syndrome, and acquired hemophilia have occurred; monitor closely for hemolysis; discontinue fludarabine if hemolysis occurs; the hemolytic effects usually recur with fludarabine rechallenge. **[U.S. Boxed Warning]: Severe bone marrow suppression (anemia, thrombocytopenia, and neutropenia) may occur;** may be cumulative. Severe myelosuppression (trilineage bone marrow hypoplasia/aplasia) has been reported (rare) with a duration of significant cytopenias ranging from 2 months to 1 year. First-line combination therapy is associated with prolonged cytopenias, with anemia lasting up to 7 months, neutropenia up to 9 months, and thrombocytopenia up to 10 months; increased age is predictive for prolonged cytopenias (Gill, 2010).

Use with caution in patients with documented infection, fever, immunodeficiency, or with a history of opportunistic infection; prophylactic anti-infectives should be considered for patients with an increased risk for developing opportunistic infections. Progressive multifocal leukoencephalopathy (PML) due to JC virus (usually fatal) has been reported with use; usually in patients who had received prior and/or other concurrent chemotherapy; onset ranges from a few weeks to 1 year; evaluate any neurological change promptly. Avoid vaccination with live vaccines during and after fludarabine treatment. May cause tumor lysis syndrome; risk is increased in patients with large tumor burden prior to treatment. Patients receiving blood products should only receive irradiated blood products due to the potential for transfusion related GVHD. Potentially significant drug-drug interactions may exist, requiring dose or frequency adjustment, additional monitoring, and/or selection of alternative therapy. **[U.S. Boxed Warnings]: Do not use in combination with pentostatin; may lead to severe, even fatal pulmonary toxicity. Should be administered under the supervision of an experienced cancer chemotherapy physician.**

Adverse Reactions

Cardiovascular: Aneurysm, angina, arrhythmia, cerebrovascular accident, CHF, deep vein thrombosis, edema, MI, phlebitis, supraventricular tachycardia, transient ischemic attack

Central nervous system: Cerebellar syndrome, chills, depression, fatigue, fever, headache, malaise, mentation impaired, pain, sleep disorder

Dermatologic: Alopecia, pruritus, rash, seborrhea

Endocrine & metabolic: Dehydration, hyperglycemia

Gastrointestinal: Anorexia, constipation, diarrhea, dysphagia, esophagitis, gastrointestinal bleeding, mucositis, nausea/vomiting, stomatitis

Genitourinary: Dysuria, hesitancy, urinary tract infection

Hematologic: Anemia, hemorrhage, myelosuppression (nadir: 10-14 days; recovery: 5-7 weeks; dose-limiting toxicity), neutropenia (nadir: ~13 days), thrombocytopenia (nadir: ~16 days)

Hepatic: Cholelithiasis, liver failure, liver function tests abnormal

Neuromuscular & skeletal: Arthralgia, myalgia, osteoporosis, paresthesia, weakness

Ocular: Visual disturbance

Otic: Hearing loss

Renal: Hematuria, proteinuria, renal failure, renal function test abnormal

Respiratory: Allergic pneumonitis, bronchitis, cough, dyspnea, epistaxis, hemoptysis, hypoxia, pharyngitis, pneumonia, sinusitis, upper respiratory infection

Miscellaneous: Anaphylaxis, diaphoresis, infection, tumor lysis syndrome

Rare but important or life-threatening: Acute respiratory distress syndrome, blindness, bone marrow fibrosis, cerebral hemorrhage, coma, Epstein-Barr virus (EBV) associated lymphoproliferation, EBV reactivation, erythema multiforme, Evans syndrome, hemolytic anemia (autoimmune), hemophilia (acquired), hemorrhagic cystitis, herpes zoster reactivation, hyperkalemia, hyperphosphatemia, hyperuricemia, hypocalcemia, interstitial pulmonary infiltrate, metabolic acidosis, myelodysplastic syndrome/acute myeloid leukemia (usually associated with prior or concurrent treatment with other anticancer agents), opportunistic infection, optic neuritis, optic neuropathy, pancytopenia, pemphigus, pericardial effusion, peripheral neuropathy, pneumonitis, progressive multifocal leukoencephalopathy (PML), pulmonary fibrosis, pulmonary hemorrhage, respiratory distress, respiratory failure, Richter's syndrome, seizure, skin cancer (new onset or exacerbation), Stevens-Johnson syndrome, thrombocytopenia (autoimmune), thrombocytopenic purpura (autoimmune), toxic epidermal necrolysis, trilineage bone marrow aplasia, trilineage bone marrow hypoplasia, urate crystalluria, wrist drop

Also observed: Neurologic syndrome characterized by cortical blindness, coma, and paralysis (onset of neurologic symptoms may be delayed for 3-4 weeks)

Drug Interactions

Metabolism/Transport Effects None known.

Avoid Concomitant Use

Avoid concomitant use of Fludarabine with any of the following: BCG; BCG (Intravesical); CloZAPine; Dipyrone; Natalizumab; Pentostatin; Pimecrolimus; Tacrolimus (Topical); Tofacitinib; Vaccines (Live)

Increased Effect/Toxicity

Fludarabine may increase the levels/effects of: CloZAPine; Leflunomide; Natalizumab; Pentostatin; Tofacitinib; Vaccines (Live)

The levels/effects of Fludarabine may be increased by: Denosumab; Dipyrone; Pentostatin; Pimecrolimus; Roflumilast; Tacrolimus (Topical); Trastuzumab

Decreased Effect

Fludarabine may decrease the levels/effects of: BCG; BCG (Intravesical); Coccidioides immitis Skin Test; Sipuleucel-T; Vaccines (Inactivated); Vaccines (Live)

The levels/effects of Fludarabine may be decreased by: Echinacea; Imatinib

Storage/Stability

IV: Store intact vials under refrigeration or at room temperature, as specified according to each manufacturer's labeling. Reconstituted solution or vials of the solution for injection that have been punctured (in use) should be used within 8 hours.

Tablet [Canadian product]: Store at 15°C to 30°C (59°F to 86°F); should be kept within packaging until use.

Mechanism of Action Fludarabine inhibits DNA synthesis by inhibition of DNA polymerase and ribonucleotide reductase; also inhibits DNA primase and DNA ligase I

Pharmacokinetics (Adult data unless noted)

Distribution: V_d: 38-96 L/m^2; widely distributed with extensive tissue binding

Protein binding: 2-fluoro-ara-A: 19% to 29%

Metabolism: IV: Fludarabine phosphate is rapidly dephosphorylated in the plasma to 2-fluoro-ara-A (active metabolite), which subsequently enters tumor cells and is phosphorylated by deoxycytidine kinase to the active triphosphate derivative (2-fluoro-ara-ATP)

Half-life: Terminal (2-fluoro-ara-A):
- Children: 12.4-19 hours
- Adults: ~20 hours

Time to peak serum concentration: Oral: 1-2 hours

Elimination: Urine (60%, 23% as 2-fluoro-ara-A) within 24 hours; clearance appears to be inversely correlated with serum creatinine

Dosing: Usual

Infants, Children, and Adolescents: Refer to individual protocols; details concerning dosing in combination regimens should also be consulted.

AML: Infants, Children, and Adolescents: Limited data available: Continuous IV infusion: 10.5 mg/m^2 bolus followed by 30.5 mg/m^2/**day** for 48 hours in combination with cytarabine and idarubicin (Lange, 2008)

ALL or AML, relapsed: Children and Adolescents: Limited data available: IV:
- Continuous IV infusion:10.5 mg/m^2 bolus followed by 30.5 mg/m^2/**day** for 48 hours in combination with cytarabine (Avramis,1998)
- Intermittent IV dosing: 25 mg/m^2/dose once daily for 5 days in combination with cytarabine and daunorubicin was used for ALL (Parker, 2010)

Stem cell transplant (allogeneic) conditioning regimen, reduced-intensity (hematologic malignancy): Children and Adolescents: Limited data available: IV: 30 mg/m^2/dose once daily for 6 doses beginning 7-10 days prior to transplant (in combination with busulfan and thymoglobulin (Pulsipher, 2009)

Adults: Refer to individual protocols; details concerning dosing in combination regimens should also be consulted.

Chronic lymphocytic leukemia (CLL): IV: 25 mg/m^2/**day** for 5 days every 28 days

Dosing adjustment in renal impairment:

Infants, Children, and Adolescents: The following guidelines have been used by some clinicians (Aronoff, 2007): IV:
- GFR >50 mL/minute/1.73 m^2: No adjustment required
- GFR 30-50 mL/minute/1.73 m^2: Administer 80% of dose.
- GFR <30 mL/minute/1.73 m^2: Not recommended.
- Hemodialysis: Administer 25% of dose
- Continuous ambulatory peritoneal dialysis (CAPD): Not recommended.
- Continuous renal replacement therapy (CRRT): Administer 80% of dose.

Adults:
- Manufacturer labeling: CLL: IV:
  - CrCl 50-79 mL/minute: Decrease dose to 20 mg/m^2
  - CrCl 30-49 mL/minute: Decrease dose to 15 mg/m^2
  - CrCl <30 mL/minute: Avoid use.
- The following guidelines have been used by some clinicians (Aronoff, 2007): IV:
  - CrCl10-50 mL/minute: Administer 75% of dose.
  - CrCl <10 mL/minute: Administer 50% of dose.
  - Hemodialysis: Administer after dialysis
  - Continuous ambulatory peritoneal dialysis (CAPD): Administer 50% of dose.
  - Continuous renal replacement therapy (CRRT): Administer 75% of dose.

Dosing adjustment for toxicity:
- Hematologic or nonhematologic toxicity (other than neurotoxicity): Consider treatment delay or dosage reduction.
- Hemolysis: Discontinue treatment.
- Neurotoxicity: Consider treatment delay or discontinuation.

Preparation for Administration Hazardous agent; use appropriate precautions for handling and disposal (NIOSH 2014 [group 1]).

Parenteral: Consult specific protocols. Reconstitute lyophilized powder with 2 mL SWFI resulting in a fludarabine phosphate concentration of 25 mg/mL; further dilute reconstituted solution or solution for injection in 100 to 125 mL D_5W or NS for intermittent infusion per the manufacturer; concentrations of 0.25 to 1 mg/mL have been used in clinical trials. For continuous IV infusion regimens, loading doses diluted in 20 mL D_5W and continuous infusions diluted in 240 mL D_5W have been used in clinical trials.

Administration Hazardous agent; use appropriate precautions for handling and disposal (NIOSH 2014 [group 1]).

Parenteral: Consult specific protocols.
- Intermittent IV infusion: Infuse over 30 minutes; a shorter infusion has been used in some protocols (Avramis 1998)
- Continuous IV infusion with loading dose (bolus):
  - Loading dose: Administer over 15 minutes (Avramis 1998)
  - Continuous IV infusion: Administer at a constant rate of 10 mL/hour

Monitoring Parameters CBC with differential, platelet count, hemoglobin, AST, ALT, creatinine, serum electrolytes, albumin, uric acid, and examination for visual changes; monitor for signs of infection and neurotoxicity

Dosage Forms Excipient information presented when available (limited, particularly for generics); consult specific product labeling.

Solution, Intravenous, as phosphate:
 Generic: 50 mg/2 mL (2 mL)

Solution Reconstituted, Intravenous, as phosphate:
 Fludara: 50 mg (1 ea)
 Generic: 50 mg (1 ea)

Solution Reconstituted, Intravenous, as phosphate [preservative free]:
 Generic: 50 mg (1 ea)

- **Fludarabine Phosphate** *see* Fludarabine *on page 888*
- **Fludarabine Phosphate for Injection (Can)** *see* Fludarabine *on page 888*
- **Fludarabine Phosphate for Injection, USP (Can)** *see* Fludarabine *on page 888*
- **Fludarabine Phosphate Injection, PPC STD. (Can)** *see* Fludarabine *on page 888*

Fludrocortisone (floo droe KOR ti sone)

Medication Safety Issues

Sound-alike/look-alike issues:

Florinef may be confused with Fioricet, Fiorinal, Floranex, Florastor

Related Information

Corticosteroids Systemic Equivalencies *on page 2260*

Brand Names: Canada Florinef®

Therapeutic Category Adrenal Corticosteroid; Corticosteroid, Systemic; Glucocorticoid; Mineralocorticoid

Generic Availability (US) Yes

Use Partial replacement therapy for primary and secondary adrenocortical insufficiency in Addison's disease; treatment of salt-losing adrenogenital syndrome (or congenital adrenal hyperplasia) (All indications: FDA approved in adults)

Pregnancy Risk Factor C

Pregnancy Considerations Animal reproduction studies have not been conducted with fludrocortisone; adverse events have been observed with corticosteroids in animal reproduction studies. Some studies have shown an association between first trimester systemic corticosteroid use and oral clefts (Park-Wyllie, 2000; Pradat, 2003). Systemic corticosteroids may also influence fetal growth (decreased birth weight); however, information is conflicting (Lunghi, 2010). Hypoadrenalism may occur in newborns following maternal use of corticosteroids in pregnancy; monitor.

When systemic corticosteroids are needed in pregnancy, it is generally recommended to use the lowest effective dose for the shortest duration of time, avoiding high doses during the first trimester (Leachman, 2006; Lunghi, 2010). Fludrocortisone may be used to treat women during pregnancy who require therapy for congenital adrenal hyperplasia (Speiser, 2010).

Breast-Feeding Considerations Corticosteroids are excreted in human milk; information specific to fludrocortisone has not been located. The manufacturer recommends that caution be exercised when administering fludrocortisone to nursing women.

Contraindications Hypersensitivity to fludrocortisone, hypersensitivity to other corticosteroids, or any component of the formulation; systemic fungal infections

Warnings/Precautions May cause hypercorticism or suppression of hypothalamic-pituitary-adrenal (HPA) axis, particularly in younger children or in patients receiving high doses for prolonged periods. HPA axis suppression may lead to adrenal crisis. Withdrawal and discontinuation of a corticosteroid should be done slowly and carefully. Fludrocortisone is primarily a mineralocorticoid agonist, but may also inhibit the HPA axis. Prolonged use may increase risk of infection, mask acute infection, prolong or exacerbate viral infections, or limit response to vaccinations. Exposure to chickenpox should be avoided. Corticosteroids should not be used to treat ocular herpes simplex, cerebral malaria, or viral hepatitis. Close observation is required in patients with latent tuberculosis (TB) and/or TB reactivity. Restrict use in active TB (only in conjunction with antituberculosis treatment). Prolonged treatment with corticosteroids has been associated with the development of Kaposi's sarcoma (case reports); if noted, discontinuation of therapy should be considered. Acute myopathy has been reported with high-dose corticosteroids, usually in patients with neuromuscular transmission disorders; may involve ocular and/or respiratory muscles; monitor creatine kinase; recovery may be delayed.

Corticosteroid use may cause psychiatric disturbances, including depression, euphoria, insomnia, mood swings, and personality changes. Preexisting psychiatric conditions may be exacerbated by corticosteroid use. Use with caution in patients with HF; use may be associated with fluid retention, edema, weight gain and hypertension. Use with caution in patients with sodium retention and potassium loss, diabetes mellitus, GI diseases (diverticulitis, peptic ulcer, ulcerative colitis), hepatic impairment, myasthenia gravis, post- myocardial infarction, osteoporosis, and/or renal impairment. Use with caution in patients with cataracts and/or glaucoma; increased intraocular pressure, open-angle glaucoma, and cataracts have occurred with prolonged use. Consider routine eye exams in chronic users. Use with caution in patients with a history of seizure disorder; seizures have been reported with adrenal crisis. Changes in thyroid status may necessitate dosage adjustments; metabolic clearance of corticosteroids increases in hyperthyroid patients and decreases in hypothyroid ones. Use with caution in the elderly. May affect growth velocity in pediatric patients. Withdraw therapy with gradual tapering of dose.

Warnings: Additional Pediatric Considerations May cause osteoporosis (at any age) or inhibition of bone growth in pediatric patients. Use with caution in patients with osteoporosis. In a population-based study of children, risk of fracture was shown to be increased with >4 courses of corticosteroids; underlying clinical condition may also impact bone health and osteoporotic effect of corticosteroids (Leonard, 2007). Hypertrophic cardiomyopathy has been reported in premature neonates.

Adverse Reactions

Cardiovascular: Cardiac enlargement, CHF, edema, hypertension

Central nervous system: Delirium, depression, emotional instability, euphoria, hallucinations, headache, insomnia, intracranial pressure increased, malaise, mood swings, nervousness, personality changes, pseudotumor cerebri, psychiatric disorders, psychoses, seizure, vertigo

Dermatologic: Acne, bruising, erythema, hirsutism, hives, hyperpigmentation, maculopapular rash, petechiae, purpura, rash, skin test reaction impaired, striae, subcutaneous fat atrophy, thin fragile skin, urticaria, wound healing (impaired)

Endocrine & metabolic: Cushing's syndrome, diabetes mellitus, glucose intolerance, growth suppression, hyperglycemia, hypokalemia, hypokalemic alkalosis, menstrual irregularities, negative nitrogen balance, pituitary-adrenal axis suppression

Gastrointestinal: Abdominal distention, esophagitis ulceration, pancreatitis, peptic ulcer

Neuromuscular & skeletal: Fractures, necrosis (femoral and humeral heads), muscle mass loss, muscle weakness, myopathy, osteoporosis, vertebral compression fractures

Ocular: Cataracts, exophthalmos, glaucoma, increased intraocular pressure

Renal: Glycosuria
Miscellaneous: Anaphylaxis (generalized), diaphoresis

Drug Interactions

Metabolism/Transport Effects None known.

Avoid Concomitant Use

Avoid concomitant use of Fludrocortisone with any of the following: Aldesleukin; BCG; BCG (Intravesical); Indium 111 Capromab Pendetide; Mifepristone; Natalizumab; Pimecrolimus; Tacrolimus (Topical); Tofacitinib

Increased Effect/Toxicity

Fludrocortisone may increase the levels/effects of: Acetylcholinesterase Inhibitors; Amphotericin B; Androgens; Ceritinib; Deferasirox; Leflunomide; Loop Diuretics; Natalizumab; Nicorandil; NSAID (COX-2 Inhibitor); NSAID (Nonselective); Quinolone Antibiotics; Thiazide Diuretics; Tofacitinib; Vaccines (Live); Warfarin

The levels/effects of Fludrocortisone may be increased by: Aprepitant; CYP3A4 Inhibitors (Strong); Denosumab; Estrogen Derivatives; Fosaprepitant; Indacaterol; Mifepristone; Neuromuscular-Blocking Agents (Nondepolarizing); Pimecrolimus; Roflumilast; Salicylates; Tacrolimus (Topical); Telaprevir; Trastuzumab

Decreased Effect

Fludrocortisone may decrease the levels/effects of: Aldesleukin; Antidiabetic Agents; BCG; BCG (Intravesical); Calcitriol (Systemic); Coccidioides immitis Skin Test; Corticorelin; Hyaluronidase; Indium 111 Capromab Pendetide; Isoniazid; Salicylates; Sipuleucel-T; Telaprevir; Urea Cycle Disorder Agents; Vaccines (Inactivated); Vaccines (Live)

The levels/effects of Fludrocortisone may be decreased by: Antacids; Bile Acid Sequestrants; CYP3A4 Inducers (Strong); Echinacea; Mifepristone; Mitotane

Storage/Stability Store at 20°C to 25°C (68°F 77°F); avoid excessive heat. The Canadian labeling recommends to store at 2°C to 8°C (36°F to 46°F).

Mechanism of Action Very potent mineralocorticoid with high glucocorticoid activity; used primarily for its mineralocorticoid effects. Promotes increased reabsorption of sodium and loss of potassium from renal distal tubules.

Pharmacodynamics Duration: 12 to 36 hours

Pharmacokinetics (Adult data unless noted)

Absorption: Rapid and complete from GI tract
Protein binding: 42%
Metabolism: Hepatic
Half-life:
Plasma: ~3.5 hours
Biological: 18-36 hours

Dosing: Neonatal Congenital adrenal hyperplasia (salt losers): Limited data available: Oral: Maintenance therapy: 0.05 to 0.2 mg daily in 1 or 2 divided doses in combination with sodium replacement therapy (AAP, 2010; Speiser, 2010)

Dosing: Usual Note: Dosing should be individualized to lowest effective dose.

Pediatric:

Adrenal insufficiency, autoimmune (aldosterone deficiency component Addison's disease); replacement therapy: Limited data available: Oral: 0.05 to 0.2 mg daily (Betterle, 2002; Kliegman, 2011)

Congenital adrenal hyperplasia (salt losers) (eg, 21-hydroxylase deficiency): Limited data available: **Note:** Use in combination with glucocorticoid therapy (eg, hydrocortisone); concurrent sodium replacement therapy may be required, particularly in young infants. Oral: Maintenance therapy:

Infants, Children, and Adolescents (actively growing): Usual range: 0.05 to 0.2 mg daily in 1 or 2 divided doses; doses as high as 0.3 mg/day may be necessary (AAP, 2000; AAP, 2010; Speiser, 2010)

Adolescents (fully grown): 0.05 to 0.2 mg once daily (AAP, 2010; Speiser, 2010)

Adult:

Addison's disease: Oral: Initial: 0.1 mg daily; if transient hypertension develops, reduce dose to 0.05 mg daily; maintenance dosage range: 0.1 mg 3 times weekly to 0.2 mg daily

Salt-losing adrenogenital syndrome (or congenital adrenal hyperplasia): Oral: 0.1 to 0.2 mg daily. The Endocrine Society recommends a maintenance dose range of 0.05 to 0.2 mg once daily (in combination with hydrocortisone) for patients with congenital adrenal hyperplasia due to 21-hydroxylase deficiency (Speiser, 2010).

Dosing adjustment in renal impairment: There are no dosage adjustments provided in the manufacturer's labeling; use with caution.

Dosing adjustment in hepatic impairment: There are no dosage adjustments provided in the manufacturer's labeling.

Administration Oral: May administer without regard to food; if GI upset, may take with food

Monitoring Parameters Monitor blood pressure and signs of edema when patient is on chronic therapy; monitor serum electrolytes (eg, potassium, sodium, calcium), glucose, plasma renin activity. Monitor intraocular pressure (if therapy >6 weeks), linear growth of pediatric patients (with chronic use), assess HPA suppression; monitor for evidence of infection

Additional Information In patients with salt-losing forms of congenital adrenogenital syndrome, use along with cortisone or hydrocortisone; fludrocortisone 0.1 mg has sodium retention activity equal to DOCA 1 mg

Dosage Forms Excipient information presented when available (limited, particularly for generics); consult specific product labeling.

Tablet, Oral, as acetate:
Generic: 0.1 mg

◆ **Fludrocortisone Acetate** *see* Fludrocortisone *on page 891*

◆ **Flulaval** *see* Influenza Virus Vaccine (Inactivated) *on page 1108*

◆ **Flulaval Quadrivalent** *see* Influenza Virus Vaccine (Inactivated) *on page 1108*

◆ **Flumadine** *see* Rimantadine *on page 1864*

◆ **Flumadine® (Can)** *see* Rimantadine *on page 1864*

Flumazenil (FLOO may ze nil)

Medication Safety Issues

Sound-alike/look-alike issues:

Flumazenil may be confused with influenza virus vaccine

Brand Names: Canada Anexate; Flumazenil Injection; Flumazenil Injection, USP; Romazicon

Therapeutic Category Antidote, Benzodiazepine

Generic Availability (US) Yes

Use Benzodiazepine antagonist; reverses sedative effects of benzodiazepines used in general anesthesia or conscious sedation; management of benzodiazepine overdose; **not indicated** for ethanol, barbiturate, general anesthetic or opioid overdose

Pregnancy Risk Factor C

Pregnancy Considerations Teratogenic effects were not seen in animal reproduction studies. Embryocidal effects were seen at large doses. Use during labor and delivery is not recommended.In general, medications used as antidotes should take into consideration the health and prognosis of the mother; antidotes should be administered to pregnant women if there is a clear indication for use and should not be withheld because of fears of teratogenicity (Bailey, 2003).

Breast-Feeding Considerations It is not known if flumazenil is excreted in breast milk. The manufacturer recommends that caution be used if administering to breast-feeding women.

Contraindications Hypersensitivity to flumazenil, benzodiazepines, or any component of the formulation; patients given benzodiazepines for control of potentially life-threatening conditions (eg, control of intracranial pressure or status epilepticus); patients who are showing signs of serious cyclic-antidepressant overdosage

Warnings/Precautions [U.S. Boxed Warning]: Benzodiazepine reversal may result in seizures; seizures may occur more frequently in patients on benzodiazepines for long-term sedation or following tricyclic antidepressant overdose. Dose should be individualized and practitioners should be prepared to manage seizures. Seizures may also develop in patients with concurrent major sedative-hypnotic drug withdrawal, recent therapy with repeated doses of parenteral benzodiazepines, myoclonic jerking or seizure activity prior to flumazenil administration. Use with caution in patients relying on a benzodiazepine for seizure control. May cause CNS depression, which may impair physical or mental abilities; patients must be cautioned about performing tasks which require mental alertness (eg, operating machinery or driving) for 24 hours after discharge.

Flumazenil may not reliably reverse respiratory depression/hypoventilation. Flumazenil is not a substitute for evaluation of oxygenation; establishing an airway and assisting ventilation, as necessary, is always the initial step in overdose management. Resedation occurs more frequently in patients where a large single dose or cumulative dose of a benzodiazepine is administered along with a neuromuscular-blocking agent and multiple anesthetic agents. Flumazenil should be used with caution in the intensive care unit because of increased risk of unrecognized benzodiazepine dependence in such settings. Should not be used to diagnose benzodiazepine-induced sedation. Reverse neuromuscular blockade before considering use. Flumazenil does not antagonize the CNS effects of other GABA agonists (such as ethanol, barbiturates, or general anesthetics); nor does it reverse opioids. Flumazenil does not consistently reverse amnesia; patient may not recall verbal instructions after procedure.

Use with caution in patients with a history of panic disorder; may provoke panic attacks. Use caution in drug and ethanol-dependent patients; these patients may also be dependent on benzodiazepines. Not recommended for treatment of benzodiazepine dependence. Use with caution in patients with a head injury; may alter cerebral blood flow or precipitate convulsions in patients receiving benzodiazepines. Use caution in patients with mixed drug overdoses; toxic effects of other drugs taken may emerge once benzodiazepine effects are reversed. Use caution in hepatic dysfunction; repeated doses of the drug should be reduced in frequency or amount.

Warnings: Additional Pediatric Considerations Pediatric patients (especially 1 to 5 years of age) may experience resedation; these patients may require repeat bolus doses or continuous infusion.

Adverse Reactions

Cardiovascular: Flushing, palpitation, vasodilation

Central nervous system: Abnormal crying, agitation, anxiety, ataxia, depersonalization, depression, dizziness, dysphoria, emotional lability, euphoria, fatigue, headache, insomnia, malaise, nervousness, paranoia, vertigo

Endocrine & metabolic: Hot flashes

Gastrointestinal: Nausea, vomiting, xerostomia

Local: Injection site reaction, pain at injection site, rash, skin abnormality, thrombophlebitis

Neuromuscular & skeletal: Hypoesthesia, paresthesia, weakness, tremor

Ocular: Abnormal vision, blurred vision, lacrimation

Respiratory: Dyspnea, hyperventilation

Miscellaneous: Diaphoresis

Rare but important or life-threatening: Abnormal hearing, altered blood pressure increased/decreased, arrhythmia, bradycardia, chest pain, confusion, coldness sensation, delirium, difficulty concentrating, dysphonia, fear, generalized seizure, hiccups, hyperacusis, hypertension, junctional tachycardia, panic attacks, rigors, seizure, shivering, somnolence, stupor, tachycardia, thick tongue, tinnitus, transient hearing impairment, ventricular tachycardia, withdrawal syndrome

Drug Interactions

Metabolism/Transport Effects None known.

Avoid Concomitant Use There are no known interactions where it is recommended to avoid concomitant use.

Increased Effect/Toxicity There are no known significant interactions involving an increase in effect.

Decreased Effect

Flumazenil may decrease the levels/effects of: Hypnotics (Nonbenzodiazepine)

Storage/Stability Store at 20°C to 25°C (68°F to 77°F). For IV use only. Once drawn up in the syringe or mixed with solution use within 24 hours. Discard any unused solution after 24 hours.

Mechanism of Action Competitively inhibits the activity at the benzodiazepine receptor site on the GABA/benzodiazepine receptor complex. Flumazenil does not antagonize the CNS effect of drugs affecting GABA-ergic neurons by means other than the benzodiazepine receptor (ethanol, barbiturates, general anesthetics) and does not reverse the effects of opioids

Pharmacodynamics

Onset of action: Benzodiazepine reversal: Within 1-3 minutes

Maximum effect: 6-10 minutes

Duration: Usually <1 hour; duration is related to dose given and benzodiazepine plasma concentrations; reversal effects of flumazenil may wear off before effects of benzodiazepine and resedation may occur

Pharmacokinetics (Adult data unless noted) Follows a two compartment open model; **Note:** Clearance and V_d per kg are similar for children and adults, but children display more variability

Distribution: Distributes extensively in the extravascular space; Adults:

Initial V_d: 0.5 L/kg

V_{dss}: 0.9-1.1 L/kg

Protein binding: ~50%; primarily to albumin

Metabolism: In the liver to the de-ethylated free acid and its glucuronide conjugate

Half-life:

Children: Terminal: 20-75 minutes (mean: 40 minutes)

Adults:

Alpha: 4-11 minutes

Terminal: 40-80 minutes

Elimination: 99% hepatically eliminated; <1% excreted unchanged in urine

Clearance: Dependent upon hepatic blood flow; Adults: 0.8-1 L/hour/kg

Dosing: Neonatal

Benzodiazepine reversal:

IV: **Note:** Minimal information available; dosing is extrapolated from experiences in pediatric patients 1-17 years; Initial dose: 0.01 mg/kg given over 15 seconds; may repeat 0.01 mg/kg after 45 seconds, and then every minute to a maximum total cumulative dose of 0.05 mg/kg

Continuous IV infusion (as an alternative to repeat bolus doses): 0.005-0.01 mg/kg/**hour**; dose based on a case report of premature neonate (GA: 32 weeks) exposed to high doses of diazepam intrapartum (Dixon, 1998)

Myoclonus, benzodiazepine-induced: IV: 0.0078 mg/kg as a single dose was effective in one full-term neonate who was receiving continuous infusion midazolam (Zaw, 2001)

Dosing: Usual

Pediatric:

Benzodiazepine reversal when used in conscious sedation or general anesthesia: Infants, Children, and Adolescents: IV: Initial dose: 0.01 mg/kg (maximum dose: 0.2 mg) given over 15 seconds; may repeat 0.01 mg/kg (maximum dose: 0.2 mg) after 45 seconds, and then every minute to a maximum total cumulative dose of 0.05 mg/kg or 1 mg, whichever is lower; usual total dose: 0.08 to 1 mg (mean: 0.65 mg)

Suspected benzodiazepine overdose: Limited data available: Infants, Children, and Adolescents: Initial dose: 0.01 mg/kg (maximum dose: 0.2 mg) with repeat doses of 0.01 mg/kg (maximum dose: 0.2 mg) given every minute to a maximum total cumulative dose of 1 mg; as an alternative to repeat bolus doses, follow up continuous infusions of 0.005-0.01 mg/kg/**hour** have been used (Clark 1995; Richard 1991; Roald 1989; Sugarman 1994)

Adult:

Benzodiazepine reversal when used in conscious sedation or general anesthesia: 0.2 mg given over 15 seconds; may repeat 0.2 mg after 45 seconds and then every 60 seconds up to a total of 1 mg, usual total dose: 0.6 to 1 mg. In event of resedation, may repeat doses at 20-minute intervals with maximum of 1 mg/dose (given at 0.2 mg/minute); maximum dose: 3 mg in 1 hour.

Management of benzodiazepine overdose: 0.2 mg over 30 seconds; may give 0.3 mg dose after 30 seconds if desired level of consciousness is not obtained; additional doses of 0.5 mg can be given over 30 seconds at 1-minute intervals up to a cumulative dose of 3 mg; usual cumulative dose: 1 to 3 mg; rarely, patients with partial response at 3 mg may require additional titration up to total dose of 5 mg; if patient has not responded 5 minutes after cumulative dose of 5 mg, the major cause of sedation is not likely due to benzodiazepines. In the event of resedation, may repeat doses at 20-minute intervals with maximum of 1 mg/dose (given at 0.5 mg/minute); maximum dose: 3 mg in 1 hour.

Dosing adjustment in hepatic impairment: Initial dose: Use normal dose; repeat doses should be decreased in size or frequency

Administration Parenteral: For IV use only; administer by rapid IV injection over 15-30 seconds via a freely running IV infusion into larger vein (to decrease chance of pain, phlebitis). Children: Do not exceed 0.2 mg/minute. Adults: Repeat doses: Do not exceed 0.2 mg/minute for reversal of general anesthesia and do not exceed 0.5 mg/minute for reversal of benzodiazepine overdose.

Monitoring Parameters Level of consciousness and resedation, blood pressure, heart rate, respiratory rate, continuous pulse oximetry; monitor for resedation for 1-2 hours after reversal of sedation in patients who receive benzodiazepine sedation

Additional Information Flumazenil is a weak lipophilic base. In one study of conscious sedation reversal in 107 pediatric patients (1-17 years of age), resedation occurred between 19-50 minutes after the start of flumazenil. Flumazenil has been used to successfully treat paradoxical reactions in children associated with midazolam use (eg, agitation, restlessness, combativeness) (Massanari, 1997).

Dosage Forms Excipient information presented when available (limited, particularly for generics); consult specific product labeling.

Solution, Intravenous:

Generic: 0.5 mg/5 mL (5 mL); 1 mg/10 mL (10 mL)

◆ **Flumazenil Injection (Can)** *see* Flumazenil *on page 892*

◆ **Flumazenil Injection, USP (Can)** *see* Flumazenil *on page 892*

◆ **FluMist** *see* Influenza Virus Vaccine (Live/Attenuated) *on page 1113*

◆ **FluMist Quadrivalent** *see* Influenza Virus Vaccine (Live/Attenuated) *on page 1113*

Flunisolide (Nasal) (floo NISS oh lide)

Medication Safety Issues

Sound-alike/look-alike issues:

Flunisolide may be confused with Flumadine®, fluocinonide

Brand Names: Canada Apo-Flunisolide®; Nasalide®; Rhinalar®

Therapeutic Category Corticosteroid, Intranasal

Generic Availability (US) Yes

Use Management of nasal symptoms associated with seasonal or perennial rhinitis (FDA approved in ages ≥6 years and adults)

Intranasal corticosteroids have also been used as an adjunct to antibiotics in empiric treatment of acute bacterial rhinosinusitis primarily in patients with history of allergic rhinitis (Chow, 2012) and in pediatric patients with mild obstructive sleep apnea syndrome who cannot undergo adenotonsillectomy or who still have symptoms after surgery (Marcus, 2012).

Pregnancy Risk Factor C

Pregnancy Considerations Adverse effects were observed in some animal reproduction studies. Intranasal corticosteroids are recommended for the treatment of rhinitis during pregnancy; the lowest effective dose should be used (NAEPP, 2005; Wallace, 2008).

Breast-Feeding Considerations Other corticosteroids have been found in breast milk. It is not known if sufficient quantities of flunisolide are absorbed following inhalation to produce detectable amounts in breast milk. The use of inhaled corticosteroids is not considered a contraindication to breast-feeding (NAEPP, 2005). The manufacturer recommends caution be used if administered to a nursing woman.

Contraindications Hypersensitivity to flunisolide or any component of the formulation; infections of the nasal mucosa

Warnings/Precautions Avoid nasal corticosteroid use in patients with recent nasal septal ulcers, nasal surgery or nasal trauma until healing has occurred.

Avoid using higher than recommended dosages; suppression of linear growth (ie, reduction of growth velocity), reduced bone mineral density, or hypercorticism (Cushing's syndrome) may occur; titrate to lowest effective dose. Reduction in growth velocity may occur when corticosteroids are administered to pediatric patients, even at recommended doses via intranasal route (monitor growth). There have been reports of systemic corticosteroid withdrawal symptoms (eg, joint/muscle pain, lassitude, depression) when withdrawing oral inhalation therapy.

Adverse Reactions

Respiratory: Nasal burning/stinging, nasal congestion, nasal dryness, nasal irritation, rhinitis, sneezing

Miscellaneous: Loss of smell

Drug Interactions

Metabolism/Transport Effects Substrate of CYP3A4 (minor); **Note:** Assignment of Major/Minor substrate status based on clinically relevant drug interaction potential

Avoid Concomitant Use There are no known interactions where it is recommended to avoid concomitant use.

Increased Effect/Toxicity

Flunisolide (Nasal) may increase the levels/effects of: Ceritinib

Decreased Effect There are no known significant interactions involving a decrease in effect.

Storage/Stability Store at 15°C to 25°C (59°F to 77°F).

Mechanism of Action Decreases inflammation by suppression of migration of polymorphonuclear leukocytes and reversal of increased capillary permeability; does not depress hypothalamus

Pharmacodynamics Clinical effects are due to a direct local effect rather than systemic absorption

Onset of action: Within a few days

Maximum effect: 1-2 weeks

Pharmacokinetics (Adult data unless noted)

Absorption: Rapid

Bioavailability: Intranasal 50%, oral 20% (due to first-pass metabolism)

Half-life: 1-2 hours

Elimination: Urine (50%, 65% to 70% as metabolite) and feces (50%)

Dosing: Usual Note: Once symptoms are controlled, the dose should be reduced to the lowest effective amount.

Children and Adolescents: **Seasonal and perennial rhinitis:** Intranasal:

Children and Adolescents 6-14 years: Initial: 100 mcg twice daily delivered as 50 mcg (2 sprays) **per nostril** twice daily **or** 50 mcg 3 times daily delivered as 25 mcg (1 spray) **per nostril** 3 times daily; maximum daily dose: 200 mcg/**day** (4 sprays **per nostril/day**); some patients may have efficacy at a lower maintenance dose as low as 50 mcg once daily delivered as 25 mcg (1 spray) **per nostril** once daily

Adolescents ≥15 years: Initial: 100 mcg twice daily delivered as 50 mcg (2 sprays) **per nostril** twice daily; if needed, increase to 100 mcg 3 times daily delivered as 50 mcg (2 sprays) **per nostril** 3 times daily; maximum daily dose: 400 mcg/**day** (8 sprays **per nostril/day**); some patients may have efficacy at a lower maintenance dose as low as 50 mcg once daily delivered as 25 mcg (1 spray) **per nostril** once daily

Adults: **Seasonal and perennial rhinitis:** Intranasal: 100 mcg twice daily delivered as 50 mcg (2 sprays) **per nostril** twice daily; if needed, increase to 100 mcg 3 times daily delivered as 50 mcg (2 sprays) **per nostril** 3 times daily; maximum daily dose: 400 mcg/**day** (8 sprays **per nostril/day**)

Dosing adjustment in renal impairment: There are no dosage adjustments provided in the manufacturer's labeling.

Dosing adjustment in hepatic impairment: There are no dosage adjustments provided in the manufacturer's labeling.

Administration Shake well prior to each use. Before first use, prime by pressing pump 5-6 times or until a fine spray appears. Repeat priming if ≥5 days between use or if dissembled for cleaning. Administer at regular intervals. Blow nose to clear nostrils. Insert applicator into nostril, keeping bottle upright, and close off the other nostril. Breathe in through nose. While inhaling, press pump to release spray. Do not spray into eyes. Discard after labeled number of doses has been used, even if bottle is not completely empty.

Monitoring Parameters Mucous membranes for signs of fungal infection, growth (pediatric patients), signs/symptoms of HPA axis suppression/adrenal insufficiency; ocular changes

Additional Information When used short term as adjunctive therapy in acute bacterial rhinosinusitis (ABRS), intranasal steroids show modest symptomatic improvement and few adverse effects; improvement is primarily due to increased sinus drainage. Use should be considered optional in ABRS; however, intranasal corticosteroids should be routinely prescribed to ABRS patients who have a history of or concurrent allergic rhinitis (Chow, 2012).

Dosage Forms Excipient information presented when available (limited, particularly for generics); consult specific product labeling. [DSC] = Discontinued product

Solution, Nasal:

Generic: 25 mcg/actuation (0.025%) (25 mL); 29 mcg/actuation (0.025%) (25 mL [DSC])

Fluocinolone (Ophthalmic) (floo oh SIN oh lone)

Medication Safety Issues

Sound-alike/look-alike issues:

Fluocinolone may be confused with fluocinonide

Brand Names: US Iluvien; Retisert

Brand Names: Canada Retisert

Therapeutic Category Corticosteroid, Ophthalmic

Generic Availability (US) No

Use Treatment of chronic, noninfectious uveitis affecting the posterior segment of the eye (FDA approved in adults)

Pregnancy Risk Factor C

Pregnancy Considerations Animal studies have not been conducted with this product; however, adverse events have been observed with corticosteroids in animal reproduction studies.

Breast-Feeding Considerations Systemic corticosteroids are excreted in human milk. It is not known if sufficient quantities of fluocinolone are absorbed following ocular administration to produce detectable amounts in breast milk; however, systemic absorption is low. The manufacturer recommends that caution be used if administered to a nursing woman.

Contraindications

Hypersensitivity to fluocinolone, other corticosteroids, or any component of the formulation; active or suspected ocular or periocular infections including most viral diseases of the cornea and conjunctiva including epithelial herpes simplex keratitis (dendritic keratitis), vaccinia, and varicella; active bacterial, mycobacterial or fungal infections of the eye.

Iluvien only: Glaucoma (in patients who have cup to disc ratios of >0.8).

Warnings/Precautions Use of corticosteroids may result in posterior subcapsular cataract formation. Long-term use may cause increased intraocular pressure and glaucoma. Use with caution in patients with glaucoma. Monitor IOP in all patients; within 3 years postimplantation, most patients will require IOP-lowering medications and/or filtering procedures to control IOP. May enhance development of secondary bacterial, fungal, or viral infections. Not recommended in patients with a history of ocular herpes simplex (potential for reactivation). Use Retisert with caution in patients with a history of bacterial, mycobacterial, fungal, or viral infections or the cornea and conjunctiva including epithelial herpes simplex keratitis (dendritic keratitis), vaccinia and varicella. In acute purulent conditions, may mask infection. Fungal and viral infections are of particular concern. If corneal ulceration persists, consider fungal infection. Intravitreal injections have been associated with endophthalmitis, eye inflammation, increased intraocular pressure, and retinal detachment. Monitor carefully after intravitreal injection. Procedure may cause optic nerve injury. Visual defects in acuity and field of vision may occur (lasting 1 to 4 weeks postoperatively). Late-onset endophthalmitis has been observed, often associated with surgical-site integrity. Complications of Retisert may also include cataract formation, choroidal detachment, hypotony, vitreous hemorrhage, vitreous loss, and wound dehiscence. With Retisert use, perforation may occur with topical steroids in diseases which thin the cornea or sclera. Steroid use may delay healing after cataract surgery and increase bleb formation incidence.

Recommend unilateral implantation only to minimize risk of postoperative infections developing in both eyes. With Retisert, due to the potential for separation of the silicone cup reservoir from the suture tab, implant integrity should be monitored during eye exams. Assure tight closure of scleral wound and integrity of overlying conjunctiva at the wound site. With Iluvien, patients in whom the posterior capsule of the lens is absent or has a tear, implant may migrate into the anterior chamber.

Adverse Reactions

Central nervous system: Dizziness, headache

Dermatologic: Skin rash

Gastrointestinal: Nausea, vomiting

Hematologic & oncologic: Anemia

Infection: Influenza

Neuromuscular & skeletal: Arthralgia, back pain, limb pain

Ophthalmic: Abnormal sensation in eyes, anterior chamber eye hemorrhage, blepharitis, blepharoptosis, blurred vision, cataract, choroidal detachment, conjunctival hemorrhage, conjunctival hyperemia, conjunctivitis, corneal edema, decreased intraocular pressure (ocular hypotony), decreased visual acuity (immediate; duration 1 to 4 weeks), diplopia, dry eye syndrome, eye discharge, eye discomfort, eye irritation, eyelid edema, eye pain, eye pruritus, foreign body sensation of eye, glaucoma, hypopyon, increased intraocular pressure, lacrimation, macular edema, maculopathy, ocular hyperemia, optic atrophy, photophobia, photopsia, posterior capsule opacification, retinal detachment, retinal exudates, retinal hemorrhage, swelling of eye, synechiae of iris, visual disturbance, vitreous hemorrhage, vitreous opacity

Renal: Renal failure

Respiratory: Cough, nasopharyngitis, pneumonia, sinusitis, upper respiratory tract infection

Miscellaneous: Fever, procedural complications (eg, cataract fragments, implant migration, wound complications)

Rare but important or life-threatening: Endophthalmitis (late onset), ophthalmic inflammation (exacerbation), secondary infection (bacterial, viral, or fungal)

Drug Interactions

Metabolism/Transport Effects None known.

Avoid Concomitant Use There are no known interactions where it is recommended to avoid concomitant use.

Increased Effect/Toxicity

Fluocinolone (Ophthalmic) may increase the levels/effects of: Ceritinib

The levels/effects of Fluocinolone (Ophthalmic) may be increased by: NSAID (Ophthalmic)

Decreased Effect There are no known significant interactions involving a decrease in effect.

Storage/Stability Store at 15°C to 25°C (59°F to 77°F). Retisert: Protect from freezing.

Mechanism of Action Inhibit phospholipase A_2 via lipocortin induction Lipocortins may control biosynthesis of prostaglandins and leukotrienes by inhibiting arachidonic acid. Arachidonic acid is released by membrane phospholipids by phospholipase A_2.

Pharmacokinetics (Adult data unless noted)

Absorption: Systemic absorption is negligible

Duration: Releases fluocinolone acetonide at a rate of 0.6 mcg/day, decreasing over 30 days to a steady-state release rate of 0.3-0.4 mcg/day for 30 months

Distribution: Aqueous and vitreous humor

Dosing: Usual Chronic uveitis: One silicone-encased tablet (0.59 mg) surgically implanted into the posterior segment of the eye is designed to release 0.6 mcg/day, decreasing over 30 days to a steady-state release rate of 0.3-0.4 mcg/day for 30 months. Recurrence of uveitis denotes depletion of tablet, requiring reimplantation.

Administration Handle only by suture tab to avoid damaging the tablet integrity and adversely affecting release characteristics. Maintain strict adherence to aseptic handling of product; do not resterilize.

Dosage Forms Excipient information presented when available (limited, particularly for generics); consult specific product labeling.

Implant, Intraocular, as acetonide:

Iluvien: 0.19 mg (1 ea)

Retisert: 0.59 mg (1 ea)

Fluocinolone (Otic) (floo oh SIN oh lone)

Medication Safety Issues

Sound-alike/look-alike issues:

Fluocinolone may be confused with fluocinonide

Brand Names: US DermOtic

Therapeutic Category Adrenal Corticosteroid; Anti-inflammatory Agent

Generic Availability (US) Yes

Use Relief of chronic eczematous external otitis

Pregnancy Risk Factor C

Pregnancy Considerations Adverse events have been observed with corticosteroids in animal reproduction studies. In general, the use of topical corticosteroids during pregnancy is not considered to have significant risk; however, intrauterine growth retardation in the infant has been reported (rare). The use of large amounts or for prolonged periods of time should be avoided.

Breast-Feeding Considerations Systemic corticosteroids are excreted in human milk. It is not known if sufficient quantities of fluocinolone are absorbed following topical administration to produce detectable amounts in breast milk.

Contraindications Hypersensitivity to fluocinolone or any component of the formulation; **Note:** Contains peanut oil

Warnings/Precautions May cause hypercorticism or suppression of hypothalamic-pituitary-adrenal (HPA) axis, particularly in younger children or in patients receiving high doses for prolonged periods. HPA axis suppression may lead to adrenal crisis. Withdrawal and discontinuation of a corticosteroid should be done slowly and carefully. Particular care is required when patients are transferred from systemic corticosteroids to inhaled products due to possible adrenal insufficiency or withdrawal from steroids, including an increase in allergic symptoms. Adult patients receiving >20 mg per day of prednisone (or equivalent) may be most susceptible. Fatalities have occurred due to adrenal insufficiency in asthmatic patients during and after transfer from systemic corticosteroids to aerosol steroids; aerosol steroids do **not** provide the systemic steroid needed to treat patients having trauma, surgery, or infections. Steroids may mask infection; prolonged use may result in secondary infections due to immunosuppression. Adverse systemic effects may occur when used on large areas of the body, denuded areas, for prolonged periods of time, or with an occlusive dressing. Infants and children may be more susceptible to systemic toxicity from equivalent doses due to larger skin surface to body mass ratio. Allergic contact dermatitis can occur, it is usually diagnosed by failure to heal rather than clinical exacerbation.

DermOtic Oil contains peanut oil; use caution in peanut-sensitive individuals.

Adverse Reactions

Dermatologic: Acneiform eruptions, allergic contact dermatitis, burning, dryness, erythema, folliculitis, irritation, itching, hypopigmentation, keratosis pilaris, miliaria, skin atrophy, striae

Otic: Ear infection

Drug Interactions

Metabolism/Transport Effects None known.

Avoid Concomitant Use There are no known interactions where it is recommended to avoid concomitant use.

Increased Effect/Toxicity There are no known significant interactions involving an increase in effect.

Decreased Effect There are no known significant interactions involving a decrease in effect.

Storage/Stability Store a controlled room temperature of 20°C to 25°C (68°F to 77°F).

Mechanism of Action A synthetic fluorinated corticosteroid of low-to-moderate potency. The mechanism of action for all topical corticosteroids is not well defined, however, is believed to be a combination of anti-inflammatory, antipruritic, and vasoconstrictive properties.

Dosing: Usual Children ≥2 years and Adults: 5 drops into the affected ear twice daily for 1-2 weeks

Additional Information DermOtic® is made with 48% refined peanut oil, NF (peanut protein is below 0.5 ppm)

Dosage Forms Excipient information presented when available (limited, particularly for generics); consult specific product labeling.

Oil, Otic, as acetonide:

DermOtic: 0.01% (20 mL) [contains isopropyl alcohol, peanut oil]

Generic: 0.01% (20 mL)

Fluocinolone (Topical) (floo oh SIN oh lone)

Medication Safety Issues

Sound-alike/look-alike issues:

Capex may be confused with Kapidex [DSC]

Fluocinolone may be confused with fluocinonide

Related Information

Topical Corticosteroids *on page 2262*

Brand Names: US Capex; Derma-Smoothe/FS Body; Derma-Smoothe/FS Scalp; Fluocinolone Acetonide Body; Fluocinolone Acetonide Scalp; Synalar; Synalar (Cream); Synalar (Ointment); Synalar TS

Brand Names: Canada Capex®; Derma-Smoothe/FS®; Synalar®

Therapeutic Category Adrenal Corticosteroid; Anti-inflammatory Agent; Corticosteroid, Topical; Glucocorticoid

Generic Availability (US) May be product dependent

Use Relief of susceptible inflammatory dermatosis

Capex™ shampoo: Adults: Treatment of seborrheic dermatitis of the scalp

Derma-Smoothe/FS®: Children ≤2 years: Moderate to severe atopic dermatitis (for use ≤4 weeks); Adults: Atopic dermatitis or psoriasis of the scalp

Pregnancy Risk Factor C

Pregnancy Considerations Adverse events have been observed with corticosteroids in animal reproduction studies. In general, the use of topical corticosteroids during pregnancy is not considered to have significant risk; however, intrauterine growth retardation in the infant has been reported (rare). The use of large amounts or for prolonged periods of time should be avoided.

Breast-Feeding Considerations Systemic corticosteroids are excreted in human milk. It is not known if sufficient quantities of fluocinolone are absorbed following topical administration to produce detectable amounts in breast milk. Hypertension in the nursing infant has been reported following corticosteroid ointment applied to the nipples. Use with caution.

Contraindications Hypersensitivity to fluocinolone or any component of the formulation; TB of skin, herpes (including varicella)

Warnings/Precautions Adverse systemic effects may occur when used on large areas of the body, denuded areas, for prolonged periods of time, or with an occlusive dressing. Infants and children may be more susceptible to systemic toxicity from equivalent doses due to larger skin surface to body mass ratio. Infants and small children may be more susceptible to adrenal axis suppression from topical corticosteroid therapy. Allergic contact dermatitis can occur, it is usually diagnosed by failure to heal rather than clinical exacerbation.

Topical: Not for oral, ophthalmic, or intravaginal use; do not apply to the face, axillae, groin, or diaper area unless directed by hea lthcare provider. Derma-Smoothe/FS and contains peanut oil; use caution in peanut-sensitive individuals.

Warnings: Additional Pediatric Considerations Topical corticosteroids may be absorbed percutaneously. The extent of absorption is dependent on several factors, including epidermal integrity (intact vs abraded skin), formulation, age of the patient, prolonged duration of use, and the use of occlusive dressings. Percutaneous absorption of topical steroids is increased in neonates (especially preterm neonates), infants, and young children. Hypothalamic-pituitary-adrenal (HPA) suppression may occur, particularly in younger children or in patients receiving high doses for prolonged periods; acute adrenal insufficiency (adrenal crisis) may occur with abrupt withdrawal after long-term therapy or with stress. Infants and small children may be more susceptible to HPA axis suppression or other systemic toxicities due to larger skin surface area to body mass ratio; use with caution in pediatric patients.

Some dosage forms may contain propylene glycol; in neonates large amounts of propylene glycol delivered orally, intravenously (eg, >3,000 mg/day), or topically have been associated with potentially fatal toxicities which can include metabolic acidosis, seizures, renal failure, and CNS depression; toxicities have also been reported in children and adults including hyperosmolality, lactic acidosis, seizures, and respiratory depression; use caution (AAP, 1997; Shehab, 2009).

Adverse Reactions

Cardiovascular: Intracranial hypertension (rare)

Central nervous system: Telangiectasia

Dermatologic: Acneiform eruptions, allergic contact dermatitis, burning, dryness, folliculitis, irritation, itching, hypertrichosis, hypopigmentation, miliaria, perioral dermatitis, skin atrophy, striae

Endocrine & metabolic: Cushing's syndrome, HPA axis suppression

Otic: Ear infection

Miscellaneous: Herpes simplex, secondary infection

Drug Interactions

Metabolism/Transport Effects None known.

Avoid Concomitant Use

Avoid concomitant use of Fluocinolone (Topical) with any of the following: Aldesleukin

Increased Effect/Toxicity

Fluocinolone (Topical) may increase the levels/effects of: Ceritinib; Deferasirox

The levels/effects of Fluocinolone (Topical) may be increased by: Telaprevir

Decreased Effect

Fluocinolone (Topical) may decrease the levels/effects of: Aldesleukin; Corticorelin; Hyaluronidase; Telaprevir

Storage/Stability Topical: Store at controlled room temperature in tightly-closed container.

Capex®: Store at 15°C to 35°C (59°F to 86°F).

Mechanism of Action Topical corticosteroids have anti-inflammatory, antipruritic, and vasoconstrictive properties. May depress the formation, release, and activity of endogenous chemical mediators of inflammation (kinins, histamine, liposomal enzymes, prostaglandins) through the induction of phospholipase A_2 inhibitory proteins (lipocortins) and sequential inhibition of the release of arachidonic acid. Fluocinolone has low to intermediate range potency (dosage-form dependent).

Pharmacokinetics (Adult data unless noted)

Absorption: Dependent on strength of preparation, amount applied, nature of skin at application site, vehicle, and use of occlusive dressing; increased in areas of skin damage, inflammation, or occlusion

Distribution: Throughout local skin; absorbed drug is distributed rapidly into muscle, liver, skin, intestines, and kidneys

Metabolism: Primarily in skin; small amount absorbed into systemic circulation is primarily hepatic to inactive compounds

Excretion: Urine (primarily as glucuronide and sulfate, also as unconjugated products); feces (small amounts)

Dosing: Usual Children and Adults: Topical: Apply thin layer 2-4 times/day

Capex™ shampoo: Adults: Thoroughly wet hair and scalp; apply ≤1 ounce to scalp area; massage well; work into lather; allow to remain on scalp for 5 minutes; then rinse hair and scalp thoroughly; repeat daily until symptoms subside; **Note:** Once patient is symptom-free, once-weekly use usually keeps itching and flaking of dandruff from returning.

Derma-Smoothe/FS®:

Children ≥2 years: Atopic dermatitis: Apply in a thin layer to moistened skin of affected area twice daily for ≤4 weeks

Adults:

Atopic dermatitis: Apply a thin layer to affected area 3 times/day

Scalp psoriasis: Thoroughly wet or dampen hair and scalp; apply to scalp in a thin layer, massage well; cover scalp with shower cap (supplied); leave for a minimum of 4 hours or overnight, then wash hair and rinse thoroughly

Preparation for Administration Capex shampoo: Prior to dispensing, the contents of the capsule (12 mg fluocinolone acetonide) should be emptied into the liquid shampoo; shake well. Discard after 3 months.

Administration Apply sparingly in a thin film; rub in lightly

Capex shampoo: Shake well before use; do not bandage, wrap, or cover treated scalp area unless directed by physician; discard shampoo after 3 months

Derma-Smoothe/FS: Do not apply to face or diaper area; avoid application to intertriginous areas (may increase local adverse effects)

Additional Information Considered a moderate-potency steroid (Derma-Smoothe/FS® and Capex™ shampoo are considered to be low to medium potency); Derma-Smoothe/FS® is made with 48% refined peanut oil, NF (peanut protein is <0.5 ppm)

Dosage Forms Excipient information presented when available (limited, particularly for generics); consult specific product labeling.

Cream, External, as acetonide:

Synalar: 0.025% (120 g) [contains cetyl alcohol, edetate disodium, methylparaben, propylene glycol, propylparaben]

Generic: 0.01% (15 g, 60 g); 0.025% (15 g, 60 g)

Kit, External, as acetonide:

Synalar (Cream): 0.025% [contains cetyl alcohol, edetate disodium, methylparaben, propylene glycol, propylparaben]

Synalar (Ointment): 0.025%

Synalar TS: 0.01% [contains propylene glycol]

Oil, External, as acetonide:

Derma-Smoothe/FS Body: 0.01% (118.28 mL) [contains isopropyl alcohol, peanut oil]

Derma-Smoothe/FS Scalp: 0.01% (118.28 mL) [contains isopropyl alcohol, peanut oil]

Fluocinolone Acetonide Body: 0.01% (118.28 mL) [contains isopropyl alcohol, peanut oil]

Fluocinolone Acetonide Scalp: 0.01% (118.28 mL) [contains isopropyl alcohol, peanut oil]

Ointment, External, as acetonide:

Synalar: 0.025% (120 g)

Generic: 0.025% (15 g, 60 g)

Shampoo, External, as acetonide:

Capex: 0.01% (120 mL)

Solution, External, as acetonide:

Synalar: 0.01% (60 mL, 90 mL) [contains propylene glycol]

Generic: 0.01% (60 mL)

- ◆ **Fluocinolone Acetonide** *see* Fluocinolone (Ophthalmic) *on page 895*
- ◆ **Fluocinolone Acetonide** *see* Fluocinolone (Otic) *on page 896*
- ◆ **Fluocinolone Acetonide** *see* Fluocinolone (Topical) *on page 897*
- ◆ **Fluocinolone Acetonide Body** *see* Fluocinolone (Topical) *on page 897*
- ◆ **Fluocinolone Acetonide Scalp** *see* Fluocinolone (Topical) *on page 897*

Fluocinonide (floo oh SIN oh nide)

Medication Safety Issues

Sound-alike/look-alike issues:

Fluocinonide may be confused with flunisolide, fluocinolone

Lidex® may be confused with Lasix®, Videx®

Related Information

Topical Corticosteroids *on page 2262*

Brand Names: US Vanos

Brand Names: Canada Lidemol®; Lidex®; Lyderm®; Tiamol®; Topactin; Topsyn®

Therapeutic Category Adrenal Corticosteroid; Anti-inflammatory Agent; Corticosteroid, Topical; Glucocorticoid

Generic Availability (US) Yes

Use Inflammation of corticosteroid-responsive dermatoses

Pregnancy Risk Factor C

Pregnancy Considerations Teratogenic effects have been observed in animals administered potent topical corticosteroids. Topical products are not recommended for extensive use, in large quantities, or for long periods of time in pregnant women.

Breast-Feeding Considerations It is not known if topical application will result in detectable quantities in breast milk.

Contraindications Hypersensitivity to fluocinonide or any component of the formulation; viral, fungal, or tubercular skin lesions, herpes simplex

Warnings/Precautions Systemic absorption of topical corticosteroids may cause hypercorticism or suppression of hypothalamic-pituitary-adrenal (HPA) axis, particularly in younger children or in patients receiving high doses for prolonged periods. HPA axis suppression may lead to adrenal crisis. Absorption of topical corticosteroids may cause manifestations of Cushing's syndrome, hyperglycemia, or glycosuria. Absorption is increased by the use of occlusive dressings, application to denuded skin, or application to large surface areas.

Allergic contact dermatitis can occur, it is usually diagnosed by failure to heal rather than clinical exacerbation. Prolonged treatment with corticosteroids has been associated with the development of Kaposi's sarcoma (case reports); if noted, discontinuation of therapy should be considered. Lower-strength cream (0.05%) may be used cautiously on face or opposing skin surfaces that may rub or touch (eg, skin folds of the groin, axilla, and breasts); higher-strength (0.1%) should not be used on the face, groin, or axillae. Use of the 0.1% cream for >2 weeks or in patients <12 years of age is not recommended. Children may absorb proportionally larger amounts after topical application and may be more prone to systemic effects. HPA axis suppression, intracranial hypertension, and Cushing's syndrome have been reported in children receiving topical corticosteroids. Prolonged use may affect growth velocity; growth should be routinely monitored in pediatric patients.

Warnings: Additional Pediatric Considerations Topical corticosteroids may be absorbed percutaneously. The extent of absorption is dependent on several factors, including epidermal integrity (intact vs abraded skin), formulation, age of the patient, prolonged duration of use, and the use of occlusive dressings. Percutaneous absorption of topical steroids is increased in neonates (especially preterm neonates), infants, and young children. Hypothalamic-pituitary-adrenal (HPA) suppression may occur, particularly in younger children or in patients receiving high doses for prolonged periods; acute adrenal insufficiency (adrenal crisis) may occur with abrupt withdrawal after long-term therapy or with stress. Infants and small children may be more susceptible to HPA axis suppression or other systemic toxicities due to larger skin surface area to body mass ratio; use with caution in pediatric patients.

Adverse Reactions

Cardiovascular: Intracranial hypertension

Dermatologic: Acne, allergic dermatitis, contact dermatitis, dry skin, folliculitis, hypertrichosis, hypopigmentation, maceration of the skin, miliaria, perioral dermatitis, pruritus, skin atrophy, striae, telangiectasia

Endocrine & metabolic: Cushing's syndrome, growth retardation, HPA axis suppression, hyperglycemia

Local: Burning, irritation

Renal: Glycosuria

Miscellaneous: Secondary infection

Drug Interactions

Metabolism/Transport Effects None known.

Avoid Concomitant Use

Avoid concomitant use of Fluocinonide with any of the following: Aldesleukin

Increased Effect/Toxicity

Fluocinonide may increase the levels/effects of: Ceritinib; Deferasirox

The levels/effects of Fluocinonide may be increased by: Telaprevir

Decreased Effect

Fluocinonide may decrease the levels/effects of: Aldesleukin; Corticorelin; Hyaluronidase; Telaprevir

Mechanism of Action Topical corticosteroids have anti-inflammatory, antipruritic, and vasoconstrictive properties. May depress the formation, release, and activity of endogenous chemical mediators of inflammation (kinins, histamine, liposomal enzymes, prostaglandins) through the induction of phospholipase A_2 inhibitory proteins (lipocortins) and sequential inhibition of the release of arachidonic acid. Fluocinonide is fluorinated corticosteroid considered to be of high potency.

Dosing: Usual Children and Adults: Topical: Apply thin layer to affected area 2-4 times/day depending on the severity of the condition

Administration Topical: Apply sparingly in a thin film; rub in lightly

Additional Information Considered to be a high potency steroid

Dosage Forms Excipient information presented when available (limited, particularly for generics); consult specific product labeling.

Cream, External:
- Vanos: 0.1% (30 g, 60 g, 120 g)
- Generic: 0.05% (15 g, 30 g, 60 g, 120 g); 0.1% (30 g, 60 g, 120 g)

Gel, External:
- Generic: 0.05% (15 g, 30 g, 60 g)

Ointment, External:
- Generic: 0.05% (15 g, 30 g, 60 g)

Solution, External:
- Generic: 0.05% (20 mL, 60 mL)

◆ **Fluohydrisone Acetate** *see* Fludrocortisone *on page 891*

◆ **Fluohydrocortisone Acetate** *see* Fludrocortisone *on page 891*

◆ **Fluorabon** *see* Fluoride *on page 899*

◆ **Fluor-A-Day** *see* Fluoride *on page 899*

Fluoride (FLOR ide)

Medication Safety Issues

Sound-alike/look-alike issues:

Phos-Flur may be confused with PhosLo

International issues:

Fluorex [France] may be confused with Flarex brand name for fluorometholone [U.S., Canada, and multiple international markets] and Fluarix brand name for influenza virus vaccine (inactivated) [U.S., and multiple international markets]

Related Information

Fluoride Varnishes *on page 2450*

Brand Names: US Act Kids [OTC]; Act Restoring [OTC]; Act Total Care [OTC]; Act [OTC]; CaviRinse; Clinpro 5000; ControlRx; ControlRx Multi; Denta 5000 Plus; DentaGel; Fluor-A-Day; Fluorabon; Fluorinse; Fluoritab; Flura-Drops; Gel-Kam Rinse; Gel-Kam [OTC]; Just For Kids [OTC]; Lozi-Flur; NeutraCare; NeutraGard Advanced; Omni Gel [OTC]; OrthoWash; PerioMed; Phos-Flur; Phos-Flur Rinse [OTC]; PreviDent; PreviDent 5000 Booster; PreviDent 5000 Booster Plus; PreviDent 5000 Dry Mouth; PreviDent 5000 Plus; Sensodyne Repair & Protect [OTC]; StanGard Perio; Stop

Brand Names: Canada Fluor-A-Day

Therapeutic Category Mineral, Oral; Mineral, Oral Topical

Generic Availability (US) Yes: Excludes lozenge

Use

Oral drops, chewable tablet: Prevention of dental caries (FDA approved in ages 6 months to 16 years; consult specific product formulations for appropriate age group)

Lozenges: Prevention of dental caries (FDA approved in ages ≥6 years and adults)

Gel, paste, oral rinse: Prevention of dental caries (Prescription and OTC products: FDA approved in ages ≥6 years and adults; consult specific product formulations for appropriate age group); reduction of tooth sensitivity (Prevident 5000 sensitive: FDA approved in ages ≥12 years and adults)

Dental varnish: Treatment of hypersensitive teeth, sensitive root surfaces, and as a cavity preparation to seal dentinal tubules (FDA approved in ages ≥3 years and adults); has also been used for prevention of dental caries

Pregnancy Risk Factor B

Pregnancy Considerations Fluoride crosses the placenta and can be found in the fetal circulation (IOM, 1997). Adverse events have not been observed in animal reproduction studies; epidemiological studies in areas with high levels of fluorinated water have not shown an increase in adverse effects. Heavy exposure *in utero* may be linked to skeletal fluorosis seen later in childhood.

Breast-Feeding Considerations Low concentrations of fluoride can be found in breast milk and the amount is not significantly affected by supplementation or concentrations in drinking water (IOM, 1997). The manufacturer recommends that caution be exercised when administering fluoride to nursing women.

Contraindications

Fluor-A-Day: When fluoride content of drinking water exceeds 0.6 ppm; patients with arthralgia, GI ulceration, chronic renal insufficiency and failure, or osteomalacia

Fluorabon: When fluoride content of drinking water exceeds 0.6 ppm

Fluoritab: Patients with dental fluorosis

Flura-Drops, Loziflur: When fluoride content of drinking water is ≥0.3 ppm

Warnings/Precautions Prolonged ingestion with excessive doses may result in dental fluorosis and osseous changes; do **not** exceed recommended dosage. Some products contain tartrazine.

Benzyl alcohol and derivatives: Some dosage forms may contain sodium benzoate/benzoic acid; benzoic acid (benzoate) is a metabolite of benzyl alcohol; large amounts of benzyl alcohol (≥99 mg/kg/day) have been associated with a potentially fatal toxicity ("gasping syndrome") in neonates; the "gasping syndrome" consists of metabolic acidosis, respiratory distress, gasping respirations, CNS dysfunction (including convulsions, intracranial hemorrhage), hypotension, and cardiovascular collapse (AAP, 1997; CDC, 1982); some data suggests that benzoate displaces bilirubin from protein binding sites (Ahlfors, 2001); avoid or use dosage forms containing benzyl alcohol derivative with caution in neonates. See manufacturer's labeling.

Polysorbate 80: Some dosage forms may contain polysorbate 80 (also known as Tweens). Hypersensitivity reactions, usually a delayed reaction, have been reported following exposure to pharmaceutical products containing polysorbate 80 in certain individuals (Isaksson, 2002; Lucente 2000; Shelley, 1995). Thrombocytopenia, ascites, pulmonary deterioration, and renal and hepatic failure have been reported in premature neonates after receiving parenteral products containing polysorbate 80 (Alade, 1986; CDC, 1984). See manufacturer's labeling.

Warnings: Additional Pediatric Considerations Supervise children <12 years of age using topical fluoride products, especially children <6 years old, to prevent repeated swallowing; swallowing should be minimized with topical products (eg, creams, gels, rinses).

Some dosage forms may contain propylene glycol; in neonates large amounts of propylene glycol delivered orally, intravenously (eg, >3,000 mg/day), or topically have been associated with potentially fatal toxicities which can include metabolic acidosis, seizures, renal failure, and CNS depression; toxicities have also been reported in children and adults including hyperosmolality, lactic acidosis, seizures, and respiratory depression; use caution (AAP, 1997; Shehab, 2009).

Adverse Reactions

Dermatologic: Skin rash

Gastrointestinal: Dental discoloration (with products containing stannous fluoride; temporary), nausea

Hypersensitivity: Hypersensitivity reaction

Drug Interactions

Metabolism/Transport Effects None known.

Avoid Concomitant Use There are no known interactions where it is recommended to avoid concomitant use.

Increased Effect/Toxicity There are no known significant interactions involving an increase in effect.

Decreased Effect There are no known significant interactions involving a decrease in effect.

Storage/Stability Store at room temperature.

Mechanism of Action Promotes remineralization of decalcified enamel; inhibits the cariogenic microbial process in dental plaque; increases tooth resistance to acid dissolution

Pharmacokinetics (Adult data unless noted)

Absorption: Oral: ~50% absorbed from GI tract (IOM, 1997); dairy products may delay absorption

Distribution: 99% in calcified tissue (IOM, 1997)

Elimination: Urine (IOM, 1997)

Dosing: Neonatal Adequate Intake (AI) (IOM, 1997): Oral: 0.01 mg/day; supplementation is not recommended in neonates

Dosing: Usual

Pediatric:

Adequate Intake (AI): (IOM, 1997): Infants, Children, and Adolescents: Oral:

- 1 to 6 months: 0.01 mg/day; additional supplementation is not recommended in infants <6 months of age
- 7 to 12 months: 0.5 mg/day
- 1 to 3 years: 0.7 mg/day
- 4 to 8 years: 1 mg/day
- 9 to 13 years: 2 mg/day
- 14 to 18 years: 3 mg/day

Dental caries, prevention:

Systemic therapy:

Drops/tablets (Fluorabon, Fluor-A-Day, Fluoritab, Flura-drops): Oral: The recommended oral daily dose of fluoride is adjusted in proportion to the fluoride content of available drinking water:

Birth to 6 months: No supplement required regardless of fluoride content of drinking water

6 months to 3 years:
- <0.3 ppm: 0.25 mg once daily
- ≥0.3 ppm: No supplement required

3 to 6 years:
- <0.3 ppm: 0.5 mg once daily
- 0.3 to 0.6 ppm: 0.25 mg once daily
- >0.6 ppm: No supplement required

6 to 16 years:
- <0.3 ppm: 1 mg once daily
- 0.3 to 0.6 ppm: 0.5 mg once daily
- >0.6 ppm: No supplement required

Lozenges (Lozi-Flur): Children ≥6 years and Adolescents: Oral: 1 lozenge daily; allow lozenge to dissolve slowly in the mouth and swallow with saliva. **Note:** For use in areas where the fluoride content of drinking water is <0.3 ppm.

Topical therapy:

Dental rinse: **Note:** Do not eat, drink, or rinse mouth for at least 30 minutes after treatment; do not swallow.

Acidulated phosphate fluoride rinse (Phos-Flur): Children ≥6 years and Adolescents: Topical: 10 mL once daily after brushing; swish between teeth for 1 minute, then spit.

Sodium fluoride: Topical:

0.02% Sodium fluoride (ACT Restoring, ACT Total Care): Children ≥6 years and Adolescents: 10 mL swish and spit twice daily after brushing

0.05% Sodium fluoride (ACT Anticavity Rinse, ACT Kids): Children ≥6 years and Adolescents: 10 mL swish and spit once daily after brushing

0.2% Neutral sodium fluoride (CaviRinse, Previ-Dent Rinse): Children ≥6 years and Adolescents: 10 mL swish and spit once **weekly**, preferably at bedtime after brushing. **Note:** CaviRinse labeling recommends children and adolescents 6 to 16 years rinse with water immediately following treatment.

Stannous fluoride 0.63% (Gel-Kam): Children ≥12 years and Adolescents: Topical: After diluting solution as directed, rinse with 15 mL for 1 minute, then spit; repeat with remaining solution. Use at least once daily.

Gel: Stannous fluoride 0.4% (Just for Kids): Children ≥6 years and Adolescents: Topical: Once daily after brushing, apply a pea-sized amount of gel to teeth and brush thoroughly. Allow gel to remain on teeth for 1 minute prior to spitting out. Do not eat or drink for 30 minutes after using.

Paste: Sodium fluoride 1.1%: Topical:

Clinpro 5000, Control Rx, Denta 5000 Plus:Children ≥6 years and Adolescents: Once daily, preferably at bedtime, in place of conventional toothpaste; brush teeth with a thin ribbon or pea-sized amount of toothpaste for at least 2 minutes; after brushing expectorate and rinse mouth thoroughly with water.

PreviDent 5000 Sensitive: Children ≥12 years and Adolescents: Twice daily, brush teeth with a 1-inch strip of toothpaste for at least 1 minute. After brushing, expectorate and rinse mouth thoroughly.

Dental varnish: 5% Sodium Fluoride (2.26% Fluoride ion): Infants (after primary tooth eruption), Children and Adolescents: Topical: Apply a thin layer of varnish to surfaces of teeth at least every 3 to 6 months (ADA [Weyant], 2013). **Note:** Must be professionally applied; USPSTF recommends dental varnish may be applied by primary care practitioners to the primary teeth of all infants and children starting at the age of primary tooth eruption through 5 years of age (USPSTF, 2014):

Adult:

Adequate Intake (AI) (IOM, 1997): Oral:

Males: 4 mg/day

Females: 3 mg/day

Dental caries, prevention:

Systemic therapy: Lozenges (Lozi-Flur): Oral: 1 lozenge daily regardless of drinking water fluoride content

Topical therapy:

Dental rinse: Topical:

Acidulated phosphate fluoride rinse (Phos-Flur): 10 mL rinse and spit once daily after brushing; do not eat, drink, or rinse mouth for at least 30 minutes after treatment; do not swallow

Sodium fluoride:

0.02% Sodium fluoride (ACT Restoring, ACT Total Care): 10 mL rinse and spit twice daily after brushing; do not eat, drink, or rinse mouth for at least 30 minutes after treatment; do not swallow

0.05% Sodium fluoride (ACT Anticavity Rinse): 10 mL rinse and spit once daily after brushing; do not eat, drink, or rinse mouth for at least 30 minutes after treatment; do not swallow

0.2% Neutral sodium fluoride (CaviRinse, PreviDent Rinse): 10 mL rinse and then spit once **weekly** after brushing; preferably at bedtime; do not swallow. For maximum benefit with PreviDent rinse, do not eat, drink, or rinse mouth for at least 30 minutes after treatment.

Paste: Topical:

Clinpro 5000 paste, Control Rx 1.1%, Denta 5000 Plus: Once daily, in place of conventional toothpaste, brush teeth with a thin ribbon or pea-sized amount of paste for at least 2 minutes. Brush teeth with cream or paste once daily regardless of fluoride content of drinking water.

Prevident 5000 Sensitive: Twice daily, brush teeth with a 1-inch strip of toothpaste for at least 1 minute. After brushing, expectorate and rinse mouth thoroughly. Brush teeth twice daily regardless of fluoride content of drinking water.

Preparation for Administration Concentrated oral rinse (stannous fluoride 0.63%): Must be diluted with water to stannous fluoride 0.1% prior to use. Pour the concentrated rinse to the 1/8 fluid ounce mark in the mixing vial (to the bottom mark). Add water to the 1 fluid ounce line and mix. This prepares a 0.1% (w/v) stannous fluoride rinse. Use immediately after preparing the rinse

Administration

Systemic therapy (Drops/solution, lozenges, tablets): Dairy products should be avoided within 1 hour of administration.

Fluorabon drops: May be administered undiluted or mixed in a nondairy food that will be totally consumed.

Fluor-A-Day: Drops may be administered in juice or water; ensure entire contents are consumed. Tablets should be dissolved in mouth or chewed prior to swallowing.

Flura-drops: May be administered undiluted or mixed with water or juice, ensure entire contents are consumed.

Lozi-Flur: Lozenge should be dissolved in mouth and swallowed with saliva.

Topical therapy:

Dental rinse: Swish or rinse in mouth then expectorate; do not swallow. Once daily products are generally used at bedtime. Do not eat, drink, or rinse mouth for at least 30 minutes after treatment. Consult specific product labeling for details.

Dental varnish: Briefly mix varnish with brush prior to application as contents may separate during storage. Dry teeth with cotton gauze immediately prior to use. Apply varnish on all surfaces of teeth. It is not necessary to use entire unit dose. Avoid eating or drinking for 30 minutes; avoid hot food and beverages; do not brush teeth until the following day (AAP [Clark], 2014). Do not apply on patients with active stomatitis or other ulcerative oral diseases. Do not use on patients with a known colophony allergy.

Paste:

Clinpro 5000 paste, Control Rx 1.1%, Denta 5000 Plus: After brushing for at least 2 minutes, adults should expectorate and children 6 to 16 years should expectorate and rinse mouth thoroughly with water.

Prevident 5000 Sensitive: After brushing for at least 1 minute, expectorate and rinse mouth thoroughly with water.

Reference Range Total plasma fluoride: 0.14-0.19 mcg/mL

Dosage Forms Excipient information presented when available (limited, particularly for generics); consult specific product labeling.

Cream, oral, as sodium [toothpaste]: 1.1% (51 g) [equivalent to fluoride 2.5 mg/dose]

Denta 5000 Plus: 1.1% (51 g) [spearmint flavor; equivalent to fluoride 2.5 mg/dose]

PreviDent 5000 Plus: 1.1% (51 g) [contains sodium benzoate; fruitastic flavor; equivalent to fluoride 2.5 mg/dose]

PreviDent 5000 Plus: 1.1% (51 g) [contains sodium benzoate; spearmint flavor; equivalent to fluoride 2.5 mg/dose]

Gel, oral, as sodium [toothpaste]:

PreviDent 5000 Booster: 1.1% (100 mL, 106 mL) [contains sodium benzoate; fruitastic flavor; equivalent to fluoride 2.5 mg/dose]

PreviDent 5000 Booster: 1.1% (100 mL, 106 mL) [contains sodium benzoate; spearmint flavor; equivalent to fluoride 2.5 mg/dose]

PreviDent 5000 Booster Plus: 1.1% (100 mL) [contains sodium benzoate; fruitastic flavor; equivalent to fluoride 2.5 mg/dose]

PreviDent 5000 Booster Plus: 1.1% (100 mL) [contains sodium benzoate; spearmint flavor; equivalent to fluoride 2.5 mg/dose]

PreviDent 5000 Dry Mouth: 1.1% (100 mL) [mint flavor; equivalent to fluoride 2.5 mg/dose]

Gel, topical, as sodium: 1.1% (56 g) [equivalent to fluoride 2 mg/dose]

DentaGel: 1.1% (56 g) [fresh mint flavor; neutral pH; equivalent to fluoride 2 mg/dose]

NeutraCare: 1.1% (60 g) [grape flavor; neutral pH]

NeutraCare: 1.1% (60 g) [mint flavor; neutral pH]

NeutraGard Advanced: 1.1% (60 g) [mint flavor; neutral pH]

NeutraGard Advanced: 1.1% (60 g) [mixed berry flavor; neutral pH]

Phos-Flur: 1.1% (51 g) [contains propylene glycol, sodium benzoate; mint flavor; equivalent to fluoride 0.5%]

PreviDent: 1.1% (56 g) [mint flavor; neutral pH; equivalent to fluoride 2 mg/dose]

PreviDent: 1.1% (56 g) [very berry flavor; neutral pH; equivalent to fluoride 2 mg/dose]

Gel, topical, as stannous fluoride:

Gel-Kam: 0.4% (129 g) [cinnamon flavor]

Gel-Kam: 0.4% (129 g) [fruit & berry flavor]

Gel-Kam: 0.4% (129 g) [mint flavor]

Just For Kids: 0.4% (122 g) [bubblegum flavor]

Just For Kids: 0.4% (122 g) [fruit-punch flavor]

Just For Kids: 0.4% (122 g) [grapey grape flavor]

Omni Gel: 0.4% (122 g) [cinnamon flavor]

Omni Gel: 0.4% (122 g) [grape flavor]

Omni Gel: 0.4% (122 g) [mint flavor]

Omni Gel: 0.4% (122 g) [natural flavor]

Omni Gel: 0.4% (122 g) [raspberry flavor]

Liquid, oral, as base:

Fluoritab: 0.125 mg/drop [dye free]

Lozenge, oral, as sodium:

Lozi-Flur: 2.21 mg (90s) [sugar free; cherry flavor; equivalent to fluoride 1 mg]

Paste, oral, as sodium [toothpaste]:

Clinpro 5000: 1.1% (113 g) [vanilla-mint flavor]

ControlRx: 1.1% (57 g) [berry flavor]

ControlRx: 1.1% (57 g) [vanilla-mint flavor]

ControlRx Multi: 1.1% (57 g) [vanilla-mint flavor]

Paste, oral, as stannous fluoride [toothpaste]:

Sensodyne Repair & Protect: 0.454% (96.4 g) [mint flavor]

Solution, oral, as fluoride [rinse]:

Act Total Care: 0.02% (1000 mL) [ethanol free; contains menthol, propylene glycol, sodium benzoate, tartrazine; fresh mint flavor; equivalent to fluoride 0.009%]

Solution, oral, as sodium [drops]: 1.1 mg/mL (50 mL) [equivalent to fluoride 0.5 mg/mL]

Fluor-A-Day: 0.278 mg/drop (30 mL) [equivalent to fluoride 0.125 mg/drop]

Fluorabon: 0.55 mg/0.6 mL (60 mL) [dye free, sugar free; equivalent to fluoride 0.25 mg/0.6 mL]

Flura-Drops: 0.55 mg/drop (24 mL) [dye free, sugar free; contains natural rubber/natural latex in packaging; equivalent to fluoride 0.25 mg/drop]

Solution, oral, as sodium [rinse]: 0.2% (473 mL)

Act: 0.05% (532 mL) [contains benzyl alcohol, propylene glycol, sodium benzoate, tartrazine; cinnamon flavor; equivalent to fluoride 0.02%]

Act: 0.05% (532 mL) [contains propylene glycol, sodium benzoate, tartrazine; mint flavor; equivalent to fluoride 0.02%]

Act Kids: 0.05% (532 mL) [ethanol free; contains benzyl alcohol, propylene glycol, sodium benzoate; bubblegum flavor; equivalent to fluoride 0.02%]

Act Kids: 0.05% (500 mL) [ethanol free; contains benzyl alcohol, propylene glycol, sodium benzoate; ocean berry flavor; equivalent to fluoride 0.02%]

Act Restoring: 0.02% (1000 mL) [contains ethanol 11%, propylene glycol, sodium benzoate; Cool Splash mint flavor; equivalent to fluoride 0.009%]

Act Restoring: 0.02% (1000 mL) [contains ethanol 11%, propylene glycol, sodium benzoate; Cool Splash spearmint flavor; equivalent to fluoride 0.009%]

Act Restoring: 0.05% (532 mL) [contains ethanol 11%, propylene glycol, sodium benzoate; Cool Splash mint flavor; equivalent to fluoride 0.02%]

Act Restoring: 0.05% (532 mL) [contains ethanol 11%, propylene glycol, sodium benzoate; Cool Splash spearmint flavor; equivalent to fluoride 0.02%]

Act Restoring: 0.05% (532 mL) [contains ethanol 11%, propylene glycol, sodium benzoate; Cool Splash vanilla-mint flavor; equivalent to fluoride 0.02%]

Act Total Care: 0.02% (1000 mL) [contains ethanol 11%, propylene glycol, sodium benzoate; icy clean mint flavor; equivalent to fluoride 0.009%]

Act Total Care: 0.05% (88 mL, 532 mL) [contains ethanol 11%, propylene glycol, sodium benzoate; icy clean mint flavor; equivalent to fluoride 0.02%]

Act Total Care: 0.05% (88 mL, 532 mL) [ethanol free; contains menthol, propylene glycol, sodium benzoate, tartrazine; fresh mint flavor; equivalent to fluoride 0.02%]

CaviRinse: 0.2% (240 mL) [mint flavor]

Fluorinse: 0.2% (480 mL) [ethanol free; cinnamon flavor]

Fluorinse: 0.2% (480 mL) [ethanol free; mint flavor]

OrthoWash: 0.044% (480 mL) [contains sodium benzoate; grape flavor]

OrthoWash: 0.044% (480 mL) [contains sodium benzoate; strawberry flavor]

Phos-Flur Rinse: 0.044% (473 mL) [ethanol free, sugar free; bubblegum flavor]

Phos-Flur Rinse: 0.044% (473 mL) [ethanol free, sugar free; gushing grape flavor]

Phos-Flur Rinse: 0.044% (500 mL) [sugar free; cool mint flavor]

PreviDent: 0.2% (473 mL) [contains benzoic acid, ethanol 6%, sodium benzoate; cool mint flavor]

Solution, oral, as stannous fluoride [concentrated rinse]: 0.63% (300 mL) [equivalent to fluoride 7 mg/30 mL dose]

Gel-Kam Rinse: 0.63% (300 mL) [mint flavor; equivalent to fluoride 7 mg/30 mL dose]

PerioMed: 0.63% (284 mL) [ethanol free; cinnamon flavor; equivalent to fluoride 7 mg/30 mL dose]

PerioMed: 0.63% (284 mL) [ethanol free; mint flavor; equivalent to fluoride 7 mg/30 mL dose]

PerioMed: 0.63% (284 mL) [ethanol free; tropical fruit flavor; equivalent to fluoride 7 mg/30 mL dose]

StanGard Perio: 0.63% (284 mL) [mint flavor]

Tablet, chewable, oral, as sodium: 0.55 mg [equivalent to fluoride 0.25 mg], 1.1 mg [equivalent to fluoride 0.5 mg], 2.2 mg [equivalent to fluoride 1 mg]

Fluor-A-Day: 0.55 mg [raspberry flavor; equivalent to fluoride 0.25 mg]

Fluor-A-Day: 1.1 mg [raspberry flavor; equivalent to fluoride 0.5 mg]

Fluor-A-Day: 2.2 mg [raspberry flavor; equivalent to fluoride 1 mg]

Fluoritab: 2.2 mg [cherry flavor; equivalent to fluoride 1 mg]

Fluoritab: 1.1 mg [dye free; cherry flavor; equivalent to fluoride 0.5 mg]

◆ **Fluorinse** *see* Fluoride *on page 899*

◆ **Fluoritab** *see* Fluoride *on page 899*

◆ **5-Fluorocytosine** *see* Flucytosine *on page 886*

◆ **9α-Fluorohydrocortisone Acetate** *see* Fludrocortisone *on page 891*

Fluorometholone (flure oh METH oh lone)

Medication Safety Issues

International issues:

Flarex [U.S., Canada, and multiple international markets] may be confused with Fluarix brand name for influenza virus vaccine (inactivated) [U.S. and multiple international markets] and Fluorex brand name for fluoride [France]

Brand Names: US Flarex; FML; FML Forte; FML Liquifilm

Brand Names: Canada Flarex®; FML Forte®; FML®; PMS-Fluorometholone

Therapeutic Category Adrenal Corticosteroid; Anti-inflammatory Agent, Ophthalmic; Corticosteroid, Ophthalmic; Glucocorticoid

Generic Availability (US) May be product dependent

Use Inflammatory conditions of the eye, including keratitis, iritis, cyclitis, and conjunctivitis

Pregnancy Risk Factor C

Pregnancy Considerations Teratogenic effects were observed in animal reproduction studies following use of ophthalmic fluorometholone. The extent of systemic absorption following topical application of the ophthalmic drops is not known.

Breast-Feeding Considerations Systemic corticosteroids are excreted in human milk. The extent of systemic absorption following topical application of the ophthalmic drops is not known.

Contraindications Hypersensitivity to fluorometholone or any component of the formulation; viral diseases of the cornea and conjunctiva (including epithelial herpes simplex keratitis, vaccinia, and varicella); mycobacterial or fungal infections of the eye; untreated eye infections which may be masked/enhanced by a steroid

Warnings/Precautions Prolonged use of corticosteroids may result in posterior subcapsular cataract formation. Use following cataract surgery may delay healing or increase the incidence of bleb formation. Corneal perforation may occur with topical steroids in diseases which cause thinning of the cornea or sclera. Use with caution in presence of glaucoma. Prolonged use of corticosteroids may result in elevated intraocular pressure (IOP); damage to the optic nerve; and defects in visual acuity and fields of vision. Monitor IOP in any patient receiving treatment for ≥10 days. May mask infection or enhance existing infection. The possibility of persistent corneal fungal infection should be considered after prolonged use. May exacerbate severity of viral infections. Use caution in patients with history of herpes simplex; re-evaluate after 2 days if symptoms have not improved; use is contraindicated in most viral diseases of the cornea and conjunctiva.

Some products contain benzalkonium chloride which may be adsorbed by contact lenses; remove contacts prior to administration and wait 15 minutes before reinserting. Initial prescription and renewal of medication >20 mL should be made by healthcare provider only after examination with the aid of magnification such as slit lamp biomicroscopy or fluorescein staining (if appropriate). Patients should be re-evaluated if symptoms fail to improve after 2 days.

Adverse Reactions

Dermatologic: Skin rash

Endocrine & metabolic: Hypercorticoidism (rare)

Gastrointestinal: Dysgeusia

Hypersensitivity: Hypersensitivity reaction

Ophthalmic: Bacterial eye infection (secondary), blurred vision, burning sensation of eyes, cataract, decreased visual acuity, erythema of eyelid, eye discharge, eye irritation, eyelid edema, eye pain, eye pruritus, foreign body sensation of eye, fungal eye infection (secondary), glaucoma, increased intraocular pressure, increased lacrimation, optic nerve damage, stinging of eyes, swelling of eye, viral eye infection (secondary), visual field defect, wound healing impairment

Drug Interactions

Metabolism/Transport Effects None known.

Avoid Concomitant Use

Avoid concomitant use of Fluorometholone with any of the following: Aldesleukin

Increased Effect/Toxicity

Fluorometholone may increase the levels/effects of: Ceritinib; Deferasirox

The levels/effects of Fluorometholone may be increased by: NSAID (Ophthalmic); Telaprevir

Decreased Effect

Fluorometholone may decrease the levels/effects of: Aldesleukin; Corticorelin; Hyaluronidase; Telaprevir

Storage/Stability

Ointment: Store at 15°C to 25°C (59°F to 77°F; avoid temperatures >40°C (104°F).

Suspension: Store at 2°C to 25°C (36°F to 77°F); do not freeze.

Mechanism of Action Corticosteroids inhibit the inflammatory response including edema, capillary dilation, leukocyte migration, and scar formation. Fluorometholone penetrates cells readily to induce the production of lipocortins. These proteins modulate the activity of prostaglandins and leukotrienes.

Pharmacokinetics (Adult data unless noted) Absorption: Into aqueous humor with slight systemic absorption

Dosing: Usual Children >2 years and Adults: Ophthalmic:

Ointment: May be applied every 4 hours in severe cases or 1-3 times/day in mild to moderate cases.

Drops: Instill 1-2 drops into conjunctival sac every hour during day, every 2 hours at night until favorable response is obtained, then use 1 drop every 4 hours; in mild or moderate inflammation: 1-2 drops into conjunctival sac 2-4 times/day.

Administration Ophthalmic: Avoid contact of medication tube or bottle tip with skin or eye; suspension: Shake well before use; apply finger pressure to lacrimal sac during and for 1-2 minutes after instillation to decrease risk of absorption and systemic effects; the preservative (benzalkonium chloride) may be absorbed by soft contact lenses; wait at least 15 minutes after administration of suspension before inserting soft contact lenses

Monitoring Parameters Intraocular pressure (if used ≥10 days)

Dosage Forms Excipient information presented when available (limited, particularly for generics); consult specific product labeling.

Ointment, Ophthalmic, as base:

FML: 0.1% (3.5 g) [contains phenylmercuric acetate]

Suspension, Ophthalmic, as acetate:

Flarex: 0.1% (5 mL)

Suspension, Ophthalmic, as base:

FML Forte: 0.25% (5 mL, 10 mL)

FML Liquifilm: 0.1% (5 mL, 10 mL)

Generic: 0.1% (5 mL, 10 mL, 15 mL)

◆ **Fluoro Uracil** *see* Fluorouracil (Systemic) *on page* 903

◆ **5-Fluorouracil** *see* Fluorouracil (Systemic) *on page* 903

Fluorouracil (Systemic) (flure oh YOOR a sil)

Medication Safety Issues

Sound-alike/look-alike issues:

Fluorouracil may be confused with floxuridine, flucytosine

High alert medication:

This medication is in a class the Institute for Safe Medication Practices (ISMP) includes among its list of

drug classes which have a heightened risk of causing significant patient harm when used in error.

Administration issues:

Continuous infusion: Serious errors have occurred when doses administered by continuous ambulatory infusion pumps have inadvertently been given over 1 to 4 hours instead of the intended extended continuous infusion duration. Depending on protocol, infusion duration may range from 46 hours to 7 days for continuous infusions of fluorouracil. Ambulatory pumps utilized for continuous infusions should have safeguards to allow for detection of programming errors. If using an elastomeric device for ambulatory continuous infusion, carefully select and double check the flow rate on the device. Appropriate prescribing (in single daily doses [not course doses] with instructions to infuse over a specific time period), appropriate training/certification/education of staff involved with dispensing and administration processes, and independent double checks should be utilized throughout dispensing and administration procedures.

Related Information

Management of Drug Extravasations *on page 2298*

Prevention of Chemotherapy-Induced Nausea and Vomiting in Children *on page 2368*

Safe Handling of Hazardous Drugs *on page 2455*

Brand Names: US Adrucil

Brand Names: Canada Fluorouracil Injection

Therapeutic Category Antineoplastic Agent, Antimetabolite

Generic Availability (US) Yes

Use Treatment of carcinoma of stomach (gastric), colon, rectum, breast, and pancreas (FDA approved in adults); has also been used for the treatment of hepatoblastoma, nasopharyngeal carcinoma, head and neck cancer, bladder cancer, and cervical cancer

Pregnancy Risk Factor D

Pregnancy Considerations Adverse effects (increased resorptions, embryolethality, and teratogenicity) have been observed in animal reproduction studies. Based on the mechanism of action, fluorouracil may cause fetal harm if administered during pregnancy (according to the manufacturer's labeling). The National Comprehensive Cancer Network (NCCN) breast cancer guidelines (v.3.2012) state that chemotherapy, if indicated, may be administered to pregnant women with breast cancer as part of a combination chemotherapy regimen (common regimens administered during pregnancy include doxorubicin, cyclophosphamide, and fluorouracil); chemotherapy should not be administered during the first trimester, after 35 weeks gestation, or within 3 weeks of planned delivery.

Breast-Feeding Considerations Based on the mechanism of action, the manufacturer's labeling recommends against breast-feeding if receiving fluorouracil.

Contraindications Hypersensitivity to fluorouracil or any component of the formulation; poor nutritional states; depressed bone marrow function; potentially serious infections

Warnings/Precautions Hazardous agent - use appropriate precautions for handling and disposal (NIOSH 2014 [group 1]). Use with caution in patients with impaired kidney or liver function. Discontinue if intractable vomiting or diarrhea, precipitous falls in leukocyte or platelet counts, gastrointestinal ulcer or bleeding, stomatitis, or esophagopharyngitis, hemorrhage, or myocardial ischemia occurs. Use with caution in poor-risk patients who have had high-dose pelvic radiation or previous use of alkylating agents and in patients with widespread metastatic marrow involvement. Palmar-plantar erythrodysesthesia (hand-foot) syndrome has been associated with use (symptoms include a tingling sensation, which may progress to pain, and then to symmetrical swelling and erythema with tenderness; desquamation may occur; with treatment interruption, generally resolves over 5-7 days).

Continuous infusion: Serious errors have occurred when doses administered by continuous ambulatory infusion pumps have inadvertently been given over 1 to 4 hours instead of the intended extended continuous infusion duration. Depending on protocol, infusion duration may range from 46 hours to 7 days for continuous infusions of fluorouracil. Ambulatory pumps utilized for continuous infusions should have safeguards to allow for detection of programming errors. If using an elastomeric device for ambulatory continuous infusion, carefully select and double check the flow rate on the device. Appropriate prescribing (in single daily doses [not course doses] with instructions to infuse over a specific time period), appropriate training/certification/education of staff involved with dispensing and administration processes, and independent double checks should be utilized throughout dispensing and administration procedures (ISMP [Smetzer 2015]).

An investigational uridine prodrug, uridine triacetate (formerly called vistonuridine), has been studied in a limited number of cases of fluorouracil overdose. Of 17 patients receiving uridine triacetate beginning within 8-96 hours after fluorouracil overdose, all patients fully recovered (von Borstel, 2009). Updated data has described a total of 28 patients treated with uridine triacetate for fluorouracil overdose (including overdoses related to continuous infusions delivering fluorouracil at rates faster than prescribed), all of whom recovered fully (Bamat, 2010).

Administration to patients with a genetic deficiency of dihydropyrimidine dehydrogenase (DPD) has been associated with prolonged clearance and increased toxicity (diarrhea, neutropenia, and neurotoxicity) following administration; rechallenge has resulted in recurrent toxicity (despite dose reduction). **[U.S. Boxed Warning]: Should be administered under the supervision of an experienced cancer chemotherapy physician; the manufacturer's labeling recommends hospitalizing patients during the first treatment course due to the potential for severe toxicity.** Potentially significant drug-drug interactions may exist, requiring dose or frequency adjustment, additional monitoring, and/or selection of alternative therapy.

Adverse Reactions Toxicity depends on duration of treatment and/or rate of administration

Cardiovascular: Angina, arrhythmia, heart failure, MI, myocardial ischemia, vasospasm, ventricular ectopy

Central nervous system: Acute cerebellar syndrome, confusion, disorientation, euphoria, headache, nystagmus, stroke

Dermatologic: Alopecia, dermatitis, dry skin, fissuring, nail changes (nail loss), palmar-plantar erythrodysesthesia syndrome, pruritic maculopapular rash, photosensitivity, Stevens-Johnson syndrome, toxic epidermal necrolysis, vein pigmentation

Gastrointestinal: Anorexia, bleeding, diarrhea, esophagopharyngitis, mesenteric ischemia (acute), nausea, sloughing, stomatitis, ulceration, vomiting

Hematologic: Agranulocytosis, anemia, leukopenia (nadir: days 9-14; recovery by day 30), pancytopenia, thrombocytopenia

Local: Thrombophlebitis

Ocular: Lacrimation, lacrimal duct stenosis, photophobia, visual changes

Respiratory: Epistaxis

Miscellaneous: Anaphylaxis, generalized allergic reactions

Drug Interactions

Metabolism/Transport Effects Inhibits CYP2C9 (strong)

Avoid Concomitant Use

Avoid concomitant use of Fluorouracil (Systemic) with any of the following: BCG; BCG (Intravesical); CloZAPine; Dipyrone; Gimeracil; Natalizumab; Pimecrolimus; Tacrolimus (Topical); Tofacitinib; Vaccines (Live)

Increased Effect/Toxicity

Fluorouracil (Systemic) may increase the levels/effects of: Bosentan; Carvedilol; CloZAPine; CYP2C9 Substrates; Diclofenac (Systemic); Dronabinol; Fosphenytoin; Lacosamide; Leflunomide; Natalizumab; Ospemifene; Parecoxib; Phenytoin; Ramelteon; Tetrahydrocannabinol; Tofacitinib; Vaccines (Live); Vitamin K Antagonists

The levels/effects of Fluorouracil (Systemic) may be increased by: Cannabis; Cimetidine; Denosumab; Dipyrone; Gemcitabine; Gimeracil; Leucovorin Calcium-Levoleucovorin; MetroNIDAZOLE (Systemic); Pimecrolimus; Roflumilast; SORAfenib; Tacrolimus (Topical); Trastuzumab

Decreased Effect

Fluorouracil (Systemic) may decrease the levels/effects of: BCG; BCG (Intravesical); Coccidioides immitis Skin Test; Sipuleucel-T; Vaccines (Inactivated); Vaccines (Live)

The levels/effects of Fluorouracil (Systemic) may be decreased by: Echinacea; SORAfenib

Storage/Stability Store intact vials at room temperature. Do not refrigerate or freeze. Protect from light. Slight discoloration may occur during storage; does not usually denote decomposition. If exposed to cold, a precipitate may form; **gentle** heating to 60°C (140°F) will dissolve the precipitate without impairing the potency. According to the manufacturer, pharmacy bulk vials should be used within 4 hours of initial entry. Solutions for infusion should be used promptly. Fluorouracil 50 mg/mL in NS was stable in polypropylene infusion pump syringes for 7 days when stored at 30°C (86°F) (Stiles, 1996). Stability of fluorouracil 1 mg/mL or 10 mg/mL in NS or D_5W in PVC bags was demonstrated for up to 14 days at 4°C (39.2°F) and 21°C (69.8°F) (Martel, 1996). Stability of undiluted fluorouracil (50 mg/mL) in ethylene-vinyl acetate ambulatory pump reservoirs was demonstrated for 3 days at 4°C (39.2°F) (precipitate formed after 3 days) and for 14 days at 33°C (91.4°F) (Martel, 1996). Stability of undiluted fluorouracil (50 mg/mL) in PVC ambulatory pump reservoirs was demonstrated for 5 days at 4°C (39.2°F) (precipitate formed after 5 days) and for 14 days at 33°C (91.4°F) (Martel, 1996).

Mechanism of Action A pyrimidine analog antimetabolite that interferes with DNA and RNA synthesis; after activation, F-UMP (an active metabolite) is incorporated into RNA to replace uracil and inhibit cell growth; the active metabolite F-dUMP, inhibits thymidylate synthetase, depleting thymidine triphosphate (a necessary component of DNA synthesis).

Pharmacokinetics (Adult data unless noted)

Distribution: Penetrates tumors, intestinal mucosa, liver, bone marrow, ascitic fluid, brain tissue, and CSF

Metabolism: Hepatic (90%); via a dehydrogenase enzyme; FU must be metabolized to be active metabolites, 5-fluoroxyuridine monophosphate (F-UMP) and 5-5-fluoro-2'-deoxyuridine-5'-O-monophosphate (F-dUMP)

Half-life: 16 minutes (range: 8-20 minutes); two metabolites, F-dUMP and F-UMP, have prolonged half-lives depending on the type of tissue

Elimination: Urine (7% to 20% as unchanged drug within 6 hours; also as metabolites within 9-10 hours); lung (as expired CO_2)

Dosing: Usual

Pediatric: **Note:** Dose, frequency, number of doses, and/or start date may vary by protocol and treatment phase. Refer to individual protocols.

Hepatoblastoma: Limited data available: Infants, Children, and Adolescents: IV: 600 mg/m²/dose every 3 weeks on day 2 or 3 (in combination with cisplatin, vincristine ± doxorubicin) (Douglas, 1993; Ortega, 2000; Watanabe, 2013)

Nasopharyngeal carcinoma: Limited data available: Children ≥8 years and Adolescents: Continuous IV infusion: 1000 mg/m²/day for 3-5 days every 3-4 weeks for 3-4 cycles (in combination with other chemotherapy agents) (Buehrlen, 2012; Casanova, 2012; Mertens, 2005; Rodriguez-Galindo, 2005)

Adult: **Note:** Utilize patient's actual body weight (full weight) for calculation of body surface area- or weight-based dosing, particularly when the intent of therapy is curative; manage regimen-related toxicities in the same manner as for nonobese patients; if a dose reduction is utilized due to toxicity, consider resumption of full weight-based dosing with subsequent cycles, especially if cause of toxicity (eg, hepatic or renal impairment) is resolved (Griggs, 2012). Details concerning dosing in combination regimens should be consulted:

Breast cancer: IV:

CEF regimen: 500 mg/m² on days 1 and 8 every 28 days (in combination with cyclophosphamide and epirubicin) for 6 cycles (Levine, 1998)

CMF regimen: 600 mg/m² on days 1 and 8 every 28 days (in combination with cyclophosphamide and methotrexate) for 6 cycles (Goldhirsch, 1998; Levine, 1998)

FAC regimen: 500 mg/m² on days 1 and 8 every 21-28 days (in combination with cyclophosphamide and doxorubicin) for 6 cycles (Assikis, 2003)

Colorectal cancer: IV:

FLOX regimen: 500 mg/m² bolus on days 1, 8, 15, 22, 29, and 36 (1 hour after leucovorin) every 8 weeks (in combination with leucovorin and oxaliplatin) for 3 cycles (Kuebler, 2007)

FOLFOX6 and mFOLFOX6 regimen: 400 mg/m² bolus on day 1, followed by 1200 mg/m²/day continuous infusion for 2 days (over 46 hours) every 2 weeks (in combination with leucovorin and oxaliplatin) until disease progression or unacceptable toxicity (Cheeseman, 2002)

FOLFIRI regimen: 400 mg/m² bolus on day 1, followed by 1200 mg/m²/day continuous infusion for 2 days (over 46 hours) every 2 weeks (in combination with leucovorin and irinotecan) until disease progression or unacceptable toxicity; after 2 cycles, may increase continuous infusion fluorouracil dose to 1500 mg/m²/day (over 46 hours) (André, 1999)

Roswell Park regimen: 500 mg/m² (bolus) on days 1, 8, 15, 22, 29, and 36 (1 hour after leucovorin) every 8 weeks (in combination with leucovorin) for 4 cycles (Haller, 2005)

Gastric cancer: IV:

CF regimen: 750-1000 mg/m²/day continuous infusion days 1-4 and 29-32 of a 35-day treatment cycle (preoperative chemoradiation; in combination with cisplatin) (NCCN Gastric Cancer Guidelines v2.2012; Tepper, 2008)

ECF regimen (resectable disease): 200 mg/m²/day continuous infusion days 1-21 every 3 weeks (in combination with epirubicin and cisplatin) for 6 cycles (3 cycles preoperatively and 3 cycles postoperatively) (Cunningham, 2006)

ECF or EOF regimen (advanced disease): 200 mg/m²/day continuous infusion days 1-21 every 3 weeks (in combination with epirubicin and either cisplatin or oxaliplatin) for a planned duration of 24 weeks (Sumpter, 2005)

TCF or DCF regimen: 750 mg/m^2/day continuous infusion days 1-5 every 3 weeks or 1000 mg/m^2/day continuous infusion days 1-5 every 4 weeks (in combination with docetaxel and cisplatin) until disease progression or unacceptable toxicity (Ajani, 2007; NCCN Gastric Cancer Guidelines v2.2012; Van Cutsem, 2006)

ToGA regimen (HER2-positive): 800 mg/m^2/day continuous infusion days 1-5 every 3 weeks (in combination with cisplatin and trastuzumab) until disease progression or unacceptable toxicity (Bang, 2010)

Pancreatic cancer: IV:

Chemoradiation therapy: 250 mg/m^2/day continuous infusion for 3 weeks prior to and then throughout radiation therapy (Regine, 2008)

Fluorouracil-Leucovorin: 425 mg/m^2/day (bolus) days 1-5 every 28 days (in combination with leucovorin) for 6 cycles (Neoptolemos, 2010)

FOLFIRINOX regimen: 400 mg/m^2 bolus on day 1, followed by 1200 mg/m^2/day continuous infusion for 2 days (over 46 hours) every 14 days (in combination with leucovorin, irinotecan, and oxaliplatin) until disease progression or unacceptable toxicity for a recommended 12 cycles (Conroy, 2011)

Dosing adjustment in renal impairment: Adult: There are no dosage adjustments provided in the manufacturer's labeling; however, extreme caution should be used in patients with renal impairment. The following adjustments have been recommended:

CrCl <50 mL/minute and continuous renal replacement therapy (CRRT): No dosage adjustment necessary (Aronoff, 2007).

Hemodialysis:

Administer standard dose following hemodialysis on dialysis days (Janus, 2010).

Administer 50% of standard dose following hemodialysis (Aronoff, 2007).

Dosing adjustment in hepatic impairment: Adult: There are no dosage adjustments provided in the manufacturer's labeling; however, extreme caution should be used in patients with hepatic impairment. The following adjustments have been recommended:

Hepatic impairment (degree not specified): Administer <50% of dose, then increase if toxicity does not occur (Koren, 1992)

Bilirubin >5 mg/dL: Avoid use (Floyd, 2006)

Preparation for Administration Hazardous agent; use appropriate precautions for handling and disposal (NIOSH 2014 [group 1]).

IV push: May dispense undiluted in a syringe

IV infusion: Further dilute in NS or D_5W for infusion.

Administration Hazardous agent; use appropriate precautions for handling and disposal (NIOSH 2014 [group 1]).

IV: Administration rate varies by protocol; refer to specific reference for protocol. May be administered undiluted by IV push, or further diluted in appropriate fluids and administered by IV bolus, or as a continuous infusion. Avoid extravasation (may be an irritant).

Vesicant/Extravasation Risk May be an irritant

Monitoring Parameters CBC with differential and platelet count, renal function tests, liver function tests; signs of palmar-plantar erythrodysesthesia syndrome, stomatitis, diarrhea, hemorrhage, or gastrointestinal ulcers or bleeding

Dosage Forms Excipient information presented when available (limited, particularly for generics); consult specific product labeling.

Solution, Intravenous:

Adrucil: 500 mg/10 mL (10 mL); 2.5 g/50 mL (50 mL); 5 g/100 mL (100 mL)

Generic: 500 mg/10 mL (10 mL); 1 g/20 mL (20 mL); 2.5 g/50 mL (50 mL); 5 g/100 mL (100 mL)

◆ **Fluorouracil Injection (Can)** *see* Fluorouracil (Systemic) *on page 903*

◆ **Fluouracil** *see* Fluorouracil (Systemic) *on page 903*

FLUoxetine (floo OKS e teen)

Medication Safety Issues

Sound-alike/look-alike issues:

FLUoxetine may be confused with DULoxetine, famotidine, Feldene, fluconazole, fluvastatin, fluvoxaMINE, fosinopril, furosemide, Loxitane [DSC], PARoxetine, thiothixene, vortioxetine

PROzac may be confused with Paxil, Prelone, PriLOSEC, Prograf, Proscar, ProSom, Provera

Sarafem may be confused with Serophene

BEERS Criteria medication:

This drug may be potentially inappropriate for use in geriatric patients with a history of falls or fractures (Quality of evidence - high [moderate for SIADH]; Strength of recommendation - strong).

International issues:

Reneuron [Spain] may be confused with Remeron brand name for mirtazapine [U.S., Canada, and multiple international markets]

Related Information

Antidepressant Agents *on page 2257*

Oral Medications That Should Not Be Crushed or Altered *on page 2476*

Brand Names: US PROzac; PROzac Weekly; Sarafem

Brand Names: Canada Apo-Fluoxetine; Ava-Fluoxetine; CO Fluoxetine; Dom-Fluoxetine; Fluoxetine Capsules BP; FXT 40; Gen-Fluoxetine; JAMP-Fluoxetine; Mint-Fluoxetine; Mylan-Fluoxetine; Novo-Fluoxetine; Nu-Fluoxetine; PHL-Fluoxetine; PMS-Fluoxetine; PRO-Fluoxetine; Prozac; Q-Fluoxetine; ratio-Fluoxetine; Riva-Fluoxetine; Sandoz-Fluoxetine; Teva-Fluoxetine; ZYM-Fluoxetine

Therapeutic Category Antidepressant, Selective Serotonin Reuptake Inhibitor (SSRI)

Generic Availability (US) Yes

Use Treatment (acute and maintenance) of major depressive disorder (FDA approved in ages ≥8 years and adults); treatment (acute and maintenance) of obsessive-compulsive disorder (FDA approved in ages ≥7 years and adults); treatment of bulimia nervosa (FDA approved in adults); treatment of panic disorder with or without agoraphobia (FDA approved in adults); treatment of premenstrual dysphoric disorder (PMDD) (Sarafem®: FDA approved in adults); has also been used for anxiety and/or selective mutism and repetitive behavior associated with an autism spectrum disorder (eg, autism, Asperger's syndrome, pervasive developmental disorders)

Medication Guide Available Yes

Pregnancy Risk Factor C

Pregnancy Considerations Adverse events have been observed in animal reproduction studies. Fluoxetine and its metabolite cross the human placenta. An increased risk of teratogenic effects, including cardiovascular defects, may be associated with maternal use of fluoxetine or other SSRIs; however, available information is conflicting. Nonteratogenic effects in the newborn following SSRI/SNRI exposure late in the third trimester include respiratory distress, cyanosis, apnea, seizures, temperature instability, feeding difficulty, vomiting, hypoglycemia, hypo- or hypertonia, hyper-reflexia, jitteriness, irritability, constant crying, and tremor. Symptoms may be due to the toxicity of the SSRIs/SNRIs or a discontinuation syndrome and may be consistent with serotonin syndrome associated with SSRI treatment. Persistent pulmonary hypertension of the newborn (PPHN) has also been reported with SSRI exposure. The long-term effects of *in utero* SSRI exposure on infant development and behavior are not known.

Due to pregnancy-induced physiologic changes, women who are pregnant may require dose adjustments of fluoxetine to achieve euthymia. The ACOG recommends that therapy with SSRIs or SNRIs during pregnancy be individualized; treatment of depression during pregnancy should incorporate the clinical expertise of the mental health clinician, obstetrician, primary healthcare provider, and pediatrician. According to the American Psychiatric Association (APA), the risks of medication treatment should be weighed against other treatment options and untreated depression. For women who discontinue antidepressant medications during pregnancy and who may be at high risk for postpartum depression, the medications can be restarted following delivery. Treatment algorithms have been developed by the ACOG and the APA for the management of depression in women prior to conception and during pregnancy.

Breast-Feeding Considerations Fluoxetine and its metabolite are excreted into breast milk and can be detected in the serum of breast-feeding infants. Concentrations in breast milk are variable. In comparison to other SSRIs, fluoxetine concentrations in breast milk are higher and adverse events have been observed in nursing infants. Maternal use of an SSRI during pregnancy may cause delayed milk secretion. Breast-feeding is not recommended by the manufacturer. Long-term effects on development and behavior have not been studied.

Contraindications Hypersensitivity to fluoxetine or any component of the formulation; use of MAO inhibitors intended to treat psychiatric disorders (concurrently, within 5 weeks of discontinuing fluoxetine, or within 2 weeks of discontinuing the MAO inhibitor); initiation of fluoxetine in a patient receiving linezolid or intravenous methylene blue; use with pimozide or thioridazine (**Note:** Thioridazine should not be initiated until 5 weeks after the discontinuation of fluoxetine)

Warnings/Precautions [U.S. Boxed Warning]: Antidepressants increase the risk of suicidal thinking and behavior in children, adolescents, and young adults (18-24 years of age) with major depressive disorder (MDD) and other psychiatric disorders; consider risk prior to prescribing. Short-term studies did not show an increased risk in patients >24 years of age and showed a decreased risk in patients ≥65 years. Closely monitor all patients for clinical worsening, suicidality, or unusual changes in behavior, particularly during the initial 1-2 months of therapy or during periods of dosage adjustments (increases or decreases); the patient's family or caregiver should be instructed to closely observe the patient and communicate condition with healthcare provider. A medication guide concerning the use of antidepressants should be dispensed with each prescription. **Fluoxetine is FDA approved for the treatment of OCD in children ≥7 years of age and MDD in children ≥8 years of age.**

The possibility of a suicide attempt is inherent in major depression and may persist until remission occurs. Use caution in high-risk patients. Worsening depression and severe abrupt suicidality that are not part of the presenting symptoms may require discontinuation or modification of drug therapy. Prescriptions should be written for the smallest quantity consistent with good patient care. The patient's family or caregiver should be alerted to monitor patients for the emergence of suicidality and associated behaviors (such as agitation, irritability, hostility, impulsivity, and hypomania) and call healthcare provider.

May worsen psychosis in some patients or precipitate a shift to mania or hypomania in patients with bipolar disorder. Patients presenting with depressive symptoms should be screened for bipolar disorder. Monotherapy in patients with bipolar disorder should be avoided. **Fluoxetine monotherapy is not FDA approved for the treatment of bipolar depression.** May cause insomnia, anxiety, nervousness, or anorexia. Use with caution in patients where weight loss is undesirable. May impair cognitive or motor performance; caution operating hazardous machinery or driving.

QT prolongation and ventricular arrhythmia including torsade de pointes has occurred. Use with caution in patients with risk factors for QT prolongation, under conditions that predispose to arrhythmias, or increased fluoxetine exposure. Consider discontinuation of fluoxetine if ventricular arrhythmia suspected and initiate cardiac evaluation. Avoid concurrent use with other medications that increase QT interval.

Potentially life-threatening serotonin syndrome (SS) has occurred with serotonergic agents (eg, SSRIs, SNRIs), particularly when used in combination with other serotonergic agents (eg, triptans, TCAs, fentanyl, lithium, tramadol, buspirone, St John's wort, tryptophan) or agents that impair metabolism of serotonin (eg, MAO inhibitors intended to treat psychiatric disorders, other MAO inhibitors [ie, linezolid and intravenous methylene blue]). Discontinue treatment (and any concomitant serotonergic agent) immediately if signs/symptoms arise. Fluoxetine use has been associated with occurrences of significant rash and allergic events, including vasculitis, lupus-like syndrome, laryngospasm, anaphylactoid reactions, and pulmonary inflammatory disease. Discontinue if underlying cause of rash cannot be identified.

Use caution in patients with a previous seizure disorder or condition predisposing to seizures such as brain damage or alcoholism. Use with caution in patients with hepatic or severe renal dysfunction and in elderly patients. Use caution in elderly patients; may be potentially inappropriate in patients with a history of falls or fractures, and may cause or exacerbate syndrome of inappropriate antidiuretic hormone secretion or hyponatremia; monitor sodium closely with initiation or dosage adjustments in older adults (Beers Criteria). May also cause agitation, sleep disturbances, and excessive CNS stimulation. May cause hyponatremia/SIADH (elderly at increased risk); volume depletion (diuretics may increase risk). May increase the risks associated with electroconvulsive treatment. Use caution with history of MI or unstable heart disease; use in these patients is limited. May alter glycemic control in patients with diabetes. Due to the long half-life of fluoxetine and its metabolites, the effects and interactions noted may persist for prolonged periods following discontinuation. May cause or exacerbate sexual dysfunction. May cause mild pupillary dilation, which in susceptible individuals can lead to an episode of narrow-angle glaucoma. Consider evaluating patients who have not had an iridectomy for narrow-angle glaucoma risk factors. Bone fractures have been associated with antidepressant treatment. Consider the possibility of a fragility fracture if an antidepressant-treated patient presents with unexplained bone pain, point tenderness, swelling, or bruising (Rabenda, 2013; Rizzoli, 2012). Potentially significant drug-drug interactions may exist, requiring dose or frequency adjustment, additional monitoring, and/or selection of alternative therapy.

Abrupt discontinuation or interruption of antidepressant therapy has been associated with a discontinuation syndrome. Symptoms arising may vary with antidepressant however commonly include nausea, vomiting, diarrhea, headaches, light-headedness, dizziness, diminished appetite, sweating, chills, tremors, paresthesias, fatigue, somnolence, and sleep disturbances (eg, vivid dreams, insomnia). Greater risks for developing a discontinuation syndrome have been associated with antidepressants with shorter half-lives, longer durations of treatment, and abrupt discontinuation. For antidepressants of short or intermediate half-lives, symptoms may emerge within 2-5 days after treatment discontinuation and last 7-14 days (APA, 2010; Fava, 2006; Haddad, 2001; Shelton, 2001; Warner, 2006).

Benzyl alcohol and derivatives: Some dosage forms may contain sodium benzoate/benzoic acid; benzoic acid (benzoate) is a metabolite of benzyl alcohol; large amounts of benzyl alcohol (≥99 mg/kg/day) have been associated with a potentially fatal toxicity ("gasping syndrome") in neonates; the "gasping syndrome" consists of metabolic acidosis, respiratory distress, gasping respirations, CNS dysfunction (including convulsions, intracranial hemorrhage), hypotension, and cardiovascular collapse (AAP, 1997; CDC, 1982); some data suggests that benzoate displaces bilirubin from protein binding sites (Ahlfors, 2001); avoid or use dosage forms containing benzyl alcohol derivative with caution in neonates. See manufacturer's labeling.

Warnings: Additional Pediatric Considerations
SSRI-associated behavioral activation (ie, restlessness, hyperkinesis, hyperactivity, agitation) is two- to threefold more prevalent in children compared to adolescents; it is more prevalent in adolescents compared to adults. Somnolence (including sedation and drowsiness) is more common in adults compared to children and adolescents (Safer, 2006). SSRI-associated vomiting is two- to threefold more prevalent in children compared to adolescents and is more prevalent in adolescents compared to adults (Safer, 2006). May cause abnormal bleeding (eg, ecchymosis, purpura, upper GI bleeding); use with caution in patients with impaired platelet aggregation and with concurrent use of aspirin, NSAIDs, or other drugs that affect coagulation. A recent report describes five children (age: 8 to 15 years) who developed epistaxis (n=4) or bruising (n=1) while receiving SSRI therapy (sertraline) (Lake, 2000). Fluoxetine may cause decreased growth (smaller increases in weight and height) in children and adolescent patients; currently, no studies directly evaluate fluoxetine's long-term effects on growth, development, and maturation of pediatric patients; periodic monitoring of height and weight in pediatric patients is recommended. Case reports of decreased growth in children receiving fluoxetine or fluvoxamine (n=4; age: 11.6 to 13.7 years) for 6 months to 5 years suggest a suppression of growth hormone secretion during SSRI therapy (Weintrob, 2002).

Adverse Reactions

Cardiovascular: Chest pain, hypertension, palpitations, vasodilation

Central nervous system: Abnormal dreams, abnormality in thinking, agitation, amnesia, anxiety, chills, confusion, dizziness, drowsiness, emotional lability, headache, insomnia, nervousness, sleep disorder, yawning

Dermatologic: Diaphoresis, pruritus, skin rash

Endocrine & metabolic: Decreased libido, hypermenorrhea, increased thirst, weight gain, weight loss

Gastrointestinal: Anorexia, constipation, diarrhea, dysgeusia, dyspepsia, flatulence, increased appetite, nausea, vomiting, xerostomia

Genitourinary: Ejaculatory disorder, impotence, urinary frequency

Neuromuscular & skeletal: Hyperkinesia, tremor, weakness

Ophthalmic: Visual disturbance

Otic: Otalgia, tinnitus

Respiratory: Epistaxis, flu-like symptoms, pharyngitis, sinusitis

<1% (Limited to important or life-threatening): Abnormal hepatic function tests, acne vulgaris, acute abdominal condition, akathisia, albuminuria, alopecia, amenorrhea, anaphylactoid reaction, anemia, angina pectoris, angle-closure glaucoma, aphthous stomatitis, aplastic anemia, arthritis, asthma, ataxia, atrial fibrillation, bruise, bruxism, bursitis, cardiac arrest, cardiac arrhythmia, cataract, cerebrovascular accident, cholelithiasis, cholestatic jaundice, colitis, congestive heart failure, dehydration, delusions, depersonalization, dyskinesia, dysphagia, dysuria, ecchymoses, edema, eosinophilic pneumonitis, equilibrium disturbance, erythema multiforme, erythema nodosum, esophagitis, euphoria, exfoliative dermatitis, extrapyramidal reaction (rare), gastritis, gastroenteritis, gastrointestinal ulcer, glossitis, gout, gynecological bleeding, gynecomastia, hallucination, hemolytic anemia (immune-related), hepatic failure, hepatic necrosis, hepatitis, hiccups, hostility, hypercholesteremia, hyperprolactinemia, hypersensitivity reaction, hypertonia, hyperventilation, hypoglycemia, hypokalemia, hyponatremia (possibly in association with SIADH), hypotension, hypothyroidism, immune thrombocytopenia, laryngeal edema, laryngospasm, leg cramps, lupus-like syndrome, malaise, melena, migraine, mydriasis, myocardial infarction, myoclonus, neuroleptic malignant syndrome (Stevens, 2008), optic neuritis, orthostatic hypotension, ostealgia, pancreatitis, pancytopenia, paranoia, petechia, priapism, prolonged Q-T interval on ECG, pulmonary embolism, pulmonary fibrosis, pulmonary hypertension, purpuric rash, renal failure, serotonin syndrome, skin photosensitivity, Stevens-Johnson syndrome, suicidal ideation, syncope, tachycardia, thrombocytopenia, toxic epidermal necrolysis, vasculitis, ventricular tachycardia (including torsades de pointes), violent behavior

Drug Interactions

Metabolism/Transport Effects **Substrate** of CYP1A2 (minor), CYP2B6 (minor), CYP2C19 (minor), CYP2C9 (major), CYP2D6 (major), CYP2E1 (minor), CYP3A4 (minor); **Note:** Assignment of Major/Minor substrate status based on clinically relevant drug interaction potential; **Inhibits** CYP1A2 (weak), CYP2B6 (weak), CYP2C19 (moderate), CYP2C9 (weak), CYP2D6 (strong)

Avoid Concomitant Use

Avoid concomitant use of FLUoxetine with any of the following: Dapoxetine; Dosulepin; Haloperidol; Highest Risk QTc-Prolonging Agents; Iobenguane I 123; Ivabradine; Linezolid; MAO Inhibitors; Mequitazine; Methylene Blue; Mifepristone; Moderate Risk QTc-Prolonging Agents; Pimozide; Propafenone; Tamoxifen; Thioridazine; Tryptophan; Urokinase; Ziprasidone

Increased Effect/Toxicity

FLUoxetine may increase the levels/effects of: Agents with Antiplatelet Properties; Anticoagulants; Antidepressants (Serotonin Reuptake Inhibitor/Antagonist); Antipsychotic Agents; Apixaban; ARIPiprazole; Aspirin; AtoMOXetine; Beta-Blockers; Blood Glucose Lowering Agents; BusPIRone; CarBAMazepine; Cilostazol; Collagenase (Systemic); CYP2C19 Substrates; CYP2D6 Substrates; Dabigatran Etexilate; Deoxycholic Acid; Desmopressin; Dextromethorphan; Dosulepin; DOXOrubicin (Conventional); Fesoterodine; Fosphenytoin; Haloperidol; Highest Risk QTc-Prolonging Agents; Ibritumomab; Mequitazine; Methylene Blue; Metoprolol; Mexiletine; Nebivolol; NIFEdipine; NiMODipine; NSAID (COX-2 Inhibitor); NSAID (Nonselective); Obinutuzumab; Phenytoin; Pimozide; Propafenone; Rivaroxaban; Salicylates; Serotonin Modulators; Tamsulosin; Thiazide Diuretics; Thioridazine; Thrombolytic Agents; TiZANidine; Tositumomab and Iodine I 131 Tositumomab; TraMADol; Tricyclic Antidepressants; Urokinase; Vitamin K Antagonists; Vortioxetine; Ziprasidone

The levels/effects of FLUoxetine may be increased by: Abiraterone Acetate; Alcohol (Ethyl); Analgesics (Opioid); Antiemetics (5HT3 Antagonists); Antipsychotic Agents; ARIPiprazole; BuPROPion; BusPIRone; Cimetidine; CNS Depressants; Cobicistat; CYP2C9 Inhibitors (Moderate); CYP2C9 Inhibitors (Strong); CYP2D6 Inhibitors (Moderate); CYP2D6 Inhibitors (Strong); Dapoxetine;

Darunavir; Fosphenytoin; Glucosamine; Herbs (Anticoagulant/Antiplatelet Properties); Ibrutinib; Ivabradine; Limaprost; Linezolid; Lithium; MAO Inhibitors; Metoclopramide; Metyrosine; Mifepristone; Moderate Risk QTc-Prolonging Agents; Multivitamins/Fluoride (with ADE); Multivitamins/Minerals (with ADEK, Folate, Iron); Multivitamins/Minerals (with AE, No Iron); Omega-3 Fatty Acids; Pentosan Polysulfate Sodium; Pentoxifylline; Propafenone; Prostacyclin Analogues; QTc-Prolonging Agents (Indeterminate Risk and Risk Modifying); Tedizolid; TraMADol; Tryptophan; Vitamin E; Ziprasidone

Decreased Effect

FLUoxetine may decrease the levels/effects of: Clopidogrel; Codeine; Hydrocodone; Iobenguane I 123; Ioflupane I 123; Tamoxifen; Thyroid Products

The levels/effects of FLUoxetine may be decreased by: CarBAMazepine; CYP2C9 Inducers (Strong); Cyproheptadine; Dabrafenib; NSAID (COX-2 Inhibitor); NSAID (Nonselective); Peginterferon Alfa-2b

Storage/Stability All dosage forms should be stored at controlled room temperature. Protect from light.

Mechanism of Action Inhibits CNS neuron serotonin reuptake; minimal or no effect on reuptake of norepinephrine or dopamine; does not significantly bind to alpha-adrenergic, histamine, or cholinergic receptors

Pharmacodynamics Maximum effect: Antidepressant: Usually occur after >4 weeks; due to long half-life, resolution of adverse reactions after discontinuation may be slow

Pharmacokinetics (Adult data unless noted) Note: Average steady-state fluoxetine serum concentrations in children (n=10; 6 to <13 years of age) were 2-fold higher than in adolescents (n=11; 13 to <18 years of age); all patients received 20 mg/day; average steady-state norfluoxetine serum concentrations were 1.5-fold higher in the children compared with adolescents; differences in weight almost entirely explained the differences in serum concentrations

Absorption: Oral: Well absorbed; enteric-coated pellets contained in Prozac® Weekly™ resist dissolution until GI pH >5.5 and therefore delay onset of absorption 1-2 hours compared to immediate release formulations

Distribution: V_d: 12-43 L/kg; widely distributed

Protein binding: ~95% (albumin and alpha$_1$-glycoprotein)

Metabolism: Hepatic, via CYP2C19 and 2D6, to norfluoxetine (activity equal to fluoxetine) and other metabolites

Bioavailability: Capsules, tablets, solution, and weekly capsules are bioequivalent

Half-life:

- Fluoxetine: Acute dosing: 1-3 days; chronic dosing: 4-6 days; cirrhosis: 7.6 days
- Norfluoxetine: Acute and chronic dosing: 4-16 days; cirrhosis: 12 days

Time to peak serum concentration: Immediate release formulation: After 6-8 hours

Elimination: Urine (10% as norfluoxetine, 2.5% to 5% as fluoxetine)

Dialysis: Not removed by hemodialysis

Note: Weekly formulation results in greater fluctuations between peak and trough concentrations of fluoxetine and norfluoxetine compared to once-daily dosing (24% daily/164% weekly; 17% daily/43% weekly, respectively). Trough concentrations are 76% lower for fluoxetine and 47% lower for norfluoxetine than the concentrations maintained by 20 mg once-daily dosing. Steady-state fluoxetine concentrations are ~50% lower following the once-weekly regimen compared to 20 mg once daily.

Dosing: Usual Note: Upon discontinuation of fluoxetine therapy, gradually taper dose. If intolerable symptoms occur following a dose reduction, consider resuming the previously prescribed dose and/or decrease dose at a more gradual rate. If used for an extended period of time, long-term usefulness of fluoxetine should be periodically re-evaluated for the individual patient.

Children and Adolescents:

Anxiety with associated phobias and panic attacks: Very limited data available: Children 2-6 years: Oral: 5 mg/dose or 0.25 mg/kg/dose once daily; adequate trial is considered to be 8-10 weeks; continuation of therapy should be evaluated at 6-9 months after initiation; dosing based on case report in a 2.5-year old child and expert recommendations (Gleason, 2007)

Bulimia nervosa adjunct therapy with cognitive behavioral therapy: Limited data available: Children ≥12 years and Adolescents: Oral: Initial: 20 mg once daily for 3 days, then 40 mg once daily for 3 days, then 60 mg once daily; dosing based on an open-label study of 10 pediatric patients (age: 12-18 years) which showed significant decrease in number of weekly purges; other reports describe use in adolescents (Gable, 2005; Kotler, 2003; Rosen, 2010)

Depression:

Manufacturer's labeling: Children ≥8 years and Adolescents:

- Lower weight Children: Oral: Initial: 10 mg once daily; usual daily dose: 10 mg/**day**; if needed, may increase dose to 20 mg once daily after several weeks; maximum daily dose: 20 mg/**day**
- Higher weight Children and Adolescents: Oral: Initial: 10-20 mg once daily; in patients started at 10 mg once daily, may increase dose to 20 mg after 1 week; maximum daily dose: 20 mg/**day**

Alternate dosing: Limited data available: Lower initial dosing has been recommended by some experts (Dopheide, 2006; Gleason, 2007):

- Children ≤11 years: Oral: Initial: 5 mg once daily; clinically, doses have been titrated up to 40 mg once daily in pediatric patients
- Children ≥12 years and Adolescents: Oral: Initial: 10 mg once daily; clinically, doses have been titrated up to 40 mg once daily in pediatric patients

Obsessive-compulsive disorder:

Children <7 years: Limited data available: Oral: Initial: 5 mg once daily (Gleason, 2007)

Children ≥7 years and Adolescents: Oral:

- Lower weight Children: Initial: 10 mg once daily; if needed, may increase dose after several weeks; usual daily dose: 20-30 mg/**day**; minimal experience with doses >20 mg/**day**; no experience with doses >60 mg/**day**
- Higher weight Children and Adolescents: Initial: 10 mg once daily; increase dose to 20 mg once daily after 2 weeks; may increase dose after several more weeks, if needed; usual daily dose: 20-60 mg/**day**

Repetitive behavior associated with autism spectrum disorders (ASD): Limited data available: Children ≥5 years and Adolescents: Oral: Initial: 2.5 mg once daily for 7 days; then may titrate at weekly intervals using weight-based dosing: 0.3 mg/kg/**day** during week 2; followed by 0.5 mg/kg/**day** during week 3, up to a maximum of 0.8 mg/kg/**day**; dosing based on a double-blind, crossover, placebo-controlled trial in 39 pediatric patients (age: 5-16 years) which showed statistically significant improvement in behavior scores compared to placebo; mean final dose: 9.9 mg/**day** (range: 2.4-20 mg/**day**) or 0.36 ± 0.116 mg/kg/**day** (Hollander, 2005)

Selective mutism: Limited data available: Children ≥5 years and Adolescents: Oral: Initial: 5 mg once daily for 7 days, then increase to 10 mg daily for 7 days, and then increase to 20 mg daily; may further titrate in 20 mg/**day** increments if needed every 2 weeks; maximum daily dose: 60 mg/**day**. Dosing is based on an open-label study of 21 pediatric patients (age: 5-14 years); positive responses were reported in 76% of patients and required a dose of at least 20 mg/**day**; mean final dose: 28.1 mg/**day** (1.1 mg/kg/**day**) (Dummitt, 1996). Weight-based dosing has been reported in a double-blind placebo-controlled trial (treatment group: n=6; placebo: n=9; age: 6-12 years) using the following titration: 0.2 mg/kg/**day** for 1 week, then 0.4 mg/kg/**day** for 1 week, then 0.6 mg/kg/**day** for 10 weeks; mean final dose: 21.4 mg/**day** (Black,1994). To fully assess therapeutic response, a therapeutic trial of at least 9-12 weeks or longer has been suggested (Black, 1994; Dummitt; 1996; Kaakeh, 2008).

Adults: **Depression, obsessive-compulsive disorder, premenstrual dysphoric disorder, bulimia:** Oral: Initial: 20 mg once daily in the morning; may increase after several weeks by 20 mg/**day** increments; maximum daily dose: 80 mg/**day**; doses >20 mg may be given once daily or divided twice daily. **Note:** Lower doses of 5-10 mg/**day** have been used for initial treatment.

Bulimia nervosa: Oral: 60 mg once daily

Depression: Oral: Initial: 20 mg once daily; may increase after several weeks if inadequate response (maximum: 80 mg/**day**). Patients maintained on Prozac® 20 mg/day may be changed to Prozac® Weekly™ 90 mg/week, starting dose 7 days after the last 20 mg/day dose

Depression associated with bipolar disorder (in combination with olanzapine): Oral: Initial: 20 mg in the evening; adjust as tolerated to usual range of 20-50 mg/**day**. See **"Note"** below.

Obsessive-compulsive disorder: Oral: Initial: 20 mg once daily; may increase after several weeks if inadequate response; recommended range: 20-60 mg/**day** (maximum daily dose: 80 mg/**day**)

Panic disorder: Oral: Initial: 10 mg once daily; after 1 week, increase to 20 mg/**day**; may increase after several weeks; doses >60 mg/**day** have not been evaluated

Premenstrual dysphoric disorder (Sarafem®): Oral: 20 mg once daily continuously **or** 20 mg once daily starting 14 days prior to menstruation and through first full day of menses (repeat with each cycle)

Treatment-resistant depression (in combination with olanzapine): Oral: Initial: 20 mg in the evening; adjust as tolerated to usual range of 20-50 mg/**day**. See **"Note"**.

Note: When using individual components of fluoxetine with olanzapine rather than fixed dose combination product (Symbyax®), approximate dosage correspondence is as follows:

- Olanzapine 2.5 mg + fluoxetine 20 mg = Symbyax® 3/25
- Olanzapine 5 mg + fluoxetine 20 mg = Symbyax® 6/25
- Olanzapine 12.5 mg + fluoxetine 20 mg = Symbyax® 12/25
- Olanzapine 5 mg + fluoxetine 50 mg = Symbyax® 6/50
- Olanzapine 12.5 mg + fluoxetine 50 mg = Symbyax® 12/50

Dosage adjustment in renal impairment: Children, Adolescents, and Adults: Adjustment not routinely needed

Single dose studies: Adults: Pharmacokinetics of fluoxetine and norfluoxetine were similar among subjects with all levels of impaired renal function, including anephric patients on chronic hemodialysis.

Chronic administration: Additional accumulation of fluoxetine or norfluoxetine may occur in patients with severely impaired renal function.

Dosage adjustment in hepatic impairment:

Children and Adolescents: Elimination half-life of fluoxetine is prolonged in patients with hepatic impairment; lower doses or less frequent administration are recommended

Adults: Elimination half-life of fluoxetine is prolonged in patients with hepatic impairment; lower doses or less frequent administration are recommended

Cirrhosis patient: Administer a lower dose or less frequent dosing interval

Compensated cirrhosis without ascites: Administer 50% of normal dose

Administration Oral: May be administered without regard to food

Indication specific:

Major depressive disorder and obsessive compulsive disorder: Take in the morning; if twice daily dosing, take at morning and noon

Bipolar I disorder and treatment-resistant depression (with concurrent olanzapine): Take in the evening

Bulimia: Take in the morning

Monitoring Parameters Liver function, weight, serum glucose; serum sodium (in volume depleted patients); monitor for rash and signs or symptoms of anaphylactoid reactions; monitor height and weight in pediatric patients periodically. Monitor patient periodically for symptom resolution; monitor for worsening depression, suicidality, and associated behaviors (especially at the beginning of therapy or when doses are increased or decreased)

Reference Range Therapeutic levels have not been well established:

Therapeutic: Fluoxetine 100-800 ng/mL (SI: 289-2314 nmol/L); norfluoxetine 100-600 ng/mL (SI: 289-1735 nmol/L)

Toxic: (Fluoxetine plus norfluoxetine): >2000 ng/mL (SI: >5784 nmol/L)

Dosage Forms Excipient information presented when available (limited, particularly for generics); consult specific product labeling.

Capsule, Oral:
- PROzac: 10 mg, 20 mg, 40 mg
- Generic: 10 mg, 20 mg, 40 mg

Capsule Delayed Release, Oral:
- PROzac Weekly: 90 mg
- Generic: 90 mg

Solution, Oral:
- Generic: 20 mg/5 mL (5 mL, 120 mL)

Tablet, Oral:
- Sarafem: 10 mg, 20 mg [contains fd&c yellow #10 aluminum lake, fd&c yellow #6 aluminum lake]
- Generic: 10 mg, 20 mg, 60 mg

Extemporaneous Preparations Note: Commercial oral solution is available (4 mg/mL)

A 1 mg/mL fluoxetine oral solution may be prepared using the commercially available preparation (4 mg/mL). In separate graduated cylinders, measure 5 mL of the commercially available fluoxetine preparation and 15 mL of Simple Syrup, NF. Mix thoroughly in incremental proportions. For a 2 mg/mL solution, mix equal proportions of both the commercially available fluoxetine preparation and Simple Syrup, NF. Label "refrigerate". Both concentrations are stable for up to 56 days.

Nahata MC, Pai VB, and Hipple TF, *Pediatric Drug Formulations*, 5th ed, Cincinnati, OH: Harvey Whitney Books Co, 2004.

◆ **Fluoxetine Capsules BP (Can)** *see* FLUoxetine *on page 906*

◆ **Fluoxetine Hydrochloride** *see* FLUoxetine *on page 906*

Fluoxymesterone (floo oks i MES te rone)

Medication Safety Issues

International issues:

Halotestin [Great Britain] may be confused with Haldol brand name for haloperidol [U.S. and multiple international markets]

Related Information
Safe Handling of Hazardous Drugs *on page 2455*
Brand Names: US Androxy [DSC]
Therapeutic Category Androgen
Generic Availability (US) No
Use Replacement of endogenous testicular hormone; in females used as palliative treatment of breast cancer, postpartum breast engorgement
Pregnancy Risk Factor X
Pregnancy Considerations Use is contraindicated in women who are or may become pregnant. May cause androgenic effects to the female fetus; clitoral hypertrophy, labial fusion, urogenital sinus defect, vaginal atresia, and ambiguous genitalia have been reported.
Breast-Feeding Considerations It is not known if fluoxymesterone is excreted in breast milk. Due to the potential for serious adverse reactions in the nursing infant, a decision should be made whether to discontinue nursing or to discontinue the drug, taking into account the importance of treatment to the mother.
Contraindications Males with carcinoma of the breast or the prostate (known or suspected); women who are or may become pregnant
Warnings/Precautions Hazardous agent - use appropriate precautions for handling and disposal (NIOSH 2014 [group 2]).

Anabolic steroids may alter serum lipid profile; use caution in patients with history of myocardial infarction or coronary artery disease. May cause gynecomastia. Prolonged use of high doses of oral androgens has been associated with serious hepatic effects (eg, peliosis, hepatitis, hepatic neoplasms, cholestatic hepatitis, jaundice). Discontinue use in patients with cholestatic hepatitis with jaundice or abnormal liver function tests. Use with caution in patients with breast cancer or immobilization; may cause hypercalcemia by stimulating osteolysis. Discontinue use if hypercalcemia occurs; may indicate bony metastasis. Use with caution in patients with diabetes mellitus; monitor carefully. Use with caution in patients with conditions influenced by edema (eg, cardiovascular disease, migraine, seizure disorder, renal impairment); may cause fluid retention. Monitor women for signs of virilization (eg, deepening of voice, hirsutism, acne, clitoromegaly, menstrual irregularities); discontinue with evidence of mild virilization to prevent irreversible symptoms. Use with caution in elderly. Use with caution in hepatic impairment. May accelerate bone maturation without producing compensatory gain in linear growth in children. In prepubertal children, perform radiographic examination of the hand and wrist every 6 months to determine the rate of bone maturation and to assess the effect of treatment on the epiphyseal centers.

Adverse Reactions
Male: Gynecomastia, oligospermia (at higher doses), priapism, prostatic carcinoma, prostatic hypertrophy, testicular atrophy
Female: Menstrual irregularities (including amenorrhea), virilism (including deepening of the voice, clitoris hypertrophy)
Cardiovascular: Edema
Central nervous system: Anxiety, depression, headache
Dermatologic: Acne, hirsutism, "male pattern" baldness
Endocrine & metabolic: Electrolyte abnormalities (sodium, chloride, calcium, potassium, and inorganic phosphate retention), hypercholesterolemia, libido changes (increased or decreased), water retention
Gastrointestinal: GI irritation, nausea, vomiting
Genitourinary: Prostatic hyperplasia
Hematologic: Clotting factor suppression, polycythemia
Hepatic: Cholestatic jaundice, hepatic coma (rare), hepatic dysfunction, hepatocellular neoplasms (rare), liver function tests abnormal, peliosis hepatitis (rare)
Neuromuscular & skeletal: Paresthesia
Miscellaneous: Hypersensitivity, nonimmunologic anaphylaxis (formerly known as anaphylactoid reaction)
Rare but important or life-threatening: Hepatotoxicity (idiosyncratic) (Chalasani, 2014)

Drug Interactions
Metabolism/Transport Effects None known.
Avoid Concomitant Use There are no known interactions where it is recommended to avoid concomitant use.
Increased Effect/Toxicity
Fluoxymesterone may increase the levels/effects of: Blood Glucose Lowering Agents; C1 inhibitors; CycloSPORINE (Systemic); Vitamin K Antagonists

The levels/effects of Fluoxymesterone may be increased by: Corticosteroids (Systemic)
Decreased Effect There are no known significant interactions involving a decrease in effect.
Storage/Stability Store between 15°C to 30°C (59°F to 86°F); protect from light.
Mechanism of Action Synthetic derivative of testosterone; responsible for the normal growth and development of male sex hormones, male sex organs, and maintenance of secondary sex characteristics; large doses suppress endogenous testosterone release
Pharmacokinetics (Adult data unless noted)
Absorption: Oral: Rapid
Protein binding: 98%
Metabolism: In the liver
Half-life: 10-100 minutes
Elimination: Enterohepatic circulation and urinary excretion (90%)
Halogenated derivative of testosterone with up to 5 times the activity of methyltestosterone
Dosing: Usual Adults: Oral:
Male:
Hypogonadism: 5-20 mg/day
Delayed puberty: 2.5-20 mg/day for 4-6 months
Female:
Inoperable breast carcinoma: 10-40 mg/day in divided doses for 1-3 months
Breast engorgement: 2.5 mg after delivery, 5-10 mg/day in divided doses for 4-5 days
Administration Hazardous agent; use appropriate precautions for handling and disposal (NIOSH 2014 [group 2]).
Monitoring Parameters Periodic radiographic exams of hand and wrist (when used in children); hemoglobin, hematocrit (if receiving high dosages or long-term therapy)
Test Interactions Decreased levels of thyroxine-binding globulin; decreased total T_4 serum levels; increased resin uptake of T_3 and T_4
Controlled Substance C-III
Dosage Forms Excipient information presented when available (limited, particularly for generics); consult specific product labeling. [DSC] = Discontinued product
Tablet, Oral:
Androxy: 10 mg [DSC] [scored]

◆ **5-Fluracil** *see* Fluorouracil (Systemic) *on page 903*
◆ **Flura-Drops** *see* Fluoride *on page 899*

Flurandrenolide (flure an DREN oh lide)

Medication Safety Issues
Sound-alike/look-alike issues:
Cordran may be confused with Cardura, codeine, Cordarone
Related Information
Topical Corticosteroids *on page 2262*
Brand Names: US Cordran
Therapeutic Category Corticosteroid, Topical
Generic Availability (US) No

Use Inflammation of corticosteroid-responsive dermatoses (FDA approved in pediatric patients [age not specified] and adults)

Pregnancy Risk Factor C

Pregnancy Considerations Adverse events have been observed with corticosteroids in animal reproduction studies. When topical corticosteroids are needed during pregnancy, low- to mid-potency preparations are preferred; higher-potency preparations should be used for the shortest time possible and fetal growth should be monitored (Chi, 2011; Chi, 2013). Topical products are not recommended for extensive use, in large quantities, or for long periods of time in pregnant women (Leachman, 2006).

Breast-Feeding Considerations Corticosteroids are excreted in human milk; information specific to flurandrenolide has not been located. It is not known if systemic absorption following topical administration results in detectable quantities in human milk. The manufacturer recommends that caution be exercised when administering flurandrenolide to nursing women. Do not apply topical corticosteroids to nipples; hypertension was noted in a nursing infant exposed to a topical corticosteroid while nursing (Leachman, 2006).

Contraindications

Hypersensitivity to flurandrenolide or any component of the formulation; not recommended for lesions exuding serum or in intertriginous areas (tape)

Documentation of allergenic cross-reactivity for corticosteroids is limited. However, because of similarities in chemical structure and/or pharmacologic actions, the possibility of cross-sensitivity cannot be ruled out with certainty.

Warnings/Precautions Avoid contact with eyes; generally not for routine use on the face, underarms, or groin area (including diaper area). Avoid use with occlusive dressing unless directed by a health care provider. If no improvement is seen within 2 weeks, reassessment of diagnosis may be necessary. Systemic absorption of topical corticosteroids may cause hypothalamic-pituitary-adrenal (HPA) axis suppression (reversible), particularly in younger children. HPA axis suppression may lead to adrenal crisis. Risk is increased when used over large surface areas, for prolonged periods, or with occlusive dressings. Patients receiving large doses of potent topical steroids should be periodically evaluated for HPA axis suppression using urinary free cortisol and ACTH stimulation tests. Withdrawal and discontinuation of a corticosteroid should be done slowly and carefully by reducing the frequency of application or substitution of a less potent steroid. Recovery is usually prompt and complete upon drug discontinuation, but may require supplemental systemic corticosteroids if signs and symptoms of steroid withdrawal occur. Allergic contact dermatitis can occur and it is usually diagnosed by failure to heal rather than clinical exacerbation; discontinue if dermatological infection persists despite appropriate antimicrobial therapy. Prolonged treatment with corticosteroids has been associated with the development of Kaposi's sarcoma (case reports); if noted, discontinuation of therapy should be considered. Adverse systemic effects, including hyperglycemia and glycosuria, may occur when used on large surface areas, for prolonged periods, or with an occlusive dressing. Use appropriate antibacterial or antifungal agents to treat concomitant skin infections; discontinue flurandrenolide treatment if infection does not resolve promptly. Chronic use of corticosteroids in children may interfere with growth and development. The tape is most effective for dry, scaling, localized lesions.

Benzyl alcohol and derivatives: Some dosage forms may contain benzyl alcohol; large amounts of benzyl alcohol (≥99 mg/kg/day) have been associated with a potentially fatal toxicity ("gasping syndrome") in neonates; the "gasping syndrome" consists of metabolic acidosis, respiratory distress, gasping respirations, CNS dysfunction (including convulsions, intracranial hemorrhage), hypotension and cardiovascular collapse (AAP, 1997; CDC, 1982); some data suggests that benzoate displaces bilirubin from protein binding sites (Ahlfors, 2001); avoid or use dosage forms containing benzyl alcohol with caution in neonates. See manufacturer's labeling.

Warnings: Additional Pediatric Considerations Some dosage forms may contain propylene glycol; in neonates large amounts of propylene glycol delivered orally, intravenously (eg, >3,000 mg/day), or topically have been associated with potentially fatal toxicities which can include metabolic acidosis, seizures, renal failure, and CNS depression; toxicities have also been reported in children and adults including hyperosmolality, lactic acidosis, seizures, and respiratory depression; use caution (AAP, 1997; Shehab, 2009).

Adverse Reactions

Central nervous system: Burning sensation

Dermatologic: Acne vulgaris, acneiform eruptions, allergic contact dermatitis, atrophic striae, folliculitis, hypopigmentation, hypertrichosis, maceration of the skin, miliaria, perioral dermatitis, pruritus, skin atrophy, xeroderma

Local: Local irritation

Infection: Secondary infection

Rare but important or life-threatening: Hypersensitivity

Drug Interactions

Metabolism/Transport Effects None known.

Avoid Concomitant Use

Avoid concomitant use of Flurandrenolide with any of the following: Aldesleukin

Increased Effect/Toxicity

Flurandrenolide may increase the levels/effects of: Ceritinib; Deferasirox

The levels/effects of Flurandrenolide may be increased by: Telaprevir

Decreased Effect

Flurandrenolide may decrease the levels/effects of: Aldesleukin; Corticorelin; Hyaluronidase; Telaprevir

Storage/Stability

Cream, lotion, ointment: Store at 20°C to 25°C (68°F to 77°F); excursions are permitted between 15°C and 30°C (59°F and 86°F). Protect from light. Protect lotion from freezing.

Tape: Store at 20°C to 25°C (68°F to 77°F).

Mechanism of Action Topical corticosteroids have anti-inflammatory, antipruritic, and vasoconstrictive properties. May depress the formation, release, and activity of endogenous chemical mediators of inflammation (kinins, histamine, liposomal enzymes, prostaglandins) through the induction of phospholipase A_2 inhibitory proteins (lipocortins) and sequential inhibition of the release of arachidonic acid. Flurandrenolide has intermediate range potency.

Pharmacokinetics (Adult data unless noted)

Absorption: Topical corticosteroids are absorbed percutaneously. The extent is dependent on several factors, including epidermal integrity (intact vs abraded skin), formulation, and the use of occlusive dressings. Repeated applications of flurandrenolide may lead to depot effects on skin, potentially resulting in enhanced percutaneous.

Metabolism: Hepatic

Elimination: Urine; feces (small amounts)

Dosing: Usual Dosage should be based on severity of disease and patient response; use smallest amount for shortest period of time to avoid HPA axis suppression. If no improvement is seen within 2 weeks of therapy initiation, reassessment of diagnosis may be necessary. **Note:** Therapy should be discontinued when control is achieved.

Pediatric: **Dermatoses (steroid-responsive, including contact/atopic dermatitis):** Infants, Children, and Adolescents: Topical:

Cream, lotion, ointment: Apply small quantity or thin film 2 to 3 times daily

Tape: Apply 1 to 2 times daily

Adult: **Inflammation of corticosteroid-responsive dermatoses:**

Topical: Apply thin film to affected area 2 to 3 times per day

Tape: Apply 1 to 2 times per day

Dosing adjustment in renal impairment: There are no dosage adjustments provided in manufacturer's labeling.

Dosing adjustment in hepatic impairment: There are no dosage adjustments provided in manufacturer's labeling.

Administration

Cream, lotion, ointment: For external use only. Apply a thin film to clean, dry skin and rub in gently. Avoid contact with eyes; generally not for routine use on the face, underarms, or groin area. Use of occlusive dressings is not recommended unless directed by the health care provider. Do not use tight-fitting diapers or plastic pants on infants and children being treated in the diaper area. Shake lotion well before use.

Tape: Apply to clean, dry skin (allow skin to dry 1 hour before applying new tape). Shave or clip hair in the treatment area to promote adherence and easy removal. Do not tear tape; always cut. Use of occlusive dressings is not recommended unless used for management of psoriasis or recalcitrant conditions. Replacement of tape every 12 hours is best tolerated, but may be left in place for 24 hours if well tolerated. May be used just at night and removed during the day.

Monitoring Parameters Growth in pediatric patients; assess HPA axis suppression (eg, ACTH stimulation test, morning plasma cortisol test, urinary free cortisol test)

Additional Information Cream, lotion, ointment, tape: Intermediate potency corticosteroid

Dosage Forms Excipient information presented when available (limited, particularly for generics); consult specific product labeling.

Cream, External:

Cordran: 0.05% (15 g, 30 g, 60 g, 120 g) [contains cetyl alcohol, propylene glycol]

Lotion, External:

Cordran: 0.05% (15 mL, 60 mL, 120 mL) [contains benzyl alcohol, cetyl alcohol, menthol]

Ointment, External:

Cordran: 0.05% (60 g) [contains cetyl alcohol]

Tape, External:

Cordran: 4 mcg/cm^2 (1 ea)

◆ **Flurandrenolone** *see* Flurandrenolide *on page 911*

Flurazepam (flure AZ e pam)

Medication Safety Issues

Sound-alike/look-alike issues:

Flurazepam may be confused with temazepam

Dalmane may be confused with Demulen®

BEERS Criteria medication:

This drug may be potentially inappropriate for use in geriatric patients (Quality of evidence - high; Strength of recommendation - strong).

Brand Names: Canada Apo-Flurazepam; Bio-Flurazepam; Dalmane; PMS-Flurazepam; Som Pam

Therapeutic Category Benzodiazepine; Hypnotic; Sedative

Generic Availability (US) Yes

Use Short-term treatment of insomnia (FDA approved in ages ≥15 years)

Medication Guide Available Yes

Pregnancy Risk Factor C

Pregnancy Considerations

Adverse events have been observed in animal reproduction studies for benzodiazepines. All benzodiazepines are assumed to cross the placenta. Teratogenic effects have been observed with some benzodiazepines; however, additional studies are needed. The incidence of premature birth and low birth weights may be increased following maternal use of benzodiazepines; hypoglycemia and respiratory problems in the neonate may occur following exposure late in pregnancy. Neonatal withdrawal symptoms may occur within days to weeks after birth and "floppy infant syndrome" (which also includes withdrawal symptoms) has been reported with some benzodiazepines (Bergman, 1992; Iqbal, 2002; Wikner, 2007). Neonatal depression has been observed, specifically following exposure to flurazepam when used maternally for 10 consecutive days prior to delivery. Serum levels of N-desalkylflurazepam were measurable in the infant during the first 4 days of life. Use of flurazepam during pregnancy is contraindicated.

Patients exposed to flurazepam during pregnancy are encouraged to enroll themselves into the North American Antiepileptic Drug (NAAED) Pregnancy Registry by calling 1-888-233-2334. Additional information is available at http://www.aedpregnancyregistry.org.

Breast-Feeding Considerations Although information specific to flurazepam has not been located, all benzodiazepines are expected to be excreted into breast milk. Drowsiness, lethargy, or weight loss in nursing infants have been observed in case reports following maternal use of some benzodiazepines (Iqbal, 2002).

Contraindications

Hypersensitivity to flurazepam, other benzodiazepines, or any component of the formulation; pregnancy

Documentation of allergenic cross-reactivity for benzodiazepines is limited. However, because of similarities in chemical structure and/or pharmacologic actions, the possibility of cross-sensitivity cannot be ruled out with certainty.

Warnings/Precautions Use with caution in elderly or debilitated patients, patients with hepatic or renal impairment, and patients with respiratory disease.

Causes CNS depression (dose related); patients must be cautioned about performing tasks which require mental alertness (eg, operating machinery or driving). Use with caution in patients receiving other CNS depressants or psychoactive agents. Benzodiazepines have been associated with falls and traumatic injury and should be used with extreme caution in patients who are at risk of these events. In older adults, benzodiazepines increase the risk of impaired cognition, delirium, falls, fractures, and motor vehicle accidents. Due to increased sensitivity in this age group and slower metabolism of long-acting agents (such as flurazepam), avoid use for treatment of insomnia, agitation, or delirium (Beers Criteria).

Use caution in patients with depression, particularly if suicidal risk may be present. Minimize risks of overdose by prescribing the least amount of drug that is feasible in suicidal patients. Worsening of depressive symptoms has also been reported with use of benzodiazepines. Abnormal thinking and behavior changes including symptoms of decreased inhibition (eg, excessive aggressiveness and extroversion), bizarre behavior, agitation, hallucinations, and depersonalization have been reported with the use of benzodiazepine hypnotics. Some evidence suggests symptoms may be dose related. Use with caution in patients with a history of drug abuse or acute alcoholism; potential for drug dependency exists. Tolerance, psychological and physical dependence may occur with prolonged use. Rebound or withdrawal symptoms may occur following abrupt discontinuation or large decreases in dose. Use caution when reducing dose or withdrawing therapy; decrease slowly and monitor for withdrawal symptoms. Flumazenil may cause withdrawal in patients receiving long-term benzodiazepine therapy.

As a hypnotic, should be used only after evaluation of potential causes of sleep disturbance. Failure of sleep disturbance to resolve after 7 to 10 days may indicate psychiatric or medical illness. A worsening of insomnia or the emergence of new abnormalities of thought or behavior may represent unrecognized psychiatric or medical illness and requires immediate and careful evaluation. Reports of hypersensitivity reactions, including anaphylaxis and angioedema, have been reported with flurazepam. Patients who develop angioedema should not be rechallenged with flurazepam. An increased risk for hazardous sleep-related activities such as sleep-driving, cooking and eating food, having sex, and making phone calls while asleep have also been noted. Concurrent use of alcohol and other CNS depressants as well as increases in dose may increase the risk of these behaviors.

Benzodiazepines have been associated with anterograde amnesia. Paradoxical reactions have been reported, particularly in adolescent/pediatric or psychiatric patients. Flurazepam is a long half-life benzodiazepine. Duration of action after a single dose is determined by redistribution rather than metabolism. Tolerance develops to the hypnotic effects (Vinkers, 2012). Chronic use of this agent may increase the perioperative benzodiazepine dose needed to achieve desired effect. Does not have analgesic, antidepressant, or antipsychotic properties. Potentially significant drug-drug interactions may exist, requiring dose or frequency adjustment, additional monitoring, and/or selection of alternative therapy.

Adverse Reactions

Cardiovascular: Chest pain, flushing, hypotension, palpitation

Central nervous system: Apprehension, ataxia, confusion, depression, dizziness, drowsiness, euphoria, faintness, falling, hallucinations, hangover effect, headache, irritability, lightheadedness, memory impairment, nervousness, paradoxical reactions, restlessness, slurred speech, staggering, talkativeness

Dermatologic: Pruritus, rash

Gastrointestinal: Appetite increased/decreased, bitter taste, constipation, diarrhea, GI pain, heartburn, nausea, salivation increased/excessive, upset stomach, vomiting, weight gain/loss, xerostomia

Hematologic: Granulocytopenia, leukopenia

Hepatic: Alkaline phosphatase increased, ALT increased, AST increased, cholestatic jaundice, total bilirubin increased

Neuromuscular & skeletal: Body/joint pain, dysarthria, reflex slowing, weakness

Ocular: Blurred vision, burning eyes, difficulty focusing

Respiratory: Apnea, dyspnea

Miscellaneous: Diaphoresis, drug dependence

Postmarketing and/or case reports: Anaphylaxis, angioedema, complex sleep-related behavior (sleep-driving, cooking or eating food, making phone calls)

Drug Interactions

Metabolism/Transport Effects Substrate of CYP3A4 (major); **Note:** Assignment of Major/Minor substrate status based on clinically relevant drug interaction potential; **Inhibits** CYP2E1 (weak)

Avoid Concomitant Use

Avoid concomitant use of Flurazepam with any of the following: Azelastine (Nasal); Conivaptan; Fusidic Acid (Systemic); Idelalisib; Methadone; OLANZapine; Orphenadrine; Paraldehyde; Sodium Oxybate; Thalidomide

Increased Effect/Toxicity

Flurazepam may increase the levels/effects of: Alcohol (Ethyl); Azelastine (Nasal); Buprenorphine; CloZAPine; CNS Depressants; Hydrocodone; Methadone; Methotrimeprazine; Metyrosine; Mirtazapine; Orphenadrine; Paraldehyde; Pramipexole; ROPINIRole; Rotigotine; Selective Serotonin Reuptake Inhibitors; Sodium Oxybate; Suvorexant; Thalidomide; Zolpidem

The levels/effects of Flurazepam may be increased by: Aprepitant; Brimonidine (Topical); Cannabis; Conivaptan; CYP3A4 Inhibitors (Moderate); CYP3A4 Inhibitors (Strong); Dasatinib; Doxylamine; Dronabinol; Droperidol; Fosamprenavir; Fosaprepitant; Fusidic Acid (Systemic); HydrOXYzine; Idelalisib; Ivacaftor; Kava Kava; Luliconazole; Magnesium Sulfate; Methotrimeprazine; Mifepristone; Nabilone; Netupitant; OLANZapine; Palbociclib; Perampanel; Ritonavir; Rufinamide; Saquinavir; Simeprevir; Stiripentol; Tapentadol; Teduglutide; Tetrahydrocannabinol

Decreased Effect

The levels/effects of Flurazepam may be decreased by: Bosentan; CYP3A4 Inducers (Moderate); CYP3A4 Inducers (Strong); Dabrafenib; Deferasirox; Mitotane; Siltuximab; St Johns Wort; Theophylline Derivatives; Tocilizumab; Yohimbine

Food Interactions Benzodiazepine serum concentrations may be increased by grapefruit juice. Management: Limit or avoid grapefruit juice (Bjornsson, 2003).

Storage/Stability Store at 20°C to 25°C (68°F to 77°F); protect from light.

Mechanism of Action Binds to stereospecific benzodiazepine receptors on the postsynaptic GABA neuron at several sites within the central nervous system, including the limbic system, reticular formation. Enhancement of the inhibitory effect of GABA on neuronal excitability results by increased neuronal membrane permeability to chloride ions. This shift in chloride ions results in hyperpolarization (a less excitable state) and stabilization. Benzodiazepine receptors and effects appear to be linked to the GABA-A receptors. Benzodiazepines do not bind to GABA-B receptors (Vinkers, 2012).

Pharmacodynamics Hypnotic effects:

Onset of action: 15-20 minutes

Maximum effect: 3-6 hours

Duration: 7-8 hours

Pharmacokinetics (Adult data unless noted)

Absorption: Rapid

Distribution: V_d: Adults: 3.4 L/kg

Protein binding: ~97%

Metabolism: Hepatic to N-desalkylflurazepam (active) and N-hydroxyethylflurazepam

Half-life: Adults:
- Flurazepam: Mean: 2.3 hours
- N-desalkylflurazepam: Single dose: 74-90 hours; multiple doses: 111-113 hours

Time to peak serum concentration:
- Flurazepam: 30–60 minutes
- N-desalkylflurazepam: 10.6 hours (range: 7.6-13.6 hours)
- N-hydroxyethylflurazepam: ~1 hour

Elimination: Urine: N-hydroxyethylflurazepam (22% to 55%); N-desalkylflurazepam (<1%)

Dosing: Usual Oral:

Children:
- <15 years: Dose not established; use not recommended by manufacturer
- ≥15 years: 15 mg at bedtime

Adults: 15-30 mg at bedtime

Administration May be administered without regard to meals; administer dose at bedtime

Controlled Substance C-IV

Dosage Forms Excipient information presented when available (limited, particularly for generics); consult specific product labeling.

Capsule, Oral, as hydrochloride:

Generic: 15 mg, 30 mg

◆ **Flurazepam Hydrochloride** *see* Flurazepam *on page 913*

Flurbiprofen (Systemic) (flure BI proe fen)

Medication Safety Issues

Sound-alike/look-alike issues:

Flurbiprofen may be confused with fenoprofen

Ansaid may be confused with Asacol, Axid

Brand Names: Canada Alti-Flurbiprofen; Ansaid; Apo-Flurbiprofen; Froben; Froben-SR; Novo-Flurprofen; Nu-Flurprofen

Therapeutic Category Analgesic, Non-narcotic; Anti-inflammatory Agent; Nonsteroidal Anti-inflammatory Drug (NSAID), Oral

Generic Availability (US) Yes

Use Management of inflammatory disease and rheumatoid disorders, dysmenorrhea, pain

Medication Guide Available Yes

Pregnancy Risk Factor C

Pregnancy Considerations Adverse events were not observed in the initial animal reproduction studies; therefore, the manufacturer classifies flurbiprofen as pregnancy category C. NSAID exposure during the first trimester is not strongly associated with congenital malformations; however, cardiovascular anomalies and cleft palate have been observed following NSAID exposure in some studies. The use of an NSAID close to conception may be associated with an increased risk of miscarriage. Nonteratogenic effects have been observed following NSAID administration during the third trimester including myocardial degenerative changes, prenatal constriction of the ductus arteriosus, fetal tricuspid regurgitation, failure of the ductus arteriosus to close postnatally; renal dysfunction or failure, oligohydramnios; gastrointestinal bleeding or perforation, increased risk of necrotizing enterocolitis; intracranial bleeding (including intraventricular hemorrhage), platelet dysfunction with resultant bleeding; pulmonary hypertension. Because they may cause premature closure of the ductus arteriosus, use of NSAIDs late in pregnancy should be avoided (use after 31 or 32 weeks gestation is not recommended by some clinicians). The chronic use of NSAIDs in women of reproductive age may be associated with infertility that is reversible upon discontinuation of the medication.

Breast-Feeding Considerations Low levels of flurbiprofen are found in breast milk. Breast-feeding is not recommended by the manufacturer. The pharmacokinetics of flurbiprofen immediately postpartum are similar to healthy volunteers.

Contraindications Hypersensitivity to flurbiprofen, aspirin, other NSAIDs, or any component of the formulation; perioperative pain in the setting of coronary artery bypass (CABG) surgery

Warnings/Precautions **[U.S. Boxed Warning]: NSAIDs are associated with an increased risk of adverse cardiovascular thrombotic events, including MI and stroke.** Risk may be increased with duration of use or preexisting cardiovascular risk factors or disease. Carefully evaluate individual cardiovascular risk profiles prior to prescribing. May cause new-onset hypertension or worsening of existing hypertension. Use caution with fluid retention. Avoid use in heart failure (ACCF/AHA [Yancy, 2013]). Concurrent administration of ibuprofen, and potentially other nonselective NSAIDs, may interfere with aspirin's cardioprotective effect. **[U.S. Boxed Warning]: Use is contraindicated for treatment of perioperative pain in the setting of coronary artery bypass graft (CABG) surgery.** Risk of MI and stroke may be increased with use following CABG surgery.

Platelet adhesion and aggregation may be decreased; may prolong bleeding time; patients with coagulation disorders or who are receiving anticoagulants should be monitored closely. Anemia may occur; patients on long-term NSAID therapy should be monitored for anemia. NSAID use may compromise existing renal function; dose-dependent decreases in prostaglandin synthesis may result from NSAID use, reducing renal blood flow which may cause renal decompensation. Patients with impaired renal function, dehydration, heart failure, liver dysfunction, those taking diuretics, and ACE inhibitors, and the elderly are at greater risk of renal toxicity. Rehydrate patient before starting therapy; monitor renal function closely. Not recommended for use in patients with advanced renal disease. Long-term NSAID use may result in renal papillary necrosis.

[U.S. Boxed Warning]: NSAIDs may increase risk of gastrointestinal irritation, inflammation, ulceration, bleeding, and perforation. These events may occur at any time during therapy and without warning. Use caution with a history of GI disease (bleeding or ulcers), concurrent therapy with aspirin, anticoagulants and/or corticosteroids, smoking, use of alcohol, the elderly, or debilitated patients. When used concomitantly with aspirin, a substantial increase in the risk of gastrointestinal complications (eg, ulcer) occurs; concomitant gastroprotective therapy (eg, proton pump inhibitors) is recommended (Bhatt, 2008).

Use the lowest effective dose for the shortest duration of time, consistent with individual patient goals, to reduce risk of cardiovascular or GI adverse events. Alternate therapies should be considered for patients at high risk.

NSAIDs may cause serious skin adverse events including exfoliative dermatitis, Stevens-Johnson syndrome (SJS), and toxic epidermal necrolysis (TEN); discontinue use at first sign of skin rash or hypersensitivity. Anaphylactoid reactions may occur, even without prior exposure; patients with "aspirin triad" (bronchial asthma, aspirin intolerance, rhinitis) may be at increased risk. Do not use in patients who experience bronchospasm, asthma, rhinitis, or urticaria with NSAID or aspirin therapy. Use caution in other forms of asthma.

Use with caution in patients with decreased hepatic function. Closely monitor patients with any abnormal LFT. Severe hepatic reactions (eg, fulminant hepatitis, liver failure) have occurred with NSAID use, rarely; discontinue if signs or symptoms of liver disease develop, or if systemic manifestations occur.

The elderly are at increased risk for adverse effects (especially peptic ulceration, CNS effects, renal toxicity) from NSAIDs even at low doses.

Withhold for at least 4-6 half-lives prior to surgical or dental procedures. Safety and efficacy have not been established in children.

Adverse Reactions

Cardiovascular: Edema

Central nervous system: Amnesia, anxiety, depression, dizziness, headache, insomnia, malaise, nervousness, somnolence, vertigo

Dermatologic: Rash

Gastrointestinal: Abdominal pain, constipation, diarrhea, dyspepsia, flatulence, GI bleeding, nausea, vomiting, weight changes

Hepatic: Liver enzymes increased

Neuromuscular & skeletal: Reflexes increased, tremor, weakness

Ocular: Vision changes
Otic: Tinnitus
Respiratory: Rhinitis
Rare but important or life-threatening: Anaphylactic reaction, anemia, angioedema, asthma, bruising, cerebrovascular ischemia, CHF, confusion, eczema, eosinophilia, epistaxis, exfoliative dermatitis, fever, gastric/peptic ulcer, hematocrit increased, hematuria, hemoglobin decreased, hepatitis, hepatotoxicity (idiosyncratic) (Chalasani, 2014), hypertension, hyperuricemia, interstitial nephritis, jaundice, leukopenia, paresthesia, parosmia, photosensitivity, pruritus, purpura, renal failure, stomatitis, thrombocytopenia, toxic epidermal necrolysis, urticaria, vasodilation

Drug Interactions

Metabolism/Transport Effects **Substrate** of CYP2C9 (minor); **Note:** Assignment of Major/Minor substrate status based on clinically relevant drug interaction potential; **Inhibits** CYP2C9 (weak)

Avoid Concomitant Use

Avoid concomitant use of Flurbiprofen (Systemic) with any of the following: Dexketoprofen; Floctafenine; Ketorolac (Nasal); Ketorolac (Systemic); Morniflumate; NSAID (COX-2 Inhibitor); Omacetaxine; Urokinase

Increased Effect/Toxicity

Flurbiprofen (Systemic) may increase the levels/effects of: 5-ASA Derivatives; Agents with Antiplatelet Properties; Aliskiren; Aminoglycosides; Anticoagulants; Apixaban; Bisphosphonate Derivatives; Collagenase (Systemic); CycloSPORINE (Systemic); Dabigatran Etexilate; Deferasirox; Deoxycholic Acid; Desmopressin; Digoxin; Drospirenone; Eplerenone; Haloperidol; Ibritumomab; Lithium; Methotrexate; Nonsteroidal Anti-Inflammatory Agents; NSAID (COX-2 Inhibitor); Obinutuzumab; Omacetaxine; PEMEtrexed; Porfimer; Potassium-Sparing Diuretics; PRALAtrexate; Quinolone Antibiotics; Rivaroxaban; Salicylates; Tacrolimus (Systemic); Tenofovir; Thrombolytic Agents; Tositumomab and Iodine I 131 Tositumomab; Urokinase; Vancomycin; Verteporfin; Vitamin K Antagonists

The levels/effects of Flurbiprofen (Systemic) may be increased by: ACE Inhibitors; Angiotensin II Receptor Blockers; Antidepressants (Tricyclic, Tertiary Amine); Corticosteroids (Systemic); CycloSPORINE (Systemic); Dasatinib; Dexketoprofen; Diclofenac (Systemic); Floctafenine; Glucosamine; Herbs (Anticoagulant/Antiplatelet Properties); Ibrutinib; Ketorolac (Nasal); Ketorolac (Systemic); Limaprost; Morniflumate; Multivitamins/Fluoride (with ADE); Multivitamins/Minerals (with ADEK, Folate, Iron); Multivitamins/Minerals (with AE, No Iron); Omega-3 Fatty Acids; Pentosan Polysulfate Sodium; Pentoxifylline; Probenecid; Prostacyclin Analogues; Selective Serotonin Reuptake Inhibitors; Serotonin/Norepinephrine Reuptake Inhibitors; Sodium Phosphates; Tipranavir; Treprostinil; Vitamin E

Decreased Effect

Flurbiprofen (Systemic) may decrease the levels/effects of: ACE Inhibitors; Aliskiren; Angiotensin II Receptor Blockers; Beta-Blockers; Eplerenone; HydrALAZINE; Loop Diuretics; Potassium-Sparing Diuretics; Prostaglandins (Ophthalmic); Salicylates; Selective Serotonin Reuptake Inhibitors; Thiazide Diuretics

The levels/effects of Flurbiprofen (Systemic) may be decreased by: Bile Acid Sequestrants; Salicylates

Food Interactions Food may decrease the rate but not the extent of absorption. Management: May administer with food, milk, or antacid to decrease GI effects.

Mechanism of Action Reversibly inhibits cyclooxygenase-1 and 2 (COX-1 and 2) enzymes, which results in decreased formation of prostaglandin precursors; has antipyretic, analgesic, and anti-inflammatory properties

Other proposed mechanisms not fully elucidated (and possibly contributing to the anti-inflammatory effect to varying degrees), include inhibiting chemotaxis, altering lymphocyte activity, inhibiting neutrophil aggregation/activation, and decreasing proinflammatory cytokine levels.

Pharmacokinetics (Adult data unless noted)

Time to peak serum concentration: Within 1.5-2 hours
Elimination: 95% in urine

Dosing: Usual Adults: Oral:

Arthritis: 200-300 mg/day in 2-4 divided doses; maximum dose: 100 mg/dose; maximum: 300 mg/day
Dysmenorrhea: 50 mg 4 times/day

Administration Administer with food, milk, or antacid to decrease GI effects.

Monitoring Parameters CBC, platelets, BUN, serum creatinine, liver enzymes, occult blood loss

Dosage Forms Excipient information presented when available (limited, particularly for generics); consult specific product labeling.

Tablet, Oral:
Generic: 50 mg, 100 mg

Flurbiprofen (Ophthalmic) (flure BI proe fen)

Medication Safety Issues

Sound-alike/look-alike issues:

Flurbiprofen may be confused with fenoprofen
Ocufen® may be confused with Ocuflox®

International issues:

Ocufen [U.S., Canada, and multiple international markets] may be confused with Ocupres brand name for timolol [India]; Ocupress brand name for dorzolamide [Brazil]

Brand Names: US Ocufen

Therapeutic Category Anti-inflammatory Agent, Ophthalmic; Nonsteroidal Anti-inflammatory Drug (NSAID), Ophthalmic

Generic Availability (US) Yes

Use For inhibition of intraoperative trauma-induced miosis; the value of flurbiprofen for the prevention and management of postoperative ocular inflammation and postoperative cystoid macular edema remains to be determined

Pregnancy Risk Factor C

Pregnancy Considerations Adverse events were observed following systemic administration of flurbiprofen in animal reproduction studies; therefore, flurbiprofen ophthalmic is classified as pregnancy category C. Information related to systemic absorption following topical application of the eye drops has not been located. Systemic absorption would be required in order for flurbiprofen to cross the placenta and reach the fetus. Refer to the Flurbiprofen (Systemic) monograph for additional information.

Breast-Feeding Considerations When administered orally, flurbiprofen enters breast milk. Refer to the Flurbiprofen (Systemic) monograph for details. Information related to systemic absorption following topical application of the eye drops has not been located. Systemic absorption would be required in order for flurbiprofen to enter breast milk. Breast-feeding is not recommended by the manufacturer.

Contraindications Hypersensitivity to flurbiprofen or any component of the formulation

Warnings/Precautions Use with caution in patients with previous sensitivity to aspirin or other NSAIDs, including patients who experience bronchospasm, asthma, rhinitis, or urticaria following NSAID or aspirin. May increase bleeding time associated with ocular surgery. Use with caution in patients with known bleeding tendencies or those receiving anticoagulants. Healing time may be slowed or delayed. To minimize the risk of infection following surgery of both eyes, two separate bottles of eye drops (one for each eye) should be used; instruct patients not to use the same bottle for both eyes.

Adverse Reactions Ocular: Bleeding tendency increased in ocular tissue (in conjunction with ocular surgery), burning (transient), fibrosis, hyperemia, hyphemia, irritation, miosis, mydriasis, stinging (transient)

Drug Interactions

Metabolism/Transport Effects None known.

Avoid Concomitant Use There are no known interactions where it is recommended to avoid concomitant use.

Increased Effect/Toxicity

Flurbiprofen (Ophthalmic) may increase the levels/effects of: Corticosteroids (Ophthalmic)

Decreased Effect There are no known significant interactions involving a decrease in effect.

Storage/Stability Store at 15°C to 25°C (59°F to 79°F).

Mechanism of Action Reversibly inhibits cyclooxygenase-1 and 2 (COX-1 and 2) enzymes, which results in decreased formation of prostaglandin precursors; has antipyretic, analgesic, and anti-inflammatory properties

Other proposed mechanisms not fully elucidated (and possibly contributing to the anti-inflammatory effect to varying degrees), include inhibiting chemotaxis, altering lymphocyte activity, inhibiting neutrophil aggregation/activation, and decreasing proinflammatory cytokine levels.

Dosing: Usual Children and Adults: Instill 1 drop every 30 minutes starting 2 hours prior to surgery (total of 4 drops to each affected eye)

Administration Instill drops into affected eye(s); avoid contact of container tip with skin or eye; apply finger pressure to lacrimal sac during and for 1-2 minutes after instillation to decrease risk of absorption and systemic effects

Monitoring Parameters Periodic eye exams

Dosage Forms Excipient information presented when available (limited, particularly for generics); consult specific product labeling.

Solution, Ophthalmic, as sodium:

Ocufen: 0.03% (2.5 mL) [contains edetate disodium, thimerosal]

Generic: 0.03% (2.5 mL)

◆ **Flurbiprofen Sodium** *see* Flurbiprofen (Ophthalmic) *on page 916*

◆ **Flurbiprofen Sodium** *see* Flurbiprofen (Systemic) *on page 915*

◆ **5-Flurocytosine** *see* Flucytosine *on page 886*

Fluticasone (Nasal) (floo TIK a sone)

Medication Safety Issues

Sound-alike/look-alike issues:

Flonase may be confused with Flovent

International issues:

Allegro: Brand name for fluticasone [Israel], but also the brand name for frovatriptan [Germany]

Allegro [Israel] may be confused with Allegra and Allegra-D brand names for fexofenadine and fexofenadine/pseudoephedrine, respectively, [US, Canada, and multiple international markets]

Brand Names: US Flonase Allergy Relief [OTC]; Flonase [DSC]; Veramyst

Brand Names: Canada Apo-Fluticasone; Avamys; Flonase; ratio-Fluticasone

Therapeutic Category Corticosteroid, Intranasal

Generic Availability (US) Yes

Use

Flonase®: Management of nasal symptoms associated with seasonal and perennial allergic rhinitis and nonallergic rhinitis (FDA approved in ages ≥4 years and adults)

Veramyst®: Management of nasal symptoms associated with seasonal and perennial allergic rhinitis (FDA approved in ages ≥2 years and adults)

Intranasal corticosteroids have also been used as an adjunct to antibiotics in empiric treatment of acute bacterial rhinosinusitis primarily in patients with history of allergic rhinitis (Chow, 2012) and in pediatric patients with mild obstructive sleep apnea syndrome who cannot undergo adenotonsillectomy or who still have symptoms after surgery (Marcus, 2012).

Pregnancy Risk Factor C

Pregnancy Considerations Adverse events have been observed in some animal reproduction studies. Hypoadrenalism may occur in newborns following maternal use of corticosteroids in pregnancy; monitor. Intranasal corticosteroids are recommended for the treatment of rhinitis during pregnancy; the lowest effective dose should be used (NAEPP 2005; Wallace 2008).

Breast-Feeding Considerations Systemic corticosteroids are excreted in human milk. It is not known if sufficient quantities of fluticasone are absorbed following inhalation to produce detectable amounts in breast milk. The manufacturer recommends caution be used if administered to nursing women. The use of inhaled corticosteroids is not considered a contraindication to breast-feeding (NAEPP 2005).

Contraindications Hypersensitivity to fluticasone or any component of the formulation

OTC labeling: When used for self-medication, do not use in children <4 years of age, for the treatment of asthma, or with current injury or surgery to nose that is not fully healed

Documentation of allergenic cross-reactivity for intranasal steroids is limited. However, because of similarities in chemical structure and/or pharmacologic actions, the possibility of cross-sensitivity cannot be ruled out with certainty.

Warnings/Precautions May cause hypercorticism or suppression of hypothalamic-pituitary-adrenal (HPA) axis, particularly in younger children or in patients receiving high doses for prolonged periods. HPA axis suppression may lead to adrenal crisis. Withdrawal and discontinuation of a corticosteroid should be done slowly and carefully. Pediatric patients may be more susceptible to systemic toxicity. Particular care is required when patients are transferred from systemic corticosteroids to inhaled products due to possible adrenal insufficiency or withdrawal from steroids, including an increase in allergic symptoms. Patients receiving ≥20 mg per day of prednisone (or equivalent) may be most susceptible. Concurrent use of ritonavir (and potentially other strong inhibitors of CYP3A4) may increase fluticasone levels and effects on HPA suppression.

Hypersensitivity reactions (including anaphylaxis, angioedema, rash, contact dermatitis, and urticaria) have been reported; discontinue for severe reactions. Prolonged use of corticosteroids may also increase the incidence of secondary infection, mask acute infection (including fungal infections), prolong or exacerbate viral infections, or limit response to vaccines. Exposure to chickenpox and/or measles should be avoided; especially if not immunized. Avoid use or use with caution in patients with latent/active tuberculosis, systemic fungal, bacterial, viral, or parasitic infections, or ocular herpes simplex. Avoid nasal corticosteroid use in patients with recent nasal septal ulcers, nasal surgery, or nasal trauma until healing has occurred. Nasal septal perforation, nasal ulceration, epistaxis, and localized *Candida albicans* infections of the nose and/or pharynx may occur. Monitor patients periodically for adverse nasal effects; discontinuation of therapy may be necessary if an infection occurs.

Use caution or avoid in patients with active or latent tuberculosis or in patients with untreated fungal, bacterial, or systemic viral infections. Do not use in untreated localized infection involving the nasal mucosa; concurrent antimicrobial therapy should be administered if bacterial infection of the sinuses is suspected/confirmed. Use with caution in patients with cataracts and/or glaucoma; increased intraocular pressure, open-angle glaucoma, and cataracts have occurred with prolonged use. Consider routine eye exams in long-term users or in patients who report visual changes.

Avoid using higher than recommended dosages; suppression of linear growth (ie, reduction of growth velocity), reduced bone mineral density, or hypercorticism (Cushing's syndrome) may occur; titrate to lowest effective dose. Reduction in growth velocity may occur when corticosteroids are administered to pediatric patients, even at recommended doses via intranasal route (monitor growth).

Prior to use, the dose and duration of treatment should be based on the risk vs benefit for each individual patient. In general, use the smallest effective dose for the shortest duration of time to minimize adverse events. There have been reports of systemic corticosteroid withdrawal symptoms (eg, joint/muscle pain, lassitude, depression) when withdrawing inhalation therapy. Discontinue OTC use and contact healthcare provider if symptoms do not begin to improve after 7 days or new symptoms occur (eg, facial pain, thick nasal discharge, nosebleeds, whistling sound from the nose). Use with caution in patients with moderate to severe hepatic impairment (accumulation may occur); monitor patients closely. Potentially significant interactions may exist, requiring dose or frequency adjustment, additional monitoring, and/or selection of alternative therapy.

Warnings: Additional Pediatric Considerations In a small pediatric study conducted over one year, no statistically significant effect on growth velocity or clinically relevant changes in bone mineral density or HPA axis function were observed in children 3 to 9 years of age receiving fluticasone propionate nasal spray (200 mcg/day; n=56) versus placebo (n=52); effects at higher doses or in susceptible pediatric patients cannot be ruled out.

Adverse Reactions

Central nervous system: Dizziness, fever, headache

Gastrointestinal: Abdominal pain, diarrhea, nausea, vomiting

Neuromuscular & skeletal: Back pain

Respiratory: Asthma symptoms, blood in nasal mucous, bronchitis, cough, epistaxis, nasal ulcer, pharyngitis, pharyngolaryngeal pain, runny nose

Miscellaneous: Aches and pains, flu-like syndrome

Rare but important or life-threatening: Alteration or loss of sense of taste and/or smell, anaphylaxis/anaphylactoid reactions, angioedema, AST increased, AV block (second degree), cataracts, conjunctivitis, glaucoma, hypersensitivity reactions, increased intraocular pressure, nasal candidiasis, nasal septal perforation (rare), psychomotor hyperactivity, skin rash, tremor, vaginal candidiasis

Drug Interactions

Metabolism/Transport Effects **Substrate** of CYP3A4 (minor); **Note:** Assignment of Major/Minor substrate status based on clinically relevant drug interaction potential

Avoid Concomitant Use

Avoid concomitant use of Fluticasone (Nasal) with any of the following: Ritonavir; Tipranavir

Increased Effect/Toxicity

Fluticasone (Nasal) may increase the levels/effects of: Ceritinib

The levels/effects of Fluticasone (Nasal) may be increased by: Cobicistat; CYP3A4 Inhibitors (Strong); Ritonavir; Telaprevir; Tipranavir

Decreased Effect There are no known significant interactions involving a decrease in effect.

Storage/Stability

Flonase: Store between 4°C to 30°C (39°F to 86°F).

Veramyst: Store between 15°C to 30°C (59°F to 86°F); do not refrigerate or freeze. Store in upright position with cap on.

Avamys [Canadian product]: Store between 4°C to 30°C (39°F to 86°F); do not refrigerate or freeze. Store in upright position with cap on.

Mechanism of Action Fluticasone belongs to a group of corticosteroids which utilizes a fluorocarbothioate ester linkage at the 17 carbon position; extremely potent vasoconstrictive and anti-inflammatory activity

Pharmacodynamics Onset of action: Variable; may occur within 24 hours

Pharmacokinetics (Adult data unless noted) Bioavailability: ≤2 %

Dosing: Usual Note: Product formulations are not interchangeable: Flonase®: One spray delivers 50 mcg; Veramyst®: One spray delivers 27.5 mcg

Children and Adolescents: **Seasonal and perennial rhinitis:** Intranasal: **Note:** For optimal effects, nasal spray should be used at regular intervals (eg, once or twice daily); however, some patients ≥12 years of age with seasonal allergic rhinitis may have effective control of symptoms with prn (as needed) use.

Flonase® (fluticasone propionate): Children ≥4 years and Adolescents: Initial: 100 mcg once daily delivered as 50 mcg (1 spray) **per nostril** once daily. If response is inadequate, increase to 200 mcg once daily given as 100 mcg (2 sprays) **per nostril** once daily. Once symptoms are controlled, reduce dose to 100 mcg once daily delivered as 50 mcg (1 spray) **per nostril** once daily.

Veramyst® (fluticasone furoate):

Children 2-11 years: Initial: 55 mcg once daily delivered as 27.5 mcg (1 spray) **per nostril** once daily; if response is inadequate, increase to 110 mcg once daily delivered as 55 mcg (2 sprays) **per nostril** once daily; once symptoms have been controlled, the dosage may be reduced to 55 mcg once daily delivered as 27.5 mcg (1 spray) **per nostril** once daily

Children ≥12 years and Adolescents: Initial: 110 mcg once daily delivered as 55 mcg (2 sprays) **per nostril** once daily; once symptoms are controlled, dosage may be reduced to 55 mcg once daily delivered as 27.5 mcg (1 spray) **per nostril** once daily

Adults: **Seasonal and perennial rhinitis:** Intranasal: **Note:** For optimal effects, nasal spray should be used at regular intervals (eg, once or twice daily); however, some adult patients with seasonal allergic rhinitis may have effective control of symptoms with prn (as needed) use.

Flonase® (fluticasone propionate): Initial: 200 mcg once daily delivered as 100 mcg (2 sprays) **per nostril** once daily; alternatively, the same total daily dosage may be divided and given as 100 mcg twice daily administered as 50 mcg (1 spray) **per nostril** twice daily. After the first few days, dosage may be reduced to 100 mcg once daily delivered as 50 mcg (1 spray) **per nostril** once daily for maintenance therapy.

Veramyst® (fluticasone furoate): Initial: 110 mcg once daily delivered as 55 mcg (2 sprays) **per nostril** once daily; once symptoms are controlled, may reduce dosage to 55 mcg once daily delivered as 27.5 mcg (1 spray) **per nostril** once daily for maintenance therapy.

Dosing adjustment in renal impairment: No adjustment required.

Dosing adjustment in hepatic impairment: There are no dosage adjustments provided in the manufacturer's labeling. Use with caution in patients with severe hepatic impairment; systemic availability of fluticasone may be increased in patients with hepatic impairment.

Administration Shake well prior to each use. Blow nose to clear nostrils before each use. Insert applicator into nostril, keeping bottle upright, and close off the other nostril. Breathe in through nose. While inhaling, press pump to release spray. Do not spray into eyes. Discard after labeled number of doses has been used, even if bottle is not completely empty.

Flonase®: Prime pump (press 6 times until fine spray appears) prior to first use or if spray unused for ≥7 days.

Veramyst®: Prime pump (press 6 times until fine spray appears) prior to first use, if spray unused for >30 days, or if cap left off bottle for ≥5 days.

Monitoring Parameters Mucous membranes for signs of fungal infection, growth (pediatric patients), signs/symptoms of HPA axis suppression/adrenal insufficiency; ocular changes

Additional Information When used short term as adjunctive therapy in acute bacterial rhinosinusitis (ABRS), intranasal steroids show modest symptomatic improvement and few adverse effects, improvement is primarily due to increased sinus drainage. Use should be considered optional in ABRS; however, intranasal corticosteroids should be routinely prescribed to ABRS patients who have a history of or concurrent allergic rhinitis (Chow, 2012).

Dosage Forms Considerations Flonase 16 g bottles and Veramyst 10 g bottles contain 120 sprays each.

Dosage Forms Excipient information presented when available (limited, particularly for generics); consult specific product labeling. [DSC] = Discontinued product

Suspension, Nasal, as furoate:

Veramyst: 27.5 mcg/spray (10 g) [contains benzalkonium chloride]

Suspension, Nasal, as propionate:

Flonase: 50 mcg/actuation (16 g [DSC]) [contains benzalkonium chloride, polysorbate 80]

Flonase Allergy Relief: 50 mcg/actuation (9.9 mL, 15.8 mL) [contains benzalkonium chloride, polysorbate 80]

Generic: 50 mcg/actuation (16 g); 50 mcg/actuation (16 g)

Fluticasone (Oral Inhalation) (floo TIK a sone)

Medication Safety Issues

Sound-alike/look-alike issues:

Flovent may be confused with Flonase

International issues:

Allegro: Brand name for fluticasone [Israel], but also the brand name for frovatriptan [Germany]

Allegro [Israel] may be confused with Allegra and Allegra-D brand names for fexofenadine and fexofenadine/pseudoephedrine, respectively [US, Canada, and multiple international markets]

Flovent [US, Canada] may be confused with Flogen brand name for naproxen [Mexico]; Flogene brand name for piroxicam [Brazil]

Related Information

Inhaled Corticosteroids *on page 2261*

Brand Names: US Arnuity Ellipta; Flovent Diskus; Flovent HFA

Brand Names: Canada Flovent Diskus; Flovent HFA

Therapeutic Category Adrenal Corticosteroid; Anti-inflammatory Agent; Antiasthmatic; Corticosteroid, Inhalant (Oral); Glucocorticoid

Generic Availability (US) No

Use Oral inhalation: Long-term (chronic) control of persistent bronchial asthma; **not** indicated for the relief of acute bronchospasm. Also used to help reduce or discontinue oral corticosteroid therapy for asthma (FDA approved in ages ≥4 years and adults)

Oral (swallowed; using metered dose inhaler): Has been used for eosinophilic esophagitis

Pregnancy Risk Factor C

Pregnancy Considerations Adverse events were observed in some animal reproduction studies. Hypoadrenalism may occur in infants born to mothers receiving corticosteroids during pregnancy. Based on available data, an overall increased risk of congenital malformations or a decrease in fetal growth has not been associated with maternal use of inhaled corticosteroids during pregnancy (Bakhireva, 2005; NAEPP, 2005; Namazy, 2004). Uncontrolled asthma is associated with adverse events in pregnancy (increased risk of perinatal mortality, pre-eclampsia, preterm birth, low birth weight infants). Inhaled corticosteroids are recommended for the treatment of asthma during pregnancy (most information available using budesonide) (ACOG, 2008; NAEPP, 2005).

Breast-Feeding Considerations Systemic corticosteroids are excreted in human milk. It is not known if sufficient quantities of fluticasone are absorbed following inhalation to produce detectable amounts in breast milk. The manufacturer recommends that caution be exercised when administering fluticasone to nursing women. The use of inhaled corticosteroids is not considered a contraindication to breast-feeding (NAEPP, 2005).

Contraindications

Hypersensitivity to fluticasone or any component of the formulation; severe hypersensitivity to milk proteins or lactose (Arnuity Ellipta and Flovent Diskus); primary treatment of status asthmaticus or other acute episodes of asthma requiring intensive measures

Documentation of allergenic cross-reactivity for corticosteroids in this class is limited. However, because of similarities in chemical structure and/or pharmacologic actions, the possibility of cross-sensitivity cannot be ruled out with certainty.

Canadian labeling: Additional contraindications (not in US labeling): Moderate-to-severe bronchiectasis; untreated fungal, bacterial or tubercular infections of the respiratory tract

Warnings/Precautions May cause hypercorticism or suppression of hypothalamic-pituitary-adrenal (HPA) axis. HPA axis suppression may lead to adrenal crisis. Withdrawal and discontinuation of a corticosteroid should be done slowly and carefully. Particular care is required when patients are transferred from systemic corticosteroids to inhaled corticosteroids due to possible adrenal insufficiency or withdrawal from steroids, including an increase in allergic symptoms. Patients receiving ≥20 mg per day of prednisone (or equivalent) may be most susceptible. Fatalities have occurred due to adrenal insufficiency in asthmatic patients during and after transfer from systemic corticosteroids to aerosol steroids; aerosol steroids do **not** provide the systemic steroid needed to treat patients having trauma, surgery, or infections. Select surgical patients on long-term, high-dose, inhaled corticosteroid (ICS), should be given stress doses of hydrocortisone intravenously during the surgical period and the dose reduced rapidly within 24 hours after surgery (NAEPP, 2007).

Bronchospasm may occur with wheezing after inhalation; if this occurs, stop steroid and treat with a fast-acting bronchodilator. Hypersensitivity reactions including, allergic dermatitis, anaphylaxis, angioedema, bronchospasm, flushing, hypotension, urticaria, and rash have been reported. Supplemental steroids (oral or parenteral) may be needed during stress or severe asthma attacks. Corticosteroid use may cause psychiatric disturbances, including depression, euphoria, insomnia, mood swings, and personality changes. Preexisting psychiatric conditions may be exacerbated by corticosteroid use. Prolonged use of corticosteroids may also increase the incidence of secondary infection, mask acute infection (including fungal infections), prolong or exacerbate viral infections, or limit response to vaccines. Avoid use if possible in patients with ocular herpes; active or quiescent tuberculosis infections of the respiratory tract; or untreated viral, fungal, parasitic or bacterial systemic infections (Canadian labeling contraindicates use with untreated respiratory infections). Exposure to chickenpox and measles should be avoided; if the patient is exposed, prophylaxis with varicella zoster immune globulin or pooled intramuscular immunoglobulin, respectively, may be indicated; if chickenpox develops, treatment with antiviral agents may be considered. Rare cases of vasculitis (Churg-Strauss syndrome) or other systemic eosinophilic conditions can occur. Prolonged treatment with corticosteroids has been associated with the development of Kaposi's sarcoma (case reports); if noted, discontinuation of therapy should be considered.

Use with caution in patients with thyroid disease, hepatic impairment, renal impairment, cardiovascular disease, diabetes, glaucoma, cataracts, myasthenia gravis, patients at risk for osteoporosis, patients at risk for seizures, or GI diseases (diverticulitis, peptic ulcer, ulcerative colitis) due to perforation risk. Use caution following acute MI (corticosteroids have been associated with myocardial rupture). When transferring to oral inhaler, previously-suppressed allergic conditions (rhinitis, conjunctivitis, eczema) may be unmasked.

Orally-inhaled corticosteroids may cause a reduction in growth velocity in pediatric patients (~1 centimeter per year [range: 0.3-1.8 cm per year] and related to dose and duration of exposure). To minimize the systemic effects of orally-inhaled corticosteroids, each patient should be titrated to the lowest effective dose. Growth should be routinely monitored in pediatric patients.

Potentially significant drug-drug interactions may exist, requiring dose or frequency adjustment, additional monitoring, and/or selection of alternative therapy. Not to be used in status asthmaticus or for the relief of acute bronchospasm. Flovent Diskus and Arnuity Ellipta contain lactose; very rare anaphylactic reactions have been reported in patients with severe milk protein allergy. Withdraw systemic corticosteroid therapy with gradual tapering of dose; consider reducing the daily prednisone dose by 2.5 to 5 mg on a weekly basis beginning at least 1 week after inhalation therapy. Monitor lung function, beta-agonist use, asthma symptoms, and for signs and symptoms of adrenal insufficiency (fatigue, lassitude, weakness, nausea and vomiting, hypotension) during withdrawal. Local yeast infections (eg, oropharyngeal candidiasis) may occur.

Adverse Reactions

Cardiovascular: Hypertension, subarachnoid hemorrhage

Central nervous system: Fatigue, headache, herniated disk, malaise, pain, procedural pain, voice disorder

Dermatologic: Skin rash, pruritus

Gastrointestinal: Abdominal pain, gastrointestinal distress, gastrointestinal pain, nausea and vomiting, oral candidiasis, oropharyngeal candidiasis, toothache, viral gastroenteritis, viral gastrointestinal infection

Hematologic & oncologic: Malignant neoplasm of breast

Infection: Abscess, influenza, viral infection

Neuromuscular & skeletal: Arthralgia, arthritis, back pain, muscle injury, musculoskeletal pain

Respiratory: Allergic rhinitis, bronchitis, cough, hoarseness, nasal congestion, nasopharyngitis, oropharyngeal pain, pharyngitis, rhinitis, sinus infection, sinusitis, throat irritation, upper respiratory tract infection, upper respiratory tract inflammation, viral respiratory infection

Miscellaneous: Accidental injury, amputation, fever

Rare but important or life-threatening: Adrenocortical insufficiency, aggressive behavior, agitation, allergic skin reaction, anxiety, aphonia, bacterial infection, bacterial reproductive infection, behavioral changes (very rare: includes hyperactivity and irritability in children), blepharoconjunctivitis, bronchospasm (immediate and delayed), bruise, burn, cataract (long-term use), change in appetite, chest tightness, cholecystitis, Churg-Strauss syndrome, conjunctivitis, cranial nerve palsy, Cushingoid appearance, decreased bone mineral density (long-term use), decreased linear skeletal growth rate (children/adolescents), dental caries, dental discoloration, depression, dermatitis, diarrhea, disturbance in fluid balance, dizziness, drug toxicity, dyspnea, ecchymoses, edema, eosinophilia, epistaxis, esophageal candidiasis, exacerbation of asthma, facial edema, folliculitis, fungal infection, gastrointestinal disease, glaucoma (long-term use), hematoma, HPA-axis suppression, hypercorticoidism, hyperglycemia, hypersensitivity reaction (immediate and delayed; includes ear, nose, and throat allergic disorders, anaphylaxis, angioedema, bronchospasm, hypotension, skin rash, urticaria), increased intraocular pressure (long-term use), inflammation (musculoskeletal), keratitis, laceration, laryngitis, migraine, mobility disorder, mood disorder, mouth disease (and tongue disease), muscle cramps, muscle rigidity (stiffness, tightness), muscle spasm, oral discomfort (and pain), oral mucosa ulcer, oral rash (and erythema), oropharyngeal edema, palpitations, paradoxical bronchospasm, paranasal sinus disease, photodermatitis, pneumonia, polyp (ear, nose, throat), pressure-induced disorder, reduced salivation, restlessness, rhinorrhea, sleep disorder, soft tissue injury, urinary tract infection, vasculitis, viral skin infection, wheezing, wound

Drug Interactions

Metabolism/Transport Effects Substrate of CYP3A4 (major); **Note:** Assignment of Major/Minor substrate status based on clinically relevant drug interaction potential

Avoid Concomitant Use

Avoid concomitant use of Fluticasone (Oral Inhalation) with any of the following: Aldesleukin; BCG; BCG (Intravesical); Cobicistat; Conivaptan; Fusidic Acid (Systemic); Idelalisib; Loxapine; Natalizumab; Pimecrolimus; Tacrolimus (Topical); Tipranavir; Tofacitinib

Increased Effect/Toxicity

Fluticasone (Oral Inhalation) may increase the levels/effects of: Amphotericin B; Deferasirox; Leflunomide; Loop Diuretics; Loxapine; Natalizumab; Thiazide Diuretics; Tofacitinib

The levels/effects of Fluticasone (Oral Inhalation) may be increased by: Aprepitant; Cobicistat; Conivaptan; CYP3A4 Inhibitors (Moderate); CYP3A4 Inhibitors (Strong); Dasatinib; Denosumab; Fosaprepitant; Fusidic Acid (Systemic); Idelalisib; Ivacaftor; Luliconazole; Mifepristone; Netupitant; Palbociclib; Pimecrolimus; Simeprevir; Stiripentol; Tacrolimus (Topical); Telaprevir; Tipranavir; Trastuzumab

Decreased Effect

Fluticasone (Oral Inhalation) may decrease the levels/effects of: Aldesleukin; BCG; BCG (Intravesical); Coccidioides immitis Skin Test; Corticorelin; Hyaluronidase; Sipuleucel-T; Telaprevir; Vaccines (Inactivated)

The levels/effects of Fluticasone (Oral Inhalation) may be decreased by: Echinacea

Storage/Stability

Arnuity Ellipta and Flovent Diskus: Store at 20°C to 25°C (68°F to 77°F); excursions are permitted from 15°C to 30°C (59°F to 86°F). Store in a dry place away from direct heat or sunlight. Discard after 6 weeks (Arnuity Ellipta and 50 mcg diskus) or after 2 months (100 mcg and 250 mcg diskus) from removal from protective foil pouch or when the dose counter reads "0" (whichever comes first); device is not reusable.

Flovent HFA: Store between 20°C and 25°C (68°F and 77°F); excursions are permitted from 15°C to 30°C (59°F to 86°F). Discard device when the dose counter reads "000". Store with mouthpiece down. Do not expose to temperatures >120°F. Do not puncture or incinerate.

Mechanism of Action Fluticasone belongs to a group of corticosteroids which utilizes a fluorocarbothioate ester linkage at the 17 carbon position; extremely potent vasoconstrictive and anti-inflammatory activity. The effectiveness of inhaled fluticasone is due to its direct local effect.

Pharmacodynamics Oral inhalation: Clinical effects are due to direct local effect rather than systemic absorption

Onset of action: Variable; may occur within 24 hours

Maximum effect: 1-2 weeks or more

Duration after discontinuation: Several days or more

Pharmacokinetics (Adult data unless noted)

Distribution: V_d: 4.2 L/kg

Protein binding: 91% to 99%

Metabolism: Via cytochrome P450 3A4 pathway to 17β-carboxylic acid (inactive)

Bioavailability: Oral inhalation: Flovent®: 30% of dose delivered from actuator; Flovent® HFA: 30% lower than Flovent®; Diskus®: 18%

Half-life: 7.8 hours

Dosing: Neonatal Inhalation: Bronchopulmonary dysplasia, treatment: See **Dosing: Usual** for dosing in infants (PNA in clinical trials >28 days)

Dosing: Usual

Oral inhalation:

Asthma: If adequate response is not seen after 2 weeks of initial dosage, increase dosage; doses should be titrated to the lowest effective dose once asthma is controlled:

Inhalation aerosol (Flovent® HFA): Manufacturer's recommendations:

Children 4-11 years: Initial: 88 mcg twice daily; maximum dose: 88 mcg twice daily

Children ≥12 years and Adults:

Patients previously treated with bronchodilators only: Initial: 88 mcg twice daily; maximum dose: 440 mcg twice daily

Patients treated with an inhaled corticosteroid: Initial: 88-220 mcg twice daily; maximum dose: 440 mcg twice daily; may start doses above 88 mcg twice daily in poorly controlled patients or in those who previously required higher doses of inhaled corticosteroids

Patients previously treated with oral corticosteroids: 440 mcg twice daily; maximum dose: 880 mcg twice daily

NIH Asthma Guidelines (NAEPP, 2007) (give in divided doses twice daily):

Children <12 years:

"Low" dose: 88-176 mcg/day (44 mcg/puff: 2-4 puffs/day)

"Medium" dose: >176-352 mcg/day (44 mcg/puff: 4-8 puffs/day or 110 mcg/puff: 2-3 puffs/day)

"High" dose: >352 mcg/day (110 mcg/puff: >3 puffs/day or 220 mcg/puff: >1 puff/day)

Children ≥12 years and Adults:

"Low" dose: 88-264 mcg/day (44 mcg/puff: 2-6 puffs/day or 110 mcg/puff: 2 puffs/day)

"Medium" dose: >264-440 mcg/day (110 mcg/puff: 2-4 puffs/day)

"High" dose: >440 mcg/day (110 mcg/puff: >4 puffs/day or 220 mcg/puff: >2 puffs/day)

Bronchopulmonary dysplasia, treatment: Infants: Some centers have used 2-4 puffs (44 mcg/puff) every 12 hours via a face mask and a spacer. One trial used fixed doses administered via a spacer and neonatal anesthesia bag (into ventilator, directly into nasopharyngeal endotracheal tube, or with a face mask) in 16 former preterm neonates (GA: ≤32 weeks; PNA: 28-60 days); chest radiograph score was improved compared to placebo; the treatment group had increased blood pressure compared to baseline; the authors conclude that the trial results do not support the use of fluticasone in oxygen-dependent patients with moderate BPD; exact dosing cannot be replicated in the U.S. with available products (Dugas, 2005)

Body weight:

0.5-1.2 kg: 125 mcg every 12 hours for 3 weeks, followed by 125 mcg once daily for the 4th week

≥1.2 kg: 250 mcg every 12 hours for 3 weeks, followed by 250 mcg once daily for the 4th week

Inhalation powder (Flovent® Diskus®): Manufacturer's recommendations:

Children 4-11 years: Patients previously treated with bronchodilators alone or inhaled corticosteroids: Initial: 50 mcg twice daily; maximum dose: 100 mcg twice daily; may start higher initial dose in poorly controlled patients or in those who previously required higher doses of inhaled corticosteroids

Adolescents and Adults:

Patients previously treated with bronchodilators alone: Initial: 100 mcg twice daily; maximum dose: 500 mcg twice daily

Patients previously treated with inhaled corticosteroids: Initial: 100-250 mcg twice daily; maximum dose: 500 mcg twice daily; may start doses above 100 mcg twice daily in poorly controlled patients or in those who previously required higher doses of inhaled corticosteroids

Patients previously treated with oral corticosteroids: Initial: 500-1000 mcg twice daily (select dose based on assessment of individual patient); maximum dose: 1000 mcg twice daily; **Note:** Inability to reduce oral corticosteroid therapy may indicate need for maximum fluticasone dose.

NIH Asthma Guidelines (NAEPP, 2007) (give in divided doses twice daily):

Children 5-11 years:

"Low" dose: 100-200 mcg/day (50 mcg/puff: 2-4 puffs/day or 100 mcg/puff: 1-2 puffs/day)

"Medium" dose: >200-400 mcg/day (50 mcg/puff: 4-8 puffs/day or 100 mcg/puff: 2-4 puffs/day)

"High" dose: >400 mcg/day (50 mcg/puff: >8 puffs/day or 100 mcg/puff: >4 puffs/day)

Children ≥12 years and Adults:

"Low" dose: 100-300 mcg/day (50 mcg/puff: 2-6 puffs/day or 100 mcg/puff: 1-3 puffs/day)

"Medium" dose: >300-500 mcg/day (50 mcg/puff: 6-10 puffs/day or 100 mcg/puff: 3-5 puffs/day)

"High" dose: >500 mcg/day (50 mcg/puff: >10 puffs/day or 100 mcg/puff: >5 puffs/day)

Oral (swallowed): Note: Patients use an oral inhaler without a spacer and swallow the medication.

Children: Eosinophilic esophagitis: Optimal dose and dosing regimen are not established. Dosing from two more recent studies is presented.

A randomized, double-blind, placebo-controlled trial (n=31) demonstrated efficacy by assessment of histologic remission (Konikoff, 2006): Children: 3-16 years: 440 mcg twice daily for 3 months

A prospective, randomized trial (n=80) compared swallowed fluticasone to oral prednisone; a greater degree of improvement in histologic response was seen in the prednisone group; however, no difference in clinical response was observed between the two groups (Schaffer, 2008):

Children: 1-10 years: 220 mcg 4 times daily for 4 weeks, 220 mcg 3 times daily for 3 weeks, 220 mcg twice daily for 3 weeks, 220 mcg daily for 2 weeks

Children and Adolescents: 11-18 years: 440 mcg 4 times daily for 4 weeks, 440 mcg 3 times daily for 3 weeks, 440 mcg twice daily for 3 weeks, 440 mcg daily for 2 weeks

Dosage adjustment in hepatic impairment: Use with caution; monitor patients closely; **Note:** Fluticasone is primarily eliminated via hepatic metabolism and serum concentrations may be elevated in patients with hepatic disease.

Administration

Oral inhalation: Rinse mouth with water (without swallowing) after inhalation to decrease chance of oral candidiasis.

Aerosol inhalation: Shake canister well for 5 seconds before each spray; use at room temperature. Inhaler must be primed before first use with four test sprays (spray into air away from face, shake well for 5 seconds between sprays) and primed again with one test spray if not used for >7 days or if dropped. Use a spacer device for children <8 years of age. Patient should contact pharmacy for refill when the dose counter reads "020." Discard device when the dose counter reads "000." Do not try to alter numbers on counter or remove the counter from the metal canister. Do not immerse canister into water (ie, do not use "float test" to determine contents).

Powder for oral inhalation: Flovent® Diskus®: Do not use with spacer device; do not exhale into Diskus®; do not wash or take apart; activate and use Diskus® in horizontal position

Oral (swallowed): **Note:** This method of administration is for treatment of eosinophilic esophagitis only. Use metered dose inhaler. Do not use a spacer. Shake canister well for 5 seconds before each spray. Prime inhaler as outlined above. Actuate inhaler and spray medication into pharynx; swallow the medication (rather than inhale). Do not eat, drink, or rinse mouth for 30 minutes following administration (Konikoff, 2006; Schaefer, 2008).

Monitoring Parameters Check mucus membranes for signs of fungal infection; monitor growth in pediatric patients; monitor IOP with therapy >6 weeks. Monitor for symptoms of asthma, FEV_1, peak flow, and/or other pulmonary function tests. Assess HPA suppression in patients using potent topical steroids applied to a large surface area or to areas under occlusion.

Additional Information Flovent® HFA does **not** contain CFCs as the propellant; Flovent® HFA is packaged in a plastic-coated, moisture-protective foil pouch that also contains a desiccant; the desiccant should be discarded when the pouch is opened

When using fluticasone oral inhalation to help reduce or discontinue oral corticosteroid therapy, begin prednisone taper after at least 1 week of fluticasone inhalation therapy; do not decrease prednisone faster than 2.5 mg/day on a weekly basis; monitor patients for signs of asthma instability and adrenal insufficiency; decrease fluticasone to lowest effective dose **after** prednisone reduction is complete. If bronchospasm with wheezing occurs after oral inhalation use, a fast-acting bronchodilator may be used; discontinue orally inhaled corticosteroid and initiate alternative chronic therapy.

Oral (swallowed) use: In the study by Schaffer that compared swallowed fluticasone to oral prednisone, systemic adverse effects occurred more frequently in the oral prednisone group; esophageal candidiasis occurred in 15% of patients using swallowed fluticasone (Schaffer, 2008).

Dosage Forms Considerations Flovent HFA 10.6 g and 12 g canisters contain 120 inhalations.

Dosage Forms Excipient information presented when available (limited, particularly for generics); consult specific product labeling.

Aerosol, Inhalation, as propionate:

Flovent HFA: 44 mcg/actuation (10.6 g); 110 mcg/actuation (12 g); 220 mcg/actuation (12 g)

Aerosol Powder Breath Activated, Inhalation, as furoate:

Arnuity Ellipta: 100 mcg/actuation (14 ea, 30 ea); 200 mcg/actuation (14 ea, 30 ea) [contains lactose monohydrate]

Aerosol Powder Breath Activated, Inhalation, as propionate:

Flovent Diskus: 50 mcg/blister (60 ea); 100 mcg/blister (28 ea, 60 ea); 250 mcg/blister (28 ea, 60 ea) [contains lactose]

Fluticasone (Topical) (floo TIK a sone)

Medication Safety Issues

Sound-alike/look-alike issues:

Cutivate® may be confused with Ultravate®

International issues:

Allegro: Brand name for fluticasone [Israel], but also the brand name for frovatriptan [Germany]

Allegro [Israel] may be confused with Allegra and Allegra-D brand names for fexofenadine and fexofenadine/pseudoephedrine, respectively, [U.S., Canada, and multiple international markets]

Related Information

Topical Corticosteroids *on page 2262*

Brand Names: US Cutivate

Brand Names: Canada Cutivate

Therapeutic Category Corticosteroid, Topical

Generic Availability (US) Yes

Use

Cream: Relief of inflammation and pruritus associated with corticosteroid-responsive dermatoses (eg, atopic dermatitis) (medium potency topical corticosteroid) (FDA approved in ages ≥3 months and adults)

Lotion: Relief of inflammation and pruritus associated with atopic dermatitis (FDA approved in ages ≥1 year and adults)

Ointment: Relief of inflammation and pruritus associated with corticosteroid-responsive dermatoses (medium potency topical corticosteroid) (FDA approved in adults)

Pregnancy Risk Factor C

Pregnancy Considerations Adverse events have been observed with systemic corticosteroids in animal reproduction studies. In general, the use of topical corticosteroids during pregnancy is not considered to have significant risk; however, intrauterine growth retardation in the infant has been reported (rare). The use of large amounts or for prolonged periods of time should be avoided.

Breast-Feeding Considerations Systemic corticosteroids are excreted in human milk. It is not known if sufficient quantities of fluticasone are absorbed following topical administration to produce detectable amounts in breast milk. Hypertension in the nursing infant has been reported following corticosteroid ointment applied to the nipples. Use with caution.

Contraindications

Cream and ointment: Hypersensitivity to fluticasone or any component of the formulation.

Lotion: There are no contraindications listed in the manufacturer's labeling.

Warnings/Precautions May cause hypercorticism or suppression of hypothalamic-pituitary-adrenal (HPA) axis, particularly in younger children or in patients receiving high doses for prolonged periods. HPA axis suppression may lead to adrenal crisis. Use appropriate antibacterial or antifungal agents to treat concomitant skin infections; discontinue treatment if infection does not resolve promptly. Lotion and cream contain imidurea, an excipient; imidurea releases trace amounts of formaldehyde which may cause irritation or allergic sensitization upon contact with skin. Discontinue if irritation occurs and institute appropriate therapy. Allergic contact dermatitis can occur and is usually diagnosed by failure to heal rather than clinical exacerbation; discontinue fluticasone if appropriate. May cause local reactions, including skin atrophy; risk increased with use under occlusion. Topical corticosteroids may be absorbed percutaneously. Absorption of topical corticosteroids may cause manifestations of Cushing syndrome, hyperglycemia, or glycosuria. Absorption is increased by the use of occlusive dressings, application to denuded skin, or application to large surface areas.

Children may absorb proportionally larger amounts after topical application and may be more prone to systemic effects. HPA axis suppression, intracranial hypertension, and Cushing syndrome have been reported in children receiving topical corticosteroids. Prolonged use may affect growth velocity; growth should be routinely monitored in pediatric patients. Safety and efficacy of lotion and cream (in children) beyond 4 weeks of use have not been established. Avoid contact with eyes; generally not for routine use on the face, underarms, or groin area (including diaper area). Avoid use with occlusive dressing unless directed by a health care provider. If no improvement is seen within 2 weeks, reassessment of diagnosis may be necessary.

Warnings: Additional Pediatric Considerations Topical corticosteroids may be absorbed percutaneously. The extent of absorption is dependent on several factors, including epidermal integrity (intact vs abraded skin), formulation, age of the patient, prolonged duration of use, and the use of occlusive dressings. Percutaneous absorption of topical steroids is increased in neonates (especially preterm neonates), infants, and young children. Hypothalamic-pituitary-adrenal (HPA) suppression may occur, particularly in younger children or in patients receiving high doses for prolonged periods; acute adrenal insufficiency (adrenal crisis) may occur with abrupt withdrawal after long-term therapy or with stress. Infants and small children may be more susceptible to HPA axis suppression or other systemic toxicities due to larger skin surface area to body mass ratio; use with caution in pediatric patients. HPA axis suppression occurred in two children (2 and 5 years of age) of 43 pediatric patients treated topically with fluticasone cream for 4 weeks; application covered at least 35% of body surface area. HPA axis suppression was not reported with use of fluticasone lotion for at least 3 to 4 weeks in young pediatric patients (4 months to <6 years) during clinical trials; however, it cannot be ruled out when topical fluticasone is used in any patient and especially with longer use.

Some dosage forms may contain propylene glycol; in neonates large amounts of propylene glycol delivered orally, intravenously (eg, >3,000 mg/day), or topically have been associated with potentially fatal toxicities which can include metabolic acidosis, seizures, renal failure, and CNS depression; toxicities have also been reported in children and adults including hyperosmolality, lactic acidosis, seizures and respiratory depression; use caution (AAP, 1997; Shehab, 2009).

Adverse Reactions

Dermatologic: Dryness, eczema infection, exacerbation of eczema, pruritus, rash (erythematous; children), skin irritation, telangiectasia (children)

Neuromuscular & skeletal: Numbness of fingers

Rare but important or life-threatening: Acneiform eruptions, atrophy, blurred vision, Cushing syndrome, dermatitis, edema, folliculitis, hemorrhage, hyperglycemia, immunosuppression, leukopenia, secondary infection, sepsis, skin discoloration, thrombocytopenia, urticaria, viral warts

Reported with other topical corticosteroids (in decreasing order of occurrence): Hypopigmentation, perioral dermatitis, allergic contact dermatitis, skin atrophy, striae, hypertrichosis, miliaria, pustular psoriasis from chronic plaque psoriasis

Drug Interactions

Metabolism/Transport Effects **Substrate** of CYP3A4 (minor); **Note:** Assignment of Major/Minor substrate status based on clinically relevant drug interaction potential

Avoid Concomitant Use

Avoid concomitant use of Fluticasone (Topical) with any of the following: Aldesleukin

Increased Effect/Toxicity

Fluticasone (Topical) may increase the levels/effects of: Ceritinib; Deferasirox

The levels/effects of Fluticasone (Topical) may be increased by: Telaprevir

Decreased Effect

Fluticasone (Topical) may decrease the levels/effects of: Aldesleukin; Corticorelin; Hyaluronidase; Telaprevir

Storage/Stability

Cream and ointment: Store at 2°C to 30°C (36°F to 86°F).

Lotion: Store at 15°C to 30°C (59°F to 86°F); do not refrigerate; keep tightly sealed.

Mechanism of Action Topical corticosteroids have anti-inflammatory, antipruritic, and vasoconstrictive properties. May depress the formation, release, and activity of endogenous chemical mediators of inflammation (kinins, histamine, liposomal enzymes, prostaglandins) through the induction of phospholipase A_2 inhibitory proteins (lipocortins) and sequential inhibition of the release of arachidonic acid. Fluticasone has intermediate range potency.

Dosing: Usual Topical: **Note:** If no improvement is seen within 2 weeks, reassessment of diagnosis may be necessary.

Infants, Children, and Adolescents: **Note:** Safety and efficacy of use >4 weeks in pediatric patients have not been established.

Atopic dermatitis:

Infants ≥3 months, Children, and Adolescents: Cream: Apply sparingly to affected area once or twice daily

Children ≥1 year and Adolescents: Lotion: Apply sparingly to affected area once daily

Corticosteroid-responsive dermatoses: Infants ≥3 months, Children, and Adolescents: Cream: Apply sparingly to affected area twice daily

Adults:

Atopic dermatitis: Cream, lotion: Apply sparingly to affected area once or twice daily

Corticosteroid-responsive dermatoses: Cream, lotion, ointment: Apply sparingly to affected area twice daily

Administration Apply sparingly to affected area, gently rub in until disappears; do not use on open skin; avoid application on face, underarms, or groin area unless directed by physician; avoid contact with eyes; do not occlude area unless directed; do not apply to diaper area

Dosage Forms Excipient information presented when available (limited, particularly for generics); consult specific product labeling.

Cream, External, as propionate:

Cutivate: 0.05% (30 g, 60 g) [contains cetyl alcohol, propylene glycol]

Generic: 0.05% (15 g, 30 g, 60 g)

Lotion, External, as propionate:

Cutivate: 0.05% (120 mL) [contains cetostearyl alcohol, methylparaben, propylene glycol, propylparaben]

Generic: 0.05% (60 mL, 120 mL)

Ointment, External, as propionate:

Cutivate: 0.005% (30 g, 60 g)

Generic: 0.005% (15 g, 30 g, 60 g)

Fluticasone and Salmeterol

(floo TIK a sone & sal ME te role)

Medication Safety Issues

Sound-alike/look-alike issues:

Advair may be confused with Adcirca, Advicor

Brand Names: US Advair Diskus; Advair HFA

Brand Names: Canada Advair; Advair Diskus

Therapeutic Category Adrenal Corticosteroid; Adrenergic Agonist Agent; Anti-inflammatory Agent; Antiasthmatic; $Beta_2$-Adrenergic Agonist; Bronchodilator; Corticosteroid, Inhalant (Oral); Glucocorticoid

Generic Availability (US) No

Use

Advair Diskus®, Advair® HFA: Maintenance treatment of asthma (Advair Diskus®: FDA approved in ages ≥4 years and adults; Advair® HFA: FDA approved in ages ≥12 years and adults); **NOT** indicated for the relief of acute bronchospasm

Advair Diskus®: Maintenance treatment of airflow obstruction in patients with COPD associated with chronic bronchitis and emphysema (FDA approved in adults); **NOT** indicated for the relief of acute bronchospasm

Medication Guide Available Yes

Pregnancy Risk Factor C

Pregnancy Considerations Adverse events were observed in animal reproduction studies using this combination. Refer to individual agents.

Breast-Feeding Considerations It is not known if fluticasone or salmeterol are excreted into breast milk. The manufacturer recommends that caution be used if administering this combination to breast-feeding women. Refer to individual agents.

Contraindications

Hypersensitivity to fluticasone, salmeterol, or any component of the formulation; status asthmaticus; acute episodes of asthma or COPD; severe hypersensitivity to milk proteins (Advair Diskus)

Documentation of allergenic cross-reactivity for corticosteroids and sympathomimetics are limited. However, because of similarities in chemical structure and/or pharmacologic actions, the possibility of cross-sensitivity cannot be ruled out with certainty.

Warnings/Precautions See individual agents.

Adverse Reactions

Cardiovascular: Cardiac arrhythmia, chest symptoms, edema, myocardial infarction, palpitations, syncope, tachycardia

Central nervous system: Dizziness, headache, migraine, mouth pain, pain, sleep disorder

Dermatologic: Dermatitis, diaphoresis, eczema, exfoliation of skin, urticaria, viral skin infection

Endocrine & metabolic: Fluid retention, hypothyroidism, weight gain

Gastrointestinal: Constipation, diarrhea, dysgeusia, gastrointestinal infection (including viral), nausea, oral candidiasis, oral mucosa ulcer, vomiting

Genitourinary: Urinary tract infection

Hematologic & oncologic: Hematoma

Hepatic: Abnormal hepatic function tests

Hypersensitivity: Hypersensitivity reaction

Infection: Bacterial infection, candidiasis, viral infection

Neuromuscular & skeletal: Arthralgia, bone disease, bone fracture, muscle cramps, muscle injury, muscle rigidity, muscle spasm, musculoskeletal pain, myalgia, ostealgia, rheumatoid arthritis, tremor

Ophthalmic: Conjunctivitis, eye redness, keratitis, xerophthalmia

Respiratory: Bronchitis, chest congestion, cough, ENT infection, epistaxis, hoarseness, laryngitis, lower respiratory signs and symptoms (hemorrhage), lower respiratory tract infection (COPD diagnosis and age >65 years increase risk), nasal signs and symptoms (irritation), pharyngitis, rhinitis, rhinorrhea, sinusitis, sneezing, throat irritation, upper respiratory tract infection, upper respiratory tract inflammation, viral respiratory tract infection

Miscellaneous: Burn, laceration, wound

Rare but important or life-threatening: Aggressive behavior, atrial fibrillation, cataract, Churg-Strauss syndrome, Cushing's syndrome, decreased linear skeletal growth rate, depression, dysmenorrhea, ecchymoses, esophageal candidiasis, exacerbation of asthma (serious and some fatal), glaucoma, hyperactivity, hyperglycemia, hypersensitivity reaction (immediate and delayed), hypertension, hypokalemia, hypothyroidism, influenza, irritability, lassitude, myositis, osteoporosis, pallor, paranasal sinus disease, paresthesia, pelvic inflammatory disease, photodermatitis, skin rash, supraventricular tachycardia, syncope, tracheitis, ventricular tachycardia, vulvovaginitis

Drug Interactions

Metabolism/Transport Effects Refer to individual components.

Avoid Concomitant Use

Avoid concomitant use of Fluticasone and Salmeterol with any of the following: Aldesleukin; BCG; BCG (Intravesical); Beta-Blockers (Nonselective); Cobicistat; Conivaptan; CYP3A4 Inhibitors (Strong); Fusidic Acid (Systemic); Idelalisib; Iobenguane I 123; Long-Acting Beta2-Agonists; Loxapine; Natalizumab; Pimecrolimus; Tacrolimus (Topical); Telaprevir; Tipranavir; Tofacitinib

Increased Effect/Toxicity

Fluticasone and Salmeterol may increase the levels/effects of: Amphotericin B; Atosiban; Deferasirox; Highest Risk QTc-Prolonging Agents; Leflunomide; Long-Acting Beta2-Agonists; Loop Diuretics; Loxapine; Moderate Risk QTc-Prolonging Agents; Natalizumab; Sympathomimetics; Thiazide Diuretics; Tofacitinib

The levels/effects of Fluticasone and Salmeterol may be increased by: Aprepitant; AtoMOXetine; Cannabinoid-Containing Products; Cobicistat; Conivaptan; CYP3A4 Inhibitors (Moderate); CYP3A4 Inhibitors (Strong); Dasatinib; Denosumab; Fosaprepitant; Fusidic Acid (Systemic); Idelalisib; Ivacaftor; Linezolid; Luliconazole; MAO Inhibitors; Mifepristone; Netupitant; Palbociclib; Pimecrolimus; Simeprevir; Stiripentol; Tacrolimus (Topical); Tedizolid; Telaprevir; Tipranavir; Trastuzumab; Tricyclic Antidepressants

Decreased Effect

Fluticasone and Salmeterol may decrease the levels/effects of: Aldesleukin; BCG; BCG (Intravesical); Coccidioides immitis Skin Test; Corticorelin; Hyaluronidase; Iobenguane I 123; Sipuleucel-T; Vaccines (Inactivated)

The levels/effects of Fluticasone and Salmeterol may be decreased by: Beta-Blockers (Beta1 Selective); Beta-Blockers (Nonselective); Betahistine; Echinacea

Storage/Stability

Advair Diskus: Store at 20°C to 25°C (68°F to 77°F). Store in a dry place out of direct heat or sunlight. Diskus device should be discarded 1 month after removal from foil pouch, or when dosing indicator reads "0" (whichever comes first); device is not reusable.

Advair HFA: Store at 20°C to 25°C (68°F to 77°F), excursions permitted from 15°C to 30°C (59°F to 86°F). Store with mouthpiece down. Discard after 120 inhalations. Discard device when the dose counter reads "000". Device is not reusable.

Mechanism of Action Combination of fluticasone (corticosteroid) and salmeterol (long-acting $beta_2$-agonist) designed to improve pulmonary function and control over what is produced by either agent when used alone. Because fluticasone and salmeterol act locally in the lung, plasma levels do not predict therapeutic effect.

Fluticasone: The mechanism of action for all topical corticosteroids is believed to be a combination of three important properties: Anti-inflammatory activity, immunosuppressive properties, and antiproliferative actions. Fluticasone has extremely potent vasoconstrictive and anti-inflammatory activity.

Salmeterol: Relaxes bronchial smooth muscle by selective action on $beta_2$-receptors with little effect on heart rate

Pharmacodynamics See individual agents.

Pharmacokinetics (Adult data unless noted) See individual agents.

Dosing: Usual

Asthma, maintenance treatment: Note: Titrate dosage to the lowest effective strength which maintains control of asthma. Dose may be increased after 2 weeks if patient does not respond adequately.

Oral powder for inhalation: Advair Diskus®:

Children 4-11 years without prior inhaled corticosteroid: Fluticasone 100 mcg/salmeterol 50 mcg (Advair™ Diskus® 100/50) 1 inhalation twice daily

Children ≥12 years and Adults without prior inhaled corticosteroid: Fluticasone 100 mcg/salmeterol 50 mcg (Advair™ Diskus® 100/50) 1 inhalation twice daily

Children ≥12 years and Adults currently receiving an inhaled corticosteroid: The starting dose is dependent upon the current steroid therapy, see table.

Oral inhalation: Metered dose inhaler: Advair® HFA:

Children ≥12 years and Adults without prior inhaled corticosteroid: 2 inhalations twice daily of either fluticasone 45 mcg/salmeterol 21 mcg (Advair® HFA 45/21) or fluticasone 115 mcg/salmeterol 21 mcg (Advair® HFA 115/21); not to exceed 2 inhalations twice daily of fluticasone 230 mcg/salmeterol 21 mcg (Advair® HFA 230/21)

Children ≥12 years and Adults currently receiving an inhaled corticosteroid: The starting dose is dependent upon the current steroid therapy; see table. Not to exceed 2 inhalations twice daily of fluticasone 230 mcg/salmeterol 21 mcg (Advair® HFA 230/21)

COPD, maintenance treatment: Oral powder for inhalation: Advair Diskus®: Adults: Fluticasone 250 mcg/salmeterol 50 mcg (Advair Diskus® 250/50) 1 inhalation twice daily

Recommended Starting Dose of Fluticasone / Salmeterol (Advair Diskus®) for Patients Currently Taking Inhaled Corticosteroids

Current Daily Dose of Inhaled Corticosteroid[1]		Advair Diskus® 1 inhalation twice daily
Beclomethasone dipropionate HFA inhalation aerosal	160 mcg	100/50
	320 mcg	250/50
	640 mcg	500/50
Budesonide inhalation aerosal	≤400 mcg	100/50
	800-1200 mcg	250/50
	1600 mcg	500/50
Flunisolide inhalation aerosal	≤1000 mcg	100/50
	1250-2000 mcg	250/50
Flunisolide HFA inhalation aerosal	≤320 mcg	100/50
	640 mcg	250/50
Fluticasone propionate HFA inhalation aerosol	≤176 mcg	100/50
	440 mcg	250/50
	660-880 mcg	500/50
Fluticasone propionate inhalation powder	≤200 mcg	100/50
	500 mcg	250/50
	1000 mcg	500/50
Mometasone furoate inhalation powder	220 mcg	100/50
	440 mcg	250/50
	880 mcg	500/50
Triamcinolone acetate inhalation aerosal	≤1000 mcg	100/50
	1100-1600 mcg	250/50

(continued)

(continued)

[1]Not for use in patients transferring from systemic corticosteroid therapy

Recommended Starting Dose of Fluticasone / Salmeterol (Advair® HFA) for Patients Currently Taking Inhaled Corticosteroids

Current Daily Dose of Inhaled Corticosteroid[1]		Advair® HFA 2 inhalations twice daily
Beclomethasone dipropionate HFA inhalation aerosal	≤160 mcg	45/21
	320 mcg	115/21
	640 mcg	230/21
Budesonide inhalation powder	≤400 mcg	45/21
	800-1200 mcg	115/21
	1600 mcg	230/21
Flunisolide CFC inhalation aerosal	≤1000 mcg	45/21
	1250-2000 mcg	115/21
Flunisolide HFA inhalation aerosal	≤320 mcg	45/21
	640 mcg	115/21
Fluticasone propionate HFA inhalation aerosol	≤176 mcg	45/21
	440 mcg	115/21
	660-880 mcg	230/21
Fluticasone propionate inhalation powder	≤200 mcg	45/21
	500 mcg	115/21
	1000 mcg	230/21
Mometasone furoate inhalation powder	220 mcg	45/21
	440 mcg	115/21
	880 mcg	230/21
Triamcinolone acetonide inhalation aerosal	≤1000 mcg	45/21
	1100-1600 mcg	115/21

[1]Not for use in patients transferring from systemic corticosteroid therapy

Administration Oral inhalation:

Advair Diskus®, powder for oral inhalation: A device containing a double-foil blister of a powder formulation for oral inhalation; each blister contains 1 complete dose of both medications; the medication is opened by activating the device, dispersed into the airstream created by the patient inhaling through the mouthpiece; it may not be used with a spacer. Follow the patient directions for use which are provided with each device; do not exhale into the Diskus® or attempt to take it apart. Always activate and use the Diskus® in a level, horizontal position. Do not wash the mouthpiece or any part of the Diskus®; it must be kept dry.

Advair® HFA, metered dose inhalation: Prime before using the first time by releasing 4 test sprays into the air away from the face, shaking well for 5 seconds before each spray. Reprime with 2 test sprays if the inhaler has been dropped or not used for more than 4 weeks; discard after

120 actuations. Never immerse canister into water. Shake well for 5 seconds before using.

Monitoring Parameters Pulmonary function tests, vital signs, CNS stimulation, serum glucose, serum potassium; check mucous membranes for signs of fungal infection; monitor growth in pediatric patients

Additional Information When fluticasone/salmeterol is initiated in patients previously receiving a short-acting beta agonist, instruct the patient to discontinue regular use of the short-acting beta agonist and to utilize the shorter-acting agent for symptomatic acute episodes only.

Dosage Forms Excipient information presented when available (limited, particularly for generics); consult specific product labeling.

Aerosol, for oral inhalation:

Advair HFA:

45/21: Fluticasone propionate 45 mcg and salmeterol 21 mcg per inhalation (8 g) [chlorofluorocarbon free; 60 metered actuations]

45/21: Fluticasone propionate 45 mcg and salmeterol 21 mcg per inhalation (12 g) [chlorofluorocarbon free; 120 metered actuations]

115/21: Fluticasone propionate 115 mcg and salmeterol 21 mcg per inhalation (8 g) [chlorofluorocarbon free; 60 metered actuations]

115/21: Fluticasone propionate 115 mcg and salmeterol 21 mcg per inhalation (12 g) [chlorofluorocarbon free; 120 metered actuations]

230/21: Fluticasone propionate 230 mcg and salmeterol 21 mcg per inhalation (8 g) [chlorofluorocarbon free; 60 metered actuations]

230/21: Fluticasone propionate 230 mcg and salmeterol 21 mcg per inhalation (12 g) [chlorofluorocarbon free; 120 metered actuations]

Powder, for oral inhalation:

Advair Diskus:

100/50: Fluticasone propionate 100 mcg and salmeterol 50 mcg (14s, 60s) [contains lactose]

250/50: Fluticasone propionate 250 mcg and salmeterol 50 mcg (14s, 60s) [contains lactose]

500/50: Fluticasone propionate 500 mcg and salmeterol 50 mcg (14s, 60s) [contains lactose]

◆ **Fluticasone Furoate** *see* Fluticasone (Nasal) *on page 917*

◆ **Fluticasone Furoate** *see* Fluticasone (Oral Inhalation) *on page 919*

◆ **Fluticasone Propionate** *see* Fluticasone (Nasal) *on page 917*

◆ **Fluticasone Propionate** *see* Fluticasone (Oral Inhalation) *on page 919*

◆ **Fluticasone Propionate** *see* Fluticasone (Topical) *on page 922*

◆ **Fluticasone Propionate and Azelastine Hydrochloride** *see* Azelastine and Fluticasone *on page 241*

◆ **Fluticasone Propionate and Salmeterol Xinafoate** *see* Fluticasone and Salmeterol *on page 923*

Fluvastatin (FLOO va sta tin)

Medication Safety Issues

Sound-alike/look-alike issues:

Fluvastatin may be confused with fluoxetine, nystatin, pitavastatin

Related Information

Oral Medications That Should Not Be Crushed or Altered *on page 2476*

Brand Names: US Lescol; Lescol XL

Brand Names: Canada Lescol; Lescol XL; Teva-Fluvastatin

Therapeutic Category Antilipemic Agent; HMG-CoA Reductase Inhibitor

Generic Availability (US) May be product dependent

Use Adjunct to dietary therapy to reduce elevated total-C, LDL-C, and apo-B levels in patients with heterozygous familial hypercholesterolemia (HFH) and if LDC-C remains ≥190 mg/dL or if ≥160 mg/dL with family history of premature cardiovascular disease or presence of ≥2 cardiovascular risk factors [FDA approved in ages 10-16 years (girls ≥1 year postmenarche)]. Adjunct to dietary therapy to reduce elevated total cholesterol (total-C), LDL-C, triglyceride, and apolipoprotein B (apo-B) levels and to increase HDL-C in primary hypercholesterolemia, and mixed dyslipidemia (Fredrickson types IIa and IIb) (FDA approved in adults); to slow the progression of coronary atherosclerosis in patients with coronary heart disease (FDA approved in adults); to reduce risk of coronary revascularization procedures in patients with coronary heart disease (FDA approved in adults)

Pregnancy Risk Factor X

Pregnancy Considerations Adverse events were not observed in animal reproduction studies. There are reports of congenital anomalies following maternal use of HMG-CoA reductase inhibitors in pregnancy; however, maternal disease, differences in specific agents used, and the low rates of exposure limit the interpretation of the available data (Godfrey 2012; Lecarpentier 2012). Cholesterol biosynthesis may be important in fetal development; serum cholesterol and triglycerides increase normally during pregnancy. The discontinuation of lipid lowering medications temporarily during pregnancy is not expected to have significant impact on the long term outcomes of primary hypercholesterolemia treatment.

Use of fluvastatin is contraindicated in pregnancy. HMG-CoA reductase inhibitors should be discontinued prior to pregnancy (ADA 2013). If treatment of dyslipidemias is needed in pregnant women or in women of reproductive age, other agents are preferred (Berglund 2012; Stone 2013). The manufacturer recommends administration to women of childbearing potential only when conception is highly unlikely and patients have been informed of potential hazards.

Breast-Feeding Considerations It is not known if fluvastatin is excreted into breast milk. Due to the potential for serious adverse reactions in a nursing infant, use while breast-feeding is contraindicated by the manufacturer.

Contraindications Hypersensitivity to fluvastatin or any component of the formulation; active liver disease; unexplained persistent elevations of serum transaminases; pregnancy; breast-feeding

Warnings/Precautions Secondary causes of hyperlipidemia should be ruled out prior to therapy. Liver function must be monitored by periodic laboratory assessment. Rhabdomyolysis with acute renal failure has occurred with fluvastatin and other HMG-CoA reductase inhibitors. Risk may be increased with concurrent use of other drugs which may cause rhabdomyolysis (including colchicine, cyclosporine, erythromycin, fibric acid derivatives, or niacin at doses ≥1 g/day). Immune-mediated necrotizing myopathy (IMNM), an autoimmune-mediated myopathy, has been reported (rarely) with HMG-CoA reductase inhibitor therapy. IMNM presents as proximal muscle weakness with elevated CPK levels, which persists despite discontinuation of HMG-CoA reductase inhibitor therapy; additionally, muscle biopsy may show necrotizing myopathy with limited inflammation; immunosuppressive therapy (eg, corticosteroids, azathioprine) may be used for treatment. The manufacturer recommends temporary discontinuation for elective major surgery, acute medical or surgical conditions, or in any patient experiencing an acute or serious condition predisposing to renal failure (eg, sepsis, hypotension, trauma, uncontrolled seizures). Based on current research and clinical guidelines (Fleisher 2009), HMG-CoA reductase inhibitors should be continued in the perioperative period. Use with caution in patients with advanced age; these patients are predisposed to myopathy. Use caution in patients with previous liver disease or heavy ethanol use.

If serious hepatotoxicity with clinical symptoms and/or hyperbilirubinemia or jaundice occurs during treatment, interrupt therapy. If an alternate etiology is not identified, do not restart fluvastatin. Liver enzyme tests should be obtained at baseline and as clinically indicated; routine periodic monitoring of liver enzymes is not necessary. Increases in HbA_{1c} and fasting blood glucose have been reported with HMG-CoA reductase inhibitors; however, the benefits of statin therapy far outweigh the risk of dysglycemia. Use caution in patients with concurrent medications or conditions which reduce steroidogenesis.

Adverse Reactions As reported with fluvastatin capsules; in general, adverse reactions reported with fluvastatin extended release tablet were similar, but the incidence was less.

Central nervous system: Fatigue, headache, insomnia
Gastrointestinal: Abdominal pain, diarrhea, dyspepsia, nausea
Genitourinary: Urinary tract infection
Neuromuscular & skeletal: Myalgia
Respiratory: Bronchitis, sinusitis
Rare but important or life-threatening (including additional class-related events - not necessarily reported with fluvastatin therapy): Alopecia, amnesia (reversible), anaphylaxis, angioedema, arthralgia, arthritis, blood glucose increased, cataracts, cholestatic jaundice, cirrhosis, cognitive impairment (reversible), confusion (reversible), CPK increased (>10x normal), depression, dermatomyositis, dyspnea, eosinophilia, erectile dysfunction, erythema multiforme, ESR increased, facial paresis, fatty liver, fever, fulminant hepatic necrosis, glycosylated hemoglobin (Hb A_{1c}) increased, gynecomastia, hemolytic anemia, hepatitis, hepatoma, hypersensitivity reaction, immune-mediated necrotizing myopathy (IMNM), impotence, interstitial lung disease, leukopenia, memory disturbance (reversible), memory impairment (reversible), muscle cramps, myopathy, nodules, ophthalmoplegia, pancreatitis, paresthesia, peripheral nerve palsy, peripheral neuropathy, photosensitivity, polymyalgia rheumatica, positive ANA, pruritus, psychic disturbance, purpura, rash, renal failure (secondary to rhabdomyolysis), rhabdomyolysis, skin discoloration, Stevens-Johnson syndrome, systemic lupus erythematosus-like syndrome, taste alteration, thrombocytopenia, thyroid dysfunction, toxic epidermal necrolysis, transaminases increased, tremor, urticaria, vasculitis, vertigo

Drug Interactions

Metabolism/Transport Effects Substrate of CYP2C9 (minor), CYP2D6 (minor), CYP3A4 (minor), SLCO1B1; **Note:** Assignment of Major/Minor substrate status based on clinically relevant drug interaction potential; **Inhibits** CYP1A2 (weak), CYP2C8 (weak), CYP2C9 (moderate), CYP2D6 (weak)

Avoid Concomitant Use

Avoid concomitant use of Fluvastatin with any of the following: Amodiaquine; Fusidic Acid (Systemic); Gemfibrozil; Red Yeast Rice

Increased Effect/Toxicity

Fluvastatin may increase the levels/effects of: Amodiaquine; ARIPiprazole; Bosentan; Cannabis; Carvedilol; CYP2C9 Substrates; DAPTOmycin; Dronabinol; PAZOPanib; Tetrahydrocannabinol; TiZANidine; Trabectedin; Vitamin K Antagonists

The levels/effects of Fluvastatin may be increased by: Acipimox; Amiodarone; Atazanavir; Bezafibrate; Boceprevir; Ciprofibrate; Colchicine; CycloSPORINE (Systemic); Cyproterone; Eltrombopag; Fenofibrate and Derivatives; Fluconazole; Fusidic Acid (Systemic); Gemfibrozil; Mifepristone; Niacin; Niacinamide; Paritaprevir; Raltegravir; Red Yeast Rice; Telaprevir; Teriflunomide

Decreased Effect

Fluvastatin may decrease the levels/effects of: Lanthanum

The levels/effects of Fluvastatin may be decreased by: Antacids; Cholestyramine Resin; Etravirine; Fosphenytoin; Phenytoin; Rifamycin Derivatives

Food Interactions Food reduces rate but not the extent of absorption. Management: Administer without regard to meals.

Storage/Stability Store at 25°C (77°F); excursions permitted to 15°C to 30°C (59°F to 86°F). Protect from light.

Mechanism of Action Acts by competitively inhibiting 3-hydroxyl-3-methylglutaryl-coenzyme A (HMG-CoA) reductase, the enzyme that catalyzes the reduction of HMG-CoA to mevalonate; this is an early rate-limiting step in cholesterol biosynthesis. HDL is increased while total, LDL, and VLDL cholesterols; apolipoprotein B; and plasma triglycerides are decreased. In addition to the ability of HMG-CoA reductase inhibitors to decrease levels of high-sensitivity C-reactive protein (hsCRP), they also possess pleiotropic properties including improved endothelial function, reduced inflammation at the site of the coronary plaque, inhibition of platelet aggregation, and anticoagulant effects (de Denus 2002; Ray 2005).

Pharmacodynamics Maximum effect: LDL-C reduction: Achieved within 4 weeks

Pharmacokinetics (Adult data unless noted)

Distribution: Adults: V_d: 0.35 L/kg
Protein binding: >98%
Metabolism: To inactive and active metabolites (oxidative metabolism via CYP2C9 [75%], 2C8 [~5%], and 3A4 [~20%] isoenzymes); active forms do not circulate systemically; extensive (saturable) first-pass hepatic extraction
Bioavailability: Absolute: Capsule: 24%; Extended release tablet: 29%
Half-life: Capsule: <3 hours; Extended release tablet: 9 hours
Time to peak serum concentration: Capsule: 1 hour; Extended release tablet: 3 hours
Elimination: Feces (90%); urine (5%)

Dosing: Usual

Children and Adolescents: **Hyperlipidemia or heterozygous familial and nonfamilial hypercholesterolemia: Note:** Begin treatment if after adequate trial of diet the following are present: LDL-C ≥190 mg/dL or LDL-C remains ≥160 mg/dL and positive family history of premature cardiovascular disease or meets NCEP classification (NHLBI, 2011). Therapy may be considered for children 8-9 years of age meeting the above criteria or for children with diabetes mellitus and LDL-C ≥130 mg/dL (Daniels, 2008).

Children and Adolescents (10-16 years): Oral:
Immediate release capsule: Initial: 20 mg once daily; may titrate dose or frequency (twice daily dosing) at 6-week intervals; maximum dose: 40 mg twice daily
Extended release tablet: Should not be used to initiate therapy; may convert patient if total daily dose is 80 mg/day

Adults: **Dyslipidemia or delay in progression of CAD:** Oral:
Patients requiring ≥25% decrease in LDL-C: 40 mg capsule once daily in the evening, 80 mg extended release tablet once daily (anytime), or 40 mg capsule twice daily
Patients requiring <25% decrease in LDL-C: Initial: 20 mg capsule once daily in the evening; may increase based on tolerability and response to a maximum daily

dose: 80 mg/**day**, given in 2 divided doses (immediate release capsule) or as a single daily dose (extended release tablet)

Dosing adjustment for fluvastatin with concomitant medications: Children, Adolescents, and Adults:

Cyclosporine, fluconazole: Do not exceed 20 mg twice daily

Dosing adjustment in renal impairment: Adults:

Mild to moderate renal impairment: No dosage adjustment needed.

Severe renal impairment: Use with caution (doses >40 mg/day have not been studied).

Dosing adjustment in hepatic impairment: There are no dosage adjustments provided in the manufacturer labeling; systemic exposure may be increased in patients with liver disease; use is contraindicated in patients with active liver disease or unexplained transaminase elevations.

Administration Fluvastatin may be taken without regard to meals.

Immediate release capsules: Do not open capsules; do not use two 40 mg capsules for an 80 mg once daily dose; extended release formulation should be used.

Extended release tablet: Do not break, chew, or crush; swallow whole.

Monitoring Parameters

Pediatric patients: Baseline: ALT, AST, and creatine phosphokinase levels (CPK); fasting lipid panel (FLP) and repeat ALT and AST should be checked after 4 weeks of therapy; if no myopathy symptoms or laboratory abnormalities, then monitor FLP, ALT, and AST every 3 to 4 months during the first year and then every 6 months thereafter (NHLBI, 2011).

Adults:

2013 ACC/AHA Blood Cholesterol Guideline recommendations (Stone, 2013):

Lipid panel (total cholesterol, HDL, LDL, triglycerides): Baseline lipid panel; fasting lipid profile within 4 to 12 weeks after initiation or dose adjustment and every 3 to 12 months (as clinically indicated) thereafter. If 2 consecutive LDL levels are <40 mg/dL, consider decreasing the dose.

Hepatic transaminase levels: Baseline measurement of hepatic transaminase levels (ie, ALT); measure hepatic function if symptoms suggest hepatotoxicity (eg, unusual fatigue or weakness, loss of appetite, abdominal pain, dark-colored urine or yellowing of skin or sclera) during therapy.

CPK: CPK should not be routinely measured. Baseline CPK measurement is reasonable for some individuals (eg, family history of statin intolerance or muscle disease, clinical presentation, concomitant drug therapy that may increase risk of myopathy). May measure CPK in any patient with symptoms suggestive of myopathy (pain, tenderness, stiffness, cramping, weakness, or generalized fatigue).

Evaluate for new-onset diabetes mellitus during therapy; if diabetes develops, continue statin therapy and encourage adherence to a heart-healthy diet, physical activity, a healthy body weight, and tobacco cessation.

If patient develops a confusional state or memory impairment, may evaluate patient for nonstatin causes (eg, exposure to other drugs), systemic and neuropsychiatric causes, and the possibility of adverse effects associated with statin therapy.

Manufacturer recommendations: Liver enzyme tests at baseline and repeated when clinically indicated. Measure CPK when myopathy is being considered. Upon initiation or titration, lipid panel should be analyzed at 4 weeks.

Dosage Forms Excipient information presented when available (limited, particularly for generics); consult specific product labeling.

Capsule, Oral:

Lescol: 20 mg, 40 mg

Generic: 20 mg, 40 mg

Tablet Extended Release 24 Hour, Oral:

Lescol XL: 80 mg

◆ **Fluviral (Can)** *see* Influenza Virus Vaccine (Inactivated) *on page 1108*

◆ **Fluvirin** *see* Influenza Virus Vaccine (Inactivated) *on page 1108*

◆ **Fluvirin Preservative Free** *see* Influenza Virus Vaccine (Inactivated) *on page 1108*

FluvoxaMINE (floo VOKS a meen)

Medication Safety Issues

Sound-alike/look-alike issues:

FluvoxaMINE may be confused with flavoxATE, FLUoxetine, fluPHENAZine

Luvox may be confused with Lasix, Levoxyl, Lovenox

BEERS Criteria medication:

This drug may be potentially inappropriate for use in geriatric patients with a history of falls or fractures (Quality of evidence - high [moderate for SIADH]; Strength of recommendation - strong).

Related Information

Antidepressant Agents *on page 2257*

Oral Medications That Should Not Be Crushed or Altered *on page 2476*

Brand Names: US Luvox CR [DSC]

Brand Names: Canada ACT-Fluvoxamine; Apo-Fluvoxamine; Ava-Fluvoxamine; Dom-Fluvoxamine; Luvox; Novo-Fluvoxamine; PHL-Fluvoxamine; PMS-Fluvoxamine; ratio-Fluvoxamine; Riva-Fluvox; Sandoz-Fluvoxamine

Therapeutic Category Antidepressant, Selective Serotonin Reuptake Inhibitor (SSRI)

Generic Availability (US) Yes

Use

Tablets: Treatment of obsessive-compulsive disorder (OCD) (FDA approved in ages ≥8 years and adults)

Extended-release capsules: Treatment of obsessive-compulsive disorder (OCD) (FDA approved in adults)

Medication Guide Available Yes

Pregnancy Risk Factor C

Pregnancy Considerations Adverse events have been observed in animal reproduction studies. Fluvoxamine crosses the human placenta. An increased risk of teratogenic effects, including cardiovascular defects, may be associated with maternal use of fluvoxamine or other SSRIs; however, available information is conflicting. Nonteratogenic effects in the newborn following SSRI/SNRI exposure late in the third trimester include respiratory distress, cyanosis, apnea, seizures, temperature instability, feeding difficulty, vomiting, hypoglycemia, hypo- or hypertonia, hyper-reflexia, jitteriness, irritability, constant crying, and tremor. Symptoms may be due to the toxicity of the SSRIs/SNRIs or a discontinuation syndrome and may be consistent with serotonin syndrome associated with SSRI treatment. Persistent pulmonary hypertension of the newborn (PPHN) has also been reported with SSRI exposure. The long-term effects of *in utero* SSRI exposure on infant development and behavior are not known.

The ACOG recommends that therapy with SSRIs or SNRIs during pregnancy be individualized; treatment of depression during pregnancy should incorporate the clinical expertise of the mental health clinician, obstetrician, primary healthcare provider, and pediatrician. According to the American Psychiatric Association (APA), the risks of medication treatment should be weighed against other treatment options and untreated depression. For women who discontinue antidepressant medications during pregnancy and who may be at high risk for postpartum depression, the medications can be restarted following delivery. Treatment algorithms have been developed by the ACOG and the APA for the management of depression in women prior to conception and during pregnancy.

Breast-Feeding Considerations Fluvoxamine is excreted in breast milk. Based on case reports, the dose the infant receives is relatively small and adverse events have not been observed. Adverse events have been reported in nursing infants exposed to some SSRIs. According to the manufacturer, the decision to continue or discontinue breast-feeding during therapy should take into account the risk of exposure to the infant and the benefits of treatment to the mother.

The long-term effects on development and behavior have not been studied; therefore, fluvoxamine should be prescribed to a mother who is breast-feeding only when the benefits outweigh the potential risks. Maternal use of an SSRI during pregnancy may cause delayed milk secretion.

Contraindications

Concurrent use with alosetron, pimozide, ramelteon, thioridazine, or tizanidine; use of MAO inhibitors intended to treat psychiatric disorders (concurrently or within 14 days of discontinuing either fluvoxamine or the MAO inhibitor); initiation of fluvoxamine in a patient receiving linezolid or intravenous methylene blue.

Canadian labeling: Additional contraindications (not in US labeling): Hypersensitivity to fluvoxamine or any component of the formulation; concurrent use with astemizole, cisapride, mesoridazine, or terfenadine.

Warnings/Precautions [US Boxed Warning]: Antidepressants increase the risk of suicidal thinking and behavior in children, adolescents, and young adults (18 to 24 years of age) with major depressive disorder (MDD) and other psychiatric disorders; consider risk prior to prescribing. Short-term studies did not show an increased risk in patients >24 years of age and showed a decreased risk in patients ≥65 years. Closely monitor patients for clinical worsening, suicidality, or unusual changes in behavior, particularly during the initial 1 to 2 months of therapy or during periods of dosage adjustments (increases or decreases); the patient's family or caregiver should be instructed to closely observe the patient and communicate condition with healthcare provider. A medication guide concerning the use of antidepressants should be dispensed with each prescription. **Fluvoxamine is FDA approved for the treatment of OCD in children ≥8 years of age.**

The possibility of a suicide attempt is inherent in major depression and may persist until remission occurs. Use caution in high-risk patients. Worsening depression and severe abrupt suicidality that are not part of the presenting symptoms may require discontinuation or modification of drug therapy. The patient's family or caregiver should be alerted to monitor patients for the emergence of suicidality and associated behaviors (such as agitation, irritability, hostility, impulsivity, and hypomania) and call healthcare provider.

May worsen psychosis in some patients or precipitate a shift to mania or hypomania in patients with bipolar disorder. Patients presenting with depressive symptoms should be screened for bipolar disorder. Monotherapy in patients with bipolar disorder should be avoided. **Fluvoxamine is not FDA approved for the treatment of bipolar depression.**

Potentially life-threatening serotonin syndrome (SS) has occurred with serotonergic agents (eg, SSRIs, SNRIs), particularly when used in combination with other serotonergic agents (eg, triptans, TCAs, fentanyl, lithium, tramadol, buspirone, St John's wort, tryptophan) or agents that impair metabolism of serotonin (eg, MAO inhibitors intended to treat psychiatric disorders, other MAO inhibitors [ie, linezolid and intravenous methylene blue]). Discontinue treatment (and any concomitant serotonergic agent) immediately if signs/symptoms arise. Fluvoxamine has a low potential to impair cognitive or motor performance; caution operating hazardous machinery or driving. Use caution in patients with a previous seizure disorder rand avoid use with unstable seizure disorder. Discontinue use if seizures occur or if seizure frequency increases. Potentially significant drug-drug interactions may exist, requiring dose or frequency adjustment, additional monitoring, and/or selection of alternative therapy. Fluvoxamine levels may be lower in patients who smoke.

Benefit/risks of combined therapy with electroconvulsive therapy have not been established. Bone fractures have been associated with antidepressant treatment. Consider the possibility of a fragility fracture if an antidepressant-treated patient presents with unexplained bone pain, point tenderness, swelling, or bruising (Rabenda, 2013; Rizzoli, 2012). Use with caution in patients with hepatic dysfunction and in elderly patients. May cause hyponatremia/ SIADH (elderly at increased risk); volume depletion (diuretics may increase risk). Use with caution in patients at risk of bleeding or receiving concurrent anticoagulant therapy, although not consistently noted, fluvoxamine may cause impairment in platelet function. May cause or exacerbate sexual dysfunction. Use caution in elderly patients; may be potentially inappropriate in patients with a history of falls or fractures, and may cause or exacerbate SIADH or hyponatremia; monitor sodium closely with initiation or dosage adjustments in older adults (Beers Criteria). May cause mild pupillary dilation which in susceptible individuals can lead to an episode of narrow-angle glaucoma. Consider evaluating patients who have not had an iridectomy for narrow-angle glaucoma risk factors. Impaired glucose control (eg, hyperglycemia, hypoglycemia) has been reported; monitor for signs/symptoms of loss of glucose control particularly in diabetic patients. Abrupt discontinuation or interruption of antidepressant therapy has been associated with a discontinuation syndrome. Symptoms arising may vary with antidepressant however commonly include nausea, vomiting, diarrhea, headaches, light-headedness, dizziness, diminished appetite, sweating, chills, tremors, paresthesias, fatigue, somnolence, and sleep disturbances (eg, vivid dreams, insomnia). Greater risks for developing a discontinuation syndrome have been associated with antidepressants with shorter half-lives, longer durations of treatment, and abrupt discontinuation. For antidepressants of short or intermediate half-lives, symptoms may emerge within 2 to 5 days after treatment discontinuation and last 7 to 14 days (APA, 2010; Fava, 2006; Haddad, 2001; Shelton, 2001; Warner, 2006).

Warnings: Additional Pediatric Considerations SSRI-associated behavioral activation (ie, restlessness, hyperkinesis, hyperactivity, agitation) is two- to threefold more prevalent in children compared to adolescents; it is more prevalent in adolescents compared to adults. Somnolence (including sedation and drowsiness) is more common in adults compared to children and adolescents (Safer, 2006). May impair cognitive or motor performance. SSRI-associated vomiting is two- to threefold more prevalent in children compared to adolescents and is more prevalent in adolescents compared to adults (Safer, 2006).

Adverse Reactions

Cardiovascular: Chest pain, edema, hypertension, hypotension, palpitations, syncope, vasodilation

Central nervous system: Abnormal dreams, abnormality in thinking, agitation, amnesia, anorgasmia, anxiety, apathy, central nervous system stimulation, chills, depression, dizziness, drowsiness, headache, hypertonia, insomnia, malaise, manic reaction, myoclonus, nervousness, pain,

paresthesia, psychoneurosis, psychotic reaction, twitching, yawning
Dermatologic: Acne vulgaris, diaphoresis, ecchymoses
Endocrine & metabolic: Decreased libido (incidence higher in males), hypermenorrhea, weight gain, weight loss
Gastrointestinal: Abdominal pain, anorexia, constipation, diarrhea, dysgeusia, dyspepsia, dysphagia, flatulence, gingivitis, nausea, vomiting, xerostomia
Genitourinary: Ejaculatory disorder, impotence, sexual disorder, urinary frequency, urinary retention, urinary tract infection
Hepatic: Abnormal hepatic function tests
Infection: Viral infection
Neuromuscular & skeletal: Hyperkinesia, hypokinesia, myalgia, tremor, weakness
Ophthalmic: Amblyopia
Renal: Polyuria
Respiratory: Bronchitis, dyspnea, epistaxis, flu-like symptoms, increased cough, laryngitis, pharyngitis, sinusitis, upper respiratory tract infection
Rare but important or life-threatening: Acute renal failure, agranulocytosis, akinesia, anaphylaxis, anemia, angina, angioedema, angle-closure glaucoma, anuria, aplastic anemia, apnea, asthma, ataxia, bradycardia, bullous skin disease, cardiac conduction delay, cardiac failure, cardiomyopathy, cardiorespiratory arrest, cerebrovascular accident, cholecystitis, cholelithiasis, colitis, coronary artery disease, decreased white blood cell count, dental caries, dental extraction, diplopia, dyskinesia, dystonia, extrapyramidal reaction, first degree atrioventricular block, gastrointestinal hemorrhage, goiter, hallucination, hematemesis, hematuria, hemoptysis, hepatitis, homicidal ideation, hypercholesterolemia, hyperglycemia, hypersensitivity reaction, hypoglycemia, hypokalemia, hyponatremia, hypothyroidism, IgA vasculitis, interstitial pulmonary disease, intestinal obstruction, jaundice, leukocytosis, leukopenia, loss of consciousness, lymphadenopathy, myasthenia, myocardial infarction, myopathy, neuroleptic malignant syndrome (Stevens, 2008), pancreatitis, paralysis, pericarditis, porphyria, prolonged Q-T interval on ECG, purpura, rhabdomyolysis, seizure, serotonin syndrome, ST segment changes on ECG, Stevens-Johnson syndrome, suicidal tendencies, supraventricular extrasystole, tachycardia, tardive dyskinesia, thrombocytopenia, thromboembolism, tooth abscess, toothache, toxic epidermal necrolysis, vasculitis, ventricular arrhythmia, ventricular tachycardia (including torsades de pointes)

Drug Interactions

Metabolism/Transport Effects Substrate of CYP1A2 (major), CYP2D6 (major); **Note:** Assignment of Major/Minor substrate status based on clinically relevant drug interaction potential; **Inhibits** CYP1A2 (strong), CYP2B6 (weak), CYP2C19 (strong), CYP2C9 (weak), CYP2D6 (weak), CYP3A4 (weak)

Avoid Concomitant Use

Avoid concomitant use of FluvoxaMINE with any of the following: Agomelatine; Alosetron; Dapoxetine; Dosulepin; DULoxetine; Iobenguane I 123; Linezolid; MAO Inhibitors; Methylene Blue; Pimozide; Pomalidomide; Ramelteon; Tasimelteon; Thioridazine; TiZANidine; Tryptophan; Urokinase

Increased Effect/Toxicity

FluvoxaMINE may increase the levels/effects of: Agents with Antiplatelet Properties; Agomelatine; Alosetron; ALPRAZolam; Anticoagulants; Antidepressants (Serotonin Reuptake Inhibitor/Antagonist); Antipsychotic Agents; Apixaban; ARIPiprazole; Asenapine; Aspirin; Bendamustine; Blood Glucose Lowering Agents; Bromazepam; BusPIRone; CarBAMazepine; Cilostazol; Citalopram; Clopidogrel; CloZAPine; Collagenase (Systemic); CYP1A2 Substrates; CYP2C19 Substrates; Dabigatran Etexilate; Deoxycholic Acid; Desmopressin; Dofetilide; Dosulepin; DULoxetine; Erlotinib; Etizolam; Fosphenytoin; Haloperidol; Hydrocodone; Ibritumomab; Lomitapide; Methadone; Methylene Blue; Mexiletine; NiMODipine; NSAID (COX-2 Inhibitor); NSAID (Nonselective); Obinutuzumab; OLANZapine; Pentoxifylline; Phenytoin; Pimozide; Pirfenidone; Pomalidomide; Propafenone; Propranolol; QuiNIDine; Ramelteon; Rivaroxaban; Roflumilast; Ropivacaine; Salicylates; Serotonin Modulators; Tasimelteon; Theophylline Derivatives; Thiazide Diuretics; Thioridazine; Thrombolytic Agents; TiZANidine; Tositumomab and Iodine I 131 Tositumomab; TraMADol; Tricyclic Antidepressants; Urokinase; Vitamin K Antagonists; Zolpidem

The levels/effects of FluvoxaMINE may be increased by: Abiraterone Acetate; Alcohol (Ethyl); Analgesics (Opioid); Antiemetics (5HT3 Antagonists); Antipsychotic Agents; BuPROPion; BusPIRone; Cimetidine; CNS Depressants; Cobicistat; CYP1A2 Inhibitors (Moderate); CYP1A2 Inhibitors (Strong); CYP2D6 Inhibitors (Moderate); CYP2D6 Inhibitors (Strong); Dapoxetine; Darunavir; Dasatinib; Deferasirox; Glucosamine; Grapefruit Juice; Herbs (Anticoagulant/Antiplatelet Properties); Ibrutinib; Limaprost; Linezolid; Lithium; MAO Inhibitors; Metoclopramide; Metyrosine; Multivitamins/Fluoride (with ADE); Multivitamins/Minerals (with ADEK, Folate, Iron); Multivitamins/Minerals (with AE, No Iron); Omega-3 Fatty Acids; Panobinostat; Peginterferon Alfa-2b; Pentosan Polysulfate Sodium; Pentoxifylline; Prostacyclin Analogues; QuiNIDine; Tedizolid; TraMADol; Tryptophan; Vemurafenib; Vitamin E

Decreased Effect

FluvoxaMINE may decrease the levels/effects of: Clopidogrel; Iobenguane I 123; Ioflupane I 123; Thyroid Products

The levels/effects of FluvoxaMINE may be decreased by: Cannabis; CarBAMazepine; CYP1A2 Inducers (Strong); Cyproheptadine; Cyproterone; NSAID (COX-2 Inhibitor); NSAID (Nonselective); Peginterferon Alfa-2b; Teriflunomide

Storage/Stability Protect from high humidity and store at controlled room temperature 25°C (77°F); excursions are permitted between 15°C and 30°C (59°F and 86°F).

Mechanism of Action Inhibits CNS neuron serotonin uptake; minimal or no effect on reuptake of norepinephrine or dopamine; does not significantly bind to alpha-adrenergic, histamine or cholinergic receptors

Pharmacodynamics

Onset of action: 1-2 weeks
Maximum effect: 8-12 weeks
Duration: 1-2 days

Pharmacokinetics (Adult data unless noted) Note: Steady-state plasma concentrations (following administration of the immediate-release product) have been noted to be 2-3 times higher in children than those in adolescents; female children demonstrated a significantly higher AUC and peak concentration than males.

Distribution: V_d, apparent: Adults: ~25 L/kg
Protein binding: ~80%, primarily to albumin
Metabolism: Extensive via the liver; major metabolic routes are oxidative demethylation and deamination; dose-dependent (nonlinear) pharmacokinetics
Bioavailability: Immediate release: 53%; extended release: 84% (compared to immediate release); bioavailability is not significantly affected by food for either formulation
Half-life: Adults: 15.6 hours
Time to peak serum concentration: 3-8 hours
Elimination: 94% of the dose is excreted in the urine, primarily as metabolites; 2% as unchanged drug
Clearance: Hepatic dysfunction: Decreased by 30%

Dosing: Usual Oral:

Obsessive compulsive disorder:

Children 8-17 years: Immediate release: Initial: 25 mg once daily at bedtime; adjust in 25 mg increments at 7- to 14-day intervals, as tolerated, to maximum therapeutic benefit; usual dosage range: 50-200 mg/day; daily doses >50 mg should be divided into 2 doses; administer larger portion at bedtime

Maximum: Children: 8-11 years: 200 mg/day; Adolescents: 300 mg/day; lower doses may be effective in female versus male patients

Note: Slower titration of dose every 2-4 weeks may minimize the risk of behavioral activation; behavioral activation associated with SSRI use increases the risk of suicidal behavior. Higher mg/kg doses are needed in children compared to adolescents.

Adults:

Immediate release: Initial: 50 mg once daily at bedtime; adjust in 50 mg increments at 4- to 7-day intervals; usual dosage range: 100-300 mg/day; daily doses >100 mg should be divided into 2 doses; administer larger portion at bedtime; maximum dose: 300 mg/day

Extended release: Initial: 100 mg once daily at bedtime; may be increased in 50 mg increments at intervals of at least 1 week; usual dosage range: 100-300 mg/day; maximum dose: 300 mg/day

Dosage adjustment in hepatic impairment: Decrease initial dose and dose titration; titrate slowly

Administration May be administered without regard to meals. Do not chew or crush extended-release capsule; swallow whole.

Monitoring Parameters Monitor patient periodically for symptom resolution; monitor for worsening depression, suicidality, and associated behaviors (especially at the beginning of therapy or when doses are increased or decreased. Monitor for anxiety, social functioning, mania, panic attacks; akathisia, weight gain or loss, nutritional intake, sleep. Monitor for signs and symptoms of serotonin syndrome or neuroleptic malignant syndrome-like reactions.

Additional Information A recent report (Lake 2000) describes five children (age 8 to 15 years) who developed epistaxis (n=4) or bruising (n=1) while receiving sertraline therapy. Another recent report describes the SSRI discontinuation syndrome in six children; the syndrome was similar to that reported in adults (Diler 2002). Due to limited long-term studies, the clinical usefulness of fluvoxamine should be periodically reevaluated in patients receiving the drug for extended intervals; effects of long term use of fluvoxamine on pediatric growth, development, and maturation have not been directly assessed. **Note:** Case reports of decreased growth in children receiving fluoxetine or fluvoxamine (n=4; age: 11.6 to 13.7 years) for 6 months to 5 years suggest a suppression of growth hormone secretion during SSRI therapy (Weintrob 2002).

Neonates born to women receiving SSRIs late during the third trimester may experience respiratory distress, apnea, cyanosis, temperature instability, vomiting, feeding difficulty, hypoglycemia, constant crying, irritability, hypotonia, hypertonia, hyper-reflexia, tremor, jitteriness, and seizures; these symptoms may be due to a direct toxic effect, withdrawal syndrome, or (in some cases) serotonin syndrome. Withdrawal symptoms occur in 30% of neonates exposed to SSRIs *in utero*; monitor newborns for at least 48 hours after birth; long-term effects of *in utero* exposure to SSRIs are unknown (Levinson-Castiel 2006).

Dosage Forms Excipient information presented when available (limited, particularly for generics); consult specific product labeling. [DSC] = Discontinued product

Capsule Extended Release 24 Hour, Oral, as maleate:

Luvox CR: 100 mg [DSC], 150 mg [DSC] [gluten free; contains fd&c blue #2 (indigotine)]

Generic: 100 mg, 150 mg

Tablet, Oral, as maleate:

Generic: 25 mg, 50 mg, 100 mg

- ◆ **Fluzone** *see* Influenza Virus Vaccine (Inactivated) *on page 1108*
- ◆ **Fluzone High-Dose** *see* Influenza Virus Vaccine (Inactivated) *on page 1108*
- ◆ **Fluzone Pediatric PF [DSC]** *see* Influenza Virus Vaccine (Inactivated) *on page 1108*
- ◆ **Fluzone Preservative Free [DSC]** *see* Influenza Virus Vaccine (Inactivated) *on page 1108*
- ◆ **Fluzone Quadrivalent** *see* Influenza Virus Vaccine (Inactivated) *on page 1108*
- ◆ **FML** *see* Fluorometholone *on page 903*
- ◆ **FML® (Can)** *see* Fluorometholone *on page 903*
- ◆ **FML Forte** *see* Fluorometholone *on page 903*
- ◆ **FML Forte® (Can)** *see* Fluorometholone *on page 903*
- ◆ **FML Liquifilm** *see* Fluorometholone *on page 903*
- ◆ **Focalin** *see* Dexmethylphenidate *on page 619*
- ◆ **Focalin XR** *see* Dexmethylphenidate *on page 619*
- ◆ **Foille [OTC]** *see* Benzocaine *on page 268*
- ◆ **Folacin** *see* Folic Acid *on page 931*
- ◆ **Folate** *see* Folic Acid *on page 931*

Folic Acid (FOE lik AS id)

Medication Safety Issues

Sound-alike/look-alike issues:

Folic acid may be confused with folinic acid (leucovorin calcium)

Brand Names: US FA-8 [OTC]

Brand Names: Canada Apo-Folic®

Therapeutic Category Nutritional Supplement; Vitamin, Water Soluble

Generic Availability (US) Yes

Use Treatment of megaloblastic and macrocytic anemias due to folate deficiency (FDA approved in all ages); has also been used as a dietary supplement to prevent neural tube defects and prevention of gingival hyperplasia due to phenytoin

Pregnancy Risk Factor A

Pregnancy Considerations Water soluble vitamins cross the placenta. Folate requirements increase during pregnancy. Folate supplementation during the periconceptual period decreases the risk of neural tube defects. Folate supplementation (doses larger than the RDA) is recommended for women who may become pregnant (IOM, 1998).

Breast-Feeding Considerations Folate is found in breast milk; concentrations are not affected by dietary intake unless the mother has a severe deficiency (IOM, 1998).

Contraindications Hypersensitivity to folic acid or any component of the formulation

Warnings/Precautions Not appropriate for monotherapy with pernicious, aplastic, or normocytic anemias when anemia is present with vitamin B_{12} deficiency. Doses >0.1 mg/day may obscure pernicious anemia with continuing irreversible nerve damage progression. Resistance to treatment may occur with depressed hematopoiesis, alcoholism, and deficiencies of other vitamins. Injection contains benzyl alcohol (1.5%) as preservative (use care in administration to neonates).

Aluminum: The parenteral product may contain aluminum; toxic aluminum concentrations may be seen with high doses, prolonged use, or renal dysfunction. Premature neonates are at higher risk due to immature renal function and aluminum intake from other parenteral sources. Parenteral aluminum exposure of >4 to 5 mcg/kg/day is associated with CNS and bone toxicity; tissue loading may occur at lower doses (Federal Register, 2002). See manufacturer's labeling.

Benzyl alcohol and derivatives: Some dosage forms may contain benzyl alcohol; large amounts of benzyl alcohol (≥99 mg/kg/day) have been associated with a potentially fatal toxicity ("gasping syndrome") in neonates; the "gasping syndrome" consists of metabolic acidosis, respiratory distress, gasping respirations, CNS dysfunction (including convulsions, intracranial hemorrhage), hypotension and cardiovascular collapse (AAP, 1997; CDC, 1982); some data suggests that benzoate displaces bilirubin from protein binding sites (Ahlfors, 2001); avoid or use dosage forms containing benzyl alcohol with caution in neonates. See manufacturer's labeling.

Adverse Reactions

Cardiovascular: Flushing (slight)
Central nervous system: Malaise (general)
Dermatologic: Erythema, pruritus, rash
Respiratory: Bronchospasm
Miscellaneous: Allergic reaction

Drug Interactions

Metabolism/Transport Effects None known.

Avoid Concomitant Use

Avoid concomitant use of Folic Acid with any of the following: Raltitrexed

Increased Effect/Toxicity There are no known significant interactions involving an increase in effect.

Decreased Effect

Folic Acid may decrease the levels/effects of: Fosphenytoin; PHENobarbital; Phenytoin; Primidone; Raltitrexed

The levels/effects of Folic Acid may be decreased by: Green Tea; SulfaSALAzine

Storage/Stability Store at 20°C to 25°C (68°F to 77°F); protect from light.

Mechanism of Action Folic acid is necessary for formation of a number of coenzymes in many metabolic systems, particularly for purine and pyrimidine synthesis; required for nucleoprotein synthesis and maintenance in erythropoiesis; stimulates WBC and platelet production in folate deficiency anemia. Folic acid enhances the metabolism of formic acid, the toxic metabolite of methanol, to nontoxic metabolites (off-label use).

Pharmacodynamics Maximum effect: Oral: Within 30-60 minutes

Pharmacokinetics (Adult data unless noted)

Absorption: In the proximal part of the small intestine
Bioavailability: Oral: Folic acid supplement: ~100%; in presence of food: 85%; Dietary folate: 50% (IOM, 1999)
Metabolism: Hepatic
Time to peak serum concentration: Oral: 1 hour
Elimination: Trace amounts of unchanged drug in urine; 90% of dose as metabolites

Dosing: Neonatal

Enteral daily recommendations; adequate intake (Vanek, 2012): Oral:
Premature neonates: 25-50 mcg/kg/day
Full-term neonates: 65 mcg/day

Parenteral nutrition, maintenance requirement of folic acid (Vanek, 2012): IV:
Premature neonates: 56 mcg/kg/day
Full-term neonates: 140 mcg/day

Dosing: Usual

Infants, Children, and Adolescents:

Adequate intake (AI): Oral: **Note:** Dosing presented as dietary folate equivalents (DFE) to adjust for ~50% decreased bioavailability of food folate compared with that of folic acid supplement.
1-6 months: 65 mcg/day
7-12 months: 80 mcg/day

Recommended daily allowance (RDA): Oral: **Note:** Dosing presented as dietary folate equivalents (DFE) to adjust for ~50% decreased bioavailability of food folate compared with that of folic acid supplement.
1-3 years: 150 mcg/day
4-8 years: 200 mcg/day
9-13 years: 300 mcg/day
Adolescents ≥14 years: 400 mcg/day

Anemia (folic acid deficiency); treatment: Oral, IM, IV, SubQ:
Infants: 0.1 mg/day
Children <4 years: Up to 0.3 mg/day
Children >4 years and Adolescents: 0.4 mg/day

Parenteral nutrition, maintenance requirement of folic acid (Vanek, 2012): IV:
Infants: 56 mcg/kg/day
Children and Adolescents ≤13 years: 140 mcg/day
Adolescents ≥14 years: 400 mcg/day

Gingival hyperplasia due to phenytoin, prevention: Limited data available: Oral: Children ≥6 years and Adolescents: 0.5 mg/day was used in a double-blind, randomized, placebo-controlled trial of 120 pediatric patients (treatment arm, n=62; age range: 6-15 years) who were started on phenytoin therapy within the last month for a seizure disorder; results showed a statistically significant difference in development of hyperplasia (treatment arm: 21% vs placebo: 88%); severity of cases less in treatment arm than placebo; study duration: 6 months (Arya, 2011)

Adults:

Recommended daily allowance (RDA): Expressed as dietary folate equivalents: Oral: 400 mcg/day
Pregnancy: 600 mcg/day
Lactation: 500 mcg/day

Anemia (folic acid deficiency); treatment: Oral, IM, IV, SubQ:
Nonpregnant and nonlactating adults: 0.4 mg/day
Pregnant and lactating women: 0.8 mg/day

Prevention of neural tube defects: Oral:
Females of childbearing potential: 400-800 mcg/day (USPSTF, 2009)
Females at high-risk or with family history of neural tube defects: 4 mg/day (ACOG, 2003)

Preparation for Administration Parenteral: IV: May further dilute doses ≤5 mg in 50 mL of NS or D_5W; maximum concentration: 0.1 mg/mL. May also be added to IV maintenance solution.

Administration

Oral: May be administered without regard to meals
Parenteral:
IM, SubQ: May administer undiluted deep IM or SubQ
IV: May administer doses ≤5 mg undiluted over ≥1 minute **or** may further dilute and infuse over 30 minutes. May also be given as an infusion when added to IV maintenance solutions.

Monitoring Parameters CBC with differential

Reference Range Total folate: Normal: 5-15 ng/mL; folate deficiency: <5 ng/mL; megaloblastic anemia: <2 ng/mL

Test Interactions Falsely low serum concentrations may occur with the *Lactobacillus casei* assay method in patients on anti-infectives (eg, tetracycline)

Additional Information Dietary folate equivalents (DFE) is used to adjust for ~50% decreased bioavailability of food folate compared with that of folic acid supplement:
1 mcg DFE = 0.6 mcg folic acid from fortified food or as a supplement taken with meals, or
1 mcg DFE of food folate = 0.5 mcg of a supplement taken on an empty stomach

As of January 1998, the FDA has required manufacturers of enriched flour, bread, corn meal, pasta, rice, and other grain products to add folic acid to their products. The intent is to help decrease the risk of neural tube defects by increasing folic acid intake. Other foods which contain folic acid include dark green leafy vegetables, citrus fruits and juices, and lentils.

Dosage Forms Excipient information presented when available (limited, particularly for generics); consult specific product labeling.

Capsule, Oral [preservative free]:
FA-8: 0.8 mg [dye free, sugar free, yeast free]
Generic: 5 mg, 20 mg

Solution, Injection, as sodium folate:
Generic: 5 mg/mL (10 mL)

Tablet, Oral:
Generic: 400 mcg, 800 mcg, 1 mg

Tablet, Oral [preservative free]:
FA-8: 800 mcg [dye free]
Generic: 400 mcg, 800 mcg

Extemporaneous Preparations A 1 mg/mL folic acid oral solution may be made with tablets. Heat 90 mL of purified water almost to boiling. Dissolve parabens (methylparaben 200 mg and propylparaben 20 mg) in the heated water; cool to room temperature. Crush one-hundred 1 mg tablets, then dissolve folic acid in the solution. Adjust pH to 8-8.5 with sodium hydroxide 10%; add sufficient quantity of purified water to make 100 mL; mix well. Stable for 30 days at room temperature (Allen, 2007).

A 0.05 mg/mL folic acid oral solution may be prepared using the injectable formulation (5 mg/mL). Mix 1 mL of injectable folic acid with 90 mL of purified water. Adjust pH to 8-8.5 with sodium hydroxide 10%; add sufficient quantity of purified water to make 100 mL; mix well. Stable for 30 days at room temperature (Nahata, 2004).

Allen LV Jr, "Folic Acid 1-mg/mL Oral Liquid," *Int J Pharm Compound*, 2007, 11(3):244.

Nahata MC, Pai VB, and Hipple TF, *Pediatric Drug Formulations*, 5th ed, Cincinnati, OH: Harvey Whitney Books Co, 2004.

◆ **Folinate Calcium** *see* Leucovorin Calcium *on page 1226*

◆ **Folinic Acid (error prone synonym)** *see* Leucovorin Calcium *on page 1226*

Fomepizole (foe ME pi zole)

Medication Safety Issues

Sound-alike/look-alike issues:

Fomepizole may be confused with omeprazole

Brand Names: US Antizol

Brand Names: Canada Antizol

Therapeutic Category Antidote, Ethylene Glycol Toxicity; Antidote, Methanol Toxicity

Generic Availability (US) Yes

Use Antidote for ethylene glycol (antifreeze) or methanol toxicity; may be useful in propylene glycol toxicity; FDA approved in ages ≥18 years

Pregnancy Risk Factor C

Pregnancy Considerations Animal reproduction studies have not been conducted. In general, medications used as antidotes should take into consideration the health and prognosis of the mother; antidotes should be administered to pregnant women if there is a clear indication for use and should not be withheld because of fears of teratogenicity (Bailey, 2003).

Breast-Feeding Considerations It is not known if fomepizole is excreted in breast milk. The manufacturer recommends that caution be exercised when administering fomepizole to nursing women.

Contraindications Hypersensitivity to fomepizole, other pyrazoles, or any component of the formulation

Warnings/Precautions Should not be given undiluted or by bolus injection. Fomepizole is metabolized in the liver and excreted in the urine; use caution with hepatic or renal impairment. Hemodialysis should be considered as an adjunct to fomepizole in patients with renal failure, significant acidosis (pH <7.25-7.3), worsening metabolic acidosis, or ethylene glycol or methanol concentrations ≥50 mg/dL. Pediatric administration is not FDA approved; however, safe and efficacious use in this patient population for ethylene glycol and methanol intoxication has been reported (Baum, 2000; Benitez, 2000; Boyer, 2001; Brown, 2001; De Brabander, 2005; Detaille, 2004; Fisher, 1998); consider consultation with a clinical toxicologist or poison control center.

Adverse Reactions

Cardiovascular: Bradycardia, facial flush, hypotension, shock, tachycardia

Central nervous system: Agitation, anxiety, dizziness, drowsiness increased, fever, headache, lightheadedness, seizure, vertigo

Dermatologic: Rash

Endocrine & metabolic: Liver function tests increased

Gastrointestinal: Abdominal pain, appetite decreased, bad/metallic taste, diarrhea, heartburn, nausea, vomiting

Hematologic: Anemia, disseminated intravascular coagulation (DIC), eosinophilia, lymphangitis

Local: Application site reaction, injection site inflammation, pain during injection, phlebitis

Neuromuscular & skeletal: Backache

Ocular: Nystagmus, transient blurred vision, visual disturbances

Renal: Anuria

Respiratory: Abnormal smell, hiccups, pharyngitis

Miscellaneous: Multiorgan failure, speech disturbances

Rare but important or life-threatening: Mild allergic reactions (mild rash, eosinophilia)

Drug Interactions

Metabolism/Transport Effects None known.

Avoid Concomitant Use There are no known interactions where it is recommended to avoid concomitant use.

Increased Effect/Toxicity There are no known significant interactions involving an increase in effect.

Decreased Effect There are no known significant interactions involving a decrease in effect.

Food Interactions Ethanol decreases the rate of fomepizole elimination by ~50%; conversely, fomepizole decreases the rate of elimination of ethanol by ~40%.

Storage/Stability Store at controlled room temperature, 20°C to 25°C (68°F to 77°F); fomepizole solidifies at temperatures <25°C (77°F). If solution becomes solid in the vial, it be should be carefully warmed by running the vial under warm water or by holding in the hand. Solidification does not affect the efficacy, safety, or stability of the drug. Diluted solution should be used within 24 hours and may be stored at room temperature or under refrigeration.

Mechanism of Action Fomepizole competitively inhibits alcohol dehydrogenase, an enzyme which catalyzes the metabolism of ethanol, ethylene glycol, and methanol to their toxic metabolites. Ethylene glycol is metabolized to glycoaldehyde, then oxidized to glycolate, glyoxylate, and oxalate. Glycolate and oxalate are responsible for metabolic acidosis and renal damage. Methanol is metabolized to formaldehyde, then oxidized to formic acid. Formic acid is responsible for metabolic acidosis and visual disturbances.

Pharmacokinetics (Adult data unless noted)

Distribution: V_d: 0.6-1.02 L/kg; rapidly distributes into total body water

Protein binding: Negligible

Metabolism: Liver; primarily to 4-carboxypyrazole; after single doses, exhibits saturable, Michaelis-Menton kinetics; with multiple dosing, fomepizole induces its own metabolism via the cytochrome P450 system; after enzyme induction elimination follows first order kinetics

Elimination: 1% to 3.5% excreted unchanged in the urine

Dialysis: Dialyzable

Dosing: Usual IV:

Children and Adults **not requiring** hemodialysis: Initial: 15 mg/kg loading dose; followed by 10 mg/kg every 12 hours for 4 doses; then 15 mg/kg every 12 hours until ethylene glycol or methanol levels have been reduced to <20 mg/dL

Children and Adults **requiring** hemodialysis: Since fomepizole is dialyzable, follow the above dose recommendations at intervals related to institution of hemodialysis and its duration:

Dose at the beginning of hemodialysis:

If <6 hours since last fomepizole dose: Do **not** administer dose

If ≥6 hours since last fomepizole dose: Administer next scheduled dose

Dose during hemodialysis: Administer every 4 hours or as continuous infusion 1-1.5 mg/kg/hour

Dose at the time hemodialysis is completed (dependent upon the time between the last dose and the end of hemodialysis):

<1 hour: Do **not** administer at the end of hemodialysis

1-3 hours: Administer 1/2 of the next scheduled dose

>3 hours: Administer the next scheduled dose

Maintenance dose off hemodialysis: Give next scheduled dose 12 hours from last dose administered

Dosage adjustment in renal impairment: Fomepizole is substantially excreted by the kidney and the risk of toxic reactions to this drug may be increased in patients with impaired renal function; no dosage recommendations for patients with impaired renal function have been established

Preparation for Administration Parenteral: Dilute in at least 100 mL NS or D_5W (<25 mg/mL). Although, it is chemically and physically stable when diluted as recommended, sterile precautions should be observed because diluents generally do not contain preservatives.

Administration Parenteral: IV: Infuse over 30 minutes; rapid infusion at a concentration of 25 mg/mL has been associated with vein irritation and phlebosclerosis.

Monitoring Parameters Vital signs, arterial blood gases, acid-base status, urinary oxalate, anion and osmolar gaps, clinical signs and symptoms of toxicity (arrhythmias, seizures, coma); serum and urinary ethylene glycol or serum methanol level depending upon the agent ingested; formic acid level (methanol ingestion)

Reference Range Ethylene glycol or methanol serum concentration: Goal: <20 mg/dL; therapeutic plasma fomepizole level: 0.8 mcg/mL

Additional Information If ethylene glycol poisoning is left untreated, the natural progression of the poisoning leads to accumulation of toxic metabolites, including glycolic and oxalic acids; these metabolites can induce metabolic acidosis, seizures, stupor, coma, calcium oxaluria, acute tubular necrosis and death; as ethylene glycol levels diminish in the blood when metabolized to glycolate, the diagnosis of this poisoning may be difficult

Dosage Forms Excipient information presented when available (limited, particularly for generics); consult specific product labeling.

Solution, Intravenous [preservative free]:

Antizol: 1 g/mL (1.5 mL)

Generic: 1 g/mL (1.5 mL); 1.5 g/1.5 mL (1.5 mL)

◆ **Foradil (Can)** *see* Formoterol *on page 934*

◆ **Foradil Aerolizer** *see* Formoterol *on page 934*

◆ **Forfivo XL** *see* BuPROPion *on page 324*

Formoterol (for MOH te rol)

Medication Safety Issues

Sound-alike/look-alike issues:

Foradil may be confused with Fortical, Toradol

Administration issues:

Foradil capsules for inhalation are for administration via Aerolizer inhaler and are **not** for oral use.

International issues:

Foradil [U.S., Canada, and multiple international markets] may be confused with Theradol brand name for tramadol [Netherlands]

Brand Names: US Foradil Aerolizer; Perforomist

Brand Names: Canada Foradil; Oxeze Turbuhaler

Therapeutic Category Adrenergic Agonist Agent; Antiasthmatic; $Beta_2$-Adrenergic Agonist; Bronchodilator; Sympathomimetic

Generic Availability (US) No

Use

Foradil® Aerolizer™: Concomitant therapy with inhaled corticosteroids for maintenance treatment of asthma and prevention of bronchospasm in patients with reversible obstructive airway disease, including patients with nocturnal symptoms (FDA approved in ≥5 years and adults); prevention of exercise-induced bronchospasm as concomitant therapy in patients with persistent asthma and as monotherapy in those without persistent asthma (FDA approved in ≥5 years and adults); **NOT** indicated for the relief of acute bronchospasm

Foradil® Aerolizer™, Perforomist™: Maintenance treatment of bronchoconstriction in COPD (FDA approved in adults); **NOT** indicated for the relief of acute bronchospasm

Medication Guide Available Yes

Pregnancy Risk Factor C

Pregnancy Considerations Adverse events were observed in some animal reproduction studies. Formoterol has the potential to affect uterine contractility if administered during labor.

Uncontrolled asthma is associated with adverse events on pregnancy (increased risk of perinatal mortality, preeclampsia, preterm birth, low birth weight infants). Although data related to its use in pregnancy is limited, formoterol may be used as an alternative agent when a long-acting beta agonist is needed to treat moderate persistent or severe persistent asthma in pregnant women (NAEPP, 2005).

Breast-Feeding Considerations It is not known if formoterol is excreted into breast milk. The manufacturer recommends that caution be exercised when administering formoterol to nursing women. The use of $beta_2$-receptor agonists are not considered a contraindication to breast-feeding (NAEPP, 2005).

Contraindications

Hypersensitivity to formoterol or any component of the formulation (Foradil Aerolizer only); treatment of status asthmaticus or other acute episodes of asthma or COPD (Foradil Aerolizer only); monotherapy in the treatment of asthma (ie, use without a concomitant long-term asthma control medication, such as an inhaled corticosteroid)

Canadian labeling: Additional contraindications (not in U.S. labeling): Presence of tachyarrhythmias

Warnings/Precautions [U.S. Boxed Warning]: Long-acting $beta_2$-agonists (LABAs) increase the risk of asthma-related deaths. Formoterol should only be used in asthma patients as adjuvant therapy in patients who are currently receiving but are not adequately controlled on a long-term asthma control medication (ie, an inhaled corticosteroid). Monotherapy with an LABA is contraindicated in the treatment of asthma. In a large, randomized, placebo-controlled U.S.

clinical trial (SMART, 2006), salmeterol was associated with an increase in asthma-related deaths (when added to usual asthma therapy); risk is considered a class effect among all LABAs. Data are not available to determine if the addition of an inhaled corticosteroid lessens this increased risk of death associated with LABA use. Assess patients at regular intervals once asthma control is maintained on combination therapy to determine if step-down therapy is appropriate and the LABA can be discontinued (without loss of asthma control), and the patient can be maintained on an inhaled corticosteroid. LABAs are not appropriate in patients whose asthma is adequately controlled on low- or medium-dose inhaled corticosteroids. Do **not** use for acute bronchospasm. Short-acting beta$_2$-agonist (eg, albuterol) should be used for acute symptoms and symptoms occurring between treatments. Do **not** initiate in patients with significantly worsening or acutely deteriorating asthma; reports of severe (sometimes fatal) respiratory events have been reported when formoterol has been initiated in this situation. Corticosteroids should not be stopped or reduced when formoterol is initiated. Formoterol is not a substitute for inhaled or systemic corticosteroids and should not be used as monotherapy. During initiation, watch for signs of worsening asthma. **[U.S. Boxed Warning] (Foradil Aerolizer): LABAs may increase the risk of asthma-related hospitalization in pediatric and adolescent patients**. In general, a combination product containing a LABA and an inhaled corticosteroid is preferred in patients <18 years of age to ensure compliance.

Because LABAs may disguise poorly controlled persistent asthma, frequent or chronic use of LABAs for exercise-induced bronchospasm is discouraged by the NIH Asthma Guidelines (NIH, 2007). The safety and efficacy of Perforomist in asthma patients have not been established and is not FDA approved for the treatment of asthma.

Do **not** use for acute episodes of COPD. Do **not** initiate in patients with significantly worsening or acutely deteriorating COPD. Data are not available to determine if LABA use increases the risk of death in patients with COPD. Increased use and/or ineffectiveness of short-acting beta$_2$-agonists may indicate rapidly deteriorating disease and should prompt re-evaluation of the patient's condition.

Immediate hypersensitivity reactions (urticaria, angioedema, rash, bronchospasm) have been reported. Do not exceed recommended dose or frequency; serious adverse events (including serious asthma exacerbations and fatalities) have been associated with excessive use of inhaled sympathomimetics. Beta$_2$-agonists may increase risk of arrhythmias, decrease serum potassium, prolong QTc interval, or increase serum glucose. These effects may be exacerbated in hypoxemia. Use caution in patients with cardiovascular disease (arrhythmia, coronary insufficiency, hypertension, HF, or aneurysm), seizures, diabetes, hyperthyroidism, pheochromocytoma, or hypokalemia. Beta-agonists may cause elevation in blood pressure and heart rate, and result in CNS stimulation/excitation. Tolerance to the bronchodilator effect, measured by FEV$_1$, has been observed in studies.

Powder for oral inhalation contains lactose; very rare anaphylactic reactions have been reported in patients with severe milk protein allergy. The contents of the Foradil Aerolizer capsules are for inhalation only via the Aerolizer device. There have been reports of incorrect administration (swallowing of the capsules).

Adverse Reactions

Cardiovascular: Chest pain, palpitation
Central nervous system: Anxiety, dizziness, dysphonia, fever, headache, insomnia
Dermatologic: Pruritus, rash
Gastrointestinal: Abdominal pain, diarrhea, dyspepsia, gastroenteritis, nausea, vomiting, xerostomia
Neuromuscular & skeletal: Muscle cramps, tremor
Respiratory: Asthma exacerbation, bronchitis, dyspnea, infection, pharyngitis, sinusitis, tonsillitis
Miscellaneous: Viral infection
Rare but important or life-threatening: Acute asthma deterioration, anaphylactic reactions (severe hypotension/angioedema), agitation, angina, arrhythmia, atrial fibrillation, bronchospasm (paradoxical), cough, fatigue, hyperglycemia, hypertension, hypokalemia, glucose intolerance, malaise, metabolic acidosis, nervousness, QTc prolongation, tachycardia, ventricular extrasystoles

Drug Interactions

Metabolism/Transport Effects Substrate of CYP2C9 (minor); **Note:** Assignment of Major/Minor substrate status based on clinically relevant drug interaction potential

Avoid Concomitant Use

Avoid concomitant use of Formoterol with any of the following: Beta-Blockers (Nonselective); Iobenguane I 123; Long-Acting Beta2-Agonists; Loxapine

Increased Effect/Toxicity

Formoterol may increase the levels/effects of: Atosiban; Highest Risk QTc-Prolonging Agents; Long-Acting Beta2-Agonists; Loop Diuretics; Loxapine; Moderate Risk QTc-Prolonging Agents; Sympathomimetics; Thiazide Diuretics

The levels/effects of Formoterol may be increased by: AtoMOXetine; Caffeine and Caffeine Containing Products; Cannabinoid-Containing Products; Inhalational Anesthetics; Linezolid; MAO Inhibitors; Mifepristone; Tedizolid; Theophylline Derivatives; Tricyclic Antidepressants

Decreased Effect

Formoterol may decrease the levels/effects of: Iobenguane I 123

The levels/effects of Formoterol may be decreased by: Beta-Blockers (Beta1 Selective); Beta-Blockers (Nonselective); Betahistine

Storage/Stability

Foradil Aerolizer: Prior to dispensing, store in refrigerator at 2°C to 8°C (36°F to 46°F). After dispensing, store at room temperature at 20°C to 25°C (68°F to 77°F). Protect from heat and moisture. Capsules should always be stored in the blister and only removed immediately before use.
Perforomist: Prior to dispensing, store in refrigerator at 2°C to 8°C (36°F to 46°F). After dispensing, store at 2°C to 25°C (36°F to 77°F) for up to 3 months. Protect from heat. Unit-dose vials should always be stored in the foil pouch and only removed immediately before use.

Mechanism of Action Relaxes bronchial smooth muscle by selective action on beta$_2$ receptors with little effect on heart rate. Formoterol has a long-acting effect.

Pharmacodynamics

Onset of action: Powder for oral inhalation: 1-3 minutes
Peak effect:
  Powder for oral inhalation: 80% of peak effect within 15 minutes
  Solution for nebulization: Median: 2 hours
Duration: Improvement in FEV$_1$ observed for 12 hours in most patients

Pharmacokinetics (Adult data unless noted)

Absorption: Rapidly into plasma
Protein binding: 61% to 64%
Metabolism: Extensive via glucuronidation and o-demethylation; CYP2D6, CYP2C8/9, CYP2C19, CYP2A6 involved in O-demethylation
Half-life:
  Powder for oral inhalation: ~10-14 hours
  Solution for nebulization: ~7 hours

Time to peak serum concentration: Inhalation: 5 minutes
Elimination:
Children 5-12 years: 7% to 9% eliminated in urine as direct glucuronide metabolites, 6% as unchanged drug
Adults: 15% to 18% eliminated in urine as direct glucuronide metabolites, 2% to 10% as unchanged drug

Dosing: Usual

Asthma, maintenance treatment: Children ≥5 years, Adolescents, and Adults: Inhalation: Foradil® Aerolizer™: 12 mcg (contents of 1 capsule aerosolized) twice daily, 12 hours apart; maximum daily dose: 24 mcg; **Note:** For long-term asthma control, long-acting $beta_2$-agonists should be used in combination with inhaled corticosteroids and **not** as monotherapy

Exercise-induced asthma, prevention: Children ≥5 years, Adolescents, and Adults: Inhalation: Foradil® Aerolizer™: 12 mcg (contents of 1 capsule aerosolized) 15 minutes prior to exercise; additional doses should not be used for 12 hours; maximum daily dose: 24 mcg; patients who are using formoterol twice daily should **not** use an additional formoterol dose prior to exercise; if twice daily use is not effective during exercise, consider other appropriate therapy; **Note:** Because long-acting $beta_2$-agonists (LABAs) may disguise poorly-controlled persistent asthma, frequent or chronic use of LABAs for exercise-induced bronchospasm is discouraged by the NAEPP Asthma Guidelines (NAEPP, 2007).

COPD, maintenance treatment: Adults: Inhalation:
Foradil® Aerolizer™: 12 mcg (contents of 1 capsule aerosolized) twice daily, 12 hours apart; maximum daily dose: 24 mcg
Perforomist™: 20 mcg (2 mL) twice daily by nebulization; maximum daily dose: 40 mcg

Administration

Foradil® Aerolizer™: Remove capsule from foil blister immediately before use. The contents of a capsule are aerosolized via a device called an Aerolizer™. Place the capsule into the Aerolizer™. The capsule is pierced by pressing and releasing the buttons on the side of the Aerolizer™. The formoterol formulation is dispersed into the air stream when the patient inhales rapidly and deeply through the mouthpiece. The patient should not exhale into the device. May not be used with spacer device.

Perforomist™: Remove unit-dose vial from foil pouch immediately before use. Solution does not require dilution prior to administration; do not mix other medications with Perforomist™ solution. Place contents of vial into the reservoir of a standard jet nebulizer connected to an air compressor; nebulize until all of the medication has been inhaled. Discard any unused medication immediately. Not for oral ingestion.

Monitoring Parameters Pulmonary function tests, vital signs, CNS stimulation, serum glucose, serum potassium

Additional Information When formoterol is initiated in patients previously receiving a short-acting beta agonist, instruct the patient to discontinue the regular use of the short-acting beta agonist and to utilize the shorter-acting agent for symptomatic or acute episodes only.

Dosage Forms Excipient information presented when available (limited, particularly for generics); consult specific product labeling.
Capsule, Inhalation, as fumarate:
Foradil Aerolizer: 12 mcg [contains milk protein]
Nebulization Solution, Inhalation, as fumarate dihydrate:
Perforomist: 20 mcg/2 mL (2 mL)

- ◆ **Formoterol and Budesonide** *see* Budesonide and Formoterol *on page 313*
- ◆ **Formoterol and Mometasone** *see* Mometasone and Formoterol *on page 1457*
- ◆ **Formoterol and Mometasone Furoate** *see* Mometasone and Formoterol *on page 1457*
- ◆ **Formoterol Fumarate** *see* Formoterol *on page 934*
- ◆ **Formoterol Fumarate Dihydrate** *see* Formoterol *on page 934*
- ◆ **Formoterol Fumarate Dihydrate and Budesonide** *see* Budesonide and Formoterol *on page 313*
- ◆ **Formoterol Fumarate Dihydrate and Mometasone** *see* Mometasone and Formoterol *on page 1457*
- ◆ **Formula E 400 [OTC]** *see* Vitamin E *on page 2188*
- ◆ **Formulex (Can)** *see* Dicyclomine *on page 645*
- ◆ **5-Formyl Tetrahydrofolate** *see* Leucovorin Calcium *on page 1226*
- ◆ **Fortamet** *see* MetFORMIN *on page 1375*
- ◆ **Fortaz** *see* CefTAZidime *on page 407*
- ◆ **Fortaz in D5W** *see* CefTAZidime *on page 407*
- ◆ **Fortesta** *see* Testosterone *on page 2025*
- ◆ **Fortical** *see* Calcitonin *on page 337*

Fosamprenavir (FOS am pren a veer)

Medication Safety Issues

Sound-alike/look-alike issues:
Lexiva may be confused with Levitra, Pexeva

High alert medication:
This medication is in a class the Institute for Safe Medication Practices (ISMP) includes among its list of drug classes that have a heightened risk of causing significant patient harm when used in error.

Related Information

Adult and Adolescent HIV *on page 2392*
Pediatric HIV *on page 2380*
Perinatal HIV *on page 2400*

Brand Names: US Lexiva

Brand Names: Canada Telzir

Therapeutic Category Antiretroviral Agent; HIV Agents (Anti-HIV Agents); Protease Inhibitor

Generic Availability (US) No

Use

Treatment of HIV infection in combination with other antiretroviral agents (boosted with ritonavir) in therapy-naïve patients (FDA approved in ages ≥4 weeks and adults); **Note:** Current guidelines **do not recommend** a boosted regimen in therapy-naïve patients <6 months due to low systemic exposure (DHHS [pediatric]; 2014)

Treatment of HIV infection in combination with other antiretroviral agents (boosted with ritonavir) in therapy-experienced patients (FDA approved in ages ≥6 months and adults)

Treatment of HIV infection in combination with other antiretroviral agents (unboosted; without ritonavir) (FDA approved in therapy-naïve patients ages ≥2 years and adults); **Note:** Current guidelines **do not recommend** an unboosted regimen in pediatric patients due to low systemic exposure (DHHS [pediatric]; 2014)

Note: HIV regimens consisting of **three** antiretroviral agents are strongly recommended.

Pregnancy Risk Factor C

Pregnancy Considerations Adverse events were observed in some animal reproduction studies. Fosamprenavir has a low level of transfer across the human placenta. A small increased risk of preterm birth has been associated with maternal use of protease inhibitor-based combination antiretroviral (ARV) therapy during pregnancy; however, the benefits of use generally outweigh this risk and protease inhibitors (PIs) should not be withheld if otherwise recommended. Hyperglycemia, new onset of diabetes mellitus, or diabetic ketoacidosis have been reported with PIs; it is not clear if pregnancy increases this risk. The DHHS Perinatal HIV Guidelines note there are insufficient data to recommend use during pregnancy; however, if used, they recommend that fosamprenavir be given with low-dose ritonavir boosting.

Regardless of CD4 count or HIV RNA copy number, all HIV-infected pregnant women should receive a combination antiretroviral ARV drug regimen. A combination of antepartum, intrapartum, and infant ARV prophylaxis is recommended. ARV therapy should be started as soon as possible in women with symptomatic infection. Although earlier initiation may be more effective in reducing the perinatal transmission of HIV, initiation may be delayed until after 12 weeks gestation in women who do not require immediate treatment after careful consideration of maternal conditions (eg, nausea and vomiting) and the potential risks of first trimester fetal exposure for specific agents A scheduled cesarean delivery at 38 weeks gestation is recommended for all women with HIV RNA >1000 copies/mL or unknown concentrations near delivery in order to decrease transmission. If ARV therapy must be interrupted for <24 hours during the peripartum period, stop then restart all medications simultaneously in order to decrease the chance of developing resistance. Long-term follow-up is recommended for all infants exposed to ARV medications. In couples who want to conceive, the HIV-infected partner should attain maximum viral suppression prior to conception.

Health care providers are encouraged to enroll pregnant women exposed to antiretroviral medications in the Antiretroviral Pregnancy Registry (1-800-258-4263 or www.-APRegistry.com). Health care providers caring for HIV-infected women and their infants may contact the National Perinatal HIV Hotline (888-448-8765) for clinical consultation (HHS [perinatal], 2014).

Breast-Feeding Considerations It is not known if fosamprenavir is excreted into breast milk. Maternal or infant antiretroviral therapy does not completely eliminate the risk of postnatal HIV transmission. In addition, multiclass-resistant virus has been detected in breast-feeding infants despite maternal therapy. Therefore, in the United States, where formula is accessible, affordable, safe, and sustainable, and the risk of infant mortality due to diarrhea and respiratory infections is low, complete avoidance of breast-feeding by HIV-infected women is recommended to decrease potential transmission of HIV (HHS [perinatal], 2014).

Contraindications Clinically-significant hypersensitivity (eg, Stevens-Johnson syndrome) to fosamprenavir, amprenavir, or any component of the formulation; concurrent therapy with CYP3A4 substrates with a narrow therapeutic window; concomitant use with alfuzosin, cisapride, delavirdine, ergot derivatives, lovastatin, midazolam, pimozide, rifampin, simvastatin, St John's wort, and triazolam; use of flecainide and propafenone with concomitant ritonavir therapy; sildenafil (when used for pulmonary artery hypertension [eg, Revatio®])

Warnings/Precautions Concomitant use of fosamprenavir with some drugs may require cautious use, may not be recommended, may require dosage adjustments, or may be contraindicated. Do not use with hormonal contraceptives. Do not coadminister colchicine in patient with renal or hepatic impairment.

Use with caution in patients with diabetes mellitus or sulfonamide allergy. Use caution with hepatic impairment (dosage adjustment required) or underlying hepatitis B or C. Redistribution of fat may occur (eg, buffalo hump, peripheral wasting, cushingoid appearance). Dosage adjustment is required for combination therapies (ritonavir and/or efavirenz); in addition, the risk of hyperlipidemia may be increased during concurrent therapy. Protease inhibitors have been associated with a variety of hypersensitivity events (some severe), including rash, anaphylaxis (rare), angioedema, bronchospasm, erythema multiforme, and/or Stevens-Johnson syndrome (rare). It is generally recommended to discontinue treatment if severe rash or moderate symptoms accompanied by other systemic symptoms occur. Acute hemolytic anemia has been reported in association with amprenavir use. Cases of nephrolithiasis have been reported in postmarketing surveillance; temporary or permanent discontinuation of therapy should be considered if symptoms develop. Spontaneous bleeding has been reported in patients with hemophilia A or B following treatment with protease inhibitors; use caution. Immune reconstitution syndrome may develop, resulting in the occurrence of an inflammatory response to an indolent or residual opportunistic infection during initial HIV treatment or activation of autoimmune disorders (eg, Graves' disease, polymyositis, Guillain-Barré syndrome) later in therapy; further evaluation and treatment may be required.

Warnings: Additional Pediatric Considerations May cause vomiting; reported in 30% of pediatric patients (regardless of causality) receiving fosamprenavir twice daily with ritonavir (compared to 10% of adults) and occurred in 56% of children 2 to 5 years of age receiving twice daily fosamprenavir without ritonavir (compared to 16% of adults).

Some dosage forms may contain propylene glycol; in neonates large amounts of propylene glycol delivered orally, intravenously (eg, >3,000 mg/day), or topically have been associated with potentially fatal toxicities which can include metabolic acidosis, seizures, renal failure, and CNS depression; toxicities have also been reported in children and adults including hyperosmolality, lactic acidosis, seizures and respiratory depression; use caution (AAP, 1997; Shehab, 2009).

Adverse Reactions

Central nervous system: Fatigue, headache

Dermatologic: Pruritus, rash (onset: ~11 days; duration: ~13 days)

Endocrine & metabolic: Hyperglycemia, hypertriglyceridemia

Gastrointestinal: Abdominal pain, diarrhea, nausea, serum lipase increased, vomiting

Hematologic: Neutropenia

Hepatic: Transaminases increased

Rare but important or life-threatening: Angioedema, hypercholesterolemia, myocardial infarction, nephrolithiasis, oral paresthesia, QT prolongation (with amprenavir), Stevens-Johnson syndrome, stroke

Frequency not defined: Diabetes mellitus, fat redistribution, and immune reconstitution syndrome have been associated with protease inhibitor therapy. Spontaneous bleeding has been reported in patients with hemophilia A or B following treatment with protease inhibitors. Acute hemolytic anemia has been reported in association with amprenavir use.

Drug Interactions

Metabolism/Transport Effects Substrate of CYP2C9 (minor), CYP2D6 (minor), CYP3A4 (major), P-glycoprotein; **Note:** Assignment of Major/Minor substrate status based on clinically relevant drug interaction potential; **Inhibits** CYP2C19 (weak)

Avoid Concomitant Use

Avoid concomitant use of Fosamprenavir with any of the following: Alfuzosin; Cisapride; Delavirdine; Ergot Derivatives; Etravirine; Flecainide; Lopinavir; Lovastatin; Midazolam; Pimozide; Propafenone; Rifampin; Simeprevir; Simvastatin; St Johns Wort; Telaprevir; Tipranavir; Triazolam

Increased Effect/Toxicity

Fosamprenavir may increase the levels/effects of: Alfuzosin; ALPRAZolam; Amiodarone; AtorvaSTATin; Bosentan; Calcium Channel Blockers (Dihydropyridine); Calcium Channel Blockers (Nondihydropyridine);

CarBAMazepine; Cisapride; Clarithromycin; Clorazepate; Colchicine; Cyclophosphamide; CycloSPORINE (Systemic); Dexamethasone (Systemic); Diazepam; Digoxin; Enfuvirtide; Ergot Derivatives; Flecainide; Flurazepam; Itraconazole; Ketoconazole (Systemic); Lovastatin; Meperidine; Midazolam; Nefazodone; Pimozide; Propafenone; Protease Inhibitors; QuiNIDine; Rifabutin; Riociguat; Rosuvastatin; Sildenafil; Simeprevir; Simvastatin; Tacrolimus (Systemic); Tacrolimus (Topical); Temsirolimus; TraZODone; Triazolam; Tricyclic Antidepressants; Voriconazole; Warfarin

The levels/effects of Fosamprenavir may be increased by: Clarithromycin; CycloSPORINE (Systemic); Delavirdine; Enfuvirtide; Etravirine; Fosphenytoin; Itraconazole; Ketoconazole (Systemic); P-glycoprotein/ABCB1 Inhibitors; Phenytoin; Posaconazole; Rifabutin; Simeprevir; Voriconazole

Decreased Effect

Fosamprenavir may decrease the levels/effects of: Abacavir; Antidiabetic Agents; Boceprevir; Clarithromycin; Contraceptives (Estrogens); Contraceptives (Progestins); Delavirdine; Dolutegravir; Fosphenytoin; Lopinavir; Meperidine; Methadone; PARoxetine; Phenytoin; Posaconazole; Raltegravir; Telaprevir; Valproic Acid and Derivatives; Zidovudine

The levels/effects of Fosamprenavir may be decreased by: Boceprevir; Bosentan; CarBAMazepine; Contraceptives (Progestins); CYP3A4 Inducers (Moderate); CYP3A4 Inducers (Strong); Dabrafenib; Deferasirox; Dexamethasone (Systemic); Efavirenz; Garlic; H2-Antagonists; Lopinavir; Methadone; Mitotane; Nevirapine; P-glycoprotein/ABCB1 Inducers; Raltegravir; Rifampin; Siltuximab; St Johns Wort; Telaprevir; Tipranavir; Tocilizumab

Storage/Stability

Lexiva®: Store tablets at 25°C (77°F); excursions permitted to 15°C to 30°C (59°F to 86°F). Store oral suspension at 5°C to 30°C (41°F to 86°F). Do not freeze.

Telzir®: Store tablets 2°C to 30°C; do not freeze and discard 25 days after opening.

Mechanism of Action Fosamprenavir is rapidly and almost completely converted to amprenavir by cellular phosphatases *in vivo*. Amprenavir binds to the site of HIV-1 protease activity and inhibits cleavage of viral Gag-Pol polyprotein precursors into individual functional proteins required for infectious HIV. This results in the formation of immature, noninfectious viral particles.

Pharmacokinetics (Adult data unless noted)

Protein binding: 90%; primarily to alpha$_1$ acid glycoprotein; concentration-dependent binding; protein binding is decreased in patients with hepatic impairment

Metabolism: Fosamprenavir is the prodrug of amprenavir; fosamprenavir is rapidly hydrolyzed to amprenavir and inorganic phosphate by cellular phosphatases in the gut epithelium as it is absorbed; amprenavir is metabolized in the liver via cytochrome P450 CYP3A4 isoenzyme system; glucuronide conjugation of oxidized metabolites also occurs

Bioavailability: Absolute oral bioavailability is not established. Similar amprenavir AUCs occurred in adults when single doses of the oral suspension versus tablets were administered in the fasted state; however, the suspension provided a 14.5% higher peak concentration.

Half-life: Amprenavir: Adults: 7.7 hours

Time to peak serum concentration: Amprenavir (single dose of fosamprenavir): Median: 2.5 hours; range: 1.5 to 4 hours

Elimination: Minimal excretion of unchanged drug in urine (1%) and feces; 75% of dose excreted as metabolites via biliary tract into feces and 14% excreted as metabolites in urine

Dosing: Neonatal Not approved for use; appropriate dose is unknown.

Dosing: Usual

Pediatric: **HIV infection, treatment:** Use in combination with other antiretroviral agents: Oral: **Note:** Maximum dose should not exceed adult dose. Once-daily dosing of fosamprenavir is **not** recommended in pediatric patients; data from a pediatric once-daily dosing study of fosamprenavir plus ritonavir were insufficient to support once-daily dosing in any pediatric patient population.

Antiretroviral-naive patients:

Ritonavir unboosted regimen:

Infants and Children <2 years: Not approved for use; appropriate dose is unknown

Children ≥2 years and Adolescents:

AIDS*info* guidelines: Do not use due to low systemic exposure (DHHS [pediatric], 2014)

Manufacturer's labeling: 30 mg/kg/dose twice daily; maximum dose 1400 mg/dose

Ritonavir boosted regimen:

Infants, Children, and Adolescents:

AIDS*info* guidelines: Do not use in infants <6 months due to low systemic exposure; do not use in former premature neonates (ie, born at <38 weeks gestation) (DHHS [pediatric], 2014)

Manufacturer's labeling: Use only in infants born at ≥38 weeks GA and who are at least 28 days PNA

<11 kg: Fosamprenavir 45 mg/kg/dose **plus** ritonavir 7 mg/kg/dose twice daily

11 to <15 kg: Fosamprenavir 30 mg/kg/dose **plus** ritonavir 3 mg/kg/dose twice daily

15 to <20 kg: Fosamprenavir 23 mg/kg/dose **plus** ritonavir 3 mg/kg/dose twice daily

≥20 kg: Fosamprenavir 18 mg/kg/dose (maximum dose: 700 mg) twice daily **plus** ritonavir 3 mg/kg/dose (maximum dose: 100 mg) twice daily

Note: When combined with ritonavir, fosamprenavir tablets may be administered to children who weigh ≥39 kg.

Antiretroviral therapy-experienced:

Ritonavir boosted regimen:

Infants <6 months: Not approved for use; appropriate dose is unknown

Infants ≥6 months, Children, and Adolescents:

<11 kg: Fosamprenavir 45 mg/kg/dose **plus** ritonavir 7 mg/kg/dose twice daily

11 to <15 kg: Fosamprenavir 30 mg/kg/dose **plus** ritonavir 3 mg/kg/dose twice daily

15 to <20 kg: Fosamprenavir 23 mg/kg/dose **plus** ritonavir 3 mg/kg/dose twice daily

≥20 kg: Fosamprenavir 18 mg/kg/dose (maximum dose: 700 mg) twice daily **plus** ritonavir 3 mg/kg/dose twice daily (maximum dose: 100 mg) twice daily

Note: When combined with ritonavir, fosamprenavir tablets may be administered to children who weigh ≥39 kg

Adult: **HIV infection, treatment: Note:** Use in combination with other antiretroviral agents: Oral:

Antiretroviral-naïve patients:

Unboosted regimen (ie, regimen without ritonavir): Fosamprenavir 1400 mg twice daily. **Note:** This regimen is not recommended due to inferior potency compared to other protease inhibitor based regimens and the potential for cross-resistance to darunavir (DHHS [adult], 2014).

Ritonavir boosted regimens:

Once-daily regimen: Fosamprenavir 1400 mg **plus** ritonavir 100 to 200 mg once daily

Twice-daily regimen: Fosamprenavir 700 mg **plus** ritonavir 100 mg twice daily

Protease inhibitor-experienced: Fosamprenavir 700 mg **plus** ritonavir 100 mg twice daily. **Note:** Once-daily dosing of fosamprenavir is not recommended in protease inhibitor-experienced patients.

Dosing adjustments for concomitant therapy: Adults:

Concomitant therapy with efavirenz: Note: Only ritonavir-boosted regimens should be used when efavirenz is used in combination with fosamprenavir.

Once-daily regimen: Protease inhibitor-naïve **only**: Fosamprenavir 1400 mg **plus** ritonavir 300 mg **plus** efavirenz 600 mg once daily

Twice-daily regimen: Fosamprenavir 700 mg **plus** ritonavir 100 mg twice daily with efavirenz 600 mg once daily. **Note:** No change in ritonavir dosage is required when patients receive efavirenz with twice-daily dosing of fosamprenavir with ritonavir.

Combination therapy with maraviroc: Fosamprenavir 700 mg **plus** ritonavir 100 mg **plus** maraviroc 150 mg all dosed twice daily

Dosing adjustment in renal impairment: No dosage adjustment required (DHHS [adult], 2014)

Dosing adjustment in hepatic impairment: Use with caution: Adults:

Mild impairment (Child-Pugh score 5 to 6): Reduce dosage of fosamprenavir to 700 mg twice daily without concurrent ritonavir (therapy-naïve) or fosamprenavir 700 mg twice daily plus ritonavir 100 mg once daily (therapy-naïve or PI-experienced)

Moderate impairment (Child-Pugh score 7 to 9): Reduce dosage of fosamprenavir to 700 mg twice daily without concurrent ritonavir (therapy-naïve) or fosamprenavir 450 mg twice daily plus ritonavir 100 mg once daily (therapy-naïve or PI-experienced)

Severe impairment (Child-Pugh score 10 to 15): Reduce dosage of fosamprenavir to 350 mg twice daily without concurrent ritonavir (therapy naïve) or use fosamprenavir 300 mg twice daily plus ritonavir 100 mg once daily (therapy naïve or protease inhibitor experienced).

Administration Oral: Do not administer concurrently with antacids or buffered formulations of other medications (separate administration by 1 hour).

Oral suspension: Administer **with** food to pediatric patients; administer **without** food to adults. Readminister dose of suspension if emesis occurs within 30 minutes after dosing. Shake suspension vigorously prior to use.

Tablets: Administer **with** food to pediatric patients and adult patients when coadministered with ritonavir; may be administered without regard to meals in adults if not taken with ritonavir (DHHS [adult, pediatric], 2014)

Monitoring Parameters Note: Monitor CD4 percentage (if <5 years of age) or CD4 count (if ≥5 years of age) at least every 3 to 4 months (DHHS [pediatric], 2014).

Prior to initiation of therapy: Genotypic resistance testing, CD4 and viral load (every 3 to 4 months), CBC with differential, LFTs, BUN, creatinine, electrolytes, glucose, lipid panel, urinalysis (every 6 to 12 months), and assessment of readiness for adherence with medication regimen. At initiation and with any change in treatment regimen: CBC with differential, electrolytes, calcium, phosphate, glucose, LFTs, bilirubin, urinalysis (at initiation), BUN, creatinine, albumin, total protein, lipid panel (at initiation), CD4, and viral load. After 1 to 2 weeks of therapy: Signs of medication toxicity and adherence. After 2 to 4 weeks of therapy: CBC with differential, viral load, signs of medication toxicity, and adherence; then every 3 to 4 months: CBC with differential, electrolytes, glucose, LFTs, bilirubin, BUN, creatinine, CD4, viral load, signs of medication toxicity, and adherence. Every 6 to 12 months: Lipid panel and urinalysis. CD4 monitoring frequency may be decreased to every 6 to 12 months in children who are adherent to therapy if the value is well above the threshold for opportunistic infections, viral suppression is sustained, and the clinical status is stable for more than 2 to 3 years (DHHS [pediatric], 2014). Monitor for growth and development, signs of HIV-specific physical conditions, HIV disease progression, opportunistic infections or hepatitis.

Reference Range Plasma trough concentration: Amprenavir: ≥400 ng/mL (DHHS [adult, pediatric], 2014)

Additional Information Oral suspension contains 50 mg/mL of fosamprenavir as fosamprenavir calcium and is equivalent to amprenavir 43 mg/mL. Fosamprenavir calcium 700 mg (1 tablet) is approximately equal to amprenavir 600 mg.

Dosage Forms Excipient information presented when available (limited, particularly for generics); consult specific product labeling.

Suspension, Oral, as calcium:

Lexiva: 50 mg/mL (225 mL) [contains methylparaben, polysorbate 80, propylene glycol, propylparaben; grape bubblegum peppermint flavor]

Tablet, Oral, as calcium:

Lexiva: 700 mg

◆ **Fosamprenavir Calcium** *see* Fosamprenavir *on page 936*

Fosaprepitant (fos a PRE pi tant)

Medication Safety Issues

Sound-alike/look-alike issues:

Fosaprepitant may be confused with aprepitant, fosamprenavir, fospropofol

Emend® for Injection (fosaprepitant) may be confused with Emend® (aprepitant) which is an oral capsule formulation.

Brand Names: US Emend

Brand Names: Canada Emend® IV

Therapeutic Category Antiemetic; Substance P/Neurokinin 1 Receptor Antagonist

Generic Availability (US) No

Use Prevention of acute and delayed nausea and vomiting associated with initial and repeat courses of moderate and highly emetogenic cancer chemotherapy (MEC & HEC) in combination with other antiemetic agents (FDA approved in adults)

Pregnancy Risk Factor B

Pregnancy Considerations Teratogenic effects were not observed in animal reproduction studies for aprepitant. Use during pregnancy only if clearly needed. Efficacy of hormonal contraceptive may be reduced; alternative or additional methods of contraception should be used both during treatment with fosaprepitant or aprepitant and for at least 1 month following the last fosaprepitant/aprepitant dose.

Breast-Feeding Considerations It is not known if fosaprepitant is excreted in breast milk. Due to the potential for serious adverse reactions in the nursing infant, a decision should be made whether to discontinue nursing or to discontinue the drug, taking into account the importance of treatment to the mother.

Contraindications Hypersensitivity to fosaprepitant, aprepitant, polysorbate 80, or any component of the formulation; concurrent use with pimozide or cisapride

Canadian labeling: Additional contraindications (not in U.S. labeling): Concurrent use with astemizole or terfenadine

Warnings/Precautions Fosaprepitant is rapidly converted to aprepitant, which has a high potential for drug interactions. Potentially significant drug-drug interactions may exist, requiring dose or frequency adjustment, additional monitoring, and/or selection of alternative therapy. Immediate hypersensitivity has been reported (rarely) with fosaprepitant; stop infusion with hypersensitivity symptoms (dyspnea, erythema, flushing, or anaphylaxis); do not reinitiate. Some dosage forms may contain polysorbate 80 (also known as Tweens). Hypersensitivity reactions, usually a delayed reaction, have been reported following exposure to pharmaceutical products containing polysorbate 80 in certain individuals (Isaksson, 2002; Lucente 2000; Shelley, 1995). Thrombocytopenia, ascites, pulmonary deterioration, and renal and hepatic failure have been reported in premature neonates after receiving parenteral products containing polysorbate 80 (Alade, 1986; CDC, 1984). See manufacturer's labeling. Use caution with hepatic impairment; has not been studied in patients with severe hepatic impairment (Child-Pugh class C). Not studied for treatment of existing nausea and vomiting. Chronic continuous administration of fosaprepitant is not recommended.

Adverse Reactions Adverse reactions reported with aprepitant and fosaprepitant (as part of a combination chemotherapy regimen) occurring at a higher frequency than standard antiemetic therapy:

Central nervous system: Fatigue, headache

Gastrointestinal: Anorexia, constipation, diarrhea, dyspepsia, eructation

Hepatic: ALT increased, AST increased

Local: Injection site reactions (includes erythema, induration, pain, pruritus, or thrombophlebitis)

Neuromuscular & skeletal: Weakness

Miscellaneous: Hiccups

Rare but important or life-threatening: Abdominal pain, alkaline phosphatase increased, anaphylactic reaction, anemia, angioedema, bradycardia, candidiasis, cardiovascular disorder, chest discomfort, chills, cognitive disorder, conjunctivitis, cough, disorientation, dizziness, duodenal ulcer (perforating), dyspnea, edema, erythema, flushing, gait disturbance, hematuria (microscopic), hyperglycemia, hyperhydrosis, hypersensitivity reaction, hypertension, hyponatremia, miosis, nausea, neutropenia, neutropenic colitis, neutropenic fever, palpitation, photosensitivity, pollakiuria, polyuria, pruritus, rash, sensory disturbance, somnolence, staphylococcal infection, Stevens-Johnson syndrome, stomatitis, subileus, tinnitus, toxic epidermal necrolysis, urticaria, visual acuity decreased, vomiting, wheezing

Drug Interactions

Metabolism/Transport Effects **Substrate** of CYP1A2 (minor), CYP2C19 (minor), CYP3A4 (major); **Note:** Assignment of Major/Minor substrate status based on clinically relevant drug interaction potential; **Inhibits** CYP2C19 (weak), CYP2C9 (weak), CYP3A4 (moderate); **Induces** CYP2C9 (weak/moderate), CYP3A4 (weak)

Avoid Concomitant Use

Avoid concomitant use of Fosaprepitant with any of the following: Astemizole; Bosutinib; Cisapride; Conivaptan; Domperidone; Fusidic Acid (Systemic); Ibrutinib; Idelalisib; Ivabradine; Lomitapide; Naloxegol; Olaparib; Pimozide; Simeprevir; Terfenadine; Tolvaptan; Trabectedin; Ulipristal

Increased Effect/Toxicity

Fosaprepitant may increase the levels/effects of: Astemizole; Avanafil; Bosentan; Bosutinib; Budesonide (Systemic, Oral Inhalation); Budesonide (Topical); Cannabis; Cilostazol; Cisapride; Colchicine; Corticosteroids (Systemic); CYP3A4 Substrates; Dapoxetine; Diltiazem; Dofetilide; Domperidone; DOXOrubicin (Conventional); Dronabinol; Eliglustat; Eplerenone; Everolimus; FentaNYL; Halofantrine; Hydrocodone; Ibrutinib; Ifosfamide; Imatinib; Ivabradine; Ivacaftor; Lomitapide; Lurasidone; Naloxegol; NiMODipine; Olaparib; OxyCODONE; Pimecrolimus; Pimozide; Propafenone; Ranolazine; Rivaroxaban; Salmeterol; Saxagliptin; Simeprevir; Sirolimus; Suvorexant; Terfenadine; Tetrahydrocannabinol; Tolvaptan; Trabectedin; Ulipristal; Vilazodone; Zopiclone; Zuclopenthixol

The levels/effects of Fosaprepitant may be increased by: Aprepitant; Conivaptan; CYP3A4 Inhibitors (Moderate); CYP3A4 Inhibitors (Strong); Dasatinib; Diltiazem; Fusidic Acid (Systemic); Idelalisib; Luliconazole; Mifepristone; Netupitant; Palbociclib; Stiripentol

Decreased Effect

Fosaprepitant may decrease the levels/effects of: ARIPiprazole; Contraceptives (Estrogens); Contraceptives (Progestins); Hydrocodone; NiMODipine; PARoxetine; Saxagliptin; TOLBUTamide; Warfarin

The levels/effects of Fosaprepitant may be decreased by: Bosentan; CYP3A4 Inducers (Moderate); CYP3A4 Inducers (Strong); Dabrafenib; Deferasirox; Mitotane; PARoxetine; Rifampin; Siltuximab; St Johns Wort; Tocilizumab

Food Interactions Aprepitant serum concentration may be increased when taken with grapefruit juice. Management: Avoid concurrent use.

Storage/Stability Store intact vials at 2°C to 8°C (36°F to 46°F). Solutions diluted to 1 mg/mL for infusion are stable for 24 hours at room temperature or at ≤25°C (≤77°F). Solutions diluted to a final volume of 250 mL (0.6 mg/mL) should be administered within 24 hours (data on file [Merck, 2013]).

Mechanism of Action Fosaprepitant is a prodrug of aprepitant, a substance P/neurokinin 1 (NK1) receptor antagonist. It is rapidly converted to aprepitant which prevents acute and delayed vomiting by inhibiting the substance P/neurokinin 1 (NK1) receptor; augments the antiemetic activity of the 5-HT_3 receptor antagonist and corticosteroid activity and inhibits chemotherapy-induced emesis.

Pharmacokinetics (Adult data unless noted)

Distribution: V_d: Fosaprepitant: ~5 L; Aprepitant: V_d: ~70 L; crosses the blood-brain barrier

Protein binding: Aprepitant: >95%

Metabolism:

Fosaprepitant: Hepatic and extrahepatic; rapidly (within 30 minutes after the end of infusion) converted to aprepitant (nearly complete conversion)

Aprepitant: Hepatic via CYP3A4 (major); CYP1A2 and CYP2C19 (minor); forms 7 weakly-active metabolites

Half-life: Fosaprepitant: ~2 minutes; Aprepitant: ~9 to 13 hours

Elimination: Urine (57%); feces (45%)

Clearance: 62 to 90 mL/minute

Dosing: Usual Adults: **Prevention of chemotherapy-induced nausea and vomiting:** IV:

Single-dose regimen (for highly emetogenic chemotherapy): 150 mg over 20 to 30 minutes ~30 minutes prior to chemotherapy on day 1 only (in combination with a 5-HT_3 antagonist on day 1 and dexamethasone on days 1 to 4)

Dosage adjustment in renal impairment:

Mild, moderate, or severe impairment: No adjustment required

Dialysis-dependent end-stage renal disease (ESRD): No adjustment required

Dosage adjustment in hepatic impairment:

Mild to moderate impairment (Child-Pugh score 5-9): No adjustment necessary

Severe impairment (Child-Pugh score >9): Use caution; no data available

Preparation for Administration Parenteral: Reconstitute vial with 5 mL NS, directing diluent down side of vial to avoid foaming; swirl gently. Further dilute in NS to a final concentration of 1 mg/mL; gently invert bag to mix. Solutions may be diluted to a final volume of 250 mL (0.6 mg/mL) (data on file [Merck 2013]).

Administration Parenteral: Infuse over 20 to 30 minutes; administer ~30 minutes prior to chemotherapy

Monitoring Parameters Immediate hypersensitivity reactions during infusion (anaphylaxis, dyspnea, erythema, or flushing). If reaction occurs, infusion should be stopped and not reinitiated.

Dosage Forms Excipient information presented when available (limited, particularly for generics); consult specific product labeling.

Solution Reconstituted, Intravenous:

Emend: 150 mg (1 ea) [contains disodium edta, polysorbate 80]

◆ **Fosaprepitant Dimeglumine** *see* Fosaprepitant *on page 939*

Foscarnet (fos KAR net)

Brand Names: US Foscavir

Brand Names: Canada Foscavir®

Therapeutic Category Antiviral Agent, Parenteral

Generic Availability (US) Yes

Use Alternative to ganciclovir for treatment of CMV infections; treatment of CMV retinitis in patients with acquired immunodeficiency syndrome (FDA approved in adults); treatment of acyclovir-resistant mucocutaneous herpes simplex virus infections in immunocompromised patients and acyclovir-resistant herpes zoster infections (FDA approved in adults)

Pregnancy Risk Factor C

Pregnancy Considerations Adverse events have been observed in animal reproductions studies. A single case report of use during the third trimester with normal infant outcome was observed. Monitoring of amniotic fluid volumes by ultrasound is recommended weekly after 20 weeks of gestation to detect oligohydramnios (DHHS [adult], 2014).

Breast-Feeding Considerations It is not known if foscarnet is excreted in breast milk. Due to the potential for serious adverse reactions in the nursing infant, the manufacturer recommends a decision be made whether to discontinue nursing or to discontinue the drug, taking into account the importance of treatment to the mother. In the United States, where formula is accessible, affordable, safe, and sustainable, and the risk of infant mortality due to diarrhea and respiratory infections is low, complete avoidance of breast-feeding by HIV-infected women is recommended to decrease potential transmission of HIV (DHHS [perinatal], 2014).

Contraindications Hypersensitivity to foscarnet or any component of the formulation

Warnings/Precautions [U.S. Boxed Warning]: Indicated only for immunocompromised patients with CMV retinitis and mucocutaneous acyclovir-resistant HSV infection. [U.S. Boxed Warning]: Renal impairment occurs to some degree in the majority of patients treated with foscarnet; renal impairment may occur at any time and is usually reversible within 1 week following dose adjustment or discontinuation of therapy, however, several patients have died with renal failure within 4 weeks of stopping foscarnet; therefore, renal function should be closely monitored. To reduce the risk of nephrotoxicity and the potential to administer a relative overdose, always calculate the creatine clearance even if serum creatinine is within the normal range. Adequate hydration may reduce the risk of nephrotoxicity; the manufacturer makes specific recommendations regarding this (see Administration).

Imbalance of serum electrolytes or minerals occurs in at least 15% of patients (hypocalcemia, low ionized calcium, hyper/hypophosphatemia, hypomagnesemia, or hypokalemia). Correct electrolytes before initiating therapy. Use caution when administering other medications that cause electrolyte imbalances. Patients who experience signs or symptoms of an electrolyte imbalance should be assessed immediately. **[U.S. Boxed Warning]: Seizures related to plasma electrolyte/mineral imbalance may occur;** incidence has been reported in up to 10% of HIV patients. Risk factors for seizures include impaired baseline renal function, low total serum calcium, and underlying CNS conditions. Due to sodium content, use with caution in patients with heart failure. May cause anemia and granulocytopenia. May cause genital/vascular tissue irritation/ulceration; adequately hydrate and administer only into vein with adequate blood flow to minimize risk. Foscarnet is deposited in teeth and bone of young, growing animals; it has adversely affected tooth enamel development in rats. Potentially significant drug-drug interactions exist, requiring dose or frequency adjustment, additional monitoring, and/or selection of alternative therapy.

Adverse Reactions

Cardiovascular: Chest pain, edema, facial edema, first degree atrioventricular block, flushing, hypertension, hypotension, palpitations, sinus tachycardia, ST segment changes on ECG

Central nervous system: Abnormal coordination, abnormal electroencephalogram, aggressive behavior, agitation, amnesia, anxiety, aphasia, ataxia, cerebrovascular disease, confusion, convulsions, dementia, depression, dizziness, fatigue, fever, hallucination, headache, hypoesthesia, insomnia, malaise, meningitis, nervousness, pain, seizures, somnolence, stupor

Dermatologic: Dermal ulcer, diaphoresis, erythematous rash, maculopapular rash, pruritus, seborrhea, skin discoloration, skin rash

Endocrine & metabolic: Abnormal albumin-Globulin ratio, acidosis, electrolyte disturbance, hyperphosphatemia, hypocalcemia, hypokalemia, hypomagnesemia, hyponatremia, hypophosphatemia, increased thirst

Gastrointestinal: Abdominal pain, anorexia, aphthous stomatitis, cachexia, candidiasis, constipation, diarrhea, dysgeusia, dyspepsia, dysphagia, flatulence, melena, nausea, pancreatitis, rectal hemorrhage, vomiting, weight loss, xerostomia

Genitourinary: Dysuria, nephrotoxicity, nocturia, urinary retention, urinary tract infection

Hematologic & oncologic: Abnormal white cell differential, altered platelet function, anemia, bone marrow suppression, granulocytopenia, leukopenia, lymphadenopathy, mineral abnormalities, neutropenia, pseudolymphoma, sarcoma, thrombocytopenia, thrombosis

Hepatic: Abnormal hepatic function tests, increased lactate dehydrogenase, increased serum alkaline phosphatase, increase serum ALT, increased serum AST

Infection: Bacterial infection, fungal infection, sepsis

Local: Abscess, inflammation at injection site, irritation at injection site, pain at injection site

Neuromuscular & skeletal: Arthralgia, back pain, leg cramps, muscle spasm, myalgia, neuropathy (peripheral), paresthesia, rigors, sensory disturbance, tremor, weakness

Ophthalmic: Conjunctivitis, eye irritation, eye pain, visual disturbance

Renal: Acute renal failure, albuminuria, decreased creatinine clearance, increased blood urea nitrogen, increased serum creatinine, polyuria, renal insufficiency

Respiratory: Bronchospasm, cough, dyspnea, flu-like symptoms, hemoptysis, pharyngitis, pneumonia, pneumothorax, pulmonary infiltrates, respiratory failure, respiratory insufficiency, rhinitis, sinusitis, stridor

Rare but important or life-threatening: Cardiac arrest, coma, diabetes insipidus (usually nephrogenic), erythema multiforme, esophageal ulcer, hematuria, hypoproteinemia, myositis, nephrolithiasis, pancytopenia, prolonged Q-T interval on ECG, renal disease (crystal-induced), renal tubular acidosis, renal tubular necrosis, rhabdomyolysis, SIADH, Stevens-Johnson syndrome, toxic epidermal necrolysis, ventricular arrhythmia

Drug Interactions

Metabolism/Transport Effects None known.

Avoid Concomitant Use
Avoid concomitant use of Foscarnet with any of the following: Acyclovir-Valacyclovir; Aminoglycosides; Amphotericin B; CycloSPORINE (Systemic); Methotrexate; Tacrolimus (Systemic)

Increased Effect/Toxicity
Foscarnet may increase the levels/effects of: Acyclovir-Valacyclovir; Aminoglycosides; Amphotericin B; CycloSPORINE (Systemic); Highest Risk QTc-Prolonging Agents; Methotrexate; Moderate Risk QTc-Prolonging Agents; Tacrolimus (Systemic)

The levels/effects of Foscarnet may be increased by: Loop Diuretics; Mifepristone; Pentamidine

Decreased Effect There are no known significant interactions involving a decrease in effect.

Storage/Stability Foscarnet injection is a clear, colorless solution. Store intact bottles at room temperature of 20°C to 25°C (68°F to 77°F) and protect from temperatures >40°C (>104°F) and from freezing. Diluted solution is stable for 24 hours at room temperature or under refrigeration.

Mechanism of Action Pyrophosphate analogue which acts as a noncompetitive inhibitor of many viral RNA and DNA polymerases as well as HIV reverse transcriptase. Similar to ganciclovir, foscarnet is a virostatic agent. Foscarnet does not require activation by thymidine kinase.

Pharmacokinetics (Adult data unless noted)
Distribution: V_d: ~0.5 L/kg; up to 28% of cumulative IV dose may be deposited in bone; CSF levels are ~2/3 of serum concentrations
Protein binding: 14% to 17%
Half-life, plasma: Adults: 2-4.5 hours
Elimination: 80% to 90% excreted unchanged in urine

Dosing: Usual
Infants and Children:
Cytomegalovirus (CMV) infection (HIV-exposed/-positive) (CDC, 2009):
CNS disease:
Treatment; induction: IV: 60 mg/kg/dose every 8 hours in combination with ganciclovir; continue until symptom improvement, followed by chronic suppressive (maintenance) therapy
Maintenance therapy: IV: 90-120 mg/kg/dose once daily
Retinitis, disseminated disease:
Treatment; induction: IV: 60 mg/kg/dose every 8 hours for 14-21 days with or without ganciclovir, followed by chronic suppressive (maintenance) therapy
Maintenance therapy: IV: 90-120 mg/kg/dose once daily
Herpes simplex virus (HSV) infection acyclovir-resistant; treatment (HIV-exposed/-positive) (CDC, 2009): IV: 40 mg/kg/dose every 8 hours or 60 mg/kg/dose every 12 hours for up to 3 weeks or until lesions heal; repeat treatment may lead to the development of resistance
Varicella zoster virus (VZ) infection (HIV-exposed/-positive) (CDC, 2009):
Chickenpox not responding to acyclovir; treatment: IV: 40-60 mg/kg/dose every 8 hours for 7-10 days
Zoster: Progressive outer retinal necrosis; treatment:
IV: 90 mg/kg/dose every 12 hours in combination with ganciclovir intravenous and intravitreal foscarnet and/or ganciclovir
Intravitreal: 1.2 mg/0.05 mL per dose twice weekly in combination with systemic foscarnet and ganciclovir and/or intravitreal ganciclovir

Adolescents:
Cytomegalovirus (CMV) retinitis (HIV-exposed/-positive) (CDC, 2009a):
Treatment; induction: IV: 60 mg/kg/dose every 8 hours for 14-21 days **or** 90 mg/kg every 12 hours for 14-21 days
Maintenance therapy: IV: 90-120 mg/kg/dose once daily
Herpes simplex virus (HSV) infection acyclovir-resistant; treatment (HIV-exposed/-positive) (CDC, 2009a): IV: 40 mg/kg/dose every 8-12 hours until clinical response
Varicella zoster virus (VZ) infection (HIV-exposed/-positive) (CDC, 2009a):
Chickenpox not responding to acyclovir; treatment: IV: 90 mg/kg/dose every 12 hours
Zoster: Progressive outer retinal necrosis; treatment:
IV: 90 mg/kg/dose every 12 hours in combination with systemic ganciclovir and intravitreal foscarnet and/or ganciclovir
Intravitreal: 1.2 mg/0.05 mL per dose twice weekly in combination with systemic foscarnet and ganciclovir and/or intravitreal ganciclovir

Adults:
Cytomegalovirus (CMV) retinitis: IV:
Treatment; induction: 60 mg/kg/dose every 8 hours for 14-21 days **or** 90 mg/kg/dose every 12 hours for 14-21 days
Maintenance therapy: 90-120 mg/kg/day as a single daily infusion
Herpes simplex virus (HSV) infection acyclovir-resistant; treatment: IV: 40 mg/kg/dose every 8-12 hours for 14-21 days

Dosing interval in renal impairment: Adults:
CMV Induction (equivalent to 60 mg/kg every 8 hours):
CrCl >1.4 mL/minute/kg: 60 mg/kg every 8 hours
CrCl >1-1.4 mL/minute/kg: 45 mg/kg every 8 hours
CrCl >0.8-1 mL/minute/kg: 50 mg/kg every 12 hours
CrCl >0.6-0.8 mL/minute/kg: 40 mg/kg every 12 hours
CrCl >0.5-0.6 mL/minute/kg: 60 mg/kg every 24 hours
CrCl ≥0.4-0.5 mL/minute/kg: 50 mg/kg every 24 hours
CrCl <0.4 mL/minute/kg: Not recommended
CMV Induction (equivalent to 90 mg/kg every 12 hours):
CrCl >1.4 mL/minute/kg: 90 mg/kg every 12 hours
CrCl >1-1.4 mL/minute/kg: 70 mg/kg every 12 hours
CrCl >0.8-1 mL/minute/kg: 50 mg/kg every 12 hours
CrCl >0.6-0.8 mL/minute/kg: 80 mg/kg every 24 hours
CrCl >0.5-0.6 mL/minute/kg: 60 mg/kg every 24 hours
CrCl ≥0.4-0.5 mL/minute/kg: 50 mg/kg every 24 hours
CrCl <0.4 mL/minute/kg: Not recommended
CMV Maintenance:
CrCl >1.4 mL/minute/kg: 90-120 mg/kg every 24 hours
CrCl >1-1.4 mL/minute/kg: 70-90 mg/kg every 24 hours
CrCl >0.8-1 mL/minute/kg: 50-65 mg/kg every 24 hours
CrCl >0.6-0.8 mL/minute/kg: 80-105 mg/kg every 48 hours
CrCl >0.5-0.6 mL/minute/kg: 60-80 mg/kg every 48 hours
CrCl ≥0.4-0.5 mL/minute/kg: 50-65 mg/kg every 48 hours
CrCl <0.4 mL/minute/kg: Not recommended
HSV Infection (equivalent to 40 mg/kg every 8 hours):
CrCl >1.4 mL/minute/kg: 40 mg/kg every 8 hours
CrCl >1-1.4 mL/minute/kg: 30 mg/kg every 8 hours
CrCl >0.8-1 mL/minute/kg: 35 mg/kg every 12 hours
CrCl >0.6-0.8 mL/minute/kg: 25 mg/kg every 12 hours
CrCl >0.5-0.6 mL/minute/kg: 40 mg/kg every 24 hours
CrCl ≥0.4-0.5 mL/minute/kg: 35 mg/kg every 24 hours
CrCl <0.4 mL/minute/kg: Not recommended
HSV Infection (equivalent to 40 mg/kg every 12 hours):
CrCl >1.4 mL/minute/kg: 40 mg/kg every 12 hours
CrCl >1-1.4 mL/minute/kg: 30 mg/kg every 12 hours

CrCl >0.8-1 mL/minute/kg: 20 mg/kg every 12 hours
CrCl >0.6-0.8 mL/minute/kg: 35 mg/kg every 24 hours
CrCl >0.5-0.6 mL/minute/kg: 25 mg/kg every 24 hours
CrCl ≥0.4-0.5 mL/minute/kg: 20 mg/kg every 24 hours
CrCl <0.4 mL/minute/kg: Not recommended

Preparation for Administration Parenteral: Foscarnet should be diluted in D_5W or NS. For peripheral line administration, foscarnet **must** be diluted to ≤12 mg/mL with D_5W or NS. For central line administration, foscarnet may be administered undiluted (24 mg/mL).

Administration Parenteral: Administer using an infusion pump at a rate **not to exceed** 60 mg/kg/dose over 1 hour or 120 mg/kg/dose over 2 hours (1 mg/kg/minute).
Hydration:
Initial: Prehydration prior to initial infusion: Children: 10 to 20 mL/kg (maximum: 1,000 mL) of age-appropriate fluid (usually NS); adults: 750 to 1,000 mL NS or D_5W
Subsequent foscarnet doses: Concurrent hydration: Children: 10 to 20 mL/kg (maximum: 1,000 mL) of age-appropriate fluid; adults: 500 to 1,000 mL NS or D_5W; concurrent hydration volume is dependent on foscarnet dose

Monitoring Parameters Serum creatinine, calcium, phosphorus, potassium, magnesium; CBC, ophthalmologic exams, clinical signs of polyuria, and polydipsia

Reference Range Therapeutic serum concentration for CMV: 150 mcg/mL

Dosage Forms Excipient information presented when available (limited, particularly for generics); consult specific product labeling. [DSC] = Discontinued product
Solution, Intravenous, as sodium:
Generic: 24 mg/mL (500 mL [DSC])
Solution, Intravenous, as sodium [preservative free]:
Foscavir: 24 mg/mL (250 mL)

◆ **Foscavir** *see* Foscarnet *on page 941*
◆ **Foscavir® (Can)** *see* Foscarnet *on page 941*

Fosinopril (foe SIN oh pril)

Medication Safety Issues
Sound-alike/look-alike issues:
Fosinopril may be confused with FLUoxetine, Fosamax®, furosemide, lisinopril
Monopril may be confused with Accupril®, minoxidil, moexipril, Monoket®, Monurol®, ramipril

Brand Names: Canada Apo-Fosinopril; Ava-Fosinopril; Jamp-Fosinopril; Mylan-Fosinopril; PMS-Fosinopril; RAN-Fosinopril; Riva-Fosinopril; Teva-Fosinopril

Therapeutic Category Angiotensin-Converting Enzyme (ACE) Inhibitor; Antihypertensive Agent

Generic Availability (US) Yes

Use Treatment of hypertension, either alone or in combination with other antihypertensive agents (FDA approved in ages ≥6 years and adults); adjunctive treatment of heart failure (FDA approved in adults)

Pregnancy Risk Factor D

Pregnancy Considerations [U.S. Boxed Warning]: Drugs that act on the renin-angiotensin system can cause injuy and death to the developing fetus. Discontinue as soon as possible once pregnancy is detected. Drugs that act on the renin-angiotensin system are associated with oligohydramnios. Oligohydramnios, due to decreased fetal renal function, may lead to fetal lung hypoplasia and skeletal malformations. Their use in pregnancy is also associated with anuria, hypotension, renal failure, skull hypoplasia, and death in the fetus/neonate. The exposed fetus should be monitored for fetal growth, amniotic fluid volume, and organ formation. Infants exposed *in utero* should be monitored for hyperkalemia, hypotension, and oliguria (exchange transfusions or dialysis may be needed). These adverse events are generally associated with maternal use in the second and third trimesters.

Untreated chronic maternal hypertension is associated with adverse events in the fetus, infant, and mother. The of use angiotensin-converting enzyme inhibitors is not recommended to treat chronic uncomplicated hypertension or heart failure in pregnant women and should generally be avoided in women of reproductive potential (ACOG, 2013; Yancy, 2013).

Breast-Feeding Considerations Fosinoprilat is excreted in breast milk. Breast-feeding is not recommended by the manufacturer.

Contraindications Hypersensitivity to fosinopril, any other ACE inhibitor, or any component of the formulation; angioedema related to previous treatment with an ACE inhibitor; concomitant use with aliskiren in patients with diabetes mellitus

Warnings/Precautions Anaphylactic reactions may occur rarely with ACE inhibitors. At any time during treatment (especially following first dose), angioedema may occur rarely with ACE inhibitors; it may involve the head and neck (potentially compromising airway) or the intestine (presenting with abdominal pain). African-Americans may be at an increased risk and patients with idiopathic or hereditary angioedema may be at an increased risk. Prolonged frequent monitoring may be required especially if tongue, glottis, or larynx are involved as they are associated with airway obstruction. Patients with a history of airway surgery may have a higher risk of airway obstruction. Aggressive early and appropriate management is critical. Use in patients with previous angioedema associated with ACE inhibitor therapy is contraindicated. Severe anaphylactoid reactions may be seen during hemodialysis (eg, CVVHD) with high-flux dialysis membranes (eg, AN69), and rarely, during low density lipoprotein apheresis with dextran sulfate cellulose. Rare cases of anaphylactoid reactions have been reported in patients undergoing sensitization treatment with hymenoptera (bee, wasp) venom while receiving ACE inhibitors.

Symptomatic hypotension with or without syncope can occur with ACE inhibitors (usually with the first several doses); effects are most often observed in volume-depleted patients; correct volume depletion prior to initiation; close monitoring of patient is required especially with initial dosing and dosing increases; blood pressure must be lowered at a rate appropriate for the patient's clinical condition. Initiation of therapy in patients with ischemic heart disease or cerebrovascular disease warrants close observation due to the potential consequences posed by falling blood pressure (eg, MI, stroke). Use with caution in hypertrophic cardiomyopathy with outflow tract obstruction and severe aortic stenosis. In patients on chronic ACE inhibitor therapy, intraoperative hypotension may occur with induction and maintenance of general anesthesia; use with caution before, during, or immediately after major surgery. Cardiopulmonary bypass, intraoperative blood loss, or vasodilating anesthesia increases endogenous renin release. Use of ACE inhibitors perioperatively will blunt angiotensin II formation and may result in hypotension. However, discontinuation of therapy prior to surgery is controversial. If continued preoperatively, avoidance of hypotensive agents during surgery is prudent (Hillis, 2011). **[U.S. Boxed Warning]: Drugs that act on the renin-angiotensin system can cause injury and death to the developing fetus. Discontinue as soon as possible once pregnancy is detected.**

Hyperkalemia may occur with ACE inhibitors; risk factors include renal dysfunction, diabetes mellitus, concomitant use of potassium-sparing diuretics, potassium supplements, and/or potassium-containing salts. Use cautiously, if at all, with these agents and monitor potassium closely.

Cough may occur with ACE inhibitors. Other causes of cough should be considered (eg, pulmonary congestion in patients with heart failure) and excluded prior to discontinuation. Use with caution in hepatic impairment; fosinopril undergoes hepatic and gut wall metabolism to its active form (fosinoprilat) and may accumulate in hepatic impairment. In patients with alcoholic or biliary cirrhosis, the rate of fosinoprilat formation was slowed, its total body clearance decreased and its AUC ~doubled.

May be associated with deterioration of renal function and/or increases in serum creatinine, particularly in patients with low renal blood flow (eg, renal artery stenosis, heart failure) whose glomerular filtration rate (GFR) is dependent on efferent arteriolar vasoconstriction by angiotensin II; deterioration may result in oliguria, acute renal failure, and progressive azotemia. Small increases in serum creatinine may occur following initiation; consider discontinuation only in patients with progressive and/or significant deterioration in renal function. Use with caution in patients with unstented unilateral/bilateral renal artery stenosis. When unstented bilateral renal artery stenosis is present, use is generally avoided due to the elevated risk of deterioration in renal function unless possible benefits outweigh risks. Potentially significant drug-drug interactions may exist, requiring dose or frequency adjustment, additional monitoring, and/or selection of alternative therapy.

Rare toxicities associated with ACE inhibitors include cholestatic jaundice (which may progress to fulminant hepatic necrosis), agranulocytosis, neutropenia or leukopenia with myeloid hypoplasia. Patients with collagen vascular diseases (especially with concomitant renal impairment) or renal impairment alone may be at increased risk for hematologic toxicity; periodically monitor CBC with differential in these patients.

Warnings: Additional Pediatric Considerations Pediatric racial differences were identified in a multicentered, prospective, double-blind, placebo-controlled trial that investigated the dose-response of fosinopril in 253 children 6 to 16 years of age; this study found that black children required a higher dose of fosinopril (per kg body weight) in order to adequately control blood pressure (Menon, 2006); the findings of this study are consistent with adult studies assessing ACE inhibitors; consider dosage adjustments in these patients.

In pediatric patients, an isolated dry hacking cough lasting >3 weeks was reported in 7 of 42 pediatric patients (17%) receiving ACE inhibitors (von Vigier, 2000); a review of pediatric randomized-controlled ACE inhibitor trials reported a lower incidence of 3.2% (Baker-Smith, 2010). Other causes of cough should be considered (eg, pulmonary congestion in patients with heart failure) and excluded prior to discontinuation.

Adverse Reactions Higher rates of adverse reactions have generally been noted in patients with CHF. However, the frequency of adverse effects associated with placebo is also increased in this population.

Cardiovascular: Orthostatic hypotension, palpitation
Central nervous system: Dizziness, fatigue, headache
Endocrine & metabolic: Hyperkalemia
Gastrointestinal: Diarrhea, nausea, vomiting
Hepatic: Transaminases increased
Neuromuscular & skeletal: Musculoskeletal pain, noncardiac chest pain, weakness
Renal: Renal function worsening (in patients with bilateral renal artery stenosis or hypovolemia), serum creatinine increased
Respiratory: Cough
Miscellaneous: Upper respiratory infection
Rare but important or life-threatening: Anaphylactoid reaction, angina, angioedema, arthralgia, bronchospasm, cerebral infarction, cerebrovascular accident, gout, hepatitis, hepatomegaly, myalgia, MI, pancreatitis, paresthesia, photosensitivity, pleuritic chest pain, pruritus, rash, renal insufficiency, shock, sudden death, syncope, TIA, tinnitus, urticaria, vertigo. In a small number of patients, a symptom complex of cough, bronchospasm, and eosinophilia has been observed with fosinopril.
Other events reported with ACE inhibitors: Acute renal failure, agranulocytosis, anemia, aplastic anemia, bullous pemphigus, cardiac arrest, eosinophilic pneumonitis, exfoliative dermatitis, gynecomastia, hemolytic anemia, hepatic failure, jaundice, neutropenia, pancytopenia, Stevens-Johnson syndrome, symptomatic hyponatremia, thrombocytopenia. In addition, a syndrome which may include arthralgia, elevated ESR, eosinophilia and positive ANA, fever, interstitial nephritis, myalgia, rash, and vasculitis has been reported for other ACE inhibitors.

Drug Interactions

Metabolism/Transport Effects None known.

Avoid Concomitant Use There are no known interactions where it is recommended to avoid concomitant use.

Increased Effect/Toxicity

Fosinopril may increase the levels/effects of: Allopurinol; Amifostine; Antihypertensives; AzaTHIOprine; Ciprofloxacin (Systemic); Drospirenone; DULoxetine; Ferric Gluconate; Gold Sodium Thiomalate; Grass Pollen Allergen Extract (5 Grass Extract); Hypotensive Agents; Iron Dextran Complex; Levodopa; Lithium; Nonsteroidal Anti-Inflammatory Agents; Obinutuzumab; Pregabalin; RisperiDONE; RiTUXimab; Sodium Phosphates

The levels/effects of Fosinopril may be increased by: Alfuzosin; Aliskiren; Angiotensin II Receptor Blockers; Barbiturates; Brimonidine (Topical); Canagliflozin; Dapoxetine; Diazoxide; DPP-IV Inhibitors; Eplerenone; Everolimus; Heparin; Heparin (Low Molecular Weight); Herbs (Hypotensive Properties); Loop Diuretics; MAO Inhibitors; Nicorandil; Pentoxifylline; Phosphodiesterase 5 Inhibitors; Potassium Salts; Potassium-Sparing Diuretics; Prostacyclin Analogues; Sirolimus; Temsirolimus; Thiazide Diuretics; TiZANidine; Tolvaptan; Trimethoprim

Decreased Effect

The levels/effects of Fosinopril may be decreased by: Antacids; Aprotinin; Herbs (Hypertensive Properties); Icatibant; Lanthanum; Methylphenidate; Nonsteroidal Anti-Inflammatory Agents; Salicylates; Yohimbine

Storage/Stability Store at 25°C (77°F); excursions permitted to 15°C to 30°C (59°F to 86°F). Protect from moisture.

Mechanism of Action Competitive inhibitor of angiotensin-converting enzyme (ACE); prevents conversion of angiotensin I to angiotensin II, a potent vasoconstrictor; results in lower levels of angiotensin II which causes an increase in plasma renin activity and a reduction in aldosterone secretion; a CNS mechanism may also be involved in hypotensive effect as angiotensin II increases adrenergic outflow from CNS; vasoactive kallikreins may be decreased in conversion to active hormones by ACE inhibitors, thus reducing blood pressure

Pharmacodynamics

Onset of action: Antihypertensive effect: 1 hour
Maximum effect: Antihypertensive effect: 2-6 hours postdose
Duration: Antihypertensive effect: 24 hours

Pharmacokinetics (Adult data unless noted)

Absorption: Slow and incomplete
Protein binding: 95%
Metabolism: Fosinopril is a prodrug (inactive) and is hydrolyzed to fosinoprilat (active) by intestinal wall and hepatic esterases; fosinopril is also metabolized to a glucuronide conjugate and a p-hydroxy metabolite of fosinoprilat
Bioavailability: 36%
Half-life: Fosinoprilat:
Children and Adolescents 6-16 years: 11-13 hours

Adults: 12 hours
Adults with CHF: 14 hours
Time to peak serum concentration: ~3 hours
Elimination: Urine and feces (as fosinoprilat and other metabolites in roughly equal proportions, 45% to 50%)

Dosing: Usual Note: Dosage must be titrated according to patient's response; use lowest effective dose.

Children ≥6 years and Adolescents: **Hypertension:** Oral:
≤50 kg: Initial: 0.1 mg/kg/dose once daily; reported range studied: 0.1-0.6 mg/kg/day; maximum daily dose: 40 mg/**day**; some patients may require a lower initial dose (Li, 2004; NHLBI, 2011)
>50 kg: Initial: 5-10 mg once daily, as monotherapy; maximum daily dose: 40 mg/**day**

Adults:
Hypertension: Oral: Initial: 10 mg once daily; usual maintenance: 20-40 mg/day. May need to divide the dose into two if trough effect is inadequate; discontinue the diuretic, if possible 2-3 days before initiation of therapy; resume diuretic therapy carefully, if needed.
Heart failure: Oral: Initial: 10 mg once daily (5 mg once daily if renal dysfunction present or if patient has been vigorously diuresed); increase dose, as needed, to a maximum of 40 mg once daily over several weeks; usual dose: 20-40 mg/day. If hypotension, orthostasis, or azotemia occurs during titration, consider decreasing concomitant diuretic dose, if any.

Dosage adjustment in renal impairment: Children, Adolescents, and Adults: None needed since hepatobiliary elimination compensates adequately for diminished renal elimination.

Dosage adjustment in hepatic impairment: Children, Adolescents, and Adults: Decrease dose and monitor effects.

Administration Oral: May be administered without regard to food.

Monitoring Parameters Blood pressure, BUN, serum creatinine, renal function, urine dipstick for protein, serum potassium, WBC with differential, especially during first 3 months of therapy for patients with renal impairment and/or collagen vascular disease; monitor for angioedema and anaphylactoid reactions; hypovolemia and postural hypotension when beginning therapy, adjusting dosage, and on a regular basis throughout

Test Interactions May cause false low serum digoxin levels with the Digi-Tab RIA kit for digoxin.

Dosage Forms Excipient information presented when available (limited, particularly for generics); consult specific product labeling.

Tablet, Oral, as sodium:
Generic: 10 mg, 20 mg, 40 mg

◆ **Fosinopril Sodium** *see* Fosinopril *on page 943*

Fosphenytoin (FOS fen i toyn)

Medication Safety Issues

Sound-alike/look-alike issues:
Cerebyx may be confused with CeleBREX, CeleXA, Cerezyme, Cervarix
Fosphenytoin may be confused with fospropofol

Administration issues:
Overdoses have occurred due to confusion between the **mg per mL concentration** of fosphenytoin (50 mg phenytoin equivalent (PE)/mL) and **total drug content per vial** (either 100 mg PE/2 mL vial or 500 mg PE/10 mL vial). ISMP recommends that the total drug content per container is identified instead of the concentration in mg per mL to avoid confusion and potential overdoses. Additionally, since most errors have occurred with overdoses in children, ISMP recommends that pediatric hospitals consider stocking only the 2 mL vial.

Related Information
Phenytoin *on page 1690*
Safe Handling of Hazardous Drugs *on page 2455*

Brand Names: US Cerebyx

Brand Names: Canada Cerebyx

Therapeutic Category Anticonvulsant, Hydantoin

Generic Availability (US) Yes

Use Management of generalized convulsive status epilepticus; short-term (≤5 days) parenteral administration of phenytoin when other routes are not possible; prevention and treatment of seizures occurring during neurosurgery (All indications: FDA approved in adults)

Pregnancy Risk Factor D

Pregnancy Considerations Fosphenytoin is the prodrug of phenytoin. Refer to Phenytoin monograph for additional information.

Breast-Feeding Considerations Fosphenytoin is the prodrug of phenytoin. It is not known if fosphenytoin is excreted in breast milk prior to conversion to phenytoin. Refer to Phenytoin monograph for additional information.

Contraindications Hypersensitivity to phenytoin, other hydantoins, or any component of the formulation; patients with sinus bradycardia, sinoatrial block, second- and third-degree AV block, or Adams-Stokes syndrome; occurrence of rash during treatment (should not be resumed if rash is exfoliative, purpuric, or bullous); treatment of absence seizures; concurrent use of delavirdine (due to loss of virologic response and possible resistance to delavirdine or other non-nucleoside reverse transcriptase inhibitors [NNRTIs])

Warnings/Precautions Hazardous agent - use appropriate precautions for handling and disposal (NIOSH 2014 [group 2]).

[U.S. Boxed Warning]: Fosphenytoin administration should not exceed 150 mg phenytoin equivalents (PE)/minute in adult patients. Hypotension and severe cardiac arrhythmias (eg, heart block, ventricular tachycardia, ventricular fibrillation) may occur with rapid administration; adverse cardiac events have been reported at or below the recommended infusion rate. In the treatment of status epilepticus, the rate of administration is 150 mg PE/minute. In a nonemergent situation, administer more slowly or use oral phenytoin. Cardiac monitoring is necessary during and after administration of intravenous fosphenytoin; reduction in rate of administration or discontinuation of infusion may be necessary.

Doses of fosphenytoin are always expressed as their phenytoin sodium equivalent (PE). 1 mg PE is equivalent to 1 mg phenytoin sodium. Do not change the recommended doses when substituting fosphenytoin for phenytoin or vice versa as they are not equivalent on a mg to mg basis. Dosing errors have also occurred due to misinterpretation of vial concentrations resulting in two- or tenfold overdoses (some fatal); ensure correct volume of fosphenytoin is withdrawn from vial. Severe burning or itching, and/or paresthesias, mostly perineal, may occur upon administration, usually at the maximum administration rate and last from minutes to hours; occurrence and intensity may be lessened by slowing or temporarily stopping the infusion. Antiepileptic drugs should not be abruptly discontinued. Acute hepatotoxicity associated with a hypersensitivity syndrome characterized by fever, skin eruptions, and lymphadenopathy has been reported to occur within the first 2 months of treatment. Discontinue if skin rash or lymphadenopathy occurs. A spectrum of hematologic effects have been reported with use (eg, neutropenia, leukopenia, thrombocytopenia, pancytopenia, and anemias). Use with caution in patients with hypotension, severe myocardial insufficiency, diabetes mellitus, porphyria, hypoalbuminemia, hypothyroidism, fever, or hepatic dysfunction. Use with caution in patients with renal impairment; also consider the phosphate load of fosphenytoin (0.0037 mmol phosphate/mg PE fosphenytoin). Effects with other sedative drugs or ethanol may be potentiated. Severe reactions, including toxic epidermal necrolysis (TEN) and Stevens-Johnson syndromes, although rarely reported, have resulted in fatalities; drug should be discontinued if there are any signs of rash and patient should be evaluated for signs and symptoms of drug reaction with eosinophilia and systemic symptoms (DRESS). Patients of Asian descent with the variant *HLA-B*1502* may be at an increased risk of developing Stevens-Johnson syndrome and/or TEN.

The "purple glove syndrome" (ie, discoloration with edema and pain of distal limb) may occur following peripheral IV administration of fosphenytoin. This syndrome may or may not be associated with drug extravasation. Symptoms may resolve spontaneously; however, skin necrosis and limb ischemia may occur. In general, fosphenytoin has significantly less venous irritation and phlebitis compared with an equimolar dose of phenytoin (Jamerson, 1994). Sedation, confusional states, or cerebellar dysfunction (loss of motor coordination) may occur at higher total serum concentrations or at lower total serum concentrations when the free fraction of phenytoin is increased.

Warnings: Additional Pediatric Considerations Safety and efficacy of fosphenytoin in pediatric patients has not been established; based on experience with parenteral fosphenytoin, consider a maximum IV infusion rate in pediatric patients of 1 to 3 mg PE/kg/minute (Hegenbarth, 2008). In a nonemergent situation, administer more slowly or use oral phenytoin.

Pediatric patients may be at increased risk for vitamin D deficiency; with chronic therapy, phenytoin may cause catabolism of vitamin D; the daily vitamin D requirement may be increased in these patients (≥400 units/day); vitamin D status should be periodically monitored with laboratory data (Misra, 2008; Wagner, 2008).

Adverse Reactions The more important adverse clinical events caused by the IV use of fosphenytoin or phenytoin are cardiovascular collapse and/or central nervous system depression. Hypotension can occur when either drug is administered rapidly by the IV route.

The adverse clinical events most commonly observed with the use of fosphenytoin in clinical trials were nystagmus, dizziness, pruritus, paresthesia, headache, somnolence, and ataxia. Paresthesia and pruritus were seen more often following fosphenytoin (versus phenytoin) administration and occurred more often with IV fosphenytoin than with IM administration. These events were dose and rate related (adult doses ≥15 mg/kg at a rate of 150 mg PE/minute). These sensations, generally described as itching, burning, or tingling are usually not at the infusion site. The location of the discomfort varied with the groin mentioned most frequently. The paresthesia and pruritus were transient events that occurred within several minutes of the start of infusion and generally resolved within 10 minutes after completion of infusion.

Transient pruritus, tinnitus, nystagmus, somnolence, and ataxia occurred 2-3 times more often at adult doses ≥15 mg/kg and rates ≥150 mg PE/minute.

IV and IM administration (as reported in clinical trials):

Cardiovascular: Facial edema, hypertension
Central nervous system: Chills, fever, intracranial hypertension, nervousness
Endocrine & metabolic: Hypokalemia
Neuromuscular & skeletal: Hyperreflexia, myasthenia

IV administration (maximum dose/rate):

Central nervous system: Ataxia, dizziness, nystagmus, somnolence
Dermatologic: Pruritus
Cardiovascular: Hypotension, tachycardia, vasodilation
Central nervous system: Agitation, brain edema, dysarthria, extrapyramidal syndrome, headache, hypoesthesia, incoordination, paresthesia, stupor, tremor, vertigo
Gastrointestinal: Dry mouth, nausea, tongue disorder, vomiting
Neuromuscular & skeletal: Back pain, muscle weakness, pelvic pain
Ocular: Amblyopia, diplopia
Otic: Deafness, tinnitus
Miscellaneous: Taste perversion

IM administration (substitute for oral phenytoin):

Central nervous system: Ataxia, dizziness, headache, incoordination, nystagmus, paresthesia, reflexes decreased, somnolence, tremor
Dermatologic: Pruritus
Gastrointestinal: Nausea, vomiting
Hematologic/lymphatic: Ecchymosis
Neuromuscular & skeletal: Muscle weakness

IV and IM administration: Rare but important or life-threatening: Acidosis, acute hepatic failure, acute hepatotoxicity, alkalosis, akathisia, amnesia, anemia, anorexia, aphasia, apnea, arthralgia, asthma, atrial flutter, Babinski sign positive, bundle branch block, cachexia, cardiac arrest, cardiomegaly, cerebral hemorrhage, cerebral infarct, CHF, circumoral paresthesia, CNS depression, cyanosis, dehydration, diabetes insipidus, dyskinesia, dysphagia, dyspnea, edema, emotional lability, encephalopathy, epistaxis, extrapyramidal symptoms, GI hemorrhage, hemiplegia, hemoptysis, hostility, hyperacusis, hyperesthesia, hyper-/hypokinesia, hyperkalemia, hyperventilation, hypochromic anemia, hypophosphatemia, hypotonia, hypoxia, ileus, injection site (edema, hemorrhage, inflammation), ketosis, leg cramps, leukocytosis, leukopenia, LFTs abnormal, malaise, migraine, myalgia, mydriasis, myopathy, neurosis, orthostatic hypotension, palpitation, paralysis, parosmia, petechia, photophobia, photosensitivity reaction, psychosis, pulmonary embolus, QT interval prolongation, rash (maculopapular or pustular), renal failure, sinus bradycardia, shock, subdural hematoma, syncope, Stevens-Johnson syndrome, tenesmus, thrombocytopenia, thrombophlebitis, tongue edema, toxic epidermal necrolysis, urticaria, ventricular extrasystoles, visual field defect

Drug Interactions

Metabolism/Transport Effects Substrate of CYP2C19 (major), CYP2C9 (major), CYP3A4 (minor); **Note:** Assignment of Major/Minor substrate status based on clinically relevant drug interaction potential; **Induces** CYP2B6 (strong), CYP2C19 (strong), CYP2C8 (strong), CYP2C9 (strong), CYP3A4 (strong), P-glycoprotein

Avoid Concomitant Use

Avoid concomitant use of Fosphenytoin with any of the following: Abiraterone Acetate; Apixaban; Apremilast; Artemether; Axitinib; Azelastine (Nasal); Bedaquiline; Boceprevir; Bortezomib; Bosutinib; Cabozantinib; Ceritinib; CloZAPine; Crizotinib; Dabigatran Etexilate; Darunavir; Dasabuvir; Delavirdine; Dienogest; Dolutegravir; Dronedarone; Eliglustat; Enzalutamide; Etravirine; Everolimus; Ibrutinib; Idelalisib; Irinotecan; Isavuconazonium Sulfate; Itraconazole; Ivabradine; Ivacaftor; Lapatinib; Ledipasvir; Lumefantrine; Lurasidone; Macitentan; Mifepristone; Naloxegol; Netupitant; NIFEdipine; Nilotinib; NiMODipine; Nintedanib; Nisoldipine; Olaparib; Ombitasvir; Orphenadrine; Palbociclib; Panobinostat; Paraldehyde; Paritaprevir; PAZOPanib; PONATinib; Praziquantel; Ranolazine; Regorafenib; Rilpivirine; Rivaroxaban; Roflumilast; RomiDEPsin; Simeprevir; Sofosbuvir; SORAfenib; Suvorexant; Tasimelteon; Telaprevir; Thalidomide; Ticagrelor; Tofacitinib; Tolvaptan; Toremifene; Trabectedin; Ulipristal; Vandetanib; Vemurafenib; VinCRIStine (Liposomal); Vorapaxar

Increased Effect/Toxicity

Fosphenytoin may increase the levels/effects of: Amiodarone; Azelastine (Nasal); Buprenorphine; Ciprofloxacin (Systemic); Clarithromycin; CNS Depressants; FLUoxetine; Fosamprenavir; Highest Risk QTc-Prolonging Agents; Hydrocodone; Lithium; Methotrexate; Methotrimeprazine; Metyrosine; Moderate Risk QTc-Prolonging Agents; Neuromuscular-Blocking Agents (Nondepolarizing); Orphenadrine; Paraldehyde; PHENobarbital; Pramipexole; QuiNIDine; ROPINIRole; Rotigotine; Selective Serotonin Reuptake Inhibitors; Thalidomide; Vitamin K Antagonists; Zolpidem

The levels/effects of Fosphenytoin may be increased by: Alcohol (Ethyl); Amiodarone; Antifungal Agents (Azole Derivatives, Systemic); Benzodiazepines; Brimonidine (Topical); Calcium Channel Blockers; Cannabis; Capecitabine; CarBAMazepine; Carbonic Anhydrase Inhibitors; CeFAZolin; Chlorpheniramine; Cimetidine; Clarithromycin; CYP2C19 Inhibitors (Moderate); CYP2C19 Inhibitors (Strong); CYP2C9 Inhibitors (Moderate); CYP2C9 Inhibitors (Strong); Delavirdine; Dexamethasone (Systemic); Dexketoprofen; Dexmethylphenidate; Disopyramide; Disulfiram; Doxylamine; Dronabinol; Droperidol; Efavirenz; Eslicarbazepine; Ethosuximide; Felbamate; Floxuridine; Fluconazole; Fluorouracil (Systemic); Fluorouracil (Topical); FLUoxetine; FluvoxaMINE; Halothane; HydrOXYzine; Isoniazid; Kava Kava; Luliconazole; Magnesium Sulfate; Methotrimeprazine; Methylphenidate; MetroNIDAZOLE (Systemic); Miconazole (Oral); Nabilone; Omeprazole; OXcarbazepine; Rufinamide; Sertraline; Sodium Oxybate; Tacrolimus (Systemic); Tapentadol; Tegafur; Telaprevir; Tetrahydrocannabinol; Ticlopidine; Topiramate; TraZODone; Trimethoprim; Vitamin K Antagonists

Decreased Effect

Fosphenytoin may decrease the levels/effects of: Abiraterone Acetate; Acetaminophen; Afatinib; Amiodarone; Antifungal Agents (Azole Derivatives, Systemic); Apixaban; Apremilast; ARIPiprazole; Artemether; Axitinib; Bazedoxifene; Bedaquiline; Boceprevir; Bortezomib; Bosutinib; Brentuximab Vedotin; Busulfan; Cabozantinib; Canagliflozin; Cannabidiol; Cannabis; CarBAMazepine; Ceritinib; Clarithromycin; CloZAPine; Cobicistat; Contraceptives (Estrogens); Contraceptives (Progestins); Corticosteroids (Systemic); Crizotinib; CycloSPORINE (Systemic); CYP2B6 Substrates; CYP2C19 Substrates; CYP2C8 Substrates; CYP2C9 Substrates; CYP3A4 Substrates; Dabigatran Etexilate; Darunavir; Dasabuvir; Dasatinib; Deferasirox; Delavirdine; Dexamethasone (Systemic); Diclofenac (Systemic); Dienogest; Disopyramide; Dolutegravir; DOXOrubicin (Conventional); Doxycycline; Dronabinol; Dronedarone; Efavirenz; Eliglustat; Elvitegravir; Enzalutamide; Erlotinib; Eslicarbazepine; Ethosuximide; Etoposide; Etoposide Phosphate; Etravirine; Everolimus; Exemestane; Ezogabine; Felbamate; FentaNYL; Flunarizine; Gefitinib; GuanFACINE; HMG-CoA Reductase Inhibitors; Hydrocortisone (Systemic); Ibrutinib; Idelalisib; Imatinib; Irinotecan; Isavuconazonium Sulfate; Itraconazole; Ivabradine; Ivacaftor; Ixabepilone; Lacosamide; LamoTRIgine; Lapatinib; Ledipasvir; Levodopa; Linagliptin; Loop Diuretics; Lopinavir; Lumefantrine; Lurasidone; Macitentan; Maraviroc; Mebendazole; Meperidine; Methadone; MethylPREDNISolone; MetroNIDAZOLE (Systemic); Metyrapone; Mexiletine; Mianserin; Mifepristone; Naloxegol; Nelfinavir; Netupitant; Neuromuscular-Blocking Agents (Nondepolarizing); NIFEdipine; Nilotinib; NiMODipine; Nintedanib; Nisoldipine; Olaparib; Ombitasvir; Omeprazole; OXcarbazepine; Palbociclib; Paliperidone; Panobinostat; Paritaprevir; PAZOPanib; Perampanel; P-glycoprotein/ABCB1 Substrates; PONATinib; Praziquantel; PrednisoLONE (Systemic); PredniSONE; Primidone; Propafenone; QUEtiapine; QuiNIDine; QuiNINE; Ranolazine; Regorafenib; Rilpivirine; Ritonavir; Rivaroxaban; Roflumilast; RomiDEPsin; Rufinamide; Saxagliptin; Sertraline; Simeprevir; Sirolimus; Sofosbuvir; SORAfenib; SUNItinib; Suvorexant; Tacrolimus (Systemic); Tadalafil; Tasimelteon; Telaprevir; Temsirolimus; Teniposide; Tetrahydrocannabinol; Theophylline Derivatives; Thyroid Products; Ticagrelor; Tipranavir; Tofacitinib; Tolvaptan; Topiramate; Topotecan; Toremifene; Trabectedin; TraZODone; Treprostinil; Trimethoprim; Ulipristal; Valproic Acid and Derivatives; Vandetanib; Vemurafenib; Vilazodone; VinCRIStine; VinCRIStine (Liposomal); Vorapaxar; Vortioxetine; Zaleplon; Zonisamide

The levels/effects of Fosphenytoin may be decreased by: Alcohol (Ethyl); CarBAMazepine; Ciprofloxacin (Systemic); CYP2C19 Inducers (Strong); CYP2C9 Inducers (Strong); Dabrafenib; Dexamethasone (Systemic); Diazoxide; Enzalutamide; Folic Acid; Fosamprenavir; Leucovorin Calcium-Levoleucovorin; Levomefolate; Lopinavir; Mefloquine; Methotrexate; Methylfolate; Mianserin; Multivitamins/Minerals (with ADEK, Folate, Iron); Nelfinavir; PHENobarbital; Platinum Derivatives; Pyridoxine; Rifampin; Ritonavir; Theophylline Derivatives; Tipranavir; Valproic Acid and Derivatives; Vigabatrin; VinCRIStine

Food Interactions

Acute use: Ethanol inhibits metabolism of phenytoin. Management: Monitor patients.

Chronic use: Ethanol stimulates metabolism of phenytoin. Management: Monitor patients.

Storage/Stability Refrigerate at 2°C to 8°C (36°F to 46°F). Do not store at room temperature for more than 48 hours. Do not use vials that develop particulate matter. Has been shown to be stable at 1, 8, and 20 mg PE/mL in normal saline or D_5W at 25°C (77°F) for 30 days in glass container and at 4°C to 20°C (39°F to 68°F) for 30 days in PVC bag. Undiluted fosphenytoin injection (50 mg PE/mL) is stable in polypropylene syringes for 30 days at 25°C, 4°C, or frozen at -20°C. Fosphenytoin at concentrations of 1, 8, and 20 mg PE/mL prepared in $D_5{}^1/_2$NS, $D_5{}^1/_2$NS with KCl 20 mEq/L, $D_5{}^1/_2$NS with 40 mEq/L, LR, D_5LR, $D_{10}W$, amino acid 10%, mannitol 20%, hetastarch 6% in NS or Plasma-Lyte® A injection is stable in polyvinyl chloride bags for 7 days when stored at 25°C (room temperature) (Fischer, 1997).

Mechanism of Action Diphosphate ester salt of phenytoin which acts as a water soluble prodrug of phenytoin; after administration, plasma esterases convert fosphenytoin to phosphate, formaldehyde (not expected to be clinically consequential [Fierro, 1996]), and phenytoin as the active moiety; phenytoin works by stabilizing neuronal membranes and decreasing seizure activity by increasing efflux or decreasing influx of sodium ions across cell membranes in the motor cortex during generation of nerve impulses

Pharmacokinetics (Adult data unless noted) The pharmacokinetics of fosphenytoin-derived phenytoin are the same as those for phenytoin. Parameters listed below are for fosphenytoin (the prodrug) unless otherwise noted. **Note:** The pharmacokinetics of intravenous fosphenytoin in pediatric patients have been evaluated in two studies (n= 49, age range: 1 day to 16.7 years; n=8, age range: 5-18 years) and found to be similar to the pharmacokinetics observed in young adults; the conversion rate of fosphenytoin to phenytoin was consistent throughout childhood (Fischer, 2003; Pellock, 1996).

Bioavailability: IM, IV: 100%

Distribution: V_d: 4.3-10.8 L; V_d of fosphenytoin increases with dose and rate of administration (Fischer, 2003)

Protein binding: 95% to 99% primarily to albumin; binding of fosphenytoin to protein is saturable (the percent bound decreases as total concentration increases); fosphenytoin displaces phenytoin from protein binding sites; during the time fosphenytoin is being converted to phenytoin, fosphenytoin may temporarily increase the free fraction of phenytoin up to 30% unbound

Metabolism: Each millimole of fosphenytoin is metabolized to 1 millimole of phenytoin, phosphate, and formaldehyde; formaldehyde is converted to formate, which is then metabolized by a folate-dependent mechanism; conversion of fosphenytoin to phenytoin increases with increasing dose and infusion rate, most likely due to a decrease in fosphenytoin protein binding

Half-life:

Conversion of fosphenytoin to phenytoin:

Pediatric patients (ages: 1 day to 16.7 years): 8.3 minutes (range: 2.5-18.5 minutes) (Fischer, 2003)

Adults: Mean range: 7-15 minutes (Fischer, 2003)

Time for complete conversion to phenytoin:

IM: 4 hours after injection

IV: 2 hours after the end of infusion

Time to peak serum concentration (phenytoin):

IV: Adults: 30-60 minutes from the beginning of fosphenytoin infusion (Fischer, 2003)

IM:

Neonates and Infants ≤6 months: 1-3 hours was reported in a case series (n=3; PNA: 15-47 days) (Fischer, 2003)

Pediatric patients >7 months: Therapeutic concentrations within 30 minutes; time to maximum serum concentration not reported (Fischer, 2003)

Adults: 3 hours

Elimination: 0% fosphenytoin excreted in urine

Dosing: Neonatal

The dose, concentration in solutions, and infusion rates for fosphenytoin are expressed as PHENYTOIN SODIUM EQUIVALENTS (PE)

Fosphenytoin should ALWAYS be prescribed and dispensed in mg of PE; otherwise, significant medication errors may occur

Note: A limited number of clinical studies have been conducted; based on pharmacokinetic studies, experts recommend the following (Fischer 2003): Use the neonatal IV phenytoin dosing guidelines to dose fosphenytoin using doses in **PE** equal to the phenytoin doses (ie, phenytoin 1 mg = fosphenytoin 1 mg **PE**). Dosage should be individualized based upon clinical response and serum concentrations.

Status epilepticus; neonatal seizures: Limited data available: Loading dose: IM, IV: 15 to 20 mg PE/kg; then begin maintenance therapy usually 12 hours after dose. **Note:** Phenobarbital is the preferred antiepileptic agent for treatment of neonatal seizures (Hegenbarth 2008).

Seizures; maintenance therapy, short-term when oral route not available or appropriate: Limited data available:

Not currently on phenytoin: **Note:** Assess if loading dose is required; calculate loading dose as above for status epilepticus.

IM or IV: Initial: 5 mg PE/kg/day in 2 divided doses; usual range: 4 to 8 mg PE/kg/day in 2 divided doses; some patients may require dosing every 8 hours; dosing based on phenytoin recommendations for this patient population; in adult patients, treatment duration >5 days has not been evaluated.

Substitution for oral phenytoin therapy: IM or IV: May be substituted for oral phenytoin sodium at the same total daily dose; due to bioavailability differences of oral phenytoin dosage forms, serum phenytoin concentrations may increase when IM or IV fosphenytoin is substituted for oral phenytoin sodium therapy; monitor serum concentrations closely when converting dosage form.

Dosing: Usual

The dose, concentration in solutions, and infusion rates for fosphenytoin are expressed as PHENYTOIN SODIUM EQUIVALENTS (PE)

Fosphenytoin should ALWAYS be prescribed and dispensed in mg of PE; otherwise significant medication errors may occur

Pediatric: IV: **Note:** A limited number of clinical studies have been conducted in pediatric patients; based on pharmacokinetic studies, experts recommend the following (Fischer, 2003): Use the pediatric IV phenytoin dosing guidelines to dose fosphenytoin using doses in **PE** equal to the phenytoin doses (ie, phenytoin 1 mg = fosphenytoin 1 mg **PE**). Dosage should be individualized based upon clinical response and serum concentrations.

Status epilepticus: Limited data available: Infants, Children, and Adolescents: Loading dose: IM, IV: 15 to 20 mg PE/kg; maximum dose: 1,000 mg PE; then begin maintenance therapy usually 12 hours after dose (Brophy 2012; Hegenbarth 2008). An additional load of 5 mg PE/kg may be given 10 minutes after initial loading infusion completed if status epilepticus is not resolved; however, some experts recommend trying another agent once a total loading dose of 20 mg PE/kg has been given (Brophy 2012).

Seizures; maintenance therapy, short-term when oral route not available or appropriate: Limited data available: Infants, Children, and Adolescents: **Note:** Dosing presented based on phenytoin recommendations for this patient population:

Not currently receiving phenytoin: **Note:** Assess if loading dose is required; calculate loading dose as above for status epilepticus.

Maintenance therapy: IM, IV: Initial 5 mg PE/kg/day divided twice daily; usual range: 4 to 8 mg PE/kg/day divided twice daily; maximum daily dose: 300 mg PE/**day**. Some experts suggest higher maintenance doses (8 to 10 mg PE/kg/day) may be necessary in infants and young children (Guerrini 2006). Dosing should be based upon ideal body weight (IBW); in adult patients, treatment duration >5 days has not been evaluated.

Substitution for oral phenytoin therapy: IM or IV: May be substituted for oral phenytoin sodium at the same total daily dose; however, Dilantin capsules are ~90% bioavailable by the oral route; phenytoin, supplied as fosphenytoin, is 100% bioavailable by both the IM and IV routes; for this reason, plasma phenytoin concentrations may increase when IM or IV fosphenytoin is substituted for oral phenytoin sodium therapy; in adult clinical trials, IM fosphenytoin was administered as a single daily dose utilizing either 1 or 2 injection sites; some patients may require more frequent dosing

Traumatic brain injury; seizure prophylaxis: Limited data available; efficacy results variable; dosing based on experience with phenytoin: Infants, Children, and Adolescents: IV: Initial: 18 mg PE/kg loading dose; followed by 6 mg PE/kg/day divided every 8 hours for 48 hours was used in a double-blind, placebo-controlled trial of 102 pediatric patients (n=46 treatment group; median age: 6.4 years) and showed no significant difference in seizure frequency between groups; however, the trial was stopped early due to a very low seizure frequency among both study groups (Young, 2004). In a retrospective trial, reduced seizure frequency with prophylactic phenytoin use was described (Lewis 1993). **Note:** Current guidelines suggest that prophylactic phenytoin may be considered to reduce the incidence of early post-traumatic seizures in pediatric patients with severe traumatic brain injuries but it does not reduce the risk of long-term seizures or improve neurologic outcome (Kochanek 2012).

Adult: **Note:** The dose, concentration in solutions, and infusion rates for fosphenytoin are expressed as phenytoin sodium equivalents (PE); fosphenytoin should always be prescribed and dispensed in phenytoin sodium equivalents (PE).

Status epilepticus: IV: Loading dose: 15-20 mg PE/kg administered at 100 to 150 mg PE/minute

Nonemergent loading and maintenance dosing:

Loading dose: IM, IV: 10 to 20 mg PE/kg; for IV administration, infuse more slowly (eg, over 30 minutes); maximum rate: 150 mg PE/minute

Initial daily maintenance dose: IM, IV: 4 to 6 mg PE/kg/day in divided doses

Substitution for oral phenytoin therapy: IM or IV: May be substituted for oral phenytoin sodium at the same total daily dose; however, Dilantin capsules are ~90% bioavailable by the oral route; phenytoin, supplied as fosphenytoin, is 100% bioavailable by both the IM and IV routes; for this reason, plasma phenytoin concentrations may increase when IM or IV fosphenytoin is substituted for oral phenytoin sodium therapy; in clinical trials, IM fosphenytoin was administered as a single daily dose utilizing either 1 or 2 injection sites; some patients may require more frequent dosing.

Dosing adjustment in renal impairment: Adults: No initial dosage adjustment necessary. Free (unbound) phenytoin serum concentrations should be monitored closely in patients with renal disease or in those with hypoalbuminemia, free phenytoin serum concentrations may be increased; furthermore, fosphenytoinconversion to phenytoin may be increased without a similar increase in phenytoin conversion in these patients leading to increase frequency and severity of adverse events.

Dosing adjustment in hepatic impairment: Adults: No initial dosage adjustment necessary. Phenytoin clearance may be substantially reduced in cirrhosis and serum concentration monitoring with dose adjustment advisable. Free (unbound) phenytoin concentrations should be monitored closely in patients with hepatic disease or in those with hypoalbuminemia; free phenytoin concentrations may be increased; furthermore, fosphenytoin conversion to phenytoin may be increased without a similar increase in phenytoin clearance in these patients leading to increased frequency and severity of adverse events.

Preparation for Administration Hazardous agent; use appropriate precautions for handling and disposal (NIOSH 2014 [group 2]).

IV: Solution for injection must be further diluted with D_5W or NS to a final concentration of 1.5 to 25 mg PE/mL.

Administration Hazardous agent; use appropriate precautions for handling and disposal (NIOSH 2014 [group 2]).

IM: May administer undiluted; the quadricep area has been recommended as an injection site; in adults, fosphenytoin has been administered as a single daily dose using 1-4 injection sites (up to 20 mL per site well tolerated in adults) (Meek 1999; Pryor 2001)

IV: Administer diluted solution as intermittent IV infusion; do not administer as a continuous infusion or IV push

Maximum rates of infusion:

Pediatric patients: Administer at **1 to 3 mg PE/kg/minute up to a maximum of 150 mg PE/minute** (Brophy 2012; Hegenbarth 2008); slower administration reduces incidence of cardiovascular events (eg, hypotension, arrhythmia) as well as severity of paresthesias and pruritus. For nonemergent situations, may administer loading dose more slowly (eg, over 30 minutes) (Fischer 2003). Highly sensitive patients (eg, patients with preexisting cardiovascular conditions) should receive fosphenytoin more slowly (Meek 1999).

Adults: **Do not exceed 150 mg PE/minute.** Slower administration reduces incidence of cardiovascular events (eg, hypotension, arrhythmia) as well as severity of paresthesias and pruritus. For nonemergent situations, may administer loading dose more slowly [eg, over 30 minutes (~33 mg PE/minute for 1,000 mg PE) **or** 50 to 100 mg PE/minute (Fischer 2003)]. Highly sensitive patients (eg, elderly, patients with preexisting cardiovascular conditions) should receive fosphenytoin more slowly (eg, 25 to 50 mg PE/minute) (Meek 1999).

Monitoring Parameters CBC with differential, platelets, serum glucose, liver function. Serum phenytoin concentrations: If available, free phenytoin concentrations should be obtained in patients with hyperbilirubinemia, renal impairment, uremia, or hypoalbuminemia; in adult patients, if free phenytoin concentrations are unavailable, the adjusted total concentration may be determined based upon equations. Trough serum concentrations are generally recommended for routine monitoring. To ensure therapeutic concentration is attained, peak serum concentrations may be measured 1 hour after the end of an IV infusion (particularly after a loading dose).

Additional monitoring with IV use: Continuous cardiac monitoring (rate, rhythm, blood pressure) and clinical observation during administration is recommended; blood pressure and pulse should be monitored every 15 minutes for 1 hour after administration with nonemergency use (Meek, 1999); emergency use may require more frequent monitoring and for a longer time after administration; infusion site reactions

Reference Range Note: Information based on experience with phenytoin.

Timing of serum samples: The apparent serum half-life varies with the dosage and the drug follows Michaelis-Menten kinetics. In adults, the average apparent half-life is about 24 hours; in pediatric patients, the apparent half-life is age-dependent (longer in neonates). Steady-state concentrations are reached in 5-10 days.

Toxicity is measured clinically and some patients may require levels outside the suggested therapeutic range.

Therapeutic range:

Total phenytoin:

Neonates: 8-15 mcg/mL

Pediatric patients ≥1 month and Adults: 10-20 mcg/mL

Concentrations of 5-10 mcg/mL may be therapeutic for some patients, but concentrations <5 mcg/mL are not likely to be effective

50% of adult patients show decreased frequency of seizures at concentrations >10 mcg/mL

86% of adult patients show decreased frequency of seizures at concentrations >15 mcg/mL

Add another anticonvulsant if satisfactory therapeutic response is not achieved with a phenytoin concentration of 20 mcg/mL.

Free phenytoin: 1-2.5 mcg/mL

Total phenytoin:

Toxic: >30 mcg/mL (SI: >119 micromole/L)

Lethal: >100 mcg/mL (SI: >400 micromole/L)

After a loading dose: If rapid therapeutic serum concentrations are needed, initial concentrations may be drawn after 1 hour (after end of IV loading dose) to aid in determining maintenance dose or need to reload.

Rapid achievement: Early assessment of serum concentrations: Draw within 2-3 days of therapy initiation to ensure that the patient's metabolism is not remarkably different from that which would be predicted by average literature-derived pharmacokinetic parameters; early serum concentrations should be used cautiously in design of new dosing regimens.

See Phenytoin monograph for further information.

Test Interactions Falsely high plasma phenytoin concentrations (due to cross-reactivity with fosphenytoin) when measured by immunoanalytical techniques (eg, TD_X®, TD_XFL_X™, Emit® 2000) prior to complete conversion of fosphenytoin to phenytoin. Phenytoin may produce falsely low results for dexamethasone or metyrapone tests.

Additional Information Dosing equivalency: Fosphenytoin sodium 1.5 mg is equivalent to phenytoin sodium 1 mg which is equivalent to fosphenytoin 1 mg **PE**

Fosphenytoin is water soluble and has a lower pH (8.8) than phenytoin (12), irritation at injection site or phlebitis is reduced.

Formaldehyde production from fosphenytoin is not expected to be clinically significant in adults with short-term use (eg, 1 week); potentially harmful amounts of phosphate and formaldehyde could occur with an overdose of fosphenytoin; fosphenytoin is more water soluble than phenytoin and, therefore, the injection does not contain propylene glycol; antiarrhythmic effects should be similar to phenytoin

Overdose may result in: Lethargy, nausea, vomiting, hypotension, syncope, tachycardia, bradycardia, asystole, cardiac arrest, hypocalcemia, and metabolic acidosis; fatalities have also been reported

Dosage Forms Excipient information presented when available (limited, particularly for generics); consult specific product labeling.

Solution, Injection, as sodium:

Cerebyx: 100 mg PE/2 mL (2 mL); 500 MG PE/10ML (2 mL, 10 mL); 500 mg PE/10 mL (10 mL)

Generic: 100 mg PE/2 mL (2 mL); 500 mg PE/10 mL (10 mL)

- ◆ **Fosphenytoin Sodium** *see* Fosphenytoin *on page 945*
- ◆ **Fresenius Propoven** *see* Propofol *on page 1786*
- ◆ **Frisium (Can)** *see* CloBAZam *on page 495*
- ◆ **Froben (Can)** *see* Flurbiprofen (Systemic) *on page 915*
- ◆ **Froben-SR (Can)** *see* Flurbiprofen (Systemic) *on page 915*
- ◆ **Fruit C [OTC]** *see* Ascorbic Acid *on page 202*
- ◆ **Fruit C 500 [OTC]** *see* Ascorbic Acid *on page 202*
- ◆ **Fruity C [OTC]** *see* Ascorbic Acid *on page 202*
- ◆ **Frusemide** *see* Furosemide *on page 951*
- ◆ **FTC** *see* Emtricitabine *on page 739*
- ◆ **FTC, TDF, and EFV** *see* Efavirenz, Emtricitabine, and Tenofovir *on page 734*
- ◆ **FU** *see* Fluorouracil (Systemic) *on page 903*
- ◆ **5-FU** *see* Fluorouracil (Systemic) *on page 903*

Fulvestrant (fool VES trant)

Related Information

Safe Handling of Hazardous Drugs *on page 2455*

Brand Names: US Faslodex

Brand Names: Canada Faslodex

Therapeutic Category Antineoplastic Agent, Estrogen Receptor Antagonist

Generic Availability (US) No

Use Treatment of hormone receptor-positive metastatic breast cancer in postmenopausal women with disease progression following antiestrogen therapy (FDA approved in adults); has also been used in treatment of McCune-Albright Syndrome (MAS) in girls associated with progressive precocious puberty

Pregnancy Risk Factor D

Pregnancy Considerations Adverse events were observed in animal reproduction studies. Fulvestrant is approved for use only in postmenopausal women. If used prior to confirmed menopause, women of reproductive potential should be advised not to become pregnant. Based on the mechanism of action, may cause fetal harm if administered during pregnancy.

Breast-Feeding Considerations Approved for use only in postmenopausal women. Because of the potential for serious adverse reactions in the nursing infant, a decision should be made to discontinue breast-feeding or the drug, taking into account the importance of treatment to the mother.

Contraindications Known hypersensitivity to fulvestrant or any component of the formulation

Warnings/Precautions Hazardous agent - use appropriate precautions for handling and disposal (NIOSH 2014 [group 1]). Exposure is increased and dosage adjustment is recommended in patients with moderate hepatic impairment. Safety and efficacy have not been established in severe hepatic impairment. Use with caution in patients with a history of bleeding disorders (including thrombocytopenia) and/or patients on anticoagulant therapy; bleeding/hematoma may occur from IM administration. Hypersensitivity reactions, including urticaria and angioedema, have been reported.

Benzyl alcohol and derivatives: Some dosage forms may contain benzyl alcohol; large amounts of benzyl alcohol (≥99 mg/kg/day) have been associated with a potentially fatal toxicity ("gasping syndrome") in neonates; the "gasping syndrome" consists of metabolic acidosis, respiratory distress, gasping respirations, CNS dysfunction (including convulsions, intracranial hemorrhage), hypotension and cardiovascular collapse (AAP, 1997; CDC, 1982); some data suggests that benzoate displaces bilirubin from protein binding sites (Ahlfors 2001); avoid or use dosage forms containing benzyl alcohol with caution in neonates. See manufacturer's labeling.

Adverse Reactions

Cardiovascular: Ischemic disorder

Central nervous system: Fatigue, headache

Endocrine & metabolic: Hot flushes

Gastrointestinal: Anorexia, constipation, nausea, vomiting, weight gain

Genitourinary: Urinary tract infection

Hepatic: Alkaline phosphatase increased, transaminases increased

Local: Injection site pain

Neuromuscular & skeletal: Arthralgia, back pain, bone pain, extremity pain, joint disorders, musculoskeletal pain, weakness

Respiratory: Cough, dyspnea

Rare but important or life-threatening (reported with 250 mg or 500 mg dose): Angioedema, hepatitis, hypersensitivity reactions, leukopenia, liver failure, osteoporosis, thrombosis, vaginal bleeding

Drug Interactions

Metabolism/Transport Effects Substrate of CYP3A4 (minor); **Note:** Assignment of Major/Minor substrate status based on clinically relevant drug interaction potential

Avoid Concomitant Use There are no known interactions where it is recommended to avoid concomitant use.

Increased Effect/Toxicity There are no known significant interactions involving an increase in effect.

Decreased Effect There are no known significant interactions involving a decrease in effect.

Storage/Stability Store in original carton at 2°C to 8°C (36°F to 46°F). Protect from light.

Mechanism of Action Estrogen receptor antagonist; competitively binds to estrogen receptors on tumors and other tissue targets, producing a nuclear complex that causes a dose-related down-regulation of estrogen receptors and inhibits tumor growth.

Pharmacodynamics Duration: IM: Steady state concentrations reached within first month, when administered with additional dose given 2 weeks following the initial dose; plasma levels maintained for at least 1 month

Pharmacokinetics (Adult data unless noted)

Distribution: V_d: ~3-5 L/kg

Protein binding: 99%; to plasma proteins (VLDL, LDL, and HDL lipoprotein fractions)

Metabolism: Hepatic via multiple biotransformation pathways (CYP3A4 substrate involved in oxidation pathway, although relative contribution to metabolism unknown); metabolites formed are either less active or have similar activity to parent compound

Half-life:

Children 1-10 years: 70.4 days (Sims, 2012)

Adults: 250 mg: ~40 days

Excretion: Feces (~90%); urine (<1%)

Clearance: Children 1-8 years: Decreased by 32% compared to adults

Dosing: Usual

Pediatric: **McCune-Albright Syndrome; progressive precocious puberty:** Limited data available: Children 1 to 10 years: IM: 4 mg/kg once monthly; dosing based on a trial in 30 girls ≤10 years of age (range: 1 to 8.5 years) who received monthly injections for 1 year; significant decrease in vaginal bleeding and reduction in rates of skeletal maturation were reported (Sims 2012)

Adult: **Breast cancer, metastatic (postmenopausal women):** IM: Initial: 500 mg on days 1, 15, and 29; Maintenance: 500 mg once monthly

Dosage adjustment in renal impairment: Adults:

CrCl ≥30 mL/minute: No dosage adjustment required.

CrCl <30 mL/minute: No dosage adjustment provided in manufacturer's labeling (has not been studied); however, renal elimination of fulvestrant is negligible.

Dosage adjustment in hepatic impairment: Adults:

Mild impairment (Child-Pugh class A): No dosage adjustment required.

Moderate impairment (Child-Pugh class B): Decrease initial and maintenance doses to 250 mg.

Severe impairment (Child-Pugh class C): Use has not been evaluated.

Administration Hazardous agent; use appropriate precautions for handling and disposal (NIOSH 2014 [group 1]). **For IM administration only; do not administer IV, SubQ, or intra-arterially.** In adults, administer 500 mg dose as two 5 mL injections (one in each buttock) slowly over 1-2 minutes per injection; depending upon final dose volume, pediatric patients may be able to receive entire dose as one injection.

Monitoring Parameters McCune-Albright syndrome: In the pediatric clinical trial (study duration: 12 months), the following were monitored: Serum estradiol, testosterone, LH, and FSH (baseline, and at 3, 6, 12 months of therapy); liver function test (baseline and at 12 months of therapy); CBC and INR at baseline; assessments of puberty status and growth at baseline and periodically during therapy [6 and 12 months: Height, weight, Tanner stage, bone age (radiographs), vaginal bleeding data, and pelvic ultrasounds] (Sims, 2012)

Dosage Forms Excipient information presented when available (limited, particularly for generics); consult specific product labeling.

Solution, Intramuscular:

Faslodex: 250 mg/5 mL (5 mL) [contains alcohol, usp, benzyl alcohol, benzyl benzoate]

- **Fungi-Guard [OTC]** *see* Tolnaftate *on page 2083*
- **Fungi-Nail® [OTC]** *see* Undecylenic Acid and Derivatives *on page 2135*
- **Fungizone (Can)** *see* Amphotericin B (Conventional) *on page 147*
- **Fungoid-D [OTC]** *see* Tolnaftate *on page 2083*
- **Fungoid Tincture [OTC]** *see* Miconazole (Topical) *on page 1431*
- **Furadantin** *see* Nitrofurantoin *on page 1521*
- **Furazosin** *see* Prazosin *on page 1752*

Furosemide (fyoor OH se mide)

Medication Safety Issues

Sound-alike/look-alike issues:

Furosemide may be confused with famotidine, finasteride, fluconazole, FLUoxetine, fosinopril, loperamide, torsemide

Lasix may be confused with Lanoxin, Lidex, Lomotil, Lovenox, Luvox, Luxiq

International issues:

Lasix [U.S., Canada, and multiple international markets] may be confused with Esidrex brand name for hydrochlorothiazide [multiple international markets]; Esidrix brand name for hydrochlorothiazide [Germany]; Losec brand name for omeprazole [multiple international markets]

Urex [Australia, Hong Kong, Turkey] may be confused with Eurax brand name for crotamiton [U.S., Canada, and multiple international markets]

Brand Names: US Lasix

Brand Names: Canada Apo-Furosemide; AVA-Furosemide; Bio-Furosemide; Dom-Furosemide; Furosemide Injection Sandoz Standard; Furosemide Injection, USP; Furosemide Special; Furosemide Special Injection; Lasix; Lasix Special; Novo-Semide; NTP-Furosemide; Nu-Furosemide; PMS-Furosemide; Teva-Furosemide

Therapeutic Category Antihypertensive Agent; Diuretic, Loop

Generic Availability (US) Yes

Use Management of edema associated with heart failure and hepatic or renal disease; used alone or in combination with antihypertensives in treatment of hypertension

Pregnancy Risk Factor C

Pregnancy Considerations Adverse events have been observed in animal reproduction studies. Furosemide crosses the placenta (Riva 1978). Furosemide has been used to treat heart failure in pregnant women (ESC 2011; Johnson-Coyle 2012). Monitor fetal growth if used during pregnancy; may increase birth weight.

Breast-Feeding Considerations Furosemide is excreted into breast milk; maternal use may suppress lactation. The U.S. manufacturer recommends that caution be used if administered to a nursing woman. Canadian labeling contraindicates use while breast-feeding.

Contraindications Hypersensitivity to furosemide or any component of the formulation; anuria

Canadian labeling: Additional contraindications (not in U.S. labeling): Hypersensitivity to sulfonamide-derived drugs; complete renal shutdown; hepatic coma and precoma; uncorrected states of electrolyte depletion, hypovolemia, or hypotension; jaundiced newborn infants or infants with disease(s) capable of causing hyperbilirubinemia and possibly kernicterus; breast-feeding. **Note:** Manufacturer labeling for Lasix® Special and Furosemide Special Injection also includes: GFR <5 mL/minute or GFR >20 mL/minute; hepatic cirrhosis; renal failure accompanied by hepatic coma and precoma; renal failure due to poisoning with nephrotoxic or hepatotoxic substances.

Warnings/Precautions [U.S. Boxed Warning]: If given in excessive amounts, furosemide, similar to other loop diuretics, can lead to profound diuresis, resulting in fluid and electrolyte depletion; close medical supervision and dose evaluation are required. Watch for and correct electrolyte disturbances; adjust dose to avoid dehydration. When electrolyte depletion is present, therapy should not be initiated unless serum electrolytes, especially potassium, are normalized. In cirrhosis, avoid electrolyte and acid/base imbalances that might lead to hepatic encephalopathy; correct electrolyte and acid/base imbalances prior to initiation when hepatic coma is present. In contrast to thiazide diuretics, a loop diuretic can also lower serum calcium concentrations. Electrolyte disturbances can predispose a patient to serious cardiac arrhythmias. Coadministration of antihypertensives may increase the risk of hypotension.

Monitor fluid status and renal function in an attempt to prevent oliguria, azotemia, and reversible increases in BUN and creatinine; close medical supervision of aggressive diuresis is required. May increase risk of contrast-induced nephropathy. Diuretic resistance may occur in some patients, despite higher doses of loop diuretic treatment. Diuretic resistance can usually be overcome by intravenous administration, the use of two diuretics together (eg, furosemide and chlorothiazide), or the use of a diuretic with a positive inotropic agent. Rapid IV administration, renal impairment, excessive doses, hypoproteinemia, and concurrent use of other ototoxins is associated with ototoxicity. Asymptomatic hyperuricemia has been reported with use; rarely, gout may precipitate. Photosensitization may occur.

Use with caution in patients with prediabetes or diabetes mellitus; may see a change in glucose control. Use with caution in patients with systemic lupus erythematosus (SLE); may cause SLE exacerbation or activation. Use with caution in patients with prostatic hyperplasia/urinary stricture; may cause urinary retention. May lead to nephrocalcinosis or nephrolithiasis in premature infants or in children <4 years of age with chronic use. May prevent closure of patent ductus arteriosus in premature infants. Chemical similarities are present among sulfonamides, sulfonylureas, carbonic anhydrase inhibitors, thiazides, and loop diuretics (except ethacrynic acid). A risk of cross-reaction exists in patients with allergy to any of these compounds; avoid use when previous reaction has been severe. Discontinue if signs of hypersensitivity are noted. Some dosage forms may contain propylene glycol; large amounts are potentially toxic and have been associated hyperosmolality, lactic acidosis, seizures, and respiratory depression; use caution. If given the morning of surgery, furosemide may render the patient volume depleted and blood pressure may be labile during general anesthesia.

Adverse Reactions

Cardiovascular: Acute hypotension, chronic aortitis, necrotizing angiitis, orthostatic hypotension, vasculitis

Central nervous system: Dizziness, fever, headache, hepatic encephalopathy, lightheadedness, restlessness, vertigo

Dermatologic: Bullous pemphigoid, cutaneous vasculitis, drug rash with eosinophilia and systemic symptoms (DRESS), erythema multiforme, exanthematous pustulosis (generalized), exfoliative dermatitis, photosensitivity, pruritus, purpura, rash, Stevens-Johnson syndrome, toxic epidermal necrolysis, urticaria

Endocrine & metabolic: Cholesterol and triglycerides increased, glucose tolerance test altered, gout, hyperglycemia, hyperuricemia, hypocalcemia, hypochloremia, hypokalemia, hypomagnesemia, hyponatremia, metabolic alkalosis

Gastrointestinal: Anorexia, constipation, cramping, diarrhea, nausea, oral and gastric irritation, pancreatitis, vomiting

Genitourinary: Urinary bladder spasm, urinary frequency

Hematological: Agranulocytosis (rare), anemia, aplastic anemia (rare), eosinophilia, hemolytic anemia, leukopenia, thrombocytopenia

Hepatic: Intrahepatic cholestatic jaundice, ischemic hepatitis, liver enzymes increased

Local: Injection site pain (following IM injection), thrombophlebitis

Neuromuscular & skeletal: Muscle spasm, paresthesia, weakness

Ocular: Blurred vision, xanthopsia

Otic: Hearing impairment (reversible or permanent with rapid IV or IM administration), tinnitus

Renal: Allergic interstitial nephritis, fall in glomerular filtration rate and renal blood flow (due to overdiuresis), glycosuria, transient rise in BUN

Miscellaneous: Anaphylaxis (rare), exacerbate or activate systemic lupus erythematosus

Drug Interactions

Metabolism/Transport Effects Substrate of OAT3

Avoid Concomitant Use

Avoid concomitant use of Furosemide with any of the following: Chloral Hydrate; Ethacrynic Acid; Mecamylamine

Increased Effect/Toxicity

Furosemide may increase the levels/effects of: ACE Inhibitors; Allopurinol; Amifostine; Aminoglycosides; Antihypertensives; Cardiac Glycosides; Chloral Hydrate; CISplatin; Dofetilide; DULoxetine; Ethacrynic Acid; Foscarnet; Hypotensive Agents; Ivabradine; Levodopa; Lithium; Mecamylamine; Methotrexate; Neuromuscular-Blocking Agents; Obinutuzumab; RisperiDONE; RiTUXimab; Salicylates; Sodium Phosphates; Topiramate

The levels/effects of Furosemide may be increased by: Alfuzosin; Analgesics (Opioid); Barbiturates; Beta2-Agonists; Brimonidine (Topical); Canagliflozin; Corticosteroids (Orally Inhaled); Corticosteroids (Systemic); CycloSPORINE (Systemic); Diazoxide; Herbs (Hypotensive Properties); Licorice; MAO Inhibitors; Methotrexate; Nicorandil; Pentoxifylline; Phosphodiesterase 5 Inhibitors; Probenecid; Prostacyclin Analogues; Teriflunomide

Decreased Effect

Furosemide may decrease the levels/effects of: Antidiabetic Agents; Lithium; Neuromuscular-Blocking Agents

The levels/effects of Furosemide may be decreased by: Aliskiren; Bile Acid Sequestrants; Fosphenytoin; Herbs (Hypertensive Properties); Methotrexate; Methylphenidate; Nonsteroidal Anti-Inflammatory Agents; Phenytoin; Probenecid; Salicylates; Sucralfate; Yohimbine

Food Interactions Furosemide serum levels may be decreased if taken with food. Management: Administer on an empty stomach.

Storage/Stability

Injection: Store at room temperature of 15°C to 30°C (59°F to 86°F). Protect from light. Exposure to light may cause discoloration; do not use furosemide solutions if they have a yellow color. Furosemide solutions are unstable in acidic media, but very stable in basic media. Refrigeration may result in precipitation or crystallization; however, resolubilization at room temperature or warming may be performed without affecting the drug's stability. Infusion solution is stable for 24 hours at room temperature.

Tablet: Store at 25°C (77°F); excursions permitted to 15°C to 30°C (59°F to 89°F). Protect from light.

Mechanism of Action Inhibits reabsorption of sodium and chloride in the ascending loop of Henle and distal renal tubule, interfering with the chloride-binding cotransport system, thus causing increased excretion of water, sodium, chloride, magnesium, and calcium

Pharmacodynamics

Onset of action:
- Oral: Within 30-60 minutes
- IM: 30 minutes
- IV: 5 minutes

Maximum effect: Oral: Within 1-2 hours

Duration:
Oral: 6-8 hours
IV: 2 hours

Pharmacokinetics (Adult data unless noted)

Absorption: 65% in patients with normal renal function, decreases to 45% in patients with renal failure
Protein binding: 98%
Half-life: Adults:
Normal renal function: 30 minutes
Renal failure: 9 hours
Elimination: 50% of oral dose and 80% of IV dose excreted unchanged in the urine within 24 hours; the remainder is eliminated by other nonrenal pathways including liver metabolism and excretion of unchanged drug in feces

Dosing: Neonatal Note: Oral and parenteral (IV, IM) doses are not interchangeable; due to differences in bioavailability, oral doses are typically higher than IV.

Edema:
Oral: Doses of 1 mg/kg/dose 1 to 2 times/day have been used
IM, IV: **Note:** Significant absorption within ECMO circuit; avoid administration directly into circuit; high doses may be required for adequate diuretic effect (Buck 2003):
GA <31 weeks: 1 mg/kg/dose every 24 hours; accumulation and increased risk of toxicity may be observed with doses >2 mg/kg or doses of 1 mg/kg given more frequently than every 24 hours (Mirochnick 1988)
GA ≥31 weeks: 1 to 2 mg/kg/dose every 12 to 24 hours
Continuous IV infusion: 0.2 mg/kg/**hour**, increase in 0.1 mg/kg/**hour** increments every 12 to 24 hours to a maximum infusion rate of 0.4 mg/kg/**hour** (Luciani 1997; Schoemaker 2002)

Pulmonary edema: Inhalation: 1 to 2 mg/kg/dose diluted in 2 mL NS as a single dose (Brion 2009)

Dosing: Usual Note: Dose equivalency for adult patients with normal renal function (approximate): Furosemide 40 mg = bumetanide 1 mg = torsemide 20 mg = ethacrynic acid 50 mg

Infants and Children: **Note:** Oral and parenteral (IV, IM) doses are not interchangeable; due to differences in bioavailability, oral doses are typically higher than IV.

Edema:
Oral: 2 mg/kg once daily; if ineffective, may increase in increments of 1 to 2 mg/kg/dose every 6 to 8 hours; not to exceed 6 mg/kg/dose. In most cases, it is not necessary to exceed individual doses of 4 mg/kg or a dosing frequency of once or twice daily
IM, IV: 1 to 2 mg/kg/dose every 6 to 12 hours
Continuous IV infusion: 0.05 mg/kg/**hour**; titrate dosage to clinical effect

Adults:

Edema, heart failure:
Oral: Initial: 20 to 80 mg/dose with the same dose repeated or increased in increments of 20 to 40 mg/dose at intervals of 6 to 8 hours; usual maintenance dose interval is once or twice daily; may be titrated up to 600 mg/day with severe edematous states. **Note:** May also be given on 2 to 4 consecutive days every week
IM, IV: 20 to 40 mg/dose; repeat in 1 to 2 hours as needed and increase by 20 mg/dose until the desired effect has been obtained; usual dosing interval: 6 to 12 hours
Continuous IV infusion: Initial IV bolus dose of 20 to 40 mg over 1 to 2 minutes, followed by continuous IV infusion doses of 10 to 40 mg/**hour**. If urine output is <1 mL/kg/**hour**, increase as necessary to a maximum of 80 to 160 mg/**hour**. The risk associated with higher infusion rates (80 to 160 mg/**hour**) must be weighed against alternative strategies. **Note:** ACC/AHA 2005 guidelines for chronic HF recommend 40 mg IV dose followed by 10 to 40 mg/**hour** infusion.

Acute pulmonary edema: IV: 40 mg over 1 to 2 minutes; if response not adequate within 1 hour, may increase dose to 80 mg; **Note:** ACC/AHA 2005 guidelines for chronic HF recommend a maximum single dose of 160 to 200 mg.

Hypertension, resistant (JNC 7): Oral: 20 to 80 mg/day in 2 divided doses

Refractory CHF: Oral, IV: Doses up to 8 g/day have been used

Dosing adjustment in renal impairment: Adults: Acute renal failure: High doses (up to 1 to 3 g/day - oral/IV) have been used to initiate desired response; avoid use in oliguric states

Dialysis: Not removed by hemo- or peritoneal dialysis; supplemental dose is not necessary

Dosing adjustment in hepatic disease: Diminished natriuretic effect with increased sensitivity to hypokalemia and volume depletion in cirrhosis; monitor effects, particularly with high doses

Usual Infusion Concentrations: Neonatal IV infusion: 2 mg/mL **or** undiluted as 10 mg/mL

Usual Infusion Concentrations: Pediatric IV infusion: 1 mg/mL **or** 2 mg/mL **or** undiluted as 10 mg/mL

Preparation for Administration Parenteral: IV: May be further diluted in NS or D_5W to a concentration of 1 to 2 mg/mL for IV infusion; maximum concentration: 10 mg/mL. ISMP and Vermont Oxford Network recommend a standard concentration of 2 or 10 mg/mL for neonates (ISMP 2011).

Administration

Oral: May administer with food or milk to decrease GI distress

Parenteral: IV: May be administered undiluted direct IV at a maximum rate of 0.5 mg/kg/minute (not to exceed 4 mg/minute); may also be diluted and infused over 10 to 15 minutes (following maximum rate as above); in adults, 20 to 40 mg undiluted solution may be administered over 1 to 2 minutes

Monitoring Parameters Serum electrolytes, renal function, blood pressure, hearing (if high dosages used)

Additional Information Single dose studies utilizing nebulized furosemide at 1-2 mg/kg/dose (diluted to a final volume of 2 mL with NS) have been shown to be effective in improving pulmonary function in preterm infants with bronchopulmonary dysplasia undergoing mechanical ventilation; no diuresis or systemic side effects were noted

Dosage Forms Excipient information presented when available (limited, particularly for generics); consult specific product labeling.

Solution, Injection:
Generic: 10 mg/mL (2 mL, 4 mL, 10 mL)
Solution, Injection [preservative free]:
Generic: 10 mg/mL (2 mL, 4 mL, 10 mL)
Solution, Oral:
Generic: 8 mg/mL (5 mL, 500 mL); 10 mg/mL (60 mL, 120 mL)
Tablet, Oral:
Lasix: 20 mg
Lasix: 40 mg, 80 mg [scored]
Generic: 20 mg, 40 mg, 80 mg

- ◆ **Furosemide Injection Sandoz Standard (Can)** *see* Furosemide *on page 951*
- ◆ **Furosemide Injection, USP (Can)** *see* Furosemide *on page 951*
- ◆ **Furosemide Special (Can)** *see* Furosemide *on page 951*
- ◆ **Furosemide Special Injection (Can)** *see* Furosemide *on page 951*
- ◆ **Fusilev** *see* LEVOleucovorin *on page 1248*
- ◆ **Fuzeon** *see* Enfuvirtide *on page 750*

- ◆ **FVIII/vWF** *see* Antihemophilic Factor/von Willebrand Factor Complex (Human) *on page 173*
- ◆ **FXT 40 (Can)** *see* FLUoxetine *on page 906*
- ◆ **Fycompa** *see* Perampanel *on page 1674*
- ◆ **GAA** *see* Alglucosidase Alfa *on page 94*

Gabapentin (GA ba pen tin)

Medication Safety Issues

Sound-alike/look-alike issues:

Neurontin may be confused with Motrin, Neoral, nitrofurantoin, Noroxin [DSC], Zarontin

Related Information

Oral Medications That Should Not Be Crushed or Altered *on page 2476*

Brand Names: US Fanatrex FusePaq; Gralise; Gralise Starter; Neurontin

Brand Names: Canada Apo-Gabapentin; Auro-Gabapentin; CO Gabapentin; Dom-Gabapentin; Gabapentin Tablets USP; GD-Gabapentin; JAMP-Gabapentin; Mylan-Gabapentin; Neurontin; PHL-Gabapentin; PMS-Gabapentin; PRO-Gabapentin; RAN-Gabapentin; ratio-Gabapentin; Riva-Gabapentin; Teva-Gabapentin

Therapeutic Category Anticonvulsant, Miscellaneous

Generic Availability (US) May be product dependent

Use Adjunct for treatment of partial seizures with or without secondary generalized seizures (Neurontin: FDA approved in ages ≥3 years and adults); management of post-herpetic neuralgia (Gralise, Neurontin: FDA approved in adults); has also been used as adjunct in the treatment of neuropathic pain

Medication Guide Available Yes

Pregnancy Risk Factor C

Pregnancy Considerations Adverse events have been observed in animal reproduction studies. Gabapentin crosses the placenta. In a small study (n=6), the umbilical/maternal plasma concentration ratio was ~1.74. Neonatal concentrations declined quickly after delivery and at 24 hours of life were ~27% of the cord blood concentrations at birth (gabapentin neonatal half-life ~14 hours) (Ohman, 2005). Outcome data following maternal use of gabapentin during pregnancy is limited (Holmes, 2012).

Patients exposed to gabapentin during pregnancy are encouraged to enroll in the North American Antiepileptic Drug (NAAED) Pregnancy Registry by calling 1-888-233-2334. Additional information is available at www.aedpregnancyregistry.org.

Breast-Feeding Considerations Gabapentin is excreted in human breast milk. Per the manufacturer, a nursed infant could be exposed to ~1 mg/kg/day of gabapentin; the effect on the child is not known. Use in breast-feeding women only if the benefits to the mother outweigh the potential risk to the infant.

In a small study of breast-feeding women (n=6), the estimated exposure of gabapentin to the nursing infants was ~1% to 4% of the weight-adjusted maternal dose (sampling occurred from 12-97 days after delivery and maternal doses ranged from 600-2100 mg daily). Gabapentin was detected in the serum of 2 nursing infants 2-3 weeks after delivery and in 1 infant after 3 months of breast-feeding. Serum concentrations were <12% of the maternal plasma concentrations and <5% of those measured in the umbilical cord. Adverse events were not reported in the breast-fed infants (Ohman, 2005).

Contraindications Hypersensitivity to gabapentin or any component of the formulation

Warnings/Precautions Antiepileptics are associated with an increased risk of suicidal behavior/thoughts with use (regardless of indication); patients should be monitored for signs/symptoms of depression, suicidal tendencies, and other unusual behavior changes during therapy and instructed to inform their healthcare provider immediately if symptoms occur. Avoid abrupt withdrawal, may precipitate seizures; Gralise should be withdrawn over ≥1 week. Use cautiously in patients with severe renal dysfunction; male rat studies demonstrated an association with pancreatic adenocarcinoma (clinical implication unknown). May cause CNS depression including somnolence and dizziness, which may impair physical or mental abilities. Patients must be cautioned about performing tasks which require mental alertness (eg, operating machinery or driving). Pediatric patients have shown increased incidence of CNS-related adverse effects, including emotional lability, hostility, changes in behavior and thinking, and hyperkinesia. Gabapentin immediate release and Gralise products are not interchangeable with each other **or** with gabapentin enacarbil (Horizant). The safety and efficacy of Gralise has not been studied in patients with epilepsy. Potentially serious, sometimes fatal multiorgan hypersensitivity (also known as drug reaction with eosinophilia and systemic symptoms [DRESS]) has been reported with some antiepileptic drugs, including gabapentin; may affect lymphatic, hepatic, renal, cardiac, and/or hematologic systems; fever, rash, and eosinophilia may also be present. Discontinue immediately if suspected.

Warnings: Additional Pediatric Considerations Neuropsychiatric adverse events, such as emotional lability (eg, behavioral problems), hostility, aggressive behaviors, thought disorders (eg, problems with concentration and school performance), and hyperkinesia (eg, hyperactivity and restlessness), have been reported in clinical trials of pediatric patients ages 3 to 12 years. Most of these pediatric neuropsychiatric adverse events are mild to moderate in terms of intensity but discontinuation of gabapentin may be required; children with mental retardation and attention-deficit disorders may be at increased risk for behavioral side effects (Lee 1996).

Adverse Reactions

Cardiovascular: Peripheral edema, vasodilatation

Central nervous system: Abnormal gait, abnormality in thinking, amnesia, ataxia, depression, dizziness (more common in adults), drowsiness (more common in adults), emotional lability (children), fatigue (more common in adults), headache, hostility (children), hyperesthesia, hyperkinesia (children), lethargy, nervousness, pain, tremor, twitching, vertigo

Dermatologic: Pruritus, skin rash

Endocrine & metabolic: Hyperglycemia, weight gain

Gastrointestinal: Abdominal pain, constipation, dental disease, diarrhea, dry throat, dyspepsia, flatulence, increased appetite, nausea and vomiting (more common in children), xerostomia

Genitourinary: Impotence, urinary tract infection

Hematologic & oncologic: Decreased white blood cell count, leukopenia

Infection: Infection, viral infection (children)

Neuromuscular & skeletal: Back pain, bone fracture, dysarthria, limb pain, myalgia, weakness

Ophthalmic: Blurred vision, conjunctivitis, diplopia, nystagmus

Otic: Otitis media

Respiratory: Bronchitis (children), cough, nasopharyngitis, pharyngitis, respiratory tract infection (children), rhinitis

Miscellaneous: Fever (children)

Rare but important or life-threatening: Acute renal failure, altered serum glucose, anemia, angina pectoris, angioedema, aphasia, aspiration pneumonia, blindness, blood coagulation disorder, bradycardia, brain disease, breast hypertrophy, cardiac arrhythmia (various), cardiac failure, cerebrovascular accident, CNS neoplasm, colitis, confusion, Cushingoid appearance, DRESS syndrome, drug abuse, drug dependence, erythema multiforme, facial paralysis, fecal incontinence, gastroenteritis, glaucoma, glycosuria, hearing loss, heart block, hematemesis, hematuria, hemiplegia, hemorrhage, hepatitis, hepatomegaly, herpes zoster, hyperlipidemia, hypertension, hyperthyroidism, hyperventilation, hyponatremia, hypotension, hypothyroidism, hypoventilation, increased creatine phosphokinase, increased liver enzymes, increased serum creatinine, jaundice, joint swelling, leukocytosis, lymphadenopathy, lymphocytosis, memory impairment, meningism, migraine, movement disorder, myocardial infarction, myoclonus (local), nephrolithiasis, nephrosis, nerve palsy, non-Hodgkin's lymphoma, ovarian failure, pancreatitis, peptic ulcer, pericardial effusion, pericardial rub, pericarditis, peripheral vascular disease, pneumonia, psychosis, pulmonary thromboembolism, purpura, retinopathy, rhabdomyolysis, seasonal allergy, skin necrosis, status epilepticus, Stevens-Johnson syndrome, subdural hematoma, suicidal ideation, suicidal tendencies, syncope, tachycardia, thrombocytopenia, thrombophlebitis, tumor growth, withdrawal syndrome

Drug Interactions

Metabolism/Transport Effects None known.

Avoid Concomitant Use

Avoid concomitant use of Gabapentin with any of the following: Azelastine (Nasal); Orphenadrine; Paraldehyde; Thalidomide

Increased Effect/Toxicity

Gabapentin may increase the levels/effects of: Alcohol (Ethyl); Azelastine (Nasal); Buprenorphine; CNS Depressants; Hydrocodone; Methotrimeprazine; Metyrosine; Mirtazapine; Orphenadrine; Paraldehyde; Pramipexole; ROPINIRole; Rotigotine; Selective Serotonin Reuptake Inhibitors; Suvorexant; Thalidomide; Zolpidem

The levels/effects of Gabapentin may be increased by: Brimonidine (Topical); Cannabis; Doxylamine; Dronabinol; Droperidol; HydrOXYzine; Kava Kava; Magnesium Salts; Methotrimeprazine; Nabilone; Perampanel; Rufinamide; Sodium Oxybate; Tapentadol; Tetrahydrocannabinol

Decreased Effect

The levels/effects of Gabapentin may be decreased by: Antacids; Magnesium Salts; Mefloquine; Mianserin; Orlistat

Food Interactions Tablet, solution (immediate release): No significant effect on rate or extent of absorption; tablet (Gralise): Increases rate and extent of absorption. Management: Administer immediate release products without regard to food. Administer Gralise with food.

Storage/Stability

Capsules and tablets: Store at 25°C (77°F); excursions permitted to 15°C to 30°C (59°F to 86°F). Use scored 600 or 800 mg tablets that are broken in half within 28 days of breaking the tablet.

Oral solution: Store refrigerated at 2°C to 8°C (36°F to 46°F).

Mechanism of Action Gabapentin is structurally related to GABA. However, it does not bind to $GABA_A$ or $GABA_B$ receptors, and it does not appear to influence synthesis or uptake of GABA. High affinity gabapentin binding sites have been located throughout the brain; these sites correspond to the presence of voltage-gated calcium channels specifically possessing the alpha-2-delta-1 subunit. This channel appears to be located presynaptically, and may modulate the release of excitatory neurotransmitters which participate in epileptogenesis and nociception.

Pharmacokinetics (Adult data unless noted)

Absorption: Variable, from proximal small bowel by L-amino transport system; saturable process; dose-dependent

Distribution: V_d: 58 ± 6 L; CSF concentrations are ~20% of plasma concentrations

Protein binding: <3% (not clinically significant)

Metabolism: Not metabolized

Bioavailability:

Immediate release: ~60% (300 mg dose given 3 times/day); bioavailability decreases with increasing doses; bioavailability is 27% with 1600 mg dose given 3 times/day

Extended release: Variable; increased with higher fat content meal

Time to peak serum concentration:

Immediate release:

Infants 1 month to Children 12 years: 2 to 3 hours

Adults: 2 to 4 hours

Extended release: 8 hours

Half-life, elimination:

Infants 1 month to Children 12 years: 4.7 hours

Adults, normal: 5 to 7 hours; increased half-life with decreased renal function; anuric adult patients: 132 hours; adults during hemodialysis: 3.8 hours

Elimination: Urine (as unchanged drug)

Clearance: Apparent oral clearance is directly proportional to CrCl: Clearance in infants is highly variable; oral clearance (per kg) in children <5 years of age is higher than in children ≥5 years of age

Dosing: Usual Note: Do not exceed 12 hours between doses with 3 times daily dosing:

Pediatric:

Seizures, partial onset; adjunctive therapy: Oral: Immediate release: **Note:** If gabapentin is discontinued or if another anticonvulsant is added to therapy, it should be done slowly over a minimum of 1 week.

Children 3 to <12 years:

Initial: 10 to 15 mg/kg/**day** divided into 3 doses daily; titrate dose upward over ~3 days

Maintenance usual dose:

Children 3 to 4 years: 40 mg/kg/**day** divided into 3 doses daily; maximum daily dose: In one long-term study, doses up to 50 mg/kg/**day** were well-tolerated

Children 5 to <12 years: 25 to 35 mg/kg/**day** divided into 3 doses daily; maximum daily dose: In one long-term study, doses up to 50 mg/kg/**day** were well-tolerated

Children ≥12 years and Adolescents: Initial: 300 mg 3 times daily; titrate dose upward if needed; usual maintenance dose: 900 to 1,800 mg/day divided into 3 doses daily; doses up to 2,400 mg/day divided into 3 doses daily are well tolerated long-term; maximum daily dose: Doses up to 3,600 mg/**day** have been tolerated in short-term studies.

Neuropathic pain: Limited data available: Oral: Immediate release: Children and Adolescents: Initial: 5 mg/kg/dose up to 300 mg at bedtime; day 2: Increase to 5 mg/kg/dose twice daily (up to 300 mg twice daily); day 3: Increase to 5 mg/kg/dose 3 times daily (up to 300 mg 3 times daily); further titrate with dosage increases (not frequency) to effect; American Pain Society (APS) recommends a lower initial dose of 2 mg/kg/**day** which may be considered if concurrent analgesics are also sedating; usual dosage range: 8 to 35 mg/kg/**day** divided into 3 doses daily (APS, 2008; Galloway, 2000); maximum daily dose: 3,600 mg/**day**

Adult:

Seizures, partial onset: Oral: Immediate release:

Initial: 300 mg 3 times daily, if necessary the dose may be gradually increased up to 1,800 mg/**day**

Maintenance: 900 to 1,800 mg/**day** administered in 3 divided doses; doses of up to 2,400 mg/**day** have been tolerated in long-term clinical studies; doses up to 3,600 mg/**day** have been tolerated in short-term studies

Note: If gabapentin is discontinued or if another anticonvulsant is added to therapy, it should be done slowly over a minimum of 1 week.

Post-herpetic neuralgia: Oral:

Immediate release: Day 1: 300 mg once; Day 2: 300 mg twice daily; Day 3: 300 mg 3 times daily; titrate dose as needed for pain relief (range: 1,800 to 3,600 mg/**day** in divided doses; doses >1,800 mg/**day** do not generally show greater benefit)

Extended release (Gralise): Day 1: 300 mg once, Day 2: 600 mg once, Days 3 to 6: 900 mg once daily, Days 7 to 10: 1,200 mg once daily, Days 11 to 14: 1,500 mg once daily, Days ≥15: 1,800 mg once daily

Dosing adjustment in renal impairment:

Immediate release:

Children <12 years: There are no dosing adjustments provided in the manufacturer's labeling (has not been studied).

Children ≥12 years, Adolescents, and Adults: See table.

Gabapentin Dosing Adjustments in Renal Impairment

Creatinine Clearance (mL/min)	Total Daily Dose Range (mg/day)	Dosage Regimens (Maintenance Doses) (mg)				
≥60	900 to 3,600	300 3 times/day	400 3 times/day	600 3 times/day	800 3 times/day	1200 tid
>30 to 59	400 to 1,400	200 twice daily	300 twice daily	400 twice daily	500 twice daily	700 twice daily
>15 to 29	200 to 700	200 daily	300 daily	400 daily	500 daily	700 daily
15[1]	100 to 300	100 daily	125 daily	150 daily	200 daily	300 daily
Hemodialysis[2]		Posthemodialysis Supplemental Dose				
		125 mg	150 mg	200 mg	250 mg	350 mg

[1]CrCl <15 mL/minute: Reduce daily dose in proportion to creatinine clearance.

[2]Supplemental dose should be administered after each 4 hours of hemodialysis (patients on hemodialysis should also receive maintenance doses based on renal function as listed in the upper portion of the table).

Extended release (Gralise): **Note:** Follow initial dose titration schedule if treatment-naive.

CrCl ≥60 mL/minute: 1,800 mg once daily

CrCl >30 to 59 mL/minute: 600 to 1,800 mg once daily; dependent on tolerability and clinical response

CrCl <30 mL/minute: Use is not recommended.

ESRD requiring hemodialysis: Use is not recommended.

Dosing adjustment in hepatic impairment: There are no dosage adjustments provided in the manufacturer's labeling; however, adjustment not necessary since gabapentin is not hepatically metabolized.

Administration

Immediate release: Capsule, tablet, oral solution: May consider administration of first dose on first day at bedtime to avoid somnolence and dizziness. May be administered without regard to meals; administration with meals may decrease adverse GI effects. Dose may be administered as combination of dosage forms; do not administer within 2 hours of magnesium- or aluminum-containing antacids. When given 3 times daily, the maximum time between doses should not exceed 12 hours. Capsule should be administered with plenty of water to ensure complete swallowing. Although the manufacturer recommends swallowing capsules whole, some centers have opened the capsules and mixed the contents in drinks (eg, orange juice) or food (eg, applesauce) when necessary (Gidal 1998; Khurana 1996). The 600 mg and 800 mg tablets are scored and may be split if a half-tablet is needed; manufacturer recommends that half tablets not used within 28 days of breaking the scored tablets should be discarded.

Extended release (Gralise): Tablet: Take once daily with evening meal. Swallow whole; do not chew, crush, or split.

Monitoring Parameters Seizure frequency and duration; renal function; weight; behavior in children; signs and symptoms of suicidality (eg, anxiety, depression, behavior changes)

Reference Range Routine monitoring of drug levels is not required; a specific target serum concentration range for antiseizure response has not been established (Lindberger 2003); a minimum effective serum concentration may be 2 mcg/mL (Krasowski 2010)

Test Interactions False positives have been reported with the Ames N-Multistix SG® dipstick test for urine protein

Additional Information Gabapentin is not effective for absence seizures; gabapentin does not induce liver enzymes

Dosage Forms Excipient information presented when available (limited, particularly for generics); consult specific product labeling.

Capsule, Oral:

Neurontin: 100 mg, 300 mg, 400 mg

Generic: 100 mg, 300 mg, 400 mg

Miscellaneous, Oral:

Gralise Starter: 300 & 600 mg (78 ea) [contains soybean lecithin]

Solution, Oral:

Neurontin: 250 mg/5 mL (470 mL) [strawberry anise flavor]

Generic: 250 mg/5 mL (5 mL, 6 mL, 470 mL, 473 mL)

Suspension, Oral:

Fanatrex FusePaq: 25 mg/mL (420 mL) [contains saccharin sodium, sodium benzoate]

Tablet, Oral:

Gralise: 300 mg [contains soybean lecithin]

Gralise: 600 mg

Neurontin: 600 mg, 800 mg [scored]

Generic: 600 mg, 800 mg

Extemporaneous Preparations Note: Commercial oral solution is available (50 mg/mL)

A 100 mg/mL suspension may be made with tablets (immediate release) and either a 1:1 mixture of Ora-Sweet® (100 mL) and Ora-Plus® (100 mL) or 1:1 mixture of methylcellulose 1% (100 mL) and Simple Syrup N.F. (100 mL). Crush sixty-seven 300 mg tablets in a mortar and reduce to a fine powder. Add small portions of the chosen vehicle and mix to a uniform paste; mix while adding the vehicle in incremental proportions to **almost** 200 mL; transfer to a calibrated bottle, rinse mortar with vehicle, and add sufficient quantity of vehicle to make 200 mL. Label "shake well" and "refrigerate". Stable for 91 days refrigerated (preferred) or 56 days at room temperature.

Nahata MC, Pai VB, and Hipple TF, *Pediatric Drug Formulations*, 5th ed, Cincinnati, OH: Harvey Whitney Books Co, 2004.

◆ **Gabapentin Tablets USP (Can)** *see* Gabapentin *on page 954*

◆ **Gabitril** *see* TiaGABine *on page 2060*

◆ **Gablofen** *see* Baclofen *on page 254*

Galsulfase (gal SUL fase)

Brand Names: US Naglazyme

Therapeutic Category Enzyme

Generic Availability (US) No

Use Treatment of mucopolysaccharidosis VI (MPS VI, Maroteaux-Lamy Syndrome) for improvement of walking and stair-climbing capacity [FDA approved in pediatric patients (age not specified) and adults ≤29 years]

Pregnancy Risk Factor B

Pregnancy Considerations Fetal harm was not reported in animal studies. There are no studies in pregnant women. Pregnant women are encouraged to enroll in the Clinical Surveillance Program.

Breast-Feeding Considerations

Breast-feeding women are encouraged to enroll in the Clinical Surveillance Program.

Contraindications

There are no contraindications listed within the manufacturer's approved labeling

Warnings/Precautions Severe hypersensitivity reactions, including anaphylactic reactions and anaphylactic shock have been reported during and within 24 hours after infusion; immediate treatment for hypersensitivity reactions should be available during administration. Discontinue treatment immediately if signs or symptoms occur; use caution with readministration. Patients should be premedicated with antihistamines and/or antipyretics prior to infusion. Infusion-related reactions have been reported; may be sporadic and/or severe; reactions may occur as late as week 146 of treatment. In case of reaction, decrease the rate of infusion, temporarily discontinue the infusion, and/or administer additional antipyretics/antihistamines and possibly corticosteroids. Evaluate airway prior to therapy (due to possible effects of antihistamine use). Severe immune-mediated reactions (eg, membranous glomerulonephritis) have occurred; monitor patients closely and consider discontinuation of treatment if signs or symptoms occur; use caution with readministration. Use with caution in patients who are at risk of fluid overload (patients <20 kg, underlying respiratory disease, or compromised cardiopulmonary function); may cause heart failure. Monitor patients closely. Use with caution in patients with sleep apnea; antihistamine pretreatment may increase the risk of apneic episodes; apnea treatment options should be readily available. Worsening and new-onset spinal/cervical cord compression (SCC) has been reported. Monitor patients for signs and symptoms of SCC (eg, back pain, limb paralysis, urinary and fecal incontinence). Consider delaying treatment in patients with an acute febrile or respiratory illness. Some dosage forms may contain polysorbate 80 (also known as Tweens). Hypersensitivity reactions, usually a delayed reaction, have been reported following exposure to pharmaceutical products containing polysorbate 80 in certain individuals (Isaksson, 2002; Lucente 2000; Shelley, 1995). Thrombocytopenia, ascites, pulmonary deterioration, and renal and hepatic failure have been reported in premature neonates after receiving parenteral products containing polysorbate 80 (Alade, 1986; CDC, 1984). See manufacturer's labeling. Excess agitation of solution prior to or after dilution may denature galsulfase rendering it inactive. Studies did not include patients >29 years of age.

A Clinical Surveillance Program has been created to monitor therapeutic response, progression of disease and adverse effects during long-term treatment, as well as, effects on pregnant women, breast-feeding, and their offspring; patients should be encouraged to register. Registry information may be obtained at http://www.naglazyme.com/en/clinical-resources/surveillance-program.aspx or by calling 800-983-4587.

Adverse Reactions

Cardiovascular: Chest pain, hypertension

Central nervous system: Absent reflexes, chills, headache, malaise, pain

Dermatologic: Pruritus, skin rash, urticaria

Gastrointestinal: Abdominal pain, gastroenteritis, nausea, vomiting

Hypersensitivity: Angioedema

Neuromuscular & skeletal: Areflexia

Ophthalmic: Conjunctivitis, corneal opacity (increased)

Otic: Auditory impairment, otalgia

Respiratory: Apnea, dyspnea, laryngeal edema, nasal congestion, pharyngitis, respiratory distress

Miscellaneous: Antibody development, fever, infusion related reaction, umbilical hernia

Rare but important or life-threatening: Anaphylaxis, bradycardia, bronchospasm, cyanosis, erythema, hypotension, hypoxia, pallor, paresthesia, renal disease (membranous), respiratory failure, shock, spinal cord compression, tachycardia, tachypnea, thrombocytopenia

Drug Interactions

Metabolism/Transport Effects None known.

Avoid Concomitant Use There are no known interactions where it is recommended to avoid concomitant use.

Increased Effect/Toxicity There are no known significant interactions involving an increase in effect.

Decreased Effect There are no known significant interactions involving a decrease in effect.

Storage/Stability Prior to use, store vials under refrigeration, 2°C to 8°C (36°F to 46°F). Do not freeze or shake. Protect from light. Following dilution, use immediately. May store under refrigeration if used within 48 hours from the time of preparation to the completion of infusion. Do not store solution for infusion at room temperature. Allow vials to reach room temperature prior to dilution. Do not keep vials at room temperature >24 hours prior to dilution. Do not heat or microwave vials.

Mechanism of Action Galsulfase is a recombinant form of N-acetylgalactosamine 4-sulfatase, produced in Chinese hamster cells. A deficiency of this enzyme leads to accumulation of the glycosaminoglycan dermatan sulfate in various tissues, causing progressive disease which includes decreased growth, skeletal deformities, upper airway obstruction, clouding of the cornea, heart disease, and coarse facial features. Replacement of this enzyme has been shown to improve mobility and physical function (measured by walking and stair-climbing).

Pharmacokinetics (Adult data unless noted) Note: Data based on mixed patient population of children ≥5 years and adults <29 years.

Half-life elimination: Week 1: Median: 9 minutes (range: 6-21 minutes); Week 24: Median: 26 minutes (range: 8-40 minutes)

Dosing: Usual Note: Premedicate with antihistamines with or without antipyretics 30-60 minutes prior to infusion.

MPS VI:

Infants: Limited data available: I.V: 1 or 2 mg/kg/dose once weekly has been used in four infants (3-12 months); similar safety results to those of older patients were reported

Children, Adolescents, and Adults: IV: 1 mg/kg/dose once weekly

Preparation for Administration Parenteral: IV: Manufacturer recommends rounding dose to the nearest whole vial to prepare infusion. Dilute in NS to a final volume (including drug volume) of 250 mL; if patient weight <20 kg or susceptible to fluid overload dose maybe diluted in 100 mL. Slowly add galsulfase to infusion bag; compatibility in glass containers has not been studied. Gently rotate to distribute. Do not shake or agitate, do not use filter needle.

Administration Parenteral: IV: Infuse via an infusion pump and PVC infusion set with in-line, low-protein-binding 0.2 micrometer filter. Pretreatment with antihistamines with or without antipyretics is recommended 30 to 60 minutes prior to infusion. Infuse over at least 4 hours; infuse 250 mL solution at 6 mL/hour for the first hour; if well-tolerated, increase rate to 80 mL/hour for the remaining 3 hours. For 100 mL infusion, use a lower rate to ensure infusion over at least 4 hours. Infusion time may be extended up to 20 hours if infusion reactions occur. If hypersensitivity or infusion-related reaction occurs, discontinue immediately.

Monitoring Parameters Vital signs; presence of infusion-related reactions (chills, pruritis, urticaria, dyspnea, rash, shortness of breath, nausea, abdominal pain); in clinical studies, tests of mobility and physical function were monitored at baseline and every 6 weeks.

Additional Information In order to better understand MPS VI disease progression and to monitor long-term effects of galsulfase, a voluntary Clinical Surveillance Program has been established. Monitoring also includes the effect of galsulfase on pregnant women and their offspring, and during lactation. For more information, visit www.naglazyme.com/en/clinical-resources/surveillance-program.aspx or call (800) 983-4587.

Dosage Forms Excipient information presented when available (limited, particularly for generics); consult specific product labeling.

Solution, Intravenous [preservative free]:

Naglazyme: 1 mg/mL (5 mL) [contains mouse protein (murine) (hamster), polysorbate 80]

- ◆ **Galzin** *see* Zinc Acetate *on page 2212*
- ◆ **GamaSTAN S/D** *see* Immune Globulin *on page 1089*
- ◆ **Gamastan S/D (Can)** *see* Immune Globulin *on page 1089*
- ◆ **Gamma Benzene Hexachloride** *see* Lindane *on page 1267*
- ◆ **Gammagard** *see* Immune Globulin *on page 1089*
- ◆ **Gammagard Liquid (Can)** *see* Immune Globulin *on page 1089*
- ◆ **Gammagard S/D [DSC]** *see* Immune Globulin *on page 1089*
- ◆ **Gammagard S/D (Can)** *see* Immune Globulin *on page 1089*
- ◆ **Gammagard S/D Less IgA** *see* Immune Globulin *on page 1089*
- ◆ **Gamma Globulin** *see* Immune Globulin *on page 1089*
- ◆ **Gammaked** *see* Immune Globulin *on page 1089*
- ◆ **Gammaphos** *see* Amifostine *on page 115*
- ◆ **Gammaplex** *see* Immune Globulin *on page 1089*
- ◆ **Gamunex (Can)** *see* Immune Globulin *on page 1089*
- ◆ **Gamunex-C** *see* Immune Globulin *on page 1089*

Ganciclovir (Systemic) (gan SYE kloe veer)

Medication Safety Issues

Sound-alike/look-alike issues:

Cytovene® may be confused with Cytosar®, Cytosar-U

Ganciclovir may be confused with acyclovir

Related Information

Safe Handling of Hazardous Drugs *on page 2455*

Brand Names: US Cytovene

Brand Names: Canada Cytovene; Ganciclovir for Injection

Therapeutic Category Antiviral Agent, Parenteral

Generic Availability (US) Yes

Use Treatment of cytomegalovirus (CMV) retinitis in immunocompromised patients, including patients with AIDS (FDA approved in adults); prevention of CMV disease in transplant recipients at risk for CMV (FDA approved in adults); has also been used in CMV GI infections and pneumonitis; ganciclovir also has antiviral activity against herpes simplex virus types 1 and 2

Pregnancy Risk Factor C

Pregnancy Considerations [U.S. Boxed Warning]: Animal studies have demonstrated carcinogenic and teratogenic effects, and inhibition of spermatogenesis. Female patients should use effective contraception during therapy; male patients should use a barrier contraceptive during and for at least 90 days after therapy.

Breast-Feeding Considerations Due to the carcinogenic and teratogenic effects observed in animal studies, the possibility of adverse events in a nursing infant is considered likely. Therefore, nursing should be discontinued during therapy. In addition, the CDC recommends **not** to breast-feed if diagnosed with HIV to avoid postnatal transmission of the virus.

Contraindications Hypersensitivity to ganciclovir, acyclovir, or any component of the formulation

Warnings/Precautions Hazardous agent - use appropriate precautions for handling and disposal (NIOSH 2014 [group 2]).

[U.S. Boxed Warning]: Granulocytopenia (neutropenia), anemia, and thrombocytopenia may occur. Dosage adjustment or interruption of ganciclovir therapy may be necessary in patients with neutropenia and/or thrombocytopenia and patients with impaired renal function. **[U.S. Boxed Warning]: Animal studies have demonstrated carcinogenic and teratogenic effects, and inhibition of spermatogenesis;** contraceptive precautions for female and male patients need to be followed during and for at least 90 days after therapy with the drug; take care to administer only into veins with good blood flow. **[U.S. Boxed Warning]: Indicated only for treatment of CMV retinitis in the immunocompromised patient and CMV prevention in transplant patients at risk.**

Adverse Reactions

Central nervous system: Chills, fever, neuropathy

Dermatologic: Pruritus

Gastrointestinal: Anorexia, diarrhea, vomiting

Hematologic: Anemia, leukopenia, neutropenia with ANC <500/mm^3, thrombocytopenia

Ocular: Retinal detachment (relationship to ganciclovir not established)

Renal: Serum creatinine increased

Miscellaneous: Diaphoresis, sepsis

Rare but important or life-threatening: Allergic reaction (including anaphylaxis), alopecia, arrhythmia, bronchospasm, cardiac arrest, cataracts, cholestasis, coma, dyspnea, edema, encephalopathy, exfoliative dermatitis, extrapyramidal symptoms, hepatitis, hepatic failure, pancreatitis, pancytopenia, pulmonary fibrosis, psychosis, rhabdomyolysis, seizure, alopecia, urticaria, eosinophilia, hemorrhage, Stevens-Johnson syndrome, torsade de pointes, renal failure, SIADH, visual loss

Drug Interactions

Metabolism/Transport Effects None known.

Avoid Concomitant Use

Avoid concomitant use of Ganciclovir (Systemic) with any of the following: Imipenem

Increased Effect/Toxicity

Ganciclovir (Systemic) may increase the levels/effects of: Imipenem; Mycophenolate; Reverse Transcriptase Inhibitors (Nucleoside); Tenofovir

The levels/effects of Ganciclovir (Systemic) may be increased by: Mycophenolate; Probenecid; Tenofovir

Decreased Effect There are no known significant interactions involving a decrease in effect.

Storage/Stability Store intact vials at temperatures below 40°C (104°F). Reconstituted solution is stable for 12 hours at room temperature, however, conflicting data indicates that reconstituted solution is stable for 60 days under refrigeration (4°C). Stability of parenteral admixture at room temperature (25°C) and at refrigeration temperature (4°C) for 35 days has been reported. However, the manufacturer recommends use within 24 hours of preparation.

Mechanism of Action Ganciclovir is phosphorylated to a substrate which competitively inhibits the binding of deoxyguanosine triphosphate to DNA polymerase resulting in inhibition of viral DNA synthesis

Pharmacokinetics (Adult data unless noted)

Distribution: Distributes to most body fluids, tissues, and organs, including the eyes and brain

V_d:
Children 9 months to 12 years: 0.64 ± 0.22 L/kg
Adults: 0.74 ± 0.15 L/kg
Protein binding: 1% to 2%
Half-life (prolonged with impaired renal function):
Neonates 2-49 days of age: 2.4 hours
Children 9 months to 12 years: 2.4 ± 0.7 hours
Adults: Mean: 2.5-3.6 hours (range: 1.7-5.8 hours)
Elimination: Majority (80% to 99%) excreted as unchanged drug in the urine
Dialysis: 40% to 50% removed by a 4-hour hemodialysis

Dosing: Neonatal IV: **Congenital CMV (symptomatic; CNS-disease); treatment (independent of HIV status):** 6 mg/kg/dose every 12 hours for 6 weeks; if neonate diagnosed as HIV-positive, a longer duration of therapy may be considered (CDC, 2009; Redbook, 2009)

Dosing: Usual IV:

CMV infection:
Congenital CMV (symptomatic; CNS-disease); treatment (independent of HIV status): 6 mg/kg/dose every 12 hours for 6 weeks; if neonate diagnosed as HIV-positive a longer duration of therapy may be considered (CDC, 2009; Redbook, 2009)
CNS infection, treatment (HIV-exposed/-positive): Infants and Children: 5 mg/kg/dose every 12 hours plus foscarnet; continue until symptoms improve, followed by chronic suppression (CDC, 2009)
Disseminated disease and retinitis, treatment:
Induction therapy:
Infants ≥3 months and Children: 5 mg/kg/dose every 12 hours for 14-21 days; may be increased to 7.5 mg/kg/dose every 12 hours (CDC, 2009)
Adults: Manufacturer's labeling: 5 mg/kg/dose every 12 hours for 14-21 days
Maintenance therapy:
Infants ≥ 3 months and Children: 5 mg/kg/dose as a single daily dose for 5-7 days/week (CDC, 2009)
Adults: Manufacturer's labeling: 5 mg/kg/dose as a single daily dose for 7 days/week or 6 mg/kg/dose for 5 days/week
Secondary prevention in HIV-exposed/-infected patients: Infants and Children: 5 mg/kg/dose once daily (CDC, 2009)
Prevention in transplant recipients: Children and Adults: Initial: 5 mg/kg/dose every 12 hours for 1-2 weeks, followed by 5 mg/kg/dose once daily 7 days/week or 6 mg/kg/dose once daily 5 days/week for 100 days
Prevention in lung/heart-lung transplant patients (CMV-positive donor with CMV-positive recipient): Children and Adults: 6 mg/kg/dose once daily for 28 days
Other CMV infections: Children and Adults: Initial: 5 mg/kg/dose every 12 hours for 14-21 days; maintenance therapy: 5 mg/kg/dose once daily for 7 days/week or 6 mg/kg/dose once daily for 5 days/week

Varicella zoster; progressive outer retinal necrosis: Infants, Children, Adolescents, and Adults: 5 mg/kg/dose every 12 hours plus systemic foscarnet and intravitreal ganciclovir or foscarnet (CDC, 2009; Kaplan, 2009)

Dosing interval in renal impairment: Adults:
Induction:
CrCl 50-69 mL/minute: Administer 2.5 mg/kg/dose every 12 hours
CrCl 25-49 mL/minute: Administer 2.5 mg/kg/dose every 24 hours
CrCl 10-24 mL/minute: Administer 1.25 mg/kg/dose every 24 hours
CrCl <10 mL/minute: Administer 1.25 mg/kg/dose 3 times/week following hemodialysis
Maintenance:
CrCl 50-69 mL/minute: Administer 2.5 mg/kg/dose every 24 hours
CrCl 25-49 mL/minute: Administer 1.25 mg/kg/dose every 24 hours
CrCl 10-24 mL/minute: Administer 0.625 mg/kg/dose every 24 hours
CrCl <10 mL/minute: Administer 0.625 mg/kg/dose 3 times/week following hemodialysis
Intermittent hemodialysis (IHD) (administer after hemodialysis on dialysis days): Dialyzable (50%): CMV Infection: IV: Induction: 1.25 mg/kg every 48-72 hours; Maintenance: 0.625 mg/kg every 48-72 hours. **Note:** Dosing dependent on the assumption of 3 times/week, complete IHD sessions.
Peritoneal dialysis (PD): Dose as for CrCl <10 mL/minute
Continuous renal replacement therapy (CRRT) (Heintz, 2009; Trotman, 2005): Drug clearance is highly dependent on the method of renal replacement, filter type, and flow rate. Appropriate dosing requires close monitoring of pharmacologic response, signs of adverse reactions due to drug accumulation, as well as drug concentrations in relation to target trough (if appropriate). The following are general recommendations only (based on dialysate flow/ultrafiltration rates of 1-2 L/hour and minimal residual renal function) and should not supersede clinical judgment: CMV infection:
CVVH: IV: Induction: 2.5 mg/kg every 24 hours; Maintenance: 1.25 mg/kg every 24 hours
CVVHD/CVVHDF: IV: Induction: 2.5 mg/kg every 12 hours; Maintenance: 2.5 mg/kg every 24 hours

Preparation for Administration Hazardous agent; use appropriate precautions for handling and disposal (NIOSH 2014 [group 2]).
Parenteral: Reconstitute 500 mg vial with 10 mL SWFI **not** bacteriostatic water because parabens may cause precipitation. Further dilute in D_5W or NS to a final concentration ≤10 mg/mL.

Administration Hazardous agent; use appropriate precautions for handling and disposal (NIOSH 2014 [group 2]). Follow same precautions utilized with antineoplastic agents when preparing and administering ganciclovir.
Parenteral: Administer by slow IV infusion over at least 1 hour; too rapid infusion can cause increased toxicity and excessive plasma levels. Flush line well with NS before and after administration. Do not administer IM or SubQ; due to high pH, may cause severe tissue irritation.

Monitoring Parameters CBC with differential and platelet count, urine output, serum creatinine, ophthalmologic exams, liver enzyme tests, blood pressure, urinalysis

Additional Information Sodium content of 1 g: 4 mEq

Dosage Forms Excipient information presented when available (limited, particularly for generics); consult specific product labeling.
Solution Reconstituted, Intravenous:
Cytovene: 500 mg (1 ea)
Generic: 500 mg (1 ea)

Ganciclovir (Ophthalmic) (gan SYE kloe veer)

Medication Safety Issues
Sound-alike/look-alike issues:
Ganciclovir may be confused with acyclovir, valGANciclovir

Related Information
Safe Handling of Hazardous Drugs *on page 2455*

Brand Names: US Zirgan

Generic Availability (US) No

Use Treatment of acute herpetic keratitis (dendritic ulcers) (FDA approved in ages ≥2 years and adults)

Pregnancy Risk Factor C

Pregnancy Considerations Adverse events were observed in animal reproduction studies conducted with systemic ganciclovir. Based on animal studies, a U.S. Boxed Warning has been added to the labeling of the systemic product and effective contraception is recommended in males and females using systemic therapy. The amount of ganciclovir available systemically following topical application of the Zirgan ophthalmic gel is significantly less in comparison to IV doses (0.1%).

Breast-Feeding Considerations The amount of ganciclovir available systemically following ophthalmic application is not known. The manufacturer recommends that caution be used with administration of the ophthalmic gel to nursing women. Nursing mothers with herpetic lesions near or on the breast should avoid breast-feeding (AAP, 2012).

Contraindications There are no contraindications listed in the manufacturer's labeling.

Warnings/Precautions Hazardous agent - use appropriate precautions for handling and disposal (NIOSH 2014 [group 2]).

For topical ophthalmic use only. Blurred vision commonly occurs; may also cause eye irritation. Contact lenses should not be worn during the course of therapy or in any patient with signs/symptoms of herpetic keratitis.

Warnings: Additional Pediatric Considerations Use with caution in children; long-term safety has not been determined; the potential long-term carcinogenic and adverse reproductive effects of ganciclovir should be considered.

Adverse Reactions Ocular: Blurred vision, conjunctival hyperemia, irritation, punctate keratitis

Drug Interactions

Metabolism/Transport Effects None known.

Avoid Concomitant Use There are no known interactions where it is recommended to avoid concomitant use.

Increased Effect/Toxicity There are no known significant interactions involving an increase in effect.

Decreased Effect There are no known significant interactions involving a decrease in effect.

Storage/Stability Store at 15°C to 25°C (59°F to 77°F). Do not freeze.

Mechanism of Action Ganciclovir is phosphorylated to a substrate, which competitively inhibits the binding of deoxyguanosine triphosphate to DNA polymerase resulting in inhibition of DNA replication by herpes simplex viruses.

Pharmacokinetics (Adult data unless noted) Absorption: Ophthalmic gel: Minimal systemic exposure due to very low dose of ophthalmic product relative to systemic products

Dosing: Usual

Pediatric: **Herpetic keratitis:** Children ≥2 years and Adolescents: Ophthalmic gel: Apply 1 drop in affected eye 5 times daily (approximately every 3 hours while awake) until corneal ulcer heals, then 1 drop 3 times daily for 7 days

Adult: **Herpetic keratitis:** Ophthalmic gel: Apply 1 drop in affected eye 5 times daily (approximately every 3 hours while awake) until corneal ulcer heals, then 1 drop 3 times daily for 7 days

Dosing adjustment in renal impairment: There are no dosage adjustments provided in the manufacturer's labeling; however, dosage adjustment unlikely due to low systemic absorption.

Dosing adjustment in hepatic impairment: There are no dosage adjustments provided in the manufacturer's labeling; however, dosage adjustment unlikely due to low systemic absorption.

Administration Hazardous agent; use appropriate precautions for handling and disposal (NIOSH 2014 [group 2]).

Ophthalmic gel: Gel is intended for topical ophthalmic use only; avoid touching tip of applicator to eye or other surfaces.

Monitoring Parameters Ophthalmologic exams

Dosage Forms Excipient information presented when available (limited, particularly for generics); consult specific product labeling.

Gel, Ophthalmic:

Zirgan: 0.15% (5 g) [contains benzalkonium chloride]

◆ **Ganciclovir for Injection (Can)** *see* Ganciclovir (Systemic) *on page 958*

◆ **GAR-936** *see* Tigecycline *on page 2065*

◆ **Garamycin** *see* Gentamicin (Ophthalmic) *on page 968*

◆ **Garamycin® (Can)** *see* Gentamicin (Ophthalmic) *on page 968*

◆ **Gardasil** *see* Papillomavirus (Types 6, 11, 16, 18) Vaccine (Human, Recombinant) *on page 1625*

◆ **Gardasil 9** *see* Papillomavirus (9-Valent) Vaccine (Human, Recombinant) *on page 1623*

◆ **Gas-X [OTC]** *see* Simethicone *on page 1927*

◆ **Gas-X Childrens [OTC]** *see* Simethicone *on page 1927*

◆ **Gas-X Extra Strength [OTC]** *see* Simethicone *on page 1927*

◆ **Gas-X Infant Drops [OTC]** *see* Simethicone *on page 1927*

◆ **Gas-X Ultra Strength [OTC]** *see* Simethicone *on page 1927*

◆ **GasAid [OTC]** *see* Simethicone *on page 1927*

◆ **Gas Free Extra Strength [OTC]** *see* Simethicone *on page 1927*

◆ **Gas Relief [OTC]** *see* Simethicone *on page 1927*

◆ **Gas Relief Extra Strength [OTC]** *see* Simethicone *on page 1927*

◆ **Gas Relief Maximum Strength [OTC]** *see* Simethicone *on page 1927*

◆ **Gas Relief Ultra Strength [OTC]** *see* Simethicone *on page 1927*

◆ **Gastrocrom** *see* Cromolyn (Systemic, Oral Inhalation) *on page 541*

Gatifloxacin (gat i FLOKS a sin)

Brand Names: US Zymaxid

Brand Names: Canada Zymar

Therapeutic Category Antibiotic, Ophthalmic; Antibiotic, Quinolone

Generic Availability (US) Yes

Use Treatment of bacterial conjunctivitis caused by susceptible organisms (FDA approved in ages ≥1 year and adults).

Pregnancy Risk Factor C

Pregnancy Considerations Adverse events were observed in some animal reproduction studies. Systemic concentrations of gatifloxacin following ophthalmic administration are below the limit of quantification. If ophthalmic agents are needed during pregnancy, the minimum effective dose should be used in combination with punctual occlusion for 3 to 5 minutes after application to decrease potential exposure to the fetus (Samples 1988).

Breast-Feeding Considerations It is not known if gatifloxacin is excreted into breast milk. The manufacturer recommends that caution be exercised when administering gatifloxacin to nursing women.

Contraindications

Zymaxid: There are no contraindications listed in the manufacturer's labeling.

Zymar: Hypersensitivity to gatifloxacin, other quinolones, or any component of the formulation

Warnings/Precautions Severe hypersensitivity reactions, including anaphylaxis, have occurred with systemic quinolone therapy. Reactions may present as typical allergic symptoms after a single dose, or may manifest as severe idiosyncratic dermatologic, vascular, pulmonary, renal, hepatic, and/or hematologic events, usually after multiple doses. Prompt discontinuation of drug should occur if skin rash or other symptoms arise. Prolonged use may result in fungal or bacterial superinfection. For topical ophthalmic use only. Do not inject ophthalmic solution subconjunctivally or introduce directly into the anterior chamber of the eye. Contact lenses should not be worn during treatment of ophthalmic infections.

Adverse Reactions

Cardiovascular: Edema

Dermatologic: Contact dermatitis, erythema

Gastrointestinal: Taste disturbance

Ocular: Conjunctival irritation, discharge, dry eye, edema, irritation, keratitis, lacrimation increased, pain, papillary conjunctivitis, visual acuity decreased

Respiratory: Rhinorrhea

Rare but important or life-threatening: Angioedema, blepharitis (allergic), chemosis, conjunctival cyst, conjunctival hemorrhage, corneal deposits, corneal disorder, corneal ulcer, dermatitis, dizziness, endophthalmitis, eye redness, iritis, keratoconjunctivitis, macular edema, nausea, paresthesia (oral), photophobia, pruritus, subepithelial opacities, tinnitus, tremor, urticaria, uveitis, vision blurred, throat sore

Drug Interactions

Metabolism/Transport Effects None known.

Avoid Concomitant Use There are no known interactions where it is recommended to avoid concomitant use.

Increased Effect/Toxicity There are no known significant interactions involving an increase in effect.

Decreased Effect There are no known significant interactions involving a decrease in effect.

Storage/Stability Store between 15°C to 25°C (59°F to 77°F); do not freeze.

Mechanism of Action Gatifloxacin is a DNA gyrase inhibitor, and also inhibits topoisomerase IV. DNA gyrase (topoisomerase II) is an essential bacterial enzyme that maintains the superhelical structure of DNA. DNA gyrase is required for DNA replication and transcription, DNA repair, recombination, and transposition; inhibition is bactericidal.

Pharmacokinetics (Adult data unless noted) Absorption: Not measurable

Dosing: Usual Children ≥1 year and Adults:

Zymar®: Days 1 and 2: Instill 1 drop into affected eye(s) every 2 hours while awake (maximum: 8 times/day). Days 3-7: Instill 1 drop into affected eye(s) up to 4 times/day while awake.

Zymaxid™: Day 1: Instill 1 drop into affected eye(s) every 2 hours while awake (maximum: 8 times/day). Days 2-7: Instill 1 drop into affected eye(s) 2-4 times/day while awake.

Administration For topical ophthalmic use only; avoid touching tip of applicator to eye, fingers, or other surfaces. Apply finger pressure to lacrimal sac during and for 1-2 minutes after instillation to decrease risk of absorption and systemic effects.

Monitoring Parameters Signs of infection

Test Interactions Some quinolones may produce a false-positive urine screening result for opioids using commercially-available immunoassay kits. This has been demonstrated most consistently for levofloxacin and ofloxacin, but other quinolones have shown cross-reactivity in certain assay kits. Confirmation of positive opioid screens by more specific methods should be considered.

Additional Information Evidence of damage to weight-bearing joints in pediatric populations with ophthalmic administration has not been shown.

Dosage Forms Excipient information presented when available (limited, particularly for generics); consult specific product labeling.

Solution, Ophthalmic:

Zymaxid: 0.5% (2.5 mL) [contains benzalkonium chloride, edetate disodium]

Generic: 0.5% (2.5 mL)

- ◆ **GaviLAX [OTC]** *see* Polyethylene Glycol 3350 *on page 1723*
- ◆ **GaviLyte-C** *see* Polyethylene Glycol-Electrolyte Solution *on page 1724*
- ◆ **GaviLyte-G** *see* Polyethylene Glycol-Electrolyte Solution *on page 1724*
- ◆ **GaviLyte-N** *see* Polyethylene Glycol-Electrolyte Solution *on page 1724*
- ◆ **G-CSF** *see* Filgrastim *on page 876*
- ◆ **G-CSF (PEG Conjugate)** *see* Pegfilgrastim *on page 1641*
- ◆ **GCV Sodium** *see* Ganciclovir (Systemic) *on page 958*
- ◆ **GD-Amlodipine (Can)** *see* AmLODIPine *on page 133*
- ◆ **GD-Atorvastatin (Can)** *see* AtorvaSTATin *on page 220*
- ◆ **GD-Azithromycin (Can)** *see* Azithromycin (Systemic) *on page 242*
- ◆ **GD-Celecoxib (Can)** *see* Celecoxib *on page 418*
- ◆ **GD-Gabapentin (Can)** *see* Gabapentin *on page 954*
- ◆ **GD-Quinapril (Can)** *see* Quinapril *on page 1820*
- ◆ **GD-Sertraline (Can)** *see* Sertraline *on page 1916*
- ◆ **GD-Sildenafil (Can)** *see* Sildenafil *on page 1921*
- ◆ **GD-Terbinafine (Can)** *see* Terbinafine (Systemic) *on page 2021*
- ◆ **GD-Topiramate (Can)** *see* Topiramate *on page 2085*
- ◆ **GD-Venlafaxine XR (Can)** *see* Venlafaxine *on page 2166*
- ◆ **Gel-Kam [OTC]** *see* Fluoride *on page 899*
- ◆ **Gel-Kam Rinse** *see* Fluoride *on page 899*
- ◆ **Gelnique** *see* Oxybutynin *on page 1588*
- ◆ **GelRite [OTC]** *see* Alcohol (Ethyl) *on page 86*
- ◆ **Gel-Stat [OTC]** *see* Alcohol (Ethyl) *on page 86*
- ◆ **Gelusil Extra Strength (Can)** *see* Aluminum Hydroxide and Magnesium Hydroxide *on page 111*

Gemcitabine (jem SITE a been)

Medication Safety Issues

Sound-alike/look-alike issues:

Gemcitabine may be confused with gemtuzumab

Gemzar may be confused with Zinecard

High alert medication:

This medication is in a class the Institute for Safe Medication Practices (ISMP) includes among its list of drug classes which have a heightened risk of causing significant patient harm when used in error.

International issues:

In Canada, gemcitabine is available as a concentrated solution for injection in different strengths (38 mg/mL and 40 mg/mL), and a powder for reconstitution (final concentration of 38 mg/mL after reconstitution). Verify product concentration prior to preparation for administration.

Related Information

Management of Drug Extravasations *on page 2298*

Prevention of Chemotherapy-Induced Nausea and Vomiting in Children *on page 2368*

Safe Handling of Hazardous Drugs *on page 2455*

Brand Names: US Gemzar

Brand Names: Canada Gemcitabine For Injection; Gemcitabine For Injection Concentrate; Gemcitabine For Injection, USP; Gemcitabine Hydrochloride For Injection; Gemcitabine Injection; Gemcitabine Sun For Injection; Gemzar

Therapeutic Category Antineoplastic Agent, Antimetabolite (Pyrimidine Antagonist)

Generic Availability (US) Yes

Use Treatment of locally advanced, inoperable (stage IIIA or IIIB), or metastatic (stage IV) non-small cell lung cancer (NSCLC), metastatic breast cancer, and advanced relapsed ovarian cancer as part of combination therapy (FDA approved in adults); treatment of locally advanced or metastatic pancreatic cancer as a single agent (FDA approved in adults); has also been used in the treatment of refractory solid tumors (including brain tumors), refractory or relapsed Hodgkin's lymphoma, and refractory germ cell tumors

Pregnancy Risk Factor D

Pregnancy Considerations Adverse events were observed in animal reproduction studies. May cause fetal harm if administered during pregnancy; adverse effects in reproduction are anticipated based on the mechanism of action.

Breast-Feeding Considerations It is not known if gemcitabine is excreted in breast milk. Due to the potential for serious adverse reactions in the nursing infant, the decision to discontinue gemcitabine or to discontinue breast-feeding should take into account the benefits of treatment to the mother.

Contraindications Hypersensitivity to gemcitabine or any component of the formulation

Warnings/Precautions Hazardous agent - use appropriate precautions for handling and disposal (NIOSH 2014 [group 1]). Gemcitabine may suppress bone marrow function (neutropenia, thrombocytopenia, and anemia); myelosuppression is usually the dose-limiting toxicity; toxicity is increased when used in combination with other chemotherapy; monitor blood counts; dosage adjustments are frequently required.

Hemolytic uremic syndrome (HUS) has been reported; may lead to renal failure and dialysis (including fatalities); monitor for evidence of anemia with microangiopathic hemolysis (elevation of bilirubin or LDH, reticulocytosis, severe thrombocytopenia, and/or renal failure) and monitor renal function at baseline and periodically during treatment. Permanently discontinue if HUS or severe renal impairment occurs; renal failure may not be reversible despite discontinuation. Serious hepatotoxicity (including liver failure and death) has been reported (when used alone or in combination with other hepatotoxic medications); use in patients with hepatic impairment (history of cirrhosis, hepatitis, or alcoholism) or in patients with hepatic metastases may lead to exacerbation of hepatic impairment. Monitor hepatic function at baseline and periodically during treatment; consider dose adjustments with elevated bilirubin; discontinue if severe liver injury develops. Capillary leak syndrome (CLS) with serious consequences has been reported, both with single-agent gemcitabine and with combination chemotherapy; discontinue if CLS develops.

Pulmonary toxicity, including adult respiratory distress syndrome, interstitial pneumonitis, pulmonary edema, and pulmonary fibrosis, has been observed; may lead to respiratory failure (some fatal) despite discontinuation. Onset for symptoms of pulmonary toxicity may be delayed up to 2 weeks beyond the last dose. Discontinue for unexplained dyspnea (with or without bronchospasm) or other evidence or pulmonary toxicity. Posterior reversible encephalopathy syndrome (PRES) has been reported, both with single-agent therapy and with combination chemotherapy. PRES may manifest with blindness, confusion, headache, hypertension, lethargy, seizure, and other visual and neurologic disturbances. If PRES diagnosis is confirmed, discontinue therapy. Not indicated for use with concurrent radiation therapy; radiation toxicity, including tissue injury, severe mucositis, esophagitis, or pneumonitis, has been reported with concurrent and non-concurrent administration; may have radiosensitizing activity when gemcitabine and radiation therapy are given ≤7 days apart; radiation recall may occur when gemcitabine and radiation therapy are given >7 days apart. Potentially significant drug-drug interactions may exist, requiring dose or frequency adjustment, additional monitoring, and/or selection of alternative therapy.

Prolongation of the infusion duration >60 minutes or more frequent than weekly dosing have been shown to alter the half-life and increase toxicity (hypotension, flu-like symptoms, myelosuppression, weakness); a fixed-dose rate (FDR) infusion rate of 10 mg/m^2/minute has been studied in adults in order to optimize the pharmacokinetics (off-label); prolonged infusion times increase the intracellular accumulation of the active metabolite, gemcitabine triphosphate (Ko, 2006; Tempero, 2003); patients who receive gemcitabine FDR experience more grade 3/4 hematologic toxicity (Ko, 2006; Poplin, 2009).

Adverse Reactions Adverse reactions reported for single-agent use of gemcitabine only; bone marrow depression is the dose-limiting toxicity.

Cardiovascular: Edema, peripheral edema

Central nervous system: Drowsiness, paresthesia

Dermatologic: Alopecia, skin rash

Gastrointestinal: Diarrhea, nausea and vomiting, stomatitis

Genitourinary: Hematuria, proteinuria

Hematologic & oncologic: Anemia, hemorrhage, neutropenia, thrombocytopenia

Hepatic: Increased serum alkaline phosphatase, increased serum ALT, increased serum AST, increased serum bilirubin

Infection: Infection

Local: Injection site reaction

Renal: Increased blood urea nitrogen, increased serum creatinine

Respiratory: Bronchospasm, dyspnea, flu-like symptoms

Miscellaneous: Fever

Rare but important or life-threatening (reported with single-agent use or with combination therapy): Adult respiratory distress syndrome (acute), anaphylactoid reaction, Budd-Chiari syndrome, bullous pemphigoid, capillary leak syndrome, cardiac arrhythmia, cardiac failure, cellulitis, cerebrovascular accident, desquamation, digital vasculitis, gangrene of skin or other tissue, hemolytic-uremic syndrome, hepatic cirrhosis, hepatic necrosis, hepatic veno-occlusive disease, hepatotoxicity (rare), hypertension, hypotension, increased gamma-glutamyl transferase, interstitial pneumonitis, myocardial infarction, neuropathy, petechiae, pulmonary edema, pulmonary fibrosis, radiation recall phenomenon, renal failure, respiratory failure, reversible posterior leukoencephalopathy syndrome, sepsis, supraventricular cardiac arrhythmia, thrombotic thrombocytopenic purpura

Drug Interactions

Metabolism/Transport Effects None known.

Avoid Concomitant Use

Avoid concomitant use of Gemcitabine with any of the following: BCG; BCG (Intravesical); CloZAPine; Dipyrone; Natalizumab; Pimecrolimus; Tacrolimus (Topical); Tofacitinib; Vaccines (Live)

Increased Effect/Toxicity

Gemcitabine may increase the levels/effects of: Bleomycin; CloZAPine; Fluorouracil (Systemic); Fluorouracil (Topical); Leflunomide; Natalizumab; Tofacitinib; Vaccines (Live); Warfarin

The levels/effects of Gemcitabine may be increased by: Denosumab; Dipyrone; Pimecrolimus; Roflumilast; Tacrolimus (Topical); Trastuzumab

Decreased Effect

Gemcitabine may decrease the levels/effects of: BCG; BCG (Intravesical); Coccidioides immitis Skin Test; Sipuleucel-T; Vaccines (Inactivated); Vaccines (Live)

The levels/effects of Gemcitabine may be decreased by: Echinacea

Storage/Stability

Lyophilized powder: Store intact vials at room temperature of 20°C to 25°C (68°F to 77°F); excursions permitted to 15°C to 30°C (59°F to 86°F). Reconstituted vials are stable for 24 hours at room temperature. Do not refrigerate (may form crystals).

Solution for injection: Store intact vials refrigerated at 2°C to 8°C (36°F to 46°F); do not freeze.

Solutions diluted for infusion in NS are stable for 24 hours at room temperature. Do not refrigerate.

Mechanism of Action A pyrimidine antimetabolite that inhibits DNA synthesis by inhibition of DNA polymerase and ribonucleotide reductase, cell cycle-specific for the S-phase of the cycle (also blocks cellular progression at G1/S-phase). Gemcitabine is phosphorylated intracellularly by deoxycytidine kinase to gemcitabine monophosphate, which is further phosphorylated to active metabolites gemcitabine diphosphate and gemcitabine triphosphate. Gemcitabine diphosphate inhibits DNA synthesis by inhibiting ribonucleotide reductase; gemcitabine triphosphate incorporates into DNA and inhibits DNA polymerase.

Pharmacokinetics (Adult data unless noted)

Distribution: Widely distributed into tissues; present in ascitic fluid

V_d:

IV infusion <70 minutes: 50 L/m^2

IV infusion 70-285 minutes: 370 L/m^2

Protein binding: Negligible

Metabolism: Intracellularly by nucleoside kinases to active di- and triphosphate metabolites; metabolized by cytidine deaminase to an inactive metabolite

Half-life:

IV infusion <70 minutes: 0.7-1.6 hours

IV infusion 70-285 minutes: 4.1-10.6 hours

Elimination: 92% to 98% excreted in the urine as gemcitabine (<10%) and inactive uracil metabolite, difluorodeoxyuridine (dFdU)

Dosing: Usual Details concerning dosing in combination regimens should also be consulted. **Note:** Prolongation of the infusion time >60 minutes and administration more frequently than once weekly have been shown to increase toxicity. Refer to individual protocols: IV:

Children and Adolescents:

Hodgkin's lymphoma, refractory or relapsed:

Children ≥10 years and Adolescents: 1000 mg/m^2/dose over 100 minutes on days 1 and 8 (in combination with vinorelbine); repeat cycle every 21 days (Cole, 2009)

Adolescents ≥17 years: 1000 mg/m^2/dose over 60 minutes on days 1, 8, and 15 (in combination with vinorelbine); repeat cycle every 28 days (Suyani, 2011) **or** 800 mg/m^2/dose on days 1 and 4 (in combination with ifosfamide and vinorelbine); repeat cycle every 21 days (Santoro, 2007)

Sarcomas, refractory or relapsed (including Ewing's sarcoma, osteosarcoma): Children ≥3 years and Adolescents: 675 **or** 1000 mg/m^2/dose over 90 minutes on days 1 and 8 (in combination with docetaxel); repeat cycle every 21 days (Mora, 2009; Navid, 2008) **or** 1000 mg/m^2/dose over 30 minutes on days 1 and 8 (in combination with oxaliplatin and irinotecan); repeat cycle every 28 days (Hartmann, 2011)

Solid tumors, refractory or relapsed: Children ≥1 year and Adolescents: 1000 mg/m^2/dose over 30 minutes on days 1 and 8 (in combination with oxaliplatin and irinotecan); repeat cycle every 28 days (Hartmann, 2011) **or** 1000 mg/m^2/dose over 100 minutes on day 1 (in combination with oxaliplatin); repeat cycle every 14 days (Geoerger, 2011)

Note: Dosage reductions for toxicity (Geoerger, 2011): 800 mg/m^2/dose over 80 minutes if grade 3/4 nonhematological toxicity, grade 4 neutropenia with documented infection or lasting >7 days, grade 3/4 thrombocytopenia lasting >7 days or requiring platelets during >7 days, or delay of next cycle ≥14 days; if necessary dose could be reduced a second time to 600 mg/m^2/dose

Germ cell tumor, refractory: Adolescents ≥16 years: 1200 mg/m^2/dose over 30 minutes on days 1, 8, and 15; repeat cycle every 28 days for up to 6 cycles (Einhorn, 1999)

Adults:

Breast cancer, metastatic (AGC should be ≥1500/mm^3 and platelets ≥100,000/mm^3 prior to each cycle): 1250 mg/m^2 over 30 minutes on days 1 and 8; repeat cycle every 21 days (in combination with paclitaxel)

Non-small cell lung cancer, locally advanced or metastatic (in combination with cisplatin): 1000 mg/m^2 over 30 minutes on days 1, 8, and 15; repeat cycle every 28 days **or** 1250 mg/m^2 over 30 minutes on days 1 and 8; repeat cycle every 21 days

Ovarian cancer, advanced (AGC should be ≥1500/mm^3 and platelets ≥100,000/mm^3 prior to each cycle): 1000 mg/m^2 over 30 minutes days 1 and 8; repeat cycle every 21 days (in combination with carboplatin)

Pancreatic cancer, locally advanced or metastatic: Initial: 1000 mg/m^2 over 30 minutes once weekly for up to 7 weeks followed by 1 week of rest; then 1000 mg/m^2 once weekly for 3 weeks out of every 4 weeks

Dose escalation: Patients who complete an entire cycle of therapy may have the dose in subsequent cycles increased by 25% as long as the absolute granulocyte count (AGC) nadir is >1500/mm^3, platelet nadir is >100,000/mm^3, and nonhematologic toxicity is less than WHO Grade 1. If the increased dose is tolerated (with the same parameters) the dose in subsequent cycles may again be increased by 20%.

Dosing adjustment for renal impairment: Adults: The manufacturer's labeling does not contain dosing adjustment guidelines; use with caution in patients with preexisting renal dysfunction. Discontinue if severe renal toxicity or hemolytic uremic syndrome (HUS) occur during gemcitabine treatment.

The following adjustments have been made by some clinicians (Janus, 2010; Li, 2007):

Mild to severe renal impairment: No adjustment required

ESRD withhemodialysis: Hemodialysis should begin 6-12 hours after gemcitabine infusion

Dosing adjustment for hepatic impairment: Adults: The manufacturer's labeling does not contain dosing adjustment guidelines; use with caution. Discontinue if severe hepatotoxicity occurs during treatment with gemcitabine. The following guidelines have been used by some clinicians:

Transaminases elevated (with normal bilirubin): No adjustment required (Venook, 2000)

Serum bilirubin >1.6 mg/dL: Use initial dose of 800 mg/m^2; may escalate if tolerated (Ecklund, 2005; Floyd, 2006; Venook, 2000)

Dosing adjustment for hematologic toxicity: Adults:

Breast cancer: Adjustments based on granulocyte and platelet counts on day 8:

AGC ≥1200/mm^3 **and** platelet count >75,000/mm^3: Administer 100% of full dose

AGC 1000-1199/mm^3 **or** platelet count 50,000-75,000/mm^3: Administer 75% of full dose
AGC 700-999/mm^3 **and** platelet count ≥50,000/mm^3: Administer 50% of full dose
AGC <700/mm^3 **or** platelet count <50,000/mm^3: Hold dose
Severe (grades 3 or 4) nonhematologic toxicity (except alopecia, nausea, and vomiting): Hold or decrease dose by 50%. Paclitaxel dose may also need adjusted.

Non-small cell lung cancer: Refer to guidelines for pancreatic cancer. Cisplatin dosage may also need adjusted.
Severe (grades 3 or 4) nonhematologic toxicity (except alopecia, nausea, and vomiting): Hold or decrease dose by 50%

Ovarian cancer:
Adjustments based on granulocyte and platelet counts on day 8:
AGC ≥1500/mm^3 **and** platelet count ≥100,000/mm^3: Administer 100% of full dose
AGC 1000-1499/mm^3 **and/or** platelet count 75,000-99,999/mm^3: Administer 50% of full dose
AGC <1000/mm^3 **and/or** platelet count <75,000/mm^3: Hold dose
Severe (grades 3 or 4) nonhematologic toxicity (except nausea and vomiting): Hold or decrease dose by 50%. Carboplatin dose may also need adjusted.
Dose adjustment for subsequent cycles:
AGC <500/mm^3 for >5 days, AGC <100/mm^3 for >3 days, febrile neutropenia, platelet count <25,000/mm^3, cycle delay >1 week due to toxicity: Reduce gemcitabine to 800 mg/m^2 on days 1 and 8
For recurrence of any of the above toxicities after initial dose reduction: Administer gemcitabine 800 mg/m2 on day 1 only for the subsequent cycle

Pancreatic cancer:
AGC ≥1000/mm^3 **and** platelet count ≥100,000/mm^3: Administer 100% of full dose
AGC 500-999/mm^3 **or** platelet count 50,000-99,999/mm^3: Administer 75% of full dose
AGC <500/mm^3 **or** platelet count <50,000/mm^3: Hold dose

Preparation for Administration Hazardous agent; use appropriate precautions for handling and disposal (NIOSH 2014 [group 1]).

IV: Reconstitute lyophilized powder with preservative free NS according to manufacturer's labeling to a final concentration of 38 mg/mL (solutions must be reconstituted to ≤40 mg/mL to completely dissolve). Gemcitabine is also supplied as a concentrated solution for injection (38 mg/mL). Further dilute gemcitabine in 50 to 500 mL NS to concentrations as low as 0.1 mg/mL.

Administration Hazardous agent; use appropriate precautions for handling and disposal (NIOSH 2014 [group 1]).

IV: Infuse over 30 minutes per manufacturer; however, for other protocols and uses, infusion times may vary (refer to specific protocols). Prolongation of the infusion time >60 minutes has been shown to prolong gemcitabine's half-life and increase toxicity in adults; gemcitabine has been administered in adults utilizing a fixed-dose rate (FDR) of 10 mg/m^2/minute; prolonged infusion times increase the accumulation of the active metabolite, gemcitabine triphosphate, optimizing the pharmacokinetics (Ko 2006; Tempero 2003); patients who receive gemcitabine FDR experience more grade 3/4 hematologic toxicity (Ko 2006; Poplin 2009).

Vesicant/Extravasation Risk May be an irritant

Monitoring Parameters CBC with differential and platelet count prior to each dose; monitor renal and hepatic function prior to initial dose and then periodically, bilirubin, LDH, and reticulocyte count; monitor serum electrolytes, including potassium, magnesium, and calcium (when in combination therapy with cisplatin)

Dosage Forms Excipient information presented when available (limited, particularly for generics); consult specific product labeling.
Solution, Intravenous:
Generic: 200 mg/5.26 mL (5.26 mL); 1 g/26.3 mL (26.3 mL); 2 g/52.6 mL (52.6 mL)
Solution Reconstituted, Intravenous:
Gemzar: 200 mg (1 ea); 1 g (1 ea)
Generic: 200 mg (1 ea); 1 g (1 ea); 2 g (1 ea)
Solution Reconstituted, Intravenous [preservative free]:
Generic: 200 mg (1 ea); 1 g (1 ea)

- **Gemcitabine For Injection (Can)** *see* Gemcitabine *on page 961*
- **Gemcitabine For Injection Concentrate (Can)** *see* Gemcitabine *on page 961*
- **Gemcitabine For Injection, USP (Can)** *see* Gemcitabine *on page 961*
- **Gemcitabine Hydrochloride** *see* Gemcitabine *on page 961*
- **Gemcitabine Hydrochloride For Injection (Can)** *see* Gemcitabine *on page 961*
- **Gemcitabine Injection (Can)** *see* Gemcitabine *on page 961*
- **Gemcitabine Sun For Injection (Can)** *see* Gemcitabine *on page 961*
- **Gemzar** *see* Gemcitabine *on page 961*
- **Genac** *see* Triprolidine and Pseudoephedrine *on page 2129*
- **Genahist [OTC]** *see* DiphenhydrAMINE (Systemic) *on page 668*
- **Genaphed [OTC]** *see* Pseudoephedrine *on page 1801*
- **Gen-Clozapine (Can)** *see* CloZAPine *on page 519*
- **Gene-Activated Human Acid-Beta-Glucosidase** *see* Velaglucerase Alfa *on page 2165*
- **Generlac** *see* Lactulose *on page 1204*
- **Gen-Fluoxetine (Can)** *see* FLUoxetine *on page 906*
- **Gengraf** *see* CycloSPORINE (Systemic) *on page 556*
- **Gen-Hydroxychloroquine (Can)** *see* Hydroxychloroquine *on page 1052*
- **Gen-Hydroxyurea (Can)** *see* Hydroxyurea *on page 1055*
- **Gen-Ipratropium (Can)** *see* Ipratropium (Oral Inhalation) *on page 1155*
- **Gen-Medroxy (Can)** *see* MedroxyPROGESTERone *on page 1339*
- **Gen-Nizatidine (Can)** *see* Nizatidine *on page 1528*
- **Genotropin** *see* Somatropin *on page 1957*
- **Genotropin GoQuick (Can)** *see* Somatropin *on page 1957*
- **Genotropin MiniQuick** *see* Somatropin *on page 1957*
- **Genpril [OTC]** *see* Ibuprofen *on page 1064*
- **Gentak** *see* Gentamicin (Ophthalmic) *on page 968*
- **Gentak® (Can)** *see* Gentamicin (Ophthalmic) *on page 968*

Gentamicin (Systemic) (jen ta MYE sin)

Medication Safety Issues

Sound-alike/look-alike issues:

Gentamicin may be confused with gentian violet, kanamycin, vancomycin

High alert medication:

The Institute for Safe Medication Practices (ISMP) includes this medication (intrathecal administration) among its list of drug classes which have a heightened risk of causing significant patient harm when used in error.

Brand Names: Canada Gentamicin Injection, USP

Therapeutic Category Antibiotic, Aminoglycoside

Generic Availability (US) Yes

Use Treatment of documented or suspected infections caused by susceptible gram-negative bacilli, including *Pseudomonas*, *E. coli*, *Proteus*, *Serratia*, and gram-positive *Staphylococcus* (FDA approved in all ages); treatment of bone infections, CNS infections, respiratory tract infections, skin and soft tissue infections, as well as abdominal and urinary tract infections, endocarditis, and septicemia; used in combination with ampicillin as empiric therapy for sepsis in newborns

Pregnancy Risk Factor D

Pregnancy Considerations Gentamicin crosses the placenta and produces detectable serum levels in the fetus. Renal toxicity has been described in two case reports following first trimester exposure. There are several reports of total irreversible bilateral congenital deafness in children whose mothers received streptomycin during pregnancy; therefore, the manufacturer classifies gentamicin as pregnancy category D. Although ototoxicity has not been reported following maternal use of gentamicin, a potential for harm exists. **[U.S. Boxed Warning]: Aminoglycosides may cause fetal harm if administered to a pregnant woman.**

Due to pregnancy induced physiologic changes, some pharmacokinetic parameters of gentamicin may be altered. Pregnant women have an average-to-larger volume of distribution which may result in lower serum peak levels than for the same dose in nonpregnant women. Serum half-life is also shorter.

Breast-Feeding Considerations Gentamicin is excreted into breast milk; however, it is not well absorbed when taken orally. This limited oral absorption may minimize exposure to the nursing infant. Nondose-related effects could include modification of bowel flora.

Contraindications Hypersensitivity to gentamicin or other aminoglycosides

Warnings/Precautions [U.S. Boxed Warning]: Aminoglycosides may cause neurotoxicity and/or nephrotoxicity; usual risk factors include pre-existing renal impairment, concomitant neuro-/nephrotoxic medications, advanced age and dehydration. Ototoxicity may be directly proportional to the amount of drug given and the duration of treatment; tinnitus or vertigo are indications of vestibular injury and impending hearing loss; renal damage is usually reversible. May cause neuromuscular blockade and respiratory paralysis; especially when given soon after anesthesia or muscle relaxants.

Not intended for long-term therapy due to toxic hazards associated with extended administration; use caution in preexisting renal insufficiency, vestibular or cochlear impairment, myasthenia gravis, hypocalcemia, conditions which depress neuromuscular transmission. Dosage modification required in patients with impaired renal function. Prolonged use may result in fungal or bacterial superinfection, including *C. difficile*-associated diarrhea (CDAD) and pseudomembranous colitis; CDAD has been observed >2 months postantibiotic treatment.

Warnings: Additional Pediatric Considerations Use with caution in pediatric patients on extracorporeal membrane oxygenation (ECMO); pharmacokinetics of aminoglycosides may be altered; dosage adjustment and close monitoring necessary. Oral use for the prevention of NEC in premature neonates may potentially increase the risk for development of resistant bacteria; routine use for this is not recommended (Bury, 2001; Reber, 2004).

Adverse Reactions

Cardiovascular: Edema, hyper/hypotension

Central nervous system: Ataxia, confusion, depression, dizziness, drowsiness, encephalopathy, fever, headache, lethargy, pseudomotor cerebri, seizures, vertigo

Dermatologic: Alopecia, erythema, itching, purpura, rash, urticaria

Endocrine & metabolic: Hypocalcemia, hypokalemia, hypomagnesemia, hyponatremia

Gastrointestinal: Anorexia, appetite decreased, *C. difficile*-associated diarrhea, enterocolitis, nausea, salivation increased, splenomegaly, stomatitis, vomiting, weight loss

Hematologic: Agranulocytosis, anemia, eosinophilia, granulocytopenia, leukopenia, reticulocytes increased/decreased, thrombocytopenia

Hepatic: Hepatomegaly, LFTs increased

Local: Injection site reactions, pain at injection site, phlebitis/thrombophlebitis

Neuromuscular & skeletal: Arthralgia, gait instability, muscle cramps, muscle twitching, muscle weakness, myasthenia gravis-like syndrome, numbness, paresthesia, peripheral neuropathy, tremor, weakness

Ocular: Visual disturbances

Otic: Hearing impairment, hearing loss (associated with persistently increased serum concentrations; early toxicity usually affects high-pitched sound), tinnitus

Renal: BUN increased, casts (hyaline, granular) in urine, creatinine clearance decreased, distal tubular dysfunction, Fanconi-like syndrome (high dose, prolonged course) (infants and adults), oliguria, renal failure (high trough serum concentrations), polyuria, proteinuria, serum creatinine increased, tubular necrosis, urine specific gravity decreased

Respiratory: Dyspnea, laryngeal edema, pulmonary fibrosis, respiratory depression

Miscellaneous: Allergic reaction, anaphylaxis, anaphylactoid reactions

Drug Interactions

Metabolism/Transport Effects None known.

Avoid Concomitant Use

Avoid concomitant use of Gentamicin (Systemic) with any of the following: Agalsidase Alfa; Agalsidase Beta; BCG; BCG (Intravesical); Foscarnet; Mannitol; Mecamylamine

Increased Effect/Toxicity

Gentamicin (Systemic) may increase the levels/effects of: AbobotulinumtoxinA; Bisphosphonate Derivatives; CARBOplatin; Colistimethate; CycloSPORINE (Systemic); Mecamylamine; Neuromuscular-Blocking Agents; OnabotulinumtoxinA; RimabotulinumtoxinB; Tenofovir

The levels/effects of Gentamicin (Systemic) may be increased by: Amphotericin B; Capreomycin; Cephalosporins (2nd Generation); Cephalosporins (3rd Generation); Cephalosporins (4th Generation); CISplatin; Foscarnet; Loop Diuretics; Mannitol; Nonsteroidal Anti-Inflammatory Agents; Tenofovir; Vancomycin

Decreased Effect

Gentamicin (Systemic) may decrease the levels/effects of: Agalsidase Alfa; Agalsidase Beta; BCG; BCG (Intravesical); BCG Vaccine (Immunization); Sodium Picosulfate; Typhoid Vaccine

The levels/effects of Gentamicin (Systemic) may be decreased by: Penicillins

Storage/Stability Gentamicin is a colorless to slightly yellow solution which should be stored between 2°C to 30°C, but refrigeration is not recommended. IV infusion solutions mixed in NS or D_5W solution are stable for 48 hours at room temperature and refrigeration (Goodwin, 1991). Premixed bag: Manufacturer expiration date; remove from overwrap stability: 30 days.

Mechanism of Action Interferes with bacterial protein synthesis by binding to 30S and 50S ribosomal subunits resulting in a defective bacterial cell membrane

Pharmacodynamics Displays concentration-dependent killing; bacteriocidal

Pharmacokinetics (Adult data unless noted)

Absorption:
- Oral: Poorly absorbed (<2%)
- Intramuscular: Rapid and complete

Distribution: Primarily in the extracellular fluid volume and in most tissues; poor penetration into CSF; drug accumulates in the renal cortex; small amounts distribute into bile, sputum, saliva, and tears
- V_d: Higher in neonates than older pediatric patients; also increased in patients with edema, ascites, fluid overload; decreased in patients with dehydration:
  - Neonates: 0.45 ± 0.1 L/kg
  - Infants: 0.4 ± 0.1 L/kg
  - Children: 0.35 ± 0.15 L/kg
  - Adolescents: 0.3 ± 0.1 L/kg
  - Adults: 0.2-0.3 L/kg

Protein binding: <30%

Half-life:
- Neonates:
  - <1 week: 3-11.5 hours
  - 1 week to 1 month: 3-6 hours
- Infants: 4 ± 1 hour
- Children: 2 ± 1 hour
- Adolescents: 1.5 ± 1 hour
- Adults with normal renal function: 1.5-3 hours
- Anuria: 36-70 hours

Time to peak serum concentration:
- IM: Within 30-90 minutes
- IV: 30 minutes after 30-minute infusion; **Note:** Distribution may be prolonged after larger doses. One study reported a 1.7-hour distribution period after a 60-minute, high-dose aminoglycoside infusion (Demczar, 1997).

Elimination: Clearance is directly related to renal function; eliminated almost completely by glomerular filtration of unchanged drug with excretion into urine
- Clearance:
  - Neonates: 0.045 ± 0.01 L/hour/kg
  - Infants: 0.1 ± 0.05 L/hour/kg
  - Children: 0.1 ± 0.03 L/hour/kg
  - Adolescents: 0.09 ± 0.03 L/hour/kg
- Dialysis: Dialyzable (50% to 100%)

Dosing: Neonatal Note: Dosage should be based on actual weight unless the patient has hydrops fetalis. Dosage should be individualized based upon serum concentration monitoring.

General dosing; susceptible infection: IV: Extended-interval dosing strategies may vary by institution as a wide variety of dosing regimens have been studied. Consider single-dose administration with serum concentration monitoring in patients with urine output <1 mL/kg/hour or serum creatinine >1.3 mg/dL rather than scheduled dosing. Consider prolongation of dosing interval when coadministered with ibuprofen or indomethacin or in neonates with history of the following: Birth depression, birth hypoxia/asphyxia, or cyanotic congenital heart disease. Some dosing based on tobramycin studies.

Age-directed dosing (de Hoog 2002; DiCenzo 2003; Hagen 2009; Hansen 2003; Ohler 2000; Serane 2009):
- GA <32 weeks: 4 to 5 mg/kg/dose every 48 hours
- GA 32-36 weeks: 4 to 5 mg/kg/dose every 36 hours
- GA ≥37 weeks: 4 to 5 mg/kg/dose every 24 hours

Note: In some trials, a fixed interval of every 24 hours was used with dosages ranging from 2.5 to 4 mg/kg/dose based on GA (ie, lower doses were used for younger GA).

Weight-directed dosing (*Red Book* 2012): IM, IV:
- Body weight <1 kg:
  - PNA ≤14 days: 5 mg/kg/dose every 48 hours
  - PNA 15 to 28 days: 4-5 mg/kg/dose every 24 to 48 hours
- Body weight 1 to 2 kg:
  - PNA ≤7 days: 5 mg/kg/dose every 48 hours
  - PNA 8-28 days: 4 to 5 mg/kg/dose every 24 to 48 hours
- Body weight >2 kg:
  - PNA ≤7 days: 4 mg/kg/dose every 24 hours
  - PNA 8-28 days: 4 mg/kg/dose every 12 to 24 hours

ECMO, initial dosing in full-term neonates: IV: Initial dose: 2.5 to 3 mg/kg/dose every 18 to 24 hours; some experts recommend a higher initial dose of 5 mg/kg/dose; subsequent doses should be individualized by monitoring serum drug concentrations; when ECMO is discontinued, dosage may require readjustment due to large shifts in body water (Buck 2003; Southgate 1989)

CNS infection (VP-shunt infection, ventriculitis): Limited information available: Intraventricular/intrathecal **(use a preservative free preparation)**: 1 mg/**day** (Tunkel 2004)

NEC, prevention: Limited data available; efficacy results variable: Oral: 2.5 mg/kg/dose every 6 hours beginning at birth and continued for 1 week was used in 22 neonates at high risk for the development of NEC (including prematurity, asphyxia, use of a UAC); results showed significant decrease in incidence of NEC with treatment group compared to placebo (Bury 2001; Grylack 1978); due to risk of resistant bacteria development, clinical benefits and risk with use should be evaluated prior to use.

Surgical prophylaxis: IV: 2.5 to 3 mg/kg as a single dose (*Red Book*, 2012)

Dosing: Usual Note: Dosage should be based on an estimate of ideal body weight. In morbidly obese children, adolescents, and adults, dosage requirement may best be estimated using a dosing weight of IBW + 0.4 (TBW - IBW). Dosage should be individualized based upon serum concentration monitoring.

Infants, Children, and Adolescents: **Note:** Some dosing is based on tobramycin studies:

General dosing:
- Conventional dosing: IM, IV: 2.5 mg/kg/dose every 8 hours; some pediatric patients may require larger doses (ie, patients undergoing continuous hemofiltration, patients with major burns, febrile granulocytopenic patients); modify dose based on individual patient requirements as determined by renal function, serum drug concentrations, and patient-specific clinical parameters
  - Manufacturer's recommendations: IM, IV:
    - Infants: 2.5 mg/kg/dose every 8 hours
    - Children: 2 to 2.5 mg/kg/dose every 8 hours
- Extended-interval dosing: IV:
  - Weight-directed: 4.5 to 7.5 mg/kg/dose every 24 hours in patients with normal renal function (Contopoulos-Ioannidis 2004; *Red Book* 2012)
  - Age-directed: Based on data from 114 patients, the following has been suggested (McDade 2010):
    - 3 months to <2 years: 9.5 mg/kg/dose every 24 hours
    - 2 to <8 years: 8.5 mg/kg/dose every 24 hours
    - ≥8 years: 7 mg/kg/dose every 24 hours

CNS infection:
Meningitis (Tunkel 2004):
Infants and Children: IV 7.5 mg/kg/**day** divided every 8 hours
Adolescents: IV: 5 mg/kg/**day** divided every 8 hours
VP-shunt infection, ventriculitis: Limited data available: Intraventricular/intrathecal **(use a preservative free preparation)** (Tunkel 2004):
Infants >3 months and Children: 1 to 2 mg/**day**
Adults: 4 to 8 mg/**day**
Cystic fibrosis, pulmonary infection:
Conventional dosing: IM, IV: 3.3 mg/kg/dose every 8 hours
Extended-interval dosing: IV: 10 to 12 mg/kg/dose every 24 hours (Flume 2009; Van Meter 2009); **Note:** The CF Foundation recommends extended-interval dosing as preferred over conventional dosing.
Endocarditis, treatment: IM, IV: 3 mg/kg/**day** divided into 1 to 3 doses in combination with other antibiotics dependent upon organism and source of infection (ie, valve-type) (Baddour 2007; Liu 2011)
Intra-abdominal infection, complicated: IV: 3 to 7.5 mg/kg/**day** divided every 8 to 24 hours (Solomkin 2010)
Peritonitis (CAPD) (Warady 2012): Intraperitoneal:
Intermittent:
Anuric: 0.6 mg/kg/dose every 24 hours in the long dwell
Nonanuric: 0.75 mg/kg/dose every 24 hours in the long dwell
Continuous: Loading dose: 8 mg per liter of dialysate; maintenance dose: 4 mg per liter
Surgical prophylaxis: IV:
AAP recommendations (*Red Book* 2012): 2 mg/kg as a single dose
ASHP recommendation, endorsed by IDSA (Bratzler 2013): Children and Adolescents: 2.5 mg/kg as a single dose
UTI: Extended-interval dosing: IV: Based on data from 179 patients, the following age-directed dosing has been suggested (Carapetis 2001):
1 month to <5 years: 7.5 mg/kg/dose every 24 hours
5 to 10 years: 6 mg/kg/dose every 24 hours
>10 years: 4.5 mg/kg/dose every 24 hours
Adult: **General dosing, susceptible infection:**
Conventional: IM, IV: 1 to 2.5 mg/kg/dose every 8 to 12 hours; to ensure adequate peak concentrations early in therapy, higher initial dosage may be considered in selected patients when extracellular water is increased (edema, septic shock, postsurgical, or trauma)
Once daily: IV: 4 to 7 mg/kg/dose once daily; some clinicians recommend this approach for all patients with normal renal function; this dose is at least as efficacious with similar, if not less, toxicity than conventional dosing

Dosing adjustment in renal impairment:
Infants, Children, and Adolescents: IM, IV:
The following adjustments have been recommended (Aronoff 2007): **Note:** Renally adjusted dose recommendations are based on doses of 2.5 mg/kg/dose every 8 hours:
GFR >50 mL/minute/1.73 m^2: No adjustment required
GFR 30 to 50 mL/minute/1.73 m^2: Administer every 12 to 18 hours
GFR 10 to 29 mL/minute/1.73 m^2: Administer every 18 to 24 hours
GFR <10 mL/minute/1.73 m^2: Administer every 48 to 72 hours
Intermittent hemodialysis: 2 mg/kg/dose; redose as indicated by serum concentration
Peritoneal dialysis (PD): 2 mg/kg/dose; redose as indicated by serum concentration
Continuous renal replacement therapy (CRRT): 2 to 2.5 mg/kg/dose every 12 to 24 hours, monitor serum concentrations
Adults:
Conventional dosing:
CrCl ≥60 mL/minute: Administer every 8 hours
CrCl 40 to 60 mL/minute: Administer every 12 hours
CrCl 20 to 40 mL/minute: Administer every 24 hours
CrCl <20 mL/minute: Loading dose, then monitor concentrations
High-dose therapy: Interval may be extended (eg, every 48 hours) in patients with moderate renal impairment (CrCl 30 to 59 mL/minute) and/or adjusted based on serum concentration determinations
Intermittent hemodialysis (IHD) (administer after hemodialysis on dialysis days) (Heintz 2009): Dialyzable (~50%; variable; dependent on filter, duration, and type of IHD); **Note:** Dosing dependent on the assumption of 3 times/week, complete IHD sessions:
Loading dose: 2 to 3 mg/kg loading dose followed by:
Mild UTI or synergy: 1 mg/kg every 48-72 hours; consider redosing for pre-HD or post-HD serum concentrations <1 mcg/mL
Moderate to severe UTI: 1 to 1.5 mg/kg every 48 to 72 hours; consider redosing for pre-HD serum concentrations <1.5 to 2 mcg/mL or post-HD concentrations <1 mcg/mL
Systemic gram-negative rod infection: 1.5 to 2 mg/kg every 48 to 72 hours; consider redosing for pre-HD serum concentrations <3 to 5 mcg/mL or post-HD concentrations <2 mcg/mL
Peritoneal dialysis (PD):
Administration via PD fluid:
Gram-positive infection (eg, synergy): 3 to 4 mg/L (3 to 4 mcg/mL) of PD fluid
Gram-negative infection: 4 to 8 mg/L (4 to 8 mcg/mL) of PD fluid
Administration via IV, IM route during PD: Dose as for CrCl <10 mL/minute and follow serum concentrations
Continuous renal replacement therapy (CRRT) (Heintz 2009; Trotman 2005): Drug clearance is highly dependent on the method of renal replacement, filter type, and flow rate. Appropriate dosing requires close monitoring of pharmacologic response, signs of adverse reactions due to drug accumulation, as well as drug concentrations in relation to target trough (if appropriate). The following are general recommendations only (based on dialysate flow/ultrafiltration rates of 1 to 2 L/hour and minimal residual renal function) and should not supersede clinical judgment:
CVVH/CVVHD/CVVHDF: Loading dose of 2 to 3 mg/kg followed by:
Mild UTI or synergy: 1 mg/kg every 24 to 36 hours (redose when serum concentration <1 mcg/mL)
Moderate to severe UTI: 1 to 1.5 mg/kg every 24 to 36 hours (redose when serum concentration <1.5 to 2 mcg/mL)
Systemic gram-negative infection: 1.5 to 2.5 mg/kg every 24 to 48 hours (redose when serum concentration <3 to 5 mcg/mL)

Preparation for Administration IV: May dilute in NS or D_5W. In adults, dilution in 50 to 200 mL is recommended; premix admixtures commercially available for some dosages. In infants and children, the volume should be less but allow for accurate measurement and administration; maximum concentration <10 mg/mL.

Administration
IM: Administer undiluted by deep IM route. Slower absorption and lower peak concentrations, probably due to poor circulation in the atrophic muscle, may occur following IM injection; in paralyzed patients, suggest IV route.

IV:
Administer as diluted solution by slow intermittent infusion over 30 to 120 minutes; usual infusion time is 30 to 60 minutes; consider longer infusion time (60 to 120 minutes) with high doses. Conventional doses may also be administered by direct injection with quicker infusion times (<30 minutes) including IV push over 5 minutes (Mendelson 1976). Avoid formulations with preservatives in neonates and infants.
Administer beta-lactams at least 1 hour before or after gentamicin; simultaneous administration may result in reduced antibacterial efficacy.

Monitoring Parameters
Urinalysis, urine output, BUN, serum creatinine, peak and trough serum gentamicin concentrations, hearing test especially for those at risk for ototoxicity or who will be receiving prolonged therapy (>2 weeks), CBC with differential
With conventional dosing, typically obtain serum concentration after the third dose; exceptions for earlier monitoring may include neonates or patients with rapidly changing renal function. With extended-interval dosing, usually obtain serum concentration after first, second, or third dose.
Not all infants and children who receive aminoglycosides require monitoring of serum aminoglycoside concentrations. Indications for use of aminoglycoside serum concentration monitoring include:
Treatment course >5 days
Patients with decreased or changing renal function
Patients with poor therapeutic response
Neonates and Infants <3 months of age
Atypical body constituency (obesity, expanded extracellular fluid volume)
Clinical need for higher doses or shorter intervals (eg, cystic fibrosis, burns, endocarditis, meningitis, critically ill patients, relatively resistant organism)
Patients on hemodialysis or chronic ambulatory peritoneal dialysis
Signs of nephrotoxicity or ototoxicity
Concomitant use of other nephrotoxic agents

Reference Range
Conventional dosing: Timing of serum samples: Draw peak 30 minutes after 30-minute infusion has been completed or 1 hour following IM injection or beginning of infusion; draw trough immediately before next dose
Therapeutic concentrations:
Peak:
Serious infections: 6-8 mcg/mL (12-17 micromole/L)
Life-threatening infections: 8-10 mcg/mL (17-21 micromole/L)
Urinary tract infections: 4-6 mcg/mL
Synergy against gram-positive organisms: 3-5 mcg/mL
Trough:
Serious infections: 0.5-1 mcg/mL
Life-threatening infections: 1-2 mcg/mL
The American Thoracic Society (ATS) recommends trough levels of <1 mcg/mL for adult patients with hospital-acquired pneumonia.
Extended-interval: Note: Pediatric therapeutic monitoring protocols have not been standardized; peak values are 2-3 times greater with extended-interval dosing regimens compared to conventional dosing
Noncystic fibrosis patients: Consider monitoring serum concentration 18-20 hours after the start of the infusion to ensure the drug-free interval does not exceed typical postantibiotic effect (PAE) duration.
Cystic fibrosis patients: Clinically two methods are utilized. Peak: 25-35 mcg/mL (some centers use 20-30 mcg/mL); 18- to 20-hour value: Detectable but <1 mcg/mL; trough: Nondetectable
Method A: Obtain two serum concentrations at least 1 half-life apart after distribution is complete (eg, obtain a serum concentration 2 hours and 10 hours after the start of the infusion), calculate elimination rate and extrapolate a C_{max} and C_{min}
Method B: Obtain a peak serum concentration 60 minutes after a 60-minute infusion and a serum concentration 18-20 hours after the start of the infusion to ensure the drug-free interval does not exceed typical postantibiotic effect (PAE) duration (4-6 hours)

Test Interactions Some penicillin derivatives may accelerate the degradation of aminoglycosides *in vitro*, leading to a potential underestimation of aminoglycoside serum concentration.

Additional Information Some penicillins (eg, carbenicillin, ticarcillin, and piperacillin) have been shown to inactivate aminoglycosides *in vitro*. This has been observed to a greater extent with tobramycin and gentamicin, while amikacin has shown greater stability against inactivation. Concurrent use of these agents may pose a risk of reduced antibacterial efficacy in vivo, particularly in the setting of profound renal impairment; however, definitive clinical evidence is lacking. If combination penicillin/aminoglycoside therapy is desired in a patient with renal dysfunction, separation of doses (if feasible), and routine monitoring of aminoglycoside levels, CBC, and clinical response should be considered.

Dosage Forms Excipient information presented when available (limited, particularly for generics); consult specific product labeling.
Solution, Injection:
Generic: 10 mg/mL (2 mL); 40 mg/mL (2 mL, 20 mL)
Solution, Injection [preservative free]:
Generic: 10 mg/mL (2 mL)
Solution, Intravenous:
Generic: 60 mg (50 mL); 70 mg (50 mL); 80 mg (50 mL, 100 mL); 90 mg (100 mL); 100 mg (50 mL, 100 mL); 120 mg (100 mL); 10 mg/mL (6 mL, 8 mL, 10 mL)

Gentamicin (Ophthalmic) (jen ta MYE sin)

Medication Safety Issues
Sound-alike/look-alike issues:
Gentamicin may be confused with gentian violet, kanamycin, vancomycin

Brand Names: US Garamycin; Gentak

Brand Names: Canada Diogent®; Garamycin®; Gentak®; Gentocin; PMS-Gentamicin

Therapeutic Category Antibiotic, Aminoglycoside; Antibiotic, Ophthalmic

Generic Availability (US) Yes

Use Topical treatment of ophthalmic infections caused by susceptible bacteria (FDA approved in ages ≥1 month and adults)

Pregnancy Risk Factor C

Pregnancy Considerations Adverse events were observed following systemic administration of gentamicin in animal reproduction studies; therefore, gentamicin ophthalmic is classified as pregnancy category C. The amount of gentamicin available systemically following application of the ophthalmic drops is below the limit of detection (<0.5 mcg/mL). Systemic absorption would be required in order for gentamicin to cross the placenta and reach the fetus. When administered IM or IV, gentamicin crosses the placenta. Refer to the Gentamicin (Systemic) monograph for details.

Breast-Feeding Considerations When administered IM, gentamicin is detected in breast milk. The portion that reaches the maternal milk would then be poorly absorbed by the infant's gastrointestinal tract. Refer to the Gentamicin (Systemic) monograph for details. The amount of gentamicin available systemically following application of the ophthalmic drops is below the limit of detection (<0.5 mcg/mL).

Contraindications Hypersensitivity to gentamicin, or other components of the formulation

Warnings/Precautions May delay corneal healing. Topical use has been associated with local sensitization (redness, irritation); discontinue if sensitization is noted. Prolonged use may result in fungal or bacterial superinfection; if purulent discharge, inflammation, or pain are increased, therapy should be re-evaluated. Not for injection into the eye. Not intended for long-term therapy.

Warnings: Additional Pediatric Considerations Ointment should not be used as routine prophylaxis for ophthalmia neonatorum due to reports of severe ocular reactions described as eyelid erythema and swelling, ocular discharge, and periocular blistering, typically reported within 48 hours after administration (Binenbaum, 2010; Nathawad, 2011).

Adverse Reactions

Ophthalmic: Burning, irritation

Rare but important or life-threatening: Allergic reaction, corneal ulceration, hallucinations, purpura, thrombocytopenia

Drug Interactions

Metabolism/Transport Effects None known.

Avoid Concomitant Use There are no known interactions where it is recommended to avoid concomitant use.

Increased Effect/Toxicity There are no known significant interactions involving an increase in effect.

Decreased Effect There are no known significant interactions involving a decrease in effect.

Storage/Stability Store at controlled room temperature of 20°C to 25°C (68°F to 77°F).

Mechanism of Action Interferes with bacterial protein synthesis by binding to 30S and 50S ribosomal subunits resulting in a defective bacterial cell membrane

Pharmacokinetics (Adult data unless noted) Absorption: Ophthalmic drops: Systemic absorption: Undetected (<0.5 mcg/mL)

Dosing: Neonatal Ophthalmic infections: Limited data available: Ophthalmic:

Ointment: Apply 2-3 times daily; **Note:** Use should be reserved for treatment of susceptible infection and not routine prophylaxis for ophthalmia neonatorum.

Solution: Instill 1-2 drops every 4 hours; up to 2 drops every hour for severe infections

Dosing: Usual

Infants, Children, and Adolescents: **Ophthalmic infections:** Ophthalmic:

Ointment: Instill 1/2 inch (1.25 cm) 2-3 times daily

Solution: Instill 1-2 drops every 4 hours; up to 2 drops every hour for severe infections

Adults: **Ophthalmic infections:** Ophthalmic:

Ointment: Instill 1/2 inch (1.25 cm) 2-3 times daily

Solution: Instill 1-2 drops every 4 hours; up to 2 drops every hour for severe infections

Dosing adjustment in renal impairment: There are no dosage adjustments provided in the manufacturer's labeling; however, dosage adjustment unlikely necessary due to low systemic absorption.

Dosing adjustment in hepatic impairment: There are no dosage adjustments provided in the manufacturer's labeling; however, dosage adjustment unlikely necessary due to low systemic absorption.

Administration Gentamicin solution is not for subconjunctival injection. Solution may be instilled into the affected eye or a small amount of ointment may be placed into the conjunctival sac. Avoid contaminating tip of the solution bottle or ointment tube.

Solution: Apply finger pressure to lacrimal sac during and for 1-2 minutes after instillation to decrease risk of absorption and systemic effects

Dosage Forms Excipient information presented when available (limited, particularly for generics); consult specific product labeling. [DSC] = Discontinued product

Ointment, Ophthalmic:

Garamycin: 0.3% (3.5 g [DSC])

Gentak: 0.3% (3.5 g) [contains methylparaben, propylparaben]

Generic: 0.3% (3.5 g)

Solution, Ophthalmic:

Garamycin: 0.3% (5 mL) [contains benzalkonium chloride]

Generic: 0.3% (5 mL, 15 mL)

Gentamicin (Topical) (jen ta MYE sin)

Medication Safety Issues

Sound-alike/look-alike issues:

Gentamicin may be confused with gentian violet, kanamycin, vancomycin

Brand Names: Canada PMS-Gentamicin; ratio-Gentamicin

Therapeutic Category Antibiotic, Aminoglycoside; Antibiotic, Topical

Generic Availability (US) Yes

Use Used to treat superficial infections of the skin including folliculitis, impetigo contagiosa, furunculosis, sycosis barbae, ecthyma, pyoderma gangrenosum, infectious eczematoid dermatitits, pustular acne, pustular psoriasis, infected seborrheic dermatitits or contact dermatitis, and infected excoriations (FDA approved for ages >1 year and adults)

Pregnancy Considerations When administered IM or IV, gentamicin crosses the placenta and produces detectable serum levels in the fetus. Refer to the Gentamicin (Systemic) monograph for details. Systemic absorption following topical application would be required in order for gentamicin to cross the placenta and reach the fetus. Gentamicin is measurable in the serum following topical application to burn patients.

Breast-Feeding Considerations When administered IM, gentamicin enters breast milk; however, it is not well absorbed when taken orally. Refer to the Gentamicin (Systemic) monograph for details.

Contraindications Hypersensitivity to gentamicin or other aminoglycosides

Warnings/Precautions Prolonged use may result in fungal or bacterial superinfection; discontinue if superinfection is noted. Topical use has been associated with local sensitization (redness, irritation); discontinue if sensitization is noted. Not intended for long-term therapy.

Adverse Reactions Dermatologic: Erythema, pruritus

Drug Interactions

Metabolism/Transport Effects None known.

Avoid Concomitant Use

Avoid concomitant use of Gentamicin (Topical) with any of the following: BCG; BCG (Intravesical)

Increased Effect/Toxicity There are no known significant interactions involving an increase in effect.

Decreased Effect

Gentamicin (Topical) may decrease the levels/effects of: BCG; BCG (Intravesical); BCG Vaccine (Immunization); Sodium Picosulfate

Storage/Stability Store at controlled room temperature of 20°C to 25°C (68°F to 77°F).

Mechanism of Action Interferes with bacterial protein synthesis by binding to 30S and 50S ribosomal subunits resulting in a defective bacterial cell membrane

Dosing: Usual Infants, Children, and Adults: Apply 3-4 times/day

Administration Apply a small amount gently to the cleansed affected area

Test Interactions Some penicillin derivatives may accelerate the degradation of aminoglycosides *in vitro*, leading to a potential underestimation of aminoglycoside serum concentration.

Dosage Forms Excipient information presented when available (limited, particularly for generics); consult specific product labeling.

Cream, External:
  Generic: 0.1% (15 g, 30 g)

Ointment, External:
  Generic: 0.1% (15 g, 30 g)

- ◆ **Gentamicin and Prednisolone** *see* Prednisolone and Gentamicin *on page 1759*
- ◆ **Gentamicin Injection, USP (Can)** *see* Gentamicin (Systemic) *on page 965*
- ◆ **Gentamicin Sulfate** *see* Gentamicin (Ophthalmic) *on page 968*
- ◆ **Gentamicin Sulfate** *see* Gentamicin (Systemic) *on page 965*
- ◆ **GenTeal PM [OTC]** *see* Artificial Tears *on page 201*

Gentian Violet (JEN shun VYE oh let)

Medication Safety Issues

Sound-alike/look-alike issues:

Gentian violet may be confused with gentamicin

Therapeutic Category Antibacterial, Topical; Antifungal Agent, Topical

Generic Availability (US) Yes

Use Treatment of cutaneous or mucocutaneous infections caused by *Candida albicans* and other superficial skin infections refractory to topical nystatin, clotrimazole, miconazole, or econazole

Breast-Feeding Considerations Due to the potential for serious adverse reactions in the nursing infant, breast-feeding is not recommended; safer alternatives for topical skin infections are available (Stoukides, 1993).

Contraindications Hypersensitivity to gentian violet or any component of the formulation; ulcerated areas

Warnings/Precautions Discontinue if sensitivity or irritation occur, or if condition worsens. Will stain skin and clothing. Application to ulcerative lesions may result in tattooing. For topical use only; avoid contact with eyes. Not for self-medication (OTC use) for serious burns or deep puncture wounds

Adverse Reactions

Dermatologic: Necrotic skin reactions, staining, vesicle formation

Gastrointestinal: Esophagitis, gastrointestinal irritation, ulceration of mucous membranes

Genitourinary: Hemorrhagic cystitis

Local: Burning, irritation

Ocular: Keratoconjunctivitis

Respiratory: Epistaxis, laryngitis, laryngeal obstruction, tracheitis

Miscellaneous: Allergic contact dermatitis, sensitivity reactions

Drug Interactions

Metabolism/Transport Effects None known.

Avoid Concomitant Use

Avoid concomitant use of Gentian Violet with any of the following: BCG; BCG (Intravesical)

Increased Effect/Toxicity There are no known significant interactions involving an increase in effect.

Decreased Effect

Gentian Violet may decrease the levels/effects of: BCG; BCG (Intravesical); BCG Vaccine (Immunization); Sodium Picosulfate

Mechanism of Action Topical antiseptic/germicide effective against some vegetative gram-positive bacteria, particularly *Staphylococcus* sp, and some yeast; it is much less effective against gram-negative bacteria and is ineffective against acid-fast bacteria

Dosing: Usual Topical: Oral candidiasis:

Infants: Apply to affected area (under tongue or on lesion) twice daily; solutions diluted to 0.25% to 0.5% may be less irritating.

Children and Adults: Apply to affected area once or twice daily; solutions diluted to 0.25% to 0.5% may be less irritating. Do not swallow.

Administration Topical: Apply to lesions with cotton; do not apply to ulcerative lesions on the face. Keep affected area dry and exposed to air.

Additional Information 0.25% or 0.5% solution is less irritating than a 1% to 2% solution and is reported to be as effective

Dosage Forms Excipient information presented when available (limited, particularly for generics); consult specific product labeling.

Solution, External:
  Generic: 1% (59 mL); 2% (59 mL, 59.14 mL)

- ◆ **Gentle Laxative [OTC]** *see* Bisacodyl *on page 289*
- ◆ **Gentocin (Can)** *see* Gentamicin (Ophthalmic) *on page 968*
- ◆ **Geodon** *see* Ziprasidone *on page 2216*
- ◆ **Geri-Dryl [OTC]** *see* DiphenhydrAMINE (Systemic) *on page 668*
- ◆ **Geri-Hydrolac™ [OTC]** *see* Lactic Acid and Ammonium Hydroxide *on page 1202*
- ◆ **Geri-Hydrolac™-12 [OTC]** *see* Lactic Acid and Ammonium Hydroxide *on page 1202*
- ◆ **Geri-kot [OTC]** *see* Senna *on page 1914*
- ◆ **Geri-Mucil [OTC]** *see* Psyllium *on page 1804*
- ◆ **Geri-Pectate [OTC]** *see* Bismuth Subsalicylate *on page 290*
- ◆ **Geri-Stool [OTC]** *see* Docusate and Senna *on page 698*
- ◆ **Geri-Tussin [OTC]** *see* GuaiFENesin *on page 988*
- ◆ **GG** *see* GuaiFENesin *on page 988*
- ◆ **GI87084B** *see* Remifentanil *on page 1843*
- ◆ **Giazo** *see* Balsalazide *on page 257*
- ◆ **Glargine Insulin** *see* Insulin Glargine *on page 1126*
- ◆ **GlcCerase** *see* Velaglucerase Alfa *on page 2165*
- ◆ **Gleevec** *see* Imatinib *on page 1078*
- ◆ **Gleostine** *see* Lomustine *on page 1286*
- ◆ **Gliadel Wafer** *see* Carmustine *on page 377*
- ◆ **Glibenclamide** *see* GlyBURIDE *on page 975*

GlipiZIDE (GLIP i zide)

Medication Safety Issues

Sound-alike/look-alike issues:

GlipiZIDE may be confused with glimepiride, glyBURIDE

Glucotrol may be confused with Glucophage, Glucotrol XL, glyBURIDE, GlycoTrol (dietary supplement)

High alert medication:

The Institute for Safe Medication Practices (ISMP) includes this medication among its list of drugs which have a heightened risk of causing significant patient harm when used in error.

Related Information

Oral Medications That Should Not Be Crushed or Altered *on page 2476*

Brand Names: US GlipiZIDE XL; Glucotrol; Glucotrol XL

Therapeutic Category Antidiabetic Agent, Oral; Antidiabetic Agent, Sulfonylurea; Hypoglycemic Agent, Oral

Generic Availability (US) Yes

Use Management of type II diabetes mellitus (noninsulin-dependent, NIDDM) when hyperglycemia cannot be managed by diet alone; may be used concomitantly with metformin or insulin to improve glycemic control

Pregnancy Risk Factor C

Pregnancy Considerations Adverse events have been observed in some animal reproduction studies. Glipizide was found to cross the placenta in vitro (Elliott 1994). Severe hypoglycemia lasting 4 to 10 days has been noted in infants born to mothers taking a sulfonylurea at the time of delivery.

In women with diabetes, maternal hyperglycemia can be associated with congenital malformations as well as adverse effects in the fetus, neonate, and the mother (ACOG 2005; ADA 2015; Kitzmiller 2008; Metzger 2007). To prevent adverse outcomes, prior to conception and throughout pregnancy maternal blood glucose and HbA_{1c} should be kept as close to target goals as possible but without causing significant hypoglycemia (ACOG 2013; ADA 2015; Blumer 2013; Kitzmiller 2008). Prior to pregnancy, effective contraception should be used until glycemic control is achieved (Kitzmiller 2008). Other agents are currently recommended to treat diabetes in pregnant women (ACOG 2013; Blumer 2013).

The manufacturer recommends if glipizide is used during pregnancy, it should be discontinued at least 1 month before the expected delivery date.

Breast-Feeding Considerations Data from two mother-infant pairs note that glipizide was not detected in breast milk (Feig 2005). According to the manufacturer, due to the potential for hypoglycemia in the nursing infant, a decision should be made whether to discontinue nursing or to discontinue the drug, taking into account the importance of treatment to the mother. Breast-feeding is encouraged for all women, including those with diabetes (ACOG 2005; Blumer 2013; Metzger 2007). A small snack (such as milk) before nursing may help decrease the risk of hypoglycemia in women with pregestational diabetes (ACOG 2005; ADA 2015; Reader 2004). All types of insulin may be used while breast-feeding and some oral agents, including glipizide, may be acceptable for use as well (Metzger, 2007).

Contraindications Hypersensitivity to glipizide or any component of the formulation; type 1 diabetes mellitus (insulin dependent, IDDM); diabetic ketoacidosis (with or without coma)

Warnings/Precautions All sulfonylurea drugs are capable of producing severe hypoglycemia. Hypoglycemia is more likely to occur when caloric intake is deficient, after severe or prolonged exercise, when ethanol is ingested, or when more than one glucose-lowering drug is used. It is also more likely in elderly patients, malnourished patients and in patients with impaired renal or hepatic function; use with caution. Autonomic neuropathy, advanced age, and concomitant use of beta-blockers or other sympatholytic agents may impair the patient's ability to recognize the signs and symptoms of hypoglycemia; use with caution.

Use with caution in patients with hepatic or renal impairment. It may be necessary to discontinue therapy and administer insulin if the patient is exposed to stress (fever, trauma, infection, surgery). Loss of efficacy may be observed following prolonged use as a result of the progression of type 2 diabetes mellitus which results in continued beta cell destruction. In patients who were previously responding to sulfonylurea therapy, consider additional factors which may be contributing to decreased efficacy (eg, inappropriate dose, nonadherence to diet and exercise regimen). If no contributing factors can be identified, consider discontinuing use of the sulfonylurea due to secondary failure of treatment. Additional antidiabetic therapy (eg, insulin) will be required.

Patients with G6PD deficiency may be at an increased risk of sulfonylurea-induced hemolytic anemia; however, cases have also been described in patients without G6PD deficiency during postmarketing surveillance. Use with caution and consider a nonsulfonylurea alternative in patients with G6PD deficiency.

Product labeling states oral hypoglycemic drugs may be associated with an increased cardiovascular mortality as compared to treatment with diet alone or diet plus insulin. Data to support this association are limited, and several studies, including a large prospective trial (UKPDS) have not supported an association. Avoid use of extended release tablets (Glucotrol XL®) in patients with known stricture/narrowing of the GI tract.

Sulfonamide ("sulfa") allergy: The FDA-approved product labeling for many medications containing a sulfonamide chemical group includes a broad contraindication in patients with a prior allergic reaction to sulfonamides. There is a potential for cross-reactivity between members of a specific class (eg, two antibiotic sulfonamides). However, concerns for cross-reactivity have previously extended to all compounds containing the sulfonamide structure (SO_2NH_2). An expanded understanding of allergic mechanisms indicates cross-reactivity between antibiotic sulfonamides and nonantibiotic sulfonamides may not occur or at the very least this potential is extremely low (Brackett 2004; Johnson 2005; Slatore 2004; Tornero 2004). In particular, mechanisms of cross-reaction due to antibody production (anaphylaxis) are unlikely to occur with nonantibiotic sulfonamides. T-cell-mediated (type IV) reactions (eg, maculopapular rash) are less well understood and it is not possible to completely exclude this potential based on current insights. In cases where prior reactions were severe (Stevens-Johnson syndrome/TEN), some clinicians choose to avoid exposure to these classes.

Adverse Reactions

Cardiovascular: Syncope

Central nervous system: Anxiety, depression, dizziness, drowsiness, headache, hypoesthesia, insomnia, nervousness, pain

Dermatologic: Eczema, erythema, maculopapular eruptions, morbilliform eruptions, pruritus, rash, urticaria

Endocrine & metabolic: Hypoglycemia

Gastrointestinal: Abdominal pain, constipation, diarrhea, dyspepsia, flatulence, nausea, vomiting

Hepatic: Alkaline phosphatase increased, AST increased, LDH increased

Neuromuscular & skeletal: Arthralgia, leg cramps, myalgia, paresthesia, tremor

Ocular: Blurred vision

Renal: Blood urea nitrogen increased, creatinine increased

Respiratory: Rhinitis

Miscellaneous: Diaphoresis

Rare but important or life-threatening: Agranulocytosis, anorexia, aplastic anemia, arrhythmia, blood in stool, cholestatic jaundice, conjunctivitis, disulfiram-like reaction, edema, gait instability, hemolytic anemia, hypertension, hypertonia, hyponatremia, jaundice, leukopenia, liver injury, migraine, pancytopenia, photosensitivity, porphyria, retinal hemorrhage, SIADH, thrombocytopenia, vertigo

Drug Interactions

Metabolism/Transport Effects Substrate of CYP2C9 (major); **Note:** Assignment of Major/Minor substrate status based on clinically relevant drug interaction potential

Avoid Concomitant Use

Avoid concomitant use of GlipiZIDE with any of the following: Mecamylamine

Increased Effect/Toxicity

GlipiZIDE may increase the levels/effects of: Alcohol (Ethyl); Carbocisteine; Hypoglycemia-Associated

Agents; Mecamylamine; Porfimer; Verteporfin; Vitamin K Antagonists

The levels/effects of GlipiZIDE may be increased by: Alpha-Lipoic Acid; Androgens; Antidiabetic Agents; Antidiabetic Agents (Thiazolidinedione); Beta-Blockers; Ceritinib; Chloramphenicol; Cimetidine; Clarithromycin; Cyclic Antidepressants; CYP2C9 Inhibitors (Moderate); CYP2C9 Inhibitors (Strong); Dexketoprofen; DPP-IV Inhibitors; Fibric Acid Derivatives; Fluconazole; GLP-1 Agonists; Herbs (Hypoglycemic Properties); MAO Inhibitors; Metreleptin; Miconazole (Oral); Mifepristone; Pegvisomant; Posaconazole; Probenecid; Quinolone Antibiotics; Ranitidine; Salicylates; Selective Serotonin Reuptake Inhibitors; SGLT2 Inhibitors; Sulfonamide Derivatives; Vitamin K Antagonists; Voriconazole

Decreased Effect

The levels/effects of GlipiZIDE may be decreased by: Colesevelam; CYP2C9 Inducers (Strong); Dabrafenib; Hyperglycemia-Associated Agents; Quinolone Antibiotics; Rifampin; Thiazide Diuretics

Food Interactions

Ethanol: May cause rare disulfiram reactions. Management: Monitor patients.

Food: A delayed release of insulin may occur if glipizide is taken with food. Management: Immediate release tablets should be administered 30 minutes before meals to avoid erratic absorption.

Storage/Stability Store below 30°C (86°F)

Mechanism of Action Stimulates insulin release from the pancreatic beta cells; reduces glucose output from the liver; insulin sensitivity is increased at peripheral target sites

Pharmacodynamics

Onset of action: Immediate release formulation: 15-30 minutes; extended release formulation: 2-3 hours

Maximum effect: Immediate release formulation: Within 2-3 hours; extended release formulation: 6-12 hours

Duration: Immediate release formulation: 12-24 hours; extended release formulation: 24 hours

Average decrease in fasting blood glucose (when used as monotherapy): 60-70 mg/dL

Pharmacokinetics (Adult data unless noted)

Absorption: Rapid and complete

Distribution: V_d: Adults: 10 L

Protein binding: 98% to 99%

Metabolism: Extensive liver metabolism to inactive metabolites

Bioavailability: 80% to 100%

Half-life: Adults: 2-5 hours

Time to peak serum concentration:

Immediate release formulation: 1-3 hours

Extended release formulation: 6-12 hours

Elimination: <10% of drug excreted into urine as unchanged drug; 90% of drug excreted as metabolites in urine and 10% excreted in feces

Dosing: Usual Adults: Oral:

Management of noninsulin-dependent diabetes mellitus in patients **previously untreated:** Initial: 5 mg/day immediate release or extended release tablets; adjust dosage in 2.5-5 mg daily increments in intervals of 3-7 days for immediate release tablets or 5 mg daily increments in intervals of at least 7 days for extended release tablets; if total daily dose for immediate release tablets is >15 mg, divide into twice daily dosage; maximum daily dose for immediate release tablets: 40 mg; maximum daily dose for extended release tablets: 20 mg

Note: Patients may be converted from immediate release tablets to extended release tablets by giving the nearest equivalent total daily dose once daily

Management of noninsulin-dependent diabetes mellitus in patients **previously maintained on insulin:**

Insulin dosage ≤20 units/day: Use recommended initial dose and abruptly discontinue insulin

Insulin dosage >20 units/day: Use recommended initial dose and reduce daily insulin dosage by 50%; continue to withdraw daily insulin dosage gradually over several days as tolerated with incremental increases of glipizide

Dosing adjustment/comments in renal impairment: CrCl <10 mL/minute: Some investigators recommend not using

Dosing adjustment in hepatic impairment: Reduce initial dosage to 2.5 mg/day

Administration Oral: Administer immediate release tablets 30 minutes before a meal; extended release tablets should be swallowed whole and administered with breakfast; do not cut, crush, or chew

Monitoring Parameters Signs and symptoms of hypoglycemia, fasting blood glucose, glycosylated hemoglobin (hemoglobin A_{1c})

Reference Range Target range:

Blood glucose: Fasting and preprandial: 80-120 mg/dL; bedtime: 100-140 mg/dL

Glycosylated hemoglobin (hemoglobin A_{1c}): <7%

Additional Information When transferring from other sulfonylurea antidiabetic agents to glyburide, with the exception of chlorpropamide, the administration of the other agent may be abruptly discontinued; due to the prolonged elimination half-life of chlorpropamide, a 2- to 3-day drug-free interval may be advisable before glipizide therapy is begun

Dosage Forms Excipient information presented when available (limited, particularly for generics); consult specific product labeling.

Tablet, Oral:

Glucotrol: 5 mg, 10 mg [scored]

Generic: 5 mg, 10 mg

Tablet Extended Release 24 Hour, Oral:

GlipiZIDE XL: 2.5 mg, 5 mg, 10 mg

Glucotrol XL: 2.5 mg, 5 mg, 10 mg

Generic: 2.5 mg, 5 mg, 10 mg

◆ **GlipiZIDE XL** *see* GlipiZIDE *on page* 970

◆ **Glivec** *see* Imatinib *on page* 1078

◆ **GlucaGen (Can)** *see* Glucagon *on page* 972

◆ **GlucaGen Diagnostic** *see* Glucagon *on page* 972

◆ **GlucaGen HypoKit** *see* Glucagon *on page* 972

Glucagon (GLOO ka gon)

Brand Names: US GlucaGen Diagnostic; GlucaGen HypoKit; Glucagon Emergency

Brand Names: Canada GlucaGen; GlucaGen HypoKit

Therapeutic Category Antihypoglycemic Agent

Generic Availability (US) No

Use Treatment of severe hypoglycemia [FDA approved in pediatric patients (age not specified) and adults]; diagnostic aid in the radiologic examination of GI tract to temporarily inhibit GI tract movement (FDA approved in adults); has also been used for prevention of hypoglycemia during illness and management of beta-blocker or calcium channel blocker toxicity

Pregnancy Risk Factor B

Pregnancy Considerations Adverse events have not been observed in animal reproduction studies.

Breast-Feeding Considerations Glucagon is not absorbed from the GI tract and therefore, it is unlikely adverse effects would occur in a breast-feeding infant.

Contraindications Known hypersensitivity to glucagon, lactose, or any component of the formulation; patients with pheochromocytoma or insulinoma

Warnings/Precautions Use of glucagon is contraindicated in insulinoma; exogenous glucagon may cause an initial rise in blood glucose followed by rebound hypoglycemia. Use of glucagon is contraindicated in pheochromocytoma; exogenous glucagon may cause the release of catecholamines, resulting in an increase in blood pressure. Use caution with prolonged fasting, starvation, adrenal insufficiency, glucagonoma, or chronic hypoglycemia; levels of glucose stores in liver may be decreased. Allergic reactions including skin rash and anaphylactic shock (with hypotension and respiratory difficulties) have been reported; reactions have generally been associated with endoscopic patients. Use with caution in patients with cardiac disease undergoing endoscopic or radiographic procedures. Use caution if using as diagnostic aid in patients with diabetes on insulin; may cause hyperglycemia. Supplemental carbohydrates should be given to patients who respond to glucagon for severe hypoglycemia to prevent secondary hypoglycemia. Monitor blood glucose levels closely.

In patients with hypoglycemia secondary to insulin or sulfonylurea overdose, dextrose should be immediately administered; if IV access cannot be established or if dextrose is not available, glucagon may be considered as alternative acute treatment until dextrose can be administered.

May contain lactose; avoid administration in hereditary galactose intolerance, Lapp lactase deficiency, or glucose-galactose malabsorption.

Warnings: Additional Pediatric Considerations Glucagon depletes glycogen stores; supplemental carbohydrates (which may include IV dextrose) should be administered as soon as physically possible. If a patient fails to respond to glucagon, IV dextrose must be administered.

Adverse Reactions Frequency not defined.

Cardiovascular: Hypertension, hypotension (up to 2 hours after GI procedures), increased blood pressure, increased pulse, tachycardia

Gastrointestinal: Nausea, vomiting (high incidence with rapid administration of high doses)

Miscellaneous: Anaphylaxis, hypersensitivity reaction

Rare but important or life-threatening: Hypoglycemia, hypoglycemic coma, respiratory distress, urticaria

Drug Interactions

Metabolism/Transport Effects None known.

Avoid Concomitant Use

Avoid concomitant use of Glucagon with any of the following: Anticholinergic Agents

Increased Effect/Toxicity

Glucagon may increase the levels/effects of: Vitamin K Antagonists

The levels/effects of Glucagon may be increased by: Anticholinergic Agents

Decreased Effect

Glucagon may decrease the levels/effects of: Antidiabetic Agents

The levels/effects of Glucagon may be decreased by: Indomethacin

Food Interactions Glucagon depletes glycogen stores.

Storage/Stability Prior to reconstitution, store at controlled room temperature of 20°C to 25°C (69°F to 77°F) up to 24 months; excursions are permitted between 15°C and 30°C (59°F and 86°F). Do not freeze. Protect from light. Use reconstituted solution immediately; discard unused portion.

Mechanism of Action Stimulates adenylate cyclase to produce increased cyclic AMP, which promotes hepatic glycogenolysis and gluconeogenesis, causing a raise in blood glucose levels; antihypoglycemic effect requires preexisting hepatic glycogen stores. Extra hepatic effects of glucagon include relaxation of the smooth muscle of the stomach, duodenum, small bowel, and colon.

Pharmacodynamics

Blood glucose increase:

Onset of action: IM: 10 minutes; IV: 1 minute

Peak effect: IM: 26-30 minutes; SubQ: 30 minutes

Duration: IM, IV: 60-90 minutes

GI tract relaxation:

Onset of action: IM: 4-10 minutes; IV: ≤1 minute

Duration: IM: 12-32 minutes; IV: 9-25 minutes

Pharmacokinetics (Adult data unless noted)

Distribution: V_d: 0.25 L/kg

Metabolism: Primarily hepatic; some inactivation occurring renally and in plasma

Half-life, plasma: IM: 45 minutes; IV: 8-18 minutes

Dosing: Neonatal

Hypoglycemia, persistent:

IM, IV, SubQ: 0.02-0.2 mg/kg/dose (maximum dose: 1 mg), may repeat dose in 20 minutes if needed (Hawdon, 1993; Mehta, 1987); **Note:** Wide variance in doses exists between manufacturer's labeling and published case reports.

Continuous IV infusion: 1 mg infused over 24 hours; doses >0.02 mg/kg/**hour** did not produce additional benefit; dosing based on a retrospective observation of 55 newborns (GA: 24-41 weeks) with hypoglycemia due to multiple causes (Miralles, 2002)

Congenital hyperinsulinism; hyperinsulinemic hypoglycemia: Continuous IV infusion: 0.005-0.02 mg/kg/**hour**; some centers use a lower dose (0.001 mg/kg/**hour**) in combination with octreotide (Aynsley-Green, 2000; Hussain, 2004, Kapoor, 2009)

Dosing: Usual

Pediatric:

Hypoglycemia, severe; treatment:

Weight-directed dosing:

Manufacturer's labeling: Infants, Children, or Adolescents weighing <20 kg: Glucagon: IM, IV, SubQ: 0.02-0.03 mg/kg; maximum dose: 0.5 mg

Alternate dosing: Infants, Children, and Adolescents:

AAP: IM, IV, SubQ: 0.03 mg/kg; maximum dose: 1 mg (Hegenbarth, 2008)

IDF-ISPAD: IM, SubQ: 0.01-0.03 mg/kg; maximum dose dependent on age: <12 years: 0.5 mg; ≥12 years: 1 mg (IDF-ISPAD, 2011)

Fixed dosing; age-directed:

Manufacturer's labeling: GlucaGen: IM, IV, SubQ:

Infants and Children <6 years: 0.5 mg

Children and Adolescents ≥6 years: 1 mg

Alternate dosing: IM, SubQ:

IDF-ISPAD (IDF-ISPAD, 2011):

Infants and Children <12 years: 0.5 mg

Children and Adolescents ≥12 years: 1 mg

CDA (Canadian Diabetes Association, 2013):

Infants and Children ≤5 years: 0.5 mg

Children and Adolescents >5 years: 1 mg

Fixed dosing; weight-directed: Infants, Children, and Adolescents: Manufacturer's labeling: IM, IV, SubQ:

Glucagon: Patient weight:

<20 kg: 0.5 mg

≥20 kg: 1 mg

GlucaGen: Patient weight:

<25 kg: 0.5 mg

≥25 kg: 1 mg

Hypoglycemia, prevention during illness (fixed dosing, mini-dose): Limited data available (Haymond, 2001; IDF-ISPAD, 2011): SubQ: **Note:** These doses are lower than hypoglycemia treatment doses and have been shown to prevent hypoglycemia for several hours during hypoglycemia-associated illness (eg, gastroenteritis, nausea/vomiting).

Infants and Children <2 years: 0.02 mg

Children and Adolescents 2-15 years: 0.01 mg per year of age
Adolescents >15 years: 0.15 mg

Beta-blocker or calcium channel blocker toxicity/overdose:
Infants and Children: Limited data available (Hegenbarth, 2008): IV:
Loading dose: 0.03-0.15 mg/kg
Continuous IV infusion: 0.07 mg/kg/hour; maximum rate: 5 mg/hour
Adolescents [Hegenbarth, 2008; PALS guidelines (Kleinman, 2010)]: IV:
Loading dose: 5-10 mg over several minutes
Continuous IV infusion: 1-5 mg/hour

Adult:
Hypoglycemia: IM, IV, SubQ: 1 mg; may repeat in 20 minutes as needed; **Note:** IV dextrose should be administered as soon as it is available; if patient fails to respond to glucagon, IV dextrose must be given.
Beta-blocker- or calcium channel blocker-induced myocardial depression (with or without hypotension) unresponsive to standard measures: IV: 3-10 mg (or 0.05-0.15 mg/kg) bolus followed by an infusion of 3-5 mg/hour (or 0.05-0.1 mg/kg/hour); titrate infusion rate to achieve adequate hemodynamic response (ACLS, 2010)
Diagnostic aid:
IM: 1-2 mg 10 minutes prior to gastrointestinal procedure
IV: 0.25-2 mg 10 minutes prior to gastrointestinal procedure
Dosing adjustments in renal impairment: There are no dosage adjustment provided in manufacturer's labeling.
Dosing adjustments in hepatic impairment: There are no dosage adjustment provided in manufacturer's labeling.

Preparation for Administration Parenteral: Reconstitute powder for injection by adding 1 mL of manufacturer-supplied sterile diluent or SWFI to a vial containing 1 unit of the drug, to provide solutions containing 1 mg of glucagon/mL. In pediatric patients, doses >2 mg should be reconstituted with SWFI instead of manufacturer supplied diluent (Hegenbarth 2008). Gently roll vial to dissolve. Solution for continuous IV infusion may be prepared with further dilution in NS or D_5W (Love 1998); in adults the usual IV infusion concentration is 0.08 mg/mL (4 mg in 50 mL D_5W).

Administration Parenteral May administer IM, IV, or SubQ. When treating beta-blocker/calcium channel blocker toxicity, initial loading dose (bolus) should be administered over 3 to 5 minutes; may also administer as a continuous IV infusion; ensure adequate supply available to continue therapy (AHA [Vanden Hoek] 2010).

Mini-dose: Inject subcutaneously using an insulin syringe (U-100); 1 unit on the syringe provides 0.01 mg of glucagon (Haymond 2001; IDF-ISPAD 2011)

Monitoring Parameters Blood glucose, blood pressure, ECG, heart rate, mentation; in pediatric patients when used for hypoglycemia prevention (mini-doses), monitor blood glucose [every 30 minutes for the first hours and then at least hourly (or more often if appropriate)] (Haymond, 2001)

Dosage Forms Excipient information presented when available (limited, particularly for generics); consult specific product labeling.
Kit, Injection:
Glucagon Emergency: 1 mg
Solution Reconstituted, Injection, as hydrochloride:
GlucaGen Diagnostic: 1 mg (1 ea)
GlucaGen HypoKit: 1 mg (1 ea)

◆ **Glucagon Emergency** *see* Glucagon *on page 972*
◆ **Glucagon Hydrochloride** *see* Glucagon *on page 972*

Glucarpidase (gloo KAR pid ase)

Brand Names: US Voraxaze
Therapeutic Category Antidote; Enzyme
Generic Availability (US) No

Use Treatment of toxic plasma methotrexate concentrations (>1 micromole/L) in patients with delayed clearance due to renal impairment (FDA approved in ages ≥1 month and adults); has also been used as a rescue agent to reduce methotrexate toxicity in patients with accidental intrathecal methotrexate overdose

Note: Due to the risk of subtherapeutic methotrexate exposure, glucarpidase is **not** indicated when methotrexate clearance is within expected range (plasma methotrexate concentration ≤2 standard deviations of mean methotrexate excretion curve specific for dose administered) **or** with normal renal function or mild renal impairment

Prescribing and Access Restrictions Voraxaze® is distributed through ASD Healthcare; procurement information is available (24 hours a day; 365 days a year) at 1-855-7-VORAXAZE (1-855-786-7292). Voraxaze® is also commercially available in the U.S. through certain pharmacy wholesalers on a drop-ship basis; orders will only be processed during business hours for overnight delivery. For additional information, refer to http://www.btgplc.com/products/specialty-pharmaceuticals/voraxaze.

Pregnancy Risk Factor C

Pregnancy Considerations Animal reproduction studies have not been conducted. If administered to a pregnant woman, the risk to the fetus is unknown; use only if clearly needed. In general, medications used as antidotes should take into consideration the health and prognosis of the mother.

Breast-Feeding Considerations Caution should be used if administered to a breast-feeding woman.

Contraindications There are no contraindications listed in the manufacturer's labeling.

Warnings/Precautions Serious allergic reactions have been reported.

Leucovorin calcium administration should be continued after glucarpidase; the same dose as was given prior to glucarpidase should be continued for the first 48 hours after glucarpidase; after 48 hours, leucovorin doses should be based on methotrexate concentrations. A single methotrexate concentration should not determine when leucovorin should be discontinued; continue leucovorin until the methotrexate concentration remains below the threshold for leucovorin treatment for ≥3 days. Leucovorin calcium is a substrate for glucarpidase and may compete with methotrexate for binding sites; **do not administer leucovorin calcium within 2 hours before or after glucarpidase.** In addition to leucovorin, glucarpidase use should be accompanied with adequate hydration and urinary alkalinization. During the first 48 hours following glucarpidase administration, the only reliable method of measuring methotrexate concentrations is the chromatographic method. DAMPA, an inactive methotrexate metabolite with a half-life of 9 hours, may interfere with immunoassay and result in the overestimation of the methotrexate concentration (when collected within 48 hours of glucarpidase administration). Glucarpidase use for intrathecal methotrexate overdose (off-label route/use) should be used in conjunction with immediate lumbar drainage; concurrent dexamethasone (4 mg IV every 6 hours for 4 doses) may minimize methotrexate-induced chemical arachnoiditis; leucovorin calcium (100 mg IV every 6 hours for 4 doses) may prevent systemic methotrexate toxicity (Widemann, 2004).

Warnings: Additional Pediatric Considerations In children, upon resolution of renal dysfunction following glucarpidase therapy, rechallenge with high-dose methotrexate therapy has been successfully completed; monitor renal function and serum methotrexate concentrations closely in these patients (Christensen, 2012). Glucarpidase for intrathecal methotrexate overdose should be used in conjunction with immediate lumbar drainage; in a case series of seven patients including four children (5 to 9 years of age) concurrent dexamethasone (4 mg IV every 6 hours for 4 doses) may minimize methotrexate-induced chemical arachnoiditis; leucovorin calcium (100 mg IV every 6 hours for 4 doses) may prevent systemic methotrexate toxicity (Widemann, 2004).

Adverse Reactions

Cardiovascular: Flushing, hypotension

Central nervous system: Headache

Gastrointestinal: Nausea/vomiting

Immunologic: Antibody development

Neuromuscular & skeletal: Paresthesia

Rare but important or life-threatening: Blurred vision, diarrhea, hypersensitivity reaction, hypertension, localized warm feeling, skin rash, throat irritation, tremor

Drug Interactions

Metabolism/Transport Effects None known.

Avoid Concomitant Use There are no known interactions where it is recommended to avoid concomitant use.

Increased Effect/Toxicity There are no known significant interactions involving an increase in effect.

Decreased Effect

Glucarpidase may decrease the levels/effects of: Leucovorin Calcium-Levoleucovorin

Storage/Stability Store intact vials refrigerated at 2°C to 8°C (36°F to 46°F); do not freeze. Reconstituted solutions should be used immediately or may be stored for up to 4 hours under refrigeration.

Mechanism of Action Recombinant enzyme which rapidly hydrolyzes the carboxyl-terminal glutamate residue from extracellular methotrexate into inactive metabolites (DAMPA and glutamate), resulting in a rapid reduction of methotrexate concentrations independent of renal function

Pharmacodynamics

Onset of action: Methotrexate toxicity: IV: Within 15 minutes a ≥97% reduction of methotrexate serum concentrations

Duration: Methotrexate toxicity: Up to 8 days a >95% of methotrexate serum concentration reduction maintained

Pharmacokinetics (Adult data unless noted)

Distribution: V_d: IV: 3.6 L; distribution restricted to plasma volume

Half-life: IV: Normal renal function: 6-9 hours; impaired renal function (CrCl <30 mL/minute): 8-10 hours (Phillips, 2008)

Dosing: Usual Pediatric:

Methotrexate toxicity: Infants, Children, and Adolescents: IV: 50 units/kg as a single dose (Buchen 2005; Widemann 1997; Widemann 2010)

Intrathecal methotrexate overdose: Limited data available: Children ≥5 years and Adolescents: Intrathecal: 2,000 units as soon as possible after accidental exposure (O'Marcaigh 1996; Widemann 2004)

Adult: **Methotrexate toxicity:** IV: 50 units/kg (Buchen 2005; Widemann 1997; Widemann 2010)

Dosing adjustment in renal impairment: Infants, Children, Adolescents, and Adults: No dosage adjustment necessary

Dosing adjustment in hepatic impairment: Infants, Children, Adolescents, and Adults: There are no dosage adjustment provided in the manufacturer's labeling; has not been studied

Preparation for Administration

IV: Reconstitute each vial (1,000 units/vial) with 1 mL NS; mix gently by rolling or tilting vial; do not shake. Upon reconstitution, solution should be clear, colorless and free of particulate matter.

Intrathecal: Reconstitute 2,000 units with 12 mL preservative-free NS (Widemann 2004)

Administration

IV: Prior to administration, flush IV line; infuse glucarpidase over 5 minutes; flush IV line after administration.

Intrathecal: Typically 2,000 units administered over 5 minutes via lumbar route, ventriculostomy, Ommaya reservoir, or lumbar and ventriculostomy (O'Marcaigh 1996; Widemann 2004); others reports of lower doses (1,000 units) have been administered through ventricular or lumbar catheter over 5 minutes (O'Marcaigh 1996)

Monitoring Parameters Serum methotrexate concentrations using chromatographic method if <48 hours from glucarpidase administration (DAMPA interferes with immunoassay results until >48 hours). CBC with differential, bilirubin, ALT, AST, serum creatinine; evaluate for signs/symptoms of methotrexate toxicity

Test Interactions Methotrexate levels: During the first 48 hours following glucarpidase administration, the only reliable method of measuring methotrexate concentrations is the chromatographic method. DAMPA, an inactive methotrexate metabolite with a half-life of 9 hours, may interfere with immunoassay and result in the overestimation of the methotrexate concentration (when collected within 48 hours of glucarpidase administration).

Additional Information Leucovorin calcium administration should be continued after glucarpidase; the same dose as was given prior to glucarpidase should be continued for the first 48 hours after glucarpidase; after 48 hours, leucovorin doses should be based on methotrexate concentrations. A single methotrexate concentration should not determine when leucovorin should be discontinued; continue leucovorin until the methotrexate concentration remains below the threshold for leucovorin treatment for ≥3 days.

Dosage Forms Excipient information presented when available (limited, particularly for generics); consult specific product labeling.

Solution Reconstituted, Intravenous [preservative free]:

Voraxaze: 1000 units (1 ea)

- ◆ **Glucobay (Can)** *see* Acarbose *on page* *43*
- ◆ **Glucophage** *see* MetFORMIN *on page* *1375*
- ◆ **Glucophage XR** *see* MetFORMIN *on page* *1375*
- ◆ **Glucose** *see* Dextrose *on page* *633*
- ◆ **Glucose Monohydrate** *see* Dextrose *on page* *633*
- ◆ **Glucose Nursette [OTC]** *see* Dextrose *on page* *633*
- ◆ **Glucotrol** *see* GlipiZIDE *on page* *970*
- ◆ **Glucotrol XL** *see* GlipiZIDE *on page* *970*
- ◆ **Glulisine Insulin** *see* Insulin Glulisine *on page* *1129*
- ◆ **Glumetza** *see* MetFORMIN *on page* *1375*
- ◆ **Glutol [OTC]** *see* Dextrose *on page* *633*
- ◆ **Glutose 15 [OTC]** *see* Dextrose *on page* *633*
- ◆ **Glutose 45 [OTC]** *see* Dextrose *on page* *633*
- ◆ **Glybenclamide** *see* GlyBURIDE *on page* *975*
- ◆ **Glybenzcyclamide** *see* GlyBURIDE *on page* *975*

GlyBURIDE (GLYE byoor ide)

Medication Safety Issues

Sound-alike/look-alike issues:

GlyBURIDE may be confused with glipiZIDE, Glucotrol

Diaβeta may be confused with Zebeta

Micronase may be confused with Microzide

High alert medication:

The Institute for Safe Medication Practices (ISMP) includes this medication among its list of drugs which have a heightened risk of causing significant patient harm when used in error.

BEERS Criteria medication:

This drug may be potentially inappropriate for use in geriatric patients (Quality of evidence - high; Strength of recommendation - strong).

Brand Names: US Diabeta; Glynase

Brand Names: Canada Apo-Glyburide; Ava-Glyburide; DiaBeta; Dom-Glyburide; Euglucon; Mylan-Glybe; PMS-Glyburide; PRO-Glyburide; ratio-Glyburide; Riva-Glyburide; Sandoz-Glyburide; Teva-Glyburide

Therapeutic Category Antidiabetic Agent, Oral; Antidiabetic Agent, Sulfonylurea; Hypoglycemic Agent, Oral

Generic Availability (US) Yes

Use Adjunct to diet and exercise for the management of type II diabetes mellitus (noninsulin-dependent, NIDDM); may be used concomitantly with metformin or insulin to improve glycemic control

Pregnancy Risk Factor B/C (manufacturer dependent)

Pregnancy Considerations Outcomes of animal reproduction studies differ by manufacturer labeling. Glyburide crosses the placenta. Some pharmacokinetic properties of glyburide may change during pregnancy (Hebert 2009).

Severe hypoglycemia lasting 4 to 10 days has been noted in infants born to mothers taking a sulfonylurea at the time of delivery. Additional adverse maternal and fetal events have been noted in some studies and may be influenced by maternal glycemic control and/or differences in study design (Bertini 2005; Ekpebegh 2007; Joy 2012; Langer 2000; Langer 2005).

In women with diabetes, maternal hyperglycemia can be associated with congenital malformations as well as adverse effects in the fetus, neonate, and the mother (ACOG 2005; ADA 2015; Kitzmiller 2008; Metzger 2007). To prevent adverse outcomes, prior to conception and throughout pregnancy maternal blood glucose and HbA_{1c} should be kept as close to target goals as possible but without causing significant hypoglycemia (ACOG 2013; ADA 2015; Blumer 2013; Kitzmiller 2008). Prior to pregnancy, effective contraception should be used until glycemic control is achieved (Kitzmiller 2008).

Glyburide may be used to treat GDM when nonpharmacologic therapy is not effective in maintaining glucose control (ACOG 2013; ADA 2015; Blumer 2013). Women with type 2 diabetes are usually treated with insulin prior to and during pregnancy (Blumer 2013). According to the manufacturer, if glyburide is used during pregnancy, it should be discontinued at least 2 weeks before the expected delivery date.

Breast-Feeding Considerations Data from initial studies note that glyburide was not detected in breast milk (Feig 2005). According to the manufacturer, due to the potential for hypoglycemia in the nursing infant, a decision should be made whether to discontinue nursing or to discontinue the drug, taking into account the importance of treatment to the mother. Current guidelines note that breast-feeding is encouraged for all women, including those with diabetes (ACOG 2005; Blumer 2013; Metzger 2007). A small snack (such as milk) before nursing may help decrease the risk of hypoglycemia in women with pregestational diabetes (ACOG 2005; ADA 2015; Reader 2004). Glyburide may be used in breast-feeding women (Blumer 2013; Metzger 2007).

Contraindications

Hypersensitivity to glyburide or any component of the formulation; type 1 diabetes mellitus or diabetic ketoacidosis, with or without coma; concomitant use with bosentan.

Canadian labeling: Additional contraindications (not in U.S. labeling): Diabetic precoma or coma, stress conditions (eg, severe infections, trauma, surgery); liver disease or frank jaundice; renal impairment; pregnancy; breast-feeding.

Documentation of allergenic cross-reactivity for sulfonylureas is limited. However, because of similarities in chemical structure and/or pharmacologic actions, the possibility of cross-sensitivity cannot be ruled out with certainty.

Warnings/Precautions All sulfonylurea drugs are capable of producing severe hypoglycemia. Hypoglycemia is more likely to occur when caloric intake is deficient, after severe or prolonged exercise, when ethanol is ingested, or when more than one glucose-lowering drug is used. It is also more likely in elderly patients, malnourished, or debilitated patients and in patients with severe renal or hepatic impairment; adrenal and/or pituitary insufficiency, use with caution.

It may be necessary to discontinue therapy and administer insulin if the patient is exposed to stress (fever, trauma, infection, surgery). Loss of efficacy may be observed following prolonged use as a result of the progression of type 2 diabetes mellitus which results in continued beta cell destruction. In patients who were previously responding to sulfonylurea therapy, consider additional factors which may be contributing to decreased efficacy (eg, inappropriate dose, nonadherence to diet and exercise regimen). If no contributing factors can be identified, consider discontinuing use of the sulfonylurea due to secondary failure of treatment. Additional antidiabetic therapy (eg, insulin) will be required.

Avoid use in elderly patients due to increased risk of prolonged hypoglycemia (Beers Criteria). If therapy is initiated, dosing should be conservative; monitor closely for hypoglycemia.

Product labeling states oral hypoglycemic drugs may be associated with an increased cardiovascular mortality as compared to treatment with diet alone or diet plus insulin. Data to support this association are limited, and several studies, including a large prospective trial (UKPDS) have not supported an association.

Patients with G6PD deficiency may be at an increased risk of sulfonylurea-induced hemolytic anemia; however, cases have also been described in patients without G6PD deficiency during postmarketing surveillance. Use with caution and consider a nonsulfonylurea alternative in patients with G6PD deficiency.

Micronized glyburide tablets are **not** bioequivalent to *conventional* glyburide tablets; retitration should occur if patients are being transferred to a different glyburide formulation (eg, micronized-to-conventional or vice versa) or from other hypoglycemic agents.

Sulfonamide ("sulfa") allergy: The FDA-approved product labeling for many medications containing a sulfonamide chemical group includes a broad contraindication in patients with a prior allergic reaction to sulfonamides. There is a potential for cross-reactivity between members of a specific class (eg, two antibiotic sulfonamides). However, concerns for cross-reactivity have previously extended to all compounds containing the sulfonamide structure (SO_2NH_2). An expanded understanding of allergic mechanisms indicates cross-reactivity between antibiotic sulfonamides and nonantibiotic sulfonamides may not occur or at the very least this potential is extremely low (Brackett 2004; Johnson 2005; Slatore 2004; Tornero 2004). In particular, mechanisms of cross-reaction due to antibody production (anaphylaxis) are unlikely to occur with nonantibiotic sulfonamides. T-cell-mediated (type IV) reactions (eg, maculopapular rash) are less well understood and it is not possible to completely exclude this potential based on current insights. In cases where prior reactions were severe (Stevens-Johnson syndrome/TEN), some clinicians choose to avoid exposure to these classes.

Adverse Reactions

Cardiovascular: Vasculitis

Central nervous system: Dizziness, headache

Dermatologic: Angioedema, erythema, maculopapular eruptions, morbilliform eruptions, photosensitivity reaction, pruritus, purpura, rash, urticaria

Endocrine & metabolic: Disulfiram-like reaction, hypoglycemia, hyponatremia (SIADH reported with other sulfonylureas)

Gastrointestinal: Anorexia, constipation, diarrhea, epigastric fullness, heartburn, nausea

Genitourinary: Nocturia

Hematologic: Agranulocytosis, aplastic anemia, hemolytic anemia, leukopenia, pancytopenia, porphyria cutanea tarda, thrombocytopenia

Hepatic: Cholestatic jaundice, hepatitis, liver failure, transaminase increased

Neuromuscular & skeletal: Arthralgia, myalgia, paresthesia

Ocular: Blurred vision

Renal: Diuretic effect (minor)

Miscellaneous: Allergic reaction

Drug Interactions

Metabolism/Transport Effects **Substrate** of CYP2C9 (major); **Note:** Assignment of Major/Minor substrate status based on clinically relevant drug interaction potential; **Inhibits** CYP2C8 (weak)

Avoid Concomitant Use

Avoid concomitant use of GlyBURIDE with any of the following: Amodiaquine; Bosentan; Mecamylamine

Increased Effect/Toxicity

GlyBURIDE may increase the levels/effects of: Alcohol (Ethyl); Amodiaquine; Bosentan; Carbocisteine; CycloSPORINE (Systemic); Hypoglycemia-Associated Agents; Mecamylamine; Porfimer; Verteporfin; Vitamin K Antagonists

The levels/effects of GlyBURIDE may be increased by: Alpha-Lipoic Acid; Androgens; Antidiabetic Agents; Antidiabetic Agents (Thiazolidinedione); Beta-Blockers; Ceritinib; Chloramphenicol; Cimetidine; Clarithromycin; Cyclic Antidepressants; CYP2C9 Inhibitors (Moderate); CYP2C9 Inhibitors (Strong); Dexketoprofen; DPP-IV Inhibitors; Fibric Acid Derivatives; Fluconazole; GLP-1 Agonists; Herbs (Hypoglycemic Properties); MAO Inhibitors; Metreleptin; Miconazole (Oral); Mifepristone; Pegvisomant; Probenecid; Quinolone Antibiotics; Ranitidine; Salicylates; Selective Serotonin Reuptake Inhibitors; SGLT2 Inhibitors; Sulfonamide Derivatives; Vitamin K Antagonists; Voriconazole

Decreased Effect

GlyBURIDE may decrease the levels/effects of: Bosentan

The levels/effects of GlyBURIDE may be decreased by: Bosentan; Colesevelam; CycloSPORINE (Systemic); CYP2C9 Inducers (Strong); Dabrafenib; Hyperglycemia-Associated Agents; Quinolone Antibiotics; Rifampin; Thiazide Diuretics

Food Interactions Ethanol may cause rare disulfiram reactions. Management: Monitor patients.

Storage/Stability

Conventional tablets (Diaβeta): Store at 25°C (77°F); excursions are permitted between 15°C and 30°C (59°F and 86°F).

Micronized tablets (Glynase PresTab): Store at 20°C to 25°C (68°F to 77°F).

Mechanism of Action Stimulates insulin release from the pancreatic beta cells; reduces glucose output from the liver; insulin sensitivity is increased at peripheral target sites

Pharmacodynamics

Onset of action: 45-60 minutes

Maximum effect: 1.5-3 hours

Duration: Conventional formulations: 16-24 hours; micronized formulations: 12-24 hours

Average decrease in fasting blood glucose (when used as monotherapy): 60-70 mg/dL

Pharmacokinetics (Adult data unless noted)

Absorption: Reliably and almost completely absorbed

Distribution: V_d: 0.125 L/kg

Metabolism: Completely metabolized to one moderately active and several inactive metabolites

Protein binding: High (>99%)

Half-life: Biphasic: Terminal elimination half-life: Average: 1.4-1.8 hours (range: 0.7-3 hours); may be prolonged with renal or hepatic insufficiency

Time to peak serum concentration: Conventional formulation: 4 hours; micronized formulation: 2-3 hours

Elimination: 30% to 50% of dose excreted in the urine as metabolites in first 24 hours; the remainder of the metabolite via biliary excretion

Dialysis: Not dialyzable

Dosing: Usual Adults: Oral: Formulations of micronized glyburide (Glynase® Prestab®) are **not** bioequivalent with conventional formulations (eg, Diaβeta®) and dosage should be retitrated when transferring patients from one formulation to the other

Management of noninsulin-dependent diabetes mellitus in patients **previously untreated**:

Tablet (Diaβeta®):

Initial: 2.5-5 mg/day; in patients who are more sensitive to hypoglycemic drugs, start at 1.25 mg/day; increase in increments of no more than 2.5 mg/day at weekly intervals

Maintenance: 1.25-20 mg/day given as single or divided doses; maximum: 20 mg/day; doses >10 mg should be divided into twice daily doses

Micronized tablets (Glynase® Prestab®):

Initial: 1.5-3 mg/day; in patients who are more sensitive to hypoglycemic drugs, start at 0.75 mg/day; increase in increments of no more than 1.5 mg/day at weekly intervals

Maintenance: 0.75-12 mg/day given as a single dose or in divided doses; maximum: 12 mg/day; doses >6 mg/day should be divided into twice daily doses

Management of noninsulin-dependent diabetes mellitus in patients **previously maintained on insulin:** Initial dosage dependent upon previous insulin dosage, see table

Previous Daily Insulin Dosage (units)	Initial Glyburide Dosage (mg conventional formulation)	Initial Glyburide Dosage (mg micronized formulation)	Insulin Dosage Change (after glyburide started)
<20	2.5-5	1.5-3	Discontinue
20-40	5	3	Discontinue
>40	5 (increase in increments of 1.25-2.5 mg every 2-10 days)	3 (increase in increments of 0.75-1.5 mg every 2-10 days)	Reduce insulin dosage by 50% (gradually taper off insulin as glyburide dosage increased)

Dosing adjustment in renal impairment: CrCl <50 mL/minute: Not recommended

Dosing adjustment in hepatic impairment: Use conservative initial and maintenance doses and avoid use in severe disease

Administration Oral: May administer with food every morning 30 minutes before breakfast or the first main meal

Monitoring Parameters Signs and symptoms of hypoglycemia, fasting blood glucose, hemoglobin A_{1c}

Reference Range Target range:

Blood glucose: Fasting and preprandial: 80-120 mg/dL; bedtime: 100-140 mg/dL

Glycosylated hemoglobin (hemoglobin A_{1c}): <7%

Additional Information When transferring from other sulfonylurea antidiabetic agents to glyburide, with the exception of chlorpropamide, the administration of the other agent may be abruptly discontinued; due to the prolonged elimination half-life of chlorpropamide, a 2- to 3-day drug-free interval may be advisable before glyburide therapy is begun

Dosage Forms Considerations Micronized formulation: Glynase

Dosage Forms Excipient information presented when available (limited, particularly for generics); consult specific product labeling.

Tablet, Oral:

Diabeta: 1.25 mg, 2.5 mg, 5 mg [scored]

Glynase: 1.5 mg, 3 mg, 6 mg [scored]

Generic: 1.25 mg, 1.5 mg, 2.5 mg, 3 mg, 5 mg, 6 mg

◆ **Glycate** *see* Glycopyrrolate *on page* 979

Glycerin (GLIS er in)

Brand Names: US Fleet Liquid Glycerin Supp [OTC]; Glycerin (Adult) [OTC]; Pedia-Lax [OTC]; Sani-Supp Adult [OTC]; Sani-Supp Pediatric [OTC]

Therapeutic Category Laxative, Osmotic

Generic Availability (US) May be product dependent

Use

Oral: Gel: Relief of symptoms of dry mouth (OTC product: FDA approved in ages ≥2 years and adults)

Rectal: Suppository: Treatment of constipation (OTC product: FDA approved in ages ≥2 years and adults)

Pregnancy Considerations Glycerin suppositories are generally considered safe to use during pregnancy (Cullen, 2007; Wald, 2003).

Warnings/Precautions Oral products are for use as an oral demulcent; do not swallow excessive amounts. Rectal products may cause rectal discomfort or a burning sensation.

Warnings: Additional Pediatric Considerations Frequent use of laxatives may lead to bowel dependence and should be avoided (Tabbers [NASPGHAN/ESPGHAN] 2014).

Suppository: Use suppository with caution in patients with abdominal pain, nausea, or vomiting; physician should be consulted prior to use. In children, if bowel movement does not occur within 1 hour of use or rectal bleeding occurs; consult a physician.

Oral gel: Should be applied topically to the oral mucosa area; swallowing of product should be avoided during application, especially in young children; if swallowing of an excessive amount of glycerin occurs, consult prescriber or a local Poison Control Center. If sore mouth symptoms associated with dry mouth do not improve within 7 days or if sore throat is severe, persists more than 2 days, or is accompanied by fever, headache, rash, nausea, or vomiting consult a physician.

Rectal: Neonatal use: Although several trials have been conducted, data supporting the use of glycerin enemas for rapid meconium evacuation or treatment of constipation in neonates is inconclusive and not supported in guidelines (Haiden 2007; Shah 2011; Tabbers [NASPGHAN/ESPGHAN] 2014)

Adverse Reactions Rectal: Gastrointestinal: Cramping pain, rectal irritation, tenesmus

Drug Interactions

Metabolism/Transport Effects None known.

Avoid Concomitant Use There are no known interactions where it is recommended to avoid concomitant use.

Increased Effect/Toxicity There are no known significant interactions involving an increase in effect.

Decreased Effect There are no known significant interactions involving a decrease in effect.

Storage/Stability Store at room temperature; protect rectal products from heat.

Mechanism of Action Osmotic dehydrating agent which increases osmotic pressure; draws fluid into colon and thus stimulates evacuation

Pharmacodynamics Onset of action: Laxative effect: Rectal: 15-30 minutes

Pharmacokinetics (Adult data unless noted) Absorption: Rectal: Poorly absorbed

Dosing: Neonatal

Infrequent stool: Limited data available; dosing regimens variable: Rectal:

Liquid suppository: 0.2 mL of the pediatric liquid suppository preparation (2.8 g/4 mL) was used in premature neonates (n=13; PNA: 0 to 35 days; weight: 0.86 to 1.9 kg) with no stool output for >24 hours and was shown to be as effective as glycerin chip (Zenk 1993). Some centers have used higher doses of 0.5 mL/kg as an enema. **Note:** Although several trials have been conducted, data supporting the use of glycerin enemas for rapid meconium evacuation or the treatment of constipation in neonates is inconclusive and not supported in guidelines (Haiden 2007; Shah 2011; Tabbers [NASPGHAN/ESPGHAN] 2014)

Solid suppository: A tip or chip of the pediatric suppository (Zenk 1993)

Dosing: Usual

Pediatric:

Fecal impaction, rapid disempaction: Limited data available: Rectal: Infants and Children <2 years: Suppository: 1 pediatric suppository once (Wyllie 2011)

Constipation: Rectal: Suppository:

Children 2 to 5 years: 1 pediatric suppository once daily as needed or as directed

Children ≥6 years and Adolescents: 1 adult suppository once daily as needed or as directed

Mouth/throat irritation: Oral: Oral gel: Children ≥2 years and Adolescents: Apply a 1-inch strip directly to tongue and oral cavity as needed

Adult:

Constipation: Rectal: 1 adult suppository once daily as needed or as directed

Mouth/throat irritation: Oral: Apply a 1-inch strip directly to tongue and oral cavity as needed

Administration

Oral: Apply oral gel topically to oral mucosa (tongue and oral cavity); do not rinse after use; avoid swallowing product.

Rectal: Insert suppository in the rectum and retain 15 minutes; suppository does not need to melt to produce response

Rectal enema: Remove protective shield; insert tip into rectum with light side to side movement; squeeze the until nearly all liquid expelled. Gently remove the unit; a small amount of liquid will remain in unit after use.

Monitoring Parameters Evacuation of stool

Dosage Forms Excipient information presented when available (limited, particularly for generics); consult specific product labeling.

Enema, Rectal:

Fleet Liquid Glycerin Supp: 5.6 g/dose (7.5 mL)

Suppository, Rectal:

Glycerin (Adult): 2 g (12 ea, 24 ea, 50 ea); 2.1 g (25 ea)

Pedia-Lax: 1 g (12 ea); 2.8 g (4 mL) [contains edetate disodium]

Sani-Supp Adult: 2 g (10 ea, 25 ea)

Sani-Supp Pediatric: 1.2 g (10 ea, 25 ea)

◆ **Glycerin (Adult) [OTC]** *see* Glycerin *on page* 978

◆ **Glycerol** *see* Glycerin *on page 978*

◆ **Glycerol Guaiacolate** *see* GuaiFENesin *on page 988*

◆ **Glyceryl Trinitrate** *see* Nitroglycerin *on page 1523*

◆ **GlycoLax [OTC]** *see* Polyethylene Glycol 3350 *on page 1723*

◆ **Glycon (Can)** *see* MetFORMIN *on page 1375*

◆ **Glycophos** *see* Sodium Glycerophosphate Pentahydrate *on page 1943*

Glycopyrrolate (glye koe PYE roe late)

Medication Safety Issues

International issues:

Robinul [U.S. and multiple international markets] may be confused with Reminyl brand name for galantamine [Canada and multiple international markets]

Brand Names: US Cuvposa; Glycate; Robinul; Robinul-Forte

Brand Names: Canada Glycopyrrolate Injection, USP; Seebri Breezhaler

Therapeutic Category Anticholinergic Agent; Antispasmodic Agent, Gastrointestinal

Generic Availability (US) Yes

Use

Oral: Adjunct in treatment of peptic ulcer disease (FDA approved in adults). **Note:** Indication listed in product labeling but currently has no place in management of peptic ulcer disease. Has also been used for control of upper airway secretions.

Oral solution (Cuvposa™): Treatment of severe chronic drooling in association with neurologic conditions (eg, cerebral palsy) (FDA approved in ages 3-16 years)

Parenteral: Used preoperatively to inhibit salivation and excessive secretions of the respiratory tract, reduce volume and acidity of gastric secretions, and blockade of cardiac vagal inhibitory reflexes during induction of anesthesia and intubation; used intraoperatively to counteract surgically, drug-induced, or vagal mediated bradyarrhythmias; reversal of the muscarinic effects of cholinergic agents, such as neostigmine and pyridostigmine, during reversal of neuromuscular blockade (FDA approved in ages ≥1 month and adults); adjunct in treatment of peptic ulcer (FDA approved in adults). **Note:** Indication of peptic ulcer listed in product labeling but currently has no place in management of peptic ulcer disease.

Pregnancy Risk Factor B (injection) / C (oral solution)

Pregnancy Considerations Teratogenic effects were not observed in animal studies. Small amounts of glycopyrrolate cross the human placenta.

Breast-Feeding Considerations May suppress lactation

Contraindications Hypersensitivity to glycopyrrolate or any component of the formulation; medical conditions that preclude use of anticholinergic medication; severe ulcerative colitis, toxic megacolon complicating ulcerative colitis, paralytic ileus, obstructive disease of GI tract (eg, pyloric stenosis), intestinal atony in the elderly or debilitated patient; unstable cardiovascular status in acute hemorrhage; narrow-angle glaucoma; acute hemorrhage; tachycardia; obstructive uropathy; myasthenia gravis

Oral solution: Additional contraindication: Concomitant use of potassium chloride in a solid oral dosage form

Seebri Breezhaler [Canadian product]: Hypersensitivity to glycopyrronium bromide or any component of the formulation

Warnings/Precautions Diarrhea may be a sign of incomplete intestinal obstruction, treatment should be discontinued if this occurs. Use caution in elderly and in patients with autonomic neuropathy, narrow-angle glaucoma, renal disease, or ulcerative colitis; may precipitate/aggravate ileus or toxic megacolon, hyperthyroidism, CAD, CHF, arrhythmias, tachycardia, BPH, bladder neck obstruction, or hiatal hernia with reflux. Use of anticholinergics in gastric ulcer treatment may cause a delay in gastric emptying. Caution should be used in individuals demonstrating decreased pigmentation (skin and iris coloration, dark versus light) since there has been some evidence that these individuals have an enhanced sensitivity to the anticholinergic response. May cause drowsiness, eye sensitivity to light, or blurred vision; caution should be used when performing tasks which require mental alertness, such as driving. The risk of heat stroke with this medication may be increased during exercise or hot weather. Seebri® Breezhaler® [Canadian product] is not indicated for the initial (rescue) treatment of acute episodes of bronchospasm or with acutely deteriorating COPD; after initiation of therapy, patients should use short-acting bronchodilators only on an as needed basis for acute symptoms. Rarely, paradoxical bronchospasm may occur with use of inhaled bronchodilating agents; discontinue use of inhaler and consider other therapy if bronchospasm occurs. Patients using Seebri® Breezhaler® should avoid getting the powder into their eyes.

Benzyl alcohol and derivatives: Some dosage forms may contain benzyl alcohol; large amounts of benzyl alcohol (≥99 mg/kg/day) have been associated with a potentially fatal toxicity ("gasping syndrome") in neonates; the "gasping syndrome" consists of metabolic acidosis, respiratory distress, gasping respirations, CNS dysfunction (including convulsions, intracranial hemorrhage), hypotension and cardiovascular collapse (AAP, 1997; CDC, 1982); some data suggests that benzoate displaces bilirubin from protein binding sites (Ahlfors, 2001); avoid or use dosage forms containing benzyl alcohol with caution in neonates. See manufacturer's labeling. Some dosage forms may contain propylene glycol; large amounts are potentially toxic and have been associated hyperosmolality, lactic acidosis, seizures, and respiratory depression; use caution (AAP, 1997; Zar, 2007).

Warnings: Additional Pediatric Considerations Infants, patients with Down syndrome, and children with spastic paralysis or brain damage may be hypersensitive to antimuscarinic effects. Paradoxical excitation may occur in infants and young children. In children treated with Cuvposa, the following adverse reactions were reported with an incidence >30%: Flushing, constipation, vomiting, xerostomia, and nasal congestion.

Some dosage forms may contain propylene glycol; in neonates large amounts of propylene glycol delivered orally, intravenously (eg, >3,000 mg/day), or topically have been associated with potentially fatal toxicities which can include metabolic acidosis, seizures, renal failure, and CNS depression; toxicities have also been reported in children and adults including hyperosmolality, lactic acidosis, seizures and respiratory depression; use caution (AAP, 1997; Shehab, 2009).

Adverse Reactions

Cardiovascular: Arrhythmias, cardiac arrest, flushing, heart block, hyper-/hypotension, malignant hyperthermia, pallor, palpitation, QTc-interval prolongation, tachycardia

Central nervous system: Aggressiveness, agitation, confusion, crying (abnormal), dizziness, drowsiness, excitement, headache, insomnia, irritability, mood changes, pain, restlessness, nervousness, seizure

Dermatologic: Dry skin, pruritus, rash, urticaria

Endocrine & metabolic: Dehydration, lactation suppression

Gastrointestinal: Abdominal distention, abdominal pain, constipation, flatulence, retching, bloated feeling, intestinal obstruction, loss of taste, nausea, pseudo-obstructio, vomiting, xerostomia

Genitourinary: Impotence, urinary hesitancy, urinary retention, urinary tract infection

Local: Injection site reactions (edema, erythema, pain)
Neuromuscular & skeletal: Weakness
Ocular: Blurred vision, cycloplegia, mydriasis, nystagmus, ocular tension increased, photophobia, sensitivity to light increased
Respiratory: Bronchial secretion (thickening), nasal congestion, nasal dryness, pneumonia, respiratory depression, sinusitis, upper respiratory tract infection
Miscellaneous: Anaphylactoid reactions, diaphoresis decreased, hypersensitivity reactions

As reported with Seebri® Breezhaler® [Canadian product]:
Central nervous system: Headache
Gastrointestinal: Dyspepsia, gastroenteritis, vomiting, xerostomia
Genitourinary: Dysuria, urinary tract infection
Neuromuscular & skeletal: Musculoskeletal pain
Respiratory: Nasopharyngitis, rhinitis
Rare but important or life-threatening: Cough, cystitis, dental caries, diabetes mellitus, epistaxis, fatigue, hypoesthesia, palpitations, rash, throat irritation, urinary retention, weakness

Drug Interactions

Metabolism/Transport Effects None known.

Avoid Concomitant Use

Avoid concomitant use of Glycopyrrolate with any of the following: Aclidinium; Eluxadoline; Glucagon; Ipratropium (Oral Inhalation); Potassium Chloride; Tiotropium; Umeclidinium

Increased Effect/Toxicity

Glycopyrrolate may increase the levels/effects of: AbobotulinumtoxinA; Analgesics (Opioid); Anticholinergic Agents; Atenolol; Cannabinoid-Containing Products; Digoxin; Eluxadoline; Glucagon; MetFORMIN; Mirabegron; OnabotulinumtoxinA; Potassium Chloride; RimabotulinumtoxinB; Thiazide Diuretics; Tiotropium; Topiramate

The levels/effects of Glycopyrrolate may be increased by: Aclidinium; Amantadine; Ipratropium (Oral Inhalation); MAO Inhibitors; Mianserin; Pramlintide; Umeclidinium

Decreased Effect

Glycopyrrolate may decrease the levels/effects of: Acetylcholinesterase Inhibitors; Haloperidol; Itopride; Levodopa; Metoclopramide; Secretin

The levels/effects of Glycopyrrolate may be decreased by: Acetylcholinesterase Inhibitors

Food Interactions Administration with a high-fat meal significantly reduced absorption. Management: Administer on an empty stomach.

Storage/Stability Store at 20°C to 25°C (68°F to 77°F).
Oral capsules for inhalation [Canadian product]: Store at 15°C to 25°C (59°F to 77°F) in blister. Capsules should be stored in the blister pack and only removed immediately before use. Once protective foil is peeled back and/or removed the capsule should be used immediately; if capsule is not used immediately, it should be discarded. Do not store capsules in Seebri® Breezhaler®. Protect from moisture.

Mechanism of Action Blocks the action of acetylcholine at parasympathetic sites in smooth muscle, secretory glands, and the CNS; indirectly reduces the rate of salivation by preventing the stimulation of acetylcholine receptors

In COPD, competitively and reversibly inhibits the action of acetylcholine at muscarinic receptor subtypes 1-3 (greater affinity for subtypes 1 and 3) in bronchial smooth muscle thereby causing bronchodilation

Pharmacodynamics
Onset of action:
Oral: Within 1 hour
IM: 15 to 30 minutes
IV: 1 minute
Maximum effect: Oral: ~1 hour; IM: 30 to 45 minutes
Duration: Vagal effect: 2 to 3 hours; inhibition of salivation Up to 7 hours; anticholinergic: Oral: 8 to 12 hours Parenteral: 7 hours

Pharmacokinetics (Adult data unless noted)
Absorption: Oral tablets: Poor (~3%); variable and erratic; Oral solution: 23% lower compared to tablet
Distribution: V_d:
Pediatric patients (1 to 14 years): Mean range: 1.3 to 1.8 L/kg
Adults: 0.2 to 0.64 L/kg
Half-life:
Infants: 22 to 130 minutes
Children: 19 to 99 minutes
Adults: ~60 to 75 minutes; Oral solution: 3 hours
Elimination: Urine (as unchanged drug, IM: 80%, IV: 85%); bile (as unchanged drug)
Clearance:
Pediatric patients (1 to 14 years): Mean range: 1 to 1.4 L/kg/hour
Adults: Mean range: 0.4 to 0.68 L/kg/hour

Dosing: Neonatal Endotracheal intubation, nonemergent: Limited data available: IV: 4 to 10 mcg/kg as a single dose (acceptable, but not preferred vagolytic) (Kumar 2010). A small study of 20 neonates used 3 to 5 mcg/kg as a single dose prior to intubation (Pokela 1994).

Dosing: Usual
Pediatric:
Chronic drooling: Children and Adolescents 3 to 16 years: Oral solution (Cuvposa): 20 mcg/kg/dose 3 times daily, titrate in increments of 20 mcg/kg/dose every 5 to 7 days as tolerated to response up to a maximum dose of 100 mcg/kg/dose 3 times daily; not to exceed 1,500 to 3,000 mcg/dose
Control of secretions (chronic): Limited data available (Nelson 1996): Children:
Oral: 40 to 100 mcg/kg/dose 3 to 4 times daily
IM, IV: 4 to 10 mcg/kg/dose every 3 to 4 hours
Reduction of secretions (preoperative):
≤2 years: IM: 4 to 9 mcg/kg/dose 30 to 60 minutes before procedure
>2 years: IM: 4 mcg/kg/dose 30 to 60 minutes before procedure
Reversal of bradycardia, vagal reflexes (intraoperative): Infants, Children, and Adolescents: IV: 4 mcg/kg/dose (maximum dose: 100 mcg/dose) at 2 to 3 minute intervals
Reversal of muscarinic effects of cholinergic agents: Infants, Children, and Adolescents: IV: 0.2 **mg** for each 1 mg of neostigmine or 5 mg of pyridostigmine administered
Adult:
Reduction of secretions (preoperative): IM: 4 mcg/kg 30 to 60 minutes before procedure
Reversal of bradycardia, vagal reflexes (intraoperative): IV: 0.1 **mg** repeated as needed at 2 to 3 minute intervals
Reversal of neuromuscular blockade: IV: 0.2 **mg** for each 1 mg of neostigmine or 5 mg of pyridostigmine administered or 5 to 15 mcg/kg glycopyrrolate with 25 to 70 mcg/kg of neostigmine or 0.1 to 0.3 mg/kg of pyridostigmine (agents usually administered simultaneously, but glycopyrrolate may be administered first if bradycardia is present)

Dosing adjustment in renal impairment: There are no dosage adjustments provided in manufacturer's labeling; however, data suggest renal impairment reduces glycopyrrolate elimination; use with caution.

Dosing adjustment in hepatic impairment: There are no dosage adjustment provided in manufacturer's labeling (has not been studied).

Preparation for Administration Parenteral: IV infusion: May further dilute in a compatible solution

Administration

Oral: Tablets: Administer without regard to meals; Oral solution: Administer on an empty stomach, 1 hour before or 2 hours after meals.

Parenteral: May be administered undiluted IM or by slow IV injection; in perioperative setting, usually administered over 1 to 2 minutes (eg, in adults: 0.2 mg over 1 to 2 minutes); for chronic pediatric uses, may consider further dilution and infusing over 20 to 30 minutes (Nelson 1996).

Monitoring Parameters Heart rate; anticholinergic effects; bowel sounds; bowel movements; effects on drooling

Dosage Forms Excipient information presented when available (limited, particularly for generics); consult specific product labeling.

Solution, Injection:

Robinul: 0.2 mg/mL (1 mL); 0.4 mg/2 mL (2 mL); 1 mg/5 mL (5 mL); 4 mg/20 mL (20 mL) [contains benzyl alcohol]

Generic: 0.2 mg/mL (1 mL); 0.4 mg/2 mL (2 mL); 1 mg/5 mL (5 mL); 4 mg/20 mL (20 mL)

Solution, Oral:

Cuvposa: 1 mg/5 mL (473 mL) [contains methylparaben, propylene glycol, propylparaben, saccharin sodium; cherry flavor]

Tablet, Oral:

Glycate: 1.5 mg [dye free]

Robinul: 1 mg [scored]

Robinul-Forte: 2 mg [scored]

Generic: 1 mg, 2 mg

Extemporaneous Preparations A 0.5 mg/mL oral suspension may be made with 1 mg tablets and a 1:1 mixture of Ora-Plus® and either Ora-Sweet® or Ora-Sweet® SF. Crush thirty 1 mg tablets in a mortar and reduce to a fine powder. Prepare diluent by mixing 30 mL of Ora-Plus® with 30 mL of either Ora-Sweet® or Ora-Sweet® SF and stir vigorously. Add 30 mL of diluent (via geometric dilution) to powder until smooth suspension is obtained. Transfer suspension to 60 mL amber bottle. Rinse contents of mortar into bottle with sufficient quantity of remaining diluent to obtain 60 mL (final volume). Label "shake well". Stable at room temperature for 90 days. Due to bitter aftertaste, chocolate syrup may be administered prior to or mixed (1:1 v/v) with suspension immediately before administration (Cober, 2011).

A 0.5 mg/mL oral solution can be made from tablets. Crush fifty 1 mg tablets in a mortar and reduce to a fine powder. Add enough distilled water to make about 90 mL, mix well. Transfer to a bottle, rinse mortar with water, and add a quantity of water sufficient to make 100 mL. Label "shake well" and "protect from light". Stable at room temperature for 25 days (Gupta, 2001).

A 0.1 mg/mL oral solution may be made using glycopyrrolate 0.2 mg/mL injection without preservatives. Withdraw 50 mL from vials with a needle and syringe, add to 50 mL of a 1:1 mixture of Ora-Sweet® and Ora-Plus® in a bottle. Label "shake well", "protect from light," and "refrigerate". Stable refrigerated for 35 days (Landry, 2005).

Cober MP, Johnson CE, Sudekum D, et al, "Stability of Extemporaneously Prepared Glycopyrrolate Oral Suspensions," *Am J Health Syst Phar*,. 2011, 68(9):843-5.

Gupta VD, "Stability of an Oral Liquid Dosage Form of Glycopyrrolate Prepared from Tablets," *IJPC* 2001, 5(6):480-1.

Landry C, "Stability and Subjective Taste Acceptability of Four Glycopyrrolate Solutions for Oral Administration," *IJPC*, 2005, 9(5):396-98.

◆ **Glycopyrrolate Injection, USP (Can)** *see* Glycopyrrolate *on page 979*

◆ **Glycopyrronium Bromide** *see* Glycopyrrolate *on page 979*

◆ **Glycosum** *see* Dextrose *on page 633*

◆ **Glydiazinamide** *see* GlipiZIDE *on page 970*

◆ **Glydo** *see* Lidocaine (Topical) *on page 1258*

◆ **Glynase** *see* GlyBURIDE *on page 975*

◆ **Gly-Oxide [OTC]** *see* Carbamide Peroxide *on page 371*

◆ **GM-CSF** *see* Sargramostim *on page 1905*

◆ **GnRH Agonist** *see* Histrelin *on page 1022*

◆ **GoLYTELY** *see* Polyethylene Glycol-Electrolyte Solution *on page 1724*

◆ **GoodSense Acid Reducer [OTC]** *see* Ranitidine *on page 1836*

◆ **GoodSense Allergy Relief [OTC]** *see* DiphenhydrAMINE (Systemic) *on page 668*

◆ **GoodSense Mucus Relief [OTC]** *see* GuaiFENesin *on page 988*

◆ **GoodSense Senna Laxative [OTC]** *see* Senna *on page 1914*

◆ **Gordofilm** *see* Salicylic Acid *on page 1894*

◆ **Gordon Boro-Packs [OTC]** *see* Aluminum Acetate *on page 110*

◆ **Gordons-Vite A [OTC]** *see* Vitamin A *on page 2186*

◆ **Gordons-Vite E [OTC]** *see* Vitamin E *on page 2188*

◆ **GP 47680** *see* OXcarbazepine *on page 1584*

◆ **GR38032R** *see* Ondansetron *on page 1564*

◆ **Gralise** *see* Gabapentin *on page 954*

◆ **Gralise Starter** *see* Gabapentin *on page 954*

Granisetron (gra NI se tron)

Medication Safety Issues

Sound-alike/look-alike issues:

Granisetron may be confused with dolasetron, ondansetron, palonosetron

Related Information

Prevention of Chemotherapy-Induced Nausea and Vomiting in Children *on page 2368*

Serotonin Syndrome *on page 2447*

Brand Names: US Granisol [DSC]; Sancuso

Brand Names: Canada Granisetron Hydrochloride Injection; Kytril

Therapeutic Category 5-HT_3 Receptor Antagonist; Antiemetic

Generic Availability (US) May be product dependent

Use

IV: Prophylaxis of nausea and/or vomiting associated with initial and repeat courses of emetogenic chemotherapy including high-dose cisplatin (FDA approved in ages 2 to 16 years and adults); has also been used for prevention of postoperative nausea and vomiting

Oral tablet: Prophylaxis of nausea and vomiting associated with emetogenic chemotherapy and radiation therapy (FDA approved in adults)

Transdermal patch: Prophylaxis of nausea and vomiting associated with moderate to high emetogenic chemotherapy (FDA approved in ages ≥18 years and adults)

Pregnancy Risk Factor B

Pregnancy Considerations Adverse events were not observed in animal reproduction studies. Injection (1 mg/mL strength) contains benzyl alcohol which may cross the placenta. The Canadian labeling does not recommend use during pregnancy.

Breast-Feeding Considerations It is not known if granisetron is excreted in breast milk. The U.S. labeling recommends that caution be exercised when administering granisetron to nursing women. The Canadian labeling does not recommend use in nursing women.

Contraindications

Hypersensitivity to granisetron or any component of the formulation

Canadian labeling: Additional contraindications (not in U.S. labeling): Concomitant use with apomorphine

Warnings/Precautions Use with caution in patients with congenital long QT syndrome or other risk factors for QT prolongation (eg, medications known to prolong QT interval, electrolyte abnormalities, and cumulative high-dose anthracycline therapy). 5-HT_3 antagonists have been associated with a number of dose-dependent increases in ECG intervals (eg, PR, QRS duration, QT/QTc, JT), usually occurring 1 to 2 hours after IV administration. In general, these changes are not clinically relevant, however, when used in conjunction with other agents that prolong these intervals, arrhythmia may occur. When used with agents that prolong the QT interval (eg, Class I and III antiarrhythmics), clinically relevant QT interval prolongation may occur resulting in torsade de pointes. IV formulations of 5-HT_3 antagonists have more association with ECG interval changes, compared to oral formulations.

Antiemetics are most effective when used prophylactically (Roila, 2010). If emesis occurs despite optimal antiemetic prophylaxis, re-evaluate emetic risk, disease, concurrent morbidities and medications to assure antiemetic regimen is optimized (Basch, 2011).

Serotonin syndrome has been reported with 5-HT_3 receptor antagonists, predominantly when used in combination with other serotonergic agents (eg, SSRIs, SNRIs, MAOIs, mirtazapine, fentanyl, lithium, tramadol, and/or methylene blue). Some of the cases have been fatal. The majority of serotonin syndrome reports due to 5-HT_3 receptor antagonist have occurred in a postanesthesia setting or in an infusion center. Serotonin syndrome has also been reported following overdose of another 5-HT_3 receptor antagonist. Monitor patients for signs of serotonin syndrome, including mental status changes (eg, agitation, hallucinations, delirium, coma); autonomic instability (eg, tachycardia, labile blood pressure, diaphoresis, dizziness, flushing, hyperthermia); neuromuscular changes (eg, tremor, rigidity, myoclonus, hyperreflexia, incoordination); gastrointestinal symptoms (eg, nausea, vomiting, diarrhea); and/or seizures. If serotonin syndrome occurs, discontinue 5-HT_3 receptor antagonist treatment and begin supportive management. Use with caution in patients allergic to other 5-HT_3 receptor antagonists; cross-reactivity has been reported. Does not stimulate gastric or intestinal peristalsis (should not be used instead of nasogastric suction); may mask progressive ileus and/or gastric distension. Application site reactions, generally mild, have occurred with transdermal patch use; if skin reaction is severe or generalized, remove patch. Cover patch application site with clothing to protect from natural or artificial sunlight exposure while patch is applied and for 10 days following removal; granisetron may potentially be affected by natural or artificial sunlight. Do not apply patch to red, irritated, or damaged skin. Potentially significant drug-drug interactions may exist, requiring dose or frequency adjustment, additional monitoring, and/or selection of alternative therapy

Benzyl alcohol and derivatives: Some dosage forms may contain benzyl alcohol; large amounts of benzyl alcohol (≥99 mg/kg/day) have been associated with a potentially fatal toxicity ("gasping syndrome") in neonates; the "gasping syndrome" consists of metabolic acidosis, respiratory distress, gasping respirations, CNS dysfunction (including convulsions, intracranial hemorrhage), hypotension and cardiovascular collapse (AAP, 1997; CDC, 1982); some data suggests that benzoate displaces bilirubin from protein binding sites (Ahlfors, 2001); avoid or use dosage forms containing benzyl alcohol with caution in neonates. See manufacturer's labeling.

Polysorbate 80: Some dosage forms may contain polysorbate 80 (also known as Tweens). Hypersensitivity reactions, usually a delayed reaction, have been reported following exposure to pharmaceutical products containing polysorbate 80 in certain individuals (Isaksson, 2002; Lucente 2000; Shelley, 1995). Thrombocytopenia, ascites, pulmonary deterioration, and renal and hepatic failure have been reported in premature neonates after receiving parenteral products containing polysorbate 80 (Alade, 1986; CDC, 1984). See manufacturer's labeling.

Adverse Reactions

Cardiovascular: Hypertension, prolonged Q-T interval on ECG (>450 milliseconds, not associated with any arrhythmias)

Central nervous system: Agitation, anxiety, central nervous system stimulation, dizziness, drowsiness, headache (more common in oral and IV), insomnia

Dermatologic: Alopecia, skin rash

Gastrointestinal: Abdominal pain, constipation (more common in oral and IV), decreased appetite, diarrhea, dysgeusia, dyspepsia, nausea, vomiting

Hematologic and oncologic: Anemia, leukopenia, thrombocytopenia

Hepatic: Increased serum ALT (>2 x ULN), increased serum AST (>2 x ULN)

Neuromuscular & skeletal: Weakness (more common in oral)

Miscellaneous: Fever

Rare but important or life-threatening: Angina pectoris, application site reactions (transdermal: allergic rash including erythematous, macular, papular rash, or pruritus), atrial fibrillation, atrioventricular block (IV), cardiac arrhythmia, ECG abnormality (IV), extrapyramidal reaction (oral), hypersensitivity reaction (includes anaphylaxis, dyspnea, hypotension, urticaria), hypotension, serotonin syndrome, sinus bradycardia (IV), ventricular ectopy (IV; includes non-sustained tachycardia)

Drug Interactions

Metabolism/Transport Effects Substrate of CYP3A4 (minor); **Note:** Assignment of Major/Minor substrate status based on clinically relevant drug interaction potential

Avoid Concomitant Use

Avoid concomitant use of Granisetron with any of the following: Apomorphine; Highest Risk QTc-Prolonging Agents; Ivabradine; Mifepristone

Increased Effect/Toxicity

Granisetron may increase the levels/effects of: Apomorphine; Highest Risk QTc-Prolonging Agents; Moderate Risk QTc-Prolonging Agents; Panobinostat; Serotonin Modulators

The levels/effects of Granisetron may be increased by: Ivabradine; Mifepristone; QTc-Prolonging Agents (Indeterminate Risk and Risk Modifying)

Decreased Effect

Granisetron may decrease the levels/effects of: Tapentadol; TraMADol

Storage/Stability

IV: Store at 15°C to 30°C (59°F to 86°F). Protect from light. Do not freeze vials. Stable when mixed in NS or D_5W for 7 days under refrigeration and for 3 days at room temperature.

Oral: Store tablet or oral solution at 15°C to 30°C (59°F to 86°F). Protect from light.

Transdermal patch: Store at 20°C to 25°C (68°F to 77°F). Keep patch in original packaging until immediately prior to use.

Mechanism of Action Selective 5-HT_3-receptor antagonist, blocking serotonin, both peripherally on vagal nerve terminals and centrally in the chemoreceptor trigger zone

Pharmacodynamics
Onset of action: IV: 1-3 minutes
Duration: IV: ≤24 hours

Pharmacokinetics (Adult data unless noted)
Absorption: Transdermal patch: ~66% over 7 days
Distribution: V_d: Mean range: 3 to 4 L/kg; widely distributed throughout the body
Protein binding: 65%
Metabolism: Hepatic via N-demethylation, oxidation, and conjugation; some metabolites may have 5-HT_3 antagonist activity
Half-life: Oral: 6 hours; IV: Mean range: 5 to 9 hours
Time to peak serum concentration: Transdermal patch: ~48 hours
Elimination: Urine (11% to 12% as unchanged drug, 48% to 49% as metabolites); feces (34% to 38% as metabolites)

Dosing: Usual
Pediatric:
Chemotherapy-induced nausea and vomiting (CINV), prevention:
IV:
Manufacturer's labeling: Children ≥2 years and Adolescents: 10 mcg/kg administered within 30 minutes prior to chemotherapy; maximum dose: 1 mg/dose (ASCO [Basch], 2011)
POGO recommendations: Infants, Children, and Adolescents: 40 mcg/kg as a single daily dose prior to chemotherapy; POGO guidelines do not recommend a maximum dose; however, one study used a maximum dose of 3 mg regardless of bodyweight (Dupuis, 2013)
Oral: *Low to moderately emetogenic chemotherapy*: Infants, Children, and Adolescents: 40 mcg/kg/dose every 12 hours (Dupuis, 2013); usual adult dose: 1 mg/dose
Transdermal: Adolescents ≥18 years: Apply 1 patch at least 24 hours prior to chemotherapy; do not apply ≥48 hours before chemotherapy. Remove patch a minimum of 24 hours after chemotherapy completion. Maximum duration: Patch may be worn up to 7 days, depending on chemotherapy regimen duration.
Postoperative nausea and vomiting, prevention: Limited data available: Children and Adolescents: IV: 40 mcg/kg as a single dose; maximum dose: 0.6 mg/dose (Gan, 2014); ideal administration time in pediatric patients is not defined; in adults, administration is recommended at the end of surgery; in a granisetron pediatric PONV trial, doses were administered before the surgical incision (Cieslak, 1996; Gan, 2014). **Note:** QT prolongation has been observed at this dose in pediatric patients 2 to 16 years of age; monitor closely.
Adult:
Chemotherapy-induced nausea and vomiting, prevention:
Oral: 2 mg once daily up to 1 hour before chemotherapy **or** 1 mg twice daily; the first 1 mg dose should be given up to 1 hour before chemotherapy. Administer only on the day(s) chemotherapy is given.
IV: 10 mcg/kg 30 minutes prior to chemotherapy; only on the day(s) chemotherapy is given
Transdermal patch: Apply 1 patch at least 24 hours prior to chemotherapy; may be applied up to 48 hours before chemotherapy. Remove patch a minimum of 24 hours after chemotherapy completion. Maximum duration: Patch may be worn up to 7 days, depending on chemotherapy regimen duration.
Prophylaxis of radiation therapy-associated emesis: Oral: 2 mg once daily within 1 hour of radiation therapy
Dosing adjustments in renal impairment: Children ≥2 years, Adolescents, and Adults: No dosage adjustment necessary.
Dosing adjustments in hepatic impairment: Children ≥2 years, Adolescents, and Adults: Pharmacokinetic studies in patients with hepatic impairment showed that total clearance was approximately halved; however, standard doses were very well tolerated, and dose adjustments are not necessary.

Preparation for Administration Parenteral: IV: May be diluted in a small volume of NS or D_5W; volumes ranging from 2 to 20 mL have been reported in trials with pediatric patients (Cieslak 1996; Hahlen 1995)

Administration
Oral: Given at least 1 hour prior to chemotherapy/radiation; may be repeated 12 hours based on dose and indication
Parenteral: IV: Infuse over 30 seconds undiluted **or** dilute in small volume NS or D_5W and administer over 5 minutes; infusions administered over 30 to 60 minutes have also been reported (Komada 1999; Miyajima1994; Wada 2001)
Transdermal (Sancuso): Apply patch to clean, dry, intact skin on upper outer arm. Do not use on red, irritated, or damaged skin. Remove patch from pouch immediately before application. Do not cut patch.

Dosage Forms Excipient information presented when available (limited, particularly for generics); consult specific product labeling. [DSC] = Discontinued product
Patch, Transdermal:
Sancuso: 3.1 mg/24 hr (1 ea)
Solution, Intravenous:
Generic: 0.1 mg/mL (1 mL); 1 mg/mL (1 mL); 4 mg/4 mL (4 mL)
Solution, Intravenous [preservative free]:
Generic: 0.1 mg/mL (1 mL); 1 mg/mL (1 mL)
Solution, Oral:
Granisol: 2 mg/10 mL (30 mL [DSC]) [contains fd&c yellow #6 (sunset yellow), sodium benzoate; orange flavor]
Tablet, Oral:
Generic: 1 mg

Extemporaneous Preparations Note: Commercial oral solution is available (0.2 mg/mL)

A 0.2 mg/mL oral suspension may be made with tablets. Crush twelve 1 mg tablets in a mortar and reduce to a fine powder. Add 30 mL distilled water, mix well, and transfer to a bottle. Rinse the mortar with 10 mL cherry syrup and add to bottle. Add sufficient quantity of cherry syrup to make a final volume of 60 mL. Label "shake well". Stable 14 days at room temperature or refrigerated (Quercia, 1997).

A 50 mcg/mL oral suspension may be made with tablets and one of three different vehicles (Ora-Sweet®, Ora-Plus®, or a mixture of methylcellulose 1% and Simple Syrup, N.F.). Crush one 1 mg tablet in a mortar and reduce to a fine powder. Add 20 mL of the chosen vehicle and mix to a uniform paste; transfer to a calibrated bottle. Label "shake well" and "refrigerate". Stable for 91 days refrigerated (Nahata, 1998).

Nahata MC, Morosco RS, and Hipple TF, "Stability of Granisetron Hydrochloride in Two Oral Suspensions," *Am J Health Syst Pharm*, 1998, 55(23):2511-3.
Quercia RA, Zhang J, Fan C, et al, "Stability of Granisetron Hydrochloride in an Extemporaneously Prepared Oral Liquid," *Am J Health Syst Pharm*, 1997, 54(12):1404-6.

◆ **Granisetron Hydrochloride Injection (Can)** *see* Granisetron *on page 981*
◆ **Granisol [DSC]** *see* Granisetron *on page 981*
◆ **Granix** *see* Filgrastim *on page 876*
◆ **Granulocyte Colony Stimulating Factor** *see* Filgrastim *on page 876*
◆ **Granulocyte Colony Stimulating Factor (PEG Conjugate)** *see* Pegfilgrastim *on page 1641*
◆ **Granulocyte-Macrophage Colony Stimulating Factor** *see* Sargramostim *on page 1905*

Grass Pollen Allergen Extract (5 Grass Extract)

(GRAS POL uhn al er juhn EK strakt five GRAS EK strakt)

Medication Safety Issues

Sound-alike/look-alike issues:

Oralair may be confused with Singulair

Grass Pollen Allergen Extract (5 Grass Extract) may be confused with Grass Pollen Allergen Extract (Timothy Grass)

Brand Names: US Oralair

Brand Names: Canada Oralair

Therapeutic Category Allergen-Specific Immunotherapy

Generic Availability (US) No

Use Immunotherapy for treatment of grass pollen-induced allergic rhinitis with or without conjunctivitis confirmed by positive skin test or *in vitro* testing for pollen specific IgE antibodies for any of the 5 grass species contained in the product (FDA approved in ages 10 to 65 years)

Medication Guide Available Yes

Pregnancy Risk Factor B

Pregnancy Considerations Adverse events have not been observed in animal reproduction studies.

Breast-Feeding Considerations It is not known if grass pollen allergen extract is excreted in breast milk. The manufacturer recommends that caution be exercised when administering to nursing women.

Contraindications

Hypersensitivity to any of the inactive ingredients (mannitol, microcrystalline cellulose, croscarmellose sodium, colloidal anhydrous silica, magnesium stearate and lactose monohydrate) contained in this product or any component of the formulation; severe, unstable or uncontrolled asthma; history of any severe systemic allergic reaction; history of any severe local reaction to sublingual allergen immunotherapy; history of eosinophilic esophagitis

Canadian labeling: Additional contraindications (not in U.S. labeling): Immunotherapy is not indicated if a patient has not demonstrated symptoms, IgE antibodies, positive skin tests, or properly controlled challenge testing; concomitant therapy with beta-blockers or ACE inhibitors; severe and/or unstable asthma (FEV_1 <70% of predicted value); severe immune deficiency or autoimmune disease; any malignant disease (eg, cancer); oral inflammation (eg, oral lichen planus, oral ulcerations, or oral mycosis)

Warnings/Precautions [U.S. Boxed Warning]: Severe, life-threatening allergic reactions, including anaphylaxis and severe laryngopharyngeal restrictions, may occur. Discontinue use if systemic allergic reactions occur. Re-evaluate patients with escalating or persistent local reactions; consider discontinuation. Increased risk of local or systemic adverse reactions may occur when given with concomitant allergen immunotherapy; the initiation of therapy during grass pollen season may increase the risk of adverse reactions. The Canadian labeling reports that diarrhea and angioneurotic edema were observed in clinical trials within the first year of treatment; use of antihistamines may be considered if moderate local adverse reactions occur.

[U.S. Boxed Warning]: Auto-injectable epinephrine should be prescribed to patients; instruct patients on appropriate use and to obtain immediate medical care upon its use. [U.S. Boxed Warning]: Use may not be suitable for patients who may be unresponsive to epinephrine or inhaled bronchodilators due to concomitant drug therapy. The effect of epinephrine may be potentiated or inhibited by the following medications: beta blockers, alpha blockers, ergot alkaloids, tricyclic antidepressants, levothyroxine, monoamine oxidase inhibitors, antihistamines, cardiac glycosides, and diuretics.

[U.S. Boxed Warning]: Use may not be suitable for patients with conditions that may reduce their ability to survive a serious allergic reaction, including but not limited to compromised lung function (either chronic or acute) and cardiovascular conditions (eg, unstable angina, recent MI, arrhythmia, and uncontrolled hypertension).

[U.S. Boxed Warning]: Do not administer to patients with severe, unstable, or uncontrolled asthma; use has not been studied in patients with moderate or severe asthma or in patients requiring daily medication. Withhold treatment if patient is experiencing an acute asthma exacerbation. Re-evaluate patients with recurrent asthma exacerbations and consider discontinuation.

Eosinophilic esophagitis has been reported with use. Discontinue therapy in patients who experience severe or persistent gastroesophageal symptoms (including dysphagia or chest pain) and consider a diagnosis of eosinophilic esophagitis. Discontinue therapy to allow for complete healing of the oral cavity due to oral inflammation (eg, oral lichen planus, mouth ulcers, or thrush) or oral wounds following oral surgery or dental extraction. After healing is complete, the Canadian labeling recommends that therapy be resumed at dose used prior to procedure; if interruption >7 days, resume therapy under medical supervision. The effect of vaccination during therapy has not been evaluated; Canadian labeling suggests that vaccines may be administered during therapy if deemed appropriate after clinical assessment of patient.

[U.S. Boxed Warning]: Monitor all patients for at least 30 minutes after initial dose in a health care setting. Each subsequent dose in pediatric patients should be done under direct adult supervision. Canadian labeling recommends monitoring pediatric patients for at least 30 minutes after each dose. Canadian labeling recommends that only physicians experienced in the treatment of adult or pediatric respiratory allergic diseases should prescribe and initiate treatment. May contain lactose; Canadian labeling recommends avoiding use in patients with hereditary problems of galactose intolerance, Lapp lactase deficiency, glucose-galactose malabsorption or significant lactose allergies.

Adverse Reactions Adverse reactions similar in adult and pediatric patients, unless otherwise noted.

Cardiovascular: Lip edema

Central nervous system: Oral hypoesthesia, oral paresthesia, voice disorder (children and adolescents 5 to 17 years)

Dermatologic: Atopic dermatitis (children and adolescents 5 to 17 years), lip pruritus (children and adolescents 5 to 17 years), pruritus of ear, tongue pruritus

Gastrointestinal: Abdominal pain, dyspepsia, dysphagia, esophageal pain, gastritis, gastroesophageal reflux disease, nausea, oral itching, stomatitis, vomiting

Hypersensitivity: Mouth edema, tongue edema

Respiratory: Asthma (children and adolescents 5 to 17 years), cough, oropharyngeal pain, pharyngeal edema, throat irritation, tonsillitis (children and adolescents 5 to 17 years), upper respiratory tract infection (children and adolescents 5 to 17 years)

Rare but important or life-threatening: Acanthoma, allergic myocarditis, aphonia, chest pain, chronic lymphocytic thyroiditis, Crohn's disease, enlargement of salivary glands, eosinophilia, eosinophilic esophagitis, extrinsic asthma (analgesic asthma syndrome), eyelid injury, food allergy (oral allergy syndrome), gastroenteritis, headache, hypersensitivity reaction, loss of consciousness, lymphadenopathy, neoplasm (plasmacytoma), oropharyngeal blistering, peripheral vascular disease, stridor, tachycardia, vascular disease, weight loss

Drug Interactions

Metabolism/Transport Effects None known.

Avoid Concomitant Use There are no known interactions where it is recommended to avoid concomitant use.

Increased Effect/Toxicity

The levels/effects of Grass Pollen Allergen Extract (5 Grass Extract) may be increased by: ACE Inhibitors; Beta-Blockers

Decreased Effect There are no known significant interactions involving a decrease in effect.

Storage/Stability Store between 20°C and 25°C (68°F and 77°F); excursions are permitted between 15°C and 30°C (59°F and 86°F). Protect from moisture.

Mechanism of Action Grass pollen allergen extract is a mix of the following 5 pollens: Sweet vernal, orchard, perennial rye, timothy, and Kentucky blue grass. While the exact mechanism has not been fully elucidated, specific immunotherapy (SIT) may act by inducing a switch from T helper 2 cell response (Th2) to T helper 1 cell (Th1) response resulting in decreased interleukin-4 (IL-4) and interleukin-5 (IL-5) and increased interleukin-10 (IL-10), production of IgG-blocking antibodies that compete with IgE antibodies for allergen binding, proliferation of regulatory T lymphocytes and cytokines, and decreases in mast cells, eosinophils, and early- and late-phase allergic responses (Leith, 2006).

Dosing: Usual Dosage strength expressed in Index of Reactivity (IR). **Note:** Initiate treatment 4 months before expected onset of each grass pollen season and continue throughout pollen season. Safety of initiating treatment during grass pollen season or restarting treatment after missing a dose have not been established.

Pediatric: **Grass pollen-induced allergic rhinitis:**

Children 5 to <10 years: Limited data available: Sublingual: Initial: Day 1: 100 IR once daily; Day 2: 200 IR once daily; Maintenance (Day 3 and thereafter): 300 IR once daily; dosing based on a large multicenter, multinational, double-blind, placebo-controlled, phase II study (n=266, age range: 5 to 17 years, including 131 patients who received treatment) that showed improvement in symptoms with only mild or moderate adverse effects; no serious adverse reactions were reported (Wahn, 2009).

Children ≥10 years and Adolescents: Sublingual: Initial: Day 1: 100 IR once daily; Day 2: 200 IR once daily; Maintenance (Day 3 and thereafter): 300 IR once daily

Adult: **Grass pollen-induced allergic rhinitis:** Adults ≤65 years: Sublingual: 300 IR once daily

Dosage adjustment in renal impairment: There are no dosage adjustments provided in the manufacturer's labeling.

Dosage adjustment in hepatic impairment: There are no dosage adjustments provided in the manufacturer's labeling.

Administration Sublingual: Administer first dose in a health care setting due to the potential for allergic reactions; monitor patient for 30 minutes after first dose. If well tolerated, subsequent doses may be taken at home; subsequent pediatric doses should be done under adult supervision. Remove sublingual tablet from blister immediately prior to administration. Place tablet(s) under tongue until completely dissolved (≥1 minute) and then swallow. Wash hands after handling tablet. Avoid food or beverage for 5 minutes following dissolution of tablet (to prevent the swallowing of allergen extract). Auto-injectable epinephrine should be made available to patients.

Monitoring Parameters Signs/symptoms of hypersensitivity; monitor patients for at least 30 minutes after administration of first dose.

Dosage Forms Excipient information presented when available (limited, particularly for generics); consult specific product labeling.

Tablet, Sublingual:

Oralair: 100 IR, 300 IR (source of grass pollen: Sweet Vernal [*Anthoxanthum odoratum* L.], Orchard [*Dactylis glomerata* L.], Perennial Rye [*Lolium perenne* L.], Timothy [*Phleum pratense* L.], Kentucky Blue Grass [*Poa pratensis* L.])

Grass Pollen Allergen Extract (Timothy Grass) (GRAS POL uhn al er juhn EK strakt TIM oh thee GRAS)

Medication Safety Issues

Sound-alike/look-alike issues:

Grass Pollen Allergen Extract (Timothy Grass) may be confused with Grass Pollen Allergen Extract (5 Grass Extract)

Brand Names: US Grastek

Brand Names: Canada Grastek

Therapeutic Category Allergen-Specific Immunotherapy

Generic Availability (US) No

Use Immunotherapy for treatment of grass pollen-induced allergic rhinitis with or without conjunctivitis confirmed by positive skin test or *in vitro* testing for pollen-specific IgE antibodies for timothy grass or cross-reactive grass pollens (FDA approved in ages 5 to 65 years)

Medication Guide Available Yes

Pregnancy Risk Factor B

Pregnancy Considerations Adverse events have not been observed in animal reproduction studies. Canadian labeling recommends not initiating therapy in pregnant women.

Breast-Feeding Considerations It is not known if grass pollen allergen extract is excreted in breast milk. The manufacturer recommends that caution be exercised when administering to nursing women.

Contraindications

Hypersensitivity to any of the inactive ingredients (gelatin, mannitol, and sodium hydroxide) contained in this product or any other component of the formulation; severe, unstable or uncontrolled asthma; history of any severe systemic allergic reaction; history of any severe local reaction to sublingual allergen immunotherapy; history of eosinophilic esophagitis

Canadian labeling: Additional contraindications (not in U.S. labeling): Unstable, severe chronic, or severe seasonal asthma (FEV_1 <70% of predicted value in adults; <80% in children); concomitant beta-blocker therapy; oral inflammation (eg, oral lichen planus, oral ulcerations, severe oral candidiasis, or dental extraction)

Warnings/Precautions [U.S. Boxed Warning]: Severe, life-threatening allergic reactions, including anaphylaxis and severe laryngopharyngeal restrictions, may occur. Local reactions in the mouth or throat may occur; consider discontinuation in patients experiencing escalating and persistent adverse reactions in the mouth or throat. Increased risk of local or systemic adverse reactions may occur when given with concomitant allergen immunotherapy.

[U.S. Boxed Warning]: Auto-injectable epinephrine should be prescribed to patients; instruct patients on appropriate use and to obtain immediate medical care upon its use. [U.S. Boxed Warning]: Use may not be suitable for patients who may be unresponsive to epinephrine or inhaled bronchodilators due to concomitant drug therapy. The effect of epinephrine may be potentiated or inhibited by the following medications: beta blockers, alpha blockers, ergot alkaloids, tricyclic antidepressants, levothyroxine, monoamine oxidase inhibitors, antihistamines, cardiac glycosides, and diuretics.

[U.S. Boxed Warning]: Use may not be suitable for patients with conditions that may reduce their ability to survive a serious allergic reaction, including but not limited to compromised lung function (either chronic or acute) and cardiovascular conditions (eg, unstable angina, recent MI, arrhythmia, and uncontrolled hypertension).

[U.S. Boxed Warning]: Do not administer to patients with severe, unstable, or uncontrolled asthma; use has not been studied in patients with moderate or severe asthma or in patients requiring daily medication. Withhold treatment if patient is experiencing an acute asthma exacerbation. Re-evaluate patients with recurrent asthma exacerbations and consider discontinuation.

Discontinue therapy to allow for complete healing of the oral cavity due to oral inflammation (eg, oral lichen planus, mouth ulcers, or thrush) or oral wounds following oral surgery or dental extraction. The effect of vaccination during therapy has not been evaluated; Canadian labeling suggests that vaccines may be administered during therapy if deemed appropriate after clinical assessment of patient. Eosinophilic esophagitis has been reported with sublingual tablet immunotherapy; discontinue therapy in patients who experience severe or persistent gastroesophageal symptoms (eg, dysphagia, chest pain). Use is contraindicated in patients with a history of eosinophilic esophagitis.

[U.S. Boxed Warning]: Monitor all patients for at least 30 minutes after initial dose in a healthcare setting under the supervision of a physician with experience in the diagnosis and treatment of allergic diseases. Each subsequent dose in pediatric patients should be done under direct adult supervision. Canadian labeling recommends monitoring pediatric patients for at least 30 minutes after each dose. Canadian labeling recommends that only physicians experienced in the treatment of adult or pediatric respiratory allergic diseases should prescribe and initiate treatment.

Adverse Reactions Adverse reactions similar in adult and pediatric patients, unless otherwise noted.

Cardiovascular: Chest discomfort, lip edema (adults)

Central nervous system: Fatigue (adults), headache, oral hypoesthesia

Dermatologic: Lip pruritus (children and adolescents 5 to 17 years), pruritus (adults), pruritus of ear, tongue pruritus, urticaria

Endocrine & metabolic: Palatal edema (adults)

Gastrointestinal: Abdominal pain (adults), dyspepsia (adults), dysphagia, gastroesophageal reflux disease (adults), glossalgia, glossitis (adults), lip swelling, nausea, oral discomfort, oral itching, oral mucosa erythema, oral paresthesia, stomatitis, swollen tongue, tongue disease (adults)

Hypersensitivity: Mouth edema

Ophthalmic: Eye pruritus (children and adolescents 5 to 17 years)

Respiratory: Constriction of the pharynx (adults), cough (children and adolescents 5 to 17 years), dry throat (adults), dyspnea, nasal congestion (children and adolescents 5 to 17 years), nasal discomfort, oropharyngeal pain, pharyngeal edema, pharyngeal erythema (children and adolescents 5 to 17 years), sneezing (children and adolescents 5 to 17 years), throat irritation

Rare but important or life-threatening: Eosinophilic esophagitis, exacerbation of asthma, exacerbation of ulcerative colitis, foreign body sensation, hypersensitivity reaction, oral mucosa ulcer, pneumonia

Drug Interactions

Metabolism/Transport Effects None known.

Avoid Concomitant Use There are no known interactions where it is recommended to avoid concomitant use.

Increased Effect/Toxicity There are no known significant interactions involving an increase in effect.

Decreased Effect There are no known significant interactions involving a decrease in effect.

Storage/Stability Store between 20°C and 25°C (68°F and 77°F); excursions are permitted between 15°C and 30°C (59°F and 86°F). Protect from moisture.

Mechanism of Action Grass pollen allergen extract contains extract from timothy grass. While the exact mechanism has not been fully elucidated, specific immunotherapy (SIT) may act by inducing a switch from T helper 2 cell response (Th2) to T helper 1 cell (Th1) response resulting in decreased interleukin-4 (IL-4) and interleukin-5 (IL-5) and increased interleukin-10 (IL-10) production of IgG-blocking antibodies that compete with IgE antibodies for allergen binding, proliferation of regulatory T lymphocytes and cytokines, and decreases in mast cells, eosinophils, and early- and late-phase allergic responses (Leith, 2006).

Dosing: Usual Dosage strength expressed in Bioequivalent Allergy Units (BAU). **Note:** Initiate treatment ≥12 weeks before expected onset of each grass pollen season and continue throughout pollen season. May be taken daily for 3 consecutive years (including intervals between grass pollen seasons). Safety and efficacy of initiating treatment during grass pollen season or restarting treatment after missing a dose have not been established. In clinical trials, treatment interruptions ≤7 days were allowed.

Pediatric: **Grass pollen-induced allergic rhinitis:** Children ≥5 years and Adolescents: Sublingual: One tablet (2800 BAU) once daily

Adult: **Grass pollen-induced allergic rhinitis:** Adults ≤65 years: Sublingual: One tablet (2800 BAU) once daily

Dosage adjustment in renal impairment:

There are no dosage adjustments provided in the manufacturer's labeling.

Dosage adjustment in hepatic impairment: There are no dosage adjustments provided in the manufacturer's labeling.

Administration Sublingual: Administer first dose in a health care setting due to the potential for allergic reactions; monitor patient for 30 minutes after first dose. If well tolerated, subsequent doses may be taken at home; subsequent pediatric doses should be done under adult supervision. Remove sublingual tablet from blister unit with dry hands immediately prior to administration. Place tablet under tongue until completely dissolved (≥1 minute) and then swallow. Wash hands after handling tablet. Avoid food or beverage for 5 minutes following dissolution of tablet (to prevent the swallowing of allergen extract). Auto-injectable epinephrine should be made available to patients.

Monitoring Parameters Signs/symptoms of hypersensitivity; monitor patients for at least 30 minutes after administration of first dose.

Dosage Forms Excipient information presented when available (limited, particularly for generics); consult specific product labeling.

Tablet Sublingual, Sublingual:

Grastek: 2800 bau [contains gelatin (fish)]

◆ **Grastek** *see* Grass Pollen Allergen Extract (Timothy Grass) *on page 985*

◆ **Gravol [OTC] (Can)** *see* DimenhyDRINATE *on page 664*

◆ **Gravol IM (Can)** *see* DimenhyDRINATE *on page 664*

◆ **Grifulvin V** *see* Griseofulvin *on page 986*

Griseofulvin (gri see oh FUL vin)

Brand Names: US Grifulvin V; Gris-PEG

Therapeutic Category Antifungal Agent, Systemic

Generic Availability (US) Yes

Use Treatment of tinea infections of the skin and hair caused by susceptible species of *Microsporum*, *Epidermophyton*, or *Trichophyton* (FDA approved in ages >2 years and adults) when lesions are unresponsive to topical antifungal therapy

Pregnancy Risk Factor X

Pregnancy Considerations Teratogenic effects have been observed in animal reproduction studies. Griseofulvin crosses the placenta (Pacifici, 2006). Because adverse events have also been observed in humans (two cases of conjoined twins), use during pregnancy is contraindicated. Effective contraception should be used during therapy and for 1 month after therapy is discontinued in women of reproductive potential. Men should avoid fathering a child for at least 6 months after therapy.

Breast-Feeding Considerations It is not known if griseofulvin is excreted in breast milk. women. Due to the potential for serious adverse reactions in the nursing infant, breast-feeding is not recommended.

Contraindications Hypersensitivity to griseofulvin or any component of the formulation; liver failure; porphyria; pregnancy

Warnings/Precautions Use for the prophylaxis of fungal infections has not been established; not effective for the treatment of tinea versicolor. Severe skin reactions (eg, Stevens-Johnson syndrome, toxic epidermal necrolysis, erythema multiforme) have been reported (may be serious or even fatal); discontinue use if severe skin reactions occur. Discontinue therapy if granulocytopenia occurs. May cause jaundice and elevated liver function tests or bilirubin (may be serious or even fatal); discontinue therapy if necessary. Avoid exposure to intense sunlight to prevent photosensitivity reactions. Hypersensitivity cross reaction between penicillins and griseofulvin is possible.

Adverse Reactions

Central nervous system: Dizziness, fatigue, headache, insomnia, mental confusion

Dermatologic: Angioneurotic edema (rare), erythema multiforme-like drug reaction, photosensitivity, rash (most common), urticaria (most common),

Gastrointestinal: Diarrhea, epigastric distress, GI bleeding, nausea, vomiting

Hematologic: Granulocytopenia, leukopenia (rare)

Hepatic: Hepatotoxicity

Neuromuscular & skeletal: Paresthesia (rare)

Renal: Nephrosis, proteinuria (rare)

Miscellaneous: Drug-induced lupus-like syndrome (rare), oral thrush

Rare but important or life-threatening: Bilirubin increased, liver transaminases increased, Stevens-Johnson syndrome, toxic epidermal necrolysis

Drug Interactions

Metabolism/Transport Effects Induces CYP1A2 (weak/moderate), CYP2C9 (weak/moderate), CYP3A4 (weak)

Avoid Concomitant Use

Avoid concomitant use of Griseofulvin with any of the following: Contraceptives (Progestins); Saccharomyces boulardii; Ulipristal

Increased Effect/Toxicity

Griseofulvin may increase the levels/effects of: Alcohol (Ethyl); Carbocisteine; Porfimer; Verteporfin

Decreased Effect

Griseofulvin may decrease the levels/effects of: ARIPiprazole; Contraceptives (Estrogens); Contraceptives (Progestins); CycloSPORINE (Systemic); Hydrocodone; NiMODipine; Saccharomyces boulardii; Saxagliptin; Ulipristal; Vitamin K Antagonists

The levels/effects of Griseofulvin may be decreased by: Barbiturates

Food Interactions

Ethanol: Concomitant use will cause a "disulfiram"-type reaction consisting of tachycardia, flushing, headache, nausea, and in some patients, vomiting and chest and/or abdominal pain. Management: Monitor patients for signs of reaction.

Food: Griseofulvin concentrations may be increased if taken with food, especially with high-fat meals. Management: Take with a fatty meal (peanuts or ice cream) to increase absorption, or with food or milk to avoid GI upset.

Storage/Stability

Suspension: Store at 20°C to 25°C (68°F to 77°F).

Ultramicrosize tablets: Store at 15°C to 30°C (59°F to 86°F)

Mechanism of Action Inhibits fungal cell mitosis at metaphase; binds to human keratin making it resistant to fungal invasion

Pharmacokinetics (Adult data unless noted)

Absorption: Ultramicrosize griseofulvin absorption is almost complete; absorption of microsize griseofulvin is variable (25% to 70% of an oral dose); absorbed from the duodenum

Distribution: Deposited in the keratin layer of skin, hair, and nails; concentrates in liver, fat, and skeletal muscles; crosses the placenta

V_d: ~1.5L (Vozeh, 1988)

Metabolism: Extensively hepatic

Half-life: 9-22 hours

Time to peak serum concentration: 4 hours

Elimination: <1% excreted unchanged in urine; also excreted in feces and perspiration

Dosing: Usual

Infants, Children, and Adolescents:

General dosing; susceptible infection (*Red Book*, 2012): Oral: Children >2 years and Adolescents:

Microsize: 10-20 mg/kg/day in single or 2 divided doses; maximum daily dose: 1000 mg/**day**

Ultramicrosize: 5-15 mg/kg/day once daily or in 2 divided doses; maximum daily dose: 750 mg/**day**

Tinea capitis: Oral:

Infants >1 month to Children ≤2 years: Limited data available: 10 mg/kg/day in single or divided doses (Higgins, 2000)

Children >2 years:

Microsize: 20-25 mg/kg/day once daily (maximum daily dose 1000 mg/day) for 6-8 weeks or until fungal cultures clear; in some cases, treatment up to 16 weeks may be necessary (Ali, 2007; Higgins, 2000, Kakourou, 2010, *Red Book*, 2012)

Ultramicrosize: 10-15 mg/kg/day once daily (maximum daily dose 750 mg/day) for 6-8 weeks or until fungal cultures clear; in some cases, treatment up to 16 weeks may be necessary (Ali, 2007; Higgins, 2000, Kakourou, 2010, *Red Book*, 2012)

Adults:

Tinea corporis:

Microsize: 500 mg daily in single or divided doses for 2-4 weeks

Ultramicrosize: 375 mg daily in single or divided doses for 2-4 weeks

Tinea cruris:

Microsize: 500 mg daily in single or divided doses 2-6 weeks (*Red Book*, 2012)

Ultramicrosize: 375 mg daily in single or divided doses 2-6 weeks (*Red Book*, 2012)

Tinea capitis:

Microsize: 500 mg daily in single or divided doses for 4-6 weeks

Ultramicrosize: 375 mg daily in single or divided doses for 4-6 weeks

Tinea pedis:

Microsize: 1000 mg daily in single or divided doses for 4-8 weeks

Ultramicrosize: 375 mg daily in single or divided doses for 4-8 weeks; doses up to 750 mg daily in divided doses have been used

Tinea unguium:
Microsize: 1000 mg daily in single or divided doses for 4-6 months or longer
Ultramicrosize: 375 mg daily in single or divided doses 4-6 months or longer; doses up to 750 mg daily in divided doses have been used

Administration Oral: Administer with a fatty meal (peanut butter or ice cream to increase absorption), or with food or milk to avoid GI upset; shake suspension well before use. Ultramicrosize tablets may be swallowed whole or crushed and sprinkled onto 1 tablespoonful of applesauce and taken immediately without chewing.

Monitoring Parameters Periodic renal, hepatic, and hematopoietic function tests

Test Interactions False-positive urinary VMA levels

Dosage Forms Considerations
Microsized formulations: Suspensions, Grifulvin V tablets
Ultramicrosize formulation: Gris-PEG tablets

Dosage Forms Excipient information presented when available (limited, particularly for generics); consult specific product labeling.
Suspension, Oral:
Generic: 125 mg/5 mL (118 mL, 120 mL)
Tablet, Oral:
Grifulvin V: 500 mg [scored]
Gris-PEG: 125 mg, 250 mg [scored]
Generic: 125 mg, 250 mg, 500 mg

- ◆ **Griseofulvin Microsize** *see* Griseofulvin *on page 986*
- ◆ **Griseofulvin Ultramicrosize** *see* Griseofulvin *on page 986*
- ◆ **Gris-PEG** *see* Griseofulvin *on page 986*
- ◆ **Growth Hormone, Human** *see* Somatropin *on page 1957*
- ◆ **GRX Hemorrhoidal [OTC]** *see* Phenylephrine (Topical) *on page 1690*
- ◆ **GRx HiCort 25** *see* Hydrocortisone (Topical) *on page 1041*
- ◆ **GSK-580299** *see* Papillomavirus (Types 16, 18) Vaccine (Human, Recombinant) *on page 1628*
- ◆ **GTN** *see* Nitroglycerin *on page 1523*
- ◆ **Guaiatussin AC** *see* Guaifenesin and Codeine *on page 990*
- ◆ **Guaicon DMS [OTC]** *see* Guaifenesin and Dextromethorphan *on page 992*

GuaiFENesin (gwye FEN e sin)

Medication Safety Issues
Sound-alike/look-alike issues:
Bidex may be confused with Videx
GuaiFENesin may be confused with guanFACINE
Mucinex may be confused with Mucinex Allergy, Mucomyst

Related Information
Oral Medications That Should Not Be Crushed or Altered *on page 2476*

Brand Names: US Altarussin [OTC]; Bidex [OTC]; Buckleys Chest Congestion [OTC]; Cough Syrup [OTC]; Diabetic Siltussin DAS-Na [OTC]; Diabetic Tussin Mucus Relief [OTC]; Diabetic Tussin [OTC]; Fenesin IR [OTC]; Geri-Tussin [OTC]; GoodSense Mucus Relief [OTC]; Iophen-NR [OTC]; Liquibid [OTC]; Liquituss GG [OTC]; Mucinex Chest Congestion Child [OTC]; Mucinex For Kids [OTC]; Mucinex Maximum Strength [OTC]; Mucinex [OTC]; Mucosa [OTC]; Mucus Relief Childrens [OTC]; Mucus Relief [OTC]; Mucus-ER [OTC]; Organ-I NR [OTC]; Q-Tussin [OTC]; Refenesen 400 [OTC]; Refenesen [OTC]; Robafen [OTC]; Robitussin Chest Congestion [OTC]; Robitussin Mucus+Chest Congest [OTC]; Scot-Tussin Expectorant [OTC]; Siltussin DAS [OTC]; Siltussin SA [OTC]; Tussin [OTC]; Xpect [OTC]

Brand Names: Canada Balminil Expectorant; Benylin® E Extra Strength; Koffex Expectorant; Robitussin®

Therapeutic Category Expectorant

Generic Availability (US) May be product dependent

Use Expectorant used for the symptomatic treatment of productive coughs (FDA approved in adults; refer to product specific information regarding FDA approval in pediatric patients). **Note:** Approved ages and uses for generic products may vary; consult labeling for specific information.

Pregnancy Considerations Based on the limited available data, an increased risk of adverse birth outcomes has not been observed following maternal use of guaifenesin in pregnancy. Alcohol may be present in some liquid formulations of guaifenesin. If consumed in sufficient quantities during pregnancy, fetal alcohol syndrome may result. Guaifenesin has been investigated as an agent to improve cervical mucus and improve fertility.

Breast-Feeding Considerations It is not known if guaifensin is excreted in breast milk. The manufacturer recommends that caution be exercised when administering guaifensin to nursing women.

Contraindications Hypersensitivity to guaifenesin or any component of the formulation

Warnings/Precautions When used for self medication (OTC) notify healthcare provider if symptoms do not improve within 7 days, or are accompanied by fever, rash, or persistent headache. Do not use for persistent or chronic cough (as with smoking, asthma, chronic bronchitis, emphysema) or if cough is accompanied by excessive phlegm unless directed to do so by healthcare provider. Not for OTC use in children <2 years of age.

Some products may contain phenylalanine.

Benzyl alcohol and derivatives: Some dosage forms may contain sodium benzoate/benzoic acid; benzoic acid (benzoate) is a metabolite of benzyl alcohol; large amounts of benzyl alcohol (≥99 mg/kg/day) have been associated with a potentially fatal toxicity ("gasping syndrome") in neonates; the "gasping syndrome" consists of metabolic acidosis, respiratory distress, gasping respirations, CNS dysfunction (including convulsions, intracranial hemorrhage), hypotension, and cardiovascular collapse (AAP, 1997; CDC, 1982); some data suggests that benzoate displaces bilirubin from protein binding sites (Ahlfors, 2001); avoid or use dosage forms containing benzyl alcohol derivative with caution in neonates. See manufacturer's labeling.

Warnings: Additional Pediatric Considerations Safety and efficacy for the use of cough and cold products in pediatric patients <4 years of age is limited; the AAP warns against the use of these products for respiratory illnesses in this age group. Serious adverse effects including death have been reported. Many of these products contain multiple active ingredients, increasing the risk of accidental overdose when used with other products. The FDA notes that there are no approved OTC uses for these products in pediatric patients <2 years of age. Health care providers are reminded to ask caregivers about the use of OTC cough and cold products in order to avoid exposure to multiple medications containing the same ingredient (AAP 2012; FDA 2012).

Some dosage forms may contain propylene glycol; in neonates large amounts of propylene glycol delivered orally, intravenously (eg, >3,000 mg/day), or topically have been associated with potentially fatal toxicities which can include metabolic acidosis, seizures, renal failure, and CNS depression; toxicities have also been reported in children and adults including hyperosmolality, lactic

acidosis, seizures and respiratory depression; use caution (AAP 1997; Shehab 2009).

Adverse Reactions

Central nervous system: Dizziness, drowsiness, headache
Dermatologic: Rash
Endocrine & metabolic: Uric acid levels decreased
Gastrointestinal: Nausea, stomach pain, vomiting
Rare but important or life-threatening: Kidney stone formation (with consumption of large quantities)

Drug Interactions

Metabolism/Transport Effects None known.

Avoid Concomitant Use There are no known interactions where it is recommended to avoid concomitant use.

Increased Effect/Toxicity There are no known significant interactions involving an increase in effect.

Decreased Effect There are no known significant interactions involving a decrease in effect.

Mechanism of Action Thought to act as an expectorant by irritating the gastric mucosa and stimulating respiratory tract secretions, thereby increasing respiratory fluid volumes and decreasing mucous viscosity

Pharmacokinetics (Adult data unless noted) Absorption: Well absorbed

Dosing: Usual

Pediatric: **Cough (expectorant):** Oral:

Liquid:

Children 2 years to <4 years: Limited data available: 50 to 100 mg every 4 hours as needed; do not exceed 6 doses in 24 hours (Kliegman 2007)
Children 4 years to <6 years: 50 to 100 mg every 4 hours as needed; do not exceed 6 doses in 24 hours.
Children 6 years to <12 years: 100 to 200 mg every 4 hours as needed; do not exceed 6 doses in 24 hours
Children ≥12 years and Adolescents: 200 to 400 mg every 4 hours as neede; do not exceed 6 doses in 24 hours

Granules:

Children 4 years to <6 years: 100 mg every 4 hours as needed; do not exceed 6 doses in 24 hours
Children 6 years to <12 years: 100 to 200 mg every 4 hours as needed; do not exceed 6 doses in 24 hours
Children ≥12 years and Adolescents: 200 to 400 mg every 4 hours as needed; do not exceed 6 doses in 24 hours

Immediate release tablet:

Children 6 years to <12 years: 200 mg every 4 hours as needed do not exceed 6 doses in 24 hours
Children ≥12 years and Adolescents: 400 mg every 4 hours as needed; do not exceed 6 doses in 24 hours

Extended release tablet: Children ≥12 years and Adolescents: 600 mg to 1,200 mg every 12 hours as needed; do not exceed 4 tablets in 24 hours

Adult: **Cough (expectorant):** Oral:

Liquid: 200 to 400 mg every 4 hours as needed
Immediate release tablet: 400 mg every 4 hours as needed
Extended release tablet: 600 to 1,200 mg every 12 hours as needed

Dosing adjustment in renal impairment: There are no dosage adjustments provided in manufacturer's labeling.

Dosing adjustment in hepatic impairment: There are no dosage adjustments provided in manufacturer's labeling.

Administration Oral: Administer with a large quantity of fluid to ensure proper action:

Extended release tablet: Do not crush or chew extended release tablet
Granules: Empty contents of packet onto tongue and swallow; for best taste, do not chew granules.

Test Interactions Possible color interference with determination of 5-HIAA and VMA; discontinue for 48 hours prior to test

Dosage Forms Excipient information presented when available (limited, particularly for generics); consult specific product labeling. [DSC] = Discontinued product

Liquid, Oral:

Buckleys Chest Congestion: 100 mg/5 mL (118 mL) [alcohol free, sugar free; contains butylparaben, menthol, propylene glycol, propylparaben]
Diabetic Siltussin DAS-Na: 100 mg/5 mL (118 mL) [alcohol free, color free, fructose free, sodium free, sorbitol free, sugar free; contains aspartame, benzoic acid, methylparaben, propylene glycol; strawberry flavor]
Diabetic Tussin: 100 mg/5 mL (118 mL) [alcohol free, dye free, fructose free, sodium free, sorbitol free, sugar free; contains aspartame, menthol, methylparaben]
Diabetic Tussin Mucus Relief: 200 mg/5 mL (118 mL) [alcohol free, dye free, fructose free, sodium free, sorbitol free, sugar free; contains aspartame, benzoic acid, menthol, polyethylene glycol, propylene glycol]
Iophen-NR: 100 mg/5 mL (473 mL) [contains propylene glycol, saccharin sodium, sodium benzoate; raspberry flavor]
Liquituss GG: 200 mg/5 mL (118 mL, 473 mL) [alcohol free, sugar free; contains methylparaben, propylene glycol, propylparaben, saccharin sodium]
Mucinex Chest Congestion Child: 100 mg/5 mL (118 mL) [alcohol free; contains brilliant blue fcf (fd&c blue #1), edetate disodium, fd&c red #40, propylene glycol, sodium benzoate; grape flavor]
Mucinex Chest Congestion Child: 100 mg/5 mL (118 mL) [alcohol free; contains brilliant blue fcf (fd&c blue #1), fd&c red #40, propylene glycol, saccharin sodium, sodium benzoate; grape flavor]
Mucus Relief Childrens: 100 mg/5 mL (118 mL) [alcohol free; contains brilliant blue fcf (fd&c blue #1), fd&c red #40, propylene glycol, saccharin sodium, sodium benzoate]
Robitussin Mucus+Chest Congest: 100 mg/5 mL (118 mL) [alcohol free; contains fd&c red #40, menthol, propylene glycol, saccharin sodium, sodium benzoate]
Scot-Tussin Expectorant: 100 mg/5 mL (30 mL, 118 mL, 240 mL, 480 mL, 3780 mL) [alcohol free, dye free, saccharin free, sodium free, sorbitol free, sugar free]
Siltussin DAS: 100 mg/5 mL (118 mL) [alcohol free, dye free, sugar free; strawberry flavor]

Packet, Oral:

Mucinex For Kids: 50 mg (12 ea [DSC]) [contains aspartame; grape flavor]
Mucinex For Kids: 100 mg (12 ea) [contains aspartame; bubble-gum flavor]

Solution, Oral:

Generic: 100 mg/5 mL (5 mL, 10 mL, 15 mL); 200 mg/10 mL (10 mL); 300 mg/15 mL (15 mL)

Syrup, Oral:

Altarussin: 100 mg/5 mL (120 mL, 236 mL, 473 mL, 3840 mL)
Altarussin: 100 mg/5 mL (120 mL, 240 mL, 480 mL, 3840 mL) [contains alcohol, usp]
Cough Syrup: 100 mg/5 mL (118 mL, 473 mL) [alcohol free; contains fd&c red #40, menthol, propylene glycol, saccharin sodium, sodium benzoate; fruit flavor]
Geri-Tussin: 100 mg/5 mL (473 mL) [alcohol free, sugar free; contains fd&c red #40, menthol, saccharin sodium, sodium benzoate]
Q-Tussin: 100 mg/5 mL (118 mL, 240 mL, 473 mL) [alcohol free; contains fd&c red #40, saccharin sodium, sodium benzoate; cherry flavor]
Robafen: 100 mg/5 mL (118 mL, 240 mL [DSC], 473 mL) [contains alcohol, usp; cherry flavor]
Robitussin Chest Congestion: 100 mg/5 mL (118 mL, 237 mL) [alcohol free; contains fd&c red #40, saccharin sodium, sodium benzoate; flavored flavor]
Siltussin SA: 100 mg/5 mL (118 mL, 237 mL, 473 mL) [strawberry flavor]

Tussin: 100 mg/5 mL (118 mL, 237 mL) [alcohol free]
Generic: 100 mg/5 mL (480 mL)

Tablet, Oral:
Bidex: 400 mg [DSC] [scored]
Bidex: 400 mg [scored; contains saccharin sodium]
Diabetic Tussin Mucus Relief: 400 mg [scored; dye free, sodium free, sugar free]
Fenesin IR: 400 mg
GoodSense Mucus Relief: 400 mg [scored]
Liquibid: 400 mg
Mucosa: 400 mg [scored]
Mucus Relief: 400 mg
Mucus Relief: 400 mg [scored; dye free]
Organ-I NR: 200 mg [scored; contains fd&c red #40 aluminum lake]
Refenesen: 200 mg [scored; contains fd&c red #40 aluminum lake]
Refenesen 400: 400 mg [scored; dye free]
Xpect: 400 mg [scored; contains saccharin sodium]
Generic: 200 mg, 400 mg

Tablet Extended Release 12 Hour, Oral:
Mucinex: 600 mg [contains fd&c blue #1 aluminum lake]
Mucinex Maximum Strength: 1200 mg [contains fd&c blue #1 aluminum lake]
Mucus-ER: 600 mg [gluten free]
Generic: 600 mg

◆ **Guaifenesin AC Liquid** *see* Guaifenesin and Codeine *on page 990*

Guaifenesin and Codeine

(gwye FEN e sin & KOE deen)

Brand Names: US Allfen CD; Allfen CDX; Codar GF; Dex-Tuss; Guaiatussin AC; Guaifenesin AC Liquid; Iophen C-NR; M-Clear; M-Clear WC; Mar-Cof CG; Robafen AC; Virtussin A/C

Therapeutic Category Antitussive; Cough Preparation; Expectorant

Generic Availability (US) Yes: Oral solution, syrup

Use Temporary control of cough due to minor throat and bronchial irritation and loosening and thinning of mucus and bronchial secretions (FDA approved in ages ≥6 years and adults)

Pregnancy Considerations See individual agents.

Breast-Feeding Considerations See individual agents.

Contraindications Hypersensitivity to guaifenesin, codeine, or any component of the formulation; asthma

Warnings/Precautions Use with caution in patients with hypersensitivity reactions to other phenanthrene derivative opioid agonists (morphine, hydrocodone, hydromorphone, levorphanol, oxycodone, oxymorphone). May cause hypotension. Use caution with respiratory diseases (including emphysema, COPD, decreased respiratory reserve), CNS depression, acute alcoholism, acute abdominal conditions, fever, hypothyroidism, Addison's disease, ulcerative colitis, prostatic hyperplasia, recent GI or urinary tract surgery, seizure disorders, head injury or increased intracranial pressure, or severe liver or renal insufficiency; tolerance or drug dependence may result from extended use. Avoid use in patients with CNS depression or coma as these patients are susceptible to intracranial effects of CO_2 retention.

Use caution in patients with two or more copies of the variant CYP2D6*2 allele; may have extensive conversion from codeine to morphine and thus increased opioid-mediated effects. Avoid the use of codeine in these patients; consider alternative analgesics such as morphine or a nonopioid agent (Crews, 2012). The occurrence of this phenotype is seen in 0.5% to 1% of Chinese and Japanese, 0.5% to 1% of Hispanics, 1% to 10% of Caucasians, 3% of African-Americans, and 16% to 28% of North Africans, Ethiopians, and Arabs.

Use with caution in the elderly; may be more sensitive to adverse effects. Use with caution in debilitated patients. Causes sedation; caution must be used in performing tasks which require alertness (eg, operating machinery or driving). Effects may be potentiated when used with other sedative drugs or ethanol. Underlying cause of cough should be determined prior to prescribing. Dose should not be increased if cough does not respond; reevaluate within 5 days for possible underlying pathology.

Some products may contain phenylalanine.

Benzyl alcohol and derivatives: Some dosage forms may contain sodium benzoate/benzoic acid; benzoic acid (benzoate) is a metabolite of benzyl alcohol; large amounts of benzyl alcohol (≥99 mg/kg/day) have been associated with a potentially fatal toxicity ("gasping syndrome") in neonates; the "gasping syndrome" consists of metabolic acidosis, respiratory distress, gasping respirations, CNS dysfunction (including convulsions, intracranial hemorrhage), hypotension, and cardiovascular collapse (AAP, 1997; CDC, 1982); some data suggests that benzoate displaces bilirubin from protein binding sites (Ahlfors, 2001); avoid or use dosage forms containing benzyl alcohol derivative with caution in neonates. See manufacturer's labeling.

Warnings: Additional Pediatric Considerations Safety and efficacy for the use of cough and cold products in pediatric patients <4 years of age is limited; the AAP warns against the use of these products for respiratory illnesses in this age group. Serious adverse effects including death have been reported. Many of these products contain multiple active ingredients, increasing the risk of accidental overdose when used with other products. Health care providers are reminded to ask caregivers about the use of OTC cough and cold products in order to avoid exposure to multiple medications containing the same ingredient (AAP 2012; FDA 2008). In July 2015, the FDA announced that it would be further evaluating the risk of serious adverse effects of codeine-containing products to treat cough and colds in pediatric patients <18 years including slowed or difficulty breathing. In April 2015, the European Medicines Agency (EMA) stated that codeine-containing medicines should not be used in children <12 years, and use is not recommended in pediatric patients 12 to 18 years who have breathing problems including asthma or other chronic breathing problems (FDA 2015).

Some dosage forms may contain propylene glycol; in neonates large amounts of propylene glycol delivered orally, intravenously (eg, >3,000 mg/day), or topically have been associated with potentially fatal toxicities which can include metabolic acidosis, seizures, renal failure, and CNS depression; toxicities have also been reported in children and adults including hyperosmolality, lactic acidosis, seizures and respiratory depression; use caution (AAP, 1997; Shehab, 2009).

Adverse Reactions See individual agents.

Drug Interactions

Metabolism/Transport Effects Refer to individual components.

Avoid Concomitant Use

Avoid concomitant use of Guaifenesin and Codeine with any of the following: Azelastine (Nasal); Eluxadoline; Mixed Agonist / Antagonist Opioids; Orphenadrine; Paraldehyde; Thalidomide

Increased Effect/Toxicity

Guaifenesin and Codeine may increase the levels/effects of: Alcohol (Ethyl); Alvimopan; Azelastine (Nasal); CNS Depressants; Desmopressin; Diuretics; Eluxadoline; Hydrocodone; Methotrimeprazine; Metyrosine;

Mirtazapine; Orphenadrine; Paraldehyde; Pramipexole; ROPINIRole; Rotigotine; Selective Serotonin Reuptake Inhibitors; Suvorexant; Thalidomide; Zolpidem

The levels/effects of Guaifenesin and Codeine may be increased by: Amphetamines; Anticholinergic Agents; Antipsychotic Agents (Phenothiazines); Brimonidine (Topical); Cannabis; Doxylamine; Dronabinol; Droperidol; HydrOXYzine; Kava Kava; Magnesium Sulfate; Methotrimeprazine; Nabilone; Perampanel; Rufinamide; Sodium Oxybate; Somatostatin Analogs; Succinylcholine; Tapentadol; Tetrahydrocannabinol

Decreased Effect

Guaifenesin and Codeine may decrease the levels/effects of: Pegvisomant

The levels/effects of Guaifenesin and Codeine may be decreased by: Ammonium Chloride; CYP2D6 Inhibitors (Moderate); CYP2D6 Inhibitors (Strong); Mixed Agonist / Antagonist Opioids; Naltrexone

Mechanism of Action

Guaifenesin may act as an expectorant by irritating the gastric mucosa and stimulating respiratory tract secretions, thereby increasing respiratory fluid volumes and decreasing phlegm viscosity

Codeine is an antitussive that controls cough by depressing the medullary cough center

Dosing: Usual Note: Dosage units vary based on product (mg, mL, capsules, or tablets); use caution when verifying dose with product formulation.

Children ≥2 years and Adolescents: **Cough (antitussive/expectorant):** Oral:

Children 2 to <6 years: Limited data available: 1-1.5 mg/kg codeine/day divided into 4 doses administered every 4-6 hours as needed; maximum total dose: Codeine: 30 mg/24 hours or guaifenesin: 600 mg/24 hours, whichever is less.

Children 6-11 years:

Capsule: Guaifenesin 200 mg and codeine 9 mg: 1 capsule every 4 hours as needed; maximum daily dose: 6 capsules/**day**

Liquid:

Guaifenesin 100 mg and codeine 6.33 mg per 5 mL: 7.5 mL every 4-6 hours as needed; maximum daily dose: 45 mL/**day**

Guaifenesin 100-200 mg and codeine 8-10 mg per 5 mL: 5 mL every 4 hours as needed; maximum daily dose: 30 mL/**day**

Guaifenesin 225 mg and codeine 7.5 mg per 5 mL: 3.75 mL every 4-6 hours as needed; maximum total dose: 22.5 mL/24 hours

Guaifenesin 300 mg and codeine 10 mg per 5 mL: 2.5 mL every 4-6 hours as needed; maximum daily dose: 20 mL/**day**

Tablet: Guaifenesin 400 mg and codeine 10-20 mg: 1/2 tablet every 4-6 hours as needed; maximum daily dose: 3 tablets/**day**

Children ≥12 years and Adolescents:

Capsule: Guaifenesin 200 mg and codeine 9 mg: 2 capsules every 4 hours as needed; maximum daily dose: 12 capsules/**day**

Liquid:

Guaifenesin 100 mg and codeine 6.33 mg per 5 mL: 15 mL every 4-6 hours as needed; maximum daily dose: 90 mL/**day**

Guaifenesin 100-200 mg and codeine 8-10 mg per 5 mL: 10 mL every 4 hours as needed; maximum daily dose: 60 mL/**day**

Guaifenesin 225 mg and codeine 7.5 mg per 5 mL: 7.5 mL every 4-6 hours as needed; maximum total dose: 45 mL/24 hours

Guaifenesin 300 mg and codeine 10 mg per 5 mL: 5 mL every 4-6 hours as needed; maximum daily dose: 40 mL/**day**

Tablet: Guaifenesin 400 mg and codeine 10-20 mg: 1 tablet every 4-6 hours as needed; maximum daily dose: 6 tablets/**day**

Adults: **Cough (antitussive/expectorant):** Oral:

Capsule: Guaifenesin 200 mg and codeine 9 mg: 2 capsules every 4 hours as needed; maximum daily dose: 12 capsules/**day**

Liquid:

Guaifenesin 100 mg and codeine 6.33 mg per 5 mL: 15 mL every 4-6 hours as needed; maximum daily dose: 90 mL/**day**

Guaifenesin 100-200 mg and codeine 8-10 mg per 5 mL: 10 mL every 4 hours as needed; maximum daily dose: 60 mL/**day**

Guaifenesin 300 mg and codeine 10 mg per 5 mL: 5 mL every 4-6 hours as needed; maximum daily dose: 40 mL/**day**

Tablet: Guaifenesin 400 mg and codeine 10-20 mg: 1 tablet every 4-6 hours as needed; maximum daily dose: 6 tablets/**day**

Administration Oral: Administer with a large quantity of fluid to ensure proper action; may administer with food to decrease nausea and GI upset from codeine

Test Interactions May cause a colorimetric interference with certain laboratory determinations of 5-hydroxy indoleacetic acid (5-HIAA) and vanillylmandelic acid (VMA)

Controlled Substance Capsule: C-V; Liquid products: C-V; Tablet: C-III

Dosage Forms Excipient information presented when available (limited, particularly for generics); consult specific product labeling.

Capsule, oral:

M-Clear: Guaifenesin 200 mg and codeine phosphate 9 mg [contains tartrazine]

Liquid, oral:

Codar GF: Guaifenesin 200 mg and codeine phosphate 8 mg per 5 mL (473 mL) [contains propylene glycol; cotton candy flavor]

Dex-Tuss: Guaifenesin 300 mg and codeine phosphate 10 mg per 5 mL (473 mL) [ethanol free, gluten free, sugar free; contains propylene glycol; grape flavor]

Iophen C-NR: Guaifenesin 100 mg and codeine phosphate 10 mg per 5 mL (473 mL) [contains propylene glycol, sodium benzoate; raspberry flavor]

M-Clear WC: Guaifenesin 100 mg and codeine phosphate 6.33 mg per 5 mL (473 mL) [contains propylene glycol; cotton candy flavor]

Solution, oral: Guaifenesin 100 mg and codeine phosphate 10 mg per 5 mL (5 mL, 10 mL, 118 mL, 473 mL)

Mar-Cof CG: Guaifenesin 225 mg and codeine phosphate 7.5 mg per 5 mL (473 mL) [ethanol free, sugar free; contains propylene glycol, sodium benzoate, sodium 6 mg/5 mL]

Virtussin A/C: Guaifenesin 100 mg and codeine phosphate 10 mg per 5 mL (118 mL, 473 mL) [sugar free; contains propylene glycol; cherry flavor]

Syrup, oral: Guaifenesin 100 mg and codeine phosphate 10 mg per 5 mL (473 mL)

Guaiatussin AC: Guaifenesin 100 mg and codeine phosphate 10 mg per 5 mL (5 mL, 10 mL, 118 mL, 473 mL) [sugar free; contains ethanol 3.5%, sodium 1 mg/5 mL, sodium benzoate; cherry flavor]

Robafen AC: Guaifenesin 100 mg and codeine phosphate 10 mg per 5 mL (120 mL, 480 mL) [contains ethanol 3.5%, sodium 4 mg/5 mL, sodium benzoate; cherry flavor]

Tablet, oral:

Allfen CD: Guaifenesin 400 mg and codeine phosphate 10 mg

Allfen CDX: Guaifenesin 400 mg and codeine phosphate 20 mg

Guaifenesin and Dextromethorphan

(gwye FEN e sin & deks troe meth OR fan)

Medication Safety Issues

Sound-alike/look-alike issues:

Benylin may be confused with Benadryl, Ventolin

Mucinex DM may be confused with Mucinex D

Related Information

Oral Medications That Should Not Be Crushed or Altered *on page 2476*

Brand Names: US Cheracol D [OTC]; Cheracol Plus [OTC]; Coricidin HBP Chest Congestion and Cough [OTC]; Diabetic Siltussin-DM DAS-Na Maximum Strength [OTC]; Diabetic Siltussin-DM DAS-Na [OTC]; Diabetic Tussin DM Maximum Strength [OTC]; Diabetic Tussin DM [OTC]; Double Tussin DM [OTC]; Fenesin DM IR [OTC]; Guaicon DMS [OTC]; Iophen DM-NR [OTC]; Kolephrin GG/DM [OTC]; Mucinex DM Maximum Strength [OTC]; Mucinex DM [OTC]; Mucinex Fast-Max DM Max [OTC]; Mucinex Kid's Cough Mini-Melts [OTC]; Mucinex Kid's Cough [OTC]; Q-Tussin DM [OTC]; Refenesen DM [OTC]; Robafen DM [OTC]; Robitussin Maximum Strength Cough + Congestion DM [OTC]; Robitussin Peak Cold Cough + Chest Congestion DM [OTC]; Robitussin Peak Cold Maximum Strength Cough + Chest Congestion DM [OTC]; Robitussin Peak Cold Sugar-Free Cough + Chest Congestion DM [OTC]; Safe Tussin DM [OTC]; Scot-Tussin Senior [OTC]; Silexin [OTC]; Siltussin DM DAS [OTC]; Siltussin DM [OTC]; Triaminic Cough & Congestion [OTC]; Vicks 44E [OTC]; Vicks DayQuil Mucus Control DM [OTC]; Vicks Nature Fusion Cough & Chest Congestion [OTC]; Vicks Pediatric Formula 44E [OTC]; Zyncof [OTC]

Brand Names: Canada Balminil DM E; Benylin DM-E

Therapeutic Category Antitussive; Cough Preparation; Expectorant

Generic Availability (US) Yes: Excludes extended release tablet

Use Temporary control of cough due to minor throat and bronchial irritation

Pregnancy Considerations See individual agents.

Breast-Feeding Considerations See individual agents.

Contraindications Hypersensitivity to guaifenesin, dextromethorphan, or any component of the formulation; use with or within 14 days of MAO inhibitor therapy

Warnings/Precautions Underlying cause of cough should be determined prior to prescribing. Use caution in patients who are sedated, debilitated or confined to a supine position; use with caution in atopic children. Not for OTC use in children <2 years of age. When used for self medication (OTC) notify healthcare provider if symptoms do not improve within 7 days, or are accompanied by fever, rash, or persistent headache.

Some products may contain phenylalanine.

Benzyl alcohol and derivatives: Some dosage forms may contain sodium benzoate/benzoic acid; benzoic acid (benzoate) is a metabolite of benzyl alcohol; large amounts of benzyl alcohol (≥99 mg/kg/day) have been associated with a potentially fatal toxicity ("gasping syndrome") in neonates; the "gasping syndrome" consists of metabolic acidosis, respiratory distress, gasping respirations, CNS dysfunction (including convulsions, intracranial hemorrhage), hypotension, and cardiovascular collapse (AAP, 1997; CDC, 1982); some data suggests that benzoate displaces bilirubin from protein binding sites (Ahlfors, 2001); avoid or use dosage forms containing benzyl alcohol derivative with caution in neonates. See manufacturer's labeling.

Warnings: Additional Pediatric Considerations Safety and efficacy for the use of cough and cold products in children <2 years of age is limited. Serious adverse effects including death have been reported. The FDA notes that there are no approved OTC uses for these products in children <2 years of age. Health care providers are reminded to ask caregivers about the use of OTC cough and cold products in order to avoid exposure to multiple medications containing the same ingredient.

Some dosage forms may contain propylene glycol; in neonates large amounts of propylene glycol delivered orally, intravenously (eg, >3,000 mg/day), or topically have been associated with potentially fatal toxicities which can include metabolic acidosis, seizures, renal failure, and CNS depression; toxicities have also been reported in children and adults including hyperosmolality, lactic acidosis, seizures and respiratory depression; use caution (AAP, 1997; Shehab, 2009).

Adverse Reactions See individual agents.

Drug Interactions

Metabolism/Transport Effects Refer to individual components.

Avoid Concomitant Use

Avoid concomitant use of Guaifenesin and Dextromethorphan with any of the following: Dapoxetine; MAO Inhibitors

Increased Effect/Toxicity

Guaifenesin and Dextromethorphan may increase the levels/effects of: Antipsychotic Agents; ARIPiprazole; Memantine; Metoclopramide; Serotonin Modulators

The levels/effects of Guaifenesin and Dextromethorphan may be increased by: Abiraterone Acetate; Antiemetics (5HT3 Antagonists); Antipsychotic Agents; Cobicistat; CYP2D6 Inhibitors (Moderate); CYP2D6 Inhibitors (Strong); Dapoxetine; Darunavir; MAO Inhibitors; Panobinostat; Parecoxib; Peginterferon Alfa-2b; QuiNIDine; Selective Serotonin Reuptake Inhibitors

Decreased Effect

The levels/effects of Guaifenesin and Dextromethorphan may be decreased by: Peginterferon Alfa-2b

Storage/Stability Store at room temperature.

Mechanism of Action

Guaifenesin is thought to act as an expectorant by irritating the gastric mucosa and stimulating respiratory tract secretions, thereby increasing respiratory fluid volumes and decreasing phlegm viscosity

Dextromethorphan is a chemical relative of morphine lacking opioid properties except in overdose; controls cough by depressing the medullary cough center

Pharmacokinetics (Adult data unless noted) Absorption: Dextromethorphan is rapidly absorbed from the GI tract

Dosing: Usual Oral (dose expressed in mg of **dextromethorphan**):

Children: 1-2 mg/kg/day divided every 6-8 hours

Children >12 years and Adults: 60-120 mg/day divided every 6-8 hours or as extended release product 30-60 mg every 12 hours; not to exceed 120 mg/day

Administration Oral: Administer without regard to meals, with a large quantity of fluid to ensure proper effect; do not crush, chew, or break extended release tablets

Test Interactions See individual agents.

Dosage Forms Excipient information presented when available (limited, particularly for generics); consult specific product labeling.

Caplet, oral:

Fenesin DM IR: Guaifenesin 400 mg and dextromethorphan hydrobromide 15 mg

Refenesen DM: Guaifenesin 400 mg and dextromethorphan hydrobromide 20 mg

Capsule, oral:

Coricidin HBP Chest Congestion and Cough: Guaifenesin 200 mg and dextromethorphan hydrobromide 10 mg

Robitussin Maximum Strength Cough + Congestion DM: Guaifenesin 200 mg and dextromethorphan hydrobromide 10 mg

Granules, oral:

Mucinex Kid's Cough Mini-Melts: Guaifenesin 100 mg and dextromethorphan hydrobromide 5 mg per packet (12s) [contains magnesium 6 mg/pack, phenylalanine 2 mg/packet, sodium 3 mg/packet; orange crème flavor]

Liquid, oral:

Diabetic Tussin DM: Guaifenesin 100 mg and dextromethorphan hydrobromide 10 mg per 5 mL (120 mL) [dye free, ethanol free, sugar free; contains phenylalanine 8.4 mg/5 mL]

Diabetic Tussin DM Maximum Strength: Guaifenesin 200 mg and dextromethorphan hydrobromide 10 mg per 5 mL (120 mL) [dye free, ethanol free, sugar free; contains phenylalanine 8.4 mg/5 mL]

Double Tussin DM: Guaifenesin 300 mg and dextromethorphan hydrobromide 20 mg per 5 mL (120 mL, 480 mL) [dye free, ethanol free, sugar free]

Iophen DM-NR: Guaifenesin 100 mg and dextromethorphan hydrobromide 10 mg per 5 mL (480 mL) [contains propylene glycol, sodium benzoate; raspberry flavor]

Kolephrin GG/DM: Guaifenesin 150 mg and dextromethorphan hydrobromide 10 mg per 5 mL (120 mL) [ethanol free; cherry flavor]

Mucinex Fast-Max DM Max: Guaifenesin 400 mg and dextromethorphan hydrobromide 20 mg per 20 mL (180 mL) [contains propylene glycol, potassium 6 mg/20 mL, sodium 13 mg/20 mL]

Mucinex Kid's Cough: Guaifenesin 100 mg and dextromethorphan hydrobromide 5 mg per 5 mL (120 mL) [contains propylene glycol, sodium 3 mg/5 mL; cherry flavor]

Robitussin Peak Cold Cough + Chest Congestion DM: Guaifenesin 100 mg and dextromethorphan hydrobromide 10 mg per 5 mL (120 mL, 240 mL) [contains menthol, propylene glycol, sodium 3.5 mg/5 mL, sodium benzoate]

Robitussin Peak Cold Sugar-Free Cough + Chest Congestion DM: Guaifenesin 100 mg and dextromethorphan hydrobromide 10 mg per 5 mL (120 mL) [sugar free; contains propylene glycol, sodium 3 mg/5 mL, sodium benzoate]

Robitussin Peak Cold Maximum Strength Cough + Chest Congestion DM: Guaifenesin 200 mg and dextromethorphan hydrobromide 10 mg per 5 mL (120 mL, 240 mL) [contains menthol, propylene glycol, sodium 5 mg/5 mL, sodium benzoate]

Safe Tussin DM: Guaifenesin 100 mg and dextromethorphan hydrobromide 15 mg per 5 mL (120 mL) [contains benzoic acid, phenylalanine 4.2 mg/5 mL, and propylene glycol; orange and mint flavors]

Scot-Tussin Senior: Guaifenesin 200 mg and dextromethorphan hydrobromide 15 mg per 5 mL (120 mL) [ethanol free, sodium free, sugar free]

Vicks 44E: Guaifenesin 200 mg and dextromethorphan hydrobromide 20 mg per 15 mL (120 mL, 235 mL) [contains ethanol, sodium 31 mg/15 mL, sodium benzoate]

Vicks DayQuil Mucus Control DM: Guaifenesin 200 mg and dextromethorphan hydrobromide 10 mg per 15 mL (295 mL) [contains propylene glycol, sodium 25 mg/15 mL, sodium benzoate; citrus blend flavor]

Vicks Nature Fusion Cough & Chest Congestion: Guaifenesin 200 mg and dextromethorphan hydrobromide 20 mg per 30 mL (236 mL) [dye free, ethanol free, gluten free; contains propylene glycol, sodium 36 mg/30 mL; honey flavor]

Vicks Pediatric Formula 44E: Guaifenesin 100 mg and dextromethorphan hydrobromide 10 mg per 15 mL (120 mL) [ethanol free; contains sodium 30 mg/15 mL, sodium benzoate; cherry flavor]

Generic: Guaifenesin 100 mg and dextromethorphan hydrobromide 10 mg per 5 mL (480 mL)

Syrup, oral:

Cheracol D: Guaifenesin 100 mg and dextromethorphan hydrobromide 10 mg per 5 mL (120 mL, 180 mL) [contains benzoic acid, ethanol 4.75%]

Cheracol Plus: Guaifenesin 100 mg and dextromethorphan hydrobromide 10 mg per 5 mL (120 mL) [contains benzoic acid, ethanol 4.75%]

Diabetic Siltussin-DM DAS-Na: Guaifenesin 100 mg and dextromethorphan hydrobromide 10 mg per 5 mL (118 mL) [ethanol free, sugar free; contains benzoic acid, phenylalanine 3 mg/5 mL, propylene glycol; strawberry flavor]

Diabetic Siltussin-DM DAS-Na Maximum Strength: Guaifenesin 200 mg and dextromethorphan hydrobromide 10 mg per 5 mL (118 mL) [ethanol free, sugar free; contains benzoic acid, phenylalanine 3 mg/5 mL, propylene glycol; strawberry flavor]

Guaicon DMS: Guaifenesin 100 mg and dextromethorphan hydrobromide 10 mg per 5 mL (10 mL) [ethanol free, sugar free]

Q-Tussin DM: Guaifenesin 100 mg and dextromethorphan hydrobromide 10 mg per 5 mL (118 mL, 237 mL, 473 mL) [ethanol free, contains sodium benzoate; cherry flavor]

Robafen DM: Guaifenesin 100 mg and dextromethorphan hydrobromide 10 mg per 5 mL (120 mL, 240 mL, 480 mL) [cherry flavor]

Silexin: Guaifenesin 100 mg and dextromethorphan hydrobromide 10 mg per 5 mL (45 mL) [ethanol free, sugar free)]

Siltussin DM: Guaifenesin 100 mg and dextromethorphan hydrobromide 10 mg per 5 mL (120 mL, 240 mL, 480 mL) [strawberry flavor]

Siltussin DM DAS: Guaifenesin 100 mg and dextromethorphan hydrobromide 10 mg per 5 mL (120 mL) [dye free, ethanol free, sugar free; strawberry flavor]

Triaminic Cough & Cold: Guaifenesin 100 mg and dextromethorphan hydrobromide 5 mg per 5 mL (118 mL) [contains propylene glycol, sodium benzoate; cherry flavor]

Zyncof: Guaifenesin 400 mg and dextromethorphan hydrobromide 20 mg per 5 mL (120 mL, 480 mL) [dye free, ethanol free, sugar free; contains propylene glycol; grape flavor]

Generic: Guaifenesin 100 mg and dextromethorphan hydrobromide 10 mg per 5 mL (5 mL, 10 mL, 120 mL, 480 mL)

Tablet, oral:

Silexin: Guaifenesin 100 mg and dextromethorphan hydrobromide 10 mg

Generic: Guaifenesin 1000 mg and dextromethorphan hydrobromide 60 mg; guaifenesin 1200 mg and dextromethorphan hydrobromide 60 mg

Tablet, extended release, oral:

Mucinex DM: Guaifenesin 600 mg and dextromethorphan hydrobromide 30 mg

Mucinex DM Maximum Strength: Guaifenesin 1200 mg and dextromethorphan hydrobromide 60 mg

Generic: Guaifenesin 1200 mg and dextromethorphan hydrobromide 60 mg

GuanFACINE (GWAHN fa seen)

Medication Safety Issues

Sound-alike/look-alike issues:

GuanFACINE may be confused with guaiFENesin, guanabenz, guanidine

Intuniv may be confused with Invega
Tenex may be confused with Entex, Xanax

BEERS Criteria medication:

This drug may be potentially inappropriate for use in geriatric patients (Quality of evidence - low; Strength of recommendation - strong).

International issues:

Tenex [U.S.] may be confused with Kinex brand name for biperiden [Mexico]

Related Information

Oral Medications That Should Not Be Crushed or Altered *on page 2476*

Brand Names: US Intuniv; Tenex

Brand Names: Canada Intuniv XR

Therapeutic Category $Alpha_2$-Adrenergic Agonist

Generic Availability (US) Yes

Use

Immediate release: Management of hypertension alone or in combination with other hypertensive agents, especially thiazide-type diuretics (FDA approved ages ≥12 years and adults); has also been used in attention-deficit/hyperactivity disorder (ADHD), including ADHD with tic disorder (or Tourette's syndrome) and ADHD with autism or pervasive developmental disorders (PDD) comorbidities

Extended release: Short-term treatment (≤9 weeks) of ADHD as monotherapy or adjunctive therapy with stimulant medication (FDA approved in ages 6-17 years); has also been used for long-term treatment (24 months) of ADHD (Biederman, 2008; Sallee, 2009)

Pregnancy Risk Factor B

Pregnancy Considerations Adverse events were not observed in animal reproduction studies except in doses that also caused maternal toxicity. Information related to guanfacine use during pregnancy is limited (Philipp, 1980). Untreated chronic maternal hypertension is associated with adverse events in the fetus, infant, and mother. If treatment for hypertension during pregnancy is needed, other agents are preferred (ACOG, 2012).

Breast-Feeding Considerations It is not known if guanfacine is excreted in breast milk. The manufacturer recommends that caution be exercised when administering guanfacine to nursing women.

Contraindications Hypersensitivity to guanfacine or any component of the formulation

Warnings/Precautions May cause atrioventricular (AV) heart block, bradycardia, hypotension, orthostasis, sinus node dysfunction, and syncope; these effects are dose-dependent and more pronounced during the first month of therapy, or may worsen especially when used with other sympatholytic drugs. Monitor vital signs frequently in patients with cardiac conduction abnormalities or those concomitantly treated with other sympatholytic drugs. Use with caution in patients with severe coronary insufficiency, recent MI, or a history of bradycardia, cardiovascular disease, heart block, hypotension, or syncope. Cautious use is also recommended in patients with cerebrovascular disease, chronic hepatic or renal impairment (dosage adjustment may be necessary in severe impairment), or conditions that predispose them to syncope (eg, orthostasis, dehydration). May cause sedation and drowsiness, which may impair physical or mental abilities; patients must be cautioned about performing tasks that require mental alertness (eg, operating machinery, driving). Skin rash with exfoliation has been reported; discontinue guanfacine and monitor patients who develop a rash. Potentially significant interactions may exist, requiring dose or frequency adjustment, additional monitoring, and/or selection of alternative therapy.

Abrupt discontinuation can result in nervousness, anxiety, and, rarely, rebound hypertension (occurs 2 to 4 days after withdrawal). To minimize these effects, taper the dose in decrements of ≤1 mg every 3 to 7 days and monitor blood pressure and pulse following dosage reduction/discontinuation. Formulations of guanfacine (immediate release versus extended release) are not interchangeable on a mg:mg basis because bioavailability, C_{max}, and T_{max} vary.

Avoid use in elderly patients because of high risk of CNS adverse effects; may also cause orthostatic hypotension and bradycardia; not recommended for routine use as an antihypertensive (Beers Criteria). Recommended to be used as part of a comprehensive treatment program for attention-deficit disorders; safety and efficacy of long-term use for the treatment of ADHD (>2 years) have not been established.

Warnings: Additional Pediatric Considerations The American Heart Association recommends that all children diagnosed with ADHD who may be candidates for medication, such as guanfacine, should have a thorough cardiovascular assessment prior to initiation of therapy. These recommendations are based upon reports of serious cardiovascular adverse events (including sudden death) in patients (both children and adults) taking usual doses of stimulant medications. Most of these patients were found to have underlying structural heart disease (eg, hypertrophic obstructive cardiomyopathy). This assessment should include a combination of thorough medical history, family history, and physical examination. An ECG is not mandatory but should be considered. **Note:** In older clinical data, ECG abnormalities and four cases of sudden cardiac death were reported in children receiving clonidine (a less selective $alpha_2$-agonist) with methylphenidate; reduce dose of methylphenidate by 40% when used concurrently with clonidine; consider ECG monitoring. However, more recent (published after 2001) multicenter trials have not reported serious cardiovascular outcomes or events in medically screened children and adolescents receiving concomitant clonidine and psychostimulant therapy; the most frequent reported adverse effects with combination therapy were drowsiness, dizziness, and somnolence (Wilens, 2012). A double-blind, placebo-controlled trial of 461 pediatric patients (age: 6 to 17 years) examining the effect of the addition of extended release guanfacine to current psychostimulant therapy did not report any cardiovascular adverse events; in this trial, the most common (>10% incidence) treatment emergent adverse effects were headache, somnolence, fatigue, and dizziness (Wilens, 2012). Further studies are needed to examine the long-term safety and efficacy of guanfacine in combination with psychostimulants.

Adverse Reactions

Cardiovascular: Atrioventricular block, bradycardia, chest pain, hypertension, hypotension (includes orthostatic), sinus arrhythmia, syncope

Central nervous system: Agitation, anxiety, convulsions, depression, dizziness, drowsiness, fatigue, headache, emotional lability, insomnia, irritability, lethargy, nightmares

Dermatologic: Pallor, pruritus, skin rash

Endocrine & metabolic: Weight gain

Gastrointestinal: Abdominal pain, constipation, decreased appetite, diarrhea, dyspepsia, nausea, stomach pain, vomiting, xerostomia

Genitourinary: Impotence, urinary frequency, urinary incontinence

Hepatic: Increased serum ALT

Hypersensitivity: Hypersensitivity reaction

Neuromuscular & skeletal: Weakness

Respiratory: Asthma

Miscellaneous: Fever (Biederman 2008)

Rare but important or life-threatening: Alopecia, amnesia, cardiac failure, cardiac fibrillation, cerebrovascular accident, dermatitis, dysphagia, exacerbation of cardiac disease (sinus node dysfunction, atrioventricular block), exfoliative dermatitis, hallucination, hypersensitivity reaction, hypokinesia, iritis, mania (immediate release; children), myocardial infarction, nocturia, palpitations, paresis, Raynaud phenomenon, rebound hypertension, renal failure, tachycardia, visual disturbance

Drug Interactions

Metabolism/Transport Effects Substrate of CYP3A4 (major); **Note:** Assignment of Major/Minor substrate status based on clinically relevant drug interaction potential

Avoid Concomitant Use

Avoid concomitant use of GuanFACINE with any of the following: Alcohol (Ethyl); Azelastine (Nasal); Ceritinib; Conivaptan; Fusidic Acid (Systemic); Idelalisib; Iobenguane I 123; Orphenadrine; Paraldehyde; Thalidomide

Increased Effect/Toxicity

GuanFACINE may increase the levels/effects of: Amifostine; Antihypertensives; Azelastine (Nasal); Beta-Blockers; Bradycardia-Causing Agents; Buprenorphine; Ceritinib; CNS Depressants; DULoxetine; Hydrocodone; Hypotensive Agents; Ivabradine; Lacosamide; Levodopa; Methotrimeprazine; Metyrosine; Obinutuzumab; Orphenadrine; Paraldehyde; Pramipexole; RisperiDONE; RiTUXimab; ROPINIRole; Rotigotine; Selective Serotonin Reuptake Inhibitors; Suvorexant; Thalidomide; Valproic Acid and Derivatives; Zolpidem

The levels/effects of GuanFACINE may be increased by: Alcohol (Ethyl); Alfuzosin; Aprepitant; Barbiturates; Beta-Blockers; Bretylium; Brimonidine (Topical); Cannabis; Conivaptan; CYP3A4 Inhibitors (Moderate); CYP3A4 Inhibitors (Strong); Dasatinib; Diazoxide; Doxylamine; Dronabinol; Droperidol; Fosaprepitant; Fusidic Acid (Systemic); Herbs (Hypotensive Properties); HydrOXYzine; Idelalisib; Ivacaftor; Kava Kava; Luliconazole; Magnesium Sulfate; MAO Inhibitors; Methotrimeprazine; Mifepristone; Nabilone; Netupitant; Nicorandil; Palbociclib; Pentoxifylline; Perampanel; Phosphodiesterase 5 Inhibitors; Prostacyclin Analogues; Rufinamide; Ruxolitinib; Simeprevir; Sodium Oxybate; Stiripentol; Tapentadol; Tetrahydrocannabinol; Tofacitinib

Decreased Effect

GuanFACINE may decrease the levels/effects of: Iobenguane I 123

The levels/effects of GuanFACINE may be decreased by: Bosentan; CYP3A4 Inducers (Moderate); CYP3A4 Inducers (Strong); Dabrafenib; Deferasirox; Herbs (Hypertensive Properties); Methylphenidate; Mirtazapine; Mitotane; Serotonin/Norepinephrine Reuptake Inhibitors; Siltuximab; St Johns Wort; Tocilizumab; Tricyclic Antidepressants; Yohimbine

Storage/Stability

Immediate release: Store at 20°C to 25°C (68°F to 77°F).

Extended release: Store at 20°C to 25°C (68°F to 77°F); excursions permitted between 15°C and 30°C (59°F and 86°F).

Mechanism of Action Guanfacine is a selective $alpha_{2A}$-adrenoreceptor agonist which reduces sympathetic nerve impulses, resulting in reduced sympathetic outflow and a subsequent decrease in vasomotor tone and heart rate. In addition, guanfacine preferentially binds postsynaptic $alpha_{2A}$-adrenoreceptors in the prefrontal cortex and has been theorized to improve delay-related firing of prefrontal cortex neurons. As a result, underlying working memory and behavioral inhibition are affected; thereby improving symptoms associated with ADHD. Guanfacine is not a CNS stimulant.

Pharmacodynamics Antihypertensive effect: Duration: 24 hours following single dose

Pharmacokinetics (Adult data unless noted) Note: When dosed at same mg dose, the extended-release product has a lower peak serum concentration (60% lower) and AUC (43% lower) compared to the immediate release formulation.

Distribution:

- Immediate release: V_d: 6.3 L/kg
- Extended release: V_d (apparent): Children: 23.7 L/kg; Adolescent: 19.9 L/kg (Boellner, 2007)

Protein binding: ~70%

Metabolism: Hepatic via CYP3A4

Bioavailability: Oral:

- Immediate release: ~80%
- Extended release (relative to immediate release): 58%

Half-life:

- Immediate release: ~17 hours (range: 10-30 hours)
- Extended release: Children: 14.4 hours; Adolescents: 18 hours (Boellner, 2007)

Time to peak serum concentration:

- Immediate release: 2.6 hours (range: 1-4 hours)
- Extended release: Children and Adolescents: 5 hours (Boellner, 2007); Adults: 4-8 hours

Elimination: ~50% (40% to 75% of dose) excreted as unchanged drug in urine; tubular secretion of the drug may occur

Dialysis: Not dialyzable in clinically significant amounts (2.4%)

Dosing: Usual Note: Immediate release and extended release products are not interchangeable on a mg-per-mg basis due to differences in pharmacokinetic profiles.

Pediatric:

Attention-deficit/hyperactivity disorder:

Immediate release product: Limited data available (Dopheide 2009; Pliszka 2007): Children ≥6 years and Adolescents:

≤45 kg: Oral: Initial: 0.5 mg once daily at bedtime; may titrate every 3 to 4 days in 0.5 mg/day increments to 0.5 mg twice daily, then 0.5 mg three times daily, then 0.5 mg four times daily; maximum daily dose: Patient weight 27 to 40.5 kg: 2 mg/**day**; 40.5 to 45 kg: 3 mg/**day**

>45 kg: Oral: Initial: 1 mg once daily at bedtime; may titrate every 3 to 4 days in 1 mg/day increments to 1 mg twice daily, then 1 mg three times daily, then 1 mg four times daily; maximum daily dose: 4 mg/**day**

Extended release product (Intuniv): Children and Adolescents 6 to 17 years: Oral: Initial: 1 mg once daily administered at the same time of day (in the morning or evening); may titrate dose by no more than 1 mg/week increments, as tolerated. Usual maintenance dose: 1 to 4 mg/day; maximum daily dose: 4 mg/**day**. In clinical monotherapy trials, initial clinical response was associated with doses of 0.05 to 0.08 mg/kg once daily; increased efficacy was seen with increasing mg/kg doses; doses up to 0.12 mg/kg once daily have shown benefit when tolerated. In adjunctive therapy trials with stimulant medication, doses of 0.0 to -0.12 mg/kg/day produced optimal clinical response in the majority of patients.

Conversion from immediate release guanfacine to the extended release product: Discontinue the immediate release product; initiate the extended release product at the doses recommended above.

Missed doses of extended release: If patient misses two or more consecutive doses, repeat titration of dose should be considered.

Discontinuation of extended release: Taper dose by no more than 1 mg every 3 to 7 days.

Dosing adjustment for concomitant CYP3A4 inhibitors/inducers: Extended release:

Strong CYP3A4 inhibitors: If initiating guanfacine while taking a strong 3A4 inhibitor, do not exceed a maximum guanfacine dose of 2 mg/day. If continuing guanfacine and adding a strong CYP3A4 inhibitor, decrease guanfacine dose by 50%. If the strong CYP3A4 inhibitor is discontinued, double the guanfacine dose (maximum daily dose: 4 mg/**day**).

Strong CYP3A4 inducers: If initiating guanfacine while taking a strong CYP3A4 inducer, may titrate guanfacine up to 8 mg/day; consider faster titration (eg, 2 mg/week). If continuing guanfacine and adding a strong CYP3A4 inducer, consider increasing guanfacine gradually over 1 to 2 weeks to double the original dose, as tolerated. If the strong CYP3A4 inducer is discontinued, decrease guanfacine dose by 50% over 1 to 2 weeks (maximum daily dose: 4 mg/**day**).

Hypertension: Children ≥12 years and Adolescents: Immediate release product: Oral: 1 mg usually at bedtime; may increase, if needed, at 3- to 4-week intervals; usual range: 0.5 to 2 mg/day; maximum daily dose: 2 mg/**day**

Pervasive developmental disorders (PDD) and ADHD: Limited data available; efficacy results variable: Children and Adolescents 5 to 14 years: Immediate release product:

<25 kg: Oral: Initial: 0.25 mg once daily, increase dose as tolerated every 4 days in 0.25 mg/day increments in 2 to 3 divided doses; maximum daily dose: 3 mg/**day** (Scahill 2006)

≥25 kg: Oral: Initial: 0.5 mg once daily, increase dose as tolerated every 4 days in 0.5 mg/day increments in 2 to 3 divided doses; maximum daily dose: 3 mg/**day** (Handen 2008; Scahill 2006)

Dosing based on a double-blind, placebo-controlled, 6-week crossover trial conducted in children with ADHD and autism or intellectual disabilities (n=11; age: 5 to 9 years); five of 11 patients showed improvement in hyperactivity scores; other patient assessment parameters did not show improvements (Handen, 2008). In an open-label 8-week pilot study in children with ADHD and PDD (n=25; mean age: 9 years; range: 5-14 years), patients showed improvement in parent- and teacher-rated hyperactivity subscale scores; increased irritability occurred in seven patients; the authors note that patients with PDD may be more sensitive to irritability-type adverse effects (Scahill 2006). A retrospective chart review of pediatric autism spectrum disorders (n=80; age: 3 to 18 years) reported ~24% of patients responded to mean dose of 2.6 mg/day; the authors noted patients with Asperger's or PDD not otherwise specified (NOS) responded more frequently than those with autistic disorder or comorbidity of mental retardation (Posey 2004).

Tic disorder and ADHD: Limited data available: Children and Adolescents 7 to 16 years: Immediate release product: Oral: Initial: 0.5 mg once daily at bedtime for 3 days, then 0.5 mg twice daily for 4 days, then 0.5 mg 3 times daily for 7 days; further upward titration based on clinical response; dosing based on a double-blind, placebo-controlled study in patients with ADHD and mild to moderate tics (n=34; mean age: 10.4 years; range: 7 to 14 years); reported final dose range: 1.5 to 3 mg/day in 3 divided doses; improvement in teacher-rated ADHD scores and tic scores after 8 weeks was reported (Scahill 2001). A small open-label trial (n=10; age range: 8 to 16 years) used similar initial doses with dose titration; final dose range: 0.75 to 3 mg/day in divided doses; 7 of 10 patients required a final dose of 1.5 mg/day in divided doses (Chappell 1995).

Adult: **Hypertension:** Immediate release: Oral: 1 mg usually at bedtime; may increase, if needed, at 3- to 4-week intervals; usual dose range (JNC 7): 0.5 to 2 mg once daily

Dosing adjustment in renal impairment:

Immediate release: Children ≥12 years and Adults: There are no dosage adjustments provided in the manufacturer's labeling; however, the lower end of the dosing range is recommended in patients with renal impairment; use with caution, as ~50% of the dose (40% to 75% of dose) is excreted as unchanged drug in urine.

Extended release (Intuniv): Children ≥6 years and Adolescents: There are no dosage adjustments provided in manufacturer's labeling (has not been studied); however, dosage adjustments may be necessary in patients with significant renal impairment.

Hemodialysis: Immediate release or extended release: Dialysis clearance is low (~15% of total clearance).

Dosing adjustment in hepatic impairment:

Immediate release: Children ≥12 years and Adults: There are no specific dosage adjustments provided in the manufacturer's labeling; however, use with caution in chronic hepatic impairment; consider dosage reduction.

Extended release (Intuniv): Children ≥6 years and Adolescents: There are no dosage adjustments provided in manufacturer's labeling (has not been studied); however, dosage adjustments may be necessary in patients with significant hepatic impairment.

Administration

Immediate release: Take at bedtime to minimize somnolence

Extended release: Take at the same time each day (either morning or evening); swallow tablet whole with water, milk, or other liquid; do not crush, break, or chew; do not administer with high-fat meal

Monitoring Parameters Heart rate, blood pressure, consider ECG monitoring in patients with history of heart disease or concurrent use of medications affecting cardiac conduction

ADHD: Evaluate patients for cardiac disease prior to initiation of therapy for ADHD with thorough medical history, family history, and physical exam; consider ECG; perform ECG and echocardiogram if findings suggest cardiac disease; promptly conduct cardiac evaluation in patients who develop chest pain, unexplained syncope, or any other symptom of cardiac disease during treatment.

Additional Information Guanfacine is a more selective alpha$_2$-agonist than clonidine; therefore, has less sedation and dizziness associated with use than clonidine; withdrawal effects less commonly occur due to its longer half-life.

Medications used to treat ADHD should be part of a total treatment program that may include other components, such as psychological, educational, and social measures. Long-term usefulness of guanfacine for the treatment of ADHD should be periodically re-evaluated in patients receiving the drug for extended periods of time.

Dosage Forms Excipient information presented when available (limited, particularly for generics); consult specific product labeling.

Tablet, Oral:

Tenex: 1 mg [contains fd&c red #40 aluminum lake]

Tenex: 2 mg [contains fd&c yellow #10 aluminum lake]

Generic: 1 mg, 2 mg

Tablet Extended Release 24 Hour, Oral:

Intuniv: 1 mg, 2 mg, 3 mg, 4 mg

Generic: 1 mg, 2 mg, 3 mg, 4 mg

◆ **Guanfacine Hydrochloride** *see* GuanFACINE *on page 993*

◆ **GUM Paroex (Can)** *see* Chlorhexidine Gluconate *on page 434*

◆ **GW506U78** *see* Nelarabine *on page 1496*

◆ **GW433908G** *see* Fosamprenavir *on page 936*

◆ **Gyne-Lotrimin [OTC]** *see* Clotrimazole (Topical) *on page 518*

◆ **Gyne-Lotrimin 3 [OTC]** *see* Clotrimazole (Topical) *on page 518*

◆ **H1N1 Influenza Vaccine** *see* Influenza Virus Vaccine (Inactivated) *on page 1108*

◆ **H1N1 Influenza Vaccine** *see* Influenza Virus Vaccine (Live/Attenuated) *on page 1113*

◆ **H_2O_2** *see* Hydrogen Peroxide *on page 1044*

Haemophilus b Conjugate and Hepatitis B Vaccine

(he MOF i lus bee KON joo gate & hep a TYE tis bee vak SEEN)

Medication Safety Issues

Sound-alike/look-alike issues:

Comvax may be confused with Recombivax [Recombivax HB]

Related Information

Centers for Disease Control and Prevention (CDC) and Other Links *on page 2424*

Immunization Administration Recommendations *on page 2411*

Immunization Schedules *on page 2416*

Brand Names: US Comvax

Therapeutic Category Vaccine; Vaccine, Inactivated Bacteria; Vaccine, Inactivated Virus

Generic Availability (US) No

Use Immunization against invasive disease caused by *H. influenzae* type b and against infection caused by all known subtypes of hepatitis B virus in patients born of HB_sAg-negative mothers (FDA approved in ages 6 weeks to 15 months)

Infants born of HB_sAg-positive mothers or mothers of unknown HB_sAg status should receive hepatitis B immune globulin and monovalent hepatitis B vaccine (recombinant) at birth and should complete the hepatitis B vaccination series

Pregnancy Risk Factor C

Pregnancy Considerations Animal reproduction studies have not been conducted. This product is not indicated for use in women of childbearing age.

Breast-Feeding Considerations This product is not indicated for use in women of childbearing age. Inactivated virus vaccines do not affect the safety of breast-feeding for the mother or the infant (NCIRD/ACIP 2011). Breast-feeding also appears to reduce the incidence of infant fever associated with routine childhood immunization (Piscane 2010). Breast-feeding infants should be vaccinated according to the recommended schedules (NCIRD/ACIP 2011).

Contraindications Hypersensitivity to *Haemophilus* b vaccine, hepatitis B vaccine, yeast, or to any component of the formulation

Warnings/Precautions Vaccination may not result in effective immunity in all patients. Response depends upon multiple factors (eg, type of vaccine, age of patient) and may be improved by administering the vaccine at the recommended dose, route, and interval. Vaccines may not be effective if administered during periods of altered immune competence (NCIRD/ACIP 2011). Infection may occur within the week of vaccination, prior to the onset of the vaccine. Use with caution in severely immunocompromised patients (eg, patients receiving chemo/radiation therapy or other immunosuppressive therapy [including high dose corticosteroids]); may have a reduced response to vaccination. May be used in patients with HIV infection. In general, household and close contacts of persons with altered immunocompetence may receive all age appropriate vaccines (IDSA [Rubin 2014]; NCIRD/ACIP 2011); inactivated vaccines should be administered ≥2 weeks prior to planned immunosuppression when feasible (IDSA [Rubin 2014]). Syncope has been reported with use of injectable vaccines and may result in serious secondary injury (eg, skull fracture, cerebral hemorrhage); typically reported in adolescents and young adults and within 15 minutes after vaccination. Procedures should be in place to avoid injuries from falling and to restore cerebral perfusion if syncope occurs (NCIRD/ACIP 2011). Apnea has occurred following intramuscular vaccine administration in premature infants; consider clinical status implications. In general, preterm infants should be vaccinated at the same chronological age as full-term infants (NCIRD/ACIP 2011). Antipyretics have not been shown to prevent febrile seizures; antipyretics may be used to treat fever or discomfort following vaccination (NCIRD/ACIP 2011). One study reported that routine prophylactic administration of acetaminophen to prevent fever prior to vaccination decreased the immune response of some vaccines; the clinical significance of this reduction in immune response has not been established (Prymula 2009).

The decision to administer or delay vaccination because of current or recent febrile illness depends on the severity of symptoms and the etiology of the disease. Consider deferring administration in patients with moderate or severe acute illness (with or without fever); vaccination should not be delayed for patients with mild acute illness (with or without fever) (NCIRD/ACIP 2011). Use caution in children with coagulation disorders (including thrombocytopenia) and patients on anticoagulant therapy; bleeding/hematoma may occur from IM administration; if the patient receives antihemophilia or other similar therapy, IM injection can be scheduled shortly after such therapy is administered (NCIRD/ACIP 2011). Immediate treatment (including epinephrine 1:1,000) for anaphylactoid and/or hypersensitivity reactions should be available during vaccine use (NCIRD/ACIP 2011).Packaging contains natural latex rubber. In order to maximize vaccination rates, the ACIP recommends simultaneous administration (ie, >1 vaccine on the same day at different anatomic sites) of all age-appropriate vaccines (live or inactivated) for which a person is eligible at a single clinic visit, unless contraindications exist. The use of combination vaccines is generally preferred over separate injections, taking into consideration provider assessment, patient preference, and adverse events. When using combination vaccines, the minimum age for administration is the oldest minimum age for any individual component; the minimum interval between dosing is the greatest minimum interval between any individual components. The ACIP prefers each dose of a specific vaccine in a series come from the same manufacturer when possible (NCIRD/ACIP 2011). Comvax is not indicated for use as the "birth dose" of hepatitis B vaccine; hepatitis B vaccine (recombinant) is indicated for all infants at birth. This combination vaccine cannot be administered to any infant <6 weeks of age or >71 months of age. Infants born of HBsAg-positive mothers or mothers of unknown HBsAg status should receive hepatitis B vaccine (recombinant) at birth and should complete the hepatitis B vaccination series given according to a particular schedule (refer to current ACIP recommendations). Infants born of HBsAg-positive mothers should also receive hepatitis B immune globulin at birth.

Adverse Reactions All serious adverse reactions must be reported to the U.S. Department of Health and Human Services (DHHS) Vaccine Adverse Event Reporting System (VAERS) at 1-800-822-7967 or online at https://vaers.hhs.gov/esub/index.

Central nervous system: Crying (unusual/high pitched), fever, irritability, somnolence

Dermatologic: Rash

Gastrointestinal: Anorexia, diarrhea, oral candidiasis, vomiting

Local: Injection site reactions: Erythema pain/soreness, swelling/induration

Otic: Otitis media

Respiratory: Cough, respiratory congestion, rhinorrhea, upper respiratory tract infection

Postmarketing and/or case reports: Anaphylaxis, angioedema, erythema multiforme, febrile seizure, seizure, thrombocytopenia, urticaria

Drug Interactions

Metabolism/Transport Effects None known.

Avoid Concomitant Use There are no known interactions where it is recommended to avoid concomitant use.

Increased Effect/Toxicity There are no known significant interactions involving an increase in effect.

Decreased Effect

The levels/effects of Haemophilus b Conjugate and Hepatitis B Vaccine may be decreased by: Belimumab; Fingolimod; Immunosuppressants

Storage/Stability Store at 2°C to 8°C (36°F to 48°F); do not freeze.

Mechanism of Action See individual agents.

Pharmacodynamics See individual agents.

Dosing: Usual Pediatric:

Primary Immunization: Infants and Children 6 weeks through 15 months: IM: 0.5 mL per dose for a total of 3 doses administered as follows: 2, 4, and 12 to 15 months of age; **Note:** If the recommended schedule cannot be followed, the interval between the first two doses should be at least 6 weeks and the interval between the second and third doses should be as close as possible to 8 to 11 months.

Modified Schedule: Children who receive one dose of hepatitis B vaccine at or shortly after birth may receive Comvax on a schedule of 2, 4, and 12 to 15 months of age

Dosing adjustment in renal impairment: There are no dosage adjustments provided in the manufacturer's labeling.

Dosing adjustment in hepatic impairment: There are no dosage adjustments provided in the manufacturer's labeling.

Administration Shake well and administer IM in either the anterolateral aspect of the thigh or deltoid muscle of the arm; not for IV or SubQ administration. US law requires that the date of administration, the vaccine manufacturer, lot number of vaccine, and the administering person's name, title, and address be entered into the patient's permanent medical record.

For patients at risk of hemorrhage following intramuscular injection, the vaccine should be administered intramuscularly if, in the opinion of the physician familiar with the patient's bleeding risk, the vaccine can be administered with by this route with reasonable safety. If the patient receives antihemophilia or other similar therapy, intramuscular vaccination can be scheduled shortly after such therapy is administered. A fine needle (23 gauge or smaller) can be used for the vaccination and firm pressure applied to the site (without rubbing) for at least 2 minutes. The patient should be instructed concerning the risk of hematoma from the injection. Patients on anticoagulant therapy should be considered to have the same bleeding risks and treated as those with clotting factor disorders (NCIRD/ACIP 2011).

Monitoring Parameters Observe for syncope for 15 minutes following administration (NCIRD/ACIP 2011). If seizure-like activity associated with syncope occurs, maintain patient in supine or Trendelenburg position to reestablish adequate cerebral perfusion.

Product Availability Production of Comvax has been discontinued by the manufacturer (Merck). As of December 31, 2014, Comvax is no longer available for direct purchase from Merck. Product may still be available from wholesalers and physician distributors. Refer to the following for additional information https://www.merckvaccines.com/is-bin/intershop.static/WFS/Merck-MerckVaccines-Site/Merck-MerckVaccines/en_US/Professional-Resources/Documents/announcements/VACC-1114028-0000.pdf.

Dosage Forms Excipient information presented when available (limited, particularly for generics); consult specific product labeling.

Injection, suspension [preservative free]:

Comvax®: *Haemophilus* b capsular polysaccharide 7.5 mcg (bound to *Neisseria meningitides* OMPC 125 mcg) and hepatitis B surface antigen 5 mcg per 0.5 mL (0.5 mL) [contains aluminum; contains natural rubber/natural latex in packaging]

◆ ***Haemophilus* B Conjugate (Hib)** *see* Diphtheria and Tetanus Toxoids, Acellular Pertussis, Poliovirus and *Haemophilus* b Conjugate Vaccine *on page 679*

Haemophilus b Conjugate Vaccine

(he MOF fi lus bee KON joo gate vak SEEN)

Related Information

Centers for Disease Control and Prevention (CDC) and Other Links *on page 2424*

Immunization Administration Recommendations *on page 2411*

Immunization Schedules *on page 2416*

Brand Names: US ActHIB; Hiberix; PedvaxHIB

Brand Names: Canada ActHIB; PedvaxHIB

Therapeutic Category Vaccine; Vaccine, Inactivated Bacteria

Generic Availability (US) No

Use Routine, full series immunization of children 2 months to 5 years of age against invasive disease caused by *H. influenzae* (ActHIB: FDA approved in ages 2 months to 5 years; PedvaxHIB: FDA approved in ages 2 to 71 months)

Routine booster only immunization of children (Hiberix: FDA approved in ages 15 months to 4 years)

The Advisory Committee on Immunization Practices (ACIP) recommends vaccination for the following (CDC/ACIP [Kim 2015]; CDC/ACIP [Strikas 2015]); CDC/ACIP [Briere 2014]):

- Routine immunization in all infants and children through 59 months
- Unimmunized* children 12 through 59 months including chemotherapy recipients, anatomic or functional asplenia (including sickle cell disease), HIV infection, immunoglobulin deficiency, or early component complement deficiency

Efficacy data are not available for use in older children and adults with chronic conditions associated with an increased risk of Hib disease; however, may be used in certain situations:

- Unimmunized* children ≥5 years, adolescents, and adults with anatomic or functional asplenia (including sickle cell disease)
- Unimmunized* children ≥5 years and adolescents with HIV infection
- Children <5 years undergoing chemotherapy or radiation treatment
- Successful hematopoietic stem cell transplant recipients
- Children ≥15 months and adolescents undergoing elective splenectomy

* Unimmunized is defined as persons who have not received a primary series and booster dose or at least 1 dose of a Hib vaccine after 14 months of age

Medication Guide Available Yes

Pregnancy Risk Factor C

Pregnancy Considerations Animal reproduction studies have not been conducted. Inactivated vaccines have not been shown to cause increased risks to the fetus (NCIRD/ACIP 2011).

Breast-Feeding Considerations Inactivated vaccines do not affect the safety of breast-feeding for the mother or the infant (NCIRD/ACIP 2011). Breast-feeding also appears to reduce the incidence of infant fever associated with routine childhood immunization (Piscane 2010). Breast-feeding infants should be vaccinated according to the recommended schedules (NCIRD/ACIP 2011).

Contraindications Hypersensitivity to *Haemophilus* b polysaccharide or any component of the formulation

Warnings/Precautions Vaccination may not result in effective immunity in all patients. Response depends upon multiple factors (eg, type of vaccine, age of patient) and may be improved by administering the vaccine at the recommended dose, route, and interval. Vaccines may not be effective if administered during periods of altered immune competence (NCIRD/ACIP 2011). Infection may occur within the week of vaccination, prior to the onset of the vaccine. Use with caution in severely immunocompromised patients (eg, patients receiving chemo/radiation therapy or other immunosuppressive therapy [including high-dose corticosteroids]); may have a reduced response to vaccination. May be used in patients with HIV infection (NCIRD/ACIP 2011). In general, household and close contacts of persons with altered immunocompetence may receive all age appropriate vaccines (IDSA [Rubin 2014]; NCIRD/ACIP 2011). inactivated vaccines should be administered ≥2 weeks prior to planned immunosuppression when feasible (IDSA [Rubin 2014]). Use of this vaccine for specific medical and/or other indications (eg, immunocompromising conditions, hepatic or kidney disease, diabetes) is also addressed in the ACIP Adult Recommended Immunization Schedule (CDC/ACIP [Kim 2015]). Specific recommendations for use of this vaccine in immunocompromised patients with asplenia, cancer, HIV infection, cerebrospinal fluid leaks, cochlear implants, hematopoietic stem cell transplant (prior to or after), sickle cell disease, solid organ transplant (prior to or after), or those receiving immunosuppressive therapy for chronic conditions are available from the IDSA (Rubin 2014).

The decision to administer or delay vaccination because of current or recent febrile illness depends on the severity of symptoms and the etiology of the disease. Consider deferring administration in patients with moderate or severe acute illness (with or without fever); vaccination should not be delayed for patients with mild acute illness (with or without fever) (NCIRD/ACIP 2011). Antipyretics have not been shown to prevent febrile seizures; antipyretics may be used to treat fever or discomfort following vaccination (NCIRD/ACIP 2011). One study reported that routine prophylactic administration of acetaminophen to prevent fever prior to vaccination decreased the immune response of some vaccines; the clinical significance of this reduction in immune response has not been established (Prymula 2009).

Use caution in children with coagulation disorders (including thrombocytopenia) and patients on anticoagulant therapy; bleeding/hematoma may occur from IM administration; if the patient receives antihemophilia or other similar therapy, IM injection can be scheduled shortly after such therapy is administered (NCIRD/ACIP 2011). Immediate treatment (including epinephrine 1:1000) for anaphylactoid and/or hypersensitivity reactions should be available during vaccine use (NCIRD/ACIP 2011). Syncope has been reported with use of injectable vaccines and may result in serious secondary injury (eg, skull fracture, cerebral hemorrhage); typically reported in adolescents and young adults and within 15 minutes after vaccination. Procedures should be in place to avoid injuries from falling and to restore cerebral perfusion if syncope occurs (NCIRD/ACIP 2011).

Apnea has occurred following intramuscular vaccine administration in premature infants; consider clinical status implications. In general, preterm infants should be vaccinated at the same chronological age as full-term infants (NCIRD/ACIP 2011).

ActHIB, Hiberix: Use with caution in patients with history of Guillain-Barré syndrome (GBS); carefully consider risks and benefits to vaccination in patients known to have experienced GBS within 6 weeks following previous influenza vaccination.

In order to maximize vaccination rates, the ACIP recommends simultaneous administration (ie, >1 vaccine on the same day at different anatomic sites) of all age-appropriate vaccines (live or inactivated) for which a person is eligible at a single clinic visit, unless contraindications exist. The use of combination vaccines is generally preferred over separate injections, taking into consideration provider assessment, patient preference, and adverse events. When using combination vaccines, the minimum age for administration is the oldest minimum age for any individual component; the minimum interval between dosing is the greatest minimum interval between any individual components. The ACIP prefers each dose of Hib containing combination vaccines in a series come from the same manufacturer when possible; monovalent Hib vaccines are interchangeable (NCIRD/ACIP 2011).

Packaging may contain latex. Some products may contain lactose.

Adverse Reactions All serious adverse reactions must be reported to the U.S. Department of Health and Human Services (DHHS) Vaccine Adverse Event Reporting System (VAERS) 1-800-822-7967 or online at https://vaers.hhs.gov/esub/index. In Canada, adverse reactions may be reported to local provincial/territorial health agencies or to the Vaccine Safety Section at Public Health Agency of Canada (1-866-844-0018).

Central nervous system: Crying (unusual, high pitched, prolonged), drowsiness, fussiness, irritability, lethargy, pain, restlessness, seizure

Dermatologic: Skin rash, urticaria

Gastrointestinal: Anorexia, diarrhea, vomiting

Hematologic & oncologic: Thrombocytopenia

Local: Injection site: Erythema, induration, pain, soreness, swelling

Neuromuscular & skeletal: Weakness

Otic: Otitis media

Respiratory: Tracheitis, upper respiratory tract infection

Miscellaneous: Fever

Rare but important or life-threatening: Abscess at injection site (sterile), anaphylaxis, anaphylactoid reaction, angioedema, apnea, febrile seizures, Guillain-Barré syndrome, hypersensitivity reaction, hypotonic/hyporesponsive episode, lymphadenopathy, mass, peripheral edema, pneumonia, swelling of the injected limb (extensive), syncope, vasodepressor syncope

Drug Interactions

Metabolism/Transport Effects None known.

Avoid Concomitant Use There are no known interactions where it is recommended to avoid concomitant use.

Increased Effect/Toxicity There are no known significant interactions involving an increase in effect.

Decreased Effect

The levels/effects of Haemophilus b Conjugate Vaccine may be decreased by: Belimumab; Fingolimod; Immunosuppressants

Storage/Stability

ActHIB: Store lyophilized powder and diluent under refrigeration at 2°C to 8°C (36°F to 46°F); do not freeze. If not used immediately after reconstitution, may store under refrigeration for up to 24 hours.

Hiberix: Prior to reconstitution, store powder under refrigeration at 2°C to 8°C (36°F to 46°F). Protect from light. Diluent may be stored under refrigeration or at room temperature; do not freeze, discard diluent if frozen. If not used immediately after reconstitution, may store under refrigeration for up to 24 hours.

PedvaxHIB: Store under refrigeration at 2°C to 8°C (36°F to 46°F); do not freeze.

Mechanism of Action Stimulates production of anticapsular antibodies and provides active immunity to *Haemophilus influenzae* type b. Vaccination provides protective antibodies in >95% of infants who are vaccinated with a 2- or 3-dose series (CDC 2012). An anti-PRP concentration of ≥1.0 mcg/mL predicts long-term protection.

Pharmacodynamics Efficacy: The initial unconjugated polysaccharide Hib vaccines produced 45% to 88% reduction in disease incidence among children at least 18 to 24 months of age. The initial protein-conjugated Hib vaccines produced >90% protection in infants after a multidose series. After the initial Hib conjugate vaccines were licensed, subsequent formulations were licensed based on noninferior antibody responses.

Onset of action: Immunity develops progressively with each dose. Immunity can be inferred ~2 weeks after the initial series is complete.

Duration: Antibody concentrations exceeding 0.15 mcg/mL correlate with clinical protection from disease. Antibody concentrations exceeding 1 mcg/mL correlate with prolonged protection from disease, generally implying several years of protection.

Dosing: Usual

Pediatric:

Primary immunization: Note: Preterm infants should be vaccinated according to their chronological age, beginning at 2 months of age; number of doses for completion of Hib series dependent upon products including some combination formulations (3 doses: ActHIB, 2 doses: PedvaxHIB) (see combination product monographs for specific dosing information)

Infants 6 weeks to 6 months: Minimum age for first dose is 6 weeks.

ActHib (PRP-T): IM: 0.5 mL per dose for a total of 3 doses administered as follows: 2, 4, and 6 months of age

PedvaxHIB (PRP-OMP): IM: 0.5 mL per dose for a total of 2 doses administered as follows: 2 and 4 months of age

Booster immunization:

ActHIB, PedvaxHIB: Children 12 to 15 months: IM: 0.5 mL as a single dose

Hiberix: Children 12 months to 4 years: IM: 0.5 mL as a single dose

Catch-up immunization (CDC/ACIP [Strikas 2015]): **Note:** Do not restart the series. If doses have been given, begin the below schedule at the applicable dose number.

Infants and Children 4 to 59 months: IM: 0.5 mL per dose for a total of 1 to 4 doses administered as follows:

First dose given on the elected date.

Second dose given at least 4 weeks after the first dose (if first dose at <12 months of age) **or** 8 weeks after the first dose (if first dose at 12 to 14 months of age); this dose is not needed if the first dose was given at ≥15 months.

Third dose:

4-week interval: Give third dose at least 4 weeks after the second dose if currently <12 months of age, first dose at <7 months of age, and at least one PRP-T (ActHib, Pentacel) or type unknown

8-week interval: Give at least 8 weeks after the first dose and at 12 to 59 months of age if:

- currently <12 months of age and first dose at 7 to 11 months of age **or**
- currently 12 to 59 months of age and first dose <12 months of age and second dose at <15 months **or**
- first two doses were PRP-OMP (PedvaxHIB, Comvax) and given at <12 months of age

Third dose is not needed if the previous dose was given at ≥15 months of age.

Fourth dose given 8 weeks after the third dose: This dose is only needed for children 12 to 59 months who received 3 doses at <12 months of age

Children ≥5 years and Adolescents; unimmunized **and** are at increased risk for invasive Hib disease due to anatomic/functional asplenia or splenectomy, HIV infection, immunoglobulin deficiency, early component complement deficiency, or chemotherapy or radiation therapy: IM: 0.5 mL as a single dose; may use any of the Hib conjugate vaccines (CDC/ACIP [Briere, 2014]). Unimmunized defined as persons who have not received a primary series and booster dose or at least 1 dose of a Hib vaccine after 14 months of age.

Repeat immunization for high-risk conditions (CDC/ACIP [Briere, 2014):

Invasive Hib disease: Infants and Children <24 months: Revaccinate with a second primary series beginning 4 weeks after onset of disease

Undergoing chemotherapy or radiation therapy: Infants and Children <60 months: If dose administered within 14 days of starting or given during therapy: Repeat the doses at least 3 months after therapy completion

Hematopoietic stem cell transplant recipient: Children and Adolescents: Revaccinate with a 3-dose regimen beginning 6 to 12 months after successful transplant, regardless of vaccination history. Doses should be administered ≥4 weeks apart.

Adult: **Immunization: Note:** Only indicated for those who have not received the childhood Hib series **and** are at increased risk for invasive Hib disease due to sickle cell disease, anatomic/functional asplenia or splenectomy: IM: 0.5 mL as a single dose; may use any of the Hib conjugate vaccines; give ≥14 days prior to elective splenectomy (CDC/ACIP [Briere 2014]; CDC/ACIP [Kim 2015])

Hematopoietic stem cell transplant: Revaccinate with a 3-dose regimen beginning 6 to 12 months after the transplant, regardless of vaccination history. Doses should be administered ≥4 weeks apart (CDC/ACIP [Briere, 2014]).

Dosing adjustment in renal impairment: There are no dosage adjustments provided in the manufacturer's labeling.

Dosing adjustment in hepatic impairment: There are no dosage adjustments provided in the manufacturer's labeling.

Preparation for Administration

IM:

ActHIB: Reconstitute lyophilized powder with 0.6 mL of provided saline diluent only (sodium chloride 0.4%); agitate vial to form a clear, colorless solution. After reconstitution, administer promptly or store refrigerated and use within 24 hours. Shake well prior to use.

Hiberix: Reconstitute with provided saline diluent only. Transfer entire contents of prefilled syringe containing diluent into the vial; with needle still inserted, shake vigorously until it becomes a clear, colorless solution. Shake well prior to use.

PedvaxHIB: Use as supplied; no reconstitution is necessary. Shake well; thorough agitation is necessary to maintain suspension of the vaccine.

Administration IM: Shake well prior to administration; must be administered within 24 hours of reconstitution. Administer IM into midlateral aspect of the thigh in infants and small children; administer in the deltoid area to older children and adults; **not for IV or SubQ administration**. Adolescents and adults should be vaccinated while seated or lying down (NCIRD/ACIP 2011). US law requires that the date of administration, the vaccine manufacturer, lot number of vaccine, and the administering person's name, title, and address be entered into the patient's permanent medical record.

For patients at risk of hemorrhage following intramuscular injection, the vaccine should be administered intramuscularly if, in the opinion of the physician familiar with the patient's bleeding risk, the vaccine can be administered by this route with reasonable safety. If the patient receives antihemophilia or other similar therapy, intramuscular vaccination can be scheduled shortly after such therapy is administered. A fine needle (23 gauge or smaller) should be used for the vaccination and firm pressure on the site (without rubbing) for at least 2 minutes. The patient should be instructed concerning the risk of hematoma from the injection. Patients on anticoagulant therapy should be considered to have the same bleeding risks and treated as those with clotting factor disorders (NCIRD/ACIP 2011).

Monitoring Parameters Observe for syncope for 15 minutes following administration (NCIRD/ACIP 2011). If seizure-like activity associated with syncope occurs, maintain patient in supine or Trendelenburg position to reestablish adequate cerebral perfusion.

Test Interactions May interfere with interpretation of urine antigen detection tests; antigenuria may occur up to 2 weeks following immunization

Additional Information If Hiberix is inadvertently administered during the primary vaccination series, the dose can be counted as a valid PRP-T dose that does not need repeated if administered according to schedule. In this case, a total of 3 doses completes the primary series (CDC 58[36] 2009).

The conjugate vaccines currently available consist of *Haemophilus influenzae* type b (Hib) capsular polysaccharide (also referred to as PRP) linked to a carrier protein. PedvaxHIB (PRP-OMP) is linked to the outer membrane protein complex from *Neisseria meningitidis*. ActHIB and Hiberix (PRP-T) use tetanus toxoid conjugate as the carrier protein.

Dosage Forms Excipient information presented when available (limited, particularly for generics); consult specific product labeling.

Injection, powder for reconstitution [preservative free]:

ActHIB *Haemophilus* b capsular polysaccharide 10 mcg [bound to tetanus toxoid 24 mcg] per 0.5 mL [contains sucrose; may be reconstituted with provided diluent (forms solution; contains natural rubber/natural latex in packaging)]

Hiberix: *Haemophilus* b capsular polysaccharide 10 mcg [bound to tetanus toxoid 25 mcg] per 0.5 mL (0.5 mL) [contains lactose 12.6 mg]

Injection, suspension:

PedvaxHIB: *Haemophilus* b capsular polysaccharide 7.5 mcg [bound to *Neisseria meningitidis* OMPC 125 mcg] per 0.5 mL (0.5 mL) [contains aluminum; natural rubber/natural latex in packaging]

◆ ***Haemophilus* b (meningococcal protein conjugate) Conjugate Vaccine** *see* *Haemophilus* b Conjugate and Hepatitis B Vaccine *on page 997*

◆ ***Haemophilus* B Polysaccharide** *see* Diphtheria and Tetanus Toxoids, Acellular Pertussis, Poliovirus and *Haemophilus* b Conjugate Vaccine *on page 679*

◆ ***Haemophilus influenzae* Type b** *see* *Haemophilus* b Conjugate Vaccine *on page 998*

◆ **Halcion** *see* Triazolam *on page 2120*

◆ **Haldol** *see* Haloperidol *on page 1002*

◆ **Haldol Decanoate** *see* Haloperidol *on page 1002*

◆ **Halfprin [OTC]** *see* Aspirin *on page 206*

Halobetasol (hal oh BAY ta sol)

Medication Safety Issues

Sound-alike/look-alike issues:

Ultravate® may be confused with Cutivate®

Related Information

Topical Corticosteroids *on page 2262*

Brand Names: US Halonate; Ultravate; Ultravate PAC [DSC]

Brand Names: Canada Ultravate®

Therapeutic Category Adrenal Corticosteroid; Anti-inflammatory Agent; Corticosteroid, Topical; Glucocorticoid

Generic Availability (US) May be product dependent

Use Relief of inflammation and pruritus associated with corticosteroid-response dermatoses

Pregnancy Risk Factor C

Pregnancy Considerations Teratogenic effects have been observed in animal reproduction studies. Topical products are not recommended for extensive use, in large quantities, or for long periods of time in pregnant women (Reed, 1997).

Breast-Feeding Considerations Systemically administered corticosteroids appear in human milk and may cause adverse effects in a nursing infant. It is not known if the systemic absorption of topical halobetasol results in detectable quantities in human milk. Use with caution while breast-feeding; do not apply to nipples (Reed, 1997).

Contraindications Hypersensitivity to halobetasol or any component of the formulation

Warnings/Precautions Topical corticosteroids may be absorbed percutaneously. Absorption of topical corticosteroids may cause manifestations of Cushing's syndrome, hyperglycemia, or glycosuria. Absorption is increased by the use of occlusive dressings, application to denuded skin, or application to large surface areas. May cause hypercorticism or suppression of hypothalamic-pituitary-adrenal (HPA) axis, particularly in younger children or in patients receiving high doses for prolonged periods. HPA axis suppression may lead to adrenal crisis. Children may absorb proportionally larger amounts of corticosteroids after topical application and may be more prone to systemic effects. HPA axis suppression, intracranial hypertension, and Cushing's syndrome have been reported in children receiving topical corticosteroids. Prolonged use may affect growth velocity; growth should be routinely monitored in pediatric patients.

Allergic contact dermatitis can occur, it is usually diagnosed by failure to heal rather than clinical exacerbation. Discontinue therapy if irritation develops. Use appropriate antibacterial or antifungal agents to treat concomitant skin infections; discontinue halobetasol treatment if infection does not resolve promptly. Prolonged treatment with corticosteroids has been associated with the development of Kaposi's sarcoma (case reports); if noted, discontinuation of therapy should be considered. Not for ophthalmic use. Topical halobetasol should not be used for the treatment of rosacea or perioral dermatitis. Not recommended for application to the face, groin, or axillae.

Warnings: Additional Pediatric Considerations The extent of percutaneous absorption is dependent on several factors, including epidermal integrity (intact vs abraded skin), formulation, age of the patient, prolonged duration of use, and the use of occlusive dressings. Percutaneous absorption of topical steroids is increased in neonates (especially preterm neonates), infants, and young children. Infants and small children may be more susceptible to HPA axis suppression, intracranial hypertension, Cushing syndrome, or other systemic toxicities due to larger skin surface area to body mass ratio.

Some dosage forms may contain propylene glycol; in neonates large amounts of propylene glycol delivered orally, intravenously (eg, >3,000 mg/day), or topically have been associated with potentially fatal toxicities which can include metabolic acidosis, seizures, renal failure, and CNS depression; toxicities have also been reported in children and adults including hyperosmolality, lactic acidosis, seizures and respiratory depression; use caution (AAP, 1997; Shehab, 2009).

Adverse Reactions

Central nervous system: Intracranial hypertension (systemic effect reported in children treated with topical corticosteroids)

Dermatologic: Acneiform eruptions, allergic contact dermatitis, dry skin, erythema, folliculitis, hypertrichosis, hypopigmentation, itching, leukoderma, miliaria, perioral dermatitis, pruritus, pustulation, rash, skin atrophy, skin infection (secondary), striae, telangiectasia, vesicles, urticaria

Endocrine: Glycosuria, HPA axis suppression, metabolic effects (hyperglycemia, hypokalemia)

Local: Burning, stinging

Neuromuscular & skeletal: Paresthesia

Drug Interactions

Metabolism/Transport Effects None known.

Avoid Concomitant Use

Avoid concomitant use of Halobetasol with any of the following: Aldesleukin

Increased Effect/Toxicity

Halobetasol may increase the levels/effects of: Ceritinib; Deferasirox

The levels/effects of Halobetasol may be increased by: Telaprevir

Decreased Effect

Halobetasol may decrease the levels/effects of: Aldesleukin; Corticorelin; Hyaluronidase; Telaprevir

Storage/Stability Store between 15°C to 30°C (59°F to 86°F).

Mechanism of Action Topical corticosteroids have anti-inflammatory, antipruritic, and vasoconstrictive properties. May depress the formation, release, and activity of endogenous chemical mediators of inflammation (kinins, histamine, liposomal enzymes, prostaglandins) through the induction of phospholipase A_2 inhibitory proteins (lipocortins) and sequential inhibition of the release of arachidonic acid. Halobetasol has high range potency.

Pharmacokinetics (Adult data unless noted)

Absorption: Percutaneous absorption varies and depends on many factors including vehicle used, integrity of epidermis, dose, and use of occlusive dressing; absorption is increased by occlusive dressings or with decreased integrity of skin (eg, inflammation or skin disease)

Cream: <6% of topically applied dose enters circulation within 96 hours following application

Metabolism: Hepatic

Elimination: Renal

Dosing: Usual

Children <12 years: Use not recommended (high risk of systemic adverse effects, eg, HPA axis suppression, Cushing's syndrome)

Children ≥12 years and Adults: Topical: Steroid-responsive dermatoses: Apply sparingly once or twice daily; maximum dose: 50 g/week; do not treat for >2 weeks. **Note:** To decrease risk of systemic effects, only treat small areas at any one time; discontinue therapy when control is achieved; reassess diagnosis if no improvement is seen in 2 weeks.

Administration Topical: Apply sparingly to affected area, gently rub in until disappears; do not use on open skin; do not apply to face, underarms, or groin area; avoid contact with eyes; do not occlude affected area.

Monitoring Parameters Assess HPA axis suppression in patients using potent topical steroids applied to a large surface area or to areas under occlusion (eg, ACTH stimulation test, morning plasma cortisol test, urinary free cortisol test)

Additional Information Considered to be a super high potency topical corticosteroid; patients with psoriasis who were treated with halobetasol cream or ointment in divided doses of 7 g/day for one week developed HPA axis suppression

Dosage Forms Excipient information presented when available (limited, particularly for generics); consult specific product labeling. [DSC] = Discontinued product

Cream, External, as propionate:

Ultravate: 0.05% (50 g) [contains cetyl alcohol]

Generic: 0.05% (15 g, 50 g)

Kit, External, as propionate:

Halonate: 0.05 & 12 % (Foam) [contains cetyl alcohol, propylene glycol, trolamine (triethanolamine)]

Ultravate PAC: 0.05 & 12 % (Cream) [DSC] [contains cetyl alcohol, methylparaben, propylene glycol, propylparaben]

Ointment, External, as propionate:

Ultravate: 0.05% (50 g) [contains propylene glycol]

Generic: 0.05% (15 g, 50 g)

◆ **Halobetasol Propionate** *see* Halobetasol *on page* 1001

◆ **Halonate** *see* Halobetasol *on page* 1001

Haloperidol (ha loe PER i dole)

Medication Safety Issues

Sound-alike/look-alike issues:

Haldol may be confused with Halcion, Halog, Stadol

BEERS Criteria medication:

This drug may be potentially inappropriate for use in geriatric patients (Quality of evidence - moderate; Strength of recommendation - strong).

International issues:

Haldol [U.S. and multiple international markets] may be confused with Halotestin brand name for fluoxymesterone [Great Britain]

Brand Names: US Haldol; Haldol Decanoate

Brand Names: Canada Apo-Haloperidol; Apo-Haloperidol LA; Haloperidol Injection, USP; Haloperidol Long Acting; Haloperidol-LA; Haloperidol-LA Omega; Novo-Peridol; PMS-Haloperidol; PMS-Haloperidol LA

Therapeutic Category Antipsychotic Agent, Typical, Butyrophenone

Generic Availability (US) Yes

Use

Oral: Tablet and solution: Management of psychotic disorders (FDA approved in ages ≥3 years and adults), control of tics and vocal utterances of Tourette's disorder (FDA approved in ages ≥3 years and adults), treatment of severe behavioral problems in children displayed by combativeness and/or explosive hyperexcitable behavior and in short-term treatment of hyperactive children (FDA approved in ages 3 to 12 years); has also been used for emergency sedation of severely agitated or delirious patients and for agitation during palliative care

Parenteral:

Injection, immediate release (lactate): Management of schizophrenia (FDA approved in adults); control of tics and vocal utterances of Tourette's disorder (FDA approved in adults); has also been used for emergency sedation of severely agitated or delirious patients

Injection, extended release (decanoate): Management of schizophrenia in patients requiring prolonged parenteral antipsychotic treatment (FDA approved in adults)

Pregnancy Risk Factor C

Pregnancy Considerations Adverse events were observed in animal reproduction studies. Haloperidol crosses the placenta in humans (Newport, 2007). Although haloperidol has not been found to be a major human teratogen, an association with limb malformations following first trimester exposure in humans cannot be ruled out (ACOG, 2008; Diav-Citrin, 2005). Antipsychotic use during the third trimester of pregnancy has a risk for abnormal muscle movements (extrapyramidal symptoms [EPS]) and withdrawal symptoms in newborns following delivery. Symptoms in the newborn may include agitation, feeding disorder, hypertonia, hypotonia, respiratory distress, somnolence, and tremor; these effects may be selflimiting or require hospitalization. If needed, the minimum effective maternal dose should be used in order to decrease the risk of EPS (ACOG, 2008).

Breast-Feeding Considerations Haloperidol is found in breast milk and has been detected in the plasma and urine of nursing infants (Whalley, 1981; Yoshida, 1999). Breast engorgement, gynecomastia, and lactation are known side effects with the use of haloperidol. Breast-feeding is not recommended by the manufacturer.

Contraindications Hypersensitivity to haloperidol or any component of the formulation; Parkinson's disease; severe CNS depression; coma

Warnings/Precautions [U.S. Boxed Warning]: Elderly patients with dementia-related psychosis treated with antipsychotics are at an increased risk of death compared to placebo. Most deaths appeared to be either cardiovascular (eg, heart failure, sudden death) or infectious (eg, pneumonia) in nature. Haloperidol is not approved for the treatment of dementia-related psychosis. Hypotension may occur, particularly with parenteral administration. Although the short-acting form (lactate) is used clinically, the IV use of the injection is not an FDA-approved route of administration; the decanoate form should never be administered intravenously.

May alter cardiac conduction and prolong QT interval; life-threatening arrhythmias have occurred with therapeutic doses of antipsychotics but risk may be increased with doses exceeding recommendations and/or intravenous administration (off-label route). Use caution or avoid use in patients with electrolyte abnormalities (eg, hypokalemia, hypomagnesemia), hypothyroidism, familial long QT syndrome, concomitant medications which may augment QT prolongation, or any underlying cardiac abnormality which may also potentiate risk. Monitor ECG closely for dose-related QT effects. Adverse effects of decanoate may be prolonged. Avoid in thyrotoxicosis.

Leukopenia, neutropenia, and agranulocytosis (sometimes fatal) have been reported in clinical trials and postmarketing reports with antipsychotic use; presence of risk factors (eg, preexisting low WBC or history of drug-induced leuko-/neutropenia) should prompt periodic blood count assessment. Discontinue therapy at first signs of blood dyscrasias or if absolute neutrophil count <1000/mm^3.

May be sedating, use with caution in disorders where CNS depression is a feature. Effects may be potentiated when used with other sedative drugs or ethanol. Caution in patients with severe cardiovascular disease, predisposition to seizures, subcortical brain damage, or renal disease. Esophageal dysmotility and aspiration have been associated with antipsychotic use - use with caution in patients at risk of pneumonia (eg, Alzheimer's disease). Use associated with increased prolactin levels; clinical significance of hyperprolactinemia in patients with breast cancer or other prolactin-dependent tumors is unknown. May alter temperature regulation or mask toxicity of other drugs due to antiemetic effects. May cause orthostatic hypotension; use with caution in patients at risk of this effect or those who would tolerate transient hypotensive episodes (cerebrovascular disease, cardiovascular disease, or other medications which may predispose). Some tablets contain tartrazine. Antipsychotics have been associated with pigmentary retinopathy.

May cause anticholinergic effects (confusion, agitation, constipation, xerostomia, blurred vision, urinary retention). Therefore, they should be used with caution in patients with decreased gastrointestinal motility, urinary retention, BPH, xerostomia, visual problems, or narrow-angle glaucoma (screening is recommended). Relative to other neuroleptics, haloperidol has a low potency of cholinergic blockade.

May cause extrapyramidal symptoms, including pseudoparkinsonism, acute dystonic reactions, akathisia, and tardive dyskinesia. Risk of dystonia (and possibly other EPS) may be greater with increased doses, use of conventional antipsychotics, males, and younger patients. Risk of tardive dyskinesia and potential for irreversibility may be increased in elderly patients (particularly women), prolonged therapy, and higher total cumulative dose; antipsychotics may also mask signs/symptoms of tardive dyskinesia. May be associated with neuroleptic malignant syndrome (NMS). Use in elderly patients with dementia is associated with an increased risk of mortality and cerebrovascular accidents; avoid antipsychotic use for behavioral problems associated with dementia unless alternative nonpharmacologic therapies have failed and patient may harm self or others. In addition, use may cause or exacerbate syndrome of inappropriate antidiuretic hormone secretion or hyponatremia; monitor sodium closely with initiation or dosage adjustments in older adults (Beers Criteria). Increased risk for developing tardive dyskinesia, particularly elderly women.

Benzyl alcohol and derivatives: Some dosage forms may contain benzyl alcohol; large amounts of benzyl alcohol (≥99 mg/kg/day) have been associated with a potentially fatal toxicity ("gasping syndrome") in neonates; the "gasping syndrome" consists of metabolic acidosis, respiratory distress, gasping respirations, CNS dysfunction (including convulsions, intracranial hemorrhage), hypotension and cardiovascular collapse (AAP, 1997; CDC, 1982); some data suggests that benzoate displaces bilirubin from protein binding sites (Ahlfors, 2001); avoid or use dosage forms containing benzyl alcohol with caution in neonates. See manufacturer's labeling.

Warnings: Additional Pediatric Considerations For the management of delirium in pediatric patients, intravenous haloperidol has been widely studied for efficacy and has been frequently used due to lower sedative effects and rapid onset of action; however, its use is associated with adverse effects including cardiac effects (eg, arrhythmias and QT prolongation, circulatory and respiratory insufficiency, extrapyramidal symptoms (eg, cogwheel rigidity, tremor, dystonia, oculogyric crisis), and neuroleptic malignant syndrome (Harrison 2006; Slooff 2014; Turkel 2014). Newer atypical antipsychotics have shown similar efficacy with less adverse effects and are being utilized more frequently. Intravenous haloperidol for delirium may be considered in patients that are unresponsive to an atypical agent or who require intravenous therapy; ECG monitoring could be considered (Turkel 2014).

Adverse Reactions

Cardiovascular: Abnormal T waves with prolonged ventricular repolarization, arrhythmia, hyper-/hypotension, QT prolongation, sudden death, tachycardia, torsade de pointes

Central nervous system: Agitation, akathisia, altered central temperature regulation, anxiety, confusion, depression, drowsiness, dystonic reactions, euphoria, extrapyramidal reactions, headache, insomnia, lethargy, neuroleptic malignant syndrome (NMS), pseudoparkinsonian signs and symptoms, restlessness, seizure, tardive dyskinesia, tardive dystonia, vertigo

Dermatologic: Alopecia, contact dermatitis, hyperpigmentation, photosensitivity (rare), pruritus, rash

Endocrine & metabolic: Amenorrhea, breast engorgement, galactorrhea, gynecomastia, hyper-/hypoglycemia, hyponatremia, lactation, mastalgia, menstrual irregularities, sexual dysfunction

Gastrointestinal: Anorexia, constipation, diarrhea, dyspepsia, hypersalivation, nausea, vomiting, xerostomia

Genitourinary: Priapism, urinary retention

Hematologic: Agranulocytosis (rare), leukopenia, leukocytosis, neutropenia, anemia, lymphomonocytosis

Hepatic: Cholestatic jaundice, obstructive jaundice

Ocular: Blurred vision

Respiratory: Bronchospasm, laryngospasm

Miscellaneous: Diaphoresis, heat stroke

Drug Interactions

Metabolism/Transport Effects Substrate of CYP1A2 (minor), CYP2D6 (major), CYP3A4 (major); **Note:** Assignment of Major/Minor substrate status based on clinically relevant drug interaction potential; **Inhibits** CYP2D6 (moderate)

Avoid Concomitant Use

Avoid concomitant use of Haloperidol with any of the following: Aclidinium; Amisulpride; Azelastine (Nasal); Conivaptan; Eluxadoline; FLUoxetine; Fusidic Acid (Systemic); Glucagon; Highest Risk QTc-Prolonging Agents; Idelalisib; Ipratropium (Oral Inhalation); Ivabradine; Metoclopramide; Mifepristone; Orphenadrine; Paraldehyde; Potassium Chloride; QuiNIDine; Sulpiride; Thalidomide; Thioridazine; Tiotropium; Umeclidinium

Increased Effect/Toxicity

Haloperidol may increase the levels/effects of: AbobotulinumtoxinA; Alcohol (Ethyl); Amisulpride; Analgesics (Opioid); Anticholinergic Agents; ARIPiprazole; Azelastine (Nasal); Buprenorphine; ChlorproMAZINE; CNS Depressants; CYP2D6 Substrates; DOXOrubicin (Conventional); Eluxadoline; Fesoterodine; Glucagon; Highest Risk QTc-Prolonging Agents; Hydrocodone; Mequitazine; Methotrimeprazine; Methylphenidate; Metoprolol; Metyrosine; Mirabegron; Mirtazapine; Moderate Risk QTc-Prolonging Agents; Nebivolol; OnabotulinumtoxinA; Orphenadrine; Paraldehyde; Potassium Chloride; QuiNIDine; RimabotulinumtoxinB; Selective Serotonin Reuptake Inhibitors; Serotonin Modulators; Sulpiride; Suvorexant; Thalidomide; Thiazide Diuretics; Thioridazine; Tiotropium; Topiramate; Zolpidem

The levels/effects of Haloperidol may be increased by: Abiraterone Acetate; Acetylcholinesterase Inhibitors (Central); Aclidinium; Aprepitant; ARIPiprazole; Brimonidine (Topical); Cannabis; ChlorproMAZINE; Conivaptan; CYP2D6 Inhibitors (Moderate); CYP2D6 Inhibitors (Strong); CYP3A4 Inhibitors (Moderate); CYP3A4 Inhibitors (Strong); Dasatinib; Doxylamine; Dronabinol; Droperidol; FLUoxetine; FluvoxaMINE; Fosaprepitant; Fusidic Acid (Systemic); HydrOXYzine; Idelalisib; Ipratropium (Oral Inhalation); Ivabradine; Ivacaftor; Kava Kava; Lithium; Luliconazole; Magnesium Sulfate; Methotrimeprazine; Methylphenidate; Metoclopramide; Metyrosine; Mianserin; Mifepristone; Nabilone; Netupitant; Nonsteroidal Anti-Inflammatory Agents; Palbociclib; Panobinostat; Peginterferon Alfa-2b; Perampanel; Pramlintide; QTc-Prolonging Agents (Indeterminate Risk and Risk Modifying); QuiNIDine; Rufinamide; Serotonin Modulators; Simeprevir; Sodium Oxybate; Stiripentol; Tapentadol; Tetrahydrocannabinol; Umeclidinium

Decreased Effect

Haloperidol may decrease the levels/effects of: Acetylcholinesterase Inhibitors; Amphetamines; Anti-Parkinson's Agents (Dopamine Agonist); Codeine; Itopride; Quinagolide; Secretin; Tamoxifen; TraMADol; Urea Cycle Disorder Agents

The levels/effects of Haloperidol may be decreased by: Acetylcholinesterase Inhibitors; Anti-Parkinson's Agents (Dopamine Agonist); ARIPiprazole; Bosentan; CarBAMazepine; CYP3A4 Inducers (Moderate); CYP3A4 Inducers (Strong); Dabrafenib; Deferasirox; Glycopyrrolate; Lithium; Mitotane; Peginterferon Alfa-2b; Siltuximab; St Johns Wort; Tocilizumab

Storage/Stability Protect oral dosage forms from light. Haloperidol lactate injection should be stored at controlled room temperature; do not freeze or expose to temperatures >40°C. Protect from light; exposure to light may cause discoloration and the development of a grayish-red precipitate over several weeks. Stability of standardized solutions is 38 days at room temperature (24°C).

Mechanism of Action Haloperidol is a butyrophenone antipsychotic which blocks postsynaptic mesolimbic dopaminergic D_1 and D_2 receptors in the brain; depresses the release of hypothalamic and hypophyseal hormones; believed to depress the reticular activating system thus affecting basal metabolism, body temperature, wakefulness, vasomotor tone, and emesis

Pharmacokinetics (Adult data unless noted)

Absorption: Oral: Well absorbed, undergoes first-pass metabolism in the liver

Distribution: Crosses the placenta; appears in breast milk

Protein binding: 92%

Metabolism: In the liver, hydroxy-metabolite is active

Bioavailability: Oral: 60%

Half-life: Adults: 20 hours; range: 13-35 hours

Elimination: Excreted in urine and feces as drug and metabolites

Dosing: Usual Note: Dosing should be individualized based on patient response. Gradually decrease dose to the lowest effective maintenance dosage once a satisfactory therapeutic response is obtained.

Pediatric: **Note:** Dosing presented as fixed (mg) dosing and weight-based (mg/**kg**) dosing; use caution when prescribing and dispensing.

Behavior disorders, nonpsychotic:

Children 3 to 12 years weighing 15 to 40 kg: Oral: Initial: 0.5 mg/day in 2 to 3 divided doses; may increase by 0.5 mg every 5 to 7 days to usual maintenance range of 0.05 to 0.075 mg/**kg**/day in 2 to 3 divided doses. Maintenance range calculates to a fixed dose of 0.75 to 3 mg/day in divided doses; maximum dose not established; children with severe, nonpsychotic disturbance may require higher doses; however, no improvement has been shown with doses >6 mg/day.

Children >40 kg and Adolescents: Limited data available: Oral: 0.5 to 15 mg/day in 2 to 3 divided doses; begin at lower end of the range and may increase as needed (no more frequently than every 5 to 7 days); maximum daily dose: 15 mg/day. **Note:** Higher doses may be necessary in severe or refractory cases (Kliegman 2011).

Delirium: Limited data available; optimal dose not established; **Note:** Reported experience in infants is very limited and suggests that lower doses may be required. Infants ≥3 months, Children, and Adolescents: IV (lactate, immediate release): Loading dose: 0.15 to 0.25 mg/dose infused slowly over 30 to 45 minutes

(Schieveld 2007); maintenance dose: 0.05 to 0.5 mg/**kg**/day in divided doses (Brown 1996; Schieveld 2007); a retrospective review of 27 patients (ages: 3 months to 17 years) using this dosing showed the signs/symptoms of delirium responded well to treatment in all patients; however, two patients experienced dystonic reactions (Schieveld 2007). In a small case-series, loading doses of 0.025 to 0.1 mg/**kg**/dose administered every 10 minutes until sedation achieved (reported total haloperidol loading dose: 0.09 to 0.25 mg/**kg** total) followed by maintenance doses of 0.06 to 0.45 mg/**kg**/day in divided doses every 6 to 8 hours were described (n=5; age range: 9 months to 16 years); infants (n=2) were noted to require lower doses (total loading dose: 0.09 to 0.1 mg/**kg** total; maintenance: 0.015 to 0.025 mg/**kg**/dose every 6 hours); one patient experienced a dystonic reaction (Harrison 2002)

Psychotic disorders:

Children 3 to 12 years weighing 15 to 40 kg: Oral: Initial: 0.5 mg/day in 2 to 3 divided doses; increase by 0.5 mg every 5 to 7 days to usual maintenance range of 0.05 to 0.15 mg/**kg**/day in 2 to 3 divided doses (maintenance range calculates to a fixed dose of 0.75 to 6 mg/day in divided doses); higher doses may be necessary in severe or refractory cases; maximum dose not established; in adolescents, the maximum daily dose is 15 mg/day (Kliegman 2011)

Children >40 kg and Adolescents: Limited data available: Oral: 0.5 to 15 mg/day in 2 to 3 divided doses; begin at lower end of the range and may increase as needed (no more frequently than every 5 to 7 days); maximum daily dose: 15 mg/day (Kliegman 2011; Willner 1969). **Note:** Higher doses may be necessary in severe or refractory cases (Kliegman 2011).

Agitation (acute); psychosis: Limited data available: Infants, Children, and Adolescents: IM, IV (lactate, immediate release): 0.05 to 0.15 mg/**kg**; may be repeated hourly as needed; maximum dose: 5 mg/dose (Hegenbarth 2008)

Agitation (palliative care): Limited data available: Children ≥3 years and Adolescents: Oral: 0.01 mg/**kg**/dose 3 times daily as needed; to manage new-onset acute episode: 0.025 to 0.05 mg/**kg** once then may repeat 0.025 mg/**kg**/dose in one hour as needed (Kliegman 2011)

Tourette syndrome:

Children 3 to 12 years weighing 15 to 40 kg: Oral:

Manufacturer's labeling: Initial: 0.5 mg/day in 2 to 3 divided doses; increase by 0.25 to 0.5 mg every 5 to 7 days to usual maintenance of 0.05 to 0.075 mg/kg/day in 2 to 3 divided doses (maintenance range calculates to a fixed dose of 0.75 to 3 mg/day in divided doses); maximum dose not established; however, no improvement has been shown with doses >6 mg/day in patients with nonpsychotic disturbances

Alternate dosing: Limited data available: Initial: 0.25 to 0.5 mg/day in 2 to 3 divided doses titrated to a usual daily dose range of 1 to 4 mg/day (Roessner 2011; Scahill 2006)

Children weighing >40 kg and Adolescents: Limited data available: Oral: 0.25 to 15 mg/day in 2 to 3 divided doses; begin at lower end of the range and may increase as needed (no more frequently than every 5 to 7 days) (Kleigman 2011; Roessner 2011); usual dose range: 1 to 4 mg/day (Roessner 2011; Scahill 2006); maximum dose not established; however, no improvement has been shown with doses >6 mg/day in patients with nonpsychotic disturbances

Adult: **Psychosis:**

Oral: 0.5 to 5 mg 2 to 3 times daily; usual maximum: 30 mg/day

IM (as lactate): 2 to 5 mg every 4 to 8 hours as needed

IM (as decanoate): Initial: 10 to 20 times the daily oral dose administered at 4-week intervals. Maintenance dose: 10 to 15 times initial oral dose; used to stabilize psychiatric symptoms

Dosing adjustment in renal impairment: Children ≥3 years, Adolescents, and Adults: There are no dosage adjustments provided in the manufacturer's labeling.

Hemodialysis/peritoneal dialysis: Supplemental dose is not necessary.

Dosing adjustment in hepatic impairment: Children ≥3 years, Adolescents, and Adults: There are no dosage adjustments provided in manufacturer's labeling.

Preparation for Administration

Oral: Oral concentrated solution: Dilute oral concentrate with ≥2 ounces of water or acidic beverage; do not mix oral concentrate with coffee or tea. Avoid skin contact with oral suspension or solution; may cause contact dermatitis.

Parenteral: IV infusion or IVPB: Lactate (Immediate release): May further dilute in D_5W solutions to a concentration <5 mg/mL; in adults, dose (0.5 to 100 mg) is usually added to 50 to 100 mL. Do not use NS solutions due to reports of decreased stability and incompatibility.

Administration

Oral: Administer with food or milk to decrease GI distress. Avoid skin contact with oral suspension or solution; may cause contact dermatitis.

Parenteral:

IM:

Lactate (immediate release): May be administered undiluted IM

Decanoate (extended release): For IM use only, do not administer decanoate IV. A 21-guage needle is recommended. The maximum volume per injection site should not exceed 3 mL. Administer in the gluteal muscle by deep IM injection; Z-track injection techniques are recommended to limit leakage after injections (Baweja 2012; Gillespie 2013; McEvoy 2006).

IV: Infusion or IVPB: Lactate (immediate release): May be administered undiluted (5 mg/mL), or diluted in D_5W. Rate of IV administration is not well defined but should be slow; in pediatric delirium patients, loading doses have been administered over 30 to 45 minutes (Schieveld 2005; Schieveld 2007); in adults, rates of a maximum of 5 mg/minute (Lerner 1979) and 0.125 mg/kg (in 10 mL NS) over 1 to 2 minutes (Magliozzi 1985) have been reported. **Note:** IV administration has been associated with QT prolongation and the manufacturer recommends ECG monitoring for QT prolongation and arrhythmias. Consult individual institutional policies and procedures prior to administration.

Monitoring Parameters Blood pressure, heart rate, CBC with differential, liver enzymes with long-term use; serum glucose, sodium, magnesium; ECG (with non-FDA approved intravenous administration); mental status, abnormal involuntary movement scale (AIMS), extrapyramidal symptoms (EPS)

Dosage Forms Excipient information presented when available (limited, particularly for generics); consult specific product labeling.

Concentrate, Oral, as lactate [strength expressed as base]:

Generic: 2 mg/mL (5 mL, 15 mL, 120 mL)

Solution, Intramuscular, as decanoate [strength expressed as base]:

Haldol Decanoate: 50 mg/mL (1 mL); 100 mg/mL (1 mL) [contains benzyl alcohol, sesame oil]

Generic: 50 mg/mL (1 mL, 5 mL); 100 mg/mL (1 mL, 5 mL)

Solution, Injection, as lactate [strength expressed as base]:

Haldol: 5 mg/mL (1 mL)

Generic: 5 mg/mL (1 mL, 10 mL)

Solution, Injection, as lactate [strength expressed as base, preservative free]:
Generic: 5 mg/mL (1 mL)
Tablet, Oral:
Generic: 0.5 mg, 1 mg, 2 mg, 5 mg, 10 mg, 20 mg

- ◆ **Haloperidol Decanoate** *see* Haloperidol *on page 1002*
- ◆ **Haloperidol Injection, USP (Can)** *see* Haloperidol *on page 1002*
- ◆ **Haloperidol-LA (Can)** *see* Haloperidol *on page 1002*
- ◆ **Haloperidol Lactate** *see* Haloperidol *on page 1002*
- ◆ **Haloperidol-LA Omega (Can)** *see* Haloperidol *on page 1002*
- ◆ **Haloperidol Long Acting (Can)** *see* Haloperidol *on page 1002*
- ◆ **Harkoseride** *see* Lacosamide *on page 1200*
- ◆ **Havrix** *see* Hepatitis A Vaccine *on page 1011*
- ◆ **HAVRIX (Can)** *see* Hepatitis A Vaccine *on page 1011*
- ◆ **H-BAT** *see* Botulism Antitoxin, Heptavalent *on page 297*
- ◆ **HBIG** *see* Hepatitis B Immune Globulin (Human) *on page 1013*
- ◆ **hCG** *see* Chorionic Gonadotropin (Human) *on page 453*
- ◆ **HCTZ (error-prone abbreviation)** *see* Hydrochlorothiazide *on page 1028*
- ◆ **HDCV** *see* Rabies Vaccine *on page 1832*
- ◆ **HealthyLax [OTC]** *see* Polyethylene Glycol 3350 *on page 1723*
- ◆ **Healthy Mama Move It Along [OTC]** *see* Docusate *on page 697*
- ◆ **Heartburn Relief [OTC]** *see* Famotidine *on page 847*
- ◆ **Heartburn Relief 24 Hour [OTC] [DSC]** *see* Lansoprazole *on page 1219*
- ◆ **Heartburn Relief Max St [OTC]** *see* Famotidine *on page 847*
- ◆ **Heartburn Treatment 24 Hour [OTC]** *see* Lansoprazole *on page 1219*
- ◆ **Heather** *see* Norethindrone *on page 1530*
- ◆ **Heavy Mineral Oil** *see* Mineral Oil *on page 1439*
- ◆ **Hecoria [DSC]** *see* Tacrolimus (Systemic) *on page 1999*
- ◆ **Helixate FS** *see* Antihemophilic Factor (Recombinant) *on page 168*
- ◆ **Hemangeol** *see* Propranolol *on page 1789*
- ◆ **Hemocyte [OTC]** *see* Ferrous Fumarate *on page 869*
- ◆ **Hemofil M** *see* Antihemophilic Factor (Human) *on page 167*
- ◆ **Hemorrhoidal [OTC]** *see* Phenylephrine (Topical) *on page 1690*
- ◆ **Hemorrhoidal HC** *see* Hydrocortisone (Topical) *on page 1041*
- ◆ **Hem-Prep [OTC]** *see* Phenylephrine (Topical) *on page 1690*
- ◆ **Hemril-30 [DSC]** *see* Hydrocortisone (Topical) *on page 1041*
- ◆ **HepA** *see* Hepatitis A Vaccine *on page 1011*
- ◆ **HepaGam B** *see* Hepatitis B Immune Globulin (Human) *on page 1013*

Heparin (HEP a rin)

Medication Safety Issues

Sound-alike/look-alike issues:

Heparin may be confused with Hespan

High alert medication:

The Institute for Safe Medication Practices (ISMP) includes this medication among its list of drugs which have a heightened risk of causing significant patient harm when used in error.

National Patient Safety Goals:

The Joint Commission (TJC) requires healthcare organizations that provide anticoagulant therapy to have a process in place to reduce the risk of anticoagulant-associated patient harm. Patients receiving anticoagulants should receive individualized care through a defined process that includes standardized ordering, dispensing, administration, monitoring and education. This does not apply to routine short-term use of anticoagulants for prevention of venous thromboembolism when the expectation is that the patient's laboratory values will remain within or close to normal values (NPSG.03.05.01).

Administration issues:

The 100 unit/mL concentration should not be used to flush heparin locks, IV lines, or intra-arterial lines in neonates or infants <10 kg (systemic anticoagulation may occur). The 10 unit/mL flush concentration may inadvertently cause systemic anticoagulation in infants <1 kg who receive frequent flushes.

Other safety concerns:

Heparin sodium injection 10,000 units/mL and Hep-Lock U/P 10 units/mL have been confused with each other. Fatal medication errors have occurred between the two whose labels are both blue. **Never rely on color as a sole indicator to differentiate product identity.**

Labeling changes: Effective May 1st, 2013, heparin labeling is required to include the total amount of heparin per vial (rather than only including the amount of heparin per mL). During the transition, hospitals should consider only stocking the newly labeled heparin to avoid potential errors and confusion with the older labeling.

Heparin lock flush solution is intended only to maintain patency of IV devices and is **not** to be used for anticoagulant therapy.

Brand Names: US Hep Flush-10

Brand Names: Canada Heparin Leo; Heparin Lock Flush; Heparin Sodium Injection, USP

Therapeutic Category Anticoagulant

Generic Availability (US) Yes

Use Prophylaxis and treatment of thromboembolic disorders [Injection: FDA approved in pediatric patients (age not specified) and adults]; **Note:** Heparin lock flush solution is intended only to maintain patency of IV devices and is not to be used for systemic anticoagulant therapy (FDA approved in adults)

Pregnancy Risk Factor C

Pregnancy Considerations Increased resorptions were observed in some animal reproduction studies. Heparin does not cross the placenta. Heparin may be used for the prevention and treatment of thromboembolism in pregnant women; however the use of low molecular weight heparin (LMWH) is preferred. Twice-daily heparin should be discontinued prior to induction of labor or a planned cesarean delivery. In pregnant women with mechanical heart valves, adjusted-dose LMWH or adjusted-dose heparin may be used throughout pregnancy or until week 13 of gestation when therapy can be changed to warfarin. LMWH or heparin should be resumed close to delivery. In women who are at a very high risk for thromboembolism (older generation prosthesis in mitral position or history of thromboembolism), warfarin can be used throughout pregnancy and replaced with LMWH or heparin near term; the use of low-dose aspirin is also recommended. When choosing therapy, fetal outcomes (ie, pregnancy loss, malformations), maternal outcomes (ie, VTE, hemorrhage), burden of therapy, and maternal preference should be considered (Guyatt, 2012).

Some products contain benzyl alcohol as a preservative; their use in pregnant women is contraindicated by some manufacturers; use of a preservative free formulation is recommended.

Breast-Feeding Considerations Heparin is not excreted into breast milk and can be used in breast-feeding women (Guyatt, 2012). Some products contain benzyl alcohol as a preservative; their use in breast-feeding women is contraindicated by some manufacturers due to the association of gasping syndrome in premature infants.

Contraindications Hypersensitivity to heparin or any component of the formulation (unless a life-threatening situation necessitates use and use of an alternative anticoagulant is not possible); severe thrombocytopenia; uncontrolled active bleeding except when due to disseminated intravascular coagulation (DIC); not for use when appropriate blood coagulation tests cannot be obtained at appropriate intervals (applies to full-dose heparin only)

Note: Some products contain benzyl alcohol as a preservative; their use in neonates, infants, or pregnant or nursing mothers is contraindicated by some manufacturers.

Warnings/Precautions Hypersensitivity reactions can occur. Only in life-threatening situations when use of an alternative anticoagulant is not possible should heparin be cautiously used in patients with a documented hypersensitivity reaction. Hemorrhage is the most common complication. Monitor for signs and symptoms of bleeding. Certain patients are at increased risk of bleeding. Risk factors for bleeding include bacterial endocarditis; congenital or acquired bleeding disorders; active ulcerative or angiodysplastic GI diseases; continuous GI tube drainage; severe uncontrolled hypertension; history of hemorrhagic stroke; or use shortly after brain, spinal, or ophthalmology surgery; patient treated concomitantly with platelet inhibitors; conditions associated with increased bleeding tendencies (hemophilia, vascular purpura); recent GI bleeding; thrombocytopenia or platelet defects; severe liver disease; hypertensive or diabetic retinopathy; renal failure; or in patients undergoing invasive procedures including spinal tap or spinal anesthesia. Many concentrations of heparin are available ranging from 1 unit/mL to 20,000 units/mL. Clinicians **must** carefully examine each prefilled syringe or vial prior to use ensuring that the correct concentration is chosen; fatal hemorrhages have occurred related to heparin overdose especially in pediatric patients. A higher incidence of bleeding has been reported in patients >60 years of age, particularly women. They are also more sensitive to the dose. Discontinue heparin if hemorrhage occurs; severe hemorrhage or overdosage may require protamine (consult Protamine monograph for dosing recommendations).

May cause thrombocytopenia; monitor platelet count closely. Patients who develop HIT may be at risk of developing a new thrombus (heparin-induced thrombocytopenia and thrombosis [HITT]). Discontinue therapy and consider alternatives if platelets are <100,000/mm^3 and/or thrombosis develops. HIT or HITT may be delayed and can occur up to several weeks after discontinuation of heparin. Use with extreme caution (for a limited duration) or avoid in patients with history of HIT, especially if administered within 100 days of HIT episode (Dager, 2007; Warkentin, 2001); monitor platelet count closely. Osteoporosis may occur with prolonged use (>6 months) due to a reduction in bone mineral density. Monitor for hyperkalemia; can cause hyperkalemia by suppressing aldosterone production. Patients >60 years of age may require lower doses of heparin.

Benzyl alcohol and derivatives: Some dosage forms may contain benzyl alcohol as a preservative. In neonates, large amounts of benzyl alcohol (≥99 mg/kg/day) have been associated with a potentially fatal toxicity ("gasping syndrome"); the "gasping syndrome" consists of metabolic acidosis, respiratory distress, gasping respirations, CNS dysfunction (including convulsions, intracranial hemorrhage), hypotension, and cardiovascular collapse (AAP, 1997; CDC, 1982); some data suggests that benzoate displaces bilirubin from protein binding sites (Ahlfors, 2001); avoid or use dosage forms containing benzyl alcohol with caution in neonates. See manufacturer's labeling. Use in neonates, infants, or pregnant or nursing mothers is contraindicated by some manufacturers; the use of preservative-free heparin is, therefore, recommended in these populations. Some preparations contain sulfite which may cause allergic reactions.

Heparin resistance may occur in patients with antithrombin deficiency, increased heparin clearance, elevations in heparin-binding proteins, elevations in factor VIII and/or fibrinogen; frequently encountered in patients with fever, thrombosis, thrombophlebitis, infections with thrombosing tendencies, MI, cancer, and in postsurgical patients; measurement of anticoagulant effects using antifactor Xa levels may be of benefit.

Warnings: Additional Pediatric Considerations Confirm the concentration of all heparin injection vials prior to administration; do not use heparin injection as a "catheter lock flush" as the injection is supplied in various concentrations including highly concentrated strengths. Fatal hemorrhages have occurred in pediatric patients when higher concentrations of heparin injection were confused with lower concentrations of heparin lock flush.

Adverse Reactions Note: Immunologically mediated heparin-induced thrombocytopenia (HIT) occurs in a small percentage of patients and is and is marked by a progressive fall in platelet counts and, in some cases, thromboembolic complications (skin necrosis, pulmonary embolism, gangrene of the extremities, stroke, or MI).

Cardiovascular: Allergic vasospastic reaction (possibly related to thrombosis), chest pain, hemorrhagic shock, shock, thrombosis

Central nervous system: Chills, fever, headache

Dermatologic: Alopecia (delayed, transient), bruising (unexplained), cutaneous necrosis, dysesthesia pedis, erythematous plaques (case reports), eczema, urticaria, purpura

Endocrine & metabolic: Adrenal hemorrhage, hyperkalemia (suppression of aldosterone synthesis), ovarian hemorrhage, rebound hyperlipidemia on discontinuation

Gastrointestinal: Constipation, hematemesis, nausea, tarry stools, vomiting

Genitourinary: Frequent or persistent erection

Hematologic: Bleeding from gums, epistaxis, hemorrhage, ovarian hemorrhage, retroperitoneal hemorrhage, thrombocytopenia (see Note)

Hepatic: Liver enzymes increased

Local: Irritation, erythema, pain, hematoma, and ulceration have been rarely reported with deep SubQ injections; IM injection (not recommended) is associated with a high incidence of these effects

Neuromuscular & skeletal: Peripheral neuropathy, osteoporosis (chronic therapy effect)

Ocular: Conjunctivitis (allergic reaction), lacrimation

Renal: Hematuria

Respiratory: Asthma, bronchospasm (case reports), hemoptysis, pulmonary hemorrhage, rhinitis

Miscellaneous: Allergic reactions, anaphylactoid reactions, heparin resistance, hypersensitivity (including chills, fever, and urticaria)

Drug Interactions

Metabolism/Transport Effects None known.

Avoid Concomitant Use

Avoid concomitant use of Heparin with any of the following: Apixaban; Corticorelin; Dabigatran Etexilate; Edoxaban; Omacetaxine; Oritavancin; Rivaroxaban; Streptokinase; Telavancin; Urokinase; Vorapaxar

Increased Effect/Toxicity

Heparin may increase the levels/effects of: ACE Inhibitors; Aliskiren; Angiotensin II Receptor Blockers; Anticoagulants; Canagliflozin; Collagenase (Systemic); Corticorelin; Deferasirox; Deoxycholic Acid; Eplerenone; Ibritumomab; Nintedanib; Obinutuzumab; Omacetaxine; Palifermin; Potassium Salts; Potassium-Sparing Diuretics; Rivaroxaban; Tositumomab and Iodine I 131 Tositumomab

The levels/effects of Heparin may be increased by: 5-ASA Derivatives; Agents with Antiplatelet Properties; Apixaban; Aspirin; Dabigatran Etexilate; Dasatinib; Edoxaban; Herbs (Anticoagulant/Antiplatelet Properties); Ibrutinib; Limaprost; Nonsteroidal Anti-Inflammatory Agents; Omega-3 Fatty Acids; Pentosan Polysulfate Sodium; Pentoxifylline; Prostacyclin Analogues; Salicylates; Streptokinase; Sugammadex; Thrombolytic Agents; Tibolone; Tipranavir; Urokinase; Vitamin E; Vorapaxar

Decreased Effect

The levels/effects of Heparin may be decreased by: Estrogen Derivatives; Nitroglycerin; Oritavancin; Progestins; Telavancin

Storage/Stability Heparin solutions are colorless to slightly yellow. Minor color variations do not affect therapeutic efficacy. Heparin should be stored at controlled room temperature. Protect from freezing and temperatures >40°C.

Stability at room temperature and refrigeration:

Prepared bag: 24-72 hours (specific to solution, concentration, and/or study conditions)

Premixed bag: After seal is broken, 4 days.

Out of overwrap stability: 30 days.

Mechanism of Action Potentiates the action of antithrombin III and thereby inactivates thrombin (as well as activated coagulation factors IX, X, XI, XII, and plasmin) and prevents the conversion of fibrinogen to fibrin; heparin also stimulates release of lipoprotein lipase (lipoprotein lipase hydrolyzes triglycerides to glycerol and free fatty acids)

Pharmacodynamics Anticoagulation effect: Onset of action:

SubQ: 20-60 minutes

IV: Immediate

Pharmacokinetics (Adult data unless noted)

Absorption: SubQ, IM: Erratic

Distribution: Does not cross the placenta; does not appear in breast milk

Metabolism: Believed to be partially metabolized in the reticuloendothelial system

Half-life: Mean: 90 minutes; range: 60-120 minutes; affected by obesity, renal function, malignancy, presence of pulmonary embolism, and infections; half-life has been reported to be dose-dependent: IV bolus: 25 units/kg: 30 minutes; 100 units/kg: 60 minutes; 400 units/kg: 150 minutes (Hirsh, 2008)

Elimination: Renal; small amount excreted unchanged in urine; **Note:** At therapeutic doses, elimination occurs rapidly via nonrenal mechanisms. With very high doses, renal elimination may play more of a role; however, dosage adjustment remains unnecessary for patients with renal impairment (Hirsh, 2008).

Dosing: Neonatal Note: Many concentrations of heparin are available and range from 1-20,000 units/mL. Carefully examine each prefilled syringe, bag, or vial prior to use to ensure that the correct concentration is chosen. Heparin lock flush solution is intended only to maintain patency of IV devices and is not to be used for anticoagulant therapy.

Line flushing: When using daily flushes of heparin to maintain patency of single and double lumen central catheters, 10 units/mL is the concentration used in neonates. Capped polyvinyl chloride catheters and peripheral heparin locks require flushing more frequently (eg, every 6-8 hours). Volume of heparin flush is usually similar to volume of catheter (or slightly greater) or may be standardized according to specific NICU policy (eg, 0.5-1 mL/flush). Dose of heparin flush used should not approach therapeutic unit per kg dose. Additional flushes should be given when stagnant blood is observed in catheter, after catheter is used for drug or blood administration, and after blood withdrawal from catheter.

TPN: Heparin 0.5-1 unit/mL (final concentration) may be added to TPN solutions, both central and peripheral. (Addition of heparin to peripheral TPN has been shown to increase duration of line patency). The final concentration of heparin used for TPN solutions may need to be decreased to 0.5 units/mL in small neonates receiving larger TPN volumes in order to avoid approaching therapeutic amounts.

Arterial lines: Heparinize with a usual final concentration of 1 unit/mL; range: 0.5-1 units/mL; in order to avoid large total doses and systemic effects, use 0.5 unit/mL in low birth weight/premature newborns and in other patients receiving multiple lines containing heparin

Peripheral arterial catheters *in situ*: Continuous IV infusion of heparin at a final concentration of 5 units/mL at 1 mL/hour (Monagle, 2008)

Umbilical artery catheter (UAC) prophylaxis: Low-dose heparin continuous IV infusion via the UAC with a heparin concentration of 0.25–1 unit/mL (Monagle, 2008)

Prophylaxis for cardiac catheterization via an artery: IV: Bolus: 100-150 units/kg; for prolonged procedures, further doses may be required (Monagle, 2008)

Systemic heparinization: IV infusion: Initial loading dose: 75 units/kg given over 10 minutes; then initial maintenance dose: 28 units/kg/hour; adjust dose to maintain APTT of 60-85 seconds (assuming this reflects an antifactor Xa level of 0.35-0.7 units/mL); see table on next page

PROTOCOL FOR SYSTEMIC HEPARIN ADJUSTMENT

To be used after initial loading dose and maintenance IV infusion dose (see above) to maintain APTT of 60-85 seconds (assuming this reflects antifactor Xa level of 0.35-0.7 units/mL)

Obtain blood for APTT 4 hours after heparin loading dose and 4 hours after every infusion rate change

Obtain daily CBC and APTT after APTT is therapeutic

APTT* (seconds)	Dosage Adjustment	Time to Repeat APTT
<50	Give 50 units/kg bolus and increase infusion rate by 10%	4 h after rate change
50-59	Increase infusion rate by 10%	4 h after rate change
60-85	Keep rate the same	Next day
86-95	Decrease infusion rate by 10%	4 h after rate change
96-120	Hold infusion for 30 minutes and decrease infusion rate by 10%	4 h after rate change
>120	Hold infusion for 60 minutes and decrease infusion rate by 15%	4 h after rate change

*Adjust heparin rate to maintain APTT of 60-85 seconds, assuming this reflects antifactor-Xa level of 0.35-0.7 units/mL (reagent specific)

Modified from Monagle P, Chalmers E, Chan A, et al, "Antithrombotic Therapy in Neonates and Children," *Chest*, 2008, 133 (6):887S-968S.

Dosing: Usual

Note: Many concentrations of heparin are available and range from 1-20,000 units/mL. Carefully examine each prefilled syringe, bag, or vial prior to use to ensure that the correct concentration is chosen. Heparin lock flush solution is intended only to maintain patency of IV devices and is not to be used for anticoagulant therapy.

Line flushing: When using daily flushes of heparin to maintain patency of single and double lumen central catheters, 10 units/mL is commonly used for younger infants (eg, <10 kg) while 100 units/mL is used for older infants, children, and adults. Capped polyvinyl chloride catheters and peripheral heparin locks require flushing more frequently (eg, every 6-8 hours). Volume of heparin flush is usually similar to volume of catheter (or slightly greater) or may be standardized according to specific hospital's policy (eg, 2-5 mL/flush). Dose of heparin flush used should not approach therapeutic unit per kg dose. Additional flushes should be given when stagnant blood is observed in catheter, after catheter is used for drug or blood administration, and after blood withdrawal from catheter.

TPN: Infants and Children: Heparin 1 unit/mL (final concentration) may be added to TPN solutions, both central and peripheral. (Addition of heparin to peripheral TPN has been shown to increase duration of line patency.) The final concentration of heparin used for TPN solutions may need to be decreased to 0.5 units/mL in small infants receiving larger TPN volumes in order to avoid approaching therapeutic amounts.

Arterial lines: Infants and Children: Heparinize with a usual final concentration of 1 unit/mL; range: 0.5-2 units/mL; in order to avoid large total doses and systemic effects, use 0.5 unit/mL in patients receiving multiple lines containing heparin

Peripheral arterial catheters *in situ*: Infants and Children: Continuous IV infusion of heparin at a final concentration of 5 units/mL at 1 mL/hour (Monagle, 2008)

Prophylaxis for cardiac catheterization via an artery: Infants and Children: IV: Bolus: 100-150 units/kg; for prolonged procedures, further doses may be required (Monagle, 2008)

Systemic heparinization:

Infants <1 year: IV infusion: Initial loading dose: 75 units/kg given over 10 minutes; then initial maintenance dose: 28 units/kg/hour; adjust dose to maintain APTT of 60-85 seconds (assuming this reflects an antifactor Xa level of 0.35-0.7 units/mL); see table.

Children >1 year:

Intermittent IV: Initial: 50-100 units/kg, then 50-100 units/kg every 4 hours (**Note:** Continuous IV infusion is preferred):

IV infusion: Initial loading dose: 75 units/kg given over 10 minutes, then initial maintenance dose: 20 units/kg/hour; adjust dose to maintain APTT of 60-85 seconds (assuming this reflects an antifactor Xa level of 0.35-0.7 units/mL); see table.

PROTOCOL FOR SYSTEMIC HEPARIN ADJUSTMENT

To be used after initial loading dose and maintenance IV infusion dose (see above) to maintain APTT of 60-85 seconds (assuming this reflects antifactor Xa level of 0.35-0.7 units/mL)

Obtain blood for APTT 4 hours after heparin loading dose and 4 hours after every infusion rate change

Obtain daily CBC and APTT after APTT is therapeutic

APTT* (seconds)	Dosage Adjustment	Time to Repeat APTT
<50	Give 50 units/kg bolus and increase infusion rate by 10%	4 h after rate change
50-59	Increase infusion rate by 10%	4 h after rate change
60-85	Keep rate the same	Next day
86-95	Decrease infusion rate by 10%	4 h after rate change
96-120	Hold infusion for 30 minutes and decrease infusion rate by 10%	4 h after rate change
>120	Hold infusion for 60 minutes and decrease infusion rate by 15%	4 h after rate change

*Adjust heparin rate to maintain APTT of 60-85 seconds, assuming this reflects antifactor-Xa level of 0.35-0.7 units/mL (reagent specific)

Modified from Monagle P, Chalmers E, Chan A, et al, "Antithrombotic Therapy in Neonates and Children," *Chest*, 2008, 133 (6):887S-968S.

Adults:

Prophylaxis (low dose heparin): SubQ: 5000 units every 8-12 hours

Intermittent IV: Initial: 10,000 units, then 50-70 units/kg/dose (5000-10,000 units) every 4-6 hours (**Note:** Continuous IV infusion is preferred)

IV infusion: Initial loading dose: 80 units/kg; initial maintenance dose: 18 units/kg/hour with dose adjusted according to APTT; usual range: 10-30 units/kg/hour

Adults: *Chest*, 2008 Recommendations (Goodman, 2008; Harrington, 2008; Kearon, 2008):

Prophylaxis of DVT and PE: SubQ: 5000 units every 8 or 12 hours or adjusted low-dose heparin

Treatment of DVT and PE:

IV: Initial (loading dose): IV bolus: 80 units/kg (or alternatively 5000 units); follow with continuous IV infusion of 18 units/kg/hour (or alternatively 1300 units/hour). Adjust dosage to achieve and maintain therapeutic APTT as determined by correlating APPT results with a therapeutic range of heparin levels as measured by antifactor Xa assay (0.3-0.7 units/mL).

SubQ:

Monitored dosing regimen: Initial: 17,500 units (or 250 units/kg) then 250 units/kg/dose every 12 hours. Adjust dosage to achieve and maintain therapeutic APTT as determined by correlating APPT results with a therapeutic range of heparin levels as measured by antifactor Xa assay (0.3-0.7 units/mL) when measured 6 hours after injection.

Unmonitored dosing regimen: Initial: 333 units/kg; followed by 250 units/kg/dose every 12 hours

Unstable angina or Non-ST-elevation myocardial infarction (NSTEMI): Initial loading dose: IV bolus: 60-70 units/kg (maximum: 5000 units), then initial maintenance dose: IV infusion: 12-15 units/kg/hour (maximum: 1000 units/hour); adjust dose to maintain therapeutic APTT of 50-75s

STEMI after thrombolytic therapy (full dose alteplase, tenecteplase, or reteplase): Initial loading dose: IV bolus: 60 units/kg (maximum: 4000 units), then initial maintenance dose: IV infusion: 12 units/kg/hour (maximum: 1000 units/hour); adjust dose to maintain therapeutic APTT of 50-70s for 48 hours

Dosage adjustment in renal impairment: No dosage adjustment required; adjust therapeutic heparin according to aPTT or anti-Xa activity

Dosage adjustment in hepatic impairment: No dosage adjustment required; adjust therapeutic heparin according to aPTT or anti-Xa activity

Usual Infusion Concentrations: Neonatal IV infusion: Maintenance of line patency: 0.5 unit/mL

Usual Infusion Concentrations: Pediatric Note: Premixed solutions available

IV infusion: 100 units/mL

Preparation for Administration Note: Many concentrations of heparin are available and range from 1 to 20,000 units/mL. Carefully examine each prefilled syringe, bag, or vial prior to use to ensure that the correct concentration is chosen. Heparin lock flush solution is intended only to maintain patency of IV devices and is not to be used for anticoagulant therapy.

Parenteral: Concentration should be determined based on indication and dose to allow for safe and accurate administration of the correct dose. After addition of heparin to the infusion solution, invert the solution at least 6 times to ensure adequate mixing and prevent pooling of heparin. Products containing benzyl alcohol or derivatives should not be used to prepare products for neonates. ISMP and Vermont Oxford Network recommend a standard concentration of 0.5 units/mL (in 0.45% NS) for maintaining line patency in neonates (ISMP 2011).

Administration Note: Many concentrations of heparin are available and range from 1 to 20,000 units/mL. Carefully examine each prefilled syringe, bag, or vial prior to use to ensure that the correct concentration is chosen.

Parenteral: Do **not** administer IM due to pain, irritation, and hematoma formation.

IV:

Continuous IV infusion: Infuse via infusion pump. IV bolus should be administered over 10 minutes

Heparin lock: Inject via injection cap using positive pressure flushing technique. Heparin lock flush solution is intended only to maintain patency of IV devices and is **not** to be used for anticoagulant therapy.

Central venous catheters: Must be flushed with heparin solution when newly inserted, daily (at the time of tubing change), after blood withdrawal or transfusion, and after an intermittent infusion through an injectable cap.

SubQ: Not all preparation intended for SubQ administration, verify product selection. Inject in subcutaneous tissue only (not muscle tissue). Injection sites should be rotated (usually left and right portions of the abdomen, above iliac crest)

Monitoring Parameters Platelet counts, signs of bleeding, hemoglobin, hematocrit, APTT; for full-dose heparin (ie, nonlow dose), the dose should be titrated according to APTT (see table). For intermittent IV injections, APTT is measured 3.5-4 hours after IV injection.

Reference Range Venous thromboembolism: Heparin: 0.3-0.7 unit/mL anti-Xa activity (by chromogenic assay) or 0.2-0.4 unit/mL (by protamine titration); APTT: 1.5-2.5 times control (usually reflects an APTT of 60-85 seconds) (Hirsh, 2008; Kearon, 2008)

When used with thrombolytic therapy in patients with MI, a lower therapeutic range corresponding to an antiXa level of 0.2-0.5 units/mL by chromogenic assay; APTT: 1.5-2 times control (or approximately an APTT of 50-70 seconds) is recommended (Goodman, 2008)

Test Interactions Increased thyroxine (competitive protein binding methods); increased PT

Aprotinin significantly increases aPTT and celite Activated Clotting Time (ACT) which may not reflect the actual degree of anticoagulation by heparin. Kaolin-based ACTs are not affected by aprotinin to the same degree as celite ACTs. While institutional protocols may vary, a minimal celite ACT of 750 seconds or kaolin-ACT of 480 seconds is recommended in the presence of aprotinin. Consult the manufacturer's information on specific ACT test interpretation in the presence of aprotinin.

Additional Information To reverse the effects of heparin, use protamine. Heparin is available from bovine lung and from porcine intestinal mucosa sources

Duration of heparin therapy (pediatric):

DVT and PE: At least 5-10 days

Note: Oral anticoagulation should be started on day 1 of heparin; oral anticoagulation should be overlapped with heparin for 5 days (or more, if INR is not >2)

Updates to the United States Pharmacopeia (USP) heparin monograph were made in response to over 200 deaths linked to contaminated heparin products in 2007-2008. Serious adverse effects (including hypersensitivity reactions) were associated with a heparin-like contaminant (oversulfated chondroitin sulfate). At the time, the available quality assurance tests did not test for oversulfated chondroitin sulfate. Effective October 1, 2009, a new reference standard for heparin and a new test to determine potency (the chromogenic antifactor IIa test) were established by USP. The updated USP heparin monograph also harmonized the USP unit with the WHO international standard (IS) unit (ie, international unit). The new standard may result in a 10% reduction in potency for heparin marketed in the United States. The FDA has requested that all manufacturers differentiate (from "old" heparin products) heparin products manufactured by the new standards. The labels of products manufactured according to the new standard will have an "N" in the lot number or following the expiration date. Additionally, products manufactured by Hospira may be identified by the number "82" or higher (eg, 83, 84) at the beginning of their lot numbers. For therapeutic use, practitioners may or may not notice that larger doses of heparin are required to achieve "therapeutic" activity of anticoagulation. The impact of this change in potency should be less significant when heparin is administered by subcutaneous injection due to low and variable bioavailability. Heparin dosing should always be individualized according to the patient-specific clinical situation. Appropriate clinical judgment is essential in determining heparin dosage (Smythe, 2010).

Dosage Forms Excipient information presented when available (limited, particularly for generics); consult specific product labeling.

Solution, Injection, as sodium:

Generic: 1000 units (500 mL); 2000 units (1000 mL); 12,500 units (250 mL); 25,000 units (250 mL, 500 mL); 1000 units/mL (1 mL, 10 mL, 30 mL); 2500 units/mL (10 mL); 5000 units/mL (1 mL, 10 mL); 10,000 units/mL (1 mL, 4 mL, 5 mL); 20,000 units/mL (1 mL)

Solution, Injection, as sodium [preservative free]:

Generic: 1000 units/mL (2 mL); 5000 units/0.5 mL (0.5 mL)

Solution, Intravenous, as sodium:

Hep Flush-10: 10 units/mL (10 mL)

Generic: 10,000 units (250 mL); 12,500 units (250 mL); 20,000 units (500 mL); 25,000 units (250 mL, 500 mL); 1 units/mL (1 mL, 2 mL, 2.5 mL, 3 mL, 5 mL, 10 mL); 2 units/mL (3 mL); 10 units/mL (1 mL, 2 mL, 2.5 mL, 3 mL, 5 mL, 10 mL, 30 mL); 100 units/mL (1 mL, 2 mL, 2.5 mL, 3 mL, 5 mL, 10 mL, 30 mL, 100 mL); 2000 units/mL (5 mL)

Solution, Intravenous, as sodium [preservative free]:

Generic: 1 units/mL (3 mL); 10 units/mL (1 mL, 3 mL, 5 mL); 100 units/mL (1 mL, 3 mL, 5 mL)

- **Heparin Calcium** *see* Heparin *on page 1006*
- **Heparinized Saline** *see* Heparin *on page 1006*
- **Heparin Leo (Can)** *see* Heparin *on page 1006*
- **Heparin Lock Flush** *see* Heparin *on page 1006*
- **Heparin Sodium** *see* Heparin *on page 1006*
- **Heparin Sodium Injection, USP (Can)** *see* Heparin *on page 1006*

Hepatitis A Vaccine (hep a TYE tis aye vak SEEN)

Medication Safety Issues

International issues:

Avaxim [Canada and multiple international markets] may be confused with Avastin brand name for bevacizumab [U.S., Canada, and multiple international markets]

Related Information

Centers for Disease Control and Prevention (CDC) and Other Links *on page 2424*

Immunization Administration Recommendations *on page 2411*

Immunization Schedules *on page 2416*

Brand Names: US Havrix; VAQTA

Brand Names: Canada Avaxim; Avaxim-Pediatric; HAV-RIX; VAQTA

Therapeutic Category Vaccine; Vaccine, Inactivated Virus

Generic Availability (US) No

Use Active immunization against disease caused by hepatitis A virus (HAV) (FDA approved in ages ≥12 months and adults)

The Advisory Committee on Immunization Practices (ACIP) recommends routine vaccination for:

- All children ≥12 months of age (CDC/ACIP [Fiore 2006])
- All unvaccinated adults requesting protection from HAV infection (CDC/ACIP [Fiore 2006])
- Unvaccinated persons with any of the following conditions: Men who have sex with men; injection and noninjection illicit drug users; persons who work with HAV-infected primates or with HAV in a research laboratory setting; persons with chronic liver disease; patients who receive clotting-factor concentrates; persons traveling to or working in countries with high or intermediate levels of endemic HAV infection (CDC/ACIP [Fiore 2006])
- Vaccination can be a component of hepatitis A outbreak response or as postexposure prophylaxis, as determined by local public health authorities (CDC/ACIP [Fiore 2006]; CDC/ACIP 56[41] 2007)
- Unvaccinated persons who anticipate close personal contact with international adoptees from a country of intermediate to high endemicity of HAV, during their first 60 days of arrival into the United States (eg, household contacts, babysitters) (CDC/ACIP 58[36] 2009)

Medication Guide Available Yes

Pregnancy Risk Factor C

Pregnancy Considerations Animal reproduction studies have not been conducted. The safety of vaccination during pregnancy has not been determined, however, the theoretical risk to the infant is expected to be low. Inactivated vaccines have not been shown to cause increased risks to the fetus (NCIRD/ACIP 2011).

Breast-Feeding Considerations It is not known if this vaccine is excreted into breast milk. The manufacturer recommends that caution be used if administered to nursing women. Inactivated vaccines do not affect the safety of breast-feeding for the mother or the infant. Breast-feeding infants should be vaccinated according to the recommended schedules (NCIRD/ACIP 2011).

Contraindications Immediate and/or severe allergic or hypersensitivity reaction to hepatitis A containing vaccines or any component of the formulation, including neomycin.

Warnings/Precautions Use with caution in patients with bleeding disorders (including thrombocytopenia) and patients on anticoagulant therapy; bleeding/hematoma may occur from IM administration; if the patient receives antihemophilia or other similar therapy, IM injection can be scheduled shortly after such therapy is administered (NCIRD/ACIP 2011). Canadian product labeling suggests that subcutaneous administration may be considered in exceptional circumstances (eg, patients with thrombocytopenia or at risk for hemorrhage; however, this may convey a higher risk for local reactions (eg, injection site nodule). In healthy adults, seroconversion following an initial subcutaneous dose of VAQTA was slower than that historically observed following intramuscular administration (Linglöf 2001).

Immediate treatment (including epinephrine 1:1,000) for anaphylactoid and/or hypersensitivity reactions should be available during vaccine use (NCIRD/ACIP 2011). The decision to administer or delay vaccination because of current or recent febrile illness depends on the severity of symptoms and the etiology of the disease. Consider deferring administration in patients with moderate or severe acute illness (with or without fever); vaccination should not be delayed for patients with mild acute illness (with or without fever) (NCIRD/ACIP 2011). Use with caution in severely immunocompromised patients (eg, patients receiving chemo/radiation therapy or other immunosuppressive therapy [including high dose corticosteroids]); may have a reduced response to vaccination. In general, household and close contacts of persons with altered immunocompetence may receive all age appropriate vaccines (IDSA [Rubin 2014]; NCIRD/ACIP 2011); inactivated vaccines should be administered ≥2 weeks prior to planned immunosuppression when feasible (IDSA [Rubin 2014]). Vaccination may not result in effective immunity in all patients. Response depends upon multiple factors (eg, type of vaccine, age of patient) and is improved by administering the vaccine at the recommended dose, route, and interval. Vaccines may not be effective if administered during periods of altered immune competence (NCIRD/ACIP 2011). Due to the long incubation period for hepatitis A (15 to 50 days), unrecognized hepatitis A infection may be present; immunization may not prevent infection in these patients. Recommended for patients with chronic liver disease; however, these patients may have decreased antibody response. Antipyretics have not been shown to prevent febrile seizures; antipyretics may be used to treat fever or discomfort following vaccination (NCIRD/ACIP 2011). One study reported that routine prophylactic administration of acetaminophen to prevent fever prior to vaccination decreased the immune response of some vaccines; the clinical significance of this reduction in immune response has not been established (Prymula 2009).

Syncope has been reported with use of injectable vaccines and may result in serious secondary injury (eg, skull fracture, cerebral hemorrhage); typically reported in adolescents and young adults and within 15 minutes after vaccination. Procedures should be in place to avoid injuries from falling and to restore cerebral perfusion if syncope occurs (NCIRD/ACIP 2011). Packaging may contain natural latex rubber; some products may contain neomycin. In order to maximize vaccination rates, the ACIP recommends simultaneous administration (ie, >1 vaccine on the same day at different anatomic sites) of all age-appropriate vaccines (live or inactivated) for which a person is eligible at a single clinic visit, unless contraindications exist. The use of combination vaccines is generally preferred over separate injections, taking into consideration provider assessment, patient preference, and adverse events. When using combination vaccines, the minimum age for administration is the oldest minimum age for any individual component; the minimum interval between dosing is the greatest minimum interval between any individual components. The ACIP prefers each dose of a specific vaccine in a series come from the same manufacturer when possible (NCIRD/ACIP 2011). Use of this vaccine for specific medical and/or other indications (eg, immunocompromising conditions, hepatic or kidney disease, diabetes) is also addressed in the ACIP Adult Recommended Immunization Schedule (CDC/ACIP [Kim 2015]). Specific recommendations for vaccination in immunocompromised patients with asplenia, cancer, HIV infection, cerebrospinal fluid leaks, cochlear implants, hematopoietic stem cell transplant (prior to or after), sickle cell disease, solid organ transplant (prior to or after), or those receiving immunosuppressive therapy for chronic conditions as well as contacts of immunocompromised patients are available from the IDSA (Rubin 2014).

Adverse Reactions All serious adverse reactions must be reported to the U.S. Department of Health and Human Services (DHHS) Vaccine Adverse Event Reporting System (VAERS) at 1-800-822-7967 or online at https://vaers.hhs.gov/esub/index. In Canada, adverse reactions may be reported to local provincial/territorial health agencies or to the Vaccine Safety Section at Public Health Agency of Canada (1-866-844-0018).

Central nervous system: Chills, drowsiness, fatigue, headache, insomnia, irritability, malaise

Dermatologic: Skin rash

Endocrine & metabolic: Menstrual disease

Gastrointestinal: Abdominal pain, anorexia, constipation, decreased appetite, diarrhea, gastroenteritis, nausea, vomiting

Local: Bruising at injection site, erythema at injection site, induration at injection site, injection site reaction (soreness, warmth), pain at injection site, swelling at injection site, tenderness at injection site

Neuromuscular & skeletal: Arm pain, back pain, myalgia, stiffness, weakness

Ophthalmic: Conjunctivitis

Otic: Otitis media

Respiratory: Asthma, cough, nasal congestion, nasopharyngitis, pharyngitis, rhinitis, rhinorrhea, upper respiratory tract infection

Miscellaneous: Excessive crying, fever (≥102°F [1-5 days postvaccination]; ≥100.4°F [1-5 days postvaccination]; >98.6°C [1-14 days postvaccination])

Rare but important or life-threatening: Anaphylaxis, angioedema, ataxia (cerebellar), bronchiolitis, bronchoconstriction, dehydration, dermatitis, encephalitis, erythema multiforme, Guillain-Barre syndrome, hematoma at injection site, hepatitis, hypersensitivity reaction, hypoesthesia, increased creatine kinase, increased serum transaminases (transient), injection site reaction (nodule), jaundice, lymphadenopathy, multiple sclerosis, myelitis, neuropathy, paresthesia, photophobia, pruritus, rash at injection site, seizure, serum sickness-like reaction, syncope, thrombocytopenia, vasculitis, wheezing

Drug Interactions

Metabolism/Transport Effects None known.

Avoid Concomitant Use There are no known interactions where it is recommended to avoid concomitant use.

Increased Effect/Toxicity There are no known significant interactions involving an increase in effect.

Decreased Effect

The levels/effects of Hepatitis A Vaccine may be decreased by: Belimumab; Fingolimod; Immunosuppressants

Storage/Stability

Store refrigerated between 2°C and 8°C (36°F and 46°F). Do not freeze; discard if the product has been frozen.

The following stability information has also been reported for Havrix: May be stored at room temperature for up to 72 hours (Cohen 2007).

VAQTA: Canadian labeling suggests that the vaccine may be used if cumulative exposure to temperatures of 0°C to 2°C (32°F to 36°F) or 8°C to 25°C (46°F to 77°F) is ≤72 hours.

Mechanism of Action As an inactivated virus vaccine, hepatitis A vaccine induces active immunity against hepatitis A virus infection

Pharmacodynamics

Onset of action: Protective antibodies develop in 95% of adults after the first dose and in 100% of adults after the second dose of the vaccine; ≥97% of children and adolescents will be seropositive within 1 month of the first dose and 100% will develop protective antibodies after receiving two doses. The efficacy of preventing hepatitis A disease in children living in highly infected areas is 94% to 100% (CDC, 2012).

Duration: Protective antibodies induced by the vaccine may persist for ≥20 years (CDC, 2012).

Dosing: Usual Note: Although it is preferred to use the vaccines according to their approved labeling, Havrix and VAQTA are considered to be interchangeable for booster doses (CDC/ACIP [Fiore 2006]).

Pediatric:

Primary immunization: Note: When used for primary immunization, the vaccine should be given at least 2 weeks prior to expected HAV exposure. When used prior to an international adoption, the vaccination series should begin when adoption is being planned, but at least ≥2 weeks prior to expected arrival of adoptee (CDC 58[36] 2009).

ACIP recommendations (CDC/ACIP [Fiore 2006]):

Children 12 to 23 months: IM: 0.5 mL per dose for a total of two doses. The series should be initiated at 12 to 23 months of age; the two doses should be separated by 6 to 18 months

Children ≥ 2 years and Adolescents (unvaccinated) if immunity against hepatitis A virus infection is desired: IM: 0.5 mL per dose for a total of two doses separated by 6 to 18 months

Manufacturer's labeling:

Havrix: Children and Adolescents: IM: 0.5 mL (720 ELISA units) per dose for a total of two doses given 6 to 12 months apart

VAQTA: Children and Adolescents: IM: 0.5 mL (25 units) per dose for a total of two doses given 6 to 18 months of age apart; **Note:** VAQTA should be given at 6 to 12 months if following the primary dose of Havrix.

Catch-up immunization: CDC (ACIP) recommendations (Strikas 2015): **Note:** Do not restart the series. If doses have been given, begin the following schedule at the applicable dose number. Children ≥2 years and Adolescents if immunity against hepatitis A virus infection is desired: IM: 0.5 mL per dose for a total of two doses separated by at least 6 months

Postexposure prophylaxis: Children and Adolescents without immunity: IM: 0.5 mL once as soon as possible following recent exposure to hepatitis A virus (during last two weeks) (CDC, 56[41], 2007)

Adult: **Primary immunization:**

Havrix: IM: 1 mL (1440 ELISA units) per dose for a total of two doses given 6 to 12 months apart

VAQTA: IM: 1 mL (50 units) per dose for a total of two doses given 6 to 18 months apart; **Note:** VAQTA should be given at 6 to 12 months if following the primary dose of Havrix

Dosing adjustment in renal impairment: There are no dosage adjustments provided in the manufacturer's labeling.

Dosing adjustment in hepatic impairment: There are no dosage adjustments provided in the manufacturer's labeling; however, data suggest patients with chronic liver disease have a lower antibody response to HAVRIX than healthy subjects.

Administration Shake well and administer IM into midlateral aspect of the thigh in infants and small children; administer in the deltoid area to older children and adults; not for IV, intradermal, or SubQ administration. Do not administer to the gluteal region; may decrease efficacy. To prevent syncope related injuries, adolescents and adults should be vaccinated while seated or lying down (NCIRD/ACIP 2011). US law requires that the date of administration, the vaccine manufacturer, lot number of vaccine, and the administering person's name, title, and address be entered into the patient's permanent medical record.

For patients at risk of hemorrhage following intramuscular injection, the vaccine should be administered intramuscularly if, in the opinion of the physician familiar with the patient's bleeding risk, the vaccine can be administered by this route with reasonable safety. If the patient receives antihemophilia or other similar therapy, intramuscular vaccination can be scheduled shortly after such therapy is administered. A fine needle (23 gauge or smaller) should be used for the vaccination and firm pressure on the site (without rubbing) for at least 2 minutes. The patient should be instructed concerning the risk of hematoma from the injection. Patients on anticoagulant therapy should be considered to have the same bleeding risks and treated as those with clotting factor disorders (NCIRD/ACIP 2011).

Monitoring Parameters Liver function tests. Observe for syncope for 15 minutes following administration (NCIRD/ACIP 2011). If seizure-like activity associated with syncope occurs, maintain patient in supine or Trendelenburg position to reestablish adequate cerebral perfusion.

Additional Information The ACIP currently recommends that immunocompromised patients, persons with underlying medical conditions (including chronic liver disease), or older adults that are vaccinated <2 weeks from departure to an area with a high or intermediate risk of hepatitis A infection also receive immune globulin (CDC/ACIP 56 [41] 2007]).

For postexposure prophylaxis, hepatitis A vaccine is preferred over immune globulin for people ages 12 months to 40 years who have recently been exposed to HAV and who have not previously received hepatitis A vaccine. Administer a single dose of hepatitis A vaccine as soon as possible. For people older than 40 years, immune globulin is preferred, although vaccine can be used if immune globulin is unavailable (CDC/ACIP 56[41] 2007])

Dosage Forms Excipient information presented when available (limited, particularly for generics); consult specific product labeling.

Injection, suspension [adult, preservative free]:

Havrix: Hepatitis A virus antigen 1440 ELISA units/mL (1 mL) [contains aluminum, neomycin (may have trace amounts); may contain natural rubber/natural latex in prefilled syringe]

VAQTA: Hepatitis A virus antigen 50 units/mL (1 mL) [contains aluminum, natural rubber/natural latex in packaging]

Injection, suspension [pediatric, preservative free]:

Havrix: Hepatitis A virus antigen 720 ELISA units/0.5 mL (0.5 mL) [contains aluminum, neomycin (may have trace amounts); may contain natural rubber/natural latex in prefilled syringe]

Injection, suspension [pediatric/adolescent, preservative free]:

VAQTA: Hepatitis A virus antigen 25 units/0.5 mL (0.5 mL) [contains aluminum, natural rubber/natural latex in packaging]

Hepatitis B Immune Globulin (Human)

(hep a TYE tis bee i MYUN GLOB yoo lin YU man)

Medication Safety Issues

Sound-alike/look-alike issues:

HBIG may be confused with BabyBIG

International issues:

Bayhep-B [Philippines, Turkey] may be confused with Bayrab which is a brand name for rabies immune globulin [Philippines, Turkey]; Bayrho-D which is brand name for Rh_oD immune globulin [Israel, Turkey]

Related Information

Centers for Disease Control and Prevention (CDC) and Other Links *on page 2424*

Immunization Administration Recommendations *on page 2411*

Immunization Schedules *on page 2416*

Brand Names: US HepaGam B; HyperHEP B S/D; Nabi-HB

Brand Names: Canada HepaGam B; HyperHEP B S/D

Therapeutic Category Immune Globulin

Generic Availability (US) No

Use Parenteral:

IM: HepaGam B®, HyperHEP B™ S/D, Nabi-HB®: Provide prophylactic post-exposure passive immunity to hepatitis B following perinatal exposure of infants born to HBsAg-positive mothers (FDA approved in neonates and infants); provide prophylactic postexposure passive immunity to hepatitis B following acute exposure to blood containing hepatitis B surface antigen (HBsAg), sexual

sure to persons with acute HBV infection (FDA approved in infants, children, and adults)

IV: HepaGam B®: Prevention of hepatitis B virus recurrence after liver transplantation in HBsAg-positive transplant patients

Note: Hepatitis B immune globulin is not indicated for treatment of active hepatitis B infection and is ineffective in the treatment of chronic active hepatitis B infection.

Pregnancy Risk Factor C

Pregnancy Considerations Animal reproduction studies have not been conducted. Use of HBIG is not contraindicated in pregnant women and may be used for postexposure prophylaxis when indicated (CDC, 2001). In addition, use of HBIG has been evaluated to reduce maternal to fetal transmission of hepatis B virus during pregnancy (ACOG, 2007)

Breast-Feeding Considerations It is not known if immune globulin from these preparations is excreted into breast milk. The manufacturer recommends that caution be used if administered to breast-feeding women. Endogenous immune globulins can be found in breast milk (Agarwal, 2011). Infants born to HBsAg-positive mothers may be breast fed (CDC, 2005). Use of HBIG is not contraindicated in breast-feeding women (CDC, 2001).

Contraindications

HepaGam B: Anaphylactic or severe systemic reaction to human globulin preparations; postexposure prophylaxis in patients with severe thrombocytopenia or other coagulation disorders which would contraindicate IM injections (administer only if benefit outweighs the risk)

HyperHEP B S/D: No contraindications listed in manufacturer's labeling

Nabi-HB: Anaphylactic or severe systemic reaction to human globulin preparations

Warnings/Precautions Hypersensitivity and anaphylactic reactions can occur; immediate treatment (including epinephrine 1:1000) should be available. Use with caution in patients with previous systemic hypersensitivity to human immunoglobulins. Use with caution in patients with thrombocytopenia or coagulation disorders; IM injections may be contraindicated. Use with caution in patients with IgA deficiency. When administered IV, do not exceed recommended infusion rates; may increase risk of adverse events. Patients should be monitored for adverse events during and after the infusion. Thrombotic events have been reported with administration of intravenous immune globulin; use with caution in patients of advanced age, with a history of atherosclerosis or cardiovascular and/or thrombotic risk factors, patients with impaired cardiac output, coagulation disorders, prolonged immobilization, or patients with known/suspected hyperviscosity. Consider a baseline assessment of blood viscosity in patients at risk for hyperviscosity. Product of human plasma; may potentially contain infectious agents which could transmit disease. Screening of donors, as well as testing and/or inactivation or removal of certain viruses, reduces the risk. Infections thought to be transmitted by this product should be reported to the manufacturer. Some products may contain maltose, which may result in falsely-elevated blood glucose readings. Some dosage forms may contain polysorbate 80 (also known as Tweens). Hypersensitivity reactions, usually a delayed reaction, have been reported following exposure to pharmaceutical products containing polysorbate 80 in certain individuals (Isaksson, 2002; Lucente 2000; Shelley, 1995). Thrombocytopenia, ascites, pulmonary deterioration, and renal and hepatic failure have been reported in premature neonates after receiving parenteral products containing polysorbate 80 (Alade, 1986; CDC, 1984). See manufacturer's labeling.

Adverse Reactions Reported with postexposure prophylaxis. Adverse events reported in liver transplant patients included tremor and hypotension, were associated with a single infusion during the first week of treatment, and did not recur with additional infusions.

Cardiovascular: Hypotension

Central nervous system: Headache, malaise

Dermatologic: Ecchymoses, erythema

Gastrointestinal: Nausea, vomiting

Hematologic & oncologic: Change in WBC count

Hepatic: Increased liver enzymes, increased serum alkaline phosphatase

Local: Pain at injection site

Neuromuscular & skeletal: Joint stiffness, myalgia

Renal: Increased serum creatinine

Rare but important or life-threatening: Anaphylactic reaction (rare), angioedema, hypersensitivity, increased serum lipase, increased serum transaminases, sinus tachycardia

Drug Interactions

Metabolism/Transport Effects None known.

Avoid Concomitant Use There are no known interactions where it is recommended to avoid concomitant use.

Increased Effect/Toxicity There are no known significant interactions involving an increase in effect.

Decreased Effect

Hepatitis B Immune Globulin (Human) may decrease the levels/effects of: Vaccines (Live)

Storage/Stability Refrigerate at 2°C to 8°C (36°F to 46°F); do not freeze. Do not shake vial; avoid foaming.

HepaGamB®; Nabi-HB®: Use within 6 hours of entering vial.

HyperHEP B™ S/D: May be exposed to room temperature for a cumulative 7 days (Cohen, 2007).

Mechanism of Action Hepatitis B immune globulin (HBIG) is a nonpyrogenic sterile solution containing immunoglobulin G (IgG) specific to hepatitis B surface antigen (HBsAg). HBIG differs from immune globulin in the amount of anti-HBs. Immune globulin is prepared from plasma that is not preselected for anti-HBs content. HBIG is prepared from plasma preselected for high titer anti-HBs. In the U.S., HBIG has an anti-HBs high titer >1:100,000 by IRA.

Pharmacodynamics Duration: Postexposure prophylaxis: 3-6 months

Pharmacokinetics (Adult data unless noted)

Absorption: IM: Slow

Half-life: 17-25 days

Time to peak serum concentration: IM: 2-10 days

Dosing: Neonatal

Perinatal exposure, prophylaxis (CDC, 2005): **Note:** HBIG may be administered at the same time (but at a different site) or up to 1 month preceding hepatitis B vaccination without impairing the active immune response:

Neonates born to HBsAg-positive mothers: IM: 0.5 mL as soon after birth as possible (within 12 hours; efficacy decreases significantly if treatment is delayed >48 hours); hepatitis B vaccine series to begin at the same time; if this series is delayed for as long as 3 months, the HBIG dose may be repeated (Saari, 2003)

Neonates born to mothers with unknown HBsAg status at birth: IM:

Birth weight <2 kg: 0.5 mL within 12 hours of birth (along with hepatitis B vaccine) if unable to determine maternal HBsAg status within that time

Birth weight ≥2 kg: 0.5 mL within 7 days of birth while awaiting maternal HBsAg results; if mother is determined to be HBsAg positive, administer dose as soon as possible.

Dosing: Usual Note: For exposure prophylaxis, HBIG may be administered at the same time (but at a different site) or up to 1 month preceding hepatitis B vaccination without impairing the active immune response.

Infants, Children, and Adolescents:

Perinatal exposure, prophylaxis (CDC, 2005): *Infants born to HBsAg-positive mothers:* IM: 0.5 mL as a repeat of birth dose if the hepatitis B vaccination series is delayed for as long as 3 months (hepatitis B vaccine should also be administered at the same time/different site)

Postexposure, prophylaxis:

Infants <12 months: IM: 0.5 mL as soon as possible after exposure (eg, mother or primary caregiver with acute HBV infection); initiate hepatitis B vaccine series

Children ≥12 months and Adolescents: IM: 0.06 mL/kg as soon as possible after exposure (ie, within 24 hours of needlestick, ocular, or mucosal exposure or within 14 days of sexual exposure); repeat at 28-30 days after exposure

Adults:

Postexposure, prophylaxis: IM: 0.06 mL/kg as soon as possible after exposure (ie, within 24 hours of needlestick, ocular, or mucosal exposure or within 14 days of sexual exposure); repeat at 28-30 days after exposure

Prevention of hepatitis B recurrence in liver transplant patients: IV: HepaGam B™: 20,000 units/dose according to the following schedule:

Anhepatic phase (initial dose): One dose given with the liver transplant

Week 1 postop: One dose daily for 7 days (days 1-7)

Weeks 2-12 postop: One dose every 2 weeks starting on day 14

Month 4 onward: One dose monthly starting on month 4

Dose adjustment: Adjust dose to reach anti-HBs levels of 500 units/L within the first week after transplantation. In patients with surgical bleeding, abdominal fluid drainage >500 mL or those undergoing plasmapheresis, administer 10,000 units/dose every 6 hours until target anti-HBs levels are reached.

Dosing adjustment in renal impairment: There are no dosage adjustments provided in the manufacturer labeling.

Dosing adjustment in hepatic impairment: There are no dosing adjustments provided in the manufacturer labeling.

Preparation for Administration IV: HepaGamB: May dilute with NS prior to IV administration if preferred; do not dilute with D_5W.

Administration

IM: Inject only in the anterolateral aspects of the upper thigh or the deltoid muscle; multiple injections may be necessary when the dosage is a large volume (postexposure prophylaxis). Do not administer hepatitis vaccine and HBIG in same syringe (vaccine will be neutralized); hepatitis vaccine may be administered at the same time at a separate site

IV:

HepaGam B: Administer at 2 mL/minute. Decrease infusion to <1 mL/minute for patient discomfort or infusion-related adverse events. Actual volume of dosage is dependent upon potency labeled on each individual vial.

Nabi-HB: Although not FDA approved for this purpose, Nabi-HB® has been administered intravenously in hepatitis B-positive liver transplant adult patients (Dickson 2006).

Monitoring Parameters Liver transplant patients: anti-HB levels; infusion-related adverse events

Test Interactions

Glucose testing: HepaGam B™ contains maltose. Falsely-elevated blood glucose levels may occur when glucose monitoring devices and test strips utilizing the glucose dehydrogenase pyrroloquinolinequinone (GDH-PQQ) based methods are used.

Serological testing: Antibodies transferred following administration of immune globulins may provide misleading positive test results (eg, Coombs' test)

Dosage Forms Excipient information presented when available (limited, particularly for generics); consult specific product labeling.

Solution, Injection [preservative free]:

HepaGam B: (1 mL, 5 mL) [contains polysorbate 80]

Solution, Intramuscular:

HyperHEP B S/D: (0.5 mL, 1 mL, 5 mL)

Nabi-HB: (1 mL, 5 mL) [thimerosal free]

◆ **Hepatitis B Inactivated Virus Vaccine (recombinant DNA)** *see* Hepatitis B Vaccine (Recombinant) *on page 1015*

Hepatitis B Vaccine (Recombinant)

(hep a TYE tis bee vak SEEN ree KOM be nant)

Medication Safety Issues

Sound-alike/look-alike issues:

Engerix-B adult may be confused with Engerix-B pediatric/adolescent

Recombivax HB may be confused with Comvax

Related Information

Centers for Disease Control and Prevention (CDC) and Other Links *on page 2424*

Immunization Administration Recommendations *on page 2411*

Immunization Schedules *on page 2416*

Brand Names: US Engerix-B; Recombivax HB

Brand Names: Canada Engerix-B; Recombivax HB

Therapeutic Category Vaccine; Vaccine, Inactivated Virus

Generic Availability (US) No

Use Active immunization against infection caused by all known subtypes of hepatitis B virus (FDA approved in all ages).

The Advisory Committee on Immunization Practices (ACIP) recommends routine vaccination for the following:

- All neonates before hospital discharge (CDC/ACIP [Mast 2005])
- All infants and children (CDC/ACIP [Mast 2005])
- All unvaccinated adults requesting protection from HBV infection (CDC/ACIP [Mast 2006])
- All unvaccinated adults at risk for HBV infection such as those with:
  - Behavioral risks: Sexually active persons with >1 partner in a 6-month period; persons seeking evaluation or treatment for a sexually transmitted disease; men who have sex with men; injection drug users (CDC/ACIP [Mast 2006])
  - Occupational risks: Healthcare and public safety workers with reasonably anticipated risk for exposure to blood or blood-contaminated body fluids (CDC/ACIP [Mast 2006])
  - Medical risks: Persons with end-stage renal disease (including predialysis, hemodialysis, peritoneal dialysis, and home dialysis); persons with HIV infection; persons with chronic liver disease (CDC/ACIP [Mast 2006]). Adults (19 to 59 years of age) with diabetes mellitus type 1 or type 2 should be vaccinated as soon as possible following diagnosis. Adults ≥60 years with diabetes mellitus may also be vaccinated at the discretion of their treating clinician based on the likelihood of acquiring HBV infection (CDC/ACIP 60 [50] 2011).
  - Other risks: Household contacts and sex partners of persons with chronic HBV infection; residents and staff of facilities for developmentally disabled persons; international travelers to regions with high or intermediate levels of endemic HBV infection (CDC/ACIP [Mast 2006])

In addition, the ACIP recommends vaccination for any persons who are wounded in bombings or similar mass casualty events who have penetrating injuries or nonintact skin exposure, or who have contact with mucous membranes (exception - superficial contact with intact skin), and who cannot confirm receipt of a hepatitis B vaccination (CDC [Chapman 2008]).

Medication Guide Available Yes

Pregnancy Risk Factor C

Pregnancy Considerations Animal reproduction studies have not been conducted. The ACIP recommends HBsAg testing for all pregnant women. Based on limited data, there is no apparent risk to the fetus when the hepatitis B vaccine is administered during pregnancy. Pregnancy itself is not a contraindication to vaccination; vaccination should be considered if otherwise indicated (CDC/ACIP [Mast 2006]).

Breast-Feeding Considerations It is not known if this vaccine is excreted into breast milk. The manufacturer recommends that caution be used if administered to a nursing woman. However, maternal vaccination is not a contraindication to breast-feeding (CDC [Schillie 2013]). Inactivated virus vaccines do not affect the safety of breast-feeding for the mother or the infant. Breast-feeding infants should be vaccinated according to the recommended schedules (NCIRD/ACIP 2011). Infants born to HBsAg-positive mothers may be breast-fed (CDC/ACIP [Mast 2005]). Female health care providers who are exposed to the hepatitis B virus do not need to discontinue nursing when the vaccine is administered as part of post exposure care (CDC [Schillie 2013]).

Contraindications Severe allergic or hypersensitivity reaction to yeast, hepatitis B vaccine, or any component of the formulation.

Warnings/Precautions Immediate treatment (including epinephrine 1:1,000) for anaphylactoid and/or hypersensitivity reactions should be available during vaccine use (NCIRD/ACIP 2011). The decision to administer or delay vaccination because of current or recent febrile illness depends on the severity of symptoms and the etiology of the disease. Consider deferring administration in patients with moderate or severe acute illness (with or without fever); vaccination should not be delayed for patients with mild acute illness (with or without fever) (NCIRD/ACIP 2011). Bleeding disorders: Use with caution in patients with bleeding disorders (including thrombocytopenia) and patients on anticoagulant therapy; bleeding/hematoma may occur from IM administration; if the patient receives antihemophilia or other similar therapy, IM injection can be scheduled shortly after such therapy is administered (NCIRD/ACIP 2011). Vaccination may not result in effective immunity in all patients. Response depends upon multiple factors (eg, type of vaccine, age of patient) and is improved by administering the vaccine at the recommended dose, route, and interval. Vaccines may not be effective if administered during periods of altered immune competence (NCIRD/ACIP 2011). Due to the long incubation period for hepatitis, unrecognized hepatitis B infection may be present prior to vaccination; immunization may not prevent infection in these patients. Patients >60 years of age may have lower response rates. Use with caution in severely immunocompromised patients (eg, patients receiving chemo/radiation therapy or other immunosuppressive therapy [including high-dose corticosteroids]); may have a reduced response to vaccination. In general, household and close contacts of persons with altered immunocompetence may receive all age appropriate vaccines (IDSA [Rubin 2014]; NCIRD/ACIP 2011); inactivated vaccines should be administered ≥2 weeks prior to planned immunosuppression when feasible (IDSA [Rubin 2014]). Use caution in multiple sclerosis patients; rare exacerbations of symptoms have been observed. Apnea has been reported following IM vaccine administration in premature infants; consider clinical status implications. In general, preterm infants should be vaccinated at the same chronological age as full-term infants (NCIRD/ACIP 2011). However, infants born to HBsAg-negative mothers and weighing <2 kg at birth may have the initial dose deferred up to 30 days of chronological age or until hospital discharge. If the mothers HBsAg status at delivery is unknown or positive, hepatitis B vaccine and hepatitis B immune globulin should be administered within 12 hours of life and the first dose of the vaccine should not be counted as part of the vaccine series.

Syncope has been reported with use of injectable vaccines and may result in serious secondary injury (eg, skull fracture, cerebral hemorrhage); typically reported in adolescents and young adults and within 15 minutes after vaccination. Procedures should be in place to avoid injuries from falling and to restore cerebral perfusion if syncope occurs (NCIRD/ACIP 2011). Some dosage packaging may contain natural latex rubber. In order to maximize vaccination rates, the ACIP recommends simultaneous administration (ie, >1 vaccine on the same day at different anatomic sites)of all age-appropriate vaccines (live or inactivated) for which a person is eligible at a single clinic visit, unless contraindications exist. The use of combination vaccines is generally preferred over separate injections, taking into consideration provider assessment, patient preference, and adverse events. When using combination vaccines, the minimum age for administration is the oldest minimum age for any individual component; the minimum interval between dosing is the greatest minimum interval between any individual components. The ACIP prefers each dose of a specific vaccine in a series come from the same manufacturer when possible (NCIRD/ACIP 2011). Antipyretics have not been shown to prevent febrile seizures; antipyretics may be used to treat fever or discomfort following vaccination (NCIRD/ACIP 2011). One study reported that routine prophylactic administration of acetaminophen to prevent fever prior to vaccination decreased the immune response of some vaccines; the clinical significance of this reduction in immune response has not been established (Prymula 2009).

Use of this vaccine for specific medical and/or other indications (eg, immunocompromising conditions, hepatic or kidney disease, diabetes) is also addressed in the ACIP Adult Recommended Immunization Schedule (CDC/ACIP [Kim 2015]). Specific recommendations for vaccination in immunocompromised patients with asplenia, cancer, HIV infection, cerebrospinal fluid leaks, cochlear implants, hematopoietic stem cell transplant (prior to or after), sickle cell disease, solid organ transplant (prior to or after), or those receiving immunosuppressive therapy for chronic conditions are available in the IDSA guidelines (Rubin 2014).

Adverse Reactions All serious adverse reactions must be reported to the U.S. Department of Health and Human Services (DHHS) Vaccine Adverse Event Reporting System (VAERS) at 1-800-822-7967 or online at https://vaers.hhs.gov/esub/index.

Cardiovascular: Flushing, hypotension

Central nervous system: Body pain, chills, dizziness, drowsiness, fatigue, headache, insomnia, irritability, malaise, paresthesia, tingling sensation, vertigo

Dermatologic: Diaphoresis, pruritus, skin rash, urticaria

Gastrointestinal: Abdominal pain, anorexia, decreased appetite, diarrhea, dyspepsia, nausea, stomach cramps, vomiting

Genitourinary: Dysuria

Hematologic & oncologic: Lymphadenopathy

Hypersensitivity: Angioedema

Infection: Influenza

Local: Bruising at injection site, erythema at injection site, induration at injection site, injection site nodule, itching at injection site, local soreness/soreness at injection site, pain at injection site, swelling at injection site, tenderness at injection site, warm sensation at injection site

Neuromuscular & skeletal: Arthralgia, back pain, myalgia, neck pain, neck stiffness, shoulder pain, weakness

Otic: Otalgia

Respiratory: Cough, pharyngitis, rhinitis, upper respiratory tract infection

Miscellaneous: Fever (≥37.5°C/100°F)

Rare but important or life-threatening: Acute exacerbations of multiple sclerosis, anaphylaxis, apnea, Bell's palsy, encephalitis, febrile seizures, Guillain-Barre syndrome, herpes zoster, hypersensitivity reaction, hypoesthesia, increased erythrocyte sedimentation rate, increased liver enzymes, keratitis, lupus-like syndrome, migraine, multiple sclerosis, myelitis, neuropathy, optic neuritis, paralysis, paresis, periarteritis nodosa, peripheral neuropathy, purpura, radiculopathy, seizure, serum-sickness like reaction (may be delayed days to weeks), Stevens-Johnson syndrome, syncope, systemic lupus erythematosus, tachycardia, thrombocytopenia, transverse myelitis, uveitis, vasculitis, visual disturbances

Drug Interactions

Metabolism/Transport Effects None known.

Avoid Concomitant Use There are no known interactions where it is recommended to avoid concomitant use.

Increased Effect/Toxicity There are no known significant interactions involving an increase in effect.

Decreased Effect

The levels/effects of Hepatitis B Vaccine (Recombinant) may be decreased by: Belimumab; Fingolimod; Immunosuppressants

Storage/Stability Refrigerate at 2°C to 8°C (36°F to 46°F); do not freeze. The following stability information has also been reported for Engerix-B®: May be stored at room temperature for up to 72 hours (Cohen 2007).

Mechanism of Action Recombinant hepatitis B vaccine is a noninfectious subunit viral vaccine, which confers active immunity via formation of antihepatitis B antibodies. The vaccine is derived from hepatitis B surface antigen (HBsAg) produced through recombinant DNA techniques from yeast cells. The portion of the hepatitis B gene which codes for HBsAg is cloned into yeast, which is then cultured to produce hepatitis B vaccine.

Pharmacodynamics Postvaccination seroprotection is found in ~95% of healthy infants, ~92% of health care personnel <40 years of age, and ~84% of health care personnel ≥40 years of age (CDC [Schillie 2013]).

Duration: Following a 3-dose series in pediatric patients, up to 50% of patients will have low or undetectable anti-HB antibody 5 to 15 years postvaccination. However, anamnestic increases in anti-HB have been shown up to 23 years later, suggesting a lifelong immune memory response (CDC/ACIP [Mast, 2005]; CDC/ACIP [Mast 2006]).

Dosing: Neonatal Although hepatitis B vaccine products differ by concentration (mcg/mL), when dosed in terms of volume (mL), the equivalent dose is the same between products (ie, 0.5 mL of Recombivax-HB is equivalent to 0.5 mL of Engerix-B). Combination vaccines should not be used for the "birth" dose but may be used to complete the immunization series after the infant is 6 weeks of age.

Primary immunization:

Manufacturer's labeling: Recombivax-HB, Engerix-B (Pediatric/Adolescent formulation): IM: 0.5 mL per dose for a total of 3 doses; the second and third dose should be given 1 and 6 months after the first dose; ideally first dose given at birth

CDC (ACIP) Recommendations (CDC/ACIP [Mast 2005]; CDC/ACIP [Strikas 2015]):

*Neonates born to HBsAg-**positive** mothers:* Administer first dose within the first 12 hours of life, even if premature and regardless of birth weight (hepatitis immune globulin should also be administered at the same time/different site); **Note:** Due to possible decreased immunogenicity, premature neonates <2 kg should receive 4 total doses at 0, 1, 2 to 3, and 6 to 7 months of chronological age.

*Neonates born to HBsAg-**negative** mothers:* First dose should be given at hospital discharge; **Note:** Premature neonates <2 kg may have the initial dose deferred up to 30 days of chronological age or at hospital discharge.

Neonates born to mothers with unknown HBsAg status at birth: Administer first dose within 12 hours of birth even if premature and regardless of birth weight, second dose following 1 to 2 months later; if HBsAg test is positive, the neonate should receive hepatitis immune globulin as soon as possible (no later than 12 hours of age if <2 kg or age 1 week if ≥2 kg). **Note:** Due to possible decreased immunogenicity, premature neonates <2 kg, who received an initial dose within 12 hours of birth, should receive 4 total doses at 0, 1, 2 to 3, and 6 to 7 months of chronological age.

Neonates with recent exposure to the virus or certain travelers to high-risk areas: Engerix-B: (Pediatric/Adolescent formulation): IM: 0.5 mL per dose for 4 doses given at 0, 1, 2, and 12 months

Dosing: Usual Although hepatitis B vaccine products differ by concentration (mcg/mL), when dosed in terms of volume (mL), the equivalent dose is the same between products (ie, 0.5 mL of Recombivax-HB is equivalent to 0.5 mL of Engerix-B). Combination vaccines may be used to complete the immunization series after the infant is 6 weeks of age. Please see combination vaccine monographs for dose and schedule details. Vaccines from different manufacturers are interchangeable during an immunization series with the exception of an adolescent (11 to 15 years) 2-dose Recombivax-HB regimen (CDC/ACIP [Mast, 2005]).

Pediatric:

Primary immunization:

CDC (ACIP) recommendations (CDC/ACIP [Mast 2005]; CDC/ACIP [Strikas 2015]):

Infants: Recombivax-HB, Engerix-B (Pediatric/Adolescent formulation): IM: 0.5 mL per dose for a total of 3 doses given as follows: Ideally first dose is given at birth, the second dose is given at 1 to 2 months of age, and a final third dose at 6 months up to 18 months; minimum age for the final (third) dose is 24 weeks

*Infants born of HBsAg-**positive** mothers:* First dose should be given within the first 12 hours of life, even if premature and regardless of birth weight (hepatitis immune globulin should also be administered at the same time/different site); the second dose is administered at 1 to 2 months of age and the third dose at 6 months of age; anti-HBs and HBsAg levels should be checked at 9 to 18 months of age (ie, next well child visit after series completion). If anti-HBs and HBsAg are negative, reimmunize with 3 doses 2 months apart and reassess. **Note:** Due to possible decreased immunogenicity, premature neonates <2 kg should receive 4 total doses at 0, 1, 2 to 3, and 6 to 7 months of chronological age.

*Infants born of HBsAg-**negative** mothers:* First dose should be given at hospital discharge; another dose is given 1 to 2 months later and a final dose at 6 to 18 months of age; 4 total doses of vaccine may be given if a "birth dose" is administered and a combination vaccine is used to complete the series. If "birth dose" not received, then full-term neonates should begin vaccine series as soon as feasible. **Note:** Premature neonates <2 kg may have the initial dose deferred up to 30 days of chronological age or at hospital discharge.

*Infants born of mothers whose HBsAg status is **unknown** at birth:* First dose given within 12 hours of birth even if premature and regardless of birth weight, second dose following 1 to 2 months later; the third dose at 6 months of age; if the mother's blood HBsAg test is positive, the infant should receive hepatitis immune globulin as soon as possible (no later than 12 hours of age if <2 kg or age 1 week if ≥2 kg). **Note:** Due to possible decreased immunogenicity, premature neonates <2 kg who received an initial dose within 12 hours of birth, should receive 4 total doses at 0, 1, 2 to 3, and 6 to 7 months of chronological age.

Note: For infants born to HBsAg-positive mothers, anti-HBs and HBsAg levels should be checked at 9 to 18 months of age (ie, next well child visit after series completion). If HBsAg negative, and anti-HBs levels <10 mIU/mL, reimmunize with 3 doses 2 months apart and reassess. Due to possible decreased immunogenicity, former premature neonates <2 kg should receive 4 total doses at 0, 1, 2 to 3, and 6 to 7 months of chronological age.

Catch-up immunization:

CDC (ACIP) recommendations (CDC/ACIP [Strikas 2015]): **Note:** Do not restart the series. If doses have been given, begin the below schedule at the applicable dose number.

Infants ≥4 months, Children, and Adolescents: Recombivax-HB, Engerix-B (Pediatric/Adolescent formulation): IM: 0.5 mL per dose for 3 total doses
First dose given on the elected date
Second dose given at least 4 weeks after the first dose
Third dose given at least 8 weeks after the second dose and at least 16 weeks after the first dose; minimum age for the final (third) dose is 24 weeks

Alternate regimen: Adolescents 11 to 15 years: Recombivax HB (Adult formulation): IM: 1 mL per dose for 2 doses; first dose given on the elected date, second dose given 4 to 6 months later if patient still ≤15 years.
Note: Refer to CDC guideline (Mast 2005) for other options. Manufacturer's labeling may include alternate immunization schedules.

Bombings or similar mass casualty events: IM: In persons without a reliable history of vaccination against hepatitis B and who have no known contraindications to the vaccine, vaccination should begin within 24 hours (but no later than 7 days) following the event (CDC [Chapman, 2008])

Adult:

Primary immunization:

Note: Adult formulations of hepatitis B vaccine products differ by concentration (mcg/mL), but when dosed in terms of volume (mL), the dose of Engerix-B and Recombivax HB are the same (both 1 mL).

Immunocompetent adults: IM: 1 mL/dose (adult formulation) for 3 total doses administered at 0, 1, and 6 months. **Note:** Refer to CDC guideline (Mast 2006) for other options. Manufacturer's labeling may include alternate immunization schedules.

Adults with immunocompromising conditions (CDC/ACIP [Kim 2015]): IM:
Engerix-B 20 mcg/mL: Administer 2 mL per dose at 0, 1, 2, and 6 months
Recombivax HB 40 mcg/mL: Administer 1 mL per dose at 0, 1, and 6 months

Bombings or similar mass casualty events: IM: In persons without a reliable history of vaccination against HepB and who have no known contraindications to the vaccine, vaccination should begin within 24 hours (but no later than 7 days) following the event (CDC [Chapman 2008]).

Postexposure management of health care personnel (HCP) (CDC [Schillie 2013]): IM:

Documented vaccine responder: If the HCP has prior documentation of ≥3 doses of a hepatitis B vaccine and a postvaccination anti-HBs ≥10 mIU/mL, then additional hepatitis B vaccine is not needed, regardless of the patient's HBsAg status. HCP is considered seroprotected.

Unvaccinated or incompletely vaccinated: The primary vaccination series should be completed regardless of the source patient's HbsAg status. If the source patient is HBsAG positive or their status is unknown, 1 dose of hepatitis B vaccine and 1 dose of hepatitis B immunoglobulin (HBIG) should be administered as soon as possible.

Vaccinated with 3 doses of hepatitis B vaccine but postvaccination anti-HBs status is unknown: Test HCP for anti-HBs. If anti-HBs ≥10 mIU/mL, additional hepatitis B vaccine is not needed. If anti-HBs <10 mIU/mL, initiate revaccination by administering a single dose of the vaccine and retesting for anti-HBs in 1 to 2 months; if needed, 2 additional doses may be given and then retest anti-HBs level. Alternately, administer 3 consecutive doses of the vaccine and then retest anti-HBs level. Minimum dosing intervals are 4 weeks between doses 1 and 2 and 8 weeks between doses 2 and 3; maximum total of 6 doses of hepatitis B vaccine (including the original series). If the source patient is HBsAG positive or their status is unknown, 1 dose of HBIG should also be administered.

Vaccinated with 6 doses of hepatitis B vaccine but documented as a nonresponder to the vaccine: No postexposure vaccination is recommended. If the source patient is HBsAG positive or unknown, administer two doses of HBIG separated by 1 month.

Dosing adjustment in renal impairment: Hemodialysis patients often respond poorly to hepatitis B vaccination; higher vaccine doses or increased number of doses may be required. The anti-HBs (antibody to hepatitis B surface antigen) response of such persons should be tested after they are vaccinated, and those who have not responded should be revaccinated with 1 to 3 additional doses. Patients with chronic renal disease should be vaccinated as early as possible, ideally before they require hemodialysis.

Chronic renal impairment: Administer dose at 0, 1 to 2, and 4 to 6 months; repeat dose depending upon annual assessment of hepatitis B surface antigen (anti-HB) level; if anti-HB <10 milli-international units/mL administer an additional dose (CDC/ACIP [Mast 2005])

Infants, Children, Adolescents, and Adults <20 years: Dialysis and predialysis patients (CrCl <60 ml/minute/1.73 m^2): Limited data available: IM: Recombivax-HB (dialysis formulation): 20 **mcg**/dose; no specific ACIP recommendations; dosing based on a multicenter trial of 78 pediatric patients (age: 1 to 18 years) using Recombivax-HB (Dialysis formulation) and showed protective levels of antibody occurring in 75% to 97% of pediatric hemodialysis patients using higher dose (CDC/ACIP [Mast 2005]; Watkins 2002)

Adults ≥20 years:
Predialysis patients: Recombivax HB 40 mcg/mL: IM: Administer 1 mL per dose at 0, 1, and 6 months
Dialysis patients: IM:
Engerix-B 20 mcg/mL: Administer 2 mL per dose at 0, 1, 2, and 6 months
Recombivax HB 40 mcg/mL: Administer 1 mL per dose at 0, 1, and 6 months

Dosing adjustment in hepatic impairment: There are no dosage adjustments provided in the manufacturer's labeling.

Administration Shake well; administer IM into midlateral aspect of the thigh in infants and small children; administer in the deltoid area to older children and adults; not for IV administration. Adolescents and adults should be vaccinated while seated or lying down (NCIRD/ACIP 2011). US law requires that the date of administration; the vaccine manufacturer; lot number of vaccine; and the administering person's name, title, and address be entered into the patient's permanent medical record.

For patients at risk of hemorrhage following intramuscular injection, hepatitis B vaccine may be administered subcutaneously although lower titers and/or increased incidence of local reactions may result. The ACIP recommends that the vaccine should be administered intramuscularly if, in the opinion of the physician familiar with the patient's bleeding risk, the vaccine can be administered by this route with reasonable safety. If the patient receives antihemophilia or other similar therapy, intramuscular vaccination can be scheduled shortly after such therapy is administered. A fine needle (23 gauge or smaller) can be used for the vaccination and firm pressure applied to the site (without rubbing) for at least 2 minutes. The patient should be instructed concerning the risk of hematoma from the injection. Patients on anticoagulant therapy should be considered to have the same bleeding risks and treated as those with clotting factor disorders (NCIRD/ACIP 2011).

Monitoring Parameters HBsAg and antibodies to HBsAg (anti-HBs) should be tested in infants born to mothers positive for HBsAg when they are 9 to 18 months of age; annual anti-HB in dialysis patients. Vaccination at the time of HBsAg testing: For persons in whom vaccination is recommended, the first dose of hepatitis B vaccine can be given after blood is drawn to test for HBsAg. Observe for syncope for 15 minutes following administration (NCIRD/ACIP 2011). If seizure-like activity associated with syncope occurs, maintain patient in supine or Trendelenburg position to reestablish adequate cerebral perfusion.

Additional Information With use of hepatitis B vaccine, hepatitis D should also be prevented since delta virus replicates only in presence of HBV infection.

Dosage Forms Excipient information presented when available (limited, particularly for generics); consult specific product labeling.

Injection, suspension [adult, preservative free]:

Engerix-B: Hepatitis B surface antigen 20 mcg/mL (1 mL) [contains aluminum, yeast protein, may contain natural rubber/natural latex in prefilled syringe]

Engerix-B: Hepatitis B surface antigen 20 mcg/mL (1 mL) [contains aluminum, yeast protein; vial]

Recombivax HB: Hepatitis B surface antigen 10 mcg/mL (1 mL) [contains aluminum, natural rubber/natural latex in packaging, yeast protein]

Injection, suspension [dialysis formulation, preservative free]:

Recombivax HB: Hepatitis B surface antigen 40 mcg/mL (1 mL) [contains aluminum, natural rubber/natural latex in packaging, yeast protein]

Injection, suspension [pediatric/adolescent, preservative free]:

Engerix-B: Hepatitis B surface antigen 10 mcg/0.5 mL (0.5 mL) [contains aluminum, yeast protein, may contain natural rubber/natural latex in prefilled syringe]

Recombivax HB: Hepatitis B surface antigen 5 mcg/0.5 mL (0.5 mL) [contains aluminum, natural rubber/natural latex in packaging, yeast protein]

◆ **Hepatitis B Vaccine (Recombinant)** *see Haemophilus* b Conjugate and Hepatitis B Vaccine *on page 997*

◆ **HepB** *see* Hepatitis B Vaccine (Recombinant) *on page 1015*

◆ **Hep Flush-10** *see* Heparin *on page 1006*

◆ **Hepsera** *see* Adefovir *on page 72*

◆ **Heptavalent Botulinum Antitoxin** *see* Botulism Antitoxin, Heptavalent *on page 297*

◆ **Heptavalent Botulism Antitoxin** *see* Botulism Antitoxin, Heptavalent *on page 297*

◆ **Heptovir (Can)** *see* LamiVUDine *on page 1205*

◆ **HES** *see* Hetastarch *on page 1019*

◆ **HES** *see* Tetrastarch *on page 2037*

◆ **HES 130/0.4** *see* Tetrastarch *on page 2037*

◆ **HES 450/0.7** *see* Hetastarch *on page 1019*

◆ **Hespan** *see* Hetastarch *on page 1019*

Hetastarch (HET a starch)

Medication Safety Issues

Sound-alike/look-alike issues:

Hespan may be confused with heparin

Brand Names: US Hespan; Hextend

Brand Names: Canada Hextend

Therapeutic Category Plasma Volume Expander

Generic Availability (US) Yes

Use Treatment of hypovolemia (Hespan® and Hextend®: FDA approved in adults); adjunctive use during leukapheresis to improve granulocyte harvesting and increase the yield of granulocytes by centrifucation (Hespan®: FDA approved in adults); **Note:** This is not a substitute for blood or plasma; does not have oxygen-carrying capacity.

Pregnancy Risk Factor C

Pregnancy Considerations Adverse events have been observed in some animal reproduction studies.

Breast-Feeding Considerations It is not known if hetastarch is excreted into breast milk. The manufacturer recommends that caution be exercised when administering hetastarch to nursing women.

Contraindications Hypersensitivity to hydroxyethyl starch or any component of the formulation; renal failure with oliguria or anuria (not related to hypovolemia); any fluid overload condition (eg, pulmonary edema, congestive heart failure); pre-existing coagulation or bleeding disorders; critically ill adult patients, including patients with sepsis, due to increased risk of mortality and renal replacement therapy; severe liver disease

Hextend is also contraindicated in the treatment of lactic acidosis and in leukapheresis

Warnings/Precautions [U.S. Boxed Warning]: HES solutions have been associated with mortality and renal injury requiring renal replacement therapy in critically-ill patients, including patients with sepsis; avoid use in critically-ill adult patients, including those with sepsis. Use should also be avoided in patients admitted to the ICU (Brunkhorst, 2008; Perel, 2011; Perner, 2012; Zarychanski, 2009). The Society of Critical Care Medicine (SCCM) also recommends against the use of HES solutions for fluid resuscitation of severe sepsis and septic shock; crystalloids (eg, sodium chloride) are recommended instead (Dellinger, 2013). If used in patients who are not critically ill, avoid use in patients with pre-existing renal dysfunction and discontinue use at the first sign of renal injury. Since the need for renal replacement therapy has been reported up to 90 days after HES administration, continue to monitor renal function in all patients for at least 90 days.

Not recommended for use as a cardiac bypass pump prime, while the patient is on cardiopulmonary bypass, or in the period immediately afterward. HES solutions have been associated with excess bleeding in these patients. Monitor the coagulation status in patients undergoing open heart surgery in association with cardiopulmonary bypass. Discontinue use of HES at the first sign of coagulopathy. May cause coagulation abnormalities in conjunction with a reversible, acquired von Willebrands-like syndrome and/or factor VIII deficiency when used over a period of days. Consider replacement therapy if a severe factor VIII deficiency is detected. Coagulopathies may take several days to resolve. When used to prevent cerebral vasospasm in patients with subarachnoid hemorrhage (off-label use), significant clinical bleeding, intracranial bleeding and death have been reported.

Large volumes of pentastarch may cause reduction in hemoglobin concentration, coagulation factors, and other plasma proteins due to hemodilution; when used for leukapheresis, frequent clinical evaluation and complete blood counts (CBC) are recommended. If leukapheresis frequency is greater than whole blood donation guidelines, consider monitoring total leukocyte and platelet counts, leukocyte differential, PT, and PTT as well. Coagulation may be impaired (eg, prolonged PT, PTT, and clotting times) and a transient prolongation of bleeding time may be observed. Use caution in severe bleeding disorders (eg, von Willebrand's disease); may increase the risk of more bleeding. Use with caution in patients with active hemorrhage. Not a substitute for red blood cells or coagulation factors.

Anaphylactoid reactions have occurred; discontinue use immediately with signs of hypersensitivity and administer appropriate therapy. Use caution in patients allergic to corn (may have cross allergy to hetastarch). Use with caution in patients at risk from overexpansion of blood volume, including the very young or elderly patients; use is contraindicated in heart failure or any pre-existing condition where volume overload is a potential concern. Use with caution in patients with thrombocytopenia; large volumes may interfere with platelet function and transiently prolong bleeding time; observe for bleeding.

Use with caution in patients with severe liver disease. Monitor liver function at baseline and periodically during treatment. Use is contraindicated in patients with severe liver disease; may result in further reduction of coagulation factors, increasing the risk of bleeding. Note electrolyte content of Hextend including calcium, lactate, and potassium; use caution in situations where electrolyte and/or acid-base disturbances may be exacerbated (renal impairment, respiratory alkalosis, metabolic alkalosis) and do not use in leukapheresis. Avoid use in patients with preexisting renal impairment; monitor fluid status, urine output, and infusion rate; discontinue use at the first sign of renal injury. Larger hetastarch molecules may leak into urine in patients with glomerular damage; may elevate urine specific gravity. Use is contraindicated with oliguria or anuria not related to hypovolemia. May cause temporarily elevated serum amylase levels and interfere with pancreatitis diagnosis. Dilutional effects (particularly with high doses) can cause decreased plasma proteins (including coagulation factors) and a decreased hematocrit.

Warnings: Additional Pediatric Considerations Hetastarch use has been associated with acute kidney injury in pediatric patients (Reinhart, 2012).

Adverse Reactions

Cardiovascular: Bradycardia, cardiac failure, circulatory overload, increased plasma volume, peripheral edema, tachycardia

Central nervous system: Chills, headache, intracranial hemorrhage

Dermatologic: Pruritus (dose dependent; may be delayed), skin rash

Endocrine & metabolic: Increased amylase (transient), metabolic acidosis

Gastrointestinal: Parotid gland enlargement, vomiting

Hematologic & oncologic: Anemia, blood coagulation disorder (Factor VIII deficiency, acquired von Willebrand's like syndrome, dilutional coagulopathy), disseminated intravascular coagulopathy (rare), hemolysis (rare), hemorrhage, prolonged bleeding time, prolonged partial thromboplastin time, prolonged prothrombin time, thrombocytopenia, wound hemorrhage

Hepatic: Increased serum bilirubin (indirect)

Hypersensitivity: Anaphylactoid reaction, hypersensitivity

Neuromuscular & skeletal: Myalgia

Respiratory: Bronchospasm, flu-like symptoms (mild), noncardiogenic pulmonary edema

Miscellaneous: Fever

Rare but important or life-threatening: Angioedema, cough, erythema multiforme, facial edema, hypotension, laryngeal edema, periorbital edema, renal insufficiency, severe hypotension, stridor, submaxillary gland enlargement, tachypnea, urticaria, ventricular fibrillation

Drug Interactions

Metabolism/Transport Effects None known.

Avoid Concomitant Use There are no known interactions where it is recommended to avoid concomitant use.

Increased Effect/Toxicity There are no known significant interactions involving an increase in effect.

Decreased Effect There are no known significant interactions involving a decrease in effect.

Storage/Stability Store at 25°C (77°F); avoid excessive heat; do not freeze. Brief exposure up to 40°C (104°F) does not adversely affect the product. Do not use if crystalline precipitate forms or is turbid deep brown. In leukapheresis, admixtures of 500-560 mL of Hespan with citrate concentrations up to 2.5% are compatible for 24 hours.

Mechanism of Action Produces plasma volume expansion by virtue of its highly colloidal starch structure

Pharmacodynamics

Onset of volume expansion: IV: Within 30 minutes

Duration: 24-36 hours

Pharmacokinetics (Adult data unless noted)

Metabolism: Molecules >50,000 daltons require enzymatic degradation by the reticuloendothelial system or amylases in the blood prior to urinary and fecal excretion

Elimination: Smaller molecular weight molecules are readily excreted in urine; ~33% of dose excreted in first 24 hours in patients with normal renal function

Dosing: Usual Note: With severe dehydration, administer crystalloid first. Dose and rate of infusion dependent on amount of blood lost, on maintenance or restoration of hemodynamics, and on amount of hemodilution. Titrate to individual colloid needs, hemodynamics, and hydration status. Do not use in critically ill patients, those undergoing open heart surgery with cardiopulmonary bypass, or those with preexisting renal dysfunction.

Children and Adolescents: **Volume expansion:** IV infusion: Very limited data available: Children ≥1 year and Adolescents: 10 mL/kg/dose; dosing based on a small randomized, double-blinded study of 38 patients (age range: 1-15.5 years) compared hetastarch (n=20) and albumin (n=18) as a postoperative volume expander in the first 24 hours after congenital heart surgery; no differences in safety compared to albumin were found at hetastarch daily doses ≤20 mL/kg/day; patients receiving doses of 20-30 mL/kg/day were noted to have an increased PT; however, there was no difference in clinical bleeding; doses >30 mL/kg have not been studied (Brutacao, 1996).

Adults:

Plasma volume expansion: IV infusion: 500-1000 mL (up to 1500 mL/day) or 20 mL/kg/day (up to 1500 mL/day)

Leukapheresis (Hespan®): IV infusion: 250-700 mL; **Note:** Citrate anticoagulant is added before use.

Dosing adjustment in renal impairment: Adults: Avoid use in patients with pre-existing renal dysfunction. Use is contraindicated in renal failure with oliguria or anuria (not related to hypovolemia). Discontinue use at the first sign of renal injury.

Dosing adjustment in hepatic impairment: Adults: No dosage adjustment provided in manufacturer's labeling; use with caution.

Administration Parenteral: IV: Administer IV only; may be administered via infusion pump or pressure infusion; if administered by pressure infusion, air should be withdrawn or expelled from bag prior to infusion to prevent air embolus. Administration rates vary depending upon the extent of blood loss, age, and clinical condition of patient but, in general, should not exceed 1.2 **g/kg/hour** (20 mL/kg/**hour**) in adults. Change IV tubing or flush copiously with normal saline before administering blood through the same line. Do not administer Hextend® with blood through the same administration set. Change IV tubing at least every 24 hours. Anaphylactoid reactions can occur; have epinephrine and resuscitative equipment available.

Monitoring Parameters

Volume expansion: Blood pressure, capillary refill time, CVP, RAP, MAP, urine output, heart rate, if pulmonary artery catheter in place, monitor cardiac index, PWCP, SVR, and PVR; hemoglobin, hematocrit, serum electrolytes, renal function (continue to monitor for at least 90 days after administration), acid-base balance, coagulation parameters, platelets

Leukapheresis, CBC, total leukocyte and platelet counts, leukocyte differential count, hemoglobin, hematocrit, prothrombin time, and partial thromboplastin time

Test Interactions

Serum amylase levels may be temporarily elevated following administration; could interfere with the diagnosis of pancreatitis.

Large hetastarch volumes may result in decreased coagulation factors, plasma proteins, and /or hematocrit due to dilutional effect.

Additional Information Hetastarch is a synthetic polymer derived from a waxy starch composed of amylopectin, average molecular weight of Hespan® is 600,000 kDa (range: 450,000-800,000 kDa), average molecular weight of Hextend® is 670,000 kDa (range: 450,000-800,000 kDa); each liter of Hespan® provides 154 mEq sodium chloride; each liter of Hextend® contains the following electrolytes: Sodium 143 mEq, chloride 124 mEq, lactate 28 mEq, calcium 5 mEq, magnesium 0.9 mEq, potassium 3 mEq, and dextrose 0.99 g

Dosage Forms Excipient information presented when available (limited, particularly for generics); consult specific product labeling.

Solution, Intravenous:

Hespan: 6% (500 mL)

Hextend: 6% (500 mL)

Generic: 6% (500 mL)

◆ **Hexachlorocyclohexane** *see* Lindane *on page 1267*

Hexachlorophene (heks a KLOR oh feen)

Medication Safety Issues

Sound-alike/look-alike issues:

pHisoHex may be confused with Fostex, pHisoDerm

Related Information

Safe Handling of Hazardous Drugs *on page 2455*

Brand Names: US Phisohex [DSC]

Brand Names: Canada pHisoHex

Therapeutic Category Antibacterial, Topical; Soap

Generic Availability (US) No

Use Surgical scrub and as a bacteriostatic skin cleanser; to control an outbreak of gram-positive staphylococcal infection when other infection control procedures have been unsuccessful

Pregnancy Risk Factor C

Pregnancy Considerations Adverse events have been observed in animal reproduction studies. Hexachlorophene is absorbed systemically when applied topically. Following use as an antiseptic for vaginal exams during labor, hexachlorophene is detectable in the maternal serum and cord blood (Strickland, 1983). Vaginal use as a pack or tampon and application to mucous membranes is contraindicated.

Breast-Feeding Considerations It is not known if hexachlorophene is excreted in breast milk. Due to the potential for serious adverse reactions in the nursing infant, a decision should be made whether to discontinue nursing or to discontinue the drug, taking into account the importance of treatment to the mother.

Contraindications Hypersensitivity to halogenated phenol derivatives or hexachlorophene; use on burned or denuded skin; use as an occlusive dressing, wetpack, or lotion; application to mucous membranes; use as a vaginal pack or tampon; routine use for prophylactic total body bathing

Warnings/Precautions Hazardous agent - use appropriate precautions for handling and disposal (EPA, U-listed). For external use only; avoid exposure to eyes. Discontinue use if signs of cerebral irritability occur; exposure of preterm infants or patients with extensive burns has been associated with apnea, convulsions, agitation and coma; do not use for bathing infants, premature infants are particularly susceptible to hexachlorophene topical absorption.

Warnings: Additional Pediatric Considerations Premature and low birth weight neonates are particularly susceptible to hexachlorophene topical absorption; irritability, generalized clonic muscular contractions, decerebrate rigidity, and brain lesions in the white matter have occurred in infants following topical use of 6% hexachlorophene; exposure of preterm infants or patients with extensive burns has been associated with apnea, convulsions, agitation, and coma.

Adverse Reactions

Central nervous system: CNS injury, irritability, seizure

Dermatologic: Dermatitis, dry skin, photosensitivity, redness

Drug Interactions

Metabolism/Transport Effects None known.

Avoid Concomitant Use

Avoid concomitant use of Hexachlorophene with any of the following: BCG; BCG (Intravesical)

Increased Effect/Toxicity There are no known significant interactions involving an increase in effect.

Decreased Effect

Hexachlorophene may decrease the levels/effects of: BCG; BCG (Intravesical); BCG Vaccine (Immunization); Sodium Picosulfate

Storage/Stability Store in nonmetallic container. Prolonged direct exposure to strong light may cause brownish surface discoloration, but this does not affect its action.

Mechanism of Action Bacteriostatic polychlorinated biphenyl which inhibits membrane-bound enzymes and disrupts the cell membrane

Pharmacokinetics (Adult data unless noted)

Absorption: Percutaneously through inflamed, excoriated and intact skin

Distribution: Crosses the placenta

Half-life, infants: 6.1-44.2 hours

Dosing: Usual Children and Adults: Topical: Apply 5 mL cleanser and water to area to be cleansed; lather and rinse thoroughly under running water; for use as a surgical scrub, a second application of 5 mL cleanser should be made and the hands and forearms scrubbed for an additional 3 minutes, rinsed thoroughly with running water and dried

Administration Topical: For external use only; rinse thoroughly after each use

Product Availability All products have been discontinued for more than 1 year.

Dosage Forms Excipient information presented when available (limited, particularly for generics); consult specific product labeling. [DSC] = Discontinued product

Liquid, External:

Phisohex: 3% (148 mL [DSC], 473 mL [DSC])

◆ **Hexamethylenetetramine** *see* Methenamine *on page 1385*

◆ **Hextend** *see* Hetastarch *on page 1019*

◆ **hGH** *see* Somatropin *on page 1957*

◆ **Hib** *see Haemophilus* b Conjugate Vaccine *on page 998*

◆ **Hib Conjugate Vaccine** *see Haemophilus* b Conjugate and Hepatitis B Vaccine *on page 997*

◆ **Hiberix** *see Haemophilus* b Conjugate Vaccine *on page 998*

◆ **Hib-HepB** *see Haemophilus* b Conjugate and Hepatitis B Vaccine *on page 997*

◆ **Hibiclens [OTC]** *see* Chlorhexidine Gluconate *on page 434*

◆ **Hibistat [OTC]** *see* Chlorhexidine Gluconate *on page 434*

- ◆ **Hib-MenCY-TT** *see* Meningococcal Polysaccharide (Groups C and Y) and *Haemophilus* b Tetanus Toxoid Conjugate Vaccine *on page 1356*
- ◆ **High-Molecular-Weight Iron Dextran (DexFerrum)** *see* Iron Dextran Complex *on page 1164*
- ◆ **Hiprex** *see* Methenamine *on page 1385*
- ◆ **Hiprex® (Can)** *see* Methenamine *on page 1385*
- ◆ **Histafed** *see* Triprolidine and Pseudoephedrine *on page 2129*
- ◆ **Histantil (Can)** *see* Promethazine *on page 1777*
- ◆ **Hist-PSE** *see* Triprolidine and Pseudoephedrine *on page 2129*

Histrelin (his TREL in)

Related Information

Safe Handling of Hazardous Drugs *on page 2455*

Brand Names: US Supprelin LA; Vantas

Brand Names: Canada Vantas

Therapeutic Category Gonadotropin Releasing Hormone Agonist

Generic Availability (US) No

Use

Supprelin® LA: Treatment of children with either neurogenic or idiopathic central precocious puberty (CPP) (FDA approved in ages ≥2 years)

Vantas®: Palliative treatment of advanced prostate cancer (FDA approved in adults)

Pregnancy Risk Factor X

Pregnancy Considerations Adverse events were observed in animal reproduction studies. May cause fetal harm or spontaneous abortion if administered during pregnancy. Histrelin is contraindicated for use during pregnancy or in women who may become pregnant.

Breast-Feeding Considerations It is not known if histrelin is excreted in breast milk. The products are not indicated for use in postpubertal women.

Contraindications Hypersensitivity to histrelin acetate, gonadotropin releasing hormone (GnRH), GnRH-agonist analogs, or any component of the formulation; females who are or may become pregnant

Warnings/Precautions Hazardous agent - use appropriate precautions for handling and disposal (meets NIOSH 2014 criteria). Proper surgical insertion technique is essential to avoid complications. Patients should keep arm dry for 24 hours and avoid heavy lifting/strenuous exertion of insertion arm for 7 days after implantation. Potentially significant drug-drug interactions may exist, requiring dose or frequency adjustment, additional monitoring, and/or selection of alternative therapy.

CPP: Transient increases in estradiol serum levels (female) or testosterone levels (female and male) may occur during the first week of use. Worsening symptoms may occur, however, manifestations of puberty should decrease within 4 weeks. If the implant breaks during removal, the remaining pieces should be removed; confirm the removal of the entire implant (refer to manufacturer's instructions for removal procedure).

Prostate cancer: Transient increases in testosterone serum levels occur during the first week of use (initial tumor flare), which may result in a worsening of disease signs and symptoms such as bone pain, hematuria, neuropathy, ureteral or bladder outlet obstruction, and spinal cord compression. Spinal cord compression may contribute to paralysis; close attention should be given during the first few weeks of therapy to both patients having metastatic vertebral lesions and/or urinary tract obstructions, and to any patients reporting weakness, paresthesias or poor urine output. Androgen-deprivation therapy (ADT) may increase the risk for cardiovascular disease (Levine, 2010); an increased risk of MI, sudden cardiac death, and stroke has been reported with GnRH agonist use in men; monitor for symptoms associated with cardiovascular disease. ADT may prolong the QT/QTc interval; consider the benefits of ADT versus the risk for QT prolongation in patients with a history of QTc prolongation, congenital long QT syndrome, heart failure, frequent electrolyte abnormalities, and in patients with medications known to prolong the QT interval, or with preexisting cardiac disease. Consider periodic monitoring of electrocardiograms and electrolytes in at-risk patients. Hyperglycemia has been reported with androgen deprivation therapy (in prostate cancer) and may manifest as diabetes or worsening of preexisting diabetes; monitor blood glucose and/or HbA_{1c}. Rare cases of pituitary apoplexy (frequently secondary to pituitary adenoma) have been observed with GnRH agonist administration (onset from 1 hour to usually <2 weeks); may present as sudden headache, vomiting, visual or mental status changes, and infrequently cardiovascular collapse; immediate medical attention required. Safety and efficacy have not been established in patients with hepatic dysfunction. In studies, the implant was not recovered in a small number of patients. Serum testosterone rose above castrate level and the implant was not palpable or visualized (via ultrasound); it was believed to have been extruded. Some patients had continued testosterone levels below castration level even though the implant was not palpable.

Adverse Reactions

CPP:

Endocrine & metabolic: Metrorrhagia

Local: Insertion site reaction (includes bruising, discomfort, itching, pain, protrusion of implant area, soreness, swelling, tingling); keloid scar, pain at the application site, post procedural pain, scar, suture-related complication

Rare but important or life-threatening: Amblyopia, breast tenderness, cold feeling, disease progression, dysmenorrhea, epistaxis, erythema, flu-like syndrome, gynecomastia, headache, infection at the implant site, menorrhagia, migraine, mood swings, pituitary adenoma, pituitary apoplexy, pruritus, seizures, weight gain

Prostate cancer:

Central nervous system: Fatigue, headache, insomnia

Endocrine & metabolic: Gynecomastia, hot flashes, libido decreased, sexual dysfunction

Gastrointestinal: Constipation, weight gain

Genitourinary: Testicular atrophy

Local: Implant site reaction (includes bruising, erythema, pain, soreness, swelling, tenderness)

Renal: Renal impairment

Rare but important or life-threatening: Abdominal discomfort, alopecia, anemia, appetite increased, arthralgia, AST increased, back pain, bone density decreased, bone pain, breast pain, breast tenderness, cold feeling, contusion, craving food, creatinine increased, depression, diaphoresis, dizziness, dyspnea (exertional), dysuria, fluid retention, flushing, genital pruritus, hematoma, hematuria, hepatic injury (severe), hypercalcemia, hypercholesterolemia, hyperglycemia, irritability, LDH increased, lethargy, limb pain, liver disorder, malaise, muscle twitching, myalgia, nausea, neck pain, night sweats, pain, palpitation, peripheral edema, prostatic acid phosphatase increased, pruritus, pituitary apoplexy, renal calculi, renal failure, stent occlusion, testosterone increased, tremor, urinary frequency, urinary retention, ventricular asystoles, weakness, weight loss

Drug Interactions

Metabolism/Transport Effects None known.

Avoid Concomitant Use

Avoid concomitant use of Histrelin with any of the following: Corifollitropin Alfa; Indium 111 Capromab Pendetide

Increased Effect/Toxicity

Histrelin may increase the levels/effects of: Corifollitropin Alfa; Highest Risk QTc-Prolonging Agents; Moderate Risk QTc-Prolonging Agents

The levels/effects of Histrelin may be increased by: Mifepristone

Decreased Effect

Histrelin may decrease the levels/effects of: Antidiabetic Agents; Choline C 11; Indium 111 Capromab Pendetide

Storage/Stability Upon delivery, separate contents of implant carton. Store implant under refrigeration at 2°C to 8°C (36°F to 46°F); excursions permitted to 25°C (77°F) for 7 days (if unused within 7 days, may return to proper refrigeration until product expiration date). Keep implant wrapped in the amber pouch for protection from light; do not freeze. The implantation insertion kit does not require refrigeration.

Mechanism of Action Potent inhibitor of gonadotropin secretion; continuous administration results in, after an initiation phase, the suppression of luteinizing hormone (LH), follicle-stimulating hormone (FSH), and a subsequent decrease in testosterone and dihydrotestosterone (males) and estrone and estradiol (premenopausal females). Testosterone levels are reduced to castrate levels in males (treated for prostate cancer) within 2 to 4 weeks. Additionally, in patients with CPP, linear growth velocity is slowed (improves chance of attaining predicted adult height).

Pharmacodynamics

Onset of action:

CPP: Within 1 month

Prostate cancer: Within 2-4 weeks

Duration: 1 year (plus a few additional weeks of histrelin release)

Pharmacokinetics (Adult data unless noted)

Distribution: V_d: ~58 L

Protein binding: 70% ± 9%

Metabolism: Hepatic via C-terminal dealkylation and hydrolysis

Bioavailability: 92%

Half-life elimination: Terminal: ~4 hours

Time to peak serum concentration: 12 hours

Dosing: Usual

Children ≥2 years: **Central precocious puberty:** SubQ: Supprelin LA: 50 mg implant surgically inserted every 12 months; discontinue at the appropriate time for the onset of puberty

Adults: **Prostate cancer, advanced:** SubQ: Vantas: 50 mg implant surgically inserted every 12 months

Dosage adjustment in renal impairment: Children ≥2 years and Adults:

Vantas: CrCl: ≥15 mL/minute: No dosage adjustment necessary.

Supprelin LA: There are no dosage adjustments provided in manufacturer's labeling.

Dosage adjustment in hepatic impairment: There are no dosage adjustments provided in manufacturer's labeling; has not been adequately studied.

Preparation for Administration Hazardous agent; use appropriate precautions for handling and disposal (meets NIOSH, 2014 criteria).

SubQ: The implant may be slightly curved when removed from refrigerator; may roll implant (in sterile-gloved hands) a few times between fingers and thumb. If resistance is felt when inserting implant into insertion tool cannula, remove and manually manipulate or roll as needed and reinsert into cannula.

Administration Hazardous agent; use appropriate precautions for handling and disposal (meets NIOSH, 2014 criteria).

SubQ: Surgical implantation within a sterile field using provided implantation device is required. Insert into the inner portion of the upper arm; it is preferable to use the patient's nondominant arm for placement; implant should be placed halfway between the shoulder and the elbow at the crease between the tricep and the bicep. Implant removal should occur after ~12 months; a replacement implant may be inserted if therapy is to be continued. For removal, palpate area of incision to locate implant; if not readily palpated, ultrasound, CT, or MRI may be necessary to locate implant; plain films are not recommended because the implant is not radiopaque. Refer to manufacturer's labeling for full insertion and removal details.

Monitoring Parameters

Central precocious puberty:

Manufacturer labeling: LH, FSH, estradiol, or testosterone serum concentration (after 1 month then every 6 months); height, bone age (every 6-12 months); Tanner staging, monitor for clinical evidence of suppression of CPP manifestations

Consensus recommendation: Tanner stage and growth (growth velocity, height) every 3-6 months and bone age periodically. Routine or random stimulated measurements of gonadotropins or sex steroids may be used, particularly if suboptimal response; however, use of FSH levels not typically used (Carel, 2009).

Prostate cancer: Serum testosterone levels, prostate specific antigen (PSA); bone mineral density; weakness, paresthesias, and urinary tract obstruction (especially during first few weeks of therapy); screen for diabetes; monitor for symptoms associated with cardiovascular disease

Test Interactions Results of diagnostic test of pituitary gonadotropic and gonadal functions may be affected during and after therapy

Dosage Forms Excipient information presented when available (limited, particularly for generics); consult specific product labeling.

Kit, Subcutaneous:

Supprelin LA: 50 mg

Vantas: 50 mg

◆ **Histrelin Acetate** *see* Histrelin *on page* 1022

◆ **Hizentra** *see* Immune Globulin *on page* 1089

◆ **HN_2** *see* Mechlorethamine (Systemic) *on page* 1335

◆ **Hold [OTC]** *see* Dextromethorphan *on page* 631

◆ **Homatropaire** *see* Homatropine *on page* 1023

Homatropine (hoe MA troe peen)

Medication Safety Issues

Sound-alike/look-alike issues:

Homatropine may be confused with Humatrope®, somatropin

Brand Names: US Homatropaire; Isopto Homatropine

Therapeutic Category Anticholinergic Agent, Ophthalmic; Ophthalmic Agent, Mydriatic

Generic Availability (US) Yes

Use Producing cycloplegia and mydriasis for refraction; treatment of acute inflammatory conditions of the uveal tract; relief of ciliary spasm; optical aid in some cases of axial lens opacities (All indications: Homatropine®: FDA approved in ages ≥3 months and adults, Isopto®-Homatropine: FDA approved in adults)

Pregnancy Risk Factor C

Pregnancy Considerations Animal reproduction studies have not been conducted.

Breast-Feeding Considerations Small amounts of homatropine are excreted into breast milk. Due to the potential for serious adverse reactions in the nursing infant, a decision should be made whether to discontinue nursing or to discontinue the drug, taking into account the importance of treatment to the mother.

Contraindications

Primary glaucoma or tendency toward glaucoma (eg, narrow anterior chamber angle); hypersensitivity to homatropine or any of the components of the formulation.

Documentation of allergenic cross-reactivity for belladonna alkaloids is limited. However, because of similarities in chemical structure and/or pharmacologic actions, the possibility of cross-sensitivity cannot be ruled out with certainty.

Warnings/Precautions Excessive use may cause CNS disturbances, including confusion, delirium, agitation and coma (rare); may occur with any age group, although children and the elderly are more susceptible. Patients should be cautioned about performing tasks which require mental alertness (eg, operating machinery, driving). Patients with Down syndrome are predisposed to angle-closure glaucoma; use with caution. Use with caution in patients with keratoconus; may result in fixed pupil dilation. Safety and efficacy have not been established in infants and young children, therefore, use with extreme caution due to susceptibility of systemic effects; avoid use during the first 3 months of life. Use with caution in the elderly. May cause sensitivity to light; appropriate eye protection should be used. Some strengths may contain benzalkonium chloride which may be adsorbed by contact lenses; remove contacts prior to administration and wait 15 minutes before reinserting. For topical ophthalmic use only; discontinue use if pain within the eye occurs. To minimize systemic absorption, apply pressure over the lacrimal sac for 1-3 minutes after instillation. To avoid contamination, do not touch dropper tip to any surface. To avoid precipitating angle closure glaucoma, an estimation of the depth of the anterior chamber angle should be made prior to use.

Adverse Reactions

Cardiovascular: Edema

Central nervous system: Burning sensation, stinging sensation

Dermatologic: Eczema

Endocrine & metabolic: Increased thirst

Gastrointestinal: Xerostomia

Local: Local irritation

Ophthalmic: Blurred vision, follicular conjunctivitis, increased intraocular pressure, ocular exudate, photophobia, vascular congestion of the eye

Drug Interactions

Metabolism/Transport Effects None known.

Avoid Concomitant Use

Avoid concomitant use of Homatropine with any of the following: Aclidinium; Eluxadoline; Glucagon; Ipratropium (Oral Inhalation); Potassium Chloride; Tiotropium; Umeclidinium

Increased Effect/Toxicity

Homatropine may increase the levels/effects of: AbobotulinumtoxinA; Analgesics (Opioid); Anticholinergic Agents; Cannabinoid-Containing Products; Eluxadoline; Glucagon; Mirabegron; OnabotulinumtoxinA; Potassium Chloride; RimabotulinumtoxinB; Thiazide Diuretics; Tiotropium; Topiramate

The levels/effects of Homatropine may be increased by: Aclidinium; Ipratropium (Oral Inhalation); Mianserin; Pramlintide; Umeclidinium

Decreased Effect

Homatropine may decrease the levels/effects of: Acetylcholinesterase Inhibitors; Itopride; Metoclopramide; Secretin

The levels/effects of Homatropine may be decreased by: Acetylcholinesterase Inhibitors

Storage/Stability

Isopto homatropine: Store at 8°C to 24°C (46°F to 75°F).
Other preparations: Store at 15°C to 30°C (59°F to 86°F).

Mechanism of Action Blocks response of iris sphincter muscle and the accommodative muscle of the ciliary body to cholinergic stimulation resulting in dilation (mydriasis) and paralysis of accommodation (cycloplegia)

Pharmacodynamics Ophthalmic:

Onset of accommodation and pupil action:

Maximum mydriatic effect: Within 10-30 minutes

Maximum cycloplegic effect: Within 30-90 minutes

Duration:

Mydriasis: Persists for 6 hours to 4 days

Cycloplegia: 10-48 hours

Dosing: Usual

Infants ≥3 months and Children:

Mydriasis and cycloplegia for refraction: Ophthalmic: 2% solution: Instill 1-2 drops immediately prior to procedure; repeat every 10-15 minutes as needed; maximum: 5 doses

Uveitis: Ophthalmic: 2% solution: Instill 1-2 drops 2-3 times daily

Adults: **Note:** Patients with heavily pigmented irides may require increased dose.

Refraction: Ophthalmic:

2% solution: 1-2 drops into eye(s); repeat every 10-15 minutes if necessary; maximum: 5 doses

5% solution: 1-2 drops into eye(s); repeat dose in 15 minutes

Uveitis: Ophthalmic: 2% or 5% solution: 1-2 drops 2-3 times daily (Alexander, 2004), may give up to every 3-4 hours for severe uveitis

Administration Ophthalmic: Wash hands before and after use. Do not touch tip of container to eye. Contact lenses should be removed before instillation; do not reinsert contact lenses within 15 minutes of drops. Finger pressure should be applied to lacrimal sac for 1-3 minutes after instillation to decrease risk of absorption and systemic reactions.

Dosage Forms Excipient information presented when available (limited, particularly for generics); consult specific product labeling.

Solution, Ophthalmic, as hydrobromide:

Homatropaire: 5% (5 mL)

Isopto Homatropine: 2% (5 mL); 5% (5 mL)

Generic: 5% (5 mL)

- ◆ **Homatropine and Hydrocodone** *see* Hydrocodone and Homatropine *on page 1036*
- ◆ **Homatropine Hydrobromide** *see* Homatropine *on page 1023*
- ◆ **Horse Antihuman Thymocyte Gamma Globulin** *see* Antithymocyte Globulin (Equine) *on page 178*
- ◆ **12 Hour Nasal Relief Spray [OTC]** *see* Oxymetazoline (Nasal) *on page 1599*
- ◆ **12 Hour Nasal Spray [OTC]** *see* Oxymetazoline (Nasal) *on page 1599*
- ◆ **HP Acthar** *see* Corticotropin *on page 536*
- ◆ **HPV2** *see* Papillomavirus (Types 16, 18) Vaccine (Human, Recombinant) *on page 1628*
- ◆ **HPV4** *see* Papillomavirus (Types 6, 11, 16, 18) Vaccine (Human, Recombinant) *on page 1625*
- ◆ **HPV9** *see* Papillomavirus (9-Valent) Vaccine (Human, Recombinant) *on page 1623*
- ◆ **HPV 16/18 L1 VLP/AS04 VAC** *see* Papillomavirus (Types 16, 18) Vaccine (Human, Recombinant) *on page 1628*
- ◆ **HPV Vaccine (Bivalent)** *see* Papillomavirus (Types 16, 18) Vaccine (Human, Recombinant) *on page 1628*
- ◆ **HPV Vaccine (Quadrivalent)** *see* Papillomavirus (Types 6, 11, 16, 18) Vaccine (Human, Recombinant) *on page 1625*
- ◆ **HRIG** *see* Rabies Immune Globulin (Human) *on page 1830*

Hyaluronidase (hye al yoor ON i dase)

Related Information

Management of Drug Extravasations *on page 2298*

Brand Names: US Amphadase; Hylenex; Vitrase

Therapeutic Category Antidote, Extravasation

Generic Availability (US) Yes

Use Adjunct therapy to increase the dispersion and absorption of other drugs; adjunct therapy to increase rate of absorption of parenteral fluids given by hypodermoclysis for hydration; adjunct therapy in subcutaneous urography for improving resorption of radiopaque agents (all indications: FDA approved in all ages); has also been used in the management of IV extravasations

Pregnancy Risk Factor C

Pregnancy Considerations Adverse events have not been observed in animal reproduction studies (not conducted with all products). Administration during labor did not cause any increase in blood loss or differences in cervical trauma. It is not known whether it affects the fetus if used during labor. Hyaluronidase has been evaluated for use prior to intracytoplasmic sperm injection (ICSI) to increase male fertility (DeVos, 2008; Evison, 2009).

Breast-Feeding Considerations It is not known if hyaluronidase is excreted in breast milk. The manufacturer recommends that caution be exercised when administering hyaluronidase to nursing women.

Contraindications Hypersensitivity to hyaluronidase or any component of the formulation

Warnings/Precautions For labeled indications, do not administer intravenously (enzyme is rapidly inactivated and desired effects will not be produced); do not inject in or around infected or inflamed areas; may spread localized infection. Do not apply directly to the cornea; not for topical use. Hyaluronidase is ineffective for extravasation management of vasoconstrictors (eg, dopamine, epinephrine, norepinephrine, phenylephrine, vasopressin) or to reduce swelling of bites or stings; do not use in these settings. Use with caution in patients with reported history of bee sting allergy; hyaluronidase is an active component in bee venom. Discontinue if sensitization occurs (a skin test may be performed to determine hypersensitivity). Some products may contain albumin; albumin carries an extremely remote risk for transmission of viral diseases, Creutzfeldt-Jakob disease (CJD) and variant CJD (vCJD). No cases of transmission of viral diseases, CJD, or vCJD have been identified for licensed albumin or albumin contained in other licensed products. Potentially significant interactions may exist, requiring dose or frequency adjustment, additional monitoring, and/or selection of alternative therapy.

Adverse Reactions

Cardiovascular: Edema

Local: Injection site reaction

Rare but important or life-threatening: Anaphylactic-like reactions (retrobulbar block or IV injections), anaphylaxis, hypersensitivity reaction

Drug Interactions

Metabolism/Transport Effects None known.

Avoid Concomitant Use

Avoid concomitant use of Hyaluronidase with any of the following: Phenylephrine (Systemic)

Increased Effect/Toxicity

Hyaluronidase may increase the levels/effects of: Alpha-/Beta-Agonists; DOPamine; Local Anesthetics; Phenylephrine (Systemic)

Decreased Effect
The levels/effects of Hyaluronidase may be decreased by: Antihistamines; Corticosteroids; Estrogen Derivatives; Salicylates

Storage/Stability
Amphadase, Hylenex: Store intact vials in refrigerator at 2°C to 8°C (36°F to 46°F); do not freeze.
Vitrase: Store intact vials in refrigerator at 2°C to 8°C (36°F to 46°F); do not freeze. Protect from light. If adding to other injectable solutions, store admixture at 15°C to 25°C (59°F to 77°F) and use within 6 hours.

Mechanism of Action Enzymatically modifies the permeability of connective tissue through hydrolysis of hyaluronic acid, one of the chief components of tissue cement which offers resistance to diffusion of liquids through tissues; hyaluronidase increases the distribution/dispersion and absorption of locally injected or extravasated substances.

Pharmacodynamics
Onset of action by the SubQ or intradermal routes for the treatment of extravasation: Immediate; when used for extravasation, there is usually a reduction in swelling within 15-30 minutes after administration (Zenk, 1981)
Duration: 24-48 hours

Dosing: Neonatal
Dehydration: Hypodermoclysis: SubQ: 15 units added to each 100 mL of replacement fluid to be administered; dosing extrapolated from experience with larger volumes (ie, in older patients, 150 units facilitates absorption of ≥1000 mL of solution). The volume of subcutaneous fluid administered is dependent upon the age, weight, and clinical condition of the patient, as well as laboratory determinations; maximum daily volume of clysis is 25 mL/kg/**day** and the rate of administration should not exceed 2 mL/minute
Extravasation: Limited data available: SubQ, intradermal: Use 5 separate 0.2 mL injections of a 15-150 units/mL solution into the extravasation site at the leading edge (Hurst, 2004; Kuensting, 2010; MacCara, 1983). **Note:** Some centers determine the concentration of hyaluronidase based upon the volume of extravasation, so for smaller extravasation volumes (<100 mL), a less concentrated solution (15 units/mL) has been used or by the medication risk of tissue toxicity (based on pH, osmolarity, known tissue toxicity); to prepare 15 units/mL solution, dilute 0.1 mL of the 150 unit/mL solution in 0.9 mL NS (MacCara, 1983).

Dosing: Usual
Infants, Children, and Adolescents:
Skin test: Intradermal: 0.02 mL (Amphadase 3 units, Hylenex 3 units, or Vitrase 4 units) of a 150 units/mL (Amphadase, Hylenex) or 200 units/mL (Vitrase) solution. Positive reaction consists of a wheal with pseudopods appearing within 5 minutes and persisting for 20-30 minutes with localized itching (transient erythema is not considered a positive reaction). Skin testing is not necessary prior to use for extravasation management.
Dehydration: Hypodermoclysis:
SubQ prior to infusion: SubQ: 150 units or 200 units, followed by subcutaneous isotonic fluid administration at a rate appropriate for age, weight, and clinical condition of the patient; 150 units facilitates absorption of ≥1000 mL of solution. If the infusion is continued greater than 24 hours, additional doses have been administered at 24 hour intervals up to a total of 3 doses (Allen, 2009)
Added to replacement solution: Dose dependent on volume to be infused; 150 units of hyaluronidase facilitates the absorption of ≥1000 mL of fluid; for patients (ie, neonates, young infants) who require smaller volumes for replacement fluid (≤100 mL), 15 units added for every 100 mL of replacement fluid has been used at some centers; maximum daily dose: 150 units/**day**
Maximum clysis volumes:
Infants and Children <3 years: Volume of a single clysis should not exceed 200 mL
Children ≥3 years and Adolescents: Rate and volume of a single clysis should not exceed those used for infusion of IV fluids
Dispersion/absorption enhancement of injected drugs: Children and Adolescents: SubQ: 50-300 units (usual dose: 150 units) either injected prior to drug administration or added to injection solution (consult compatibility reference prior to mixing)
Extravasation: Limited data available: SubQ, intradermal: Use 5 separate 0.2 mL injections of a 150 units/mL solution into the extravasation site at the leading edge as soon as possible (preferably within 1 hour) after extravasation is recognized (Hurst, 2004; Wiegand, 2010). **Note:** Some centers may determine concentration of hyaluronidase based upon the medication risk of tissue toxicity (risk determined by pH, osmolarity, known tissue toxicity) or by volume of extravasation so for smaller volumes (<100 mL), a less concentrated solution (15 units/mL) has been used (Hurst, 2004; MacCara, 1983; Sokol, 1998; Wiegand, 2010); to prepare 15 units/mL solution, dilute 0.1 mL of the 150 unit/mL solution in 0.9 mL NS (MacCara, 1983)
Urography, subcutaneous: SubQ: 75 units over each scapula followed by injection of contrast medium at the same site; patient should be in the prone position during drug administration
Adults: **Dehydration: Hypodermoclysis:**
Dehydration: Hypodermoclysis: SubQ: 150 or 200 units followed by subcutaneous isotonic fluid administration ≥1000 mL **or** may be added to small volumes (≤200 mL) of subcutaneous replacement fluid. Rate and volume of a single clysis should not exceed those used for infusion of IV fluids.
Dispersion/absorption enhancement of injected drugs: SubQ: 50-300 units (usual dose: 150 units) either injected prior to drug administration or added to injection solution (consult compatibility reference prior to mixing)
Dosage adjustment in renal impairment: All patients: There are no dosage adjustments provided in the manufacturer's labeling; hyaluronidase exerts its effects locally and is rapidly inactivated in the blood; adverse effects would not be expected.
Dosage adjustment in hepatic impairment: All patients: There are no dosage adjustments provided in the manufacturer's labeling; hyaluronidase exerts its effects locally and is rapidly inactivated in the blood; adverse effects would not be expected.

Preparation for Administration Extravasation management: To make a 15 units/mL concentration, mix 0.1 mL (of 150 units/mL) with 0.9 mL NS (MacCara 1983).

Administration
Parenteral: Do not administer IV (enzyme is rapidly inactivated and desired effects will not be produced)
Extravasation management: May administer undiluted (150 units/mL) or dilutions may be used for smaller volumes of extravasation. Infiltrate area of extravasation with 5 small injections at the leading edge; use 27- or 30-gauge needles and change needle between each skin entry to prevent bacterial contamination and minimize pain.

Monitoring Parameters Observe appearance of lesion for induration, swelling, discoloration, blanching, and blister formation every 15 minutes for ~2 hours

Dosage Forms Excipient information presented when available (limited, particularly for generics); consult specific product labeling. [DSC] = Discontinued product
Solution, Injection:
Amphadase: 150 units/mL (1 mL) [contains edetate disodium, thimerosal]

Solution, Injection [preservative free]:
  Hylenex: 150 units/mL (1 mL [DSC]) [contains albumin human, edetate disodium]
  Hylenex: 150 units/mL (1 mL) [contains albumin human, polysorbate 80]
  Vitrase: 200 units/mL (1.2 mL)
  Generic: 150 units/mL (1 mL)

◆ **Hycamptamine** *see* Topotecan *on page 2092*

◆ **Hycamtin** *see* Topotecan *on page 2092*

◆ **hycet®** *see* Hydrocodone and Acetaminophen *on page 1032*

◆ **Hycodan** *see* Hydrocodone and Homatropine *on page 1036*

◆ **Hycort™ (Can)** *see* Hydrocortisone (Topical) *on page 1041*

◆ **Hydeltra T.B.A. (Can)** *see* PrednisoLONE (Systemic) *on page 1755*

◆ **Hyderm (Can)** *see* Hydrocortisone (Topical) *on page 1041*

HydrALAZINE (hye DRAL a zeen)

Medication Safety Issues

Sound-alike/look-alike issues:

HydrALAZINE may be confused with hydrOXYzine

Brand Names: Canada Apo-Hydralazine; Apresoline; Novo-Hylazin; Nu-Hydral

Therapeutic Category Antihypertensive Agent; Vasodilator

Generic Availability (US) Yes

Use Management of moderate to severe hypertension (FDA approved in pediatric patient [age not specified] and adults); has also been used for hypertensive emergency/urgency and hypertension secondary to preeclampsia/eclampsia

Pregnancy Risk Factor C

Pregnancy Considerations Adverse events were observed in some animal reproduction studies. Hydralazine crosses the placenta (Liedholm, 1982). Intravenous hydralazine is recommended for use in the management of acute onset, severe hypertension (systolic BP ≥160 mm Hg or diastolic BP ≥110 mm Hg) with preeclampsia or eclampsia in pregnant and postpartum women. Untreated chronic maternal hypertension is associated with adverse events in the fetus, infant, and mother. If treatment for chronic hypertension in pregnancy is needed, other oral agents are preferred as initial therapy (ACOG, 2013; Magee, 2014).

Breast-Feeding Considerations Hydralazine is excreted into breast milk. In a case report, following a maternal dose of hydralazine 50 mg three times daily, exposure to the infant was calculated to be 0.013 mg per 75 mL breast milk (Liedholm, 1982). The manufacturer recommends that caution be used if administered to a nursing woman.

Contraindications Hypersensitivity to hydralazine or any component of the formulation; mitral valve rheumatic heart disease

Warnings/Precautions May cause peripheral neuritis or a drug-induced lupus-like syndrome (more likely on larger doses, longer duration). Discontinue hydralazine in patients who develop SLE-like syndrome or positive ANA. Use with caution in patients with severe renal disease or cerebral vascular accidents or with known or suspected coronary artery disease; monitor blood pressure closely with IV use. Slow acetylators, patients with decreased renal function, and patients receiving >200 mg/day (chronically) are at higher risk for SLE. Titrate dosage cautiously to patient's response. Hypotensive effect after IV administration may be delayed and unpredictable in some patients. Usually administered with diuretic and a beta-blocker to counteract side effects of sodium and water retention and reflex tachycardia.

Adjust dose in severe renal dysfunction. Use with caution in CAD (increase in tachycardia may increase myocardial oxygen demand). Use with caution in pulmonary hypertension (may cause hypotension). Patients may be poorly compliant because of frequent dosing. Hydralazine-induced fluid and sodium retention may require addition or increased dosage of a diuretic.

Adverse Reactions

Cardiovascular: Angina pectoris, flushing, orthostatic hypotension, palpitations, paradoxical hypertension, peripheral edema, tachycardia, vascular collapse

Central nervous system: Anxiety, chills, depression, disorientation, dizziness, fever, headache, increased intracranial pressure (IV; in patient with pre-existing increased intracranial pressure), psychotic reaction

Dermatologic: Pruritus, rash, urticaria

Gastrointestinal: Anorexia, constipation, diarrhea, nausea, paralytic ileus, vomiting

Genitourinary: Dysuria, impotence

Hematologic: Agranulocytosis, eosinophilia, erythrocyte count reduced, hemoglobin decreased, hemolytic anemia, leukopenia, thrombocytopenia (rare)

Neuromuscular & skeletal: Muscle cramps, peripheral neuritis, rheumatoid arthritis, tremor, weakness

Ocular: Conjunctivitis, lacrimation

Respiratory: Dyspnea, nasal congestion

Miscellaneous: Diaphoresis, drug-induced lupus-like syndrome (dose related; fever, arthralgia, splenomegaly, lymphadenopathy, asthenia, myalgia, malaise, pleuritic chest pain, edema, positive ANA, positive LE cells, maculopapular facial rash, positive direct Coombs' test, pericarditis, pericardial tamponade)

Drug Interactions

Metabolism/Transport Effects None known.

Avoid Concomitant Use There are no known interactions where it is recommended to avoid concomitant use.

Increased Effect/Toxicity

HydrALAZINE may increase the levels/effects of: Amifostine; Antihypertensives; DULoxetine; Hypotensive Agents; Levodopa; Obinutuzumab; RisperiDONE; RiTUXimab

The levels/effects of HydrALAZINE may be increased by: Alfuzosin; Barbiturates; Brimonidine (Topical); Dapoxetine; Diazoxide; Herbs (Hypotensive Properties); MAO Inhibitors; Nicorandil; Pentoxifylline; Phosphodiesterase 5 Inhibitors; Prostacyclin Analogues

Decreased Effect

The levels/effects of HydrALAZINE may be decreased by: Herbs (Hypertensive Properties); Methylphenidate; Nonsteroidal Anti-Inflammatory Agents; Yohimbine

Food Interactions Food enhances bioavailability of hydralazine. Management: Administer without regard to food, but keep consistent.

Storage/Stability Intact ampuls/vials of hydralazine should not be stored under refrigeration because of possible precipitation or crystallization.

Mechanism of Action Direct vasodilation of arterioles (with little effect on veins) with decreased systemic resistance

Pharmacodynamics

Onset of action:
  Oral: 20-30 minutes
  IV: 5-20 minutes

Duration:
  Oral: 2-4 hours
  IV: 2-6 hours

Pharmacokinetics (Adult data unless noted)

Distribution: Crosses placenta; appears in breast milk

Protein-binding: 85% to 90%
Metabolism: Acetylated in the liver
Bioavailability: 30% to 50%; large first-pass effect orally
Half-life, adults: 2-8 hours; half-life varies with genetically determined acetylation rates
Elimination: 14% excreted unchanged in urine

Dosing: Usual

Pediatric:

Hypertension: Children and Adolescents: Oral: Initial: 0.75 mg/kg/day in 2 to 4 divided doses, maximum initial dose: 10 mg/dose; may increase gradually over 3 to 4 weeks up to a maximum of 7.5 mg/kg/day in 2 to 4 divided doses not to exceed 200 mg/**day** (NHBPEP 2005; NHLBI 2012; Parks 2014)

Hypertensive emergency/urgency: Children and Adolescents: IM, IV: Initial: 0.1 to 0.2 mg/kg/**dose**; increase as required to suggested usual range: 0.2 to 0.6 mg/kg/**dose** every 4 to 6 hours as needed; maximum dose: 20 mg/dose (NHBPEP 2005; Parks 2014; Thomas 2011); manufacturer labeling suggests a dose range of 1.7 to 3.5 mg/kg/day divided in 4 to 6 doses

Adult:

Hypertension: Oral: Initial: 10 mg 4 times daily for the first 2 to 4 days; increase to 25 mg 4 times daily for the balance of the first week; further increase by 10 to 25 mg/dose gradually (every 2 to 5 days) to 50 mg 4 times daily (maximum: 300 mg daily in divided doses)

Hypertensive emergency: Note: Use is generally not recommended due to unpredictable and prolonged antihypertensive effects (Marik 2007): IM, IV: 10 to 20 mg/dose every 4 to 6 hours as needed (Rhoney 2009)

Hypertensive emergency in pregnancy (systolic BP ≥160 mm Hg or diastolic BP ≥110 mm Hg): IM, IV: Initial: 5 or 10 mg; may repeat dose in 20 to 40 minutes with 5 to 10 mg if blood pressure continues to exceed thresholds (ACOG 2015; Magee 2014; Too 2013). Also refer to administration protocols developed by the American College of Obstetricians and Gynecologists (ACOG 2015). A maximum total cumulative dose of 20 mg (IV) or 30 mg (IM) is recommended (Magee 2014). **Note:** After the initial dose, may initiate a continuous infusion of 0.5 to 10 mg/hour instead of intermittent dosing (Magee 2014).

Dosing adjustment in renal impairment:

Children and Adolescents: There are no dosage adjustments provided in the manufacturer's labeling; however, the following adjustments have been recommended (Aronoff 2007). **Note:** Renally adjusted dose recommendations are based on doses: Oral: 0.75 to 1 mg/kg/day divided every 6 to 12 hours; maximum daily dose: 200 mg/day; IV: 0.1 to 0.2 mg/kg/**dose** every 6 hours; maximum dose: 20 mg/dose

GFR >50 mL/minute/1.73 m^2: No adjustment necessary
GFR 10 to 50 mL/minute/1.73 m^2: Administer every 8 hours
GFR <10 mL/minute/1.73 m^2: Administer every 12 to 24 hours
Intermittent hemodialysis: Administer every 12 to 24 hours
Peritoneal dialysis (PD): Administer every 12 to 24 hours
Continuous renal replacement therapy (CRRT): Administer every 8 hours

Adults:

CrCl 10 to 50 mL/minute: Administer every 8 hours
CrCl <10 mL/minute: Administer every 8 to 16 hours in fast acetylators and every 12 to 24 hours in slow acetylators
Hemodialysis effects: Supplemental dose is not necessary
Peritoneal dialysis effects: Supplemental dose is not necessary

Dosing adjustment in hepatic impairment: There are no dosage adjustments provided in the manufacturer's labeling; however, hydralazine undergoes extensive hepatic metabolism.

Preparation for Administration Parenteral: IV: Manufacturer does not recommend dilution. If further dilution is desired hydralazine should be diluted in NS for IVPB administration due to decreased stability in D_5W. Stability of IVPB solution in NS is 4 days at room temperature.

Administration

Oral: Administer with food

Parenteral:

IM: Administer undiluted as IM injection
IV: Administer undiluted (20 mg/mL) as slow IV push over 1 to 2 minutes (Artman 1984; Beekman 1982); maximum rate: 5 mg/minute (Klaus 1989)

Monitoring Parameters Heart rate, blood pressure, ANA titer

Additional Information Slow acetylators, patients with decreased renal function and patients receiving >200 mg/day (chronically) are at higher risk for SLE. Titrate dosage to patient's response. Usually administered with diuretic and a beta-blocker to counteract hydralazine's side effects of sodium and water retention and reflex tachycardia.

Dosage Forms Excipient information presented when available (limited, particularly for generics); consult specific product labeling.

Solution, Injection, as hydrochloride:
Generic: 20 mg/mL (1 mL)
Tablet, Oral, as hydrochloride:
Generic: 10 mg, 25 mg, 50 mg, 100 mg

Extemporaneous Preparations A 4 mg/mL oral suspension may be made with tablets and a 1:1 mixture of Ora-Sweet SF and Ora-Plus. Crush four 100 mg tablets in a mortar and reduce to a fine powder. Add 15 mL of the vehicle and mix to a uniform paste; mix while adding the vehicle in incremental proportions to **almost** 100 mL; transfer to a calibrated bottle, rinse mortar with vehicle, and add quantity of vehicle sufficient to make 100 mL. Label "Shake Well", "Protect From Light", "Store in a Refrigerator". Stable for 2 days when stored in amber plastic prescription bottles in the dark and refrigerated (Allen, 1998).

Note: Stability reduced to 24 hours if Ora-Sweet is substituted for Ora-Sweet SF.

Allen LV Jr, Erickson MA 3rd. Stability of alprazolam, chloroquine phosphate, cisapride, enalapril maleate, and hydralazine hydrochloride in extemporaneously compounded oral liquids. *Am J Health-Syst Pharm*. 1998;55(18):1915-1920.

◆ **Hydralazine Hydrochloride** *see* HydrALAZINE *on page 1027*
◆ **Hydrated Chloral** *see* Chloral Hydrate *on page 429*
◆ **Hydrea** *see* Hydroxyurea *on page 1055*
◆ **Hydrisalic [OTC] [DSC]** *see* Salicylic Acid *on page 1894*

Hydrochlorothiazide (hye droe klor oh THYE a zide)

Medication Safety Issues

Sound-alike/look-alike issues:

HCTZ is an error-prone abbreviation (mistaken as hydrocortisone)
Hydrochlorothiazide may be confused with hydrocortisone, Viskazide
Microzide may be confused with Maxzide, Micronase

International issues:

Esidrex [multiple international markets] may be confused with Lasix brand name for furosemide [U.S., Canada, and multiple international markets]

Esidrix [Germany] may be confused with Lasix brand name for furosemide [U.S., Canada, and multiple international markets]

Brand Names: US Microzide

Brand Names: Canada Apo-Hydro; Ava-Hydrochlorothiazide; Bio-Hydrochlorothiazide; PMS-Hydrochlorothiazide; Teva-Hydrochlorothiazide; Urozide

Therapeutic Category Antihypertensive Agent; Diuretic, Thiazide

Generic Availability (US) Yes

Use Oral:

Capsules: Management of hypertension alone or in combination with other antihypertensive agents (FDA approved in adults); **Note:** Use in pregnancy should be reserved for those cases causing extreme discomfort and unrelieved by rest; should not be routinely used during pregnancy.

Tablets: Treatment of edema due to heart failure, hepatic cirrhosis, estrogen, or corticosteroid therapy (FDA approved in infants, children, and adults); treatment of various forms of renal dysfunction, including nephrotic syndrome, acute glomerulonephritis, and chronic renal failure (FDA approved in infants, children, and adults); management of hypertension either alone or in combination with other antihypertensive agents (FDA approved in infants, children, and adults); has also been used for bronchopulmonary dysplasia (BPD), idiopathic hypercalcuria, and congenital nephrogenic diabetes insipidus. **Note:** Use in pregnancy should be reserved for those cases causing extreme discomfort and unrelieved by rest; should not be routinely used during pregnancy.

Pregnancy Risk Factor B

Pregnancy Considerations Adverse events were not observed in animal reproduction studies. Thiazide diuretics cross the placenta and are found in cord blood. Maternal use may cause may cause fetal or neonatal jaundice, thrombocytopenia, or other adverse events observed in adults. Use of thiazide diuretics to treat edema during normal pregnancies is not appropriate; use may be considered when edema is due to pathologic causes (as in the nonpregnant patient); monitor. Untreated chronic maternal hypertension is associated with adverse events in the fetus, infant, and mother (ACOG, 2013). Women who required thiazide diuretics for the treatment of hypertension prior to pregnancy may continue their use (ACOG, 2013).

Breast-Feeding Considerations Thiazide diuretics are found in breast milk. Following a single oral maternal dose of hydrochlorothiazide 50 mg, the mean breast milk concentration was 80 ng/mL (samples collected over 24 hours) and hydrochlorothiazide was not detected in the blood of the breast-feeding infant (limit of detection 20 ng/mL) (Miller, 1982). Peak plasma concentrations reported in adults following hydrochlorothiazide 12.5-100 mg are 70-490 ng/mL. Due to the potential for serious adverse reactions in the nursing infant, the manufacturer recommends a decision be made whether to discontinue nursing or to discontinue the drug, taking into account the importance of treatment to the mother (Canadian labeling contraindicates use in nursing women). Diuretics have the potential to decrease milk volume and suppress lactation.

Contraindications

Hypersensitivity to hydrochlorothiazide, any component of the formulation, or sulfonamide-derived drugs; anuria

Note: Although the FDA approved product labeling states this medication is contraindicated with other sulfonamide-containing drug classes, the scientific basis of this statement has been challenged. See "Warnings/Precautions" for more detail.

Canadian labeling: Additional contraindications (not in U.S. labeling): Increasing azotemia and oliguria during treatment of severe progressive renal disease; breast-feeding

Warnings/Precautions Hypersensitivity reactions may occur with hydrochlorothiazide. Risk is increased in patients with a history of allergy or bronchial asthma. Avoid in severe renal disease (ineffective as a diuretic). Electrolyte disturbances (hypokalemia, hypochloremic alkalosis, hypomagnesemia, hyponatremia) can occur. Development of electrolyte disturbances can be minimized when used in combination with other electrolyte sparing antihypertensives (eg, ACE inhibitors or angiotensin receptor blockers). (Sica, 2011) Use with caution in severe hepatic dysfunction; hepatic encephalopathy can be caused by electrolyte disturbances. Gout may be precipitated in certain patients with a history of gout, a familial predisposition to gout, or chronic renal failure. Thiazide diuretics reduce calcium excretion; pathologic changes in the parathyroid glands with hypercalcemia and hypophosphatemia have been observed with prolonged use. Should be discontinued prior to testing for parathyroid function. Use with caution in patients with prediabetes and diabetes; may alter glucose control. May cause SLE exacerbation or activation. Use with caution in patients with moderate or high cholesterol concentrations. Photosensitization may occur. Correct hypokalemia before initiating therapy. Thiazide diuretics may decrease renal calcium excretion; consider avoiding use in patients with hypercalcemia. May cause acute transient myopia and acute angle-closure glaucoma, typically occurring within hours to weeks following initiation; discontinue therapy immediately in patients with acute decreases in visual acuity or ocular pain. Risk factors may include a history of sulfonamide or penicillin allergy. Cumulative effects may develop, including azotemia, in patients with impaired renal function. If given the morning of surgery, hydrochlorothiazide may render the patient volume depleted and blood pressure may be labile during general anesthesia.

Sulfonamide ("sulfa") allergy: The FDA-approved product labeling for many medications containing a sulfonamide chemical group includes a broad contraindication in patients with a prior allergic reaction to sulfonamides. There is a potential for cross-reactivity between members of a specific class (eg, two antibiotic sulfonamides). However, concerns for cross-reactivity have previously extended to all compounds containing the sulfonamide structure (SO_2NH_2). An expanded understanding of allergic mechanisms indicates cross-reactivity between antibiotic sulfonamides and nonantibiotic sulfonamides may not occur or at the very least this potential is extremely low (Brackett 2004; Johnson 2005; Slatore 2004; Tornero 2004). In particular, mechanisms of cross-reaction due to antibody production (anaphylaxis) are unlikely to occur with nonantibiotic sulfonamides. T-cell-mediated (type IV) reactions (eg, maculopapular rash) are less well understood and it is not possible to completely exclude this potential based on current insights. In cases where prior reactions were severe (Stevens-Johnson syndrome/TEN), some clinicians choose to avoid exposure to these classes.

Adverse Reactions The occurrence of adverse events are dose related, with the majority occurring with doses ≥25 mg.

Cardiovascular: Hypotension, necrotizing angiitis, orthostatic hypotension

Central nervous system: Dizziness, headache, paresthesia, restlessness, vertigo

Dermatologic: Alopecia, erythema multiforme, exfoliative dermatitis, skin photosensitivity, skin rash, Stevens-Johnson syndrome, toxic epidermal necrolysis, urticaria

Endocrine & metabolic: Glycosuria, hypercalcemia, hyperglycemia, hyperuricemia, hypochloremic alkalosis, hypokalemia, hypomagnesemia, hyponatremia

Gastrointestinal: Abdominal cramps, anorexia, constipation, diarrhea, gastric irritation, nausea, pancreatitis, sialadenitis, vomiting

Genitourinary: Impotence

Hematologic & oncologic: Agranulocytosis, aplastic anemia, hemolytic anemia, leukopenia, purpura, thrombocytopenia
Hepatic: Jaundice
Hypersensitivity: Anaphylaxis
Neuromuscular & skeletal: Muscle spasm, weakness
Ophthalmic: Blurred vision (transient), xanthopsia
Renal: Interstitial nephritis, renal failure, renal insufficiency
Respiratory: Respiratory distress, pneumonitis, pulmonary edema
Miscellaneous: Fever
Rare but important or life-threatening: Allergic myocarditis, eosinophilic pneumonitis, hepatic insufficiency, lip cancer (Friedman, 2012), systemic lupus erythematosus

Drug Interactions

Metabolism/Transport Effects None known.

Avoid Concomitant Use

Avoid concomitant use of Hydrochlorothiazide with any of the following: Dofetilide; Mecamylamine

Increased Effect/Toxicity

Hydrochlorothiazide may increase the levels/effects of: ACE Inhibitors; Allopurinol; Amifostine; Antihypertensives; Benazepril; Calcium Salts; CarBAMazepine; Cardiac Glycosides; Cyclophosphamide; Diazoxide; Dofetilide; DULoxetine; Hypotensive Agents; Ivabradine; Levodopa; Lithium; Mecamylamine; Multivitamins/Minerals (with ADEK, Folate, Iron); Multivitamins/Minerals (with AE, No Iron); Obinutuzumab; OXcarbazepine; Porfimer; RisperiDONE; RiTUXimab; Sodium Phosphates; Topiramate; Toremifene; Valsartan; Verteporfin; Vitamin D Analogs

The levels/effects of Hydrochlorothiazide may be increased by: Alcohol (Ethyl); Alfuzosin; Analgesics (Opioid); Anticholinergic Agents; Barbiturates; Beta2-Agonists; Brimonidine (Topical); Corticosteroids (Orally Inhaled); Corticosteroids (Systemic); Dexketoprofen; Diazoxide; Herbs (Hypotensive Properties); Licorice; MAO Inhibitors; Multivitamins/Fluoride (with ADE); Nicorandil; Pentoxifylline; Phosphodiesterase 5 Inhibitors; Prostacyclin Analogues; Selective Serotonin Reuptake Inhibitors; Valsartan

Decreased Effect

Hydrochlorothiazide may decrease the levels/effects of: Antidiabetic Agents

The levels/effects of Hydrochlorothiazide may be decreased by: Benazepril; Bile Acid Sequestrants; Herbs (Hypertensive Properties); Methylphenidate; Nonsteroidal Anti-Inflammatory Agents; Yohimbine

Storage/Stability Store at 20°C to 25°C (68°F to 77°F) (USP Controlled Room Temperature). Protect from light and moisture.

Mechanism of Action Inhibits sodium reabsorption in the distal tubules causing increased excretion of sodium and water as well as potassium and hydrogen ions

Pharmacodynamics

Onset of action: Diuresis: Oral:
Infants: 2-6 hours (Chemtob, 1989)
Adults: Within 2 hours
Maximum effect: Diuresis: Within 4-6 hours
Duration: Diuresis:
Infants: 8 hours (Chemtob, 1989)
Adults: 6-12 hours

Pharmacokinetics (Adult data unless noted)

Absorption: Oral: ~50% to 80%
Distribution: V_d: 3.6-7.8 L/kg
Protein binding: 68%
Half-life: 5.6-14.8 hours
Time to peak serum concentration: 1-2.5 hours
Elimination: Urine (as unchanged drug)

Dosing: Neonatal Bronchopulmonary dysplasia (BPD) diuresis, hypertension: Oral: 1-2 mg/kg/dose every 12 hours (Albersheim, 1989; Chemtob, 1989; Engelhardt, 1989)

Dosing: Usual

Infants, Children, and Adolescents:

Bronchopulmonary dysplasia: Infants: Oral 3-4 mg/kg/day in 2 divided doses (Albersheim, 1989; Engelhardt, 1989)

Edema (diuresis):

Manufacturer labeling:
Infants 2-6 months: Oral: 1-3 mg/kg/day in 1-2 divided doses
Infants >6 months, Children, and Adolescents: Oral 1-2 mg/kg/day in 1-2 divided doses
Maximum daily dose:
Infants and Children < 2 years: 37.5 mg/**day**
Children 2-12 years: 100 mg/**day**
Adolescents: 200 mg/**day**

Hypertension: Oral: Initial: 1 mg/kg/day once daily; may increase to maximum 3 mg/kg/day; not to exceed 50 mg/day (NHBPEP, 2004; NHLBI, 2011)
Maximum daily dose:
Infants and Children <2 years: 37.5 mg/**day**
Children 2-12 years: 100 mg/**day**
Adolescents: 200 mg/**day**

Hypercalciuria: Limited data available: Oral: Initial: 1-2 mg/kg/day once daily; titrate until goal urinary calcium excretion goals reached and symptoms resolve; treatment usually continued for 1 year; maximum daily dose: 100 mg/**day** (Copelovitch, 2012).

Nephrogenic diabetes insipidus; congenital: Limited data available: Oral: 2-3 mg/kg/day in combination with amiloride; dosing based on a retrospective descriptive analysis (n=30, age range 1 month to 40 years) and a pediatric case-series (n=4). (Kirchlechner, 1999; Van Lieburg, 1999)

Adults:

Edema (diuresis): Oral: 25-100 mg/day in 1-2 doses; maximum: 200 mg/day

Hypertension: Oral: 12.5-50 mg/day; minimal increase in response and more electrolyte disturbances are seen with doses >50 mg/day

Dosage adjustment in renal impairment: CrCl <10 mL/minute: Avoid use.

Note: ACC/AHA 2009 Adult Heart Failure guidelines suggest that thiazides lose their efficacy when CrCl <40 mL/minute.

Administration Oral: May administer with food or milk; administer early in day to avoid nocturia; if multiple daily dosing, the last dose should not be administered later than 6 PM unless instructed otherwise.

Monitoring Parameters Serum electrolytes, BUN, creatinine, blood pressure, fluid balance, body weight, urinary electrolytes (if applicable); serum glucose levels

Test Interactions May interfere with parathyroid function tests and may decrease serum iodine (protein bound) without signs of thyroid disturbance.

Dosage Forms Excipient information presented when available (limited, particularly for generics); consult specific product labeling.

Capsule, Oral:
Microzide: 12.5 mg
Generic: 12.5 mg
Tablet, Oral:
Generic: 12.5 mg, 25 mg, 50 mg

Hydrochlorothiazide and Spironolactone

(hye droe klor oh THYE a zide & speer on oh LAK tone)

Medication Safety Issues

Sound-alike/look-alike issues:

Aldactazide may be confused with Aldactone

Brand Names: US Aldactazide

Brand Names: Canada Aldactazide 25; Aldactazide 50; Teva-Spironolactone/HCTZ

Therapeutic Category Antihypertensive Agent, Combination; Diuretic, Combination

Generic Availability (US) Yes

Use Treatment of edematous conditions associated with heart failure, cirrhosis of the liver, and nephrotic syndrome when other diuretics are inappropriate (eg, hypokalemia) or lacked adequate response (FDA approved in adults); treatment of primary hypertension (FDA approved in adults). **Note:** Use in pregnancy should be reserved for those cases causing extreme discomfort and unrelieved by rest; should not be routinely used during pregnancy.

Pregnancy Risk Factor C

Pregnancy Considerations Animal reproduction studies have not been conducted with this combination product. See individual agents.

Breast-Feeding Considerations The active metabolite of spironolactone (canrenone) and thiazide diuretics are found in breast milk. Due to the potential for serious adverse reactions in the nursing infant, the manufacturer recommends a decision be made whether to discontinue nursing or to discontinue the drug, taking into account the importance of treatment to the mother. See individual agents.

Contraindications

Hypersensitivity to spironolactone, hydrochlorothiazide or any component of the formulation, thiazides, or sulfonamide-derived drugs; acute renal insufficiency; anuria; renal decompensation; significant impairment of renal excretory function; hypercalcemia; hyperkalemia; Addison's disease; acute or severe hepatic impairment

Note: Although the FDA approved product labeling states this medication is contraindicated with other sulfonamide-containing drug classes, the scientific basis of this statement has been challenged. See "Warnings/Precautions" for more detail.

Canadian labeling: Additional contraindications (not in U.S. labeling): Concomitant use with eplerenone, heparin, or low molecular weight heparin

Warnings/Precautions See individual agents.

Adverse Reactions See individual agents.

Drug Interactions

Metabolism/Transport Effects None known.

Avoid Concomitant Use

Avoid concomitant use of Hydrochlorothiazide and Spironolactone with any of the following: AMILoride; CycloSPORINE (Systemic); Dofetilide; Mecamylamine; Tacrolimus (Systemic); Triamterene

Increased Effect/Toxicity

Hydrochlorothiazide and Spironolactone may increase the levels/effects of: ACE Inhibitors; Allopurinol; Amifostine; Ammonium Chloride; Antihypertensives; Benazepril; Calcium Salts; CarBAMazepine; Cardiac Glycosides; Ciprofloxacin (Systemic); Cyclophosphamide; CycloSPORINE (Systemic); Diazoxide; Digoxin; Dofetilide; DULoxetine; Hypotensive Agents; Ivabradine; Levodopa; Lithium; Mecamylamine; Multivitamins/Minerals (with ADEK, Folate, Iron); Multivitamins/Minerals (with AE, No Iron); Neuromuscular-Blocking Agents (Nondepolarizing); Obinutuzumab; OXcarbazepine; Porfimer; RisperiDONE; RiTUXimab; Sodium Phosphates; Tacrolimus (Systemic); Topiramate; Toremifene; Valsartan; Verteporfin; Vitamin D Analogs

The levels/effects of Hydrochlorothiazide and Spironolactone may be increased by: Alcohol (Ethyl); Alfuzosin; AMILoride; Analgesics (Opioid); Angiotensin II Receptor Blockers; Anticholinergic Agents; AtorvaSTATin; Barbiturates; Beta2-Agonists; Brimonidine (Topical); Canagliflozin; Corticosteroids (Orally Inhaled); Corticosteroids (Systemic); Dexketoprofen; Diazoxide; Drospirenone; Eplerenone; Heparin; Heparin (Low Molecular Weight); Herbs (Hypotensive Properties); Licorice; MAO Inhibitors; Multivitamins/Fluoride (with ADE); Nicorandil; Nitrofurantoin; Nonsteroidal Anti-Inflammatory Agents; Pentoxifylline; Phosphodiesterase 5 Inhibitors; Potassium Salts; Prostacyclin Analogues; Selective Serotonin Reuptake Inhibitors; Tolvaptan; Triamterene; Trimethoprim; Valsartan

Decreased Effect

Hydrochlorothiazide and Spironolactone may decrease the levels/effects of: Abiraterone Acetate; Alpha-/Beta-Agonists; Antidiabetic Agents; Cardiac Glycosides; Mitotane; QuiNIDine

The levels/effects of Hydrochlorothiazide and Spironolactone may be decreased by: Benazepril; Bile Acid Sequestrants; Herbs (Hypertensive Properties); Methylphenidate; Nonsteroidal Anti-Inflammatory Agents; Yohimbine

Food Interactions Excessive potassium intake may cause hyperkalemia. Management: Avoid food with high potassium content and potassium-containing salt substitutes.

Storage/Stability Store below 25°C (77°F).

Pharmacokinetics (Adult data unless noted) See individual agents.

Dosing: Usual Note: Product is a fixed combination of equal **mg proportions of components**; the following dosage represents mg of each component (spironolactone and hydrochlorothiazide).

Infants, Children, and Adolescents: **Hypertension, diuresis:**

Infants: Limited data available: Oral: 1-3 mg/kg/day in divided doses once or twice daily (Engelhardt, 1989)

Children and Adolescents: Oral: Initial: 1 mg/kg/day in divided doses once or twice daily, may titrate up to maximum daily dose: 3-3.3 mg/kg/**day** or 100 mg/**day** of spironolactone (NHBPEP, 2004; NHLBI, 2011)

Adults: **Hypertension, edema:** Oral: 12.5-50 mg/day; manufacturer labeling states hydrochlorothiazide maximum 200 mg/day; however, usual dose in JNC-7 is 12.5-50 mg/day

Dosing adjustment in renal impairment: Adults: Efficacy of hydrochlorothiazide is limited in patients with CrCl <30 mL/minute; contraindicated in patients with anuria

Administration Oral: Administer in the morning; administer the last dose of multiple doses before 6 PM unless instructed otherwise

Monitoring Parameters Serum electrolytes, BUN, creatinine, blood pressure, fluid balance, body weight

Test Interactions See individual agents.

Dosage Forms Excipient information presented when available (limited, particularly for generics); consult specific product labeling.

Tablet: Hydrochlorothiazide 25 mg and spironolactone 25 mg

Aldactazide:

25/25: Hydrochlorothiazide 25 mg and spironolactone 25 mg

50/50: Hydrochlorothiazide 50 mg and spironolactone 50 mg

Extemporaneous Preparations An oral suspension containing hydrochlorothiazide 5 mg and spironolactone 5 mg per mL may be made with tablets. Crush twenty-four 25 mg hydrochlorothiazide and twenty-four 25 mg spironolactone tablets and reduce to a fine powder. Add small portions of a 1:1 mixture of Ora-Sweet and Ora-Plus and mix to a uniform paste; mix while adding the vehicle in equal proportions to **almost** 120 mL; transfer to a calibrated bottle, rinse mortar with vehicle, and add sufficient quantity of vehicle to make 120 mL. Label "shake well". Stable 60 days under refrigeration or at room temperature.

Allen LV and Erickson MA, "Stability of Extemporaneously Prepared Pediatric Formulations Using Ora-Plus With Ora-Sweet and Ora-Sweet SF – Part II," *Secundum Artem*, Volume 6 (1). Available at: www.paddocklabs.com.

Hydrocodone and Acetaminophen

(hye droe KOE done & a seet a MIN oh fen)

Medication Safety Issues

Sound-alike/look-alike issues:

Hydrocodone and Acetaminophen may be confused with Oxycodone and Acetaminophen

Lorcet may be confused with Fioricet

Lortab may be confused with Cortef

Vicodin may be confused with Hycodan, Indocin

Zydone may be confused with Vytone

High alert medication:

The Institute for Safe Medication Practices (ISMP) includes this medication among its list of drug classes which have a heightened risk of causing significant patient harm when used in error.

Other safety concerns:

Duplicate therapy issues: This product contains acetaminophen, which may be a component of other combination products. Do not exceed the maximum recommended daily dose of acetaminophen.

Related Information

Opioid Conversion Table *on page 2285*

Brand Names: US hycet®; Lorcet® 10/650 [DSC]; Lorcet® Plus [DSC]; Lortab®; Maxidone [DSC]; Norco; Stagesic [DSC]; Verdrocet; Vicodin ES; Vicodin HP; Vicodin®; Xodol 10/300; Xodol 5/300; Xodol 7.5/300; Zamicet [DSC]; Zolvit [DSC]; Zydone [DSC]

Therapeutic Category Analgesic, Narcotic; Antitussive; Cough Preparation

Generic Availability (US) Yes: Oral solution, tablet

Use Relief of moderate to moderately severe pain (Oral solution or oral elixir: FDA approved in ages ≥2 years and adults; Capsules and tablets: FDA approved in adults)

Pregnancy Risk Factor C

Pregnancy Considerations Animal reproduction studies have not been conducted with this combination product. See individual agents.

Breast-Feeding Considerations Acetaminophen and hydrocodone are excreted in breast milk. Due to the potential for serious adverse reactions in the nursing infant, the manufacturer recommends a decision be made whether to discontinue nursing or to discontinue the drug, taking into account the importance of treatment to the mother. See individual agents.

Contraindications Hypersensitivity to hydrocodone, acetaminophen, or any component of the formulation; CNS depression; severe respiratory depression

Warnings/Precautions Use with caution in patients with hypersensitivity reactions to other phenanthrene derivative opioid agonists (morphine, hydromorphone, levorphanol, oxycodone, oxymorphone); tolerance or drug dependence may result from extended use. Concurrent use of agonist/antagonist analgesics may precipitate withdrawal symptoms and/or reduced analgesic efficacy in patients following prolonged therapy with mu opioid agonists. Abrupt discontinuation following prolonged use may also lead to withdrawal symptoms.

Respiratory depression may occur even at therapeutic dosages; use with extreme caution in children. Respiratory depressant effects may be increased with head injuries. Use caution with acute abdominal conditions; clinical course may be obscured. Use caution with adrenal insufficiency, biliary tract impairment, pancreatitis, morbidly obese patients, toxic psychosis, thyroid dysfunction, prostatic hyperplasia, respiratory disease, hepatic or renal disease, and in the debilitated or elderly. Hydrocodone may cause constipation which may be problematic in patients with unstable angina and patients post-myocardial infarction. Causes sedation; caution must be used in performing tasks which require alertness (eg, operating machinery or driving). Effects may be potentiated when used with other sedative drugs or ethanol. May cause hypotension.

Rarely, acetaminophen may cause serious and potentially fatal skin reactions such as acute generalized exanthematous pustulosis, Stevens-Johnson syndrome (SJS), and toxic epidermal necrolysis (TEN). Discontinue treatment if severe skin reactions develop.

Due to the role of CYP2D6 in the metabolism of hydrocodone to hydromorphone (an active metabolite with higher binding affinity to mu-opioid receptors compared to hydrocodone), patients with genetic variations of CYP2D6, including "poor metabolizers" or "extensive metabolizers," may have decreased or increased hydromorphone formation, respectively. Variable effects in positive and negative opioid effects have been reported in these patients; however, limited data exists to determine if clinically significant differences of analgesia and toxicity can be predicted based on CYP2D6 phenotype (Hutchinson, 2004; Otton, 1993; Zhou, 2009).

[U.S. Boxed Warning]: Acetaminophen may cause severe hepatotoxicity, potentially requiring liver transplant or resulting in death; hepatotoxicity is usually associated with excessive acetaminophen intake (>4 g/day in adults). Risk is increased with alcohol use, preexisting liver disease, and intake of more than one source of acetaminophen-containing medications. Chronic daily dosing in adults has also resulted in liver damage in some patients. Hypersensitivity and anaphylactic reactions have been reported with acetaminophen use; discontinue immediately if symptoms of allergic or hypersensitivity reactions occur. Use caution in patients with known G6PD deficiency.

Some dosage forms may contain propylene glycol; large amounts are potentially toxic and have been associated hyperosmolality, lactic acidosis, seizures and respiratory depression; use caution (AAP, 1997; Zar, 2007).

Warnings: Additional Pediatric Considerations Infants born to women physically dependent on opioids will also be physically dependent and may experience respiratory difficulties or opioid withdrawal symptoms (neonatal abstinence syndrome [NAS]). Onset, duration, and severity of NAS depend upon the drug used (maternal), duration of use, maternal dose, and rate of drug elimination by the newborn. Symptoms of opioid withdrawal may include excessive crying, diarrhea, fever, hyper-reflexia, irritability, tremors, or vomiting or failure to gain weight. Opioid withdrawal syndrome in the neonate may be life-threatening and should be promptly treated.

Some dosage forms may contain propylene glycol; in neonates large amounts of propylene glycol delivered orally, intravenously (eg, >3,000 mg/day), or topically have been associated with potentially fatal toxicities which can include metabolic acidosis, seizures, renal failure, and CNS depression; toxicities have also been reported in children and adults including hyperosmolality, lactic acidosis, seizures and respiratory depression; use caution (AAP, 1997; Shehab, 2009).

Adverse Reactions

Cardiovascular: Bradycardia, cardiac arrest, circulatory shock, hypotension

Central nervous system: Anxiety, clouding of consciousness, coma, dizziness, drowsiness, drug dependence,

dysphoria, euphoria, fear, lethargy, malaise, mental deficiency, mood changes, sedation, stupor
Dermatologic: Cold and clammy skin, diaphoresis, pruritus, skin rash
Endocrine & metabolic: Hypoglycemic coma
Gastrointestinal: Abdominal pain, constipation, gastric distress, heartburn, nausea, occult blood in stools, peptic ulcer, vomiting
Genitourinary: Nephrotoxicity, ureteral spasm, urinary retention
Hematologic & oncologic: Agranulocytosis, hemolytic anemia, iron deficiency anemia, prolonged bleeding time, thrombocytopenia
Hepatic: Hepatic necrosis, hepatitis
Hypersensitivity: Hypersensitivity reaction
Neuromuscular & skeletal: Vesicle sphincter spasm
Otic: Hearing loss (chronic overdose)
Renal: Renal tubular necrosis
Respiratory: Airway obstruction, apnea, dyspnea, respiratory depression (dose related)
Rare but important or life-threatening: Hypogonadism (Brennan, 2013; Debono, 2011)

Drug Interactions

Metabolism/Transport Effects Refer to individual components.

Avoid Concomitant Use

Avoid concomitant use of Hydrocodone and Acetaminophen with any of the following: Alcohol (Ethyl); Azelastine (Nasal); Conivaptan; Eluxadoline; Fusidic Acid (Systemic); Idelalisib; MAO Inhibitors; Mixed Agonist / Antagonist Opioids; Orphenadrine; Paraldehyde; Thalidomide

Increased Effect/Toxicity

Hydrocodone and Acetaminophen may increase the levels/effects of: Alvimopan; Azelastine (Nasal); Busulfan; Dasatinib; Desmopressin; Diuretics; Eluxadoline; Imatinib; Methotrimeprazine; Metyrosine; Mipomersen; Orphenadrine; Paraldehyde; Phenylephrine (Systemic); Pramipexole; Prilocaine; ROPINIRole; Rotigotine; Selective Serotonin Reuptake Inhibitors; Sodium Nitrite; SORAfenib; Suvorexant; Thalidomide; Vitamin K Antagonists; Zolpidem

The levels/effects of Hydrocodone and Acetaminophen may be increased by: Alcohol (Ethyl); Amphetamines; Anticholinergic Agents; Aprepitant; Brimonidine (Topical); Cannabis; Ceritinib; CNS Depressants; Conivaptan; CYP3A4 Inhibitors (Moderate); CYP3A4 Inhibitors (Strong); CYP3A4 Inhibitors (Weak); Dasatinib; Dronabinol; Droperidol; Fosaprepitant; Fusidic Acid (Systemic); Idelalisib; Isoniazid; Ivacaftor; Kava Kava; Luliconazole; Magnesium Sulfate; MAO Inhibitors; Methotrimeprazine; Metyrapone; Mifepristone; Nabilone; Netupitant; Nitric Oxide; Palbociclib; Perampanel; Probenecid; Rufinamide; Simeprevir; Sodium Oxybate; SORAfenib; Stiripentol; Succinylcholine; Tapentadol; Tetrahydrocannabinol

Decreased Effect

Hydrocodone and Acetaminophen may decrease the levels/effects of: Pegvisomant

The levels/effects of Hydrocodone and Acetaminophen may be decreased by: Ammonium Chloride; Bosentan; Cholestyramine Resin; CYP2D6 Inhibitors (Strong); CYP3A4 Inducers (Moderate); CYP3A4 Inducers (Strong); CYP3A4 Inducers (Weak); Dabrafenib; Deferasirox; Mitotane; Mixed Agonist / Antagonist Opioids; Naltrexone; QuiNIDine; Siltuximab; St Johns Wort; Tocilizumab

Mechanism of Action Hydrocodone, as with other opioid analgesics, blocks pain perception in the cerebral cortex by binding to specific receptor molecules (opiate receptors) within the neuronal membranes of synapses. This binding results in a decreased synaptic chemical transmission throughout the CNS thus inhibiting the flow of pain sensations into the higher centers. Mu and kappa are the two subtypes of the opiate receptor which hydrocodone binds to cause analgesia.

Acetaminophen inhibits the synthesis of prostaglandins in the CNS and peripherally blocks pain impulse generation; produces antipyresis from inhibition of hypothalamic heat-regulating center.

Pharmacodynamics Opioid analgesia:
Onset of action: Within 10-20 minutes
Duration: 4-6 hours

Pharmacokinetics (Adult data unless noted) Hydrocodone:
Metabolism: Hepatic; O-demethylation via primarily CYP2D6 to hydromorphone (major, active metabolite with 10- to 33-fold higher or as much as a >100-fold higher binding affinity for the mu-opioid receptor than hydrocodone); N-demethylation via CYP3A4 to norhydrocodone (major metabolite); ~40% of metabolism/clearance occurs via non-CYP pathways, including 6-ketosteroid reduction to 6-alpha-hydrocol and 6-beta-hydrocol, and other elimination pathways (eg, fecal, biliary, intestinal, renal) (Hutchinson, 2004; Volpe, 2011; Zhou, 2009)
Half-life elimination: ~4 hours
Time to peak serum concentration: 1-1.6 hours
Elimination: Urine (26% of single dose in 72 hours, with ~12% as unchanged drug, 5% as norhydrocodone, 4% as conjugated hydrocodone, 3% as 6-hydrocodol, and 0.1% as conjugated 6-hydromorphol) (Zhou, 2009)

Dosing: Usual Note: Doses based on hydrocodone; titrate to appropriate analgesic effect.
Infants, Children, and Adolescents: Analgesic; opioid-naive patients (American Pain Society, 2008; Kleigman, 2011): Limited data available in infants and children <2 years: **Note:** Maximum daily dose of acetaminophen should be limited to ≤75 mg/kg/**day** in ≤5 divided doses and not to exceed 4000 mg/**day** (and possibly less in patients with hepatic impairment or ethanol use).
Patient weight:
<50 kg: Oral: Usual initial dose: Hydrocodone 0.1-0.2 mg/kg/dose every 4-6 hours; in infants, reduced doses and close monitoring should be considered due to possible increased sensitivity to respiratory depressant effects; use with caution in infants.
≥50 kg: Oral: Usual initial dose: Hydrocodone 5-10 mg every 4-6 hours
Adults: **Analgesic:** Oral: Average starting dose in opioid-naive patients: Hydrocodone 5-10 mg 4 times daily; maximum daily dose of acetaminophen should be limited to ≤4000 mg/day (and possibly less in patients with hepatic impairment or ethanol use).
Dosage ranges (based on specific product labeling): Hydrocodone 2.5-10 mg every 4-6 hours; maximum dose of hydrocodone may be limited by the acetaminophen content of specific product

Administration Oral: May administer with food or milk to decrease GI distress

Monitoring Parameters Pain relief; respiratory rate; mental status; blood pressure; signs of misuse, abuse, and addiction

Test Interactions Acetaminophen may cause false-positive urinary 5-hydroxyindoleacetic acid.

Controlled Substance C-II

Dosage Forms Excipient information presented when available (limited, particularly for generics); consult specific product labeling. [DSC] = Discontinued product
Capsule, oral:
Stagesic™: Hydrocodone bitartrate 5 mg and acetaminophen 500 mg [DSC]
Elixir, oral:
Lortab®: Hydrocodone bitartrate 7.5 mg and acetaminophen 500 mg per 15 mL (480 mL) [contains ethanol 7%, propylene glycol; tropical fruit punch flavor] [DSC]

Lortab®: Hydrocodone bitartrate 10 mg and acetaminophen 300 mg per 15 mL (480 mL) [contains ethanol 7%, propylene glycol; tropical fruit punch flavor] [DSC]

Solution, oral: Hydrocodone bitartrate 7.5 mg and acetaminophen 325 mg per 15 mL; hydrocodone bitartrate 7.5 mg and acetaminophen 500 mg per 15 mL (5 mL [DSC], 10 mL [DSC], 15 mL [DSC], 118 mL [DSC], 473 mL [DSC])

hycet®: Hydrocodone bitartrate 7.5 mg and acetaminophen 325 mg per 15 mL (473 mL) [contains ethanol 7%, propylene glycol; tropical fruit punch flavor]

Zamicet™: Hydrocodone bitartrate 10 mg and acetaminophen 325 mg per 15 mL (473 mL) [contains ethanol 6.7%, propylene glycol; fruit flavor] [DSC]

Zolvit®: Hydrocodone bitartrate 10 mg and acetaminophen 300 mg per 15 mL (480 mL) [contains ethanol 7%, propylene glycol; tropical fruit punch flavor] [DSC]

Tablet, oral:

Hydrocodone bitartrate 2.5 mg and acetaminophen 325 mg

Hydrocodone bitartrate 2.5 mg and acetaminophen 500 mg [DSC]

Hydrocodone bitartrate 5 mg and acetaminophen 300 mg

Hydrocodone bitartrate 5 mg and acetaminophen 325 mg

Hydrocodone bitartrate 5 mg and acetaminophen 500 mg [DSC]

Hydrocodone bitartrate 7.5 mg and acetaminophen 300 mg

Hydrocodone bitartrate 7.5 mg and acetaminophen 325 mg

Hydrocodone bitartrate 7.5 mg and acetaminophen 500 mg [DSC]

Hydrocodone bitartrate 7.5 mg and acetaminophen 650 mg [DSC]

Hydrocodone bitartrate 7.5 mg and acetaminophen 750 mg DSC]

Hydrocodone bitartrate 10 mg and acetaminophen 300 mg

Hydrocodone bitartrate 10 mg and acetaminophen 325 mg

Hydrocodone bitartrate 10 mg and acetaminophen 500 mg [DSC]

Hydrocodone bitartrate 10 mg and acetaminophen 650 mg DSC]

Hydrocodone bitartrate 10 mg and acetaminophen 750 mg [DSC]

Lorcet® 10/650: Hydrocodone bitartrate 10 mg and acetaminophen 650 mg [DSC]

Lorcet® Plus: Hydrocodone bitartrate 7.5 mg and acetaminophen 650 mg [DSC]

Lortab®:

5/500: Hydrocodone bitartrate 5 mg and acetaminophen 500 mg [DSC]

7.5/500: Hydrocodone bitartrate 7.5 mg and acetaminophen 500 mg [DSC]

10/500: Hydrocodone bitartrate 10 mg and acetaminophen 500 mg [DSC]

Maxidone®: Hydrocodone bitartrate 10 mg and acetaminophen 750 mg [DSC]

Norco®:

Hydrocodone bitartrate 5 mg and acetaminophen 325 mg

Hydrocodone bitartrate 7.5 mg and acetaminophen 325 mg

Hydrocodone bitartrate 10 mg and acetaminophen 325 mg

Verdrocet: Hydrocodone bitartrate 2.5 mg and acetaminophen 325 mg

Vicodin®: Hydrocodone bitartrate 5 mg and acetaminophen 300 mg

Vicodin ES®: Hydrocodone bitartrate 7.5 mg and acetaminophen 300 mg

Vicodin HP®: Hydrocodone bitartrate 10 mg and acetaminophen 300 mg

Xodol®:

5/300: Hydrocodone bitartrate 5 mg and acetaminophen 300 mg

7.5/300: Hydrocodone bitartrate 7.5 mg and acetaminophen 300 mg

10/300: Hydrocodone bitartrate 10 mg and acetaminophen 300 mg

Zydone®:

Hydrocodone bitartrate 5 mg and acetaminophen 400 mg [DSC]

Hydrocodone bitartrate 7.5 mg and acetaminophen 400 mg [DSC]

Hydrocodone bitartrate 10 mg and acetaminophen 400 mg [DSC]

Hydrocodone and Chlorpheniramine

(hye droe KOE done & klor fen IR a meen)

Medication Safety Issues

Sound-alike/look-alike issues:

Tussionex represents a different product in the U.S. than it does in Canada. In the U.S., Tussionex (Pennkinetic) contains hydrocodone and chlorpheniramine, while in Canada the product bearing this name contains hydrocodone and phenyltoloxamine.

High alert medication:

The Institute for Safe Medication Practices (ISMP) includes this medication among its list of drug classes which have a heightened risk of causing significant patient harm when used in error.

Brand Names: US TussiCaps; Tussionex Pennkinetic; Vituz

Therapeutic Category Antihistamine; Antitussive; Cough Preparation

Generic Availability (US) Yes: Extended release suspension

Use Symptomatic relief of cough and upper respiratory symptoms associated with cold and allergy (Extended release: Capsules, Suspension: FDA approved in ages ≥6 years and adults; Immediate release: Oral solution: FDA approved in ages ≥18 years and adults)

Pregnancy Risk Factor C

Pregnancy Considerations Animal reproduction studies have not been conducted with this combination product. See individual agents.

Breast-Feeding Considerations Hydrocodone and chlorpheniramine are excreted into breast milk. Due to the potential for serious adverse reactions in the nursing infant, the manufacturer recommends a decision be made whether to discontinue nursing or to discontinue the drug, taking into account the importance of treatment to the mother. See individual agents.

Contraindications Hypersensitivity to hydrocodone, chlorpheniramine, or any component of the formulation

ER capsule and ER suspension: Additional contraindications: Use in children <6 years of age due to the risk of fatal respiratory depression

Solution: Additional contraindications: Concurrent use during or within 14 days of MAO inhibitor therapy, narrow angle glaucoma, urinary retention, severe hypertension, severe coronary artery disease

Warnings/Precautions See individual agents.

Warnings: Additional Pediatric Considerations Do not use to make an infant or child sleep.

Safety and efficacy for the use of cough and cold products in pediatric patients <4 years of age is limited; the AAP warns against the use of these products for respiratory illnesses in this age group. Serious adverse effects including death have been reported. Many of these products contain multiple active ingredients, increasing the risk of accidental overdose when used with other products. Health care providers are reminded to ask caregivers about the use of OTC cough and cold products in order to avoid exposure to multiple medications containing the same ingredient (AAP 2012; FDA 2008).

Some dosage forms may contain propylene glycol; in neonates large amounts of propylene glycol delivered orally, intravenously (eg, >3,000 mg/day), or topically have been associated with potentially fatal toxicities which can include metabolic acidosis, seizures, renal failure, and CNS depression; toxicities have also been reported in children and adults including hyperosmolality, lactic acidosis, seizures and respiratory depression; use caution (AAP 1997; Shehab 2009).

Adverse Reactions Also refer to Chlorpheniramine monograph.

Cardiovascular: Chest tightness

Central nervous system: Agitation, anxiety, confusion, decreased mental acuity, dizziness, drowsiness, drug dependence, dysphoria, euphoria, fear, headache, irritability, lethargy, mood changes, sedation

Dermatologic: Diaphoresis, erythema, pruritus, skin rash, urticaria

Gastrointestinal: Abdominal distention, abdominal pain, acute pancreatitis, constipation, decreased appetite, dyspepsia, epigastric distress, nausea, vomiting, xerostomia

Genitourinary: Dysuria, ureteral spasm, urinary frequency, urinary hesitancy, urinary retention

Neuromuscular & skeletal: Facial dyskinesia, tremor, vesicle sphincter spasm

Ophthalmic: Blurred vision, diplopia, visual disturbance

Respiratory: Dry throat, dyspnea, laryngismus, respiratory depression, wheezing

Rare but important or life-threatening: Hypogonadism (Brennan, 2013; Debono, 2011)

Drug Interactions

Metabolism/Transport Effects Refer to individual components.

Avoid Concomitant Use

Avoid concomitant use of Hydrocodone and Chlorpheniramine with any of the following: Aclidinium; Alcohol (Ethyl); Azelastine (Nasal); Conivaptan; Eluxadoline; Fusidic Acid (Systemic); Glucagon; Idelalisib; Ipratropium (Oral Inhalation); MAO Inhibitors; Mixed Agonist / Antagonist Opioids; Orphenadrine; Paraldehyde; Potassium Chloride; Thalidomide; Tiotropium; Umeclidinium

Increased Effect/Toxicity

Hydrocodone and Chlorpheniramine may increase the levels/effects of: AbobotulinumtoxinA; Alvimopan; Anticholinergic Agents; Azelastine (Nasal); Desmopressin; Diuretics; Eluxadoline; Glucagon; Hydrocodone; Methotrimeprazine; Metyrosine; Mirabegron; OnabotulinumtoxinA; Orphenadrine; Paraldehyde; Potassium Chloride; Pramipexole; RimabotulinumtoxinB; ROPINIRole; Rotigotine; Selective Serotonin Reuptake Inhibitors; Suvorexant; Thalidomide; Thiazide Diuretics; Thioridazine; Tiotropium; Zolpidem

The levels/effects of Hydrocodone and Chlorpheniramine may be increased by: Abiraterone Acetate; Aclidinium; Alcohol (Ethyl); Amphetamines; Anticholinergic Agents; Aprepitant; Brimonidine (Topical); Cannabis; Ceritinib; CNS Depressants; Cobicistat; Conivaptan; CYP2D6 Inhibitors (Moderate); CYP2D6 Inhibitors (Strong); CYP3A4 Inhibitors (Moderate); CYP3A4 Inhibitors (Strong); CYP3A4 Inhibitors (Weak); Darunavir; Dasatinib; Dronabinol; Droperidol; Fosaprepitant; Fusidic Acid (Systemic); Idelalisib; Ipratropium (Oral Inhalation); Ivacaftor; Kava Kava; Luliconazole; Magnesium Sulfate; MAO Inhibitors; Methotrimeprazine; Mifepristone; Nabilone; Netupitant; Palbociclib; Panobinostat; Peginterferon Alfa-2b; Perampanel; Pramlintide; Rufinamide; Simeprevir; Sodium Oxybate; Stiripentol; Succinylcholine; Tapentadol; Tetrahydrocannabinol; Thioridazine; Umeclidinium

Decreased Effect

Hydrocodone and Chlorpheniramine may decrease the levels/effects of: Acetylcholinesterase Inhibitors; Benzylpenicilloyl Polylysine; Betahistine; Hyaluronidase; Itopride; Metoclopramide; Pegvisomant; Secretin

The levels/effects of Hydrocodone and Chlorpheniramine may be decreased by: Acetylcholinesterase Inhibitors; Ammonium Chloride; Amphetamines; Bosentan; CYP3A4 Inducers (Moderate); CYP3A4 Inducers (Strong); CYP3A4 Inducers (Weak); Dabrafenib; Deferasirox; Mitotane; Mixed Agonist / Antagonist Opioids; Naltrexone; Peginterferon Alfa-2b; Siltuximab; St Johns Wort; Tocilizumab

Storage/Stability Store at 20°C to 25°C (68°F to 77°F); protect from light.

Mechanism of Action

Hydrocodone binds to opiate receptors in the CNS, altering the perception of and response to pain; suppresses cough in medullary center; produces generalized CNS depression

Chlorpheniramine competes with histamine for H_1-receptor sites on effector cells in the gastrointestinal tract, blood vessels, and respiratory tract

Pharmacodynamics

Onset of action: Chlorpheniramine: 6 hours

Duration: Chlorpheniramine: 24 hours

Pharmacokinetics (Adult data unless noted)

Distribution: V_d: Chlorpheniramine:

- Children: 3.8 L/kg
- Adults: 2.5-3.2 L/kg

Protein binding: Chlorpheniramine: 69% to 72%

Metabolism:

- Chlorpheniramine: Substantial metabolism in GI mucosa and on first pass through liver
- Hydrocodone: O-demethylation via primarily CYP2D6 to hydromorphone (major, active metabolite with ~10- to 33-fold higher or as much as a >100-fold higher binding affinity for the mu-opioid receptor than hydrocodone); N-demethylation via CYP3A4 to norhydrocodone (major metabolite); and ~40% of metabolism/clearance occurs via other non-CYP pathways, including 6-ketosteroid reduction to 6-alpha-hydrocol and 6-beta-hydrocol, and other elimination pathways (eg, fecal, biliary, intestinal, renal) (Hutchinson, 2004; Volpe, 2011; Zhou, 2009)

Half-life elimination:

- Chlorpheniramine:
  - Children: Average: 9.6-13.1 hours (range: 5.2-23.1 hours)
  - Adults: 12-43 hours
- Hydrocodone: ~4 hours

Time to peak serum concentration:

- Extended release suspension:
  - Chlorpheniramine: 6.3 hours
  - Hydrocodone: 3.4 hours
- Immediate release oral solution:
  - Chlorpheniramine: 3.5 hours
  - Hydrocodone: 1.4 hours

Elimination:

- Chlorpheniramine: 35% excreted in 48 hours
- Hydrocodone: Urine (26% of single dose in 72 hours, with ~12% as unchanged drug, 5% as norhydrocodone, 4% as conjugated hydrocodone, 3% as 6-hydrocodol, and 0.21% as conjugated 6-hydromorphol) (Zhou, 2009)

Dosing: Usual Note: Dosage units vary based on product (mg, mL, capsules, or tablets); use caution when verifying dose with product formulation.

Pediatric: **Cough (antitussive/antihistamine):** Oral:
Note: Immediate release oral solution is **NOT** indicated for patients <18 years.
Children 6 to <12 years: Extended release:
Capsules (hydrocodone 5 mg and chlorpheniramine 4 mg per capsule): One capsule every 12 hours; maximum daily dose: 2 capsules/24 hours
Suspension (hydrocodone 10 mg and chlorpheniramine 8 mg per 5 mL): 2.5 mL every 12 hours; maximum daily dose: 5 mL/24 hours
Children ≥12 years and Adolescents: Extended release:
Capsules (hydrocodone 10 mg and chlorpheniramine 8 mg per capsule): One capsule every 12 hours; maximum daily dose: 2 capsules/24 hours
Suspension: (hydrocodone 10 mg and chlorpheniramine 8 mg per 5 mL): 5 mL every 12 hours; maximum daily dose: 10 mL/24 hours
Adult: **Cough (antitussive/antihistamine):** Oral:
Immediate release: Oral solution: 5 mL every 4-6 hours as needed; maximum daily dose: 20 mL/24 hours
Extended release:
Capsules (hydrocodone 10 mg and chlorpheniramine 8 mg per capsule): One capsule every 12 hours; maximum daily dose: 2 capsules/24 hours
Suspension: 5 mL every 12 hours; maximum daily dose: 10 mL/24 hours

Dosing adjustment in renal impairment: There are no dosage adjustments provided in the manufacturer's labeling; use with caution.

Dosing adjustment in hepatic impairment: There are no dosage adjustments provided in the manufacturer's labeling; use with caution.

Administration
Extended release:
Capsules: Administer without regard to meals. Do not dilute with fluid or mix with other medications. Do not give more frequently than every 12 hours.
Suspension: Shake well before using. Do not dilute with fluid or mix with other medications. Use calibrated oral syringe to measure doses. Do not give more frequently than every 12 hours.
Immediate release: Oral solution: To prevent overdose, use calibrated oral syringe to measure doses.

Test Interactions Chlorpheniramine: May suppress the wheal and flare reactions to skin test antigens.

Controlled Substance C-II

Dosage Forms Excipient information presented when available (limited, particularly for generics); consult specific product labeling.
Capsule, extended release, oral:
TussiCaps® 5/4: Hydrocodone polistirex [equivalent to hydrocodone bitartrate 5 mg] and chlorpheniramine polistirex [equivalent to chlorpheniramine maleate 4 mg]
TussiCaps® 10/8: Hydrocodone polistirex [equivalent to hydrocodone bitartrate 10 mg] and chlorpheniramine polistirex [equivalent to chlorpheniramine maleate 8 mg]
Solution, oral:
Vituz®: Hydrocodone bitartrate 5 mg and chlorpheniramine maleate 4 mg per 5 mL (480 mL) [contains propylene glycol; grape flavor]
Suspension, extended release, oral: Hydrocodone polistirex [equivalent to hydrocodone bitartrate 10 mg] and chlorpheniramine polistirex [equivalent to chlorpheniramine maleate 8 mg] per 5 mL (480 mL)
Tussionex® Pennkinetic®: Hydrocodone polistirex [equivalent to hydrocodone bitartrate 10 mg] and chlorpheniramine polistirex [equivalent to chlorpheniramine maleate 8 mg] per 5 mL (115 mL, 480 mL [DSC]) [contains propylene glycol]

Hydrocodone and Homatropine

(hye droe KOE done & hoe MA troe peen)

Medication Safety Issues
Sound-alike/look-alike issues:
Hycodan may be confused with Vicodin
High alert medication:
The Institute for Safe Medication Practices (ISMP) includes this medication among its list of drug classes which have a heightened risk of causing significant patient harm when used in error.

Brand Names: US Hydromet; Tussigon

Therapeutic Category Antitussive; Cough Preparation

Generic Availability (US) Yes

Use Symptomatic relief of cough (FDA approved in ages ≥6 years and adults)

Pregnancy Risk Factor C

Pregnancy Considerations Animal reproduction studies have not been conducted with this combination. See individual agents.

Breast-Feeding Considerations Hydrocodone and homatropine are excreted in breast milk. Due to the potential for serious adverse reactions in the nursing infant, the manufacturer recommends a decision be made whether to discontinue nursing or to discontinue the drug, taking into account the importance of treatment to the mother. See individual agents.

Contraindications
Hypersensitivity to hydrocodone, homatropine, or any component of the formulation.
Documentation of allergenic cross-reactivity for drugs in these classes is limited. However, because of similarities in chemical structure and/or pharmacologic actions, the possibility of cross-sensitivity cannot be ruled out with certainty.

Warnings/Precautions Causes sedation; caution must be used in performing tasks which require alertness (eg, operating machinery or driving). Effects may be potentiated when used with other sedative drugs or ethanol. Use with caution in patients with hypersensitivity reactions to other phenanthrene-derivative opioid agonists (morphine, codeine, hydromorphone, levorphanol, oxycodone, oxymorphone); should be used with caution in debilitated patients, and those with severe impairment of hepatic or renal function, prostatic hyperplasia, or urethral stricture. Also use caution in patients with head injury, increased intracranial pressure, acute abdomen, Addison's disease, glaucoma, or impaired thyroid function. Hydrocodone causes respiratory depression; caution should be exercised in patients with pulmonary diseases (including asthma, emphysema, COPD). Tolerance or drug dependence may result from extended use; use caution in patients with history of substance abuse. Underlying cause of cough should be determined prior to prescribing.

Due to the role of CYP2D6 in the metabolism of hydrocodone to hydromorphone (an active metabolite with higher binding affinity to mu-opioid receptors compared to hydrocodone), patients with genetic variations of CYP2D6, including "poor metabolizers" or "extensive metabolizers," may have decreased or increased hydromorphone formation, respectively. Variable effects in positive and negative opioid effects have been reported in these patients; however, limited data exists to determine if clinically significant differences of analgesia and toxicity can be predicted based on CYP2D6 phenotype (Hutchinson, 2004; Otton, 1993; Zhou, 2009).

Respiratory depression may occur even at therapeutic dosages; use with extreme caution in children. Per the Beers Criteria, homatropine is highly anticholinergic and should be avoided in older adults.

Benzyl alcohol and derivatives: Some dosage forms may contain sodium benzoate/benzoic acid; benzoic acid (benzoate) is a metabolite of benzyl alcohol; large amounts of benzyl alcohol (≥99 mg/kg/day) have been associated with a potentially fatal toxicity ("gasping syndrome") in neonates; the "gasping syndrome" consists of metabolic acidosis, respiratory distress, gasping respirations, CNS dysfunction (including convulsions, intracranial hemorrhage), hypotension, and cardiovascular collapse (AAP, 1997; CDC, 1982); some data suggests that benzoate displaces bilirubin from protein binding sites (Ahlfors, 2001); avoid or use dosage forms containing benzyl alcohol derivative with caution in neonates. See manufacturer's labeling.

Propylene glycol: Some dosage forms may contain propylene glycol; large amounts are potentially toxic and have been associated hyperosmolality, lactic acidosis, seizures and respiratory depression; use caution (AAP, 1997; Zar, 2007).

Adverse Reactions

Central nervous system: Anxiety, dizziness, drowsiness, dysphoria, fear, lethargy, mental clouding, mental impairment, mood changes, sedation

Dermatologic: Pruritus, rash

Gastrointestinal: Constipation, nausea, vomiting, xerostomia

Genitourinary: Urinary retention, urinary tract spasm

Respiratory: Respiratory depression

Miscellaneous: Physical and psychological dependence with prolonged use

Rare but important or life-threatening: Cardiorespiratory arrest

Drug Interactions

Metabolism/Transport Effects Refer to individual components.

Avoid Concomitant Use

Avoid concomitant use of Hydrocodone and Homatropine with any of the following: Aclidinium; Alcohol (Ethyl); Azelastine (Nasal); Conivaptan; Eluxadoline; Fusidic Acid (Systemic); Glucagon; Idelalisib; Ipratropium (Oral Inhalation); MAO Inhibitors; Mixed Agonist / Antagonist Opioids; Orphenadrine; Paraldehyde; Potassium Chloride; Thalidomide; Tiotropium; Umeclidinium

Increased Effect/Toxicity

Hydrocodone and Homatropine may increase the levels/effects of: AbobotulinumtoxinA; Alvimopan; Analgesics (Opioid); Anticholinergic Agents; Azelastine (Nasal); Desmopressin; Diuretics; Eluxadoline; Glucagon; Methotrimeprazine; Metyrosine; Mirabegron; OnabotulinumtoxinA; Orphenadrine; Paraldehyde; Potassium Chloride; Pramipexole; RimabotulinumtoxinB; ROPINIRole; Rotigotine; Selective Serotonin Reuptake Inhibitors; Suvorexant; Thalidomide; Thiazide Diuretics; Tiotropium; Zolpidem

The levels/effects of Hydrocodone and Homatropine may be increased by: Aclidinium; Alcohol (Ethyl); Amphetamines; Anticholinergic Agents; Aprepitant; Brimonidine (Topical); Cannabis; Ceritinib; CNS Depressants; Conivaptan; CYP3A4 Inhibitors (Moderate); CYP3A4 Inhibitors (Strong); CYP3A4 Inhibitors (Weak); Dasatinib; Dronabinol; Droperidol; Fosaprepitant; Fusidic Acid (Systemic); Idelalisib; Ipratropium (Oral Inhalation); Ivacaftor; Kava Kava; Luliconazole; Magnesium Sulfate; MAO Inhibitors; Methotrimeprazine; Mifepristone; Nabilone; Netupitant; Palbociclib; Perampanel; Pramlintide; Rufinamide; Simeprevir; Sodium Oxybate; Stiripentol; Succinylcholine; Tapentadol; Tetrahydrocannabinol; Umeclidinium

Decreased Effect

Hydrocodone and Homatropine may decrease the levels/effects of: Acetylcholinesterase Inhibitors; Itopride; Metoclopramide; Pegvisomant; Secretin

The levels/effects of Hydrocodone and Homatropine may be decreased by: Acetylcholinesterase Inhibitors; Ammonium Chloride; Bosentan; CYP2D6 Inhibitors (Strong); CYP3A4 Inducers (Moderate); CYP3A4 Inducers (Strong); CYP3A4 Inducers (Weak); Dabrafenib; Deferasirox; Mitotane; Mixed Agonist / Antagonist Opioids; Naltrexone; QuiNIDine; Siltuximab; St Johns Wort; Tocilizumab

Storage/Stability Store at 15°C to 30°C (59°F to 86°F). Dispense in a tight, light-resistant container.

Mechanism of Action

Hydrocodone binds to opiate receptors in the CNS, altering the perception of and response to pain; suppresses cough in medullary center; produces generalized CNS depression.

Homatropine is an anticholinergic agent, present in a subtherapeutic amount to discourage deliberate overdose.

Pharmacokinetics (Adult data unless noted) Hydrocodone:

Metabolism: Hepatic; O-demethylation via primarily CYP2D6 to hydromorphone (major, active metabolite with ~10- to 33-fold higher or as much as a >100-fold higher binding affinity for the mu-opioid receptor than hydrocodone); N-demethylation via CYP3A4 to norhydrocodone (major metabolite); and ~40% of metabolism/clearance occurs via other non-CYP pathways, including 6-ketosteroid reduction to 6-alpha-hydrocol and 6-beta-hydrocol, and other elimination pathways (eg, fecal, biliary, intestinal, renal) (Hutchinson, 2004; Volpe, 2011; Zhou, 2009)

Half-life elimination: ~4 hours

Time to peak serum concentration: 1.3 ± 0.3 hours

Elimination: Urine (26% of single dose in 72 hours, with ~12% as unchanged drug, 5% as norhydrocodone, 4% as conjugated hydrocodone, 3% as 6-hydrocodol, and 0.21% as conjugated 6-hydromorphol) (Zhou, 2009)

Dosing: Usual

Pediatric: **Cough (antitussive):** Oral:

Tablet (Hydrocodone 5 mg and homatropine 1.5 mg per tablet):

Children 6-12 years: One-half (1/2) tablet every 4-6 hours as needed; maximum daily dose: 3 tablets/24 hours

Adolescents: One tablet every 4-6 hours as needed; maximum daily dose: 6 tablets/24 hours

Syrup (Hydrocodone 5 mg and homatropine 1.5 mg per 5 mL):

Children 6-12 years: 2.5 mL every 4-6 hours as needed; maximum daily dose: 15 mL/24 hours

Adolescents: 5 mL every 4-6 hours as needed; maximum daily dose: 30 mL/24 hours

Adult: **Cough (antitussive):** Oral:

Tablet (Hydrocodone 5 mg and homatropine 1.5 mg): One tablet every 4-6 hours as needed; maximum daily dose: 6 tablets/24 hours

Syrup: 5 mL every 4-6 hours as needed; maximum daily dose: 30 mL/24 hours

Dosing adjustment in renal impairment: There are no dosage adjustments provided in the manufacturer's labeling.

Dosing adjustment in hepatic impairment: There are no dosage adjustments provided in the manufacturer's labeling.

Administration To prevent overdose, administer syrup with an accurate measuring device (not a household teaspoon).

Test Interactions Increased ALT, AST

Controlled Substance C-II

Dosage Forms Excipient information presented when available (limited, particularly for generics); consult specific product labeling. [DSC] = Discontinued product

Syrup:

Hydromet: Hydrocodone bitartrate 5 mg and homatropine methylbromide 1.5 mg per 5 mL (480 mL) [cherry flavor]

Generic: Hydrocodone bitartrate 5 mg and homatropine methylbromide 1.5 mg per 5 mL (473 mL)

Tablet:

Tussigon: Hydrocodone bitartrate 5 mg and homatropine methylbromide 1.5 mg

Generic: Hydrocodone bitartrate 5 mg and homatropine methylbromide 1.5 mg

◆ **Hydrocodone Bitartrate and Homatropine Methylbromide** *see* Hydrocodone and Homatropine *on page 1036*

◆ **Hydrocodone Polistirex and Chlorpheniramine Polistirex** *see* Hydrocodone and Chlorpheniramine *on page 1034*

Hydrocortisone (Systemic)

(hye droe KOR ti sone)

Medication Safety Issues

Sound-alike/look-alike issues:

Hydrocortisone may be confused with hydrocodone, hydroxychloroquine, hydrochlorothiazide

Cortef may be confused with Coreg, Lortab

HCT (occasional abbreviation for hydrocortisone) is an error-prone abbreviation (mistaken as hydrochlorothiazide)

Solu-CORTEF may be confused with Solu-MEDROL

Related Information

Corticosteroids Systemic Equivalencies *on page 2260*

Prevention of Chemotherapy-Induced Nausea and Vomiting in Children *on page 2368*

Brand Names: US A-Hydrocort; Cortef; Solu-CORTEF

Brand Names: Canada Cortef; Solu-Cortef

Therapeutic Category Adrenal Corticosteroid; Anti-inflammatory Agent; Antiasthmatic; Corticosteroid, Systemic; Glucocorticoid

Generic Availability (US) May be product dependent

Use Anti-inflammatory or immunosuppressant agent in the treatment of a variety of diseases, including those of allergic, hematologic, dermatologic, gastrointestinal, ophthalmic, neoplastic, rheumatic, autoimmune, nervous system, renal, and respiratory origin [FDA approved in pediatric patients (age not specified) and adults]; primary or secondary adrenocorticoid deficiency (drug of choice) [FDA approved in pediatric patients (age not specified) and adults]; has also been used for management of septic shock and in neonates for treatment of hypotension and prevention of bronchopulmonary dysplasia

Pregnancy Risk Factor C

Pregnancy Considerations Adverse events have been observed with corticosteroids in animal reproduction studies. Some studies have shown an association between first trimester systemic corticosteroid use and oral clefts (Park-Wyllie, 2000; Pradat, 2003). Systemic corticosteroids may also influence fetal growth (decreased birth weight); however, information is conflicting (Lunghi, 2010). Hypoadrenalism may occur in newborns following maternal use of corticosteroids in pregnancy (monitor). When systemic corticosteroids are needed in pregnancy, it is generally recommended to use the lowest effective dose for the shortest duration of time, avoiding high doses during the first trimester (Leachman, 2006; Lunghi, 2010; Makol, 2011; Østensen, 2009).

Breast-Feeding Considerations Corticosteroids are excreted in breast milk. The manufacturer notes that when used systemically, maternal use of corticosteroids have the potential to cause adverse events in a nursing infant (eg, growth suppression, interfere with endogenous corticosteroid production). If there is concern about exposure to the infant, some guidelines recommend waiting 4 hours after the maternal dose of an oral systemic corticosteroid before breast-feeding in order to decrease potential exposure to the nursing infant (based on a study using prednisolone) (Bae, 2011; Leachman, 2006; Makol, 2011; Ost, 1985).

Contraindications Hypersensitivity to hydrocortisone or any component of the formulation; systemic fungal infections; serious infections, except septic shock or tuberculous meningitis; viral, fungal, or tubercular skin lesions; IM administration contraindicated in idiopathic thrombocytopenia purpura; intrathecal administration of injection

Warnings/Precautions Corticosteroids are not approved for epidural injection. Serious neurologic events (eg, spinal cord infarction, paraplegia, quadriplegia, cortical blindness, stroke), some resulting in death, have been reported with epidural injection of corticosteroids, with and without use of fluoroscopy. Avoid injection or leakage into the dermis; dermal and/or subdermal skin depression may occur at the site of injection. Avoid deltoid muscle injection; subcutaneous atrophy may occur.

Use with caution in patients with thyroid disease, hepatic impairment, renal impairment, heart failure, hypertension, diabetes, glaucoma, cataracts, myasthenia gravis, osteoporosis, seizures, or GI diseases (diverticulitis, intestinal anastomoses, peptic ulcer, ulcerative colitis) due to perforation risk. Avoid ethanol may enhance gastric mucosal irritation. Use caution following acute MI (corticosteroids have been associated with myocardial rupture). Because of the risk of adverse effects, systemic corticosteroids should be used cautiously in the elderly in the smallest possible effective dose for the shortest duration. May affect growth velocity; growth should be routinely monitored in pediatric patients. Withdraw therapy with gradual tapering of dose. Patients may require higher doses when subject to stress (ie, trauma, surgery, severe infection).

May cause hypercorticism or suppression of hypothalamic-pituitary-adrenal (HPA) axis, particularly in younger children or in patients receiving high doses for prolonged periods. HPA axis suppression may lead to adrenal crisis. Withdrawal and discontinuation of a corticosteroid should be done slowly and carefully. Particular care is required when patients are transferred from systemic corticosteroids to inhaled products due to possible adrenal insufficiency or withdrawal from steroids, including an increase in allergic symptoms. Adult patients receiving >20 mg per day of prednisone (or equivalent) may be most susceptible. Fatalities have occurred due to adrenal insufficiency in asthmatic patients during and after transfer from systemic corticosteroids to aerosol steroids; aerosol steroids do not provide the systemic steroid needed to treat patients having trauma, surgery, or infections.

Acute myopathy has been reported with high dose corticosteroids, usually in patients with neuromuscular transmission disorders; may involve ocular and/or respiratory muscles; monitor creatine kinase; recovery may be delayed. Corticosteroid use may cause psychiatric disturbances, including depression, euphoria, insomnia, mood swings, and personality changes. Preexisting psychiatric conditions may be exacerbated by corticosteroid use. Prolonged use of corticosteroids may increase the incidence of secondary infection, mask acute infection (including fungal infections), prolong or exacerbate viral infections, or limit response to vaccines. Exposure to chickenpox should be avoided; corticosteroids should not be used to treat ocular herpes simplex. Corticosteroids should not be used for cerebral malaria, fungal infections, or viral hepatitis. Oral steroid treatment is not recommended for the treatment of acute optic neuritis. Close observation is required in patients with latent tuberculosis and/or TB reactivity; restrict use in active TB (only fulminating or disseminated TB in conjunction with antituberculosis treatment). Amebiasis should be ruled out in any patient with recent travel to tropic climates or unexplained diarrhea prior to initiation of corticosteroids. Prolonged treatment with corticosteroids has been associated with the development of Kaposi sarcoma (case reports); if noted, discontinuation of therapy should be considered. High-dose corticosteroids should not be used to manage acute head injury. Potentially significant drug-drug interactions may exist, requiring dose or frequency adjustment, additional monitoring, and/or selection of alternative therapy.

Benzyl alcohol and derivatives: Diluent for injection may contain benzyl alcohol and some dosage forms may contain sodium benzoate/benzoic acid; benzoic acid (benzoate) is a metabolite of benzyl alcohol; large amounts of benzyl alcohol (≥99 mg/kg/day) have been associated with a potentially fatal toxicity ("gasping syndrome") in neonates; the "gasping syndrome" consists of metabolic acidosis, respiratory distress, gasping respirations, CNS dysfunction (including convulsions, intracranial hemorrhage), hypotension and cardiovascular collapse (AAP, 1997; CDC, 1982); some data suggests that benzoate displaces bilirubin from protein binding sites (Ahlfors, 2001); avoid or use dosage forms containing benzyl alcohol and/or benzyl alcohol derivative with caution in neonates. See manufacturer's labeling.

Warnings: Additional Pediatric Considerations May cause osteoporosis (at any age) or inhibition of bone growth in pediatric patients. Use with caution in patients with osteoporosis. In a population-based study of children, risk of fracture was shown to be increased with >4 courses of corticosteroids; underlying clinical condition may also impact bone health and osteoporotic effect of corticosteroids (Leonard, 2007). In premature neonates, reports of gastrointestinal perforation in the hydrocortisone treatment arm have resulted in the closure of two large BPD clinical trials (Peltoniemi, 2005; Watterberg, 2004); concomitant use with indomethacin or ibuprofen may increase the risk and should be avoided in this population (Seri, 2006). Increased IOP may occur especially with prolonged use; in children, increased IOP has been shown to be dose dependent and produce a greater IOP in children <6 years than older children treated with ophthalmic dexamethasone (Lam, 2005). Hypertrophic cardiomyopathy has been reported in premature neonates.

Adverse Reactions

Cardiovascular: Arrhythmias, bradycardia, cardiac arrest, cardiomegaly, circulatory collapse, congestive heart failure, edema, fat embolism, hypertension, hypertrophic cardiomyopathy (premature infants), myocardial rupture (post MI), syncope, tachycardia, thromboembolism, vasculitis

Central nervous system: Delirium, depression, emotional instability, euphoria, hallucinations, headache, insomnia, intracranial pressure increased, malaise, mood swings, nervousness, neuritis, neuropathy, personality changes, pseudotumor cerebri, psychic disorders, psychoses, seizure, vertigo

Dermatologic: Acne, allergic dermatitis, alopecia, bruising, burning/tingling, dry scaly skin, edema, erythema, hirsutism, hyper-/hypopigmentation, impaired wound healing, petechiae, rash, skin atrophy, skin test reaction impaired, sterile abscess, striae, urticaria

Endocrine & metabolic: Adrenal suppression, alkalosis, amenorrhea, carbohydrate intolerance increased, Cushing's syndrome, diabetes mellitus, glucose intolerance, growth suppression, hyperglycemia, hyperlipidemia, hypokalemia, hypokalemic alkalosis, menstrual irregularities, negative nitrogen balance, pituitary-adrenal axis suppression, potassium loss, protein catabolism, sodium and water retention, sperm motility increased/decreased, spermatogenesis increased/decreased

Gastrointestinal: Abdominal distention, appetite increased, bowel dysfunction (intrathecal administration), indigestion, nausea, pancreatitis, peptic ulcer, gastrointestinal perforation, ulcerative esophagitis, vomiting, weight gain

Genitourinary: Bladder dysfunction (intrathecal administration)

Hematologic: Leukocytosis (transient)

Hepatic: Hepatomegaly, transaminases increased

Local: Atrophy (at injection site), postinjection flare (intra-articular use), thrombophlebitis

Neuromuscular & skeletal: Arthralgia, necrosis (femoral and humoral heads), Charcot-like arthropathy, fractures, muscle mass loss, muscle weakness, myopathy, osteoporosis, tendon rupture, vertebral compression fractures

Ocular: Cataracts, exophthalmoses, glaucoma, intraocular pressure increased

Miscellaneous: Abnormal fat deposits, anaphylaxis, avascular necrosis, diaphoresis, hiccups, hypersensitivity reactions, infection, secondary malignancy

Drug Interactions

Metabolism/Transport Effects **Substrate** of CYP3A4 (minor), P-glycoprotein; **Note:** Assignment of Major/Minor substrate status based on clinically relevant drug interaction potential; **Induces** CYP3A4 (weak)

Avoid Concomitant Use

Avoid concomitant use of Hydrocortisone (Systemic) with any of the following: Aldesleukin; BCG; BCG (Intravesical); Indium 111 Capromab Pendetide; Mifepristone; Natalizumab; Pimecrolimus; Tacrolimus (Topical); Tofacitinib

Increased Effect/Toxicity

Hydrocortisone (Systemic) may increase the levels/effects of: Acetylcholinesterase Inhibitors; Amphotericin B; Androgens; Ceritinib; Deferasirox; Leflunomide; Loop Diuretics; Natalizumab; Nicorandil; NSAID (COX-2 Inhibitor); NSAID (Nonselective); Quinolone Antibiotics; Thiazide Diuretics; Tofacitinib; Vaccines (Live); Warfarin

The levels/effects of Hydrocortisone (Systemic) may be increased by: Aprepitant; CYP3A4 Inhibitors (Strong); Denosumab; Estrogen Derivatives; Fosaprepitant; Indacaterol; Mifepristone; Neuromuscular-Blocking Agents (Nondepolarizing); P-glycoprotein/ABCB1 Inhibitors; Pimecrolimus; Roflumilast; Salicylates; Tacrolimus (Topical); Telaprevir; Trastuzumab

Decreased Effect

Hydrocortisone (Systemic) may decrease the levels/effects of: Aldesleukin; Antidiabetic Agents; ARIPiprazole; BCG; BCG (Intravesical); Calcitriol (Systemic); Coccidioides immitis Skin Test; Corticorelin; Hyaluronidase; Hydrocodone; Indium 111 Capromab Pendetide; Isoniazid; NiMODipine; Salicylates; Saxagliptin; Sipuleucel-T; Telaprevir; Urea Cycle Disorder Agents; Vaccines (Inactivated); Vaccines (Live)

The levels/effects of Hydrocortisone (Systemic) may be decreased by: Antacids; Bile Acid Sequestrants; CYP3A4 Inducers (Strong); Echinacea; Mifepristone; Mitotane; P-glycoprotein/ABCB1 Inducers

Storage/Stability Store at controlled room temperature 20°C to 25°C (68°F to 77°F). Protect from light. Hydrocortisone sodium phosphate and hydrocortisone sodium succinate are clear, light yellow solutions which are heat labile.

Sodium succinate: After initial reconstitution, hydrocortisone sodium succinate solutions are stable for 3 days at room temperature or under refrigeration when protected from light. Stability of parenteral admixture (Solu-Cortef®) at room temperature (25°C) and at refrigeration temperature (4°C) is concentration-dependent:

Stability of concentration 1 mg/mL: 24 hours

Stability of concentration 2 mg/mL to 60 mg/mL: At least 4 hours

Mechanism of Action Short-acting corticosteroid with minimal sodium-retaining potential; decreases inflammation by suppression of migration of polymorphonuclear leukocytes and reversal of increased capillary permeability

Pharmacodynamics Anti-inflammatory effects:

Maximum effect:

Oral: 12-24 hours

IV: 4-6 hours

Duration: 8-12 hours

Pharmacokinetics (Adult data unless noted)

Absorption: Rapid

Metabolism: In the liver

Half-life, biologic: 8-12 hours

Elimination: Renally, mainly as 17-hydroxysteroids and 17-ketosteroids

Dosing: Neonatal Dose should be based on severity of disease and patient response.

Bronchopulmonary dysplasia, prevention (preterm neonates with prenatal inflammatory exposure): PNA ≤48 hours: IV: 1 mg/kg/day divided every 12 hours for 9 or 12 days followed by 0.5 mg/kg/day divided every 12 hours for 3 days; low-dose (ie, physiologic replacement) has been shown to be effective at improving survival without BPD in chorioamnionitis-exposed ELBW neonates (birth weight: 500-999 g) (Watterberg, 1999; Watterberg, 2004; Watterberg, 2010); of note, a higher incidence of gastrointestinal perforation in the treatment arm resulted in early study closure of the largest trial (Watterberg, 2004). In another trial of VLBW neonates (PNA ≤36 hours, GA <30 weeks, birth weight: 500-1250 g), higher dosages (ie, stress dose): 2 mg/kg/day divided every 8 hours for 2 days followed by 1.5 mg/kg/day divided every 8 hours for 2 days followed by 0.75 mg/kg/day divided every 12 hours for 6 days showed a trend in the treatment arm of decreased severity of respiratory failure, shorten length of oxygen therapy and promotion of PDA closure; this trial was closed early due to higher incidence of gastrointestinal perforation in the treatment arm versus placebo (Peltoniemi, 2005). **Note:** The AAP suggests that for neonates with prenatal inflammatory exposure, low-dose hydrocortisone therapy (1 mg/kg/day) during the first 2 weeks of life may improve survival without BPD and without adverse neurodevelopmental outcomes (Watterberg, 2010).

Congenital adrenal hyperplasia: Oral [tablets (crushed)]: Initial: 10-15 mg/m^2/day in 3 divided doses; higher initial doses (20 mg/m^2/day) may be required to achieve initial target hormone serum concentrations. Administer morning dose as early as possible. Due to uneven distribution of the drug in the liquid, use of oral suspension is **not** recommended [AAP, 2000; Speiser (Endocrine Society), 2010]

Hypoglycemia, refractory (refractory to continuous glucose infusion of >12-15 mg/kg/minute): Oral, IV: 5 mg/kg/day divided every 8-12 hours or 1-2 mg/kg/**dose** every 6 hours

Hypotension, refractory; shock: IV: Limited data available; dosage regimens variable (Brierley, 2009; Higgins, 2010): 3 mg/kg/day divided every 8 hours for 5 days; dosing based on the largest, prospective, randomized, placebo-controlled trial of 48 hypotensive, VLBW neonates (PNA: <7 days; GA: <32 weeks; birth weight: <1500 g) who were also receiving dopamine at doses ≥10 mcg/kg/minute (Ng, 2006); other smaller trials have used 2 mg/kg/day divided every 12 hours for 1-3 days (Seri, 2001) or 2 mg/kg once, followed by 2 mg/kg/day divided every 12 hours for 4 doses (Noori, 2006)

Dosing: Usual Dose should be based on severity of disease and patient response.

Infants, Children, and Adolescents:

Adrenal insufficiency (acute): IM, IV:

Infants and young Children: 1-2 mg/kg/**dose** IV bolus, then 25-150 mg/day in divided doses every 6-8 hours

Older Children: 1-2 mg/kg/**dose** IV bolus, then 150-250 mg/day in divided doses every 6-8 hours

Anti-inflammatory or immunosuppressive:

Infants and Children:

Oral: 2.5-10 mg/kg/day or 75-300 mg/m^2/day divided every 6-8 hours

IM, IV: 1-5 mg/kg/day or 30-150 mg/m^2/day divided every 12-24 hours

Adolescents: Oral, IM, IV, SubQ: 15-240 mg every 12 hours

Congenital adrenal hyperplasia: Oral (tablets): AAP Recommendations: **Note:** Administer morning dose as early as possible. Tablets may result in more reliable serum concentrations than oral liquid formulation; use of oral suspension is not recommended. Individualize dose by monitoring growth, hormone levels, and bone age; mineralocorticoid (eg, fludrocortisone) and sodium supplement may be required in salt losers (AAP, 2000; AAP, 2010; Endocrine Society, 2010)

Initial: 10-15 mg/m^2/day in 3 divided doses; higher initial doses (20 mg/m^2/day) may be required to achieve initial target hormone serum concentrations (AAP, 2010; Endocrine Society, 2010).

Maintenance dose: Usual requirement:

Infants: 2.5-5 mg/**dose** 3 times/day

Children: 5-10 mg/**dose** 3 times/day;

Physiologic replacement: Infants and Children: Oral: 8-10 mg/m^2/day divided every 8 hours; up to 12 mg/m^2/day in some patients (Ahmet, 2011; Gupta, 2008; Maguire, 2007).

Septic shock: Infants, Children, and Adolescents: IV: Initial: 1-2 mg/kg/day (intermittent or as continuous IV infusion); doses may be titrated up to 50 mg/kg/day if necessary for shock reversal (Brierley, 2009); alternative dosing suggests 50 mg/m^2/day (Dellinger, 2008); **Note:** Use recommended only in catecholamine-resistant shock and suspected or proven adrenal insufficiency

Adults:

Adrenal insufficiency (acute): IM, IV: 100 mg IV bolus, then 300 mg/day in divided doses every 8 hours or as a continuous infusion for 48 hours; once patient is stable, change to oral, 50 mg every 8 hours for 6 doses, then taper to 30-50 mg/day in divided doses

Adrenal insufficiency (chronic), physiologic replacement: Oral: 15-25 mg/day in 2-3 divided doses. **Note:** Studies suggest administering one-half to two-thirds of the daily dose in the morning in order to mimic the physiological cortisol secretion pattern. If the twice-daily regimen is utilized, the second dose should be administered 6-8 hours following the first dose (Arlt, 2003).

Anti-inflammatory or immunosuppressive: Oral, IM, IV: 15-240 mg every 12 hours

Congenital adrenal hyperplasia: Oral: 15-25 mg/day in 2-3 divided doses (Speiser, 2010)

Septic shock: IV: 50 mg every 6 hours (Annane, 2002; Marik, 2008); not to exceed 300 mg/day (Dellinger, 2008). Practice guidelines also recommend alternative dosing of 100 mg bolus, followed by continuous infusion of 10 mg/hour (240 mg/day). Taper slowly (for total of 11 days) and do not stop abruptly. **Note:** Fludrocortisone is optional with use of hydrocortisone.

Status asthmaticus: IV: 1-2 mg/kg/dose every 6 hours for 24 hours, then maintenance of 0.5-1 mg/kg every 6 hours

Stress dosing (surgery) in patients known to be adrenally-suppressed or on chronic systemic steroids: IV:

Minor stress (ie, inguinal herniorrhaphy): 25 mg/day for 1 day

Moderate stress (ie, joint replacement, cholecystectomy): 50-75 mg/day (25 mg every 8-12 hours) for 1-2 days

Major stress (pancreatoduodenectomy, esophagogastrectomy, cardiac surgery): 100-150 mg/day (50 mg every 8-12 hours) for 2-3 days

Preparation for Administration

Parenteral: Reconstitute vial with appropriate diluent, either bacteriostatic water or NS (see manufacturer's labeling for details). For the commonly used 100 mg vial, reconstitute with a volume of diluent not to exceed 2 mL resulting in a concentration ≥ 50 mg/mL. Act-O-Vial (self-contained powder for injection plus diluent [preservative free SWFI]) may be reconstituted by pressing the activator to force diluent into the powder compartment. Following gentle agitation, solution may be withdrawn via syringe through a needle inserted into the center of the stopper. May be administered (IV or IM) without further dilution.

Intermittent IV infusion: Reconstituted solutions may be further diluted in an appropriate volume of compatible solution for infusion. Concentration should generally not exceed 1 mg/mL. In pediatric patients, a concentration of 5 mg/mL has been used (Miller 1980). The manufacturer suggests, in cases where administration of a small volume of fluid is desirable, concentrations up to 60 mg/mL (100 to 3,000 mg in 50 mL of D_5W or NS; stability limited to 4 hours) may be used.

Administration

Oral: Administer with food or milk to decrease GI upset

Parenteral: Hydrocortisone sodium succinate may be administered by IM or IV routes. Dermal and/or subdermal skin depression may occur at the site of injection.

IM: Avoid injection into deltoid muscle (high incidence of SubQ atrophy)

IV bolus: Administer undiluted over at least 30 seconds; for large doses (≥500 mg), administer over 10 minutes

Intermittent IV infusion: Further dilute in a compatible fluid and administer over 20 to 30 minutes (Miller 1980)

Monitoring Parameters Blood pressure; weight; serum glucose; electrolytes; growth in pediatric patients; presence of infection, bone mineral density; assess HPA axis suppression (eg, ACTH stimulation test, morning plasma cortisol test, urinary free cortisol test). Monitor IOP with therapy >6 weeks.

Reference Range Hydrocortisone (normal endogenous morning levels): 4-30 mcg/mL

Test Interactions Interferes with skin tests

Additional Information Cortef oral suspension was reformulated in July 1998; the suspending agent was changed from tragacanth to xanthan gum; this suspension was found **not** to be bioequivalent to hydrocortisone tablets in the treatment of children with congenital adrenal hyperplasia; children required higher doses of the suspension (19.6 mg/m^2/day) compared to the tablets (15.2 mg/m^2/day); based on these findings, Cortef suspension was voluntarily recalled from the market on July 18, 2000 (Merke 2001).

In premature neonates, the use of high-dose dexamethasone (approximately >0.5 mg/kg/day) for the prevention or treatment of BPD has been associated with adverse neurodevelopmental outcomes, including higher rates of cerebral palsy without additional clinical benefit over lower doses; current data does not support use of high doses. Data specific to hydrocortisone use in this population has shown that use <7 days of therapy does not appear to be associated with adverse neurodevelopmental outcomes (Needelman 2010).

Hydrocortisone has been studied in children with cystic fibrosis and an ongoing lower respiratory tract infection using 2.5 mg/kg/**dose** every 6 hours for 10 days in addition to standard therapies. A double-blind, placebo- controlled trial of 22 infants and children (age: <18 months; mean: 8.8 to 9.5 months) showed no significant difference in pulmonary function on day 10 of therapy between treatment and placebo groups; however, at 1 to 2 months after discharge, follow-up testing showed significant, sustained improvement of pulmonary function in the hydrocortisone group compared to placebo (Tepper 1997). Hydrocortisone is not recommended for routine use in current cystic fibrosis guidelines (Flume 2009).

Dosage Forms Excipient information presented when available (limited, particularly for generics); consult specific product labeling.

Solution Reconstituted, Injection, as sodium succinate [strength expressed as base]:
- A-Hydrocort: 100 mg (1 ea)
- Solu-CORTEF: 100 mg (1 ea)

Solution Reconstituted, Injection, as sodium succinate [strength expressed as base, preservative free]:
- Solu-CORTEF: 100 mg (1 ea); 250 mg (1 ea); 500 mg (1 ea); 1000 mg (1 ea)

Tablet, Oral, as base:
- Cortef: 5 mg, 10 mg, 20 mg [scored]
- Generic: 5 mg, 10 mg, 20 mg

Extemporaneous Preparations A 2.5 mg/mL oral suspension may be made with either tablets or powder and a vehicle containing sodium carboxymethylcellulose (1 g), syrup BP (10 mL), hydroxybenzoate 0.1% preservatives (0.1 g), polysorbate 80 (0.5 mL), citric acid (0.6 g), and water. To make the vehicle, dissolve the hydroxybenzoate, citric acid, and syrup BP in hot water. Cool solution and add the carboxymethylcellulose; leave overnight. Crush twelve-and-one-half 20 mg hydrocortisone tablets (or use 250 mg of powder) in a mortar and reduce to a fine powder while adding polysorbate 80. Add small portions of vehicle and mix to a uniform paste; mix while adding the vehicle in incremental proportions to **almost** 100 mL; transfer to a calibrated bottle, rinse mortar with vehicle, and add sufficient quantity of vehicle to make 100 mL. Label "shake well" and "refrigerate". Stable for 90 days.

Fawcett JP, Boulton DW, Jiang R, et al, "Stability of Hydrocortisone Oral Suspensions Prepared From Tablets and Powder," *Ann Pharmacother*, 1995, 29(10):987-90.

Hydrocortisone (Topical) (hye droe KOR ti sone)

Medication Safety Issues

Sound-alike/look-alike issues:

Hydrocortisone may be confused with hydrocodone, hydroxychloroquine, hydrochlorothiazide

Anusol® may be confused with Anusol-HC®, Aplisol®, Aquasol®

Cortizone® may be confused with cortisone

HCT (occasional abbreviation for hydrocortisone) is an error-prone abbreviation (mistaken as hydrochlorothiazide)

Hytone® may be confused with Vytone®

Proctocort® may be confused with ProctoCream®

International issues:

Nutracort [multiple international markets] may be confused with Nitrocor brand name of nitroglycerin [Italy, Russia, and Venezuela]

Related Information

Topical Corticosteroids *on page 2262*

Brand Names: US Ala Cort; Ala Scalp; Anti-Itch Maximum Strength [OTC]; Anucort-HC; Anusol-HC; Aquanil HC [OTC]; Beta HC [OTC]; Colocort; Cortaid Maximum Strength [OTC]; CortAlo; Cortenema; Corticool [OTC]; Cortifoam; Dermasorb HC; First-Hydrocortisone; GRx HiCort 25; Hemril-30 [DSC]; Hydro Skin Maximum

Strength [OTC]; Hydrocortisone Max St [OTC]; Hydrocortisone Max St/12 Moist [OTC]; HydroSKIN [OTC]; Instacort 10 [OTC]; Instacort 5 [OTC]; Locoid; Locoid Lipocream; Med-Derm Hydrocortisone [OTC]; Medi-First Hydrocortisone [OTC]; NuCort; NuZon [DSC]; Pandel; Pediaderm HC; Preparation H Hydrocortisone [OTC]; Procto-Pak; Proctocort; Proctosol HC; Proctozone-HC; Recort Plus [OTC]; Rectacort-HC; Rederm [OTC]; Sarnol-HC [OTC]; Scalacort; Scalacort DK; Scalpicin Maximum Strength [OTC]; Texacort; TheraCort [OTC]; Westcort

Brand Names: Canada Aquacort®; Cortamed®; Cortenema®; Cortifoam™; Emo-Cort®; Hycort™; Hyderm; HydroVal®; Locoid®; Prevex® HC; Sarna® HC; Westcort®

Therapeutic Category Anti-inflammatory Agent; Anti-inflammatory Agent, Rectal; Corticosteroid, Rectal; Corticosteroid, Topical; Glucocorticoid

Generic Availability (US) May be product dependent

Use Relief of inflammation and pruritus associated with corticosteroid-responsive dermatoses; adjunctive treatment of ulcerative colitis

Pregnancy Risk Factor C

Pregnancy Considerations Adverse events have been observed with corticosteroids in animal reproduction studies. Topical products are not recommended for extensive use, in large quantities, or for long periods of time in pregnant women (Reed, 1997).

Breast-Feeding Considerations Systemically administered corticosteroids are excreted in breast milk and endogenous hydrocortisone is also found in human milk. It is not known if systemic absorption following topical administration results in detectable quantities in human milk. Use with caution while breast-feeding; do not apply to nipples (Reed, 1997).

Contraindications Hypersensitivity to any component of the formulation.

Rectal enema: Systemic fungal infections; ileocolostomy during the immediate or early postoperative period

Cortifoam® is also contraindicated with obstruction, abscess, perforation, peritonitis, fresh intestinal anastomoses, extensive fistulas and sinus tracts (other enemas are labeled to be used with caution).

Warnings/Precautions May cause hypercorticism or suppression of hypothalamic-pituitary-adrenal (HPA) axis, particularly in younger children or in patients receiving high doses for prolonged periods. HPA axis suppression may lead to adrenal crisis. Withdrawal and discontinuation of a corticosteroid should be done slowly and carefully. Children may absorb proportionally larger amounts after topical application and may be more prone to systemic effects. HPA axis suppression, intracranial hypertension, and Cushing's syndrome have been reported in children receiving topical corticosteroids. Prolonged use may affect growth velocity; growth should be routinely monitored in pediatric patients. Rare cases of anaphylactoid reactions have been observed in patients receiving corticosteroids.

Prolonged use of corticosteroids may increase the incidence of secondary infection, mask acute infection (including fungal infections), prolong or exacerbate viral infections, or limit response to vaccines. Exposure to chickenpox should be avoided. Close observation is required in patients with latent tuberculosis and/or TB reactivity; restrict use in active TB (only in conjunction with antituberculosis treatment). Prolonged treatment with corticosteroids has been also associated with the development of Kaposi's sarcoma (case reports); if noted, discontinuation of therapy should be considered. Prolonged use of corticosteroids may produce cataracts or glaucoma and may enhance the establishment of secondary ocular infections Use caution with ocular herpes simplex.

Acute myopathy has been reported with high-dose corticosteroids, usually in patients with neuromuscular transmission disorders; may involve ocular and/or respiratory muscles; monitor creatine kinase; recovery may be delayed. Corticosteroid use may cause psychiatric disturbances, including depression, euphoria, insomnia, mood swings, and personality changes. Preexisting psychiatric conditions may be exacerbated by corticosteroid use.

Use with caution in patients with hypertension, GI diseases (diverticulitis, peptic ulcer), hepatic impairment (including cirrhosis), osteoporosis, myasthenia gravis, osteoporosis, renal impairment, or thyroid disease. In patients with severe ulcerative colitis, it may be hazardous to delay surgery while waiting for response to treatment.

Topical corticosteroids may be absorbed percutaneously. Absorption is increased by the use of occlusive dressings, application to denuded skin, or application to large surface areas. Avoid use of topical preparations with occlusive dressings or on weeping or exudative lesions. Topical use has been associated with local sensitization (redness, irritation); discontinue if sensitization is noted. Because of the risk of adverse effects associated with systemic absorption, topical corticosteroids should be used cautiously in the elderly in the smallest possible effective dose for the shortest duration.

Benzyl alcohol and derivatives: Some dosage forms may contain benzyl alcohol; large amounts of benzyl alcohol (≥99 mg/kg/day) have been associated with a potentially fatal toxicity ("gasping syndrome") in neonates; the "gasping syndrome" consists of metabolic acidosis, respiratory distress, gasping respirations, CNS dysfunction (including convulsions, intracranial hemorrhage), hypotension, and cardiovascular collapse (AAP, 1997; CDC, 1982); some data suggests that benzoate displaces bilirubin from protein binding sites (Ahlfors, 2001); avoid or use dosage forms containing benzyl alcohol with caution in neonates. See manufacturer's labeling.

Rectal enema: Damage to the rectal wall may occur from improper or careless insertion of the enema tip.

Self-medication (OTC use): Contact healthcare provider if condition worsens, symptoms persist for >7 days, or rectal bleeding occurs. Consult with healthcare provider prior to use if needed for diaper rash.

Warnings: Additional Pediatric Considerations The extent of percutaneous absorption is dependent on several factors, including epidermal integrity (intact vs abraded skin), formulation, age of the patient, prolonged duration of use, and the use of occlusive dressings. Percutaneous absorption of topical steroids is increased in neonates (especially preterm neonates), infants, and young children. Infants and small children may be more susceptible to HPA axis suppression, intracranial hypertension, Cushing syndrome, or other systemic toxicities due to larger skin surface area to body mass ratio.

Some dosage forms may contain propylene glycol; in neonates large amounts of propylene glycol delivered orally, intravenously (eg, >3,000 mg/day), or topically have been associated with potentially fatal toxicities which can include metabolic acidosis, seizures, renal failure, and CNS depression; toxicities have also been reported in children and adults including hyperosmolality, lactic acidosis, seizures and respiratory depression; use caution (AAP, 1997; Shehab, 2009).

Adverse Reactions Local adverse events presented. Adverse events similar to those observed with systemic absorption are also observed, especially following rectal use. Refer to the Hydrocortisone (Systemic) monograph for details.

Cream, ointment: Acneiform eruptions, burning, dryness, folliculitis, hypertrichosis, hypopigmentation, irritation, itching, maceration of skin, miliaria, perioral dermatitis, secondary infection, skin atrophy, striae

Enema: Burning, pain, rectal bleeding

Suppositories: Allergic contact dermatitis, burning, dryness, folliculitis, hypopigmentation, itching, secondary infection

Drug Interactions

Metabolism/Transport Effects **Substrate** of CYP3A4 (minor); **Note:** Assignment of Major/Minor substrate status based on clinically relevant drug interaction potential

Avoid Concomitant Use

Avoid concomitant use of Hydrocortisone (Topical) with any of the following: Aldesleukin

Increased Effect/Toxicity

Hydrocortisone (Topical) may increase the levels/effects of: Ceritinib; Deferasirox

The levels/effects of Hydrocortisone (Topical) may be increased by: Telaprevir

Decreased Effect

Hydrocortisone (Topical) may decrease the levels/effects of: Aldesleukin; Corticorelin; Hyaluronidase; Telaprevir

Storage/Stability Store at controlled room temperature.

Mechanism of Action Topical corticosteroids have anti-inflammatory, antipruritic, and vasoconstrictive properties. May depress the formation, release, and activity of endogenous chemical mediators of inflammation (kinins, histamine, liposomal enzymes, prostaglandins) through the induction of phospholipase A_2 inhibitory proteins (lipocortins) and sequential inhibition of the release of arachidonic acid. Hydrocortisone has low to intermediate range potency (dosage-form dependent).

Pharmacokinetics (Adult data unless noted)

Absorption: Topical corticosteroids are absorbed percutaneously. The extent is dependent on several factors, including epidermal integrity (intact vs abraded skin), formulation, age of the patient, and the use of occlusive dressings. Percutaneous absorption of topical steroids is increased in neonates (especially preterm neonates), infants, and young children. Rectal absorption is more substantial than most topical preparations; therefore, systemic effects are more common.

Metabolism: In the liver

Half-life, biologic: 8-12 hours

Elimination: Renally, mainly as 17-hydroxysteroids and 17-ketosteroids

Dosing: Usual

Topical: Children and Adults: Usual: Apply 2-3 times/day (depending on severity); may be applied up to 4 times/day

Rectal: Adolescents and Adults: Insert 1 application 1-2 times/day for 2-3 weeks

Ulcerative colitis: One enema nightly for 21 days, or until remission occurs; clinical symptoms should subside within 3-5 days; discontinue use if no improvement within 2-3 weeks; some patients may require 2-3 months of therapy; if therapy lasts >21 days, discontinue slowly by decreasing use to every other night for 2-3 weeks

Administration

Rectal: Patient should lie on left side during administration and for 30 minutes after; retain enema for at least 1 hour, preferably all night

Topical: Apply a thin film to clean, dry skin and rub in gently; avoid contact with eyes. Do not apply to face, underarms, or groin unless directed by physician. Do not wrap or bandage affected area unless directed by physician. Do not apply to diaper areas because diapers or plastic pants may be occlusive.

Monitoring Parameters Growth in pediatric patients; assess HPA axis suppression in patients using topical steroids applied to a large surface area or to areas under occlusion (eg, ACTH stimulation test, morning plasma cortisol test, urinary free cortisol test).

Additional Information To facilitate retention of enema, prior antidiarrheal medication or sedation may be required (especially when beginning therapy)

Dosage Forms Excipient information presented when available (limited, particularly for generics); consult specific product labeling. [DSC] = Discontinued product

Cream, External, as acetate:
- Hydrocortisone Max St: 1% (28.4 g)

Cream, External, as base:
- Ala Cort: 1% (28.4 g, 85.2 g) [contains cetyl alcohol, propylene glycol]
- Anti-Itch Maximum Strength: 1% (28 g) [contains cetyl alcohol, methylparaben]
- Anti-Itch Maximum Strength: 1% (28 g) [contains cetyl alcohol, methylparaben, propylene glycol, propylparaben]
- Cortaid Maximum Strength: 1% (14 g, 28 g) [contains cetyl alcohol, disodium edta, ethylparaben, methylparaben, propylparaben]
- Hydrocortisone Max St/12 Moist: 1% (28.4 g) [contains cetearyl alcohol, methylparaben, propylene glycol, propylparaben]
- HydroSKIN: 1% (28 g) [contains benzyl alcohol]
- Instacort 5: 0.5% (28.4 g)
- Med-Derm Hydrocortisone: 0.5% (30 g); 1% (30 g)
- Medi-First Hydrocortisone: 1% (1 ea) [contains trolamine (triethanolamine)]
- Preparation H Hydrocortisone: 1% (26 g)
- Recort Plus: 1% (30 g)
- Generic: 0.5% (15 g, 28.35 g, 28.4 g, 30 g); 1% (1 g, 1.5 g, 14.2 g, 20 g, 28 g, 28.35 g, 28.4 g, 30 g, 120 g, 453.6 g, 454 g); 2.5% (20 g, 28 g, 28.35 g, 30 g, 453.6 g)

Cream, Rectal, as base:
- Anusol-HC: 2.5% (30 g)
- Procto-Pak: 1% (28.4 g)
- Proctocort: 1% (28.35 g) [contains cetyl alcohol, propylene glycol]
- Proctosol HC: 2.5% (28.35 g)
- Proctozone-HC: 2.5% (30 g)

Cream, External, as butyrate:
- Locoid: 0.1% (15 g, 45 g) [contains butylparaben, propylparaben]
- Locoid Lipocream: 0.1% (15 g [DSC])
- Locoid Lipocream: 0.1% (45 g, 60 g) [contains butylparaben, cetostearyl alcohol, propylparaben]
- Generic: 0.1% (15 g, 45 g, 60 g)

Cream, External, as probutate:
- Pandel: 0.1% (15 g, 45 g, 80 g) [contains butylparaben, methylparaben, propylene glycol]

Cream, External, as valerate:
- Generic: 0.2% (15 g, 45 g, 60 g)

Enema, Rectal, as base:
- Colocort: 100 mg/60 mL (60 mL)
- Cortenema: 100 mg/60 mL (60 mL) [contains methylparaben, polysorbate 80]
- Generic: 100 mg/60 mL (60 mL)

Foam, Rectal, as acetate:
- Cortifoam: 90 mg (15 g) [contains cetyl alcohol, methylparaben, propylene glycol, propylparaben, trolamine (triethanolamine)]

Gel, External, as acetate:
- CortAlo: 2% (43 g) [contains benzyl alcohol, menthol, trolamine (triethanolamine)]
- NuZon: 2% (43 g [DSC]) [contains menthol, trolamine (triethanolamine)]
- Generic: 2% (43 g [DSC])

Gel, External, as base:
- Corticool: 1% (42.53 g) [contains cremophor el, propylene glycol]
- First-Hydrocortisone: 10% (60 g) [contains propylene glycol, simethicone]
- Instacort 10: 1% (30 g)

Kit, External, as base:
Dermasorb HC: 2% [contains menthol, methylparaben, propylene glycol, propylparaben]
Pediaderm HC: 2% [contains benzalkonium chloride, cetyl alcohol, isopropyl alcohol, methylparaben, propylene glycol, propylparaben]
Scalacort DK: Hydrocortisone lotion 2% and Sal Acid 2% and sulfur 2% [contains benzalkonium chloride, isopropyl alcohol, methylparaben, propylene glycol, propylparaben, soybean lecithin]
Lotion, External, as acetate:
NuCort: 2% (60 g) [contains benzyl alcohol, cetyl alcohol, menthol, trolamine (triethanolamine)]
Lotion, External, as base:
Ala Scalp: 2% (29.6 mL) [contains benzalkonium chloride, isopropyl alcohol, propylene glycol]
Aquanil HC: 1% (120 mL)
Beta HC: 1% (60 mL)
Hydro Skin Maximum Strength: 1% (118 mL) [contains benzyl alcohol]
Rederm: 1% (120 mL)
Sarnol-HC: 1% (59 mL)
Scalacort: 2% (29.6 mL) [contains benzalkonium chloride, isopropyl alcohol, propylene glycol]
TheraCort: 1% (118 mL) [contains methylparaben, propylene glycol, propylparaben, trolamine (triethanolamine)]
Generic: 1% (114 g); 2.5% (59 mL, 118 mL)
Lotion, External, as butyrate:
Locoid: 0.1% (59 mL, 118 mL) [contains butylparaben, cetostearyl alcohol, propylparaben]
Ointment, External, as base:
Generic: 0.5% (28.35 g, 30 g); 1% (25 g, 28 g, 28.35 g, 28.4 g, 30 g, 110 g, 430 g, 453.6 g); 2.5% (20 g, 28.35 g, 453.6 g, 454 g)
Ointment, External, as butyrate:
Locoid: 0.1% (15 g, 45 g)
Generic: 0.1% (15 g, 45 g)
Ointment, External, as valerate:
Westcort: 0.2% (15 g, 45 g, 60 g) [contains propylene glycol]
Generic: 0.2% (15 g, 45 g, 60 g)
Solution, External, as base:
Scalpicin Maximum Strength: 1% (44 mL) [contains disodium edta, menthol, propylene glycol]
Texacort: 2.5% (30 mL) [lipid free, paraben free; contains alcohol, usp]
Solution, External, as butyrate:
Locoid: 0.1% (60 mL) [contains isopropyl alcohol]
Generic: 0.1% (20 mL, 60 mL)
Suppository, Rectal, as acetate:
Anucort-HC: 25 mg (12 ea, 24 ea, 100 ea)
Anusol-HC: 25 mg (12 ea, 24 ea)
GRx HiCort 25: 25 mg (12 ea)
Hemril-30: 30 mg (12 ea [DSC], 24 ea [DSC])
Proctocort: 30 mg (12 ea)
Rectacort-HC: 25 mg (12 ea, 24 ea)
Generic: 25 mg (12 ea, 24 ea); 30 mg (12 ea)

◆ **Hydrocortisone Acetate** *see* Hydrocortisone (Topical) *on page 1041*

◆ **Hydrocortisone, Acetic Acid, and Propylene Glycol Diacetate** *see* Acetic Acid, Propylene Glycol Diacetate, and Hydrocortisone *on page 56*

◆ **Hydrocortisone and Acyclovir** *see* Acyclovir and Hydrocortisone *on page 66*

◆ **Hydrocortisone and Ciprofloxacin** *see* Ciprofloxacin and Hydrocortisone *on page 470*

◆ **Hydrocortisone, Bacitracin, Neomycin, and Polymyxin B** *see* Bacitracin, Neomycin, Polymyxin B, and Hydrocortisone *on page 253*

◆ **Hydrocortisone Butyrate** *see* Hydrocortisone (Topical) *on page 1041*

◆ **Hydrocortisone Max St [OTC]** *see* Hydrocortisone (Topical) *on page 1041*

◆ **Hydrocortisone Max St/12 Moist [OTC]** *see* Hydrocortisone (Topical) *on page 1041*

◆ **Hydrocortisone, Neomycin, and Polymyxin B** *see* Neomycin, Polymyxin B, and Hydrocortisone *on page 1503*

◆ **Hydrocortisone Probutate** *see* Hydrocortisone (Topical) *on page 1041*

◆ **Hydrocortisone Sodium Succinate** *see* Hydrocortisone (Systemic) *on page 1038*

◆ **Hydrocortisone Valerate** *see* Hydrocortisone (Topical) *on page 1041*

◆ **Hydrodiuril** *see* Hydrochlorothiazide *on page 1028*

◆ **Hydrogen Dioxide** *see* Hydrogen Peroxide *on page 1044*

Hydrogen Peroxide (HYE droe jen per OKS ide)

Therapeutic Category Antibacterial, Otic; Antibacterial, Topical; Antibiotic, Oral Rinse

Generic Availability (US) Yes

Use Cleanse wounds, suppurating ulcers, and local infections; used in the treatment of inflammatory conditions of the external auditory canal and as a mouthwash or gargle; hydrogen peroxide concentrate (30%) has been used as a hair bleach and as a tooth bleaching agent

Contraindications Should not be used in abscesses

Mechanism of Action Antiseptic oxidant that slowly releases oxygen and water upon contact with serum or tissue catalase

Pharmacodynamics Duration: Only while bubbling action occurs

Dosing: Usual Children and Adults:
Mouthwash or gargle: Dilute the 3% solution with an equal volume of water; swish around in the mouth over the affected area for at least 1 minute and then expel; use up to 4 times/day (after meals and at bedtime)
Topical:
1.5% to 3% solution for cleansing wounds
1.5% gel for cleansing wounds or mouth/gum irritations: Apply a small amount to the affected area for at least 1 minute, then expectorate; use up to 4 times/day (after meals and at bedtime)

Administration Topical: Do not inject or instill into closed body cavities from which released oxygen cannot escape; strong solutions (30.5%) of hydrogen peroxide should not be applied undiluted to tissues

Dosage Forms Excipient information presented when available (limited, particularly for generics); consult specific product labeling.
Solution, External:
Generic: 3% (237 mL)

◆ **Hydromet** *see* Hydrocodone and Homatropine *on page 1036*

◆ **Hydromorph Contin (Can)** *see* HYDROmorphone *on page 1044*

HYDROmorphone (hye droe MOR fone)

Medication Safety Issues
Sound-alike/look-alike issues:
Dilaudid may be confused with Demerol, Dilantin
HYDROmorphone may be confused with morphine; significant overdoses have occurred when hydromorphone products have been inadvertently administered instead of morphine sulfate. Commercially available prefilled syringes of both products looks similar and are often

stored in close proximity to each other. **Note:** Hydromorphone 1 mg oral is approximately equal to morphine 4 mg oral; hydromorphone 1 mg IV is approximately equal to morphine 5 mg IV

High alert medication:

The Institute for Safe Medication Practices (ISMP) includes this medication among its list of drug classes which have a heightened risk of causing significant patient harm when used in error.

Administration issues:

Dilaudid, Dilaudid-HP: Extreme caution should be taken to avoid confusing the highly-concentrated (Dilaudid-HP) injection with the less-concentrated (Dilaudid) injectable product.

Exalgo: Extreme caution should be taken to avoid confusing the extended release Exalgo 8 mg tablets with immediate release hydromorphone 8 mg tablets.

Significant differences exist between oral and IV dosing. Use caution when converting from one route of administration to another.

Related Information

Opioid Conversion Table *on page 2285*

Oral Medications That Should Not Be Crushed or Altered *on page 2476*

Patient Information for Disposal of Unused Medications *on page 2453*

Brand Names: US Dilaudid; Dilaudid-HP; Exalgo

Brand Names: Canada Apo-Hydromorphone; Dilaudid; Dilaudid-HP; Hydromorph Contin; Hydromorphone HP; Hydromorphone HP 10; Hydromorphone HP 20; Hydromorphone HP 50; Hydromorphone HP Forte; Hydromorphone Hydrochloride Injection, USP; Jurnista; PMS-Hydromorphone; Teva-Hydromorphone

Therapeutic Category Analgesic, Narcotic

Generic Availability (US) May be product dependent

Use

Oral (immediate release): Management of moderate to severe pain (FDA approved in adults)

Oral (extended release; Exalgo): For once-daily administration for the management of moderate to severe pain in **opioid-tolerant** patients who require continuous, around-the-clock analgesia for an extended period of time (FDA approved in adults). Should **NOT** be used as an as-needed analgesic or for management of acute or post-operative pain.

Parenteral: Injection: Management of moderate to severe pain (FDA approved in adults)

Concentrated; Dilaudid-HP injection: Use in **opioid-tolerant** patients who require larger than usual doses of opioids for pain relief (FDA approved in adults)

Rectal: Management of moderate to severe pain (FDA approved in adults)

Note: Patients are considered to be opioid-tolerant if they have been taking oral morphine ≥60 mg/day, fentanyl transdermal ≥25 mcg/hour, oral oxycodone ≥30 mg/day, oral hydromorphone ≥8 mg/day, oral oxymorphone ≥25 mg/day, or an equianalgesic dose of another opioid for ≥1 week

Prescribing and Access Restrictions Exalgo: As a requirement of the REMS program, healthcare providers who prescribe Exalgo need to receive training on the proper use and potential risks of Exalgo. For training, please refer to http://www.exalgorems.com. Prescribers will need retraining every 2 years or following any significant changes to the Exalgo REMS program.

Medication Guide Available Yes

Pregnancy Risk Factor C

Pregnancy Considerations Adverse events have been observed in some animal reproduction studies. Hydromorphone crosses the placenta. Some dosage forms are specifically contraindicated for use in obstetrical analgesia. The Canadian labeling contraindicates use of some dosage forms during pregnancy and/or labor and delivery.

When used for pain relief during labor, opioids may temporarily affect the heart rate of the fetus (ACOG 2002). Monitor the neonate for respiratory depression if hydromorphone is used during labor.

[US Boxed Warning]: Prolonged maternal use of opioids during pregnancy can cause neonatal withdrawal syndrome in the newborn, which may be life-threatening if not recognized and treated according to protocols developed by neonatology experts. If prolonged opioid therapy is required in a pregnant woman, ensure treatment is available and warn patient of risk to the neonate. If chronic opioid exposure occurs in pregnancy, adverse events in the newborn (including withdrawal) may occur; monitoring of the neonate is recommended. The minimum effective dose should be used if opioids are needed (Chou 2009). Neonatal abstinence syndrome following opioid exposure may present with autonomic (eg, fever, temperature instability), GI (eg, diarrhea, vomiting, poor feeding/weight gain), or neurologic (eg, high-pitched crying, increased muscle tone, irritability, seizure, tremor) symptoms (Dow 2012; Hudak 2012). Long-term opioid use may cause secondary hypogonadism, which may lead to sexual dysfunction or infertility (Brennan 2013).

Breast-Feeding Considerations Low concentrations of hydromorphone can be found in breast milk. Withdrawal symptoms may be observed in breast-feeding infants when opioid analgesics are discontinued. The US labeling does not recommend use in breast-feeding women. The Canadian labeling contraindicates use. Parenteral opioids used during labor have the potential to interfere with a newborn's natural reflex to nurse within the first few hours after birth. Breast-feeding infants exposed to large doses of opioids should be monitored for apnea and sedation (Montgomery, 2012).

Contraindications

US labeling: Hypersensitivity to hydromorphone, or any component of the formulation; acute or severe asthma, respiratory depression (in absence of resuscitative equipment or ventilatory support)

Additional product-specific contraindications:

Dilaudid liquid and tablets: Obstetrical analgesia

Dilaudid injection, Dilaudid-HP injection: Opioid-nontolerant patients (Dilaudid-HP injection only); patients with risk of developing GI obstruction, especially paralytic ileus

Exalgo: Opioid-nontolerant patients, paralytic ileus (known or suspected), preexisting GI surgery and/or diseases resulting in narrowing of GI tract, blind loops in the GI tract, or GI obstruction

Suppository: Intracranial lesion associated with increased intracranial pressure; whenever ventilatory function is depressed (eg, COPD, cor pulmonale, emphysema, kyphoscoliosis, status asthmaticus)

Canadian labeling: Hypersensitivity to hydromorphone or any component of the formulation

Dilaudid, Hydromorph Contin, Jurnista: Known or suspected mechanical GI obstruction (eg, bowel obstruction or strictures) or any disease that affects bowel transit (eg, ileus of any type); suspected surgical abdomen (eg, acute appendicitis or pancreatitis); mild, intermittent, or short-duration pain that can be managed with other pain medications; acute asthma or other obstructive airway and status asthmaticus; acute respiratory depression, hypercarbia and cor pulmonale; acute alcoholism, delirium tremens, and convulsive disorders; severe CNS depression, increased cerebrospinal or intracranial pressure, and head injury; coadministration with monoamine oxidase inhibitors (concomitant use or within 14 days); women during pregnancy, labor and delivery, or breast-feeding

Hydromorphone HP, Hydromorphone HP Forte: Patients not already receiving high doses or high concentrations of opioids; respiratory depression in the absence of resuscitative equipment; severe CNS depression; status asthmaticus; obstetrical analgesia; mild or moderate pain

Suppository, syrup: Respiratory depression in the absence of resuscitative equipment; status asthmaticus

Additional product-specific contraindications:

Dilaudid: Hypersensitivity to other opioid analgesics

Hydromorph Contin: Hypersensitivity to other opioid analgesics; management of acute pain, including use in outpatient or day surgeries; management of perioperative pain

Jurnista: Prior surgical procedures and/or underlying disease that may result in narrowing of the GI tract, blind loops of the GI tract, or GI obstruction; management of acute or perioperative pain

Warnings/Precautions Use with caution in patients with hypersensitivity reactions to other phenanthrene derivative opioid agonists (codeine, hydrocodone, levorphanol, oxycodone, oxymorphone). Hydromorphone shares toxic potential of opioid agonists, including CNS depression and respiratory depression. Precautions associated with opioid agonist therapy should be observed. May cause CNS depression, which may impair physical or mental abilities; patients must be cautioned about performing tasks that require mental alertness (eg, operating machinery or driving). Myoclonus and seizures have been reported with high doses; use with caution in patients with a history of seizure disorder. Use with caution in patients with cardiovascular disease, morbid obesity, adrenocortical insufficiency, hypothyroidism, acute alcoholism, delirium tremens, toxic psychoses, prostatic hyperplasia and/or urinary stricture, or severe liver or renal failure. Use with caution and monitor for respiratory depression in patients with significant chronic obstructive pulmonary disease or cor pulmonale, and patients having a substantially decreased respiratory reserve, hypoxia, hypercarbia, or preexisting respiratory depression, particularly when initiating therapy and titrating with hydromorphone; even therapeutic doses may decrease respiratory drive to the point of apnea. Consider the use of alternative nonopioid analgesics in these patients. Avoid use in patients with CNS depression or coma, as these patients are susceptible to intracranial effects of CO_2 retention. Use with caution in patients with biliary tract dysfunction. Hydromorphone may increase biliary tract pressure following spasm in sphincter of Oddi. Use caution in patients with inflammatory or obstructive bowel disorder, acute pancreatitis secondary to biliary tract disease, and patients undergoing biliary surgery. Use extreme caution in patients with head injury, intracranial lesions, or elevated intracranial pressure (ICP); exaggerated elevation of ICP may occur (in addition, hydromorphone may complicate neurologic evaluation due to pupillary dilation and CNS depressant effects). Use with caution in patients with depleted blood volume or drugs which may exaggerate hypotensive effects (including phenothiazines or general anesthetics). May obscure diagnosis or clinical course of patients with acute abdominal conditions. Effects may be potentiated when used with other CNS depressants (eg, sedatives, anxiolytics, hypnotics, neuroleptics, other opioids). Potentially significant interactions may exist, requiring dose or frequency adjustment, additional monitoring, and/or selection of alternative therapy.

An opioid-containing analgesic regimen should be tailored to each patient's needs and based upon the type of pain being treated (acute versus chronic), the route of administration, degree of tolerance for opioids (naive versus chronic user), age, weight, and medical condition. The optimal analgesic dose varies widely among patients. Doses should be titrated to pain relief/prevention. IM use may result in variable absorption and a lag time to peak effect. Concurrent use of mixed agonist/antagonist analgesics (eg, pentazocine, nalbuphine, butorphanol) or partial agonist (eg, buprenorphine) analgesics may precipitate withdrawal symptoms and/or reduced analgesic efficacy in patients following prolonged therapy with mu opioid agonists. Abrupt discontinuation following prolonged use may also lead to withdrawal symptoms. May cause constipation. Consider preventive measures to reduce the potential for constipation. Use with extreme caution in patients with chronic constipation. Use immediate-release formulations with caution in the perioperative setting; severe pain may antagonize the respiratory depressant effects of hydromorphone. The Canadian labeling (immediate-release formulations) recommends withholding hydromorphone within 24 hours of procedures that interfere with pain transmission pathways (eg, cordotomy); the Canadian labeling for extended-release formulations contraindicates use in the perioperative setting.

Dosage form specific warnings:

Some dosage forms may contain trace amounts of sodium metabisulfite, which may cause allergic reactions, including anaphylactic symptoms and life-threatening or less severe asthmatic episodes in susceptible individuals. Some formulations may contain lactose; consider lactose content prior to initiating therapy in patients with hereditary diseases of galactose intolerance (eg, galactosemia, glucose-galactose malabsorption).

Immediate-release formulations: **[US Boxed Warning]: High potential for abuse and risk of producing respiratory depression. Alcohol, other opioids, and CNS depressants potentiate the respiratory depressant effects of hydromorphone, increasing the risk of respiratory depression that might result in death.**

Injection: Vial stoppers of single-dose injectable vials may contain latex. **[US Boxed Warning]: Dilaudid-HP: Extreme caution should be taken to avoid confusing the highly concentrated (Dilaudid-HP) injection with the less-concentrated (Dilaudid) injectable product.** Dilaudid-HP should only be used in patients who are opioid tolerant. Highly concentrated products available in Canada (Hydromorphone HP and Hydromorphone HP Forte) are for use only in opioid-tolerant patients with severe pain.

Extended-release tablets: **[US Boxed Warning]: May cause serious, life-threatening, or fatal respiratory depression. Monitor closely for respiratory depression, especially during initiation or dose escalation. Patients should swallow tablets whole; crushing, chewing, or dissolving can cause rapid release and a potentially fatal dose.** Carbon dioxide retention from opioid-induced respiratory depression can exacerbate the sedating effects of opioids. **[US Boxed Warning]: Users are exposed to the risks of addiction, abuse, and misuse, potentially leading to overdose and death. Assess each patient's risk prior to prescribing; monitor all patients regularly for development of these behaviors or conditions.** Risk of opioid abuse is increased in patients with a history or family history of alcohol or drug abuse or mental illness. Tolerance or drug dependence may result from extended use; however, concerns for abuse should not prevent effective management of pain. In general, abrupt discontinuation of therapy in dependent patients should be avoided. **[US Boxed Warning]: Prolonged maternal use of opioids during pregnancy can cause neonatal withdrawal syndrome in the**

newborn, which may be life-threatening if not recognized and treated according to protocols developed by neonatology experts. If prolonged opioid therapy is required in a pregnant woman, ensure treatment is available and warn patient of risk to the neonate. Signs and symptoms include irritability, hyperactivity and abnormal sleep pattern, high-pitched cry, tremor, vomiting, diarrhea, and failure to gain weight. Onset, duration, and severity depend on the drug used, duration of use, maternal dose, and rate of drug elimination by the newborn. Therapy should only be prescribed by health care professionals familiar with the use of potent opioids for chronic pain. Exalgo and Jurnista [Canadian product] tablets are nondeformable; do not administer to patients with preexisting severe GI narrowing (eg, esophageal motility, small bowel inflammatory disease, short gut syndrome, history of peritonitis, cystic fibrosis, chronic intestinal pseudo-obstruction, Meckel's diverticulum); obstruction may occur. Tablets may be visible on abdominal x-rays, especially when digital enhancing techniques are used. The tablet shell may appear in the excreted stool.

Warnings: Additional Pediatric Considerations Prolonged use of any hydromorphone product during pregnancy can result in neonatal opioid withdrawal syndrome, which may be life-threatening if not recognized and treated, and requires management according to protocols developed by neonatology experts.

Adverse Reactions

Cardiovascular: Bradycardia, extrasystoles, flushing (facial), hypertension, hypotension, palpitations, peripheral edema, peripheral vasodilation, syncope, tachycardia

Central nervous system: Abnormal dreams, abnormal gait, abnormality in thinking, aggressive behavior, agitation, apprehension, ataxia, brain disease, burning sensation of skin (Exalgo), central nervous system depression, chills, cognitive dysfunction, confusion, decreased body temperature (Exalgo), depression, disruption of body temperature regulation (Exalgo), dizziness, drowsiness, drug dependence, dysarthria, dysphoria, equilibrium disturbance, euphoria, fatigue, hallucination, headache, hyperesthesia, hyperreflexia, hypoesthesia, hypothermia, increased intracranial pressure, insomnia, lack of concentration, lethargy, malaise, memory impairment, mood changes, myoclonus, nervousness, painful defecation, panic attack, paranoia, paresthesia, psychomotor agitation, restlessness, sedation, seizure, sleep disorder (Exalgo), suicidal ideation, uncontrolled crying, vertigo

Dermatologic: Diaphoresis, erythema (Exalgo), hyperhidrosis, pruritus, skin rash, urticaria

Endocrine & metabolic: Antidiuretic effect, decreased amylase, decreased libido, decreased plasma testosterone, dehydration, fluid retention, hyperuricemia, hypokalemia, weight loss

Gastrointestinal: Abdominal distention, anal fissure, anorexia, bezoar formation (Exalgo), biliary tract spasm, constipation, decreased appetite, decreased gastrointestinal motility (Exalgo), delayed gastric emptying, diarrhea, diverticulitis, diverticulosis, duodenitis, dysgeusia, dysphagia, eructation, flatulence, gastroenteritis, gastroesophageal reflux disease (aggravated; Exalgo), hematochezia, increased appetite, intestinal perforation (large intestine; Exalgo), nausea, paralytic ileus, stomach cramps, vomiting, xerostomia

Genitourinary: Bladder spasm, decreased urine output, difficulty in micturition, dysuria, erectile dysfunction, hypogonadism, sexual disorder, ureteral spasm, urinary frequency, urinary hesitancy, urinary retention

Hematologic & oncologic: Oxygen desaturation

Hepatic: Increased liver enzymes

Hypersensitivity: Histamine release

Local: Pain at injection site, post-injection flare

Neuromuscular & skeletal: Arthralgia, dyskinesia, laryngospasm, muscle rigidity, muscle spasm, myalgia, tremor, weakness

Ophthalmic: Blurred vision, diplopia, dry eye syndrome, miosis, nystagmus

Otic: Tinnitus

Respiratory: Apnea, bronchospasm, dyspnea, flu-like symptoms (Exalgo), hyperventilation, hypoxia, respiratory depression, respiratory distress, rhinorrhea

Rare but important or life-threatening: Angioedema, hypersensitivity

Drug Interactions

Metabolism/Transport Effects None known.

Avoid Concomitant Use

Avoid concomitant use of HYDROmorphone with any of the following: Azelastine (Nasal); Eluxadoline; MAO Inhibitors; Mixed Agonist / Antagonist Opioids; Orphenadrine; Paraldehyde; Thalidomide

Increased Effect/Toxicity

HYDROmorphone may increase the levels/effects of: Alcohol (Ethyl); Alvimopan; Azelastine (Nasal); CNS Depressants; Desmopressin; Diuretics; Eluxadoline; Hydrocodone; Methotrimeprazine; Metyrosine; Mirtazapine; Orphenadrine; Paraldehyde; Pramipexole; ROPINIRole; Rotigotine; Selective Serotonin Reuptake Inhibitors; Suvorexant; Thalidomide; Zolpidem

The levels/effects of HYDROmorphone may be increased by: Amphetamines; Anticholinergic Agents; Antipsychotic Agents (Phenothiazines); Brimonidine (Topical); Cannabis; Doxylamine; Dronabinol; Droperidol; HydrOXYzine; Kava Kava; Magnesium Sulfate; MAO Inhibitors; Methotrimeprazine; Nabilone; Perampanel; Rufinamide; Sodium Oxybate; Succinylcholine; Tapentadol; Tetrahydrocannabinol

Decreased Effect

HYDROmorphone may decrease the levels/effects of: Pegvisomant

The levels/effects of HYDROmorphone may be decreased by: Ammonium Chloride; Mixed Agonist / Antagonist Opioids; Naltrexone

Storage/Stability

Injection: Store at 15°C to 30°C (59°F to 86°F). Protect from light. A slightly yellowish discoloration has not been associated with a loss of potency. Stable for at least 24 hours when protected from light and stored at 25°C in most common large volume parenteral solutions.

Oral dosage forms: Store at 25°C (77°F); excursions permitted from 15°C to 30°C (59°F to 86°F). Protect tablets from light.

Suppository:

US labeling: Store in refrigerator. Protect from light.

Canadian labeling: Store at 15°C to 30°C (59°F to 86°F). Protect from light.

Mechanism of Action Binds to opioid receptors in the CNS, causing inhibition of ascending pain pathways, altering the perception of and response to pain; causes cough suppression by direct central action in the medulla; produces generalized CNS depression

Pharmacodynamics Analgesic effects:

Onset of action:

Oral: Immediate release formulations: Within 15 to 30 minutes

IV: Within 5 minutes

Maximum effect:

Oral: Immediate release formulations: Within 30 to 90 minutes

IV: 10 to 20 minutes

Duration: Oral: Immediate release formulations, IV: 4 to 5 hours; suppository may provide longer duration of effect

Pharmacokinetics (Adult data unless noted)

Absorption:

IM: Variable

Oral: Rapidly absorbed; extensive first-pass effect

Distribution: V_d: 4 L/kg

Protein binding: ~8% to 19%

Metabolism: Primarily in the liver via glucuronidation to inactive metabolites; >95% is metabolized to hydromorphone-3-glucuronide; minor amounts as 6-hydroxy reduction metabolites

Bioavailability: Oral: 62%

Half-life: 2-3 hours; Exalgo: Apparent half-life: ~11 hours

Time to peak serum concentration: Oral: Immediate release: 30 to 60 minutes; Exalgo: 12 to 16 hours

Elimination: In urine, principally as glucuronide conjugates; minimal unchanged drug is excreted in urine (~7%) and feces (1%)

Dosing: Usual

Pediatric:

Acute pain, moderate to severe: Limited data available: **Note:** Doses should be titrated to appropriate analgesic effects, while minimizing adverse effects; when changing routes of administration, note that oral doses are less than one-half as effective as parenteral doses (may be only 1/5 as effective):

Infants >6 months weighing >10 kg (Friedrichsdorf 2007; Zernikow 2009):

Oral: Immediate release: Usual initial: 0.03 mg/kg/dose every 4 hours as needed; usual range: 0.03 to 0.06 mg/kg/dose

IV: Usual initial: 0.01 mg/kg/dose every 3 to 6 hours as needed

Continuous IV infusion: Usual initial: 0.003 to 0.005 mg/kg/**hour**

Children weighing <50 kg and Adolescents weighing <50 kg:

Oral: Immediate release: 0.03 to 0.08 mg/kg/dose every 3 to 4 hours as needed; **Note:** The American Pain Society (2008) recommends an initial oral dose of 0.06 mg/kg for severe pain in children.

IV: 0.015 mg/kg/dose every 3 to 6 hours as needed

Continuous IV infusion: Usual initial: 0.003 to 0.005 mg/kg/**hour** (maximum: 0.2 mg/**hour**) (Friedrichsdorf 2007; Zernikow 2009)

Children weighing ≥50 kg and Adolescents weighing ≥50 kg:

Oral: Immediate release: Initial: Opioid-naive: 1 to 2 mg/dose every 3 to 4 hours as needed; patients with prior opioid exposure may tolerate higher initial doses; usual adult dose: 2 to 4 mg/dose; doses up to 8 mg have been used in adults

IV: Initial: Opioid-naive: 0.2 to 0.6 mg/dose every 2 to 4 hours as needed; patients with prior opioid exposure may tolerate higher initial doses

IM, SubQ: **Note**: IM use may result in variable absorption and a lag time to peak effect. Initial: Opioid-naive: 0.8 to 1 mg every 4 to 6 hours as needed; patients with prior opioid exposure may require higher initial doses; usual dosage range: 1 to 2 mg every 3 to 6 hours as needed

Rectal: 3 mg (1 suppository) every 4 to 8 hours as needed

Patient-controlled analgesia (PCA): Limited data available: Opioid-naïve: **Note:** PCA has been used in children as young as 5 years of age; however, clinicians need to assess children 5 to 8 years of age to determine if they are able to use the PCA device correctly. All patients should receive an initial loading dose of an analgesic (to attain adequate control of pain) before starting PCA for maintenance. Adjust doses, lockouts, and limits based on required loading dose, age, state of health, and presence of opioid tolerance. Use lower end of dosing range for opioid-naive; a continuous (basal) infusion is not recommended in opioid-naive patients (ISMP 2009). Assess patient and pain control at regular intervals and adjust settings if needed (American Pain Society 2008):

Children ≥5 years weighing <50 kg and Adolescents weighing <50 kg:

Usual concentration: 0.2 mg/mL

Demand dose: Usual initial: 0.003 to 0.004 mg/kg/dose; usual range: 0.003 to 0.005 mg/kg/dose

Lockout: Usual initial: 5 doses/hour

Lockout interval: Range: 6 to 10 minutes

Usual basal rate: 0 to 0.004 mg/kg/**hour**

Children weighing ≥50 kg and Adolescents weighing ≥50 kg:

Usual concentration: 0.2 mg/mL

Demand dose: Usual initial: 0.1 to 0.2 mg; usual range: 0.05 to 0.4 mg

Lockout interval: Usual initial: 6 minutes; usual range: 5 to 10 minutes

Adult:

Acute pain (moderate to severe): Note: These are guidelines and do not represent the maximum doses that may be required in all patients. Doses should be titrated to provide adequate pain relief. When changing routes of administration, oral doses and parenteral doses are **NOT** equivalent; parenteral doses are up to 5 times more potent. Therefore, when administered parenterally, one-fifth of the oral dose will provide similar analgesia.

Oral: Immediate release: Initial: Opioid-naive: 2 to 4 mg every 4 to 6 hours as needed; elderly/debilitated patients may require lower doses; patients with prior opioid exposure may require higher initial doses. **Note:** In adults with severe pain, the American Pain Society recommends an initial dose of 4 to 8 mg.

IV: Initial: Opioid-naive: 0.2 to 1 mg every 2 to 3 hours as needed; patients with prior opioid exposure may require higher initial doses.

Patient-controlled analgesia (PCA): (*American Pain Society* 2008): **Note:** Opioid-naive: Consider lower end of dosing range. A continuous (basal) infusion is not recommended in opioid-naive patients (ISMP 2009):

Usual concentration: 0.2 mg/mL

Demand dose: Usual: 0.1 to 0.2 mg; range: 0.05 to 0.4 mg

Lockout interval: 5 to 10 minutes

Epidural PCA (de Leon-Casasola 1996; Liu 2010; Smith 2009):

Usual concentration: 0.01 mg/mL

Bolus dose: 0.4 to 1 mg

Infusion rate: 0.03 to 0.3 mg/**hour**

Demand dose: 0.02 to 0.05 mg

Lockout interval: 10 to 15 minutes

IM, SubQ: **Note:** IM use may result in variable absorption and lag time to peak effect; IM route not recommended for use (American Pain Society 2008).

Initial: Opioid-naive: 0.8 to 1 mg every 3 to 4 hours as needed; patients with prior opioid exposure may require higher initial doses.

Rectal: 3 mg every 6 to 8 hours as needed

Chronic pain: **Note:** Patients taking opioids chronically may become tolerant and require doses higher than the usual dosage range to maintain the desired effect. Tolerance can be managed by appropriate dose titration. There is no optimal or maximal dose for hydromorphone in chronic pain. The appropriate dose is one that relieves pain throughout its dosing interval without causing unmanageable side effects.

Extended release formulation (Exalgo): Oral: **Note:** For use in opioid-tolerant patients only. Patients considered opioid tolerant are those who are receiving, for 1 week or longer, at least 60 mg oral morphine daily, 25 mcg transdermal fentanyl per hour, 30 mg oral oxycodone daily, 8 mg oral hydromorphone daily, 25 mg oral oxymorphone daily, or an equianalgesic dose of another opioid.

Opioid-tolerant patients: Discontinue or taper all other extended release opioids when starting therapy.

Individualization of dose: Suggested recommendations for converting to Exalgo from other analgesics are presented, but when selecting the initial dose, other characteristics (eg, patient status, degree of opioid tolerance, concurrent medications, type of pain, risk factors for addiction, abuse, and misuse) should also be considered. Pain relief and adverse events should be assessed frequently.

Conversion from other oral hydromorphone formulations to Exalgo: Start with the equivalent total daily dose of immediate release hydromorphone administered once daily.

Conversion from other opioids to Exalgo: Discontinue all other around-the-clock opioids when therapy is initiated. Substantial interpatient variability exists in relative potency. Therefore, it is safer to underestimate a patient's daily oral hydromorphone requirement and provide breakthrough pain relief with rescue medication (eg, immediate release opioid) than to overestimate requirements. In general, start Exalgo at 50% of the calculated total daily dose every 24 hours (see Conversion Factors to Exalgo). The following conversion ratios may be used to convert from oral opioid therapy to Exalgo.

Conversion factors to Exalgo (see table): Select the opioid, sum the current total daily dose, multiply by the conversion factor on the table to calculate the approximate oral hydromorphone daily dose, then calculate the approximate starting dose for Exalgo at 50% of the calculated oral hydromorphone daily does; administer every 24 hours. Round down, if necessary, to the nearest strength available. For patients on a regimen of more than one opioid, calculate the approximate oral hydromorphone dose for each opioid and sum the totals to obtain the approximate total hydromorphone daily dose. For patients on a regimen of fixed-ratio opioid/nonopioid analgesic medications, only the opioid component of these medications should be used in the conversion. **Note:** The conversion factors in this conversion table are only to be used for the conversion from current oral opioid therapy to Exalgo. Conversion factors in this table cannot be used to convert from Exalgo to another oral opioid (doing so may lead to fatal overdose due to overestimation of the new opioid). This is not a table of equianalgesic doses.

Conversion Factors to Exalgo[1]

Previous Oral Opioid	Oral Conversion Factor
Hydromorphone	1
Codeine	0.06
Hydrocodone	0.4
Methadone[2]	0.6
Morphine	0.2
Oxycodone	0.4
Oxymorphone	0.6

[1]Conversion factors for the conversion from one of the listed current oral opioid agents to Exalgo.

[2]Monitor closely; ratio between methadone and other opioid agonists may vary widely as a function of previous drug exposure. Methadone has a long half-life and may accumulate in the plasma.

Conversion from transdermal fentanyl to Exalgo: Treatment with Exalgo can be started 18 hours after the removal of the transdermal fentanyl patch. For every fentanyl 25 mcg/hour transdermal dose, the equianalgesic dose of Exalgo is 12 mg every 24 hours. An appropriate starting dose is 50% of the calculated total daily dose given every 24 hours. If necessary, round down to the appropriate Exalgo tablet strength available.

Titration and maintenance: Dose adjustments in 4 to 8 mg increments may occur every 3 to 4 days. In patients experiencing breakthrough pain, consider increasing the dose of Exalgo or providing rescue medication of an immediate release analgesic at an appropriate dose. Do not administer Exalgo more frequently than every 24 hours.

Discontinuing Exalgo: Taper by gradually decreasing the dose by 25% to 50% every 2 to 3 days to a dose of 8 mg every 24 hours before discontinuing therapy.

Dosing adjustment in renal impairment: Adults:

Oral (immediate release), injectable: Initiate with 25% to 50% of the usual starting dose depending on the degree of impairment. Monitor closely for respiratory and CNS depression.

Oral (extended release; Exalgo):

Moderate impairment (CrCl 30 to 60 mL/minute): Initiate with 50% of the usual starting dose for patients with normal renal function; monitor closely for respiratory and CNS depression.

Severe impairment (CrCl <30 mL/minute): Initiate with 25% of the usual starting dose for patients with normal renal function; monitor closely for respiratory and CNS depression. Consider use of an alternate analgesic with better dosing flexibility.

Dosing adjustment in hepatic impairment: Adults:

Oral (immediate release), injectable:

Moderate impairment: Initiate with 25% to 50% of the usual starting dose for patients with normal hepatic function.

Severe impairment: Has not been studied; initial dose should be more conservative as compared to those with moderate impairment; use with caution.

Oral (extended release; Exalgo):

Moderate impairment: Initiate with 25% of the usual starting dose for patients with normal hepatic function; monitor closely for respiratory and CNS depression.

Severe impairment: Use alternate analgesic.

Administration

Oral: **Note:** Hydromorphone is available in an 8 mg immediate release tablet and an 8 mg extended release tablet. Extreme caution should be taken to avoid confusing dosage forms.

Immediate release: Administer with food or milk to decrease GI upset.

Extended release tablets (Exalgo): Tablets should be swallowed whole; do not crush, break, chew, dissolve, or inject. May be taken with or without food.

Parenteral:

IV: Administer via slow IV injection over at least 2 to 3 minutes; rapid IV administration has been associated with an increase in side effects, especially respiratory depression and hypotension.

IM: May be administered IM, but not recommended due to variable absorption and a lag time to peak effect (APS 2008).

Rectal: Insert suppository rectally and retain

Monitoring Parameters Respiratory rate; oxygen saturation; mental status; blood pressure; heart rate; pain relief; signs of misuse, abuse, and addiction; level of sedation

Test Interactions Some quinolones may produce a false-positive urine screening result for opioids using commercially-available immunoassay kits. This has been demonstrated most consistently for levofloxacin and ofloxacin, but other quinolones have shown cross-reactivity in certain assay kits. Confirmation of positive opioid screens by more specific methods should be considered.

Additional Information Equianalgesic doses: Morphine 10 mg IM = hydromorphone 1.5 mg IM

Controlled Substance C-II

Dosage Forms Excipient information presented when available (limited, particularly for generics); consult specific product labeling. [DSC] = Discontinued product

Liquid, Oral, as hydrochloride:

Dilaudid: 1 mg/mL (473 mL) [contains methylparaben, propylparaben, sodium metabisulfite; sweet flavor]

Generic: 1 mg/mL (473 mL)

Solution, Injection, as hydrochloride:

Dilaudid: 1 mg/mL (1 mL [DSC]); 2 mg/mL (1 mL); 4 mg/mL (1 mL)

Dilaudid-HP: 10 mg/mL (1 mL, 5 mL, 50 mL)

Generic: 1 mg/mL (0.5 mL, 1 mL); 2 mg/mL (1 mL, 20 mL); 4 mg/mL (1 mL); 10 mg/mL (1 mL); 50 mg/5 mL (5 mL); 500 mg/50 mL (50 mL)

Solution, Injection, as hydrochloride [preservative free]:

Generic: 10 mg/mL (1 mL); 50 mg/5 mL (5 mL); 500 mg/50 mL (50 mL)

Solution Reconstituted, Injection, as hydrochloride:

Dilaudid-HP: 250 mg (1 ea)

Suppository, Rectal, as hydrochloride:

Generic: 3 mg (6 ea)

Tablet, Oral, as hydrochloride:

Dilaudid: 2 mg, 4 mg [contains fd&c yellow #10 aluminum lake, sodium metabisulfite]

Dilaudid: 8 mg [scored; contains sodium metabisulfite]

Generic: 2 mg, 4 mg, 8 mg

Tablet ER 24 Hour Abuse-Deterrent, Oral, as hydrochloride:

Exalgo: 8 mg, 12 mg, 16 mg, 32 mg [contains sodium metabisulfite]

Generic: 8 mg, 12 mg, 16 mg, 32 mg

◆ **Hydromorphone HP (Can)** *see* HYDROmorphone *on page 1044*

◆ **Hydromorphone HP 10 (Can)** *see* HYDROmorphone *on page 1044*

◆ **Hydromorphone HP 20 (Can)** *see* HYDROmorphone *on page 1044*

◆ **Hydromorphone HP 50 (Can)** *see* HYDROmorphone *on page 1044*

◆ **Hydromorphone HP Forte (Can)** *see* HYDROmorphone *on page 1044*

◆ **Hydromorphone Hydrochloride** *see* HYDROmorphone *on page 1044*

◆ **Hydromorphone Hydrochloride Injection, USP (Can)** *see* HYDROmorphone *on page 1044*

◆ **HydroSKIN [OTC]** *see* Hydrocortisone (Topical) *on page 1041*

◆ **Hydro Skin Maximum Strength [OTC]** *see* Hydrocortisone (Topical) *on page 1041*

◆ **HydroVal® (Can)** *see* Hydrocortisone (Topical) *on page 1041*

Hydroxocobalamin (hye droks oh koe BAL a min)

Brand Names: US Cyanokit

Brand Names: Canada Cyanokit

Therapeutic Category Antidote, Cyanide; Nutritional Supplement; Vitamin, Water Soluble

Generic Availability (US) May be product dependent

Use

IM injection: Treatment of pernicious anemia and other vitamin B_{12} deficiency states; dietary supplement particularly in conditions of increased requirements (eg, pregnancy, thyrotoxicosis, hemorrhage, malignancy, liver or kidney disease) [FDA approved in pediatric patients (all ages) and adults]

IV infusion (Cyanokit®): Treatment of cyanide poisoning (FDA approved in adults)

Pregnancy Risk Factor C

Pregnancy Considerations Animal studies are insufficient to determine the effect, if any, on pregnancy or fetal development. There are no adequate and well-controlled studies in pregnant women. Data on the use of hydroxocobalamin in pregnancy for the treatment of cyanide poisoning and cobalamin defects are limited. In general medications used as antidotes should take into consideration the health and prognosis of the mother; antidotes should be administered to pregnant women if there is a clear indication for use and should not be withheld because of fears of teratogenicity (Bailey, 2003).

Breast-Feeding Considerations It is not known if hydroxocobalamin is excreted in breast milk. Hydroxocobalamin may be administered in life-threatening situations; therefore, use in a breast-feeding woman is not contraindicated. Because of the unknown potential for adverse reactions in nursing infants, the patient should discontinue nursing.

Contraindications

IM: Hypersensitivity to hydroxocobalamin or any component of the formulation

IV (Cyanokit®): There are no contraindications listed in the manufacturer's labeling.

Warnings/Precautions

Solution for IM injection: Treatment of severe vitamin B_{12} megaloblastic anemia may result in thrombocytosis and severe hypokalemia, sometimes fatal, due to intracellular potassium shift upon anemia resolution. Use caution in folic acid deficient megaloblastic anemia; administration of vitamin B_{12} alone is not a substitute for folic acid and might mask true diagnosis. Vitamin B_{12} deficiency masks signs of polycythemia vera; vitamin B_{12} administration may unmask this condition. Neurologic manifestations of vitamin B_{12} deficiency will not be prevented with folic acid unless vitamin B_{12} is also given; spinal cord degeneration might also occur when folic acid is used as a substitute for vitamin B_{12} in anemia prevention. Blunted therapeutic response to vitamin B_{12} may occur in certain conditions (eg, infection, uremia, concurrent iron or folic acid deficiency) or in patients on medications with bone marrow suppressant properties (eg, chloramphenicol). Approved for use as IM injection only.

Cyanokit®: Use caution or consider alternatives in patients known to be allergic to, or who have experienced anaphylaxis,with hydroxocobalamin or cyanocobalamin. Increased blood pressure (≥180 mm Hg systolic or ≥110 mm Hg diastolic) may occur with infusion; elevations usually noted at the beginning of the infusion, peak toward the end of the infusion and return to baseline within 4 hours of the infusion. May offset hypotension induced by nitrite administration or cyanide. Collection of pretreatment blood cyanide concentrations does not preclude administration and should not delay administration in the emergency management of suspected or confirmed cyanide toxicity. Pretreatment cyanide concentrations may be useful as post infusion concentrations may be inaccurate. Treatment of cyanide poisoning should include external decontamination and supportive therapy. Fire victims may present with both cyanide and carbon monoxide poisoning. In this scenario, hydroxocobalamin is the agent of choice for cyanide intoxication. Hydroxocobalamin can discolor the skin and exudates, complicating the assessment of burn severity. Use caution with concurrent use of other cyanide antidotes; safety has not been established. Hydroxocobalamin may interfere with and/or trip alarms in patients who use hemodialysis machines that rely on colorimetric technology. Photosensitivity is a potential concern; avoid direct sunlight while skin remains discolored.

Adverse Reactions

IM injection:

Dermatologic: Exanthema (transient), itching

Gastrointestinal: Diarrhea (mild, transient)

Local: Injection site pain

Miscellaneous: Anaphylaxis, feeling of swelling of the entire body

IV infusion (Cyanokit®):

Cardiovascular: Blood pressure increased, chest discomfort, hot flashes, peripheral edema

Central nervous system: Dizziness, headache, memory impairment, restlessness

Dermatologic: Angioneurotic edema (postmarketing reports), erythema (may last up to 2 weeks), pruritus, rash (predominantly acneiform; can appear 7-28 days after administration and usually resolves within a few weeks), urticaria

Gastrointestinal: Abdominal discomfort, diarrhea, dyspepsia, dysphagia, hematochezia, nausea, vomiting

Genitourinary: Chromaturia (may last up to 5 weeks after administration)

Hematologic: Lymphocytes decreased

Local: Infusion site reaction

Ocular: Irritation, redness, swelling

Respiratory: Dry throat, dyspnea, throat tightness

Miscellaneous: Allergic reaction (including anaphylaxis)

Drug Interactions

Metabolism/Transport Effects None known.

Avoid Concomitant Use There are no known interactions where it is recommended to avoid concomitant use.

Increased Effect/Toxicity There are no known significant interactions involving an increase in effect.

Decreased Effect

The levels/effects of Hydroxocobalamin may be decreased by: Chloramphenicol

Storage/Stability

Solution for IM injection: Store at 20°C to 25°C (68°F to 77°F). Protect from light.

IV infusion (Cyanokit®): Prior to reconstitution, store at 25°C (77°F): excursions permitted to 15°C to 30°C (59°F to 86°F).

Temperature variation exposure allowed for transport of lyophilized form:

Usual transport: ≤15 days at 5°C to 40°C (41°F to 104°F)

Desert transport: ≤4 days at 5°C to 60°C (41°F to 140°F)

Freezing/defrosting cycles: ≤15 days at -20°C to 40°C (-4°F to 104°F)

Following reconstitution, store up to 6 hours at ≤40°C (104°F); do not freeze. Discard any remaining solution after 6 hours.

Mechanism of Action Hydroxocobalamin (vitamin B_{12a}) is a precursor to cyanocobalamin (vitamin B_{12}). Cyanocobalamin acts as a coenzyme for various metabolic functions, including fat and carbohydrate metabolism and protein synthesis, used in cell replication and hematopoiesis. In the presence of cyanide, each hydroxocobalamin molecule can bind one cyanide ion by displacing it for the hydroxo ligand linked to the trivalent cobalt ion, forming cyanocobalamin, which is then excreted in the urine.

Pharmacodynamics Onset of action: IM: Megaloblastic anemia: Increased reticulocytes: 2-5 days

Pharmacokinetics (Adult data unless noted)

Distribution: Principally stored in the liver; also stored in the kidneys and adrenals

Protein binding: IM solution: Bound to transcobalamin II; IV: Cyanokit®: Significant; forms various cobalamin-(III) complexes

Half-life: IV: 26-31 hours

Metabolism: Converted in the tissues to active coenzymes methylcobalamin and deoxyadenosylcobalamin

Time to peak serum concentration: 2 hours

Elimination: Urine (50% to 60% within initial 72 hours)

Dosing: Neonatal IM:

Congenital transcobalamin deficiency: 1000 **mcg** twice weekly

Cobalamin C disease: 1000 **mcg**/dose once daily was used in a single full-term neonate in conjunction with carnitine and folinic acid (Kind, 2002)

Dosing: Usual

Infants, Children, and Adolescents: **Note:** Due to large difference in dose for different indications; pediatric dosage may be presented in mg or **mcg**; verify dosing units.

Cyanide poisoning: Cyanokit®: Limited data available: **Note**: If cyanide poisoning is suspected, antidotal therapy must be given immediately: IV: 70 mg/kg as a single infusion; maximum dose: 5000 mg; may repeat a second dose of 35 mg/kg (maximum dose: 2500 mg) depending on the severity of poisoning and clinical response (Shepherd, 2008)

Vitamin B_{12} deficiency (pernicious anemia); treatment (uncomplicated disease): IM:

Manufacturer labeling: Initial: 100 **mcg**/day for ≥2 weeks total dose range: 1000-5000 **mcg**; maintenance: 30-50 **mcg**/month

Alternate dosing: Initial: 1000 **mcg**/day for 7 days, then 100 **mcg** once weekly for 1 month; then maintenance: 100 **mcg**/month

Adults:

Cyanide poisoning: (Cyanokit®): **Note:** If cyanide poisoning is suspected, antidotal therapy must be given immediately. IV: Initial: 5 g as single infusion; may repeat a second 5 g dose depending on the severity of poisoning and clinical response: maximum cumulative dose: 10 g

Vitamin B_{12} deficiency (pernicious anemia); treatment: IM: Initial: 30 **mcg** once daily for 5-10 days; maintenance: 100-200 **mcg** once per month. **Note:** Larger doses may be required in critically ill patients or if patient has neurologic disease, an infectious disease, or hyperthyroidism.

Dosing adjustment in renal impairment: There are no dosage adjustments provided in manufacturer's labeling (has not been studied).

Dosing adjustment in hepatic impairment: There are no dosage adjustments provided in manufacturer's labeling (has not been studied).

Preparation for Administration Parenteral: IV (Cyanokit): Reconstitute each 5 g vial with 200 mL of NS using provided sterile transfer spike. If NS is unavailable, may use LR or D_5W. Invert or rock each vial for 60 seconds prior to infusion; do not shake. Discard if solution is **not** dark red.

Administration Parenteral:

IM: Administer 1000 mcg/mL injection IM only; do not administer SubQ

IV: Cyanokit: Administer as IV infusion over 15 minutes; if second dose is needed, administer second dose over 15 minutes to 2 hours depending upon the patient's clinical state. Hydroxocobalamin is chemically incompatible with sodium thiosulfate and sodium nitrite and separate IV lines must be used if concomitant administration is desired **(the safety of coadministration is not established)**.

Monitoring Parameters

Vitamin B_{12}, hematocrit, hemoglobin, reticulocyte count, red blood cell counts, folate and iron levels should be obtained prior to treatment and periodically during treatment.

Cyanide poisoning: Blood pressure and heart rate during and after infusion, serum lactate levels, venous-arterial PO_2gradient. Pretreatment cyanide levels may be useful as post infusion levels may be inaccurate.

Megaloblastic anemia: In addition to normal hematological parameters, serum potassium and platelet counts should be monitored during therapy, particularly in the first 48 hours of treatment.

Reference Range

Vitamin B_{12}: Normal: 200-900 pg/mL; vitamin B_{12} deficiency: <200 pg/mL; megaloblastic anemia: <100 pg/mL

Cyanide poisoning: Blood cyanide levels may be used for diagnosis confirmation; however, reliable levels require prompt testing and proper storage conditions

Cyanide levels related to clinical symptomatology:

- Tachycardia/flushing: 0.5-1 mg/L
- Obtundation: 1-2.5 mg/L
- Coma: 2.5-3 mg/L
- Death: >3 mg/L

Test Interactions The following values may be affected, *in vitro*, following hydroxocobalamin 5 g dose. Interference following hydroxocobalamin 10 g dose can be expected to last up to an additional 24 hours. **Note:** Extent and duration of interference dependent on analyzer used and patient variability.

Falsely elevated:

- Basophils, hemoglobin, MCH, and MCHC [duration: 12-16 hours]
- Albumin, alkaline phosphatase, cholesterol, creatinine, glucose, total protein, and triglycerides [duration: 24 hours]
- Bilirubin [duration: up to 4 days]
- Urinalysis: Glucose, protein, erythrocytes, leukocytes, ketones, bilirubin, urobilinogen, nitrite [duration: 2-8 days]

Falsely decreased: ALT and amylase [duration: 24 hours]

Unpredictable:

- AST, CK, CKMB, LDH, phosphate, and uric acid [duration: 24 hours]
- PT (quick or INR) and aPTT [duration: 24-48 hours]
- Urine pH [duration: 2-8 days]

May also interfere with colorimetric tests and cause hemodialysis machines to shut down due to false detection of a blood leak from the blood-like appearance of the solution.

Additional Information Cyanocobalamin is preferred over hydroxocobalamin as a treatment agent for anemia due to reports of antibody formation to the hydroxocobalamin-transcobalamin complex. Cyanide is a clear colorless gas or liquid with a faint bitter almond odor. Cyanide reacts with trivalent ions in cytochrome oxidase in the mitochondria leading to histotoxic hypoxia and lactic acidosis. Signs and symptoms of cyanide toxicity include headache, altered mental status, dyspnea, mydriasis, chest tightness, nausea, vomiting, tachycardia/hypertension (initially), bradycardia/hypotension (later), seizures, cardiovascular collapse, or coma. Expert advice from a regional poison control center for appropriate use may be obtained (1-800-222-1222). Guidelines suggest that at least 10 **g** be stocked. This is enough to treat 1 patient weighing 100 kg for an initial 8- to 24-hour period (Dart, 2009).

Dosage Forms Excipient information presented when available (limited, particularly for generics); consult specific product labeling.

Solution, Intramuscular:

Generic: 1000 mcg/mL (30 mL)

Solution Reconstituted, Intravenous:

Cyanokit: 5 g (1 ea)

◆ **Hydroxycarbamide** *see* Hydroxyurea *on page 1055*

Hydroxychloroquine (hye droks ee KLOR oh kwin)

Medication Safety Issues

Sound-alike/look-alike issues:

Hydroxychloroquine may be confused with hydrocortisone

Plaquenil may be confused with Platinol

Brand Names: US Plaquenil

Brand Names: Canada Apo-Hydroxyquine; Gen-Hydroxychloroquine; Mylan-Hydroxychloroquine; Plaquenil; PRO-Hydroxyquine

Therapeutic Category Antimalarial Agent; Antirheumatic, Disease Modifying

Generic Availability (US) Yes

Use Suppression or treatment of malaria caused by susceptible *P. vivax*, *P. ovale*, *P. malariae*, and some strains of *P. falciparum* (not effective against chloroquine-resistant strains of *P. falciparum*; not active against pre-erythrocytic or exoerythrocytic tissue stages of *Plasmodium*); treatment of systemic lupus erythematosus (SLE) and acute or chronic rheumatoid arthritis

Pregnancy Considerations Hydroxychloroquine can be detected in the cord blood at delivery in concentrations similar to those in the maternal serum (Costedoat-Chalumeau, 2002). In animal reproduction studies with chloroquine, accumulation in fetal ocular tissues was observed and remained for several months following drug elimination from the rest of the body. Based on available human data, an increased risk of fetal ocular toxicity has not been observed following maternal use of hydroxychloroquine, but additional studies are needed to confirm (Osadchy, 2011).

Maternal lupus is associated with adverse maternal and fetal events; however, pregnancy outcomes may be improved if conception does not occur until the disease has been inactive for ≥6 months. Hydroxychloroquine is one of the medications recommended for the management of lupus and lupus nephritis in pregnant women. If pregnancy is detected during therapy, it should not be stopped (could precipitate a flare in maternal disease and exposure to the fetus will still continue for 6-8 weeks due to tissue binding) (Baer, 2011; Bertsias, 2012; Hahn, 2012; Levy, 2001). Maternal use of hydroxychloroquine may also decrease the incidence of cardiac malformations associated with neonatal lupus (Izmirly, 2012).

Malaria infection in pregnant women may be more severe than in nonpregnant women and has a high risk of maternal and perinatal morbidity and mortality. Therefore, pregnant women and women who are likely to become pregnant are advised to avoid travel to malaria-risk areas. Hydroxychloroquine is recommended as an alternative treatment of pregnant women for uncomplicated malaria in chloroquine-sensitive regions (refer to current guidelines) (CDC, 2011).

Women exposed to hydroxychloroquine for the treatment of rheumatoid arthritis or systemic lupus erythematosus during pregnancy may be enrolled in the Organization of Teratology Information Specialists (OTIS) Autoimmune Diseases Study pregnancy registry (877-311-8972).

Breast-Feeding Considerations Hydroxychloroquine is excreted into breast milk in low concentrations (Costedoat-Chalumeau, 2002; Ostensen, 1985). In a case report, hydroxychloroquine concentrations were ~100 ng/mL in the maternal serum and 3.2 ng/mL in breast milk 15-24 hours after an initial maternal dose of 200 mg twice daily; the highest milk concentration was 10.6 ng/mL when measured 39-48 hours into the dosing regimen (Østensen, 1985)

Contraindications Hypersensitivity to hydroxychloroquine, 4-aminoquinoline derivatives, or any component of the formulation; retinal or visual field changes attributable to 4-aminoquinolines; long-term use in children

Warnings/Precautions May cause ophthalmic adverse effects (risk factors include daily doses >6.5 mg/kg lean body weight) or neuromyopathy; perform baseline and periodic (every 3 months) ophthalmologic examinations; test periodically for muscle weakness. Rare cardiomyopathy has been associated with long-term use of hydroxychloroquine. Aminoquinolines have been associated with rare hematologic reactions, including agranulocytosis, aplastic anemia, and thrombocytopenia; monitoring (CBC) is recommended in prolonged therapy. Use with caution in patients with hepatic disease, G6PD deficiency, psoriasis, and porphyria. Use caution in children due to increased sensitivity to adverse effects (long-term use in children is contraindicated). Not effective in the treatment of malaria caused by chloroquine resistant *P. falciparum.* **[U.S. Boxed Warning]: Should be prescribed by physicians familiar with its use.**

Adverse Reactions

Cardiovascular: Cardiomyopathy (rare, relationship to hydroxychloroquine unclear)

Central nervous system: Ataxia, dizziness, emotional disturbance, headache, irritability, lassitude, nerve deafness, nervousness, nightmares, psychosis, seizure, suicidal tendencies (children may be more susceptible), vertigo

Dermatologic: Alopecia, bleaching of hair, bullous rash (including erythema multiforme, Stevens-Johnson syndrome, toxic epidermal necrolysis, photosensitivity, exfoliative dermatitis), dyschromia (skin and mucosal; black-blue color), exacerbation of psoriasis (nonlight sensitive), pruritus, urticaria

Endocrine & metabolic: Exacerbation of porphyria, weight loss

Gastrointestinal: Anorexia, diarrhea, nausea, stomach cramps, vomiting

Hematologic & oncologic: Agranulocytosis, anemia, aplastic anemia, hemolysis (in patients with glucose-6-phosphate deficiency), leukopenia, thrombocytopenia

Hepatic: Hepatic insufficiency (hepatic failure; isolated cases)

Hypersensitivity: Angioedema

Neuromuscular & skeletal: Myopathy (including palsy or neuromyopathy, leading to progressive weakness and atrophy of proximal muscle groups; may be associated with mild sensory changes, loss of deep tendon reflexes, and abnormal nerve conduction)

Ophthalmic: Accommodation disturbance, corneal changes (transient edema, punctate to lineal opacities, decreased sensitivity, deposits, visual disturbances, blurred vision, photophobia [reversible on discontinuation]), decreased visual acuity, epithelial keratopathy, macular degeneration, macular edema, maculopathy, nystagmus, optic disk disorder (pallor/atrophy), retinal pigment changes, retinal vascular disease (attenuation of arterioles), retinitis pigmentosa, retinopathy (early changes reversible [may progress despite discontinuation if advanced]), scotoma, vision color changes, visual field defect

Otic: Tinnitus

Respiratory: Bronchospasm, respiratory failure (myopathy-related)

Postmarketing and/or case reports: Hypoglycemia (Cansu, 2008; Unübol, 2011), keratopathy (Dosso, 2007)

Drug Interactions

Metabolism/Transport Effects None known.

Avoid Concomitant Use

Avoid concomitant use of Hydroxychloroquine with any of the following: Artemether; Lumefantrine; Mefloquine

Increased Effect/Toxicity

Hydroxychloroquine may increase the levels/effects of: Antipsychotic Agents (Phenothiazines); Beta-Blockers; Cardiac Glycosides; Dapsone (Systemic); Dapsone (Topical); Lumefantrine; Mefloquine

The levels/effects of Hydroxychloroquine may be increased by: Artemether; Dapsone (Systemic); Mefloquine

Decreased Effect

Hydroxychloroquine may decrease the levels/effects of: Anthelmintics

Storage/Stability Store tablets at room temperature; protect from light.

Mechanism of Action Interferes with digestive vacuole function within sensitive malarial parasites by increasing the pH and interfering with lysosomal degradation of hemoglobin; inhibits locomotion of neutrophils and chemotaxis of eosinophils; impairs complement-dependent antigen-antibody reactions

Pharmacodynamics Onset of action for JRA: 2-4 months, up to 6 months

Pharmacokinetics (Adult data unless noted)

Absorption: Highly variable (31% to 100%)

Distribution: Extensive distribution to most body fluids and tissues; excreted into breast milk; crosses the placenta

Metabolism: In the liver

Bioavailability: Increased when administered with food

Elimination: Metabolites and unchanged drug slowly excreted in the urine

Dosing: Usual Oral:

Children:

Chemoprophylaxis of malaria: 5 mg/kg **(base)** once weekly; do not exceed the recommended adult dose; begin 2 weeks before exposure; continue for 4 weeks after leaving endemic area

Uncomplicated acute attack of malaria: 10 mg/kg **(base)** initial dose; followed by 5 mg/kg **(base)** in 6-8 hours on day 1; 5 mg/kg **(base)** as a single dose on day 2 and on day 3

JRA or SLE: 3-5 mg/kg/day **(as sulfate)** divided 1-2 times/day to a maximum of 400 mg/day **(as sulfate)**; not to exceed 7 mg/kg/day

Adults:

Chemoprophylaxis of malaria: 310 mg **(base)** once weekly on same day each week; begin 2 weeks before exposure; continue for 4 weeks after leaving endemic area

Uncomplicated acute attack of malaria: 620 mg **(base)** first dose day one; 310 mg **(base)** in 6-8 hours day one; 310 mg **(base)** as a single dose day 2; and 310 mg **(base)** as a single dose on day 3

Rheumatoid arthritis: 400-600 mg/day **(as sulfate)** once daily to start; increase dose until optimum response level is reached; usually after 4-12 weeks dose should be reduced by 50% and a maintenance dose given of 200-400 mg/day **(as sulfate)** divided 1-2 times/day

Lupus erythematosus: 400 mg **(as sulfate)** every day or twice daily for several weeks depending on response; 200-400 mg/day **(as sulfate)** for prolonged maintenance therapy

Administration Oral: Administer with food or milk to decrease GI distress

Monitoring Parameters Ophthalmologic examination at baseline and every 3 months with prolonged therapy (including visual acuity, slit-lamp, fundoscopic, and visual field exam), CBC with differential and platelet count; check for muscular weakness with prolonged therapy

Dosage Forms Excipient information presented when available (limited, particularly for generics); consult specific product labeling.

Tablet, Oral, as sulfate:

Plaquenil: 200 mg

Generic: 200 mg

Extemporaneous Preparations A 25 mg/mL hydroxychloroquine sulfate oral suspension may be made with tablets. With a towel moistened with alcohol, remove the coating from fifteen 200 mg hydroxychloroquine sulfate tablets. Crush tablets in a mortar and reduce to a fine powder. Add 15 mL of Ora-Plus® and mix to a uniform paste; add an additional 45 mL of vehicle and mix until uniform. Mix while adding sterile water for irrigation in incremental proportions to **almost** 120 mL; transfer to a calibrated bottle, rinse mortar with sterile water, and add sufficient quantity of sterile water to make 120 mL. Label "shake well". A 30-day expiration date is recommended, although stability testing has not been performed.

Pesko LJ, "Compounding: Hydroxychloroquine," *Am Druggist*, 1993, 207(4):57.

- ◆ **Hydroxychloroquine Sulfate** *see* Hydroxychloroquine *on page 1052*
- ◆ **Hydroxydaunomycin Hydrochloride** *see* DOXOrubicin (Conventional) *on page 713*
- ◆ **Hydroxyethylcellulose** *see* Artificial Tears *on page 201*
- ◆ **Hydroxyethyl Starch** *see* Hetastarch *on page 1019*
- ◆ **Hydroxyethyl Starch** *see* Tetrastarch *on page 2037*
- ◆ **Hydroxyldaunorubicin Hydrochloride** *see* DOXOrubicin (Conventional) *on page 713*

Hydroxyprogesterone Caproate

(hye droks ee proe JES te rone CAP ro ate)

Medication Safety Issues

Sound-alike/look-alike issues:

Hydroxyprogesterone caproate may be confused with medroxyPROGESTERone

Related Information

Safe Handling of Hazardous Drugs *on page 2455*

Brand Names: US Makena

Therapeutic Category Progestin

Generic Availability (US) No

Use To reduce the risk of preterm birth in women with singleton pregnancies who have a history of spontaneous preterm birth (delivery <37 weeks gestation) with previous singleton pregnancies (FDA approved in ages ≥16 years and adults). **Note:** Not for use in women with multiple gestations or other risk factors for preterm birth; not intended to stop active preterm labor.

Prescribing and Access Restrictions The Makena Care Connection™ is a comprehensive program for patients and healthcare providers which provides administrative support (including insurance benefit investigation and prescription fulfillment); financial and co-pay assistance for eligible patients; and treatment support (including educational information, home health care service and scheduled treatment reminders). The Makena Care Connection™ is available by calling 1-800-847-3418, Monday-Friday, 8 AM to 9 PM EST.

Pregnancy Risk Factor B

Pregnancy Considerations Teratogenic events were not observed in animal reproduction studies; embryolethality was observed in some species. Teratogenic effects were not observed in human studies following second or third trimester exposure; first trimester data not available.

Maternal serum concentrations of hydroxyprogesterone caproate are widely variable and may be decreased in women with increased BMI. Hydroxyprogesterone is metabolized by the placenta and reaches the fetal circulation. In one study, the cord:maternal concentration ratio averaged 0.2. Hydroxyprogesterone caproate was detected in cord blood when delivery occurred ≥44 days after the last injection (Cartitis, 2012; Hemauer, 2008).

Breast-Feeding Considerations Progestins have been detected in milk and have not been found to adversely affect breast-feeding, health, growth, or development of the infant. Use of hydroxyprogesterone caproate is not indicated following delivery.

Contraindications Current or history of thrombosis or thromboembolic disorders; hepatic impairment, hepatic tumors or cholestatic jaundice of pregnancy; carcinoma of the breast (known or suspected) or other hormone sensitive cancers; undiagnosed vaginal bleeding unrelated to pregnancy; uncontrolled hypertension

Warnings/Precautions Hazardous agent - use appropriate precautions for handling and disposal (NIOSH 2014 [group 2]).

Not for use in women with multiple gestations or other risk factors for preterm birth. Clinical benefits related to improved neonatal mortality or morbidity following maternal use have not been demonstrated. Not intended to stop active preterm labor. May have adverse effects on glucose tolerance; use caution in women with diabetes. Use with caution in patients with depression; discontinue if depression occurs. Use with caution in patients with diseases which may be exacerbated by fluid retention, including asthma, epilepsy, migraine, diabetes, pre-eclampsia, cardiac or renal dysfunction. Specific studies have not been conducted in patients with hepatic impairment (use is contraindicated); elimination may be decreased. Monitor women who develop hypertension during therapy; consider risk versus benefit of continuation. Use is contraindicated with uncontrolled hypertension. Monitor women who develop jaundice during therapy; consider risk versus benefit of continuation. Use is contraindicated in women with cholestatic jaundice of pregnancy. Discontinue if arterial thrombosis, DVT, or thromboembolic events occur. Use is contraindicated with current or history of thrombosis or thromboembolic disorders. Limited numbers of pregnant women between 16 and 18 years of age were included in clinical trials. Contains castor oil. Discontinue if allergic reactions (eg urticaria, pruritus, angioedema) occur.

Benzyl alcohol and derivatives: Some dosage forms may contain benzyl alcohol; large amounts of benzyl alcohol (≥99 mg/kg/day) have been associated with a potentially fatal toxicity ("gasping syndrome") in neonates; the "gasping syndrome" consists of metabolic acidosis, respiratory distress, gasping respirations, CNS dysfunction (including convulsions, intracranial hemorrhage), hypotension, and cardiovascular collapse (AAP, 1997; CDC, 1982); some data suggests that benzoate displaces bilirubin from protein binding sites (Ahlfors, 2001); avoid or use dosage forms containing benzyl alcohol with caution in neonates. See manufacturer's labeling.

Warnings: Additional Pediatric Considerations Clinical benefits related to neonatal mortality and morbidity following use have not been demonstrated. Long-term effects of hydroxyprogesterone in utero exposure were evaluated in a follow-up safety study of 278 children (mean age: 48 months) whose mothers were part of an earlier hydroxyprogesterone-placebo efficacy trial; no significant differences in physical development, neurodevelopment, and health status were reported between the treatment and placebo groups (Northen, 2007).

Adverse Reactions

Cardiovascular: Preeclampsia

Dermatologic: Pruritus, urticaria

Endocrine & metabolic: Gestational diabetes

Gastrointestinal: Diarrhea, nausea

Genitourinary: Oligohydramnios, preterm labor (admission), spontaneous abortion, stillborn infant

Local: Local pruritus, pain at injection site, swelling at injection site

Miscellaneous: Nodule

Rare but important or life-threatening: Angioedema, cellulitis at injection site, cervical dilation, cervical shortening, decreased glucose tolerance, depression, fluid retention, headache, hypersensitivity reaction, hypertension, hot flash, jaundice, premature rupture of membranes, pulmonary embolism, skin rash, thromboembolic complications, urinary tract infection

Drug Interactions

Metabolism/Transport Effects Substrate of CYP3A4 (major); **Note:** Assignment of Major/Minor substrate status based on clinically relevant drug interaction potential; **Induces** CYP1A2 (weak/moderate), CYP2A6 (strong), CYP2B6 (weak/moderate)

Avoid Concomitant Use

Avoid concomitant use of Hydroxyprogesterone Caproate with any of the following: Conivaptan; Fusidic Acid (Systemic); Idelalisib; Ulipristal

Increased Effect/Toxicity

Hydroxyprogesterone Caproate may increase the levels/effects of: C1 inhibitors

The levels/effects of Hydroxyprogesterone Caproate may be increased by: Aprepitant; Conivaptan; CYP3A4 Inhibitors (Moderate); CYP3A4 Inhibitors (Strong); Dasatinib; Fosaprepitant; Fusidic Acid (Systemic); Herbs (Progestogenic Properties); Idelalisib; Ivacaftor; Luliconazole; Mifepristone; Netupitant; Palbociclib; Simeprevir; Stiripentol

Decreased Effect

Hydroxyprogesterone Caproate may decrease the levels/effects of: Anticoagulants; Antidiabetic Agents; CYP2A6 Substrates; Ulipristal

The levels/effects of Hydroxyprogesterone Caproate may be decreased by: Bosentan; CYP3A4 Inducers (Moderate); CYP3A4 Inducers (Strong); Dabrafenib; Deferasirox; Mitotane; Siltuximab; St Johns Wort; Tocilizumab; Ulipristal

Storage/Stability Store upright at controlled room temperature of 15°C to 30°C (59°F to 86°F); protect from light. Discard within 5 weeks of first use.

Mechanism of Action Hydroxyprogesterone is a synthetic progestin. The mechanism by which hydroxyprogesterone reduces the risk of recurrent preterm birth is not known.

Pharmacokinetics (Adult data unless noted)

Distribution: Extensively bound to albumin and corticosteroid-binding globulins

Metabolism: Hepatic via CYP3A4 and 3A5; forms metabolites

Half-life elimination: ~8 days

Time to peak, serum concentration: 3-7 days

Elimination: Urine (~30%) and feces (~50%); primarily as metabolites

Dosing: Usual

Reduce the risk of preterm birth: Adolescents ≥16 years and Adults: IM: 250 mg every 7 days; treatment should be initiated between 16 weeks 0 days and 20 weeks 6 days of gestation, can be continued up to 37 weeks gestation (ie, 36 weeks 6 days) or until delivery, whichever occurs first.

Administration Hazardous agent; use appropriate precautions for handling and disposal (NIOSH 2014 [group 2]).

IM: Withdraw dose using an 18-gauge needle; inject dose using a 21-gauge 1 1/2-inch needle. Administer by slow injection (≥1 minute) into the upper outer quadrant of the gluteus maximus by a healthcare professional. Solution is viscous and oily; do not use if solution is cloudy or contains solid particles. Apply pressure to injection site to decrease bruising and swelling.

Monitoring Parameters Signs and symptoms of thromboembolic disorders; signs or symptoms of depression; signs and symptoms of jaundice; glucose in patients with diabetes; or blood pressure

Dosage Forms Excipient information presented when available (limited, particularly for generics); consult specific product labeling.

Oil, Intramuscular:

Makena: 250 mg/mL (5 mL) [contains benzyl alcohol, benzyl benzoate]

◆ **9-hydroxy-risperidone** *see* Paliperidone *on page 1604*

Hydroxyurea (hye droks ee yoor EE a)

Medication Safety Issues

Sound-alike/look-alike issues:

Hydrea may be confused with Lyrica

Hydroxyurea may be confused with hydrOXYzine

High alert medication:

This medication is in a class the Institute for Safe Medication Practices (ISMP) includes among its list of drug classes which have a heightened risk of causing significant patient harm when used in error.

International issues:

Hydrea [US, Canada, and multiple international markets] may be confused with Hydra brand name for isoniazid [Japan]

Related Information

Oral Medications That Should Not Be Crushed or Altered *on page 2476*

Prevention of Chemotherapy-Induced Nausea and Vomiting in Children *on page 2368*

Safe Handling of Hazardous Drugs *on page 2455*

Brand Names: US Droxia; Hydrea

Brand Names: Canada Apo-Hydroxyurea; Gen-Hydroxyurea; Hydrea; Mylan-Hydroxyurea

Therapeutic Category Antineoplastic Agent, Miscellaneous

Generic Availability (US) Yes

Use Treatment of refractory chronic myelocytic leukemia (CML), melanoma, and recurrent, metastatic or inoperable ovarian carcinoma (Hydrea: FDA approved in adults); treatment of primary squamous cell carcinomas of the head and neck with radiation (excluding lip cancer) (Hydrea: FDA approved in adults); management of sickle cell anemia in patients who have had at least three painful crises in the previous 12 months (to reduce frequency of these crises and the need for blood transfusions) (Droxia: FDA approved in adults)

Pregnancy Risk Factor D

Pregnancy Considerations Animal reproduction studies have demonstrated teratogenicity and embryotoxicity at doses lower than the usual human dose (based on BSA). Hydroxyurea may cause fetal harm if administered during pregnancy. Women of childbearing potential should be advised to avoid becoming pregnant during treatment and should use effective contraception.

Breast-Feeding Considerations Hydroxyurea is excreted in breast milk. Due to the potential for serious adverse reactions in the nursing infant, the decision to discontinue hydroxyurea or to discontinue breast-feeding should take into account the importance of treatment to the mother.

Contraindications Hypersensitivity to hydroxyurea or any component of the formulation

Hydrea: Marked bone marrow suppression (WBC <2500/mm^3 or platelet count <100,000/mm^3) or severe anemia

Warnings/Precautions Hazardous agent - use appropriate precautions for handling and disposal (NIOSH 2014 [group 1]); to decrease risk of exposure, wear gloves when handling and wash hands before and after contact. Leukopenia and neutropenia commonly occur (thrombocytopenia and anemia are less common); leukopenia/neutropenia occur first. Hematologic toxicity reversible (rapid) with treatment interruption. Correct severe anemia prior to initiating treatment. Hydrea use is contraindicated in marked bone marrow suppression; Droxia should not be used in sickle cell anemia with severe bone marrow suppression (neutrophils <2,000/mm^3, platelets <80,000/mm^3, hemoglobin <4.5 g/dL, or reticulocytes <80,000/mm^3 when hemoglobin <9 g/dL per manufacturer's labeling). Use with caution in patients with a history of prior chemotherapy or radiation therapy; myelosuppression is more common. Patients with a history of radiation therapy are also at risk for exacerbation of post irradiation erythema. Self-limiting megaloblastic erythropoiesis may be seen early in treatment (may resemble pernicious anemia, but is unrelated to vitamin B_{12} or folic acid deficiency). Plasma iron clearance may be delayed and iron utilization rate (by erythrocytes) may be reduced. Potentially significant drug-drug interactions may exist, requiring dose or frequency adjustment, additional monitoring, and/or selection of alternative therapy. When treated concurrently with hydroxyurea and antiretroviral agents (including didanosine and stavudine), HIV-infected patients are at higher risk for potentially fatal pancreatitis, hepatotoxicity, hepatic failure, and severe peripheral neuropathy; discontinue immediately if signs of these toxicities develop. Hyperuricemia may occur with antineoplastic treatment; adequate hydration and initiation or dosage adjustment of uricosuric agents (eg, allopurinol) may be necessary.

In patients with sickle cell anemia, Droxia is not recommended if neutrophils <2,000/mm^3, platelets <80,000/mm^3, hemoglobin <4.5 g/dL, or reticulocytes <80,000/mm^3 when hemoglobin <9 g/dL per manufacturer's labeling. May cause macrocytosis, which can mask folic acid deficiency; prophylactic folic acid supplementation is recommended. **[US Boxed Warning]: Hydroxyurea is mutagenic and clastogenic; causes cellular transformation resulting in tumorigenicity; also considered genotoxic and may be carcinogenic. Treatment of myeloproliferative disorders (eg, polycythemia vera, thrombocythemia) with long-term hydroxyurea is associated with secondary leukemia;** it is unknown if this is drug-related or disease-related. Skin cancer has been reported with long-term hydroxyurea use. Cutaneous vasculitic toxicities (vasculitic ulceration and gangrene) have been reported with hydroxyurea treatment, most often in patients with a history of or receiving concurrent interferon therapy; discontinue hydroxyurea and consider alternate cytoreductive therapy if cutaneous vasculitic toxicity develops. Use caution with renal dysfunction; may require dose reductions. Elderly patients may be more sensitive to the effects of hydroxyurea; may require lower doses. **[US Boxed Warning]: Should be administered under the supervision of a physician experienced in the treatment of sickle cell anemia** or in cancer chemotherapy.

Adverse Reactions

Cardiovascular: Edema, hypersensitivity angiitis

Central nervous system: Chills, disorientation, dizziness, drowsiness (dose-related), hallucination, headache, malaise, peripheral neuropathy (HIV-infected patients), seizure, vasculitic ulcerations

Dermatologic: Alopecia, atrophy of nail, changes in nails, dermal ulcer, dermatomyositis-like skin changes, desquamation, eczema, erythema (peripheral), facial erythema, gangrene of skin or other tissue, hyperpigmentation, leg ulcer, maculopapular rash, nail discoloration, papule (violet), skin atrophy, skin carcinoma

Endocrine & metabolic: Increased uric acid

Gastrointestinal: Acute mucocutaneous toxicity, anorexia, BSP abnormality (retention), constipation, diarrhea, gastric distress, gastrointestinal irritation (potentiated with radiation therapy), mucositis (potentiated with radiation therapy), nausea, oral mucosa ulcer, pancreatitis (HIV-infected patients), stomatitis, vomiting

Genitourinary: Dysuria

Hematologic & oncologic: Abnormal erythropoiesis (megaloblastic; self-limiting), bone marrow depression (neutropenia, thrombocytopenia; hematologic recovery: within 2 weeks), leukemia (secondary; long-term use), leukopenia, macrocytosis, reticulocytopenia

Hepatic: Hepatic failure (HIV-infected patients), hepatotoxicity, increased liver enzymes

Neuromuscular & skeletal: Panniculitis, weakness

Renal: Increased blood urea nitrogen, increased serum creatinine, renal tubular disease

Respiratory: Asthma, dyspnea, pulmonary fibrosis (rare), pulmonary infiltrates (diffuse, rare)

Rare but important or life-threatening: Actinic keratosis (Antonioli 2012), basal cell carcinoma (Antonioli 2012), hyperkeratosis (Antonioli 2012), lesion (dyschromic [Antonioli 2012]), malignant neoplasm (Wong 2014), mucous membrane lesion (Antonioli 2012), pneumonitis (Antonioli 2012), squamous cell carcinoma (Antonioli 2012)

Drug Interactions

Metabolism/Transport Effects None known.

Avoid Concomitant Use

Avoid concomitant use of Hydroxyurea with any of the following: BCG; BCG (Intravesical); CloZAPine; Didanosine; Dipyrone; Natalizumab; Pimecrolimus; Stavudine; Tacrolimus (Topical); Tofacitinib; Vaccines (Live)

Increased Effect/Toxicity

Hydroxyurea may increase the levels/effects of: CloZAPine; Didanosine; Leflunomide; Natalizumab; Stavudine; Tofacitinib; Vaccines (Live)

The levels/effects of Hydroxyurea may be increased by: Denosumab; Didanosine; Dipyrone; Pimecrolimus; Roflumilast; Stavudine; Tacrolimus (Topical); Trastuzumab

Decreased Effect

Hydroxyurea may decrease the levels/effects of: BCG; BCG (Intravesical); Coccidioides immitis Skin Test; Sipuleucel-T; Vaccines (Inactivated); Vaccines (Live)

The levels/effects of Hydroxyurea may be decreased by: Echinacea

Storage/Stability Store at room temperature of 25°C (77°F); excursions permitted between 15°C and 30°C (59°F and 86°F).

Mechanism of Action Antimetabolite which selectively inhibits ribonucleoside diphosphate reductase, preventing the conversion of ribonucleotides to deoxyribonucleotides, halting the cell cycle at the G1/S phase and therefore has radiation sensitizing activity by maintaining cells in the G_1 phase and interfering with DNA repair. In sickle cell anemia, hydroxyurea increases red blood cell (RBC) hemoglobin F levels, RBC water content, deformability of sickled cells, and alters adhesion of RBCs to endothelium.

Pharmacodynamics

Onset: Sickle cell anemia: Fetal hemoglobin increase: 4 to 12 weeks

Maximum effect: Sickle cell anemia: 6 to 18 months

Pharmacokinetics (Adult data unless noted) Note: In pediatric patients, large interpatient variability and phenotypic differences have been reported (Ware 2011).

Absorption: Relatively rapid (Rodriguez 1998)

Distribution: Distributes widely into tissues (including into the brain); concentrates in leukocytes and erythrocytes; estimated volume of distribution approximating total body water (Gwilt 1998)

V_d:

Children: ~12 L (range: 2.5 to 52) (Ware 2011)

Adults: ~20 L/m^2 (Rodriguez 1998)

Metabolism: 60% via hepatic metabolism and urease found in intestinal bacteria

Bioavailability: ~100% (Rodriguez 1998)

Half-life:

Children: 1.7 hours (range: 0.65 to 3.05 hours) (Ware 2011)

Adults: 1.9 to 3.9 hours (Gwilt 1998)

Time to peak serum concentration:

Children: "Fast" phenotype: 15 to 30 minutes; "Slow" phenotype: 60 to 120 minutes (Ware 2011)

Adults: 1 to 4 hours

Elimination: Urine (sickle cell anemia: 40% of administered dose)

Clearance:

Children: ~7 L/hour (range: 1.6 to 22) (Ware 2011)

Adults: ~7.5 L/hour (Rodriguez 1998)

Dosing: Usual Note: Doses should be based on ideal or actual body weight, whichever is less (per manufacturer).

Pediatric: **Sickle cell anemia:** Limited data available: Infants ≥6 months, Children, and Adolescents: Oral: 20 mg/kg/dose once daily; increase by 5 mg/kg/**day** every 8 weeks until mild myelosuppression (neutrophils 2,000 to 4,000/mm^3) is achieved up to a maximum of 35 mg/kg/**day** (Hankins 2005; NHLBI 2014; Strouse 2012). If myelosuppression occurs (platelets <80,000/mm^3, neutrophils <2,000/mm^3; younger patients with lower baseline counts may safely tolerate ANC down to 1,250/mm^3), hold therapy until counts recover (monitor weekly); reinitiate at a dose 5 mg/kg/day lower than the dose given prior to onset of cytopenias (NHLBI 2014); some have recommended reinitiating at a dose 2.5 mg/kg/day lower (Hankins 2005; Heeney 2008; Wang 2001; Wang 2011; Zimmerman 2004). **Note:** A clinical response to treatment may take 3 to 6 months; a 6 month trial on the maximum tolerated dose is recommended prior to considering discontinuation due to treatment failure; effectiveness of hydroxyurea depends upon daily dosing adherence. For patients who have a clinical response, long-term hydroxyurea therapy is indicated (NHLBI 2014)

Adult:

Antineoplastic uses: Titrate dose to patient response; if WBC count falls to <2,500/mm^3, or the platelet count to <100,000/mm^3, therapy should be stopped for at least 3 days and resumed when values rise toward normal.

ASCO guidelines for chemotherapy dosing in obese adults with cancer: Utilize patient's actual body weight (full weight) for calculation of body surface area- or weight-based dosing, particularly when the intent of therapy is curative; manage regimen-related toxicities in the same manner as for nonobese patients; if a dose reduction is utilized due to toxicity, consider resumption of full weight-based dosing with subsequent cycles, especially if cause of toxicity (eg, hepatic or renal impairment) is resolved (Griggs 2012). **Note:** The manufacturer recommends dosing based on ideal or actual body weight, whichever is less.

Chronic myelocytic leukemia (resistant): Oral: Continuous therapy: 20 to 30 mg/kg/dose once daily

Solid tumors (head and neck cancer, melanoma, ovarian cancer): Oral:

Intermittent therapy: 80 mg/kg as a single dose every third day

Continuous therapy: 20 to 30 mg/kg/dose once daily

Concomitant therapy with irradiation (head and neck cancer): 80 mg/kg as a single dose every third day starting at least 7 days before initiation of irradiation

Sickle cell anemia:

Manufacturer's labeling: Initial: 15 mg/kg/day as a single dose; if blood counts are in an acceptable range, may increase by 5 mg/kg/day every 12 weeks until the maximum tolerated dose of 35 mg/kg/day is achieved or the dose that does not produce toxic effects (do not increase dose if blood counts are between acceptable and toxic ranges). Monitor for toxicity every 2 weeks; if toxicity occurs, withhold treatment until the bone marrow recovers, then restart with a dose reduction of 2.5 mg/kg/day; if no toxicity occurs over the next 12 weeks, then the subsequent dose may be increased by 2.5 mg/kg/day every 12 weeks to a maximum tolerated dose (dose which does not produce hematologic toxicity for 24 consecutive weeks). If hematologic toxicity recurs a second time at a specific dose, do not retry that dose.

Acceptable hematologic ranges: Neutrophils ≥2,500/mm^3; platelets ≥95,000/mm^3; hemoglobin >5.3 g/dL, and reticulocytes ≥95,000/mm^3 if the hemoglobin concentration is <9 g/dL

Toxic hematologic ranges: Neutrophils <2,000/mm^3; platelets <80,000/mm^3; hemoglobin <4.5 g/dL; and reticulocytes <80,000/mm^3 if the hemoglobin concentration is <9 g/dL

Alternate recommendations: Initial: 15 mg/kg/day; if dosage escalation is warranted based on clinical/laboratory findings, may increase by 5 mg/kg/day increments every 8 weeks. Monitor for toxicity at least every 4 weeks when adjusting dose; aim for a target absolute neutrophils ≥2,000/mm^3 (younger patients with lower baseline counts may safely tolerate absolute neutrophils down to 1,250/mm^3; maintain platelet count ≥80,000/mm^3. Give until mild myelosuppression is achieved (absolute neutrophils: 2,000/mm^3 to 4,000/mm^3), up to a maximum dose of 35 mg/kg/day. If toxicity occurs (neutropenia or thrombocytopenia), withhold treatment until the bone marrow recovers (monitor weekly), then restart at a dose 5 mg/kg/day lower than the dose given prior to onset of cytopenias (NHLBI 2014). **Note:** A clinical response to treatment may take 3 to 6 months; a 6 month trial on the maximum tolerated dose is recommended prior to considering discontinuation due to treatment failure; effectiveness of hydroxyurea depends upon daily dosing adherence. For patients who have a clinical response, long-term hydroxyurea therapy is indicated (NHLBI 2014).

Dosing adjustment for toxicity: Adults:

Cutaneous vasculitic ulcerations: Discontinue

Gastrointestinal toxicity (severe nausea, vomiting, anorexia): Temporarily interrupt treatment

Mucositis (severe): Temporarily interrupt treatment

Pancreatitis: Discontinue permanently

Hematologic toxicity:

Antineoplastic uses (CML, head and neck cancer, melanoma, ovarian cancer): WBC <2,500/mm^3 or platelets <100,000/mm^3: Interrupt treatment (for at least 3 days), may resume when values rise toward normal

Sickle cell anemia:

Manufacturer's labeling: Neutrophils <2,000/mm^3, platelets <80,000/mm^3, hemoglobin <4.5 g/dL, or reticulocytes <80,000/mm^3 with hemoglobin <9 g/dL: Interrupt treatment; following recovery, may resume with a dose reduction of 2.5 mg/kg/day. If no toxicity occurs over the next 12 weeks, subsequent dose may be increased by 2.5 mg/kg/day every 12 weeks to a dose which does not produce hematologic toxicity for 24 consecutive weeks. If hematologic toxicity recurs a second time at a specific dose, do not retry that dose.

Alternate recommendations: Absolute neutrophils <2,000/mm^3 (younger patients with lower baseline counts may safely tolerate absolute neutrophils down to 1,250/mm^3), platelets <80,000/mm^3: Interrupt treatment; following recovery, may restart at a dose 5 mg/kg/day lower than the dose given prior to onset of cytopenias (NHLBI 2014).

Dosing adjustment in renal impairment:

Infants, Children, and Adolescents: The following guidelines have been used by some clinicians: Reduce initial dose to 15 mg/kg/dose once daily (Heeney 2008)

Adult:

Manufacturer labeling:

Sickle cell anemia:

CrCl ≥60 mL/minute: No adjustment (of initial dose) required

CrCl <60 mL/minute: Reduce initial dose to 7.5 mg/kg/day (Yan 2005); titrate to response/avoidance of toxicity (refer to usual dosing)

ESRD: Reduce initial dose to 7.5 mg/kg/dose (administer after dialysis on dialysis days); titrate to response/avoidance of toxicity

Other approved indications: It is recommended to reduce the initial dose; however, no specific guidelines are available.

The following guidelines have been used by some clinicians:

Aronoff 2007: Adults:

CrCl >50 mL/minute: No dosage adjustment necessary.

CrCl 10 to 50 mL/minute: Administer 50% of dose

CrCl <10 mL/minute: Administer 20% of dose

Hemodialysis: Administer dose after dialysis on dialysis days

Continuous renal replacement therapy (CRRT): Administer 50% of dose

NHLBI 2014: Sickle cell anemia: Adults: Chronic kidney disease: Initial 5 to 10 mg/kg/day

Kintzel 1995:

CrCl 46 to 60 mL/minute: Administer 85% of dose

CrCl 31 to 45 mL/minute: Administer 80% of dose

CrCl <30 mL/minute: Administer 75% of dose

Dosing adjustment in hepatic impairment: Adults: There are no dosage adjustments provided in the manufacturer's labeling; closely monitor for bone marrow toxicity.

Administration Hazardous agent; use appropriate precautions for handling and disposal (NIOSH 2014 [group 1]).

Oral: The manufacturer does not recommend opening the capsules; observe proper handling procedures (eg, wear gloves). Doses rounded to the nearest 100 mg when using capsules allows for dosing accuracy within ~2 mg/kg/day (Heeney 2008). For patients unable to swallow capsules, an oral solution may be prepared.

Monitoring Parameters

General: CBC with differential, liver function tests and renal function should be checked at baseline and then periodically throughout therapy; serum uric acid, signs and symptoms of pancreatitis

Sickle cell anemia: Monitor hemoglobin F levels. During dose escalation, monitor for toxicity every 2 weeks (neutrophils, platelets, hemoglobin, reticulocytes) per manufacturer's labeling, or at least every 4 weeks when adjusting the dose (CBC with WBC differential, reticulocytes) [NHLBI 2014]). Once on a stable dose, may monitor CBC with differential, reticulocyte count and platelets every 2 to 3 months (NHLBI 2014). Monitor RBC, MCV (mean corpuscular volume) and HbF (fetal hemoglobin) levels for evidence of consistent or progressive laboratory response (NHLBI 2014).

Test Interactions False-negative triglyceride measurement by a glycerol oxidase method. An analytical interference between hydroxyurea and enzymes (lactate dehydrogenase, urease, and uricase) may result in false elevations of lactic acid, urea, and uric acid.

Dosage Forms Excipient information presented when available (limited, particularly for generics); consult specific product labeling.

Capsule, Oral:

Droxia: 200 mg, 300 mg, 400 mg

Hydrea: 500 mg

Generic: 500 mg

Extemporaneous Preparations Hazardous agent: Use appropriate precautions for handling and disposal (NIOSH 2014 [group 1]). When manipulating capsules, NIOSH recommends double gloving, a protective gown, and preparation in a controlled device; if not prepared in a controlled device, respiratory and eye protection as well as ventilated engineering controls are recommended (NIOSH 2014).

A 40 mg/mL oral suspension may be prepared with capsules and either a 1:1 mixture of Ora-Sweet® and Ora-Plus® or a 1:1 mixture of methylcellulose 1% and simple syrup NF. Empty the contents of eight 500 mg capsules into a mortar. Add small portions of chosen vehicle and mix to a uniform paste; mix while incrementally adding the vehicle to **almost** 100 mL; transfer to a calibrated bottle, rinse mortar with vehicle, and add sufficient quantity of vehicle to make 100 mL. Label "shake well" and "refrigerate". Store in plastic prescription bottles. Stable for 14 days at room temperature or refrigerated (preferred) (Nahata 2003).

A 100 mg/mL oral solution may be prepared with capsules. Mix the contents of twenty 500 mg capsules with enough room temperature sterile water (~50 mL) to initially result in a 200 mg/mL concentration. Stir vigorously using a magnetic stirrer for several hours, then filter to remove insoluble contents. Add 50 mL Syrpalta® (flavored syrup, HUMCO) to filtered solution, resulting in 100 mL of a 100 mg/mL hydroxyurea solution. Stable for 1 month at room temperature in amber plastic bottle (Heeney 2004).

Heeney MM, Whorton MR, Howard TA, et al, "Chemical and Functional Analysis of Hydroxyurea Oral Solutions," *J Pediatr Hematol Oncol* 2004, 26(3):179-84.

Nahata MC, Morosco RS, Boster EA, et al, "Stability of Hydroxyurea in Two Extemporaneously Prepared Oral Suspensions Stored at Two Temperatures," 2003, 38:P-161(E) [abstract from 2003 ASHP Midyear Clinical Meeting].

HydrOXYzine (hye DROKS i zeen)

Medication Safety Issues

Sound-alike/look-alike issues:

HydrOXYzine may be confused with hydrALAZINE, hydroxyurea

Atarax may be confused with Ativan

Vistaril may be confused with Restoril, Versed, Zestril®

BEERS Criteria medication:

This drug may be potentially inappropriate for use in geriatric patients (Quality of evidence - high; Strength of recommendation - strong).

International issues:

Vistaril [U.S. and Turkey] may be confused with Vastarel brand name for trimetazidine [multiple international markets]

Related Information

Management of Drug Extravasations *on page 2298*

Brand Names: US Vistaril

Brand Names: Canada Apo-Hydroxyzine; Atarax; Hydroxyzine Hydrochloride Injection, USP; Novo-Hydroxyzin; Nu-Hydroxyzine; PMS-Hydroxyzine; Riva-Hydroxyzine

Therapeutic Category Antianxiety Agent; Antiemetic; Antihistamine; Sedative

Generic Availability (US) Yes

Use

Oral: Treatment of anxiety and pruritus; preoperative sedation [FDA approved in pediatric patients (age not specified) and adults]

Parenteral: Treatment of anxiety and pruritus; perioperative sedation; antiemetic [FDA approved in infants, children, adolescents, and adults]

Pregnancy Considerations Adverse events were observed in animal reproduction studies. Hydroxyzine crosses the placenta. Maternal hydroxyzine use has generally not resulted in an increased risk of birth defects. Use of hydroxyzine early in pregnancy is contraindicated but hydroxyzine is approved for pre- and postpartum adjunctive therapy to reduce opioid dosage, treat anxiety, and control emesis. Antihistamines are recommended for the treatment pruritus with rash in pregnant women (although second generation antihistamines may be preferred). Antihistamines are not recommended for treatment of pruritus associated with intrahepatic cholestasis in pregnancy. Possible withdrawal symptoms have been observed in neonates following chronic maternal use of hydroxyzine during pregnancy.

Breast-Feeding Considerations It is not known if hydroxyzine is excreted in breast milk. Breast-feeding is not recommended by the manufacturer. Antihistamines may decrease maternal serum prolactin concentrations when administered prior to the establishment of nursing.

Contraindications Hypersensitivity to hydroxyzine or any component of the formulation; early pregnancy; SubQ, intra-arterial, or IV injection

Warnings/Precautions Causes sedation, caution must be used in performing tasks which require alertness (eg, operating machinery or driving). Sedative effects of CNS depressants or ethanol are potentiated. Use with caution with narrow-angle glaucoma, prostatic hyperplasia, bladder neck obstruction, asthma, or COPD. In the elderly, avoid use of this potent anticholinergic agent due to increased risk of confusion, dry mouth, constipation, and other anticholinergic effects; clearance decreases in patients of advanced age (Beers Criteria).

For IM use only. Subcutaneous, IV, and intra-arterial routes of administration are contraindicated. Intravascular hemolysis, thrombosis, and digital gangrene have been reported with IV or intra-arterial administration (Baumgartner, 1979); SubQ administration may result in significant tissue damage. If inadvertent IV administration results in extravasation, stop infusion immediately and disconnect (leave cannula/needle in place); gently aspirate extravasated solution (do **NOT** flush the line); remove needle/cannula; elevate extremity.

Benzyl alcohol and derivatives: Some dosage forms may contain benzyl alcohol and/or sodium benzoate/benzoic acid; benzoic acid (benzoate) is a metabolite of benzyl alcohol; large amounts of benzyl alcohol (≥99 mg/kg/day) have been associated with a potentially fatal toxicity ("gasping syndrome") in neonates; the "gasping syndrome" consists of metabolic acidosis, respiratory distress, gasping respirations, CNS dysfunction (including convulsions, intracranial hemorrhage), hypotension and cardiovascular collapse (AAP, 1997; CDC, 1982); some data suggests that benzoate displaces bilirubin from protein binding sites (Ahlfors, 2001); avoid or use dosage forms containing benzyl alcohol and/or benzyl alcohol derivative with caution in neonates. See manufacturer's labeling.

Warnings: Additional Pediatric Considerations Neonatal withdrawal symptoms, including seizures, have been reported following long-term maternal use or the use of large doses near term (Serreau, 2005).

Adverse Reactions

Central nervous system: Dizziness, drowsiness (transient), fatigue, involuntary movements

Gastrointestinal: Xerostomia

Hypersensitivity: Hypersensitivity reaction

Ophthalmic: Blurred vision

Respiratory: Respiratory depression (at higher than recommended doses)

Rare but important or life-threatening: Fixed drug eruption, hallucination, seizure (at considerably higher than recommended doses), skin rash, tremor (at considerably higher than recommended doses)

Drug Interactions

Metabolism/Transport Effects **Inhibits** CYP2D6 (weak)

Avoid Concomitant Use

Avoid concomitant use of HydrOXYzine with any of the following: Aclidinium; Azelastine (Nasal); Eluxadoline; Glucagon; Ipratropium (Oral Inhalation); Orphenadrine; Paraldehyde; Potassium Chloride; Thalidomide; Tiotropium; Umeclidinium

Increased Effect/Toxicity

HydrOXYzine may increase the levels/effects of: AbobotulinumtoxinA; Alcohol (Ethyl); Anticholinergic Agents; ARIPiprazole; Azelastine (Nasal); Barbiturates; Buprenorphine; CNS Depressants; Eluxadoline; Glucagon; Highest Risk QTc-Prolonging Agents; Hydrocodone; Meperidine; Methotrimeprazine; Metyrosine; Mirabegron; Mirtazapine; Moderate Risk QTc-Prolonging Agents; OnabotulinumtoxinA; Orphenadrine; Paraldehyde; Potassium Chloride; Pramipexole; RimabotulinumtoxinB; ROPINIRole; Rotigotine; Selective Serotonin Reuptake Inhibitors; Suvorexant; Thalidomide; Thiazide Diuretics; Tiotropium; Topiramate; Zolpidem

The levels/effects of HydrOXYzine may be increased by: Aclidinium; Brimonidine (Topical); Cannabis; Doxylamine; Dronabinol; Droperidol; Ipratropium (Oral Inhalation); Kava Kava; Magnesium Sulfate; Methotrimeprazine; Mianserin; Mifepristone; Nabilone; Perampanel; Pramlintide; Rufinamide; Sodium Oxybate; Tapentadol; Tetrahydrocannabinol; Umeclidinium

Decreased Effect

HydrOXYzine may decrease the levels/effects of: Acetylcholinesterase Inhibitors; Benzylpenicilloyl Polylysine; Betahistine; Hyaluronidase; Itopride; Metoclopramide; Secretin

The levels/effects of HydrOXYzine may be decreased by: Acetylcholinesterase Inhibitors; Amphetamines

Storage/Stability

Injection: Store at 20°C to 25°C (68°F to 77°F); excursions permitted to 15°C to 30°C (59°F to 86°F). Protect from light.

Capsules: Store below 30°C (86°F); protect from light.

Solution (hydrochloride salt): Store at 15°C to 30°C (59°F to 86°F); protect from light.

Tablets: Store at 20°C to 25°C (68°F to 77°F).

Mechanism of Action Competes with histamine for H_1-receptor sites on effector cells in the gastrointestinal tract, blood vessels, and respiratory tract. Possesses skeletal muscle relaxing, bronchodilator, antihistamine, antiemetic, and analgesic properties.

Pharmacodynamics

Onset of action: Oral: Within 15-30 minutes; IM: Rapid

Maximum effect: Suppression of antihistamine-induced wheal and flare: 6-12 hours (Simons, 1984a)

Duration: Decreased histamine-induced wheal and flare areas: 2 to ≥36 hours; Suppression of pruritus: 1-12 hours (Simons, 1984a)

Pharmacokinetics (Adult data unless noted)

Absorption: Oral: Well absorbed

Distribution: V_d, apparent:

Children and Adolescents 1-14 years: 18.5 ± 8.6 L/kg (Simons, 1984)

Adults: 16 ± 3 L/kg (Simons, 1984a)

Metabolism: Hepatic to multiple metabolites, including cetirizine (active) (Simons, 1989)

Half-life:

Children and Adolescents 1-14 years (mean age: 6.1 ± 4.6 years): 7.1 ± 2.3 hours; **Note:** Half-life increased with increasing age and was 4 hours in patients 1-year old and 11 hours in a 14-year old patient (Simons, 1984)

Adults: 3 hours; one study reported a terminal half-life of 20 hours (Simons, 1984a)

Time to peak serum concentration: Oral: 2 hours

Elimination: Active metabolite (cetirizine) is renally eliminated (Simons, 1994)

Dosing: Usual

Infants, Children, and Adolescents:

Antiemetic: IM: 1.1 mg/kg/dose; maximum single dose: 100 mg

Anxiety:

Manufacturer's labeling: Oral:

Children <6 years: 50 mg/day in 4 divided doses

Children and Adolescents ≥6 years: 50-100 mg/day in 4 divided doses

Alternate dosing:

Oral: Children and Adolescents: 2 mg/kg/day divided every 6-8 hours as needed; **Note:** Some experts have recommended lower initial doses. Maximum single dose is age-dependent: Age <6 years: 12.5 mg; age 6-12 years: 25 mg; age >12 years: 100 mg

IM: Children and Adolescents: 0.5-1 mg/kg/**dose** every 4-6 hours as needed; maximum single dose: 100 mg

Pruritus; associated with allergic conditions or chronic urticaria: Oral:

Manufacturer's labeling:

Children <6 years: 50 mg/day in 4 divided doses as needed

Children and Adolescents ≥6 years: 50-100 mg/day in 4 divided doses as needed

Alternate dosing: Children and Adolescents: Oral:

Patient weight ≤40 kg: 2 mg/kg/day divided every 6-8 hours as needed (Simons, 1994); **Note:** Some experts have recommended lower doses; maximum single dose: 25 mg

Patient weight >40 kg: 25-50 mg once daily at bedtime or twice daily (Simons, 1994)

Pruritus; associated with opioid use: Children and Adolescents: Limited data available: IM, Oral: 0.5 mg/kg/dose every 6 hours as needed; maximum single dose: 50 mg (Berde, 1990)

Sedation; procedural, pre-/postoperative:

Manufacturer's labeling:

Oral: Children and Adolescents: 0.6 mg/kg/**dose**; maximum single dose: 100 mg

IM: Infants, Children, and Adolescents: 1.1 mg/kg/**dose**; maximum single dose: 100 mg

Alternate dosing: Oral: Children 2-5 years: 1 mg/kg/**dose** as a single dose 30-45 minutes prior to procedure in combination with other sedatives (eg, midazolam, chloral hydrate) has been used in preschool children prior to dental procedures or echocardiograms (Chowdhury, 2005; Roach, 2010)

Adults:

Antiemetic: IM: 25-100 mg/dose

Anxiety:

Oral: 50-100 mg 4 times daily

IM: 50–100 mg every 4-6 hours as needed

Preoperative sedation:

Oral: 50-100 mg

IM: 25-100 mg

Pruritus: Oral: 25 mg 3-4 times daily

Psychiatric emergency: IM: 50-100 mg immediately; repeat every 4-6 hours as needed

Dosing adjustment in renal impairment: There are no dosage adjustments provided in the manufacturer's labeling; active metabolite (cetirizine) is renally eliminated (Simons, 1994)

Dosing adjustment in hepatic impairment: Adults: In patients with primary biliary cirrhosis, change dosing interval to every 24 hours (Simons, 1989)

Administration

Oral: May be administered without regard to food

Parenteral: Subcutaneous, intra-arterial, and IV administration are contraindicated and **not** recommended under any circumstances; intravascular hemolysis, thrombosis, and digital gangrene can occur; extravasation can result in sterile abscess and marked tissue induration. Administer IM deep in large muscle. For IM administration in children, injections should be made into the midlateral muscles of the thigh. In the very rare instance that IV administration may be necessary, slow IV injection through a central venous line has been used in pediatric oncology patients (Berde, 1990).

Vesicant; the manufacturer considers IV administration a contraindication; however, if IV administration is necessary ensure proper needle or catheter placement prior to and during IV infusion. Avoid extravasation. If extravasation occurs, stop infusion immediately and disconnect (leave cannula/needle in place); gently aspirate extravasated solution (do **NOT** flush the line); remove needle/cannula; elevate extremity.

Vesicant/Extravasation Risk Vesicant (IV administration is contraindicated)

Monitoring Parameters Relief of symptoms, mental status, blood pressure

Test Interactions May cause false-positive serum TCA screen.

Dosage Forms Excipient information presented when available (limited, particularly for generics); consult specific product labeling. [DSC] = Discontinued product

Capsule, Oral, as pamoate:

Vistaril: 25 mg, 50 mg

Generic: 25 mg, 50 mg, 100 mg

Solution, Intramuscular, as hydrochloride:

Generic: 25 mg/mL (1 mL [DSC]); 50 mg/mL (1 mL [DSC], 2 mL [DSC], 10 mL [DSC])

Solution, Oral, as hydrochloride:

Generic: 10 mg/5 mL (473 mL)

Syrup, Oral, as hydrochloride:

Generic: 10 mg/5 mL (25 mL, 118 mL, 473 mL)

Tablet, Oral, as hydrochloride:

Generic: 10 mg, 25 mg, 50 mg

- ◆ **Hydroxyzine Hydrochloride** *see* HydrOXYzine *on page 1058*
- ◆ **Hydroxyzine Hydrochloride Injection, USP (Can)** *see* HydrOXYzine *on page 1058*
- ◆ **Hydroxyzine Pamoate** *see* HydrOXYzine *on page 1058*
- ◆ **Hydurea** *see* Hydroxyurea *on page 1055*
- ◆ **Hygroton** *see* Chlorthalidone *on page 446*
- ◆ **Hylenex** *see* Hyaluronidase *on page 1025*
- ◆ **HyoMax-SL** *see* Hyoscyamine *on page 1061*
- ◆ **Hyoscine Butylbromide** *see* Scopolamine (Systemic) *on page 1907*

◆ **Hyoscine Hydrobromide** *see* Scopolamine (Ophthalmic) *on page 1909*

Hyoscyamine (hye oh SYE a meen)

Medication Safety Issues

Sound-alike/look-alike issues:

Anaspaz may be confused with Anaprox, Antispas

Levbid may be confused with Enbrel, Lithobid, Lopid, Lorabid

Levsin/SL may be confused with Levaquin

BEERS Criteria medication:

This drug may be potentially inappropriate for use in geriatric patients (Quality of evidence - moderate; Strength of recommendation - strong).

Related Information

Oral Medications That Should Not Be Crushed or Altered *on page 2476*

Brand Names: US Anaspaz; Ed-Spaz; HyoMax-SL; Hyosyne; Levbid; Levsin; Levsin/SL; NuLev; Oscimin; Oscimin SR; Symax Duotab; Symax FasTabs; Symax-SL; Symax-SR

Brand Names: Canada Levsin

Therapeutic Category Anticholinergic Agent; Antispasmodic Agent, Gastrointestinal

Generic Availability (US) May be product dependent

Use Treatment of GI tract disorders caused by spasm; adjunctive therapy for peptic ulcers and hypermotility disorders of lower urinary tract; infant colic

Pregnancy Risk Factor C

Pregnancy Considerations Crosses the placenta, effects to the fetus not known; use during pregnancy only if clearly needed.

Breast-Feeding Considerations Excreted in breast milk in trace amounts. May also suppress lactation. Breast-feeding is not recommended.

Contraindications Hypersensitivity to belladonna alkaloids or any component of the formulation; glaucoma; obstructive uropathy; myasthenia gravis; obstructive GI tract disease, paralytic ileus, intestinal atony of elderly or debilitated patients, severe ulcerative colitis, toxic megacolon complicating ulcerative colitis; unstable cardiovascular status; myocardial ischemia. **Note:** Some extended release products are not recommended in children <12 years of age; refer to manufacturer's labeling.

Warnings/Precautions Heat prostration may occur in hot weather. Diarrhea may be a sign of incomplete intestinal obstruction, especially in patients with ileostomy or colostomy; treatment should be discontinued if this occurs. May produce side effects as seen with other anticholinergic medications including drowsiness, dizziness, blurred vision, or psychosis. Prolonged use may lead to development of dental caries, periodontal disease, oral candidiasis, or discomfort due to decreased salivation. Children and the elderly may be more susceptible to these effects. Use with caution in children with spastic paralysis or brain damage; may be more susceptible to anticholinergic effects. Use with caution in patients with autonomic neuropathy, coronary heart disease (contraindicated in patients with unstable cardiovascular status or myocardial ischemia), CHF, cardiac arrhythmias, prostatic hyperplasia, hyperthyroidism, hypertension, renal disease, and hiatal hernia associated with reflux esophagitis. Avoid use in the elderly due to potent anticholinergic adverse effects and uncertain effectiveness (Beers Criteria).

Benzyl alcohol and derivatives: Some dosage forms may contain sodium benzoate/benzoic acid; benzoic acid (benzoate) is a metabolite of benzyl alcohol; large amounts of benzyl alcohol (≥99 mg/kg/day) have been associated with a potentially fatal toxicity ("gasping syndrome") in neonates; the "gasping syndrome" consists of metabolic acidosis, respiratory distress, gasping respirations, CNS dysfunction (including convulsions, intracranial hemorrhage), hypotension, and cardiovascular collapse (AAP, 1997; CDC, 1982); some data suggests that benzoate displaces bilirubin from protein binding sites (Ahlfors, 2001); avoid or use dosage forms containing benzyl alcohol derivative with caution in neonates. See manufacturer's labeling.

Adverse Reactions

Cardiovascular: Flushing, palpitations, tachycardia

Central nervous system: Amnesia (short-term), ataxia, confusion (more common in elderly), dizziness, drowsiness, excitement (more common in elderly), fatigue, hallucination, headache, insomnia, nervousness, psychosis, speech disturbance

Dermatologic: Hypohidrosis, urticaria

Gastrointestinal: Abdominal pain, ageusia, bloating, constipation, diarrhea, dysgeusia, dysphagia, heartburn, nausea, vomiting, xerostomia

Genitourinary: Decreased lactation, impotence, urinary hesitancy, urinary retention

Hypersensitivity: Hypersensitivity reaction

Neuromuscular & skeletal: Weakness

Ophthalmic: Blurred vision, cycloplegia, increased intraocular pressure, mydriasis

Miscellaneous: Fever

Drug Interactions

Metabolism/Transport Effects None known.

Avoid Concomitant Use

Avoid concomitant use of Hyoscyamine with any of the following: Aclidinium; Eluxadoline; Glucagon; Ipratropium (Oral Inhalation); Potassium Chloride; Tiotropium; Umeclidinium

Increased Effect/Toxicity

Hyoscyamine may increase the levels/effects of: AbobotulinumtoxinA; Analgesics (Opioid); Anticholinergic Agents; Cannabinoid-Containing Products; Eluxadoline; Glucagon; Mirabegron; OnabotulinumtoxinA; Potassium Chloride; RimabotulinumtoxinB; Thiazide Diuretics; Tiotropium; Topiramate

The levels/effects of Hyoscyamine may be increased by: Aclidinium; Ipratropium (Oral Inhalation); Mianserin; Pramlintide; Umeclidinium

Decreased Effect

Hyoscyamine may decrease the levels/effects of: Acetylcholinesterase Inhibitors; Itopride; Metoclopramide; Secretin

The levels/effects of Hyoscyamine may be decreased by: Acetylcholinesterase Inhibitors; Antacids

Storage/Stability Store at 20°C to 25°C (68°F to 77°F); excursions are permitted between 15°C and 30°C (59°F and 86°F).

Mechanism of Action Blocks the action of acetylcholine at parasympathetic sites in smooth muscle, secretory glands, and the CNS; increases cardiac output, dries secretions, antagonizes histamine and serotonin

Pharmacodynamics

Onset of action:

- Oral: 20-30 minutes
- Sublingual: 5-20 minutes
- IV: 2-3 minutes

Duration: 4-6 hours

Pharmacokinetics (Adult data unless noted)

Absorption: Well absorbed from the GI tract

Distribution: Crosses the placenta; small amounts appear in breast milk

Protein binding: 50%

Metabolism: In the liver

Half-life: 3.5 hours

Elimination: 30% to 50% eliminated unchanged in urine within 12 hours

Dosing: Usual

GI tract disorders:

Infants and Children <2 years: Oral: The following table lists the hyoscyamine dosage using the drop formulation; hyoscyamine drops are dosed every 4 hours as needed

Hyoscyamine Drops Dosage

Weight (kg)	Dose (drops)	Maximum Daily Dose (drops)
2.3	3	18
3.4	4	24
5	5	30
7	6	36
10	8	48
15	11	66

Oral, S.L.:

Children 2-12 years: 0.0625-0.125 mg every 4 hours as needed; maximum daily dosage 0.75 mg **or** timed release 0.375 mg every 12 hours; maximum daily dosage 0.75 mg

Children >12 years to Adults: 0.125-0.25 mg every 4 hours as needed; maximum daily dosage 1.5 mg **or** timed release 0.375-0.75 mg every 12 hours; maximum daily dosage 1.5 mg

IV, IM, SubQ: Children >12 years to Adults: 0.25-0.5 mg at 4-hour intervals for 1-4 doses

Adjunct to anesthesia: IM, IV, SubQ: Children >2 years to Adults: 5 mcg/kg given 30-60 minutes prior to induction of anesthesia

Hypermotility of lower urinary tract: Oral, S.L.: Adults: 0.15-0.3 mg four times daily; timed release: 0.375 mg every 12 hours

Reversal of neuromuscular blockage: IV, IM, SubQ: 0.2 mg for every 1 mg neostigmine

Administration

Oral: Administer before meals; timed release tablets are scored and may be cut for easier dosage titration; S.L.: Place under the tongue

Parenteral: May be administered IM, IV, and SubQ; no information is available for IV administration rate or dilution

Monitoring Parameters Pulse, anticholinergic effects, urine output, GI symptoms

Dosage Forms Excipient information presented when available (limited, particularly for generics); consult specific product labeling.

Elixir, Oral, as sulfate:
- Hyosyne: 0.125 mg/5 mL (473 mL) [contains alcohol, usp; lemon flavor]
- Generic: 0.125 mg/5 mL (473 mL)

Solution, Injection, as sulfate:
- Levsin: 0.5 mg/mL (1 mL) [contains benzyl alcohol]

Solution, Oral, as sulfate:
- Hyosyne: 0.125 mg/mL (15 mL) [lemon flavor]
- Generic: 0.125 mg/mL (15 mL)

Tablet, Oral, as sulfate:
- Levsin: 0.125 mg
- Oscimin: 0.125 mg [peppermint flavor]
- Generic: 0.125 mg

Tablet Dispersible, Oral, as sulfate:
- Anaspaz: 0.125 mg [scored]
- Ed-Spaz: 0.125 mg [scored]
- NuLev: 0.125 mg [peppermint flavor]
- Oscimin: 0.125 mg [peppermint flavor]
- Symax FasTabs: 0.125 mg [mint flavor]
- Generic: 0.125 mg

Tablet Extended Release, Oral, as sulfate:
- Symax Duotab: 0.375 mg [contains brilliant blue fcf (fd&c blue #1)]

Tablet Extended Release 12 Hour, Oral, as sulfate:
- Levbid: 0.375 mg
- Oscimin SR: 0.375 mg
- Symax-SR: 0.375 mg [scored]
- Generic: 0.375 mg

Tablet Sublingual, Sublingual, as sulfate:
- HyoMax-SL: 0.125 mg
- Levsin/SL: 0.125 mg
- Oscimin: 0.125 mg [peppermint flavor]
- Symax-SL: 0.125 mg [mint flavor]
- Generic: 0.125 mg

Hyoscyamine, Atropine, Scopolamine, and Phenobarbital

(hye oh SYE a meen, A troe peen, skoe POL a meen, & fee noe BAR bi tal)

Medication Safety Issues

Sound-alike/look-alike issues:

Donnatal® may be confused with Donnagel, Donnatal Extentabs®

BEERS Criteria medication:

This drug may be potentially inappropriate for use in geriatric patients (Quality of evidence - moderate; Strength of recommendation - strong).

Related Information

Oral Medications That Should Not Be Crushed or Altered *on page 2476*

Brand Names: US Donnatal Extentabs®; Donnatal®

Therapeutic Category Anticholinergic Agent; Antispasmodic Agent, Gastrointestinal

Generic Availability (US) No

Use Adjunct in treatment of peptic ulcer disease, irritable bowel, spastic colitis, spastic bladder, and renal colic

Pregnancy Risk Factor C

Pregnancy Considerations Reproduction studies with this combination have not been done; refer to individual monographs.

Breast-Feeding Considerations Refer to individual monographs.

Contraindications Hypersensitivity to hyoscyamine, atropine, scopolamine, phenobarbital, or any component of the formulation; narrow-angle glaucoma; GI and GU obstruction; myasthenia gravis; paralytic ileus; intestinal atony; unstable cardiovascular status in acute hemorrhage; severe ulcerative colitis (especially complicated by toxic megacolon); hiatal hernia associated with reflux esophagitis; acute intermittent porphyria; restlessness and/or excitement caused by phenobarbital

Warnings/Precautions Heat prostration may occur in hot weather and during exercise. Use with caution in patients with hepatic or renal disease, hyperthyroidism, autonomic neuropathy. Use with caution in patients with coronary artery disease, arrhythmias, tachycardia, heart failure, or hypertension. Use of anticholinergics in gastric ulcer treatment may cause a delay in gastric emptying due to antral statis. Use caution in patients with ileostomy or colostomy; diarrhea may occur and may be an early symptom of incomplete intestinal obstruction. May causes sedation or blurred vision, caution must be used in performing tasks which require alertness (eg, operating machinery or driving). Effects may be potentiated when used with other sedative drugs or ethanol. Use with caution in patients with a history of drug abuse or acute alcoholism; potential for drug dependency exists. Tolerance, psychological and physical dependence may occur with prolonged use. Should not be discontinued abruptly because of the possibility of increased seizure frequency (due to phenobarbital component); therapy should be withdrawn gradually to minimize the potential of increased seizure frequency, unless safety concerns require a more rapid withdrawal. Avoid long-term use in the elderly due to anticholinergic adverse effects and uncertain effectiveness (Beers Criteria). Use with caution in patients on anticoagulant therapy. Use has not been shown to prevent or treat duodenal ulcers.

Adverse Reactions

Cardiovascular: Palpitation, tachycardia

Central nervous system: Dizziness, drowsiness, excitement, headache, insomnia, nervousness

Dermatologic: Urticaria

Endocrine & metabolic: Lactation suppressed

Gastrointestinal: Bloating, constipation, nausea, taste loss, vomiting, xerostomia

Genitourinary: Impotence, urinary hesitancy, urinary retention

Neuromuscular & skeletal: Musculoskeletal pain, weakness

Ocular: Blurred vision, cycloplegia, mydriasis, ocular tension increased

Miscellaneous: Allergic reaction (may be severe), anaphylaxis, sweating decreased

Drug Interactions

Metabolism/Transport Effects Refer to individual components.

Avoid Concomitant Use

Avoid concomitant use of Hyoscyamine, Atropine, Scopolamine, and Phenobarbital with any of the following: Abiraterone Acetate; Aclidinium; Apixaban; Apremilast; Artemether; Axitinib; Azelastine (Nasal); Bedaquiline; Boceprevir; Bortezomib; Bosutinib; Cabozantinib; Ceritinib; CloZAPine; Crizotinib; Dabigatran Etexilate; Dasabuvir; Dienogest; Dolutegravir; Dronedarone; Eliglustat; Eluxadoline; Enzalutamide; Etravirine; Everolimus; Glucagon; Ibrutinib; Idelalisib; Ipratropium (Oral Inhalation); Irinotecan; Isavuconazonium Sulfate; Itraconazole; Ivabradine; Ivacaftor; Lapatinib; Ledipasvir; Lumefantrine; Lurasidone; Macitentan; Mianserin; Mifepristone; Naloxegol; Netupitant; NIFEdipine; Nilotinib; NiMODipine; Nintedanib; Nisoldipine; Olaparib; Ombitasvir; Orphenadrine; Palbociclib; Panobinostat; Paraldehyde; Paritaprevir; PAZOPanib; Perampanel; Pirfenidone; PONATinib; Potassium Chloride; Praziquantel; Ranolazine; Regorafenib; Rilpivirine; Rivaroxaban; Roflumilast; RomiDEPsin; Simeprevir; Sofosbuvir; Somatostatin Acetate; SORAfenib; Stiripentol; Suvorexant; Tasimelteon; Telaprevir; Thalidomide; Ticagrelor; Tiotropium; Tofacitinib; Tolvaptan; Toremifene; Trabectedin; Ulipristal; Umeclidinium; Vandetanib; Vemurafenib; VinCRIStine (Liposomal); Vorapaxar; Voriconazole

Increased Effect/Toxicity

Hyoscyamine, Atropine, Scopolamine, and Phenobarbital may increase the levels/effects of: AbobotulinumtoxinA; Alcohol (Ethyl); Analgesics (Opioid); Anticholinergic Agents; Azelastine (Nasal); Buprenorphine; Clarithromycin; CNS Depressants; Eluxadoline; Glucagon; Hydrocodone; Hypotensive Agents; Meperidine; Methotrimeprazine; Metyrosine; Mirabegron; OnabotulinumtoxinA; Orphenadrine; Paraldehyde; Potassium Chloride; Pramipexole; Prilocaine; QuiNIDine; RimabotulinumtoxinB; Rotigotine; Selective Serotonin Reuptake Inhibitors; Sodium Nitrite; Thalidomide; Thiazide Diuretics; Tiotropium; Topiramate; Zolpidem

The levels/effects of Hyoscyamine, Atropine, Scopolamine, and Phenobarbital may be increased by: Aclidinium; Brimonidine (Topical); Cannabis; Chloramphenicol; Clarithromycin; Cosyntropin; CYP2C19 Inhibitors (Moderate); CYP2C19 Inhibitors (Strong); Dexmethylphenidate; Doxylamine; Dronabinol; Droperidol; Felbamate; Fosphenytoin; HydrOXYzine; Ipratropium (Oral Inhalation); Kava Kava; Luliconazole; Magnesium Sulfate; Methotrimeprazine; Methylphenidate; Mianserin; Nabilone; Nitric Oxide; OXcarbazepine; Phenytoin; Pramlintide; Primidone; QuiNINE; Rufinamide; Sodium Oxybate; Somatostatin Acetate; Tapentadol; Tetrahydrocannabinol; Umeclidinium; Valproic Acid and Derivatives

Decreased Effect

Hyoscyamine, Atropine, Scopolamine, and Phenobarbital may decrease the levels/effects of: Abiraterone Acetate; Acetaminophen; Acetylcholinesterase Inhibitors; Afatinib; Albendazole; Apixaban; Apremilast; ARIPiprazole; Artemether; Axitinib; Bazedoxifene; Bedaquiline; Bendamustine; Beta-Blockers; Boceprevir; Bortezomib; Bosutinib; Brentuximab Vedotin; Cabozantinib; Calcium Channel Blockers; Canagliflozin; Cannabidiol; Cannabis; Ceritinib; Chloramphenicol; Clarithromycin; CloZAPine; Cobicistat; Contraceptives (Estrogens); Contraceptives (Progestins); Corticosteroids (Systemic); Crizotinib; CycloSPORINE (Systemic); CYP1A2 Substrates; CYP2A6 Substrates; CYP2B6 Substrates; CYP2C8 Substrates; CYP2C9 Substrates; CYP3A4 Substrates; Dabigatran Etexilate; Dasabuvir; Dasatinib; Deferasirox; Dexamethasone (Systemic); Diclofenac (Systemic); Dienogest; Disopyramide; Dolutegravir; DOXOrubicin (Conventional); Doxycycline; Dronabinol; Dronedarone; Eliglustat; Elvitegravir; Enzalutamide; Erlotinib; Eslicarbazepine; Etoposide; Etravirine; Everolimus; Exemestane; Felbamate; FentaNYL; Fosphenytoin; Gefitinib; Griseofulvin; GuanFACINE; Hydrocortisone (Systemic); Ibrutinib; Idelalisib; Imatinib; Irinotecan; Isavuconazonium Sulfate; Itopride; Itraconazole; Ivabradine; Ivacaftor; Ixabepilone; Lacosamide; LamoTRIgine; Lapatinib; Ledipasvir; Linagliptin; Lopinavir; Lumefantrine; Lurasidone; Macitentan; Maraviroc; Methadone; MethylPREDNISolone; Metoclopramide; MetroNIDAZOLE (Systemic); Mianserin; Mifepristone; Naloxegol; Netupitant; NIFEdipine; Nilotinib; NiMODipine; Nintedanib; Nisoldipine; Olaparib; Ombitasvir; OXcarbazepine; Palbociclib; Paliperidone; Panobinostat; Paritaprevir; PAZOPanib; Perampanel; P-glycoprotein/ABCB1 Substrates; Phenytoin; Pirfenidone; PONATinib; Praziquantel; PrednisoLONE (Systemic); PredniSONE; Propafenone; QUEtiapine; QuiNIDine; QuiNINE; Ranolazine; Regorafenib; Rilpivirine; Rivaroxaban; Roflumilast; RomiDEPsin; Rufinamide; Saxagliptin; Secretin; Simeprevir; Sofosbuvir; SORAfenib; Stiripentol; SUNItinib; Suvorexant; Tadalafil; Tasimelteon; Telaprevir; Teniposide; Tetrahydrocannabinol; Ticagrelor; Tipranavir; Tofacitinib; Tolvaptan; Toremifene; Trabectedin; Treprostinil; Tricyclic Antidepressants; Ulipristal; Valproic Acid and Derivatives; Vandetanib; Vemurafenib; Vilazodone; VinCRIStine (Liposomal); Vitamin K Antagonists; Vorapaxar; Voriconazole; Vortioxetine; Zaleplon; Zonisamide; Zuclopenthixol

The levels/effects of Hyoscyamine, Atropine, Scopolamine, and Phenobarbital may be decreased by: Acetylcholinesterase Inhibitors; Amphetamines; Antacids; Cholestyramine Resin; CYP2C19 Inducers (Strong); Dabrafenib; Darunavir; Folic Acid; Leucovorin Calcium-Levoleucovorin; Levomefolate; Mefloquine; Methylfolate; Mianserin; Multivitamins/Minerals (with ADEK, Folate, Iron); Orlistat; Pyridoxine; Rifamycin Derivatives; Tipranavir

Storage/Stability Store at controlled room temperature 20°C to 25°C (68°F to 77°F). Protect from light and moisture. Avoid freezing (elixir).

Mechanism of Action Anticholinergic agents (hyoscyamine, atropine, and scopolamine) inhibit the muscarinic actions of acetylcholine at the postganglionic parasympathetic neuroeffector sites including smooth muscle, secretory glands, and CNS sites; specific anticholinergic responses are dose-related.

Pharmacokinetics (Adult data unless noted) Absorption: Well absorbed from the GI tract

Dosing: Usual Oral:

Children: Donnatal®: 0.1 mL/kg/dose every 4 hours; maximum dose: 5 mL **or** see table for alternative.

Donnatal® Dosage

Weight (kg)	Dose (mL)	
	Every 4 Hours	Every 6 Hours
4.5	0.5	0.75
10	1	1.5
14	1.5	2
23	2.5	3.8
34	3.8	5
≥45	5	7.5

Adults: Donnatal®: 1-2 tablets or capsules 3-4 times/day **or** 5-10 mL 3-4 times/day or 1 extended release tablet every 12 hours (may increase to every 8 hours if needed)

Administration Oral: Administer 30-60 minutes before meals; do not crush or chew extended release tablets

Controlled Substance C-IV or nonscheduled (DEA exemption status dependent)

Dosage Forms Considerations Elixir contains ethanol (up to 23.8%).

Dosage Forms Excipient information presented when available (limited, particularly for generics); consult specific product labeling.

Elixir:

Donnatal®: Hyoscyamine sulfate 0.1037 mg, atropine sulfate 0.0194 mg, scopolamine hydrobromide 0.0065 mg, and phenobarbital 16.2 mg per 5 mL (120 mL, 480 mL) [contains ethanol <23.8%; grape flavor]

Donnatal®: Hyoscyamine sulfate 0.1037 mg, atropine sulfate 0.0194 mg, scopolamine hydrobromide 0.0065 mg, and phenobarbital 16.2 mg per 5 mL (120 mL, 480 mL) [contains ethanol <23.8%, tartrazine; mint flavor]

Tablet:

Donnatal®: Hyoscyamine sulfate 0.1037 mg, atropine sulfate 0.0194 mg, scopolamine hydrobromide 0.0065 mg, and phenobarbital 16.2 mg

Tablet, extended release:

Donnatal Extentabs®: Hyoscyamine sulfate 0.3111 mg, atropine sulfate 0.0582 mg, scopolamine hydrobromide 0.0195 mg, and phenobarbital 48.6 mg

- ◆ **Hyoscyamine Sulfate** *see* Hyoscyamine *on page* 1061
- ◆ **Hyosyne** *see* Hyoscyamine *on page* 1061
- ◆ **HyperHEP B S/D** *see* Hepatitis B Immune Globulin (Human) *on page* 1013
- ◆ **HyperRAB S/D** *see* Rabies Immune Globulin (Human) *on page* 1830
- ◆ **HyperRHO S/D** *see* Rh_o(D) Immune Globulin *on page* 1847
- ◆ **HyperSal** *see* Sodium Chloride *on page* 1938
- ◆ **HyperTET S/D** *see* Tetanus Immune Globulin (Human) *on page* 2031
- ◆ **Hypertonic Saline** *see* Sodium Chloride *on page* 1938
- ◆ **HypoTears [OTC]** *see* Artificial Tears *on page* 201
- ◆ **HyQvia** *see* Immune Globulin *on page* 1089
- ◆ **Hyqvia** *see* Immune Globulin *on page* 1089
- ◆ **Hytrin** *see* Terazosin *on page* 2020
- ◆ **Ibavyr (Can)** *see* Ribavirin *on page* 1851
- ◆ **Ibenzmethyzin** *see* Procarbazine *on page* 1772
- ◆ **Ibidomide Hydrochloride** *see* Labetalol *on page* 1197
- ◆ **IBU-200 [OTC]** *see* Ibuprofen *on page* 1064

Ibuprofen (eye byoo PROE fen)

Medication Safety Issues

Sound-alike/look-alike issues:

Haltran may be confused with Halfprin

Motrin may be confused with Neurontin

BEERS Criteria medication:

This drug may be potentially inappropriate for use in geriatric patients (Quality of evidence - moderate; Strength of recommendation - strong).

Administration issues:

Injectable formulations: Both ibuprofen and ibuprofen lysine are available for parenteral use. Ibuprofen lysine is **only** indicated for closure of a clinically-significant patent ductus arteriosus.

Related Information

Oral Medications That Should Not Be Crushed or Altered *on page* 2476

Brand Names: US Addaprin [OTC]; Advil Junior Strength [OTC]; Advil Migraine [OTC]; Advil [OTC]; Caldolor; Childrens Advil [OTC]; Childrens Ibuprofen [OTC]; Childrens Motrin Jr Strength [OTC]; Childrens Motrin [OTC]; Dyspel [OTC]; EnovaRX-Ibuprofen; Genpril [OTC]; I-Prin [OTC]; IBU-200 [OTC]; Ibuprofen Childrens [OTC]; Ibuprofen Comfort Pac; Ibuprofen Junior Strength [OTC]; Infants Advil [OTC]; Infants Ibuprofen [OTC]; KS Ibuprofen [OTC]; Motrin IB [OTC]; Motrin Infants Drops [OTC]; Motrin Junior Strength [OTC]; Motrin [OTC]; NeoProfen; Provil [OTC]

Brand Names: Canada Advil; Advil Pediatric Drops; Apo-Ibuprofen; Caldolor; Children's Advil; Children's Europrofen; Ibuprofen Muscle and Joint; Jamp-Ibuprofen; Motrin; Motrin (Children's); Motrin IB; Novo-Profen; Pamprin Ibuprofen Formula; PMS-Ibuprofen; Super Strength Motrin IB Liquid Gel Capsules

Therapeutic Category Analgesic, Non-narcotic; Anti-inflammatory Agent; Antipyretic; Nonsteroidal Anti-inflammatory Drug (NSAID), Oral; Nonsteroidal Anti-inflammatory Drug (NSAID), Parenteral

Generic Availability (US) May be product dependent

Use

Oral:

OTC products:

Infant drops, suspension, and chewable tablets: Relief of minor aches and pains due to the common cold, flu, sore throat, headaches, and toothaches; reduction of fever (All indications: OTC products: FDA approved in ages 6 months to 11 years; consult specific product formulation for appropriate age group)

Capsule/Tablet: Relief of minor aches and pains due to the common cold, headaches, minor pain of arthritis, backache, menstrual cramps, muscle aches, and toothaches (All indications: OTC products: FDA approved in ages ≥12 years and adults)

Capsule (Advil Migraine): Treatment of migraines (OTC products: FDA approved in adults)

Prescription strength (400, 600, and 800 mg tablets): Relief of mild to moderate pain; relief of signs and symptoms of osteoarthritis and rheumatoid arthritis; treatment of primary dysmenorrhea (All indications: FDA approved in adults)

Oral ibuprofen has also been used for juvenile idiopathic arthritis (JIA), cystic fibrosis, migraine pain, gout, and for PDA closure.

Parenteral:

Ibuprofen injection (Caldolor): Management of mild to moderate pain, management of moderate to severe pain when used concurrently with an opioid analgesic, reduction of fever (All indications: FDA approved in ages ≥17 years and adults)

Ibuprofen lysine injection (NeoProfen): Treatment (ie, closure) of a clinically significant PDA when usual treatments are ineffective (FDA approved in premature neonates ≤32 weeks gestational age and weighing 500-1500 g). **Note:** The prophylactic use of ibuprofen is not currently indicated nor recommended (Ohlsson, 2011).

Medication Guide Available Yes

Pregnancy Risk Factor C/D ≥30 weeks gestation

Pregnancy Considerations Adverse events were not observed in the initial animal reproduction studies; therefore, the manufacturer classifies ibuprofen as pregnancy category C (category D: ≥30 weeks' gestation). NSAID exposure during the first trimester is not strongly associated with congenital malformations; however, cardiovascular anomalies and cleft palate have been observed following NSAID exposure in some studies. The use of a NSAID close to conception may be associated with an increased risk of miscarriage. Nonteratogenic effects have been observed following NSAID administration during the third trimester including: Myocardial degenerative changes, prenatal constriction of the ductus arteriosus, fetal tricuspid regurgitation, failure of the ductus arteriosus to close postnatally; renal dysfunction or failure, oligohydramnios; gastrointestinal bleeding or perforation, increased risk of necrotizing enterocolitis; intracranial bleeding (including intraventricular hemorrhage), platelet dysfunction with resultant bleeding; pulmonary hypertension. Because they may cause premature closure of the ductus arteriosus, use of NSAIDs late in pregnancy should be avoided (use after 31 or 32 weeks' gestation is not recommended by some clinicians). US labeling for Caldolor specifically notes that use at ≥30 weeks' gestation should be avoided and therefore classifies ibuprofen as pregnancy category D at this time. Canadian labeling contraindicates use of ibuprofen (IV and oral) during the third trimester. The chronic use of NSAIDs in women of reproductive age may be associated with infertility that is reversible upon discontinuation of the medication. A registry is available for pregnant women exposed to autoimmune medications including ibuprofen. For additional information contact the Organization of Teratology Information Specialists, OTIS Autoimmune Diseases Study, at 877-311-8972.

Breast-Feeding Considerations Based on limited data, only very small amounts of ibuprofen are excreted into breast milk. Adverse events have not been reported in nursing infants. Because there is a potential for adverse events to occur in nursing infants, the manufacturer does not recommend the use of ibuprofen while breast-feeding. Use with caution in nursing women with hypertensive disorders of pregnancy or pre-existing renal disease.

Contraindications

Hypersensitivity to ibuprofen; history of asthma, urticaria, or allergic-type reaction to aspirin or other NSAIDs; aspirin triad (eg, bronchial asthma, aspirin intolerance, rhinitis); perioperative pain in the setting of coronary artery bypass graft (CABG) surgery

Ibuprofen lysine (NeoProfen): Preterm neonates: With proven or suspected infection that is untreated; congenital heart disease in whom patency of the PDA is necessary for satisfactory pulmonary or systemic blood flow (eg, pulmonary atresia, severe coarctation of the aorta, severe tetralogy of Fallot); bleeding (especially those with active intracranial hemorrhage or GI bleeding); thrombocytopenia; coagulation defects; proven or suspected necrotizing enterocolitis; or significant renal function impairment.

Canadian labeling: Additional contraindications (not in US labeling): Cerebrovascular bleeding or other bleeding disorders; active gastric/duodenal/peptic ulcer, active GI bleeding; inflammatory bowel disease; uncontrolled heart failure; moderate [IV formulation only] to severe renal impairment (creatinine clearance [CrCl] <30 mL/minute); deteriorating renal disease; moderate [IV formulation only] to severe hepatic impairment; active hepatic disease; hyperkalemia; third trimester of pregnancy; breast-feeding; patients <18 years of age [IV formulation only]; patients <12 years of age [oral formulation only]; systemic lupus erythematosus [oral formulation only]

OTC labeling: When used for self-medication, do not use if previous allergic reaction to any other pain reliever/fever reducer; prior to or following cardiac surgery.

Warnings/Precautions [U.S. Boxed Warning]: NSAIDs are associated with an increased risk of adverse cardiovascular thrombotic events, including fatal MI and stroke. Risk may be increased with duration of use or preexisting cardiovascular risk factors or disease. Carefully evaluate individual cardiovascular risk profiles prior to prescribing. May cause new-onset hypertension or worsening of existing hypertension. Response to ACE inhibitors, thiazides, or loop diuretics may be impaired with concurrent use of NSAIDs. Use caution with fluid retention. Avoid use in heart failure (ACCF/AHA [Yancy, 2013]). Concurrent administration of ibuprofen, and potentially other nonselective NSAIDs, may interfere with aspirin's cardioprotective effect. **[U.S. Boxed Warning]: Use is contraindicated for treatment of perioperative pain in the setting of coronary artery bypass graft (CABG) surgery.** Risk of MI and stroke may be increased with use following CABG surgery.

May increase the risk of aseptic meningitis, especially in patients with systemic lupus erythematosus (SLE) and mixed connective tissue disorders. Platelet adhesion and aggregation may be decreased; may prolong bleeding time; patients with coagulation disorders or who are receiving anticoagulants should be monitored closely. Anemia may occur; patients on long-term NSAID therapy should be monitored for anemia. Rarely, NSAID use may cause severe blood dyscrasias (eg, agranulocytosis, aplastic anemia, thrombocytopenia).

NSAID use may compromise existing renal function; dose-dependent decreases in prostaglandin synthesis may result from NSAID use, reducing renal blood flow which may cause renal decompensation. NSAID use may increase the risk for hyperkalemia. Patients with impaired renal function, dehydration, heart failure, liver dysfunction, those taking diuretics, and ACE inhibitors, and the elderly are at greater risk of renal toxicity and hyperkalemia. Rehydrate patient before starting therapy; monitor renal function closely. The Canadian labeling contraindicates use in moderate (IV only) to severe renal impairment, with deteriorating renal disease and in patients with hyperkalemia. Use of ibuprofen lysine (NeoProfen) is contraindicated in preterm infants with significant renal impairment. Long-term NSAID use may result in renal papillary necrosis.

NSAIDs may increase risk of gastrointestinal irritation, inflammation, ulceration, bleeding, and perforation. These events can be fatal and may occur at any time during therapy and without warning. Elderly patients are at increased risk for serious adverse events. Use caution with a history of GI disease (bleeding or ulcers), concurrent therapy with aspirin, anticoagulants and/or corticosteroids, smoking, use of ethanol, the elderly or debilitated patients. When used concomitantly with aspirin, a substantial increase in the risk of gastrointestinal complications (eg, ulcer) occurs; concomitant gastroprotective therapy (eg, proton pump inhibitors) is recommended (Bhatt, 2008). The Canadian labeling contraindicates use in patients with active GI disease (eg, peptic ulcer) or GI bleeding and inflammatory bowel disease.

Use the lowest effective dose for the shortest duration of time, consistent with individual patient goals, to reduce risk of cardiovascular or GI adverse events. Alternate therapies should be considered for patients at high risk.

NSAIDs may cause serious skin adverse events including exfoliative dermatitis, Stevens-Johnson Syndrome (SJS) and toxic epidermal necrolysis (TEN); discontinue use at first sign of skin rash or hypersensitivity. Anaphylactoid reactions may occur, even without prior exposure; patients with "aspirin triad" (bronchial asthma, aspirin intolerance, rhinitis) may be at increased risk. Do not use in patients who experience bronchospasm, asthma, rhinitis, or urticaria with NSAID or aspirin therapy. Use caution in other forms of asthma.

NSAIDS may cause drowsiness, dizziness, blurred vision and other neurologic effects which may impair physical or mental abilities; patients must be cautioned about performing tasks which require mental alertness (eg, operating machinery or driving). Monitor vision with long-term therapy. Blurred/diminished vision, scotomata, and changes in color vision have been reported. Discontinue use with altered vision and perform ophthalmologic exam.

Use with caution in patients with decreased hepatic function. Closely monitor patients with any abnormal LFT. Severe hepatic reactions (eg, fulminant hepatitis, jaundice, liver necrosis, liver failure) have occurred with NSAID use, rarely; discontinue if signs or symptoms of liver disease develop, or if systemic manifestations occur. The Canadian labeling contraindicates use in moderate (IV only) to severe impairment and with active hepatic disease.

In the elderly, avoid chronic use (unless alternative agents ineffective and patient can receive concomitant gastroprotective agent); nonselective oral NSAID use is associated with an increased risk of GI bleeding and peptic ulcer disease in older adults in high risk category (eg, >75 years or age or receiving concomitant oral/parenteral corticosteroids, anticoagulants, or antiplatelet agents) (Beers Criteria). Potentially significant drug interactions may exist, requiring dose or frequency adjustment, additional monitoring, and/or selection of alternative therapy.

Withhold for at least 4-6 half-lives prior to surgical or dental procedures.

Ibuprofen injection (Caldolor) must be diluted prior to administration; hemolysis can occur if not diluted.

Ibuprofen lysine injection (NeoProfen): Hold second or third doses if urinary output is <0.6 mL/kg/hour. May alter signs of infection. May inhibit platelet aggregation; monitor for signs of bleeding. May displace bilirubin; use caution when total bilirubin is elevated. Long-term evaluations of neurodevelopment, growth, or diseases associated with prematurity following treatment have not been conducted. A second course of treatment, alternative pharmacologic therapy or surgery may be needed if the ductus arteriosus fails to close or reopens following the initial course of therapy.

Benzyl alcohol and derivatives: Some dosage forms may contain sodium benzoate/benzoic acid; benzoic acid (benzoate) is a metabolite of benzyl alcohol; large amounts of benzyl alcohol (≥99 mg/kg/day) have been associated with a potentially fatal toxicity ("gasping syndrome") in neonates; the "gasping syndrome" consists of metabolic acidosis, respiratory distress, gasping respirations, CNS dysfunction (including convulsions, intracranial hemorrhage), hypotension, and cardiovascular collapse (AAP, 1997; CDC, 1982); some data suggests that benzoate displaces bilirubin from protein binding sites (Ahlfors, 2001); avoid or use dosage forms containing benzyl alcohol derivative with caution in neonates. See manufacturer's labeling.

Propylene glycol: Some dosage forms may contain propylene glycol; large amounts are potentially toxic and have been associated hyperosmolality, lactic acidosis, seizures and respiratory depression; use caution (AAP, 1997; Zar, 2007).

Polysorbate 80: Some dosage forms may contain polysorbate 80 (also known as Tweens). Hypersensitivity reactions, usually a delayed reaction, have been reported following exposure to pharmaceutical products containing polysorbate 80 in certain individuals (Isaksson, 2002; Lucente 2000; Shelley, 1995). Thrombocytopenia, ascites, pulmonary deterioration, and renal and hepatic failure have been reported in premature neonates after receiving parenteral products containing polysorbate 80 (Alade, 1986; CDC, 1984). See manufacturer's labeling.

Phenylalanine: Some products may contain phenylalanine.

Self medication (OTC use): Prior to self-medication, patients should contact healthcare provider if they have had recurring stomach pain or upset, ulcers, bleeding problems, high blood pressure, heart or kidney disease, other serious medical problems, are currently taking a diuretic, aspirin, anticoagulant, or are ≥60 years of age. If patients are using for migraines, they should also contact healthcare provider if they have not had a migraine diagnosis by healthcare provider, a headache that is different from usual migraine, worst headache of life, fever and neck stiffness, headache from head injury or coughing, first headache at ≥50 years of age, daily headache, or migraine requiring bed rest. Recommended dosages should not be exceeded, due to an increased risk of GI bleeding. Stop use and consult a healthcare provider if symptoms get worse, newly appear, fever lasts for >3 days or pain lasts >3 days (children) and >10 days (adults). Do not give for >10 days unless instructed by healthcare provider. Consuming ≥3 alcoholic beverages/day or taking longer than recommended may increase the risk of GI bleeding.

Warnings: Additional Pediatric Considerations A single-center, 10-year, retrospective review of pediatric patients diagnosed with acute kidney injury (AKI) (n=1015; ages: ≤18 years) reported NSAIDS as a potential cause of AKI in 2.7% of patients (n=27); a higher incidence (6.6%) was reported when additional exclusion factors were included in the data analysis. Dosing information was available for 74% of the NSAID-associated AKI cases (n=20); dosing was within the recommended range in 75% (n=15) of these cases. The median age of children with NSAID-associated AKI was 14.7 years (range: 0.5 to 17.7 years) and 15% of patients were <5 years and more likely to require dialysis than the older patients. Some experts suggest the incidence of NSAID-associated AKI found in this study is conservative due to aggressive exclusion criteria (eg, concurrent aminoglycoside or other nephrotoxic therapy) and the actual incidence may be higher (Brophy, 2013; Misurac, 2013).

In neonates, pulmonary hypertension has occurred following use for treatment of PDA; ten cases have been reported; three following early (prophylactic) administration of tromethamine ibuprofen (not available in U.S.) and seven cases following L-lysine ibuprofen therapy (Bellini, 2006; Gournay, 2002; Ohlsson, 2013). Avoid extravasation of ibuprofen lysine injection (NeoProfen); IV solution may be irritating to tissues. Use with caution in neonates with controlled infection or those at risk for infection; ibuprofen may alter the usual signs of infection. Use with caution in neonates when total bilirubin is elevated; ibuprofen may displace bilirubin from albumin-binding sites. Intraventricular hemorrhage has been reported; overall incidence: 29%, grade 3/4: 15%. Long-term evaluations of neurodevelopmental outcome, growth, or diseases associated with prematurity (eg, chronic lung disease, retinopathy of prematurity) following treatment have not been conducted.

Some dosage forms may contain propylene glycol; in neonates large amounts of propylene glycol delivered orally, intravenously (eg, >3,000 mg/day), or topically have been associated with potentially fatal toxicities which can include metabolic acidosis, seizures, renal failure, and CNS depression; toxicities have also been reported in children and adults including hyperosmolality, lactic acidosis, seizures and respiratory depression; use caution (AAP, 1997; Shehab, 2009).

Adverse Reactions

Oral:

Cardiovascular: Edema

Central nervous system: Dizziness, headache, nervousness

Dermatologic: Pruritus, skin rash

Endocrine & metabolic: Fluid retention

Gastrointestinal: Abdominal pain, constipation, decreased appetite, diarrhea, dyspepsia, epigastric pain, flatulence, heartburn, nausea, vomiting

Otic: Tinnitus

Rare but important or life-threatening: Abnormal liver function tests, acute renal failure, agranulocytosis, anaphylaxis, aplastic anemia, azotemia, blurred vision, bone marrow depression, confusion, decreased creatinine clearance, decreased hematocrit, decreased hemoglobin, decreased platelet aggregation, duodenal ulcer, eosinophilia, epistaxis, erythema multiforme, gastric ulcer, gastrointestinal hemorrhage, gastrointestinal ulcer, hallucination, hearing loss, hematuria, hemolytic anemia, hepatitis, hepatotoxicity (idiosyncratic) (Chalasani, 2014), hypertension, jaundice, leukopenia, melena, neutropenia, pancreatitis, skin photosensitivity, Stevens-Johnson syndrome, thrombocytopenia, toxic amblyopia, toxic epidermal necrolysis, urticaria, vesiculobullous dermatitis, visual disturbance

Injection: Ibuprofen (Caldolor):

Cardiovascular: Edema, hypertension

Central nervous system: Dizziness, headache

Dermatologic: Pruritus

Endocrine & metabolic: Hypernatremia, hypokalemia

Gastrointestinal: Abdominal pain, dyspepsia, flatulence, nausea, vomiting

Genitourinary: Urinary retention

Hematologic & oncologic: Anemia, hemorrhage, neutropenia

Renal: Increased blood urea nitrogen

Respiratory: Cough

Rare but important or life-threatening: Hepatotoxicity (idiosyncratic) (Chalasani, 2014)

Injection: Ibuprofen lysine (NeoProfen):

Cardiovascular: Cardiac failure, edema, hypotension, tachycardia

Central nervous system: Intraventricular hemorrhage, seizure

Dermatologic: Skin irritation

Endocrine & metabolic: Adrenocortical insufficiency, hyperglycemia, hypernatremia, hypocalcemia, hypoglycemia

Gastrointestinal: Abdominal distension, cholestasis, gastritis, gastroesophageal reflux disease, gastrointestinal disease (non NEC), intestinal obstruction, inguinal hernia

Genitourinary: Decreased urine output (small decrease reported on days 2 to 6 with compensatory increase in output on day 9), uremia, urinary tract infection

Hematologic & oncologic: Anemia, neutropenia, thrombocytopenia

Hepatic: Jaundice

Infection: Sepsis, infection

Local: Injection site reaction

Renal: Increased serum creatinine, renal insufficiency, renal failure

Respiratory: Apnea, atelectasis, respiratory failure, respiratory tract infection

Miscellaneous: Reduced intake of food/fluids

Rare but important or life-threatening: Gastrointestinal perforation, hepatotoxicity (idiosyncratic) (Chalasani, 2014), necrotizing enterocolitis

Drug Interactions

Metabolism/Transport Effects Substrate of CYP2C19 (minor), CYP2C9 (minor); **Note:** Assignment of Major/Minor substrate status based on clinically relevant drug interaction potential; **Inhibits** CYP2C9 (weak)

Avoid Concomitant Use

Avoid concomitant use of Ibuprofen with any of the following: Dexketoprofen; Floctafenine; Ketorolac (Nasal); Ketorolac (Systemic); Morniflumate; NSAID (COX-2 Inhibitor); Omacetaxine; Urokinase

Increased Effect/Toxicity

Ibuprofen may increase the levels/effects of: 5-ASA Derivatives; Agents with Antiplatelet Properties; Aliskiren; Aminoglycosides; Anticoagulants; Apixaban; Bisphosphonate Derivatives; Collagenase (Systemic); CycloSPORINE (Systemic); Dabigatran Etexilate; Deferasirox; Deoxycholic Acid; Desmopressin; Digoxin; Drospirenone; Eplerenone; Haloperidol; Ibritumomab; Lithium; Methotrexate; Nonsteroidal Anti-Inflammatory Agents; NSAID (COX-2 Inhibitor); Obinutuzumab; Omacetaxine; PEMEtrexed; Porfimer; Potassium-Sparing Diuretics; PRALAtrexate; Quinolone Antibiotics; Rivaroxaban; Salicylates; Tacrolimus (Systemic); Tenofovir; Thrombolytic Agents; Tositumomab and Iodine I 131 Tositumomab; Urokinase; Vancomycin; Verteporfin; Vitamin K Antagonists

The levels/effects of Ibuprofen may be increased by: ACE Inhibitors; Angiotensin II Receptor Blockers; Antidepressants (Tricyclic, Tertiary Amine); Corticosteroids (Systemic); CycloSPORINE (Systemic); Dasatinib; Dexketoprofen; Diclofenac (Systemic); Floctafenine; Glucosamine; Herbs (Anticoagulant/Antiplatelet Properties); Ibrutinib; Ketorolac (Nasal); Ketorolac (Systemic); Limaprost; Morniflumate; Multivitamins/Fluoride (with ADE); Multivitamins/Minerals (with ADEK, Folate, Iron); Multivitamins/Minerals (with AE, No Iron); Omega-3 Fatty Acids; Pentosan Polysulfate Sodium; Pentoxifylline; Probenecid; Prostacyclin Analogues; Selective Serotonin Reuptake Inhibitors; Serotonin/Norepinephrine Reuptake Inhibitors; Sodium Phosphates; Tipranavir; Treprostinil; Vitamin E; Voriconazole

Decreased Effect

Ibuprofen may decrease the levels/effects of: ACE Inhibitors; Aliskiren; Angiotensin II Receptor Blockers; Beta-Blockers; Eplerenone; HydrALAZINE; Imatinib; Loop Diuretics; Potassium-Sparing Diuretics; Prostaglandins (Ophthalmic); Salicylates; Selective Serotonin Reuptake Inhibitors; Thiazide Diuretics

The levels/effects of Ibuprofen may be decreased by: Bile Acid Sequestrants; Salicylates

Food Interactions Ibuprofen peak serum levels may be decreased if taken with food. Management: Administer with food.

Storage/Stability

Ibuprofen injection (Caldolor): Store intact vials at room temperature of 20°C to 25°C (68°F to 77°F). Must be diluted prior to use. Diluted solutions stable for 24 hours at room temperature.

Ibuprofen lysine injection (NeoProfen): Store at 20°C to 25°C (68°F to 77°F); excursions are permitted between 15°C and 30°C (59°F and 86°F). Protect from light. Store vials in carton until use. After first withdrawal from vial, discard remaining solution (preservative free). Following dilution, use within 30 minutes.

Suspension: Store at controlled room temperature of 15°C to 30°C (59°F to 86°F).

Tablet: Store at controlled room temperature of 20°C to 25°C (68°F to 77°F).

Mechanism of Action Reversibly inhibits cyclooxygenase-1 and 2 (COX-1 and 2) enzymes, which results in decreased formation of prostaglandin precursors; has antipyretic, analgesic, and anti-inflammatory properties

Other proposed mechanisms not fully elucidated (and possibly contributing to the anti-inflammatory effect to varying degrees), include inhibiting chemotaxis, altering lymphocyte activity, inhibiting neutrophil aggregation/activation, and decreasing proinflammatory cytokine levels.

Pharmacodynamics

Fever reduction:

Onset of action (single oral dose 8 mg/kg) (Kauffman, 1992):

Infants ≤1 year: 69 ± 22 minutes

Children ≥6 years: 109 ± 64 minutes

Maximum effect: 2-4 hours

Duration: 6-8 hours (dose-related)

Pharmacokinetics (Adult data unless noted)

Absorption: Oral: Rapid (85%)

Distribution: V_d:

Oral:

Febrile children <11 years: 0.2 L/kg

Adults: 0.12 L/kg

IV: Ibuprofen lysine: Premature neonates, GA <32 weeks: Variable results observed: 0.32 L/kg, others have reported: a central compartment V_d that decreases with increasing PNA and ductal closure (Van Overmeire, 2001) and a V_d, apparent: 0.062 L/kg in 21 premature neonates (GA <32 weeks, PNA: <1 day) (Aranda, 1997); a 2-compartment open model was observed

Protein binding: 90% to 99%

Metabolism: Oxidized in the liver; **Note:** Ibuprofen is a racemic mixture of R and S isomers; the R isomer (thought to be inactive) is slowly and incompletely (~60%) converted to the S isomer (active) in adults; the amount of conversion in children is not known, but it is thought to be similar to adults; a study in preterm neonates estimated the conversion to be 61% after prophylactic ibuprofen use and 86% after curative treatment (Gregoire, 2004).

Half-life:

Oral:

Infants and Children 3 months to 10 years: Oral suspension: 1.6 ± 0.7 hours (Kauffman, 1992)

Adults: 1.8-2 hours; end-stage renal disease: Unchanged

IV:

Ibuprofen (Caldor): 2.22-2.44 hours

Ibuprofen lysine (Neoprofen):

Premature neonates, GA < 32 weeks: Reported data highly variable.

R-enantiomer: 10 hours; S-enantiomer: 25.5 hours (Gregoire, 2004)

Age-based observations:

PNA < 1 day: 30.5 ± 4.2 hours (Aranda, 1997)

PNA 3 days: 43.1 ± 26.1 hours (Van Overmeire, 2001)

PNA 5 days: 26.8 ± 23.6 hours (Van Overmeire, 2001)

Time to peak serum concentration: Tablets: 1-2 hours; suspension: 1 hour

Children with cystic fibrosis (Scott, 1999):

Suspension (n=22): 0.74 ± 0.43 hours (median: 30 minutes)

Chewable tablet (n=4): 1.5 ± 0.58 hours (median: 1.5 hours)

Tablet (n=12): 1.33 ± 0.95 hours (median: 1 hour)

Elimination: Urine [primarily as metabolites (45% to 80%); ~1% as unchanged drug and 14% as conjugated]; some biliary excretion

Dosing: Neonatal **PDA closure: Note:** Use birth weight to calculate all doses; monitor urine output; a decrease in urine output may require dose adjustment or holding of therapy.

IV:

Manufacturer's labeling: Ibuprofen lysine (NeoProfen): GA ≤32 weeks weighing 500 to 1,500 g at birth: Initial dose: 10 mg/kg, followed by two doses of 5 mg/kg/dose at 24 and 48 hours after the initial dose. A second course of treatment, alternative pharmacologic therapy, or surgery may be needed if the ductus arteriosus fails to close or reopens following the initial course of therapy.

Alternate dosing: Ibuprofen lysine: Reported dosing approach variable (standard or high-dose therapy):

Standard-dose therapy: Limited data available: GA >32 weeks: Initial dose: 10 mg/kg, followed by two doses of 5 mg/kg/dose administered at 24 hour intervals (Hirt 2008; Meißner 2012)

High-dose therapy: Limited data available: GA 24 to <40 weeks: Initial dose: 20 mg/kg, followed by two doses of 10 mg/kg/dose administered at 24-hour intervals has been evaluated in a total of 58 neonates in two studies (GA: 24 to 39 weeks, PNA ≤5 days for majority of patients). In comparison to the standard dose, these studies found a higher rate of PDA closure using high dose therapy without an increase in adverse effects (Dani 2012; Meißner 2012). Pharmacokinetic data suggest that clearance increases with postnatal age; therefore, doses at the higher end of the dosage range may be necessary in older neonates (Hirt 2008; Van Overmeire 2001).

Oral suspension: Limited data available: GA <34 weeks weighing <1500 g at birth: Initial dose: 10 mg/kg, followed by two doses of 5 mg/kg/dose at 24 and 48 hours after the initial dose; doses were administered undiluted through a feeding tube and immediately followed with a flush (~1 mL) of distilled water; this dosing regimen has been used in several trials and has been shown to be safe and as effective as IV ibuprofen and IV indomethacin (Erdeve 2012; Heyman 2003; Lee 2012); in one retrospective study, oral ibuprofen (n=52) was associated with lower rates of elevated serum creatinine compared to IV indomethacin (n=88) (Lee 2012).

Dosing adjustment in renal impairment: IV: Ibuprofen lysine (Neoprofen): If anuria or marked oliguria (urinary output <0.6 mL/kg/hour) is evident at the scheduled time of the second or third dose, hold dose until renal function returns to normal. Use is contraindicated in preterm infants with significant renal impairment.

Dosing: Usual **Note:** To reduce the risk of adverse cardiovascular and GI effects, use the lowest effective dose for the shortest period of time:

Pediatric:

Analgesic:

IV: Ibuprofen injection (Caldolor): Adolescents ≥17 years: 400 to 800 mg every 6 hours as needed; maximum daily dose: 3,200 mg/**day**. **Note:** Patients should be well hydrated prior to administration.

Oral:

Weight-directed dosing: Infants and Children <50 kg: Limited data available in infants <6 months: 4 to 10 mg/kg/dose every 6 to 8 hours; maximum single dose: 400 mg; maximum daily dose: 40 mg/kg/**day** (APS 2008; Berde 1990; Berde 2002; Kliegman 2011)

Fixed dosing:

Infants and Children 6 months to 11 years: See table based upon manufacturer's labeling; use of weight to select dose is preferred; if weight is not available, then use age; doses may be repeated every 6 to 8 hours; maximum: 4 doses/day; treatment of sore throat for >2 days or use in infants and children <3 years of age with sore throat is not recommended, unless directed by health care provider.

Ibuprofen Dosing

Weight (preferred)[1]		Age	Dosage (mg)
lbs	kg		
12 to 17	5.4 to 8.1	6 to 11 months	50
18 to 23	8.2 to 10.8	12 to 23 months	75
24 to 35	10.9 to 16.3	2 to 3 years	100
36 to 47	16.4 to 21.7	4 to 5 years	150
48 to 59	21.8 to 27.2	6 to 8 years	200
60 to 71	27.3 to 32.6	9 to 10 years	250
72 to 95	32.7 to 43.2	11 years	300

[1]Manufacturer's recommendations are based on weight in pounds (OTC labeling); weight in kg listed here is derived from pounds and rounded; kg weight listed also is adjusted to allow for continuous weight ranges in kg.

Children ≥12 years and Adolescents: Oral: 200 mg every 4 to 6 hours as needed; if pain does not respond may increase to 400 mg; maximum daily dose: 1,200 mg/**day**; treatment of pain for >10 days is not recommended, unless directed by health care provider

Antipyretic:

IV: Ibuprofen injection (Caldolor): Adolescents ≥17 years: Initial: 400 mg, then 400 mg every 4 to 6 hours or 100 to 200 mg every 4 hours as needed; maximum daily dose: 3,200 mg/**day**. **Note:** Patients should be well hydrated prior to administration.

Oral:

Weight-directed dosing: Infants ≥6 months, Children, and Adolescents: 5 to 10 mg/kg/dose every 6 to 8 hours; maximum single dose: 400 mg; maximum daily dose: 40 mg/kg/**day** up to 1200 mg, unless directed by physician; under physician supervision daily doses ≤2,400 mg may be used (Kliegman 2011; Litalien 2001; Sullivan 2011)

Fixed dosing:

Infants and Children 6 months to 11 years: Oral: See table based upon manufacturer's labeling; use of weight to select dose is preferred; if weight is not available, then use age; doses may be repeated every 6 to 8 hours; maximum: 4 doses/day; treatment for >3 days is not recommended unless directed by health care provider

Weight (preferred)[1]		Age	Dosage (mg)
lbs	kg		
12 to 17	5.4 to 8.1	6 to 11 months	50
18 to 23	8.2 to 10.8	12 to 23 months	75
24 to 35	10.9 to 16.3	2 to 3 years	100
36 to 47	16.4 to 21.7	4 to 5 years	150
48 to 59	21.8 to 27.2	6 to 8 years	200
60 to 71	27.3 to 32.6	9 to 10 years	250
72 to 95	32.7 to 43.2	11 years	300

[1]Manufacturer's recommendations are based on weight in pounds (OTC labeling); weight in kg listed here is derived from pounds and rounded; kg weight listed also is adjusted to allow for continuous weight ranges in kg.

Cystic fibrosis, mild disease (to slow lung disease progression): Limited data available: Children and Adolescents 6 to 17 years with FEV_1 >60% predicted (Mogayzel 2013): Oral: Initial: 20 to 30 mg/kg/dose twice daily; titrate to achieve peak plasma concentrations of 50 to 100 mcg/mL; should not eat or take pancreatic enzymes for 2 hours after the ibuprofen dose. Dosing based on a study of 41 patients (ages: 5 to 39 years); mean required dose: ~25 mg/kg/dose twice daily, reported range: 16.2 to 31.6 mg/kg/dose every 12 hours required to achieve target concentration; results showed that chronic ibuprofen use (over 4 years) slowed the rate of decline in FEV_1; patients 5 to 13 years old with mild lung disease were observed to have greatest benefit; (Konstan 1995). A follow up observational study (n=1,365; ages: 6 to 17 years) under noncontrolled conditions (real world) showed significant improvement in the rate of decline of lung disease progression with chronic ibuprofen therapy (Konstan 2007). **Note:** Timing of blood sampling post-dose is based on dosage form: Oral suspension: Obtain blood samples at 30, 45, and 60 minutes postdose; tablets: Obtain blood samples at 1, 2, and 3 hours postdose (Litalien 2001; Scott 1999).

Juvenile idiopathic arthritis (JIA): Children and Adolescents: Usual range: 30 to 40 mg/kg/**day** in 3 to 4 divided doses; start at lower end of dosing range and titrate; patients with milder disease may be treated with 20 mg/kg/**day**; patients with more severe disease may require up to 50 mg/kg/**day**; maximum single dose: 800 mg; maximum daily dose: 2,400 mg/**day** (Giannini 1990; Kliegman 2011; Litalien 2001)

Adult:

Inflammatory disease: Oral: 400 to 800 mg/dose 3 to 4 times daily; maximum daily dose: 3,200 mg/**day**

Analgesia/pain/fever/dysmenorrhea: Oral: 200 to 400 mg/dose every 4 to 6 hours; maximum daily dose: 1,200 mg/**day**, unless directed by physician; under physician supervision daily doses ≤2,400 mg may be used

Analgesic: IV (Caldolor): 400 to 800 mg every 6 hours as needed; maximum daily dose: 3,200 mg/**day**. **Note:** Patients should be well hydrated prior to administration.

Antipyretic: IV (Caldolor): Initial: 400 mg, then 400 mg every 4 to 6 hours or 100 to 200 mg every 4 hours as needed; maximum daily dose: 3,200 mg/**day**. **Note:** Patients should be well hydrated prior to administration.

OTC labeling:

Analgesia/Antipyretic: Oral: 200 mg every 4 to 6 hours as needed; if no relief may increase to 400 mg every 4 to 6 hours as needed; maximum daily dose: 1200 mg/24 hours; treatment for >10 days as an analgesic or >3 days as an antipyretic is not recommended unless directed by health care provider

Migraine: Oral: 400 mg at onset of symptoms; maximum daily dose: 400 mg/24 hours unless directed by health care provider

Dosing adjustment in renal impairment:

Infants, Children, and Adolescents: Oral: There are no dosage adjustments provided in the manufacturer's labeling; however, the 2012 KDIGO guidelines provide the following recommendations for NSAIDs:

eGFR 30 to <60 mL/minute/1.73 m^2: Avoid use in patients with intercurrent disease that increases risk of acute kidney injury

eGFR <30 mL/minute/1.73 m^2: Avoid use

Adults: Oral, IV: There are no dosage adjustments provided in the manufacturer's labeling; however, the 2012 KDIGO guidelines provide the following recommendations for NSAIDs:

eGFR 30 to <60 mL/minute/1.73 m^2: Avoid use in patients with intercurrent disease that increases risk of acute kidney injury

eGFR <30 mL/minute/1.73 m^2: Avoid use

Dosing adjustment in hepatic impairment: Adults: Oral, IV: There are no dosage adjustments provided in the manufacturer's labeling; use caution and discontinue if hepatic function worsens.

Preparation for Administration IV:

Ibuprofen injection (Caldolor): Must be diluted prior to use. Dilute with D_5W, NS or LR to a final concentration ≤4 mg/mL.

Ibuprofen lysine injection (NeoProfen): Dilute with dextrose or saline to an appropriate volume.

Administration

Oral: Administer with food or milk to decrease GI upset; shake suspension well before use

IV:

Ibuprofen injection (Caldolor): For IV administration only; infuse over at least 30 minutes

Ibuprofen lysine injection (NeoProfen): For IV administration only; administration via umbilical arterial line has not been evaluated. Infuse over 15 minutes through IV port closest to insertion site. Avoid extravasation. Do not administer simultaneously via same line with TPN. If needed, interrupt TPN for 15 minutes prior to and after ibuprofen administration, keeping line open with dextrose or saline.

Monitoring Parameters CBC, serum electrolytes, occult blood loss, liver enzymes; urine output, serum BUN, and creatinine in patients receiving IV ibuprofen, concurrent diuretics, those with decreased renal function, or in patients on chronic therapy. Monitor preterm neonates for signs of bleeding and infection; serum electrolytes, glucose, calcium and bilirubin; vital signs; monitor IV site for signs of extravasation. Patients receiving long-term therapy for JIA should receive periodic ophthalmological exams.

Reference Range Plasma concentrations >200 mcg/mL may be associated with severe toxicity; cystic fibrosis: therapeutic peak plasma concentration: 50-100 mcg/mL

Test Interactions May interfere with urine detection of phencyclidine, cannabinoids, and barbiturates (false-positives) (Marchei, 2007; Rollins, 1990)

Additional Information Motrin suspension contains sucrose 0.3 g/mL and 1.6 calories/mL. Due to its effects on platelet function, ibuprofen should be withheld for at least 4-6 half-lives prior to surgical or dental procedures.

There is currently no scientific evidence to support alternating acetaminophen with ibuprofen in the treatment of fever (Mayoral, 2000)

IV ibuprofen is as effective as IV indomethacin for the treatment of PDA in preterm neonates, but is less likely to cause adverse effects on renal function (eg, oliguria, increased serum creatinine) (Aranda, 2006; Lago, 2002; Ohlsson, 2013; Van Overmeire, 2000). Ibuprofen (compared to indomethacin) also has been shown to decrease the risk of developing NEC (Ohlsson, 2013).

Dosage Forms Considerations EnovaRX-Ibuprofen cream is compounded from a kit. Refer to manufacturer's labeling for compounding instructions.

Dosage Forms Excipient information presented when available (limited, particularly for generics); consult specific product labeling.

Capsule, Oral:

Advil: 200 mg

Advil Migraine: 200 mg

KS Ibuprofen: 200 mg [contains fd&c blue #2 (indigotine)]

Generic: 200 mg

Cream, External:

EnovaRX-Ibuprofen: 10% (60 g, 120 g) [contains cetearyl alcohol]

Kit, Combination:

Ibuprofen Comfort Pac: 800 mg [contains methylparaben, trolamine (triethanolamine)]

Solution, Intravenous:

Caldolor: 400 mg/4 mL (4 mL); 800 mg/8 mL (8 mL)

Solution, Intravenous, as lysine [preservative free]:

NeoProfen: 10 mg/mL (2 mL)

Suspension, Oral:

Childrens Advil: 100 mg/5 mL (120 mL) [fruit flavor]

Childrens Advil: 100 mg/5 mL (120 mL) [contains edetate disodium, fd&c red #40, polysorbate 80, propylene glycol, sodium benzoate]

Childrens Advil: 100 mg/5 mL (120 mL) [alcohol free; grape flavor]

Childrens Advil: 100 mg/5 mL (120 mL) [alcohol free; contains brilliant blue fcf (fd&c blue #1), edetate disodium, fd&c red #40, polysorbate 80, propylene glycol, sodium benzoate; grape flavor]

Childrens Advil: 100 mg/5 mL (120 mL) [alcohol free; contains brilliant blue fcf (fd&c blue #1), propylene glycol, sodium benzoate; blue raspberry flavor]

Childrens Advil: 100 mg/5 mL (30 mL, 120 mL) [alcohol free, dye free; contains edetate disodium, polysorbate 80, propylene glycol, sodium benzoate; white grape flavor]

Childrens Advil: 100 mg/5 mL (120 mL) [alcohol free, dye free, sugar free; contains edetate disodium, polysorbate 80, propylene glycol, sodium benzoate; berry flavor]

Childrens Ibuprofen: 100 mg/5 mL (118 mL) [alcohol free; contains brilliant blue fcf (fd&c blue #1), fd&c red #40, polysorbate 80, sodium benzoate; grape flavor]

Childrens Ibuprofen: 100 mg/5 mL (120 mL) [alcohol free; contains butylparaben, fd&c red #40, polysorbate 80, propylene glycol, sodium benzoate; bubble-gum flavor]

Childrens Ibuprofen: 100 mg/5 mL (5 mL, 118 mL, 237 mL, 240 mL) [alcohol free; contains fd&c red #40, fd&c yellow #10 (quinoline yellow), polysorbate 80, sodium benzoate; berry flavor]

Childrens Ibuprofen: 100 mg/5 mL (118 mL) [alcohol free; contains fd&c red #40, polysorbate 80, sodium benzoate]

Childrens Ibuprofen: 40 mg/mL (15 mL) [alcohol free; berry flavor]

Childrens Ibuprofen: 100 mg/5 mL (118 mL) [alcohol free, dye free; contains polysorbate 80, sodium benzoate]

Childrens Ibuprofen: 100 mg/5 mL (118 mL) [alcohol free, gluten free; contains brilliant blue fcf (fd&c blue #1), fd&c red #40, polysorbate 80, sodium benzoate; grape flavor]

Childrens Motrin: 40 mg/mL (15 mL) [berry flavor]

Childrens Motrin: 100 mg/5 mL (120 mL) [alcohol free]

Childrens Motrin: 100 mg/5 mL (60 mL, 120 mL) [alcohol free; contains fd&c red #40, fd&c yellow #10 (quinoline yellow), polysorbate 80, sodium benzoate; berry flavor]

Childrens Motrin: 100 mg/5 mL (120 mL) [alcohol free; contains fd&c red #40, fd&c yellow #10 (quinoline yellow), sodium benzoate; berry flavor]

Childrens Motrin: 100 mg/5 mL (120 mL) [alcohol free; contains fd&c red #40, polysorbate 80, sodium benzoate]
Childrens Motrin: 100 mg/5 mL (120 mL) [alcohol free; contains fd&c red #40, sodium benzoate]
Childrens Motrin: 100 mg/5 mL (120 mL) [alcohol free; contains fd&c red #40, sodium benzoate; bubble-gum flavor]
Childrens Motrin: 100 mg/5 mL (120 mL) [alcohol free; contains fd&c red #40, sodium benzoate; tropical punch flavor]
Childrens Motrin: 100 mg/5 mL (120 mL) [alcohol free, dye free; contains polysorbate 80, sodium benzoate]
Childrens Motrin: 100 mg/5 mL (120 mL) [alcohol free, dye free; contains sodium benzoate; berry flavor]
Ibuprofen Childrens: 100 mg/5 mL (120 mL) [alcohol free; contains butylparaben, fd&c red #40, fd&c yellow #6 (sunset yellow), polysorbate 80, propylene glycol, sodium benzoate; fruit flavor]
Ibuprofen Childrens: 100 mg/5 mL (120 mL) [alcohol free, gluten free; contains brilliant blue fcf (fd&c blue #1), fd&c red #40, polysorbate 80, sodium benzoate; grape flavor]
Ibuprofen Childrens: 100 mg/5 mL (120 mL, 240 mL) [alcohol free, gluten free; contains fd&c red #40, fd&c yellow #10 (quinoline yellow), polysorbate 80, sodium benzoate; berry flavor]
Ibuprofen Childrens: 100 mg/5 mL (118 mL) [alcohol free, gluten free; contains fd&c red #40, polysorbate 80, sodium benzoate; bubble-gum flavor]
Infants Advil: 50 mg/1.25 mL (30 mL) [alcohol free, dye free; contains edetate disodium, polysorbate 80, propylene glycol, sodium benzoate]
Infants Advil: 50 mg/1.25 mL (15 mL) [alcohol free, dye free; contains edetate disodium, polysorbate 80, propylene glycol, sodium benzoate; white grape flavor]
Infants Ibuprofen: 50 mg/1.25 mL (15 mL) [alcohol free; contains butylparaben, fd&c red #40, polysorbate 80, propylene glycol, sodium benzoate; berry flavor]
Infants Ibuprofen: 50 mg/1.25 mL (15 mL, 30 mL) [alcohol free, dye free; contains polysorbate 80, sodium benzoate; berry flavor]
Infants Ibuprofen: 50 mg/1.25 mL (15 mL) [alcohol free, gluten free; contains butylparaben, fd&c red #40, polysorbate 80, propylene glycol, sodium benzoate; berry flavor]
Motrin: 40 mg/mL (15 mL) [alcohol free, dye free; berry flavor]
Motrin Infants Drops: 50 mg/1.25 mL (15 mL) [alcohol free; contains fd&c red #40, polysorbate 80, sodium benzoate; berry flavor]
Motrin Infants Drops: 50 mg/1.25 mL (15 mL, 30 mL) [alcohol free, dye free; contains polysorbate 80, sodium benzoate]
Generic: 100 mg/5 mL (5 mL, 118 mL, 120 mL, 473 mL)

Tablet, Oral:
Addaprin: 200 mg
Advil: 200 mg
Advil Junior Strength: 100 mg
Dyspel: 200 mg
Genpril: 200 mg
I-Prin: 200 mg
IBU-200: 200 mg
Motrin IB: 200 mg
Motrin IB: 200 mg [contains fd&c yellow #6 (sunset yellow)]
Motrin Junior Strength: 100 mg [scored]
Provil: 200 mg
Generic: 200 mg, 400 mg, 600 mg, 800 mg

Tablet Chewable, Oral:
Advil Junior Strength: 100 mg [scored; contains aspartame, fd&c blue #2 aluminum lake; grape flavor]
Childrens Motrin: 50 mg [scored; contains aspartame, fd&c yellow #6 (sunset yellow); orange flavor]
Childrens Motrin Jr Strength: 100 mg [scored; contains aspartame, brilliant blue fcf (fd&c blue #1); grape flavor]
Ibuprofen Junior Strength: 100 mg [contains aspartame, fd&c yellow #6 (sunset yellow), soybean oil, whey protein]
Motrin Junior Strength: 100 mg [contains aspartame, brilliant blue fcf (fd&c blue #1)]
Motrin Junior Strength: 100 mg [scored; contains aspartame, fd&c yellow #6 (sunset yellow); orange flavor]

- **Ibuprofen and Pseudoephedrine** *see* Pseudoephedrine and Ibuprofen *on page 1803*
- **Ibuprofen Childrens [OTC]** *see* Ibuprofen *on page 1064*
- **Ibuprofen Comfort Pac** *see* Ibuprofen *on page 1064*
- **Ibuprofen Junior Strength [OTC]** *see* Ibuprofen *on page 1064*
- **Ibuprofen Lysine** *see* Ibuprofen *on page 1064*
- **Ibuprofen Muscle and Joint (Can)** *see* Ibuprofen *on page 1064*
- **IC51** *see* Japanese Encephalitis Virus Vaccine (Inactivated) *on page 1184*
- **ICI-182,780** *see* Fulvestrant *on page 950*
- **ICI-204,219** *see* Zafirlukast *on page 2203*
- **ICI-46474** *see* Tamoxifen *on page 2005*
- **ICL670** *see* Deferasirox *on page 594*
- **ICRF-187** *see* Dexrazoxane *on page 622*
- **Idamycin PFS** *see* IDArubicin *on page 1071*

IDArubicin (eye da ROO bi sin)

Medication Safety Issues

Sound-alike/look-alike issues:
IDArubicin may be confused with DOXOrubicin, DAUNOrubicin, epirubicin, idelalisib
Idamycin PFS may be confused with Adriamycin

High alert medication:
This medication is in a class the Institute for Safe Medication Practices (ISMP) includes among its list of drug classes which have a heightened risk of causing significant patient harm when used in error.

Related Information
Management of Drug Extravasations *on page 2298*
Prevention of Chemotherapy-Induced Nausea and Vomiting in Children *on page 2368*
Safe Handling of Hazardous Drugs *on page 2455*

Brand Names: US Idamycin PFS

Brand Names: Canada Idamycin PFS; Idarubicin Hydrochloride Injection

Therapeutic Category Antineoplastic Agent, Anthracycline; Antineoplastic Agent, Topoisomerase II Inhibitor

Generic Availability (US) Yes

Use Used in combination with other antineoplastic agents for treatment of acute myeloid leukemia (AML) (FDA approved in adults)

Pregnancy Risk Factor D

Pregnancy Considerations Adverse events were observed in animal reproduction studies. Fetal fatality was noted in a case report following second trimester exposure in a pregnant woman. The manufacturer recommends that women of childbearing potential avoid pregnancy.

Breast-Feeding Considerations It is not known if idarubicin is excreted in breast milk. Due to the potential for serious adverse reactions in the nursing infant, breast-feeding is not recommended by the manufacturer.

Contraindications Bilirubin >5 mg/dL

Documentation of allergenic cross-reactivity for drugs in this class is limited. However, because of similarities in chemical structure and/or pharmacologic actions, the possibility of cross-sensitivity cannot be ruled out with certainty.

Warnings/Precautions Hazardous agent - use appropriate precautions for handling and disposal (NIOSH 2014 [group 1]). **[US Boxed Warning]: May cause myocardial toxicity; may lead to heart failure. Cardiotoxicity is more common in patients who have previously received anthracyclines or have preexisting cardiac disease.** The risk of myocardial toxicity is also increased in patients with concomitant or prior mediastinal/pericardial irradiation, patients with anemia, bone marrow depression, infections, leukemic pericarditis or myocarditis. Patients with active or dormant cardiovascular disease, concurrent administration of cardiotoxic drugs, prior therapy with other anthracyclines or anthracenediones are also at increased risk for cardiotoxicity. Potentially fatal heart failure, acute arrhythmias (may be life-threatening) or other cardiomyopathies may also occur. Regular monitoring of LVEF and discontinuation at the first sign of impairment is recommended, especially in patients with cardiac risk factors or impaired cardiac function. The half-life of other cardiotoxic agents (eg, trastuzumab) must be considered. Avoid the use of anthracycline-based therapy for at least 5 half-lives after discontinuation of the cardiotoxic agent. Monitor cardiac function during treatment. Patients >60 years who were undergoing induction therapy experienced heart failure, serious arrhythmias, chest pain, MI, and asymptomatic declines in LVEF more frequently than younger patients.

[US Boxed Warning]: Vesicant; may cause severe local tissue damage and necrosis if extravasation occurs. For IV administration only. NOT for IM or SubQ administration. Administer through a rapidly flowing IV line. Ensure proper needle or catheter placement prior to and during infusion. Avoid extravasation.

[US Boxed Warning]: May cause severe myelosuppression when used at therapeutic doses. Patients are at risk of developing infection and bleeding (may be fatal) due to neutropenia and thrombocytopenia, respectively. Monitor blood counts frequently. Do not use in patients with preexisting bone marrow suppression unless the benefit outweighs the risk. **[US Boxed Warning]: Dosage reductions are recommended in patients with renal or hepatic impairment.** Do not use if bilirubin >5 mg/dL. Rapid lysis of leukemic cells may lead to hyperuricemia. Ensure adequate hydration and consider use of antihyperuricemic prophylaxis. Systemic infections should be controlled prior to initiation of treatment. **[US Boxed Warning]: Should be administered under the supervision of an experienced cancer chemotherapy physician.** Use in facilities with laboratory and supportive resources adequate to monitor drug tolerance and protect and maintain a patient compromised by drug toxicity. The physician and institution must be capable of responding rapidly and completely to severe hemorrhagic conditions and/or overwhelming infection. Idarubicin is associated with a moderate emetic potential; antiemetics are recommended to prevent nausea and vomiting (Basch, 2011; Dupuis, 2011; Roila, 2010). Abdominal pain, diarrhea, and mucositis may commonly occur. Potentially significant drug-drug interactions may exist, requiring dose or frequency adjustment, additional monitoring, and/or selection of alternative therapy.

Adverse Reactions

Cardiovascular: CHF (dose related), transient ECG abnormalities (supraventricular tachycardia, S-T wave changes, atrial or ventricular extrasystoles) are generally asymptomatic and self-limiting. The relative cardiotoxicity of idarubicin compared to doxorubicin is unclear. Some investigators report no increase in cardiac toxicity for adults at cumulative oral idarubicin doses up to 540 mg/m^2; other reports suggest a maximum cumulative intravenous dose of 150 mg/m^2.

Central nervous system: Headache, seizure

Dermatologic: Alopecia, radiation recall, skin rash, urticaria

Gastrointestinal: Diarrhea, GI hemorrhage, nausea, vomiting, stomatitis

Emetic potential: Moderate (30% to 60%)

Genitourinary: Discoloration of urine (darker yellow)

Hematologic: Myelosuppression (nadir: 10-15 days; recovery: 21-28 days), primarily leukopenia; thrombocytopenia and anemia. Effects are generally less severe with oral dosing.

Hepatic: Bilirubin increased, transaminases increased

Neuromuscular & skeletal: Peripheral neuropathy

Local: Tissue necrosis upon extravasation, erythematous streaking

Rare but important or life-threatening: Cardiomyopathy, hyperuricemia, myocarditis, neutropenic typhlitis

Drug Interactions

Metabolism/Transport Effects Substrate of P-glycoprotein

Avoid Concomitant Use

Avoid concomitant use of IDArubicin with any of the following: BCG; BCG (Intravesical); CloZAPine; Dipyrone; Natalizumab; Pimecrolimus; Tacrolimus (Topical); Tofacitinib; Vaccines (Live)

Increased Effect/Toxicity

IDArubicin may increase the levels/effects of: CloZAPine; Leflunomide; Natalizumab; Tofacitinib; Vaccines (Live)

The levels/effects of IDArubicin may be increased by: Bevacizumab; Cyclophosphamide; Denosumab; Dipyrone; P-glycoprotein/ABCB1 Inhibitors; Pimecrolimus; Roflumilast; Tacrolimus (Topical); Taxane Derivatives; Trastuzumab

Decreased Effect

IDArubicin may decrease the levels/effects of: BCG; BCG (Intravesical); Cardiac Glycosides; Coccidioides immitis Skin Test; Sipuleucel-T; Vaccines (Inactivated); Vaccines (Live)

The levels/effects of IDArubicin may be decreased by: Cardiac Glycosides; Echinacea; P-glycoprotein/ABCB1 Inducers

Storage/Stability Store intact vials of solution refrigerated at 2°C to 8°C (36°F to 46°F). Protect from light.

Mechanism of Action Similar to daunorubicin, idarubicin inhibits DNA and RNA synthesis by intercalation between DNA base pairs and by steric obstruction. Although the exact mechanism is unclear, it appears that direct binding to DNA (intercalation) and inhibition of DNA repair (topoisomerase II inhibition) result in blockade of DNA and RNA synthesis and fragmentation of DNA.

Pharmacokinetics (Adult data unless noted)

Distribution: V_d: Large volume of distribution due to extensive tissue binding; distributes into CSF

Protein binding:

Idarubicin: 97%

Idarubicinol: 94%

Metabolism: Hepatic to idarubicinol (active metabolite)

Half-life:

Children: Children ≥1 year and adolescents: 17.6 ± 6.8 hours (range: 8.3 to 29.6 hours) (Reid, 1990)

Adults: 22 hours (range: 4 to 48 hours)

Idarubicinol: >45 hours

Elimination: Primarily by biliary excretion; minor amount eliminated renally

Dosing: Usual Note: Dose, frequency, number of doses, and start date may vary by protocol and/or treatment phase; refer to specific protocol. Idarubicin is associated with a moderate emetic potential; antiemetics are recommended to prevent nausea and vomiting (Basch 2011; Dupuis 2011; Roila 2010).

Pediatric: **Acute myeloid leukemia (AML):** Limited data available: Infants, Children, and Adolescents:

New diagnosis (CCG-2961) (Lange 2008):

Induction: IV: IdaDCTER: Idarubicin 5 mg/m^2/dose daily for 4 days on days 0 to 3 in combination with cytarabine, etoposide, thioguanine, and dexamethasone

Consolidation: IV:

IdaDCTER: Idarubicin 5 mg/m^2/dose daily for 4 days on days 0 to 3 in combination with cytarabine, etoposide, thioguanine, and dexamethasone

OR

Idarubicin 12 mg/m^2/dose daily for 3 days on days 0 to 2 in combination with fludarabine and cytarabine

Relapsed/refractory: IV: Children and Adolescents: 12 mg/m^2 once daily for 3 days in combination with fludarabine and cytarabine (Dinndorf 1997; Leahey 1997)

Adult: Utilize patient's actual body weight (full weight) for calculation of body surface area- or weight-based dosing, particularly when the intent of therapy is curative; manage regimen-related toxicities in the same manner as for nonobese patients; if a dose reduction is utilized due to toxicity, consider resumption of full weight-based dosing with subsequent cycles, especially if cause of toxicity (eg, hepatic or renal impairment) is resolved (Griggs 2012).

Acute myeloid leukemia (AML): IV: Induction: 12 mg/m^2/day for 3 days (in combination with cytarabine); a second induction cycle may be administered if necessary

Dosing adjustment in renal impairment: There are no specific dosasge adjustments provided in the manufacturer's labeling; however, it does recommend that dosage reductions be made. Patients with Scr ≥2 mg/dL did not receive treatment in many clinical trials. The following adjustments have also been recommended (Aronoff, 2007):

Infants, Children, and Adolescents:

GFR >50 mL/minute/1.73 m^2: No adjustment necessary

GFR ≤50 mL/minute/1.73 m^2: Administer 75% of dose

Intermittent hemodialysis: Administer 75% of dose

Peritoneal dialysis (PD): Administer 75% of dose

Continuous renal replacement therapy (CRRT): Administer 75% of dose

Adults:

CrCl 10 to 50 mL/minute: Administer 75% of dose

CrCl <10 mL/minute: Administer 50% of dose

Hemodialysis: Supplemental dose not needed

Continuous ambulatory peritoneal dialysis (CAPD): Supplemental dose not needed

Dosing adjustment in hepatic impairment: There are no specific dosage adjustments provided in the manufacturer's labeling; however, it does recommend that dosage reductions be made. Avoid use if bilirubin is >5 mg/dL. Dosage should be reduced by 50% if bilirubin is 2.6 to 5 mg/dL (Perry 2012).

Administration Hazardous agent; use appropriate precautions for handling and disposal (NIOSH, 2012).

Idarubicin is associated with a moderate emetic potential; antiemetics are recommended to prevent nausea and vomiting (Basch 2011; Dupuis 2011; Roila 2010).

For IV administration only. Do not administer IM or SubQ; administer as slow push over 3 to 5 minutes, preferably into the side of a freely-running saline or dextrose infusion or as intermittent infusion over 10 to 15 minutes into a free-flowing IV solution of NS or D_5W.

Vesicant; ensure proper needle or catheter placement prior to and during infusion; avoid extravasation. If extravasation occurs, stop infusion immediately and disconnect (leave cannula/needle in place); gently aspirate extravasated solution (do **NOT** flush the line); remove needle/cannula; elevate extremity. Initiate antidote (dimethyl sulfate [DMSO] or dexrazoxane [adult]) (see Management of Drug Extravasations for more details). Apply dry cold compresses for 20 minutes 4 times daily for 1 to 2 days (Pérez Fidalgo 2012); withhold cooling beginning 15 minutes before dexrazoxane infusion; continue withholding cooling until 15 minutes after infusion is completed. Topical DMSO should not be administered in combination with dexrazoxane; may lessen dexrazoxane efficacy.

Vesicant/Extravasation Risk Vesicant

Monitoring Parameters CBC with differential, platelet count, ECHO, ECG, serum electrolytes, creatinine, uric acid, ALT, AST, bilirubin, signs of extravasation

Dosage Forms Excipient information presented when available (limited, particularly for generics); consult specific product labeling.

Solution, Intravenous, as hydrochloride [preservative free]:

Idamycin PFS: 5 mg/5 mL (5 mL); 10 mg/10 mL (10 mL); 20 mg/20 mL (20 mL)

Generic: 5 mg/5 mL (5 mL); 10 mg/10 mL (10 mL); 20 mg/20 mL (20 mL)

◆ **Idarubicin Hydrochloride** *see* IDArubicin *on page 1071*

◆ **Idarubicin Hydrochloride Injection (Can)** *see* IDArubicin *on page 1071*

◆ **IDEC-C2B8** *see* RiTUXimab *on page 1875*

◆ **IDR** *see* IDArubicin *on page 1071*

Idursulfase (eye dur SUL fase)

Medication Safety Issues

Sound-alike/look-alike issues:

Elaprase may be confused with Elspar

Brand Names: US Elaprase

Brand Names: Canada Elaprase

Therapeutic Category Enzyme

Generic Availability (US) No

Use Replacement therapy in mucopolysaccharidosis II (MPS II, Hunter syndrome) (FDA approved in ages ≥5 years and adults)

Pregnancy Risk Factor C

Pregnancy Considerations Animal reproduction studies have not been conducted.

Breast-Feeding Considerations It is not known if idursulfase is excreted in breast milk. The manufacturer recommends that caution be exercised when administering idursulfase to nursing women.

Contraindications There are no contraindications listed in the manufacturer's labeling.

Warnings/Precautions [U.S. Boxed Warning]: Serious hypersensitivity reactions, including life-threatening anaphylactic reactions, have been reported during and within 24 hours after infusion. Anaphylaxis may present as respiratory distress, hypoxia, hypotension, urticaria, and/or tongue/throat angioedema. Monitor closely during and after infusion. Appropriate medical support should be readily available. Patients with compromised respiratory function or acute respiratory disease are at risk of respiratory disease exacerbation due to hypersensitivity; additional monitoring may be required. Discontinue immediately if anaphylactic or acute reaction occurs. Patients experiencing initial severe or refractory reactions may need prolonged monitoring. Antihistamines, corticosteroids and/or decreased infusion rates may be used to manage subsequent infusions.

Use with caution in patients at risk for fluid overload or in conditions where fluid restriction is indicated (eg, acute underlying respiratory illness, compromised cardiac and/or respiratory function); conditions may be exacerbated during infusion. Extended observation may be necessary for some patients. Use with caution in patients with severe genetic mutations (eg, complete gene deletion, large gene rearrangement, nonsense, frameshift or splice site mutations); may increase risk of hypersensitivity reactions, serious adverse reactions, and antibody development. Use caution and consider delaying treatment in patients with compromised respiratory function or acute febrile or respiratory illness; may be at increased risk for life-threatening complications from hypersensitivity reactions. Development of anti-idursulfase IgG antibodies has been reported in 51% of patients; may increase incidence of hypersensitivity reactions. Patients and healthcare providers are encouraged to participate in the Hunter Outcome Survey, intended to monitor disease progression, patient outcomes, and long-term effects of therapy. For more information, refer to www.elaprase.com or call OnePath[sm] at 1-866-888-0660.

Warnings: Additional Pediatric Considerations Per the manufacturer, a small, open-labeled evaluation of the safety and efficacy of 53 weeks of therapy in 28 pediatric patients ≤5 years of age showed enzyme replacement with idursulfase reduced splenic volume similar to older pediatric patients but data did not support improvement in other disease-related symptoms (which were undefined) or long-term clinical outcomes (which were undefined). **Note:** Proving clinical benefit of therapy for disease-related symptoms in this population is challenging due to age-related compliance with evaluation techniques (eg, walking capacity evaluations, FEV) (Muenzer 2011). A larger observation trial (n=124) of patients <6 years (including infants) showed weekly administration of idursulfase produced a significant decrease in hepatic volume and a reduction in urine GAG levels similar to that in older pediatric patients (Muenzer 2011). Guidelines suggest the initiation of idursulfase therapy at the time of diagnosis to delay the development of permanent life-threatening disease manifestations (Scarpa 2011)

When compared to pediatric patients >7 years, the patients ≤7 years of age were shown to have more frequent development of anti-idursulfase IgG antibodies (68% vs 51%) and neutralizing antibodies (79% vs 41%). In patients <5 years of age, an association between the presence of antibodies and reduced systemic idursulfase exposure has been observed; this has not been reported in older pediatric patients (≥5 years of age). Younger pediatric patients have also been shown to develop neutralizing antibodies earlier in therapy (at week 9 vs 27) and at higher titers.

Adverse Reactions

Cardiovascular: Atrial abnormality, flushing, hypertension, tachycardia

Central nervous system: Anxiety, chills, dizziness, fatigue, headache, irritability, malaise

Dermatologic: Erythema, nausea, pruritic rash, pruritus, skin disorder, skin rash, urticaria

Gastrointestinal: Diarrhea, dyspepsia, vomiting

Hypersensitivity: Anaphylaxis, hypersensitivity reaction

Immunologic: Antibody development (neutralizing), development of IgG antibodies

Local: Abscess, infusion site edema

Neuromuscular & skeletal: Arthralgia, chest wall musculoskeletal pain, limb pain, musculoskeletal dysfunction, musculoskeletal pain

Ophthalmic: Visual disturbance

Otic: Otitis (children 16 months to 4 years)

Respiratory: Cough, pneumonia (children 16 months to 4 years), wheezing

Miscellaneous: Antibody development, fever, infusion reactions, superficial injury

Rare but important or life-threatening: Angioedema, cardiac arrhythmia, cardiac failure, cardiorespiratory arrest, cyanosis, hypotension, infection, loss of consciousness, pulmonary embolism, respiratory distress, respiratory failure, seizure

Drug Interactions

Metabolism/Transport Effects None known.

Avoid Concomitant Use There are no known interactions where it is recommended to avoid concomitant use.

Increased Effect/Toxicity There are no known significant interactions involving an increase in effect.

Decreased Effect There are no known significant interactions involving a decrease in effect.

Storage/Stability Store vials under refrigeration at 2°C to 8°C (36°F to 46°F). Protect from light, do not freeze or shake. Should be used immediately after dilution. However, solution for infusion may be stored under refrigeration for up to 24 hours.

Mechanism of Action Idursulfase is a recombinant form of iduronate-2-sulfatase, an enzyme needed to hydrolyze the mucopolysaccharides dermatan sulfate and heparan sulfate in various cells. Accumulation of these polysaccharides can lead to various manifestations of disease, including physical changes, CNS involvement, cardiac, respiratory, and mobility dysfunction. Replacement of this enzyme has been shown to improve walking capacity in patients with a deficiency.

Pharmacokinetics (Adult data unless noted)

Distribution: Varies dependent upon age and presence of antibodies (particularly patients <7.5 years): V_{dss}:

Children 16 months to <7.5 years: Week 1: 394 ± 423 mL/kg; Week 27: Antibody negative: 272 ± 112 mL/kg; antibody positive: 829 ± 636 mL/kg

Children ≥7.5 years, Adolescents, and Adults <27 years: Mean range: 213 to 254 mL/kg

Half-life elimination: Varies dependent upon age and presence of antibodies (particularly patients <7.5 years)

Children 16 months to <7.5 years: Week 1: 160 ± 69 minutes; Week 27: Antibody negative: 134 ± 19 minutes; antibody positive: 84 ±46 minutes

Children ≥7.5 years, Adolescents, and Adults <27 years: Mean range: 44 to 48 minutes

Dosing: Usual

Pediatric: **Mucopolysaccharidosis type II (MPS II, Hunter syndrome): Note:** Current consensus opinion recommends initiation of therapy as early as possible following diagnosis (Scarpa 2011):

Children 16 months to <5 years: Limited data available: IV: 0.5 mg/kg once weekly (Muenzer 2011; Scarpa 2011)

Children ≥5 years and Adolescents: IV: 0.5 mg/kg once weekly

Adult: **Mucopolysaccharidosis type II (MPS II, Hunter syndrome):** IV: 0.5 mg/kg once weekly

Dosing adjustment in renal impairment: There are no dosage adjustments provided in the manufacturer's labeling.

Dosing adjustment in hepatic impairment: There are no dosage adjustments provided in the manufacturer's labeling.

Preparation for Administration IV: Allow vials to reach room temperature prior to preparation. Dilute dose in NS 100 mL. Mix gently; do not shake.

Administration IV: Administer using an infusion set containing a 0.2 micron low protein-binding inline filter. Infuse at an initial rate of 8 mL/hour for the first 15 minutes. If tolerated, may increase rate by 8 mL/hour increments every 15 minutes up to maximum infusion rate of 100 mL/hour. Rate may be decreased, temporarily stopped, or discontinued based on tolerance. Initial infusion should be over 3 hours; if tolerated, subsequent infusions may be gradually reduced to a 1-hour infusion. Total infusion time should not exceed 8 hours. **Note:** For subsequent doses, current guidelines suggest that shortened infusion time of 1 hour is not desirable and increased the risk of infusion-related reaction; extra precautions should be used (Scarpa 2011).

Monitoring Parameters Monitor for infusion-related and hypersensitivity reactions; pulmonary function, oxygen saturation; blood pressure

Dosage Forms Excipient information presented when available (limited, particularly for generics); consult specific product labeling.

Solution, Intravenous [preservative free]:

Elaprase: 6 mg/3 mL (3 mL)

◆ **IDV** *see* Indinavir *on page 1098*

◆ **iFerex 150 [OTC]** *see* Polysaccharide-Iron Complex *on page 1728*

◆ **Ifex** *see* Ifosfamide *on page 1075*

Ifosfamide (eye FOSS fa mide)

Medication Safety Issues

Sound-alike/look-alike issues:

Ifosfamide may be confused with cyclophosphamide

High alert medication:

This medication is in a class the Institute for Safe Medication Practices (ISMP) includes its list of drug classes which have a heightened risk of causing significant patient harm when used in error.

Related Information

Management of Drug Extravasations *on page 2298*

Prevention of Chemotherapy-Induced Nausea and Vomiting in Children *on page 2368*

Safe Handling of Hazardous Drugs *on page 2455*

Brand Names: US Ifex

Brand Names: Canada Ifex

Therapeutic Category Antineoplastic Agent, Alkylating Agent

Generic Availability (US) Yes

Use Treatment of germ cell testicular cancer in combination with other antineoplastic agents (FDA approved in adults); **Note:** Should be used in combination with mesna for prophylaxis of hemorrhagic cystitis; has also been used in the treatment of Hodgkin and non-Hodgkin's lymphoma, Ewing sarcoma, osteosarcoma, and soft tissue sarcomas

Pregnancy Risk Factor D

Pregnancy Considerations Embryotoxic and teratogenic effects have been observed in animal reproduction studies. Fetal growth retardation and neonatal anemia have been reported with exposure to ifosfamide-containing regimens during human pregnancy. Male and female fertility may be affected (dose and duration dependent). Ifosfamide interferes with oogenesis and spermatogenesis; amenorrhea, azoospermia, and sterility have been reported and may be irreversible. Avoid pregnancy during treatment; male patients should not father a child for at least 6 months after completion of therapy.

Breast-Feeding Considerations Breast-feeding should be avoided during ifosfamide treatment. According to the manufacturer, the decision to discontinue ifosfamide or discontinue breast-feeding should take into account the risk of exposure to the infant and the benefits of treatment to the mother.

Contraindications Hypersensitivity to ifosfamide or any component of the formulation; urinary outflow obstruction

Canadian labeling: Additional contraindications (not in U.S. labeling): Severe myelosuppression; severe renal or hepatic impairment; active infection (bacterial, fungal, viral); severe immunosuppression; urinary tract disease (eg, cystitis); advanced cerebral arteriosclerosis

Warnings/Precautions Hazardous agent: Use appropriate precautions for handling and disposal (NIOSH 2014 [group 1]). **[U.S. Boxed Warning]: Hemorrhagic cystitis may occur; concomitant mesna reduces the risk of hemorrhagic cystitis.** Hydration (at least 2 L/day in adults), dose fractionation, and/or mesna administration will reduce the incidence of hematuria and protect against hemorrhagic cystitis. Obtain urinalysis prior to each dose; if microscopic hematuria is detected, withhold until complete resolution. Exclude or correct urinary tract obstructions prior to treatment. Use with caution (if at all) in patients with active urinary tract infection. Hemorrhagic cystitis is dose-dependent and is increased with high single doses (compared with fractionated doses); past or concomitant bladder radiation or busulfan treatment may increase the risk for hemorrhagic cystitis. **[U.S. Boxed Warning]: May cause severe nephrotoxicity, resulting in renal failure.** Acute and chronic renal failure as well as renal parenchymal and tubular necrosis (including acute) have been reported; tubular damage may be delayed and may persist. Renal manifestations include decreased glomerular rate, increased creatinine, proteinuria, enzymuria, cylindruria, aminoaciduria, phosphaturia, and glycosuria. Syndrome of inappropriate antidiuretic hormone (SIADH), renal rickets, and Fanconi syndrome have been reported. Evaluate renal function prior to and during treatment; monitor urine for erythrocytes and signs of urotoxicity.

[U.S. Boxed Warning]: May cause CNS toxicity which may be severe, resulting in encephalopathy and death; monitor for CNS toxicity; discontinue for encephalopathy. Symptoms of CNS toxicity (somnolence, confusion, dizziness, disorientation, hallucinations, cranial nerve dysfunction, psychotic behavior, extrapyramidal symptoms, seizures, coma blurred vision, and/or incontinence) have been observed within a few hours to a few days after initial dose and generally resolve within 2-3 days of treatment discontinuation (although may persist longer); maintain supportive care until complete resolution. Risk factors may include hypoalbuminemia, renal dysfunction, and prior history of ifosfamide-induced encephalopathy. Concomitant centrally-acting medications may result in additive CNS effects. Peripheral neuropathy has been reported.

[U.S. Boxed Warning]: Severe bone marrow suppression may occur (dose-limiting toxicity); monitor blood counts before and after each cycle. Leukopenia, neutropenia, thrombocytopenia and anemia are associated with ifosfamide. Myelosuppression is dose dependent, increased with single high doses (compared to fractionated doses) and increased with decreased renal function. Severe myelosuppression may occur when administered in combination with other chemotherapy agents or radiation therapy. Use with caution in patients with compromised bone marrow reserve. Unless clinically necessary, avoid administering to patients with WBC <2000/mm^3 and platelets <50,000/mm^3. Antimicrobial prophylaxis may be necessary in some neutropenic patients; Administer antibiotics and/or antifungal agents for neutropenic fever. May cause significant suppression of the immune responses; may lead to serious infection, sepsis or septic shock; reported infections have included bacterial, viral, fungal, and parasitic; latent infections may be reactivated; use with caution with other immunosuppressants or in patients with infection.

Arrhythmias, ST-segment or T-wave changes, cardiomyopathy, pericardial effusion, pericarditis, and epicardial fibrosis have been observed; the risk for cardiotoxicity is dose-dependent; concomitant cardiotoxic agents (eg, anthracyclines), irradiation of the cardiac region, and renal impairment may also increase the risk; use with caution in patients with cardiac risk factors or pre-existing cardiac disease. Interstitial pneumonitis, pulmonary fibrosis, and pulmonary toxicity leading to respiratory failure have been reported; monitor for signs and symptoms of pulmonary toxicity.

Anaphylactic/anaphylactoid reactions have been associated with ifosfamide; cross sensitivity with similar agents may occur. Hepatic sinusoidal obstruction syndrome (SOS), formerly called veno-occlusive disease (VOD), has been reported with ifosfamide-containing regimens. Secondary malignancies may occur; the risk for myelodysplastic syndrome (which may progress to acute leukemia) is increased with treatment. May interfere with wound healing. Use with caution in patients with prior radiation therapy. Ifosfamide is associated with a moderate emetic potential; antiemetics are recommended to prevent nausea and vomiting (Basch, 2011; Dupuis, 2011; Roila, 2010).

Adverse Reactions

Central nervous system: CNS toxicity or encephalopathy, fever

Dermatologic: Alopecia

Endocrine & metabolic: Metabolic acidosis

Gastrointestinal: Anorexia, nausea/vomiting

Hematologic: Anemia, leukopenia, neutropenic fever, thrombocytopenia

Hepatic: Bilirubin increased, liver dysfunction, transaminases increased

Local: Phlebitis

Renal: Hematuria (reduced with mesna), renal impairment

Miscellaneous: Infection

Rare but important or life-threatening: Acute respiratory distress syndrome, acute tubular necrosis, agranulocytosis, alkaline phosphatase increased, allergic reaction, alveolitis (allergic), amenorrhea, aminoaciduria, amnesia, anaphylactic reaction, angina, angioedema, anuria, arrhythmia, arthralgia, asterixis, atrial ectopy, atrial fibrillation/flutter, azoospermia, bladder irritation, bleeding, blurred vision, bone marrow failure, bradycardia, bradyphrenia, bronchospasm, bundle branch block, BUN increased, capillary leak syndrome, cardiac arrest, cardiogenic shock, cardiomyopathy, cardiotoxicity, catatonia, cecitis, chest pain, cholestasis, coagulopathy, colitis, conjunctivitis, creatinine clearance decreased/increased, creatinine increased, cylindruria, cytolytic hepatitis, delirium, delusion, dermatitis, diarrhea, DIC, DVT, dysesthesia, dyspnea, dysuria, echolalia, edema, ejection fraction decreased, enterocolitis, enuresis, enzymuria, erythema, extrapyramidal disorder, facial swelling, Fanconi syndrome, fatigue, gait disturbance, GGT increased, GI hemorrhage, glycosuria, gonadotropin increased, granulocytopenia, growth retardation (children), hemolytic anemia, hemolytic uremic syndrome, hemorrhagic cystitis, hepatic failure, hepatic sinusoidal obstruction syndrome (SOS; formerly veno-occlusive disease [VOD]), hepatitis fulminant, hepatitis (viral), hepatorenal syndrome, herpes zoster, hyperglycemia, hyper-/hypotension, hypersensitivity reactions, hypocalcemia, hypokalemia, hyponatremia, hypophosphatemia, hypoxia, ileus, immunosuppression, infertility, infusion site reactions (erythema, inflammation, pain, pruritus, swelling, tenderness), interstitial lung disease, jaundice, LDH increased, leukoencephalopathy, lymphopenia, malaise, mania, mental status change, methemoglobinemia, MI, mucosal inflammation/ulceration, multiorgan failure, mutism, myocardial hemorrhage, myocarditis, nephrogenic diabetes insipidus, neuralgia, neutropenia, oligospermia, oliguria, osteomalacia (adults), ovarian failure, ovulation disorder, palmar-plantar erythrodysesthesia syndrome, pancreatitis, pancytopenia, panic attack, paranoia, paresthesia, pericardial effusion, pericarditis, peripheral neuropathy, petechiae, phosphaturia, pleural effusion, *Pneumocystis jiroveci* pneumonia, pneumonia, pneumonitis, pollakiuria, polydipsia, polyneuropathy, polyuria, portal vein thrombosis, premature atrial contractions, premature menopause, progressive multifocal leukoencephalopathy, proteinuria, pruritus, pulmonary edema, pulmonary embolism, pulmonary fibrosis, pulmonary hypertension, QRS complex abnormal, radiation recall dermatitis, rash (including macular and papular), renal failure, renal parenchymal damage, renal tubular acidosis, respiratory failure, reversible posterior leukoencephalopathy syndrome (RPLS), rhabdomyolysis, rickets, salivation, secondary malignancy, seizure, sepsis, septic shock, SIADH, skin necrosis, spermatogenesis impaired, status epilepticus, sterility, Stevens-Johnson syndrome, stomatitis, ST segment abnormal, supraventricular extrasystoles, tachycardia, tinnitus, toxic epidermal necrolysis, tubulointerstitial nephritis, tumor lysis syndrome, T-wave inversion, uremia, urticaria, vasculitis, ventricular extrasystoles/fibrillation/tachycardia, ventricular failure, vertigo, visual impairment, wound healing impairment

Drug Interactions

Metabolism/Transport Effects Substrate of CYP2B6 (major), CYP2C19 (minor), CYP2C8 (minor), CYP2C9 (minor), CYP3A4 (minor); **Note:** Assignment of Major/Minor substrate status based on clinically relevant drug interaction potential; **Induces** CYP2C9 (weak/moderate)

Avoid Concomitant Use

Avoid concomitant use of Ifosfamide with any of the following: BCG; BCG (Intravesical); CloZAPine; Dipyrone; Natalizumab; Pimecrolimus; Tacrolimus (Topical); Tofacitinib; Vaccines (Live)

Increased Effect/Toxicity

Ifosfamide may increase the levels/effects of: CloZAPine; Leflunomide; Natalizumab; Tofacitinib; Vaccines (Live); Vitamin K Antagonists

The levels/effects of Ifosfamide may be increased by: Aprepitant; Busulfan; CYP2B6 Inhibitors (Moderate); CYP3A4 Inducers (Moderate); CYP3A4 Inducers (Strong); Denosumab; Dipyrone; Fosaprepitant; Pimecrolimus; Quazepam; Roflumilast; Tacrolimus (Topical); Trastuzumab

Decreased Effect

Ifosfamide may decrease the levels/effects of: BCG; BCG (Intravesical); Coccidioides immitis Skin Test; Sipuleucel-T; Vaccines (Inactivated); Vaccines (Live)

The levels/effects of Ifosfamide may be decreased by: CYP2B6 Inducers (Strong); CYP3A4 Inducers (Moderate); CYP3A4 Inducers (Strong); CYP3A4 Inhibitors (Moderate); CYP3A4 Inhibitors (Strong); Dabrafenib; Echinacea

Storage/Stability Store intact vials of powder for injection at room temperature of 20°C to 25°C (68°F to 77°F); avoid temperatures >30°C (86°F). Store intact vials of solution under refrigeration at 2°C to 8°C (36°F to 46°F). Reconstituted solutions and solutions diluted for administration are stable for 24 hours refrigerated.

Mechanism of Action Causes cross-linking of strands of DNA by binding with nucleic acids and other intracellular structures; inhibits protein synthesis and DNA synthesis

Pharmacokinetics (Adult data unless noted) Note: Pharmacokinetics are dose-dependent.

Distribution: Approximates total body water; unchanged ifosfamide penetrates CNS but not in therapeutic concentrations

Protein binding: Neglible

Metabolism: Hepatic to active metabolites isofosforamide mustard, 4-hydroxy-ifosfamide, acrolein, and inactive dichloroethylated and carboxy metabolites; acrolein is the agent implicated in development of hemorrhagic cystitis

Half-life: Terminal:

Low dose (1600 to 2400 mg/m^2): ~7 hours

High dose (3800 to 5000 mg/m^2): ~15 hours

Elimination:

Low dose (1600 to 2400 mg/m^2): Urine (12% to 18% as unchanged drug)

High dose (5000 mg/m^2): Urine (70% to 86%; 61% as unchanged drug)

Dosing: Usual Refer to individual protocols; details concerning dosing in combination regimens should also be consulted. **Note:** To prevent bladder toxicity, combination therapy with mesna (urinary protectant) and hydration, in adults: At least 2 L/day of oral or IV fluid; specific protocols should be consulted for hydration recommendation in pediatric patients; some centers have used 2 times maintenance.

Pediatric:

Ewing sarcoma: Limited data available; dosing regimens and combinations variable: Children and Adolescents:

IE regimen: IE component: IV: 1800 mg/m^2/day for 5 days in combination with mesna and etoposide every 3 weeks for 12 cycles; or may alternate with VAC (vincristine, doxorubicin, and cyclophosphamide) every 3 weeks for a total of 17 courses (Grier, 2003; Miser, 1987)

ICE regimen: IV: 1800 mg/m^2/day for 5 days every 3 to 4 weeks for up to 12 cycles in combination with carboplatin, etoposide, and mesna; or may follow with 2 courses of CAV (cyclophosphamide, doxorubicin, and vincristine) (Milano, 2006; van Winkle, 2005)

VAIA regimen: IV: 3000 mg/m^2/day on days 1, 2, 22, 23, 43, and 44 for 4 courses in combination with vincristine, doxorubicin, dactinomycin, and mesna (Paulussen, 2001) **or** 2000 mg/m^2/day for 3 days every 3 weeks for 14 courses in combination with vincristine, doxorubicin, and dactinomycin (Paulussen, 2008)

VIDE regimen: IV: 3000 mg/m^2/day over 1 to 3 hours for 3 days every 3 weeks for 6 courses in combination with vincristine, doxorubicin, etoposide, and mesna (Juergens, 2006)

Lymphoma, Hodgkin (HL) and Non-Hodgkin (NHL), recurrent/refractory: Limited data available; dosing regimens and combinations variable:

IE regimen: Children and Adolescents: IV: 1800 mg/m^2/day for 5 days alternating in combination with etoposide and mesna; alternate at 3-week intervals with DECAL [dexamethasone, etoposide, cisplatin, cytarabine (high-dose ara-C)], and L-asparaginase for 4 cycles; in the trial, all patients were <21 years of age, the median age for NHL: 11 years; median age for HL: 15 years (Kobrinsky, 2001)

ICE regimen:

Cairo, 2004: Children and Adolescents: IV: 1800 mg/m^2/day for 5 days every 3 weeks for 6 courses in combination with etoposide, carboplatin, and mesna; in the trial, although the minimum age for inclusion was 1 year of age, the reported patient age range was 8 months to 26 years (median: 10.5 years)

Moskowitz, 2001: Children ≥12 years and Adolescents: IV: 5000 mg/m^2 (over 24 hours) beginning on day 2 every 2 weeks for 2 cycles (in combination with mesna, carboplatin, and etoposide)

MIED regimen: Children and Adolescents:

Sandlund, 2011: IV: 2000 mg/m^2/day over 2 hours on days 2 to 4 in combination with high dose methotrexate, etoposide, and dexamethasone (and mesna); patients with NHL also received intrathecal methotrexate, hydrocortisone, and cytarabine

Griffin, 2009: IV: 3000 mg/m^2/day over 2 hours on days 3 to 5 in combination with rituximab and ICE (carboplatin, etoposide, and mensa) every 23 days for up to 3 courses has been used in NHL patients

Osteosarcoma: Limited data available; dosing regimens and combinations variable:

IE regimen: Children and Adolescents: IV: 3000 mg/m^2/day over 3 hours for 4 days every 3 to 4 weeks in combination with etoposide and mesna has been used in children and adolescents 7 to 19 years of age (Gentet, 1997)

ICE regimen: Children and Adolescents: IV: 1800 mg/m^2/day for 5 days every 3 weeks for up to 12 cycles in combination with carboplatin, etoposide, and mesna (van Winkle, 2005)

Ifosfamide/cisplatin/doxorubicin/HDMT: Children and Adolescents: IV: 3000 mg/m^2/day continuous infusion for 5 days (total dose: 15 g/m^2) during weeks 4 and 10 (preop) and during weeks 16, 25, and 34 (postop) in combination with cisplatin, doxorubicin, methotrexate (high-dose), and mesna has been used in patients 6 to 39 years (median: 18.1 years) with newly diagnosed high-grade osteosarcoma of the extremity with metastases (Bacci, 2003)

Ifosfamide/cisplatin/epirubicin regimen: Adolescents: IV: 2000 mg/m^2/day over 4 hours for 3 days (days 2, 3, and 4) every 3 weeks for 3 cycles (preop) and every 4 weeks for 3 cycles (postop) in combination with cisplatin, epirubicin, and mesna has been used in patients 15 to 41 years (median: 22 years) (Basaran, 2007)

Ifosfamide/HDMT/etoposide regimen: Children and Adolescents: IV: 3000 mg/m^2/day over 3 hours for 4 days during weeks 4 and 9 (three additional postop courses were administered in good responders) in combination with methotrexate (high-dose), etoposide, and mesna has been used in patients 5 to 19 years (median: 13.3 years) (Le Deley, 2007)

Adult: **Testicular cancer:** IV: 1200 mg/m^2/day for 5 days in combination with other chemotherapy agents and mesna every 3 weeks or after hematologic recovery

Dosing adjustments in renal impairment:

Infants, Children, and Adolescents: The following adjustments have been recommended (Aronoff, 2007):

GFR ≥10 mL/minute/1.73 m^2: No dosage adjustment necessary

GFR <10 mL/minute/1.73 m^2: Administer 75% of dose

Hemodialysis: 1000 mg/m^2 followed by hemodialysis 6 to 8 hours later

Continuous renal replacement therapy (CRRT): No dosage adjustment necessary

Adults: Manufacturer's labeling: There are no dosage adjustments provided in the manufacturer's labeling (has not been studied); ifosfamide (and metabolites) are excreted renally and may accumulate in patients with renal dysfunction. Dose reductions may be necessary.

The following adjustments have been recommended:

Aronoff, 2007:

CrCl ≥10 mL/minute: No dosage adjustment necessary

CrCl <10 mL/minute: Administer 75% of dose

Hemodialysis: No supplemental dose needed

Kintzel, 1995:

CrCl >60 mL/minute: No dosage adjustment necessary.

CrCl 46 to 60 mL/minute: Administer 80% of dose

CrCl 31 to 45 mL/minute: Administer 75% of dose

CrCl ≤30 mL/minute: Administer 70% of dose

Dosing adjustments in hepatic impairment: Adults: There are no dosage adjustments provided in the manufacturer's labeling; however, ifosfamide is extensively metabolized in the liver to both active and inactive metabolites; use with caution. The following adjustments have been recommended (Floyd, 2006): Bilirubin >3 mg/dL: Administer 25% of dose.

Preparation for Administration Hazardous agent; use appropriate precautions for handling and disposal (NIOSH 2014 [group 1]).

IV: Reconstitute powder with SWFI or bacteriostatic SWFI (1,000 mg in 20 mL or 3,000 mg in 60 mL) to a concentration of 50 mg/mL. Further dilute in D_5W, NS, or LR to a final concentration of 0.6 to 20 mg/mL (per manufacturer). In ambulatory infusion cassettes, higher concentrations have been prepared (20 mg/mL, 40 mg/mL, and 80 mg/mL) (Muñoz 1992).

Administration Hazardous agent; use appropriate precautions for handling and disposal (NIOSH 2014 [group 1]).

IV: Administer as a slow IV intermittent infusion or continuous infusion; infusion times may vary by protocol; usually over at least 30 minutes; in most pediatric trials, usual infusion time was 2 hours or administer as a 24-hour infusion.

Vesicant/Extravasation Risk May be an irritant

Monitoring Parameters CBC with differential (prior to each dose), urine output, urinalysis (prior to each dose), liver and renal function tests, serum electrolytes, CNS changes, signs and symptoms of pulmonary toxicity, signs and symptoms of hemorrhagic cystitis

Dosage Forms Excipient information presented when available (limited, particularly for generics); consult specific product labeling.

Solution, Intravenous:
  Generic: 1 g/20 mL (20 mL); 3 g/60 mL (60 mL)
Solution, Intravenous [preservative free]:
  Generic: 1 g/20 mL (20 mL); 3 g/60 mL (60 mL)
Solution Reconstituted, Intravenous:
  Ifex: 1 g (1 ea); 3 g (1 ea)
  Generic: 1 g (1 ea); 3 g (1 ea)

- ◆ **IG** *see* Immune Globulin *on page 1089*
- ◆ **IGIM** *see* Immune Globulin *on page 1089*
- ◆ **IGIV** *see* Immune Globulin *on page 1089*
- ◆ **IGIVnex (Can)** *see* Immune Globulin *on page 1089*
- ◆ **IGSC** *see* Immune Globulin *on page 1089*
- ◆ **IIV** *see* Influenza Virus Vaccine (Inactivated) *on page 1108*
- ◆ **IIV3** *see* Influenza Virus Vaccine (Inactivated) *on page 1108*
- ◆ **IIV4** *see* Influenza Virus Vaccine (Inactivated) *on page 1108*
- ◆ **IL-1Ra** *see* Anakinra *on page 165*
- ◆ **IL-2** *see* Aldesleukin *on page 89*
- ◆ **IL-11** *see* Oprelvekin *on page 1570*
- ◆ **Ilaris** *see* Canakinumab *on page 356*
- ◆ **Ilotycin** *see* Erythromycin (Ophthalmic) *on page 782*
- ◆ **Iluvien** *see* Fluocinolone (Ophthalmic) *on page 895*

Imatinib (eye MAT eh nib)

Medication Safety Issues

Sound-alike/look-alike issues:

Imatinib may be confused with axitinib, dasatinib, erlotinib, gefitinib, ibrutinib, idelalisib, nilotinib, nintedanib, PONATinib, SORAfenib, SUNItinib, vandetanib

High alert medication:

This medication is in a class the Institute for Safe Medication Practices (ISMP) includes among its list of drug classes which have a heightened risk of causing significant patient harm when used in error.

Related Information

Oral Medications That Should Not Be Crushed or Altered *on page 2476*

Prevention of Chemotherapy-Induced Nausea and Vomiting in Children *on page 2368*

Safe Handling of Hazardous Drugs *on page 2455*

Brand Names: US Gleevec

Brand Names: Canada ACT-Imatinib; Apo-Imatinib; Gleevec; Teva-Imatinib

Therapeutic Category Antineoplastic Agent, BCR-ABL Tyrosine Kinase Inhibitor; Antineoplastic Agent, Tyrosine Kinase Inhibitor

Generic Availability (US) No

Use

Treatment of newly diagnosed Philadelphia chromosome-positive (Ph+) acute lymphoblastic leukemia (ALL) in combination with chemotherapy (FDA approved in ages ≥1 year); treatment of newly diagnosed Ph+ chronic myeloid leukemia (CML) in chronic phase (FDA approved in ages ≥1 year and adults)

Treatment of (the following indications: FDA approved in adults): Ph+ acute lymphoblastic leukemia (ALL) (relapsed or refractory), gastrointestinal stromal tumors (GIST) kit-positive (CD117), including unresectable and/or metastatic malignant and adjuvant treatment following complete resection, aggressive systemic mastocytosis (ASM) without D816V c-Kit mutation (or c-Kit mutation status unknown), dermatofibrosarcoma protuberans (DFSP) (unresectable, recurrent, and/or metastatic), hypereosinophilic syndrome (HES) and/or chronic eosinophilic leukemia (CEL), myelodysplastic/myeloproliferative disease (MDS/MPD) associated with platelet-derived growth factor receptor (PDGFR) gene rearrangements

Has also been used in the treatment of desmoid tumors (soft tissue sarcoma); poststem cell transplant (allogeneic) follow-up treatment in CML

Pregnancy Risk Factor D

Pregnancy Considerations Adverse events have been observed in animal reproduction studies. Women of childbearing potential are advised not to become pregnant (female patients and female partners of male patients); highly effective contraception is recommended. The Canadian labeling recommends women of childbearing potential have a negative pregnancy test (urine or serum) with a sensitivity of at least 25 mIU/mL within 1 week prior to therapy initiation. Case reports of pregnancies while on therapy (both males and females) include reports of spontaneous abortion, minor abnormalities (hypospadias, pyloric stenosis, and small intestine rotation) at or shortly after birth, and other congenital abnormalities including skeletal malformations, hypoplastic lungs, exomphalos, kidney abnormalities, hydrocephalus, cerebellar hypoplasia, and cardiac defects.

Retrospective case reports of women with CML in complete hematologic response (CHR) with cytogenic response (partial or complete) who interrupted imatinib therapy due to pregnancy, demonstrated a loss of response in some patients while off treatment. At 18 months after treatment reinitiation following delivery, CHR was again achieved in all patients and cytogenic response was achieved in some patients. Cytogenetic response rates may not be at as high as compared to patients with 18 months of uninterrupted therapy (Ault, 2006; Pye, 2008).

Breast-Feeding Considerations Imatinib and its active metabolite are found in human breast milk; the milk/plasma ratio is 0.5 for imatinib and 0.9 for the active metabolite. Based on body weight, up to 10% of a therapeutic maternal dose could potentially be received by a breast-fed infant. Due to the potential for serious adverse reactions in the breast-feeding infant, the manufacturer recommends a decision be made to discontinue breast-feeding or to discontinue the drug, taking into account the importance of treatment to the mother.

Contraindications

There are no contraindications listed in the manufacturer's US labeling.

Canadian labeling: Hypersensitivity to imatinib or any component of the formulation

Warnings/Precautions Hazardous agent - use appropriate precautions for handling and disposal (NIOSH 2014 [group 1]). Often associated with fluid retention, weight gain, and edema (risk increases with higher doses and age >65 years); occasionally serious and may lead to significant complications, including pleural effusion, pericardial effusion, pulmonary edema, and ascites. Monitor regularly for rapid weight gain or other signs/symptoms of fluid retention. Use with caution in patients where fluid accumulation may be poorly tolerated, such as in cardiovascular disease (heart failure [HF] or hypertension) and pulmonary disease. Severe HF and left ventricular dysfunction (LVD) have been reported occasionally, usually in patients with comorbidities and/or risk factors; carefully monitor patients with preexisting cardiac disease or risk factors for HF or history of renal failure. With initiation of imatinib treatment, cardiogenic shock and/or LVD have been reported in patients with hypereosinophilic syndrome and cardiac involvement (reversible with systemic steroids, circulatory support and temporary cessation of imatinib). Patients with high eosinophil levels and an abnormal echocardiogram or abnormal serum troponin level may benefit from prophylactic systemic steroids (for 1 to 2 weeks) with the initiation of imatinib.

Severe bullous dermatologic reactions (including erythema multiforme and Stevens-Johnson syndrome) have been reported; recurrence has been described with rechallenge. Case reports of successful resumption at a lower dose (with corticosteroids and/or antihistamine) have been described; however, some patients may experience recurrent reactions. Drug reaction with eosinophilia and systemic symptoms (DRESS) has been reported; if DRESS occurs, interrupt therapy and consider permanent discontinuation.

Hepatotoxicity may occur (may be severe); fatal hepatic failure and severe hepatic injury requiring liver transplantation have been reported with both short- and long-term use; monitor liver function prior to initiation and monthly or as needed thereafter; therapy interruption or dose reduction may be necessary. Transaminase and bilirubin elevations, and acute liver failure have been observed with imatinib in combination with chemotherapy. Use with caution in patients with preexisting hepatic impairment; dosage adjustment recommended in patients with severe impairment. Use with caution in renal impairment; dosage adjustment recommended for moderate and severe impairment. Tumor lysis syndrome (TLS), including fatalities, has been reported in patients with acute lymphoblastic leukemia (ALL), chronic myeloid leukemia (CML) eosinophilic leukemias, and gastrointestinal stromal tumors (GIST); risk for TLS is higher in patients with a high tumor burden or high proliferation rate; monitor closely; correct clinically significant dehydration and treat high uric acid levels prior to initiation of imatinib.

Imatinib is associated with a moderate emetic potential; antiemetics may be recommended to prevent nausea and vomiting (Dupuis, 2011; Roila, 2010). May cause GI irritation, severe hemorrhage (grades 3 and 4; including GI hemorrhage and/or tumor hemorrhage; hemorrhage incidence is higher in patients with GIST [GI tumors may have been hemorrhage source; gastric antral vascular ectasia has also been reported]), or hematologic toxicity (anemia, neutropenia, and thrombocytopenia; usually occurring within the first several months of treatment). Monitor blood counts weekly for the first month, biweekly for the second month, and as clinically necessary thereafter; median duration of neutropenia is 2 to 3 weeks; median duration of thrombocytopenia is 3 to 4 weeks. In CML, cytopenias are more common in accelerated or blast phase than in chronic phase. Hypothyroidism has been reported in patients who were receiving thyroid hormone replacement therapy prior to the initiation of imatinib; monitor thyroid function; the average onset for imatinib-induced hypothyroidism is 2 weeks; consider doubling levothyroxine doses upon initiation of imatinib (Hamnvik, 2011). Potentially significant drug-drug interactions may exist, requiring dose or frequency adjustment, additional monitoring, and/or selection of alternative therapy. Imatinib exposure may be reduced in patients who have had gastric surgery (eg, bypass, major gastrectomy, or resection); monitor imatinib trough concentrations (Liu, 2011; Pavlovsky, 2009; Yoo, 2010). Growth retardation has been reported in children receiving imatinib for the treatment of CML; generally where treatment was initiated in prepubertal children; growth velocity was usually restored as pubertal age was reached (Shima, 2011); monitor growth closely. The incidence of edema was increased with age older than 65 years in CML and GIST studies. Reports of accidents have been received but it is unclear if imatinib has been the direct cause in any case; advise patients regarding side effects such as dizziness, blurred vision, or somnolence; use caution when driving/operating motor vehicles and heavy machinery.

Warnings: Additional Pediatric Considerations Growth retardation has been reported in prepubescent children receiving imatinib for the treatment of CML (Bansal, 2012; Rastogi, 2012; Shima, 2011); the majority of the preliminary data reported statistically significant decreases in height-SD (standard deviation) scores; less commonly reported are decreases in weight-SD scores or decreased BMI; incidence and extent of growth retardation as well as other related risk factors have not been fully characterized; reported incidence from reports is highly variable (48% to 71%), with onset during the first year of therapy and persisting with treatment. One report suggests that growth velocity was restored as pubertal age was reached; however, in other reports, patients did not have improvement in height velocity and genetically predicted adult heights were not achieved. Monitor growth closely.

Adverse Reactions Adverse reactions listed as a composite of data across many trials, except where noted for a specific indication.

Cardiovascular: Cardiac failure, chest pain, edema (includes aggravated edema, anasarca, ascites, pericardial effusion, peripheral edema, pulmonary edema, and superficial edema), facial edema, flushing, hypertension, hypotension, palpitations, pleural effusion

Central nervous system: Anxiety, cerebral hemorrhage, chills, depression, dizziness, fatigue, headache, hypoesthesia, insomnia, pain, paresthesia, peripheral neuropathy, rigors, taste disorder

Dermatologic: Alopecia, dermatitis (GIST), diaphoresis (GIST), erythema, nail disease, night sweats (CML), pruritus, skin photosensitivity, skin rash, xeroderma

Endocrine & metabolic: decreased serum albumin, fluid retention (Ph+ CML, pleural effusion, pericardial effusion, ascites, or pulmonary edema), hyperkalemia, hyperglycemia, hypocalcemia, hypokalemia (more common in Ph+ ALL [pediatric] grades 3/4), hypophosphatemia, increased lactate dehydrogenase, weight gain, weight loss

Gastrointestinal: abdominal distension, abdominal pain, anorexia, constipation, decreased appetite, diarrhea, dyspepsia, flatulence, gastritis, gastroenteritis, gastroesophageal reflux, gastrointestinal hemorrhage, increased serum lipase (CML grades 3/4), nausea, stomatitis, vomiting, xerostomia

Hematologic & oncologic: Anemia, eosinophilia, febrile neutropenia, hemorrhage, hypoproteinemia, leukopenia (GIST), lymphocytopenia, neutropenia, pancytopenia, purpura, thrombocytopenia

Hepatic: Increased alkaline phosphatase, increased serum ALT, increased serum AST, increased serum bilirubin, increased serum transaminases

Infection: Infection (more common in Ph+ ALL [pediatric] grades 3/4), influenza (Ph+ CML)

Neuromuscular & skeletal: arthralgia, back pain, joint swelling, limb pain, muscle cramps, musculoskeletal pain (more common in adults), myalgia, ostealgia, weakness

Ophthalmic: Blurred vision, conjunctival hemorrhage, conjunctivitis, dry eyeseyelid edema (Ph+ CML), increased lacrimation (DFSP, GIST), periorbital edema

Renal: Increased serum creatinine

Respiratory: cough, dyspnea, epistaxis, flu-like symptoms, hypoxia, nasopharyngitis, oropharyngeal pain (Ph+ CML), pharyngitis (CML), pharyngolaryngeal pain, pneumonia (CML), pneumonitis (Ph+ ALL [pediatric] grades 3/4), rhinitis (DFSP), sinusitis, upper respiratory tract infection,

Miscellaneous: Fever

Rare but important or life-threatening: Actinic keratosis, acute generalized exanthematous pustulosis, anaphylactic shock, angina pectoris, angioedema, aplastic anemia, arthritis, ascites, atrial fibrillation, avascular necrosis of bones, bullous rash, cardiac arrest, cardiac arrhythmia, cardiac tamponade, cardiogenic shock, cataract, cellulitis, cerebral edema, decreased linear skeletal growth rate (children), diverticulitis, DRESS syndrome, dyschromia, embolism, erythema multiforme, exfoliative dermatitis, fungal infection, gastric ulcer, gastrointestinal obstruction, gastrointestinal perforation, glaucoma, gout, hearing loss, hematemesis, hematoma, hematuria, hemolytic anemia, hepatic failure, hepatic necrosis, hepatitis, hepatotoxicity, herpes simplex infection, herpes zoster, hypercalcemia, hyperkalemia, hypersensitivity angiitis, hyperuricemia, hypomagnesemia, hyponatremia, hypophosphatemia, hypothyroidism, IgA vasculitis, increased intracranial pressure, inflammatory bowel disease, interstitial pneumonitis, interstitial pulmonary disease, intestinal obstruction, left ventricular dysfunction, lichen planus, lower respiratory tract infection, lymphadenopathy, macular edema, melena, memory impairment, migraine, myocardial infarction, myopathy, optic neuritis, osteonecrosis (hip), ovarian cyst (hemorrhagic), palmar-plantar erythrodysesthesia, pancreatitis, papilledema, pericarditis, psoriasis, pulmonary fibrosis, pulmonary hemorrhage, pulmonary hypertension, Raynauds phenomenon, renal failure, respiratory failure, restless leg syndrome, retinal hemorrhage, rhabdomyolysis, ruptured corpus luteal cyst, sciatica, seizure, sepsis, Stevens-Johnson syndrome, subconjunctival hemorrhage, subdural hematoma, Sweet syndrome, syncope, tachycardia, telangiectasia (gastric antral), thrombocythemia, thrombosis, toxic epidermal necrolysis, tumor hemorrhage (GIST), tumor lysis syndrome, urinary tract infection, vitreous hemorrhage

Drug Interactions

Metabolism/Transport Effects Substrate of CYP1A2 (minor), CYP2C19 (minor), CYP2C8 (minor), CYP2C9 (minor), CYP2D6 (minor), CYP3A4 (major), P-glycoprotein; **Note:** Assignment of Major/Minor substrate status based on clinically relevant drug interaction potential; **Inhibits** BCRP, CYP2C9 (weak), CYP2D6 (weak), CYP3A4 (moderate), P-glycoprotein

Avoid Concomitant Use

Avoid concomitant use of Imatinib with any of the following: BCG; BCG (Intravesical); Bosutinib; CloZAPine; Dipyrone; Domperidone; Ibrutinib; Ivabradine; Lomitapide; Naloxegol; Natalizumab; Olaparib; PAZOPanib; Pimecrolimus; Pimozide; Simeprevir; Tacrolimus (Topical); Tofacitinib; Tolvaptan; Trabectedin; Ulipristal; Vaccines (Live)

Increased Effect/Toxicity

Imatinib may increase the levels/effects of: ARIPiprazole; Avanafil; Bosentan; Bosutinib; Budesonide (Systemic, Oral Inhalation); Budesonide (Topical); Cannabis; Cilostazol; CloZAPine; Colchicine; CycloSPORINE (Systemic); CYP3A4 Substrates; Dapoxetine; Dofetilide; Domperidone; DOXOrubicin (Conventional); Dronabinol; Eliglustat; Eplerenone; Everolimus; FentaNYL; Halofantrine; Hydrocodone; Ibrutinib; Ivabradine; Ivacaftor; Leflunomide; Lomitapide; Lurasidone; Naloxegol; Natalizumab; NiMODipine; Olaparib; OxyCODONE; PAZOPanib; Pimozide; Propafenone; Ranolazine; Rivaroxaban; Salmeterol; Saxagliptin; Simeprevir; Simvastatin; Suvorexant; Tetrahydrocannabinol; Tofacitinib; Tolvaptan; Topotecan; Trabectedin; Ulipristal; Vaccines (Live); Vilazodone; Warfarin; Zopiclone; Zuclopenthixol

The levels/effects of Imatinib may be increased by: Acetaminophen; CYP3A4 Inhibitors (Moderate); CYP3A4 Inhibitors (Strong); Denosumab; Dipyrone; Lansoprazole; P-glycoprotein/ABCB1 Inhibitors; Pimecrolimus; Roflumilast; Tacrolimus (Topical); Trastuzumab

Decreased Effect

Imatinib may decrease the levels/effects of: BCG; BCG (Intravesical); Coccidioides immitis Skin Test; Fludarabine; Ifosfamide; Sipuleucel-T; Vaccines (Inactivated); Vaccines (Live)

The levels/effects of Imatinib may be decreased by: Bosentan; CYP3A4 Inducers (Moderate); CYP3A4 Inducers (Strong); Dabrafenib; Deferasirox; Dexamethasone (Systemic); Echinacea; Gemfibrozil; Ibuprofen; Mitotane; P-glycoprotein/ABCB1 Inducers; Rifamycin Derivatives; Siltuximab; St Johns Wort; Tocilizumab

Food Interactions Food may reduce GI irritation. Grapefruit juice may increase imatinib plasma concentration. Management: Take with a meal and a large glass of water. Avoid grapefruit juice. Maintain adequate hydration, unless instructed to restrict fluid intake.

Storage/Stability Store at 25°C (77°F); excursions permitted between 15°C to 30°C (59°F to 86°F). Protect from moisture.

Mechanism of Action Inhibits Bcr-Abl tyrosine kinase, the constitutive abnormal gene product of the Philadelphia chromosome in chronic myeloid leukemia (CML). Inhibition of this enzyme blocks proliferation and induces apoptosis in Bcr-Abl positive cell lines as well as in fresh leukemic cells in Philadelphia chromosome positive CML. Also inhibits tyrosine kinase for platelet-derived growth factor (PDGF), stem cell factor (SCF), c-Kit, and cellular events mediated by PDGF and SCF.

Pharmacokinetics (Adult data unless noted)

Absorption: Rapid

Protein binding: ~95% to albumin and alpha$_1$-acid glycoprotein (parent drug and metabolite)

Metabolism: Hepatic via CYP3A4 (minor metabolism via CYP1A2, CYP2D6, CYP2C9, CYP2C19); primary metabolite (active): N-demethylated piperazine derivative (CGP74588); severe hepatic impairment (bilirubin >3-10 times ULN) increases AUC by 45% to 55% for imatinib and its active metabolite, respectively

Bioavailability: 98%; may be decreased in patients who have had gastric surgery (eg, bypass, total or partial resection)

Half-life elimination:

Children: Parent drug: ~15 hours

Adults: Parent drug: ~18 hours; N-desmethyl metabolite: ~40 hours

Time to peak serum concentration: 2-4 hours (adults and children)

Elimination: Feces (68% primarily as metabolites, 20% as unchanged drug); urine (≤13% primarily as metabolites, 5% as unchanged drug)

Dosing: Usual Note: Treatment may be continued until disease progression or unacceptable toxicity. The optimal duration of therapy for CML in complete remission is not yet determined. Discontinuing CML treatment is not recommended unless part of a clinical trial (Baccarani, 2009; NCCN CML guidelines v.3.2013).

Children and Adolescents:

Ph+ ALL (newly diagnosed): Oral: 340 mg/m^2/day administered once daily; in combination with chemotherapy; maximum daily dose: 600 mg/**day**

Ph+ CML (chronic phase, newly diagnosed): Oral: 340 mg/m^2/day; may administer once daily or in 2 divided doses; maximum daily dose: 600 mg/**day**

Adults: **Note:** Doses ≤600 mg should be administered once daily; 800 mg doses should be administered as 400 mg/dose twice a day

ASM with eosinophilia: Oral: Initiate at 100 mg once daily; titrate up to a maximum of 400 mg once daily (if tolerated) for insufficient response to lower dose

ASM without D816V c-Kit mutation or c-Kit mutation status unknown: Oral: 400 mg once daily

GIST (adjuvant treatment following complete resection): Oral: 400 mg once daily; recommended treatment duration: 3 years

GIST (unresectable and/or metastatic malignant): Oral: 400 mg/day; may be increased up to 800 mg/day (400 mg/dose twice daily), if tolerated, for disease progression; **Note:** Significant improvement (progression-free survival, objective response rate) was demonstrated in patients with KIT exon 9 mutation with 800 mg (versus 400 mg), although overall survival (OS) was not impacted. The higher dose did not demonstrate a difference in time to progression or OS patients with Kit exon 11 mutation or wild-type status (Debiec-Rychter, 2006; Heinrich, 2008).

DFSP: Oral: 400 mg twice daily

HES/CEL: Oral: 400 mg once daily

HES/CEL with FIP1L1-PDGFRα fusion kinase: Oral: Initiate at 100 mg once daily; titrate up to a maximum of 400 mg once daily (if tolerated) if insufficient response to lower dose

MDS/MPD: Oral: 400 mg once daily

Ph+ ALL (relapsed or refractory): Oral: 600 mg once daily

Ph+ CML: Oral

Chronic phase: 400 mg once daily; may be increased to 600 mg daily, if tolerated, for disease progression, lack of hematologic response after 3 months, lack of cytogenetic response after 6-12 months, or loss of previous hematologic or cytogenetic response; ranges up to 800 mg/day (400 mg twice daily) are included in the NCCN CML guidelines (v.3.2013)

Accelerated phase or blast crisis: 600 mg once daily; may be increased to 800 mg daily (400 mg/dose twice daily), if tolerated, for disease progression, lack of hematologic response after 3 months, lack of cytogenetic response after 6-12 months, or loss of previous hematologic or cytogenetic response

Dosing adjustment with concomitant strong CYP3A4 inducers: Children, Adolescents, and Adults: Avoid concomitant use of strong CYP3A4 inducers (eg, dexamethasone, carbamazepine, phenobarbital, phenytoin, rifabutin, rifampin); if concomitant use cannot be avoided, increase imatinib dose by at least 50% with careful monitoring.

Dosing adjustment for renal impairment:

Mild impairment (CrCl 40-59 mL/minute): Adults: Maximum recommended dose: 600 mg/day

Moderate impairment (CrCl 20-39 mL/minute): Children, Adolescents, and Adults: Decrease recommended starting dose by 50%; dose may be increased as tolerated; maximum recommended dose: 400 mg/day

Severe impairment (CrCl <20 mL/minute): Use caution; in adults with severe impairment, a dose of 100 mg/day has been tolerated (Gibbons, 2008)

Dosing adjustment for hepatic impairment: Children, Adolescents, and Adults:

Baseline:

Mild to moderate impairment: No adjustment necessary

Severe impairment: Reduce dose by 25%

During therapy (hepatotoxicity): Withhold treatment until toxicity resolves; may resume if appropriate (depending on initial severity of adverse event)

If elevations of bilirubin >3 times ULN or liver transaminases >5 times ULN occur, withhold treatment until bilirubin <1.5 times ULN and transaminases <2.5 times ULN. Resume treatment at a reduced dose as follows:

Children, Adolescents, and Adults: If current dose 340 mg/m^2/day, reduce dose to 260 mg/m^2/day; maximum dose range: 300-400 mg

Adults:

If initial dose 400 mg, reduce dose to 300 mg

If initial dose 600 mg, reduce dose to 400 mg

If initial dose 800 mg, reduce dose to 600 mg

Dosing adjustment for other nonhematologic adverse reactions: Withhold treatment until toxicity resolves; may resume if appropriate (depending on initial severity of adverse event)

Dosing adjustment for hematologic adverse reactions:

Chronic phase CML (Initial dose: Children: 340 mg/m^2/day ***or*** *Adults: 400 mg/day), ASM, MDS/MPD, and HES/CEL (initial dose: 400 mg/day), or GIST (initial dose: 400 mg):* If ANC <1 x 10^9/L and/or platelets <50 x 10^9/L: Withhold until ANC ≥1.5 x 10^9/L and platelets ≥75 x 10^9/L; resume treatment at previous dose. For recurrent neutropenia and/or thrombocytopenia, withhold until recovery and reinstitute treatment at a reduced dose as follows:

Children and Adolescents: If initial dose 340 mg/m^2/day, reduce dose to 260 mg/m^2/day

Adults: If initial dose 400 mg/day, reduce dose to 300 mg/day

CML (accelerated phase or blast crisis) and PH+ ALL: Adults (initial dose: 600 mg): If ANC <0.5 x 10^9/L and/or platelets <10 x 10^9/L, establish whether cytopenia is related to leukemia (bone marrow aspirate or biopsy). If unrelated to leukemia, reduce dose to 400 mg/day. If cytopenia persists for an additional 2 weeks, further reduce dose to 300 mg/day. If cytopenia persists for 4 weeks and is still unrelated to leukemia, withhold treatment until ANC ≥1 x 10^9/L and platelets ≥20 x 10^9/L, then resume treatment at 300 mg/day.

ASM-associated with eosinophilia and HES/CEL with FIP1L1-PDGFRα fusion kinase (starting dose: 100 mg/day): Adults: If ANC <1 x 10^9/L and/or platelets <50 x 10^9/L: Withhold until ANC ≥1.5 x 10^9/L and platelets ≥75 x 10^9/L; resume treatment at previous dose.

DFSP (initial dose: 800 mg/day): Adults: If ANC <1 x 10^9/L and/or platelets <50 x 10^9/L, withhold until ANC ≥1.5 x 10^9/L and platelets ≥75 x 10^9/L; resume treatment at reduced dose of 600 mg/day. For recurrent neutropenia and/or thrombocytopenia, withhold until recovery and reinstitute treatment with a further dose reduction to 400 mg/day.

Administration Hazardous agent; use appropriate precautions for handling and disposal (NIOSH 2014 [group 1]). Should be administered orally with a meal and a large glass of water. Do not crush tablets; tablets may be dispersed in water or apple juice (using ~50 mL for 100 mg tablet, ~200 mL for 400 mg tablet); stir until tablet dissolves and administer immediately. Dosing in children may be once or twice daily when treating CML and once daily for Ph+ ALL. In adults, doses ≤600 mg may be given once daily; 800 mg dose should be administered as 400 mg twice daily. For daily dosing ≥800 mg, the 400 mg tablets should be used to reduce iron exposure (tablets are coated with ferric oxide).

Monitoring Parameters CBC (weekly for first month, biweekly for second month, then periodically thereafter), liver function tests [at baseline and monthly or as clinically indicated; more frequently (at least weekly) in patients with moderate to severe hepatic impairment (Ramanathan, 2008)], renal function, serum electrolytes (including calcium, phosphorus, potassium, and sodium levels); bone marrow cytogenetics (in CML; at 6, 12, and 18 months); fatigue, weight, and edema/fluid status; consider echocardiogram and serum troponin levels in patients with HES/CEL, and in patients with MDS/MPD or ASM with high eosinophil levels; in pediatric patients, also monitor serum glucose, albumin, and growth parameters (height, weight, BMI)

Gastric surgery (eg, bypass, major gastrectomy, or resection) patients: Monitor imatinib trough concentrations (Liu, 2011; Pavlovsky, 2009, Yoo, 2010)

Thyroid function testing (Hamnvik, 2011):

Preexisting levothyroxine therapy: Obtain baseline TSH levels, then monitor every 4 weeks until levels and levothyroxine dose are stable, then monitor every 2 months

Without preexisting thyroid hormone replacement: TSH at baseline, then every 4 weeks for 4 months, then every 2-3 months

Monitor for signs/symptoms of CHF in patients at risk for cardiac failure or patients with preexisting cardiac disease; some suggest a baseline evaluation of left ventricular ejection fraction prior to initiation of imatinib therapy in all patients with known underlying heart disease or in elderly patients. Monitor for signs/symptoms of gastrointestinal irritation or perforation and dermatologic toxicities.

Dosage Forms Excipient information presented when available (limited, particularly for generics); consult specific product labeling.

Tablet, Oral:

Gleevec: 100 mg, 400 mg [scored]

Extemporaneous Preparations Hazardous agent: Use appropriate precautions for handling and disposal (NIOSH 2014 [group 1]). When manipulating tablets, NIOSH recommends double gloving, a protective gown, and preparation in a controlled device; if not prepared in a controlled device, respiratory and eye protection as well as ventilated engineering controls are recommended (NIOSH, 2014).

An oral suspension may be prepared by placing tablets (whole, do not crush) in a glass of water or apple juice. Use ~50 mL for 100 mg tablet, or ~200 mL for 400 mg tablet. Stir until tablets are disintegrated, then administer immediately. To ensure the full dose is administered, rinse the glass and administer residue.

Gleevec (imatinib) [prescribing information]. East Hanover, NJ: Novartis Pharmaceuticals; January 2015.

◆ **Imatinib Mesylate** *see* Imatinib *on page* 1078
◆ **Imferon** *see* Iron Dextran Complex *on page* 1164
◆ **IMI 30** *see* IDArubicin *on page* 1071
◆ **Imidazole Carboxamide** *see* Dacarbazine *on page* 572
◆ **Imidazole Carboxamide Dimethyltriazene** *see* Dacarbazine *on page* 572
◆ **IMIG** *see* Immune Globulin *on page* 1089

Imiglucerase (i mi GLOO ser ace)

Medication Safety Issues

Sound-alike/look-alike issues:

Cerezyme may be confused with Cerebyx, Ceredase

Brand Names: US Cerezyme

Brand Names: Canada Cerezyme

Therapeutic Category Enzyme, Glucocerebrosidase; Gaucher's Disease, Treatment Agent

Generic Availability (US) No

Use Long-term enzyme replacement therapy for patients with Type 1 Gaucher's disease

Pregnancy Risk Factor C

Pregnancy Considerations Animal reproduction studies have not been conducted; however, imiglucerase has been used safely during pregnancy based on available data (Sherer, 2003; Zimran, 2009). Doses of imiglucerase should be based on prepregnancy weight and adjusted as clinically indicated (Granovsky-Grisaru, 2011).

Breast-Feeding Considerations It is not known if imiglucerase is excreted in breast milk. The manufacturer recommends that caution be exercised when administering imiglucerase to nursing women. A case report described a small amount of imiglucerase excreted into breast milk. The maximum amount of enzyme activity was obtained in the first milk at the end of the imiglucerase infusion; enzyme activity rapidly declined to preinfusion levels (Sekijima, 2010). Enzyme ingested by a nursing infant would likely degrade in their digestive system (Zimran, 2009). The benefits of nursing to the infant should be weighed against the potential for additional bone loss in the mother (Granovsky-Grisaru, 2011; Zimran, 2009).

Contraindications

U.S. labeling: There are no known contraindications in the manufacturer's labeling.

Canadian labeling: Severe hypersensitivity to imiglucerase or any component of the formulation

Warnings/Precautions Anaphylactoid reactions have been reported (<1%). Most patients have continued treatment with pretreatment (antihistamines and/or corticosteroids) and a slower rate of infusion. Discontinue immediately for severe reactions and initiate appropriate medical treatment. Development of IgG antibodies has been reported in ~15% of patients and has been observed within 6 months from the onset of therapy; antibody formation is rare after 12 months of therapy; may increase risk of hypersensitivity reactions. Use caution in patients with previous hypersensitivity to, previously treated with, or who have developed antibodies to alglucerase. Canadian labeling contraindicates use in patients with severe hypersensitivity to imiglucerase. Pulmonary hypertension and pneumonia have been observed during treatment; causal relationship has not been established as this is a complication of Gaucher disease. Afebrile patients with respiratory symptoms should be assessed for pulmonary hypertension. Some dosage forms may contain polysorbate 80 (also known as Tweens). Hypersensitivity reactions, usually a delayed reaction, have been reported following exposure to pharmaceutical products containing polysorbate 80 in certain individuals (Isaksson, 2002; Lucente 2000; Shelley, 1995). Thrombocytopenia, ascites, pulmonary deterioration, and renal and hepatic failure have been reported in premature neonates after receiving parenteral products containing polysorbate 80 (Alade, 1986; CDC, 1984). See manufacturer's labeling.

Should be administered under the supervision of a physician experienced in treatment of Gaucher disease. A registry has been established and all patients with Gaucher disease, and physicians who treat Gaucher disease are encouraged to participate. Information on the International Collaborative Gaucher Group (ICGG) Gaucher Registry may be obtained at https://www.registrynxt.com, or by calling 1-800-745-4447 (ext.15500).

Adverse Reactions

Cardiovascular: Tachycardia

Central nervous system: Chills, dizziness, fatigue, fever, headache

Dermatologic: Pruritus, rash

Gastrointestinal: Abdominal discomfort, diarrhea, nausea, vomiting

Neuromuscular & skeletal: Backache

Miscellaneous: Hypersensitivity reaction (symptoms may include pruritus, flushing, urticaria, angioedema, chest discomfort, dyspnea, coughing, cyanosis, hypotension, paresthesia)

Rare but important or life-threatening: Anaphylactoid reactions; cyanosis, injection site burning, swelling, or sterile abscess; peripheral edema, pneumonia, pulmonary hypertension, rigors

Drug Interactions

Metabolism/Transport Effects None known.

Avoid Concomitant Use There are no known interactions where it is recommended to avoid concomitant use.

Increased Effect/Toxicity There are no known significant interactions involving an increase in effect.

Decreased Effect There are no known significant interactions involving a decrease in effect.

Storage/Stability Prior to reconstitution, store at 2°C to 8°C (36°F to 46°F). Reconstituted solution is stable for 12 hours at 25°C (77°F) and at 2°C to 8°C (36°F to 46°F) resulting in a concentration of 40 units/mL. Slight flocculation (thin translucent fibers) may appear; however, do not use if discolored or contains opaque particles. Solution diluted for infusion further diluted in NS is stable for up to 24 hours when stored at 2°C to 8°C (36°F to 46°F). Contains no preservatives; reconstituted vials should not be stored for future use.

Mechanism of Action Imiglucerase is an analogue of glucocerebrosidase; it is produced by recombinant DNA technology using mammalian cell culture. Glucocerebrosidase is an enzyme deficient in Gaucher's disease. It is needed to catalyze the hydrolysis of glucocerebroside to glucose and ceramide.

Pharmacodynamics

Onset of significant improvement in symptoms:

Hepatosplenomegaly and hematologic abnormalities: Within 6 months

Improvement in bone mineralization: Noted at 80-104 weeks of therapy

Pharmacokinetics (Adult data unless noted)

Distribution: V_d: 0.09-0.15 L/kg

Half-life, elimination: 3.6-10.4 minutes

Clearance: 9.8-20.3 mL/minute/kg

Dosing: Usual IV: Children and Adults: 30-60 units/kg every 2 weeks; range in dosage: 2.5 units/kg 3 times/week to 60 units/kg once weekly to every 4 weeks. Initial dose should be based on disease severity and rate of progression. Children at high risk for complications from Gaucher's disease (one or more of the following: symptomatic disease including manifestations of abdominal or bone pain, fatigue, exertional limitations, weakness, and cachexia; growth failure; evidence of skeletal involvement; platelet count ≤60,000 mm^3 and/or documented abnormal bleeding episode(s); Hgb ≥2.0 g/dL below lower limit for age and sex; impaired quality of life) should receive an initial dose of 60 units/kg; failure to respond to treatment within 6 months indicates the need for a higher dosage.

Maintenance: After patient response is well established a reduction in dosage may be attempted; progressive reductions may be made at intervals of 3-6 months; assess dosage frequently to maintain consistent dosage per kg body weight

Preparation for Administration Parenteral: Reconstitute 200 unit vial with 5.1 mL SWFI or 400 unit vial with 10.2 mL SWFI resulting in a 40 units/mL concentration; visually inspect the solution following reconstitution for particulate matter. Withdraw appropriate volume of reconstituted solution and further dilute in NS to a final volume of 100 to 200 mL.

Administration Parenteral: Infuse over 1 to 2 hours; may filter diluted solution through an in-line low protein-binding 0.2 micron filter during administration; do not administer products with visualized particulate matter.

Monitoring Parameters CBC, platelets, liver function tests, MRI or CT scan (spleen and liver volume), skeletal x-rays

Dosage Forms Excipient information presented when available (limited, particularly for generics); consult specific product labeling.

Solution Reconstituted, Intravenous:

Cerezyme: 200 units (1 ea); 400 units (1 ea)

◆ **Imipemide** *see* Imipenem and Cilastatin *on page* 1083

Imipenem and Cilastatin

(i mi PEN em & sye la STAT in)

Medication Safety Issues

Sound-alike/look-alike issues:

Imipenem may be confused with ertapenem, meropenem

Primaxin may be confused with Premarin, Primacor

Brand Names: US Primaxin® I.V.

Brand Names: Canada Imipenem and Cilastatin for Injection; Imipenem and Cilastatin for Injection, USP; Primaxin; RAN-Imipenem-Cilastatin

Therapeutic Category Antibiotic, Carbapenem

Generic Availability (US) Yes

Use Treatment of documented multidrug-resistant gram-negative infection of the lower respiratory tract, urinary tract, intra-abdominal, gynecologic, bone and joint, septicemias, endocarditis, and skin and skin structure due to organisms proven or suspected to be susceptible to imipenem/cilastatin (FDA approved in all ages); treatment of multiple organism infection in which other agents have an insufficient spectrum of activity or are contraindicated due to toxic potential; therapeutic alternative for treatment of gram-negative sepsis in immunocompromised patients

Pregnancy Risk Factor C

Pregnancy Considerations Teratogenic events have not been observed in animal reproduction studies. Due to pregnancy induced physiologic changes, some pharmacokinetic parameters of imipenem/cilastatin may be altered. Pregnant women have a larger volume of distribution resulting in lower serum peak levels than for the same dose in nonpregnant women. Clearance is also increased.

Breast-Feeding Considerations Imipenem is excreted in human milk. The low concentrations and low oral bioavailability suggest minimal exposure risk to the infant. The manufacturer recommends that caution be exercised when administering imipenem/cilastatin to nursing women. Nondose-related effects could include modification of bowel flora.

Contraindications Hypersensitivity to imipenem/cilastatin or any component of the formulation

Warnings/Precautions Dosage adjustment required in patients with impaired renal function; elderly patients often require lower doses (adjust to renal function). Prolonged use may result in fungal or bacterial superinfection, including *C. difficile*-associated diarrhea (CDAD) and pseudomembranous colitis; CDAD has been observed >2 months postantibiotic treatment. Carbapenems have been associated with CNS adverse effects, including confusional states and seizures (myoclonic); use caution with CNS disorders (eg, brain lesions and history of seizures) and adjust dose in renal impairment to avoid drug accumulation, which may increase seizure risk. Use with caution in patients with hypersensitivity to beta-lactams (including penicillins or cephalosporins); patients with impaired renal function are at increased risk of seizures if not properly dose adjusted. May decrease divalproex sodium/valproic acid concentrations leading to breakthrough seizures; concomitant use is not recommended. Not recommended in pediatric CNS infections due to seizure risk. Serious hypersensitivity reactions, including anaphylaxis, have been reported (some without a history of previous allergic reactions to beta-lactams).

Adverse Reactions

Cardiovascular: Phlebitis, tachycardia

Central nervous system: Seizure

Dermatologic: Skin rash

Gastrointestinal: Diarrhea, gastroenteritis, nausea, oral candidiasis, vomiting

Genitourinary: Oliguria, proteinuria, urine discoloration

Hematologic & oncologic: Decreased hematocrit (more common in infants and children 3 months to 12 years), decreased hemoglobin, decreased platelet count, eosinophilia, increased hematocrit, neutropenia, thrombocythemia,

Hepatic: Decreased serum bilirubin, increased serum alkaline phosphatase, increased serum ALT, increased serum AST (more common in infants and children 3 months to 12 years), increased serum bilirubin

Local: Irritation at injection site

Renal: Increased serum creatinine

Rare but important or life-threatening: Acute renal failure, agranulocytosis, back pain (thoracic spinal), basophilia, bilirubinuria, bone marrow depression, brain disease, candidiasis, casts in urine, change in prothrombin time, *Clostridium difficile* associated diarrhea, confusion, cyanosis, decreased serum sodium, dental discoloration, drug fever, dyskinesia, erythema multiforme, hallucination, hearing loss, heartburn, hematuria, hemolytic anemia, hemorrhagic colitis, hepatic failure, hepatitis (including fulminant onset), hyperchloremia, hypersensitivity, hyperventilation, hypotension, increased blood urea nitrogen, increased lactate dehydrogenase, increased serum potassium, increased urinary urobilinogen, injection site infection, jaundice, leukocytosis, leukocyturia, leukopenia, lymphocytosis, myoclonus, neutropenia, pancytopenia, positive direct Coombs' test, pseudomembranous colitis, pseudomonas infection (resistant *P. aeruginosa*), psychiatric disturbances, Stevens-Johnson syndrome, thrombocytopenia, toxic epidermal necrolysis

Drug Interactions

Metabolism/Transport Effects None known.

Avoid Concomitant Use

Avoid concomitant use of Imipenem and Cilastatin with any of the following: BCG; BCG (Intravesical); Ganciclovir-Valganciclovir

Increased Effect/Toxicity

Imipenem and Cilastatin may increase the levels/effects of: CycloSPORINE (Systemic)

The levels/effects of Imipenem and Cilastatin may be increased by: CycloSPORINE (Systemic); Ganciclovir-Valganciclovir; Probenecid

Decreased Effect

Imipenem and Cilastatin may decrease the levels/effects of: BCG; BCG (Intravesical); BCG Vaccine (Immunization); CycloSPORINE (Systemic); Sodium Picosulfate; Typhoid Vaccine; Valproic Acid and Derivatives

Storage/Stability Imipenem/cilastatin powder for injection should be stored at <25°C (77°F).

IV: Reconstituted IV solutions are stable for 4 hours at room temperature and 24 hours when refrigerated. Do not freeze.

Mechanism of Action Inhibits bacterial cell wall synthesis by binding to one or more of the penicillin-binding proteins (PBPs); which in turn inhibits the final transpeptidation step of peptidoglycan synthesis in bacterial cell walls, thus inhibiting cell wall biosynthesis. Bacteria eventually lyse due to ongoing activity of cell wall autolytic enzymes (autolysins and murein hydrolases) while cell wall assembly is arrested. Cilastatin prevents renal metabolism of imipenem by competitive inhibition of dehydropeptidase along the brush border of the renal tubules.

Pharmacokinetics (Adult data unless noted)

Distribution: Rapidly and widely to most tissues and fluids including sputum, pleural fluid, peritoneal fluid, interstitial fluid, bile, aqueous humor, and bone; highest concentrations in pleural fluid, interstitial fluid, and peritoneal fluid; only low concentrations penetrate into CSF

Protein binding:

- Imipenem: 20%
- Cilastatin: 40%

Metabolism: Imipenem is metabolized in the kidney by dehydropeptidase; cilastatin prevents imipenem metabolism by this enzyme; cilastatin is partially metabolized in the kidneys

Half-life, both drugs: Prolonged with renal insufficiency

- Neonates (Freij, 1985):
  - Imipenem: 1.7-2.4 hours
  - Cilastatin: 3.9-6.3 hours
- Infants and Children: Imipenem: 1.2 hours (Blumer, 1996)
- Adults, both drugs: 1 hour

Elimination: When imipenem is given with cilastatin, urinary excretion of unchanged imipenem increases to 70%; 70% to 80% of a cilastatin dose is excreted unchanged in the urine

Dosing: Neonatal Note: Dosage recommendations are based on **imipenem** component; not the preferred carbapenem for preterm infants due to cilastatin accumulation and possible seizures (Blumer, 1996; Freij, 1985; *Red Book*, 2012; Reed, 1990); not recommended for CNS infections

General dosing, susceptible infection (*Red Book*, 2012): IV:

- Body weight <1 kg:
  - PNA ≤14 days: 20 mg/kg/dose every 12 hours
  - PNA 15-28 days: 25 mg/kg/dose every 12 hours
- Body weight 1-2 kg:
  - PNA ≤7 days: 20 mg/kg/dose every 12 hours
  - PNA 8-28 days: 25 mg/kg/dose every 12 hours
- Body weight >2 kg:
  - PNA ≤7 days: 25 mg/kg/dose every 12 hours
  - PNA 8-28 days: 25 mg/kg/dose every 8 hours

Dosing: Usual Note: Dosage recommendations are based on **imipenem** component.

Infants, Children, and Adolescents:

General dosing, susceptible infection (*Red Book*, 2012): IV: Serious infections: 60-100 mg/kg/**day** divided every 6 hours; maximum daily dose: 4000 mg/**day**

***Burkholderia pseudomallei* (melioidosis):** IV: Initial: 60-100 mg/kg/**day** divided every 6-8 hours for at least 10 days; maximum daily dose: 4000 mg/**day**; continue parenteral therapy until clinical improvement, then switch to oral therapy if tolerated and/or appropriate (Currie, 2003; White, 2003)

Intra-abdominal infection, complicated: IV: 60-100 mg/kg/**day** divided every 6 hours; maximum dose: 500 mg (Solomkin, 2010)

Peritonitis (CAPD): Intraperitoneal: Continuous: Loading dose: 250 mg per liter of dialysate; maintenance dose: 50 mg per liter (Warady, 2012)

Pulmonary exacerbation, cystic fibrosis: IV: 100 mg/kg/**day** divided every 6 hours; maximum daily dose: 4000 mg/**day**; efficacy may be limited due to rapid development of resistance (Doring, 2009; Zobell, 2012)

Adults:

Usual dosage range: Weight ≥70 kg: IV: 250-1000 mg every 6-8 hours; maximum: 4000 mg/day. **Note:** For adults weighing <70 kg, refer to Dosing Adjustment in Renal Impairment.

Indication-specific dosing:

Mild infections: Note: Rarely a suitable option in mild infections; normally reserved for moderate-severe cases: IV:

Fully susceptible organisms: 250 mg every 6 hours

Moderately susceptible organisms: 500 mg every 6 hours

Moderate infections: IV:

Fully susceptible organisms: 500 mg every 6-8 hours

Moderately susceptible organisms: 500 mg every 6 hours or 1000 mg every 8 hours

Severe infections: IV:

Fully susceptible organisms: 500 mg every 6 hours

Moderately susceptible organisms: 1000 mg every 6-8 hours

Maximum daily dose should not exceed 50 mg/kg or 4000 mg/day, whichever is lower

***Pseudomonas* infections:** IV: 500 mg every 6 hours; **Note:** Higher doses may be required based on organism sensitivity.

Urinary tract infection, uncomplicated: IV: 250 mg every 6 hours

Urinary tract infection, complicated: IV: 500 mg every 6 hours

Dosing adjustment in renal impairment:

Infants, Children, and Adolescents: IV:

Manufacturer's labeling: Patient weight <30 kg and impaired renal function (not defined): Use not recommended

The following adjustments have been recommended (Aronoff, 2007): **Note:** Renally adjusted dose recommendations are based on doses of 60-100 mg/kg/day divided every 6 hours.

GFR 30-50 mL/minute/1.73 m^2: Administer 7-13 mg/kg/dose every 8 hours

GFR 10-29 mL/minute/1.73 m^2: Administer 7.5-12.5 mg/kg/dose every 12 hours

GFR <10 mL/minute/1.73 m^2: Administer 7.5-12.5 mg/kg/dose every 24 hours

Intermittent hemodialysis (IHD): Dialysis: Moderately dialyzable (20% to 50%): 7.5-12.5 mg/kg/dose every 24 hours (administer after hemodialysis on dialysis days)

Peritoneal dialysis (PD): 7.5-12.5 mg/kg/dose every 24 hours

Continuous renal replacement therapy (CRRT): 7-13 mg/kg/dose every 8 hours

Adults: Manufacturer's labeling: Reduce dose based on creatinine clearance and/or body weight:

Imipenem and Cilastatin Dosage in Renal Impairment

Reduced IV Dosage Regimen Based on Creatinine Clearance (mL/minute/1.73 m^2) and/or Body Weight <70 kg					
	Body Weight (kg)				
	≥70	60	50	40	30
Total daily dose for normal renal function: 1000 mg/day					
CrCl ≥71	250 mg q6h	250 mg q8h	125 mg q6h	125 mg q6h	125 mg q8h
CrCl 41-70	250 mg q8h	125 mg q6h	125 mg q6h	125 mg q8h	125 mg q8h
CrCl 21-40	250 mg q12h	250 mg q12h	125 mg q8h	125 mg q12h	125 mg q12h
CrCl 6-20	250 mg q12h	125 mg q12h	125 mg q12h	125 mg q12h	125 mg q12h
Total daily dose for normal renal function: 1500 mg/day					
CrCl ≥71	500 mg q8h	250 mg q6h	250 mg q6h	250 mg q8h	125 mg q6h
CrCl 41-70	250 mg q6h	250 mg q8h	250 mg q8h	125 mg q6h	125 mg q8h
CrCl 21-40	250 mg q8h	250 mg q8h	250 mg q12h	125 mg q8h	125 mg q8h
CrCl 6-20	250 mg q12h	250 mg q12h	250 mg q12h	125 mg q12h	125 mg q12h
Total daily dose for normal renal function: 2000 mg/day					
CrCl ≥71	500 mg q6h	500 mg q8h	250 mg q6h	250 mg q6h	250 mg q8h
CrCl 41-70	500 mg q8h	250 mg q6h	250 mg q6h	250 mg q8h	125 mg q6h
CrCl 21-40	250 mg q6h	250 mg q8h	250 mg q8h	250 mg q12h	125 mg q8h
CrCl 6-20	250 mg q12h	250 mg q12h	250 mg q12h	250 mg q12h	125 mg q12h
Total daily dose for normal renal function: 3000 mg/day					
CrCl ≥71	1000 mg q8h	750 mg q8h	500 mg q6h	500 mg q8h	250 mg q6h
CrCl 41-70	500 mg q6h	500 mg q8h	500 mg q8h	250 mg q6h	250 mg q8h
CrCl 21-40	500 mg q8h	500 mg q8h	250 mg q6h	250 mg q8h	250 mg q8h
CrCl 6-20	500 mg q12h	500 mg q12h	250 mg q12h	250 mg q12h	250 mg q12h
Total daily dose for normal renal function: 4000 mg/day					
CrCl ≥71	1000 mg q6h	1000 mg q8h	750 mg q8h	500 mg q6h	500 mg q8h
CrCl 41-70	750 mg q8h	750 mg q8h	500 mg q6h	500 mg q8h	250 mg q6h
CrCl 21-40	500 mg q6h	500 mg q8h	500 mg q8h	250 mg q6h	250 mg q8h
CrCl 6-20	500 mg q12h	500 mg q12h	500 mg q12h	250 mg q12h	250 mg q12h

Patients with a CrCl ≤5 mL/minute/1.73 m^2 should not receive imipenem/cilastatin unless hemodialysis is instituted within 48 hours.

Patients weighing <30 kg with impaired renal function should not receive imipenem/cilastatin.

Intermittent hemodialysis (IHD) (administer after hemodialysis on dialysis days): Dialysis: Moderately dialyzable (20% to 50%): Use the dosing recommendation for patients with a CrCl 6-20 mL/minute; administer dose after dialysis session and every 12 hours thereafter **or** 250-500 mg every 12 hours (Heintz, 2009). **Note:** Dosing dependent on the assumption of 3 times/week, complete IHD sessions.

Peritoneal dialysis: Dose as for CrCl 6-20 mL/minute (Somani, 1988)

Continuous renal replacement therapy (CRRT) (Heintz, 2009; Trotman, 2005): Drug clearance is highly dependent on the method of renal replacement, filter type, and flow rate. Appropriate dosing requires close monitoring of pharmacologic response, signs of adverse reactions due to drug accumulation, as well as drug concentrations in relation to target trough (if appropriate). The following are general recommendations only (based on dialysate flow/ultrafiltration rates of 1-2 L/hour and minimal residual renal function) and should not supersede clinical judgment:

CVVH: Loading dose of 1000 mg followed by either 250 mg every 6 hours **or** 500 mg every 8 hours

CVVHD: Loading dose of 1000 mg followed by either 250 mg every 6 hours **or** 500 mg every 6-8 hours

CVVHDF: Loading dose of 1000 mg followed by either 250 mg every 6 hours **or** 500 mg every 6 hours

Note: Data suggest that 500 mg every 8-12 hours may provide sufficient time above MIC to cover organisms with MIC values ≤2 mg/L; however, a higher dose of 500 mg every 6 hours is recommended for resistant organisms (particularly *Pseudomonas* spp) with MIC ≥4 mg/L or deep-seated infections (Fish, 2005).

Dosing adjustment in hepatic impairment: There are no dosage adjustments provided in the manufacturer's labeling.

Preparation for Administration IV: Dilute dose in a compatible solution to a final concentration not to exceed 5 mg/mL; concentrations >5 mg/mL may have shortened stability; a final admixture of imipenem-cilastatin 10 mg/mL in NS was shown to maintain solubility for 4 hours at room temperature however, an 8 mg/mL solution showed > 90% stability for <3 hours (Trissel 1999; Viaene 2002). Imipenem is inactivated at acidic or alkaline pH.

Administration IV: Administer by IV intermittent infusion; doses ≤500 mg may be infused over 15 to 30 minutes; doses >500 mg should be infused over 40 to 60 minutes. If nausea and/or vomiting occur during administration, decrease the rate of IV infusion.

Monitoring Parameters Periodic renal, hepatic, and hematologic function tests; bowel movement frequency

Test Interactions Interferes with urinary glucose determination using Clinitest®; positive Coombs' [direct]

Additional Information Sodium content: 250 mg vial contains 0.8 mEq; 500 mg vial contains 1.6 mEq

Dosage Forms Excipient information presented when available (limited, particularly for generics); consult specific product labeling.

Injection, powder for reconstitution: Imipenem 250 mg and cilastatin 250 mg; imipenem 500 mg and cilastatin 500 mg

Primaxin® I.V.: Imipenem 250 mg and cilastatin 250 mg [contains sodium 18.8 mg (0.8 mEq)]; imipenem 500 mg and cilastatin 500 mg [contains sodium 37.5 mg (1.6 mEq)]

◆ **Imipenem and Cilastatin for Injection (Can)** *see* Imipenem and Cilastatin *on page 1083*

◆ **Imipenem and Cilastatin for Injection, USP (Can)** *see* Imipenem and Cilastatin *on page 1083*

Imipramine (im IP ra meen)

Medication Safety Issues

Sound-alike/look-alike issues:

Imipramine may be confused with amitriptyline, desipramine, Norpramin

BEERS Criteria medication:

This drug may be potentially inappropriate for use in geriatric patients (Quality of evidence - high [moderate for SIADH]; Strength of recommendation - strong).

Related Information

Antidepressant Agents *on page 2257*

Brand Names: US Tofranil; Tofranil-PM

Brand Names: Canada Impril; Novo-Pramine; PMS Imipramine

Therapeutic Category Antidepressant, Tricyclic (Tertiary Amine)

Generic Availability (US) Yes

Use Treatment of childhood enuresis (Tofranil®: FDA approved in ages ≥6 years); treatment of depression (Tofranil®: FDA approved in adolescents and adults, Tofranil-PM®: FDA approved in adults); has also been used for attention-deficit/hyperactivity disorder (ADHD) and as analgesic for certain chronic and neuropathic pain

Medication Guide Available Yes

Pregnancy Considerations Animal reproduction studies are inconclusive. Congenital abnormalities have been reported in humans; however, a causal relationship has not been established. Tricyclic antidepressants may be associated with irritability, jitteriness, and convulsions (rare) in the neonate (Yonkers, 2009). Due to pregnancy-induced physiologic changes, women who are pregnant may require dose adjustments late in pregnancy to achieve euthymia (Altshuler, 1996).

The ACOG recommends that therapy for depression during pregnancy be individualized; treatment should incorporate the clinical expertise of the mental health clinician, obstetrician, primary healthcare provider, and pediatrician (ACOG, 2008). According to the American Psychiatric Association (APA), the risks of medication treatment should be weighed against other treatment options and untreated depression. For women who discontinue antidepressant medications during pregnancy and who may be at high risk for postpartum depression, the medications can be restarted following delivery (APA, 2010). Treatment algorithms have been developed by the ACOG and the APA for the management of depression in women prior to conception and during pregnancy (Yonkers, 2009).

Breast-Feeding Considerations Imipramine and its active metabolite (desipramine) are excreted into breast milk (Sovner, 1979). Concentrations of imipramine may be similar to those in the maternal plasma. Based on information from five mother/infant pairs, following maternal use of imipramine 75-200 mg/day, the estimated exposure to the breast-feeding infant would be 0.1% to 7.5% of the weight-adjusted maternal dose. Although adverse events were not reported, infants should be monitored for signs of adverse events (Fortinguerra, 2009). Imipramine can also be detected in the urine of nursing infants (Yoshida, 1997). Breast-feeding is not recommended by the manufacturer.

Contraindications Hypersensitivity to imipramine (cross-reactivity with other dibenzodiazepines may occur) or any component of the formulation; in a patient during acute recovery phase of MI; use of MAO inhibitors intended to treat psychiatric disorders (concurrently or within 14 days of discontinuing either imipramine or the MAO inhibitor); initiation of imipramine in a patient receiving linezolid or intravenous methylene blue

Warnings/Precautions [U.S. Boxed Warning]: Antidepressants increase the risk of suicidal thinking and behavior in children, adolescents, and young adults (18-24 years of age) with major depressive disorder (MDD) and other psychiatric disorders; consider risk prior to prescribing. Short-term studies did not show an increased risk in patients >24 years of age and showed a decreased risk in patients ≥65 years. Closely monitor for clinical worsening, suicidality, or unusual changes in behavior, particularly during the initial 1-2 months of therapy or during periods of dosage adjustments (increases or decreases); the patient's family or caregiver should be instructed to closely observe the patient and communicate condition with healthcare provider. A medication guide should be dispensed with each prescription. **Imipramine is FDA approved for the treatment of nocturnal enuresis in children ≥6 years of age.**

The possibility of a suicide attempt is inherent in major depression and may persist until remission occurs. Worsening depression and severe abrupt suicidality that are not part of the presenting symptoms may require discontinuation or modification of drug therapy. The patient's family or caregiver should be alerted to monitor patients for the emergence of suicidality and associated behaviors (such as agitation, irritability, hostility, impulsivity, and hypomania) and notify healthcare provider.

May worsen psychosis in some patients or precipitate a shift to mania or hypomania in patients with bipolar disorder. Patients presenting with depressive symptoms should be screened for bipolar disorder. Monotherapy in patients with bipolar disorder should be avoided. **Imipramine is not FDA approved for the treatment of bipolar depression.**

Potentially life-threatening serotonin syndrome (SS) has occurred with serotonergic agents (eg, SSRIs, SNRIs), particularly when used in combination with other serotonergic agents (eg, triptans, TCAs, fentanyl, lithium, tramadol, buspirone, St John's wort, tryptophan) or agents that impair metabolism of serotonin (eg, MAO inhibitors intended to treat psychiatric disorders, other MAO inhibitors such as linezolid and intravenous methylene blue). Discontinue treatment (and any concomitant serotonergic agent) immediately if signs/symptoms arise. TCAs may rarely cause bone marrow suppression; monitor for any signs of infection and obtain CBC if symptoms (eg, fever, sore throat) evident. The degree of sedation, anticholinergic effects, orthostasis, and conduction abnormalities are high relative to other antidepressants. Imipramine often causes drowsiness/sedation, resulting in impaired performance of tasks requiring alertness (eg, operating machinery or driving). Use with caution in patients with a history of cardiovascular disease (including previous MI, stroke, tachycardia, or conduction abnormalities). Use with caution in patients with urinary retention, benign prostatic hyperplasia, increased intraocular pressure, angle-closure glaucoma, xerostomia, visual problems, constipation, or a history of bowel obstruction.

Consider discontinuing, when possible, prior to elective surgery. Therapy should not be abruptly discontinued in patients receiving high doses for prolonged periods. May lower seizure threshold - use caution in patients with a previous seizure disorder or condition predisposing to seizures such as brain damage, alcoholism, or concurrent therapy with other drugs which lower the seizure threshold. May increase the risks associated with electroconvulsive therapy. Bone fractures have been associated with antidepressant treatment. Consider the possibility of a fragility fracture if an antidepressant-treated patient presents with unexplained bone pain, point tenderness, swelling, or bruising (Rabenda, 2013; Rizzoli, 2012). Use with caution in patients with diabetes mellitus; may alter glucose regulation. Use with caution in patients with hepatic or renal dysfunction and in elderly patients. May cause mild pupillary dilation which in susceptible individuals can lead to an episode of narrow-angle glaucoma. Consider evaluating patients who have not had an iridectomy for narrow-angle glaucoma risk factors. Pharmacokinetics of imipramine may be altered in smokers and patients with chronic alcohol use disorder. Has been associated with photosensitization. Potentially significant interactions may exist, requiring dose or frequency adjustment, additional monitoring, and/or selection of alternative therapy.

A dose of 2.5 mg/kg/day of imipramine hydrochloride should not be exceeded in childhood. ECG changes of unknown significance have been reported in pediatric patients with doses twice this amount. Avoid use in the elderly due to its potent anticholinergic and sedative properties, and potential to cause orthostatic hypotension. In addition, may also cause or exacerbate syndrome of inappropriate antidiuretic hormone secretion or hyponatremia; monitor sodium closely with initiation or dosage adjustments in older adults (Beers Criteria). Lower doses may be required in elderly patients due to pharmacokinetic changes.

Warnings: Additional Pediatric Considerations The American Heart Association recommends that all children diagnosed with ADHD who may be candidates for medication, such as imipramine, should have a thorough cardiovascular assessment prior to initiation of therapy. These recommendations are based upon reports of serious cardiovascular adverse events (including sudden death) in patients (both children and adults) taking usual doses of stimulant medications. Most of these patients were found to have underlying structural heart disease (eg, hypertrophic obstructive cardiomyopathy). This assessment should include a combination of thorough medical history, family history, and physical examination. An ECG is not mandatory but should be considered. Use with caution in patients with a history of cardiovascular disease (including previous MI, stroke, tachycardia, or conduction abnormalities); the risk of conduction abnormalities with this agent is high relative to other antidepressants. Baseline and periodic ECG assessment is recommended with use of higher dosages; should also be considered in patients with preexisting cardiovascular disease.

Use of capsules is generally not recommended in children due to high mg strength and increased potential for acute overdose. Safety of imipramine for long-term chronic use in the treatment of enuresis has not been established; long-term usefulness should be periodically reevaluated for the individual patient; medication should be tapered off gradually to achieve drug-free period for reassessment; children who relapse with enuresis during drug-free period do not always respond to subsequent courses of therapy.

Adverse Reactions Reported for tricyclic antidepressants in general.

Cardiovascular: Cardiac arrhythmia, cardiac failure, cerebrovascular accident, ECG changes, heart block, hypertension, myocardial infarction, orthostatic hypotension, palpitations, tachycardia

Central nervous system: Agitation, anxiety, ataxia, confusion, delusions, disorientation, dizziness, drowsiness, EEG pattern changes, extrapyramidal reaction, falling, fatigue, hallucination, headache, hypomania, insomnia, nightmares, numbness, paresthesia, peripheral neuropathy, psychosis, restlessness, seizure, taste disorder, tingling sensation

Dermatologic: Alopecia, diaphoresis, pruritus, skin photosensitivity, skin rash, urticaria

Endocrine & metabolic: Decreased libido, decreased serum glucose, galactorrhea, gynecomastia, increased libido, increased serum glucose, SIADH, weight gain, weight loss

Gastrointestinal: Abdominal cramps, anorexia, constipation, diarrhea, epigastric distress, intestinal obstruction, melanoglossia, nausea, stomatitis, sublingual adenitis, vomiting, xerostomia

Genitourinary: Breast hypertrophy, impotence, testicular swelling, urinary hesitancy, urinary retention, urinary tract dilation

Hematologic & oncologic: Agranulocytosis, eosinophilia, petechia, purpura, thrombocytopenia

Hepatic: Cholestatic jaundice, increased serum transaminases

Hypersensitivity: Hypersensitivity (eg, drug fever, edema)

Neuromuscular & skeletal: Tremor, weakness

Ophthalmic: Accommodation disturbance, angle-closure glaucoma, blurred vision, mydriasis

Otic: Tinnitus

Drug Interactions

Metabolism/Transport Effects **Substrate** of CYP1A2 (minor), CYP2B6 (minor), CYP2C19 (major), CYP2D6 (major), CYP3A4 (minor); **Note:** Assignment of Major/Minor substrate status based on clinically relevant drug interaction potential; **Inhibits** CYP1A2 (weak), CYP2C19 (weak), CYP2D6 (moderate), CYP2E1 (weak)

Avoid Concomitant Use

Avoid concomitant use of Imipramine with any of the following: Aclidinium; Azelastine (Nasal); Dapoxetine; Eluxadoline; Glucagon; Iobenguane I 123; Ipratropium (Oral Inhalation); Linezolid; MAO Inhibitors; Methylene Blue; Moxonidine; Orphenadrine; Paraldehyde; Potassium Chloride; Thalidomide; Thioridazine; Tiotropium; Umeclidinium

Increased Effect/Toxicity

Imipramine may increase the levels/effects of: AbobotulinumtoxinA; Alcohol (Ethyl); Alpha-/Beta-Agonists (Direct-Acting); Alpha1-Agonists; Amphetamines; Analgesics (Opioid); Anticholinergic Agents; Antipsychotic Agents; ARIPiprazole; Aspirin; Azelastine (Nasal); Beta2-Agonists; Buprenorphine; Citalopram; CNS Depressants; CYP2D6 Substrates; Desmopressin; DOXOrubicin (Conventional); Eliglustat; Eluxadoline; Escitalopram; Fesoterodine; Glucagon; Highest Risk QTc-Prolonging Agents; Hydrocodone; Methotrimeprazine; Methylene Blue; Metoprolol; Metyrosine; Mirabegron; Moderate Risk QTc-Prolonging Agents; Nebivolol; Nicorandil; NSAID (COX-2 Inhibitor); NSAID (Nonselective); OnabotulinumtoxinA; Orphenadrine; Paraldehyde; Potassium Chloride; Pramipexole; QuiNIDine; RimabotulinumtoxinB; ROPINIRole; Rotigotine; Serotonin Modulators; Sodium Phosphates; Sulfonylureas; Suvorexant; Thalidomide; Thiazide Diuretics; Thioridazine; Tiotropium; TiZANidine; Topiramate; TraMADol; Vitamin K Antagonists; Yohimbine; Zolpidem

The levels/effects of Imipramine may be increased by: Abiraterone Acetate; Aclidinium; Altretamine; Antiemetics (5HT3 Antagonists); Antipsychotic Agents; Brimonidine (Topical); BuPROPion; Cannabis; Cimetidine; Cinacalcet; Citalopram; Cobicistat; CYP2C19 Inhibitors (Moderate); CYP2C19 Inhibitors (Strong); CYP2D6 Inhibitors (Moderate); CYP2D6 Inhibitors (Strong); Dapoxetine; Darunavir; Dexmethylphenidate; Doxylamine; Dronabinol; Droperidol; DULoxetine; Escitalopram; FLUoxetine; FluvoxaMINE; HydrOXYzine; Ipratropium (Oral Inhalation); Kava Kava; Linezolid; Lithium; Luliconazole; Magnesium Sulfate; MAO Inhibitors; Methotrimeprazine; Methylphenidate; Metoclopramide; Metyrosine; Mianserin; Mifepristone; Nabilone; Panobinostat; PARoxetine; Peginterferon Alfa-2b; Perampanel; Pramlintide; Propafenone; Protease Inhibitors; QuiNIDine; Rufinamide; Sertraline; Sodium Oxybate; Tapentadol; Tedizolid; Terbinafine (Systemic); Tetrahydrocannabinol; Thyroid Products; TraMADol; Umeclidinium; Valproic Acid and Derivatives

Decreased Effect

Imipramine may decrease the levels/effects of: Acetylcholinesterase Inhibitors; Alpha1-Agonists; Alpha2-Agonists; Alpha2-Agonists (Ophthalmic); Codeine; Iobenguane I 123; Itopride; Moxonidine; Secretin; Tamoxifen

The levels/effects of Imipramine may be decreased by: Acetylcholinesterase Inhibitors; Barbiturates; CYP2C19 Inducers (Strong); Dabrafenib; Peginterferon Alfa-2b; St Johns Wort

Storage/Stability Capsules, tablets: Store between 20°C to 25°C (68°F to 77°F).

Mechanism of Action Traditionally believed to increase the synaptic concentration of serotonin and/or norepinephrine in the central nervous system by inhibition of their reuptake by the presynaptic neuronal membrane. However, additional receptor effects have been found including desensitization of adenyl cyclase, down regulation of beta-adrenergic receptors, and down regulation of serotonin receptors.

Pharmacodynamics Maximum antidepressant effects usually occur after ≥2 weeks

Pharmacokinetics (Adult data unless noted)

Absorption: Oral: Well absorbed

Distribution:

V_d: Children: 14.5 L/kg; Adults: ~17 L/kg

Protein binding: >90% (primarily to $alpha_1$ acid glycoprotein and lipoproteins; to a lesser extent albumin)

Metabolism: Hepatic, primarily via CYP2D6 to desipramine (active) and other metabolites; significant first-pass effect

Bioavailability: 20% to 80%

Half-life: Range: 6-18 hours

Mean: Children: 11 hours; Adults: 16-17 hours

Desipramine (active metabolite): 22-28 hours

Time to peak serum concentration: Within 1-2 hours

Elimination: Urine

Dosing: Usual

Children and Adolescents: **Note:** Dosing presented is based on hydrochloride salt.

Attention-deficit/hyperactivity disorder: Children ≥6 years and Adolescents: Oral: Limited data available: Initial: 1 mg/kg/day in 1-3 divided doses; titrate as needed; maximum daily dose: 4 mg/kg/**day** or 200 mg/**day**; for doses >2 mg/kg/day, monitor serum concentrations (target: ≤200 ng/mL) (Himpel, 2005; Pliszka, 2007). **Note:** Manufacturer's labeling warns against use of doses >2.5 mg/kg/day in pediatric patients; ECG changes (of unknown significance) have been reported in pediatric patients who received twice this amount.

Depression: Oral: Limited data available: **Note:** Controlled clinical trials have not shown tricyclic antidepressants to be superior to placebo for the treatment of depression in children and adolescents; not recommended as first line medication; may be beneficial for patient with comorbid conditions (ADHD, enuresis) (Birmaher, 2007; Dopheide, 2006; Wagner, 2005).

Children: 1.5 mg/kg/day in 2-3 divided doses; titrate as needed in increments of 1 mg/kg every 3-4 days; maximum daily doses of 5 mg/kg/**day** has been used by some centers; monitor carefully especially with doses ≥3.5 mg/kg/day; manufacturer's labeling warns against use of doses >2.5 mg/kg/day in pediatric patients; ECG changes (of unknown significance) have been reported in pediatric patients who received twice this amount

Adolescents: Initial: 25-50 mg/day; increase gradually; maximum daily dose: 100 mg/**day** in single or divided doses

Enuresis: Children ≥4 years and Adolescents: Oral: Initial: 10-25 mg at bedtime, if inadequate response still seen after 1 week of therapy, increase by 25 mg/day; maximum daily dose: The lesser of: 2.5 mg/kg/**day** or 50 mg/**day** if 6 to <12 years old; and 75 mg/**day** if ≥12 years old; for early night bedwetters, drug has been shown to be more effective if given earlier and in divided amounts (eg, 25 mg in midafternoon and repeated at bedtime). **Note:** Due to the risk of serious side effects (eg, arrhythmias, heart block, seizures), imipramine is considered third-line treatment for enuresis (Deshpande, 2012).

Neuropathic pain: Note: Not the preferred TCA; amitriptyline or nortriptyline recommended as first-line TCAs. Limited data available: Initial: 0.2-0.4 mg/kg at bedtime; dose may be increased by 50% every 2-3 days up to 1-3 mg/kg/dose at bedtime (Berde, 1990). **Note:** Manufacturer labeling warns against use of doses >2.5 mg/kg/**day** in pediatric patients; ECG changes (of unknown significance) have been reported in pediatric patients who received twice this amount.

Adults: **Depression:** Oral:

Outpatients: Initial: 75 mg/day; may increase gradually to 150 mg/day. May be given in divided doses or as a single bedtime dose; maximum daily dose: 200 mg/**day**

Inpatients: Initial: 100-150 mg/day; may increase gradually to 200 mg/day; if no response after 2 weeks, may further increase to 250-300 mg/day. May be given in divided doses or as a single bedtime dose; maximum daily dose: 300 mg/**day**

Note: Maximum antidepressant effect may not be seen for 2 or more weeks after initiation of therapy.

Dosing adjustment in renal impairment: There are no dosage adjustments provided in manufacturer's labeling; use with caution.

Dosing adjustment in hepatic impairment: There are no dosage adjustments provided in manufacturer's labeling; use with caution.

Administration Oral: May administer with food to decrease GI distress. For treatment of enuresis, administer dose 1 hour before bedtime; for early night bedwetters, drug has been shown to be more effective if given earlier and in divided amounts (eg, 25 mg in midafternoon and repeated at bedtime)

Monitoring Parameters Heart rate, ECG, supine and standing blood pressure (especially in children), liver enzymes, CBC, serum drug concentrations. Obtain ECG before initiation of therapy and at appropriate intervals in patients with any evidence of cardiovascular disease and in all patients who will receive doses that are larger than usual. Monitor patient periodically for symptom resolution; monitor for worsening depression, suicidality, and associated behaviors (especially at the beginning of therapy or when doses are increased or decreased). Monitor for signs/symptoms of serotonin syndrome.

ADHD: Evaluate patients for cardiac disease prior to initiation of therapy for ADHD with thorough medical history, family history, and physical exam; consider ECG; perform ECG and echocardiogram if findings suggest cardiac disease; promptly conduct cardiac evaluation in patients who develop chest pain, unexplained syncope, or any other symptom of cardiac disease during treatment.

Reference Range Note: Utility of serum concentration monitoring controversial.

Therapeutic: Imipramine and desipramine 150-250 ng/mL (SI: 530-890 nmol/L); desipramine 150-300 ng/mL (SI: 560-1125 nmol/L)

Potentially toxic: >300 ng/mL (SI: >1070 nmol/L)

Toxic: >1000 ng/mL (SI: >3570 nmol/L)

Dosage Forms Excipient information presented when available (limited, particularly for generics); consult specific product labeling.

Capsule, Oral, as pamoate:

Tofranil-PM: 75 mg, 100 mg, 125 mg, 150 mg

Generic: 75 mg, 100 mg, 125 mg, 150 mg

Tablet, Oral, as hydrochloride:

Tofranil: 10 mg, 25 mg, 50 mg

Generic: 10 mg, 25 mg, 50 mg

- ◆ **Imipramine Hydrochloride** *see* Imipramine *on page 1086*
- ◆ **Imipramine Pamoate** *see* Imipramine *on page 1086*
- ◆ **Imitrex** *see* SUMAtriptan *on page 1995*
- ◆ **Imitrex DF (Can)** *see* SUMAtriptan *on page 1995*
- ◆ **Imitrex Injection (Can)** *see* SUMAtriptan *on page 1995*
- ◆ **Imitrex Nasal Spray (Can)** *see* SUMAtriptan *on page 1995*
- ◆ **Imitrex STATdose Refill** *see* SUMAtriptan *on page 1995*
- ◆ **Imitrex STATdose System** *see* SUMAtriptan *on page 1995*

Immune Globulin (i MYUN GLOB yoo lin)

Medication Safety Issues

Sound-alike/look-alike issues:

Gamimune N may be confused with CytoGam

Immune globulin (intravenous) may be confused with hepatitis B immune globulin

Privigen (immune globulin) may be confused with Albuminar-25 (albumin) due to similar packaging

Related Information

Centers for Disease Control and Prevention (CDC) and Other Links *on page 2424*

Immune Globulin Product Comparison *on page 2264*

Immunization Administration Recommendations *on page 2411*

Immunization Schedules *on page 2416*

Brand Names: US Bivigam; Carimune NF; Flebogamma DIF; Flebogamma [DSC]; GamaSTAN S/D; Gammagard; Gammagard S/D Less IgA; Gammagard S/D [DSC]; Gammaked; Gammaplex; Gamunex-C; Hizentra; Hyqvia; Octagam; Privigen

Brand Names: Canada Gamastan S/D; Gammagard Liquid; Gammagard S/D; Gamunex; Hizentra; IGIVnex; Octagam 10%; Privigen

Therapeutic Category Blood Product Derivative; Immune Globulin

Generic Availability (US) No

Use Treatment of primary humoral immunodeficiency syndromes (may include but not limited to: Congenital agammaglobulinemia, severe combined immunodeficiency syndromes [SCIDS], common variable immunodeficiency, X-linked immunodeficiency, Wiskott-Aldrich syndrome); acute and chronic immune thrombocytopenia (ITP); chronic inflammatory demyelinating polyneuropathy (CIDP); and multifocal motor neuropathy. Prevention of coronary artery aneurysms associated with Kawasaki syndrome (in combination with aspirin).

Adjunctive treatment of bacterial infection in patients with hypogammaglobulinemia and/or recurrent bacterial infections with B-cell chronic lymphocytic leukemia (CLL); and serious infection in immunoglobulin deficiency (select agammaglobulinemias).

To provide passive immunity for prophylaxis in the following susceptible individuals: Hepatitis A (pre-exposure and postexposure [within 14 days and prior to manifestation of disease]); measles (postexposure [within 6 days] in an unvaccinated or nonimmune person); rubella (postexposure during early pregnancy); and varicella zoster (immunosuppressed patients when varicella zoster immune globulin is unavailable).

See table for product specific indications, FDA approved age ranges, and routes of administration.

Product	Indication	FDA Approval Ages	Route(s)
Bivigam	Primary immunodeficiency (treatment)	≥6 years and adults	Intravenous
Carimune NF	Primary immunodeficiency (treatment)	Pediatric patients (age not specified) and adults	Intravenous
	Acute and chronic ITP (treatment)		
Flebogamma 5% DIF	Primary immunodeficiency (treatment)	Adults	Intravenous
Flebogamma 10% DIF	Primary immunodeficiency (treatment)	Adults	Intravenous
GamaSTAN S/D	Passive immunity - Hepatitis A	Pediatric patients (age not specified) and adults	Intramuscular
	Passive immunity - Measles		
	Passive immunity - Rubella	Adults	
	Passive immunity - Varicella	Pediatric patients (age not specified) and adults	
Gammagard Liquid	Primary immunodeficiency (treatment)	≥2 years and adults	Intravenous, Subcutaneous
	Multifocal motor neuropathy (MMN)	Adults	Intravenous
Gammagard S/D	Primary immunodeficiency (treatment)	≥2 years and adults	Intravenous
	B-cell chronic lymphocytic leukemia (CLL)	Adults	
	Chronic ITP (treatment)	Adults	
	Kawasaki syndrome	Pediatric patients (age not specified)	
Gammaked	Primary immunodeficiency (treatment)	0 to 16 years	Intravenous
		Adults	Intravenous, Subcutaneous
	Acute ITP (treatment)	Pediatric patients (age not specified) and adults	Intravenous
	Chronic inflammatory demyelinating polyneuropathy (CIDP)	Adults	Intravenous
Gammaplex	Primary immunodeficiency (treatment)	Adults	Intravenous
	Chronic ITP (treatment)	Adults	

(continued)

(continued)

Product	Indication	FDA Approval Ages	Route(s)
Gamunex-C	Primary immunodeficiency (treatment)	0 to 16 years	Intravenous
		Adults	Intravenous, Subcutaneous
	Acute and chronic ITP (treatment)	Pediatric patients (age not specified) and adults	Intravenous
	Chronic inflammatory demyelinating polyneuropathy (CIDP)	Adults	Intravenous
Hizentra	Primary immunodeficiency (treatment)	≥2 years and adults	Subcutaneous
Octagam	Primary immunodeficiency (treatment)	6 to 16 years and adults	Intravenous
Privigen	Primary immunodeficiency (treatment)	≥3 years and adults	Intravenous
	Chronic ITP (treatment)	≥15 years and adults	Intravenous

Has also been used for acute disseminated encephalomyelitis (ADEM), acute myocarditis, chronic *Clostridium difficile* colitis, Guillain-Barré syndrome, hematopoietic stem cell transplantation with hypogammaglobulinemia, isoimmune hemolytic disease (Rh-incompatibility), multiple sclerosis, myasthenia gravis, neonatal sepsis, pediatric HIV infection and associated thrombocytopenia, refractory dermatomyositis, Stevens-Johnson syndrome (SJS)/toxic epidermal necrolysis (TEN), and refractory polymyositis.

Pregnancy Risk Factor C

Pregnancy Considerations Animal reproduction studies have not been conducted. Immune globulins cross the placenta in increased amounts after 30 weeks gestation. Intravenous immune globulin has been recommended for use in fetal-neonatal alloimmune thrombocytopenia and pregnancy-associated ITP (Anderson, 2007). Intravenous immune globulin is recommended to prevent measles in nonimmune women exposed during pregnancy (CDC, 2013). May also be used in postexposure prophylaxis for rubella to reduce the risk of infection and fetal damage in exposed pregnant women who will not consider therapeutic abortion (per GamaSTAN S/D product labeling; use for postexposure rubella prophylaxis is not currently recommended [CDC, 2013]).

HyQvia: Women who become pregnant during treatment are encouraged to enroll in the HyQvia Pregnancy Registry (1-866-424-6724).

Breast-Feeding Considerations It is not known if immune globulin from these preparations is excreted in breast milk. The manufacturer recommends that caution be exercised when administering immune globulin to nursing women. The manufacturer of HyQvia recommends administration to nursing women only if clearly indicated.

Contraindications Hypersensitivity to immune globulin or any component of the formulation; IgA deficiency (with anti-IgA antibodies and history of hypersensitivity); hyperprolinemia (Hizentra, Privigen); isolated IgA deficiency (GamaSTAN S/D); severe thrombocytopenia or coagulation disorders where IM injections are contraindicated (GamaSTAN S/D); hypersensitivity to corn (Octagam); hereditary intolerance to fructose; infants/neonates for whom sucrose or fructose tolerance has not been established (Gammaplex); hypersensitivity to hyaluronidase or recombinant human hyaluronidase (HyQvia)

Warnings/Precautions [U.S. Boxed Warning]: IV administration only: Acute renal dysfunction (increased serum creatinine, oliguria, acute renal failure, osmotic nephrosis) can rarely occur and has been associated with fatalities; usually within 7 days of use (more likely with products stabilized with sucrose). Use with caution in the elderly, patients with renal disease, diabetes mellitus, volume depletion, sepsis, paraproteinemia, and nephrotoxic medications due to risk of renal dysfunction. In patients at risk of renal dysfunction, ensure adequate hydration prior to administration; the rate of infusion and concentration of solution should be minimized. Discontinue if renal function deteriorates.

[U.S. Boxed Warning]: Thrombosis may occur with immune globulin products even in the absence of risk factors for thrombosis. For patients at risk of thrombosis (eg, advanced age, history of atherosclerosis, impaired cardiac output, prolonged immobilization, hypercoagulable conditions, history of venous or arterial thrombosis, use of estrogens, indwelling central vascular catheters, hyperviscosity, and cardiovascular risk factors), administer at the minimum dose and infusion rate practicable. Ensure adequate hydration before administration. Monitor for signs and symptoms of thrombosis and assess blood viscosity in patients at risk for hyperviscosity such as those with cryoglobulins, fasting chylomicronemia/severe hypertriglyceridemia, or monoclonal gammopathies.

High-dose regimens (1 g/kg for 1 to 2 days) are not recommended for individuals with fluid overload or where fluid volume may be of concern. Hypersensitivity and anaphylactic reactions can occur (some severe); patients with anti-IgA antibodies are at greater risk; a severe fall in blood pressure may rarely occur with anaphylactic reaction; immediate treatment (including epinephrine 1:1000) should be available. Product of human plasma; may potentially contain infectious agents which could transmit disease, including unknown or emerging viruses and other pathogens. Screening of donors, as well as testing and/or inactivation or removal of certain viruses, reduces the risk. Infections thought to be transmitted by this product should be reported to the manufacturer. Aseptic meningitis may occur with high doses (≥1 g/kg) and/or rapid infusion; syndrome usually appears within several hours to 2 days following treatment; usually resolves within several days after product is discontinued; patients with a migraine history may be at higher risk for AMS. Increased risk of hypersensitivity, especially in patients with anti-IgA antibodies; use is contraindicated in patients with IgA deficiency (with antibodies against IgA and history of hypersensitivity) or isolated IgA deficiency (GamaSTAN S/D). Increased risk of hematoma formation when administered subcutaneously for the treatment of ITP.

Intravenous immune globulin has been associated with antiglobulin hemolysis (acute or delayed); monitor for signs of hemolytic anemia. Cases of hemolysis-related renal dysfunction/failure or disseminated intravascular coagulation (DIC) have been reported. Risk factors include high doses (≥2 g/kg) and non-O blood type (FDA, 2012). In chronic ITP, assess risk versus benefit of high-dose regimen in patients with increased risk of thrombosis, hemolysis, acute kidney injury, or volume overload.

Patients should be adequately hydrated prior to initiation of therapy. Hyperproteinemia, increased serum viscosity and hyponatremia may occur; distinguish hyponatremia from pseudohyponatremia to prevent volume depletion, a further increase in serum viscosity, and a higher risk of thrombotic events. Patients should be monitored for adverse events during and after the infusion. Stop administration with signs of infusion reaction (fever, chills, nausea, vomiting, and rarely shock). Risk may be increased with initial treatment, when switching brands of immune globulin, and with treatment interruptions of >8 weeks. Monitor for transfusion-related acute lung injury (TRALI); noncardiogenic pulmonary edema has been reported with immune globulin use. TRALI is characterized by severe respiratory distress, pulmonary edema, hypoxemia, and fever (in the presence of normal left ventricular function) and usually occurs within 1-6 hours after infusion. Response to live vaccinations may be impaired. Some clinicians may administer intravenous immune globulin products as a subcutaneous infusion based on patient tolerability and clinical judgment. SubQ infusion should begin 1 week after the last IV dose; dose should be individualized based on clinical response and serum IgG trough concentrations; consider premedicating with acetaminophen and diphenhydramine.

Some products may contain maltose, which may result in falsely elevated blood glucose readings; maltose-containing products may be contraindicated in patients with an allergy to corn. Some products may contain sodium and/or sucrose. Some dosage forms may contain polysorbate 80 (also known as Tweens). Hypersensitivity reactions, usually a delayed reaction, have been reported following exposure to pharmaceutical products containing polysorbate 80 in certain individuals (Isaksson, 2002; Lucente 2000; Shelley, 1995). Thrombocytopenia, ascites, pulmonary deterioration, and renal and hepatic failure have been reported in premature neonates after receiving parenteral products containing polysorbate 80 (Alade, 1986; CDC, 1984). See manufacturer's labeling. Some products may contain sorbitol; do not use in patients with fructose intolerance. Hizentra and Privigen contain the stabilizer L-proline and are contraindicated in patients with hyperprolinemia. Packaging of some products may contain natural latex/natural rubber; skin testing should not be performed with GamaSTAN S/D as local irritation can occur and be misinterpreted as a positive reaction.

Adverse Reactions Adverse effects are reported as class effects rather than for specific products.

Cardiovascular: Chest tightness, edema, facial flushing, hypertension, hypotension, palpitations, tachycardia

Central nervous system: Anxiety, aseptic meningitis, chills, dizziness, drowsiness, fatigue, headache, lethargy, malaise, migraine, pain, rigors

Dermatologic: Dermatitis, diaphoresis, eczema, erythema, hyperhidrosis, pruritus, skin rash, urticaria

Endocrine & metabolic: Dehydration, increased lactate dehydrogenase

Gastrointestinal: Abdominal cramps, abdominal pain, diarrhea, dyspepsia, gastroenteritis, gastrointestinal distress, nausea, sore throat, toothache, vomiting

Genitourinary: Anuria, oliguria, osmotic nephrosis, proximal tubular nephropathy

Hematologic & oncologic: Anemia, bruise, decreased hematocrit, hematoma, hemolysis (mild), hemolytic anemia, hemorrhage, petechia, purpura, thrombocytopenia

Hepatic: Increased serum bilirubin

Hypersensitivity: Anaphylaxis, angioedema, hypersensitivity reaction

Local: Infusion site reaction (including erythema at injection site, irritation at injection site, itching at injection site, pain at injection site, swelling at injection site, warm sensation at injection site)

Neuromuscular & skeletal: Arthralgia, back pain, leg cramps, limb pain, muscle cramps, muscle spasm, myalgia, neck pain, weakness

Ophthalmic: Conjunctivitis

Otic: Otalgia

Renal: Acute renal failure, increased blood urea nitrogen, increased serum creatinine, renal tubular necrosis

Respiratory: Bronchitis, cough, dyspnea, epistaxis, exacerbation of asthma, flu-like symptoms, nasal congestion, oropharyngeal pain, pharyngitis, rhinitis, rhinorrhea, sinusitis, upper respiratory tract infection, wheezing

Miscellaneous: Fever, infusion related reaction

Rare but important or life-threatening): Antibody development (nonneutralizing antibodies to recombinant human hyaluronidase), blurred vision, bronchospasm, burning sensation, cardiac failure, cerebrovascular accident, chest pain, circulatory shock, coma, cyanosis, decreased serum alkaline phosphatase, disseminated intravascular coagulation, epidermolysis, erythema multiforme, exacerbation of autoimmune pure red cell aplasia, hepatic insufficiency, insomnia, pancytopenia, positive direct Coombs test, pulmonary edema, pulmonary embolism, renal insufficiency, respiratory distress, seizure, Stevens-Johnson syndrome, syncope, thromboembolism, transfusion-related acute lung injury, transient ischemic attack, tremor

Drug Interactions

Metabolism/Transport Effects None known.

Avoid Concomitant Use There are no known interactions where it is recommended to avoid concomitant use.

Increased Effect/Toxicity

The levels/effects of Immune Globulin may be increased by: Estrogen Derivatives

Decreased Effect

Immune Globulin may decrease the levels/effects of: Vaccines (Live)

Storage/Stability Stability is dependent upon the manufacturer and brand. Do not freeze (do not use if previously frozen). Do not shake. Do not heat (do not use if previously heated).

Bivigam: Store under refrigeration at 2°C to 8°C (36°F to 46°F). Dilution is not recommended.

Carimune NF: Prior to reconstitution, store at or below 30°C (86°F). Reconstitute with NS, D_5W, or SWFI. Following reconstitution in a sterile laminar air flow environment, store under refrigeration. Begin infusion within 24 hours.

Flebogamma DIF: Store at 2°C to 25°C (36°F to 77°F).

GamaSTAN S/D: Store under refrigeration at 2°C to 8°C (36°F to 46°F). The following stability information has also been reported for GamaSTAN S/D: May be exposed to room temperature for a cumulative 7 days (Cohen, 2007).

Gammagard Liquid: Prior to use, store at 2°C to 8°C (36°F to 46°F). May store at room temperature of 25°C (77°F) within the first 24 months of manufacturing. Storage time at room temperature varies with length of time previously refrigerated; refer to product labeling for details.

Gammagard S/D: Store at ≤25°C (≤77°F). May store diluted solution under refrigeration at 2°C to 8°C (36°F to 46°F) for up to 24 hours if originally prepared in a sterile laminar air flow environment.

Gammaked: Store at 2°C to 8°C (36°F to 46°F); may be stored at ≤25°C (≤77°F) for up to 6 months.

Gammaplex: Store at 2°C to 25°C (36°F to 77°F). Protect from light.

Gamunex-C: Store at 2°C to 8°C (36°F to 46°F); may be stored at ≤25°C (≤77°F) for up to 6 months.

Hizentra: Store at ≤25°C (≤77°F). Keep in original carton to protect from light.

HyQvia: Store at 2°C to 8°C (36°F to 46°F) for up to 36 months; may store at ≤25°C (≤77°F) for up to 3 months during the first 24 months from the date of manufacture (after 3 months at room temperature, discard); do not return vial to refrigerator after it has been stored at room temperature.

Octagam 5%: Store at 2°C to 25°C (36°F to 77°F).

Octagam 10%: Store at 2°C to 8°C (36°F to 46°F) for 24 months from the date of manufacture; within these first 12 months, may store up to 6 months at ≤25°C (77°F); after storage at ≤25°C (77°F), the product must be used or discarded.

Privigen: Store at ≤25°C (≤77°F). Protect from light.

Mechanism of Action Replacement therapy for primary and secondary immunodeficiencies, and IgG antibodies against bacteria, viral, parasitic and mycoplasma antigens; interference with F_c receptors on the cells of the reticuloendothelial system for autoimmune cytopenias and ITP; provides passive immunity by increasing the antibody titer and antigen-antibody reaction potential

Pharmacodynamics

Onset of action: IV: Provides immediate antibody levels

Duration: IM, IV: Immune effect: 3 to 4 weeks (variable)

Pharmacokinetics (Adult data unless noted) Note: Consult manufacturers' labeling for additional product-specific information.

Half-life: IM: 23 days; IV: IgG concentrations variable: Healthy subjects: 14 to 24 days; patients with congenital humoral immunodeficiencies: 26 to 40 days; decreased half-life has been reported to coincide with fever and infection, may be due to hypermetabolism.

Time to peak serum concentration: IM: Within 48 hours; SubQ: 2.5 to 2.9 days

Dosing: Neonatal Note: Not all products are interchangeable with regards to route of administration; consult manufacturers' labeling for additional information. Consider osmolarity and concentration during product selection; infuse as slowly as indication and stability allow (see "Immune Globulin Product Comparison" section in Appendix for details). Dosage expressed as mg/kg or mL/kg dependent upon route of administration; use extra precaution to ensure accuracy.

Immune thrombocytopenia (ITP): IV: 400 to 1000 mg/kg/day for 2 to 5 consecutive days (total dose: 2000 mg/kg); maintenance dose: 400 to 1000 mg/kg/dose every 3 to 6 weeks based on clinical response and platelet count

Isoimmune hemolytic disease (Rh-incompatibility): IV: GA ≥35 weeks: 500 to 1000 mg/kg/dose once over 2 hours; if needed, dose may be repeated in 12 hours; most effective when administered as soon as possible after diagnosis (AAP Subcommittee on Hyperbilirubinemia, 2004; Girish, 2008; Gottstein, 2003; Miqdad, 2004)

Measles, prophylaxis (CDC, 2013):

Pre-exposure prophylaxis (eg, during an outbreak, travel to endemic area): Immunocompromised patients: IV: ≥400 mg/kg/dose within 3 weeks before anticipated exposure

Postexposure prophylaxis: Any neonate without evidence of measles immunity:

IM: 0.5 **mL**/kg/dose within 6 days of exposure; **Note:** Not all immune globulin preparations may be administered by the IM route; of the products currently available on the market, GamaSTAN S/D may be given IM; consult product labeling for additional information as market availability may change.

IV: 400 mg/kg/dose within 6 days of exposure

Myasthenia gravis (severe exacerbation): IV: 400 to 1000 mg/kg/dose once daily over 2 to 5 days for a total dose of 2000 mg/kg; if additional therapy required, dose should be based on clinical response and titrated to minimum effective dose (Bassan, 1998; Feasby, 2007)

Myocarditis, acute: IV: 2000 mg/kg as a single dose. A cohort study of 21 young patients, including neonates, showed improvement in LVF recovery and survival at 1 year as compared to untreated historical cohort (Drucker, 1994); efficacy results are variable (English, 2004; Hia, 2004; Klugman, 2010); the largest data analysis did not show clear clinical benefit nor positive impact on survival (Klugman, 2010).

Sepsis, adjunctive treatment: IV: Limited data available; efficacy results variable: Usual dose: 500 to 1000 mg/kg/dose once daily for 1 to 3 days (Jenson, 1997; Ohlsson,

2010). The largest trial, INIS (n=3493), reported no difference in outcomes (including incidence of subsequent sepsis, death, or major disability at 2 years) between treatment and control groups using 500 mg/kg/day for 2 days (INIS Collaborative Group, 2011).

Dosing: Usual Note: Not all products are interchangeable with regards to route of administration; consult manufacturers' labeling for additional information. Product-specific dosing is provided where applicable; some clinicians use ideal body weight or an adjusted ideal body weight in morbidly-obese patients to calculate an IVIG dose (Siegel, 2010, Wimperis, 2011). Dosage expressed as mg/kg or mL/kg and is dependent upon route of administration; use extra precaution to ensure accuracy.

Pediatric:

Acute disseminated encephalomyelitis (ADEM): Limited data available: Children and Adolescents: IV: 1000 mg/kg/dose once daily for 2 days (Feasby, 2007)

Colitis due to *Clostridium difficile*, chronic: Limited data available: Infants and Children: IV: 400 mg/kg/dose every 3 weeks resulted in resolution of colitis symptoms during treatment; duration of therapy was unclear (n=5; age range: 6 to 37 months) (Abougergi, 2011; Leung, 1991; McFarland, 2000)

Dermatomyositis, refractory: Limited data available: Children: IV: 1000 mg/kg/dose once daily for 2 days; **Note:** If maintenance therapy is required, the dose and frequency should be based on clinical response and doses should not exceed 2000 mg/kg per treatment course (Feasby, 2007).

Guillain-Barré syndrome: Various regimens have been used: Limited data available: Children: IV: 1000 mg/kg/dose once daily for 2 days (Feasby, 2007; Korinthenberg, 2005) **or** 400 mg/kg/dose once daily for 5 days (El-Bayoumi 2011; Korinthenberg, 2005)

Hematopoietic cell transplantation (HCT) with hypogammaglobulinemia (IgG <400 mg/dL), prevention of bacterial infection (Tomblyn, 2009): **Note:** Increase dose or frequency to maintain IgG concentration >400 mg/dL.

Within first 100 days after HCT:

Infants and Children (Allogeneic HCT recipients): IV: 400 mg/kg/dose once monthly

Adolescents: IV: 500 mg/kg/dose once weekly

>100 days after HCT: Infants, Children, and Adolescents: IV: 500 mg/kg/dose every 3 to 4 weeks

Hepatitis A, prophylaxis: Infants, Children, and Adolescents: **Note:** Hepatitis A vaccine preferred for patients 12 months to 40 years (CDC, 2007): GamaSTAN S/D: **Note:** In adults, total dose volumes >10 mL should be split into multiple injections given at different sites; in pediatric patients, consider splitting doses <10 mL based on patient size.

Pre-exposure prophylaxis upon travel into endemic areas:

Anticipated duration of risk <3 months: IM:0.02 **mL**/kg/dose as a single dose

Anticipated duration of risk ≥3 months: IM:0.06 **mL**/kg/dose once every 4 to 6 months if exposure continues

Postexposure prophylaxis: IM: 0.02 **mL**/kg/dose as a single dose given within 14 days of exposure and prior to manifestation of disease; not needed if at least 1 dose of hepatitis A vaccine was given at ≥1 month before exposure (CDC, 2006)

HIV infection (DHHS [pediatric], 2013): Infants and Children:

Primary prophylaxis for serious bacterial infection in patients with hypogammaglobulinemia (IgG <400 mg/dL): IV: 400 mg/kg/dose every 2 to 4 weeks

Secondary prophylaxis for invasive bacterial infections: Should only be used if subsequent infections are frequent severe infections (>2 infections during a 1-year period): IV: 400 mg/kg/dose every 2 to 4 weeks

Immune thrombocytopenia (ITP):

General dosing: **Note:** Dosing regimens variable, consult product specific information if available: Infants, Children, and Adolescents:

Acute therapy: IV: 400 to 1000 mg/kg/dose once daily for 2 to 5 consecutive days for a total cumulative dose of 2000 mg/kg; in some cases, cumulative doses up to 3000 mg/kg have been used

Chronic therapy: IV: 400 to 1000 mg/kg/dose every 3 to 6 weeks based on clinical response and platelet count

Manufacturer's labeling:

Carimune NF: Infants, Children, and Adolescents:

Acute therapy: IV: 400 mg/kg/dose once daily for 2 to 5 days to maintain platelet count ≥30,000/mm^3 and/or to control significant bleeding

Chronic therapy: IV: 400 mg/kg/dose as a single infusion; may increase to 800 to 1000 mg/kg/dose to maintain platelet count ≥30,000/mm^3 and/or to control significant bleeding

Gammaked: Infants, Children, and Adolescents: Acute therapy: IV: 400 to 1000 mg/kg/dose once daily for 2 to 5 consecutive days for a total cumulative dose of 2000 mg/kg; if an adequate platelet response is observed after the initial 1000 mg/kg/dose, then the subsequent dose may be held

Gamunex-C: Infants, Children, and Adolescents: Acute or chronic therapy: IV: 1000 mg/kg/dose once daily for 1 to 2 days based on patient response and/or platelet response or for fluid-restricted patients or other conditions sensitive to volume: 400 mg/kg once daily for 5 days

Privigen: Adolescents ≥15 years: Chronic therapy: IV: 1000 mg/kg/dose once daily for 2 days

Kawasaki disease: Infants and Children: IV: 2000 mg/kg as a single dose within 10 days of disease onset; must be used in combination with aspirin; if signs and symptoms persist ≥36 hours after completion of the infusion, retreatment with a second 2000 mg/kg infusion should be considered (Newburger, 2004)

Measles, prophylaxis:

Pre-exposure prophylaxis (eg, during an outbreak, travel to endemic area):

Manufacturer's labeling: Patients with primary humoral immunodeficiency:

IV: Gammaked, Gamunex-C (Infants, Children, and Adolescents), Octagam (Children and Adolescents, 6 to 16 years): ≥400 mg/kg/dose immediately before expected exposure; **Note:** Should only administer to patients whose routine dose is <400 mg/kg/dose.

SubQ infusion: Hizentra: Children ≥2 years and Adolescents:

Weekly dosing: ≥200 mg/kg/dose once weekly for 2 consecutive weeks

Biweekly dosing: ≥400 mg/kg for 1 dose

Alternate dosing: ACIP recommendations (CDC, 2013): Immunocompromised patients: Infants, Children, and Adolescents:

IV: ≥400 mg/kg/dose within 3 weeks before anticipated exposure

SubQ: 200 mg/kg/dose once weekly for 2 consecutive weeks prior to anticipated exposure (CDC, 2013); **Note:** Not all immune globulin preparations may be administered by the SubQ route; Hizentra is the only product currently approved for this indication that may be administered SubQ; consult product labeling for additional information as market availability may change

Postexposure prophylaxis:
Manufacturer's labeling: Patients with primary humoral immunodeficiency:
IV: Gammaked, Gamunex-C (Infants, Children, and Adolescents), Octgam (Children and Adolescent, 6 to 16 years): 400 mg/kg/dose administered as soon as possible after exposure
SubQ infusion: Hizentra: Children ≥2 years and Adolescents:
Weekly dosing: ≥200 mg/kg/dose as soon as possible following exposure
Biweekly dosing: ≥400 mg/kg as soon as possible following exposure
Alternate dosing: ACIP guidelines (CDC, 2013): Any person without evidence of measles immunity: Infants, Children, and Adolescents:
IM: 0.5 **mL**/kg/dose; maximum dose: 15 mL within 6 days of exposure; in adults, doses >10 mL should be split into multiple injections and administered at different sites; in pediatric patients, may also split doses <10 mL based on patient size. **Note:** Not all immune globulin preparations may be administered by the IM route; of the products currently available on the market, GamaSTAN S/D may be given IM; consult product labeling for additional information as market availability may change. GamaSTAN S/D manufacturer labeling suggests a lower IM dose of 0.25 **mL**/kg; however, this dosing was based on previous immune globulin donor potency concentrations; recent data indicates that potency from current donor populations has decreased (ie, measles immunity now from vaccinations instead of immunity from disease) requiring a higher IM immune globulin dose (0.5 **mL**/kg) in all patients without evidence of measles immunity to ensure adequate serum titers.
IV: 400 mg/kg/dose within 6 days of exposure

Multiple sclerosis (relapsing-remitting, when other therapies cannot be used): Limited data available: Children and Adolescents: Dosage regimen variable; optimal dose not established: IV: 1000 mg/kg/dose once monthly, with or without an induction of 400 mg/kg/day for 5 days (Feasby, 2007)

Myasthenia gravis, severe exacerbation: Limited data available: Children: IV: 400 to 1000 mg/kg/dose once daily over 2 to 5 days for a total dose of 2000 mg/kg; if additional therapy required, dose should be based on clinical response and titrated to minimum effective dose (Feasby, 2007)

Myocarditis, acute: Limited data available: Infants, Children, and Adolescents: IV: 2000 mg/kg as a single dose. A cohort study of 21 children showed improvement in LVF recovery and survival at 1 year as compared to untreated historical cohort (Drucker, 1994); efficacy results are variable (English, 2004; Hia, 2004; Klugman, 2010); the largest data analysis did not show clear clinical benefit nor positive impact on survival (Klugman, 2010)

Primary immunodeficiency disorders: Adjust dose/frequency based on desired IgG concentration and clinical response; a trough IgG concentration of ≥500 mg/dL has been recommended by some experts (Bonilla, 2005); consult product specific labeling for appropriate age groups.
IV:
General dosing: Infants, Children, and Adolescents: 200 to 800 mg/kg/dose every 3 to 4 weeks
Manufacturer's labeling:
Carimune NF: Infants, Children, and Adolescents: 400 to 800 mg/kg/dose every 3 to 4 weeks
Gammagard Liquid, Gammagard S/D (Children ≥2 years and Adolescents), Gammaked, Gamunex-C (Infants, Children, and Adolescents), Octagam (Children and Adolescents 6 to 16 years): 300 to 600 mg/kg/dose every 3 to 4 weeks
Bivigam: Children ≥6 years and Adolescents: 300 to 800 mg/kg/dose every 3 to 4 weeks
Privigen: Children ≥3 years and Adolescents: 200 to 800 mg/kg/dose every 3 to 4 weeks
SubQ infusion:
Gammagard Liquid: Children ≥ 2 years and Adolescents: Begin 1 week after last IV dose. Use the following equation to calculate initial dose:
Initial weekly dose: Dose (grams) = (1.37 x IV dose [grams]) divided by (IV dose interval [weeks]); **Note:** For subsequent doses, refer to product labeling.
Hizentra: Children ≥2 years and Adolescents: For weekly dosing, begin 1 week after last IV infusion. For biweekly dosing, begin 1 or 2 weeks after last IV infusion or 1 week after the last Hizentra weekly infusion. **Note:** Patient should have received an IV immune globulin routinely for at least 3 months before switching to SubQ. Use the following equation to calculate initial dose:
Initial **weekly** dose: Dose (grams) = (Previous IV dose [grams]) divided by (IV dose interval [weeks]) then multiply by 1.53; **Note:** To convert the dose (in grams) to mL, multiply the calculated dose (in grams) by 5.
Initial **biweekly** dose: Dose (grams) = Multiply the calculated weekly dose by 2
Note: For subsequent doses refer to product labeling.

Rubella, prophylaxis during pregnancy (postexposure): GamaSTAN S/D: Adolescents: IM: 0.55 **mL**/kg/dose as a single dose within 72 hours of exposure (Watson, 1998); **Note:** Not recommended for routine use; may reduce, but not eliminate, risk for rubella. In adults, total dose volumes >10 mL should be split into multiple injections given at different sites.

Stevens-Johnson syndrome (SJS)/toxic epidermal necrolysis (TEN): Limited data available: Infants, Children, and Adolescents: IV: Usual dose: 1500 to 2000 mg/kg total dose as a single dose or divided over 2 to 4 days; dosing based on retrospective reviews and case reports; efficacy results are variable (Koh, 2010; Morci 2000; Tristani-Firouzi, 2002)

Varicella-zoster, postexposure prophylaxis (independent of HIV-status): Infants, Children, and Adolescents: **Note:** Use only if varicella-zoster immune globulin is unavailable.
IV: 400 mg/kg as a single infusion as soon as possible and within 10 days of exposure; ideally within 96 hours of exposure (DHHS [pediatric], 2013; *Red Book* [AAP], 2012)
IM: GamaSTAN S/D: 0.6 to 1.2 **mL**/kg/dose as a single dose within 72 hours of exposure; **Note:** In adults, injections >10 mL should be split into multiple injections given at different sites; in pediatric patients, consider splitting doses <10 mL based on patient size.

Adult:

B-cell chronic lymphocytic leukemia (CLL): Gammagard S/D: IV: 400 mg/kg/dose every 3 to 4 weeks

Chronic inflammatory demyelinating polyneuropathy (CIDP): Gammaked, Gammunex-C: IV: Loading dose: 2000 mg/kg (given in divided doses over 2 to 4 consecutive days); Maintenance: 1000 mg/kg every 3 weeks. Alternatively, administer 500 mg/kg/day for 2 consecutive days every 3 weeks.

Hepatitis A: GamaSTAN S/D: IM:
Preexposure prophylaxis upon travel into endemic areas (hepatitis A vaccine preferred):
0.02 **mL**/kg for anticipated risk of exposure <3 months

0.06 **mL**/kg for anticipated risk of exposure ≥3 months; repeat every 4 to 6 months.

Postexposure prophylaxis: 0.02 **mL**/kg given within 14 days of exposure and/or prior to manifestation of disease; not needed if at least 1 dose of hepatitis A vaccine was given at ≥1 month before exposure

Immunoglobulin deficiency: GamaSTAN S/D: IM: 0.66 **mL**/kg (minimum dose should be 100 mg/kg) every 3 to 4 weeks. Administer a double dose at onset of therapy; some patients may require more frequent injections.

Immune thrombocytopenia (ITP):

Carimune NF: IV: Initial: 400 mg/kg/day for 2 to 5 days; Maintenance: 400 mg/kg as needed to maintain platelet count ≥30,000/mm^3 and/or to control significant bleeding; may increase dose if needed (range: 800 to 1000 mg/kg)

Gammagard S/D: IV: 1000 mg/kg; up to 3 additional doses may be given based on patient response and/or platelet count. **Note:** Additional doses should be given on alternate days.

Gammaked, Gamunex-C: IV: 1000 mg/kg/day for 2 consecutive days (second dose may be withheld if adequate platelet response in 24 hours) **or** 400 mg/kg once daily for 5 consecutive days

Gammaplex, Privigen: IV: 1000 mg/kg/day for 2 consecutive days

Measles:

GamaSTAN S/D: IM:

Immunocompetent: 0.25 **mL**/kg given within 6 days of exposure

Postexposure prophylaxis, any nonimmune person: 0.5 **mL**/kg (maximum dose: 15 **mL**) within 6 days of exposure (CDC, 2013)

Gammaked, Gamunex-C, Octagam: IV:

Prophylaxis in patients with primary humoral immunodeficiency (**ONLY** if routine dose is <400 mg/kg): ≥400 mg/kg immediately before expected exposure

Treatment in patients with primary immunodeficiency: 400 mg/kg administered as soon as possible after exposure

Postexposure prophylaxis, any nonimmune person: 400 mg/kg within 6 days of exposure (CDC, 2013)

Hizentra: SubQ infusion: Measles exposure in patients with primary humoral immunodeficiency: Weekly dose: ≥200 mg/kg for 2 consecutive weeks for patients at risk of measles exposure (eg, during an outbreak; travel to endemic area). Biweekly dose: ≥400 mg/kg single infusion. In patients who have been exposed to measles, administer the minimum dose as soon as possible following exposure.

ACIP recommendations: The Advisory Committee on Immunization Practices (ACIP) recommends postexposure prophylaxis with immune globulin (IG) to any nonimmune person exposed to measles. The following patient groups are at risk for severe measles complications and should receive IG therapy: Infants <12 months of age, pregnant women without evidence of immunity; severely compromised persons (eg, persons with severe primary immunodeficiency; some bone marrow transplant patients; some ALL patients; and some patients with AIDS or HIV infection [refer to guidelines for additional details]). IGIM is recommended for infants <12 months of age. IGIV is recommended for pregnant women and immunocompromised persons. Although prophylaxis may be given to any nonimmune person, priority should be given to those at greatest risk for measles complications and also to persons exposed in settings with intense, prolonged, close contact (eg, households, daycare centers, classrooms). Following IG administration, any nonimmune person should then receive the measles mumps and rubella (MMR) vaccine if the person is ≥12 months of age at the time of vaccine administration and the vaccine is not otherwise contraindicated. MMR should not be given until 6 months following IGIM or 8 months following IGIV administration. If a person is already receiving IGIV therapy, a dose of 400 mg/kg IV within 3 weeks prior to exposure (or 200 mg/kg SubQ for 2 consecutive weeks prior to exposure if previously on SubQ therapy) should be sufficient to prevent measles infection. IG therapy is not indicated for any person who already received one dose of a measles-containing vaccine at ≥12 months of age unless they are severely immunocompromised (CDC, 2013).

Multifocal motor neuropathy: Gammagard Liquid: IV: 500 to 2400 mg/kg/month based upon response

Primary humoral immunodeficiency disorders:

IV infusion dosing:

Bivigam, Gammaplex: IV: 300 to 800 mg/kg every 3 to 4 weeks; dose adjusted based on monitored trough serum IgG concentrations and clinical response

Carimune NF: IV: 400 to 800 mg/kg every 3 to 4 weeks

Flebogamma DIF, Gammagard Liquid, Gammagard S/D, Gammaked, Gamunex-C, Octagam: IV: 300 to 600 mg/kg every 3 to 4 weeks; dose adjusted based on monitored trough serum IgG concentrations and clinical response

Privigen: IV: 200 to 800 mg/kg every 3 to 4 weeks; dose adjusted based on monitored trough serum IgG concentrations and clinical response

Switching to weekly subcutaneous infusion dosing:

Gammagard Liquid, Gammaked, Gamunex-C: SubQ infusion: Begin 1 week after last IV dose. Use the following equation to calculate initial dose:

Initial weekly dose (g) = (1.37 x IGIV dose [g]) divided by (IV dose interval [weeks])

Note: For subsequent dose adjustments, refer to product labeling.

Hizentra: SubQ infusion: For weekly dosing, begin 1 week after last IV infusion. For biweekly dosing, begin 1 or 2 weeks after last IV infusion or 1 week after the last Hizentra weekly infusion. **Note:** Patient should have received an IV immune globulin routinely for at least 3 months before switching to SubQ. Use the following equation to calculate initial weekly dose:

Initial weekly dose (g) = (Previous IGIV dose [g]) divided by (IV dose interval [eg, 3 or 4 weeks]) then multiply by 1.53. To convert the dose (in g) to mL, multiply the calculated dose (in g) by 5.

Initial biweekly dose (g) = Multiply the calculated weekly dose by 2.

Note: For subsequent dose adjustments, refer to product labeling.

Rubella: GamaSTAN S/D: IM: Prophylaxis during pregnancy: 0.55 **mL**/kg

Varicella: GamaSTAN S/D: IM: Prophylaxis: 0.6 to 1.2 **mL**/kg (varicella zoster immune globulin preferred) within 72 hours of exposure

Preparation for Administration Dilution is dependent upon the manufacturer and brand. Gently swirl; do not shake; avoid foaming. Do not heat. Do not mix products from different manufacturers together. Discard unused portion of vials.

Bivigam: Dilution is not recommended.

Carimune NF: In a sterile laminar air flow environment, reconstitute with NS, D_5W, or SWFI. Complete dissolution may take up to 20 minutes. Begin infusion within 24 hours.

Flebogamma DIF: Dilution is not recommended.

Gammagard Liquid: May dilute in D_5W only.

Gammagard S/D: Reconstitute with SWFI.

Gammaked: May dilute in D_5W only.

Gamunex-C: May dilute in D_5W only.

Privigen: If necessary to further dilute, D_5W may be used.

Administration Note: If plasmapheresis employed for treatment of condition, administer immune globulin **after** completion of plasmapheresis session.

IV: Infuse over 2 to 24 hours with initial infusion administered slowly and titrated as tolerated; administer in separate infusion line from other medications; if using primary line, flush with NS or D_5W (product specific; consult product prescribing information) prior to administration. Decrease dose, rate, and/or concentration of infusion in patients who may be at risk of renal failure. Decreasing the rate or stopping the infusion may help relieve some adverse effects (flushing, changes in pulse rate, changes in blood pressure). Epinephrine should be available during administration.

For initial treatment or in the elderly, a lower concentration and/or a slower rate of infusion should be used. Initial rate of administration and titration is specific to each IVIG product. Refrigerated product should be warmed to room temperature prior to infusion. Some products require filtration; refer to individual product labeling. Antecubital veins should be used, especially with concentrations ≥10% to prevent injection site discomfort.

Bivigam 10%: Primary humoral immunodeficiency: Initial (first 10 minutes): 0.5 mg/kg/minute (0.3 **mL**/kg/**hour**); Maintenance: Increase every 20 minutes (if tolerated) by 0.8 mg/kg/minute (0.48 **mL**/kg/**hour**) up to 6 mg/kg/minute (3.6 **mL**/kg/**hour**)

Carimune NF: Initial: 0.5 mg/kg/minute; Maintenance: Increase in 30 minutes (if tolerated) to 1 mg/kg/minute, if tolerated after 30 minutes, may increase gradually up to 3 mg/kg/minute; rate in mL/kg/hour varies based on concentration; refer to product labeling

Flebogamma DIF 10%: Primary humoral immunodeficiency: Initial: 1 mg/kg/minute (0.6 **mL**/kg/**hour**); Maintenance: Increase slowly (if tolerated) up to 8 mg/kg/minute (4.8 **mL**/kg/**hour**)

Gammagard Liquid 10%:

Multifocal motor neuropathy (MMN): Initial: 0.8 mg/kg/minute (0.5 **mL**/kg/**hour**); Maintenance: Increase gradually (if tolerated) up to 9 mg/kg/minute (5.4 **mL**/kg/**hour**)

Primary humoral immunodeficiency: Initial (first 30 minutes): 0.8 mg/kg/minute (0.5 **mL**/kg/**hour**); Maintenance: Increase every 30 minutes (if tolerated) up to 8 mg/kg/minute (5 **mL**/kg/**hour**)

Gammagard S/D: 5% solution: Initial: 0.5 **mL**/kg/**hour**; may increase (if tolerated) to a maximum rate of 4 **mL**/kg/**hour**. If 5% solution is tolerated at maximum rate, may administer 10% solution with an initial rate of 0.5 **mL**/kg/**hour**; may increase (if tolerated) to a maximum rate of 8 **mL**/kg/**hour**.

Gammaked 10%:

CIDP: Initial (first 30 minutes): 2 mg/kg/minute (1.2 **mL**/kg/**hour**); Maintenance: Increase gradually (if tolerated) up to 8 mg/kg/minute (4.8 **mL**/kg/**hour**)

Primary humoral immunodeficiency or ITP: Initial (first 30 minutes): 1 mg/kg/minute (0.6 **mL**/kg/**hour**); Maintenance: Increase gradually (if tolerated) up to 8 mg/kg/minute (4.8 **mL**/kg/**hour**)

Gammaplex 5%: Primary humoral immunodeficiency or ITP: Initial (first 15 minutes): 0.5 mg/kg/minute (0.6 **mL**/kg/**hour**); Maintenance: Increase every 15 minutes (if tolerated) up to 4 mg/kg/minute (4.8 **mL**/kg/**hour**)

Gamunex-C 10%:

CIDP: Initial (first 30 minutes): 2 mg/kg/minute (1.2 **mL**/kg/**hour**); Maintenance: Increase gradually (if tolerated) up to 8 mg/kg/minute (4.8 **mL**/kg/**hour**)

Primary humoral immunodeficiency or ITP: Initial (first 30 minutes): 1 mg/kg/minute (0.6 **mL**/kg/**hour**); Maintenance: Increase gradually (if tolerated) up to 8 mg/kg/minute (4.8 **mL**/kg/**hour**)

Octagam 5%: Primary humoral immunodeficiency: Initial (first 30 minutes): 0.5 mg/kg/minute (0.6 **mL**/kg/**hour**); Maintenance: Double infusion rate (if tolerated) every 30 minutes up to a maximum rate of <3.33 mg/kg/minute (4.2 **mL**/kg/**hour**)

Privigen 10%:

ITP: Initial: 0.5 mg/kg/minute (0.3 **mL**/kg/**hour**); Maintenance: Increase gradually (if tolerated) up to 4 mg/kg/minute (2.4 **mL**/kg/**hour**)

Primary humoral immunodeficiency: Initial: 0.5 mg/kg/minute (0.3 **mL**/kg/**hour**); Maintenance: Increase gradually (if tolerated) up to 8 mg/kg/minute (4.8 **mL**/kg/**hour**)

IM: Administer IM in the anterolateral aspects of the upper thigh or deltoid muscle of the upper arm. Avoid gluteal region due to risk of injury to sciatic nerve. Divide doses >10 mL (adult) and inject in multiple sites; in pediatric patients, consider splitting doses <10 mL based on patient size.

SubQ infusion: Initial dose should be administered in a healthcare setting capable of providing monitoring and treatment in the event of hypersensitivity. Using aseptic technique, follow the infusion device manufacturer's instructions for filling the reservoir and preparing the pump. Remove air from administration set and needle by priming. Appropriate injection sites include the abdomen, thigh, upper arm, lateral hip, and/or lower back; dose may be infused into multiple sites (spaced ≥2 inches apart) simultaneously. After administration sites are clean and dry, attach infusion device (eg, primed needle and administration set); ensure blood vessel has not been inadvertently accessed; if blood is present, remove and discard needle and tubing; repeat process using a new needle and tubing and different injection site. Repeat for each administration site; deliver the dose following instructions for the infusion device. Rotate the site(s) weekly. Treatment may be transitioned to the home/home care setting in the absence of adverse reactions.

Gammagard Liquid:

Injection sites: ≤8 simultaneous injection sites

Recommended infusion rate:

<40 kg (<88 lbs): Initial infusion: 15 mL/hour per injection site; subsequent infusions: 15 to 20 mL/hour per injection site; maximum: 160 mL/hour for all simultaneous sites combined

≥40 kg (≥88 lbs): Initial infusion: 20 mL/hour per injection site; subsequent infusions: 20 to 30 mL/hour per injection site; maximum: 240 mL/hour for all simultaneous sites combined

Maximum infusion volume:

<40 kg (<88 lbs): 20 mL per injection site

≥40 kg (≥88 lbs): 30 mL per injection site

Gammaked, Gamunex-C:

Injection sites: ≤8 simultaneous injection sites

Recommended infusion rate: 20 mL/hour per injection site

Hizentra:

Injection sites:

Weekly dosing: ≤4 simultaneous injection sites **or** ≤12 sites consecutively per infusion

Biweekly dosing: Increase the number of injection sites as needed

Maximum infusion rate: First infusion: 15 mL/hour per injection site; subsequent infusions: 25 mL/hour per injection site

Maximum infusion volume: First 4 infusions: 15 mL per injection site; subsequent infusions: 20 mL per injection site; maximum: 25 mL per site as tolerated

Monitoring Parameters Renal function, urine output, IgG concentrations, hemoglobin and hematocrit, platelets (in patients with ITP); infusion- or injection-related adverse reactions, anaphylaxis, signs and symptoms of hemolysis; blood viscosity (in patients at risk for hyperviscosity); presence of antineutrophil antibodies (if TRALI is suspected); volume status; neurologic symptoms (if aseptic meningitis syndrome suspected); clinical response (as defined by disease state)

For patients at high risk of hemolysis (dose ≥2000 mg/kg, given as a single dose or divided over several days, and non-O blood type): Hemoglobin or hematocrit prior to and 36 to 96 hours postinfusion

SubQ infusion: Monitor IgG trough levels every 2 to 3 months before/after conversion from IV; subcutaneous infusions provide more constant IgG levels than usual IV immune globulin treatments

Test Interactions Octagam 5% and Octagam 10% contain maltose. Falsely elevated blood glucose levels may occur when glucose monitoring devices and test strips utilizing the glucose dehydrogenase pyrroloquinolinequinone (GDH-PQQ) based methods are used. Glucose monitoring devices and test strips which utilize the glucose-specific method are recommended. Passively transferred antibodies may yield false-positive serologic testing results; may yield false-positive direct and indirect Coombs' test. Skin testing should not be performed with GamaSTAN S/D because local chemical irritation can occur and be misinterpreted as a positive reaction.

Additional Information

IM: When administering immune globulin for hepatitis A prophylaxis, use should be considered for the following close contacts of persons with confirmed hepatitis A: Unvaccinated household and sexual contacts, persons who have shared illicit drugs, regular babysitters, staff and attendees of child care centers, food handlers within the same establishment (CDC, 2006).

DIF: Dual inactivation plus nanofiltration

NF: Nanofiltered

S/D: Solvent detergent treated

Octagam contains sodium 30 mmol/L.

IgA content:

Bivigam: ≤200 mcg/mL

Carimune NF: Manufacturer's labeling: Trace amounts; others have reported 1000-2000 mcg/mL in a 6% solution (Siegel, 2011)

Flebogamma 5% DIF: <50 mcg/mL

Flebogamma 10% DIF: <100 mcg/mL

Gammagard Liquid: 37 mcg/mL

Gammagard S/D 5% solution: <1 mcg/mL or <2.2 mcg/mL (product dependent) (see **Note**)

Gammaked: 46 mcg/mL

Gammaplex: <10 mcg/mL

Gamunex-C: 46 mcg/mL

Hizentra: ≤50 mcg/mL

Octagam: ≤200 mcg/mL

Privigen: ≤25 mcg/mL

Note: Manufacturer has discontinued Gammagard S/D 5% solution; however, the lower IgA product will remain available by special request for patients with known reaction to IgA or IgA deficiency with antibodies.

Dosage Forms Considerations

Carimune NF may contain a significant amount of sodium and also contains sucrose.

Gammagard S/D may contain a significant amount of sodium and also contains glucose.

Octagam contains maltose.

Hyqvia Kit is supplied with a Hyaluronidase (Human Recombinant) component intended for injection prior to Immune Globulin administration to improve dispersion and absorption of the Immune Globulin.

Dosage Forms Excipient information presented when available (limited, particularly for generics); consult specific product labeling. [DSC] = Discontinued product

Injectable, Intramuscular [preservative free]:

GamaSTAN S/D: 15% to 18% [150 to 180 mg/mL] (2 mL, 10 mL)

Kit, Subcutaneous:

Hyqvia: 2.5 g/25 mL, 5 g/50 mL, 10 g/100 mL, 20 g/200 mL, 30 g/300 mL [contains albumin human, edetate disodium dihydrate, mouse protein (murine) (hamster)]

Solution, Injection [preservative free]:

Gammagard: 1 g/10 mL (10 mL); 2.5 g/25 mL (25 mL); 5 g/50 mL (50 mL); 10 g/100 mL (100 mL); 20 g/200 mL (200 mL); 30 g/300 mL (300 mL) [latex free]

Gammaked: 1 g/10 mL (10 mL); 2.5 g/25 mL (25 mL); 5 g/50 mL (50 mL); 10 g/100 mL (100 mL); 20 g/200 mL (200 mL) [latex free]

Gamunex-C: 1 g/10 mL (10 mL); 2.5 g/25 mL (25 mL); 5 g/50 mL (50 mL); 10 g/100 mL (100 mL); 20 g/200 mL (200 mL); 40 g/400 mL (400 mL) [latex free]

Solution, Intravenous [preservative free]:

Bivigam: 5 g/50 mL (50 mL); 10 g/100 mL (100 mL) [sugar free; contains polysorbate 80]

Flebogamma: 0.5 g/10 mL (10 mL [DSC])

Flebogamma DIF: 0.5 g/10 mL (10 mL); 2.5 g/50 mL (50 mL); 5 g/50 mL (50 mL); 5 g/100 mL (100 mL); 10 g/100 mL (100 mL); 10 g/200 mL (200 mL); 20 g/200 mL (200 mL); 20 g/400 mL (400 mL) [contains polyethylene glycol]

Gammaplex: 2.5 g/50 mL (50 mL); 5 g/100 mL (100 mL); 10 g/200 mL (200 mL); 20 g/400 mL (400 mL) [contains polysorbate 80]

Octagam: 1 g/20 mL (20 mL); 2 g/20 mL (20 mL); 2.5 g/50 mL (50 mL); 5 g/50 mL (50 mL); 5 g/100 mL (100 mL); 10 g/100 mL (100 mL); 10 g/200 mL (200 mL); 20 g/200 mL (200 mL); 25 g/500 mL (500 mL) [sucrose free]

Privigen: 5 g/50 mL (50 mL); 10 g/100 mL (100 mL); 20 g/200 mL (200 mL); 40 g/400 mL (400 mL)

Solution, Subcutaneous [preservative free]:

Hizentra: 1 g/5 mL (5 mL); 2 g/10 mL (10 mL); 4 g/20 mL (20 mL); 10 g/50 mL (50 mL) [contains polysorbate 80]

Solution Reconstituted, Intravenous:

Gammagard S/D: 2.5 g (1 ea [DSC]); 5 g (1 ea [DSC]); 10 g (1 ea [DSC])

Solution Reconstituted, Intravenous [preservative free]:

Carimune NF: 3 g (1 ea [DSC]); 6 g (1 ea); 12 g (1 ea)

Gammagard S/D Less IgA: 5 g (1 ea); 10 g (1 ea)

- ◆ **Immune Globulin Subcutaneous (Human)** *see* Immune Globulin *on page 1089*
- ◆ **Immune Serum Globulin** *see* Immune Globulin *on page 1089*
- ◆ **Immunine VH (Can)** *see* Factor IX (Human) *on page 838*
- ◆ **Imodium® (Can)** *see* Loperamide *on page 1288*
- ◆ **Imodium A-D [OTC]** *see* Loperamide *on page 1288*
- ◆ **Imogam Rabies-HT** *see* Rabies Immune Globulin (Human) *on page 1830*
- ◆ **Imogam Rabies Pasteurized (Can)** *see* Rabies Immune Globulin (Human) *on page 1830*
- ◆ **Imovax Polio (Can)** *see* Poliovirus Vaccine (Inactivated) *on page 1721*
- ◆ **Imovax Rabies** *see* Rabies Vaccine *on page 1832*
- ◆ **Impril (Can)** *see* Imipramine *on page 1086*
- ◆ **Imuran** *see* AzaTHIOprine *on page 236*
- ◆ **Inactivated Influenza Vaccine, Quadrivalent** *see* Influenza Virus Vaccine (Inactivated) *on page 1108*
- ◆ **Inactivated Influenza Vaccine, Trivalent** *see* Influenza Virus Vaccine (Inactivated) *on page 1108*
- ◆ **Increlex** *see* Mecasermin *on page 1334*

◆ **Inderal (Can)** *see* Propranolol *on page 1789*
◆ **Inderal XL** *see* Propranolol *on page 1789*
◆ **Inderal LA** *see* Propranolol *on page 1789*

Indinavir (in DIN a veer)

Medication Safety Issues

Sound-alike/look-alike issues:

Indinavir may be confused with Denavir

High alert medication:

This medication is in a class the Institute for Safe Medication Practices (ISMP) includes among its list of drug classes that have a heightened risk of causing significant patient harm when used in error.

Related Information

Adult and Adolescent HIV *on page 2392*
Oral Medications That Should Not Be Crushed or Altered *on page 2476*
Pediatric HIV *on page 2380*
Perinatal HIV *on page 2400*

Brand Names: US Crixivan

Brand Names: Canada Crixivan

Therapeutic Category Antiretroviral Agent; HIV Agents (Anti-HIV Agents); Protease Inhibitor

Generic Availability (US) No

Use Treatment of HIV infection in combination with other antiretroviral agents; **Note:** HIV regimens consisting of **three** antiretroviral agents are strongly recommended (FDA approved in adults)

Pregnancy Risk Factor C

Pregnancy Considerations Adverse events were observed in some animal reproduction studies. Placental passage in humans is minimal. No increased risk of overall birth defects has been observed according to data collected by the antiretroviral pregnancy registry. A small increased risk of preterm birth has been associated with maternal use of protease inhibitor-based combination antiretroviral (ARV) therapy during pregnancy; however, the benefits of use generally outweigh this risk and protease inhibitors (PIs) should not be withheld if otherwise recommended. Hyperglycemia, new onset of diabetes mellitus, or diabetic ketoacidosis have been reported with PIs; it is not clear if pregnancy increases this risk. Hyperbilirubinemia may occur in neonates following *in utero* exposure to indinavir. Plasma concentrations of unboosted indinavir are decreased during pregnancy. Until optimal dosing during pregnancy has been established, the manufacturer does not recommend indinavir use in pregnant patients. The DHHS Perinatal HIV Guidelines do not recommend indinavir for initial therapy in antiretroviral-naïve pregnant women due to concerns regarding maternal kidney stones or neonatal hyperbilirubinemia; if needed, must be used in combination with low-dose ritonavir boosting during pregnancy.

Regardless of CD4 count or HIV RNA copy number, all HIV-infected pregnant women should receive a combination antiretroviral ARV drug regimen. A combination of antepartum, intrapartum, and infant ARV prophylaxis is recommended. ARV therapy should be started as soon as possible in women with symptomatic infection. Although earlier initiation may be more effective in reducing the perinatal transmission of HIV, initiation may be delayed until after 12 weeks gestation in women who do not require immediate treatment after careful consideration of maternal conditions (eg, nausea and vomiting) and the potential risks of first trimester fetal exposure for specific agents. A scheduled cesarean delivery at 38 weeks gestation is recommended for all women with HIV RNA >1000 copies/mL or unknown concentrations near delivery in order to decrease transmission. If ARV therapy must be interrupted for <24 hours during the peripartum period, stop then restart all medications simultaneously in order to decrease the chance of developing resistance. Long-term follow-up is recommended for all infants exposed to ARV medications. In couples who want to conceive, the HIV-infected partner should attain maximum viral suppression prior to conception.

Healthcare providers are encouraged to enroll pregnant women exposed to antiretroviral medications in the Antiretroviral Pregnancy Registry (1-800-258-4263 or www.APRegistry.com). Healthcare providers caring for HIV-infected women and their infants may contact the National Perinatal HIV Hotline (888-448-8765) for clinical consultation (HHS [perinatal], 2014).

Breast-Feeding Considerations It is not known if indinavir is excreted into breast milk. Maternal or infant antiretroviral therapy does not completely eliminate the risk of postnatal HIV transmission. In addition, multiclass-resistant virus has been detected in breast-feeding infants despite maternal therapy. Therefore, in the United States, where formula is accessible, affordable, safe, and sustainable, and the risk of infant mortality due to diarrhea and respiratory infections is low, complete avoidance of breast-feeding by HIV-infected women is recommended to decrease potential transmission of HIV (HHS [perinatal], 2014).

Contraindications Hypersensitivity to indinavir or any component of the formulation; concurrent use of alfuzosin, alprazolam, amiodarone, cisapride, ergot alkaloids, lovastatin, midazolam (oral), pimozide, simvastatin, St John's wort, or triazolam; sildenafil (when used for pulmonary artery hypertension [eg, Revatio®])

Warnings/Precautions Because indinavir may cause nephrolithiasis/urolithiasis the drug should be discontinued if signs and symptoms occur. Adequate hydration is recommended. May cause tubulointerstitial nephritis (rare); severe asymptomatic leukocyturia may warrant evaluation. Indinavir has a high potential for drug interactions; concomitant use of indinavir with some drugs may require cautious use, may not be recommended, may require dosage adjustments, or may be contraindicated.

Patients with hepatic insufficiency due to cirrhosis should have dose reduction. Warn patients about fat redistribution that can occur. Indinavir has been associated with hemolytic anemia (discontinue if diagnosed), hepatitis, hyperbilirubinemia, and hyperglycemia (exacerbation or new-onset diabetes).

Patients may develop immune reconstitution syndrome resulting in the occurrence of an inflammatory response to an indolent or residual opportunistic infection during initial HIV treatment or activation of autoimmune disorders (eg, Graves' disease, polymyositis, Guillain-Barré syndrome) later in therapy; further evaluation and treatment may be required.

Use caution in patients with hemophilia; spontaneous bleeding has been reported.

Warnings: Additional Pediatric Considerations Incidence of nephrolithiasis and urolithiasis is higher in children than adults, 29% vs 12.4%, respectively. Indirect hyperbilirubinemia (incidence: ~14%) and elevated serum transaminases may occur. Not recommended for use in neonates due to risk of hyperbilirubinemia and kernicterus (DHHS [pediatric], 2014).

Adverse Reactions

Central nervous system: Dizziness, drowsinesss, fatigue, headache, malaise

Dermatologic: Pruritus, skin rash

Gastrointestinal: Abdominal pain, anorexia, diarrhea, dysgeusia, dyspepsia, gastroesophageal reflux disease, increased appetite, increased serum amylase, nausea, vomiting

Genitourinary: Dysuria

Hematologic & oncologic: Anemia, neutropenia
Hepatic: Hyperbilirubinemia (dose dependent), increased serum transaminases, jaundice
Neuromuscular & skeletal: Back pain, weakness
Renal: Hydronephrosis, nephrolithiasis (including flank pain with/without hematuria; more common in pediatric patients), urolithiasis (including flank pain with/without hematuria; more common in pediatric patients)
Respiratory: Cough
Miscellaneous: Fever
Rare but important or life-threatening: Abdominal distention, alopecia, anaphylactoid reaction, cerebrovascular disease, depression, diabetes mellitus, erythema multiforme, hemolytic anemia, hemorrhage (spontaneous in patients with hemophilia A or B), hepatic failure, immune reconstitution syndrome, increased serum cholesterol, interstitial nephritis (with medullary calcification and cortical atrophy), leukocyturia (severe and asymptomatic), myocardial infarction, pancreatitis, paronychia, periarthritis, pharyngitis, pyelonephritis, redistribution of body fat, renal failure, Stevens-Johnson syndrome, thrombocytopenia, torsades de pointes, upper respiratory tract infection, vasculitis

Drug Interactions

Metabolism/Transport Effects Substrate of CYP2D6 (minor), CYP3A4 (major), P-glycoprotein; **Note:** Assignment of Major/Minor substrate status based on clinically relevant drug interaction potential; **Inhibits** CYP2C19 (weak), CYP2C9 (weak), CYP2D6 (weak), CYP3A4 (strong), UGT1A1

Avoid Concomitant Use

Avoid concomitant use of Indinavir with any of the following: Ado-Trastuzumab Emtansine; Alfuzosin; ALPRAZolam; Amiodarone; Apixaban; Astemizole; Atazanavir; Avanafil; Axitinib; Barnidipine; Bosutinib; Cabozantinib; Ceritinib; Cisapride; Conivaptan; Crizotinib; Dapoxetine; Domperidone; Dronedarone; Eplerenone; Ergot Derivatives; Everolimus; Halofantrine; Ibrutinib; Irinotecan; Isavuconazonium Sulfate; Ivabradine; Lapatinib; Lercanidipine; Lomitapide; Lovastatin; Lurasidone; Macitentan; Midazolam; Naloxegol; Nilotinib; NiMODipine; Nisoldipine; Olaparib; Palbociclib; Pimozide; Ranolazine; Red Yeast Rice; Regorafenib; Rifampin; Rivaroxaban; Salmeterol; Silodosin; Simeprevir; Simvastatin; St Johns Wort; Suvorexant; Tamsulosin; Terfenadine; Ticagrelor; Tipranavir; Tolvaptan; Toremifene; Trabectedin; Triazolam; Ulipristal; Vemurafenib; VinCRIStine (Liposomal); Vorapaxar

Increased Effect/Toxicity

Indinavir may increase the levels/effects of: Ado-Trastuzumab Emtansine; Alfuzosin; Almotriptan; Alosetron; ALPRAZolam; Amiodarone; Apixaban; ARIPiprazole; Astemizole; Atazanavir; AtorvaSTATin; Avanafil; Axitinib; Barnidipine; Bedaquiline; Bortezomib; Bosentan; Bosutinib; Brentuximab Vedotin; Brinzolamide; Budesonide (Nasal); Budesonide (Systemic, Oral Inhalation); Budesonide (Topical); Cabazitaxel; Cabozantinib; Calcium Channel Blockers (Dihydropyridine); Calcium Channel Blockers (Nondihydropyridine); Cannabis; CarBAMazepine; Ceritinib; Cilostazol; Cisapride; Clarithromycin; Colchicine; Conivaptan; Corticosteroids (Orally Inhaled); Corticosteroids (Systemic); Crizotinib; Cyclophosphamide; CycloSPORINE (Systemic); CYP3A4 Substrates; Dapoxetine; Dasatinib; Dienogest; Digoxin; Dofetilide; Domperidone; DOXOrubicin (Conventional); Dronabinol; Dronedarone; Drospirenone; Dutasteride; Eliglustat; Enfuvirtide; Eplerenone; Ergot Derivatives; Erlotinib; Etizolam; Everolimus; FentaNYL; Fesoterodine; Fluticasone (Nasal); Fluticasone (Oral Inhalation); GuanFACINE; Halofantrine; Hydrocodone; Ibrutinib; Idelalisib; Iloperidone; Imatinib; Imidafenacin; Irinotecan; Isavuconazonium Sulfate; Itraconazole; Ivabradine; Ivacaftor; Ixabepilone; Ketoconazole (Systemic); Lacosamide; Lapatinib; Lercanidipine; Levobupivacaine; Levomilnacipran; Lomitapide; Lovastatin; Lumefantrine; Lurasidone; Macitentan; Maraviroc; MedroxyPROGESTERone; Meperidine; MethylPREDNISolone; Midazolam; Mifepristone; Naloxegol; Nefazodone; Nilotinib; NiMODipine; Nisoldipine; Olaparib; Ospemifene; Oxybutynin; OxyCODONE; Palbociclib; Panobinostat; Parecoxib; Paricalcitol; PAZOPanib; Pimecrolimus; Pimozide; PONATinib; Pranlukast; PrednisoLONE (Systemic); PredniSONE; Propafenone; Protease Inhibitors; QUEtiapine; QuiNIDine; Ramelteon; Ranolazine; Red Yeast Rice; Regorafenib; Repaglinide; Retapamulin; Rifabutin; Rilpivirine; Riociguat; Rivaroxaban; RomiDEPsin; Rosuvastatin; Ruxolitinib; Salmeterol; Saxagliptin; Sildenafil; Silodosin; Simeprevir; Simvastatin; SORAfenib; Suvorexant; Tacrolimus (Systemic); Tacrolimus (Topical); Tadalafil; Tamsulosin; Tasimelteon; Temsirolimus; Terfenadine; Tetrahydrocannabinol; Ticagrelor; Tofacitinib; Tolterodine; Tolvaptan; Toremifene; Trabectedin; TraMADol; TraZODone; Triazolam; Tricyclic Antidepressants; Ulipristal; Vardenafil; Vemurafenib; Vilazodone; VinCRIStine (Liposomal); Vorapaxar; Zopiclone; Zuclopenthixol

The levels/effects of Indinavir may be increased by: Atazanavir; Clarithromycin; CycloSPORINE (Systemic); Delavirdine; Enfuvirtide; Etravirine; Itraconazole; Ketoconazole (Systemic); P-glycoprotein/ABCB1 Inhibitors; Simeprevir

Decreased Effect

Indinavir may decrease the levels/effects of: Abacavir; Antidiabetic Agents; Boceprevir; Clarithromycin; Delavirdine; Etravirine; Ifosfamide; Meperidine; Prasugrel; Ticagrelor; Valproic Acid and Derivatives; Zidovudine

The levels/effects of Indinavir may be decreased by: Atovaquone; Boceprevir; Bosentan; CarBAMazepine; CYP3A4 Inducers (Moderate); CYP3A4 Inducers (Strong); Dabrafenib; Deferasirox; Didanosine; Efavirenz; Garlic; H2-Antagonists; Mitotane; Nevirapine; Proton Pump Inhibitors; Rifabutin; Rifampin; Siltuximab; St Johns Wort; Tipranavir; Tocilizumab; Venlafaxine

Food Interactions Indinavir bioavailability may be decreased if taken with food. Meals high in calories, fat, and protein result in a significant decrease in drug levels. Management: Administer with water 1 hour before or 2 hours after a meal. May also be administered with other liquids (eg, skim milk, juice, coffee, tea) or a light meal (eg, toast, corn flakes). Administer around-the-clock to avoid significant fluctuation in serum levels. Drink at least 48 oz of water daily. May be taken with food when administered in combination with ritonavir.

Storage/Stability Medication should be stored at 15°C to 30°C (59°F to 86°F), and used in the original container and the desiccant should remain in the bottle. Capsules are sensitive to moisture.

Mechanism of Action Binds to the site of HIV-1 protease activity and inhibits cleavage of viral Gag-Pol polyprotein precursors into individual functional proteins required for infectious HIV. This results in the formation of immature, noninfectious viral particles.

Pharmacokinetics (Adult data unless noted)

Absorption: Rapid (in the fasted state); presence of food high in calories, fat, and protein significantly decreases the extent of absorption
Protein binding: 60%
Metabolism: Hepatic via CYP3A4 to inactive metabolites; 6 oxidative and 1 glucuronide conjugate metabolites have been identified
Bioavailability: Wide interpatient variability in children: 15% to 50%
Half-life:
Children 4 to 17 years (n=18): 1.1 hours
Adults: 1.8 ± 0.4 hours

Adults with mild to moderate hepatic dysfunction: 2.8 ± 0.5 hours
Time to peak serum concentration: 0.8 ± 0.3 hours
Elimination: 83% in feces as unabsorbed drug and metabolites; ~10% excreted in urine as unchanged drug

Dosing: Usual

Pediatric: **HIV infection, treatment:** Oral: Use in combination with other antiretroviral agents:

Children: Limited data available; optimal dose not established: Ritonavir-boosted: Indinavir 400 mg/m²/dose (maximum: 800 mg) every 12 hour **plus** ritonavir 100 to 125 mg/m²/dose (maximum 100 mg) every 12 hours; in clinical trials, this dose produced AUCs similar to adult exposure of indinavir 800 mg/ritonavir 100 mg twice daily; however, studies report high rates of interindividual variability and toxicity in pediatric patients; several other ritonavir-boosted dosing regimens have been evaluated with supratherapeutic (indinavir 500 mg/m²/dose every 12 hours) and subtherapeutic (indinavir 234 to 250 mg/m²/dose every 12 hours) indinavir serum concentrations reported (DHHS [pediatric], 2014).

Adolescents:

Unboosted: 800 mg/dose every 8 hours (DHHS [adult, 2014)

Ritonavir-boosted: Indinavir 800 mg **plus** ritonavir 100 to 200 mg twice daily (DHHS [adult, pediatric] 2014)

Adult: **HIV infection, treatment:** Oral: **Note:** Use in combination with other antiretroviral agents (DHHS [adult], 2014):

Unboosted: 800 mg/dose every 8 hours

Ritonavir-boosted: Indinavir 800 mg **plus** ritonavir 100 to 200 mg twice daily

Dosing adjustment for concomitant therapy: Adolescents and Adults: The following are manufacturer labeling recommendations for adults and should also be considered in adolescent patients receiving adult dose (DHHS [adult], 2014)

Concomitant therapy with delavirdine, itraconazole, or ketoconazole: Adolescents and Adults: Reduce indinavir dose to 600 mg every 8 hours

Concomitant therapy with efavirenz or nevirapine: Adolescents and Adults: Increase indinavir dose to 1000 mg every 8 hours

Concomitant therapy with lopinavir and ritonavir (Kaletra): Adolescents and Adults: Reduce indinavir dose to 600 mg twice daily

Concomitant therapy with nelfinavir: Adolescents and Adults: Increase indinavir dose to 1200 mg twice daily

Concomitant therapy with rifabutin: Adolescents and Adults: Increase dose of indinavir to 1000 mg every 8 hours and reduce dose of rifabutin to 1/2 the standard dose

Dosing adjustment in renal impairment: There are no dosage adjustments provided in the manufacturer's labeling; has not been studied.

Dosing adjustment in hepatic impairment:

Children: No dosing information is available (DHHS [pediatric], 2014)

Adults:

Mild to moderate hepatic impairment: Decrease to 600 mg every 8 hours

Severe hepatic impairment: There are no dosage adjustments provided in the manufacturer's labeling; has not been studied.

Administration Administer with water on an empty stomach or with a light snack 1 hour before or 2 hours after a meal; may administer with other liquids (ie, skim milk, coffee, tea, juice) or a light snack (ie, dry toast with jelly or cornflakes with skim milk). May administer with food if taken in combination with ritonavir (ie, meal restrictions are not required). If coadministered with didanosine, give at least 1 hour apart on an empty stomach. Administer every 8 hours around-the-clock to avoid significant fluctuation in serum levels.

Monitoring Parameters Note: Monitor CD4 percentage (if <5 years of age) or CD4 count (if ≥5 years of age) at least every 3 to 4 months (DHHS [pediatric], 2014).

Prior to initiation of therapy: Genotypic resistance testing, CD4 and viral load (every 3 to 4 months), CBC with differential, LFTs, BUN, creatinine, electrolytes, glucose, urinalysis (every 6 to 12 months), and assessment of readiness for adherence with medication regimen. At initiation and with any change in treatment regimen: CBC with differential, electrolytes, calcium, phosphate, glucose, LFTs, bilirubin, urinalysis (at initiation), BUN, creatinine, albumin, total protein, lipid panel (at initiation), CD4, and viral load. After 1 to 2 weeks of therapy: Signs of medication toxicity and adherence. After 2 to 4 weeks of therapy: CBC with differential, viral load, signs of medication toxicity, and adherence; then every 3 to 4 months: CBC with differential, electrolytes, glucose, LFTs, bilirubin, BUN, creatinine, CD4, viral load, medication toxicity, and adherence. Every 6 to 12 months: Lipid panel and urinalysis. CD4 monitoring frequency may be decreased to every 6 to 12 months in children who are adherent to therapy if the value is well above the threshold for opportunistic infections, viral suppression is sustained, and the clinical status is stable for more than 2 to 3 years (DHHS [pediatric], 2014). Monitor for growth and development, signs of HIV-specific physical conditions, HIV disease progression, opportunistic infections, kidney stones, or pancreatitis.

Reference Range Trough concentration: ≥0.1 mg/L (DHHS [adult, pediatric], 2014)

Additional Information One study in children 4 to 17 years of age (n=18), adjusted the indinavir dose and dosing interval to maintain trough plasma concentrations. A mean daily dose of 2043 mg/m² was required with 9 of 18 children requiring doses every 6 hours (Fletcher, 2000). Other pediatric studies have also suggested that every 6 hour dosing may be needed in some children (Gatti, 2000) and that a wide range of doses (1250 to 2450 mg/m²/day) may be required (van Rossum, 2000a). However, it should be noted that the higher incidence of renal toxicity observed in children versus adults, may preclude studying higher doses of unboosted indinavir.

Two small studies assessed the use of indinavir in combination with ritonavir. One study used doses of indinavir 500 mg/m²/dose **plus** ritonavir 100 mg/m²/dose twice daily (n=4; 1 to 10 years of age); one patient attained high concentrations of both drugs and developed renal toxicity (van Rossum, 2000). Another study used doses of indinavir 400 mg/m²/dose **plus** ritonavir 125 mg/m²/dose twice daily in children (n=14); AUC and trough concentrations were similar to adults receiving ritonavir boosted doses; however, peak concentrations were slightly decreased (Bergshoeff, 2004). A pediatric clinical trial that used these same doses demonstrated good virologic efficacy; however, 4 of 21 patients developed nephrolithiasis; a high rate of overall side effects and intolerance to the dosing regimen was observed (Fraaij, 2007). Further studies are needed.

Dosage Forms Excipient information presented when available (limited, particularly for generics); consult specific product labeling.

Capsule, Oral:

Crixivan: 200 mg, 400 mg

Extemporaneous Preparations A 10 mg/mL oral solution may be prepared using capsules. First, prepare a

100 mg/mL indinavir concentrate by adding the contents of fifteen 400 mg capsules and 60 mL purified water to a 100 mL amber glass bottle. Place bottle in an ultrasonic bath filled with water at 37°C for 60 minutes, stirring the solution every 10 minutes. Filter solution; wash bottle and filter with 6 mL purified water; cool solution to room temperature. Add 50 mL of 100 mg/mL indinavir concentrate to 360 mL viscous sweet base, 90 mL simple syrup, 1.8 g citric acid, 45 mg azorubine, 0.1M sodium hydroxide solution to pH 3, and 12 drops of lemon oil, to make a final volume of 500 mL. Mix to a uniform solution. Label "refrigerate". Stable for 2 weeks refrigerated.

Hugen PW, Burger DM, ter Hofstede HJ, et al, "Development of an Indinavir Oral Liquid for Children," *Am J Health Syst Pharm*, 2000, 57 (14):1332-9.

◆ **Indinavir Sulfate** *see* Indinavir *on page 1098*

◆ **Indocin** *see* Indomethacin *on page 1101*

◆ **Indometacin** *see* Indomethacin *on page 1101*

Indomethacin (in doe METH a sin)

Medication Safety Issues

Sound-alike/look-alike issues:

Indocin may be confused with Imodium, Lincocin, Minocin, Vicodin

BEERS Criteria medication:

This drug may be potentially inappropriate for use in geriatric patients (Quality of evidence - moderate; Strength of recommendation - strong).

Related Information

Oral Medications That Should Not Be Crushed or Altered *on page 2476*

Brand Names: US Indocin; Tivorbex

Brand Names: Canada Apo-Indomethacin; Novo-Methacin; Pro-Indo; ratio-Indomethacin; Sandoz-Indomethacin

Therapeutic Category Analgesic, Non-narcotic; Anti-inflammatory Agent; Antipyretic; Nonsteroidal Anti-inflammatory Drug (NSAID), Oral; Nonsteroidal Anti-inflammatory Drug (NSAID), Parenteral

Generic Availability (US) May be product dependent

Use

Oral, Rectal: Management of inflammatory conditions (ie, moderate to severe ankylosing spondylitis, bursitis, and/or tendinitis of the shoulder) and moderate to severe rheumatoid arthritis and osteoarthritis (immediate release oral capsule [excluding Tivorbex], extended release oral capsule, oral suspension, rectal: FDA approved in ages ≥15 and adults); acute gouty arthritis (immediate release oral capsule, oral suspension, rectal: FDA approved in ages ≥15 years and adults); mild to moderate pain (oral capsule: Tivorbex only: FDA approved in adults)

Parenteral: Closure of hemodynamically significant patent ductus arteriosus (PDA) (FDA approved in premature neonates weighing 0.5 to 1.75 kg); has also been used for prophylaxis of PDA and prevention of intraventricular hemorrhage in VLBW neonates

Medication Guide Available Yes

Pregnancy Risk Factor C (<30 weeks gestation); C/D (≥30 weeks gestation [manufacturer specific])

Pregnancy Considerations Adverse events have been observed in animal reproduction studies; studies in pregnant women have demonstrated risk to the fetus if administered at ≥30 weeks gestation. Indomethacin crosses the placenta and can be detected in fetal plasma and amniotic fluid. Indomethacin exposure during the first trimester is not strongly associated with congenital malformations; however, cardiovascular anomalies and cleft palate have been observed following NSAID exposure in some studies. The use of an NSAID close to conception may be associated with an increased risk of miscarriage. Nonteratogenic effects have been observed following NSAID administration during the third trimester, including myocardial degenerative changes, prenatal constriction of the ductus arteriosus, failure of the ductus arteriosus to close postnatally, and fetal tricuspid regurgitation; renal dysfunction or failure, oligohydramnios; gastrointestinal bleeding or perforation, increased risk of necrotizing enterocolitis; intracranial bleeding (including intraventricular hemorrhage), platelet dysfunction with resultant bleeding; and pulmonary hypertension. The risk of fetal ductal constriction following maternal use of indomethacin is increased with gestational age and duration of therapy. Because they may cause premature closure of the ductus arteriosus, use of NSAIDs late in pregnancy should be avoided (use after 31 or 32 weeks gestation is not recommended by some clinicians). Indomethacin has been used for a short duration (eg, ≤48 hours) in the management of preterm labor. Indomethacin should be used with caution in pregnant women with hypertension. The chronic use of NSAIDs in women of reproductive age may be associated with infertility that is reversible upon discontinuation of the medication.

Breast-Feeding Considerations Indomethacin is excreted into breast milk and low amounts have been measured in the plasma of nursing infants. Seizures in a nursing infant were observed in one case report, although adverse events have not been noted in other cases. Breast-feeding is not recommended by most manufacturers; Tivorbex may be used with caution during breast-feeding. (The therapeutic use of indomethacin is contraindicated in neonates with significant renal failure.) Hypertensive crisis and psychiatric side effects have been noted in case reports following use of indomethacin for analgesia in postpartum women. Use with caution in nursing women with hypertensive disorders of pregnancy or pre-existing renal disease.

Contraindications

Hypersensitivity (eg, anaphylactic reactions and serious skin reactions) to indomethacin, aspirin, other NSAIDs, or any component of the formulation; perioperative pain in the setting of coronary artery bypass graft (CABG) surgery;history of asthma, urticaria, or allergic-type reactions after taking aspirin or other NSAID agents (severe, even fatal, anaphylactic-like reactions have been reported); patients with a history of proctitis or recent rectal bleeding (suppositories)

Neonates: Necrotizing enterocolitis; impaired renal function; active bleeding (including intracranial hemorrhage and gastrointestinal bleeding), thrombocytopenia, coagulation defects; untreated infection; congenital heart disease where patent ductus arteriosus is necessary

Warnings/Precautions [U.S. Boxed Warning]: NSAIDs are associated with an increased risk of adverse cardiovascular thrombotic events, including MI and stroke. Risk may be increased with duration of use or pre-existing cardiovascular risk factors or disease. May cause new-onset hypertension or worsening of existing hypertension. Monitor blood pressure closely during initiation of treatment and throughout the course of therapy. Use caution in patients with fluid retention. Avoid use in heart failure (ACCF/AHA [Yancy, 2013]). Concurrent administration of ibuprofen, and potentially other nonselective NSAIDs, may interfere with aspirin's cardioprotective effect. **[U.S. Boxed Warning]: Use is contraindicated for treatment of perioperative pain in the setting of coronary artery bypass graft (CABG) surgery.** Risk of MI and stroke may be increased with use following CABG surgery.

Platelet adhesion and aggregation may be decreased; may prolong bleeding time; patients with coagulation disorders or who are receiving anticoagulants should be monitored closely. Anemia may occur; patients on long-term NSAID therapy should be monitored for anemia.

Rarely, NSAID use may cause severe blood dyscrasias (eg, agranulocytosis, aplastic anemia, thrombocytopenia).

NSAID use may compromise existing renal function; dose-dependent decreases in prostaglandin synthesis may result from NSAID use, reducing renal blood flow which may cause renal decompensation. NSAID use may increase the risk for hyperkalemia. Patients with impaired renal function, dehydration, heart failure, liver dysfunction, those taking diuretics, and ACE inhibitors are at greater risk of renal toxicity and hyperkalemia. Rehydrate patient before starting therapy; monitor renal function closely. Not recommended for use in patients with advanced renal disease. Long-term NSAID use may result in renal papillary necrosis.

[U.S. Boxed Warning]: NSAIDs may increase risk of gastrointestinal irritation, inflammation, ulceration, bleeding, and perforation. Use caution with a history of GI disease (bleeding or ulcers), concurrent therapy with aspirin, anticoagulants and/or corticosteroids, smoking, use of alcohol, the elderly or debilitated patients. When used concomitantly with aspirin, a substantial increase in the risk of gastrointestinal complications (eg, ulcer) occurs; concomitant gastroprotective therapy (eg, proton pump inhibitors) is recommended (Bhatt, 2008).

Use the lowest effective dose for the shortest duration of time, consistent with individual patient goals, to reduce risk of cardiovascular or GI adverse events. Alternate therapies should be considered for patients at high risk.

NSAIDS may cause drowsiness, dizziness, blurred vision and other neurologic effects which may impair physical or mental abilities; patients must be cautioned about performing tasks which require mental alertness (eg, operating machinery or driving). Discontinue use with blurred or diminished vision and perform ophthalmologic exam. Monitor vision with long-term therapy. Headache may occur; cessation of therapy required if headache persists after dosage reduction.

NSAIDs may cause potentially fatal serious skin adverse events including exfoliative dermatitis, Stevens-Johnson syndrome (SJS) and toxic epidermal necrolysis (TEN); discontinue use at first sign of skin rash or hypersensitivity. Anaphylactoid reactions may occur, even without prior exposure; patients with "aspirin triad" (bronchial asthma, aspirin intolerance, rhinitis) may be at increased risk. Use is contraindicated in patients who experience bronchospasm, asthma, rhinitis, or urticaria with NSAID or aspirin therapy. Use caution in other forms of asthma.

Use with caution in patients with decreased hepatic function. Closely monitor patients with any abnormal LFT. Severe hepatic reactions (eg, jaundice, fulminant hepatitis, liver necrosis, liver failure) have occurred with NSAID use, rarely; discontinue if signs or symptoms of liver disease develop, or if systemic manifestations occur. The elderly are at increased risk for adverse effects (especially peptic ulceration, CNS effects, renal toxicity) from NSAIDs even at low doses. Prolonged use may cause corneal deposits and retinal disturbances; discontinue if visual changes are observed. Use caution with depression, epilepsy, or Parkinson's disease.

Withhold for at least 4-6 half-lives prior to surgical or dental procedures. Potentially significant drug-drug interactions may exist, requiring dose or frequency adjustment, additional monitoring, and/or selection of alternative therapy. Consult drug interactions database for more detailed information.

Elderly: Nonselective oral NSAID use is associated with an increased risk of GI bleeding and peptic ulcer disease in older adults in high risk category (eg, >75 years or age or receiving concomitant oral/parenteral corticosteroids, anticoagulants, or antiplatelet agents). Risk of adverse events may be higher with indomethacin compared to other NSAIDs; avoid use in this age group (Beers Criteria). Indomethacin may cause confusion or, rarely, psychosis; remain alert to the possibility of such adverse reactions in elderly patients.

Oral: Hepatotoxicity has been reported in younger children treated for juvenile idiopathic arthritis (JIA). Closely monitor if use is needed in children ≥2 years of age.

Adverse Reactions

Cardiovascular: Presyncope, syncope

Central nervous system: Depression, dizziness, drowsiness, fatigue, headache, malaise, vertigo

Dermatologic: Hyperhidrosis, pruritus, skin rash

Endocrine & metabolic: Hot flash

Gastrointestinal: Abdominal pain, constipation, decreased appetite, diarrhea, dyspepsia, epigastric pain, heartburn, nausea, rectal irritation (suppository), tenesmus (suppository), vomiting

Hematologic & oncologic: Postoperative hemorrhage

Otic: Tinnitus

Miscellaneous: Swelling (postprocedural)

Rare but important or life-threatening: Acute respiratory distress, agranulocytosis, anaphylaxis, anemia, angioedema, aphthous stomatitis, aplastic anemia, aseptic meningitis, asthma, bone marrow depression, cardiac arrhythmia, cardiac failure, cerebrovascular accident, chest pain, cholestatic jaundice, coma, confusion, convulsions, corneal deposits, depersonalization, depression, diplopia, disseminated intravascular coagulation, dysarthria, edema, erythema multiforme, erythema nodosum, exacerbation of epilepsy, exacerbation of Parkinson's disease, exfoliative dermatitis, fluid retention, gastritis, gastroenteritis, gastrointestinal hemorrhage, gastrointestinal perforation (rare), gastrointestinal ulcer, glycosuria, gynecomastia, hearing loss, hematuria, hemodynamic deterioration (patients with severe heart failure and hyponatremia), hemolytic anemia, hepatic failure, hepatic necrosis, hepatitis (including fatal cases), hepatotoxicity (idiosyncratic) (Chalasani, 2014), hyperglycemia, hyperkalemia, hypersensitivity reaction, hypertension, hypotension, immune thrombocytopenia, interstitial nephritis, intestinal obstruction, intestinal stenosis, involuntary muscle movements, jaundice, leukopenia, maculopathy, myocardial infarction, necrotizing fasciitis, nephrotic syndrome, oliguria, peripheral neuropathy, proctitis, psychosis, pulmonary edema, purpura, rectal hemorrhage, regional ileitis, renal failure, renal insufficiency, retinal disturbance, shock, significant cardiovascular event, Stevens-Johnson syndrome, stomatitis, syncope, thrombocytopenia, thrombophlebitis, toxic amblyopia, toxic epidermal necrolysis, ulcerative colitis, vaginal hemorrhage

Drug Interactions

Metabolism/Transport Effects Substrate of CYP2C19 (minor), CYP2C9 (minor); **Note:** Assignment of Major/Minor substrate status based on clinically relevant drug interaction potential; **Inhibits** CYP2C19 (weak), CYP2C9 (weak)

Avoid Concomitant Use

Avoid concomitant use of Indomethacin with any of the following: Dexketoprofen; Floctafenine; Ketorolac (Nasal); Ketorolac (Systemic); Morniflumate; NSAID (COX-2 Inhibitor); Omacetaxine; Urokinase

Increased Effect/Toxicity

Indomethacin may increase the levels/effects of: 5-ASA Derivatives; Agents with Antiplatelet Properties; Aliskiren; Aminoglycosides; Anticoagulants; Apixaban; Bisphosphonate Derivatives; Collagenase (Systemic); CycloSPORINE (Systemic); Dabigatran Etexilate; Deferasirox; Deoxycholic Acid; Desmopressin; Digoxin; Drospirenone; Eplerenone; Haloperidol; Ibritumomab; Lithium;

Methotrexate; Nonsteroidal Anti-Inflammatory Agents; NSAID (COX-2 Inhibitor); Obinutuzumab; Omacetaxine; PEMEtrexed; Porfimer; Potassium-Sparing Diuretics; PRALAtrexate; Quinolone Antibiotics; Rivaroxaban; Salicylates; Tacrolimus (Systemic); Tenofovir; Thrombolytic Agents; Tiludronate; Tositumomab and Iodine I 131 Tositumomab; Triamterene; Urokinase; Vancomycin; Verteporfin; Vitamin K Antagonists

The levels/effects of Indomethacin may be increased by: ACE Inhibitors; Angiotensin II Receptor Blockers; Antidepressants (Tricyclic, Tertiary Amine); Corticosteroids (Systemic); CycloSPORINE (Systemic); Dasatinib; Dexketoprofen; Diclofenac (Systemic); Floctafenine; Glucosamine; Herbs (Anticoagulant/Antiplatelet Properties); Ibrutinib; Ketorolac (Nasal); Ketorolac (Systemic); Limaprost; Morniflumate; Multivitamins/Fluoride (with ADE); Multivitamins/Minerals (with ADEK, Folate, Iron); Multivitamins/Minerals (with AE, No Iron); Omega-3 Fatty Acids; Pentosan Polysulfate Sodium; Pentoxifylline; Probenecid; Prostacyclin Analogues; Selective Serotonin Reuptake Inhibitors; Serotonin/Norepinephrine Reuptake Inhibitors; Sodium Phosphates; Tipranavir; Treprostinil; Vitamin E

Decreased Effect

Indomethacin may decrease the levels/effects of: ACE Inhibitors; Aliskiren; Angiotensin II Receptor Blockers; Beta-Blockers; Eplerenone; Glucagon; HydrALAZINE; Loop Diuretics; Potassium-Sparing Diuretics; Prostaglandins (Ophthalmic); Salicylates; Selective Serotonin Reuptake Inhibitors; Thiazide Diuretics

The levels/effects of Indomethacin may be decreased by: Bile Acid Sequestrants; Salicylates

Food Interactions Food may decrease the rate but not the extent of absorption. Indomethacin peak serum levels may be delayed if taken with food. Management: Administer with food or milk to minimize GI upset.

Storage/Stability

Capsules: Store at 15°C to 30°C (59°F to 86°F). Protect from light. Protect ER capsules from moisture.

Tivorbex: Store Tivorbex capsules at 25°C (77°F); excursions permitted to 15°C to 30°C (59°F to 86°F). Store in the original container; protect from moisture and light.

IV: Store below 30°C (86°F). Protect from light.

Suppositories: Store refrigerated at 2°C to 8°C (36°F to 46°F).

Suspension: Store below 30°C (86°F). Avoid temperatures above 50°C (122°F). Protect from freezing.

Mechanism of Action Reversibly inhibits cyclooxygenase-1 and 2 (COX-1 and 2) enzymes, which results in decreased formation of prostaglandin precursors; has antipyretic, analgesic, and anti-inflammatory properties

Other proposed mechanisms not fully elucidated (and possibly contributing to the anti-inflammatory effect to varying degrees), include inhibiting chemotaxis, altering lymphocyte activity, inhibiting neutrophil aggregation/activation, and decreasing proinflammatory cytokine levels.

Pharmacokinetics (Adult data unless noted)

Absorption: Oral:

Immediate Release:

Neonates: Formulation specific

Adults: Rapid and well absorbed

Extended Release: Adults: 90% over 12 hours (**Note:** 75 mg product is designed to initially release 25 mg and then 50 mg over an extended period of time)

Distribution:

Neonates: PDA: 0.36 L/kg

Post-PDA closure: 0.26 L/kg

Adults: 0.34-1.57 L/kg

Protein binding: 99%

Metabolism: In the liver via glucuronide conjugation and other pathways

Bioavailability: Oral:

Neonates, premature: Percent bioavailability reported in the literature is highly variable and may be influenced by formulation components and indomethacin physicochemical properties (Scanlon, 1982); some have suggested that aqueous formulations are less bioavailable compared to ethanol based formulations (Mrongovious, 1982; Scanlon, 1982); aqueous suspension (in saline): 13% to 20% (Mrongovious, 1982; Sharma, 2003); ethanol based (96% v/v) suspension: 98.6% (Al Za'abi, 2007)

Adults: ~100%

Half-life:

Neonates:

Postnatal age (PNA) <2 weeks: ~20 hours

PNA >2 weeks: ~11 hours

Adults: 2.6-11.2 hours

Elimination: Significant enterohepatic recycling; 33% excreted in feces as demethylated metabolites with 1.5% as unchanged drug; 60% eliminated in urine as drug and metabolites

Clearance: Preterm neonates: ~19 mL/hour/kg (range: 4.7-45.5 mL/hour/kg) (Al Za'abi, 2007)

Dosing: Neonatal

Patent ductus arteriosus:

Treatment: IV: Initial: 0.2 mg/kg/dose, followed by 2 doses depending on postnatal age (PNA):

PNA **at time of first dose** <48 hours: 0.1 mg/kg at 12- to 24-hour intervals

PNA **at time of first dose** 2-7 days: 0.2 mg/kg at 12- to 24-hour intervals

PNA **at time of first dose** >7 days: 0.25 mg/kg at 12- to 24-hour intervals

Note: In general, may use 12-hour dosing interval if urine output >1 mL/kg/hour after prior dose; use 24-hour dosing interval if urine output is <1 mL/kg/hour but >0.6 mL/kg/hour; doses should be withheld if patient has oliguria (urine output <0.6 mL/kg/hour) or anuria

Prophylaxis: Limited data available: Preterm neonates: Various regimens have been evaluated in VLBW neonates with first dose administered within the first 12 to 24 hours of life. Typical dosing: IV: Initial: 0.1 to 0.2 mg/kg/dose followed by 0.1 mg/kg/dose every 12 to 24 hours for 2 additional doses (Fowlie 2010)

Intraventricular hemorrhage (IVH), prevention: Limited data available: Preterm neonates weighing <1.25 kg: IV: Initial: 0.1 mg/kg administered within 6 to 12 hours of birth, followed by 2 additional doses of 0.1 mg/kg every 24 hours for a total of 3 doses (Ment 1994; Mirza 2013)

Note: Due to potential adverse effects with indomethacin therapy, one study protocol discontinued indomethacin if any of the following occurred: Excessive bleeding from IV sites or GI or pulmonary systems; grade 3 or 4 IVH; platelets < 50,000/mm^3; evidence of NEC; SCr >1.8 mg/dL; urine output <0.5 mL/kg/hour; serum K >7 mEq/L with EKG changes and/or Na <120 or >150 mEq/L (Ment 1994).

Dosing based on a prospective, randomized placebo controlled trial (treatment group: n=209) in which a decrease in the incidence and severity of IVH occurred with prophylactic indomethacin compared to placebo (Ment 1994); similar short-term findings were confirmed through meta-analysis of 19 trials (Fowlie 2003). Timing of the initial dose corroborated in a large retrospective cohort study (n=868) which showed administration at <6 hours of birth did not lower the incidence of IVH (Mirza 2013). The reported effects of indomethacin on long-term neurologic outcome and development have been variable (neutral to somewhat positive) and dependent on endpoints used; a meta-analysis reported that long-term neurologic outcome and development do not appear to be affected (Fowlie 2010); however, one study reported improved cognitive vocabulary skills and less mental retardation at 54 months corrected age in indomethacin treatment group compared to the placebo group (Ment 2000).

Dosing: Usual

Pediatric: **Inflammatory/rheumatoid disorders: Note:** Use lowest effective dose: Children ≥2 years and Adolescents (Limited data available in ages <15 years): Oral: Initial: 1 to 2 mg/kg/day in 2 to 4 divided doses; usual initial adult dose range: 25 to 50 mg; maximum daily dose: 4 mg/kg/**day** or 200 mg/**day**, whichever is less (Kliegman 2007)

Adult:

Inflammatory/rheumatoid disorders: (Use lowest effective dose): Oral (excluding Tivorbex), rectal: 25 to 50 mg/dose 2 to 3 times/day; maximum dose: 200 mg/day; extended release capsule should be given on a 1 to 2 times/day schedule (maximum dose for extended release: 150 mg daily). In patients with arthritis and persistent night pain and/or morning stiffness, may give the larger portion (up to 100 mg) of the total daily dose at bedtime.

Bursitis/tendonitis: Oral (excluding Tivorbex), rectal: Initial dose: 75 to 150 mg daily in 3 to 4 divided doses or 1 to 2 divided doses for extended release; usual treatment is 7 to 14 days

Acute gouty arthritis: Oral (excluding extended release capsule and Tivorbex), rectal: 50 mg 3 times daily until pain is tolerable, then reduce dose; usual treatment <3 to 5 days

Acute pain (mild to moderate): Oral (Tivorbex only): 20 mg 3 times daily or 40 mg 2 or 3 times daily

Preparation for Administration Parenteral: IV: Reconstitute with 1 to 2 mL preservative free NS or SWFI just prior to administration, resulting concentration will be 0.5 to 1 mg/mL. Discard any unused portion. Do not use preservative-containing diluents for reconstitution.

Administration

Oral: Administer with food, milk, or antacids to decrease GI adverse effects; extended release capsules must be swallowed whole, do not crush or chew

Parenteral: IV: Administer over 20 to 30 minutes

Note: Do **not** administer via IV bolus or IV infusion via an umbilical catheter into vessels near the superior mesenteric artery, as these may cause vasoconstriction and can compromise blood flow to the intestines. Do not administer intra-arterially.

Monitoring Parameters BUN, serum creatinine, potassium, liver enzymes, CBC with differential; in addition, in neonates treated for PDA: heart rate, heart murmur, blood pressure, urine output, echocardiogram, serum sodium and glucose, platelet count, and serum concentrations of concomitantly administered drugs which are renally eliminated (eg, aminoglycosides, digoxin); periodic ophthalmic exams with chronic use

Test Interactions False-negative dexamethasone suppression test

Additional Information Indomethacin may mask signs and symptoms of infections; fatalities in children have been reported, due to unrecognized overwhelming sepsis. Drowsiness, lethargy, nausea, vomiting, seizures, paresthesia, headache, dizziness, tinnitus, GI bleeding, cerebral edema, and cardiac arrest have been reported with overdoses

Dosage Forms Excipient information presented when available (limited, particularly for generics); consult specific product labeling.

Capsule, Oral:

Tivorbex: 20 mg, 40 mg [contains brilliant blue fcf (fd&c blue #1), fd&c blue #2 (indigotine), fd&c red #40]

Generic: 25 mg, 50 mg

Capsule Extended Release, Oral:

Generic: 75 mg

Solution Reconstituted, Intravenous:

Indocin: 1 mg (1 ea)

Generic: 1 mg (1 ea)

Solution Reconstituted, Intravenous [preservative free]:

Generic: 1 mg (1 ea)

Suppository, Rectal:

Indocin: 50 mg (30 ea)

Suspension, Oral:

Indocin: 25 mg/5 mL (237 mL) [contains alcohol, usp; pineapple-coconut-mint flavor]

- **Indomethacin Sodium Trihydrate** *see* Indomethacin *on page 1101*
- **INF-alpha 2** *see* Interferon Alfa-2b *on page 1148*
- **Infanrix** *see* Diphtheria and Tetanus Toxoids, and Acellular Pertussis Vaccine *on page 681*
- **Infanrix-IPV/HIB (Can)** *see* Diphtheria and Tetanus Toxoids, Acellular Pertussis, Poliovirus and *Haemophilus* b Conjugate Vaccine *on page 679*
- **Infants Advil [OTC]** *see* Ibuprofen *on page 1064*
- **Infants Gas Relief [OTC]** *see* Simethicone *on page 1927*
- **Infants Ibuprofen [OTC]** *see* Ibuprofen *on page 1064*
- **Infants Simethicone [OTC]** *see* Simethicone *on page 1927*
- **Infasurf** *see* Calfactant *on page 355*
- **Infed** *see* Iron Dextran Complex *on page 1164*
- **Inflectra (Can)** *see* InFLIXimab *on page 1104*

InFLIXimab (in FLIKS e mab)

Medication Safety Issues

Sound-alike/look-alike issues:

InFLIXimab may be confused with riTUXimab

Remicade may be confused with Renacidin, Rituxan

High alert medication:

This medication is in a class the Institute for Safe Medication Practices (ISMP) includes among its list of drug classes that have a heightened risk of causing significant patient harm when used in error.

Brand Names: US Remicade

Brand Names: Canada Inflectra; Remicade; Remsima

Therapeutic Category Antirheumatic, Disease Modifying; Gastrointestinal Agent, Miscellaneous; Immunosuppressant Agent; Monoclonal Antibody; Tumor Necrosis Factor (TNF) Blocking Agent

Generic Availability (US) No

Use Reduction of signs and symptoms of Crohn's disease in patients with moderate to severely active disease who have had an inadequate response to conventional therapy (FDA approved in children ≥6 years and adults); reduction of signs and symptoms of ulcerative colitis in patients with moderate to severely active disease who have had an inadequate response to conventional therapy (FDA approved in children ≥6 years and adults); in combination with methotrexate for reducing signs and symptoms, inhibiting progression of structural damage, and improving physical function in patients with moderate to severe rheumatoid arthritis (FDA approved in adults); reduction of signs and symptoms of ankylosing spondylitis (FDA approved in adults); treatment of psoriatic arthritis (to reduce signs/symptoms of active arthritis and inhibit progression of structural damage and improve physical function) (FDA approved in adults); treatment of chronic severe plaque psoriasis (FDA approved in adults)

Medication Guide Available Yes

Pregnancy Risk Factor B

Pregnancy Considerations Animal reproduction studies have not been conducted. Infliximab crosses the placenta and can be detected in the serum of infants for up to 6 months following *in utero* exposure. The safety of administering live or live-attenuated vaccines to exposed infants is not known. If a biologic agent such as infliximab is needed to treat inflammatory bowel disease during pregnancy, it is recommended to hold therapy after 30 weeks gestation (Habal, 2012). The Canadian labeling recommends that women of childbearing potential use effective contraception during therapy and for at least 6 months after discontinuation.

Healthcare providers are also encouraged to enroll women exposed to infliximab during pregnancy in the Mother-ToBaby Autoimmune Diseases Study by contacting the Organization of Teratology Information Specialists (OTIS) (877-311-8972).

Breast-Feeding Considerations Small amounts of infliximab have been detected in breast milk. Information is available from three postpartum women who were administered infliximab 5 mg/kg 1-24 weeks after delivery. Infliximab was detected within 12 hours and the highest milk concentrations (0.09-0.105 mcg/mL) were seen 2-3 days after the dose. Corresponding maternal serum concentrations were 18-64 mcg/mL (Ben-Horin, 2011). Due to the potential for serious adverse reactions in the nursing infant, the manufacturer recommends a decision be made whether to discontinue nursing or to discontinue the drug, taking into account the importance of treatment to the mother.

Contraindications

Hypersensitivity to infliximab, murine proteins or any component of the formulation; doses >5 mg/kg in patients with moderate or severe heart failure (NYHA Class III/IV)

Canadian labeling: Additional contraindications (not in US labeling): Severe infections (eg, sepsis, abscesses, tuberculosis, and opportunistic infections); use in patients with moderate or severe heart failure (NYHA Class III/IV)

Warnings/Precautions [US Boxed Warning]: Patients receiving infliximab are at increased risk for serious infections which may result in hospitalization and/or fatality; infections usually developed in patients receiving concomitant immunosuppressive agents (eg, methotrexate or corticosteroids) and may present as disseminated (rather than local) disease. Active tuberculosis (or reactivation of latent tuberculosis), invasive fungal (including aspergillosis, blastomycosis, candidiasis, coccidioidomycosis, histoplasmosis, and pneumocystosis) and bacterial, viral or other opportunistic infections (including legionellosis and listeriosis) have been reported. Monitor closely for signs/symptoms of infection. Discontinue for serious infection or sepsis. Consider risks versus benefits prior to use in patients with a history of chronic or recurrent infection. Consider empiric antifungal therapy in patients who are at risk for invasive fungal infection and develop severe systemic illness. Caution should be exercised when considering use the elderly or in patients with conditions that predispose them to infections (eg, diabetes) or residence/travel from areas of endemic mycoses (blastomycosis, coccidioidomycosis, histoplasmosis), or with latent or localized infections. Do not initiate infliximab therapy in patients with an active infection, including clinically important localized infection. Patients who develop a new infection while undergoing treatment should be monitored closely. Potentially significant drug interactions may exist, requiring dose or frequency adjustment, additional monitoring, and/or selection of alternative therapy.

[US Boxed Warning]: Infliximab treatment has been associated with active tuberculosis (may be disseminated or extrapulmonary) or reactivation of latent infections; evaluate patients for tuberculosis risk factors and latent tuberculosis infection (with a tuberculin skin test) prior to and during therapy; treatment of latent tuberculosis should be initiated before use. Patients with initial negative tuberculin skin tests should receive continued monitoring for tuberculosis throughout treatment. Most cases of reactivation have been reported within the first couple months of treatment. Caution should be exercised when considering the use of infliximab in patients who have been exposed to tuberculosis.

Patients should be brought up to date with all immunizations before initiating therapy. Live vaccines should not be given concurrently; there is no data available concerning secondary transmission of live vaccines in patients receiving therapy. Use caution when administering live vaccines to infants born to female patients who received infliximab therapy while pregnant; infliximab crosses the placenta and has been detected in infants' serum for up to 6 months. Reactivation of hepatitis B virus (HBV) has occurred in chronic virus carriers (may be fatal); use with caution; evaluate prior to initiation and during treatment.

[US Boxed Warning]: Lymphoma and other malignancies (may be fatal) have been reported in children and adolescent patients receiving TNF-blocking agents including infliximab. Half the cases are lymphomas (Hodgkin's and non-Hodgkin's). **[US Boxed Warning]: Postmarketing cases of hepatosplenic T-cell lymphoma have been reported in patients treated with infliximab. Almost all patients had received and concurrent or prior treatment with azathioprine or mercaptopurine at or prior to diagnosis and the majority of reported cases occurred in adolescent and young adult males with Crohn disease or ulcerative colitis.** Malignancies occurred after a median of 30 months (range 1 to 84 months) after the first dose of TNF blocker therapy; most patients were receiving concomitant immunosuppressants. The impact of infliximab on the development and course of malignancies is not fully defined. As compared to the general population, an increased risk of lymphoma has been noted in clinical trials; however, rheumatoid arthritis alone has been previously associated with an increased rate of lymphoma. Use caution in patients with a history of COPD, higher rates of malignancy were reported in COPD patients treated with infliximab. Psoriasis patients with a history of phototherapy had a higher incidence of nonmelanoma skin cancers. Melanoma and Merkel cell carcinoma have been reported in patients receiving TNF-blocking agents including infliximab. Perform periodic skin examinations in all patients during therapy, particularly those at increased risk for skin cancer.

Severe hepatic reactions (including hepatitis, jaundice, acute hepatic failure, and cholestasis) have been reported during treatment; reactions occurred between 2 weeks to >1 year after initiation of therapy and some cases were fatal or necessitated liver transplantation; discontinue with jaundice and/or marked increase in liver enzymes (≥5 times ULN). Use caution with heart failure; if a decision is made to use with heart failure, monitor closely and discontinue if exacerbated or new symptoms occur. Doses >5 mg/kg should not be administered in patients with moderate to severe heart failure (HF) (NYHA Class III/IV). The Canadian labeling contraindicates use in moderate or severe HF. Use caution with history of hematologic abnormalities; hematologic toxicities (eg, leukopenia, neutropenia, thrombocytopenia, pancytopenia) have been reported (may be fatal); discontinue if significant abnormalities occur. Positive antinuclear antibody titers have been detected in patients (with negative baselines). Rare cases of autoimmune disorder, including lupus-like syndrome, have been reported; monitor and discontinue if symptoms develop. Rare cases of optic neuritis and demyelinating disease (including multiple sclerosis, systemic vasculitis, and Guillain-Barré syndrome) have been reported; use with caution in patients with pre-existing or recent onset CNS demyelinating disorders, or seizures; discontinue if significant CNS adverse reactions develop.

Acute infusion reactions may occur. Hypersensitivity reaction may occur within 2 hours of infusion. Medication and equipment for management of hypersensitivity reaction should be available for immediate use. Interruptions and/or reinstitution at a slower rate may be required (consult protocols). Pretreatment may be considered, and may be warranted in all patients with prior infusion reactions. Serum sickness-like reactions have occurred; may be associated with a decreased response to treatment. The development of antibodies to infliximab may increase the risk of hypersensitivity and/or infusion reactions; concomitant use of immunosuppressants may lessen the development of anti-infliximab antibodies. The risk of infusion reactions may be increased with re-treatment after an interruption or discontinuation of prior maintenance therapy. Re-treatment in psoriasis patients should be resumed as a scheduled maintenance regimen without any induction doses; use of an induction regimen should be used cautiously for re-treatment of all other patients.

Some dosage forms may contain polysorbate 80 (also known as Tweens). Hypersensitivity reactions, usually a delayed reaction, have been reported following exposure to pharmaceutical products containing polysorbate 80 in certain individuals (Isaksson, 2002; Lucente 2000; Shelley, 1995). Thrombocytopenia, ascites, pulmonary deterioration, and renal and hepatic failure have been reported in premature neonates after receiving parenteral products containing polysorbate 80 (Alade, 1986; CDC, 1984). See manufacturer's labeling.

Efficacy was not established in a study to evaluate infliximab use in juvenile idiopathic arthritis (JIA).

Warnings: Additional Pediatric Considerations In an analysis of children and adolescents who had received TNF-blockers (etanercept and infliximab), the FDA identified 48 cases of malignancy. Of the 48 cases, ~50% were lymphomas (eg, Hodgkin and non-Hodgkin lymphoma). Other malignancies, such as leukemia, melanoma, Merkel cell carcinoma, and solid organ tumors, were reported; malignancies rarely seen in children (eg, leiomyosarcoma, hepatic malignancies, and renal cell carcinoma) were also observed. Of note, most of these cases (88%) were receiving other immunosuppressive medications (eg, azathioprine and methotrexate). As compared to the general population, an increased risk of lymphoma has been noted in clinical trials; however, rheumatoid arthritis has been previously associated with an increased rate of lymphoma. The role of TNF-blockers in the development of malignancies in children cannot be excluded. The FDA also reviewed 147 postmarketing reports of leukemia (including acute myeloid leukemia, chronic lymphocytic leukemia, and chronic myeloid leukemia) in patients (children and adults) using TNF blockers. Average onset time to development of leukemia was within the first 1 to 2 years of TNF-blocker initiation. Although most patients were receiving other immunosuppressive agents, the role of TNF blockers in the development of leukemia could not be excluded. The FDA concluded that there is a possible association with the development of leukemia and the use of TNF-blockers.

The risk of infusion-related reactions may be increased with retreatment after an interruption or discontinuation of prior maintenance dose. A retrospective study of 57 children receiving 361 infliximab infusions reported that the rate of infusion-related reactions in children was similar to that in adults (9.7% incidence reported). Female gender, immunosuppressive use for <4 months, and prior infusion reactions were risk factors for subsequent infusion reactions in children (Crandall, 2003).

Adverse Reactions

Reported in adults with rheumatoid arthritis:

Cardiovascular: Bradycardia, cardiac arrest, cardia arrhythmia, cardiac failure, cerebral infarction, circulator shock, edema, hypertension, hypotension, myocardia infarction, pulmonary embolism, syncope, tachycardia thrombophlebitis (deep)

Central nervous system: Confusion, dizziness, fatigue headache, meningitis, neuritis, pain, peripheral neuro pathy, seizure, suicidal tendencies

Dermatologic: Cellulitis, diaphoresis, pruritus, skin rash

Endocrine & metabolic: Dehydration, menstrual disease

Gastrointestinal: Abdominal pain (more common in Crohn's patients), biliary colic, cholecystitis, cholelithia sis, constipation, diarrhea, dyspepsia, gastrointestina hemorrhage, intestinal obstruction, intestinal perforation intestinal stenosis, nausea, pancreatitis, peritonitis, rec tal pain

Genitourinary: Urinary tract infection

Hematologic & oncologic: Anemia, basal cell carcinoma hemolytic anemia, leukopenia, lymphadenopathy, malig nant lymphoma, malignant neoplasm, malignant neo plasm of breast, pancytopenia, sarcoidosis thrombocytopenia

Hepatic: Hepatitis, increased serum ALT (risk increase with concomitant methotrexate)

Hypersensitivity: Delayed hypersensitivity (plaque psoria sis), hypersensitivity reaction, serum sickness

Immunologic: Antibody development (anti-infliximab Mayer, 2006), antibody development (double-strande DNA), increased ANA titer

Infection: Abscess (including Crohn's patients with fistuliz ing disease), candidiasis, infection, sepsis

Neuromuscular & skeletal: Arthralgia, back pain, herniate disk, lupus-like syndrome, myalgia, tendon disease

Renal: Nephrolithiasis, renal failure

Respiratory: Adult respiratory distress syndrome, bronchi tis, cough, dyspnea, pharyngitis, pleural effusion pleurisy, pulmonary edema, respiratory insufficiency, rhi nitis, sinusitis, upper respiratory tract infection

Miscellaneous: Fever, ulcer

The following adverse events were reported in chil dren with Crohn's disease and were more common in children than adults:

Cardiovascular: Flushing

Gastrointestinal: Bloody stools

Hepatic: Increased liver enzymes

Hematologic & oncologic: Anemia, leukopenia, neutro penia

Hypersensitivity: Hypersensitivity reaction (respiratory)

Immunologic: Antibody development (anti-infliximab)

Infection: Bacterial infection, infection (more common with every 8-week vs every 12-week infusions), viral infection

Neuromuscular & skeletal: Bone fracture

Rare but important or life-threatening (adults or chil dren): Agranulocytosis, anaphylactic shock, anaphylaxis angina pectoris, angioedema, autoimmune hepatitis, car diac failure (worsening), cholestasis, demyelinating dis ease of the central nervous system (eg, multiple sclerosis, optic neuritis), demyelinating disease (periph eral; eg, Guillain-Barré syndrome, chronic inflammatory demyelinating polyneuropathy, multifocal motor neuro pathy), dysgeusia, erythema multiforme, hepatic carci noma, hepatic failure, hepatic injury, hepatitis B (reactivation), hepatotoxicity (idiosyncratic) (Chalasani 2014), Hodgkin lymphoma, immune thrombocytopenia interstitial fibrosis, interstitial pneumonitis, jaundice, leu kemia, liver function tests increased, lupus-like syndrome (drug-induced), malignant lymphoma (hepatosplenic T-cell [HSTCL]), malignant melanoma, malignant neoplasm (leiomyosarcoma), Merkel cell carcinoma, neuropathy opportunistic infection, pericardial effusion, pneumonia psoriasis (including new onset, palmoplantar, pustular, or exacerbation), reactivated tuberculosis, renal cell carcinoma, seizure, Stevens-Johnson syndrome, thrombotic thrombocytopenia purpura, toxic epidermal necrolysis, transverse myelitis, tuberculosis, vasculitis (systemic and cutaneous)

Drug Interactions

Metabolism/Transport Effects None known.

Avoid Concomitant Use

Avoid concomitant use of InFLIXimab with any of the following: Abatacept; Adalimumab; Anakinra; BCG; BCG (Intravesical); Belimumab; Canakinumab; Certolizumab Pegol; Etanercept; Golimumab; Natalizumab; Pimecrolimus; Rilonacept; Tacrolimus (Topical); Tocilizumab; Tofacitinib; Ustekinumab; Vaccines (Live); Vedolizumab

Increased Effect/Toxicity

InFLIXimab may increase the levels/effects of: Abatacept; Anakinra; Belimumab; Canakinumab; Certolizumab Pegol; Leflunomide; Natalizumab; Rilonacept; Tofacitinib; Vaccines (Live); Vedolizumab

The levels/effects of InFLIXimab may be increased by: Adalimumab; Denosumab; Etanercept; Golimumab; Pimecrolimus; Roflumilast; Tacrolimus (Topical); Tocilizumab; Trastuzumab; Ustekinumab

Decreased Effect

InFLIXimab may decrease the levels/effects of: BCG; BCG (Intravesical); Coccidioides immitis Skin Test; Sipuleucel-T; Vaccines (Inactivated); Vaccines (Live)

The levels/effects of InFLIXimab may be decreased by: Echinacea

Storage/Stability Store vials at 2°C to 8°C (36°F to 46°F).

Mechanism of Action Infliximab is a chimeric monoclonal antibody that binds to human tumor necrosis factor alpha (TNFα), thereby interfering with endogenous TNFα activity. Elevated TNFα levels have been found in involved tissues/fluids of patients with rheumatoid arthritis, ankylosing spondylitis, psoriatic arthritis, plaque psoriasis, Crohn disease and ulcerative colitis. Biological activities of TNFα include the induction of proinflammatory cytokines (interleukins), enhancement of leukocyte migration, activation of neutrophils and eosinophils, and the induction of acute phase reactants and tissue degrading enzymes. Animal models have shown TNFα expression causes polyarthritis, and infliximab can prevent disease as well as allow diseased joints to heal.

Pharmacodynamics

Onset:

Crohn's disease: 1-2 weeks

Rheumatoid arthritis: 3-7 days

Duration:

Crohn's disease: 8-48 weeks

Rheumatoid arthritis: 6-12 weeks

Pharmacokinetics (Adult data unless noted) Note: Pharmacokinetic data in pediatric patients (6-17 years) reported to be similar to adult values.

Distribution: Within the vascular compartment

V_d: 3-6 L (Klotz, 2007)

Half-life, terminal: 7-12 days (Klotz, 2007)

Dosing: Usual Note: Premedication with antihistamines (H_1-antagonist and/or H_2-antagonist), acetaminophen and/or corticosteroids may be considered to prevent and/or manage infusion-related reactions:

Children and Adolescents:

Crohn's disease: Children ≥6 years and Adolescents: IV: Initial: 5 mg/kg/dose at 0, 2, and 6 weeks, followed by maintenance: 5 mg/kg/dose every 8 weeks thereafter. **Note:** If the response is incomplete, dose has been increased up to 10 mg/kg (Rufo, 2012; Stephens, 2003); in adult patients with Crohn's disease, it has been observed that patients who do not respond by week 14 are unlikely to respond with continued dosing; consider therapy discontinuation in these patients.

Juvenile idiopathic arthritis; refractory to conventional disease modifying drugs: Limited data available: Children ≥4 years and Adolescents: IV: Initial: 3 mg/kg at 0, 2, and 6 weeks; then 3-6 mg/kg/dose every 8 weeks thereafter, in combination with methotrexate during induction and maintenance (Ruperto, 2010). Alternatively, some studies used 6 mg/kg/dose starting at week 14 of a methotrexate induction regimen (weeks 0-13); repeat dose (6 mg/kg/dose) at week 16 and 20, then every 8 weeks thereafter (Ruperto, 2007; Ruperto, 2010; Visvanathan, 2012).

Ulcerative colitis: Children ≥6 years and Adolescents: IV: Initial: 5 mg/kg/dose at 0, 2, and 6 weeks, followed by maintenance: 5 mg/kg/dose every 8 weeks thereafter. **Note:** If the response is incomplete, dose has been increased up to 10 mg/kg (Rufo, 2012; Stephens, 2003)

Adults:

Crohn's disease: IV: 5 mg/kg at 0, 2, and 6 weeks, followed by 5 mg/kg every 8 weeks thereafter; dose may be increased to 10 mg/kg in patients who respond but then lose their response. If no response by week 14, consider discontinuing therapy.

Rheumatoid arthritis (in combination with methotrexate): IV: Initial: 3 mg/kg at 0, 2, and 6 weeks, followed by 3 mg/kg every 8 weeks thereafter; doses have ranged from 3-10 mg/kg repeated at 4- to 8-week intervals

Ankylosing spondylitis: IV: Initial: 5 mg/kg; repeat 5 mg/kg/dose at 2 and 6 weeks after the first infusion, then every 6 weeks thereafter

Plaque psoriasis: IV: Initial: 5 mg/kg at 0, 2, and 6 weeks, then every 8 weeks thereafter

Psoriatic arthritis (with or without methotrexate): IV: Initial: 5 mg/kg at 0, 2, and 6 weeks, followed by 5 mg/kg every 8 weeks thereafter

Ulcerative colitis: IV: Initial: 5 mg/kg at 0, 2, and 6 weeks, then every 8 weeks thereafter

Dosage adjustment with heart failure (HF): Adults: Weigh risk versus benefits for individual patient: Moderate to severe (NYHA Class III or IV): ≤5 mg/kg

Dosing adjustment in renal impairment: There are no dosage adjustments provided in manufacturer's labeling.

Dosing adjustment in hepatic impairment: There are no dosage adjustments provided in manufacturer's labeling.

Preparation for Administration Parenteral: Reconstitute vials with 10 mL SWFI. Swirl vial gently to dissolve powder; do not shake. Allow solution to stand for 5 minutes. Total dose of reconstituted product should be further diluted in NS to a final concentration of 0.4 to 4 mg/mL (usually dose added to 250 mL NS). Infusion of dose should begin within 3 hours of preparation.

Administration Parenteral: The infusion should begin within 3 hours of preparation. Administer by IV infusion through an in-line, sterile, nonpyrogenic, low-protein-binding filter with pore size of ≤1.2 micrometers; do not infuse in the same IV line as other agents. Infuse over at least 2 hours; a rate titration schedule may be used to prevent acute infusion reactions. Temporarily discontinue or decrease infusion rate with infusion-related reactions. Antihistamines (H_1-antagonist ± H_2-antagonist), acetaminophen and/or corticosteroids may be used to manage reactions. Infusion may be reinitiated at a lower rate upon resolution of mild to moderate symptoms.

Adults: Guidelines for the treatment and prophylaxis of infusion reactions: Data limited to adult patients and dosages used in Crohn's; prospective data for other populations (pediatrics, other indications/dosing) are not available. A protocol for the treatment of infusion reactions, as well as prophylactic therapy for repeat infusions, has been published (Mayer, 2006).

Treatment of infusion reactions: Medications for the treatment of hypersensitivity reactions should be available for immediate use. For mild reactions, the rate of infusion should be decreased to 10 mL/hour. Initiate a NS infusion (500-1000 mL/hour) and appropriate symptomatic treatment (eg, acetaminophen and diphenhydramine); monitor vital signs every 10 minutes until normal. After 20 minutes, the infliximab infusion may be increased at 15-minute intervals, as tolerated, to completion [initial increase to 20 mL/hour, then 40 mL/hour, then 80 mL/hour, etc (maximum of 125 mL/hour)]. For moderate reactions, the infusion should be stopped or slowed. Initiate a NS (500-1000 mL/hour) and appropriate symptomatic treatment. Monitor vital signs every 5 minutes until normal. After 20 minutes, the infliximab infusion may be reinstituted at 10 mL/hour; then increased at 15-minute intervals, as tolerated, to completion [initial increase 20 mL/hour, then 40 mL/hour, then 80 mL/hour, etc (maximum of 125 mL/hour)]. For severe reactions, the infusion should be stopped with administration of appropriate symptomatic treatment (eg, hydrocortisone/methylprednisolone, diphenhydramine and epinephrine) and frequent monitoring of vitals. Retreatment after a severe reaction should only be done if the benefits outweigh the risks and with appropriate prophylaxis. Delayed infusion reactions typically occur 1 to 7 days after an infusion. Treatment should consist of appropriate symptomatic treatment (eg, acetaminophen, antihistamine, methylprednisolone).

Prophylaxis of infusion reactions: Premedication with acetaminophen and diphenhydramine 90 minutes prior to infusion may be considered in all patients with prior infusion reactions, and in patients with severe reactions corticosteroid administration is recommended. Steroid dosing may be oral (prednisone 50 mg orally every 12 hours for 3 doses prior to infusion) or intravenous (a single dose of hydrocortisone 100 mg or methylprednisolone 20 to 40 mg administered 20 minutes prior to the infusion). On initiation of the infusion, begin with a test dose at 10 mL/hour of infliximab for 15 minutes. Thereafter, the infusion may be increased at 15-minute intervals, as tolerated, to completion (initial increase 20 mL/hour, then 40 mL/hour, then 80 mL/hour, etc). A maximum rate of 125 mL/hour is recommended in patients who experienced prior mild-moderate reactions and 100 mL/hour is recommended in patients who experienced prior severe reactions. In patients with cutaneous flushing, aspirin may be considered (Becker, 2004). For delayed infusion reactions, premedicate with acetaminophen and diphenhydramine 90 minutes prior to infusion. On initiation of the infusion, begin with a test dose at 10 mL/hour for 15 minutes. Thereafter, the infusion may be increased to infuse over 3 hours. Postinfusion therapy with acetaminophen for 3 days and an antihistamine for 7 days is recommended. **Note:** In a trial of pediatric patients, premedication with acetaminophen (20 mg/kg; maximum single dose: 1000 mg) and cetirizine (0.3 mg/kg if <5 years, 10 mg if ≥5 years) did not significantly impact incidence of infusion-related reactions; patients should be monitored closely (Lahdenne, 2010).

Monitoring Parameters Monitor improvement of symptoms and physical function assessments. During infusion, if reaction is noted, monitor vital signs every 2-10 minutes, depending on reaction severity, until normal. Latent TB screening prior to initiating and during therapy; signs/symptoms of infection (prior to, during, and following therapy); CBC with differential; signs/symptoms/worsening of heart failure; HBV screening prior to initiating (all patients), HBV carriers (during and for several months following therapy); signs and symptoms of hypersensitivity reaction; symptoms of lupus-like syndrome; LFTs (discontinue if >5 times ULN); signs and symptoms of malignancy (eg, splenomegaly, hepatomegaly, abdominal pain, persistent fever, night sweats, weight loss).

Dosage Forms Considerations Remicade contains sucrose 500 mg per vial

Dosage Forms Excipient information presented when available (limited, particularly for generics); consult specific product labeling.

Solution Reconstituted, Intravenous [preservative free]:

Remicade: 100 mg (1 ea) [contains polysorbate 80]

◆ **Infliximab, Recombinant** *see* InFLIXimab *on page 1104*

◆ **Influenza Vaccine** *see* Influenza Virus Vaccine (Inactivated) *on page 1108*

◆ **Influenza Vaccine** *see* Influenza Virus Vaccine (Live/Attenuated) *on page 1113*

Influenza Virus Vaccine (Inactivated)

(in floo EN za VYE rus vak SEEN, in ak ti VAY ted)

Medication Safety Issues

Sound-alike/look-alike issues:

Fluarix may be confused with Flarex

FluMist may be confused with flumazenil

Influenza virus vaccine may be confused with perflutren lipid microspheres

Influenza virus vaccine may be confused with tetanus toxoid and tuberculin products. Medication errors have occurred when tuberculin skin tests (PPD) have been inadvertently administered instead of tetanus toxoid products and influenza virus vaccine. These products are refrigerated and often stored in close proximity to each other.

International issues:

Fluarix [US, Canada, and multiple international markets] may be confused with Flarex brand name for fluorometholone [US and multiple international markets] and Fluorex brand name for fluoride [France]

Related Information

Centers for Disease Control and Prevention (CDC) and Other Links *on page 2424*

Immunization Administration Recommendations *on page 2411*

Immunization Schedules *on page 2416*

Brand Names: US Afluria; Afluria Preservative Free; Fluarix; Fluarix Quadrivalent; Flucelvax; Flulaval; Flulaval Quadrivalent; Fluvirin; Fluvirin Preservative Free; Fluzone; Fluzone High-Dose; Fluzone Pediatric PF [DSC]; Fluzone Preservative Free [DSC]; Fluzone Quadrivalent; Medical Provider EZ Flu; Medical Provider EZ Flu PF; Medical Provider EZ Flu Shot; Physicians EZ Use Flu

Brand Names: Canada Agriflu; Fluad; Fluviral; Fluzone; Fluzone Quadrivalent; Influvac; Intanza; Vaxigrip

Therapeutic Category Vaccine; Vaccine, Inactivated Virus

Generic Availability (US) May be product dependent

Use Active immunization against influenza disease caused by influenza virus subtypes A and type B contained in the vaccine

Trade Name	Manufacturer	Approval age
Fluzone, Fluzone Quadrivalent	Sanofi Pasteur	≥6 months
Fluarix, Fluarix Quadrivalent	GlaxoSmithKline	≥3 years
FluLaval, FluLaval Quadrivalent	ID Biomedical Corporation of Quebec	≥ 3 years
Fluvirin	Novartis vaccine	≥4 years
Afluria	CSL Biotherapies	≥5 years*
Flucelvax	Novartis vaccine	≥18 years
Fluzone Intradermal Fluzone Intradermal Quadrivalent	Sanofi Pasteur	18 to 64 years
Fluzone High-Dose	Sanofi Pasteur	≥65 years

***Note:** Due to an increased incidence of fever and febrile seizures in infants and children <5 years of age observed with the use of the 2010 Southern Hemisphere formulation of Afluria®, the Advisory Committee on Immunization Practices (ACIP) recommends that Afluria® should not be used in infants and children 6 months through 8 years of age, although use in 5 to 8 years of age is reserved for patients if no other age-appropriate vaccine is available (CDC/ACIP [Grohskopf 2014]).

Recommendations for annual seasonal influenza vaccination: The Advisory Committee on Immunization Practices (ACIP) recommends routine annual vaccination with the seasonal influenza vaccine for all persons ≥6 months of age who do not otherwise have contraindications to the vaccine (CDC/ACIP [Grohskopf 2014]).

The ACIP recommends use of any age and risk factor appropriate product and does not have a preferential recommendation for use of the trivalent inactivated influenza vaccine (IIV3) or the quadrivalent inactivated influenza vaccine (IIV4). In addition to the IIV products, other alternative products are available for certain patient populations: Healthy nonpregnant persons aged 2 to 49 years may receive vaccination with the live attenuated influenza vaccine (LAIV); persons ≥18 may receive vaccination with the recombinant influenza vaccine (RIV) (CDC/ACIP [Grohskopf 2014]).

When vaccine supply is limited, target groups for vaccination (those at higher risk of complications from influenza infection and their close contacts) include the following (CDC/ACIP 62[07] 2013):

- All infants ≥6 months and children 12 to 59 months of age
- Persons ≥50 years of age
- Residents of nursing homes and other long-term care facilities
- Patients with chronic pulmonary disorders (including asthma) or cardiovascular system disorders (except hypertension), renal, hepatic, neurologic, or metabolic disorders (including diabetes mellitus)
- Persons who have immunosuppression (including immunosuppression caused by medications or HIV)
- Infants, children, and adolescents (6 months to 18 years of age) who are receiving long-term aspirin therapy and therefore, may be at risk for developing Reye's syndrome after influenza
- Women who are or will be pregnant during influenza season
- Healthy household contacts (including children) and caregivers of neonates, infants, and children aged 0 to 59 months (particularly neonates and infants <6 months) and adults ≥50 years
- Household contacts (including children) and caregivers of persons with medical conditions which put them at high risk of complications from influenza infection
- Healthcare personnel
- American Indians/Alaska Natives
- Morbidly obese (BMI ≥40)

Medication Guide Available Yes

Pregnancy Risk Factor B/C (manufacturer specific)

Pregnancy Considerations Adverse events were not observed in animal reproduction studies. Inactivated influenza vaccine has not been shown to cause fetal harm when given to pregnant women, although information related to use in the first trimester is limited (CDC/ACIP 62[07] 2013). Following maternal immunization with the inactivated influenza virus vaccine, vaccine specific antibodies are observed in the newborn (Englund, 1993; Steinhoff 2010; Zaman 2008; Zuccotti 2010). Vaccination of pregnant women protects infants from influenza infection, including infants <6 months of age who are not able to be vaccinated (CDC/ACIP 62[07] 2013).

Pregnant women are at an increased risk of complications from influenza infection (Rasmussen 2008). Influenza vaccination with the inactivated influenza vaccine (IIV) is recommended for all women who are or will become pregnant during the influenza season and who do not otherwise have contraindications to the vaccine (CDC/ACIP 62[07] 2013). Pregnant women should observe the same precautions as nonpregnant women to reduce the risk of exposure to influenza and other respiratory infections (CDC 2010). When vaccine supply is limited, focus on delivering the vaccine should be given to women who are pregnant or will be pregnant during the flu season, as well as mothers of newborns and contacts or caregivers of children <5 years of age (CDC/ACIP 62[07] 2013)

Healthcare providers are encouraged to refer women exposed to the influenza vaccine during pregnancy to the Vaccines and Medications in Pregnancy Surveillance System (VAMPSS) by contacting The Organization of Teratology Information Specialists (OTIS) at (877) 311-8972.

Women exposed to Flulaval, Flulaval Quadrivalent, Fluarix, or Fluarix Quadrivalent vaccine during pregnancy or their healthcare provider may also contact the GlaxoSmithKline registry at 888-452-9622.

Healthcare providers may enroll women exposed to Fluzone Intradermal or Fluzone Quadrivalent during pregnancy in the Sanofi Pasteur vaccination registry at 800-822-2463.

Breast-Feeding Considerations It is not known if inactivated influenza vaccine is excreted into breast milk. The manufacturers recommend that caution be used if administered to nursing women. Anti-influenza IgA antibodies can be detected in breast milk following maternal vaccination with the trivalent IIV vaccine (Schlaudecker 2013). Inactivated vaccines do not affect the safety of breastfeeding for the mother or the infant (NCIRD/ACIP 2011). Postpartum women may be vaccinated with either IIV or LAIV (CDC/ACIP 62[07] 2013). When vaccine supply is limited, focus on delivering the vaccine should be given to women who are pregnant or will be pregnant during the flu season, as well as mothers of newborns and contacts or caregivers of children <5 years of age (CDC/ACIP 62[07] 2013). Breast-feeding infants should be vaccinated according to the recommended schedules (NCIRD/ACIP 2011).

Contraindications Severe allergic reaction (eg, anaphylaxis) to a previous influenza vaccination; hypersensitivity to any component of the formulation

Additional manufacturer contraindications for Afluria, Fluarix, Fluarix Quadrivalent, FluLaval, FluLaval

Quadrivalent, Fluvirin, Fluzone, Fluzone High-Dose, Fluzone Intradermal, Fluzone Intradermal Quadrivalent, Fluzone Quadrivalent: History of severe allergic reaction (eg, anaphylaxis) to egg protein

Fluviral (not available in US): Canadian labeling: Additional contraindications: Presence of acute respiratory infection, other active infections, or serious febrile illness

Warnings/Precautions Immediate treatment (including epinephrine 1:1000) for anaphylactoid and/or hypersensitivity reactions should be available during vaccine use (NCIRD/ACIP 2011). Oculorespiratory syndrome (ORS) is an acute, self-limiting reaction to IIV with one or more of the following symptoms appearing within 2 to 24 hours after the dose: Chest tightness, cough, difficulty breathing, facial swelling, red eyes, sore throat, or wheezing. Symptoms resolve within 48 hours of onset. The cause of ORS has not been established, but studies have suggested that it is not IgE-mediated. However, because ORS symptoms may be similar to those of an IgE-mediated hypersensitivity reaction, health care providers unsure of etiology of symptoms should seek advice from an allergist/immunologist when determining whether a patient may be revaccinated in subsequent seasons (CDC/ACIP 62[07] 2013).

Most products are manufactured with chicken egg protein (expressed as ovalbumin content when content is disclosed on prescribing information). The ovalbumin content may vary from season to season and lot to lot of vaccine. Allergy to eggs must be distinguished from allergy to the vaccine. Recommendations are available from the ACIP and NACI regarding influenza vaccination to persons who report egg allergies; however, ACIP states a prior severe allergic reaction to influenza vaccine, regardless of the component suspected, is a contraindication to vaccination. Patients with a history of egg allergy who have experienced only hives following egg exposure should receive influenza vaccine using IIV (egg- or cell-culture based) or RIV, if otherwise appropriate; however, the vaccine should only be administered by a health care provider familiar with the manifestations of egg allergy and patients be monitored for at least 30 minutes after vaccination (CDC/ACIP [Grohskopf 2014]). NACI does not consider an egg allergy as a contraindication to vaccination (NACI July 2014). Flucelvax (ccIIV$_3$) is an inactivated influenza vaccine manufactured using cell culture technology and provides an alternative to vaccines cultured with chicken egg protein but should not be considered egg free. It may be used in persons with a mild egg allergy if age appropriate and there are no other contraindications; appropriate precautions should be observed (CDC/ACIP [Grohskopf 2014]). Some products are manufactured with gentamicin, kanamycin, neomycin, polymyxin or thimerosal; some packaging may contain natural latex rubber.

Some dosage forms may contain polysorbate 80 (also known as Tweens). Hypersensitivity reactions, usually a delayed reaction, have been reported following exposure to pharmaceutical products containing polysorbate 80 in certain individuals (Isaksson 2002; Lucente 2000; Shelley, 1995). Thrombocytopenia, ascites, pulmonary deterioration, and renal and hepatic failure have been reported in premature neonates after receiving parenteral products containing polysorbate 80 (Alade, 1986; CDC, 1984). See manufacturer's labeling.

The decision to administer or delay vaccination because of current or recent febrile illness depends on the severity of symptoms and the etiology of the disease. Consider deferring administration in patients with moderate or severe acute illness (with or without fever); vaccination should not be delayed for patients with mild acute illness (with or without fever) (NCIRD/ACIP 2011). Postmarketing reports of increased incidence of fever and febrile seizures in children <5 years of age has been observed with the use of the 2010 Southern Hemisphere formulation of the Afluri[a] vaccine. Febrile events have also been reported in childre[n] 5 to <9 years of age. Based on information from the CDC an increased rate of febrile seizures has been reported i[n] young children 6 months to 4 years who received vacc[i]nation with inactivated influenza vaccine (IIV) and the 13-valent pneumococcal conjugate vaccine (PCV13) simulta[-]neously. However, due to the risks associated with delay[-]ing either vaccine, administering them at separate visits o[r] deviating from the recommended vaccine schedule is no[t] currently recommended. The ACIP does not recommen[d] use of Afluria in children <9 years of age (CDC 62[07] 2013, CDC/ACIP [Grohskopf 2014]). Antipyretics have no[t] been shown to prevent febrile seizures; antipyretics ma[y] be used to treat fever or discomfort following vaccinatio[n] (NCIRD/ACIP 2011). One study reported that routine pro[-]phylactic administration of acetaminophen to prevent feve[r] prior to vaccination decreased the immune response [o]f some vaccines; the clinical significance of this reduction i[n] immune response has not been established (Pry[-]mula 2009).

Syncope has been reported with use of injectable vaccine[s] and may result in serious secondary injury (eg, sku[ll] fracture, cerebral hemorrhage); typically reported in ado[-]lescents and young adults and within 15 minutes afte[r] vaccination. Procedures should be in place to avoid inju[-]ries from falling and to restore cerebral perfusion if syn[-]cope occurs (NCIRD/ACIP 2011).

Use with caution in patients with history of Guillain-Barr[é] syndrome (GBS); patients with history of GBS have [a] greater likelihood of developing GBS than those withou[t]. As a precaution, the ACIP recommends that patients wit[h] a history of GBS and who are at low risk for sever[e] influenza complications, and patients known to have expe[-]rienced GBS within 6 weeks following previous vaccinatio[n] should generally not be vaccinated (consider influenz[a] antiviral chemoprophylaxis in these patients). The benefit of vaccination may outweigh the potential risks in person[s] with a history of GBS who are also at high risk fo[r] complications of influenza (CDC/ACIP 62[07] 2013). Recent studies of patients who received the trivalen[t] inactivated influenza vaccine or the monovalent H1N[1] influenza vaccine have shown the risk of GBS is lowe[r] with vaccination than with influenza infection (Baxter 2013; Greene 2013; Kwong 2013). Some Canadian produc[t] labeling recommends delaying therapy in patients wit[h] active neurologic disorders.

Use with caution in severely immunocompromised patient[s] (eg, patients receiving chemo/radiation therapy or othe[r] immunosuppressive therapy [including high-dose cortico[-]steroid]); may have a reduced response to vaccination. Inactivated vaccine (IIV or RIV) is preferred over live viru[s] vaccine for household members, healthcare workers an[d] others coming in close contact with severely-immunosup[-]pressed persons requiring care in a protected environmen[t] (CDC/ACIP [Grohskopf 2014]; NCIRD/ACIP 2011). In gen[-]eral, inactivated vaccines should be administered ≥[2] weeks prior to planned immunosuppression when feasibl[e] (IDSA [Rubin 2014]). Antigenic response may not be a[s] great as expected in HIV-infected persons with CD4 cell[s] <100/mm^3 and viral copies of HIV type 1 >30,000/mL, an[d] a second dose does not improve immune response i[n] these persons (CDC/ACIP 62[07] 2013). Antibod[y] responses may be lower and decline faster in older adult[s] ≥65 years compared to younger adults, especially by [6] months postvaccination; however, deferral to later in th[e] season may result in missed vaccination opportunities o[r] early season infection (CDC/ACIP [Grohskopf 2014]). Us[e] of this vaccine for specific medical and/or other indication[s] (eg, immunocompromising conditions, hepatic or kidne[y] disease, diabetes) is also addressed in the ACIP

Recommended Adult Immunization Schedule (CDC/ACIP [Kim 2015]). Specific recommendations for use of this vaccine in immunocompromised patients with asplenia, cancer, HIV infection, cerebrospinal fluid leaks, cochlear implants, hematopoietic stem cell transplant (prior to or after), sickle cell disease, solid organ transplant (prior to or after), or those receiving immunosuppressive therapy for chronic conditions are available from the IDSA (Rubin 2014).

Use with caution in patients with a history of bleeding disorders (including thrombocytopenia) and/or patients on anticoagulant therapy; bleeding/hematoma may occur from IM administration; if the patient receives antihemophilia or other similar therapy, IM injection can be scheduled shortly after such therapy is administered (NCIRD/ACIP 2011). In order to maximize vaccination rates, the ACIP, as well as the Canadian National Advisory Committee on Immunization (NACI), recommends simultaneous administration (ie, >1 vaccine on the same day at different anatomic sites) of all age-appropriate vaccines (live or inactivated) for which a person is eligible at a single clinic visit, unless contraindications exist. The ACIP prefers each dose of a specific vaccine in a series come from the same manufacturer when possible (NACI July 2014; NCIRD/ACIP 2011). Vaccination may not result in effective immunity in all patients. Response depends upon multiple factors (eg, type of vaccine, age of patient) and may be improved by administering the vaccine at the recommended dose, route, and interval. Vaccines may not be effective if administered during periods of altered immune competence (NCIRD/ACIP 2011). Influenza vaccines from previous seasons must not be used (CDC/ACIP 62[07] 2013).

Warnings: Additional Pediatric Considerations Use with caution in patients with history of febrile convulsions.

Adverse Reactions All serious adverse reactions must be reported to the US Department of Health and Human Services (DHHS) Vaccine Adverse Event Reporting System (VAERS) 1-800-822-7967 or online at https://vaers.hhs.gov/esub/index. In Canada, adverse reactions may be reported to local provincial/territorial health agencies or to the Vaccine Safety Section at Public Health Agency of Canada (1-866-844-0018).

Adverse reactions in adults ≥65 years of age may be greater using the high-dose vaccine, but are typically mild and transient.

Cardiovascular: Chest tightness, hypertension

Central nervous system: Chills, drowsiness, fatigue, headache, irritability, malaise, migraine, shivering

Dermatologic: Diaphoresis, ecchymoses

Gastrointestinal: Decreased appetite, diarrhea, gastroenteritis, nausea, sore throat, upper abdominal pain, vomiting

Infection: Infection, varicella

Local: Injection site reactions (including bruising, erythema, induration, inflammation, itching at injection site, pain, soreness, swelling at injection site, tenderness at injection site)

Neuromuscular & skeletal: Arthralgia, back pain, myalgia (may start within 6 to 12 hours and last 1 to 2 days; incidence generally equal to placebo in adults; occurs more frequently than placebo in children)

Ophthalmic: Eye redness

Respiratory: Bronchitis, cough, dyspnea, nasal congestion, nasopharyngitis, oropharyngeal pain, pharyngitis, pharyngolaryngeal pain, respiratory congestion (upper), rhinitis, rhinorrhea, upper respiratory tract infection, wheezing

Miscellaneous: Crying (infants and children 6 to 35 months), fever

Rare but important or life-threatening: Bell's palsy, erythema multiforme, febrile seizures, Guillain-Barre syndrome, hypersensitivity reaction (including oculorespiratory syndrome, an acute, self-limited reaction with ocular and respiratory symptoms) (CDC 62[07] 2013), IgA vasculitis, limb paralysis, lymphadenopathy, maculopapular rash, microscopic polyangiitis (vasculitis), myelitis (including encephalomyelitis), neuralgia, optic neuritis, optic neuropathy, paralysis (including limb), photophobia, seizure, serum sickness, Stevens-Johnson syndrome, syncope, tachycardia, thrombocytopenia, transverse myelitis, vasculitis, vesicobullous rash

Drug Interactions

Metabolism/Transport Effects None known.

Avoid Concomitant Use There are no known interactions where it is recommended to avoid concomitant use.

Increased Effect/Toxicity There are no known significant interactions involving an increase in effect.

Decreased Effect

Influenza Virus Vaccine (Inactivated) may decrease the levels/effects of: Pneumococcal Conjugate Vaccine (13-Valent)

The levels/effects of Influenza Virus Vaccine (Inactivated) may be decreased by: Belimumab; Fingolimod; Immunosuppressants; Pneumococcal Conjugate Vaccine (13-Valent)

Storage/Stability Store all products between 2°C to 8°C (36°F to 46°F). Potency is destroyed by freezing; do not use if product has been frozen.

Afluria: Discard multiple dose vials 28 days after initial entry. Between uses, the multiple dose vial should be stored at 2°C to 8°C (36°F to 46°F).

Fluarix, Fluarix Quadrivalent, Flucelvax: Protect from light.

Agriflu, Fluad: Protect from light. May be used if exposed to temperatures between 8°C to 25°C for less than 2 hours.

FluLaval, Fluviral: Discard multiple dose vials 28 days after initial entry. Protect from light.

Flulaval Quadrivalent: Between uses, the multiple dose vial should be stored at 2°C to 8°C (36°F to 46°F). Protect from light. Discard multiple dose vials 28 days after initial entry.

Fluvirin: Between uses, the multiple dose vial should be stored at 2°C to 8°C (36°F to 46°F). Protect from light.

Fluzone: Between uses, the multiple dose vial should be stored at 2°C to 8°C (36°F to 46°F).

Vaxigrip: Between uses, the multiple dose vial should be stored at 2°C to 8°C (36°F to 46°F). Discard 7 days after initial entry. Protect from light.

Mechanism of Action Promotes immunity to seasonal influenza virus by inducing specific antibody production. Each year the formulation is standardized according to the US Public Health Service. Preparations from previous seasons must not be used.

Pharmacodynamics

Onset of action: Most adults have antibody protection within 2 weeks of vaccination (CDC 62[07] 2013)

Duration: ≥6 to 8 months when vaccine is antigenically similar to circulating virus (CDC 62[07] 2013); response may be diminished in persons ≥65 years and limited evidence suggests titers may decline significantly 6 months following vaccination in this population (CDC/ACIP [Grohskopf 2014])

Dosing: Usual Influenza seasons vary in their timing and duration from year to year. In general, vaccination should begin soon after the vaccine becomes available (and, if possible, by October) and prior to onset of influenza activity in the community; however, vaccination should continue throughout the influenza season as long as vaccine is available. Unless noted, the ACIP does not have a preference for any given inactivated influenza vaccine (IIV) formulation when used within their specified age indications.

Pediatric:

Immunization:

Note: In infants and children <9 years, the number of doses needed per flu season is dependent upon vaccination history (see below). Additional dosing considerations are provided when vaccination history is available prior to the 2010 to 2011 season; see current guidelines for additional information (CDC/ACIP [Grohskopf 2014]).

A single dose for the 2014 to 2015 season if either of the following:

- If patient received ≥1 dose of seasonal influenza vaccine for the 2013 to 2014 season
- If patient received a total of ≥2 doses of seasonal influenza vaccine since July 1, 2010

Two doses for the 2014 to 2015 needed (separated by ≥4 weeks) if any of the following:

- Total of ≤1 dose of seasonal vaccine since July 1, 2010 (including no previous vaccination) unless the patient received the 2013 to 2014 seasonal influenza vaccine
- Vaccination status cannot be determined

Fluzone, Fluzone Quadrivalent: IM:

Infants and Children 6 to 35 months: 0.25 mL per dose for a total of 1 or 2 doses per season, dependent upon vaccination history (see **Note**)

Children 3 to 8 years: 0.5 mL per dose for a total of 1 or 2 doses per season, dependent upon vaccination history (see **Note**)

Children ≥9 years and Adolescents: 0.5 mL per dose as a single dose per season

Fluarix, Fluarix Quadrivalent, FluLaval, FluLaval Quadrivalent: IM:

Children 3 to 8 years: 0.5 mL per dose for a total of 1 or 2 doses per season, dependent upon vaccination history (see **Note**)

Children ≥9 years and Adolescents: 0.5 mL per dose as a single dose per season

Fluvirin: IM:

Children 4 to 8 years: 0.5 mL per dose for a total of 1 or 2 doses per season, dependent upon vaccination history (see **Note**)

Children ≥9 years and Adolescents: 0.5 mL per dose as a single dose per season

Afluria: **Note:** Although approved for use in children ≥5 years of age, the ACIP does not recommend use of Afluria in infants or children <9 years of age due to an increased incidence of fever and febrile seizures noted during the 2010 to 2011 influenza season. However, if other age appropriate vaccines are not available, children 5 to 8 years of age who are also considered at risk for influenza complications may be given Afluria after benefits and risks are discussed with parents or caregivers (AAP 2014; CDC/ACIP [Grohskopf 2014]).

Children 5 to 8 years: IM: 0.5 mL per dose for a total of 1 or 2 doses per season, dependent upon vaccination history (see **Note**)

Children ≥9 years and Adolescents <18 years: IM: 0.5 mL per dose as a single dose per season

Adolescents ≥18 years: IM or via PharmaJet Stratis Needle-Free Injection System: 0.5 mL per dose as a single dose per season

Fluzone Intradermal, Fluzone Intradermal Quadrivalent: Intradermal: Adolescents ≥18 years 0.1 mL per dose as a single dose per season

Flucelvax: IM: Adolescents ≥18 years: 0.5 mL per dose as a single dose per season

Adult:

Immunization:

Afluria:

≤64 years: IM or via PharmaJet Stratis Needle-Free Injection System: 0.5 mL per dose as a single dose per season

>64 years: IM: 0.5 mL per dose as a single dose per season

Fluarix, Fluarix Quadrivalent, Flucelvax, FluLaval, FluLaval Quadrivalent, Fluvirin, Fluzone, Fluzone Quadrivalent: IM: 0.5 mL per dose as a single dose per season

Fluzone Intradermal, Fluzone Intradermal Quadrivalent: Age ≤64 years: Intradermal: 0.1 mL per dose as a single dose per season

Fluzone High-Dose: IM: Adults ≥65 years: 0.5 mL per dose as a single dose per season

Dosing adjustment in renal impairment: There are no dosage adjustments provided in manufacturer's labeling.

Dosing adjustment in hepatic impairment: There are no dosage adjustments provided in manufacturer's labeling.

Administration To prevent syncope related injuries, adolescents and adults should be vaccinated while seated or lying down (NCIRD/ACIP 2011). US law requires that the date of administration; the vaccine manufacturer; lot number of vaccine; the administering person's name, title, and address; and documentation of the vaccine information statement (VIS; date on VIS and date given to patient) be entered into the patient's permanent medical record.

Intradermal: Fluzone Intradermal, Fluzone Intradermal Quadravalent: For intradermal administration over the deltoid muscle only. Shake gently prior to use. Hold system using the thumb and middle finger (do not place fingers on windows). Insert needle perpendicular to the skin; inject using index finger to push on plunger. Do not aspirate.

Intramuscular: Afluria, Fluarix, Fluarix Quadrivalent, FluLaval, FluLaval Quadrivalent, Flucelvax, Fluvirin, Fluzone, Fluzone High-Dose, Fluzone Quadrivalent: For IM administration only. Inspect for particulate matter and discoloration prior to administration. Shake suspension well prior to use. Jet injectors should not be used to administer inactivated influenza vaccines unless otherwise indicated in product labeling. Currently Afluria is the only influenza vaccine in the US that can be given IM by a jet-injector device.

Infants: IM injection in the anterolateral aspect of the thigh using a 1-inch needle length; do not inject into the gluteal region or areas where there may be a major nerve trunk

Children and Adults: IM injection in the deltoid muscle using a ≥1-inch needle length; children with adequate deltoid muscle mass should be vaccinated using a 1-inch needle, in some young children (1 to 2 years) a 5/8-inch needle may be adequate (NCIRD/ACIP 2011)

Afluria via PharmaJet Stratis Needle-Free Injection System: For IM administration only. For detailed instructions on preparation and administration of a dose, refer to the "Instructions For Use" available online at www.-pharmajet.com.

Patients at risk of bleeding (eg, patient receiving antihemophilic factor): For patients at risk of hemorrhage following intramuscular injection, the vaccine should be administered intramuscularly if, in the opinion of the physician familiar with the patient's bleeding risk, the vaccine can be administered by this route with reasonable safety. If the patient receives antihemophilia or other similar therapy, intramuscular vaccination can be scheduled shortly after such therapy is administered. A fine needle (23-gauge or smaller) can be used for the vaccination and firm pressure applied to the site (without rubbing) for at least 2 minutes. The patient should be instructed concerning the risk of hematoma from the injection. Patients on anticoagulant therapy should be considered to have the same bleeding risks and treated as those with clotting factor disorders (NCIRD/ACIP 2011).

If a pediatric vaccine (0.25 mL) is inadvertently administered to an adult an additional 0.25 mL should be administered to provide the full adult dose (0.5 mL). If the error is discovered after the patient has left, an adult dose should be given as soon as the patient can return. If an adult vaccine (0.5 mL) is inadvertently given to a child, no action needs to be taken (CDC 62[07] 2013).

Monitoring Parameters Observe for syncope for 15 minutes following administration (NCIRD/ACIP 2011). If seizure-like activity associated with syncope occurs, maintain patient in supine or Trendelenburg position to reestablish adequate cerebral perfusion. For those individuals who report a history of egg allergy but it is determined that the inactivated vaccine can be used, observe vaccine recipient for at least 30 minutes after receipt of vaccine (CDC/ACIP [Grohskopf 2014]).

Additional Information Pharmacies will stock the formulation(s) standardized according to the USPHS requirements for the season. Influenza vaccines from previous seasons must not be used. Seasonal quadrivalent influenza vaccines contain two subtype A strains and two subtype B strains; trivalent influenza vaccines contain two subtype A strains and one subtype B strain.

Dosage Forms Excipient information presented when available (limited, particularly for generics); consult specific product labeling. [DSC] = Discontinued product

Kit, Intramuscular:
- Physicians EZ Use Flu: [contains egg white (egg protein), neomycin, thimerosal]

Kit, Intramuscular [preservative free]:
- Medical Provider EZ Flu Shot: 0.5 mL [contains egg white (egg protein)]

Prefilled Syringe Kit, Intramuscular:
- Medical Provider EZ Flu: 0.5 mL (1 ea) [contains polysorbate 80]

Prefilled Syringe Kit, Intramuscular [preservative free]:
- Medical Provider EZ Flu PF: 0.5 mL (1 ea) [contains egg white (egg protein), neomycin]
- Medical Provider EZ Flu Shot: 0.5 mL (1 ea) [contains egg white (egg protein)]

Suspension, Intramuscular:
- Afluria: (5 mL) [contains egg white (egg protein), neomycin sulfate, thimerosal]
- Flulaval: (5 mL) [contains egg white (egg protein), polysorbate 80, thimerosal]
- Flulaval: (5 mL [DSC]) [contains egg white (egg protein), thimerosal]
- Flulaval Quadrivalent: (5 mL) [contains egg white (egg protein), polysorbate 80, thimerosal]
- Fluvirin: (5 mL) [contains egg white (egg protein), neomycin, thimerosal]
- Fluzone: (5 mL) [contains egg white (egg protein), formaldehyde solution, gelatin (pork), thimerosal]
- Fluzone: (5 mL [DSC]) [contains egg white (egg protein), gelatin (pork), thimerosal]
- Fluzone Quadrivalent: (5 mL) [contains egg white (egg protein), formaldehyde solution, thimerosal]
- Fluzone Quadrivalent: (5 mL [DSC]) [contains egg white (egg protein), polysorbate 80, thimerosal]

Suspension, Intramuscular [preservative free]:
- Fluzone Preservative Free: (0.5 mL [DSC]) [contains egg white (egg protein), gelatin (pork)]
- Fluzone Quadrivalent: 0.5 mL (0.5 mL) [contains egg white (egg protein)]
- Fluzone Quadrivalent: 0.5 mL (0.5 mL) [contains egg white (egg protein), formaldehyde solution]

Suspension Pen-injector, Intradermal [preservative free]:
- Fluzone: 9 mcg/strain (0.1 mL [DSC]) [contains egg white (egg protein)]
- Fluzone Quadrivalent: 9 mcg/strain (0.1 mL) [contains egg white (egg protein), formaldehyde solution]

Suspension Prefilled Syringe, Intramuscular:
- Fluarix Quadrivalent: 0.5 mL (0.5 mL [DSC]) [contains egg white (egg protein)]
- Fluarix Quadrivalent: 0.5 mL (0.5 mL) [contains egg white (egg protein), polysorbate 80]

Suspension Prefilled Syringe, Intramuscular [preservative free]:
- Afluria Preservative Free: 0.5 mL (0.5 mL) [contains egg white (egg protein), neomycin sulfate]
- Fluarix: 0.5 mL (0.5 mL) [contains egg white (egg protein), polysorbate 80]
- Fluarix Quadrivalent: 0.5 mL (0.5 mL) [contains egg white (egg protein), formaldehyde solution, polysorbate 80]
- Flucelvax: 0.5 mL (0.5 mL) [contains polysorbate 80]
- Flulaval Quadrivalent: 0.5 mL (0.5 mL) [contains egg white (egg protein), polysorbate 80]
- Fluvirin Preservative Free: 0.5 mL (0.5 mL) [contains egg white (egg protein), neomycin]
- Fluzone High-Dose: 0.5 mL (0.5 mL [DSC]) [contains egg white (egg protein)]
- Fluzone High-Dose: 0.5 mL (0.5 mL) [contains egg white (egg protein), formaldehyde solution, gelatin (pork), thimerosal]
- Fluzone Pediatric PF: 0.25 mL (0.25 mL [DSC]) [contains egg white (egg protein), gelatin (pork)]
- Fluzone Preservative Free: 0.5 mL (0.5 mL [DSC]) [contains egg white (egg protein), gelatin (pork)]
- Fluzone Quadrivalent: 0.25 mL (0.25 mL [DSC]) [contains egg white (egg protein)]
- Fluzone Quadrivalent: 0.25 mL (0.25 mL) [contains egg white (egg protein), formaldehyde solution]
- Fluzone Quadrivalent: 0.5 mL (0.5 mL [DSC]) [contains egg white (egg protein)]
- Fluzone Quadrivalent: 0.5 mL (0.5 mL) [contains egg white (egg protein), formaldehyde solution]

Influenza Virus Vaccine (Live/Attenuated)

(in floo EN za VYE rus vak SEEN live ah TEN yoo aye ted)

Medication Safety Issues

Sound-alike/look-alike issues:

FluMist may be confused with flumazenil

Related Information

Centers for Disease Control and Prevention (CDC) and Other Links *on page 2424*

Immunization Administration Recommendations *on page 2411*

Immunization Schedules *on page 2416*

Brand Names: US FluMist; FluMist Quadrivalent

Brand Names: Canada FluMist

Therapeutic Category Vaccine; Vaccine, Live (Viral); Vaccine, Live/Attenuated

Generic Availability (US) No

Use Active immunization against influenza disease caused by influenza virus subtypes A and type B contained in the vaccine (FDA approved in ages 2 to 49 years)

The Advisory Committee on Immunization Practices (ACIP) recommends routine annual vaccination with seasonal influenza vaccine for all persons ≥6 months who do not otherwise have contraindications to the vaccine. ACIP recommends use of any age- and risk factor-appropriate product. Healthy, nonpregnant persons aged 2 to 49 years may receive vaccination with the seasonal live, attenuated influenza vaccine (LAIV) (nasal spray). In addition, other alternative products are available for certain patient populations: Persons ≥6 months of age may receive the trivalent inactivated influenza vaccine (IIV3) or the quadrivalent inactivated influenza vaccine (IIV4); persons ≥18 years may receive vaccination with the recombinant influenza vaccine (RIV) (CDC/ACIP [Grohskopf 2014]).

Medication Guide Available Yes

Pregnancy Risk Factor B

Pregnancy Considerations Adverse events were not observed in animal reproduction studies. LAIV is not recommended for use during pregnancy. Influenza vaccination with the inactivated influenza vaccine (IIV) is recommended for all women who are or will become pregnant during the influenza season and who do not otherwise have contraindications to the vaccine (CDC 62[07] 2013).

Healthy pregnant women do not need to avoid contact with persons vaccinated with LAIV (CDC 62[07] 2013). The nasal vaccine contains the same strains of influenza A and B found in the injection. Information specific to the use of LAIV in pregnancy is limited.

Health care providers are encouraged to refer women exposed to the influenza vaccine during pregnancy to the Vaccines and Medications in Pregnancy Surveillance System (VAMPSS) by contacting The Organization of Teratology Information Specialists (OTIS) at (877) 311-8972.

Breast-Feeding Considerations It is not known if the vaccine is excreted into breast milk. LAIV should be used with caution in breast-feeding women (per manufacturer) due to the possibility of virus excretion into breast milk; however, LAIV may be administered to breast-feeding women unless contraindicated due to other reasons (per CDC). Postpartum women may be vaccinated with either IIV or LAIV. When vaccine supply is limited, focus on delivering the vaccine should be given to mothers of newborns and contacts or caregivers of children <5 years of age (CDC 62[07] 2013).

Contraindications Severe allergic reaction (eg, anaphylaxis) to previous influenza vaccination; hypersensitivity to any component of the formulation, including egg protein; children and adolescents through 17 years of age receiving aspirin therapy

Warnings/Precautions Immediate treatment (including epinephrine 1:1000) for anaphylactoid and/or hypersensitivity reactions should be available during vaccine use (NCIRD/ACIP 2011). Manufactured with chicken egg protein. Allergy to eggs must be distinguished from allergy to the vaccine. Recommendations are available from the CDC regarding influenza vaccination to persons who report egg allergies; however, a prior severe allergic reaction to influenza vaccine, regardless of the component suspected, is a contraindication to vaccination. ACIP recommends use of IIV or RIV (if RIV is age appropriate) over LAIV when considering vaccination in persons reporting an egg allergy (due to lack of data of LAIV use in this setting) (CDC/ACIP [Grohskopf 2014]). Also manufactured with arginine, gelatin, and gentamicin.

Use with caution in patients with history of Guillain-Barré syndrome (GBS); patients with history of GBS have a greater likelihood of developing GBS than those without. As a precaution, the ACIP recommends that patients with a history of GBS and who are at low risk for severe influenza complications, and patients known to have experienced GBS within 6 weeks following previous vaccination should generally not be vaccinated (consider influenza antiviral chemoprophylaxis in these patients). Based on limited data, the benefits of vaccinating persons with a history of GBS who are also at high risk for complications of influenza may outweigh the risks (CDC 62[07] 2013). Recent studies of patients who received the trivalent inactivated influenza vaccine or the monovalent H1N1 influenza vaccine have shown the risk of GBS is lower with vaccination than with influenza infection (Baxter 2013; Greene 2013; Kwong 2013).

Data on the use of the nasal spray in immunocompromised patients is limited. **Avoid contact with severely immunocompromised individuals for at least 7 days following vaccination (at least 14 days per Canadian labeling).** ACIP does not recommend the use of LAIV in immunosuppressed patients (CDC/ACIP [Grohskopf 2014]). ACIP does not recommend the use of LAIV for persons who care for severely immunocompromised individuals who require a protective environment due to the theoretical risk of transmitting the live virus from the vaccine. Persons who care for the severely immunocompromised should receive either IIV or RIV. Persons who have received LAIV should avoid contact with severely immunocompromised individuals for at least 7 days following vaccination (at least 14 days per Canadian labeling) (CDC 62[07] 2013). In general, live vaccines should be administered ≥4 weeks prior to planned immunosuppression and avoided within 2 weeks of immunosuppression when feasible (IDSA [Rubin 2014]).

Per the US prescribing information, the nasal spray should not be used in patients with asthma or children <5 years of age with recurrent wheezing; risk of wheezing following vaccination is increased. Patients with severe asthma or active wheezing were not included in clinical trials. Children <24 months of age had increased wheezing and hospitalizations following administration in clinical trials; use of the nasal spray is not approved in this age group. ACIP does not recommend the use of LAIV in patients with chronic pulmonary disorders including asthma and children 2-4 years of age who have had asthma or wheezing episodes within the past year (CDC/ACIP [Grohskopf 2014]). The safety of LAIV has not been established in individuals with underlying medical conditions that may predispose them to complications following wild-type influenza infection.

The decision to administer or delay vaccination because of current or recent febrile illness depends on the severity of symptoms and the etiology of the disease. Consider deferring administration in patients with moderate or severe acute illness (with or without fever); vaccination should not be delayed for patients with mild acute illness (with or without fever) (NCIRD/ACIP 2011). ACIP does not recommend the use of LAIV in patients with chronic disorders of the cardiovascular system (except isolated hypertension), chronic metabolic diseases, hematologic disorders and hemoglobinopathies, hepatic disease, persons with HIV, neurologic or neuromuscular disorders, renal disease, or pregnant women (CDC/ACIP [Grohskopf 2014]). Use of this vaccine for specific medical and/or other indications (eg, immunocompromising conditions, hepatic or kidney disease, diabetes) is also addressed in the ACIP Recommended Adult Immunization Schedule (CDC/ACIP [Kim 2015]). Specific recommendations for use of this vaccine in immunocompromised patients with asplenia, cancer, HIV infection, cerebrospinal fluid leaks, cochlear implants, hematopoietic stem cell transplant (prior to or after), sickle cell disease, solid organ transplant (prior to or after), or those receiving immunosuppressive therapy for chronic conditions as well as contacts of immunocompromised patients are available from the IDSA (Rubin 2014).

Defer immunization if nasal congestion is present which may impede delivery of vaccine (CDC 62[07] 2013). In order to maximize vaccination rates, the ACIP recommends simultaneous administration (ie, >1 vaccine on the same day at different anatomic sites) of all age-appropriate vaccines (live or inactivated) for which a person is eligible at a single clinic visit, unless contraindications exist. The ACIP prefers each dose of a specific vaccine in a series come from the same manufacturer when possible (NCIRD/ACIP 2011).

Studies conducted in children using trivalent IIV and LAIV have shown significantly greater efficacy of LAIV in younger children. Information is not yet available for the quadrivalent LAIV vaccine (CDC 62[07] 2013). The safety and efficacy of the nasal spray have not been established in adults ≥50 years of age (US labeling) or ≥60 years of age (Canadian labeling). Vaccination may not result in effective immunity in all patients. Response depends upon multiple factors (eg, type of vaccine, age of patient) and may be improved by administering the vaccine at the recommended dose, route, and interval. Vaccines may not be effective if administered during periods of altered immune competence (NCIRD/ACIP 2011). Influenza vaccines from previous seasons must not be used (CDC 62 [07] 2013).

Adverse Reactions All serious adverse reactions must be reported to the U.S. Department of Health and Human Services (DHHS) Vaccine Adverse Event Reporting System (VAERS) 1-800-822-7967 or online at https://vaers.hhs.gov/esub/index. In Canada, adverse reactions may be reported to local provincial/territorial health agencies or to the Vaccine Safety Section at Public Health Agency of Canada (1-866-844-0018).

Central nervous system: Chills, fever, headache, irritability, lethargy

Gastrointestinal: Abdominal pain, appetite decreased

Neuromuscular & skeletal: Muscle aches, tiredness/ weakness

Otic: Otitis media

Respiratory: Sinusitis, sneezing

Respiratory: Cough, nasal congestion/ runny nose, wheezing

Rare but important or life-threatening: Anaphylactic reactions, asthma exacerbations, Bell's palsy, encephalitis (vaccine associated), epistaxis, Guillain-Barré syndrome, hypersensitivity reaction, meningitis (including eosinophilic meningitis), mitochondrial encephalomyopathy (Leigh syndrome) exacerbation, pericarditis

Drug Interactions

Metabolism/Transport Effects None known.

Avoid Concomitant Use

Avoid concomitant use of Influenza Virus Vaccine (Live/ Attenuated) with any of the following: Belimumab; Fingolimod; Immunosuppressants; Salicylates

Increased Effect/Toxicity

Influenza Virus Vaccine (Live/Attenuated) may increase the levels/effects of: Salicylates

The levels/effects of Influenza Virus Vaccine (Live/Attenuated) may be increased by: AzaTHIOprine; Belimumab; Corticosteroids (Systemic); Dimethyl Fumarate; Fingolimod; Immunosuppressants; Leflunomide; Mercaptopurine; Methotrexate

Decreased Effect

Influenza Virus Vaccine (Live/Attenuated) may decrease the levels/effects of: Tuberculin Tests

The levels/effects of Influenza Virus Vaccine (Live/Attenuated) may be decreased by: Antiviral Agents (Influenza A and B); AzaTHIOprine; Corticosteroids (Systemic); Dimethyl Fumarate; Fingolimod; Immunosuppressants; Leflunomide; Mercaptopurine; Methotrexate

Storage/Stability Store in refrigerator at 2°C to 8°C (35°F to 46°F). **Do not freeze.** The vaccine may be exposed to temperatures of up to 25°C for up to 12 hours without adverse impact; return to refrigerator as soon as possible; only a single excursion outside of the recommended storage conditions is permitted.

Mechanism of Action The vaccine contains live attenuated viruses which infect and replicate within the cells lining the nasopharynx. Promotes immunity to seasonal influenza virus by inducing specific antibody production. Each year the formulation is standardized according to the US Public Health Service. Preparations from previous seasons must not be used.

Pharmacodynamics

Onset of action: Adults: Most adults have antibody protection within 2 weeks of vaccination (CDC 62[07] 2013)

Duration: ≥6 to 8 months when vaccine is antigenically similar to circulating virus (CDC 62[07] 2013); response may be diminished in persons ≥65 years and limited evidence suggests titers may decline significantly 6 months following vaccination in this population (CDC/ ACIP [Grohskopf 2014])

Pharmacokinetics (Adult data unless noted) Distribution: Following nasal administration, vaccine is distributed in the nasal cavity (~90%), stomach (~3%), brain (~2%), and lung (0.4%)

Dosing: Usual Administer vaccine prior to exposure to influenza. It is important to note that influenza seasons vary in their timing and duration from year to year. In general, vaccination should begin soon after the vaccine becomes available (and, if possible, by October) and prior to onset of influenza activity in the community; however, vaccination should continue throughout the influenza season as long as vaccine is available (CDC/ACIP [Grohskopf 2014]).

Pediatric: **Immunization:**

Note: In infants and children <9 years, the number of doses needed per flu season is dependent upon vaccination history (see below). Additional dosing considerations are provided when vaccination history is available prior to the 2010 to 2011 season; see current guidelines for additional information (CDC/ACIP [Grohskopf 2014]).

A single dose for the 2014 to 2015 season if either of the following:

- If patient received ≥ 1 dose of seasonal influenza vaccine for the 2013 to 2014 season
- If patient received a total of ≥2 doses of seasonal influenza vaccine since July 1, 2010

Two doses for the 2014 to 2015 needed (separated by ≥4 weeks) if any of the following:

- Total of ≤1 dose of seasonal vaccine since July 1, 2010 (including no previous vaccination) unless the patient received the 2013 to 2014 seasonal influenza vaccine
- Vaccination status cannot be determined

Children 2 to 8 years: Intranasal: 0.2 mL per dose (half dose per nostril); 1 or 2 doses per season, dependent upon vaccination history (see **Note**)

Children and Adolescents 9 to 18 years: Intranasal: 0.2 mL per dose (half dose per nostril (1 dose per season)

Adult: **Immunization:** Adults ≤49 years: Intranasal: 0.2 mL per dose (half dose per nostril) (1 dose per season)

Dosing adjustment in renal impairment: There are no dosage adjustments provided in manufacturer's labeling.

Dosing adjustment in hepatic impairment: There are no dosage adjustments provided in manufacturer's labeling.

Administration Intranasal: For intranasal administration only; do not inject. Administer 0.1 mL (half of the dose from a single sprayer) into each nostril while the recipient is in an upright position. Place the tip of the sprayer inside the nostril and depress plunger as rapidly as possible to deliver the dose. Remove dose divider clip and repeat into opposite nostril. The patient does not need to inhale during administration (may breath normally). If recipient sneezes following administration, the dose should not be repeated (CDC/ACIP 62[07] 2013).

U.S. law requires that the date of administration, name of the vaccine manufacturer, lot number of vaccine, and the administering person's name, title, and address and documentation of the vaccine information statement (VIS; date on VIS, and date given to patient) be entered into the patient's permanent medical record.

Test Interactions Administration of the intranasal influenza virus vaccine (live, LAIV) may cause a positive result on the rapid influenza diagnostic test for the 7 days after vaccine administration; for a person with influenza-like illness during this time, the positive test could be caused by either the live attenuated vaccine or wild-type influenza virus (Ali 2004).

Additional Information Seasonal quadrivalent influenza vaccines contain two subtype A strains and two subtype B strains; trivalent influenza vaccines contain two subtype A strains and one subtype B strain.

When vaccine supply is limited, target groups for influenza vaccination (those at higher risk of complications from influenza infection and their close contacts) include the following (CDC/ACIP 62[07] 2013): **Note:** Only use LAIV if appropriate:

- All Infants and Children 6 to 59 months of age
- Persons ≥50 years of age
- Residents of nursing homes and other long-term care facilities
- Adults and children with chronic pulmonary disorders (including asthma) or cardiovascular systems disorders (except hypertension), renal, hepatic, neurologic, or metabolic disorders (including diabetes mellitus)
- Persons who have immunosuppression (including immunosuppression caused by medications or HIV)
- Infants, children, and adolescents (6 months to 18 years of age) who are receiving long-term aspirin therapy, and therefore, may be at risk for developing Reye's syndrome after influenza
- Women who are or will be pregnant during the influenza season
- Health care personnel
- Household contacts (including children) and caregivers of neonates, infants, and children <5 years (particularly children <6 months) and adults ≥50 years
- Household contacts (including children) and caregivers of persons with medical conditions which put them at high risk of complications from influenza infection
- American Indians/Alaska Natives
- Morbidly obese (BMI ≥40)

Dosage Forms Excipient information presented when available (limited, particularly for generics); consult specific product labeling. [DSC] = Discontinued product

Liquid, Nasal [preservative free]:

FluMist: (1 ea) [contains egg white (egg protein), gelatin (pork)]

Suspension, Nasal [preservative free]:

FluMist Quadrivalent: (1 ea [DSC]) [latex free; contains egg white (egg protein), gelatin (pork)]

FluMist Quadrivalent: (1 ea) [contains egg white (egg protein), gelatin (pork)]

◆ **Influenza Virus Vaccine (Purified Surface Antigen)** *see* Influenza Virus Vaccine (Inactivated) *on page 1108*

Influenza Virus Vaccine (Recombinant)

(in floo EN za VYE rus vak SEEN ree KOM be nant)

Medication Safety Issues

Sound-alike/look-alike issues:

Influenza virus vaccine may be confused with perflutren lipid microspheres

Influenza virus vaccine may be confused with tetanus toxoid and tuberculin products. Medication errors have occurred when tuberculin skin tests (PPD) have been inadvertently administered instead of tetanus toxoid products and influenza virus vaccine. These products are refrigerated and often stored in close proximity to each other.

Related Information

Centers for Disease Control and Prevention (CDC) and Other Links *on page 2424*

Immunization Administration Recommendations *on page 2411*

Immunization Schedules *on page 2416*

Brand Names: US Flublok

Therapeutic Category Vaccine; Vaccine, Recombinant

Generic Availability (US) No

Use Active immunization against influenza disease caused by influenza virus subtypes A and type B contained in the vaccine (FDA approved in ages ≥18 years)

The Advisory Committee on Immunization Practices (ACIP) recommends routine annual vaccination with seasonal influenza vaccine for all persons ≥6 months who do not otherwise have contraindications to the vaccine. ACIP recommends use of any age- and risk factor-appropriate product. Persons ≥18 years may receive vaccination with the recombinant influenza vaccine (RIV). In addition to RIV, other products are available for certain patient populations: Healthy nonpregnant persons aged 2 to 49 years may receive vaccination with the live attenuated influenza vaccine (LAIV). Persons ≥6 months of age may receive the trivalent inactivated influenza vaccine (IIV3) or the quadrivalent inactivated influenza vaccine (IIV4) (CDC/ACIP [Grohskopf 2014]).

Pregnancy Risk Factor B

Pregnancy Considerations Adverse events were not observed in animal reproduction studies. Information specific to the use of RIV in pregnancy has not been located.

Pregnant women are at an increased risk of complications from influenza infection (Rasmussen 2008). Influenza vaccination with the inactivated influenza vaccine (IIV) is recommended for all women who are or will become pregnant during the influenza season and who do not otherwise have contraindications to the vaccine (CDC 62 [07] 2013). Pregnant women should observe the same precautions as nonpregnant women to reduce the risk of exposure to influenza and other respiratory infections (CDC 2010). When vaccine supply is limited, focus on delivering the vaccine should be given to women who are pregnant or will be pregnant during the flu season, as well as mothers of newborns and contacts or caregivers of children <5 years of age (CDC 62[07] 2013).

Health care providers are encouraged to refer women exposed to the influenza vaccine during pregnancy to the *Vaccines and Medications in Pregnancy Surveillance System* (VAMPSS) by contacting The Organization of Teratology Information Specialists (OTIS) at (877) 311-8972. Women exposed to this vaccine during pregnancy may also contact the Flublock pregnancy registry at 888-855-7871.

Breast-Feeding Considerations It is not known if this vaccine is excreted into breast milk. The manufacturer recommends that caution be used if administered to breast-feeding women. Recombinant vaccines do not affect the safety of breast-feeding for the mother or the infant. Breast-feeding infants should be vaccinated according to the recommended schedules (NCIRD/ACIP 2011). When vaccine supply is limited, focus on delivering the vaccine should be given to women who are pregnant or will be pregnant during the flu season, as well as mothers of newborns and contacts or caregivers of children <5 years of age (CDC 62[07] 2013).

Contraindications Severe allergic reaction (eg, anaphylaxis) to any component of the vaccine

Warnings/Precautions Immediate treatment (including epinephrine 1:1000) for anaphylactoid and/or hypersensitivity reactions should be available during vaccine use (NCIRD/ACIP 2011). Syncope has been reported with use of injectable vaccines and may result in serious secondary injury (eg, skull fracture, cerebral hemorrhage); typically reported in adolescents and young adults and within 15 minutes after vaccination. Procedures should be in place to avoid injuries from falling and to restore cerebral perfusion if syncope occurs (NCIRD/ACIP 2011). The decision to administer or delay vaccination because of current or recent febrile illness depends on the severity of symptoms and the etiology of the disease. Consider deferring administration in patients with moderate or severe acute illness (with or without fever); vaccination should not be delayed for patients with mild acute illness (with or without fever) (NCIRD/ACIP 2011). Use with caution in patients with a history of bleeding disorders (including thrombocytopenia) and/or patients on anticoagulant therapy; bleeding/hematoma may occur from IM administration; if the patient receives antihemophilia or other similar therapy, IM injection can be scheduled shortly after such therapy is administered (NCIRD/ACIP 2011). Use with caution in patients with history of Guillain-Barré syndrome (GBS); patients with history of GBS have a greater likelihood of developing GBS than those without. As a precaution, the ACIP recommends that patients with a history of GBS and who are at low risk for severe influenza complications, and patients known to have experienced GBS within 6 weeks following previous vaccination should generally not be vaccinated (consider influenza antiviral chemoprophylaxis in these patients). The benefits of vaccination may outweigh the potential risks in persons with a history of GBS who are also at high risk for complications of influenza. Influenza infection itself may cause Guillain-Barré syndrome (CDC 62[07] 2013). Recent studies of patients who received the trivalent inactivated influenza vaccine or the monovalent H1N1 influenza vaccine have shown the risk of GBS is lower with vaccination than with influenza infection (Baxter 2013; Greene 2013; Kwong 2013). Use with caution in severely-immunocompromised patients (eg, patients receiving chemo/radiation therapy or other immunosuppressive therapy [including high-dose corticosteroid]); may have a reduced response to vaccination. Inactivated vaccine (IIV or RIV) is preferred over live virus vaccine for household members, healthcare workers and others coming in close contact with severely immunosuppressed persons requiring care in a protected environment (CDC/ACIP [Grohskopf 2014]; NCIRD/ACIP 2011); inactivated vaccines should be administered ≥2 weeks prior to planned immunosuppression when feasible (IDSA [Rubin 2014]).

In a clinical trial of infants and children 6 months through 3 years of age, a decreased response to Flublok was reported compared to currently licensed US influenza vaccine for this population, suggesting that it would not be effective in children ≤3 years; safety and efficacy in older pediatric patients have not been established; use has not been studied. Flublok is a trivalent influenza vaccine produced using continuous insect cell lines. It is a recombinant hemagglutinin (rHA) vaccine; it does not use the influenza virus or eggs in its production process. ACIP states it may be used in persons with an egg allergy of any severity if otherwise appropriate (CDC/ACIP [Grohskopf 2014]).

In order to maximize vaccination rates, the ACIP recommends simultaneous administration (ie, >1 vaccine on the same day at different anatomic sites) of all age-appropriate vaccines (live or inactivated) for which a person is eligible at a single clinic visit, unless contraindications exist. The ACIP prefers each dose of a specific vaccine in a series come from the same manufacturer when possible (NCIRD/ACIP 2011). Vaccination may not result in effective immunity in all patients. Response depends upon multiple factors (eg, type of vaccine, age of patient) and may be improved by administering the vaccine at the recommended dose, route, and interval. Vaccines may not be effective if administered during periods of altered immune competence (NCIRD/ACIP 2011). Influenza vaccines from previous seasons must not be used (CDC 62 [07] 2013). Use of this vaccine for specific medical and/or other indications (eg, immunocompromising conditions, hepatic or kidney disease, diabetes) is also addressed in the ACIP Recommended Adult Immunization Schedule (Kim 2015).

Adverse Reactions All serious adverse reactions must be reported to the U.S. Department of Health and Human Services (DHHS) Vaccine Adverse Event Reporting System (VAERS) 1-800-822-7967 or online at https://vaers.hhs.gov/esub/index. In Canada, adverse reactions may be reported to local provincial/territorial health agencies or to the Vaccine Safety Section at Public Health Agency of Canada (1-866-844-0018).

Central nervous system: Chills, fatigue, headache (more common in older adults)

Gastrointestinal: Nausea

Local: Injection site reactions (includes redness, swelling and firmness), pain at injection site

Neuromuscular & skeletal: Arthralgia, myalgia

Respiratory: Cough, nasal congestion, nasopharyngitis, pharyngolaryngeal pain, rhinorrhea, upper respiratory tract infection

Rare but important or life-threatening: Hypersensitivity reaction, pleuropericarditis

Storage/Stability Store between 2°C to 8°C (36°F to 46°F). Protect from light. Do not freeze. Discard if frozen.

Mechanism of Action Promotes immunity to seasonal influenza virus by inducing specific antibody production. Each year the formulation is standardized according to the US Public Health Service. Preparations from previous seasons must not be used.

Pharmacodynamics

Onset of action: Most adults have antibody protection within 2 weeks of vaccination (CDC 62[07] 2013)

Duration: ≥6 to 8 months when vaccine is antigenically similar to circulating virus (CDC 62[07] 2013); response may be diminished in persons ≥65 years and limited evidence suggests titers may decline significantly 6 months following vaccination in this population (CDC/ACIP [Grohskopf 2014])

Dosing: Usual Influenza seasons vary in their timing and duration from year to year. In general, vaccination should begin soon after the vaccine becomes available (if possible, by October) and prior to onset of influenza activity in the community; however, vaccination should continue throughout the influenza season as long as vaccine is available (CDC/ACIP [Grohskopf 2014]).

Immunization: Adolescents ≥18 years and Adults: IM: 0.5 mL per dose as a single dose per season.

Dosing adjustment in renal impairment: There are no dosage adjustments provided in manufacturer's labeling.

Dosing adjustment in hepatic impairment: There are no dosage adjustments provided in manufacturer's labeling.

Administration To prevent syncope related injuries, adolescents and adults should be vaccinated while seated or lying down (NCIRD/ACIP 2011). US law requires that the date of administration; the vaccine manufacturer; lot number of vaccine; the administering person's name, title, and address; and documentation of the vaccine information statement (VIS; date on VIS and date given to patient) be entered into the patient's permanent medical record.

For IM administration only. Shake gently prior to use; inspect for particulate matter and discoloration prior to administration; avoid use if visible particles are present in the solution after shaking. Administer IM in the deltoid muscle; do not inject into the gluteal region or areas where there may be a major nerve trunk. Jet injectors should not be used to administer inactivated influenza vaccines unless otherwise indicated in product labeling (CDC 62 [07] 2013). Currently Afluria is the only influenza vaccine in the US that can be given by a jet-injector device.

For patients at risk of hemorrhage following intramuscular injection, the vaccine should be administered intramuscularly if, in the opinion of the physician familiar with the patient's bleeding risk, the vaccine can be administered by this route with reasonable safety. If the patient receives antihemophilia or other similar therapy, intramuscular vaccination can be scheduled shortly after such therapy is administered. A fine needle (23 gauge or smaller) can be used for the vaccination and firm pressure applied to the site (without rubbing) for at least 2 minutes. The patient should be instructed concerning the risk of hematoma from the injection. Patients on anticoagulant therapy should be considered to have the same bleeding risks and treated as those with clotting factor disorders (NCIRD/ACIP 2011).

Monitoring Parameters Monitor for syncope for 15 minutes following administration (NCIRD/ACIP 2011). If seizure-like activity associated with syncope occurs, maintain patient in supine or Trendelenburg position to reestablish adequate cerebral perfusion.

Additional Information Pharmacies will stock the formulation(s) standardized according to the USPHS requirements for the season. Influenza vaccines from previous seasons must not be used.

Seasonal quadrivalent influenza vaccines contain two subtype A strains and two subtype B strains; trivalent influenza vaccines contain two subtype A strains and one subtype B strain.

Dosage Forms Excipient information presented when available (limited, particularly for generics); consult specific product labeling.

Solution, Intramuscular [preservative free]:

Flublok: (0.5 mL) [no egg protein]

◆ **Influenza Virus Vaccine (Split-Virus)** *see* Influenza Virus Vaccine (Inactivated) *on page 1108*

◆ **Influenza Virus Vaccine (Trivalent, Live)** *see* Influenza Virus Vaccine (Live/Attenuated) *on page 1113*

◆ **Influvac (Can)** *see* Influenza Virus Vaccine (Inactivated) *on page 1108*

◆ **Infufer (Can)** *see* Iron Dextran Complex *on page 1164*

◆ **Infumorph 200** *see* Morphine (Systemic) *on page 1461*

◆ **Infumorph 500** *see* Morphine (Systemic) *on page 1461*

◆ **INH** *see* Isoniazid *on page 1168*

◆ **InnoPran XL** *see* Propranolol *on page 1789*

◆ **Inova** *see* Benzoyl Peroxide *on page 270*

◆ **Instacort 5 [OTC]** *see* Hydrocortisone (Topical) *on page 1041*

◆ **Instacort 10 [OTC]** *see* Hydrocortisone (Topical) *on page 1041*

◆ **Insta-Glucose [OTC]** *see* Dextrose *on page 633*

Insulin Aspart (IN soo lin AS part)

Medication Safety Issues

Sound-alike/look-alike issues:

NovoLOG® may be confused with HumaLOG®, HumuLIN® R, Nimbex®, NovoLIN® N, NovoLIN® R, NovoLOG® Mix 70/30

High alert medication:

The Institute for Safe Medication Practices (ISMP) includes this medication among its list of drugs which have a heightened risk of causing significant patient harm when used in error. ***Due to the number of insulin preparations, it is essential to identify/clarify the type of insulin to be used.***

Other safety concerns:

Cross-contamination may occur if insulin pens are shared among multiple patients. Steps should be taken to prohibit sharing of insulin pens.

Related Information

Insulin Products *on page 2319*

Brand Names: US NovoLOG; NovoLOG FlexPen; NovoLOG PenFill

Brand Names: Canada NovoRapid®

Therapeutic Category Antidiabetic Agent, Parenteral; Insulin, Rapid-Acting

Generic Availability (US) No

Use Treatment of type 1 diabetes mellitus (insulin dependent, IDDM); type 2 diabetes mellitus (noninsulin dependent, NIDDM) to control hyperglycemia

Pregnancy Risk Factor B

Pregnancy Considerations Dose-related adverse effects were observed in animal reproduction studies. Insulin aspart can be detected in cord blood (Pettitt, 2007).

In women with diabetes, maternal hyperglycemia can be associated with congenital malformations as well as adverse effects in the fetus, neonate, and the mother (ACOG 2005; ADA 2015; Kitzmiller 2008; Metzger 2007). To prevent adverse outcomes, prior to conception and throughout pregnancy maternal blood glucose and HbA_{1c} should be kept as close to target goals as possible but without causing significant hypoglycemia (ACOG 2013; ADA 2015; Blumer 2013; Kitzmiller 2008; Lambert 2013). Prior to pregnancy, effective contraception should be used until glycemic control is achieved (Kitzmiller 2008).

Insulin requirements tend to fall during the first trimester of pregnancy and increase in the later trimesters, peaking at 28 to 32 weeks of gestation. Following delivery, insulin requirements decrease rapidly (ACOG 2005). Insulin aspart may be used to treat diabetes in pregnant women (ACOG 2013; Blumer 2013; Kitzmiller 2008; Lambert 2013).

Breast-Feeding Considerations In a study using insulin aspart, both exogenous and endogenous insulin were excreted into breast milk (Whitmore 2012). Breast-feeding is encouraged for all women, including those with type 1, type 2, or GDM (ACOG 2005; Blumer 2013; Metzger 2007). A small snack (such as milk) before nursing may help decrease the risk of hypoglycemia in women with pregestational diabetes (ACOG 2005; ADA 2015; Reader 2004). The manufacturer considers the use of insulin aspart to be compatible with breast-feeding, although adjustments of the mothers insulin dose may be needed.

Contraindications Hypersensitivity to insulin aspart or any component of the formulation; during episodes of hypoglycemia

Warnings/Precautions Hypoglycemia is the most common adverse effect of insulin. The timing of hypoglycemia differs among various insulin formulations. Hypoglycemia may result from increased work or exercise without eating; use of long-acting insulin preparations (eg, insulin detemir, insulin glargine) may delay recovery from hypoglycemia. Profound and prolonged episodes of hypoglycemia may result in convulsions, unconsciousness, temporary or permanent brain damage, or even death. Insulin requirements may be altered during illness, emotional disturbances, or other stressors. Instruct patients to use caution with ethanol; may increase risk of hypoglycemia. Insulin may produce hypokalemia which, if left untreated, may result in respiratory paralysis, ventricular arrhythmia, and even death. Use with caution in patients at risk for hypokalemia (eg, IV insulin use). Use with caution in renal or hepatic impairment. In the elderly, avoid use of sliding scale insulin in this population due to increased risk of hypoglycemia without benefits in management of hyperglycemia regardless of care setting (Beers Criteria).

Due to the short duration of action of insulin aspart, a longer acting insulin or CSII via an external insulin pump is needed to maintain adequate glucose control in patients with type 1 diabetes mellitus. In both type 1 and type 2 diabetes, preprandial administration of insulin aspart should be immediately followed by a meal within 5-10 minutes. May also be administered via CSII; do not dilute or mix with other insulin formulations when using an external insulin pump. Rule out pump failure if unexplained hyperglycemia or ketosis occurs; temporary SubQ insulin administration may be required until the problem is identified and corrected. Insulin aspart may also be administered IV in selected clinical situations to control hyperglycemia; close monitoring of blood glucose and serum potassium as well as medical supervision is required. According to the Centers for Disease Control and Prevention (CDC), pen-shaped injection devices should never be used for more than one person (even when the needle is changed) because of the risk of infection. The injection device should be clearly labeled with individual patient information to ensure that the correct pen is used (CDC, 2012).

The general objective of exogenous insulin therapy is to approximate the physiologic pattern of insulin secretion which is characterized by two distinct phases. Phase 1 insulin secretion suppresses hepatic glucose production and phase 2 insulin secretion occurs in response to carbohydrate ingestion; therefore, exogenous insulin therapy may consist of basal insulin (eg, intermediate- or long-acting insulin or via continuous subcutaneous insulin infusion [CSII]) and/or preprandial insulin (eg, short- or rapid-acting insulin [eg, insulin aspart]) (see Related Information: Insulin Products). Patients with type 1 diabetes do not produce endogenous insulin; therefore, these patients require both basal and preprandial insulin administration. Patients with type 2 diabetes retain some beta-cell function in the early stages of their disease; however, as the disease progresses, phase 1 insulin secretion may become completely impaired and phase 2 insulin secretion becomes delayed and/or inadequate in response to meals. Therefore, patients with type 2 diabetes may be treated with oral antidiabetic agents, basal insulin, and/or preprandial insulin depending on the stage of disease and current glycemic control. Since treatment regimens often consist of multiple agents, dosage adjustments must address the specific phase of insulin release that is primarily contributing to the patient's impaired glycemic control. Diabetes self-management education (DSME) is essential to maximize the effectiveness of therapy. Treatment and monitoring regimens must be individualized.

Potentially significant drug-drug interactions may exist, requiring dose or frequency adjustment, additional monitoring, and/or selection of alternative therapy.

Adverse Reactions Primarily symptoms of hypoglycemia

Cardiovascular: Pallor, palpitation, tachycardia

Central nervous system: Fatigue, headache, hypothermia, loss of consciousness, mental confusion

Dermatologic: Redness, urticaria

Endocrine & metabolic: Hypoglycemia, hypokalemia

Gastrointestinal: Hunger, nausea, numbness of mouth

Local: Atrophy or hypertrophy of SubQ fat tissue; edema, itching, pain or warmth at injection site; stinging

Neuromuscular & skeletal: Muscle weakness, paresthesia, tremor

Ocular: Transient presbyopia or blurred vision

Miscellaneous: Anaphylaxis, diaphoresis, local and/or systemic hypersensitivity reactions

Drug Interactions

Metabolism/Transport Effects None known.

Avoid Concomitant Use

Avoid concomitant use of Insulin Aspart with any of the following: Rosiglitazone

Increased Effect/Toxicity

Insulin Aspart may increase the levels/effects of: Hypoglycemia-Associated Agents; Rosiglitazone

The levels/effects of Insulin Aspart may be increased by: Alpha-Lipoic Acid; Androgens; Antidiabetic Agents; Beta-Blockers; DPP-IV Inhibitors; Edetate CALCIUM Disodium; Edetate Disodium; GLP-1 Agonists; Herbs (Hypoglycemic Properties); Liraglutide; MAO Inhibitors; Metreleptin; Pegvisomant; Pioglitazone; Pramlintide; Quinolone Antibiotics; Salicylates; Selective Serotonin Reuptake Inhibitors; SGLT2 Inhibitors

Decreased Effect

The levels/effects of Insulin Aspart may be decreased by: Hyperglycemia-Associated Agents; Quinolone Antibiotics; Thiazide Diuretics

Storage/Stability Unopened vials, cartridges, and prefilled pens may be stored under refrigeration between 2°C and 8°C (36°F to 46°F) until the expiration date or at room temperature <30°C (<86°F) for 28 days; do not freeze; keep away from heat and sunlight. Once punctured (in use), vials may be stored under refrigeration or at room temperature <30°C (<86°F); use within 28 days. Cartridges and prefilled pens that have been punctured (in use) should be stored at temperatures <30°C (<86°F) and used within 28 days; do not freeze or refrigerate. When used for CSII, insulin aspart contained within an external insulin pump reservoir should be replaced at least every 6 days; discard if exposed to temperatures >37°C (>98.6°F).

For SubQ administration: *NovoLog® vials:* According to the manufacturer, diluted insulin should be stored at temperatures <30°C (<86°F) and used within 28 days.

For IV infusion: Stable for 24 hours at room temperature.

Mechanism of Action Insulin acts via specific membrane-bound receptors on target tissues to regulate metabolism of carbohydrate, protein, and fats. Target organs for insulin include the liver, skeletal muscle, and adipose tissue.

Within the liver, insulin stimulates hepatic glycogen synthesis. Insulin promotes hepatic synthesis of fatty acids, which are released into the circulation as lipoproteins. Skeletal muscle effects of insulin include increased protein synthesis and increased glycogen synthesis. Within adipose tissue, insulin stimulates the processing of circulating lipoproteins to provide free fatty acids, facilitating triglyceride synthesis and storage by adipocytes; it also directly inhibits the hydrolysis of triglycerides. In addition, insulin stimulates the cellular uptake of amino acids and increases cellular permeability to several ions, including potassium, magnesium, and phosphate. By activating sodium-potassium ATPases, insulin promotes the intracellular movement of potassium.

Normally secreted by the pancreas, insulin products are manufactured for pharmacologic use through recombinant DNA technology using either *E. coli* or *Saccharomyces cerevisiae*. Insulins are categorized based on the onset, peak, and duration of effect (eg, rapid-, short-, intermediate-, and long-acting insulin). Insulin aspart is a rapid-acting insulin analog.

Pharmacodynamics Onset and duration of hypoglycemic effects depend upon the route of administration (adsorption and onset of action are more rapid after deeper IM injections than after SubQ), site of injection (onset and duration are progressively slower with SubQ injection into the abdomen, arm, buttock, or thigh respectively), volume and concentration of injection, and the preparation administered; local heat and massage also increase the rate of absorption.

Onset of action: 0.17-0.33 hours
Maximum effect: 1-3 hours
Duration: 3-5 hours

Pharmacokinetics (Adult data unless noted)
Protein binding: 0% to 9%
Half-life: Adults: 81 minutes
Time to peak serum concentration: 40-50 minutes
Elimination: Urine
Clearance: Adults: 1.22 L/hour/kg

Dosing: Usual Insulin aspart is a rapid-acting insulin analog which is normally administered SubQ as a premeal component of the insulin regimen or as a continuous SubQ infusion and should be used with intermediate- or long-acting insulin. When compared to insulin regular, insulin aspart has a more rapid onset and shorter duration of activity. In carefully controlled clinical settings with close medical supervision and monitoring of blood glucose and potassium, insulin aspart may also be administered IV in some situations. Insulin requirements vary dramatically between patients and dictate frequent monitoring and close medical supervision. See Insulin Regular for additional information.

General insulin dosing:

Type 1 diabetes mellitus: Children, Adolescents, and Adults: **Note:** Multiple daily doses or continuous subcutaneous infusions guided by blood glucose monitoring are the standard of diabetes care. Combinations of insulin formulations are commonly used. The daily doses presented below are expressed as the **total units/kg/day of all insulin formulations combined**.

Initial total insulin dose: SubQ: 0.2-0.6 units/kg/day in divided doses. Conservative initial doses of 0.2-0.4 units/kg/day are often recommended to avoid the potential for hypoglycemia. A rapidly acting insulin may be the only insulin formulation used initially.

Usual maintenance range: SubQ: 0.5-1 unit/kg/day in divided doses. An estimate of anticipated needs may be based on body weight and/or activity factors as follows:
Nonobese: 0.4-0.6 units/kg/day
Obese: 0.8-1.2 units/kg/day
Pubescent Children and Adolescents: During puberty, requirements may substantially increase to >1 unit/kg/day and in some cases up to 2 units/kg/day (IDF/ISPAD, 2011)

Adjustment of dose: Dosage must be titrated to achieve glucose control and avoid hypoglycemia. Adjust dose to maintain premeal and bedtime glucose in target range. Since combinations of agents are frequently used, dosage adjustment must address the individual component of the insulin regimen which most directly influences the blood glucose value in question, based on the known onset and duration of the insulin component.

Continuous SubQ insulin infusion (insulin pump): A combination of a "basal" continuous insulin infusion rate with preprogrammed, premeal bolus doses which are patient controlled. When converting from multiple daily SubQ doses of maintenance insulin, it is advisable to reduce the basal rate to less than the equivalent of the total daily units of longer acting insulin (eg, NPH); divide the total number of units by 24 to get the basal rate in units/hour. Do not include the total units of regular insulin or other rapid-acting insulin formulations in this calculation. The same premeal regular insulin dosage may be used.

Type 2 diabetes mellitus: Augmentation therapy (patients for which diet, exercise, weight reduction, and oral hypoglycemic agents have not been adequate): Adults: SubQ: Initial dosage of 0.2 units/kg/day or 10 units/day of an intermediate-acting (eg, NPH) or long-acting insulin administered at bedtime has been recommended. As an alternative, regular insulin or rapid-acting insulin formulations administered before meals have also been used. Dosage must be carefully adjusted.

Dosing adjustment in renal impairment: There are no dosage adjustments provided in manufacturer's labeling; insulin requirements are reduced due to changes in insulin clearance or metabolism; monitor blood glucose closely.

Dosing adjustment in hepatic impairment: There are no dosage adjustments provided in manufacturer's labeling; insulin requirements may be reduced due to changes in insulin clearance or metabolism; monitor blood glucose closely.

Preparation for Administration Parenteral:
SubQ: NovoLog vials: May be diluted with Insulin Diluting Medium for NovoLog to a concentration of 10 units/mL (U-10) or 50 units/mL (U-50). Do not dilute insulin contained in a cartridge, prefilled pen, or external insulin pump. May be mixed in the same syringe with NPH insulin. When mixing insulin aspart with NPH insulin, aspart should be drawn into the syringe first.
IV: May be diluted in NS, D_5W, or $D_{10}W$ to concentrations of 0.05 to 1 unit/mL.

Administration Parenteral: Do not use if solution is viscous or cloudy; use only if clear and colorless.
SubQ: Administration is usually made into the subcutaneous fat of the thighs, arms, buttocks, or abdomen, with sites rotated; cold injections should be avoided. May be mixed in the same syringe with NPH insulin. When mixing insulin aspart with NPH insulin, aspart should be drawn into the syringe first. Administer immediately before meals (within 5 to 10 minutes of the start of a meal).
Continuous SubQ insulin infusion (insulin pump): Do not use if solution is viscous or cloudy; use only if clear and colorless. Patients should be trained in the proper use of their external insulin pump and in intensive insulin therapy. Infusion sets and infusion set insertion sites should be changed at least every 3 days; rotate infusion sites. Do not dilute or mix other insulin formulations with insulin aspart that is to be used in an external insulin pump.
IV: Insulin aspart may be administered IV in selected clinical situations to control hyperglycemia. Closely monitor blood glucose and serum potassium; appropriate medical supervision is required. Do not administer insulin mixtures intravenously.
To minimize insulin adsorption to IV tubing: Flush the IV tubing with a priming infusion of 20 mL from the insulin infusion, whenever a new IV tubing set is added to the insulin infusion container (Jacobi 2012; Thompson 2012). Also refer to institution-specific protocols where appropriate.
Because of insulin adsorption to IV tubing or infusion bags, the actual amount of insulin being administered via IV infusion could be substantially less than the apparent amount. Therefore, adjustment of the IV infusion rate should be based on effect and not solely on the apparent insulin dose. The apparent dose may be used as a starting point for determining the subsequent SubQ dosing regimen (Moghissi 2009); however, the transition to SubQ administration requires continuous medical supervision, frequent monitoring of blood glucose, and careful adjustment of therapy. In addition, SubQ insulin should be given 1 to 4 hours prior to the discontinuation of IV insulin to prevent hyperglycemia (Moghissi 2009).

Monitoring Parameters Urine sugar and acetone, serum glucose, electrolytes, Hb A_{1c}, lipid profile; when used intravenously, close monitoring of serum glucose and potassium are required to avoid hypoglycemia and/or hypokalemia

Reference Range

Plasma Blood Glucose and Hgb A_{1c} Goals for Type 1 Diabetes (ADA, 2013): Note: Goals should be individualized based on individual needs/circumstances (eg, patients who experience severe hypoglycemia, patients with hypoglycemic unawareness); lower goals may be reasonable if they can be achieved without excessive hypoglycemia. **Note:** Postprandial blood glucose should be measured when there is a discrepancy between preprandial blood glucose concentrations and Hb A_{1c} values and to help assess glycemia for patients who receive basal/bolus regimens. It is usually drawn 1-2 hours after starting meal and is considered to be the "peak."

Toddlers/Preschoolers (0-6 years):
- Preprandial glucose: 100-180 mg/dL
- Bedtime/overnight glucose: 110-200 mg/dL
- Hb A_{1c}: <8.5%

School age (6-12 years):
- Preprandial glucose: 90-180 mg/dL
- Bedtime/overnight glucose: 100-180 mg/dL
- Hb A_{1c}: <8%

Adolescents/Young Adults (13-19 years):
- Preprandial glucose: 90-130 mg/dL
- Bedtime/overnight glucose: 90-150 mg/dL
- Hb A_{1c}: <7.5%

Adults, nonpregnant:
- Preprandial glucose: 70-130 mg/dL
- Postprandial glucose: <180 mg/dL
- Hb A_{1c}: <7%

Criteria for diagnosis of DKA:

Serum glucose:
- Children: >200 mg/dL
- Adults: >250 mg/dL

Arterial pH:
- Children: <7.3
- Adults: <7-7.24

Bicarbonate:
- Children: <15 mEq/L
- Adults: <10-15 mEq/L

Moderate ketonuria or ketonemia

Additional Information

Division of daily insulin requirement ("conventional therapy"): Generally, 50% to 75% of the daily insulin dose is given as an intermediate- or long-acting form of insulin (in 1-2 daily injections). The remaining portion of the 24-hour insulin requirement is divided and administered as either regular insulin or a rapid-acting form (eg, insulin aspart) of insulin at the same time before breakfast and dinner.

Division of daily insulin requirement ("intensive therapy"): Basal insulin delivery with 1 or 2 doses of intermediate- or long-acting insulin formulations superimposed with doses of rapid- or very rapid-acting insulin (eg, insulin aspart) formulations 3 or more times daily.

Dosage Forms Excipient information presented when available (limited, particularly for generics); consult specific product labeling.

Solution, Subcutaneous:
- NovoLOG: 100 units/mL (10 mL) [contains metacresol, phenol]

Solution Cartridge, Subcutaneous:
- NovoLOG PenFill: 100 units/mL (3 mL) [contains metacresol, phenol]

Solution Pen-injector, Subcutaneous:
- NovoLOG FlexPen: 100 units/mL (3 mL) [contains metacresol, phenol]

◆ **Insulin Aspart and Insulin Aspart Protamine** *see* Insulin Aspart Protamine and Insulin Aspart *on page 1121*

Insulin Aspart Protamine and Insulin Aspart (IN soo lin AS part PROE ta meen & IN soo lin AS part)

Medication Safety Issues

Sound-alike/look-alike issues:

NovoLOG® Mix 70/30 may be confused with HumaLOG® Mix 75/25™, HumuLIN® 70/30, NovoLIN® 70/30, NovoLOG®

High alert medication:

The Institute for Safe Medication Practices (ISMP) includes this medication among its list of drugs which have a heightened risk of causing significant patient harm when used in error. ***Due to the number of insulin preparations, it is essential to identify/clarify the type of insulin to be used.***

Other safety concerns:

Cross-contamination may occur if insulin pens are shared among multiple patients. Steps should be taken to prohibit sharing of insulin pens.

Related Information

Insulin Products *on page 2319*

Brand Names: US NovoLOG® Mix 70/30; NovoLOG® Mix 70/30 FlexPen®

Brand Names: Canada NovoMix® 30

Therapeutic Category Antidiabetic Agent, Parenteral; Insulin, Combination

Generic Availability (US) No

Use Treatment of type 1 diabetes mellitus (insulin dependent, IDDM); type 2 diabetes mellitus (noninsulin dependent, NIDDM) to control hyperglycemia (FDA approved in adults)

Pregnancy Risk Factor B

Pregnancy Considerations Animal reproduction studies have not been conducted. Biphasic insulin aspart (insulin aspart protamine suspension 70% [intermediate acting] and insulin aspart solution 30% [rapid acting]) was found to be comparable to biphasic human insulin (Insulin NPH suspension 70% [intermediate acting] and insulin regular solution 30% [short acting]) in initial studies of women with gestational diabetes mellitus (Balaji 2010; Balaji 2012).

In women with diabetes, maternal hyperglycemia can be associated with congenital malformations as well as adverse effects in the fetus, neonate, and the mother (ACOG 2005; ADA 2015; Kitzmiller 2008; Metzger 2007). To prevent adverse outcomes, prior to conception and throughout pregnancy maternal blood glucose and HbA_{1c} should be kept as close to target goals as possible but without causing significant hypoglycemia (ACOG 2013; ADA 2015; Blumer 2013; Kitzmiller 2008; Lambert 2013). Prior to pregnancy, effective contraception should be used until glycemic control is achieved (Kitzmiller 2008).

Insulin requirements tend to fall during the first trimester of pregnancy and increase in the later trimesters, peaking at 28 to 32 weeks of gestation. Following delivery, insulin requirements decrease rapidly (ACOG 2005).

Breast-Feeding Considerations In a study using insulin aspart, both exogenous and endogenous insulin were excreted into breast milk (Whitmore 2012). Breast-feeding is encouraged for all women, including those with type 1, type 2, or GDM (ACOG 2005; Blumer 2013; Metzger 2007). A small snack (such as milk) before nursing may help decrease the risk of hypoglycemia in women with pregestational diabetes (ACOG 2005; ADA 2015; Reader 2004). The manufacturer notes that adjustments of the mothers insulin dose may be needed.

Contraindications Hypersensitivity to any component of the formulation; during episodes of hypoglycemia

Warnings/Precautions Hypoglycemia is the most common adverse effect of insulin. The timing of hypoglycemia differs among various insulin formulations. Hypoglycemia may result from increased work or exercise without eating. Profound and prolonged episodes of hypoglycemia may result in convulsions, unconsciousness, temporary or permanent brain damage or even death. Insulin requirements may be altered during illness, emotional disturbances or other stressors. Instruct patients to use caution with ethanol; may increase risk of hypoglycemia. Insulin may produce hypokalemia which, if left untreated, may result in respiratory paralysis, ventricular arrhythmia, and even death. Use with caution in renal or hepatic impairment.

Any change of insulin should be made cautiously; changing manufacturers, type, and/or method of manufacture may result in the need for a change of dosage. Insulin aspart protamine and insulin aspart premixed combination products are **NOT** intended for IV or IM administration. According to the Centers for Disease Control and Prevention (CDC), pen-shaped injection devices should never be used for more than one person (even when the needle is changed) because of the risk of infection. The injection device should be clearly labeled with individual patient information to ensure that the correct pen is used (CDC, 2012).

The general objective of exogenous insulin therapy is to approximate the physiologic pattern of insulin secretion which is characterized by two distinct phases. Phase 1 insulin secretion suppresses hepatic glucose production and phase 2 insulin secretion occurs in response to carbohydrate ingestion; therefore, exogenous insulin therapy may consist of basal insulin (eg, intermediate- or long-acting insulin or via continuous subcutaneous insulin infusion [CSII]) and/or preprandial insulin (eg, short- or rapid-acting insulin). Patients with type 1 diabetes do not produce endogenous insulin; therefore, these patients require both basal and preprandial insulin administration. Patients with type 2 diabetes retain some beta-cell function in the early stages of their disease; however, as the disease progresses, phase 1 insulin secretion may become completely impaired and phase 2 insulin secretion becomes delayed and/or inadequate in response to meals. Therefore, patients with type 2 diabetes may be treated with oral antidiabetic agents, basal insulin, and/or preprandial insulin depending on the stage of disease and current glycemic control. Since treatment regimens often consist of multiple agents, dosage adjustments must address the specific phase of insulin release that is primarily contributing to the patient's impaired glycemic control. Diabetes self-management education (DSME) is essential to maximize the effectiveness of therapy. Treatment and monitoring regimens must be individualized.

Potentially significant drug-drug interactions may exist, requiring dose or frequency adjustment, additional monitoring, and/or selection of alternative therapy.

Adverse Reactions

Cardiovascular: Palpitation, pallor, peripheral edema, tachycardia

Central nervous system: Fatigue, headache, hypothermia, loss of consciousness, mental confusion

Dermatologic: Pruritus, rash, redness, urticaria

Endocrine & metabolic: Hypoglycemia, hypokalemia

Gastrointestinal: Hunger, nausea, numbness of mouth, weight gain

Local: Injection site reaction (including edema, itching, pain or warmth, stinging), lipoatrophy, lipodystrophy

Neuromuscular & skeletal: Muscle weakness, paresthesia, tremor

Ocular: Transient presbyopia or blurred vision

Miscellaneous: Anaphylaxis, antibodies to insulin (no change in efficacy), diaphoresis, local allergy, systemic allergic symptoms

Drug Interactions

Metabolism/Transport Effects None known.

Avoid Concomitant Use

Avoid concomitant use of Insulin Aspart Protamine and Insulin Aspart with any of the following: Rosiglitazone

Increased Effect/Toxicity

Insulin Aspart Protamine and Insulin Aspart may increase the levels/effects of: Hypoglycemia-Associated Agents; Rosiglitazone

The levels/effects of Insulin Aspart Protamine and Insulin Aspart may be increased by: Alpha-Lipoic Acid; Androgens; Antidiabetic Agents; Beta-Blockers; DPP-IV Inhibitors; Edetate CALCIUM Disodium; Edetate Disodium; GLP-1 Agonists; Herbs (Hypoglycemic Properties); Liraglutide; MAO Inhibitors; Metreleptin; Pegvisomant; Pioglitazone; Pramlintide; Quinolone Antibiotics; Salicylates; Selective Serotonin Reuptake Inhibitors; SGLT2 Inhibitors

Decreased Effect

The levels/effects of Insulin Aspart Protamine and Insulin Aspart may be decreased by: Hyperglycemia-Associated Agents; Quinolone Antibiotics; Thiazide Diuretics

Storage/Stability Unopened vials and prefilled pens may be stored under refrigeration between 2°C and 8°C (36°F to 46°F) until the expiration date or at room temperature <30°C (<86°F) for 14 days (prefilled pens) or 28 days (vials); do not freeze; keep away from heat and sunlight. Once punctured (in use), vials may be stored under refrigeration or at room temperature <30°C (<86°F); use within 28 days. Prefilled pens that have been punctured (in use) should be stored at room temperature <30°C (<86°F) and used within 14 days; do not freeze or refrigerate.

Mechanism of Action Insulin aspart protamine and insulin aspart is an intermediate-acting combination insulin product with a more rapid onset and similar duration of action as compared to that of insulin NPH and insulin regular combination products. Insulin acts via specific membrane-bound receptors on target tissues to regulate metabolism of carbohydrate, protein, and fats. Target organs for insulin include the liver, skeletal muscle, and adipose tissue.

Within the liver, insulin stimulates hepatic glycogen synthesis. Insulin promotes hepatic synthesis of fatty acids, which are released into the circulation as lipoproteins. Skeletal muscle effects of insulin include increased protein synthesis and increased glycogen synthesis. Within adipose tissue, insulin stimulates the processing of circulating lipoproteins to provide free fatty acids, facilitating triglyceride synthesis and storage by adipocytes; also directly inhibits the hydrolysis of triglycerides. In addition, insulin stimulates the cellular uptake of amino acids and increases cellular permeability to several ions, including potassium, magnesium, and phosphate. By activating sodium-potassium ATPases, insulin promotes the intracellular movement of potassium.

Normally secreted by the pancreas, insulin products are manufactured for pharmacologic use through recombinant DNA technology using either *E. coli* or *Saccharomyces cerevisiae*. Insulins are categorized based on the onset, peak, and duration of effect (eg, rapid-, short-, intermediate-, and long-acting insulin).

Pharmacodynamics

Onset of action: 10-20 minutes

Maximum effect: 1-4 hours

Duration: 18-24 hours

Pharmacokinetics (Adult data unless noted)

Protein binding: ≤9%

Half-life: 8-9 hours (mean)

Time to peak serum concentration: 1-1.5 hours

Elimination: Urine

Dosing: Usual Insulin aspart protamine is an intermediate-acting insulin and insulin aspart is a rapid-acting insulin administered by SubQ injection. Insulin aspart protamine and insulin aspart combination products are approximately equipotent to insulin NPH and insulin regular combination products with a similar duration of activity, but with a more rapid onset. With combination insulin products, the proportion of rapid-acting to long-acting insulin is fixed; basal vs prandial dose adjustments cannot be made. Fixed ratio insulins (such as insulin aspart protamine and insulin aspart combination) are typically administered as 2 daily doses with each dose intended to cover two meals and a snack. Because of variability in the peak effect and individual patient variability in activities, meals, etc, it may be more difficult to achieve complete glycemic control using fixed combinations of insulins; frequent monitoring and close medical supervision may be necessary. See Insulin Regular for additional information.

General insulin dosing:

Type 1 diabetes mellitus: Children, Adolescents, and Adults: **Note:** Multiple daily doses are utilized and guided by blood glucose monitoring. Combinations of different insulin formulations are commonly used. The daily doses presented below are expressed as the **total units/kg/day of all insulin formulations combined**. Insulin aspart protamine and insulin aspart combination product is **not** intended for initial therapy; basal insulin requirements should be established **first** to direct dosing of combination insulin products.

Usual maintenance range: SubQ: 0.5-1 unit/kg/day in divided doses. An estimate of anticipated needs may be based on body weight and/or activity factors as follows:

Nonobese: 0.4-0.6 units/kg/day

Obese: 0.8-1.2 units/kg/day

Pubescent Children and Adolescents: During puberty, requirements may substantially increase to >1 unit/kg/day and in some cases up to 2 units/kg/day (IDF/ISPAD, 2011)

Adjustment of dose: Dosage must be titrated to achieve glucose control and avoid hypoglycemia. Adjust dose to maintain premeal and bedtime glucose in target range. Since combinations of agents are frequently used, dosage adjustment must address the individual component of the insulin regimen which most directly influences the blood glucose value in question, based on the known onset and duration of the insulin component.

Type 2 diabetes mellitus: Augmentation therapy (patients for which diet, exercise, weight reduction, and oral hypoglycemic agents have not been adequate): Adults: SubQ: **Note:** Insulin aspart protamine and insulin aspart combination product is **not** intended for initial therapy; basal insulin requirements should be established **first** to direct dosing of combination insulin products. Dosage must be carefully adjusted.

Dosing adjustment in renal impairment: There are no dosage adjustments provided in manufacturer's labeling; insulin requirements are reduced due to changes in insulin clearance or metabolism; monitor blood glucose closely.

Dosing adjustment in hepatic impairment: There are no dosage adjustments provided in manufacturer's labeling; insulin requirements may be reduced due to changes in insulin clearance or metabolism; monitor blood glucose closely.

Administration Parenteral: SubQ: Gently roll vial or pen in the palms of the hands to resuspend before use; administer into the subcutaneous fat of the thighs, arms, buttocks, or abdomen, with sites rotated. Cold injections should be avoided. Administer within 15 minutes before a meal (type 1 diabetes) or 15 minutes before or after a meal (type 2 diabetes) (eg, before breakfast and supper). Do not mix or dilute with other insulins. **Not for IV administration** or use in an insulin infusion pump.

Monitoring Parameters Urine sugar and acetone, serum glucose, electrolytes, Hb A_{1c}, lipid profile

Reference Range

Plasma Blood Glucose and Hgb A_{1c} Goals for Type 1 Diabetes (ADA, 2013): Note: Goals should be individualized based on individual needs/circumstances (eg, patients who experience severe hypoglycemia, patients with hypoglycemic unawareness); lower goals may be reasonable if they can be achieved without excessive hypoglycemia. **Note:** Postprandial blood glucose should be measured when there is a discrepancy between preprandial blood glucose concentrations and Hb A_{1c} values and to help assess glycemia for patients who receive basal/bolus regimens. It is usually drawn 1-2 hours after starting meal and is considered to be the "peak."

Toddlers/Preschoolers (0-6 years):
- Preprandial glucose: 100-180 mg/dL
- Bedtime/overnight glucose: 110-200 mg/dL
- Hb A_{1c}: <8.5%

School age (6-12 years):
- Preprandial glucose: 90-180 mg/dL
- Bedtime/overnight glucose: 100-180 mg/dL
- Hb A_{1c}: <8%

Adolescents/Young Adults (13-19 years):
- Preprandial glucose: 90-130 mg/dL
- Bedtime/overnight glucose: 90-150 mg/dL
- Hb A_{1c}: <7.5%

Adults, nonpregnant:
- Preprandial glucose: 70-130 mg/dL
- Postprandial glucose: <180 mg/dL
- Hb A_{1c}: <7%

Criteria for diagnosis of DKA:

Serum glucose:
- Children: >200 mg/dL
- Adults: >250 mg/dL

Arterial pH:
- Children: <7.3
- Adults: <7-7.24

Bicarbonate:
- Children: <15 mEq/L
- Adults: <10-15 mEq/L

Moderate ketonuria or ketonemia

Additional Information

Division of daily insulin requirement ("conventional therapy"): Generally, 50% to 75% of the daily insulin dose is given as an intermediate- or long-acting form of insulin (in 1-2 daily injections). The remaining portion of the 24-hour insulin requirement is divided and administered as either regular insulin or a rapid-acting form of insulin at the same time before breakfast and dinner.

Division of daily insulin requirement ("intensive therapy"): Basal insulin delivery with 1 or 2 doses of intermediate- or long-acting insulin formulations superimposed with doses of rapid- or very rapid-acting insulin formulations 3 or more times daily.

Dosage Forms Excipient information presented when available (limited, particularly for generics); consult specific product labeling.

Injection, suspension:

NovoLOG® Mix 70/30: Insulin aspart protamine suspension 70% [intermediate acting] and insulin aspart solution 30% [rapid acting]: 100 units/mL (10 mL)

NovoLOG® Mix 70/30 FlexPen®: Insulin aspart protamine suspension 70% [intermediate acting] and insulin aspart solution 30% [rapid acting]: 100 units/mL (3 mL)

Insulin Detemir (IN soo lin DE te mir)

Medication Safety Issues

Sound-alike/look-alike issues:

Levemir may be confused with Lovenox

High alert medication:

The Institute for Safe Medication Practices (ISMP) includes this medication among its list of drugs which have a heightened risk of causing significant patient harm when used in error. ***Due to the number of insulin preparations, it is essential to identify/clarify the type of insulin to be used.***

Administration issues:

Insulin detemir is a clear solution, but it is NOT intended for IV or IM administration.

Other safety concerns:

Cross-contamination may occur if insulin pens are shared among multiple patients. Steps should be taken to prohibit sharing of insulin pens.

Related Information

Insulin Products *on page 2319*

Brand Names: US Levemir; Levemir FlexPen [DSC]; Levemir FlexTouch

Brand Names: Canada Levemir®

Therapeutic Category Antidiabetic Agent, Parenteral; Insulin, Long-Acting

Generic Availability (US) No

Use Treatment of type 1 diabetes mellitus (insulin dependent, IDDM) to improve glycemic control (FDA approved in ages ≥2 years and adults); treatment of type 2 diabetes mellitus (noninsulin dependent, NIDDM) to improve glycemic control (FDA approved in adults)

Pregnancy Risk Factor B

Pregnancy Considerations Dose-related adverse events were observed in animal reproduction studies. Insulin detemir has been detected in cord blood. An increased risk of fetal abnormalities has not been observed following the use of insulin detemir in pregnancy; pregnancy outcomes are similar following maternal use of insulin detemir and NPH insulin.

In women with diabetes, maternal hyperglycemia can be associated with congenital malformations as well as adverse effects in the fetus, neonate, and the mother (ACOG 2005; ADA 2015; Kitzmiller 2008; Metzger 2007). To prevent adverse outcomes, prior to conception and throughout pregnancy maternal blood glucose and HbA_{1c} should be kept as close to target goals as possible but without causing significant hypoglycemia (ACOG 2013; ADA 2015; Blumer 2013; Kitzmiller 2008; Lambert 2013). Prior to pregnancy, effective contraception should be used until glycemic control is achieved (Kitzmiller 2008).

Insulin requirements tend to fall during the first trimester of pregnancy and increase in the later trimesters, peaking at 28 to 32 weeks of gestation. Following delivery, insulin requirements decrease rapidly (ACOG 2005). Women who are stable on insulin detemir prior to conception may continue it during pregnancy. Pregnant women may also be switched to insulin detemir during pregnancy when therapy with NPH insulin is not adequate (Blumer 2013).

Breast-Feeding Considerations Both exogenous and endogenous insulin are excreted into breast milk (study not conducted with this preparation) (Whitmore 2012). Breast-feeding is encouraged for all women, including those with type 1, type 2, or GDM (ACOG 2005; Blumer 2013; Metzger 2007). A small snack (such as milk) before nursing may help decrease the risk of hypoglycemia in women with pregestational diabetes (ACOG 2005; ADA 2015; Reader 2004). The manufacturer recommends that caution be used in nursing women; adjustments of the mothers insulin dose may be needed.

Contraindications Hypersensitivity to insulin detemir or any component of the formulation

Warnings/Precautions Hypoglycemia is the most common adverse effect of insulin. The timing of hypoglycemia differs among various insulin formulations. Hypoglycemia may result from increased work or exercise without eating; use of long-acting insulin preparations (eg, insulin detemir, insulin glargine) may delay recovery from hypoglycemia. Profound and prolonged episodes of hypoglycemia may result in convulsions, unconsciousness, temporary or permanent brain damage or even death. Insulin requirements may be altered during illness, emotional disturbances or other stressors. Instruct patients to use caution with ethanol; may increase risk of hypoglycemia. Insulin may produce hypokalemia which, if left untreated, may result in respiratory paralysis, ventricular arrhythmia and even death. Use with caution in renal or hepatic impairment.

The duration of action of insulin detemir is dose-dependent; consider this factor during dosage adjustment and titration. Insulin detemir, although a clear solution, is **NOT** intended for IV or IM administration. According to the Centers for Disease Control and Prevention (CDC), pen-shaped injection devices should never be used for more than one person (even when the needle is changed) because of the risk of infection. The injection device should be clearly labeled with individual patient information to ensure that the correct pen is used (CDC, 2012).

The general objective of exogenous insulin therapy is to approximate the physiologic pattern of insulin secretion which is characterized by two distinct phases. Phase 1 insulin secretion suppresses hepatic glucose production and phase 2 insulin secretion occurs in response to carbohydrate ingestion; therefore, exogenous insulin therapy may consist of basal insulin (eg, intermediate- or long-acting insulin or via continuous subcutaneous insulin infusion [CSII]) and/or preprandial insulin (eg, short- or rapid-acting insulin) (see Related Information: Insulin Products). Patients with type 1 diabetes do not produce endogenous insulin; therefore, these patients require both basal and preprandial insulin administration. Patients with type 2 diabetes retain some beta-cell function in the early stages of their disease; however, as the disease progresses, phase 1 insulin secretion may become completely impaired and phase 2 insulin secretion becomes delayed and/or inadequate in response to meals. Therefore, patients with type 2 diabetes may be treated with oral antidiabetic agents, basal insulin, and/or preprandial insulin depending on the stage of disease and current glycemic control. Since treatment regimens often consist of multiple agents, dosage adjustments must address the specific phase of insulin release that is primarily contributing to the patient's impaired glycemic control. Diabetes self-management education (DSME) is essential to maximize the effectiveness of therapy. Treatment and monitoring regimens must be individualized.

Potentially significant drug-drug interactions may exist, requiring dose or frequency adjustment, additional monitoring, and/or selection of alternative therapy.

Adverse Reactions Primarily symptoms of hypoglycemia

Cardiovascular: Pallor, palpitation, tachycardia

Central nervous system: Fatigue, headache, hypothermia, loss of consciousness, mental confusion

Dermatologic: Redness, urticaria

Endocrine & metabolic: Hypoglycemia, hypokalemia

Gastrointestinal: Hunger, nausea, numbness of mouth

Local: Atrophy or hypertrophy of SubQ fat tissue; edema, itching, pain or warmth at injection site; stinging

Neuromuscular & skeletal: Muscle weakness, paresthesia tremor

Ocular: Transient presbyopia or blurred vision

Miscellaneous: Anaphylaxis, diaphoresis, local and/or systemic hypersensitivity reactions

Drug Interactions

Metabolism/Transport Effects None known.

Avoid Concomitant Use

Avoid concomitant use of Insulin Detemir with any of the following: Rosiglitazone

Increased Effect/Toxicity

Insulin Detemir may increase the levels/effects of: Hypoglycemia-Associated Agents; Rosiglitazone

The levels/effects of Insulin Detemir may be increased by: Alpha-Lipoic Acid; Androgens; Antidiabetic Agents; Beta-Blockers; DPP-IV Inhibitors; Edetate CALCIUM Disodium; Edetate Disodium; GLP-1 Agonists; Herbs (Hypoglycemic Properties); Liraglutide; MAO Inhibitors; Metreleptin; Pegvisomant; Pioglitazone; Pramlintide; Quinolone Antibiotics; Salicylates; Selective Serotonin Reuptake Inhibitors; SGLT2 Inhibitors

Decreased Effect

The levels/effects of Insulin Detemir may be decreased by: Hyperglycemia-Associated Agents; Quinolone Antibiotics; Thiazide Diuretics

Storage/Stability Unopened vials, cartridges, and prefilled pens may be stored under refrigeration between 2°C and 8°C (36°F to 46°F) until the expiration date or at room temperature <30°C (<86°F) for 42 days; do not freeze; keep away from heat and sunlight. Once punctured (in use), vials may be stored under refrigeration or at room temperature <30°C (<86°F); use within 42 days. Cartridges and prefilled pens that have been punctured (in use) should be stored at temperatures <30°C (<86°F) and used within 42 days; do not freeze or refrigerate.

Mechanism of Action Insulin acts via specific membrane-bound receptors on target tissues to regulate metabolism of carbohydrate, protein, and fats. Target organs for insulin include the liver, skeletal muscle, and adipose tissue.

Within the liver, insulin stimulates hepatic glycogen synthesis. Insulin promotes hepatic synthesis of fatty acids, which are released into the circulation as lipoproteins. Skeletal muscle effects of insulin include increased protein synthesis and increased glycogen synthesis. Within adipose tissue, insulin stimulates the processing of circulating lipoproteins to provide free fatty acids, facilitating triglyceride synthesis and storage by adipocytes; also directly inhibits the hydrolysis of triglycerides. In addition, insulin stimulates the cellular uptake of amino acids and increases cellular permeability to several ions, including potassium, magnesium, and phosphate. By activating sodium-potassium ATPases, insulin promotes the intracellular movement of potassium.

Normally secreted by the pancreas, insulin products are manufactured for pharmacologic use through recombinant DNA technology using either *E. coli* or *Saccharomyces cerevisiae*. Insulins are categorized based on the onset, peak, and duration of effect (eg, rapid-, short-, intermediate-, and long-acting insulin).

Pharmacodynamics

Onset of action: 3-4 hours

Maximum effect: 3-9 hours (Plank, 2005)

Duration: 6-23 hours (dose dependent); **Note:** Duration is dose-dependent. At lower dosages (0.1-0.2 units/kg), mean duration is variable (5.7-12.1 hours). At 0.4 units/kg, the mean duration was 19.9 hours. At high dosages (≥0.8 units/kg) the duration is longer and less variable (mean: 22-23 hours) (Plank, 2005).

Pharmacokinetics (Adult data unless noted)

Distribution: V_d: 0.1 L/kg

Protein binding: >98% (albumin)

Bioavailability: 60%

Half-life: SubQ: 5-7 hours (dose dependent)

Time to peak serum concentration: 6-8 hours

Elimination: Urine

Dosing: Usual Note: Insulin detemir is a long-acting insulin administered by SubQ injection. When compared to insulin NPH, insulin detemir has slower, more prolonged absorption; duration of activity is dose-dependent. Insulin detemir may be given once or twice daily when used as the basal insulin component of therapy. Changing the basal insulin component from another insulin to insulin detemir can be done on a unit-to-unit basis. Insulin requirements vary dramatically between patients and dictate frequent monitoring and close medical supervision. See Insulin Regular for additional information.

Pediatric:

General insulin dosing: Type 1 diabetes mellitus (DM): Infants, Children, and Adolescents: **Note:** Insulin regimens should be individualized to achieve glycemic goals without causing hypoglycemia. Multiple daily doses are utilized and guided by blood glucose monitoring. Combinations of insulin formulations are commonly used. The daily doses presented below are expressed as the **total units/kg/day of all insulin formulations combined**.

Usual maintenance range: SubQ: 0.5 to 1 unit/kg/day in divided doses; doses must be individualized; however, an estimate can be determined based on phase of diabetes and level of maturity (ISPAD [Couper 2014]; ISPAD [Danne 2014]).

Partial remission phase (Honeymoon phase): <0.5 units/kg/day

Prepubertal children (not in partial remission): 0.7 to 1 units/kg/day

Pubescent Children and Adolescents: During puberty, requirements may substantially increase to >1.2 unit/kg/day and in some cases up to 2 units/kg/day

Adjustment of dose: Dosage must be titrated to achieve glucose control and avoid hypoglycemia. Adjust dose to maintain premeal and bedtime glucose in target range. Since combinations of agents are frequently used, dosage adjustment must address the individual component of the insulin regimen which most directly influences the blood glucose value in question, based on the known onset and duration of the insulin component.

Insulin detemir-specific dosing:

Type 1 diabetes mellitus: Children ≥2 years and Adolescents: SubQ: Initial dose: Approximately one-third of the total daily insulin requirement; a rapid-acting or short-acting insulin should also be used. If administered once daily, doses are generally administered with evening meals or at bedtime.

Conversion from insulin glargine or NPH insulin: SubQ: May be substituted on an equivalent unit-per-unit basis; in one Type 2 diabetes clinical trial, higher doses of insulin detemir were required than insulin NPH.

Adult:

General insulin dosing:

Diabetes mellitus, type 1: SubQ: **Note:** Multiple daily doses are utilized and guided by blood glucose monitoring. Combinations of insulin formulations are commonly used. The daily doses presented below are expressed as the **total units/kg/day of all insulin formulations combined**.

Usual maintenance range: 0.5 to 1 units/kg/day in divided doses. An estimate of anticipated needs may be based on body weight and/or activity factors as follows:

Nonobese: 0.4 to 0.6 units/kg/day

Obese: 0.8 to 1.2 units/kg/day

Division of daily insulin requirement ("conventional therapy"): Generally, 50% to 75% of the total daily dose (TDD) is given as an intermediate-acting or a long-acting form of insulin (in 1 to 2 daily injections). The remaining portion of the TDD is then divided and administered before or at mealtimes (depending on the formulation) as a rapid-acting or short-acting form of insulin.

Division of daily insulin requirement ("intensive therapy"): Basal insulin delivery with 1 or 2 doses of intermediate-acting or long-acting insulin formulations superimposed with doses of short- or rapid-acting insulin formulations 3 or more times daily

Adjustment of dose: Dosage must be titrated to achieve glucose control and avoid hypoglycemia. Adjust dose to maintain premeal and bedtime glucose in target range. Since combinations of agents are frequently used, dosage adjustment must address the individual component of the insulin regimen which most directly influences the blood glucose value in question, based on the known onset and duration of the insulin component. Treatment and monitoring regimens must be individualized.

Insulin detemir-specific dosing: Manufacturer's labeling:

Diabetes mellitus, type 1: SubQ: Initial dose: Approximately one-third of the total daily insulin requirement administered in 1 to 2 divided doses. A rapid- or short-acting insulin should be used to complete the balance (~2/3) of the total daily insulin requirement.

Conversion from insulin glargine or NPH insulin: May be substituted on an equivalent unit-per–unit basis; in one Type 2 diabetes clinical trial, higher doses of insulin detemir were required than insulin NPH.

Diabetes mellitus, type 2: SubQ: Initial:

Inadequately controlled on oral antidiabetic agents: 10 units (or 0.1 to 0.2 units/kg) once daily in the evening; may also administer total daily dose in 2 divided doses.

Inadequately controlled on GLP-1 receptor agonist: 10 units once daily in the evening.

Conversion from insulin glargine or NPH insulin: May be substituted on an equivalent unit-per-unit basis; in one Type 2 diabetes clinical trial, higher doses of insulin detemir were required than insulin NPH.

Dosing adjustment in renal impairment: There are no dosage adjustments provided in manufacturer's labeling; insulin requirements are reduced due to changes in insulin clearance or metabolism; monitor blood glucose closely.

Dosing adjustment in hepatic impairment: There are no dosage adjustments provided in manufacturer's labeling; insulin requirements may be reduced due to changes in insulin clearance or metabolism; monitor blood glucose closely.

Administration Parenteral: SubQ: Administer into the thighs, deltoids, or abdomen, with sites rotated. Cold injections should be avoided. **Not for IV infusion** or use in insulin infusion pumps. Do not use if solution is viscous or cloudy; use only if clear and colorless with no visible particles. May not be diluted or mixed with other insulins or solutions. When treated once daily, administer with evening meal or at bedtime. When treated twice daily, administer evening dose with evening meal, at bedtime, or 12 hours following the morning dose.

Monitoring Parameters Plasma glucose, electrolytes, Hb A_{1c}

Reference Range Type I DM: Plasma Blood Glucose and HbA_{1c} Goals (ADA 2015): **Note:** Goals should be individualized based on individual needs/circumstances (eg, patients who experience severe hypoglycemia, patients with hypoglycemic unawareness); lower goals may be reasonable if they can be achieved without excessive hypoglycemia. **Note:** Postprandial blood glucose should be measured when there is a discrepancy between preprandial blood glucose concentrations and HbA_{1c} values and to help assess glycemia for patients who receive basal/bolus regimens. It is usually drawn 1 to 2 hours after starting meal and is considered to be the "peak."

Infants, Children, and Adolescents:

Preprandial glucose: 90 to 130 mg/dL

Bedtime/overnight glucose: 90 to 150 mg/dL

HbA_{1c}: <7.5%

Adults, nonpregnant:

Preprandial glucose: 80 to 130 mg/dL

Postprandial glucose: <180 mg/dL

HbA_{1c}: <7%

Additional Information

Division of daily insulin requirement ("conventional therapy"): Generally, 50% to 75% of the daily insulin dose is given as an intermediate or long-acting form of insulin (in 1 to 2 daily injections; dependent upon insulin type). The remaining portion of the 24-hour insulin requirement is divided and administered as either regular insulin or a rapid-acting form of insulin at the same time before breakfast and dinner.

Division of daily insulin requirement ("intensive therapy"): Basal insulin delivery with 1 or 2 doses of intermediate or long acting form of insulin (number of daily injections dependent upon insulin type) superimposed with doses of rapid- or very rapid-acting insulin formulations 3 or more times daily.

Dosage Forms Excipient information presented when available (limited, particularly for generics); consult specific product labeling. [DSC] = Discontinued product

Solution, Subcutaneous:

Levemir: 100 units/mL (10 mL) [contains metacresol, phenol]

Solution Pen-injector, Subcutaneous:

Levemir FlexPen: 100 units/mL (3 mL [DSC]) [contains metacresol, phenol]

Levemir FlexTouch: 100 units/mL (3 mL) [contains metacresol, phenol]

Insulin Glargine (IN soo lin GLAR jeen)

Medication Safety Issues

Sound-alike/look-alike issues:

Insulin glargine may be confused with insulin glulisine

Lantus may be confused with latanoprost, Latuda, Xalatan

High alert medication:

The Institute for Safe Medication Practices (ISMP) includes this medication among its list of drugs which have a heightened risk of causing significant patient harm when used in error. ***Due to the number of insulin preparations, it is essential to identify/clarify the type of insulin to be used.***

Administration issues:

Insulin glargine is a clear solution, but it is NOT intended for IV or IM administration.

Other safety concerns:

Cross-contamination may occur if insulin pens are shared among multiple patients. Steps should be taken to prohibit sharing of insulin pens.

International issues:

Lantus [U.S., Canada, and multiple international markets] may be confused with Lanvis brand name for thioguanine [Canada and multiple international markets]

Related Information

Insulin Products *on page 2319*

Brand Names: US Lantus; Lantus SoloStar; Toujeo SoloStar

Brand Names: Canada Lantus; Lantus OptiSet

Therapeutic Category Antidiabetic Agent, Parenteral; Insulin, Long-Acting

Generic Availability (US) No

Use Treatment of type 1 diabetes mellitus (insulin dependent, IDDM); type 2 diabetes mellitus (noninsulin dependent, NIDDM) requiring basal (long-acting) insulin to control hyperglycemia

Pregnancy Risk Factor C

Pregnancy Considerations In animal reproduction studies, outcomes were similar to those observed with regular insulin. In women with diabetes, maternal hyperglycemia can be associated with congenital malformations as well as adverse effects in the fetus, neonate, and the mother (ACOG 2005; ADA 2015; Kitzmiller 2008; Metzger 2007). To prevent adverse outcomes, prior to conception and throughout pregnancy maternal blood glucose and HbA_{1c} should be kept as close to target goals as possible but without causing significant hypoglycemia (ACOG 2013; ADA 2015; Blumer 2013; Kitzmiller 2008; Lambert 2013). Prior to pregnancy, effective contraception should be used until glycemic control is achieved (Kitzmiller 2008).

Insulin requirements tend to fall during the first trimester of pregnancy and increase in the later trimesters, peaking at 28 to 32 weeks of gestation. Following delivery, insulin requirements decrease rapidly (ACOG 2005).

Because insulin glargine has an increased affinity to the insulin-like growth factor (IGF-I) receptor, there are theoretical concerns that it may contribute to adverse events when used during pregnancy (Jovanovic 2007; Lambert 2013), although this has not been observed in available studies (Lambert 2013). Available data is insufficient to evaluate the use of insulin glargine during pregnancy (Lambert 2013). Women who are stable on insulin glargine prior to conception may continue it during pregnancy. Theoretical concerns of insulin glargine should be discussed prior to conception (Blumer 2013).

Breast-Feeding Considerations In a study using insulin glargine, both exogenous and endogenous insulin were excreted into breast milk (Whitmore 2012). Breast-feeding is encouraged for all women, including those with type 1, type 2, or GDM (ACOG 2005; Blumer 2013; Metzger 2007). A small snack (such as milk) before nursing may help decrease the risk of hypoglycemia in women with pregestational diabetes (ACOG 2005; ADA 2015; Reader 2004). The manufacturer considers the use of insulin glargine to be compatible with breast-feeding, although adjustments of the mothers insulin dose may be needed.

Contraindications

Hypersensitivity to insulin glargine or any component of the formulation; during episodes of hypoglycemia (Toujeo only)

Documentation of allergenic cross-reactivity for insulin is limited. However, because of similarities in chemical structure and/or pharmacologic actions, the possibility of cross-sensitivity cannot be ruled out with certainty.

Warnings/Precautions Severe, life-threatening allergic reactions, including anaphylaxis, may occur. If hypersensitivity reactions occur, discontinue therapy. Hypoglycemia is the most common adverse effect of insulin. The timing of hypoglycemia differs among various insulin formulations. Hypoglycemia may result from increased work or exercise without eating; use of long-acting insulin preparations (eg, insulin detemir, insulin glargine) may delay recovery from hypoglycemia. Profound and prolonged episodes of hypoglycemia may result in convulsions, unconsciousness, temporary or permanent brain damage or even death. Insulin requirements may be altered during illness, emotional disturbances or other stressors. Instruct patients to use caution with ethanol; may increase risk of hypoglycemia. Insulin may produce hypokalemia which, if left untreated, may result in respiratory paralysis, ventricular arrhythmia and even death. Use with caution in renal or hepatic impairment.

Insulin glargine is a clear solution, but it is **NOT** intended for IV or IM administration or via an insulin pump. According to the Centers for Disease Control and Prevention (CDC), pen-shaped injection devices should never be used for more than one person (even when the needle is changed) because of the risk of infection. The injection device should be clearly labeled with individual patient information to ensure that the correct pen is used (CDC 2012).

The general objective of exogenous insulin therapy is to approximate the physiologic pattern of insulin secretion which is characterized by two distinct phases. Phase 1 insulin secretion suppresses hepatic glucose production and phase 2 insulin secretion occurs in response to carbohydrate ingestion; therefore, exogenous insulin therapy may consist of basal insulin (eg, intermediate- or long-acting insulin [eg, insulin glargine] or via continuous subcutaneous insulin infusion [CSII]) and/or preprandial insulin (eg, short- or rapid-acting insulin) (see Related Information: Insulin Products). Patients with type 1 diabetes do not produce endogenous insulin; therefore, these patients require both basal and preprandial insulin administration. Patients with type 2 diabetes retain some beta-cell function in the early stages of their disease; however, as the disease progresses, phase 1 insulin secretion may become completely impaired and phase 2 insulin secretion becomes delayed and/or inadequate in response to meals. Therefore, patients with type 2 diabetes may be treated with oral antidiabetic agents, basal insulin, and/or preprandial insulin depending on the stage of disease and current glycemic control. Since treatment regimens often consist of multiple agents, dosage adjustments must address the specific phase of insulin release that is primarily contributing to the patient's impaired glycemic control. Diabetes self-management education (DSME) is essential to maximize the effectiveness of therapy. Treatment and monitoring regimens must be individualized.

Potentially significant drug-drug interactions may exist, requiring dose or frequency adjustment, additional monitoring, and/or selection of alternative therapy. Concurrent use with peroxisome proliferator-activated receptor (PPAR)-gamma agonists, including thiazolidinediones (TZDs) may cause dose-related fluid retention and lead to or exacerbate heart failure. If PPAR-gamma agonists are prescribed, monitor for signs and symptoms of heart failure. If heart failure develops, consider PPAR-gamma agonist dosage reduction or therapy discontinuation.

Adverse Reactions Primarily symptoms of hypoglycemia

Cardiovascular: Retinal vascular disease

Central nervous system: Depression, headache

Endocrine & metabolic: Hypoglycemia (more common in Type I on combination regimens)

Gastrointestinal: Diarrhea

Genitourinary: Urinary tract infection

Immunologic: Antibody development (effect on therapy not reported)

Infection: Infection, influenza

Local: Pain at injection site

Neuromuscular & skeletal: Arthralgia, back pain, limb pain

Ophthalmic: Cataract, retinopathy

Respiratory: Bronchitis, cough, nasopharyngitis, pharyngitis (children & adolescents), rhinitis (children & adolescents), sinusitis, upper respiratory tract infection (more common in adults)

Miscellaneous: Accidental injury

Rare but imporant or life-threatening: Hyperglycemia, hypersensitivity reaction, injection site reaction (including redness, itching, urticaria, edema, inflammation, erythema, and pruritus), lipoatrophy, lipodystrophy, lipohypertrophy, skin rash, weight gain

Drug Interactions

Metabolism/Transport Effects None known.

Avoid Concomitant Use

Avoid concomitant use of Insulin Glargine with any of the following: Rosiglitazone

Increased Effect/Toxicity

Insulin Glargine may increase the levels/effects of: Hypoglycemia-Associated Agents; Rosiglitazone

The levels/effects of Insulin Glargine may be increased by: Alpha-Lipoic Acid; Androgens; Antidiabetic Agents; Beta-Blockers; DPP-IV Inhibitors; Edetate CALCIUM Disodium; Edetate Disodium; GLP-1 Agonists; Herbs (Hypoglycemic Properties); Liraglutide; MAO Inhibitors; Metreleptin; Pegvisomant; Pioglitazone; Pramlintide; Quinolone Antibiotics; Salicylates; Selective Serotonin Reuptake Inhibitors; SGLT2 Inhibitors

Decreased Effect

The levels/effects of Insulin Glargine may be decreased by: Hyperglycemia-Associated Agents; Quinolone Antibiotics; Thiazide Diuretics

Storage/Stability

Lantus: Store unopened vials, cartridges, and prefilled pens refrigerated at 2°C to 8°C (36°F to 46°F) until the expiration date or at room temperature <30°C (<86°F) for 28 days; do not freeze; keep away from heat and sunlight. Once punctured (in use), store vials refrigerated or at room temperature <30°C (<86°F) and use within 28 days. Store cartridges within the OptiClik system and prefilled pens (SoloStar) that have been punctured (in use) at temperatures <30°C (<86°F) and use within 28 days; do not freeze or refrigerate.

Toujeo: Store unopened prefilled pen (SoloStar) at 2°C to 8°C (36°F to 46°F) until the expiration date; do not freeze. Store prefilled pens (SoloStar) that have been punctured (in use) at temperatures <30°C (<86°F) and use within 28 days; do not freeze or refrigerate.

Mechanism of Action Insulin acts via specific membrane-bound receptors on target tissues to regulate metabolism of carbohydrate, protein, and fats. Target organs for insulin include the liver, skeletal muscle, and adipose tissue.

Within the liver, insulin stimulates hepatic glycogen synthesis. Insulin promotes hepatic synthesis of fatty acids, which are released into the circulation as lipoproteins. Skeletal muscle effects of insulin include increased protein synthesis and increased glycogen synthesis. Within adipose tissue, insulin stimulates the processing of circulating lipoproteins to provide free fatty acids, facilitating triglyceride synthesis and storage by adipocytes; also directly inhibits the hydrolysis of triglycerides. In addition, insulin stimulates the cellular uptake of amino acids and increases cellular permeability to several ions, including potassium, magnesium, and phosphate. By activating sodium-potassium ATPases, insulin promotes the intracellular movement of potassium.

Normally secreted by the pancreas, insulin products are manufactured for pharmacologic use through recombinant DNA technology using either *E. coli* or *Saccharomyces cerevisiae*. Insulins are categorized based on the onset, peak, and duration of effect (eg, rapid-, short-, intermediate-, and long-acting insulin). Insulin glargine is a long-acting insulin analog.

Pharmacodynamics

Onset of action: 3-4 hours

Duration: 24 hours

Pharmacokinetics (Adult data unless noted)

Absorption: Slow; after injection it forms microprecipitates in the skin which allow small amounts to release over time

Metabolism: Partially metabolized in the skin to form two active metabolites

Time to peak serum concentration: No pronounced peak

Elimination: Urine

Dosing: Usual Insulin glargine is a long-acting insulin administered by SubQ injection. Insulin glargine is approximately equipotent to human insulin, but has a slower onset, no pronounced peak, and a longer duration of activity. Changing the basal insulin component from another insulin to insulin glargine can be done on a unit-to-unit basis. Insulin requirements vary dramatically between patients and dictates frequent monitoring and close medical supervision. See Insulin Regular for additional information.

General insulin dosing:

Type 1 diabetes mellitus: Children, Adolescents, and Adults: **Note:** Multiple daily doses are utilized and guided by blood glucose monitoring. Combinations of insulin formulations are commonly used. The daily doses presented below are expressed as the **total units/kg/day of all insulin formulations** used. Insulin glargine must be used in combination with a short-acting insulin.

Usual maintenance range: SubQ: 0.5-1 unit/kg/day in divided doses. An estimate of anticipated needs may be based on body weight and/or activity factors as follows:

Nonobese: 0.4-0.6 units/kg/day

Obese: 0.8-1.2 units/kg/day

Pubescent Children and Adolescents: During puberty, requirements may substantially increase to >1 unit/kg/day and in some cases up to 2 units/kg/day (IDF/ISPAD, 2011)

Adjustment of dose: Dosage must be titrated to achieve glucose control and avoid hypoglycemia. Adjust dose to maintain premeal and bedtime glucose in target range. Since combinations of agents are frequently used, dosage adjustment must address the individual component of the insulin regimen which most directly influences the blood glucose value in question, based on the known onset and duration of the insulin component.

Insulin glargine-specific dosing:

Type 1 diabetes mellitus: Children ≥6 years, Adolescents, and Adults: SubQ: Initial dose: Approximately one-third of the total daily insulin requirement; a rapid-acting or short-acting insulin should also be used.

Type 2 diabetes mellitus: Adults: SubQ: Initial basal insulin dose: 10 units (**or** 0.2 units/kg) once daily in the evening; may also administer total daily dose in 2 divided doses

Type 1 or type 2 diabetes; previously receiving basal insulin plus bolus insulin (eg, NPH + regular insulin):

Children <6 years: SubQ: Limited data available: 40% of the established total daily insulin requirement; this resulted in a reduction in hypoglycemic episodes in 35 nonobese preschool-aged children (age range: 2.6-6.3 years) when used in conjunction with a rapid-acting insulin prior to meals (Alemzadeh, 2005).

Children ≥6 years and Adults: SubQ:

Converting from once-daily NPH insulin: May be substituted on an equivalent unit-per-unit basis

Converting from twice-daily NPH insulin: Initial dose: Use 80% of the total daily dose of NPH (eg, 20% reduction); administer once daily; adjust dosage according to patient response

Dosing adjustment in renal impairment: There are no dosage adjustments provided in manufacturer's labeling;

insulin requirements are reduced due to changes in insulin clearance or metabolism; monitor blood glucose closely.

Dosing adjustment in hepatic impairment: There are no dosage adjustments provided in manufacturer's labeling; insulin requirements may be reduced due to changes in insulin clearance or metabolism; monitor blood glucose closely.

Administration Parenteral: SubQ: Administer into the subcutaneous fat of the thighs, arms, buttocks, or abdomen, with sites rotated. Cold injections should be avoided. Administer once daily, at any time of day, but at the same time each day. Do not mix with any other insulin or solution.

Monitoring Parameters Urine sugar and acetone, serum glucose, electrolytes, Hb A_{1c}, lipid profile

Reference Range

Plasma Blood Glucose and Hgb A_{1c} Goals for Type 1 Diabetes (ADA, 2013): Note: Goals should be individualized based on individual needs/circumstances (eg, patients who experience severe hypoglycemia, patients with hypoglycemic unawareness); lower goals may be reasonable if they can be achieved without excessive hypoglycemia. **Note:** Postprandial blood glucose should be measured when there is a discrepancy between preprandial blood glucose concentrations and Hb A_{1c} values and to help assess glycemia for patients who receive basal/bolus regimens. It is usually drawn 1-2 hours after starting meal and is considered to be the "peak."

Toddlers/Preschoolers (0-6 years):
- Preprandial glucose: 100-180 mg/dL
- Bedtime/overnight glucose: 110-200 mg/dL
- Hb A_{1c}: <8.5%

School age (6-12 years):
- Preprandial glucose: 90-180 mg/dL
- Bedtime/overnight glucose: 100-180 mg/dL
- Hb A_{1c}: <8%

Adolescents/Young Adults (13-19 years):
- Preprandial glucose: 90-130 mg/dL
- Bedtime/overnight glucose: 90-150 mg/dL
- Hb A_{1c}: <7.5%

Adults, nonpregnant:
- Preprandial glucose: 70-130 mg/dL
- Postprandial glucose: <180 mg/dL
- Hb A_{1c}: <7%

Criteria for diagnosis of DKA:

Serum glucose:
- Children: >200 mg/dL
- Adults: >250 mg/dL

Arterial pH:
- Children: <7.3
- Adults: <7-7.24

Bicarbonate:
- Children: <15 mEq/L
- Adults: <10-15 mEq/L

Moderate ketonuria or ketonemia

Additional Information

Division of daily insulin requirement ("conventional therapy"): Generally, 50% to 75% of the daily insulin dose is given as an intermediate- or long-acting form (eg, insulin glargine) of insulin (in 1-2 daily injections). The remaining portion of the 24-hour insulin requirement is divided and administered as either regular insulin or a rapid-acting form of insulin at the same time before breakfast and dinner.

Division of daily insulin requirement ("intensive therapy"): Basal insulin delivery with 1 or 2 doses of intermediate- or long-acting insulin (eg, insulin glargine) formulations superimposed with doses of rapid- or very rapid-acting insulin formulations 3 or more times daily.

Dosage Forms Excipient information presented when available (limited, particularly for generics); consult specific product labeling.

Solution, Subcutaneous:
- Lantus: 100 units/mL (10 mL) [contains metacresol]

Solution Pen-injector, Subcutaneous:
- Lantus SoloStar: 100 units/mL (3 mL)
- Toujeo SoloStar: 300 units/mL (1.5 mL) [contains metacresol]

Insulin Glulisine (IN soo lin gloo LIS een)

Medication Safety Issues

Sound-alike/look-alike issues:
- Apidra may be confused with Spiriva
- Insulin glulisine may be confused with insulin glargine

High alert medication:

The Institute for Safe Medication Practices (ISMP) includes this medication among its list of drugs which have a heightened risk of causing significant patient harm when used in error. ***Due to the number of insulin preparations, it is essential to identify/clarify the type of insulin to be used.***

Other safety concerns:

Cross-contamination may occur if insulin pens are shared among multiple patients. Steps should be taken to prohibit sharing of insulin pens.

Related Information

Insulin Products *on page 2319*

Brand Names: US Apidra; Apidra SoloStar

Brand Names: Canada Apidra®

Therapeutic Category Insulin, Rapid-Acting

Generic Availability (US) No

Use Treatment of type 1 diabetes mellitus (insulin dependent, IDDM); type 2 diabetes mellitus (noninsulin dependent, NIDDM) to control hyperglycemia

Pregnancy Risk Factor C

Pregnancy Considerations In animal reproduction studies, outcomes were similar to those observed with regular insulin.

In women with diabetes, maternal hyperglycemia can be associated with congenital malformations as well as adverse effects in the fetus, neonate, and the mother (ACOG 2005; ADA 2015; Kitzmiller 2008; Metzger 2007). To prevent adverse outcomes, prior to conception and throughout pregnancy maternal blood glucose and Hb A_{1c} should be kept as close to target goals as possible but without causing significant hypoglycemia (ACOG 2013; ADA 2015; Blumer 2013; Kitzmiller 2008; Lambert 2013). Prior to pregnancy, effective contraception should be used until glycemic control is achieved (Kitzmiller 2008)

Insulin requirements tend to fall during the first trimester of pregnancy and increase in the later trimesters, peaking at 28 to 32 weeks of gestation. Following delivery, insulin requirements decrease rapidly (ACOG 2005).

Due to lack of clinical data, insulin glulisine is not currently recommended for use in pregnant women (Blumer 2013).

Breast-Feeding Considerations Both exogenous and endogenous insulin are excreted into breast milk (study not conducted with this preparation) (Whitmore 2012). Breast-feeding is encouraged for all women, including those with type 1, type 2, or GDM (ACOG 2005; Blumer 2013; Metzger 2007). A small snack (such as milk) before nursing may help decrease the risk of hypoglycemia in women with pregestational diabetes (ACOG 2005; ADA 1015; Reader 2004).

All types of insulin may be used while breast-feeding (Metzger 2007). The manufacturer recommends that caution be used in nursing women; adjustments of the mothers insulin dose may be needed.

Contraindications Hypersensitivity to insulin glulisine or any component of the formulation; during episodes of hypoglycemia

Warnings/Precautions Hypoglycemia is the most common adverse effect of insulin. The timing of hypoglycemia differs among various insulin formulations. Hypoglycemia may result from increased work or exercise without eating; use of long-acting insulin preparations (eg, insulin detemir, insulin glargine) may delay recovery from hypoglycemia. Profound and prolonged episodes of hypoglycemia may result in convulsions, unconsciousness, temporary or permanent brain damage or even death. Insulin requirements may be altered during illness, emotional disturbances or other stressors. Instruct patients to use caution with ethanol; may increase risk of hypoglycemia. Insulin may produce hypokalemia which, if left untreated, may result in respiratory paralysis, ventricular arrhythmia and even death. Use with caution in patients at risk for hypokalemia (eg, IV insulin use). Use with caution in renal or hepatic impairment. In the elderly, avoid use of sliding scale insulin in this population due to increased risk of hypoglycemia without benefits in management of hyperglycemia regardless of care setting (Beers Criteria).

Due to the short duration of action of insulin glulisine, a longer acting insulin or CSII via an external insulin pump is needed to maintain adequate glucose control in patients with type 1 diabetes mellitus. In both type 1 and type 2 diabetes, preprandial administration of insulin glulisine should be immediately followed by a meal within 15 minutes. May also be administered via CSII; do not dilute or mix with other insulin formulations when using an external insulin pump. Rule out pump failure if unexplained hyperglycemia or ketosis occurs; temporary SubQ insulin administration may be required until the problem is identified and corrected. Insulin glulisine may also be administered IV in selected clinical situations to control hyperglycemia; close monitoring of blood glucose and serum potassium as well as medical supervision is required. According to the Centers for Disease Control and Prevention (CDC), pen-shaped injection devices should never be used for more than one person (even when the needle is changed) because of the risk of infection. The injection device should be clearly labeled with individual patient information to ensure that the correct pen is used (CDC, 2012).

The general objective of exogenous insulin therapy is to approximate the physiologic pattern of insulin secretion which is characterized by two distinct phases. Phase 1 insulin secretion suppresses hepatic glucose production and phase 2 insulin secretion occurs in response to carbohydrate ingestion; therefore, exogenous insulin therapy may consist of basal insulin (eg, intermediate- or long-acting insulin or via continuous subcutaneous insulin infusion [CSII]) and/or preprandial insulin (eg, short- or rapid-acting insulin [eg, insulin glulisine]) (see Related Information: Insulin Products). Patients with type 1 diabetes do not produce endogenous insulin; therefore, these patients require both basal and preprandial insulin administration. Patients with type 2 diabetes retain some beta-cell function in the early stages of their disease; however, as the disease progresses, phase 1 insulin secretion may become completely impaired and phase 2 insulin secretion becomes delayed and/or inadequate in response to meals. Therefore, patients with type 2 diabetes may be treated with oral antidiabetic agents, basal insulin, and/or preprandial insulin depending on the stage of disease and current glycemic control. Since treatment regimens often consist of multiple agents, dosage adjustments must address the specific phase of insulin release that is primarily contributing to the patient's impaired glycemic control. Diabetes self-management education (DSME) is essential to maximize the effectiveness of therapy. Treatment and monitoring regimens must be individualized.

Potentially significant drug-drug interactions may exist, requiring dose or frequency adjustment, additional monitoring, and/or selection of alternative therapy.

Adverse Reactions Primarily symptoms of hypoglycemia

Cardiovascular: Pallor, palpitation, tachycardia

Central nervous system: Fatigue, headache, hypothermia, loss of consciousness, mental confusion

Dermatologic: Redness, urticaria

Endocrine & metabolic: Hypoglycemia, hypokalemia

Gastrointestinal: Hunger, nausea, numbness of mouth

Local: Atrophy or hypertrophy of SubQ fat tissue; edema, itching, pain or warmth at injection site; stinging

Neuromuscular & skeletal: Muscle weakness, paresthesia, tremor

Ocular: Transient presbyopia or blurred vision

Miscellaneous: Anaphylaxis, diaphoresis, local and/or systemic hypersensitivity reactions

Drug Interactions

Metabolism/Transport Effects None known.

Avoid Concomitant Use

Avoid concomitant use of Insulin Glulisine with any of the following: Rosiglitazone

Increased Effect/Toxicity

Insulin Glulisine may increase the levels/effects of: Hypoglycemia-Associated Agents; Rosiglitazone

The levels/effects of Insulin Glulisine may be increased by: Alpha-Lipoic Acid; Androgens; Antidiabetic Agents; Beta-Blockers; DPP-IV Inhibitors; Edetate CALCIUM Disodium; Edetate Disodium; GLP-1 Agonists; Herbs (Hypoglycemic Properties); Liraglutide; MAO Inhibitors; Metreleptin; Pegvisomant; Pioglitazone; Pramlintide; Quinolone Antibiotics; Salicylates; Selective Serotonin Reuptake Inhibitors; SGLT2 Inhibitors

Decreased Effect

The levels/effects of Insulin Glulisine may be decreased by: Hyperglycemia-Associated Agents; Quinolone Antibiotics; Thiazide Diuretics

Storage/Stability Unopened vials, cartridges, and prefilled pens may be stored under refrigeration between 2°C and 8°C (36°F to 46°F) until the expiration date or at room temperature for 28 days; do not freeze; keep away from heat and sunlight. Once punctured (in use), vials may be stored under refrigeration or at room temperature ≤25°C (≤77°F); use within 28 days. Cartridges and prefilled pens that have been punctured (in use) should be stored at temperatures ≤25°C (≤77°F) and used within 28 days; do not freeze or refrigerate. When used for CSII, insulin glulisine contained within an external insulin pump reservoir should be replaced every 48 hours; discard if exposed to temperatures >37°C (>98.6°F).

For IV infusion: Stable for 48 hours at room temperature.

Mechanism of Action Insulin acts via specific membrane-bound receptors on target tissues to regulate metabolism of carbohydrate, protein, and fats. Target organs for insulin include the liver, skeletal muscle, and adipose tissue.

Within the liver, insulin stimulates hepatic glycogen synthesis. Insulin promotes hepatic synthesis of fatty acids which are released into the circulation as lipoproteins. Skeletal muscle effects of insulin include increased protein synthesis and increased glycogen synthesis. Within adipose tissue, insulin stimulates the processing of circulating lipoproteins to provide free fatty acids, facilitating triglyceride synthesis and storage by adipocytes; also directly inhibits the hydrolysis of triglycerides. In addition, insulin stimulates the cellular uptake of amino acids and increases cellular permeability to several ions, including potassium, magnesium, and phosphate. By activating sodium-potassium ATPases, insulin promotes the intracellular movement of potassium.

Normally secreted by the pancreas, insulin products are manufactured for pharmacologic use through recombinant DNA technology using either *E. coli* or *Saccharomyces cerevisiae*. Insulins are categorized based on the onset, peak, and duration of effect (eg, rapid-, short-, intermediate-, and long-acting insulin). Insulin glulisine is a rapid-acting insulin analog.

Pharmacodynamics Onset and duration of hypoglycemic effects depend upon the route of administration (adsorption and onset of action are more rapid after deeper IM injections than after SubQ), site of injection (onset and duration are progressively slower with SubQ injection into the abdomen, arm, buttock, or thigh respectively), volume and concentration of injection, and the preparation administered; local heat and massage also increase the rate of absorption.

Onset of action: 5-15 minutes

Maximum effect: 45-75 minutes

Duration: 2-4 hours

Pharmacokinetics (Adult data unless noted)

Distribution: V_d: Adults: 13 L

Bioavailability: SubQ: ~70%

Half-life:

SubQ: 42 minutes

IV: 13 minutes

Time to peak serum concentration: SubQ: 60 minutes (range: 40-120 minutes)

Elimination: Urine

Dosing: Usual Insulin glulisine is a rapid-acting insulin analog which is normally administered SubQ as a premeal component of the insulin regimen or as a continuous SubQ infusion and should be used with an intermediate- or long-acting insulin. Insulin glulisine is equipotent to insulin regular, but has a more rapid onset and shorter duration of activity. In carefully controlled clinical settings with close medical supervision and monitoring of blood glucose and potassium, insulin glulisine may be administered IV in some situations. Insulin requirements vary dramatically between patients and dictate frequent monitoring and close medical supervision. See Insulin Regular for additional information.

General insulin dosing:

Type 1 diabetes mellitus: Children, Adolescents, and Adults: **Note:** Multiple daily doses or continuous subcutaneous infusions guided by blood glucose monitoring are utilized. Combinations of insulin formulations are commonly used. The daily doses presented below are expressed as the **total units/kg/day of all insulin formulations combined**.

Initial dose: SubQ: 0.2-0.6 units/kg/day in divided doses. Conservative initial doses of 0.2-0.4 units/kg/day are often recommended to avoid the potential for hypoglycemia. A rapidly acting insulin may be the only insulin formulation used initially.

Usual maintenance range: SubQ: 0.5-1 unit/kg/day in divided doses. An estimate of anticipated needs may be based on body weight and/or activity factors as follows:

Nonobese: 0.4-0.6 units/kg/day

Obese: 0.8-1.2 units/kg/day

Pubescent Children and Adolescents: During puberty, requirements may substantially increase to >1 unit/kg/day and in some cases up to 2 units/kg/day (IDF/ISPAD, 2011)

Adjustment of dose: Dosage must be titrated to achieve glucose control and avoid hypoglycemia. Adjust dose to maintain premeal and bedtime glucose in target range. Since combinations of agents are frequently used, dosage adjustment must address the individual component of the insulin regimen which most directly influences the blood glucose value in question, based on the known onset and duration of the insulin component.

Continuous SubQ insulin infusion (insulin pump): A combination of a "basal" continuous insulin infusion rate with preprogrammed premeal bolus doses which are patient controlled. When converting from multiple daily SubQ doses of maintenance insulin, it is advisable to reduce the basal rate to less than the equivalent of the total daily units of longer-acting insulin (eg, NPH); divide the total number of units by 24 to get the basal rate in units/hour. Do not include the total units of regular insulin or other rapid-acting insulin formulations in this calculation. The same premeal regular insulin dosage may be used.

Type 2 diabetes mellitus: Augmentation therapy (patients for which diet, exercise, weight reduction, and oral hypoglycemic agents have not been adequate): Adults: SubQ: Initial dosage of 0.2 units/kg/day or 10 units/day of an intermediate- or long-acting insulin administered at bedtime has been recommended. As an alternative, regular insulin or rapid-acting insulin (eg, insulin glulisine) formulations administered before meals have also been used. Dosage must be carefully adjusted.

Dosing adjustment in renal impairment: There are no dosage adjustments provided in manufacturer's labeling; insulin requirements are reduced due to changes in insulin clearance or metabolism; monitor blood glucose closely.

Dosing adjustment in hepatic impairment: There are no dosage adjustments provided in manufacturer's labeling; insulin requirements may be reduced due to changes in insulin clearance or metabolism; monitor blood glucose closely.

Preparation for Administration Parenteral:

SubQ: May be mixed in the same syringe with NPH insulin. When mixing insulin glulisine with NPH insulin, glulisine should be drawn into the syringe first.

IV: May be diluted in NS to concentrations of 0.05 to 1 unit/mL.

Administration Parenteral: Do not use if solution is viscous or cloudy; use only if clear and colorless. May be administered IV with close monitoring of blood glucose and serum potassium; appropriate medical supervision is required. Do not administer insulin mixtures intravenously.

SubQ: Administration is usually made into the subcutaneous fat of the thighs, arms, buttocks, or abdomen, with sites rotated; cold injections should be avoided. May be mixed in the same syringe with NPH insulin. When mixing insulin glulisine with NPH insulin, glulisine should be drawn into the syringe first. Administer 15 minutes before meals or within 20 minutes after starting a meal.

Continuous SubQ insulin infusion (Insulin pump): Do not use if solution is viscous or cloudy; use only if clear and colorless. Patients should be trained in the proper use of their external insulin pump and in intensive insulin therapy. Infusion sets, reservoirs, and infusion set insertion sites should be changed every 48 hours; rotate infusion sites. Do not dilute or mix other insulin formulations with insulin glulisine that is to be used in an external insulin pump.

IV: Further dilute and administer using polyvinyl chloride infusion bags into a dedicated infusion line (the use of other bags and tubing has not been studied). Closely monitor blood glucose and serum potassium; appropriate medical supervision is required. Do not administer insulin mixtures intravenously.

To minimize insulin adsorption to IV tubing: Flush the IV tubing with a priming infusion of 20 mL from the insulin infusion, whenever a new IV tubing set is added to the insulin infusion container (Jacobi 2012; Thompson 2012). Also refer to institution-specific protocols where appropriate

Because of insulin adsorption to IV tubing or infusion bags, the actual amount of insulin being administered via IV infusion could be substantially less than the apparent amount. Therefore, adjustment of the IV infusion rate should be based on effect and not solely on the apparent insulin dose. The apparent dose may be used as a starting point for determining the subsequent SubQ dosing regimen (Moghissi 2009); however, the transition to SubQ administration requires continuous medical supervision, frequent monitoring of blood glucose, and careful adjustment of therapy. In addition, SubQ insulin should be given 1 to 4 hours prior to the discontinuation of IV insulin to prevent hyperglycemia (Moghissi 2009).

Monitoring Parameters Urine sugar and acetone, serum glucose, electrolytes, Hb A_{1c}, lipid profile

Reference Range

Plasma Blood Glucose and Hgb A_{1c} Goals for Type 1 Diabetes (ADA, 2013): Note: Goals should be individualized based on individual needs/circumstances (eg, patients who experience severe hypoglycemia, patients with hypoglycemic unawareness); lower goals may be reasonable if they can be achieved without excessive hypoglycemia. **Note:** Postprandial blood glucose should be measured when there is a discrepancy between preprandial blood glucose concentrations and Hb A_{1c} values and to help assess glycemia for patients who receive basal/bolus regimens. It is usually drawn 1-2 hours after starting meal and is considered to be the "peak."

Toddlers/Preschoolers (0-6 years):
- Preprandial glucose: 100-180 mg/dL
- Bedtime/overnight glucose: 110-200 mg/dL
- Hb A_{1c}: <8.5%

School age (6-12 years):
- Preprandial glucose: 90-180 mg/dL
- Bedtime/overnight glucose: 100-180 mg/dL
- Hb A_{1c}: <8%

Adolescents/Young Adults (13-19 years):
- Preprandial glucose: 90-130 mg/dL
- Bedtime/overnight glucose: 90-150 mg/dL
- Hb A_{1c}: <7.5%

Adults, nonpregnant:
- Preprandial glucose: 70-130 mg/dL
- Postprandial glucose: <180 mg/dL
- Hb A_{1c}: <7%

Criteria for diagnosis of DKA:

Serum glucose:
- Children: >200 mg/dL
- Adults: >250 mg/dL

Arterial pH:
- Children: <7.3
- Adults: <7-7.24

Bicarbonate:
- Children: <15 mEq/L
- Adults: <10-15 mEq/L

Moderate ketonuria or ketonemia

Additional Information

Division of daily insulin requirement ("conventional therapy"): Generally, 50% to 75% of the daily insulin dose is given as an intermediate- or long-acting form of insulin (in 1-2 daily injections). The remaining portion of the 24-hour insulin requirement is divided and administered as either regular insulin or a rapid-acting (eg, insulin glulisine) form of insulin at the same time before breakfast and dinner.

Division of daily insulin requirement ("intensive therapy"): Basal insulin delivery with 1 or 2 doses of intermediate- or long-acting insulin formulations superimposed with doses of rapid- or very rapid-acting insulin (eg, insulin glulisine) formulations 3 or more times daily.

Dosage Forms Excipient information presented when available (limited, particularly for generics); consult specific product labeling.

Solution, Injection:
- Apidra: 100 units/mL (10 mL) [contains metacresol]

Solution Pen-injector, Subcutaneous:
- Apidra SoloStar: 100 units/mL (3 mL) [contains metacresol]

Insulin Lispro (IN soo lin LYE sproe)

Medication Safety Issues

Sound-alike/look-alike issues:
- HumaLOG may be confused with HumaLOG Mix 50/50, Humira, HumuLIN N, HumuLIN R, NovoLOG
- Humapen Memoir (used with HumaLOG) may be confused with the Humira Pen

High alert medication:

The Institute for Safe Medication Practices (ISMP) includes this medication among its list of drugs which have a heightened risk of causing significant patient harm when used in error. ***Due to the number of insulin preparations, it is essential to identify/clarify the type and strength of insulin to be used.***

Other safety concerns:

Cross-contamination may occur if insulin pens are shared among multiple patients. Steps should be taken to prohibit sharing of insulin pens.

Related Information

Insulin Products *on page 2319*

Brand Names: US HumaLOG; HumaLOG KwikPen

Brand Names: Canada Humalog; HumaLOG KwikPen

Therapeutic Category Antidiabetic Agent, Parenteral; Insulin, Rapid-Acting

Generic Availability (US) No

Use Treatment of type 1 diabetes mellitus (insulin dependent, IDDM); type 2 diabetes mellitus (noninsulin dependent, NIDDM) to control hyperglycemia

Pregnancy Risk Factor B

Pregnancy Considerations Adverse events have not been observed in animal reproduction studies. Insulin lispro has not been shown to cross the placenta at standard clinical doses (Boskovic 2003; Holcberg 2004; Jovanovic 1999).

In women with diabetes, maternal hyperglycemia can be associated with congenital malformations as well as adverse effects in the fetus, neonate, and the mother (ACOG 2005; ADA 2015; Kitzmiller 2008; Metzger 2007). To prevent adverse outcomes, prior to conception and throughout pregnancy maternal blood glucose and HbA_{1c} should be as kept close to target goals as possible but without causing significant hypoglycemia (ACOG 2013; ADA 2015; Blumer 2013; Kitzmiller 2008; Lambert 2013). Prior to pregnancy, effective contraception should be used until glycemic control is achieved (Kitzmiller 2008)

Insulin requirements tend to fall during the first trimester of pregnancy and increase in the later trimesters, peaking at 28 to 32 weeks of gestation. Following delivery, insulin requirements decrease rapidly (ACOG 2005). Insulin lispro may be used to treat diabetes in pregnant women (ACOG 2013; Blumer 2013; Kitzmiller 2008; Lambert 2013)

Breast-Feeding Considerations Both exogenous and endogenous insulin are excreted into breast milk (study not conducted with this preparation) (Whitmore 2012). Breast-feeding is encouraged for all women, including those with type 1, type 2, or GDM (ACOG 2005; Blumer 2013; Metzger 2007). A small snack (such as milk) before nursing may help decrease the risk of hypoglycemia in women with pregestational diabetes (ACOG 2005; ADA

2015; Reader 2004). All types of insulin may be used while breast-feeding (Metzger 2007). The manufacturer considers the use of insulin lispro to be compatible with breast-feeding, although adjustments of the mothers insulin dose may be needed.

Contraindications Hypersensitivity to insulin lispro or any component of the formulation; during episodes of hypoglycemia

Warnings/Precautions Hypersensitivity reactions (serious, life-threatening and anaphylaxis) have occurred. If hypersensitivity reactions occur, discontinue administration and initiate supportive care measures. Hypoglycemia is the most common adverse effect of insulin. The timing of hypoglycemia differs among various insulin formulations. Hypoglycemia may result from changes in meal pattern (eg, macronutrient content or timing of meals), changes in the level of physical activity, increased work or exercise without eating or changes to coadministered medications. Hyperglycemia is also a concern; may occur with CSII pump or infusion set malfunctions or insulin degradation; hyper- or hypoglycemia may result from changes in insulin strength, manufacturer, type or administration method. Use of long-acting insulin preparations (eg, insulin detemir, insulin glargine) may delay recovery from hypoglycemia. Patients with renal or hepatic impairment may be at a higher risk. Symptoms differ in patients and may change over time in the same patient; awareness may be less pronounced in those with long standing diabetes, diabetic nerve disease, patients taking beta-blockers or in those who experience recurrent hypoglycemia. Profound and prolonged episodes of hypoglycemia may result in convulsions, unconsciousness, temporary or permanent brain damage, or even death. Insulin requirements may be altered during illness, emotional disturbances, or other stressors. Instruct patients to use caution with ethanol; may increase risk of hypoglycemia. Insulin may produce hypokalemia which, if left untreated, may result in respiratory paralysis, ventricular arrhythmia, and even death. Use with caution in patients at risk for hypokalemia (eg, IV insulin use). Use with caution in renal or hepatic impairment; patients may require more frequent dose adjustment and glucose monitoring. In the elderly, avoid use of sliding scale insulin in this population due to increased risk of hypoglycemia without benefits in management of hyperglycemia regardless of care setting (Beers Criteria).

Due to the short duration of action of insulin lispro, a longer acting insulin or CSII via an external insulin pump is needed to maintain adequate glucose control in patients with type 1 diabetes mellitus. In both type 1 and type 2 diabetes, preprandial administration of insulin lispro should be immediately followed by a meal within 15 minutes. May also be administered via CSII; do not dilute or mix with other insulin formulations when using an external insulin pump. Rule out pump failure if unexplained hyperglycemia or ketosis occurs; temporary SubQ insulin administration may be required until the problem is identified and corrected. Insulin lispro may also be administered IV in selected clinical situations to control hyperglycemia; close monitoring of blood glucose and serum potassium as well as medical supervision is required. According to the Centers for Disease Control and Prevention (CDC), pen-shaped injection devices should never be used for more than one person (even when the needle is changed) because of the risk of infection. The injection device should be clearly labeled with individual patient information to ensure that the correct pen is used (CDC, 2012). Do not perform dose conversion when using KwikPen devices; the dose window shows the number of units to be delivered and no conversion is needed. Do not transfer product from the KwikPen U 200 to a syringe for administration; do not mix with other insulins, administer in a CSII pump, or administer IV. Only insulin lispro U 100 (eg, 100 units/mL) is approved for use in children ≥3 years by CSII pump.

The general objective of exogenous insulin therapy is to approximate the physiologic pattern of insulin secretion which is characterized by two distinct phases. Phase 1 insulin secretion suppresses hepatic glucose production and phase 2 insulin secretion occurs in response to carbohydrate ingestion; therefore, exogenous insulin therapy may consist of basal insulin (eg, intermediate- or long-acting insulin or via continuous subcutaneous insulin infusion [CSII]) and/or preprandial insulin (eg, short- or rapid-acting insulin [insulin lispro]) (see Related Information: Insulin Products). Patients with type 1 diabetes do not produce endogenous insulin; therefore, these patients require both basal and preprandial insulin administration. Patients with type 2 diabetes retain some beta-cell function in the early stages of their disease; however, as the disease progresses, phase 1 insulin secretion may become completely impaired and phase 2 insulin secretion becomes delayed and/or inadequate in response to meals. Therefore, patients with type 2 diabetes may be treated with oral antidiabetic agents, basal insulin, and/or preprandial insulin depending on the stage of disease and current glycemic control. Since treatment regimens often consist of multiple agents, dosage adjustments must address the specific phase of insulin release that is primarily contributing to the patient's impaired glycemic control. Diabetes self-management education (DSME) is essential to maximize the effectiveness of therapy. Treatment and monitoring regimens must be individualized.

Potentially significant drug-drug interactions may exist, requiring dose or frequency adjustment, additional monitoring, and/or selection of alternative therapy.

Adverse Reactions Primarily symptoms of hypoglycemia

Cardiovascular: Pallor, palpitation, tachycardia

Central nervous system: Fatigue, headache, hypothermia, loss of consciousness, mental confusion

Dermatologic: Redness, urticaria

Endocrine & metabolic: Hypoglycemia, hypokalemia

Gastrointestinal: Hunger, nausea, numbness of mouth

Local: Atrophy or hypertrophy of SubQ fat tissue; edema, itching, pain or warmth at injection site; stinging

Neuromuscular & skeletal: Muscle weakness, paresthesia, tremor

Ocular: Transient presbyopia or blurred vision

Miscellaneous: Anaphylaxis, diaphoresis, local and/or systemic hypersensitivity reactions

Drug Interactions

Metabolism/Transport Effects None known.

Avoid Concomitant Use

Avoid concomitant use of Insulin Lispro with any of the following: Rosiglitazone

Increased Effect/Toxicity

Insulin Lispro may increase the levels/effects of: Hypoglycemia-Associated Agents; Rosiglitazone

The levels/effects of Insulin Lispro may be increased by: Alpha-Lipoic Acid; Androgens; Antidiabetic Agents; Beta-Blockers; DPP-IV Inhibitors; Edetate CALCIUM Disodium; Edetate Disodium; GLP-1 Agonists; Herbs (Hypoglycemic Properties); Liraglutide; MAO Inhibitors; Metreleptin; Pegvisomant; Pioglitazone; Pramlintide; Quinolone Antibiotics; Salicylates; Selective Serotonin Reuptake Inhibitors; SGLT2 Inhibitors

Decreased Effect

The levels/effects of Insulin Lispro may be decreased by: Hyperglycemia-Associated Agents; Quinolone Antibiotics; Thiazide Diuretics

Storage/Stability Unopened vials, cartridges, and prefilled pens may be stored under refrigeration between 2°C and 8°C (36°F to 46°F) until the expiration date or at room temperature <30°C (<86°F) for 28 days; do not freeze;

keep away from heat and sunlight. Once punctured (in use), vials may be stored under refrigeration or at room temperature <30°C (<86°F); use within 28 days. Cartridges and prefilled pens that have been punctured (in use) should be stored at temperatures <30°C (<86°F) and used within 28 days; do not freeze or refrigerate. When used for CSII, insulin lispro contained within an external insulin pump reservoir should be changed every 7 days and insulin lispro contained within a 3 mL cartridge should be discarded after 7 days; discard if exposed to temperatures >37°C (>98.6°F).

For SubQ administration: *Humalog vials:* According to the manufacturer, diluted insulin lispro should be stored at 30°C (86°F) and used within 14 days or 5°C (41°F) and used within 28 days.

For IV infusion: Stable for 48 hours when stored under refrigeration between 2°C and 8°C (36°F to 46°F); may then be used at room temperature for an additional 48 hours.

Mechanism of Action Insulin acts via specific membrane-bound receptors on target tissues to regulate metabolism of carbohydrate, protein, and fats. Target organs for insulin include the liver, skeletal muscle, and adipose tissue.

Within the liver, insulin stimulates hepatic glycogen synthesis. Insulin promotes hepatic synthesis of fatty acids, which are released into the circulation as lipoproteins. Skeletal muscle effects of insulin include increased protein synthesis and increased glycogen synthesis. Within adipose tissue, insulin stimulates the processing of circulating lipoproteins to provide free fatty acids, facilitating triglyceride synthesis and storage by adipocytes; also directly inhibits the hydrolysis of triglycerides. In addition, insulin stimulates the cellular uptake of amino acids and increases cellular permeability to several ions, including potassium, magnesium, and phosphate. By activating sodium-potassium ATPases, insulin promotes the intracellular movement of potassium.

Normally secreted by the pancreas, insulin products are manufactured for pharmacologic use through recombinant DNA technology using either *E. coli* or *Saccharomyces cerevisiae*. Insulins are categorized based on the onset, peak, and duration of effect (eg, rapid-, short-, intermediate-, and long-acting insulin). Insulin lispro is a rapid-acting insulin analog.

Pharmacodynamics Onset and duration of hypoglycemic effects depend upon the route of administration (adsorption and onset of action are more rapid after deeper IM injections than after SubQ), site of injection (onset and duration are progressively slower with SubQ injection into the abdomen, arm, buttock, or thigh respectively), volume and concentration of injection, and the preparation administered; local heat, and massage also increase the rate of absorption.

Onset of action: 15-30 minutes

Maximum effect: 0.5-2.5 hours

Duration: 3-6.5 hours

Pharmacokinetics (Adult data unless noted)

Distribution: V_d: 0.26-0.36 L/kg

Bioavailability: 55% to 77%

Half-life: SubQ: 1 hour

Excretion: Urine

Dosing: Usual Insulin lispro is a rapid-acting insulin analog which is normally administered SubQ as a premeal component of the insulin regimen or as a continuous SubQ infusion and should be used with intermediate- or long-acting insulin. When compared to insulin regular, insulin lispro has a more rapid onset and shorter duration of activity. In carefully controlled clinical settings with close medical supervision and monitoring of blood glucose and potassium, insulin lispro may also be administered IV in some situations; insulin requirements vary dramatically between patients and dictate frequent monitoring and close medical supervision. See Insulin Regular for additional information.

General insulin dosing:

Type 1 diabetes mellitus: Children, Adolescents, and Adults: **Note:** Multiple daily doses or continuous subcutaneous infusions guided by blood glucose monitoring are the standard of diabetes care. Combinations of insulin formulations are commonly used. The daily doses presented below are expressed as the **total units/kg/day of all insulin formulations combined**.

Initial dose: SubQ: 0.2-0.6 units/kg/day in divided doses. Conservative initial doses of 0.2-0.4 units/kg/day are often recommended to avoid the potential for hypoglycemia. Regular insulin may be the only insulin formulation used initially.

Usual maintenance range: SubQ: 0.5-1 unit/kg/day in divided doses. An estimate of anticipated needs may be based on body weight and/or activity factors as follows:

Nonobese: 0.4-0.6 units/kg/day

Obese: 0.8-1.2 units/kg/day

Pubescent Children and Adolescents: During puberty, requirements may substantially increase to >1 unit/kg/day and in some cases up to 2 units/kg/day (IDF/ISPAD, 2011)

Adjustment of dose: Dosage must be titrated to achieve glucose control and avoid hypoglycemia. Adjust dose to maintain premeal and bedtime glucose in target range. Since combinations of agents are frequently used, dosage adjustment must address the individual component of the insulin regimen which most directly influences the blood glucose value in question, based on the known onset and duration of the insulin component.

Continuous SubQ insulin infusion (insulin pump): A combination of a "basal" continuous insulin infusion rate with preprogrammed, premeal bolus doses which are patient controlled. When converting from multiple daily SubQ doses of maintenance insulin, it is advisable to reduce the basal rate to less than the equivalent of the total daily units of longer-acting insulin (eg, NPH); divide the total number of units by 24 to get the basal rate in units/hour. Do not include the total units of regular insulin or other rapid-acting insulin formulations in this calculation. The same premeal regular insulin dosage may be used.

Type 2 diabetes mellitus: Augmentation therapy (patients for which diet, exercise, weight reduction, and oral hypoglycemic agents have not been adequate): Adults: SubQ: Initial dosage of 00.2 units/kg/day or 10 units/day of an intermediate- or long-acting insulin administered at bedtime has been recommended. As an alternative, regular insulin or rapid-acting insulin (eg, insulin lispro) formulations administered before meals have also been used. Dosage must be carefully adjusted.

Dosing adjustment in renal impairment: Insulin requirements are reduced due to changes in insulin clearance or metabolism; monitor blood glucose closely. There are no dosage adjustments provided in manufacturer's labeling; however, the following adjustments have been used by some clinicians (Aronoff, 2007): Adults:

CrCl >50 mL/minute: No adjustment necessary

CrCl 10-50 mL/minute: Administer at 75% of recommended dose

CrCl <10 mL/minute: Administer at 50% of recommended dose and monitor glucose closely

Hemodialysis: Because of a large molecular weight (6000 daltons), insulin is not significantly removed by either peritoneal or hemodialysis; supplemental dose is not necessary

Peritoneal dialysis: Supplemental dose is not necessary

Continuous renal replacement therapy: Administer at 75% of recommended dose

Dosing adjustment in hepatic impairment: There are no dosage adjustments provided in manufacturer's labeling; insulin requirements may be reduced due to changes in insulin clearance or metabolism; monitor blood glucose closely.

Preparation for Administration Parenteral:

SubQ: *Humalog vials:* May be diluted with the universal diluent, Sterile Diluent for Humalog, Humulin N, Humulin R, Humulin 70/30, and Humulin R U-500, to a concentration of 10 units/mL (U-10) or 50 units/mL (U-50). Do not dilute insulin contained in a cartridge, prefilled pen, or external insulin pump. May be mixed in the same syringe with NPH insulin. When mixing insulin lispro with NPH insulin, lispro should be drawn into the syringe first; administer immediately after mixing.

IV: May be diluted in NS to concentrations of 0.1 to 1 units/mL.

Administration Parenteral:

SubQ: Administration is usually made into the subcutaneous fat of the thighs, arms, buttocks, or abdomen, with sites rotated; cold injections should be avoided. Administer 15 minutes before meals or immediately after. May be mixed in the same syringe with NPH insulin. When mixing insulin lispro with NPH insulin, lispro should be drawn into the syringe first; administer immediately after mixing.

Continuous SubQ insulin infusion (Insulin pump): Do not use if solution is viscous or cloudy; use only if clear and colorless. Patients should be trained in the proper use of their external insulin pump and in intensive insulin therapy. Infusion sets and infusion set insertion sites should be changed every 3 days; rotate infusion sites. Insulin in reservoir should be changed every 7 days. Do not dilute or mix other insulin formulations with insulin lispro contained in an external insulin pump.

IV: Do not use if solution is viscous or cloudy; use only if clear and colorless. Further dilute with NS. May be administered IV with close monitoring of blood glucose and serum potassium; appropriate medical supervision is required. Do not administer insulin mixtures intravenously.

To minimize adsorption to IV solution bag: **Note:** Refer to institution-specific protocols where appropriate.

*If new tubing is **not** needed:* Wait a minimum of 30 minutes between the preparation of the solution and the initiation of the infusion.

If new tubing is needed: After receiving the insulin drip solution, the administration set should be attached to the IV container and the entire line should be flushed with a priming infusion of 20 to 50 mL of the insulin solution (Goldberg 2006; Hirsch 2006). Wait 30 minutes, and then flush the line again with the insulin solution prior to initiating the infusion.

Because of adsorption, the actual amount of insulin being administered via IV infusion could be substantially less than the apparent amount. Therefore, adjustment of the IV infusion rate should be based on effect and not solely on the apparent insulin dose. The apparent dose may be used as a starting point for determining the subsequent SubQ dosing regimen (Moghissi 2009); however, the transition to SubQ administration requires continuous medical supervision, frequent monitoring of blood glucose, and careful adjustment of therapy. In addition, SubQ insulin should be given 1 to 4 hours prior to the discontinuation of IV insulin to prevent hyperglycemia (Moghissi 2009).

Monitoring Parameters Urine sugar and acetone, serum glucose, electrolytes, Hb A_{1c}, lipid profile

Reference Range

Plasma Blood Glucose and Hgb A_{1c} Goals for Type 1 Diabetes (ADA, 2013): Note: Goals should be individualized based on individual needs/circumstances (eg, patients who experience severe hypoglycemia, patients with hypoglycemic unawareness); lower goals may be reasonable if they can be achieved without excessive hypoglycemia. **Note:** Postprandial blood glucose should be measured when there is a discrepancy between preprandial blood glucose concentrations and Hb A_{1c} values and to help assess glycemia for patients who receive basal/bolus regimens. It is usually drawn 1-2 hours after starting meal and is considered to be the "peak."

Toddlers/Preschoolers (0-6 years):
- Preprandial glucose: 100-180 mg/dL
- Bedtime/overnight glucose: 110-200 mg/dL
- Hb A_{1c}: <8.5%

School age (6-12 years):
- Preprandial glucose: 90-180 mg/dL
- Bedtime/overnight glucose: 100-180 mg/dL
- Hb A_{1c}: <8%

Adolescents/Young Adults (13-19 years):
- Preprandial glucose: 90-130 mg/dL
- Bedtime/overnight glucose: 90-150 mg/dL
- Hb A_{1c}: <7.5%

Adults, nonpregnant:
- Preprandial glucose: 70-130 mg/dL
- Postprandial glucose: <180 mg/dL
- Hb A_{1c}: <7%

Criteria for diagnosis of DKA:

Serum glucose:
- Children: >200 mg/dL
- Adults: >250 mg/dL

Arterial pH:
- Children: <7.3
- Adults: <7-7.24

Bicarbonate:
- Children: <15 mEq/L
- Adults: <10-15 mEq/L

Moderate ketonuria or ketonemia

Additional Information

Division of daily insulin requirement ("conventional therapy"): Generally, 50% to 75% of the daily insulin dose is given as an intermediate- or long-acting form of insulin (in 1-2 daily injections). The remaining portion of the 24-hour insulin requirement is divided and administered as either regular insulin or a rapid-acting form of insulin (eg, insulin lispro) at the same time before breakfast and dinner.

Division of daily insulin requirement ("intensive therapy"): Basal insulin delivery with 1 or 2 doses of intermediate- or long-acting insulin formulations superimposed with doses of rapid- or very rapid-acting insulin (eg, insulin lispro) formulations 3 or more times daily.

Product Availability Humalog 200 units/mL KwikPen: FDA approved May 2015; availability anticipated in July 2015. Consult prescribing information for additional information.

Dosage Forms Excipient information presented when available (limited, particularly for generics); consult specific product labeling.

Solution, Subcutaneous:
- HumaLOG: 100 units/mL (3 mL, 10 mL) [contains metacresol, phenol]

Solution Pen-injector, Subcutaneous:
- HumaLOG KwikPen: 100 units/mL (3 mL); 200 units/mL (3 mL) [contains metacresol, phenol]

◆ **Insulin Lispro and Insulin Lispro Protamine** *see* Insulin Lispro Protamine and Insulin Lispro *on page 1136*

Insulin Lispro Protamine and Insulin Lispro

(IN soo lin LYE sproe PROE ta meen & IN soo lin LYE sproe)

Medication Safety Issues

Sound-alike/look-alike issues:

HumaLOG® Mix 50/50™ may be confused with HumaLOG®

HumaLOG® Mix 75/25™ may be confused with HumuLIN® 70/30, NovoLIN® 70/30, and NovoLOG® Mix 70/30

High alert medication:

The Institute for Safe Medication Practices (ISMP) includes this medication among its list of drugs which have a heightened risk of causing significant patient harm when used in error. ***Due to the number of insulin preparations, it is essential to identify/clarify the type of insulin to be used.***

Other safety concerns:

Cross-contamination may occur if insulin pens are shared among multiple patients. Steps should be taken to prohibit sharing of insulin pens.

Related Information

Insulin Products *on page 2319*

Brand Names: US HumaLOG® Mix 50/50™; HumaLOG® Mix 50/50™ KwikPen™; HumaLOG® Mix 75/25™; HumaLOG® Mix 75/25™ KwikPen™

Brand Names: Canada Humalog Mix 25; Humalog Mix 50

Therapeutic Category Antidiabetic Agent, Parenteral; Insulin, Combination

Generic Availability (US) No

Use Treatment of type 1 diabetes mellitus (insulin dependent, IDDM); type 2 diabetes mellitus (noninsulin dependent, NIDDM) to control hyperglycemia

Pregnancy Risk Factor B

Pregnancy Considerations Adverse events have not been observed in animal reproduction studies. Insulin lispro has not been shown to cross the placenta at standard clinical doses (Boskovic 2003; Holcberg 2004; Jovanovic 1999).

In women with diabetes, maternal hyperglycemia can be associated with congenital malformations as well as adverse effects in the fetus, neonate, and the mother (ACOG 2005; ADA 2015; Kitzmiller 2008; Metzger 2007). To prevent adverse outcomes, prior to conception and throughout pregnancy maternal blood glucose and HbA_{1c} should be kept as close to target goals as possible but without causing significant hypoglycemia (ACOG 2013; ADA 2015; Blumer 2013; Kitzmiller 2008; Lambert 2013). Prior to pregnancy, effective contraception should be used until glycemic control is achieved (Kitzmiller 2008).

Insulin requirements tend to fall during the first trimester of pregnancy and increase in the later trimesters, peaking at 28 to 32 weeks of gestation. Following delivery, insulin requirements decrease rapidly (ACOG 2005).

Prior to pregnancy, women with diabetes who are trying to conceive should be treated with multiple daily doses of insulin or continuous subcutaneous insulin infusion (CSII) as opposed to split-dose, premixed insulin therapy. This is to allow for better glucose control and flexibility during pregnancy (Blumer 2013).

Breast-Feeding Considerations Both exogenous and endogenous insulin are excreted into breast milk (study not conducted with this preparation) (Whitmore 2012). Breast-feeding is encouraged for all women, including those with type 1, type 2, or GDM (ACOG 2005; Blumer 2013; Metzger 2007). A small snack (such as milk) before nursing may help decrease the risk of hypoglycemia in women with pregestational diabetes (ACOG 2005; ADA 2015; Reader 2004). The manufacturer recommends that caution be used in nursing women; adjustments of the mothers insulin dose may be needed.

Contraindications Hypersensitivity to any component of the formulation; during episodes of hypoglycemia

Warnings/Precautions Hypoglycemia is the most common adverse effect of insulin. The timing of hypoglycemia differs among various insulin formulations. Hypoglycemia may result from increased work or exercise without eating; use of long-acting insulin preparations (eg, insulin detemir, insulin glargine) may delay recovery from hypoglycemia. Profound and prolonged episodes of hypoglycemia may result in convulsions, unconsciousness, temporary or permanent brain damage or even death. Insulin requirements may be altered during illness, emotional disturbances or other stressors. Instruct patients to use caution with ethanol; may increase risk of hypoglycemia. Insulin may produce hypokalemia which, if left untreated, may result in respiratory paralysis, ventricular arrhythmia and even death. Use with caution in renal or hepatic impairment.

Insulin lispro protamine and insulin lispro premixed combination products are **NOT** intended for IV or IM administration. According to the Centers for Disease Control and Prevention (CDC), pen-shaped injection devices should never be used for more than one person (even when the needle is changed) because of the risk of infection. The injection device should be clearly labeled with individual patient information to ensure that the correct pen is used (CDC, 2012).

The general objective of exogenous insulin therapy is to approximate the physiologic pattern of insulin secretion which is characterized by two distinct phases. Phase 1 insulin secretion suppresses hepatic glucose production and phase 2 insulin secretion occurs in response to carbohydrate ingestion; therefore, exogenous insulin therapy may consist of basal insulin (eg, intermediate- [insulin lispro protamine and insulin lispro] or long-acting insulin or via continuous subcutaneous insulin infusion [CSII]) and/or preprandial insulin (eg, short- or rapid-acting insulin) (see Related Information: Insulin Products). Patients with type 1 diabetes do not produce endogenous insulin; therefore, these patients require both basal and preprandial insulin administration. Patients with type 2 diabetes retain some beta-cell function in the early stages of their disease; however, as the disease progresses, phase 1 insulin secretion may become completely impaired and phase 2 insulin secretion becomes delayed and/or inadequate in response to meals. Therefore, patients with type 2 diabetes may be treated with oral antidiabetic agents, basal insulin, and/or preprandial insulin depending on the stage of disease and current glycemic control. Since treatment regimens often consist of multiple agents, dosage adjustments must address the specific phase of insulin release that is primarily contributing to the patient's impaired glycemic control. Diabetes self-management education (DSME) is essential to maximize the effectiveness of therapy. Treatment and monitoring regimens must be individualized.

Potentially significant drug-drug interactions may exist, requiring dose or frequency adjustment, additional monitoring, and/or selection of alternative therapy.

Adverse Reactions Primarily symptoms of hypoglycemia

Cardiovascular: Pallor, palpitation, tachycardia

Central nervous system: Fatigue, headache, hypothermia, loss of consciousness, mental confusion

Dermatologic: Redness, urticaria

Endocrine & metabolic: Hypoglycemia, hypokalemia

Gastrointestinal: Hunger, nausea, numbness of mouth

Local: Atrophy or hypertrophy of SubQ fat tissue; edema, itching, pain or warmth at injection site; stinging

Neuromuscular & skeletal: Muscle weakness, paresthesia, tremor

Ocular: Transient presbyopia or blurred vision

Miscellaneous: Anaphylaxis, diaphoresis, local and/or systemic hypersensitivity reactions

Drug Interactions

Metabolism/Transport Effects None known.

Avoid Concomitant Use

Avoid concomitant use of Insulin Lispro Protamine and Insulin Lispro with any of the following: Rosiglitazone

Increased Effect/Toxicity

Insulin Lispro Protamine and Insulin Lispro may increase the levels/effects of: Hypoglycemia-Associated Agents; Rosiglitazone

The levels/effects of Insulin Lispro Protamine and Insulin Lispro may be increased by: Alpha-Lipoic Acid; Androgens; Antidiabetic Agents; Beta-Blockers; DPP-IV Inhibitors; Edetate CALCIUM Disodium; Edetate Disodium; GLP-1 Agonists; Herbs (Hypoglycemic Properties); Liraglutide; MAO Inhibitors; Metreleptin; Pegvisomant; Pioglitazone; Pramlintide; Quinolone Antibiotics; Salicylates; Selective Serotonin Reuptake Inhibitors; SGLT2 Inhibitors

Decreased Effect

The levels/effects of Insulin Lispro Protamine and Insulin Lispro may be decreased by: Hyperglycemia-Associated Agents; Quinolone Antibiotics; Thiazide Diuretics

Storage/Stability Unopened vials and prefilled pens may be stored under refrigeration between 2°C and 8°C (36°F to 46°F) until the expiration date or at room temperature <30°C (<86°F) for 10 days (prefilled pens) or 28 days (vials); do not freeze; keep away from heat and sunlight. Once punctured (in use), vials may be stored under refrigeration or at room temperature <30°C (<86°F); use within 28 days. Prefilled pens that have been punctured (in use) should be stored at room temperature <30°C (<86°F) and used within 10 days; do not freeze or refrigerate.

Mechanism of Action Insulin acts via specific membrane-bound receptors on target tissues to regulate metabolism of carbohydrate, protein, and fats. Target organs for insulin include the liver, skeletal muscle, and adipose tissue.

Within the liver, insulin stimulates hepatic glycogen synthesis. Insulin promotes hepatic synthesis of fatty acids, which are released into the circulation as lipoproteins. Skeletal muscle effects of insulin include increased protein synthesis and increased glycogen synthesis. Within adipose tissue, insulin stimulates the processing of circulating lipoproteins to provide free fatty acids, facilitating triglyceride synthesis and storage by adipocytes; also directly inhibits the hydrolysis of triglycerides. In addition, insulin stimulates the cellular uptake of amino acids and increases cellular permeability to several ions, including potassium, magnesium, and phosphate. By activating sodium-potassium ATPases, insulin promotes the intracellular movement of potassium.

Normally secreted by the pancreas, insulin products are manufactured for pharmacologic use through recombinant DNA technology using either *E. coli* or *Saccharomyces cerevisiae*. Insulins are categorized based on the onset, peak, and duration of effect (eg, rapid-, short-, intermediate-, and long-acting insulin). Insulin lispro protamine and insulin lispro is an intermediate-acting combination product with a more rapid onset and similar duration of action as compared to that of insulin NPH and insulin regular combination products.

Pharmacodynamics

Onset of action: 0.25-0.5 hours

Maximum effect: 2 hours

Duration: 18-24 hours

Pharmacokinetics (Adult data unless noted)

Time to peak serum concentration: 1 hour (median; range: 0.5-4 hours)

Elimination: Urine

Dosing: Usual Lispro protamine is an intermediate-acting insulin and lispro is a rapid-acting insulin administered by SubQ injection. Insulin lispro protamine and insulin lispro combination products are approximately equipotent to insulin NPH and insulin regular combination products with a similar duration of activity but a more rapid onset. With combination insulin products, the proportion of rapid-acting to long-acting insulin is fixed; basal vs prandial dose adjustments cannot be made. Fixed ratio insulins (such as insulin lispro protamine and insulin lispro combination) are typically administered as 2 daily doses with each dose intended to cover two meals and a snack. Because of variability in the peak effect and individual patient variability in activities, meals, etc, it may be more difficult to achieve complete glycemic control using fixed combinations of insulins; frequent monitoring and close medical supervision may be necessary. See Insulin Regular for additional information.

General insulin dosing:

Type 1 diabetes mellitus: Children, Adolescents, and Adults: **Note:** Multiple daily doses are utilized and guided by blood glucose monitoring. Combinations of insulin formulations are commonly used. The daily doses presented below are expressed as the **total units/kg/day of all insulin formulations combined**. Insulin lispro protamine and insulin lispro combination product is **not** intended for initial therapy; basal insulin requirements should be established **first** to direct dosing.

Usual maintenance range: SubQ: 0.5-1 unit/kg/day in divided doses. An estimate of anticipated needs may be based on body weight and/or activity factors as follows:

Nonobese: 0.4-0.6 units/kg/day

Obese: 0.8-1.2 units/kg/day

Pubescent Children and Adolescents: During puberty, requirements may substantially increase to >1 unit/kg/day and in some cases up to 2 units/kg/day (IDF/ISPAD, 2011)

Adjustment of dose: Dosage must be titrated to achieve glucose control and avoid hypoglycemia. Adjust dose to maintain premeal and bedtime glucose in target range. Since combinations of agents are frequently used, dosage adjustment must address the individual component of the insulin regimen which most directly influences the blood glucose value in question, based on the known onset and duration of the insulin component.

Type 2 diabetes mellitus: Augmentation therapy (patients for which diet, exercise, weight reduction, and oral hypoglycemic agents have not been adequate): Adults: SubQ: **Note:** Insulin lispro protamine and insulin lispro combination product is **not** intended for initial therapy; basal insulin requirements should be established **first** to direct dosing. Dosage must be carefully adjusted.

Dosing adjustment in renal impairment: There are no dosage adjustments provided in manufacturer's labeling; insulin requirements are reduced due to changes in insulin clearance or metabolism; monitor blood glucose closely.

Dosing adjustment in hepatic impairment: There are no dosage adjustments provided in manufacturer's labeling; insulin requirements may be reduced due to changes in insulin clearance or metabolism; monitor blood glucose closely.

Administration Parenteral: SubQ: Gently roll vial or pen in the palms of the hands to resuspend before use; administer into the subcutaneous fat of the thighs, arms, buttocks, or abdomen, with sites rotated. Cold injections should be avoided. Administer within 15 minutes before a meal (breakfast and supper). Do not mix or dilute with other insulins. **Not for IV administration** or use in an insulin infusion pump.

Monitoring Parameters Urine sugar and acetone, serum glucose, electrolytes, Hb A_{1c}, lipid profile

Reference Range

Plasma Blood Glucose and Hgb A_{1c} Goals for Type 1 Diabetes (ADA, 2013): Note: Goals should be individualized based on individual needs/circumstances (eg, patients who experience severe hypoglycemia, patients with hypoglycemic unawareness); lower goals may be reasonable if they can be achieved without excessive hypoglycemia. **Note:** Postprandial blood glucose should be measured when there is a discrepancy between preprandial blood glucose concentrations and Hb A_{1c} values and to help assess glycemia for patients who receive basal/bolus regimens. It is usually drawn 1-2 hours after starting meal and is considered to be the "peak."

- Toddlers/Preschoolers (0-6 years):
  - Preprandial glucose: 100-180 mg/dL
  - Bedtime/overnight glucose: 110-200 mg/dL
  - Hb A_{1c}: <8.5%
- School age (6-12 years):
  - Preprandial glucose: 90-180 mg/dL
  - Bedtime/overnight glucose: 100-180 mg/dL
  - Hb A_{1c}: <8%
- Adolescents/Young Adults (13-19 years):
  - Preprandial glucose: 90-130 mg/dL
  - Bedtime/overnight glucose: 90-150 mg/dL
  - Hb A_{1c}: <7.5%
- Adults, nonpregnant:
  - Preprandial glucose: 70-130 mg/dL
  - Postprandial glucose: <180 mg/dL
  - Hb A_{1c}: <7%

Criteria for diagnosis of DKA:

- Serum glucose:
  - Children: >200 mg/dL
  - Adults: >250 mg/dL
- Arterial pH:
  - Children: <7.3
  - Adults: <7-7.24
- Bicarbonate:
  - Children: <15 mEq/L
  - Adults: <10-15 mEq/L
- Moderate ketonuria or ketonemia

Additional Information

Division of daily insulin requirement ("conventional therapy"): Generally, 50% to 75% of the daily insulin dose is given as an intermediate- or long-acting form of insulin (in 1-2 daily injections). The remaining portion of the 24-hour insulin requirement is divided and administered as either regular insulin or a rapid-acting form of insulin at the same time before breakfast and dinner.

Division of daily insulin requirement ("intensive therapy"): Basal insulin delivery with 1 or 2 doses of intermediate- or long-acting insulin formulations superimposed with doses of rapid- or very rapid-acting insulin formulations 3 or more times daily.

Dosage Forms Excipient information presented when available (limited, particularly for generics); consult specific product labeling.

Injection, suspension:

HumaLOG® Mix 50/50™: Insulin lispro protamine suspension 50% [intermediate acting] and insulin lispro solution 50% [rapid acting]: 100 units/mL (10 mL)

HumaLOG® Mix 50/50™ KwikPen™: Insulin lispro protamine suspension 50% [intermediate acting] and insulin lispro solution 50% [rapid acting]: 100 units/mL (3 mL)

HumaLOG® Mix 75/25™: Insulin lispro protamine suspension 75% [intermediate acting] and insulin lispro solution 25% [rapid acting]: 100 units/mL (10 mL)

HumaLOG® Mix 75/25™ KwikPen™: Insulin lispro protamine suspension 75% [intermediate acting] and insulin lispro solution 25% [rapid acting]: 100 units/mL (3 mL)

Insulin NPH (IN soo lin N P H)

Medication Safety Issues

Sound-alike/look-alike issues:

HumuLIN N may be confused with HumuLIN R, HumaLOG, Humira

NovoLIN N may be confused with NovoLIN R, NovoLOG

High alert medication:

The Institute for Safe Medication Practices (ISMP) includes this medication among its list of drugs which have a heightened risk of causing significant patient harm when used in error. ***Due to the number of insulin preparations, it is essential to identify/clarify the type of insulin to be used.***

Other safety concerns:

Cross-contamination may occur if insulin pens are shared among multiple patients. Steps should be taken to prohibit sharing of insulin pens.

Related Information

Insulin Products *on page 2319*

Brand Names: US HumuLIN N KwikPen [OTC]; HumuLIN N Pen [OTC] [DSC]; HumuLIN N [OTC]; NovoLIN N ReliOn [OTC]; NovoLIN N [OTC]

Brand Names: Canada Humulin® N; Novolin® ge NPH

Therapeutic Category Antidiabetic Agent, Insulin; Insulin, Intermediate-Acting

Generic Availability (US) No

Use Treatment of type 1 diabetes mellitus (insulin dependent, IDDM); type 2 diabetes mellitus (noninsulin dependent, NIDDM) to control hyperglycemia

Pregnancy Risk Factor B

Pregnancy Considerations Animal reproduction studies have not been conducted; however, use provides maternal and fetal benefits.

In women with diabetes, maternal hyperglycemia can be associated with congenital malformations as well as adverse effects in the fetus, neonate, and the mother (ACOG 2005; ADA 2015; Kitzmiller 2008; Metzger 2007). To prevent adverse outcomes, prior to conception and throughout pregnancy maternal blood glucose and HbA_{1c} should be kept as close to target goals as possible but without causing significant hypoglycemia (ACOG 2013; ADA 2015; Blumer 2013; Kitzmiller 2008; Lambert 2013). Prior to pregnancy, effective contraception should be used until glycemic control is achieved (Kitzmiller 2008).

Insulin requirements tend to fall during the first trimester of pregnancy and increase in the later trimesters, peaking at 28 to 32 weeks of gestation. Following delivery, insulin requirements decrease rapidly (ACOG 2005). NPH insulin may be used to treat diabetes in pregnant women (Blumer 2013; Kitzmiller 2008; Lambert 2013)

Breast-Feeding Considerations Both exogenous and endogenous insulin are excreted into breast milk (study not conducted with this preparation) (Whitmore 2012). Breast-feeding is encouraged for all women, including those with type 1, type 2, or GDM (ACOG 2005; Blumer 2013; Metzger 2007). A small snack (such as milk) before nursing may help decrease the risk of hypoglycemia in women with pregestational diabetes (ACOG 2005; ADA 2015; Reader 2004). All types of insulin may be used while breast-feeding (Metzger 2007). Adverse events have not been reported in nursing infants following maternal use of NPH insulin; adjustments of the mothers insulin dose may be needed.

Contraindications Hypersensitivity to insulin NPH or any component of the formulation

Warnings/Precautions Hypoglycemia is the most common adverse effect of insulin. The timing of hypoglycemia differs among various insulin formulations. Hypoglycemia may result from increased work or exercise without eating; use of long-acting insulin preparations (eg, insulin detemir, insulin glargine) may delay recovery from hypoglycemia. Profound and prolonged episodes of hypoglycemia may result in convulsions, unconsciousness, temporary or permanent brain damage or even death. Insulin requirements may be altered during illness, emotional disturbances or other stressors. Instruct patients to use caution with ethanol; may increase risk of hypoglycemia. Insulin may produce hypokalemia which, if left untreated, may result in respiratory paralysis, ventricular arrhythmia and even death. Use with caution in renal or hepatic impairment.

Insulin NPH is **NOT** intended for IV or IM administration. According to the Centers for Disease Control and Prevention (CDC), pen-shaped injection devices should never be used for more than one person (even when the needle is changed) because of the risk of infection. The injection device should be clearly labeled with individual patient information to ensure that the correct pen is used (CDC, 2012).

The general objective of exogenous insulin therapy is to approximate the physiologic pattern of insulin secretion which is characterized by two distinct phases. Phase 1 insulin secretion suppresses hepatic glucose production and phase 2 insulin secretion occurs in response to carbohydrate ingestion; therefore, exogenous insulin therapy may consist of basal insulin (eg, intermediate- [insulin NPH] or long-acting insulin or via continuous subcutaneous insulin infusion [CSII]) and/or preprandial insulin (eg, short- or rapid-acting insulin) (see Related Information: Insulin Products). Patients with type 1 diabetes do not produce endogenous insulin; therefore, these patients require both basal and preprandial insulin administration. Patients with type 2 diabetes retain some beta-cell function in the early stages of their disease; however, as the disease progresses, phase 1 insulin secretion may become completely impaired and phase 2 insulin secretion becomes delayed and/or inadequate in response to meals. Therefore, patients with type 2 diabetes may be treated with oral antidiabetic agents, basal insulin, and/or preprandial insulin depending on the stage of disease and current glycemic control. Since treatment regimens often consist of multiple agents, dosage adjustments must address the specific phase of insulin release that is primarily contributing to the patient's impaired glycemic control. Diabetes self-management education (DSME) is essential to maximize the effectiveness of therapy. Treatment and monitoring regimens must be individualized.

Potentially significant drug-drug interactions may exist, requiring dose or frequency adjustment, additional monitoring, and/or selection of alternative therapy.

Adverse Reactions Frequency not defined.

Cardiovascular: Peripheral edema

Endocrine & metabolic: Hypoglycemia, hypokalemia, weight gain

Hypersensitivity: Hypersensitivity reaction

Immunologic: Immunogenicity

Local: Atrophy at injection site, hypertrophy at injection site, injection site reaction (including redness, swelling, and itching)

Neuromuscular & skeletal: Swelling of extremities

Ophthalmic: Visual disturbance

Drug Interactions

Metabolism/Transport Effects None known.

Avoid Concomitant Use

Avoid concomitant use of Insulin NPH with any of the following: Rosiglitazone

Increased Effect/Toxicity

Insulin NPH may increase the levels/effects of: Hypoglycemia-Associated Agents; Rosiglitazone

The levels/effects of Insulin NPH may be increased by: Alpha-Lipoic Acid; Androgens; Antidiabetic Agents; Beta-Blockers; DPP-IV Inhibitors; Edetate CALCIUM Disodium; Edetate Disodium; GLP-1 Agonists; Herbs (Hypoglycemic Properties); Liraglutide; MAO Inhibitors; Metreleptin; Pegvisomant; Pioglitazone; Pramlintide; Quinolone Antibiotics; Salicylates; Selective Serotonin Reuptake Inhibitors; SGLT2 Inhibitors

Decreased Effect

The levels/effects of Insulin NPH may be decreased by: Hyperglycemia-Associated Agents; Quinolone Antibiotics; Thiazide Diuretics

Storage/Stability

Humulin® N vials: Store unopened vials in refrigerator between 2°C and 8°C (36°F to 46°F; do not freeze; keep away from heat and sunlight. Once punctured (in use), vials may be stored for up to 31 days in the refrigerator between 2°C and 8°C (36°F to 46°F) or at room temperature ≤30°C (≤86°F)

Humulin® N pens and cartridges: Store unopened pens and unused cartridges in the refrigerator between 2°C and 8°C (36°F to 46°F); do not freeze; keep away from heat and sunlight. Once punctured (in use), cartridge/pen should be stored at room temperature 15°C to 30°C (59°F to 86°F) for up to 14 days.

Novolin® N vials: Store unopened vials in refrigerator between 2°C and 8°C (36°F to 46°F) until product expiration date or at room temperature ≤25°C (≤77°F) for up to 42 days; do not freeze; keep away from heat and sunlight. Once punctured (in use), store vials at room temperature ≤25°C (≤77°F) for up to 42 days (this includes any days stored at room temperature prior to opening vial); refrigeration of in-use vials is not recommended.

Canadian labeling (not in U.S. labeling): All products: Unopened vials, cartridges, and pens should be stored under refrigeration between 2°C and 8°C (36°F to 46°F) until the expiration date; do not freeze; keep away from heat and sunlight. Once punctured (in use), Humulin® vials, cartridges and pens should be stored at room temperature <25°C (<77°F) for up to 4 weeks. Once punctured (in use), Novolin® ge vials, cartridges, and pens may be stored for up to 1 month at room temperature <25°C (<77°F) for vials or <30°C (<86°F) for pens/cartridges; do not refrigerate.

For SubQ administration: *Humulin® N vials:* According to the manufacturer, storage and stability information are not available for diluted Humulin® N.

Mechanism of Action Insulin acts via specific membrane-bound receptors on target tissues to regulate metabolism of carbohydrate, protein, and fats. Target organs for insulin include the liver, skeletal muscle, and adipose tissue.

Within the liver, insulin stimulates hepatic glycogen synthesis. Insulin promotes hepatic synthesis of fatty acids, which are released into the circulation as lipoproteins. Skeletal muscle effects of insulin include increased protein synthesis and increased glycogen synthesis. Within adipose tissue, insulin stimulates the processing of circulating lipoproteins to provide free fatty acids, facilitating triglyceride synthesis and storage by adipocytes; also directly inhibits the hydrolysis of triglycerides. In addition, insulin stimulates the cellular uptake of amino acids and increases cellular permeability to several ions, including potassium, magnesium, and phosphate. By activating sodium-potassium ATPases, insulin promotes the intracellular movement of potassium.

Normally secreted by the pancreas, insulin products are manufactured for pharmacologic use through recombinant DNA technology using either *E. coli* or *Saccharomyces cerevisiae*. Insulins are categorized based on the onset, peak, and duration of effect (eg, rapid-, short-, intermediate-, and long-acting insulin). Insulin NPH, an isophane suspension of human insulin, is an intermediate-acting insulin.

Pharmacodynamics

Onset of action: 1-2 hours

Maximum effect: 6-14 hours

Duration: 18 to >24 hours

Pharmacokinetics (Adult data unless noted) Elimination: Urine

Dosing: Usual Insulin NPH is an intermediate-acting insulin formulation which is usually administered subcutaneously once or twice daily. When compared to insulin regular, insulin NPH has a slower onset and longer duration of activity. Insulin requirements vary dramatically between patients and dictate frequent monitoring and close medical supervision. See Insulin Regular for additional information.

Type 1 diabetes mellitus: Children, Adolescents, and Adults: **Note:** Multiple daily doses are utilized and guided by blood glucose monitoring. Combinations of insulin formulations are commonly used. The daily doses presented below are expressed as the **total units/kg/day of all insulin formulations combined**. Insulin NPH is **not** intended for initial therapy; basal insulin requirements should be established **first** to direct dosing.

Usual maintenance range: SubQ: 0.5-1 unit/kg/day in divided doses. An estimate of anticipated needs may be based on body weight and/or activity factors as follows:

Nonobese: 0.4-0.6 units/kg/day

Obese: 0.8-1.2 units/kg/day

Pubescent Children and Adolescents: During puberty, requirements may substantially increase to >1 unit/kg/day and in some cases up to 2 units/kg/day (IDF/ISPAD, 2011)

Adjustment of dose: Dosage must be titrated to achieve glucose control and avoid hypoglycemia. Adjust dose to maintain premeal and bedtime glucose in target range. Since combinations of agents are frequently used, dosage adjustment must address the individual component of the insulin regimen which most directly influences the blood glucose value in question, based on the known onset and duration of the insulin component.

Type 2 diabetes mellitus: Augmentation therapy (patients for which diet, exercise, weight reduction, and oral hypoglycemic agents have not been adequate): Adults: SubQ: Initial dosage of 0.2 units/kg/day or 10 units/day of an intermediate-acting (eg, NPH) or long-acting insulin administered at bedtime has been recommended. As an alternative, regular insulin or rapid-acting insulin formulations administered before meals have also been used. Dosage must be carefully adjusted.

Dosing adjustment in renal impairment: There are no dosage adjustments provided in manufacturer's labeling; insulin requirements are reduced due to changes in insulin clearance or metabolism; monitor blood glucose closely.

Dosing adjustment in hepatic impairment: There are no dosage adjustments provided in manufacturer's labeling; insulin requirements may be reduced due to changes in insulin clearance or metabolism; monitor blood glucose closely.

Preparation for Administration Parenteral: SubQ:

Humulin N vials: May be diluted with the universal diluent, Sterile Diluent for Humalog, Humulin N, Humulin R, Humulin 70/30, and Humulin R U-500. Do not dilute insulin contained in a cartridge or prefilled pen.

Novolin N: Insulin Diluting Medium for NovoLog is not intended for use with Novolin N or any insulin product other than insulin aspart.

May be mixed with regular insulin, insulin aspart, insulin lispro, and insulin glulisine; always add NPH insulin last.

Administration Parenteral: SubQ: In order to properly resuspend the insulin, vials should be carefully shaken or rolled several times, prefilled pens should be rolled between the palms ten times and inverted 180° ten times, and cartridges should be inverted 180° at least ten times. Properly resuspended insulin NPH should look uniformly cloudy or milky; do not use if any white insulin substance remains at the bottom of the container, if any clumps are present, or if white particles are stuck to the bottom or wall of the container. Administer into the subcutaneous fat of the thighs, arms, buttocks, or abdomen, with sites rotated. Cold injections should be avoided. Administer within 15 minutes before a meal (before breakfast and supper). When mixing insulin NPH with other preparations of insulin (eg, insulin aspart, insulin glulisine, insulin lispro, insulin regular), insulin NPH should be drawn into the syringe after the other insulin preparations. Do not dilute or mix other insulin formulations with insulin NPH contained in a cartridge or prefilled pen. Insulin NPH is **NOT** recommended **for IV administration** or use in external SubQ insulin infusion pump.

Monitoring Parameters Urine sugar and acetone, serum glucose, electrolytes, Hb A_{1c}, lipid profile

Reference Range

Plasma Blood Glucose and Hgb A_{1c} Goals for Type 1 Diabetes (ADA, 2013): Note: Goals should be individualized based on individual needs/circumstances (eg, patients who experience severe hypoglycemia, patients with hypoglycemic unawareness); lower goals may be reasonable if they can be achieved without excessive hypoglycemia. **Note:** Postprandial blood glucose should be measured when there is a discrepancy between preprandial blood glucose concentrations and Hb A_{1c} values and to help assess glycemia for patients who receive basal/bolus regimens. It is usually drawn 1-2 hours after starting meal and is considered to be the "peak."

Toddlers/Preschoolers (0-6 years):

Preprandial glucose: 100-180 mg/dL

Bedtime/overnight glucose: 110-200 mg/dL

Hb A_{1c}: <8.5%

School age (6-12 years):

Preprandial glucose: 90-180 mg/dL

Bedtime/overnight glucose: 100-180 mg/dL

Hb A_{1c}: <8%

Adolescents/Young Adults (13-19 years):

Preprandial glucose: 90-130 mg/dL

Bedtime/overnight glucose: 90-150 mg/dL

Hb A_{1c}: <7.5%

Adults, nonpregnant:

Preprandial glucose: 70-130 mg/dL

Postprandial glucose: <180 mg/dL

Hb A_{1c}: <7%

Criteria for diagnosis of DKA:

Serum glucose:

Children: >200 mg/dL

Adults: >250 mg/dL

Arterial pH:

Children: <7.3

Adults: <7-7.24

Bicarbonate:

Children: <15 mEq/L

Adults: <10-15 mEq/L

Moderate ketonuria or ketonemia

Additional Information

Division of daily insulin requirement ("conventional therapy"): Generally, 50% to 75% of the daily insulin dose is given as an intermediate-acting (eg, NPH) or long-acting form of insulin (in 1-2 daily injections). The remaining portion of the 24-hour insulin requirement is divided and administered as either regular insulin or a rapid-acting form of insulin at the same time before breakfast and dinner.

Division of daily insulin requirement ("intensive therapy"): Basal insulin delivery with 1 or 2 doses of intermediate-acting (eg, NPH) or long-acting insulin formulations superimposed with doses of rapid- or very rapid-acting insulin formulations 3 or more times daily.

Dosage Forms Excipient information presented when available (limited, particularly for generics); consult specific product labeling. [DSC] = Discontinued product

Suspension, Subcutaneous:

HumuLIN N: 100 units/mL (3 mL, 10 mL) [contains metacresol, phenol]

NovoLIN N: 100 units/mL (10 mL) [contains metacresol, phenol]

NovoLIN N ReliOn: 100 units/mL (10 mL) [contains metacresol, phenol]

Suspension Pen-injector, Subcutaneous:

HumuLIN N KwikPen: 100 units/mL (3 mL) [contains metacresol, phenol]

HumuLIN N Pen: 100 units/mL (3 mL [DSC]) [contains metacresol, phenol]

Insulin NPH and Insulin Regular

(IN soo lin N P H & IN soo lin REG yoo ler)

Medication Safety Issues

Sound-alike/look-alike issues:

HumuLIN 70/30 may be confused with HumaLOG Mix 75/25, HumuLIN R, NovoLIN 70/30, NovoLOG Mix 70/30

NovoLIN 70/30 may be confused with HumaLOG Mix 75/25, HumuLIN 70/30, HumuLIN R, NovoLIN R, and NovoLOG Mix 70/30

High alert medication:

The Institute for Safe Medication Practices (ISMP) includes this medication among its list of drugs which have a heightened risk of causing significant patient harm when used in error. ***Due to the number of insulin preparations, it is essential to identify/clarify the type of insulin to be used.***

Other safety concerns:

Cross-contamination may occur if insulin pens are shared among multiple patients. Steps should be taken to prohibit sharing of insulin pens.

Related Information

Insulin Products *on page 2319*

Brand Names: US HumuLIN 70/30; HumuLIN 70/30 KwikPen; NovoLIN 70/30

Brand Names: Canada Humulin 20/80; Humulin 70/30; Novolin ge 30/70; Novolin ge 40/60; Novolin ge 50/50

Therapeutic Category Antidiabetic Agent, Parenteral; Insulin, Combination

Generic Availability (US) No

Use Treatment of type 1 diabetes mellitus (insulin dependent, IDDM); type 2 diabetes mellitus (noninsulin dependent, NIDDM) to control hyperglycemia

Pregnancy Risk Factor B

Pregnancy Considerations Animal reproduction studies have not been conducted, however use provides maternal and fetal benefits.

In women with diabetes, maternal hyperglycemia can be associated with congenital malformations as well as adverse effects in the fetus, neonate, and the mother (ACOG 2005; ADA 2015; Kitzmiller 2008; Metzger 2007). To prevent adverse outcomes, prior to conception and throughout pregnancy maternal blood glucose and HbA_{1c} should be kept as close to target goals as possible but without causing significant hypoglycemia (ACOG 2013; ADA 2015; Blumer 2013; Kitzmiller 2008; Lambert 2013). Prior to pregnancy, effective contraception should be used until glycemic control is achieved (Kitzmiller 2008).

Insulin requirements tend to fall during the first trimester of pregnancy and increase in the later trimesters, peaking at 28 to 32 weeks of gestation. Following delivery, insulin requirements decrease rapidly (ACOG 2005).

Prior to pregnancy, women with diabetes who are trying to conceive should be treated with multiple daily doses of insulin or continuous subcutaneous insulin infusion (CSII) as opposed to split-dose, premixed insulin therapy. This is to allow for better glucose control and flexibility during pregnancy (Blumer 2013).

Breast-Feeding Considerations Both exogenous and endogenous insulin are excreted into breast milk (study not conducted with this preparation) (Whitmore 2012). Breast-feeding is encouraged for all women, including those with type 1, type 2, or GDM (ACOG, 2005; Blumer 2013; Metzger 2007). A small snack (such as milk) before nursing may help decrease the risk of hypoglycemia in women with pregestational diabetes (ACOG 2005; ADA 2015; Reader 2004). All types of insulin may be used while breast-feeding (Metzger 2007). Adverse events have not been reported in nursing infants following maternal use of insulin; adjustments of the mothers insulin dose may be needed.

Contraindications Hypersensitivity to any component of the formulation; during episodes of hypoglycemia

Warnings/Precautions Hypoglycemia is the most common adverse effect of insulin. The timing of hypoglycemia differs among various insulin formulations. Hypoglycemia may result from increased work or exercise without eating; use of long-acting insulin preparations (eg, insulin detemir, insulin glargine) may delay recovery from hypoglycemia. Profound and prolonged episodes of hypoglycemia may result in convulsions, unconsciousness, temporary or permanent brain damage or even death. Insulin requirements may be altered during illness, emotional disturbances or other stressors. Instruct patients to use caution with ethanol; may increase risk of hypoglycemia. Insulin may produce hypokalemia which, if left untreated, may result in respiratory paralysis, ventricular arrhythmia and even death. Use with caution in renal or hepatic impairment.

Insulin NPH and insulin regular combination products are **NOT** intended for IV or IM administration. According to the Centers for Disease Control and Prevention (CDC), pen-shaped injection devices should never be used for more than one person (even when the needle is changed) because of the risk of infection. The injection device should be clearly labeled with individual patient information to ensure that the correct pen is used (CDC, 2012). The general objective of exogenous insulin therapy is to approximate the physiologic pattern of insulin secretion which is characterized by two distinct phases. Phase 1 insulin secretion suppresses hepatic glucose production and phase 2 insulin secretion occurs in response to carbohydrate ingestion; therefore, exogenous insulin therapy may consist of basal insulin (eg, intermediate- [insulin NPH and insulin regular] or long-acting insulin or via continuous subcutaneous insulin infusion [CSII]) and/or preprandial insulin (eg, short- or rapid-acting insulin) (see Related Information: Insulin Products). Patients with type 1 diabetes do not produce endogenous insulin; therefore, these patients require both basal and preprandial insulin administration. Patients with type 2 diabetes retain some beta-cell function in the early stages of their disease; however, as the disease progresses, phase 1 insulin secretion may become completely impaired and phase 2 insulin secretion becomes delayed and/or inadequate in response to meals. Therefore, patients with type 2 diabetes may be treated with oral antidiabetic agents, basal insulin, and/or preprandial insulin depending on the stage of disease and current glycemic control. Since treatment regimens often consist of multiple agents, dosage adjustments must address the specific phase of insulin release that is primarily contributing to the patient's impaired glycemic control. Diabetes self-management education (DSME) is essential to maximize the effectiveness of therapy. Treatment and monitoring regimens must be individualized.

Potentially significant drug-drug interactions may exist, requiring dose or frequency adjustment, additional monitoring, and/or selection of alternative therapy.

Adverse Reactions See individual agents. Frequency not defined.

Cardiovascular: Peripheral edema

Dermatologic: Pruritus

Endocrine & metabolic: Hypoglycemia, hypokalemia, weight gain

Hypersensitivity: Hypersensitivity reaction

Immunologic: Immunogenicity

Local: Hypertrophy at injection site, lipoatrophy at injection site

Drug Interactions

Metabolism/Transport Effects None known.

Avoid Concomitant Use

Avoid concomitant use of Insulin NPH and Insulin Regular with any of the following: Rosiglitazone

Increased Effect/Toxicity

Insulin NPH and Insulin Regular may increase the levels/effects of: Hypoglycemia-Associated Agents; Rosiglitazone

The levels/effects of Insulin NPH and Insulin Regular may be increased by: Alpha-Lipoic Acid; Androgens; Antidiabetic Agents; Beta-Blockers; DPP-IV Inhibitors; Edetate CALCIUM Disodium; Edetate Disodium; GLP-1 Agonists; Herbs (Hypoglycemic Properties); Liraglutide; MAO Inhibitors; Metreleptin; Pegvisomant; Pioglitazone; Pramlintide; Quinolone Antibiotics; Salicylates; Selective Serotonin Reuptake Inhibitors; SGLT2 Inhibitors

Decreased Effect

The levels/effects of Insulin NPH and Insulin Regular may be decreased by: Hyperglycemia-Associated Agents; Quinolone Antibiotics; Thiazide Diuretics

Storage/Stability

Humulin 70/30 vials: Store unopened vials in refrigerator between 2°C and 8°C (36°F to 46°F); do not freeze; keep away from heat and sunlight. Once punctured (in use), vials may be stored for up to 31 days in the refrigerator between 2°C and 8°C (36°F to 46°F) or at room temperature ≤30°C (≤86°F).

Humulin 70/30 pens and cartridges: Store unopened pen and unused cartridges in refrigerator between 2°C and 8°C (36°F to 46°F); do not freeze; keep away from heat and sunlight. Once punctured (in use), cartridge/pen should be stored at room temperature 15°C to 30°C (59°F to 86°F) for up to 10 days.

Novolin 70/30 vials: Store unopened vials in refrigerator between 2°C and 8°C (36°F to 46°F) until product expiration date or at room temperature ≤25°C (≤77°F) for up to 42 days; do not freeze; keep away from heat and sunlight. Once punctured (in use), store vials at room temperature ≤25°C (≤77°F) for up to 42 days (this includes any days stored at room temperature prior to opening vial); refrigeration of in-use vials is not recommended.

Canadian labeling (not in U.S. labeling): All products: Unopened vials, cartridges, and pens should be stored under refrigeration between 2°C and 8°C (36°F to 46°F) until the expiration date; do not freeze; keep away from heat and sunlight. Once punctured (in use), Humulin vials, cartridges, and pens should be stored at room temperature <25°C (<77°F) for up to 4 weeks. Once punctured (in use), Novolin ge vials, cartridges, and pens may be stored for up to 1 month at room temperature <25°C (<77°F) for vials or <30°C (<86°F) for pens/cartridges; do not refrigerate.

For SubQ administration: *Humulin 70/30:* According to the manufacturer, storage and stability information are not available for diluted Humulin 70/30.

Mechanism of Action Insulin acts via specific membrane-bound receptors on target tissues to regulate metabolism of carbohydrate, protein, and fats. Target organs for insulin include the liver, skeletal muscle, and adipose tissue.

Within the liver, insulin stimulates hepatic glycogen synthesis. Insulin promotes hepatic synthesis of fatty acids, which are released into the circulation as lipoproteins. Skeletal muscle effects of insulin include increased protein synthesis and increased glycogen synthesis. Within adipose tissue, insulin stimulates the processing of circulating lipoproteins to provide free fatty acids, facilitating triglyceride synthesis and storage by adipocytes; also directly inhibits the hydrolysis of triglycerides. In addition, insulin stimulates the cellular uptake of amino acids and increases cellular permeability to several ions, including potassium, magnesium, and phosphate. By activating sodium-potassium ATPases, insulin promotes the intracellular movement of potassium.

Normally secreted by the pancreas, insulin products are manufactured for pharmacologic use through recombinant DNA technology using either *E. coli* or *Saccharomyces cerevisiae*. Insulins are categorized based on the onset, peak, and duration of effect (eg, rapid-, short-, intermediate-, and long-acting insulin). Insulin NPH and insulin regular is an intermediate-acting combination insulin product with a more rapid onset than that of insulin NPH alone.

Pharmacodynamics

Onset of action: Novolin® 70/30, Humulin® 70/30: 0.5 hours

Maximum effect: Novolin® 70/30, Humulin® 70/30: 1.5-12 hours

Duration: Novolin® 70/30, Humulin® 70/30: Up to 24 hours

Pharmacokinetics (Adult data unless noted)

Elimination: Urine

Dosing: Usual Insulin NPH is an intermediate-acting insulin and regular insulin is a short-acting insulin administered by SubQ injection. When compared to insulin NPH, the combination product (insulin NPH and insulin regular) has a shorter onset of action and a similar duration of action. With combination insulin products, the proportion of short-acting to long-acting insulin is fixed in the combination products; basal vs prandial dose adjustments cannot be made. Fixed ratio insulins (such as insulin NPH and insulin regular combination) are typically administered as 2 daily doses with each dose intended to cover two meals and a snack. Because of variability in the peak effect and individual patient variability in activities, meals, etc, it may be more difficult to achieve complete glycemic control using fixed combinations of insulins; frequent monitoring and close medical supervision may be necessary. See Insulin Regular for additional information.

General insulin dosing:

Type 1 diabetes mellitus: Children, Adolescents, and Adults: **Note:** Multiple daily doses are utilized and guided by blood glucose monitoring. Combinations of insulin formulations are commonly used. The daily doses presented below are expressed as the **total units/kg/day of all insulin formulations combined.** Insulin NPH and insulin regular combination product is **not** intended for initial therapy; basal insulin requirements should be established **first** to direct dosing.

Usual maintenance range: SubQ: 0.5-1 unit/kg/day in divided doses. An estimate of anticipated needs may be based on body weight and/or activity factors as follows:

Nonobese: 0.4-0.6 units/kg/day

Obese: 0.8-1.2 units/kg/day

Pubescent Children and Adolescents: During puberty, requirements may substantially increase to >1 unit/kg/day and in some cases up to 2 units/kg/day (IDF/ISPAD, 2011)

Adjustment of dose: Dosage must be titrated to achieve glucose control and avoid hypoglycemia. Adjust dose to maintain premeal and bedtime glucose in target range. Since combinations of agents are frequently used, dosage adjustment must address the individual component of the insulin regimen which most directly influences the blood glucose value in question, based on the known onset and duration of the insulin component.

Type 2 diabetes mellitus: Augmentation therapy (patients for which diet, exercise, weight reduction, and oral hypoglycemic agents have not been adequate): Adults: SubQ: **Note:** Insulin NPH and insulin regular combination product is **not** intended for initial therapy; basal insulin requirements should be established **first** to direct dosing. Dosage must be carefully adjusted.

Dosing adjustment in renal impairment: There are no dosage adjustments provided in manufacturer's labeling; insulin requirements are reduced due to changes in insulin clearance or metabolism; monitor blood glucose closely.

Dosing adjustment in hepatic impairment: There are no dosage adjustments provided in manufacturer's labeling; insulin requirements may be reduced due to changes in insulin clearance or metabolism; monitor blood glucose closely.

Preparation for Administration

Parenteral: SubQ:

Humulin 70/30: May be diluted with the universal diluent, Sterile Diluent for Humalog, Humulin N, Humulin R, Humulin 70/30, and Humulin R U-500. Do not dilute insulin contained in a cartridge or prefilled pen.

Novolin 70/30: Insulin Diluting Medium for NovoLog is not intended for use with Novolin 70/30 or any insulin product other than insulin aspart.

Administration Parenteral: SubQ: In order to properly resuspend the insulin, vials should be carefully shaken or rolled several times, prefilled pens should be rolled between the palms ten times and inverted 180° ten times, and cartridges should be inverted 180° at least ten times. Properly resuspended insulin should look uniformly cloudy or milky; do not use if any white insulin substance remains at the bottom of the container, if any clumps are present, if the insulin remains clear after adequate mixing, or if white particles are stuck to the bottom or wall of the container. Administer into the subcutaneous fat of the thighs, arms, buttocks, or abdomen, with sites rotated. Cold injections should be avoided. Administer within 30 minutes before a meal (before breakfast and supper). Do not mix or dilute with other insulins. **Not for IV administration** or use in an insulin infusion pump.

Monitoring Parameters Urine sugar and acetone, serum glucose, electrolytes, Hb A_{1c}, lipid profile

Reference Range

Plasma Blood Glucose and Hgb A_{1c} Goals for Type 1 Diabetes (ADA, 2013): Note: Goals should be individualized based on individual needs/circumstances (eg, patients who experience severe hypoglycemia, patients with hypoglycemic unawareness); lower goals may be reasonable if they can be achieved without excessive hypoglycemia. **Note:** Postprandial blood glucose should be measured when there is a discrepancy between preprandial blood glucose concentrations and Hb A_{1c} values and to help assess glycemia for patients who receive basal/bolus regimens. It is usually drawn 1-2 hours after starting meal and is considered to be the "peak."

Toddlers/Preschoolers (0-6 years):
- Preprandial glucose: 100-180 mg/dL
- Bedtime/overnight glucose: 110-200 mg/dL
- Hb A_{1c}: <8.5%

School age (6-12 years):
- Preprandial glucose: 90-180 mg/dL
- Bedtime/overnight glucose: 100-180 mg/dL
- Hb A_{1c}: <8%

Adolescents/Young Adults (13-19 years):
- Preprandial glucose: 90-130 mg/dL
- Bedtime/overnight glucose: 90-150 mg/dL
- Hb A_{1c}: <7.5%

Adults, nonpregnant:
- Preprandial glucose: 70-130 mg/dL
- Postprandial glucose: <180 mg/dL
- Hb A_{1c}: <7%

Criteria for diagnosis of DKA:

Serum glucose:
- Children: >200 mg/dL
- Adults: >250 mg/dL

Arterial pH:
- Children: <7.3
- Adults: <7-7.24

Bicarbonate:
- Children: <15 mEq/L
- Adults: <10-15 mEq/L

Moderate ketonuria or ketonemia

Additional Information

Division of daily insulin requirement ("conventional therapy"): Generally, 50% to 75% of the daily insulin dose is given as an intermediate-acting or long-acting form of insulin (in 1-2 daily injections). The remaining portion of the 24-hour insulin requirement is divided and administered as either regular insulin or a rapid-acting form of insulin at the same time before breakfast and dinner.

Division of daily insulin requirement ("intensive therapy"): Basal insulin delivery with 1 or 2 doses of intermediate-acting or long-acting insulin formulations superimposed with doses of rapid- or very rapid-acting insulin formulations 3 or more times daily.

Dosage Forms Excipient information presented when available (limited, particularly for generics); consult specific product labeling.

Injection, suspension:

HumuLIN 70/30: Insulin NPH suspension 70% [intermediate acting] and insulin regular solution 30% [short acting]: 100 units/mL (3 mL, 10 mL) [vial]

HumuLIN 70/30 KwikPen: Insulin NPH suspension 70% [intermediate acting] and insulin regular solution 30% [short acting]: 100 units/mL (3 mL)

NovoLIN 70/30: Insulin NPH suspension 70% [intermediate acting] and insulin regular solution 30% [short acting]: 100 units/mL (10 mL) [vial]

Insulin Regular (IN soo lin REG yoo ler)

Medication Safety Issues

Sound-alike/look-alike issues:

HumuLIN R may be confused with HumaLOG, Humira, HumuLIN 70/30, HumuLIN N, NovoLIN 70/30, NovoLIN R, NovoLOG

NovoLIN R may be confused with HumuLIN R, NovoLIN 70/30, NovoLIN N, NovoLOG

High alert medication:

The Institute for Safe Medication Practices (ISMP) includes this medication among its list of drugs which have a heightened risk of causing significant patient harm when used in error. ***Due to the number of insulin preparations, it is essential to identify/clarify the type of insulin to be used.***

BEERS Criteria medication:

This drug may be potentially inappropriate for use in geriatric patients (Quality of evidence - moderate; Strength of recommendation - strong).

Administration issues:

Concentrated solutions (eg, U-500) should not be available in patient care areas. U-500 regular insulin should be stored, dispensed, and administered separately from U-100 regular insulin. For patients who receive U-500 insulin in the hospital setting, highlighting the strength prominently on the patient's medical chart and medication record may help to reduce dispensing errors.

Other safety concerns:

Cross-contamination may occur if insulin pens are shared among multiple patients. Steps should be taken to prohibit sharing of insulin pens.

Related Information

Insulin Products *on page 2319*

Brand Names: US HumuLIN R U-500 (CONCENTRATED); HumuLIN R [OTC]; NovoLIN R ReliOn [OTC]; NovoLIN R [OTC]

Brand Names: Canada Humulin R; Novolin ge Toronto

Therapeutic Category Antidiabetic Agent, Parenteral; Antidote; Hyperkalemia, Adjunctive Treatment Agent; Insulin, Short-Acting

Generic Availability (US) No

Use Treatment of diabetes mellitus (type 1 or type 2) to improve glycemic control (FDA approved in children and adults); has also been used for treatment of diabetic ketoacidosis (DKA) and hyperosmolar hyperglycemic state (HHS) and treatment of hyperkalemia (used in combination with glucose to cause intracellular shift of potassium and lower serum potassium levels)

Pregnancy Risk Factor B

Pregnancy Considerations Recombinant human insulin for injection is identical to endogenous insulin; therefore, animal reproduction studies have not been conducted. Minimal amounts of endogenous insulin cross the placenta. Exogenous insulin bound to anti-insulin antibodies can be detected in cord blood (Menon 1990)

In women with diabetes, maternal hyperglycemia can be associated with congenital malformations as well as adverse effects in the fetus, neonate, and the mother (ACOG 2005; ADA 2015; Kitzmiller 2008; Metzger 2007). To prevent adverse outcomes, prior to conception and throughout pregnancy maternal blood glucose and HbA_{1c} should be kept as close to target goals as possible but without causing significant hypoglycemia (ACOG 2013; ADA 2015; Blumer 2013; Kitzmiller 2008; Lambert 2013). Prior to pregnancy, effective contraception should be used until glycemic control is achieved (Kitzmiller 2008).

Insulin requirements tend to fall during the first trimester of pregnancy and increase in the later trimesters, peaking at 28 to 32 weeks of gestation. Following delivery, insulin requirements decrease rapidly (ACOG 2005).

Rapid acting insulins, such as insulin aspart or insulin lispro may be preferred over regular human insulin in women trying to conceive (Blumer 2013); however, there is no need to switch a pregnant woman who is well controlled on injectable human insulin to a short acting analogue (Lambert 2013).

Breast-Feeding Considerations Both exogenous and endogenous insulin are excreted into breast milk (study not conducted with this preparation) (Whitmore 2012). Breast-feeding is encouraged for all women, including those with type 1, type 2, or GDM (ACOG 2005; Blumer 2013; Metzger 2007). A small snack (such as milk) before nursing may help decrease the risk of hypoglycemia in women with pregestational diabetes (ACOG 2005; ADA 2015; Reader 2004).

Adverse events have not been reported in nursing infants following use of regular insulin for injection; adjustments of the mothers insulin dose may be needed.

Contraindications

Hypersensitivity to regular insulin or any component of the formulation; during episodes of hypoglycemia.

Documentation of allergenic cross-reactivity for insulin is limited. However, because of similarities in chemical structure and/or pharmacologic actions, the possibility of cross-sensitivity cannot be ruled out with certainty.

Warnings/Precautions Hypoglycemia is the most common adverse effect of insulin. The timing of hypoglycemia differs among various insulin formulations. Hypoglycemia may result from increased work or exercise without eating; use of long-acting insulin preparations (eg, insulin detemir, insulin glargine) may delay recovery from hypoglycemia. Profound and prolonged episodes of hypoglycemia may result in convulsions, unconsciousness, temporary or permanent brain damage or even death. Insulin requirements may be altered during illness, emotional disturbances or other stressors. Instruct patients to use caution with ethanol; may increase risk of hypoglycemia. Insulin may produce hypokalemia which, if left untreated, may result in respiratory paralysis, ventricular arrhythmia and even death. Use with caution in patients at risk for hypokalemia (eg, IV insulin use). Severe, life-threatening, generalized allergic reactions, including anaphylaxis, may occur. If hypersensitivity reactions occur, discontinue therapy, treat the patient with supportive care and monitor until signs and symptoms resolve. Use with caution in renal or hepatic impairment. In the elderly, avoid use of sliding scale injectable insulin in this population due to increased risk of hypoglycemia without benefits in management of hyperglycemia regardless of care setting (Beers Criteria).

Human insulin differs from animal-source insulin. Any change of insulin should be made cautiously; changing manufacturers, type, and/or method of manufacture may result in the need for a change of dosage. U-500 regular insulin is a concentrated insulin formulation which contains 500 units of insulin per mL; for SubQ administration only using a U-100 insulin syringe or tuberculin syringe; **not for IV administration**. To avoid dosing errors when using a U-100 insulin syringe, the prescribed dose should be written in actual insulin units and as unit markings on the U-100 insulin syringe (eg, 50 units [10 units on a U-100 insulin syringe]). To avoid dosing errors when using a tuberculin syringe, the prescribed dose should be written in actual insulin units and as a volume (eg, 50 units [0.1 mL]). Mixing U-500 regular insulin with other insulin formulations is not recommended.

Regular insulin may be administered IV or IM in selected clinical situations; close monitoring of blood glucose and serum potassium, as well as medical supervision, is required.

The general objective of exogenous insulin therapy is to approximate the physiologic pattern of insulin secretion which is characterized by two distinct phases. Phase 1 insulin secretion suppresses hepatic glucose production and phase 2 insulin secretion occurs in response to carbohydrate ingestion; therefore, exogenous insulin therapy may consist of basal insulin (eg, intermediate- or long-acting insulin or via continuous subcutaneous insulin infusion [CSII]) and/or preprandial insulin (eg, short- or rapid-acting insulin) (see Related Information: Insulin Products). Patients with type 1 diabetes do not produce endogenous insulin; therefore, these patients require both basal and preprandial insulin administration. Patients with type 2 diabetes retain some beta-cell function in the early stages of their disease; however, as the disease progresses, phase 1 insulin secretion may become completely impaired and phase 2 insulin secretion becomes delayed and/or inadequate in response to meals. Therefore, patients with type 2 diabetes may be treated with oral antidiabetic agents, basal insulin, and/or preprandial insulin depending on the stage of disease and current glycemic control. Since treatment regimens often consist of multiple agents, dosage adjustments must address the specific phase of insulin release that is primarily contributing to the patient's impaired glycemic control. Diabetes self-management education (DSME) is essential to maximize the effectiveness of therapy. Treatment and monitoring regimens must be individualized. Exclusive use of a sliding scale insulin regimen to manage persistent hyperglycemia in the hospital is discouraged. An effective insulin regimen will achieve the goal glucose range without the risk of severe hypoglycemia (ADA 2015).

Potentially significant drug-drug interactions may exist, requiring dose or frequency adjustment, additional monitoring, and/or selection of alternative therapy. In particular, concurrent use with peroxisome proliferator-activated receptor (PPAR)-gamma agonists, including thiazolidinediones (TZDs) may cause dose-related fluid retention and lead to or exacerbate heart failure.

Adverse Reactions

Cardiovascular: Peripheral edema

Dermatologic: Erythema at injection site, injection site pruritus

Endocrine & metabolic: Hypoglycemia, hypokalemia, weight gain

Hypersensitivity: Anaphylaxis, hypersensitivity, hypersensitivity reaction

Local: Hypertrophy at injection site, lipoatrophy at injection site

Drug Interactions

Metabolism/Transport Effects None known.

Avoid Concomitant Use

Avoid concomitant use of Insulin Regular with any of the following: Rosiglitazone

Increased Effect/Toxicity

Insulin Regular may increase the levels/effects of: Hypoglycemia-Associated Agents; Rosiglitazone

The levels/effects of Insulin Regular may be increased by: Alpha-Lipoic Acid; Androgens; Antidiabetic Agents; Beta-Blockers; DPP-IV Inhibitors; Edetate CALCIUM Disodium; Edetate Disodium; GLP-1 Agonists; Herbs (Hypoglycemic Properties); Liraglutide; MAO Inhibitors; Metreleptin; Pegvisomant; Pioglitazone; Pramlintide; Quinolone Antibiotics; Salicylates; Selective Serotonin Reuptake Inhibitors; SGLT2 Inhibitors

Decreased Effect

The levels/effects of Insulin Regular may be decreased by: Hyperglycemia-Associated Agents; Quinolone Antibiotics; Thiazide Diuretics

Storage/Stability

Humulin R, Humulin R U-500: Store unopened vials in refrigerator between 2°C and 8°C (36°F to 46°F); do not freeze; keep away from heat and sunlight. Once punctured (in use), vials may be stored for up to 31 days in the refrigerator between 2°C and 8°C (36°F to 46°F) or at room temperature of ≤30°C (≤86°F).

Novolin R: Store unopened vials in refrigerator between 2°C and 8°C (36°F to 46°F) until product expiration date or at room temperature ≤25°C (≤77°F) for up to 42 days; do not freeze; keep away from heat and sunlight. Once punctured (in use), store vials at room temperature ≤25°C (≤77°F) for up to 42 days (this includes any days stored at room temperature prior to opening vial); refrigeration of in-use vials is not recommended.

Canadian labeling (not in U.S. labeling): All products: Unopened vials, cartridges, and pens should be stored under refrigeration between 2°C and 8°C (36°F to 46°F) until the expiration date; do not freeze; keep away from heat and sunlight. Once punctured (in use), Humulin vials, cartridges, and pens should be stored at room temperature <25°C (<77°F) for up to 4 weeks. Once punctured (in use), Novolin ge vials, cartridges, and pens may be stored for up to 1 month at room temperature <25°C (<77°F) for vials or <30°C (<86°F) for pens/cartridges; do not refrigerate.

For SubQ administration:

Humulin R: According to the manufacturer, diluted insulin should be stored at 30°C (86°F) and used within 14 days **or** at 5°C (41°F) and used within 28 days.

For IV infusion:

Humulin R: Stable for 48 hours at room temperature or for 48 hours under refrigeration followed by 48 hours at room temperature.

Novolin R: Stable for 24 hours at room temperature

Mechanism of Action Insulin acts via specific membrane-bound receptors on target tissues to regulate metabolism of carbohydrate, protein, and fats. Target organs for insulin include the liver, skeletal muscle, and adipose tissue.

Within the liver, insulin stimulates hepatic glycogen synthesis. Insulin promotes hepatic synthesis of fatty acids, which are released into the circulation as lipoproteins. Skeletal muscle effects of insulin include increased protein synthesis and increased glycogen synthesis. Within adipose tissue, insulin stimulates the processing of circulating lipoproteins to provide free fatty acids, facilitating triglyceride synthesis and storage by adipocytes; also directly inhibits the hydrolysis of triglycerides. In addition, insulin stimulates the cellular uptake of amino acids and increases cellular permeability to several ions, including potassium, magnesium, and phosphate. By activating sodium-potassium ATPases, insulin promotes the intracellular movement of potassium.

Normally secreted by the pancreas, insulin products are manufactured for pharmacologic use through recombinant DNA technology using either *E. coli* or *Saccharomyces cerevisiae*. Insulins are categorized based on the onset, peak, and duration of effect (eg, rapid-, short-, intermediate-, and long-acting insulin).

Pharmacodynamics Note: Rate of absorption, onset, and duration of activity may be affected by site administration, exercise, presence of lipodystrophy, local blood supply, and/or temperature.

Onset of action: U-100: IV: 10 to 15 minutes; SubQ: 30 minutes

Maximum effect: SubQ: ~3 hours (range: 20 minutes to 7 hours)

Duration:

IV: U-100: 2 to 6 hours

SubQ: U-100: 4 to 12 hours (may increase with dose); U-500: Up to 24 hours

Pharmacokinetics (Adult data unless noted)

Distribution: V_d: 0.26-0.36 L/kg

Half-life: IV: ~0.5 to 1 hour (dose-dependent); SubQ: 1.5 hours

Time to peak plasma concentration: SubQ: 0.8 to 2 hours

Elimination: Urine

Dosing: Neonatal

Hyperglycemia: Limited data available (Cloherty 2012): **Note:** Neonates are extremely sensitive to the effects of insulin; initiate therapy at the lower end of infusion rate and monitor closely; routine use in neonates is not recommended: IV:

Intermittent IV infusion: 0.05 to 0.1 units/kg infused over 15 minutes every 4 to 6 hours as needed; **Note:** Should be used as initial management; monitor blood glucose every 30 minutes to 1 hour following doses

Continuous IV infusion: Initial rate: 0.05 units/kg/**hour**, monitor blood glucose every 30 minutes and titrate in 0.01 units/kg/**hour** increments, usual range: 0.01 to 0.2 units/kg/**hour**

Hyperkalemia: Limited data available:

IV: 0.1 units/kg with 400 mg/kg of glucose; **Note:** Ratio of 1 unit of insulin for every 4 g of glucose (Hegenbarth 2008)

Continuous IV infusion: Initial bolus: 0.05 units/kg with 2 **mL**/kg of $D_{10}W$ followed by continuous IV infusion of insulin at 0.1 unit/kg/**hour** in combination with $D_{10}W$ infusion at 2 to 4 **mL**/kg/hour (Cloherty 2012); insulin infusions as low as 0.05 units/kg/**hour** in conjunction with dextrose infusion have been used in premature neonates (GA: <28 weeks) (Malone 1991).

Dosing: Usual The general objective of insulin replacement therapy is to approximate the physiologic pattern of insulin secretion. This requires a basal level of insulin throughout the day, supplemented by additional insulin at mealtimes. Since combinations using different types of insulins are frequently used, dosage adjustment must address the individual component of the insulin regimen which most directly influences the blood glucose value in question, based on the known onset and duration of the insulin component. The frequency of doses and monitoring must be individualized in consideration of the patient's ability to manage therapy.

Pediatric:

Type 1 diabetes mellitus: Infants (Limited data available), Children, and Adolescents: **Note:** Insulin regimens should be individualized to achieve glycemic goals without causing hypoglycemia. Multiple daily doses or continuous subcutaneous infusion guided by blood glucose monitoring are the standard of diabetes care. The daily doses presented are expressed as the total units/kg/day **of all insulin formulations combined.**

Initial dose: SubQ: 0.2 to 0.6 units/kg/day in divided doses. Conservative initial doses of 0.2 to 0.4 units/kg/day are often recommended to avoid the potential for hypoglycemia.

Division of daily insulin requirement ("conventional therapy"): Generally, 50% to 75% of the daily insulin dose is given as an intermediate- or long-acting form of insulin (in 1 to 2 daily injections). The remaining portion of the 24-hour insulin requirement is divided and administered as either regular insulin or a rapid-acting form of insulin at the same time before breakfast and dinner.

Division of daily insulin requirement ("intensive therapy"): Basal insulin delivery with 1 or 2 doses of intermediate- or long-acting insulin formulations superimposed with doses of rapid- or very rapid-acting insulin formulations 3 or more times daily.

Adjustment of dose: Dosage must be titrated to achieve glucose control and avoid hypoglycemia. Adjust dose to maintain premeal and bedtime glucose in target range. Since combinations of agents are frequently used, dosage adjustment must address the individual component of the insulin regimen which most directly influences the blood glucose value in question, based on the known onset and duration of the insulin component.

Usual maintenance range: 0.5 to 1 unit/kg/day in divided doses; doses must be individualized; however an estimate can be determined based on phase of diabetes and level of maturity (ISPAD [Danne 2014])

Partial remission phase (Honeymoon phase): <0.5 units/kg/day

Prepubertal children (not in partial remission): 0.7 to 1 units/kg/day

Pubescent Children and Adolescents: During puberty, requirements may substantially increase to >1.2 unit/kg/day and in some cases up to 2 units/kg/day

Continuous SubQ insulin infusion (insulin pump): A combination of a "basal" continuous insulin infusion rate with preprogrammed, premeal bolus doses which are patient controlled. When converting from multiple daily SubQ doses of maintenance insulin, it is advisable to reduce the basal rate to less than the equivalent of the total daily units of longer acting insulin (eg, NPH). Divide the total number of units by 24 to get the basal rate in units/hour. Do not include the total units of regular insulin or other rapid-acting insulin formulations in this calculation. The same premeal regular insulin dosage may be used.

Type 2 diabetes mellitus: Children ≥10 years and Adolescents: SubQ: The goal of therapy is to achieve an HbA_{1c} <6.5% as quickly as possible using the safe titration of medications. Initial therapy in metabolically unstable patients (eg, plasma glucose ≥ 250 mg/dL, HbA_{1c} >9% and symptoms excluding acidosis) may include once daily intermediate-acting insulin or basal insulin in combination with lifestyle changes and metformin. In patients who fail to achieve glycemic goals with metformin and basal insulin, may consider initiating prandial insulin (regular insulin or rapid acting insulin) and titrate to achieve goals. Once initial goal reached, insulin should be slowly tapered and the patient transitioned to lowest effective doses or metformin monotherapy if able (AAP [Copeland 2013]; ISPAD [Zeitler 2014]). **Note:** Patients who are ketotic or present with ketoacidosis require aggressive management as indicated.

Diabetic ketoacidosis (DKA): Limited data available: Infants, Children, and Adolescents: **Note:** Only IV regular insulin should be used for treatment of DKA; the rare exception where the use of SubQ rapid-acting insulin analogs (eg, aspart, lispro) may be appropriate is for patients with uncomplicated DKA in whom peripheral circulation is adequate and continuous IV regular insulin administration is not possible. Treatment should continue until resolution of acid-base abnormalities (eg, pH >7.3, serum HCO3 >15 mEq/L, and/or closure of anion gap); serum glucose is not a direct indicator of these abnormalities, and may decrease more rapidly than correction of the metabolic abnormalities. As part of overall DKA management, dextrose should be added to IV fluids to prevent hypoglycemia, usually once serum glucose is between 250 to 300 mg/dL but it may be required sooner if serum glucose has decreased precipitously. Generally, only dextrose 5% is necessary and is added to NS or ½NS; however, dextrose 10% or 12.5% may be necessary in some cases (ADA [Wolfsdorf 2006]; ISPAD [Wolfsdorf 2014]). Refer to institution-specific protocols where appropriate.

Continuous IV infusion:

Initial: 0.05 to 0.1 units/kg/**hour**; continue the rate at 0.05 to 0.1 units/kg/hour if tolerated until resolution of ketoacidosis (pH >7.3; bicarbonate >15 mEq/L and/or closure of anion gap); **Note:** Some patients (eg, some young children with DKA, or older children with established diabetes) may have marked sensitivity to insulin requiring lower infusion rates; these lower infusion rates should only be used provided that resolution of the acidosis continues (ADA [Wolfsdorf 2006]; ISPAD [Wolfsdorf 2014]).

After resolution of DKA: Once ketoacidosis has resolved and oral intake is tolerated, transition to a SubQ insulin regimen. An overlap between discontinuation of IV insulin and administration of SubQ insulin is recommended to ensure adequate plasma insulin levels; timing of SubQ insulin administration prior to infusion discontinuation is dependent on type of insulin used; for SubQ regular insulin: 1 to 2 hours, or for rapid-acting insulin: 15 to 30 minutes (IPSAD [Wolfsdorf 2014]).

Hyperkalemia: Limited data available: Infants, Children, and Adolescents: IV: 0.1 unit/kg with 400 mg/kg of glucose; usual ratio of combination therapy of insulin to glucose is 1 unit of insulin for every 4 g of glucose (Hegenbarth 2008). An alternate approach is glucose 1 g/kg followed by 0.2 units of insulin/g of glucose administered over 15 to 30 minutes then infused continuously as a similar amount per hour (Fuhrman 2011). In adults, the usual dose is 10 units of insulin mixed with 25 g of dextrose (50 mL of $D_{50}W$) administered over 15 to 30 minutes (ACLS [Vanden Hoek 2010]).

Hyperosmolar hyperglycemic state (HHS): Limited data available: Children and Adolescents: **Note:** Only regular IV insulin should be used. Insulin administration should be initiated when serum glucose concentration is no longer declining at a rate ≥50 mg/dL per hour with fluid administration alone; earlier initiation may be required in patients with severe ketosis and acidosis. Infusion should continue until reversal of mental status changes and hyperosmolality. Serum glucose is not a direct indicator of these abnormalities, and may decrease more rapidly than correction of the metabolic abnormalities. Refer to institution-specific protocols where appropriate.

Continuous IV infusion: Initial: 0.025 to 0.05 units/kg/**hour**; titrate dose to achieve a decrease in serum glucose concentration at a rate of 50 to 75 mg/dL per hour; higher rates of decline may be required in some patients; however, if rate of decline exceeds 100 mg/dL per hour discontinue infusion (ISPAD [Wolfsdorf 2014]; Zeitler 2011)

Adult:

Diabetes mellitus: SubQ: **Note:** Insulin requirements vary dramatically between patients and therapy requires dosage adjustments with careful medical supervision. Specific formulations may require distinct administration procedures; please see individual agents.

Diabetes mellitus, type 1: **Note:** Multiple daily injections (MDI) guided by blood glucose monitoring or the use of continuous subcutaneous insulin infusions (CSII) is the standard of care for patients with type 1 diabetes. Combinations of insulin formulations are commonly used.

Initial dose: 0.5 to 1 units/kg/day in divided doses. Conservative initial doses of 0.2 to 0.4 units/kg/day may be recommended to avoid the potential for hypoglycemia.

Division of daily insulin requirement: Generally, 50% to 75% of the total daily dose (TDD) is given as an intermediate or long-acting form of insulin (in 1 to 2 daily injections). The remaining portion of the TDD is then divided and administered before or at mealtimes (depending on the formulation) as a rapid-acting or short-acting form of insulin.

Adjustment of dose: Dosage must be titrated to achieve glucose control and avoid hypoglycemia. Adjust dose to maintain preprandial plasma glucose between 70 to 130 mg/dL for most patients. Since treatment regimens often consist of multiple formulations, dosage adjustments must address the specific phase of insulin release that is primarily contributing to the patient's impaired glycemic control. Treatment and monitoring regimens must be individualized.

Usual maintenance range: 0.5 to 1.2 units/kg/day in divided doses. Insulin requirements are patient-specific and may vary based on age, body weight, and/or activity factors

Diabetes mellitus, type 2: The goal of therapy is to achieve an HbA_{1c} <7% as quickly as possible using the safe titration of medications. According to a consensus statement by the ADA and European Association for the Study of Diabetes (EASD), basal insulin therapy (eg, intermediate- or long-acting insulin) should be considered in patients with type 2 diabetes who fail to achieve glycemic goals with lifestyle interventions and metformin ± a sulfonylurea. Pioglitazone or a GLP-1 agonist may also be considered prior to initiation of basal insulin therapy. In patients who continue to fail to achieve glycemic goals despite the addition of basal insulin, intensification of insulin therapy should be considered; this generally consists of multiple daily injections with a combination of insulin formulations (Nathan 2009).

Intensification of therapy: Add a second injection of a short-, rapid-, or intermediate-acting insulin as needed based on blood glucose monitoring; the timing of administration and type of insulin added for intensification of therapy depends on the blood glucose level that is consistently out of the target range (eg, preprandial glucose levels before lunch or dinner, postprandial glucose levels, and/or bedtime glucose levels). Additional injections and subsequent dosage adjustments must address the specific phase of insulin release that is primarily contributing to the patient's impaired glycemic control. Intensification of therapy can usually begin with a second injection of ~4 units/day followed by adjustments of ~2 units/day every 3 days until the targeted blood glucose is within range (Nathan 2009).

In the setting of glucose toxicity (loss of beta-cell sensitivity to glucose concentrations), insulin therapy may be used for short-term management to restore sensitivity of beta-cells; in these cases, the dose may need to be rapidly reduced/withdrawn when sensitivity is reestablished.

Dosing adjustment in renal impairment: Insulin requirements are reduced due to changes in insulin clearance or metabolism; there are no dosage adjustments provided in manufacturer's labeling; however, the following adjustments have been used by some clinicians (Aronoff 2007): Adults:

CrCl >50 mL/minute: No adjustment necessary.

CrCl 10 to 50 mL/minute: Administer at 75% of normal dose and monitor glucose closely.

CrCl <10 mL/minute: Administer at 50% of normal dose and monitor glucose closely.

Hemodialysis: Because of a large molecular weight (6,000 daltons), insulin is not significantly removed by hemodialysis; supplemental dose is not necessary.

Peritoneal dialysis: Because of a large molecular weight (6,000 daltons), insulin is not significantly removed by peritoneal dialysis; supplemental dose is not necessary.

Continuous renal replacement therapy: Administer at 75% of normal dose and monitor glucose closely; supplemental dose is not necessary.

Dosing adjustment in hepatic impairment: There are no dosage adjustments provided in manufacturer's labeling; insulin requirements may be reduced due to changes in insulin clearance or metabolism; monitor blood glucose closely.

Usual Infusion Concentrations: Neonatal IV Infusion: 0.1 unit/mL **or** 0.5 unit/mL

Usual Infusion Concentrations: Pediatric IV infusion: 0.1 unit/mL, 0.5 unit/mL, **or** 1 unit/mL

Preparation for Administration

Parenteral:

SubQ:

Humulin R: May be diluted with the universal diluent, Sterile Diluent for Humalog, Humulin N, Humulin R,

Humulin 70/30, and Humulin R U-500, to a concentration of 10 units/mL (U-10) or 50 units/mL (U-50).

Novolin R: Insulin Diluting Medium for NovoLog is **not** intended for use with Novolin R or any insulin product other than insulin aspart.

Regular Insulin may be mixed with other insulins; when mixing regular insulin with other insulin preparations, regular insulin should be drawn into syringe first.

IV: Only use U-100 preparations.

Humulin R: May be diluted in NS or D_5W to concentrations of 0.1 to 1 unit/mL.

Novolin R: May be diluted in NS, D_5W, **or** $D_{10}W$ with 40 mEq/L potassium chloride at concentrations of 0.05 to 1 unit/mL.

Note: ISMP and Vermont Oxford Network recommend a standard concentration of 0.1 or 0.5 units/mL for neonates (ISMP 2011).

Administration Parenteral: Do not use if solution is viscous or cloudy; use only if clear and colorless.

SubQ: Administer 30 to 60 minutes before meals. Cold injections should be avoided. Administration is usually made into the subcutaneous fat of the thighs, arms, buttocks, or abdomen, with sites rotated. When mixing regular insulin with other insulin preparations, regular insulin should be drawn into the syringe first. While not preferred, regular insulin may be infused SubQ by external insulin pump (eg, when rapid-acting insulin not available) (Danne [ISPAD], 2014); however, when used in an external pump, it is not recommended to be diluted with other solutions.

IM: May be administered IM in selected clinical situations; close monitoring of blood glucose and serum potassium as well as medical supervision is required.

IV: Regular U-100 insulin is the preferred insulin formulation approved for IV administration; requires close monitoring of blood glucose and serum potassium; appropriate medical supervision. If possible, do not administer mixtures of insulin formulations intravenously. IV administration of U-500 regular insulin is not recommended.

Continuous IV Infusion: To minimize insulin adsorption to IV tubing: Flush the IV tubing with a priming infusion of 20 mL from the insulin infusion, whenever a new IV tubing set is added to the insulin infusion container (Jacobi 2012; Thompson 2012). **Note:** Also refer to institution-specific protocols where appropriate.

If insulin is required prior to the availability of the insulin drip, regular insulin should be administered by IV push injection.

Because of adsorption to IV tubing or infusion bags, the actual amount of insulin being administered could be substantially less than the apparent amount. Therefore, adjustment of the IV infusion rate should be based on the effect and not solely on the apparent insulin dose. The apparent dose may be used as a starting point for determining the subsequent SubQ dosing regimen (Moghissi 2009); however, the transition to SubQ administration requires continuous medical supervision, frequent monitoring of blood glucose, and careful adjustment of therapy. In addition, SubQ insulin should be given 1 to 4 hours prior to the discontinuation of IV insulin to prevent hyperglycemia (Moghissi 2009)

Monitoring Parameters

Diabetes: Plasma glucose, electrolytes, HbA_{1c}

DKA/HHS: Vital signs, arterial blood gases (initial), venous pH, CBC with differential, urinalysis, serum glucose BUN, creatinine, electrolytes, calcium, magnesium, phosphate, anion gap, fluid status blood β-hydroxybutyrate (β-OH) concentration; neurological observations; mental status (ISPAD [Wolfsdorf 2014]).

Hyperkalemia: Serum potassium and glucose must be closely monitored to avoid hypoglycemia and/or hypokalemia.

Reference Range

Type I DM: Plasma Blood Glucose and HbA_{1c} Goals (ADA 2015): **Note:** Goals should be individualized based on individual needs/circumstances (eg, patients who experience severe hypoglycemia, patients with hypoglycemic unawareness); lower goals may be reasonable if they can be achieved without excessive hypoglycemia. **Note:** Postprandial blood glucose should be measured when there is a discrepancy between preprandial blood glucose concentrations and HbA_{1c} values and to help assess glycemia for patients who receive basal/bolus regimens. It is usually drawn 1 to 2 hours after starting meal and is considered to be the "peak."

Infants, Children, and Adolescents:

Preprandial glucose: 90 to 130 mg/dL

Bedtime/overnight glucose: 90 to 150 mg/dL

HbA_{1c}: <7.5%

Adults, nonpregnant:

Preprandial glucose: 80 to 130 mg/dL

Postprandial glucose: <180 mg/dL

HbA_{1c}: <7%

Type 2 DM: Indicators optimal glycemic control: Children and Adolescents: **Note:** Targets must be adjusted based on individual needs/circumstances (eg, patients who experience severe hypoglycemia, patients with hypoglycemic unawareness):

HbA_{1c}: <6.5 to 7% (AAP [Copeland 2013]; ADA 2000; IPSAD [Zeitler 2014])

Fasting glucose: 70 to 130 mg/dL (AAP [Copeland 2013])

Dosage Forms Excipient information presented when available (limited, particularly for generics); consult specific product labeling.

Solution, Injection:

HumuLIN R: 100 units/mL (3 mL, 10 mL) [contains metacresol, phenol]

NovoLIN R: 100 units/mL (10 mL) [contains metacresol]

NovoLIN R ReliOn: 100 units/mL (10 mL) [contains metacresol]

Solution, Subcutaneous:

HumuLIN R U-500 (CONCENTRATED): 500 units/mL (20 mL) [contains metacresol]

- **Insulin Regular and Insulin NPH** *see* Insulin NPH and Insulin Regular *on page* 1141
- **Intanza (Can)** *see* Influenza Virus Vaccine (Inactivated) *on page* 1108
- **Intelence** *see* Etravirine *on page* 823
- **Intelence® (Can)** *see* Etravirine *on page* 823
- **α-2-interferon** *see* Interferon Alfa-2b *on page* 1148
- **Interferon Alfa-2a (PEG Conjugate)** *see* Peginterferon Alfa-2a *on page* 1642
- **Interferon Alfa-2b (PEG Conjugate)** *see* Peginterferon Alfa-2b *on page* 1646

Interferon Alfa-2b (in ter FEER on AL fa too bee)

Medication Safety Issues

Sound-alike/look-alike issues:

Interferon alfa-2b may be confused with interferon alfa-2a, interferon alfa-n3, pegylated interferon alfa-2b, peginterferon beta-1a

Intron A may be confused with PEG-Intron

International issues:

Interferon alfa-2b may be confused with interferon alpha multi-subtype which is available in international markets

Related Information

Prevention of Chemotherapy-Induced Nausea and Vomiting in Children *on page* 2368

Brand Names: US Intron A

Brand Names: Canada Intron A

Therapeutic Category Antineoplastic Agent, Biologic Response Modulator; Biological Response Modulator; Immunomodulator, Systemic; Interferon

Generic Availability (US) No

Use Treatment of chronic hepatitis B (FDA approved in ages ≥1 year and adults); chronic hepatitis C (in combination with ribavirin) (FDA approved in ages ≥3 years and adults); chronic hepatitis C (without ribavirin) (FDA approved in adults); hairy cell leukemia (FDA approved in adults); treatment of AIDS-related Kaposi's sarcoma (FDA approved in adults); condylomata acuminata (FDA approved in adults); adjuvant therapy of malignant melanoma following surgical excision (FDA approved in adults); and follicular non-Hodgkin's lymphoma (FDA approved in adults)

Other uses include hemangiomas of infancy, cutaneous ulcerations of Behçet's disease, neuroendocrine tumors (including carcinoid syndrome and islet cell tumor), cutaneous T-cell lymphoma, desmoid tumor, hepatitis D, chronic myelogenous leukemia (CML), non-Hodgkin's lymphomas (other than follicular lymphoma, see approved use), multiple myeloma, renal cell carcinoma, West Nile virus

Medication Guide Available Yes

Pregnancy Risk Factor C / X in combination with ribavirin

Pregnancy Considerations Animal reproduction studies have demonstrated abortifacient effects. Disruption of the normal menstrual cycle was also observed in animal studies; therefore, the manufacturer recommends that reliable contraception is used in women of childbearing potential. Alfa interferon is endogenous to normal amniotic fluid. *In vitro* administration studies have reported that when administered to the mother, it does not cross the placenta. Case reports of use in pregnant women are limited. The Perinatal HIV Guidelines Working Group does not recommend that interferon-alfa be used during pregnancy. Interferon alfa-2b monotherapy should only be used in pregnancy when the potential benefit to the mother justifies the possible risk to the fetus. Combination therapy with ribavirin is contraindicated in pregnancy (refer to Ribavirin monograph); two forms of contraception should be used during combination therapy and patients should have monthly pregnancy tests. A pregnancy registry has been established for women inadvertently exposed to ribavirin while pregnant (800-593-2214).

Breast-Feeding Considerations Breast milk samples obtained from a lactating mother prior to and after administration of interferon alfa-2b showed that interferon alfa is present in breast milk and administration of the medication did not significantly affect endogenous levels. Breast-feeding is not linked to the spread of hepatitis C virus; however, if nipples are cracked or bleeding, breast-feeding is not recommended. Mothers coinfected with HIV are discouraged from breast-feeding to decrease potential transmission of HIV.

Contraindications

Hypersensitivity to interferon alfa or any component of the formulation; decompensated liver disease; autoimmune hepatitis

Combination therapy with interferon alfa-2b and ribavirin is also contraindicated in women who are pregnant, in males with pregnant partners; in patients with hemoglobinopathies (eg, thalassemia major, sickle-cell anemia); creatinine clearance <50 mL/minute; or hypersensitivity to ribavirin or any component of the formulation

Documentation of allergenic cross-reactivity for interferons is limited. However, because of similarities in chemical structure and/or pharmacologic actions, the possibility of cross-sensitivity cannot be ruled out with certainty.

Warnings/Precautions [US Boxed Warning]: May cause or aggravate fatal or life-threatening autoimmune disorders, neuropsychiatric symptoms (including depression and/or suicidal thoughts/behaviors), ischemic, and/or infectious disorders; monitor closely with clinical and laboratory evaluations (periodic); discontinue treatment for severe persistent or worsening symptoms; some cases may resolve with discontinuation.

Neuropsychiatric disorders: May cause neuropsychiatric events, including depression, psychosis, mania, suicidal behavior/ideation, attempts and completed suicides and homicidal ideation; may occur in patients with or without previous psychiatric symptoms. Effects are usually rapidly reversible upon therapy discontinuation, but have persisted up to three weeks. If psychiatric symptoms persist or worsen, or suicidal or homicidal ideation or aggressive behavior towards others is identified, discontinue treatment, and follow the patient closely. Careful neuropsychiatric monitoring is recommended during and for 6 months after treatment in patients who develop psychiatric disorders (including clinical depression). New or exacerbated neuropsychiatric or substance abuse disorders are best managed with early intervention. Use with caution in patients with a history of psychiatric disorders. Drug screening and periodic health evaluation (including monitoring of psychiatric symptoms) is recommended if initiating treatment in patients with coexisting psychiatric condition or substance abuse disorders. Suicidal ideation or attempts may occur more frequently in pediatric patients (eg, adolescents) when compared to adults. Higher doses, usually in elderly patients, may result in increased CNS toxicity (eg, obtundation and coma).

Hepatic disease: May cause hepatotoxicity; monitor closely if abnormal liver function tests develop. A transient increase in ALT (≥2 times baseline) may occur in patients treated with interferon alfa-2b for chronic hepatitis B. Therapy generally may continue; monitor. Worsening and potentially fatal liver disease, including jaundice, hepatic encephalopathy, and hepatic failure have been reported in patients receiving interferon alfa for chronic hepatitis B and C with decompensated liver disease, autoimmune hepatitis, history of autoimmune disease, and immunosuppressed transplant recipients; avoid use in these patients; use is contraindicated in decompensated liver disease. Patients with cirrhosis are at increased risk of hepatic decompensation. Therapy should be discontinued for any patient developing signs and symptoms of liver failure. Permanently discontinue for severe (grade 3) hepatic injury or hepatic decompensation (Child-Pugh class B and C [score >6]). Chronic hepatitis B or C patients with a history of autoimmune disease or who are immunosuppressed transplant recipients should not receive interferon alfa-2b.

Bone marrow suppression: Causes bone marrow suppression, including potentially severe cytopenias, and very rarely, aplastic anemia. Discontinue treatment for severe neutropenia (ANC <500/mm^3) or thrombocytopenia (platelets <25,000/mm^3). Hemolytic anemia (hemoglobin <10 g/dL) was observed when combined with ribavirin; anemia occurred within 1 to 2 weeks of initiation of therapy. Use caution in patients with pre-existing myelosuppression and in patients with concomitant medications which cause myelosuppression.

Autoimmune disorders: Avoid use in patients with history of autoimmune disorders; development of autoimmune disorders (thrombocytopenia, vasculitis, Raynaud's disease, rheumatoid arthritis, lupus erythematosus and rhabdomyolysis) has been associated with use. Monitor closely; consider discontinuing. Worsening of psoriasis and sarcoidosis (and the development of new sarcoidosis) have been reported; use extreme caution.

Cardiovascular disease/coagulation disorders: Use caution and monitor closely in patients with cardiovascular disease (ischemic or thromboembolic), arrhythmias, hypertension, and in patients with a history of MI or prior therapy with cardiotoxic drugs. Patients with preexisting cardiac disease and/or advanced cancer should have baseline and periodic ECGs. May cause hypotension (during administration or delayed up to 2 days), arrhythmia, tachycardia (≥150 bpm), cardiomyopathy (~2% in AIDS-related Kaposi Sarcoma patients), and/or MI. Some experiencing cardiovascular adverse effects had no prior history of cardiac disease. Supraventricular arrhythmias occur rarely, and are associated with preexisting cardiac disease or prior therapy with cardiotoxic agents. Dose modification, discontinuation, and/or additional therapies may be necessary. Hemorrhagic cerebrovascular events have been observed with therapy. Use caution in patients with coagulation disorders.

Endocrine disorders: Thyroid disorders (possibly reversible) have been reported; use caution in patients with preexisting thyroid disease. TSH levels should be within normal limits prior to initiating interferon. Treatment should not be initiated in patients with preexisting thyroid disease who cannot be maintained in normal ranges by medication. Discontinue interferon use in patients who develop thyroid abnormalities during treatment and in patients with thyroid disease who subsequently cannot maintain normal ranges with thyroid medication. Discontinuation of interferon therapy may or may not reverse thyroid dysfunction. Diabetes mellitus has been reported; discontinue if cannot effectively manage with medication. Use with caution in patients with a history of diabetes mellitus, particularly if prone to DKA. Hypertriglyceridemia has been reported; discontinue if persistent and severe, and/or combined with symptoms of pancreatitis.

Pulmonary disease: Dyspnea, pulmonary infiltrates, pulmonary hypertension, interstitial pneumonitis, pneumonia, bronchiolitis obliterans, and sarcoidosis may be induced or aggravated by treatment, sometimes resulting in respiratory failure or fatality. Has been reported more in patients being treated for chronic hepatitis C, although has also occurred with use for oncology indications. Patients with fever, cough, dyspnea or other respiratory symptoms should be evaluated with a chest x-ray; monitor closely and consider discontinuing treatment with evidence of impaired pulmonary function. Use with caution in patients with a history of pulmonary disease.

Ophthalmic disorders: Decreased or loss of vision, macular edema, optic neuritis, retinal hemorrhages, cotton wool spots, papilledema, retinal detachment (serous), and retinal artery or vein thrombosis have occurred (or been aggravated) in patients receiving alpha interferons. Use caution in patients with pre-existing eye disorders; monitor closely; a complete eye exam should be done promptly in patients who develop ocular symptoms; discontinue with new or worsening ophthalmic disorders.

Dental and periodontic disorders: In patients receiving combination interferon and ribavirin therapy, dental and periodontal disorders have been reported; additionally, dry mouth can damage teeth and mouth mucous membranes during chronic therapy.

Commonly associated with fever and flu-like symptoms; rule out other causes/infection with persistent fever; use with caution in patients with debilitating conditions. Acute hypersensitivity reactions (eg, urticaria, angioedema, bronchoconstriction, anaphylaxis) have been reported (rarely) with alfa interferons. If an acute reaction develops, discontinue therapy immediately; transient rashes have occurred in some patients following injection, but have not necessitated treatment interruption. Do not treat patients with visceral AIDS-related Kaposi sarcoma associated with rapidly-progressing or life-threatening disease. Some formulations contain albumin, which may carry a remote risk of viral transmission. Due to differences in dosage, patients should not change brands of interferons without the concurrence of their healthcare provider. Combination therapy with ribavirin is associated with birth defects and/or fetal mortality and hemolytic anemia. Do not use combination therapy with ribavirin in patients with CrCl <50 mL/minute. Interferon alfa-2b at doses ≥10 million units/m^2 is associated with a moderate emetic potential; antiemetics may be recommended to prevent nausea and vomiting. Potentially significant drug-drug interactions may exist, requiring dose or frequency adjustment, additional monitoring, and/or selection of alternative therapy.

Benzyl alcohol and derivatives: Diluent for injection may contain benzyl alcohol; large amounts of benzyl alcohol (≥99 mg/kg/day) have been associated with a potentially fatal toxicity ("gasping syndrome") in neonates; the "gasping syndrome" consists of metabolic acidosis, respiratory distress, gasping respirations, CNS dysfunction (including convulsions, intracranial hemorrhage), hypotension, and cardiovascular collapse (AAP 1997; CDC 1982); some data suggests that benzoate displaces bilirubin from protein binding sites (Ahlfors 2001); avoid or use dosage forms containing benzyl alcohol with caution in neonates.

Some dosage forms may contain polysorbate 80 (also known as Tweens). Hypersensitivity reactions, usually a delayed reaction, have been reported following exposure to pharmaceutical products containing polysorbate 80 in certain individuals (Isaksson, 2002; Lucente 2000; Shelley 1995). Thrombocytopenia, ascites, pulmonary deterioration, and renal and hepatic failure have been reported in premature neonates after receiving parenteral products containing polysorbate 80 (Alade 1986; CDC 1984). See manufacturer's labeling.

Adverse Reactions Note: In a majority of patients, a flu-like symptom (fever, chills, tachycardia, malaise, myalgia, headache), occurs within 1-2 hours of administration; may last up to 24 hours and may be dose limiting.

Cardiovascular: Chest pain, edema, hypertension

Central nervous system: Agitation, amnesia, anxiety, chills, confusion, depression, dizziness, drowsiness, fatigue, headache, hypoesthesia, insomnia, irritability, lack of concentration, malaise, pain, paresthesia, right upper quadrant pain, rigors, vertigo

Dermatologic: Alopecia, dermatitis, diaphoresis, pruritus, skin rash, xeroderma

Endocrine & metabolic: Amenorrhea, decreased libido, weight loss

Gastrointestinal: Abdominal pain, anorexia, constipation, diarrhea, dysgeusia, dyspepsia, gingivitis, loose stools, nausea, vomiting (more common in children), xerostomia

Genitourinary: Urinary tract infection

Hematologic & oncologic: Anemia, leukopenia, neutropenia, purpura, thrombocytopenia

Hepatic: Increased serum alkaline phosphatase, increased serum ALT, increased serum AST

Infection: Candidiasis, infection, herpes virus infection

Local: Injection site reaction

Neuromuscular & skeletal: Arthralgia, back pain, myalgia, skeletal pain, weakness

Renal: Increased blood urea nitrogen, increased serum creatinine, polyuria

Respiratory: Bronchitis, cough, dyspnea, epistaxis, flu-like symptoms, nasal congestion, pharyngitis, sinusitis

Miscellaneous: Fever (more common in children)

Rare but important or life-threatening: Abnormal hepatic function tests, aggressive behavior, albuminuria, alcohol intolerance, amyotrophy, anaphylaxis, angina pectoris, angioedema, aphasia, aplastic anemia (rarely), ascites, asthma, atrial fibrillation, Bell's palsy, bradycardia, bronchiolitis obliterans, bronchoconstriction, bronchospasm, cardiac arrhythmia, cardiac failure, cardiomegaly, cardiomyopathy, cellulitis, cerebrovascular accident, colitis, coma, conjunctivitis, coronary artery disease, cyanosis, cystitis, dehydration, diabetes mellitus, dysphasia, dysuria, eczema, epidermal cyst, erythema, erythema multiforme, erythematous rash, exacerbation of psoriasis, exacerbation of sarcoidosis, extrapyramidal reaction, extrasystoles, gastrointestinal hemorrhage, granulocytopenia, hallucination, hearing loss, heart valve disease, hematuria, hemolytic anemia, hemoptysis, hepatic encephalopathy, hepatic failure, hepatitis, hepatotoxicity, hot flash, homicidal ideation, hyperbilirubinemia, hypercalcemia, hyperglycemia, hypermenorrhea, hypersensitivity reaction (acute), hypertriglyceridemia, hyperthyroidism, hypochromic anemia, hypotension, hypothermia, hypothyroidism, hypoventilation, immune thrombocytopenia, impotence, increased lactate dehydrogenase, interstitial pneumonitis, jaundice, leukorrhea, lupus erythematosus, lymphadenitis, lymphadenopathy, lymphocytopenia, lymphocytosis, macular edema, maculopapular rash, migraine, myocardial infarction, myositis, nephrotic syndrome, neuralgia, neuropathy, nystagmus, optic neuritis, palpitations, pancreatitis, pancytopenia, papilledema, paranoia, peripheral ischemia, peripheral neuropathy, photophobia, pituitary insufficiency, pleural effusion, pneumonia, psychoneurosis, pneumothorax, proteinuria, psychosis, pulmonary embolism, pulmonary fibrosis, pulmonary hypertension, pulmonary infiltrates, pure red cell aplasia, Raynaud's phenomenon, reduced ejection fraction, renal failure, renal insufficiency, respiratory insufficiency, retinal detachment (serous), retinal thrombosis, retinal cotton-wool spot, retinal vein occlusion, rhabdomyolysis, seizure, sepsis, sexual disorder, skin photosensitivity, Stevens-Johnson syndrome, stomatitis, suicidal ideation, syncope, systemic lupus erythematosus, tachycardia, tendonitis, tissue necrosis at injection site, thrombotic thrombocytopenic purpura, thrombosis, toxic epidermal necrolysis, upper respiratory tract infection, urinary incontinence, urticaria, uterine hemorrhage, vasculitis, Vogt-Koyanagi-Harada syndrome, wheezing

Drug Interactions

Metabolism/Transport Effects Inhibits CYP1A2 (weak)

Avoid Concomitant Use

Avoid concomitant use of Interferon Alfa-2b with any of the following: BCG (Intravesical); CloZAPine; Dipyrone; Telbivudine

Increased Effect/Toxicity

Interferon Alfa-2b may increase the levels/effects of: Aldesleukin; CloZAPine; Methadone; Ribavirin; Telbivudine; Theophylline Derivatives; TiZANidine; Zidovudine

The levels/effects of Interferon Alfa-2b may be increased by: Dipyrone

Decreased Effect

Interferon Alfa-2b may decrease the levels/effects of: BCG (Intravesical)

Storage/Stability Store intact vials under refrigeration at 2°C to 8°C (36°F to 46°F); do not freeze. After reconstitution of powder for injection, product should be used immediately, but may be stored under refrigeration for ≤24 hours.

Mechanism of Action Binds to a specific receptor on the cell wall to initiate intracellular activity; multiple effects can be detected including induction of gene transcription. Inhibits cellular growth, alters the state of cellular differentiation, interferes with oncogene expression, alters cell surface antigen expression, increases phagocytic activity of macrophages, and augments cytotoxicity of lymphocytes for target cells

Pharmacokinetics (Adult data unless noted)

Metabolism: Majority of dose is thought to be metabolized in the kidney, filtered and absorbed at the renal tubule

Bioavailability:
- IM: 83%
- SubQ: 90%

Half-life, elimination:
- IM, IV: 2 hours
- SubQ: 3 hours

Time to peak serum concentration: IM, SubQ: ~3 to 8 hours

Dosing: Usual Note: Consider premedication with acetaminophen to reduce the incidence of some adverse reactions. Not all dosage forms and strengths are appropriate for all indications; refer to product labeling for details.

Pediatric:

Hemangiomas: Infants, Children, and Adolescents: Limited data available: SubQ: 3 million units/m^2/dose once daily (Garmendia, 2001)

Hepatitis B, chronic: Children and Adolescents: SubQ: 3 million units/m^2/dose 3 times/week for 1 week; then 6 million units/m^2/dose 3 times/week; maximum dose: 10 million units/dose; total duration of therapy is 24 weeks. Higher doses may be used for retreatment or failed lower-dose therapy: 10 million units/m^2/dose 3 times/week for 6 months; dosing may also be used in infants in the setting of HIV-exposure/-infection (DHHS [pediatric], 2013).

Hepatitis C, chronic: Children ≥3 years and Adolescents: SubQ: 3 to 5 million units/m^2/dose 3 times/week

Adult:

AIDS-related Kaposi's sarcoma: IM, SubQ: 30 million units/m^2/dose 3 times/week; continue until disease progression or until maximal response has been achieved after 16 weeks

Condylomata acuminata: Intralesionally: 1 million units/lesion 3 times/week (on alternate days) for 3 weeks; not to exceed 5 million units per treatment (maximum dose: 5 lesions at one time) (use only the 10 million units vial); may administer a second course at 12-16 weeks

Hairy cell leukemia: IM, SubQ: 2 million units/m^2/dose 3 times/week for up to 6 months (may continue treatment with sustained treatment response); discontinue for disease progression or failure to respond after 6 months

Hepatitis B, chronic: IM, SubQ: 5 million units/dose given once daily **or** 10 million units/dose given 3 times/week for 4 months

Hepatitis C, chronic: IM, SubQ: 3 million units/dose 3 times/week for 16 weeks. In patients with normalization of ALT at 16 weeks, continue treatment for 18-24 months; consider discontinuation if normalization does not occur at 16 weeks. **Note:** May be used in combination therapy with ribavirin in previously untreated patients or in patients who relapse following alpha interferon therapy.

Lymphoma (follicular): SubQ: 5 million units/dose 3 times/week for ≤18 months

Malignant melanoma adjuvant therapy:
- Induction: IV: 20 million units/m^2/dose 5 days/week for 4 weeks
- Maintenance: SubQ: 10 million units/m^2/dose 3 days/week for 48 weeks

Dosage adjustment for toxicity:

Hematologic toxicity (also refer to indication specified adjustments below): ANC <500/mm^3 or platelets <25,000/mm^3: Discontinue treatment.

Hypersensitivity reaction (acute, serious), ophthalmic disorders (new or worsening), thyroid abnormality development (which cannot be normalized with medication), signs or symptoms of liver failure: Discontinue treatment.

Liver function abnormality, pulmonary infiltrate development, evidence of pulmonary function impairment, or autoimmune disorder development, triglycerides >1000 mg/dL in adults: Monitor closely and discontinue if appropriate.

Neuropsychiatric disorders (during treatment): Children, Adolescents, and Adults:

Clinical depression or other psychiatric problem: Monitor closely during and for 6 months after treatment.

Severe depression or other psychiatric disorder: Discontinue treatment.

Persistent or worsening psychiatric symptoms, suicidal ideation, aggression towards others: Discontinue treatment and follow with appropriate psychiatric intervention.

Indication-specific, manufacturer-recommended adjustments:

Lymphoma (follicular): Adults:

Neutrophils >1000/mm^3 to <1500/mm^3: Reduce dose by 50%; may re-escalate to starting dose when neutrophils return to >1500/mm^3

Severe toxicity (neutrophils <1000/mm^3 or platelets <50,000/mm^3): Temporarily withhold.

AST >5 times ULN or serum creatinine >2 mg/dL: Permanently discontinue.

Hairy cell leukemia: Adults:

Platelet count <50,000/mm^3: Do not administer intramuscularly (administer SubQ instead).

Severe toxicity: Reduce dose by 50% or temporarily withhold and resume with 50% dose reduction; permanently discontinue if persistent or recurrent severe toxicity is noted.

Chronic hepatitis B: Children, Adolescents, and Adults:

WBC <1500/mm^3, granulocytes <750/mm^3, or platelet count <50,000/mm^3, or other laboratory abnormality or severe adverse reaction: Reduce dose by 50%; may re-escalate to starting dose upon resolution of hematologic toxicity. Discontinue for persistent intolerance.

WBC <1000/mm^3, granulocytes <500/mm^3, or platelet count <25,000/mm^3: Permanently discontinue.

Hepatitis C, chronic: Children, Adolescents, and Adults: Severe toxicity: Reduce dose by 50% or temporarily withhold until subsides; permanently discontinue for persistent toxicities after dosage reduction.

AIDS-related Kaposi's sarcoma: Adults: Severe toxicity: Reduce dose by 50% or temporarily withhold; may resume at reduced dose with toxicity resolution; permanently discontinue for persistent/recurrent toxicities.

Malignant melanoma (induction and maintenance): Adults:

Severe toxicity, including neutrophils >250/mm^3 to <500/mm^3 or ALT/AST >5-10 times ULN: Temporarily withhold; resume with a 50% dose reduction when adverse reaction abates.

Neutrophils <250/mm^3, ALT/AST >10 times ULN, or severe/persistent adverse reactions: Permanently discontinue.

Preparation for Administration Parenteral: Powder for injection: The manufacturer recommends reconstituting vial with the diluent provided (SWFI). When reconstituted with 1 mL SWFI, the 10 million unit vial concentration is 10 million units/mL, the 18 million unit vial concentration is 18 million units/mL, and the 50 million unit vial concentration is 50 million units/mL. Swirl gently to mix. To prepare solution for infusion, further dilute appropriate dose in 100 mL NS. Final concentration should be ≥10 million units/100 mL.

Administration Parenteral: Not all dosage forms are recommended for all administration routes; refer to manufacturer's labeling. Allow product to reach room temperature prior to injection.

IM: Administer dose in the evening (if possible) to enhance tolerability. Rotate injection sites. Some patients may be appropriate for self-administration with appropriate training. In hairy cell leukemia treatment, if platelets are <50,000/mm^3, do not administer intramuscularly (administer SubQ instead).

IV: Infuse over ~20 minutes. Administer dose in the evening (if possible) to enhance tolerability.

SubQ: Suggested for those who are at risk for bleeding or are thrombocytopenic. Rotate SubQ injection site. Administer dose in the evening (if possible) to enhance tolerability. Patient should be well hydrated. Some patients may be appropriate for self-administration with appropriate training.

Intralesional: Inject dose at an angle nearly parallel to the plane of the skin, directing the needle to center of the base of the wart to infiltrate the lesion core and cause a small wheal. Only infiltrate the keratinized layer; avoid administration which is too deep or shallow.

Monitoring Parameters CBC with differential (baseline and periodic during treatment), liver function tests (baseline and periodic), electrolytes (baseline and periodic), serum creatinine (baseline), albumin, prothrombin time, triglycerides, thyroid-stimulating hormone (TSH) baseline and periodically during treatment (in patients with preexisting thyroid disorders, repeat TSH at 3 months and 6 months); chest x-ray (baseline), weight; ophthalmic exam (baseline and periodic, or with new ocular symptoms); ECG (baseline and during treatment; in patients with preexisting cardiac abnormalities or in advanced stages of cancer); neuropsychiatric changes during and for 6 months after therapy

Hepatitis B, chronic: CBC with differential and platelets and liver function tests: Baseline, weeks 1, 2, 4, 8, 12, and 16, at the end of treatment, and then 3 and 6 months posttreatment

Hepatitis C, chronic:

CBC with differential and platelets: Baseline, weeks 1 and 2, then monthly

Liver function: Every 3 months

TSH: Baseline and periodically during treatment; in patients with pre-existing thyroid disorders also repeat at 3 months and 6 months

Malignant melanoma: CBC with differential and platelets and liver function tests: Weekly during induction phase, then monthly during maintenance

Oncology patients: Thyroid function monitoring (Hamnvik, 2011): TSH and anti-TPO antibodies at baseline; if TPO antibody positive, monitor TSH every 2 months; if TPO antibody negative, monitor TSH every 6 months

Dosage Forms Excipient information presented when available (limited, particularly for generics); consult specific product labeling.

Solution, Injection:

Intron A: 6,000,000 units/mL (3.8 mL); 10,000,000 units/mL (3.2 mL) [contains edetate disodium, metacresol, polysorbate 80]

Solution Reconstituted, Injection [preservative free]:

Intron A: 10,000,000 units (1 ea); 18,000,000 units (1 ea); 50,000,000 units (1 ea) [contains albumin human]

- ◆ **Interferon Alpha-2b** *see* Interferon Alfa-2b *on page 1148*
- ◆ **Interleukin-1 Receptor Antagonist** *see* Anakinra *on page 165*
- ◆ **Interleukin 2** *see* Aldesleukin *on page 89*
- ◆ **Interleukin-11** *see* Oprelvekin *on page 1570*
- ◆ **Intermezzo** *see* Zolpidem *on page 2220*
- ◆ **Intralipid** *see* Fat Emulsion (Plant Based) *on page 850*
- ◆ **Intravenous Fat Emulsion** *see* Fat Emulsion (Plant Based) *on page 850*
- ◆ **Intron A** *see* Interferon Alfa-2b *on page 1148*
- ◆ **Intropin** *see* DOPamine *on page 704*

- ◆ **Intuniv** *see* GuanFACINE *on page 993*
- ◆ **Intuniv XR (Can)** *see* GuanFACINE *on page 993*
- ◆ **INVanz** *see* Ertapenem *on page 777*
- ◆ **Invanz (Can)** *see* Ertapenem *on page 777*
- ◆ **Invega** *see* Paliperidone *on page 1604*
- ◆ **Invega Sustenna** *see* Paliperidone *on page 1604*
- ◆ **Invega Trinza** *see* Paliperidone *on page 1604*
- ◆ **Invirase** *see* Saquinavir *on page 1902*

Iodine (EYE oh dyne)

Medication Safety Issues

Sound-alike/look-alike issues:

Iodine may be confused with codeine, Iopidine, Lodine

Therapeutic Category Topical Skin Product

Generic Availability (US) Yes

Use Used topically as an antiseptic in the management of minor, superficial skin wounds and has been used to disinfect the skin preoperatively

Pregnancy Considerations An adequate amount of iodine intake is essential for thyroid function. Iodine crosses the placenta and requirements are increased during pregnancy. Iodine deficiency in pregnancy can lead to neurologic damage in the newborn; an extreme form, cretinism, is characterized by gross mental retardation, short stature, deaf mutism, and spasticity. Large amounts of iodine during pregnancy can cause fetal goiter or hyperthyroidism. Transient hypothyroidism in the newborn has also been reported following topical or vaginal use prior to delivery.

Breast-Feeding Considerations Iodine is excreted in breast milk and is a source of iodine for the nursing infant. Actual levels are variable, but have been reported as 113-270 mcg/L in American women. Application of topical iodine antiseptic solutions can be absorbed in amounts which may affect levels in breast milk. Exposure to excess iodine may cause thyrotoxicosis. Skin rash in the nursing infant has been reported with maternal intake of potassium iodide.

Contraindications Hypersensitivity to iodine or any component of the formulation

Iodosorb®, Iodoflex™: Hashimoto thyroiditis, history of Grave's disease, or nontoxic nodular goiter; pregnancy; breast-feeding

Warnings/Precautions Not for application to large areas of the body or for use with tight or air-excluding bandages. When used as a topical antiseptic, improper use may lead to product contamination. Although infrequent, product contamination has been associated with reports of localized and systemic infections. To reduce the risk of infection, ensure antiseptic products are used according to the labeled instructions; avoid diluting products after opening; and apply single-use containers only one time to one patient and discard any unused solution (FDA Drug Safety Communication, 2013). Use caution with renal dysfunction. When used for self-medication (OTC), do not use on deep wounds, puncture wounds, animal bites, or serious burns without consulting with health care provider. Notify healthcare provider if condition does not improve within 7 days. Iodosorb is for use as topical application to wet wounds only.

Warnings: Additional Pediatric Considerations The extent of percutaneous absorption is dependent on several factors, including epidermal integrity (intact vs abraded skin) and age of the patient. Percutaneous absorption of iodine is increased in neonates (especially preterm neonates); risk of systemic absorption and adverse effects higher in neonates due to larger skin surface area to body mass ratio.

Adverse Reactions

Reactions reported following topical application:

Endocrine & metabolic: TSH increased
Local: Eczema, edema, irritation, pain, redness
Miscellaneous: Allergic reaction

Reactions reported more likely observed following large doses or chronic iodine intoxication; frequency not defined:

Central nervous system: Fever, headache
Dermatologic: Skin rash, angioedema, urticaria, acne
Endocrine & metabolic: Hypothyroidism
Gastrointestinal: Metallic taste, diarrhea
Hematologic: Eosinophilia, hemorrhage (mucosal)
Neuromuscular & skeletal: Arthralgia
Ocular: Swelling of eyelids
Respiratory: Pulmonary edema
Miscellaneous: Ioderma, lymph node enlargement

Drug Interactions

Metabolism/Transport Effects None known.

Avoid Concomitant Use There are no known interactions where it is recommended to avoid concomitant use.

Increased Effect/Toxicity There are no known significant interactions involving an increase in effect.

Decreased Effect There are no known significant interactions involving a decrease in effect.

Storage/Stability Store at room temperature.

Mechanism of Action Iodine is required for thyroid hormone synthesis. Iodine is also known to be a powerful broad spectrum germicidal agent effective against a wide range of bacteria, viruses, fungi, protozoa, and spores. Iodosorb® and Iodoflex™ contain iodine in hydrophilic beads of cadexomer which allows a slow release of iodine into the wound and absorption of fluid, bacteria, and other substances from the wound

Pharmacokinetics (Adult data unless noted)

Absorption: Topical: Amount absorbed systemically depends upon the iodine concentration and skin characteristics

Metabolism: Degraded by amylases normally present in wound fluid

Excretion: Urine (>90%)

Dosing: Usual Children and Adults:

Antiseptic for minor cuts, scrapes: Apply small amount to affected area 1-3 times/day

Cleaning wet ulcers and wounds (Iodosorb®, Iodoflex™): Apply to clean wound; maximum: 50 g/application and 150 g/week. Change dressing ~3 times/week; reduce applications as exudate decreases. Do not use for >3 months; discontinue when wound is free of exudate.

Administration Topical: Apply to affected areas; avoid tight bandages because iodine may cause burns on occluded skin.

Iodosorb®: Apply 1/8" to 1/4" thickness to dry sterile gauze, then place prepared gauze onto clean wound. Change dressing when gel changes color from brown to yellow/gray (~3 times/week). Remove with sterile water, saline, or wound cleanser; gently blot fluid from surface leaving wound slightly moist before reapplying gel.

Test Interactions Large amounts from excessive absorption may alter thyroid function tests.

Additional Information Sodium thiosulfate inactivates iodine and is an effective chemical antidote for iodine poisoning; solutions of sodium thiosulfate may be used to remove iodine stains from skin and clothing

Dosage Forms Excipient information presented when available (limited, particularly for generics); consult specific product labeling.

Tincture, External:

Generic: 2% (30 mL, 473 mL, 20000 mL); 7% (30 mL, 59 mL, 480 mL); (30 mL)

◆ **Iodine and Potassium Iodide** *see* Potassium Iodide and Iodine *on page 1742*

Iodixanol (EYE oh dix an ole)

Medication Safety Issues

High alert medication:

This medication is in a class the Institute for Safe Medication Practices (ISMP) includes among its list of drug classes that have a heightened risk of causing significant patient harm when used in error.

Administration issues:

Not for intrathecal use.

Brand Names: US Visipaque

Brand Names: Canada Visipaque

Therapeutic Category Radiological/Contrast Media, Nonionic

Generic Availability (US) No

Use Nonionic contrast media for radiological use intra-arterially: Digital subtraction angiography; angiocardiography (left ventriculography and selective coronary arteriography), peripheral arteriography, visceral arteriography, and cerebralarteriography. Intravenously: Contrast enhanced computed tomography (CECT) imaging of the head and body, excretory urography, and peripheral venography

Pregnancy Risk Factor B

Pregnancy Considerations Fetal harm was not observed in animal studies. There are no adequate and well-controlled studies in pregnant women. In general, iodinated contrast media agents are avoided during pregnancy unless essential for diagnosis.

Breast-Feeding Considerations Due to the potential for adverse reactions, temporary discontinuation of breast-feeding should be considered.

Contraindications Hypersensitivity to iodixanol or any component of the formulation; not intended for intrathecal use

In pediatric population: Prolonged fasting or laxative administration prior to iodixanol administration

Refer to product labeling for procedure-specific contraindications.

Warnings/Precautions For IV or intra-arterial use only. **[U.S. Boxed Warning]: May be fatal if given intrathecally.** May cause serious thromboembolic events including MI and stroke. Use caution with renal or hepatic dysfunction or cardiovascular disease. May worsen renal insufficiency in multiple myeloma patients. Use caution with thyroid disease; thyroid storm has been reported in patients with history of hyperthyroidism. Minimize exposure of iodixanol and monitor blood pressure closely in patients with pheochromocytoma. May promote sickling in patients with sickle cell disease. Use caution with iodine or contrast dye allergy; may cause serious and potentially fatal anaphylactoid reactions. May cause delayed reaction; monitor for 30 to 60 minutes after injection. Vesicant; ensure proper needle/catheter/line placement prior to and during administration. Avoid extravasation, particularly in patients with severe arterial or venous disease. Use with caution in elderly patients with age-related renal impairment. Children may have an increased risk of adverse effects, especially patients with asthma, sensitivity to allergens or medications, heart disease, or renal dysfunction. Clotting has been reported when blood remains in contact with syringes containing ioxilan; use of plastic syringes in place of glass syringes has been reported to decrease, but not eliminate, the likelihood of in vitro clotting.

Warnings: Additional Pediatric Considerations Use with caution in pediatric patients with asthma, hypersensitivity to other medication and/or allergens, cyanotic and acyanotic heart disease, CHF, serum creatinine >1.5 mg/dL, and neonates (immature renal function) due to an increased risk of adverse effects with iodixanol. Dehydration, particularly in children, may also increase the risk of adverse effects. Patients should be adequately hydrated both prior to and after iodixanol administration. In pediatric patients, apnea, arrhythmias (AV block, bundle branch block), cardiac failure, disseminated intravascular coagulation, and taste perversion have been reported.

Adverse Reactions

Cardiovascular: Angina/chest pain

Central nervous system: Headache/migraine, vertigo

Dermatologic: Nonurticarial rash/erythema, pruritus

Gastrointestinal: Nausea, taste perversion,

Local: Injection site reactions (discomfort/pain/warmth)

Neuromuscular & skeletal: Paresthesia

Respiratory: Parosoma

Rare but important or life-threatening: Acute renal failure, anaphylactoid reaction, anaphylaxis, apnea (children only), arrhythmia (children only), asthma, AV block (children only), back pain, bundle branch block (children only), cardiac arrest, cardiac failure (children only), cerebral vascular disorder, disseminated intravascular coagulation (children only), hematoma, hemorrhage, hypersensitivity, hypertension, hypoglycemia, hypotensive collapse, peripheral ischemia, pharyngeal edema, pulmonary edema, pulmonary embolism, respiratory depression, seizure, shock

Drug Interactions

Metabolism/Transport Effects None known.

Avoid Concomitant Use There are no known interactions where it is recommended to avoid concomitant use.

Increased Effect/Toxicity

Iodixanol may increase the levels/effects of: MetFORMIN

The levels/effects of Iodixanol may be increased by: Aldesleukin

Decreased Effect There are no known significant interactions involving a decrease in effect.

Storage/Stability Store in protective foil at room temperature of 15°C to 30°C (59°F to 86°F); do not freeze. Do not use if inadvertently frozen. Protect from light. Vials, glass and polymer bottles (**not** flexible containers) may be stored for up to 1 month at 37°C (98.6°F) in contrast agent warmer.

Mechanism of Action Opacifies vessels in the path of flow permitting radiographic imaging of internal structures.

Pharmacodynamics Following administration, the increase in tissue density is related to blood flow, the concentration of the iodixanol solution used, and the extraction of iodixanol by various interstitial tissues. The degree of enhancement is directly related to the iodine content in an administered dose.

Kidney:

Visualization: Renal parenchyma: 30-60 seconds; calyces and pelves (normal renal function): 1-3 minutes

Optimum contrast: 5-15 minutes

Pharmacokinetics (Adult data unless noted)

Distribution: V_d: Adults: 0.26 L/kg

Metabolism: Metabolites have not been identified.

Time to peak level: IV: Children: 0.75-1.25 hours

Half-life:

Newborns to Infants <2 months: 4.1 ± 1.4 hours

Infants 2-6 months: 2.8 ± 0.6 hours

Infants 6-12 months: 2.4 ± 0.4 hours

Children 1 to <3 years: 2.2 ± 0.5 hours

Children 3 to <12 years: 2.3 ± 0.5 hours

Adults: 2.1 ± 0.1 hours

Elimination: 97% excreted unchanged in the urine within 24 hours; <2% excreted in feces

Clearance: Adults: 110 mL/minute

Dialysis: Dialyzable (36% to 49% depending upon the membrane)

Dosing: Usual The concentration and volume of iodixanol to be used should be individualized depending upon age, weight, size of vessel, and rate of blood flow within the vessel.

Children >1 year:

Intra-arterial: Cerebral, cardiac chambers and related major arteries, and visceral studies: **320 mg iodine/mL**: 1-2 mL/kg; not to exceed 4 mL/kg

IV: Contrast-enhanced computerized tomography or excretory urography: **270 mg iodine/mL**: 1-2 mL/kg; not to exceed 2 mL/kg

Children >12 years and Adults: Maximum recommended total dose of iodine: 80 g

Intra-arterial: Iodixanol **320 mg iodine/mL**: Dose individualized based on injection site and study type; refer to product labeling

IV: Iodixanol **270 mg and 320 mg iodine/mL**: concentration and dose vary based on study type; refer to product labeling.

Dosage adjustment in renal impairment: Not studied; use caution

Administration IV or intra-arterial: Administer without further dilution. **Not for intrathecal administration** . Avoid extravasation.

Vesicant/Extravasation Risk Vesicant

Monitoring Parameters Monitor signs and symptoms of hypersensitivity reactions

Test Interactions Thyroid function tests (protein bound and radioactive iodine uptake studies) may be inaccurate for up to 16 days after administration; may cause false positive urine protein test using Multistix®; may affect urine specific gravity

Dosage Forms Excipient information presented when available (limited, particularly for generics); consult specific product labeling.

Solution, Intravenous:

Visipaque: 320 mg/mL (50 mL, 100 mL, 150 mL, 200 mL, 500 mL) [contains edetate calcium disodium]

Visipaque: 270 mg/mL (50 mL, 100 mL, 150 mL, 200 mL) [pyrogen free; contains edetate calcium disodium, trolamine (triethanolamine)]

Solution, Intravenous [preservative free]:

Visipaque: 320 mg/mL (50 mL) [pyrogen free; contains edetate calcium disodium]

◆ **Iodoflex** *see* Iodine *on page 1153*

Iodoquinol (eye oh doe KWIN ole)

Brand Names: US Yodoxin

Brand Names: Canada Diodoquin®

Therapeutic Category Amebicide

Generic Availability (US) No

Use Treatment of acute and chronic intestinal amebiasis due to *Entamoeba histolytica*; asymptomatic cyst passers; *Blastocystis hominis* infections; iodoquinol alone is ineffective for amebic hepatitis or hepatic abscess

Pregnancy Considerations There is very limited data on the use of iodoquinol during pregnancy and safety has not been established.

Breast-Feeding Considerations It is unknown if iodoquinol is excreted in human milk and safety during lactation has not been established.

Contraindications Hypersensitivity to iodine or iodoquinol or any component of the formulation; hepatic damage

Warnings/Precautions Discontinue use if hypersensitivity reactions occur. Optic neuritis, optic atrophy, and peripheral neuropathy have occurred following prolonged use of high doses; avoid long-term therapy. Use with caution in patients with thyroid abnormalities.

Adverse Reactions

Central nervous system: Chills, fever, headache, vertigo

Dermatologic: Pruritus, rash, skin eruptions, urticaria

Endocrine & metabolic: Thyroid gland enlargement

Gastrointestinal: Abdominal cramps, anal itching, diarrhea, nausea, vomiting

Neuromuscular & skeletal: Peripheral neuropathy

Ocular: Optic atrophy, optic neuritis

Drug Interactions

Metabolism/Transport Effects None known.

Avoid Concomitant Use There are no known interactions where it is recommended to avoid concomitant use.

Increased Effect/Toxicity There are no known significant interactions involving an increase in effect.

Decreased Effect There are no known significant interactions involving a decrease in effect.

Storage/Stability Store at 20°C to 25°C (68°F to 77°F)

Mechanism of Action Contact amebicide that works in the lumen of the intestine by an unknown mechanism

Pharmacokinetics (Adult data unless noted)

Absorption: Oral: Poor and irregular

Metabolism: In the liver

Elimination: In feces; metabolites appear in urine

Dosing: Usual Oral:

Children: 30-40 mg/kg/day in 3 divided doses for 20 days; not to exceed 1.95 g/day

Adults: 650 mg 3 times/day after meals for 20 days; not to exceed 2 g/day

Administration Oral: Administer medication after meals; tablets may be crushed and mixed with applesauce or chocolate syrup

Monitoring Parameters Ophthalmologic exam

Test Interactions May increase protein-bound serum iodine concentrations reflecting a decrease in ^{131}I uptake; false-positive ferric chloride test for phenylketonuria

Dosage Forms Excipient information presented when available (limited, particularly for generics); consult specific product labeling.

Tablet, Oral:

Yodoxin: 210 mg, 650 mg

◆ **Iodosorb** *see* Iodine *on page 1153*

◆ **Ionil [OTC]** *see* Salicylic Acid *on page 1894*

◆ **Ionil-T [OTC]** *see* Coal Tar *on page 523*

◆ **Ionsys** *see* FentaNYL *on page 857*

◆ **Iophen C-NR** *see* Guaifenesin and Codeine *on page 990*

◆ **Iophen DM-NR [OTC]** *see* Guaifenesin and Dextromethorphan *on page 992*

◆ **Iophen-NR [OTC]** *see* GuaiFENesin *on page 988*

◆ **IPOL** *see* Poliovirus Vaccine (Inactivated) *on page 1721*

Ipratropium (Oral Inhalation)

(i pra TROE pee um)

Medication Safety Issues

Sound-alike/look-alike issues:

Atrovent may be confused with Alupent, Serevent

Ipratropium may be confused with tiotropium

Brand Names: US Atrovent HFA

Brand Names: Canada Atrovent HFA; Gen-Ipratropium; Mylan-Ipratropium Sterinebs; Novo-Ipramide; Nu-Ipratropium; PMS-Ipratropium; ratio-Ipratropium UDV; Teva-Ipratropium Sterinebs

Therapeutic Category Antiasthmatic; Anticholinergic Agent; Bronchodilator

Generic Availability (US) May be product dependent

Use

Nebulization: Maintenance treatment of bronchospasm associated with chronic obstructive pulmonary disease (COPD), including chronic bronchitis and emphysema alone or in combination with bronchodilators (FDA approved in ages ≥12 years and adults); has also been used to treat bronchospasm associated with asthma and as a bronchodilating agent in bronchopulmonary dysplasia and neonatal respiratory distress syndrome

Oral inhalation: Atrovent HFA: Maintenance treatment of bronchospasm associated with chronic obstructive pulmonary disease (COPD), including chronic bronchitis and emphysema (FDA approved in adults); has also been used to treat bronchospasm associated with asthma and as a bronchodilating agent in bronchopulmonary dysplasia and neonatal respiratory distress syndrome

Pregnancy Risk Factor B

Pregnancy Considerations Teratogenic effects were not observed in animal studies. Inhaled ipratropium is recommended for use as additional therapy for pregnant women with severe asthma exacerbations.

Breast-Feeding Considerations It is not known if ipratropium (oral inhalation) is excreted in breast milk. The manufacturer recommends that caution be exercised when administering ipratropium (oral inhalation) to nursing women.

Contraindications Hypersensitivity to ipratropium, atropine (and its derivatives), or any component of the formulation

Warnings/Precautions Immediate hypersensitivity reactions (urticaria, angioedema, rash, bronchospasm) have been reported. Rarely, paradoxical bronchospasm may occur with use of inhaled bronchodilating agents; this should be distinguished from inadequate response. Not indicated for the initial treatment of acute episodes of bronchospasm where rescue therapy is required for rapid response. Should only be used in acute exacerbations of asthma in conjunction with short-acting beta-adrenergic agonists for acute episodes (NAEPP 2007). Use with caution in patients with myasthenia gravis, narrow-angle glaucoma, benign prostatic hyperplasia (BPH), or bladder neck obstruction

Adverse Reactions

Central nervous system: Dizziness, headache

Gastrointestinal: Dyspepsia, nausea, taste perversion, xerostomia

Genitourinary: Urinary tract infection

Neuromuscular & skeletal: Back pain

Respiratory: Bronchitis, COPD exacerbation, cough, dyspnea, rhinitis, sinusitis, upper respiratory infection

Miscellaneous: Flu-like syndrome

Rare but important or life-threatening: Accommodation disorder, anaphylactic reaction, angioedema, bronchospasm, corneal edema, eye pain (acute), glaucoma, hypersensitivity reactions, hypotension, intraocular pressure increased, laryngospasm, palpitations, stomatitis, tachycardia, urinary retention

Drug Interactions

Metabolism/Transport Effects None known.

Avoid Concomitant Use

Avoid concomitant use of Ipratropium (Oral Inhalation) with any of the following: Aclidinium; Anticholinergic Agents; Eluxadoline; Glucagon; Loxapine; Potassium Chloride; Tiotropium; Umeclidinium

Increased Effect/Toxicity

Ipratropium (Oral Inhalation) may increase the levels/effects of: AbobotulinumtoxinA; Analgesics (Opioid); Anticholinergic Agents; Cannabinoid-Containing Products; Eluxadoline; Glucagon; Loxapine; Mirabegron; OnabotulinumtoxinA; Potassium Chloride; RimabotulinumtoxinB; Thiazide Diuretics; Tiotropium; Topiramate

The levels/effects of Ipratropium (Oral Inhalation) may be increased by: Aclidinium; Mianserin; Pramlintide; Umeclidinium

Decreased Effect

Ipratropium (Oral Inhalation) may decrease the levels/effects of: Acetylcholinesterase Inhibitors; Itopride; Metoclopramide; Secretin

The levels/effects of Ipratropium (Oral Inhalation) may be decreased by: Acetylcholinesterase Inhibitors

Storage/Stability

Aerosol: Store at controlled room temperature of 25°C (77°F). Do not store near heat or open flame.

Solution: Store at 15°C to 30°C (59°F to 86°F). Protect from light.

Mechanism of Action Blocks the action of acetylcholine at parasympathetic sites in bronchial smooth muscle causing bronchodilation; local application to nasal mucosa inhibits serous and seromucous gland secretions.

Pharmacodynamics Bronchodilation:

Onset of action: Within 15-30 minutes

Maximum effect: Within 1-2 hours

Duration: Oral inhalation: 2-4 hours; Nebulization: 4-5 hours, up to 7-8 hours in some patients

Pharmacokinetics (Adult data unless noted)

Absorption: Not readily absorbed into the systemic circulation from the surface of the lung or from the GI tract; ~7% absorbed after nebulization of a 2 mg dose

Distribution: Following inhalation, 15% of dose reaches the lower airways

Metabolism: Partially metabolized to inactive ester hydrolysis products

Half-life: 1.6-2 hours

Elimination: Urine (50%)

Dosing: Neonatal

Bronchopulmonary dysplasia/Respiratory distress syndrome (RDS), ventilated patients: Very limited data available; optimal dose not established.

Nebulization:

Weight-based dosing: 25 mcg/kg/dose 3 times daily. Dosing based on a placebo controlled, comparative trial in 17 preterm infants (ipratropium group, n=5; EGA 25-29 weeks; PNA 19-103 days) with BPD and reported a significant decrease in respiratory resistance (Wilkie, 1987).

Fixed-dosing: Some centers have used 175 mcg/dose 3 times daily administered through the ventilator circuit; dosing based on a dose range study of 10 preterm infants with BPD (EGA 24-28 weeks, PNA 18-34 days) which showed significant reduction in respiratory resistance; additional benefit observed when administered after albuterol (Brundage, 1990).

Inhalation, MDI: 4 puffs/dose every 6-8 hours delivered as either a single dose or 2 puffs every 20 minutes for 2 inhalations. In a randomized, placebo-controlled trial in preterm neonates (n=10, PNA: 1 week; EGA: 26-34 weeks) with RDS which evaluated a single 72 mcg dose [4 puffs (18 mcg/puff product used; not currently available in the U.S.)] and reported beneficial effects on blood gases and ventilator efficiency. In another trial, which was a crossover, randomized, controlled, double-blind trial of preterm neonates (n=21, PNA: 20 ± 9 days; EGA: 27.3 ± 1.6 weeks) with RDS, a significant reduction in respiratory resistance was reported in 38% of patients after a total dose of 80 mcg [40 mcg every 20 minutes for 2 doses (20 mcg/puff product used; not currently available in the U.S.)]; higher doses [120 mcg (6 puffs)] were not shown to have additional benefit (Fayon, 2007; Lee, 1994).

Dosing: Usual

Infants, Children, and Adolescents:

Bronchospasm, wheezing: Limited data available; efficacy results variable: Infants: Nebulization: 0.125-0.25 mg (125-250 mcg) every 4 hours has been found helpful in some infants with chronic or recurrent wheezing, and some patients with bronchiolitis;

however, most bronchiolitis data suggests ipratropium is not effective (Hodges, 1981; Prendiville, 1987; Schuh, 1992; Stokes, 1983; Wang, 1992).

Asthma, acute exacerbation: Limited data available: **Note:** Ipratropium has not been shown to provide further benefit once the patient is hospitalized (NIH guidelines, 2007):

Children:

Nebulization: 0.25-0.5 mg (250-500 mcg) every 20 minutes for 3 doses, then as needed

Metered-dose inhaler: 4-8 puffs every 20 minutes as needed for up to 3 hours

Adolescents:

Nebulization: 0.5 mg (500 mcg) every 20 minutes for 3 doses, then as needed

Metered-dose inhaler: 8 puffs every 20 minutes as needed for up to 3 hours

Asthma, maintenance (nonacute): Limited data available: **Note:** Evidence is lacking that ipratropium provides added benefit to beta$_2$-agonists in long-term control asthma therapy (GINA; 2012; NIH Guidelines, 2007):

Children <12 years:

Nebulization: 0.25-0.5 mg (250-500 mcg) every 6-8 hours

Metered-dose inhaler: 1-2 inhalations every 6 hours; not to exceed 12 inhalations/day

Children ≥12 years and Adolescents:

Nebulization: 0.25 mg (250 mcg) every 6 hours

Metered-dose inhaler: 2-3 inhalations every 6 hours; maximum daily dose: 12 inhalations/**day**

Bronchospasm associated with chronic pulmonary conditions: Children ≥12 years and Adolescents: Nebulization: 0.5 mg (500 mcg, one unit-dose vial) 3-4 times daily with doses 6-8 hours apart

Adults:

Asthma exacerbation, acute (NIH Asthma Guidelines, 2007):

Nebulization: 0.5 mg (500 mcg, 1 unit dose vial) every 20 minutes for 3 doses, then as needed. **Note:** Should be given in combination with a short acting beta-adrenergic agonist.

Metered-dose inhaler: 8 inhalations every 20 minutes as needed for up to 3 hours. **Note:** Should be given in combination with a short acting beta-adrenergic agonist.

Bronchospasm associated with COPD:

Nebulization: 0.5 mg (500 mcg, one unit-dose vial) 3-4 times daily, with doses 6-8 hours apart

Metered-dose inhaler: 2 inhalations 4 times daily; maximum daily dose: 12 inhalations/**day**

Dosing adjustment in renal impairment: There are no dosage adjustments provided in the manufacturer's labeling (not studied); however, dosage adjustment unlikely necessary due to low systemic absorption.

Dosing adjustment in hepatic impairment: There are no dosage adjustments provided in the manufacturer's labeling (not studied); however, dosage adjustment unlikely necessary due to low systemic absorption.

Administration

Nebulization: May be administered with or without dilution in NS; use of a nebulizer with a mouth piece, rather than a face mask, may be preferred to prevent contact with eyes

Oral Inhalation (metered-dose inhaler): Atrovent HFA: Prior to initial use, prime inhaler by releasing 2 test sprays into the air. If the inhaler has not been used for >3 days, reprime. Avoid spraying into the eyes. Use spacer device in children <8 years; use spacer device and face mask for children ≤4 years.

Additional Information Atrovent® HFA does not contain soya lecithin or any soy ingredients like the previous formulation did. Atrovent HFA supplies 21 mcg/puff from the valve and 17 mcg/puff from the mouthpiece.

Dosage Forms Considerations Atrovent HFA 12.9 g canister contains 200 inhalations.

Dosage Forms Excipient information presented when available (limited, particularly for generics); consult specific product labeling.

Aerosol Solution, Inhalation, as bromide:

Atrovent HFA: 17 mcg/actuation (12.9 g) [contains alcohol, usp]

Solution, Inhalation, as bromide:

Generic: 0.02% (2.5 mL)

Solution, Inhalation, as bromide [preservative free]:

Generic: 0.02% (2.5 mL)

Ipratropium (Nasal) (i pra TROE pee um)

Medication Safety Issues

Sound-alike/look-alike issues:

Atrovent® may be confused with Alupent, Serevent®

Ipratropium may be confused with tiotropium

Brand Names: US Atrovent

Brand Names: Canada Alti-Ipratropium; Apo-Ipravent®; Atrovent®; Mylan-Ipratropium Solution

Therapeutic Category Anticholinergic Agent

Generic Availability (US) Yes

Use Symptomatic relief of rhinorrhea associated with allergic and nonallergic rhinitis

Pregnancy Risk Factor B

Pregnancy Considerations Teratogenic effects were not observed in animal studies.

Breast-Feeding Considerations It is not known if ipratropium (nasal) is excreted in breast milk. The manufacturer recommends that caution be exercised when administering ipratropium (nasal) to nursing women.

Contraindications Hypersensitivity to ipratropium, atropine (and its derivatives), or any component of the formulation

Warnings/Precautions Immediate hypersensitivity reactions (urticaria, angioedema, rash, bronchospasm) have been reported. Use with caution in patients with myasthenia gravis, narrow-angle glaucoma, benign prostatic hyperplasia (BPH), or bladder neck obstruction

Adverse Reactions

Central nervous system: Headache

Gastrointestinal: Diarrhea, nausea, taste perversion, xerostomia

Respiratory: Epistaxis, pharyngitis, nasal congestion, nasal dryness, nasal irritation, upper respiratory tract infection

Rare but important or life-threatening: Anaphylactic reaction, angioedema, blurred vision, conjunctivitis, cough, dizziness, hoarseness, laryngospasm, nasal burning, ocular irritation, palpitation, rash, tachycardia, thirst, tinnitus, urticaria

Drug Interactions

Metabolism/Transport Effects None known.

Avoid Concomitant Use

Avoid concomitant use of Ipratropium (Nasal) with any of the following: Aclidinium; Eluxadoline; Glucagon; Ipratropium (Oral Inhalation); Potassium Chloride; Tiotropium; Umeclidinium

Increased Effect/Toxicity

Ipratropium (Nasal) may increase the levels/effects of: AbobotulinumtoxinA; Analgesics (Opioid); Anticholinergic Agents; Cannabinoid-Containing Products; Eluxadoline; Glucagon; Mirabegron; OnabotulinumtoxinA; Potassium Chloride; RimabotulinumtoxinB; Thiazide Diuretics; Tiotropium; Topiramate

The levels/effects of Ipratropium (Nasal) may be increased by: Aclidinium; Ipratropium (Oral Inhalation); Mianserin; Pramlintide; Umeclidinium

Decreased Effect

Ipratropium (Nasal) may decrease the levels/effects of: Acetylcholinesterase Inhibitors; Itopride; Metoclopramide; Secretin

The levels/effects of Ipratropium (Nasal) may be decreased by: Acetylcholinesterase Inhibitors

Storage/Stability Store at controlled room temperature of 25°C (77°F). Do not store near heat or open flame.

Mechanism of Action Local application to nasal mucosa inhibits serous and seromucous gland secretions.

Dosing: Usual

Children >6 years and Adults: 0.03%: 2 sprays in each nostril 2-3 times/day

Children >5 years and Adults: 0.06%: 2 sprays in each nostril 3-4 times/day

Administration Pump must be primed before usage by 7 actuations into the air away from the face; if not used for >24 hours, pump must be reprimed with 2 actuations; if not used >7 days, reprime with 7 actuations

Dosage Forms Considerations Atrovent 0.03% (21 mcg/spray) nasal solution 30 mL bottles contain 345 sprays, and the 0.06% (42 mcg/spray) 15 mL bottles contain 165 sprays.

Dosage Forms Excipient information presented when available (limited, particularly for generics); consult specific product labeling.

Solution, Nasal, as bromide:

Atrovent: 0.03% (30 mL); 0.06% (15 mL)

Generic: 0.03% (30 mL); 0.06% (15 mL)

◆ **Ipratropium Bromide** *see* Ipratropium (Nasal) *on page 1157*

◆ **Ipratropium Bromide** *see* Ipratropium (Oral Inhalation) *on page 1155*

◆ **I-Prin [OTC]** *see* Ibuprofen *on page 1064*

◆ **Iproveratril Hydrochloride** *see* Verapamil *on page 2170*

◆ **IPV** *see* Poliovirus Vaccine (Inactivated) *on page 1721*

Irbesartan (ir be SAR tan)

Medication Safety Issues

Sound-alike/look-alike issues:

Avapro may be confused with Anaprox

Brand Names: US Avapro

Brand Names: Canada ACT-Irbesartan; Apo-Irbesartan; Auro-Irbesartan; Ava-Irbesartan; Avapro; Dom-Irbesartan; JAMP-Irbesartan; Mylan-Irbesartan; PMS-Irbesartan; RAN-Irbesartan; ratio-Irbesartan; Sandoz-Irbesartan; Teva-Irbesartan

Therapeutic Category Angiotensin II Receptor Blocker; Antihypertensive Agent

Generic Availability (US) Yes

Use Treatment of hypertension alone or in combination with other antihypertensives (FDA approved in adults); treatment of diabetic nephropathy in patients with type 2 diabetes mellitus (noninsulin dependent, NIDDM) and hypertension (FDA approved in adults); has also been used to reduce proteinuria in children with chronic kidney disease either as monotherapy or in addition to ACE inhibitor therapy

Pregnancy Risk Factor D

Pregnancy Considerations **[U.S. Boxed Warning]: Drugs that act on the renin-angiotensin system can cause injury and death to the developing fetus. Discontinue as soon as possible once pregnancy is detected.** The use of drugs which act on the renin-angiotensin system are associated with oligohydramnios. Oligohydramnios, due to decreased fetal renal function, may lead to fetal lung hypoplasia and skeletal malformations. Use is also associated with anuria, hypotension, renal failure, skull hypoplasia, and death in the fetus/neonate. The exposed fetus should be monitored for fetal growth, amniotic fluid volume, and organ formation. Infants exposed *in utero* should be monitored for hyperkalemia, hypotension, and oliguria (exchange transfusions or dialysis may be needed). These adverse events are generally associated with maternal use in the second and third trimesters.

Untreated chronic maternal hypertension is also associated with adverse events in the fetus, infant, and mother. The use of angiotensin II receptor blockers is not recommended to treat chronic uncomplicated hypertension in pregnant women and should generally be avoided in women of reproductive potential (ACOG, 2013).

Breast-Feeding Considerations It is not known if irbesartan is excreted into breast milk. Due to the potential for serious adverse reactions in the nursing infant, the manufacturer recommends a decision be made whether to discontinue nursing or to discontinue the drug, taking into account the importance of treatment to the mother.

Contraindications

Hypersensitivity to irbesartan or any component of the formulation; concomitant use with aliskiren in patients with diabetes mellitus

Documentation of allergenic cross-reactivity for drugs in this class is limited. However, because of similarities in chemical structure and/or pharmacologic actions, the possibility of cross-sensitivity cannot be ruled out with certainty.

Canadian labeling: Additional contraindications (not in U.S. labeling): Concomitant use with aliskiren in patients with moderate to severe renal impairment (GFR <60 mL/minute/1.73 m^2)

Warnings/Precautions **[U.S. Boxed Warning]: Drugs that act on the renin-angiotensin system can cause injury and death to the developing fetus. Discontinue as soon as possible once pregnancy is detected.** May cause hyperkalemia; avoid potassium supplementation unless specifically required by health care provider. May be associated with deterioration of renal function and/or increases in serum creatinine, particularly in patients with low renal blood flow (eg, renal artery stenosis, heart failure) whose glomerular filtration rate (GFR) is dependent on efferent arteriolar vasoconstriction by angiotensin II. Avoid use or use a much smaller dose in patients who are intravascularly volume-depleted; use caution in patients with unstented unilateral or bilateral renal artery stenosis. When unstented bilateral renal artery stenosis is present, use is generally avoided due to the elevated risk of deterioration in renal function unless possible benefits outweigh risks. AUCs of irbesartan (not the active metabolite) are about 50% greater in patients with CrCl <30 mL/minute and are doubled in hemodialysis patients. In surgical patients on chronic angiotensin receptor blocker (ARB) therapy, intraoperative hypotension may occur with induction and maintenance of general anesthesia.

Potentially significant drug interactions may exist, requiring dose or frequency adjustment, additional monitoring, and/or selection of alternative therapy.

Angioedema has been reported rarely with some angiotensin II receptor antagonists (ARBs) and may occur at any time during treatment (especially following first dose). It may involve the head and neck (potentially compromising airway) or the intestine (presenting with abdominal pain). Patients with idiopathic or hereditary angioedema or previous angioedema associated with ACE-inhibitor therapy may be at an increased risk. Prolonged frequent monitoring may be required, especially if tongue, glottis, or larynx are involved, as they are associated with airway obstruction. Patients with a history of airway surgery may have a higher risk of airway obstruction. Discontinue therapy immediately if angioedema occurs. Aggressive early management is critical. Intramuscular (IM) administration of epinephrine may be necessary. Do not readminister to patients who have had angioedema with ARBs.

Adverse Reactions

Cardiovascular: Orthostatic hypotension

Central nervous system: Dizziness, fatigue

Endocrine & metabolic: Hyperkalemia

Gastrointestinal: Diarrhea, dyspepsia

Respiratory: Cough, upper respiratory infection

Rare but important or life-threatening: Anemia (case report; Simonetti, 2007), angina, angioedema, arrhythmia, cardiopulmonary arrest, conjunctivitis, depression, dyspnea, ecchymosis, epistaxis, gout, heart failure, hepatitis, hypotension, jaundice, libido decreased, MI, orthostatic hypotension, paresthesia, renal failure, renal function impaired, sexual dysfunction, stroke, thrombocytopenia, transaminases increased, urticaria

Drug Interactions

Metabolism/Transport Effects **Substrate** of CYP2C9 (minor); **Note:** Assignment of Major/Minor substrate status based on clinically relevant drug interaction potential; **Inhibits** CYP2C8 (moderate), CYP2C9 (moderate), CYP2D6 (weak)

Avoid Concomitant Use

Avoid concomitant use of Irbesartan with any of the following: Amodiaquine

Increased Effect/Toxicity

Irbesartan may increase the levels/effects of: ACE Inhibitors; Amifostine; Amodiaquine; Antihypertensives; ARIPiprazole; Bosentan; Cannabis; Carvedilol; Ciprofloxacin (Systemic); CycloSPORINE (Systemic); CYP2C8 Substrates; CYP2C9 Substrates; Dronabinol; Drospirenone; DULoxetine; Hypotensive Agents; Levodopa; Lithium; Nonsteroidal Anti-Inflammatory Agents; Obinutuzumab; Potassium-Sparing Diuretics; RisperiDONE; RiTUXimab; Sodium Phosphates; Tetrahydrocannabinol

The levels/effects of Irbesartan may be increased by: Alfuzosin; Aliskiren; Barbiturates; Brimonidine (Topical); Canagliflozin; Dapoxetine; Diazoxide; Eplerenone; Heparin; Heparin (Low Molecular Weight); Herbs (Hypotensive Properties); MAO Inhibitors; Nicorandil; Pentoxifylline; Phosphodiesterase 5 Inhibitors; Potassium Salts; Prostacyclin Analogues; Tolvaptan; Trimethoprim

Decreased Effect

The levels/effects of Irbesartan may be decreased by: Herbs (Hypertensive Properties); Methylphenidate; Nonsteroidal Anti-Inflammatory Agents; Yohimbine

Storage/Stability Store at 25°C (77°F); excursions are permitted between 15°C and 30°C (59°F and 86°F).

Mechanism of Action Irbesartan is an angiotensin receptor antagonist. Angiotensin II acts as a vasoconstrictor. In addition to causing direct vasoconstriction, angiotensin II also stimulates the release of aldosterone. Once aldosterone is released, sodium as well as water are reabsorbed. The end result is an elevation in blood pressure. Irbesartan binds to the AT1 angiotensin II receptor. This binding prevents angiotensin II from binding to the receptor thereby blocking the vasoconstriction and the aldosterone secreting effects of angiotensin II.

Pharmacodynamics Antihypertensive effect:

Onset of action: 1-2 hours

Maximum effect: 3-6 hours postdose; with chronic dosing maximum effect: ~2 weeks

Duration: >24 hours

Pharmacokinetics (Adult data unless noted)

Absorption: Rapid and almost complete

Distribution: V_d: Adults: 53-93 L

Protein binding: 90%, primarily to albumin and $alpha_1$ acid gylcoprotein

Metabolism: Hepatic, via glucuronide conjugation and oxidation; oxidation occurs primarily by cytochrome P450 isoenzyme CYP2C9

Bioavailability: 60% to 80%

Half-life, elimination: Adults: 11-15 hours

Time to peak serum concentration: 1.5-2 hours

Elimination: Excreted via biliary and renal routes; feces (80%); urine (20%)

Dialysis: Not removed by hemodialysis

Dosing: Usual Note: Use a lower starting dose of 50% of the recommended initial dose in volume- and salt-depleted patients.

Children and Adolescents:

Hypertension: Limited data available (NHBPEP, 2004; NHLBI, 2011; Sakarcan, 2001): Oral:

Children 6-12 years: Initial: 75 mg once daily; may be titrated to a maximum dose of 150 mg once daily

Adolescents ≥13 years: Initial: 150 mg once daily; may be titrated to a maximum dose of 300 mg once daily

Proteinuria reduction in children with chronic kidney disease: Limited data available: Oral: Children and Adolescents 4-18 years: Studies utilized a fixed dosage based on weight categories (see below); initial doses were approximately 2 mg/kg once daily; doses were increased after 3-5 weeks and after 8-12 weeks if needed, according to specific blood pressure criteria; median final dose in the largest study (n=44; median age: 10 years): 4 mg/kg once daily (Franscini, 2002; Gartenmann, 2003; von Vigier, 2000)

10-20 kg: Initial: 37.5 mg once daily

21-40 kg: Initial: 75 mg once daily

>40 kg: Initial: 150 mg once daily

Adults:

Hypertension: Oral: Initial: 150 mg once daily; may be titrated to a maximum dose of 300 mg once daily; **Note:** Use a starting dose of 75 mg once daily in volume- or salt-depleted patients.

Nephropathy with type 2 diabetes and hypertension: Oral: Target dose: 300 mg once daily

Dosing adjustment in renal impairment: No dosage adjustment necessary with mild-to-severe impairment unless the patient is also volume depleted.

Dosing adjustment in hepatic impairment: No dosage adjustment is needed.

Administration May be administered without regard to food. Capsules may be opened and mixed with small amount of applesauce prior to administration (Sakaran, 2001).

Monitoring Parameters Blood pressure, BUN, serum creatinine, renal function, baseline and periodic serum electrolytes, urinalysis

Dosage Forms Excipient information presented when available (limited, particularly for generics); consult specific product labeling.

Tablet, Oral:

Avapro: 75 mg, 150 mg, 300 mg

Generic: 75 mg, 150 mg, 300 mg

Irinotecan (eye rye no TEE kan)

Medication Safety Issues

Sound-alike/look-alike issues:

Irinotecan may be confused with topotecan

High alert medication:

This medication is in a class the Institute for Safe Medication Practices (ISMP) includes among its list of drug classes which have a heightened risk of causing significant patient harm when used in error.

Related Information

Management of Drug Extravasations *on page 2298*

Prevention of Chemotherapy-Induced Nausea and Vomiting in Children *on page 2368*

Safe Handling of Hazardous Drugs *on page 2455*

Brand Names: US Camptosar

Brand Names: Canada Camptosar; Irinotecan For Injection; Irinotecan Hydrochloride Trihydrate Injection

Therapeutic Category Antineoplastic Agent, Camptothecin; Antineoplastic Agent, Topoisomerase I Inhibitor

Generic Availability (US) Yes

Use Treatment of metastatic carcinoma of the colon or rectum (FDA approved in adults); has also been used in the treatment of advanced non-small cell lung cancer, extensive state small cell lung cancer, recurrent or metastatic cervical cancer, esophageal cancer, metastatic or locally advanced gastric cancer, recurrent ovarian cancer, advanced pancreatic cancer, brain tumors (recurrent glioblastoma), and in children to treat recurrent or progressive Ewing's sarcoma, rhabdomyosarcoma, neuroblastoma, and other refractory solid tumors (IV and oral)

Pregnancy Risk Factor D

Pregnancy Considerations Adverse events were observed in animal reproduction studies. May cause fetal harm if administered during pregnancy. Women of childbearing potential should avoid becoming pregnant while receiving treatment.

Breast-Feeding Considerations It is not known if irinotecan is excreted in breast milk. Due to the potential for serious adverse reactions in the nursing infant, the manufacturer recommends a decision be made to discontinue nursing or to discontinue the drug, taking into account the importance of treatment to the mother.

Contraindications Hypersensitivity to irinotecan or any component of the formulation

Warnings/Precautions Hazardous agent - use appropriate precautions for handling and disposal (NIOSH 2014 [group 1]). Severe hypersensitivity reactions (including anaphylaxis) have occurred. Monitor closely; discontinue therapy if hypersensitivity occurs. Irinotecan is an irritant; avoid extravasation. If extravasation occurs, the manufacturer recommends flushing the external site with sterile water and applying ice.

[U.S. Boxed Warning]: Severe diarrhea may be dose-limiting and potentially fatal; early-onset and late-onset diarrhea may occur. Early diarrhea occurs during or within 24 hours of receiving irinotecan and is characterized by cholinergic symptoms; may be prevented or treated with atropine. Late diarrhea may be life-threatening and should be promptly treated with loperamide. Antibiotics may be necessary if patient develops ileus, fever, or severe neutropenia. Interrupt treatment and reduce subsequent doses for severe diarrhea. Early diarrhea is generally transient and rarely severe; cholinergic symptoms may include increased salivation, rhinitis, miosis, diaphoresis, flushing, abdominal cramping, and lacrimation; bradycardia may also occur. Cholinergic symptoms may occur more frequently with higher irinotecan doses. Late diarrhea occurs more than 24 hours after treatment, which may lead to dehydration, electrolyte imbalance, or sepsis. Late diarrhea may be complicated by colitis, ulceration, bleeding, ileus, obstruction, or infection; cases of megacolon and intestinal perforation have been reported. The median time to onset for late diarrhea is 5 days with every-3-week irinotecan dosing and 11 days with weekly dosing. Advise patients to have loperamide readily available for the treatment of late diarrhea. Patients with diarrhea should be carefully monitored and treated promptly; may require fluid and electrolyte therapy. Bowel function should be returned to baseline for at least 24 hours prior to resumption of weekly irinotecan dosing. Avoid diuretics and laxatives in patients experiencing diarrhea. Patients >65 years of age are at greater risk for early and late diarrhea. A dose reduction is recommended for patients ≥70 years of age receiving the every-3-week regimen. Irinotecan is associated with a moderate emetic potential; antiemetics are recommended to prevent nausea and vomiting (Basch, 2011; Dupuis, 2011; Roila, 2010).

[U.S. Boxed Warning]: May cause severe myelosuppression. Deaths due to sepsis following severe neutropenia have been reported. Complications due to neutropenia should be promptly managed with antibiotics. Therapy should be temporarily withheld if neutropenic fever occurs or if the absolute neutrophil count is <1,000/mm^3; reduce the dose upon recovery to an absolute neutrophil count ≥1,000/mm^3. Patients who have previously received pelvic/abdominal radiation therapy have an increased risk of severe bone marrow suppression; the incidence of grade 3 or 4 neutropenia was higher in patients receiving weekly irinotecan who have previously received pelvic/abdominal radiation therapy. Concurrent radiation therapy is not recommended with irinotecan (based on limited data). Fatal cases of interstitial pulmonary disease (IPD)-like events have been reported with single-agent and combination therapy. Risk factors for pulmonary toxicity include preexisting lung disease, use of pulmonary toxic medications, radiation therapy, and colony-stimulating factors. Patients with risk factors should be monitored for respiratory symptoms before and during irinotecan treatment. Promptly evaluate progressive changes in baseline pulmonary symptoms or any new-onset pulmonary symptoms (eg, dyspnea, cough, fever). Discontinue all chemotherapy if IPD is diagnosed.

Patients with even modest elevations in total serum bilirubin levels (1 to 2 mg/dL) have a significantly greater likelihood of experiencing first-course grade 3 or 4 neutropenia than those with bilirubin levels that were <1 mg/dL. Patients with abnormal glucuronidation of bilirubin, such as those with Gilbert's syndrome, may also be at greater risk of myelosuppression when receiving therapy with irinotecan. Use caution when treating patients with known hepatic dysfunction or hyperbilirubinemia exposure to the active metabolite (SN-38) is increased; toxicities may be increased. Dosage adjustments should be considered.

Patients homozygous for the UGT1A1*28 allele are at increased risk of neutropenia; initial one-level dose reduction should be considered for both single-agent and combination regimens. Heterozygous carriers of the UGT1A1*28 allele may also be at increased neutropenic risk; however, most patients have tolerated normal starting doses. A test is available for clinical determination of UGT phenotype, although a dose reduction is already recommended in patients who have experienced toxicity.

Renal impairment and acute renal failure have been reported, possibly due to dehydration secondary to diarrhea. Use with caution in patients with renal impairment; not recommended in patients on dialysis. Patients with bowel obstruction should not be treated with irinotecan until resolution of obstruction. Contains sorbitol; do not use in patients with hereditary fructose intolerance. Thromboembolic events have been reported. Higher rates of hospitalization, neutropenic fever, thromboembolism, first-cycle discontinuation, and early mortality were observed in patients with a performance status of 2 than in patients with a performance status of 0 or 1. Except as part of a clinical trial, use in combination with fluorouracil and leucovorin administered for 4 or 5 consecutive days ("Mayo Clinic" regimen) is not recommended due to increased toxicity. Potentially significant interactions may exist, requiring dose or frequency adjustment, additional monitoring, and/or selection of alternative therapy.

CYP3A4 enzyme inducers may decrease exposure to irinotecan and SN-38 (active metabolite); enzyme inhibitors may increase exposure; for use in patients with CNS tumors (off-label use), selection of antiseizure medications that are not enzyme inducers is preferred.

Warnings: Additional Pediatric Considerations In pediatric patients, provide antibiotic support if patient develops persistent diarrhea (grade 3 or 4), ileus, fever, sepsis, or severe neutropenia; cefixime (8 mg/kg/day, maximum dose: 400 mg) has been used in children as prophylaxis for diarrhea beginning 5 days prior to irinotecan therapy and continued throughout course (Wagner, 2008); cefpodoxime (10 mg/kg/day divided twice daily, maximum dose: 200 mg) has also been used (McNall-Knapp, 2010; Wagner, 2010).

Adverse Reactions

Cardiovascular: Edema, hypotension, thromboembolic events, vasodilation

Central nervous system: Chills, cholinergic toxicity (includes rhinitis, increased salivation, miosis, lacrimation, diaphoresis, flushing and intestinal hyperperistalsis); confusion, dizziness, fever, headache, insomnia, pain, somnolence

Dermatologic: Alopecia, rash

Endocrine & metabolic: Dehydration

Gastrointestinal: Abdominal fullness/pain, anorexia, constipation, cramps, diarrhea (early/late), dyspepsia, flatulence, mucositis, nausea, stomatitis, vomiting, weight loss

Hematologic: Anemia, hemorrhage, leukopenia, neutropenia, neutropenic fever/infection, thrombocytopenia

Hepatic: Alkaline phosphatase increased, ascites and/or jaundice, AST increased, bilirubin increased

Neuromuscular & skeletal: Back pain, weakness

Respiratory: Cough, dyspnea, pneumonia, rhinitis

Miscellaneous: Diaphoresis

Rare but important or life-threatening: ALT increased, amylase increased, anaphylactoid reaction, anaphylaxis, angina, arterial thrombosis, bleeding, bradycardia, cardiac arrest, cerebral infarct, cerebrovascular accident, circulatory failure, colitis, dysrhythmia, embolus, gastrointestinal bleeding, gastrointestinal obstruction, hepatomegaly, hyperglycemia, hypersensitivity, hyponatremia, ileus, interstitial pulmonary disease (IPD), intestinal perforation, ischemic colitis, lipase increased, lymphocytopenia, megacolon, MI, myocardial ischemia, neutropenic typhlitis, pancreatitis, paresthesia, peripheral vascular disorder, pulmonary embolus; pulmonary toxicity (dyspnea, fever, reticulonodular infiltrates on chest x-ray); renal failure (acute), renal impairment, thrombocytopenia (immune mediated), thrombophlebitis, thrombosis, typhlitis, ulcerative colitis

Note: In limited pediatric experience, dehydration (often associated with severe hypokalemia and hyponatremia) was among the most significant grade 3/4 adverse events.

Drug Interactions

Metabolism/Transport Effects Substrate of CYP2B6 (major), CYP3A4 (major), P-glycoprotein, SLCO1B1, UGT1A1; **Note:** Assignment of Major/Minor substrate status based on clinically relevant drug interaction potential

Avoid Concomitant Use

Avoid concomitant use of Irinotecan with any of the following: BCG; BCG (Intravesical); CloZAPine; Conivaptan; CYP3A4 Inducers (Strong); CYP3A4 Inhibitors (Strong); Dipyrone; Fusidic Acid (Systemic); Gemfibrozil; Grapefruit Juice; Idelalisib; Natalizumab; Pimecrolimus; St Johns Wort; Tacrolimus (Topical); Tofacitinib; UGT1A1 Inhibitors; Vaccines (Live)

Increased Effect/Toxicity

Irinotecan may increase the levels/effects of: CloZAPine; Leflunomide; Natalizumab; Tofacitinib; Vaccines (Live)

The levels/effects of Irinotecan may be increased by: Aprepitant; Bevacizumab; Conivaptan; CYP2B6 Inhibitors (Moderate); CYP3A4 Inhibitors (Moderate); CYP3A4 Inhibitors (Strong); Dasatinib; Denosumab; Dipyrone; Fosaprepitant; Fusidic Acid (Systemic); Gemfibrozil; Grapefruit Juice; Idelalisib; Ivacaftor; Luliconazole; Mifepristone; Netupitant; Palbociclib; P-glycoprotein/ABCB1 Inhibitors; Pimecrolimus; Quazepam; Regorafenib; Roflumilast; Simeprevir; SORAfenib; Stiripentol; Tacrolimus (Topical); Teriflunomide; Trastuzumab; UGT1A1 Inhibitors

Decreased Effect

Irinotecan may decrease the levels/effects of: BCG; BCG (Intravesical); Coccidioides immitis Skin Test; Sipuleucel-T; Vaccines (Inactivated); Vaccines (Live)

The levels/effects of Irinotecan may be decreased by: Bosentan; CYP2B6 Inducers (Strong); CYP3A4 Inducers (Moderate); CYP3A4 Inducers (Strong); Dabrafenib; Deferasirox; Echinacea; P-glycoprotein/ABCB1 Inducers; Siltuximab; St Johns Wort; Tocilizumab

Storage/Stability Store intact vials at 15°C to 30°C (59°F to 86°F). Protect from light; retain vials in original carton until use. Solutions diluted in NS may precipitate if refrigerated. Solutions diluted in D_5W are stable for 24 hours at room temperature or 48 hours under refrigeration at 2°C to 8°C (36°F to 46°F), although the manufacturer recommends use within 24 hours if refrigerated, or within 4 to 12 hours (manufacturer dependent; refer to specific prescribing information) at room temperature (including infusion time) only if prepared under strict aseptic conditions (eg, laminar flow hood). Do not freeze. Undiluted commercially available injectable solution prepared in oral syringes is stable for 21 days under refrigeration (Wagner, 2010).

Mechanism of Action Irinotecan and its active metabolite (SN-38) bind reversibly to topoisomerase I-DNA complex preventing religation of the cleaved DNA strand. This results in the accumulation of cleavable complexes and double-strand DNA breaks. As mammalian cells cannot efficiently repair these breaks, cell death consistent with S-phase cell cycle specificity occurs, leading to termination of cellular replication.

Pharmacokinetics (Adult data unless noted)

Distribution:
- Children and Adolescents: ~37 L/m^2 (range: 15.2-77 L/m^2) (Ma, 2000); distributes to pleural fluid, sweat, and saliva
- Adults: 33-150 L/m^2

Protein binding:
- Irinotecan: 30% to 68%
- SN-38 (active metabolite): 95%

Bioavailability: Median: 9%; increased in presence of gefitinib (median: 42%) (Furman, 2009)

Half-life, terminal:
- Children and Adolescents (Ma, 2000):
  - Irinotecan: 2.66 hours (range: 1.82-4.47 hours)
  - SN-38 (active metabolite): 1.58 hours (range: 0.29-8.28 hours)
- Adults:
  - Irinotecan: 6-12 hours
  - SN-38 (active metabolite): 10-20 hours

Time to peak serum concentration:
- Irinotecan: Oral: Children and Adolescents: 3 hours (Wagner, 2010a)
- SN-38: IV: ~1 hour following a 90-minute infusion

Metabolism: Irinotecan is converted to its active metabolite SN-38 by carboxylesterase-mediated cleavage of the carbamate bond. SN-38 undergoes conjugation by the enzyme UDP-glucuronosyl transferase 1A1 (UGT1A1) to a glucuronide metabolite in the liver. Irinotecan also undergoes oxidation by cytochrome P450 3A4 to yield to 2 inactive metabolites.

Elimination: 11% to 20% of irinotecan and <1% SN-38 is excreted in the urine; clearance in children comparable to adult rates although greater interpatient variability in pediatric patients has been reported (Ma, 2000)

Dosing: Usual Note: A reduction in the starting dose by one dose level should be considered for prior pelvic/ abdominal radiotherapy, performance status of 2, or known homozygosity for UGT1A1*28 allele. Consider premedication of atropine IV or SubQ in patients with cholinergic symptoms (eg, increased salivation, diaphoresis, abdominal cramping) or diarrhea. Details concerning dosage in combination regimens should also be consulted.

Infants, Children, and Adolescents:

Ewing's sarcoma, recurrent or progressive: Children ≥2 years and Adolescents: IV: 10-20 mg/m²/dose once daily on days 1-5 (5 doses) and days 8-12 (5 doses) every 3 weeks; in combination with temozolomide (Casey, 2009; Wagner, 2007)

Neuroblastoma, refractory or palliative: IV:

Single-agent: 50 mg/m²/dose once daily on days 1-5 (5 doses); repeat cycle every 21 days (Kushner, 2005)

Combination therapy: 10 mg/m²/dose once daily on days 1-5 (5 doses) and days 8-12 (5 doses) ever 3 weeks with temozolomide; may repeat up to 6 cycles (Bagatell, 2010)

Refractory solid tumor or CNS tumor (low-dose, protracted schedule): IV:

Single-agent: 15-20 mg/m²/dose once daily on days 1-5 (5 doses) and days 8-12 (5 doses) every 3 weeks; higher doses may be tolerated (30 mg/m²/dose) with concurrent cefpodoxime therapy (Cosetti, 2002; McGregor, 2011)

Combination therapy:

With temozolomide: Irinotecan dose: 10 mg/m²/dose once daily on days 1-5 (5 doses) and days 8-12 (5 doses) ever 3 weeks; may repeat up to 6 cycles (Bagatell, 2010)

With temozolomide and vincristine: Irinotecan dose: 15 mg/m²/dose once daily on days 1-5 (5 doses) and days 8-12 (5 doses) of a 28-day treatment cycle; may repeat cycle if tolerated (McNall-Knapp, 2010)

Refractory solid tumor or CNS tumor: Children and Adolescents:

IV:

Single-agent: 50 mg/m²/dose once daily on days 1-5 (5 doses); repeat cycle every 21 days (Kushner, 2005)

Weekly regimen (Bomgaars, 2006):

Heavily pretreated patients: 125 mg/m²/dose once weekly for 4 weeks over 90 minutes, repeat cycle every 6 weeks

Less-heavily pretreated patients: 160 mg/m²/dose once weekly for 4 weeks over 90 minutes, repeat cycle every 6 weeks

Oral: Combination therapy: 90 mg/m²/dose once daily on days 1-5 (5 doses) repeat every 3 weeks; in combination with vincristine and temozolomide (Wagner, 2010a)

Rhabdomyosarcoma, refractory or metastatic: IV:

Single-agent (Vassal, 2007):

<10 kg: 20 mg/**kg**/dose once every 3 weeks; if dosage reduction necessary, next cycle was 17 mg/kg/dose; if further dosage reduction necessary due to toxicity, subsequent cycles were 14 mg/kg/dose

≥10 kg: 600 mg/m²/dose once every 3 weeks; if dosage reduction necessary, next cycle was 500 mg/m²/dose; if further dosage reduction necessary due to toxicity, subsequent cycles were 420 mg/m²/dose

Combination therapy with vincristine:

High-dose, short schedule: 50 mg/m²/dose once daily for 5 days on weeks 1 and 4 (Mascarenhas, 2010)

Low-dose, protracted schedule: 20 mg/m²/dose once daily for 5 days followed by 2 days of rest then 20 mg/m²/dose once daily for 5 days on weeks 0, 1, 3, and 4; maximum dose: 40 mg (Pappo, 2007)

Adults:

Colorectal cancer, metastatic (single-agent therapy): IV:

Weekly regimen: 125 mg/m² over 90 minutes on days 1, 8, 15, and 22 of a 6-week treatment cycle (may adjust upward to 150 mg/m² if tolerated)

Adjusted dose level -1: 100 mg/m²

Adjusted dose level -2: 75 mg/m²

Further adjust to 50 mg/m² (in decrements of 25-50 mg/m²) if needed

Once-every-3-week regimen: 350 mg/m² over 90 minutes, once every 3 weeks

Adjusted dose level -1: 300 mg/m²

Adjusted dose level -2: 250 mg/m²

Further adjust to 200 mg/m² (in decrements of 25-50 mg/m²) if needed

Colorectal cancer, metastatic (in combination with fluorouracil and leucovorin): IV: Six-week (42-day) cycle:

Regimen 1: 125 mg/m² over 90 minutes on days 1, 8, 15, and 22; to be given in combination with bolus leucovorin and fluorouracil (leucovorin administered immediately following irinotecan; fluorouracil immediately following leucovorin)

Adjusted dose level -1: 100 mg/m²

Adjusted dose level -2: 75 mg/m²

Further adjust if needed in decrements of ~20%

Regimen 2: 180 mg/m² over 90 minutes on days 1, 15, and 29; to be given in combination with infusional leucovorin and bolus/infusion fluorouracil (leucovorin administered immediately following irinotecan; fluorouracil immediately following leucovorin)

Adjusted dose level -1: 150 mg/m²

Adjusted dose level -2: 120 mg/m²

Further adjust if needed in decrements of ~20%

Dosing adjustment in renal impairment: Adults:

Renal impairment: No dosage adjustment provided in manufacturer's labeling (has not been studied); use with caution.

Dialysis: Use in patients with dialysis is not recommended by the manufacturer; however, literature suggests reducing weekly dose from 125 mg/m² to 50 mg/m² and administering after hemodialysis or on nondialysis days (Janus, 2010).

Dosing adjustment in hepatic impairment:

Liver metastases with normal hepatic function: No adjustment required.

Bilirubin >ULN to ≤2 mg/dL: Consider reducing initial dose by one dose level.

Bilirubin >2 mg/dL: Use is not recommended.

The following guidelines have been used by some clinicians: Bilirubin 1.5-3 mg/dL: Administer 75% of dose (Floyd, 2006).

Dosing adjustment for toxicity: It is recommended that new courses begin only after the granulocyte count recovers to ≥1500/mm³, the platelet counts recover to ≥100,000/mm³, and treatment-related diarrhea has fully resolved. Depending on the patient's ability to tolerate therapy, adult doses should be adjusted in increments of 25-50 mg/m². Treatment should be delayed 1-2 weeks to allow for recovery from treatment-related toxicities. If the patient has not recovered after a 2-week delay, consider discontinuing irinotecan. See table for adult dosage recommendations.

Colorectal Cancer: Single-Agent Schedule: Recommended Adult Dosage Modifications[1]

Toxicity NCI Grade[2] (Value)	During a Cycle of Therapy	At Start of Subsequent Cycles of Therapy (After Adequate Recovery), Compared to Starting Dose in Previous Cycle[1]	
	Weekly	**Weekly**	**Once Every 3 Weeks**
No toxicity	Maintain dose level	↑ 25 mg/m² up to a maximum dose of 150 mg/m²	Maintain dose level
Neutropenia			
1 (1500-1999/mm³)	Maintain dose level	Maintain dose level	Maintain dose level
2 (1000-1499/mm³)	↓ 25 mg/m²	Maintain dose level	Maintain dose level
3 (500-999/mm³)	Omit dose until resolved to ≤ grade 2, then ↓ 25 mg/m²	↓ 25 mg/m²	↓ 50 mg/m²
4 (<500/mm³)	Omit dose until resolved to ≤ grade 2, then ↓ 50 mg/m²	↓ 50 mg/m²	↓ 50 mg/m²
Neutropenic Fever (grade 4 neutropenia and ≥ grade 2 fever)	Omit dose until resolved, then ↓ 50 mg/m²	↓ 50 mg/m²	↓ 50 mg/m²
Other Hematologic Toxicities	Dose modifications for leukopenia, thrombocytopenia, and anemia during a course of therapy and at the start of subsequent courses of therapy are also based on NCI toxicity criteria and are the same as recommended for neutropenia above.		
Diarrhea			
1 (2-3 stools/day > pretreatment)	Maintain dose level	Maintain dose level	Maintain dose level
2 (4-6 stools/day > pretreatment)	↓ 25 mg/m²	Maintain dose level	Maintain dose level
3 (7-9 stools/day > pretreatment)	Omit dose until resolved to ≤ grade 2, then ↓ 25 mg/m²	↓ 25 mg/m²	↓ 50 mg/m²
4 (≥10 stools/day > pretreatment)	Omit dose until resolved to ≤ grade 2, then ↓ 50 mg/m²	↓ 50 mg/m²	↓ 50 mg/m²
Other Nonhematologic Toxicities[3]			
1	Maintain dose level	Maintain dose level	Maintain dose level
2	↓ 25 mg/m²	↓ 25 mg/m²	↓ 50 mg/m²
3	Omit dose until resolved to ≤ grade 2, then ↓ 25 mg/m²	↓ 25 mg/m²	↓ 50 mg/m²
4	Omit dose until resolved to ≤ grade 2, then ↓ 50 mg/m²	↓ 50 mg/m²	↓ 50 mg/m²

[1]All dose modifications should be based on the worst preceding toxicity.

[2]National Cancer Institute Common Toxicity Criteria (version 1.0).

[3]Excludes alopecia, anorexia, asthenia.

Preparation for Administration Hazardous agent; use appropriate precautions for handling and disposal (NIOSH 2014 [group 1]).

Oral: In clinical pediatric trials, doses were prepared using commercially available injectable solution (20 mg/mL); doses were drawn up in oral syringes and refrigerated until ready for use; for administration, dose was mixed with cranberry grape juice (Wagner 2010; Wagner 2010a)

Parenteral: IV infusion: Dilute in D_5W (preferred) or NS to a final concentration of 0.12 to 2.8 mg/mL.

Administration Hazardous agent; use appropriate precautions for handling and disposal (NIOSH 2014 [group 1]).

Parenteral: IV infusion: Infuse usually over 90 minutes dependent upon specific protocol. Higher incidence of cholinergic symptoms have been reported with more rapid infusion rates; consider premedication with atropine and oral cephalosporin antibiotics.

Vesicant/Extravasation Risk May be an irritant

Monitoring Parameters Signs of diarrhea and dehydration, serum electrolytes, serum BUN and creatinine; infusion site for signs of inflammation; CBC with differential and platelet count, hemoglobin, liver function tests, and serum bilirubin

A test is available for genotyping of UGT1A1; however, guidelines for use are not established and not recommended in patients who have experienced toxicity as a dose reduction is already recommended (NCCN Colon Cancer Guidelines v.1.2011)

Additional Information Loperamide dosing for treatment of late diarrhea: Oral:

8-10 kg: 1 mg after the first loose bowel movement followed by 0.5 mg every 3 hours until a normal pattern of bowel movement returns. Take 0.75 mg every 4 hours during the night rather than every 3 hours.

10.1-20 kg: 1 mg after the first loose bowel movement followed by 1 mg every 3 hours until a normal pattern of bowel movement returns. Take 1 mg every 4 hours during the night rather than every 3 hours.

20.1-30 kg: 2 mg after the first loose bowel movement followed by 1 mg every 3 hours until a normal pattern of bowel movement returns. Take 2 mg every 4 hours during the night rather than every 3 hours.

30.1-43 kg: 2 mg after the first loose bowel movement followed by 1 mg every 2 hours until a normal pattern of bowel movement returns. Take 2 mg every 4 hours during the night rather than every 2 hours.

>43 kg: 4 mg after the first loose bowel movement followed by 2 mg every 2 hours until the patient is diarrhea free for 12 hours. Take 4 mg every 4 hours during the night rather than every 2 hours.

Dosage Forms Excipient information presented when available (limited, particularly for generics); consult specific product labeling.

Solution, Intravenous, as hydrochloride:

Camptosar: 40 mg/2 mL (2 mL); 100 mg/5 mL (5 mL); 300 mg/15 mL (15 mL)

Generic: 40 mg/2 mL (2 mL); 100 mg/5 mL (5 mL); 500 mg/25 mL (25 mL)

Solution, Intravenous, as hydrochloride [preservative free]:

Generic: 40 mg/2 mL (2 mL); 100 mg/5 mL (5 mL)

- ◆ **Irinotecan For Injection (Can)** *see* Irinotecan *on page 1159*
- ◆ **Irinotecan HCl** *see* Irinotecan *on page 1159*
- ◆ **Irinotecan Hydrochloride** *see* Irinotecan *on page 1159*
- ◆ **Irinotecan Hydrochloride Trihydrate Injection (Can)** *see* Irinotecan *on page 1159*
- ◆ **Iron Dextran** *see* Iron Dextran Complex *on page 1164*

Iron Dextran Complex

(EYE ern DEKS tran KOM pleks)

Medication Safety Issues

Sound-alike/look-alike issues:

Dexferrum may be confused with Desferal

Iron dextran complex may be confused with ferumoxytol

Brand Names: US Dexferrum [DSC]; Infed

Brand Names: Canada Dexiron; Infufer

Therapeutic Category Iron Salt, Parenteral; Mineral, Parenteral

Generic Availability (US) No

Use Treatment of iron deficiency when oral iron administration is infeasible or ineffective (FDA approved in children ≥4 months and adults)

Pregnancy Risk Factor C

Pregnancy Considerations Adverse events have been observed in animal reproduction studies. It is not known if iron dextran (as iron dextran) crosses the placenta. It is recommended that pregnant women meet the dietary requirements of iron with diet and/or supplements in order to prevent adverse events associated with iron deficiency anemia in pregnancy. Treatment of iron deficiency anemia in pregnant women is the same as in nonpregnant women and in most cases, oral iron preparations may be used. Except in severe cases of maternal anemia, the fetus achieves normal iron stores regardless of maternal concentrations.

Breast-Feeding Considerations Trace amounts of iron dextran (as iron dextran) are found in human milk. Iron is normally found in breast milk. Breast milk or iron fortified formulas generally provide enough iron to meet the recommended dietary requirements of infants. The amount of iron in breast milk is generally not influenced by maternal iron status.

Contraindications Hypersensitivity to iron dextran or any component of the formulation; any anemia not associated with iron deficiency

Warnings/Precautions **[U.S. Boxed Warning]: Deaths associated with parenteral administration following anaphylactic-type reactions have been reported (use only where resuscitation equipment and personnel are available). A test dose should be administered to all patients prior to the first therapeutic dose. Fatal reactions have occurred even in patients who tolerated the test dose. Monitor patients for signs/symptoms of anaphylactic reactions during any iron dextran administration; fatalities have occurred with the test dose. A history of drug allergy (including multiple drug allergies) and/or the concomitant use of an ACE inhibitor may increase the risk of anaphylactic-type reactions.** Adverse events (including life-threatening) associated with iron dextran usually occur with the high-molecular-weight formulation (Dexferrum), compared to low-molecular-weight (INFeD) (Chertow, 2006). Delayed (1-2 days) infusion reaction (including arthralgia, back pain, chills, dizziness, and fever) may occur with large doses (eg, total dose infusion) of IV iron dextran; usually subsides within 3-4 days. Delayed reaction may also occur (less commonly) with IM administration; subsiding within 3-7 days. Use with caution in patients with a history of significant allergies, asthma, serious hepatic impairment, pre-existing cardiac disease (may exacerbate cardiovascular complications), and rheumatoid arthritis (may exacerbate joint pain and swelling). Avoid use during acute kidney infection.

In patients with chronic kidney disease (CKD) requiring iron supplementation, the IV route is preferred for hemodialysis patients; either oral iron or IV iron may be used for nondialysis and peritoneal dialysis CKD patients. In patients with cancer-related anemia (either due to cancer or chemotherapy-induced) requiring iron supplementation, the IV route is superior to oral therapy; IM administration is not recommended for parenteral iron supplementation.

[U.S. Boxed Warning]: Use only in patients where the iron deficient state is not amenable to oral iron therapy. Discontinue oral iron prior to initiating parenteral iron therapy. Exogenous hemosiderosis may result from excess iron stores; patients with refractory anemias and/or hemoglobinopathies may be prone to iron overload with unwarranted iron supplementation. Anemia in the elderly is often caused by "anemia of chronic disease" or associated with inflammation rather than blood loss. Iron stores are usually normal or increased, with a serum ferritin >50 ng/mL and a decreased total iron binding capacity. IV administration of iron dextran is often preferred over IM in the elderly secondary to a decreased muscle mass and the need for daily injections. Intramuscular injections of iron-carbohydrate complexes may have a risk of delayed injection site tumor development. Iron dextran products differ in chemical characteristics. The high-molecular-weight formulation (Dexferrum) and the low-molecular-weight formulation (INFeD) are not clinically interchangeable. Intramuscular iron dextran use in neonates may be associated with an increased incidence of gram-negative sepsis.

Warnings: Additional Pediatric Considerations Use parenteral iron products with caution in premature neonates; necrotizing enterocolitis has been reported; however, no causal relationship established.

Adverse Reactions Adverse event risk is reported to be higher with the high-molecular-weight iron dextran formulation.

Cardiovascular: Arrhythmia, bradycardia, cardiac arrest, chest pain, chest tightness, cyanosis, flushing, hyper-/hypotension, shock, syncope, tachycardia

Central nervous system: Chills, disorientation, dizziness, fever, headache, malaise, seizure, unconsciousness, unresponsiveness

Dermatologic: Pruritus, purpura, rash, urticaria

Gastrointestinal: Abdominal pain, diarrhea, nausea, taste alteration, vomiting

Genitourinary: Discoloration of urine

Hematologic: Leukocytosis, lymphadenopathy

Local: Injection site reactions (cellulitis, inflammation, pain, phlebitis, soreness, swelling), muscle atrophy/fibrosis (with IM injection), skin/tissue staining (at the site of IM injection), sterile abscess

Neuromuscular & skeletal: Arthralgia, arthritis/arthritis exacerbation, back pain, myalgia, paresthesia, weakness

Respiratory: Bronchospasm, dyspnea, respiratory arrest, wheezing

Renal: Hematuria

Miscellaneous: Anaphylactic reactions (sudden respiratory difficulty, cardiovascular collapse), diaphoresis

Postmarketing and/or case reports: Angioedema, tumor formation (at former injection site)

Drug Interactions

Metabolism/Transport Effects None known.

Avoid Concomitant Use

Avoid concomitant use of Iron Dextran Complex with any of the following: Dimercaprol

Increased Effect/Toxicity

The levels/effects of Iron Dextran Complex may be increased by: ACE Inhibitors; Dimercaprol

Decreased Effect There are no known significant interactions involving a decrease in effect.

Storage/Stability Store at 20°C to 25°C (68°F to 77°F); excursions permitted to 15°C to 30°C (59°F to 86°F).

Mechanism of Action The released iron, from the plasma, eventually replenishes the depleted iron stores in the bone marrow where it is incorporated into hemoglobin

Pharmacodynamics

Onset of action: Hematologic response to either oral or parenteral iron salts is essentially the same; red blood cell form and color changes within 3-10 days

Maximum effect: Peak reticulocytosis occurs in 5-10 days, and hemoglobin values increase within 2-4 weeks; serum ferritin peak: 7-9 days after IV dose

Pharmacokinetics (Adult data unless noted)

Absorption: IM: 60% absorbed after 3 days; 90% after 1-3 weeks, the balance is slowly absorbed over months

Note: Following IV doses, the uptake of iron by the reticuloendothelial system appears to be constant at about 40-60 mg/hour

Half-life: 48 hours

Elimination: By the reticuloendothelial system and excreted in urine and feces (via bile)

Dialysis: Not dialyzable

Dosing: Neonatal IV (Dexferrum®, INFeD®): **Note: Multiple forms for parenteral iron exist; close attention must be paid to the specific product when ordering and administering**; incorrect selection or substitution of one form for another without proper dosage adjustment may result in serious over- or underdosing; test doses are recommended before starting therapy.

Anemia of prematurity: 0.2-1 mg/kg/day or 20 mg/kg/week with epoetin alfa therapy

Dosing: Usual

Multiple forms for parenteral iron exist; close attention must be paid to the specific product when ordering and administering; incorrect selection or substitution of one form for another without proper dosage adjustment may result in serious over- or underdosing; test doses are recommended before starting therapy.

Iron deficiency anemia:

IM (INFeD®), IV (Dexferrum®, INFeD®): Test dose (given 1 hour prior to starting iron dextran therapy):

Infants <10 kg: 10 mg (0.2 mL)

Children 10-20 kg: 15 mg (0.3 mL)

Children >20 kg, Adolescents, and Adults: 25 mg (0.5 mL)

Total replacement dosage of iron dextran for iron deficiency anemia:

(mL) = 0.0442 x LBW (kg) x (Hb_n - Hb_o) + [0.26 x LBW (kg)]

LBW = lean body weight

Hb_n = desired hemoglobin (g/dL) = 12 if <15 kg or 14.8 if >15 kg

Hb_o = measured hemoglobin (g/dL)

Acute blood loss; total iron replacement dosage: Assumes 1 mL of normocytic, normochromic red cells = 1 mg elemental iron

Iron dextran (mL) = 0.02 x blood loss (mL) x hematocrit (expressed as a decimal fraction)

Note: Total dose infusions have been used safely and are the preferred method of administration

IM, IV: Maximum daily dose: Injected in daily or less frequent increments:

Infants <5 kg: 25 mg (0.5 mL)

Children 5-10 kg: 50 mg (1 mL)

Children >10 kg and Adults: 100 mg (2 mL)

Anemia of chronic renal failure: IV: National Kidney Foundation DOQI Guidelines: **Note:** Initiation of iron therapy, determination of dose, and duration of therapy should be guided by results of iron status tests combined with the Hb level and the dose of the erythropoietin stimulating agent. See Reference Range for target levels. There is insufficient evidence to recommend IV iron if ferritin level >500 ng/mL.

Infants and Children: Predialysis or peritoneal dialysis: As a single dose repeated as often as necessary:

<10 kg: 125 mg

10-20 kg: 250 mg

>20 kg: 500 mg

Infants and Children: Hemodialysis: Given during each dialysis for 10 doses:

<10 kg: 25 mg

10-20 kg: 50 mg

>20 kg: 100 mg

Adults: Initial: 100 mg at every dialysis for 10 doses; maintenance: 25-100 mg once, twice, or three times/week for 10 weeks (should provide 250-1000 mg total dose within 12 weeks)

Cancer-associated anemia: Adults: IV: 25 mg slow IV push test dose, followed 1 hour later by 100 mg over 5 minutes; larger doses, up to total dose infusion (over several hours) may be administered

Preparation for Administration Parenteral: IV: May dilute large or total replacement doses in 250 to 1,000 mL NS (Burns 1995; Silverstein 2004); volumes as low as 50 mL have been used in pediatric patients (Reed 1981). Avoid dilution in dextrose due to an increased incidence of local pain and phlebitis.

Administration

Parenteral: **Note:** A test dose should be administered on the first day of therapy; observe the patient for at least 1 hour for hypersensitivity reaction, then the remainder of the day's dose (dose minus the test dose) should be administered. Resuscitation equipment, medication, and trained personnel should be available. An uneventful test dose does not ensure an anaphylactic-type reaction will not occur during administration of the therapeutic dose.

IM: Use Z-track technique for IM administration (deep into the upper outer quadrant of buttock); alternate buttocks with subsequent injections; administer test dose at same recommended site using the same technique.

IV: Test dose: Infuse test dose over at least 30 seconds (INFeD) or 5 minutes (Dexferum); doses may be injected undiluted at a rate not to exceed 50 mg/minute; large or total replacement doses may be diluted and infused over 1 to 6 hours at a maximum rate of 50 mg/minute (Silverstein 2004)

Monitoring Parameters Vital signs and other symptoms of anaphylactoid reactions (during IV infusion); reticulocyte count, serum ferritin, hemoglobin, serum iron concentrations, and transferrin saturation (TSAT). Ferritin and TSAT may be inaccurate if measured within 14 days of receiving a large single dose (1000 mg in adults).

Reference Range

Serum iron:

Newborns: 110-270 mcg/dL

Infants: 30-70 mcg/dL

Children: 55-120 mcg/dL

Adults: Male: 75-175 mcg/dL; female: 65-165 mcg/dL

Total iron binding capacity:

Newborns: 59-175 mcg/dL

Infants: 100-400 mcg/dL

Children and Adults: 230-430 mcg/dL

Transferrin: 204-360 mg/dL

Percent transferrin saturation (TSAT): 20% to 50%

Iron levels >300 mcg/dL may be considered toxic; should be treated as an overdosage

Ferritin: 13-300 ng/mL

Chronic kidney disease (CKD): Targets for iron therapy (KDOQI Guidelines, 2007) to maintain Hgb 11-12 g/dL:

Children: Nondialysis CKD, hemodialysis, or peritoneal dialysis: Ferritin: >100 ng/mL and TSAT >20%

Adults: Nondialysis (CKD) or peritoneal dialysis: Ferritin: >100 ng/mL and TSAT >20%

Hemodialysis: Ferritin >200 ng/mL and TSAT >20% or CHr (content of hemoglobin in reticulocytes) >29 pg/cell

Test Interactions May cause falsely elevated values of serum bilirubin and falsely decreased values of serum calcium. Residual iron dextran may remain in reticuloendothelial cells; may affect accuracy of examination of bone marrow iron stores. Bone scans with 99m Tc-labeled bone seeking agents may show reduced bony uptake, marked renal activity, and excess blood pooling and soft tissue accumulation following IV iron dextran infusion or with high serum ferritin levels. Following IM iron dextran, bone scans with 99m Tc-diphosphonate may show dense activity in the buttocks.

Additional Information Iron storage may lag behind the appearance of normal red blood cell morphology; use periodic hematologic determination to assess therapy

Dosage Forms Considerations Strength of iron dextran complex is expressed as elemental iron.

Dosage Forms Excipient information presented when available (limited, particularly for generics); consult specific product labeling. [DSC] = Discontinued product

Solution, Injection:

Dexferrum: 50 mg/mL (1 mL [DSC], 2 mL [DSC])

Infed: 50 mg/mL (2 mL)

◆ **Iron Fumarate** *see* Ferrous Fumarate *on page* 869

◆ **Iron Gluconate** *see* Ferrous Gluconate *on page* 870

◆ **Iron-Polysaccharide Complex** *see* Polysaccharide-Iron Complex *on page* 1728

Iron Sucrose (EYE ern SOO krose)

Medication Safety Issues

Sound-alike/look-alike issues:

Iron sucrose may be confused with ferumoxytol

Brand Names: US Venofer

Brand Names: Canada Venofer

Therapeutic Category Iron Salt, Parenteral; Mineral, Parenteral

Generic Availability (US) No

Use Treatment of iron deficiency anemia in hemodialysis-dependent chronic kidney disease (HDD-CKD) (FDA approved in ages ≥2 years and adults); treatment of iron deficiency anemia with concurrent erythropoietin therapy in peritoneal dialysis-dependent (PDD) CKD and nondialysis-dependent (NDD) CKD (FDA approved in ages ≥2 years); treatment of iron deficiency anemia in PDD-CKD and NDD-CKD (FDA approved in adults); has also been used for treatment of nonrenal iron deficiency anemia and supplementation of iron in patients for which oral therapy is neither effective nor tolerated (eg, long-term TPN)

Pregnancy Risk Factor B

Pregnancy Considerations Teratogenic effects were not observed in animal studies. There are no adequate and well-controlled studies in pregnant women. Based on limited data, iron sucrose may be effective for the treatment of iron-deficiency anemia in pregnancy. It is recommended that pregnant women meet the dietary requirements of iron with diet and/or supplements in order to prevent adverse events associated with iron deficiency anemia in pregnancy. Treatment of iron deficiency anemia in pregnant women is the same as in nonpregnant women and in most cases, oral iron preparations may be used. Except in severe cases of maternal anemia, the fetus achieves normal iron stores regardless of maternal concentrations.

Breast-Feeding Considerations Iron is normally found in breast milk. Breast milk or iron fortified formulas generally provide enough iron to meet the recommended dietary requirements of infants. The amount of iron in breast milk is generally not influenced by maternal iron status.

Contraindications Known hypersensitivity to iron sucrose or any component of the formulation

Warnings/Precautions Hypersensitivity reactions, including rare postmarketing anaphylactic and anaphylactoid reactions (some fatal), have been reported; monitor patients during and for ≥30 minutes postadministration; discontinue immediately for signs/symptoms of a hypersensitivity reaction (shock, hypotension, loss of consciousness). Equipment for resuscitation and trained personnel experienced in handling medical emergencies should always be immediately available. Significant hypotension has been reported frequently in hemodialysis-dependent patients. Hypotension has also been reported in peritoneal dialysis and nondialysis patients. Hypotension may be related to total dose or rate of administration (avoid rapid IV injection), follow recommended guidelines. Withhold iron in the presence of tissue iron overload; periodic monitoring of hemoglobin, hematocrit, serum ferritin, and transferrin saturation is recommended.

Warnings: Additional Pediatric Considerations Use parenteral iron products with caution in premature neonates; necrotizing enterocolitis has been reported; however, no causal relationship established.

Adverse Reactions Events are associated with use in adults unless otherwise specified.

Cardiovascular: Arteriovenous fistula thrombosis (children), chest pain, hyper-/hypotension, peripheral edema

Central nervous system: Dizziness, fever, headache

Dermatologic: Pruritus

Endocrine & metabolic: Fluid overload, gout, hyper-/hypoglycemia

Gastrointestinal: Abdominal pain, diarrhea, nausea, peritonitis (children), vomiting, taste perversion

Local: Injection site reaction

Neuromuscular & skeletal: Arthralgia, back pain, extremity pain, muscle cramps, myalgia, weakness

Ocular: Conjunctivitis

Otic: Ear pain

Respiratory: Cough, dyspnea, nasal congestion, nasopharyngitis, pharyngitis, sinusitis, upper respiratory infection

Miscellaneous: Graft complication, sepsis

Rare but important or life-threatening: Anaphylactic shock, anaphylactoid reactions, angioedema, bradycardia, cardiovascular collapse, hypersensitivity (including wheezing), loss of consciousness, necrotizing enterocolitis (reported in premature infants, no causal relationship established), seizure, shock, urine discoloration

Drug Interactions

Metabolism/Transport Effects None known.

Avoid Concomitant Use

Avoid concomitant use of Iron Sucrose with any of the following: Dimercaprol

Increased Effect/Toxicity

The levels/effects of Iron Sucrose may be increased by: Dimercaprol

Decreased Effect There are no known significant interactions involving a decrease in effect.

Storage/Stability Store intact vials at controlled room temperature of 20°C to 25°C (68°F to 77°F); excursions permitted to 15°C to 30°C (59°F to 86°F); do not freeze. Iron sucrose is stable for 7 days at room temperature (23°C to 27°C [73°F to 81°F]) or under refrigeration (2°C to 6°C [36°F to 43°F]) when undiluted in a plastic syringe or following dilution in normal saline in a plastic syringe (concentration 2-10 mg/mL) or for 7 days at room temperature (23°C to 27°C [73°F to 81°F]) following dilution in normal saline in an IV bag (concentration 1-2 mg/mL).

Mechanism of Action Iron sucrose is dissociated by the reticuloendothelial system into iron and sucrose. The released iron increases serum iron concentrations and is incorporated into hemoglobin.

Pharmacodynamics

Onset of action: Hematologic response to either oral or parenteral iron salts is essentially the same; red blood cell form and color changes within 3-10 days

Maximum effect: Peak reticulocytosis occurs in 5-10 days, and hemoglobin values increase within 2-4 weeks

Pharmacokinetics (Adult data unless noted) Following IV doses, the uptake of iron by the reticuloendothelial system appears to be constant at about 40-60 mg/hour

Distribution: V_{dss}: Healthy adults: 7.9 L

Metabolism: Dissociated into iron and sucrose by the reticuloendothelial system

Half-life: Adolescents (nondialysis-dependent): 8 hours; adults: 6 hours

Elimination: Healthy adults: Urine (5%) within 24 hours

Dialysis: Not dialyzable

Dosing: Neonatal Multiple forms for parenteral iron exist; close attention must be paid to the specific product when ordering and administering; incorrect selection or substitution of one form for another without proper dosage adjustment may result in serious over- or under-dosing. Doses are expressed as mg of **elemental iron**.

Anemia of prematurity: Limited data available: IV: 1 mg/kg/**day** infused over 2 hours; dosing based on results of a small comparative trial with oral iron therapy and erythropoietin which included 29 premature neonates (GA <31 weeks; treatment group, n=10) who at the time of treatment initiation had a mean age of 23.3 ± 2.9 days, and mean weight of 1266 ± 81 g; higher reticulocyte counts and fewer transfusions were observed in the parenteral iron group compared to the oral treatment arm; due to potential oxidative injury risk in smaller, less stable premature neonates, the authors suggest that lower doses should be considered (Pollock, 2001; Pollock, 2001a).

Dosing: Usual Multiple forms for parenteral iron exist; close attention must be paid to the specific product when ordering and administering; incorrect selection or substitution of one form for another without proper dosage adjustment may result in serious over- or underdosing. Doses are expressed as mg of **elemental iron**. **Note:** Per National Kidney Foundation DOQI Guidelines, initiation of iron therapy, determination of dose, and duration of therapy should be guided by results of iron status tests combined with the Hb level and the dose of the erythropoietin stimulating agent. See Reference Range for target levels. There is insufficient evidence to recommend IV iron if ferritin level >500 ng/mL.

Infants, Children, and Adolescents:

Iron deficiency anemia in CKD:

Repletion treatment: Limited data available: Children ≥2 years and Adolescents <15 years: IV: 1 mg/kg/dialysis; dosing based on a dose-finding trial in 14 pediatric patients and successfully increased ferritin therapeutic levels; iron overload (serum ferritin >400 ng/mL) was reported with the higher dose used in the study (3 mg/kg/dialysis) (Leijn, 2004)

Maintenance therapy: Children ≥2 years and Adolescents: IV:

Hemodialysis-dependent CKD: 0.5 mg/kg/dose (maximum dose: 100 mg) every 2 weeks for 12 weeks (6 doses); may repeat if clinically indicated

Peritoneal dialysis-dependent CKD; concurrent erythropoietin therapy: 0.5 mg/kg/dose (maximum dose: 100 mg) every 4 weeks for 12 weeks (3 doses); may repeat if clinically indicated

Nondialysis-dependent CKD; concurrent erythropoietin therapy: 0.5 mg/kg/dose (maximum dose: 100 mg) every 4 weeks for 12 weeks (3 doses); may repeat if clinically indicated

Nonrenal iron deficiency anemia; treatment in patients refractory to oral therapy (eg, long-term TPN, GI malabsorption): Limited data available (Norman, 2011; Pinsk, 2008):

Calculate Iron Deficit: Total replacement dose (mg of iron) = 0.6 x weight (kg) x [100 - (actual Hgb /12 x 100)]; **Note:** In this equation, 12 is the desired target Hgb concentration; in some patients, a different target may be required.

Initial dose: IV: 5-7 mg/kg; maximum dose: 100 mg

Maintenance dose: IV: 5-7 mg/kg every 1-7 days until total replacement dose achieved; maximum single dose: 300 mg

Adults: **Iron deficiency anemia in CKD:** IV:

Hemodialysis-dependent CKD: 100 mg administered during consecutive dialysis sessions to a cumulative total dose of 1000 mg (10 doses); may repeat treatment if clinically indicated

Peritoneal dialysis-dependent CKD: Two infusions of 300 mg administered 14 days apart, followed by a single 400 mg infusion 14 days later (total cumulative dose of 1000 mg in 3 divided doses); may repeat treatment if clinically indicated

Nonhemodialysis-dependent CKD: 200 mg administered on 5 different occasions within a 14-day period; cumulative total dose: 1000 mg in 14-day period. **Note:** Dosage has also been administered as two infusions of 500 mg in a maximum of 250 mL normal saline infused over 3.5-4 hours on day 1 and day 14 (limited experience); may repeat treatment if clinically indicated

Preparation for Administration Parenteral: Avoid dilution in dextrose containing solutions due to an increased incidence of local pain and phlebitis.

Premature neonates: Infusion: Dilute dose to 2 mg/mL in NS (Pollak 2001)

Infants, Children, and Adolescents: Dependent upon indication:

CKD treatment of iron deficiency anemia: May administer undiluted or diluted in 25 mL of NS. Do not dilute to concentrations <1 mg/mL.

Nonrenal treatment of iron deficiency anemia: One trial reported dilution of iron dose to a final concentration of 1 mg/mL in NS (Pinsk 2008)

Others suggest the following recommendations (Norman 2011):

For doses ≤100 mg, dilute dose in 100 mL NS

For doses >100 mg and ≤200 mg, dilute dose in 200 mL NS

For doses >200 mg and ≤300 mg, dilute dose in 250 mL NS

Adults: Doses ≤200 mg may be administered undiluted or diluted in a maximum of 100 mL NS. Doses >200 mg should be diluted in a maximum of 250 mL NS. Do not dilute to concentrations <1 mg/mL.

Administration Parenteral: May administer IV; not for IM use.

Pediatric patients:

Premature neonates: Infusion: Infuse over at least 2 hours (Pollak 2001)

Infants, Children, and Adolescents: Dependent upon indication:

CKD treatment of iron deficiency anemia:

Slow IV injection: Administer undiluted over 5 minutes

Infusion: Dilute and infuse over 5 to 60 minutes

Nonrenal treatment of iron deficiency anemia: One trial reported infusion of a diluted 1 mg/mL solution at 1 to 1.3 mL/minute (Pinsk 2008)

Others suggest the following recommendations (Norman 2011):

For doses ≤100 mg, infuse over at least 30 minutes

For doses >100 mg and ≤200 mg, infuse over at least 60 minutes

For doses >200 mg and ≤300 mg, infuse over at least 90 minutes

Adults:

Slow IV injection: May administer doses ≤200 mg undiluted by slow IV injection over 2 to 5 minutes; when administering to hemodialysis-dependent patients, give iron sucrose early during the dialysis session

Infusion: Infuse diluted doses ≤200 mg over at least 15 minutes; infuse diluted 300 mg dose over 1.5 hours; infuse diluted 400 mg dose over 2.5 hours; infuse diluted 500 mg dose over 3.5 to 4 hours (limited experience). When administering to hemodialysis-dependent patients, give iron sucrose early during the dialysis session.

Monitoring Parameters Hematocrit, hemoglobin, serum ferritin, transferrin, percent transferrin saturation, TIBC; takes about 4 weeks of treatment to see increased serum iron and ferritin, and decreased TIBC. Serum iron concentrations should be drawn ≥48 hours after last dose (due to rapid increase in values following administration); signs/ symptoms of hypersensitivity reactions (during and ≥30 minutes following infusion); hypotension (following infusion).

Reference Range

Serum iron:
- Newborns: 110-270 mcg/dL
- Infants: 30-70 mcg/dL
- Children: 55-120 mcg/dL
- Adults: Male: 75-175 mcg/dL; female: 65-165 mcg/dL

Total iron binding capacity:
- Newborns: 59-175 mcg/dL
- Infants: 100-400 mcg/dL
- Children and Adults: 230-430 mcg/dL

Transferrin: 204-360 mg/dL

Percent transferrin saturation (TSAT): 20% to 50%

Iron levels >300 mcg/dL may be considered toxic; should be treated as an overdosage

Ferritin: 13-300 ng/mL

Chronic kidney disease (CKD): Targets for iron therapy (KDOQI Guidelines, 2007) to maintain Hgb 11-12 g/dL:
- Children: Nondialysis CKD, hemodialysis, or peritoneal dialysis: Ferritin: >100 ng/mL and TSAT >20%
- Adults: Nondialysis (CKD) or peritoneal dialysis: Ferritin: >100 ng/mL and TSAT >20%
  - Hemodialysis: Ferritin >200 ng/mL and TSAT >20% or CHr (content of hemoglobin in reticulocytes) >29 pg/cell

Additional Information Contains sucrose: 300 mg/mL

Dosage Forms Considerations Strength of iron sucrose is expressed as elemental iron.

Dosage Forms Excipient information presented when available (limited, particularly for generics); consult specific product labeling.

Solution, Intravenous [preservative free]:
- Venofer: 20 mg/mL (2.5 mL, 5 mL, 10 mL)

- ◆ **Iron Sulfate** *see* Ferrous Sulfate *on page 871*
- ◆ **Iron Supplement Childrens [OTC]** *see* Ferrous Sulfate *on page 871*
- ◆ **Isagel [OTC]** *see* Alcohol (Ethyl) *on page 86*
- ◆ **Isentress** *see* Raltegravir *on page 1833*
- ◆ **ISG** *see* Immune Globulin *on page 1089*
- ◆ **Isoamyl Nitrite** *see* Amyl Nitrite *on page 162*

Isoniazid (eye soe NYE a zid)

Medication Safety Issues

International issues:

Hydra [Japan] may be confused with Hydrea brand name for hydroxyurea [U.S., Canada, and multiple international markets]

Brand Names: Canada Dom-Isoniazid; Isotamine; PDP-Isoniazid

Therapeutic Category Antitubercular Agent

Generic Availability (US) Yes

Use Treatment of susceptible mycobacterial infection due to *M. tuberculosis* and prophylactically to those individuals exposed to tuberculosis (FDA approved in infant, children, and adults)

Pregnancy Risk Factor C

Pregnancy Considerations Adverse events were observed in some animal reproduction studies. Isoniazid crosses the human placenta. Due to the risk of tuberculosis to the fetus, treatment is recommended when the probability of maternal disease is moderate to high. The CDC recommends isoniazid as part of the initial treatment regimen. Pyridoxine supplementation is recommended (25 mg/day) (CDC, 2003). Due to biologic changes during pregnancy and early postpartum, pregnant women may have increased susceptibility to tuberculosis infection or reactivation of latent disease (Mathad, 2012).

Breast-Feeding Considerations Small amounts of isoniazid are excreted in breast milk; concentrations are considered nontoxic and not therapeutic to the nursing infant. Women with tuberculosis taking isoniazid should not be discouraged from breast-feeding. Pyridoxine supplementation is recommended for the mother and infant (CDC, 2003). Women with tuberculosis mastitis should breast-feed using the unaffected breast (Mathad, 2012). In the United States, breast-feeding is not recommended for women with tuberculosis who are also coinfected with HIV (DHHS [adult], 2014).

Contraindications Hypersensitivity to isoniazid or any component of the formulation, including drug-induced hepatitis; acute liver disease; previous history of hepatic injury during isoniazid therapy; previous severe adverse reaction (drug fever, chills, arthritis) to isoniazid

Warnings/Precautions Use with caution in patients with severe renal impairment and liver disease. **[U.S. Boxed Warning]: Severe and sometimes fatal hepatitis may occur; usually occurs within the first 3 months of treatment, although may develop even after many months of treatment.** The risk of developing hepatitis is age-related, although isoniazid-induced hepatotoxicity has been reported in children; daily ethanol consumption, chronic liver disease, or injection drug use may also increase the risk. Contraindicated in patients with acute liver disease or previous isoniazid-associated hepatic injury. Fatal hepatitis associated with isoniazid may be increased in women (particularly black and Hispanic and in any woman in the postpartum period). Closer monitoring may be considered in these groups. Patients given isoniazid must be monitored carefully and interviewed at monthly intervals. Patients must report any prodromal symptoms of hepatitis, such as fatigue, paresthesias of hands and feet, weakness, dark urine, rash, anorexia, nausea, fever >3 days' duration, and/or abdominal pain (especially right upper quadrant discomfort), icterus, or vomiting. Patients should be instructed to immediately hold therapy if any of these symptoms occur, and contact their prescriber. If abnormalities of liver function exceed 3 to 5 times the upper limit of normal (ULN), strongly consider discontinuation of isoniazid. If isoniazid must be reinstituted, wait for symptoms and laboratory abnormalities to resolve and use very small and gradual increasing doses, withdrawing therapy immediately if an indication of recurrent hepatic involvement. Treatment with isoniazid for latent tuberculosis infection should be deferred in patients with acute hepatic diseases. Periodic ophthalmic examinations are recommended even when usual symptoms do not occur. Potentially significant drug interactions may exist, requiring dose or frequency adjustment, additional monitoring, and/or selection of alternative therapy. Use should be carefully monitored in the following groups: Daily users of alcohol, active chronic liver disease, severe renal dysfunction, age >35 years, concurrent use of any chronically administered drug, history of previous isoniazid discontinuation, existence of or conditions predisposing to peripheral neuropathy, pregnancy, injection drug use, women in minority groups (particularly postpartum), HIV seropositive patients. AST and ALT should be obtained at baseline and at least monthly during LTBI use. Discontinue temporarily or permanently if liver function tests >3 to 5 times ULN. Pyridoxine (10 to 50 mg/day) is recommended in individuals at risk for development of peripheral neuropathies (eg, HIV infection, nutritional deficiency, diabetes, pregnancy). Children with low milk and low meat intake should receive concomitant pyridoxine therapy. Multidrug regimens should be utilized for the treatment of active tuberculosis to prevent the emergence of drug resistance.

Adverse Reactions

Cardiovascular: Hypertension, palpitation, tachycardia, vasculitis

Central nervous system: Depression, dizziness, encephalopathy, fever, lethargy, memory impairment, psychosis, seizure, slurred speech, toxic encephalopathy

Dermatologic: Flushing, rash (morbilliform, maculopapular, pruritic, or exfoliative)

Endocrine & metabolic: Gynecomastia, hyperglycemia, metabolic acidosis, pellagra, pyridoxine deficiency

Gastrointestinal: Anorexia, epigastric distress, nausea, stomach pain, vomiting

Hematologic: Agranulocytosis, anemia (sideroblastic, hemolytic, or aplastic), eosinophilia, thrombocytopenia

Hepatic: Bilirubinuria, hepatic dysfunction, hepatitis (may involve progressive liver damage; risk increases with age), hyperbilirubinemia, jaundice, LFTs mildly increased

Neuromuscular & skeletal: Arthralgia, hyper-reflexia, paresthesia, peripheral neuropathy (dose-related incidence), weakness

Ocular: Blurred vision, loss of vision, optic neuritis/atrophy

Miscellaneous: Lupus-like syndrome, lymphadenopathy, rheumatic syndrome

Drug Interactions

Metabolism/Transport Effects Substrate of CYP2E1 (major); **Note:** Assignment of Major/Minor substrate status based on clinically relevant drug interaction potential; **Inhibits** CYP1A2 (weak), CYP2A6 (moderate), CYP2C19 (moderate), CYP2C9 (weak), CYP2D6 (moderate), CYP2E1 (moderate), CYP3A4 (weak); **Induces** CYP2E1 (weak/moderate)

Avoid Concomitant Use

Avoid concomitant use of Isoniazid with any of the following: Artesunate; Pimozide; Tegafur; Thioridazine

Increased Effect/Toxicity

Isoniazid may increase the levels/effects of: Acetaminophen; ARIPiprazole; Artesunate; CarBAMazepine; Chlorzoxazone; Cilostazol; Citalopram; CycloSERINE; CYP2A6 Substrates; CYP2C19 Substrates; CYP2D6 Substrates; CYP2E1 Substrates; Dofetilide; DOXOrubicin (Conventional); Eliglustat; Fesoterodine; Fosphenytoin; Hydrocodone; Lomitapide; Metoprolol; Nebivolol; NiMODipine; Phenytoin; Pimozide; Theophylline Derivatives; Thioridazine; TiZANidine

The levels/effects of Isoniazid may be increased by: Disulfiram; Ethionamide; Propafenone; Rifamycin Derivatives

Decreased Effect

Isoniazid may decrease the levels/effects of: Artesunate; Clopidogrel; Codeine; Itraconazole; Ketoconazole (Systemic); Levodopa; Tamoxifen; Tegafur; TraMADol

The levels/effects of Isoniazid may be decreased by: Antacids; Corticosteroids (Systemic); Cyproterone

Food Interactions

Isoniazid may decrease folic acid absorption and alters pyridoxine metabolism. Management: Increase dietary intake of folate, niacin, and magnesium.

Tyramine-containing food: Isoniazid has weak monoamine oxidase inhibiting activity and may potentially inhibit tyramine metabolism. Several case reports of mild reactions (flushing, palpitations, headache, mild increase in blood pressure, diaphoresis) after ingestion of certain types of cheese or red wine, have been reported (Self, 1999; Toutoungi, 1985). Management: Manufacturer's labeling recommends avoiding tyramine-containing foods (eg, aged or matured cheese, air-dried or cured meats including sausages and salamis; fava or broad bean pods, tap/draft beers, Marmite concentrate, sauerkraut, soy sauce, and other soybean condiments). However, the clinical relevance of the tyramine reaction for the vast majority of patients receiving isoniazid has been questioned due to isoniazid's weak MAO inhibition and the relatively few published case reports of the interaction. Although not fully investigated, it has been proposed that the reaction has a genetic component and may only be significant in poor or intermediate acetylators since isoniazid is primarily inactivated by acetylation (DiMartini, 1995; Toutoungi, 1985).

Histamine-containing food: Isoniazid may also inhibit diamine oxidase resulting in headache, sweating, palpitations, flushing, diarrhea, itching, wheezing, dyspnea or hypotension to histamine-containing foods (eg, skipjack, tuna, saury, other tropical fish). Management: Manufacturer's labeling recommends avoiding histamine-containing foods; corticosteroids and antihistamines may be administered if histamine intoxication occurs (Miki, 2005).

Storage/Stability

Tablet: Store at 20°C to 25°C (68°F to 77°F). Protect from light.

Oral solution: Store at 15°C to 30°C (59°F to 86°F). Protect from light.

Injection: Store at 20°C to 25°C (68°F to 77°F). Protect from light. Isoniazid injection may crystallize at low temperatures. If this occurs, warm the vial to room temperature before use to redissolve the crystals.

Mechanism of Action Isoniazid inhibits the synthesis of mycoloic acids, an essential component of the bacterial cell wall. At therapeutic levels isoniazid is bacteriocidal against actively growing intracellular and extracellular *Mycobacterium tuberculosis* organisms.

Pharmacokinetics (Adult data unless noted)

Absorption: Oral, IM: Rapid and complete; food reduces rate and extent of absorption

Distribution: Crosses the placenta; distributes into most body tissues and fluids, including the CSF

Protein binding: 10% to 15%

Metabolism: By the liver to acetylisoniazid with decay rate determined genetically by acetylation phenotype; undergoes further hydrolysis to isonicotinic acid and acetylhydrazine

Half-life: May be prolonged in patients with impaired hepatic function or severe renal impairment

- Fast acetylators: 30-100 minutes
- Slow acetylators: 2-5 hours

Time to peak serum concentration: Oral: Within 1-2 hours

Elimination: 75% to 95% excreted in urine as unchanged drug and metabolites; small amounts excreted in feces and saliva

Dialysis: Dialyzable (50% to 100%)

Dosing: Usual Oral, IM; **Note:** Recommendations often change due to resistant strains and newly developed information; consult *MMWR* for current CDC recommendations. Intramuscular injection is available for patients who are unable to either take or absorb oral therapy.

Infants, Children <40 kg, and Adolescents ≤14 years and <40 kg:

Treatment of active TB infection: CDC Recommendations: 10-15 mg/kg/day once daily (maximum dose: 300 mg/day) **or** 20-30 mg/kg/dose (maximum dose: 900 mg) twice weekly as part of a multidrug regimen (*MMWR*, 2003)

Treatment of latent TB infection (LTBI): 10-20 mg/kg/day given once daily (maximum dose: 300 mg/day) **or** 20-40 mg/kg/dose (maximum dose: 900 mg) twice weekly; treatment duration: 9 months

Primary prophylaxis for TB in HIV-exposed/positive patients: 10-15 mg/kg/day once daily (maximum dose: 300 mg/day) **or** 20-30 mg/kg/dose (maximum dose: 900 mg) twice weekly; treatment duration: 9 months

Children and Adolescents >40 kg or Adolescents ≥15 years: See Adult Dosing

Adults:

Treatment of latent tuberculosis infection (LTBI): Oral, IM: CDC recommendations: 5 mg/kg (maximum: 300 mg/dose) once daily or 15 mg/kg (maximum: 900 mg/dose) twice weekly by directly observed therapy (DOT) for 6-9 months in patients who do not have HIV infection (9 months is optimal, 6 months may be considered to reduce costs of therapy) and 9 months in patients who have HIV infection. Extend to 12 months of therapy if interruptions in treatment occur (*MMWR*, 2000)

Treatment of active TB infection (drug susceptible): Oral, IM:

Daily therapy: CDC recommendations: 5 mg/kg/day once daily (usual dose: 300 mg/day) (*MMWR*, 2003)

Directly observed therapy (DOT): CDC recommendations: 15 mg/kg (maximum: 900 mg/dose) twice weekly or 3 times/week; **Note:** CDC guidelines state that once-weekly therapy (15 mg/kg/dose) may be considered, but only after the first 2 months of initial therapy in HIV-negative patients, and only in combination with rifapentine (*MMWR*, 2003).

Note: Treatment may be defined by the number of doses administered (eg, "6-month" therapy involves 182 doses of INH and rifampin, and 56 doses of pyrazinamide). Six months is the shortest interval of time over which these doses may be administered, assuming no interruption of therapy.

Note: Concomitant administration of 10-50 mg/day pyridoxine is recommended in malnourished patients or those prone to neuropathy (eg, alcoholics, patients with diabetes).

Dosing adjustment in renal impairment: No dosage adjustment needed in patients with renal impairment.

Administration

Oral: Administer 1 hour before or 2 hours after meals with water; administration of isoniazid syrup has been associated with diarrhea

Parenteral: IM: Administer IM when oral therapy is not possible; injection solution pH: 6-7

Monitoring Parameters Periodic liver function tests; monitor for prodromal signs of hepatitis; ophthalmologic exam; chest x-ray

LTBI therapy: American Thoracic Society/Centers for Disease Control (ATS/CDC) recommendations: Monthly clinical evaluation, including brief physical exam for adverse events. Baseline serum AST or ALT and bilirubin should be considered for patients at higher risk for adverse events (eg, history of liver disease, chronic ethanol use, HIV-infected patients, women who are pregnant or postpartum ≤3 months, older adults with concomitant medications or diseases). Routine, periodic monitoring is recommended for any patient with an abnormal baseline or at increased risk for hepatoxicity.

Test Interactions False-positive urinary glucose with Clinitest®

Additional Information

Prophylactic use is recommended for patients with ≥5 mm positive tuberculin skin test reaction who are HIV-positive or persons with risk factors for HIV infection; close contacts of newly diagnosed person with infectious tuberculosis; persons with fibrotic changes on chest XR suggestive of previous tuberculosis or inadequate treatment; persons with organ transplants or receiving immunosuppressive therapy

Prophylactic use is recommended for patients with ≥10 mm positive tuberculin skin test reaction who recently arrived (<5 years) from endemic areas; substance abusers; residents/employees of healthcare, correctional, or long-term care facilities; children <4 years; children and adolescents exposed to high-risk adults; persons at high-risk due to certain medical conditions like silicosis, diabetes mellitus, leukemia, end-stage renal disease, chronic malabsorption syndrome, cancer of head and neck, intestinal bypass or gastrectomy, and low body weight

Dosage Forms Excipient information presented when available (limited, particularly for generics); consult specific product labeling.

Solution, Injection:

Generic: 100 mg/mL (10 mL)

Syrup, Oral:

Generic: 50 mg/5 mL (473 mL)

Tablet, Oral:

Generic: 100 mg, 300 mg

Extemporaneous Preparations Note: Commercial oral solution is available (50 mg/mL)

A 10 mg/mL oral suspension may be made with tablets, purified water, and sorbitol. Crush ten 100 mg tablets in a mortar and reduce to a fine powder. Add 10 mL of purified water and mix to a uniform paste. Mix while adding sorbitol in incremental proportions to **almost** 100 mL; transfer to a graduated cylinder, rinse mortar with sorbitol, and add quantity of sorbitol sufficient to make 100 mL (do not use sugar-based solutions). Label "shake well" and "refrigerate". Stable for 21 days refrigerated.

Nahata MC, Pai VB, and Hipple TF, *Pediatric Drug Formulations*, 5th ed, Cincinnati, OH: Harvey Whitney Books Co, 2004.

◆ **Isonicotinic Acid Hydrazide** *see* Isoniazid *on page 1168*

◆ **Isonipecaine Hydrochloride** *see* Meperidine *on page 1359*

◆ **Isophane Insulin** *see* Insulin NPH *on page 1138*

◆ **Isophane Insulin and Regular Insulin** *see* Insulin NPH and Insulin Regular *on page 1141*

◆ **Isophosphamide** *see* Ifosfamide *on page 1075*

Isoproterenol (eye soe proe TER e nole)

Medication Safety Issues

Sound-alike/look-alike issues:

Isuprel® may be confused with Disophrol®, Isordil®

High alert medication:

The Institute for Safe Medication Practices (ISMP) includes this medication among its list of drugs which have a heightened risk of causing significant patient harm when used in error.

Related Information

Emergency Drip Calculations *on page 2229*

Brand Names: US Isuprel

Therapeutic Category Adrenergic Agonist Agent; Antiasthmatic; $Beta_1$ & $Beta_2$-Adrenergic Agonist Agent; Bronchodilator; Sympathomimetic

Generic Availability (US) No

Use Treatment of asthma or COPD (reversible airway obstruction); ventricular arrhythmias due to A-V nodal block; hemodynamically compromised bradyarrhythmias or atropine-resistant bradyarrhythmias, temporary use in third degree A-V block until pacemaker insertion; low cardiac output or vasoconstrictive shock states

Pregnancy Risk Factor C

Pregnancy Considerations Animal reproduction studies have not been conducted by the manufacturer. Use of isoproterenol may interfere with uterine contractions at term (Mahon, 1967).

Breast-Feeding Considerations It is not known if isoproterenol is excreted in breast milk. The manufacturer recommends that caution be exercised when administering isoproterenol to nursing women.

Contraindications Angina, pre-existing ventricular arrhythmias, tachyarrhythmias; cardiac glycoside intoxication

Warnings/Precautions Use with extreme caution; not currently a treatment of choice; use with caution in elderly patients, patients with diabetes, cardiovascular disease, or hyperthyroidism; excessive or prolonged use may result in decreased effectiveness. Contains sulfites; may cause allergic reaction in susceptible individuals.

Adverse Reactions

Cardiovascular: Angina, flushing, hyper-/hypotension, pallor, palpitation, paradoxical bradycardia (with tilt table testing), premature ventricular beats, Stokes-Adams attacks, tachyarrhythmia, ventricular arrhythmia

Central nervous system: Dizziness, headache, nervousness, restlessness, Stokes-Adams seizure

Endocrine & metabolic: Hypokalemia, serum glucose increased

Gastrointestinal: Nausea, vomiting

Neuromuscular & skeletal: Tremor, weakness

Ocular: Blurred vision

Respiratory: Dyspnea, pulmonary edema

Miscellaneous: Diaphoresis

Drug Interactions

Metabolism/Transport Effects Substrate of COMT

Avoid Concomitant Use

Avoid concomitant use of Isoproterenol with any of the following: Inhalational Anesthetics; Iobenguane I 123

Increased Effect/Toxicity

Isoproterenol may increase the levels/effects of: Highest Risk QTc-Prolonging Agents; Moderate Risk QTc-Prolonging Agents; Sympathomimetics

The levels/effects of Isoproterenol may be increased by: AtoMOXetine; Cannabinoid-Containing Products; COMT Inhibitors; Inhalational Anesthetics; Linezolid; Mifepristone; Tedizolid

Decreased Effect

Isoproterenol may decrease the levels/effects of: Iobenguane I 123; Theophylline Derivatives

Storage/Stability Store undiluted solution at 20°C to 25°C (68°F to 77°F). Solution should not be used if a color or precipitate is present. Exposure to air, light, or increased temperature may cause a pink to brownish pink color to develop. Stability of parenteral admixture at room temperature (25°C) or at refrigeration (4°C) is 24 hours.

Mechanism of Action Stimulates $beta_1$- and $beta_2$-receptors resulting in relaxation of bronchial, GI, and uterine smooth muscle, increased heart rate and contractility, vasodilation of peripheral vasculature

Pharmacodynamics

Onset of action: IV: Immediately

Duration: IV (single dose): Few minutes

Pharmacokinetics (Adult data unless noted)

Metabolism: By conjugation in many tissues including the liver and lungs

Half-life: 2.5-5 minutes

Elimination: In urine principally as sulfate conjugates

Dosing: Neonatal Bradyarrhythmias: Continuous IV infusion: 0.05-2 mcg/kg/minute; titrate to effect

Dosing: Usual Bradyarrhythmias, AV nodal block, or refractory torsade de pointes: Continuous IV infusion:

Infants and Children: 0.05-2 mcg/kg/minute; titrate to effect

Adults: 2-20 mcg/minute; titrate to effect

Usual Infusion Concentrations: Pediatric IV infusion: 20 **mcg**/mL

Preparation for Administration Parenteral: For continuous infusions, dilute in dextrose or NS to a maximum concentration of 20 mcg/mL; concentrations as high as 64 mcg/mL have been used by some institutions in patients needing extreme fluid restriction (Sinclair-Pingel 2006)

Administration Parenteral: Administer by continuous IV infusion; requires the use of an infusion pump

Monitoring Parameters Heart rate, blood pressure, respiratory rate, arterial blood gases, central venous pressure, ECG

Additional Information Hypotension is more common in hypovolemic patients

Dosage Forms Excipient information presented when available (limited, particularly for generics); consult specific product labeling. [DSC] = Discontinued product

Solution, Injection, as hydrochloride:

Isuprel: 0.2 mg/mL (1 mL, 5 mL) [contains disodium edta]

Isuprel: 0.2 mg/mL (1 mL [DSC], 5 mL [DSC]) [contains sodium metabisulfite]

◆ **Isoproterenol Hydrochloride** *see* Isoproterenol *on page 1170*

◆ **Isoptin SR** *see* Verapamil *on page 2170*

◆ **Isopto Atropine** *see* Atropine *on page 227*

◆ **Isopto® Atropine (Can)** *see* Atropine *on page 227*

◆ **Isopto Carpine** *see* Pilocarpine (Ophthalmic) *on page 1701*

◆ **Isopto® Carpine (Can)** *see* Pilocarpine (Ophthalmic) *on page 1701*

◆ **Isopto Homatropine** *see* Homatropine *on page 1023*

◆ **Isopto Hyoscine** *see* Scopolamine (Ophthalmic) *on page 1909*

◆ **Isotamine (Can)** *see* Isoniazid *on page 1168*

ISOtretinoin (eye soe TRET i noyn)

Medication Safety Issues

Sound-alike/look-alike issues:

Accutane may be confused with Accolate, Accupril

Claravis may be confused with Cleviprex

ISOtretinoin may be confused with tretinoin

Other safety concerns:

Isotretinoin may be confused with tretinoin (which is also called all-*trans* retinoic acid, or ATRA); while both products may have uses in cancer treatment, they are **not** interchangeable.

Related Information

Oral Medications That Should Not Be Crushed or Altered *on page 2476*

Safe Handling of Hazardous Drugs *on page 2455*

Brand Names: US Absorica; Amnesteem; Claravis; Myorisan; Zenatane

Brand Names: Canada Accutane; Clarus; Epuris

Therapeutic Category Acne Products; Antineoplastic Agent, Retinoic Acid Derivatives; Retinoic Acid Derivative; Vitamin A Derivative

Generic Availability (US) No

Use Treatment of severe recalcitrant nodular acne unresponsive to conventional therapy, including systemic antibiotics (FDA approved in ages ≥12 years and adults); has also been used for the treatment of moderate acne and high-risk neuroblastoma

Prescribing and Access Restrictions As a requirement of the REMS program, access to this medication is restricted. All patients (male and female), prescribers, wholesalers, and dispensing pharmacists must register and be active in the iPLEDGE™ risk management program, designed to eliminate fetal exposures to isotretinoin. This program covers all isotretinoin products (brand and generic). The iPLEDGE™ program requires that all patients meet qualification criteria and monthly program requirements (eg, pregnancy testing). Healthcare providers can only prescribe a maximum 30-day supply at each monthly visit and must counsel patients on the iPLEDGE™ program requirements and confirm counseling via the iPLEDGE™ automated system. Registration, activation, and additional information are provided at www.-ipledgeprogram.com or by calling 866-495-0654.

Medication Guide Available Yes

Pregnancy Risk Factor X

Pregnancy Considerations Isotretinoin and its metabolites can be detected in fetal tissue following maternal use during pregnancy (Benifla, 1995; Kraft, 1989). **[U.S. Boxed Warnings]: Use of isotretinoin is contraindicated in females who are or may become pregnant. Birth defects (facial, eye, ear, skull, central nervous system, cardiovascular, thymus and parathyroid gland abnormalities) have been noted following isotretinoin exposure during pregnancy and the risk for severe birth defects is high, with any dose or even with short treatment duration. Low IQ scores have also been reported. The risk for spontaneous abortion and premature births is increased. Because of the high likelihood of teratogenic effects, all patients (male and female), prescribers, wholesalers, and dispensing pharmacists must register and be active in the iPLEDGE™ risk evaluation and mitigation strategy (REMS) program; do not prescribe isotretinoin for women who are or who are likely to become pregnant while using the drug. If pregnancy occurs during therapy, isotretinoin should be discontinued immediately and the patient referred to an obstetrician-gynecologist specializing in reproductive toxicity.** This medication is contraindicated in females of childbearing potential unless they are able to comply with the guidelines of the iPLEDGE™ pregnancy prevention program. Females of childbearing potential must have two negative pregnancy tests with a sensitivity of at least 25 mIU/mL prior to beginning therapy and testing should continue monthly during therapy. Females of childbearing potential should not become pregnant during therapy or for 1 month following discontinuation of isotretinoin. Upon discontinuation of treatment, females of childbearing potential should have a pregnancy test after their last dose and again one month after their last dose. Two forms of contraception should be continued during this time. Any pregnancies should be reported to the iPLEDGE™ program (www.-ipledgeprogram.com or 866-495-0654) and the FDA through MedWatch (800-FDA-1088).

Breast-Feeding Considerations It is not known if isotretinoin is excreted in breast milk. A case report describes a green discharge from the breast of a nonlactating woman which was determined to be iatrogenic galactorrhea due to isotretinoin (Larsen, 1985). Due to the potential for serious adverse reactions in the nursing infant, the manufacturer recommends a decision be made whether to discontinue nursing or to discontinue the drug, taking into account the importance of treatment to the mother.

Contraindications Hypersensitivity to isotretinoin or any component of the formulation; sensitivity to parabens, vitamin A, or other retinoids; pregnant women or those who may become pregnant

Warnings/Precautions Hazardous agent - use appropriate precautions for handling and disposal (meets NIOSH 2014 criteria). This medication should only be prescribed by prescribers competent in treating severe recalcitrant nodular acne and experienced with the use of systemic retinoids. Anaphylaxis and other types of allergic reactions, including cutaneous reactions and allergic vasculitis, have been reported. **[U.S. Boxed Warnings]: Birth defects (facial, eye, ear, skull, central nervous system, cardiovascular, thymus and parathyroid gland abnormalities) have been noted following isotretinoin exposure during pregnancy and the risk for severe birth defects is high, with any dose or even with short treatment duration. Low IQ scores have also been reported. The risk for spontaneous abortion and premature births is increased. Because of the high likelihood of teratogenic effects, all patients (male and female), prescribers, wholesalers, and dispensing pharmacists must register and be active in the iPLEDGE™ risk evaluation and mitigation strategy (REMS) program; do not prescribe isotretinoin for women who are or who are likely to become pregnant while using the drug. If pregnancy occurs during therapy, isotretinoin should be discontinued immediately and the patient referred to an obstetrician-gynecologist specializing in reproductive toxicity (see Additional Information for details).** Women of childbearing potential must be capable of complying with effective contraceptive measures. Patients must select and commit to two forms of contraception. Therapy is begun after two negative pregnancy tests; effective contraception must be used for at least 1 month before beginning therapy, during therapy, and for 1 month after discontinuation of therapy. Prescriptions should be written for no more than a 30-day supply, and pregnancy testing and counseling should be repeated monthly.

May cause depression, psychosis, aggressive or violent behavior, and changes in mood; use with extreme caution in patients with psychiatric disorders. Rarely, suicidal thoughts and actions have been reported during isotretinoin usage. All patients should be observed closely for symptoms of depression or suicidal thoughts. Discontinuation of treatment alone may not be sufficient, further evaluation may be necessary. Cases of pseudotumor cerebri (benign intracranial hypertension) have been reported, some with concomitant use of tetracycline (avoid using together). Patients with papilledema, headache, nausea, vomiting, and visual disturbances should be referred to a neurologist and treatment with isotretinoin discontinued. Hearing impairment, which can continue after therapy is discontinued, may occur. Clinical hepatitis, elevated liver enzymes, inflammatory bowel disease, skeletal hyperostosis, premature epiphyseal closure, vision impairment, corneal opacities, decreased tolerance to contact lenses (due to dry eyes), and decreased night vision have also been reported with the use of isotretinoin. Rare postmarketing cases of severe skin reactions (eg, Stevens-Johnson syndrome, erythema multiforme) have been reported with use.

Use with caution in patients with diabetes mellitus; impaired glucose control has been reported. Use caution in patients with hypertriglyceridemia; acute pancreatitis and fatal hemorrhagic pancreatitis (rare) have been reported. Instruct patients to avoid or limit ethanol; may increase triglyceride levels if taken in excess. Bone mineral density may decrease; use caution in patients with a genetic predisposition to bone disorders (ie, osteoporosis, osteomalacia) and with disease states or concomitant medications that can induce bone disorders. Patients may be at risk when participating in activities with repetitive impact (such as sports). Patients should be instructed not to donate blood during therapy and for 1 month following discontinuation of therapy due to risk of donated blood being given to a pregnant female. Safety of long-term use is not established and is not recommended.

Absorica™: Absorption is ~83% greater than Accutane® when administered under fasting conditions; they are bioequivalent when taken with a high-fat meal. Absorica™ is **not** interchangeable with other generic isotretinoin products. Isotretinoin and tretinoin (which is also known as all-*trans* retinoic acid, or ATRA) may be confused, while both products may be used in cancer treatment, they are **not** interchangeable; verify product prior to dispensing and administration to prevent medication errors.

Warnings: Additional Pediatric Considerations Children may experience a higher frequency of some adverse effects including arthralgia (22%) and back pain (29%).

Adverse Reactions

Cardiovascular: Chest pain, edema, flushing, palpitation, stroke, syncope, tachycardia, vascular thrombotic disease

Central nervous system: Aggressive behavior, depression, dizziness, drowsiness, emotional instability, fatigue, headache, insomnia, lethargy, malaise, nervousness, paresthesia, pseudotumor cerebri, psychosis, seizure, stroke, suicidal ideation, suicide attempts, suicide, violent behavior

Dermatologic: Abnormal wound healing acne fulminans, alopecia, bruising, cheilitis, cutaneous allergic reactions, dry nose, dry skin, eczema, eruptive xanthomas, facial erythema, fragility of skin, hair abnormalities, hirsutism, hyperpigmentation, hypopigmentation, increased sunburn susceptibility, nail dystrophy, paronychia, peeling of palms, peeling of soles, photoallergic reactions, photosensitizing reactions, pruritus, purpura, rash

Endocrine & metabolic: Abnormal menses, blood glucose increased, cholesterol increased, HDL decreased, hyperuricemia, triglycerides increased

Gastrointestinal: Bleeding and inflammation of the gums, colitis, esophagitis, esophageal ulceration, inflammatory bowel disease, nausea, nonspecific gastrointestinal symptoms, pancreatitis, weight loss, xerostomia

Genitourinary: Nonspecific urogenital findings

Hematologic: Agranulocytosis (rare), anemia, neutropenia, pyogenic granuloma, thrombocytopenia

Hepatic: Alkaline phosphatase increased, ALT increased, AST increased, GGTP increased, hepatitis, LDH increased

Neuromuscular & skeletal: Arthralgia, arthritis, back pain, bone abnormalities, bone mineral density decreased, calcification of tendons and ligaments, CPK increased, myalgia, premature epiphyseal closure, skeletal hyperostosis, tendonitis, weakness

Ocular: Blepharitis, cataracts, chalazion, color vision disorder, conjunctivitis, corneal opacities, eyelid inflammation, hordeolum, keratitis, night vision decreased, optic neuritis, photophobia, visual disturbances

Otic: Hearing impairment, tinnitus

Renal: Glomerulonephritis, hematuria, proteinuria, pyuria, vasculitis

Respiratory: Bronchospasms, epistaxis, respiratory infection, voice alteration, Wegener's granulomatosis

Miscellaneous: Allergic reactions, anaphylactic reactions, disseminated herpes simplex, diaphoresis, infection, lymphadenopathy

Rare but important or life-threatening: Abnormal meibomian gland secretion, erythema multiforme, meibomian gland atrophy, myopia, pseudotumor cerebri, rhabdomyolysis, Stevens-Johnson syndrome, toxic epidermal necrolysis, visual acuity decreased

Drug Interactions

Metabolism/Transport Effects None known.

Avoid Concomitant Use

Avoid concomitant use of ISOtretinoin with any of the following: Multivitamins/Fluoride (with ADE); Multivitamins/Minerals (with ADEK, Folate, Iron); Multivitamins/Minerals (with AE, No Iron); Tetracycline Derivatives; Vitamin A

Increased Effect/Toxicity

ISOtretinoin may increase the levels/effects of: Mipomersen; Porfimer; Verteporfin

The levels/effects of ISOtretinoin may be increased by: Alcohol (Ethyl); Multivitamins/Fluoride (with ADE); Multivitamins/Minerals (with ADEK, Folate, Iron); Multivitamins/Minerals (with AE, No Iron); Tetracycline Derivatives; Vitamin A

Decreased Effect

ISOtretinoin may decrease the levels/effects of: Contraceptives (Estrogens); Contraceptives (Progestins)

Food Interactions Isotretinoin bioavailability increased if taken with food or milk. Management: Administer orally with a meal (except Absorica™ which may be taken without regard to meals).

Storage/Stability Store at 20°C to 25°C (68°F to 77° F); excursions permitted between 15°C to 30°C (59°F to 86°F). Protect from light.

Mechanism of Action Reduces sebaceous gland size and reduces sebum production in acne treatment; in neuroblastoma, decreases cell proliferation and induces differentiation

Pharmacokinetics (Adult data unless noted) Note: Pharmacokinetic parameters in adolescents (12-15 years) are similar to adults.

Absorption: Enhanced with a high-fat meal; Absorica™ absorption is ~83% greater than Accutane® when administered under fasting conditions; they are bioequivalent when taken with a high-fat meal

Protein binding: 99% to 100%; primarily albumin

Metabolism: Hepatic via CYP2B6, 2C8, 2C9, 2D6, 3A4; forms metabolites; major metabolite: 4-oxo-isotretinoin (active)

Half-life, terminal: Parent drug: 21 hours; Metabolite: 21-24 hours

Time to peak serum concentration: Fasting conditions: Within 3 hours

Elimination: Urine and feces (equal amounts)

Dosing: Usual

Children and Adolescents:

Acne vulgaris, severe recalcitrant nodular: Children ≥12 years and Adolescents: Oral: 0.5-1 mg/kg/day in 2 divided doses; for severe cases (involving trunk, nuchal region, lower back, buttocks, thighs) may require higher doses up to 2 mg/kg/day in 2 divided doses. Duration of therapy is typically 15-20 weeks or until the total cyst count decreases by 70%, whichever is sooner; an alternate reported approach is continuation until a total cumulative dose of 120 mg/kg (eg, 1 mg/kg/day for 120 days). An initial dose of ≤0.5 mg/kg/day may be used to minimize initial flaring (Strauss, 2007)

Acne vulgaris, moderate: Limited data available: Children ≥12 years and Adolescents: 20 mg/day (~0.3-0.5 mg/kg/day) continued for 6-12 months to cumulative dose 120 mg/kg has been shown effective (Amichai, 2006)

Neuroblastoma, maintenance: Children ≥1 year and Adolescents: Oral: 160 mg/m^2/day in 2 divided doses for 14 consecutive days in a 28-day cycle for 6 cycles; begin after continuation chemotherapy or transplantation (Matthay, 1999)

Adults: **Acne vulgaris:** Oral: 0.5-1 mg/kg/day in 2 divided doses for 15-20 weeks or until the total cyst count decreases by 70%, whichever is sooner. Adults with very severe disease/scarring or primarily involves the trunk may require dosage adjustment up to 2 mg/kg/day. A second course of therapy may be initiated after a period of ≥2 months of therapy. An initial dose of ≤0.5 mg/kg/day may be used to minimize initial flaring (Strauss, 2007).

Dosing adjustment in renal impairment: There are no dosage adjustments provided in the manufacturer's labeling.

Dosing adjustment in hepatic impairment: Children, Adolescents, and Adults:

Hepatic impairment prior to treatment: There are no dosage adjustments provided in the manufacturer's labeling.

Hepatotoxicity during treatment: Liver enzymes may normalize with dosage reduction or with continued treatment; discontinue if normalization does not readily occur or if hepatitis is suspected.

Preparation for Administration Hazardous agent; use appropriate precautions for handling and disposal (meets NIOSH, 2014 criteria).

Administration Hazardous agent; use appropriate precautions for handling and disposal (meets NIOSH, 2014 criteria).

Oral: Administer orally with a meal (except Absorica™ which may be taken without regard to meals). According to the manufacturers' labeling, capsules should be swallowed whole with a full glass of liquid. For patients unable to swallow capsule whole, an oral liquid may be prepared; may irritate esophagus if contents are removed from the capsule.

Monitoring Parameters CBC with differential and platelet count, baseline sedimentation rate, glucose, CPK; signs of depression, mood alteration, psychosis, aggression, severe skin reactions

Pregnancy test (for all female patients of childbearing potential): Two negative tests with a sensitivity of at least 25 mIU/mL prior to beginning therapy (the second performed at least 19 days after the first test and performed during the first 5 days of the menstrual period immediately preceding the start of therapy); monthly tests to rule out pregnancy prior to refilling prescription

Lipids: Prior to treatment and at weekly or biweekly intervals until response to treatment is established. Test should not be performed <36 hours after consumption of ethanol.

Liver function tests: Prior to treatment and at weekly or biweekly intervals until response to treatment is established.

Dosage Forms Excipient information presented when available (limited, particularly for generics); consult specific product labeling.

Capsule, Oral:

- Absorica: 10 mg, 20 mg [contains soybean oil]
- Absorica: 25 mg [contains brilliant blue fcf (fd&c blue #1), fd&c yellow #6 (sunset yellow), soybean oil, tartrazine (fd&c yellow #5)]
- Absorica: 30 mg [contains soybean oil]
- Absorica: 35 mg [contains fd&c blue #2 (indigotine), soybean oil]
- Absorica: 40 mg [contains soybean oil]
- Amnesteem: 10 mg, 20 mg, 40 mg [contains soybean oil]
- Claravis: 10 mg [contains fd&c yellow #6 (sunset yellow), soybean oil]
- Claravis: 20 mg [contains soybean oil]
- Claravis: 30 mg
- Claravis: 40 mg [contains fd&c yellow #6 (sunset yellow), soybean oil]
- Myorisan: 10 mg, 20 mg [contains soybean oil]
- Myorisan: 40 mg [contains fd&c yellow #6 (sunset yellow), soybean oil]
- Zenatane: 10 mg [contains brilliant blue fcf (fd&c blue #1), edetate disodium, fd&c yellow #10 (quinoline yellow), methylparaben, propylparaben, soybean oil]
- Zenatane: 20 mg [contains edetate disodium, methylparaben, propylparaben, soybean oil]
- Zenatane: 30 mg [contains edetate disodium, fd&c blue #2 aluminum lake, fd&c yellow #10 (quinoline yellow), methylparaben, propylparaben, soybean oil]
- Zenatane: 40 mg [contains brilliant blue fcf (fd&c blue #1), edetate disodium, fd&c blue #2 (indigotine), fd&c yellow #10 (quinoline yellow), methylparaben, propylparaben, soybean oil]

Extemporaneous Preparations Hazardous agent: Use appropriate precautions for handling and disposal of teratogenic capsule contents (meets NIOSH 2014 criteria).

For patients unable to swallow the capsules whole, an oral liquid may be prepared with softgel capsules (not recommended by the manufacturers) by one of the following methods:

- Place capsules (softgel formulations only) in small container and add warm (~37°C [97°F]) water or milk to cover capsule(s); wait 2-3 minutes until capsule is softened and then drink the milk or water with the softened capsule, or swallow softened capsule.
- Puncture capsule (softgel formulations only) with needle or cut with scissors; squeeze capsule contents into 5-10 mL of milk or tube feed formula; draw mixture up into oral syringe and administer via feeding tube; flush feeding tube with ≥30 mL additional milk or tube feeding formula.
- Puncture capsule (softgel formulations only) with needle or cut with scissors and draw contents into oral syringe; add 1-5 mL of medium chain triglyceride, soybean, or safflower oil to the oral syringe; mix gently and administer via feeding tube; flush feeding tube with ≥30 mL milk or tube feeding formula.

Lam MS, "Extemporaneous Compounding of Oral Liquid Dosage Formulations and Alternative Drug Delivery Methods for Anticancer Drugs," *Pharmacotherapy*, 2011, 31(2):164-92.

◆ **Isotretinoinum** *see* ISOtretinoin *on page 1171*

Isradipine (iz RA di peen)

Therapeutic Category Antihypertensive Agent; Calcium Channel Blocker; Calcium Channel Blocker, Dihydropyridine

Generic Availability (US) Yes

Use Treatment of hypertension alone or in combination with thiazide-type diuretics (FDA approved in adults)

Pregnancy Risk Factor C

Pregnancy Considerations Adverse events were not observed in animal reproduction studies when using doses that were not maternally toxic. Isradipine crosses the human placenta (Lunell, 1993). Untreated chronic maternal hypertension is associated with adverse events in the fetus, infant, and mother. If treatment for hypertension during pregnancy is needed, other agents are preferred (ACOG, 2013).

Breast-Feeding Considerations It is not known if isradipine is excreted into breast milk. Due to the potential for serious adverse reactions in the nursing infant, the manufacturer recommends a decision be made whether to discontinue nursing or to discontinue the drug, taking into account the importance of treatment to the mother.

Contraindications Hypersensitivity to isradipine or any component of the formulation

Warnings/Precautions Increased angina and/or MI has occurred with initiation or dosage titration of dihydropyridine calcium channel blockers. Reflex tachycardia may occur, resulting in angina and/or MI in patients with obstructive coronary disease, especially in the absence of concurrent beta-blockade. A common side effect is peripheral edema (dose-dependent); may begin within 2-3 weeks of starting therapy. Symptomatic hypotension with or without syncope can rarely occur; blood pressure must be lowered at a rate appropriate for the patient's clinical condition. Use with extreme caution in patients with severe aortic stenosis; may reduce coronary perfusion, resulting in ischemia. Use with caution in patients with hypertrophic cardiomyopathy (HCM) and outflow tract obstruction since reduction in afterload may worsen symptoms associated with this condition. The ACCF/AHA heart failure guidelines recommend to avoid use in patients with heart failure due to lack of benefit and/or worse outcomes with calcium channel blockers in general (ACCF/AHA [Yancy, 2013]).

Adverse Reactions

Cardiovascular: Chest pain, edema (dose related), flushing (dose related), palpitations (dose related), tachycardia

Central nervous system: Dizziness, fatigue (dose related), headache (dose related)

Dermatologic: Skin rash

Gastrointestinal: Abdominal distress, diarrhea, nausea, vomiting

Neuromuscular & skeletal: Weakness

Renal: Urinary frequency

Respiratory: Dyspnea

Rare but important or life-threatening: Atrial fibrillation, cardiac failure, cerebrovascular accident, cough, decreased libido, depression, foot cramps, hyperhidrosis, hypotension, impotence, increased liver enzymes, insomnia, leg cramps, leukopenia, myocardial infarction, nocturia, numbness, paresthesia, pruritus, sore throat, syncope, transient ischemic attacks, urticaria, ventricular fibrillation, visual disturbance

Drug Interactions

Metabolism/Transport Effects Substrate of CYP3A4 (major); **Note:** Assignment of Major/Minor substrate status based on clinically relevant drug interaction potential

Avoid Concomitant Use

Avoid concomitant use of Isradipine with any of the following: Conivaptan; Fusidic Acid (Systemic); Idelalisib

Increased Effect/Toxicity

Isradipine may increase the levels/effects of: Amifostine; Antihypertensives; Atosiban; Calcium Channel Blockers (Nondihydropyridine); DULoxetine; Fosphenytoin; Highest Risk QTc-Prolonging Agents; Hypotensive Agents; Levodopa; Magnesium Salts; Moderate Risk QTc-Prolonging Agents; Neuromuscular-Blocking Agents (Nondepolarizing); Nitroprusside; Obinutuzumab; Phenytoin; RisperiDONE; RiTUXimab; Tacrolimus (Systemic)

The levels/effects of Isradipine may be increased by: Alfuzosin; Alpha1-Blockers; Antifungal Agents (Azole Derivatives, Systemic); Aprepitant; Barbiturates; Brimonidine (Topical); Calcium Channel Blockers (Nondihydropyridine); Cimetidine; Conivaptan; CycloSPORINE (Systemic); CYP3A4 Inhibitors (Moderate); CYP3A4 Inhibitors (Strong); Dapoxetine; Dasatinib; Diazoxide; Fluconazole; Fosaprepitant; Fusidic Acid (Systemic); Herbs (Hypotensive Properties); Idelalisib; Ivacaftor; Luliconazole; Macrolide Antibiotics; Magnesium Salts; MAO Inhibitors; Mifepristone; Netupitant; Nicorandil; Palbociclib; Pentoxifylline; Phosphodiesterase 5 Inhibitors; Prostacyclin Analogues; Protease Inhibitors; Simeprevir; Stiripentol

Decreased Effect

Isradipine may decrease the levels/effects of: Clopidogrel

The levels/effects of Isradipine may be decreased by: Barbiturates; Bosentan; Calcium Salts; CarBAMazepine; CYP3A4 Inducers (Moderate); CYP3A4 Inducers (Strong); Dabrafenib; Deferasirox; Efavirenz; Herbs (Hypertensive Properties); Melatonin; Methylphenidate; Mitotane; Nafcillin; Rifamycin Derivatives; Siltuximab; St Johns Wort; Tocilizumab; Yohimbine

Food Interactions Administration with food delays absorption, but does not affect availability. Management: Administer without regard to meals.

Storage/Stability Store at 20°C to 25°C (68°F to 77°F) in a tight container, protected from moisture, humidity, and light.

Mechanism of Action Inhibits calcium ion from entering the "slow channels" or select voltage-sensitive areas of vascular smooth muscle and myocardium during depolarization, producing relaxation of vascular smooth muscle, resulting in coronary vasodilation and reduced blood pressure; increases myocardial oxygen delivery in patients with vasospastic angina

Pharmacodynamics

Onset of action: 2-3 hours; **Note:** Full hypotensive effect may not occur for 2-4 weeks.

Duration: >12 hours

Pharmacokinetics (Adult data unless noted)

Absorption: 90% to 95%, but large first-pass effect

Distribution: V_d (apparent): 3 L/kg

Protein binding: 95%

Metabolism: Extensive first-pass effect; hepatically metabolized via cytochrome P450 isoenzyme CYP3A4; major metabolic pathways include oxidation and ester cleavage; six inactive metabolites have been identified

Bioavailability: 15% to 24%

Mild renal impairment (CrCl 30-80 mL/minute): Increased by 45%

Severe renal impairment (CrCl <10 mL/minute); concurrent hemodialysis: Decreased by 20% to 50%

Hepatic impairment: Increased by 52%

Half-life: Alpha half-life: 1.5-2 hours; terminal half-life: 8 hours

Time to peak serum concentration: 1.5 hours

Elimination: Urine (60% to 65% as metabolites; no unchanged drug detected); feces: 25% to 30%

Dosing: Usual

Children and Adolescents: Limited data available: **Hypertension:** Oral: Initial: 0.15-0.2 mg/kg/day divided 3 or 4 times daily; titrate upwards at 2- to 4-week intervals; maximum daily dose: 0.8 mg/kg/**day** or 20 mg/**day** (whichever is lower) (NHBPEP, 2004; NHLBI, 2011). Based on retrospective observations, higher initial doses (0.05-0.15 mg/kg/dose) administered 3-4 times daily have been suggested especially in patients with secondary hypertension and severe hypertension; usual daily dose: 0.3-0.4 mg/kg/day divided every 8 hours (range: 0.04-1.2 mg/kg/day) (Flynn, 2002; Flynn, 2009; Johnson, 1997; Strauser, 2000). **Note:** Most adult patients show no improvement with doses >10 mg daily and adverse reaction rate increases.

Adults: **Hypertension:** Oral: 2.5 mg twice daily; antihypertensive response occurs in 2-3 hours; maximal response in 2-4 weeks; increase dose at 2- to 4-week intervals at 2.5-5 mg increments; usual dose range (JNC 7): 2.5-10 mg daily in 2 divided doses. **Note:** Most patients show no improvement with doses >10 mg daily, except adverse reaction rate increases; therefore, maximal dose in older adults should be 10 mg daily.

Dosing adjustment in renal impairment: There are no dosage adjustments provided in manufacturer's labeling; however, bioavailability is increased with mild renal impairment; trend is reversed with further renal function deterioration. Other sources recommend that no initial dosage adjustment is required in pediatric and adult patients (Aronoff, 2007). Isradipine is not removed by hemodialysis; therefore, supplemental doses after hemodialysis are not necessary (Schönholzer, 1992).

Dosing adjustment in hepatic impairment: Adults: There are no dosage adjustments provided in manufacturer's labeling; however, peak serum concentrations are increased by 32% and bioavailability is increased by 52%.

Administration Oral: May be administered without regard to meals.

Monitoring Parameters Blood pressure, heart rate, liver and renal function

Dosage Forms Excipient information presented when available (limited, particularly for generics); consult specific product labeling.

Capsule, Oral:

Generic: 2.5 mg, 5 mg

Extemporaneous Preparations A 1 mg/mL oral suspension may be made from isradipine capsules; glycerin, USP; and Simple Syrup, N.F. Empty the contents of ten 5 mg isradipine capsules into a glass mortar. Add a small portion of glycerin, USP and mix to a fine paste; mix while adding 15 mL of simple syrup and transfer contents to a 60 mL amber glass prescription bottle. Rinse mortar with 10 mL simple syrup, NF and transfer to the prescription bottle; repeat, and add quantity of vehicle sufficient to make 50 mL. Label "protect from light", "refrigerate", and "shake well". Stable for 35 days when stored in amber glass prescription bottles in the dark and refrigerated.

MacDonald JL, Johnson CE, and Jacobson P, "Stability of Isradipine in Extemporaneously Compounded Oral Liquids," *Am J Hosp Pharm*, 1994, 51(19):2409-11.

◆ **Istalol** *see* Timolol (Ophthalmic) *on page 2067*

◆ **Isuprel** *see* Isoproterenol *on page 1170*

◆ **Itch Relief [OTC]** *see* DiphenhydrAMINE (Topical) *on page 672*

Itraconazole (i tra KOE na zole)

Medication Safety Issues

Sound-alike/look-alike issues:

Itraconazole may be confused with fluconazole, posaconazole, voriconazole

Sporanox may be confused with Suprax, Topamax

Brand Names: US Onmel; Sporanox; Sporanox Pulsepak

Brand Names: Canada Sporanox

Therapeutic Category Antifungal Agent, Systemic

Generic Availability (US) May be product dependent

Use Treatment of susceptible systemic fungal infections in immunocompromised and nonimmunocompromised patients including blastomycosis, coccidioidomycosis, paracoccidioidomycosis, histoplasmosis, and aspergillosis in patients who do not respond to or cannot tolerate amphotericin B (Capsules: FDA approved in adults); treatment of onchomycosis of the toenail in nonimmunocompromised patients (Tablet: FDA approved in adults); treatment of oropharyngeal or esophageal candidiasis (Oral solution: FDA approved in adults)

Pregnancy Risk Factor C

Pregnancy Considerations Dose related adverse events were observed in animal reproduction studies. Use is contraindicated for the treatment of onychomycosis during pregnancy. If used for the treatment of onychomycosis in women of reproductive potential, effective contraception should be used during treatment and for 2 months following treatment. Therapy should begin on the second or third day following menses. Congenital abnormalities have been reported during postmarketing surveillance, but a causal relationship has not been established. The Canadian labeling contraindicates use in the treatment of onychomycosis or dermatomycoses (tinea corporis, tinea cruris, tinea pedis, pityriasis versicolor) in women who are pregnant or intend to become pregnant.

Breast-Feeding Considerations Itraconazole is excreted in breast milk. According to the manufacturer, the decision to continue or discontinue breast-feeding during therapy should take into account the risk of exposure to the infant and the benefits of treatment to the mother.

Contraindications

Hypersensitivity to itraconazole or any component of the formulation; concurrent administration with cisapride, disopyramide, dofetilide, dronedarone, eplerenone, ergot derivatives, felodipine, irinotecan, lovastatin, lurasidone, methadone, midazolam (oral), nisoldipine, pimozide, quinidine, ranolazine, simvastatin, ticagrelor, or triazolam; concurrent administration with colchicine, fesoterodine, telithromycin, and solifenacin in patients with varying degrees of renal or hepatic impairment; treatment of onychomycosis (or other non-life-threatening indications) in patients with evidence of ventricular dysfunction, such as congestive heart failure (CHF) or a history of CHF; treatment of onychomycosis in women who are pregnant or intend to become pregnant

Canadian labeling: Additional contraindications (not in US labeling): Concurrent administration with domperidone, eletriptan, fesoterodine in patients with moderate to severe renal or hepatic impairment, or solifenacin in patients with severe renal impairment or moderate to severe hepatic impairment (capsule, oral solution); Concurrent administration with the following drugs (none of which are available in Canada): Astemizole, bepridil, halofantrine, ivabradine, lercanidipine, levacetylmethadol, mizolastine, telithromycin (in patients with severe renal or hepatic impairment), sertindole, terfenadine (capsule, oral solution); treatment of dermatomycosis (tinea pedis, tinea cruris, tinea corporis, pityriasis versicolor) in women who are pregnant or intend to become pregnant (capsule)

Warnings/Precautions [US Boxed Warning]: Negative inotropic effects have been observed following intravenous administration. Discontinue or reassess use if signs or symptoms of HF (heart failure) occur during treatment. [US Boxed Warning]: Use is contraindicated for treatment of onychomycosis in patients with ventricular dysfunction or a history of HF. Cases of HF, peripheral edema, and pulmonary edema have occurred in patients treated for onychomycosis. HF has been reported, particularly in patients receiving a total daily oral dose of 400 mg. Use with caution in patients with risk factors for HF (COPD, renal failure, edematous disorders, ischemic or valvular disease). Discontinue if signs or symptoms of HF or neuropathy occur during treatment. Due to potential toxicity, the manufacturer recommends confirmation of diagnosis testing of nail specimens prior to treatment of onychomycosis. The Canadian labeling contraindicates use in the treatment of dermatomycoses (tinea corporis, tinea cruris, tinea pedis, pityriasis versicolor) in patients with evidence of ventricular dysfunction or a history of HF.

[US Boxed Warning]: Coadministration with itraconazole can cause elevated plasma concentrations of certain drugs and can lead to QT prolongation and ventricular tachyarrhythmias, including torsades de pointes. Coadministration with methadone, disopyramide, dofetilide, dronedarone, quinidine, ergot alkaloids, irinotecan, lurasidone, oral midazolam, pimozide, triazolam, felodipine, nisoldipine, ranolazine, eplerenone, cisapride, lovastatin, simvastatin, ticagrelor and, in subjects with vaying degrees of renal or hepatic impairment, colchicine, fesoterodine, telithromycin, and solifencacin is contraindicated. Additional potentially significant interactions may exist, requiring dose or frequency adjustment, additional monitoring, and/or selection of alternative therapy.

May cause CNS depression, which may impair physical or mental abilities; patients must be cautioned about performing tasks that require mental alertness (eg, operating machinery, driving). Use with caution in patients with renal impairment; dosage adjustment may be needed. Use caution in patients with a history of hypersensitivity to other azoles. Rare cases of serious hepatotoxicity (including liver failure and death) have been reported (including some cases occurring within the first week of therapy); hepatotoxicity was reported in some patients without pre-existing liver disease or risk factors. Use with caution in patients with pre-existing hepatic impairment; monitor liver function closely. Not recommended for use in patients with active liver disease, elevated liver enzymes, or prior hepatotoxic reactions to other drugs unless the expected benefit exceeds the risk of hepatotoxicity. Discontinue treatment if signs or symptoms of hepatotoxicity develop. Transient or permanent hearing loss has been reported. Quinidine (a contraindicated drug) was used concurrently in several of these cases. Hearing loss usually resolves after discontinuation, but may persist in some patients.

Large differences in itraconazole pharmacokinetic parameters have been observed in cystic fibrosis patients receiving the solution; if a patient with cystic fibrosis does not respond to therapy, alternate therapies should be considered. Due to differences in bioavailability, oral capsules and oral solution cannot be used interchangeably. Only the oral solution has proven efficacy for oral and esophageal candidiasis. Initiation of treatment with oral solution is not recommended in patients at immediate risk for systemic candidiasis (eg, patients with severe neutropenia). Absorption of itraconazole capsules is reduced when gastric acidity is reduced; administer capsules or tablets with an acidic beverage (eg, cola) in patients with reduced gastric acidity and separate administration from acid suppressive therapy. Some dosage forms may contain propylene glycol; large amounts are potentially toxic and have been associated hyperosmolality, lactic acidosis, seizures and respiratory depression; use caution (AAP, 1997; Zar, 2007). The Canadian labeling contraindicates use in the treatment of dermatomycoses (tinea corporis, tinea cruris, tinea pedis, pityriasis versicolor) in women who are pregnant or intend to become pregnant.

Adverse Reactions

Cardiovascular: Chest pain, edema, hypertension

Central nervous system: Abnormal dreams, anxiety, depression, dizziness, fatigue, headache, malaise, pain

Dermatologic: Diaphoresis, pruritus, skin rash

Endocrine & metabolic: Hypertriglyceridemia, hypokalemia

Gastrointestinal: Abdominal pain, aphthous stomatitis, constipation, diarrhea, dyspepsia, flatulence, gastritis, gastroenteritis, gastrointestinal disease, gingivitis, increased appetite, nausea, vomiting

Genitourinary: Cystitis, urinary tract infection

Hepatic: Abnormal hepatic function tests, increased liver enzymes

Infection: Herpes zoster

Neuromuscular & skeletal: Bursitis, myalgia, tremor, weakness

Respiratory: Cough, dyspnea, increased bronchial secretions, pharyngitis, pneumonia, rhinitis, sinusitis, upper respiratory tract infection

Miscellaneous: Fever

Rare but important or life-threatening: Abnormal urinalysis, acute generalized exanthematous pustulosis, adrenal insufficiency, albuminuria, anaphylactoid reaction, anaphylaxis, angioedema, cardiac arrhythmia, cardiac failure, confusion, congestive heart failure, dehydration, dysphagia, erythema multiforme, erythematous rash, exfoliative dermatitis, gastrointestinal disease, gynecomastia, hearing loss, hematuria, hepatic failure, hepatitis, hepatotoxicity, hyperbilirubinemia, hyperglycemia, hyperhidrosis, hyperkalemia, hypersensitivity angiitis, hypersensitivity reaction, hypomagnesemia, increased blood urea nitrogen, increased creatine phosphokinase, increased gamma-glutamyl transferase, increased lactate dehydrogenase, increased serum alkaline phosphatase, increased serum ALT, increased serum AST, left heart failure, leukopenia, menstrual disease, mucosal inflammation, neutropenia, orthostatic hypotension, pancreatitis, paresthesia, peripheral edema, pollakiuria, pulmonary edema, renal insufficiency, rigors, serum sickness, sinus bradycardia, Stevens-Johnson syndrome, tachycardia, thrombocytopenia, toxic epidermal necrolysis, vasculitis, voice disorder

Drug Interactions

Metabolism/Transport Effects Substrate of CYP3A4 (major); **Note:** Assignment of Major/Minor substrate status based on clinically relevant drug interaction potential; **Inhibits** CYP3A4 (strong), P-glycoprotein

Avoid Concomitant Use

Avoid concomitant use of Itraconazole with any of the following: Ado-Trastuzumab Emtansine; Alfuzosin; Aliskiren; ALPRAZolam; Apixaban; Astemizole; Avanafil; Axitinib; Barnidipine; Bosutinib; Cabozantinib; Ceritinib; Cisapride; Conivaptan; Crizotinib; CYP3A4 Inducers (Strong); Dapoxetine; Dihydroergotamine; Disopyramide; Dofetilide; Domperidone; Dronedarone; Efavirenz; Eletriptan; Eplerenone; Ergoloid Mesylates; Ergonovine; Ergotamine; Estazolam; Everolimus; Felodipine; Fusidic Acid (Systemic); Halofantrine; Ibrutinib; Idelalisib; Irinotecan; Isavuconazonium Sulfate; Ivabradine; Lapatinib; Lercanidipine; Lomitapide; Lovastatin; Lurasidone; Macitentan; Methadone; Methylergonovine; Midazolam; Naloxegol; Nevirapine; Nilotinib; NiMODipine; Nisoldipine; Olaparib; Palbociclib; PAZOPanib; Pimozide; QuiNIDine; Ranolazine; Red Yeast Rice; Regorafenib; Rivaroxaban; Saccharomyces boulardii; Salmeterol; Silodosin; Simeprevir; Simvastatin; Suvorexant; Tamsulosin; Telithromycin; Terfenadine; Ticagrelor; Tolvaptan; Topotecan; Toremifene; Trabectedin; Triazolam; Ulipristal; Vemurafenib; VinCRIStine (Liposomal); Vorapaxar

Increased Effect/Toxicity

Itraconazole may increase the levels/effects of: Ado-Trastuzumab Emtansine; Afatinib; Alfuzosin; Aliskiren; Almotriptan; Alosetron; ALPRAZolam; Apixaban; ARIPiprazole; Astemizole; AtorvaSTATin; Avanafil; Axitinib; Barnidipine; Bedaquiline; Boceprevir; Bortezomib; Bosentan; Bosutinib; Brentuximab Vedotin; Brinzolamide; Budesonide (Nasal); Budesonide (Systemic, Oral Inhalation); Budesonide (Topical); BusPIRone; Busulfan; Cabazitaxel; Cabozantinib; Calcium Channel Blockers; Cannabis; Cardiac Glycosides; Ceritinib; Cilostazol; Cisapride; Cobicistat; Colchicine; Conivaptan; Corticosteroids (Orally Inhaled); Corticosteroids (Systemic); Crizotinib; CycloSPORINE (Systemic); CYP3A4 Substrates; Dabigatran Etexilate; Dapoxetine; Darunavir; Dasatinib; Dienogest; Dihydroergotamine; Disopyramide; DOCEtaxel; Dofetilide; Domperidone; DOXOrubicin (Conventional); Dronabinol; Dronedarone; Drospirenone; Dutasteride; Edoxaban; Eletriptan; Eliglustat; Elvitegravir; Eplerenone; Ergoloid Mesylates; Ergonovine; Ergotamine; Erlotinib; Estazolam; Etizolam; Etravirine; Everolimus; Felodipine; FentaNYL; Fesoterodine; Fexofenadine; Fluticasone (Nasal); Fluticasone (Oral Inhalation); Fosamprenavir; GuanFACINE; Halofantrine; Highest Risk QTc-Prolonging Agents; Hydrocodone; Ibrutinib; Iloperidone; Imatinib; Imidafenacin; Indinavir; Irinotecan; Isavuconazonium Sulfate; Ivabradine; Ivacaftor; Ixabepilone; Lacosamide; Lapatinib; Ledipasvir; Lercanidipine; Levobupivacaine; Levomilnacipran; Lomitapide; Losartan; Lovastatin; Lurasidone; Macitentan; Maraviroc; MedroxyPROGESTERone; Methadone; Methylergonovine; MethylPREDNISolone; Midazolam; Mifepristone; Moderate Risk QTc-Prolonging Agents; Naloxegol; Nilotinib; NiMODipine; Nintedanib; Nisoldipine; Olaparib; Ospemifene; Oxybutynin; OxyCODONE; Palbociclib; Paliperidone; Panobinostat; Parecoxib; Paricalcitol; PAZOPanib; P-glycoprotein/ABCB1 Substrates; Pimecrolimus; Pimozide; PONATinib; Pranlukast; Pravastatin; PrednisoLONE (Systemic); PredniSONE; Propafenone; Prucalopride; QUEtiapine; QuiNIDine; Ramelteon; Ranolazine; Red Yeast Rice; Regorafenib; Repaglinide; Retapamulin; Rifaximin; Rilpivirine; Riociguat; Rivaroxaban; RomiDEPsin; Rosuvastatin; Ruxolitinib; Salmeterol; Saquinavir; Saxagliptin; Sildenafil; Silodosin; Simeprevir; Simvastatin; Sirolimus; Solifenacin; SORAfenib; SUNItinib; Suvorexant; Tacrolimus (Systemic); Tacrolimus (Topical); Tadalafil; Tamsulosin; Tasimelteon; Telaprevir; Telithromycin; Temsirolimus; Terfenadine; Tetrahydrocannabinol; Ticagrelor; Tofacitinib; Tolterodine; Tolvaptan;

Topotecan; Toremifene; Trabectedin; TraMADol; Triazolam; Ulipristal; Vardenafil; Vemurafenib; Vilazodone; VinBLAStine; VinCRIStine; VinCRIStine (Liposomal); Vinorelbine; Vitamin K Antagonists; Vorapaxar; Zolpidem; Zopiclone; Zuclopenthixol

The levels/effects of Itraconazole may be increased by: Boceprevir; Cobicistat; Conivaptan; CYP3A4 Inhibitors (Moderate); CYP3A4 Inhibitors (Strong); Darunavir; Etravirine; Fosamprenavir; Fusidic Acid (Systemic); Grapefruit Juice; Idelalisib; Indinavir; Lopinavir; Luliconazole; Mifepristone; Netupitant; Ritonavir; Saquinavir; Stiripentol; Telaprevir; Telithromycin; Tipranavir

Decreased Effect

Itraconazole may decrease the levels/effects of: Amphotericin B; Ifosfamide; Meloxicam; Prasugrel; Saccharomyces boulardii; Ticagrelor

The levels/effects of Itraconazole may be decreased by: Antacids; Bosentan; CYP3A4 Inducers (Moderate); CYP3A4 Inducers (Strong); Dabrafenib; Deferasirox; Didanosine; Efavirenz; Etravirine; Grapefruit Juice; H2-Antagonists; Isoniazid; Nevirapine; Proton Pump Inhibitors; Siltuximab; St Johns Wort; Sucralfate; Tocilizumab

Food Interactions

Capsules: Absorption enhanced by food and possibly by gastric acidity. Cola drinks have been shown to increase the absorption of the capsules in patients with achlorhydria or those taking H_2-receptor antagonists or other gastric acid suppressors. Grapefruit/grapefruit juice may increase serum levels. Management: Take capsules immediately after meals. Avoid grapefruit juice.

Solution: Food decreases the bioavailability and increases the time to peak concentration. Management: Take solution on an empty stomach 1 hour before or 2 hours after meals.

Storage/Stability

Capsule: Store at room temperature of 15°C to 25°C (59°F to 77°F). Protect from light and moisture.

Oral solution: Store at ≤25°C (77°F); do not freeze.

Tablet: Store at room temperature 15°C to 25°C (59°F to 77°F); excursions are permitted between 15°C and 30°C (59°F and 86°F). Protect from light and moisture.

Mechanism of Action Interferes with cytochrome P450 activity, decreasing ergosterol synthesis (principal sterol in fungal cell membrane) and inhibiting cell membrane formation

Pharmacokinetics (Adult data unless noted)

Absorption: Requires gastric acidity; capsule and tablet better absorbed with food; solution better absorbed on empty stomach

Distribution: V_d: 10 L/kg; highly lipophilic and tissue concentrations are higher than plasma concentrations. High affinity for tissues (liver, lung, kidney, adipose tissue, brain, vagina, dermis, epidermis); poor penetration into CSF, eye fluid, saliva; distributes into bronchial exudate and sputum

Protein binding: 99.8%; metabolite hydroxy-itraconazole: 99.6%

Metabolism: Extensively hepatic via CYP3A4 into >30 metabolites including hydroxy-itraconazole (major metabolite); appears to have *in vitro* antifungal activity. Main metabolic pathway is oxidation; may undergo saturation metabolism with multiple dosing.

Bioavailability: Variable, ~55% (oral solution) in one small study; **Note:** Oral solution has a higher degree of bioavailability (149% ± 68%) relative to oral capsules; should not be interchanged

Half-life:

Pediatric patients (6 months to 12 years): Oral solution: ~36 hours; metabolite hydroxy-itraconazole: ~18 hours

Adults: Oral: Single dose: 16 to 28 hours, Multiple doses: 34 to 42 hours; cirrhosis (single dose): 37 hours (range: 20 to 54 hours)

Time to peak serum concentration: Capsules/tablets: 2 to [illegible] hours; Oral solution: 2.5 hours

Elimination: Urine (<0.03% active drug, 35% as inactive metabolites); feces (54%; ~3% to 18% as unchanged drug)

Dialysis: Nondialyzable

Dosing: Neonatal Tinea capitis (*Microsporum canis*) Very limited data available: Oral: Oral solution: 5 mg/kg/dose once daily for 6 weeks was used in a single, full-term neonate as part of a larger open-label pilot study of seven infants (age: 3-46 weeks) who received therapy for 3-6 weeks (Binder, 2009)

Dosing: Usual Oral:

Infants and Children:

General dosing: Limited data available: Usual reported range: 3-5 mg/kg/dose once daily; doses as high as 5-10 mg/kg/**day** divided every 12-24 hours have been used in 32 patients with chronic granulomatous disease for prophylaxis against Aspergillus infection; doses of 6-8 mg/kg/**day** have been used in the treatment of disseminated histoplasmosis

***Candidiasis* (HIV-exposed/-positive)** (CDC, 2009):

Oropharyngeal, treatment: Oral solution: 2.5 mg/kg/dose twice daily for 7-14 days (maximum daily dose: 200 mg/**day** or 400 mg/**day** if fluconazole-refractory)

Esophageal, treatment: Oral solution: 5 mg/kg/**day** divided once or twice daily for 4-21 days

***Coccidioidomycosis*, disseminated, non-CNS (HIV-exposed/-positive)** (CDC, 2009):

Treatment: Oral: 5-10 mg/kg/dose twice daily for 3 days followed by 2-5 mg/kg/dose twice daily (maximum daily dose: 400 mg/**day**); product formulation not specified

Relapse prevention: 2-5 mg/kg/dose twice daily (maximum daily dose: 400 mg/**day**); product formulation not specified

***Crypotococcus* (HIV-exposed/-positive)** (CDC, 2009):

Treatment, consolidation therapy: Oral solution (preferred): Initial load: 2.5-5 mg/kg/dose 3 times daily (maximum daily dose: 600 mg/**day**) for 3 days (9 doses) followed by 5-10 mg/kg/**day** divided once or twice daily (maximum daily dose: 400 mg/**day**) for a minimum of 8 weeks

Relapse prevention: Oral solution: 5 mg/kg/dose once daily (maximum daily dose: 200 mg/**day**)

***Histoplasmosis* (HIV-exposed/-positive)** (CDC, 2009):

Treatment, mild disseminated disease: Oral solution: 2-5 mg/kg/dose 3 times daily for 3 days (9 doses) followed by 2-5 mg/kg/dose twice daily for 12 months (maximum dose: 200 mg/dose)

Consolidation treatment for moderate-severe to severe disseminated disease, including CNS infection (following appropriate induction therapy): Oral solution: 2-5 mg/kg/dose 3 times daily for 3 days (9 doses) followed by 2-5 mg/kg/dose (maximum dose: 200 mg/dose) twice daily for 12 months for non-CNS disseminated disease or for ≥12 months for CNS infection as determined by clinical response.

Relapse prevention: Oral solution: 5 mg/kg/dose twice daily (maximum daily dose: 400 mg/**day**)

Tinea capitis (*Microsporum canis*): Oral solution or capsules: 5 mg/kg/dose once daily for 3-6 weeks was used in a small open-label pilot study of seven infants (age: 3-46 weeks); if capsules were used, they were opened and sprinkled on main meal of the day (Binder, 2009)

Adolescents:

General dosing: 100-600 mg/**day**; doses >200 mg/**day** are usually given in 2 divided doses; length of therapy varies from 1 day to >6 months depending on the condition and mycological response

Candidiasis **(HIV-exposed/-positive)** (CDC, 2009a):

Oropharyngeal, treatment: Oral solution: 200 mg once daily for 7-14 days

Esophageal, treatment: Oral solution: 200 mg once daily for 14-21 days

Vulvovaginal, uncomplicated: Oral solution: 200 mg once daily for 3-7 days

Coccidioidomycosis **(HIV-exposed/-positive)** (CDC, 2009a):

Mild infection, treatment (eg, focal pneumonia): 200 mg 3 times daily for 3 days followed by 200 mg twice daily

Meningitis:

Treatment: 200 mg 3 times daily for 3 days followed by 200 mg twice daily

Maintenance therapy: 200 mg twice daily

Prevention of first episode: 200 mg twice daily

Crypotococcus **(CNS disease, meningitis) (HIV-exposed/-positive)** (CDC, 2009a):

Consolidation therapy: 200 mg twice daily for 8 weeks or as determined by target CD4+ counts; may be initiated after at least 2 weeks of successful induction therapy (eg, significant clinical improvement and negative CSF culture)

Maintenance therapy: 200 mg once daily

Histoplasmosis **(HIV-exposed/-positive)** (CDC, 2009a): **Note:** Monitoring of serum concentrations recommended to ensure adequate absorption.

Mild disseminated disease, treatment: Oral solution (preferred): 200 mg 3 times/day for 3 days, then 200 mg twice daily for at least 12 months

Moderate to severe non-CNS disease, maintenance therapy: Oral solution (preferred): 200 mg 3 times/day for 3 days, then 200 mg twice daily following amphotericin B induction therapy

Meningitis, maintenance therapy: Oral solution (preferred): 200 mg twice daily or 3 times/day for ≥1 year following liposomal amphotericin B induction therapy

Long-term suppression therapy: Oral solution (preferred): 200 mg once daily

Prevention of first episode: Oral solution (preferred): 200 mg once daily

Microsporidiosis**, treatment disseminated disease (HIV-exposed/-positive)** (CDC, 2009a): 400 mg once daily in conjunction with albendazole

Penicilliosis (HIV-exposed/-positive) (CDC, 2009a):

Acute infection (severely ill), maintenance therapy: 400 mg once daily for 10 weeks; initiate after completion of 2 weeks induction therapy with amphotericin B

Mild disease, treatment: 400 mg once daily for 8 weeks

Maintenance therapy: 200 mg once daily

Adult: **Note:** Doses >200 mg/**day** should be given in 2 divided doses.

Aspergillosis: Oral capsule: 200 to 400 mg daily. **Note:** For life-threatening infections, the US labeling recommends administering a loading dose of 200 mg 3 times daily (total: 600 mg daily) for the first 3 days of therapy. Continue treatment for at least 3 months and until clinical and laboratory evidence suggest that infection has resolved.

Blastomycosis:

Manufacturer's labeling: Oral capsule: Initial: 200 mg once daily; if no clinical improvement or evidence of progressive infection, may increase dose in increments of 100 mg up to maximum of 400 mg daily. **Note:** For life-threatening infections, the US labeling recommends administering a loading dose of 200 mg 3 times daily (total: 600 mg daily) for the first 3 days of therapy. Continue treatment for at least 3 months and until clinical and laboratory evidence suggest that infection has resolved.

Alternate dosing: Oral capsule: 200 mg 3 times daily for 3 days, then 200 mg twice daily for 6 to 12 months; in moderately severe to severe infection, therapy should be initiated with ~2 weeks of amphotericin B (Chapman 2008).

Candidiasis: Oral:

Esophageal: Oral solution: 100 to 200 mg once daily for a minimum of 3 weeks; continue dosing for 2 weeks after resolution of symptoms

Oropharyngeal: Oral solution: 200 mg once daily for 1 to 2 weeks; in patients unresponsive or refractory to fluconazole: 100 mg twice daily (clinical response expected in 2 to 4 weeks)

Histoplasmosis:

Manufacturer's labeling: Oral capsule: Initial: 200 mg once daily; if no clinical improvement or evidence of progressive infection, may increase dose in increments of 100 mg up to maximum of 400 mg daily. **Note:** For life-threatening infections, the US labeling recommends administering a loading dose of 200 mg 3 times daily (total: 600 mg daily) for the first 3 days of therapy. Continue treatment for at least 3 months and until clinical and laboratory evidence suggest that infection has resolved.

Alternative dosing: Oral capsule: 200 mg 3 times daily for 3 days, then 200 mg twice daily (or once daily in mild to moderate disease) for 6 to 12 weeks in mild to moderate disease or ≥12 months in progressive disseminated or chronic cavitary pulmonary histoplasmosis; in moderately severe to severe infection, therapy should be initiated with ~2 weeks of a lipid formation of amphotericin B (Wheat 2007).

Onychomycosis (fingernail involvement only): Oral capsule: 200 mg twice daily for 1 week; repeat 1-week course after 3-week off-time

Onychomycosis (toenails due to *Trichophyton rubrum* or *T. mentagrophytes*): Oral tablet: 200 mg once daily for 12 consecutive weeks.

Onychomycosis (toenails with or without fingernail involvement): Oral capsule: 200 mg once daily for 12 consecutive weeks

Dosing adjustment in renal impairment: The FDA-approved labeling states to use with caution in patients with renal impairment. The following guidelines have been used by some clinicians: Adults (Aronoff 2007):

CrCl >10 mL/minute: No adjustment recommended.

CrCl <10 mL/minute: Administer 50% of normal dose.

Poorly dialyzed; no supplemental dose or dosage adjustment necessary, including patients on intermittent hemodialysis, peritoneal dialysis, or continuous renal replacement therapy (eg, CVVHD).

Dosing adjustment in hepatic impairment: Use caution.

Administration Oral: Doses >200 mg/day are given in 2 divided doses; do not administer with antacids. **Capsule and oral solution formulations are not bioequivalent and thus are not interchangeable.** Capsule absorption is best if taken with food, therefore, it is best to administer itraconazole after meals; solution should be taken on an empty stomach. When treating oropharyngeal and esophageal candidiasis, solution should be swished vigorously in mouth, then swallowed.

Monitoring Parameters Liver function in patients with pre-existing hepatic dysfunction, and in all patients being treated for longer than 1 month; serum concentrations particularly for oral therapy (due to erratic bioavailability with capsule formulation); renal function; serum potassium; monitor for prodromal signs of hepatitis; signs/symptoms of CHF

Reference Range

Serum concentrations may be performed to assure therapeutic levels. Itraconazole plus the metabolite hydroxyitraconazole concentrations should be >1 mcg/mL (not to exceed 10 mcg/mL).

Timing of serum samples: Obtain level after ~2 weeks of therapy, level may be drawn anytime during the dosing interval.

Dosage Forms Excipient information presented when available (limited, particularly for generics); consult specific product labeling.

Capsule, Oral:

Sporanox: 100 mg [contains brilliant blue fcf (fd&c blue #1), d&c red #22 (eosine), fd&c blue #2 (indigotine)]

Sporanox Pulsepak: 100 mg [contains brilliant blue fcf (fd&c blue #1), d&c red #22 (eosine), fd&c blue #2 (indigotine)]

Generic: 100 mg

Solution, Oral:

Sporanox: 10 mg/mL (150 mL)

Tablet, Oral:

Onmel: 200 mg

Extemporaneous Preparations Note: Commercial oral solution is available (10 mg/mL)

A 20 mg/mL oral suspension may be made with capsules. Empty the contents of forty 100 mg capsules and add 15 mL of Alcohol, USP. Let stand for 5 minutes. Crush the beads in a mortar and reduce to a fine powder. Mix while adding a 1:1 mixture of Ora-Sweet and Ora-Plus in incremental proportions to **almost** 200 mL; transfer to a calibrated bottle, rinse mortar with vehicle, and add quantity of vehicle sufficient to make 200 mL. Label "shake well" and "refrigerate". Stable for 56 days refrigerated.

Nahata MC, Pai VB, and Hipple TF, *Pediatric Drug Formulations*, 5th ed, Cincinnati, OH: Harvey Whitney Books Co, 2004.

Ivacaftor (eye va KAF tor)

Brand Names: US Kalydeco

Brand Names: Canada Kalydeco

Therapeutic Category Cystic Fibrosis Transmembrane Conductance Regulator Potentiator

Generic Availability (US) No

Use Treatment of cystic fibrosis (CF) in patients who have one of the following mutations in the cystic fibrosis transmembrane conductance regulator (CFTR) gene: G551D, G1244E, G1349D, G178R, G551S, R117H, S1251N, S1255P, S549N, or S549R (FDA approved in ages ≥2 years and adults); **Note:** If the patient's genotype is unknown, a US Food and Drug Administration-cleared cystic fibrosis mutation test should be used to detect the presence of a CFTR mutation followed by verification with bidirectional sequencing when recommended by the mutation test instructions for use. Has not been shown effective in CF patients who are homozygous for the F508del mutation in the CFTR gene

Pregnancy Risk Factor B

Pregnancy Considerations Adverse events have not been observed in animal reproduction studies.

Breast-Feeding Considerations Although unknown, the manufacturer suggests that excretion of ivacaftor in breast milk is probable; caution is recommended when administering ivacaftor to nursing women.

Contraindications There are no contraindications listed in the manufacturer's U.S. labeling.

Canadian labeling: Hypersensitivity to ivacaftor or any component of the formulation

Warnings/Precautions May increase hepatic transaminases. Monitor liver function; increased monitoring may be necessary in patients with a history of elevated hepatic transaminases. Temporarily discontinue treatment if ALT or AST >5 times ULN. Use with caution in patients with moderate or severe hepatic impairment; dosage adjustment recommended. Noncongenital lens opacities and cataracts have been reported in pediatric patients treated with ivacaftor; other risk factors were present in some cases (eg, corticosteroid use, exposure to radiation), but a possible risk related to ivacaftor cannot be excluded. Baseline and follow-up ophthalmological examinations are recommended in pediatric patients. Potentially significant drug-drug interactions may exist, requiring dose or frequency adjustment, additional monitoring, and/or selection of alternative therapy.

Adverse Reactions

Central nervous system: Dizziness, headache

Dermatologic: Acne vulgaris, Skin rash

Gastrointestinal: Abdominal pain, diarrhea, nausea

Endocrine & metabolic: Hypoglycemia, increased serum glucose

Hepatic: Increased liver enzymes, increased serum ALT

Neuromuscular & skeletal: Arthralgia, musculoskeletal chest pain, myalgia

Ophthalmic: Cataract (children)

Respiratory: Change in bronchial secretions (bacteria present), nasal congestion, nasopharyngitis, oropharyngeal pain, pharyngeal erythema, pleuritic chest pain, rhinitis, sinus congestion, sinus headache, upper respiratory tract infection, wheezing

Miscellaneous: Bacteria in sputum

Drug Interactions

Metabolism/Transport Effects Substrate of CYP3A4 (major); **Note:** Assignment of Major/Minor substrate status based on clinically relevant drug interaction potential. **Inhibits** CYP2C8 (weak), CYP2C9 (weak), CYP3A4 (weak), P-glycoprotein

Avoid Concomitant Use

Avoid concomitant use of Ivacaftor with any of the following: Amodiaquine; Bitter Orange; Bosutinib; Conivaptan; CYP3A4 Inducers (Strong); Fusidic Acid (Systemic); Grapefruit Juice; Idelalisib; PAZOPanib; Pimozide; Silodosin; St Johns Wort; Topotecan; VinCRIStine (Liposomal)

Increased Effect/Toxicity

Ivacaftor may increase the levels/effects of: Afatinib; Amodiaquine; ARIPiprazole; Bosutinib; Brentuximab Vedotin; Colchicine; CYP3A4 Substrates; Dabigatran Etexilate; Dofetilide; DOXOrubicin (Conventional); Edoxaban; Everolimus; Hydrocodone; Ledipasvir; Lomitapide; Naloxegol; NiMODipine; PAZOPanib; P-glycoprotein/ABCB1 Substrates; Pimozide; Prucalopride; Rifaximin; Rivaroxaban; Silodosin; Topotecan; VinCRIStine (Liposomal)

The levels/effects of Ivacaftor may be increased by: Bitter Orange; Conivaptan; CYP3A4 Inhibitors (Moderate); CYP3A4 Inhibitors (Strong); Dasatinib; Fusidic Acid (Systemic); Grapefruit Juice; Idelalisib; Luliconazole; Mifepristone; Palbociclib; Simeprevir; Stiripentol

Decreased Effect

The levels/effects of Ivacaftor may be decreased by: Bosentan; CYP3A4 Inducers (Moderate); CYP3A4 Inducers (Strong); Dabrafenib; Deferasirox; Siltuximab; St Johns Wort; Tocilizumab

Food Interactions Ivacaftor serum concentrations may be increased when taken with grapefruit or Seville oranges. Management: Avoid concurrent use.

Storage/Stability Store at 20°C to 25°C (68°F to 77°F); excursions permitted to 15°C to 30°C (59°F to 86°F); after mixing the granules, the product is stable for 1 hour.

Mechanism of Action Potentiates epithelial cell chloride ion transport of defective (G551D mutant) cell-surface CFTR protein thereby improving the regulation of salt and water absorption and secretion in various tissues (eg, lung, gastrointestinal tract).

Pharmacodynamics Onset of action: FEV_1 increased, sweat chloride decreased within ~2 weeks

Pharmacokinetics (Adult data unless noted)

Absorption: Variable; increased (by two- to fourfold) with fatty foods

Distribution: V_d: 353 L ± 122 L

Protein binding: ~99%; primarily to alpha$_1$ acid glycoprotein, albumin

Metabolism: Hepatic; extensive via CYP3A4; forms 2 major metabolites [M1 (active; 1/6 potency) and M6 (inactive)]

Half-life: ~12 hours

Time to peak serum concentration: ~4 hours

Elimination: Feces (88%, 65% of administered dose as metabolites); urine (minimal, as unchanged drug)

Dosing: Usual

Pediatric: **Cystic Fibrosis:**

Children 2 to < 6 years: Oral granules:

<14 kg: 50 mg granule packet every 12 hours

≥14 kg: 75 mg granule packet every 12 hours

Children ≥6 years and Adolescents: Oral tablet: 150 mg every 12 hours

Dosage adjustment for concomitant therapy:

Coadministration with CYP3A4 strong inhibitors (eg, ketoconazole, itraconazole, posaconazole, voriconazole, clarithromycin, telithromycin):

Children 2 to < 6 years: Oral granules:

<14 kg: 50 mg granule packet twice **weekly**

≥14 kg: 75 mg granule packet twice **weekly**

Children ≥6 years and Adolescents: Oral tablet: 150 mg twice **weekly**

Coadministration with CYP3A4 moderate inhibitors (eg, erythromycin, fluconazole):

Children 2 to <6 years: Oral granules:

<14 kg: 50 mg granule packet once daily

≥14 kg: 75 mg granule packet once daily

Children ≥6 years and Adolescents: Oral tablet: 150 mg once daily

Adult: **Cystic Fibrosis:** Oral tablet: 150 mg every 12 hours

Dosage adjustment for concomitant therapy:

Coadministration with CYP3A4 strong inhibitors (eg, ketoconazole, itraconazole, posaconazole, voriconazole, clarithromycin, telithromycin): Oral tablet: 150 mg twice **weekly**

Coadministration with CYP3A4 moderate inhibitors (eg, erythromycin, fluconazole): Oral tablet: 150 mg once daily

Dosing adjustment for toxicity; elevation of aminotransferases: Children ≥2 years, Adolescents, and Adults: ALT or AST >5 times ULN: Oral: Hold ivacaftor; may resume if elevated transaminases resolved and after assessing benefits vs risks of continued treatment

Dosing adjustment in renal impairment: Children ≥2 years, Adolescents, and Adults:

CrCl >30 mL/minute: No dosage adjustment necessary

CrCl ≤30 mL/minute: There are no dosage adjustments provided in manufacturer's labeling (not studied); use with caution

End-stage renal disease (ESRD): There are no dosage adjustments provided in manufacturer's labeling (not studied); use with caution.

Dosing adjustment in hepatic impairment: Children ≥2 years, Adolescents, and Adults:

Mild impairment (Child-Pugh class A): No dosage adjustment necessary

Moderate impairment (Child-Pugh class B): Oral: Administer usual dose once daily

Severe impairment (Child-Pugh class C): Oral: Administer usual dose once daily or less frequently; use with caution

Administration

Oral granules: Administer before or after high-fat-containing foods (eg, butter, cheese pizza, eggs, peanut butter, whole milk dairy products [eg, whole milk, cheese, yogurt]). Mix entire packet of granules with a teaspoon of soft food (eg, pureed fruits or vegetables, yogurt, applesauce) or 5 mL of liquid (eg, water, milk, juice); food or liquid should be at or below room temperature. Granule mixture should be completely consumed within 1 hour.

Oral tablet: Administer with high-fat-containing foods (eg, butter, cheese pizza, eggs, peanut butter).

Monitoring Parameters CF mutation test (prior to therapy initiation if G551D mutation status unknown); ALT/AST at baseline, every 3 months for 1 year, then annually thereafter or as clinically indicated (consider more frequent monitoring in patients with a history of elevated hepatic transaminases); FEV$_1$; baseline and follow-up ophthalmological exams in pediatric patients

Dosage Forms Excipient information presented when available (limited, particularly for generics); consult specific product labeling.

Packet, Oral:

Kalydeco: 50 mg (56 ea); 75 mg (56 ea)

Tablet, Oral:

Kalydeco: 150 mg [contains fd&c blue #2 (indigotine)]

Ivermectin (Systemic) (eye ver MEK tin)

Brand Names: US Stromectol

Therapeutic Category Anthelmintic; Anti-ectoparasitic Agent

Generic Availability (US) Yes

Use Treatment of intestinal strongyloidiasis (FDA approved in pediatric patients ≥15 kg and adults); treatment of onchocerciasis due to the immature form of *Onchocerca volvulus* (FDA approved in pediatric patients ≥15 kg and adults). Has also been used for the treatment of other parasitic infections including but not limited to: *Ancylostoma braziliense*, *Ascaris lumbricoides*, *Gnathostoma spinigerum*, *Mansonella ozzardi*, *Mansonella streptocerca*, *Pediculus humanus capitis*, *Pediculus humanus corporis*, *Phthirus pubis*, *Trichuris trichiura*, *Sarcoptes scabiei*, *Wucheria bancrofti*

Pregnancy Risk Factor C

Pregnancy Considerations Teratogenic effects have been observed in animal reproduction studies; therefore, the manufacturer classifies ivermectin as pregnancy category C. Ivermectin is not recommended for use in pregnancy. Although studies during pregnancy are limited, several mass treatment programs have not identified an increased risk of adverse fetal, neonatal, or maternal outcomes following ivermectin use in the first and second trimesters.

Breast-Feeding Considerations Ivermectin is measurable in low concentrations in breast milk and is less than maternal plasma concentrations. Peak concentrations of ivermectin in breast milk may occur 4-12 hours after the oral dose. In one study, the calculated infant daily dose was 2.75 mcg/kg in a 1-month-old infant and would not be expected to cause adverse effects in the infant. The manufacturer and the CDC do not have safety data in children <15 kg and the CDC does not recommend the use of ivermectin in lactating women.

Contraindications Hypersensitivity to ivermectin or any component of the formulation

Warnings/Precautions Data have shown that antihelmintic drugs like ivermectin may cause cutaneous and/or systemic reactions (Mazzoti reaction) of varying severity including ophthalmological reactions in patients with onchocerciasis. These reactions are probably due to allergic and inflammatory responses to the death of microfilariae. Patients with hyper-reactive onchodermatitis may be more likely than others to experience severe adverse reactions, especially edema and aggravation of the onchodermatitis. Repeated treatment may be required in immunocompromised patients (eg, HIV); control of extraintestinal strongyloidiasis may necessitate suppressive (once monthly) therapy. Pretreatment assessment for *Loa loa* infection is recommended in any patient with significant exposure to endemic areas (West and Central Africa); serious and/or fatal encephalopathy has been reported (rarely) during treatment in patients with loiasis. Ivermectin has no activity against adult *Onchocerca volvulus* parasites.

Warnings: Additional Pediatric Considerations Avoid use or use with extreme caution in pediatric patients <2 years or <15 kg; the American Academy of Pediatrics (AAP) cautions against using ivermectin in these patients due to a less developed blood-brain barrier compared to older pediatric patients and an increased risk for CNS effects (ie, encephalopathy); monitor patients closely.

Adverse Reactions

Cardiovascular: Facial edema, orthostatic hypotension, peripheral edema, tachycardia

Central nervous system: Dizziness

Dermatologic: Pruritus

Gastrointestinal: Diarrhea, nausea

Hematologic: Eosinophilia, hemoglobin increased, leukocytes decreased

Hepatic: ALT increased, AST increased

Miscellaneous: Mazzotti-type reaction (with onchocerciasis): Arthralgia/synovitis, fever, lymph node enlargement/tenderness, pruritus, skin involvement (edema/urticarial rash)

Rare but important or life-threatening: Abdominal distention, abdominal pain, anemia, anorexia, anterior uveitis, asthma exacerbation, back pain, bilirubin increased, chest discomfort, chorioretinitis, choroiditis, coma, confusion, conjunctival hemorrhage (associated with onchocerciasis), conjunctivitis, constipation, dyspnea, encephalopathy (rare; associated with loiasis), eyelid edema, eye sensation abnormal, fatigue, fecal incontinence, headache, hepatitis, hypotension, INR increased (with concomitant warfarin), keratitis, lethargy, leukopenia, mental status changes, myalgia, neck pain, rash, red eye, seizure, somnolence, standing/walking difficulty, Stevens-Johnson syndrome, stupor, toxic epidermal necrolysis, tremor, urinary incontinence, urticaria, vertigo, vision loss (transient), vomiting, weakness

Drug Interactions

Metabolism/Transport Effects Substrate of CYP3A4 (minor), P-glycoprotein; **Note:** Assignment of Major/Minor substrate status based on clinically relevant drug interaction potential

Avoid Concomitant Use

Avoid concomitant use of Ivermectin (Systemic) with any of the following: BCG; BCG (Intravesical)

Increased Effect/Toxicity

Ivermectin (Systemic) may increase the levels/effects of: Vitamin K Antagonists

The levels/effects of Ivermectin (Systemic) may be increased by: Azithromycin (Systemic); P-glycoprotein/ABCB1 Inhibitors

Decreased Effect

Ivermectin (Systemic) may decrease the levels/effects of: BCG; BCG (Intravesical); BCG Vaccine (Immunization); Sodium Picosulfate; Typhoid Vaccine

The levels/effects of Ivermectin (Systemic) may be decreased by: P-glycoprotein/ABCB1 Inducers

Food Interactions Bioavailability is increased 2.5-fold when administered following a high-fat meal. Management: Administer on an empty stomach.

Storage/Stability Store at <30°C (86°F).

Mechanism of Action Ivermectin is a semisynthetic anthelminthic agent; it binds selectively and with strong affinity to glutamate-gated chloride ion channels which occur in invertebrate nerve and muscle cells. This leads to increased permeability of cell membranes to chloride ions then hyperpolarization of the nerve or muscle cell, and death of the parasite.

Pharmacokinetics (Adult data unless noted)

Absorption: Well absorbed

Distribution: V_d: 3.1-3.5 L/kg; High concentration in the liver and adipose tissue; excreted in breast milk in low concentrations; does not readily cross the blood-brain barrier in patients >15 kg or >2 years

Protein binding: 93% primarily to albumin

Half-life: 18 hours (range: 16-35 hours)

Time to peak serum concentration: 4 hours

Metabolism: >97% in the liver by CYP3A4; substrate of the p-glycoprotein transport system

Elimination: <1% in urine; feces

Dosing: Usual Oral: Children ≥15 kg, Adolescents, and Adults:

Onchocerciasis: 150 mcg/kg/dose as a single dose; may repeat every 3-12 months until asymptomatic

Strongyloidiasis: Manufacturer recommendations: 200 mcg/kg as a single dose; perform follow-up stool examinations; Alternative dosing: 200 mcg/kg/day once daily for 2 days (*Red Book*, 2009). In immunocompromised patients or patients with disseminated disease, may need to repeat therapy at 2-week intervals.

Ascariasis: 150-200 mcg/kg/dose as a single dose

Cutaneous larva migran due to *Ancylostoma braziliense*: 200 mcg/kg once daily for 1-2 days

Gnathostomiasis due to *Gnathostoma spinigerum*: 200 mcg/kg once daily for 2 days

Filariasis due to *Mansonella streptocerca*: 150 mcg/kg/dose as a single dose

Filariasis due to *Mansonella ozzardi*: 200 mcg/kg/dose as a single dose

Pediculosis: 400 mcg/kg/dose as a single dose on days 1 and 8 (Chosidow, 2010); alternatively, 200 mcg/kg/dose every 7 days for 3 doses (Foucault, 2006) **or** 200 mcg/kg/dose repeated once after 10 days (Jones, 2003) have been shown to be effective

Scabies due to *Sarcoptes scabiei*: 200 mcg/kg/dose as a single dose; may need to repeat in 10-14 days

Trichuriasis due to *Trichuris trichiura*: 200 mcg/kg once daily for 3 days

Filariasis due to *Wucheria bancrofti*: 200 mcg/kg/dose as a single dose given in combination with albendazole

Alternatively, the following weight-based dosing can be used: See tables.

Weight-Based Dosage to Provide ~150 mcg/kg

Patient Weight (kg)	Single Oral Dose
15-25	3 mg
26-44	6 mg
45-64	9 mg
65-84	12 mg
≥85	150 mcg/kg

Weight-Based Dosage to Provide ~200 mcg/kg

Patient Weight (kg)	Single Oral Dose
15-24	3 mg
25-35	6 mg
36-50	9 mg
51-65	12 mg
66-79	15 mg
≥80	200 mcg/kg

Administration Oral: Administer on an empty stomach with water

Monitoring Parameters Skin and eye microfilarial counts, periodic ophthalmologic exams; follow up stool examinations

Dosage Forms Excipient information presented when available (limited, particularly for generics); consult specific product labeling.

Tablet, Oral:

Stromectol: 3 mg

Generic: 3 mg

Ivermectin (Topical) (eye ver MEK tin)

Brand Names: US Sklice; Soolantra

Therapeutic Category Antiparasitic Agent, Topical; Pediculocide

Generic Availability (US) No

Use

Lotion (Sklice): Treatment of head lice *(Pediculus capitis)* infestation (FDA approved in ages ≥6 months and adults)

Cream (Soolantra): Treatment of inflammatory lesions of rosacea (FDA approved in adults)

Pregnancy Risk Factor C

Pregnancy Considerations Teratogenic effects have been observed in animal reproduction studies following oral administration. Refer to the Ivermectin (Systemic) monograph for additional information. Systemic absorption is less following topical application than with oral administration.

Breast-Feeding Considerations Following oral administration, ivermectin is measurable in low concentrations in breast milk. Refer to Ivermectin (Systemic) monograph for additional information. Systemic absorption is less following topical application than with oral administration.

Contraindications There are no contraindications listed in the manufacturer's labeling.

Warnings/Precautions Lotion is for topical use on scalp and scalp hair only; avoid contact with eyes. Cream is not for oral, ophthalmic, or vaginal use; avoid contact with eyes and lips. For lotion or cream, wash hands after application.

Warnings: Additional Pediatric Considerations In infants <6 months, systemic absorption may be increased due to higher skin surface area to body mass ratio and immature skin barrier; risk for ivermectin toxicity potentially increased; avoid use in these patients.

Adverse Reactions

Central nervous system: Localized burning

Dermatologic: Skin irritation

Rare but important or life-threatening: Conjunctivitis, eye irritation, ocular hyperemia, seborrheic dermatitis of scalp, xeroderma

Drug Interactions

Metabolism/Transport Effects None known.

Avoid Concomitant Use There are no known interactions where it is recommended to avoid concomitant use.

Increased Effect/Toxicity There are no known significant interactions involving an increase in effect.

Decreased Effect There are no known significant interactions involving a decrease in effect.

Storage/Stability Store at 20°C to 25°C (68°F to 77°F); excursions permitted between 15°C to 30°C (59°F to 86°F). Lotion: do not freeze.

Mechanism of Action In pediculosis capitus treatment, ivermectin is a semisynthetic anthelminthic agent; it binds selectively and with strong affinity to glutamate-gated chloride ion channels which occur in invertebrate nerve and muscle cells. This leads to increased permeability of cell membranes to chloride ions then hyperpolarization of the nerve or muscle cell, and death of the parasite.

In rosacea treatment, the mechanism of action is unknown.

Dosing: Usual

Pediatric: **Head lice:** Topical: Lotion (Sklice): Infants ≥6 months, Children, and Adolescents: Apply sufficient amount (up to 1 tube) to completely cover dry hair and scalp; for single use only

Adult:

Head lice: Topical: Lotion (Sklice): Apply sufficient amount (up to 1 tube) to completely cover dry scalp and hair; for single-dose use only

Rosacea: Topical: Cream (Soolanta): Apply to each affected area (eg, forehead, chin, nose, each cheek) once daily

Dosing adjustment in renal impairment: All patients: There are no dosing adjustments provided in the manufacturer's labeling.

Dosing adjustment in hepatic impairment: All patients: There are no dosing adjustments provided in the manufacturer's labeling.

Administration

Head lice: Topical Lotion: For external use only. Apply to dry scalp and hair closest to scalp first, then apply outward towards ends of hair; completely covering scalp and hair. Leave on for 10 minutes (start timing treatment after the scalp and hair have been completely covered). The hair should then be rinsed thoroughly with warm water. Avoid contact with the eyes. Nit combing is not required, although a fine-tooth comb may be used to remove treated lice and nits. Lotion is for one-time use; discard any unused portion.

Ivermectin should be a portion of a whole lice removal program, which should include washing or dry cleaning all clothing, hats, bedding, and towels recently worn or used by the patient and washing combs, brushes, and hair accessories in hot, soapy water.

Rosacea: Topical cream: For external use only. Not for use in the eye, mouth or vagina. Wash hands with soap and water prior to application and after application. Apply a pea-size amount as a thin layer on each affected area (eg, forehead, chin, nose, each cheek).

Dosage Forms Excipient information presented when available (limited, particularly for generics); consult specific product labeling.

Cream, External:

Soolantra: 1% (30 g) [contains cetyl alcohol, edetate disodium, methylparaben, propylene glycol, propylparaben]

Lotion, External:

Sklice: 0.5% (117 g) [contains methylparaben, propylparaben]

◆ **Ivermectin Cream** *see* Ivermectin (Topical) *on page 1183*

◆ **Ivermectin Lotion** *see* Ivermectin (Topical) *on page 1183*

◆ **IVIG** *see* Immune Globulin *on page 1089*

◆ **IV Immune Globulin** *see* Immune Globulin *on page 1089*

◆ **Ivy-Rid [OTC]** *see* Benzocaine *on page 268*

◆ **Ixiaro** *see* Japanese Encephalitis Virus Vaccine (Inactivated) *on page 1184*

◆ **Ixinity** *see* Factor IX (Recombinant) *on page 842*

◆ **JAA-Aminophylline (Can)** *see* Aminophylline *on page 122*

◆ **Jadenu** *see* Deferasirox *on page 594*

◆ **JAMP-Allopurinol (Can)** *see* Allopurinol *on page 96*

◆ **JAMP-Amlodipine (Can)** *see* AmLODIPine *on page 133*

◆ **JAMP-Atenolol (Can)** *see* Atenolol *on page 215*

◆ **JAMP-Atorvastatin (Can)** *see* AtorvaSTATin *on page 220*

- ◆ **JAMP-Candesartan (Can)** *see* Candesartan *on page 358*
- ◆ **JAMP-Carvedilol (Can)** *see* Carvedilol *on page 380*
- ◆ **JAMP-Celecoxib (Can)** *see* Celecoxib *on page 418*
- ◆ **JAMP-Ciprofloxacin (Can)** *see* Ciprofloxacin (Systemic) *on page 463*
- ◆ **JAMP-Citalopram (Can)** *see* Citalopram *on page 476*
- ◆ **JAMP-Clopidogrel (Can)** *see* Clopidogrel *on page 513*
- ◆ **Jamp-Colchicine (Can)** *see* Colchicine *on page 528*
- ◆ **JAMP-Cyclobenzaprine (Can)** *see* Cyclobenzaprine *on page 548*
- ◆ **Jamp-Dicyclomine (Can)** *see* Dicyclomine *on page 645*
- ◆ **Jamp-Dimenhydrinate [OTC] (Can)** *see* DimenhyDRINATE *on page 664*
- ◆ **Jamp-Docusate [OTC] (Can)** *see* Docusate *on page 697*
- ◆ **JAMP-Escitalopram (Can)** *see* Escitalopram *on page 786*
- ◆ **JAMP-Ezetimibe (Can)** *see* Ezetimibe *on page 832*
- ◆ **JAMP-Fluoxetine (Can)** *see* FLUoxetine *on page 906*
- ◆ **Jamp-Fosinopril (Can)** *see* Fosinopril *on page 943*
- ◆ **JAMP-Gabapentin (Can)** *see* Gabapentin *on page 954*
- ◆ **Jamp-Ibuprofen (Can)** *see* Ibuprofen *on page 1064*
- ◆ **JAMP-Irbesartan (Can)** *see* Irbesartan *on page 1158*
- ◆ **Jamp-Lactulose (Can)** *see* Lactulose *on page 1204*
- ◆ **JAMP-Letrozole (Can)** *see* Letrozole *on page 1224*
- ◆ **JAMP-Levetiracetam (Can)** *see* LevETIRAcetam *on page 1234*
- ◆ **JAMP-Lisinopril (Can)** *see* Lisinopril *on page 1280*
- ◆ **JAMP-Losartan (Can)** *see* Losartan *on page 1302*
- ◆ **JAMP-Metformin (Can)** *see* MetFORMIN *on page 1375*
- ◆ **JAMP-Metformin Blackberry (Can)** *see* MetFORMIN *on page 1375*
- ◆ **JAMP-Methotrexate (Can)** *see* Methotrexate *on page 1390*
- ◆ **JAMP-Metoprolol-L (Can)** *see* Metoprolol *on page 1418*
- ◆ **Jamp-Montelukast (Can)** *see* Montelukast *on page 1459*
- ◆ **JAMP-Mycophenolate (Can)** *see* Mycophenolate *on page 1473*
- ◆ **JAMP-Olanzapine ODT (Can)** *see* OLANZapine *on page 1546*
- ◆ **JAMP-Omeprazole DR (Can)** *see* Omeprazole *on page 1555*
- ◆ **JAMP-Ondansetron (Can)** *see* Ondansetron *on page 1564*
- ◆ **Jamp-Oxcarbazepine (Can)** *see* OXcarbazepine *on page 1584*
- ◆ **JAMP-Pantoprazole (Can)** *see* Pantoprazole *on page 1618*
- ◆ **JAMP-Paroxetine (Can)** *see* PARoxetine *on page 1634*
- ◆ **JAMP-Pravastatin (Can)** *see* Pravastatin *on page 1749*
- ◆ **JAMP-Quetiapine (Can)** *see* QUEtiapine *on page 1815*
- ◆ **JAMP-Risperidone (Can)** *see* RisperiDONE *on page 1866*
- ◆ **JAMP-Rizatriptan (Can)** *see* Rizatriptan *on page 1879*
- ◆ **JAMP-Rizatriptan IR (Can)** *see* Rizatriptan *on page 1879*
- ◆ **Jamp-Rosuvastatin (Can)** *see* Rosuvastatin *on page 1886*
- ◆ **JAMP-Sertraline (Can)** *see* Sertraline *on page 1916*
- ◆ **Jamp-Sildenafil (Can)** *see* Sildenafil *on page 1921*
- ◆ **JAMP-Simvastatin (Can)** *see* Simvastatin *on page 1928*
- ◆ **JAMP-Terbinafine (Can)** *see* Terbinafine (Systemic) *on page 2021*
- ◆ **JAMP-Tobramycin (Can)** *see* Tobramycin (Systemic, Oral Inhalation) *on page 2073*
- ◆ **JAMP-Vancomycin (Can)** *see* Vancomycin *on page 2151*
- ◆ **Jantoven** *see* Warfarin *on page 2195*

Japanese Encephalitis Virus Vaccine (Inactivated)

(jap a NEESE en sef a LYE tis VYE rus vak SEEN, in ak ti VAY ted)

Related Information

Centers for Disease Control and Prevention (CDC) and Other Links *on page 2424*

Immunization Administration Recommendations *on page 2411*

Immunization Schedules *on page 2416*

Brand Names: US Ixiaro

Brand Names: Canada Ixiaro

Therapeutic Category Vaccine; Vaccine, Inactivated Virus

Generic Availability (US) No

Use Provide active immunity to Japanese encephalitis virus (Ixiaro®: FDA approved in ages ≥2 months and adults).

Japanese encephalitis vaccine is not recommended for all persons traveling to or residing in Asia. The Advisory Committee on Immunization Practices (ACIP) recommends vaccination for (CDC, 2010):

- Persons spending ≥1 month in endemic areas during transmission season.
- Research laboratory workers who may be exposed to the Japanese encephalitis virus.

Vaccination may also be considered for the following:

- Travel to areas with an ongoing outbreak
- Travelers planning to go outside of urban areas during transmission season and have an increased risk of exposure. For example, high-risk activities include extensive outdoor activity in rural areas especially at night; extensive outdoor activities such as camping, hiking, etc; staying in accommodations without air conditioning, screens or bed nets
- Travelers to endemic areas who are unsure of specific destination, activities, or duration of travel

Medication Guide Available Yes

Pregnancy Risk Factor B

Pregnancy Considerations Adverse events were not observed in animal reproduction studies. Risks of vaccine administration should be carefully considered and in general, pregnant women should only be vaccinated if they are at high risk for exposure. Infection from Japanese encephalitis during the first or second trimesters of pregnancy may increase risk of miscarriage. Intrauterine transmission of the Japanese encephalitis virus has been reported (CDC, 2010). To report inadvertent use of Ixiaro® during pregnancy, contact Novartis Vaccines (877-683-4732).

Breast-Feeding Considerations It is not known if the vaccine is excreted into breast milk; however, the ACIP does not consider breast-feeding to be a contraindication to (CDC, 2010). The manufacturer recommends that caution be used if administered to nursing women.

Contraindications

U.S. labeling: Severe allergic reaction to a previous dose of the vaccine, any other Japanese encephalitis virus vaccine, or any component of the vaccine, including protamine sulfate

Canadian labeling: Hypersensitivity to a previous dose of the vaccine or to any component of the formulation; acute severe febrile conditions

Warnings/Precautions Because of the potential for severe adverse reactions, Japanese encephalitis vaccine is not recommended for all persons traveling to or residing in Asia. Use is not recommended for short-term travelers (<30 days) who will not be outside of an urban area or when the visit is outside of a well-defined Japanese encephalitis virus transmission season. Risk of exposure to the Japanese encephalitis virus may vary from year to year for a particular area. Immediate treatment for anaphylactic/anaphylactoid reaction should be available during vaccine use (CDC, 2010).

Use of vaccine should also include other means to reduce the risk of mosquito exposure (bed nets, insect repellents, protective clothing, avoidance of travel in endemic areas, and avoidance of outdoor activity during twilight and evening periods) (CDC, 2010).

May contain protamine sulfate which may cause hypersensitivity reactions in certain individuals. Immunization should be completed ≥7 days prior to potential exposure.

In general, the decision to administer or delay vaccination because of current or recent febrile illness depends on the severity of symptoms and the etiology of the disease. Immunocompromised patients may have a reduced response to vaccines; information not available specific to this vaccine. In general, household and close contacts of persons with altered immunocompetence may receive all age appropriate vaccines. Vaccination may not result in effective immunity in all patients. Response depends upon multiple factors (eg, type of vaccine, age of patient) and may be improved by administering the vaccine at the recommended dose, route, and interval. Vaccines may not be effective if administered during periods of altered immune competence (CDC 60[2], 2011). In order to maximize vaccination rates, the ACIP recommends simultaneous administration of all age-appropriate vaccines (live or inactivated) for which a person is eligible at a single clinic visit, unless contraindications exist (CDC 60[2], 2011); inactivated vaccines should be administered ≥2 weeks prior to planned immunosuppression when feasible (Rubin, 2014). Canadian labeling recommends avoiding IM administration in patients with bleeding disorders (eg, thrombocytopenia, hemophilia) and suggests that SubQ administration may be considered in these patients. Clinical efficacy data regarding this route is lacking and the U.S. labeling does not recommend SubQ administration.

Warnings: Additional Pediatric Considerations Routine prophylactic administration of acetaminophen to prevent fever due to vaccines has been shown to decrease the immune response of some vaccines; the clinical significance of this reduction in immune response has not been established (Prymula, 2009).

Adverse Reactions Report allergic or unusual adverse reactions to the Vaccine Adverse Event Reporting System (VAERS) 1-800-822-7967 or online at https://vaers.hhs.gov/esub/index. In Canada, adverse reactions may be reported to local provincial/territorial health agencies or to the Vaccine Safety Section at Public Health Agency of Canada (1-866-844-0018).

Central nervous system: Fatigue (more common in adults), headache (more common in adults), irritability (infants, children, and adolescents; more common in infants and children <3 years)

Dermatologic: Skin rash (more common in infants and children <3 years)

Gastrointestinal: Decreased appetite (infants, children, and adolescents), diarrhea (more common in infants and children <3 years), nausea (more common in adults), vomiting (more common in infants and children <3 years)

Infection: Influenza (adults)

Local: Erythema at injection site (more common in infants and children <3 years), induration at injection site (more common in adults), itching at injection site (more common in adults), pain at injection site (more common in adults), swelling at injection site, tenderness at injection site (more common in adults)

Neuromuscular & skeletal: Back pain (adults), myalgia (more common in adults)

Respiratory: Cough (adults), flu-like symptoms (more common in adults), nasopharyngitis (adults), pharyngolaryngeal pain (adults), rhinitis (adults), sinusitis (adults), upper respiratory tract infection (adults)

Miscellaneous: Febrile seizures (children <3 years), fever (more common in infants and children <3 years)

Rare but important or life-threatening: Appendicitis, cerebral infarction, chest pain, dermatomyositis, disseminated intravascular coagulation, encephalitis, epilepsy, herpes zoster, iritis, labyrinthitis, limb abscess, limb pain, musculoskeletal injury, neuritis, oropharyngeal spasm, ovarian torsion, paresthesia, rectal hemorrhage, rupture of ovarian cyst, seizure, syncope

Drug Interactions

Metabolism/Transport Effects None known.

Avoid Concomitant Use There are no known interactions where it is recommended to avoid concomitant use.

Increased Effect/Toxicity There are no known significant interactions involving an increase in effect.

Decreased Effect

The levels/effects of Japanese Encephalitis Virus Vaccine (Inactivated) may be decreased by: Belimumab; Fingolimod; Immunosuppressants

Storage/Stability Store in original packaging under refrigeration at 2°C to 8°C (35°F to 46°F); do not freeze. Protect from light.

Mechanism of Action This vaccine induces antibodies to neutralize the Japanese encephalitis virus. Antibody response is measured using a 50% plaque-reduction neutralization antibody test ($PRNT_{50}$); a threshold of ≥1:10 is considered protective immunity.

Pharmacokinetics (Adult data unless noted) Onset of action: Protective immunity was observed in 96% to 100% of pediatric patients (2 months to 17 years) and ~21% of adults 10 days after the first vaccine dose and adults 28 days after the second vaccine dose

Dosing: Usual

Infants ≥2 months, Children, and Adolescents:

Primary immunization schedule:

Infants 2 months to Children <3 years: IM: 0.25 mL/dose on days 0 and 28 for a total of 2 doses; series should be completed at least 1 week prior to potential exposure.

Children ≥3 years and Adolescents: IM: 0.5 mL/dose on days 0 and 28 for a total of 2 doses; series should be completed at least 1 week prior to potential exposure.

Booster dose: Adolescents ≥17 years: 0.5 mL/dose may be given prior to potential re-exposure if the primary series was completed >1 year previously; **Note:** The safety and immunogenicity of booster doses in pediatric patients <17 years has not been evaluated.

Adults:

Primary immunization schedule: IM: 0.5 mL/dose; a total of 2 doses given on days 0 and 28. Series should be completed at least 1 week prior to potential exposure.

Booster dose: Booster dose may be given prior to potential re-exposure if the primary series was completed >1 year previously.

Dosage adjustment in renal impairment: There are no dosage adjustments provided in manufacturer's labeling.

Dosage adjustment in hepatic impairment: There are no dosage adjustments provided in manufacturer's labeling.

Administration For IM injection; do not inject IV, SubQ, or intradermally. Shake well prior to use to form a homogeneous suspension. Do not use if discolored or if particulate matter remains.

Ixiaro is available only in a prefilled syringe containing 0.5 mL. In order to administer a 0.25 mL dose in children 2 months to <3 years, first shake the syringe to form a homogenous suspension. Attach a sterile needle to the prefilled syringe and while holding the syringe upright, discard 0.25 mL of the suspension. Attach a new sterile needle prior to administration.

Administration site (preferred):

Infants 2 to <12 months: Anterolateral aspect of the thigh

Children 1 to <3 years: Anterolateral aspect of the thigh or deltoid muscle may be used (if mass is adequate)

Children ≥3 years, Adolescents, and Adults: Deltoid muscle

U.S. law requires that the date of administration, name of manufacturer, lot number, and administering person's name, title and address be entered into patient's permanent medical record.

Additional Information Ixiaro® is a purified Japanese encephalitis vaccine made from the SA_{14}-14-2 strain grown in Vero cells (JE-VC). It was developed due to neurologic side effects observed with Je-Vax®, a vaccine derived from mice-brain cells (JE-MB) that contains additives which may contribute to the adverse effects. Studies are currently planned to determine the need for booster doses following initial vaccination with Ixiaro®. Adults who previously received Je-Vax® vaccine and require further immunization against Japanese encephalitis should be administered a 2-dose primary series of Ixiaro® [CDC 60 (20), 2011].

Dosage Forms Excipient information presented when available (limited, particularly for generics); consult specific product labeling.

Suspension, Intramuscular:

Ixiaro: (0.5 mL) [latex free; contains albumin bovine, protamine sulfate, sodium metabisulfite]

- ◆ **Jencycla** *see* Norethindrone *on page 1530*
- ◆ **JE-VC (Ixiaro)** *see* Japanese Encephalitis Virus Vaccine (Inactivated) *on page 1184*
- ◆ **Jock Itch Spray [OTC]** *see* Tolnaftate *on page 2083*
- ◆ **Jolivette** *see* Norethindrone *on page 1530*
- ◆ **J-Tan D PD [OTC]** *see* Brompheniramine and Pseudoephedrine *on page 305*
- ◆ **Jurnista (Can)** *see* HYDROmorphone *on page 1044*
- ◆ **Just For Kids [OTC]** *see* Fluoride *on page 899*
- ◆ **K-10 (Can)** *see* Potassium Chloride *on page 1736*
- ◆ **K-99 [OTC]** *see* Potassium Gluconate *on page 1739*
- ◆ **Kadian** *see* Morphine (Systemic) *on page 1461*
- ◆ **Kala® [OTC]** *see Lactobacillus on page 1203*
- ◆ **Kalbitor** *see* Ecallantide *on page 726*
- ◆ **Kaletra** *see* Lopinavir and Ritonavir *on page 1291*
- ◆ **Kalexate** *see* Sodium Polystyrene Sulfonate *on page 1953*
- ◆ **Kalydeco** *see* Ivacaftor *on page 1180*
- ◆ **Kank-A Mouth Pain [OTC]** *see* Benzocaine *on page 268*
- ◆ **Kaote DVI** *see* Antihemophilic Factor (Human) *on page 167*
- ◆ **Kao-Tin [OTC]** *see* Bismuth Subsalicylate *on page 290*
- ◆ **Kao-Tin [OTC]** *see* Docusate *on page 697*
- ◆ **Kapvay** *see* CloNIDine *on page 508*
- ◆ **Karbinal™ ER** *see* Carbinoxamine *on page 372*
- ◆ **Karbinal ER** *see* Carbinoxamine *on page 372*
- ◆ **Kayexalate** *see* Sodium Polystyrene Sulfonate *on page 1953*
- ◆ **Kayexalate® (Can)** *see* Sodium Polystyrene Sulfonate *on page 1953*
- ◆ **KCl** *see* Potassium Chloride *on page 1736*
- ◆ **Kdur** *see* Potassium Chloride *on page 1736*
- ◆ **K-Dur (Can)** *see* Potassium Chloride *on page 1736*
- ◆ **Kedbumin** *see* Albumin *on page 79*
- ◆ **Keep Alert [OTC]** *see* Caffeine *on page 335*
- ◆ **Keflex** *see* Cephalexin *on page 422*
- ◆ **Kefzol** *see* CeFAZolin *on page 388*
- ◆ **Kemsol (Can)** *see* Dimethyl Sulfoxide *on page 667*
- ◆ **Kenalog** *see* Triamcinolone (Systemic) *on page 2112*
- ◆ **Kenalog** *see* Triamcinolone (Topical) *on page 2117*
- ◆ **Kenalog® (Can)** *see* Triamcinolone (Topical) *on page 2117*
- ◆ **Keppra** *see* LevETIRAcetam *on page 1234*
- ◆ **Keppra XR** *see* LevETIRAcetam *on page 1234*
- ◆ **Keralyt** *see* Salicylic Acid *on page 1894*
- ◆ **Keralyt Scalp** *see* Salicylic Acid *on page 1894*
- ◆ **Kerr Insta-Char [OTC]** *see* Charcoal, Activated *on page 425*
- ◆ **Kerr Insta-Char in Sorbitol [OTC]** *see* Charcoal, Activated *on page 425*
- ◆ **Ketalar** *see* Ketamine *on page 1186*

Ketamine (KEET a meen)

Medication Safety Issues

Sound-alike/look-alike issues:

Ketalar may be confused with Kenalog, ketorolac

High alert medication:

The Institute for Safe Medication Practices (ISMP) includes this medication among its list of drugs which have a heightened risk of causing significant patient harm when used in error.

Related Information

Preprocedure Sedatives in Children *on page 2444*

Brand Names: US Ketalar

Brand Names: Canada Ketalar; Ketamine Hydrochloride Injection, USP

Therapeutic Category General Anesthetic

Generic Availability (US) Yes

Use Anesthesia, short surgical procedures, dressing changes

Pregnancy Considerations Adverse events have not been observed in animal reproduction studies. Ketamine crosses the placenta and can be detected in fetal tissue. Ketamine produces dose dependent increases in uterine contractions; effects may vary by trimester. The plasma clearance of ketamine is reduced during pregnancy. Dose related neonatal depression and decreased APGAR scores have been reported with large doses administered at delivery (Ghoneim 1977; Little 1972; White 1982).

Breast-Feeding Considerations It is not known if ketamine is excreted in breast milk.

Contraindications

Hypersensitivity to ketamine or any component of the formulation; conditions in which an increase in blood pressure would be hazardous

Additional absolute contraindications according to the American College of Emergency Physicians (ACEP [Green 2011]): Infants <3 months of age; known or suspected schizophrenia (even if currently stable or controlled with medications)

Warnings/Precautions The American College of Emergency Physicians considers the use of ketamine in patients with known or suspected schizophrenia (even if currently stable or controlled with medications) an absolute contraindication and relatively contraindicated for major procedures involving the posterior pharynx (eg, endoscopy), for patients with an active pulmonary infection or disease (including upper respiratory disease or asthma), history of airway instability, tracheal surgery, or tracheal stenosis, in patients with CNS masses, CNS abnormalities, or hydrocephalus, glaucoma, acute globe injury, porphyria, thyroid disorder, or receiving a thyroid medication (ACEP [Green 2011]). Use with caution in patients with coronary artery disease, catecholamine depletion, hypertension, and tachycardia. Cardiac function should be continuously monitored in patients with increased blood pressure or cardiac decompensation. Ketamine increases blood pressure, heart rate, and cardiac output thereby increasing myocardial oxygen demand. The use of concurrent benzodiazepine, inhaled anesthetics, and propofol or administration of ketamine as a continuous infusion may reduce these cardiovascular effects (Miller 2010). The American College of Emergency Physicians recommends avoidance in patients who are already hypertensive and in older adults with risk factors for coronary artery disease (ACEP [Green 2011]). Rapid IV administration or overdose may cause respiratory depression, apnea, and enhanced pressor response. Resuscitative equipment should be available during use.

Use with caution in patients with increased intraocular pressure and avoid use in patients with an open eye injury or other ophthalmologic disorder where an increase in intraocular pressure would prove to be detrimental; ketamine may further increase intraocular pressure (Cunningham 1986; Miller 2010; Nagdeve 2006). Postanesthetic emergence reactions which can manifest as vivid dreams, hallucinations, and/or frank delirium occur; these reactions are less common in patients <15 years of age and >65 years and when given intramuscularly. Emergence reactions, confusion, or irrational behavior may occur up to 24 hours postoperatively and may be reduced by pretreatment with a benzodiazepine and the use of ketamine at the lower end of the dosing range. Avoid use in patients with schizophrenia (Lahti 1995; Malhotra 1997). Use with caution in patients with CSF pressure elevation, the chronic alcoholic or acutely alcohol-intoxicated. May cause dependence (withdrawal symptoms on discontinuation) and tolerance with prolonged use. May cause CNS depression, which may impair physical or mental abilities; patients must be cautioned about performing tasks which require mental alertness (eg, operating machinery or driving). When used for outpatient surgery, the patient be accompanied by a responsible adult. Should be administered under the supervision of a physician experienced in administering general anesthetics.

Warnings: Additional Pediatric Considerations May reduce postanesthetic emergence reactions minimization of verbal, tactile, and visual patient stimulation during recovery, or by pretreatment with a benzodiazepine (using lower recommended doses of ketamine). Severe emergent reactions may require treatment with a small hypnotic dose of a short or ultrashort acting barbiturate. Animal data suggests that exposure of the developing brain to anesthetics like ketamine (especially during the critical time of synaptogenesis) may result in long-term impairment of cognitive function (Patel, 2009).

Adverse Reactions Frequency not always defined.

Cardiovascular: Bradycardia, cardiac arrhythmia, hypotension, increased blood pressure, increased pulse

Central nervous system: Drug dependence, hypertonia (tonic-clonic movements sometimes resembling seizures), increased cerebrospinal fluid pressure, prolonged emergence from anesthesia (includes confusion, delirium, dreamlike state, excitement, hallucinations, irrational behavior, vivid imagery)

Dermatologic: Erythema (transient), morbilliform rash (transient), rash at injection site

Endocrine & metabolic: Central diabetes insipidus (Hatab 2014)

Gastrointestinal: Anorexia, nausea, sialorrhea (Hatab 2014), vomiting

Genitourinary (adverse reactions can be severe in patients with a history of chronic ketamine use/abuse): Cystitis, irritable bladder, urethritis, urinary tract irritation

Hypersensitivity: Anaphylaxis

Local: Pain at injection site

Neuromuscular & skeletal: Laryngospasm

Ophthalmic: Diplopia, increased intraocular pressure, nystagmus

Respiratory: Airway obstruction, apnea, respiratory depression

Drug Interactions

Metabolism/Transport Effects Substrate of CYP2B6 (major), CYP2C9 (major), CYP3A4 (major); **Note:** Assignment of Major/Minor substrate status based on clinically relevant drug interaction potential

Avoid Concomitant Use

Avoid concomitant use of Ketamine with any of the following: Azelastine (Nasal); Conivaptan; Fusidic Acid (Systemic); Idelalisib; Orphenadrine; Paraldehyde; Thalidomide

Increased Effect/Toxicity

Ketamine may increase the levels/effects of: Alcohol (Ethyl); Azelastine (Nasal); Buprenorphine; CNS Depressants; Hydrocodone; Memantine; Methotrimeprazine; Metyrosine; Mirtazapine; Orphenadrine; Paraldehyde; Pramipexole; ROPINIRole; Rotigotine; Selective Serotonin Reuptake Inhibitors; Suvorexant; Thalidomide; Thiopental; Zolpidem

The levels/effects of Ketamine may be increased by: Brimonidine (Topical); Cannabis; Conivaptan; CYP2B6 Inhibitors (Moderate); CYP2C9 Inhibitors (Moderate); CYP2C9 Inhibitors (Strong); CYP3A4 Inhibitors (Moderate); CYP3A4 Inhibitors (Strong); Dasatinib; Doxylamine; Dronabinol; Droperidol; Fosaprepitant; Fusidic Acid (Systemic); HydrOXYzine; Idelalisib; Ivacaftor; Kava Kava; Luliconazole; Magnesium Sulfate; Methotrimeprazine; Mifepristone; Nabilone; Netupitant; Palbociclib; Perampanel; Quazepam; Rufinamide; Simeprevir; Sodium Oxybate; Stiripentol; Tapentadol; Tetrahydrocannabinol

Decreased Effect

The levels/effects of Ketamine may be decreased by: CYP2C9 Inducers (Strong); Dabrafenib

Storage/Stability Store at 20°C to 25°C (68°F to 77°F). Protect from light.

Mechanism of Action Produces a cataleptic-like state in which the patient is dissociated from the surrounding environment by direct action on the cortex and limbic system. Ketamine is a noncompetitive NMDA receptor antagonist that blocks glutamate. Low (subanesthetic) doses produce analgesia, and modulate central sensitization, hyperalgesia and opioid tolerance. Reduces polysynaptic spinal reflexes.

Pharmacodynamics

Onset of action:
- Anesthesia:
  - IM: 3-4 minutes
  - IV: Within 30 seconds
- Analgesia:
  - Oral: Within 30 minutes
  - IM: Within 10-15 minutes

Duration: Following single dose:
- Anesthesia:
  - IM: 12-25 minutes
  - IV: 5-10 minutes

Analgesia: IM: 15-30 minutes
Recovery:
IM: 3-4 hours
IV: 1-2 hours

Pharmacokinetics (Adult data unless noted)
Metabolism: In the liver via N-dealkylation, hydroxylation of cyclohexone ring, glucuronide conjugation, and dehydration of hydroxylated metabolites
Half-life:
Alpha: 10-15 minutes
Terminal: 2.5 hours

Dosing: Neonatal Note: Some neonatal experts do not recommend the use of ketamine in neonates; an increase in neuronal apoptosis has been observed in neonatal animal studies (Patel 2009). Individualize dose and titrate to effect.

Adjunct to anesthesia: Limited data available: IV: 0.5 to 2 mg/kg/dose has been reported. A study of 23 patients [mean age: 3.2 years (9 days to 7 years)] undergoing MRI received a fixed dose of 0.5 mg/kg of ketamine prior to propofol bolus and infusion. A single case report describes ketamine (1 to 2 mg/kg) adjunct use with sevoflurane in a one-day old neonate (GA: 33 weeks) undergoing pacemaker placement (Castilla 2004; Tomatir 2004).

Procedural sedation/analgesia: Limited data available: Full-term neonates: IV: 0.2 to 1 mg/kg/dose; may repeat 0.5 mg/kg/dose as needed; use most frequently reported in cardiac catheterization and ROP corrective procedures (Jobeir 2003; Lyon 2008; Pees 2003)

Dosing: Usual Note: Titrate dose to effect.
Children:
Oral: 6 to 10 mg/kg for 1 dose (mixed in cola or other beverage) given 30 minutes before the procedure
IM: 3 to 7 mg/kg
IV: Range: 0.5 to 2 mg/kg, use smaller doses (0.5 to 1 mg/kg) for sedation for minor procedures; usual induction dosage: 1 to 2 mg/kg
Continuous IV infusion: Sedation: 5 to 20 mcg/kg/minute; start at lower dosage listed and titrate to effect
Adults:
IM: 3 to 8 mg/kg
IV: Range: 1 to 4.5 mg/kg; usual induction dosage: 1 to 2 mg/kg
Children and Adults: Maintenance: Supplemental doses of $1/3$ to $1/2$ of initial dose

Preparation for Administration Note: Three concentrations are available (10 mg/mL, 50 mg/mL and 100 mg/mL); preparation information may be product specific.
Oral (using parenteral dosage form): Use the 100 mg/mL IV solution and mix the appropriate dose in 0.2 to 0.3 mL/kg of cola or other beverage (Gutstein 1992; Tobias 1992)
Parenteral:
IV push: If using the 100 mg/mL concentration, must further dilute with an equal volume of SWFI, NS, or D_5W; maximum concentration: 50 mg/mL
IV infusion: The 50 mg/mL and 100 mg/mL vials may be further diluted in D_5W or NS to a final concentration of 1 mg/mL; in fluid restricted patients a concentration of 2 mg/mL may be used
Note: Do not mix with barbiturates or diazepam (precipitation may occur).

Administration
Oral (using parenteral dosage form): Use the 100 mg/mL IV solution and mix the appropriate dose in 0.2 to 0.3 mL/kg of cola or other beverage (Gutstein 1992; Tobias 1992)
Parenteral:
IV push: May administer the 10 mg/mL and 50 mg/mL undiluted. Administer slowly over 60 seconds, do not exceed 0.5 mg/kg/minute; more rapid administration may result in respiratory depression and enhanced pressor response. Some experts suggest administration over 2 to 3 minutes (Miller 2010).
IV infusion: May be administered as a continuous IV infusion

Monitoring Parameters Cardiovascular effects, heart rate, blood pressure, respiratory rate, transcutaneous O_2 saturation

Test Interactions May interfere with urine detection of phencyclidine (false-positive).

Additional Information Used in combination with anticholinergic agents to decrease hypersalivation; should not be used for sedation for procedures that require a total lack of movement (eg, MRI, radiation therapy) due to association with purposeless movements

Controlled Substance C-III

Dosage Forms Excipient information presented when available (limited, particularly for generics); consult specific product labeling.
Solution, Injection:
Ketalar: 10 mg/mL (20 mL); 50 mg/mL (10 mL); 100 mg/mL (5 mL)
Generic: 10 mg/mL (20 mL); 50 mg/mL (10 mL); 100 mg/mL (5 mL, 10 mL)

◆ **Ketamine Hydrochloride** *see* Ketamine *on page 1186*

◆ **Ketamine Hydrochloride Injection, USP (Can)** *see* Ketamine *on page 1186*

Ketoconazole (Systemic) (kee toe KOE na zole)

Medication Safety Issues
Sound-alike/look-alike issues:
Nizoral may be confused with Nasarel, Neoral, Nitrol

Brand Names: Canada Apo-Ketoconazole; Teva-Ketoconazole

Therapeutic Category Antifungal Agent, Systemic

Generic Availability (US) Yes

Use Treatment of susceptible fungal infections, including blastomycosis, coccidioidomycosis, histoplasmosis, paracoccidioidomycosis, and chromomycosis in patients who have failed or who are intolerant to other antifungal therapies (FDA approved in ages ≥2 years of age and adults). **Note:** Due to serious adverse effects (hepatotoxicity) and significant drug interactions, ketoconazole is seldom used in pediatric patients (*Red Book* [AAP], 2012); use should be reserved for patients who have failed or are intolerant to other antifungal therapies.

Medication Guide Available Yes

Pregnancy Risk Factor C

Pregnancy Considerations Adverse effects were noted in animal reproduction studies.

Breast-Feeding Considerations In a case report, ketoconazole in concentrations of ≤0.22 mcg/mL were detected in the breast milk of a woman 1 month postpartum. She had been taking oral ketoconazole 200 mg/day for 5 days at the time of sampling. The maximum milk concentration occurred 3.25 hours after the dose and concentrations were undetectable 24 hours after the dose. Based on the highest milk concentration, the estimated dose to the nursing infant was 1.4% of the maternal dose. Breast-feeding is not recommended by the manufacturer.

Contraindications
Hypersensitivity to ketoconazole or any component of the formulation; acute or chronic liver disease; coadministration with alprazolam, cisapride, colchicine, disopyramide, dofetilide, dronedarone, eplerenone, ergot alkaloids (eg, dihydroergotamine, ergometrine, ergotamine, methylergometrine), felodipine, HMG-CoA reductase inhibitors (eg, lovastatin, simvastatin), irinotecan, lurasidone,

methadone, oral midazolam, nisoldipine, pimozide, quinidine, ranolazine, tolvaptan, triazolam

Canadian labeling: Additional contraindications (not in U.S. labeling): Women of childbearing potential unless effective forms of contraception are used; coadministration with astemizole or terfenadine

Warnings/Precautions [U.S. Boxed Warning]: Use only when other effective antifungal therapy is unavailable or not tolerated and the benefits of ketoconazole treatment are considered to outweigh the risks. Ketoconazole has poor penetration into cerebral-spinal fluid and should not be used to treat fungal meningitis.

[U.S. Boxed Warning]: Ketoconazole has been associated with hepatotoxicity, including fatal cases and cases requiring liver transplantation; some patients had no apparent risk factors for hepatic disease. Patients should be advised of the hepatotoxicity risks and monitored closely. Toxicity was observed after a median duration of therapy of ~4 weeks but has also been noted after as little as 3 days; may occur when patients receive high doses for short durations or low doses for long durations. Most cases have been observed in the treatment of onychomycosis. Use with caution in patients with pre-existing hepatic impairment, those on prolonged therapy and/or taking other hepatotoxic drugs concurrently. Hepatic dysfunction is typically (but not always) reversible upon discontinuation. Obtain liver function tests at baseline and frequently throughout therapy; serum ALT should be monitored weekly throughout therapy. Discontinue therapy for elevated hepatic enzymes that persist or worsen or if accompanied by signs/symptoms (eg, jaundice, nausea/vomiting, dark urine) of hepatic injury.

High doses of ketoconazole may depress adrenocortical function; returns to baseline upon discontinuation of therapy. Recommended maximum dosing should not be exceeded. Monitor adrenal function as clinically necessary, particularly in patients with adrenal insufficiency and in patients under prolonged stress (eg, intensive care, major surgery). In European clinical trials of men with metastatic prostate cancer, fatalities were reported in a small number of study participants within 14 days of initiating high-dose ketoconazole (1200 mg daily); a causal effect has not been established. In animal studies, increased long bone fragility with cases of fracture has been observed with high-dose ketoconazole. Careful dose selection may be advisable for patients susceptible to bone fragility (eg, postmenopausal women, elderly). Cases of hypersensitivity reactions (including rare cases of anaphylaxis) have been reported; some reactions occurred after the initial dose.

[U.S. Boxed Warning]: Concomitant use with cisapride, disopyramide, dofetilide, dronedarone, methadone, pimozide, quinidine, and ranolazine is contraindicated due to the possible occurrence of life-threatening ventricular arrhythmias such as torsade de pointes. Concomitant use with HMG-CoA reductase inhibitors (eg, lovastatin, simvastatin) or with oral midazolam, triazolam, and alprazolam is contraindicated. Absorption is reduced in patients with achlorhydria; administer with acidic liquids (eg, soda pop). Avoid concomitant use of drugs that decrease gastric acidity (eg, proton pump inhibitors, antacids, H_2-blockers). Other potentially significant interactions may exist, requiring dose or frequency adjustment, additional monitoring, and/or selection of alternative therapy.

Adverse Reactions

Cardiovascular: Orthostatic hypotension, peripheral edema

Central nervous system: Fatigue, insomnia, malaise, nervousness, paresthesia

Dermatologic: Alopecia, dermatitis, erythema, erythema multiforme, pruritus, skin rash, urticaria, xeroderma

Endocrine & metabolic: Hot flash, hyperlipidemia, menstrual disease

Gastrointestinal: Abdominal pain, anorexia, constipation, dysgeusia, dyspepsia, flatulence, increased appetite, nausea, tongue discoloration, upper abdominal pain, vomiting, xerostomia

Hematologic & oncologic: Decreased platelet count

Hepatic: Jaundice

Hypersensitivity: Anaphylactoid reaction

Neuromuscular & skeletal: Myalgia, weakness

Respiratory: Epistaxis

Miscellaneous: Alcohol intolerance

Rare but important or life-threatening: Acute generalized exanthematous pustulosis, adrenocortical insufficiency (≥400 mg/day), anaphylactic shock, anaphylaxis, angioedema, azoospermia, bulging fontanel (infants), cholestatic hepatitis, cirrhosis, decreased plasma testosterone (impaired at 800 mg/day), depression, erectile dysfunction (doses >200-400 mg/day), gynecomastia, hemolytic anemia, hepatic failure, hepatic necrosis, hepatitis, hepatotoxicity, hypertriglyceridemia, hypersensitivity reaction, impotence, increased intracranial pressure (reversible), leukopenia, myopathy, papilledema, photophobia, prolonged Q-T interval on ECG, skin photosensitivity, suicidal tendencies, thrombocytopenia

Drug Interactions

Metabolism/Transport Effects Substrate of CYP3A4 (major); **Note:** Assignment of Major/Minor substrate status based on clinically relevant drug interaction potential; **Inhibits** CYP1A2 (weak), CYP2A6 (moderate), CYP2B6 (weak), CYP2C19 (moderate), CYP2C8 (weak), CYP2C9 (moderate), CYP2D6 (moderate), CYP3A4 (strong), P-glycoprotein, UGT1A1

Avoid Concomitant Use

Avoid concomitant use of Ketoconazole (Systemic) with any of the following: Ado-Trastuzumab Emtansine; Alfuzosin; ALPRAZolam; Amodiaquine; Apixaban; Artesunate; Astemizole; Avanafil; Axitinib; Barnidipine; Bosutinib; Cabozantinib; Ceritinib; Cisapride; Conivaptan; Crizotinib; Dapoxetine; Dihydroergotamine; Disopyramide; Dofetilide; Domperidone; Dronedarone; Efavirenz; Eletriptan; Eplerenone; Ergoloid Mesylates; Ergonovine; Ergotamine; Estazolam; Everolimus; Felodipine; Halofantrine; Ibrutinib; Indium 111 Capromab Pendetide; Irinotecan; Isavuconazonium Sulfate; Ivabradine; Lapatinib; Lercanidipine; Lomitapide; Lovastatin; Lurasidone; Macitentan; Methadone; Methylergonovine; Midazolam; Naloxegol; Nevirapine; Nilotinib; NiMODipine; Nisoldipine; Olaparib; Palbociclib; PAZOPanib; Pimozide; QuiNIDine; Ranolazine; Red Yeast Rice; Regorafenib; Rivaroxaban; Saccharomyces boulardii; Salmeterol; Silodosin; Simeprevir; Simvastatin; Suvorexant; Tamsulosin; Tegafur; Telithromycin; Terfenadine; Thioridazine; Ticagrelor; Tolvaptan; Topotecan; Toremifene; Trabectedin; Triazolam; Ulipristal; Vemurafenib; VinCRIStine (Liposomal); Vorapaxar

Increased Effect/Toxicity

Ketoconazole (Systemic) may increase the levels/effects of: Ado-Trastuzumab Emtansine; Afatinib; Alcohol (Ethyl); Alfuzosin; Aliskiren; Almotriptan; Alosetron; ALPRAZolam; Amodiaquine; Apixaban; ARIPiprazole; Artesunate; Astemizole; AtorvaSTATin; Avanafil; Axitinib; Barnidipine; Bedaquiline; Boceprevir; Bortezomib; Bosentan; Bosutinib; Brentuximab Vedotin; Brinzolamide; Budesonide (Nasal); Budesonide (Systemic, Oral Inhalation); Budesonide (Topical); BusPIRone; Busulfan; Cabazitaxel; Cabozantinib; Calcium Channel Blockers; Cannabis; Carbocisteine; Carvedilol; Ceritinib; Cilostazol; Cisapride; Citalopram; Cobicistat; Colchicine; Conivaptan; Corticosteroids (Orally Inhaled); Corticosteroids (Systemic); Crizotinib; CycloSPORINE (Systemic);

CYP2A6 Substrates; CYP2C19 Substrates; CYP2C9 Substrates; CYP2D6 Substrates; CYP3A4 Substrates; Dabigatran Etexilate; Dapoxetine; Darunavir; Dasatinib; Dienogest; Dihydroergotamine; Disopyramide; DOCEtaxel; Dofetilide; Domperidone; DOXOrubicin (Conventional); Dronabinol; Dronedarone; Drospirenone; Dutasteride; Edoxaban; Eletriptan; Eliglustat; Elvitegravir; Eplerenone; Ergoloid Mesylates; Ergonovine; Ergotamine; Erlotinib; Estazolam; Etizolam; Etravirine; Everolimus; Felodipine; FentaNYL; Fesoterodine; Fexofenadine; Fimasartan; Fingolimod; Fluticasone (Nasal); Fluticasone (Oral Inhalation); Fosamprenavir; Fosphenytoin; GuanFACINE; Halofantrine; Highest Risk QTc-Prolonging Agents; Hydrocodone; Ibrutinib; Idelalisib; Iloperidone; Imatinib; Imidafenacin; Indinavir; Irinotecan; Isavuconazonium Sulfate; Ivabradine; Ivacaftor; Ixabepilone; Lacosamide; Lapatinib; Ledipasvir; Lercanidipine; Levobupivacaine; Levomilnacipran; Lomitapide; Lopinavir; Losartan; Lovastatin; Lurasidone; Macitentan; Maraviroc; MedroxyPROGESTERone; Methadone; Methylergonovine; MethylPREDNISolone; Metoprolol; Midazolam; Mifepristone; Mirabegron; Moderate Risk QTc-Prolonging Agents; Naloxegol; Nebivolol; Nilotinib; NiMODipine; Nintedanib; Nisoldipine; Olaparib; Ospemifene; Oxybutynin; OxyCODONE; Palbociclib; Panobinostat; Parecoxib; Paricalcitol; PAZOPanib; P-glycoprotein/ABCB1 Substrates; Phenytoin; Pimecrolimus; Pimozide; PONATinib; Pranlukast; Praziquantel; PrednisoLONE (Systemic); PredniSONE; Propafenone; Proton Pump Inhibitors; Prucalopride; QUEtiapine; QuiNIDine; Ramelteon; Ranolazine; Red Yeast Rice; Regorafenib; Repaglinide; Retapamulin; Rifamycin Derivatives; Rifaximin; Rilpivirine; Riociguat; Rivaroxaban; RomiDEPsin; Ruxolitinib; Salmeterol; Saquinavir; Saxagliptin; Sildenafil; Silodosin; Simeprevir; Simvastatin; Sirolimus; Solifenacin; SORAfenib; SUNItinib; Suvorexant; Tacrolimus (Systemic); Tacrolimus (Topical); Tadalafil; Tamsulosin; Tasimelteon; Telaprevir; Telithromycin; Temsirolimus; Terfenadine; Tetrahydrocannabinol; Thioridazine; Ticagrelor; TiZANidine; Tofacitinib; Tolterodine; Tolvaptan; Topotecan; Toremifene; Trabectedin; TraMADol; Triazolam; Ulipristal; Vardenafil; Vemurafenib; Vilazodone; VinCRIStine (Liposomal); Vitamin K Antagonists; Vorapaxar; Zolpidem; Zopiclone; Zuclopenthixol

The levels/effects of Ketoconazole (Systemic) may be increased by: AtorvaSTATin; Boceprevir; Cobicistat; Darunavir; Etravirine; Fosamprenavir; Indinavir; Lopinavir; Mifepristone; Propafenone; Ritonavir; Saquinavir; Telaprevir; Telithromycin; Tipranavir

Decreased Effect

Ketoconazole (Systemic) may decrease the levels/effects of: Amphotericin B; Artesunate; Choline C 11; Clopidogrel; Codeine; Ifosfamide; Indium 111 Capromab Pendetide; Prasugrel; Saccharomyces boulardii; Tamoxifen; Tegafur; Ticagrelor; TraMADol

The levels/effects of Ketoconazole (Systemic) may be decreased by: Antacids; Bosentan; CYP3A4 Inducers (Moderate); CYP3A4 Inducers (Strong); Dabrafenib; Deferasirox; Didanosine; Efavirenz; Etravirine; Fosphenytoin; H2-Antagonists; Isoniazid; Mitotane; Nevirapine; Phenytoin; Proton Pump Inhibitors; Rifamycin Derivatives; Rilpivirine; Siltuximab; St Johns Wort; Sucralfate; Tocilizumab

Food Interactions Ketoconazole peak serum levels may be prolonged if taken with food. Management: May administer with food or milk to decrease GI adverse effects.

Storage/Stability Store at 15°C to 25°C (59°F to 77°F). Protect from light and moisture.

Mechanism of Action Alters the permeability of the cell wall by blocking fungal cytochrome P450; inhibits biosynthesis of triglycerides and phospholipids by fungi; inhibits several fungal enzymes that results in a build-up of toxic concentrations of hydrogen peroxide; for management of prostate cancer, ketoconazole inhibits androgen synthesis

Pharmacokinetics (Adult data unless noted)

Distribution: Well into inflamed joint fluid, saliva, bile, urine, sebum, cerumen, feces, tendons, skin and soft tissue, and testes; crosses blood-brain barrier poorly; only negligible amounts reach CSF

Protein binding: ~99% (mainly albumin)

Metabolism: Partially hepatic via CYP3A4 to inactive metabolites

Bioavailability: Decreases as pH of the gastric contents increases

Half-life, biphasic:

Initial: 2 hours

Terminal: 8 hours

Time to peak serum concentration: Within 1-2 hours

Elimination: Primarily in feces (57%) with smaller amounts excreted in urine (~13%)

Dosing: Usual

Pediatric: **Fungal infections:** Children ≥2 years and Adolescents: Oral: 3.3 to 6.6 mg/kg/day once daily; maximum daily dose: 400 mg/**day**; duration of therapy variable; continue therapy until active fungal infection has resolved (based on clinical and laboratory parameters); some infections may require at least 6 months of therapy. **Note:** Due to serious adverse effects (hepatotoxicity) and significant drug interactions, ketoconazole is seldom used in pediatric patients (*Red Book* [AAP], 2012); use should be reserved for patients who have failed or are intolerant to other antifungal therapies.

Adult: **Fungal infections:** Oral: 200 to 400 mg once daily; continue therapy until active fungal infection has resolved (based on clinical and laboratory parameters); some infections may require at least 6 months of therapy

Dosing adjustment in renal impairment: No dosage adjustment provided in manufacturer's labeling. Some clinicians suggest that no dosage adjustment is necessary in mild to severe impairment (Aronoff, 2007). Not dialyzable.

Dosing adjustment in hepatic impairment: Children ≥2 years, Adolescents, and Adults:

Baseline hepatic impairment: No dosage adjustment provided in manufacturer's labeling; use with extreme caution due to risks of hepatotoxicity; use is contraindicated with acute or chronic liver disease.

Hepatotoxicity during treatment: If ALT >ULN or 30% above baseline (or if patient is symptomatic), interrupt therapy and obtain full hepatic function panel. Upon normalization of liver function, may consider resuming therapy if benefit outweighs risk (hepatotoxicity has been reported on rechallenge).

Administration Administer oral tablets 2 hours prior to antacids to prevent decreased absorption due to the high pH of gastric contents. Patients with achlorhydria should administer with acidic liquid (eg, soda pop).

Monitoring Parameters Hepatic function tests (baseline and frequently during therapy), including weekly ALT for the duration of treatment, adrenal function (as clinically necessary)

Dosage Forms Excipient information presented when available (limited, particularly for generics); consult specific product labeling.

Tablet, Oral:

Generic: 200 mg

Extemporaneous Preparations A 20 mg/mL oral suspension may be made with tablets and one of three different vehicles (a 1:1 mixture of Ora-Sweet® and Ora-Plus®, a 1:1 mixture of Ora-Sweet® SF and Ora-Plus®, or a 1:4 mixture of cherry syrup and Simple Syrup, NF). Crush twelve 200 mg tablets in a mortar and reduce to a fine powder. Add 20 mL of chosen vehicle and mix to a uniform paste; mix while adding the vehicle in incremental proportions to **almost** 120 mL; transfer to a calibrated bottle, rinse mortar with vehicle, and add quantity of vehicle sufficient to make 120 mL. Label "shake well" and "refrigerate". Stable for 60 days.

Nahata MC, Pai VB, and Hipple TF, *Pediatric Drug Formulations*, 5th ed, Cincinnati, OH: Harvey Whitney Books Co, 2004.

Ketoconazole (Topical) (kee toe KOE na zole)

Medication Safety Issues

Sound-alike/look-alike issues:

Nizoral may be confused with Nasarel, Neoral, Nitrol

Brand Names: US Extina; Ketodan; Nizoral; Nizoral A-D [OTC]; Xolegel

Brand Names: Canada Ketoderm; Nizoral

Therapeutic Category Antifungal Agent, Topical

Generic Availability (US) May be product dependent

Use

Cream: Topical treatment of tinea corporis, tinea cruris, tinea pedis, tinea versicolor, and cutaneous candidiasis (FDA approved in adults)

Foam (Extina®); gel (Xolegel®): Topical treatment of seborrheic dermatitis in immunocompetent patients (FDA approved in ages ≥12 years and adults)

Shampoo:

1% shampoo (Nizoral® A-D): Control flaking, scaling, and itching associated with dandruff (OTC product: FDA approved in ages ≥12 years and adults)

2% shampoo (Nizoral®): Topical treatment of tinea versicolor (FDA approved in adults)

Pregnancy Risk Factor C

Pregnancy Considerations Adverse effects were noted in animal reproduction studies with oral ketoconazole. Ketoconazole is not detectable in the plasma following chronic use of the shampoo.

Breast-Feeding Considerations Ketoconazole has been detected in breast milk following oral dosing. Although it is not detected in the plasma following chronic use of the shampoo, and concentrations in the plasma following application of the gel are <250 times those observed with oral dosing, the manufacturers recommend that caution be used when administering to a nursing woman.

Contraindications Hypersensitivity to ketoconazole or any component of the formulation

Warnings/Precautions Cases of hypersensitivity reactions (including rare cases of anaphylaxis) have been reported. Formulations may contain sulfites. Avoid exposure of gel to open flames or smoking during or immediately after application. Foam formulation contains alcohol and propane/butane; do not expose to open flame or smoking during or immediately after application; do not puncture or incinerate container. Use of shampoo may remove curl from permanently wavy hair, cause hair discoloration, and changes in hair texture; avoid contact with eyes. Discontinue use if irritation occurs.

Warnings: Additional Pediatric Considerations Some dosage forms may contain propylene glycol; in neonates large amounts of propylene glycol delivered orally, intravenously (eg, >3,000 mg/day), or topically have been associated with potentially fatal toxicities which can include metabolic acidosis, seizures, renal failure, and CNS depression; toxicities have also been reported in children and adults including hyperosmolality, lactic acidosis, seizures and respiratory depression; use caution (AAP, 1997; Shehab, 2009).

Adverse Reactions

Topical cream/gel: Acne, allergic reaction, contact dermatitis (possibly related to sulfites or propylene glycol), discharge, dizziness, dryness, erythema, facial swelling, headache, impetigo, keratoconjunctivitis sicca, local burning, nail discoloration, ocular irritation/swelling, pain, paresthesia, pruritus, pustules, pyogenic granuloma, severe irritation, stinging

Topical foam: Application site burning, application site reaction, contact sensitization, dryness, erythema, pruritus, rash

Shampoo: Abnormal hair texture, alopecia, anaphylaxis, angioedema, application site reaction, burning sensation, contact dermatitis, dry skin, hair discoloration, hair loss increased, hypersensitivity, irritation, itching, oiliness/dryness of hair, pruritus, rash, scalp pustules, urticaria

Drug Interactions

Metabolism/Transport Effects None known.

Avoid Concomitant Use There are no known interactions where it is recommended to avoid concomitant use.

Increased Effect/Toxicity There are no known significant interactions involving an increase in effect.

Decreased Effect There are no known significant interactions involving a decrease in effect.

Storage/Stability

Cream: Store at <25°C (<77°F).

Foam: Store at 20°C to 25°C (68°F to 77°F). Do not refrigerate. Do not store in direct sunlight. Contents are flammable.

Gel: Store at <25°C (<77°F); excursions permitted to 15°C to 30°C (59°F to 86°F). Contents are flammable.

Shampoo:

Nizoral®: Store at ≤25°C (≤77°F). Protect from light.

Nizoral® A-D:Store between 2°C to 30°C (35°F to 86°F); protect from freezing. Protect from light.

Mechanism of Action Alters the permeability of the cell wall by blocking fungal cytochrome P450; inhibits biosynthesis of triglycerides and phospholipids by fungi; inhibits several fungal enzymes that results in a build-up of toxic concentrations of hydrogen peroxide; also inhibits androgen synthesis

Dosing: Usual

Children and Adolescents:

Dandruff (flaking, scaling, and itching; OTC labeling): Children ≥12 years and Adolescents: Topical: Shampoo (ketoconazole 1%): Shampoo every 3-4 days for up to 8 weeks; then use only as needed to control dandruff

Seborrheic dermatitis: Children ≥12 years and Adolescents: Topical:

Foam: Apply to affected area twice daily for 4 weeks

Gel: Apply to affected area once daily for 2 weeks

Adults:

Fungal infections: Topical:

Cream: Rub gently into the affected and immediate surrounding area once daily. Duration of treatment: Candidial infection or tinea corporis, cruris, or vesicolor: 2 weeks; tinea pedis: 6 weeks

Shampoo (ketoconazole 2%): Tinea versicolor: Apply to damp skin of the affected area and a wide margin surrounding this area, lather, leave on 5 minutes, and rinse (one application should be sufficient)

Seborrheic dermatitis: Topical:

Foam: Apply to affected area twice daily for 4 weeks

Gel: Apply to affected area once daily for 2 weeks

Shampoo (ketoconazole 1%; OTC labeling): Shampoo every 3-4 days for up to 8 weeks; then use only as needed to control dandruff

Dosing adjustment in renal impairment: There are no dosage adjustments provided in manufacturer's labeling; however, dosage adjustment unlikely necessary due to low systemic absorption.

Administration For external use only; not for ophthalmic, oral, or intravaginal use. Avoid contact with eyes and other mucous membranes.

Cream: Apply to cover the affected and immediate surrounding area.

Foam (Extina®): Hold the container upright and dispense foam into cap or other cool surface; do not dispense into hands as foam will begin to melt immediately upon contact with warm skin. If fingers are warm, rinse in cold water and dry thoroughly; pick up small amounts of foam with the fingers, and gently massage into the affected area(s) until foam disappears. For hair-bearing areas, part the hair, so foam may be applied directly to skin (rather than on the hair). Avoid fire, flame, and/or smoking during and immediately following application.

Gel (Xolegel®): Apply thin layer on affected skin; wait at least 3 hours after application before washing area(s). Avoid fire, flame, and/or smoking during and immediately following application.

Shampoo:

1%: Apply to wet hair, lather and rinse hair thoroughly; repeat

2%: Apply to damp skin, covering affected area and a wide margin surrounding the area, lather, leave on 5 minutes, and rinse

Dosage Forms Excipient information presented when available (limited, particularly for generics); consult specific product labeling. [DSC] = Discontinued product

Cream, External:

Generic: 2% (15 g, 30 g, 60 g)

Foam, External:

Extina: 2% (50 g, 100 g) [contains alcohol, usp, cetyl alcohol, propylene glycol]

Ketodan: 2% (100 g) [contains alcohol, usp, cetyl alcohol, propylene glycol]

Generic: 2% (50 g [DSC], 100 g [DSC])

Gel, External:

Xolegel: 2% (45 g) [contains alcohol, usp, fd&c yellow #10 (quinoline yellow), fd&c yellow #6 (sunset yellow), propylene glycol]

Kit, External:

Ketodan: 2% [contains cetyl alcohol, edetate disodium, propylene glycol]

Shampoo, External:

Nizoral: 2% (120 mL) [contains fd&c red #40]

Nizoral A-D: 1% (125 mL, 200 mL)

Generic: 2% (120 mL)

◆ **Ketodan** *see* Ketoconazole (Topical) *on page 1191*

◆ **Ketoderm (Can)** *see* Ketoconazole (Topical) *on page 1191*

Ketorolac (Systemic) (KEE toe role ak)

Medication Safety Issues

Sound-alike/look-alike issues:

Ketorolac may be confused with Ketalar, methadone

Toradol may be confused with Foradil, Inderal, TEGretol, traMADol, tromethamine

BEERS Criteria medication:

This drug may be potentially inappropriate for use in geriatric patients (Quality of evidence - high; Strength of recommendation - strong).

International issues:

Toradol [Canada and multiple international markets] may be confused with Theradol brand name for tramadol [Netherlands]

Brand Names: Canada Apo-Ketorolac Injectable®; Apo-Ketorolac®; Ketorolac Tromethamine Injection, USP; Novo-Ketorolac; Toradol®; Toradol® IM

Therapeutic Category Analgesic, Non-narcotic; Anti-inflammatory Agent; Antipyretic; Nonsteroidal Anti-inflammatory Drug (NSAID), Oral; Nonsteroidal Anti-inflammatory Drug (NSAID), Parenteral

Generic Availability (US) Yes

Use

IM, IV: Single-dose administration for moderately severe acute pain (FDA approved in ages ≥2 years and adults). Short-term (≤5 days) management of moderate to severe pain, usually postoperative pain (FDA approved in adults); has also been used to treat visceral pain associated with cancer, pain associated with trauma

Oral: Short-term (≤5 days) management of moderate to severe pain, usually postoperative pain, and only as continuation therapy of IM or IV ketorolac (FDA approved in adults); the combined duration of oral and parenteral ketorolac should not be >5 days due to the increased risk of serious adverse effects

Medication Guide Available Yes

Pregnancy Risk Factor C

Pregnancy Considerations Adverse events were observed in some animal reproduction studies. Ketorolac crosses the placenta (Walker, 1988). NSAID exposure during the first trimester is not strongly associated with congenital malformations; however, cardiovascular anomalies and cleft palate have been observed following NSAID exposure in some studies (Ericson, 2001). The use of an NSAID close to conception may be associated with an increased risk of miscarriage (Li, 2003; Nielsen, 2001). Nonteratogenic effects have been observed following NSAID administration during the third trimester, including myocardial degenerative changes, prenatal constriction of the ductus arteriosus, fetal tricuspid regurgitation, failure of the ductus arteriosus to close postnatally; renal dysfunction or failure, oligohydramnios; gastrointestinal bleeding or perforation, increased risk of necrotizing enterocolitis; intracranial bleeding (including intraventricular hemorrhage), platelet dysfunction with resultant bleeding; pulmonary hypertension (Van den Veyver, 1993). Because they may cause premature closure of the ductus arteriosus, use of NSAIDs late in pregnancy should be avoided (use after 31 or 32 weeks gestation is not recommended by some clinicians) (Moise, 1993). **[U.S. Boxed Warning]: Ketorolac is contraindicated during labor and delivery (may inhibit uterine contractions and adversely affect fetal circulation).** The chronic use of NSAIDs in women of reproductive age may be associated with infertility that is reversible upon discontinuation of the medication.

Breast-Feeding Considerations Low concentrations of ketorolac are found in breast milk (milk concentrations were <1% of the weight-adjusted maternal dose in one study [Wischnik, 1989]). The manufacturer recommends that caution be used if administered to nursing women.

Contraindications Hypersensitivity to ketorolac, aspirin, other NSAIDs, or any component of the formulation; active or history of peptic ulcer disease; recent or history of GI bleeding or perforation; patients with advanced renal disease or risk of renal failure (due to volume depletion); prophylaxis before major surgery; suspected or confirmed cerebrovascular bleeding; hemorrhagic diathesis, incomplete hemostasis, or high risk of bleeding; concurrent use with ASA, other NSAIDs, probenecid or pentoxifylline; epidural or intrathecal administration; perioperative pain in the setting of coronary artery bypass graft (CABG) surgery; labor and delivery

Warnings/Precautions [U.S. Boxed Warning]: Inhibits platelet function; contraindicated in patients with cerebrovascular bleeding (suspected or confirmed), hemorrhagic diathesis, incomplete hemostasis and patients at high risk for bleeding. Effects on platelet adhesion and aggregation may prolong bleeding time. Anemia may occur; patients on long-term NSAID therapy should be monitored for anemia. Rarely, NSAID use has been associated with potentially severe blood dyscrasias (eg, agranulocytosis, thrombocytopenia, aplastic anemia).

[U.S. Boxed Warning]: NSAIDs are associated with an increased risk of adverse cardiovascular thrombotic events, including MI and stroke. Risk may be increased with duration of use or pre-existing cardiovascular risk factors or disease. Carefully evaluate individual cardiovascular risk profiles prior to prescribing. May cause new-onset hypertension or worsening of existing hypertension.

Use caution with fluid retention. Avoid use in heart failure (ACCF/AHA [Yancy, 2013]). Concurrent use of aspirin has not been shown to consistently reduce thromboembolic events. **[U.S. Boxed Warning]: Use is contraindicated as prophylactic analgesic before any major surgery and is contraindicated for treatment of perioperative pain in the setting of coronary artery bypass graft (CABG) surgery.** Risk of MI and stroke may be increased with use following CABG surgery. Wound bleeding and postoperative hematomas have been associated with ketorolac use in the perioperative setting.

[U.S. Boxed Warning]: Ketorolac is contraindicated in patients with advanced renal impairment and in patients at risk for renal failure due to volume depletion. NSAID use may compromise existing renal function; dose-dependent decreases in prostaglandin synthesis may result from NSAID use, reducing renal blood flow which may cause renal decompensation. NSAID use may increase the risk for hyperkalemia. Patients with impaired renal function, dehydration, heart failure, liver dysfunction, those taking diuretics and ACE inhibitors, and the elderly are at greater risk of renal toxicity. Use with caution in patients with impaired renal function or history of kidney disease; dosage adjustment is required in patients with moderate elevation in serum creatinine. Monitor renal function closely. Acute renal failure, interstitial nephritis, and nephrotic syndrome have been reported with ketorolac use; papillary necrosis and renal injury have been reported with the use of NSAIDs. Use of NSAIDs can compromise existing renal function. Rehydrate patient before starting therapy.

[U.S. Boxed Warning]: NSAIDs may increase risk of gastrointestinal irritation, inflammation, ulceration, bleeding, and perforation. These events may occur at any time during therapy and without warning. Use is contraindicated in patients with active/history of peptic ulcer disease and recent/history of GI bleeding or perforation. Use caution with a history of inflammatory bowel disease, concurrent therapy with anticoagulants, and/or corticosteroids, smoking, use of alcohol, the elderly, or debilitated patients.

[U.S. Boxed Warning]: Ketorolac injection is contraindicated in patients with prior hypersensitivity reaction to aspirin or NSAIDs. NSAIDs may cause serious skin adverse events including exfoliative dermatitis, Stevens-Johnson syndrome (SJS), and toxic epidermal necrolysis (TEN); discontinue use at first sign of skin rash or hypersensitivity. Hypersensitivity or anaphylactoid reactions may occur, even without prior exposure; patients with "aspirin triad" (bronchial asthma, aspirin intolerance, rhinitis) may be at increased risk. Do not use in patients who experience bronchospasm, asthma, rhinitis, or urticaria with NSAID or aspirin therapy. Use caution in other forms of asthma.

Use with caution in patients with hepatic impairment or a history of liver disease. Closely monitor patients with any abnormal LFT. Rarely, severe hepatic reactions (eg, fulminant hepatitis, hepatic necrosis, liver failure) have occurred with NSAID use; discontinue if signs or symptoms of liver disease develop, or if systemic manifestations occur.

[U.S. Boxed Warning]: Dosage adjustment is required for patients ≥65 years of age. Avoid use in older adults; use is associated with an increased risk of GI bleeding and peptic ulcer disease in older adults in high risk category (eg, >75 years or age or receiving concomitant oral/parenteral corticosteroids, anticoagulants, or antiplatelet agents) (Beers Criteria). **[U.S. Boxed Warning]: Dosage adjustment is required for patients weighing <50 kg (<110 pounds). [U.S. Boxed Warning]: Ketorolac is contraindicated during labor and delivery (may inhibit uterine contractions and adversely affect fetal circulation). [U.S. Boxed Warning]: Concurrent use of ketorolac with aspirin or other NSAIDs is contraindicated due to the increased risk of adverse reactions.**

[U.S. Boxed Warning]: Contraindicated for epidural or intrathecal administration (formulation contains alcohol). [U.S. Boxed Warning]: Systemic ketorolac is indicated for short term (≤5 days) use in adults for treatment of moderately severe acute pain requiring opioid-level analgesia. Low doses of opioids may be needed for breakthrough pain. **[U.S. Boxed Warning]: Oral therapy is only indicated for use as continuation treatment, following parenteral ketorolac and is not indicated for minor or chronic painful conditions. Do not exceed maximum daily recommended doses; does not improve efficacy but may increase the risk of serious adverse effects.** The combined therapy duration (oral and parenteral) should not exceed 5 days. Use the lowest effective dose for the shortest duration of time, consistent with individual patient goals, to reduce risk of cardiovascular or GI adverse events. Alternate therapies should be considered for patients at high risk. **[U.S. Boxed Warning]: Ketorolac is not indicated for use in children.**

Potentially significant drug-drug interactions may exist, requiring dose or frequency adjustment, additional monitoring, and/or selection of alternative therapy.

NSAIDS may cause drowsiness, dizziness, blurred vision and other neurologic effects which may impair physical or mental abilities; patients must be cautioned about performing tasks which require mental alertness (eg, operating machinery or driving). Discontinue use with blurred or diminished vision and perform ophthalmologic exam.

Adverse Reactions

Cardiovascular: Edema, hypertension

Central nervous system: Dizziness, drowsiness, headache

Dermatologic: Diaphoresis, pruritus, skin rash

Gastrointestinal: Constipation, diarrhea, dyspepsia, flatulence, gastrointestinal fullness, gastrointestinal hemorrhage, gastrointestinal pain, gastrointestinal perforation, gastrointestinal ulcer, heartburn, nausea, stomatitis, vomiting

Hematologic & oncologic: Anemia, prolonged bleeding time, purpura

Hepatic: Increased liver enzymes

Local: Pain at injection site

Otic: Tinnitus

Renal: Renal function abnormality

Rare but important or life-threatening: Abnormality in thinking, acute pancreatitis, acute renal failure, agranulocytosis, alopecia, anaphylactoid reaction, anaphylaxis, angioedema, aplastic anemia, aseptic meningitis, asthma, azotemia, bradycardia, bronchospasm, bruise, cardiac arrhythmia, cholestatic jaundice, coma, confusion, congestive heart failure, conjunctivitis, cough, cystitis, depression, dysuria, eosinophilia, epistaxis, eructation, erythema multiforme, euphoria, exacerbation of urinary frequency, exfoliative dermatitis, extrapyramidal reaction, flank pain, gastritis, glossitis, hallucination, hearing loss, hematemesis, hematuria, hemolytic anemia, hemolytic-uremic syndrome, hepatic failure, hepatitis, hepatotoxicity (idiosyncratic) (Chalasani, 2014), hyperglycemia, hyperkalemia, hyperkinesis, hypersensitivity reaction, hyponatremia, hypotension, increased susceptibility to infection, increased thirst, infertility, inflammatory bowel disease, insomnia, interstitial nephritis, jaundice, lack of concentration, laryngeal edema, leukopenia, lymphadenopathy, maculopapular rash, melena, myocardial infarction, nephritis, oliguria, palpitations, pancytopenia, paresthesia, pneumonia, polyuria, proteinuria, psychosis, pulmonary edema, rectal hemorrhage, renal failure, respiratory depression, rhinitis, seizure, sepsis, skin photosensitivity, Stevens-Johnson syndrome, stomatitis (ulcerative), stupor, syncope, tachycardia, thrombocytopenia, tongue edema, toxic epidermal necrolysis, urinary retention, urticaria, vasculitis, weight gain, wound hemorrhage (postoperative)

Drug Interactions

Metabolism/Transport Effects None known.

Avoid Concomitant Use

Avoid concomitant use of Ketorolac (Systemic) with any of the following: Aspirin; Dexketoprofen; Floctafenine; Ketorolac (Nasal); Morniflumate; Nonsteroidal Anti-Inflammatory Agents; Omacetaxine; Pentoxifylline; Probenecid; Urokinase

Increased Effect/Toxicity

Ketorolac (Systemic) may increase the levels/effects of: 5-ASA Derivatives; Agents with Antiplatelet Properties; Aliskiren; Aminoglycosides; Anticoagulants; Apixaban; Aspirin; Bisphosphonate Derivatives; Collagenase (Systemic); CycloSPORINE (Systemic); Dabigatran Etexilate; Deferasirox; Deoxycholic Acid; Desmopressin; Digoxin; Drospirenone; Eplerenone; Haloperidol; Ibritumomab; Lithium; Methotrexate; Neuromuscular-Blocking Agents (Nondepolarizing); Nonsteroidal Anti-Inflammatory Agents; Obinutuzumab; Omacetaxine; PEMEtrexed; Pentoxifylline; Porfimer; Potassium-Sparing Diuretics; PRALAtrexate; Quinolone Antibiotics; Rivaroxaban; Salicylates; Tacrolimus (Systemic); Tenofovir; Thrombolytic Agents; Tositumomab and Iodine I 131 Tositumomab; Urokinase; Vancomycin; Verteporfin; Vitamin K Antagonists

The levels/effects of Ketorolac (Systemic) may be increased by: ACE Inhibitors; Angiotensin II Receptor Blockers; Antidepressants (Tricyclic, Tertiary Amine); Corticosteroids (Systemic); CycloSPORINE (Systemic); Dasatinib; Dexketoprofen; Floctafenine; Glucosamine; Herbs (Anticoagulant/Antiplatelet Properties); Ibrutinib; Ketorolac (Nasal); Limaprost; Morniflumate; Multivitamins/Fluoride (with ADE); Multivitamins/Minerals (with ADEK, Folate, Iron); Multivitamins/Minerals (with AE, No Iron); Omega-3 Fatty Acids; Pentosan Polysulfate Sodium; Probenecid; Prostacyclin Analogues; Selective Serotonin Reuptake Inhibitors; Serotonin/Norepinephrine Reuptake Inhibitors; Sodium Phosphates; Tipranavir; Treprostinil; Vitamin E

Decreased Effect

Ketorolac (Systemic) may decrease the levels/effects of: ACE Inhibitors; Aliskiren; Angiotensin II Receptor Blockers; Aspirin; Beta-Blockers; Eplerenone; HydrALAZINE; Loop Diuretics; Potassium-Sparing Diuretics; Prostaglandins (Ophthalmic); Salicylates; Selective Serotonin Reuptake Inhibitors; Thiazide Diuretics

The levels/effects of Ketorolac (Systemic) may be decreased by: Bile Acid Sequestrants; Salicylates

Food Interactions High-fat meals may delay time to peak (by ~1 hour) and decrease peak concentrations. Management: Administer tablet with food or milk to decrease gastrointestinal distress.

Storage/Stability

Injection: Store at room temperature of 15°C to 30°C (59°F to 86°F). Protect from light. Injection is clear and has a slight yellow color. Precipitation may occur at relatively low pH values.

Tablet: Store at room temperature of 15°C to 30°C (59°F to 86°F).

Mechanism of Action Reversibly inhibits cyclooxygenase-1 and 2 (COX-1 and 2) enzymes, which results in decreased formation of prostaglandin precursors; has antipyretic, analgesic, and anti-inflammatory properties

Other proposed mechanisms not fully elucidated (an possibly contributing to the anti-inflammatory effect t varying degrees), include inhibiting chemotaxis, alterin lymphocyte activity, inhibiting neutrophil aggregation/acti vation, and decreasing proinflammatory cytokine levels.

Pharmacodynamics Analgesia:

Onset of action:
- Oral: 30-60 minutes
- IM, IV: ~30 minutes

Maximum effect:
- Oral: 1.5-4 hours
- IM, IV: 2-3 hours

Duration: 4-6 hours

Pharmacokinetics (Adult data unless noted)

Absorption:
- Oral: Well-absorbed; 100%
- IM: Rapid and complete

Distribution: Crosses placenta, crosses into breast milk poor penetration into CSF; follows two-compartmen model

V_d beta:
- Children 4-8 years: 0.19-0.44 L/kg (mean: 0.26 L/kg)
- Adults: 0.11-0.33 L/kg (mean: 0.18 L/kg)

Protein binding: 99%

Metabolism: In the liver; undergoes hydroxylation an glucuronide conjugation; in children 4-8 years, V_{dss} an plasma clearance were twice as high as adults

Bioavailability: Oral, IM: 100%

Half-life, terminal:
- Infants 6-18 months of age (n=25): S-enantiomer: 0.83 ± 0.7 hours; R-enantiomer: 4 ± 0.8 hours (Lynn, 2007)
- Children:
  - 1-16 years (n=36): Mean: 3 ± 1.1 hours (Dsida, 2002)
  - 3-18 years (n=24): Mean: 3.8 ± 2.6 hours
  - 4-8 years (n=10): Mean: 6 hours; range: 3.5-10 hours
- Adults: Mean: ~5 hours; range: 2-9 hours [S-enantiome ~2.5 hours (biologically active); R-enantiomer ~5 hours
  - With renal impairment: Scr 1.9-5 mg/dL: Mean: ~1 hours; range: 4-19 hours
  - Renal dialysis patients: Mean: ~14 hours; range: 8-4 hours

Time to peak serum concentration:
- Oral: ~45 minutes
- IM: 30-45 minutes
- IV: 1-3 minutes

Elimination: Renal excretion: 60% in urine as unchange drug with 40% as metabolites; 6% of dose excreted i feces

Dosing: Neonatal Note: Due to a lack of substantia evidence, NSAIDs are **not** recommended for use in neo nates as an adjunct to postoperative analgesia (AAP 2006).

Full-term neonates: Multiple-dose treatment: IV: Dose nc established; limited data available; one retrospective study (n=10; mean PNA: 3 ± 4 weeks) recommend 0.5 mg/kg/dose every 8 hours for up to 1-2 days post operatively; do not exceed 48 hours of treatment (Burd 2002); **Note:** To reduce the risk of adverse cardiovascu lar and GI effects, use the lowest effective dose for the shortest period of time.

Dosing: Usual Note: To reduce the risk of adverse car diovascular and GI effects, use the lowest effective dose for the shortest period of time.

Infants ≥1 month and Children <2 years: Multiple-dose treatment: IV: 0.5 mg/kg every 6-8 hours, not to excee 48-72 hours of treatment (Burd, 2002; Dawkins, 2009 Gupta, 2004; Moffett, 2006)

Children 2-16 years and Children >16 years who are <50 kg: Do not exceed adult doses

Single-dose treatment:

Manufacturer's recommendations:
- IM: 1 mg/kg as a single dose; maximum dose: 30 mg
- IV: 0.5 mg/kg as a single dose; maximum dose: 15 mg

Alternative dosing:

IM, IV: 0.4-1 mg/kg as a single dose; **Note:** Limited information exists. Single IV doses of 0.5-1 mg/kg have been studied in children 2-16 years of age for postoperative analgesia. In one study (Maunuksela, 1992), the median required single IV dose was 0.4 mg/kg.

Oral: One study used 1 mg/kg as a single dose for analgesia in 30 children (mean ± SD age: 3 ± 2.5 years) undergoing bilateral myringotomy.

Multiple-dose treatment:

IM, IV: 0.5 mg/kg every 6 hours, not to exceed 5 days of treatment (Buck, 1994; Dsida, 2002; Gupta, 2004; Gupta, 2005)

Oral: No pediatric studies exist.

Children >16 years and >50 kg and Adults <65 years:

Single-dose treatment:

IM: 60 mg as a single dose

IV: 30 mg as a single dose

Multiple-dose treatment:

IM, IV: 30 mg every 6 hours; maximum dose: 120 mg/day

Oral: Initial: 20 mg, then 10 mg every 4-6 hours; maximum dose: 40 mg/day

Adults ≥65 years, renally impaired, or <50 kg:

Single-dose treatment:

IM: 30 mg as a single dose

IV: 15 mg as a single dose

Multiple-dose treatment:

IM, IV: 15 mg every 6 hours; maximum dose: 60 mg/day

Oral: 10 mg every 4-6 hours; maximum dose: 40 mg/day

Administration

Oral: May administer with food or milk to decrease GI upset

Parenteral:

IM: Administer slowly and deeply into muscle; 60 mg/2 mL vial is for IM use only

IV bolus: Administer undiluted over at least 15 seconds; in children, ketorolac has been infused over 1 to 5 minutes (Buck 1994)

Monitoring Parameters Signs of pain relief (eg, increased appetite and activity); BUN, serum creatinine, liver enzymes, CBC, serum electrolytes, occult blood loss, urinalysis, urine output; signs and symptoms of GI bleeding

Reference Range Serum concentration:

Therapeutic: 0.3-5 mcg/mL

Toxic: >5 mcg/mL

Additional Information 30 mg provides analgesia comparable to 12 mg of morphine or 100 mg of meperidine; ketorolac may possess an opioid-sparing effect; diarrhea, pallor, vomiting, and labored breathing may occur with overdose

Dosage Forms Excipient information presented when available (limited, particularly for generics); consult specific product labeling.

Solution, Injection, as tromethamine:

Generic: 15 mg/mL (1 mL); 30 mg/mL (1 mL); 60 mg/2 mL (2 mL); 300 mg/10 mL (10 mL)

Solution, Injection, as tromethamine [preservative free]:

Generic: 15 mg/mL (1 mL); 30 mg/mL (1 mL); 60 mg/2 mL (2 mL)

Solution, Intramuscular, as tromethamine:

Generic: 60 mg/2 mL (2 mL)

Tablet, Oral, as tromethamine:

Generic: 10 mg

Ketorolac (Ophthalmic) (KEE toe role ak)

Medication Safety Issues

Sound-alike/look-alike issues:

Acular® may be confused with Acthar®, Ocular

Ketorolac may be confused with Ketalar®

Brand Names: US Acular; Acular LS; Acuvail

Brand Names: Canada Acular LS®; Acular®; Apo-Ketorolac® Ophthalmic; ratio-Ketorolac

Therapeutic Category Anti-inflammatory Agent; Nonsteroidal Anti-inflammatory Drug (NSAID), Ophthalmic

Generic Availability (US) Yes

Use

Acular®: Treatment of ocular itch associated with seasonal allergic conjunctivitis; postoperative inflammation following cataract extraction (FDA approved in ages ≥3 years and adults)

Acular LS™: Reduction of ocular pain, burning, and stinging after corneal refractive surgery (FDA approved in ages ≥3 years and adults)

Acuvail®: Treatment of postoperative pain and inflammation following cataract surgery (FDA approved in adults)

Pregnancy Risk Factor C

Pregnancy Considerations Adverse events have been observed in animal studies; therefore, the manufacturer classifies ketorolac ophthalmic as pregnancy category C. When administered IM, ketorolac crosses the placenta. Refer to the Ketorolac (Systemic) monograph for details. The amount of ketorolac available systemically following topical application of the ophthalmic drops is significantly less in comparison to oral doses. Because they may cause premature closure of the ductus arteriosus, the use of NSAIDs late in pregnancy (including ketorolac ophthalmic drops) should be avoided.

Breast-Feeding Considerations When administered orally, ketorolac enters breast milk. The use of systemic ketorolac is contraindicated in breast-feeding women. Refer to the Ketorolac (Systemic) monograph for details. The amount of ketorolac available systemically following topical application of the ophthalmic drops is significantly less in comparison to oral doses. The manufacturer recommends that caution be used when administering ketorolac ophthalmic to breast-feeding women.

Contraindications Hypersensitivity to ketorolac or any component of the formulation

Warnings/Precautions May increase bleeding time associated with ocular surgery. Use with caution in patients with known bleeding tendencies or those receiving anticoagulants. Healing time may be slowed or delayed. Concurrent use of ocular corticosteroids may increase risk of delayed healing. Corneal thinning, erosion, or ulceration have been reported with topical NSAIDs; discontinue if corneal epithelial breakdown occurs. Use caution with complicated ocular surgery, corneal denervation, corneal epithelial defects, diabetes, rheumatoid arthritis, ocular surface disease, or ocular surgeries repeated within short periods of time; risk of corneal epithelial breakdown (leading to possible loss of vision) may be increased. Use for >24 hours prior to or for >14 days following surgery also increases risk of corneal adverse effects. Use with caution in patients with sensitivity to acetylsalicylic acid, phenylacetic acid derivatives, or other nonsteroidal anti-inflammatory agents; bronchospasm or exacerbation of asthma may occur. May contain benzalkonium chloride which may be absorbed by contact lenses; contact lenses should not be worn during treatment. Allow at least 5 minutes between applications with other eye drops. To avoid contamination, do not touch tip of container to any surface. The safety and efficacy of Acular LS® have not been established in postcataract surgery patients. To minimize the risk of infection following surgery of both eyes, two separate bottles of eye drops (one for each eye) should be used; instruct patients not to use the same bottle for both eyes.

Adverse Reactions

Central nervous system: Headache

Hypersensitivity: Hypersensitivity reaction

Ophthalmic: Blurred vision, burning sensation of eyes (transient), conjunctival hyperemia, corneal edema, corneal infiltrates, eye irritation,eye pain, increased intraocular pressure, iritis, lacrimation, ocular edema, ophthalmic inflammation, superficial eye infection, superficial keratitis

Rare but important or life-threatening: Corneal erosion, corneal perforation, corneal thinning (including corneal melt), corneal ulcer, dry eye syndrome, epithelial keratopathy (breakdown), keratitis (ulcerative)

Drug Interactions

Metabolism/Transport Effects None known.

Avoid Concomitant Use There are no known interactions where it is recommended to avoid concomitant use.

Increased Effect/Toxicity

Ketorolac (Ophthalmic) may increase the levels/effects of: Corticosteroids (Ophthalmic)

Decreased Effect There are no known significant interactions involving a decrease in effect.

Storage/Stability

Acular®, Acular LS®: Store at room temperature 15°C to 25°C (59°F to 77°F). Protect from light.

Acuvail®: Store at room temperature 15°C to 30°C(59°F to 86°F). Store in pouch with ends folded; protect from light.

Mechanism of Action Reversibly inhibits cyclooxygenase-1 and 2 (COX-1 and 2) enzymes, which results in decreased formation of prostaglandin precursors; has anti-inflammatory properties

Other proposed mechanisms not fully elucidated (and possibly contributing to the anti-inflammatory effect to varying degrees), include inhibiting chemotaxis, altering lymphocyte activity, inhibiting neutrophil aggregation/activation, and decreasing proinflammatory cytokine levels.

Dosing: Usual

Children and Adolescents:

Seasonal allergic conjunctivitis: Acular®: Children ≥3 years, Adolescents: Ophthalmic: Instill 1 drop in eye(s) 4 times daily

Postoperative inflammation following cataract extracation: Acular®: Children ≥3 years, Adolescents: Ophthalmic: Instill 1 drop in affected eye(s) 4 times daily starting 24 hours after cataract surgery and through 14 days after surgery

Postoperative pain, burning, and stinging following corneal refractive surgery: Acular LS™: Children ≥3 years, Adolescents: Ophthalmic: Instill 1 drop in affected eye 4 times daily as needed for up to 4 days after corneal refractive surgery

Adults:

Seasonal allergic conjunctivitis (relief of ocular itching): Acular®: Ophthalmic: Instill 1 drop 4 times daily

Inflammation following cataract extraction:

Acular®: Ophthalmic: Instill 1 drop to affected eye(s) 4 times daily beginning 24 hours after surgery; continue for 2 weeks

Acuvail®: Ophthalmic: Instill 1 drop twice daily into affected eye; begin treatment 1 day prior to cataract surgery and continue on day of surgery, and for 2 weeks postoperatively

Pain following corneal refractive surgery: Acular LS®: Ophthalmic: Instill 1 drop 4 times daily as needed to affected eye for up to 4 days

Administration May contain benzalkonium chloride which may be absorbed by contact lenses; contact lenses should not be worn during treatment. Instill drops into affected eye(s); avoid contact of container tip with skin or eyes; apply finger pressure to lacrimal sac during and for 1-2 minutes after instillation to decrease risk of absorption and systemic effects; wait at least 5 minutes before administering other ophthalmic drops. To minimize the risk of infection following surgery of both eyes, two separate bottles of eye drops (one for each eye) should be used; instruct patients not to use the same bottle for both eyes.

Dosage Forms Excipient information presented when available (limited, particularly for generics); consult specific product labeling.

Solution, Ophthalmic, as tromethamine:

Acular: 0.5% (5 mL) [contains benzalkonium chloride, edetate disodium]

Acular LS: 0.4% (5 mL) [contains benzalkonium chloride, edetate disodium]

Generic: 0.4% (5 mL); 0.5% (3 mL, 5 mL, 10 mL)

Solution, Ophthalmic, as tromethamine [preservative free]:

Acuvail: 0.45% (30 ea)

◆ **Ketorolac Tromethamine** *see* Ketorolac (Ophthalmic) *on page 1195*

◆ **Ketorolac Tromethamine** *see* Ketorolac (Systemic) *on page 1192*

◆ **Ketorolac Tromethamine Injection, USP (Can)** *see* Ketorolac (Systemic) *on page 1192*

Ketotifen (Ophthalmic) (kee toe TYE fen)

Medication Safety Issues

Sound-alike/look-alike issues:

Claritin Eye (ketotifen) may be confused with Claritin (loratadine)

Ketotifen may be confused with ketoprofen

ZyrTEC Itchy Eye (ketotifen) may be confused with ZyrTEC (cetirizine)

Brand Names: US Alaway Childrens Allergy [OTC]; Alaway [OTC]; Claritin Eye [OTC]; Zaditor [OTC]; ZyrTEC Itchy Eye [OTC]

Brand Names: Canada Zaditor®

Therapeutic Category Antiallergic, Ophthalmic; Histamine H_1 Antagonist, Ophthalmic

Generic Availability (US) Yes

Use Temporary relief of eye itching due to allergic conjunctivitis (FDA approved in children ≥3 years and adults)

Pregnancy Risk Factor C

Pregnancy Considerations Topical ocular administration has not been studied.

Breast-Feeding Considerations Ketotifen has been identified in rat breast milk. It is not known whether detectable levels of ketotifen would appear in human breast milk following topical ocular administration.

Contraindications Hypersensitivity to ketotifen or any component of the formulation

Warnings/Precautions Ophthalmic solution should not be used to treat contact lens-related irritation. After ketotifen use, soft contact lens wearers should wait at least 10 minutes before reinserting contact lenses. Do not wear contact lenses if eyes are red. Do not contaminate dropper tip or solution when placing drops in eyes.

When using ophthalmic solution for self-medication (OTC), notify healthcare provider if symptoms worsen or do not improve within 3 days. Contact healthcare provider if change in vision, eye pain, or redness occur. Do not use if solution is cloudy or changes color.

Adverse Reactions

Ocular: Allergic reactions, burning or stinging, conjunctivitis, discharge, dry eyes, eye pain, eyelid disorder, itching, keratitis, lacrimation disorder, mydriasis, photophobia, rash

Respiratory: Pharyngitis

Miscellaneous: Flu syndrome

Drug Interactions

Metabolism/Transport Effects None known.

Avoid Concomitant Use

Avoid concomitant use of Ketotifen (Ophthalmic) with any of the following: Aclidinium; Azelastine (Nasal); Eluxadoline; Glucagon; Ipratropium (Oral Inhalation); Orphenadrine; Paraldehyde; Potassium Chloride; Thalidomide; Umeclidinium

Increased Effect/Toxicity

Ketotifen (Ophthalmic) may increase the levels/effects of: AbobotulinumtoxinA; Alcohol (Ethyl); Analgesics (Opioid); Anticholinergic Agents; Azelastine (Nasal); Buprenorphine; CNS Depressants; Eluxadoline; Glucagon; Hydrocodone; Methotrimeprazine; Metyrosine; Mirabegron; Mirtazapine; OnabotulinumtoxinA; Orphenadrine; Paraldehyde; Potassium Chloride; Pramipexole; RimabotulinumtoxinB; ROPINIRole; Rotigotine; Selective Serotonin Reuptake Inhibitors; Suvorexant; Thalidomide; Thiazide Diuretics; Topiramate; Zolpidem

The levels/effects of Ketotifen (Ophthalmic) may be increased by: Aclidinium; Brimonidine (Topical); Cannabis; Doxylamine; Dronabinol; Droperidol; HydrOXYzine; Ipratropium (Oral Inhalation); Kava Kava; Magnesium Sulfate; Methotrimeprazine; Mianserin; Nabilone; Perampanel; Pramlintide; Rufinamide; Sodium Oxybate; Tapentadol; Tetrahydrocannabinol; Umeclidinium

Decreased Effect

Ketotifen (Ophthalmic) may decrease the levels/effects of: Acetylcholinesterase Inhibitors; Benzylpenicilloyl Polylysine; Betahistine; Hyaluronidase; Itopride; Metoclopramide; Secretin

The levels/effects of Ketotifen (Ophthalmic) may be decreased by: Acetylcholinesterase Inhibitors; Amphetamines

Storage/Stability Store at 4°C to 25°C (39°F to 77°F).

Mechanism of Action Exhibits noncompetitive H_1-receptor antagonist and mast cell stabilizer properties. Efficacy in conjunctivitis likely results from a combination of anti-inflammatory and antihistaminergic actions including interference with chemokine-induced migration of eosinophils into inflamed conjunctiva.

Pharmacodynamics

Onset of action: 5-15 minutes

Duration: 5-8 hours

Dosing: Usual Ophthalmic: Children ≥3 years and Adults: Instill 1 drop into lower conjunctival sac of affected eye(s) twice daily, every 8-12 hours

Administration Ophthalmic: Instill into conjunctival sac avoiding contact of bottle tip with skin or eye; apply finger pressure to lacrimal sac during and for 1-2 minutes after instillation to decrease risk of absorption and systemic effects. Administer other topical ophthalmic medications at least 5 minutes apart.

Monitoring Parameters Improvement in symptomatology (eg, reduction in itching, tearing, and hyperaemia)

Dosage Forms Excipient information presented when available (limited, particularly for generics); consult specific product labeling.

Solution, Ophthalmic:

Alaway: 0.025% (10 mL) [contains benzalkonium chloride]

Alaway Childrens Allergy: 0.025% (5 mL) [contains benzalkonium chloride]

Claritin Eye: 0.025% (5 mL) [contains benzalkonium chloride]

Zaditor: 0.025% (5 mL) [contains benzalkonium chloride]

ZyrTEC Itchy Eye: 0.025% (5 mL) [contains benzalkonium chloride]

Generic: 0.025% (5 mL)

- ◆ **Ketotifen Fumarate** *see* Ketotifen (Ophthalmic) *on page 1196*
- ◆ **Khloditan** *see* Mitotane *on page 1446*
- ◆ **KI** *see* Potassium Iodide *on page 1740*
- ◆ **Kineret** *see* Anakinra *on page 165*
- ◆ **Kinrix** *see* Diphtheria and Tetanus Toxoids, Acellular Pertussis, and Poliovirus Vaccine *on page 677*
- ◆ **Kionex** *see* Sodium Polystyrene Sulfonate *on page 1953*
- ◆ **Kitabis Pak** *see* Tobramycin (Systemic, Oral Inhalation) *on page 2073*
- ◆ **Kitabis Pak** *see* Tobramycin (Systemic, Oral Inhalation) *on page 2073*
- ◆ **Kivexa (Can)** *see* Abacavir and Lamivudine *on page 36*
- ◆ **Klaron** *see* Sulfacetamide (Topical) *on page 1982*
- ◆ **Klean-Prep (Can)** *see* Polyethylene Glycol-Electrolyte Solution *on page 1724*
- ◆ **KlonoPIN** *see* ClonazePAM *on page 506*
- ◆ **Klor-Con** *see* Potassium Chloride *on page 1736*
- ◆ **Klor-Con 10** *see* Potassium Chloride *on page 1736*
- ◆ **Klor-Con M10** *see* Potassium Chloride *on page 1736*
- ◆ **Klor-Con M15** *see* Potassium Chloride *on page 1736*
- ◆ **Klor-Con M20** *see* Potassium Chloride *on page 1736*
- ◆ **Koate-DVI** *see* Antihemophilic Factor (Human) *on page 167*
- ◆ **Koffex Expectorant (Can)** *see* GuaiFENesin *on page 988*
- ◆ **Kogenate FS** *see* Antihemophilic Factor (Recombinant) *on page 168*
- ◆ **Kogenate FS Bio-Set** *see* Antihemophilic Factor (Recombinant) *on page 168*
- ◆ **Kolephrin GG/DM [OTC]** *see* Guaifenesin and Dextromethorphan *on page 992*
- ◆ **Konakion (Can)** *see* Phytonadione *on page 1698*
- ◆ **Konsyl [OTC]** *see* Psyllium *on page 1804*
- ◆ **Konsyl-D [OTC]** *see* Psyllium *on page 1804*
- ◆ **K-Phos Neutral** *see* Potassium Phosphate and Sodium Phosphate *on page 1746*
- ◆ **K-Phos No. 2** *see* Potassium Phosphate and Sodium Phosphate *on page 1746*
- ◆ **Kristalose** *see* Lactulose *on page 1204*
- ◆ **KS Ibuprofen [OTC]** *see* Ibuprofen *on page 1064*
- ◆ **K-Sol** *see* Potassium Chloride *on page 1736*
- ◆ **KS Stool Softener [OTC]** *see* Docusate *on page 697*
- ◆ **K-Tab** *see* Potassium Chloride *on page 1736*
- ◆ **Kuvan** *see* Sapropterin *on page 1900*
- ◆ **K-Vescent** *see* Potassium Chloride *on page 1736*
- ◆ **Kwell** *see* Lindane *on page 1267*
- ◆ **Kwellada-P [OTC] (Can)** *see* Permethrin *on page 1675*
- ◆ **Kynesia (Can)** *see* Benztropine *on page 272*
- ◆ **Kytril** *see* Granisetron *on page 981*
- ◆ **L-749,345** *see* Ertapenem *on page 777*
- ◆ **L-758,298** *see* Fosaprepitant *on page 939*
- ◆ **L 754030** *see* Aprepitant *on page 186*

Labetalol (la BET a lole)

Medication Safety Issues

Sound-alike/look-alike issues:

Labetalol may be confused with betaxolol, lamoTRIgine, Lipitor

Normodyne may be confused with Norpramin

Trandate may be confused with traMADol, TRENtal

High alert medication:

The Institute for Safe Medication Practices (ISMP) includes this medication among its list of drugs which have a heightened risk of causing significant patient harm when used in error.

Administration issues:

Significant differences exist between oral and IV dosing. Use caution when converting from one route of administration to another.

Brand Names: US Trandate

Brand Names: Canada Apo-Labetalol; Labetalol Hydrochloride Injection, USP; Normodyne; Trandate

Therapeutic Category Alpha-/Beta- Adrenergic Blocker; Antihypertensive Agent

Generic Availability (US) Yes

Use

Oral: Treatment of hypertension alone or in combination (particularly with thiazide or loop diuretics) (FDA approved in adults)

Parenteral: Treatment of severe hypertension (FDA approved in adults)

Pregnancy Risk Factor C

Pregnancy Considerations Adverse events have been observed in some animal reproduction studies. Labetalol crosses the placenta and can be detected in cord blood and infant serum after delivery (Haraldsson, 1989; Rogers, 1990). Fetal/neonatal bradycardia, hypoglycemia, hypotension, and/or respiratory depression have been observed following in utero exposure to labetalol. Adequate facilities for monitoring infants at birth should be available.

Untreated chronic maternal hypertension and preeclampsia are also associated with adverse events in the fetus, infant, and mother. Oral labetalol is considered an appropriate agent for the treatment of chronic hypertension in pregnancy (ACOG, 2013; Magee, 2014). Intravenous labetalol is recommended for use in the management of acute onset, severe hypertension (systolic BP ≥160 mm Hg or diastolic BP ≥110 mm Hg) with preeclampsia or eclampsia in pregnant and postpartum women. In general, avoid use of labetalol in women with asthma or heart failure (ACOG, 2015; Magee, 2014).

Breast-Feeding Considerations Low amounts of labetalol are found in breast milk and can be detected in the serum of nursing infants. The manufacturer recommends that caution be exercised when administering labetalol to nursing women.

Contraindications Hypersensitivity to labetalol or any component of the formulation; severe bradycardia; heart block greater than first degree (except in patients with a functioning artificial pacemaker); cardiogenic shock; bronchial asthma; uncompensated cardiac failure; conditions associated with severe and prolonged hypotension

Warnings/Precautions Consider pre-existing conditions such as sick sinus syndrome before initiating. Symptomatic hypotension with or without syncope may occur with labetalol; close monitoring of patient is required especially with initial dosing and dosing increases; blood pressure must be lowered at a rate appropriate for the patient's clinical condition. Initiation with a low dose and gradual up-titration may help to decrease the occurrence of hypotension or syncope. Patients should be advised to avoid driving or other hazardous tasks during initiation of therapy due to the risk of syncope. Orthostatic hypotension may occur with IV administration; patient should remain supine during and for up to 3 hours after IV administration. Use with caution in impaired hepatic function; bioavailability is increased due to decreased first-pass metabolism. Severe hepatic injury including some fatalities have also been rarely reported with use: periodically monitor LFTs with prolonged use. Use with caution in patients with diabetes mellitus; may potentiate hypoglycemia and/or mask signs and symptoms. Bradycardia may be observed more frequently in elderly patients (>65 years of age); dosage reductions may be necessary. May also reduce release of insulin in response to hyperglycemia; dosage of antidiabetic agents may need to be adjusted. May mask signs of hyperthyroidism (eg, tachycardia); if hyperthyroidism is suspected, carefully manage and monitor; abrupt withdrawal may exacerbate symptoms of hyperthyroidism or precipitate thyroid storm. Elimination of labetalol is reduced in elderly patients; lower maintenance doses may be required.

Use only with extreme caution in compensated heart failure and monitor for a worsening of the condition. Beta-blocker therapy should not be withdrawn abruptly (particularly in patients with CAD), but gradually tapered to avoid acute tachycardia, hypertension, and/or ischemia. Chronic beta-blocker therapy should not be routinely withdrawn prior to major surgery. Use caution with concurrent use of digoxin, verapamil, or diltiazem; bradycardia or heart block can occur. Use with caution in patients receiving inhaled anesthetic agents known to depress myocardial contractility. Patients with bronchospastic disease should not receive beta-blockers; if used at all, should be used cautiously with close monitoring. Use with caution in patients with myasthenia gravis or psychiatric disease (may cause or exacerbate CNS depression). Can precipitate or aggravate symptoms of arterial insufficiency in patients with PVD and Raynaud's disease; use with caution and monitor for progression of arterial obstruction. If possible, obtain diagnostic tests for pheochromocytoma prior to use. May induce or exacerbate psoriasis. Labetalol has been shown to be effective in lowering blood pressure and relieving symptoms in patients with pheochromocytoma. However, some patients have experienced paradoxical hypertensive responses; use with caution in patients with pheochromocytoma. Additional alpha-blockade may be required during use of labetalol. Use caution with history of severe anaphylaxis to allergens; patients taking beta-blockers may become more sensitive to repeated challenges. Treatment of anaphylaxis (eg, epinephrine) in patients taking beta-blockers may be ineffective or promote undesirable effects.

Intraoperative floppy iris syndrome has been observed in cataract surgery patients who were on or were previously treated with $alpha_1$-blockers; causality has not been established and there appears to be no benefit in discontinuing alpha-blocker therapy prior to surgery. Instruct patients to inform ophthalmologist of labetalol use when considering eye surgery.

Benzyl alcohol and derivatives: Some dosage forms may contain sodium benzoate/benzoic acid; benzoic acid (benzoate) is a metabolite of benzyl alcohol; large amounts of benzyl alcohol (≥99 mg/kg/day) have been associated with a potentially fatal toxicity ("gasping syndrome") in neonates; the "gasping syndrome" consists of metabolic acidosis, respiratory distress, gasping respirations, CNS dysfunction (including convulsions, intracranial hemorrhage), hypotension, and cardiovascular collapse (AAP, 1997; CDC, 1982); some data suggests that benzoate displaces bilirubin from protein binding sites (Ahlfors, 2001); avoid or use dosage forms containing benzyl alcohol derivative with caution in neonates. See manufacturer's labeling.

Warnings: Additional Pediatric Considerations In children, two cases of reversible myopathy have been reported (Willis, 1990).

Adverse Reactions

Cardiovascular: Edema, flushing, hypotension, orthostatic hypotension (IV use), ventricular arrhythmia (IV use)

Central nervous system: Dizziness, fatigue, headache, somnolence, vertigo
Dermatologic: Pruritus, rash, scalp tingling
Gastrointestinal: Dyspepsia, nausea, taste disturbance, vomiting
Genitourinary: Ejaculatory failure, impotence
Hepatic: Transaminases increased
Neuromuscular & skeletal: Paresthesia, weakness
Ocular: Vision abnormal
Renal: BUN increased
Respiratory: Dyspnea, nasal congestion
Miscellaneous: Diaphoresis
Rare but important or life-threatening: Alopecia (reversible), anaphylactoid reaction, ANA positive, angioedema, bradycardia, bronchospasm, cholestatic jaundice, CHF, diabetes insipidus, heart block, hepatic necrosis, hepatitis, hypersensitivity, Peyronie's disease, psoriaform rash, Raynaud's syndrome, syncope, systemic lupus erythematosus, toxic myopathy, urinary retention, urticaria
Other adverse reactions noted with beta-adrenergic blocking agents include agranulocytosis, catatonia, emotional lability, intensification of pre-existing AV block, ischemic colitis. laryngospasm, mental depression, mesenteric artery thrombosis, nonthrombocytopenic purpura, respiratory distress, short-term memory loss, and thrombocytopenic purpura.

Drug Interactions

Metabolism/Transport Effects None known.

Avoid Concomitant Use

Avoid concomitant use of Labetalol with any of the following: Beta2-Agonists; Ceritinib; Floctafenine; Methacholine; Rivastigmine

Increased Effect/Toxicity

Labetalol may increase the levels/effects of: Alpha-/Beta-Agonists (Direct-Acting); Alpha1-Blockers; Alpha2-Agonists; Amifostine; Antihypertensives; Antipsychotic Agents (Phenothiazines); Bradycardia-Causing Agents; Bupivacaine; Cardiac Glycosides; Ceritinib; Cholinergic Agonists; Disopyramide; DULoxetine; Ergot Derivatives; Fingolimod; Grass Pollen Allergen Extract (5 Grass Extract); Hypotensive Agents; Insulin; Ivabradine; Lacosamide; Levodopa; Lidocaine (Systemic); Lidocaine (Topical); Mepivacaine; Methacholine; Midodrine; Obinutuzumab; RisperiDONE; RiTUXimab; Sulfonylureas

The levels/effects of Labetalol may be increased by: Acetylcholinesterase Inhibitors; Alpha2-Agonists; Aminoquinolines (Antimalarial); Amiodarone; Anilidopiperidine Opioids; Antipsychotic Agents (Phenothiazines); Barbiturates; Bretylium; Brimonidine (Topical); Calcium Channel Blockers (Nondihydropyridine); Diazoxide; Dipyridamole; Disopyramide; Dronedarone; Floctafenine; Herbs (Hypotensive Properties); MAO Inhibitors; Nicorandil; NIFEdipine; Pentoxifylline; Phosphodiesterase 5 Inhibitors; Propafenone; Prostacyclin Analogues; Regorafenib; Reserpine; Rivastigmine; Ruxolitinib; Tofacitinib

Decreased Effect

Labetalol may decrease the levels/effects of: Beta2-Agonists; Theophylline Derivatives

The levels/effects of Labetalol may be decreased by: Barbiturates; Herbs (Hypertensive Properties); Methylphenidate; Nonsteroidal Anti-Inflammatory Agents; Rifamycin Derivatives; Yohimbine

Food Interactions Labetalol serum concentrations may be increased if taken with food. Management: Administer with food.

Storage/Stability

Tablets: Store at room temperature (refer to manufacturer's labeling for detailed storage requirements). Protect from light and excessive moisture.
Injectable: Store at room temperature (refer to manufacturer's labeling for detailed storage requirements); do not freeze. Protect from light. The solution is clear to slightly yellow.
Parenteral admixture: Stability of parenteral admixture at room temperature (25°C) and refrigeration temperature (4°C): 3 days.

Mechanism of Action Blocks alpha-, beta$_1$-, and beta$_2$-adrenergic receptor sites; elevated renins are reduced. The ratios of alpha- to beta-blockade differ depending on the route of administration: 1:3 (oral) and 1:7 (IV).

Pharmacodynamics

Onset of action:
  Oral: 20 minutes to 2 hours
  IV: 2-5 minutes
Maximum effect:
  Oral: 1-4 hours
  IV: 5-15 minutes
Duration:
  Oral: 8-24 hours (dose dependent)
  IV: 2-4 hours

Pharmacokinetics (Adult data unless noted)

Distribution: Crosses the placenta; small amounts in breast milk
V_d: 3-16 L/kg; mean: 9.4 L/kg
Protein-binding: 50%
Metabolism: Hepatic via primarily glucuronide conjugation; extensive first-pass effect
Bioavailability: Oral: 25%; increased bioavailability with liver disease, elderly
Time to peak serum concentration: Oral: 1-2 hours
Half-life: 5-8 hours
Elimination: Urine (55% to 60%, primarily as glucuronide conjugates, <5% as unchanged drug); possible decreased clearance in neonates and infants
Dialysis: Not removed by hemo- or peritoneal dialysis; supplemental dose is not necessary

Dosing: Usual Note: Use care with labetalol continuous IV infusions; the rate of administration is different for pediatric patients (mg/kg/hour) versus adult patients (mg/minute).

Infants, Children, and Adolescents:

Hypertension: Children and Adolescents: Limited data available:
  Oral: Initial: 1-3 mg/kg/**day** in 2 divided doses; maximum daily dose: 10-12 mg/kg/**day**, up to 1200 mg/day (NHLBI, 2011)
  IV (intermittent bolus): 0.2-1 mg/kg/dose; maximum dose: 40 mg; use should be reserved for severe hypertension (NHBPEP, 2004)

Hypertensive emergency: Infants, Children, and Adolescents: Continuous IV infusion: 0.25-3 mg/kg/**hour**; initiate at lower end of range, and titrate up slowly (NHBPEP, 2004). One retrospective study in infants and children ≤24 months of age observed reductions in blood pressure at doses up to 0.59 mg/kg/hour with little additional benefit at higher doses (Thomas, 2011).

Adults:

Hypertension: Oral: Initial: 100 mg twice daily, may increase as needed every 2-3 days by 100 mg twice daily (titration increments not to exceed 200 mg twice daily) until desired response is obtained; usual dose: 100-400 mg twice daily (JNC 7); may require up to 2400 mg/day

Acute hypertension (hypertensive emergency/urgency):
  IV bolus: Manufacturer's labeling: Initial: 20 mg IV push over 2 minutes; may administer 40-80 mg at 10-minute intervals, up to 300 mg total cumulative dose; as appropriate, follow with oral antihypertensive regimen

IV infusion (acute loading): Manufacturer's labeling: Initial: 2 mg/minute; titrate to response up to 300 mg total cumulative dose (eg, discontinue after 2.5 hours of 2 mg/minute); usual total dose required: 50-200 mg; as appropriate, follow with oral antihypertensive regimen

Note: There is limited documentation of prolonged continuous IV infusions (ie, >300 mg/day). In rare clinical situations, higher continuous IV infusion doses up to 6 mg/minute have been used in the critical care setting (eg, aortic dissection) and up to 8 mg/minute (eg, hypertension with ongoing acute ischemic stroke). At the other extreme, continuous infusions at relatively low doses (0.03-0.1 mg/minute) have been used in some settings (following loading infusion in patients who are unable to be converted to oral regimens or in some cases as a continuation of outpatient oral regimens). These prolonged infusions should not be confused with loading infusions. Because of wide variation in the use of infusions, an awareness of institutional policies and practices is extremely important. Careful clarification of orders and specific infusion rates/units is required to avoid confusion. Due to the prolonged duration of action, careful monitoring should be extended for the duration of the infusion and for several hours after the infusion. Excessive administration may result in prolonged hypotension and/or bradycardia.

IV to oral conversion: Upon discontinuation of IV infusion, may initiate oral dose of 200 mg followed in 6-12 hours with an additional dose of 200-400 mg. Thereafter, dose patients with 400-2400 mg/day in divided doses depending on blood pressure response.

Dosage adjustment in hepatic impairment: Dosage reduction may be necessary.

Usual Infusion Concentrations: Pediatric IV infusion: 1 mg/mL

Preparation for Administration Parenteral: Continuous IV infusion: Further dilute in a compatible solution to a concentration of 0.67 to 1 mg/mL; in adults, higher concentrations (2 mg/mL) are typical and per the manufacturer a final concentration of 3.75 mg/mL has been shown to be compatible.

Administration

Oral: May administer with food but should be administered in a consistent manner with regards to meals

Parenteral:

IV bolus: May administer undiluted over 2 minutes; maximum: 10 mg/minute

Continuous IV infusion: Administer as a continuous IV infusion with the use of an infusion pump; adjust infusion rate to effect.

Monitoring Parameters Blood pressure, heart rate, pulse, ECG; **Note:** IV use: Monitor closely; due to the prolonged duration of action, careful monitoring should be extended for the duration of the infusion and for several hours after the infusion; excessive administration may result in prolonged hypotension and/or bradycardia

Test Interactions False-positive urine catecholamines, vanillylmandelic acid (VMA) if measured by fluorometric or photometric methods; use HPLC or specific catecholamine radioenzymatic technique; false-positive amphetamine if measured by thin-layer chromatography or radioenzymatic assay (gas chromatographic-mass spectrometer technique should be used)

Dosage Forms Excipient information presented when available (limited, particularly for generics); consult specific product labeling.

Solution, Intravenous, as hydrochloride:

Generic: 5 mg/mL (4 mL, 20 mL, 40 mL)

Tablet, Oral, as hydrochloride:

Trandate: 100 mg, 200 mg, 300 mg [scored]

Generic: 100 mg, 200 mg, 300 mg

Extemporaneous Preparations A 40 mg/mL labetalol hydrochloride oral suspension may be made with tablets and one of three different vehicles (cherry syrup, a 1:1 mixture of Ora-Sweet® and Ora-Plus®, or a 1:1 mixture of Ora-Sweet® SF and Ora-Plus®). Crush sixteen 300 mg tablets in a mortar and reduce to a fine powder. Add 20 mL of the chosen vehicle and mix to a uniform paste; mix while adding the vehicle in incremental proportions to **almost** 120 mL; transfer to a calibrated bottle, rinse mortar with vehicle, and add quantity of vehicle sufficient to make 120 mL. Label "shake well" and "protect from light". Stable for 60 days when stored in amber plastic prescription bottles in the dark at room temperature or refrigerated (Allen, 1996).

Extemporaneously prepared solutions of labetalol hydrochloride (approximate concentrations 7-10 mg/mL) prepared in distilled water, simple syrup, apple juice, grape juice, and orange juice were stable for 4 weeks when stored in amber glass or plastic prescription bottles at room temperature or refrigerated (Nahata, 1991).

Allen LV Jr and Erickson MA 3rd, "Stability of Labetalol Hydrochloride, Metoprolol Tartrate, Verapamil Hydrochloride, and Spironolactone with Hydrochlorothiazide in Extemporaneously Compounded Oral Liquids," *Am J Health Syst Pharm*, 1996, 53(19):2304-9.

Nahata MC, "Stability of Labetalol Hydrochloride in Distilled Water, Simple Syrup, and Three Fruit Juices," *DICP*, 1991, 25(5):465-9.

◆ **Labetalol Hydrochloride** *see* Labetalol *on page 1197*

◆ **Labetalol Hydrochloride Injection, USP (Can)** *see* Labetalol *on page 1197*

◆ **Lac-Hydrin®** *see* Lactic Acid and Ammonium Hydroxide *on page 1202*

◆ **Lac-Hydrin® Five [OTC]** *see* Lactic Acid and Ammonium Hydroxide *on page 1202*

◆ **LAClotion™** *see* Lactic Acid and Ammonium Hydroxide *on page 1202*

Lacosamide (la KOE sa mide)

Medication Safety Issues

Sound-alike/look-alike issues:

Lacosamide may be confused with zonisamide

Vimpat may be confused with Vimovo

Brand Names: US Vimpat

Brand Names: Canada Vimpat

Therapeutic Category Anticonvulsant, Miscellaneous

Generic Availability (US) No

Use

Oral: Solution, tablets: Adjunctive therapy in the treatment of partial-onset seizures (FDA approved in ages ≥17 years and adults)

Parenteral: Short-term adjunctive therapy in the treatment of partial-onset seizures when oral therapy is not feasible (FDA approved in ages ≥17 years and adults)

Medication Guide Available Yes

Pregnancy Risk Factor C

Pregnancy Considerations Adverse events were observed in animal reproduction studies. Available information related to use in pregnancy is limited; if inadvertent exposure occurs during pregnancy, close monitoring of the mother and fetus/newborn is recommended (Hoeltzenbein, 2011). A registry is available for women exposed to lacosamide during pregnancy: Pregnant women may contact the North American Antiepileptic Drug (AED) Pregnancy Registry (888-233-2334 or http://www.aedpregnancyregistry.org).

Breast-Feeding Considerations It is unknown if lacosamide is excreted in human milk. The manufacturer recommends a decision be made whether to discontinue nursing or to discontinue the drug, taking into account the importance of treatment to the mother.

Contraindications

U.S. labeling: There are no contraindications listed in manufacturer's labeling.

Canadian labeling: Hypersensitivity to lacosamide or any component of the formulation; second- or third-degree atrioventricular (AV) block (current or history of).

Warnings/Precautions Antiepileptics are associated with an increased risk of suicidal behavior/thoughts with use (regardless of indication); patients should be monitored for signs/symptoms of depression, suicidal tendencies, and other unusual behavior changes during therapy and instructed to inform their healthcare provider immediately if symptoms occur. CNS effects may occur; patients should be cautioned about performing tasks which require alertness (eg, operating machinery or driving). Lacosamide may prolong PR interval; second degree and complete AV block has also been reported. Use caution in patients with conduction problems (eg, first/second degree atrioventricular block and sick sinus syndrome without pacemaker), sodium channelopathies (eg, Brugada Syndrome), myocardial ischemia, heart failure, structural heart disease, or if concurrent use with other drugs that prolong the PR interval; ECG is recommended prior to initiating therapy and when at the steady state maintenance dose. Monitor closely with IV lacosamide administration; bradycardia and AV block have occurred during infusions. Instruct patients to contact their healthcare provider if signs or symptoms of conduction problems occur (eg, low or irregular pulse, feeling of lightheadedness and fainting). During short-term trials, atrial fibrillation/flutter, or syncope occurred slightly more often in patients with diabetic neuropathy and/or cardiovascular disease. In addition, in open-label studies, syncope has been associated with a history of cardiac disease risk factors and use of drugs that slow AV conduction. Use caution with renal or hepatic impairment and if these patients are taking strong inhibitors of CYP3A4 and CYP2C9; dosage adjustment may be necessary. Multiorgan hypersensitivity reactions can occur (rare); monitor patient and discontinue therapy if necessary. Withdraw therapy gradually (≥1 week) to minimize the potential of increased seizure frequency. Blurred vision and diplopia may occur during therapy. If visual disturbances persist, further assessment may be necessary. Consider increased monitoring in patients with known vision-related issues or ocular conditions. Effects with ethanol may be potentiated. Some products may contain phenylalanine. Some dosage forms may contain propylene glycol; large amounts are potentially toxic and have been associated hyperosmolality, lactic acidosis, seizures and respiratory depression; use caution (AAP, 1997; Zar, 2007).

Warnings: Additional Pediatric Considerations *In vitro* data has shown lacosamide interferes with CRMP-2, a protein involved with neuronal differentiation and control of axonal outgrowth; potential effect on CNS development cannot be excluded. Lacosamide administered to neonatal and juvenile rats resulted in decreased brain weights and long-term neurobehavioral changes including learning and memory deficits. Studies of the effects of lacosamide on human CNS development are needed before this medication can be recommended for routine use in pediatric patients.

Some dosage forms may contain propylene glycol; in neonates large amounts of propylene glycol delivered orally, intravenously (eg, >3,000 mg/day), or topically have been associated with potentially fatal toxicities which can include metabolic acidosis, seizures, renal failure, and CNS depression; toxicities have also been reported in children and adults including hyperosmolality, lactic acidosis, seizures and respiratory depression; use caution (AAP, 1997; Shehab, 2009).

Adverse Reactions

Cardiovascular: Syncope (adults; dose-related: >400 mg/day)

Central nervous system: Abnormal gait, ataxia, depression, dizziness, drowsiness, equilibrium disturbance, fatigue, headache, memory impairment, vertigo

Dermatologic: Pruritus

Gastrointestinal: Diarrhea, nausea, vomiting

Hematologic & oncologic: Bruise

Hepatic: Increased serum ALT

Local: Local irritation, pain at injection site

Neuromuscular & skeletal: Tremor, weakness

Ophthalmic: Blurred vision, diplopia, nystagmus

Miscellaneous: Laceration

Rare but important or life-threatening: Abnormal hepatic function tests, acute psychosis, aggressive behavior, agitation, agranulocytosis, anemia, angioedema, atrial fibrillation, atrial flutter, atrioventricular block, bradycardia, cerebellar syndrome, cognitive dysfunction, disturbance in attention, DRESS syndrome, euphoria, falling, hallucination, hepatitis, insomnia, nephritis, neutropenia, Stevens-Johnson syndrome, toxic epidermal necrolysis, urticaria

Drug Interactions

Metabolism/Transport Effects Substrate of CYP2C19 (minor); **Note:** Assignment of Major/Minor substrate status based on clinically relevant drug interaction potential; **Inhibits** CYP2C19 (weak)

Avoid Concomitant Use There are no known interactions where it is recommended to avoid concomitant use.

Increased Effect/Toxicity

The levels/effects of Lacosamide may be increased by: Bradycardia-Causing Agents; CarBAMazepine; CYP2C9 Inhibitors (Strong); CYP3A4 Inhibitors (Strong); Delavirdine; NiCARdipine

Decreased Effect

The levels/effects of Lacosamide may be decreased by: CarBAMazepine; Fosphenytoin; Mefloquine; Mianserin; Orlistat; PHENobarbital; Phenytoin

Storage/Stability

Injection: Store at 20°C to 25°C (68°F to 77°F); excursions are permitted between 15°C and 30°C (59°F and 86°F). Do not freeze. Stable when mixed with compatible diluents (NS, LR, D_5W) for up to 4 hours at room temperature [Canadian labeling indicates the admixture in glass or polyvinyl chloride (PVC) bags is stable for at least 24 hours at 15°C to 30°C]. Discard any unused portion.

Oral solution, tablets: Store at 20°C to 25°C (68°F to 77°F); excursions are permitted between 15°C and 30°C (59°F and 86°F). Do not freeze oral solution. Discard any unused portion of oral solution after 7 weeks.

Mechanism of Action *In vitro* studies have shown that lacosamide stabilizes hyperexcitable neuronal membranes and inhibits repetitive neuronal firing by enhancing the slow inactivation of sodium channels (with no effects on fast inactivation of sodium channels).

Pharmacokinetics (Adult data unless noted)

Absorption: Oral: Completely

Distribution: V_d: ~0.6 L/kg

Protein binding: <15%

Metabolism: Hepatic (CYP2C19 substrate); forms metabolite, O-desmethyl-lacosamide (inactive)

Bioavailability: ~100%

Half-life elimination: 13 hours

Time to peak plasma concentration: Oral: 1-4 hours

Excretion: Urine (95%; 40% as unchanged drug, 30% as inactive metabolite, 20% as uncharacterized metabolite); feces (<0.5%)

Dialysis: Effectively removed by hemodialysis; AUC decreased by 50% following 4-hour HD session; supplemental dose recommended

Dosing: Usual
Pediatric: **Partial onset seizure:**
Children ≥3 years and Adolescents ≤16 years: Limited data available: Oral: Initial: 1 mg/kg/day divided twice daily (maximum dose: 50 mg); increased at weekly intervals by 1 mg/kg/day up to 10 mg/kg/day (mean: 6.34 mg/kg/day; range: 1.7 to 10 mg/kg/day); dosing based on an open-label, prospective trial of 18 patients (mean age: 10.6 years; range: 3 to 18 years) with refractory partial seizures (Gavatha 2011). A retrospective study of 16 patients (mean age: 15 years; range: 8 to 21 years) with refractory partial seizures reported a mean initial dose of 1.3 mg/kg/day and titrated to a mean maintenance dose of 4.9 mg/kg/day; maximum daily dose: 400 mg/day (Guilhoto 2011).
Adolescents ≥17 years: Oral, IV:
Initial: 50 mg twice daily; may be increased at weekly intervals by 100 mg/day
Maintenance dose: 200 to 400 mg/day in two divided doses
Note: When switching from oral to IV formulations, the total daily dose and frequency should be the same; IV therapy should only be used temporarily. Clinical study experience of IV lacosamide is limited to 5 days of consecutive treatment.
Adult:
Partial onset seizure:
Monotherapy: Oral, IV:
Initial: 100 mg twice daily; may be increased at weekly intervals by 50 mg twice daily based on response and tolerability.
Alternative initial dosage: Loading dose: 200 mg followed approximately 12 hours later by 100 mg twice daily for 1 week; may be increased at weekly intervals by 50 mg twice daily based on response and tolerability. **Note:** Administer loading doses under medical supervision because of the increased incidence of CNS adverse reactions.
Maintenance: 150 to 200 mg twice daily. **Note:** For patients already on a single antiepileptic and converting to lacosamide monotherapy, maintain the maintenance dose for 3 days before beginning withdrawal of the concomitant antiepileptic drug. Gradually taper the concomitant antiepileptic drug over ≥6 weeks.
Adjunctive therapy: Oral, IV:
Initial: 50 mg twice daily; may be increased at weekly intervals by 50 mg twice daily based on response and tolerability.
Alternative initial dosage: Loading dose of 200 mg followed approximately 12 hours later by 100 mg twice daily for 1 week; may be increased at weekly intervals by 50 mg twice daily based on response and tolerability. **Note:** Administer loading doses under medical supervision because of the increased incidence of CNS adverse reactions.
Maintenance dose: 100 to 200 mg twice daily
Switching from oral to IV dosing: When switching from oral to IV formulations, the total daily dose and frequency should be the same; IV therapy should only be used temporarily. Clinical study experience of IV lacosamide is limited to 5 days of consecutive treatment.

Dosing adjustment in renal impairment: Adolescents ≥17 years and Adults: Titrate dose with caution.
Mild to moderate renal impairment: No dose adjustment necessary
Severe renal impairment (CrCl ≤30 mL/minute): Maximum dose: 300 mg/day
Hemodialysis: Removed by hemodialysis; after 4-hour HD treatment, a supplemental dose of up to 50% should be considered.

Dosing adjustment in hepatic impairment: Adolescents ≥17 years and Adults: Titrate dose with caution.
Mild to moderate hepatic impairment: Maximum dose: 300 mg/day
Severe hepatic impairment: Use is not recommended

Preparation for Administration IV: May be further diluted with NS, LR, or D_5W in glass or PVC.

Administration
IV: Administer over 30 to 60 minutes. May be administered undiluted or may be further diluted with a compatible diluent
Oral: Solution, tablets: May be administered with or without food. Oral solution should be administered with a calibrated measuring device (not a household teaspoon or tablespoon).

Monitoring Parameters Seizure frequency, duration, and severity; patients with conduction problems or severe cardiac disease should have ECG tracing prior to start of therapy and when at steady-state; monitor hepatic and renal function; suicidality (eg, suicidal thoughts, depression, behavioral changes)

Additional Information Twice daily IV infusions have been used for up to 5 days.

Controlled Substance C-V

Dosage Forms Excipient information presented when available (limited, particularly for generics); consult specific product labeling.
Solution, Intravenous:
Vimpat: 200 mg/20 mL (20 mL)
Solution, Oral:
Vimpat: 10 mg/mL (200 mL, 465 mL) [contains aspartame, methylparaben, polyethylene glycol, propylene glycol; strawberry flavor]
Tablet, Oral:
Vimpat: 50 mg [contains fd&c blue #2 aluminum lake]
Vimpat: 100 mg, 150 mg
Vimpat: 200 mg [contains fd&c blue #2 aluminum lake]

◆ **LaCrosse Complete [OTC]** *see* Sodium Phosphates *on page 1949*

Lactic Acid and Ammonium Hydroxide
(LAK tik AS id & a MOE nee um hye DROKS ide)

Brand Names: US AmLactin® [OTC]; Geri-Hydrolac™ [OTC]; Geri-Hydrolac™-12 [OTC]; Lac-Hydrin®; Lac-Hydrin® Five [OTC]; LAClotion™

Therapeutic Category Topical Skin Product

Generic Availability (US) Yes

Use Topical humectant used in the treatment of ichthyosis vulgaris, ichthyosis xerosis, and dry skin conditions

Pregnancy Risk Factor B

Pregnancy Considerations Lactic acid is a normal component in blood and tissues. Topical application in animals has not shown fetal harm.

Breast-Feeding Considerations It is not known how this medication affects normal levels of lactic acid in human milk. Because studies have not been done in nursing women, use with caution when needed.

Contraindications Hypersensitivity to lactic acid, ammonium hydroxide, or any component of the formulation

Warnings/Precautions For external use only; not for use on eyes, lips, or mucous membranes; use with caution to facial area (may be more sensitive to irritation). May cause burning or stinging upon application to abraded skin. May cause photosensitivity; minimize exposure to the sun of areas being treated.

Adverse Reactions Dermatologic: Burning/stinging, dry skin, itching, rash (including erythema and irritation)

Drug Interactions
Metabolism/Transport Effects None known.

Avoid Concomitant Use There are no known interactions where it is recommended to avoid concomitant use.

Increased Effect/Toxicity There are no known significant interactions involving an increase in effect.

Decreased Effect There are no known significant interactions involving a decrease in effect.

Storage/Stability Lac-Hydrin® cream/lotion: Store at 15°C to 30°C (59°F to 86°F).

Mechanism of Action Exact mechanism of action unknown; lactic acid is a normal component in blood and tissues. When applied topically to the skin, acts as a humectant.

Pharmacodynamics Onset of action: Ichthyosis xerosis: 3-7 days

Pharmacokinetics (Adult data unless noted) Bioavailability: 6%

Dosing: Usual Infants, Children, and Adults: Topical: Apply twice daily

Administration Topical: Apply a small amount to the affected area(s) and rub in thoroughly; avoid contact with eyes, lips, or mucous membranes; shake lotion well before use

Monitoring Parameters Physical examination of skin condition

Dosage Forms Excipient information presented when available (limited, particularly for generics); consult specific product labeling.

Cream, topical: Lactic acid 12% with ammonium hydroxide (140 g, 280 g, 385 g)

AmLactin®: Lactic acid 12% with ammonium hydroxide (140 g)

Lac-Hydrin®: Lactic acid 12% with ammonium hydroxide (280 g, 385 g)

Lotion, topical: Lactic acid 12% with ammonium hydroxide (225 g, 400 g)

AmLactin®, Lac-Hydrin®, LAClotion™: Lactic acid 12% with ammonium hydroxide (225 g, 400 g)

Geri-Hydrolac™, Lac-Hydrin® Five: Lactic acid 5% with ammonium hydroxide (120 mL, 240 mL)

Geri-Hydrolac™-12: Lactic acid 12% with ammonium hydroxide (120 mL, 240 mL)

◆ **Lactinex™ [OTC]** *see Lactobacillus on page 1203*

Lactobacillus (lak toe ba SIL us)

Medication Safety Issues

Sound-alike/look-alike issues:

Floranex may be confused with Florinef

Brand Names: US Advanced Probiotic [OTC]; Bacid® [OTC]; Culturelle® [OTC]; Dofus [OTC]; Flora-Q™ [OTC]; Floranex™ [OTC]; Kala® [OTC]; Lactinex™ [OTC]; Lacto-Bifidus [OTC]; Lacto-Key [OTC]; Lacto-Pectin [OTC]; Lacto-TriBlend [OTC]; Megadophilus® [OTC]; MoreDophilus® [OTC]; RisaQuad®-2 [OTC]; RisaQuad™ [OTC]; Superdophilus® [OTC]; VSL #3® [OTC]; VSL #3®-DS

Brand Names: Canada Bacid; Bio-K+; Fermalac

Therapeutic Category Antidiarrheal

Generic Availability (US) Yes

Use Treatment of uncomplicated diarrhea particularly that caused by antibiotic therapy; re-establish normal physiologic and bacterial flora of the intestinal tract

Contraindications Hypersensitivity to any component of the formulation

Warnings/Precautions *Lactobacillus* species have been studied for various gastrointestinal disorders including diarrhea, inflammatory bowel disease, gastrointestinal infection. Effectiveness may be dependent upon actual species used; studies are ongoing. Currently, there are no FDA-approved disease-prevention or therapeutic indications for these products.

Adverse Reactions Gastrointestinal: Bloating (intestinal), flatulence

Drug Interactions

Metabolism/Transport Effects None known.

Avoid Concomitant Use There are no known interactions where it is recommended to avoid concomitant use.

Increased Effect/Toxicity There are no known significant interactions involving an increase in effect.

Decreased Effect There are no known significant interactions involving a decrease in effect.

Storage/Stability

Bacid®: Store at room temperature.

Flora-Q™: Store at or below room temperature; do not store in bathroom.

Kala®, MoreDophilus®: Refrigeration recommended after opening.

Lactinex™, Dofus: Store in refrigerator.

VSL #3®, VSL #3®-DS: Store in refrigerator; may be stored at room temperature for up to 1 week without loss in potency

Mechanism of Action Helps re-establish normal intestinal flora; suppresses the growth of potentially pathogenic microorganisms by producing lactic acid which favors the establishment of an aciduric flora.

Pharmacokinetics (Adult data unless noted)

Absorption: Not orally absorbed

Distribution: Locally, primarily in the colon

Elimination: In feces

Dosing: Usual Children and Adults: Oral:

Capsule: 1-2 capsules 2-4 times/day

Granules: 1 packet added to or taken with cereal, food, milk, fruit juice, or water 3-4 times/day

Powder: 1/4-1 teaspoon 1-3 times/day with liquid

Tablet, chewable: 4 tablets 3-4 times/day; may follow each dose with a small amount of milk, fruit juice, or water

Recontamination protocol for BMT unit: 1 packet 3 times/day for 6 doses for those patients who refuse yogurt

Administration Oral: Granules, powder, or contents of capsules may be added to or administered with cereal, food, milk, fruit juice, or water

Dosage Forms Excipient information presented when available (limited, particularly for generics); consult specific product labeling.

Capsule:

Advanced Probiotic: *L. acidophilus, L. casei, L. delbrueckii,* and *L. rhamnosus* GG 10 billion live cultures [also includes *Bifidobacterium lactis*, and *B. longum*]

Culturelle®: *L. rhamnosus* GG 10 billion colony-forming units [contains casein and whey]

Dofus: *L. acidophilus* and *L. bifidus* 10:1 ratio [beet root powder base]

Flora-Q™: *L. acidophilus* and *L. paracasei* ≥8 billion colony-forming units [also contains *Bifidobacterium* and *S. thermophilus*]

Lacto-Key:

100: *L. acidophilus* 1 billion colony-forming units [milk, soy, and yeast free; rice derived]

600: *L. acidophilus* 6 billion colony-forming units [milk, soy, and yeast free; rice derived]

Lacto-Bifidus:

100: *L. bifidus* 1 billion colony-forming units [milk, soy, and yeast free; rice derived]

600: *L. bifidus* 6 billion colony-forming units [milk, soy, and yeast free; rice derived]

Lacto-Pectin: *L. acidophilus* and *L. casei* ≥5 billion colony-forming units [also contains *Bifidobacterium lactis* and citrus pectin cellulose complex]

Lacto-TriBlend:

100: *L. acidophilus, L. bifidus,* and *L. bulgaricus* 1 billion colony-forming units [milk, soy and yeast free; rice derived]

600: *L. acidophilus, L. bifidus,* and *L. bulgaricus* 6 billion colony-forming units [milk, soy and yeast free; rice derived]

Megadophilus®, Superdophilus®: *L. acidophilus* 2 billion units [available in dairy based or dairy free formulations]

RisaQuad™: *L. acidophilus* and *L. paracasei* 8 billion colony-forming units [also includes *Bifidobacterium* and *Streptococcus thermophilus*]

RisaQuad®-2: *L. acidophilus* and *L. paracasei* 16 billion colony-forming units [gluten free; also includes *Bifidobacterium* and *Streptococcus thermophilus*]

VSL #3®: *L. acidophilus, L. plantarum, L. paracasei, L. bulgaricus* 112 billion live cells [also contains *Bifidobacterium breve, B. longum, B. infantis,* and *Streptococcus thermophilus*]

Caplet:

Bacid®: *L. acidophilus* and *L. bulgaricus* [also contains *Bifidobacterium biffidum* and *Streptococcus thermophilus*

Granules:

Floranex™: *L. acidophilus* and *L. bulgaricus* 100 million live cells per 1 g packet (12s) [contains milk, sodium 5 mg/packet, soy]

Lactinex™: *L. acidophilus* and *L. bulgaricus* 100 million live cells per 1 g packet (12s) [gluten free; contains calcium 5 mg/packet, lactose 380 mg/packet, potassium 20 mg/packet, sodium 5 mg/packet, sucrose 34 mg/packet, whey, evaporated milk, and soy peptone]

Powder:

Lacto-TriBlend: *L. acidophilus, L. bifidus,* and *L. bulgaricus* 10 billion colony-forming units per ¼ teaspoon (60 g) [milk, soy, and yeast free; rice derived]

Megadophilus®, Superdophilus®: *L. acidophilus* 2 billion units per half-teaspoon (49 g, 70 g, 84 g, 126 g) [available in dairy based or dairy free (garbanzo bean) formulations]

MoreDophilus®: *L. acidophilus* 12.4 billion units per teaspoon (30 g, 120 g) [dairy free, yeast free; soy and carrot derived]

VSL #3®: *L. acidophilus, L. plantarum, L. paracasei, L. bulgaricus* 450 billion live cells per sachet (10s, 30s) [gluten free; also contains *Bifidobacterium breve, B. longum, B. infantis,* and *Streptococcus thermophilus*; lemon cream flavor and unflavored]

VSL #3®-DS: *L. acidophilus, L. plantarum, L. paracasei, L. bulgaricus* 900 billion live cells per packet (20s,) [gluten free; also contains *Bifidobacterium breve, B. longum, B. infantis,* and *Streptococcus thermophilus*]

Tablet: *L. acidophilus* 35 million and *L. sporogenes* 25 million

Floranex™: *L. acidophilus* and *L. bulgaricus* 1 million colony-forming units [contains lactose, nonfat dried milk, whey]

Kala®: *L. acidophilus* 200 million units [dairy free, yeast free; soy based]

Tablet, chewable: *L. reuteri* 100 million organisms

Lactinex™: *L. acidophilus* and *L. bulgaricus* 1 million live cells [gluten free; contains calcium 5.2 mg/4 tablets, lactose 960 mg/4 tablets, potassium 20 mg/4 tablets, sodium 5.6 mg/4 tablets, and sucrose 500 sucrose/4 tablets; contains whey, evaporated milk, and soy peptone]

Wafer: *L. acidophilus* 90 mg and *L. bifidus* 25 mg (100s) [provides 1 billion organisms/wafer at time of manufacture; milk free]

- ◆ ***Lactobacillus acidophilus*** *see* Lactobacillus *on page 1203*
- ◆ ***Lactobacillus bifidus*** *see* Lactobacillus *on page 1203*
- ◆ ***Lactobacillus bulgaricus*** *see* Lactobacillus *on page 1203*
- ◆ ***Lactobacillus casei*** *see* Lactobacillus *on page 1203*
- ◆ ***Lactobacillus paracasei*** *see* Lactobacillus *on page 1203*
- ◆ ***Lactobacillus plantarum*** *see* Lactobacillus *on page 1203*
- ◆ ***Lactobacillus reuteri*** *see* Lactobacillus *on page 1203*
- ◆ ***Lactobacillus rhamnosus* GG** *see* Lactobacillus *on page 1203*
- ◆ **Lacto-Bifidus [OTC]** *see* Lactobacillus *on page 1203*
- ◆ **Lactoflavin** *see* Riboflavin *on page 1856*
- ◆ **Lacto-Key [OTC]** *see* Lactobacillus *on page 1203*
- ◆ **Lacto-Pectin [OTC]** *see* Lactobacillus *on page 1203*
- ◆ **Lacto-TriBlend [OTC]** *see* Lactobacillus *on page 1203*

Lactulose (LAK tyoo lose)

Medication Safety Issues

Sound-alike/look-alike issues:

Lactulose may be confused with lactose

Brand Names: US Constulose; Enulose; Generlac; Kristalose

Brand Names: Canada Apo-Lactulose; Euro-Lac; Jamp-Lactulose; PMS-Lactulose; Ratio-Lactulose; Teva-Lactulose

Therapeutic Category Ammonium Detoxicant; Hyperammonemia Agent; Laxative, Miscellaneous

Generic Availability (US) May be product dependent

Use Prevention and treatment of portal-systemic encephalopathy (PSE) (Enulose: FDA approved in infants, children, adolescents, and adults); treatment of constipation (FDA approved in adults)

Pregnancy Risk Factor B

Pregnancy Considerations Adverse events have not been observed in animal reproduction studies. Lactulose is poorly absorbed following oral administration. Use of dietary fiber or bulk-forming laxatives along with increased fluid intake is generally considered first line therapy for treating constipation in pregnant women. Short-term use of lactulose is also considered to be safe/low risk when therapy is needed; however, side effects may limit its use (Cullen, 2007; Mahadevan, 2006; Prather, 2004; Wald, 2003).

Breast-Feeding Considerations It is not known if lactulose is excreted into breast milk; however, lactulose is poorly absorbed following oral administration. The manufacturer recommends that caution be used if administered to a nursing woman.

Contraindications Use in patients requiring a low galactose diet

Warnings/Precautions Use with caution in patients with diabetes mellitus; solution contains galactose and lactose. Monitor periodically for electrolyte imbalance when lactulose is used >6 months or in patients predisposed to electrolyte abnormalities (eg, elderly). Hepatic disease may predispose patients to electrolyte imbalance. Infants receiving lactulose may develop hyponatremia and dehydration. Patients receiving lactulose and an oral anti-infective agent should be monitored for possible inadequate response to lactulose. During proctoscopy or colonoscopy procedures involving electrocautery, a theoretical risk of reaction between H_2 gas accumulation and electrical spark may exist; thorough bowel cleansing with a nonfermentable solution is recommended.

Warnings: Additional Pediatric Considerations Electrolyte imbalances may occur with chronic use or in patients predisposed to electrolyte imbalances including infants; infants may also develop dehydration with hyponatremia.

Adverse Reactions

Endocrine & metabolic: Dehydration, hypernatremia, hypokalemia

Gastrointestinal: Abdominal discomfort, abdominal distention, belching, cramping, diarrhea (excessive dose), flatulence, nausea, vomiting

Drug Interactions

Metabolism/Transport Effects None known.

Avoid Concomitant Use There are no known interactions where it is recommended to avoid concomitant use.

Increased Effect/Toxicity There are no known significant interactions involving an increase in effect.

Decreased Effect There are no known significant interactions involving a decrease in effect.

Storage/Stability Store at room temperature; do not freeze. Protect from light. Discard solution if cloudy or very dark. Prolonged exposure to cold temperatures will cause thickening which will return to normal upon warming to room temperature.

Mechanism of Action The bacterial degradation of lactulose resulting in an acidic pH inhibits the diffusion of NH_3 into the blood by causing the conversion of NH_3 to NH_4^+; also enhances the diffusion of NH_3 from the blood into the gut where conversion to NH_4^+ occurs; produces an osmotic effect in the colon with resultant distention promoting peristalsis; reduces blood ammonia concentration to reduce the degree of portal systemic encephalopathy

Pharmacodynamics Onset of action:

Constipation: Up to 24-48 hours to produce a normal bowel movement

Encephalopathy: At least 24-48 hours

Pharmacokinetics (Adult data unless noted)

Absorption: Oral: Not absorbed appreciably

Metabolism: By colonic flora to lactic acid and acetic acid

Elimination: Primarily in feces; urine (≤3%)

Dosing: Usual

Pediatric: **Note:** Doses in pediatric patients may be expressed in volume (mL) or weight (g); use extra precaution.

Constipation; chronic: Limited data available: Infants, Children, and Adolescents: Oral: 1 to 2 g/kg/day (1.5 to 3 mL/kg/day) divided once or twice daily (NASPGHAN [Tabbers 2014]); maximum daily dose: 60 mL/day in adults

Constipation, palliative care: Limited data available: Children and Adolescents: Oral: 2 to 30 mL every 6 to 24 hours (Johnston 2005), others have suggested 5 to 10 mL every 2 hours until bowel movement (Kliegman 2011)

Fecal impaction, slow disimpaction: Limited data available: Infants, Children, and Adolescents: Oral: 1.33 g/kg/dose (2 mL/kg) twice daily for 7 days (Wyllie 2011; Pashankar 2005)

Portal systemic encephalopathy, prevention: Oral liquid:

Infants: 1.7 to 6.7 g/day (2.5 to 10 mL/day) in divided doses; adjust dosage to produce 2 to 3 stools/day

Children and Adolescents: 26.7 to 60 g/day (40 to 90 mL/day) in divided doses; adjust dosage to produce 2 to 3 stools/day

Adult:

Constipation: Oral: 10 to 20 g (15 to 30 mL) daily; may increase to 40 g (60 mL) daily if necessary

Portal systemic encephalopathy, prevention: Oral: 20 to 30 g (30 to 45 mL) 3 to 4 times/day; adjust dose every 1 to 2 days to produce 2 to 3 soft stools/day

Portal systemic encephalopathy, treatment:

Oral: 20 to 30 g (30 to 45 mL) every 1 hour to induce rapid laxation; reduce to 20 to 30 g (30 to 45 mL) 3 to 4 times/day after laxation is achieved; titrate to produce 2 to 3 soft stools/day

Rectal administration (retention enema): 200 g (300 mL) diluted with 700 mL of water or NS via rectal balloon catheter; retain for 30 to 60 minutes; may repeat every 4 to 6 hours; transition to oral treatment prior to discontinuing rectal administration

Dosing adjustment in renal impairment: There are no dosage adjustments provided in manufacturer's labeling.

Dosing adjustment in hepatic impairment: There are no dosage adjustments provided in manufacturer's labeling.

Administration

Oral:

Oral solution: May mix with fruit juice, water, or milk

Crystals for oral solution: Dissolve contents of packet in 120 mL water

Rectal: Adults: Mix with water or normal saline; administer as retention enema using a rectal balloon catheter; retain for 30 to 60 minutes. Transition to oral lactulose when appropriate (able to take oral medication and no longer a risk for aspiration) prior to discontinuing rectal administration.

Monitoring Parameters Serum ammonia, serum electrolytes, fluid status, stool output

Additional Information Upon discontinuation of therapy, allow 24 to 48 hours for resumption of normal bowel movements

Dosage Forms Excipient information presented when available (limited, particularly for generics); consult specific product labeling.

Packet, Oral:

Kristalose: 10 g (30 ea); 20 g (30 ea)

Solution, Oral:

Constulose: 10 g/15 mL (237 mL, 946 mL) [unflavored flavor]

Enulose: 10 g/15 mL (473 mL) [unflavored flavor]

Generlac: 10 g/15 mL (473 mL, 1892 mL) [unflavored flavor]

Generic: 10 g/15 mL (15 mL, 30 mL, 236 mL, 237 mL, 473 mL, 500 mL, 946 mL, 1892 mL); 20 g/30 mL (30 mL)

- **Ladakamycin** *see* AzaCITIDine *on page 233*
- **LAIV** *see* Influenza Virus Vaccine (Live/Attenuated) *on page 1113*
- **LAIV$_4$** *see* Influenza Virus Vaccine (Live/Attenuated) *on page 1113*
- **L-AmB** *see* Amphotericin B (Liposomal) *on page 153*
- **LaMICtal** *see* LamoTRIgine *on page 1211*
- **Lamictal (Can)** *see* LamoTRIgine *on page 1211*
- **LaMICtal ODT** *see* LamoTRIgine *on page 1211*
- **LaMICtal Starter** *see* LamoTRIgine *on page 1211*
- **LaMICtal XR** *see* LamoTRIgine *on page 1211*
- **LamISIL** *see* Terbinafine (Systemic) *on page 2021*
- **Lamisil (Can)** *see* Terbinafine (Systemic) *on page 2021*
- **Lamisil (Can)** *see* Terbinafine (Topical) *on page 2023*
- **LamISIL Advanced [OTC]** *see* Terbinafine (Topical) *on page 2023*
- **LamISIL AF Defense [OTC]** *see* Tolnaftate *on page 2083*
- **LamISIL AT [OTC]** *see* Terbinafine (Topical) *on page 2023*
- **LamISIL AT Jock Itch [OTC]** *see* Terbinafine (Topical) *on page 2023*
- **LamISIL AT Spray [OTC]** *see* Terbinafine (Topical) *on page 2023*
- **LamISIL Spray** *see* Terbinafine (Topical) *on page 2023*

LamiVUDine (la MI vyoo deen)

Medication Safety Issues

Sound-alike/look-alike issues:

LamiVUDine may be confused with lamoTRIgine

Epivir may be confused with Combivir

High alert medication:

This medication is in a class the Institute for Safe Medication Practices (ISMP) includes among its list of drug classes that have a heightened risk of causing significant patient harm when used in error.

Related Information

Adult and Adolescent HIV *on page 2392*
Pediatric HIV *on page 2380*
Perinatal HIV *on page 2400*

Brand Names: US Epivir; Epivir HBV

Brand Names: Canada 3TC; Apo-Lamivudine; Apo-Lamivudine HBV; Heptovir

Therapeutic Category Antiretroviral Agent; HIV Agents (Anti-HIV Agents); Nucleoside Reverse Transcriptase Inhibitor (NRTI)

Generic Availability (US) Yes

Use

Epivir: Treatment of HIV-1 infection in combination with other antiretroviral agents (FDA approved in ages ≥3 months and adults); **Note:** HIV regimens consisting of three antiretroviral agents are strongly recommended; has also been used for chemoprophylaxis after occupational exposure to HIV and prevention of maternal-fetal transmission of HIV infection.

Epivir-HBV: Management of chronic hepatitis B infection associated with evidence of hepatitis B viral replication and active liver inflammation (FDA approved in ages ≥2 years and adults)

Pregnancy Risk Factor C

Pregnancy Considerations Adverse events were observed in some animal reproduction studies. Lamivudine has a high level of transfer across the human placenta. No increased risk of overall birth defects has been observed following first trimester exposure according to data collected by the antiretroviral pregnancy registry. The pharmacokinetics of lamivudine during pregnancy are not significantly altered and dosage adjustment is not required. Cases of lactic acidosis/hepatic steatosis syndrome related to mitochondrial toxicity have been reported in pregnant women with prolonged use of nucleoside analogues. It is not known if pregnancy itself potentiates this known side effect; however, women may be at increased risk of lactic acidosis and liver damage. In addition, these adverse events are similar to other rare but life-threatening syndromes which occur during pregnancy (eg, HELLP syndrome). Hepatic enzymes and electrolytes should be monitored in women receiving nucleoside analogues and clinicians should watch for early signs of the syndrome. In addition, mitochondrial dysfunction may develop in infants following in utero exposure. The DHHS Perinatal HIV Guidelines consider lamivudine in combination with either abacavir, tenofovir, or zidovudine to be a preferred NRTI backbone for antiretroviral-naïve pregnant women. The DHHS Perinatal HIV Guidelines also consider lamivudine plus tenofovir a recommended dual NRTI/NtRTI backbone for HIV/HBV coinfected pregnant women. Use caution with hepatitis B coinfection; hepatitis B flare may occur if lamivudine is discontinued postpartum.

Regardless of CD4 count or HIV RNA copy number, all HIV-infected pregnant women should receive a combination antiretroviral (ARV) drug regimen. A combination of antepartum, intrapartum, and infant ARV prophylaxis is recommended. ARV therapy should be started as soon as possible in women with symptomatic infection. Although earlier initiation may be more effective in reducing the perinatal transmission of HIV, initiation may be delayed until after 12 weeks gestation in women who do not require immediate treatment after careful consideration of maternal conditions (eg, nausea and vomiting) and the potential risks of first trimester fetal exposure for specific agents. A scheduled cesarean delivery at 38 weeks gestation is recommended for all women with HIV RNA >1000 copies/mL or unknown concentrations near delivery in order to decrease transmission. If ARV therapy must be interrupted for <24 hours during the peripartum period, stop then restart all medications simultaneously in order to decrease the chance of developing resistance. Long-term follow-up is recommended for all infants exposed to ARV medications. In couples who want to conceive, the HIV-infected partner should attain maximum viral suppression prior to conception.

Health care providers are encouraged to enroll pregnant women exposed to antiretroviral medications in the Antiretroviral Pregnancy Registry (1-800-258-4263 or www.APRegistry.com). Health care providers caring for HIV-infected women and their infants may contact the National Perinatal HIV Hotline (888-448-8765) for clinical consultation (HHS [perinatal], 2014).

Breast-Feeding Considerations Lamivudine is excreted into breast milk and can be detected in the serum of nursing infants.

Maternal or infant antiretroviral therapy does not completely eliminate the risk of postnatal HIV transmission. In addition, multiclass-resistant virus has been detected in breast-feeding infants despite maternal therapy. Therefore, in the United States, where formula is accessible, affordable, safe, and sustainable, and the risk of infant mortality due to diarrhea and respiratory infections is low, complete avoidance of breast-feeding by HIV-infected women is recommended to decrease potential transmission of HIV (HHS [perinatal], 2014).

Contraindications Clinically significant hypersensitivity (eg, anaphylaxis) to lamivudine or any component of the formulation

Warnings/Precautions Use caution with renal impairment; dosage reduction recommended. Use with extreme caution in children with history of pancreatitis or risk factors for development of pancreatitis. Pancreatitis has been reported, particularly in HIV-infected children with a history of nucleoside use. Do not use as monotherapy in treatment of HIV. Lamivudine combined with emtricitabine is not recommended as a dual-NRTI combination due to similar resistance patterns and negligible additive antiviral activity; lamivudine and abacavir or tenofovir combination is recommended as the NRTIs in a fully suppressive antiretroviral regimen (HHS [adult], 2014). Treatment of HBV in patients with unrecognized/untreated HIV may lead to rapid HIV resistance. In addition, treatment of HIV in patients with unrecognized/untreated HBV may lead to rapid HBV resistance. Use with caution in combination with interferon alfa with or without ribavirin in HIV/HBV coinfected patients; monitor closely for hepatic decompensation, anemia, or neutropenia; dose reduction or discontinuation of interferon and/or ribavirin may be required if toxicity evident. In HIV/HBV coinfection, lamivudine and tenofovir are a recommended NRTI backbone in a fully suppressive antiretroviral regimen to provide activity against both HIV and HBV (HHS [adult], 2014). **[US Boxed Warning]: Do not use Epivir HBV tablets or Epivir HBV oral solution for the treatment of HIV.** Potentially significant drug-drug interactions may exist, requiring dose or frequency adjustment, additional monitoring, and/or selection of alternative therapy. Some dosage forms may contain propylene glycol; large amounts are potentially toxic and have been associated hyperosmolality, lactic acidosis, seizures and respiratory depression; use caution (AAP, 1997; Zar, 2007).

[US Boxed Warning]: Lactic acidosis and severe hepatomegaly with steatosis have been reported, including fatal cases. Use caution in hepatic impairment. Pregnancy, obesity, and/or prolonged therapy may increase the risk of lactic acidosis and liver damage.

Immune reconstitution syndrome may develop resulting in the occurrence of an inflammatory response to an indolent or residual opportunistic infection during initial HIV treatment or activation of autoimmune disorders (eg, Graves' disease, polymyositis, Guillain-Barré syndrome) later in therapy. May be associated with fat redistribution. Concomitant use of other lamivudine-containing products should be avoided.

[US Boxed Warning]: Monitor patients closely for several months following discontinuation of therapy for chronic hepatitis B; clinical exacerbations may occur, including fatal cases. **Monitor hepatic function with clinical and laboratory follow up for at least several months after hepatitis B treatment discontinuation. Initiate antihepatitis B (HBV) medications if clinically appropriate. [US Boxed Warning]: HIV-1 resistance may emerge in chronic hepatitis B-infection patients with unrecognized or untreated HIV-1 infection. Counseling and (HIV) testing should be offered to all patients before beginning treatment with lamivudine for hepatitis B and then periodically during treatment. Lamivudine dosing for hepatitis B is subtherapeutic if used for HIV-1 infection treatment. Lamivudine monotherapy is not appropriate for HIV-1 infection treatment.** Lamivudine resistant HIV-1 can develop rapidly and limit treatment options if used in unrecognized or untreated HIV-1 infection or if a patient becomes coinfected during HBV treatment. Lamivudine dosing for hepatitis B is also subtherapeutic if used for HIV-1/HBV coinfection treatment. If lamivudine is chosen as part of a HIV-1 treatment regimen in coinfected patients, the higher lamivudine dosage indicated for HIV-1 therapy should be used, with other drugs, in an appropriate combination regimen.

Not recommended as first-line therapy of chronic HBV due to high rate of resistance. Consider use only if other anti-HBV antiviral regimens with more favorable resistance patterns cannot be used. May be appropriate for short-term treatment of acute HBV (Lok, 2009). Potential compliance problems, frequency of administration, and adverse effects should be discussed with patients before initiating therapy to help prevent the emergence of resistance.

Warnings: Additional Pediatric Considerations The major clinical toxicity of lamivudine in pediatric patients is pancreatitis which has occurred in 14% of patients in one open-label, uncontrolled study; discontinue lamivudine therapy if clinical signs, symptoms, or laboratory abnormalities suggestive of pancreatitis occur. Use with extreme caution and only if there is no satisfactory alternative therapy in pediatric patients with a history of pancreatitis or other significant risk factors for the development of pancreatitis. Infants receiving lamivudine in combination with nelfinavir (powder no longer available in the US) and zidovudine for prevention of maternal-fetal transmission experienced a higher rate of neutropenia compared to zidovudine/nevirapine combination or zidovudine alone (27.5% vs 15%). Other studies in infants reported significantly higher rates of anemia and neutropenia when lamivudine was administered in combination with zidovudine (HHS [perinatal] 2014).

Some dosage forms may contain propylene glycol; in neonates large amounts of propylene glycol delivered orally, intravenously (eg, >3,000 mg/day), or topically have been associated with potentially fatal toxicities which can include metabolic acidosis, seizures, renal failure, and CNS depression; toxicities have also been reported in children and adults including hyperosmolality, lactic acidosis, seizures and respiratory depression; use caution (AAP 1997; Shehab 2009).

Adverse Reactions

Central nervous system: Chills, depression, dizziness, fatigue, fever, headache, insomnia

Dermatologic: Rash

Gastrointestinal: Abdominal pain, amylase increased, anorexia, diarrhea, dyspepsia, heartburn, lipase increased, nausea, pancreatitis, vomiting

Hematologic: Hemoglobinemia, neutropenia, thrombocytopenia

Hepatic: Transaminases increased

Neuromuscular & skeletal: Arthralgia, creatine phosphokinase increased, musculoskeletal pain, myalgia, neuropathy

Miscellaneous: Infections (includes ear, nose, and throat)

Rare but important or life-threatening: Alopecia, anaphylaxis, anemia, body fat redistribution, hepatitis B exacerbation, hepatomegaly, hyperbilirubinemia, hyperglycemia, immune reconstitution syndrome, lactic acidosis, lymphadenopathy, muscle weakness, paresthesia, peripheral neuropathy, pruritus, red cell aplasia, rhabdomyolysis, splenomegaly, steatosis, stomatitis, urticaria, weakness, wheezing

Drug Interactions

Metabolism/Transport Effects None known.

Avoid Concomitant Use

Avoid concomitant use of LamiVUDine with any of the following: Emtricitabine

Increased Effect/Toxicity

LamiVUDine may increase the levels/effects of: Emtricitabine

The levels/effects of LamiVUDine may be increased by: Ganciclovir-Valganciclovir; Ribavirin; Trimethoprim

Decreased Effect There are no known significant interactions involving a decrease in effect.

Food Interactions Food decreases the rate of absorption and C_{max}; however, there is no change in the systemic AUC. Management: Administer with or without food.

Storage/Stability

Oral solution:

Epivir: Store at 25°C (77°F) tightly closed.

Epivir HBV: Store at 20°C to 25°C (68°F to 77°F) tightly closed.

Tablet: Store at 25°C (77°F); excursions are permitted between 15°C and 30°C (59°F and 86°F).

Mechanism of Action Lamivudine is a cytosine analog. *In vitro*, lamivudine is triphosphorylated, the principle mode of action is inhibition of HIV reverse transcription via viral DNA chain termination; inhibits RNA- and DNA-dependent DNA polymerase activities of reverse transcriptase. In hepatitis B, the monophosphate form of lamivudine is incorporated into the viral DNA by hepatitis B virus polymerase, resulting in DNA chain termination.

Pharmacokinetics (Adult data unless noted)

Absorption: Oral: Rapid

Distribution: Into extravascular spaces

Children (n=38): CSF concentrations were 14.2 ± 7.9% of the serum concentration

V_d: 1.3 ± 0.4 L/kg

Protein binding: <36%

Metabolism: Converted intracellularly to the active triphosphate form

Bioavailability:

Children: Oral solution: 66% ± 26%

Adolescents and Adults:

150 mg tablet: 86% ± 16%

Oral solution: 87% ± 13%

Half-life:

Intracellular: 10 to 15 hours

Elimination:

Children 4 months to 14 years: 2 ± 0.6 hours

Adults with normal renal function: 5 to 7 hours

Time to peak serum concentration:
Pediatric patients 0.5 to 17 years: Median: 1.5 hours (range: 0.5 to 4 hours) (Lewis, 1996)
Adolescents 13 to 17 years: 0.5 to 1 hour
Adults: Fasting state: 0.9 hours; Fed state: 3.2 hours
Elimination: Urine (70%, unchanged); weight-corrected oral clearance is highest at age 2 years, then declines from age 2 to 12 years, where values then remain comparable to adult values

Dosing: Neonatal

HIV infection, treatment: Use in combination with other antiretroviral agents: Oral: 2 mg/kg/dose twice daily (HHS [pediatric] 2015)

Perinatal transmission, prevention: Note: Consider for infants of mothers who received no antiretroviral therapy prior to or during labor, infants born to mothers with only intrapartum antiretroviral therapy, infants born to mothers with suboptimal viral suppression at delivery, or infants born to mothers with known antiretroviral drug-resistant virus. However, the recommended regimen for prophylaxis in these patients is zidovudine plus nevirapine (HHS [perinatal] 2014); HHS [pediatric] 2015).
AIDS*info* recommendation: Oral: 2 mg/kg/dose twice daily; duration typically ranges from 1 to 2 weeks and is used in combinations with a 6-week-course of zidovudine, usually in combination with a 3-dose-course of nevirapine (HHS [perinatal] 2014; HHS [pediatric] 2015).

Dosing adjustment in renal impairment for HIV: Insufficient data exist to recommend specific dosing adjustments for renal impairment; consider reducing the dose or increasing the dosing interval; use with caution; monitor closely; drug is renally eliminated

Dosing: Usual

Pediatric:

HIV infection, treatment: Use in combination with other antiretroviral agents:
Infants 1 month to <3 months: Oral solution: 4 mg/kg/dose twice daily (HHS [pediatric], 2015; Tremoulet, 2007)
Infants ≥3 months, Children, and Adolescents <16 years:
Twice daily dosing:
Oral solution: 4 mg/kg/dose twice daily; maximum dose: 150 mg/dose
Oral tablet: Weight-band dosing for patients ≥14 kg who are able to swallow tablets (using scored 150 mg tablets):
Manufacturer's labeling:
14 to <20 kg: 75 mg (1/2 tablet) twice daily
20 to <25 kg: 75 mg (1/2 tablet) in the morning and 150 mg (1 tablet) in the evening
≥25 kg: 150 mg (1 tablet) twice daily
Alternate dosing (HHS [pediatric] 2015):
14 to 21 kg: 75 mg (1/2 tablet) twice daily
>21 kg to <30 kg: 75 mg (1/2 tablet) in the morning and 150 mg (1 tablet) in the evening
≥30 kg: 150 mg (1 tablet) twice daily
Once daily dosing: **Note:** Not recommended as initial therapy. Efficacy of once daily dosing has only been demonstrated in patients who transitioned from twice daily dosing after 36 weeks of treatment. Some experts recommend reserving once daily therapy for use as a component of a once-daily regimen in clinically stable patients ≥ 3 years of age who have undetectable viral loads and stable CD4 counts (HHS [pediatric] 2015).
Oral solution:
Manufacturer's labeling: 8 mg/kg/dose once daily; maximum dose: 300 mg/dose
Alternate dosing (HHS [pediatric] 2015): 8 to 10 mg/kg/dose once daily; maximum dose: 300 mg/dose
Oral tablet: Weight-band dosing for patients ≥14 kg who are able to swallow tablets (scored 150 mg tablets):
14 to < 20 kg: 150 mg (1 tablet) once daily
20 to <25 kg: 225 mg (1 + 1/2 tablet) once daily
≥25 kg: 300 mg (2 tablets) once daily
Adolescents ≥16 years (HHS [pediatric] 2015): Oral:
Body weight <50 kg: 4 mg/kg/dose twice daily; maximum dose: 150 mg/dose
Body weight ≥50 kg: 150 mg twice daily **or** 300 mg once daily

HIV postexposure, prophylaxis: Adolescents ≥16 years: Oral: 150 mg twice daily or 300 mg once daily in combination with zidovudine, tenofovir, stavudine, or didanosine, with or without a protease inhibitor depending on risk (CDC, 2005)

Hepatitis B, treatment (Epivir-HBV) (non-HIV-exposed/-positive): Note: Use in HBV treatment is discouraged due to rapid resistance development; consider use only if other anti-HBV antiviral regimens with more favorable resistance patterns cannot be used. Children ≥2 years and Adolescents: Oral: 3 mg/kg/dose once daily; maximum daily dose: 100 mg/**day**
AASLD practice guidelines (Lok, 2009): Treatment duration:
Hepatitis Be antigen (HBeAg) positive chronic hepatitis: Treat ≥1 year until HBeAg confirmed seroconversion and undetectable serum HBV DNA; continue therapy for ≥6 months after HBeAg seroconversion
HBeAg negative chronic hepatitis: Treat >1 year until hepatitis B surface antigen (HBsAg) clearance
Note: Patients not achieving <2 log decrease in serum HBV DNA after at least 6 months of therapy should either receive additional treatment or be switched to an alternative therapy (Lok, 2009)

Hepatitis B/HIV coinfection, treatment of both infections: Epivir: Infants, Children, and Adolescents: Oral: 4 mg/kg/dose twice daily; maximum dose: 150 mg/dose; in combination with other antiretrovirals in a HAART regimen; **Note:** The formulation and dosage of Epivir-HBV are not appropriate to treat patients infected with both HBV and HIV (DHHS [pediatric] 2013).

Adult:

HIV infection, treatment: Use with at least two other antiretroviral agents:
Weight <50 kg: Oral: 4 mg/kg twice daily; maximum dose: 150 mg/dose (HHS [pediatric] 2015)
Weight ≥50 kg: Oral: 150 mg twice daily **or** 300 mg once daily

HIV postexposure, prophylaxis: Oral: 150 mg twice daily or 300 mg once daily in combination with zidovudine, tenofovir, stavudine, or didanosine, with or without a protease inhibitor depending on risk (CDC, 2005).

Hepatitis B, treatment (Epivir-HBV) (non-HIV-exposed/-positive): Note: Use in HBV treatment is discouraged due to rapid resistance development; consider use only if other anti-HBV antiviral regimens with more favorable resistance patterns cannot be used. Oral: 100 mg once daily

Hepatitis B/HIV coinfection, treatment of both infections: Epivir: Oral: 150 mg twice daily or 300 mg once daily, in combination with other antiretrovirals in a HAART regimen. **Note:** The formulation and dosage of Epivir-HBV are not appropriate for patients infected with both HBV and HIV. Tenofovir and lamivudine are a preferred NRTI backbone in a fully suppressive antiretroviral regimen for the treatment of HIV/HBV coinfection (DHHS [adult], 2014).

Dosing adjustment in renal impairment for HIV:
Manufacturer labeling:
Infants, Children, and Adolescents <25 kg: There are no dosage adjustments provided in the manufacturer's

labeling; consider reducing the dose or increasing the dosing interval; use with caution; monitor closely

Children and Adolescents ≥25 kg and Adults:

CrCl ≥50 mL/minute: No adjustment necessary

CrCl 30 to 49 mL/minute: 150 mg once daily

CrCl 15 to 29 mL/minute: 150 mg first dose, then 100 mg once daily

CrCl 5 to 14 mL/minute: 150 mg first dose, then 50 mg once daily

CrCl <5 mL/minute: 50 mg first dose, then 25 mg once daily

Note: On dialysis days, take dose after dialysis; additional dose of lamivudine after routine (4 hour) peritoneal or hemodialysis is not required (HHS [adult], 2014).

Alternate dosing: The following dosage adjustments have been recommended (Aronoff, 2007):

Infants, Children, and Adolescents:

GFR >50 mL/minute/1.73 m^2: No adjustment necessary

GFR 30 to 50 mL/minute/1.73 m^2: 4 mg/kg/dose once daily

GFR 10 to 29 mL/minute/1.73 m^2: 2 mg/kg/dose once daily

GFR <10 mL/minute/1.73 m^2: 1 mg/kg/dose once daily

Intermittent hemodialysis (IHD): 1 mg/kg/dose once daily

Peritoneal dialysis (PD): 1 mg/kg/dose once daily

Continuous renal replacement therapy (CRRT): 4 mg/kg/dose once daily

Dosing adjustment in renal impairment for chronic hepatitis B (Epivir-HBV):

Children ≥2 years and Adolescents: There are no dosage adjustments provided in the manufacturer's labeling; reduction in the dose should be considered; use with caution; monitor closely

Adults:

CrCl ≥50 mL/minute: No adjustment necessary

CrCl 30 to 49 mL/minute: 100 mg first dose, then 50 mg once daily

CrCl 15 to 29 mL/minute: 100 mg first dose, then 25 mg once daily

CrCl 5 to 14 mL/minute: 35 mg first dose, then 15 mg once daily

CrCl <5 mL/minute: 35 mg first dose, then 10 mg once daily

Note: Additional dose of lamivudine after routine (4 hour) peritoneal or hemodialysis is not required

Dosing adjustment in hepatic impairment: No dosage adjustments required; use with caution in patients with decompensated liver disease; safety and efficacy not established with these patients.

Administration Oral: May be administered without regard to meals

Monitoring Parameters

Hepatitis B: Screen for HIV before starting lamivudine; monitor LFTs prior to, periodically during, and for at least several months after discontinuation; monitor HBV DNA levels periodically during treatment

HIV: **Note:** The absolute CD4 cell count is currently recommended to monitor immune status in children of all ages; CD4 percentage can be used as an alternative. This recommendation is based on the use of absolute CD4 cell counts in the current pediatric HIV infection stage classification and as thresholds for initiation of antiretroviral treatment (HHS [pediatric] 2015).

Screen for hepatitis B before starting lamivudine. Also prior to initiation of therapy: Genotypic resistance testing, CD4 and viral load (every 3 to 4 months), CBC with differential, LFTs, BUN, creatinine, electrolytes, glucose, urinalysis (every 6 to 12 months), and assessment of readiness for adherence with medication regimen. At initiation and with any change in treatment regimen: CBC with differential, electrolytes, calcium, phosphate, glucose, LFTs, bilirubin, urinalysis (at initiation), BUN, creatinine, albumin, total protein, lipid panel (at initiation), CD4, and viral load, and screen for hepatitis B. After 1 to 2 weeks of therapy: Signs of medication toxicity and adherence. After 2 to 4 weeks of therapy: CBC with differential, viral load, signs of medication toxicity, and adherence; then every 3 to 4 months: CBC with differential, electrolytes, glucose, LFTs, bilirubin, BUN, creatinine, CD4, viral load, signs of medication toxicity, and adherence. Lipid panel and urinalysis every 6 to 12 months. CD4 monitoring frequency may be decreased to every 6 to 12 months in children who are adherent to therapy if the value is well above the threshold for opportunistic infections, viral suppression is sustained, and the clinical status is stable for more than 2 to 3 years (HHS [pediatric] 2015). Monitor for growth and development, signs of HIV-specific physical conditions, HIV disease progression opportunistic infections, pancreatitis, or lactic acidosis. Infants receiving lamivudine for prevention of maternal-fetal HIV transmission: Hemoglobin and neutrophil counts at 4 weeks after initiation of prophylaxis.

Dosage Forms Excipient information presented when available (limited, particularly for generics); consult specific product labeling.

Solution, Oral:

Epivir: 10 mg/mL (240 mL) [contains methylparaben, propylene glycol, propylparaben; strawberry-banana flavor]

Epivir HBV: 5 mg/mL (240 mL) [contains methylparaben, propylene glycol, propylparaben; strawberry-banana flavor]

Generic: 10 mg/mL (240 mL)

Tablet, Oral:

Epivir: 150 mg [scored]

Epivir: 300 mg

Epivir HBV: 100 mg

Generic: 100 mg, 150 mg, 300 mg

◆ **Lamivudine, Abacavir, and Zidovudine** *see* Abacavir, Lamivudine, and Zidovudine *on page* 38

◆ **Lamivudine and Abacavir** *see* Abacavir and Lamivudine *on page* 36

Lamivudine and Zidovudine

(la MI vyoo deen & zye DOE vyoo deen)

Medication Safety Issues

Sound-alike/look-alike issues:

Combivir may be confused with Combivent, Epivir

High alert medication:

This medication is in a class the Institute for Safe Medication Practices (ISMP) includes among its list of drug classes that have a heightened risk of causing significant patient harm when used in error.

Other safety concerns:

AZT is an error-prone abbreviation (mistaken as azaTHIOprine, aztreonam)

Related Information

Adult and Adolescent HIV *on page* 2392

Pediatric HIV *on page* 2380

Perinatal HIV *on page* 2400

Brand Names: US Combivir

Brand Names: Canada Combivir; Teva-Lamivudine/Zidovudine

Therapeutic Category Antiretroviral Agent; HIV Agents (Anti-HIV Agents); Nucleoside Reverse Transcriptase Inhibitor (NRTI)

Generic Availability (US) Yes

Use Treatment of HIV-1 infection in combination with at least one other antiretroviral agent (FDA approved in children ≥30 kg, adolescents ≥30 kg, and adults). **Note:** HIV regimens consisting of **three** antiretroviral agents are strongly recommended.

Pregnancy Risk Factor C

Pregnancy Considerations Adverse events were observed in animal reproduction studies. See individual agents. The DHHS Perinatal HIV Guidelines consider lamivudine in combination with zidovudine as one of the preferred NRTI backbones for antiretroviral-naïve pregnant women. Although use of this combination has the most experience for in pregnant women, it has an increased potential for hematologic toxicity (HHS [perinatal], 2014).

Breast-Feeding Considerations Lamivudine and zidovudine are both excreted into breast milk. See individual agents.

Contraindications Hypersensitivity to lamivudine, zidovudine, or any component of the formulation

Warnings/Precautions [U.S. Boxed Warning]: Zidovudine is associated with hematologic toxicity including neutropenia and severe anemia. Use with caution in patients with bone marrow compromise (granulocytes <1000 cells/mm^3 or hemoglobin <9.5 mg/dL).

[U.S. Boxed Warning]: Lactic acidosis and severe hepatomegaly with steatosis (including fatal cases) have been reported with the use of nucleoside analogues. Use with caution in patients with risk factors for liver disease (risk may be increased in women, obese patients, and/or prolonged exposure) and suspend treatment in any patient who develops clinical or laboratory findings suggestive of lactic acidosis (transaminase elevation may/may not accompany hepatomegaly and steatosis). Use caution in combination with interferon alfa with or without ribavirin in HIV/HBV coinfected patients; monitor closely for hepatic decompensation, anemia, or neutropenia. Combivir® is not recommended for use in patients with renal (CrCl <50 mL/minute) or hepatic impairment.

[U.S. Boxed Warning]: Monitor closely for chronic hepatitis B for several months following discontinuation of therapy in patients coinfected with HBV and HIV; clinical exacerbations may occur and may warrant anti-hepatitis B therapy.

[U.S. Boxed Warning]: Prolonged use of zidovudine has been associated with symptomatic myopathy and myositis. Immune reconstitution syndrome may develop resulting in the occurrence of an inflammatory response to an indolent or residual opportunistic infection during initial HIV treatment or activation of autoimmune disorders (eg, Graves' disease, polymyositis, Guillain-Barré syndrome) later in therapy; further evaluation and treatment may be required. May be associated with fat redistribution (buffalo hump, increased abdominal girth, breast engorgement, facial atrophy, and dyslipidemia).

Concomitant use of other zidovudine- or lamivudine-containing products with the fixed dose combination product should be avoided. Concomitant use of emtricitabine-containing products should be avoided; cross-resistance may develop.

Warnings: Additional Pediatric Considerations The major clinical toxicity of lamivudine in pediatric patients is pancreatitis which has occurred in 14% of patients in one open-label, uncontrolled study; discontinue lamivudine therapy if clinical signs, symptoms, or laboratory abnormalities suggestive of pancreatitis occur. Use with extreme caution and only if there is no satisfactory alternative therapy in pediatric patients with a history of pancreatitis or other significant risk factors for the development of pancreatitis. Use of the fixed-dose combination product is not recommended for patients who need a dosage reduction, including children <30 kg, patients with renal or hepatic impairment, or those patients experiencing dose-limiting adverse effects (use individual antiretroviral agents to appropriately adjust dosages).

Adverse Reactions See individual agents.

Drug Interactions

Metabolism/Transport Effects Refer to individual components.

Avoid Concomitant Use

Avoid concomitant use of Lamivudine and Zidovudine with any of the following: Amodiaquine; BCG (Intravesical); CloZAPine; Dipyrone; Emtricitabine; Stavudine

Increased Effect/Toxicity

Lamivudine and Zidovudine may increase the levels/effects of: Amodiaquine; CloZAPine; Emtricitabine; Ribavirin

The levels/effects of Lamivudine and Zidovudine may be increased by: Acyclovir-Valacyclovir; Clarithromycin; Dexketoprofen; Dipyrone; DOXOrubicin (Conventional); DOXOrubicin (Liposomal); Fluconazole; Ganciclovir-Valganciclovir; Interferons; Methadone; Probenecid; Raltegravir; Teriflunomide; Trimethoprim; Valproic Acid and Derivatives

Decreased Effect

Lamivudine and Zidovudine may decrease the levels/effects of: BCG (Intravesical); Stavudine

The levels/effects of Lamivudine and Zidovudine may be decreased by: Clarithromycin; DOXOrubicin (Conventional); DOXOrubicin (Liposomal); Protease Inhibitors; Rifamycin Derivatives

Storage/Stability Store between 2°C and 30°C (36°F and 86°F).

Mechanism of Action The combination of zidovudine and lamivudine is believed to act synergistically to inhibit reverse transcriptase via DNA chain termination after incorporation of the nucleoside analogue as well as to delay the emergence of mutations conferring resistance

Pharmacokinetics (Adult data unless noted) One Combivir tablet is bioequivalent to one lamivudine 150 mg tablet plus one zidovudine 300 mg tablet; see individual agents

Dosing: Usual Note: Use in combination with at least one other antiretroviral agent.

Pediatric: **HIV Treatment:**

Children and Adolescents weighing 30 kg: Not intended for use; product is a fixed-dose combination; safety and efficacy have not been established in these patients

Children and Adolescents weighing ≥30 kg: Oral: One tablet twice daily

Adult: **HIV Treatment:** Oral: One tablet twice daily

Dosing adjustment in renal impairment: All patients: CrCl <50 mL/minute: Use not recommended; use individual agents for reduction in lamivudine and zidovudine dosage.

Dosing adjustment in hepatic impairment: Use not recommended; use individual antiretroviral agents to reduce dosage.

Administration Oral: May be administered without regard to meals

Monitoring Parameters Note: Monitor CD4 percentage (if <5 years of age) or CD4 count (if ≥5 years of age) at least every 3-4 months (DHHS [pediatric], 2014).

Screen for hepatitis B before starting. Prior to initiation of therapy: Genotypic resistance testing, CD4 and viral load (every 3 to 4 months), CBC with differential, LFTs, BUN, creatinine, electrolytes, glucose, urinalysis (every 6 to 12 months), and assessment of readiness for adherence with medication regimen. At initiation and with any change in treatment regimen: CBC with differential, electrolytes, calcium, phosphate, glucose, LFTs, bilirubin, urinalysis (at initiation), BUN, creatinine, albumin, total protein, lipid panel (at initiation), CD4, and viral load. After 1 to 2 weeks of therapy: Signs of medication toxicity and adherence.

After 2 to 4 weeks of therapy: CBC with differential, viral load, signs of medication toxicity, and adherence; then every 3 to 4 months: CBC with differential, electrolytes, glucose, LFTs, bilirubin, BUN, creatinine, CD4, viral load, signs of medication toxicity, and adherence. Lipid panel and urinalysis every 6 to 12 months. CD4 monitoring frequency may be decreased to every 6 to 12 months in children who are adherent to therapy if the value is well above the threshold for opportunistic infections, viral suppression is sustained, and the clinical status is stable for more than 2 to 3 years (DHHS [pediatric], 2014). Monitor for growth and development, signs of HIV-specific physical conditions, HIV disease progression, opportunistic infections, hepatotoxicity, pancreatitis, anemia, or lactic acidosis.

Dosage Forms Excipient information presented when available (limited, particularly for generics); consult specific product labeling.

Tablet, oral: Lamivudine 150 mg and zidovudine 300 mg

Combivir: Lamivudine 150 mg and zidovudine 300 mg [scored]

LamoTRIgine (la MOE tri jeen)

Medication Safety Issues

Sound-alike/look-alike issues:

LamoTRIgine may be confused with labetalol, LamISIL, lamiVUDine, levETIRAcetam, levothyroxine, Lomotil

LaMICtal may be confused with LamISIL, Lomotil

Administration issues:

Potential exists for medication errors to occur among different formulations of LaMICtal (tablets, extended release tablets, orally disintegrating tablets, and chewable/dispersible tablets). Patients should be instructed to visually inspect tablets dispensed to verify receiving the correct medication and formulation. The medication guide includes illustrations to aid in tablet verification.

International issues:

Lamictal [US, Canada, and multiple international markets] may be confused with Ludiomil brand name for maprotiline [multiple international markets]

Lamotrigine [US, Canada, and multiple international markets] may be confused with Ludiomil brand name for maprotiline [multiple international markets]

Related Information

Oral Medications That Should Not Be Crushed or Altered *on page 2476*

Brand Names: US LaMICtal; LaMICtal ODT; LaMICtal Starter; LaMICtal XR

Brand Names: Canada Apo-Lamotrigine; Auro-Lamotrigine; Lamictal; Mylan-Lamotrigine; PMS-Lamotrigine; ratio-Lamotrigine; Teva-Lamotrigine

Therapeutic Category Anticonvulsant, Miscellaneous

Generic Availability (US) May be product dependent

Use

Tablets, chewable dispersible tablets, and orally disintegrating tablets: Adjunctive treatment of generalized seizures of Lennox-Gastaut syndrome, primary generalized tonic-clonic seizures, and partial seizures (FDA approved in ages ≥2 years and adults); monotherapy of partial seizures in patients who are converted from valproic acid or a single enzyme-inducing AED (specifically, carbamazepine, phenytoin, phenobarbital, or primidone) (FDA approved in ages ≥16 years and adults); maintenance treatment of bipolar disorder (FDA approved in ages ≥18 years and adults); has also been used as adjunctive treatment of partial seizures in ages <24 months and monotherapy for absence seizures

Extended-release tablets: Adjunctive treatment of primary generalized tonic-clonic seizures and partial onset seizures with or without secondary generalization (FDA approved in ages ≥13 years and adults); monotherapy of partial seizures in patients who are converted from a single AED (FDA approved in ages ≥13 years and adults)

Has also been used as add-on therapy for atypical absence, atonic, tonic, and myoclonic seizures; and as monotherapy in adults and adolescents for idiopathic generalized tonic-clonic seizures

Medication Guide Available Yes

Pregnancy Risk Factor C

Pregnancy Considerations Adverse events have been observed in animal reproduction studies. Lamotrigine crosses the human placenta and can be measured in the plasma of exposed newborns (Harden and Pennell, 2009; Ohman, 2000). An overall increase in major congenital malformations has not been observed in available studies; however, an increased risk for cleft lip or cleft palate has not been ruled out (Cunnington, 2011; Hernández-Díaz, 2012; Holmes, 2012). An increased risk of malformations following maternal lamotrigine use may be associated with larger doses (Cunnington, 2007; Tomson, 2011). Polytherapy may increase the risk of congenital malformations; monotherapy with the lowest effective dose is recommended (Harden and Meader, 2009).

Due to pregnancy-induced physiologic changes, women who are pregnant may require dose adjustments of lamotrigine in order to maintain clinical response; monitoring during pregnancy should be considered (Harden and Pennell, 2009). For women with epilepsy who are planning a pregnancy in advance, baseline serum concentrations should be measured once or twice prior to pregnancy during a period when seizure control is optimal. Monitoring can then be continued up to once a month during pregnancy and every second day during the first week postpartum (Patsalos, 2008). In women taking lamotrigine who are trying to avoid pregnancy, potentially significant interactions may exist with hormone-containing contraceptives; consult drug interactions database for more detailed information.

Pregnancy registries are available for women who have been exposed to lamotrigine. Patients may enroll themselves in the North American Antiepileptic Drug (NAAED) Pregnancy Registry by calling (888) 233-2334. Additional information is available at www.aedpregnancyregistry.org.

Breast-Feeding Considerations Lamotrigine is excreted in breast milk and may be as high as 50% of the maternal serum concentration. Adverse events observed in breast-feeding infants include apnea, drowsiness, and poor sucking. The manufacturer recommends that caution be exercised when administering lamotrigine to nursing women and to monitor the nursing infant.

Contraindications Hypersensitivity (eg, rash, angioedema, acute urticaria, extensive pruritus, mucosal ulceration) to lamotrigine or any component of the formulation

Warnings/Precautions [US Boxed Warning]: Serious skin rashes requiring hospitalization and discontinuation of treatment have been reported; incidence of serious rash is higher in pediatric patients than adults; risk may be increased by coadministration with valproic acid, higher than recommended initial doses, exceeding recommended initial dose titration, or exceeding the recommended dose escalation for lamotrigine. One rash-related death was reported in a pediatric patients taking lamotrigine immediate-release as adjunctive therapy. Nearly all cases of life-threatening rashes associated with lamotrigine have occurred within 2 to 8 weeks of treatment initiation; however, isolated cases may occur after prolonged treatment (eg, 6 months) or in patients without these risk factors; discontinue at first sign of rash and do not reinitiate therapy unless rash is clearly not drug related. Rare cases of toxic epidermal necrolysis and/or rash-related death have been reported. Discontinuation of treatment may not prevent a rash from

becoming life-threatening or permanently disabling or disfiguring.

Antiepileptics are associated with an increased risk of suicidal behavior/thoughts with use (regardless of indication); patients should be monitored for signs/symptoms of depression, suicidal tendencies, and other unusual behavior changes during therapy and instructed to inform their healthcare provider immediately if symptoms occur.

A spectrum of hematologic effects have been reported with use (eg, neutropenia, leukopenia, thrombocytopenia, pancytopenia, anemias, and rarely, aplastic anemia and pure red cell aplasia); patients with a previous history of adverse hematologic reaction to any drug may be at increased risk. Early detection of hematologic change is important; advise patients of early signs and symptoms including fever, sore throat, mouth ulcers, infections, easy bruising, petechial or purpuric hemorrhage. May be associated with hypersensitivity syndrome (eg, anticonvulsant hypersensitivity syndrome). Multiorgan hypersensitivity reactions (drug reaction with eosinophilia and systemic symptoms [DRESS]) have been reported. Symptoms may include fever, rash, and/or lymphadenopathy; monitor for signs and symptoms of possible disparate manifestations associated with lymphatic, hepatic, renal, and/or hematologic organ systems. Evaluate patient with fever and lymphadenopathy, even if rash is not present; discontinuation and conversion to alternate therapy may be required. Increased risk of developing aseptic meningitis has been reported; symptoms (eg, headache, nuchal rigidity, fever, nausea/vomiting, rash, photophobia) have generally occurred within 1 to 45 days following therapy initiation. Use caution in patients with renal or hepatic impairment. Avoid abrupt cessation, taper over at least 2 weeks if possible.

May cause CNS depression, which may impair physical or mental abilities. Patients must be cautioned about performing tasks which require mental alertness (eg, operating machinery or driving). Effects with other sedative drugs or ethanol may be potentiated. Binds to melanin and may accumulate in the eye and other melanin-rich tissues; the clinical significance of this is not known. Safety and efficacy for the treatment of epilepsy have not been established for use as initial monotherapy, conversion to monotherapy from antiepileptic drugs (AED) other than carbamazepine, phenytoin, phenobarbital, primidone or valproic acid or conversion to monotherapy from two or more AEDs. Patients treated for bipolar disorder should be monitored closely for clinical worsening or suicidality; reassess patients to determine the need for maintenance treatment if on therapy >16 weeks. Prescriptions should be written for the smallest quantity consistent with good patient care. Treatment of acute manic or mixed episodes is not recommended; efficacy in the acute treatment of mood episodes has not been established. Children are at increased risk for developing serious skin rashes during therapy; lower starting doses and slower dose escalations may decrease the risk of rash. Potentially significant drug-drug interactions may exist, requiring dose or frequency adjustment, additional monitoring, and/or selection of alternative therapy. There is a potential for medication errors with similar-sounding medications and among different lamotrigine formulations; medication errors have occurred.

Some dosage forms may contain polysorbate 80 (also known as Tweens). Hypersensitivity reactions, usually a delayed reaction, have been reported following exposure to pharmaceutical products containing polysorbate 80 in certain individuals (Isaksson, 2002; Lucente, 2000; Shelley, 1995). Thrombocytopenia, ascites, pulmonary deterioration, and renal and hepatic failure have been reported in premature neonates after receiving parenteral products containing polysorbate 80 (Alade, 1986; CDC, 1984). See manufacturer's labeling.

Warnings: Additional Pediatric Considerations Incidence of serious rash is higher in pediatric patients than adults. Serious skin rashes (including Stevens-Johnson syndrome) occur in 0.8% of pediatric epilepsy patients (2 to 16 years of age) and 0.3% of adult epilepsy patients and in up to 0.13% of adult patients treated for bipolar and other mood disorders; rare cases of toxic epidermal necrolysis and angioedema have been reported; rash-related deaths have occurred in pediatric and adult patients. In addition to pediatric age, the risk of rash may be increased in patients receiving valproic acid, high initial doses, or with rapid dosage increases; however, rash has been reported in patients without risk factors. Rash usually appears in the first 2 to 8 weeks of therapy, but may occur after prolonged treatment (eg, 6 months). Benign rashes may occur, but one cannot predict which rashes will become serious or life-threatening; the manufacturer recommends (ordinarily) discontinuation of lamotrigine at the first sign of rash (unless rash is clearly not drug related); discontinuation of lamotrigine may not prevent rash from becoming life-threatening or permanently disfiguring or disabling. Risk of nonserious rash may also be increased when the initial recommended dose or dose escalation rate is exceeded in patients with a history of rash or allergy to other AEDs.

Do not abruptly discontinue; when discontinuing therapy, gradually reduce the dose by ~50% per week and taper over at least 2 weeks unless safety concerns require a more rapid withdrawal. Lamotrigine should not be restarted in patients who discontinued therapy due to lamotrigine-associated rash, unless benefits clearly outweigh risks; if restarting lamotrigine after withholding for >5 half-lives, use the initial dosing recommendations and titrate dosage accordingly (ie, do not restart at the previous maintenance dose).

A small randomized, double-blind, placebo-controlled study in pediatric patients 1 to 24 months of age did not demonstrate safety and efficacy of immediate release lamotrigine when used as adjunctive treatment for partial seizures; lamotrigine was associated with an increased risk for infectious and respiratory adverse reactions.

Adverse Reactions

Cardiovascular: Chest pain, edema, peripheral edema

Central nervous system: Abnormal dreams, abnormality in thinking, agitation, amnesia, anxiety, ataxia, confusion, depression, dizziness, drowsiness, dyspraxia, emotional lability, fatigue, hyperreflexia, hypoesthesia, hyporeflexia, insomnia, irritability, migraine, pain, paresthesia, suicidal ideation

Dermatologic: Skin rash (nonserious is more common), dermatitis, diaphoresis, xeroderma

Endocrine & metabolic: Dysmenorrhea, weight gain, weight loss

Gastrointestinal: Abdominal pain, anorexia, constipation, dyspepsia, flatulence, peptic ulcer, vomiting, xerostomia

Gastrointestinal: Nausea

Genitourinary: Increased libido, urinary frequency

Hematologic & oncologic: Rectal hemorrhage

Infection: Infection

Neuromuscular & skeletal: Arthralgia, back pain, myalgia, neck pain, weakness

Ophthalmic: Amblyopia, nystagmus, visual disturbance

Respiratory: Bronchitis, cough, dyspnea, epistaxis, nasopharyngitis, pharyngitis, rhinitis, sinusitis, upper respiratory tract infection

Miscellaneous: Fever

Rare but important or life-threatening: Abnormal hepatic function tests, abnormal lacrimation, accommodation disturbance, acne vulgaris, acute renal failure, ageusia, agranulocytosis, akathisia, alcohol intolerance, alopecia, altered sense of smell, amyotrophy, anemia, anorgasmia, apathy, aphasia, apnea, arthritis, aseptic meningitis, blepharoptosis, breast abscess, breast neoplasm, bursitis, central nervous system depression, cerebellar syndrome, conjunctivitis, cystitis, deafness, decreased fibrin, decreased libido, decreased serum fibrinogen, deep vein thrombophlebitis, delirium, delusions, depersonalization, depression, dermatitis (exfoliative, fungal), disseminated intravascular coagulation, DRESS syndrome, dry eye syndrome, dysphagia, dysphoria, dysuria, ecchymosis, ejaculatory disorder, eosinophilia, epididymitis, eructation, erythema multiforme, esophagitis, exacerbation of Parkinson disease, extrapyramidal reaction, gastritis, gastrointestinal hemorrhage, gingival hemorrhage, gingival hyperplasia, gingivitis, glossitis, hallucination, hemiplegia, hemorrhage, hepatitis, hepatotoxicity (idiosyncratic) (Chalasani, 2014), herpes zoster, hirsutism, hostility, hot flash, hyperalgesia, hyperbilirubinemia, hyperesthesia, hyperglycemia, hypermenorrhagia, hypersensitivity reaction, hypertension, hyperventilation, hypokinesia, hypothyroidism, hypotonia, immunosuppression (progressive), impotence, increased appetite, increased gamma glutamyl transpeptidase, increased serum alkaline phosphatase, increased serum ALT, increased serum AST, lactation, leg cramps, leukocytosis, leukoderma, leukopenia, lupus-like syndrome, lymphadenopathy, lymphocytosis, maculopapular rash, malaise, manic depressive reaction, memory impairment, multiorgan failure, muscle spasm, myasthenia, myoclonus, neuralgia, neutropenia, nightmares, oral mucosa ulcer, orthostatic hypotension, oscillopsia, otalgia, palpitations, pancreatitis, pancytopenia, panic attack, paralysis, paranoid reaction, pathological fracture, peripheral neuritis, personality disorder, petechia, photophobia, polyuria, psychosis, pure red cell aplasia, pustular rash, racing mind, renal pain, rhabdomyolysis, sialorrhea, skin discoloration, sleep disorder, status epilepticus, Stevens-Johnson syndrome, strabismus, suicidal tendencies, syncope, tachycardia, tendinous contracture, thrombocytopenia, tics, tinnitus, tonic-clonic seizures (exacerbation), urinary incontinence, urinary retention, urinary urgency, uveitis, vasculitis, vasodilation, vesiculobullous dermatitis, visual field defect, withdrawal seizures

Drug Interactions

Metabolism/Transport Effects Inhibits OCT2

Avoid Concomitant Use

Avoid concomitant use of LamoTRIgine with any of the following: Azelastine (Nasal); Dofetilide; Orphenadrine; Paraldehyde; Thalidomide

Increased Effect/Toxicity

LamoTRIgine may increase the levels/effects of: Alcohol (Ethyl); Azelastine (Nasal); Buprenorphine; CarBAMazepine; CNS Depressants; Desmopressin; Dofetilide; Hydrocodone; MetFORMIN; Methotrimeprazine; Metyrosine; Mirtazapine; OLANZapine; Orphenadrine; Paraldehyde; Pramipexole; Procainamide; ROPINIRole; Rotigotine; Selective Serotonin Reuptake Inhibitors; Suvorexant; Thalidomide; Zolpidem

The levels/effects of LamoTRIgine may be increased by: Brimonidine (Topical); Cannabis; Doxylamine; Dronabinol; Droperidol; HydrOXYzine; Kava Kava; Magnesium Sulfate; Methotrimeprazine; Nabilone; Perampanel; Rufinamide; Sodium Oxybate; Tapentadol; Tetrahydrocannabinol; Valproic Acid and Derivatives

Decreased Effect

LamoTRIgine may decrease the levels/effects of: Contraceptives (Progestins)

The levels/effects of LamoTRIgine may be decreased by: Atazanavir; Barbiturates; CarBAMazepine; Contraceptives (Estrogens); Ezogabine; Fosphenytoin; Mefloquine; Mianserin; Orlistat; Phenytoin; Primidone; Rifampin; Ritonavir

Food Interactions Food has no effect on absorption.

Storage/Stability Store at 15°C to 30°C (59°F to 86°F). Protect from light.

Mechanism of Action A triazine derivative which inhibits release of glutamate (an excitatory amino acid) and inhibits voltage-sensitive sodium channels, which stabilizes neuronal membranes. Lamotrigine has weak inhibitory effect on the 5-HT_3 receptor; *in vitro* inhibits dihydrofolate reductase.

Pharmacokinetics (Adult data unless noted)

Absorption: Oral: Immediate release: Rapid, 97.6% absorbed; **Note:** Orally disintegrating tablets (either swallowed whole with water or disintegrated in the mouth) are equivalent to regular tablets (swallowed whole with water) in terms of rate and extent of absorption.

Distribution: V_d: 1.1 L/kg; range: 0.9 to 1.3 L/kg

Protein binding: 55% (primarily albumin)

Metabolism: Hepatic; >75% metabolized via glucuronidation; autoinduction may occur

Bioavailability: Immediate release: 98%; **Note:** AUCs were similar for immediate release and extended release preparations in patients receiving nonenzyme-inducing AEDs. In subjects receiving concomitant enzyme-inducing AEDs, bioavailability of extended release product was ~21% lower than immediate-release product; in some of these subjects, a decrease in AUC of up to 70% was observed when switching from immediate-release to extended-release tablets.

Half-life:

- Infants and Children:
  - With enzyme-inducing AEDs (ie, phenytoin, phenobarbital, carbamazepine, primidone):
    - Infants and Children 10 months to 5.3 years: 7.7 hours (range: 6 to 11 hours)
    - Children 5 to 11 years: 7 hours (range: 4 to 10 hours)
  - With enzyme-inducing AED and valproic acid (VPA): Children 5 to 11 years: 19 hours (range: 7 to 31 hours)
  - With VPA:
    - Infants and Children 10 months to 5.3 years: 45 hours (range: 30 to 52 hours)
    - Children 5 to 11 years: 66 hours (range: 50 to 74 hours)
  - With no enzyme-inducing AED: Infants and Children 10 months to 5.3 years: 19 hours (range: 13 to 27 hours)
- Adults:
  - Normal: Single dose: 33 hours; multiple dose: ~25 hours (range: 12 to 62 hours)
  - With enzyme-inducing AEDs: Single dose: 14 hours; multiple dose: 13 hours (range: 8 to 23 hours)
  - With enzyme-inducing AED and VPA: Single dose: ~27 hours (range: 11 to 52 hours)
  - With VPA: Single dose: 59 hours (range: 30 to 89 hours)
  - Hepatic dysfunction: Child-Pugh classification:
    - Mild liver impairment: 46 ± 20 hours
    - Moderate liver impairment: 72 ± 44 hours
    - Severe liver impairment without ascites: 67± 11 hours
    - Severe liver impairment with ascites: 100 ± 48 hours
  - Chronic renal impairment (CrCl mean: 13 mL/minute): ~43 hours
  - Severe renal dysfunction (requiring hemodialysis):
    - Between dialysis sessions: 57.4 hours
    - During dialysis: 13 hours

Time to peak serum concentration: Oral:

- Immediate release: 1.4 to 4.8 hours
- Extended release: 4 to 11 hours (dependent on adjunct therapy)

Elimination: ~94% in urine (86% excreted as glucuronide metabolites and 10% as unchanged drug); feces (2%)

Dosing: Neonatal Note: Dosage depends on patient's concomitant medications (ie, valproic acid; enzyme-inducing AEDs [specifically phenytoin, phenobarbital, carbamazepine, and primidone]; or AEDs other than carbamazepine, phenytoin, phenobarbital, primidone, or valproic acid). Patients receiving concomitant rifampin or other drugs that induce lamotrigine glucuronidation and increase clearance should follow the same dosing regimen as that used with anticonvulsants that have this effect (eg, phenytoin, phenobarbital, carbamazepine, and primidone).

Anticonvulsant: Adjunctive (add-on) therapy for refractory seizures: Limited data available: Oral: PNA 14 to 28 days: Immediate release: Initial: 2 mg/kg/dose once daily; may increase by 2 mg/kg/day at intervals of at least 7 days to a maximum dose of 10 mg/kg/day; this dosing was described in a prospective, open-label trial that included five neonates (GA not reported) in the study population; all patients had previously received enzyme-inducing agents, such as phenytoin, phenobarbital, and/or carbamazepine; patients were treated with lamotrigine for 3 months (Mikati 2002)

Dosing: Usual Note: Tablets should not be split to achieve dose; whole tablets should be used for dosing; round calculated dose down to the nearest whole tablet. Alternatively, a suspension may be prepared using immediate release tablets (see Extemporaneous Preparations). Dosage depends on patient's concomitant medications [ie, valproic acid; enzyme-inducing AEDs (specifically phenytoin, phenobarbital, carbamazepine, and primidone); or other AEDs not previously mentioned. Patients receiving concomitant rifampin or other drugs that induce lamotrigine glucuronidation and increase clearance should follow the same dosing regimen as that used with anticonvulsants that have similar effects (eg, phenytoin, phenobarbital, carbamazepine, and primidone).

Pediatric:

Anticonvulsant: Lennox-Gastaut syndrome, primary generalized tonic-clonic seizures, or partial seizures; adjunctive (add-on) therapy: Oral:

Immediate release formulations:

Infants and Children <24 months: Adjunctive therapy; partial seizures: Limited data available (Piña-Garza, 2008; Piña-Garza, 2008a): **Note:** As reported in the trials, initial doses were administered every other day if necessary due to limited strengths of commercially available products; use of an extemporaneously compounded suspension may allow for more frequent dosing; usually, daily doses are divided into 1 to 2 doses per day; daily doses in these trials were divided 3 times daily once sufficiently large enough to utilize commercially available products; this was done due to the possible increased clearance of lamotrigine in this age group.

Patients receiving AED regimens ***containing valproic acid or nonenzyme-inducing*** *AEDs:* **Note:** Studies excluded patients <6.7 kg:

Weeks 1 and 2: 0.15 mg/kg/day

Weeks 3 and 4: 0.3 mg/kg/day

Maintenance dose: Titrate dose to effect; after week 4, increase dose every week by no more than 0.3 mg/kg/day; maximum maintenance dose: 5.1 mg/kg/day in 3 divided doses not to exceed 200 mg/day; mean final dose required in open-label phase of trial was 3.1 mg/kg/day; n=51 (Piña-Garza, 2008a)

Patients receiving ***enzyme-inducing*** *AED regimens (eg, carbamazepine, phenytoin, phenobarbital, or primidone)* ***without valproic acid****:*

Weeks 1 and 2: 0.6 mg/kg/day

Weeks 3 and 4: 1.2 mg/kg/day

Maintenance dose: Titrate dose to effect; after week 4, increase dose every week by no more than 1.2 mg/kg/day; maximum maintenance dose: 15.6 mg/kg/day in 3 divided doses not to exceed 400 mg/day; mean final dose required in open-label phase of trial was 8.9 mg/kg/day; n=126 (Piña-Garza, 2008a)

Children 2 to 12 years: **Note: Only whole tablets should be used for dosing**; children 2 to 6 years will likely require maintenance doses at the higher end of recommended range; patients weighing <30 kg may need as much as a 50% increase in maintenance dose compared with patients weighing >30 kg; titrate dose to clinical effect

Patients receiving AEDs ***other than carbamazepine, phenytoin, phenobarbital, primidone, or valproic acid:***

Weeks 1 and 2: 0.3 mg/kg/day in 1 to 2 divided doses; round dose down to the nearest whole tablet

Weeks 3 and 4: 0.6 mg/kg/day in 2 divided doses; round dose down to the nearest whole tablet

Maintenance dose: Titrate dose to effect; after week 4, increase dose every 1 to 2 weeks by a calculated increment; calculate increment as 0.6 mg/kg/day rounded down to the nearest whole tablet; add this amount to the previously administered daily dose; usual maintenance: 4.5 to 7.5 mg/kg/day in 2 divided doses; maximum daily dose: 300 mg/day

Patients receiving AED regimens ***containing valproic acid****:*

Weeks 1 and 2: 0.15 mg/kg/day in 1 to 2 divided doses; round dose down to the nearest whole tablet; use 2 mg every other day for patients weighing >6.7 kg and <14 kg

Weeks 3 and 4: 0.3 mg/kg/day in 1 to 2 divided doses; round dose down to the nearest whole tablet

Maintenance dose: Titrate dose to effect; after week 4, increase dose every 1 to 2 weeks by a calculated increment; calculate increment as 0.3 mg/kg/day rounded down to the nearest whole tablet; add this amount to the previously administered daily dose; usual maintenance: 1 to 5 mg/kg/day in 1 to 2 divided doses; maximum daily dose: 200 mg/day. **Note:** Usual maintenance dose in children adding lamotrigine to valproic acid **alone**: 1 to 3 mg/kg/day

Patients receiving ***enzyme-inducing*** *AED regimens (eg, carbamazepine, phenytoin, phenobarbital, or primidone)* ***without valproic acid****:*

Weeks 1 and 2: 0.6 mg/kg/day in 2 divided doses; round dose down to the nearest whole tablet

Weeks 3 and 4: 1.2 mg/kg/day in 2 divided doses; round dose down to the nearest whole tablet

Maintenance dose: Titrate dose to effect; after week 4, increase dose every 1 to 2 weeks by a calculated increment; calculate increment as 1.2 mg/kg/day rounded down to the nearest whole tablet; add this amount to the previously administered daily dose; usual maintenance: 5 to 15 mg/kg/day in 2 divided doses; maximum daily dose: 400 mg/day

Adolescents:

Patients receiving AEDs ***other than carbamazepine, phenytoin, phenobarbital, primidone, or valproic acid:***

Weeks 1 and 2: 25 mg every day

Weeks 3 and 4: 50 mg every day

Maintenance dose: Titrate dose to effect; after week 4, increase dose every 1 to 2 weeks by 50 mg/day; usual maintenance: 225 to 375 mg/day in 2 divided doses

Patients receiving AED regimens ***containing valproic acid****:*

Weeks 1 and 2: 25 mg every other day

Weeks 3 and 4: 25 mg every day

Maintenance dose: Titrate dose to effect; after week 4, increase dose every 1 to 2 weeks by 25 to 50 mg/day; usual maintenance in patients receiving valproic acid and other drugs that induce glucuronidation: 100 to 400 mg/day in 1 to 2 divided doses; usual maintenance in patients adding lamotrigine to valproic acid **alone**: 100 to 200 mg/day

*Patients receiving **enzyme-inducing** AED regimens (eg, carbamazepine, phenytoin, phenobarbital, or primidone) **without valproic acid**:*

Weeks 1 and 2: 50 mg/day

Weeks 3 and 4: 100 mg/day in 2 divided doses

Maintenance dose: Titrate dose to effect; after week 4, increase dose every 1 to 2 weeks by 100 mg/day; usual maintenance: 300 to 500 mg/day in 2 divided doses; doses as high as 700 mg/day in 2 divided doses have been used

Extended release formulation: Adolescents: **Note:** Dose increases after week 8 should not exceed 100 mg/day at weekly intervals

*Regimens **not containing** carbamazepine, phenytoin, phenobarbital, primidone, or valproic acid:* Initial: Weeks 1 and 2: 25 mg once daily; Weeks 3 and 4: 50 mg once daily; Week 5: 100 mg once daily; Week 6: 150 mg once daily; Week 7: 200 mg once daily; Maintenance: 300 to 400 mg once daily

*Regimens **containing** valproic acid:* Initial: Weeks 1 and 2: 25 mg every other day; Weeks 3 and 4: 25 mg once daily; Week 5: 50 mg once daily; Week 6: 100 mg once daily; Week 7: 150 mg once daily; Maintenance: 200 to 250 mg once daily

*Regimens **containing** carbamazepine, phenytoin, phenobarbital, or primidone and **without** valproic acid:* Initial: Weeks 1 and 2: 50 mg once daily; Weeks 3 and 4: 100 mg once daily; Week 5: 200 mg once daily; Week 6: 300 mg once daily; Week 7: 400 mg once daily; Maintenance: 400 to 600 mg once daily

Conversion from immediate release to extended release (Lamictal XR): Initial dose of the extended release tablet (given once daily) should match the total daily dose of the immediate release formulation; monitor for seizure control, especially in patients on AED agents. Adjust dose as needed within the recommended dosing guidelines.

Anticonvulsant: Partial seizures; monotherapy: Oral:

Immediate release formulations: Adolescents ≥16 years:

*Conversion from adjunctive therapy with a **single enzyme-inducing** AED (eg, carbamazepine, phenytoin, phenobarbital, or primidone and **not valproate**) to lamotrigine immediate release monotherapy:* **Note:** First add lamotrigine and titrate it (as outlined below) to the recommended maintenance monotherapy dose (500 mg/day in 2 divided doses), while maintaining the enzyme-inducing AED at a fixed level; then gradually taper the enzyme-inducing AED by 20% decrements each week to fully withdraw over a 4-week period.

Weeks 1 and 2: 50 mg/day

Weeks 3 and 4: 100 mg/day in 2 divided doses

Maintenance dose: After week 4, increase dose every 1 to 2 weeks by 100 mg/day; recommended maintenance monotherapy dose: 500 mg/day in 2 divided doses

*Conversion from adjunctive therapy with **valproate** to lamotrigine immediate release monotherapy:* **Note:** This is a 4-step conversion process to achieve the lamotrigine recommended monotherapy dose (500 mg/day in 2 divided doses).

First: Add lamotrigine and titrate it to a dose of 200 mg/day as follows (if not already receiving 200 mg/day), while maintaining the valproate dose at a fixed level:

Weeks 1 and 2: 25 mg every other day

Weeks 3 and 4: 25 mg every day

Then increase dose every 1 to 2 weeks by 25 to 50 mg/day

Second: Keep lamotrigine dose at 200 mg/day; slowly taper valproate dose in decrements of ≤500 mg/day per week, to a dose of 500 mg/day; maintain this dose for one week

Third: Increase lamotrigine to 300 mg/day and decrease valproate to 250 mg/day; maintain this dose for one week

Fourth: Discontinue valproate and increase lamotrigine by 100 mg/day at weekly intervals to achieve recommended maintenance monotherapy dose of 500 mg/day in 2 divided doses

Conversion from adjunctive therapy with AEDs other than enzyme-inducing AEDs or valproate to lamotrigine immediate release monotherapy: No specific guidelines available

Extended release formulation: Adolescents:

*Conversion from adjunctive therapy with AEDs **other than** enzyme-inducing AEDs or valproate to lamotrigine extended release monotherapy:* First add lamotrigine and titrate it (as outlined below) to a recommended lamotrigine dose of 250 to 300 mg once daily, while maintaining the concomitant AED at a fixed level; then gradually taper the concomitant AED by 20% decrements each week to fully withdraw over a 4-week period.

Weeks 1 and 2: 25 mg once daily

Weeks 3 and 4: 50 mg once daily

Week 5: 100 mg once daily

Week 6: 150 mg once daily

Week 7: 200 mg once daily

Maintenance: 250 to 300 mg once daily

*Conversion from adjunctive therapy with **valproate** to lamotrigine extended release monotherapy:* **Note:** This is a 4-step conversion process to achieve the lamotrigine recommended extended release monotherapy dose (250 to 300 mg once daily).

First: Add lamotrigine and titrate it to a dose of 150 mg/day as follows (if not already receiving 150 mg/day), while maintaining the valproate dose at a fixed level:

Weeks 1 and 2: 25 mg every other day

Weeks 3 and 4: 25 mg once daily

Week 5: 50 mg once daily

Week 6: 100 mg once daily

Week 7: 150 mg once daily

Second: Keep lamotrigine dose at 150 mg/day; slowly taper valproate dose in decrements of ≤500 mg/day per week, to a dose of 500 mg/day; maintain this dose for 1 week

Third: Increase lamotrigine to 200 mg/day and decrease valproate to 250 mg/day; maintain this dose for 1 week

Fourth: Discontinue valproate and increase lamotrigine to a maintenance dose of 250 to 300 mg/day

*Conversion from adjunctive therapy with a **single enzyme-inducing** AED (eg, carbamazepine, phenytoin, phenobarbital, or primidone and **not valproate**) to lamotrigine extended release monotherapy in patients with partial seizures:* **Note:** First add lamotrigine and titrate it (as outlined below) to a recommended lamotrigine dose of 500 mg/day, while maintaining the enzyme-inducing AED at a fixed level; then gradually taper the enzyme-inducing AED by 20% decrements each week to fully withdraw over a 4-week period. Two weeks following withdrawal of the enzyme-inducing AED, the dosage of lamotrigine extended release may be tapered in decrements of ≤100 mg/day at intervals of 1 week to achieve a maintenance dosage range of 250 to 300 mg/day

Weeks 1 and 2: 50 mg once daily

Weeks 3 and 4: 100 mg once daily

Maintenance: After week 4, increase dose every 1 week by 100 mg/day to a lamotrigine dose of 500 mg once daily

Anticonvulsant: Absence seizures; monotherapy: Oral: Limited data available; efficacy results variable, optimal dose and titration not defined:

Immediate release formulations: Children and Adolescents 2.5 to 13 years: Initial: 0.3 mg/kg/day in 2 divided doses for 2 weeks; then 0.6 mg/kg/day for 2 weeks; titrate weekly to effect/tolerability to a maximum daily dose of 12 mg/kg/day or 600 mg/day (whichever is less) (Glauser, 2010; Glauser, 2013). Multiple titration strategies have been reported. In the largest trial (n=453), the efficacy of lamotrigine (n=149) was compared with valproic acid (n=148) and ethosuximide (n=156); the initial lamotrigine dose was 0.3 mg/kg/day for 2 weeks, followed by 0.6 mg/kg/day for 2 weeks, then the dose was increased at weekly intervals until efficacy or intolerability in 0.6 mg/kg/day increments up to 3 mg/kg/day for 1 week (week 8), then increased to 4.5 mg/kg/day for 2 weeks, then 7 mg/kg/day for 2 weeks, then 9 mg/kg/day for 2 weeks, and then finally 12 mg/kg/day (week 15); mean final dose reported was 9.7 ± 6.3 mg/kg/day. Results showed the lamotrigine treatment arm had a treatment failure rate of 71%, compared to 47% failure with ethosuximide and 42% failure with valproic acid; the superior efficacy of valproic acid and ethosuximide persisted at 12 months (Glauser, 2010; Glauser, 2013). Another titration strategy based on two smaller studies used a higher initial dose of 0.5 mg/kg/day in 2 divided doses for 2 weeks, increased to 1 mg/kg/day for 2 weeks, then increased by 1 mg/kg/day increments every 5 days (or as clinically indicated) to a maximum of 12 mg/kg/day (Coppola, 2004; Frank, 1999). In one dose-escalation trial of 45 patients (2 to 15 years old), the median effective dose required was 5 mg/kg/day (range: 2 to 15 mg/kg/day) (Frank, 1999). The other study was an open-label trial comparing lamotrigine (n=19) to valproic acid (n=19) in 3 to 13 year olds; the mean lamotrigine dose required at 3 months was 6.5 mg/kg/day (range: 2 to 11.5 mg/kg/day) (Coppola, 2004).

Bipolar disorder: Oral: Immediate release formulation: Adolescents ≥18 years:

*Patients **not** receiving enzyme-inducing drugs (eg, carbamazepine, phenytoin, phenobarbital, primidone, rifampin) or valproate:*

Weeks 1 and 2: 25 mg/day

Weeks 3 and 4: 50 mg/day

Week 5: 100 mg/day

Week 6 and thereafter: 200 mg/day

*Patients receiving **valproate**:*

Weeks 1 and 2: 25 mg every other day

Weeks 3 and 4: 25 mg/day

Week 5: 50 mg/day

Week 6 and thereafter: 100 mg/day

Note: If valproate is discontinued, increase daily lamotrigine dose in 50 mg increments at weekly intervals until dosage of 200 mg/day is attained.

*Patients receiving **enzyme-inducing drugs** (eg, carbamazepine, phenytoin, phenobarbital, primidone, rifampin) **without valproate**:*

Weeks 1 and 2: 50 mg/day

Weeks 3 and 4: 100 mg/day in divided doses

Week 5: 200 mg/day in divided doses

Week 6: 300 mg/day in divided doses

Week 7 and thereafter: May increase to 400 mg/day in divided doses

Note: If carbamazepine (or other enzyme-inducing drug) is discontinued, maintain current lamotrigine dose for 1 week, then decrease daily lamotrigine dose in 100 mg increments at weekly intervals until dosage of 200 mg/day is attained.

Adult:

Lennox-Gastaut (adjunctive): Oral: Immediate release formulation:

*Regimens **not containing** carbamazepine, phenytoin, phenobarbital, primidone, or valproic acid:* Initial: Weeks 1 and 2: 25 mg once daily; Weeks 3 and 4: 50 mg once daily; Week 5 and beyond: Increase by 50 mg daily every 1 to 2 weeks; Usual maintenance: 225 to 375 mg daily in 2 divided doses

*Regimens **containing** valproic acid:* Initial: Weeks 1 and 2: 25 mg every other day; Weeks 3 and 4: 25 mg once daily; Week 5 and beyond: Increase by 25 to 50 mg daily every 1 to 2 weeks; Usual maintenance: 100 to 200 mg daily (valproic acid alone) or 100 to 400 mg daily (valproic acid and other drugs that induce glucuronidation) in 1 or 2 divided doses

*Regimens **containing** carbamazepine, phenytoin, phenobarbital, or primidone and without valproic acid:* Initial: Weeks 1 and 2: 50 mg once daily; Weeks 3 and 4: 100 mg daily in 2 divided doses; Week 5 and beyond: Increase by 100 mg daily every 1 to 2 weeks; Usual maintenance: 300 to 500 mg daily in 2 divided doses; maximum daily dose: 700 mg/**day**

Partial seizures (adjunctive) and primary generalized tonic-clonic seizures (adjunctive): Oral:

Immediate release formulation:

*Regimens **not containing** carbamazepine, phenytoin, phenobarbital, primidone, or valproic acid:* Initial: Weeks 1 and 2: 25 mg once daily; Weeks 3 and 4: 50 mg once daily; Week 5 and beyond: Increase by 50 mg daily every 1 to 2 weeks; Usual maintenance: 225 to 375 mg daily in 2 divided doses

*Regimens **containing** valproic acid:* Initial: Weeks 1 and 2: 25 mg every other day; Weeks 3 and 4: 25 mg once daily; Week 5 and beyond: Increase by 25 to 50 mg daily every 1 to 2 weeks; Usual maintenance: 100 to 200 mg daily (valproic acid alone) or 100 to 400 mg daily (valproic acid and other drugs that induce glucuronidation) in 1 or 2 divided doses

*Regimens **containing** carbamazepine, phenytoin, phenobarbital, or primidone and without valproic acid:* Initial: Weeks 1 and 2: 50 mg once daily; Weeks 3 and 4: 100 mg daily in 2 divided doses; Week 5 and beyond: Increase by 100 mg daily every 1 to 2 weeks; Usual maintenance: 300 to 500 mg daily in 2 divided doses; maximum daily dose: 700 mg

Extended release formulation:

*Regimens **not containing** carbamazepine, phenytoin, phenobarbital, primidone, or valproic acid:* Initial: Weeks 1 and 2: 25 mg once daily; Weeks 3 and 4: 50 mg once daily; Week 5: 100 mg once daily; Week 6: 150 mg once daily; Week 7: 200 mg once daily; Week 8 and beyond: Dose increases should not exceed 100 mg daily at weekly intervals; Usual maintenance: 300 to 400 mg once daily

*Regimens **containing** valproic acid:* Initial: Weeks 1 and 2: 25 mg every other day; Weeks 3 and 4: 25 mg once daily; Week 5: 50 mg once daily; Week 6: 100 mg once daily; Week 7: 150 mg once daily; Week 8 and beyond: Dose increases should not exceed 100 mg daily at weekly intervals; Usual maintenance: 200 to 250 mg once daily

*Regimens **containing** carbamazepine, phenytoin, phenobarbital, or primidone and without valproic acid:* Initial: Weeks 1 and 2: 50 mg once daily; Weeks 3 and 4: 100 mg once daily; Week 5: 200 mg once daily; Week 6: 300 mg once daily; Week 7: 400 mg once daily; Week 8 and beyond: Dose increases should not exceed 100 mg daily at weekly intervals; Usual maintenance: 400 to 600 mg once daily

Conversion strategy from adjunctive therapy with valproic acid to monotherapy with lamotrigine:

Immediate release formulation:

- Initiate and titrate as per escalation recommendations for adjunctive therapy to a lamotrigine dose of 200 mg daily.
- Then taper valproic acid dose in decrements of not >500 mg/day/week to a valproic acid dosage of 500 mg daily; this dosage should be maintained for 1 week. The lamotrigine dosage should then be increased to 300 mg daily while valproic acid is simultaneously decreased to 250 mg daily; this dosage should be maintained for 1 week.
- Valproic acid may then be discontinued, while the lamotrigine dose is increased by 100 mg daily at weekly intervals to achieve a lamotrigine maintenance dose of 500 mg daily in 2 divided doses.

Extended release formulation:

- Initiate and titrate as per escalation recommendations for adjunctive therapy to a lamotrigine dose of 150 mg daily.
- Then taper valproic acid dose in decrements of not >500 mg/day/week to a valproic acid dose of 500 mg daily; this dosage should be maintained for 1 week. The lamotrigine dosage should then be increased to 200 mg daily while valproic acid is simultaneously decreased to 250 mg daily; this dosage should be maintained for 1 week.
- Valproic acid may then be discontinued, while the lamotrigine dose is increased to achieve a maintenance dosage range of 250 to 300 mg once daily.

Conversion strategy from adjunctive therapy with carbamazepine, phenytoin, phenobarbital, or primidone to monotherapy with lamotrigine: Immediate release formulation and extended release formulation:

- Initiate and titrate as per escalation recommendations for adjunctive therapy to a lamotrigine dose of 500 mg daily.
- Concomitant enzyme-inducing AED should then be withdrawn by 20% decrements each week over a 4-week period.
- Two weeks after withdrawal of the enzyme-inducing AED, the dosage of lamotrigine extended release may be tapered in decrements of not >100 mg/day at intervals of 1 week to achieve a maintenance dosage range of 250 to 300 mg once daily; no further dosage reduction is required for lamotrigine immediate release.

Conversion strategy from adjunctive therapy with AED other than carbamazepine, phenytoin, phenobarbital, primidone or valproic acid to monotherapy with lamotrigine:

Immediate release formulation: No specific guidelines available

Extended release formulation: Initiate and titrate as per escalation recommendations for adjunctive therapy to a lamotrigine dose of 250 to 300 mg daily. Concomitant AED should then be withdrawn by 20% decrements each week over a 4-week period.

Conversion from immediate release to extended release (Lamictal XR): Initial dose of the extended release tablet should match the total daily dose of the immediate release formulation. Adjust dose as needed within the recommended dosing guidelines.

Bipolar disorder: Oral: Immediate release formulation:

*Regimens **not containing** carbamazepine, phenytoin, phenobarbital, primidone, or valproic acid:* Initial: Weeks 1 and 2: 25 mg once daily; Weeks 3 and 4: 50 mg once daily; Week 5: 100 mg once daily; Week 6 and maintenance: 200 mg once daily

*Regimens **containing** valproic acid:* Initial: Weeks 1 and 2: 25 mg every other day; Weeks 3 and 4: 25 mg once daily; Week 5: 50 mg once daily; Week 6 and maintenance: 100 mg once daily

*Regimens **containing** carbamazepine, phenytoin, phenobarbital, or primidone and without valproic acid:* Initial: Weeks 1 and 2: 50 mg once daily; Weeks 3 and 4: 100 mg daily in divided doses; Week 5: 200 mg daily in divided doses; Week 6: 300 mg daily in divided doses; Maintenance: Up to 400 mg daily in divided doses

Adjustment following discontinuation of psychotropic medication:

Discontinuing valproic acid with current dose of lamotrigine 100 mg daily: 150 mg daily for week 1, then increase to 200 mg daily beginning week 2

Discontinuing carbamazepine, phenytoin, phenobarbital, primidone, or rifampin with current dose of lamotrigine 400 mg daily: 400 mg daily for week 1, then decrease to 300 mg daily for week 2, then decrease to 200 mg daily beginning week 3

Dosing adjustment with concomitant estrogen-containing oral contraceptives: Adolescents and Adults: Follow initial lamotrigine dosing guidelines, maintenance dose should be adjusted as follows:

*Patients **taking** concomitant carbamazepine, phenytoin, phenobarbital, primidone, or other drugs, such as rifampin, that induce lamotrigine glucuronidation:* No dosing adjustment required

*Patients **not taking** concomitant carbamazepine, phenytoin, phenobarbital, primidone, or other drugs, such as rifampin, that induce lamotrigine glucuronidation:* If already taking estrogen-containing oral contraceptives, the maintenance dose of lamotrigine may need to be increased by as much as twofold over the target maintenance dose listed above. If already taking a stable dose of lamotrigine and starting an oral contraceptive agent, the lamotrigine maintenance dose may need to be increased by as much as twofold. Dose increases should start when contraceptive agent is started and titrated to clinical response increasing no more rapidly than 50 to 100 mg/day every week. Gradual increases of lamotrigine plasma levels may occur during the inactive "pill-free" week and will be greater when dose increases are made the week before. If increased adverse events consistently occur during "pill-free" week, overall dose adjustments may be required. Dose adjustments during "pill-free" week are not recommended. When discontinuing combination hormonal contraceptive, dose of lamotrigine may need decreased by as much as 50%; do not decrease by more than 25% of total daily dose over a 2-week period unless clinical response or plasma levels indicate otherwise.

Additional considerations:

Discontinuing therapy: Children ≥2 years, Adolescents, and Adults: Do not abruptly discontinue; when discontinuing lamotrigine therapy, gradually decrease the dose by ~50% per week and taper over at least 2 weeks unless safety concerns require a more rapid withdrawal. **Note:** If discontinuing other anticonvulsants and maintaining lamotrigine therapy, keep in mind that discontinuing carbamazepine, phenytoin, phenobarbital, primidone, or other drugs, such as rifampin, that induce lamotrigine glucuronidation should prolong the half-life of lamotrigine; discontinuing valproic acid should shorten the half-life of lamotrigine; monitor patient closely; dosage change may be needed.

Restarting therapy after discontinuation: Children ≥2 years, Adolescents, and Adults: If lamotrigine has been withheld for >5 half-lives, restart according to initial dosing recommendations. **Note:** Concomitant medications may affect the half-life of lamotrigine; consider pharmacokinetic interactions when restarting therapy.

Dosing adjustment in renal impairment: Use with caution; has not been adequately studied; base initial dose on patient's AED regimen; decreased maintenance dosage may be effective in patients with significant renal impairment; during a 4-hour hemodialysis period, ~20% is removed

Dosing adjustment in hepatic impairment: Note: Adjust escalation and maintenance doses by clinical response.

Mild hepatic impairment: No dosage adjustment required

Moderate and severe hepatic impairment without ascites: Reduce initial, escalation, and maintenance doses by ~25%

Severe hepatic impairment with ascites: Reduce initial, escalation, and maintenance doses by 50%

Preparation for Administration Oral: Chewable, dispersible tablet: To disperse, add tablets to a small amount of liquid (~5 mL or enough to cover the medication); tablets should be completely dispersed in about 1 minute.

Administration Oral: Doses should be rounded down to the nearest whole tablet. May be administered without regard to food. If medication is received in blisterpack, examine blisterpack before use; do not use if blisters are broken, torn, or missing.

Regular tablet: Do not chew, as a bitter taste may result; swallow tablet whole

Chewable, dispersible tablet: Only whole tablets should be administered (tablets should not be cut or divided); may swallow whole, chew, or disperse in water or diluted fruit juice; if chewed, administer a small amount of water or diluted fruit juice to help in swallowing. If dispersed in a small amount of liquid, swirl the solution after tablet completely dispersed and administer entire amount immediately. Do not attempt to administer partial quantities of dispersed tablets.

Extended-release tablet (Lamictal XR): May be administered without regard to meals. Swallow tablet whole; do not chew, crush, or break.

Orally disintegrating tablet (Lamictal ODT): Place tablet on tongue and move around in the mouth. Tablet will dissolve rapidly and can be swallowed with or without food or water.

Monitoring Parameters All patients: Monitor for hypersensitivity reactions, especially rash; CBC with differential; liver and renal function

Epilepsy: Seizure frequency, duration, and severity; serum levels of concurrent anticonvulsants; signs and symptoms of suicidality (eg, anxiety, depression, behavior changes)

Bipolar disorder: Clinical worsening of depressive symptoms or suicidality, especially with initiation of therapy or dosage changes

Reference Range The clinical value of monitoring lamotrigine plasma concentrations has not been established. Dosing should be based on therapeutic response. Proposed therapeutic range: 1-5 mcg/mL. Lamotrigine plasma concentrations of 0.25-29.1 mcg/mL have been reported in the literature.

Test Interactions May interfere with some rapid urine drug screens, particularly phencyclidine (false-positives).

Additional Information Low water solubility. Does **not** induce P450 microsomal enzymes. The clinical usefulness of lamotrigine should be periodically re-evaluated in patients with bipolar disorder who are receiving the drug for extended intervals (ie, >16 weeks).

The extended-release tablets contain a modified-release eroding formulation as the core of the tablet. The clear enteric coating has an aperture drilled through it on both sides of the tablet; this allows an extended release of the medication in the acidic environment within the stomach. The design of the table controls the dissolution rate of the medication over a 12-15 hour period.

Three different lamotrigine "Starter Kits" are available for adult patients for three different dosage forms (tablets, extended release tablets, and orally disintegrating tablets); each starter kit contains a blisterpack with a certain number and mg strength of tablets that are specific for initiating doses in different patient populations.

Dosage Forms Considerations

LaMICtal Kits are available as follows:

Blue - for patients already taking valproate

LaMICtal Starter: 25 mg (35s)

LaMICtal ODT (Titration): 25 mg (21s) and 50 mg (7s)

LaMICtal XR (Titration): 25 mg (21s) and 50 mg (7s)

Green- for patients already taking carbamazepine, phenytoin, phenobarbital, or primidone, and **not** taking valproate

LaMICtal Starter: 25 mg (84s) and 100 mg (14s)

LaMICtal ODT (Titration): 50 mg (42s) and 100 mg (14s)

LaMICtal XR (Titration): 50 mg (14s) and 100 mg (14s) and 200 mg (7s)

Orange - for patients not taking carbamazepine, phenytoin, phenobarbital, primidone, or valproate

LaMICtal Starter: 25 mg (42s) and 100 mg (7s)

LaMICtal ODT (Titration): 25 mg (14s) and 50 mg (14s) and 100 mg (7s)

LaMICtal XR (Titration): 25 mg (14s) and 50 mg (14s) and 100 mg (7s)

Dosage Forms Excipient information presented when available (limited, particularly for generics); consult specific product labeling. [DSC] = Discontinued product

Kit, Oral:

LaMICtal ODT: Blue Kit: 25 mg (21s) & 50 mg (7s), Orange Kit: 25 mg (14s) & 50 mg (14s) & 100 mg (7s), Green Kit: 50 mg (42s) & 100 mg (14s)

LaMICtal Starter: Blue Kit: 25 mg (35s)

LaMICtal Starter: Green Kit: 25 mg (84s) & 100 mg (14s), Orange Kit: 25 mg (42s) & 100 mg (7s) [contains fd&c yellow #6 aluminum lake]

LaMICtal XR: Green Kit: 50 mg (14s) & 100 mg (14s) & 200 mg (7s) [contains fd&c blue #2 aluminum lake, polysorbate 80]

LaMICtal XR: Blue Kit: 25 mg (21s) & 50 mg (7s), Orange Kit: 25 mg (14s) & 50 mg (14s) & 100 mg (7s) [contains polysorbate 80]

Tablet, Oral:

LaMICtal: 25 mg, 100 mg, 150 mg, 200 mg [scored]

Generic: 25 mg, 100 mg, 150 mg, 200 mg

Tablet Chewable, Oral:

LaMICtal: 2 mg [DSC] [contains saccharin sodium]

LaMICtal: 5 mg [scored; berry flavor]

LaMICtal: 25 mg [berry flavor]

Generic: 5 mg, 25 mg

Tablet Dispersible, Oral:

LaMICtal ODT: 25 mg, 50 mg, 100 mg, 200 mg

Generic: 25 mg, 50 mg, 100 mg, 200 mg

Tablet Extended Release 24 Hour, Oral:

LaMICtal XR: 25 mg, 50 mg, 100 mg [contains polysorbate 80]

LaMICtal XR: 200 mg [contains fd&c blue #2 aluminum lake, polysorbate 80]

LaMICtal XR: 250 mg [contains fd&c blue #2 aluminum lake]

LaMICtal XR: 300 mg [contains polysorbate 80]
Generic: 25 mg, 50 mg, 100 mg, 200 mg, 250 mg, 300 mg

Extemporaneous Preparations A 1 mg/mL oral suspension may be made with tablets and one of two different vehicles (a 1:1 mixture of Ora-Sweet and Ora-Plus or a 1:1 mixture of Ora-Sweet SF and Ora-Plus). Crush one 100 mg tablet in a mortar and reduce to a fine powder. Add small portions of the chosen vehicle and mix to a uniform paste; mix while adding the vehicle in incremental proportions to **almost** 100 mL; transfer to a graduated cylinder, rinse mortar with vehicle, and add quantity of vehicle sufficient to make 100 mL. Label "shake well" and "protect from light". Stable for 91 days when stored in amber plastic prescription bottles in the dark at room temperature or refrigerated.

Nahata M, Morosco R, Hipple T. "Stability of Lamotrigine in Two Extemporaneously Prepared Oral Suspensions at 4 and 25 Degrees C," *Am J Health Syst Pharm*, 1999, 56(3):240-2.

◆ **Lanoxin** *see* Digoxin *on page 652*

◆ **Lanoxin Pediatric** *see* Digoxin *on page 652*

Lansoprazole (lan SOE pra zole)

Medication Safety Issues

Sound-alike/look-alike issues:

Lansoprazole may be confused with aripiprazole, dexlansoprazole

Prevacid may be confused with Pravachol, Prevpac, PriLOSEC, Prinivil

Related Information

Oral Medications That Should Not Be Crushed or Altered *on page 2476*

Brand Names: US First-Lansoprazole; Heartburn Relief 24 Hour [OTC] [DSC]; Heartburn Treatment 24 Hour [OTC]; Prevacid; Prevacid 24HR [OTC]; Prevacid SoluTab

Brand Names: Canada Apo-Lansoprazole; Mylan-Lansoprazole; PMS-Lansoprazole; Prevacid; Prevacid FasTab; Q-Lansoprazole; RAN-Lansoprazole; Riva-Lansoprazole; Sandoz-Lansoprazole; Teva-Lansoprazole

Therapeutic Category Gastric Acid Secretion Inhibitor; Gastrointestinal Agent, Gastric or Duodenal Ulcer Treatment; Proton Pump Inhibitor

Generic Availability (US) May be product dependent

Use Short-term treatment of symptomatic gastroesophageal reflux disease (GERD) (FDA approved in ages ≥1 year and adults); short-term treatment (up to 8 weeks) for healing and symptomatic relief of all grades of erosive esophagitis (FDA approved in ages ≥1 year and adults); maintenance of healed erosive esophagitis (FDA approved in adults); short-term treatment (up to 8 weeks) of active benign gastric ulcer (FDA approved in adults); short-term treatment (≤4 weeks) for healing and symptomatic relief of active duodenal ulcer (FDA approved in adults); maintenance treatment of healed duodenal ulcers (FDA approved in adults); treatment of pathological hypersecretory conditions, including Zollinger-Ellison syndrome (FDA approved in adults); adjuvant therapy in the treatment of duodenal ulcers associated with *Helicobacter pylori* (FDA approved in adults); prevention (for patients at high risk) and treatment of NSAID-associated gastric ulcers (FDA approved in adults); relief of frequent heartburn (≥2 days/week) (OTC product: FDA approved in adults)

Medication Guide Available Yes

Pregnancy Risk Factor B

Pregnancy Considerations Adverse events have not been observed in animal reproduction studies. An increased risk of hypospadias was reported following maternal use of proton pump inhibitors (PPIs) during pregnancy (Anderka, 2012), but this was based on a small number of exposures and the same association was not found in another study (Erichsen, 2012). Most available studies have not shown an increased risk of major birth defects following maternal use of PPIs during pregnancy (Diav-Citrin, 2005; Matok, 2012; Pasternak, 2010). When treating GERD in pregnancy, PPIs may be used when clinically indicated (Katz, 2013).

Breast-Feeding Considerations It is not known if lansoprazole is excreted in breast milk. Due to the potential for serious adverse reactions in the nursing infant, the manufacturer recommends a decision be made whether to discontinue nursing or to discontinue the drug, taking into account the importance of treatment to the mother.

Contraindications Hypersensitivity (eg, anaphylaxis, angioedema, anaphylactic shock, angioedema, bronchospasm, acute interstitial nephritis, urticaria) to lansoprazole, other substituted benzimidazole proton pump inhibitors, or any component of the formulation

Warnings/Precautions Use of proton pump inhibitors (PPIs) may increase the risk of gastrointestinal infections (eg, *Salmonella, Campylobacter*). Relief of symptoms does not preclude the presence of a gastric malignancy. Atrophic gastritis (by biopsy) has been noted with long-term omeprazole therapy; this may also occur with lansoprazole. No reports of enterochromaffin-like (ECL) cell carcinoids, dysplasia, or neoplasia have occurred. Use of proton pump inhibitors (PPIs) may increase risk of CDAD, especially in hospitalized patients; consider CDAD diagnosis in patients with persistent diarrhea that does not improve. Use the lowest dose and shortest duration of PPI therapy appropriate for the condition being treated. Severe liver dysfunction may require dosage reductions. Decreased *H. pylori* eradication rates have been observed with short-term (≤7 days) combination therapy. The American College of Gastroenterology recommends 10-14 days of therapy (triple or quadruple) for eradication of *H. pylori* (Chey, 2007).

PPIs may diminish the therapeutic effect of clopidogrel thought to be due to reduced formation of the active metabolite of clopidogrel. The manufacturer of clopidogrel recommends either avoidance of both omeprazole (even when scheduled 12 hours apart) and esomeprazole or use of a PPI with comparatively less effect on the active metabolite of clopidogrel (eg, pantoprazole). Although lansoprazole exhibits the most potent CYP2C19 inhibition *in vitro* (Li, 2004; Ogilvie, 2011), an *in vivo* study of extensive CYP2C19 metabolizers showed less reduction of the active metabolite of clopidogrel by lansoprazole/dexlansoprazole compared to esomeprazole/omeprazole (Frelinger, 2012). The manufacturer of lansoprazole states that no dosage adjustment is necessary for clopidogrel when used concurrently. In contrast to these warnings, others have recommended the continued use of PPIs, regardless of the degree of inhibition, in patients with a history of GI bleeding or multiple risk factors for GI bleeding who are also receiving clopidogrel since no evidence has established clinically meaningful differences in outcome; however, a clinically-significant interaction cannot be excluded in those who are poor metabolizers of clopidogrel (Abraham, 2010; Levine, 2011). Additionally, concomitant use of lansoprazole with some drugs may require cautious use, may not be recommended, or may require dosage adjustments.

Increased incidence of osteoporosis-related bone fractures of the hip, spine, or wrist may occur with PPI therapy. Patients on high-dose or long-term therapy should be monitored. Use the lowest effective dose for the shortest duration of time, use vitamin D and calcium supplementation, and follow appropriate guidelines to reduce risk of fractures in patients at risk. Acute interstitial nephritis has been observed in patients taking PPIs; may occur at any time during therapy and is generally due to an idiopathic hypersensitivity reaction. Discontinue if acute interstitial nephritis develops. Lansoprazole has been shown to be ineffective for the treatment of symptomatic GERD in children 1 month to <1 year.

Hypomagnesemia, reported rarely, usually with prolonged PPI use of >3 months (most cases >1 year of therapy); may be symptomatic or asymptomatic; severe cases may cause tetany, seizures, and cardiac arrhythmias. Consider obtaining serum magnesium concentrations prior to beginning long-term therapy, especially if taking concomitant digoxin, diuretics, or other drugs known to cause hypomagnesemia; and periodically thereafter. Hypomagnesemia may be corrected by magnesium supplementation, although discontinuation of lansoprazole may be necessary; magnesium levels typically return to normal within 1 week of stopping.

Prolonged treatment (≥2 years) may lead to vitamin B_{12} malabsorption and subsequent vitamin B_{12} deficiency. The magnitude of the deficiency is dose-related and the association is stronger in females and those younger in age (<30 years); prevalence is decreased after discontinuation of therapy (Lam, 2013).

Benzyl alcohol and derivatives: Some dosage forms may contain benzyl alcohol; large amounts of benzyl alcohol (≥99 mg/kg/day) have been associated with a potentially fatal toxicity ("gasping syndrome") in neonates; the "gasping syndrome" consists of metabolic acidosis, respiratory distress, gasping respirations, CNS dysfunction (including convulsions, intracranial hemorrhage), hypotension, and cardiovascular collapse (AAP, 1997; CDC, 1982); some data suggests that benzoate displaces bilirubin from protein binding sites (Ahlfors, 2001); avoid or use dosage forms containing benzyl alcohol with caution in neonates. See manufacturer's labeling.

When used for self-medication, patients should be instructed not to use if they have difficulty swallowing, are vomiting blood, or have bloody or black stools. Prior to use, patients should contact healthcare provider if they have liver disease, heartburn for >3 months, heartburn with dizziness, lightheadedness, or sweating, MI symptoms, frequent chest pain, frequent wheezing (especially with heartburn), unexplained weight loss, nausea/vomiting, stomach pain, or are taking antifungals, atazanavir, digoxin, tacrolimus, theophylline, or warfarin. Patients should stop use and consult a healthcare provider if heartburn continues or worsens, or if they need to take for >14 days or more often than every 4 months. Patients should be informed that it may take 1-4 days for full effect to be seen; should not be used for immediate relief.

Adverse Reactions

Central nervous system: Dizziness, headache

Gastrointestinal: Abdominal pain, constipation, diarrhea, nausea

Rare but important or life-threatening: Abdomen enlarged, abnormal dreams, abnormal menses, abnormal stools, abnormal vision, agitation, agranulocytosis, albuminuria, allergic reaction, alkaline phosphatase increased, ALT increased, alopecia, amblyopia, amnesia, anaphylactoid reaction, anemia, angina, anorexia, anxiety, aplastic anemia, appetite increased, arrhythmia, AST increased, arthralgia, arthritis, asthma, avitaminosis, bezoar, bilirubinemia, blepharitis, blurred vision, bradycardia, breast enlargement, breast pain, breast tenderness, bronchitis, candidiasis, carcinoma, cardiospasm, cataract, cerebrovascular accident, cerebral infarction, chest pain, chills, cholelithiasis, cholesterol increased/decreased, *Clostridium difficile*-associated diarrhea (CDAD), colitis, confusion, conjunctivitis, cough increased, creatinine increased, deafness, dehydration, dementia, depersonalization, depression, diabetes mellitus, diaphoresis, diplopia, dry eyes, dry skin, dyspepsia, dysphagia, dyspnea, dysmenorrhea, dysuria, edema, electrolyte imbalance, emotional lability, enteritis, eosinophilia, epistaxis, eructation, erythema multiforme, esophageal stenosis, esophageal ulcer, esophagitis, fecal discoloration, fever, fixed eruption, flatulence, flu-like syndrome, fracture, fundic gland polyps, gastric nodules, gastrin level increased, gastritis, gastroenteritis, gastrointestinal anomaly, gastrointestinal hemorrhage, GGTP increased/decreased, glaucoma, glucocorticoid levels increased, glossitis, glycosuria, goiter, gout, gum hemorrhage, gynecomastia, halitosis, hallucinations, hematemesis, hematuria, hemiplegia, hemolysis, hemolytic anemia, hemoptysis, hepatotoxicity, hostility aggravated, hyper-/hypoglycemia, hyperkinesia, hyperlipemia, hypertonia, hypoesthesia, hyper-/hypotension, hypomagnesemia, hypothyroidism, impotence, infection, insomnia, interstitial nephritis, kidney calculus, laryngeal neoplasia, LDH increased, leg cramps, leukopenia, leukorrhea, libido decreased/increased, liver function test abnormal, lung fibrosis, lymphadenopathy, maculopapular rash, malaise, melena, menorrhagia, migraine, moniliasis (oral), mouth ulceration, musculoskeletal pain, myalgia, myasthenia, myositis, MI, nervousness, neurosis, neutropenia, pain, palpitation, pancreatitis, pancytopenia, paresthesia, parosmia, pelvic pain, peripheral edema, pharyngitis, photophobia, platelet abnormalities, pneumonia, polyuria, pruritus, ptosis, rash, rectal hemorrhage, retinal degeneration, rhinitis, salivation increased, seizure, shock, sinusitis, skin carcinoma, sleep disorder, somnolence, speech disorder, Stevens-Johnson syndrome, stomatitis, stridor, syncope, synovitis, tachycardia, taste loss, taste perversion, tenesmus, thirst, thrombocytopenia, thrombotic thrombocytopenic purpura, tinnitus, tremor, tongue disorder, toxic epidermal necrolysis, ulcerative colitis, ulcerative stomatitis, upper respiratory inflammation, upper respiratory infection, urethral pain, urinary frequency/urgency, urination impaired, urinary retention, urinary tract infection, urticaria, vaginitis, vasodilation, vertigo, visual field defect, vomiting, weakness, WBC abnormal, weight gain/loss, xerostomia

Drug Interactions

Metabolism/Transport Effects Substrate of CYP2C19 (major), CYP2C9 (minor), CYP3A4 (major); **Note:** Assignment of Major/Minor substrate status based on clinically relevant drug interaction potential; **Inhibits** CYP2C19 (weak), CYP2C9 (weak), CYP2D6 (weak); **Induces** CYP1A2 (weak/moderate)

Avoid Concomitant Use

Avoid concomitant use of Lansoprazole with any of the following: Dasatinib; Delavirdine; Erlotinib; Nelfinavir; PAZOPanib; Rilpivirine; Risedronate

Increased Effect/Toxicity

Lansoprazole may increase the levels/effects of: Amphetamine; ARIPiprazole; Dexmethylphenidate; Dextroamphetamine; Imatinib; Methotrexate; Methylphenidate; Raltegravir; Risedronate; Saquinavir; Tacrolimus (Systemic); Vitamin K Antagonists; Voriconazole

The levels/effects of Lansoprazole may be increased by: Fluconazole; Ketoconazole (Systemic); Voriconazole

Decreased Effect

Lansoprazole may decrease the levels/effects of: Atazanavir; Bisphosphonate Derivatives; Bosutinib; Cefditoren; Clopidogrel; Dabigatran Etexilate; Dabrafenib; Dasatinib; Delavirdine; Erlotinib; Gefitinib; Indinavir; Iron Salts; Itraconazole; Ketoconazole (Systemic); Ledipasvir; Mesalamine; Multivitamins/Minerals (with ADEK, Folate, Iron); Mycophenolate; Nelfinavir; Nilotinib; PAZOPanib; Posaconazole; Rilpivirine; Riociguat; Risedronate

The levels/effects of Lansoprazole may be decreased by: Bosentan; CYP2C19 Inducers (Strong); CYP3A4 Inducers (Moderate); CYP3A4 Inducers (Strong); Dabrafenib; Deferasirox; Mitotane; Siltuximab; St Johns Wort; Tipranavir; Tocilizumab

Food Interactions Prolonged treatment (≥2 years) may lead to malabsorption of dietary vitamin B_{12} and subsequent vitamin B_{12} deficiency (Lam, 2013).

Storage/Stability

Capsules, orally disintegrating tablets: Store at 25°C (77°F); excursions permitted to 15°C to 30°C (59°F to 86°F). Protect from light and moisture.

Powder for suspension (First® compounding kit): Prior to compounding, store at 15°C to 30°C (59°F to 86°F). Once compounded, the product is stable for 30 days at room temperature and under refrigeration; manufacturer recommendation is for the compounded product to be stored under refrigeration; protect from freezing. Protect from light.

Mechanism of Action Decreases acid secretion in gastric parietal cells through inhibition of (H+, K+)-ATPase enzyme system, blocking the final step in gastric acid production.

Pharmacodynamics

Duration of antisecretory activity: ≥24 hours

Relief of symptoms:

- Gastric or duodenal ulcers: 1 week
- Reflux esophagitis: 1-4 weeks

Ulcer healing:

- Duodenal: 2 weeks
- Gastric: 4 weeks

Pharmacokinetics (Adult data unless noted)

Absorption: Extremely acid labile and will degrade in acid pH of stomach; enteric coated granules improve bioavailability (80%)

Distribution: V_d:

- Children: 0.61-0.9 L/kg
- Adults: 15.7 ± 1.9 L

Protein binding: 97%

Metabolism: Hepatic via CYP2C19 and 3A4 to inactive metabolites, and in parietal cells to two active metabolites that are not present in systemic circulation

Bioavailability: 80% (reduced by 50% to 70% if given 30 minutes after food)

Half-life:

- Children: 1.2-1.5 hours
- Adults: 1.5 ± 1 hour

Time to peak serum concentration: 1.7 hours

Elimination: Biliary excretion is major route of elimination; feces (67%); urine (33%; 14% to 25% as metabolites and <1% as unchanged drug)

Clearance:

- Children: 0.57-0.71 L/hour/kg
- Adults: 11.1 ± 3.8 L/hour
- Adults: Hepatic impairment: 3.2-7.2 hours

Dosing: Neonatal GERD: Oral: Limited data available; dose not established; ideal dose-response not established: 0.5 to 1.5 mg/kg/day as a single dose or divided twice daily has been shown to be well tolerated and improve gastric pH; 0.5 to 1 mg/kg administered once daily was evaluated in 24 neonates (mean PNA: 3.7 ± 4 weeks, mean weight: 3.015 ± 0.893 kg); this regimen resulted in increased gastric pH and was associated with a decreased frequency of GERD symptoms (Springer, 2008). In another study, 10 VLBW premature neonates (mean PNA: 3.6 ± 1.49 weeks, mean weight: 1.13 ± 0.03 kg) received 1.5 mg/kg/day divided twice daily; although gastric pH increased it was not adequate to protect from esophagitis (Tham, 2012). A pharmacokinetic study showed patients <10 weeks of age had substantially decreased clearance and suggests a lower dose should be used (~0.2 mg/kg/day) (Zhang, 2008).

Dosing: Usual

Pediatric:

GERD, symptomatic:

Weight-based dosing:

Infants: 1 to 2 mg/kg/day (Orenstein, 2009; Springer, 2008; Zhang, 2008). **Note:** A pharmacokinetic study showed patients <10 weeks of age had substantially decreased clearance and suggests a lower dose should be used (~0.2 mg/kg/day) (Zhang, 2008).

Children: 0.7 to 3 mg/kg/day (AAP [Lightdale], 2013)

Fixed dosing:

Infants ≥3 months: 7.5 mg twice daily **or** 15 mg once daily was shown to provide better symptom relief compared to dietary management in 68 patients (Khoshoo, 2008)

Children 1 to 11 years:

- ≤30 kg: 15 mg once daily for up to 12 weeks
- >30 kg: 30 mg once daily for up to 12 weeks

Children ≥12 years and Adolescents: Oral: 15 mg once daily for up to 8 weeks

Erosive esophagitis:

Children 1-11 years:

- ≤30 kg: 15 mg once daily for up to 12 weeks
- >30 kg: 30 mg once daily for up to 12 weeks

Children ≥12 years and Adolescents: Oral: 30 mg once daily for up to 8 weeks

Adult:

Duodenal ulcer: Oral: 15 mg once daily for 4 weeks; maintenance therapy: 15 mg once daily

Erosive esophagitis: Oral: 30 mg once daily for up to 8 weeks; additional 8 weeks may be tried in those patients who failed to respond or for a recurrence of esophagitis; maintenance: 15 mg once daily

Gastric ulcer: Oral: 30 mg once daily for up to 8 weeks

GERD, symptomatic: Oral: 15 mg once daily for up to 8 weeks

Hypersecretory conditions: Oral: Initial: 60 mg once daily; adjust dosage based upon patient response and to reduce acid secretion to <10 mEq/hour (5 mEq/hour in patients with prior gastric surgery); doses of 90 mg twice daily have been used; administer doses >120 mg/day in divided doses

***Helicobacter pylori* eradication:** Oral: 30 mg twice daily for 2 weeks (in combination with amoxicillin and clarithromycin). Alternatively, in patients allergic to or intolerant of clarithromycin or in whom resistance to clarithromycin is known or suspected, lansoprazole 30 mg every 8 hours may be given for 2 weeks (in combination with amoxicillin)

NSAID-associated gastric ulcer: Oral:

- Healing: 30 mg once daily for up to 8 weeks
- Prevention: 15 mg once daily for up to 12 weeks

Heartburn: OTC labeling: Oral: 15 mg once daily for 14 days; may repeat 14 days of therapy every 4 months. Do not take for >14 days or more often than every 4 months, unless instructed by healthcare provider.

Dosing adjustment in renal impairment: Children, Adolescents, and Adults: No dosage adjustments are recommended

Dosing adjustment in hepatic impairment: Children, Adolescents, and Adults: Bioavailability increased in hepatic impairment; consider dose reduction for severe impairment

Administration Oral: Administer before eating; best if taken 30 minutes before a meal (Lightdale 2013); intact granules should not be chewed or crushed

Capsules: Swallow whole; do not chew or crush. For patients with difficulty swallowing the capsule, capsules may be opened and the intact granules sprinkled on 1 tablespoon of applesauce, Ensure pudding, cottage cheese, yogurt, or strained pears; the mixture should be swallowed immediately. Capsules may also be opened and emptied into ~60 mL of apple juice, orange juice, or tomato juice; mix and swallow immediately. Rinse the glass with additional juice and swallow to assure complete delivery of the dose.

For nasogastric tube ≥16 French: Capsule can be opened, the granules mixed (not crushed) with 40 mL of apple juice and then injected through the NG tube into the stomach, then flush tube with additional apple juice. Do not mix with other liquids based on manufacturer labeling; additional information may be available for NG administration; contact manufacturer to obtain current recommendations.

Tablet, orally-disintegrating: Should not be swallowed whole, broken, cut, or chewed. Place the tablet on the tongue and allow to disintegrate with or without water until the particles can be swallowed.

Administration via an oral syringe: Place the 15 mg tablet in an oral syringe and draw up ~4 mL water, or place the 30 mg tablet in an oral syringe and draw up ~10 mL water. Shake gently. After tablet has dispersed, administer within 15 minutes. Refill the syringe with water (2 mL for the 15 mg tablet; 5 mL for the 30 mg tablet), shake gently, then administer any remaining contents.

For nasogastric tube ≥8 French: Place a 15 mg tablet in a syringe and draw up ~4 mL water, or place the 30 mg tablet in a syringe and draw up ~10 mL water. Shake gently. After tablet has dispersed, administer within 15 minutes. Refill the syringe with ~5 mL water, shake gently, and then flush the nasogastric tube.

Monitoring Parameters Patients with Zollinger-Ellison syndrome should be monitored for gastric acid output, which should be maintained at 10 mEq/hour or less during the last hour before the next lansoprazole dose; lab monitoring should include CBC, liver function, renal function, and serum gastrin levels

Dosage Forms Excipient information presented when available (limited, particularly for generics); consult specific product labeling. [DSC] = Discontinued product

Capsule Delayed Release, Oral:

Heartburn Relief 24 Hour: 15 mg [DSC] [sodium free; contains brilliant blue fcf (fd&c blue #1), fd&c red #40, fd&c yellow #10 (quinoline yellow)]

Heartburn Treatment 24 Hour: 15 mg [sodium free; contains brilliant blue fcf (fd&c blue #1), fd&c yellow #10 (quinoline yellow)]

Prevacid: 15 mg, 30 mg [contains brilliant blue fcf (fd&c blue #1), fd&c red #40]

Prevacid 24HR: 15 mg [sodium free; contains brilliant blue fcf (fd&c blue #1), fd&c red #40]

Generic: 15 mg, 30 mg

Suspension, Oral:

First-Lansoprazole: 3 mg/mL (90 mL, 150 mL, 300 mL) [contains benzyl alcohol, fd&c red #40, saccharin sodium; strawberry flavor]

Tablet Dispersible, Oral:

Prevacid SoluTab: 15 mg, 30 mg [contains aspartame]

Extemporaneous Preparations A 3 mg/mL oral solution (Simplified Lansoprazole Solution [SLS]) may be made with capsules and sodium bicarbonate. Empty the contents of ten lansoprazole 30 mg capsules into a beaker. Add 100 mL sodium bicarbonate 8.4% and gently stir until dissolved (about 15 minutes). Transfer solution to an amber-colored syringe or bottle. A prior study showed that SLS was stable for 8 hours at room temperature or for 14 days refrigerated (DiGiancinto, 2000). However, a more recent study, demonstrated SLS to be stable for 48 hours at room temperature in oral syringes and for only 7 days when refrigerated (Morrison, 2013).

Note: A more palatable lansoprazole (3 mg/mL) suspension is commercially available as a compounding kit (First-Lansoprazole).

DiGiancinto JL, Olsen KM, Bergman KL, et al, "Stability of Suspension Formulations of Lansoprazole and Omeprazole Stored in Amber-Colored Plastic Oral Syringes," *Ann Pharmacother*, 2000, 34(5):600-5

Morrison JT, Lugo RA, Thigpen JC, et al, "Stability of Extemporaneously Prepared Lansoprazole Suspension at Two Temperatures," *J Pediatr Pharmacol Ther*, 2013, 18(2):122-7.

Sharma V, "Comparison of 24-hour Intragastric pH Using Four Liquid Formulations of Lansoprazole and Omeprazole," *Am J Health Syst Pharm*, 1999, 56(Suppl 4):18-21.

Sharma VK, Vasudeva R, and Howden CW, "Simplified Lansoprazole Suspension - Liquid Formulations of Lansoprazole - Effectively Suppresses Intragastric Acidity When Administered Through a Gastrostomy," *Am J Gastroenterol*, 1999, 94(7):1813-7.

◆ **Lantus** *see* Insulin Glargine *on page* 1126

◆ **Lantus OptiSet (Can)** *see* Insulin Glargine *on page* 1126

◆ **Lantus SoloStar** *see* Insulin Glargine *on page* 1126

◆ **Lanvis® (Can)** *see* Thioguanine *on page* 2049

◆ **L-Arginine** *see* Arginine *on page* 190

◆ **L-Arginine Hydrochloride** *see* Arginine *on page* 190

Laronidase (lair OH ni days)

Brand Names: US Aldurazyme

Brand Names: Canada Aldurazyme®

Therapeutic Category Enzyme; Mucopolysaccharidosis I (MPS I) Disease, Treatment Agent

Generic Availability (US) No

Use Treatment of patients with Hurler and Hurler-Scheie forms of mucopolysaccharidosis I (MPS I), and patients with the Scheie form who have moderate to severe symptoms (FDA approved in ages ≥6 months and adults)

Pregnancy Risk Factor B

Pregnancy Considerations Teratogenic effects were not observed in animal reproduction studies. Patients are encouraged to enroll in the MPS I registry (800-745-4447 or www.MPSIregistry.com).

Breast-Feeding Considerations It is not known if laronidase is excreted in breast milk. The manufacturer recommends that caution be exercised when administering laronidase to nursing women.

Contraindications

There are no contraindications listed within the manufacturer's U.S. labeling.

Canadian labeling: Severe hypersensitivity to laronidase or any component of the formulation

Warnings/Precautions [U.S. Boxed Warning]: Anaphylactic reactions have been observed during infusion, immediate treatment for hypersensitivity reactions should be available during administration. Additional monitoring may be required in patients with compromised respiratory function or acute respiratory disease; may be at increased risk for acute exacerbation of respiratory symptoms due to infusion reaction. Reactions, which may include airway obstruction, bradycardia, bronchospasm, hypotension, hypoxia, respiratory distress/failure, stridor, tachypnea, and urticaria, may be severe and tend to occur during or within 3 hours after administration. Immediately discontinue infusion if severe reactions occur; medical support should be available during administration. Risks and benefits should be carefully considered prior to readministration following a severe hypersensitivity reaction. Patients who initially experience severe reactions may require prolonged monitoring. In the case of anaphylaxis, caution should be used if epinephrine is being considered; many patients with MPS I have pre-existing heart disease.

Infusion reactions may occur; use caution and consider delaying treatment in patients with acute febrile/respiratory illness; may result in increased risk for infusion-related reactions. Pretreatment with antipyretics and antihistamines is recommended. Decrease infusion rate, temporarily discontinue infusion, and/or administer additional antipyretics and antihistamines to manage infusion reactions.

Use with caution in patients at risk for fluid overload or in conditions where fluid restriction is indicated (eg, acute underlying respiratory illness, compromised cardiac and/or respiratory function); conditions may be exacerbated during infusion. Extended observation may be necessary for some patients. Use with caution in patients with sleep apnea; evaluate patients prior to initiation of therapy. Apnea treatment options should be readily available (eg, CPAP or supplemental oxygen) during infusion or with use of sedating antihistamines.

Use has not been studied in patients with mild symptoms of the Scheie form of MPS I. Not indicated for the CNS manifestations of the disorder. A patient registry has been established and all patients are encouraged to participate. Registry information may be obtained at www.-MPSIregistry.com or by calling 800-745-4447.

Some dosage forms may contain polysorbate 80 (also known as Tweens). Hypersensitivity reactions, usually a delayed reaction, have been reported following exposure to pharmaceutical products containing polysorbate 80 in certain individuals (Isaksson, 2002; Lucente 2000; Shelley, 1995). Thrombocytopenia, ascites, pulmonary deterioration, and renal and hepatic failure have been reported in premature neonates after receiving parenteral products containing polysorbate 80 (Alade, 1986; CDC, 1984). See manufacturer's labeling.

Adverse Reactions

Cardiovascular: Chest pain, edema, facial edema, flushing, hyper-/hypotension, pallor, poor venous access, tachycardia

Central nervous system: Chills, fever, headache

Dermatologic: Hyperhidrosis, pruritus, rash, urticaria

Gastrointestinal: Abdominal pain/discomfort, diarrhea, vomiting

Hematologic: Thrombocytopenia

Hepatic: Bilirubinemia

Immunologic: Antibody development

Local: Abscess, injection site pain, injection site reaction

Neuromuscular & skeletal: Arthralgia, back pain, hyperreflexia, musculoskeletal pain, paresthesia, tremor

Ocular: Corneal opacity

Otic: Otitis media

Respiratory: Bronchospasm, cough, crepitations, dyspnea, oxygen saturation decreased, respiratory distress, upper respiratory tract infection, wheezing

Miscellaneous: Allergic reaction, feeling warm/cold, infusion reactions

Rare but important or life-threatening: Anaphylaxis, angioedema, cardiac failure, cardiorespiratory arrest, cyanosis, erythema, extravasation, pneumonia, respiratory failure

Drug Interactions

Metabolism/Transport Effects None known.

Avoid Concomitant Use There are no known interactions where it is recommended to avoid concomitant use.

Increased Effect/Toxicity There are no known significant interactions involving an increase in effect.

Decreased Effect There are no known significant interactions involving a decrease in effect.

Storage/Stability Store vials under refrigeration at 2°C to 8°C (36°F to 46°F); do not freeze. Protect from light. Do not shake. Following dilution, solution for infusion should be used immediately; however, if not used immediately, diluted solutions should be refrigerated at 2°C to 8°C (36°F to 46°F) for up to 36 hours.

Mechanism of Action Laronidase is a recombinant (replacement) form of α-L-iduronidase derived from Chinese hamster cells. α-L-iduronidase is an enzyme needed to break down endogenous glycosaminoglycans (GAGs) within lysosomes. A deficiency of α-L-iduronidase leads to an accumulation of GAGs, causing cellular, tissue, and organ dysfunction as seen in MPS I. Improved pulmonary function and walking capacity have been demonstrated with the administration of laronidase to patients with Hurler, Hurler-Scheie, or Scheie (with moderate-to-severe symptoms) forms of MPS.

Pharmacokinetics (Adult data unless noted)

Distribution:

Infants and Children 6 months to 5 years: V_d: 0.12 to 0.56 L/kg

Children ≥6 years and Adults: V_d: 0.24 to 0.6 L/kg

Half-life:

Infants and Children 6 months to 5 years: 0.3 to 1.9 hours

Children ≥6 years and Adults: 1.5 to 3.6 hours

Clearance:

Infants and Children 6 months to 5 years: 2.2 to 7.7 mL/minute/kg

Children ≥6 years and Adults: 1.7 to 2.7 mL/minute/kg; during the first 12 weeks of therapy the clearance of laronidase increases proportionally to the amount of antibodies a given patient develops against the enzyme. However, with long-term use (≥26 weeks), antibody titers have no effect on laronidase clearance.

Dosing: Usual Note: Premedicate with antipyretic and/or antihistamines 1 hour prior to start of infusion.

Pediatric: **Mucopolysaccharidosis I (Hurler syndrome, Hurler-Scheie, and Scheie forms):** Infants ≥6 months, Children, and Adolescents: IV: 0.58 mg/kg/dose once weekly; dose should be rounded up to the nearest whole vial

Adult: **Mucopolysaccharidosis I (Hurler syndrome, Hurler-Scheie, and Scheie forms):** IV: 0.58 mg/kg/dose once weekly; dose should be rounded up to the nearest whole vial

Dosing adjustment in renal impairment: There are no dosing adjustments provided in the manufacturer's labeling.

Dosing adjustment in hepatic impairment: There are no dosing adjustments provided in the manufacturer's labeling.

Preparation for Administration IV infusion: Determine the number of vials to dilute by calculating the required dose and rounding up to the nearest whole vial. Allow vials to come to room temperature prior to admixture. Do not use if the solution is discolored or contains particulate matter. Prepare the infusion using a low protein-binding container (there is no compatability information of diluted laronidase in glass containers). Total volume of infusion is determined by body weight. For patients weighing ≤20 kg (or weighing up to 30 kg and with cardiac or respiratory compromise), dilute the required dose in 100 mL NS; for patients weighing >20 kg, dilute required dose in 250 mL NS. Remove and discard a volume of NS from the infusion bag equal to the volume of the calculated dose of laronidase. Slowly withdraw from vial(s) and slowly add laronidase to the NS; avoid excessive agitation as it denatures the enzyme, do not use filter needle. Gently rotate infusion bag to mix (do not shake).

Administration IV infusion:

Determine the number of vials to be diluted. Remove vials from the refrigerator and allow them to reach room temperature. Do not use if the solution is discolored or contains particulate matter. Determine the total infusion volume based on the patient's weight; for patients weighing ≤20 kg (or weighing up to 30 kg and with cardiac or respiratory compromise), dilute the required dose in 100 mL NS; for patients weighing >20 kg, dilute required dose in 250 mL NS.

From an NS infusion bag, remove and discard volume of NS equal to volume of laronidase injection solution to be added to the infusion bag. Add laronidase; do not agitate solution as it denatures the enzyme.

Administer using an infusion set with low protein-binding 0.2 micrometer in-line filter. Antipyretics and/or antihistamines should be administered 60 minutes prior to infusion. Volume and infusion rate are based on body weight; deliver infusion over ~3 to 4 hours. An initial 10 mcg/kg/hour infusion rate may be incrementally increased every 15 minutes during the first hour if tolerated (see below); increase to a maximum infusion rate of 200 mcg/kg/hour which is maintained for the remainder of the infusion (approximately 3 hours). Vital signs should be monitored every 15 minutes, if stable; in case of infusion-related reaction in any patient, decrease the rate of infusion, temporarily discontinue the infusion, and/or administer additional antipyretics/antihistamines. Manufacturer provides the following infusion rate information for patients receiving usual preparation:

≤20 kg: Total infusion volume: 100 mL
- 2 mL/hour for 15 minutes
- 4 mL/hour for 15 minutes
- 8 mL/hour for 15 minutes
- 16 mL/hour for 15 minutes
- 32 mL/hour for remainder of infusion (~3 hours)

>20 kg: Total infusion volume: 250 mL
- 5 mL/hour for 15 minutes
- 10 mL/hour for 15 minutes
- 20 mL/hour for 15 minutes
- 40 mL/hour for 15 minutes
- 80 mL/hour for remainder of infusion (~3 hours)

Note: A total infusion volume of 100 mL NS and slower infusion rate may be considered for patients with cardiac or respiratory compromise who weigh up to 30 kg.

Monitoring Parameters Vital signs, FVC, height, weight, range of motion, serum antibodies to α-L-iduronidase, urine levels of glycosaminoglycans (GAG), change in liver size

Dosage Forms Excipient information presented when available (limited, particularly for generics); consult specific product labeling.

Solution, Intravenous:

Aldurazyme: 2.9 mg/5 mL (5 mL) [contains mouse protein (murine) (hamster), polysorbate 80]

◆ **Lasix** *see* Furosemide *on page* *951*

◆ **Lasix Special (Can)** *see* Furosemide *on page* *951*

◆ **L-asparaginase (*Erwinia*)** *see* Asparaginase (*Erwinia*) *on page* *204*

◆ **L-asparaginase with Polyethylene Glycol** *see* Pegaspargase *on page* *1639*

◆ **Lassar's Zinc Paste** *see* Zinc Oxide *on page* *2214*

◆ ***Latrodectus* Antivenin** *see* Antivenin (*Latrodectus mactans*) *on page* *181*

◆ ***Latrodectus* Antivenom** *see* Antivenin (*Latrodectus mactans*) *on page* *181*

◆ ***Latrodectus mactans* Antivenin** *see* Antivenin (*Latrodectus mactans*) *on page* *181*

◆ ***Latrodectus mactans* Antivenom** *see* Antivenin (*Latrodectus mactans*) *on page* *181*

◆ **Lavacol [OTC]** *see* Alcohol (Ethyl) *on page* *86*

◆ **Lavoclen-4 Acne Wash** *see* Benzoyl Peroxide *on page* *270*

◆ **Lavoclen-4 Creamy Wash** *see* Benzoyl Peroxide *on page* *270*

◆ **Lavoclen-8 Acne Wash** *see* Benzoyl Peroxide *on page* *270*

◆ **Lavoclen-8 Creamy Wash** *see* Benzoyl Peroxide *on page* *270*

◆ **Laxa Basic [OTC]** *see* Docusate *on page* *697*

◆ **Laxative [OTC]** *see* Bisacodyl *on page* *289*

◆ **Lazanda** *see* FentaNYL *on page* *857*

◆ ***l*-Bunolol Hydrochloride** *see* Levobunolol *on page* *1238*

◆ **LC-4 Lidocaine [OTC]** *see* Lidocaine (Topical) *on page* *1258*

◆ **LC-5 Lidocaine [OTC]** *see* Lidocaine (Topical) *on page* *1258*

◆ **L-Carnitine** *see* LevOCARNitine *on page* *1239*

◆ **LCD** *see* Coal Tar *on page* *523*

◆ **LCM** *see* Lacosamide *on page* *1200*

◆ **Lederle Leucovorin (Can)** *see* Leucovorin Calcium *on page* *1226*

◆ **Lepargylic Acid** *see* Azelaic Acid *on page* *238*

◆ **Lescol** *see* Fluvastatin *on page* *926*

◆ **Lescol XL** *see* Fluvastatin *on page* *926*

Letrozole (LET roe zole)

Medication Safety Issues

Sound-alike/look-alike issues:

Femara may be confused with Famvir, femhrt, Provera

Letrozole may be confused with anastrozole

International issues:

Letaris, a formerly marketed Dutch brand name product for letrozole, may be confused with Letairis, a U.S. brand name for ambrisentan.

Related Information

Safe Handling of Hazardous Drugs *on page* *2455*

Brand Names: US Femara

Brand Names: Canada ACH-Letrozole; Apo-Letrozole; Auro-Letrozole; Bio-Letrozole; Femara; JAMP-Letrozole; Mar-Letrozole; MED-Letrozole; Myl-Letrozole; Nat-Letrozole; PMS-Letrozole; RAN-Letrozole; Riva-Letrozole; Sandoz-Letrozole; Teva-Letrozole; Van-Letrozole; Zinda-Letrozole

Therapeutic Category Antineoplastic Agent, Aromatase Inhibitor

Generic Availability (US) Yes

Use Adjuvant treatment of hormone receptor positive early breast cancer, extended adjuvant treatment of early breast cancer after 5 years of tamoxifen, first-line treatment of hormone receptor positive or hormone receptor unknown, locally advanced or metastatic breast cancer; treatment of advanced breast cancer with disease progression following antiestrogen therapy (All indications: FDA approved in postmenopausal women); has also been used in treatment of precocious puberty associated with McCune-Albright Syndrome (MAS) in girls; constitutional delay of growth and puberty (not due to growth hormone deficiency) and idiopathic short stature in boys

Pregnancy Risk Factor X

Pregnancy Considerations Adverse events were observed in animal reproduction studies. Letrozole is FDA approved for postmenopausal women only (no clinical benefit for breast cancer has been demonstrated in premenopausal women). Use in women who are or who may become pregnant is contraindicated. Women who are perimenopausal or recently postmenopausal should use adequate contraception until postmenopausal status is fully established.

Breast-Feeding Considerations It is not known if letrozole is excreted in breast milk. Due to the potential for serious adverse reactions in the nursing infant, a decision should be made whether to discontinue nursing or to discontinue the drug, taking into account the importance of treatment to the mother. Use in nursing women is contraindicated in the Canadian labeling.

Contraindications Use in women who are or may become pregnant

Canadian labeling: Additional contraindications (not in U.S. labeling): Hypersensitivity to letrozole, other aromatase inhibitors, or any component of the formulation; use in patients <18 years of age; breast-feeding

Warnings/Precautions Hazardous agent - use appropriate precautions for handling and disposal (NIOSH 2014 [group 1]). Not generally indicated for known hormone-receptor negative disease. Use caution with hepatic impairment; dose adjustment recommended in patients with cirrhosis or severe hepatic dysfunction. May cause dizziness, fatigue, and somnolence; patients should be cautioned before performing tasks which require mental alertness (eg, operating machinery or driving). May increase total serum cholesterol; in patients treated with adjuvant therapy and cholesterol levels within normal limits, an increase of ≥1.5 x ULN in total cholesterol has been demonstrated in 8.2% of letrozole-treated patients (25% requiring lipid-lowering medications) vs 3.2% of tamoxifen-treated patients (16% requiring medications); monitor cholesterol panel; may require antihyperlipidemics. May cause decreases in bone mineral density (BMD); a decrease in hip BMD by 3.8% from baseline in letrozole-treated patients vs 2% in placebo at 2 years has been demonstrated; however, there was no statistical difference in changes to the lumbar spine BMD scores; monitor BMD. Potentially significant drug-drug interactions may exist, requiring dose or frequency adjustment, additional monitoring, and/or selection of alternative therapy.

Warnings: Additional Pediatric Considerations In males treated for idiopathic short stature, trabecular bone and vertebral-body deformities were observed; consider prior to therapy initiation, and monitor patients closely (Palmert, 2012).

Adverse Reactions

Cardiovascular: Angina; cerebrovascular accident including hemorrhagic stroke, thrombotic stroke; chest pain, hypertension, MI, peripheral edema; thromboembolic event including venous thrombosis, thrombophlebitis, portal vein thrombosis, pulmonary embolism; transient ischemic attack

Central nervous system: Anxiety, depression, dizziness, fatigue, headache, insomnia, pain, somnolence, vertigo

Dermatologic: Alopecia, pruritus, rash

Endocrine & metabolic: Breast pain, hot flashes, hypercholesterolemia, hypercalcemia

Gastrointestinal: Abdominal pain, anorexia, constipation, diarrhea, dyspepsia, nausea, vomiting, weight gain, weight loss

Genitourinary: Urinary tract infection, vaginal bleeding, vaginal dryness, vaginal hemorrhage, vaginal irritation

Neuromuscular & skeletal: Arthralgia, arthritis, back pain, bone fracture, bone mineral density decreased, bone pain, limb pain, musculoskeletal pain, myalgia, osteoporosis, weakness

Ocular: Cataract

Renal: Renal disorder

Respiratory: Cough, dyspnea, pleural effusion

Miscellaneous: Diaphoresis, infection, influenza, night sweats, secondary malignancy, viral infection

Rare but important or life-threatening: Anaphylactic reaction, angioedema, arterial thrombosis, cardiac failure, carpal tunnel syndrome, endometrial cancer, endometrial hyperplasia, endometrial proliferation, erythema multiforme, hepatitis, leukopenia, memory impairment, stomatitis, tachycardia, thrombocytopenia, toxic epidermal necrolysis, trigger finger

Drug Interactions

Metabolism/Transport Effects **Substrate** of CYP2A6 (minor), CYP3A4 (minor); **Note:** Assignment of Major/Minor substrate status based on clinically relevant drug interaction potential; **Inhibits** CYP2A6 (strong), CYP2C19 (weak)

Avoid Concomitant Use

Avoid concomitant use of Letrozole with any of the following: Artesunate; Tegafur

Increased Effect/Toxicity

Letrozole may increase the levels/effects of: Artesunate; CYP2A6 Substrates; Methadone

Decreased Effect

Letrozole may decrease the levels/effects of: Artesunate; Tegafur

The levels/effects of Letrozole may be decreased by: Tamoxifen

Storage/Stability Store at room temperature of 25°C (77°F); excursions permitted to 15°C to 30°C (59°F to 86°F).

Mechanism of Action Nonsteroidal competitive inhibitor of the aromatase enzyme system which binds to the heme group of aromatase, a cytochrome P450 enzyme which catalyzes conversion of androgens to estrogens (specifically, androstenedione to estrone and testosterone to estradiol). This leads to inhibition of the enzyme and a significant reduction in plasma estrogen (estrone, estradiol and estrone sulfate) levels. Does not affect synthesis of adrenal or thyroid hormones, aldosterone, or androgens.

Pharmacodynamics Maximum effect: Plasma estradiol, estrone and estrone sulfate suppression: 2-3 days

Pharmacokinetics (Adult data unless noted)

Absorption: Rapid and well absorbed; not affected by food

Distribution: V_d: ~1.9 L/kg

Protein binding: Weak

Metabolism: Hepatic via CYP3A4 and CYP2A6 to an inactive carbinol metabolite

Half-life elimination: Terminal: ~2 days

Time to steady state serum concentration: 2-6 weeks; steady state serum concentrations are 1.5-2 times higher than single-dose values. In girls 3-9 years, steady state concentrations were 25% to 67% that of the mean adult values (Feuillan, 2007)

Half-life elimination: Terminal: ~2 days

Elimination: Urine (90%; 6% as unchanged drug, 75% as glucuronide carbinol metabolite; 9% as unidentified metabolites)

Dosing: Usual

Pediatric:

Delayed puberty and growth [CDGP (constitutional delay of growth and puberty)] (males): Very limited data available: Adolescents ≥14 years: Oral: 2.5 mg once daily in combination with testosterone therapy; dosing from a double-blind placebo-controlled trial of 33 adolescent males (treatment group: n=11); during the 12 months of therapy, bone maturation was delayed, predicted adult height values were significantly increased and markers of puberty progressed (Palmert; 2012; Wickman, 2001).

McCune-Albright syndrome; precocious puberty (females): Very limited data available: Children >2-10 years at time of treatment initiation: Oral: Initial: 0.5 mg/m²/day divided every 12 hours for days 1-7, then 1 mg/m²/day divided every 12 hours on days 8-14, then 1.5 mg/m²/day divided every 12 hours beginning on day 15; if needed, may further increase to 2 mg/m²/day if markers of precocious puberty including serum estradiol levels progress. Dosing based on a pilot study of nine girls (3-8 years at time of therapy initiation) which showed long-term therapy (up to 36 months) decreased rates of growth and bone maturation; although ovarian volume decreased during the first 6 months of treatment, the mean ovarian volume increased over 1-2 years of therapy with cyst redevelopment in some patients. During the pilot study, dosing was divided twice daily to alleviate GI discomfort; however, pharmacokinetic analysis showed once daily dosing would be appropriate for young children if tolerated (Feuillan, 2007). In a case series (n=3, age range at treatment: 3-7 years), a fixed dose of 2.5 mg once daily was used for 5-19 months duration (Bercaw-Pratt, 2012).

Short-stature; idiopathic (males): Limited data available: Children and Adolescents 9-16 years: Oral: 2.5 mg once daily; dosing based experience in a double-blind, placebo-controlled trial of 30 males (treatment group: n=16; age range: 9-14 years) and a retrospective observation (n= 24; age range: 9-16 years); the duration of letrozole therapy was up to 2 years (range: 4-24 months); bone maturation delay with increases in predicted adult height values were observed with treatment (Hero, 2005; Karmazin, 2005; Shulman, 2008)

Adults: Females: Postmenopausal:

Breast cancer, advanced (first- or second-line treatment): Oral: 2.5 mg once daily; continue until tumor progression

Breast cancer, early (adjuvant treatment): Oral: 2.5 mg once daily; optimal duration unknown, duration in clinical trial is 5 years; discontinue at relapse

Breast cancer, early (extended adjuvant treatment): Oral: 2.5 mg once daily; optimal duration unknown, duration in clinical trials is 5 years (after 5 years of tamoxifen); discontinue at relapse. In clinical trials, letrozole was initiated within 3 months of discontinuing tamoxifen (Goss, 2003; Jin, 2012).

Dosing adjustment in renal impairment: Adults: CrCl ≥10 mL/minute: No dosage adjustment is required.

Dosing adjustment in hepatic impairment: Adults:

Mild to moderate impairment (Child-Pugh class A or B): No adjustment recommended

Severe impairment (Child-Pugh class C) or cirrhosis: 2.5 mg every other day

Administration Hazardous agent; use appropriate precautions for handling and disposal (NIOSH 2014 [group 1]). May administer without regard to meals.

Monitoring Parameters Monitor periodically during therapy: Complete blood counts, thyroid function tests; serum electrolytes, cholesterol, transaminases, and creatinine; blood pressure; bone density

Delayed puberty and short stature: In the pediatric clinical trials (study durations: 1-2 years) the following were monitored (at baseline, and then typically 2 months, 5 months, 12 months, and 18 months): Growth indices (height, adult height predictions, bone age, lumbar and femoral bone mineral density), Tanner stage and serum concentration of key hormones, and other biochemical markers (eg, 17-B estradiol, LH, FSH, testosterone), lipid profile (Hero, 2005; Shulman, 2008; Wickman, 2001)

McCune-Albright syndrome: In the pediatric clinical trial (study duration: 12-36 months), the following were monitored (baseline, every 6 months): Rates of growth and bone age advance, levels of indices of bone metabolism (eg, osteocalcin and alkaline phosphatase); and urinary markers of steroid metabolism (eg, hydroxyproline, pyridinoline, etc.), mean ovarian volume, episodes of vaginal bleeding and serum concentrations of estradiol. (Feuillan, 2007)

Dosage Forms Excipient information presented when available (limited, particularly for generics); consult specific product labeling.

Tablet, Oral:

Femara: 2.5 mg

Generic: 2.5 mg

◆ **Leucovorin** *see* Leucovorin Calcium *on page 1226*

Leucovorin Calcium (loo koe VOR in KAL see um)

Medication Safety Issues

Sound-alike/look-alike issues:

Leucovorin may be confused with Leukeran, Leukine, LEVOleucovorin

Folinic acid may be confused with folic acid

Folinic acid is an error prone synonym and should not be used

Brand Names: Canada Lederle Leucovorin; Leucovorin Calcium Injection; Leucovorin Calcium Injection USP

Therapeutic Category Antidote, Methotrexate; Folic Acid Derivative

Generic Availability (US) Yes

Use

Oral: Rescue agent to diminish the toxicity and counteract the effects of impaired methotrexate elimination or as an antidote for folic acid antagonist overdosage (FDA approved in pediatric patients [age not specified] and adults)

Parenteral: Rescue agent after high-dose methotrexate treatment in osteosarcoma and to diminish the toxicity and counteract the effects of impaired methotrexate elimination and of inadvertent overdosage of folic acid antagonists; treatment of megaloblastic anemias due to folic acid deficiency (when oral therapy is not feasible) (FDA approved in pediatric patients [age not specified] and adults); treatment of advanced colorectal cancer (palliative) in combination with fluorouracil (FDA approved in adults); has also been used as rescue agent after high-dose methotrexate treatment in treatment of other cancers; as adjunctive cofactor therapy in methanol toxicity, adjunctive treatment with sulfadiazine and pyrimethamine to prevent hematologic toxicity

Pregnancy Risk Factor C

Pregnancy Considerations Animal reproduction studies have not been conducted. Leucovorin is a biologically active form of folic acid. Adequate amounts of folic acid are recommended during pregnancy. Refer to Folic Acid monograph.

Breast-Feeding Considerations Leucovorin is a biologically active form of folic acid. Adequate amounts of folic acid are recommended in breast-feeding women. Refer to Folic Acid monograph.

Contraindications Pernicious anemia and other megaloblastic anemias secondary to vitamin B_{12}-deficiency

Warnings/Precautions When used for the treatment of accidental folic acid antagonist overdose, administer as soon as possible. When used for the treatment of a methotrexate overdose, administer IV leucovorin as soon as possible. Monitoring of the serum methotrexate concentration is essential to determine the optimal dose/duration of leucovorin; however, do not wait for the results of a methotrexate level before initiating therapy. It is important to adjust the leucovorin dose once a methotrexate level is known. When used for methotrexate rescue therapy, methotrexate serum concentrations should be monitored to determine dose and duration of leucovorin therapy. The dose may need to be increased or administration prolonged in situations where methotrexate excretion may be delayed (eg, ascites, pleural effusion, renal insufficiency, inadequate hydration); **never administer leucovorin intrathecally**. Parenteral administration may be preferred to oral if vomiting or malabsorption is likely. Potentially significant drug-drug interactions may exist, requiring dose or frequency adjustment, additional monitoring, and/or selection of alternative therapy. Combination of leucovorin and sulfamethoxazole-trimethoprim for the acute treatment of PCP in patients with HIV infection has been reported to cause increased rates of treatment failure. Leucovorin may increase the toxicity of 5-fluorouracil; deaths from severe enterocolitis, diarrhea, and dehydration have been reported (in elderly patients); granulocytopenia and fever have also been reported. Hypersensitivity, including allergic reactions, anaphylactoid reactions, and urticaria have been reported with leucovorin.

Leucovorin is inappropriate treatment for pernicious anemia and other megaloblastic anemias secondary to a lack of vitamin B_{12}; a hematologic remission may occur while neurologic manifestations progress. Leucovorin is excreted renally; the risk for toxicities may be increased in patients with renal impairment.

Benzyl alcohol and derivatives: When doses >10 mg/m^2 are required using the powder for injection, reconstitute using sterile water for injection, not a solution containing benzyl alcohol; large amounts of benzyl alcohol (≥99 mg/kg/day) have been associated with a potentially fatal toxicity ("gasping syndrome") in neonates; the "gasping syndrome" consists of metabolic acidosis, respiratory distress, gasping respirations, CNS dysfunction (including convulsions, intracranial hemorrhage), hypotension, and cardiovascular collapse (AAP, 1997; CDC, 1982); some data suggests that benzoate displaces bilirubin from protein binding sites (Ahlfors, 2001); avoid or use dosage forms containing benzyl alcohol with caution in neonates. See manufacturer's labeling.

Injection: Due to calcium content, do not administer IV solutions at a rate >160 mg/minute. Not intended for intrathecal use.

Adverse Reactions

Dermatologic: Rash, pruritus, erythema, urticaria
Hematologic: Thrombocytosis
Respiratory: Wheezing
Miscellaneous: Allergic reactions, anaphylactoid reactions

Drug Interactions

Metabolism/Transport Effects None known.

Avoid Concomitant Use

Avoid concomitant use of Leucovorin Calcium with any of the following: Raltitrexed; Trimethoprim

Increased Effect/Toxicity

Leucovorin Calcium may increase the levels/effects of: Capecitabine; Fluorouracil (Systemic); Fluorouracil (Topical); Tegafur

Decreased Effect

Leucovorin Calcium may decrease the levels/effects of: Fosphenytoin; PHENobarbital; Phenytoin; Primidone; Raltitrexed; Trimethoprim

The levels/effects of Leucovorin Calcium may be decreased by: Glucarpidase

Storage/Stability

Powder for injection: Store at room temperature of 25°C (77°F). Protect from light. Solutions reconstituted with bacteriostatic water for injection U.S.P., must be used within 7 days. Solutions reconstituted with SWFI must be used immediately. Parenteral admixture is stable for 24 hours stored at room temperature (25°C) and for 4 days when stored under refrigeration (4°C).
Solution for injection: Prior to dilution, store vials under refrigeration at 2°C to 8°C (36°F to 46°F). Protect from light.
Tablet: Store at room temperature of 15°C to 30°C (59°F to 86°F).

Mechanism of Action A reduced form of folic acid, leucovorin supplies the necessary cofactor blocked by methotrexate. Leucovorin actively competes with methotrexate for transport sites, displaces methotrexate from intracellular binding sites, and restores active folate stores required for DNA/RNA synthesis. Stabilizes the binding of 5-dUMP and thymidylate synthetase, enhancing the activity of fluorouracil. When administered with pyrimethamine for the treatment of opportunistic infections, leucovorin reduces the risk for hematologic toxicity (DHHS, 2013).

Methanol toxicity treatment: Formic acid (methanol's toxic metabolite) is normally metabolized to carbon dioxide and water by 10-formyltetrahydrofolate dehydrogenase after being bound to tetrahydrofolate. Administering a source of tetrahydrofolate may aid the body in eliminating formic acid (Barceloux, 2002).

Pharmacodynamics Onset of action:
Oral: Within 30 minutes
IV: Within 5 minutes

Pharmacokinetics (Adult data unless noted)

Absorption: Oral, IM: Well absorbed (doses <25 mg; absorption decreases with doses ≥25 mg)
Metabolism: Rapidly converted to (5MTHF) 5-methyl-tetrahydrofolate (active) in the intestinal mucosa and by the liver
Bioavailability:
Oral absorption is saturable in doses >25 mg; apparent bioavailability:
Tablet, 25 mg: 97%
Tablet, 50 mg: 75%
Tablet, 100 mg: 37%
Injection solution, when administered orally, provides equivalent bioavailability
Half-life: ~4 to 8 hours
Time to peak serum concentration:
Oral: ~2 hours
IV: Total folates: 10 minutes; 5MTHF: ~1 hour
IM: Total folates: 52 minutes; 5MTHF: 2.8 hours
Elimination: Primarily in urine (80% to 90%) with small losses appearing in feces (5% to 8%)

Dosing: Neonatal

Pyrimethamine hematologic toxicity, prevention (Congenital toxoplasmosis): Note: Leucovorin is administered in combination with pyrmethamine and sulfadiazine in the treatment of congenital toxoplasmosis; leucovorin should continue for 1 week after pyrimethamine is discontinued (DHHS [pediatric], 2013).
HIV-exposed/-positive: IM, Oral: 10 mg with every pyrimethamine dose; treatment duration: 12 months (DHHS [pediatric], 2013)
Non-HIV-exposed/-positive: IM, Oral: 10 mg three times weekly for 12 months (McAuley, 2008)

Dosing: Usual

Pediatric: **Note:** Dosing in pediatric patients presented in mg, mg/m^2 and mg/kg; use caution. Consider parenteral administration instead of oral in patients with GI toxicity, nausea, vomiting, or when individual doses are >25 mg.

Folic acid antagonist (eg, pyrimethamine, trimethoprim) overdose: Infant, Children, and Adolescents: Oral: 5 to 15 mg daily

Megaloblastic anemia secondary to folate deficiency: Infants, Children, and Adolescents: IM, IV: ≤1 mg/day

High-dose methotrexate rescue: Infants, Children, and Adolescents: Initial: Oral, IM, IV: 15 mg (~10 mg/m^2) every 6 hours; start 24 hours after beginning of methotrexate infusion (based on a methotrexate dose of 12 to 15 **g**/m^2 IV over 4 hours). Leucovorin (and hydration and urinary alkalinization) should be continued and/or adjusted until the methotrexate level is <0.05 micromolar (5 x 10^{-8} M). Adjust dose as follows:

Normal methotrexate elimination (serum methotrexate level ~10 micromolar at 24 hours after administration, 1 micromolar at 48 hours, and <0.2 micromolar at 72 hours): Oral, IM, IV: 15 mg every 6 hours for 10 doses beginning 24 hours after the start of methotrexate infusion

Delayed late methotrexate elimination (serum methotrexate level remaining >0.2 micromolar at 72 hours and >0.05 micromolar at 96 hours after administration): Oral, IM, IV: Continue leucovorin calcium 15 mg every 6 hours until methotrexate level is <0.05 micromolar

Delayed early methotrexate elimination and/or acute renal injury (serum methotrexate level ≥50 micromolar at 24 hours, or ≥5 micromolar at 48 hours, or a doubling of serum creatinine level at 24 hours after methotrexate administration): IV: 150 mg every 3 hours until methotrexate level is <1 micromolar, then

15 mg every 3 hours until methotrexate level is <0.05 micromolar

High-dose methotrexate overexposure: Limited data available: Infants, Children, and Adolescents: Oral, IM, IV: Leucovorin nomogram dosing for high-dose methotrexate overexposure (generalized dosing derived from reference nomogram figures, refer to each reference (Bleyer, 1978; Bleyer, 1981; Widemann, 2006) or protocol-specific nomogram for details):

At 24 hours:

For methotrexate levels of ≥100 micromolar at ~24 hours, leucovorin is initially dosed at 1,000 mg/m^2 every 6 hours

For methotrexate levels of ≥10 to <100 micromolar at 24 hours, leucovorin is initially dosed at 100 mg/m^2 every 3 or 6 hours

For methotrexate levels of ~1 to 10 micromolar at 24 hours, leucovorin is initially dosed at 10 mg/m^2 every 3 or 6 hours

At 48 hours:

For methotrexate levels of ≥100 micromolar at 48 hours, leucovorin is dosed at 1,000 mg/m^2 every 6 hours

For methotrexate levels of ≥10 to <100 micromolar at 48 hours, leucovorin is dosed at 100 mg/m^2 every 3 hours

For methotrexate levels of ~1 to 10 micromolar at 48 hours, leucovorin is dosed at 100 mg/m^2 every 6 hours **or** 10 to 100 mg/m^2 every 3 hours

At 72 hours:

For methotrexate levels of ≥10 micromolar at 72 hours, leucovorin is dosed at 100 to 1,000 mg/m^2 every 3 to 6 hours

For methotrexate levels of ~1 to 10 micromolar at 72 hours, leucovorin is dosed at 10 to 100 mg/m^2 every 3 hours

For methotrexate levels of ~0.1 to 1 micromolar at 72 hours, leucovorin is dosed at 10 mg/m^2 every 3 to 6 hours

If serum creatinine is increased more than 50% above baseline, increase the standard leucovorin dose to 100 mg/m^2 every 3 hours, then adjust according to methotrexate levels above.

Follow methotrexate levels daily, leucovorin may be discontinued when methotrexate level is <0.1 micromolar; some have suggested <0.08 micromolar (8 x 10^{-8} M) is preferable (Bleyer, 1978)

Methotrexate overdose (inadvertent) (begin as soon as possible after overdose): Infants, Children, and Adolescents: Oral, IM, IV: 10 mg/m^2/dose every 6 hours until the methotrexate level is <0.01 micromolar. If serum creatinine is increased more than 50% above baseline 24 hours after methotrexate administration, if 24 hour methotrexate level is >5 micromolar, or if 48 hour methotrexate level is >0.9 micromolar, increase leucovorin dose to 100 mg/m^2 IV every 3 hours until the methotrexate level is <0.01 micromolar.

Note: Do not administer leucovorin intrathecally; use of intrathecal leucovorin is not advised (Jardine, 1996; Smith, 2008).

Megaloblastic anemia secondary to congenital deficiency of dihydrofolate reductase; treatment: Infants, Children, and Adolescents: IM, Oral: 3 to 6 mg/day (Nelson, 1996)

Pyrimethamine hematologic toxicity, prevention: Leucovorin is administered in combination with pyrimethamine and other medications in the treatment of toxoplasmosis; dosing varies with disease process and regimen; consult pyrimethamine specific monograph for additional details; duration of therapy varies based on disease state; however, leucovorin should continue for 1 week after pyrimethamine is discontinued (DHHS [pediatric], 2013); usual regimens include:

Toxoplasmosis (*Toxoplasma gondii*):

Treatment:

Congenital toxoplasmosis: Infants:

HIV-exposed/-positive: IM, Oral: 10 mg with every pyrimethamine dose; treatment duration: 12 months (DHHS [pediatric], 2013)

Non-HIV-exposed/-positive: IM, Oral: 10 mg three times weekly for 12 months (McAuley, 2008)

Acquired infection:

HIV-exposed/-positive: Infants, Children, and Adolescents: Acute induction: Oral: 10 to 25 mg once daily for ≥6 weeks (DHHS, 2014; DHHS [pediatric], 2013). **Note:** In adolescents, leucovorin may be increased to 50 to100 mg/day in divided doses in cases of pyrimethamine toxicity (rash, nausea, bone marrow suppression) (DHHS, 2014)

Non-HIV-exposed/-positive: Chorioretinitis: Infants, Children, and Adolescents: Oral: 10 to 20 mg three times weekly (McAuley, 2008)

Prophylaxis:

Primary:

HIV-exposed/-positive:

Infants and Children: Oral: 5 mg once every 3 days (DHHS [pediatric], 2013)

Adolescents: Oral: 25 mg once weekly (with pyrimethamine and dapsone) **or** 10 mg once daily (with pyrimethamine and atovaquone) (DHHS, 2014)

Hematopoietic cell transplantation recipients:

Children: Oral: 5 mg every 3 days; initiate after engraftment and administer as long as the patient remains on immunosuppressive therapy (Tomblyn, 2009)

Adolescents: Oral: 10 to 25 mg once daily; initiate after engraftment and administer as long as the patient remains on immunosuppressive therapy (Tomblyn, 2009)

Secondary: HIV-exposed/-positive:

Infants and Children: Oral: 5 mg once every 3 days (DHHS [pediatric], 2013)

Adolescents: Oral: 10 to 25 mg once daily **or** 10 mg once daily (DHHS, 2014)

Pneumocystis jirovecii pneumonia (PCP): Prophylaxis (primary and secondary): Adolescents: Oral: 25 mg once weekly **or** 10 mg once daily (DHHS, 2014)

Isosporiasis (*Isospora* belli):

Treatment, acute infection: Infants, Children, and Adolescents: Oral: 10 to 25 mg once daily (DHHS, 2014; DHHS [pediatric], 2013)

Prophylaxis, secondary:

Infants and Children: Oral: 10 to 25 mg once daily (DHHS [pediatric], 2013)

Adolescents: Oral: 5 to10 mg once daily (DHHS, 2014)

Methanol toxicity; cofactor therapy: Limited data available: Infants, Children, and Adolescents: IV: 1 mg/kg (maximum dose: 50 mg) over 30 to 60 minutes every 4 to 6 hours. Therapy should continue until methanol and formic acid have been completely eliminated (Barceloux, 2002).

Adult: **Note:** Consider parenteral administration instead of oral in patients with GI toxicity, nausea, vomiting, or when individual doses are >25 mg.

Colorectal cancer: IV: 200 mg/m²/day over at least 3 minutes for 5 days every 4 weeks for 2 cycles, then every 4 to 5 weeks (in combination with fluorouracil) **or** 20 mg/m²/day for 5 days every 4 weeks for 2 cycles, then every 4 to 5 weeks (in combination with fluorouracil)

Folic acid antagonist (eg, trimethoprim, pyrimethamine) overdose: Oral: 5 to 15 mg once daily

Folate-deficient megaloblastic anemia: IM, IV: ≤1 mg once daily

High-dose methotrexate-rescue: Initial: Oral, IM, IV: 15 mg (~10 mg/m²); start 24 hours after beginning methotrexate infusion; continue every 6 hours for 10 doses, until methotrexate level is <0.05 micromolar. Adjust dose as follows:

Normal methotrexate elimination (serum methotrexate level ~10 micromolar at 24 hours after administration, 1 micromolar at 48 hours, and <0.2 micromolar at 72 hours): Oral, IM, IV: 15 mg every 6 hours for 60 hours (10 doses) beginning 24 hours after the start of methotrexate infusion

Delayed late methotrexate elimination (serum methotrexate level remaining >0.2 micromolar at 72 hours and >0.05 micromolar at 96 hours after administration): Continue leucovorin calcium 15 mg (oral, IM, or IV) every 6 hours until methotrexate level is <0.05 micromolar

Delayed early methotrexate elimination and/or acute renal injury (serum methotrexate level ≥50 micromolar at 24 hours, or ≥5 micromolar at 48 hours, or a doubling of serum creatinine level at 24 hours after methotrexate administration): IV: 150 mg every 3 hours until methotrexate level is <1 micromolar, then 15 mg every 3 hours until methotrexate level is <0.05 micromolar

Methotrexate overdose (inadvertent) (begin as soon as possible after overdose): Oral, IM, IV: 10 mg/m² every 6 hours until the methotrexate level is <0.01 micromolar. If serum creatinine is increased more than 50% above baseline 24 hours after methotrexate administration, if 24 hour methotrexate level is >5 micromolar, or if 48 hour methotrexate level is >0.9 micromolar, increase leucovorin dose to 100 mg/m² IV every 3 hours until the methotrexate level is <0.01 micromolar.

Note: Do not administer leucovorin intrathecally; the use of intrathecal leucovorin is not advised (Jardine, 1996; Smith, 2008).

Dosing adjustment in renal impairment: Infants, Children, Adolescents, and Adults: There are no dosage adjustments provided in manufacturer's labeling.

Dosing adjustment in hepatic impairment: Infants, Children, Adolescents, and Adults: There are no dosage adjustments provided in manufacturer's labeling.

Preparation for Administration

Parenteral:

For doses ≤10 mg/m²: Reconstitute with SWFI or bacteriostatic water for injection; further dilute in D_5W or NS for infusion; maximum concentration: 20 mg/mL

For doses >10 mg/m² **or** neonatal patients: Reconstitute using SWFI; avoid using solutions containing benzyl alcohol

For methanol toxicity, dilute in D_5W (Barceloux 2002).

Administration

Oral: **This drug should be given parenterally instead of orally in patients with GI toxicity, nausea, vomiting, and when individual doses are >25 mg.**

Parenteral: Due to calcium content, do not administer IV solutions at a rate >160 mg/minute; **not intended for intrathecal use.**

Refer to individual protocols. Should be administered IM, IV push, or IV infusion (15 minutes to 2 hours). Leucovorin should not be administered concurrently with methotrexate. It is commonly initiated 24 hours after the start of methotrexate. Toxicity to normal tissues may be irreversible if leucovorin is not initiated by ~40 hours after the start of methotrexate.

As a rescue after folate antagonists: Administer by IV bolus, IM, or orally

Combination therapy with fluorouracil: Fluorouracil is usually given after, or at the midpoint, of the leucovorin infusion. Leucovorin is usually administered by IV bolus injection or short (10 to 120 minutes) IV infusion. Other administration schedules have been used; refer to individual protocols.

For the treatment of methanol toxicity, infuse over 30 to 60 minutes (Barceloux 2002)

Monitoring Parameters High-dose methotrexate therapy: CBC with differential; serum creatinine; plasma methotrexate concentrations. Leucovorin is continued until the plasma methotrexate concentration is <0.1 micromolar (1 x 10^{-7} molar) or <0.05 micromolar (0.5 x 10^{-7} molar) in situations of delayed methotrexate clearance. With 4- to 6-hour high-dose methotrexate infusions, plasma drug values in excess of 50 micromolar (5 x 10^{-5} M) and 1 micromolar (10^{-6} M) at 24 and 48 hours after starting the infusion, respectively, are often predictive of delayed methotrexate clearance. Monitor fluid and electrolyte status in patients with delayed methotrexate elimination (likely to experience renal toxicity).

When used with fluorouracil: CBC with differential, platelets, LFTs, electrolytes

Dosage Forms Excipient information presented when available (limited, particularly for generics); consult specific product labeling.

Solution, Injection [strength expressed as base]:
Generic: 300 mg/30 mL (30 mL)

Solution Reconstituted, Injection [strength expressed as base]:
Generic: 100 mg (1 ea); 200 mg (1 ea); 350 mg (1 ea); 500 mg (1 ea)

Solution Reconstituted, Injection [strength expressed as base, preservative free]:
Generic: 50 mg (1 ea); 100 mg (1 ea); 200 mg (1 ea); 350 mg (1 ea)

Tablet, Oral [strength expressed as base]:
Generic: 5 mg, 10 mg, 15 mg, 25 mg

Extemporaneous Preparations A 5 mg/mL oral suspension may be prepared with tablets, Cologel, and a 2:1 mixture of simple syrup and wild cherry syrup. Crush twenty-four 25 mg tablets in a glass mortar and reduce to a fine powder; transfer powder to amber bottle. Add 30 mL Cologel and shake mixture thoroughly. Add a quantity of syrup mixture sufficient to make 120 mL. Label "shake well" and "refrigerate". Stable for 28 days refrigerated.

Lam MS. Extemporaneous Compounding of Oral Liquid Dosage Formulations and Alternative Drug Delivery Methods for Anticancer Drugs. *Pharmacotherapy*. 2011;31(2):164-192.

◆ **Leucovorin Calcium Injection (Can)** *see* Leucovorin Calcium *on page 1226*

◆ **Leucovorin Calcium Injection USP (Can)** *see* Leucovorin Calcium *on page 1226*

◆ **Leukeran** *see* Chlorambucil *on page 430*

◆ **Leukeran® (Can)** *see* Chlorambucil *on page 430*

◆ **Leukine** *see* Sargramostim *on page 1905*

Leuprolide (loo PROE lide)

Medication Safety Issues

Sound-alike/look-alike issues:

Lupron Depot (1-month or 3-month formulation) may be confused with Lupron Depot-Ped (1-month or 3-month formulation)

Lupron Depot-Ped is available in two formulations, a 1-month formulation and a 3-month formulation. Both formulations offer an 11.25 mg strength which may further add confusion.

Related Information

Safe Handling of Hazardous Drugs *on page 2455*

Brand Names: US Eligard; Lupron Depot; Lupron Depot-Ped

Brand Names: Canada Eligard; Lupron; Lupron Depot

Therapeutic Category Antineoplastic Agent, Hormone (Gonadotropin Hormone-Releasing Analog); Luteinizing Hormone-Releasing Hormone Analog

Generic Availability (US) Yes

Use Treatment of precocious puberty (FDA approved in females ages <8 years and males ages <9 years); palliative treatment of advanced prostate carcinoma (FDA approved in adults); treatment of anemia caused by uterine leiomyomata (fibroids) (FDA approved in adults); management of endometriosis (FDA approved in adults); has also been used in the treatment of breast cancer, infertility, and as a gonadotropin-releasing hormone analog (GnRHa) stimulation test

Pregnancy Risk Factor X

Pregnancy Considerations Adverse events were observed in animal reproduction studies. Pregnancy must be excluded prior to the start of treatment. Although leuprolide usually inhibits ovulation and stops menstruation, contraception is not ensured and a nonhormonal contraceptive should be used. Use is contraindicated in pregnant women.

Breast-Feeding Considerations It is not known if leuprolide is excreted into breast milk; use is contraindicated in nursing women.

Contraindications

Hypersensitivity to leuprolide, GnRH, GnRH-agonist analogs, or any component of the formulation; undiagnosed abnormal vaginal bleeding (Lupron Depot 3.75 mg [monthly] and Lupron Depot 11.25 mg [3-month]); pregnancy; breast-feeding (Lupron Depot 3.75 mg [monthly] and Lupron Depot 11.25 mg [3-month])

Lupron Depot 22.5 mg, 30 mg, and 45 mg are also not indicated for use in women

Warnings/Precautions Hazardous agent - use appropriate precautions for handling and disposal (NIOSH 2014 [group 1]). Transient increases in testosterone serum levels (~50% above baseline) occur at the start of treatment. Androgen-deprivation therapy (ADT) may increase the risk for cardiovascular disease (Levine, 2010); sudden cardiac death and stroke have been reported in men receiving GnRH agonists; ADT may prolong the QT/QTc interval; consider the benefits of ADT versus the risk for QT prolongation in patients with a history of QTc prolongation, congenital long QT syndrome, heart failure, frequent electrolyte abnormalities, and in patients with medications known to prolong the QT interval, or with preexisting cardiac disease. Consider periodic monitoring of electrocardiograms and electrolytes in at-risk patients. Tumor flare, bone pain, neuropathy, urinary tract obstruction, and spinal cord compression have been reported when used for prostate cancer; closely observe patients for weakness, paresthesias, hematuria, and urinary tract obstruction in first few weeks of therapy. Observe patients with metastatic vertebral lesions or urinary obstruction closely. Exacerbation of endometriosis or uterine leiomyomata may occur initially. Decreased bone density has been reported when used for ≥6 months; use caution in patients with additional risk factors for bone loss (eg, chronic alcohol use, corticosteroid therapy). In patients with prostate cancer, androgen deprivation therapy may increase the risk for cardiovascular disease, diabetes, insulin resistance, obesity, alterations in lipids, and fractures; monitor as clinically necessary. Use caution in patients with a history of psychiatric illness; alteration in mood, memory impairment, and depression have been associated with use. Rare cases of pituitary apoplexy (frequently secondary to pituitary adenoma) have been observed with GnRH agonist administration (onset from 1 hour to usually <2 weeks); may present as sudden headache, vomiting, visual or mental status changes, and infrequently cardiovascular collapse; immediate medical attention required. Convulsions have been observed in postmarketing reports; patients affected included both those with and without a history of cerebrovascular disorders, central nervous system anomalies or tumors, epilepsy, seizures, and those on concomitant medications which may lower the seizure threshold. If seizures occur, manage accordingly. Females treated for precocious puberty may experience menses or spotting during the first 2 months of treatment; notify healthcare provider if bleeding continues after the second month.

Benzyl alcohol and derivatives: Some dosage forms may contain benzyl alcohol; large amounts of benzyl alcohol (≥99 mg/kg/day) have been associated with a potentially fatal toxicity ("gasping syndrome") in neonates; the "gasping syndrome" consists of metabolic acidosis, respiratory distress, gasping respirations, CNS dysfunction (including convulsions, intracranial hemorrhage), hypotension, and cardiovascular collapse (AAP, 1997; CDC, 1982); some data suggests that benzoate displaces bilirubin from protein binding sites (Ahlfors, 2001); avoid or use dosage forms containing benzyl alcohol with caution in neonates.

Some dosage forms may contain polysorbate 80 (also known as Tweens). Hypersensitivity reactions, usually a delayed reaction, have been reported following exposure to pharmaceutical products containing polysorbate 80 in certain individuals (Isaksson, 2002; Lucente 2000; Shelley, 1995). Thrombocytopenia, ascites, pulmonary deterioration, and renal and hepatic failure have been reported in premature neonates after receiving parenteral products containing polysorbate 80 (Alade, 1986; CDC, 1984). See manufacturer's labeling.

Vehicle used in depot injectable formulations (polylactide-co-glycolide microspheres) has rarely been associated with retinal artery occlusion in patients with abnormal arteriovenous anastomosis. Due to different release properties, combinations of dosage forms or fractions of dosage forms should not be interchanged.

Warnings: Additional Pediatric Considerations An increase in pubertal signs and symptoms may occur in the first 2 to 4 weeks of therapy due to the initial stimulatory effect of leuprolide before suppression occurs.

Adverse Reactions

Children (based on 1-month and 3-month pediatric formulations combined)

Cardiovascular: Vasodilation

Central nervous system: Emotional lability, headache, mood changes, pain

Dermatologic: Acne vulgaris, seborrhea, skin rash (including erythema multiforme)

Endocrine & metabolic: Weight gain

Genitourinary: Vaginal discharge, vaginal hemorrhage, vaginitis

Local: Injection site reaction, pain at injection site

Rare but important or life-threatening: Abnormal gait, alopecia, arthralgia, asthma, body odor, bradycardia, cervix disease, decreased visual acuity, depression, dysmenorrhea, dysphagia, epistaxis, excessive crying, feminization, gingivitis, goiter, growth suppression, gynecomastia, hirsutism, hyperhidrosis, hyperkinesia, hypersensitivity reaction, hypertension, infection, leukoderma, myopathy, obesity, peripheral edema, personality disorder, precocious puberty, purpura, skin striae, syncope, urinary incontinence

Adults: Note: For prostate cancer treatment, an initial rise in serum testosterone concentrations may cause "tumor flare" or worsening of symptoms, including bone pain, neuropathy, hematuria, or ureteral or bladder outlet obstruction during the first 2 weeks. Similarly, an initial increase in estradiol levels, with a temporary worsening of symptoms, may occur in women treated with leuprolide.

Delayed release formulations:

Cardiovascular: Angina pectoris, atrial fibrillation, bradycardia, cardiac arrhythmia, cardiac failure, edema, hypertension, hypotension, palpitations, syncope, tachycardia, thrombophlebitis (deep)

Central nervous system: Agitation, anxiety, confusion, delusions, dementia, depression, dizziness, fatigue, fever, headache, insomnia, nervousness, neuropathy, ostealgia, pain, paralysis, paresthesia, seizure

Dermatologic: Acne vulgaris, allergic skin reaction, alopecia, cellulitis, diaphoresis, hair disease, pruritus, skin rash

Endocrine & metabolic: Decreased libido, decreased serum bicarbonate, dehydration, gynecomastia, hirsutism, hot flash, hypercholesterolemia, hyperglycemia, hyperlipidemia, hyperuricemia, hypoalbuminemia, hypocholesterolemia, hypoproteinemia, increased lactate dehydrogenase, increased prostatic acid phosphatase, menstrual disorder, weight changes

Gastrointestinal: Anorexia, change in bowel habits, constipation, diarrhea, dysphagia, eruction, gastric ulcer, gastroenteritis, gastrointestinal disease, gastrointestinal hemorrhage, intestinal obstruction, nausea and vomiting, peptic ulcer

Genitourinary: Balanitis, bladder spasm, dysuria, erectile dysfunction, genitourinary complaint, hematuria, impotence, lactation, mastalgia, nocturia, penile disease, testicular atrophy, testicular disease, testicular pain, urinary incontinence, urinary retention, urinary tract infection, urinary urgency, vaginitis

Hematologic & oncologic: Anemia, bruise, change in platelet count (increased), decreased hemocrit, decreased hemoglobin, decreased prostatic acid phosphatase, ecchymoses, eosinophilia, leukopenia, lymphadenopathy, neoplasm

Hepatic: Abnormal hepatic function tests, hepatomegaly, increased serum AST, prolonged partial thromboplastin time, prolonged prothrombin time

Hypersensitivity: Hypersensitivity reaction

Infection: Infection

Local: Burning sensation at injection site (transient), erythema at injection site, injection site reaction, pain at injection site

Neuromuscular & skeletal: Arthralgia, arthropathy, myalgia, neuromuscular disease, pathological fracture, weakness

Renal: Decreased urine specific gravity, increased blood urea nitrogen, increased serum creatinine, increased urine specific gravity, polyuria

Respiratory: Cough, dyspnea, emphysema, epistaxis, flu-like symptoms, hemoptysis, increased bronchial secretions, pleural effusion, pulmonary edema, respiratory tract disease

Miscellaneous: Fever

Immediate release formulation:

Cardiovascular: Angina pectoris, cardiac arrhythmia, cardiac failure, ECG changes, heart murmur, hypertension, myocardial infarction, peripheral edema, pulmonary embolism, syncope, thrombophlebitis

Central nervous system: Anxiety, depression, dizziness, headache, insomnia, fatigue, fever, nervousness, ostealgia, pain, peripheral neuropathy

Endocrine & metabolic: decreased libido, diabetes mellitus, goiter, gynecomastia, hot flash, hypercalcemia, hypoglycemia

Dermatologic: Alopecia, dermatitis, hyperpigmentation, pruritus, skin lesion

Gastrointestinal: Anorexia, constipation, diarrhea, dysphagia, diarrhea, dysphagia, gastrointestinal hemorrhage, nausea and vomiting, peptic ulcer, rectal polyps

Genitourinary: Bladder spasm, decreased testicular size, dysuria, hematuria, impotence, incontinence, mastalgia, testicular pain, urinary frequency, urinary tract infection, urinary tract obstruction

Hematologic & oncologic: Anemia, bruise

Infection: Infection

Local: Injection site reaction

Neuromuscular & skeletal: Weakness

Ophthalmic: Blurred vision

Renal: Hematuria, increased blood urea nitrogen, increased serum creatinine

Respiratory: Cough, dyspnea, pneumonia, pulmonary fibrosis

Miscellaneous: Fever, inflammation

Children and Adults: *Any formulations:* Rare but important or life-threatening: Abscess at injection site, anaphylaxis, anaphylactoid reaction, asthma, bone fracture (spine), cerebrovascular accident, convulsions, coronary artery disease, decreased white blood cell count, diabetes mellitus, fibromyalgia syndrome (arthralgia/myalgia, headaches, GI distress), hemoptysis, hepatic injury, hepatic insufficiency, hepatotoxicity, hyperuricemia, hypokalemia, hypoproteinemia, induration at injection site, interstitial pulmonary disease, leukocytosis, myocardial infarction, osteopenia, paralysis, penile swelling, peripheral neuropathy, pituitary apoplexy (cardiovascular collapse, mental status altered, ophthalmoplegia, sudden headache, visual changes, vomiting), prolonged QT interval on ECG, prostate pain, pulmonary embolism, pulmonary infiltrates, retroperitoneal fibrosis (pelvic), seizure, skin photosensitivity, suicidal ideation (rare), tenosynovitis (symptoms), thrombocytopenia, transient ischemic attacks

Drug Interactions

Metabolism/Transport Effects None known.

Avoid Concomitant Use

Avoid concomitant use of Leuprolide with any of the following: Corifollitropin Alfa; Highest Risk QTc-Prolonging Agents; Indium 111 Capromab Pendetide; Ivabradine; Mifepristone

Increased Effect/Toxicity

Leuprolide may increase the levels/effects of: Corifollitropin Alfa; Highest Risk QTc-Prolonging Agents; Moderate Risk QTc-Prolonging Agents

The levels/effects of Leuprolide may be increased by: Ivabradine; Mifepristone; QTc-Prolonging Agents (Indeterminate Risk and Risk Modifying)

Decreased Effect

Leuprolide may decrease the levels/effects of: Antidiabetic Agents; Choline C 11; Indium 111 Capromab Pendetide

Storage/Stability

Eligard: Store at 2°C to 8°C (36°F to 46°F). Allow to reach room temperature prior to using; once mixed, must be administered within 30 minutes.

Lupron Depot, Lupron Depot-Ped: Store at room temperature of 25°C (77°F); excursions permitted to 15°C to 30°C (59°F to 86°F). Upon reconstitution, the suspension does not contain a preservative and should be used immediately; discard if not used within 2 hours.

Leuprolide acetate 5 mg/mL solution: Store at 20°C to 25°C (68°F to 77°F); excursions permitted to 15°C to 30°C (59°F to 86°F). Protect from light and store vial in carton until use. Do not freeze.

Mechanism of Action Leuprolide, is an agonist of gonadotropin releasing hormone (GnRH). Acting as a potent inhibitor of gonadotropin secretion; continuous administration results in suppression of ovarian and testicular steroidogenesis due to decreased levels of LH and FSH with subsequent decrease in testosterone (male) and estrogen (female) levels. In males, testosterone levels are reduced to below castrate levels. Leuprolide may also have a direct inhibitory effect on the testes, and act by a different mechanism not directly related to reduction in serum testosterone.

Pharmacodynamics

Onset of action: Serum testosterone levels first increase within 3 days of therapy, then decrease after 2-4 weeks with continued therapy

Onset of therapeutic suppression for precocious puberty:

Leuprolide: 2-4 weeks

Leuprolide depot: 1 month

Pharmacokinetics (Adult data unless noted)

Absorption: Requires parenteral administration since it is rapidly destroyed within the GI tract

Protein binding: 43% to 49%

Bioavailability: SubQ: 94%

Half-life: 3 hours

Elimination: Not well defined

Dosing: Usual

Children: **Precocious puberty: Note:** Initiate for girls <8 years or boys <9 years; consider discontinuing leuprolide therapy in girls by age 11 and boys by age 12.

IM:

Lupron Depot-Ped® (monthly formulation):

Manufacturer's labeling: Initial:

≤25 kg: 7.5 mg every 4 weeks; titrate dose in 3.75 mg increments every 4 weeks until clinical or laboratory tests indicate adequate suppression

>25-37.5 kg: 11.25 mg every 4 weeks; titrate dose in 3.75 mg increments every 4 weeks until clinical or laboratory tests indicate adequate suppression

>37.5 kg: 15 mg every 4 weeks; titrate dose in 3.75 mg increments every 4 weeks until clinical or laboratory tests indicate adequate suppression

Alternative dosing: Initial: 0.2-0.3 mg/kg/dose every 4 weeks (Carel, 2009)

Lupron Depot-Ped® (3-month formulation): 11.25 mg or 30 mg every 12 weeks

SubQ (Leuprolide acetate 5 mg/mL solution): Initial: 50 **mcg**/kg/dose once daily; may titrate dose upward by 10 **mcg**/kg/day if suppression of ovarian or testicular steroidogenesis is not achieved. **Note:** Higher **mcg**/kg doses may be required in younger children.

Leuprolide (GNrHa) Stimulation Test (Female): SubQ (Leuprolide acetate 5 mg/mL solution): 20 **mcg**/kg once; measure LH and FSH at baseline and after administration (usually two spaced measurements ≤120 minutes [eg, 30 and 60 minutes **or** 60 and 120 minutes]) (Houk, 2008; Sathasivam, 2010; Sathasivam, 2011)

Adults:

Advanced prostate cancer:

IM:

Lupron Depot® 7.5 mg (monthly): 7.5 mg every month **or**

Lupron Depot® 22.5 mg (3 month): 22.5 mg every 12 weeks **or**

Lupron Depot® 30 mg (4 month): 30 mg every 16 weeks **or**

Lupron Depot® 45 mg (6 month): 45 mg every 24 weeks

SubQ:

Eligard®: 7.5 mg monthly **or** 22.5 mg every 3 months **or** 30 mg every 4 months **or** 45 mg every 6 months

Leuprolide acetate 5 mg/mL solution: 1 mg/day

Endometriosis: IM: Initial therapy may be with leuprolide alone or in combination with norethindrone; if retreatment for an additional 6 months is necessary, concomitant norethindrone should be used. Retreatment is not recommended for longer than one additional 6-month course.

Lupron Depot®: 3.75 mg every month for up to 6 months **or**

Lupron Depot®-3 month: 11.25 mg every 3 months for up to 2 doses (6 months total duration of treatment)

Uterine leiomyomata (fibroids): IM (in combination with iron):

Lupron Depot®: 3.75 mg every month for up to 3 months **or**

Lupron Depot®-3 month: 11.25 mg as a single injection

Preparation for Administration Hazardous agent; use appropriate precautions for handling and disposal (NIOSH 2014 [group 1]).

Parenteral:

IM (Lupron Depot, Lupron Depot-Ped): Reconstitute only with diluent provided; upon reconstitution, a milky suspension is formed

SubQ: Eligard: Packaged in two syringes; one contains the Atrigel polymer system and the second contains leuprolide acetate powder; allow product to come to room temperature; follow package instructions for mixing; once mixed product must administered within 30 minutes.

Administration Hazardous agent; use appropriate precautions for handling and disposal (NIOSH 2014 [group 1]).

Parenteral: Do not administer IV

IM (Lupron Depot, Lupron Depot-Ped): Administer as a single injection; rotate administration site periodically. Reconstituted solution does not contain preservatives and should be used immediately.

SubQ:

Leuprolide acetate 5 mg/mL solution: Administer undiluted into areas on the arm, thigh, or abdomen; rotate injection site. If an alternate syringe from the manufacturer-provided syringe is required, insulin syringes should be used

Eligard: Vary injection site; choose site with adequate subcutaneous tissue (eg, upper or midabdomen, upper buttocks); avoid areas that may be compressed or rubbed (eg, belt or waistband)

Monitoring Parameters Precocious puberty: Height, weight, bone age, Tanner staging test, GnRH testing (blood LH and FSH levels), testosterone in males and estradiol in females; closely monitor patients with prostatic carcinoma for plasma testosterone, acid phosphatase, and signs of weakness, paresthesias, and urinary tract obstruction during the first few weeks of therapy

Test Interactions Interferes with pituitary gonadotropic and gonadal function tests during and up to 3 months after monthly administration of leuprolide therapy.

Dosage Forms Excipient information presented when available (limited, particularly for generics); consult specific product labeling.

Kit, Injection, as acetate:

Generic: 1 mg/0.2 mL

Kit, Intramuscular, as acetate:

Lupron Depot: 7.5 mg, 45 mg [latex free; contains polysorbate 80]

Kit, Intramuscular, as acetate [preservative free]:

Lupron Depot: 3.75 mg, 11.25 mg, 22.5 mg, 30 mg [latex free; contains polysorbate 80]

Lupron Depot-Ped: 7.5 mg, 11.25 mg, 15 mg, 30 mg (Ped), 11.25 mg (Ped) [latex free; contains polysorbate 80]

Kit, Subcutaneous, as acetate:

Eligard: 7.5 mg, 22.5 mg, 30 mg, 45 mg

◆ **Leuprolide Acetate** *see* Leuprolide *on page 1229*

◆ **Leuprorelin Acetate** *see* Leuprolide *on page 1229*

◆ **Leurocristine Sulfate** *see* VinCRIStine *on page 2178*

◆ **Leustatin** *see* Cladribine *on page 480*

Levalbuterol (leve al BYOO ter ole)

Medication Safety Issues

Sound-alike/look-alike issues:

Xopenex may be confused with Xanax

Brand Names: US Xopenex; Xopenex Concentrate; Xopenex HFA

Therapeutic Category Adrenergic Agonist Agent; Antiasthmatic; Beta$_2$-Adrenergic Agonist; Bronchodilator; Sympathomimetic

Generic Availability (US) May be product dependent

Use Treatment and prevention of bronchospasm in patients with reversible obstructive airway disease

Pregnancy Risk Factor C

Pregnancy Considerations Adverse events were not observed in animal reproduction studies. Congenital anomalies (cleft palate, limb defects) have rarely been reported following maternal use of racemic albuterol during pregnancy. Multiple medications were used in most cases, no specific pattern of defects has been reported, and no relationship to racemic albuterol has been established. Beta-agonists may interfere with uterine contractility if administered during labor.

Uncontrolled asthma is associated with adverse events on pregnancy (increased risk of perinatal mortality, pre-eclampsia, preterm birth, low birth weight infants). Other beta$_2$-receptor agonists are currently preferred for the treatment of asthma during pregnancy (NAEPP, 2005).

Breast-Feeding Considerations It is not known whether levalbuterol is excreted in human milk. According to the manufacturer, the decision to continue or discontinue breast-feeding during therapy should take into account the risk of exposure to the infant and the benefits of treatment to the mother. The use of beta$_2$-receptor agonists are not considered a contraindication to breast-feeding (NAEPP, 2005).

Contraindications Hypersensitivity to levalbuterol, albuterol, or any component of the formulation

Warnings/Precautions Optimize anti-inflammatory treatment before initiating maintenance treatment with levalbuterol. Do not use as a component of chronic therapy without an anti-inflammatory agent. Only the mildest form of asthma (Step 1 and/or exercise-induced) would not require concurrent use based upon asthma guidelines (NAEPP, 2007). If patients need more doses than usual, this may be a sign of asthma destabilization; patient should be reevaluated. Patient must be instructed to seek medical attention in cases where acute symptoms are not relieved or a previous level of response is diminished. The need to increase frequency of use may indicate deterioration of asthma, and treatment must not be delayed.

Use caution in patients with cardiovascular disease (arrhythmia or hypertension or HF), convulsive disorders, diabetes, glaucoma, hyperthyroidism, or hypokalemia. Beta-agonists may cause elevation in blood pressure, heart rate, and result in CNS stimulation/excitation. Beta$_2$-agonists may increase risk of arrhythmia, increase serum glucose, or decrease serum potassium.

Immediate hypersensitivity reactions (urticaria, angioedema, rash, bronchospasm, anaphylaxis, oropharyngeal edema) have been reported. Do not exceed recommended dose; serious adverse events including fatalities, have been associated with excessive use of inhaled sympathomimetics. Rarely, paradoxical bronchospasm may occur with use of inhaled bronchodilating agents; this should be distinguished from inadequate response. Potentially significant interactions may exist, requiring dose or frequency adjustment, additional monitoring, and/or selection of alternative therapy.

Adverse Reactions

Cardiovascular: Tachycardia

Central nervous system: Anxiety, dizziness, headache, migraine, nervousness, weakness

Dermatologic: Rash

Endocrine & metabolic: Serum glucose increased, serum potassium decreased

Gastrointestinal: Diarrhea, dyspepsia

Neuromuscular & skeletal: Leg cramps, tremor

Respiratory: Asthma, cough, nasal edema, pharyngitis, rhinitis, sinusitis, viral infection

Miscellaneous: Accidental injury, flu-like syndrome, viral infection,

Rare but important or life-threatening: Abnormal ECG, acne, anaphylaxis, angina, angioedema, arrhythmia, atrial fibrillation, chest pain, dysmenorrhea, epistaxis, extrasystole, gastroenteritis, gastroesophageal reflux disease, hematuria, hypertension, hypoesthesia (hand), hypokalemia, lymphadenopathy, metabolic acidosis, myalgia, nausea, oropharyngeal dryness, paresthesia, supraventricular arrhythmia, syncope, vaginal moniliasis

Note: Immediate hypersensitivity reactions have occurred (including angioedema, oropharyngeal edema, urticaria, and anaphylaxis).

Drug Interactions

Metabolism/Transport Effects None known.

Avoid Concomitant Use

Avoid concomitant use of Levalbuterol with any of the following: Beta-Blockers (Nonselective); Iobenguane I 123; Loxapine

Increased Effect/Toxicity

Levalbuterol may increase the levels/effects of: Atosiban; Highest Risk QTc-Prolonging Agents; Loop Diuretics; Loxapine; Moderate Risk QTc-Prolonging Agents; Sympathomimetics; Thiazide Diuretics

The levels/effects of Levalbuterol may be increased by: AtoMOXetine; Cannabinoid-Containing Products; Linezolid; MAO Inhibitors; Mifepristone; Tedizolid; Tricyclic Antidepressants

Decreased Effect

Levalbuterol may decrease the levels/effects of: Iobenguane I 123

The levels/effects of Levalbuterol may be decreased by: Beta-Blockers (Beta1 Selective); Beta-Blockers (Nonselective); Betahistine

Storage/Stability

Aerosol: Store at 20°C to 25°C (68°F to 77°F); protect from freezing and direct sunlight. Store with mouthpiece down. Discard after 200 actuations (15 g canister) or 80 actuations (8.4 g canister). Do not puncture or incinerate.

Solution for nebulization: Store in protective foil pouch at 20°C to 25°C (68°F to 77°F). Protect from light and excessive heat. Vials should be used within 2 weeks after opening protective pouch. Use within 1 week and protect from light if removed from pouch. Vials of concentrated solution should be used immediately after removing from protective pouch.

Mechanism of Action Relaxes bronchial smooth muscle by action on beta$_2$-receptors with little effect on heart rate

Pharmacodynamics

Onset of action: Nebulized: 10-17 minutes; aerosol: 5.5-10 minutes

Maximum effect: Nebulized: 1.5 hours; aerosol: 77 minutes

Duration: Nebulized: 5-6 hours; aerosol: 3-6 hours

Pharmacokinetics (Adult data unless noted) Nebulization:

Distribution: V_d: Adults: 1900 L

Metabolism: In the liver to an inactive sulfate

Half-life: 3.3-4.0 hours

Time to peak serum concentration: 0.2-1.8 hours

Elimination: 3% to 6% excreted unchanged in urine

Dosing: Neonatal Note: May consider using half of the albuterol dose; albuterol is a 1:1 racemic mixture and levalbuterol is the active isomer; limited data available. **Dosage expressed in terms of mg levalbuterol.**

Bronchodilation: Nebulization: 0.31 mg/dose every 8 hours was administered to 31 VLBW neonates (mean GA: 28.1 weeks; mean birth weight: 1127 g) for >2 weeks; no untoward hemodynamic effects were noted (Mhanna 2009)

Dosing: Usual Note: Dosage expressed in terms of mg levalbuterol.

Acute asthma exacerbation (NAEPP 2007):

Nebulization:

Children: 0.075 mg/kg (minimum dose: 1.25 mg) every 20 minutes for 3 doses then 0.075 to 0.15 mg/kg (not to exceed 5 mg) every 1 to 4 hours as needed

Adults: 1.25 to 2.5 mg every 20 minutes for 3 doses then 1.25 to 5 mg every 1 to 4 hours as needed

Inhalation: MDI: 45 mcg/spray:

Children: 4 to 8 puffs every 20 minutes for 3 doses then every 1 to 4 hours

Adults: 4 to 8 puffs every 20 minutes for up to 4 hours then every 1 to 4 hours as needed

Maintenance therapy (nonacute) (NAEPP 2007): Not recommended for long-term, daily maintenance treatment; regular use exceeding 2 days/week for symptom control indicates the need for additional long-term control therapy

Nebulization:

Children 0 to 4 years: 0.31 to 1.25 mg every 4 to 6 hours as needed

Children ≥5 years and Adults: 0.31 to 0.63 mg every 8 hours as needed

Inhalation: MDI: 45 mcg/spray:

Children <5 years: Not FDA approved

Children ≥5 years and Adults: 2 inhalations every 4 to 6 hours as needed

Preparation for Administration Oral inhalation: Nebulization: Concentrated solution should be diluted with NS prior to use, typically 2.5 mL; however, prescriber may determine amount based on patient needs.

Administration Oral Inhalation: In children <4 years, a face mask with either the metered dose inhaler or nebulizer is recommended (GINA 2014; NAEPP 2007)

Nebulization: Dilution required for concentrated solution. Safety and efficacy were established when administered with the following nebulizers: PARI LC Jet, PARI LC Plus, as well as the following compressors: PARI Master, Dura-Neb 2000, and Dura-Neb 3000. Blow-by administration is not recommended, use a mask device if patient unable to hold mouthpiece in mouth for administration.

Inhalation, aerosol (metered dose inhaler): Shake well before use. Prime the inhaler (before first use or if it has not been used for more than 2 weeks) by releasing 4 test sprays into the air away from the face.

Monitoring Parameters Serum potassium, oxygen saturation, heart rate, pulmonary function tests, respiratory rate, use of accessory muscles during respiration, suprasternal retractions; arterial or capillary blood gases (if patient's condition warrants)

Additional Information Levalbuterol administered in 1/2 the mg dose of albuterol (eg, 0.63 mg levalbuterol to 1.25 mg albuterol) provides comparable efficacy and safety. Levalbuterol has not been evaluated by continuous nebulization (NIH Guidelines, 2007).

Dosage Forms Considerations Xopenex HFA 15 g canisters contain 200 inhalations and 8.4 g canisters contain 80 inhalations.

Dosage Forms Excipient information presented when available (limited, particularly for generics); consult specific product labeling.

Aerosol, Inhalation, as tartrate [strength expressed as base]:

Xopenex HFA: 45 mcg/actuation (15 g)

Nebulization Solution, Inhalation, as hydrochloride [strength expressed as base]:

Xopenex: 0.63 mg/3 mL (3 mL); 1.25 mg/3 mL (3 mL)

Generic: 0.63 mg/3 mL (3 mL)

Nebulization Solution, Inhalation, as hydrochloride [strength expressed as base, preservative free]:

Xopenex: 0.31 mg/3 mL (3 mL)

Xopenex Concentrate: 1.25 mg/0.5 mL (1 ea, 30 ea)

Generic: 0.31 mg/3 mL (3 mL); 0.63 mg/3 mL (3 mL); 1.25 mg/3 mL (3 mL); 1.25 mg/0.5 mL (1 ea, 30 ea)

- ◆ **Levalbuterol Hydrochloride** *see* Levalbuterol *on page 1233*
- ◆ **Levalbuterol Tartrate** *see* Levalbuterol *on page 1233*
- ◆ **Levaquin** *see* Levofloxacin (Systemic) *on page 1243*
- ◆ **Levaquin in 5% Dextrose Injection (Can)** *see* Levofloxacin (Systemic) *on page 1243*
- ◆ **Levarterenol Bitartrate** *see* Norepinephrine *on page 1529*
- ◆ **Levate (Can)** *see* Amitriptyline *on page 131*
- ◆ **Levatio** *see* Capsaicin *on page 362*
- ◆ **Levbid** *see* Hyoscyamine *on page 1061*
- ◆ **Levemir** *see* Insulin Detemir *on page 1124*
- ◆ **Levemir® (Can)** *see* Insulin Detemir *on page 1124*
- ◆ **Levemir FlexPen [DSC]** *see* Insulin Detemir *on page 1124*
- ◆ **Levemir FlexTouch** *see* Insulin Detemir *on page 1124*

LevETIRAcetam (lee va tye RA se tam)

Medication Safety Issues

Sound-alike/look-alike issues:

Keppra may be confused with Keflex, Keppra XR

LevETIRAcetam may be confused with lamoTRIgine, levOCARNitine, levofloxacin

Potential for dispensing errors between Keppra and Kaletra (lopinavir/ritonavir)

Related Information

Oral Medications That Should Not Be Crushed or Altered *on page 2476*

Brand Names: US Keppra; Keppra XR

Brand Names: Canada Abbott-Levetiracetam; ACT Levetiracetam; Apo-Levetiracetam; Auro-Levetiracetam; Dom-Levetiracetam; JAMP-Levetiracetam; Keppra; PHL-Levetiracetam; PMS-Levetiracetam; PRO-Levetiracetam; RAN-Levetiracetam

Therapeutic Category Anticonvulsant, Miscellaneous

Generic Availability (US) Yes

Use

Oral:

Oral solution and immediate release tablets: Adjunctive therapy in the treatment of partial onset seizures (FDA approved in ages ≥1 month and adults); adjunctive therapy in the treatment of juvenile myoclonic epilepsy (FDA approved in ages ≥12 years) and myoclonic seizures (FDA approved in adults); adjunctive therapy in the treatment of primary generalized tonic-clonic seizures (FDA approved in ages ≥6 years and adults); has also been used for treatment of neonatal seizures, as adjunctive therapy for the treatment of generalized epilepsy with photosensitivity and Lennox-Gastaut syndrome, monotherapy for the treatment of various seizures types, treatment of tics in patients with Tourette syndrome, prophylaxis in pediatric migraine, and bipolar disorder

Extended release tablets: Adjunctive therapy in the treatment of partial onset seizures (FDA approved in ages ≥16 years and adults)

IV: Adjunctive therapy in the treatment of partial onset seizures (FDA approved in ages ≥16 years and adults); adjunctive therapy in the treatment of myoclonic seizures in patients with juvenile myoclonic epilepsy (FDA approved in ages ≥16 years and adults); adjunctive therapy in the treatment of primary generalized tonic-clinic seizures in patients with idiopathic generalized epilepsy (FDA approved in ages ≥16 years and adults); temporary use in patients in whom oral administration is not feasible (FDA approved in ages ≥16 years and adults); has also been used for treatment of refractory status epilepticus or acute repetitive seizure activity

Medication Guide Available Yes

Pregnancy Risk Factor C

Pregnancy Considerations Developmental toxicities were observed in animal reproduction studies. Levetiracetam crosses the placenta and can be detected in the neonate at birth. Concentrations in the umbilical cord at delivery are similar to those in the maternal plasma. Serum concentrations of levetiracetam may decrease as pregnancy progresses; monitor carefully throughout pregnancy and postpartum (Tomson, 2007).

A registry is available for women exposed to levetiracetam during pregnancy: Pregnant women may enroll themselves into the North American Antiepileptic Drug (AED) Pregnancy Registry (888-233-2334 or http://www.aedpregnancyregistry.org/).

The North American AED registry has published data collected from pregnant women taking levetiracetam monotherapy from 1997 to 2011 (n=450). Eleven major malformations were diagnosed within 12 weeks of birth. The relative risk of major malformations was not increased in comparison to women with epilepsy not taking AEDs (n=442; RR 2.2, 95% CI 0.8 to 6.4) or in comparison to women using lamotrigine monotherapy (n=1,562; RR 1.2, 95% CI 0.6 to 2.5) (Hernández-Díaz, 2012).

Breast-Feeding Considerations Levetiracetam can be detected in breast milk. Using data from 11 women collected 4-23 days after delivery, the estimated exposure of levetiracetam to the breast-feeding infant would be ~2 mg/kg/day (relative infant dose 7.9% of the weight-adjusted maternal dose). Adverse events were not reported in the nursing infants (Tomson, 2007). Due to the potential for serious adverse reactions in the nursing infant, the manufacturer recommends a decision be made whether to discontinue nursing or to discontinue the drug, taking into account the importance of treatment to the mother.

Contraindications

There are no contraindications listed in the U.S. manufacturer's labeling.

Canadian labeling: Hypersensitivity to levetiracetam or any component of the formulation

Warnings/Precautions Antiepileptics are associated with an increased risk of suicidal behavior/thoughts with use (regardless of indication); patients should be monitored for signs/symptoms of depression, suicidal tendencies, and other unusual behavior changes during therapy and instructed to inform their health care provider immediately if symptoms occur.

Severe reactions, including toxic epidermal necrolysis (TEN) and Stevens-Johnson syndrome (SJS), have been reported in adults and children. Onset is usually within ~2 weeks of treatment initiation, but may be delayed (>4 months); recurrence following rechallenge has been reported. Levetiracetam should be discontinued if there are any signs of a hypersensitivity reaction or unspecified rash; if signs or symptoms suggest SJS or TEN, do not resume therapy and consider alternative treatment.

Psychosis, paranoia, hallucinations, and behavioral symptoms (including aggression, agitation, anger, anxiety, apathy, confusion, depersonalization, depression, emotional lability, hostility, hyperkinesias, irritability, nervousness, neurosis, and personality disorder) may occur; incidence may be increased in children. Dose reduction or discontinuation may be required. Levetiracetam should be withdrawn gradually, when possible, to minimize the potential of increased seizure frequency. Use caution with renal impairment; dosage adjustment may be necessary. In patients with ESRD requiring hemodialysis, it is recommended that immediate-release formulations be used instead of ER formulations. Elepsia XR is not recommended in patients with moderate or severe renal impairment (CrCl <50 mL/minute/1.73 m^2). May cause CNS depression (impaired coordination, ataxia, abnormal gait, fatigue, weakness, dizziness, and somnolence), which may impair physical or mental abilities. Symptoms occur most commonly during the first month of therapy. Patients must be cautioned about performing tasks that require mental alertness (eg, operating machinery or driving). Decreases in red blood cell counts, hemoglobin, hematocrit, white blood cell counts and neutrophils have been observed. Cases of eosinophilia, agranulocytosis, and lymphocytosis have also been reported. Isolated elevations in diastolic blood pressure measurements have been reported in children <4 years of age; however, no observable differences were noted in mean diastolic measurements of children receiving levetiracetam vs placebo. Similar effects have not been observed in older children and adults. Potentially significant drug-drug interactions may exist, requiring dose or frequency adjustment, additional monitoring, and/or selection of alternative therapy.

Warnings: Additional Pediatric Considerations Incidence of behavioral abnormalities is higher in children (37.6%) than adults (13.3%); dosage reductions may be required. Isolated elevations in diastolic blood pressure measurements have been reported in infants and children 1 month to <4 years of age receiving levetiracetam; however, no difference was noted in mean diastolic measurements of these patients vs placebo group. Similar effects have not been observed in older children and adults. In pediatric clinical trials, the most frequently reported adverse reactions in pediatric patients 4 to <16 years of age were fatigue, aggression, nasal congestion, decreased appetite, and irritability and in younger pediatric patients (1 month to <4 years of age) were somnolence and irritability; additionally, children may experience a higher frequency of certain adverse effects than adults, including the following: Behavioral abnormalities (37.6% vs 13.3%), aggression/hostility (10% vs 2%), vomiting (reported in children only, 15%), and cough (9% vs 2%).

Adverse Reactions

Information given for all indications and populations (adults and children) unless otherwise specified.

Cardiovascular: Increased blood pressure (diastolic; infants and children)

Central nervous system: Aggressive behavior (children and adolescents), agitation (children and adolescents), amnesia, anxiety, ataxia (partial-onset seizures; includes abnormal gait, incoordination), behavioral problems (includes aggression, agitation, anger, anxiety, apathy, depersonalization, depression, dizziness, emotional lability, irritability, neurosis), confusion, depression, dizziness, drowsiness, emotional lability, falling (children and adolescents), fatigue, headache, hostility, insomnia (children and adolescents), irritability (infants, children and adolescents), lethargy (children and adolescents), mood changes (children and adolescents), nervousness, pain, paranoia (children and adolescents), paresthesia, psychotic symptoms, sedation (children and adolescents), vertigo

Gastrointestinal: Anorexia, constipation (children and adolescents), decreased appetite (children and adolescents), diarrhea, gastroenteritis (children and adolescents), nausea, upper abdominal pain (children and adolescents), vomiting (children and adolescents)

Hematologic & oncologic: Bruise (children and adolescents), decreased neutrophils, decreased white blood cell count, eosinophilia (children and adolescents)

Infection: Infection, influenza

Neuromuscular & skeletal: Arthralgia (children and adolescents), joint sprain (children and adolescents), neck pain, weakness

Ophthalmic: Conjunctivitis (children and adolescents), diplopia

Otic: Otalgia (children and adolescents)

Respiratory: Cough, nasal congestion (children and adolescents), nasopharyngitis, pharyngolaryngeal pain (children and adolescents), pharyngitis, rhinitis, sinusitis

Miscellaneous: Head trauma (children and adolescents)

Rare but important or life-threatening: Agranulocytosis, decreased red blood cells, dyskinesia, DRESS syndrome, eczema, equilibrium disturbance, erythema multiforme, hepatic failure, hepatitis, hyperkinesia, hyponatremia, memory impairment, myalgia, myasthenia, pancreatitis, pancytopenia (with bone marrow suppression in some cases), panic attack, personality disorder, psychosis, Stevens-Johnson syndrome, suicidal tendencies, thrombocytopenia, toxic epidermal necrolysis

Drug Interactions

Metabolism/Transport Effects None known.

Avoid Concomitant Use

Avoid concomitant use of LevETIRAcetam with any of the following: Azelastine (Nasal); Orphenadrine; Paraldehyde; Thalidomide

Increased Effect/Toxicity

LevETIRAcetam may increase the levels/effects of: Alcohol (Ethyl); Azelastine (Nasal); Buprenorphine; CNS Depressants; Hydrocodone; Methotrimeprazine; Metyrosine; Mirtazapine; Orphenadrine; Paraldehyde; Pramipexole; ROPINIRole; Rotigotine; Selective Serotonin Reuptake Inhibitors; Suvorexant; Thalidomide; Zolpidem

The levels/effects of LevETIRAcetam may be increased by: Brimonidine (Topical); Cannabis; Doxylamine; Dronabinol; Droperidol; HydrOXYzine; Kava Kava; Magnesium Sulfate; Methotrimeprazine; Nabilone; Perampanel; Rufinamide; Sodium Oxybate; Tapentadol; Tetrahydrocannabinol

Decreased Effect

The levels/effects of LevETIRAcetam may be decreased by: Mefloquine; Mianserin; Orlistat

Food Interactions Food may delay, but does not affect the extent of absorption. Management: Administer without regard to meals.

Storage/Stability

Oral solution, tablets: Store at 25°C (77°F); excursions permitted to 15°C to 30°C (59°F to 86°F).

Premixed solution for infusion: Store at 20°C to 25°C (68°F to 77°F).

Vials for injection: Store at 25°C (77°F); excursions permitted to 15°C to 30°C (59°F to 86°F). Admixed solution is stable for 24 hours in PVC bags kept at room temperature.

Mechanism of Action The precise mechanism by which levetiracetam exerts its antiepileptic effect is unknown. However, several studies have suggested the mechanism may involve one or more of the following central pharmacologic effects: inhibition of voltage-dependent N-type calcium channels; facilitation of GABA-ergic inhibitory transmission through displacement of negative modulators; reduction of delayed rectifier potassium current; and/or binding to synaptic proteins which modulate neurotransmitter release.

Pharmacokinetics (Adult data unless noted)

Absorption: Oral: Rapid and complete

Distribution: V_d: Approximates volume of intracellular and extracellular water; V_d:

Infants and Children <4 years: 0.63 ± 0.08 L/kg (Glauser, 2007)

Children 6-12 years: 0.72 ± 0.12 L/kg (Pellock, 2001)

Adults: 0.5-0.7 L/kg

Protein binding: <10%

Metabolism: Not extensive; 24% of dose is metabolized by enzymatic hydrolysis of acetamide group (major metabolic pathway; hydrolysis occurs primarily in the blood, not cytochrome P450 dependent); two minor metabolites (one via hydroxylation of 2-oxo-pyrrolidine ring and one via opening of the 2-oxo-pyrrolidine ring in position 5) are also formed; metabolites are inactive and renally excreted

Bioavailability: Oral: 100%; bioavailability of extended release tablets is similar to immediate release tablets; tablets, oral solution, and injection are bioequivalent

Half-life: Increased in patients with renal dysfunction:

Infants and Children <4 years: 5.3 ± 1.3 hours (Glauser, 2007)

Children 4-12 years: 6 ± 1.1 hours (Pellock, 2001)

Adults: 6-8 hours

Time to peak serum concentration: Oral:

Oral solution: Fasting infants and children <4 years: 1.4 ± 0.9 hours

Immediate release: Fasting adults and children: 1 hour

Extended release: 4 hours; median time to peak is 2 hours longer in the fed state

Elimination: 66% excreted in urine as unchanged drug and 27% as inactive metabolites; undergoes glomerular filtration and subsequent partial tubular reabsorption

Clearance: Correlated with creatinine clearance; clearance is decreased in patients with renal dysfunction

Infants <6 months: 1.23 mL/minute/kg (Glauser, 2007)

Infants and Children 6 months-4 years: 1.57 mL/minute/kg (Glauser, 2007)

Children 6-12 years: 1.43 mL/min/kg; 30% to 40% higher than adults on a per kg basis (Pellock, 2001)

Dialysis: Hemodialysis: Standard 4-hour treatment removes ~50% of the drug from the body; supplemental doses after dialysis are recommended

Dosing: Neonatal Neonatal Seizures:

IV: Limited data available: 10 mg/kg/day divided twice daily; increase dosage by 10 mg/kg over 3 days to 30 mg/kg/day; additional increases up to 45-60 mg/kg/day have been used with persistent seizure activity or clinical EEG findings. Dosing based on an open-label study of 38 patients [n=19 premature neonates GA <28 weeks (birth weight: 0.41-1.33 kg); n=6 premature neonates GA: 28-36 weeks (birth weight: 1.25-1.89 kg); n=13 term neonates] which reported a decrease in seizure frequency (ie, after 1 week of therapy, 30/38 patients were seizure-free). The investigators noted that patients with extensive intracerebral hemorrhage tended to be less responsive to therapy (Ramantani, 2011). For treatment of status epilepticus, loading doses of 20-30 mg/kg/dose have been used by some centers (Abend, 2009).

Oral: Dose not established, limited data available: Initial: 10 mg/kg/day in 1-2 divided doses; increase daily by 10 mg/kg to 30 mg/kg/day (maximum reported dose: 60 mg/kg/day). Dosing based on two prospective, open-label studies [n=38 (n=19, GA: <28 weeks; n=6, GA: 28-36 weeks, n=13 term); n=6, GA: >30 weeks], a case series (n=3, 2 days to 3 months) which showed levetiracetam was effective at increasing seizure-free interval, and a report of pediatric neurologists' NICU experience

(Fürwentsches, 2010; Ramantani, 2011; Shoemaker, 2007; Silverstein, 2008).

Dosing: Usual Note: When switching from oral to IV formulation, the total daily dose should be the same.

Infants, Children, and Adolescents <16 years: **Note:** Use oral solution in infants and children ≤20 kg; either oral solution or immediate release tablets may be used in children and adolescents >20 kg.

Myoclonic seizures: Children ≥12 years and Adolescents <16 years: Oral (immediate release: tablets or solution): Initial 500 mg twice daily; increase dosage every 2 weeks by 500 mg/dose twice daily, to the recommended dose of 1500 mg twice daily. Efficacy of doses other than 3000 mg/day has not been established.

Partial onset seizures:

Infants 1 to <6 months: Oral (immediate release: solution): Initial: 7 mg/kg/dose twice daily; increase dosage every 2 weeks by 7 mg/kg/dose twice daily as tolerated, to the recommended dose of 21 mg/kg/dose twice daily; effectiveness of lower doses has not been established; during clinical trials, the mean daily dose was 35 mg/kg/**day**

Infants ≥6 months and Children <4 years: Oral [immediate release: solution or tablets (patient weight >20 kg)]: Initial: 10 mg/kg/dose twice daily; increase dosage every 2 weeks by 10 mg/kg/dose twice daily, as tolerated, to the recommended dose of 25 mg/kg/dose twice daily; may reduce daily dose if not tolerated; during clinical trials, the mean daily dose was 47 mg/kg/**day**

Children ≥4 years and Adolescents <16 years: Oral (immediate release):

Oral solution: Initial: 10 mg/kg/dose twice daily; increase dosage every 2 weeks by 10 mg/kg/dose twice daily, as tolerated, to a maximum of 30 mg/kg/dose twice daily; maximum daily dose: 3000 mg/**day**; may reduce daily dose if not tolerated; during clinical trials, the mean daily dose was 44 mg/kg/**day**

Tablets: Fixed-dosing:

20-40 kg: Initial: 250 mg twice daily, increase every 2 weeks by 250 mg twice daily to the maximum recommended dose of 750 mg twice daily

>40 kg: Initial: 500 mg twice daily, increase every 2 weeks by 500 mg twice daily to the maximum recommended dose of 1500 mg twice daily

Primary generalized tonic-clonic seizures: Children 6 to <16 years: Oral [immediate release: solution or tablets (patient weight >20kg)]: Initial: 10 mg/kg/dose twice daily; increase dosage every 2 weeks by 10 mg/kg/dose given twice daily, to the recommended dose of 30 mg/kg/dose twice daily. Efficacy of doses other than 60 mg/kg/day has not been established.

Status epilepticus or acute repetitive seizure activity: Limited data available: IV: Loading dose: 50 mg/kg/dose (maximum dose: 2500 mg); followed by IV or oral maintenance dosing determined by clinical response; reported IV maintenance dose: 30-55 mg/kg/day divided twice daily (Kirmani, 2009; Ng, 2010). Dosing based on a prospective study (n=30, 6 months to <15 years), several retrospective observations, and case reports (n >100; youngest patient: 1 day old; reported loading dose range: 6.5-89 mg/kg) (Abend, 2009; Gallentine, 2009; Goraya, 2008; Kirmani, 2009; Ng, 2010; Reiter, 2010).

Adolescents ≥16 years and Adults:

Myoclonic seizures:

Oral: Immediate release: 500 mg twice daily; may increase every 2 weeks by 500 mg/dose to the recommended dose of 1500 mg twice daily. Efficacy of doses other than 3000 mg/**day** has not been established.

IV: Initial: 500 mg twice daily; increase dosage every 2 weeks by 500 mg/dose given twice daily, to the recommended dose of 1500 mg twice daily. Efficacy of doses other than 3000 mg/day has not been established.

Partial onset seizures:

Oral:

Immediate release: Initial: 500 mg twice daily; may increase every 2 weeks by 500 mg/dose given twice daily, if tolerated, to a maximum of 1500 mg twice daily. Doses >3000 mg/**day** have been used in trials; however, there is no evidence of increased benefit.

Extended release: Initial: 1000 mg once daily; may increase every 2 weeks by 1000 mg/day to a maximum of 3000 mg once daily

IV: Initial: 500 mg twice daily; may increase every 2 weeks by 500 mg/dose given twice daily, if tolerated, to a maximum of 1500 mg twice daily. Oral doses >3000 mg/day have been used in trials; however, there is no evidence of increased benefit.

Primary generalized tonic-clonic seizures:

Oral: Immediate release: Initial: 500 mg twice daily; increase dosage every 2 weeks by 500 mg/dose given twice daily, to the recommended dose of 1500 mg twice daily. Efficacy of doses other than 3000 mg/**day** has not been established.

IV: Initial: 500 mg twice daily; increase dosage every 2 weeks by 500 mg/dose given twice daily, to the recommended dose of 1500 mg twice daily. Efficacy of doses other than 3000 mg/**day** has not been established.

Dosing adjustment in renal impairment:

Infants, Children, and Adolescents <16 years (Aronoff, 2007):

GFR <50 mL/minute/1.73 m^2: Administer 50% of the dose

Hemodialysis: Administer 50% of normal dose every 24 hours; a supplemental dose after hemodialysis is recommended

CAPD: Administer 50% of normal dose

CRRT: Administer 50% of normal dose

Adolescents ≥16 years and Adults:

Immediate release and IV formulations:

CrCl >80 mL/minute/1.73 m^2: 500-1500 mg every 12 hours

CrCl 50-80 mL/minute/1.73 m^2: 500-1000 mg every 12 hours

CrCl 30-50 mL/minute/1.73 m^2: 250-750 mg every 12 hours

CrCl <30 mL/minute/1.73 m^2: 250-500 mg every 12 hours

End-stage renal disease patients using dialysis: 500-1000 mg every 24 hours; a supplemental dose of 250-500 mg following dialysis is recommended

Peritoneal dialysis (PD): 500-1000 mg every 24 hours (Aronoff, 2007)

Continuous renal replacement therapy (CRRT): 250-750 mg every 12 hours (Arnoff, 2007)

Extended release tablets: Adults:

CrCl >80 mL/minute/1.73 m^2: 1000-3000 mg every 24 hours

CrCl 50-80 mL/minute/1.73 m^2: 1000-2000 mg every 24 hours

CrCl 30-50 mL/minute/1.73 m^2: 500-1500 mg every 24 hours

CrCl <30 mL/minute/1.73 m^2: 500-1000 mg every 24 hours

End-stage renal disease patients using dialysis: Use immediate release product

Dosing adjustment in hepatic impairment: No dosage adjustment necessary

Preparation for Administration Parenteral: IV: Vials:
Pediatric patients <16 years: Dilute dose from vial in NS to final concentration 15 mg/mL (Ng 2010). A 1:1 dilution of drug from vial with D_5W or NS has also been safely used in patients ≥4 years (Wheless 2009)
Adolescents ≥16 years and Adults: Dilute dose in 100 mL of NS, LR, or D_5W. A 1:1 dilution of drug from vial with D_5W or NS has also been used in patients 4 to 32 years of age (Wheless 2009).

Administration
Oral: May be administered without regard to meals; swallow tablets (both immediate release and extended release) whole; do not break, crush, or chew. Oral solution should be administered with calibrated measuring device (not household teaspoon or tablespoon).
Parenteral: IV: Vials must be diluted prior to use. Do not use if solution contains particulate matter or is discolored. Discard unused portions; does not contain preservative.
Pediatric patients <16 years: Infuse over 15 minutes (Ng 2010)
Adolescents ≥16 years and Adults: Infuse over 15 minutes
Others have safely used a 1:1 dilution infused over 5 to 6 minutes (with doses up to 60 mg/kg) through a peripheral site in patients 4 to 32 years of age (Wheless 2009).

Monitoring Parameters Seizure frequency, duration, and severity; behavioral abnormalities and neuropsychiatric adverse events; renal function; CBC; signs and symptoms of suicidality (eg, anxiety, depression, behavior changes)

Reference Range Therapeutic range and benefit of therapeutic drug monitoring have not been established; concentrations of 6-20 mg/L (35-120 micromol/L) were attained in adult study patients receiving doses of 1000-3000 mg/day

Additional Information A recent, small, retrospective study used a rapid dosage titration of levetiracetam in 8 children, 19 months to 17 years of age (mean age: 8.6 years). Full maintenance doses of levetiracetam were achieved over a titration period of 2-14 days (mean: 10 days). The drug was effective and well-tolerated; however, one patient developed adverse behavioral effects. Further studies are needed before rapid titration of levetiracetam can be routinely recommended (Vaisleib, 2008).

In a preliminary report, levetiracetam-associated behavioral abnormalities were successfully treated with pyridoxine in 5 of 6 children, 2-10 years of age; further studies are needed before this treatment can be recommended (Miller, 2002). Levetiracetam- induced psychosis (including visual and auditory hallucinations and persecutive delusions) has been reported in pediatric patients (Kossoff, 2001).

Product Availability Elepsia XR: FDA approved March 2015; anticipated availability is currently unknown.

Dosage Forms Excipient information presented when available (limited, particularly for generics); consult specific product labeling.
Solution, Intravenous:
Keppra: 500 mg/5 mL (5 mL)
Generic: 500 mg/100 mL (100 mL); 1000 mg/100 mL (100 mL); 1500 mg/100 mL (100 mL); 500 mg/5 mL (5 mL)
Solution, Intravenous [preservative free]:
Generic: 500 mg/5 mL (5 mL)
Solution, Oral:
Keppra: 100 mg/mL (473 mL) [gluten free, lactose free; contains acesulfame potassium, methylparaben, propylparaben; grape flavor]
Generic: 100 mg/mL (5 mL, 473 mL, 500 mL)
Tablet, Oral:
Keppra: 250 mg [scored; contains fd&c blue #2 (indigotine)]
Keppra: 500 mg [scored]
Keppra: 750 mg [scored; contains fd&c yellow #6 (suns[...] yellow)]
Keppra: 1000 mg [scored]
Generic: 250 mg, 500 mg, 750 mg, 1000 mg
Tablet Extended Release 24 Hour, Oral:
Keppra XR: 500 mg, 750 mg
Generic: 500 mg, 750 mg

Levobunolol (lee voe BYOO noe lole)

Medication Safety Issues
Sound-alike/look-alike issues:
Levobunolol may be confused with levocabastine
Betagan® may be confused with Betadine®, Betoptic® [...]

Brand Names: US Betagan

Brand Names: Canada Apo-Levobunolol®; Betagan®[...] Novo-Levobunolol; PMS-Levobunolol; Ratio-Levobunolo[...] Sandoz-Levobunolol

Therapeutic Category Beta-Adrenergic Blocker, Ophthalmic

Generic Availability (US) Yes

Use To lower intraocular pressure in chronic open-angle glaucoma or ocular hypertension

Pregnancy Risk Factor C

Pregnancy Considerations Adverse events have been observed in some animal reproduction studies. If ophthalmic agents are needed for the treatment of glaucoma during pregnancy, the minimum effective dose should be used in combination with punctual occlusion to decrease potential exposure to the fetus (Johnson, 2001; Samples 1988)

Breast-Feeding Considerations It is not known if levobunolol is excreted in breast milk; however, systemic beta blockers and topical timolol are excreted in breast milk. The manufacturer recommends that caution be exercised when administering levobunolol to nursing women. The minimum effective dose should be used in combination with punctual occlusion to decrease potential exposure to the nursing infant (Johnson, 2001; Samples, 1988).

Contraindications Hypersensitivity to levobunolol or any component of the formulation; bronchial asthma, severe COPD, sinus bradycardia, second- or third-degree AV block, overt cardiac failure, cardiogenic shock

Warnings/Precautions Consider pre-existing conditions such as sick sinus syndrome before initiating. Use with caution in patients with compensated HF, diabetes mellitus, bronchospastic disease, cerebrovascular insufficiency myasthenia gravis, peripheral vascular disease, psychiatric disease, and thyroid disease. Should not be used alone in angle-closure glaucoma (has no effect on pupillary constriction). Because systemic absorption may occur with ophthalmic administration, the elderly with other disease states or syndromes that may be affected by a beta-blocker (HF, COPD, etc) should be monitored closely; absorption may lead to respiratory and cardiovascular effects (including bradycardia and/or hypotension).

Potentially significant drug interactions may exist. Consult drug interactions database for more information. Concomitant use with other topical beta-blockers should generally be avoided; monitor for increased effects. Use caution with history of severe anaphylaxis to allergens; patients taking beta-blockers may become more sensitive to repeated challenges. Treatment of anaphylaxis (eg, epinephrine) in patients taking beta-blockers may be ineffective or promote undesirable effects. Product contains benzalkonium chloride which may be absorbed by soft contact lenses; do not administer while wearing soft contact lenses. Ophthalmic solutions contain metabisulfite, which may cause allergic reactions in some people.

Adverse Reactions
Cardiovascular: Arrhythmia, bradycardia, cardiac arrest cerebral ischemia, cerebrovascular accident, chest pain,

congestive heart failure, heart block, hypotension, palpitation, syncope
Central nervous system: Ataxia (transient), confusion, depression, dizziness, headache, lethargy
Dermatologic: Alopecia, erythema, pruritus, rash, Stevens-Johnson syndrome, urticaria
Endocrine & metabolic: Hypoglycemia masked
Gastrointestinal: Diarrhea, nausea
Genitourinary: Impotence
Neuromuscular & skeletal: Myasthenia gravis exacerbation, paresthesia, weakness
Ocular: Blepharoconjunctivitis, blepharoptosis, conjunctivitis, corneal sensitivity decreased, diplopia, iridocyclitis, keratitis, ptosis, stinging/burning, visual disturbances
Respiratory: Bronchospasm, dyspnea, nasal congestion, respiratory failure
Miscellaneous: Hypersensitivity

Drug Interactions

Metabolism/Transport Effects None known.

Avoid Concomitant Use

Avoid concomitant use of Levobunolol with any of the following: Beta2-Agonists; Ceritinib; Floctafenine; Methacholine; Rivastigmine

Increased Effect/Toxicity

Levobunolol may increase the levels/effects of: Alpha-/Beta-Agonists (Direct-Acting); Bradycardia-Causing Agents; Bupivacaine; Ceritinib; Cholinergic Agonists; DULoxetine; Ergot Derivatives; Fingolimod; Grass Pollen Allergen Extract (5 Grass Extract); Hypotensive Agents; Ivabradine; Lacosamide; Levodopa; Lidocaine (Systemic); Lidocaine (Topical); Mepivacaine; Methacholine; Midodrine; RisperiDONE

The levels/effects of Levobunolol may be increased by: Anilidopiperidine Opioids; Barbiturates; Bretylium; Dronedarone; Floctafenine; MAO Inhibitors; Nicorandil; NIFEdipine; Regorafenib; Reserpine; Rivastigmine; Ruxolitinib; Tofacitinib

Decreased Effect

Levobunolol may decrease the levels/effects of: Beta2-Agonists; Theophylline Derivatives

Storage/Stability Store at 15°C to 30°C (59°F to 86°F). Protect from light.

Mechanism of Action A nonselective beta-adrenergic blocking agent that lowers intraocular pressure by reducing aqueous humor production and possibly increases the outflow of aqueous humor

Pharmacodynamics

Onset of action: Following ophthalmic instillation, decreases in intraocular pressure can be noted within 1 hour
Maximum effect: Within 2-6 hours
Maximal effectiveness: 2-3 weeks
Duration: 1-7 days

Pharmacokinetics (Adult data unless noted)

Absorption: May be absorbed systemically and produce systemic side effects
Metabolism: Extensively metabolized into several metabolites; primary metabolite (active) dihydrolevobunolol
Elimination: Not well defined

Dosing: Usual Adults: 1-2 drops of 0.5% solution in eye(s) once daily or 1-2 drops of 0.25% solution twice daily; may increase to 1 drop of 0.5% solution twice daily

Administration Intraocular: Apply drops into conjunctival sac of affected eye(s); avoid contacting bottle tip with skin; apply gentle pressure to lacrimal sac during and immediately following instillation (1-2 minutes) to decrease systemic absorption; see manufacturer's information regarding proper usage of C Cap (compliance cap)

Monitoring Parameters Intraocular pressure

Dosage Forms Excipient information presented when available (limited, particularly for generics); consult specific product labeling.

Solution, Ophthalmic, as hydrochloride:
Betagan: 0.5% (5 mL, 10 mL, 15 mL)
Generic: 0.25% (5 mL, 10 mL); 0.5% (5 mL, 10 mL, 15 mL)

◆ **Levobunolol Hydrochloride** *see* Levobunolol *on page 1238*

LevOCARNitine (lee voe KAR ni teen)

Medication Safety Issues

Sound-alike/look-alike issues:

LevOCARNitine may be confused with levETIRAcetam, levocabastine

Brand Names: US Carnitor; Carnitor SF

Brand Names: Canada Carnitor

Therapeutic Category Nutritional Supplement

Generic Availability (US) Yes

Use

Oral: Solution, tablets: Treatment of primary or secondary carnitine deficiency (FDA approved infants, children, and adults); has also been used in cyclic vomiting syndrome for the prevention of episodes
Parenteral: Treatment of secondary carnitine deficiency and prevention and treatment of carnitine deficiency in patients undergoing dialysis for end-stage renal disease (ESRD) [FDA approved in pediatric patients (age not specified) and adults]; has also been used for treatment of valproic acid toxicity

Pregnancy Risk Factor B

Pregnancy Considerations Teratogenic effects were not observed in animal studies. There are no adequate and well-controlled studies in pregnant women. However, carnitine is a naturally occurring substance in mammalian metabolism.

Breast-Feeding Considerations In breast-feeding women, use must be weighed against the potential exposure of the infant to increased carnitine intake.

Contraindications There are no contraindications listed in the manufacturer's labeling.

Warnings/Precautions Risk factors for carnitine deficiency include: Age (infants and young children are deficient in the enzyme that activates carnitine), chronic valproic acid administration, concomitant neurologic disorders, congenital metabolic disorders, hepatic cirrhosis, renal failure, critical care patients (burns, sepsis, trauma, organ failure), use of multiple antiepileptic drugs and other drugs (chemotherapy agents, antinucleoside analogues) (Katiyar, 2007).

Caution in patients with seizure disorders or in those at risk of seizures (CNS mass or medications which may lower seizure threshold). Both new-onset seizure activity as well as an increased frequency of seizures has been observed. Safety and efficacy of oral carnitine have not been established in ESRD. Chronic administration of high oral doses to patients with severely compromised renal function or ESRD patients on dialysis may result in accumulation of potentially toxic metabolites.

Warnings: Additional Pediatric Considerations Routine prophylactic use of carnitine in children receiving valproic acid to avoid carnitine deficiency and hepatotoxicity is probably not indicated (Freeman, 1994).

Adverse Reactions

Intravenous: Noted with hemodialysis patients.

Cardiovascular: Atrial fibrillation, chest pain, ECG abnormality, hypertension, palpitation, peripheral edema, tachycardia, vascular disorder
Central nervous system: Depression, dizziness, fever, headache, seizures, vertigo
Dermatologic: Rash
Endocrine & metabolic: Hypercalcemia, parathyroid disorder

Gastrointestinal: Abdominal pain, anorexia, diarrhea, gastritis, gastrointestinal disorder, melena, nausea, taste perversion, vomiting, weight gain/loss
Hematologic: Anemia, hemorrhage
Neuromuscular & skeletal: Paresthesia, weakness
Ocular: Amblyopia, eye disorder
Respiratory: Bronchitis, cough, rhinitis
Miscellaneous: Accidental injury, allergic reaction, body odor, drug dependence, infection

Oral:
Central nervous system: Seizures
Gastrointestinal: Abdominal cramps, diarrhea, nausea, vomiting
Miscellaneous: Body odor

Rare but important or life-threatening: Myasthenic syndrome (uremic patients)

Drug Interactions

Metabolism/Transport Effects None known.

Avoid Concomitant Use There are no known interactions where it is recommended to avoid concomitant use.

Increased Effect/Toxicity
LevOCARNitine may increase the levels/effects of: Vitamin K Antagonists

Decreased Effect There are no known significant interactions involving a decrease in effect.

Storage/Stability Store at 25°C (77°F).
IV solution is stable for 24 hours when mixed in NS or LR in PVC bags and stored at 25°C (77°F).

Mechanism of Action Carnitine is a naturally occurring metabolic compound which functions as a carrier molecule for long-chain fatty acids within the mitochondria, facilitating energy production. Carnitine deficiency is associated with accumulation of excess acyl CoA esters and disruption of intermediary metabolism. Carnitine supplementation increases carnitine plasma concentrations. The effects on specific metabolic alterations have not been evaluated. ESRD patients on maintenance hemodialysis may have low plasma carnitine levels because of reduced intake of meat and dairy products, reduced renal synthesis, and dialytic losses. Certain clinical conditions (malaise, muscle weakness, cardiomyopathy and arrhythmias) in hemodialysis patients may be related to carnitine deficiency.

In patients with valproic acid toxicity, administration of exogenous carnitine shifts the metabolism of valproic acid towards β-oxidation and away from ω-oxidation and potentially hepatotoxic metabolite production.

Pharmacokinetics (Adult data unless noted)

Protein binding: Does not bind
Metabolism: Hepatic to trimethylamine and trimethylamine-N-oxide
Bioavailability:
Tablet: 15.1% ± 5.3%
Solution: 15.9% ± 4.9%
Half-life, terminal: 17.4 hours
Time to peak serum concentration: Oral: 3.3 hours
Elimination: Urine (76%, 4% to 9% as unchanged drug); feces (<1% as unchanged drug)

Dosing: Neonatal

Carnitine deficiency, treatment: Limited data available: **Note:** Dosage should be individualized based upon patient response and serum carnitine concentrations.
Primary deficiency: Oral: Initial: 50 mg/kg/**day** in divided doses every 3-4 hours; titrate slowly as needed to 50-100 mg/kg/**day** in divided doses
Secondary deficiency (other inborn errors of metabolism):
Oral: Initial: 50 mg/kg/**day** in divided doses every 3-4 hours; titrate slowly as needed to 50-100 mg/kg/**day** in divided doses; some conditions may require higher daily doses (eg, 300 mg/kg/day) (Kölker, 2011; Sutton, 2012)
IV: 50 mg/kg as a single dose; titrate based on patient response. In patients with severe metabolic crisis, a 50 mg/kg loading dose followed by an equivalent dose given over the next 24 hours divided every 3-6 hours may be required; some conditions may require higher daily doses (eg, 300 mg/kg/day) (Sutton, 2012)

Supplement to parenteral nutrition: Limited data available: Premature neonates GA <34 weeks: IV: Initial 8-10 mg/kg/**day** in parenteral nutrition solution; may increase up to 20 mg/kg/**day** based on free and total plasma carnitine concentrations (ASPEN Pediatric Nutrition Support Core Curriculum, 2010)

Dosing: Usual

Infants, Children, and Adolescents:

Carnitine deficiency, treatment: Note: Dosage should be individualized based upon patient response and serum carnitine concentrations.
Primary deficiency: Oral: Initial: 50 mg/kg/**day** in divided doses; may titrate slowly as needed to 100 mg/kg/**day** in divided doses; maximum daily dose: 3000 mg/**day**
Dosing interval (product specific):
Oral solution: Divided doses at evenly spaced intervals with or during meals (every 3-4 hours)
Tablets: Divide daily dose into 2-3 doses
Secondary deficiency:
Oral: Initial: 50 mg/kg/**day** in divided doses; may titrate slowly as needed to 100 mg/kg/**day** in divided doses; some conditions may require higher daily doses (eg, 300 mg/kg/**day**); maximum daily dose: 3000 mg/**day** (Kölker, 2011; Sutton, 2012)
Dosing interval (product specific):
Oral solution: Divided doses at evenly spaced intervals with or during meals (every 3-4 hours)
Tablets: Divide daily dose into 2-3 doses
IV: 50 mg/kg as a single dose; titrate based on patient response. In patients with severe metabolic crisis, a 50 mg/kg loading dose followed by an equivalent dose given over the next 24 hours divided every 3-6 hours, may be required; maximum daily dose: 300 mg/kg/**day**

ESRD patients on hemodialysis: Limited data available: Children and Adolescents: IV: 10-20 mg/kg dry body weight after each dialysis session; evaluate clinical response at 3-month intervals and titrate to the lowest effective dose. Therapy should be discontinued if no improvement after 9-12 months of therapy. **Note:** Current guidelines do not support the routine use of levocarnitine in dialysis patients (KDOQI Guidelines, 2006; KDOQI Work Group, 2009); however, the National Kidney Foundation indicates levocarnitine therapy in patients with hyporesponsiveness to erythropoietin-based products, symptomatic intradialytic hypotension, NYHA functional class III-IV or ACC/AHA stage C-D heart failure or symptomatic cardiomyopathy, or muscle weakness and fatigability affecting quality of life which are unresponsive to standard medical therapy (Eknoyan, 2003).

Valproic acid toxicity, acute: Children and Adolescents: Limited data available; dosing based on level of hepatic involvement:
No hepatotoxicity: IV: 100 mg/kg/**day** divided every 6 hours until serum ammonia and valproic acid concentrations begin to decrease and clinical improvement is evident; maximum dose: 3000 mg (Russell, 2007)
Symptomatic hyperammonemia or hepatotoxicity: Reported dosing regimens variable: IV: Loading dose: 100 mg/kg, maximum loading dose: 6 **g**; followed by 50 mg/kg/dose every 8 hours or 15 mg/kg/dose every 4 hours, maximum dose: 3000 mg; continue treatment until serum ammonia concentrations begin to decrease and clinical improvement is evident; patients may require several days of therapy (Perrott, 2010; Russell, 2007)

Cyclic vomiting syndrome, prevention: Limited data available: Children and Adolescents: Oral: 50-100 mg/kg/**day** in divided doses 2-3 times daily; maximum dose: 1000 mg (Li, 2008)

Adults:

Primary carnitine deficiency:

Oral solution: Initial: 1000 mg daily in divided doses (spaced every 3-4 hours throughout the day); titrate slowly as needed to 1000-3000 mg per day in divided doses; higher doses may be needed in some patients

Tablets: Oral: 990 mg 2-3 times daily

IV: 50 mg/kg; titrate based on patient response. In patients with severe metabolic crisis, a 50 mg/kg loading dose followed by an equivalent dose given over the next 24 hours (divided every 3 or 4 hours, never less than every 6 hours) may be required. Maximum daily dose: 300 mg/kg/**day**

ESRD patients on hemodialysis: IV: 20 mg/kg after each dialysis session; evaluate clinical response at 3-month intervals and titrate to the lowest effective dose. Therapy should be discontinued if no improvement after 9-12 months of therapy. **Note:** Current guidelines do not support the routine use of levocarnitine in dialysis patients (KDOQI guidelines, 2000); however, the National Kidney Foundation indicates levocarnitine therapy in patients with hyporesponsiveness to erythropoietin-based products, symptomatic intradialytic hypotension, NYHA functional class III-IV or ACC/AHA stage C-D heart failure or symptomatic cardiomyopathy, or muscle weakness and fatigability affecting quality of life which are unresponsive to standard medical therapy (Eknoyan, 2003).

Note: Safety and efficacy of oral carnitine have not been established in ESRD. Chronic administration of high **oral** doses to patients with severely compromised renal function or ESRD patients on dialysis may result in accumulation of **potentially toxic** metabolites.

Preparation for Administration Parenteral: Dependent upon use: Carnitine deficiency or valproic acid toxicity: IV infusion (intermittent or continuous): May be further diluted in LR or NS to a final concentration of 0.5 to 8 mg/mL

Administration

Oral solution: May be taken directly or diluted in either beverages or liquid food; consume slowly; doses should be spaced evenly throughout the day, preferably during or following meals (every 3 to 4 hours) to improve tolerance

Parenteral: Dependent upon use:

Carnitine deficiency: May be administered undiluted (200 mg/mL) as IV push over 2 to 3 minutes **or** further dilute and administered as an intermittent IV infusion typically over 30 minutes **or** as a continuous infusion

ESRD on hemodialysis: May be administered undiluted (200 mg/mL) IV push over 2 to 3 minutes into the venous return line

Valproic acid toxicity: May be administered undiluted (200 mg/mL) IV push over 2 to 3 minutes or further dilute and administered by intermittent infusion over 30 minutes

Monitoring Parameters

Carnitine serum concentrations should be obtained at baseline and subsequently monitored weekly to monthly. In metabolic disorders: Blood chemistry, vital signs, and plasma carnitine concentration. In ESRD patients on dialysis: National Kidney Foundation guidelines recommend basing treatment on clinical signs and symptoms; evaluate response at 3-month intervals and discontinue if no clinical improvement noted within 9-12 months (Eknoyan, 2003).

Valproic acid toxicity: Serum valproic acid concentrations (every 4-6 hours until a downward trend is observed), electrolytes, blood gases, mental status, hepatic function, serum ammonia concentration, serum lactate, and platelets

Reference Range Plasma free carnitine level: >20 micromoles/L; plasma total carnitine level 30-60 micromoles/L; to evaluate for carnitine deficiency determine the plasma acylcarnitine/free carnitine ratio (A/F ratio)

A/F ratio = [plasma total carnitine - free carnitine] divided by free carnitine

Normal plasma A/F ratio = 0.25; in carnitine deficiency A/F ratio >0.4

Dosage Forms Excipient information presented when available (limited, particularly for generics); consult specific product labeling.

Capsule, Oral:
- Generic: 250 mg

Capsule, Oral [preservative free]:
- Generic: 250 mg

Solution, Intravenous:
- Carnitor: 200 mg/mL (5 mL)
- Generic: 200 mg/mL (5 mL, 12.5 mL)

Solution, Intravenous [preservative free]:
- Generic: 200 mg/mL (5 mL)

Solution, Oral:
- Carnitor: 1 g/10 mL (118 mL) [contains methylparaben, propylparaben; cherry flavor]
- Carnitor SF: 1 g/10 mL (118 mL) [sugar free; contains methylparaben, propylparaben, saccharin sodium; cherry flavor]
- Generic: 1 g/10 mL (118 mL)

Tablet, Oral:
- Carnitor: 330 mg
- Generic: 250 mg, 330 mg

Levocetirizine (LEE vo se TI ra zeen)

Medication Safety Issues

Sound-alike/look-alike issues:

Levocetirizine may be confused with cetirizine

Brand Names: US Xyzal

Therapeutic Category Antihistamine

Generic Availability (US) Yes

Use Relief of symptoms associated with perennial allergic rhinitis (FDA approved in ages ≥6 months and adults), seasonal allergic rhinitis (FDA approved in ages ≥2 years and adults), and treatment of the uncomplicated skin manifestations of chronic idiopathic urticaria (FDA approved in ages ≥6 months and adults)

Pregnancy Risk Factor B

Pregnancy Considerations Adverse events have not been observed in animal reproduction studies; therefore, the manufacturer classifies levocetirizine as pregnancy category B. The use of antihistamines for the treatment of rhinitis during pregnancy is generally considered to be safe at recommended doses. Information related to the use of levocitirizine during pregnancy is limited; therefore, other agents are preferred. Levocetirizine is the active enantiomer of cetirizine; refer to the Cetirizine monograph for additional information.

Breast-Feeding Considerations It is not known if levocetirizine is excreted in breast milk. Breast-feeding is not recommended by the manufacturer.

Contraindications Hypersensitivity to levocetirizine, cetirizine, or any component of the formulation; end-stage renal disease (CrCl <10 mL/minute); hemodialysis; infants and children 6 months to 11 years of age with renal impairment

Warnings/Precautions Use with caution in adults with mild-to-moderate renal impairment; dosage adjustments may be needed. Use is contraindicated in end-stage renal disease (CrCl <10 mL/minute), patients undergoing hemodialysis, and in children 6 months to 11 years of age with renal impairment (levocetirizine is excreted primarily by the kidneys). Use with caution in the elderly and patients with prostatic hyperplasia and/or GU obstruction. May cause drowsiness; use caution performing tasks which require alertness (eg, operating machinery or driving). Effects may be potentiated when used with other sedative drugs or ethanol.

Warnings: Additional Pediatric Considerations Safety and efficacy for the use of cough and cold products in pediatric patients <4 years of age is limited; the AAP warns against the use of these products for respiratory illnesses in this age group. Serious adverse effects including death have been reported. Many of these products contain multiple active ingredients, increasing the risk of accidental overdose when used with other products. Health care providers are reminded to ask caregivers about the use of OTC cough and cold products in order to avoid exposure to multiple medications containing the same ingredient (AAP 2012; FDA 2008).

Adverse Reactions

Central nervous system: Drowsiness, fatigue

Gastrointestinal: Constipation, diarrhea, vomiting, xerostomia

Neuromuscular & skeletal: Weakness

Otic: Otitis media

Respiratory: Cough, epistaxis, nasopharyngitis, pharyngitis

Miscellaneous: Fever (children 4%)

Rare but important or life-threatening: Aggressive behavior, agitation, anaphylaxis, angioedema, dysuria, fixed-drug eruption, hepatitis, hypersensitivity, increased serum bilirubin, increased serum transaminases, movement disorder (including dystonia and oculogyric crisis), myalgia, nausea, palpitations, paresthesia, pruritus, skin rash, seizure, suicidal ideation, syncope, urinary retention, urticaria, visual disturbances, weight gain

Drug Interactions

Metabolism/Transport Effects None known.

Avoid Concomitant Use

Avoid concomitant use of Levocetirizine with any of the following: Aclidinium; Azelastine (Nasal); Eluxadoline; Glucagon; Ipratropium (Oral Inhalation); Orphenadrine; Paraldehyde; Potassium Chloride; Thalidomide; Tiotropium; Umeclidinium

Increased Effect/Toxicity

Levocetirizine may increase the levels/effects of: AbobotulinumtoxinA; Alcohol (Ethyl); Analgesics (Opioid); Anticholinergic Agents; Azelastine (Nasal); Buprenorphine; CNS Depressants; Eluxadoline; Glucagon; Hydrocodone; Methotrimeprazine; Metyrosine; Mirabegron; Mirtazapine; OnabotulinumtoxinA; Orphenadrine; Paraldehyde; Potassium Chloride; Pramipexole; RimabotulinumtoxinB; ROPINIRole; Rotigotine; Selective Serotonin Reuptake Inhibitors; Suvorexant; Thalidomide; Thiazide Diuretics; Tiotropium; Topiramate; Zolpidem

The levels/effects of Levocetirizine may be increased by: Aclidinium; Brimonidine (Topical); Cannabis; Doxylamine; Dronabinol; Droperidol; HydrOXYzine; Ipratropium (Oral Inhalation); Kava Kava; Magnesium Sulfate; Methotrimeprazine; Mianserin; Nabilone; Perampanel; Pramlintide; Rufinamide; Sodium Oxybate; Tapentadol; Tetrahydrocannabinol; Umeclidinium

Decreased Effect

Levocetirizine may decrease the levels/effects of: Acetylcholinesterase Inhibitors; Benzylpenicilloyl Polylysine; Betahistine; Hyaluronidase; Itopride; Metoclopramide; Secretin

The levels/effects of Levocetirizine may be decreased by: Acetylcholinesterase Inhibitors; Amphetamines

Storage/Stability Store at room temperature of 20°C to 25°C (68°F to 77°F); excursions permitted to 15°C to 30°C (59°F to 86°F).

Mechanism of Action Levocetirizine is an antihistamine which selectively competes with histamine for H_1-receptor sites on effector cells in the gastrointestinal tract, blood vessels, and respiratory tract. Levocetirizine, the active enantiomer of cetirizine, has twice the binding affinity at the H_1-receptor compared to cetirizine.

Pharmacodynamics Duration: 24 hours

Pharmacokinetics (Adult data unless noted)

Absorption: Well absorbed from the GI tract

Distribution: V_d:

- Children: 0.4 L/kg
- Adults: 0.4 L/kg

Protein binding: 91% to 92%

Metabolism: Limited hepatic metabolism (~14% of a dose); metabolic pathways include aromatic oxidation, N- and O-dealkylation, and taurine conjugation

Half-life:

- Children 1-2 years: ~4 hours
- Children 6-11 years: ~6 hours (24% less than adult half-life)
- Adults: 8 hours

Time to peak serum concentration:

- Children: 1.2 hours
- Adults: Oral solution: 0.5 hours; Tablet: 0.9 hours

Elimination: 85.4% excreted unchanged in urine; 12.9% in feces

- Clearance:
  - Children 1-2 years: 1 mL/kg/minute
  - Children 6-11 years: 0.82 mL/kg/minute
  - Adults: 0.63 mL/kg/minute

Dialysis: <10% removed during hemodialysis

Dosing: Usual

Pediatric:

Allergic rhinitis, perennial: Oral:

- Infants and Children 6 months to 5 years: 1.25 mg once daily (in the evening); maximum daily dose: 1.25 mg/**day**
- Children 6-11 years: 2.5 mg once daily (in the evening); maximum: 2.5 mg/**day**
- Children ≥12 years and Adolescents: 5 mg once daily (in the evening); some patients may experience relief of symptoms with 2.5 mg once daily

Allergic rhinitis, seasonal: Oral:

- Children 2-5 years: 1.25 mg once daily (in the evening); maximum: 1.25 mg/**day**
- Children 6-11 years: 2.5 mg once daily (in the evening); maximum: 2.5 mg/**day**
- Children ≥12 years and Adolescents: 5 mg once daily (in the evening); some patients may experience relief of symptoms with 2.5 mg once daily

Urticaria, chronic: Oral:

- Infants and Children 6 months to 5 years: 1.25 mg once daily (in the evening); maximum daily dose: 1.25 mg/**day**
- Children 6-11 years: 2.5 mg once daily (in the evening); maximum: 2.5 mg/**day**
- Children ≥12 years and Adolescents: 5 mg once daily (in the evening); some patients may experience relief of symptoms with 2.5 mg once daily

Adult: **Allergic rhinitis, chronic urticaria:** Oral: 5 mg once daily (in the evening); some patients may experience relief of symptoms with 2.5 mg once daily

Dosing adjustment in renal impairment:

Infants and Children 6 months to 11 years: Contraindicated

Children ≥12 years, Adolescents, and Adults:

- CrCl 50-80 mL/minute: 2.5 mg once daily
- CrCl 30-50 mL/minute: 2.5 mg once every other day
- CrCl 10-30 mL/minute: 2.5 mg twice weekly (every 3 or 4 days)
- CrCl <10 mL/minute or on hemodialysis: Contraindicated

Dosing adjustment in hepatic impairment: No dosage adjustment necessary.

Administration Administer without regard to food in the evening.

Dosage Forms Excipient information presented when available (limited, particularly for generics); consult specific product labeling.

Solution, Oral, as dihydrochloride:

Xyzal: 2.5 mg/5 mL (148 mL) [contains methylparaben, propylparaben, saccharin]

Generic: 2.5 mg/5 mL (118 mL, 148 mL)

Tablet, Oral, as dihydrochloride:

Xyzal: 5 mg [scored]

Generic: 5 mg

◆ **Levocetirizine Dihydrochloride** *see* Levocetirizine *on page 1241*

Levofloxacin (Systemic) (lee voe FLOKS a sin)

Medication Safety Issues

Sound-alike/look-alike issues:

Levaquin may be confused with Levoxyl, Levsin/SL, Lovenox

Levofloxacin may be confused with levETIRAcetam, levodopa, Levophed, levothyroxine

International issues:

Levaquin [Argentina, Brazil, U.S., Venezuela] may be confused with Lariam brand name for mefloquine [multiple international markets]

Brand Names: US Levaquin

Brand Names: Canada ACT Levofloxacin; APO-Levofloxacin; Levaquin; Levaquin in 5% Dextrose Injection; Mylan-Levofloxacin; Novo-Levofloxacin; PMS-Levofloxacin; Sandoz-Levofloxacin

Therapeutic Category Antibiotic, Quinolone

Generic Availability (US) Yes

Use Treatment of plague and postexposure prevention of inhalational anthrax (FDA approved for ages ≥6 months and adults); treatment of acute bacterial sinusitis, pneumonia (nosocomial and community-acquired), acute bacterial exacerbation of chronic bronchitis, skin and skin structure infections (uncomplicated or complicated), chronic bacterial prostatitis, urinary tract infections (uncomplicated or complicated), and acute pyelonephritis due to multidrug-resistant organisms susceptible to levofloxacin (FDA approved in ages ≥18 years and adults). Has also been used to treat pulmonary exacerbations in cystic fibrosis and multidrug-resistant tuberculosis.

Medication Guide Available Yes

Pregnancy Risk Factor C

Pregnancy Considerations Adverse events have been observed in some animal reproduction studies. Levofloxacin crosses the placenta and can be detected in the amniotic fluid and cord blood (Ozyüncü and Beksac 2010; Ozyuncu and Nemutl, 2010). Information specific to levofloxacin use during pregnancy is limited (Padberg 2014).

Breast-Feeding Considerations Based on data from a case report, small amounts of levofloxacin are excreted in breast milk (Cahill 2005). Due to the potential for serious adverse reactions in the nursing infant, the manufacturer recommends a decision be made whether to discontinue nursing or to discontinue the drug, taking into account the importance of treatment to the mother.

Contraindications Hypersensitivity to levofloxacin, any component of the formulation, or other quinolones

Canadian labeling: Additional contraindications (not in U.S. labeling): History of tendonitis or tendon rupture associated with use of any quinolone antimicrobial agent

Warnings/Precautions **[U.S. Boxed Warning]: There have been reports of tendon inflammation and/or rupture with quinolone antibiotics; risk may be increased with concurrent corticosteroids, organ transplant recipients, and in patients >60 years of age.** Rupture of the Achilles tendon sometimes requiring surgical repair has been reported most frequently; but other tendon sites (eg, rotator cuff, biceps) have also been reported. Strenuous physical activity, rheumatoid arthritis, and renal impairment may be an independent risk factor for tendonitis. Discontinue at first sign of tendon inflammation or pain. May occur even after discontinuation of therapy. Use with caution in patients with rheumatoid arthritis; may increase risk of tendon rupture. Safety of use in pediatric patients for >14 days of therapy has not been studied; increased incidence of musculoskeletal disorders (eg, arthralgia, tendon rupture) has been observed in children. CNS effects may occur (toxic psychoses, tremor, restlessness, anxiety, lightheadedness, paranoia, depression, nightmares, confusion, and very rarely hallucinations increased intracranial pressure (including pseudotumor cerebri, seizures, or toxic psychosis). Potential for seizures, although very rare, may be increased with concomitant NSAID therapy. Use with caution in individuals at risk of seizures, with known or suspected CNS disorders or renal dysfunction. Avoid excessive sunlight and take precautions to limit exposure (eg, loose fitting clothing, sunscreen); may cause moderate-to-severe phototoxicity reactions. Discontinue use if photosensitivity occurs.

Rare cases of torsade de pointes have been reported in patients receiving levofloxacin. Use caution in patients with known prolongation of QT interval, bradycardia, hypokalemia, hypomagnesemia, or in those receiving concurrent therapy with Class Ia or Class III antiarrhythmics.

Severe hypersensitivity reactions, including anaphylaxis, have occurred with quinolone therapy. Reactions may present as typical allergic symptoms after a single dose, or may manifest as severe idiosyncratic dermatologic, vascular, pulmonary, renal, hepatic, and/or hematologic events, usually after multiple doses. Prompt discontinuation of drug should occur if skin rash or other symptoms arise. Prolonged use may result in fungal or bacterial superinfection, including *C. difficile*-associated diarrhea (CDAD) and pseudomembranous colitis; CDAD has been observed >2 months postantibiotic treatment. Peripheral neuropathy has been reported (rare); may occur soon after initiation of therapy and may be irreversible; discontinue if symptoms of sensory or sensorimotor neuropathy occur. **[U.S. Boxed Warning]: Quinolones may exacerbate myasthenia gravis; avoid use (rare, potentially life-threatening weakness of respiratory muscles may occur).** Unrelated to hypersensitivity, severe hepatotoxicity (including acute hepatitis and fatalities) has been reported. Elderly patients may be at greater risk. Discontinue therapy immediately if signs and symptoms of hepatitis occur. Hemolytic reactions may (rarely) occur with quinolone use in patients with latent or actual G6PD deficiency.

Fluoroquinolones have been associated with the development of serious, and sometimes fatal, hypoglycemia, most often in elderly diabetics, but also in patients without diabetes. This occurred most frequently with gatifloxacin (no longer available systemically) but may occur at a lower frequency with other quinolones.

Benzyl alcohol and derivatives: Some dosage forms may contain benzyl alcohol; large amounts of benzyl alcohol (≥99 mg/kg/day) have been associated with a potentially fatal toxicity ("gasping syndrome") in neonates; the "gasping syndrome" consists of metabolic acidosis, respiratory distress, gasping respirations, CNS dysfunction (including convulsions, intracranial hemorrhage), hypotension, and cardiovascular collapse (AAP, 1997; CDC, 1982); some data suggests that benzoate displaces bilirubin from ▶

protein binding sites (Ahlfors, 2001); avoid or use dosage forms containing benzyl alcohol with caution in neonates. See manufacturer's labeling.

Warnings: Additional Pediatric Considerations Increased osteochondrosis in immature rats and dogs was observed with levofloxacin and fluoroquinolones have caused arthropathy with erosions of the cartilage in weight-bearing joints of immature animals. In a pooled safety data analysis of more than 2500 pediatric patients (6 months to 16 years), musculoskeletal events (eg, tendinopathy [inflammation or tendon rupture], arthritis [joint inflammation with redness and/or swelling], arthralgia [pain], or gait abnormality [limping, refusal to walk]) were observed more frequently at 2 months and 12 months after treatment with levofloxacin than comparative treatment; the most frequently reported event was joint pain (85%). No physical joint abnormalities were observed; however, cumulative long-term (up to 5 years) outcomes showed musculoskeletal adverse events (including ongoing arthropathy; peripheral neuropathy; abnormal bone development; scoliosis; walking difficulty; myalgia; tendon disorder; hypermobility syndrome; or pain in the spine, shoulder, or hip) were slightly higher in the comparator group than levofloxacin. Safety of use in pediatric patients for >14 days of therapy has not reported; in available pediatric safety data, the typical duration of therapy was approximately 10 days (CAP, AOM) (Bradley, 2011).

In pediatric patients, fluoroquinolones are not routinely first-line therapy, but after assessment of risks and benefits, can be considered a reasonable alternative for situations where no safe and effective substitute is available [eg, resistance (common CF pathogens, multidrug resistant-tuberculosis)] or in situations where the only alternative is parenteral therapy and levofloxacin offers an oral therapy option (eg, acute otitis media/sinusitis [*S. pneumoniae*, *H. influenzae*]; pneumonia [*S. pneumoniae*, *Mycoplasma pneumonia*]) (Bradley, 2011).

Some dosage forms may contain propylene glycol; in neonates large amounts of propylene glycol delivered orally, intravenously (eg, >3,000 mg/day), or topically have been associated with potentially fatal toxicities which can include metabolic acidosis, seizures, renal failure, and CNS depression; toxicities have also been reported in children and adults including hyperosmolality, lactic acidosis, seizures and respiratory depression; use caution (AAP, 1997; Shehab, 2009).

Adverse Reactions

Cardiovascular: Chest pain, edema

Central nervous system: Dizziness, headache, insomnia

Dermatologic: Pruritus, skin rash

Gastrointestinal: Abdominal pain, constipation, diarrhea, dyspepsia, nausea, vomiting

Genitourinary: Vaginitis

Infection: Candidiasis

Local: Injection site reaction

Respiratory: Dyspnea

Rare but important or life-threatening: Abnormal electroencephalogram, abnormal gait, acute renal failure, ageusia, agranulocytosis, anaphylactoid reaction, anemia (including aplastic and hemolytic), anorexia, anosmia, brain disease (rare), cardiac arrest, cardiac arrhythmia (including ventricular tachycardia/fibrillation and torsade de pointes), casts in urine, *Clostridium difficile*-associated diarrhea, confusion, convulsions, crystalluria, depression, elevation in serum levels of skeletal-muscle enzymes, eosinophilia, epistaxis, erythema multiforme, esophagitis, exacerbation of myasthenia gravis, gastritis (including gastroenteritis), glossitis, granulocytopenia, hallucination, hepatic failure (some fatal), hepatic insufficiency, hepatitis, hepatotoxicity (idiosyncratic) (Chalasani, 2014), hyperglycemia, hyperkalemia, hyperkinesias, hypersensitivity reaction (including anaphylaxis, angioedema, rash, pneumonitis, and seru sickness), hypertension, hypertonia, hypoacusis, hyp glycemia, hypotension, increased INR, increased intr cranial pressure, increased serum alkaline phosphatas increased serum transaminases, interstitial nephriti intestinal obstruction, jaundice, leukocytosis, leukopeni leukorrhea, lymphadenopathy, multiorgan failure, musc injury, muscle spasm, pancreatitis, pancytopenia, paral sis, paranoia, peripheral neuropathy (may be irrevers ble), phlebitis, phototoxicity, prolonged prothrombin tim prolonged Q-T interval on ECG, pseudotumor cereb psychosis, renal function abnormality, rhabdomyolysi rupture of tendon, scotoma, seizure, skeletal pain, sk photosensitivity, sleep disorder (including abnorm dreams and nightmares), Stevens-Johnson syndrom stomatitis, suicidal ideation, syncope, tachycardia, tend nitis, toxic epidermal necrolysis, toxic psychosis, thron bocytopenia (including thrombotic thrombocytopen purpura), uveitis, vasculitis (leukocytoclastic), vasodilat tion, visual disturbances(including diplopia), voice dis order

Drug Interactions

Metabolism/Transport Effects None known.

Avoid Concomitant Use

Avoid concomitant use of Levofloxacin (Systemic) wit any of the following: BCG; BCG (Intravesical); Highe Risk QTc-Prolonging Agents; Ivabradine; Mifepriston Strontium Ranelate

Increased Effect/Toxicity

Levofloxacin (Systemic) may increase the levels/effect of: Blood Glucose Lowering Agents; Highest Risk QT Prolonging Agents; Moderate Risk QTc-Prolongin Agents; Porfimer; Tacrolimus (Systemic); Varenicline Verteporfin; Vitamin K Antagonists

The levels/effects of Levofloxacin (Systemic) may b increased by: Corticosteroids (Systemic); Ivabradine Mifepristone; Nonsteroidal Anti-Inflammatory Agents Probenecid; QTc-Prolonging Agents (Indeterminate Ris and Risk Modifying)

Decreased Effect

Levofloxacin (Systemic) may decrease the levels/effect of: BCG; BCG (Intravesical); BCG Vaccine (Immuniza tion); Blood Glucose Lowering Agents; Didanosine Mycophenolate; Sodium Picosulfate; Typhoid Vaccine

The levels/effects of Levofloxacin (Systemic) may b decreased by: Antacids; Calcium Salts; Didanosine; Iro Salts; Lanthanum; Magnesium Salts; Multivitamins/Min erals (with ADEK, Folate, Iron); Multivitamins/Mineral (with AE, No Iron); Quinapril; Sevelamer; Strontiu Ranelate; Sucralfate; Zinc Salts

Storage/Stability

Solution for injection:

Vial: Store at room temperature. Protect from light Diluted solution (5 mg/mL) is stable for 72 hours whe stored at room temperature; stable for 14 days whe stored under refrigeration. When frozen, stable for 6 months; do not refreeze. Do not thaw in microwave o by bath immersion.

Premixed: Store at ≤25°C (77°F); do not freeze. Brie exposure to 40°C (104°F) does not affect product Protect from light.

Tablet, oral solution: Store at 25°C (77°F); excursion permitted to 15°C to 30°C (59°F to 86°F).

Mechanism of Action As the S(-) enantiomer of the fluoroquinolone, ofloxacin, levofloxacin, inhibits DNA-gyrase in susceptible organisms thereby inhibits relaxation of supercoiled DNA and promotes breakage of DNA strands. DNA gyrase (topoisomerase II), is an essential bacterial enzyme that maintains the superhelical structure of DNA and is required for DNA replication and transcription, DNA repair, recombination, and transposition.

Pharmacokinetics (Adult data unless noted) Levofloxacin absorption (as indicated by C_{max} and t_{max}) and distribution in children are not age-dependent and are comparable to those in adults.

Absorption: Well-absorbed; levofloxacin oral tablet and solution formulations are bioequivalent

Distribution: Widely distributed in the body, including blister fluid, skin tissue, macrophages, prostate, and lung tissue; CSF concentrations ~15% of serum concentrations

V_d: IV (Chien, 2005):

Infants ≥6 months, Children, and Adolescents ≤16 years: Mean range: 1.44-1.57 L/kg; reported values not statistically different between pediatric age subgroups; distribution not age-dependent

Adults: 1.27 L/kg

Protein binding: 24% to 38%, primarily to albumin

Bioavailability: Oral: 99%

Half-life:

Infants ≥6 months and Children ≤5 years: ~4 hours (Chien, 2005)

Children 5-10 years: 4.8 hours (Chien, 2005)

Children 10-12 years: 5.4 hours (Chien, 2005)

Children 12-16 years: 6 hours (Chien, 2005)

Adults: 6-8 hours

Time to peak serum concentration: Oral: Within 1-2 hours

Elimination: 87% excreted unchanged in urine over 48 hours by tubular secretion and glomerular filtration; 4% in feces

Clearance: IV: (Chien, 2005):

Infants and Children 6 months to 2 years: 0.35 ± 0.13 L/hour/kg

Children 2-5 years: 0.32 ± 0.08 L/hour/kg

Children 5-10 years: 0.25 ± 0.05 L/hour/kg

Children 10-12 years: 0.19 ± 0.05 L/hour/kg

Children 12-16 years: 0.18 ± 0.03 L/hour/kg

Adults: 0.15 ± 0.02 L/hour/kg

Dosing: Usual

Pediatric: **Note:** In pediatric patients, fluoroquinolones are not routinely first-line therapy, but after assessment of risks and benefits, can be considered a reasonable alternative for situations where no safe and effective substitute is available [eg, resistance (cystic fibrosis)] or in situations where the only alternative is parenteral therapy and levofloxacin offers an oral therapy option (Bradley, 2011). Use of levofloxacin in infants <6 months has not been studied.

General dosing, susceptible infection (Bradley, 2011): Infants ≥6 months, Children, and Adolescents:

Oral, IV:

<5 years: 8-10 mg/kg/dose twice daily

≥5 years: 10 mg/kg/dose once daily; maximum dose: 750 mg/**day**

Anthrax, postexposure (inhalation): Infants ≥6 months, Children, and Adolescents: Oral, IV: **Note:** Begin as soon as possible after exposure:

<50 kg: 8 mg/kg/dose every 12 hours for 60 days; maximum dose: 250 mg

≥50 kg: 500 mg every 24 hours for 60 days

Cystic fibrosis pulmonary exacerbation: Limited data available (Bradley, 2011): Infants ≥6 months, Children, and Adolescents: Oral, IV: Some centers have used:

<5 years: 10 mg/kg/dose twice daily

≥5 years: 10 mg/kg/dose once daily; maximum dose 750 mg/**day**

Peritoneal dialysis; tunnel or exit site infection: Limited data available: Oral: 10 mg/kg/dose every 48 hours; maximum initial dose: 500 mg; maximum subsequent doses: 250 mg (Warady, 2012)

Plague *(Yersinia pestis)*, prophylaxis or treatment: Infants ≥6 months, Children, and Adolescents: Oral, IV: **Note:** Begin as soon as possible after exposure:

<50 kg: 8 mg/kg/dose every 12 hours for 10-14 days; maximum dose: 250 mg

≥50 kg: 500 mg every 24 hours for 10-14 days

Pneumonia, community-acquired (CAP) (Bradley-IDSA/PIDS, 2011a): **Note:** May consider addition of vancomycin or clindamycin to empiric therapy if community-acquired MRSA suspected. In children ≥5 years, a macrolide antibiotic should be added if atypical pneumonia cannot be ruled out.

Typical pathogens:

Haemophilus influenzae:

Mild infection/step down therapy: Oral:

Infants ≥6 months and Children <5 years: 8-10 mg/kg/dose every 12 hours; maximum daily dose: 750 mg/**day**

Children ≥5 years and Adolescents ≤16 years: 8-10 mg/kg/dose once every 24 hours; maximum daily dose: 750 mg/**day**

Severe infections: IV:

Infants ≥6 months and Children <5 years: 8-10 mg/kg/dose every 12 hours; maximum daily dose: 750 mg/**day**

Children ≥5 years and Adolescents ≤16 years: 8-10 mg/kg/dose once every 24 hours; maximum daily dose: 750 mg/**day**

Streptococcus pneumoniae:

Penicillin-sensitive: Mild infection/step down therapy: Oral: **Note:** Levofloxacin is not recommended for routine use for the treatment of mild to moderate infection (*Red Book*, 2012)

Infants ≥6 months and Children <5 years: 8-10 mg/kg/dose every 12 hours; maximum daily dose: 750 mg/**day**

Children ≥5 years and Adolescents ≤16 years: 8-10 mg/kg/dose once every 24 hours; maximum daily dose: 750 mg/**day**

Penicillin-resistant: Mild infection/step-down therapy: Oral: **Note:** Levofloxacin is not recommended for routine use for the treatment of mild to moderate infection (*Red Book*, 2012)

Infants ≥6 months and Children <5 years: 8-10 mg/kg/dose every 12 hours; maximum daily dose: 750 mg/**day**

Children ≥5 years and Adolescents ≤16 years: 8-10 mg/kg/dose once every 24 hours; maximum daily dose: 750 mg/**day**

Severe infections: IV:

Infants ≥6 months and Children <5 years: 8-10 mg/kg/dose every 12 hours; maximum daily dose: 750 mg/**day**

Children ≥5 years and Adolescents ≤16 years: 8-10 mg/kg/dose once every 24 hours; maximum daily dose: 750 mg/**day**

Atypical pathogens (*Mycoplasma pneumonia* or *Chlamydia ssp*):

Mild infection/step-down therapy: Oral: Adolescents with skeletal maturity: 500 mg/dose once daily

Severe infections: IV:

Infants ≥6 months and Children <5 years: 8-10 mg/kg/dose every 12 hours; maximum daily dose: 750 mg/day

Children ≥5 years and Adolescents ≤16 years: 8-10 mg/kg/dose once every 24 hours; maximum daily dose: 750 mg/day

Rhinosinusitis, acute bacterial: Note: Recommended in the following types of patients: Type I penicillin allergy, after failure of initial therapy or in patients at risk for antibiotic resistance (eg, daycare attendance, age <2 years, recent hospitalization, antibiotic use within the past month) (Chow, 2012). Children and Adolescents: Oral, IV: 10-20 mg/kg/**day** divided every 12-24 hours for 10-14 days; maximum daily dose: 500 mg/**day**

Surgical prophylaxis: Children and Adolescents: IV: 10 mg/kg as a single dose 120 minutes prior to procedure; maximum dose: 500 mg; **Note:** While fluoroquinolones have been associated with an increased risk of tendinitis/tendon rupture in all ages, use of these agents for single-dose prophylaxis is generally safe (Bratzler, 2013).

Tuberculosis, multidrug-resistant: Limited data available: **Note:** Use in combination with at least 2-3 additional anti-TB agents (overall multidrug regimen dependent upon susceptibility profile/patterns) (Seddon, 2012): Oral:

Infants and Children <5 years: 7.5-10 mg/kg/dose every 12 hours; maximum daily dose: 750 mg/day

Children ≥ 5 years and Adolescents: 7.5-10 mg/kg/dose every 24 hours; maximum daily dose: 750 mg/day

Adult:

Anthrax, postexposure (inhalation): Oral, IV: 500 mg every 24 hours for 60 days beginning as soon as possible after exposure

Bronchitis, chronic: Oral, IV: 500 mg every 24 hours for at least 7 days

***Chlamydia trachomatis* sexually transmitted infections:** Oral: 500 mg every 24 hours for 7 days (CDC, 2010)

Epididymitis, nongonococcal: Oral: 500 mg once daily for 10 days (CDC, 2010)

Intra-abdominal infection, complicated, community-acquired (in combination with metronidazole): IV: 750 mg once daily for 4-7 days (provided source controlled). **Note:** Avoid using in settings where *E. coli* susceptibility to fluoroquinolones is <90% (Solomkin, 2010).

Pelvic inflammatory disease: Oral: 500 mg once daily for 14 days with or without concomitant metronidazole; **Note:** The CDC recommends use as an alternative therapy only if standard parenteral cephalosporin therapy is not feasible and community prevalence of quinolone-resistant gonococcal organisms is low. Culture sensitivity must be confirmed (CDC, 2010).

Plague *(Yersinia pestis)*, prophylaxis or treatment: Oral, IV: 500 mg every 24 hours for 10-14 days, beginning as soon as possible after exposure

Pneumonia: Oral, IV:

Community-acquired: 500 mg every 24 hours for 7-14 days or 750 mg every 24 hours for 5 days (efficacy of 5-day regimen for multidrug resistant *S. Pneumoniae* not established)

Nosocomial: 750 mg every 24 hours for 7-14 days

Prostatitis, chronic bacterial: Oral, IV: 500 mg every 24 hours for 28 days

Rhinosinusitis, acute bacterial: Oral, IV:

Manufacturer's recommendations: 500 mg every 24 hours for 10-14 days or 750 mg every 24 hours for 5 days

Alternate recommendations: 500 mg every 24 hours for 5-7 days (Chow, 2012)

Skin and skin structure infections: Oral, IV:

Complicated: 750 mg every 24 hours for 7-14 days

Uncomplicated: 500 mg every 24 hours for 7-10 days

Urethritis, nongonococcal: Oral: 500 mg every 24 hours for 7 days (CDC, 2010)

Urinary tract infection (UTI): Oral, IV:

Complicated or acute pyelonephritis: 250 mg every 24 hours for 10 days or 750 mg every 24 hours for 5 days

Uncomplicated: 250 mg every 24 hours for 3 days

Dosing interval in renal impairment:

Infants, Children, and Adolescents: The following adjustments have been recommended (Aronoff, 2007). **Note:** Renally adjusted dose recommendations are based on doses of 5-10 mg/kg/dose every 12 hours for children ≤5 years and 5-10 mg/kg/dose every 24 hours for children >5 years.

GFR ≥30 mL/minute/1.73 m^2: No adjustment necessary

GFR 10-29 mL/minute/1.73 m^2: 5-10 mg/kg/dose every 24 hours

GFR <10 mL/minute/1.73 m^2: 5-10 mg/kg/dose every 48 hours

Intermittent hemodialysis: 5-10 mg/kg/dose every 48 hours; not removed by hemodialysis; supplemental levofloxacin doses are not required

Peritoneal dialysis (PD): 5-10 mg/kg/dose every 48 hours; not removed by peritoneal dialysis; supplemental levofloxacin doses are not required

Continuous renal replacement therapy (CRRT) 10 mg/kg/dose every 24 hours

Adults:

Normal renal function dosing of 250 mg/day:

CrCl 20-49 mL/minute: No dosage adjustment required

CrCl 10-19 mL/minute: Administer 250 mg every 48 hours (except in uncomplicated UTI, where no dosage adjustment is required)

Hemodialysis (administer after hemodialysis on dialysis days)/peritoneal dialysis (PD): No information available

Normal renal function dosing of 500 mg/day:

CrCl 20-49 mL/minute: Administer 500 mg initial dose, followed by 250 mg every 24 hours

CrCl 10-19 mL/minute: Administer 500 mg initial dose, followed by 250 mg every 48 hours

Hemodialysis (administer after hemodialysis on dialysis days)/peritoneal dialysis (PD): Administer 500 mg initial dose, followed by 250 mg every 48 hours; not removed by hemodialysis or peritoneal dialysis; supplemental levofloxacin doses are not required

Normal renal function dosing of 750 mg/day:

CrCl 20-49 mL/minute: Administer 750 mg every 48 hours

CrCl 10-19 mL/minute: Administer 750 mg initial dose, followed by 500 mg every 48 hours

Hemodialysis (administer after hemodialysis on dialysis days)/peritoneal dialysis (PD): Administer 750 mg initial dose, followed by 500 mg every 48 hours; not removed by hemodialysis or peritoneal dialysis; supplemental levofloxacin doses are not required

Normal renal function dosing of 750 or 1000 mg daily (treatment of tuberculosis **only**) (CDC, 2003): CrCl <30 mL/minute: Administer 750 or 1000 mg 3 times per week (in hemodialysis patients administer after dialysis on dialysis days)

Continuous renal replacement therapy (CRRT) (Heintz, 2009; Trotman, 2005): Drug clearance is highly dependent on the method of renal replacement, filter type, and flow rate. Appropriate dosing requires close monitoring of pharmacologic response, signs of adverse reactions due to drug accumulation, as well as drug concentrations in relation to target trough (if appropriate). The following are general recommendations only (based on dialysate flow/ultrafiltration rates of 1-2 L/hour and minimal residual renal function) and should not supersede clinical judgment:

CVVH: Loading dose of 500-750 mg followed by 250 mg every 24 hours

CVVHD: Loading dose of 500-750 mg followed by 250-500 mg every 24 hours

CVVHDF: Loading dose of 500-750 mg followed by 250-750 mg every 24 hours

Dosing adjustment in hepatic impairment: There are no dosage adjustments provided in the manufacturer's labeling; has not been studied.

Preparation for Administration Parenteral: Vials must be further diluted in compatible solution to a final concentration not to exceed 5 mg/mL prior to infusion.

Administration

Oral: Tablets may be administered with or without food; oral solution should be administered 1 hour before or 2 hours after eating; avoid antacid use within 2 hours of administration

Parenteral: Administer by slow IV infusion over 60 to 90 minutes (250 to 500 mg over 60 minutes; 750 mg over 90 minutes); avoid rapid or bolus IV infusion due to risk of hypotension; maintain adequate hydration to prevent crystalluria or cylinduria; not for IM, SubQ, or intrathecal administration

Monitoring Parameters Evaluation of organ system functions (renal, hepatic, and hematopoietic) is recommended periodically during therapy; the possibility of crystalluria should be assessed; WBC and signs of infection; number and type of stools/day for diarrhea; hydration status; patients receiving concurrent levofloxacin and theophylline should have serum levels of theophylline monitored; monitor INR in patients receiving warfarin; monitor blood glucose in patients receiving antidiabetic agents or patients with a history of diabetes

Test Interactions Some quinolones may produce a false-positive urine screening result for opioids using commercially-available immunoassay kits. This has been demonstrated most consistently for levofloxacin and ofloxacin, but other quinolones have shown cross-reactivity in certain assay kits. Confirmation of positive opioid screens by more specific methods should be considered.

Additional Information A nebulized formulation is currently under investigation in clinical trials; Levofloxacin 240 mg inhalation over ~5 minutes once daily for 7 days was well tolerated in cystic fibrosis (CF) patients (n=10, age 33.6 ± 16.4 years). In another study, CF patients were given one of three doses (120 mg once daily, 240 mg once daily, 240 mg twice daily) or placebo for 28 days (n=114 treated, 37 placebo, age 28.7 ± 9 years). All three doses were well tolerated and resulted in decreased *Pseudomonas aeruginosa* density in sputum (Geller 2011; Geller 2011a).

Dosage Forms Excipient information presented when available (limited, particularly for generics); consult specific product labeling. [DSC] = Discontinued product

Solution, Intravenous [preservative free]:

- Levaquin: 250 mg/50 mL (50 mL [DSC]); 500 mg/100 mL (100 mL); 750 mg/150 mL (150 mL)
- Generic: 250 mg/50 mL (50 mL); 500 mg/100 mL (100 mL); 750 mg/150 mL (150 mL); 25 mg/mL (20 mL, 30 mL)

Solution, Oral:

- Levaquin: 25 mg/mL (480 mL) [contains propylene glycol]
- Generic: 25 mg/mL (10 mL, 20 mL, 100 mL, 200 mL, 480 mL)

Tablet, Oral:

- Levaquin: 250 mg, 500 mg, 750 mg
- Generic: 250 mg, 500 mg, 750 mg

Extemporaneous Preparations Note: Commercial oral solution is available (25 mg/mL)

A 50 mg/mL oral suspension may be made with tablets and a 1:1 mixture of Ora-Plus® and strawberry syrup NF. Crush six 500 mg levofloxacin tablets in a mortar and reduce to a fine powder. Add small portions of the vehicle and mix to a uniform paste; mix while adding the vehicle in incremental proportions to **almost** 60 mL; transfer to a graduated cylinder, rinse mortar with vehicle, and add quantity of vehicle sufficient to make 60 mL. Label "shake well". Stable for 57 days when stored in amber plastic prescription bottles at room temperature or refrigerated.

VandenBussche HL, Johnson CE, and Fontana EM, et al, "Stability of Levofloxacin in an Extemporaneously Compounded Oral Liquid," *Am J Health Syst Pharm*, 1999, 56(22):2316-8.

Levofloxacin (Ophthalmic) (lee voe FLOKS a sin)

Medication Safety Issues

Sound-alike/look-alike issues:

Levofloxacin may be confused with levETIRAcetam, levodopa, levothyroxine

Therapeutic Category Antibiotic, Ophthalmic; Antibiotic, Quinolone

Generic Availability (US) Yes

Use Used ophthalmically for treatment of bacterial conjunctivitis due to *S. aureus* (methicillin-susceptible strains), *S. epidermidis*, *S. pneumoniae*, *Streptococcus* (groups C/F), *Streptococcus* (group G), Viridans group *Streptococci*, *Corynebacterium* spp, *H. influenzae*, *Acinetobacter*

Pregnancy Risk Factor C

Pregnancy Considerations Adverse events have been observed in some animal reproduction studies. When administered orally or IV, levofloxacin crosses the placenta (Ozyüncü and Beksac 2010; Ozyüncü and Nemutlu 2010). The amount of levofloxacin available systemically following topical application of the ophthalmic drops is significantly less in comparison to oral or IV doses. If ophthalmic agents are needed during pregnancy, the minimum effective dose should be used in combination with punctual occlusion for 3 to 5 minutes after application to decrease potential exposure to the fetus (Samples 1988).

Breast-Feeding Considerations When administered orally or IV, levofloxacin enters breast milk (Cahill 2005). The amount of levofloxacin available systemically following topical application of the ophthalmic drops is significantly less in comparison to oral or IV doses. The manufacturer recommends that caution be exercised when administering levofloxacin ophthalmic drops to nursing women.

Contraindications Hypersensitivity to levofloxacin, other quinolones, or to any component of the formulation.

Warnings/Precautions For topical use only. Do not inject subconjunctivally or introduce into anterior chamber of the eye. Contact lenses should not be worn during treatment for bacterial conjunctivitis. Serious hypersensitivity reactions, including anaphylaxis, have been reported with systemic quinolone therapy. Prompt discontinuation of drug should occur if skin rash or other symptoms arise. Prolonged use may lead to overgrowth of nonsusceptible organisms, including fungi. Discontinue use and institute appropriate alternative therapy if superinfection is suspected.

Adverse Reactions

1% to 10%:

- Central nervous system: Headache
- Ophthalmic: Burning sensation of eyes (transient), eye pain, foreign body sensation of eye, photophobia, vision loss (transient)
- Respiratory: Pharyngitis
- Miscellaneous: Fever

Rare but important or life-threatening: Hypersensitivity reaction

Drug Interactions

Metabolism/Transport Effects None known.

Avoid Concomitant Use There are no known interactions where it is recommended to avoid concomitant use.

Increased Effect/Toxicity There are no known significant interactions involving an increase in effect.

Decreased Effect There are no known significant interactions involving a decrease in effect.

Storage/Stability Store at 20°C to 25°C (68°F to 77°F).

Mechanism of Action Levofloxacin is the L-isomer of ofloxacin. Levofloxacin inhibits DNA-gyrase and topoisomerase IV in susceptible organisms and thereby inhibits relaxation of supercoiled DNA and promotes breakage of DNA strands. DNA gyrase (topoisomerase II), is an essential bacterial enzyme that maintains the superhelical structure of DNA and is required for DNA replication, transcription, repair, and recombination.

Pharmacokinetics (Adult data unless noted) Absorption: Only small amounts are absorbed systemically after ophthalmic instillation.

Dosing: Usual

Children ≥1 year and Adults: Bacterial conjunctivitis: 0.5% solution:

Treatment day 1 and day 2: Instill 1-2 drops into affected eye(s) every 2 hours while awake, up to 8 times/day

Treatment day 3-7: Instill 1-2 drops into affected eye(s) every 4 hours while awake, up to 4 times/day

Children ≥6 years and Adults: Bacterial corneal ulcer: 1.5% solution:

Treatment days 1-3: Instill 1-2 drops into affected eye(s) every 30 minutes to 2 hours while awake and ~4 and 6 hours after retiring

Treatment day 4 through treatment completion: Instill 1-2 drops into affected eye(s) every 1-4 hours while awake

Administration Not for subconjunctival injection or for use into anterior chamber of the eye. Contact lenses should not be worn during treatment. Instill drops into conjunctival sac of affected eye(s); apply finger pressure to lacrimal sac during and for 1-2 minutes after instillation to decrease risk of absorption and systemic effects; avoid contacting bottle tip with skin

Dosage Forms Excipient information presented when available (limited, particularly for generics); consult specific product labeling.

Solution, Ophthalmic:

Generic: 0.5% (5 mL)

◆ **Levo-folinic Acid** *see* LEVOleucovorin *on page 1248*

LEVOleucovorin (lee voe loo koe VOR in)

Medication Safety Issues

Sound-alike/look-alike issues:

LEVOleucovorin may be confused with leucovorin calcium, Leukeran, Leukine

Brand Names: US Fusilev

Therapeutic Category Antidote; Chemotherapy Modulating Agent; Rescue Agent (Chemotherapy)

Generic Availability (US) May be product dependent

Use Rescue agent after high-dose methotrexate therapy in osteosarcoma, antidote for impaired methotrexate elimination, and for inadvertent overdosage of folic acid antagonists (FDA approved in pediatric patients [age not specified] and adults); treatment of advanced, metastatic colorectal cancer (palliative) in combination with fluorouracil (FDA approved in adults)

Pregnancy Risk Factor C

Pregnancy Considerations Animal reproduction studies have not been conducted. Levoleucovorin is the levo isomeric form of racemic leucovorin, a biologically active form of folic acid. Adequate amounts of folic acid are recommended during pregnancy. Refer to Folic Acid monograph.

Breast-Feeding Considerations It is not known if levoleucovorin is excreted in breast milk. Due to the potential for serious adverse reactions in the nursing infant, a decision should be made to discontinue breast-feeding or to discontinue levoleucovorin, taking into account the importance of treatment to the mother. Levoleucovorin is the levo isomeric form of racemic leucovorin, a biologically active form of folic acid. Adequate amounts of folic acid are recommended in breast-feeding women. Refer to Folic Acid monograph.

Contraindications Previous allergic reaction to folic acid or leucovorin calcium (folinic acid)

Warnings/Precautions For IV administration only; do not administer intrathecally. Due to calcium content, do not administer IV solutions at a rate >160 mg levoleucovorin/minute. Methotrexate serum concentrations should be monitored to determine dose and duration of levoleucovorin therapy; dose may need to be increased or administration prolonged in situations where methotrexate excretion may be delayed (eg, ascites, pleural effusion, renal insufficiency, inadequate hydration). When used for the treatment of accidental folic acid antagonist overdose, administer as soon as possible.

Levoleucovorin and leucovorin calcium enhance the toxicity of fluorouracil. Deaths due to severe enterocolitis, diarrhea, and dehydration have been reported in elderly patients receiving weekly leucovorin calcium in combination with fluorouracil. Levoleucovorin is indicated in combination with fluorouracil for the palliative treatment of colorectal cancer; when administered together, the fluorouracil dose is reduced (compared to fluorouracil dosing without levoleucovorin). The typical fluorouracil gastrointestinal toxicities (eg, diarrhea, stomatitis) may be of greater severity or longer duration with fluorouracil and levoleucovorin combination therapy. Symptoms of gastrointestinal toxicity should be completely resolved prior to treatment. Elderly and/or debilitated patients are at higher risk for severe gastrointestinal toxicity. Concomitant use of leucovorin calcium and sulfamethoxazole-trimethoprim for the acute treatment of PCP in patients with HIV infection has been associated with increased rates of treatment failure and morbidity; may also occur with levoleucovorin. Seizures and/or syncope have been reported with leucovorin calcium; generally in patients with CNS metastases or other underlying risk factors. Potentially significant drug-drug interactions may exist, requiring dose or frequency adjustment, additional monitoring, and/or selection of alternative therapy.

Adverse Reactions Note: Adverse reactions reported with levoleucovorin either as a part of combination chemotherapy or following chemotherapy.

Central nervous system: Confusion, fatigue

Dermatologic: Alopecia, dermatitis

Gastrointestinal: Abdominal pain, anorexia/appetite decreased, diarrhea, dyspepsia, nausea, stomatitis, taste perversion, typhlitis, vomiting

Neuromuscular & skeletal: Neuropathy, weakness/malaise

Renal: Renal function abnormal

Respiratory: Dyspnea

Rare but important or life-threatening: Allergic reactions, pruritus, rash, rigors, temperature changes

Drug Interactions

Metabolism/Transport Effects None known.

Avoid Concomitant Use

Avoid concomitant use of LEVOleucovorin with any of the following: Raltitrexed; Trimethoprim

Increased Effect/Toxicity

LEVOleucovorin may increase the levels/effects of: Capecitabine; Fluorouracil (Systemic); Fluorouracil (Topical); Tegafur

Decreased Effect

LEVOleucovorin may decrease the levels/effects of: Fosphenytoin; PHENobarbital; Phenytoin; Primidone; Raltitrexed; Trimethoprim

The levels/effects of LEVOleucovorin may be decreased by: Glucarpidase

Storage/Stability

Lyophilized powder: Prior to reconstitution, store intact vials at 25°C (77°F); excursions permitted from 15°C to 30°C (59°F to 86°F). Protect from light. Initial reconstituted solution in the vial may be stored for 12 hours at room temperature. Solutions further diluted for infusion in NS are stable for 12 hours at room temperature. Solutions further diluted for infusion in D_5W are stable for 4 hours at room temperature.

Injection solution: Store intact vials between 2°C and 8°C (36°F and 46°F). Protect from light. Store in carton until contents are used. Solutions further diluted for infusion in NS or D_5W are stable for up to 4 hours at room temperature.

Mechanism of Action Levoleucovorin counteracts the toxic (and therapeutic) effects of folic acid antagonists (eg, methotrexate) which act by inhibiting dihydrofolate reductase. Levoleucovorin is the levo isomeric and pharmacologic active form of leucovorin (levoleucovorin does not require reduction by dihydrofolate reductase). A reduced derivative of folic acid, leucovorin supplies the necessary cofactor blocked by methotrexate.

Leucovorin enhances the activity (and toxicity) of fluorouracil by stabilizing the binding of 5-fluoro-2'-deoxyuridine-5'-monophosphate (FdUMP; a fluorouracil metabolite) to thymidylate synthetase resulting in inhibition of this enzyme.

Pharmacokinetics (Adult data unless noted)

Metabolism: Converted to the active reduced form of folate, 5-methyl-tetrahydrofolate (5-methyl-THF; active)

Half-life, elimination: 5 to 7 hours

Time to peak serum concentration: 0.9 hours

Dosing: Usual Note: Levoleucovorin, when substituted in place of leucovorin calcium (the racemic form), is dosed at **one-half** the usual dose of leucovorin calcium.

Pediatric:

High-dose methotrexate rescue: Children and Adolescents: IV: 7.5 mg (~5 mg/m^2) every 6 hours, beginning 24 hours after the start of the methotrexate infusion (based on a methotrexate dose of 12 **g**/m^2 IV over 4 hours). Levoleucovorin (and hydration and urinary alkalinization) should be continued and/or adjusted until the methotrexate level is <0.05 micromolar (5 x 10^{-8} M). In trials, the youngest reported patients were 4 to 6 years of age (Goorin, 1995; Jaffe, 1993). The dosage and frequency should be determined based on methotrexate elimination and serum level:

Normal methotrexate elimination (serum methotrexate levels ~10 micromolar at 24 hours post administration, 1 micromolar at 48 hours, and <0.2 micromolar at 72 hours post infusion): 7.5 mg IV every 6 hours for 10 doses

Delayed late methotrexate elimination (serum methotrexate levels >0.2 micromolar at 72 hours and >0.05 micromolar at 96 hours post-methotrexate infusion): Continue 7.5 mg IV every 6 hours until methotrexate level is <0.05 micromolar

Delayed early methotrexate elimination and/or evidence of acute renal injury (serum methotrexate level ≥50 micromolar at 24 hours, ≥5 micromolar at 48 hours, or a doubling or more of the serum creatinine level at 24 hours post-methotrexate infusion): 75 mg IV every 3 hours until methotrexate level is <1 micromolar, followed by 7.5 mg IV every 3 hours until methotrexate level is <0.05 micromolar

Significant clinical toxicity in the presence of less severe abnormalities in methotrexate elimination or renal function (as described above): Extend levoleucovorin treatment for an additional 24 hours (total of 14 doses) in subsequent treatment cycles.

Delayed methotrexate elimination due to third space fluid accumulation, renal insufficiency, or inadequate hydration: May require higher levoleucovorin doses or prolonged administration.

Methotrexate overdose (inadvertent): Children and Adolescents: 7.5 mg (~5 mg/m^2) every 6 hours; continue until the methotrexate level is <0.01 micromolar (10^{-8} M). Initiate treatment as soon as possible after methotrexate overdose. Increase the levoleucovorin dose to 50 mg/m^2 IV every 3 hours if the 24 hour serum creatinine has increased 50% over baseline, or if the 24-hour methotrexate level is >5 micromolar (5 x 10^{-6} M), or if the 48-hour methotrexate level is >0.9 micromolar (9 x 10^{-7} M); continue levoleucovorin until the methotrexate level is <0.01 micromolar (10^{-8} M). Hydration (aggressive) and urinary alkalinization (with sodium bicarbonate; goal urine pH ≥7) should also be maintained.

Adult:

Colorectal cancer: IV: The following regimens have been used (in combination with fluorouracil; fluorouracil doses may need to be adjusted for toxicity; no adjustment required for the levoleucovorin dose): 10 mg/m^2/day **or** 100 mg/m^2/day (followed by fluorouracil) for 5 days every 4 weeks for 2 cycles, then every 4 to 5 weeks depending on recovery from toxicities

Alternative dosing: Levoleucovorin, when substituted in place of leucovorin calcium within a chemotherapy regimen, is dosed at **one-half** the usual dose of leucovorin calcium (Goldberg, 1997; NCCN colon cancer guidelines v.2.2013).

High-dose methotrexate rescue: IV: Usual dose: 7.5 mg (~5 mg/m^2) every 6 hours for 10 doses, beginning 24 hours after the start of the methotrexate infusion (based on a methotrexate dose of 12 **g**/m^2 IV over 4 hours). Levoleucovorin (and hydration and urinary alkalinization) should be continued and/or adjusted until the methotrexate level is <0.05 micromolar (5 x 10^{-8} M) as follows:

Normal methotrexate elimination (serum methotrexate levels ~10 micromolar at 24 hours post administration, 1 micromolar at 48 hours and <0.2 micromolar at 72 hours post infusion): 7.5 mg IV every 6 hours for 10 doses

Delayed late methotrexate elimination (serum methotrexate levels >0.2 micromolar at 72 hours and >0.05 micromolar at 96 hours post-methotrexate infusion): Continue 7.5 mg IV every 6 hours until methotrexate level is <0.05 micromolar

Delayed early methotrexate elimination and/or evidence of acute renal injury (serum methotrexate level ≥50 micromolar at 24 hours, ≥5 micromolar at 48 hours or a doubling or more of the serum creatinine level at 24 hours post methotrexate infusion): 75 mg IV every 3 hours until methotrexate level is <1 micromolar, followed by 7.5 mg IV every 3 hours until methotrexate level is <0.05 micromolar

Significant clinical toxicity in the presence of less severe abnormalities in methotrexate elimination or renal function (as described above): Extend levoleucovorin treatment for an additional 24 hours (total of 14 doses) in subsequent treatment cycles.

Delayed methotrexate elimination due to third space fluid accumulation, renal insufficiency, or inadequate hydration: May require higher levoleucovorin doses or prolonged administration.

Methotrexate overdose (inadvertent): IV: 7.5 mg (~5 mg/m^2) every 6 hours; continue until the methotrexate level is <0.01 micromolar (10^{-8} M). Initiate treatment as soon as possible after methotrexate overdose. Increase the levoleucovorin dose to 50 mg/m^2 IV every 3 hours if the 24 hour serum creatinine has increased 50% over baseline, or if the 24-hour methotrexate level is >5 micromolar (5 x 10^{-6} M), or if the 48-hour methotrexate level is >0.9 micromolar (9 x 10^{-7} M); continue levoleucovorin until the methotrexate level is <0.01 micromolar (10^{-8} M). Hydration (aggressive) and urinary alkalinization (with sodium bicarbonate) should also be maintained.

Dosing adjustment in renal impairment: Children, Adolescents, and Adults: There are no dosage adjustments provided in the manufacturer's labeling.

Dosing adjustment in hepatic impairment: Children, Adolescents, and Adults: There are no dosage adjustments provided in the manufacturer's labeling.

Preparation for Administration Lyophilized powder: Reconstitute the 50 mg vial with 5.3 mL NS (preservative free) to a concentration of 10 mg/mL. Do not use if solution appears cloudy or contains a precipitate. May further dilute for infusion in NS or D_5W to a final concentration of 0.5 to 5 mg/mL. Do not prepare with other products in the same admixture; may cause precipitation.

Administration For IV administration only; do not administer intrathecally. Administer by slow IV push or infusion over at least 3 minutes, not to exceed 160 mg/minute (due to calcium content).

For colorectal cancer: Adults: Levoleucovorin has also been administered as IV infusion over 2 hours (Comella 2000; Tournigand 2006). Administer levoleucovorin and fluorouracil separately to avoid precipitation.

Monitoring Parameters High-dose methotrexate therapy or methotrexate overdose (inadvertent): Serum methotrexate and creatinine levels at least once daily. Monitor fluid and electrolyte status in patients with delayed methotrexate elimination (likely to experience renal toxicity).

Dosage Forms Excipient information presented when available (limited, particularly for generics); consult specific product labeling.

Solution, Intravenous:
Generic: 175 mg/17.5 mL (17.5 mL)

Solution Reconstituted, Intravenous:
Fusilev: 50 mg (1 ea)

- **Levo-leucovorin** *see* LEVOleucovorin *on page* 1248
- **Levoleucovorin Calcium Pentahydrate** *see* LEVOleucovorin *on page* 1248
- **Levophed** *see* Norepinephrine *on page* 1529
- **Levophed® (Can)** *see* Norepinephrine *on page* 1529
- **Levosalbutamol** *see* Levalbuterol *on page* 1233
- **Levothroid [DSC]** *see* Levothyroxine *on page* 1250

Levothyroxine (lee voe thye ROKS een)

Medication Safety Issues

Sound-alike/look-alike issues:

Levothyroxine may be confused with lamoTRIgine, Lanoxin, levofloxacin, liothyronine

Levoxyl may be confused with Lanoxin, Levaquin, Luvox

Synthroid may be confused with Symmetrel

Administration issues:

Significant differences exist between oral and IV dosing. Use caution when converting from one route of administration to another.

Other safety concerns:

To avoid errors due to misinterpretation of a decimal point, always express dosage in mcg (**not** mg).

Brand Names: US Levothroid [DSC]; Levoxyl; Synthroid; Tirosint; Unithroid; Unithroid Direct

Brand Names: Canada Eltroxin; Levothyroxine Sodium; Levothyroxine Sodium for Injection; Synthroid

Therapeutic Category Thyroid Product

Generic Availability (US) May be product dependent

Use

Oral:

Tablets: Replacement or supplemental therapy in congenital or acquired hypothyroidism of any etiology (FDA approved in all ages); pituitary TSH suppressant for the treatment or prevention of various types of euthyroid goiter, thyroid nodules, thyroiditis, multinodular goiter, and thyroid cancer (FDA approved in adults); **Note:** Not indicated for treatment of transient hypothyroidism associated with subacute thyroiditis

Capsules (Tirosint®): Replacement or supplemental therapy in congenital or acquired hypothyroidism of any etiology (FDA approved in older children and adults); pituitary TSH suppressant for the treatment or prevention of various types of euthyroid goiter, thyroid nodules, thyroiditis, multinodular goiter, and thyroid cancer (FDA approved in adults); **Note:** Not indicated for treatment of transient hypothyroidism associated with subacute thyroiditis

Parenteral: Treatment of myxedema coma (FDA approved in adults); has also been used for organ donor management

Pregnancy Risk Factor A

Pregnancy Considerations Endogenous thyroid hormones minimally cross the placenta; the fetal thyroid becomes active around the end of the first trimester. Levothyroxine has not been shown to increase the risk of congenital abnormalities.

Uncontrolled maternal hypothyroidism may result in adverse neonatal outcomes (eg, premature birth, low birth weight, and respiratory distress) and adverse maternal outcomes (eg, spontaneous abortion, pre-eclampsia, stillbirth, and premature delivery). To prevent adverse events, normal maternal thyroid function should be maintained prior to conception and throughout pregnancy. Levothyroxine is considered the treatment of choice for the control of hypothyroidism during pregnancy. Due to alterations of endogenous maternal thyroid hormones, the levothyroxine dose may need to be increased during pregnancy and the dose usually needs to be decreased after delivery.

Breast-Feeding Considerations Endogenous thyroid hormones are minimally found in breast milk. The amount of endogenous thyroxine found in breast milk does not influence infant plasma thyroid values. Levothyroxine was not found to cause adverse events to the infant or mother during breast-feeding. Adequate thyroid hormone concentrations are required to maintain normal lactation. Appropriate levothyroxine doses should be continued during breast-feeding.

Contraindications

Hypersensitivity to levothyroxine sodium or any component of the formulation; acute MI; thyrotoxicosis of any etiology; uncorrected adrenal insufficiency

Capsule: Additional contraindication: Inability to swallow capsules (eg, infants, small children)

Injection:

US labeling: There are no contraindications listed in the manufacturer's labeling when used for labeled indication (treatment of myxedema coma); consider contraindications for oral therapy if using as a temporary substitute for oral treatment (off-label use) in patients with chronic hypothyroidism.

Canadian labeling: Hypersensitivity to levothyroxine sodium or any component of the formulation; acute MI; thyrotoxicosis of any etiology; uncorrected adrenal insufficiency.

Warnings/Precautions [US Boxed Warning]: Thyroid supplements are ineffective and potentially toxic when used for the treatment of obesity or for weight reduction, especially in euthyroid patients. High doses may produce serious or even life-threatening toxic effects particularly when used with some anorectic drugs (eg, sympathomimetic amines). Levothyroxine, either alone or with other concomitant therapeutic agents, should not be used for the treatment of obesity or for weight loss. Routine use of T_4 for TSH suppression is not recommended in patients with benign thyroid nodules. In patients deemed appropriate candidates, treatment should never be fully suppressive (TSH <0.1 mIU/L). Use with caution and reduce dosage in patients with cardiovascular disease, including heart failure; patients with developing or worsening cardiac symptoms should have their dose reduced or therapy withheld for 7 days then resumed at a reduced dose. Use cautiously in the elderly; suppressed TSH levels may increase risk of atrial fibrillation and mortality secondary to cardiovascular disease (Gharib 2010; Parle 2001). Increase dose slowly in the elderly and monitor for signs/symptoms of angina (ATA/AACE [Garber 2012]). Patients with adrenal insufficiency, myxedema, diabetes mellitus and insipidus may have symptoms exaggerated or aggravated. Use is contraindicated in patients with uncorrected adrenal insufficiency. Treatment with glucocorticoids should precede levothyroxine therapy in patients with adrenal insufficiency (ATA/AACE [Garber 2012]). Chronic hypothyroidism predisposes patients to coronary artery disease. Long-term therapy can decrease bone mineral density. Levoxyl may rapidly swell and disintegrate causing choking or gagging (should be administered with a full glass of water); use caution in patients with dysphagia or other swallowing disorders.

Warnings: Additional Pediatric Considerations Overtreatment may result in craniosynostosis in infants and premature closure of epiphyses in children; monitor use closely. In neonates and infants, cardiac overload, arrhythmias, and aspiration from avid suckling may occur during initiation of therapy (eg, first 2 weeks); monitor closely.

Adverse Reactions

Cardiovascular: Angina pectoris, cardiac arrest, cardiac arrhythmia, congestive heart failure, flushing, hypertension, increased pulse, myocardial infarction, palpitations, tachycardia

Central nervous system: Anxiety, choking sensation (Levoxyl), emotional lability, fatigue, headache, heat intolerance, hyperactivity, insomnia, irritability, myasthenia, nervousness, pseudotumor cerebri (children), seizure (rare)

Dermatologic: Alopecia, diaphoresis

Endocrine & metabolic: Menstrual disease, weight loss

Gastrointestinal: Abdominal cramps, diarrhea, dysphagia (Levoxyl), gag reflex (Levoxyl), increased appetite, vomiting

Genitourinary: Infertility

Hepatic: Increased liver enzymes

Hypersensitivity: Hypersensitivity (to inactive ingredients; symptoms include urticaria, pruritus, rash, flushing, angioedema, GI symptoms, fever, arthralgia, serum sickness, wheezing)

Neuromuscular & skeletal: Decreased bone mineral density, slipped capital femoral epiphysis (children), tremor

Respiratory: Dyspnea

Miscellaneous: Fever

Drug Interactions

Metabolism/Transport Effects None known.

Avoid Concomitant Use

Avoid concomitant use of Levothyroxine with any of the following: Sodium Iodide I131; Sucroferric Oxyhydroxide

Increased Effect/Toxicity

Levothyroxine may increase the levels/effects of: Tricyclic Antidepressants; Vitamin K Antagonists

The levels/effects of Levothyroxine may be increased by: Piracetam

Decreased Effect

Levothyroxine may decrease the levels/effects of: Sodium Iodide I131; Theophylline Derivatives

The levels/effects of Levothyroxine may be decreased by: Aluminum Hydroxide; Bile Acid Sequestrants; Calcium Polystyrene Sulfonate; Calcium Salts; CarBAMazepine; Ciprofloxacin (Systemic); Estrogen Derivatives; Fosphenytoin; Iron Salts; Lanthanum; Magnesium Salts; Multivitamins/Minerals (with ADEK, Folate, Iron); Orlistat; Phenytoin; Polaprezinc; Raloxifene; Rifampin; Selective Serotonin Reuptake Inhibitors; Sevelamer; Sodium Polystyrene Sulfonate; Sucralfate; Sucroferric Oxyhydroxide

Food Interactions Taking levothyroxine with enteral nutrition may cause reduced bioavailability and may lower serum thyroxine levels leading to signs or symptoms of hypothyroidism. Soybean flour (infant formula), soy, grapefruit juice, espresso coffee, cottonseed meal, walnuts, and dietary fiber may interfere with absorption of levothyroxine from the GI tract. Management: Take in the morning on an empty stomach at least 30 minutes before food. Consider an increase in dose if taken with enteral tube feed.

Storage/Stability

Capsules and tablets: Store at 25°C (77°F); excursions are permitted between 15°C and 30°C (59°F and 86°F). Protect from light and moisture.

Injection: Store at 20°C to 25°C (68°F to 77°F). Protect from light.

Additional stability data:

Stability in polypropylene syringes (100 mcg/mL in NS) at 5°C ± 1°C is 7 days (Gupta 2000).

Stability in latex-free, PVC minibags protected from light and stored at 15°C to 30°C (59°F to 86°F) was 12 hours for a 2 mcg/mL concentration or 18 hours for a 0.4 mcg/mL concentration in NS. May be exposed to light; however, stability time is significantly reduced, especially for the 2 mcg/mL concentration (Strong 2010).

Mechanism of Action Levothyroxine (T_4) is a synthetic form of thyroxine, an endogenous hormone secreted by the thyroid gland. T_4 is converted to its active metabolite, L-triiodothyronine (T_3). Thyroid hormones (T_4 and T_3) then bind to thyroid receptor proteins in the cell nucleus and exert metabolic effects through control of DNA transcription and protein synthesis; involved in normal metabolism, growth, and development; promotes gluconeogenesis, increases utilization and mobilization of glycogen stores, and stimulates protein synthesis, increases basal metabolic rate

Pharmacodynamics

Onset of action: Therapeutic:

Oral: 3-5 days

IV: Within 6-8 hours

Maximum effect: 4-6 weeks

Pharmacokinetics (Adult data unless noted)

Absorption: Oral: Erratic (40% to 80%, per manufacturer); decreases with age

Bioavailability: Oral tablets: 64% (nonfasting state) to 79% to 81% (fasting state) (Dickerson, 2010; Fish, 1987)

Protein binding: >99%; bound to plasma proteins, including thyroxine-binding globulin, thyroxine-binding prealbumin, and albumin

Metabolism: Hepatic to triiodothyronine (T_3; active); ~80% T_4 deiodinated in kidney and periphery; glucuronidation/conjugation also occurs; undergoes enterohepatic recirculation

Half-life: Euthyroid: 6-7 days; Hypothyroid: 9-10 days; Hyperthyroid: 3-4 days

Time to peak serum concentration: 2-4 hours

Elimination: Urine (major route of elimination; decreases with age); feces (~20%)

Dosing: Neonatal Note: Doses should be adjusted based on clinical response and laboratory parameters; on a weight basis, dosing is higher in neonates, infants, and children than adults due to the higher metabolic clearance.

Congenital hypothyroidism:

Oral: 10 to 15 mcg/kg once daily; titrate as rapidly as possible (<2 weeks after initiation of therapy) to achieve target serum T_4 concentration (>10 mcg/dL); in full-size, term infants, some have suggested an initial dose of 50 mcg/day. If patient at risk for development of cardiac failure, begin with a lower dose (25 mcg/day). In severe cases of hypothyroidism (serum T_4 <5 mcg/dL), begin treatment at a higher dosage of ~50 mcg/day (12 to 17 mcg/kg/dose) (AAP, 2006; Selva, 2002).

IV, IM: 50% to 75% of the oral dose

Organ donor management in brain-dead patients (hormone replacement therapy): IV: Initial: 5 mcg/kg bolus dose, followed by 1.4 mcg/kg/**hour** infusion (Zuppa, 2004)

Dosing: Usual Note: Doses should be adjusted based on clinical response and laboratory parameters; on a weight basis, dosing is higher in infants and children than adults due to the higher metabolic clearance.

Pediatric:

Hypothyroidism (acquired or congenital): Note: Hyperactivity in older children may be minimized by starting at one-quarter (25%) of the recommended dose and increasing each week by that amount until the full dose is achieved (4 weeks). Children with severe or chronic hypothyroidism should be started at 25 mcg/day; adjust dose by 25 mcg every 2 to 4 weeks.

Oral:

1 to 3 months: 10 to 15 mcg/kg once daily; if the infant is at risk for development of cardiac failure, use a lower starting dose of ~25 mcg/day; if the initial serum T_4 is very low (<5 mcg/dL), begin treatment at a higher dosage of ~50 mcg/day (12 to 17 mcg/kg/day) (AAP, 2006; Selva, 2002)

3 to 6 months: 8 to 10 mcg/kg once daily

6 to 12 months: 6 to 8 mcg/kg once daily

1 to 5 years: 5 to 6 mcg/kg once daily

6 to 12 years: 4 to 5 mcg/kg once daily

>12 years with incomplete growth and puberty: 2 to 3 mcg/kg once daily

Adolescents with growth and puberty complete: 1.7 mcg/kg once daily

IV, IM: Infants, Children, and Adolescents: 50% to 75% of the oral dose; alternatively, some clinicians administer up to 80% of the oral dose in adults patients. **Note:** Bioavailability of the oral formulation is highly variable, but absorption has been measured to be ~80%, when the oral tablet formulation was administered in the recommended fasting state (Dickerson, 2010; Fish, 1987).

Organ donor management in brain-dead patients (hormone replacement therapy) (Nakagawa, 2008; Zuppa, 2004): IV:

Infants <6 months: Initial: 5 mcg/kg bolus dose, followed by 1.4 mcg/kg/**hour** infusion

Infants 6 to 12 months: Initial: 4 mcg/kg bolus dose, followed by 1.3 mcg/kg/**hour** infusion

Children 1 to 5 years: Initial: 3 mcg/kg bolus dose, followed by 1.2 mcg/kg/**hour** infusion

Children 6 to 12 years: Initial: 2.5 mcg/kg bolus dose, followed by 1 mcg/kg/**hour** infusion

Children ≥12 years and Adolescents ≤16 years: Initial: 1.5 mcg/kg bolus dose, followed by 0.8 mcg/kg/**hour** infusion

Adolescents >16 years: Initial: 0.8 mcg/kg bolus dose, followed by 0.8 mcg/kg/**hour** infusion

Adult:

Hypothyroidism: Adults <50 years of age and older adults who have been recently treated for hyperthyroidism or who have been hypothyroid for only a few months:

Oral: ~1.7 mcg/kg/day usual doses are ≤200 mcg/day [range: 100 to 125 mcg/day (70 kg adult)]; doses ≥300 mcg/day are rare (consider poor compliance, malabsorption, and/or drug interactions). Titrate dose every 6 weeks.

Note: Patients with combined hypothyroidism and cardiac disease should be monitored carefully for changes in stability.

IV, IM: 50% of the oral dose; alternatively, some clinicians administer up to 80% of the oral dose. **Note:** Bioavailability of the oral formulation is highly variable, but absorption has been measured to be ~80%, when the oral tablet formulation was administered in the recommended fasting state (Dickerson, 2010; Fish, 1987).

Severe hypothyroidism: Oral: Initial: 12.5 to 25 mcg/day; adjust dose by 25 mcg/day every 2 to 4 weeks as appropriate

Subclinical hypothyroidism (if treated): Oral: 1 mcg/kg once daily

Myxedema coma or stupor: IV: 200 to 500 mcg one time then 100 to 300 mcg the next day if necessary; smaller doses should be considered in patients with cardiovascular disease

TSH suppression: Oral:

Well-differentiated thyroid cancer: Highly individualized; doses >2 mcg/kg/day may be needed to suppress TSH to <0.1 mIU/L in intermediate- to high-risk tumors. Low risk tumors may be maintained at or slightly below the lower limit of normal (0.1 to 0.5 mIU/L) (Cooper, 2009)

Benign nodules and nontoxic multinodular goiter: Routine use of T_4 for TSH suppression is not recommended in patients with benign thyroid nodules. In patients deemed appropriate candidates, treatment should never be fully suppressive (TSH <0.1 mIU/L) (Cooper 2009; Gharib, 2010). Avoid use if TSH is already suppressed.

Preparation for Administration Parenteral: Reconstitute vial for injection with 5 mL NS. Final concentration is dependent upon vial size; concentrations for the 100 mcg, 200 mcg, and 500 mcg vials are 20 mcg/mL, 40 mcg/mL, and 100 mcg/mL, respectively. Shake well and use immediately after reconstitution (manufacturer labeling suggests reconstituted vial is stable for 4 hours); discard any unused portions.

Administration

Oral:

Capsules: Must be swallowed whole; do not cut, crush, or attempt to dissolve capsules in water to prepare a suspension

Tablets: Administer on an empty stomach 30 to 60 minutes prior to breakfast with a full glass of water to prevent gagging. If administration on an empty stomach poses a challenge, particularly in infants and small children, it may be administered with food to improve adherence and consistency of administration. For infants, crush tablet and mix with breast-milk, non-soy-based formula, or water and use immediately (Zeitler, 2010).

Parenteral: Administer IV over 2 to 3 minutes; may administer IM

Monitoring Parameters T_4, TSH, heart rate, blood pressure, clinical signs of hypo- and hyperthyroidism; growth, bone development (children); TSH is the most reliable guide for evaluating adequacy of thyroid replacement dosage. TSH may be elevated during the first few months of thyroid replacement despite patients being clinically euthyroid. In cases where T_4 remains low and TSH is within normal limits, an evaluation of "free" (unbound) T_4 is needed to evaluate further increase in dosage.

In congenital hypothyroidism, adequacy of replacement should be determined using both TSH and total- or free-T_4. During the first 3 years of life, total- or free-T_4 should be maintained in the upper 1/2 of the normal range; this should result in normalization of the TSH. In some patients, TSH may not normalize due to a resetting of the pituitary-thyroid feedback as a result of *in utero* hypothyroidism. Monitor closely for cardiac overload, arrhythmias, and aspiration from avid suckling.

Pediatric patients: Monitor closely for under/overtreatment. Undertreatment may decrease intellectual development and linear growth and lead to poor school performance due to impaired concentration and slowed mentation. Overtreatment may adversely affect brain maturation and accelerate bone age (leading to premature closure of the epiphyses and reduced adult height); craniosynostosis has been reported in infants. Perform routine clinical examinations at regular intervals (to assess mental and physical growth and development). Monitor TSH and total or free T_4 at 2 and 4 weeks after starting treatment, every 1-2 months during the first year of life, every 2-3 months between ages 1-3 years, and every 3-12 months thereafter until growth is completed; repeat tests two weeks after any change in dosage.

Adults: Monitor TSH every 6-8 weeks until normalized, 8-12 weeks after dosage changes, and every 6-12 months throughout therapy.

Reference Range

Thyroid Function Tests

Lab Parameters	Age	Normal Range
T_4 (thyroxine) serum concentration	1-7 days	10.1-20.9 mcg/dL
	8-14 days	9.8-16.6 mcg/dL
	1 month to 1 year	5.5-16.0 mcg/dL
	>1 year	4.0-12.0 mcg/dL
Free thyroxine index (FTI)	1-3 days	9.3-26.6
	1-4 weeks	7.6-20.8
	1-4 months	7.4-17.9
	4-12 months	5.1-14.5
	1-6 years	5.7-13.3
	>6 years	4.8-14.0
T_3 serum concentration	Newborns	100-470 ng/dL
	1-5 years	100-260 ng/dL
	5-10 years	90-240 ng/dL
	10 years to Adult	70-210 ng/dL
T_3 uptake		35%-45%
TSH serum concentration	Cord	3-22 micro international units/mL
	1-3 days	<40 micro international units/mL
	3-7 days	<25 micro international units/mL
	>7 days	0-10 micro international units/mL

Test Interactions

T_4-binding globulin (TBG): Factors that alter binding in serum (ATA/AACE [Garber 2012]):

Note: T_4 is ~99.97% protein bound. Factors that alter protein binding will affect serum total T_4 levels; however, measurement of serum free T_4 (the metabolically active moiety) has largely replaced serum total T_4 for thyroid status assessment.

Conditions/states that increase TBG binding: Pregnancy, hepatitis, porphyria, neonatal state

Medications that increase TBG binding: Estrogens, 5-fluorouracil, heroin, methadone, mitotane, perphenazine, selective estrogen receptor modulators (eg, tamoxifen, raloxifene)

Conditions/states that decrease TBG binding: Hepatic failure, nephrosis, severe illness.

Medications that decrease TBG binding: Androgens, anabolic steroids, glucocorticoids, L-asparaginase, nicotinic acid

Thyroxine (T_4) and triiodothyronine (T3): Serum binding inhibitors (ATA/AACE [Garber 2012]):

Medications that inhibit T_4 and T_3 binding: Carbamazepine, furosemide, free fatty acids, heparin, NSAIDS (variable, transient), phenytoin, salicylates

Thyroid gland hormone: Interference with production and secretion (ATA/AACE [Garber 2012]):

Medications affecting iodine uptake: Amiodarone, iodinated contrast agents, iodine, ethionamide

Medications affecting hormone production: Amiodarone, ethionamide, iodinated contrast agents, iodine, sulfonylureas, sulfonamides, thionamides (carbimazole, methimazole, propylthiouracil),

Medications affecting secretion: Amiodarone, iodinated contrast agents, iodine, lithium

Medications inducing thyroiditis: Alemtuzumab, amiodarone, antiangiogenic agents (lenalidomide, thalidomide), denileukin diftitoxin, interferon alpha, interleukins, lithium, tyrosine kinase inhibitors (sunitinib, sorafenib)

Medications potentially causing the development of Graves': Alemtuzumab, interferon alpha, highly active antiretroviral therapy

Medications potentially ameliorating thyroiditis (if autoimmune) or Graves': Glucocorticoids

Hypothalamic-pituitary axis and TSH: Interference with secretion (ATA/AACE [Garber 2012]):

Medications decreasing TSH secretion: Bexarotene, dopamine, dopaminergic agonists (bromocriptine, cabergoline), glucocorticoids, interleukin-6, metformin, opiates, somatostatin analogues (octreotide, lanreotide), thyroid hormone analogues

Mediations increasing TSH secretion: Amphetamine, interleukin 2, metoclopramide, ritonavir, St John's wort

Medications potentially causing hypophysitis: Ipilimumab

Additional Information Equivalent doses: The following statement on relative potency of thyroid products is included in a joint statement by American Thyroid Association (ATA), American Association of Clinical Endocrinologists (AACE) and The Endocrine Society (TES): For purposes of conversion, levothyroxine sodium (T_4) 100 mcg is usually considered equivalent to desiccated thyroid 60 mg, thyroglobulin 60 mg, or liothyronine sodium (T_3) 25 mcg. However, these are rough guidelines only and do not obviate the careful re-evaluation of a patient when switching thyroid hormone preparations, including a change from one brand of levothyroxine to another. Joint position statement is available at http://www.thyroid.org/professionals/advocacy/04_12_08_thyroxine.html.

Note: Several medications have effects on thyroid production or conversion. The impact in thyroid replacement has not been specifically evaluated, but patient response should be monitored:

Methimazole: Decreases thyroid hormone secretion, while propylthiouracil decrease thyroid hormone secretion and decreases conversion of T_4 to T_3.

Beta-adrenergic antagonists: Decrease conversion of T_4 to T_3 (dose related, propranolol ≥160 mg/day); patients may be clinically euthyroid.

Iodide, iodine-containing radiographic contrast agents may decrease thyroid hormone secretion; may also increase thyroid hormone secretion, especially in patients with Graves' disease.

Other agents reported to impact on thyroid production/conversion include aminoglutethimide, amiodarone, chloral hydrate, diazepam, ethionamide, interferon-alpha, interleukin-2, lithium, lovastatin (case report), glucocorticoids (dose-related), mercaptopurine, sulfonamides, thiazide diuretics, and tolbutamide.

In addition, a number of medications have been noted to cause transient depression in TSH secretion, which may complicate interpretation of monitoring tests for levothyroxine, including corticosteroids, octreotide, and dopamine. Metoclopramide may increase TSH secretion

Dosage Forms Excipient information presented when available (limited, particularly for generics); consult specific product labeling. [DSC] = Discontinued product

Capsule, Oral, as sodium:
Tirosint: 13 mcg, 25 mcg, 50 mcg, 75 mcg, 88 mcg, 100 mcg, 112 mcg, 125 mcg, 137 mcg, 150 mcg
Solution Reconstituted, Intravenous, as sodium [preservative free]:
Generic: 100 mcg (1 ea); 200 mcg (1 ea); 500 mcg (1 ea)
Tablet, Oral, as sodium:
Levothroid: 25 mcg [DSC] [scored; contains fd&c yellow #6 aluminum lake]
Levothroid: 50 mcg [DSC] [scored]
Levothroid: 75 mcg [DSC] [scored; contains fd&c blue #2 aluminum lake, fd&c red #40 aluminum lake]
Levothroid: 88 mcg [DSC] [scored; contains fd&c blue #1 aluminum lake, fd&c yellow #10 aluminum lake, fd&c yellow #6 aluminum lake]
Levothroid: 100 mcg [DSC] [scored; contains fd&c yellow #10 aluminum lake, fd&c yellow #6 aluminum lake]
Levothroid: 112 mcg [DSC] [scored]
Levothroid: 125 mcg [DSC] [scored; contains fd&c blue #1 aluminum lake, fd&c red #40 aluminum lake, fd&c yellow #6 aluminum lake]
Levothroid: 137 mcg [DSC] [scored; contains fd&c blue #1 aluminum lake]
Levothroid: 150 mcg [DSC] [scored; contains fd&c blue #2 aluminum lake]
Levothroid: 175 mcg [DSC] [scored; contains fd&c blue #1 aluminum lake]
Levothroid: 200 mcg [DSC] [scored; contains fd&c red #40 aluminum lake]
Levothroid: 300 mcg [DSC] [scored; contains fd&c blue #1 aluminum lake, fd&c yellow #10 (quinoline yellow), fd&c yellow #6 aluminum lake]
Levoxyl: 25 mcg [scored; contains fd&c yellow #6 aluminum lake]
Levoxyl: 50 mcg [scored]
Levoxyl: 75 mcg [scored; contains fd&c blue #1 aluminum lake]
Levoxyl: 88 mcg [scored; contains fd&c blue #1 aluminum lake, fd&c yellow #10 aluminum lake, fd&c yellow #6 aluminum lake]
Levoxyl: 100 mcg [scored; contains fd&c yellow #10 aluminum lake, fd&c yellow #6 aluminum lake]
Levoxyl: 112 mcg [scored; contains fd&c red #40 aluminum lake, fd&c yellow #6 aluminum lake]
Levoxyl: 125 mcg [scored; contains fd&c red #40 aluminum lake, fd&c yellow #10 aluminum lake]
Levoxyl: 137 mcg, 150 mcg [scored; contains fd&c blue #1 aluminum lake]
Levoxyl: 175 mcg [scored; contains fd&c blue #1 aluminum lake, fd&c yellow #10 aluminum lake]
Levoxyl: 200 mcg [scored; contains fd&c yellow #10 aluminum lake]
Synthroid: 25 mcg [scored; contains fd&c yellow #6 aluminum lake]
Synthroid: 50 mcg [scored]
Synthroid: 75 mcg [scored; contains fd&c blue #2 aluminum lake, fd&c red #40 aluminum lake]
Synthroid: 88 mcg [scored; contains fd&c blue #1 aluminum lake, fd&c yellow #10 aluminum lake, fd&c yellow #6 aluminum lake]
Synthroid: 100 mcg [scored; contains fd&c yellow #10 aluminum lake, fd&c yellow #6 aluminum lake]
Synthroid: 112 mcg [scored]
Synthroid: 125 mcg [scored; contains fd&c blue #1 aluminum lake, fd&c red #40 aluminum lake, fd&c yellow #6 aluminum lake]
Synthroid: 137 mcg [scored; contains fd&c blue #1 aluminum lake]
Synthroid: 150 mcg [scored; contains fd&c blue #2 aluminum lake]
Synthroid: 175 mcg [scored; contains fd&c blue #1 aluminum lake]
Synthroid: 200 mcg [scored; contains fd&c red #40 aluminum lake]
Synthroid: 300 mcg [scored; contains fd&c blue #1 aluminum lake, fd&c yellow #10 aluminum lake, fd&c yellow #6 aluminum lake]
Unithroid: 25 mcg [contains fd&c yellow #6 aluminum lake]
Unithroid: 25 mcg [DSC] [scored; contains fd&c yellow #6 aluminum lake]
Unithroid: 50 mcg
Unithroid: 50 mcg [DSC], 75 mcg [DSC] [scored]
Unithroid: 75 mcg [contains fd&c blue #2 aluminum lake, fd&c red #40 aluminum lake]
Unithroid: 88 mcg [DSC] [scored]
Unithroid: 88 mcg [contains fd&c blue #1 aluminum lake, fd&c yellow #10 aluminum lake, fd&c yellow #6 aluminum lake]
Unithroid: 100 mcg [contains fd&c yellow #10 aluminum lake, fd&c yellow #6 aluminum lake]
Unithroid: 100 mcg [DSC] [scored; contains fd&c yellow #10 aluminum lake, fd&c yellow #6 aluminum lake]
Unithroid: 112 mcg
Unithroid: 112 mcg [DSC] [scored]
Unithroid: 125 mcg [contains fd&c blue #1 aluminum lake, fd&c red #40 aluminum lake, fd&c yellow #6 aluminum lake]
Unithroid: 125 mcg [DSC] [scored; contains fd&c blue #1 aluminum lake, fd&c red #40 aluminum lake, fd&c yellow #6 aluminum lake]
Unithroid: 137 mcg [contains fd&c blue #1 aluminum lake]
Unithroid: 150 mcg [contains fd&c blue #2 aluminum lake]
Unithroid: 150 mcg [DSC] [scored; contains fd&c blue #2 aluminum lake]
Unithroid: 175 mcg [DSC] [scored]
Unithroid: 175 mcg [contains fd&c blue #1 aluminum lake]
Unithroid: 200 mcg [DSC] [scored]
Unithroid: 200 mcg [contains fd&c red #40 aluminum lake]
Unithroid: 300 mcg [contains fd&c blue #1 aluminum lake, fd&c yellow #10 (quinoline yellow), fd&c yellow #6 aluminum lake]
Unithroid: 300 mcg [DSC] [scored; contains fd&c blue #1 aluminum lake, fd&c yellow #10 aluminum lake, fd&c yellow #6 aluminum lake]
Unithroid Direct: 25 mcg [scored; contains fd&c yellow #6 aluminum lake]
Unithroid Direct: 50 mcg [scored]
Unithroid Direct: 75 mcg, 88 mcg [scored; contains fd&c blue #1 aluminum lake, fd&c blue #2 aluminum lake, fd&c red #40 aluminum lake, fd&c yellow #10 aluminum lake, fd&c yellow #6 aluminum lake]
Unithroid Direct: 100 mcg [scored; contains fd&c yellow #10 aluminum lake, fd&c yellow #6 aluminum lake]
Unithroid Direct: 112 mcg [scored]
Unithroid Direct: 125 mcg [scored; contains fd&c blue #1 aluminum lake, fd&c red #40 aluminum lake, fd&c yellow #6 aluminum lake]
Unithroid Direct: 150 mcg [scored; contains fd&c blue #2 aluminum lake]
Unithroid Direct: 175 mcg [scored; contains fd&c blue #1 aluminum lake]
Unithroid Direct: 200 mcg [scored; contains fd&c red #40 aluminum lake]
Unithroid Direct: 300 mcg [scored; contains fd&c blue #1 aluminum lake, fd&c yellow #10 aluminum lake, fd&c yellow #6 aluminum lake]
Generic: 25 mcg, 50 mcg, 75 mcg, 88 mcg, 100 mcg, 112 mcg, 125 mcg, 137 mcg, 150 mcg, 175 mcg, 200 mcg, 300 mcg

Extemporaneous Preparations A 25 mcg/mL oral suspension may be made with tablets and 40 mL glycerol. Crush twenty-five 0.1 mg levothyroxine tablets in a mortar and reduce to a fine powder. Add small portions of glycerol and mix to a uniform suspension. Transfer to a calibrated 100 mL amber bottle; rinse the mortar with about 10 mL of glycerol and pour into the bottle; repeat until all 40 mL of glycerol is used. Add quantity of water sufficient to make 100 mL. Label "shake well" and "refrigerate". Stable for 8 days refrigerated.

Boulton DW, Fawcett JP, and Woods DJ, "Stability of an Extemporaneously Compounded Levothyroxine Sodium Oral Liquid," *Am J Health Syst Pharm*, 1996, 53(10):1157-61.

- **Levothyroxine and Liothyronine** *see* Liotrix *on page 1276*
- **Levothyroxine and Liothyronine** *see* Thyroid, Desiccated *on page 2058*
- **Levothyroxine Sodium** *see* Levothyroxine *on page 1250*
- **Levothyroxine Sodium for Injection (Can)** *see* Levothyroxine *on page 1250*
- **Levoxyl** *see* Levothyroxine *on page 1250*
- **Levsin** *see* Hyoscyamine *on page 1061*
- **Levsin/SL** *see* Hyoscyamine *on page 1061*
- **Lexapro** *see* Escitalopram *on page 786*
- **Lexiva** *see* Fosamprenavir *on page 936*
- **LH-RH Agonist** *see* Histrelin *on page 1022*
- ***l*-Hyoscyamine Sulfate** *see* Hyoscyamine *on page 1061*
- **Lialda** *see* Mesalamine *on page 1368*
- **Lidemol® (Can)** *see* Fluocinonide *on page 898*
- **Lidex** *see* Fluocinonide *on page 898*
- **Lidex® (Can)** *see* Fluocinonide *on page 898*

Lidocaine (Systemic) (LYE doe kane)

Medication Safety Issues

High alert medication:

The Institute for Safe Medication Practices (ISMP) includes this medication (epidural administration; IV formulation) among its list of drugs which have a heightened risk of causing significant patient harm when used in error.

International issues:

Lidosen [Italy] may be confused with Lincocin brand name for lincomycin [U.S., Canada, and multiple international markets]; Lodosyn brand name for carbidopa [U.S.]

Brand Names: US Xylocaine; Xylocaine (Cardiac); Xylocaine-MPF

Brand Names: Canada Xylocard

Therapeutic Category Antiarrhythmic Agent, Class I-B; Local Anesthetic, Injectable

Generic Availability (US) Yes

Use Treatment of ventricular arrhythmias (FDA approved in adults); local or regional anesthetic [FDA approved in pediatric patients (age not specified) and adults]

PALS guidelines recommend lidocaine when amiodarone is not available for cardiac arrest with pulseless VT or VF (unresponsive to defibrillation, CPR, and epinephrine administration); consider in patients with cocaine overdose to prevent arrhythmias secondary to MI

ACLS guidelines recommend lidocaine when amiodarone is not available for cardiac arrest with pulseless VT or VF (unresponsive to defibrillation, CPR, and vasopressor administration); it is not considered to be the drug of choice but may be considered for stable monomorphic VT (in patients with preserved ventricular function) and for polymorphic VT (with normal baseline or prolonged QT interval).

Pregnancy Risk Factor B

Pregnancy Considerations Adverse events were not observed in animal reproduction studies. Lidocaine and its metabolites cross the placenta and can be detected in the fetal circulation following injection (Cavalli, 2004; Mitani, 1987). Adverse reactions in the fetus/neonate may affect the CNS, heart, or peripheral vascular tone. Fetal heart monitoring is recommended. Lidocaine injection is approved for obstetric analgesia. Lidocaine administered by local infiltration is used to provide analgesia prior to episiotomy and during repair of obstetric lacerations (ACOG, 2002). Administration by the perineal route may result in greater absorption than administration by the epidural route (Cavalli, 2004). Cumulative exposure from all routes of administration should be considered. When used as an antiarrhythmic, ACLS guidelines recommend using the same dose that would be used in a nonpregnant woman (Vanden Hoek, 2010).

Breast-Feeding Considerations Lidocaine is excreted into breast milk. The manufacturer recommends that caution be used when administered to a nursing woman. When administered by injection for dental or obstetric analgesia, small amounts are detected in breast milk; oral bioavailability to the nursing infant is expected to be low and the amount of lidocaine available to the nursing infant would not be expected to cause adverse events (Lebedevs, 1993; Ortega, 1999). Cumulative exposure from all routes of administration should be considered.

Contraindications Hypersensitivity to lidocaine or any component of the formulation; hypersensitivity to another local anesthetic of the amide type; Adam-Stokes syndrome; Wolff-Parkinson-White syndrome; severe degrees of SA, AV, or intraventricular heart block (except in patients with a functioning artificial pacemaker); premixed injection may contain corn-derived dextrose and its use is contraindicated in patients with allergy to corn or corn-related products

Warnings/Precautions Use caution in patients with severe hepatic dysfunction or pseudocholinesterase deficiency; may have increased risk of lidocaine toxicity.

Intravenous: Constant ECG monitoring is necessary during IV administration. Use cautiously in hepatic impairment, HF, marked hypoxia, severe respiratory depression, hypovolemia, history of malignant hyperthermia, or shock. Increased ventricular rate may be seen when administered to a patient with atrial fibrillation. Correct electrolyte disturbances, especially hypokalemia or hypomagnesemia, prior to use and throughout therapy. Use is contraindicated in patients with Wolff-Parkinson-White syndrome and severe degrees of SA, AV, or intraventricular heart block (except in patients with a functioning artificial pacemaker). Correct any underlying causes of ventricular arrhythmias. Monitor closely for signs and symptoms of CNS toxicity. The elderly may be prone to increased CNS and cardiovascular side effects. Reduce dose in hepatic dysfunction and CHF.

Benzyl alcohol and derivatives: Some dosage forms may contain benzyl alcohol; large amounts of benzyl alcohol (≥99 mg/kg/day) have been associated with a potentially fatal toxicity ("gasping syndrome") in neonates; the "gasping syndrome" consists of metabolic acidosis, respiratory distress, gasping respirations, CNS dysfunction (including convulsions, intracranial hemorrhage), hypotension, and cardiovascular collapse (AAP, 1997; CDC, 1982); some data suggests that benzoate displaces bilirubin from protein binding sites (Ahlfors, 2001); avoid or use dosage forms containing benzyl alcohol with caution in neonates. See manufacturer's labeling.

Injectable anesthetic: Follow appropriate administration techniques so as not to administer any intravascularly. Continuous intra-articular infusion of local anesthetics after arthroscopic or other surgical procedures is **not** an approved use; chondrolysis (primarily in the shoulder joint) has occurred following infusion, with some cases requiring arthroplasty or shoulder replacement. Solutions containing antimicrobial preservatives should not be used for epidural or spinal anesthesia. Some solutions contain a bisulfite; avoid in patients who are allergic to bisulfite. Resuscitative equipment, medicine and oxygen should be available in case of emergency. Use products containing epinephrine cautiously in patients with significant vascular disease, compromised blood flow, or during or following general anesthesia (increased risk of arrhythmias). Adjust the dose for the elderly, pediatric, acutely ill, and debilitated patients.

Adverse Reactions Effects vary with route of administration. Many effects are dose related.

Cardiovascular: Arrhythmia, bradycardia, arterial spasms, cardiovascular collapse, defibrillator threshold increased, edema, flushing, heart block, hypotension, sinus node supression, vascular insufficiency (periarticular injections)

Central nervous system: Agitation, anxiety, apprehension, coma, confusion, disorientation, dizziness, drowsiness, euphoria, hallucinations, headache, hyperesthesia, hypoesthesia, lethargy, lightheadedness, nervousness, psychosis, seizure, slurred speech, somnolence, unconsciousness

Gastrointestinal: Metallic taste, nausea, vomiting

Local: Thrombophlebitis

Intradermal system: Application site reactions: Bruising/burning/contusion/hemorrhage/pain, edema, erythema, petechiae, pruritus

Neuromuscular & skeletal: Paresthesia, transient radicular pain (subarachnoid administration), tremor, twitching, weakness

Otic: Tinnitus

Respiratory: Bronchospasm, dyspnea, respiratory depression or arrest

Miscellaneous: Allergic reactions, anaphylactic reaction, anaphylactoid reaction, sensitivity to temperature extremes

Following spinal anesthesia: Cauda equina syndrome, double vision, hypotension, nausea, peripheral nerve symptoms, positional headache, respiratory inadequacy, shivering

Rare but important or life-threatening: Asystole, confusion, disorientation, flushing, headache, hyper-/hypoesthesia, hypersensitivity, methemoglobinemia, nervousness, skin reaction, weakness

Drug Interactions

Metabolism/Transport Effects **Substrate** of CYP1A2 (major), CYP2A6 (minor), CYP2B6 (minor), CYP2C9 (minor), CYP3A4 (major); **Note:** Assignment of Major/Minor substrate status based on clinically relevant drug interaction potential; **Inhibits** CYP1A2 (weak)

Avoid Concomitant Use

Avoid concomitant use of Lidocaine (Systemic) with any of the following: Conivaptan; Fusidic Acid (Systemic); Idelalisib; Saquinavir

Increased Effect/Toxicity

Lidocaine (Systemic) may increase the levels/effects of: Prilocaine; Sodium Nitrite; TiZANidine

The levels/effects of Lidocaine (Systemic) may be increased by: Abiraterone Acetate; Amiodarone; Aprepitant; Beta-Blockers; Conivaptan; CYP1A2 Inhibitors (Moderate); CYP1A2 Inhibitors (Strong); CYP3A4 Inhibitors (Moderate); CYP3A4 Inhibitors (Strong); Dasatinib; Deferasirox; Disopyramide; Fosaprepitant; Fusidic Acid (Systemic); Hyaluronidase; Idelalisib; Ivacaftor; Luliconazole; Mifepristone; Netupitant; Nitric Oxide; Palbociclib; Peginterferon Alfa-2b; Saquinavir; Simeprevir; Stiripentol; Telaprevir; Vemurafenib

Decreased Effect

Lidocaine (Systemic) may decrease the levels/effects of: Technetium Tc 99m Tilmanocept

The levels/effects of Lidocaine (Systemic) may be decreased by: Bosentan; Cannabis; CYP1A2 Inducers (Strong); CYP3A4 Inducers (Moderate); CYP3A4 Inducers (Strong); Cyproterone; Dabrafenib; Deferasirox; Etravirine; Mitotane; Siltuximab; St Johns Wort; Teriflunomide; Tocilizumab

Storage/Stability Injection: Stable at room temperature. Stability of parenteral admixture at room temperature (25°C) is the expiration date on premixed bag; out of overwrap stability is 30 days.

Mechanism of Action Class Ib antiarrhythmic; suppresses automaticity of conduction tissue, by increasing electrical stimulation threshold of ventricle, His-Purkinje system, and spontaneous depolarization of the ventricles during diastole by a direct action on the tissues; blocks both the initiation and conduction of nerve impulses by decreasing the neuronal membrane's permeability to sodium ions, which results in inhibition of depolarization with resultant blockade of conduction

Pharmacodynamics Antiarrhythmic effect:

Onset of action (single IV bolus dose): 45-90 seconds

Duration: 10-20 minutes

Pharmacokinetics (Adult data unless noted)

Distribution: Crosses blood-brain and placental barriers; distributes into breast milk; breast milk to plasma ratio: 0.4

V_d: 1.5 ± 0.6 L/kg; range: 0.7-2.7 L/kg; V_d alterable by many patient factors; decreased in CHF and liver disease

Protein binding: 60% to 80%; binds to alpha$_1$-acid glycoprotein

Metabolism: 90% in the liver; active metabolites monoethylglycinexylidide (MEGX) and glycinexylidide (GX) can accumulate and may cause CNS toxicity

Half-life, biphasic:

Alpha: 7-30 minutes

Beta, terminal: Infants, premature: 3.2 hours; Adults: 1.5-2 hours

CHF, liver disease, shock, severe renal disease: Prolonged half-life

Elimination: <10% excreted unchanged in urine; ~90% as metabolite

Dialysis: Dialyzable (0% to 5%)

Dosing: Neonatal Antiarrhythmic: Ventricular tachycardia, ventricular fibrillation: IV, I.O.:

Loading dose: 1 mg/kg/dose; follow with continuous infusion; may repeat bolus; **Note:** Neonates with reduced hepatic function or decreased hepatic blood flow (eg, CHF or postcardiac surgery) should receive 1/2 the usual loading dose.

Continuous IV infusion: 20-50 mcg/kg/minute; use lower dose for neonates with shock, hepatic disease, cardiac arrest, or CHF

Dosing: Usual

Antiarrhythmic:

Infants, Children, and Adolescents (PALS, 2010):

IV, I.O.: (**Note:** Use if amiodarone is not available, for pulseless VT or VF; give after defibrillation attempts, CPR, and epinephrine):

Loading dose: 1 mg/kg/dose; follow with continuous IV infusion (PALS, 2010); may administer second bolus of 0.5-1 mg/kg/dose if delay between bolus and start of infusion is >15 minutes (PALS, 2010); **Note:** Patients with reduced hepatic function or decreased hepatic blood flow (eg, CHF or postcardiac surgery) should receive 1/2 the usual loading dose.

Continuous IV infusion: 20-50 mcg/kg/minute. Per manufacturer, use a maximum of 20 mcg/kg/minute in patients with shock, hepatic disease, cardiac arrest, or CHF

E.T.: 2-3 mg/kg/dose; flush with 5 mL of NS and follow with 5 assisted manual ventilations

Adults (ACLS, 2010):

VF or pulseless VT (after defibrillation attempts, CPR, and vasopressor administration) if amiodarone is not available:

IV, I.O.: Initial: 1-1.5 mg/kg. If refractory VF or pulseless VT, repeat 0.5-0.75 mg/kg bolus every 5-10 minutes (maximum cumulative dose: 3 mg/kg). Follow with continuous infusion (1-4 mg/minute) after return of perfusion. Reappearance of arrhythmia during constant infusion: 0.5 mg/kg bolus and reassessment of infusion (Zipes, 1999)

E.T. (loading dose only): 2-3.75 mg/kg (2-2.5 times the recommended IV dose); dilute in 5-10 mL NS or sterile water. **Note:** Absorption is greater with sterile water and results in less impairment of PaO_2.

Hemodynamically stable monomorphic VT: IV: 1-1.5 mg/kg; repeat with 0.5-0.75 mg/kg every 5-10 minutes as necessary (maximum cumulative dose: 3 mg/kg). Follow with continuous infusion of 1-4 mg/minute or 30-50 mcg/kg/minute

Note: Dose reduction (eg, of maintenance infusion) necessary in patients with CHF, shock, or hepatic disease.

Anesthesia, local injectable: Children and Adults: Dose varies with procedure, degree of anesthesia needed, vascularity of tissue, duration of anesthesia required, and physical condition of patient; maximum dose: 4.5 mg/kg not to exceed 300 mg.

Usual Infusion Concentrations: Pediatric Note: Premixed solutions available

IV infusion: 8000 **mcg**/mL

Preparation for Administration

Endotracheal: Pediatric patients: May dilute in 1 to 5 mL NS based on patient size (Hegenbarth 2008). Adults: Dilute in 5 to 10 mL NS or sterile water prior to E.T. administration (ACLS [Neumar] 2010.) In adults, it has been reported that absorption is greater with sterile water and results in less impairment of PaO2 (Hähnel 1990).

Parenteral:

IV

Bolus: Preparation dependent upon product; solutions containing 40 to 200 mg/mL must be diluted prior to use to a concentration not to exceed 20 mg/mL. The injectable solution of 20 mg/mL may be administered undiluted.

Continuous IV infusion:Dilute in D_5W or other compatible solution to a concentration of 1,000 to 8,000 mcg/mL (1 to 8 mg/mL) (Klaus 1989; Murray 2014; Phillips 2011); premix solution available for 4,000 and 8,000 mcg/mL (4 and 8 mg/mL).

Local infiltration: Buffered lidocaine for injectable local anesthetic may be prepared: Add 2 mL of sodium bicarbonate 8.4% to 18 mL of lidocaine 1% (Christoph 1988).

Administration

Endotracheal:

Infants, Children, and Adolescents: May administer dose undiluted, followed by flush with 5 mL of NS after E.T. administration or may further dilute prior to administration; follow with 5 assisted manual ventilations (PALS [Kleinman 2010]; Hegenbarth 2008)

Adults: Dilute in NS or sterile water prior to E.T. administration. Absorption is greater with sterile water and results in less impairment of PaO2 (Hähnel 1990). Flush with 5 mL of NS and follow immediately with several quick insufflations and continue chest compressions.

Parenteral: IV:

IV push: The manufacturer recommends that the rate of administration should not exceed 0.7 mg/kg/minute or 50 mg/minute, whichever is less; however, during acute situations (eg, pulseless VT or VF), administration by rapid IV push has been used by some clinicians in practice.

Continuous IV infusion: Administer via an infusion pump.

Monitoring Parameters Monitor ECG continuously; serum concentrations with continuous infusion; IV site (local thrombophlebitis may occur with prolonged infusions)

Reference Range

Therapeutic: 1.5-5 mcg/mL (SI: 6-21 micromoles/L)

Potentially toxic: >6 mcg/mL (SI: >26 micromoles/L)

Toxic: >9 mcg/mL (SI: >38 micromoles/L)

Dosage Forms Excipient information presented when available (limited, particularly for generics); consult specific product labeling.

Solution, Injection, as hydrochloride:

Xylocaine: 0.5% (50 mL); 1% (20 mL, 50 mL); 2% (10 mL, 20 mL, 50 mL) [contains methylparaben]

Xylocaine-MPF: 0.5% (50 mL); 1% (2 mL, 5 mL, 10 mL, 30 mL); 1.5% (10 mL, 20 mL); 2% (2 mL, 5 mL, 10 mL); 4% (5 mL) [methylparaben free]

Generic: 0.5% (50 mL); 1% (2 mL, 5 mL, 10 mL, 20 mL, 30 mL, 50 mL); 1.5% (20 mL); 2% (2 mL, 5 mL, 20 mL, 50 mL)

Solution, Injection, as hydrochloride [preservative free]:

Generic: 0.5% (50 mL); 1% (2 mL, 5 mL, 30 mL); 1.5% (20 mL); 2% (2 mL, 5 mL, 10 mL); 4% (5 mL)

Solution, Intravenous, as hydrochloride:

Xylocaine (Cardiac): 20 mg/mL (5 mL)

Generic: 10 mg/mL (5 mL); 20 mg/mL (5 mL); 0.4% [4 mg/mL] (250 mL, 500 mL); 0.8% [8 mg/mL] (250 mL); 2% (5 mL); 5% [50 mg/mL] (2 mL)

Solution, Intravenous, as hydrochloride [preservative free]:

Generic: 10 mg/mL (5 mL); 20 mg/mL (5 mL)

Lidocaine (Ophthalmic) (LYE doe kane)

Brand Names: US Akten

Therapeutic Category Local Anesthetic, Ophthalmic

Generic Availability (US) No

Use Local anesthetic for ophthalmic procedures (FDA approved in adults; refer to product specific information regarding FDA approval in pediatric patients)

Pregnancy Risk Factor B

Pregnancy Considerations Adverse events were not observed in animal reproduction studies. Although systemic exposure is not expected following application of the ophthalmic gel, cumulative exposure from all routes of administration should be considered.

Breast-Feeding Considerations When administered by injection for dental or obstetric analgesia, small amounts of lidocaine are detected in breast milk (Lebedevs, 1993; Ortega, 1999). Although systemic exposure is not expected following application of the ophthalmic gel, cumulative exposure from all routes of administration should be considered.

Contraindications There are no contraindications listed in the manufacturer's labeling

Warnings/Precautions For ophthalmic use only; not for injection. Prolonged use may cause permanent corneal ulceration and/or opacification with loss of vision.

Adverse Reactions

Local: Burning

Ocular: Conjunctival hyperemia, corneal epithelial changes, diplopia, visual changes

Drug Interactions

Metabolism/Transport Effects None known.

Avoid Concomitant Use There are no known interactions where it is recommended to avoid concomitant use.

Increased Effect/Toxicity There are no known significant interactions involving an increase in effect.

Decreased Effect There are no known significant interactions involving a decrease in effect.

Storage/Stability Store at 15°C to 25°C (59°F to 77°F). Protect from light. Discard after use.

Mechanism of Action Local anesthetics block both the initiation and conduction of nerve impulses by decreasing the neuronal membrane's permeability to sodium ions, which results in inhibition of depolarization with resultant blockade of conduction.

Pharmacodynamics Local anesthetic effect:

Onset of action: 20 seconds to 5 minutes (median: 40 seconds)

Duration: 5-30 minutes (mean: 15 minutes)

Dosing: Usual Anesthesia, ocular: Ophthalmic gel (Akten®): Children and Adults: Apply 2 drops to ocular surface in area where procedure to occur; may reapply to maintain effect

Dosage Forms Excipient information presented when available (limited, particularly for generics); consult specific product labeling.

Gel, Ophthalmic [preservative free]:

Akten: 3.5% (1 mL)

Lidocaine (Topical) (LYE doe kane)

Brand Names: US AneCream [OTC]; AneCream5 [OTC]; EnovaRX-Lidocaine HCl; Glydo; LC-4 Lidocaine [OTC]; LC-5 Lidocaine [OTC]; Lidocin; Lidoderm; Lidopin; LidoRx; Lidovex; Lidovin; Lidozol; LMX 4 Plus [OTC]; LMX 4 [OTC]; LMX 5 [OTC]; LTA 360 Kit; Predator [OTC]; Premium Lidocaine; Prozena; Prozena [OTC]; RectiCare [OTC]; Tecnu First Aid [OTC]; Topicaine 5 [OTC]; Topicaine [OTC]; Xolido XP [OTC]; Xylocaine; Zingo

Brand Names: Canada Betacaine; Lidodan; Lidoderm; Maxilene; Xylocaine

Therapeutic Category Analgesic, Topical; Local Anesthetic, Topical; Local Anesthetic, Transdermal

Generic Availability (US) May be product dependent

Use In general, local anesthetic for oral mucous membrane; laser/cosmetic surgeries; minor burns, cuts, and abrasions of the skin; specific uses will vary based on product formulation (FDA approved in adults; refer to product specific information regarding FDA approval in pediatric patients)

Product-specific indications:

Cream: Temporary relief of pain and itching due to minor cuts, scrapes, burns, sunburn, minor skin irritations, and insect bites (OTC use: Lidovex 3.75%: FDA approved in pediatric patients [age not specified] and adults; LMX 4: FDA approved in ages ≥2 years and adults); liposomal cream (LMX 4) has also been used as topical anesthetic for minor dermal procedures (eg, venipuncture, peripheral IV cannulation)

Intradermal injection (Zingo): Topical local analgesia prior to peripheral intravenous (IV) cannulation (FDA approved in ages 3 through 18 years) and topical local analgesia prior to venipuncture (FDA approved in ages ≥3 years and adults)

Topical patch (Lidoderm): Relief of allodynia (painful hypersensitivity) and postherpetic neuralgia (FDA approved in adults)

Rectal (LMX 5): Temporary relief of pain and itching due to anorectal disorders (FDA approved in ages ≥12 years and adults)

Oral solution (2% viscous): Topical anesthesia of irritated oral mucous membranes and pharyngeal tissue (FDA approved in infants, children, and adults); **Note:** Not approved for relief of teething pain and discomfort in infants and children; serious adverse (toxic) effects have been reported (AAP, 2011; AAPD, 2012; ISMP, 2014)

Topical solution (4%): Topical anesthesia of accessible mucous membranes of the oral and nasal cavities and proximal portions of the digestive tract (FDA approved in children [age not specified] and adults); **Note:** Not approved for relief of teething pain and discomfort in infants and children; serious adverse (toxic) effects have been reported (AAP, 2011; AAPD, 2012; ISMP, 2014).

Pregnancy Risk Factor B

Pregnancy Considerations Adverse events were not observed in animal reproduction studies using the systemic injection. Lidocaine and its metabolites cross the placenta and can be detected in the fetal circulation following injection (Cavalli, 2004; Mitani, 1987). The amount of lidocaine absorbed topically (and therefore available systemically to potentially reach the fetus) varies by dose administered, duration of exposure, and site of application. Cumulative exposure from all routes of administration should be considered.

Breast-Feeding Considerations Lidocaine is excreted into breast milk. The manufacturer recommends caution be used when administering lidocaine to nursing women. When administered by injection for dental or obstetric analgesia, small amounts are detected in breast milk; oral bioavailability to the nursing infant is expected to be low. The amount of lidocaine available to the nursing infant would not be expected to cause adverse events (Lebedevs, 1993; Ortega, 1999). Cumulative exposure from all routes of administration should be considered.

Contraindications Hypersensitivity to lidocaine or any component of the formulation; hypersensitivity to another local anesthetic of the amide type; traumatized mucosa, bacterial infection at the site of application (lotion and Lidovex only).

Warnings/Precautions Use with caution in patients with known drug sensitivities. Allergic reactions (cutaneous lesions, urticaria, edema, or anaphylactoid reactions) may be a result of sensitivity to lidocaine (rare) or preservatives used in formulations. Patients allergic to para-aminobenzoic acid (PABA) derivatives (eg, procaine, tetracaine, benzocaine) have not shown cross sensitivity to lidocaine. Potentially life-threatening side effects (eg, irregular heart beat, seizures, coma, respiratory depression, death) have occurred when used prior to cosmetic procedures. Excessive dosing for any indication (eg, application to large areas, use above recommended dose, application to denuded or inflamed skin, or wearing of device for longer than recommended), smaller patients, and/or impaired elimination may lead to increased absorption and systemic toxicity; patient should adhere strictly to recommended dosage and administration guidelines; serious adverse effects may require the use of supportive care and resuscitative equipment. Use caution in patients with severe hepatic disease and/or pseudocholinesterase deficiency due to diminished ability to metabolize systemically-absorbed lidocaine. Elderly or debilitated patients should be given reduced doses commensurate with their age and physical status. Use intradermal injection with caution in patients with bleeding tendencies/platelet disorders; may have a higher risk of superficial dermal bleeding.

When topical anesthetics are used prior to cosmetic or medical procedures, the lowest amount of anesthetic necessary for pain relief should be applied. High systemic levels and toxic effects (eg, methemoglobinemia, irregular heart beats, respiratory depression, seizures, death) have been reported in patients who (without supervision of a trained professional) have applied topical anesthetics in large amounts (or to large areas of the skin), left these products on for prolonged periods of time, or have used wraps/dressings to cover the skin following application. Irritation, sensitivity and/or infection may occur at the site of application; discontinue use and institute appropriate therapy if local effects occur. Potentially significant interactions may exist, requiring dose or frequency adjustment, additional monitoring, and/or selection of alternative therapy.

Topical cream, liquid, lotion, gel, and ointment: Do not leave on large body areas for >2 hours. Not for ophthalmic use. Some products are not recommended for use on mucous membranes; consult specific product labeling.

Intradermal injection: Only use on skin locations where an adequate seal can be maintained. Do not use on body orifices, mucous membranes, around the eyes, or on areas with a compromised skin barrier.

Topical oral solution/viscous: **[US Boxed Warning]: Life-threatening and fatal events in infants and young children:** Postmarketing cases of seizures, cardiopulmonary arrest, and death in patients <3 years have been reported with use of lidocaine 2% viscous solution when it was not administered in strict adherence to the dosing and administration recommendations. Lidocaine 2% viscous solution should generally not be used for teething pain. For other conditions, the use of lidocaine 2% viscous solution in patients <3 years should be limited to those situations where safer alternatives are not available or have been tried but failed. To decrease the risk of serious adverse events, instruct caregivers to strictly adhere to the prescribed dose and frequency of administration, and store the prescription bottle safely out of reach of children. Multiple cases of seizures (including fatalities) have occurred in pediatric patients using viscous lidocaine for oral discomfort, including teething pain and stomatitis (Curtis, 2009; Giard, 1983; Gonzalez del Ray, 1994; Hess, 1988; Mofenson, 1983; Puczynski, 1985; Rothstein, 1982; Smith, 1992). The FDA recommends against using topical OTC medications for teething pain as some products may cause harm. The American Academy of Pediatrics (AAP) recommends managing teething pain with a chilled (not frozen) teething ring or gently rubbing/massaging with the caregiver's finger.

When used in mouth or throat, topical anesthesia may impair swallowing and increase aspiration risk. Avoid food for ≥60 minutes following oral or throat application. This is especially important in the pediatric population. Numbness may increase the danger of tongue/buccal biting trauma; ingesting food or chewing gum should be avoided while mouth or throat is anesthetized. Excessive doses or frequent application may result in high plasma levels and serious adverse effects; strictly adhere to dosing instructions. Use measuring devices to measure the correct volume, if applicable, to ensure accuracy of dose.

Use of topical anesthetics for teething is discouraged by the AAP, the American Academy of Pediatric Dentistry, and the ISMP (AAP, 2012; AAPD, 2012; ISMP, 2014).

Topical patch: Apply only on intact skin. Do not use around or in the eyes. To avoid accidental ingestion by children, store and dispose of products out of the reach of children. Avoid exposing application site to external heat sources (eg, heating pad, electric blanket, heat lamp, hot tub).

Benzyl alcohol and derivatives: Some dosage forms may contain benzyl alcohol; large amounts of benzyl alcohol (≥99 mg/kg/day) have been associated with a potentially fatal toxicity ("gasping syndrome") in neonates; the "gasping syndrome" consists of metabolic acidosis, respiratory distress, gasping respirations, CNS dysfunction (including convulsions, intracranial hemorrhage), hypotension, and cardiovascular collapse (AAP, 1997; CDC, 1982); some data suggests that benzoate displaces bilirubin from protein binding sites (Ahlfors, 2001); avoid or use dosage forms containing benzyl alcohol with caution in neonates.

Some dosage forms may contain polysorbate 80 (also known as Tweens). Hypersensitivity reactions, usually a delayed reaction, have been reported following exposure to pharmaceutical products containing polysorbate 80 in certain individuals (Isaksson, 2002; Lucente 2000; Shelley, 1995). Thrombocytopenia, ascites, pulmonary deterioration, and renal and hepatic failure have been reported in premature neonates after receiving parenteral products containing polysorbate 80 (Alade, 1986; CDC, 1984). See manufacturer's labeling.

Warnings: Additional Pediatric Considerations In infants and children, seizures (some fatal) have been reported following topical lidocaine ingestion at serum concentrations within the therapeutic range of 1 to 5 mcg/mL (Curtis 2009); others have reported toxic effects with excessive doses or frequent application of topical oral lidocaine solution that resulted in high plasma concentrations. Multiple cases of seizures, including fatalities, have occurred in pediatric patients using viscous lidocaine for oral discomfort (eg, teething pain, herpetic gingivostomatitis) (Curtis 2009; Giard 1983; Gonzalez del Rey 1994; Hess 1988; Mofenson 1983; Puczynski 1985; Rothstein 1982; Smith 1992). Lidocaine oral solution is not approved for treatment of teething pain or discomfort; off-label use is strongly discouraged and should be avoided. When used for oral irritation, the solution should not be swallowed, but should be applied topically with a cotton swab to individual lesions or the excess should be expectorated (swish and spit). Toxicology data suggests that in infants and children<6 years, ingestion of as little as 5 mL of lidocaine may result in serious toxicity and emergency care should be sought (Curtis 2009). Additionally, the FDA recommends against using topical OTC medications for teething pain as some products may cause harm; the use of OTC topical anesthetics (eg, benzocaine) for teething pain is also discouraged by AAP, and The American Academy of Pediatric Dentistry (AAP 2011; AAPD 2012). The AAP recommends managing teething pain with a chilled (not frozen) teething ring or gently rubbing/massaging with the caregiver's finger.

Topical patches (both used and unused) may cause toxicities in children; used patches still contain large amounts of lidocaine; store and dispose patches out of the reach of children; efficacy of patches in pediatric patients has not been evaluated due to safety concerns.

Some dosage forms may contain propylene glycol; in neonates large amounts of propylene glycol delivered orally, intravenously (eg, >3,000 mg/day), or topically have been associated with potentially fatal toxicities which can include metabolic acidosis, seizures, renal failure, and CNS depression; toxicities have also been reported in children and adults including hyperosmolality, lactic acidosis, seizures, and respiratory depression; use caution (AAP 1997; Shehab 2009).

Adverse Reactions Note: Adverse effects vary with formulation and extent of systemic absorption; children may be at increased risk.

Cardiovascular: Bradycardia, edema (intradermal powder)

Central nervous system: Apprehension, confusion, dizziness, drowsiness, paresthesia

Dermatologic: dermatitis, erythema (intradermal powder), exacerbation of pain (topical patch), petechia (intradermal powder), pruritus (intradermal powder), skin depigmentation (topical patch), skin edema (topical patch), skin rash, urticaria

Gastrointestinal: Nausea (intradermal powder), vomiting (intradermal powder)

Hematologic and oncologic: Bruise (topical patch), methemoglobinemia

Hypersensitivity: Anaphylactoid reaction, angioedema, hypersensitivity reaction
Local: Local irritation (topical patch)
Neuromuscular & skeletal: Weakness

Drug Interactions

Metabolism/Transport Effects **Substrate** of CYP1A2 (major), CYP2A6 (minor), CYP2B6 (minor), CYP2C9 (minor), CYP3A4 (major); **Note:** Assignment of Major/Minor substrate status based on clinically relevant drug interaction potential; **Inhibits** CYP1A2 (weak)

Avoid Concomitant Use

Avoid concomitant use of Lidocaine (Topical) with any of the following: Conivaptan; Fusidic Acid (Systemic); Idelalisib

Increased Effect/Toxicity

Lidocaine (Topical) may increase the levels/effects of: Antiarrhythmic Agents (Class III); Prilocaine; Sodium Nitrite; TiZANidine

The levels/effects of Lidocaine (Topical) may be increased by: Abiraterone Acetate; Antiarrhythmic Agents (Class III); Aprepitant; Beta-Blockers; Conivaptan; CYP1A2 Inhibitors (Moderate); CYP1A2 Inhibitors (Strong); CYP3A4 Inhibitors (Moderate); CYP3A4 Inhibitors (Strong); Dasatinib; Deferasirox; Disopyramide; Fosaprepitant; Fusidic Acid (Systemic); Idelalisib; Ivacaftor; Luliconazole; Mifepristone; Netupitant; Nitric Oxide; Palbociclib; Peginterferon Alfa-2b; Simeprevir; Stiripentol; Vemurafenib

Decreased Effect There are no known significant interactions involving a decrease in effect.

Storage/Stability All formulations: Store at room temperature; see product-specific labeling for any additional storage requirements. Store and dispose of products out of the reach of children and pets.

Mechanism of Action Blocks both the initiation and conduction of nerve impulses by decreasing the neuronal membrane's permeability to sodium ions, which results in inhibition of depolarization with resultant blockade of conduction

Pharmacodynamics Local anesthetic effect:
Onset of action:
Jelly: 3 to 5 minutes
Patch (5%): ~4 hours (Davies 2004)

Pharmacokinetics (Adult data unless noted)

Absorption: Extent and rate variable; dependent upon concentration, dose, application site, and duration of exposure.
Topical patch (5%): 3% ± 2% is expected to be absorbed with recommended doses
Metabolism: 90% hepatic; active metabolites monoethylglycinexylidide (MEGX) and glycinexylidide (GX) can accumulate and may cause CNS toxicity
Time to peak serum concentration: Topical patch (5%): 11 hours (following application of 3 patches)
Elimination: Urine (<10% as unchanged drug)

Dosing: Neonatal **Note:** Smaller areas of treatment are recommended in younger or smaller patients (<12 months or <10 kg) or those with impaired elimination (Fein 2012); use lowest effective dose.

Circumcision; anesthetic: Topical: Cream: LMX 4 (lidocaine 4%): Full-term neonates: Apply 2 **g** of cream to foreskin and penis; occlude with plastic wrap; leave on for 20 to 30 minutes minutes prior to circumcision (AAP 2012; Lehr 2005)

Dosing: Usual

Pediatric: **Note:** Smaller areas of treatment are recommended in younger or smaller patients (<12 months or <10 kg) or those with impaired elimination (Fein 2012); use lowest effective dose

Anesthetic: Topical:
Cream:
Lidovex (lidocaine 3.75%): Infants, Children, and Adolescents: Dose varies with age, weight, and physical condition; apply a thin film to affected area 2 to 3 times daily as needed; maximum dose: 4.5 mg/kg
LMX 4 (lidocaine 4%, liposomal): Children > 2 years and Adolescents: Dose varies with age and weight; apply a thin film to affected area 3 to 4 times daily as needed; maximum dose: 4.5 mg/kg
Gel, ointment: Children ≥2 years and Adolescents: Dose varies with age and weight; apply to affected area up to 3 to 4 times daily as needed; maximum dose: 4.5 mg/kg; not to exceed 300 mg
Jelly: Children and Adolescents: Dose varies with age and weight; maximum dose: 4.5 mg/kg not to exceed 600 mg in a 12-hour period

Minor dermal procedures [eg, peripheral IV cannulation, venipuncture, lumbar puncture, abscess drainage, joint aspiration]; anesthetic: Limited data available:
Intradermal injection: Zingo: Venipuncture or peripheral IV catheter insertion: Children ≥3 years and Adolescents: Apply one intradermal lidocaine (0.5 mg) device to the site planned for venipuncture, administer 1 to 3 minutes prior to the IV needle insertion; perform procedure within 10 minutes of application
Topical: Cream LMX 4 (lidocaine 4%):
Infants and Children <4 years: 1 **g** applied to site 30 minutes prior to procedure; (Fein, 2012; Taddio, 2004)
Children ≥4 years and Adolescents ≤17 years: 1 to 2.5 **g** applied to site 30 minutes prior to procedure (Eichenfield 2002; Fein 2012; Koh 2004; Luhman 2004; Taddio 2004)
Note: For peripheral IV cannulation, some have recommended application to 6.25 cm^2 of skin (Sobanko 2012).

Oral inflammation or irritation: Topical: **Note:** Not approved for relief of teething pain and discomfort in infants and children; serious adverse (toxic) effects have been reported; AAP, AAPD, and ISMP strongly discourage use (AAP 2011; AAPD 2012; ISMP 2014).
Oral solution (2% viscous): Dose should be adjusted according to patient's age, weight, and physical condition:
Infants and Children <3 years: 25 mg/dose (1.25 mL) applied to area with a cotton-tipped applicator no more frequently than every 3 hours; maximum: 4 doses per 12-hour period; should not be swallowed
Children ≥3 years and Adolescents: Do not exceed 4.5 mg/kg/dose; maximum single dose: 300 mg; swished in the mouth and spit out no more frequently than every 3 hours; maximum: 4 doses per 12-hour period
Topical solution (4%): **Note:** For use on mucous membranes of the oral and nasal cavities and proximal portions of the digestive tract; use lowest effective dose. Children and Adolescents: Do not exceed 4.5 mg/kg/dose; maximum single dose: 300 mg; applied with cotton applicator, cotton pack, or via spray; should not be swallowed

Rectal pain, itching: Topical: Cream: LMX 5 (lidocaine 5%): Children ≥12 years and Adolescents: Apply to affected area up to 6 times daily

Skin irritation: Topical: Cream: LMX 4 (lidocaine 4%): Children ≥2 years and Adolescents: Apply up to 3 to 4 times daily to intact skin

Adult: **Anesthetic, topical:**
Cream:
LidaMantle, Lidovex: Skin irritation: Apply a thin film to affected area 2 to 3 times daily as needed

LMX 4: Skin irritation: Apply up to 3 to 4 times daily to intact skin

LMX 5: Relief of anorectal pain and itching: Apply to affected area up to 6 times/day

Gel, ointment: Apply to affected area ≤4 times/day as needed (maximum dose: 4.5 mg/kg, not to exceed 300 mg)

Intradermal injection: Apply one intradermal lidocaine (0.5 mg) device to the site planned for venipuncture, 1 to 3 minutes prior to needle insertion

Jelly: Maximum dose: 30 mL (600 mg) in any 12-hour period:

Anesthesia of male urethra: 5 to 30 mL (100 to 600 mg)

Anesthesia of female urethra: 3 to 5 mL (60 to 100 mg)

Oral topical solution (2% viscous):

Anesthesia of the mouth: 15 mL swished in the mouth and spit out no more frequently than every 3 hours (maximum: 4.5 mg/kg [or 300 mg/dose]; 8 doses per 24-hour period)

Anesthesia of the pharynx: 15 mL gargled no more frequently than every 3 hours (maximum: 4.5 mg/kg [or 300 mg/dose]; 8 doses per 24-hour period); may be swallowed

Topical patch:

Lidoderm: Postherpetic neuralgia: Apply patch to most painful area. Up to 3 patches may be applied in a single application. Patch(es) may remain in place for up to 12 hours in any 24-hour period.

LidoPatch: Pain (localized): Apply patch to painful area. Patch may remain in place for up to 12 hours in any 24-hour period. No more than 1 patch should be used in a 24-hour period.

Topical solution (4%): **Note:** For use in mucous membranes of oral and nasal cavities and proximal GI tract; use lowest effective dose. Apply 1 to 5 mL (40 to 200 mg) to affected area (maximum dose: 4.5 mg/kg, not to exceed 300 mg/dose)

Administration

Cream: Apply to affected area; occlusive dressing may be applied.

LMX-4: Minor dermal procedure (peripheral IV cannulation, venipuncture): Infants and Children: Apply to skin at least 30 minutes before procedure; in most trials, occlusion of the application site was used (Koh 2004; Luhman 2004; Taddio 2004) while another trial showed that occlusion was not required (Eichenfiled 2002); however, occlusion of the site may be helpful in active infants and children to hold cream in place

Gel (Topicaine): Apply a moderately thick layer to affected area (~1/8" thick). Allow time for numbness to develop (~20 to 60 minutes after application). When used prior to laser surgery, avoid mucous membranes; remove prior to laser treatment.

Intradermal injection: Refer to manufacturer's labeling for administration technique. Apply intradermal lidocaine 1 to 3 minutes prior to needle insertion; perform procedure within 10 minutes following application. Application of **one** additional intradermal lidocaine at a new location is acceptable after a failed attempt at peripheral IV cannulation; multiple administrations of intradermal lidocaine at the same location are not recommended. Only use on intact skin and on skin locations where an adequate seal can be maintained. Do not use on body orifices, mucous membranes, around the eyes, or on areas with a compromised skin barrier. When removing the device from the pouch, be careful not to touch the purple outlet (open end) to avoid contamination; do not use if the device has been dropped or the pouch is damaged or torn.

Oral solution (2% viscous):

Mouth irritation or inflammation: Have patient swish medication around mouth and then spit it out. In children <3 years, apply small amount to affected area with cotton-tipped applicator.

Pharyngeal anesthesia: Adults: Patient should gargle and may swallow medication.

Topical patch:

Lidoderm: Apply to intact skin to cover most painful area immediately after removal from protective envelope. May be cut (with scissors, prior to removal of release liner) to appropriate size. Clothing may be worn over application area. After removal from skin, fold used patches so the adhesive side sticks to itself; avoid contact with eyes. Remove immediately if burning sensation occurs. Wash hands after application. Avoid exposing application site to external heat sources (eg, heating pad, electric blanket, heat lamp, hot tub). Dispose of patch properly and keep out of reach of children.

LidoPatch: Remove protective film and apply to painful area. Avoid contact with eyes or mucous membranes. Do not apply to open wounds or sensitive skin and do not bandage tightly. Wash hands after application. Avoid exposing application site to external heat sources (eg, heating pad, electric blanket, heat lamp, hot tub).

Dosage Forms Considerations EnovaRX-Lidocaine cream is compounded from a kit. Refer to manufacturer's package insert for compounding instructions.

Dosage Forms Excipient information presented when available (limited, particularly for generics); consult specific product labeling.

Cream, External:

AneCream: 4% (5 g, 15 g, 30 g) [contains benzyl alcohol, polysorbate 80, propylene glycol, trolamine (triethanolamine)]

AneCream5: 5% (15 g, 30 g) [contains benzyl alcohol, polysorbate 80, propylene glycol, trolamine (triethanolamine)]

LC-4 Lidocaine: 4% (45 g) [contains cetyl alcohol]

LC-5 Lidocaine: 5% (45 g) [contains cetyl alcohol]

Lidovex: 3.75% (60 g) [contains cetyl alcohol, methylparaben, propylparaben]

Lidovin: 3.95% (60 g) [contains peg-40 castor oil]

Lidozol: 3.75% (60 g) [contains peg-40 castor oil]

LMX 4: 4% (5 g, 15 g, 30 g) [contains benzyl alcohol]

LMX 5: 5% (15 g, 30 g) [contains benzyl alcohol]

RectiCare: 5% (15 g, 30 g) [contains benzyl alcohol, polysorbate 80, propylene glycol, trolamine (triethanolamine)]

Generic: 4% (5 g, 15 g, 30 g)

Cream, External, as hydrochloride:

EnovaRX-Lidocaine HCl: 5% (60 g, 120 g); 10% (60 g, 120 g) [contains cetyl alcohol]

Lidopin: 3% (28 g, 85 g); 3.25% (28 g, 85 g) [contains cetyl alcohol, methylparaben, propylparaben]

Predator: 4% (63 g) [contains propylene glycol, trolamine (triethanolamine)]

Xolido XP: 4% (118 mL) [contains methylisothiazolinone]

Generic: 3% (28.3 g, 28.35 g, 85 g)

Device, Intradermal, as hydrochloride:

Zingo: 0.5 mg (1 ea)

Gel, External:

Topicaine: 4% (10 g, 30 g, 113 g) [contains benzyl alcohol, disodium edta]

Topicaine 5: 5% (10 g, 30 g, 113 g) [contains benzyl alcohol, disodium edta]

Gel, External, as hydrochloride:

Lidocin: 3% (120 g, 240 g) [contains brilliant blue fcf (fd&c blue #1), polysorbate 80, tartrazine (fd&c yellow #5), trolamine (triethanolamine)]

LidoRx: 3% (10 mL, 30 mL) [contains isopropyl alcohol, trolamine (triethanolamine)]

Tecnu First Aid: 0.2-2.5 % (56.7 g) [contains disodium edta]

Generic: 2% (5 mL, 20 mL, 30 mL)

Gel, External, as hydrochloride [preservative free]:

Glydo: 2% (6 mL, 11 mL) [pvc free]

Generic: 2% (5 mL, 10 mL)
Kit, External:
AneCream: 4% [contains benzyl alcohol, polysorbate 80, propylene glycol, trolamine (triethanolamine)]
LMX 4 Plus: 4% [contains benzyl alcohol]
Generic: 4%
Lotion, External, as hydrochloride:
Generic: 3% (118 mL, 177 mL)
Ointment, External:
Premium Lidocaine: 5% (50 g)
Premium Lidocaine: 5% (50 g) [contains polyethylene glycol]
Generic: 5% (30 g, 35.44 g, 50 g)
Patch, External:
Lidoderm: 5% (1 ea, 30 ea) [contains disodium edta, methylparaben, propylene glycol, propylparaben]
Prozena: 4% (5 ea, 15 ea, 30 ea)
Generic: 5% (1 ea, 30 ea)
Solution, External, as hydrochloride:
Xylocaine: 4% (50 mL) [contains methylparaben]
Generic: 4% (50 mL)
Solution, Mouth/Throat, as hydrochloride:
Generic: 2% (15 mL, 100 mL)
Solution, Mouth/Throat, as hydrochloride [preservative free]:
LTA 360 Kit: 4% (4 mL)
Generic: 4% (4 mL)

Lidocaine and Epinephrine

(LYE doe kane & ep i NEF rin)

Brand Names: US Lignospan® Forte; Lignospan® Standard; Xylocaine® MPF With Epinephrine; Xylocaine® With Epinephrine

Brand Names: Canada Xylocaine® With Epinephrine

Therapeutic Category Local Anesthetic, Injectable

Generic Availability (US) Yes

Use Local infiltration anesthesia [FDA approved in pediatric patients (age not specified) and adults]

Pregnancy Risk Factor B

Pregnancy Considerations See individual agents.

Breast-Feeding Considerations Refer to Lidocaine (Systemic) and Epinephrine (Systemic) monographs.

Contraindications Hypersensitivity to lidocaine, epinephrine, or any component of the formulation; hypersensitivity to other local anesthetics of the amide type; myasthenia gravis; shock; cardiac conduction disease; angle-closure glaucoma

Warnings/Precautions Aspirate the syringe (injection solution for infiltration formulation) after tissue penetration and before injection to minimize chance of direct vascular injection. Use caution in endocrine, hepatic, or thyroid disease. Use with caution in the elderly, debilitated, acutely ill and pediatric patients. Avoid use in presence of flammable anesthetics. Avoid in patients with uncontrolled hyperthyroidism. Use minimal amounts in patients with significant cardiovascular problems (eg, significant hypertension); sympathomimetic or sympathomimetic-containing combination products may increase blood pressure. Careful and constant monitoring of the patient's state of consciousness should be done following each local anesthetic injection; at such times, restlessness, anxiety, tinnitus, dizziness, blurred vision, tremors, depression, or drowsiness may be early warning signs of CNS toxicity. Treatment is primarily symptomatic and supportive. Continuous intra-articular infusion of local anesthetics after arthroscopic or other surgical procedures is **not** an approved use; chondrolysis (primarily in the shoulder joint) has occurred following infusion, with some cases requiring arthroplasty or shoulder replacement. Local anesthetics have been associated with rare occurrences of sudden respiratory arrest, seizures, and cardiac arrest. May contain sodium metabisulfite; use caution in patients with a sulfite allergy. Dental practitioners and/or clinicians using local anesthetic agents should be well trained in diagnosis and management of emergencies that may arise from the use of these agents. Resuscitative equipment, oxygen and other resuscitative drugs should be available for immediate use.

Adverse Reactions Degree of adverse effects in the central nervous system and cardiovascular system are directly related to the blood levels of lidocaine. The effects below are more likely to occur after systemic administration rather than infiltration.

Cardiovascular: Myocardial effects include a decrease in contraction force as well as a decrease in electrical excitability and myocardial conduction rate resulting in bradycardia and reduction in cardiac output.
Central nervous system: High blood levels result in anxiety, confusion, disorientation, dizziness, restlessness, seizure, and tremor. This is followed by depression of CNS resulting in somnolence, unconsciousness and possible respiratory arrest. In some cases, symptoms of CNS stimulation may be absent and the primary CNS effects are somnolence and unconsciousness.
Gastrointestinal: Nausea, vomiting
Hypersensitivity reactions: Extremely rare, but may be manifest as dermatologic reactions and edema at injection site. Asthmatic syndromes have occurred. Patients may exhibit hypersensitivity to bisulfites contained in local anesthetic solution to prevent oxidation of epinephrine. In general, patients reacting to bisulfites have a history of asthma and their airways are hyper-reactive to asthmatic syndrome.
Psychogenic reactions: It is common to misinterpret psychogenic responses to local anesthetic injection as an allergic reaction. Intraoral injections are perceived by many patients as a stressful procedure in dentistry. Common symptoms to this stress are diaphoresis, generalized pallor, fainting feeling, hyperventilation, palpitation.

Drug Interactions

Metabolism/Transport Effects Refer to individual components.

Avoid Concomitant Use

Avoid concomitant use of Lidocaine and Epinephrine with any of the following: Ergot Derivatives; Iobenguane I 123; Lurasidone

Increased Effect/Toxicity

Lidocaine and Epinephrine may increase the levels/effects of: Lurasidone; Sympathomimetics

The levels/effects of Lidocaine and Epinephrine may be increased by: AtoMOXetine; Beta-Blockers; Cannabinoid-Containing Products; COMT Inhibitors; Ergot Derivatives; Hyaluronidase; Inhalational Anesthetics; Linezolid; MAO Inhibitors; Serotonin/Norepinephrine Reuptake Inhibitors; Tedizolid; Tricyclic Antidepressants

Decreased Effect

Lidocaine and Epinephrine may decrease the levels/effects of: Antidiabetic Agents; Benzylpenicilloyl Polylysine; Iobenguane I 123

The levels/effects of Lidocaine and Epinephrine may be decreased by: Alpha1-Blockers; Promethazine; Spironolactone

Storage/Stability Solutions with epinephrine should be protected from light.

Mechanism of Action Lidocaine blocks both the initiation and conduction of nerve impulses via decreased permeability of sodium ions; epinephrine increases the duration of action of lidocaine by causing vasoconstriction (via alpha effects) which slows the vascular absorption of lidocaine

Pharmacodynamics

Maximum effect: Within 5 minutes

Duration: 2-6 hours, dependent on dose and anesthetic procedure

Dosing: Usual Dosage varies with the anesthetic procedure

Children: Use lidocaine concentrations of 0.5% or 1% (or even more dilute) to decrease possibility of toxicity; lidocaine dose (when using combination product of lidocaine and epinephrine) should not exceed 7 mg/kg/dose; do not repeat within 2 hours

Administration Local injection: Before injecting, withdraw syringe plunger to make sure that injection is not into vein or artery; do not administer IV or intra-arterially

Additional Information Use preservative free solutions for epidural or caudal use

Dosage Forms Excipient information presented when available (limited, particularly for generics); consult specific product labeling. [DSC] = Discontinued product

Injection, solution:

0.5% / 1:200,000: Lidocaine hydrochloride 0.5% [5 mg/mL] and epinephrine 1:200,000 (50 mL)

1% / 1:100,000: Lidocaine hydrochloride 1% [10 mg/mL] and epinephrine 1:100,000 (20 mL, 30 mL, 50 mL)

2% / 1:100,000: Lidocaine hydrochloride 2% [20 mg/mL] and epinephrine 1:100,000 (30 mL, 50 mL)

Xylocaine® with Epinephrine:

0.5% / 1:200,000: Lidocaine hydrochloride 0.5% [5 mg/mL] and epinephrine 1:200,000 (50 mL) [contains methylparaben]

1% / 1:100,000: Lidocaine hydrochloride 1% [10 mg/mL] and epinephrine 1:100,000 (10 mL, 20 mL, 50 mL) [contains methylparaben]

2% / 1:100,000: Lidocaine hydrochloride 2% [20 mg/mL] and epinephrine 1:100,000 (10 mL, 20 mL, 50 mL) [contains methylparaben]

Injection, solution [preservative free]:

1.5% / 1:200,000: Lidocaine hydrochloride 1.5% [15 mg/mL] and epinephrine 1:200,000 (5 mL, 30 mL)

2% / 1:200,000: Lidocaine hydrochloride 2% [20 mg/mL] and epinephrine 1:200,000 (20 mL)

Xylocaine®-MPF with Epinephrine:

1% / 1:200,000: Lidocaine hydrochloride 1% [10 mg/mL] and epinephrine 1:200,000 (5 mL, 10 mL, 30 mL) [contains sodium metabisulfite]

1.5% / 1:200,000: Lidocaine hydrochloride 1.5% [15 mg/mL] and epinephrine 1:200,000 (5 mL, 10 mL, 30 mL) [contains sodium metabisulfite]

2% / 1:200,000: Lidocaine hydrochloride 2% [20 mg/mL] and epinephrine 1:200,000 (5 mL, 10 mL, 20 mL) [contains sodium metabisulfite]

Injection, solution [for dental use]:

2% / 1:50,000: Lidocaine hydrochloride 2% [20 mg/mL] and epinephrine 1:50,000 (1.7 mL, 1.8 mL)

2% / 1:100,000: Lidocaine hydrochloride 2% [20 mg/mL] and epinephrine 1:100,000 (1.7 mL, 1.8 mL)

Lignospan® Forte: 2% / 1:50,000: Lidocaine hydrochloride 2% [20 mg/mL] and epinephrine 1:50,000 (1.7 mL) [contains edetate disodium, potassium metabisulfite]

Lignospan® Standard: 2% / 1:100,000: Lidocaine hydrochloride 2% [20 mg/mL] and epinephrine 1:100,000 (1.7 mL) [contains edetate disodium, potassium metabisulfite]

Xylocaine® Dental with Epinephrine:

2% / 1:50,000: Lidocaine hydrochloride 2% [20 mg/mL] and epinephrine 1:50,000 (1.7 mL; 1.8 mL [DSC]) [contains sodium metabisulfite]

2% / 1:100,000: Lidocaine hydrochloride 2% [20 mg/mL] and epinephrine 1:100,000 (1.7 mL; 1.8 mL [DSC]) [contains sodium metabisulfite]

Lidocaine and Prilocaine

(LYE doe kane & PRIL oh kane)

Brand Names: US EMLA; Oraqix; Relador Pak

Brand Names: Canada EMLA; Oraqix

Therapeutic Category Analgesic, Topical; Antipruritic, Topical; Local Anesthetic, Topical

Generic Availability (US) Yes: Cream

Use

Cream: Topical anesthetic for use on normal intact skin to provide local analgesia for minor procedures such as IV cannulation or venipuncture; topical anesthetic for superficial minor surgery of genital mucous membranes and as an adjunct for local infiltration anesthesia in genital mucous membranes [FDA approved in neonates (full-term), pediatric, and adult patients]; has also been used for painful procedures, such as lumbar puncture and skin graft harvesting

Periodontal gel: Topical anesthetic for use in periodontal pockets during scaling or root planing procedures (FDA approved in adults)

Pregnancy Risk Factor B

Pregnancy Considerations Animal reproduction studies have not been conducted with this combination. Lidocaine and prilocaine cross the placenta. Their use is not contraindicated during labor and delivery. Refer to individual agents.

Breast-Feeding Considerations Lidocaine is excreted in breast milk; excretion of prilocaine in breast milk unknown; however, systemic absorption following topical application is expected to be low. The manufacturer recommends that caution be exercised when administering to nursing women. Refer to individual agents.

Contraindications

Hypersensitivity to local anesthetics of the amide type or any component of the formulation

Canadian labeling: Additional contraindications (not in US labeling): Congenital or idiopathic methemoglobinemia.

Cream and patch only: Infants ≤12 months of age who require treatment with methemoglobin-inducing agents; preterm infants (gestational age <37 weeks); procedures requiring large amounts over a large body area that are not conducted in a facility with health care professionals trained in the diagnosis and management of dose-related toxicity and other acute emergencies, and with appropriate resuscitative treatments and equipment.

Warnings/Precautions Methemoglobinemia has been reported in infants and children; associated with large doses, larger-than-recommended areas of application, neonates and infants <3 months of age, and concomitant use of methemoglobinemia-inducing agents (eg, acetaminophen, benzocaine, chloroquine, dapsone, nitrofurantoin, nitroglycerin, nitroprusside, phenobarbital, phenytoin, quinine, sulfonamides). Neonates and infants up to 3 months of age should be monitored for methemoglobinemia. Do not use in preterm neonates (gestational age <37 weeks), infants <12 months of age requiring treatment with methemoglobinemia-inducing agents, or in patients with congenital or idiopathic methemoglobinemia. Patients with glucose-6-phosphate dehydrogenase (G6PD) deficiency may be more susceptible to drug-induced methemoglobinemia. Allergic and anaphylactic reactions may occur. Patients allergic to paraaminobenzoic acid derivatives (eg, procaine, tetracaine, benzocaine) have not shown cross sensitivity to lidocaine and/or prilocaine; use with caution in patients with a history of drug sensitivities.

Although the incidence of systemic adverse reactions with use of the cream is very low, caution should be exercised, particularly when applying over large areas and leaving on for longer than 2 hours. When used prior to cosmetic or medical procedures, the smallest amount of cream necessary for pain relief should be applied. High systemic levels and toxic effects (eg, methemoglobinemia, irregular heartbeats, respiratory depression, seizures, death) have been reported in patients who (without supervision of a trained professional) have applied topical anesthetics in large amounts (or to large areas of the skin), left these products on for a prolonged time, or have used wraps/dressings to cover the skin following application. Do not apply to broken or inflamed skin, open wounds or near the eyes. Avoid use in situations where penetration or migration past the tympanic membrane into the middle ear is possible; ototoxicity has been observed in animal studies. Avoid inadvertent trauma to the treated area (eg, scratching, rubbing, exposure to extreme hot or cold temperatures) until complete sensation has returned.

Use with caution in patients with severe hepatic impairment; smaller treatment area may be required due to risk of increased systemic exposure. Use with caution in patients with severe impairment of impulse initiation and conduction in the heart (eg, grade II and III AV block, pronounced bradycardia). Use with caution in patients with atopic dermatitis; rapid and greater absorption through the skin is observed in these patients; a shorter application time should be used. Use with caution in the debilitated or acutely ill patients and elderly patients; smaller treatment area may be required. Potentially significant drug-drug interactions may exist, requiring dose or frequency adjustment, additional monitoring, and/or selection of alternative therapy.

Do not use periodontal gel with standard dental syringes; only use with the supplied blunt-tipped applicator.

Warnings: Additional Pediatric Considerations Adjust dose in patients with increased risk for methemoglobinemia; use smaller areas for application in small children (especially infants <3 months of age). In small infants and children, an occlusive bandage may prevent the child from placing the cream in his/her mouth or smearing the cream on the eyes.

Adverse Reactions

Cream/patch:

Dermatologic: Hyperpigmentation, urticaria

Genitourinary: Blistering of foreskin (rare)

Local: Burning, edema, erythema, itching, pallor, petechia, purpura, stinging

Miscellaneous: Alteration in temperature sensation (local)

Rare but important or life-threatening: Anaphylactic shock, angioedema, central nervous system depression, central nervous system stimulation, central nervous system toxicity (high dose), circulatory shock (high dose), hypersensitivity reactions, hypotension, methemoglobinemia (high dose)

Periodontal gel:

Central nervous system: Fatigue

Gastrointestinal: Bitter taste, nausea

Local: Application site reaction (includes abscess, edema, irritation, numbness, pain, ulceration, vesicles)

Respiratory: Infection

Miscellaneous: Allergic reactions, flu-like syndrome

Drug Interactions

Metabolism/Transport Effects Refer to individual components.

Avoid Concomitant Use

Avoid concomitant use of Lidocaine and Prilocaine with any of the following: Conivaptan; Fusidic Acid (Systemic); Idelalisib

Increased Effect/Toxicity

Lidocaine and Prilocaine may increase the levels/effects of: Antiarrhythmic Agents (Class III); Prilocaine; Sodium Nitrite; TiZANidine

The levels/effects of Lidocaine and Prilocaine may be increased by: Abiraterone Acetate; Antiarrhythmic Agents (Class III); Aprepitant; Beta-Blockers; Conivaptan; CYP1A2 Inhibitors (Moderate); CYP1A2 Inhibitors (Strong); CYP3A4 Inhibitors (Moderate); CYP3A4 Inhibitors (Strong); Dasatinib; Deferasirox; Disopyramide; Fosaprepitant; Fusidic Acid (Systemic); Hyaluronidase; Idelalisib; Ivacaftor; Luliconazole; Methemoglobinemia Associated Agents; Mifepristone; Netupitant; Nitric Oxide; Palbociclib; Peginterferon Alfa-2b; Simeprevir; Stiripentol; Vemurafenib

Decreased Effect

Lidocaine and Prilocaine may decrease the levels/effects of: Technetium Tc 99m Tilmanocept

Storage/Stability

Cream:

US labeling: Store between 20°C to 25°C (68°F to 77°F).

Canadian labeling: Store between 15°C to 30°C (59°F to 86°F).

Patch (Canadian availability; not available in the US): Store between 15°C to 30°C (59°F to 86°F); do not freeze.

Periodontal gel: Store at 25°C (77°F); excursions permitted between 15°C and 30°C (59°F and 86°F); do not freeze. May turn opaque at temperature of ≤5°C. Do not use dental cartridge warmers; heat will cause product to gel prematurely (product is a microemulsion that is intended to form a gel in the periodontal pocket).

Mechanism of Action Local anesthetic action occurs by stabilization of neuronal membranes and inhibiting the ionic fluxes required for the initiation and conduction of impulses

Pharmacodynamics

Cream:

Onset of action: Dermal analgesia: 1 hour; genital mucosal analgesia: 5-10 minutes

Maximum effect: Dermal analgesia: 2-3 hours; genital mucosal analgesia: 15-20 minutes

Duration: 1-2 hours after removal of the cream

Periodontal gel:

Onset of action: 30 seconds

Duration: ~20 minutes

Pharmacokinetics (Adult data unless noted) Note: Unless specified, data refers to the topical cream product formulation.

Absorption: Related to the duration of application and to the area over which it is applied

3-hour application: 3.6% lidocaine and 6.1% prilocaine were absorbed

24-hour application: 16.2% lidocaine and 33.5% prilocaine were absorbed

Distribution: Both cross the blood-brain barrier

V_d:

Lidocaine: 1.1-2.1 L/kg

Prilocaine: 0.7-4.4 L/kg

Protein binding:

Lidocaine: 70%

Prilocaine: 55%

Metabolism:

Lidocaine: Metabolized by the liver to inactive and active metabolites

Prilocaine: Metabolized in both the liver and kidneys

Half-life:

Cream:

Lidocaine: 65-150 minutes, prolonged in cardiac or hepatic dysfunction

Prilocaine: 10-150 minutes, prolonged in hepatic or renal dysfunction

Periodontal gel:

Lidocaine: 2.2-6.5 hours, prolonged in hepatic dysfunction

Prilocaine: 2-5.7 hours, prolonged in hepatic dysfunction

Dosing: Neonatal Note: Smaller areas of treatment recommended in younger or smaller patients or those with impaired elimination; decreasing the duration of application may decrease analgesic effect; however, maximum application duration times should not be exceeded.

Circumcision (major dermal procedure): GA ≥37 weeks: Topical cream: Apply 1 to 2 g to prepuce and cover with occlusive dressing for 60 to 90 minutes prior to procedure (Weise, 2005)

Topical local anesthetic (minor dermal procedures [eg, IM injection, IV access, venipuncture]):

GA <37 weeks: Limited data available: Topical: 0.5 g per site has been most frequently reported (Weise, 2005). One study of 30 preterm neonates (GA: ≥30 weeks) showed application to the heel for 1 hour resulted in no measurable changes in methemoglobin levels; others have reported similar findings; monitor patients closely with use (Taddio, 1995; Weise, 2005)

GA ≥37 weeks and weighing <5 kg: Topical cream: Apply up to 1 g per site (typically 10 cm^2 area) cover with an occlusive dressing for usual duration of application of 60 minutes prior to procedure; maximum total dose (for all sites combined): 1 g; maximum application area: 10 cm^2; maximum application time: 1 hour

Dosing: Usual Note: Smaller areas of treatment recommended in smaller or debilitated patients or patients with impaired elimination; decreasing the duration of application may decrease analgesic effect, however maximum application duration times should not be exceeded.

Pediatric:

Minor dermal procedures (eg, intravenous access, venipuncture, intramuscular injection); anesthetic: Topical cream: General dosing information provided, dose should be individualized based on procedure and area to be anesthetized.

Infants and Children: Dosing based on patient weight:

<5 kg Topical cream: Apply up to 1 g per 10 cm^2 area cover with an occlusive dressing for usual duration of application of 60 minutes prior to procedure. Maximum dosing information for a 24-hour period: Maximum total dose (for all sites combined): 1 g; maximum application area: 10 cm^2; maximum application time: 1 hour

≥5 kg to ≤10 kg: Topical cream: Apply 1 to 2 g per 10 cm^2 area; cover with occlusive dressing for at least 60 minutes,; maximum dosing information for a 24-hour period: Maximum total dose (for all sites combined): 2 g; maximum application area: 20 cm^2; maximum application time: 4 hours

>10 kg to ≤ 20 kg: Topical cream: Apply 1 to 2 g per 10 cm^2 area; cover with occlusive dressing for at least 60 minutes; maximum dosing information for a 24-hour period: Maximum total dose (for all sites combined): 10 g; maximum application area: 100 cm^2; maximum application time: 4 hours

>20 kg: Topical cream: Apply 1 to 2 g per 10 cm^2 area; cover with occlusive dressing for at least 60 minutes; maximum dosing information for a 24-hour period: Maximum total dose (for all sites combined): 20 g; maximum application area: 200 cm^2; maximum application time: 4 hours

Adolescents: Apply 2.5 g of cream (1/2 of the 5 g tube) over 20 to 25 cm^2 of skin surface area for at least 1 hour

Major dermal procedures (eg, more painful dermatological procedures involving a larger skin area such as split thickness skin graft harvesting); anesthetic: Topical cream: Adolescents: Apply 2 g of cream per 10 cm^2 of skin and allow to remain in contact with the skin for at least 2 hours

Male genital skin (eg, pretreatment prior to local anesthetic infiltration): Apply a thick layer of cream (1 g/10 cm^2) to the skin surface for 15 minutes. Local anesthetic infiltration should be performed immediately after removal of cream.

Female genital mucous membranes: Minor procedures (eg, removal of condylomata acuminata, pretreatment for local anesthetic infiltration): Apply 5 to 10 g (thick layer) of cream for 5 to 10 minutes

Adult:

Anesthetic: Topical cream: Apply a thick layer to intact skin and cover with an occlusive dressing; **Note:** Dermal analgesia can be expected to increase for up to 3 hours under occlusive dressing and persist for 1-2 hours after removal of the cream.

Minor dermal procedures (eg, IV cannulation or venipuncture): Topical cream: Apply 2.5 g of cream (1/2of the 5 g tube) over 20-25 cm^2 of skin surface area for at least 1 hour.

Major dermal procedures (eg, more painful dermatological procedures involving a larger skin area such as split thickness skin graft harvesting): Topical cream: Apply 2 g of cream per 10 cm^2 of skin and allow to remain in contact with the skin for at least 2 hours.

Adult male genital skin (eg, pretreatment prior to local anesthetic infiltration): Apply a thick layer of cream (1 g/10 cm^2) to the skin surface for 15 minutes. Local anesthetic infiltration should be performed immediately after removal of cream.

Adult female genital mucous membranes: Minor procedures (eg, removal of condylomata acuminata, pretreatment for local anesthetic infiltration): Apply 5-10 g (thick layer) of cream for 5-10 minutes

Periodontal gel (Oraqix®): Apply on gingival margin around selected teeth using the blunt-tipped applicator included in package. Wait 30 seconds, then fill the periodontal pockets using the blunt-tipped applicator until gel becomes visible at the gingival margin. Wait another 30 seconds before starting treatment. May reapply if anesthesia starts to wear off; maximum recommended dose per treatment session: 5 cartridges (8.5 g)

Administration Topical:

Cream: For external use only. Avoid application to open wounds or near the eyes. Avoid use in situations where penetration or migration past the tympanic membrane into the middle ear is possible. In small infants and children, observe patient to prevent accidental ingestion of cream or dressing. To obtain 1 g of cream, squeeze narrow strip ~1.5 inches long and 0.2 inches wide from tube. Repeat as necessary to obtain quantity needed for dose (eg, 2 strips = 2 g dose). Apply a thick layer of cream to designated site of intact skin. Cover site with occlusive dressing. Mark the time on the dressing. Allow at least 1 hour (mild dermatologic procedures) or at least 2 hours (major dermal procedures) for optimum therapeutic effect. Remove the dressing and wipe off excess cream (gloves should be worn). Smaller areas of treatment are recommended for small children, debilitated patients, or patients with severe hepatic impairment

Periodontal gel: Oraqix is a viscous liquid: Make sure it is in the liquid form before administration; if semisolid gel forms, refrigerate until becomes liquid again. Do not use dental cartridge warmers; heat will cause product to gel prematurely (product is a microemulsion which is intended to form a gel in the periodental pocket). Apply slowly and evenly on gingival margin around selected teeth. Not to be used with standard dental syringes; use Oraqix Dispenser to apply.

Monitoring Parameters Serum methemoglobin before, during, and after use in neonates and infants up to 3 months of age

Dosage Forms Excipient information presented when available (limited, particularly for generics); consult specific product labeling.

Cream, topical: Lidocaine 2.5% and prilocaine 2.5% (5 g, 30 g)
EMLA: Lidocaine 2.5% and prilocaine 2.5% (5 g, 30 g)
Relador Pak: Lidocaine 2.5% and prilocaine 2.5% (30 g) [packaged with occlusive dressing]
Gel, periodontal:
Oraqix: Lidocaine 2.5% and prilocaine 2.5% (1.7 g)

Lidocaine and Tetracaine

(LYE doe kane & TET ra kane)

Medication Safety Issues

Other safety concerns:

Transdermal patch may contain conducting metal (eg, iron); remove patch prior to MRI.

Brand Names: US Pliaglis; Synera

Therapeutic Category Analgesic, Topical; Local Anesthetic, Topical

Generic Availability (US) Yes: cream

Use Topical anesthetic for use on intact skin to provide local analgesia for superficial venous access, including venipuncture, and for superficial dermatological procedures, including excision, electrodesiccation, and shave biopsy of skin lesions.

Pregnancy Risk Factor B

Pregnancy Considerations Adverse effects have not been observed in animal reproduction studies with this combination. Systemic absorption following topical application is expected to be low. Systemic absorption would be required in order for lidocaine and tetracaine to cross the placenta and reach the fetus. Refer to Lidocaine (Systemic), Lidocaine (Topical), and Tetracaine (Systemic) monographs.

Breast-Feeding Considerations Lidocaine is excreted in breast milk; it is not known if tetracaine is excreted in breast milk. Systemic absorption following topical application is expected to be low; according to the manufacturer, the small amount ingested by a nursing infant would not be expected to cause adverse events. The manufacturer recommends that caution be exercised if administered to nursing women. Refer to Lidocaine (Systemic) Lidocaine (Topical), and Tetracaine (Systemic) monographs.

Contraindications Hypersensitivity to lidocaine, tetracaine, amide or ester-type anesthetic agents, para-aminobenzoic acid (PABA), or any other component of the formulation

Warnings/Precautions Hypersensitivity or anaphylactic reactions may occur. Use with caution in patients who may be sensitive to systemic effects (eg, acutely ill, debilitated, elderly). If being used with other products containing local anesthetic, consider potential for additive effects. Avoid contact with eye; loss of protective reflexes may predispose to corneal irritation and/or abrasion. Application to broken or inflamed skin or mucous membranes may lead to increased systemic absorption. Use caution in patients with severe hepatic disease or pseudocholinesterase deficiency. Not for use at home. Methemoglobinemia has been reported with local anesthetics including tetracaine. Use caution in patients with congenital or idiopathic methemoglobinemia, children <12 months of age, concurrent use with methemoglobin-inducing medications, or in those patients with glucose-6-phosphate dehydrogenase deficiencies.

Application of patch for longer duration than recommended, or simultaneous or sequential application of multiple patches is not recommended because of the risk for increased drug absorption and possible adverse reactions. May contain conducting metal (eg, iron); remove patch prior to MRI. Proper storage and disposal of used patches are essential to prevent accidental exposures, especially in children; accidental exposure may result in serious adverse effects.

Application of cream for longer duration than recommended, or application over larger surface areas is not recommended because of the risk for increased drug absorption and possible adverse reactions.

Adverse Reactions Also see individual agents.

Central nervous system: Dizziness, drowsiness, headache
Dermatologic: Acne vulgaris, application site dermatitis, application site rash, ecchymosis, erythema, local discoloration, localized blanching, maculopapular rash, skin edema, xeroderma
Gastrointestinal: Nausea, vomiting
Hematologic & oncologic: Petechial rash
Rare but important or life-threatening: Anaphylactoid reaction, blepharitis, burning sensation of skin, dehydration, diaphoresis, euphoria, hyperventilation, infection, loss of consciousness, nervousness, pain, paresthesia, pharyngitis, pruritus, stupor, syncope, twitching, urticaria, vesiculobullous dermatitis

Drug Interactions

Metabolism/Transport Effects Refer to individual components.

Avoid Concomitant Use

Avoid concomitant use of Lidocaine and Tetracaine with any of the following: Conivaptan; Fusidic Acid (Systemic); Idelalisib

Increased Effect/Toxicity

Lidocaine and Tetracaine may increase the levels/effects of: Antiarrhythmic Agents (Class III); Prilocaine; Sodium Nitrite; TiZANidine

The levels/effects of Lidocaine and Tetracaine may be increased by: Abiraterone Acetate; Antiarrhythmic Agents (Class III); Aprepitant; Beta-Blockers; Conivaptan; CYP1A2 Inhibitors (Moderate); CYP1A2 Inhibitors (Strong); CYP3A4 Inhibitors (Moderate); CYP3A4 Inhibitors (Strong); Dasatinib; Deferasirox; Disopyramide; Fosaprepitant; Fusidic Acid (Systemic); Idelalisib; Ivacaftor; Luliconazole; Mifepristone; Netupitant; Nitric Oxide; Palbociclib; Peginterferon Alfa-2b; Simeprevir; Stiripentol; Vemurafenib

Decreased Effect There are no known significant interactions involving a decrease in effect.

Storage/Stability

Cream: Store refrigerated at 2°C to 8°C (36°F to 46°F); do not freeze. Stable at room temperature for up to 3 months.
Patch: Store at 25°C (77°F); excursions are permitted between 15°C and 30°C (59°F and 86°F).

Mechanism of Action Local anesthetic action occurs by stabilization of neuronal membranes and inhibiting the sodium ion fluxes required for the initiation and conduction of impulses.

Pharmacodynamics Onset of action: 20 minutes

Pharmacokinetics (Adult data unless noted)

Distribution: Lidocaine crosses the placental and blood-brain barriers; lidocaine is excreted in breast milk
V_d: Lidocaine:
Neonates: 2.75 L/kg
Adults: 1.1 L/kg
Protein binding: Lidocaine: 70%
Metabolism:
Lidocaine: Metabolized in the liver by cytochrome P450 CYP1A2 and partially by CYP3A4 to inactive and active metabolites monoethylglycinexylidide (MEGX) and glycinexylidide (GX)
Tetracaine: Hydrolysis by plasma esterases to primary metabolites para-aminobenzoic acid and diethylaminoethanol
Half-life: Lidocaine: Adults: 1.8 hours
Elimination: Lidocaine: Excreted in urine as metabolites and parent drug

Dosing: Usual Topical: Children ≥3 years and Adults:

Venipuncture or IV cannulation: Apply to intact skin for 20-30 minutes before venous access

Superficial dermatologic procedures: Apply to intact skin for 30 minutes before procedure

Note: Maximum dose: Current patch removed and one additional patch applied at a new location to facilitate venous access is acceptable after a failed attempt. Otherwise, simultaneous or sequential application of multiple patches is **not recommended**.

Administration Topical: Do not use on mucous membranes or the eyes; apply to **intact skin** immediately after opening the pouch. Do **not** cut or remove the top cover of the patch as this could result in **thermal injury**. Do not cover the holes on the top of the patch as this could cause the patch to not heat up. Avoid contact with the eyes due to potential irritation or abrasion. If contact occurs, immediately wash out the eye with water or saline, and protect the eye until sensation returns. Wash hands after handling patch. The adhesive sides of a used patch should be folded together; used patch should be disposed of immediately.

Monitoring Parameters Pain assessment

Additional Information Contains CHADD® self-warming heating element which facilitates drug delivery (when used appropriately, the patch is designed to increase skin temperature by <5°C); patch is latex free. A used patch will still contain large amounts of lidocaine and tetracaine (at least 90% of the initial amount).

Dosage Forms Excipient information presented when available (limited, particularly for generics); consult specific product labeling.

Cream, external:

Pliaglis: Lidocaine 7% and tetracaine 7% (30 g, 100 g) [contains methylparaben, propylparaben]

Generic: Lidocaine 7% and tetracaine 7% (30 g)

Patch, transdermal:

Synera: Lidocaine 70 mg and tetracaine 70 mg (10s) [contains heating component, metal; each patch is ~50 cm^2]

- ◆ **Lidocaine Hydrochloride** *see* Lidocaine (Ophthalmic) *on page* 1257
- ◆ **Lidocaine Hydrochloride** *see* Lidocaine (Systemic) *on page* 1255
- ◆ **Lidocaine Hydrochloride** *see* Lidocaine (Topical) *on page* 1258
- ◆ **Lidocaine Patch** *see* Lidocaine (Topical) *on page* 1258
- ◆ **Lidocin** *see* Lidocaine (Topical) *on page* 1258
- ◆ **Lidodan (Can)** *see* Lidocaine (Topical) *on page* 1258
- ◆ **Lidoderm** *see* Lidocaine (Topical) *on page* 1258
- ◆ **Lidopin** *see* Lidocaine (Topical) *on page* 1258
- ◆ **LidoRx** *see* Lidocaine (Topical) *on page* 1258
- ◆ **Lidovex** *see* Lidocaine (Topical) *on page* 1258
- ◆ **Lidovin** *see* Lidocaine (Topical) *on page* 1258
- ◆ **Lidozol** *see* Lidocaine (Topical) *on page* 1258
- ◆ **LID-Pack® (Can)** *see* Bacitracin and Polymyxin B *on page* 252
- ◆ **Lignocaine Hydrochloride** *see* Lidocaine (Ophthalmic) *on page* 1257
- ◆ **Lignocaine Hydrochloride** *see* Lidocaine (Systemic) *on page* 1255
- ◆ **Lignocaine Hydrochloride** *see* Lidocaine (Topical) *on page* 1258
- ◆ **Lignospan® Forte** *see* Lidocaine and Epinephrine *on page* 1262
- ◆ **Lignospan® Standard** *see* Lidocaine and Epinephrine *on page* 1262

Lindane (LIN dane)

Related Information

Safe Handling of Hazardous Drugs *on page* 2455

Therapeutic Category Antiparasitic Agent, Topical; Pediculocide; Scabicidal Agent; Shampoos

Generic Availability (US) Yes

Use

Lotion: Second-line treatment of scabies (*Sarcoptes scabiei*) in patients intolerant to or who have failed other treatment options [FDA approved in pediatric patients (age not specified) and adults]

Shampoo: Second-line treatment of *Pediculus humanus capitis* (head lice), and *Pthirus pubis* (crab lice) and their ova in patients intolerant to or who have failed other treatment options [FDA approved in pediatric patients (age not specified) and adults]

Medication Guide Available Yes

Pregnancy Risk Factor C

Pregnancy Considerations Adverse events have been observed in animal reproduction studies. Animal studies suggest possible neurologic abnormalities due to the increased susceptibility of drug and the immature central nervous system of the fetus. Lindane is lipophilic and may accumulate in the placenta. Use in pregnant women is contraindicated in some guidelines (CDC, 2010).

Breast-Feeding Considerations Lindane is excreted in breast milk. Nursing mothers should interrupt breast-feeding, express and discard milk for at least 24 hours following use. In addition, skin-to-skin contact between the infant and affected area should be avoided. Use in nursing women is contraindicated in some guidelines (CDC, 2010).

Contraindications Hypersensitivity to lindane or any component of the formulation; premature infants; uncontrolled seizure disorders; crusted (Norwegian) scabies or other skin conditions (eg, atopic dermatitis, psoriasis) which may increase systemic absorption

Warnings/Precautions Hazardous agent - use appropriate precautions for handling and disposal (EPA, U-listed). **[U.S. Boxed Warning]: Not a drug of first choice; use only in patients who have failed or cannot tolerate first-line agents. Instruct patients on proper use, including the amount to apply, how long to leave on, and to avoid re-treatment. Itching may occur as a result of killing lice and does not necessarily indicate treatment failure or need for re-treatment.** Because of the potential for systemic absorption and CNS side effects, lindane should be used with caution; consider permethrin or crotamiton agent first. Oil-based hair dressing may increase toxic potential. For external use only; avoid contact with face, eyes, mucous membranes, and urethral meatus. For treatment only; not to be used to prevent infestation. Should be used as a part of an overall lice management program.

[U.S. Boxed Warning]: May be associated with severe neurologic toxicities. Seizures and death have been reported with use (may occur with prolonged, repeated, or single use). Use is contraindicated in patients with uncontrolled seizure disorders and in premature infants. Use with caution in infants, small children, the elderly, patients with other skin conditions, patients weighing <50 kg, or patients with a history of seizures, head trauma, or HIV infection; use caution with conditions which may increase risk of seizures or medications which decrease seizure threshold.

[U.S. Boxed Warning]: Use is contraindicated in premature infants; the skin of premature infants may be more permeable and their liver enzymes may not be fully developed when compared to full-term infants. Use with caution in patients with hepatic impairment.

Warnings: Additional Pediatric Considerations Risk of neurologic toxicities increased in infants, children, and patients <50 kg compared to the elderly. Use is contraindicated in premature infants and patients with uncontrolled seizure disorders. Premature infants may have increased systemic exposure due to increased permeability of skin, larger skin surface area to volume ratio, and immature hepatic development compared to full-term infants. Use with caution in patients with a history of seizures, head trauma, HIV infection, or with conditions which may increase risk of seizures or medications which decrease seizure threshold. When lotion is used in small infants and young children, cover hands to prevent accidental lindane ingestion from thumbsucking; consider alternative therapy for the treatment of scabies in infants and young children <2 years of age (ie, permethrin). Due to availability of other effective treatments, lindane is no longer recommended for the treatment of scabies or lice in pediatric patients (Frankowski, 2010; *Red Book* [AAP], 2012).

Adverse Reactions

Central nervous system: Ataxia, dizziness, localized burning, neurotoxicity (risk greater in patients <110 lbs [50 kg]), restlessness, seizure, stinging sensation

Dermatologic: Contact dermatitis, eczematous rash

Hematologic & oncologic: Aplastic anemia (CDC, 2010)

Rare but important or life-threatening: Alopecia, dermatitis, headache, pain, paresthesia, pruritus, urticaria

Drug Interactions

Metabolism/Transport Effects None known.

Avoid Concomitant Use There are no known interactions where it is recommended to avoid concomitant use.

Increased Effect/Toxicity There are no known significant interactions involving an increase in effect.

Decreased Effect There are no known significant interactions involving a decrease in effect.

Storage/Stability Store at 20°C to 25°C (68°F to 77°F).

Mechanism of Action Directly absorbed by parasites and ova through the exoskeleton; stimulates the nervous system resulting in seizures and death of parasitic arthropods

Pharmacokinetics (Adult data unless noted)

Absorption: Topical: ~10% systemically; absorption higher when applied to weeping or excoriated skin (Ginsburg, 1977)

Metabolism: Hepatic

Half-life: Infants ≥5 months and Children ≤8 years (Ginsburg, 1977):

Healthy skin: 21.4 hours

Infected skin: 17.9 hours

Time to peak serum concentration: Infants ≥5 months and Children: Topical: 6 hours

Elimination: In urine and feces

Dosing: Usual

Infants, Children, and Adolescents: **Note:** The AAP no longer recommends lindane as a treatment option for head lice or scabies in pediatric patients due to safety concerns (*Red Book*, 2012); use extreme caution in infants, children, and adolescents weighing < 50 kg.

Head lice: Shampoo: Topical: Apply shampoo to dry hair and massage into hair for 4 minutes. Add small amounts of water to form lather, then immediately rinse lather away. Amount of shampoo needed is based on length and density of hair; most patients require ≤30 mL; maximum dose: 60 mL. Do not retreat.

Scabies: Lotion: Topical: Apply a thin layer of lotion and massage it on skin from the neck to the toes. Most patients require ≤30 mL; maximum dose: 60 mL. Do not retreat. Do not leave on for more than 12 hours.

Infants and Children: Wash off 6 hours after application (Pramanik, 1979)

Adults:

Head lice, crab lice: Topical: Apply shampoo to dry hair and massage into hair for 4 minutes; add small quantities of water to hair until lather forms, then rinse hair thoroughly and comb with a fine tooth comb to remove nits. Amount of shampoo needed is based on length and density of hair; most patients will require 30 mL (maximum: 60 mL). Do not retreat.

Scabies: Topical: Apply a thin layer of lotion and massage it on skin from the neck to the toes; after 8-12 hours; bathe and remove the drug; most patients will require 30 mL; larger adults may require up to 60 mL. Do not retreat. Do not leave on for more than 12 hours.

Dosing adjustment in renal impairment: There are no dosage adjustments provided in the manufacturer's labeling.

Dosing adjustment in hepatic impairment: There are no dosage adjustments provided in the manufacturer's labeling.

Administration Shake well prior to use. For topical use only; never administer orally. Caregivers should apply with gloves (avoid natural latex, may be permeable to lindane). Rinse off with warm (not hot) water.

Lotion: Apply to dry, cool skin; do not apply to face or eyes. In infants when treating scabies, medication should be applied head to toe since those areas may also be affected (CDC, 2010; *Red Book*, 2012). Before application, wait at least 1 hour after bathing or showering (wet or warm skin increases absorption). Skin should be clean and free of any other lotions, creams, or oil prior to lindane application. Do not use on open wounds or sores. Do not use occlusive dressings (eg, diaper). Trim nails prior to use and apply under fingernails.

Shampoo: Apply to clean, dry hair. Wait at least 1 hour after washing and drying hair before applying lindane shampoo. Hair should be washed with a shampoo not containing a conditioner; hair and skin of head and neck should be free of any lotions, oils, or creams prior to lindane application. Do not cover with shower cap or towel.

Hazardous agent; use appropriate precautions for handling and disposal (EPA, U-listed).

Additional Information Excessive absorption may result in overdose with signs and symptoms which include nausea, vomiting, seizures, headaches, arrhythmias, apnea, pulmonary edema, hematuria, hepatitis, coma, and even death (Pramanik, 1979; Singal, 2006)

Dosage Forms Excipient information presented when available (limited, particularly for generics); consult specific product labeling.

Lotion, External:

Generic: 1% (60 mL)

Shampoo, External:

Generic: 1% (60 mL)

Linezolid (li NE zoh lid)

Medication Safety Issues

Sound-alike/look-alike issues:

Zyvox may be confused with Zosyn, Zovirax

Brand Names: US Zyvox

Brand Names: Canada Apo-Linezolid; Linezolid Injection; Sandoz-Linezolid; Zyvoxam

Therapeutic Category Antibiotic, Oxazolidinone

Generic Availability (US) May be product dependent

Use Treatment of community-acquired pneumonia, hospital-acquired pneumonia, uncomplicated and complicated skin and soft tissue infections (including diabetic foot infections without concomitant osteomyelitis), and bacteremia caused by susceptible organisms, such as vancomycin-resistant *Enterococcus faecium* (VREF), *Streptococcus pneumoniae* including multidrug resistant strains, *Staphylococcus aureus* including MRSA, *Streptococcus pyogenes*, or *Streptococcus agalactiae* (FDA approved in all ages). **Note:** There have been reports of vancomycin-resistant *E. faecium* and *S. aureus* (methicillin-resistant) developing resistance to linezolid during its clinical use.

Pregnancy Risk Factor C

Pregnancy Considerations Adverse effects were observed in some animal reproduction studies at doses that were also maternally toxic. Information related to linezolid use during pregnancy is limited.

Breast-Feeding Considerations Linezolid is excreted into breast milk. The manufacturer advises caution if administering linezolid to a breast-feeding woman. Non-dose-related effects could include modification of bowel flora.

Contraindications Hypersensitivity to linezolid or any other component of the formulation; concurrent use or within 2 weeks of MAO inhibitors

Warnings/Precautions Myelosuppression has been reported and may be dependent on duration of therapy (generally >2 weeks of treatment); use with caution in patients with pre-existing myelosuppression, in patients receiving other drugs which may cause bone marrow suppression, or in chronic infection (previous or concurrent antibiotic therapy). Weekly CBC monitoring is recommended. Consider discontinuation in patients developing myelosuppression (or in whom myelosuppression worsens during treatment).

Lactic acidosis has been reported with use. Linezolid exhibits mild MAO inhibitor properties and has the potential to have the same interactions as other MAO inhibitors; use with caution and monitor closely in patients with uncontrolled hypertension, pheochromocytoma, carcinoid syndrome, or untreated hyperthyroidism; do not use in the absence of close monitoring. Hypoglycemic episodes have been reported; use with caution and closely monitor glucose in diabetic patients. Dose reductions/discontinuation of concurrent hypoglycemic agents or discontinuation of linezolid may be required. Symptoms of agitation, confusion, hallucinations, hyper-reflexia, myoclonus, shivering, and tachycardia may occur with concomitant proserotonergic drugs (eg, SSRIs/SNRIs, tricyclic antidepressants, triptans, meperidine, bupropion) or agents which reduce linezolid's metabolism; these medications should not be used concurrently unless patient is closely monitored for signs/symptoms of serotonin syndrome or neuroleptic malignant syndrome-like reactions. Patients maintained on proserotonergic drugs requiring urgent treatment with linezolid may receive linezolid if the other proserotonergic drug is discontinued promptly and the benefits of linezolid outweigh risks; monitor for 2 weeks (5 weeks for fluoxetine) after discontinuation of maintenance drug or 24 hours after last linezolid dose, whichever comes first. Unnecessary use may lead to the development of resistance to linezolid; consider alternatives before initiating outpatient treatment.

Peripheral and optic neuropathy (with vision loss) has been reported in adults and children and may occur primarily with extended courses of therapy >28 days; any symptoms of visual change or impairment warrant immediate ophthalmic evaluation and possible discontinuation of therapy. Seizures have been reported; use with caution in patients with a history of seizures. Prolonged use may result in fungal or bacterial superinfection, including *C. difficile*-associated diarrhea (CDAD) and pseudomembranous colitis; CDAD has been observed >2 months post-antibiotic treatment.

Due to inconsistent concentrations in the CSF, empiric use in pediatric patients with CNS infections is not recommended by the manufacturer; however, there are multiple case reports describing successful treatment of documented VRE and *Staphylococcus aureus* CNS and shunt infections in the literature. Linezolid should not be used in the empiric treatment of catheter-related bloodstream infection (CRBSI), but may be appropriate for targeted therapy (Mermel, 2009).

Benzyl alcohol and derivatives: Some dosage forms may contain sodium benzoate/benzoic acid; benzoic acid (benzoate) is a metabolite of benzyl alcohol; large amounts of benzyl alcohol (≥99 mg/kg/day) have been associated with a potentially fatal toxicity ("gasping syndrome") in neonates; the "gasping syndrome" consists of metabolic acidosis, respiratory distress, gasping respirations, CNS dysfunction (including convulsions, intracranial hemorrhage), hypotension, and cardiovascular collapse (AAP, 1997; CDC, 1982); some data suggests that benzoate displaces bilirubin from protein binding sites (Ahlfors, 2001); avoid or use dosage forms containing benzyl alcohol derivative with caution in neonates. See manufacturer's labeling.

Oral suspension contains phenylalanine.

Adverse Reactions

Central nervous system: Dizziness, headache, insomnia, vertigo (children)

Dermatologic: Pruritus (children), skin rash

Endocrine & metabolic: Increased amylase, increased lactate dehydrogenase

Gastrointestinal: Abdominal pain, constipation, diarrhea, dysgeusia, increased serum lipase, loose stools (children), nausea, oral candidiasis, pancreatitis, tongue discoloration, vomiting

Genitourinary: Vulvovaginal candidiasis

Hematologic & oncologic: Anemia, decreased hemoglobin, eosinophilia (children), leukopenia (more common in children), neutropenia (more common in children), thrombocytopenia

Hepatic: Abnormal hepatic function tests, increased serum alkaline phosphatase, increased serum ALT, increased serum AST (adults), increased serum bilirubin (more common in children)

Infection: Fungal infection

Renal: Increased blood urea nitrogen, increased serum creatinine

Miscellaneous: Fever

Rare but important or life-threatening: Anaphylaxis, angioedema, bullous skin disease, *Clostridium difficile*-associated diarrhea, convulsions, hypertension, hypoglycemia, lactic acidosis, optic neuropathy, pancytopenia, peripheral neuropathy, rhabdomyolysis, seizures, serotonin syndrome (with concurrent use of other serotonergic agents), Stevens-Johnson syndrome, vision loss

Drug Interactions

Metabolism/Transport Effects Inhibits Monoamine Oxidase

Avoid Concomitant Use

Avoid concomitant use of Linezolid with any of the following: Alcohol (Ethyl); Anilidopiperidine Opioids; Apraclonidine; AtoMOXetine; Atropine (Ophthalmic); BCG; BCG (Intravesical); Bezafibrate; Buprenorphine; BuPROPion; BusPIRone; CarBAMazepine; CloZAPine; Cyclobenzaprine; Cyproheptadine; Dapoxetine; Dexmethylphenidate; Dextromethorphan; Diethylpropion; Dipyrone; Hydrocodone; HYDROmorphone; Isometheptene; Levonordefrin; MAO Inhibitors; Maprotiline; Meperidine; Mequitazine; Methyldopa; Methylene Blue; Methylphenidate; Mianserin; Mirtazapine; Morphine (Liposomal); Morphine (Systemic); Nefazodone; Oxymorphone; Pholcodine; Pizotifen; Selective Serotonin Reuptake Inhibitors; Serotonin 5-HT1D Receptor Agonists; Serotonin/Norepinephrine Reuptake Inhibitors; Tapentadol; Tetrabenazine; Tetrahydrozoline (Nasal); TraZODone; Tricyclic Antidepressants; Tryptophan

Increased Effect/Toxicity

Linezolid may increase the levels/effects of: Antipsychotic Agents; Apraclonidine; AtoMOXetine; Atropine (Ophthalmic); Betahistine; Bezafibrate; Blood Glucose Lowering Agents; Brimonidine (Ophthalmic); Brimonidine (Topical); BuPROPion; CloZAPine; Cyproheptadine; Dexmethylphenidate; Dextromethorphan; Diethylpropion; Domperidone; Doxylamine; Hydrocodone; HYDROmorphone; Isometheptene; Levonordefrin; Lithium; Meperidine; Mequitazine; Methadone; Methyldopa; Methylene Blue; Methylphenidate; Metoclopramide; Mianserin; Mirtazapine; Morphine (Liposomal); Morphine (Systemic); Nefazodone; OxyCODONE; Pizotifen; Reserpine; Selective Serotonin Reuptake Inhibitors; Serotonin 5-HT1D Receptor Agonists; Serotonin Modulators; Serotonin/Norepinephrine Reuptake Inhibitors; Sympathomimetics; Tetrahydrozoline (Nasal); TraZODone; Tricyclic Antidepressants

The levels/effects of Linezolid may be increased by: Alcohol (Ethyl); Anilidopiperidine Opioids; Antiemetics (5HT3 Antagonists); Antipsychotic Agents; Buprenorphine; BusPIRone; CarBAMazepine; COMT Inhibitors; Cyclobenzaprine; Dapoxetine; Dipyrone; Levodopa; MAO Inhibitors; Maprotiline; Oxymorphone; Pholcodine; Tapentadol; Tetrabenazine; TraMADol; Tryptophan

Decreased Effect

Linezolid may decrease the levels/effects of: BCG; BCG (Intravesical); BCG Vaccine (Immunization); Domperidone; Sodium Picosulfate; Typhoid Vaccine

The levels/effects of Linezolid may be decreased by: Cyproheptadine; Domperidone

Food Interactions Concurrent ingestion of foods rich in tyramine, dopamine, tyrosine, phenylalanine, tryptophan, or caffeine may cause sudden and severe high blood pressure (hypertensive crisis or serotonin syndrome). Beverages containing tyramine (eg, hearty red wine and beer) may increase toxic effects. Management: Avoid tyramine-containing foods (aged or matured cheese, air-dried or cured meats including sausages and salamis; fava or broad bean pods, tap/draft beers, Marmite concentrate, sauerkraut, soy sauce, and other soybean condiments). Food's freshness is also an important concern; improperly stored or spoiled food can create an environment in which tyramine concentrations may increase. Avoid foods containing dopamine, tyrosine, phenylalanine, tryptophan, or caffeine. Avoid beverages containing tyramine.

Storage/Stability

Infusion: Store at 25°C (77°F); excursions permitted to 15°C to 30°C (59°F to 86°F). Protect from light. Keep infusion bags in overwrap until ready for use. Protect infusion bags from freezing.

Oral suspension: Following reconstitution, store at 25°C (77°F); excursions permitted to 15°C to 30°C (59°F to 86°F). Use reconstituted suspension within 21 days. Protect from light.

Tablet: Store at 25°C (77°F); excursions permitted to 15°C to 30°C (59°F to 86°F). Protect from light; protect from moisture.

Mechanism of Action Inhibits bacterial protein synthesis by binding to bacterial 23S ribosomal RNA of the 50S subunit. This prevents the formation of a functional 70S initiation complex that is essential for the bacterial translation process. Linezolid is bacteriostatic against enterococci and staphylococci and bactericidal against most strains of streptococci.

Pharmacokinetics (Adult data unless noted)

Absorption: Well absorbed orally

Distribution: Well-perfused tissues

V_d:

- Preterm neonates <1 week: 0.81 L/kg
- Full-term neonates <1 week: 0.78 L/kg
- Full-term neonates ≥1 week to ≤28 days: 0.66 L/kg
- Infants >28 days to <3 months: 0.79 L/kg
- Infants and Children 3 months to 11 years: 0.69 L/kg
- Adolescents: 0.61 L/kg
- Adults: 0.65 L/kg

Protein binding: 31%

Metabolism: Hepatic via oxidation of the morpholine ring, resulting in two inactive metabolites (aminoethoxyacetic acid, hydroxyethyl glycine); minimally metabolized; may be mediated by cytochrome P450

Bioavailability: 100%

Half-life:

- Preterm neonates <1 week: 5.6 hours
- Full-term neonates <1 week: 3 hours
- Full-term neonates ≥1 week to ≤28 days: 1.5 hours
- Infants >28 days to <3 months: 1.8 hours
- Infants and Children 3 months to 11 years: 2.9 hours
- Adolescents: 4.1 hours
- Adults: 4.9 hours

Time to peak serum concentration: Oral: 1-2 hours

Elimination: Urine (~30% of total dose as parent drug, ~50% of total dose as metabolites); two metabolites of linezolid may accumulate in patients with severe renal impairment; feces (~9% of total dose as metabolites); Nonrenal clearance accounts for ~65% of the total clearance

Clearance:

- Preterm neonates <1 week: 2 mL/minute/kg
- Full-term neonates <1 week: 3.8 mL/minute/kg
- Full-term neonates ≥1 week to ≤28 days: 5.1 mL/minute/kg
- Infants >28 days to <3 months: 5.4 mL/minute/kg
- Infants and Children 3 months to 11 years: 3.8 mL/minute/kg
- Adolescents: 2.1 mL/minute/kg
- Adults: 1.7 mL/minute/kg

Dialysis: 30% removed in a 3-hour hemodialysis session (linezolid dose should be given after hemodialysis)

Dosing: Neonatal

General dosing, susceptible infection (*Red Book* 2012): IV:

- Body weight <1 kg:
  - PNA ≤14 days: 10 mg/kg/dose every 12 hours
  - PNA 15 to 28 days: 10 mg/kg/dose every 8 hours
- Body weight 1 to 2 kg:
  - PNA ≤7 days: 10 mg/kg/dose every 12 hours
  - PNA 8 to 28 days: 10 mg/kg/dose every 8 hours
- Body weight >2 kg: 10 mg/kg/dose every 8 hours

Bacteremia: Oral, IV: **Note:** Treatment should continue for 10 to 28 days depending on the organism

- GA <34 weeks:
  - PNA <7 days: 10 mg/kg/dose every 12 hours
  - PNA ≥7 days: 10 mg/kg/dose every 8 hours
- GA ≥34 weeks and PNA 0 to 28 days: 10 mg/kg/dose every 8 hours

Pneumonia, community- or hospital-acquired: Oral, IV: **Note:** Treatment should continue for 10 to 14 days

- GA <34 weeks:
  - PNA <7 days: 10 mg/kg/dose every 12 hours
  - PNA ≥7 days: 10 mg/kg/dose every 8 hours
- GA ≥34 weeks and PNA 0 to 28 days: 10 mg/kg/dose every 8 hours

Skin and skin structure infections, complicated and uncomplicated: Oral, IV: **Note:** Treatment should continue for 10 to 14 days; reserve IV use for complicated infections only.

- GA <34 weeks:
  - PNA <7 days: 10 mg/kg/dose every 12 hours
  - PNA ≥7 days: 10 mg/kg/dose every 8 hours
- GA ≥34 weeks and PNA 0 to 28 days: 10 mg/kg/dose every 8 hours

Vancomycin-resistant *Enterococcus faecium* (VREF) infection: Oral, IV: **Note:** Treatment should continue for 14 to 28 days.

GA <34 weeks:
PNA <7 days: 10 mg/kg/dose every 12 hours
PNA ≥7 days: 10 mg/kg/dose every 8 hours
GA ≥34 weeks and PNA 0 to 28 days: 10 mg/kg/dose every 8 hours
Note: Case reports describe the use of higher doses up to 12 to 15 mg/kg/dose every 8 hours to treat VRE endocarditis and meningitis/ventriculitis in former premature neonates (n=2; GA: 26, 35 weeks; age at treatment: Term) (Ang 2003; Kumar 2007).

Dosing: Usual

Pediatric:

General dosing, susceptible infection (mild, moderate, or severe) (*Red Book* 2012): Oral, IV:
Infants and Children <12 years: 10 mg/kg/dose every 8 hours, maximum dose: 600 mg
Children ≥12 years and Adolescents: 600 mg every 12 hours

Bacteremia: Oral, IV: **Note:** Treatment should continue for 10 to 28 days depending on the organism.
Infants and Children <12 years: 10 mg/kg/dose every 8 hours; maximum dose: 600 mg
Children ≥12 years and Adolescents: 600 mg every 12 hours

Bone and joint infection (Liu 2011):
Osteomyelitis [*S. aureus* (methicillin-resistant)]: Oral, IV: **Note:** Treatment should continue for a minimum of 4 to 6 weeks.
Infants and Children <12 years: 10 mg/kg/dose every 8 hours; maximum dose: 600 mg
Children ≥12 years and Adolescents: 600 mg every 12 hours
Septic arthritis [*S. aureus* (methicillin-resistant)]: Oral, IV: **Note:**Treatment should continue for a minimum of 3 to 4 weeks.
Infants and Children <12 years: 10 mg/kg/dose every 8 hours; maximum dose: 600 mg
Children ≥12 years and Adolescents: 600 mg every 12 hours

Catheter-related infections, Staphylococcal (methicillin-resistant) or enterococcal (resistant) (confirmed infection): Oral, IV: **Note:** Not recommended use for empiric treatment (Mermel 2009).
Infants and Children <12 years: 10 mg/kg/dose every 8 hours; maximum dose: 600 mg
Children ≥12 years and Adolescents: 10 mg/kg/dose every 12 hours; maximum dose: 600 mg

CNS infection:
Brain abscess, subdural empyema, spinal epidural abscess [*S. aureus* (methicillin-resistant)]: Oral, IV: **Note:** Treatment should continue for 4 to 6 weeks (Liu 2011). **Note:** The manufacturer does not recommend the use of linezolid for empiric treatment of pediatric CNS infections since therapeutic linezolid concentrations are not consistently achieved or maintained in the CSF of patients with ventriculoperitoneal shunts.
Infants and Children <12 years: 10 mg/kg/dose every 8 hours; maximum dose: 600 mg
Children ≥12 years and Adolescents: 600 mg every 12 hours
Meningitis [*S. aureus* (methicillin-resistant)]: Oral, IV: **Note:** Treatment should continue for 2 weeks (Liu 2011; Tunkel 2004).
Infants and Children <12 years: 10 mg/kg/dose every 8 hours; maximum dose: 600 mg
Children ≥12 years and Adolescents: 600 mg every 12 hours

Endocarditis, treatment [*E. faecium* (vancomycin-resistant)]: Oral, IV: **Note:** Treatment should continue for at least 8 weeks (Baddour 2005).
Infants and Children <12 years: 10 mg/kg/dose every 8 hours; maximum dose: 600 mg
Children ≥12 years and Adolescents: 600 mg every 12 hours

Pneumonia
Community- or hospital-acquired (non-MRSA): Oral, IV: **Note:** Treatment should continue for 10 to 14 days.
Infants and Children <12 years: 10 mg/kg/dose every 8 hours; maximum dose: 600 mg
Children ≥12 years and Adolescents: 600 mg every 12 hours
S. aureus (methicillin-resistant): Oral, IV: **Note:** Treatment should continue for 7 to 21 days depending on severity (Liu 2011).
Infants and Children <12 years: 10 mg/kg/dose every 8 hours; maximum dose: 600 mg
Children ≥12 years and Adolescents: 600 mg every 12 hours

Septic thrombosis of cavernous or dural venous sinus [*S. aureus* (methicillin-resistant)]: Oral, IV: **Note:** Treatment should continue for 4 to 6 weeks (Liu 2011).
Infants and Children <12 years: 10 mg/kg/dose every 8 hours; maximum dose: 600 mg
Children ≥12 years and Adolescents: 600 mg every 12 hours

Skin and skin structure infections: Note: Treatment should continue for 10 to 14 days.
Uncomplicated:
Infants and Children <5 years: Oral: 10 mg/kg/dose every 8 hours
Children 5 to 11 years: Oral: 10 mg/kg/dose every 12 hours; maximum dose: 600 mg
Children ≥12 years and Adolescents: Oral: 600 mg every 12 hours
Complicated:
Infants and Children <12 years: Oral, IV: 10 mg/kg/dose every 8 hours; maximum dose: 600 mg
Children ≥12 years and Adolescents: Oral, IV: 600 mg every 12 hours

Tuberculosis, multidrug-resistant: Limited data available: Oral: **Note:** Experience in pediatric patients reflects extrapolation of dosing approach used in adult patients which includes a lower daily dose to decrease risk of adverse effects due to the anticipated long duration of therapy and if toxicity does occur, further dosage reductions (a 25% to 50% dose decrease or increased dosing interval have been used); reported treatment duration dependent upon clinical course; reported range: 13 to 36 months in pediatric patients. All reports describe linezolid as part of a multidrug antimycobacterial regimen; other reported agents within the combination therapy were variable, dependent upon specific organism sensitivities, and generally included 3 to 5 other agents.
Infants ≥4 months and Children: 10 to 12 mg/kg/dose twice daily; maximum dose: 600 mg; dosing based on case reports describing successful treatment in infants and a young child (n=3; ages: 4.5 months, 11 months, and 23 months) (Pinon 2010; Schaaf 2009). Use has also been reported in a 10-year old child, treatment was successfully completed with dosing of 600 mg once daily (Condos 2008).
Adolescents: 600 mg once daily was reported in a retrospective review of 30 patients (n= four adolescents) and a case report (patient age: 14 years) (Dauby 2011; Schecter 2010). In another case series, 600 mg twice daily dosing was used for the initial 2 weeks of therapy and then decreased to once daily dosing; at reduced dosage, patients seemed to have decreased hematologic toxicity while neurotoxicity remained unchanged (Park 2006).

Vancomycin-resistant *Enterococcus faecium* (VREF) infections: Oral, IV: **Note:** Treatment should continue for 14 to 28 days.

Infants and Children <12 years: 10 mg/kg/dose every 8 hours, maximum dose: 600 mg

Children ≥12 years and Adolescents: Oral, IV: 600 mg every 12 hours

Adult:

Usual dosage: Oral, IV: 600 mg every 12 hours

Indication-specific dosing:

MRSA infections (Liu 2011): Oral, IV: 600 mg every 12 hours; duration of therapy dependent upon site of infection and clinical response

Pneumonia, community- or hospital-acquired: Oral, IV: 600 mg every 12 hours for 10 to 14 days. **Note:** In contrast to the manufacturer's recommendations, current guidelines for the treatment of community-acquired, healthcare-, hospital-, and ventilator-associated pneumonia recommend that the duration of therapy be reduced to as short as 7 days (vs 10-14 days) in patients who demonstrate good clinical response (ATS/IDSA 2005; ATS/IDSA 2011).

Skin and skin structure infections

Complicated: Oral, IV: 600 mg every 12 hours for 10 to 14 days. **Note:** For diabetic foot infections, initial treatment duration is up to 4 weeks depending on severity of infection and response to therapy (Lipsky 2012).

Uncomplicated: Oral: 400 mg every 12 hours for 10 to 14 days. **Note:** 400 mg dose is recommended in the product labeling; however, 600 mg dose is commonly employed clinically; consider 5- to 10-day treatment course as opposed to the manufacturer recommended 10 to 14 days (Liu 2011; Stevens 2005). For diabetic foot infections, may extend treatment duration up to 4 weeks if slow to resolve (Lipsky 2012).

VREF infections, including concurrent bacteremia: Oral, IV: 600 mg every 12 hours for 14 to 28 days

Dosage adjustment in renal impairment: No adjustment is recommended. The two primary metabolites may accumulate in patients with renal impairment but the clinical significance is unknown. Weigh the risk of accumulation of metabolites versus the benefit of therapy.

Infants, Children, and Adolescents: The following adjustments have been recommended (Aronoff 2007): **Note:** Renally adjusted dose recommendations are based on doses of 10 mg/kg/dose every 8 hours (for ages <5 years) or every 12 hours (for ages 5 to 11 years).

Intermittent hemodialysis: 10 mg/kg/dose every 12 hours

Peritoneal dialysis (PD): 10 mg/kg/dose every 12 hours

Continuous renal replacement therapy (CRRT): No adjustment necessary

Adults: Intermittent hemodialysis (administer after hemodialysis on dialysis days): Dialyzable (~30% removed during 3-hour dialysis session): If administration time is not immediately after dialysis session, may consider administration of a supplemental dose especially early in the treatment course to maintain levels above the MIC (Brier 2003). Others have recommended no supplemental dose or dosage adjustment for patients on intermittent hemodialysis, peritoneal dialysis, or continuous renal replacement therapy (eg, CVVHD) (Heintz 2009; Trotman 2005).

Dosage adjustment in hepatic impairment:

Mild to moderate impairment (Child Pugh class A or B): No adjustment is recommended.

Severe hepatic impairment (Child Pugh Class C): Use has not been adequately evaluated.

Preparation for Administration Oral suspension: Reconstitute with 123 mL of distilled water (in 2 portions); shake vigorously. Concentration is 100 mg/5 mL. Prior to administration mix gently by inverting bottle; do not shake.

Administration

Oral: Administer with or without food. With reconstituted suspension, gently invert bottle 3-5 times before use. Do not shake.

Parenteral: IV: Check infusion bag for minute leaks and solution for particulate matter prior to administration. Administer without further dilution over 30 to 120 minutes. Do not mix or infuse with other medications. When the same intravenous line is used for sequential infusion of other medications, flush line with D_5W, NS, or LR before and after infusing linezolid. The yellow color of the injection may intensify over time without affecting potency.

Monitoring Parameters CBC (weekly), particularly in patients at increased risk for bleeding, patients with preexisting thrombocytopenia or myelosuppression, patients with chronic infection who have received or who are on concomitant antibiotics, or concomitant medications that decrease platelet count or function or produce bone marrow suppression, and inpatients requiring >2 weeks of therapy; number and type of stools/day for diarrhea; visual function in patients requiring ≥3 months of therapy or in patients reporting new visual symptoms

Dosage Forms Excipient information presented when available (limited, particularly for generics); consult specific product labeling.

Solution, Intravenous:

Zyvox: 2 mg/mL (100 mL, 300 mL)

Generic: 2 mg/mL (300 mL)

Suspension Reconstituted, Oral:

Zyvox: 100 mg/5 mL (150 mL) [orange flavor]

Tablet, Oral:

Zyvox: 600 mg

Generic: 600 mg

◆ **Linezolid Injection (Can)** *see* Linezolid *on page* 1268

◆ **Lioresal** *see* Baclofen *on page* 254

◆ **Lioresal D.S. (Can)** *see* Baclofen *on page* 254

◆ **Lioresal Intrathecal (Can)** *see* Baclofen *on page* 254

Liothyronine (lye oh THYE roe neen)

Medication Safety Issues

Sound-alike/look-alike issues:

Liothyronine may be confused with levothyroxine

Other safety concerns:

T3 is an error-prone abbreviation (mistaken as acetaminophen and codeine [ie, Tylenol® #3])

Brand Names: US Cytomel; Triostat

Brand Names: Canada Cytomel

Therapeutic Category Thyroid Product

Generic Availability (US) Yes

Use Replacement or supplemental therapy in congenital or acquired hypothyroidism, treatment or prevention of euthyroid goiters including thyroid nodules and chronic lymphocytic thyroiditis; as a diagnostic aid in suppression tests to differentiate suspected mild hyperthyroidism or thyroid gland autonomy

Pregnancy Risk Factor A

Pregnancy Considerations Endogenous thyroid hormones minimally cross the placenta; the fetal thyroid becomes active around the end of the first trimester. Liothyronine has not been found to increase the risk of teratogenic or adverse effects following maternal use during pregnancy.

Uncontrolled maternal hypothyroidism may result in adverse neonatal and maternal outcomes. To prevent adverse events, normal maternal thyroid function should be maintained prior to conception and throughout pregnancy. Levothyroxine is considered the treatment of choice for the control of hypothyroidism during pregnancy.

Breast-Feeding Considerations Endogenous thyroid hormones are minimally found in breast milk.

Contraindications Hypersensitivity to liothyronine sodium or any component of the formulation; undocumented or uncorrected adrenal insufficiency; recent myocardial infarction or thyrotoxicosis; artificial rewarming (injection)

Warnings/Precautions [US Boxed Warning]: Ineffective and potentially toxic for weight reduction. High doses may produce serious or even life-threatening toxic effects particularly when used with some anorectic drugs. Use with extreme caution in patients with angina pectoris or other cardiovascular disease (including hypertension) or coronary artery disease. Use with caution in elderly patients since they may be more likely to have compromised cardiovascular function. Increase dose slowly in the elderly and monitor for signs/symptoms of angina (ATA/AACE [Garber 2012]). Patients with adrenal insufficiency, myxedema, diabetes mellitus and insipidus may have symptoms exaggerated or aggravated. Treatment with glucocorticoids should precede thyroid replacement therapy in patients with adrenal insufficiency (ATA/AACE [Garber 2012]). Thyroid replacement requires periodic assessment of thyroid status. Chronic hypothyroidism predisposes patients to coronary artery disease.

Warnings: Additional Pediatric Considerations May cause transient alopecia in children during first few months of therapy.

Adverse Reactions

Cardiovascular: Arrhythmia, cardiopulmonary arrest, hypotension, MI, tachycardia

Rare but important or life-threatening: Allergic skin reactions, angina, CHF, fever, hypertension, phlebitis, twitching

Drug Interactions

Metabolism/Transport Effects None known.

Avoid Concomitant Use

Avoid concomitant use of Liothyronine with any of the following: Sodium Iodide I131

Increased Effect/Toxicity

Liothyronine may increase the levels/effects of: Tricyclic Antidepressants; Vitamin K Antagonists

The levels/effects of Liothyronine may be increased by: Piracetam

Decreased Effect

Liothyronine may decrease the levels/effects of: Sodium Iodide I131; Theophylline Derivatives

The levels/effects of Liothyronine may be decreased by: Bile Acid Sequestrants; Calcium Polystyrene Sulfonate; Calcium Salts; CarBAMazepine; Ciprofloxacin (Systemic); Estrogen Derivatives; Fosphenytoin; Lanthanum; Phenytoin; Rifampin; Selective Serotonin Reuptake Inhibitors; Sodium Polystyrene Sulfonate

Storage/Stability Vials must be stored under refrigeration at 2°C to 8°C (36°F to 46°F). Store tablets at 15°C to 30°C (59°F to 86°F).

Mechanism of Action Exact mechanism of action is unknown; however, it is believed the thyroid hormone exerts its many metabolic effects through control of DNA transcription and protein synthesis; involved in normal metabolism, growth, and development; promotes gluconeogenesis, increases utilization and mobilization of glycogen stores, and stimulates protein synthesis, increases basal metabolic rate

Pharmacodynamics IV, Oral:

Onset of action: Within a few hours

Maximum effect: Within 48 hours

Duration: Up to 72 hours

Pharmacokinetics (Adult data unless noted)

Absorption: Oral: Well absorbed (~85% to 90%)

Metabolism: In the liver to inactive compounds

Half-life: 0.75 hours (Brent, 2011)

Elimination: 76% to 83% In urine

Dosing: Neonatal

Congenital hypothyroidism: Oral: 5 mcg/day; increase by 5 mcg every 3 days to a maximum dosage of 20 mcg/day; **Note:** AAP recommends levothyroxine over liothyronine for treatment of hypothyroidism in neonates (AAP 2006)

Postcardiac surgery replacement: Very limited data available: Continuous IV infusion: 0.05 to 0.15 mcg/kg/**hour** adjusted to maintain a serum T_3 concentration 80 to 200 ng/dL; dosing based on experience in five neonates who, on postoperative days 0 to 2, required mechanical ventilation and exhibited total serum T_3 <60 ng/dL (Chowdhury 2001; Dimmick 2008)

Dosing: Usual

Congenital hypothyroidism: Infants and Children <3 years: Oral: 5 mcg/day; increase by 5 mcg every 3 days to a maximum dosage of 20 mcg/day for infants, 50 mcg/day for children 1 to 3 years of age

Hypothyroidism:

Children: Oral: 5 mcg/day increase in 5 mcg/day increments every 3 to 4 days

Usual maintenance dose:

Infants: 20 mcg/day

Children 1 to 3 years: 50 mcg/day

Children >3 years: Full adult dosage may be necessary

Adults: Oral: 25 mcg/day increase in 12.5 to 25 mcg/day increments every 1 to 2 weeks to a maximum of 100 mcg/day

Goiter, nontoxic:

Children: Oral: 5 mcg/day increase in 5 mcg/day increments every 1 to 2 weeks; usual maintenance dose 15 to 20 mcg/day

Adults: Oral: 5 mcg/day; increase in 5 to 10 mcg/day increments every 1 to 2 weeks; when 25 mcg is reached, increase dosage in 12.5 to 25 mcg increments every 1 to 2 weeks; usual maintenance dosage: 75 mcg/day

T_3 suppression test: Adults: Oral: 75 to 100 mcg/day for 7 days

Myxedema coma: Adults:

IV: 25 to 50 mcg; reduce dosage in patients with known or suspected cardiovascular disease to 10 to 20 mcg

Note: Normally, at least 4 hours should be allowed between IV doses to adequately assess therapeutic response and no more than 12 hours should elapse between doses to avoid fluctuations in hormone levels.

Oral (**Note:** Due to potential poor oral absorption in the acute phase of myxedema, oral therapy should be avoided until the clinical situation has been stabilized): 5 mcg/day; increase in 5 to 10 mcg/day increments every 1 to 2 weeks; when 25 mcg/day is reached; increase by 5 to 25 mcg/day increments every 1 to 2 weeks; usual maintenance dose: 50 to 100 mcg/day

Administration

Oral: Administer on an empty stomach

Parenteral: Adults: IV: For IV use only; **do not administer SubQ or IM** Administer at a rate of 10 mcg/minute. Administer doses at least 4 hours, and no more than 12 hours, apart. Resume oral therapy as soon as the clinical situation has been stabilized and the patient is able to take oral medication. If **levothyroxine** is used for oral therapy, there is a delay of several days in the onset of activity; therefore, discontinue IV therapy gradually.

Monitoring Parameters T_3, TSH, heart rate, blood pressure, clinical signs of hypo- and hyperthyroidism; TSH is the most reliable guide for evaluating adequacy of thyroid replacement dosage. TSH may be elevated during the first few months of thyroid replacement despite patients being clinically euthyroid.

Suggested frequency for monitoring thyroid function tests in children: Every 1-2 months during the first year of life, every 2-3 months between ages 1-3 years, and every 3-12 months thereafter until growth is completed; repeat tests two weeks after any change in dosage.

Reference Range

Thyroid Function Tests

Lab Parameters	Age	Normal Range
T_4 (thyroxine) serum concentration	1-7 days	10.1-20.9 mcg/dL
	8-14 days	9.8-16.6 mcg/dL
	1 month to 1 year	5.5-16.0 mcg/dL
	>1 year	4.0-12.0 mcg/dL
Free thyroxine index (FTI)	1-3 days	9.3-26.6
	1-4 weeks	7.6-20.8
	1-4 months	7.4-17.9
	4-12 months	5.1-14.5
	1-6 years	5.7-13.3
	>6 years	4.8-14.0
T_3 serum concentration	Newborns	100-470 ng/dL
	1-5 years	100-260 ng/dL
	5-10 years	90-240 ng/dL
	10 years to Adult	70-210 ng/dL
T_3 uptake		35%-45%
TSH serum concentration	Cord	3-22 micro international units/mL
	1-3 days	<40 micro international units/mL
	3-7 days	<25 micro international units/mL
	>7 days	0-10 micro international units/mL

Test Interactions

T_4-binding globulin (TBG): Factors that alter binding in serum (ATA/AACE [Garber 2012]):

Note: T_4 is ~99.97% protein bound. Factors that alter protein binding will affect serum total T_4 levels; however, measurement of serum free T4 (the metabolically active moiety) has largely replaced serum total T_4 for thyroid status assessment.

Conditions/states that increase TBG binding: Pregnancy, hepatitis, porphyria, neonatal state

Medications that increase TBG binding: Estrogens, 5-fluorouracil, heroin, methadone, mitotane, perphenazine, selective estrogen receptor modulators (eg, tamoxifen, raloxifene)

Conditions/states that decrease TBG binding: Hepatic failure, nephrosis, severe illness

Medications that decrease TBG binding: Androgens, anabolic steroids, glucocorticoids, L-asparaginase, nicotinic acid

Thyroxine (T_4) and Triiodothyronine (T_3): Serum binding inhibitors (ATA/AACE [Garber 2012]):

Medications that inhibit T_4 and T_3 binding: Carbamazepine, furosemide, free fatty acids, heparin, NSAIDS (variable, transient), phenytoin, salicylates

Thyroid gland hormone: Interference with production and secretion (ATA/AACE [Garber 2012]):

Medications affecting iodine uptake: Amiodarone, iodinated contrast agents, iodine, ethionamide

Medications affecting hormone production: Amiodarone, ethionamide, iodinated contrast agents, iodine, sulfonylureas, sulfonamides, thionamides (carbimazole, methimazole, propylthiouracil)

Medications affecting secretion: Amiodarone, iodinated contrast agents, iodine, lithium

Medications inducing thyroiditis: Alemtuzumab, amiodarone, antiangiogenic agents (lenalidomide, thalidomide), denileukin diftitoxin, interferon alpha, interleukins, lithium, tyrosine kinase inhibitors (sunitinib, sorafenib)

Medications potentially causing the development of Graves': Alemtuzumab, interferon alpha, highly active antiretroviral therapy

Medications potentially ameliorating thyroiditis (if autoimmune) or Graves': Glucocorticoids

Hypothalamic-pituitary axis and TSH: Interference with secretion (ATA/AACE [Garber 2012]):

Medications decreasing TSH secretion: Bexarotene, dopamine, dopaminergic agonists (bromocriptine, cabergoline), glucocorticoids, interleukin-6, metformin, opiates, somatostatin analogues (octreotide, lanreotide), thyroid hormone analogues

Mediations increasing TSH secretion: Amphetamine, interleukin 2, metoclopramide, ritonavir, St John's wort

Medications potentially causing hypophysitis: Ipilimumab

Additional Information Equivalent doses: The following statement on relative potency of thyroid products is included in a joint statement by American Thyroid Association (ATA), American Association of Clinical Endocrinologists (AACE) and The Endocrine Society (TES): For purposes of conversion, levothyroxine sodium (T_4) 100 mcg is usually considered equivalent to desiccated thyroid 60 mg, thyroglobulin 60 mg, or liothyronine sodium (T_3) 25 mcg. However, these are rough guidelines only and do not obviate the careful re-evaluation of a patient when switching thyroid hormone preparations, including a change from one brand of levothyroxine to another. Joint position statement is available at http://www.thyroid.org/professionals/advocacy/04_12_08_thyroxine.html.

A synthetic form of *L*-Triiodothyronine (T_3) can be used in patients allergic to products derived from pork or beef.

Note: Several medications have effects on thyroid production or conversion. The impact in thyroid replacement has not been specifically evaluated, but patient response should be monitored:

Methimazole: Decreases thyroid hormone secretion, while propylthiouracil decrease thyroid hormone secretion and decreases conversion of T_4 to T_3.

Beta-adrenergic antagonists: Decrease conversion of T_4 to T_3 (dose related, propranolol ≥160 mg/day); patients may be clinically euthyroid.

Iodide, iodine-containing radiographic contrast agents may decrease thyroid hormone secretion; may also increase thyroid hormone secretion, especially in patients with Graves' disease.

Other agents reported to impact on thyroid production/conversion include aminoglutethimide, amiodarone, chloral hydrate, diazepam, ethionamide, interferon-alpha, interleukin-2, lithium, lovastatin (case report), glucocorticoids (dose-related), mercaptopurine, sulfonamides, thiazide diuretics, and tolbutamide.

In addition, a number of medications have been noted to cause transient depression in TSH secretion, which may complicate interpretation of monitoring tests for thyroid hormones, including corticosteroids, octreotide, and dopamine. Metoclopramide may increase TSH secretion.

Dosage Forms Excipient information presented when available (limited, particularly for generics); consult specific product labeling.

Solution, Intravenous:

Triostat: 10 mcg/mL (1 mL) [contains alcohol, usp]

Generic: 10 mcg/mL (1 mL)

Tablet, Oral:

Cytomel: 5 mcg

Cytomel: 25 mcg, 50 mcg [scored]

Generic: 5 mcg, 25 mcg, 50 mcg

◆ **Liothyronine and Levothyroxine** *see* Liotrix *on page 1276*

◆ **Liothyronine Sodium** *see* Liothyronine *on page 1272*

Liotrix (LYE oh triks)

Medication Safety Issues

Sound-alike/look-alike issues:

Liotrix may be confused with Klotrix

Thyrolar may be confused with Thyrogen

Brand Names: US Thyrolar

Brand Names: Canada Thyrolar

Therapeutic Category Thyroid Product

Generic Availability (US) No

Use Replacement or supplemental therapy in hypothyroidism of any etiology (FDA approved in all ages); pituitary TSH suppressant for the prevention or treatment of various types of euthyroid goiter, thyroid nodules, thyroiditis (Hashimoto's), multinodular goiter, and thyroid cancer (FDA approved in adults); diagnostic agent in suppression tests to diagnose suspected mild hyperthyroidism or to demonstrate thyroid gland autonomy (FDA approved in adults); **Note:** Not indicated for treatment of transient hypothyroidism associated with subacute thyroiditis

Pregnancy Risk Factor A

Pregnancy Considerations Endogenous thyroid hormones minimally cross the placenta; the fetal thyroid becomes active around the end of the first trimester. Liotrix has not been found to increase the risk of adverse effects following maternal use during pregnancy.

Uncontrolled maternal hypothyroidism may result in adverse neonatal and maternal outcomes. To prevent adverse events, normal maternal thyroid function should be maintained prior to conception and throughout pregnancy. Levothyroxine is considered the treatment of choice for the control of hypothyroidism during pregnancy.

Breast-Feeding Considerations Endogenous thyroid hormones are minimally found in breast milk and are not associated with adverse events.

Contraindications Hypersensitivity to liotrix or any component of the formulation; uncorrected adrenal insufficiency; untreated thyrotoxicosis

Warnings/Precautions [US Boxed Warning]: In euthyroid patients, thyroid supplements are ineffective and potentially toxic for weight reduction (unapproved use); high doses may produce serious or even life-threatening toxic effects, particularly when used with some anorectic drugs. Use is not justified for the treatment of male or female infertility in euthyroid patients (unapproved use). Use with caution and reduce dosage in the elderly since they may be more likely to have compromised cardiovascular function and in patients with angina pectoris or other cardiovascular disease (chronic hypothyroidism predisposes patients to coronary artery disease). Suppressed TSH levels in the elderly may increase risk of atrial fibrillation and mortality secondary to cardiovascular disease (Gharib 2010; Parle 2001). Increase dose slowly in the elderly and monitor for signs/symptoms of angina (ATA/AACE [Garber 2012]). Use with caution in patients with adrenal insufficiency, diabetes mellitus or insipidus, and myxedema; symptoms may be exaggerated or aggravated; initial dosage reduction is recommended in patients with long-standing myxedema. Treatment with glucocorticoids should precede thyroid replacement therapy in patients with adrenal insufficiency (ATA/AACE [Garber 2012]).

Warnings: Additional Pediatric Considerations Overtreatment may result in craniosynostosis in infants and premature closure of epiphyses in children; monitor use closely. May cause transient alopecia in children during first few months of therapy. In neonates and infants, cardiac overload, arrhythmias, and aspiration from avid suckling may occur during initiation of therapy (eg, first 2 weeks); monitor closely.

Adverse Reactions

Cardiovascular: Blood pressure increased, cardiac arrhythmia, chest pain, palpitation, tachycardia

Central nervous system: Anxiety, ataxia, fever, headache insomnia, nervousness

Dermatologic: Alopecia, hyperhydrosis, pruritus, urticaria

Endocrine & metabolic: Changes in menstrual cycle increased appetite, weight loss

Gastrointestinal: Abdominal cramps, constipation, diarrhea, nausea, vomiting

Neuromuscular & skeletal: Hand tremor, myalgia, tremor

Respiratory: Dyspnea

Miscellaneous: Allergic skin reactions (rare), diaphoresis

Drug Interactions

Metabolism/Transport Effects None known.

Avoid Concomitant Use

Avoid concomitant use of Liotrix with any of the following: Sodium Iodide I131

Increased Effect/Toxicity

Liotrix may increase the levels/effects of: Tricyclic Antidepressants; Vitamin K Antagonists

The levels/effects of Liotrix may be increased by: Piracetam

Decreased Effect

Liotrix may decrease the levels/effects of: Sodium Iodide I131; Theophylline Derivatives

The levels/effects of Liotrix may be decreased by: Bile Acid Sequestrants; Calcium Polystyrene Sulfonate; Calcium Salts; CarBAMazepine; Ciprofloxacin (Systemic); Estrogen Derivatives; Fosphenytoin; Lanthanum; Phenytoin; Rifampin; Selective Serotonin Reuptake Inhibitors; Sodium Polystyrene Sulfonate

Storage/Stability Store at 2°C to 8°C (36°F to 46°F). Protect from light.

Mechanism of Action The primary active compound is T_3 (triiodothyronine), which may be converted from T_4 (thyroxine) and then circulates throughout the body to influence growth and maturation of various tissues. Liotrix is uniform mixture of synthetic T_4 and T_3 in 4:1 ratio; exact mechanism of action is unknown; however, it is believed the thyroid hormone exerts its many metabolic effects through control of DNA transcription and protein synthesis; involved in normal metabolism, growth, and development; promotes gluconeogenesis, increases utilization and mobilization of glycogen stores and stimulates protein synthesis, increases basal metabolic rate

Pharmacodynamics Onset of action: T_3: ~3 hours

Pharmacokinetics (Adult data unless noted)

Absorption: T_4: 40% to 80%; T_3: 95%

Protein binding: T_4: >99% bound to plasma proteins including thyroxine-binding globulin, thyroxine-binding prealbumin, and albumin

Metabolism: Hepatic to triiodothyronine (active); ~80% T_4 deiodinated in kidney and periphery; glucuronidation/conjugation also occurs; undergoes enterohepatic recirculation

Half-life elimination:

T_4: Euthyroid: 6-7 days; Hyperthyroid: 3-4 days; Hypothyroid: 9-10 days

T_3: 2.5 days

Time to peak serum concentration: T_4: 2-4 hours; T_3: 2-3 days

Elimination: Urine (major route of elimination); partially feces

Dosing: Neonatal Note: Doses should be adjusted based on clinical response and laboratory parameters

Congenital hypothyroidism: Note: AAP recommends levothyroxine as the preferred treatment for hypothyroidism in neonates (AAP, 2006). Neonates should have therapy initiated at full doses. Oral: Usual daily dosage range: Liothyronine (T_3): 3.1-6.25 mcg; levothyroxine (T_4): 12.5-25 mcg once daily

Dosing: Usual Note: Doses should be adjusted based on clinical response and laboratory parameters

Infants, Children, and Adolescents:

Congenital hypothyroidism: Note: Infants should have therapy initiated at full doses. Oral: Usual daily dosage range:

Infants 1-6 months: Liothyronine (T_3): 3.1-6.25 mcg/Levothyroxine (T_4): 12.5-25 mcg once daily

Infants >6-12 months: Liothyronine (T_3): 6.25-9.35 mcg/Levothyroxine (T_4): 25-37.5 mcg once daily

Children 1-5 years: Liothyronine (T_3): 9.35-12.5 mcg/Levothyroxine (T_4): 37.5-50 mcg once daily

Children 6-12 years: Liothyronine (T_3): 12.5-18.75 mcg/Levothyroxine (T_4): 50-75 mcg once daily

Adolescents: Typical doses > Liothyronine (T_3): 18.75 mcg; levothyroxine (T_4): 75 mcg once daily

Adults:

Hypothyroidism: Oral: Initial: Liothyronine (T_3) 6.25 mcg/Levothyroxine (T_4) 25 mcg once daily; may increase by liothyronine 3.1 mcg/Levothyroxine 12.5 mcg every 2-3 weeks. A lower initial dose (liothyronine 3.1 mcg/Levothyroxine 12.5 mcg) is recommended in patients with long-standing myxedema, especially if cardiovascular impairment coexists. If angina occurs, reduce dose (usual maintenance dose: Liothyronine 12.5-25 mcg/Levothyroxine 50-100 mcg)

Monitoring Parameters T_4, TSH, heart rate, blood pressure, clinical signs of hypo- and hyperthyroidism; TSH is the most reliable guide for evaluating adequacy of thyroid replacement dosage. TSH may be elevated during the first few months of thyroid replacement despite patients being clinically euthyroid. In cases where T_4 remains low and TSH is within normal limits, an evaluation of "free" (unbound) T_4 is needed to evaluate further increase in dosage.

In congenital hypothyroidism, adequacy of replacement should be determined using both TSH and total- or free-T_4. During the first 3 years of life, total- or free-T_4 should be maintained in the upper 1/2 of the normal range; this should result in normalization of TSH. In some patients, TSH may not normalize due to a resetting of the pituitary-thyroid feedback as a result of *in utero* hypothyroidism. Monitor closely for cardiac overload, arrhythmias, and aspiration from avid suckling.

Pediatric patients: Monitor closely for under/overtreatment. Undertreatment may decrease intellectual development and linear growth, and lead to poor school performance due to impaired concentration and slowed mentation. Overtreatment may adversely affect brain maturation, accelerate bone age (leading to premature closure of the epiphyses and reduced adult height); craniosynostosis has been reported in infants. Perform routine clinical examinations at regular intervals (to assess mental and physical growth and development). Suggested frequency for monitoring thyroid function tests: Every 1-2 months during the first year of life, every 2-3 months between ages 1-3 years, and every 3-12 months thereafter until growth is completed; repeat tests 2 weeks after any change in dosage.

Reference Range

Thyroid Function Tests

Lab Parameters	Age	Normal Range
T_4 (thyroxine) serum concentration	1-7 days	10.1-20.9 mcg/dL
	8-14 days	9.8-16.6 mcg/dL
	1 month to 1 year	5.5-16.0 mcg/dL
	>1 year	4.0-12.0 mcg/dL
Free thyroxine index (FTI)	1-3 days	9.3-26.6
	1-4 weeks	7.6-20.8
	1-4 months	7.4-17.9
	4-12 months	5.1-14.5
	1-6 years	5.7-13.3
	>6 years	4.8-14.0
T_3 serum concentration	Newborns	100-470 ng/dL
	1-5 years	100-260 ng/dL
	5-10 years	90-240 ng/dL
	10 years to Adult	70-210 ng/dL
T_3 uptake		35%-45%
TSH serum concentration	Cord	3-22 micro international units/mL
	1-3 days	<40 micro international units/mL
	3-7 days	<25 micro international units/mL
	>7 days	0-10 micro international units/mL

Test Interactions

T_4-binding globulin (TBG): factors that alter binding in serum (ATA/AACE [Garber 2012]):

Note: T_4 is ~99.97% protein bound. Factors that alter protein binding will affect serum total T_4 levels; however, measurement of serum free T_4 (the metabolically active moiety) has largely replaced serum total T_4 for thyroid status assessment.

Conditions/states that increase TBG binding: Pregnancy, hepatitis, porphyria, neonatal state

Medications that increase TBG binding: Estrogens, 5-fluorouracil, heroin, methadone, mitotane, perphenazine, selective estrogen receptor modulators (eg, tamoxifen, raloxifene)

Conditions/states that decrease TBG binding: Hepatic failure, nephrosis, severe illness

Medications that decrease TBG binding: Androgens, anabolic steroids, glucocorticoids, L-asparaginase, nicotinic acid

Thyroxine (T_4) and Triiodothyronine (T_3): Serum binding inhibitors (ATA/AACE [Garber 2012]):

Medications that inhibit T_4 and T_3 binding: Carbamazepine, furosemide, free fatty acids, heparin, NSAIDS (variable, transient), phenytoin, salicylates

Thyroid gland hormone: Interference with production and secretion (ATA/AACE [Garber 2012]):

Medications affecting iodine uptake: Amiodarone, iodinated contrast agents, iodine, ethionamide

Medications affecting hormone production: Amiodarone, ethionamide, iodinated contrast agents, iodine, sulfonylureas, sulfonamides, thionamides (carbimazole, methimazole, propylthiouracil)

Medications affecting secretion: Amiodarone, iodinated contrast agents, iodine, lithium

Medications inducing thyroiditis: Alemtuzumab, amiodarone, antiangiogenic agents (lenalidomide, thalidomide), denileukin diftitoxin, interferon alpha, interleukins, lithium, tyrosine kinase inhibitors (sunitinib, sorafenib)

Medications potentially causing the development of Graves': Alemtuzumab, interferon alpha, highly active antiretroviral therapy

Medications potentially ameliorating thyroiditis (if autoimmune) or Graves': Glucocorticoids

Hypothalamic-pituitary axis and TSH: Interference with secretion (ATA/AACE [Garber 2012]):

Medications decreasing TSH secretion: Bexarotene, dopamine, dopaminergic agonists (bromocriptine, cabergoline), glucocorticoids, interleukin-6, metformin, opiates, somatostatin analogues (octreotide, lanreotide), thyroid hormone analogues

Mediations increasing TSH secretion: Amphetamine, interleukin 2, metoclopramide, ritonavir, St John's wort

Medications potentially causing hypophysitis: Ipilimumab

Additional Information Equivalent doses: The following statement on relative potency of thyroid products is included in a joint statement by American Thyroid Association (ATA), American Association of Clinical Endocrinologists (AACE) and The Endocrine Society (TES): For purposes of conversion, levothyroxine sodium (T_4) 100 mcg is usually considered equivalent to desiccated thyroid 60 mg, thyroglobulin 60 mg, or liothyronine sodium (T_3) 25 mcg. However, these are rough guidelines only and do not obviate the careful re-evaluation of a patient when switching thyroid hormone preparations, including a change from one brand of levothyroxine to another. Joint position statement is available at http://www.thyroid.org/professionals/advocacy/04_12_08_thyroxine.html.

Dosage Forms Excipient information presented when available (limited, particularly for generics); consult specific product labeling.

Tablet, oral:

Thyrolar: 1/4 [levothyroxine sodium 12.5 mcg and liothyronine sodium 3.1 mcg]

Thyrolar: 1/2 [levothyroxine sodium 25 mcg and liothyronine sodium 6.25 mcg]

Thyrolar: 1 [levothyroxine sodium 50 mcg and liothyronine sodium 12.5 mcg]

Thyrolar: 2 [levothyroxine sodium 100 mcg and liothyronine sodium 25 mcg]

Thyrolar: 3 [levothyroxine sodium 150 mcg and liothyronine sodium 37.5 mcg]

- **Lipancreatin** *see* Pancrelipase *on page 1614*
- **Lipase, Protease, and Amylase** *see* Pancrelipase *on page 1614*
- **Lipitor** *see* AtorvaSTATin *on page 220*
- **Liposomal Amphotericin** *see* Amphotericin B (Liposomal) *on page 153*
- **Liposomal Amphotericin B** *see* Amphotericin B (Liposomal) *on page 153*
- **Liposyn III** *see* Fat Emulsion (Plant Based) *on page 850*
- **Liquibid [OTC]** *see* GuaiFENesin *on page 988*
- **Liquid Antidote** *see* Charcoal, Activated *on page 425*
- **Liquid Paraffin** *see* Mineral Oil *on page 1439*
- **Liquigen [OTC]** *see* Medium Chain Triglycerides *on page 1338*
- **Liquituss GG [OTC]** *see* GuaiFENesin *on page 988*

Lisdexamfetamine (lis dex am FET a meen)

Medication Safety Issues

Sound-alike/look-alike issues:

Vyvanse may be confused with Glucovance, Visanne, ViVAXIM, Vytorin, Vivactil

Brand Names: US Vyvanse

Brand Names: Canada Vyvanse

Therapeutic Category Amphetamine; Central Nervous System Stimulant

Generic Availability (US) No

Use Treatment of attention-deficit/hyperactivity disorder (ADHD) (FDA approved in ages ≥6 years and adults)

Medication Guide Available Yes

Pregnancy Risk Factor C

Pregnancy Considerations Adverse effects have not been observed in animal reproduction studies. Lisdexamfetamine is converted to dextroamphetamine. The majority of human data is based on illicit amphetamine/methamphetamine exposure and not from therapeutic maternal use (Golub, 2005). Use of amphetamines during pregnancy may lead to an increased risk of premature birth and low birth weight; newborns may experience symptoms of withdrawal. Behavioral problems may also occur later in childhood (LaGasse, 2012).

Breast-Feeding Considerations The majority of human data is based on illicit amphetamine/methamphetamine exposure and not from therapeutic maternal use (Golub, 2005). Amphetamines are excreted into breast milk and use may decrease milk production. Increased irritability, agitation, and crying have been reported in nursing infants (ACOG, 2011). According to the manufacturer, the decision to continue or discontinue breast-feeding during therapy should take into account the risk of exposure to the infant and the benefits of treatment to the mother.

Contraindications

Hypersensitivity to amphetamine products or any component of the formulation; concurrent use of MAO inhibitor, or within 14 days of the last MAO inhibitor dose.

Canadian labeling: Additional contraindications (not in U.S. labeling): Known hypersensitivity or idiosyncrasy to sympathomimetic amines; advanced arteriosclerosis; symptomatic cardiovascular disease; moderate-to-severe hypertension; hyperthyroidism; glaucoma; agitated states; history of drug abuse

Warnings/Precautions Sudden death, stroke, and myocardial infarction have been reported in adults receiving the recommended doses of CNS stimulants. In children and adolescents with preexisting structural cardiac abnormalities or other serious heart problems, sudden death has been reported while receiving the recommended doses of CNS stimulants for ADHD. These products should be avoided in the patients with known serious structural cardiac abnormalities, cardiomyopathy, serious heart rhythm abnormalities, coronary artery disease (adults), or other serious cardiac problems that could increase the risk of sudden death. Patients should be carefully evaluated for these cardiac disorders prior to initiation of therapy. Patients who develop exertional chest pain, unexplained syncope, or arrhythmias during therapy should be evaluated promptly. CNS stimulants may increase heart rate (mean increase: 3 to 6 bpm) and blood pressure (mean increase: 2 to 4 mm Hg); monitor for adverse events related to tachycardia or hypertension. Stimulants are associated with peripheral vasculopathy, including Raynaud phenomenon; signs/symptoms are usually mild and intermittent, and generally improve with dose reduction or discontinuation. Digital ulceration and/or soft tissue breakdown have been observed rarely; monitor for digital changes during therapy and seek further evaluation (eg, rheumatology) if necessary.

Use with caution in patients with preexisting psychosis or bipolar disorder (may induce mixed/manic episode). May exacerbate symptoms of behavior and thought disorder in psychotic patients; new onset psychosis or mania may occur in children or adolescents with stimulant use. Patients should be screened for bipolar disorder prior to treatment; consider discontinuation if such symptoms (eg, delusional thinking, hallucinations, or mania) occur. May be associated with aggressive behavior or hostility (causal relationship not established); monitor for development or worsening of these behaviors. Use with caution in patients with Tourette syndrome; stimulants may exacerbate tics (motor and phonic) and Tourette syndrome. Evaluate for tics and Tourette syndrome prior to therapy initiation. **[U.S. Boxed Warning]: CNS stimulants (including lisdexamfetamine) have a high potential for abuse and dependence; assess for abuse potential prior to use and monitor for signs of abuse and dependence while on therapy.** Use with caution in patients with history of ethanol or drug abuse (Canadian labeling contraindicates use if history of drug abuse). Prescriptions should be written for the smallest quantity consistent with good patient care to minimize possibility of overdose. Abrupt discontinuation following high doses or for prolonged periods may result in symptoms for withdrawal (eg, depression, extreme fatigue). Canadian labeling recommends discontinuing therapy if improvement is not observed after 1 month of dosage titration. Lisdexamfetamine is not recommended for weight loss; safety and efficacy not established for treatment of obesity.

Elderly patients may have decreased renal, hepatic or cardiac function or other concomitant disease or drug therapy; initiate dose at the low end of the dosing range. Appetite suppression may occur; particularly in children. Use of stimulants has been associated with weight loss and slowing of growth rate; monitor growth rate and weight during treatment. Treatment interruption may be necessary in patients who are not increasing in height or gaining weight as expected. Hypersensitivity, including anaphylaxis, Stevens-Johnson syndrome, angioedema, and urticaria have been observed. Potentially significant drug-drug interactions may exist, requiring dose or frequency adjustment, additional monitoring, and/or selection of alternative therapy.

Warnings: Additional Pediatric Considerations The American Heart Association recommends that all children diagnosed with ADHD who may be candidates for medication, such as lisdexamfetamine, should have a thorough cardiovascular assessment prior to initiation of therapy. This assessment should include a combination of medical history, family history, and physical examination focusing on cardiovascular disease risk factors. An ECG is not mandatory but should be considered. If a child displays symptoms of cardiovascular disease, including chest pain, dyspnea, or fainting, parents should seek immediate medical care for the child. In a recent retrospective study on the possible association between stimulant medication use and sudden death in children, 564 previously healthy children who died suddenly in motor vehicle accidents were compared to a group of 564 previously healthy children who died suddenly. Two of the 564 (0.4%) children in motor vehicle accidents were taking stimulant medications compared to 10 of 564 (1.8%) children who died suddenly. While the authors of this study conclude there may be an association between stimulant use and sudden death in children, there were a number of limitations to the study and the FDA cannot conclude this information impacts the overall risk:benefit profile of these medications (Gould, 2009). In a large retrospective cohort study involving 1,200,438 children and young adults (aged 2 to 24 years), none of the currently available stimulant medications or atomoxetine were shown to increase the risk of serious cardiovascular events (ie, acute MI, sudden cardiac death, or stroke) in current (adjusted hazard ratio: 0.75; 95% CI: 0.31 to 1.85) or former (adjusted hazard ratio: 1.03; 95% CI: 0.57 to 1.89) users compared to nonusers. It should be noted that due to the upper limit of the 95% CI, the study could not rule out a doubling of the risk, albeit low (Cooper, 2011).

Long-term effects in pediatric patients have not been determined. Use of stimulants in children has been associated with growth suppression; in pediatric clinical trials after 4 weeks of therapy, higher lisdexamfetamine doses were associated with greater weight loss; adolescents may experience larger weight loss than children; monitor growth; treatment interruption may be needed.

Adverse Reactions

Cardiovascular: Increased blood pressure (adults), increased heart rate (adults)

Central nervous system: Agitation (adults), anxiety (adults), dizziness (children), drowsiness (children), emotional lability (children), increased energy (adults), insomnia, irritability (children), jitteriness (adults), nightmares (adults), paresthesia (adults), restlessness (adults), tics (children)

Dermatologic: Hyperhidrosis (adults), pruritus (adults), skin rash (children)

Endocrine & metabolic: Decreased libido (adults), weight loss (more common in children and adolescents)

Gastrointestinal: Anorexia (adults), appetite decreased (more common in children and adolescents), constipation (adults), diarrhea (adults), gastroenteritis (adults), nausea, upper abdominal pain (more common in children), xerostomia (more common in adults)

Genitourinary: Erectile dysfunction (adults)

Neuromuscular & skeletal: Tremor (adults)

Respiratory: Dyspnea (adults), oropharyngeal pain

Miscellaneous: Fever (children)

Rare but important or life-threatening: Accommodation disturbance, bruxism, cardiomyopathy, cerebrovascular accident, decreased linear skeletal growth rate, depression, dermatillomania, diplopia, exacerbation of tics, excoriation, frequent erections, hallucination, headache, hepatitis (eosinophilic), hypersensitivity, hypertension, incoherent speech, mania, mydriasis, myocardial infarction, overstimulation, peripheral vascular insufficiency, prolonged erection, psychotic reaction, Raynaud's phenomenon, seizure, Stevens-Johnson syndrome, suicidal tendencies, tachycardia

Drug Interactions

Metabolism/Transport Effects None known.

Avoid Concomitant Use

Avoid concomitant use of Lisdexamfetamine with any of the following: Iobenguane I 123; MAO Inhibitors

Increased Effect/Toxicity

Lisdexamfetamine may increase the levels/effects of: Analgesics (Opioid); Sympathomimetics

The levels/effects of Lisdexamfetamine may be increased by: Alkalinizing Agents; Antacids; AtoMOXetine; Cannabinoid-Containing Products; Carbonic Anhydrase Inhibitors; Linezolid; MAO Inhibitors; Tedizolid; Tricyclic Antidepressants

Decreased Effect

Lisdexamfetamine may decrease the levels/effects of: Antihistamines; Ethosuximide; Iobenguane I 123; Ioflupane I 123; PHENobarbital; Phenytoin

The levels/effects of Lisdexamfetamine may be decreased by: Ammonium Chloride; Antipsychotic Agents; Ascorbic Acid; Gastrointestinal Acidifying Agents; Lithium; Methenamine; Multivitamins/Fluoride (with ADE); Multivitamins/Minerals (with ADEK, Folate, Iron); Multivitamins/Minerals (with AE, No Iron); Urinary Acidifying Agents

Food Interactions High-fat meal prolongs T_{max} by ~1 hour. Management: Administer without regard to meals.

Storage/Stability Store at 20°C to 25°C (68°F to 77°F); excursions are permitted between 15°C and 30°C (59°F and 86°F). Protect from light.

Mechanism of Action Lisdexamfetamine dimesylate is a prodrug that is converted to the active component dextroamphetamine (a noncatecholamine, sympathomimetic amine). Amphetamines are noncatecholamine, sympathomimetic amines that cause release of catecholamines (primarily dopamine and norepinephrine) from their storage sites in the presynaptic nerve terminals. A less significant mechanism may include their ability to block the reuptake of catecholamines by competitive inhibition.

Pharmacodynamics

Onset of action: 1 hour (AAP, 2011)

Duration of action: 10-12 hours (AAP, 2011)

Pharmacokinetics (Adult data unless noted)

Absorption: Rapid

Distribution: Dextroamphetamine: V_d: 3.5-4.6 L/kg; distributes into CNS; mean CSF concentrations are 80% of plasma

Metabolism: Metabolized in the blood by hydrolytic activity of red blood cells to dextroamphetamine and l-lysine; not metabolized by CYP P450

Half-life elimination: Lisdexamfetamine: <1 hour; dextroamphetamine: 10-13 hours

Time to peak serum concentration:

Lisdexamfetamine: Children 6-12 years: 1 hour (fasting)

Dextroamphetamine:

Children 6-12 years: 3.5 hours (fasting)

Adults: 3.8 hours (fasting), 4.7 hours (after a high-fat meal)

Elimination: Urine (96%; 42% of dose as amphetamine, 2% as lisdexamfetamine, 25% as hippuric acid); feces (minimal)

Dosing: Usual

Children ≥6 years and Adolescents: **Attention-deficit/hyperactivity disorder: Note:** Individualize dosage based on patient need and response to therapy. Administer at the lowest effective dose.

Manufacturer's labeling: Oral: Initial: 30 mg once daily in the morning; may increase in increments of 10 mg or 20 mg/day at weekly intervals until optimal response is obtained; maximum daily dose: 70 mg/**day**

Alternate dosing: Oral: Initial: 20 mg once daily; may increase in increments of 10 or 20 mg/day at 3-7 day intervals until optimal response is obtained; maximum daily dose: 70 mg/**day** (AAP, 2011)

Adults: **Attention-deficit/hyperactivity disorder: Note:** Individualize dosage based on patient need and response to therapy. Administer at the lowest effective dose. Oral: Initial: 30 mg once daily in the morning; may increase in increments of 10 mg or 20 mg/day at weekly intervals until optimal response is obtained; maximum daily dose: 70 mg/**day**

Administration Administer in the morning with or without food; avoid afternoon doses to prevent insomnia. Swallow capsule whole, do not chew; capsule may be opened and the entire contents dissolved in glass of water; stir until dispersed completely and consume the resulting solution immediately; do not store solution; do not divide capsule; do not take less than 1 capsule daily.

Monitoring Parameters Evaluate patients for cardiac disease prior to initiation of therapy with thorough medical history, family history, and physical exam; consider ECG; perform ECG and echocardiogram if findings suggest cardiac disease; promptly conduct cardiac evaluation in patients who develop chest pain, unexplained syncope, or any other symptom of cardiac disease during treatment. Monitor CNS activity; blood pressure and heart rate (baseline, following dose increases, and periodically during treatment), sleep, appetite, abnormal movements, height, weight, BMI, growth in children. Patients should be re-evaluated at appropriate intervals to assess continued need of the medication. Observe for signs/symptoms of aggression or hostility, or depression. Monitor for visual disturbances. Monitor for signs of misuse, abuse, and addiction.

Test Interactions Amphetamines may elevate plasma corticosteroid levels; may interfere with urinary steroid determinations.

Additional Information Treatment for ADHD should include "drug holiday" or periodic discontinuation in order to assess the patient's requirements, decrease tolerance, and limit suppression of linear growth and weight. Medications used to treat ADHD should be part of a total treatment program that may include other components such as psychological, educational, and social measures.

Controlled Substance C-II

Dosage Forms Excipient information presented when available (limited, particularly for generics); consult specific product labeling.

Capsule, Oral, as dimesylate:

Vyvanse: 10 mg [contains brilliant blue fcf (fd&c blue #1), fd&c yellow #6 (sunset yellow)]

Vyvanse: 20 mg, 30 mg, 40 mg, 50 mg, 60 mg, 70 mg [contains brilliant blue fcf (fd&c blue #1), fd&c red #40, fd&c yellow #10 (quinoline yellow)]

◆ **Lisdexamfetamine Dimesylate** *see* Lisdexamfetamine *on page 1278*

◆ **Lisdexamphetamine** *see* Lisdexamfetamine *on page 1278*

Lisinopril (lyse IN oh pril)

Medication Safety Issues

Sound-alike/look-alike issues:

Lisinopril may be confused with fosinopril, Lioresal, Lipitor, RisperDAL

Prinivil may be confused with Plendil, Pravachol, Prevacid, PriLOSEC, Proventil

Zestril may be confused with Desyrel, Restoril, Vistaril, Zegerid, Zerit, Zetia, Zostrix, ZyPREXA

International issues:

Acepril [Malaysia] may be confused with Accupril which is a brand name for quinapril [US]

Acepril: Brand name for lisinopril [Malaysia], but also the brand name for captopril [Great Britain]; enalapril [Hungary, Switzerland]

Brand Names: US Prinivil; Zestril

Brand Names: Canada Apo-Lisinopril; Auro-Lisinopril; CO Lisinopril; Dom-Lisinopril; JAMP-Lisinopril; Mylan-Lisinopril; PMS-Lisinopril; Prinivil; PRO-Lisinopril; RAN-Lisinopril; Riva-Lisinopril; Sandoz-Lisinopril; Teva-Lisinopril (Type P); Teva-Lisinopril (Type Z); Zestril

Therapeutic Category Angiotensin-Converting Enzyme (ACE) Inhibitor; Antihypertensive Agent

Generic Availability (US) Yes

Use Treatment of hypertension, either alone or in combination with other antihypertensive agents (FDA approved in ages 6-16 years and adults); adjunctive therapy in treatment of heart failure (HF) (FDA approved in adults); treatment of acute myocardial infarction (MI) within 24 hours in hemodynamically-stable patients to improve survival (FDA approved in adults); has also been used for the treatment of proteinuria associated with IgA nephropathy and for its reno-protective effects in patients with diabetes mellitus and renal parenchymal disease

Pregnancy Risk Factor D

Pregnancy Considerations **[US Boxed Warning]: Drugs that act on the renin-angiotensin system can cause injury and death to the developing fetus. Discontinue as soon as possible once pregnancy is detected.** Lisinopril crosses the placenta; teratogenic effects may occur following maternal use during pregnancy. Drugs that act on the renin-angiotensin system are associated with oligohydramnios. Oligohydramnios, due to decreased fetal renal function, may lead to fetal lung hypoplasia and skeletal malformations. Their use in pregnancy is also associated with anuria, hypotension, renal failure, skull hypoplasia, and death in the fetus/neonate. Chronic maternal hypertension itself is also associated with adverse events in the fetus/infant. ACE inhibitors are not recommended during pregnancy to treat maternal hypertension or heart failure. Use of an ACE inhibitor should also be avoided in any woman of reproductive age. Women who are planning a pregnancy should be considered for other medication options if an ACE inhibitor is currently prescribed or the ACE inhibitor should be discontinued as soon as possible once pregnancy is detected. The exposed fetus should be monitored for fetal growth, amniotic fluid volume, and organ formation. Infants exposed to an ACE inhibitor *in utero* should be monitored for hyperkalemia, hypotension, and oliguria (exchange transfusions or dialysis may be needed). These adverse events are generally associated with maternal use in the second and third trimesters.

Untreated chronic maternal hypertension is also associated with adverse events in the fetus, infant, and mother. The use of ACE inhibitors is not recommended to treat chronic uncomplicated hypertension in pregnant women and should generally be avoided in women of reproductive potential (ACOG, 2013).

Breast-Feeding Considerations It is not known if lisinopril is excreted in breast milk. The manufacturer recommends discontinuing use of lisinopril or discontinuing breast-feeding taking into account the importance of therapy to the mother.

Contraindications

Hypersensitivity to lisinopril, any component of the formulation, or other ACE inhibitors; angioedema related to previous treatment with an ACE inhibitor; patients with idiopathic or hereditary angioedema; concomitant use with aliskiren in patients with diabetes mellitus

Documentation of allergenic cross-reactivity for ACE inhibitors is limited. However, because of similarities in chemical structure and/or pharmacologic actions, the possibility of cross-sensitivity cannot be ruled out with certainty.

Canadian labeling: Additional contraindications (not in US labeling): Concomitant use with aliskiren-containing drugs in patients with moderate-to-severe renal impairment (GFR <60 mL/minute/1.73 m^2)

Warnings/Precautions Anaphylactic reactions may occur rarely with ACE inhibitors. At any time during treatment (especially following first dose), angioedema may occur rarely with ACE inhibitors; it may involve the head and neck (potentially compromising airway) or the intestine (presenting with abdominal pain). African-Americans may be at an increased risk. Prolonged frequent monitoring may be required especially if tongue, glottis, or larynx are involved as they are associated with airway obstruction. Patients with a history of airway surgery may have a higher risk of airway obstruction. Aggressive early and appropriate management is critical. Use in patients with idiopathic or hereditary angioedema or previous angioedema associated with ACE inhibitor therapy is contraindicated. Severe anaphylactoid reactions may be seen during hemodialysis (eg, CVVHD) with high-flux dialysis membranes (eg, AN69), and rarely, during low density lipoprotein apheresis with dextran sulfate cellulose. Rare cases of anaphylactoid reactions have been reported in patients undergoing sensitization treatment with hymenoptera (bee, wasp) venom while receiving ACE inhibitors.

Symptomatic hypotension with or without syncope can occur with ACE inhibitors (usually with the first several doses). Effects are most often observed in volume depleted patients; correct volume depletion prior to initiation. Other patients at risk include those with heart failure and systolic blood pressure <100 mm Hg, ischemic heart disease, cerebrovascular disease, renal dialysis, hyponatremia, high-dose diuretic therapy, severe aortic stenosis, or hypertrophic cardiomyopathy. Close monitoring of patient is required especially within the first few weeks of initial dosing and with dosing increases; blood pressure must be lowered at a rate appropriate for the patient's clinical condition. Initiation of therapy in patients with ischemic heart disease or cerebrovascular disease warrants close observation due to the potential consequences posed by falling blood pressure (eg, MI, stroke). Avoid use in hemodynamically unstable patients after acute MI. Use with caution in hypertrophic cardiomyopathy with outflow tract obstruction and severe aortic stenosis. In patients on chronic ACE inhibitor therapy, intraoperative hypotension may occur with induction and maintenance of general anesthesia; use with caution before, during, or immediately after major surgery. Cardiopulmonary bypass, intraoperative blood loss, or vasodilating anesthesia increases endogenous renin release. Use of ACE inhibitors perioperatively will blunt angiotensin II formation and may result in hypotension. However, discontinuation of therapy prior to surgery is controversial. If continued preoperatively, avoidance of hypotensive agents during surgery is prudent (Hillis, 2011). **[US Boxed Warning]: Drugs that act on the renin-angiotensin system can cause injury and death to the developing fetus. Discontinue as soon as possible once pregnancy is detected.**

Hyperkalemia may occur with ACE inhibitors; risk factors include renal dysfunction, diabetes mellitus, concomitant use of potassium-sparing diuretics, potassium supplements, and/or potassium-containing salts. Use cautiously, if at all, with these agents and monitor potassium closely. Cough may occur with ACE inhibitors. Other causes of cough should be considered (eg, pulmonary congestion in patients with heart failure) and excluded prior to discontinuation.

May be associated with deterioration of renal function and/or increases in serum creatinine, particularly in patients with low renal blood flow (eg, renal artery stenosis, heart failure) whose glomerular filtration rate (GFR) is dependent on efferent arteriolar vasoconstriction by angiotensin II; deterioration may result in oliguria, acute renal failure, and progressive azotemia. Small increases in serum creatinine may occur following initiation; consider discontinuation only in patients with progressive and/or significant deterioration in renal function. Use with caution in patients with unstented unilateral/bilateral renal artery stenosis. When unstented bilateral renal artery stenosis is present, use is generally avoided due to the elevated risk of deterioration in renal function unless possible benefits outweigh risks. In acute myocardial infarction, the Canadian labeling does not recommend initiating therapy if serum creatinine >177 micromol/L and/or proteinuria >500 mg/24 hour and recommends considering discontinuing therapy if serum creatinine >265 micromol/L or doubles from baseline during therapy. In a retrospective cohort study of elderly patients (≥65 years) with myocardial infarction and impaired left ventricular function, administration of an ACE inhibitor was associated with a survival benefit, including patients with serum creatinine concentrations >3 mg/dL (265 micromol/L) (Frances, 2000).

Potentially significant drug-drug interactions may exist, requiring dose or frequency adjustment, additional monitoring, and/or selection of alternative therapy. Use with caution in patients with preexisting hepatic impairment; consider baseline hepatic function tests prior to initiating therapy. Rare toxicities associated with ACE inhibitors include cholestatic jaundice or hepatitis (which may progress to fulminant hepatic necrosis), agranulocytosis, neutropenia, or leukopenia with myeloid hypoplasia. Patients with collagen vascular diseases (especially with concomitant renal impairment) or renal impairment alone may be at increased risk for hematologic toxicity; periodically monitor CBC with differential in these patients.

Warnings: Additional Pediatric Considerations In pediatric patients, an isolated dry hacking cough lasting >3 weeks was reported in 7 of 42 pediatric patients (17%) receiving ACE inhibitors (von Vigier, 2000); a review of pediatric randomized controlled ACE inhibitor trials reported a lower incidence of 3.2% (Baker-Smith, 2010). Other causes of cough should be considered (eg, pulmonary congestion in patients with heart failure) and excluded prior to discontinuation.

Adverse Reactions Note: Higher rates of adverse reactions have generally been noted in patients with heart failure. However, the frequency of adverse effects associated with placebo is also increased in this population.

Cardiovascular: Chest pain, flushing, hypotension, orthostatic effect, syncope

Central nervous system: Altered sense of smell, dizziness, fatigue, headache

Dermatologic: Alopecia, diaphoresis, erythema, pruritus, skin photosensitivity, Stevens-Johnson syndrome, toxic epidermal necrolysis, urticaria

Endocrine & metabolic: Diabetes mellitus, gout, hyperkalemia, increased nonprotein nitrogen, SIADH

Gastrointestinal: Constipation, diarrhea, dysgeusia, flatulence, pancreatitis, xerostomia

Genitourinary: Impotence

Hematologic & oncologic: Bone marrow depression, decreased hematocrit (small), decreased hemoglobin (small), hemolytic anemia, leukopenia, neutropenia, thrombocytopenia

Infection: Common cold

Neuromuscular & skeletal: Weakness

Ophthalmic: Blurred vision, diplopia, photophobia, vision loss

Otic: Tinnitus

Renal: Increased blood urea nitrogen, increased serum creatinine (often transient), renal insufficiency (in patients with acute myocardial infarction)

Respiratory: Cough

Rare but important or life-threatening: Acute renal failure, anaphylactoid reactions, angioedema, anuria, arthralgia, arthritis, asthma, ataxia, azotemia, bronchitis, bronchospasm, cardiac arrest, cardiac arrhythmia, cerebrovascular accident (possibly secondary to excessive hypotension in high risk patients), chills, confusion, cutaneous pseudolymphoma, dehydration, drowsiness, dyspepsia, dyspnea, dysuria, eosinophilia, eosinophilic pneumonitis, epistaxis, facial edema, fever, gastritis, hallucination, heartburn, hemoptysis, hepatic necrosis, hepatitis (hepatocellular jaundice or cholestatic jaundice), herpes zoster, hypersomnia, hypervolemia, hypoglycemia (diabetic patients on oral antidiabetic agents or insulin), hyponatremia, increased erythrocyte sedimentation rate, insomnia, intestinal angioedema, irritability, laryngitis, leukocytosis, malaise, malignant neoplasm of lung, mastalgia, memory impairment, mood changes (including depressive symptoms), muscle spasm, musculoskeletal pain, myalgia, myocardial infarction (possibly secondary to excessive hypotension in high risk patients), oliguria, orthopnea, orthostatic hypotension, palpitations, paresthesia, paroxysmal nocturnal dyspnea, pemphigus, peripheral edema, peripheral neuropathy, pharyngitis, pleural effusion, pneumonia, positive ANA titer, psoriasis, pulmonary embolism, pulmonary infarct, pulmonary infiltrates, pyelonephritis, rhinitis, rhinorrhea, sinusitis, skin infection, skin lesion, skin rash, sore throat, systemic lupus erythematosus, transient ischemic attacks, tremor, uremia, urinary tract infection, vasculitis, vertigo, viral infection, visual hallucination (Doane, 2013), weight gain, weight loss, wheezing

Drug Interactions

Metabolism/Transport Effects None known.

Avoid Concomitant Use There are no known interactions where it is recommended to avoid concomitant use.

Increased Effect/Toxicity

Lisinopril may increase the levels/effects of: Allopurinol; Amifostine; Antihypertensives; AzaTHIOprine; Ciprofloxacin (Systemic); Drospirenone; DULoxetine; Ferric Gluconate; Gold Sodium Thiomalate; Grass Pollen Allergen Extract (5 Grass Extract); Hypotensive Agents; Iron Dextran Complex; Levodopa; Lithium; Nonsteroidal Anti-Inflammatory Agents; Obinutuzumab; Pregabalin; RisperiDONE; RiTUXimab; Sodium Phosphates

The levels/effects of Lisinopril may be increased by: Alfuzosin; Aliskiren; Angiotensin II Receptor Blockers; Barbiturates; Brimonidine (Topical); Canagliflozin; Dapoxetine; Diazoxide; DPP-IV Inhibitors; Eplerenone; Everolimus; Heparin; Heparin (Low Molecular Weight); Herbs (Hypotensive Properties); Loop Diuretics; MAO Inhibitors; Nicorandil; Pentoxifylline; Phosphodiesterase 5 Inhibitors; Potassium Salts; Potassium-Sparing Diuretics; Prostacyclin Analogues; Sirolimus; Temsirolimus; Thiazide Diuretics; TiZANidine; Tolvaptan; Trimethoprim

Decreased Effect

The levels/effects of Lisinopril may be decreased by: Aprotinin; Herbs (Hypertensive Properties); Icatibant; Lanthanum; Methylphenidate; Nonsteroidal Anti-Inflammatory Agents; Salicylates; Yohimbine

Storage/Stability Store at controlled room temperature. Protect from moisture, freezing, and excessive heat.

Mechanism of Action Competitive inhibitor of angiotensin-converting enzyme (ACE); prevents conversion of angiotensin I to angiotensin II, a potent vasoconstrictor; results in lower levels of angiotensin II which causes an increase in plasma renin activity and a reduction in aldosterone secretion; a CNS mechanism may also be involved in hypotensive effect as angiotensin II increases adrenergic outflow from CNS; vasoactive kallikreins may be decreased in conversion to active hormones by ACE inhibitors, thus reducing blood pressure

Pharmacodynamics

Onset of action: Antihyptensive effect: 1 hour

Maximum effect: Antihypertensive effect: 6-8 hours

Duration: 24 hours

Pharmacokinetics (Adult data unless noted)

Absorption: Oral:

- Pediatric patients:
  - 2-15 years: 20% to 36% (Hogg, 2007)
  - 6-16 years: 28%
- Adults: 25% (range: 6% to 60%)

Protein binding: 25%

Half-life: 11-13 hours; half-life increases with renal dysfunction

Time to peak serum concentration:

- Pediatric patients 6 months to 15 years: Median (range): 5-6 hours (Hogg, 2007)
- Adults: Within 7 hours

Elimination: Primarily urine as unchanged drug

Dialysis: Removable by hemodialysis

Dosing: Usual

Pediatric:

Hypertension: Note: Dosage must be titrated according to patient's response; **reduce dose by 50% in patients with hyponatremia, hypovolemia, severe CHF, decreased renal function, or receiving diuretics**. If possible, discontinue diuretics 2 to 3 days prior to initiating lisinopril; restart diuretic, if needed, after blood pressure is stable:

Infants: Limited data available: Oral: Initial: 0.07 to 0.1 mg/kg/dose once daily; may increase at ≥2 weeks intervals; maximum daily dose: 0.5 mg/kg/**day**; dosing based on a retrospective study of pediatric patients (n=123; 59 with hypertension; age range: 2 months to 18 years) which initiated therapy in the hospital to allow for close observation; median maximum dose in patients 1 month to <2 years (n=13): 0.159 mg/kg/day (Raes 2007).

Children <6 years: Limited data available: Oral: Initial: 0.07 to 0.1 mg/kg/dose once daily; maximum initial daily dose: 5 mg/**day**; increase dose at 1- to 2-week intervals; maximum daily dose: 0.6 mg/kg/**day** or 40 mg/**day** (NHBPEP 2004; NHLBI 2011; Raes 2007)

Children ≥6 years and Adolescents: Oral: Initial: 0.07 to 0.1 mg/kg/dose once daily; maximum initial daily dose: 5 mg/**day**; increase dose at 1- to 2-week intervals; maximum daily dose: 0.6 mg/kg/**day** or 40 mg/**day**

Proteinuria (mild IgA nephropathy): Limited data available: Children ≥4 years and Adolescents: Oral: Initial: 0.2 mg/kg/dose once daily (maximum initial dose: 10 mg) for 7 days, then increase to 0.4 mg/kg/dose once daily (maximum dose: 20 mg); dosing based on a pilot study of 40 pediatric patients (mean age: 11.4 years; range: 4 to 15 years) who during a 2-year treatment period showed statistically significant resolution of proteinuria in 82% of patients; five patients developed dizziness during treatment period and four of them required dosage reduction (50% to 75%) (Nakanishi 2008).

Renal protection (diabetes mellitus or renal parenchymal disease): Limited data available: Infants, Children, and Adolescents: Oral: Initial: 0.1 mg/kg/dose once daily; maximum initial daily dose: 5 mg/day; dosing based on a retrospective study of pediatric patients (n=123 of which 60 had either DM or renal parenchymal disease; age range: 2 months to 18 years); the protocol included therapy initiation within the hospital to allow for close observation initially; median maximum dose: 0.135 mg/kg/day (Raes 2007).

Adult:

Heart failure: Oral: Initial: 2.5 to 5 mg once daily; then increase by no more than 10 mg increments at intervals no less than 2 weeks to a maximum daily dose of 40 mg. Usual maintenance: 5 to 40 mg/day as a single dose. Target dose: 20 to 40 mg once daily (ACC/AHA 2009 Heart Failure Guidelines). **Note:** If patient has hyponatremia (serum sodium <130 mEq/L) or renal impairment (CrCl <30 mL/minute or creatinine >3 mg/dL), then initial dose should be 2.5 mg/day.

Hypertension: Oral: Usual dosage range (JNC 7): 10 to 40 mg/day

Not maintained on diuretic: Initial: 10 mg/day

Maintained on diuretic: Initial: 5 mg/day

Note: Antihypertensive effect may diminish toward the end of the dosing interval especially with doses of 10 mg/day. An increased dose may aid in extending the duration of antihypertensive effect. Doses up to 80 mg/day have been used, but do not appear to give greater effect.

Patients taking diuretics should have them discontinued 2 to 3 days prior to initiating lisinopril if possible. Restart diuretic after blood pressure is stable if needed. If diuretic cannot be discontinued prior to therapy, begin with 5 mg with close supervision until stable blood pressure. In patients with hyponatremia (<130 mEq/L), start dose at 2.5 mg/day.

Acute myocardial infarction (within 24 hours in hemodynamically stable patients): Oral: 5 mg immediately, then 5 mg at 24 hours, 10 mg at 48 hours, and 10 mg every day thereafter for 6 weeks. Patients should continue to receive standard treatments such as thrombolytics, aspirin, and beta-blockers.

Dosing adjustment in renal impairment:

Infants, Children, and Adolescents:

Manufacturer's labeling: Children ≥6 years and Adolescents ≤16 years: CrCl <30 mL/minute/1.73 m^2: Use is not recommended

Alternate dosing (Aronoff 2007):

GFR >50 mL/minute/1.73 m^2: No dosage adjustment necessary

GFR 10-50 mL/minute/1.73 m^2: Administer 50% of usual dose

GFR <10 mL/minute/1.73 m^2: Administer 25% of usual dose

Intermittent hemodialysis: Administer 25% of usual dose

Peritoneal dialysis (PD): Administer 25% of usual dose

Continuous renal replacement therapy (CRRT): Administer 50% of usual dose

Adults: Manufacturer's labeling:

Heart failure: CrCl <30 mL/minute or serum creatinine >3 mg/dL: Initial: 2.5 mg/day

Hypertension: Initial doses should be modified and upward titration should be cautious, based on response (maximum: 40 mg/day)

CrCl >30 mL/minute: Initial: 10 mg/day

CrCl 10 to 30 mL/minute: Initial: 5 mg/day

Hemodialysis: Initial: 2.5 mg/day; dialyzable (50%)

Administration Oral: May be administered without regard to food

Monitoring Parameters Blood pressure, BUN, serum creatinine, renal function, urine dipstick for protein, serum potassium, WBC with differential, especially during first 3 months of therapy for patients with renal impairment and/or collagen vascular disease; monitor for angioedema and anaphylactoid reactions; hypovolemia and postural hypotension when beginning therapy, adjusting dosage, and on a regular basis throughout

Dosage Forms Excipient information presented when available (limited, particularly for generics); consult specific product labeling.

Tablet, Oral:

Prinivil: 5 mg, 10 mg, 20 mg [scored]

Zestril: 2.5 mg

Zestril: 5 mg [scored]

Zestril: 10 mg, 20 mg, 30 mg, 40 mg

Generic: 2.5 mg, 5 mg, 10 mg, 20 mg, 30 mg, 40 mg

Extemporaneous Preparations A 1 mg/mL lisinopril oral suspension may be made with tablets and a mixture of Bicitra and Ora-Sweet SF. Place ten 20 mg tablets into an 8 ounce amber polyethylene terephthalate (PET) bottle and then add 10 mL purified water and shake for at least 1 minute. Gradually add 30 mL of Bicitra and 160 mL of Ora-Sweet SF to the bottle and gently shake after each addition to disperse the contents. Store resulting suspension at ≤25°C (77°F) for up to 4 weeks. Label bottle "shake well" (Prinivil prescribing information, 2013; Thompson, 2003).

A 1 mg/mL lisinopril oral suspension may be made with tablets and a 1:1 mixture of Ora-Plus® and Ora-Sweet®. Crush ten 10 mg tablets in a mortar and reduce to a fine powder. Add small portions of the vehicle and mix to a uniform paste; mix while adding the vehicle in incremental proportions to **almost** 100 mL; transfer to a graduated cylinder; rinse mortar with vehicle, and add quantity of vehicle sufficient to make 100 mL. Store in amber plastic prescription bottles; label "shake well". Stable for 13 weeks at room temperature or refrigerated (Nahata, 2004).

A 1 mg/mL lisinopril oral suspension also be made with tablets, methylcellulose 1% with parabens, and simple syrup NF. Crush ten 10 mg tablets in a mortar and reduce to a fine powder. Add 7.7 mL of methylcellulose gel and mix to a uniform paste; mix while adding the simple syrup in incremental proportions to **almost** 100 mL; transfer to a graduated cylinder; rinse mortar with vehicle, and add quantity of vehicle sufficient to make 100 mL. Store in amber plastic prescription bottles; label "shake well".

Stable for 13 weeks refrigerated or 8 weeks at room temperature (Nahata, 2004).

A 2 mg/mL lisinopril syrup may be made with powder (Sigma Chemical Company, St. Louis, MO) and simple syrup. Dissolve 1 g of lisinopril powder in 30 mL of distilled water. Mix while adding simple syrup in incremental proportions in a quantity sufficient to make 500 mL. Label "shake well" and "refrigerate". Stable for 30 days when stored in amber plastic prescription bottles at room temperature or refrigerated. **Note:** Although no visual evidence of microbial growth was observed, the authors recommend refrigeration to inhibit microbial growth (Webster, 1997).

Nahata MC and Morosco RS, "Stability of Lisinopril in Two Liquid Dosage Forms," *Ann Pharmacother*, 2004, 38(3):396-9.
Prinivil (lisinopril) [prescribing information]. Whitehouse Station, NJ: Merck & Co., Inc; February 2013.
Thompson KC, Zhao Z, Mazakas JM, et al, "Characterization of an Extemporaneous Liquid Formulation of Lisinopril," *Am J Health Syst Pharm*, 2003, 60(1):69-74.
Webster AA, English BA, and Rose DJ, "The Stability of Lisinopril as an Extemporaneous Syrup," *Intr J Pharmaceut Compound*, 1997, 1:352-3.

◆ **Lispro Insulin** *see* Insulin Lispro *on page 1132*
◆ **Lithane (Can)** *see* Lithium *on page 1284*

Lithium (LITH ee um)

Medication Safety Issues

Sound-alike/look-alike issues:

Eskalith may be confused with Estratest
Lithium may be confused with lanthanum, Ultram
Lithobid may be confused with Levbid, Lithostat

Other safety concerns:

Do not confuse **mEq** (milliequivalent) with **mg** (milligram). **Note:** 300 mg lithium carbonate or citrate contain 8 mEq lithium. Dosage should be written in **mg** (milligrams) to avoid confusion.

Check prescriptions for unusually high volumes of the syrup for dosing errors.

Related Information

Oral Medications That Should Not Be Crushed or Altered *on page 2476*

Brand Names: US Lithobid

Brand Names: Canada Apo-Lithium Carbonate; Carbolith; Lithane; Lithmax; PMS-Lithium Carbonate; PMS-Lithium Citrate

Therapeutic Category Antidepressant, Miscellaneous; Antimanic Agent

Generic Availability (US) Yes

Use Management of acute manic episodes (FDA approved in ages ≥12 years and adults); maintenance treatment of mania in individuals with bipolar disorder (maintenance treatment decreases frequency and diminishes intensity of subsequent manic episodes) (FDA approved in ages ≥12 years and adults); has also been used as adjunct treatment for depression; used investigationally to treat severe aggression in children and adolescents with conduct disorder

Pregnancy Risk Factor D

Pregnancy Considerations Adverse events have been observed in animal reproduction studies. Lithium crosses the placenta in concentrations similar to those in the maternal plasma (Newport, 2005). Cardiac malformations in the infant, including Ebstein's anomaly, are associated with use of lithium during the first trimester of pregnancy. Other adverse events including polyhydramnios, fetal/neonatal cardiac arrhythmias, hypoglycemia, diabetes insipidus, changes in thyroid function, premature delivery, floppy infant syndrome, or neonatal lithium toxicity are associated with lithium exposure when used later in pregnancy (ACOG, 2008). The incidence of adverse events may be associated with higher maternal doses (Newport 2005).

Due to pregnancy-induced physiologic changes, women who are pregnant may require dose adjustments of lithium to achieve euthymia and avoid toxicity (ACOG, 2008; Grandjean, 2009; Yonkers, 2011).

For planned pregnancies, use of lithium during the first trimester should be avoided if possible (Grandjean, 2009). If lithium is needed during pregnancy, the minimum effective dose should be used, maternal serum concentrations should be monitored, and consideration should be given to start therapy after the period of organogenesis; lithium should be suspended 24 to 48 hours prior to delivery or at the onset of labor when delivery is spontaneous, then restarted when the patient is medically stable after delivery (ACOG, 2008; Grandjean, 2009; Newport, 2005). Fetal echocardiography should be considered if first trimester exposure occurs (ACOG, 2008).

Breast-Feeding Considerations Lithium is excreted into breast milk and serum concentrations of nursing infants may be 10% to 50% of the maternal serum concentration (Grandjean, 2009). Hypotonia, hypothermia, cyanosis, electrocardiogram changes, and lethargy have been reported in nursing infants (ACOG, 2008). It is generally recommended that breast-feeding be avoided during maternal use of lithium; however, treatment may be continued in appropriately selected patients (Grandjean, 2009; Sharma, 2009; Viguera, 2007). The hydration status of the nursing infant and maternal serum concentrations of lithium should be monitored (ACOG, 2008). In addition, monitor the infant for lethargy, growth, and feeding problems; obtain infant serum concentrations only if clinical concerns arise (Bogen, 2012; Yonkers, 2011). Long-term effects on development and behavior have not been studied (ACOG, 2008; Grandjean, 2009).

Contraindications Hypersensitivity to lithium or any component of the formulation; avoid use in patients with severe cardiovascular or renal disease, or with severe debilitation, dehydration, or sodium depletion

Warnings/Precautions [US Boxed Warning]: Lithium toxicity is closely related to serum levels and can occur at therapeutic doses; serum lithium determinations are required to monitor therapy. Use with caution in patients with mild-moderate renal impairment mild-moderate cardiovascular disease, debilitated patients, and elderly patients due to an increased risk of lithium toxicity. Likewise, use caution in patients in patients with significant fluid loss (protracted sweating, diarrhea, or prolonged fever); temporary reduction or cessation of therapy may be warranted. Lithium may unmask Brugada syndrome; avoid use in patients with or suspected of having Brugada Syndrome. Consult with a cardiologist if a patient is suspected of having Brugada syndrome or has risk factors for Brugada syndrome (eg, unexplained syncope, a family history of Brugada syndrome, a family history of sudden death before the age of 45 years), or if unexplained syncope or palpitations develop after starting therapy. Use with caution in patients with thyroid disease; hypothyroidism may occur with treatment. Hypercalcemia with or without hyperparathyroidism has been reported. Risks are greater in women and possibly in older patients; symptom onset does not appear to be related therapy duration (Lehman, 2013). Serum calcium levels typically range from slightly above normal to over 15 mg/dL and PTH levels may range from high normal to several times the upper limit of normal (Lehman, 2013); magnesium levels are often elevated; serum phosphate levels may be either normal or low (Grandjean, 2009). Monitor calcium and PTH levels as clinically indicated. Consider discontinuation if clinical manifestations of hypercalcemia are present (fatigue, weakness, abdominal pain, constipation, nephrolithiasis,bone pain) or if calcium levels are

>11.4 mg/dL. Following discontinuation check serum calcium levels weekly for one month for return to baseline. Changes are usually reversible if lithium is discontinued; however, sustained hypercalcemia and parathyroid gland enlargement has been reported (Lehman, 2013). Chronic therapy results in diminished renal concentrating ability (nephrogenic diabetes insipidus); this is usually reversible when lithium is discontinued. Changes in renal function should be monitored, and re-evaluation of treatment may be necessary. Use caution in patients at risk of suicide (suicidal thoughts or behavior) by drug overdose; lithium has a narrow therapeutic index. Lithium may impair the patient's alertness, affecting the ability to operate machinery or driving a vehicle. Neuromuscular-blocking agents should be administered with caution; the response may be prolonged. Higher serum concentrations may be required and tolerated during an acute manic phase; however, the tolerance decreases when symptoms subside. Normal fluid and salt intake must be maintained during therapy.

Benzyl alcohol and derivatives: Some dosage forms may contain benzyl alcohol; large amounts of benzyl alcohol (≥99 mg/kg/day) have been associated with a potentially fatal toxicity ("gasping syndrome") in neonates; the "gasping syndrome" consists of metabolic acidosis, respiratory distress, gasping respirations, CNS dysfunction (including convulsions, intracranial hemorrhage), hypotension, and cardiovascular collapse (AAP, 1997; CDC, 1982); some data suggests that benzoate displaces bilirubin from protein binding sites (Ahlfors, 2001); avoid or use dosage forms containing benzyl alcohol with caution in neonates. See manufacturer's labeling.

Adverse Reactions

Cardiovascular: Abnormal T waves on ECG, bradycardia, cardiac arrhythmia, chest tightness, circulatory shock, cold extremities, edema, hypotension, myxedema, sinus node dysfunction, startled response, syncope

Central nervous system: Ataxia, blackout spells, cogwheel rigidity, coma, confusion, dizziness, drowsiness, dystonia, EEG pattern changes, extrapyramidal reaction, fatigue, hallucination, headache, hyperactive deep tendon reflex, hypertonia, involuntary choreoathetoid movements, lethargy, local anesthesia, memory impairment, loss of consciousness, metallic taste, myasthenia gravis (rare), pseudotumor cerebri, psychomotor retardation, reduced intellectual ability, restlessness, salty taste, sedation, seizure, slowed intellectual functioning, slurred speech, stupor, tics, vertigo, worsening of organic brain syndromes

Dermatologic: Acne vulgaris, alopecia, blue-gray skin pigmentation, dermal ulcer, dry or thinning of hair, exacerbation of psoriasis, folliculitis, pruritus, psoriasis, skin rash, xerosis

Endocrine & metabolic: Albuminuria, dehydration, diabetes insipidus, euthyroid goiter, glycosuria, hypercalcemia (secondary to hyperparathyroidism [McKnight 2012]), hyperglycemia, hyperparathyroidism, hyperthyroidism, hypothyroidism, increased radioactive iodine uptake, increased thirst, polydipsia, weight gain, weight loss

Gastrointestinal: Abdominal pain, anorexia, dental caries, diarrhea, dysgeusia, dyspepsia, excessive salivation, flatulence, gastritis, nausea, sialadenitis, sialorrhea, swelling of lips, vomiting, xerostomia

Genitourinary: Impotence, incontinence, oliguria

Hematologic & oncologic: Leukocytosis

Hypersensitivity: Angioedema

Neuromuscular & skeletal: Joint swelling, muscle hyperirritability, neuromuscular excitability, polyarthralgia, tremor

Ophthalmic: Blurred vision, exophthalmos, nystagmus, transient scotoma

Otic: Tinnitus

Renal: Decreased creatinine clearance, polyuria

Miscellaneous: Fever

Drug Interactions

Metabolism/Transport Effects None known.

Avoid Concomitant Use

Avoid concomitant use of Lithium with any of the following: Dapoxetine

Increased Effect/Toxicity

Lithium may increase the levels/effects of: Antipsychotic Agents; Highest Risk QTc-Prolonging Agents; Metoclopramide; Moderate Risk QTc-Prolonging Agents; Neuromuscular-Blocking Agents; Selective Serotonin Reuptake Inhibitors; Serotonin Modulators; Tricyclic Antidepressants

The levels/effects of Lithium may be increased by: ACE Inhibitors; Angiotensin II Receptor Blockers; Antiemetics (5HT3 Antagonists); Calcium Channel Blockers (Nondihydropyridine); CarBAMazepine; Dapoxetine; Desmopressin; Eplerenone; Fosphenytoin; Loop Diuretics; MAO Inhibitors; Methyldopa; Mifepristone; Nonsteroidal Anti-Inflammatory Agents; Phenytoin; Potassium Iodide; Thiazide Diuretics; Topiramate

Decreased Effect

Lithium may decrease the levels/effects of: Amphetamines; Antipsychotic Agents; Desmopressin

The levels/effects of Lithium may be decreased by: Caffeine and Caffeine Containing Products; Calcitonin; Calcium Polystyrene Sulfonate; Carbonic Anhydrase Inhibitors; Loop Diuretics; Sodium Bicarbonate; Sodium Chloride; Sodium Polystyrene Sulfonate; Theophylline Derivatives

Storage/Stability Store between 15°C and 30°C (59°F to 86°F). Protect tablets and capsules from moisture.

Mechanism of Action The precise mechanism of action in mood disorders is unknown. Traditionally thought to alter cation transport across cell membranes in nerve and muscle cells, influence the reuptake of serotonin and/or norepinephrine, and inhibit second messenger systems involving the phosphatidylinositol cycle (Ward, 1994). May also provide neuroprotective effects by increasing glutamate clearance, inhibiting apoptoctic glycogen synthase kinase activity, increasing the levels of antiapoptotic protein Bcl-2 and, enhancing the expression of neurotropic factors, including brain-derived neurotrophic factor (Sanacora, 2008).

Pharmacokinetics (Adult data unless noted)

Distribution: Crosses the placenta; appears in breast milk at 35% to 50% of the concentrations in serum

Adults:

V_d: Initial: 0.3-0.4 L/kg

V_{dss}: 0.7-1 L/kg

Half-life, terminal: Adults: 18-24 hours, can increase to more than 36 hours in patients with renal impairment

Time to peak serum concentration (immediate release product): Within 0.5-2 hours

Elimination: 90% to 98% of a dose is excreted in the urine as unchanged drug; other excretory routes include feces (1%) and sweat (4% to 5%)

Dialysis: Dialyzable (50% to 100%)

Dosing: Usual Oral: **Note:** Monitor serum concentrations and clinical response (efficacy and toxicity) to determine proper dose. Each 5 mL of lithium citrate oral solution contains 8 mEq of lithium ion, equivalent to the amount of lithium in 300 mg of lithium carbonate immediate release capsules/tablets.

Bipolar Disorder:

Children 6 to 12 years: 15 to 60 mg/kg/day in 3 to 4 divided doses (immediate release); dose not to exceed usual adult dosage; initiate at lower dose and adjust dose weekly based on serum concentrations

Adolescents: 600 to 1,800 mg/day in 3 to 4 divided doses (immediate release) or 2 divided doses for extended release tablets

Adults: 300 mg 3 to 4 times/day (immediate release) or 450 to 900 mg of extended release tablets twice daily; usual maximum maintenance dose: 2.4 g/day

Dosing adjustment in renal impairment:

CrCl 10 to 50 mL/minute: Administer 50% to 75% of normal dose

CrCl <10 mL/minute: Administer 25% to 50% of normal dose

Administration Oral: Administer with meals to decrease GI upset. Do not crush or chew extended release dosage form; swallow whole

Monitoring Parameters Serum lithium concentration every 3-4 days during initial therapy; once patient is clinically stable and serum concentrations are stable, serum lithium may be obtained every 1-2 months; obtain lithium serum concentrations 8-12 hours postdose (ie, just before next dose). Monitor renal, hepatic, thyroid and cardiovascular function; CBC with differential, urinalysis, serum sodium, calcium, potassium

Reference Range

Timing of serum samples: Draw trough just before next dose (8-12 hours after previous dose)

Therapeutic: Acute mania: 0.6-1.2 mEq/L (SI: 0.6-1.2 mmol/L); protection against future episodes in most patients with bipolar disorder: 0.8-1 mEq/L (SI: 0.8-1 mmol/L). A higher rate of relapse is described in subjects who are maintained <0.4 mEq/L (SI: <0.4 mmol/L)

Toxic: >1.5 mEq/L (SI: >1.5 mmol/L)

Concentration-related adverse effects:

GI complaints/tremor: 1.5-2 mEq/L

Confusion/somnolence: 2-2.5 mEq/L

Seizures/death: >2.5 mEq/L

Additional Information In terms of efficacy, the results of studies using lithium to treat severe aggression in children and adolescents with conduct disorders, are mixed. A double-blind, placebo-controlled trial in patients 10-17 years of age (n=40) demonstrated efficacy for lithium in reducing aggressive behavior in psychiatrically hospitalized patients with conduct disorder and severe aggression. Lithium was initiated at 600 mg/day and titrated upwards by 300 mg/day. Final lithium carbonate doses ranged from 900-2100 mg/day divided into 3 doses/day (mean ± SD: 1425 ± 321 mg/day); serum lithium concentrations ranged from 0.78-1.55 mmol/L (mean ± SD: 1.07 ± 0.19 mmol/L) (Malone, 2000). In an earlier double-blind, placebo-controlled study in 50 children 5-12 years of age (mean ± SD: 9.4 ± 1.8 years), lithium was also initiated at 600 mg/day in 3 divided doses. Doses were titrated upwards in 300 mg/day increments. The mean optimal lithium dose was 1248 mg/day (range: 600-1800 mg/day); serum lithium concentrations ranged from 0.53-1.79 mmol/L (mean: 1.12 mmol/L). Doses >1500 mg/day and serum concentrations >1.13 mmol/L did not provide additional benefit (Campbell, 1995). Several other studies have not demonstrated efficacy; further studies are needed.

Dosage Forms Excipient information presented when available (limited, particularly for generics); consult specific product labeling.

Capsule, Oral, as carbonate:

Generic: 150 mg, 300 mg, 600 mg

Solution, Oral, as citrate:

Generic: 8 mEq/5 mL (5 mL, 500 mL)

Tablet, Oral, as carbonate:

Generic: 300 mg

Tablet Extended Release, Oral, as carbonate:

Lithobid: 300 mg [contains fd&c blue #2 aluminum lake, fd&c red #40 aluminum lake, fd&c yellow #6 aluminum lake]

Generic: 300 mg, 450 mg

- ◆ **Lithium Carbonate** *see* Lithium *on page* *1284*
- ◆ **Lithium Citrate** *see* Lithium *on page* *1284*
- ◆ **Lithmax (Can)** *see* Lithium *on page* *1284*
- ◆ **Lithobid** *see* Lithium *on page* *1284*
- ◆ **Little Colds Cough Formula [OTC]** *see* Dextromethorphan *on page* *631*
- ◆ **Little Colds Decongestant [OTC]** *see* Phenylephrine (Systemic) *on page* *1685*
- ◆ **Little Fevers [OTC]** *see* Acetaminophen *on page* *44*
- ◆ **Live Attenuated Influenza Vaccine** *see* Influenza Virus Vaccine (Live/Attenuated) *on page* *1113*
- ◆ **Live Attenuated Influenza Vaccine (Quadrivalent)** *see* Influenza Virus Vaccine (Live/Attenuated) *on page* *1113*
- ◆ **L-leucovorin** *see* LEVOleucovorin *on page* *1248*
- ◆ **10% LMD** *see* Dextran *on page* *624*
- ◆ **LMD in D5W** *see* Dextran *on page* *624*
- ◆ **LMD in NaCl** *see* Dextran *on page* *624*
- ◆ **LMX 4 [OTC]** *see* Lidocaine (Topical) *on page* *1258*
- ◆ **LMX 4 Plus [OTC]** *see* Lidocaine (Topical) *on page* *1258*
- ◆ **LMX 5 [OTC]** *see* Lidocaine (Topical) *on page* *1258*
- ◆ **Locoid** *see* Hydrocortisone (Topical) *on page* *1041*
- ◆ **Locoid® (Can)** *see* Hydrocortisone (Topical) *on page* *1041*
- ◆ **Locoid Lipocream** *see* Hydrocortisone (Topical) *on page* *1041*
- ◆ **Lodalis (Can)** *see* Colesevelam *on page* *530*
- ◆ **Lodine** *see* Etodolac *on page* *816*
- ◆ **Lodrane D [OTC]** *see* Brompheniramine and Pseudoephedrine *on page* *305*
- ◆ **LoHist PSB [OTC] [DSC]** *see* Brompheniramine and Pseudoephedrine *on page* *305*
- ◆ **L-OHP** *see* Oxaliplatin *on page* *1578*
- ◆ **Lomotil** *see* Diphenoxylate and Atropine *on page* *673*

Lomustine (loe MUS teen)

Medication Safety Issues

Sound-alike/look-alike issues:

Lomustine may be confused with bendamustine, carmustine

High alert medication:

This medication is in a class the Institute for Safe Medication Practices (ISMP) includes among its list of drug classes which have a heightened risk of causing significant patient harm when used in error.

Administration issues:

Lomustine should only be administered as a single dose once every 6 weeks; serious and fatal adverse events have occurred when lomustine was inadvertently administered daily. The manufacturer and the Institute for Safe Medication Practices (ISMP) recommend dispensing only enough capsules for a single dose (ISMP, 2014).

Related Information

Oral Medications That Should Not Be Crushed or Altered *on page* *2476*

Prevention of Chemotherapy-Induced Nausea and Vomiting in Children *on page* *2368*

Safe Handling of Hazardous Drugs *on page* *2455*

Brand Names: US Gleostine

Brand Names: Canada CeeNU

Therapeutic Category Antineoplastic Agent, Alkylating Agent; Antineoplastic Agent, Alkylating Agent (Nitrosourea)

Generic Availability (US) Yes

Use Treatment of primary or metastatic brain tumors (after surgery and/or radiation therapy) [FDA approved in pediatric patients (age not specified) and adults]; treatment of relapsed or refractory Hodgkin's disease (as part of a combination chemotherapy regimen) [FDA approved in pediatric patients (age not specified) and adults]; has also been used in the treatment of medulloblastoma

Pregnancy Risk Factor D

Pregnancy Considerations Adverse effects have been observed in animal reproduction studies. May cause fetal harm when administered to a pregnant woman. Women of childbearing potential should be advised to avoid pregnancy during treatment with lomustine.

Breast-Feeding Considerations It is not known if lomustine is excreted in breast milk. Due to the potential for serious adverse reactions in the nursing infant, the decision to discontinue lomustine or to discontinue breast-feeding should take into account the importance of treatment to the mother.

Contraindications Hypersensitivity to lomustine or any component of the formulation

Warnings/Precautions Hazardous agent - use appropriate precautions for handling and disposal (NIOSH 2014 [group 1]). **[U.S. Boxed Warnings]: Bone marrow suppression, particularly thrombocytopenia and leukopenia commonly occur and may be severe; may lead to bleeding and overwhelming infections in an already compromised patient. Hematologic toxicity may be delayed; monitor blood counts for at least 6 weeks after a dose. Do not administer courses more frequently than every 6 weeks due to delayed myelotoxicity. Because bone marrow toxicity is cumulative; dose adjustments should be based on nadir counts from prior dose.** Bone marrow suppression is dose-related. The onset of hematologic toxicity is ~4 to 6 weeks after administration; thrombocytopenia occurs at ~4 weeks and leukopenia occurs at 5 to 6 weeks; both persist for 1 to 2 weeks. Anemia may also be observed. Use with caution in patients with depressed platelet, leukocyte or erythrocyte counts.

May cause delayed pulmonary toxicity (infiltrates and/or fibrosis) which is rare and usually related to cumulative doses >1100 mg/m^2. May be delayed (may occur 6 months or later after treatment and has been reported up to 17 years after childhood administration in combination with radiation therapy). Patients with baseline below 70% of predicted forced vital capacity or carbon monoxide diffusing capacity are in increased risk. Long-term survivors who received nitrosoureas may have late reduction in pulmonary function; this fibrosis may be slowly progressive and has been fatal in some patients. Monitor pulmonary function tests at baseline and frequently throughout treatment. Lomustine is associated with a moderate emetic potential; antiemetics are recommended to prevent nausea and vomiting (Dupuis, 2011). Nausea and omitting may occur 3 to 6 hours after administration and the duration is generally <24 hours; may be reduced if administered on an empty stomach. Stomatitis has also been reported. Reversible hepatotoxicity (transaminase, alkaline phosphatase and bilirubin elevations) has been reported; periodically monitor liver function tests. Renal abnormalities, including azotemia (progressive), decreased kidney size, and renal failure have been reported with large cumulative doses and long-term use. Renal damage has also been observed with lower cumulative doses. Use with caution in patients with renal impairment; may require dosage adjustment; monitor renal function periodically during treatment.

Lomustine should only be administered as a single dose once every 6 weeks; serious and fatal adverse events have occurred when lomustine was inadvertently administered daily. The Institute for Safe Medication Practices (ISMP) recommends that prescribers only prescribe one dose at a time and pharmacies dispense only enough capsules for a single dose; in addition, patients should receive both verbal counseling and written instructions regarding proper dose and administration (ISMP, 2014). Long-term use of nitrosoureas may be associated with the development of secondary malignancies. Acute leukemias and bone marrow dysplasias have been reported follow chronic therapy. Potentially significant drug-drug interactions may exist, requiring dose or frequency adjustment, additional monitoring, and/or selection of alternative therapy. **[U.S. Boxed Warning]: Should be administered under the supervision of an experienced cancer chemotherapy physician.**

Adverse Reactions

Central nervous system: Ataxia, disorientation, lethargy

Dermatologic: Alopecia, skin rash

Gastrointestinal: Stomatitis; nausea and vomiting, usually within 3-6 hours after oral administration. Administration of the dose at bedtime, with an antiemetic, significantly reduces both the incidence and severity of nausea.

Hematologic: Anemia, bone marrow dysplasia, leukemia (acute)

Myelosuppression, common, dose-limiting, may be cumulative and irreversible; leukopenia (nadir: 5-6 weeks; recovery 6-8 weeks); thrombocytopenia (nadir: 4 weeks; recovery 5-6 weeks)

Hepatic: Alkaline phosphatase increased, bilirubin increased, hepatotoxicity, kidney size decreased, transaminases increased

Neuromuscular & skeletal: Dysarthria

Ocular: Blindness, optic atrophy, visual disturbances

Renal: Azotemia (progressive), renal damage, renal failure

Respiratory: Pulmonary fibrosis, pulmonary infiltrates

Drug Interactions

Metabolism/Transport Effects Substrate of CYP2D6 (minor); **Note:** Assignment of Major/Minor substrate status based on clinically relevant drug interaction potential; **Inhibits** CYP2D6 (weak)

Avoid Concomitant Use

Avoid concomitant use of Lomustine with any of the following: BCG; BCG (Intravesical); CloZAPine; Dipyrone; Natalizumab; Pimecrolimus; Tacrolimus (Topical); Tofacitinib; Vaccines (Live)

Increased Effect/Toxicity

Lomustine may increase the levels/effects of: ARIPiprazole; CloZAPine; Leflunomide; Natalizumab; Tofacitinib; Vaccines (Live)

The levels/effects of Lomustine may be increased by: Denosumab; Dipyrone; Pimecrolimus; Roflumilast; Tacrolimus (Topical); Trastuzumab

Decreased Effect

Lomustine may decrease the levels/effects of: BCG; BCG (Intravesical); Coccidioides immitis Skin Test; Sipuleucel-T; Vaccines (Inactivated); Vaccines (Live)

The levels/effects of Lomustine may be decreased by: Echinacea

Storage/Stability Store at room temperature of 25°C (77°F); excursions permitted between 15°C and 30°C (59°F and 86°F). Avoid excessive heat (over 40°C [104°F]). Keep container closed tightly.

Mechanism of Action Inhibits DNA and RNA synthesis via carbamylation of DNA polymerase, alkylation of DNA, and alteration of RNA, proteins, and enzymes

Pharmacokinetics (Adult data unless noted)

Absorption: Rapid and complete absorption from the GI tract (30-60 minutes)

Distribution: Widely distributed; lomustine and/or its metabolites penetrate into the CNS; CSF level is ≥50% of plasma concentration

Metabolism: Rapidly hepatic via hydroxylation producing at least two active metabolites; enterohepatically recycled

Half-life (metabolites): 16-48 hours

Time to peak serum concentration (of active metabolite): Within 3 hours

Elimination: Urine (~50%, as metabolites); feces (<5%); expired air (<10%)

Dosing: Usual Note: At FDA approved dosages, lomustine should only be dispensed and administered as a single dose once every 6 weeks due to delayed myelotoxicity; serious errors have occurred when lomustine was inadvertently administered daily. Repeat courses should only be administered after adequate recovery of leukocytes to >4000/mm^3 and platelets to >100,000/mm^3. Details concerning dosage in combination regimens should also be consulted; dose, frequency, number of doses, and start date may vary by protocol and treatment phase.

Pediatric:

Brain tumors:

General dosing: Manufacturer's labeling: Infants, Children, and Adolescents: Oral: Initial: 130 mg/m^2 as a single dose every 6 weeks (dosage reductions may be recommended for combination chemotherapy regimens)

Compromised marrow function: Reduce initial dose to 100 mg/m^2 as a single dose once every 6 weeks; **Note:** Subsequent doses may require adjustment after initial treatment according to platelet and leukocyte counts.

Medulloblastoma: Children ≥3 years and Adolescents: Limited data available: Oral: 75 mg/m^2 on day 0 of each chemotherapy cycle in combination with cisplatin, vincristine, and radiotherapy (Packer, 2006; Packer, 2013)

Gliomas: Infants, Children, and Adolescents: Limited data available: Oral: 110 mg/m^2 on day 3 of a 6-week cycle in combination with thioguanine, vincristine, and procarbazine for up to 8 cycles for low grade, nonoperable (usually) gliomas (including astrocytomas) (Ater, 2012; Lancaster, 2003; Levin, 2000). For treatment of high grade glioma, 90 mg/m^2 on day 1 every 4 weeks (or repeated when counts recovered) in combination with temozolamide and radiotherapy was used in a Phase I trial of children ≥4 years and adolescents (Jackaki, 2008).

Hodgkin's lymphoma: Infants, Children, and Adolescents: Initial: 130 mg/m^2 as a single dose every 6 weeks (dosage reductions may be recommended for combination chemotherapy regimens): **Note:** Subsequent doses may require adjustment after initial treatment according to platelet and leukocyte counts.

Compromised marrow function: Reduce initial dose to 100 mg/m^2 as a single dose once every 6 weeks

Adult: **Note:** Utilize patient's actual body weight (full weight) for calculation of body surface area- or weight-based dosing, particularly when the intent of therapy is curative; manage regimen-related toxicities in the same manner as for nonobese patients; if a dose reduction is utilized due to toxicity, consider resumption of full weight-based dosing with subsequent cycles, especially if cause of toxicity (eg, hepatic or renal impairment) is resolved (Griggs, 2012).

Brain tumors, Hodgkin's lymphoma: Oral: 130 mg/m^2 as a single dose once every 6 weeks (dosage reductions may be recommended for combination chemotherapy regimens)

Compromised marrow function: Reduce dose to 100 mg/m^2 as a single dose once every 6 weeks

Dosage adjustment based on hematologic response (nadir) for subsequent cycles: Pediatric and Adult patients:

Leukocytes ≥3000/mm^3, platelets ≥75,000/mm^3: No adjustment required

Leukocytes 2000-2999/mm^3, platelets 25,000-74,999/mm^3: Administer 70% of prior dose

Leukocytes <2000/mm^3, platelets <25,000/mm^3 Administer 50% of prior dose

Dosing adjustment in renal impairment: There are no dosage adjustments provided in manufacturer's labeling. The following adjustments have been recommended:

Adults:

Aronoff, 2007:

CrCl >50 mL/minute: No adjustment necessary

CrCl 10-50 mL/minute: Administer 75% of dose

CrCl <10 mL/minute: Administer 25% to 50% of dose

Hemodialysis: Supplemental dose is not necessary

Peritoneal dialysis (PD): Administer 25% to 50% of dose

Kintzel, 1995:

CrCl 46-60 mL/minute: Administer 75% of normal dose

CrCl 31-45 mL/minute: Administer 70% of normal dose

CrCl ≤30 mL/minute: Avoid use

Dosing adjustment in hepatic impairment: There are no dosage adjustments provided in manufacturer's labeling; however, lomustine is hepatically metabolized and caution should be used in patients with hepatic dysfunction.

Administration Hazardous agent; use appropriate precautions for handling and disposal (NIOSH 2014 [group 1]). Do not break capsules; wear impervious gloves when handling; avoid exposure to broken capsules.

Oral: Administer with fluids on an empty stomach and at bedtime; do not administer food or drink for 2 hours after lomustine administration to decrease incidence of nausea and vomiting. Standard antiemetics may be administered prior to lomustine if needed. Varying strengths of capsules may be required to obtain necessary dose.

Monitoring Parameters CBC with differential and platelet count (for at least 6 weeks after dose), hepatic and renal function tests (periodically), pulmonary function tests (baseline and periodically)

Dosage Forms Excipient information presented when available (limited, particularly for generics); consult specific product labeling.

Capsule, Oral:

Gleostine: 10 mg, 40 mg, 100 mg

Generic: 10 mg, 40 mg, 100 mg

- **Lomustinum** *see* Lomustine *on page 1286*
- **Longastatin** *see* Octreotide *on page 1539*
- **Long Lasting Nasal Spray [OTC]** *see* Oxymetazoline (Nasal) *on page 1599*
- **Loniten (Can)** *see* Minoxidil (Systemic) *on page 1443*
- **Loperacap (Can)** *see* Loperamide *on page 1288*

Loperamide (loe PER a mide)

Medication Safety Issues

Sound-alike/look-alike issues:

Imodium® A-D may be confused with Indocin®

Loperamide may be confused with furosemide, Lomotil®

International issues:

Indiaral [France] may be confused with Inderal and Inderal LA brand names for propranolol [U.S., Canada, and multiple international markets]

Lomotil: Brand name for loperamide [Mexico, Philippines], but also the brand name for diphenoxylate [U.S., Canada, and multiple international markets]

Lomotil [Mexico, Phillipines] may be confused with Ludiomil brand name for maprotiline [multiple international markets]

Brand Names: US Anti-Diarrheal [OTC]; Diamode [OTC]; Imodium A-D [OTC]; Loperamide A-D [OTC]

Brand Names: Canada Apo-Loperamide®; Diarr-Eze; Dom-Loperamide; Imodium®; Loperacap; Novo-Loperamide; PMS-Loperamine; Rhoxal-loperamide; Rho®-Loperamine; Riva-Loperamide; Sandoz-Loperamide

Therapeutic Category Antidiarrheal

Generic Availability (US) May be product dependent

Use Treatment of acute diarrhea including traveler's diarrhea (FDA approved in ages ≥2 years and adults; OTC use: FDA approved in ages ≥6 years and adults); treatment of chronic diarrhea associated with inflammatory bowel disease (FDA approved in adults); has also been used for chronic functional diarrhea (idiopathic), chronic diarrhea caused by short bowel syndrome or organic lesions; to decrease the volume of ileostomy discharge; management of antiretroviral-induced diarrhea and irinotecan-induced (late-onset) diarrhea

Pregnancy Risk Factor C

Pregnancy Considerations Teratogenic effects were not observed in animal reproduction studies. Information related to loperamide use in pregnancy is limited and data is conflicting (Einarson, 2000; Källén, 2008). For acute diarrhea in pregnant women, some clinicians recommend oral rehydration and dietary changes; loperamide in small amounts may be used only if symptoms are disabling (Wald, 2003).

Breast-Feeding Considerations Small amounts of loperamide are excreted in human breast milk (information is based on studies using loperamide oxide, the prodrug of loperamide [Nikodem, 1992]). The manufacturer does not recommend use in nursing women.

Contraindications Hypersensitivity to loperamide or any component of the formulation; abdominal pain without diarrhea; children <2 years of age

Avoid use as primary therapy in patients with acute dysentery (bloody stools and high fever), acute ulcerative colitis, bacterial enterocolitis (caused by *Salmonella, Shigella*, and *Campylobacter*), pseudomembranous colitis associated with broad-spectrum antibiotic use

Warnings/Precautions Loperamide is a symptom-directed treatment; if an underlying diagnosis is made, other disease-specific treatment may be indicated. Rare cases of anaphylaxis and anaphylactic shock have been reported. Use is contraindicated if diarrhea is accompanied by high fever or blood in stool. Use caution in young children as response may be variable because of dehydration; contraindicated in children <2 years of age. Concurrent fluid and electrolyte replacement is often necessary in all age groups depending upon severity of diarrhea. Should not be used when inhibition of peristalsis is undesirable or dangerous. Discontinue promptly if constipation, abdominal pain, abdominal distension, blood in stool, or ileus develop. Do not use when peristalsis inhibition should be avoided due to potential for ileus, megacolon, and/or toxic megacolon. Stop therapy in AIDS patients at the first sign of abdominal distention; cases of toxic megacolon have occurred in AIDS patients with infectious colitis (due to viral or bacterial pathogens). Use caution in patients with hepatic impairment due to reduced first-pass metabolism; monitor for signs of CNS toxicity. May cause drowsiness or dizziness, which may impair physical or mental abilities; patients must be cautioned about performing tasks which require mental alertness (eg, operating machinery or driving). Discontinue use and consult health care provider if diarrhea lasts longer than 2 days, symptoms worsen, or abdominal swelling or bulging develops.

Benzyl alcohol and derivatives: Some dosage forms may contain sodium benzoate/benzoic acid; benzoic acid (benzoate) is a metabolite of benzyl alcohol; large amounts of benzyl alcohol (≥99 mg/kg/day) have been associated with a potentially fatal toxicity ("gasping syndrome") in neonates; the "gasping syndrome" consists of metabolic acidosis, respiratory distress, gasping respirations, CNS dysfunction (including convulsions, intracranial hemorrhage), hypotension, and cardiovascular collapse (AAP, 1997; CDC, 1982); some data suggests that benzoate displaces bilirubin from protein binding sites (Ahlfors, 2001); avoid or use dosage forms containing benzyl alcohol derivative with caution in neonates. See manufacturer's labeling.

Warnings: Additional Pediatric Considerations When managing acute dysentary, concurrent fluid and electrolyte replacement is often necessary in all age groups depending upon severity of diarrhea; young pediatric patients are particularly susceptible to dehydration and electrolyte imbalances. Antidiarrheal agents are not recommended as part of the management of acute gastroenteritis in infants and children because they do not address the underlying cause (ie, do not treat the infection) and have a risk of serious adverse events (CDC, 2003). A metaanalysis evaluating the use of loperamide for adjunct treatment of acute bacterial gastroenteritis in pediatric patients identified that infants and children <3 years, malnourished, moderately to severely dehydrated, or those with bloody diarrhea have a higher risk of serious adverse events (ileus, lethargy, death) even at therapeutic doses (≤0.25 mg/kg/day of loperamide) and that the potential benefit of loperamide therapy does not outweigh risks; use should be avoided in this subset of pediatric patients (Li, 2007). The manufacturer recommends to avoid use in infants and children <2 years. Older children with milder infection and adolescents may see benefit from loperamide therapy including decreased duration of diarrhea and stool counts; monitor closely for adverse effects or worsening of infection (CDC, 2003; Li, 2007).

Some dosage forms may contain propylene glycol; in neonates large amounts of propylene glycol delivered orally, intravenously (eg, >3,000 mg/day), or topically have been associated with potentially fatal toxicities which can include metabolic acidosis, seizures, renal failure, and CNS depression; toxicities have also been reported in children and adults including hyperosmolality, lactic acidosis, seizures, and respiratory depression; use caution (AAP, 1997; Shehab, 2009).

Adverse Reactions

Central nervous system: Dizziness

Gastrointestinal: Abdominal cramping, constipation, nausea

Postmarketing and/or case reports: Abdominal distention, abdominal pain, allergic reactions, anaphylactic shock, anaphylactoid reactions, angioedema, bullous eruption (rare), drowsiness, dyspepsia, erythema multiforme (rare), fatigue, flatulence, hypersensitivity, paralytic ileus, megacolon, pruritus, rash, Stevens-Johnson syndrome (rare), toxic epidermal necrolysis (rare), toxic megacolon, urinary retention, urticaria, vomiting, xerostomia

Drug Interactions

Metabolism/Transport Effects **Substrate** of P-glycoprotein

Avoid Concomitant Use There are no known interactions where it is recommended to avoid concomitant use.

Increased Effect/Toxicity

The levels/effects of Loperamide may be increased by: P-glycoprotein/ABCB1 Inhibitors

Decreased Effect

The levels/effects of Loperamide may be decreased by: P-glycoprotein/ABCB1 Inducers

Storage/Stability Store at 20°C to 25°C (68°F to 77°F).

Mechanism of Action Acts directly on circular and longitudinal intestinal muscles, through the opioid receptor, to inhibit peristalsis and prolong transit time; reduces fecal volume, increases viscosity, and diminishes fluid and electrolyte loss; demonstrates antisecretory activity. Loperamide increases tone on the anal sphincter

Pharmacodynamics Onset of action: Within 30-60 minutes

Pharmacokinetics (Adult data unless noted)

Absorption: Rapid; poor; extensive first-pass

Protein binding: 97%

Bioavailability: 0.3%

Metabolism: Hepatic via oxidative N-demethylation to inactive metabolites; primary pathways include CYP2C8, CYP2D6, and CYP3A4

Half-life: Mean range: 14-20 hours

Time to peak serum concentration: Mean range: 4-6 hours

Elimination: Feces (15% to 33%; unchanged drug); urine (1.3%; unchanged drug or metabolites)

Dosing: Usual

Infants, Children, and Adolescents:

Acute diarrhea: Oral: Children ≥2 years and Adolescents: **Note:** For patients small for chronological age, may consider dosing according to weight range and not by age group. Use lowest effective dose for shortest duration.

Children:

2-5 years weighing 13 to <21 kg: Initial: 1 mg with first loose stool followed by 1 mg/dose after each subsequent loose stool; maximum daily dose: 3 mg/**day**

6-8 years weighing 21-27 kg: Initial: 2 mg with first loose stool followed by 1 mg/dose after each subsequent loose stool; maximum daily dose: 4 mg/**day**

9-11 years weighing 27.1-43 kg: Initial: 2 mg with first loose stool followed by 1 mg/dose after each subsequent loose stool; maximum daily dose: 6 mg/**day**

Children ≥12 years and Adolescents: Initial: 4 mg with first loose stool followed by 2 mg/dose after each subsequent loose stool; maximum daily dose: 8 mg/**day**

Chronic diarrhea; secondary to intestinal failure, short-bowel syndrome, or other noninfectious causes: Limited data available; dosing regimens variable: Oral: Infants ≥2 months and Children: 0.08-0.24 mg/kg/day divided 2-3 times/day was reported in a case series of 10 pediatric patients (age range: 2-52 months) (Buts, 1975). In a case-series of six infants and young children, higher dosing was described: Initial: 1-1.5 mg/kg/day in 4 divided doses with subsequent dose decreased as stool output and diet tolerance improved and patient weight increased. Reported final dose range of 0.25-0.5 mg/kg/day in 2 divided doses was used long-term until patient achieved target weight and dietary goals; reported duration of therapy: 6 months to ~2 years (Sandhu, 1983); maximum single dose: 2 mg

Irinotecan-induced (delayed) diarrhea: Limited data available; consult individual protocols; some organizations have used the following:

Fixed dosing (Children's Oncology Group recommendation):

Children ≥2-12 years:

<13 kg: Initial: 0.5 mg after the first loose bowel movement, followed by 0.5 mg every 3 hours while awake; during the night, may administer every 4 hours; maximum daily dose: 4 mg/**day**

13 kg to <20 kg: Initial: 1 mg after the first loose bowel movement, followed by 1 mg every 4 hours; maximum daily dose: 6 mg/**day**

20 kg to <30 kg: Initial: 2 mg after the first loose bowel movement, followed by 1 mg every 3 hours while awake; during the night, may administer every 4 hours; maximum daily dose: 8 mg/**day**

30 kg to <43 kg: Initial: 2 mg after the first loose bowel movement, followed by 1 mg every 2 hours while awake; during the night, may administer every 4 hours; maximum daily dose: 12 mg/**day**

Adolescents weighing ≥43 kg: Initial: 4 mg after the first loose bowel movement, followed by 2 mg after each loose stool; maximum daily dose: 16 mg/**day**

Weight-based dosing: Children and Adolescents 2 to <15 years (Vassal, 2007):

Grade 1 or 2: 0.03 mg/kg/dose every 4 hours

Grade 3 or 4: 0.06 mg/kg/dose every 4 hours

Maximum single dose dependent upon weight

<13 kg: 0.5 mg

13 to <20 kg: 1 mg

20 to <43 kg: Initial: 2 mg; subsequent doses: 1 mg

≥43 kg: Initial: 4 mg; subsequent doses: 2 mg

Adults:

Acute diarrhea: Oral: Initial: 4 mg, followed by 2 mg after each loose stool, up to 16 mg/day

Chronic diarrhea: Oral: Initial: Follow acute diarrhea; maintenance dose should be slowly titrated downward to minimum required to control symptoms (typically, 4-8 mg/day in divided doses)

Traveler's diarrhea: Oral: Initial: 4 mg after first loose stool, followed by 2 mg after each subsequent stool (maximum dose: 8 mg/day)

Dosing adjustment in renal impairment: No adjustment required.

Dosing adjustment in hepatic impairment: There are no dosage adjustments provided in the manufacturer labeling. Due to possible effects on first-pass metabolism, use with caution and monitor closely for signs of CNS toxicity.

Administration Oral: Drink plenty of fluids to help prevent dehydration

Dosage Forms Excipient information presented when available (limited, particularly for generics); consult specific product labeling.

Capsule, Oral, as hydrochloride:

Generic: 2 mg

Liquid, Oral, as hydrochloride:

Imodium A-D: 1 mg/7.5 mL (120 mL, 240 mL) [contains brilliant blue fcf (fd&c blue #1), fd&c yellow #10 (quinoline yellow), propylene glycol, sodium benzoate]

Imodium A-D: 1 mg/7.5 mL (30 mL, 120 mL, 240 mL, 360 mL) [contains brilliant blue fcf (fd&c blue #1), fd&c yellow #10 (quinoline yellow), propylene glycol, sodium benzoate; mint flavor]

Generic: 1 mg/5 mL (5 mL, 10 mL, 118 mL)

Suspension, Oral, as hydrochloride:

Generic: 1 mg/7.5 mL (120 mL)

Tablet, Oral, as hydrochloride:

Anti-Diarrheal: 2 mg

Anti-Diarrheal: 2 mg [scored]

Anti-Diarrheal: 2 mg [contains brilliant blue fcf (fd&c blue #1), fd&c yellow #10 (quinoline yellow)]

Anti-Diarrheal: 2 mg [scored; contains brilliant blue fcf (fd&c blue #1), fd&c yellow #10 (quinoline yellow)]

Anti-Diarrheal: 2 mg [contains fd&c blue #1 aluminum lake, fd&c yellow #10 (quinoline yellow)]

Diamode: 2 mg [scored]

Imodium A-D: 2 mg [scored; contains brilliant blue fcf (fd&c blue #1), fd&c yellow #10 (quinoline yellow)]

Imodium A-D: 2 mg [scored; contains fd&c blue #1 aluminum lake, fd&c yellow #10 aluminum lake]

Loperamide A-D: 2 mg

Tablet Chewable, Oral, as hydrochloride:

Imodium A-D: 2 mg [contains fd&c blue #1 aluminum lake, fd&c yellow #10 aluminum lake; cool mint flavor]

◆ **Loperamide A-D [OTC]** *see* Loperamide *on page 1288*

◆ **Loperamide Hydrochloride** *see* Loperamide *on page 1288*

Lopinavir and Ritonavir

(loe PIN a veer & ri TOE na vir)

Medication Safety Issues

Sound-alike/look-alike issues:

Potential for dispensing errors between Kaletra and Keppra (levETIRAcetam)

High alert medication:

This medication is in a class the Institute for Safe Medication Practices (ISMP) includes among its list of drug classes that have a heightened risk of causing significant patient harm when used in error.

Administration issues:

Children's doses are based on weight and calculated by milligrams of lopinavir. Care should be taken to accurately calculate the dose. The oral solution contains lopinavir 80 mg and ritonavir 20 mg per one mL. Children <12 years of age (and ≤40 kg) who are not taking certain concomitant antiretroviral medications will receive <5 mL of solution per dose.

Related Information

Adult and Adolescent HIV *on page 2392*

Oral Medications That Should Not Be Crushed or Altered *on page 2476*

Pediatric HIV *on page 2380*

Perinatal HIV *on page 2400*

Brand Names: US Kaletra

Brand Names: Canada Kaletra

Therapeutic Category Antiretroviral Agent; HIV Agents (Anti-HIV Agents); Protease Inhibitor

Generic Availability (US) No

Use Treatment of HIV infection in combination with other antiretroviral agents (FDA approved in ages ≥14 days and adults); **Note:** HIV regimens consisting of three antiretroviral agents are strongly recommended.

Medication Guide Available Yes

Pregnancy Considerations Adverse events were not seen in animal reproduction studies, except at doses which were also maternally toxic. Lopinavir/ritonavir has a low level of transfer across the human placenta. Based on information collected by the Antiretroviral Pregnancy Registry, an increased risk of teratogenic effects has not been observed in humans. A small increased risk of preterm birth has been associated with maternal use of protease inhibitor-based combination antiretroviral (ARV) therapy during pregnancy; however, the benefits of use generally outweigh this risk and protease inhibitors (PIs) should not be withheld if otherwise recommended. Hyperglycemia, new onset of diabetes mellitus, or diabetic ketoacidosis have been reported with PIs; it is not clear if pregnancy increases this risk.

The HHS Perinatal HIV Guidelines consider lopinavir/ritonavir to be a preferred protease inhibitor for use in antiretroviral-naive pregnant women. Lopinavir/ritonavir is not recommended for use in pregnant women with lopinavir-resistance-associated amino acid substitutions. In addition, once-daily dosing is not recommended during pregnancy and use of the oral solution should be avoided (due to alcohol and propylene glycol content).

Regardless of CD4 count or HIV RNA copy number, all HIV-infected pregnant women should receive a combination antiretroviral ARV drug regimen. A combination of antepartum, intrapartum, and infant ARV prophylaxis is recommended. ARV therapy should be started as soon as possible in women with symptomatic infection. Although earlier initiation may be more effective in reducing the perinatal transmission of HIV, initiation may be delayed until after 12 weeks gestation in women who do not require immediate treatment after careful consideration of maternal conditions (eg, nausea and vomiting) and the potential risks of first trimester fetal exposure for specific agents. A scheduled cesarean delivery at 38 weeks gestation is recommended for all women with HIV RNA >1000 copies/mL or unknown concentrations near delivery in order to decrease transmission. If ARV therapy must be interrupted for <24 hours during the peripartum period, stop then restart all medications simultaneously in order to decrease the chance of developing resistance. Long-term follow-up is recommended for all infants exposed to ARV medications. In couples who want to conceive, the HIV-infected partner should attain maximum viral suppression prior to conception.

Health care providers are encouraged to enroll pregnant women exposed to antiretroviral medications in the Antiretroviral Pregnancy Registry (1-800-258-4263 or www.APRegistry.com). Health care providers caring for HIV-infected women and their infants may contact the National Perinatal HIV Hotline (888-448-8765) for clinical consultation (HHS [perinatal], 2014).

Breast-Feeding Considerations Lopinavir/ritonavir concentrations are very low to undetectable in breast milk and undetectable in the serum of nursing infants. Maternal or infant antiretroviral therapy does not completely eliminate the risk of postnatal HIV transmission. In addition, multiclass-resistant virus has been detected in breast-feeding infants despite maternal therapy. Therefore, in the United States, where formula is accessible, affordable, safe, and sustainable, and the risk of infant mortality due to diarrhea and respiratory infections is low, complete avoidance of breast-feeding by HIV-infected women is recommended to decrease potential transmission of HIV (HHS [perinatal], 2014).

Contraindications

Hypersensitivity (eg, toxic epidermal necrolysis, Stevens-Johnson syndrome, erythema multiforme, urticaria, angioedema) to lopinavir, ritonavir, or any component of the formulation; coadministration with drugs that are highly dependent on CYP3A for clearance and for which elevated plasma concentrations are associated with serious and/or life-threatening reactions; coadministration with the potent CYP3A inducers (where significantly decreased lopinavir levels may be associated with a potential for loss of virologic response and resistance and cross-resistance to develop): Alfuzosin, cisapride, ergot derivatives (eg, dihydroergotamine, ergotamine, methylergonovine), lovastatin, oral midazolam, pimozide, rifampin, sildenafil (when used to treat pulmonary arterial hypertension), simvastatin, St John's wort, and triazolam.

Canadian labeling: Additional contraindications (not in US labeling): Coadministration with fusidic acid, midazolam, salmeterol, vardenafil, astemizole (not available in Canada), terfenadine (not available in Canada)

Warnings/Precautions Potentially significant drug-drug interactions may exist, requiring dose or frequency adjustment, additional monitoring, and/or selection of alternative therapy. Cases of pancreatitis, some fatal, have been associated with lopinavir/ritonavir; use caution in patients with a history of pancreatitis or advanced HIV-1 disease (may be at increased risk). Patients with signs or symptoms of pancreatitis should be evaluated and therapy suspended as clinically appropriate. May alter cardiac conduction and prolong the QTc and/or PR interval; second and third degree AV block and torsade de pointes have been observed. Possible higher risk of myocardial infarction associated with the cumulative use of lopinavir/ritonavir. Use with caution in patients with underlying structural heart disease, preexisting conduction system abnormalities, ischemic heart disease or cardiomyopathies. Avoid use in combination with QTc- or PR-interval prolonging drugs or in patients with hypokalemia or congenital long QT syndrome.

Changes in glucose tolerance, hyperglycemia, exacerbation of diabetes, DKA, and new-onset diabetes mellitus have been reported in patients receiving protease inhibitors. May cause hepatitis or exacerbate pre-existing hepatic dysfunction; use with caution in patients with hepatitis B or C and in hepatic disease; patients with hepatitis or elevations in transaminases prior to the start of therapy may be at increased risk for further increases in transaminases or hepatic dysfunction (rare fatalities reported postmarketing). Consider more frequent liver function test monitoring during therapy initiation in patients with pre-existing hepatic dysfunction. Large increases in total cholesterol and triglycerides have been reported; screening should be done prior to therapy and periodically throughout treatment. Increased bleeding may be seen in patients with hemophilia A or B who are taking protease inhibitors. Redistribution or accumulation of body fat has been observed in patients using antiretroviral therapy. Patients may develop immune reconstitution syndrome resulting in the occurrence of an inflammatory response to an indolent or residual opportunistic infection during initial HIV treatment or activation of autoimmune disorders (eg, Graves' disease, polymyositis, Guillain-Barré syndrome) later in therapy; further evaluation and treatment may be required.

The oral solution is highly concentrated and contains large amounts of alcohol. Monitor patients with renal impairment or with decreased ability to metabolize propylene glycol (eg, patients of Asian origin) for propylene glycol toxicity. Health care providers should pay special attention to accurate calculation, measurement, and administration of dose. Overdose in a child may lead to lethal ethanol or propylene glycol toxicity. Oral solution also contains fructose; consider fructose content in patients with fructose intolerance. Once-daily dosing is not recommended in patients with ≥3 lopinavir-resistance-associated substitutions; those receiving efavirenz, nevirapine, or nelfinavir, carbamazepine, phenobarbital, phenytoin, or in children <18 years of age. Safety, efficacy, and pharmacokinetic profiles of lopinavir and ritonavir have not been established for neonates <14 days of age. Neonates <14 days of age, particularly preterm neonates, are at risk for developing propylene glycol toxicity with use of the lopinavir/ritonavir oral solution. Oral solution contains ethanol and propylene glycol; ethanol competitively inhibits propylene glycol metabolism. Postmarketing reports in preterm neonates following use of the oral solution include cardiotoxicity (complete AV block, bradycardia, cardiomyopathy), lactic acidosis, CNS depression, respiratory complications, acute renal failure, and death. The oral solution should not be used in the immediate postnatal period, including full term neonates age <14 days or preterm neonates until 14 days after their due date, unless the infant is closely monitored and benefits clearly outweigh risk.

Warnings: Additional Pediatric Considerations Serious cardiac, renal, CNS, or respiratory problems have been reported in preterm neonates receiving lopinavir/ritonavir oral solution. The oral solution contains 42.4% ethanol (v/v) and 15.3% propylene glycol (w/v). Ethanol competitively inhibits propylene glycol metabolism, which may lead to propylene glycol toxicity due to impaired elimination in neonates. Preterm neonates are at an increased risk of adverse events from propylene glycol toxicity, including cardiotoxicity (complete AV block, bradycardia, cardiomyopathy), lactic acidosis, CNS depression, respiratory complications, acute renal failure, and death. Do not use oral solution in neonates if the patient is either PNA <14 days old or PMA <42 weeks. Toxicities have been reported with the use of products containing propylene glycol in all ages, including hyperosmolality, lactic acidosis, seizures, and respiratory depression. Due to concentration of ethanol in oral solution, an overdose in a child may cause potentially lethal alcohol toxicity. Treatment for overdose should be supportive and include general poisoning management; activated charcoal may help remove unabsorbed medication; dialysis unlikely to be of benefit; however, dialysis can remove alcohol and propylene glycol. In neonates and infants 14 days to 6 months of age, the total amounts of ethanol and propylene glycol delivered from all medications should be considered to avoid toxicity. Neonates and young infants should be closely monitored for increases in serum osmolality, serum creatinine, and other signs of propylene glycol toxicity (eg CNS depression, seizures, cardiac arrhythmias, hemolysis); in neonates particularly, symptoms should be distinguished from sepsis.

A fatal accidental overdose occurred in a 2.1 kg, 44-day old infant (born at 30 weeks gestational age) with HIV who received a single dose of 6.5 mL of lopinavir/ritonavir oral solution. The infant died of cardiogenic shock 9 days later. Health care providers are reminded that lopinavir/ritonavir oral solution is highly concentrated. To minimize the risk for medication errors, health care providers should pay special attention to accurate calculation of the dose, transcription of the medication order, dispensing information, dosing instructions, and proper measurement of the dose. New pediatric tablets containing lopinavir 100 mg and ritonavir 25 mg (ie, 12 the amount in regular tablets) are now available; caution should be taken so that dosing and dispensing errors do not occur.

May cause diarrhea (5% to 28%; children: 12%); in one adult study, incidence of diarrhea was higher in patients receiving once-daily dosing compared to twice-daily dosing. Children may have a higher incidence of vomiting (21% vs ≤6%). May cause taste perversion in children (incidence: 22%).

Adverse Reactions Data presented for short- and long-term combination antiretroviral therapy in both protease inhibitor experienced and naïve patients.

Cardiovascular: Vasodilation

Central nervous system: Anxiety, fatigue (including weakness), headache, insomnia

Dermatologic: Skin infection (including cellulitis, folliculitis, furuncle), skin rash (more common in children)

Endocrine & metabolic: Alteration in sodium (children), hypercholesterolemia, hyperglycemia, hypertriglyceridemia, hyperuricemia, increased gamma-glutamyl transferase, increased serum triglycerides, weight loss

Gastrointestinal: Abdominal pain, diarrhea, dysgeusia (more common in children), dyspepsia, flatulence, gastroenteritis, increased serum amylase, increased serum lipase, nausea, vomiting (more common in children)

Hematologic & oncologic: Neutropenia, thrombocytopenia (children)

Hepatic: Hepatitis (including increased AST, ALT, and gamma-glutamyl transferase), increased serum ALT, increased serum AST, increased serum bilirubin (more common in children)

Hypersensitivity: Hypersensitivity (including urticaria and angioedema)

Neuromuscular & skeletal: Musculoskeletal pain, weakness

Respiratory: Lower respiratory tract infection, upper respiratory tract infection

Rare but important or life-threatening: Acne vulgaris, alopecia, amenorrhea, amnesia, anemia, anorexia, asthma, atherosclerotic disease, atrial fibrillation, atrioventricular block (second and third degree), atrophic striae, bacterial infection, benign neoplasm, bradycardia, brain disease, breast hypertrophy, bronchitis, cerebral infarction, cerebrovascular accident, cholangitis, cholecystitis, confusion, Cushing's syndrome, cyst, decreased creatine clearance, decreased glucose tolerance, deep vein thrombosis, dehydration, depression, dermal ulcer, diabetes mellitus, duodenitis, dyskinesia, eczema, edema, enteritis, enterocolitis, erythema multiforme, exfoliative dermatitis, extrapyramidal reaction, facial paralysis, fecal incontinence, first degree atrioventricular block, gastritis, gastroesophageal reflux disease, gastrointestinal hemorrhage, gastrointestinal ulcer, gynecomastia, hematuria, hemorrhagic colitis, hemorrhoids, hepatic insufficiency, hepatomegaly, hyperacusis, hyperhidrosis, hypermenorrhea, hypersensitivity reaction, hypertension, hypertonia, hypogonadism (males), hypophosphatemia, hypothyroidism, immune reconstitution syndrome, impotence, jaundice, lactic acidosis, leukopenia, lipoma, liver steatosis, liver tenderness, lymphadenopathy, maculopapular rash, migraine, myocardial infarction, neoplasm, nephritis, neuropathy, obesity, oral mucosa ulcer, orthostatic hypotension, osteonecrosis, otitis media, pancreatitis, periodontitis, peripheral edema, peripheral neuropathy, prolonged Q-T interval on ECG, propylene glycol toxicity (preterm neonates [includes cardiomyopathy, lactic acidosis, acute renal failure, respiratory complications]), pulmonary edema, rectal hemorrhage, redistribution of body fat (including facial wasting), renal failure, rhabdomyolysis, seborrhea, seizure, sialadenitis, skin discoloration, splenomegaly, Stevens-Johnson syndrome, stomatitis, thrombophlebitis, torsades de pointes, tricuspid regurgitation, vasculitis, viral infection, vitamin deficiency, weight gain

Drug Interactions

Metabolism/Transport Effects Refer to individual components.

Avoid Concomitant Use

Avoid concomitant use of Lopinavir and Ritonavir with any of the following: Ado-Trastuzumab Emtansine; Alfuzosin; Amiodarone; Amodiaquine; Apixaban; Astemizole; Atovaquone; Avanafil; Axitinib; Barnidipine; Bosutinib; Cabozantinib; Ceritinib; Cisapride; Clarithromycin; Conivaptan; Crizotinib; Dapoxetine; Darunavir; Dasabuvir; Disulfiram; Domperidone; Dronedarone; Enzalutamide; Eplerenone; Ergot Derivatives; Etravirine; Everolimus; Flecainide; Fluticasone (Nasal); Fosamprenavir; Fusidic Acid (Systemic); Halofantrine; Highest Risk QTc-Prolonging Agents; Ibrutinib; Irinotecan; Isavuconazonium Sulfate; Ivabradine; Lapatinib; Lercanidipine; Lomitapide; Lovastatin; Lurasidone; Macitentan; Mequitazine; Methadone; MetroNIDAZOLE (Systemic); Midazolam; Mifepristone; Moderate Risk QTc-Prolonging Agents; Naloxegol; Nilotinib; NiMODipine; Nisoldipine; Olaparib; Palbociclib; PAZOPanib; Pimozide; Propafenone; QuiNIDine; QuiNINE; Ranolazine; Red Yeast Rice; Regorafenib; Rifampin; Rivaroxaban; Salmeterol; Saquinavir; Silodosin; Simeprevir; Simvastatin; St Johns Wort; Suvorexant; Tamoxifen; Tamsulosin; Telaprevir; Terfenadine; Thioridazine; Ticagrelor; Tipranavir; Tolvaptan; Topotecan; Toremifene; Trabectedin; TraZODone; Triazolam; Ulipristal; Vemurafenib; VinCRIStine (Liposomal); Vorapaxar; Voriconazole

Increased Effect/Toxicity

Lopinavir and Ritonavir may increase the levels/effects of: Ado-Trastuzumab Emtansine; Afatinib; Alfuzosin; Almotriptan; Alosetron; ALPRAZolam; Amiodarone; Amodiaquine; Apixaban; ARIPiprazole; Astemizole; AtoMOXetine; AtorvaSTATin; Avanafil; Axitinib; Barnidipine; Bosentan; Bosutinib; Brentuximab Vedotin; Brinzolamide; Budesonide (Nasal); Budesonide (Systemic, Oral Inhalation); Budesonide (Topical); Cabazitaxel; Cabozantinib; Calcium Channel Blockers (Dihydropyridine); Calcium Channel Blockers (Nondihydropyridine); Cannabis; Ceritinib; Cilostazol; Cisapride; Clarithromycin; Colchicine; Conivaptan; Contraceptives (Progestins); Corticosteroids (Orally Inhaled); Corticosteroids (Systemic); Crizotinib; Cyclophosphamide; CycloSPORINE (Systemic); CYP2C8 Substrates; CYP2D6 Substrates; CYP3A4 Substrates; Dabigatran Etexilate; Dapoxetine; Dasabuvir; Dasatinib; Digoxin; Disulfiram; Domperidone; DOXOrubicin (Conventional); Dronabinol; Dronedarone; Dutasteride; Edoxaban; Eluxadoline; Elvitegravir; Enfuvirtide; Enzalutamide; Eplerenone; Ergot Derivatives; Erlotinib; Estazolam; Etizolam; Everolimus; FentaNYL; Fesoterodine; Flecainide; Fluticasone (Nasal); Fluticasone (Oral Inhalation); Fusidic Acid (Systemic); GuanFACINE; Halofantrine; Highest Risk QTc-Prolonging Agents; Hydrocodone; Ibrutinib; Idelalisib; Imatinib; Imidafenacin; Irinotecan; Isavuconazonium Sulfate; Itraconazole; Ivabradine; Ivacaftor; Ixabepilone; Ketoconazole (Systemic); Lacosamide; Lapatinib; Ledipasvir; Lercanidipine; Levobupivacaine; Levomilnacipran; Linagliptin; Lomitapide; Lovastatin; Lurasidone; Macitentan; Maraviroc; Meperidine; Mequitazine; MethylPREDNISolone; Metoprolol; MetroNIDAZOLE (Systemic); Midazolam; Naloxegol; Nebivolol; Nefazodone; Nelfinavir; Nilotinib; NiMODipine; Nintedanib; Nisoldipine; Olaparib; Ospemifene; Oxybutynin; OxyCODONE; Palbociclib; Parecoxib; Paricalcitol; PAZOPanib; P-glycoprotein/ABCB1 Substrates; Pimecrolimus; Pimozide; Pioglitazone; PONATinib; Pranlukast; PrednisoLONE (Systemic); PredniSONE; Propafenone; Protease Inhibitors; Prucalopride; QuiNIDine; QuiNINE; Ramelteon; Ranolazine; Red Yeast Rice; Regorafenib; Retapamulin; Rifabutin; Rifaximin; Rilpivirine; Riociguat; Rivaroxaban; Rosuvastatin; Ruxolitinib; Salmeterol; Saxagliptin; Sildenafil; Silodosin; Simeprevir; Simvastatin; Suvorexant; Tacrolimus (Systemic); Tacrolimus (Topical); Tadalafil; Tamsulosin; Tasimelteon; Temsirolimus; Tenofovir; Terfenadine; Tetrahydrocannabinol; Thioridazine; Ticagrelor; Tofacitinib; Tolterodine; Tolvaptan; Topotecan; Toremifene; Trabectedin; TraMADol; TraZODone; Treprostinil; Triamcinolone (Systemic); Triazolam; Ulipristal; Vardenafil; Vemurafenib; Vilazodone; VinBLAStine; VinCRIStine; VinCRIStine (Liposomal); Vorapaxar; Vortioxetine; Zopiclone

The levels/effects of Lopinavir and Ritonavir may be increased by: ARIPiprazole; Clarithromycin; Delavirdine; Enfuvirtide; Fusidic Acid (Systemic); Ivabradine; Ketoconazole (Systemic); Methadone; MetroNIDAZOLE (Topical); Mifepristone; Moderate Risk QTc-Prolonging Agents; P-glycoprotein/ABCB1 Inhibitors; QTc-Prolonging Agents (Indeterminate Risk and Risk Modifying); QuiNINE; Rifabutin; Rifampin; Saquinavir; Simeprevir

Decreased Effect

Lopinavir and Ritonavir may decrease the levels/effects of: Abacavir; Antidiabetic Agents; Atovaquone; Boceprevir; BuPROPion; Canagliflozin; Clarithromycin; Codeine; Contraceptives (Estrogens); Contraceptives (Progestins); CYP2C19 Substrates; Darunavir; Deferasirox; Delavirdine; Didanosine; Etravirine; Fosamprenavir; Fosphenytoin; Hydrocodone; Ifosfamide; LamoTRIgine; Meperidine; Methadone; Phenytoin; Prasugrel; Proguanil; QuiNINE; Tamoxifen; Telaprevir; Ticagrelor; TraMADol; Valproic Acid and Derivatives; Voriconazole; Warfarin; Zidovudine

The levels/effects of Lopinavir and Ritonavir may be decreased by: Boceprevir; Bosentan; CarBAMazepine; CYP3A4 Inducers (Moderate); CYP3A4 Inducers (Strong); Dabrafenib; Efavirenz; Fosamprenavir; Fosphenytoin; Garlic; Mitotane; Nelfinavir; Nevirapine; PHENobarbital; Phenytoin; Rifampin; Siltuximab; St Johns Wort; Tipranavir; Tocilizumab

Food Interactions Moderate- to high-fat meals increase the C_{max} and AUC of lopinavir/ritonavir oral solution; no significant changes observed with oral tablets. Management: Take oral solution with food; take tablet with or without food.

Storage/Stability

Oral solution: Store at 2°C to 8°C (36°F to 46°F). Avoid exposure to excessive heat. If stored at room temperature (25°C or 77°F), use within 2 months.

Tablet: Store at USP controlled room temperature of 20°C to 25°C (68°F to 77°F). Exposure to high humidity outside of the original container for >2 weeks is not recommended.

Mechanism of Action A coformulation of lopinavir and ritonavir. The lopinavir component binds to the site of HIV-1 protease activity and inhibits the cleavage of viral Gag-Pol polyprotein precursors into individual functional proteins required for infectious HIV. This results in the formation of immature, noninfectious viral particles. The ritonavir component inhibits the CYP3A metabolism of lopinavir, allowing increased plasma levels of lopinavir.

Pharmacokinetics (Adult data unless noted) Information below refers to Lopinavir; see Ritonavir for additional information.

Protein binding: 98% to 99%; binds to both $alpha_1$ - acid glycoprotein and albumin; higher affinity for $alpha_1$-acid glycoprotein; decreased protein binding in patients with mild to moderate hepatic impairment

Metabolism: Primarily oxidative, via cytochrome P450 CYP3A isoenzyme; 13 oxidative metabolites identified; may induce its own metabolism

Bioavailability: Absolute bioavailability not established; AUC for oral solution was 22% lower than capsule when given under fasting conditions; concentrations were similar under nonfasting conditions

Half-life: Mean: 5 to 6 hours

Elimination: 2.2% of dose eliminated unchanged in urine; 83% of dose eliminated in feces

Clearance: (Apparent oral): 6 to 7 L/hour

Dialysis: Unlikely to remove significant amounts of drug (due to high protein binding)

Dosing: Neonatal HIV infection, treatment: Oral: Use in combination with other antiretroviral agents: **Note:** Dosage is based on patient body weight or surface area and is presented here based on lopinavir component. **Once daily dosing has not been studied in neonates, and therefore, is not recommended.**

PNA <14 days or PMA <42 weeks: Do not use due to potential toxicity from excipients; no data about appropriate dose or safety exists (DHHS [pediatric], 2014)

PNA ≥14 days and PMA ≥42 weeks:

Patients receiving concomitant antiretroviral therapy ***without efavirenz, fosamprenavir, nelfinavir, or nevirapine:***

Manufacturer's labeling: Lopinavir 16 mg/kg/dose or 300 mg/m²/dose twice daily

AIDS*Info* guidelines (DHHS [pediatric], 2014): Lopinavir 300 mg/m²/dose twice daily

Note: Neonates who receive the 300 mg/m²/dose twice daily may have lower serum trough concentrations compared to adults; evaluate neonates and adjust dose for incremental growth at frequent intervals (DHHS [pediatric], 2014).

Patients receiving concomitant antiretroviral therapy ***with efavirenz, fosamprenavir, nelfinavir, or nevirapine:*** Dosage information does not exist; lopinavir/ritonavir is not recommended in neonates who are receiving these agents.

Dosing: Usual

Pediatric: **HIV infection, treatment:** Oral: Use in combination with other antiretroviral agents: **Note:** Pediatric dosage is based on patient body weight or surface area and is presented here based on lopinavir component. **Do not exceed recommended adult dose.** Use of tablets in patients <15 kg or <0.6 m² is **not** recommended (use oral solution). **Once daily dosing in pediatric patients is not recommended**; in a study of treatment experienced children, once daily dosing resulted in a lower trough concentration and less virological control (Foissac, 2011)

Infants 1 to 6 months:

Patients receiving concomitant antiretroviral therapy ***without efavirenz, fosamprenavir, nelfinavir, or nevirapine:*** Lopinavir 16 mg/kg/dose or 300 mg/m²/dose twice daily. **Note:** Infants who receive 300 mg/m²/dose twice daily may have lower trough concentrations compared to adults; evaluate infants and adjust dose for incremental growth at frequent intervals (DHHS [pediatric], 2014).

Patients receiving concomitant antiretroviral therapy ***with efavirenz, fosamprenavir, nelfinavir, or nevirapine:*** Dosage information does not exist; lopinavir/ritonavir is not recommended in infants ≤6 months of age who are receiving these agents.

Infants >6 months, Children, and Adolescents:

Patients receiving concomitant antiretroviral therapy ***without efavirenz, fosamprenavir, nelfinavir, or nevirapine:***

BSA-directed dosing:

Manufacturer's labeling: Lopinavir 230 mg/m²/dose twice daily; maximum dose: 400 mg/dose

Alternate fixed dosing for patients who are able to swallow tablets:

BSA ≥0.6 to <0.9 m²: Lopinavir 200 mg twice daily

BSA ≥0.9 to <1.4 m²: Lopinavir 300 mg twice daily

BSA ≥1.4 m²: Lopinavir 400 mg twice daily

AIDS*Info* guidelines (DHHS [pediatric], 2014):

Infants >6 to 12 months: Lopinavir 300 mg/m²/dose twice daily; **Note:** Infants who receive 300 mg/m²/dose twice daily may have lower trough concentrations compared to adults; evaluate infants and adjust dose for incremental growth at frequent intervals

Children and Adolescents >12 months to 18 years:

Antiretroviral-naïve: Lopinavir 230 mg/m²/dose (maximum dose: 400 mg) twice daily; others have suggested 300 mg/m²/dose twice daily if the oral solution is used. **Note:** For patients already receiving lopinavir and ritonavir, an immediate dosage reduction at 12 months of age is **not** recommended; patients are allowed to "grow into" the 230 mg/m²/dose dosage as they gain weight over time.

Antiretroviral-experienced or suspected decreased sensitivity to lopinavir: Lopinavir 300 mg/m²/dose (maximum dose: 400 mg) twice daily

Weight-directed dosing:

<15 kg: Lopinavir 12 mg/kg/dose twice daily

≥15 to 40 kg: Lopinavir 10 mg/kg/dose twice daily

>40 kg: Lopinavir 400 mg twice daily

Fixed dosing for patients who are able to swallow tablets: AIDS*Info* guidelines (DHHS [pediatric], 2014):

Antiretroviral-naïve: Weight band dosing to give ~230 mg/m²/dose:

≥15 to 25 kg: Lopinavir 200 mg twice daily

>25 to 35 kg: Lopinavir 300 mg twice daily

>35 kg: Lopinavir 400 mg twice daily

Antiretroviral-experienced or suspected decreased sensitivity to lopinavir: Weight band dosing to give ~300 mg/m²/dose:

15 to 20 kg: 200 mg twice daily

>20 to 30 kg: 300 mg twice daily

>30 to 45 kg: 400 mg twice daily

>45 kg: 400 mg or 500 mg twice daily

Patients receiving concomitant antiretroviral therapy ***with efavirenz, fosamprenavir, nelfinavir, or nevirapine*** *(or treatment-experienced patients not receiving these agents who have suspected decreased susceptibility to lopinavir):*

BSA-directed dosing:

Manufacturer's labeling: Lopinavir 300 mg/m²/dose twice daily; maximum single lopinavir dose: Oral solution: 533 mg; Tablet: 500 mg

Alternative dosing for patients who are able to swallow tablets:

BSA ≥0.6 to <0.8 m^2: Lopinavir 200 mg twice daily

BSA ≥0.8 to < 1.2 m^2: Lopinavir 300 mg twice daily

BSA ≥1.2 to < 1.7 m^2: Lopinavir 400 mg twice daily

BSA ≥1.7 m^2: Lopinavir 500 mg twice daily; **Note:** Therapy-experienced patients in whom decreased susceptibility to lopinavir is suspected or confirmed may receive lopinavir 600 mg twice daily (DHHS [pediatric], 2014).

AIDS*Info* guidelines (DHHS [pediatric], 2014): Lopinavir 300 mg/m^2/dose twice daily; maximum single lopinavir dose: Oral solution: 533 mg; Tablet: 500 mg

Weight-directed dosing:

<15 kg: Lopinavir 13 mg/kg/dose twice daily

≥15 to 45 kg: Lopinavir 11 mg/kg/dose twice daily

>45 kg:

Oral solution: Lopinavir 533 mg (6.5 mL) twice daily

Tablets: Lopinavir 500 mg twice daily

Fixed dosing for patients who are able to swallow tablets:

≥15 to 20 kg: Lopinavir 200 mg twice daily

>20 to 30 kg: Lopinavir 300 mg twice daily

>30 to 45 kg: Lopinavir 400 mg twice daily

>45 kg: Lopinavir 400 mg or 500 mg twice daily; **Note:** Therapy-experienced patients in whom decreased susceptibility to lopinavir is suspected or confirmed may receive lopinavir 600 mg twice daily (DHHS [pediatric], 2014).

Adult: **HIV infection, treatment:** Oral: Use in combination with other antiretroviral agents:

*Patients receiving concomitant antiretroviral therapy **without efavirenz, fosamprenavir, nelfinavir, or nevirapine:***

Therapy-naïve or therapy-experienced: Lopinavir 400 mg/ritonavir 100 mg twice daily.

Once-daily dosing: **Antiretroviral-naïve patients or experienced patients with <3 lopinavir resistance-associated amino acid substitutions in protease enzyme**: Lopinavir 800 mg/ritonavir 200 mg once daily

Note: Once daily dosing is **not** recommended for antiretroviral-experienced patients with ≥3 lopinavir-resistance-associated substitutions (L10F/I/R/V, K20M/N/R, L24I, L33F, M36I, I47V, G48V, I54L/T/V, V82A/C/F/S/T, and I84V), or for patients receiving efavirenz, fosamprenavir, nelfinavir, nevirapine, carbamazepine, phenobarbital, or phenytoin; once daily dosing has not been evaluated with concurrent use of indinavir or saquinavir

*Dosing adjustment for combination therapy **with efavirenz, fosamprenavir, nelfinavir, or nevirapine: Note:*** Once daily dosing is **not** recommended:

Oral solution: Lopinavir 533 mg/ritonavir 133 mg (6.5 mL) twice daily

Tablets: Lopinavir 500 mg/ritonavir 125 mg twice daily

Dosing adjustment in renal impairment: Has not been studied in patients with renal impairment; however, a decrease in clearance is not expected. Avoid once daily dosing in patients on hemodialysis (DHHS [adult], 2014).

Dosing adjustment in hepatic impairment: Lopinavir AUC may be increased ~30% in patients with mild to moderate hepatic impairment; use with caution. No data available in patients with severe impairment.

Administration Oral:

Oral solution: Administer with food to enhance bioavailability and decrease kinetic variability; use a calibrated oral dosing syringe to measure and administer the oral solution; **Note:** Dose must be accurately measured and administered to pediatric patients as oral solution is very concentrated and a fatal accidental overdose has been reported

Methods to improve poor palatability of the oral solution include numbing the taste buds with ice chips before or after drug administration, or administering the medication with sweet or tangy foods, chocolate syrup, or peanut butter to help mask the taste; flavoring the solution prior to dispensing may also help improve palatability (DHHS [pediatric], 2014).

Tablets: May be administered without regard to meals; swallow tablets whole, do not crush, break, or chew; crushing tablets was shown to decrease AUC of lopinavir and ritonavir by 45% and 47%, respectively (Best, 2011)

Monitoring Parameters Note: Monitor CD4 percentage (if <5 years of age) or CD4 count (if ≥5 years of age) at least every 3 to 4 months (DHHS [pediatric], 2014).

Prior to initiation of therapy: Genotypic resistance testing, CD4 and viral load (every 3 to 4 months), CBC with differential, LFTs, BUN, creatinine, electrolytes, glucose, urinalysis (every 6 to 12 months), and assessment of readiness for adherence with medication regimen. At initiation and with any change in treatment regimen: CBC with differential, electrolytes, calcium, phosphate, glucose, LFTs, bilirubin, urinalysis (at initiation), BUN, creatinine, albumin, total protein, lipid panel (at initiation), CD4, and viral load. After 1 to 2 weeks of therapy: Signs of medication toxicity and adherence. After 2 to 4 weeks of therapy: CBC with differential, viral load, signs of medication toxicity, and adherence; then every 3 to 4 months: CBC with differential, electrolytes, glucose, LFTs, bilirubin, BUN, creatinine, CD4, viral load, signs of medication toxicity, and adherence. Every 6 to 12 months: Lipid panel and urinalysis. CD4 monitoring frequency may be decreased to every 6 to 12 months in children who are adherent to therapy if the value is well above the threshold for opportunistic infections, viral suppression is sustained, and the clinical status is stable for more than 2 to 3 years (DHHS [pediatric], 2014). Monitor for growth and development, signs of HIV-specific physical conditions, HIV disease progression, opportunistic infections or pancreatitis.

Due to potential toxicity from excipients in the oral solution, in pediatric patients 14 days to 6 months of age, the total amounts of ethanol and propylene glycol delivered from all medications should be monitored to avoid toxicity. Neonates and young infants should be closely monitored for increases in serum osmolality, serum creatinine, and other signs of propylene glycol toxicity (eg, CNS depression, seizures, cardiac arrhythmias, hemolysis); in neonates particularly, symptoms should be distinguished from sepsis.

Reference Range Plasma trough concentration: Lopinavir: ≥1000 ng/mL (DHHS [adult, pediatric], 2014)

Additional Information Preliminary studies have reported response rates (defined as viral loads <400 copies/mL) of 91%, 81%, and 33% for patients with 0 to 5, 6 to 7, and 8 to 10 protease mutations at baseline, respectively (Hurst, 2000).

Dosage Forms Excipient information presented when available (limited, particularly for generics); consult specific product labeling.

Solution, oral:

Kaletra: Lopinavir 80 mg and ritonavir 20 mg per 1 mL (160 mL) [contains ethanol 42.4%, menthol, propylene glycol; cotton candy flavor]]

Tablet:

Kaletra:

Lopinavir 100 mg and ritonavir 25 mg

Lopinavir 200 mg and ritonavir 50 mg

◆ **Lopresor (Can)** *see* Metoprolol *on page 1418*

- ◆ **Lopresor SR (Can)** *see* Metoprolol *on page 1418*
- ◆ **Lopressor** *see* Metoprolol *on page 1418*
- ◆ **Loprox** *see* Ciclopirox *on page 458*
- ◆ **Loradamed [OTC]** *see* Loratadine *on page 1296*

Loratadine (lor AT a deen)

Medication Safety Issues

Sound-alike/look-alike issues:

Claritin may be confused with clarithromycin

Claritin (loratadine) may be confused with Claritin Eye (ketotifen)

Lorcaserin hydrochloride may be confused with lorcaserin hydrochloride

BEERS Criteria medication:

This drug may be potentially inappropriate for use in geriatric patients (Quality of evidence - varies based on comorbidity; Strength of recommendation - varies based on comorbidity)

Brand Names: US Alavert [OTC]; Allergy Relief For Kids [OTC]; Allergy Relief [OTC]; Allergy [OTC]; Childrens Loratadine [OTC]; Claritin Reditabs [OTC]; Claritin [OTC]; Loradamed [OTC]; Loratadine Childrens [OTC]; Loratadine Hives Relief [OTC]; QlearQuil 24 Hour Relief [OTC]; Triaminic Allerchews [OTC]

Brand Names: Canada Apo-Loratadine; Claritin®; Claritin® Kids

Therapeutic Category Antihistamine

Generic Availability (US) May be product dependent

Use Symptomatic relief of nasal and non-nasal symptoms of allergic rhinitis (OTC product: FDA approved in ages ≥2 years and adults); has also been used for the treatment of chronic idiopathic urticaria

Pregnancy Considerations Maternal use of loratadine has not been associated with an increased risk of major malformations. The use of antihistamines for the treatment of rhinitis during pregnancy is generally considered to be safe at recommended doses. Although safety data is limited, loratadine may be the preferred second generation antihistamine for the treatment of rhinitis or urticaria during pregnancy.

Breast-Feeding Considerations Small amounts of loratadine and its active metabolite, desloratadine, are excreted into breast milk.

Contraindications Hypersensitivity to loratadine or any component of the formulation

Warnings/Precautions Use with caution in patients with liver or renal impairment. Hepatic impairment increases systemic exposure. Some products may contain phenylalanine. May be inappropriate in older adults depending on comorbidities (eg, dementia, delirium) due to its potent anticholinergic effects (Beers Criteria). Effects may be potentiated when used with other sedative drugs or ethanol.

Benzyl alcohol and derivatives: Some dosage forms may contain sodium benzoate/benzoic acid; benzoic acid (benzoate) is a metabolite of benzyl alcohol; large amounts of benzyl alcohol (≥99 mg/kg/day) have been associated with a potentially fatal toxicity ("gasping syndrome") in neonates; the "gasping syndrome" consists of metabolic acidosis, respiratory distress, gasping respirations, CNS dysfunction (including convulsions, intracranial hemorrhage), hypotension, and cardiovascular collapse (AAP, 1997; CDC, 1982); some data suggests that benzoate displaces bilirubin from protein binding sites (Ahlfors, 2001); avoid or use dosage forms containing benzyl alcohol derivative with caution in neonates. See manufacturer's labeling.

Warnings: Additional Pediatric Considerations Safety and efficacy for the use of cough and cold products in pediatric patients <4 years of age is limited; the AAP warns against the use of these products for respirator illnesses in this age group. Serious adverse effects includ ing death have been reported. Many of these product contain multiple active ingredients, increasing the risk c accidental overdose when used with other products. Th FDA notes that there are no approved OTC uses for thes products in pediatric patients <2 years of age. Health car providers are reminded to ask caregivers about the use o OTC cough and cold products in order to avoid exposur to multiple medications containing the same ingredien (AAP 2012; FDA 2008).

Adverse Reactions

Central nervous system: Fatigue, headache, malaise nervousness, somnolence

Dermatologic: Rash

Gastrointestinal: Abdominal pain, stomatitis, xerostomia

Neuromuscular & skeletal: Hyperkinesia

Ocular: Conjunctivitis

Respiratory: Dysphonia, epistaxis, pharyngitis, upper respiratory infection, wheezing

Miscellaneous: Flu-like syndrome, viral infection

Rare but important or life-threatening: Abnormal hepatic function, agitation, alopecia, altered lacrimation, altered micturition, altered salivation, altered taste, amnesia anaphylaxis, angioneurotic edema, anorexia, arthralgia, back pain, blepharospasm, blurred vision, breast enlargement, breast pain, bronchospasm, chest pain, confusion, depression, dizziness, dysmenorrhea, dyspnea, erythema multiforme, hemoptysis, hepatic necrosis, hepatitis, hypotension, impaired concentration, impotence, insomnia, irritability, jaundice, menorrhagia, migraine, nausea, palpitation, paresthesia, paroniria, peripheral edema, photosensitivity, pruritus, purpura, rigors, seizure, supraventricular tachyarrhythmia, syncope, tachycardia, tremor, urinary discoloration, urticaria, thrombocytopenia, vaginitis, vertigo, vomiting, weight gain

Drug Interactions

Metabolism/Transport Effects Substrate of CYP2D6 (minor), CYP3A4 (minor), P-glycoprotein; **Note:** Assignment of Major/Minor substrate status based on clinically relevant drug interaction potential; **Inhibits** CYP2C19 (weak), CYP2C8 (weak), CYP2D6 (weak)

Avoid Concomitant Use

Avoid concomitant use of Loratadine with any of the following: Aclidinium; Amodiaquine; Azelastine (Nasal); Eluxadoline; Glucagon; Ipratropium (Oral Inhalation); Orphenadrine; Paraldehyde; Potassium Chloride; Thalidomide; Tiotropium; Umeclidinium

Increased Effect/Toxicity

Loratadine may increase the levels/effects of: AbobotulinumtoxinA; Alcohol (Ethyl); Amodiaquine; Analgesics (Opioid); Anticholinergic Agents; ARIPiprazole; Azelastine (Nasal); Buprenorphine; CNS Depressants; Eluxadoline; Glucagon; Hydrocodone; Methotrimeprazine; Metyrosine; Mirabegron; Mirtazapine; OnabotulinumtoxinA; Orphenadrine; Paraldehyde; Potassium Chloride; Pramipexole; RimabotulinumtoxinB; ROPINIRole; Rotigotine; Selective Serotonin Reuptake Inhibitors; Suvorexant; Thalidomide; Thiazide Diuretics; Tiotropium; Topiramate; Zolpidem

The levels/effects of Loratadine may be increased by: Aclidinium; Amiodarone; Brimonidine (Topical); Cannabis; Doxylamine; Dronabinol; Droperidol; HydrOXYzine; Ipratropium (Oral Inhalation); Kava Kava; Magnesium Sulfate; Methotrimeprazine; Mianserin; Nabilone; Perampanel; P-glycoprotein/ABCB1 Inhibitors; Pramlintide; Rufinamide; Sodium Oxybate; Tapentadol; Tetrahydrocannabinol; Umeclidinium

Decreased Effect

Loratadine may decrease the levels/effects of: Acetylcholinesterase Inhibitors; Benzylpenicilloyl Polylysine;

Betahistine; Hyaluronidase; Itopride; Metoclopramide; Secretin

The levels/effects of Loratadine may be decreased by: Acetylcholinesterase Inhibitors; Amphetamines; P-glycoprotein/ABCB1 Inducers

Food Interactions Food increases bioavailability and delays peak. Management: Administer without regard to meals.

Storage/Stability Store at 20°C to 25°C (68°F to 77°F).
Rapidly-disintegrating tablets: Use within 6 months of opening foil pouch, and immediately after opening individual tablet blister. Store in a dry place.

Mechanism of Action Long-acting tricyclic antihistamine with selective peripheral histamine H_1-receptor antagonistic properties

Pharmacodynamics
Onset of action: Within 1 to 3 hours (Claritin prescribing information 2000)
Maximum effect: 8 to 12 hours (Claritin prescribing information 2000)
Duration: >24 hours (Claritin prescribing information 2000)

Pharmacokinetics (Adult data unless noted) Note: The pharmacokinetic profile of children 2 to 12 years is similar to that of adults (Claritin prescribing information 2000)
Absorption: Rapid; food increases total bioavailability (AUC) by 40% to 48% (Claritin prescribing information 2000)
Distribution: Vd: 119 L/kg (Haria 1994); binds preferentially to peripheral nervous system H_1 receptors; no appreciable entry into CNS (Claritin prescribing information 2000)
Protein binding: 97% to 99% (loratadine), 73% to 76% (metabolite) (Haria 1994)
Metabolism: Extensive first-pass metabolism by cytochrome P450 system (3A4) to an active metabolite (descarboethoxyloratadine) (Claritin prescribing information 2000)
Half-life: 8.4 hours (range 3 to 20 hours) (loratadine), 28 hours (range 8.8 to 92 hours) (metabolite) (Claritin prescribing information 2000)
Time to peak serum concentration: Loratadine: 1.3 hours (loratadine), 2.3 hours (metabolite) (Claritin prescribing information 2000)
Elimination: 80% eliminated via urine & feces as metabolic products (Claritin prescribing information 2000)

Dosing: Usual
Pediatric:
Allergic symptoms/rhinitis: Oral
Children 2 to <6 years: Oral liquid or chewable tablet: 5 mg once daily
Children ≥6 years and Adolescents:
Oral liquid, capsule, tablet, or chewable tablet: 10 mg once daily
Dispersible tablet: 5 mg twice daily or 10 mg once daily
Chronic idiopathic urticaria: Limited data available (Kliegman 2011; Simons 1994):
Children 2 to 12 years: 5 mg once daily
Adolescents: 10 mg once daily
Adult:
Allergic symptoms/rhinitis: Oral:
Oral liquid, capsule, tablet, or chewable tablet: 10 mg daily once daily
Dispersible tablet: 5 mg twice daily or 10 mg once daily
Dosing adjustment in renal impairment: There are no dosage adjustments provided in manufacturer's labeling; however, the following recommendations have been recommended (Aronoff 2007):
Children ≥2 years and Adolescents: No dosage adjustment necessary for any degree of renal impairment.
Adults:
CrCl >50 mL/minute: No adjustment necessary
CrCl 10 to 50 mL/minute: 10 mg every 24 to 48 hours.
CrCl <10 mL/minute: 10 mg every 48 hours.
Continuous renal replacement therapy (CRRT): No dosage adjustment necessary if clearance is 2,000 mL/minute.
Dosing adjustment in hepatic impairment: There are no dosage adjustments provided in manufacturer's labeling.

Administration Oral: Administer without regard to meals
Rapidly disintegrating tablet: Place rapidly disintegrating tablet) on the tongue; tablet disintegration occurs rapidly; may administer with or without water

Monitoring Parameters Improvement in signs and symptoms of allergic rhinitis or chronic idiopathic urticaria

Test Interactions May suppress the wheal and flare reactions to skin test antigens

Dosage Forms Excipient information presented when available (limited, particularly for generics); consult specific product labeling.
Capsule, Oral:
Claritin: 10 mg [contains brilliant blue fcf (fd&c blue #1)]
Solution, Oral:
Childrens Loratadine: 5 mg/5 mL (120 mL) [alcohol free, dye free, sugar free; contains propylene glycol, sodium benzoate; grape flavor]
Loratadine Childrens: 5 mg/5 mL (120 mL) [alcohol free, dye free, sugar free; contains propylene glycol, sodium benzoate; fruit flavor]
Loratadine Hives Relief: 5 mg/5 mL (120 mL) [alcohol free, dye free, sugar free; contains propylene glycol, sodium benzoate; grape flavor]
Syrup, Oral:
Allergy Relief: 5 mg/5 mL (236 mL) [alcohol free; contains propylene glycol, sodium benzoate]
Allergy Relief For Kids: 5 mg/5 mL (120 mL) [contains propylene glycol, sodium benzoate; fruit flavor]
Childrens Loratadine: 5 mg/5 mL (120 mL) [fruit flavor]
Childrens Loratadine: 5 mg/5 mL (120 mL) [alcohol free, dye free; contains propylene glycol, sodium benzoate, sodium metabisulfite; grape flavor]
Claritin: 5 mg/5 mL (60 mL, 120 mL, 150 mL) [alcohol free, color free, dye free, sugar free; contains edetate disodium, propylene glycol, sodium benzoate; grape flavor]
Loratadine Childrens: 5 mg/5 mL (120 mL) [sugar free; contains polyethylene glycol, propylene glycol, sodium benzoate, sodium metabisulfite; grape flavor]
Tablet, Oral:
Alavert: 10 mg
Allergy: 10 mg
Allergy Relief: 10 mg
Claritin: 10 mg
Loradamed: 10 mg
QlearQuil 24 Hour Relief: 10 mg
Generic: 10 mg
Tablet Chewable, Oral:
Claritin: 5 mg [contains aspartame, fd&c blue #2 aluminum lake; grape flavor]
Tablet Dispersible, Oral:
Alavert: 10 mg [contains aspartame]
Alavert: 10 mg [contains aspartame; bubble-gum flavor]
Alavert: 10 mg [contains aspartame; citrus flavor]
Allergy: 10 mg [contains aspartame; fruit flavor]
Allergy Relief: 10 mg [contains aspartame]
Allergy Relief: 10 mg [contains aspartame; fruit flavor]
Claritin Reditabs: 5 mg, 10 mg
Triaminic Allerchews: 10 mg

◆ **Loratadine-D 12 Hour [OTC]** *see* Loratadine and Pseudoephedrine *on page 1298*

Loratadine and Pseudoephedrine

(lor AT a deen & soo doe e FED rin)

Medication Safety Issues

Sound-alike/look-alike issues:

Claritin-D® may be confused with Claritin-D® 24

Claritin-D® 24 may be confused with Claritin-D®

Related Information

Oral Medications That Should Not Be Crushed or Altered *on page 2476*

Brand Names: US Alavert™ Allergy and Sinus [OTC]; Claritin-D® 12 Hour Allergy & Congestion [OTC]; Claritin-D® 24 Hour Allergy & Congestion [OTC]; Loratadine-D 12 Hour [OTC]

Brand Names: Canada Chlor-Tripolon ND®; Claritin® Extra; Claritin® Liberator

Therapeutic Category Antihistamine/Decongestant Combination

Generic Availability (US) Yes

Use Symptomatic relief of symptoms of seasonal allergic rhinitis and nasal congestion (OTC product: FDA approved in ages ≥12 years and adults). **Note:** Approved ages and uses for generic products may vary; consult labeling for specific information.

Contraindications Hypersensitivity to loratadine, pseudoephedrine, or any component of the formulation; use with or within 14 days of MAO inhibitors

Warnings/Precautions Use with caution in hypertension, diabetes mellitus, ischemic heart disease, increased intraocular pressure, hyperthyroidism, and prostatic hyperplasia. Use with caution in the elderly; may be more sensitive to adverse effects. Patients with swallowing difficulties (eg, upper GI narrowing or abnormal esophageal peristalsis) should not use Claritin-D® 24-Hour. Use caution with hepatic or renal impairment; dose adjustment may be required. When used for self medication (OTC), notify healthcare provider if symptoms do not improve within 7 days or are accompanied by fever. Discontinue and contact healthcare provider if nervousness, dizziness or sleeplessness occur. Effects may be potentiated when used with other sedative drugs or ethanol.

Warnings: Additional Pediatric Considerations Safety and efficacy for the use of cough and cold products in pediatric patients <4 years of age is limited; the AAP warns against the use of these products for respiratory illnesses in this age group. Serious adverse effects including death have been reported (in some cases, high blood concentrations of pseudoephedrine were found). Many of these products contain multiple active ingredients, increasing the risk of accidental overdose when used with other products. The FDA notes that there are no approved OTC uses for these products in pediatric patients <2 years of age. Health care providers are reminded to ask caregivers about the use of OTC cough and cold products in order to avoid exposure to multiple medications containing the same ingredient (AAP 2012; FDA 2008).

Adverse Reactions See individual agents.

Drug Interactions

Metabolism/Transport Effects Refer to individual components.

Avoid Concomitant Use

Avoid concomitant use of Loratadine and Pseudoephedrine with any of the following: Aclidinium; Amodiaquine; Azelastine (Nasal); Eluxadoline; Ergot Derivatives; Glucagon; Iobenguane I 123; Ipratropium (Oral Inhalation); MAO Inhibitors; Orphenadrine; Paraldehyde; Potassium Chloride; Thalidomide; Tiotropium; Umeclidinium

Increased Effect/Toxicity

Loratadine and Pseudoephedrine may increase the levels/effects of: AbobotulinumtoxinA; Alcohol (Ethyl); Amodiaquine; Analgesics (Opioid); Anticholinergic Agents; ARIPiprazole; Azelastine (Nasal); Buprenorphine; CNS Depressants; Eluxadoline; Glucagon; Hydrocodone; Methotrimeprazine; Metyrosine; Mirabegron; Mirtazapine; OnabotulinumtoxinA; Orphenadrine; Paraldehyde; Potassium Chloride; Pramipexole; RimabotulinumtoxinB; ROPINIRole; Rotigotine; Selective Serotonin Reuptake Inhibitors; Suvorexant; Sympathomimetics; Thalidomide; Thiazide Diuretics; Tiotropium; Topiramate; Zolpidem

The levels/effects of Loratadine and Pseudoephedrine may be increased by: Aclidinium; Alkalinizing Agents; Amiodarone; AtoMOXetine; Brimonidine (Topical); Cannabis; Carbonic Anhydrase Inhibitors; Doxylamine; Dronabinol; Droperidol; Ergot Derivatives; HydrOXYzine; Ipratropium (Oral Inhalation); Kava Kava; Linezolid; Magnesium Sulfate; MAO Inhibitors; Methotrimeprazine; Mianserin; Nabilone; Perampanel; P-glycoprotein/ABCB1 Inhibitors; Pramlintide; Rufinamide; Serotonin/Norepinephrine Reuptake Inhibitors; Sodium Oxybate; Tapentadol; Tedizolid; Tetrahydrocannabinol; Umeclidinium

Decreased Effect

Loratadine and Pseudoephedrine may decrease the levels/effects of: Acetylcholinesterase Inhibitors; Benzylpenicilloyl Polylysine; Betahistine; FentaNYL; Hyaluronidase; Iobenguane I 123; Itopride; Metoclopramide; Secretin

The levels/effects of Loratadine and Pseudoephedrine may be decreased by: Acetylcholinesterase Inhibitors; Alpha1-Blockers; Amphetamines; P-glycoprotein/ABCB1 Inducers; Spironolactone; Urinary Acidifying Agents

Food Interactions See individual agents.

Pharmacokinetics (Adult data unless noted) See individual agents.

Dosing: Usual

Pediatric: **Seasonal allergic rhinitis/nasal decongestion:** Oral: Children ≥12 years and Adolescents:

12-hour formulation (loratadine 5 mg and pseudoephedrine 120 mg): 1 tablet every 12 hours

24-hour formulation (loratadine 10 mg and pseudoephedrine 240 mg): 1 tablet once daily

Adult: **Seasonal allergic rhinitis/nasal congestion:** Oral:

12-hour formulation (loratadine 5 mg and pseudoephedrine 120 mg): 1 tablet every 12 hours

24-hour formulation (loratadine 10 mg and pseudoephedrine 240 mg): 1 tablet once daily

Dosing adjustment in renal impairment: Children ≥12 years, Adolescents, and Adults: Recommended dosing from previous FDA approved labeling (Claritin D prescribing information 1998)

CrCl ≥30 mL/minute: No adjustment necessary

CrCl <30 mL/minute

12-hour formulation: 1 tablet every 24 hours

24-hour formulation: 1 tablet every other day

Dosing adjustment in hepatic impairment: There are no dosage adjustments provided in manufacturer's labeling; however, hepatic impairment increases loratadine systemic exposure; use with caution and dosage adjustment should be considered. Previous FDA approved labeling recommended to avoid use in patients with hepatic impairment (Claritin D prescribing information 1998).

Administration Oral: Administer on an empty stomach or before meals; swallow extended release tablets whole, do not chew or crush

Monitoring Parameters Improvement in signs and symptoms of allergic rhinitis or nasal congestion

Test Interactions See individual agents.

Dosage Forms Excipient information presented when available (limited, particularly for generics); consult specific product labeling.

Tablet, extended release: Loratadine 10 mg and pseudoephedrine sulfate 240 mg

Alavert™ Allergy and Sinus: Loratadine 5 mg and pseudoephedrine sulfate 120 mg
Claritin-D® 12 Hour Allergy & Congestion: Loratadine 5 mg and pseudoephedrine sulfate 120 mg [contains calcium 30 mg/tablet]
Claritin-D® 24 Hour Allergy & Congestion: Loratadine 10 mg and pseudoephedrine sulfate 240 mg [contains calcium 25 mg/tablet]
Loratadine-D 12 Hour: Loratadine 5 mg and pseudoephedrine sulfate 120 mg

◆ **Loratadine Childrens [OTC]** *see* Loratadine *on page 1296*

◆ **Loratadine Hives Relief [OTC]** *see* Loratadine *on page 1296*

LORazepam (lor A ze pam)

Medication Safety Issues

Sound-alike/look-alike issues:

LORazepam may be confused with ALPRAZolam, clonazePAM, diazepam, KlonoPIN, Lovaza, temazepam, zolpidem

Ativan may be confused with Ambien, Atarax, Atgam, Avitene

BEERS Criteria medication:

This drug may be potentially inappropriate for use in geriatric patients (Quality of evidence - high; Strength of recommendation - strong).

Administration issues:

Injection dosage form contains propylene glycol. Monitor for toxicity when administering continuous lorazepam infusions.

Related Information

Preprocedure Sedatives in Children *on page 2444*

Prevention of Chemotherapy-Induced Nausea and Vomiting in Children *on page 2368*

Brand Names: US Ativan; LORazepam Intensol

Brand Names: Canada Apo-Lorazepam; Ativan; Dom-Lorazepam; Lorazepam Injection, USP; PHL-Lorazepam; PMS-Lorazepam; PRO-Lorazepam; Teva-Lorazepam

Therapeutic Category Antianxiety Agent; Anticonvulsant, Benzodiazepine; Antiemetic; Benzodiazepine; Hypnotic; Sedative

Generic Availability (US) Yes

Use

Oral: Management of anxiety disorders, short-term relief of symptoms of anxiety, anxiety associated with depressive symptoms (All indications: FDA approved in ages ≥12 years and adults); has also been used for preprocedure sedation

Parenteral: Treatment of status epilepticus (FDA approved in adults); preoperative sedation, anxiolytic and amnestic (FDA approved in adults); has also been used for breakthrough nausea and vomiting associated with chemotherapy

Pregnancy Risk Factor D

Pregnancy Considerations Teratogenic effects have been observed in some animal reproduction studies. Lorazepam and its metabolite cross the human placenta. Teratogenic effects in humans have been observed with some benzodiazepines (including lorazepam); however, additional studies are needed. The incidence of premature birth and low birth weights may be increased following maternal use of benzodiazepines; hypoglycemia and respiratory problems in the neonate may occur following exposure late in pregnancy. Neonatal withdrawal symptoms may occur within days to weeks after birth and "floppy infant syndrome" (which also includes withdrawal symptoms) have been reported with some benzodiazepines (including lorazepam). Elimination of lorazepam in the newborn infant is slow; following *in utero* exposure, term infants may excrete lorazepam for up to 8 days (Bergman 1992; Iqbal 2002; Wikner 2007).

Breast-Feeding Considerations Lorazepam can be detected in breast milk. Drowsiness, lethargy, or weight loss in nursing infants have been observed in case reports following maternal use of some benzodiazepines (Iqbal 2002). Breast-feeding is not recommended by the manufacturer.

Contraindications

Hypersensitivity to lorazepam, any component of the formulation, or other benzodiazepines (cross-sensitivity with other benzodiazepines may exist); acute narrow-angle glaucoma; sleep apnea (parenteral); intra-arterial injection of parenteral formulation; severe respiratory insufficiency (except during mechanical ventilation)

Canadian labeling: Additional contraindications (not in U.S. labeling): Myasthenia gravis

Warnings/Precautions Use with caution in elderly or debilitated patients, patients with hepatic disease (including alcoholics) or renal impairment. In older adults, benzodiazepines increase the risk of impaired cognition, delirium, falls, fractures, and motor vehicle accidents. Due to increased sensitivity in this age group, avoid use for treatment of insomnia, agitation, or delirium. (Beers Criteria). Use with caution in patients with respiratory disease (COPD or sleep apnea) or limited pulmonary reserve, or impaired gag reflex. Initial doses in elderly or debilitated patients should be at the lower end of the dosing range. May worsen hepatic encephalopathy.

Causes CNS depression (dose-related) resulting in sedation, dizziness, confusion, or ataxia which may impair physical and mental capabilities. Patients must be cautioned about performing tasks which require mental alertness (eg, operating machinery or driving). Effects may be potentiated when used with other sedative drugs or ethanol. Potentially significant drug-drug interactions may exist, requiring dose or frequency adjustment, additional monitoring, and/or selection of alternative therapy. Benzodiazepines have been associated with falls and traumatic injury and should be used with extreme caution in patients who are at risk of these events.

Lorazepam may cause anterograde amnesia. Paradoxical reactions, including hyperactive or aggressive behavior have been reported with benzodiazepines, particularly in adolescent/pediatric or psychiatric patients. Does not have analgesic, antidepressant, or antipsychotic properties.

Preexisting depression may worsen or emerge during therapy. Not recommended for use in primary depressive or psychotic disorders. Should not be used in patients at risk for suicide without adequate antidepressant treatment. Risk of dependence increases in patients with a history of alcohol or drug abuse and those with significant personality disorders; use with caution in these patients. Tolerance, psychological and physical dependence may also occur with higher dosages and prolonged use. The risk of dependence is decreased with short-term treatment (2 to 4 weeks); evaluate the need for continued treatment prior to extending therapy duration. Benzodiazepines have been associated with dependence and acute withdrawal symptoms on discontinuation or reduction in dose. Acute withdrawal, including seizures, may be precipitated after administration of flumazenil to patients receiving long-term benzodiazepine therapy. Lorazepam is a short half-life benzodiazepine. Tolerance develops to the sedative, hypnotic, and anticonvulsant effects. It does not develop to the anxiolytic effects (Vinkers 2012). Chronic use of this agent may increase the perioperative benzodiazepine dose needed to achieve desired effect.

As a hypnotic agent, should be used only after evaluation of potential causes of sleep disturbance. Failure of sleep disturbance to resolve after 7 to 10 days may indicate psychiatric or medical illness. A worsening of insomnia or the emergence of new abnormalities of thought or behavior may represent unrecognized psychiatric or medical illness and requires immediate and careful evaluation.

Status epilepticus should not be treated with injectable benzodiazepines alone; requires close observation and management and possibly ventilatory support. When used as a component of preanesthesia, monitor for heavy sedation and airway obstruction; equipment necessary to maintain airway and ventilatory support should be available. Parenteral formulation of lorazepam contains polyethylene glycol which has resulted in toxicity during high-dose and/or longer-term infusions. Parenteral formulation also contains propylene glycol (PG); may be associated with dose-related toxicity and can occur ≥48 hours after initiation of lorazepam. Limited data suggest increased risk of PG accumulation at doses of ≥6 mg/hour for 48 hours or more (Nelson 2008). Monitor for signs of toxicity which may include acute renal failure, lactic acidosis, and/or osmol gap. May consider using enteral delivery of lorazepam tablets to decrease the risk of PG toxicity (Lugo 1999).

Benzyl alcohol and derivatives: Some dosage forms may contain benzyl alcohol; large amounts of benzyl alcohol (≥99 mg/kg/day) have been associated with a potentially fatal toxicity ("gasping syndrome") in neonates; the "gasping syndrome" consists of metabolic acidosis, respiratory distress, gasping respirations, CNS dysfunction (including convulsions, intracranial hemorrhage), hypotension, and cardiovascular collapse (AAP 1997; CDC 1982); some data suggests that benzoate displaces bilirubin from protein binding sites (Ahlfors 2001); avoid or use dosage forms containing benzyl alcohol with caution in neonates. See manufacturer's labeling.

Warnings: Additional Pediatric Considerations Use with caution in neonates, especially in preterm infants; several cases of neurotoxicity and myoclonus (rhythmic myoclonic jerking) have been reported. Paradoxical reactions, including hyperactive or aggressive behavior, have been reported with benzodiazepines, particularly in pediatric/adolescent or psychiatric patients; discontinue drug if this occurs.

Some dosage forms may contain propylene glycol; in neonates large amounts of propylene glycol delivered orally, intravenously (eg, >3,000 mg/day), or topically have been associated with potentially fatal toxicities which can include metabolic acidosis, seizures, renal failure, and CNS depression; toxicities have also been reported in children and adults including hyperosmolality, lactic acidosis, seizures, and respiratory depression; use caution (AAP, 1997; Shehab, 2009).

Adverse Reactions

Cardiovascular: Hypotension

Central nervous system: Aggressive behavior, agitation, akathisia, amnesia, anxiety, central nervous system stimulation, coma, disinhibition, disorientation, dizziness, drowsiness, dysarthria, euphoria, excitement, extrapyramidal reaction, fatigue, headache, hostility, hypothermia, irritability, mania, memory impairment, outbursts of anger, psychosis, sedation, seizures, sleep apnea (exacerbation), sleep disturbances, slurred speech, stupor, suicidal behavior, suicidal ideation, unsteadiness, vertigo

Dermatologic: Alopecia, skin rash

Gastrointestinal: Changes in appetite, constipation

Endocrine & metabolic: Change in libido, hyponatremia, SIADH

Genitourinary: Impotence, orgasm disturbance

Hematologic & oncologic: Agranulocytosis, pancytopenia, thrombocytopenia

Hepatic: Increased serum alkaline phosphatase, increased serum bilirubin, increased serum transaminases, jaundice

Hypersensitivity: Anaphylaxis, anaphylactoid reaction, hypersensitivity reaction

Local: Erythema at injection site, pain at injection site

Neuromuscular & skeletal: Weakness

Ophthalmic: Visual disturbances (including diplopia and blurred vision)

Respiratory: Apnea, exacerbation of obstructive pulmonary disease, hypoventilation, nasal congestion, respiratory depression, respiratory failure, worsening of sleep apnea

Rare but important or life-threatening: Abnormal gait, abnormal hepatic function tests, abnormality in thinking, acidosis, cardiac arrhythmia, ataxia, blood coagulation disorder, bradycardia, cardiac arrest, cardiac failure, cerebral edema, confusion, convulsions, cystitis, decreased mental acuity, delirium, depression, drug dependence (with prolonged use), drug toxicity (polyethylene glycol or propylene glycol poisoning [prolonged IV infusion]), excessive crying, gastrointestinal hemorrhage, hallucinations, hearing loss, heart block, hematologic abnormality, hepatotoxicity, hypertension, hyperventilation, hyporeflexia, infection, injection site reaction, myoclonus, neuroleptic malignant syndrome, paralysis, pericardial effusion, pheochromocytoma (aggravation), pneumothorax, pulmonary edema, pulmonary hemorrhage, pulmonary hypertension, seizure, tachycardia, urinary incontinence, ventricular arrhythmia, withdrawal syndrome

Drug Interactions

Metabolism/Transport Effects None known.

Avoid Concomitant Use

Avoid concomitant use of LORazepam with any of the following: Azelastine (Nasal); Methadone; OLANZapine; Orphenadrine; Paraldehyde; Sodium Oxybate; Thalidomide

Increased Effect/Toxicity

LORazepam may increase the levels/effects of: Alcohol (Ethyl); Azelastine (Nasal); Buprenorphine; CloZAPine; CNS Depressants; Fosphenytoin; Hydrocodone; Methadone; Methotrimeprazine; Metyrosine; Mirtazapine; Orphenadrine; Paraldehyde; Phenytoin; Pramipexole; ROPINIRole; Rotigotine; Selective Serotonin Reuptake Inhibitors; Sodium Oxybate; Suvorexant; Thalidomide; Zolpidem

The levels/effects of LORazepam may be increased by: Brimonidine (Topical); Cannabis; Doxylamine; Dronabinol; Droperidol; HydrOXYzine; Kava Kava; Loxapine; Magnesium Sulfate; Methotrimeprazine; Nabilone; OLANZapine; Perampanel; Probenecid; Rufinamide; Tapentadol; Teduglutide; Tetrahydrocannabinol; Valproic Acid and Derivatives

Decreased Effect

The levels/effects of LORazepam may be decreased by: Theophylline Derivatives; Yohimbine

Storage/Stability

Parenteral: Intact vials should be refrigerated (room temperature storage information may be available; contact product manufacturer to obtain current recommendations). Protect from light. Do not use discolored or precipitate-containing solutions. Parenteral admixture is stable at room temperature (25°C) for 24 hours.

Oral concentrate: Store at colder room temperature or refrigerate at 2°C to 8°C (36°F to 46°F). Discard open bottle after 90 days.

Oral tablet: Store at 25°C (77°F); excursions are permitted between 15°C and 30°C (59°F and 86°F).

Sublingual tablet [Canadian product]: Store at 15°C to 25°C (59°F to 77°F). Protect from light.

Mechanism of Action Binds to stereospecific benzodiazepine receptors on the postsynaptic GABA neuron at several sites within the central nervous system, including the limbic system, reticular formation. Enhancement of the inhibitory effect of GABA on neuronal excitability results by increased neuronal membrane permeability to chloride ions. This shift in chloride ions results in hyperpolarization (a less excitable state) and stabilization. Benzodiazepine receptors and effects appear to be linked to the GABA-A receptors. Benzodiazepines do not bind to GABA-B receptors.

Pharmacodynamics

Onset of action:

Anticonvulsant: IV: Within 10 minutes

Hypnosis: IM: 20 to 30 minutes

Sedation: IV: Within 2 to 3 minutes (Greenblatt 1983)

Maximum effect:

Amnesia: IV: Within 15 to 20 minutes; I.M.: Within 2 hours

Duration: Hypnosis/Sedation: Up to 8 hours

Pharmacokinetics (Adult data unless noted)

Absorption: IM: Rapid, complete; Oral: Readily absorbed

Distribution: Crosses the blood brain barrier

V_d:

Neonates: 0.76 ± 0.37 L/kg (range: 0.14 to 1.3 L/kg) (McDermott 1992)

Pediatric patients (Chamberlain 2012):

5 months to < 3 years: 1.62 L/kg (range: 0.67 to 3.4 L/kg)

3 to <13 years: 1.5 L/kg (range: 0.49 to 3 L/kg)

13 to <18 years: 1.27 L/kg (range: 1 to 1.54 L/kg)

Adults: 1.3 L/kg

Protein binding: ~85% to 91%

Metabolism: Hepatic; primarily by glucuronide conjugation to an inactive metabolite (lorazepam glucuronide)

Bioavailability: Oral: 90%

Half-life:

Full-term neonates: 40.2 ± 16.5 hours; range: 18 to 73 hours (McDermott 1992)

Pediatric patients (Chamberlain, 2012):

5 months to <3 years: 15.8 hours (range: 5.9 to 28.4 hours)

3 to <13 years: 16.9 hours (range: 7.5 to 40.6 hours)

13 to <18 years: 17.8 hours (range: 8.2 to 42 hours)

Adults: Oral: ~12 hours; IV: 14 hours

Time to peak serum concentration: Oral: 2 hours; IM: Within 3 hours

Elimination: Urine (88%, primarily as the glucuronide conjugate), feces (7%)

Dosing: Neonatal

Sedation: Limited data available: IV: 0.05 to 0.1 mg/kg/dose every 4 to 6 hours as needed (Cloherty 2012; Kliegman 2007)

Status epilepticus: Limited data available: IV: 0.05 to 0.1 mg/kg slow IV over 2 to 5 minutes; may repeat in 10 to 15 minutes (AAP [Hegenbarth 2008]; Kleigman 2011)

Dosing: Usual

Pediatric:

Chemotherapy-induced nausea and vomiting, anticipatory: Limited data available: Infants, Children, and Adolescents: Oral: 0.04 to 0.08 mg/kg/dose; maximum dose: 2 mg/dose; administer a dose the night before chemotherapy and again the next day prior to chemotherapy administration (Dupuis 2014)

Chemotherapy-associated nausea and vomiting, breakthrough: Limited data available: Children and Adolescents: IV: 0.025 to 0.05 mg/kg/dose every 6 hours as needed; maximum dose: 2 mg/dose (Dupuis 2003)

Anxiety, acute:

Infants and Children <12 years: Limited data available: Oral, IV: Usual: 0.05 mg/kg/dose (maximum dose: 2 mg/dose) every 4 to 8 hours; range: 0.02 to 0.1 mg/kg/dose (Kleigman 2007)

Children ≥12 years and Adolescents: Oral: 0.25 to 2 mg/dose 2 or 3 times daily; maximum dose: 2 mg/dose (Kleigman 2011)

Insomnia due to anxiety or stress: Children ≥12 years and Adolescents: Oral: Usual: 2 mg at bedtime; maximum: 4 mg/dose

Sedation (preprocedure): Limited data available: Children and Adolescents: Oral: Usual: 0.05 mg/kg; range: 0.02 to 0.09 mg/kg; usual maximum: 4 mg/dose (Henry 1991)

Status epilepticus: Limited data available: Infants, Children, and Adolescents:

IV: 0.05 to 0.1 mg/kg (maximum: 4 mg/dose) slow IV over 2 to 5 minutes; may repeat in 5 to 15 minutes if needed (AAP [Hegenbarth 2008]; NCS [Brophy 2012]; Kleigman 2007); usual total maximum dose: 8 mg (Crawford 1987; NICE 2012). **Note:** May be administered IM if IV not possible (Hegenbarth 2008).

Intranasal: **Note:** Reserve for patients without IV access: 0.1 mg/kg/dose; maximum dose: 4 mg/dose (Ahmad 2006; Arya 2011; Kleigman 2011)

Adult:

Anxiety disorder: Oral: 1 to 10 mg daily in 2 to 3 divided doses; usual dose: 2 to 6 mg daily in divided doses

Insomnia due to anxiety or stress: Oral: 2 to 4 mg at bedtime

Premedication for anesthesia:

IM: 0.05 mg/kg administered 2 hours before surgery; maximum dose: 4 mg/dose

IV: 0.044 mg/kg administered 15 to 20 minutes before surgery; usual dose: 2 mg; maximum dose: 4 mg/dose. **Note:** Doses >2 mg should generally not be exceeded in patients >50 years.

Status epilepticus: IV: 4 mg slow IV; may repeat in 5 to 10 minutes (Brophy, 2012). May be given IM, but IV preferred.

Dosing adjustment for lorazepam with concomitant medications: Probenecid or valproic acid: Reduce lorazepam dose by 50%

Dosing adjustment in renal impairment:

Oral: Children ≥12 years, Adolescents, and Adults: There are no dosage adjustments provided in the manufacturer's labeling; however, some clinicians recommend no dosage adjustments are necessary (Aronoff, 2007).

IV: Adults: No dosage adjustment necessary for acute doses. Use repeated doses with caution; may increase the risk of propylene glycol toxicity. Monitor closely if using for prolonged periods of time or at high doses.

Dialysis: 8% as intact lorazepam and 40% as lorazepam glucuronide removed during a 6-hour session

Dosing adjustment in hepatic impairment: Children ≥12 years, Adolescents, and Adults: No dosage adjustment necessary. For severe hepatic disease, use with caution; benzodiazepines may worsen hepatic encephalopathy.

Preparation for Administration Parenteral: IV: Dilute dose prior to use with an equal volume of compatible diluent (D_5W, NS, SWFI).

Neonates: Since both concentrations of the injection contain 2% benzyl alcohol, some experts recommend using the 4 mg/mL product for dilution with preservative free SWFI to make a 0.4 mg/mL dilution (in order to decrease the amount of benzyl alcohol delivered to the neonate); however, the stability of this dilution has not been studied.

Administration

Oral: May administer with food to decrease GI distress; dilute oral solution in water, juice, soda, or semisolid food (eg, applesauce, pudding).

Intranasal: Administer undiluted (injectable formulation) into one nostril using a needleless syringe or nasal atomizer (Ahmad 2006; Anya 2011)

Parenteral:

IV: Dilute prior to administration. Do not exceed 2 mg/minute or 0.05 mg/kg over 2 to 5 minutes; administer IV using repeated aspiration with slow IV injection, to make sure the injection is not intra-arterial and that perivascular extravasation has not occurred.

IM: Administer undiluted by deep injection into muscle mass

Monitoring Parameters Respiratory rate, blood pressure, heart rate; CBC with differential and liver function with long-term use; symptoms of anxiety; clinical signs of propylene glycol toxicity (for continuous high-dose and/or long duration intravenous use) including serum creatinine, BUN, serum lactate, and osmol gap

Controlled Substance C-IV

Dosage Forms Excipient information presented when available (limited, particularly for generics); consult specific product labeling.

Concentrate, Oral:

LORazepam Intensol: 2 mg/mL (30 mL) [alcohol free, dye free, sugar free; unflavored flavor]

Generic: 2 mg/mL (30 mL)

Solution, Injection:

Ativan: 2 mg/mL (1 mL, 10 mL); 4 mg/mL (1 mL, 10 mL) [contains benzyl alcohol, polyethylene glycol, propylene glycol]

Generic: 2 mg/mL (1 mL, 10 mL); 4 mg/mL (1 mL, 10 mL)

Tablet, Oral:

Ativan: 0.5 mg

Ativan: 1 mg, 2 mg [scored]

Generic: 0.5 mg, 1 mg, 2 mg

Extemporaneous Preparations Note: Commercial oral solution is available (2 mg/mL)

Two different 1 mg/mL oral suspensions may be made from different generic lorazepam tablets (Mylan Pharmaceuticals or Watson Laboratories), sterile water, Ora-Sweet, and Ora-Plus.

Mylan tablets: Place one-hundred-eighty 2 mg tablets in a 12-ounce amber glass bottle; add 144 mL of sterile water to disperse the tablets; shake until slurry is formed. Add 108 mL Ora-Plus in incremental proportions; then add a quantity of Ora-Sweet sufficient to make 360 mL. Label "shake well" and "refrigerate". Stable for 91 days when stored in amber glass prescription bottles at room temperature or refrigerated (preferred).

Watson tablets: Place one-hundred-eighty 2 mg tablets in a 12-ounce amber glass bottle; add 48 mL sterile water to disperse the tablets; shake until slurry is formed. Add 156 mL of Ora-Plus in incremental proportions; then add a quantity of Ora-Sweet sufficient to make 360 mL. Label "shake well" and "refrigerate". Store in amber glass prescription bottles. Stable for 63 days at room temperature or 91 days refrigerated.

Lee ME, Lugo RA, Rusho WJ, et al, "Chemical Stability of Extemporaneously Prepared Lorazepam Suspension at Two Temperatures," *J Pediatr Pharmacol Ther*, 2004, 9(4):254-58.

◆ **Lorazepam Injection, USP (Can)** *see* LORazepam *on page* 1299

◆ **LORazepam Intensol** *see* LORazepam *on page* 1299

◆ **Lorcet® 10/650 [DSC]** *see* Hydrocodone and Acetaminophen *on page* 1032

◆ **Lorcet® Plus [DSC]** *see* Hydrocodone and Acetaminophen *on page* 1032

◆ **Lortab®** *see* Hydrocodone and Acetaminophen *on page* 1032

◆ **Lorzone** *see* Chlorzoxazone *on page* 447

Losartan (loe SAR tan)

Medication Safety Issues

Sound-alike/look-alike issues:

Cozaar may be confused with Colace, Coreg, Hyzaar, Zocor

Losartan may be confused with locaserin, valsartan

Brand Names: US Cozaar

Brand Names: Canada ACT Losartan; Apo-Losartan; Auro-Losartan; Cozaar; JAMP-Losartan; Mint-Losartan; Mylan-Losartan; PMS-Losartan; RAN-Losartan; Sandoz Losartan; Septa Losartan; Teva-Losartan

Therapeutic Category Angiotensin II Receptor Blocker; Antihypertensive Agent

Generic Availability (US) Yes

Use Treatment of hypertension alone or in combination with other antihypertensive agents (FDA approved in ages 6-16 years and adults); treatment of diabetic nephropathy in patients with type 2 diabetes mellitus (noninsulin dependent, NIDDM) and hypertension (FDA approved in adults); reduction of the risk of stroke in patients with hypertension and left ventricular hypertrophy (FDA approved in adults); has also been used to reduce proteinuria in children with chronic kidney disease, either as monotherapy or in addition to ACE inhibitor therapy, and in Marfan's Syndrome to slow the rate of progression of aortic-root dilation

Pregnancy Risk Factor D

Pregnancy Considerations [U.S. Boxed Warning]: Drugs that act on the renin-angiotensin system can cause injury and death to the developing fetus. Discontinue as soon as possible once pregnancy is detected. The use of drugs which act on the renin-angiotensin system are associated with oligohydramnios. Oligohydramnios, due to decreased fetal renal function, may lead to fetal lung hypoplasia and skeletal malformations. Use is also associated with anuria, hypotension, renal failure, skull hypoplasia, and death in the fetus/neonate. The exposed fetus should be monitored for fetal growth, amniotic fluid volume, and organ formation. Infants exposed *in utero* should be monitored for hyperkalemia, hypotension, and oliguria (exchange transfusions or dialysis may be needed). These adverse events are generally associated with maternal use in the second and third trimesters.

Untreated chronic maternal hypertension is also associated with adverse events in the fetus, infant, and mother. The use of angiotensin II receptor blockers is not recommended to treat chronic uncomplicated hypertension in pregnant women and should generally be avoided in women of reproductive potential (ACOG, 2013).

Breast-Feeding Considerations It is not known if losartan is found in breast milk. Due to the potential for serious adverse reactions in the nursing infant, the manufacturer recommends a decision be made whether to discontinue nursing or to discontinue the drug, taking into account the importance of treatment to the mother.

Contraindications

Hypersensitivity to losartan or any component of the formulation; concomitant use with aliskiren in patients with diabetes mellitus

Documentation of allergenic cross-reactivity for angiotensin receptor blockers is limited. However, because of similarities in chemical structure and/or pharmacologic actions, the possibility of cross-sensitivity cannot be ruled out with certainty.

Canadian labeling: Additional contraindications (not in U.S. labeling): Concomitant use with aliskiren in patients with moderate-to-severe renal impairment (GFR <60 mL/minute/1.73 m^2)

Warnings/Precautions [U.S. Boxed Warning]: Drugs that act on the renin-angiotensin system can cause injury and death to the developing fetus. Discontinue as soon as possible once pregnancy is detected. Avoid use or use a much smaller dose in patients who are volume-depleted; correct depletion first. Use with caution in patients with significant aortic/mitral stenosis. May cause hyperkalemia; avoid potassium supplementation unless specifically required by healthcare provider. May be associated with deterioration of renal function and/or increases in serum creatinine, particularly in patients with low renal blood flow (eg, renal artery stenosis, heart failure) whose glomerular filtration rate (GFR) is dependent on efferent arteriolar vasoconstriction by angiotensin II. Use caution in patients with unstented unilateral/bilateral renal artery stenosis. When unstented bilateral renal artery stenosis is present, use is generally avoided due to the elevated risk of deterioration in renal function unless possible benefits outweigh risks. Use with caution with preexisting renal insufficiency. AUCs of losartan (not the active metabolite) are about 50% greater in patients with CrCl <30 mL/minute and are doubled in hemodialysis patients. Potentially significant drug interactions may exist, requiring dose or frequency adjustment, additional monitoring, and/or selection of alternative therapy. In surgical patients on chronic angiotensin receptor blocker (ARB) therapy, intraoperative hypotension may occur with induction and maintenance of general anesthesia.

Angioedema has been reported rarely with some angiotensin II receptor antagonists (ARBs) and may occur at any time during treatment (especially following first dose). It may involve the head and neck (potentially compromising airway) or the intestine (presenting with abdominal pain). Patients with idiopathic or hereditary angioedema or previous angioedema associated with ACE-inhibitor therapy may be at an increased risk. Prolonged frequent monitoring may be required, especially if tongue, glottis, or larynx are involved, as they are associated with airway obstruction. Patients with a history of airway surgery may have a higher risk of airway obstruction. Discontinue therapy immediately if angioedema occurs. Aggressive early management is critical. Intramuscular (IM) administration of epinephrine may be necessary. Do not readminister to patients who have had angioedema with ARBs.

When used to reduce the risk of stroke in patients with HTN and LVH, may not be effective in the black population. Use caution with hepatic dysfunction, dose adjustment may be needed.

Warnings: Additional Pediatric Considerations Not recommended for use in children <6 years of age or in children with GFR <30 mL/minute/1.73m^2 (no data exists).

Adverse Reactions

Cardiovascular: Chest pain, hypotension, orthostatic hypotension, first-dose hypotension (dose related)

Central nervous system: Dizziness, fatigue, fever, hypoesthesia, insomnia

Dermatology: Cellulitis

Endocrine: Hyperkalemia, hypoglycemia

Gastrointestinal: Abdominal pain, diarrhea, dyspepsia, gastritis, nausea, weight gain

Genitourinary: Urinary tract infection

Hematologic: Anemia

Neuromuscular & skeletal: Back pain, knee pain, leg pain, muscle cramps, muscular weakness, myalgia, weakness

Respiratory: Bronchitis, cough, nasal congestion, sinusitis upper respiratory infection

Miscellaneous: Flu-like syndrome, infection

Frequency ≤ placebo: Abdominal pain, edema, headache, nausea, pharyngitis

Rare but important or life-threatening: Acute psychosis with paranoid delusions, ageusia, allergic reaction, alopecia, anaphylactic reactions, anemia, angina, angioedema, anorexia, anxiety, arrhythmia, arthralgia, arthritis, ataxia, AV block (second degree), bilirubin increased, blurred vision, bradycardia, bronchitis, BUN increased, confusion, conjunctivitis, constipation, CVA, depression, dermatitis, dysgeusia, dyspnea, ecchymosis, epistaxis, erythroderma, erythema, facial edema, fever, flatulence, flushing, gastritis, gout, hematocrit decreased, hemoglobin decreased, Henoch-Schönlein purpura (IgA vasculitis), hepatitis, hyponatremia, hypotension, impotence, joint swelling, maculopapular rash, malaise, memory impairment, MI, migraine, muscle weakness, myositis, neoplasm, nervousness, orthostatic effects, pancreatitis, paresthesia, peripheral neuropathy, pharyngitis, photosensitivity, pruritus, rash, rhabdomyolysis, rhinitis, serum creatinine increased, sleep disorder, somnolence, syncope, tachycardia, taste perversion, thrombocytopenia, tinnitus, transaminases increased, tremor, urinary frequency, urticaria, vasculitis, ventricular arrhythmia, vertigo, visual acuity decreased, vomiting, xerostomia

Drug Interactions

Metabolism/Transport Effects Substrate of CYP2C9 (major), CYP3A4 (major); **Note:** Assignment of Major/Minor substrate status based on clinically relevant drug interaction potential; **Inhibits** CYP1A2 (weak), CYP2C19 (weak), CYP2C8 (moderate), CYP2C9 (moderate)

Avoid Concomitant Use

Avoid concomitant use of Losartan with any of the following: Amodiaquine

Increased Effect/Toxicity

Losartan may increase the levels/effects of: ACE Inhibitors; Amifostine; Amodiaquine; Antihypertensives; Bosentan; Cannabis; Carvedilol; Ciprofloxacin (Systemic); CycloSPORINE (Systemic); CYP2C8 Substrates; CYP2C9 Substrates; Dronabinol; Drospirenone; DULoxetine; Hypotensive Agents; Levodopa; Lithium; Nonsteroidal Anti-Inflammatory Agents; Obinutuzumab; Potassium-Sparing Diuretics; RisperiDONE; RiTUXimab; Sodium Phosphates; Tetrahydrocannabinol; TiZANidine

The levels/effects of Losartan may be increased by: Alfuzosin; Aliskiren; Antifungal Agents (Azole Derivatives, Systemic); Barbiturates; Brimonidine (Topical); Canagliflozin; Ceritinib; CYP2C9 Inhibitors (Moderate); CYP2C9 Inhibitors (Strong); Dapoxetine; Diazoxide; Eplerenone; Heparin; Heparin (Low Molecular Weight); Herbs (Hypotensive Properties); MAO Inhibitors; Mifepristone; Nicorandil; Pentoxifylline; Phosphodiesterase 5 Inhibitors; Potassium Salts; Prostacyclin Analogues; Tolvaptan; Trimethoprim

Decreased Effect

The levels/effects of Losartan may be decreased by: Bosentan; CYP2C9 Inducers (Strong); CYP3A4 Inducers (Moderate); CYP3A4 Inducers (Strong); Dabrafenib; Deferasirox; Fluconazole; Herbs (Hypertensive Properties); Methylphenidate; Mitotane; Nonsteroidal Anti-Inflammatory Agents; Rifampin; Siltuximab; St Johns Wort; Tocilizumab; Yohimbine

Storage/Stability Store at 25°C (77°F); excursions are permitted to 15°C to 30°C (59°F to 86°F). Protect from light.

Mechanism of Action As a selective and competitive, nonpeptide angiotensin II receptor antagonist, losartan blocks the vasoconstrictor and aldosterone-secreting effects of angiotensin II; losartan interacts reversibly at the AT1 and AT2 receptors of many tissues and has slow dissociation kinetics; its affinity for the AT1 receptor is 1000 times greater than the AT2 receptor. Angiotensin II receptor antagonists may induce a more complete inhibition of the renin-angiotensin system than ACE inhibitors, they do not affect the response to bradykinin, and are less likely to be associated with nonrenin-angiotensin effects (eg, cough and angioedema). Losartan increases urinary flow rate and in addition to being natriuretic and kaliuretic, increases excretion of chloride, magnesium, uric acid, calcium, and phosphate.

Pharmacodynamics Antihypertensive effect:

Maximum effect: 6 hours postdose; with chronic dosing, substantial hypotensive effects are seen within 1 week; maximum effect: 3-6 weeks

Duration: 24 hours

Pharmacokinetics (Adult data unless noted) Note: No significant differences in pharmacokinetic parameters have been identified across studied pediatric age groups (6-16 years) and adult population.

Absorption: Oral: Well-absorbed

Distribution: V_d: Adults:

- Losartan: ~34 L
- E-3174: ~12 L

Protein binding: Highly bound, >98%; primarily to albumin

Metabolism: Extensive first-pass effect; metabolized in the liver via CYP2C9 and 3A4 to active carboxylic metabolite, E-3174 (14% of dose; 40 times more potent than losartan) and several inactive metabolites

Bioavailability: Oral: 33%; AUC of E-3174 is four times greater than that of losartan; extemporaneously prepared suspension and tablet have similar bioavailability of losartan and E-3174

Half-life elimination:

- Losartan:
  - Children 6-16 years: 2.3 ± 0.8 hours
  - Adults: 2.1 ± 0.7 hours
- E-3174:
  - Children 6-16 years: 5.6 ± 1.2 hours
  - Adults: 7.4 ± 2.4 hours

Time to peak serum concentration:

- Losartan:
  - Children: 2 hours
  - Adults: 1 hour
- E-3174:
  - Children: 4 hours
  - Adults: 3.5 hours

Excretion: Biliary excretion plays a role in the elimination of parent drug and metabolites; 35% of an oral dose is eliminated in the urine and 60% in the feces; 4% of dose is eliminated as unchanged drug in the urine; 6% as E-3174

- Clearance: Adults:
  - Plasma:
    - Losartan: 600 mL/minute
    - E-3174: 50 mL/minute
  - Renal:
    - Losartan: 75 mL/minute
    - E-3174: 25 mL/minute

Dialysis: Losartan and E-3174: Not removed by hemodialysis

Dosing: Usual

Pediatric:

Hypertension:

Children and Adolescents 6 to 16 years: Oral: Initial: 0.7 mg/kg once daily (maximum dose: 50 mg); titrate to desired effect up to a maximum dose of 1.4 mg/kg/day or 100 mg/day; may be administered once daily or divided twice daily (NHBPEP 2004; NHLBI 2011); **Note:** Doses >1.4 mg/kg/day (or >100 mg/day) have not been studied (Shahinfar 2005).

Adolescents ≥17 years: Oral: Initial: 50 mg once daily; increase dose to achieve desired effect; total daily dosage range: 25 to 100 mg/day; can be administered once or twice daily; **Note:** Patients receiving diuretics or with intravascular volume depletion: Initial dose: 25 mg once daily

Proteinuria reduction in children with chronic kidney disease: Limited data available: Children ≥4 years and Adolescents: Oral: Initial: 0.4 to 0.8 mg/kg/day; increase dose if no adverse effects occur and blood pressure remains >90th percentile or proteinuria does not fall <50% of baseline excretion; doses can be increased slowly up to 1 mg/kg/day (maximum 50 mg/day); dosing based on experience from three retrospective clinical trials (Chandar 2007; Ellis 2003; Ellis 2004)

Marfan's syndrome aortic-root dilation: Limited data available: Children and Adolescents 14 months to 16 years: Oral: Initial: 0.6 mg/kg/day for 3 weeks (while assessing for adverse events); then gradually increase dose to 1.4 mg/kg/day (maximum: 100 mg/day); dosing based on preliminary results of a small (n=18), nonrandomized, retrospective, clinical study (Brooke 2008)

Adult:

Hypertension: Oral: Initial: 50 mg once daily; can be administered once or twice daily; increase dose to achieve desired effect; total daily dosage range: 25 to 100 mg/day; **Note:** Patients receiving diuretics or with intravascular volume depletion: Initial dose: 25 mg once daily

Nephropathy in patients with type 2 diabetes and hypertension: Oral: Initial: 50 mg once daily; can be increased to 100 mg once daily based on blood pressure response

Stroke reduction (HTN with LVH): Oral: Initial: 50 mg once daily (maximum daily dose: 100 mg); may be used in combination with a thiazide diuretic

Dosing adjustment in renal impairment:

Children: Use is not recommended if CrCl <30 mL/minute/1.73 m^2

Adults: No initial dosage adjustment necessary

Dosing adjustment in hepatic impairment:

Children: No specific dosing recommendations provided by manufacturer; however, it is advisable to initiate at a reduced dosage.

Adults: Reduce initial dose to 25 mg/day

Administration May be administered with or without food.

Monitoring Parameters Blood pressure, BUN, serum creatinine, renal function, baseline and periodic serum electrolytes, urinalysis

Additional Information Potassium content: 25 mg tablets: 2.12 mg (0.054 mEq); 50 mg tablets: 4.24 mg (0.108 mEq); 100 mg tablets: 8.48 mg (0.216 mEq)

Evidence from the LIFE study (Dahlöf, 2002) suggests that when used to reduce the risk of stroke in patients with HTN and LVH, losartan may not be effective in the African-American population.

Dosage Forms Excipient information presented when available (limited, particularly for generics); consult specific product labeling.

Tablet, Oral, as potassium:

- Cozaar: 25 mg
- Cozaar: 50 mg [scored]
- Cozaar: 100 mg
- Generic: 25 mg, 50 mg, 100 mg

Extemporaneous Preparations A 2.5 mg/mL losartan oral suspension may be made with tablets and a 1:1 mixture of Ora-Plus® and Ora-Sweet® SF. Combine 10 mL of purified water and ten losartan 50 mg tablets in an 8-ounce amber polyethylene terephthalate bottle. Shake well for at least 2 minutes. Allow concentrate to stand for 1 hour, then shake for 1 minute. Separately, prepare 190 mL of a 1:1 mixture of Ora-Plus® and Ora-Sweet® SF; add to tablet and water mixture in the bottle and shake for 1 minute. Label "shake well" and "refrigerate". Return promptly to refrigerator after each use. Stable for 4 weeks when stored in amber polyethylene terephthalate prescription bottles and refrigerated (Cozaar prescribing information, 2014).

Cozaar prescribing information, Merck & Co, Inc, Whitehouse Station, NJ, 2014.

◆ **Losartan Potassium** *see* Losartan *on page* 1302

◆ **Losec (Can)** *see* Omeprazole *on page 1555*

◆ **Lotensin** *see* Benazepril *on page 265*

◆ **Lotrimin AF [OTC]** *see* Clotrimazole (Topical) *on page 518*

◆ **Lotrimin AF [OTC]** *see* Miconazole (Topical) *on page 1431*

◆ **Lotrimin AF Deodorant Powder [OTC]** *see* Miconazole (Topical) *on page 1431*

◆ **Lotrimin AF For Her [OTC]** *see* Clotrimazole (Topical) *on page 518*

◆ **Lotrimin AF Jock Itch Powder [OTC]** *see* Miconazole (Topical) *on page 1431*

◆ **Lotrimin AF Powder [OTC]** *see* Miconazole (Topical) *on page 1431*

Lovastatin (LOE va sta tin)

Medication Safety Issues

Sound-alike/look-alike issues:

Lovastatin may be confused with atorvaSTATin, Leustatin, Livostin, Lotensin, nystatin, pitavastatin

Mevacor may be confused with Benicar, Lipitor

International issues:

Lovacol [Chile and Finland] may be confused with Levatol brand name for penbutolol [U.S.]

Lovastin [Malaysia, Poland, and Singapore] may be confused with Livostin brand name for levocabastine [multiple international markets]

Mevacor [U.S., Canada, and multiple international markets} may be confused with Mivacron brand name for mivacurium [multiple international markets]

Related Information

Oral Medications That Should Not Be Crushed or Altered *on page 2476*

Brand Names: US Altoprev; Mevacor

Brand Names: Canada Apo-Lovastatin; Ava-Lovastatin; CO Lovastatin; Dom-Lovastatin; Mevacor; Mylan-Lovastatin; PHL-Lovastatin; PMS-Lovastatin; PRO-Lovastatin; Riva-Lovastatin; Sandoz-Lovastatin; Teva-Lovastatin

Therapeutic Category Antilipemic Agent; HMG-CoA Reductase Inhibitor

Generic Availability (US) May be product dependent

Use Treatment of heterozygous familial hypercholesterolemia as adjunct to dietary therapy to decrease elevated serum total and low density lipoprotein and apolipoprotein B levels [immediate release tablets: FDA approved in males and postmenarcheal (>1 year) females ages 10-17 years]

Treatment of primary hypercholesterolemia as adjunct to dietary therapy to decrease elevated serum total and low density lipoprotein cholesterol (LDL-C) (immediate and extended release tablets: FDA approved in adults); to reduce the risk of myocardial infarction, unstable angina, and coronary revascularization procedures in patients without symptomatic disease with average to moderately elevated total and LDL-C and below average HDL-cholesterol (primary prevention) and slow progression of coronary atherosclerosis in patients with coronary heart disease (immediate and extended release tablets: FDA approved in adults)

Pregnancy Risk Factor X

Pregnancy Considerations Adverse events were observed in animal reproduction studies. There are reports of congenital anomalies following maternal use of HMG-CoA reductase inhibitors in pregnancy; however, maternal disease, differences in specific agents used, and the low rates of exposure limit the interpretation of the available data (Godfrey 2012; Lecarpentier 2012). Cholesterol biosynthesis may be important in fetal development; serum cholesterol and triglycerides increase normally during pregnancy. The discontinuation of lipid lowering medications temporarily during pregnancy is not expected to have significant impact on the long term outcomes of primary hypercholesterolemia treatment.

Use of lovastatin is contraindicated in pregnancy. HMG-CoA reductase inhibitors should be discontinued prior to pregnancy (ADA 2013). If treatment of dyslipidemias is needed in pregnant women or in women of reproductive age, other agents are preferred (Berglund 2012; Stone 2013). The manufacturer recommends administration to women of childbearing potential only when conception is highly unlikely and patients have been informed of potential hazards.

Breast-Feeding Considerations It is not known if lovastatin is excreted into breast milk. Due to the potential for serious adverse reactions in a nursing infant, use while breast-feeding is contraindicated by the manufacturer.

Contraindications

Hypersensitivity to lovastatin or any component of the formulation; active liver disease; unexplained persistent elevations of serum transaminases; concomitant use of strong CYP3A4 inhibitors (eg, clarithromycin, erythromycin, itraconazole, ketoconazole, nefazodone, posaconazole, voriconazole, protease inhibitors [including boceprevir and telaprevir], telithromycin, cobicistat-containing products); pregnancy; breast-feeding

Canadian labeling: Additional contraindications (not in US labeling): Concomitant use of cyclosporine

Warnings/Precautions Secondary causes of hyperlipidemia should be ruled out prior to therapy. Liver enzyme tests should be obtained at baseline and as clinically indicated; routine periodic monitoring of liver enzymes is not necessary. Use with caution in patients who consume large amounts of ethanol or have a history of liver disease; use is contraindicated with active liver disease and with unexplained transaminase elevations. Rhabdomyolysis with or without acute renal failure has occurred. Risk of rhabdomyolysis is dose-related and increased with concurrent use of lipid-lowering agents which may also cause rhabdomyolysis (fibric acid derivatives or niacin at doses ≥1 g/day) or during concurrent use with potent CYP3A4 inhibitors. Use is contraindicated in patients taking strong CYP3A4 inhibitors. Concomitant use of lovastatin with some drugs may require cautious use, may not be recommended, may require dosage adjustments, or may be contraindicated. Increases in HbA_{1c} and fasting blood glucose have been reported with HMG-CoA reductase inhibitors; however, the benefits of statin therapy far outweigh the risk of dysglycemia. Monitor closely if used with other drugs associated with myopathy (eg, colchicine). Patients should be instructed to report unexplained muscle pain or weakness; lovastatin should be discontinued if myopathy is suspected/confirmed. Immune-mediated necrotizing myopathy (IMNM), an autoimmune-mediated myopathy, has been reported (rarely) with HMG-CoA reductase inhibitor therapy. IMNM presents as proximal muscle weakness with elevated CPK levels, which persists despite discontinuation of HMG-CoA reductase inhibitor therapy; additionally, muscle biopsy may show necrotizing myopathy with limited inflammation; immunosuppressive therapy (eg, corticosteroids, azathioprine) may be used for treatment. The manufacturer recommends temporary discontinuation for elective major surgery, acute medical or surgical conditions, or in any patient experiencing an acute or serious condition predisposing to renal failure (eg, sepsis, hypotension, trauma, uncontrolled seizures). Based on current research and clinical guidelines (Fleisher 2009), HMG-CoA reductase inhibitors should be continued in the perioperative period. Use with caution in patients with advanced age; these patients are predisposed to myopathy.

Adverse Reactions

Central nervous system: Dizziness, headache

Dermatologic: Rash

Gastrointestinal: Abdominal pain, constipation, diarrhea, dyspepsia, flatulence, nausea

Neuromuscular & skeletal: Increased CPK (>2x normal), muscle cramps, myalgia, weakness

Ocular: Blurred vision

Rare but important or life-threatening: Acid regurgitation, alopecia, amnesia (reversible), arthralgia, blood glucose increased, chest pain, cognitive impairment (reversible), confusion (reversible), dermatomyositis, diabetes mellitus (new onset), eye irritation, glycosylated hemoglobin (Hb A_{1c}) increased, insomnia, leg pain, memory disturbance (reversible), memory impairment (reversible), paresthesia, pruritus, vomiting, xerostomia

Additional class-related events or case reports (not necessarily reported with lovastatin therapy): Alkaline phosphatase increased, alteration in taste, anaphylaxis, angioedema, anorexia, anxiety, arthritis, cataracts, chills, cholestatic jaundice, cirrhosis, depression, dryness of skin/mucous membranes, dyspnea, eosinophilia, erectile dysfunction, erythema multiforme, ESR increased, facial paresis, fatty liver, fever, flushing, fulminant hepatic necrosis, GGT increased, gynecomastia, hemolytic anemia, hepatic failure (fatal and nonfatal), hepatitis, hepatoma, hyperbilirubinemia, hypersensitivity reaction, immune-mediated necrotizing myopathy (IMNM), impaired extraocular muscle movement, impotence, interstitial lung disease, leukopenia, libido decreased, malaise, myopathy, nail changes, nodules, ophthalmoplegia, pancreatitis, peripheral nerve palsy, peripheral neuropathy, photosensitivity, polymyalgia rheumatica, positive ANA, psychic disturbance, purpura, renal failure (secondary to rhabdomyolysis), rhabdomyolysis, skin discoloration, Stevens-Johnson syndrome, systemic lupus erythematosus-like syndrome, thrombocytopenia, thyroid dysfunction, toxic epidermal necrolysis, transaminases increased, tremor, urticaria, vasculitis, vertigo

Drug Interactions

Metabolism/Transport Effects **Substrate** of CYP3A4 (major), P-glycoprotein; **Note:** Assignment of Major/Minor substrate status based on clinically relevant drug interaction potential; **Inhibits** CYP2C9 (weak)

Avoid Concomitant Use

Avoid concomitant use of Lovastatin with any of the following: Boceprevir; Clarithromycin; Conivaptan; CycloSPORINE (Systemic); CYP3A4 Inhibitors (Strong); Erythromycin (Systemic); Fusidic Acid (Systemic); Gemfibrozil; Idelalisib; Lomitapide; Mifepristone; Protease Inhibitors; Red Yeast Rice; Telaprevir; Telithromycin

Increased Effect/Toxicity

Lovastatin may increase the levels/effects of: DAPTOmycin; Diltiazem; PAZOPanib; Trabectedin; Vitamin K Antagonists

The levels/effects of Lovastatin may be increased by: Acipimox; Amiodarone; Aprepitant; Azithromycin (Systemic); Bezafibrate; Boceprevir; Ciprofibrate; Clarithromycin; Colchicine; Conivaptan; CycloSPORINE (Systemic); CYP3A4 Inhibitors (Moderate); CYP3A4 Inhibitors (Strong); Cyproterone; Danazol; Dasatinib; Diltiazem; Dronedarone; Erythromycin (Systemic); Fenofibrate and Derivatives; Fluconazole; Fosaprepitant; Fusidic Acid (Systemic); Gemfibrozil; Grapefruit Juice; Idelalisib; Ivacaftor; Lomitapide; Luliconazole; Mifepristone; Netupitant; Niacin; Niacinamide; Palbociclib; P-glycoprotein/ABCB1 Inhibitors; Protease Inhibitors; QuiNINE; Raltegravir; Ranolazine; Red Yeast Rice; Sildenafil; Simeprevir; Stiripentol; Telaprevir; Telithromycin; Ticagrelor; Verapamil

Decreased Effect

Lovastatin may decrease the levels/effects of: Lanthanum

The levels/effects of Lovastatin may be decreased by: Antacids; Bosentan; CYP3A4 Inducers (Moderate); CYP3A4 Inducers (Strong); Dabrafenib; Deferasirox; Efavirenz; Etravirine; Fosphenytoin; Mitotane; P-glycoprotein/ABCB1 Inducers; Phenytoin; Rifamycin Derivatives; Siltuximab; St Johns Wort; Tocilizumab

Food Interactions Food decreases the bioavailability of lovastatin extended release tablets and increases the bioavailability of lovastatin immediate release tablets. Lovastatin serum concentrations may be increased if taken with grapefruit juice. Management: Avoid concurrent intake of large quantities (>1 quart/day) of grapefruit juice.

Storage/Stability

Tablet, immediate release: Store at 20°C to 25°C (68°F to 77°F). Protect from light

Tablet, extended release: Store at 20°C to 25°C (68°F to 77°F); excursions permitted between 15°C to 30°C (59°F to 86°F). Avoid excessive heat and humidity.

Mechanism of Action Lovastatin acts by competitively inhibiting 3-hydroxyl-3-methylglutaryl-coenzyme A (HMG-CoA) reductase, the enzyme that catalyzes the rate-limiting step in cholesterol biosynthesis. In addition to the ability of HMG-CoA reductase inhibitors to decrease levels of high-sensitivity C-reactive protein (hsCRP), they also possess pleiotropic properties including improved endothelial function, reduced inflammation at the site of the coronary plaque, inhibition of platelet aggregation, and anticoagulant effects (de Denus 2002; Ray 2005).

Pharmacodynamics

Onset of action: LDL-cholesterol reduction: 3 days

Maximum effect: LDL-cholesterol reduction: 4-6 weeks

LDL-C reduction: 40 mg/day: 31% (for each doubling of this dose, LDL-C is lowered by ~6%)

Average HDL-C increase: 5% to 15%

Average triglyceride reduction: 7% to 30%

Pharmacokinetics (Adult data unless noted)

Absorption: Oral: 30% absorbed but less than 5% reaches the systemic circulation due to an extensive first-pass effect; absorption increased with extended release tablets

Protein binding: 95%

Half-life: 1.1-1.7 hours

Time to peak serum concentration:

Immediate release: 2-4 hours

Extended release: 12-14 hours

Elimination: ~80% to 85% of dose excreted in feces and 10% in urine

Dosing: Usual

Children and Adolescents:

Heterozygous familial hypercholesterolemia: Note: Begin treatment if after adequate trial of diet the following are present: LDL-C >189 mg/dL or LDL-C remains >160 mg/dL and positive family history of premature cardiovascular disease or meets NCEP classification. Females must be ≥1 year postmenarche.

Children and Adolescents 10-17 years: Oral: Immediate release tablet:

LDL reduction <20%: Initial: 10 mg once daily with evening meal

LDL reduction ≥20%: Initial: 20 mg once daily with evening meal

Usual range: 10-40 mg once daily with evening meal; may titrate at 4-week intervals; maximum daily dose: 40 mg/**day**

Adults: **Dyslipidemia and primary prevention of CAD: Note:** Doses should be individualized according to the baseline LDL-cholesterol levels, the recommended goal of therapy, and patient response. For patients requiring smaller reductions in cholesterol, the use of the extended release tablet is not recommended; consider use of immediate release formulation.

Immediate release tablet: Oral: Initial: 20 mg once daily with evening meal; adjust dosage at 4-week intervals; maximum daily dose: 80 mg/**day**

Extended release tablet: Oral: Initial: 20, 40, or 60 mg once daily at bedtime; adjust dosage at 4-week intervals; maximum daily dose: 60 mg/**day**

Dosage adjustment in patients who are concomitantly receiving amiodarone: Adults: Dose should not exceed 40 mg/day

Dosage adjustment in patients who are concomitantly receiving danazol, diltiazem, or verapamil: Adults: Initial: 10 mg once daily, not to exceed 20 mg/day

Dosage adjustment in renal impairment: CrCl <30 mL/minute:

Immediate release: Children ≥10 years, Adolescents, and Adults: Doses exceeding 20 mg/day should be carefully considered and implemented cautiously

Extended release: Adults: Initial: 20 mg once daily at bedtime; doses exceeding 20 mg/day should be carefully considered and implemented cautiously

Dosage adjustment in hepatic impairment: There are no dosage adjustment provided in manufacturer's labeling (has not been studied); use is contraindicated in active liver disease or unexplained transaminase elevations.

Administration Oral:

Immediate release tablets: Take with the evening meal.

Extended release tablets: Take at bedtime; do not crush or chew.

Monitoring Parameters

Pediatric patients: Baseline: ALT, AST, and creatine phosphokinase levels (CPK); fasting lipid panel (FLP) and repeat ALT and AST should be checked after 4 weeks of therapy; if no myopathy symptoms or laboratory abnormalities, then monitor FLP, ALT, and AST every 3 to 4 months during the first year and then every 6 months thereafter (NHLBI, 2011).

Adults:

2013 ACC/AHA Blood Cholesterol Guideline recommendations (Stone, 2013):

Lipid panel (total cholesterol, HDL, LDL, triglycerides): Baseline lipid panel; fasting lipid profile within 4 to 12 weeks after initiation or dose adjustment and every 3 to 12 months (as clinically indicated) thereafter. If 2 consecutive LDL levels are <40 mg/dL, consider decreasing the dose.

Hepatic transaminase levels: Baseline measurement of hepatic transaminase levels (ie, ALT); measure hepatic function if symptoms suggest hepatotoxicity (eg, unusual fatigue or weakness, loss of appetite, abdominal pain, dark-colored urine or yellowing of skin or sclera) during therapy.

CPK: CPK should not be routinely measured. Baseline CPK measurement is reasonable for some individuals (eg, family history of statin intolerance or muscle disease, clinical presentation, concomitant drug therapy that may increase risk of myopathy). May measure CPK in any patient with symptoms suggestive of myopathy (pain, tenderness, stiffness, cramping, weakness, or generalized fatigue).

Evaluate for new-onset diabetes mellitus during therapy; if diabetes develops, continue statin therapy and encourage adherence to a heart-healthy diet, physical activity, a healthy body weight, and tobacco cessation.

If patient develops a confusional state or memory impairment, may evaluate patient for nonstatin causes (eg, exposure to other drugs), systemic and neuropsychiatric causes, and the possibility of adverse effects associated with statin therapy.

Manufacturer recommendations: Liver enzyme tests at baseline and repeated when clinically indicated. Measure CPK when myopathy is being considered or may measure CPK periodically in patients starting therapy or when dosage increase is necessary. Analyze lipid panel at intervals of 4 weeks or more.

Dosage Forms Excipient information presented when available (limited, particularly for generics); consult specific product labeling.

Tablet, Oral:

Mevacor: 20 mg, 40 mg

Generic: 10 mg, 20 mg, 40 mg

Tablet Extended Release 24 Hour, Oral:

Altoprev: 20 mg, 40 mg, 60 mg [contains fd&c yellow #6 (sunset yellow)]

- ◆ **Lovenox** *see* Enoxaparin *on page 752*
- ◆ **Lovenox HP (Can)** *see* Enoxaparin *on page 752*
- ◆ **Lovenox With Preservative (Can)** *see* Enoxaparin *on page 752*
- ◆ **Low-Molecular-Weight Iron Dextran (INFeD)** *see* Iron Dextran Complex *on page 1164*
- ◆ **Lozi-Flur** *see* Fluoride *on page 899*
- ◆ **L-PAM** *see* Melphalan *on page 1348*
- ◆ **L-Phenylalanine Mustard** *see* Melphalan *on page 1348*
- ◆ **L-Sarcolysin** *see* Melphalan *on page 1348*
- ◆ **LTA 360 Kit** *see* Lidocaine (Topical) *on page 1258*
- ◆ **LTG** *see* LamoTRIgine *on page 1211*
- ◆ ***L*-Thyroxine Sodium** *see* Levothyroxine *on page 1250*
- ◆ **Lu-26-054** *see* Escitalopram *on page 786*

Lucinactant (loo sin AK tant)

Brand Names: US Surfaxin

Therapeutic Category Lung Surfactant

Generic Availability (US) No

Use Prevention of respiratory distress syndrome (RDS) in premature neonates at high risk for RDS (FDA approved in neonates)

Contraindications There are no contraindications listed within the FDA-approved labeling.

Warnings/Precautions For endotracheal administration only. Rapidly affects oxygenation and lung compliance; restrict use to a highly-supervised clinical setting with immediate availability of clinicians experienced in intubation and ventilatory management of premature infants. Transient episodes of bradycardia, decreased oxygen saturation, endotracheal tube blockage, or reflux of lucinactant into endotracheal tube may occur. Interrupt dosing procedure and initiate measures to stabilize infant's condition; may reinstitute after the patient is stable. Produces rapid improvements in lung oxygenation and compliance that may require frequent adjustments to oxygen delivery and ventilator settings. In clinical trials of lucinactant in adults with acute respiratory distress syndrome (ARDS), an increased incidence of sepsis, pneumothorax, pulmonary embolism, hypotension, sepsis, and death was observed; therapy is not appropriate in the treatment of ARDS in adults.

Adverse Reactions Events observed during the dosing procedure:

Cardiovascular: Bradycardia

Local: Endotracheal tube obstruction, endotracheal tube reflux

Respiratory: Oxygen desaturation

Drug Interactions

Metabolism/Transport Effects None known.

Avoid Concomitant Use

Avoid concomitant use of Lucinactant with any of the following: Ceritinib

Increased Effect/Toxicity

Lucinactant may increase the levels/effects of: Bradycardia-Causing Agents; Ceritinib; Ivabradine; Lacosamide

The levels/effects of Lucinactant may be increased by: Bretylium; Ruxolitinib; Tofacitinib

Decreased Effect There are no known significant interactions involving a decrease in effect.

Storage/Stability Store intact vials refrigerated at 2°C to 8°C (36°F to 46°F); do not freeze. Protect from light.

Mechanism of Action Surfactant administration replaces deficient or ineffective endogenous lung surfactant in neonates at risk of developing RDS. Surfactant prevents the alveoli from collapsing during expiration by lowering surface tension between air and alveolar surfaces. Lucinactant, a synthetic surfactant containing phospholipids, also contains sinapultide (KL4 peptide) which resembles and is believed to mimic the action of one of the human surfactant proteins (SPs), namely SP-B.

Dosing: Neonatal Respiratory distress syndrome, prophylaxis: Premature neonates: Endotracheal: 5.8 mL/kg/dose; may repeat for up to 3 subsequent doses (total of 4 doses) at ≥6 hour intervals within the first 48 hours of life. **Note:** Use in neonates with birthweight >1250 g has not been evaluated.

Preparation for Administration Endotracheal: Prior to administration, warm by placing vial in a preheated dry block heater set at 44°C (111°F) for 15 minutes. After warming, shake vial vigorously until a uniform, free-flowing, and opaque white to off-white suspension appears. If not used immediately, may store protected from light for up to 2 hours at room temperature after warming; do not return to refrigerator. Discard vial or any unused part if not used within 2 hours.

Administration For endotracheal administration only.

Prior to administration, verify that the suspension has been properly warmed; shake vial vigorously; visually inspect to ensure the suspension is uniform, free-flowing, and opaque white to off-white. Vials are for single use only; discard any unused portion. If not used immediately after warming, may store protected from light for up to 2 hours at room temperature; do not return to refrigerator after warming. Discard warmed vial if not used within 2 hours.

Slowly draw up the appropriate amount of lucinactant into a single, appropriately sized syringe (depending on total dose volume) using a 16- or 18-gauge needle. Neonate may be suctioned prior to administration; allow neonate to stabilize prior to administration. Administer endotracheally by instilling through a 5-French end-hole catheter inserted into the endotracheal tube. Administer in four aliquots of 1.45 mL/kg each (1/4 of total volume) alternating positions between right and left lateral decubitus. Each aliquot is instilled as a bolus with continued positive pressure ventilation; evaluate neonate's respiratory status and allow for stabilization between aliquots; oxygen saturation and heart rate should be ≥90% and >120 bpm, respectively, prior to administering the next aliquot. Following administration of one full dose (four aliquots), withhold suctioning for 1 hour unless signs of significant airway obstruction occur and keep the neonate's bed elevated ≥10° for at least 1 to 2 hours.

Monitoring Parameters Continuous heart rate and transcutaneous O_2 saturation; ventilator settings; frequent ABG sampling is necessary to prevent postdosing hyperoxia and hypocarbia.

Additional Information Each mL contains 30 mg phospholipids (22.5 mg dipalmitoylphosphatidylcholine and 7.5 mg palmitoyloleoyl-phosphatidylglycerol, sodium salt), 4.05 mg palmitic acid, and 0.862 mg sinapultide.

Dosage Forms Excipient information presented when available (limited, particularly for generics); consult specific product labeling.

Suspension, Inhalation:
Surfaxin: 30 mg/mL (8.5 mL)

- **Lugol's Solution** *see* Potassium Iodide and Iodine *on page 1742*
- **Lumefantrine and Artemether** *see* Artemether and Lumefantrine *on page 200*
- **Luminal Sodium** *see* PHENobarbital *on page 1679*
- **Lumizyme** *see* Alglucosidase Alfa *on page 94*
- **Lupron (Can)** *see* Leuprolide *on page 1229*
- **Lupron Depot** *see* Leuprolide *on page 1229*
- **Lupron Depot-Ped** *see* Leuprolide *on page 1229*
- **Luvox** *see* FluvoxaMINE *on page 928*
- **Luvox CR [DSC]** *see* FluvoxaMINE *on page 928*
- **Luxiq** *see* Betamethasone (Topical) *on page 280*
- **LY139603** *see* AtoMOXetine *on page 217*
- **LY146032** *see* DAPTOmycin *on page 582*
- **LY170053** *see* OLANZapine *on page 1546*
- **LY-188011** *see* Gemcitabine *on page 961*
- **Lyderm® (Can)** *see* Fluocinonide *on page 898*
- **Lymphocyte Immune Globulin** *see* Antithymocyte Globulin (Equine) *on page 178*
- **Lymphocyte Mitogenic Factor** *see* Aldesleukin *on page 89*
- **Lysodren** *see* Mitotane *on page 1446*
- **Lysteda** *see* Tranexamic Acid *on page 2101*
- **Lyza** *see* Norethindrone *on page 1530*
- **Maalox [OTC]** *see* Calcium Carbonate *on page 343*
- **Maalox Childrens [OTC]** *see* Calcium Carbonate *on page 343*
- **MaC Patch** *see* Capsaicin *on page 362*
- **Macrobid** *see* Nitrofurantoin *on page 1521*
- **Macrodantin** *see* Nitrofurantoin *on page 1521*
- **Macrogol** *see* Polyethylene Glycol 3350 *on page 1723*

Mafenide (MA fe nide)

Brand Names: US Sulfamylon

Therapeutic Category Antibiotic, Topical

Generic Availability (US) May be product dependent

Use

Topical:

Cream: Adjunct in the treatment of second and third degree burns (FDA approved in pediatric patients [age not specified] and adults)

Solution: Adjunctive antibacterial agent for use under moist dressings over meshed autografts on excised burn wounds (FDA approved in ages ≥3 months and adults)

Pregnancy Risk Factor C

Pregnancy Considerations Adverse events were not observed in animal reproduction studies using an oral preparation. The manufacturer does not recommended use in women of childbearing potential unless the burn area covers >20% of the total body surface or when benefits of treatment outweigh possible risks to the fetus.

Breast-Feeding Considerations It is not known if mafenide is excreted in breast milk. Due to the potential for serious adverse reactions in the nursing infant, a decision should be made whether to discontinue nursing or to discontinue the drug, taking into account the importance of treatment to the mother.

Contraindications Hypersensitivity to mafenide or any component of the formulation

Warnings/Precautions Mafenide and its metabolite inhibit carbonic anhydrase; metabolic acidosis may occur.

Symptoms may include compensatory hyperventilation; risk is increased in patients with impaired renal function. Some patients experience masked hyperventilation and respiratory alkalosis; etiology is unknown. Monitor acid-base balance, especially in patients with extensive second-degree or partial-thickness burns and in patients with pulmonary or renal dysfunction. Use with caution in burn patients with acute renal impairment; accumulation of parent drug and metabolite may enhance carbonic anhydrase inhibition and increase risk of metabolic acidosis. Use caution in patients with G6PD deficiency; hemolytic anemia with DIC (including fatalities) has been reported with use, presumably related to G6PD deficiency. Prolonged use may result in fungal or bacterial superinfection, including *C. difficile*-associated diarrhea (CDAD) and pseudomembranous colitis; CDAD has been observed >2 months postantibiotic treatment.

Chemical similarities are present among sulfonamides, sulfonylureas, carbonic anhydrase inhibitors, thiazides, and loop diuretics (except ethacrynic acid). Use in patients with sulfonamide allergy is specifically contraindicated in product labeling, however, a risk of cross-reaction exists in patients with allergy to any of these compounds; avoid use when previous reaction has been severe. Some dosage forms contain sulfites which may cause allergic-type reactions (including anaphylaxis) as well as life-threatening or less severe asthmatic episodes in certain individuals; consider discontinuation of therapy if allergic reactions occur. Potentially significant drug-drug interactions may exist, requiring dose or frequency adjustment, additional monitoring, and/or selection of alternative therapy.

Adverse Reactions

Cardiovascular: Edema, facial edema

Dermatologic: Erythema, maceration, pruritus, rash, urticaria

Endocrine & metabolic: Hyperchloremia, metabolic acidosis

Gastrointestinal: Diarrhea (following accidental ingestion)

Hematologic: Bleeding, bone marrow suppression, DIC, eosinophilia, hemolytic anemia, porphyria

Local: Blisters, burning sensation, excoriation, pain

Respiratory: Dyspnea, hyperventilation, pCO_2 decreased, tachypnea

Miscellaneous: Hypersensitivity

Drug Interactions

Metabolism/Transport Effects None known.

Avoid Concomitant Use

Avoid concomitant use of Mafenide with any of the following: BCG; BCG (Intravesical)

Increased Effect/Toxicity

Mafenide may increase the levels/effects of: Prilocaine; Sodium Nitrite

The levels/effects of Mafenide may be increased by: Nitric Oxide

Decreased Effect

Mafenide may decrease the levels/effects of: BCG; BCG (Intravesical); BCG Vaccine (Immunization); Sodium Picosulfate

Storage/Stability

Cream: Avoid exposure to excessive heat (>40°C [>104°F]).

Powder for solution: Prior to reconstitution, store powder at 15°C to 30°C (59°F to 86°F). Store prepared solution at 20°C to 25°C (68°F to 77°F); excursions permitted between 15°C and 30°C (59°F and 86°F). May store at 15°C to 30°C (59°F to 86°F) for limited periods. Solution may be stored in unopened containers for up to 28 days; once container is open, discard unused portion within 48 hours.

Mechanism of Action As a sulfonamide, mafenide interferes with bacterial folic acid synthesis through competitive inhibition of para-aminobenzoic acid. Spectrum of activity encompasses both gram positive and negative organisms, including *Pseudomonas* and some anaerobes.

Pharmacokinetics (Adult data unless noted)

Absorption: Diffuses through devascularized areas and is rapidly absorbed from burned surface

Metabolism: To para-carboxybenzene sulfonamide which is a carbonic anhydrase inhibitor

Time to peak serum concentration: Topical: 2-4 hours

Elimination: In urine as metabolites

Dosing: Usual

Pediatric: **Burns:** Topical:

Cream: Infants, Children, and Adolescents: Apply once or twice daily with a sterile-gloved hand; apply to a thickness of approximately 1/16 inch; the burned area should be covered with cream at all times.

Solution (5%): Infants ≥3 months, Children, and Adolescents: Cover graft area with 1 layer of fine mesh gauze. Wet an 8-ply burn dressing with mafenide solution and cover graft area. Keep dressing wet using syringe or irrigation tubing every 4 hours (or as necessary), or by moistening dressing every 6 to 8 hours (or as necessary). Irrigation dressing should be secured with bolster dressing and wrapped as appropriate. May leave dressings in place for up to 5 days.

Adult: **Burns:** Topical:

Cream: Apply once or twice daily with a sterile-gloved hand; apply to a thickness of approximately 1/16 inch; the burned area should be covered with cream at all times.

Solution (5%): Cover graft area with 1 layer of fine mesh gauze. Wet an 8-ply burn dressing with mafenide solution and cover graft area. Keep dressing wet using syringe or irrigation tubing every 4 hours (or as necessary), or by moistening dressing every 6 to 8 hours (or as necessary). Irrigation dressing should be secured with bolster dressing and wrapped as appropriate. May leave dressings in place for up to 5 days.

Preparation for Administration Topical: Solution: To prepare a 5% topical solution, add 50 g mafenide powder packet to 1,000 mL of NS for irrigation or sterile water for irrigation. Mix until completely dissolved.

Administration

Topical:

Cream: Apply to cleansed, debrided, burned area with a sterile-gloved hand. Keep burn area covered with cream at all times.

Solution: Cover affected area with gauze and the dressing wetted with mafenide solution; wound dressing may be left undisturbed for up to 5 days.

Monitoring Parameters Acid base balance, improvement of wound healing

Dosage Forms Excipient information presented when available (limited, particularly for generics); consult specific product labeling. [DSC] = Discontinued product

Cream, External, as acetate [strength expressed as base]:

Sulfamylon: 85 mg/g (56.7 g, 113.4 g, 453.6 g) [contains methylparaben, propylparaben, sodium metabisulfite]

Packet, External, as acetate:

Sulfamylon: 50 g (1 ea, 5 ea)

Generic: 50 g (1 ea [DSC], 5 ea [DSC])

◆ **Mafenide Acetate** *see* Mafenide *on page* 1308

◆ **Mag-200 [OTC]** *see* Magnesium Oxide *on page* 1316

◆ **Mag-Al [OTC]** *see* Aluminum Hydroxide and Magnesium Hydroxide *on page* 111

◆ **Mag Citrate** *see* Magnesium Citrate *on page* 1311

◆ **Mag-Delay [OTC]** *see* Magnesium Chloride *on page* 1310

◆ **Mag-G [OTC]** *see* Magnesium Gluconate *on page* 1312

◆ **Maginex™ [OTC]** *see* Magnesium L-aspartate Hydrochloride *on page 1315*

◆ **Maginex™ DS [OTC]** *see* Magnesium L-aspartate Hydrochloride *on page 1315*

◆ **Magnesia Magma** *see* Magnesium Hydroxide *on page 1313*

Magnesium Chloride (mag NEE zhum KLOR ide)

Related Information

Oral Medications That Should Not Be Crushed or Altered *on page 2476*

Brand Names: US Chloromag; Mag-Delay [OTC]; Mag-SR Plus Calcium [OTC]; Mag-SR [OTC]; Slow Magnesium/ Calcium [OTC]; Slow-Mag [OTC]

Therapeutic Category Electrolyte Supplement, Oral; Electrolyte Supplement, Parenteral; Magnesium Salt

Generic Availability (US) Yes

Use Treatment and prevention of hypomagnesemia; dietary supplement (All indications: FDA approved in adults)

Pregnancy Risk Factor C

Pregnancy Considerations Animal reproduction studies have not been conducted. Magnesium crosses the placenta; serum levels in the fetus correlate with those in the mother (Idama, 1998; Osada, 2002).

Breast-Feeding Considerations Magnesium is found in breast milk; concentrations remain constant during the first year of lactation and are not influenced by dietary intake under normal conditions. Magnesium requirements are the same in lactating and non-lactating females (IOM, 1997).

Contraindications Hypersensitivity to any component of the formulation; renal impairment; myocardial disease; coma

Warnings/Precautions Use with caution in patients with impaired renal function (accumulation of magnesium may lead to magnesium intoxication). Monitor serum magnesium level, respiratory rate, blood pressure, deep tendon reflex, and renal function when administered parenterally. Use with extreme caution in patients with myasthenia gravis or other neuromuscular disease. Vigilant monitoring and safe administration techniques (ISMP Medication Safety Alert, 2005) recommended to avoid potential for errors resulting in toxicity when used in obstetrics; monitor patient and fetal status, and serum magnesium levels closely.

Aluminum: The parenteral product may contain aluminum; toxic aluminum concentrations may be seen with high doses, prolonged use, or renal dysfunction. Premature neonates are at higher risk due to immature renal function and aluminum intake from other parenteral sources. Parenteral aluminum exposure of >4 to 5 mcg/kg/day is associated with CNS and bone toxicity; tissue loading may occur at lower doses (Federal Register, 2002). See manufacturer's labeling. Concurrent hypokalemia or hypocalcemia can accompany a magnesium deficit.

Benzyl alcohol and derivatives: Some dosage forms may contain benzyl alcohol; large amounts of benzyl alcohol (≥99 mg/kg/day) have been associated with a potentially fatal toxicity ("gasping syndrome") in neonates; the "gasping syndrome" consists of metabolic acidosis, respiratory distress, gasping respirations, CNS dysfunction (including convulsions, intracranial hemorrhage), hypotension, and cardiovascular collapse (AAP, 1997; CDC, 1982); some data suggests that benzoate displaces bilirubin from protein binding sites (Ahlfors, 2001); avoid or use dosage forms containing benzyl alcohol with caution in neonates. See manufacturer's labeling.

Warnings: Additional Pediatric Considerations Multiple salt forms of magnesium exist; close attention must be paid to the salt form when ordering and administering magnesium; incorrect selection or substitution of one salt for another without proper dosage adjustment may result in serious over- or underdosing.

Adverse Reactions Gastrointestinal: Diarrhea (excessive oral doses)

Drug Interactions

Metabolism/Transport Effects None known.

Avoid Concomitant Use

Avoid concomitant use of Magnesium Chloride with any of the following: Raltegravir

Increased Effect/Toxicity

Magnesium Chloride may increase the levels/effects of: Calcium Channel Blockers; Gabapentin; Neuromuscular-Blocking Agents

The levels/effects of Magnesium Chloride may be increased by: Alfacalcidol; Calcitriol (Systemic); Calcium Channel Blockers

Decreased Effect

Magnesium Chloride may decrease the levels/effects of: Alpha-Lipoic Acid; Bisphosphonate Derivatives; Deferiprone; Dolutegravir; Eltrombopag; Gabapentin; Levothyroxine; Multivitamins/Fluoride (with ADE); Mycophenolate; Phosphate Supplements; Quinolone Antibiotics; Raltegravir; Tetracycline Derivatives; Trientine

The levels/effects of Magnesium Chloride may be decreased by: Alpha-Lipoic Acid; Trientine

Storage/Stability Injection: Prior to reconstitution, store at controlled room temperature of 15°C to 30°C (59°F to 86°F).

Mechanism of Action Magnesium is important as a cofactor in many enzymatic reactions in the body involving protein synthesis and carbohydrate metabolism (at least 300 enzymatic reactions require magnesium). Actions on lipoprotein lipase have been found to be important in reducing serum cholesterol and on sodium/potassium ATPase in promoting polarization (eg, neuromuscular functioning).

Pharmacokinetics (Adult data unless noted)

Absorption: Oral: Up to 30%

Elimination: Renal with unabsorbed drug excreted in feces

Dosing: Neonatal Note: Dosing presented in mg and mEq, verify dosing units; 1 g magnesium chloride = elemental magnesium 120 mg = magnesium 9.85 mEq = magnesium 4.93 mmol

Adequate intake (AI): Dose expressed as **elemental magnesium:** Oral: 30 mg daily; requirements may vary based on prematurity, postnatal age, and other clinical factors; serum magnesium concentrations should be monitored closely to determine patient-specific needs (IOM 1997)

Hypomagnesemia: Limited data available: **Note:** Dose depends on clinical condition and serum magnesium concentration; monitor closely. Dose expressed as **elemental magnesium:** IM, IV: 2.5 to 5 mg/kg/dose every 8 to 12 hours for 2 to 3 doses; dosing based on experience with magnesium sulfate salt which is preferred (Kliegman 2011)

Parenteral nutrition, maintenance requirement: Limited data available: Dose expressed as **elemental magnesium:** IV: 0.3 to 0.5 mEq/kg/day (Mirtallo 2004)

Dosing: Usual Note: Dosing presented in mg and mEq, verify dosing units; 1 g magnesium chloride = elemental magnesium 120 mg = magnesium 9.85 mEq = magnesium 4.93 mmol; serum magnesium is poor reflection of repletional status as the majority of magnesium is intracellular; serum concentrations may be transiently normal for a few hours after a dose is given; therefore, aim for consistently high normal serum concentrations in patients with normal renal function for most efficient repletion.

Pediatric:

Adequate intake (AI) (IOM 1997): Dose expressed in terms of **elemental magnesium:**

1 to 6 months: 30 mg daily

7 to 12 months: 75 mg daily

Recommended daily allowance (RDA) (IOM 1997): Dose expressed in terms of **elemental magnesium;** during pregnancy and lactation, requirements may change:

1 to 3 years: 80 mg daily

4 to 8 years: 130 mg daily

9 to 13 years: 240 mg daily

14 to 18 years:

Male: 410 mg daily

Female: 360 mg daily

Hypomagnesemia: Limited data available: Infants, Children and Adolescents: Dose expressed as **elemental magnesium:**

IV: 2.5 to 5 mg/kg/dose every 6 hours for 2 to 3 doses; dosing based on experience with magnesium sulfate salt which is preferred (Kliegman 2011)

Oral: **Note:** Achieving optimal magnesium levels using oral therapy may be difficult due to the propensity for magnesium to cause diarrhea; IV replacement may be more appropriate particularly in situations of severe deficit: 10 to 20 mg/kg/dose up to 4 times daily (Kliegman 2007)

Parenteral nutrition, maintenance requirement (Mirtallo 2004): **Note:** Dose expressed as **elemental magnesium:** IV:

Infants and Children ≤50 kg: 0.3 to 0.5 **mEq**/kg/day

Children >50 kg and Adolescents: 10 to 30 **mEq**/kg/day

Adult:

Recommended daily allowance (RDA) (IOM 1997):

Adults 19 to 30 years:

Females: 310 mg elemental magnesium daily

Pregnant females: 350 mg elemental magnesium daily

Breast-feeding females: 310 mg elemental magnesium daily

Males: 400 mg elemental magnesium daily

Adults ≥31 years:

Females: 320 mg elemental magnesium daily

Pregnant females: 360 mg elemental magnesium daily

Breast-feeding females: 320 mg elemental magnesium daily

Males: 420 mg elemental magnesium daily

Dietary supplement: Oral (Mag 64, Mag Delay, Slow-Mag): 2 tablets once daily

Parenteral nutrition, maintenance requirement: IV: 8 to 20 mEq **elemental magnesium** daily (Mirtallo 2004)

Dosing adjustment in renal impairment: According to the manufacturer, use is contraindicated in patients with renal impairment.

Dosing adjustment in hepatic impairment: There are no dosage adjustments provided in the manufacturer's labeling.

Preparation for Administration Parenteral: Intermittent IV infusion: Per the manufacturer dilute magnesium chloride 4,000 mg in 250 mL D_5W (resultant concentration: 16 mg/mL of magnesium chloride).

Administration

Oral: Tablet: Take with full glass of water; do not chew or crush sustained release formulations

Parenteral: Intermittent IV infusion: After dilution (concentration: 16 mg/mL magnesium chloride), infuse slowly at a rate not to exceed 48 mg/minute of magnesium chloride

Monitoring Parameters Serum magnesium, deep tendon reflexes, respiratory rate, renal function, blood pressure, stool output (laxative use)

Reference Range

Pediatric: 1.5 to 2.5 mEq/L

Adult: 1.6 to 2.5 mEq/L

Additional Information

Elemental Magnesium Content of Magnesium Salts

Magnesium Salt	Elemental Magnesium (mg/500 mg salt)	Magnesium (mEq/500 mg salt)
Magnesium chloride	60	4.93
Magnesium gluconate	27	2.25
Magnesium L-aspartate	49.6	4.05
Magnesium oxide	300	24.88
Magnesium sulfate	49.3	4.06

Adverse effects associated with elevated serum magnesium concentrations may include:

>3 mg/dL: Blocked peripheral neuromuscular transmission leading to anticonvulsant effects, depressed CNS

>5 mg/dL: Depressed deep tendon reflexes, flushing, somnolence

>12 mg/dL: Complete heart block, respiratory paralysis

Dosage Forms Considerations

1 g magnesium chloride = elemental magnesium 120 mg = magnesium 9.85 mEq = magnesium 4.93 mmol

Elemental magnesium 64 mg = magnesium 5.26 mEq = magnesium 2.62 mmol

Dosage Forms Excipient information presented when available (limited, particularly for generics); consult specific product labeling.

Solution, Injection, as hexahydrate:

Chloromag: 200 mg/mL (50 mL) [contains benzyl alcohol]

Generic: 200 mg/mL (50 mL)

Tablet Delayed Release, Oral:

Mag-SR Plus Calcium: 64-106 MG [starch free, sugar free]

Slow Magnesium/Calcium: 64-106 MG

Slow-Mag: 71.5-119 MG [contains fd&c blue #2 aluminum lake]

Tablet Extended Release, Oral:

Mag-Delay: 535 (64 Mg) MG

Mag-SR: 535 (64 Mg) MG [starch free, sugar free]

Magnesium Citrate (mag NEE zhum SIT rate)

Brand Names: US Citroma [OTC]

Brand Names: Canada Citro-Mag

Therapeutic Category Laxative, Osmotic; Magnesium Salt

Generic Availability (US) Yes

Use Short-term treatment of constipation

Pregnancy Considerations Magnesium crosses the placenta; serum concentrations in the fetus are similar to those in the mother (Idama, 1998; Osada, 2002). The American Gastroenterological Association considers the use of magnesium citrate as a laxative to be low risk in pregnancy, but long term use should be avoided (not the preferred treatment of chronic constipation) (Mahadevan, 2006).

Breast-Feeding Considerations Magnesium is found in breast milk; concentrations remain constant during the first year of lactation and are not influenced by dietary intake under normal conditions (IOM, 1997).

Contraindications OTC labeling: When used for self-medication, do not use if on low salt diet

Warnings/Precautions Use with caution in patients with impaired renal function (accumulation of magnesium may lead to magnesium intoxication) or in patients with myasthenia gravis or other neuromuscular disease.

Constipation (self-medication, OTC use): Appropriate use: For occasional use only; serious side effects may occur with prolonged use. For use only under the supervision of a physician in patients with kidney dysfunction, sodium- or magnesium-restricted diets, abdominal pain/nausea/vomiting, with a sudden change in bowel habits which has persisted for >2 weeks, or use of a laxative for >1 week. If rectal bleeding develops or a bowel movement does not occur after use, discontinue use and consult a healthcare provider.

Warnings: Additional Pediatric Considerations Multiple salt forms of magnesium exist; close attention must be paid to the salt form when ordering and administering magnesium; incorrect selection or substitution of one salt for another without proper dosage adjustment may result in serious over- or underdosing.

Adverse Reactions Gastrointestinal: Abdominal pain, diarrhea, gas formation, nausea, vomiting

Drug Interactions

Metabolism/Transport Effects None known.

Avoid Concomitant Use

Avoid concomitant use of Magnesium Citrate with any of the following: Calcium Polystyrene Sulfonate; Raltegravir; Sodium Polystyrene Sulfonate

Increased Effect/Toxicity

Magnesium Citrate may increase the levels/effects of: Aluminum Hydroxide; Calcium Channel Blockers; Calcium Polystyrene Sulfonate; Gabapentin; Neuromuscular-Blocking Agents; Sodium Polystyrene Sulfonate

The levels/effects of Magnesium Citrate may be increased by: Alfacalcidol; Calcitriol (Systemic); Calcium Channel Blockers

Decreased Effect

Magnesium Citrate may decrease the levels/effects of: Alpha-Lipoic Acid; Bisphosphonate Derivatives; Deferiprone; Dolutegravir; Eltrombopag; Gabapentin; Levothyroxine; Multivitamins/Fluoride (with ADE); Mycophenolate; Phosphate Supplements; Quinolone Antibiotics; Raltegravir; Tetracycline Derivatives; Trientine

The levels/effects of Magnesium Citrate may be decreased by: Alpha-Lipoic Acid; Trientine

Storage/Stability Store at controlled room temperature of 15°C to 30°C (59°F to 86°F).

Oral solution: Discard remaining medication within 24 hours of opening.

Mechanism of Action Promotes bowel evacuation by causing osmotic retention of fluid which distends the colon with increased peristaltic activity

Pharmacodynamics Onset of action: Laxative: Oral: 4-8 hours

Pharmacokinetics (Adult data unless noted)

Absorption: Oral: Up to 30%

Elimination: Renal with unabsorbed drug excreted in feces

Dosing: Usual Cathartic: Oral:

Children <6 years: 2-4 mL/kg/dose given once or in divided doses

Children 6-12 years: 100-150 mL/dose given once or in divided doses

Children >12 years and Adults: 150-300 mL/dose given once or in divided doses

Dosing adjustment in renal impairment: Patients in severe renal failure should not receive magnesium due to toxicity from accumulation. Patients with a CrCl <25 mL/minute receiving magnesium should have serum magnesium levels monitored.

Administration Oral:

Solution: Mix with water and administer on an empty stomach.

Tablet: Take with full glass of water.

Monitoring Parameters Stool output

Test Interactions Increased magnesium; decreased protein, decreased calcium (S), decreased potassium (S)

Dosage Forms Considerations 1 g magnesium citrate elemental magnesium 160 mg = magnesium 13 mEq magnesium 6.5 mmol

Dosage Forms Excipient information presented when available (limited, particularly for generics); consult specific product labeling.

Solution, Oral:

Citroma: 1.745 g/30 mL (296 mL) [contains polyethylene glycol, saccharin sodium; lemon flavor]

Citroma: 1.745 g/30 mL (296 mL) [low sodium; lemon flavor]

Citroma: 1.745 g/30 mL (296 mL) [low sodium; contains fd&c red #40, saccharin sodium; cherry flavor]

Generic: 1.745 g/30 mL (296 mL)

Tablet, Oral:

Generic: 100 mg

Magnesium Gluconate

(mag NEE zhum GLOO koe nate)

Brand Names: US Mag-G [OTC]; Magonate [OTC]

Therapeutic Category Electrolyte Supplement, Oral; Magnesium Salt

Generic Availability (US) May be product dependent

Use Treatment and prevention of hypomagnesemia; dietary supplement

Pregnancy Considerations Magnesium crosses the placenta; serum concentrations in the fetus are similar to those in the mother (Idama, 1998; Osada, 2002).

Breast-Feeding Considerations Magnesium is found in breast milk; concentrations remain constant during the first year of lactation and are not influenced by dietary intake under normal conditions. Magnesium requirements are the same in lactating and nonlactating females (IOM, 1997).

Contraindications Hypersensitivity to any component of the formulation

Warnings/Precautions Use magnesium with caution in patients with impaired renal function (accumulation of magnesium may lead to magnesium intoxication). Use with extreme caution in patients with myasthenia gravis or other neuromuscular disease.

Constipation (self-medication, OTC use): For occasional use only; serious side effects may occur with prolonged use. For use only under the supervision of a healthcare provider in patients with kidney dysfunction, or with a sudden change in bowel habits which persist for >2 weeks. Do not use if abdominal pain, nausea, or vomiting are present.

Benzyl alcohol and derivatives: Some dosage forms may contain sodium benzoate/benzoic acid; benzoic acid (benzoate) is a metabolite of benzyl alcohol; large amounts of benzyl alcohol (≥99 mg/kg/day) have been associated with a potentially fatal toxicity ("gasping syndrome") in neonates; the "gasping syndrome" consists of metabolic acidosis, respiratory distress, gasping respirations, CNS dysfunction (including convulsions, intracranial hemorrhage), hypotension, and cardiovascular collapse (AAP, 1997; CDC, 1982); some data suggests that benzoate displaces bilirubin from protein binding sites (Ahlfors, 2001); avoid or use dosage forms containing benzyl alcohol derivative with caution in neonates. See manufacturer's labeling.

Warnings: Additional Pediatric Considerations Multiple salt forms of magnesium exist; close attention must be paid to the salt form when ordering and administering magnesium; incorrect selection or substitution of one salt for another without proper dosage adjustment may result in serious over- or underdosing.

Adverse Reactions Gastrointestinal: Diarrhea (excessive oral doses)

Drug Interactions

Metabolism/Transport Effects None known.

Avoid Concomitant Use

Avoid concomitant use of Magnesium Gluconate with any of the following: Raltegravir

Increased Effect/Toxicity

Magnesium Gluconate may increase the levels/effects of: Calcium Channel Blockers; Gabapentin; Neuromuscular-Blocking Agents

The levels/effects of Magnesium Gluconate may be increased by: Alfacalcidol; Calcitriol (Systemic); Calcium Channel Blockers

Decreased Effect

Magnesium Gluconate may decrease the levels/effects of: Alpha-Lipoic Acid; Bisphosphonate Derivatives; Deferiprone; Dolutegravir; Eltrombopag; Gabapentin; Levothyroxine; Multivitamins/Fluoride (with ADE); Mycophenolate; Phosphate Supplements; Quinolone Antibiotics; Raltegravir; Tetracycline Derivatives; Trientine

The levels/effects of Magnesium Gluconate may be decreased by: Alpha-Lipoic Acid; Trientine

Mechanism of Action Magnesium is important as a cofactor in many enzymatic reactions in the body involving protein synthesis and carbohydrate metabolism (at least 300 enzymatic reactions require magnesium). Actions on lipoprotein lipase have been found to be important in reducing serum cholesterol and on sodium/potassium ATPase in promoting polarization (eg, neuromuscular functioning).

Pharmacokinetics (Adult data unless noted)

Absorption: Oral: Up to 30%

Elimination: Renal with unabsorbed drug excreted in feces

Dosing: Neonatal Recommended daily allowance of magnesium: Oral: 40 mg/day

Dosing: Usual Oral: **Note:** Achieving optimal magnesium levels using oral therapy may be difficult due to the propensity for magnesium to cause diarrhea: IV replacement may be more appropriate particularly in situations of severe deficit.

Recommended daily allowance of magnesium: See table.

Magnesium – Recommended Daily Allowance (RDA) and Estimated Average Requirement (EAR) (in terms of elemental magnesium)

Age	RDA (mg/day)	EAR (mg/day)
1 to <6 mo	40	30
6 to <12 mo	60	75
1-3 y	80	65
4-8 y	130	110
Male		
9-13 y	240	200
14-18 y	410	340
Female		
9-13 y	240	200
14-18 y	360	300

Prevention and treatment of hypomagnesemia:

Children: 10-20 mg/kg **elemental** magnesium per dose up to 4 times/day

Adults: 500-1000 mg 3 times/day

Dosing adjustment in renal impairment: Patients in severe renal failure should not receive magnesium due to toxicity from accumulation. Patients with a CrCl <25 mL/minute receiving magnesium should have serum magnesium levels monitored.

Administration Oral:

Solution: Mix with water and administer on an empty stomach.

Tablet: Take with full glass of water.

Additional Information Magnesium gluconate 500 mg = 27 mg **elemental** magnesium = 2.4 mEq magnesium

Elemental Magnesium Content of Magnesium Salts

Magnesium Salt	Elemental Magnesium (mg/500 mg salt)	Magnesium (mEq/500 mg salt)
Magnesium chloride	59	4.9
Magnesium gluconate	27	2.4
Magnesium L-aspartate	49.6	4.1
Magnesium oxide	302	25
Magnesium sulfate	49.3	4.1

Adverse effects associated with elevated serum magnesium concentrations may include:

>3 mg/dL: Blocked peripheral neuromuscular transmission leading to anticonvulsant effects, depressed CNS

>5 mg/dL: Depressed deep tendon reflexes, flushing, somnolence

>12 mg/dL: Complete heart block, respiratory paralysis

Dosage Forms Considerations 1 g magnesium gluconate = elemental magnesium 54 mg = magnesium 4.5 mEq = magnesium 2.25 mmol

Dosage Forms Excipient information presented when available (limited, particularly for generics); consult specific product labeling.

Liquid, Oral:

Magonate: Magnesium carbonate equivalent to magnesium gluconate 1000 mg (54 mg elemental magnesium) per 5 mL (355 mL) [contains sodium benzoate; mixed melon flavor]

Tablet, Oral:

Mag-G: 500 mg (27 mg elemental magnesium)

Magonate: 500 mg (27 mg elemental magnesium) [scored]

Magonate: 500 mg (27 mg elemental magnesium) [scored; contains fd&c yellow #6 aluminum lake]

Generic: Elemental magnesium 27.5 mg

Tablet, Oral [preservative free]:

Generic: 500 mg (27 mg elemental magnesium)

Magnesium Hydroxide

(mag NEE zhum hye DROKS ide)

Brand Names: US Dulcolax Milk of Magnesia [OTC]; Milk of Magnesia Concentrate [OTC]; Milk of Magnesia [OTC]; Pedia-Lax [OTC]

Therapeutic Category Antacid; Laxative, Osmotic

Generic Availability (US) May be product dependent

Use Relief of occasional constipation (OTC products: FDA approved in ages ≥2 years and adults); relief of heartburn, sour stomach, acid indigestion, and upset stomach associated with these conditions (OTC products: Phillips chewable tablet: FDA approved in ages ≥12 years and adults). **Note:** Refer to product labeling for specific information on uses and approval in pediatric patients.

Pregnancy Considerations Magnesium crosses the placenta; serum concentrations in the fetus are similar to those in the mother (Idama, 1998; Osada, 2002). The American Gastroenterological Association considers the use of magnesium containing antacids to be low risk in pregnancy (Mahadevan, 2006).

Breast-Feeding Considerations Magnesium is found in breast milk; concentrations remain constant during the first year of lactation and are not influenced by dietary intake under normal conditions (IOM, 1997).

Contraindications Hypersensitivity to magnesium hydroxide or any component of the formulation

Warnings/Precautions Use magnesium with caution in patients with impaired renal function (accumulation of magnesium may lead to magnesium intoxication). Use with extreme caution in patients with myasthenia gravis or other neuromuscular disease.

For self-medication (OTC use): For occasional use only; serious side effects may occur with prolonged use. For use only under the supervision of a healthcare provider in patients with kidney dysfunction, or with a sudden change in bowel habits which persist for >2 weeks. Patients should notify healthcare provider of any sudden change in bowel habits which last >14 days, stomach pain, nausea, or vomiting or if use is needed for >1 week. Not for OTC use in children <2 years of age.

Warnings: Additional Pediatric Considerations Multiple salt forms of magnesium exist; close attention must be paid to the salt form when ordering and administering magnesium; incorrect selection or substitution of one salt for another without proper dosage adjustment may result in serious over- or underdosing.

Some dosage forms may contain propylene glycol; in neonates large amounts of propylene glycol delivered orally, intravenously (eg, >3,000 mg/day), or topically have been associated with potentially fatal toxicities which can include metabolic acidosis, seizures, renal failure, and CNS depression; toxicities have also been reported in children and adults including hyperosmolality, lactic acidosis, seizures, and respiratory depression; use caution (AAP, 1997; Shehab, 2009).

Drug Interactions

Metabolism/Transport Effects None known.

Avoid Concomitant Use

Avoid concomitant use of Magnesium Hydroxide with any of the following: Calcium Polystyrene Sulfonate; QuiNINE; Raltegravir; Sodium Polystyrene Sulfonate

Increased Effect/Toxicity

Magnesium Hydroxide may increase the levels/effects of: Amphetamines; Calcium Channel Blockers; Calcium Polystyrene Sulfonate; Dexmethylphenidate; Gabapentin; Methylphenidate; Misoprostol; Neuromuscular-Blocking Agents; QuiNIDine; Sodium Polystyrene Sulfonate

The levels/effects of Magnesium Hydroxide may be increased by: Alfacalcidol; Calcitriol (Systemic); Calcium Channel Blockers

Decreased Effect

Magnesium Hydroxide may decrease the levels/effects of: Allopurinol; Alpha-Lipoic Acid; Antipsychotic Agents (Phenothiazines); Atazanavir; Bisacodyl; Bismuth Subcitrate; Bisphosphonate Derivatives; Bosutinib; Captopril; Cefditoren; Cefpodoxime; Cefuroxime; Chloroquine; Corticosteroids (Oral); Dabigatran Etexilate; Dabrafenib; Dasatinib; Deferiprone; Delavirdine; Dolutegravir; Eltrombopag; Elvitegravir; Erlotinib; Fexofenadine; Fosinopril; Gabapentin; HMG-CoA Reductase Inhibitors; Hyoscyamine; Iron Salts; Isoniazid; Itraconazole; Ketoconazole (Systemic); Ledipasvir; Levothyroxine; Mesalamine; Methenamine; Multivitamins/Fluoride (with ADE); Multivitamins/Minerals (with ADEK, Folate, Iron); Mycophenolate; Nilotinib; PAZOPanib; PenicillAMINE; Phosphate Supplements; Potassium Acid Phosphate; QuiNINE; Quinolone Antibiotics; Raltegravir; Rilpivirine; Riociguat; Sotalol; Strontium Ranelate; Sulpiride; Tetracycline Derivatives; Trientine

The levels/effects of Magnesium Hydroxide may be decreased by: Alpha-Lipoic Acid; Trientine

Mechanism of Action Promotes bowel evacuation by causing osmotic retention of fluid which distends the colon with increased peristaltic activity; reacts with hydrochloric acid in stomach to form magnesium chloride

Pharmacokinetics (Adult data unless noted)

Absorption: Oral: Up to 30%

Elimination: Renal with unabsorbed drug excreted in feces

Dosing: Usual

Pediatric: **Note:** Dose expressed as mg of magnesium hydroxide.

Antacid: Oral: Children ≥12 years and Adolescents (Phillips 311 mg chewable tablet): 2 to 4 tablets every 4 hours up to 4 times per day. Do not exceed 4 doses in 24 hours.

Constipation, chronic: Oral: Infants, Children, and Adolescents: Limited data available: 80 to 240 mg/kg/day divided once or twice daily (Wyllie 2011); usual adult dose is 2,400 to 4,800 mg/day

Constipation, occasional: Oral:

Children 2 to <6 years: 400 to 1,200 mg/day in single or divided doses. Maximum daily dose: 1,200 mg/**day**

Children 6 to <12 years: 1,200 to 2,400 mg/day in single or divided doses. Maximum daily dose: 2,400 mg/**day**

Children ≥12 years and Adolescents: 2,400 to 4,800 mg/day in single or divided doses. Maximum daily dose: 4,800 mg/**day**

Fecal impaction, slow disimpaction: Limited data available: Oral: Children and Adolescents: 160 mg/kg twice daily for 7 days (Pashankar 2005; Wyllie 2011)

Adult:

Antacid: OTC labeling: Oral:

Liquid: Magnesium hydroxide 400 mg per 5 mL: 5 to 15 mL as needed up to 4 times/day

Tablet: Magnesium hydroxide 311 mg per tablet: 2 to 4 tablets every 4 hours up to 4 times/day

Laxative: OTC labeling: Oral:

Liquid:

Magnesium hydroxide 400 mg per 5 mL: 30 to 60 mL/day once daily at bedtime or in divided doses

Magnesium hydroxide 800 mg per 5 mL: 15 to 30 mL/day once daily at bedtime or in divided doses

Tablet: Magnesium hydroxide 311 mg/tablet: 8 tablets/day once daily at bedtime or in divided doses

Dosing adjustment in renal impairment: Patients in severe renal failure should not receive magnesium due to toxicity from accumulation. Patients with a CrCl <30 mL/minute receiving magnesium should have serum magnesium levels monitored.

Dosing adjustment in hepatic impairment: There are no dosage adjustments provided in manufacturer's labeling.

Administration Oral: Liquid doses may be diluted with a small amount of water prior to administration. All doses should be followed by 8 ounces of water in patients ≥2 years of age.

Test Interactions Increased magnesium; decreased protein, calcium (S), decreased potassium (S)

Dosage Forms Excipient information presented when available (limited, particularly for generics); consult specific product labeling. [DSC] = Discontinued product

Suspension, Oral:

Dulcolax Milk of Magnesia: 400 mg/5 mL (355 mL) [sugar free; unflavored flavor]

Dulcolax Milk of Magnesia: 400 mg/5 mL (355 mL) [sugar free; contains saccharin sodium; mint flavor]

Milk of Magnesia: 400 mg/5 mL (355 mL, 480 mL); 1200 mg/15 mL (355 mL)

Milk of Magnesia: 1200 mg/15 mL (355 mL) [mint flavor]

Milk of Magnesia: 7.75% (360 mL, 480 mL)

Milk of Magnesia: 7.75% (355 mL, 473 mL) [mint flavor]

Milk of Magnesia: 7.75% (30 mL) [spearmint flavor]

Milk of Magnesia: 400 mg/5mL (473 mL [DSC])

Milk of Magnesia: 1200 mg/15 mL (355 mL) [gluten free, stimulant free, sugar free; contains saccharin sodium]

Milk of Magnesia: 400 mg/5 mL (355 mL, 473 mL) [low sodium, sugar free]

Milk of Magnesia: 400 mg/5 mL (473 mL, 769 mL); 1200 mg/15 mL (355 mL) [stimulant free, sugar free]
Milk of Magnesia: 1200 mg/15 mL (355 mL) [stimulant free, sugar free; contains saccharin sodium]
Milk of Magnesia: 400 mg/5 mL (473 mL); 1200 mg/15 mL (355 mL) [sugar free]
Milk of Magnesia Concentrate: 2400 mg/10 mL (100 mL, 400 mL) [lemon flavor]
Milk of Magnesia Concentrate: 2400 mg/10 mL (10 mL) [contains methylparaben, propylene glycol, propylparaben, saccharin sodium; lemon flavor]
Tablet Chewable, Oral:
Pedia-Lax: 400 mg [scored; stimulant free; contains fd&c red #40 aluminum lake; watermelon flavor]

◆ **Magnesium Hydroxide and Aluminum Hydroxide** *see* Aluminum Hydroxide and Magnesium Hydroxide *on page 111*

Magnesium L-aspartate Hydrochloride

(mag NEE zhum el as PAR tate hye droe KLOR ide)

Brand Names: US Maginex™ DS [OTC]; Maginex™ [OTC]

Therapeutic Category Electrolyte Supplement, Oral; Magnesium Salt

Generic Availability (US) No

Use Magnesium supplement

Pregnancy Considerations Magnesium crosses the placenta; serum concentrations in the fetus are similar to those in the mother (Idama, 1998; Osada, 2002).

Breast-Feeding Considerations Magnesium is found in breast milk; concentrations remain constant during the first year of lactation and are not influenced by dietary intake under normal conditions. Magnesium requirements are the same in lactating and nonlactating females (IOM, 1997).

Contraindications There are no contraindications in the manufacturer's labeling.

Warnings/Precautions Use magnesium with caution in patients with impaired renal function (accumulation of magnesium may lead to magnesium intoxication). Use with extreme caution in patients with myasthenia gravis or other neuromuscular disease.

Constipation (self-medication, OTC use): Appropriate use: For occasional use only; serious side effects may occur with prolonged use. For use only under the supervision of a physician in patients with kidney dysfunction, sodium or magnesium restricted diets, abdominal pain/nausea/vomiting, or with a sudden change in bowel habits which has persisted for >2 weeks. If rectal bleeding develops or a bowel movement does not occur after use, discontinue use and consult a healthcare provider.

Warnings: Additional Pediatric Considerations Multiple salt forms of magnesium exist; close attention must be paid to the salt form when ordering and administering magnesium; incorrect selection or substitution of one salt for another without proper dosage adjustment may result in serious over- or underdosing.

Adverse Reactions Gastrointestinal: Abdominal cramps, diarrhea (excessive oral doses), gas formation

Drug Interactions

Metabolism/Transport Effects None known.

Avoid Concomitant Use

Avoid concomitant use of Magnesium L-aspartate Hydrochloride with any of the following: Raltegravir

Increased Effect/Toxicity

Magnesium L-aspartate Hydrochloride may increase the levels/effects of: Calcium Channel Blockers; Gabapentin; Neuromuscular-Blocking Agents

The levels/effects of Magnesium L-aspartate Hydrochloride may be increased by: Alfacalcidol; Calcitriol (Systemic); Calcium Channel Blockers

Decreased Effect

Magnesium L-aspartate Hydrochloride may decrease the levels/effects of: Alpha-Lipoic Acid; Bisphosphonate Derivatives; Deferiprone; Dolutegravir; Eltrombopag; Gabapentin; Levothyroxine; Multivitamins/Fluoride (with ADE); Mycophenolate; Phosphate Supplements; Quinolone Antibiotics; Raltegravir; Tetracycline Derivatives; Trientine

The levels/effects of Magnesium L-aspartate Hydrochloride may be decreased by: Alpha-Lipoic Acid; Trientine

Storage/Stability Store at room temperature in a cool, dry place.

Mechanism of Action Magnesium is important as a cofactor in many enzymatic reactions in the body involving protein synthesis and carbohydrate metabolism (at least 300 enzymatic reactions require magnesium). Actions on lipoprotein lipase have been found to be important in reducing serum cholesterol and on sodium/potassium ATPase in promoting polarization (eg, neuromuscular functioning).

Pharmacokinetics (Adult data unless noted)
Absorption: Oral: Up to 30%
Elimination: Renal with unabsorbed drug excreted in feces

Dosing: Neonatal Recommended daily allowance of magnesium: Oral: 40 mg/day

Dosing: Usual Oral:
Recommended daily allowance of magnesium: See table.

Magnesium – Recommended Daily Allowance (RDA) and Estimated Average Requirement (EAR) (in terms of elemental magnesium)

Age	RDA (mg/day)	EAR (mg/day)
1 to <6 mo	40	30
6 to <12 mo	60	75
1-3 y	80	65
4-8 y	130	110
Male		
9-13 y	240	200
14-18 y	410	340
Female		
9-13 y	240	200
14-18 y	360	300

Hypomagnesemia: **Note:** Achieving optimal magnesium levels using oral therapy may be difficult due to the propensity for magnesium to cause diarrhea: IV replacement may be more appropriate particularly in situations of severe deficit:
Children: 10-20 mg/kg elemental magnesium per dose up to 4 times/day
Dietary supplement: Adults: 1230 mg up to 3 times/day

Dosing adjustment in renal impairment: Patients in severe renal failure should not receive magnesium due to toxicity from accumulation. Patients with a CrCl <25 mL/minute receiving magnesium should have serum magnesium levels monitored.

Preparation for Administration Oral: Granules: Mix each packet in 4 ounces of water or juice prior to administration.

Administration
Oral:
Granules: Mix each packet prior to administration
Tablet: Take with full glass of water

Additional Information Magnesium L-aspartate 500 mg = 49.6 mg **elemental** magnesium = 4.1 mEq magnesium

Elemental Magnesium Content of Magnesium Salts

Magnesium Salt	Elemental Magnesium (mg/500 mg salt)	Magnesium (mEq/500 mg salt)
Magnesium chloride	59	4.9
Magnesium gluconate	27	2.4
Magnesium L-aspartate	49.6	4.1
Magnesium oxide	302	25
Magnesium sulfate	49.3	4.1

Dosage Forms Considerations 1 g magnesium L-aspartate Hydrochloride ≈ elemental magnesium 100 mg = magnesium 8.1 mEq = magnesium 4.05 mmol

Dosage Forms Excipient information presented when available (limited, particularly for generics); consult specific product labeling.

Granules for solution, oral [preservative free]:

Maginex™ DS: 1230 mg/packet (30s) [sugar free; lemon flavor; equivalent to elemental magnesium 122 mg]

Tablet, enteric coated, oral [preservative free]:

Maginex™: 615 mg [sugar free; equivalent to elemental magnesium 61 mg]

Magnesium Oxide (mag NEE zhum OKS ide)

Brand Names: US Mag-200 [OTC]; Maox [OTC]; Uro-Mag [OTC]

Therapeutic Category Electrolyte Supplement, Oral; Laxative, Osmotic; Magnesium Salt

Generic Availability (US) May be product dependent

Use Magnesium supplement; short-term treatment of constipation; treatment of hyperacidity symptoms

Pregnancy Considerations Magnesium crosses the placenta; serum concentrations in the fetus are similar to those in the mother (Idama, 1998; Osada, 2002)

Breast-Feeding Considerations Magnesium is found in breast milk; concentrations remain constant during the first year of lactation and are not influenced by dietary intake under normal conditions. Magnesium requirements are the same in lactating and nonlactating females (IOM,1997).

Contraindications There are no contraindications in the manufacturer's labeling

Warnings/Precautions Use magnesium with caution in patients with impaired renal function (accumulation of magnesium may lead to magnesium intoxication). Use with extreme caution in patients with myasthenia gravis or other neuromuscular disease.

Acid indigestion/upset stomach (self-medication, OTC use): For occasional use only; serious side effects may occur with prolonged use. For use only under the supervision of a physician in patients with kidney dysfunction or who are pregnant or breastfeeding. Unless directed by a physician, do not use for >2 weeks or exceed the recommended daily dose.

Constipation (self-medication, OTC use): For occasional use only; serious side effects may occur with prolonged use. For use only under the supervision of a physician in patients with kidney dysfunction, sodium or magnesium restricted diets, abdominal pain/nausea/vomiting,a sudden change in bowel habits which has persisted for >2 weeks, or who are pregnant or breastfeeding. If rectal bleeding develops or a bowel movement does not occur after use, discontinue use and consult healthcare provider.

Warnings: Additional Pediatric Considerations Multiple salt forms of magnesium exist; close attention must be paid to the salt form when ordering and administerin magnesium; incorrect selection or substitution of one sa for another without proper dosage adjustment may result i serious over- or underdosing.

Adverse Reactions Gastrointestinal: Diarrhea (excessiv oral doses)

Drug Interactions

Metabolism/Transport Effects None known.

Avoid Concomitant Use

Avoid concomitant use of Magnesium Oxide with any o the following: Calcium Polystyrene Sulfonate; Raltegra vir; Sodium Polystyrene Sulfonate

Increased Effect/Toxicity

Magnesium Oxide may increase the levels/effects o Calcium Channel Blockers; Calcium Polystyrene Sulfo nate; Gabapentin; Neuromuscular-Blocking Agents Sodium Polystyrene Sulfonate

The levels/effects of Magnesium Oxide may be increase by: Alfacalcidol; Calcitriol (Systemic); Calcium Channe Blockers

Decreased Effect

Magnesium Oxide may decrease the levels/effects o Alpha-Lipoic Acid; Bisphosphonate Derivatives; Deferi prone; Dolutegravir; Eltrombopag; Gabapentin; Levothyr oxine; Multivitamins/Fluoride (with ADE); Mycophenolate Phosphate Supplements; Quinolone Antibiotics; Ralte gravir; Tetracycline Derivatives; Trientine

The levels/effects of Magnesium Oxide may be decreased by: Alpha-Lipoic Acid; Trientine

Storage/Stability Store at controlled room temperature Protect from moisture.

Mechanism of Action Magnesium is important as a cofactor in many enzymatic reactions in the body involvin protein synthesis and carbohydrate metabolism (at leas 300 enzymatic reactions require magnesium). Actions o lipoprotein lipase have been found to be important in reducing serum cholesterol and on sodium/potassium ATPase in promoting polarization (eg, neuromuscular func tioning).

Pharmacokinetics (Adult data unless noted)

Absorption: Oral: Up to 30%

Elimination: Renal with unabsorbed drug excreted in feces

Dosing: Neonatal Recommended daily allowance of mag nesium: Oral: 40 mg/day

Dosing: Usual Oral:

Recommended daily allowance of magnesium: See table

Magnesium – Recommended Daily Allowance (RDA) and Estimated Average Requirement (EAR) (in terms of elemental magnesium)

Age	RDA (mg/day)	EAR (mg/day)
1 to <6 mo	40	30
6 to <12 mo	60	75
1-3 y	80	65
4-8 y	130	110
Male		
9-13 y	240	200
14-18 y	410	340
Female		
9-13 y	240	200
14-18 y	360	300

Antacid: Adults: 140 mg 3-4 times/day or 400-840 mg/day

Cathartic: Adults: 2-4 g at bedtime

Hypomagnesemia: **Note:** Achieving optimal magnesium levels using oral therapy may be difficult due to the propensity for magnesium to cause diarrhea: IV replacement may be more appropriate particularly in situations of severe deficit.

Children: 10-20 mg/kg elemental magnesium per dose up to 4 times/day

Dosing adjustment in renal impairment: Patients in severe renal failure should not receive magnesium due to toxicity from accumulation. Patients with a CrCl <25 mL/minute receiving magnesium should have serum magnesium levels monitored.

Administration Oral: Tablet: Take with full glass of water.

Reference Range

Neonates and Infants: 1.5-2.3 mEq/L

Children: 1.5-2.0 mEq/L

Adults: 1.4-2.0 mEq/L

Additional Information Magnesium oxide 500 mg = 302 mg **elemental** magnesium = 25 mEq magnesium

Elemental Magnesium Content of Magnesium Salts

Magnesium Salt	Elemental Magnesium (mg/500 mg salt)	Magnesium (mEq/500 mg salt)
Magnesium chloride	59	4.9
Magnesium gluconate	27	2.4
Magnesium L-aspartate	49.6	4.1
Magnesium oxide	302	25
Magnesium sulfate	49.3	4.1

Adverse effects associated with elevated serum magnesium concentrations may include:

>3 mg/dL: Blocked peripheral neuromuscular transmission leading to anticonvulsant effects, depressed CNS

>5 mg/dL: Depressed deep tendon reflexes, flushing, somnolence

>12 mg/dL: Complete heart block, respiratory paralysis

Dosage Forms Considerations 400 mg magnesium oxide = elemental magnesium 240 mg = magnesium 19.9 mEq = magnesium 9.85 mmol

Dosage Forms Excipient information presented when available (limited, particularly for generics); consult specific product labeling.

Capsule, Oral:

Uro-Mag: 140 mg

Tablet, Oral:

Mag-200: 200 mg [contains para-aminobenzoic acid]

Maox: 420 mg [contains tartrazine (fd&c yellow #5)]

Generic: 250 mg, 400 mg, 420 mg

Tablet, Oral [preservative free]:

Generic: 400 mg, 500 mg

Magnesium Sulfate (mag NEE zhum SUL fate)

Medication Safety Issues

Sound-alike/look-alike issues:

Magnesium sulfate may be confused with manganese sulfate, morphine sulfate

$MgSO_4$ is an error-prone abbreviation (mistaken as morphine sulfate)

High alert medication:

The Institute for Safe Medication Practices (ISMP) includes this medication (IV formulation) among its list of drugs which have a heightened risk of causing significant patient harm when used in error.

Brand Names: US Epsom Salt [OTC]

Therapeutic Category Anticonvulsant; Electrolyte Supplement, Oral; Electrolyte Supplement, Parenteral; Magnesium Salt

Generic Availability (US) Yes

Use

Oral: Laxative for the relief of occasional constipation (OTC product: FDA approved in ages ≥6 years and adults)

Parenteral: Treatment and prevention of hypomagnesemia (FDA approved in all ages); prevention and treatment of seizures in severe preeclampsia or eclampsia (FDA approved in pregnant females); has also been used IV and as an oral nebulization for adjunctive treatment of asthma exacerbation (severe, life-threatening) unresponsive to 1 hour of intensive conventional treatment and IV for treatment of torsade de pointes or VF/pulseless VT associated with torsade de pointes

Topical: Soaking aid for minor sprains and bruises (OTC product: FDA approved in adults)

Pregnancy Risk Factor D

Pregnancy Considerations Magnesium crosses the placenta; serum concentrations in the fetus are similar to those in the mother (Idama, 1998; Osada, 2002). Continuous maternal use for >5-7 days (in doses such as those used for preterm labor, an off-label use) may cause fetal hypocalcemia and bone abnormalities, as well as fractures in the neonate. Magnesium sulfate injection is used for the prevention and treatment of seizures in pregnant or postpartum women with severe pre-eclampsia or eclampsia (ACOG, 2013). Magnesium sulfate may also be used prior to early preterm delivery to reduce the risk of cerebral palsy (ACOG, 2010; Reeves, 2011). Tocolytics may be used for the short-term (48 hour) prolongation of pregnancy to allow for the administration of antenatal steroids and should not be used prior to fetal viability or when the risks of use to the fetus or mother are greater than the risk of preterm birth; maintenance therapy with tocolytics is ineffective and not recommended. Magnesium sulfate injection may be used in conjunction with tocolytics for neuroprotection (it is not preferred for use as a tocolytic); however, an increased risk of maternal complications may be observed when used in combination with some tocolytic agents (ACOG, 2012).

Breast-Feeding Considerations Magnesium is found in breast milk; concentrations remain constant during the first year of lactation and are not influenced by dietary intake under normal conditions. Magnesium requirements are the same in lactating and nonlactating females (IOM, 1997). When magnesium sulfate is used in the intrapartum management of eclampsia, breast milk concentrations are generally increased for only ~24 hours after the end of treatment (Idama, 1998). The manufacturer recommends that caution be used if administered to nursing women.

Contraindications Hypersensitivity to any component of the formulation; heart block; myocardial damage; IV use for pre-eclampsia/eclampsia during the 2 hours prior to delivery

Warnings/Precautions Use magnesium with caution in patients with impaired renal function (accumulation of magnesium may lead to magnesium intoxication). Use with extreme caution in patients with myasthenia gravis or other neuromuscular disease. Magnesium toxicity can lead to fatal cardiovascular arrest and/or respiratory paralysis. The parenteral product may contain aluminum; toxic aluminum concentrations may be seen with high doses, prolonged use, or renal dysfunction. Premature neonates are at higher risk due to immature renal function and aluminum intake from other parenteral sources. Parenteral aluminum exposure of >4 to 5 mcg/kg/day is associated with CNS and bone toxicity; tissue loading may occur at lower doses (Federal Register, 2002). See manufacturer's labeling. Concurrent hypokalemia or hypocalcemia can accompany a magnesium deficit. Unlikely to effectively terminate irregular/polymorphic VT (with normal baseline QT interval) (Neumar, 2010).

Obstetric use: Vigilant monitoring and safe administration techniques (ISMP, 2005) recommended to avoid potential for errors resulting in toxicity. Monitor mother and fetus closely. Use longer than 5-7 days may cause adverse fetal events.

Self-medication (OTC Use): When used as a soaking aid, patients should not use if there is evidence of infection or prompt relief is not obtained. When used as a laxative, patients should consult a healthcare provider prior to use if they have: kidney disease; are on a magnesium-restricted diet; have abdominal pain, nausea, or vomiting; change in bowel habits lasting >2 weeks; have already used a laxative for >1 week

Warnings: Additional Pediatric Considerations Multiple salt forms of magnesium exist; close attention must be paid to the salt form when ordering and administering magnesium; incorrect selection or substitution of one salt for another without proper dosage adjustment may result in serious over- or underdosing.

Adverse Reactions Adverse effects on neuromuscular function may occur at lower concentrations in patients with neuromuscular disease (eg, myasthenia gravis).

Cardiovascular: Flushing (IV; dose related), hypotension (IV; rate related), vasodilation (IV; rate related)

Endocrine & metabolic: Hypermagnesemia

Drug Interactions

Metabolism/Transport Effects None known.

Avoid Concomitant Use

Avoid concomitant use of Magnesium Sulfate with any of the following: Calcium Polystyrene Sulfonate; Raltegravir; Sodium Polystyrene Sulfonate

Increased Effect/Toxicity

Magnesium Sulfate may increase the levels/effects of: Calcium Channel Blockers; Calcium Polystyrene Sulfonate; CNS Depressants; Gabapentin; Neuromuscular-Blocking Agents; Sodium Polystyrene Sulfonate

The levels/effects of Magnesium Sulfate may be increased by: Alfacalcidol; Calcitriol (Systemic); Calcium Channel Blockers

Decreased Effect

Magnesium Sulfate may decrease the levels/effects of: Alpha-Lipoic Acid; Bisphosphonate Derivatives; Deferiprone; Dolutegravir; Eltrombopag; Gabapentin; Levothyroxine; Multivitamins/Fluoride (with ADE); Mycophenolate; Phosphate Supplements; Quinolone Antibiotics; Raltegravir; Tetracycline Derivatives; Trientine

The levels/effects of Magnesium Sulfate may be decreased by: Alpha-Lipoic Acid; Trientine

Food Interactions Increased alcohol intake can deplete magnesium stores (IOM, 1997).

Storage/Stability Prior to use, store at room temperature of 20°C to 25°C (68°F to 77°F). Do not freeze. Refrigeration of solution may result in precipitation or crystallization.

Mechanism of Action When taken orally, magnesium promotes bowel evacuation by causing osmotic retention of fluid which distends the colon with increased peristaltic activity; parenterally, magnesium decreases acetylcholine in motor nerve terminals and acts on myocardium by slowing rate of S-A node impulse formation and prolonging conduction time. Magnesium is necessary for the movement of calcium, sodium, and potassium in and out of cells, as well as stabilizing excitable membranes.

Intravenous magnesium may improve pulmonary function in patients with asthma; causes relaxation of bronchial smooth muscle independent of serum magnesium concentration.

Pharmacodynamics

Onset of action:

Anticonvulsant:

IM: 60 minutes

IV: Immediately

Laxative: Oral: 0.5 to 6 hours

Duration: Anticonvulsant:

IM: 3 to 4 hours

IV: 30 minutes

Pharmacokinetics (Adult data unless noted)

Absorption: Oral: Slow and poor (approximately one-third absorbed)

Distribution: Bone (50% to 60%); extracellular fluid (1% to 2%) (IOM 1997)

Protein binding: 30% to albumin

Elimination: Renal with unabsorbed drug excreted in feces

Dosing: Neonatal Note: 1,000 mg of magnesium sulfate = 98.6 mg **elemental** magnesium = 8.12 mEq magnesium = 4.06 mmol magnesium

Adequate intake (AI): Dose expressed as **elemental** magnesium: Oral: 30 mg daily; requirements may vary based on prematurity, postnatal age, and other clinical factors; serum magnesium concentrations should be monitored closely to determine patient-specific needs (IOM 1997)

Hypomagnesemia: Note: Dose depends on clinical condition and serum magnesium concentration; monitor closely.

General dosing:

Dose expressed as **magnesium sulfate:** IM, IV: 25 to 50 mg/kg/dose every 8 to 12 hours for 2 to 3 doses (Kliegman 2011)

Dose expressed as **elemental magnesium:** IM, IV: 2.5 to 5 mg/kg/dose every 8 to 12 hours for 2 to 3 doses (Kliegman 2011)

Severe (<1.6 mg/dL or in presence of seizure due to neonatal hypocalcemia): Dose expressed as **magnesium sulfate**: IV: 50 to 100 mg/kg/dose over 1 to 2 hours; may repeat dose in 12 hours if necessary (Cloherty 2012)

Parenteral nutrition, maintenance requirement: Dose expressed as **elemental magnesium:** IV: 0.3 to 0.5 mEq/kg/day (Mirtallo 2004)

Torsades de pointes, ventricular tachycardia: Dose expressed as **magnesium sulfate**: IV, IO: 25 to 50 mg/kg/dose; if pulseless, administer as a bolus; if pulse, administer over 10 to 20 minutes (Hegenbarth 2008; PALS [Kleinman 2010])

Dosing: Usual Note: 1,000 mg of magnesium sulfate = 98.6 mg **elemental** magnesium = 8.12 mEq magnesium = 4.06 mmol magnesium. **Note:** Serum magnesium is poor reflection of repletion status as the majority of magnesium is intracellular; serum concentrations may be transiently normal for a few hours after a dose is given, therefore, aim for consistently high normal serum concentrations in patients with normal renal function for most efficient repletion.

Pediatric:

Adequate intake (AI) (IOM 1997): Dose expressed as **elemental** magnesium. Oral:

1 to 6 months: 30 mg daily

7 to 12 months: 75 mg daily

Recommended daily allowance (RDA) (IOM 1997): Dose expressed as **elemental** magnesium; during pregnancy and lactation, requirements may change: Oral:

1 to 3 years: 80 mg daily

4 to 8 years: 130 mg daily

9 to 13 years: 240 mg daily

14 to 18 years:

Male: 410 mg daily

Female: 360 mg daily

Hypomagnesemia: Infants, Children, and Adolescents: **Note:** Dose depends on clinical condition and serum magnesium concentration.

Dose expressed as **magnesium sulfate:** IV, IO: 25 to 50 mg /kg/dose every 6 hours for 2 to 3 doses, then recheck serum concentration; maximum dose: 2,000 mg/dose (Hegenbarth 2008; Kliegman 2011; PALS [Kleinman 2010])

Dose expressed as **elemental magnesium:** IV: 2.5 to 5 mg/kg/dose every 6 hours for 2 to 3 doses (Kliegman 2011)

Constipation, occasional: Oral: **Note**: With OTC use, should not exceed recommended treatment duration (7 days) unless directed by health care provider.

Children 6 to <12 years: 1 to 2 level teaspoons of granules dissolved in 8 ounces of water; may repeat in 4 to 6 hours. Do not exceed 2 doses per day.

Children ≥12 years and Adolescents: 2 to 4 level teaspoons of granules dissolved in 8 ounces of water; may repeat in 4 to 6 hours. Do not exceed 2 doses per day.

Parenteral nutrition, maintenance requirement (Mirtallo 2004): Dose expressed as **elemental** magnesium: IV:

Infants and Children <50 kg: 0.3 to 0.5 **mEq/kg**/day

Children >50 kg and Adolescents: 10 to 30 **mEq/**day

Torsade de pointes or VF/pulseless VT associated with torsade de pointes: Dose expressed as **magnesium sulfate:** IV: Infants, Children, and Adolescents: IV, IO: 25 to 50 mg/kg/dose; maximum dose: 2,000 mg /dose (PALS [Kleinman 2010])

Asthma, acute refractory status: Limited data available: Dose expressed as **magnesium sulfate**.

IV: Infants, Children, and Adolescents: 25 to 75 mg/kg/ dose as a single dose; maximum dose: 2,000 mg/ dose; recommended as adjunctive therapy in severe acute asthma for patients who have life-threatening exacerbations and in those whose exacerbations remain in the severe category after 1 hour of intensive conventional therapy (GINA 2014; Hegenbarth 2008; NAEPP 2007). Efficacy results variable. Two trials (Ciarallo 1996; Ciarallo 2000) showed significant improvement in pulmonary function in children who received a single dose of 25 mg/kg or 40 mg/kg magnesium sulfate vs. placebo; in another trial, pulmonary index scores after magnesium sulfate 75 mg/kg (maximum dose: 2,500 mg/dose) vs. placebo were not statistically different in 54 children between 1 to 18 years of age (Scarfone 2000).

Oral inhalation: Nebulization (prepared from injectable formulation); given with a nebulized beta2-agonist (eg. albuterol): Limited data available: Optimal dose not established; efficacy results variable:

Mild to moderate asthma: Single dose: Children ≥5 years and Adolescents: 2.5 mL isotonic magnesium sulfate solution mixed with albuterol 2.5 mg (0.5 mL) as a single dose. Magnesium was supplied as a 6.3% solution of magnesium heptahydrate, which is equivalent to anhydrous magnesium sulfate 3.18%. Doses were nebulized with 8 to 10 L/min of oxygen. Magnesium was found to have an additive effect on albuterol response (Mahajan 2004).

Moderate to severe asthma: Three-dose series: Children ≥2 years and Adolescents ≤16 years: 151 mg isotonic magnesium sulfate mixed with albuterol and ipratropium was administered every 20 minutes for 3 doses to patients with severe acute asthma who did not respond to standard inhalation treatment. In this large randomized, placebo-controlled trial (n=508, including 252 who received magnesium sulfate treatment; ages: 2 to 16 years) improvement was statistically significant, but clinically significant changes were only observed in the most severe patients (SaO2 <92%) (Powell 2013). **Note:** Higher doses 500 mg magnesium sulfate mixed with albuterol (1 mL of 500 mg/mL parenteral solution and albuterol 1 mL nebulization solution mixed with 8 mL of distilled water; total volume: 10 mL) have been described for use in adolescents; however, the addition of magnesium showed no therapeutic benefit compared to albuterol alone (Aggarwal 2006).

Adult: Dose represented as magnesium sulfate unless stated otherwise.

RDA (IOM 1997): Oral:

Adults 19 to 30 years:

Females: 310 mg elemental magnesium daily

Pregnant females: 350 mg elemental magnesium daily

Breast-feeding females: 310 mg elemental magnesium daily

Males: 400 mg elemental magnesium daily

Adults ≥31 years:

Females: 320 mg elemental magnesium daily

Pregnant females: 360 mg elemental magnesium daily

Breast-feeding females: 320 mg elemental magnesium daily

Males: 420 mg elemental magnesium daily

Constipation, occasional: Oral: 2 to 6 teaspoons of granules dissolved in water once daily

Hypomagnesemia: Note: Treatment depends on severity and clinical status. In asymptomatic patients (when oral route is available), oral replacement therapy is a better replacement method than IV administration.

Mild deficiency: IM: Manufacturer's labeling: 1,000 mg every 6 hours for 4 doses, or as indicated by serum magnesium concentrations

Mild to moderate (serum concentration 1 to 1.5 mg/dL): IV: 1,000 to 4,000 mg (up to 125 mg/kg), administer at ≤1,000 mg/hour if asymptomatic; do not exceed 12 **g** over 12 hours (Kraft 2005). **Note:** Additional supplementation may be required after the initial dose with replenishment occurring over several days.

Severe deficiency:

IM: Manufacturer's labeling: Up to 250 mg/kg within a 4-hour period

IV:

Severe (<1 mg/dL): 4,000 mg to 8 **g** (up to 0.1875 g/ kg), administer at ≤1,000 mg/hour if asymptomatic; in symptomatic patients, may administer ≤4,000 mg over 4 to 5 minutes (Kraft 2005)

With polymorphic VT (including torsade de pointes): IV push: 1,000 to 2,000 mg (ACLS [Neumar 2010])

Obesity: Weight >130% of ideal body weight (IBW) or body mass index (BMI) ≥30 kg/m^2: When determining maximum per kg dose for replacement, some clinicians suggest using adjusted body weight (AdjBW) (Kraft 2005).

AdjBW (men) = ([wt (kg) -IBW (kg)] x 0.3) + IBW

AdjBW (women) = ([wt (kg) -IBW (kg)] x 0.25) + IBW

Eclampsia/preeclampsia (severe):

Manufacturer's labeling: IV: An initial total dose of 10 to 14 **g** administered as follows: 4,000 mg infusion with simultaneous IM injections of 4,000 to 5,000 mg in each buttock. After the initial IV/IM doses, may administer a 1,000 to 2,000 mg/hour continuous infusion or may follow with IM doses of 4,000 to 5,000 mg into alternate buttocks every 4 hours as necessary; maximum: 40 **g**/24 hours. IV use for preeclampsia/eclampsia is contraindicated during the 2 hours prior to delivery.

Alternate dosing: IV: 4,000 mg to 6 **g** loading dose followed by 1,000 to 2,000 mg/hour continuous infusion for at least 24 hours (ACOG 2013)

Parenteral nutrition supplementation: IV: 8 to 24 **mEq elemental** magnesium daily

Soaking aid: Topical: Dissolve 2 cupfuls of granules per gallon of warm water

Asthma: IV: 2,000 mg (NAEPP 2007)

Torsade de pointes or VF/pulseless VT associated with torsade de pointes: IV, I.O.: 1,000 to 2,000 mg (ACLS [Neumar, 2010])

Dosing adjustment in renal impairment:
Hypomagnesemia:
Infants, Children, and Adolescents: Use with caution; monitor closely for hypermagnesemia
Adults: Reduce dose by 50% (Kraft 2005). Use with caution; monitor for hypermagnesemia
Preeclampsia/eclampsia: Severe renal impairment: Per the manufacturer, do not exceed 20 grams during a 48-hour period.
Dosing adjustment in hepatic impairment: No dosage adjustment necessary.

Preparation for Administration
Oral: Dissolve granules in 8 ounces of water prior to administration.
Oral inhalation: Limited data available: Nebulizer solution: Use injectable solution to prepare dose and add to albuterol solution for nebulization; see Dosing-Usual for details (Aggarwal 2006; Mahajan 2004; Powell 2013)
Parenteral:
IM:
Infants and Children: Dilute to a maximum concentration of 20% (ie, 200 mg/mL of **magnesium sulfate** or 1.6 mEq/mL of magnesium) prior to administration
Adults: May dilute to a concentration of 25%
IV: Dilute in an appropriate fluid to a usual concentration of 0.5 mEq/mL of magnesium (ie, 60 mg/mL of **magnesium sulfate**); maximum concentration: 20% (ie, 200 mg/mL of **magnesium sulfate** or 1.6 mEq/mL of magnesium)
Topical: Dissolve 2 cups of granules per gallon of warm water to use as a soaking aid

Administration
Oral: Must dissolve granules prior to administration. When used as a laxative, the patient should drink a full 8 ounces of liquid following each dose. Lemon juice may be added to the initial solution to improve the taste. **Note:** Most effective when taken on an empty stomach.
Oral inhalation: Nebulization: Mix injectable solution with albuterol ± ipratropium and administer over 10 to 20 minutes (Aggarwal 2006; Mahajan 2004; Powell 2013)
Parenteral:
IM:
Infants and Children: Dilute prior to injection
Adults: May administer undiluted (50%) or may further dilute in a compatible fluid
IV: Dilute in an appropriate fluid prior to administration. Rate of infusion dependent upon use:
For general replacement therapy:
Pediatric patients: Infuse slowly generally over 1 to 4 hours; in asymptomatic patients, a rate of ≤0.1 mEq/kg/hour may be considered (in adults, the usual rate is ≤1,000 mg/hour of **magnesium sulfate**); faster rates could be used up to a maximum infusion rate: 1 mEq/kg/hour (125 mg/kg/hour of **magnesium sulfate**); rate should be slowed if patient experiences diaphoresis, flushing or a warm sensation (Corkins 2010; Kliegman 2007)
Adults: Up to 50% of an IV dose may be eliminated in the urine; therefore, slower administration may improve retention. If severely symptomatic, may administer ≤4,000 mg over 4 to 5 minutes. For doses <6 **g**, infuse over 8 to 12 hours and for larger doses, infuse over 24 hours if patient asymptomatic (Kraft 2005); maximum rate: 150 mg/minute
Acute/emergent therapy:
Pediatric patients:
Pulseless torsades or VT: May administer as a bolus (Hegenbarth 2008)
Hypomagnesemia or torsades with pulses: 10 to 20 minutes (Hegenbarth 2008)
Status asthmaticus: 15 to 30 minutes (Ciarallo 1996; Ciarallo 2000; Hegenbarth 2008)
Adults: Should generally be given no faster tha 150 mg/minute; ACLS guidelines recommen administration over 15 minutes in patients with to sade de pointes (ACLS [Neumar 2010]). In cases c severe eclampsia with seizures, or persistent pulse less VT or VF with known hypomagnesemia faste rates (ie, over 1 to 2 minutes) may be necessar (Dager 2006). In patients not in cardiac arrest, hypc tension and asystole may occur with rapid admin istration.
Continuous IV infusion: After dilution, administer via a infusion pump
Topical: Adult: Dissolve granules in warm water prior t use; may use as a soaking aid or for a compress. T make a compress, use a towel to apply as a we dressing.

Monitoring Parameters
Oral: Stool output (laxative use)
IV: Rapid administration: ECG monitoring, vital signs, dee tendon reflexes; magnesium concentrations if frequent c prolonged dosing required particularly in patients wit renal dysfunction, calcium, and potassium concentra tions; renal function
Obstetrics: Patient status including vital signs, oxyge saturation, deep tendon reflexes, level of conscious ness, fetal heart rate, maternal uterine activity

Reference Range Typical values: Total magnesium: 1.5 t 2.5 mEq/L

Additional Information

Elemental Magnesium Content of Magnesium Salts

Magnesium Salt	Elemental Magnesium (mg/500 mg salt)	Magnesium (mEq/500 mg salt)
Magnesium chloride	59	4.9
Magnesium gluconate	27	2.4
Magnesium L-aspartate	49.6	4.1
Magnesium oxide	302	25
Magnesium sulfate	49.3	4.1

Dosage Forms Considerations 1 g of magnesium sul fate = elemental magnesium 98.6 mg = magnesium 8.12 mEq = magnesium 4.06 mmol

Magnesium sulfate 1% [10 mg/mL] in Dextrose 5% injec tion is equivalent to elemental magnesium 0.081 mEq/mL.
Magnesium sulfate 2% [20 mg/mL] in Dextrose 5% injec tion is equivalent to elemental magnesium 0.162 mEq/mL.
Magnesium sulfate 4% [40 mg/mL] in Water injection is equivalent to elemental magnesium 0.325 mEq/mL.
Magnesium sulfate 8% [80 mg/mL] in Water injection is equivalent to elemental magnesium 0.65 mEq/mL.
Magnesium sulfate 50% injection is equivalent to elemental magnesium 4 mEq/mL.

Dosage Forms Excipient information presented wher available (limited, particularly for generics); consult specific product labeling.
Capsule, Oral:
Generic: 70 mg
Granules, Oral:
Epsom Salt: (454 g, 1810 g, 1816 g)
Solution, Injection:
Generic: 40 mg/mL (50 mL, 100 mL, 500 mL, 1000 mL); 80 mg/mL (50 mL); 50% (2 mL, 10 mL, 20 mL, 50 mL)
Solution, Intravenous:
Generic: 10 mg/mL (100 mL); 20 mg/mL (500 mL)

◆ **Magonate [OTC]** *see* Magnesium Gluconate *on page 1312*

◆ **Mag Oxide** *see* Magnesium Oxide *on page 1316*

◆ **Mag-SR [OTC]** *see* Magnesium Chloride *on page 1310*

◆ **Mag-SR Plus Calcium [OTC]** *see* Magnesium Chloride *on page 1310*

◆ **MAH** *see* Magnesium L-aspartate Hydrochloride *on page 1315*

◆ **Makena** *see* Hydroxyprogesterone Caproate *on page 1054*

◆ **Malarone®** *see* Atovaquone and Proguanil *on page 224*

◆ **Malarone® Pediatric (Can)** *see* Atovaquone and Proguanil *on page 224*

Malathion (mal a THYE on)

Brand Names: US Ovide

Therapeutic Category Antiparasitic Agent, Topical; Pediculocide; Scabicidal Agent

Generic Availability (US) Yes

Use Treatment of *Pediculus capitis* (head lice and their ova) (FDA approved in ages ≥6 years and adults)

Pregnancy Risk Factor B

Pregnancy Considerations Adverse events have not been observed in animal reproduction studies

Breast-Feeding Considerations It is not known if the malathion 0.5% lotion formulation is excreted in breast milk. Use with caution if administered to or handled by breast-feeding mothers.

Contraindications Hypersensitivity to malathion or any component of the formulation; use in neonates and/or infants

Warnings/Precautions For topical use on scalp hair only; leave hair uncovered after application (allow hair to dry naturally). Avoid contact with eyes; flush immediately with water if eye contact occurs. Wash hands immediately after application. Lotion is flammable; do not expose lotion or hair wetted with malathion to open flames or electric heat sources (eg, hair dryer, curling iron, flat iron). Do not smoke while applying lotion or while hair is wet. Chemical burns, including second-degree burns, and stinging sensations may occur; discontinue use temporarily if skin irritation occurs.

Warnings: Additional Pediatric Considerations Systemic absorption may be increased in infants and neonates due to higher skin surface area to body mass ratio and immature skin barrier; risk for malathion toxicity potentially increased; use is contraindicated in these patients.

Adverse Reactions

Dermatologic: Chemical burns (including second-degree burns), skin/scalp irritation, stinging sensations

Ocular: Conjunctivitis (following contact with eyes)

Drug Interactions

Metabolism/Transport Effects None known.

Avoid Concomitant Use There are no known interactions where it is recommended to avoid concomitant use.

Increased Effect/Toxicity There are no known significant interactions involving an increase in effect.

Decreased Effect There are no known significant interactions involving a decrease in effect.

Storage/Stability Store at room temperature 20°C to 25°C (68°F to 77°F). Do not expose to heat and open flames.

Mechanism of Action Organophosphate that acts as a pediculicide by inhibiting cholinesterase activity in *Pediculus humanus capitis* (head lice and their ova)

Dosing: Usual

Children ≥2 years and Adolescents:

Head lice: Children ≥6 years and Adolescents: Topical: Apply sufficient amount to cover and thoroughly moisten dry hair and scalp, leave on for 8-12 hours (typically overnight application); may shampoo upon completion; during clinical trials, a maximum dose of 2 fl oz was used. **Note:** In a blinded-comparative trial with permethrin; a shorter application time of 20 minutes was shown effective (AAP, 2010; Meinking, 2004). Further treatment is generally not necessary.

Head lice resistant to permethrin/pyrethrins or previously failed courses: Children 2-5 years: Limited data available: Topical: Apply sufficient amount to cover and thoroughly moisten dry hair and scalp, leave on for 8-12 hours (typically overnight application); may shampoo upon completion; during clinical trials, a maximum dose of 2 fl oz was used (AAP, 2010)

Adults: **Head lice:** Topical: Apply sufficient amount to cover and thoroughly moisten dry hair and scalp; shampoo after 8-12 hours. If required, repeat with second application in 7-9 days. Further treatment is generally not necessary.

Administration Topical: For external use only; avoid contact with eyes. Apply to dry hair and scalp and rub gently until thoroughly moistened; pay special attention to the back of the head and neck. Allow hair to dry naturally; do not use heat; leave hair uncovered; after 8-12 hours, wash hair with a nonmedicated shampoo; rinse and use a fine-toothed (nit) comb to remove dead lice and eggs. Wash hands immediately after use.

Malathion should be a portion of a whole lice removal program, which should include washing or dry cleaning all clothing, hats, bedding, and towels recently worn or used by the patient and washing combs, brushes, and hair accessories in hot, soapy water.

Dosage Forms Excipient information presented when available (limited, particularly for generics); consult specific product labeling.

Lotion, External:

Ovide: 0.5% (59 mL) [contains isopropyl alcohol]

Generic: 0.5% (59 mL)

◆ **Mandelamine® (Can)** *see* Methenamine *on page 1385*

◆ **Mandrake** *see* Podophyllum Resin *on page 1720*

◆ **Manganese** *see* Trace Elements *on page 2097*

Mannitol (MAN i tole)

Medication Safety Issues

Sound-alike/look-alike issues:

Osmitrol® may be confused with esmolol

Related Information

Management of Drug Extravasations *on page 2298*

Brand Names: US Aridol; Osmitrol; Resectisol

Brand Names: Canada Osmitrol®

Therapeutic Category Diuretic, Osmotic

Generic Availability (US) May be product dependent

Use

Injection: Reduction of increased intracranial pressure (ICP) associated with cerebral edema and increased intraocular pressure (IOP) [FDA approved in pediatric patients (age not specified) and adults]; promotion of urinary excretion of toxic substances and diuresis in the prevention and/or treatment of oliguria or anuria due to acute renal failure [FDA approved in pediatric patients (age not specified) and adults]. **Note:** Although FDA-labeled indications, the use of mannitol for the prevention of acute renal failure and/or promotion of diuresis is not routinely recommended (Kellum, 2008).

Irrigation solution, genitourinary: Irrigation in transurethral prostatic resection or other transurethral surgical procedures (FDA approved in adults)

Oral inhalation powder: Assessment of bronchial hyperresponsiveness (FDA approved in ages ≥6 years and adults)

Pregnancy Risk Factor C

Pregnancy Considerations Reproduction studies have not been conducted.

Breast-Feeding Considerations It is not known if mannitol is excreted in breast milk. The manufacturer recommends that caution be exercised when administering mannitol to nursing women.

Contraindications

Injection: Hypersensitivity to mannitol or any component of the formulation; severe renal disease (anuria); severe dehydration; active intracranial bleeding except during craniotomy; progressive heart failure, pulmonary congestion, or renal dysfunction after mannitol administration; severe pulmonary edema or congestion

Genitourinary irrigation solution: Anuria

Powder for inhalation: Hypersensitivity to mannitol, gelatin, or any component of the formulation; conditions that may be compromised by induced bronchospasm or repeated spirometry (eg, aortic or cerebral aneurysm, uncontrolled hypertension, recent MI or cerebral vascular accident)

Warnings/Precautions Should not be administered until adequacy of renal function and urine flow is established; use 1-2 test doses to assess renal response. Excess amounts can lead to profound diuresis with fluid and electrolyte loss; close medical supervision and dose evaluation are required. Watch for and correct electrolyte disturbances; adjust dose to avoid dehydration. May cause renal dysfunction especially with high doses; use caution in patients taking other nephrotoxic agents, with sepsis or preexisting renal disease. To minimize adverse renal effects, adjust to keep serum osmolality less than 320 mOsm/L. Discontinue if evidence of acute tubular necrosis.

In patients being treated for cerebral edema, mannitol may accumulate in the brain (causing rebound increases in intracranial pressure) if circulating for long periods of time as with continuous infusion; intermittent boluses preferred. Cardiovascular status should also be evaluated; do not administer electrolyte-free mannitol solutions with blood. If hypotension occurs monitor cerebral perfusion pressure to ensure adequate. Vesicant (at concentrations >5%); ensure proper catheter or needle position prior to and during IV infusion; avoid extravasation of IV infusions.

Powder for inhalation (Aridol): **[U.S. Boxed Warning] Use may result in severe bronchospasm; use only for bronchial challenge testing. Testing should only be done by trained professionals. Not for use in patients with asthma or very low baseline pulmonary function. Medications (eg, short-acting inhaled beta-agonist) and equipment for the treatment of severe bronchospasm should be readily available.** Use with caution in patients with conditions that may increase sensitivity to bronchoconstriction (eg, severe cough, ventilatory impairment, spirometry-induced bronchoconstriction, hemoptysis of unknown origin, pneumothorax, recent abdominal, thoracic, or intraocular surgery, unstable angina, active upper or lower respiratory tract infection). Patients who have ≥10% reduction in FEV_1 on administration of the 0 mg capsule, patients with a positive response to bronchial challenge testing, or patients who develop significant respiratory symptoms should receive short acting inhaled beta-agonist; monitor until full recovery to baseline. Bronchial challenge testing should not be performed in children <6 years of age as these patients are unable to provide reliable spirometric results.

Warnings: Additional Pediatric Considerations Mannitol may increase cerebral blood flow, increase the risk of postoperative bleeding in neurosurgical patients, and worsen intracranial hypertension in children who develop generalized cerebral hyperemia during the first 24 to 48 hours after traumatic brain injury.

Adverse Reactions

Inhalation:

Cardiovascular: Chest discomfort

Central nervous system: Dizziness, headache

Gastrointestinal: Nausea, retching, throat irritation

Respiratory: Cough, dyspnea, pharyngolaryngeal pain rhinorrhea, wheezing

Rare but important or life-threatening: FEV_1 decreased gagging

Injection:

Cardiovascular: Chest pain, CHF, circulatory overload, hyper-/hypotension, peripheral edema, tachycardia

Central nervous system: Chills, convulsions, dizziness, fever, headache

Dermatologic: Bullous eruption, urticaria

Endocrine & metabolic: Fluid and electrolyte imbalance, dehydration and hypovolemia secondary to rapid diuresis, hyperglycemia, hypernatremia, hyponatremia (dilutional), hyperosmolality-induced hyperkalemia, metabolic acidosis (dilutional), osmolar gap increased, water intoxication

Gastrointestinal: Nausea, vomiting, xerostomia

Genitourinary: Dysuria, polyuria

Local: Pain, thrombophlebitis, tissue necrosis

Ocular: Blurred vision

Renal: Acute renal failure, acute tubular necrosis (adult dose >200 g/day; serum osmolality >320 mOsm/L)

Respiratory: Pulmonary edema, rhinitis

Miscellaneous: Allergic reactions

Drug Interactions

Metabolism/Transport Effects None known.

Avoid Concomitant Use

Avoid concomitant use of Mannitol with any of the following: Aminoglycosides

Increased Effect/Toxicity

Mannitol may increase the levels/effects of: Amifostine; Aminoglycosides; Antihypertensives; DULoxetine; Hypotensive Agents; Levodopa; Obinutuzumab; RisperiDONE; RiTUXimab; Sodium Phosphates

The levels/effects of Mannitol may be increased by: Alfuzosin; Analgesics (Opioid); Barbiturates; Brimonidine (Topical); Diazoxide; Herbs (Hypotensive Properties); MAO Inhibitors; Nicorandil; Pentoxifylline; Phosphodiesterase 5 Inhibitors; Prostacyclin Analogues

Decreased Effect

The levels/effects of Mannitol may be decreased by: Herbs (Hypertensive Properties); Methylphenidate; Yohimbine

Storage/Stability

Injection: Should be stored at room temperature of 15°C to 30°C (59°F to 86°F); do not freeze. In concentrations ≥15%, crystallization may occur at low temperatures; do not use solutions that contain crystals. Heating in a hot water bath and vigorous shaking may be utilized for resolubilization. Cool solutions to body temperature before using.

Irrigation: Store at room temperature of 25°C (77°F); excursions permitted up to 40°C. Avoid excessive heat; do not warm above 150°F (66°C). Do not freeze.

Powder for inhalation: Store at <25°C (<77°F); excursions permitted between 15°C to 30°C (59°F to 86°F). Do not freeze.

Mechanism of Action Produces an osmotic diuresis by increasing the osmotic pressure of glomerular filtrate, which inhibits tubular reabsorption of water and electrolytes and increases urinary output. Mechanism of action in reduction of intracranial pressure (ICP) is controversial. However, it is thought that mannitol reduces ICP by reducing blood viscosity which transiently increases cerebral blood flow and oxygen transport. This in turn reduces cerebral blood volume and ICP. Furthermore, mannitol reduces ICP by withdrawing water from the brain parenchyma and excretes water in the urine (Allen, 1998; Bratton, 2007; Miller, 2010).

Pharmacodynamics

Onset of action:

Bronchospasm, challenge: Inhalation: Within 1 minute if positive response

Diuresis: IV: Within 1-3 hours

ICP reduction: IV: Within 15 minutes

Duration: ICP reduction: IV: 3-6 hours

Pharmacokinetics (Adult data unless noted)

Distribution: 34.3 L; remains confined to extracellular space; does not penetrate blood-brain barrier except in very high concentrations or with acidosis

Metabolism: Minimal amounts in the liver to glycogen

Bioavailability: Inhalation: Absolute: 59% (relative to oral administration: 96%)

Half-life:

Injection: 0.25-1.7 hours; 6-36 hours in renal failure

Inhalation: 4.7 hours

Time to peak serum concentration: Inhalation: 1.5 hours

Elimination: Urine (~55% to 87% as unchanged drug by glomerular filtration)

Dosing: Neonatal Acute renal failure: IV: 0.5-1 g/kg/dose (Andreoli, 2004); some experts recommend against routine use due to the risk of IVH in low birth weight neonates (solution is hypertonic) or the precipitation of CHF if a lack of response occurs (Andreoli, 2004; Chua, 2005)

Dosing: Usual

Infants, Children, and Adolescents: **Note:** The manufacturer's labeling recommends a test dose prior to starting IV mannitol therapy in patients with marked oliguria or suspected renal insufficiency.

Acute renal failure (oliguria): IV: Initial: 0.5-1 g/kg/dose infused over 2-6 hours; usual range: 0.25-2 g/kg/dose; may repeat dose every 4-6 hours; do not repeat dose if oliguria persists. **Note:** Although FDA-labeled indications, the use of mannitol for the prevention of acute renal failure and/or promotion of diuresis is not routinely recommended (Kellum, 2008).

Test dose (to assess adequate renal function): IV: 0.2 g/kg (maximum dose: 12.5 g) over 3-5 minutes to produce a urine flow of at least 1 mL/kg/hour for 1-3 hours

Bronchial hyper-responsiveness assessment: Children ≥6 years and Adolescents: Oral inhalation: Administer in a stepwise fashion (measuring FEV_1 in duplicate at baseline and after each administration) until the patient has a positive response or 635 mg of mannitol has been administered (whichever comes first).

Positive test: 15% reduction in FEV_1 from baseline or 10% incremental reduction in FEV_1 between consecutive doses

Negative test: Administration of full dose (635 mg) without reduction in FEV_1 sufficient to meet criteria for a positive test

Administration should be as follows:

Stepwise Administration Schedule

Dose #	Dose (mg)	Cumulative Dose (mg)	Capsules/Dose
1	0	0	1
2	5	5	1
3	10	15	1
4	20	35	1
5	40	75	1
6	80	155	2 x 40 mg caps
7	160	315	4 x 40 mg caps
8	160	475	4 x 40 mg caps
9	160	635	4 x 40 mg caps

Intracranial pressure (ICP), reduction: IV: Usual range: 0.25-1 g/kg/dose infused over 20-30 minutes; repeat as needed to maintain serum osmolality <300-320 mOsm/kg (Bratton, 2007; Hegenbarth, 2008; Kochanek, 2012). **Note:** The manufacturer's labeling allows for higher single doses up to 2 g/kg/dose.

Intraocular pressure (IOP), reduction: IV: 1-2 g/kg/dose **or** 30-60 g/m²/dose infused over 30-60 minutes administered 1-1.5 hours prior to surgery

IOP (traumatic hyphema), reduction: IV: 1.5 g/kg/dose infused over 45 minutes twice daily for IOP >35 mm Hg; may administer every 8 hours in patients with extremely high pressure (Crouch, 1999)

Adults:

Bronchial hyper-responsiveness, assessment: Inhalation: Administer in a stepwise fashion (measuring FEV_1 in duplicate at baseline and after each administration) until the patient has a positive response or 635 mg of mannitol has been administered (whichever comes first).

Positive test: 15% reduction in FEV_1 from baseline or 10% incremental reduction in FEV_1 between consecutive doses

Negative test: Administration of full dose (635 mg) without reduction in FEV_1 sufficient to meet criteria for a positive test

Administration should be as follows:

Stepwise Administration Schedule

Dose #	Dose (mg)	Cumulative Dose (mg)	Capsules/Dose
1	0	0	1
2	5	5	1
3	10	15	1
4	20	35	1
5	40	75	1
6	80	155	2 x 40 mg caps
7	160	315	4 x 40 mg caps
8	160	475	4 x 40 mg caps
9	160	635	4 x 40 mg caps

Increased intracranial pressure (ICP), cerebral edema: IV: 0.25-1 g/kg/dose; may repeat every 6-8 hours as needed (Bratton, 2007; Kochanek, 2012); maintain serum osmolality <300-320 mOsm/kg (Kochanek, 2012; Rabinstein, 2006)

Intraocular pressure (IOP), reduction: IV: 0.25-2 g/kg infused over 30-60 minutes administered 1-1.5 hours prior to surgery

IOP (traumatic hyphema), reduction: IV: 1.5 g/kg infused over 45 minutes twice daily for IOP >35 mm Hg; may administer every 8 hours in patients with extremely high pressure (Crouch, 1999)

Transurethral irrigation: Topical: Use 5% urogenital solution as required for irrigation.

Dosage adjustment for renal impairment: Contraindicated in severe renal impairment. Use with caution in patients with underlying renal disease. May be used to reduce the incidence of acute tubular necrosis when administered prior to revascularization during kidney transplantation.

Dosage adjustment for hepatic impairment: No adjustment required.

Administration

Irrigation: For irrigation only; not for injection: Administer using only the appropriate transurethral urologic instrumentation. Do not warm above 66°C (150°F).

IV: Do not administer IM or SubQ. In-line filter set (≤5 micron) should always be used for mannitol infusion with concentrations ≥20%; maximum concentration for administration: 25%. Inspect for crystals prior to administration; if crystals are present, redissolve by warming solution. Do not administer with blood; crenation and agglutination of red blood cells may occur. Infusion rate is dependent upon indication:

Acute renal failure: Administer over 2 to 6 hours

Cerebral edema or increased intracranial pressure: Administer over 20 to 30 minutes

Test dose (for oliguria): Administer over 3 to 5 minutes

Vesicant (at concentrations >5%); ensure proper catheter or needle position prior to and during IV infusion. Avoid extravasation of IV infusions. If extravasation occurs, stop infusion immediately and disconnect (leave needle/cannula in place); gently aspirate extravasated solution (do **NOT** flush the line); initiate hyaluronidase antidote (see Management of Drug Extravasations for more details); remove needle/cannula; apply dry cold compresses (Hurst, 2004); elevate extremity.

Oral inhalation (Aridol): Administer using supplied single patient use inhaler; do not puncture capsule more than once; do not swallow capsules. A nose clip may be used if preferred. The patient should exhale completely, followed by a controlled rapid deep inspiration from the device; hold breath for 5 seconds and exhale through the mouth. Measure FEV_1 in duplicate 60 seconds after inhalation; repeat process until positive response or full dose (635 mg) has been administered.

Vesicant/Extravasation Risk Vesicant (at concentrations >5%)

Monitoring Parameters

Renal function, daily fluid intake and output, serum electrolytes, serum and urine osmolality; for treatment of elevated intracranial pressure, maintain serum osmolality <300-320 mOsm/kg

Bronchial challenge test: Standard spirometry prior to bronchial challenge test; FEV_1 in duplicate 60 seconds after administration of each step of test

Additional Information Approximate osmolarity: Mannitol 20%: 1100 mOsm/L; mannitol 25%: 1375 mOsm/L

Bronchial challenge testing: The dose of inhaled mannitol which causes a 15% reduction in FEV_1 is expressed as PD_{15}

Dosage Forms Excipient information presented when available (limited, particularly for generics); consult specific product labeling.

Kit, Inhalation:
- Aridol:

Solution, Intravenous:
- Osmitrol: 5% (1000 mL); 10% (500 mL); 15% (500 mL); 20% (250 mL, 500 mL)
- Generic: 5% (1000 mL); 10% (1000 mL); 15% (500 mL); 20% (250 mL, 500 mL); 25% (50 mL)

Solution, Intravenous [preservative free]:
- Generic: 25% (50 mL)

Solution, Irrigation:
- Resectisol: 5% (2000 mL)

◆ **Maox [OTC]** *see* Magnesium Oxide *on page 1316*

◆ **Mapap [OTC]** *see* Acetaminophen *on page 44*

◆ **Mapap Arthritis Pain [OTC]** *see* Acetaminophen *on page 44*

◆ **Mapap Children's [OTC]** *see* Acetaminophen *on page 44*

◆ **Mapap Extra Strength [OTC]** *see* Acetaminophen *on page 44*

◆ **Mapap Infant's [OTC]** *see* Acetaminophen *on page 44*

◆ **Mapezine (Can)** *see* CarBAMazepine *on page 367*

◆ **Mar-Allopurinol (Can)** *see* Allopurinol *on page 96*

◆ **Mar-Amlodipine (Can)** *see* AmLODIPine *on page 133*

Maraviroc (mah RAV er rock)

Medication Safety Issues

High alert medication:

This medication is in a class the Institute for Safe Medication Practices (ISMP) includes among its list of drug classes that have a heightened risk of causing significant patient harm when used in error.

Related Information

Adult and Adolescent HIV *on page 2392*

Pediatric HIV *on page 2380*

Perinatal HIV *on page 2400*

Brand Names: US Selzentry

Brand Names: Canada Celsentri

Therapeutic Category Antiretroviral Agent; Antiretroviral CCR5 Antagonist (Anti-HIV); CCR5 Antagonist; HIV Agents (Anti-HIV Agents)

Generic Availability (US) No

Use Treatment of CCR5-tropic HIV-1 infection, in combination with other antiretroviral agents (FDA approved in ages ≥16 years and adults); **Note:** HIV regimens consisting of **three** antiretroviral agents are strongly recommended.

Medication Guide Available Yes

Pregnancy Risk Factor B

Pregnancy Considerations Adverse effects have not been observed in animal reproduction studies. Maraviroc has minimal to low transfer across the human placenta. The DHHS Perinatal HIV Guidelines note there are insufficient data to recommend use in pregnancy.

Regardless of CD4 count or HIV RNA copy number, all HIV-infected pregnant women should receive a combination antiretroviral (ARV) drug regimen. A combination of antepartum, intrapartum, and infant ARV prophylaxis is recommended. ARV therapy should be started as soon as possible in women with symptomatic infection. Although earlier initiation may be more effective in reducing the perinatal transmission of HIV, initiation may be delayed until after 12 weeks gestation in women who do not require immediate treatment after careful consideration of maternal conditions (eg, nausea and vomiting) and the potential risks of first trimester fetal exposure for specific agents. A scheduled cesarean delivery at 38 weeks gestation is recommended for all women with HIV RNA >1000 copies/mL or unknown concentrations near delivery in order to decrease transmission. If ARV therapy must be interrupted for <24 hours during the peripartum period, stop then restart all medications simultaneously in order to decrease the chance of developing resistance. Long-term follow-up is recommended for all infants exposed to ARV medications. In couples who want to conceive, the HIV-infected partner should attain maximum viral suppression prior to conception.

Health care providers are encouraged to enroll pregnant women exposed to antiretroviral medications in the Antiretroviral Pregnancy Registry (1-800-258-4263 or www.-APRegistry.com). Health care providers caring for HIV-infected women and their infants may contact the National Perinatal HIV Hotline (888-448-8765) for clinical consultation (HHS [perinatal], 2014).

Breast-Feeding Considerations It is not known if maraviroc is excreted in breast milk. Maternal or infant antiretroviral therapy does not completely eliminate the risk of postnatal HIV transmission. In addition, multiclass-resistant virus has been detected in breast-feeding infants despite maternal therapy. Therefore, in the United States, where formula is accessible, affordable, safe, and sustainable, and the risk of infant mortality due to diarrhea and respiratory infections is low, complete avoidance of breast-feeding by HIV-infected women is recommended to decrease potential transmission of HIV (HHS [perinatal], 2014).

Contraindications

Patients with severe renal impairment (CrCl <30 mL/minute) or end-stage renal disease (ESRD) who are taking potent CYP3A inhibitors or inducers

Canadian labeling: Additional contraindications (not in U.S. labeling): Hypersensitivity to maraviroc or any component of the formulation

Warnings/Precautions [U.S. Boxed Warning] Possible drug-induced hepatotoxicity with allergic type features has been reported; hepatotoxicity (usually after 1 month of treatment) may be preceded by allergic type reactions (eg, pruritic rash, eosinophilia, fever or increased IgE, excluding rash alone or Stevens-Johnson syndrome (HHS [adult], 2014) and/or hepatic adverse events (transaminase increases or signs/symptoms of hepatitis); some cases have been life-threatening; immediately evaluate patients with signs and symptoms of allergic reaction or hepatitis. Use with caution in patients with pre-existing hepatic dysfunction or coinfection with HBV and/or HCV, however symptoms have occurred in the absence of pre-existing hepatic conditions. Monitor hepatic function at baseline and as clinically indicated during treatment. Consider discontinuation in any patient with possible hepatitis or with elevated transaminases combined with systemic allergic events. Rechallenge with maraviroc is not recommended (HHS [pediatric], 2014).

Severe and life-threatening skin and hypersensitivity reactions, including Stevens-Johnson syndrome, toxic epidermal necrolysis and drug rash with eosinophilia with systemic symptoms (DRESS), have been reported with use, predominately in patients also receiving concomitant agents associated with these reactions. Rash and constitutional findings (eg, fever, muscle aches, conjunctivitis, oral lesions), with or without organ dysfunction, have also accompanied these reports. Discontinue maraviroc and any other suspected agent immediately if symptoms or signs of hypersensitivity occur. Monitor liver function tests and clinical status as appropriate.

Patients may develop immune reconstitution syndrome resulting in the occurrence of an inflammatory response to an indolent or residual opportunistic infection during initial HIV treatment or activation of autoimmune disorders (eg, Graves' disease, polymyositis, Guillain-Barré syndrome) later in therapy; further evaluation and treatment may be required. May cause dizziness. If this occurs, patients should avoid driving or operating machinery. Monitor closely for signs/symptoms of developing infections; use associated with a small increase of certain upper respiratory tract infections and herpes virus infections during clinical trials. Use with caution in patients with cardiovascular disease or cardiac risk factors,. in patients with a history of or current cardiac risk factors for postural hypotension, or receiving concomitant medication known to lower blood pressure. Patients who have cardiovascular comorbidities could be at risk for cardiac adverse events prompted by postural hypotension. During trials, a small increase in cardiovascular events (myocardial ischemia and/or infarction) occurred in treated patients compared to placebo, although a contributory relationship relative to therapy is unknown. Symptomatic postural hypotension has occurred; use caution in patients at risk for postural hypotension due to concomitant medication or history of condition. An increased risk of postural hypotension may occur in patients with severe renal impairment or in those with ESRD. Patients with severe renal dysfunction or ESRD who experience postural hypotension should have dose reduced. Do not use maraviroc in patients with severe renal impairment or ESRD who are receiving CYP3A inhibitors or inducers unless no alternative treatment options are available. An increased risk of postural hypotension may occur in patients with severe renal insufficiency or in those with ESRD. Reduce dose in patients with severe renal dysfunction or ESRD if postural hypotension experienced. Renal impairment may increase maraviroc concentrations. Use with caution in patients with mild-to-moderate renal impairment.

Use caution in patients with mild-to-moderate hepatic impairment; maraviroc concentrations are increased; no dosage adjustment recommended. Maraviroc concentrations are further increased in patients with moderate hepatic impairment receiving concomitant potent CYP3A inhibitors; monitor closely for adverse events. May affect immune surveillance and lead to an increased risk of malignancy due to pharmacologic mechanism of action. No increase in malignancy has been observed. Long term follow up needed to assess this risk. Potentially significant interactions may exist, requiring dose or frequency adjustment, additional monitoring, and/or selection of alternative therapy. Prior to therapy, coreceptor tropism testing should be performed for presence of CCR5-tropic only virus HIV-1 infection. Therapy not recommended for use in patients with CXCR4- or dual/mixed tropic HIV-1 infection; efficacy not demonstrated in this population. In studies with treatment-naive patients, virologic failure and emergent lamivudine resistance was more common in maraviroc-treated patients compared to patients receiving efavirenz.

Adverse Reactions

Cardiovascular: Vascular hypertensive disorder

Central nervous system: Amnesia, anxiety, depression, dizziness (including postural dizziness), fever, impaired consciousness, insomnia, pain, paresthesia, peripheral neuropathy, sensory disturbance

Dermatologic: Acne vulgaris, alopecia, erythema, folliculitis, pruritus, skin neoplasm (benign), skin rash, tinea

Endocrine & metabolic: Lipodystrophy

Gastrointestinal: Change in appetite, constipation, decreased gastrointestinal motility

Genitourinary: Genitourinary complaint (urinary tract/bladder symptoms), warts (genital)

Hematologic & oncologic: Neutropenia (grades 3/4)

Hepatic: Increased serum ALT (grades 3/4), increased serum AST (grades 3/4), increased serum bilirubin (grades 3/4)

Infection: Bacterial infection, herpes infection, *Neisseria*

Neuromuscular & skeletal: Arthralgia, myalgia

Ophthalmic: Conjunctivitis, eye infection

Otic: Otitis media

Respiratory: Bronchitis, cough, irregular breathing, lower respiratory tract infections, nasal congestion, paranasal sinus disease, sinusitis, upper respiratory tract infection

Miscellaneous: Flu-like symptoms, sweat gland disturbances

Rare but important or life-threatening: Anal cancer, angina pectoris, basal cell carcinoma, bile duct neoplasm, bone marrow depression, carcinoma *in situ* of esophagus, cardiac failure, cerebrovascular accident, cholestatic jaundice, coronary artery disease, coronary artery occlusion, endocarditis, endocrine neoplasm, hepatic cirrhosis, hepatic failure, hepatotoxicity, hypoplastic anemia, immune reconstitution syndrome, increased creatine kinase, ischemic heart disease, liver metastases, lymphoma, meningitis (viral), multiorgan hypersensitivity, myocardial infarction, myositis, osteonecrosis, pneumonia, portal vein thrombosis, rhabdomyolysis, seizure, septic shock, squamous cell carcinoma, Stevens-Johnson syndrome, syncope, T-cell lymphoma, tongue neoplasm, toxic epidermal necrolysis, tremor

Drug Interactions

Metabolism/Transport Effects **Substrate** of CYP3A4 (major), P-glycoprotein; **Note:** Assignment of Major/Minor substrate status based on clinically relevant drug interaction potential

Avoid Concomitant Use

Avoid concomitant use of Maraviroc with any of the following: Conivaptan; Fusidic Acid (Systemic); Idelalisib; St Johns Wort

Increased Effect/Toxicity

The levels/effects of Maraviroc may be increased by: Aprepitant; Conivaptan; CYP3A4 Inhibitors (Moderate); CYP3A4 Inhibitors (Strong); Dasatinib; Fosaprepitant; Fusidic Acid (Systemic); Idelalisib; Ivacaftor; Luliconazole; Mifepristone; Netupitant; Palbociclib; Simeprevir; Stiripentol

Decreased Effect

The levels/effects of Maraviroc may be decreased by: Bosentan; CYP3A4 Inducers (Moderate); CYP3A4 Inducers (Strong); Dabrafenib; Deferasirox; Efavirenz; Etravirine; Mitotane; Siltuximab; St Johns Wort; Tocilizumab

Storage/Stability Store at 25°C (77°F); excursions permitted to 15°C to 30°C (59°F to 86°F).

Mechanism of Action Maraviroc, a CCR5 antagonist, selectively and reversibly binds to the chemokine (C-C motif receptor 5 [CCR5]) coreceptors located on human CD4 cells. CCR5 antagonism prevents interaction between the human CCR5 coreceptor and the gp120 subunit of the viral envelope glycoprotein, thereby inhibiting gp120 conformational change required for CCR5-tropic HIV-1 fusion with the CD4 cell and subsequent cell entry.

Pharmacokinetics (Adult data unless noted)

Distribution: V_d: ~194 L

Protein binding: ~76%

Metabolism: Hepatic, via CYP3A to inactive metabolites

Bioavailability: 23% to 33% (maraviroc is a substrate for the efflux transporter P-gp)

Half-life elimination: 14 to 18 hours

Time to peak, plasma: 0.5 to 4 hours

Elimination: Urine (~20%, 8% as unchanged drug); feces (76%, 25% as unchanged drug)

Dosing: Usual

Pediatric: **HIV infection, treatment:** Use in combination with other antiretroviral agents: Adolescents ≥16 years: Oral: 300 mg twice daily (DHHS [pediatric], 2014)

Adult: **HIV infection, treatment:** Use in combination with other antiretroviral agents: Oral: 300 mg twice daily (DHHS [adult], 2014)

Dosing adjustment for concomitant CYP3A4 inhibitors/inducers: Adolescents ≥16 years and Adults:

CYP3A inhibitors (with or without a CYP3A4 inducer): 150 mg twice daily; dose recommended when maraviroc administered concomitantly with strong CYP3A inhibitors including (but not limited to) protease inhibitors (excluding tipranavir/ritonavir), boceprevir, delavirdine, ketoconazole, itraconazole, clarithromycin, nefazodone, telaprevir, and telithromycin.

CYP3A inducers (without a strong CYP3A4 inhibitor): 600 mg twice daily; dose recommended when maraviroc administered concomitantly with CYP3A inducers including (but not limited to) efavirenz, etravirine, rifampin, carbamazepine, phenobarbital, and phenytoin.

Dosing adjustment in renal impairment: Adolescents ≥16 years and Adults (DHHS [adults], 2013):

CrCl ≥30 mL/minute: No adjustment required

CrCl <30 mL/minute:

CrCl <30 mL/minute or ESRD and concomitant potent CYP3A inhibitors (with or without a CYP3A4 inducer) or concomitant potent CYP3A4 inducer (without a CYP3A4 inhibitor): Use is contraindicated

CrCl <30 mL/minute or ESRD and concomitant medications (eg, tipranavir/ritonavir, nevirapine, raltegravir, all NRTIs, and enfuvirtide): 300 mg twice daily. If postural hypotension occurs, reduce dose to 150 mg twice daily.

CrCl <30 mL/minute and experiencing postural hypotension: Reduce dose to 150 mg twice daily

Hemodialysis has minimal effect on clearance

Dosing adjustment in hepatic impairment: Adolescents ≥16 years and Adults:

Mild to moderate impairment: Use with caution; maraviroc concentrations are increased although dosage adjustment is not recommended

Moderate impairment (with concomitant strong CYP3A4 inhibitor): Use with caution; monitor closely for adverse events

Severe impairment: Patient population has not been studied

Administration May administer without regards to meals.

Monitoring Parameters **Note:** Monitor CD4 percentage (if <5 years of age) or CD4 count (if ≥5 years of age) at least every 3 to 4 months (DHHS [pediatric], 2014).

Prior to initiation of therapy: Genotypic resistance testing, CD4 and viral load (every 3 to 4 months), CBC with differential, LFTs, BUN, creatinine, tropism testing, electrolytes, glucose, and urinalysis (every 6 to 12 months), and assessment of readiness for adherence with medication regimen. At initiation and with any change in treatment regimen: CBC with differential, electrolytes, calcium, phosphate, glucose, LFTs, bilirubin, urinalysis (at initiation), BUN, creatinine, albumin, total protein, lipid panel (at initiation), CD4, and viral load. After 1 to 2 weeks of therapy: Signs of medication toxicity and adherence. After 2 to 4 weeks of therapy: CBC with differential, viral load, signs of medication toxicity, and adherence; then every 3 to 4 months: CBC with differential, electrolytes, glucose, LFTs, bilirubin, BUN, creatinine, CD4, viral load, signs of medication toxicity, and adherence. Every 6 to 12 months: Lipid panel and urinalysis. CD4 monitoring frequency may be decreased to every 6 to 12 months in children who are adherent to therapy if the value is well above the threshold for opportunistic infections, viral suppression is sustained, and the clinical status is stable for more than 2 to 3 years (DHHS [pediatric], 2014). Monitor for growth and development, signs of HIV-specific physical conditions, HIV disease progression, opportunistic infections, postural hypotension, or hepatitis.

Reference Range Plasma trough concentration: ≥50 ng/mL (DHHS [adult, pediatric], 2014)

Dosage Forms Excipient information presented when available (limited, particularly for generics); consult specific product labeling.

Tablet, Oral:

Selzentry: 150 mg, 300 mg [contains fd&c blue #2 aluminum lake, soybean lecithin]

◆ **Marcaine** *see* Bupivacaine *on page 316*

◆ **Marcaine® (Can)** *see* Bupivacaine *on page 316*

Measles, Mumps, and Rubella Virus Vaccine (MEE zels, mumpz & roo BEL a VYE rus vak SEEN)

Medication Safety Issues

Sound-alike/look-alike issues:

MMR (measles, mumps and rubella virus vaccine) may be confused with MMRV (measles, mumps, rubella, and varicella) vaccine

Related Information

Centers for Disease Control and Prevention (CDC) and Other Links *on page 2424*

Immunization Administration Recommendations *on page 2411*

Immunization Schedules *on page 2416*

Brand Names: US M-M-R II

Brand Names: Canada M-M-R II; Priorix

Therapeutic Category Vaccine; Vaccine, Live (Viral)

Generic Availability (US) No

Use Provide active immunity to measles, mumps, and rubella viruses (FDA approved in ages ≥12 months and adults)

The Advisory Committee on Immunization Practices (ACIP) recommends routine vaccination for the following (CDC/ACIP [McLean, 2013]):

- All children (first dose given at 12 to 15 months of age)
- Adults born 1957 or later (without evidence of immunity or documentation of vaccination). Vaccine may be given to adults born prior to 1957 if they do not have contraindications to the MMR vaccine.
- Adults at higher risk for exposure to and transmission of measles, mumps, and rubella should receive special consideration for vaccination, unless an acceptable evidence of immunity exists. This includes international travelers, persons attending colleges and other post high school education, and persons working in healthcare facilities.

Medication Guide Available Yes

Pregnancy Risk Factor C

Pregnancy Considerations Animal reproduction studies have not been conducted. It is not known whether this vaccine can cause fetal harm or affect reproduction capacity. Based on information collected following inadvertent administration during pregnancy, adverse events have not been observed following use of rubella vaccine. However, theoretical risks cannot be ruled out; use of this vaccine is contraindicated in pregnant females and should not be administered to women trying to conceive. The manufacturer recommends that pregnancy be avoided for 3 months after vaccine administration. The Advisory Committee on Immunization Practices (ACIP) recommends that pregnancy should be avoided for 28 days following vaccination. The risk of congenital rubella syndrome following vaccination is significantly less than the risk associated following infection therefore inadvertent administration of MMR during pregnancy is not considered an indication to terminate pregnancy.

Adverse events have been reported following natural infection in unvaccinated pregnant women. Measles infection during pregnancy may increase the risk of premature labor, preterm delivery, spontaneous abortion and low birth weights. Rubella infection during the first trimester may lead to miscarriages, stillbirths, and congenital rubella syndrome (includes auditory, ophthalmic, cardiac and neurologic defects; intrauterine and postnatal growth retardation); fetal rubella infection can occur during any trimester of pregnancy. Maternal mumps infection during the first trimester may increase the risk of spontaneous abortion or intrauterine fetal death. Sterility in males and infertility in prepubescent females may also occur with natural mumps infection.

Prenatal screening is recommended for all pregnant women who lack evidence of rubella immunity. Women of childbearing age without documentation of rubella vaccination or serologic evidence of immunity should be vaccinated (for women of childbearing potential, birth prior to 1957 is not acceptable evidence of immunity to rubella). Women who are pregnant should be vaccinated upon completion or termination of pregnancy, prior to discharge. Household contacts of pregnant women may be vaccinated (CDC/ACIP [McLean 2013]).

Breast-Feeding Considerations Lactating women may secrete the rubella component of the vaccine into breast milk. Evidence of rubella infection has occurred in breastfed infants following maternal immunization, most without severe disease. It is not known if the measles or mumps components of the vaccine are found in breast milk. The manufacturer recommends that caution be used if administered to nursing women. Breast-feeding is not a contraindication to vaccination. Breast-feeding infants should be vaccinated according to the recommended schedules (NCIRD/ACIP 2011).

Contraindications Hypersensitivity to measles, mumps, and/or rubella vaccine or any component of the formulation (including neomycin); current febrile respiratory illness or other febrile infection; patients receiving immunosuppressive therapy (does not include corticosteroids as replacement therapy); primary and acquired immunodeficiency states; individuals with blood dyscrasias, leukemia, lymphomas, or other malignant neoplasms affecting the bone marrow or lymphatic systems; family history of congenital or hereditary immunodeficiency (until immune competence in the vaccine recipient is demonstrated); pregnancy

Warnings/Precautions Use caution with history of cerebral injury, seizures, or other conditions where stress due to fever should be avoided. Antipyretics have not been shown to prevent febrile seizures; antipyretics may be used to treat fever or discomfort following vaccination (NCIRD/ACIP 2011). One study reported that routine prophylactic administration of acetaminophen to prevent fever prior to vaccination decreased the immune response of some vaccines; the clinical significance of this reduction in immune response has not been established (Prymula 2009). Immediate treatment (including epinephrine 1:1000) for anaphylactoid and/or hypersensitivity reactions should be available during vaccine use (NCIRD/ACIP 2011). Use caution in patients with thrombocytopenia and those who develop thrombocytopenia after first dose; thrombocytopenia may worsen. May consider deferring administration in patients with moderate or severe acute illness (with or without fever). Although fever is a contraindication per the manufacturer, current guidelines allow for administration to patients with mild acute illness (without fever) (CDC/ACIP [McLean 2013]; NCIRD/ACIP 2011).

Vaccination may not result in effective immunity in all patients. Response depends upon multiple factors (eg, type of vaccine, age of patient) and may be improved by administering the vaccine at the recommended dose, route, and interval. Vaccines may not be effective if administered during periods of altered immune competence (NCIRD/ACIP 2011). Use is contraindicated in severely immunocompromised patients. The ACIP does not recommend vaccination for persons with primary or acquired immunodeficiency (including immunosuppression associated with cellular immunodeficiency, hypogammaglobulinemia, dysgammaglobulinemia and AIDs, or severe immunosuppression associated with HIV); persons with blood dyscrasia, leukemia, lymphoma, or other malignant neoplasms which affect the bone marrow or lymphatic system; persons with a family history of congenital or hereditary immunodeficiency in first degree relatives (unless immunocompetence can be established); persons taking systemic corticosteroid therapy for ≥2 weeks in doses of corticosteroids ≥2 mg/kg of body weight or prednisone (or equivalent) ≥20 mg/day for persons who weigh >10 kg. Patients with HIV infection, who are asymptomatic and not severely immunosuppressed may be vaccinated (severe immunosuppression is defined as CD4+ T-lymphocyte <15% at any age or CD4 count <200 lymphocytes/mm^3 for persons >5 years) (CDC/ACIP [McLean 2013]). Patients with leukemia who are in remission and who have not received chemotherapy for at least 3 months may be vaccinated. In general, household and close contacts of persons with altered immunocompetence may receive all age appropriate vaccines (NCIRD/ACIP 2011). Recent administration of blood or blood products may interfere with immune response.

Syncope has been reported with use of injectable vaccines and may result in serious secondary injury (eg, skull fracture, cerebral hemorrhage); typically reported in adolescents and young adults and within 15 minutes after vaccination. Procedures should be in place to avoid injuries from falling and to restore cerebral perfusion if syncope occurs (NCIRD/ACIP 2011).

Therapy to treat tuberculosis should be started prior to administering vaccine to patients with active tuberculosis. Patients with untreated, active tuberculosis should not receive vaccine. Exposure to measles is not a contraindication to vaccine; use within 72 hours of exposure may provide some protection. Postexposure vaccination has not been shown to prevent or alter disease following rubella or mumps exposure (CDC/ACIP [McLean 2013]). Vaccine contains trace amounts of chick embryo antigen. Use caution in patients with history of immediate hypersensitivity/anaphylactic reactions following egg ingestion. Generally, the MMR vaccine can be safely administered to persons with an egg allergy (NCIRD/ACIP 2011). Manufactured with neomycin. Patients with history of anaphylaxis should not receive vaccine; contact dermatitis to neomycin is not a contraindication to the vaccine. Contains gelatin; contraindicated if known hypersensitivity to gelatin. Safety and efficacy of measles vaccine has not been established in children <6 months of age and safety and efficacy of mumps and rubella vaccines have not been established in <12 months of age. Local health departments may recommend vaccine to children 6 to 12 months of age in outbreak situations, but this would not count towards their immunization series.

In order to maximize vaccination rates, the ACIP recommends simultaneous administration (ie, >1 vaccine on the same day at different anatomic sites) of all age-appropriate vaccines (live or inactivated) for which a person is eligible at a single clinic visit, unless contraindications exist. The use of combination vaccines is generally preferred over separate injections, taking into consideration provider assessment, patient preference, and potential adverse events. When using combination vaccines, the minimum age for administration is the oldest minimum age for any individual component; the minimum interval between dosing is the greatest minimum interval between any individual components. The ACIP prefers each dose of a specific vaccine in a series come from the same manufacturer when possible (NCIRD/ACIP 2011). Acceptable evidence of immunity is recommended healthcare workers, students entering post high school educational institutions, and travelers to endemic areas. Use of this vaccine for specific medical and/or other indications (eg, immunocompromising conditions, hepatic or kidney disease, diabetes) is also addressed in the ACIP Recommended Adult Immunization Schedule (CDC/ACIP [Kim 2015]). Specific recommendations for vaccination in immunocompromised patients with asplenia, cancer, HIV infection, cerebrospinal fluid leaks, cochlear implants, hematopoietic stem cell transplant (prior to or after), sickle cell disease, solid organ transplant (prior to or after), or those receiving immunosuppressive therapy for chronic conditions as well as contacts of immunocompromised patients are available from the IDSA (Rubin 2014).

Adverse Reactions All serious adverse reactions must be reported to the U.S. Department of Health and Human Services (DHHS) Vaccine Adverse Event Reporting System (VAERS) 1-800-822-7967 or online at https://vaers.hhs.gov/esub/index. In Canada, adverse reactions may be reported to local provincial/territorial health agencies or to the Vaccine Safety Section at Public Health Agency of Canada (1-866-844-0018).

Cardiovascular: Syncope, vasculitis

Central nervous system: Acute disseminated encephalomyelitis, ataxia, brain disease, dizziness, encephalitis, Guillain-Barré syndrome, headache, irritability, malaise, measles inclusion body encephalitis, paresthesia, polyneuropathy, retrobulbar neuritis, seizure, subacute sclerosing panencephalitis, transverse myelitis

Dermatologic: Erythema multiforme, morbilliform rash, pruritus, rash, Stevens-Johnson syndrome, urticaria

Endocrine & metabolic: Diabetes mellitus

Gastrointestinal: Diarrhea, nausea, pancreatitis, parotitis, sore throat, vomiting

Genitourinary: Epididymitis, orchitis

Hematologic & oncologic: Leukocytosis, purpura, thrombocytopenia

Hypersensitivity: Anaphylactoid reaction, anaphylaxis, angioedema

Local: Injection site reaction (including burning, induration, redness, stinging, swelling, tenderness, vesiculation, wheal and flare)

Neuromuscular & skeletal: Arthropathy (arthralgia/arthritis: Women 12% to 26%; children ≤3%), myalgia

Ophthalmic: Conjunctivitis, oculomotor nerve paralysis, optic neuritis, optic papillitis, retinitis

Otic: Nerve deafness, otitis media

Respiratory: Bronchospasm, cough, pneumonia, pneumonitis, rhinitis

Miscellaneous: Atypical measles, febrile seizures, fever, panniculitis, lymphadenopathy (regional)

Rare but important or life-threatening: Aseptic meningitis (associated with Urabe strain of mumps vaccine)

Drug Interactions

Metabolism/Transport Effects None known.

Avoid Concomitant Use

Avoid concomitant use of Measles, Mumps, and Rubella Virus Vaccine with any of the following: Belimumab; Fingolimod; Immunosuppressants

Increased Effect/Toxicity

The levels/effects of Measles, Mumps, and Rubella Virus Vaccine may be increased by: AzaTHIOprine; Belimumab; Corticosteroids (Systemic); Dimethyl Fumarate; Fingolimod; Immunosuppressants; Leflunomide; Mercaptopurine; Methotrexate

Decreased Effect

Measles, Mumps, and Rubella Virus Vaccine may decrease the levels/effects of: Tuberculin Tests

The levels/effects of Measles, Mumps, and Rubella Virus Vaccine may be decreased by: AzaTHIOprine; Corticosteroids (Systemic); Dimethyl Fumarate; Fingolimod; Immune Globulins; Immunosuppressants; Leflunomide; Mercaptopurine; Methotrexate

Storage/Stability To maintain potency, the lyophilized vaccine must be stored between -50°C to 8°C (-58°F to 46°F). Temperatures below -50°C (-58°F) may occur if stored in dry ice. Prior to reconstitution, store the powder at 2°C to 8°C (36°F to 46°F). Protect from light. Diluent may be stored in refrigerator or at room temperature. Do not freeze diluent. Use as soon as possible following reconstitution, may be stored under refrigeration for up to 8 hours.

Mechanism of Action As a live, attenuated vaccine, MMR vaccine offers active immunity to disease caused by the measles, mumps, and rubella viruses.

Pharmacodynamics

Onset of action: The median seroconversion after 1 vaccine dose is 96% (measles), 99% (rubella), mumps (94%) (CDC/ACIP [McLean, 2013])

Duration of action: The median duration of immunity after 2 doses is ≥15 years for all components of the vaccine (CDC/ACIP [McLean, 2013])

Dosing: Usual Note: The minimum interval between two doses of MMR vaccine is 28 days (CDC/ACIP [McLean 2013]). Refer to Additional Information for a description of acceptable evidence of immunity.

Pediatric:

Primary immunization: Children ≥12 months: SubQ: 0.5 mL per dose for a total of 2 doses given as follows: 12 to 15 months of age and the second dose at 4 to 6 years of age; the second dose is recommended prior to entering kindergarten or first grade. The second dose may be administered at any time provided at least 28 days have elapsed since the first dose (CDC/ACIP [McLean 2013]).

Catch-up immunization (CDC/ACIP [Strikas 2015]): School-aged Children and Adolescents: Ensure that 2 doses have been given at least 28 days apart

Measles outbreak without acceptable evidence of immunity and at risk for exposure: Note: Should be administered within 72 hours postexposure.

Infants 6 to 11 months: SubQ: 0.5 mL per dose as a single dose (CDC/ACIP [McLean 2013]). Children should be vaccinated at ≥12 months with standard 2-dose series

Children 1 to 4 years: Children who received 1 dose (0.5 mL IM) of MMR should be considered for a second dose if the outbreak involves preschool-aged children (CDC/ACIP [McLean 2013]).

Mumps outbreak without acceptable evidence of immunity and at risk for exposure: Children 1 to 4 years: Children who received 1 dose of MMR should be considered for a second dose (0.5 mL IM) if the outbreak involves preschool-aged children (CDC/ACIP [McLean 2013])

Household/close contacts of immunocompromised persons without acceptable evidence of immunity: Children ≥12 months and Adolescents: SubQ: 0.5 mL per dose for a total of 2 doses administered at least 28 days apart unless they have acceptable evidence of immunity (CDC/ACIP [McLean 2013])

HIV infection without evidence of MMR immunity: Children ≥12 months and Adolescents: SubQ: 0.5 mL per dose. Children and adolescents with HIV infection and without evidence of severe immunosuppression should have 2 additional doses of MMR; those with perinatal HIV infection who were vaccinated prior to effective ART should have 2 additional doses of MMR once ART is established (CDC/ACIP [McLean 2013]).

International travel, without evidence of immunity (CDC [Strikas 2015]; CDC/ACIP [McLean, 2013]):

Infants 6 to 11 months: SubQ: 0.5 mL per dose. Administer 1 dose of MMR before departure from the United States; these infants should be revaccinated with 2 doses of MMR with the first dose between 12 to 15 months of age (and at least 28 days after the previous dose; target 12 months of age if child remains in area where disease risk if high) and the second dose at least 28 days later.

Children ≥12 months and Adolescents: SubQ: 0.5 mL per dose. Administer 2 doses of MMR before departure from the United States with the second dose at least 28 days later.

Adult: **Primary immunization:** SubQ: 0.5 mL per dose for a total of 1 or 2 doses administered at least 28 days apart based upon the following criteria (CDC/ACIP [McLean 2013]):

Adults born in or after 1957 should be vaccinated unless they have acceptable evidence of immunity

Adults born prior to 1957 are considered immune to measles, mumps, and rubella but may be vaccinated with 1 dose if they do not have contraindications to the vaccine. Pregnant adults born prior to 1957 are not considered immune to rubella.

Healthcare personnel: Persons born during or after 1957 should have 2 doses of vaccine unless they have acceptable evidence of immunity. Unvaccinated persons born prior to 1957 should also consider vaccination with 2 doses unless they have laboratory evidence or laboratory confirmation of disease.

HIV infection (without severe immunosuppression): 2 doses of MMR unless there is acceptable evidence of immunity

Household/close contacts of immunocompromised persons: 2 doses of MMR unless there is acceptable evidence of immunity

International travelers: 2 doses of MMR prior to travel unless there is acceptable evidence of immunity

Measles, mumps, or rubella outbreak (community): Adults who received one dose of MMR should be considered for a second dose if the outbreak involves measles or mumps in adults. Vaccination should also be considered for persons born prior to 1957 without evidence of immunity who may be exposed to mumps. A single dose of a rubella-containing vaccine is considered adequate vaccination during a rubella outbreak

Measles, mumps, or rubella outbreak (healthcare facility): Unvaccinated health care personnel without evidence of immunity regardless of birth year should receive 2 doses during a measles or mumps outbreak and one dose during a rubella outbreak

Students: Persons entering post high school educational facilities should receive 2 doses of MMR unless they have acceptable evidence of immunity prior to enrollment

Women of childbearing potential: 1 dose of MMR unless they have acceptable evidence of immunity. Vaccination should not be given during pregnancy and pregnancy should be avoided for 28 days after vaccine administration

Dosing adjustment in renal impairment: There are no dosage adjustments provided in manufacturer's labeling.

Dosing adjustment in hepatic impairment: There are no dosage adjustments provided in manufacturer's labeling.

Preparation for Administration SubQ: Reconstitute with entire contents of the provided diluent. Gently agitate to mix thoroughly. Discard if powder does not dissolve. Administer as soon as possible following reconstitution; discard if not used within 8 hours.

Administration SubQ: Administer as soon as possible following reconstitution; administer subcutaneously into the anterolateral aspect of the thigh or arm; not for IV administration. To prevent syncope related injuries, adolescents and adults should be vaccinated while seated or lying down (NCIRD/ACIP 2011). US law requires that the date of administration, the vaccine manufacturer, lot number of vaccine, and the administering person's name, title, and address be entered into the patient's permanent medical record.

Monitoring Parameters Observe for syncope for 15 minutes following administration (NCIRD/ACIP 2011). If seizure-like activity associated with syncope occurs, maintain patient in supine or Trendelenburg position to reestablish adequate cerebral perfusion.

Test Interactions Temporary suppression of tuberculin skin test reactivity. Tuberculin test may be given prior to vaccination, simultaneously at separate sites on the same day as measles-containing vaccine, or 4 to 6 weeks later (CDC/ACIP [McLean 2013]).

Additional Information Using separate sites and syringes, MMR may be administered concurrently with DTaP or *Haemophilus* b conjugate vaccine (PedvaxHIB®). Varicella vaccine may be administered with MMR using separate sites and syringes; however, if not administered simultaneously, doses should be separated by at least 30 days. Unless otherwise specified, MMR should be given 1 month before or 1 month after live viral vaccines.

Acceptable presumptive evidence of immunity includes one of the following (CDC/ACIP [McLean 2013]):

1. Documentation of adequate vaccination (for measles, mumps, and rubella). Adequate vaccination for mumps and measles is defined as 1 dose of a live virus vaccine for preschool children and adults not at high risk and 2 doses of a live virus vaccine for school-aged children and high-risk adults. Healthcare personnel (paid and unpaid workers with potential exposure), international travelers, and students in institutions of post high school education are considered high-risk adults.

2. Laboratory evidence of immunity or laboratory confirmation of disease (for measles, mumps, and rubella)

3. Birth prior to 1957 (measles, mumps, and rubella); for women of childbearing potential, birth prior to 1957 is not acceptable evidence of immunity to rubella.

4. Documentation of physician-diagnosed disease (for measles, mumps, or rubella) is not acceptable evidence of immunity.

Previous vaccination:

Measles: Persons who received a measles vaccine of unknown type, an inactivated measles vaccine, or further attenuated measles vaccine accompanied by immune globulin or high-titer immune globulin should be considered unvaccinated (CDC/ACIP [McLean 2013]).

Mumps: Persons vaccinated prior to 1979 with either killed mumps vaccine or a mumps vaccine of unknown type and who are at high risk for infection should be considered for revaccination with 2 doses of MMR vaccine (CDC/ACIP [McLean 2013]).

Dosage Forms Excipient information presented when available (limited, particularly for generics); consult specific product labeling.

Injection, powder for reconstitution [preservative free]:

M-M-R II: Measles virus ≥1000 $TCID_{50}$, mumps virus ≥20,000 $TCID_{50}$, and rubella virus ≥1000 $TCID_{50}$ [contains albumin (human), bovine serum, chicken egg protein, gelatin, neomycin, sorbitol, and sucrose 1.9 mg/vial; supplied with diluent]

Measles, Mumps, Rubella, and Varicella Virus Vaccine

(MEE zels, mumpz, roo BEL a, & var i SEL a VYE rus vak SEEN)

Medication Safety Issues

Sound-alike/look-alike issues:

MMRV (measles, mumps, rubella, and varicella) vaccine may be confused with MMR (measles, mumps and rubella virus) vaccine.

Related Information

Centers for Disease Control and Prevention (CDC) and Other Links *on page 2424*

Immunization Administration Recommendations *on page 2411*

Immunization Schedules *on page 2416*

Brand Names: US ProQuad
Brand Names: Canada Priorix-Tetra
Therapeutic Category Vaccine; Vaccine, Live Virus
Generic Availability (US) No
Use To provide active immunity to measles, mumps, rubella, and varicella viruses (FDA approved in ages 12 months to 12 years)

The Advisory Committee on Immunization Practices (ACIP) recommends routine vaccination against measles, mumps, rubella, and varicella in healthy children; the first dose should be given at 12 to 15 months of age and the second dose at 4 to 6 years of age. For children receiving their first dose at 12 to 47 months of age, either the MMRV combination vaccine or separate MMR and varicella vaccines can be used. The ACIP prefers administration of separate MMR and varicella vaccines as the first dose in this age group particularly for children with a personal or family history of seizures (CDC/ACIP [Marin 2010]) unless the parent or caregiver expresses preference for the MMRV combination. For children receiving the first dose at ≥48 months or their second dose at any age, use of MMRV is preferred.

Medication Guide Available Yes

Pregnancy Considerations Animal reproduction studies have not been conducted. Use is contraindicated in pregnant females and pregnancy should be avoided for 3 months (per manufacturer labeling) following vaccination. The ACIP recommends that pregnancy should be avoided for 1 month following vaccination with any of the individual components of this vaccine.

Refer to the Varicella Virus Vaccine monograph and the Measles, Mumps, and Rubella Virus Vaccine monograph for additional information.

Breast-Feeding Considerations Lactating women may secrete the rubella component of the vaccine into breast milk. It is not known if the measles, mumps, or varicella components of the vaccine are found in breast milk. The manufacturer recommends that caution be used if administered to nursing women. Breast-feeding is not a contraindication to vaccination. Breast-feeding infants should be vaccinated according to the recommended schedules (NCIRD/ACIP 2011). Refer to the Varicella Virus Vaccine monograph and the Measles, Mumps, and Rubella Virus Vaccine monograph for additional information.

Contraindications Hypersensitivity to this vaccine, measles, mumps, rubella, and/or varicella-containing vaccines, or any component of the formulation, including gelatin; history of anaphylactic reactions to neomycin; individuals with blood dyscrasias, leukemia, lymphomas, or other malignant neoplasms affecting the bone marrow or lymphatic systems; those receiving immunosuppressive therapy (including high-dose systemic corticosteroids); primary and acquired immunodeficiency states (including AIDs or symptomatic HIV; cellular immune deficiencies; hypogammaglobulinemic and dysgammaglobulinemic states); family history of congenital or hereditary immunodeficiency (until immune competence in the vaccine recipient is demonstrated); active untreated tuberculosis; current febrile illness with fever >38.5°C (>101.3°F); pregnancy

Warnings/Precautions Use caution with history of cerebral injury, seizures, or other conditions where stress due to fever should be avoided. Children 12 to 23 months of age have been reported to have a higher risk of developing febrile seizures with the use of the combination product (MMRV) compared to administration of MMR and varicella separately. Because it is uncommon for a child to have their first febrile seizure after 4 years of age, the ACIP recommends the use of the combination MMRV vaccine for children receiving their first dose at ≥48 months or their second dose at any age. The ACIP recommends that children with a personal or family history of seizures be vaccinated with separate MMR and varicella vaccines, as opposed to the MMRV combination vaccine. For children receiving their first dose at 12 to 47 months of age, either the MMRV combination vaccine or separate MMR and varicella vaccines can be used. The ACIP prefers administration of separate MMR and varicella vaccines as the first dose in this age group unless the parent or caregiver expresses preference for the MMRV combination. Parents and caregivers should be provided with the benefits and risks of both options (CDC/ACIP [Marin 2010]). Antipyretics have not been shown to prevent febrile seizures; antipyretics may be used to treat fever or discomfort following vaccination (NCIRD/ACIP 2011). One study reported that routine prophylactic administration of acetaminophen to prevent fever prior to vaccination decreased the immune response of some vaccines; the clinical significance of this reduction in immune response has not been established (Prymula 2009).

Vaccination may not result in effective immunity in all patients. Response depends upon multiple factors (eg, type of vaccine, age of patient) and may be improved by administering the vaccine at the recommended dose, route, and interval. Vaccines may not be effective if administered during periods of altered immune competence (NCIRD/ACIP 2011); use is contraindicated in patients with immunosuppression, including those receiving immunosuppressive therapy (including high-dose systemic corticosteroids). In general, live vaccines should be administered ≥4 weeks prior to planned immunosuppression and avoided within 2 weeks of immunosuppression when feasible (IDSA [Rubin 2014]). The safety and efficacy of this combination vaccine has not been established for postexposure prophylaxis.

Syncope has been reported with use of injectable vaccines and may result in serious secondary injury (eg, skull fracture, cerebral hemorrhage); typically reported in adolescents and young adults and within 15 minutes after vaccination. Procedures should be in place to avoid injuries from falling and to restore cerebral perfusion if syncope occurs (NCIRD/ACIP 2011).

Immediate treatment (including epinephrine 1:1,000) for anaphylactoid and/or hypersensitivity reactions should be available during vaccine use (NCIRD/ACIP 2011). Use extreme caution in patients with immediate-type hypersensitivity reactions to gelatin, eggs, or neomycin; patients with history of anaphylaxis should not receive the vaccine. Products may contain albumin. Contact dermatitis to neomycin is not a contraindication to the vaccine. Generally, the vaccine can be safely administered to persons with an egg allergy (NCIRD/ACIP 2011). Use caution in patients with thrombocytopenia and those who develop thrombocytopenia after first dose; thrombocytopenia may worsen. Vaccinated individuals should not have close association with susceptible high-risk individuals for 6 weeks following vaccination. High-risk individuals susceptible to the varicella virus include immunocompromised persons, pregnant women without evidence of immunity to varicella, newborns of mothers without evidence of varicella immunity, and infants born <28 weeks gestation (regardless of maternal immunity); transmission of varicella virus may occur. Avoid use of salicylates for 6 weeks following vaccination; varicella may increase the risk of Reye's syndrome. Safety and efficacy of this combination vaccine have not been established in patients with HIV infection; use is contraindicated in patients with AIDS or symptomatic HIV. Defer treatment in patients with active untreated tuberculosis. Recent administration of blood products or immune globulins may interfere with immune response. Guidelines with suggested administration intervals are available (NCIRD/ACIP 2011). The decision to administer or delay vaccination because of current or recent febrile illness depends on the severity of symptoms and the etiology of the disease. Consider deferring administration in patients with moderate or severe acute illness (with or without fever); vaccination should not be delayed for patients with mild acute illness (with or without fever) (NCIRD/ACIP 2011). Use is contraindicated with fever >38.5°C (>101.3°F).

In order to maximize vaccination rates, the ACIP recommends simultaneous administration (ie, >1 vaccine on the same day at different anatomic sites) of all age-appropriate vaccines (live or inactivated) for which a person is eligible at a single clinic visit, unless contraindications exist. The use of combination vaccines is generally preferred over separate injections, taking into consideration provider assessment, patient preference, and potential adverse events. When using combination vaccines, the minimum age for administration is the oldest minimum age for any individual component; the minimum interval between dosing is the greatest minimum interval between any individual component. The ACIP prefers each dose of a specific vaccine in a series come from the same manufacturer when possible (NCIRD/ACIP 2011).

Warnings: Additional Pediatric Considerations Safety and efficacy of this combination vaccine have not been established in patients with HIV infection. Use is contraindicated in patients with AIDS or symptomatic HIV. MMR and varicella individual vaccines have been recommended in children with HIV infection who are asymptomatic and not immunosuppressed (CDC immunologic category 1).

MMR and MMRV vaccines are both associated with febrile seizures which may occur during the first 2 weeks following vaccination. Based on preliminary information, fever ≥102°F occurs more often with MMRV (21.5%) compared to separate MMR and varicella vaccines (14.9%) in children 12 to 23 months of age. Measles-like rash also occurs more often with MMRV (3%) than with separate MMR and varicella vaccines (2.1%) in this age group. Most cases resolve spontaneously. The risk of febrile seizures may be increased twofold in children receiving MMRV at age 12 to 23 months in comparison to separate MMR and varicella vaccines (risk is highest 5 to 12 days after first dose). This is not observed in older children (≥47 months of age). Immunization with either MMRV or separate MMR and varicella vaccines offers equivalent immunity with the first dose. Using the combination vaccine provides the child with one less injection. Parents and/or caregivers should be provided with information related to the benefits and risks of both options. The ACIP prefers administration of separate MMR and varicella vaccines as the first dose in this age group unless the parent or caregiver expresses preference for the MMRV combination. Children with a personal or family history of seizures should be vaccinated with separate MMR and varicella vaccines, as opposed to the MMRV combination vaccine (CDC/ACIP [Marin 2010]). Results from a larger study confirm that children who were 12 to 23 months of age when receiving their first dose of MMRV vaccine were at an increased risk of fevers and seizures within 7 to 10 days after vaccination. Healthcare visits for fever and seizures were associated with both MMRV and separate MMR and varicella vaccines; however, the relative risk for seizures following vaccination was most significant with the MMRV vaccine. Seizures occurred most often 8 to 10 days following MMRV vaccination (RR 7.6, p <0.0001), 7 to 10 days following separate MMR and varicella vaccination (RR 4.0, p<0.0001), and 7 to 11 days following MMR vaccination (RR 3.7, p<0.0001); no peak in seizures was observed following varicella vaccine alone. Healthcare visits due to fever also clustered between 7 to 10 days after vaccination with any measles-containing vaccine (MMRV RR 6.1, MMR and varicella RR 4.4, MMR RR 4.3). Following a chart review for verification of seizure type, the rate of febrile seizures was 87% following both MMRV and separate MMR and varicella vaccine administration (Klein 2010).

Adverse Reactions All serious adverse reactions must be reported to the U.S. Department of Health and Human Services (DHHS) Vaccine Adverse Event Reporting System (VAERS) 1-800-822-7967 or online at https://vaers.hhs.gov/esub/index. In Canada, adverse reactions may be reported to local provincial/territorial health agencies or to the Vaccine Safety Section at Public Health Agency of Canada (1-866-844-0018).

Also refer to Measles, Mumps, and Rubella Vaccines (Combined) (M-M-R II) and Varicella Virus Vaccine (Varivax) monographs for additional adverse reactions reported with those agents. Percentages reported following one dose of ProQuad at 12-23 months of age.

Central nervous system: Drowsiness, irritability

Dermatologic: Erythema, morbilliform rash, rash at injection site, skin rash, varicella-like rash, viral exanthem

Gastrointestinal: Diarrhea, vomiting

Local: Bruising at injection site, pain at injection site (pain/tenderness/soreness), swelling at injection site

Respiratory: Rhinorrhea, upper respiratory tract infection

Miscellaneous: Fever

Rare but important or life-threatening: Acute disseminated encephalomyelitis, febrile seizures

Drug Interactions

Metabolism/Transport Effects None known.

Avoid Concomitant Use

Avoid concomitant use of Measles, Mumps, Rubella, and Varicella Virus Vaccine with any of the following: Belimumab; Fingolimod; Immunosuppressants

Increased Effect/Toxicity

The levels/effects of Measles, Mumps, Rubella, and Varicella Virus Vaccine may be increased by: 5-ASA Derivatives; AzaTHIOprine; Belimumab; Corticosteroids (Systemic); Dimethyl Fumarate; Fingolimod; Immunosuppressants; Leflunomide; Mercaptopurine; Methotrexate; Salicylates

Decreased Effect

Measles, Mumps, Rubella, and Varicella Virus Vaccine may decrease the levels/effects of: Tuberculin Tests

The levels/effects of Measles, Mumps, Rubella, and Varicella Virus Vaccine may be decreased by: AzaTHIOprine; Corticosteroids (Systemic); Dimethyl Fumarate; Fingolimod; Immune Globulins; Immunosuppressants; Leflunomide; Mercaptopurine; Methotrexate

Storage/Stability

ProQuad:

Before reconstitution, store the lyophilized vaccine between -50°C and -15°C (-58°F and 5°F) for up to 18 months. Use of dry ice may subject the vaccine to temperatures colder than -50°C (-58°F).

May store at 2°C to 8°C (36°F to 46° F) for up to 72 hours prior to reconstitution. Discard any vaccine stored at 2°C to 8°C (36°F to 46°F) that is not used within 72 hours of removal from -15°C (5°F) storage.

Protect the vaccine from light at all times.

Store diluent separately at room temperature (20°C to 25°C [68°F to 77° F]), or in a refrigerator (2°C to 8°C [36°F to 46° F]).

Discard reconstituted vaccine if it is not used within 30 minutes. Do not freeze reconstituted vaccine.

Priorix-Tetra [CAN; not available in US]: Store at 2°C to 8°C (36°F to 46°F). Do not freeze. Protect from light. Following reconstitution with provided diluent, administer vaccine as soon as possible; reconstituted vaccine may be stored up to 8 hours in refrigerator 2°C to 8°C (36°F to 46°F).

Mechanism of Action A live, attenuated virus vaccine that induces active immunity to disease caused by the measles, mumps, rubella, and varicella-zoster viruses.

Pharmacodynamics

Onset of action: At 6 weeks postvaccination of a single dose, the antibody response rate in healthy children 12 to 23 months of age was ~91% to 99%. Following a second dose to children <3 years of age, the observed antibody response rate was ~98% to 99%.

Duration of action: Antibody levels persist 10 years or longer in most healthy recipients. Refer to the Varicella Virus Vaccine monograph and the Measles, Mumps, and Rubella Virus Vaccine monograph for details.

Dosing: Usual

Pediatric:

Primary immunization: Children 12 months to 12 years: ProQuad: SubQ: 0.5 mL per dose. A complete immunization series for measles, mumps, rubella, and varicella requires 2 doses of all components, administered as either the combination product (MMRV-Proquad) or as separate MMR and varicella vaccines. The first dose is usually administered at 12 to 15 months of age. The second dose is administered at 4 to 6 years of age; second dose may be administered before age 4 if needed, as long as ≥3 months have elapsed since the first dose.

CDC (ACIP) recommendations: For children receiving their first dose at 12 to 47 months of age, either the MMRV combination vaccine or separate MMR and varicella vaccines can be used; however, the ACIP prefers administration of separate MMR and varicella vaccines as the first dose in this age group unless the parent or caregiver expresses preference for the MMRV combination. For children receiving the first dose at ≥48 months or their second dose at any age, use of MMRV is preferred. The ACIP recommends that children with a personal or family history of seizures be vaccinated with separate MMR and varicella vaccines, as opposed to the MMRV combination vaccine (CDC/ACIP [Marin 2010]).

Allow at least 1 month between administering a dose of a measles-containing vaccine (eg, M-M-R II) and ProQuad.

Allow at least 3 months between administering a varicella-containing vaccine (eg, Varivax) and ProQuad.

Dosing adjustment in renal impairment: There are no dosage adjustments provided in the manufacturer's labeling.

Dosing adjustment in hepatic impairment: There are no dosage adjustments provided in the manufacturer's labeling.

Preparation for Administration Parenteral: SubQ: Reconstitute with total volume of diluent provided. Gently agitate to dissolve powder. Discard if powder does not dissolve. Must be administered within 30 minutes of reconstitution.

Administration

Parenteral: **Note:** Disinfectants (eg, alcohol) may inactivate the attenuated viruses in the vaccine. Allow disinfectant adequate time to evaporate from skin prior to administration.

SubQ: Administer within 30 minutes of reconstitution. Administer subcutaneously into the anterolateral aspect of the thigh or deltoid region of arm; not for IV administration. US law requires that the date of administration, name of manufacturer, lot number, and administering person's name, title, and address be entered into patient's permanent medical record.

Monitoring Parameters Rash, fever; observe for syncope for 15 minutes following administration (NCIRD/ACIP 2011). If seizure-like activity associated with syncope occurs, maintain patient in supine or Trendelenburg position to re-establish adequate cerebral perfusion.

Test Interactions May interfere with sensitivity to tuberculin skin test; administer at separate sites before, simultaneously with, or at least 4-6 weeks after vaccine.

Dosage Forms Excipient information presented when available (limited, particularly for generics); consult specific product labeling.

Injection, powder for reconstitution [preservative free]:

ProQuad: Measles virus ≥3.00 log_{10} $TCID_{50}$, mumps virus ≥4.3 log_{10} $TCID_{50}$, rubella virus ≥3.00 log_{10} $TCID_{50}$, and varicella virus ≥3.99 log_{10} PFU [contains albumin (human), bovine serum, chicken egg protein, gelatin, neomycin, sorbitol, and sucrose (≤21 mg/vial)]

Mebendazole (me BEN da zole)

Medication Safety Issues

Sound-alike/look-alike issues:

Mebendazole may be confused with metroNIDAZOLE

Brand Names: Canada Vermox

Therapeutic Category Anthelmintic

Generic Availability (US) May be product dependent

Use Treatment of enterobiasis (pinworm infection), trichuriasis (whipworm infection), ascariasis (roundworm infection), and hookworm infections caused by *Necator americanus* or *Ancylostoma duodenale*; drug of choice in the treatment of capillariasis

Pregnancy Risk Factor C

Pregnancy Considerations Adverse events have been observed in animal reproduction studies; adverse pregnancy outcomes have not been observed following use in pregnancy (Diav-Citrin, 2003; Gyorkos, 2006). Treatment of pinworm in pregnancy may be considered; however, the CDC suggests postponing therapy until the third trimester when possible (CDC, 2010).

Breast-Feeding Considerations Since only 2% to 10% of mebendazole is absorbed, it is unlikely that it is excreted in breast milk in significant quantities (CDC, 2010)

Contraindications Hypersensitivity to mebendazole or any component of the formulation

Warnings/Precautions Use with caution in hepatic impairment; systemic exposure may be increased. Not effective for hydatid disease. Neutropenia and agranulocytosis have been reported with high doses and prolonged use. Concomitant use with metronidazole should be avoided; may increase the risk of adverse events including Stevens-Johnson syndrome and toxic epidermal necrolysis. Experience with use in children <2 years of age is limited; convulsions in infants <1 year have been reported (rare) postmarketing.

Adverse Reactions

Central nervous system: Dizziness, drowsiness, headache, seizure

Dermatologic: Alopecia, angioedema, exanthema, itching, rash, Stevens-Johnson syndrome, toxic epidermal necrolysis, urticaria

Gastrointestinal: Abdominal pain, diarrhea, vomiting

Hematologic: Agranulocytosis, eosinophilia, hemoglobin decreased, leukopenia, neutropenia

Hepatic: Alkaline phosphatase increased, ALT increased, AST increased, GGT increased, hepatitis

Renal: BUN increased, cylindruria, glomerulonephritis, hematuria

Miscellaneous: Hypersensitivity reactions (anaphylactic, anaphylactoid)

Drug Interactions

Metabolism/Transport Effects None known.

Avoid Concomitant Use

Avoid concomitant use of Mebendazole with any of the following: MetroNIDAZOLE (Systemic)

Increased Effect/Toxicity

Mebendazole may increase the levels/effects of: MetroNIDAZOLE (Systemic)

The levels/effects of Mebendazole may be increased by: Cimetidine

Decreased Effect

The levels/effects of Mebendazole may be decreased by: Aminoquinolines (Antimalarial); CarBAMazepine; Fosphenytoin; Phenytoin

Food Interactions Mebendazole serum levels may be increased if taken with food. Management: Administer without regard to meals.

Storage/Stability Store at 15°C to 30°C (59°F to 86°F). Protect from light.

Mechanism of Action Inhibits the formation of helminth microtubules; selectively and irreversibly blocks glucose uptake and other nutrients in susceptible adult intestine-dwelling helminths

Pharmacokinetics (Adult data unless noted)

Absorption: Oral: 2% to 10%

Distribution: To liver, fat, muscle, plasma, and hepatic cysts

Protein binding: 95%

Metabolism: Extensive in the liver

Half-life: 2.8-9 hours

Time to peak serum concentration: Variable (0.5-7 hours)

Elimination: Primarily in feces as inactive metabolites with 5% to 10% eliminated in urine

Dialysis: Not dialyzable

Dosing: Usual Children and Adults: Oral:

Pinworms: Single chewable tablet (100 mg); may need to repeat after 2 weeks

Whipworms, roundworms, hookworms: 100 mg twice daily, morning and evening on 3 consecutive days; if patient is not cured within 3-4 weeks, a second course of treatment may be administered

Capillariasis: 200 mg twice daily for 20 days

Administration Oral: Administer with food; tablet can be crushed and mixed with food, swallowed whole, or chewed

Monitoring Parameters For treatment of trichuriasis, ascariasis, hookworm, or mixed infections, check for helminth ova in the feces within 3-4 weeks following the initial therapy

Product Availability Not available in the US

Mecasermin (mek a SER min)

Brand Names: US Increlex

Therapeutic Category Growth Hormone

Generic Availability (US) No

Use Treatment of growth failure in children with severe primary insulin-like growth factor-1 deficiency (IGF-1 deficiency; primary IGFD), or with growth hormone (GH) gene deletions who have developed neutralizing antibodies to GH (FDA approved in children ≥2 years)

Pregnancy Risk Factor C

Pregnancy Considerations Teratogenic effects were not observed in animal studies

Breast-Feeding Considerations It is not known if mecasermin is excreted in breast milk. The manufacturer recommends that caution be exercised when administering mecasermin to nursing women.

Contraindications Hypersensitivity to mecasermin or any component of the formulation; patients with closed epiphyses; active or suspected neoplasia; intravenous administration

Warnings/Precautions Hypersensitivity reactions (localized skin reactions to anaphylaxis) have been reported. If hypersensitivity is suspected; discontinue and instruct patient to seek immediate medical attention. Correct thyroid or nutritional deficiencies prior to therapy. May cause hypoglycemic effects, especially in small children (due to inconsistent oral intake); patients should avoid high-risk activities (eg, driving) within 2 or 3 hours after dosing, particularly at initiation of treatment, until a tolerated dose is established. Use with caution in patients with diabetes. Do not administer on days a patient cannot or will not eat; should be administered with a meal or a snack. Intracranial hypertension has been reported with growth hormone products and reverses after interruption of dosing; funduscopic examinations are recommended at initiation of therapy and periodically thereafter. Lymphoid hypertrophy has been reported and may lead to complications such as snoring, sleep apnea, and chronic middle-ear effusions. Progression of scoliosis and slipped capital femoral epiphyses may occur in children experiencing rapid growth. Not intended for use in patients with secondary forms of IGF-1 deficiency (GH deficiency, malnutrition, hypothyroidism, chronic anti-inflammatory steroid therapy).

Benzyl alcohol and derivatives: Some dosage forms may contain benzyl alcohol; large amounts of benzyl alcohol (≥99 mg/kg/day) have been associated with a potentially fatal toxicity ("gasping syndrome") in neonates; the "gasping syndrome" consists of metabolic acidosis, respiratory distress, gasping respirations, CNS dysfunction (including convulsions, intracranial hemorrhage), hypotension, and cardiovascular collapse (AAP, 1997; CDC, 1982); some data suggests that benzoate displaces bilirubin from protein binding sites (Ahlfors, 2001); avoid or use dosage forms containing benzyl alcohol with caution in neonates. See manufacturer's labeling.

Adverse Reactions

Cardiovascular: Heart murmur

Central nervous system: Dizziness, headache, seizure

Endocrine & metabolic: Hypoglycemia, lipohypertrophy (injection site), thymus hypertrophy

Gastrointestinal: Vomiting

Local: Bruising at injection site

Neuromuscular & skeletal: Arthralgia, limb pain, muscular atrophy

Otic: Abnormal tympanometry, fluid in ear (middle ear), hypoacusis, otalgia, otitis media, serous otitis media

Respiratory: Snoring, tonsillar hypertrophy

Rare but important or life-threatening: Anaphylaxis, cardiomegaly, heart valve disease, hypercholesterolemia, hypersensitivity, hypertriglyceridemia, hypoglycemic seizure, increased lactate dehydrogenase, increased serum ALT, increased serum AST, intracranial hypertension, obstructive sleep apnea syndrome, osteonecrosis (occasionally associated with slipped capital femoral epiphysis)

Drug Interactions

Metabolism/Transport Effects None known.

Avoid Concomitant Use There are no known interactions where it is recommended to avoid concomitant use.

Increased Effect/Toxicity

Mecasermin may increase the levels/effects of: Hypoglycemia-Associated Agents

The levels/effects of Mecasermin may be increased by: Androgens; Antidiabetic Agents; Herbs (Hypoglycemic Properties); MAO Inhibitors; Pegvisomant; Quinolone Antibiotics; Salicylates; Selective Serotonin Reuptake Inhibitors

Decreased Effect

The levels/effects of Mecasermin may be decreased by: Quinolone Antibiotics

Storage/Stability Store vials under refrigeration at 2°C to 8°C (35°F to 46°F); keep refrigerated and use within 30 days of initial vial entry. Do not freeze. Protect from direct light.

Mechanism of Action Mecasermin is an insulin-like growth factor (IGF-1) produced using recombinant DNA technology to replace endogenous IGF-1. Endogenous IGF-1 circulates predominately bound to insulin-like growth factor-binding protein-3 (IGFBP-3) and a growth hormone-dependent acid-labile subunit (ALS). Acting at receptors in the liver and other tissues, endogenous growth hormone

(GH) stimulates the synthesis and secretion of IGF-1. In patients with primary severe IGF-1 deficiency, growth hormone receptors in the liver are unresponsive to GH, leading to reduced endogenous IGF-I concentrations and decreased growth (skeletal, cell, and organ). Endogenous IGF-1 also suppresses liver glucose production, stimulates peripheral glucose utilization, and has an inhibitory effect on insulin secretion.

Pharmacokinetics (Adult data unless noted)

Distribution: V_d: Severe primary IGFD: 0.184-0.33 L/kg

Protein binding: >80% bound to IGFBP-3 and an acid-labile subunit (IGFBP-3 reduced with severe primary IGFD)

Metabolism: Hepatic and renal

Bioavailability: 100% (healthy subjects)

Half-life: Severe primary IGFD: 5.8 hours

Time to peak serum concentration: 2 hours

Dosing: Usual Children and Adolescents:

Primary IGFD: Increlex®: Children ≥2 years and Adolescents: SubQ: Initial: 0.04-0.08 mg/kg/dose twice daily; if tolerated for 7 days, may increase by 0.04 mg/kg/dose; maximum dose: 0.12 mg/kg given twice daily. **Note:** Must be administered within 20 minutes of a meal or snack; omit dose if patient is unable to eat. Reduce dose if hypoglycemia occurs despite adequate food intake; dose should not be increased to make up for ≥1 omitted dose.

Dosage adjustment in renal impairment: Children ≥2 years and Adolescents: No dosage adjustments are provided in the manufacturer's labeling; has not been studied.

Dosage adjustment in hepatic impairment: Children ≥2 years and Adolescents: No dosage adjustments are provided in the manufacturer's labeling; has not been studied.

Administration SubQ: Must be administered within 20 minutes of a meal or snack. May cause hypoglycemic effects; patients should avoid high-risk activities within 2-3 hours of dosing until a tolerated dose is established. If patient is unable to eat, omit dose and do not make up for omitted dose. Rotate injection site.

Monitoring Parameters Preprandial glucose during treatment initiation and dose adjustment; hypersensitivity reactions; facial features; lymphoid tissue; funduscopic examination; growth; new onset of a limp or complaints of hip or knee pain; progression of scoliosis. Monitor small children closely due to potentially erratic food intake.

Reference Range

Severe primary IGFD is defined as follows:

Height standard deviation score ≤ -3.0 **and**

Basal IGF-1 standard deviation score ≤ -3.0 **and**

Growth hormone: Normal or increased

Additional Information If using syringes that measure dose in units, doses in mg/kg must be converted to units using the following formula:

Weight (kg) × Dose (mg/kg) × 1 mL/10 mg × 100 units/1 mL = units/injection

Dosage Forms Excipient information presented when available (limited, particularly for generics); consult specific product labeling.

Solution, Subcutaneous:

Increlex: 40 mg/4 mL (4 mL) [contains benzyl alcohol]

◆ **Mecasermin (rDNA Origin)** *see* Mecasermin *on page 1334*

Mechlorethamine (Systemic)

(me klor ETH a meen)

Medication Safety Issues

High alert medication:

This medication is in a class the Institute for Safe Medication Practices (ISMP) includes among its list of drug classes which have a heightened risk of causing significant patient harm when used in error.

Related Information

Management of Drug Extravasations *on page 2298*

Prevention of Chemotherapy-Induced Nausea and Vomiting in Children *on page 2368*

Safe Handling of Hazardous Drugs *on page 2455*

Brand Names: US Mustargen

Therapeutic Category Antineoplastic Agent, Alkylating Agent; Antineoplastic Agent, Alkylating Agent (Nitrogen Mustard)

Generic Availability (US) No

Use Palliative treatment of Hodgkin lymphoma and of effusions from metastatic carcinomas (FDA approved in adults); treatment of lymphosarcoma, chronic myelocytic or chronic lymphocytic leukemia, polycythemia vera, mycosis, fungoides, and bronchogenic carcinoma (FDA approved in adults); **Note:** While FDA approved for several oncologic uses, use in practice is limited.

Pregnancy Risk Factor D

Pregnancy Considerations Adverse events have been observed in animal reproduction studies. Women of child-bearing potential are advised not to become pregnant during treatment. **[U.S. Boxed Warning]: Avoid exposure during pregnancy.**

Breast-Feeding Considerations It is not known if mechlorethamine is excreted in human breast milk. Due to the potential for serious adverse reactions in the nursing infant, the decision to discontinue mechlorethamine or to discontinue breast-feeding should take into account the importance of treatment to the mother.

Contraindications Hypersensitivity to mechlorethamine or any component of the formulation; presence of known infection

Warnings/Precautions Hazardous agent; use appropriate precautions for handling and disposal (NIOSH 2014 [group 1]). **[U.S. Boxed Warning]: Mechlorethamine is a highly toxic nitrogen mustard; avoid inhalation of vapors or dust; review and follow special handling procedures.** Avoid dust or vapor contact with skin or eyes. If accidental skin exposure occurs, wash/irrigate thoroughly with water for at least 15 minutes, followed by 2% sodium thiosulfate solution; remove and destroy any contaminated clothing. If exposure to eye(s) occurs, promptly irrigate for at least 15 minutes with copious amounts of water, normal saline, or balanced salt ophthalmic irrigating solution; obtain ophthalmology consultation. The manufacturer recommends neutralizing remaining unused mechlorethamine, empty or partial vials, gloves, tubing, glassware, etc., after mechlorethamine administration; soak in an aqueous solution containing equal volumes of sodium thiosulfate (5%) and sodium bicarbonate (5%) for 45 minutes; rinse with water; dispose of properly.

[U.S. Boxed Warning]: Mechlorethamine is a potent vesicant; extravasation results in painful inflammation with induration and sloughing. If extravasation occurs, promptly manage by infiltrating area with 1/6 molar sodium thiosulfate solution, followed by dry cold compresses for 6-12 hours. Ensure proper needle or catheter placement prior to and during infusion. Avoid extravasation.

Bone marrow suppression: May cause lymphopenia, leukopenia, granulocytopenia, thrombocytopenia and anemia. Agranulocytopenia may occur (rare); persistent pancytopenia has been reported. Monitor blood counts. Bleeding due to thrombocytopenia may occur. Use with caution in patients where neoplasm has bone marrow involvement or in those who have received prior myelosuppressive chemotherapy; marrow function may be further compromised (possibly fatal). Bone marrow function should recover after mechlorethamine administration prior to initiating radiation therapy or other chemotherapy regimens.

Hyperuricemia may occur, especially with lymphomas; ensure adequate hydration; consider antihyperuricemic therapy if appropriate. Mechlorethamine is associated with a high emetic potential (Basch, 2011; Dupuis, 2011; Roila, 2010); antiemetics are recommended to prevent nausea and vomiting. Hypersensitivity reactions, including anaphylaxis, have been reported. Mechlorethamine has immunosuppressant properties; may predispose patients to infections (bacterial, viral, or fungal). Alkylating agents, including mechlorethamine, are associated with in increased incidence of secondary malignancies; concurrent radiation therapy or combination chemotherapy may increase the risk. Potentially significant drug-drug interactions may exist, requiring dose or frequency adjustment, additional monitoring, and/or selection of alternative therapy.

[U.S. Boxed Warning]: Avoid exposure during pregnancy. Impaired spermatogenesis, azoospermia, and total germinal aplasia may occur in male patients treated with mechlorethamine, particularly when used in combination with other chemotherapy agents. Delayed menses, oligomenorrhea, or temporary or permanent amenorrhea may be observed in female patients treated with mechlorethamine.

Bone marrow failure and other toxicities are more common in chronic lymphocytic leukemia (CLL); in general, mechlorethamine is no longer used in the treatment of CLL. Bone and nervous system tumors typically respond poorly to treatment with mechlorethamine. The routine use of mechlorethamine in widely disseminated tumors is discouraged. **[U.S. Boxed Warning]: Should be administered under the supervision of an experienced cancer chemotherapy physician.**

Adverse Reactions

Central nervous system: Drowsiness, encephalopathy (high dose), fever, headache, lethargy, sedation, vertigo
Dermatologic: Alopecia, erythema multiforme, maculopapular rash, petechiae, rash
Endocrine & metabolic: Amenorrhea, hyperuricemia, oligomenorrhea, spermatogenesis decreased
Gastrointestinal: Anorexia, diarrhea, metallic taste, mucositis, nausea, vomiting
Hepatic: Jaundice
Hematologic: Agranulocytosis, granulocytopenia (onset 6-8 days, recovery 10-21 days), hemolytic anemia, leukopenia, lymphocytopenia, pancytopenia, secondary leukemias, thrombocytopenia
Local: Thrombophlebitis, tissue necrosis (extravasation)
Neuromuscular & skeletal: Weakness
Ocular: Lacrimation
Otic: Deafness, tinnitus
Miscellaneous: Anaphylaxis, diaphoresis, herpes zoster infection, hypersensitivity reactions

Drug Interactions

Metabolism/Transport Effects None known.

Avoid Concomitant Use

Avoid concomitant use of Mechlorethamine (Systemic) with any of the following: BCG; BCG (Intravesical); CloZAPine; Dipyrone; Natalizumab; Pimecrolimus; Tacrolimus (Topical); Tofacitinib; Vaccines (Live)

Increased Effect/Toxicity

Mechlorethamine (Systemic) may increase the levels/effects of: CloZAPine; Leflunomide; Natalizumab; Tofacitinib; Vaccines (Live)

The levels/effects of Mechlorethamine (Systemic) may be increased by: Denosumab; Dipyrone; Pimecrolimus; Roflumilast; Tacrolimus (Topical); Trastuzumab

Decreased Effect

Mechlorethamine (Systemic) may decrease the levels/effects of: BCG; BCG (Intravesical); Coccidioides immitis Skin Test; Sipuleucel-T; Vaccines (Inactivated); Vaccines (Live)

The levels/effects of Mechlorethamine (Systemic) may be decreased by: Echinacea

Storage/Stability Store intact vials at room temperature of 15°C to 30°C (59°F to 86°F). Protect from light. Protect from humidity. **Must be prepared immediately before use;** degradation begins shortly after dilution.

Mechanism of Action Bifunctional alkylating agent that inhibits DNA and RNA synthesis via formation of carbonium ions; produces interstrand and intrastrand cross-links in DNA resulting in miscoding, breakage, and failure of replication. Although not cell phase-specific *per se*, mechlorethamine effect is most pronounced in the S phase, and cell proliferation is arrested in the G_2 phase.

Pharmacokinetics (Adult data unless noted)

Metabolism: Rapid hydrolysis in the plasma to active metabolites (Perry, 2012)
Half-life elimination: 15 to 20 minutes (Perry, 2012)

Dosing: Usual Note: Dosing and frequency may vary by protocol and/or treatment phase; refer to specific protocol.

Pediatric: **Hodgkin lymphoma:**

MOPP regimen: **Note:** The MOPP (with or without ABVD) regimen is generally no longer used due to improved toxicity profiles with other combination regimens used in the treatment of Hodgkin lymphoma (Kelly, 2012). Children and Adolescents: IV: 6 mg/m^2 on days 1 and 8 of a 28-day cycle in combination with vincristine, procarbazine, and prednisone, may or may not alternate with doxorubicin, bleomycin, vinblastine, dacarbazine (MOPP/ABVD) (Kung, 2006; Longo, 1986)

Stanford V regimen: Adolescents ≥16 years: IV: 6 mg/m^2 as a single dose on day 1 in weeks 1, 5, and 9 (Horning, 2000; Horning, 2002; Metzger, 2012)

Adult: **Note:** Dosage should be based on ideal dry weight (evaluate the presence of edema or ascites so that dosage is based on actual weight unaugmented by edema/ascites).

Hodgkin lymphoma: IV:

MOPP regimen: 6 mg/m^2 on days 1 and 8 of a 28-day treatment cycle for 6 to 8 cycles (Canellos, 1992; Devita, 1970)

Stanford V regimen: 6 mg/m^2 as a single dose on day 1 in weeks 1, 5, and 9 (Horning, 2000; Horning, 2002)

Malignant effusion: Intracavitary: 0.4 mg/kg as a single dose; although 0.2 mg/kg (10 to 20 mg) as a single dose has been used by the *intrapericardial* route

Dosing adjustment in renal impairment: There are no dosage adjustments provided in manufacturer's labeling.

Dosing adjustment in hepatic impairment: There are no dosage adjustments provided in manufacturer's labeling.

Preparation for Administration Hazardous agent; use appropriate precautions for handling and disposal (NIOSH 2014 [group 1]).

Parenteral: **Must be prepared immediately before use;** degradation begins shortly after dilution. Dilute powder with 10 mL SWFI or NS to a final concentration of 1 mg/mL.

Intracavitary: Dilute powder with 10 mL SWFI or NS to a final concentration of 1 mg/mL; may then be further diluted in 50 to 100 mL NS.

Administration Hazardous agent; use appropriate precautions for handling and disposal (NIOSH 2014 [group 1]).

Parenteral: **Must be prepared immediately prior to administration.** Administer IV push over 1 to 5 minutes into a free-flowing IV solution. **DO NOT ADMINISTER IM or SubQ**. Mechlorethamine is associated with a high emetic potential (Basch 2011; Dupuis 2011; Roila

2010); antiemetics are recommended to prevent nausea and vomiting.

Vesicant; ensure proper needle or catheter placement prior to and during infusion; avoid extravasation. If extravasation occurs, stop infusion immediately and disconnect (leave cannula/needle in place); gently aspirate extravasated solution (do **NOT** flush the line); remove needle/cannula; initiate sodium thiosulfate antidote (see Management of Drug Extravasations for more details); elevate extremity.

Intracavitary: Adults: Prepare immediately prior to administration; rotate patient position every 5 to 10 minutes for 1 hour after administration to obtain uniform distribution

Vesicant/Extravasation Risk Vesicant

Monitoring Parameters CBC with differential and platelet count, renal and hepatic function; signs/symptoms of hypersensitivity reactions, infection, and extravasation

Product Availability Mustargen: Mustargen was acquired by Recordati Rare Diseases in 2013; availability information is currently unknown.

Dosage Forms Excipient information presented when available (limited, particularly for generics); consult specific product labeling.

Solution Reconstituted, Injection, as hydrochloride:

Mustargen: 10 mg (1 ea)

◆ **Mechlorethamine Hydrochloride** *see* Mechlorethamine (Systemic) *on page 1335*

Meclizine (MEK li zeen)

Medication Safety Issues

Sound-alike/look-alike issues:

Antivert® may be confused with Anzemet®, Axert®

BEERS Criteria medication:

This drug may be potentially inappropriate for use in geriatric patients (Quality of evidence - varies based on comorbidity; Strength of recommendation - varies based on comorbidity)

Brand Names: US Dramamine Less Drowsy [OTC]; Medi-Meclizine [OTC]; Motion-Time [OTC]; Travel Sickness [OTC]; UniVert; Vertin-32 [OTC] [DSC]

Therapeutic Category Antiemetic; Antihistamine

Generic Availability (US) Yes

Use Prevention and treatment of motion sickness; management of vertigo

Pregnancy Risk Factor B

Pregnancy Considerations Adverse events have been observed in animal reproduction studies; however, an increased risk of fetal abnormalities has not been observed following maternal use of meclizine during pregnancy.

Breast-Feeding Considerations

It is not known if meclizine is excreted into breast milk.

Contraindications Hypersensitivity to meclizine or any component of the formulation

Warnings/Precautions Use with caution in patients with asthma, angle-closure glaucoma, prostatic hyperplasia, pyloric or duodenal obstruction, or bladder neck obstruction. May be inappropriate in older adults depending on comorbidities (eg, dementia, delirium, etc) due to its potent anticholinergic effects (Beers Criteria). Use with caution in the elderly; may be more sensitive to adverse effects. If vertigo does not respond in 1-2 weeks, it is advised to discontinue use. May be sedating, use with caution in disorders where CNS depression is a feature; patients must be cautioned about performing tasks which require mental alertness (eg, operating machinery or driving). Effects may be potentiated when used with other sedative drugs or ethanol.

Adverse Reactions

Central nervous system: Drowsiness, fatigue, headache

Gastrointestinal: Vomiting, xerostomia

Ocular: Blurred vision

Miscellaneous: Anaphylactoid reaction

Drug Interactions

Metabolism/Transport Effects Substrate of CYP2D6 (minor); **Note:** Assignment of Major/Minor substrate status based on clinically relevant drug interaction potential

Avoid Concomitant Use

Avoid concomitant use of Meclizine with any of the following: Aclidinium; Azelastine (Nasal); Eluxadoline; Glucagon; Ipratropium (Oral Inhalation); Orphenadrine; Paraldehyde; Potassium Chloride; Thalidomide; Tiotropium; Umeclidinium

Increased Effect/Toxicity

Meclizine may increase the levels/effects of: AbobotulinumtoxinA; Alcohol (Ethyl); Analgesics (Opioid); Anticholinergic Agents; Azelastine (Nasal); Buprenorphine; CNS Depressants; Eluxadoline; Glucagon; Hydrocodone; Methotrimeprazine; Metyrosine; Mirabegron; Mirtazapine; OnabotulinumtoxinA; Orphenadrine; Paraldehyde; Potassium Chloride; Pramipexole; RimabotulinumtoxinB; ROPINIRole; Rotigotine; Selective Serotonin Reuptake Inhibitors; Suvorexant; Thalidomide; Thiazide Diuretics; Tiotropium; Topiramate; Zolpidem

The levels/effects of Meclizine may be increased by: Aclidinium; Brimonidine (Topical); Cannabis; Doxylamine; Dronabinol; Droperidol; HydrOXYzine; Ipratropium (Oral Inhalation); Kava Kava; Magnesium Sulfate; Methotrimeprazine; Mianserin; Nabilone; Perampanel; Pramlintide; Rufinamide; Sodium Oxybate; Tapentadol; Tetrahydrocannabinol; Umeclidinium

Decreased Effect

Meclizine may decrease the levels/effects of: Acetylcholinesterase Inhibitors; Benzylpenicilloyl Polylysine; Betahistine; Hyaluronidase; Itopride; Metoclopramide; Secretin

The levels/effects of Meclizine may be decreased by: Acetylcholinesterase Inhibitors; Amphetamines

Mechanism of Action Has central anticholinergic action by blocking chemoreceptor trigger zone; decreases excitability of the middle ear labyrinth and blocks conduction in the middle ear vestibular-cerebellar pathways

Pharmacodynamics

Onset of action: Oral: 30-60 minutes

Duration: 12-24 hours

Pharmacokinetics (Adult data unless noted)

Metabolism: In the liver

Half-life: 6 hours

Elimination: As metabolites in urine and as unchanged drug in feces

Dosing: Usual Children >12 years and Adults: Oral:

Motion sickness: 25-50 mg 1 hour before travel, repeat dose every 24 hours if needed

Vertigo: 25-100 mg/day in divided doses

Administration Oral: Administer with food to decrease GI distress

Dosage Forms Excipient information presented when available (limited, particularly for generics); consult specific product labeling. [DSC] = Discontinued product

Tablet, Oral, as hydrochloride:

Dramamine Less Drowsy: 25 mg [contains fd&c yellow #10 (quinoline yellow)]

Dramamine Less Drowsy: 25 mg [contains fd&c yellow #10 aluminum lake]

Medi-Meclizine: 25 mg

UniVert: 32 mg [scored; contains brilliant blue fcf (fd&c blue #1), fd&c yellow #10 (quinoline yellow)]

Vertin-32: 32 mg [DSC] [contains brilliant blue fcf (fd&c blue #1), fd&c yellow #10 (quinoline yellow)]

Generic: 12.5 mg, 25 mg

Tablet Chewable, Oral, as hydrochloride:
Motion-Time: 25 mg [scored; contains fd&c red #40 aluminum lake, saccharin sodium; raspberry flavor]
Travel Sickness: 25 mg [contains aspartame, fd&c red #40 aluminum lake]
Travel Sickness: 25 mg [DSC] [scored; contains aspartame, fd&c red #40 aluminum lake; raspberry flavor]
Generic: 25 mg

- ♦ **Meclizine Hydrochloride** *see* Meclizine *on page 1337*
- ♦ **Meclozine Hydrochloride** *see* Meclizine *on page 1337*
- ♦ **Med-Derm Hydrocortisone [OTC]** *see* Hydrocortisone (Topical) *on page 1041*
- ♦ **Medical Provider EZ Flu** *see* Influenza Virus Vaccine (Inactivated) *on page 1108*
- ♦ **Medical Provider EZ Flu PF** *see* Influenza Virus Vaccine (Inactivated) *on page 1108*
- ♦ **Medical Provider EZ Flu Shot** *see* Influenza Virus Vaccine (Inactivated) *on page 1108*
- ♦ **Medicinal Carbon** *see* Charcoal, Activated *on page 425*
- ♦ **Medicinal Charcoal** *see* Charcoal, Activated *on page 425*
- ♦ **Medi-First Anti-Fungal [OTC]** *see* Tolnaftate *on page 2083*
- ♦ **Medi-First Hydrocortisone [OTC]** *see* Hydrocortisone (Topical) *on page 1041*
- ♦ **Medi-Meclizine [OTC]** *see* Meclizine *on page 1337*
- ♦ **Medi-Phenyl [OTC]** *see* Phenylephrine (Systemic) *on page 1685*
- ♦ **Mediplast [OTC]** *see* Salicylic Acid *on page 1894*
- ♦ **Mediproxen [OTC]** *see* Naproxen *on page 1489*

Medium Chain Triglycerides

(mee DEE um chane trye GLIS er ides)

Brand Names: US Betaquik [OTC]; Liquigen [OTC]; MCT Oil [OTC]

Brand Names: Canada MCT Oil

Therapeutic Category Caloric Agent; Nutritional Supplement

Generic Availability (US) No

Use Nutritional supplement for those who cannot digest long chain fats; malabsorption associated with disorders such as pancreatic insufficiency, bile salt deficiency, or bacterial overgrowth of the small bowel (MCT Oil: Dietary supplement labeled for adults); has also been used to induce ketosis as a prevention for seizures

Warnings/Precautions Avoid use in patients with uncontrolled diabetic ketoacidosis. Use with caution in patients with hepatic cirrhosis; large amounts of medium chain triglycerides (MCT) may elevate blood and spinal fluid levels of medium chain fatty acids (MCFA) due to impaired hepatic clearance of MCFA (Gracey, 1970; Morgan, 1974). These products are medical foods and should be used under medical supervision. Medium chain triglycerides are not intended as a sole source of nutrition; they do not provide the recommended daily dosage of essential fatty acids. Not for parenteral use.

Adverse Reactions

Endocrine & metabolic: HDL serum levels decreased and triglycerides serum levels increased (>6 months daily use)

Gastrointestinal: Abdominal pain, bloating, cramping, diarrhea, nausea

Storage/Stability

MCT Oil: Store in a cool, dry place; protect from light. Must be stored in a glass container.

Liquigen: Store between 4°C to 25°C (39°F to 77°F). After opening, refrigerate and use within 14 days.

Betaquik: Store in a cool dry place. Once opened, refrigerate and use within 48 hours.

Mechanism of Action MCTs are saturated fatty acids in chains of 6-12 carbon atoms. They are water soluble and can pass directly through intestinal cell membranes into portal venous blood. Unlike long chain fats, MCTs do not require the presence of bile acids and pancreatic lipase for absorption. MCTs provide a source of calories while reducing the amount of malabsorbed fat remaining in stool (Gracey, 1970; Ruppin, 1980).

Pharmacodynamics Onset of action: Octanoic acid appeared in each subject by 30 minutes following ingestion; effect on seizures in children: Within 6 weeks

Pharmacokinetics (Adult data unless noted)

Absorption: Up to 30% of dose can be absorbed unchanged as a triglyceride in the mucosal cell

Metabolism: Almost entirely oxidized by the liver to acetyl CoA fragments and to carbon dioxide; little deposited in adipose tissue or elsewhere

Elimination: As much as 20% of oral dose of MCT, recovered in expired CO_2 in 50 minutes; <10% elimination of medium chain fatty acids in feces

Dosing: Neonatal Nutritional Supplement, increase caloric content: Oral: MCT oil: **Note:** Dose should be individualized to patient caloric needs, current nutritional/fluid status, and other clinical parameters. Initial: 0.5 mL every other feeding, then advance to every feeding, then increase in increments of 0.25 to 0.5 mL/feeding at intervals of 2 to 3 days as tolerated (Kliegman 2007); lower initial doses may be used depending upon caloric needs; product formulation provides 115 calories/15 mL

Dosing: Usual

Pediatric:

Nutritional supplement: Infants: Oral: MCT oil: Initial: 0.5 mL every other feeding, then advance to every feeding, then increase in increments of 0.25 to 0.5 mL/feeding at intervals of 2 to 3 days as tolerated (Kliegman 2007)

Cystic fibrosis: Children and Adolescents: Oral: MCT oil: 45 mL/day in divided doses (Kliegman 2007)

Ketogenic diet: Children and Adolescents: Oral: MCT oil: About 40 mL with each meal or 50% to 70% (800 to 1,120 kcal) of total calories (1,600 kcal) as the oil will induce the ketosis necessary for seizure control (Kliegman 2007)

Adult:

Cystic fibrosis: Oral: MCT oil: 45 mL daily in divided doses

Dietary supplement: Oral: MCT oil: 15 to 20 mL per dose (maximum daily dose: 100 mL)

Preparation for Administration Oral: Dilute with at least an equal volume of water or mix with some other beverage (eg, juice, milk) (should not be cold; flavoring may be added); may also be mixed into sauces, salad dressings, or other foods (Ruppin 1980).

Administration Oral:

Dilute prior to administration with at least an equal volume of water or mix with some other beverage (eg, juice, milk) (should not be cold; flavoring may be added); mixture should be sipped slowly; administer no more than 15 to 20 mL at any one time (up to 100 mL may be administered in divided doses in a 24-hour period) (Ruppin 1980). For administration of MCT oil through a feeding tube in adults, administer 15 mL via syringe through tube; flush with 30 mL of water after administration.

Possible GI side effects from medication can be prevented if therapy is initiated with small supplements at meals and gradually increased according to patient's tolerance (Gracey 1970; Ruppin 1980)

Monitoring Parameters

Nutritional supplement and malabsorption: Weight gain, height, stool output

Seizure treatment: Reduction in seizures, urine ketones

Additional Information Does not provide any essential fatty acids; contains only saturated fats; supplementation with safflower, corn oil, or other polyunsaturated vegetable oil must be given to provide the patient with the essential fatty acids; caloric content: 8.3 calories/g; 115 calories/15 mL

Dosage Forms Excipient information presented when available (limited, particularly for generics); consult specific product labeling.

Emulsion, Oral:

Betaquik: (250 mL)

Liquigen: (250 mL)

Oil, Oral:

MCT Oil: (946 mL)

◆ **MED-Letrozole (Can)** *see* Letrozole *on page 1224*

◆ **Medrol** *see* MethylPREDNISolone *on page 1409*

◆ **Medrol Dose Pack** *see* MethylPREDNISolone *on page 1409*

◆ **Medrol (Pak)** *see* MethylPREDNISolone *on page 1409*

◆ **Med-Rosuvastatin (Can)** *see* Rosuvastatin *on page 1886*

◆ **Medroxy (Can)** *see* MedroxyPROGESTERone *on page 1339*

MedroxyPROGESTERone

(me DROKS ee proe JES te rone)

Medication Safety Issues

Sound-alike/look-alike issues:

Depo-Provera may be confused with depo-subQ provera 104

MedroxyPROGESTERone may be confused with hydroxyprogesterone caproate, methylPREDNISolone, methylTESTOSTERone

Provera may be confused with Covera, Femara, Parlodel, Premarin, Proscar, PROzac

Administration issues:

The injectable dosage form is available in different formulations. Carefully review prescriptions to assure the correct formulation and route of administration.

Related Information

Contraceptive Comparison Table *on page 2309*

Safe Handling of Hazardous Drugs *on page 2455*

Brand Names: US Depo-Provera; Depo-SubQ Provera 104; Provera

Brand Names: Canada Alti-MPA; Apo-Medroxy; Depo-Prevera; Depo-Provera; Dom-Medroxyprogesterone; Gen-Medroxy; Medroxy; Medroxyprogesterone Acetate Injectable Suspension USP; Novo-Medrone; PMS-Medroxyprogesterone; Provera; Provera-Pak; Teva-Medroxyprogesterone

Therapeutic Category Contraceptive, Progestin Only; Progestin

Generic Availability (US) Yes

Use Secondary amenorrhea or abnormal uterine bleeding due to hormonal imbalance; prevention of pregnancy; reduction of endometrial hyperplasia in nonhysterectomized postmenopausal women receiving conjugated estrogens; endometrial carcinoma; management of endometriosis-associated pain (FDA approved in adults)

Pregnancy Risk Factor X (tablet)

Pregnancy Considerations Most products are contraindicated in women who are pregnant, suspected to be pregnant or as a diagnostic test for pregnancy. In general, there is not an increased risk of birth defects following inadvertent use of the injectable medroxyprogesterone acetate (MPA) contraceptives early in pregnancy. Hypospadias has been reported in male babies and clitoral enlargement and labial fusion have been reported in female babies exposed to MPA during the first trimester of pregnancy. High doses impair fertility. Ectopic pregnancies have been reported with use of the MPA contraceptive injection. Median time to conception/return to ovulation following discontinuation of MPA contraceptive injection is 10 months following the last injection and is unrelated to the duration of use.

Breast-Feeding Considerations Medroxyprogesterone acetate (MPA) is excreted in breast milk. Composition, quality, and quantity of breast milk are not affected; adverse developmental and behavioral effects have not been noted following exposure of infant to MPA while breast-feeding. The manufacturer does not recommend the use of MPA tablets in breast-feeding mothers; however, guidelines note that the injectable MPA contraceptives can be initiated immediately postpartum in women who are nursing (CDC, 2010; CDC, 2011; CDC, 2013). The manufacturer recommends medroxyprogesterone 400 mg/mL be used with caution in women who are nursing.

Contraindications

Angioedema, anaphylactic reaction, or hypersensitivity to medroxyprogesterone or any component of the formulation

Additional contraindications:

Injection (104 mg/0.65 mL): Active thrombophlebitis; venous thromboembolic disorders or cerebral vascular disease (current or history of); undiagnosed genital bleeding; breast cancer (known, suspected or history of); significant hepatic impairment or disease; pregnancy

Injection (150 mg/mL): Active thrombophlebitis; venous thromboembolic disorders or cerebral vascular disease (current or history of); undiagnosed genital bleeding; breast cancer (known, suspected or history of); significant hepatic impairment or disease; pregnancy; diagnostic test for pregnancy

Injection (400 mg/mL): Active thrombophlebitis; venous thromboembolic disorders or cerebral vascular disease (current or history of)

Tablet: DVT or PE (current or history of); active or history of arterial thromboembolic disease (eg, stroke, MI); estrogen or progesterone dependent tumor (known or suspected); undiagnosed abnormal genital bleeding; breast cancer (known, suspected or history of); hepatic impairment or disease; pregnancy

Warnings/Precautions Hazardous agent - use appropriate precautions for handling and disposal (NIOSH 2014 [group 2]).

Anaphylaxis or anaphylactoid reactions have been reported with use of the injection; medication for the treatment of hypersensitivity reactions should be available for immediate use.

[US Boxed Warning]: Prolonged use of medroxyprogesterone contraceptive injection may result in a loss of bone mineral density (BMD). It is not known if use during adolescence or early adulthood will decrease peak bone mass accretion or increase the risk for osteoporotic fractures later in life. Loss is related to the duration of use, may not be completely reversible on discontinuation of the drug, and incidence is not significantly different between the SubQ and IM dosage forms. The impact on peak bone mass in adolescents should be weighed against the potential for unintended pregnancies in treatment decision. Consider alternative contraceptive methods in patients at risk for osteoporosis (eg, metabolic bone disease, chronic alcohol and/or tobacco use, anorexia nervosa, strong family history of osteoporosis, chronic use of medications associated with osteoporosis such as anticonvulsants or corticosteroids). All patients should have adequate calcium and Vitamin D intake. Consider evaluating bone mineral density in patients receiving high doses of medroxyprogesterone for long term endometrial cancer. **[US Boxed Warning]: Long-term use (ie, >2 years) should be limited to situations where other birth control methods are inadequate.** When used for endometrial carcinoma, the effects of long term use on adrenal, hepatic, ovarian, pituitary, and uterine function is not known. **[US Boxed Warning]: Inform patients that injectable contraceptives do not protect against HIV infection or other sexually-transmitted diseases.**

[US Boxed Warning]: Based on data from the Women's Health Initiative (WHI) studies, an increased risk of invasive breast cancer was observed in postmenopausal women using conjugated estrogens (CE) in combination with medroxyprogesterone acetate (MPA). This risk may be associated with duration of use and declines once combined therapy is discontinued (Chlebowski, 2009). The risk of invasive breast cancer was decreased in postmenopausal women with a hysterectomy using CE only, regardless of weight. However, the risk was not significantly decreased in women at high risk for breast cancer (family history of breast cancer, personal history of benign breast disease) (Anderson, 2012). Women who used depo-medroxyprogesterone within the previous 5 years and for a duration of 12 months or longer were found to have an increased risk of breast cancer. An increase in abnormal mammogram findings has also been reported with estrogen alone or in combination with progestin therapy. Most products are contraindicated in patients with known or suspected breast cancer. Use of medroxyprogesterone for the treatment of endometrial carcinoma is not recommended in women with known or suspected breast cancer and women with a strong family history of breast cancer should be carefully monitored.

[US Boxed Warning]: Estrogens with or without progestin should not be used to prevent dementia. In the Women's Health Initiative Memory Study (WHIMS), an increased incidence of probable dementia was observed in women ≥65 years of age taking CE alone or in combination with MPA.

[US Boxed Warning]: Estrogens with progestin should not be used to prevent cardiovascular disease. Using data from the Women's Health Initiative (WHI) studies, an increased risk of deep vein thrombosis (DVT), and stroke, has been reported with CE and an increased risk of DVT, stroke, pulmonary emboli (PE) and myocardial infarction (MI) has been reported with CE with MPA in postmenopausal women 50 to 79 years of age. Additional risk factors include diabetes mellitus, hypercholesterolemia, hypertension, SLE, obesity, tobacco use, and/or history of venous thromboembolism (VTE). Risk factors should be managed appropriately; discontinue use if adverse cardiovascular events occur or are suspected. Use is contraindicated in women with active DVT, PE, active arterial thromboembolic disease or a history of these conditions. If thrombosis develops with contraceptive treatment, discontinue treatment (unless no other acceptable contraceptive alternative).

[US Boxed Warning]: Estrogens with progestin should be used for the shortest duration possible at the lowest effective dose consistent with treatment goals and risks for the individual woman. Patients should be reevaluated as clinically appropriate to determine if treatment is still necessary. Available data related to treatment risks are from Women's Health Initiative (WHI) studies, which evaluated oral CE 0.625 mg with or without MPA 2.5 mg relative to placebo in postmenopausal women. Other combinations and dosage forms of estrogens and progestins were not studied. **Outcomes reported from clinical trials using CE with or without MPA should be assumed to be similar for other doses and other dosage forms of estrogens and progestins until comparable data becomes available.** Women who are early in menopause, who are in good cardiovascular health, and who are at low risk for adverse cardiovascular events can be considered candidates for estrogen with or without progestin therapy for the relief of menopausal symptoms (ACOG 565 2013). MPA is used to reduce the risk of endometrial hyperplasia in nonhysterectomized postmenopausal women receiving conjugated estrogens. The use of unopposed estrogen in women with a uterus is associated with an increased risk of endometrial cancer. The addition of a progestin to estrogen therapy may decrease the risk of endometrial hyperplasia, a precursor to endometrial cancer. Adequate diagnostic measures, including endometrial sampling if indicated, should be performed to rule out malignancy in postmenopausal women with undiagnosed abnormal vaginal bleeding. There is no evidence that the use of natural estrogens results in a different endometrial risk profile than synthetic estrogens at equivalent estrogen doses. The risk of endometrial cancer is dose and duration dependent; risk appears to be greatest with use ≥5 years and may persist following discontinuation of therapy.

Use with caution in patients with migraine, or a history of depression. Use with caution in patients with diseases which may be exacerbated by fluid retention, including cardiac, or renal dysfunction. Discontinue pending examination in cases of sudden partial or complete vision loss, sudden onset of proptosis, diplopia, or migraine; discontinue permanently if papilledema or retinal vascular lesions are observed on examination. Unscheduled bleeding/spotting may occur. Presentation of irregular, unresolving vaginal bleeding following previously regular cycles warrants further evaluation including endometrial sampling, if indicated, to rule out malignancy. Potentially significant interactions may exist, requiring dose or frequency adjustment, additional monitoring, and/or selection of alternative therapy. Not for use prior to menarche. Whenever possible, progestins in combination with estrogens should be discontinued at least 4-6 weeks prior to surgery associated with an increased risk of thromboembolism or during periods of prolonged immobilization.

Postmenopausal estrogen therapy and combined estrogen/progesterone therapy may increase the risk of ovarian cancer; however, the absolute risk to an individual woman is small. Although results from various studies are not consistent, risk does not appear to be significantly associated with the duration, route, or dose of therapy. In one study, the risk decreased after 2 years following discontinuation of therapy (Mørch, 2009). Although the risk of ovarian cancer is rare, women who are at an increased risk (eg, family history) should be counseled about the association (NAMS, 2012). In women using estrogen plus progesterone therapy, triglycerides may be increased in women with preexisting hypertriglyceridemia; discontinue if pancreatitis occurs. Estrogen plus progestin therapy may have adverse effects on glucose tolerance; use caution in women with diabetes. Use estrogen plus progestin therapy with caution in patients with asthma, epilepsy, hepatic hemangiomas, porphyria, or SLE; may exacerbate disease. Use estrogen plus progestin therapy with caution in patients with hypoparathyroidism; estrogen-induced hypocalcemia may occur.

Estrogens plus progestins are poorly metabolized in patients with hepatic dysfunction. Use caution with a history of cholestatic jaundice associated with prior estrogen use or pregnancy. Discontinue if jaundice develops or if acute or chronic hepatic disturbances occur. Most products are contraindicated with hepatic impairment or disease. Use of medroxyprogesterone for the treatment of endometrial carcinoma is not recommended in women with significant hepatic dysfunction and should be discontinued if liver dysfunction occurs. The use of estrogens and/or progestins may change the results of some laboratory tests (eg, coagulation factors, lipids, glucose tolerance, binding proteins). The dose, route, and the specific estrogen/progestin influences these changes. In addition, personal risk factors (eg, cardiovascular disease, smoking, diabetes, age) also contribute to adverse events; use of specific products may be contraindicated in women with certain risk factors.

When used for contraception, the possibility of ectopic pregnancy should be considered in patients with severe abdominal pain. Contraceptive therapy with medroxyprogesterone commonly results in an average weight gain of ~3.7 kg after 2 years of treatment.

May cause suppression of hypothalamic-pituitary-adrenal (HPA) axis, resulting in decreased plasma cortisol concentrations, decreased cortisol secretion, and low plasma ACTH concentrations. Cushingoid symptoms may occur.

Use may mask the onset of menopause in women treated for endometrial cancer.

Some dosage forms may contain polysorbate 80 (also known as Tweens). Hypersensitivity reactions, usually a delayed reaction, have been reported following exposure to pharmaceutical products containing polysorbate 80 in certain individuals (Isaksson, 2002; Lucente 2000; Shelley, 1995). Thrombocytopenia, ascites, pulmonary deterioration, and renal and hepatic failure have been reported in premature neonates after receiving parenteral products containing polysorbate 80 (Alade, 1986; CDC, 1984). See manufacturer's labeling.

Adverse Reactions Adverse effects as reported with any dosage form

Cardiovascular: Edema

Central nervous system: Depression, dizziness, fatigue, headache, insomnia, nervousness

Dermatologic: Acne, alopecia, rash

Endocrine & metabolic: Breast pain, hot flashes, libido decreased, menstrual irregularities (includes bleeding, amenorrhea, or both)

Gastrointestinal: Abdominal pain/discomfort, bloating, nausea, weight gain (>10 lbs at 24 months)

Genitourinary: Cervical smear abnormal, leukorrhea, menometrorrhagia, menorrhagia, pelvic pain, urinary tract infection, vaginitis

Genitourinary: Dysmenorrhea, leukorrhea, vaginitis

Local: Injection site reaction (SubQ administration): Atrophy, induration, pain

Rare but important or life-threatening: Allergic reaction, anaphylaxis, anaphylactoid reactions, angioedema, asthma, blood dyscrasia, bone mineral density decreased, breast cancer, breast changes, cervical cancer, chest pain, chloasma, cholestatic jaundice, deep vein thrombosis, diaphoresis, dyspnea, facial palsy, galactorrhea, glucose tolerance decreased, hirsutism, hoarseness, injection site reactions, jaundice, lack of return to fertility, lactation decreased, melasma, nipple bleeding, optic neuritis, osteoporosis, osteoporotic fractures, paralysis, paresthesia, pulmonary embolus, rectal bleeding, retinal thrombosis, scleroderma, seizure, syncope, tachycardia, thrombophlebitis, urticaria

Drug Interactions

Metabolism/Transport Effects **Substrate** of CYP3A4 (major); **Note:** Assignment of Major/Minor substrate status based on clinically relevant drug interaction potential; **Induces** CYP3A4 (weak)

Avoid Concomitant Use

Avoid concomitant use of MedroxyPROGESTERone with any of the following: Griseofulvin; Indium 111 Capromab Pendetide; Tranexamic Acid; Ulipristal

Increased Effect/Toxicity

MedroxyPROGESTERone may increase the levels/effects of: C1 inhibitors; Selegiline; Thalidomide; Tranexamic Acid; Voriconazole

The levels/effects of MedroxyPROGESTERone may be increased by: Atazanavir; Boceprevir; Cobicistat; CYP3A4 Inhibitors (Strong); Herbs (Progestogenic Properties); Lopinavir; Metreleptin; Mifepristone; Tipranavir; Voriconazole

Decreased Effect

MedroxyPROGESTERone may decrease the levels/effects of: Anticoagulants; Antidiabetic Agents; ARIPiprazole; Choline C 11; Fosamprenavir; Hydrocodone; Indium 111 Capromab Pendetide; NiMODipine; Saxagliptin; Ulipristal; Vitamin K Antagonists

The levels/effects of MedroxyPROGESTERone may be decreased by: Acitretin; Aprepitant; Artemether; Barbiturates; Bexarotene (Systemic); Bile Acid Sequestrants; Bosentan; CarBAMazepine; CloBAZam; CYP3A4 Inducers (Moderate); CYP3A4 Inducers (Strong); Dabrafenib; Darunavir; Deferasirox; Efavirenz; Eslicarbazepine; Felbamate; Fosamprenavir; Fosaprepitant; Fosphenytoin; Griseofulvin; LamoTRIgine; Lopinavir; Metreleptin; Mifepristone; Mitotane; Mycophenolate; Nelfinavir; Nevirapine; OXcarbazepine; Perampanel; Phenytoin; Primidone; Prucalopride; Retinoic Acid Derivatives; Rifamycin Derivatives; Saquinavir; Siltuximab; St Johns Wort; Sugammadex; Telaprevir; Tocilizumab; Topiramate; Ulipristal

Food Interactions Bioavailability of the oral tablet is increased when taken with food; half-life is unchanged. Management: Administer without regard to food.

Storage/Stability Store at 20°C to 25°C (68°F to 77°F).

Mechanism of Action Medroxyprogesterone acetate (MPA) transforms a proliferative endometrium into a secretory endometrium. When administered with conjugated estrogens, MPA reduces the incidence of endometrial hyperplasia and risk of adenocarcinoma. When used as an injection for contraception (doses of 150 mg IM or 104 mg SubQ), MPA inhibits secretion of pituitary gonadotropins, which prevents follicular maturation and ovulation and causes endometrial thinning. Progestogens, such as medroxyprogesterone when used for endometriosis, lead to atrophy of the endometrial tissue. They may also suppress new growth and implantation. Pain associated with endometriosis is decreased (ASRM, 2014).

Pharmacodynamics Time to ovulation (after last injection): 10 months (range: 6 to 12 months)

Pharmacokinetics (Adult data unless noted)

Absorption: IM: Slow

Protein binding: 86% to 90% primarily to albumin; does not bind to sex hormone-binding globulin

Metabolism: Extensively hepatic via hydroxylation and conjugation; forms metabolites

Bioavailability: 0.6% to 10%

Half-life:
- Oral: 12 to 17 hours
- IM (Depo-Provera Contraceptive): ~50 days
- SubQ: ~40 days

Time to peak serum concentration:
- Oral: 2 to 4 hours
- IM (Depo-Provera Contraceptive): ~3 weeks
- SubQ (depo-subQ provera 104): 1 week

Elimination: Urine

Dosing: Usual

Adolescents and Adults:

Abnormal uterine bleeding: Oral: 5 to 10 mg for 5 to 10 days starting on day 16 or day 21 of menstrual cycle

Amenorrhea: Oral: 5 to 10 mg/day for 5 to 10 days

Contraception: First dose to be given only during first 5 days of normal menstrual period; only within 5 days postpartum if not breast-feeding, or only at sixth postpartum week if exclusively breast-feeding. When switching from other contraceptive methods, depo-subQ provera 104 should be administered within 7 days after the last day of using the last method (pill, ring, patch).

IM (Depo-Provera): 150 mg every 3 months (every 13 weeks)

SubQ (depo-subQ provera 104): 104 mg every 3 months (every 12 to 14 weeks)

Endometriosis-associated pain: SubQ (depo-subQ provera 104): 104 mg every 3 months; treatment longer than 2 years is not recommended due to impact of long-term use on bone mineral density

Adults:

Accompanying cyclic estrogen therapy (postmenopausal): Oral: 5 to 10 mg for 12 to 14 consecutive days each month, starting on day 1 or day 16 of cycle; lower doses may be used if given with estrogen continuously throughout the cycle

Endometrial carcinoma, recurrent or metastatic: IM (Depo-Provera): 400 to 1000 mg/week

Dosing adjustment in hepatic impairment: Use is contraindicated with severe impairment. Discontinue with jaundice or if liver function disturbances occur. Consider lower dose or less frequent administration with mild to moderate impairment. Use of the contraceptive injection has not been studied in patients with hepatic impairment; consideration should be given to not readminister if jaundice develops.

Administration Hazardous agent; use appropriate precautions for handling and disposal (NIOSH 2014 [group 2]).

Oral: Administer with food

Parenteral:

IM: (Depo-Provera Contraceptive): Shake suspension vigorously; administer by deep IM injection in the gluteal or deltoid muscle

SubQ (depo-subQ provera 104): Shake vigorously for at least 1 minute; administer by subQ injection slowly over 5 to 7 seconds in the anterior thigh or abdomen; avoid boney areas and the umbilicus. Do not rub the injection area; not for IM or IV use.

Monitoring Parameters Before starting therapy, a physical exam with reference to the breasts and pelvis are recommended, including a Papanicolaou smear. Exam may be deferred if appropriate prior to administration of MPA contraceptive injection; pregnancy should be ruled out prior to use. Monitor patient closely for loss of vision; sudden onset of proptosis, diplopia, or migraine; signs and symptoms of thromboembolic disorders; signs and symptoms of depression; glucose in patients with diabetes; or blood pressure. BMD with long-term use.

Adequate diagnostic measures, including endometrial sampling, if indicated, should be performed to rule out malignancy in all cases of undiagnosed abnormal vaginal bleeding.

Dosage Forms Excipient information presented when available (limited, particularly for generics); consult specific product labeling.

Suspension, Intramuscular, as acetate:

Depo-Provera: 150 mg/mL (1 mL)

Depo-Provera: 150 mg/mL (1 mL) [contains methylparaben, polyethylene glycol, polysorbate 80, propylparaben]

Depo-Provera: 400 mg/mL (2.5 mL)

Generic: 150 mg/mL (1 mL)

Suspension, Subcutaneous, as acetate:

Depo-SubQ Provera 104: 104 mg/0.65 mL (0.65 mL) [contains methylparaben, propylparaben]

Tablet, Oral, as acetate:

Provera: 2.5 mg, 5 mg, 10 mg [scored]

Generic: 2.5 mg, 5 mg, 10 mg

◆ **Medroxyprogesterone Acetate** *see* MedroxyPROGESTERone *on page 1339*

◆ **Medroxyprogesterone Acetate Injectable Suspension USP (Can)** *see* MedroxyPROGESTERone *on page 1339*

◆ **Med-Sotalol (Can)** *see* Sotalol *on page 1963*

Mefloquine (ME floe kwin)

Medication Safety Issues

International issues:

Lariam [multiple international markets] may be confused with Levaquin [Argentina, Brazil, U.S., Venezuela]

Therapeutic Category Antimalarial Agent

Generic Availability (US) Yes

Use Treatment of acute malarial infections due to *Plasmodium vivax* and *Plasmodium flaciparum* (including chloroquine-resistant strains) (FDA approved in ages ≥6 months and adults); prevention of malaria due to *Plasmodium vivax* and *Plasmodium falciparum* (including chloroquine-resistant strains) (FDA approved in pediatric patients weighing ≥20 kg and adults)

Medication Guide Available Yes

Pregnancy Risk Factor B

Pregnancy Considerations Adverse events have been observed in animal reproduction studies. Mefloquine crosses the placenta; however, clinical experience with mefloquine has not shown adverse effects in pregnant women. Use with caution during pregnancy if travel to endemic areas cannot be postponed. Malaria infection in pregnant women may be more severe than in nonpregnant women and may increase the risk of adverse pregnancy outcomes. Nonpregnant women of childbearing potential are advised to use contraception and avoid pregnancy during malaria prophylaxis and for 3 months thereafter. In case of an unplanned pregnancy, treatment with mefloquine is not considered a reason for pregnancy termination. CDC treatment guidelines are available for the use of mefloquine in the treatment of malaria during pregnancy (CDC, 2013b).

Breast-Feeding Considerations Mefloquine is excreted in breast milk in small quantities (~3% to 4% of a 250 mg dose). The manufacturer recommends that caution be exercised when administering mefloquine to nursing women. Exposure to small amounts of mefloquine from breast milk is considered safe for infants (CDC, 2014).

Contraindications Hypersensitivity to mefloquine, related compounds (eg, quinine and quinidine), or any component of the formulation; prophylactic use in patients with a history of seizures or psychiatric disorder (including active or recent history of depression, generalized anxiety disorder, psychosis, schizophrenia, or other major psychiatric disorders)

Warnings/Precautions [U.S. Boxed Warning]: May cause neuropsychiatric adverse effects that can persist after mefloquine has been discontinued. During prophylactic use, if symptoms occur, discontinue therapy and substitute an alternative medication. Should not be prescribed for prophylaxis in patients with major psychiatric disorders. Use with caution in patients with a previous history of depression. Symptoms may develop early in the course of therapy. Due to the difficulty in identifying these symptoms in infants and children, monitor closely especially in pediatric patients. Psychiatric symptoms may include anxiety, paranoia, depression, hallucinations, and psychosis. Suicidal ideation and suicide have also been reported. Neurologic symptoms of dizziness or vertigo, tinnitus, and loss of balance may also occur and have been reported to be permanent in some cases. During prophylactic use, the occurrence of psychiatric symptoms such as acute anxiety, depression, restlessness, or confusion may be a prodrome to more serious neuropsychiatric adverse reactions. Use caution in activities requiring alertness and fine motor coordination (eg, driving, piloting planes, operating machinery) with neurologic symptoms.

Mefloquine may cause alterations in the ECG including sinus bradycardia, sinus arrhythmia, first-degree AV block, QT-interval prolongation, and abnormal T waves. Use caution or avoid concomitant use of agents known to cause QT interval prolongation (eg, halofantrine, quinine, quinidine). Use caution in patients with significant cardiac disease, hepatic impairment, or seizure disorder (WHO, 2010). If mefloquine is to be used for a prolonged period, periodic evaluations including liver function tests, evaluations for neuropsychiatric effects, and ophthalmic examinations should be performed. (Retinal abnormalities have not been observed with mefloquine in humans; however, abnormalities have been reported with long-term administration to rats.) Hypersensitivity reactions ranging from mild skin reactions to anaphylaxis have occurred. Agranulocytosis and aplastic anemia have been reported with use.

In cases of life-threatening, serious, or overwhelming malaria infections due to *Plasmodium falciparum*, patients should be treated with intravenous antimalarial drug. Mefloquine may be given orally to complete the course. In cases of acute *Plasmodium vivax* infection treated with mefloquine, patients should subsequently be treated with an 8-aminoquinoline derivative (eg, primaquine) to avoid relapse. Potentially significant drug-drug interactions may exist, requiring dose or frequency adjustment, additional monitoring, and/or selection of alternative therapy. Concurrent use with chloroquine may increase risk of seizures (WHO, 2010). Early vomiting leading to treatment failure in children has been reported in some studies; consider alternate therapy if a second dose is not tolerated.

Not recommended for the treatment of malaria acquired in Southeast Asia due to drug resistance (CDC, 2013b).

Adverse Reactions

Central nervous system: Chills, dizziness, fatigue, fever, headache

Dermatologic: Rash

Gastrointestinal: Abdominal pain, appetite decreased, diarrhea, nausea, vomiting

Neuromuscular & skeletal: Myalgia

Otic: Tinnitus

Rare but important or life-threatening: Abnormal dreams, abnormal T waves, ataxia, aggressive behavior, agitation, anxiety, arrhythmia, arthralgia, AV block, cardiac arrest (with concomitant use of propranolol), chest pain, conduction abnormalities (transient), confusion, depression, diaphoresis increased, dyspepsia, dyspnea, edema, encephalopathy, erythema, erythema multiforme, exanthema, flushing, forgetfulness, hallucinations, hearing impairment, hematocrit decreased, hyper-/hypotension, insomnia, irregular pulse, leukocytosis, leukopenia, liver function tests increased, loss of balance, malaise, mood changes, muscle cramps/weakness, palpitation, panic attacks, paranoia, paresthesia, pneumonitis (allergic etiology), psychosis, QT prolongation, restlessness, somnolence, Stevens-Johnson syndrome, suicidal ideation and behavior (causal relationship not established), tachycardia, thrombocytopenia, tremor, urticaria, vertigo, visual disturbances

Drug Interactions

Metabolism/Transport Effects Substrate of CYP3A4 (major); **Note:** Assignment of Major/Minor substrate status based on clinically relevant drug interaction potential; **Inhibits** CYP2D6 (weak), P-glycoprotein

Avoid Concomitant Use

Avoid concomitant use of Mefloquine with any of the following: Aminoquinolines (Antimalarial); Artemether; Bosutinib; Conivaptan; Fusidic Acid (Systemic); Halofantrine; Idelalisib; Lumefantrine; PAZOPanib; QuiNIDine; QuiNINE; Silodosin; Topotecan; VinCRIStine (Liposomal)

Increased Effect/Toxicity

Mefloquine may increase the levels/effects of: Afatinib; Aminoquinolines (Antimalarial); Antipsychotic Agents (Phenothiazines); ARIPiprazole; Bosutinib; Brentuximab Vedotin; Colchicine; Dabigatran Etexilate; Dapsone (Systemic); Dapsone (Topical); DOXOrubicin (Conventional); Edoxaban; Everolimus; Halofantrine; Highest Risk QTc-Prolonging Agents; Ledipasvir; Lumefantrine; Moderate Risk QTc-Prolonging Agents; Naloxegol; PAZOPanib; P-glycoprotein/ABCB1 Substrates; Prucalopride; QuiNINE; Rifaximin; Rivaroxaban; Silodosin; Topotecan; VinCRIStine (Liposomal)

The levels/effects of Mefloquine may be increased by: Aminoquinolines (Antimalarial); Amodiaquine; Aprepitant; Artemether; Conivaptan; CYP3A4 Inhibitors (Moderate); CYP3A4 Inhibitors (Strong); Dapsone (Systemic); Dasatinib; Fosaprepitant; Fusidic Acid (Systemic); Idelalisib; Ivacaftor; Luliconazole; Mifepristone; Netupitant; Palbociclib; QuiNIDine; QuiNINE; Simeprevir; Stiripentol

Decreased Effect

Mefloquine may decrease the levels/effects of: Anticonvulsants

The levels/effects of Mefloquine may be decreased by: Bosentan; CYP3A4 Inducers (Moderate); CYP3A4 Inducers (Strong); Dabrafenib; Deferasirox; Mitotane; Siltuximab; St Johns Wort; Tocilizumab

Food Interactions Food increases bioavailability by ~40%. Management: Take with food and at least 8 ounces of water. Maintain adequate nutrition and hydration, unless instructed to restrict fluid intake.

Storage/Stability Store at 20°C to 25°C (68°F to 77°F).

Mechanism of Action Mefloquine is a quinoline-methanol compound structurally similar to quinine; mefloquine's effectiveness in the treatment and prophylaxis of malaria is due to the destruction of the asexual blood forms of the malarial pathogens that affect humans, *Plasmodium falciparum, P. vivax*

Pharmacokinetics (Adult data unless noted)

Absorption: Well absorbed; interpatient variability with rate observed (WHO, 2010); more complete absorption when administered as a suspension compared with tablets

Distribution: Distributes into tissues, erythrocytes, blood, urine, CSF

V_d:

Children 4-10 years: Mean: ~18-19 L/kg (Price, 1999)

Adults: ~20 L/kg

Protein binding: ~98%

Metabolism: Extensively hepatic (primarily by CYP3A4) to 2,8-bis-trifluoromethyl-4-quinoline carboxylic acid (inactive) and other metabolites

Half-life:

Children 4-10 years: Mean range: 11.6-13.6 days (range: 6.5-33 days) (Price, 1999)

Adults: ~3 weeks (range: 2-4 weeks); may be decreased during infection (2 weeks) (WHO, 2010)

Time to peak serum concentration: Median: ~17 hours (range: 6-24 hours)

Elimination: Primarily bile and feces; urine (9% of total dose as unchanged drug, 4% of total dose as primary metabolite)

Dosing: Usual Note: Dose is expressed in terms of the salt, mefloquine hydrochloride.

Infants, Children, and Adolescents: **Note:** Due to limited clinical experience and dosage form availability, WHO Guidelines exclude patients weighing <5 kg from antimalarial dosage recommendations (WHO, 2010); however, other recommendations do not exclude these patients (CDC, 2009).

Malaria, treatment (independent of HIV-status), chloroquine-sensitive: Oral: Infants ≥6 months, Children, and Adolescents:

Manufacturer's labeling: 20-25 mg/kg/day in 2 divided doses, taken 6-8 hours apart (maximum total dose: 1250 mg)

Alternate dosing: CDC Guidelines (CDC, 2009; CDC, 2013): 15 mg/kg (maximum dose: 750 mg) followed in 6-12 hours with 10 mg/kg (maximum dose: 500 mg); if clinical improvement is not seen within 48-72 hours, an alternative therapy should be used for retreatment

Malaria, treatment; uncomplicated, chloroquine-resistant *P. vivax* (independent of HIV-status): Oral: Infants ≥6 months, Children, and Adolescents: 15 mg/kg (maximum dose: 750 mg) followed in 6-12 hours with 10 mg/kg/dose (maximum dose: 500 mg) with concomitant primaquine; not recommended unless other options not available (CDC, 2009; CDC, 2013)

Malaria; chemoprophylaxis: Oral: **Note:** Begin 2 weeks before arrival in endemic area, continue weekly during travel, and for 4 weeks after leaving endemic area. Prophylaxis may begin >2 weeks prior to travel to ensure tolerance (CDC, 2014).

Weight-based dosing: 5 mg/kg/dose once weekly; maximum dose: 250 mg

Fixed dosing:

≤9 kg: 5 mg/kg/dose once weekly

>9-19 kg: 62.5 mg (1/4 of 250 mg tablet) once weekly

>19-30 kg: 125 mg (1/2 of 250 mg tablet) once weekly

>30-45 kg: 187.5 mg (3/4 of a 250 mg tablet) once weekly

>45 kg: 250 mg once weekly

Adults:

Malaria treatment (mild to moderate infection): 1250 mg as a single dose or 750 mg followed 6-12 hours later by 500 mg (CDC, 2011). If clinical improvement is not seen within 48-72 hours, an alternative therapy should be used for retreatment.

Malaria prophylaxis: 250 mg once weekly on the same day each week, starting 1 week (CDC, 2012: ≥2 weeks) before arrival in endemic area, continuing weekly during travel, and for 4 weeks after leaving endemic area. **Note:** Prophylaxis may begin 2-3 weeks prior to travel to ensure tolerance in patients on multiple medications.

Dosing adjustment in renal impairment: No dosage adjustment necessary; only a small amount of mefloquine is renally eliminated; not removed by hemodialysis.

Dosing adjustment in hepatic impairment: There are no dosage adjustment provided in manufacturer's labeling; however, half-life may be prolonged and plasma levels may be higher in patients with hepatic impairment.

Administration Oral: Administer with food and an ample amount of water, at least 8 oz of water for adults. If vomiting occurs within 30 minutes after a dose, repeat dose. If vomiting occurs within 30-60 minutes after a dose, an additional half-dose should be administered. If vomiting recurs, monitor closely and consider alternative treatment. Administering mefloquine on a full stomach may minimize nausea and vomiting. For patients unable to swallow tablets or unable to tolerate its bitter taste, crush tablets and mix with a small amount of water, milk, applesauce, chocolate syrup, jelly, or food immediately before administration. Pulverized dose of mefloquine can be enclosed in a gelatin capsule to mask bitter taste. When used for malaria prophylaxis, dose should be taken once weekly on the same day each week.

Monitoring Parameters Sequential blood smears for percent parasitemia; periodic hepatic function tests, ophthalmologic exam

Additional Information Information on recommendations for travelers can be accessed by contacting the Centers for Disease Control and Prevention (CDC) Malaria Hotline (770-488-7788) or visit the CDC website: http://www.cdc.gov/travel/diseases.htm#malaria.

Dosage Forms Excipient information presented when available (limited, particularly for generics); consult specific product labeling.

Tablet, Oral, as hydrochloride:

Generic: 250 mg

- **Mefloquine Hydrochloride** *see* Mefloquine *on page 1342*
- **Mefoxin** *see* CefOXitin *on page 402*
- **Mega-C/A Plus** *see* Ascorbic Acid *on page 202*
- **Megace ES** *see* Megestrol *on page 1344*
- **Megace Oral** *see* Megestrol *on page 1344*
- **Megace OS (Can)** *see* Megestrol *on page 1344*
- **Megadophilus® [OTC]** *see Lactobacillus on page 1203*

Megestrol (me JES trole)

Medication Safety Issues

Sound-alike/look-alike issues:

Megace may be confused with Reglan

Megestrol may be confused with mesalamine

BEERS Criteria medication:

This drug may be potentially inappropriate for use in geriatric patients (Quality of evidence - moderate; Strength of recommendation - strong).

Related Information

Safe Handling of Hazardous Drugs *on page 2455*

Brand Names: US Megace ES; Megace Oral

Brand Names: Canada Megace OS; Megestrol

Therapeutic Category Antineoplastic Agent, Miscellaneous; Progestin

Generic Availability (US) Yes

Use Appetite stimulation and promotion of weight gain in cachexia (particularly in HIV patients) which is unresponsive to nutritional supplementation; palliative treatment of breast and endometrial carcinomas

Pregnancy Risk Factor D (tablet) / X (suspension)

Pregnancy Considerations Adverse events were demonstrated in animal reproduction studies. May cause fetal harm if administered to a pregnant woman. Use during pregnancy is contraindicated (suspension) and appropriate contraception is recommended in women who may become pregnant. In clinical studies, megestrol was shown to cause breakthrough vaginal bleeding in women.

Breast-Feeding Considerations Megestrol is excreted into breast milk. Information is available from five nursing women, ~8 weeks postpartum, who were administered megestrol 4 mg in combination with ethinyl estradiol 50 mcg daily for contraception. Maternal serum and milk samples were obtained over 5 days, beginning 10 days after therapy began. The highest concentrations of megestrol were found at the samples taken 3 hours after the maternal dose. Mean concentrations of megestrol were 6.5 ng/mL (maternal serum; range: 3.7 to 10.8 ng/mL), 4.6 ng/mL (foremilk; range: 1.1 to 12.7 ng/mL), and 5.6 ng/mL (hindmilk; range: 1.2 to 18.5 ng/mL) (Nilsson, 1977). Due to the potential for adverse reaction in the newborn, the manufacturer recommends discontinuing breast-feeding while receiving megestrol. In addition, in the United States, where formula is accessible, affordable, safe, and sustainable, and the risk of infant mortality due to diarrhea and respiratory infections is low, complete avoidance of breast-feeding by HIV-infected women is recommended to decrease potential transmission of HIV (DHHS [perinatal], 2012).

Contraindications Hypersensitivity to megestrol or any component of the formulation; known or suspected pregnancy (suspension)

Warnings/Precautions Hazardous agent - use appropriate precautions for handling and disposal (NIOSH 2014 [group 1]). May suppress hypothalamic-pituitary-adrenal (HPA) axis during chronic administration; consider the possibility of adrenal suppression in any patient receiving or being withdrawn from chronic therapy when signs/symptoms suggestive of hypoadrenalism are noted (during stress or in unstressed state). Laboratory evaluation and replacement/stress doses of rapid-acting glucocorticoid should be considered. Cushing syndrome has been reported with long-term use. New-onset diabetes and exacerbation of pre-existing diabetes have been reported with long-term use. Use with caution in patients with a history of thromboembolic disease. Avoid use in older adults due to minimal effect on weight, and an increased risk of thrombosis and possibly death (Beers Criteria). Vaginal bleeding or discharge may occur in females. The effects on HIV viral replications are unknown in patients with AIDS-related cachexia. Potentially significant drug-drug interactions may exist, requiring dose or frequency adjustment, additional monitoring, and/or selection of alternative therapy.

Megace ES suspension is not equivalent to other formulations on a mg per mg basis; Megace ES suspension 625 mg/5 mL is equivalent to megestrol acetate suspension 800 mg/20 mL.

Benzyl alcohol and derivatives: Some dosage forms may contain sodium benzoate/benzoic acid; benzoic acid (benzoate) is a metabolite of benzyl alcohol; large amounts of benzyl alcohol (≥99 mg/kg/day) have been associated with a potentially fatal toxicity ("gasping syndrome") in neonates; the "gasping syndrome" consists of metabolic acidosis, respiratory distress, gasping respirations, CNS dysfunction (including convulsions, intracranial hemorrhage), hypotension, and cardiovascular collapse (AAP, 1997; CDC, 1982); some data suggests that benzoate displaces bilirubin from protein binding sites (Ahlfors, 2001); avoid or use dosage forms containing benzyl alcohol derivative with caution in neonates. See manufacturer's labeling.

Adverse Reactions

Cardiovascular: Cardiac failure, cardiomyopathy, chest pain, edema, hypertension, palpitations, peripheral edema

Central nervous system: Abnormality in thinking, carpal tunnel syndrome, confusion, convulsions, depression, headache, hypoesthesia, insomnia, lethargy, malaise, mood change, neuropathy, pain (similar to placebo), paresthesia

Dermatologic: Alopecia, dermatological disease, diaphoresis, pruritus, skin rash, vesicobullous dermatitis

Endocrine & metabolic: Adrenocortical insufficiency, albuminuria, amenorrhea, Cushing's syndrome, decreased libido, diabetes mellitus, gynecomastia, hot flash, HPA-axis suppression, hypercalcemia, hyperglycemia, increased lactate dehydrogenase, weight gain (not attributed to edema or fluid retention)

Gastrointestinal: Abdominal pain, constipation, diarrhea (similar to placebo), dyspepsia, flatulence, nausea, oral moniliasis, sialorrhea, vomiting, xerostomia

Genitourinary: Breakthrough bleeding, impotence, urinary frequency, urinary incontinence, urinary tract infection

Hematologic & oncologic: Leukopenia, sarcoma, tumor flare

Hepatic: Hepatomegaly

Infection: Candidiasis, herpes virus infection, infection

Neuromuscular & skeletal: Weakness

Ophthalmic: Amblyopia

Respiratory: Cough, dyspnea, hyperventilation, pharyngitis, pneumonia, pulmonary disorder

Miscellaneous: Fever

Rare but important or life-threatening: Decreased glucose tolerance, thromboembolic phenomena (including deep vein thrombosis, pulmonary embolism, thrombophlebitis)

Drug Interactions

Metabolism/Transport Effects None known.

Avoid Concomitant Use

Avoid concomitant use of Megestrol with any of the following: Dofetilide; Indium 111 Capromab Pendetide; Ulipristal

Increased Effect/Toxicity

Megestrol may increase the levels/effects of: C1 inhibitors; Dofetilide

The levels/effects of Megestrol may be increased by: Herbs (Progestogenic Properties)

Decreased Effect

Megestrol may decrease the levels/effects of: Anticoagulants; Antidiabetic Agents; Choline C 11; Indium 111 Capromab Pendetide; Ulipristal

The levels/effects of Megestrol may be decreased by: Ulipristal

Storage/Stability

Suspension: Store at 15°C to 25°C (59°F to 77°F); protect from heat. Store/dispense in a tight container.

Tablet: Store at 20°C to 25°C (68°F to 77°F); protect from light.

Mechanism of Action A synthetic progestin with antiestrogenic properties which disrupt the estrogen receptor cycle. Megestrol interferes with the normal estrogen cycle and results in a lower LH titer. May also have a direct effect on the endometrium. Megestrol is an antineoplastic progestin thought to act through an antileutenizing effect mediated via the pituitary. May stimulate appetite by antagonizing the metabolic effects of catabolic cytokines.

Pharmacodynamics Onset of action:

Antineoplastic: 2 months of continuous therapy

Weight gain: 2-4 weeks

Pharmacokinetics (Adult data unless noted)

Absorption: Well absorbed

Metabolism: In the liver

Half-life: Adults: 10-120 hours

Time to peak serum concentration:

Tablet: 2-3 hours

Suspension: 3-5 hours

Elimination: In urine (57% to 78%) and feces (8% to 30%) within 10 days

Dosing: Usual Oral: **Note:** Megace® ES is not equivalent mg per mg with other megestrol formulations (625 mg Megace® ES is equivalent to 800 mg megestrol tablets or suspension).

Appetite stimulant in cachexia: Titrate dosage to response; decrease dose if weight gain is excessive:

Children: Limited data has been reported in cachectic children with cystic fibrosis, HIV, and solid tumors: Megestrol (tablets or 40 mg/mL suspension): 7.5-10 mg/kg/day in 1-4 divided doses; not to exceed 800 mg/day or 15 mg/kg/day

Adolescents and Adults:

Megestrol (tablets or 40 mg/mL suspension): 800 mg/day in 1-4 divided doses; titrate dose to response; doses between 400-800 mg/day have been clinically effective

Megace® ES: 625 mg once daily

Breast carcinoma: Female Adults: Megestrol (tablets or 40 mg/mL suspension): 40 mg 4 times/day

Endometrial carcinoma: Female Adults: Megestrol (tablets or 40 mg/mL suspension): 40-320 mg/day in divided doses; not to exceed 800 mg/day

Uterine bleeding: Female Adults: Megestrol (tablets or 40 mg/mL suspension): 40 mg 2-4 times/day

Administration Hazardous agent; use appropriate precautions for handling and disposal (NIOSH 2014 [group 1]).

Oral: Shake oral suspension well before administering; administer without regard to food

Monitoring Parameters Monitor for signs of thromboembolic phenomena and adrenal axis suppression

Appetite stimulation: Weight, caloric intake, basal cortisol level

Antineoplastic: Tumor response

Dosage Forms Excipient information presented when available (limited, particularly for generics); consult specific product labeling.

Suspension, Oral, as acetate:

Megace ES: 625 mg/5 mL (150 mL) [contains alcohol, usp, sodium benzoate; lemon-lime flavor]

Megace Oral: 40 mg/mL (240 mL) [lemon-lime flavor]

Generic: 40 mg/mL (10 mL, 240 mL, 480 mL); 400 mg/10 mL (10 mL)

Tablet, Oral, as acetate:

Generic: 20 mg, 40 mg

◆ **Megestrol Acetate** *see* Megestrol *on page 1344*

◆ **Mellaril** *see* Thioridazine *on page 2051*

Meloxicam (mel OKS i kam)

Medication Safety Issues

BEERS Criteria medication:

This drug may be potentially inappropriate for use in geriatric patients (Quality of evidence - moderate; Strength of recommendation - strong).

Brand Names: US Meloxicam Comfort Pac; Mobic

Brand Names: Canada Apo-Meloxicam; Auro-Meloxicam; Ava-Meloxicam; CO Meloxicam; Dom-Meloxicam; Mobicox; Mylan-Meloxicam; PHL-Meloxicam; PMS-Meloxicam; ratio-Meloxicam; Teva-Meloxicam

Therapeutic Category Analgesic, Non-narcotic; Anti-inflammatory Agent; Nonsteroidal Anti-inflammatory Drug (NSAID), Oral

Generic Availability (US) May be product dependent

Use Relief of signs and symptoms of pauciarticular or polyarticular juvenile idiopathic arthritis (JIA) (FDA approved in ages ≥2 years); relief of signs and symptoms of osteoarthritis and rheumatoid arthritis (FDA approved in adults)

Medication Guide Available Yes

Pregnancy Risk Factor C / D ≥30 weeks gestation

Pregnancy Considerations Adverse events were not observed in the initial animal reproduction studies; therefore, the manufacturer classifies meloxicam as pregnancy category C (category D: ≥30 weeks gestation). Meloxicam crosses the placenta. NSAID exposure during the first trimester is not strongly associated with congenital malformations; however, cardiovascular anomalies and cleft palate have been observed following NSAID exposure in some studies. The use of an NSAID close to conception may be associated with an increased risk of miscarriage. Nonteratogenic effects have been observed following NSAID administration during the third trimester including myocardial degenerative changes, prenatal constriction of the ductus arteriosus, fetal tricuspid regurgitation, failure of the ductus arteriosus to close postnatally; renal dysfunction or failure, oligohydramnios; gastrointestinal bleeding or perforation, increased risk of necrotizing enterocolitis; intracranial bleeding (including intraventricular hemorrhage), platelet dysfunction with resultant bleeding; pulmonary hypertension. Because they may cause premature closure of the ductus arteriosus, use of NSAIDs late in pregnancy should be avoided (use after 31 or 32 weeks gestation is not recommended by some clinicians). Product labeling for Mobic specifically notes that use at ≥30 weeks gestation should be avoided and therefore classifies meloxicam as pregnancy category D at this time. The chronic use of NSAIDs in women of reproductive age may be associated with infertility that is reversible upon discontinuation of the medication.

Breast-Feeding Considerations It is not known whether meloxicam is excreted in human milk. Breast-feeding is not recommended by the manufacturer.

Contraindications Hypersensitivity (eg, asthma, urticaria, allergic-type reactions) to meloxicam, aspirin, other NSAIDs, or any component of the formulation; perioperative pain in the setting of coronary artery bypass graft (CABG) surgery

Warnings/Precautions [U.S. Boxed Warning]: NSAIDs are associated with an increased risk of adverse cardiovascular thrombotic events, including MI and stroke. Risk may be increased with duration of use or pre-existing cardiovascular risk factors or disease. Carefully evaluate individual cardiovascular risk profiles prior to prescribing. May cause new-onset hypertension or worsening of existing hypertension. Use caution with fluid retention. Avoid use in heart failure (ACCF/AHA [Yancy, 2013]). Concurrent administration of ibuprofen, and potentially other nonselective NSAIDs, may interfere with aspirin's cardioprotective effect. **[U.S. Boxed Warning]: Use is contraindicated for treatment of perioperative pain in the setting of coronary artery bypass graft (CABG) surgery.** Risk of MI and stroke may be increased with use within the first 10-14 days following CABG surgery.

Platelet adhesion and aggregation may be decreased; may prolong bleeding time; patients with coagulation disorders or who are receiving anticoagulants should be monitored closely. Anemia may occur; patients on long-term NSAID therapy should be monitored for anemia. Rarely, NSAID use may cause severe blood dyscrasias (eg, agranulocytosis, aplastic anemia, thrombocytopenia).

NSAID use may compromise existing renal function; dose-dependent decreases in prostaglandin synthesis may result from NSAID use, reducing renal blood flow which may cause renal decompensation. NSAID use may increase the risk for hyperkalemia. Patients with impaired renal function, dehydration, heart failure, liver dysfunction, those taking diuretics, and ACE inhibitors, and the elderly are at greater risk of renal toxicity and hyperkalemia. Rehydrate patient before starting therapy; monitor renal function closely. Not recommended for use in patients with advanced renal disease. Long-term NSAID use may result in renal papillary necrosis.

[U.S. Boxed Warning]: NSAIDs may increase risk of gastrointestinal irritation, inflammation, ulceration, bleeding, and perforation. These events may occur at any time during therapy and without warning. Use caution with a history of GI disease (bleeding or ulcers), concurrent therapy with aspirin, anticoagulants and/or corticosteroids, smoking, use of alcohol, the elderly or debilitated patients. When used concomitantly with aspirin, a substantial increase in the risk of gastrointestinal complications (eg, ulcer) occurs; concomitant gastroprotective therapy (eg, proton pump inhibitors) is recommended (Bhatt, 2008).

Use the lowest effective dose for the shortest duration of time, consistent with individual patient goals, to reduce risk of cardiovascular or GI adverse events. Alternate therapies should be considered for patients at high risk.

NSAIDs may cause serious skin adverse events including exfoliative dermatitis, Stevens-Johnson syndrome (SJS) and toxic epidermal necrolysis (TEN); discontinue use at first sign of skin rash or hypersensitivity. Anaphylactoid reactions may occur, even without prior exposure; patients with "aspirin triad" (bronchial asthma, aspirin intolerance, rhinitis) may be at increased risk. Do not use in patients who experience bronchospasm, asthma, rhinitis, or urticaria with NSAID or aspirin therapy. Use caution in other forms of asthma.

Use with caution in patients with decreased hepatic function. Closely monitor patients with any abnormal LFT. Severe hepatic reactions (eg, fulminant hepatitis, liver failure) have occurred with NSAID use, rarely; discontinue if signs or symptoms of liver disease develop, or if systemic manifestations occur.

NSAIDS may cause drowsiness, dizziness, blurred vision and other neurologic effects which may impair physical or mental abilities; patients must be cautioned about performing tasks which require mental alertness (eg, operating machinery or driving). Discontinue use with blurred or diminished vision and perform ophthalmologic exam. Monitor vision with long-term therapy.

In the elderly, avoid chronic use (unless alternative agents ineffective and patient can receive concomitant gastroprotective agent); nonselective oral NSAID use is associated with an increased risk of GI bleeding and peptic ulcer disease in older adults in high risk category (eg, >75 years or age or receiving concomitant oral/parenteral corticosteroids, anticoagulants, or antiplatelet agents) (Beers Criteria).

Oral suspension formulation may contain sorbitol. Concomitant use with sodium polystyrene sulfonate (Kayexalate®) may cause intestinal necrosis (including fatal cases); combined use should be avoided. Withhold for at least 4-6 half-lives prior to surgical or dental procedures.

Benzyl alcohol and derivatives: Some dosage forms may contain sodium benzoate/benzoic acid; benzoic acid (benzoate) is a metabolite of benzyl alcohol; large amounts of benzyl alcohol (≥99 mg/kg/day) have been associated with a potentially fatal toxicity ("gasping syndrome") in neonates; the "gasping syndrome" consists of metabolic acidosis, respiratory distress, gasping respirations, CNS dysfunction (including convulsions, intracranial hemorrhage), hypotension, and cardiovascular collapse (AAP, 1997; CDC, 1982); some data suggests that benzoate displaces bilirubin from protein binding sites (Ahlfors, 2001); avoid or use dosage forms containing benzyl alcohol derivative with caution in neonates. See manufacturer's labeling.

Warnings: Additional Pediatric Considerations Pediatric patients ≥2 years may experience a higher frequency of some adverse effects than adults, including the following: Abdominal pain, diarrhea, fever, headache, and vomiting.

Adverse Reactions

Cardiovascular: Edema

Central nervous system: Dizziness, headache

Dermatologic: Pruritus, rash

Gastrointestinal: Abdominal pain, diarrhea, dyspepsia, flatulence, nausea

Genitourinary: Micturition, urinary tract infection

Respiratory: Cough, pharyngitis, upper respiratory infection

Miscellaneous: Falls, flu-like syndrome

Rare but important or life-threatening: Abnormal dreams, abnormal vision, agranulocytosis, albuminuria, allergic reaction, alopecia, anaphylactoid reactions, angina, angioedema, anxiety, appetite increased, arrhythmia, asthma, bilirubinemia, bronchospasm, bullous eruption, BUN increased, cardiac failure, colitis, confusion, conjunctivitis, creatinine increased, dehydration, depression, diaphoresis, duodenal perforation, duodenal ulcer, dyspnea, edema (facial), eructation, erythema multiforme, esophagitis, exfoliative dermatitis, fatigue, fever, gastric perforation, gastric ulcer, gastritis, gastroesophageal reflux, gastrointestinal hemorrhage, GGT increased, hematemesis, hematuria, hepatic failure, hepatitis, hot flushes, hyper-/hypotension, interstitial nephritis, intestinal perforation, jaundice, leukopenia, malaise, melena, MI, mood alterations, nervousness, palpitation, pancreatitis, paresthesia, photosensitivity reaction, pruritus, purpura, renal failure, seizure, shock, somnolence, Stevens-Johnson syndrome, syncope, tachycardia, taste perversion, thrombocytopenia, tinnitus, toxic epidermal necrolysis, transaminases increased, tremor, ulcerative stomatitis, urinary retention (acute), urticaria, vasculitis, vertigo, xerostomia, weight gain/loss

Drug Interactions

Metabolism/Transport Effects **Substrate** of CYP2C9 (major), CYP3A4 (minor); **Note:** Assignment of Major/Minor substrate status based on clinically relevant drug interaction potential

Avoid Concomitant Use

Avoid concomitant use of Meloxicam with any of the following: Calcium Polystyrene Sulfonate; Dexketoprofen; Floctafenine; Ketorolac (Nasal); Ketorolac (Systemic); Morniflumate; NSAID (COX-2 Inhibitor); Omacetaxine; Sodium Polystyrene Sulfonate; Urokinase

Increased Effect/Toxicity

Meloxicam may increase the levels/effects of: 5-ASA Derivatives; Agents with Antiplatelet Properties; Aliskiren; Aminoglycosides; Anticoagulants; Apixaban; Bisphosphonate Derivatives; Calcium Polystyrene Sulfonate; Collagenase (Systemic); CycloSPORINE (Systemic); Dabigatran Etexilate; Deferasirox; Deoxycholic Acid; Desmopressin; Digoxin; Drospirenone; Eplerenone; Haloperidol; Ibritumomab; Lithium; Methotrexate; Nonsteroidal Anti-Inflammatory Agents; NSAID (COX-2 Inhibitor); Obinutuzumab; Omacetaxine; PEMEtrexed; Porfimer; Potassium-Sparing Diuretics; PRALAtrexate; Quinolone Antibiotics; Rivaroxaban; Salicylates; Sodium Polystyrene Sulfonate; Tacrolimus (Systemic); Tenofovir; Thrombolytic Agents; Tositumomab and Iodine I 131 Tositumomab; Urokinase; Vancomycin; Verteporfin; Vitamin K Antagonists

The levels/effects of Meloxicam may be increased by: ACE Inhibitors; Angiotensin II Receptor Blockers; Antidepressants (Tricyclic, Tertiary Amine); Ceritinib; Corticosteroids (Systemic); CycloSPORINE (Systemic); CYP2C9 Inhibitors (Moderate); CYP2C9 Inhibitors (Strong); Dasatinib; Dexketoprofen; Diclofenac (Systemic); Floctafenine; Glucosamine; Herbs (Anticoagulant/Antiplatelet Properties); Ibrutinib; Ketorolac (Nasal); Ketorolac (Systemic); Limaprost; Mifepristone; Morniflumate; Multivitamins/Fluoride (with ADE); Multivitamins/Minerals (with ADEK, Folate, Iron); Multivitamins/Minerals (with AE, No Iron); Omega-3 Fatty Acids; Pentosan Polysulfate Sodium; Pentoxifylline; Probenecid; Prostacyclin Analogues; Selective Serotonin Reuptake Inhibitors; Serotonin/Norepinephrine Reuptake Inhibitors; Sodium Phosphates; Tipranavir; Treprostinil; Vitamin E; Voriconazole

Decreased Effect

Meloxicam may decrease the levels/effects of: ACE Inhibitors; Aliskiren; Angiotensin II Receptor Blockers; Beta-Blockers; Eplerenone; HydrALAZINE; Loop Diuretics; Potassium-Sparing Diuretics; Prostaglandins (Ophthalmic); Salicylates; Selective Serotonin Reuptake Inhibitors; Thiazide Diuretics

The levels/effects of Meloxicam may be decreased by: Bile Acid Sequestrants; CYP2C9 Inducers (Strong); Dabrafenib; Itraconazole; Salicylates

Storage/Stability Store at 20°C to 25°C (68°F to 77°F). Protect tablets from moisture.

Mechanism of Action Reversibly inhibits cyclooxygenase-1 and 2 (COX-1 and 2) enzymes, which results in decreased formation of prostaglandin precursors; has antipyretic, analgesic, and anti-inflammatory properties

Other proposed mechanisms not fully elucidated (and possibly contributing to the anti-inflammatory effect to varying degrees), include inhibiting chemotaxis, altering lymphocyte activity, inhibiting neutrophil aggregation/activation, and decreasing proinflammatory cytokine levels.

Pharmacokinetics (Adult data unless noted)

Distribution:

Children 2-6 years (n=7): Apparent V_d: 0.19 L/kg (Burgos-Vargas, 2004)

Children and Adolescents 7-16 years (n=11): Apparent V_d: 0.13 L/kg (Burgos-Vargas, 2004)

Adults: Vd_{ss}: 10 L

Protein binding: ~99.4% bound, primarily albumin; **Note:** Free fraction was higher in adult patients with renal failure who were receiving chronic dialysis.

Metabolism: Extensive in the liver via CYP2C9 and CYP3A4 (minor); significant biliary and or enteral secretion occurs

Bioavailability: 89%; suspension is bioequivalent to tablets

Half-life elimination:

Children 2-6 years (n=7): 13.4 hours (Burgos-Vargas, 2004)

Children and Adolescents 7-16 years (n=11): 12.7 hours (Burgos-Vargas, 2004)

Adults: 15-20 hours

Time to peak serum concentration:

Children and Adolescents 2-16 years (n=18): Suspension: Initial: 1-3 hours; secondary: 6-12 hours (Burgos-Vargas, 2004)

Adults: Initial: 4-5 hours; secondary: 12-14 hours

Elimination: Urine and feces (as inactive metabolites); <1% excreted unchanged in urine

Clearance:

Children 2-6 years (n=7): 0.17 mL/minute/kg (Burgos-Vargas, 2004)

Children and Adolescents 7-16 years (n=11): 0.12 mL/minute/kg (Burgos-Vargas, 2004)

Adults: 7-9 mL/minute

Dosing: Usual Note: To reduce the risk of adverse cardiovascular and GI effects, use the lowest effective dose for the shortest period of time; adjust dose to specific patient's clinical needs.

Children ≥2 years and Adolescents: **Juvenile idiopathic arthritis (JIA):** Oral: 0.125 mg/kg once daily; maximum daily dose: 7.5 mg/**day**; higher doses (up to 0.375 mg/kg/**day**) have not demonstrated additional benefit in clinical trials.

Adults: **Osteoarthritis, rheumatoid arthritis:** Initial: 7.5 mg once daily; some patients may receive additional benefit from an increased dose of 15 mg once daily; maximum daily dose: 15 mg/**day**

Dosing adjustment in renal impairment:

Mild to moderate impairment: Children ≥2 years, Adolescents and Adults: No dosage adjustments are recommended.

Significant impairment (CrCl <20 mL/minute): Children ≥2 years, Adolescents, and Adults: Use is not recommended (has not been studied).

Hemodialysis: Not dialyzable; additional doses are not required after dialysis: Adults: Maximum daily dose: 7.5 mg/**day**

Dosing adjustment in hepatic impairment: Children ≥2 years, Adolescents, and Adults:

Mild to moderate impairment (Child-Pugh class A or B): No dosage adjustments are recommended.

Severe impairment: There are no dosage adjustments provided in the manufacturer's labeling (has not been studied); use with caution; meloxicam is significantly metabolized in the liver.

Administration May be taken with or without meals; administer with food or milk to minimize gastrointestinal irritation. Oral suspension: Shake gently prior to use.

Monitoring Parameters Periodic CBC, liver enzymes, serum BUN and creatinine, signs and symptoms of GI bleeding

Dosage Forms Considerations Meloxicam Comfort Pa[c] is a kit containing meloxicam oral tablets 15 mg, an[d] Duraflex topical gel.

Dosage Forms Excipient information presented whe[n] available (limited, particularly for generics); consult specifi[c] product labeling.

Kit, Combination:

Meloxicam Comfort Pac: 15 mg [contains methylparaben, trolamine (triethanolamine)]

Suspension, Oral:

Mobic: 7.5 mg/5 mL (100 mL) [contains saccharin sodium, sodium benzoate; raspberry flavor]

Generic: 7.5 mg/5 mL (100 mL)

Tablet, Oral:

Mobic: 7.5 mg, 15 mg

Generic: 7.5 mg, 15 mg

◆ **Meloxicam Comfort Pac** *see* Meloxicam *on page 134*

Melphalan (MEL fa lan)

Medication Safety Issues

Sound-alike/look-alike issues:

Melphalan may be confused with Mephyton, Myleran

Alkeran may be confused with Alferon, Leukeran, Myleran

High alert medication:

This medication is in a class the Institute for Safe Medication Practices (ISMP) includes among its list of drug classes which have a heightened risk of causing significant patient harm when used in error.

Related Information

Management of Drug Extravasations *on page 2298*

Prevention of Chemotherapy-Induced Nausea and Vomiting in Children *on page 2368*

Safe Handling of Hazardous Drugs *on page 2455*

Brand Names: US Alkeran

Brand Names: Canada Alkeran

Therapeutic Category Antineoplastic Agent, Alkylating Agent; Antineoplastic Agent, Alkylating Agent (Nitrogen Mustard)

Generic Availability (US) May be product dependent

Use

Oral: Palliative treatment of multiple myeloma and nonresectable epithelial ovarian carcinoma (FDA approved in adults)

Parenteral: Palliative treatment of multiple myeloma for whom oral therapy is not appropriate (FDA approved in adults); has also been used as part of a conditioning regimen for autologous hematopoietic stem cell transplantation

Pregnancy Risk Factor D

Pregnancy Considerations Animal studies have demonstrated embryotoxicity and teratogenicity. Therapy may suppress ovarian function leading to amenorrhea. There are no adequate and well-controlled studies in pregnant women. May cause fetal harm if administered during pregnancy. Women of childbearing potential should be advised to avoid pregnancy while on melphalan therapy.

Breast-Feeding Considerations According to the manufacturer, melphalan should not be administered if breast-feeding.

Contraindications Hypersensitivity to melphalan or any component of the formulation; patients whose disease was resistant to prior melphalan therapy

Warnings/Precautions Hazardous agent; use appropriate precautions for handling and disposal (NIOSH 2014 [group 1]).

[U.S. Boxed Warning]: Bone marrow suppression is common; may be severe and result in infection or bleeding; has been demonstrated more with the IV

formulation (compared to oral); myelosuppression is dose-related. Monitor blood counts; may require treatment delay or dose modification for thrombocytopenia or neutropenia. Use with caution in patients with prior bone marrow suppression, impaired renal function (consider dose reduction), or who have received prior (or concurrent) chemotherapy or irradiation. Myelotoxicity is generally reversible, although irreversible bone marrow failure has been reported. In patients who are candidates for autologous transplantation, avoid melphalan-containing regimens prior to transplant (due to the effects on stem cell reserve). Signs of infection, such as fever and WBC rise, may not occur; lethargy and confusion may be more prominent signs of infection.

[U.S. Boxed Warning]: Hypersensitivity reactions (including anaphylaxis) have occurred in ~2% of patients receiving IV melphalan, usually after multiple treatment cycles. Discontinue infusion and treat symptomatically. Hypersensitivity may also occur (rarely) with oral melphalan. Do not readminister (oral or IV) in patients who experience hypersensitivity to melphalan.

Gastrointestinal toxicities, including nausea, vomiting, diarrhea and mucositis, are common. When administering high-dose melphalan in autologous transplantation, cryotherapy is recommended to prevent oral mucositis (Lalla, 2014). Melphalan is associated with a moderate emetic potential (depending on dose and/or administration route); antiemetics may be recommended to prevent nausea and vomiting (Dupuis, 2011). Abnormal liver function tests may occur; hepatitis and jaundice have also been reported; hepatic sinusoidal obstruction syndrome (SOS; formerly called veno-occlusive disease) has been reported with IV melphalan. Pulmonary fibrosis (some fatal) and interstitial pneumonitis have been observed with treatment. Dosage reduction is recommended with IV melphalan in patients with renal impairment; reduced initial doses may also be recommended with oral melphalan. Closely monitor patients with azotemia.

[U.S. Boxed Warning]: Produces chromosomal changes and is leukemogenic and potentially mutagenic; secondary malignancies (including acute myeloid leukemia, myeloproliferative disease, and carcinoma) have been reported reported (some patients were receiving combination chemotherapy or radiation therapy); the risk is increased with increased treatment duration and cumulative doses. Suppresses ovarian function and produces amenorrhea; may also cause testicular suppression.

Extravasation may cause local tissue damage; administration by slow injection into a fast running IV solution into an injection port or via a central line is recommended; do not administer directly into a peripheral vein. Some dosage forms may contain propylene glycol; large amounts are potentially toxic and have been associated hyperosmolality, lactic acidosis, seizures and respiratory depression; use caution (AAP, 1997; Zar, 2007). **[U.S. Boxed Warning]: Should be administered under the supervision of an experienced cancer chemotherapy physician.** Avoid vaccination with live vaccines during treatment if immunocompromised. Toxicity may be increased in elderly; start with lowest recommended adult doses. Potentially significant drug-drug interactions may exist, requiring dose or frequency adjustment, additional monitoring, and/or selection of alternative therapy.

Warnings: Additional Pediatric Considerations Some dosage forms may contain propylene glycol; in neonates large amounts of propylene glycol delivered orally, intravenously (eg, >3,000 mg/day), or topically have been associated with potentially fatal toxicities which can include metabolic acidosis, seizures, renal failure, and CNS depression; toxicities have also been reported in children and adults including hyperosmolality, lactic acidosis, seizures, and respiratory depression; use caution (AAP, 1997; Shehab, 2009).

Adverse Reactions

Gastrointestinal: Nausea, diarrhea, oral ulceration, vomiting

Hematologic: Anemia, leukopenia (nadir: 14-21 days; recovery: 28-35 days), myelosuppression, thrombocytopenia (nadir: 14-21 days; recovery: 28-35 days)

Miscellaneous: Hypersensitivity (includes bronchospasm, dyspnea, edema, hypotension, pruritus, rash, tachycardia, urticaria); secondary malignancy (cumulative dose and duration dependent, includes acute myeloid leukemia, myeloproliferative syndrome, carcinoma)

Rare by important or life-threatening: Agranulocytosis, allergic reactions, alopecia, amenorrhea, anaphylaxis (rare), bleeding (with high-dose therapy),, bone marrow failure (irreversible), BUN increased, cardiac arrest, cardiotoxicity (angina, arrhythmia, hypertension, MI; with high-dose therapy), encephalopathy, hemolytic anemia, hemorrhagic cystitis, hepatic sinusoidal obstruction syndrome (SOS; veno-occlusive disease; high-dose IV melphalan), hepatitis, infection, injection site reactions (ulceration, necrosis), interstitial pneumonitis, jaundice, mucositis (with high-dose therapy), ovarian suppression, paralytic ileus (with high-dose therapy), pruritus, pulmonary fibrosis, radiation myelopathy, rash (maculopapular), renal toxicity (with high-dose therapy), seizure (with high-dose therapy), sepsis, SIADH, skin hypersensitivity, sterility, stomatitis, testicular suppression, tingling sensation, transaminases increased, vasculitis, warmth sensation

Drug Interactions

Metabolism/Transport Effects None known.

Avoid Concomitant Use

Avoid concomitant use of Melphalan with any of the following: BCG; BCG (Intravesical); CloZAPine; Dipyrone; Nalidixic Acid; Natalizumab; Pimecrolimus; Tacrolimus (Topical); Tofacitinib; Vaccines (Live)

Increased Effect/Toxicity

Melphalan may increase the levels/effects of: Carmustine; CloZAPine; CycloSPORINE (Systemic); Leflunomide; Natalizumab; Tofacitinib; Vaccines (Live)

The levels/effects of Melphalan may be increased by: Denosumab; Dipyrone; Nalidixic Acid; Pimecrolimus; Roflumilast; Tacrolimus (Topical); Trastuzumab

Decreased Effect

Melphalan may decrease the levels/effects of: BCG; BCG (Intravesical); Coccidioides immitis Skin Test; Sipuleucel-T; Vaccines (Inactivated); Vaccines (Live)

The levels/effects of Melphalan may be decreased by: Echinacea

Food Interactions Food interferes with oral absorption. Management: Administer on an empty stomach.

Storage/Stability

Tablet: Store in refrigerator at 2°C to 8°C (36°F to 46°F). Protect from light.

Injection: Store intact vials at 20°C to 25°C (68°F to 77°F). Protect from light. The manufacturer recommends administration be completed within 60 minutes of reconstitution; **immediately** dilute dose in NS. Do not refrigerate solution; precipitation occurs.

Mechanism of Action Alkylating agent which is a derivative of mechlorethamine that inhibits DNA and RNA synthesis via formation of carbonium ions; cross-links strands of DNA; acts on both resting and rapidly dividing tumor cells.

Pharmacokinetics (Adult data unless noted)

Absorption: Oral: Variable and incomplete

Distribution: V_{dss}: 0.5 L/kg; Low penetration into CSF

Protein binding: 53% to 92%; primarily to albumin, 40% to 60% and α_1-acid glycoprotein (20%)

Metabolism: Hepatic; chemical hydrolysis to mono- or dihydroxymelphalan

Bioavailability: Oral: Variable; ranges from 56% to 93% depending on the presence of food (exposure is reduced with a high-fat meal)

Half-life, terminal: IV: 75 minutes; Oral: 1 to 2 hours

Time to peak serum concentration: Oral: Within 2 hours

Elimination: Oral: Feces (20% to 50%); urine (~10% as unchanged drug)

Dosing: Usual Refer to individual protocols; details concerning dosing in combination regimens should also be consulted; adjust dose based on patient response and weekly blood counts.

Pediatric: **Hematopoietic stem cell transplantation, conditioning regimen for autologous HSCT:** Infants, Children, and Adolescents:

Cantete, 2009, Oberlin 2006: IV: 140 mg/m^2 2 days prior to transplantation (combined with busulfan)

Pritchard, 2005: IV: 180 mg/m^2 (with pre- and posthydration) 12 to 30 hours prior to transplantation

Berthold, 2005: IV: 45 mg/m^2/day for 4 days starting 8 days prior to transplantation (combined with busulfan or etoposide and carboplatin)

Adult:

Multiple myeloma (palliative treatment): Note: Response is gradual; may require repeated courses to realize benefit:

Oral:

6 mg (3 tablets) once daily for 2 to 3 weeks initially, followed by up to 4 weeks rest (melphalan-free period); then a maintenance dose of 2 mg once daily as hematologic recovery begins **or**

0.15 mg/kg/day for 7 days with a 2- to 6-week rest (melphalan-free period); followed by a maintenance dose of ≤0.05 mg/kg/day as hematologic recovery begins **or**

0.25 mg/kg/day for 4 days (or 0.2 mg/kg/day for 5 days); repeat at 4- to 6-week intervals as ANC and platelet counts return to normal **or**

10 mg once daily for 7 to 10 days, institute 2 mg once daily maintenance dose after WBC >4000 cells/mm^3 and platelets >100,000 cells/mm^3 (~4 to 8 weeks); titrate maintenance dose to hematologic response

IV: 16 mg/m^2/dose every 2 weeks for 4 doses, then repeat at 4-week intervals after adequate hematologic recovery

Ovarian carcinoma: Oral: 0.2 mg/kg once daily for 5 days, repeat every 4 to 5 weeks

Dosing adjustment in renal impairment: Adults:

Manufacturer's labeling:

Oral: Moderate to severe renal impairment: Consider a reduced dose initially

IV: BUN ≥30 mg/dL: Reduce dose by 50%

The following guidelines have been used by some clinicians:

Aronoff, 2007 (based on a 6 mg once daily dose):

CrCl >50 mL/minute: No dosage adjustment required

CrCl 10 to 50 mL/minute: Administer 75% of dose

CrCl <10 mL/minute: Administer 50% of dose

Hemodialysis: Administer dose after hemodialysis.

Continuous ambulatory peritoneal dialysis (CAPD): Administer 50% of dose.

Continuous renal replacement therapy (CRRT): Administer 75% of dose.

Kintzel, 1995:

Oral: Adjust dose in the presence of hematologic toxicity

IV:

CrCl 46 to 60 mL/minute: Administer 85% of normal dose.

CrCl 31 to 45 mL/minute: Administer 75% of normal dose.

CrCl <30 mL/minute: Administer 70% of normal dose.

Dosing adjustment in hepatic impairment: Adults There are no dosage adjustments provided in the manufacturer's labeling; however, dosage adjustment does not appear to be necessary (King, 2001).

Dosing adjustment for toxicity:

Oral:

WBC <3000/mm^3: Withhold treatment until recovery

Platelets <100,000/mm^3: Withhold treatment until recovery

Parenteral: IV: Adjust dose based on nadir blood cell counts

Preparation for Administration Hazardous agent; use appropriate precautions for handling and disposal (NIOSH 2014 [group 1]).

Parenteral: IV: Stability is limited; must be prepared fresh. **The time between reconstitution/dilution and administration of parenteral melphalan must be kept to a minimum (manufacturer recommends <60 minutes) because reconstituted and diluted solutions are unstable.** Reconstitute 50 mg vial for injection initially with 10 mL of supplied diluent to a concentration of 5 mg/mL; shake immediately and vigorously to dissolve. **Immediately** dilute dose in NS to a final concentration ≤0.45 mg/mL (manufacturer recommended concentration). Do not refrigerate solution; precipitation occurs. The manufacturer recommends administration within 60 minutes of reconstitution.

Administration Hazardous agent; use appropriate precautions for handling and disposal (NIOSH 2014 [group 1]).

Oral: Administer on an empty stomach (Schmidt 2002)

Parenteral: IV: **Note:** Stability is limited; must be prepared fresh; the time between reconstitution/dilution and administration of parenteral melphalan must be kept to a minimum (manufacturer recommends completing infusion within <60 minutes) because reconstituted and diluted solutions are unstable.

Administer by IV infusion typically over 15 to 20 minutes and some centers suggest at a rate not to exceed 10 mg/minute; complete administration of IV dose should occur within 60 minutes of reconstitution.

Extravasation may cause local tissue damage; administration by slow injection into a fast running IV solution into an injection port or via a central line is recommended; do not administer by direct injection into a peripheral vein.

Vesicant/Extravasation Risk May be an irritant

Monitoring Parameters CBC with differential and platelet count (at the start of therapy and prior to each subsequent dose), serum electrolytes; serum uric acid; monitor infusion site for redness and irritation

Test Interactions False-positive Coombs' test [direct]

Dosage Forms Excipient information presented when available (limited, particularly for generics); consult specific product labeling.

Solution Reconstituted, Intravenous:

Alkeran: 50 mg (1 ea) [contains alcohol, usp, propylene glycol]

Generic: 50 mg (1 ea)

Tablet, Oral:

Alkeran: 2 mg

◆ **Menactra** *see* Meningococcal (Groups A / C / Y and W-135) Diphtheria Conjugate Vaccine *on page 1352*

◆ **MenACWY** *see* Meningococcal (Groups A / C / Y and W-135) Diphtheria Conjugate Vaccine *on page 1352*

◆ **MenACWY-D (Menactra)** *see* Meningococcal (Groups A / C / Y and W-135) Diphtheria Conjugate Vaccine *on page 1352*

◆ **MenACWY-CRM (Menveo)** *see* Meningococcal (Groups A / C / Y and W-135) Diphtheria Conjugate Vaccine *on page 1352*

◆ **MenB** *see* Meningococcal Group B Vaccine *on page 1351*

◆ **MenB-4C** *see* Meningococcal Group B Vaccine *on page 1351*

◆ **MenB-FHbp** *see* Meningococcal Group B Vaccine *on page 1351*

◆ **Menhibrix** *see* Meningococcal Polysaccharide (Groups C and Y) and *Haemophilus* b Tetanus Toxoid Conjugate Vaccine *on page 1356*

◆ **Meningococcal Conjugate Vaccine** *see* Meningococcal (Groups A / C / Y and W-135) Diphtheria Conjugate Vaccine *on page 1352*

Meningococcal Group B Vaccine

me NIN joe kok al groop bee vak SEEN)

Related Information

Centers for Disease Control and Prevention (CDC) and Other Links *on page 2424*

Immunization Administration Recommendations *on page 2411*

Immunization Schedules *on page 2416*

Brand Names: US Bexsero; Trumenba

Brand Names: Canada Bexsero

Therapeutic Category Vaccine; Vaccine, Inactivated Bacteria

Generic Availability (US) No

Use Active immunization against invasive meningococcal disease caused by N. meningitidis serogroup B (FDA approved in ages 10 to 25 years).

Pregnancy Risk Factor B

Pregnancy Considerations Adverse events were not observed in animal reproduction studies. The manufacturer notes that vaccination should not be withheld in pregnant women at clear risk for infection. Inactivated vaccines have not been shown to cause increased risks to the fetus (NCIRD/ACIP 2011).

Health care providers are encouraged to enroll women exposed to Bexsero during pregnancy (1-877-683-4732).

Breast-Feeding Considerations It is not known if this vaccine is excreted into breast milk. The manufacturer recommends that caution be used if administered to nursing women. Inactivated vaccines do not affect the safety of breast-feeding for the mother or the infant (NCIRD/ACIP 2011).

Contraindications Severe hypersensitivity to the meningococcal group B vaccine or any component of the formulation

Warnings/Precautions Immediate treatment (including epinephrine 1:1000) for anaphylactoid and/or hypersensitivity reactions should be available during vaccine use (NCIRD/ACIP 2011). Syncope has been reported with use of injectable vaccines and may result in serious secondary injury (e.g. skull fracture, cerebral hemorrhage); typically reported in adolescents and young adults and within 15 minutes after vaccination. Procedures should be in place to avoid injuries from falling and to restore cerebral perfusion if syncope occurs (NCIRD/ACIP 2011).

The decision to administer or delay vaccination because of current or recent febrile illness depends on the severity of symptoms and the etiology of the disease. Consider deferring administration in patients with moderate or severe acute illness (with or without fever); vaccination should not be delayed for patients with mild acute illness (with or without fever) (NCIRD/ACIP 2011). Use with caution in patients with bleeding disorders (including thrombocytopenia) and patients on anticoagulant therapy; bleeding/hematoma may occur from IM administration; if the patient receives antihemophilia or other similar therapy, IM injection can be scheduled shortly after such therapy is administered (NCIRD/ACIP 2011). Use with caution in severely immunocompromised patients (eg, patients receiving chemo/radiation therapy or other immunosuppressive therapy [including high-dose corticosteroids]); may have a reduced response to vaccination. In general, household and close contacts of persons with altered immunocompetence may receive all age appropriate vaccines (IDSA [Rubin 2014]; NCIRD/ACIP 2011); inactivated vaccines should be administered ≥2 weeks prior to planned immunosuppression when feasible (IDSA [Rubin 2014]). Vaccination may not result in effective immunity in all patients. Response depends on multiple factors (eg, type of vaccine, age of patient) and may be improved by administering the vaccine at the recommended dose, route, and interval. Vaccines may not be effective if administered during periods of altered immune competence (NCIRD/ACIP 2011). Not to be used to treat meningococcal infections or to provide immunity against N. meningitidis serogroups A, C, W-135, or Y. In addition, vaccine does not provide protection against all circulating meningococcal group B strains. Antipyretics have not been shown to prevent febrile seizures; antipyretics may be used to treat fever or discomfort following vaccination (NCIRD/ACIP 2011). One study reported that routine prophylactic administration of acetaminophen to prevent fever prior to vaccination decreased the immune response of some vaccines; the clinical significance of this reduction in immune response has not been established (Prymula 2009).

In order to maximize vaccination rates, the ACIP recommends simultaneous administration (ie, >1 vaccine on the same day at different anatomic sites) of all age-appropriate vaccines (live or inactivated) for which a person is eligible at a single clinic visit, unless contraindications exist. The ACIP prefers each dose of a specific vaccine in a series come from the same manufacturer when possible (NCIRD/ACIP 2011). Product may contain kanamycin. The packaging (needle cover of prefilled syringe) may contain latex. Some dosage forms may contain polysorbate 80 (also known as Tweens). Hypersensitivity reactions, usually a delayed reaction, have been reported following exposure to pharmaceutical products containing polysorbate 80 in certain individuals (Isaksson 2002; Lucente 2000; Shelley 1995). Thrombocytopenia, ascites, pulmonary deterioration, and renal and hepatic failure have been reported in premature neonates after receiving parenteral products containing polysorbate 80 (Alade 1986; CDC 1984). See manufacturer's labeling.

Warnings: Additional Pediatric Considerations Clinical studies of infants <12 months of age using a lower dosage than indicated for older children resulted in fever in most patients (90%).

Adverse Reactions All serious adverse reactions must be reported to the U.S. Department of Health and Human Services (DHHS) Vaccine Adverse Event Reporting System (VAERS) 1-800-822-7967 or online at https://vaers.hhs.gov/esub/index. In Canada, adverse reactions may be reported to local provincial/territorial health agencies or to the Vaccine Safety Section at Public Health Agency of Canada (1-866-844-0018). Frequencies reported may include concomitant administration with routine pediatric vaccines or other vaccines. Adverse reactions listed below are reflective of both the U.S. and Canadian product information.

Central nervous system: Chills (children and adolescents 11 to 17 years), drowsiness (infants and children ≤10 years), excessive crying (infants and children ≤10 years), fatigue (children ≥10 years, adolescents, and adults), headache (more common in 10 to 25 years), irritability (infants and children ≤10 years), malaise (children and adolescents 11 to 17 years and adults)

Dermatologic: Skin rash (children 2 to 10 years), urticaria (infants and children <2 years)

Gastrointestinal: Change in appetite (infants and children ≤10 years), diarrhea (infants, children, and adolescents ≤17 years), nausea (children ≥10 years, adolescents, and adults), vomiting (infants, children, and adolescents ≤17 years)

Local: Erythema at injection site, induration at injection site, pain at injection site (children ≥2 years, adolescents, and adults), swelling at injection site (infants, children, and adolescents ≤17 years), tenderness at injection site (more common in children 2 to 10)

Neuromuscular & skeletal: Arthralgia (children and adolescents 2 to 17 years and adults), myalgia (children and adolescents 11 to 17 years and adults)

Respiratory: Nasopharyngitis (children ≥10 years, adolescents, and adults), upper respiratory tract infection (infants ≤7 months; mostly considered unrelated to vaccination)

Miscellaneous: Fever (more common in children 2 to 10 years, ≥40°C [104°F])

Rare but important or life-threatening: Febrile seizures, Kawasaki syndrome (rare), seizure

Drug Interactions

Metabolism/Transport Effects None known.

Avoid Concomitant Use There are no known interactions where it is recommended to avoid concomitant use.

Increased Effect/Toxicity There are no known significant interactions involving an increase in effect.

Decreased Effect

The levels/effects of Meningococcal Group B Vaccine may be decreased by: Belimumab; Fingolimod; Immunosuppressants

Storage/Stability

Bexsero: Store between 2°C to 8°C (36°F to 46°F). Do not freeze; discard if frozen. Protect from light.

Trumenba: Store between 2°C to 8°C (36°F to 46°F). Do not freeze; discard if frozen. Store syringes in the refrigerator horizontally (laying flat on the shelf) to minimize the redispersion time.

Mechanism of Action

Bexsero: Induces immunity against meningococcal disease caused by serogroup B *Neisseria meningitidis* (MenB) via the formation of antibodies directed toward the recombinant protein antigens combined together with outer membrane vesicles (OMV) from a group B strain.

Trumenba: Protection against invasive meningococcal disease is conferred mainly by complement-mediated antibody-dependent killing of *N. meningitidis*.

Efficacy:

Bexsero: Composite hSBA titer response one month after the second dose: 63% to 88%

Trumenba: 84% of adolescents had a ≥4-fold rise in hSBA titer and composite response after the third dose.

Dosing: Usual

Pediatric: **Meningococcal disease prevention:** Children ≥10 years and Adolescents:

Bexsero: IM: 0.5 mL per dose for a total of two doses administered at least 1 month apart

Trumenba: IM: 0.5 mL per dose for a total of 3 doses administered as follows: Initial dose followed by a second and third dose at 2 months and 6 months, respectively

Adult: **Meningococcal disease prevention:** Adults ≤ 2 years:

Bexsero: IM: 0.5 mL per dose for a total of two doses administered at least 1 month apart

Trumenba: IM: 0.5 mL per dose for a total of 3 doses administered as follows: Initial dose followed by a second and third dose at 2 months and 6 months, respectively

Dosing adjustment in renal impairment: There are no dosage adjustments provided in the manufacturer's labeling.

Dosing adjustment in hepatic impairment: There are no dosage adjustments provided in the manufacturer's labeling.

Administration Shake vigorously to ensure that a homogenous white suspension is obtained. Do not use the vaccine if it cannot be resuspended. Administer by IM injection into upper deltoid region; **not for intradermal, subcutaneous, or IV administration**. To prevent syncope related injuries, adolescents and adults should be vaccinated while seated or lying down (NCIRD/ACIP 2011). US law requires that the date of administration, the vaccine manufacturer, lot number of vaccine, and the administering person's name, title, and address be entered into the patient's permanent medical record.

For patients at risk of hemorrhage, the vaccine should be administered intramuscularly if, in the opinion of a physician familiar with the patient's bleeding risk, the vaccine can be administered by this route with reasonable safety. If the patient receives antihemophilia or other similar therapy, intramuscular vaccination can be scheduled shortly after such therapy is administered. A fine needle (23-gauge or smaller) can be used for the vaccination and firm pressure applied to the site (without rubbing) for at least 2 minutes. The patient or family should be instructed concerning the risk of hematoma from the injection. Patients on anticoagulant therapy should be considered to have the same bleeding risks and treated as those with clotting factor disorders (NCIRD/ACIP 2011).

Monitoring Parameters Observe for syncope for 15 minutes following administration (NCIRD/ACIP 2011). If seizure-like activity associated with syncope occurs, maintain patient in supine or Trendelenburg position to reestablish adequate cerebral perfusion.

Product Availability Bexsero: Approved January 2015; anticipated availability is currently unknown. Consult prescribing information for additional information.

Dosage Forms Excipient information presented when available (limited, particularly for generics); consult specific product labeling.

Suspension Prefilled Syringe, Intramuscular:

Bexsero: (0.5 mL)

Trumenba: (0.5 mL) [contains polysorbate 80]

Meningococcal (Groups A / C / Y and W-135) Diphtheria Conjugate Vaccine

(me NIN joe kok al groops aye, see, why & dubl yoo won thur tee fyve dif THEER ee a KON joo gate vak SEEN)

Medication Safety Issues

Administration issue:

Menactra (MCV4) should be administered by intramuscular (IM) injection only. Inadvertent subcutaneous (SubQ) administration has been reported; possibly due to confusion of this product with Menomune (MPSV4), also a meningococcal polysaccharide vaccine, which is administered by the SubQ route.

Related Information

Centers for Disease Control and Prevention (CDC) and Other Links *on page 2424*

Immunization Administration Recommendations *on page 2411*

Immunization Schedules *on page 2416*

Brand Names: US Menactra; Menveo

Brand Names: Canada Menactra; Menveo

Therapeutic Category Vaccine; Vaccine, Inactivated Bacteria

Generic Availability (US) No

Use Provide active immunization against invasive meningococcal disease caused by *N. meningitidis* serogroups A, C, Y, and W-135 (Menactra: FDA approved 9 months to 55 years; Menveo: FDA approved in ages 2 months to 55 years).

The Advisory Committee on Immunization Practices (ACIP) (CDC/ACIP [Cohn 2013]; CDC/ACIP [MacNeil 2014]) recommends routine vaccination of:

- Children and adolescents aged 11 to 18 years of age
- Persons ≥2 months of age who are at increased risk of meningococcal disease
- Persons (in all recommended age groups) at increased risk who are part of outbreaks caused by vaccine preventable serogroups

Those at increased risk of meningococcal disease include:

- Persons ≥2 months of age with medical conditions such as anatomic or functional asplenia (including sickle cell disease) or persistent complement component deficiencies (eg, C3, C5-C9, properdin, factor H, or factor D)
- Persons ≥2 months of age that travel to or reside in countries where meningococcal disease is hyperendemic or epidemic, especially if contact with the local population will be prolonged
- Unvaccinated or incompletely vaccinated first year college students living in residence halls
- Military recruits
- Microbiologists with occupational exposure

Medication Guide Available Yes

Pregnancy Risk Factor B/C (manufacturer dependent)

Pregnancy Considerations Animal reproduction studies have not been conducted with Menactra. Limited information is available following inadvertent use of Menactra during pregnancy (Zheteyeva 2013). Patients should contact the Sanofi Pasteur Inc vaccine registry at 1-800-822-2463 if they are pregnant or become aware they were pregnant at the time of Menactra vaccination.

Adverse events were not observed in animal reproduction studies conducted with Menveo. Limited information is available following inadvertent use of Menveo during pregnancy. Patients should contact the Novartis Vaccines and Diagnostics Inc. pregnancy registry at 1-877-311-8972 if they are pregnant or become aware they were pregnant at the time of Menveo vaccination.

Inactivated bacterial vaccines have not been shown to cause increased risks to the fetus (NCIRD/ACIP 2011). Pregnancy should not preclude vaccination if indicated (CDC/ACIP [Cohn 2013]).

Breast-Feeding Considerations It is not known if this vaccine is found in breast milk. The manufacturer recommends that caution be used if administered to a nursing woman. Inactivated vaccines do not affect the safety of breast-feeding for the mother or the infant. Breast-feeding infants should be vaccinated according to the recommended schedules (NCIRD/ACIP 2011).

Contraindications Hypersensitivity to other meningococcal-containing vaccines or any component of the formulation including diphtheria toxoid or CRM_{197} (a diphtheria toxin carrier protein)

Warnings/Precautions Use with caution in patients with a history of bleeding disorders (including thrombocytopenia) and/or patients on anticoagulant therapy; bleeding/hematoma may occur from IM administration; if the patient receives antihemophilia or other similar therapy, IM injection can be scheduled shortly after such therapy is administered (NCIRD/ACIP 2011). The decision to administer or delay vaccination because of current or recent febrile illness depends on the severity of symptoms and the etiology of the disease. Consider deferring administration in patients with moderate or severe acute illness (with or without fever); vaccination should not be delayed for patients with mild acute illness (with or without fever) (NCIRD/ACIP 2011). Apnea has been reported following IM vaccine administration in premature infants; consider risk versus benefit in infants born prematurely. In general, preterm infants should be vaccinated at the same chronological age as full-term infants (NCIRD/ACIP 2011).

Vaccination may not result in effective immunity in all patients. Response depends upon multiple factors (eg, type of vaccine, age of patient) and may be improved by administering the vaccine at the recommended dose, route, and interval. Vaccines may not be effective if administered during periods of altered immune competence (NCIRD/ACIP 2011). Not to be used to treat meningococcal infections or to provide immunity against *N. meningitidis* serogroup B or diphtheria. Syncope has been reported with use of injectable vaccines and may result in serious secondary injury (eg, skull fracture, cerebral hemorrhage); typically reported in adolescents and young adults and within 15 minutes after vaccination. Procedures should be in place to avoid injuries from falling and to restore cerebral perfusion if syncope occurs. (NCIRD/ACIP 2011). Use with caution in severely immunocompromised patients (eg, patients receiving chemo/radiation therapy or other immunosuppressive therapy [including high-dose corticosteroids]); may have a reduced response to vaccination. In general, household and close contacts of persons with altered immunocompetence may receive all age appropriate vaccines (NCIRD/ACIP 2011); inactivated vaccines should be administered ≥2 weeks prior to planned immunosuppression when feasible (Rubin 2014). Risk of developing Guillain-Barré syndrome (GBS) may be increased following vaccination in persons previously diagnosed with GBS. The risk of developing GBS was evaluated in a study of healthcare claims of persons 11-18 years of age (n= ~9,600,000; 15% were vaccinated with Menactra); 72 cases of GBS were confirmed and none received the vaccine within 42 days prior to symptoms; 129 reported cases of GBS could not be confirmed or excluded. Data not currently available to assess possible risk of GBS following use of Menveo. Individuals with a previous history of GBS should only receive Menactra after an assessment of risks and benefits.

Immediate treatment (including epinephrine 1:1,000) for anaphylactoid and/or hypersensitivity reactions should be available during vaccine use (NCIRD/ACIP 2011). In order to maximize vaccination rates, the ACIP recommends simultaneous administration (ie, >1 vaccine on the same day at different anatomic sites) of all age-appropriate vaccines (live or inactivated) for which a person is eligible at a single clinic visit, unless contraindications exist. The ACIP prefers each dose of a specific vaccine in a series come from the same manufacturer when possible (NCIRD/ACIP 2011). Use of this vaccine for specific medical and/or other indications (eg, immunocompromising conditions, hepatic or kidney disease, diabetes) is also addressed in the ACIP Recommended Immunization Schedule (CDC/ACIP [Kim 2015]). Specific recommendations for use of this vaccine in immunocompromised patients with asplenia, cancer, HIV infection, cerebrospinal fluid leaks, cochlear implants, hematopoietic stem cell transplant (prior to or after), sickle cell disease, solid organ transplant (prior to or after), or those receiving immunosuppressive therapy for chronic conditions are available from the IDSA (Rubin 2014). Antipyretics have not been shown to prevent febrile seizures; antipyretics may be used to treat fever or discomfort following vaccination (NCIRD/ACIP 2011). One study reported that routine prophylactic administration of acetaminophen to prevent fever prior to vaccination decreased the immune response of some vaccines; the clinical significance of this reduction in immune response has not been established (Prymula 2009).

Warnings: Additional Pediatric Considerations Children may have higher incidence of local adverse effects (erythema, swelling, tenderness).

Adverse Reactions All serious adverse reactions must be reported to the U.S. Department of Health and Human Services (DHHS) Vaccine Adverse Event Reporting System (VAERS) 1-800-822-7967 or online at https://vaers.hhs.gov/esub/index. In Canada, adverse reactions may be reported to local provincial/territorial health agencies or to the Vaccine Safety Section at Public Health Agency of Canada (1-866-844-0018).

May vary by product and age group:

Central nervous system: Chills, drowsiness, excessive crying, fatigue, headache, irritability, malaise

Dermatologic: Skin rash

Gastrointestinal: Anorexia, change in appetite, diarrhea, nausea, vomiting

Local: Erythema at injection site, induration at injection site, pain at injection site, swelling at injection site, tenderness at injection site

Neuromuscular & skeletal: Arthralgia, myalgia

Miscellaneous: Fever

Rare but important or life-threatening: Acute disseminated encephalomyelitis, anaphylactoid reaction, anaphylaxis, apnea (premature infants), appendicitis, auditory impairment, Bell's palsy, blepharoptosis, convulsions (including tonic), Cushing's syndrome, dehydration, depression, equilibrium disturbance, exfoliation of skin, facial paresis, falling, febrile seizures, gastroenteritis, Guillain-Barre syndrome, hypersensitivity, hypotension, increased serum ALT, inflammation at injection site, injection site cellulitis, Kawasaki Syndrome, ostealgia, pelvic inflammatory disease, pneumonia, pruritus at injection site, seizure, simple partial seizures, staphylococcal infection, suicidal tendencies, syncope (including vasovagal), transverse myelitis, varicella, vertebral disc disease, vestibular disturbance

Drug Interactions

Metabolism/Transport Effects None known.

Avoid Concomitant Use There are no known interactions where it is recommended to avoid concomitant use.

Increased Effect/Toxicity There are no known significant interactions involving an increase in effect.

Decreased Effect

The levels/effects of Meningococcal (Groups A / C / Y and W-135) Diphtheria Conjugate Vaccine may be decreased by: Belimumab; Fingolimod; Immunosuppressants

Storage/Stability

Menactra: Store between 2°C to 8°C (35°F to 46°F); do not freeze. Discard product exposed to freezing.

Menveo: Prior to reconstitution, store between 2°C to 8°C (36°F to 46°F); do not freeze. Protect from light. Discard product exposed to freezing. Use immediately after reconstitution but may be stored at ≤25°C (77°F) for up to 8 hours.

Mechanism of Action Induces immunity against meningococcal disease via the formation of bactericidal antibodies directed toward the polysaccharide capsular components of *Neisseria meningitidis* serogroups A, C, Y and W-135.

Dosing: Usual Note: Use of the abbreviation, MenACWY refers to either meningococcal quadrivalent polysaccharide vaccine. MenACWY-CRM refers specifically to Menveo; MenACWY-D refers specifically to Menactra.

Pediatric:

Primary immunization:

Manufacturer's labeling: General dosing:

Menactra:

Infants ≥9 months and Children <2 years: IM: 0.5 mL per dose for a total of 2 doses given 3 months apart

Children ≥2 years and Adolescents: IM: 0.5 mL per dose as a single dose

Menveo:

Infants 2 to <7 months: IM: 0.5 mL per dose for a total of 4 doses administered as follows: 2, 4, 6, and 12 months of age

Infants and Children 7 to 23 months: IM: 0.5 mL per dose for a total of 2 doses. The second dose should be given during the second year of life and at least 3 months after the first dose.

Children 2 to <6 years: IM: 0.5 mL per dose as a single dose; for children at continued high risk of meningococcal disease, may consider an additional dose given 2 months after the first dose

Children ≥6 years and Adolescents: IM: 0.5 mL per dose as a single dose

CDC (ACIP) recommendations (CDC/ACIP [Cohn 2013]; CDC/ACIP [MacNeil 2014]; CDC/ACIP [Striker 2015]):

*Primary vaccination for patients **NOT** at increased risk for meningococcal disease:*

Infants and Children <11 years: Not routinely recommended; see dosing for persons at increased risk

Children 11 to 12 years: IM: 0.5 mL per dose as a single dose. Children not at increased risk for meningococcal disease who may have been previously vaccinated with Hib-MenCY-TT (MenHibrix) or MenACWY (Menactra or Menveo) prior to their 10th birthday; should receive the routinely recommended dose of MenACWY at 11 to 12 years; **Note:** Patients who are HIV positive should receive 2 doses 2 months apart.

Adolescents: IM: 0.5 mL per dose as a single dose if not previously vaccinated; **Note:** Patients 11 to 18 years who are HIV positive should receive 2 doses 2 months apart.

Primary vaccination for patients at increased risk for meningococcal disease:

Infants ≥2 months and Children <2 years:

Anatomic or functional asplenia (including sickle cell disease): Dosing based on age at initial dose:

Infants 8 weeks to 6 months: MenACWY-CRM (Menveo): IM: 0.5 mL per dose for a total of 4 doses administered at 2, 4, 6, and 12 months of age

Children 7 to 23 months (incomplete vaccination): MenACWY-CRM (Menveo): IM: 0.5 mL per dose for a total of 2 doses given at least 3 months apart; the second dose should be given at age ≥12 months and at least 12 weeks after the first dose.

Persistent complement component deficiency: Dosing based on age at first dose:

Infants 8 weeks to 6 months: MenACWY-CRM (Menveo): IM: 0.5 mL per dose for a total of 4 doses administered at 2, 4, 6, and 12 months of age

Infants and Children 7 to 23 months:

MenACWY-CRM (Menveo): Infants and Children 7 to 23 months: IM: 0.5 mL per dose for a total of 2 doses; the second dose should be given at age ≥12 months and at least 12 weeks after the first dose

MenACWY-D (Menactra): Infants and Children 9 to 23 months: IM: 0.5 mL per dose for a total of 2 doses; the second dose should be given at least 3 months after the first dose. May be given as early as 8 weeks apart if needed prior to travel.

Community outbreak (due to vaccine serogroup): Infants ≥2 months to Children 23 months: Initiate or complete an age appropriate series of MenACWY-CRM (Menveo) or MenACWY-D (Menactra); see Primary immunization on previous page for dosing.

Travel to or residence in countries with hyperendemic or epidemic meningococcal disease: Infants 2 months to Children 23 months: Initiate or complete an age appropriate series of MenACWY-CRM (Menveo) or MenACWY-D (Menactra); see Primary immunization on previous page for dosing.

Children ≥2 years and Adolescents, not previously vaccinated and who have persistent complement deficiencies, functional or anatomic asplenia, or who have HIV infection plus another indication for vaccination: IM: 0.5 mL per dose for a total of 2 doses given 8 to12 weeks apart. If using MenACWY-D (Menactra), administer ≥4 weeks after completion of all PCV doses.

Children ≥2 years and Adolescents not previously vaccinated and who are either: First year college students ≤21 years of age living in residential housing, traveling to or residents of areas where meningococcal disease is endemic/hyperendemic, at risk during a community outbreak, or microbiologists routinely exposed to *Neisseria meningitidis*: IM: 0.5 mL as a single dose. If using MenACWY-D (Menactra), administer ≥4 weeks after completion of all PCV doses. College students ≤21 years should have documentation of a vaccination not more than 5 years before enrollment (preferably a dose on their 16th birthday). **Note:** Patients who are HIV positive should receive 2 doses 2 months apart.

Booster dose: (CDC/ACIP [Cohn 2013]):

*Booster vaccination for patients **NOT** at increased risk for meningococcal disease:* IM: 0.5 mL as a single dose. If primary vaccination was at 11 to 12 years, the booster dose should be given at age 16. If the primary vaccination was given at 13 to 15 years, the booster dose should be given at age 16 to 18. Minimum interval between MenACWY (Menveo or Menactra) doses is 8 weeks. A booster dose is not needed if the primary dose was given after the 16th birthday unless the person becomes at increased risk for meningococcal disease.

Booster vaccination for patients at increased risk for meningococcal disease:

If first dose received at 2 months to 6 years of age: Repeat dose 3 years after primary vaccination and every 5 years thereafter if the person remains at increased risk.

If first dose received at ≥7 years of age: Repeat dose 5 years after primary vaccination and every 5 years thereafter if the person remains at increased risk.

Adult:

Primary immunization:

Manufacturer's labeling: Adults ≤55 years: Menactra, Menveo: IM: 0.5 mL as a single dose

CDC (ACIP) recommendations (CDC/ACIP [Cohn 2013]):

*Primary vaccination for persons **NOT** at increased risk for meningococcal disease:*

19 to 21 years: Not routinely recommended; may receive one 0.5 mL dose as a catch-up vaccination if no dose was received after the 16th birthday. **Note:** Patients who are HIV positive should receive 2 doses 2 months apart.

≥22 years: Not routinely recommended; see dosing for persons at increased risk

Primary vaccination for persons at increased risk for meningococcal disease:

Adults ≤55 years not previously vaccinated and who have persistent complement deficiencies, functional or anatomic asplenia, or who have HIV infection plus another indication for vaccination: IM: 0.5 mL per dose for a total of two doses given 8 to 12 weeks apart. If using MenACWY-D (Menactra), administer ≥4 weeks after completion of all PCV doses

Adults ≤55 years not previously vaccinated and who are either: First year college students ≤21 years of age living in residential housing, traveling to or residents of areas where meningococcal disease is endemic/hyperendemic, at risk during a community outbreak, or microbiologists routinely exposed to *Neisseria meningitidis*: IM: 0.5 mL as a single dose. If using MenACWY-D (Menactra), administer ≥4 weeks after completion of all PCV doses. College students ≤21 years should have documentation of a vaccination not more than 5 years before enrollment (preferably a dose on their 16th birthday). **Note:** Patients who are HIV positive should receive 2 doses 2 months apart.

Adults ≥56 years: Meningococcal polysaccharide vaccine (MPSV4, Menomune) is preferred for meningococcal vaccine naïve persons in this age group who require a single dose. If multiple doses are anticipated, see booster dosing for persons at increased risk.

Booster dose:

*Booster vaccination for persons **NOT** at increased risk for meningococcal disease:* Adults ≤21 years: IM: 0.5 mL as a single dose if the first dose was given prior to the 16th birthday. A booster dose is not needed if the primary dose was given after the 16th birthday unless the person becomes at increased risk for meningococcal disease.

Booster vaccination for persons at increased risk for meningococcal disease:

Adults ≤55 years: Repeat dose every 5 years if the person remains at increased risk

Adults ≥56 years: Persons previously vaccinated with MenACWY (Menveo or Menactra) and who require revaccination or for whom multiple doses are anticipated, MenACWY (Menveo or Menactra) is preferred. Otherwise, meningococcal polysaccharide vaccine (MPSV4, Menomune) is preferred for meningococcal vaccine naïve persons in this age group who require a single dose.

Dosing adjustment in renal impairment: There are no dosage adjustments provided in manufacturer's labeling.

Dosing adjustment in hepatic impairment: There are no dosage adjustments provided in manufacturer's labeling.

Preparation for Administration

IM:

Menveo: Prior to use, remove liquid contents from vial of MenCYW-135 and inject into vial containing MenA powder. Invert and shake well until dissolved. The resulting solution should be clear and colorless. A small amount of liquid will remain in the vial after withdrawing the 0.5 mL dose. Use immediately after reconstitution but may be stored at ≤25°C (77°F) for up to 8 hours. Do not mix with other vaccines in the same syringe.

Menactra: Use as supplied; no reconstitution is necessary.

Administration IM: Administer by IM injection into midlateral aspect of the thigh in infants and small children; administer in the deltoid area to older children and adults; not for intradermal, subcutaneous, or IV administration; must administer dose within 8 hours after reconstitution. To prevent syncope-related injuries, adolescents and adults should be vaccinated while seated or lying down (NCIRD/ACIP 2011). US law requires that the date of administration, the vaccine manufacturer, lot number of vaccine, and the administering person's name, title, and address be entered into the patient's permanent medical record.

Monitoring Parameters Observe for syncope for 15 minutes following administration (NCIRD/ACIP 2011). If seizure-like activity associated with syncope occurs, maintain patient in supine or Trendelenburg position to reestablish adequate cerebral perfusion.

Additional Information Two meningococcal (Groups A/C/Y and W-135) diphtheria conjugate vaccines are available. Menveo uses oligosaccharides of the *N. meningitidis* serogroups linked to CRM_{197} (a nontoxic diphtheria toxin carrier protein) and Menactra uses polysaccharides from the serogroups linked to diphtheria toxoid.

Dosage Forms Excipient information presented when available (limited, particularly for generics); consult specific product labeling.

Injection, solution [preservative free]:

Menactra: 4 mcg each of polysaccharide antigen groups A, C, Y, and W-135 [bound to diphtheria toxoid 48 mcg] per 0.5 mL [MCV4 or MenACWY-D]

Menveo: MenA oligosaccharide 10 mcg, MenC oligosaccharide 5 mcg, MenY oligosaccharide 5 mcg, and MenW-135 oligosaccharide 5 mcg [bound to CRM_{197} protein 32.7-64.1 mcg] per 0.5 mL (0.5 mL) [MenACWY-CRM; supplied in two vials, one containing MenA powder and one containing MenCYW-135 liquid]

Meningococcal Polysaccharide (Groups C and Y) and *Haemophilus* b Tetanus Toxoid Conjugate Vaccine

(me NIN joe kok al pol i SAK a ride groops see & why & he MOF i lus bee TET a nus TOKS oyd KON joo gate vak SEEN)

Medication Safety Issues

Sound-alike/look-alike issues:

MenHibrix (Meningococcal Polysaccharide (Groups C and Y) and *Haemophilus* b Tetanus Toxoid Conjugate Vaccine) may be confused with Hiberix (*Haemophilus* b Conjugate Vaccine)

Related Information

Centers for Disease Control and Prevention (CDC) and Other Links *on page 2424*

Immunization Administration Recommendations *on page 2411*

Immunization Schedules *on page 2416*

Brand Names: US Menhibrix

Therapeutic Category Vaccine; Vaccine, Inactivated Bacteria

Generic Availability (US) No

Use Provide active immunization against *Neisseria meningitidis* serogroups C and Y and *Haemophilus influenzae* type b (FDA approved in ages 6 weeks to 18 months)

The Advisory Committee on Immunization Practices (ACIP) (CDC/ACIP [Cohn 2013)] recommends vaccination only for infants and children 2 to 18 months of age who are at increased risk for meningococcal disease, including those with:

- Persistent complement pathway deficiencies
- Anatomic or functional asplenia, including sickle cell disease
- Living in communities with serogroups C and Y meningococcal disease outbreaks

The ACIP does not recommend routine vaccination for infants not at increased risk for meningococcal disease. In addition, infants traveling to certain areas (eg, meningitis belt of sub-Saharan Africa) will require a meningococcal vaccine with serogroups A and W135; vaccination with Hib-MenCY-TT is not adequate (CDC/ACIP [Cohn 2013]).

Pregnancy Risk Factor C

Pregnancy Considerations Animal reproduction studies have not been conducted.

Contraindications Severe allergic reaction to any meningococcal, *H. influenza* type B, or tetanus toxoid-containing vaccine, or any component of the vaccine

Warnings/Precautions Use with caution in patients with history of bleeding disorders (including thrombocytopenia) and/or patients on anticoagulant therapy; bleeding/hematoma may occur from IM administration; if the patient receives antihemophilia or other similar therapy, IM injection can be scheduled shortly after such therapy is administered (NCIRD/ACIP 2011). The decision to administer or delay vaccination because of current or recent febrile illness depends on the severity of symptoms and the etiology of the disease. Immunization should be delayed during the course of an acute febrile illness. Vaccination may not result in effective immunity in all patients. Response depends upon multiple factors (eg, type of vaccine, age of patient) and is improved by administering the vaccine at the recommended dose, route, and interval. Vaccines may not be effective if administered during periods of altered immune competence (NCIRD/ACIP 2011). Has not been evaluated for use in immunosuppressed children. In general, severely immunocompromised patients (eg, patients receiving chemo/radiation therapy or other immunosuppressive therapy [including high-dose corticosteroids]) may have a reduced response to vaccination; household and close contacts of persons with altered immunocompetence may receive all age appropriate vaccines (IDSA [Rubin 2014]; NCIRD/ACIP 2011). In general, inactivated vaccines should be administered ≥2 weeks prior to planned immunosuppression when feasible (IDSA [Rubin 2014]). Syncope has been reported with use of injectable vaccines and may result in serious secondary injury (eg, skull fracture, cerebral hemorrhage); typically reported in adolescents and young adults and within 15 minutes after vaccination. Procedures should be in place to avoid injuries from falling and to restore cerebral perfusion if syncope occurs (NCIRD/ACIP 2011). Use with caution in patients with history of GBS; carefully consider risks and benefits to vaccination in patients known to have experienced GBS within 6 weeks following previous influenza vaccination. Immediate treatment (including epinephrine 1:1000) for anaphylactoid and/or hypersensitivity reactions should be available during vaccine use (NCIRD/ACIP 2011). In order to maximize vaccination rates, the ACIP recommends simultaneous administration (ie, >1 vaccine on the same day at different anatomic sites) of all age-appropriate vaccines (live or inactivated) for which a person is eligible at a single clinic visit, unless contraindications exist. The use of combination vaccines is generally preferred over separate injections, taking into consideration provider assessment, patient preference, and adverse events. When using combination vaccines, the minimum age for administration is the oldest minimum age for any individual component; the minimum interval between dosing is the greatest minimum interval between any individual components. The ACIP prefers each dose of a specific vaccine in a series come from the same manufacturer when possible (NCIRD/ACIP 2011). Not a substitute for routine tetanus immunization. Apnea has occurred following intramuscular vaccine administration in premature infants; consider clinical status implications. In general, preterm infants should be vaccinated at the same chronological age as full-term infants (NCIRD/ACIP 2011). Antipyretics have not been shown to prevent febrile seizures; antipyretics may be used to treat fever or discomfort following vaccination (NCIRD/ACIP 2011). One study reported that routine prophylactic administration of acetaminophen to prevent fever prior to vaccination decreased the immune response of some vaccines; the clinical significance of this reduction in immune response has not been established (Prymula, 2009).

Adverse Reactions All serious adverse reactions must be reported to the U.S. Department of Health and Human Services (DHHS) Vaccine Adverse Event Reporting System (VAERS) 1-800-822-7967 or online at https://vaers.hhs.gov/esub/index. In Canada, adverse reactions may be reported to local provincial/territorial health agencies or to the Vaccine Safety Section at Public Health Agency of Canada (1-866-844-0018).

Central nervous system: Fever ≥100.4°F (38°C), drowsiness, irritability
Gastrointestinal: Appetite decreased
Local: Injection site reactions: Pain, redness, swelling
Rare but important or life-threatening: Allergic reactions, anaphylactic/anaphylactoid reactions, angioedema, apnea, hypotonic-hyporesponsive episode, injection site induration, rash, somnolence, seizures (with or without fever), swelling of vaccinated limb (extensive), syncope, urticaria, vasovagal response

Drug Interactions

Metabolism/Transport Effects None known.

Avoid Concomitant Use There are no known interactions where it is recommended to avoid concomitant use.

Increased Effect/Toxicity There are no known significant interactions involving an increase in effect.

Decreased Effect

The levels/effects of Meningococcal Polysaccharide (Groups C and Y) and Haemophilus b Tetanus Toxoid Conjugate Vaccine may be decreased by: Belimumab; Fingolimod; Immunosuppressants

Storage/Stability Prior to use, store lyophilized vaccine under refrigeration at 2°C to 8°C (36°F to 46°F). Protect from light. Diluent may be stored under refrigeration or at room temperature; do not freeze; discard if frozen.

Mechanism of Action Provides active immunity against meningococcal disease via the formation of bactericidal antibodies directed toward the polysaccharide capsular components of *Neisseria meningitidis* serogroups C and Y; stimulates production of anticapsular antibodies and to *Haemophilus influenzae* type b

Pharmacodynamics Onset of action: Antibody response to the components of the vaccine occurs in ≥95% of infants following the third dose and ≥98% following the fourth dose

Dosing: Usual

Pediatric: **Primary Immunization:** Infants and Children 6 weeks to 18 months: IM: 0.5 mL per dose for a total of 4 doses administered as follows: 2, 4, 6, and 12 to 15 months of age; first dose may be administered as early as 6 weeks of age and last dose in series as late as 18 months of age

Note: If an infant at increased risk is behind on Hib vaccine doses, Hib-MenCY-TT may be used to catch up using the current Hib schedule. If the first dose of Hib-MenCY-TT is given ≥12 months of age, 2 doses should be given 8 weeks apart. If infants have/will receive a different Hib vaccine, a 2-dose series of a quadrivalent meningococcal vaccine is recommended (Menactra for ages 9 to 23 months; Menactra or Menveo for ages >23 months) (CDC/ACIP [Cohn 2013]).

Dosing adjustment in renal impairment: There are no dosage adjustments provided in the manufacturer's labeling.

Dosing adjustment in hepatic impairment: There are no dosage adjustments provided in the manufacturer's labeling.

Preparation for Administration IM: Reconstitute with 0.6 mL of provided diluent only; shake well. Final solution should be clear and colorless. Use immediately after reconstitution.

Administration IM: Administer immediately after reconstitution; in infants administer to the anterolateral aspect of the thigh; in children ≥12 months to ≤18 months, the deltoid muscle of the arm may be used. Do not administer IV or SubQ. Do not coadminister with other Hib-containing vaccines (CDC/ACIP [Cohn 2013]). US law requires that the date of administration; the vaccine manufacturer; lot number of vaccine; and the administering person's name, title, and address be entered into the patient's permanent medical record.

For patients at risk of hemorrhage following intramuscular injection, the vaccine should be administered intramuscularly if, in the opinion of the physician familiar with the patient's bleeding risk, the vaccine can be administered by this route with reasonable safety. If the patient receives antihemophilia or other similar therapy, intramuscular vaccination can be scheduled shortly after such therapy is administered. A fine needle (23 gauge or smaller) can be used for the vaccination and firm pressure applied to the site (without rubbing) for at least 2 minutes. The patient should be instructed concerning the risk of hematoma from the injection. Patients on anticoagulant therapy should be considered to have the same bleeding risks and treated as those with clotting factor disorders (NCIRD/ACIP 2011).

Monitoring Parameters Observe for syncope for 15 minutes following administration (NCIRD/ACIP 2011). If seizure-like activity associated with syncope occurs, maintain patient in supine or Trendelenburg position to reestablish adequate cerebral perfusion.

Test Interactions *H. influenzae* type b from the vaccine may be detected in the urine; urine antigen tests may not be diagnostic for *H. influenzae* type b infection within 1-2 weeks of vaccination

Dosage Forms Excipient information presented when available (limited, particularly for generics); consult specific product labeling.

Solution Reconstituted, Intramuscular [preservative free]:
Menhibrix: 5 mcg each of polysaccharide antigen groups C and Y, and 2.5 mcg Haemophilus b capsular polysaccharide per 0.5 mL dose (1 ea) [contains tetanus toxoid]

◆ **Meningococcal Polysaccharide Vaccine** *see* Meningococcal Polysaccharide Vaccine (Groups A / C / Y and W-135) *on page 1357*

Meningococcal Polysaccharide Vaccine (Groups A / C / Y and W-135)

(me NIN joe kok al pol i SAK a ride vak SEEN groops aye, see, why & dubl yoo won thur tee fyve)

Medication Safety Issues

Administration issue:

Menomune (MPSV4) should be administered by subcutaneous (SubQ) injection. Menactra (MCV4), also a meningococcal polysaccharide vaccine, is to be administered by intramuscular (IM) injection only.

Related Information

Centers for Disease Control and Prevention (CDC) and Other Links *on page 2424*
Immunization Administration Recommendations *on page 2411*
Immunization Schedules *on page 2416*

Brand Names: US Menomune-A/C/Y/W-135

Brand Names: Canada Menomune-A/C/Y/W-135

Therapeutic Category Vaccine; Vaccine, Inactivated Bacteria

Generic Availability (US) No

Use Active immunization to meningococcal serogroups contained in the vaccine (FDA approved in ages ≥2 years and adults).

The Advisory Committee on Immunization Practices (ACIP) recommends routine vaccination for persons at increased risk for meningococcal disease. Meningococcal quadrivalent conjugate vaccine (MenACWY) is preferred; meningococcal polysaccharide vaccine (MPSV4) is preferred in meningococcal vaccine naïve adults ≥56 years of age requiring only a single vaccination (CDC/ACIP [Coh, 2013]).

Those at increased risk of meningococcal disease include:

- Persons ≥2 months of age with medical conditions such as anatomical or functional asplenia or persistent complement component deficiencies (eg, C5-C9, properdin, factor H, or factor D)
- Persons ≥9 months of age that travel to or reside in countries where meningococcal disease is hyperendemic or epidemic, especially if contact with the local population will be prolonged
- Unvaccinated or incompletely vaccinated first year college students living in residence halls
- Military recruits
- Microbiologists with occupational exposure
- Persons (in all recommended age groups) at risk who are part of outbreaks caused by vaccine preventable serogroups

Pregnancy Risk Factor C

Pregnancy Considerations Animal reproduction studies have not been conducted. Inactivated bacterial vaccines have not been shown to cause increased risks to the fetus (NCIRD/ACIP 2011). Pregnancy should not preclude vaccination if indicated (CDC/ACIP [Cohn 2013]).

Breast-Feeding Considerations It is not known if this vaccine is present in breast milk. The manufacturer recommends that caution be used if administered to a nursing woman. Inactivated vaccines do not affect the safety of breast-feeding for the mother or the infant. Breast-feeding infants should be vaccinated according to the recommended schedules (NCIRD/ACIP 2011).

Contraindications Hypersensitivity to any component of the formulation

Warnings/Precautions Immediate treatment (including epinephrine 1:1,000) for anaphylactoid and/or hypersensitivity reactions should be available during vaccine use (NCIRD/ACIP 2011). Use with caution in severely immunocompromised patients (eg, patients receiving chemo/radiation therapy or other immunosuppressive therapy [including high-dose corticosteroids]); may have a reduced response to vaccination. In general, household and close contacts of persons with altered immunocompetence may receive all age-appropriate vaccines (IDSA [Rubin 2014]; NCIRD/ACIP 2011); inactivated vaccines should be administered ≥2 weeks prior to planned immunosuppression when feasible (IDSA [Rubin 2014]). Not to be used to treat meningococcal infections or to provide immunity against *N. meningitidis* serogroup B. The decision to administer or delay vaccination because of current or recent febrile illness depends on the severity of symptoms and the etiology of the disease. Consider deferring administration in patients with moderate or severe acute illness (with or without fever); vaccination should not be delayed for patients with mild acute illness (with or without fever) (NCIRD/ACIP 2011). Vaccination may not result in effective immunity in all patients. Response depends upon multiple factors (eg, type of vaccine, age of patient) and may be improved by administering the vaccine at the recommended dose, route, and interval. Vaccines may not be effective if administered during periods of altered immune competence (NCIRD/ACIP 2011). Syncope has been reported with use of injectable vaccines and may result in serious secondary injury (eg, skull fracture, cerebral hemorrhage); typically reported in adolescents and young adults and within 15 minutes after vaccination. Procedures should be in place to avoid injuries from falling and to restore cerebral perfusion if syncope occurs (NCIRD/ACIP 2011). Use with caution in patients with latex sensitivity; the stopper to the vial contains dry, natural latex rubber. Some dosage forms contain thimerosal. In order to maximize vaccination rates, the ACIP recommends simultaneous administration (ie, >1 vaccine on the same day at different anatomic sites) of all age-appropriate vaccines (live or inactivated) for which a person is eligible at a single clinic visit, unless contraindications exist. The use of combination vaccines is generally preferred over separate injections, taking into consideration provider assessment, patient preference, and adverse events. When using combination vaccines, the minimum age for administration is the oldest minimum age for any individual component; the minimum interval between dosing is the greatest minimum interval between any individual components. The ACIP prefers each dose of a specific vaccine in a series come from the same manufacturer when possible (NCIRD/ACIP 2011). Use of this vaccine for specific medical and/or other indications (eg, immunocompromising conditions, hepatic or kidney disease, diabetes) is also addressed in the ACIP Recommended Adult Immunization Schedule (CDC/ACIP [Kim 2015]). Specific recommendations for use of this vaccine in immunocompromised patients with asplenia, cerebrospinal fluid leaks, cochlear implants, or sickle cell disease are available from the IDSA (Rubin 2014). Antipyretics have not been shown to prevent febrile seizures; antipyretics may be used to treat fever or discomfort following vaccination (NCIRD/ACIP 2011). One study reported that routine prophylactic administration of acetaminophen to prevent fever prior to vaccination decreased the immune response of some vaccines; the clinical significance of this reduction in immune response has not been established (Prymula 2009).

Warnings: Additional Pediatric Considerations Children may have higher incidence of local adverse effects (erythema, swelling, tenderness).

Adverse Reactions All serious adverse reactions must be reported to the U.S. Department of Health and Human Services (DHHS) Vaccine Adverse Event Reporting System (VAERS) 1-800-822-7967 or online at https://vaers.hhs.gov/esub/index. In Canada, adverse reactions may be reported to local provincial/territorial health agencies or to the Vaccine Safety Section at Public Health Agency of Canada (1-866-844-0018).

Central nervous system: Chills, drowsiness, fatigue, fever, headache, irritability, malaise

Dermatologic: Rash

Gastrointestinal: Anorexia, diarrhea, vomiting

Local: Injection site: Induration, pain, redness, swelling

Neuromuscular & skeletal: Arthralgia

Rare but important or life-threatening: Dizziness, Guillain-Barré syndrome, hypersensitivity (angioedema, dyspnea, pruritus, rash, urticaria), myalgia, nausea, paresthesia, vasovagal syncope, weakness

Drug Interactions

Metabolism/Transport Effects None known.

Avoid Concomitant Use There are no known interactions where it is recommended to avoid concomitant use.

Increased Effect/Toxicity There are no known significant interactions involving an increase in effect.

Decreased Effect

The levels/effects of Meningococcal Polysaccharide Vaccine (Groups A / C / Y and W-135) may be decreased by: Belimumab; Fingolimod; Immunosuppressants

Storage/Stability Prior to and following reconstitution, store vaccine and diluent at 2°C to 8°C (35°F to 46°F); do not freeze.

Mechanism of Action Induces the formation of bactericidal antibodies to meningococcal antigens; the presence of these antibodies is strongly correlated with immunity to meningococcal disease caused by *Neisseria meningitidis* groups A, C, Y and W-135.

Pharmacodynamics

Onset of action: Antibody levels: 7 to 10 days

Duration: Antibodies against group A and C polysaccharides decline markedly (to prevaccination levels) over the first 3 years following a single dose of vaccine, especially in children <4 years of age

Dosing: Usual

Pediatric: **Immunization:** Children ≥2 years and Adolescents: SubQ: 0.5 mL as a single dose. Per the CDC/ACIP, this meningococcal vaccine is not routinely recommended for use in pediatric patients (CDC/ACIP [Cohn 2013])

Adult: **Immunization:** SubQ: 0.5 mL as a single dose

CDC/ACIP recommendations:

Adults <56 years: This meningococcal vaccine is not routinely recommended.

Adults ≥56 years: Meningococcal polysaccharide vaccine (MPSV4, Menomune) is preferred for meningococcal vaccine naïve persons in this age group who are at increased risk of meningococcal infection and require a single dose (eg, travelers or during a community outbreak). Persons previously vaccinated with a quadrivalent meningococcal conjugate vaccine (MenACWY, Menveo, or Menactra) and who require revaccination or for whom multiple doses are anticipated, MenACWY is preferred (eg, persons with asplenia or microbiologists).

Dosing adjustment in renal impairment: There are no dosage adjustments provided in the manufacturer's labeling.

Dosing adjustment in hepatic impairment: There are no dosage adjustments provided in the manufacturer's labeling.

Preparation for Administration SubQ: Reconstitute using provided diluent only; shake well. Use single-dose vial immediately after reconstitution. Use multidose vial within 35 days of reconstitution.

Administration SubQ: Shake well; administer by SubQ injection into the deltoid region of the upper arm; not for intradermal, IM, or IV administration. To prevent syncope-related injuries, adolescents and adults should be vaccinated while seated or lying down (NCIRD/ACIP 2011). US law requires that the date of administration, the vaccine manufacturer, lot number of vaccine, and the administering person's name, title and address be entered into the patient's permanent medical record.

Monitoring Parameters Observe for syncope for 15 minutes following administration (NCIRD/ACIP 2011). If seizure-like activity associated with syncope occurs, maintain patient in supine or Trendelenburg position to reestablish adequate cerebral perfusion.

Dosage Forms Excipient information presented when available (limited, particularly for generics); consult specific product labeling.

Injection, powder for reconstitution [MPSV4]:

Menomune-A/C/Y/W-135: 50 mcg each of polysaccharide antigen groups A, C, Y, and W-135 per 0.5 mL dose [contains lactose 2.5-5 mg/0.5 mL, natural rubber/natural latex in packaging, thimerosal in diluent for multi-dose vial]

◆ **Menomune-A/C/Y/W-135** *see* Meningococcal Polysaccharide Vaccine (Groups A / C / Y and W-135) *on page 1357*

◆ **Menostar** *see* Estradiol (Systemic) *on page 795*

◆ **Menveo** *see* Meningococcal (Groups A / C / Y and W-135) Diphtheria Conjugate Vaccine *on page 1352*

Meperidine (me PER i deen)

Medication Safety Issues

Sound-alike/look-alike issues:

Meperidine may be confused with meprobamate

Demerol may be confused with Demulen, Desyrel, Dilaudid, Pamelor

High alert medication:

The Institute for Safe Medication Practices (ISMP) includes this medication among its list of drug classes which have a heightened risk of causing significant patient harm when used in error.

BEERS Criteria medication:

This drug may be potentially inappropriate for use in geriatric patients (Quality of evidence - high; Strength of recommendation - strong).

Other safety concerns:

Avoid the use of meperidine for pain control, especially in elderly and renally-compromised patients because of the risk of neurotoxicity (American Pain Society, 2008; Institute for Safe Medication Practices [ISMP], 2007)

Related Information

Opioid Conversion Table *on page 2285*

Patient Information for Disposal of Unused Medications *on page 2453*

Preprocedure Sedatives in Children *on page 2444*

Brand Names: US Demerol; Meperitab

Brand Names: Canada Demerol

Therapeutic Category Analgesic, Narcotic

Generic Availability (US) Yes

Use

Oral: Relief of moderate to severe pain [FDA approved in pediatric patients (age not specified) and adults]

Parenteral: Relief of moderate to severe pain, preoperative medication, support of anesthesia, obstetrical analgesia [FDA approved in pediatric patients (age not specified) and adults]

Has also been used to reduce postoperative shivering and to reduce rigors from conventional amphotericin B

Pregnancy Risk Factor C

Pregnancy Considerations Animal reproduction studies have not been conducted by the manufacturer. Meperidine crosses the placenta; meperidine and its active metabolite accumulate in the fetus. Respiratory or CNS depression should be expected to occur in the newborn if maternal IM administration occurs within a few hours of delivery (Mattingly, 2003). When used for pain relief during labor, opioids may temporarily affect the heart rate of the fetus. Due to the prolonged half-life of the active metabolite, dose-dependent sedation in the neonate may be observed for 2-3 days following delivery. Meperidine has been used for the management of pain during labor; however, due to adverse maternal and fetal effects, other opioids may be preferred. Meperidine should also be avoided following delivery when postoperative analgesia is needed (ACOG, 2002).

If chronic opioid exposure occurs in pregnancy, adverse events in the newborn (including withdrawal) may occur; monitoring of the neonate is recommended. The minimum effective dose should be used if opioids are needed (Chou, 2009). Neonatal abstinence syndrome following opioid exposure may present with autonomic (eg, fever, temperature instability), gastrointestinal (eg, diarrhea, vomiting, poor feeding/weight gain), or neurologic (eg, high-pitched crying, increased muscle tone, irritability, seizure, tremor) symptoms (Dow, 2012; Hudak, 2012).

Breast-Feeding Considerations Meperidine is excreted in breast milk and may cause CNS and/or respiratory depression in the nursing infant. Due to the potential for serious adverse reactions in the nursing infant, the manufacturer recommends a decision be made whether to discontinue nursing or to discontinue the drug, taking into account the importance of treatment to the mother.

Small concentrations of meperidine are excreted into breast milk following single doses. With multiple doses, concentrations of meperidine and the active metabolite may increase and both are slowly eliminated by a nursing infant (Spigset, 2000). Parenteral opioids used during labor have the potential to interfere with a newborns natural reflex to nurse within the first few hours after birth. Nursing infants exposed to large doses of opioids should be monitored for apnea and sedation. If treatment for pain in nursing women is needed, other agents are preferred (Montgomery, 2012)

Contraindications Hypersensitivity to meperidine or any component of the formulation; use with or within 14 days of MAO inhibitors; severe respiratory insufficiency

Warnings/Precautions Oral meperidine is not recommended for acute/chronic pain management. Meperidine should not be used for acute/cancer pain because of the risk of neurotoxicity. Normeperidine (an active metabolite and CNS stimulant) may accumulate and precipitate anxiety, tremors, or seizures; risk increases with CNS or renal dysfunction, prolonged use (>48 hours), and cumulative dose (>600 mg/24 hours in adults). The Institute for Safe Medication Practice recommends avoiding the use of meperidine for pain control, especially in the elderly and renally impaired (ISMP, 2007). In the elderly; meperidine is not an effective oral analgesic at commonly used doses; may cause neurotoxicity; other agents are preferred in the elderly (Beers Criteria).

May cause CNS depression, which may impair physical or mental abilities; patients must be cautioned about performing tasks which require mental alertness (eg, operating machinery or driving). Potentially significant drug interactions may exist, requiring dose or frequency adjustment, additional monitoring, and/or selection of alternative therapy. Effects (eg, sedation, respiratory depression, hypotension) may be potentiated when used with other sedative/hypnotic drugs, general anesthetics, phenothiazines, or ethanol; consider reduced dose of meperidine if using concomitantly. Use only with extreme caution (if at all) in patients with head injury or increased intracranial pressure (ICP). Avoid use in patients with CNS depression or coma as these patients are susceptible to intracranial effects of CO_2 retention. Use caution with pulmonary, hepatic, or renal disorders, supraventricular tachycardias (including atrial flutter), acute abdominal conditions, biliary tract dysfunction, pancreatitis, delirium tremens, hypothyroidism, myxedema, toxic psychosis, kyphoscoliosis, morbid obesity, adrenal insufficiency, Addison's disease, seizure disorders, pheochromocytoma, BPH, or urethral stricture. May cause hypotension (including orthostatic hypotension); use with caution in patients with depleted blood volume or drugs which may exaggerate hypotensive effects (including phenothiazines or general anesthetics).

In patients with sickle cell anemia, use with caution and decrease initial dose; normeperidine (active metabolite) may accumulate and induce seizures in these patients; **Note:** Meperidine recommended for use in sickle cell patients by the American Pain Society (APS, 2008) and should only be used in sickle cell patients with a vaso-occlusive crisis (VOC) if it is the only effective opioid for an individual patient (NHLBI, 2014).

An opioid-containing analgesic regimen should be tailored to each patient's needs and based upon the type of pain being treated (acute versus chronic), the route of administration, degree of tolerance for opioids (naive versus chronic user), age, weight, and medical condition. The optimal analgesic dose varies widely among patients. Some preparations contain sulfites which may cause allergic reaction. Tolerance or drug dependence may result from extended use. Healthcare provider should be alert to problems of abuse, misuse, and diversion. Concurrent use of agonist/antagonist analgesics may precipitate withdrawal symptoms and/or reduced analgesic efficacy in patients following prolonged therapy with mu opioid agonists. Abrupt discontinuation following prolonged use may also lead to withdrawal symptoms. Avoid use in the elderly.

After chronic maternal exposure to opioids, neonatal withdrawal syndrome may occur in the newborn; monitor neonate closely. Signs and symptoms include irritability, hyperactivity and abnormal sleep pattern, high-pitched cry, tremor, vomiting, diarrhea, and failure to gain weight. Onset, duration and severity depend on the drug used, duration of use, maternal dose, and rate of drug elimination by the newborn. Opioid withdrawal syndrome in the neonate, unlike in adults, may be life-threatening and should be treated according to protocols developed by neonatology experts.

Benzyl alcohol and derivatives: Some dosage forms may contain sodium benzoate/benzoic acid; benzoic acid (benzoate) is a metabolite of benzyl alcohol; large amounts of benzyl alcohol (≥99 mg/kg/day) have been associated with a potentially fatal toxicity ("gasping syndrome") in neonates; the "gasping syndrome" consists of metabolic acidosis, respiratory distress, gasping respirations, CNS dysfunction (including convulsions, intracranial hemorrhage), hypotension, and cardiovascular collapse (AAP, 1997; CDC, 1982); some data suggests that benzoate displaces bilirubin from protein binding sites (Ahlfors, 2001); avoid or use dosage forms containing benzyl alcohol derivative with caution in neonates. See manufacturer's labeling.

Warnings: Additional Pediatric Considerations Due to decreased elimination rate, neonates and young infants may be at higher risk for adverse effects, especially respiratory depression; use with extreme caution and in reduced doses in this age group. In patients with sickle cell anemia, use with caution and decrease initial dose; normeperidine (active metabolite) may accumulate and induce seizures in these patients.

Adverse Reactions

Cardiovascular: Bradycardia, cardiac arrest, circulatory depression, flushing, hypotension, palpitations, shock, syncope, tachycardia

Central nervous system: Agitation, confusion, delirium, depression, disorientation, dizziness, drowsiness, drug dependence (physical dependence), dysphoria, euphoria, fatigue, habituation, hallucination, headache, increased intracranial pressure, malaise, myoclonus, nervousness, paradoxical central nervous system stimulation, restlessness, sedation, seizure (associated with metabolite accumulation), serotonin syndrome

Dermatologic: Diaphoresis, pruritus, skin rash, urticaria

Gastrointestinal: Abdominal cramps, anorexia, biliary colic, constipation, nausea, paralytic ileus, spasm of sphincter of Oddi, vomiting, xerostomia

Genitourinary: Ureteral spasm, urinary retention

Hypersensitivity: Anaphylaxis, histamine release, hypersensitivity reaction

Local: Injection site reaction (including pain, wheal, and flare)

Neuromuscular & skeletal: Muscle twitching, tremor, weakness

Ophthalmic: Visual disturbance

Respiratory: Dyspnea, respiratory arrest, respiratory depression

Rare but important or life-threatening: Hypogonadism (Brennan, 2013; Debono, 2011)

Drug Interactions

Metabolism/Transport Effects None known.

Avoid Concomitant Use

Avoid concomitant use of Meperidine with any of the following: Azelastine (Nasal); Dapoxetine; Eluxadoline; MAO Inhibitors; Mixed Agonist / Antagonist Opioids; Orphenadrine; Paraldehyde; Thalidomide

Increased Effect/Toxicity

Meperidine may increase the levels/effects of: Alcohol (Ethyl); Alvimopan; Antipsychotic Agents; Azelastine (Nasal); CNS Depressants; Desmopressin; Diuretics; Eluxadoline; Hydrocodone; Methotrimeprazine; Metoclopramide; Metyrosine; Orphenadrine; Paraldehyde; Pramipexole; ROPINIRole; Rotigotine; Serotonin Modulators; Suvorexant; Thalidomide; Zolpidem

The levels/effects of Meperidine may be increased by: Amphetamines; Anticholinergic Agents; Antiemetics (5HT3 Antagonists); Antipsychotic Agents; Antipsychotic Agents (Phenothiazines); Barbiturates; Brimonidine (Topical); Cannabis; Dapoxetine; Doxylamine; Dronabinol; Droperidol; HydrOXYzine; Kava Kava; Magnesium Sulfate; MAO Inhibitors; Methotrimeprazine; Nabilone; Perampanel; Protease Inhibitors; Rufinamide; Sodium Oxybate; Succinylcholine; Tapentadol; Tetrahydrocannabinol

Decreased Effect

Meperidine may decrease the levels/effects of: Pegvisomant

The levels/effects of Meperidine may be decreased by: Ammonium Chloride; Fosphenytoin; Mixed Agonist / Antagonist Opioids; Naltrexone; Phenytoin; Protease Inhibitors

Storage/Stability

Injection solution: Store at 20°C to 25°C (68°F to 77°F); excursions permitted to 15°C to 30°C (59°F to 86°F).

Tablets: Store at 25°C (77°F); excursions permitted to 15°C to 30°C (59°F to 86°F).

Mechanism of Action Binds to opioid receptors in the CNS, causing inhibition of ascending pain pathways, altering the perception of and response to pain; produces generalized CNS depression

Pharmacodynamics Analgesia:

Onset of action:
- Oral, IM, SubQ: Within 10-15 minutes
- IV: Within 5 minutes

Maximum effect:
- Oral, IM, SubQ: Within 1 hour
- IV: 5-7 minutes

Duration:
- Oral, IM, SubQ: 2-4 hours
- IV: 2-3 hours

Pharmacokinetics (Adult data unless noted)

Absorption: Oral: Erratic and highly variable

Distribution:

V_{dss}:
- Neonates: Preterm 1-7 days: 8.8 L/kg; term 1-7 days: 5.6 L/kg
- Infants: 1 week to 2 months: 8 L/kg; 3-18 months: 5 L/kg; 5-8 years: 2.8 L/kg
- Adults: 3-4 L/kg

Protein binding: (to $alpha_1$-acid glycoprotein)
- Neonates: 52%
- Infants: 3-18 months: 85%
- Adults: ~60% to 80%

Metabolism: Hepatic via hydrolysis and N-demethylation to meperidinic acid (inactive); also undergoes N-demethylation to normeperidine (active, has 1/2 the analgesic effect and 2-3 times the CNS effect of meperidine)

Bioavailability: ~50% to 60%, increased bioavailability with liver disease

Half-life, terminal:
- Preterm infants 3.6-65 days of age: 11.9 hours (range: 3.3-59.4 hours)
- Term infants:
  - 0.3-4 days of age: 10.7 hours (range: 4.9-16.8 hours)
  - 26-73 days of age: 8.2 hours (range: 5.7-31.7 hours)
- Neonates: 23 hours (range: 12-39 hours)
- Infants 3-18 months: 2.3 hours
- Children 5-8 years: 3 hours
- Adults: 2.5-4 hours
- Adults with liver disease: 7-11 hours
- Normeperidine (active metabolite): Neonates: 30-85 hours; Adults: 8-16 hours; normeperidine half-life is dependent on renal function and can accumulate with high doses or in patients with decreased renal function; normeperidine may precipitate tremors or seizures

Elimination: ~5% meperidine eliminated unchanged in urine

Dosing: Usual Doses should be titrated to appropriate analgesic effect; when changing route of administration, note that oral doses are about half as effective as parenteral dose.

Note: The American Pain Society (2008) and ISMP (2007) do not recommend meperidine use as an analgesic. If use for acute pain (in patients without renal or CNS disease) cannot be avoided, treatment should be limited to ≤48 hours and doses should not exceed 600 mg/24 hours in adults. Oral route is not recommended for treatment of acute or chronic pain. If IV route is required, consider a reduced dose. Patients with prior opioid exposure may require higher initial doses.

Infants, Children, and Adolescents:

Acute pain (analgesic) (Berde, 2002): Initial:
- Infants ≤6 months:
  - IM, IV, SubQ: 0.2-0.25 mg/kg/dose every 2-3 hours
  - Oral: 0.5-0.75 mg/kg/dose every 3-4 hours
- Infants >6 months, Children, and Adolescents:
  - IM, IV, or SubQ; intermittent dosing:
    - Patient weight <50 kg: 0.8-1 mg/kg/dose every 2-3 hours as needed; maximum dose: 75 mg
    - Patient weight ≥50 kg: 50-75 mg every 2-3 hours as needed
  - Oral:
    - Patient weight <50 kg: 2-3 mg/kg/dose every 3-4 hours as needed; maximum dose: 150 mg
    - Patient weight ≥50 kg: 100-150 mg every 3-4 hours as needed

Analgesia for minor procedures/sedation; preoperative:
- IM, IV, SubQ: 0.5-1 mg/kg given 30-90 minutes before the beginning of anesthesia; maximum dose: 2 mg/kg or 150 mg/dose (Zeltzer, 1990)
- Oral: 2-4 mg/kg given 30-90 minutes before the beginning of anesthesia; maximum dose: 150 mg/dose

Sickle cell disease, acute crisis (NHLBI, 2002): Note: Not recommended for first-line use; reserve for brief treatment episodes in patients who have previously benefited from meperidine therapy, or in patients who have allergies or are intolerant to other opioids (eg, morphine, hydromorphone): Initial:
- Patient weight <50 kg:
  - IV: 0.75-1 mg/kg every 3-4 hours as needed; maximum dose: 1.75 mg/kg/dose or 100 mg
  - Oral: 1.1-1.75 mg/kg every 3-4 hours as needed; maximum dose: 1.75 mg/kg/dose or 150 mg
- Patient weight ≥50 kg:
  - IV: 50-150 mg every 3 hours as needed
  - Oral: 50-150 mg every 3-4 hours as needed

Adults: **Pain (analgesic):** Oral, IM, SubQ: 50-150 mg every 3-4 hours as needed

Preoperatively: IM, SubQ: 50-150 mg given 30-90 minutes before the beginning of anesthesia

Obstetrical analgesia: IM, SubQ: 50-100 mg when pain becomes regular; may repeat at every 1-3 hours

Dosing adjustment in renal impairment: The manufacturer recommends to use with caution and reduce dose;

accumulation of meperidine and its active metabolite (normeperidine) may occur. The American Pain Society and ISMP recommend to avoid use in renal impairment. (American Pain Society, 2008; ISMP, 2007).

Dosing adjustment in hepatic impairment: Use with caution and reduce dose; accumulation of meperidine and its active metabolite (normeperidine) may occur.

Preparation for Administration

Oral: Oral solution: Dilute dose in 1/2 glass of water prior to use

Parenteral:

Slow IV push: Dilute solution to ≤10 mg/mL

Intermittent IV infusion: Dilute to 1 mg/mL

Administration

Oral: Oral solution: Dilute dose in water prior to administration; undiluted solution may cause topical anesthetic effect on mucous membranes

Parenteral:

IM: Preferred route; inject undiluted into a large muscle

IV:

Slow IV push: Do not administer rapid IV, dilute and administer over at least 5 minutes

Intermittent IV infusion: Dilute and administer over 15 to 30 minutes

SubQ: Suitable for occasional use; when repeated doses are required, the IM route of administration is preferred; administer undiluted

Monitoring Parameters Respiratory rate; oxygen saturation; mental status; blood pressure; relief of pain, level of sedation

Test Interactions Increased amylase (S), increased BSP retention, increased CPK (IM injections)

Additional Information Equianalgesic doses: morphine 10 mg IM = meperidine 75-100 mg IM. **Note**: Although meperidine has been used in combination with chlorpromazine and promethazine as a premedication ("Lytic Cocktail"), this combination may have a higher rate of adverse effects compared to alternative sedatives and analgesics (AAP Committee on Drugs, 1995)

Controlled Substance C-II

Dosage Forms Excipient information presented when available (limited, particularly for generics); consult specific product labeling.

Solution, Injection, as hydrochloride:

Demerol: 25 mg/mL (1 mL); 25 mg/0.5 mL (0.5 mL); 50 mg/mL (1 mL, 30 mL); 75 mg/1.5 mL (1.5 mL); 100 mg/2 mL (2 mL); 75 mg/mL (1 mL); 100 mg/mL (1 mL, 20 mL)

Generic: 10 mg/mL (30 mL); 25 mg/mL (1 mL); 50 mg/mL (1 mL); 100 mg/mL (1 mL)

Solution, Oral, as hydrochloride:

Generic: 50 mg/5 mL (500 mL)

Tablet, Oral, as hydrochloride:

Demerol: 50 mg [scored]

Demerol: 100 mg

Meperitab: 50 mg [scored]

Meperitab: 100 mg

Generic: 50 mg, 100 mg

◆ **Meperidine Hydrochloride** *see* Meperidine *on page 1359*

◆ **Meperitab** *see* Meperidine *on page 1359*

◆ **Mephyton®** *see* Phytonadione *on page 1698*

Mepivacaine (me PIV a kane)

Medication Safety Issues

Sound-alike/look-alike issues:

Mepivacaine may be confused with bupivacaine

Polocaine® may be confused with prilocaine

High alert medication:

The Institute for Safe Medication Practices (ISMP) includes this medication (epidural administration) among its list of drug classes which have a heightened risk of causing significant patient harm when used in error.

Brand Names: US Carbocaine; Carbocaine Preservative Free; Polocaine; Polocaine-MPF

Brand Names: Canada Carbocaine®; Polocaine®

Therapeutic Category Local Anesthetic, Injectable

Generic Availability (US) Yes

Use Local or regional analgesia; anesthesia by local infiltration, peripheral and central neural techniques including epidural and caudal blocks; **not** for use in spinal anesthesia

Pregnancy Risk Factor C

Pregnancy Considerations Animal reproduction studies have not been conducted. Mepivacaine has been used in obstetrical analgesia.

Breast-Feeding Considerations It is not known if mepivacaine is excreted in breast milk. The manufacturer recommends that caution be exercised when administering mepivacaine to nursing women.

Contraindications Hypersensitivity to mepivacaine, other amide-type local anesthetics, or any component of the formulation

Warnings/Precautions Careful and constant monitoring of the patient's state of consciousness should be done following each local anesthetic injection; at such times, restlessness, anxiety, tinnitus, dizziness, blurred vision, tremors, depression, or drowsiness may be early warning signs of CNS toxicity; treatment is primarily symptomatic and supportive. Continuous intra-articular infusion of local anesthetics after arthroscopic or other surgical procedures is **not** an approved use; chondrolysis (primarily in the shoulder joint) has occurred following infusion, with some cases requiring arthroplasty or shoulder replacement. Use with caution in patients with cardiac disease, hepatic or renal disease, or hyperthyroidism. Local anesthetics have been associated with rare occurrences of sudden respiratory arrest; convulsions due to systemic toxicity leading to cardiac arrest have been reported presumably due to intravascular injection. A test dose is recommended prior to epidural administration and all reinforcing doses with continuous catheter technique. Do not use solutions containing preservatives for caudal or epidural block. Use caution in debilitated, elderly, or acutely-ill patients; dose reduction may be required. Resuscitative equipment, oxygen, and other resuscitative drugs should be available for immediate use.

Adverse Reactions

Cardiovascular: Bradycardia, cardiac arrest, cardiac output decreased, heart block, hyper-/hypotension, myocardial depression, syncope, tachycardia, ventricular arrhythmias

Central nervous system: Anxiety, chills, convulsions, depression, dizziness, excitation, restlessness, tremors

Dermatologic: Angioneurotic edema, diaphoresis, erythema, pruritus, urticaria

Gastrointestinal: Fecal incontinence, nausea, vomiting

Genitourinary: Incontinence, urinary retention

Neuromuscular & skeletal: Chondrolysis (continuous intra-articular administration), paralysis

Ocular: Blurred vision, pupil constriction

Otic: Tinnitus

Respiratory: Apnea, hypoventilation, sneezing

Miscellaneous: Allergic reaction, anaphylactoid reaction

Drug Interactions

Metabolism/Transport Effects None known.

Avoid Concomitant Use There are no known interactions where it is recommended to avoid concomitant use.

Increased Effect/Toxicity
The levels/effects of Mepivacaine may be increased by: Beta-Blockers; Hyaluronidase

Decreased Effect
Mepivacaine may decrease the levels/effects of: Technetium Tc 99m Tilmanocept

Storage/Stability Store at controlled room temperature of 15°C to 30°C (59°F to 86°F). Brief exposure up to 40°C (104°F) does not adversely affect the product. Solutions may be sterilized.

Mechanism of Action Mepivacaine is an amide local anesthetic similar to lidocaine; like all local anesthetics, mepivacaine acts by preventing the generation and conduction of nerve impulses

Pharmacodynamics Route and dose dependent:
Onset of action: Range: 3-20 minutes
Duration: 2-2.5 hours

Pharmacokinetics (Adult data unless noted)
Protein binding: ~75%
Metabolism: Primarily hepatic via N-demethylation, hydroxylation, and glucuronidation
Half-life:
Neonates: 8.7-9 hours
Adults: 1.9-3 hours
Elimination: Urine (95% as metabolites)

Dosing: Usual Injectable local anesthetic: Dose varies with procedure, degree of anesthesia needed, vascularity of tissue, duration of anesthesia required, and physical condition of patient. The smaller dose/concentration (0.5%) will produce more superficial blockade, a higher dose (1%) will block sensory and sympathetic conduction without loss of motor function, a higher dose (1.5%) will provide extensive and often complete motor blockade, and 2% will produce complete sensory and motor blockade. The smallest dose and concentration required to produce the desired effect should be used.

Children: Maximum dose: 5-6 mg/kg; only concentrations <2% should be used in children <3 years or <14 kg (30 lbs)
Adults: Maximum dose: 400 mg; do not exceed 1000 mg/24 hours
Cervical, brachial, intercostal, pudendal nerve block: 5-40 mL of a 1% solution (maximum: 400 mg) **or** 5-20 mL of a 2% solution (maximum: 400 mg). For pudendal block: Inject 1/2 the total dose each side.
Transvaginal block (paracervical plus pudendal): Up to 30 mL (both sides) of a 1% solution (maximum: 300 mg). Inject 1/2 the total dose into each side.
Paracervical block: Up to 20 mL (both sides) of a 1% solution (maximum: 200 mg). Inject 1/2 the total dose into each side. This is the maximum recommended dose per 90-minute procedure; inject slowly with 5 minutes between sides.
Caudal and epidural block (**preservative free solutions only**): 15-30 mL of a 1% solution (maximum: 300 mg) **or** 10-25 mL of a 1.5% solution (maximum: 375 mg) **or** 10-20 mL of a 2% solution (maximum: 400 mg)
Infiltration: Up to 40 mL of a 1% solution (maximum: 400 mg)
Therapeutic block (pain management): 1-5 mL of a 1% solution (maximum: 50 mg) **or** 1-5 mL of a 2% solution (maximum: 100 mg)

Administration Parenteral: Administer in small incremental doses; when using continuous intermittent catheter techniques, use frequent aspirations before and during the injection to avoid intravascular injection

Monitoring Parameters Blood pressure, heart rate, respiration, signs of CNS toxicity (lightheadedness, dizziness, tinnitus, restlessness, tremors, twitching, drowsiness, circumoral paresthesia)

Dosage Forms Excipient information presented when available (limited, particularly for generics); consult specific product labeling.
Solution, Injection, as hydrochloride:
Carbocaine: 1% (50 mL); 2% (50 mL) [contains methylparaben]
Polocaine: 1% (50 mL); 2% (50 mL) [contains methylparaben]
Generic: 3% (1.8 mL)
Solution, Injection, as hydrochloride [preservative free]:
Carbocaine Preservative-Free: 1% (30 mL); 1.5% (30 mL); 2% (20 mL)
Polocaine-MPF: 1% (30 mL); 1.5% (30 mL); 2% (20 mL) [methylparaben free]

◆ **Mepivacaine Hydrochloride** *see* Mepivacaine *on page 1362*
◆ **Mepron** *see* Atovaquone *on page 222*
◆ **Mercaptoethane Sulfonate** *see* Mesna *on page 1371*

Mercaptopurine (mer kap toe PURE een)

Medication Safety Issues
Sound-alike/look-alike issues:
Mercaptopurine may be confused with methotrexate
Purinethol [DSC] may be confused with propylthiouracil
High alert medication:
This medication is in a class the Institute for Safe Medication Practices (ISMP) includes among its list of drug classes which have a heightened risk of causing significant patient harm when used in error.
Other safety concerns:
To avoid potentially serious dosage errors, the terms "6-mercaptopurine" or "6-MP" should be avoided; use of these terms has been associated with sixfold overdosages.
Azathioprine is metabolized to mercaptopurine; concurrent use of these commercially-available products has resulted in profound myelosuppression.

Related Information
Oral Medications That Should Not Be Crushed or Altered *on page 2476*
Prevention of Chemotherapy-Induced Nausea and Vomiting in Children *on page 2368*
Safe Handling of Hazardous Drugs *on page 2455*

Brand Names: US Purinethol [DSC]; Purixan
Brand Names: Canada Purinethol
Therapeutic Category Antineoplastic Agent, Antimetabolite; Antineoplastic Agent, Purine
Generic Availability (US) May be product dependent
Use Maintenance treatment of acute lymphoblastic leukemia (ALL) in combination with other agents (eg, methotrexate) [FDA approved in pediatric patients (age not specified) and adults]; has also been used to treat inflammatory bowel disease, autoimmune hepatitis, and maintenance treatment in acute promyelocytic leukemia (APL)
Prescribing and Access Restrictions Distribution of Purixan is provided by the specialty pharmacy, AnovoRx. For ordering information, call 888-470-0904.
Pregnancy Risk Factor D
Pregnancy Considerations May cause fetal harm if administered during pregnancy. Case reports of fetal loss have been noted with mercaptopurine administration during the first trimester; adverse effects have also been noted with second and third trimester use. Women of child bearing potential should avoid becoming pregnant during treatment.
Breast-Feeding Considerations Mercaptopurine is the active metabolite of azathioprine. Following administration of azathioprine, mercaptopurine can be detected in breast milk (Gardiner 2006). It is not known if/how much mercaptopurine is found in breast milk following oral

administration. According to the manufacturer, the decision to discontinue mercaptopurine or discontinue breast-feeding during therapy should take into account the benefits of treatment to the mother.

Contraindications Hypersensitivity to mercaptopurine or any component of the formulation; patients whose disease showed prior resistance to mercaptopurine

Warnings/Precautions Hazardous agent - use appropriate precautions for handling and disposal (NIOSH 2014 [group 1]).

Hepatotoxicity has been reported, including jaundice, ascites, hepatic necrosis (may be fatal), intrahepatic cholestasis, parenchymal cell necrosis, and/or hepatic encephalopathy; may be due to direct hepatic cell damage or hypersensitivity. While hepatotoxicity or hepatic injury may occur at any dose, dosages exceeding the recommended dose are associated with a higher incidence. Signs of jaundice generally appear early in treatment, after ~1 to 2 months (range: 1 week to 8 years) and may resolve following discontinuation; recurrence with rechallenge has been noted. Monitor liver function tests, including transaminases, alkaline phosphatase, and bilirubin weekly with treatment initiation, then monthly thereafter (monitor more frequently if used in combination with other hepatotoxic drugs or in patients with pre-existing hepatic impairment). Consider a reduced dose in patients with baseline hepatic impairment; monitor closely for toxicity. Withhold treatment for clinical signs of jaundice (hepatomegaly, anorexia, tenderness), deterioration in liver function tests, toxic hepatitis, or biliary stasis until hepatotoxicity is ruled out.

Dose-related leukopenia, thrombocytopenia, and anemia are common; however, may be indicative of disease progression. Hematologic toxicity may be delayed. Bone marrow may appear hypoplastic (could also appear normal). Monitor blood counts; dose may require adjusting for severe neutropenia or thrombocytopenia. Monitor for bleeding (due to thrombocytopenia) or infection (due to neutropenia). Profound severe or repeated hematologic toxicity may be indicative of TPMT deficiency. Patients with homozygous genetic defect of thiopurine methyltransferase (TPMT) are more sensitive to myelosuppressive effects; generally associated with rapid myelosuppression. Significant mercaptopurine dose reductions will be necessary (possibly with continued concomitant chemotherapy at normal doses). Patients who are heterozygous for TPMT defects will have intermediate activity; may have increased toxicity (primarily myelosuppression) although will generally tolerate normal mercaptopurine doses. Consider TPMT testing for severe toxicities/excessive myelosuppression. A germline variant in nucleoside diphophate-linked moiety X-type motif 15 (*NUDT15*) is strongly correlated with mercaptopurine intolerance in children receiving treatment for acute lymphoblastic leukemia (ALL). A genome-wide association study was performed in two prospective clinical childhood ALL trials, and showed that patients homozygous for the TT genotype were extremely sensitive to mercaptopurine, and achieved an average dose intensity of only 8.3%. The *NUDT15* genetic variant is most common in East Asian and Hispanic patients. In patients homozygous for either TPMT or *NUDT15* (or heterozygous for both), mercaptopurine dose reductions of ≥50% were required in 100% of patients (Yang 2015). Potentially significant drug-drug interactions may exist, requiring dose or frequency adjustment, additional monitoring, and/or selection of alternative therapy. Because azathioprine is metabolized to mercaptopurine, concomitant use with azathioprine may result in a significant increase in hematologic toxicity and profound myelosuppression; avoid concurrent use. Hematologic toxicity may be exacerbated by other medications which inhibit TPMT (eg, mesalamine, olsalazine, sulfasalazine) or by other myelosuppressive drugs.

Immunosuppressive agents, including mercaptopurine, a associated with the development of lymphoma and oth malignancies including hepatosplenic T-cell lymphon (HSTCL). Mercaptopurine is immunosuppressive; immu responses to infections may be impaired and the risk infection is increased; common signs of infection, such fever and leukocytosis may not occur; lethargy and co fusion may be more prominent signs of infection. Immu response to vaccines may be diminished; live virus va cines impose a risk for infection. Consider adjusting do age in patients with renal impairment. Some renal adver effects may be minimized with hydration and prophylac antihyperuricemic therapy. To avoid potentially serio dosage errors, the terms "6-mercaptopurine" or "6-M should be avoided; use of these terms has been asso ated with six-fold overdosages.

Warnings: Additional Pediatric Considerations Th development of secondary hemophagocytic lymphohisti cytosis (HLH), a rare and frequently fatal activation macrophages which causes phagocytosis of all bon marrow blood cell lines, is increased (100-fold) in pediat patients diagnosed with inflammatory bowel disease; th risk is further increased with concomitant thiopurine (i azathioprine or mercaptopurine) therapy, Epstein-Ba virus, or other possible infections; if patient presents wi fever (at least 5 days), cervical lymphadenopathy, an lymphopenia, discontinue immunosuppressive therap and further diagnostic evaluation for HLH should be pe formed; diagnostic delay associated with increased morta ity (Biank, 2011).

Adverse Reactions

Central nervous system: Drug fever, malaise

Dermatologic: Alopecia, hyperpigmentation, skin rash, ur caria

Endocrine & metabolic: Hyperuricemia

Gastrointestinal: Anorexia, cholestasis, diarrhea, mucos tis, oral lesion, nausea (minimal), pancreatitis, sprue-lik symptoms, stomach pain, ulcerative bowel lesion, vom ing (minimal)

Genitourinary: Oligospermia, renal toxicity, uricosuria

Hematologic: Anemia, bone marrow depression (ons 7-10 days; nadir 14 days; recovery: 21 days), granulocy topenia, hemorrhage, hepatosplenic T-cell lymphoma leukopenia, lymphocytopenia, metastases, neutropeni thrombocytopenia

Hepatic: Ascites, hepatic encephalopathy, hepatic fibrosis hepatic injury, hepatic necrosis, hepatomegaly, hepato toxicity, hyperbilirubinemia, increased serum transam nases, intrahepatic cholestasis, jaundice, toxic hepatitis

Immunologic: Immunosuppression

Infection: Infection

Respiratory: Pulmonary fibrosis

Drug Interactions

Metabolism/Transport Effects None known.

Avoid Concomitant Use

Avoid concomitant use of Mercaptopurine with any of th following: AzaTHIOprine; BCG; BCG (Intravesical); Clo ZAPine; Dipyrone; Febuxostat; Natalizumab; Pimecroli mus; Tacrolimus (Topical); Tofacitinib

Increased Effect/Toxicity

Mercaptopurine may increase the levels/effects of: Clo ZAPine; Leflunomide; Natalizumab; Tofacitinib; Vaccine (Live)

The levels/effects of Mercaptopurine may be increase by: 5-ASA Derivatives; Allopurinol; AzaTHIOprine; Deno sumab; Dipyrone; DOXOrubicin (Conventional); Febuxo stat; Pimecrolimus; Roflumilast; Sulfamethoxazole Tacrolimus (Topical); Trastuzumab; Trimethoprim

Decreased Effect

Mercaptopurine may decrease the levels/effects of: BCG BCG (Intravesical); Coccidioides immitis Skin Test

Sipuleucel-T; Vaccines (Inactivated); Vaccines (Live); Vitamin K Antagonists

The levels/effects of Mercaptopurine may be decreased by: Echinacea

Food Interactions Absorption is variable with food. Management: Take on an empty stomach at the same time each day 1 hour before or 2 hours after a meal. Maintain adequate hydration, unless instructed to restrict fluid intake.

Storage/Stability

Tablets: Store at 15°C to 25°C (59°F to 77°F). Store in a dry place.

Suspension: Store at 15°C to 25°C (59°F to 77°F). Do not store above 25°C (77°F). Store in a dry place. Use within 6 weeks after opening.

Mechanism of Action Mercaptopurine is a purine antagonist which inhibits DNA and RNA synthesis; acts as false metabolite and is incorporated into DNA and RNA, eventually inhibiting their synthesis; specific for the S phase of the cell cycle

Pharmacokinetics (Adult data unless noted)

Absorption: Variable and incomplete (~50%)

Distribution: V_d > total body water; CNS penetration is negligible

Protein binding: ~19%

Metabolism: Hepatic and in GI mucosa; hepatically via xanthine oxidase and methylation via TPMT to sulfate conjugates, 6-thiouric acid, and other inactive compounds; first-pass effect

Half-life:

Children: 21 minutes

Adults: 47 minutes

Time to peak serum concentration: Within 2 hours

Elimination: Urine (46% as mercaptopurine and metabolites)

Dosing: Usual

Children and Adolescents:

Acute lymphoblastic leukemia (ALL): Refer to individual protocols.

Manufacturer's labeling: Maintenance therapy: Oral: 1.5-2.5 mg/kg/dose once daily, combined with other agents

Alternate dosing: Adolescents ≥15 years: Multiple dosage regimens reported:

Consolidation phase: Oral: 60 mg/m²/day days 0-27 days (5-week course) **or** 60 mg/m²/day days 0-13 and days 28-41 (9-week course) (Stock, 2008)

Early intensification (two 4-week courses): Oral: 60 mg/m²/day on days 1-14 (Larson, 1995; Larson, 1998; Stock, 2008)

Interim maintenance: Oral: 60 mg/m²/day on days 0-41 (8-week course) **or** 60 mg/m²/day days 1-70 (12-week course) (Larson, 1995; Larson, 1998; Stock, 2008)

Maintenance (prolonged): Oral: 50 mg 3 times daily for 2 years (Kantarjian, 2000; Thomas, 2004) **or** 60 mg/m²/day for 2 years from diagnosis (Larson, 1995; Larson, 1998; Stock, 2008) **or** 75 mg/m²/day for 2 years (girls) or 3 years (boys) from first interim maintenance (Stock, 2008)

Acute promyelocytic leukemia (APL): Limited data available: Adolescents ≥15 years: Oral: 60 mg/m²/day for 1 year; in combination with tretinoin and methotrexate (Powell, 2010)

Autoimmune hepatitis: Very limited data available: Oral: 1.5 mg/kg/day in combination with prednisone; not considered first-line, typically used for patient who do not tolerate azathioprine (Manns, 2010)

Inflammatory bowel disease (eg, Crohn's disease, ulcerative colitis): Limited data available: 1-1.5 mg/kg/day (Markowitz, 2000; Punati, 2011; Sandhu, 2010). Some data suggest that pediatric patients ≤6 years may require higher doses to achieve remission; a median dose of 1.68 mg/kg/day (maximum daily dose: 2.4 mg/kg/day) was reported to induce remission in 62% of patients vs 17% of those receiving lower doses (<1.5 mg/kg/day study group; median dose: 1.18 mg/kg/day) (Grossman, 2008; Sandborn, 2001)

Adults: **Acute lymphoblastic leukemia (ALL):** Maintenance: Oral: 1.5-2.5 mg/kg/dose once daily; also consult guidelines for details on combination regimens

Dosing adjustment with concurrent allopurinol: Children, Adolescents, and Adults: Reduce mercaptopurine dosage to 25% to 33% of the usual dose

Dosing adjustment in TPMT-deficiency: Children, Adolescents, and Adults: Dosing not established; substantial reductions are generally required only in homozygous deficiency; however, some experts also recommend dosage reduction with intermediate activity or heterozygous phenotype (Sandborn, 2001)

Dosing adjustment in renal impairment: Children and Adolescents: The manufacturer's labeling recommends starting with reduced doses in patients with renal impairment to avoid accumulation; however, no specific dosage adjustment is provided. The following adjustments have been used by some clinicians (Aronoff, 2007):

GFR >50 mL/minute/1.73m²: No adjustment required

GFR ≤50 mL/minute/1.73m²: Administer every 48 hours

Hemodialysis: Administer every 48 hours

Continuous ambulatory peritoneal dialysis (CAPD): Administer every 48 hours

Continuous renal replacement therapy (CRRT): Administer every 48 hours

Dosing adjustment in hepatic impairment: Children, Adolescents, and Adults: The manufacturer's labeling recommends considering a reduced dose in patients with hepatic impairment; however, no specific dosage adjustment is provided.

Administration Hazardous agent; use appropriate precautions for handling and disposal (NIOSH 2014 [group 1]).

Oral: Preferably on an empty stomach (1 hour before or 2 hours after meals). Shake oral suspension well for at least 30 seconds to ensure suspension is mixed thoroughly (suspension is viscous). Measure dose with an oral dosing syringe to assure proper dose is administered. If oral syringe is intended to be re-used, wash with warm soapy water and rinse well (hold syringe under water and move plunger several times to ensure inside of syringe is clean); allow to dry completely. Use within 6 weeks after opening.

For the treatment of ALL in children: Administration of doses in the evening has demonstrated superior outcome; administration with food did not significantly affect outcome (Schmiegelow 1997).

Monitoring Parameters CBC with differential (weekly initially, although clinical status may require increased frequency), bone marrow exam (to evaluate marrow status), liver function tests (weekly initially, then monthly; monitor more frequently if on concomitant hepatotoxic agents), renal function, urinalysis; consider TPMT genotyping to identify TPMT defect (if severe toxicity occurs)

For use in inflammatory bowel disease, monitor CBC with differential weekly for 1 month, then biweekly for 1 month, followed by monitoring every 1-2 months throughout the course of therapy. LFTs should be assessed every 3 months. Monitor for signs/symptoms of malignancy (eg, splenomegaly, hepatomegaly, abdominal pain, persistent fever, night sweats, weight loss) (Sandhu, 2010).

Test Interactions TPMT testing: Recent transfusions may result in a misinterpretation of the actual TPMT activity. Concomitant drugs may influence TPMT activity in the blood.

Dosage Forms Excipient information presented when available (limited, particularly for generics); consult specific product labeling. [DSC] = Discontinued product

Suspension, Oral:

Purixan: 2000 mg/100 mL (100 mL) [contains aspartame, methylparaben, propylparaben]

Tablet, Oral:

Purinethol: 50 mg [DSC] [scored]

Generic: 50 mg

Extemporaneous Preparations Hazardous agent: Use appropriate precautions for handling and disposal (NIOSH 2014 [group 1]). When manipulating tablets, NIOSH recommends double gloving, a protective gown, and preparation in a controlled device; if not prepared in a controlled device, respiratory and eye protection as well as ventilated engineering controls are recommended (NIOSH 2014).

A 50 mg/mL oral suspension may be prepared in a vertical flow hood with tablets and a mixture of sterile water for injection (SWFI), simple syrup, and cherry syrup. Crush thirty 50 mg tablets in a mortar and reduce to a fine powder. Add ~5 mL SWFI and mix to a uniform paste; then add ~10 mL simple syrup; mix while continuing to add cherry syrup to make a final volume of 30 mL; transfer to a calibrated bottle. Label "shake well" and "caution chemotherapy". Stable for 35 days at room temperature.

Aliabadi HM, Romanick M, Desai, S, et al, "Effect of Buffer and Antioxidant on Stability of a Mercaptopurine Suspension," *Am J Health Syst Pharm* 2008, 65(5):441-7.

◆ **6-Mercaptopurine (error-prone abbreviation)** *see* Mercaptopurine *on page 1363*

◆ **Mercapturic Acid** *see* Acetylcysteine *on page 57*

Meropenem (mer oh PEN em)

Medication Safety Issues

Sound-alike/look-alike issues:

Meropenem may be confused with ertapenem, imipenem, metroNIDAZOLE

Brand Names: US Merrem

Brand Names: Canada Meropenem For Injection; Merrem

Therapeutic Category Antibiotic, Carbapenem

Generic Availability (US) Yes

Use Treatment of complicated appendicitis and peritonitis caused by viridans group streptococci, *E. coli*, *Klebsiella pneumoniae*, *P. aeruginosa*, *B. fragilis*, *B. thetaiotaomicron*, and *Peptostreptococcus* species (FDA approved in all ages); treatment of bacterial meningitis caused by *Streptococcus pneumoniae*, *Haemophilus influenzae*, and *Neisseria meningitides* (FDA approved in pediatric patients ages ≥3 months); treatment of complicated skin and skin structure infections caused by *Staphylococcus aureus* (methicillin-susceptible isolates only), *Streptococcus pyogenes*, *S. agalactiae*, viridans group streptococci, *Enterococcus faecalis* (vancomycin-susceptible isolates only), *Pseudomonas aeruginosa*, *Escherichia coli*, *Proteus mirabilis*, *Bacteroides fragilis*, and *Peptostreptococcus* species (FDA approved in ages ≥3 months and adults); has also been used for treatment of lower respiratory tract infections, acute pulmonary exacerbations in cystic fibrosis, urinary tract infections, empiric treatment of febrile neutropenia, and sepsis

Pregnancy Risk Factor B

Pregnancy Considerations Adverse events were not observed in animal reproduction studies. Incomplete transplacental transfer of meropenem was found using an *ex vivo* human perfusion model.

Breast-Feeding Considerations Small amounts of meropenem are excreted into breast milk (case report). The manufacturer recommends that caution be exercised when administering meropenem to breast-feeding women. Nondose-related effects could include modification of bowel flora.

Contraindications Hypersensitivity to meropenem, other drugs in the same class, or any component of the formulation; patients who have experienced anaphylactic reactions to beta-lactams

Warnings/Precautions Serious hypersensitivity reactions, including anaphylaxis, have been reported (some without a history of previous allergic reactions to beta-lactams). Carbapenems have been associated with CNS adverse effects, including confusional states and seizures (myoclonic); use caution with CNS disorders (eg, brain lesions and history of seizures) and adjust dose in renal impairment to avoid drug accumulation, which may increase seizure risk. Outpatient use may result in paresthesias, seizures, or headaches that can impair neuromotor function and alertness; patients should not operate machinery or drive until it is established that meropenem is well tolerated. Prolonged use may result in fungal or bacterial superinfection, including *C. difficile*-associated diarrhea (CDAD) and pseudomembranous colitis; CDAD has been observed >2 months postantibiotic treatment. Use with caution in patients with renal impairment; dosage adjustment required in patients with moderate-to-severe renal dysfunction. Thrombocytopenia has been reported in patients with renal dysfunction. Lower doses (based upon renal function) are often required in the elderly. Potentially significant drug-drug interactions may exist, requiring dose or frequency adjustment, additional monitoring, and/or selection of alternative therapy.

Adverse Reactions

Cardiovascular: bradycardia, cardiac arrest, cardiac failure, chest pain, hypertension, hypotension, myocardial infarction, peripheral edema, peripheral vascular disease, pulmonary embolism, shock, syncope, tachycardia

Central nervous system: agitation, anxiety, chills, confusion, convulsions (neonates and infants <3 months), delirium, depression, dizziness, drowsiness, hallucination, headache, insomnia, nervousness, pain, paresthesia, seizure

Dermatologic: Dermal ulcer, diaphoresis, pruritus, skin rash (includes diaper-area moniliasis in infants), urticaria

Endocrine & metabolic: Hypervolemia, hypoglycemia

Gastrointestinal: abdominal pain, anorexia, constipation, diarrhea, dyspepsia, enlargement of abdomen, flatulence, gastrointestinal disesase, glossitis, intestinal obstruction, nausea, oral candidiasis, vomiting

Genitourinary: Dysuria, pelvic pain, urinary incontinence, vulvovaginal candidiasis

Hematologic & oncologic: Anemia, hypochromic anemia

Local: Inflammation at the injection site, injection site reaction, phlebitis/thrombophlebitis

Respiratory: Apnea, pharyngitis, pneumonia

Miscellaneous: Sepsis, shock

Hepatic: Cholestatic jaundice, hepatic failure, hyperbilirubinemia (conjugated; neonates and infants <3 months), jaundice

Infection: Sepsis

Local: Inflammation at injection site

Neuromuscular & skeletal: Back pain, weakness

Renal: Renal failure

Respiratory: Apnea, asthma, cough, dyspnea, hypoxia, pharyngitis, pleural effusion, pneumonia, pulmonary edema, respiratory tract disease

Miscellaneous: Accidental injury, fever

Rare but important or life-threatening: Agranulocytosis, angioedema, anorexia, asthma, bradycardia, cardiac arrest, cardiac failure, change in platelet count, cholestatic jaundice, *Clostridium difficile* associated diarrhea, confusion, decreased hematocrit, decreased hemoglobin, decreased partial thromboplastin time, decreased prothrombin time, decreased white blood cell count, delirium, depression, dermal ulcer, eosinophilia, erythema multiforme, gastrointestinal hemorrhage, hallucination, hematuria, hemolytic anemia, hemoperitoneum, hepatic failure, hypertension, hypervolemia, hypochromic anemia, hypokalemia, hypotension, hypoxia, increased blood urea nitrogen, increased lactate dehydrogenase, increased serum alkaline phosphatase, increased serum ALT, increased serum AST, increased serum bilirubin, increased serum creatinine, ileus, intestinal obstruction, jaundice, leukocytosis, leukopenia, myocardial infarction, neutropenia, peripheral edema, pleural effusion, positive direct Coombs test, pulmonary edema, pulmonary embolism, renal failure, seizure, Stevens-Johnson syndrome, tachycardia, toxic epidermal necrolysis, urinary incontinence, vulvovaginal candidiasis

Drug Interactions

Metabolism/Transport Effects None known.

Avoid Concomitant Use

Avoid concomitant use of Meropenem with any of the following: BCG; BCG (Intravesical); Probenecid

Increased Effect/Toxicity

The levels/effects of Meropenem may be increased by: Probenecid

Decreased Effect

Meropenem may decrease the levels/effects of: BCG; BCG (Intravesical); BCG Vaccine (Immunization); Sodium Picosulfate; Typhoid Vaccine; Valproic Acid and Derivatives

Storage/Stability Freshly prepared solutions should be used. However, constituted solutions maintain satisfactory potency under the conditions described below. Solutions should not be frozen.

Store intact vials and unactivated Duplex containers at 20°C to 25°C (68°F to 77°F). Unactivated duplex units with foil strip removed from the drug chamber must be protected from light and used within 7 days at room temperature. Once activated, must be used within 1 hour if stored at room temperature or within 15 hours if stored under refrigeration. Do not freeze.

Dry powder should be stored at controlled room temperature 20°C to 25°C (68°F to 77°F).

Injection reconstitution: Stability in vial when constituted (up to 50 mg/mL) with:

SWFI:

U.S. labeling: Stable for up to 3 hours at up to 25°C (77°F) or for up to 13 hours at up to 5°C (41°F).

Canadian labeling: Stable for up to 3 hours at 15°C to 25°C (59°F to 77°F) or for up to 16 hours at 2°C to 8°C (36°F to 46°F).

Infusion admixture (1 to 20 mg/mL): Solution is stable when diluted in NS for 1 hour at up to 25°C (77°F) or 15 hours at up to 5°C (41°F). Solutions constituted with dextrose injection 5% should be used immediately. **Note:** Meropenem stability (admixed with NS at a concentration of 20 mg/mL) at room temperature for >1 hour or under refrigeration for >15 hours is not supported by the manufacturer. Data exist supporting stability (admixed with NS at a concentration of 20 mg/mL) at room temperature for ≤4 hours and under refrigeration ≤24 hours (Patel, 1997).

Mechanism of Action Inhibits bacterial cell wall synthesis by binding to several of the penicillin-binding proteins, which in turn inhibit the final transpeptidation step of peptidoglycan synthesis in bacterial cell walls, thus inhibiting cell wall biosynthesis; bacteria eventually lyse due to ongoing activity of cell wall autolytic enzymes (autolysins and murein hydrolases) while cell wall assembly is arrested

Pharmacokinetics (Adult data unless noted)

Distribution: Penetrates into most tissues and body fluids including urinary tract, peritoneal fluid, bone, bile, lung, bronchial mucosa, muscle tissue, heart valves, and CSF (CSF penetration: Neonates and Infants ≤3 months: 70%)

V_d:

Neonates and Infants ≤3 months: Median: ~0.47 L/kg (Smith, 2011)

Children: 0.3-0.4 L/kg (Blumer, 1995)

Adults: 15-20 L

Protein binding: 2%

Metabolism: 20% is hydrolyzed in plasma to an inactive metabolite

Half-life:

Neonates and Infants ≤3 months: Median: 2.7 hours; range: 1.6- 3.8 hours (Smith, 2011)

Infants and Children 3 months to 2 years: 1.5 hours

Children 2-12 years and Adults: 1 hour

Time to peak tissue and fluid concentrations: 1 hour after the start of infusion except in bile, lung, muscle, and CSF which peak at 2-3 hours

Elimination: Cleared by the kidney with 70% excreted unchanged in urine

Clearance:

Neonates and Infants ≤3 months: 0.12 L/hour/kg (Smith, 2011)

Infants and Children: 0.26-0.37 L/hour/kg (Blumer, 1995)

Dosing: Neonatal

General dosing, susceptible infection (non-CNS), treatment (Bradley 2014): Limited data available: For organisms highly susceptible to meropenem, MIC <4 mcg/mL:

Body weight ≤2 kg:

PNA ≤14 days: IV: 20 mg/kg/dose every 12 hours

PNA 15 to 28 days: IV: 20 mg/kg/dose every 8 hours

PNA 29 to 60 days: IV: 30 mg/kg/dose every 8 hours

Body weight >2 kg:

PNA ≤14 days: IV: 20 mg/kg/dose every 8 hours

PNA 15 to 60 days: IV: 30 mg/kg/dose every 8 hours

Moderately resistant infection (non-CNS), treatment: For organisms with MIC 4 to 8 mcg/mL: Limited data available: GA >30 weeks, PNA >7 days: 40 mg/kg/dose every 8 hours, some suggest as a 4-hour infusion; dosing based on a single-dose pharmacokinetic study (n=38) (van den Anker 2009)

Intra-abdominal infection, complicated:

GA <32 weeks:

PNA <14 days: IV: 20 mg/kg/dose every 12 hours

PNA ≥14 days: IV: 20 mg/kg/dose every 8 hours

GA ≥32 weeks:

PNA <14 days: IV: 20 mg/kg/dose every 8 hours

PNA ≥14 days: IV: 30 mg/kg/dose every 8 hours

Meningitis: Limited data available: IV: 40 mg/kg/dose every 8 hours (Bradley 2014). An evaluation of CSF concentrations in six patients using the dosing for susceptible infection [see Susceptible infection (non-CNS) dosing] reported levels to be above the target of 4 mcg/mL and highly variable (4.1 to 34.6 mcg/mL) at 0.3 to 7.9 hours (Smith 2011); other suggest using the upper end of the dosing range (van den Anker 2009); recommended duration of therapy dependent upon pathogen: *N. meningitides*, *H. influenza*: 7 days; *S. pneumoniae*: 10 to 14 days; aerobic gram-negative bacilli: Either 2 weeks beyond the first sterile CSF culture or >3 weeks, whichever is longer (Tunkel 2004)

Dosing: Usual

Pediatric:

General dosing, susceptible infection (Bradley 2014): Infants, Children, and Adolescents: Severe infections (non-CNS): IV: 20 mg/kg/dose every 8 hours; maximum dose: 1,000 mg/dose

Cystic fibrosis, pulmonary exacerbation: Limited data available: Infants, Children, and Adolescents: IV: 40 mg/kg/dose every 8 hours; maximum dose: 2,000 mg/dose (Zobell 2012)

Fever/neutropenia empiric treatment: Infants, Children, and Adolescents: IV: 20 mg/kg/dose every 8 hours; maximum dose: 1,000 mg/dose

Intra-abdominal infection, complicated: Note: IDSA guidelines recommend treatment duration of 4 to 7 days (Solomkin 2010)

Infants 1 to <3 months:

GA <32 weeks: IV: 20 mg/kg/dose every 8 hours

GA ≥32 weeks: IV: 30 mg/kg/dose every 8 hours

Infants ≥3 months, Children, and Adolescents: IV: 20 mg/kg/dose every 8 hours; maximum dose: 1,000 mg/dose

Meningitis: Infants (Limited data available <3 months of age), Children, and Adolescents: IV: 40 mg/kg/dose every 8 hours; maximum dose: 2,000 mg/dose (Bradley 2014); duration of therapy dependent upon pathogen: *N. meningitides*, *H. influenza:* 7 days; *S. pneumoniae*: 10 to 14 days; aerobic gram-negative bacilli: 21 days (Tunkel 2004)

Skin and skin structure infection, complicated: Infants ≥3 months, Children, and Adolescents: IV: 10 mg/kg/dose every 8 hours; maximum dose: 500 mg/dose

Adult:

General dosing, susceptible infection: IV: 500 to 2,000 mg every 8 hours

Colangitis, intra-abdominal infections, complicated: IV: 1,000 mg every 8 hours; **Note:** 2010 IDSA guidelines recommend treatment duration of 4 to 7 days (provided source controlled). Not recommended for mild to moderate, community-acquired intra-abdominal infections due to risk of toxicity and the development of resistant organisms (Solomkin 2010).

Meningitis: IV: 2,000 mg every 8 hours; duration of therapy dependent upon pathogen: *N. meningitides*, *H. influenza:* 7 days; *S. pneumoniae:* 10 to 14 days; aerobic gram-negative bacilli: 21 days (Tunkel 2004)

Skin and skin structure infection, complicated: IV:

Pseudomonas aeruginosa-suspected or confirmed: 1,000 mg every 8 hours

Pseudomonas aeruginosa not suspected: 500 mg every 8 hours

Dosing adjustment in renal impairment:

Infants, Children, and Adolescents: There are no dosage adjustments provided in the manufacturer's labeling. Some clinicians have used the following (Aronoff 2007): **Note:** Renally adjusted dose recommendations are based on doses of 20-40 mg/kg/dose every 8 hours:

GFR >50 mL/minute/1.73 m^2: No adjustment required.

GFR 30 to 50 mL/minute/1.73 m^2: Administer 20 to 40 mg/kg/dose every 12 hours

GFR 10 to 29 mL/minute/1.73 m^2: Administer 10 to 20 mg/kg/dose every 12 hours

GFR <10 mL/minute/1.73 m^2: Administer 10 to 20 mg/kg/dose every 24 hours

Intermittent hemodialysis (IHD): Meropenem and metabolite are readily dialyzable: 10 to 20 mg/kg/dose every 24 hours; on dialysis days give dose **after** hemodialysis

Peritoneal dialysis (PD): 10 to 20 mg/kg/dose every 24 hours

Continuous renal replacement therapy (CRRT): 20 to 40 mg/kg/dose every 12 hours

Adult:

CrCl >50 mL/minute: No adjustment required.

CrCl 26 to 50 mL/minute: Administer recommended dose based on indication every 12 hours

CrCl 10 to 25 mL/minute: Administer one-half recommended dose based on indication every 12 hours

CrCl <10 mL/minute: Administer one-half recommended dose based on indication every 24 hours

Intermittent hemodialysis (IHD) (administer after hemodialysis on dialysis days): Meropenem and its metabolites are readily dialyzable: 500 mg every 24 hours. **Note:** Dosing dependent on the assumption of 3 times weekly, complete IHD sessions (Heintz 2009).

Peritoneal dialysis: Administer recommended dose (based on indication) every 24 hours (Aronoff 2007).

Continuous renal replacement therapy (CRRT) (Heintz 2009; Trotman 2005): Drug clearance is highly dependent on the method of renal replacement, filter type, and flow rate. Appropriate dosing requires close monitoring of pharmacologic response, signs of adverse reactions due to drug accumulation, as well as drug concentrations in relation to target trough (if appropriate). The following are general recommendations only (based on dialysate flow/ultrafiltration rates of 1 to 2 L/hour and minimal residual renal function) and should not supersede clinical judgment:

CVVH: Loading dose of 1,000 mg followed by either 500 mg every 8 hours or 1,000 mg every 12 hours

CVVHD/CVVHDF: Loading dose of 1,000 mg followed by either 500 mg every 6 to 8 hours or 1,000 mg every 8 to 12 hours

Note: Consider giving patients receiving CVVHDF dosages of 750 mg every 8 hours or 1500 mg every 12 hours (Heintz 2009). Substantial variability exists in various published recommendations, ranging from 1,000 to 3,000 mg/**day** in 2 to -3 divided doses. One gram every 12 hours achieves a target trough of ~4 mg/L.

Dosing adjustment in hepatic impairment: No adjustment necessary.

Preparation for Administration Parenteral: Reconstitute meropenem 500 mg and 1 g vials with 10 mL and 20 mL SWFI respectively to yield a concentration of 50 mg/mL. For IV infusion, may further dilute with D_5W or NS to a final concentration ranging from 1 to 20 mg/mL.

Administration

Parenteral:

IV push: Pediatric patients ≥3 months and Adults: Administer reconstituted solution (up to 1 g) over 3 to 5 minutes; safety data is limited with 40 mg/kg doses up to a maximum of 2 g

Intermittent IV infusion: Further dilute reconstituted solution prior to administration

Infants <3 months: Administer as an IV infusion over 30 minutes

Infants ≥3 months, Children, Adolescents, and Adults: Administer IV infusion over 15 to 30 minutes

Note: Some studies have demonstrated enhanced pharmacodynamic effects when extending intermittent infusions to 4 hours (van den Anker 2009)

Monitoring Parameters Periodic renal, hepatic, and hematologic function tests. Observe for changes in bowel frequency. Monitor for signs of anaphylaxis during first dose.

Test Interactions Positive Coombs' [direct]

Dosage Forms Excipient information presented when available (limited, particularly for generics); consult specific product labeling.

Solution Reconstituted, Intravenous:

Merrem: 500 mg (1 ea); 1 g (1 ea)

Generic: 500 mg (1 ea); 1 g (1 ea)

◆ **Meropenem For Injection (Can)** *see* Meropenem *on page 1366*

◆ **Merrem** *see* Meropenem *on page 1366*

Mesalamine (me SAL a meen)

Medication Safety Issues

Sound-alike/look-alike issues:

Mesalamine may be confused with mecamylamine, megestrol, memantine, metaxalone, methenamine

Apriso may be confused with Apri

Asacol may be confused with Ansaid, Os-Cal [DSC]
Lialda may be confused with Aldara
Pentasa may be confused with Pancrease, Pangestyme

Related Information

Oral Medications That Should Not Be Crushed or Altered *on page 2476*

Brand Names: US Apriso; Asacol HD; Canasa; Delzicol; Lialda; Pentasa; Rowasa; SfRowasa

Brand Names: Canada Asacol; Asacol 800; Mesasal; Mezavant; Pentasa; Salofalk; Teva-5 ASA

Therapeutic Category 5-Aminosalicylic Acid Derivative; Anti-inflammatory Agent; Anti-inflammatory Agent, Rectal

Generic Availability (US) May be product dependent

Use Treatment and maintenance of remission of ulcerative colitis (UC); treatment of proctosigmoiditis and proctitis (FDA approved in adults; see manufacturer's labeling for specific indications); has also been used for Crohn's disease

Pregnancy Risk Factor B/C (product specific)

Pregnancy Considerations Adverse events were not observed in animal reproduction studies. Dibutyl phthalate (DBP) is an inactive ingredient in the enteric coating of Asacol and Asacol HD; adverse effects in male rats were noted at doses greater than the recommended human dose. Mesalamine is known to cross the placenta. An increased rate of congenital malformations has not been observed in human studies. Preterm birth, still birth and decreased birth weight have been observed; however, these events may also be due to maternal disease. When treatment for inflammatory bowel disease is needed during pregnancy, mesalamine may be used, although products with DBP should be avoided (Habal, 2012; Mottet, 2009).

Breast-Feeding Considerations Low concentrations of the parent drug (undetectable to 0.11 mg/L) and higher concentrations of the N-acetyl metabolite of the parent drug (5-18 mg/L) have been detected in human breast milk following oral or rectal maternal doses of 500 mg to 3 g daily. Adverse effects (diarrhea) in a nursing infant have been reported while the mother received rectal administration of mesalamine within 12 hours after the first dose (Nelis, 1989). The manufacturer recommends that caution be used if administered to a nursing woman. Other sources consider use of mesalamine to be safe while breast-feeding (Habal, 2012; Mottet, 2009).

Contraindications

U.S. labeling: Hypersensitivity to mesalamine, aminosalicylates, salicylates, or any component of the formulation (including suppository vehicle of vegetable fatty acid esters)

Canadian labeling: Hypersensitivity to mesalamine, salicylates, or any component of the formulation; severe renal impairment (GFR <30 mL/minute/1.73 m^2); severe hepatic impairment

Additional contraindications per specific Canadian product labeling: Existing gastric or duodenal ulcer, urinary tract obstruction, use in children <2 years of age (Asacol, Asacol 800, Mesasal, Pentasa, Salofalk); hemorrhagic diathesis (Mesasal); patients unable to swallow intact tablet (Asacol, Asacol 800); renal parenchymal disease (Pentasa)

Warnings/Precautions May cause an acute intolerance syndrome (cramping, acute abdominal pain, bloody diarrhea; sometimes fever, headache, rash); discontinue if this occurs. Use caution in patients with active peptic ulcers. Patients with pyloric stenosis or other gastrointestinal obstructive disorders may have prolonged gastric retention of tablets, delaying the release of mesalamine in the colon. Pericarditis or myocarditis (mesalamine-induced cardiac hypersensitivity reactions) should be considered in patients with chest pain; use with caution in patients predisposed to these conditions. Pancreatitis should be considered in patients with new abdominal discomfort. Symptomatic worsening of colitis/IBD may occur following initiation of therapy. Oligospermia (rare, reversible) has been reported in males. Use caution in patients with sulfasalazine hypersensitivity. Use caution in patients with impaired hepatic function; hepatic failure has been reported. Canadian labeling contraindicates use in severe hepatic impairment. Renal disease (including minimal change nephropathy, acute/chronic interstitial nephritis, nephrotic syndrome, and rarely renal failure) has been reported; use caution with other medications converted to mesalamine. An evaluation of renal function is recommended prior to initiation of mesalamine products and periodically during treatment. Use caution in patients with renal impairment. Canadian labeling contraindicates use in severe renal impairment GFR <30 mL/minute/1.73 m^2; urinary tract obstruction and renal parenchymal disease are also included as contraindications in specific Canadian labels (refer to Contraindications). Use caution with other medications converted to mesalamine. Postmarketing reports suggest an increased incidence of blood dyscrasias in patients >65 years of age. In addition, elderly may have difficulty administering and retaining rectal suppositories or may have decreased renal function; use with caution and monitor.

Apriso contains phenylalanine. The Asacol HD 800 mg tablet has not been shown to be bioequivalent to two Asacol 400 mg tablets [Canadian product] or two Delzicol 400 mg capsules. Canasa suppositories contain saturated vegetable fatty acid esters (contraindicated in patients with allergy to these components). Rowasa, Salofalk [Canadian product] and Pentasa [Canadian product] enema contain metabisulfite salts that may cause severe hypersensitivity reactions (ie, anaphylaxis) in patients with sulfite allergies.

Adverse Reactions Adverse effects vary depending upon dosage form.

Cardiovascular: Chest pain, hypertension, peripheral edema, vasodilation

Central nervous system: Anxiety, chills, dizziness, fatigue, headache (more common in adults), insomnia, malaise, migraine, nervousness, pain, paresthesia, vertigo

Dermatologic: Acne vulgaris, alopecia, diaphoresis, pruritus, skin rash

Endocrine & metabolic: Increased serum triglycerides, weight loss (children and adolescents)

Gastrointestinal: Abdominal distention, abdominal pain, abnormal stools, anorectal pain (on insertion of enema tip), bloody diarrhea (children and adolescents), constipation, diarrhea, dyspepsia, eructation, exacerbation of ulcerative colitis (more common in children and adolescents), flatulence, gastroenteritis, gastrointestinal hemorrhage, hemorrhoids, intolerance syndrome, nausea, pancreatitis (children and adolescents), rectal hemorrhage, rectal pain, sclerosing cholangitis (children and adolescents), tenesmus, vomiting

Genitourinary: Polyuria

Hematologic & oncologic: Hematocrit/hemoglobin decreased

Hepatic: Abnormal hepatic function tests, cholestatic hepatitis, increased serum ALT increased, increased serum transaminases

Hypersensitivity: Anaphylaxis

Infection: Infection, viral infection (adenovirus; children and adolescents)

Neuromuscular & skeletal: Arthralgia, arthritis, back pain, hypertonia, musculoskeletal pain (leg/joint), myalgia, weakness

Ophthalmic: Conjunctivitis, visual disturbance

Otic: Otalgia, tinnitus

Renal: Decreased creatinine clearance, hematuria

Respiratory: Bronchitis, cough, dyspnea, flu-like symptoms, nasopharyngitis (more common in children and adolescents), pharyngitis, rhinitis, sinusitis (more common in children and adolescents)

Miscellaneous: Fever

Rare but important or life-threatening: Abdominal distention, abnormal T waves on ECG, agranulocytosis, albuminuria, alopecia, anemia, angioedema, aplastic anemia, cholecystitis, cholestatic jaundice, DRESS syndrome, drug fever, dysuria, edema, eosinophilia, eosinophilic pneumonitis, erythema nodosum, exacerbation of asthma, fecal discoloration, frequent bowel movements, granulocytopenia, Guillain-Barré syndrome, hepatic failure, hepatic injury, hepatic necrosis, hepatitis, hepatotoxicity, hypersensitivity pneumonitis, hypersensitivity reactions, idiopathic nephrotic syndrome, increased blood urea nitrogen, increased serum bilirubin, increased serum creatinine, interstitial nephritis, interstitial pneumonitis, jaundice, Kawasaki-like syndrome, leukopenia, lupus-like syndrome, lymphadenopathy, mucus stools, myocarditis, nephrotoxicity, neutropenia, oligospermia, painful defecation, palpitations, pancytopenia, paresthesia, perforated peptic ulcer, perianal skin irritation, pericardial effusion, pericarditis, peripheral neuropathy, pharyngolaryngeal pain, pleurisy, pneumonitis, pruritus, pulmonary interstitial fibrosis, pyoderma gangrenosum, rectal discharge, rectal polyp, renal disease, renal failure, skin photosensitivity, Stevens-Johnson syndrome, systemic lupus erythematosus, tachycardia, tenesmus, thrombocythemia, thrombocytopenia, transverse myelitis, vasodilation

Drug Interactions

Metabolism/Transport Effects None known.

Avoid Concomitant Use There are no known interactions where it is recommended to avoid concomitant use.

Increased Effect/Toxicity

Mesalamine may increase the levels/effects of: Heparin; Heparin (Low Molecular Weight); Thiopurine Analogs; Varicella Virus-Containing Vaccines

The levels/effects of Mesalamine may be increased by: Nonsteroidal Anti-Inflammatory Agents

Decreased Effect

Mesalamine may decrease the levels/effects of: Cardiac Glycosides

The levels/effects of Mesalamine may be decreased by: Antacids; H2-Antagonists; Proton Pump Inhibitors

Storage/Stability

Capsule:

Apriso: Store between 20°C to 25°C (68°F to 77°F)

Delzicol: Store between 20°C to 25°C (68°F to 77°F); excursions permitted between 15°C and 30°C (59°F and 86°F).

Pentasa: Store between 15°C to 30°C (59°F to 86°F). Protect from light.

Enema: Store at room temperature. Use promptly once foil wrap is removed. Contents may darken with time (do not use if dark brown).

Suppository: Store below 25°C (below 77°F). May store under refrigeration; do not freeze. Protect from direct heat, light, and humidity.

Tablet: Store at room temperature:

Asacol HD: 20°C to 25°C (68°F to 77°F); excursions permitted between 15°C and 30°C (59°F and 86°F).

Asacol, Asacol 800 [Canadian products]: 15°C to 30°C (59°F to 86°F)

Lialda: 15°C to 30°C (59°F to 86°F)

Mezavant [Canadian product]: 15°C to 25°C (59°F to 77°F)

Mechanism of Action Mesalamine (5-aminosalicylic acid) is the active component of sulfasalazine; the specific mechanism of action of mesalamine is unknown; however, it is thought that it modulates local chemical mediators of the inflammatory response, especially leukotrienes, and is also postulated to be a free radical scavenger or an inhibitor of tumor necrosis factor (TNF); action appears topical rather than systemic

Pharmacokinetics (Adult data unless noted)

Absorption:

Oral: Capsule: ~20% to 40%; Tablet: 20% to 28%

Rectal: Variable and dependent upon retention time, underlying GI disease, and colonic pH

Protein binding: Mesalamine (5-ASA): ~43%; N-acetyl-5-ASA: ~78%

Metabolism: Hepatic and via GI tract to N-acetyl-5-aminosalicylic acid

Half-life:

5-ASA: 0.5-15 hours

N-acetyl-5-ASA: 2-15 hours

Time to peak serum concentration:

Oral: Capsule: Apriso™: ~4 hours; Pentasa®: 3 hours

Tablet: Asacol® HD: 10-16 hours; Lialda®: 9-12 hours

Rectal: 4-7 hours

Elimination: Most metabolites are excreted in urine (<8% as unchanged drug); feces (<2%)

Dosing: Usual

Children and Adolescents:

Crohn's disease; treatment (mild to moderate disease); maintenance of remission: Limited data available: Oral: 50-100 mg/kg/day divided every 6-12 hours (Fish, 2004); maximum dose: 1 **g**/dose

Ulcerative colitis (including proctitis); treatment (mild to moderate disease); induction and maintenance of remission: Limited data available: Usual course of therapy is 3-8 weeks: Oral: 30-60 mg/kg/day divided every 6-12 hours; doses as high as 100 mg/kg/day have been used; maximum daily dose: 4 **g**/day (Baldassano, 1999; Fish, 2004; Leichtner, 1995; Tomomasa, 2004)

Older Children and Adolescents: Rectal:

Enema (Rowasa): 4 **g** once daily at bedtime (Baldassano, 1999)

Suppository (Rowasa): 500 mg once daily at bedtime; some have used twice daily (Baldassano, 1999; Heyman, 2010)

Adults:

Ulcerative colitis:

Treatment: Oral: Usual course of therapy is 3-8 weeks:

Capsule (Pentasa®): 1 **g** 4 times daily; **Note:** Apriso™ capsules are approved for maintenance of remission only.

Tablet: Initial:

Asacol® HD: 1.6 **g** 3 times daily for 6 weeks

Lialda®: 2.4-4.8 **g** once daily for up to 8 weeks

Maintenance of remissions: Oral:

Capsule:

Apriso™: 1.5 **g** once daily in the morning

Pentasa®: 1 **g** 4 times daily

Tablet: Lialda®: 2.4 **g** once daily

Note: Asacol® HD tablets are approved for treatment only.

Distal ulcerative colitis, proctosigmoiditis, or proctitis (mild to moderate), treatment: Retention enema: Adults: 60 mL (4 **g**) at bedtime, retained overnight, ~8 hours

Ulcerative proctitis, treatment: Rectal suppository (Canasa®): Adults: Insert 1 suppository (1000 mg) in rectum once daily at bedtime; retained for at least 1-3 hours to achieve maximum benefit

Note: Duration of rectal therapy is 3-6 weeks; some patients may require rectal and oral therapy concurrently.

Administration

Oral: Swallow tablets or capsules whole; do not break, chew, or crush

Capsule:

Apriso™: Administer with or without food; do not administer with antacids. The capsule should be swallowed whole per the manufacturer's labeling; however, opening the capsule and placing the contents (delayed release granules) on food with a pH <6 is not expected to affect the release of mesalamine once ingested (data on file, Salix Pharmaceuticals Medical Information). There is no safety/efficacy information regarding this practice. The contents of the capsules should not be chewed or crushed.

Pentasa®: If a patient is unable to swallow the capsule, some clinicians support opening the capsules and placing the contents (controlled release beads) on yogurt or peanut butter (Crohn's & Colitis Foundation of America). There are currently no published data evaluating the safety/efficacy of this practice. The contents of the capsules should not be chewed or crushed.

Tablet: Do not break outer coating of Asacol® HD or Lialda® tablets; Lialda®: Should be administered with a meal.

Rectal:

Enema: Shake well before use; retain enema for 8 hours or as long as practical

Suppository: Avoid excessive handling; retain suppository for at least 1-3 hours for maximum benefit

Test Interactions May cause falsely-elevated urinary normetanephrine levels when measured by liquid chromatography with electrochemical detection (due to similarity in the chromatograms of normetanephrine and mesalamine's main metabolite, N-acetylaminosalicylic acid).

Dosage Forms Excipient information presented when available (limited, particularly for generics); consult specific product labeling.

Capsule Delayed Release, Oral:

Delzicol: 400 mg

Capsule Extended Release, Oral:

Pentasa: 250 mg [contains brilliant blue fcf (fd&c blue #1), fd&c yellow #10 (quinoline yellow)]

Pentasa: 500 mg [contains brilliant blue fcf (fd&c blue #1)]

Capsule Extended Release 24 Hour, Oral:

Apriso: 0.375 g [contains aspartame]

Enema, Rectal:

SfRowasa: 4 g/60 mL (60 mL) [sulfite free; contains edetate disodium, sodium benzoate]

Generic: 4 g (60 mL)

Kit, Rectal:

Rowasa: 4 g [contains edetate disodium, potassium metabisulfite, sodium benzoate]

Generic: 4 g

Suppository, Rectal:

Canasa: 1000 mg (30 ea, 42 ea)

Tablet Delayed Release, Oral:

Asacol HD: 800 mg

Lialda: 1.2 g

◆ **Mesalazine** *see* Mesalamine *on page 1368*

◆ **Mesasal (Can)** *see* Mesalamine *on page 1368*

M-Eslon (Can) *see* Morphine (Systemic) *on page 1461*

Mesna (MES na)

Brand Names: US Mesnex

Brand Names: Canada Mesna for injection; Uromitexan

Therapeutic Category Antidote; Antidote, Cyclophosphamide-induced Hemorrhagic Cystitis; Antidote, Ifosfamide-induced Hemorrhagic Cystitis; Chemoprotectant Agent

Generic Availability (US) May be product dependent

Use Detoxifying agent used as a protectant against ifosfamide-induced hemorrhagic cystitis (Oral: FDA approved in adults; parenteral: FDA approved in pediatric patients [age not specified] and adults); has also been used as a protectant against cyclophosphamide-induced hemorrhagic cystitis

Pregnancy Risk Factor B

Pregnancy Considerations Adverse effects were not observed in animal reproduction studies. Use during pregnancy only if clearly needed.

Breast-Feeding Considerations It is not known if mesna is excreted in breast milk. Benzyl alcohol, a component in some formulations, does enter breast milk and may be absorbed by a nursing infant. Due to the potential for adverse reactions in the nursing infant, a decision should be made to discontinue breast-feeding or to discontinue mesna, taking into account the importance of treatment to the mother.

Contraindications Hypersensitivity to mesna or any component of the formulation

Warnings/Precautions Monitor urine for hematuria. Severe hematuria despite utilization of mesna may require ifosfamide dose reduction or discontinuation. Examine morning urine specimen for hematuria prior to ifosfamide or cyclophosphamide treatment; if hematuria (>50 RBC/HPF) develops, reduce the ifosfamide/cyclophosphamide dose or discontinue the drug; will not prevent hemorrhagic cystitis in all patients. Mesna will not reduce the risk of hematuria related to thrombocytopenia. Patients should receive adequate hydration during treatment. Mesna is intended for the prevention of hemorrhagic cystitis and will not prevent or alleviate other toxicities associated with ifosfamide or cyclophosphamide.

Hypersensitivity reactions have been reported; symptoms ranged from mild hypersensitivity to systemic anaphylactic reactions and may include fever, hypotension, tachycardia, acute renal impairment, hypoxia, respiratory distress, urticaria, angioedema, signs of disseminated intravascular coagulation, hematologic abnormalities, increased liver enzymes, nausea, vomiting, arthralgia, and myalgia. Reactions may occur with the first exposure, or after several months of treatment. Monitor for signs/symptoms of reactions. May require discontinuation. Patients with autoimmune disorders receiving cyclophosphamide and mesna may be at increased risk. Mesna is a thiol compound; it is unknown if the risk for reaction is increased in patients who have had a reaction to other thiol compounds (eg, amifostine). Drug rash with eosinophilia and systemic symptoms and bullous/ulcerative skin and mucosal reactions consistent with Stevens-Johnson syndrome (SJS) or toxic epidermal necrolysis (TEN) have been reported. The skin and mucosal reactions may be characterized by rash, pruritus, urticaria, erythema, burning sensation, angioedema, periorbital edema, flushing, and stomatitis. Reactions may occur with the first exposure, or after several months of treatment. May require discontinuation.

Benzyl alcohol and derivatives: Some dosage forms may contain benzyl alcohol; large amounts of benzyl alcohol (≥99 mg/kg/day) have been associated with a potentially fatal toxicity ("gasping syndrome") in neonates; the "gasping syndrome" consists of metabolic acidosis, respiratory distress, gasping respirations, CNS dysfunction (including convulsions, intracranial hemorrhage), hypotension, and cardiovascular collapse (AAP, 1997; CDC, 1982); some data suggests that benzoate displaces bilirubin from protein binding sites (Ahlfors, 2001); avoid or use dosage forms containing benzyl alcohol with caution in neonates. See manufacturer's labeling.

Adverse Reactions

Mesna alone (frequency not defined):

Cardiovascular: Flushing

Central nervous system: Dizziness, fever, headache, hyperesthesia, somnolence

Dermatologic: Rash

Gastrointestinal: Anorexia, constipation, diarrhea, flatulence, nausea, taste alteration/bad taste (with oral administration), vomiting

Local: Injection site reactions

Neuromuscular: Arthralgia, back pain, rigors

Ocular: Conjunctivitis

Respiratory: Cough, pharyngitis, rhinitis

Miscellaneous: Flu-like syndrome

Mesna alone or in combination: Rare but important or life-threatening: Allergic reaction, anaphylactic reaction, hypersensitivity, hyper-/hypotension, injection site erythema, injection site pain, limb pain, malaise, myalgia, platelets decreased, ST-segment increased, tachycardia, tachypnea, transaminases increased

Drug Interactions

Metabolism/Transport Effects None known.

Avoid Concomitant Use There are no known interactions where it is recommended to avoid concomitant use.

Increased Effect/Toxicity There are no known significant interactions involving an increase in effect.

Decreased Effect There are no known significant interactions involving a decrease in effect.

Storage/Stability Store intact vials and tablets at room temperature of 20°C to 25°C (68°F to 77°F); excursions are permitted between 15°C and 30°C (59°F and 86°F). Opened multidose vials may be stored and used for use up to 8 days after initial puncture. Solutions diluted for infusion stored at room temperature should be used within 24 hours. According to the manufacturer, mesna and ifosfamide may be mixed in the same bag if the final ifosfamide concentration is ≤50 mg/mL. Solutions of mesna and ifosfamide (1:1) in NS at a concentration of up to 20 mg/mL are stable for 14 days in PVC bags (Zhang, 2014). Solutions of mesna (0.5 to 3.2 mg/mL) and cyclophosphamide (1.8 to 10.8 mg/mL) in D_5W are stable for 48 hours refrigerated or 6 hours at room temperature (Menard, 2003). Mesna injection prepared for oral administration is stable for at least 9 days undiluted in polypropylene syringes and stored at 5°C, 24°C, 35°C; for 7 days when diluted 1:2 or 1:5 with syrups and stored at 24°C in capped tubes; or for 24 hours at 5°C when diluted to 1:2, 1:10, and 1:100 in orange or apple juice, milk, or carbonated beverages (Goren, 1991).

Mechanism of Action In blood, mesna is oxidized to dimesna which in turn is reduced in the kidney back to mesna, supplying a free thiol group which binds to and inactivates acrolein, the urotoxic metabolite of ifosfamide and cyclophosphamide

Pharmacokinetics (Adult data unless noted)

Distribution: 0.65 ± 0.24 L/kg; distributed to total body water

Protein binding: 69% to 75%

Metabolism: Rapidly oxidized to mesna disulfide (dimesna) in the intravascular compartment. Mesna and dimesna do not undergo hepatic metabolism.

Bioavailability: Oral: Free mesna: 58% (range: 45% to 71%); not affected by food

Half-life: Mesna: ~22 minutes; Dimesna: ~70 minutes

Elimination: Urine (32% as mesna; 33% as dimesna); majority of IV dose excreted within 4 hours

Dosing: Usual

Pediatric: **Note:** Dose, frequency, number of doses, and start date may vary by protocol and treatment phase. Refer to individual protocols.

Prevention of ifosfamide-induced hemorrhagic cystitis: Mesna dosing schedule should be repeated each day ifosfamide is received according to protocol. If ifosfamide dose is adjusted (decreased or increased), the mesna dose should also be modified to maintain the mesna-to-ifosfamide ratio

Infants, Children, and Adolescents:

Standard-dose ifosfamide: **Note:** ASCO defin standard-dose ifosfamide IV as <2500 mg/m²/d (Hensley, 2009); other pediatric oncology expe suggest ≤2000 mg/m²/day in protocols. ASC defines standard-dose ifosfamide oral ≤2000 mg/m²/day (Hensley, 2009; Schuchter, 200

Manufacturer's labeling: IV: Mesna dose is equal 20% of the ifosfamide dose given for 3 doses: W the ifosfamide dose (hour 0), at hour 4, and at hc 8 after the ifosfamide dose (total daily mesna do is 60% of the ifosfamide dose). **Note:** Safety a efficacy not established for ifosfamide dos >2000 mg/m²/day.

Alternate dosing: Limited data available:

IV:

Short IV infusion (intermittent): ASCO guidelin Mesna dose equal to 60% of the ifosfamide do given in 3 divided doses (20% each) 15 minut before the ifosfamide dose and at 4 and 8 hou after the start of ifosfamide (Hensley, 2009)

Continuous IV infusion: Dosing regimens variab ASCO guidelines: Mesna dose (as an IV bolu equal to 20% of the ifosfamide dose, followed a continuous IV infusion of mesna at 40% of t ifosfamide dose; continue mesna infusion for to 24 hours after completion of ifosfamide inf sion (Hensley, 2009). Some centers have used mesna dose equal to 60% to 100% of t ifosfamide dose as a continuous IV infusi beginning 15 to 30 minutes before the fi ifosfamide dose and completed at least 8 hou after the end of the ifosfamide infusion (Mosk witz, 2001).

Oral: ASCO guidelines: Total mesna dose equal 100% of the ifosfamide dose, begin with IV do equal to 20% for initial dose followed by oral do at 40% of the ifosfamide dose at 2 and 6 hou after start of ifosfamide (Hensley, 2009); **Not** Typically, oral doses of mesna are twice t IV dose.

High-dose ifosfamide: **Note:** ASCO defines high do as ifosfamide dosage ≥2500 mg/m²/day (Hensle 2009); other pediatric oncology experts sugge ≥2000 mg/m²/day in protocols: Limited data ava able; dosing regimens variable: IV: ASCO conside evidence for use inadequate and dosing recomme dations are not established; more frequent and pr longed mesna administration regimens may b required (Hensley, 2009). Some centers have use a mesna dose equal to 100% of the ifosfamide do as a short IV infusions 5 divided doses (0, 3, 6, 9 ar 12) hours after the start of ifosfamide) (Kliegma 2007) or as a continuous IV infusion beginning 15 30 minutes before the first ifosfamide dose ar completed at least 12 hours after the end of t ifosfamide infusion.

Other dosing strategies have been used in combin tion with ifosfamide for specific regimens/protocol Limited data available:

Mesna continuous IV infusion: Children and Adole cents: IV: 1800 mg/m²/day to 5000 mg/m²/day as continuous infusion (100% of the ifosfamide dose repeated each day ifosfamide is received; se protocols for specific details (Bacci, 2003; Kol 2003; Moskowitz, 2001)

Mesna IV bolus followed by continuous IV infusio Children and Adolescents: IV: 1000 mg/m² 1 ho prior to ifosfamide on day 1, followed b 3000 mg/m²/day continuous infusion (continuou infusion is 100% of the ifosfamide dose) on da 1, 2, and 3 (with sufficient hydration); administ with subsequent ifosfamide doses (Juergens, 2006)

Mesna (20% higher than ifosfamide) continuous IV infusion: Children and Adolescents: IV: 3600 mg/m^2/day continuous infusion for 4 days (mesna dose is 20% higher than ifosfamide), with hydration, administer with subsequent ifosfamide doses (Le Deley, 2007)

Prevention of cyclophosphamide-induced hemorrhagic cystitis: Limited data available: **Note:** Specific protocols should be consulted for combination regimens with cyclophosphamide. Mesna dosing schedule is typically repeated with each day cyclophosphamide is received; mesna dosing should be adjusted if cyclophosphamide dose is adjusted (decreased or increased) to maintain the mesna-to-cyclophosphamide ratio for the protocol.

Infants, Children, and Adolescents:

Standard (low)-dose cyclophosphamide: **Note:** Some pediatric oncology experts have defined as cyclophosphamide dose <1800 mg/m^2/day in protocols.

IV: Reported regimens variable: Mesna doses equivalent usually 60% to 100% of the cyclophosphamide daily dose although some protocols have used up to 160%.

Short IV infusion (intermittent): Mesna dose equal to 60% of the cyclophosphamide dose given in 3 divided doses (0, 4, and 8 hours after the start of cyclophosphamide) has been used by some centers; others have used a mesna dose equal to 100% of the cyclophosphamide dose as short IV infusions in 5 divided doses (0, 3, 6, 9, and 12 hours after the start of cyclophosphamide) (Kliegman, 2007)

Continuous IV infusion: Some centers have used a mesna dose equal to 60% of the cyclophosphamide dose as a continuous IV infusion beginning 15 to 30 minutes before the first cyclophosphamide dose and completed at least 8 hours after the end of the cyclophosphamide infusion.

Oral: Some centers have used a total mesna dose equal to 100% of the cyclophosphamide dose, begin with IV dose equal to 20% for initial dose followed by oral dose at 40% of the cyclophosphamide dose at 2 and 6 hours after start of cyclophosphamide; **Note:** Typically, oral doses of mesna are twice the IV dose.

High-dose cyclophosphamide: **Note:** Some pediatric oncology experts have defined cyclophosphamide dose ≥1800 mg/m^2/day in protocols: IV: Some centers have used a mesna dose equal to 100% of the cyclophosphamide dose as short IV infusions in 5 divided doses (0, 3, 6, 9, and 12 hours after the start of) (Kliegman, 2007) or as a continuous IV infusion beginning 15 to 30 minutes before the first cyclophosphamide dose

Other dosing strategies have been used in combination with cyclophosphamide for specific regimens/protocols: Limited data available: HDCAV/IE regimen for Ewing sarcoma: Children and Adolescents: IV: 2100 mg/m^2/day continuous infusion (mesna dose is equivalent to the cyclophosphamide dose) for 2 days with cyclophosphamide infusion during cycles 1, 2, 3, and 6 (Kolb, 2003)

Adult: **Note:** Mesna dosing schedule should be repeated each day ifosfamide is received. If ifosfamide dose is adjusted (decreased or increased), the mesna dose should also be modified to maintain the mesna-to-ifosfamide ratio.

Prevention of ifosfamide-induced hemorrhagic cystitis:

Standard-dose ifosfamide (manufacturer's labeling): IV: Mesna dose is equal to 20% of the ifosfamide dose given for 3 doses: With the ifosfamide dose, hour 4, and at hour 8 after of the ifosfamide dose (total daily mesna dose is 60% of the ifosfamide dose)

Oral mesna (following I.V mesna; for ifosfamide doses ≤2 g/m^2/day): Mesna dose (IV) is equal to 20% of the ifosfamide dose at hour 0, followed by mesna dose (orally) equal to 40% of the ifosfamide dose given 2 and 6 hours after the ifosfamide dose (total daily mesna dose is 100% of the ifosfamide dose). **Note:** If the oral mesna dose is vomited within 2 hours of administration, repeat the dose or administer IV mesna.

Short infusion standard dose ifosfamide (<2.5 g/m^2/day): ASCO guidelines: IV: Total mesna dose is equal to 60% of the ifosfamide dose, in 3 divided doses (each mesna dose as 20% of ifosfamide dose), given 15 minutes before the ifosfamide dose, and 4 and 8 hours after each dose of ifosfamide (Hensley, 2009)

Continuous infusion standard dose ifosfamide (<2.5 g/m2/day): ASCO guidelines: IV: Mesna dose (as a bolus) is equal to 20% of the ifosfamide dose, followed by a continuous infusion of mesna at 40% of the ifosfamide dose; continue mesna infusion for 12 to 24 hours after completion of ifosfamide infusion (Hensley, 2009)

High-dose ifosfamide (>2.5 g/m^2/day): ASCO guidelines: Evidence for use is inadequate; more frequent and prolonged mesna administration regimens may be required (Hensley, 2009)

Dosing adjustment in renal impairment: There are no dosage adjustments provided in the manufacturer's labeling (has not been studied).

Dosing adjustment in hepatic impairment: There are no dosage adjustments provided in the manufacturer's labeling (has not been studied).

Preparation for Administration

Oral: In patients not able to swallow tablets, a solution may be prepared with parenteral solution for injection by diluting in syrup, juice (grape, apple, tomato, orange), carbonate beverages, or milk (including chocolate) (most palatable in chilled grape juice) (Goren, 1991); see Extemporaneous Preparations section.

Parenteral: IV: Further dilute in D_5W, NS, $D_5{}^1/_4NS$, $D_5{}^1/_3NS$, $D_5{}^1/_2NS$, or LR to a final concentration ≤20 mg/mL.

Administration

Oral: Administer orally in tablet form or dilute mesna injection solution for oral use before oral administration to decrease sulfur odor; see Extemporaneously Preparation section. Patients who vomit within 2 hours after taking oral mesna should repeat the dose or receive IV mesna.

Parenteral: Administer as an IV bolus (per manufacturer); current guidelines suggest administration by short IV infusion over 15 to 30 minutes, or by continuous IV infusion (maintain continuous infusion for 12 to 24 after completion of ifosfamide infusion) (Hensley 2009); in some trials, a shorter duration (eg, 8 hours) has been reported (Moskowitz 2001); refer to specific protocol for administration rate and details.

Monitoring Parameters Urinalysis, urine color; monitor for hypersensitivity reactions

Test Interactions

Urinary ketones: False-positive tests for urinary ketones may occur in patients receiving mesna with the use of nitroprusside-based urine tests, including dipstick tests.

CPK activity: Mesna may interfere with enzymatic creatine kinase (CPK) activity tests which use a thiol compound (eg, N-acetylcysteine) for CPK reactivation; may result in a falsely low CPK level.

Ascorbic acid: Mesna may result in false-positive reactions in Tillman's reagent-based urine screening tests for ascorbic acid.

Additional Information A preservative-free formulation of Mesnex injection may be obtained directly from the manufacturer. It is restricted for use in infants and children <2 years and others who are sensitive to benzyl alcohol. Contact the manufacturer (Bristol-Meyers Squibb) for additional information.

Dosage Forms Excipient information presented when available (limited, particularly for generics); consult specific product labeling.

Solution, Intravenous:

Mesnex: 100 mg/mL (10 mL) [contains benzyl alcohol, edetate disodium]

Generic: 100 mg/mL (10 mL)

Tablet, Oral:

Mesnex: 400 mg [scored]

Extemporaneous Preparations An oral solution may be prepared from mesna solution for injection. Dilute solution for injection to 20 mg/mL or 50 mg/mL with orange or grape syrup. Prior to administration, syrup-diluted solutions may be diluted to a final concentration of 1, 10, or 50 mg/mL with any of the following: carbonated beverages, apple juice, orange juice, or milk. Mesna injection prepared for oral administration is stable for at least 9 days undiluted in polypropylene syringes and stored at 5°C, 24°C, 35°C; for 7 days when diluted 1:2 or 1:5 with syrups and stored at 24°C in capped tubes; or for 24 hours at 5°C when diluted to 1:2, 1:10, and 1:100 in orange or apple juice, milk, or carbonated beverages. Dilution of mesna with diet or sugar-free preparations has not been evaluated.

Goren MP, Lyman BA, Li JT. The stability of mesna in beverages and syrup for oral administration. *Cancer Chemother Pharmacol*. 1991;28 (4):298-301.

- **Mesna for injection (Can)** *see* Mesna *on page 1371*
- **Mesnex** *see* Mesna *on page 1371*
- **Mestinon** *see* Pyridostigmine *on page 1808*
- **Mestinon-SR (Can)** *see* Pyridostigmine *on page 1808*
- **Metadate CD** *see* Methylphenidate *on page 1402*
- **Metadate ER** *see* Methylphenidate *on page 1402*
- **Metadol (Can)** *see* Methadone *on page 1379*
- **Metadol-D (Can)** *see* Methadone *on page 1379*
- **Metamucil® (Can)** *see* Psyllium *on page 1804*
- **Metamucil MultiHealth Fiber [OTC]** *see* Psyllium *on page 1804*

Metaproterenol (met a proe TER e nol)

Medication Safety Issues

Sound-alike/look-alike issues:

Metaproterenol may be confused with metipranolol, metoprolol

Alupent may be confused with Atrovent®

Brand Names: Canada Apo-Orciprenaline®; ratio-Orciprenaline®; Tanta-Orciprenaline®

Therapeutic Category Adrenergic Agonist Agent; Antiasthmatic; Beta$_2$-Adrenergic Agonist; Bronchodilator; Sympathomimetic

Generic Availability (US) Yes

Use Bronchodilator in reversible airway obstruction due to asthma or COPD (FDA approved in ages ≥6 years and adults)

Pregnancy Risk Factor C

Pregnancy Considerations Adverse events were observed in some animal reproduction studies. Beta agonists, including metaproterenol, may interfere with uterine contractility if administered during labor; maternal and fetal tachycardia have been observed (Baillie, 1970; Tyack, 1971).

Uncontrolled asthma is associated with adverse events on pregnancy (increased risk of perinatal mortality, preeclampsia, preterm birth, low birth weight infants). Oral beta$_2$-receptor agonists are not recommended to treat asthma during pregnancy (NAEPP, 2005).

Breast-Feeding Considerations It is not known if metaproterenol is excreted into breast milk. Although breast-feeding is not recommended by the manufacturer, the use of beta$_2$-receptor agonists are not considered a contraindication to breast-feeding (NAEPP, 2005).

Contraindications Hypersensitivity to metaproterenol or any component of the formulation; pre-existing cardiac arrhythmias associated with tachycardia

Warnings/Precautions Use beta$_2$-agonists with caution in patients with cardiovascular disease (arrhythmia or hypertension or HF), convulsive disorders, diabetes, glaucoma, hyperthyroidism, or hypokalemia. Beta-agonists may cause elevation in blood pressure, heart rate, and result in CNS stimulation/excitation. Beta$_2$-agonists may increase risk of arrhythmia, increase serum glucose, or decrease serum potassium. Immediate hypersensitivity reactions (urticaria, angioedema, rash, bronchospasm) have been reported.

Asthma: Appropriate use: Metaproterenol (a less selective beta$_2$-agonist) is not recommended in the management of asthma due to potential for excessive cardiac stimulation (NAEPP, 2007). Oral systemic agents (eg, tablets, syrup) should be avoided due to increased risk of adverse effects (eg, excessive cardiac stimulation).

Chronic obstructive lung disease (COPD): Appropriate use: Inhaled bronchodilators are preferred therapy for COPD exacerbations; oral systemic agents (eg, tablets, syrup) should be avoided due to increased risk of adverse effects (eg, excessive cardiac stimulation).

Benzyl alcohol and derivatives: Some dosage forms may contain sodium benzoate/benzoic acid; benzoic acid (benzoate) is a metabolite of benzyl alcohol; large amounts of benzyl alcohol (≥99 mg/kg/day) have been associated with a potentially fatal toxicity ("gasping syndrome") in neonates; the "gasping syndrome" consists of metabolic acidosis, respiratory distress, gasping respirations, CNS dysfunction (including convulsions, intracranial hemorrhage), hypotension, and cardiovascular collapse (AAP, 1997; CDC, 1982); some data suggests that benzoate displaces bilirubin from protein binding sites (Ahlfors, 2001); avoid or use dosage forms containing benzyl alcohol derivative with caution in neonates. See manufacturer's labeling.

Adverse Reactions

Cardiovascular: Palpitation, tachycardia

Central nervous system: Dizziness, fatigue, headache, insomnia, nervousness

Neuromuscular & skeletal: Tremor

Gastrointestinal: Diarrhea, nausea

Respiratory: Asthma exacerbation

Rare but important or life-threatening: Chest pain, diaphoresis, edema, facial/finger edema, hives, hypertension, laryngeal changes, spasms, syncope, vomiting, weakness

Drug Interactions

Metabolism/Transport Effects None known.

Avoid Concomitant Use

Avoid concomitant use of Metaproterenol with any of the following: Beta-Blockers (Nonselective); Iobenguane I 123; Loxapine

Increased Effect/Toxicity

Metaproterenol may increase the levels/effects of: Atosiban; Loop Diuretics; Loxapine; Sympathomimetics; Thiazide Diuretics

The levels/effects of Metaproterenol may be increased by: AtoMOXetine; Cannabinoid-Containing Products; Linezolid; MAO Inhibitors; Tedizolid; Tricyclic Antidepressants

Decreased Effect

Metaproterenol may decrease the levels/effects of: Iobenguane I 123

The levels/effects of Metaproterenol may be decreased by: Beta-Blockers (Beta1 Selective); Beta-Blockers (Nonselective); Betahistine

Storage/Stability Store at room temperature; protect from light. Protect tablets from moisture.

Mechanism of Action Stimulates $beta_2$-receptors which increases the conversion of adenosine triphosphate (ATP) to 3'-5'-cyclic adenosine monophosphate (cAMP), resulting in bronchial smooth muscle relaxation

Pharmacodynamics

Onset of bronchodilation: Within 30 minutes

Maximum effect: Within 1 hour

Duration: (~1-5 hours) regardless of route administered

Pharmacokinetics (Adult data unless noted)

Absorption: Oral: Well absorbed

Metabolism: Extensive first-pass in the liver (~40% of oral dose is available)

Elimination: Mainly as glucuronic acid conjugates

Dosing: Usual

Oral:

Infants and Children:

<2 years: 0.4 mg/kg/dose 3-4 times daily; in infants, the dose can be given every 8-12 hours

2-5 years: 1.3-2.6 mg/kg/**day** divided every 6-8 hours; maximum: 10 mg/dose

Children ≥6 years and Adolescents:

<27 kg: 10 mg 3-4 times daily

≥27 kg: 20 mg 3-4 times daily

Adults: 20 mg 3-4 times daily

Administration Administer with food to decrease GI distress

Monitoring Parameters Heart rate, respiratory rate, blood pressure, arterial or capillary blood gases if applicable, pulmonary function tests

Dosage Forms Excipient information presented when available (limited, particularly for generics); consult specific product labeling.

Syrup, Oral, as sulfate:

Generic: 10 mg/5 mL (473 mL)

Tablet, Oral, as sulfate:

Generic: 10 mg, 20 mg

◆ **Metaproterenol Sulfate** *see* Metaproterenol *on page 1374*

MetFORMIN (met FOR min)

Medication Safety Issues

Sound-alike/look-alike issues:

MetFORMIN may be confused with metroNIDAZOLE

Glucophage may be confused with Glucotrol, Glutofac

High alert medication:

The Institute for Safe Medication Practices (ISMP) includes this medication among its list of drugs that have a heightened risk of causing significant patient harm when used in error.

International issues:

Dianben [Spain] may be confused with Diovan brand name for valsartan [U.S., Canada, and multiple international markets].

Glucon brand name for metformin [Malaysia, Singapore] is also the brand name for glucosamine [Singapore]

Related Information

Oral Medications That Should Not Be Crushed or Altered *on page 2476*

Brand Names: US Fortamet; Glucophage; Glucophage XR; Glumetza; Riomet

Brand Names: Canada ACT-Metformin; Apo-Metformin; Auro-Metformin; Ava-Metformin; Dom-Metformin; ECL-Metformin; Glucophage; Glumetza; Glycon; JAMP-Metformin; JAMP-Metformin Blackberry; Mar-Metformin; Metformin FC; Mint-Metformin; Mylan-Metformin; PHL-Metformin; PMS-Metformin; PRO-Metformin; Q-Metformin; RAN-Metformin; ratio-Metformin; Riva-Metformin; Sandoz-Metformin FC; Septa-Metformin; Teva-Metformin

Therapeutic Category Antidiabetic Agent, Biguanide; Antidiabetic Agent, Oral; Hypoglycemic Agent, Oral

Generic Availability (US) May be product dependent

Use Management of type 2 diabetes mellitus (noninsulin-dependent, NIDDM) when hyperglycemia cannot be managed with diet and exercise alone (Immediate release [tablets, oral solution]: FDA approved in ages ≥10 years and adults; extended release: Fortamet, Glucophage XR: FDA approved in ages ≥17 years and adults; Glumetza: FDA approved in ages ≥18 years and adults); has also been used for weight loss in pediatric patients with severe obesity and insulin resistance in conjunction with a comprehensive lifestyle weight management program.

Note: If not contraindicated and if tolerated, metformin is the preferred initial pharmacologic agent for type 2 diabetes management (ADA 2000; ADA 2014; AAP [Copeland 2013]).

Pregnancy Risk Factor B

Pregnancy Considerations Adverse events have not been observed in animal reproduction studies. Metformin has been found to cross the placenta in concentrations which may be comparable to those found in the maternal plasma. Pharmacokinetic studies suggest that clearance of metformin may increase during pregnancy and dosing may need adjusted in some women when used during the third trimester (Charles 2006; de Oliveira Baraldi 2011; Eyal 2010; Gardiner 2003; Hughes 2006; Vanky 2005).

An increased risk of birth defects or adverse fetal/neonatal outcomes has not been observed following maternal use of metformin for GDM or type 2 diabetes when glycemic control is maintained (Balani 2009; Coetzee 1979; Coetzee 1984; Ekpebegh 2007; Niromanesh 2012; Rowan 2008; Rowan 2010; Tertti 2008). In women with diabetes, maternal hyperglycemia can be associated with congenital malformations as well as adverse effects in the fetus, neonate, and the mother (ACOG 2005; ADA 2015; Kitzmiller 2008; Metzger 2007). To prevent adverse outcomes, prior to conception and throughout pregnancy maternal blood glucose and HbA_{1c} should be kept as close to target goals as possible but without causing significant hypoglycemia (ACOG 2013; ADA 2015; Blumer 2013; Kitzmiller 2008). Prior to pregnancy, effective contraception should be used until glycemic control is achieved (Kitzmiller 2008).

Metformin may be used to treat GDM when nonpharmacologic therapy is not effective in maintaining glucose control (ACOG 2013). Metformin or lifestyle intervention may also be used in women with a history of GDM who later develop prediabetes in order to prevent or delay type 2 diabetes (ADA 2015).

Metformin is recommended to treat insulin resistance associated with PCOS; however, its use may also restore spontaneous ovulation. Women with PCOS who do not desire to become pregnant should use effective contraception. Although studied for use in women with anovulatory PCOS, there is no evidence that it improves live birth rates or decreases pregnancy complications. Routine use to treat infertility related to PCOS is not currently recommended (ACOG 2009; Fauser 2012).

Breast-Feeding Considerations Low amounts of metformin (generally ≤1% of the weight-adjusted maternal dose) are excreted into breast milk. Small amounts of metformin have been detected in the serum of nursing infants. Because breast milk concentrations of metformin stay relatively constant, avoiding nursing around peak plasma concentrations in the mother would not be helpful in reducing metformin exposure to the infant (Briggs 2005; Eyal 2010; Gardiner 2003; Hale 2002).

According to the manufacturer, due to the potential for hypoglycemia in the nursing infant, a decision should be made whether to discontinue nursing or to discontinue the drug, taking into account the importance of treatment to the mother. Breast-feeding is encouraged for all women, including those with diabetes (ACOG 2005; Blumer 2013; Metzger 2007). Small snacks before feeds may help decrease the risk of hypoglycemia in women with pregestational diabetes (ACOG 2005; Reader 2004); metformin may be used in breast-feeding women (Blumer 2013).

Contraindications

US labeling: Hypersensitivity to metformin or any component of the formulation; renal disease or renal dysfunction (serum creatinine ≥1.5 mg/dL in males or ≥1.4 mg/dL in females) or abnormal creatinine clearance from any cause, including shock, acute myocardial infarction, or septicemia; acute or chronic metabolic acidosis with or without coma (including diabetic ketoacidosis)

Canadian labeling: Hypersensitivity to metformin or any component of the formulation; renal function unknown, renal impairment, and serum creatinine levels above the upper limit of normal range; renal disease or renal dysfunction (serum creatinine ≥136 micromol/L in males or ≥124 micromol/L in females or abnormal creatinine clearance <60 mL/minute) which may result from conditions such as cardiovascular collapse (shock), acute myocardial infarction, and septicemia; unstable and/or insulin-dependent (type I) diabetes mellitus; history of ketoacidosis with or without coma; history of lactic acidosis (regardless of precipitating factors); excessive alcohol intake (acute or chronic); severe hepatic dysfunction or clinical or laboratory evidence of hepatic disease; cardiovascular collapse and disease states associated with hypoxemia including cardiorespiratory insufficiency, which are often associated with hyperlactacidemia; stress conditions (eg, severe infection, trauma, surgery and postoperative recovery phase); severe dehydration; pregnancy; breast-feeding

Note: The manufacturer recommends to temporarily discontinue metformin in patients undergoing radiologic studies in which intravascular iodinated contrast media are utilized.

Warnings/Precautions [US Boxed Warning]: Lactic acidosis is a rare, but potentially severe consequence of therapy with metformin that requires urgent care and hospitalization. The risk is increased in patients with acute congestive heart failure, dehydration, excessive alcohol intake, hepatic or renal impairment, or sepsis. Symptoms may be nonspecific (eg, abdominal distress, malaise, myalgia, respiratory distress, somnolence); low pH, increased anion gap and elevated blood lactate may be observed. Discontinue immediately if acidosis is suspected. Lactic acidosis should be suspected in any patient with diabetes receiving metformin with evidence of acidosis but without evidence of ketoacidosis. Discontinue metformin in patients with conditions associated with dehydration, sepsis, or hypoxemia. The risk of accumulation and lactic acidosis increases with the degree of impairment of renal function. Use caution in patients with congestive heart failure requiring pharmacologic management, particularly in patients with unstable or acute CHF; risk of lactic acidosis may be increased secondary to hypoperfusion.

Metformin is substantially excreted by the kidney. The risk of accumulation and lactic acidosis increases with the degree of impairment of renal function. Patients with renal function below the limit of normal for their age should not receive metformin. Metformin should be withheld in patients with prerenal azotemia. In elderly patients, renal function should be monitored regularly; do not initiate in patients ≥80 years of age unless normal renal function is confirmed; risk of lactic acidosis may be increased. Use of concomitant medications that may affect renal function (ie, affect tubular secretion) may also affect metformin disposition. Therapy should be suspended for any surgical procedures (Canadian labeling recommends discontinuing use 48 hours prior to surgical procedures excluding minor procedures not associated with restricted food and fluid intake). Restart only after normal oral intake resumed and normal renal function is verified. Due to the risk of acute alteration in renal function, the manufacturer's labeling states to temporarily discontinue metformin prior to or at the time of intravascular administration of iodinated contrast media, withhold for 48 hours after the radiologic study and restart only after renal function has been confirmed as normal. The American College of Radiology (ACR) guidelines also recommend to temporarily discontinue metformin at the time of contrast injection but only for certain patients: Patients with known renal dysfunction (and withhold until renal function monitoring assures safe reinstitution) and patients with normal renal function, but with multiple comorbidities (liver dysfunction, alcohol abuse, cardiac failure, myocardial/peripheral muscle ischemia, sepsis, severe infection) (and withhold for 48 hours). In patients with normal renal function and no known comorbidities, ACR states that discontinuation of metformin is not necessary (ACR 2013). It may be necessary to discontinue metformin and administer insulin if the patient is exposed to stress (fever, trauma, infection, surgery).

Use with caution in patients with impaired liver function. Patient must be instructed to avoid excessive acute or chronic ethanol use; ethanol may potentiate metformin's effect on lactate metabolism. May impair vitamin B_{12} absorption, particularly in those with inadequate vitamin B_{12} or calcium intake/absorption; very rarely associated with anemia. Rapid reversal of vitamin B12 deficiency may be observed with discontinuation of therapy or supplementation. Monitor vitamin B_{12} serum concentrations periodically with long-term therapy. Administration of oral antidiabetic drugs has been reported to be associated with increased cardiovascular mortality; metformin does not appear to share this risk. Potentially significant interactions may exist, requiring dose or frequency adjustment, additional monitoring, and/or selection of alternative therapy. Insoluble tablet shell of Glumetza 1,000 mg extended release tablet may remain intact and be visible in the stool. Other extended released tablets (Fortamet, Glucophage XR, Glumetza 500 mg) may appear in the stool as a soft mass resembling the tablet. Diabetes self-management education (DSME) is essential to maximize the effectiveness of therapy. Not indicated for use in patients with insulin-dependent diabetes mellitus (IDDM) (type 1) or for the treatment of diabetic ketoacidosis.

Warnings: Additional Pediatric Considerations Vitamin B_{12} serum concentrations may decrease to suboptimal levels with metformin use; although clinical manifestations do not usually appear, in very rare instances anemia has occurred; anemia is rapidly reversed with vitamin B_{12} supplementation or discontinuation of metformin.

Adverse Reactions

Cardiovascular: Chest discomfort, flushing, palpitation

Central nervous system: Chills, dizziness, headache, lightheadedness

Dermatologic: Rash
Endocrine & metabolic: Hypoglycemia
Gastrointestinal: Abdominal discomfort, abdominal distention, abnormal stools, constipation, diarrhea, dyspepsia, flatulence, heartburn, indigestion, nausea, taste disorder, vomiting
Neuromuscular & skeletal: Myalgia, weakness
Respiratory: Dyspnea, upper respiratory tract infection
Miscellaneous: Decreased vitamin B_{12} levels, flu-like syndrome, increased diaphoresis, nail disorder
Rare but important or life-threatening: Lactic acidosis, leukocytoclastic vasculitis, megaloblastic anemia, pneumonitis

Drug Interactions

Metabolism/Transport Effects **Substrate** of OCT2

Avoid Concomitant Use

Avoid concomitant use of MetFORMIN with any of the following: Alcohol (Ethyl)

Increased Effect/Toxicity

MetFORMIN may increase the levels/effects of: Dalfampridine; Dofetilide; Hypoglycemia-Associated Agents

The levels/effects of MetFORMIN may be increased by: Alcohol (Ethyl); Alpha-Lipoic Acid; Androgens; BuPROPion; Carbonic Anhydrase Inhibitors; Cephalexin; Cimetidine; Dalfampridine; Dolutegravir; Glycopyrrolate; Iodinated Contrast Agents; LamoTRIgine; MAO Inhibitors; Pegvisomant; Quinolone Antibiotics; Ranolazine; Salicylates; Selective Serotonin Reuptake Inhibitors; Topiramate; Trimethoprim; Vandetanib

Decreased Effect

MetFORMIN may decrease the levels/effects of: Trospium

The levels/effects of MetFORMIN may be decreased by: Hyperglycemia-Associated Agents; Quinolone Antibiotics; Thiazide Diuretics; Verapamil

Food Interactions Food decreases the extent and slightly delays the absorption. Management: Administer with a meal.

Storage/Stability

Oral solution: Store at 15°C to 30°C (59°F to 86°F).
Tablets: Store at 20°C to 25°C (68°F to 77°F); excursion permitted to 15°C to 30°C (59°F to 86°F). Protect from light and moisture.

Mechanism of Action Decreases hepatic glucose production, decreasing intestinal absorption of glucose and improves insulin sensitivity (increases peripheral glucose uptake and utilization)

Pharmacodynamics Onset of action: Within days, maximum effects up to 2 weeks

Pharmacokinetics (Adult data unless noted)

Distribution: V_d: 654 ± 358 L; partitions into erythrocytes
Protein binding: Plasma: Negligible
Metabolism: Not metabolized by the liver
Bioavailability: Absolute: Fasting: 50% to 60%
Half-life elimination: Plasma: 6.2 hours; blood ~17.6 hours
Time to peak serum concentration: Immediate release: 2 to 3 hours; extended release: Median: 7 hours (range: 4 to 8 hours)
Elimination: Urine (90% as unchanged drug; active secretion)

Dosing: Usual

Pediatric:

Diabetes mellitus, type 2; treatment: Note: Allow 1 to 2 weeks between dose titrations. Generally, clinically significant responses are not seen at doses less than 1,500 mg/day to 2,000 mg/day (AAP [Copeland 2013]); however, a lower recommended starting dose with a gradual increase in dosage is recommended to minimize gastrointestinal symptoms

Oral:

Immediate release tablet or solution:

Manufacturer's labeling:

Children and Adolescents 10 to 16 years: Initial: 500 mg twice daily; increase dose in increments of 500 mg at weekly intervals; maximum daily dose: 2,000 mg/**day**.

Adolescents: ≥17 years:

Twice daily regimen: Initial: 500 mg twice daily; increase daily dose in increments of 500 mg/day in 2 divided doses at weekly intervals; may also titrate from 500 mg twice a day to 850 mg twice a day after 2 weeks; recommended maximum daily dose: 2,550 mg/**day**; if a dose >2,000 mg daily is required, it may be better tolerated if given in 3 divided doses

Once daily regimen: Initial: 850 mg once daily; increase daily dose in increments of 850 mg/day every other week; maximum daily dose: 2,550 mg/**day**

Alternate dosing: Children and Adolescents 10 to <18 years: Initial: 500 mg once daily for 7 days, then increase in 500 mg increments at 1- to 2-week intervals to a target dose of 1,000 mg twice daily (AAP [Copeland 2013]; ISPAD [Zeitzler 2014])

Extended-release tablets: **Note:** If glycemic control is not achieved at maximum dose, may divide dose and administer twice daily.

Children and Adolescents 10 to 16 years: Limited data available: Initial: 500 mg once daily; dosage may be increased by 500 mg at 1- to 2-week intervals; maximum daily dose: 2,000 mg/**day** (AAP [Copeland 2013]; ISPAD [Zeitzler 2014])

Adolescents ≥17 years:

Fortamet: Adolescents ≥17 years: Initial: 500 to 1,000 mg once daily; dosage may be increased by 500 mg weekly; maximum daily dose: 2,500 mg/**day**

Glucophage XR: Adolescents ≥17 years: Initial: 500 mg once daily; dosage may be increased by 500 mg weekly; maximum daily dose: 2,000 mg/**day**

Glumetza: Adolescents ≥18 years: Initial: 1,000 mg once daily; dosage may be increased by 500 mg weekly; maximum daily dose: 2,000 mg/**day**

Obesity: Severe, adjunct therapy with lifestyle interventions: Limited data available; data has shown modest efficacy (BMI reduction ~3%); optimal treatment duration not established; most trials 6 to 12 months in duration with largest BMI change usually observed in the first 3 to 4 months of therapy; a daily multivitamin supplement may be considered with therapy (AHA [Kelly 2013]; Matson 2012; McDonagh 2014): Oral:

Immediate release: Dosing regimens variable: Children ≥6 years and Adolescents: Initial: 500 mg once **or** twice daily, titrate upward at weekly intervals by 500 mg/day increments to a target dose of 1,000 mg administered in the morning and 500 mg in the evening or 1000 mg twice daily (Kendall 2013; Yanovski 2011); several other trials have reported doses of 500 mg twice daily dosing (Matson 2012)

Extended release: Metformin XR: Adolescents: Initial: 500 mg once daily with dinner for 2 weeks; increase to 1,000 mg once daily for 2 weeks, and then 2,000 mg once daily; may slow titration if adverse gastrointestinal effects; treatment continued for 4 months (Glaser Pediatric Research Network [Wilson 2010])

Adult:

Management of type 2 diabetes mellitus: Note: Allow 1 to 2 weeks between dose titrations: Generally, clinically significant responses are not seen at doses <1,500 mg daily; however, a lower recommended starting dose and gradual increased dosage is recommended to minimize gastrointestinal symptoms. Oral:

Immediate release tablet or solution: Initial: 500 mg twice daily or 850 mg once daily; titrate in increments of 500 mg weekly or 850 mg every other week; may also titrate from 500 mg twice a day to 850 mg twice a day after 2 weeks. If a dose >2,000 mg daily is required, it may be better tolerated in 3 divided doses; maximum daily dose: 2,550 mg/day

Extended release tablet: **Note**: If glycemic control is not achieved at maximum dose, may divide dose and administer twice daily.

Fortamet: Initial: 500 to 1,000 mg once daily; dosage may be increased by 500 mg weekly; maximum daily dose: 2,500 mg/**day**

Glucophage XR: Initial: 500 mg once daily; dosage may be increased by 500 mg weekly; maximum daily dose: 2,000 mg/**day**

Glumetza: Initial: 1,000 mg once daily; dosage may be increased by 500 mg weekly; maximum daily dose: 2,000 mg/**day**

Transfer from other antidiabetic agents: No transition period is generally necessary except when transferring from chlorpropamide. When transferring from chlorpropamide, care should be exercised during the first 2 weeks because of the prolonged retention of chlorpropamide in the body, leading to overlapping drug effects and possible hypoglycemia.

Concomitant metformin and oral sulfonylurea therapy: If patients have not responded to 4 weeks of the maximum dose of metformin monotherapy, consider a gradual addition of an oral sulfonylurea, even if prior primary or secondary failure to a sulfonylurea has occurred. Continue metformin at the maximum dose. If adequate response has not occurred following 3 months of metformin and sulfonylurea combination therapy, consider switching to insulin with or without metformin.

Failed sulfonylurea therapy: Patients with prior failure on glyburide may be treated by gradual addition of metformin. Initiate with glyburide 20 mg and metformin 500 mg daily. Metformin dosage may be increased by 500 mg/day at weekly intervals, up to a maximum metformin dose (dosage of glyburide maintained at 20 mg daily).

Concomitant metformin and insulin therapy: Initial: 500 mg metformin once daily, continue current insulin dose; increase by 500 mg metformin weekly until adequate glycemic control is achieved

Maximum daily metformin dose: Immediate release and solution: 2,550 mg/**day**; Extended release: 2,000 to 2,500 mg/**day** (varies by product)

Decrease insulin dose 10% to 25% when FPG <120 mg/dL; monitor and make further adjustments as needed

Dosing adjustment in renal impairment:

Children ≥10 years and Adolescents:

Serum creatinine (S_{cr}) ≥1.5 mg/dL (males) or ≥1.4 mg/dL (females): Use is contraindicated.

Abnormal CrCl: Use is contraindicated.

Adults:

Manufacturer's labeling:

Serum creatinine (S_{cr}) ≥1.5 mg/dL (males) or ≥1.4 mg/dL (females): Use is contraindicated.

Abnormal CrCl: Use is contraindicated.

Alternate dosing: **Note:** The United Kingdom National Institute for Health and Clinical Excellence (NICE) Guidelines recommends prescribing metformin with caution in those patients who are at risk of sudden deterioration in renal function and at risk of an estimated glomerular filtration rate (eGFR) <45 mL/minute/1.73 m^2 (National Collaborating Centre [NICE 2008]). Some evidence suggests that use of metformin is unsafe when eGFR <30 ml/minute/1.73 m^2 (calculated using MDRD) (Shaw 2007). A review of the available data by members of the American Diabetes Association proposed the following recommendations based on eGFR (Lipska 2011):

eGFR ≥60 mL/minute/1.73 m^2: No contraindications; monitor renal function annually

eGFR ≥45 to <60 mL/minute/1.73 m^2: Continue use; monitor renal function every 3 to 6 months

eGFR ≥30 to <45 mL/minute/1.73 m^2: In patients currently receiving metformin, use with caution, consider dosage reduction (eg, 50% reduction or 50% of maximal dose), monitor renal function every 3 months. Do not initiate therapy in patients with eGFR <45 mL/minute/1.73 m^2

eGFR <30 mL/minute/1.73 m^2: Discontinue use.

Dosing adjustment in hepatic impairment: Children ≥10 years, Adolescents, and Adults: Avoid metformin; liver disease is a risk factor for the development of lactic acidosis during metformin therapy.

Administration Administer with a meal (to decrease GI upset).

Immediate release: Glucophage, Riomet: Administer in divided doses with meals

Extended release: Fortamet, Glucophage XR, Glumetza: Administer with evening meal; swallow whole; do not cut, crush, or chew; Fortamet should also be administered with a full glass of water

Monitoring Parameters Blood glucose (frequency based on patient-specific factors), hemoglobin A_{1c} (every 3 months; AAP [Copeland 2013]) and fructosamine, initial and periodic monitoring of hemoglobin, hematocrit, and red blood cell indices; renal function (baseline and annually); urine for glucose and ketones. While megaloblastic anemia has been rarely seen with metformin, if suspected, vitamin B_{12} deficiency should be excluded.

Reference Range Indicators of optimal glycemic control: **Note:** Targets must be adjusted based on individual needs/circumstances (eg, patients who experience severe hypoglycemia, patients with hypoglycemic unawareness):

Children ≥10 years and Adolescents:

Blood glucose, fasting and preprandial:

Children 10 to <12 years: <126 mg/dL (ADA 2000)

Children ≥12 years and Adolescents: 70 to 130 mg/dL (AAP [Copeland AAP 2013])

Glycosylated hemoglobin (hemoglobin A_{1c}): <6.5 to 7%; individual goals may be targeted based on patient-specific characteristics (ADA 2000; AAP [Copeland 2013]; ISPAD [Zeitzler 2014])

Adult (ADA 2014):

Blood glucose: Fasting and preprandial: 70 to 130 mg/dL; Peak postprandial capillary blood glucose: <180 mg/dL

Glycosylated hemoglobin (hemoglobin A_{1c}): <7% (a more aggressive [<6.5%] or less aggressive [<8%] HbA_{1c} goal may be targeted based on patient-specific characteristics)

Additional Information In a significant trial, Treatment Options for Type 2 Diabetes in Adolescents and Youth (TODAY) results showed that metformin monotherapy is inadequate at maintaining durable glycemic control in the majority of pediatric patients 10 to 17 years; metformin combined with rosiglitazone was superior than metformin monotherapy and metformin along with intensive lifestyle changes was intermediate (AAP [Copeland 2013];

Narasimhan 2014; TODAY Study Group 2013). Pediatric patients may require early aggressive therapy that is not defined at present (AAP [Copeland 2013]). Rosiglitazone therapy is associated with severe cardiovascular effects in adult patients.

Dosage Forms Considerations Extended release tablets utilize differing release mechanisms: Glucophage XR uses dual hydrophilic polymer matrix systems, Fortamet uses single-composition osmotic technology, and Glumetza uses gastric retention technology.

Dosage Forms Excipient information presented when available (limited, particularly for generics); consult specific product labeling.

Solution, Oral, as hydrochloride:
- Riomet: 500 mg/5 mL (118 mL, 473 mL) [contains propylene glycol; strawberry flavor]
- Riomet: 500 mg/5 mL (118 mL, 473 mL) [contains saccharin calcium; cherry flavor]

Tablet, Oral, as hydrochloride:
- Glucophage: 500 mg, 850 mg
- Glucophage: 1000 mg [scored]
- Generic: 500 mg, 850 mg, 1000 mg

Tablet Extended Release 24 Hour, Oral, as hydrochloride:
- Fortamet: 500 mg, 1000 mg
- Glucophage XR: 500 mg, 750 mg
- Glumetza: 500 mg, 1000 mg
- Generic: 500 mg, 750 mg, 1000 mg

◆ **Metformin FC (Can)** *see* MetFORMIN *on page 1375*

◆ **Metformin Hydrochloride** *see* MetFORMIN *on page 1375*

Methadone (METH a done)

Medication Safety Issues

Sound-alike/look-alike issues:

Methadone may be confused with dexmethylphenidate, ketorolac, Mephyton, methylphenidate, Metadate CD, Metadate ER, metolazone, morphine

High alert medication:

The Institute for Safe Medication Practices (ISMP) includes this medication among its list of drug classes which have a heightened risk of causing significant patient harm when used in error.

Related Information

Opioid Conversion Table *on page 2285*

Patient Information for Disposal of Unused Medications *on page 2453*

Brand Names: US Dolophine; Methadone HCl Intensol; Methadose; Methadose Sugar-Free

Brand Names: Canada Metadol; Metadol-D; Methadose

Therapeutic Category Analgesic, Narcotic

Generic Availability (US) Yes

Use Management of moderate to severe pain unresponsive to nonopioids; used in opioid detoxification maintenance programs and for the treatment of iatrogenic opioid dependency

Prescribing and Access Restrictions When used for treatment of opioid addiction: May only be dispensed in accordance to guidelines established by the Substance Abuse and Mental Health Services Administration's (SAMHSA) Center for Substance Abuse Treatment (CSAT). Regulations regarding methadone use may vary by state and/or country. Obtain advice from appropriate regulatory agencies and/or consult with pain management/palliative care specialists.

Note: Regulatory Exceptions to the General Requirement to Provide Opioid Agonist Treatment (per manufacturer's labeling):

1. During inpatient care, when the patient was admitted for any condition other than concurrent opioid addiction, to facilitate the treatment of the primary admitting diagnosis.
2. During an emergency period of no longer than 3 days while definitive care for the addiction is being sought in an appropriately licensed facility.

Medication Guide Available Yes

Pregnancy Risk Factor C

Pregnancy Considerations Adverse events were observed in animal reproduction studies. Methadone crosses the placenta and can be detected in cord blood, amniotic fluid, and newborn urine.

Methadone is considered the standard of care when treating opioid addiction in pregnant women. Women receiving methadone for the treatment of addiction should be maintained on their daily dose of methadone in addition to receiving the same pain management options during labor and delivery as opioid-naïve women; maintenance doses of methadone will not provide adequate pain relief. Narcotic agonist-antagonists should be avoided for the treatment of labor pain in women maintained on methadone due to the risk of precipitating acute withdrawal (ACOG, 2012; Dow, 2012).

Data is available related to fetal/neonatal outcomes following maternal use of methadone during pregnancy. Information collected by the Teratogen Information System is complicated by maternal use of illicit drugs, nutrition, infection, and psychosocial circumstances. However, pregnant women in methadone treatment programs are reported to have improved fetal outcomes compared to pregnant women using illicit drugs. Fetal growth, birth weight, length, and/or head circumference may be decreased in infants born to opioid-addicted mothers treated with methadone during pregnancy. Growth deficits do not appear to persist; however, decreased performance on psychometric and behavioral tests has been found to continue into childhood. Abnormal fetal nonstress tests have also been reported.

[U.S. Boxed Warning]: Prolonged maternal use of opioids during pregnancy can cause neonatal withdrawal syndrome in the newborn, which may be life-threatening if not recognized and treated according to protocols developed by neonatology experts. If prolonged opioid therapy is required in a pregnant woman, ensure treatment is available and warn patient of risk to the neonate. Withdrawal symptoms in the neonate may be observed up to 2 to 4 weeks after delivery and should be expected (ACOG, 2012). Neonatal abstinence syndrome following opioid exposure may present with autonomic (eg, fever, temperature instability), gastrointestinal (eg, diarrhea, vomiting, poor feeding/weight gain), or neurologic (eg, high-pitched crying, increased muscle tone, irritability, seizure, tremor) symptoms (Dow, 2012; Hudak, 2012). Monitoring is recommended for neonates born to mothers receiving methadone for neonatal abstinence syndrome (Chou, 2014).

Methadone clearance in pregnant women is increased and half-life is decreased during the 2nd and 3rd trimesters of pregnancy; the dosage of methadone may need increased or dosing interval decreased during pregnancy to avoid withdrawal symptoms in the mother. Dosage may need decreased following delivery (ACOG, 2012).

Long-term opioid use may cause secondary hypogonadism, which may lead to sexual dysfunction or infertility (Brennan, 2013). Amenorrhea may also develop secondary to substance abuse; pregnancy may occur following the initiation of buprenorphine or methadone maintenance treatment. Contraception counseling is recommended to prevent unplanned pregnancies (Dow, 2012).

Breast-Feeding Considerations Methadone is excreted into breast milk; the dose to a nursing infant has been calculated to be 2% to 3% of the maternal dose (following oral doses of 10 to 80 mg/day). Peak methadone levels appear in breast milk 4 to 5 hours after an oral dose. Methadone has been detected in the plasma of some breast-fed infants whose mothers are taking methadone. Sedation and respiratory depression have been reported in nursing infants. The manufacturer recommends that women monitor their nursing infants for sedation and that they should be instructed as to when to contact their healthcare provider for emergency care. In addition, the manufacturer recommends slowly weaning to prevent withdrawal symptoms in the nursing infant.

When methadone is used to treat opioid addiction in nursing women, guidelines do not contraindicate breastfeeding as long as the infant is tolerant to the dose and other contraindications do not exist (ACOG, 2012). If additional illicit substances are being abused, women treated with methadone should pump and discard breast milk until sobriety is established (ACOG, 2012; Dow, 2012).

Contraindications

Hypersensitivity to methadone or any component of the formulation; significant respiratory depression; acute or severe bronchial asthma (in the absence of resuscitative equipment or in an unmonitored setting) or hypercarbia; known or suspected paralytic ileus; concurrent use of selegiline (Emsam product labeling)

Methadone is not to be used on an as-needed basis; it is not for pain that is mild or not expected to persist; it is not for acute pain or postoperative pain.

Canadian labeling: Additional contraindications (not in U.S. labeling): Diarrhea associated with pseudomembranous colitis or caused by poisoning until toxic material has been eliminated from the gastrointestinal tract

Warnings/Precautions The optimal analgesic dose varies widely among patients. Doses should be titrated to pain relief/prevention. Patients maintained on stable doses of methadone may need rescue doses of a immediate release analgesic in case of acute pain (eg, postoperative pain, physical trauma). Methadone is ineffective for the relief of anxiety. May cause CNS depression, which may impair physical or mental abilities. Patients must be cautioned about performing tasks which require mental alertness (eg, operating machinery or driving). Effects may be potentiated when used with other CNS depressants (eg, sedatives, anxiolytics, hypnotics, neuroleptics, other opioids). Contraindicated in patients with respiratory depression and in those with conditions that increase the risk of life-threatening respiratory depression. Use with caution and monitor for respiratory depression in patients with significant chronic obstructive pulmonary disease or cor pulmonale, and patients having a substantially decreased respiratory reserve, hypoxia, hypercarbia, or preexisting respiratory depression, particularly when initiating therapy and titrating with methadone; even therapeutic doses may decrease respiratory drive to the point of apnea. Consider the use of alternative nonopioid analgesics in these patients. Use with caution in patients with depression or suicidal tendencies, or in patients with a history of drug or ethanol abuse. Avoid use of methadone in patients with CNS depression or coma as these patients are susceptible to intracranial effects of CO_2 retention. Use with caution in patients with head injury or increased intracranial pressure; reduced respiratory drive and resultant CO_2 retention may increase intracranial pressure. Elderly may be more susceptible to adverse effects (eg, CNS, respiratory, gastrointestinal). Decrease initial dose and use caution in the elderly, debilitated or cachectic; with hyper/hypothyroidism, morbid obesity, adrenal insufficiency, prostatic hyperplasia, or urethral stricture; or with severe renal or hepatic failure. Should only be prescribed by healthcare professionals who are knowledgeable in the use of potent opioids for chronic pain management.

[U.S. Boxed Warning]: QTc interval prolongation and serious arrhythmias (eg, torsades de pointes) have occurred during treatment. Closely monitor patients during initiation and titration for changes in cardiac rhythm. Patients should be informed of the potential arrhythmia risk, evaluated for any history of structural heart disease, arrhythmia, syncope, and for existence of potential drug interactions including drugs that possess QTc interval-prolonging properties, promote hypokalemia, hypomagnesemia, or hypocalcemia, or reduce elimination of methadone (eg, CYP3A4 inhibitors). Obtain baseline ECG for all patients and risk stratify according to QTc interval; QTc interval prolongation and torsades de pointes may be associated with doses >200 mg/day, but have also been observed with lower doses. Other agents should be used in patients with a baseline QTc interval ≥500 msecs (Chou, 2014).

Potentially significant drug-drug interactions may exist requiring dose or frequency adjustment, additional monitoring, and/or selection of alternative therapy. May cause severe hypotension; use caution with severe volume depletion or other conditions which may compromise maintenance of normal blood pressure. Use caution with cardiovascular disease or patients predisposed to dysrhythmias. Concurrent use of mixed agonist/antagonist analgesics (eg, pentazocine, nalbuphine, butorphanol) or partial agonist (eg, buprenorphine) analgesics may precipitate withdrawal symptoms and/or reduced analgesic efficacy in patients following prolonged therapy with mu opioid agonists. Abrupt discontinuation following prolonged use may also lead to withdrawal symptoms. Abrupt cessation may precipitate withdrawal symptoms. Gradually taper dose. **[U.S. Boxed Warning]: When used for treatment of opioid addiction:** May only be dispensed by certified opioid treatment programs. Exceptions include inpatient treatment of other conditions and emergency period (not >3 days) while definitive substance abuse treatment is being sought.

Benzyl alcohol and derivatives: Some dosage forms may contain sodium benzoate/benzoic acid; benzoic acid (benzoate) is a metabolite of benzyl alcohol; large amounts of benzyl alcohol (≥99 mg/kg/day) have been associated with a potentially fatal toxicity ("gasping syndrome") in neonates; the "gasping syndrome" consists of metabolic acidosis, respiratory distress, gasping respirations, CNS dysfunction (including convulsions, intracranial hemorrhage), hypotension, and cardiovascular collapse (AAP, 1997; CDC, 1982); some data suggests that benzoate displaces bilirubin from protein binding sites (Ahlfors, 2001); avoid or use dosage forms containing benzyl alcohol derivative with caution in neonates. See manufacturer's labeling.

Oral formulations:

[U.S. Boxed Warning]: May cause serious, life-threatening, or fatal respiratory depression. Monitor closely for respiratory depression, especially during initiation or dose escalation. Carbon dioxide retention from opioid-induced respiratory depression can exacerbate the sedating effects of opioids. Peak respiratory depressant effect of methadone occurs later and persists longer than the peak analgesic effect, particularly during the initial dosing phase. Misuse or abuse (chewing, swallowing, snorting, or injecting the dissolved product) causes uncontrolled medication delivery resulting in a significant risk of overdose and death. Incomplete cross tolerance may occur; patients tolerant to other mu opioid agonists may not be tolerant to methadone.

[U.S. Boxed Warning]: Prolonged maternal use of opioids during pregnancy can cause neonatal withdrawal syndrome in the newborn which may be life-threatening if not recognized and treated according to protocols developed by neonatology experts. If prolonged opioid therapy is required in a pregnant woman, ensure treatment is available and warn patient of risk to the neonate. Signs and symptoms include irritability, hyperactivity and abnormal sleep pattern, high pitched cry, tremor, vomiting, diarrhea, and failure to gain weight. Onset, duration, and severity depend on the drug used, duration of use, maternal dose, and rate of drug elimination by the newborn. **[U.S. Boxed Warning]: Users are exposed to the risks of addiction, abuse, and misuse, potentially leading to overdose and death. Assess each patient's risk prior to prescribing; monitor all patients regularly for development of these behaviors or conditions.** Risk of opioid abuse is increased in patients with a history or family history of alcohol or drug abuse or mental illness. **[U.S. Boxed Warning]: Accidental ingestion of even one dose, especially in children, can result in a fatal overdose of methadone.** Use with caution in patients with biliary tract dysfunction including acute pancreatitis; may cause constriction of sphincter of Oddi. May obscure diagnosis or clinical course of patients with acute abdominal conditions. Avoid use in gastrointestinal obstruction.

Soluble tablets (diskets): **[U.S. Boxed Warning]: For oral administration only;** excipients to deter use by injection are contained in tablets.

Adverse Reactions During prolonged administration, adverse effects may decrease over several weeks; however, constipation and sweating may persist.

Cardiovascular: Bigeminy, bradycardia, cardiac arrest, cardiac arrhythmia, cardiac failure, cardiomyopathy, ECG changes, edema, extrasystoles, flushing, hypotension, inversion T wave on ECG, orthostatic hypotension, palpitations, peripheral vasodilation, phlebitis, prolonged Q-T interval on ECG, shock, syncope, tachycardia, torsades de pointes, ventricular fibrillation, ventricular tachycardia

Central nervous system: Agitation, confusion, disorientation, dizziness, drowsiness, drug dependence (physical dependence), dysphoria, euphoria, habituation, hallucination, headache, insomnia, sedation, seizure

Dermatologic: Diaphoresis, hemorrhagic urticaria (can occur locally with intravenous administration [rare]), localized erythema (intravenous/subcutaneous), pruritus, rash at injection site (intravenous), skin rash, urticaria, urticaria at injection site (intravenous)

Endocrine & metabolic: Amenorrhea, antidiuretic effect, decreased libido, hypokalemia, hypomagnesemia, weight gain

Gastrointestinal: Abdominal pain, anorexia, biliary tract spasm, constipation, glossitis, nausea, stomach cramps, vomiting, xerostomia

Genitourinary: Impotence, urinary hesitancy, urinary retention

Hematologic: Thrombocytopenia (reversible, reported in patients with chronic hepatitis)

Local: Local pruritus (intravenous), local pain (intravenous/subcutaneous), local swelling (intravenous/subcutaneous)

Neuromuscular & skeletal: Weakness

Ophthalmic: Miosis, visual disturbance

Respiratory: Pulmonary edema, respiratory arrest, respiratory depression

Rare but important or life-threatening): Hypogonadism (Brennan, 2013; Debono, 2011)

Drug Interactions

Metabolism/Transport Effects Substrate of CYP2B6 (major), CYP2C19 (minor), CYP2C9 (minor), CYP2D6 (minor), CYP3A4 (major); **Note:** Assignment of Major/Minor substrate status based on clinically relevant drug interaction potential; **Inhibits** CYP2D6 (moderate)

Avoid Concomitant Use

Avoid concomitant use of Methadone with any of the following: Alcohol (Ethyl); Azelastine (Nasal); Benzodiazepines; Conivaptan; Dapoxetine; Eluxadoline; Fusidic Acid (Systemic); Highest Risk QTc-Prolonging Agents; Idelalisib; Itraconazole; Ivabradine; Ketoconazole (Systemic); Lopinavir; Mifepristone; Mixed Agonist / Antagonist Opioids; Orphenadrine; Paraldehyde; Posaconazole; QUEtiapine; Thalidomide; Thioridazine

Increased Effect/Toxicity

Methadone may increase the levels/effects of: Alvimopan; Antipsychotic Agents; ARIPiprazole; Azelastine (Nasal); CNS Depressants; CYP2D6 Substrates; Desmopressin; Diuretics; DOXOrubicin (Conventional); Eluxadoline; Fesoterodine; Highest Risk QTc-Prolonging Agents; Hydrocodone; Lopinavir; Mequitazine; Methotrimeprazine; Metoclopramide; Metoprolol; Metyrosine; Moderate Risk QTc-Prolonging Agents; Nebivolol; Orphenadrine; Paraldehyde; Pramipexole; QUEtiapine; ROPINIRole; Rotigotine; Saquinavir; Serotonin Modulators; Suvorexant; Thalidomide; Thioridazine; Zidovudine; Zolpidem

The levels/effects of Methadone may be increased by: Alcohol (Ethyl); Amphetamines; Anticholinergic Agents; Antiemetics (5HT3 Antagonists); Antipsychotic Agents; Antipsychotic Agents (Phenothiazines); Aprepitant; ARIPiprazole; Aromatase Inhibitors; Benzodiazepines; Boceprevir; Brimonidine (Topical); Cannabis; Cobicistat; Conivaptan; CYP2B6 Inhibitors (Moderate); CYP3A4 Inhibitors (Moderate); CYP3A4 Inhibitors (Strong); Dapoxetine; Dasatinib; Doxylamine; Dronabinol; Droperidol; Fluconazole; Fosaprepitant; Fusidic Acid (Systemic); HydrOXYzine; Idelalisib; Interferons (Alfa); Itraconazole; Ivabradine; Ivacaftor; Kava Kava; Ketoconazole (Systemic); Luliconazole; Magnesium Sulfate; MAO Inhibitors; Methotrimeprazine; Mifepristone; Nabilone; Netupitant; Palbociclib; Perampanel; Posaconazole; QTc-Prolonging Agents (Indeterminate Risk and Risk Modifying); QUEtiapine; Rufinamide; Selective Serotonin Reuptake Inhibitors; Simeprevir; Sodium Oxybate; Stiripentol; Succinylcholine; Tapentadol; Tetrahydrocannabinol; Voriconazole

Decreased Effect

Methadone may decrease the levels/effects of: Abacavir; Codeine; Didanosine; Fosamprenavir; Lubiprostone; Pegvisomant; Tamoxifen

The levels/effects of Methadone may be decreased by: Abacavir; Ammonium Chloride; Boceprevir; Bosentan; CarBAMazepine; CYP3A4 Inducers (Moderate); CYP3A4 Inducers (Strong); Dabrafenib; Darunavir; Deferasirox; Etravirine; Fosamprenavir; Fosphenytoin; Lopinavir; Mitotane; Mixed Agonist / Antagonist Opioids; Naltrexone; Nelfinavir; PHENobarbital; Phenytoin; Primidone; Reverse Transcriptase Inhibitors (Non-Nucleoside); Rifamycin Derivatives; Ritonavir; Saquinavir; Siltuximab; St Johns Wort; Telaprevir; Tipranavir; Tocilizumab

Food Interactions Grapefruit/grapefruit juice may increase levels of methadone. Management: Avoid concurrent use of grapefruit juice.

Storage/Stability

Injection: Store at 15°C to 30°C (59°F to 86°F). Protect from light.

Oral concentrate, oral solution, tablet: Store at 25°C (77°F); excursions are permitted between 15°C and 30°C (59°F and 86°F).

Mechanism of Action Binds to opiate receptors in the CNS, causing inhibition of ascending pain pathways, altering the perception of and response to pain; produces generalized CNS depression. Methadone has also been shown to have weak N-methyl-D-aspartate (NMDA) receptor antagonism (Callahan, 2004).

Pharmacodynamics Analgesia:

Onset of action:

Oral: Within 30-60 minutes

Parenteral: Within 10-20 minutes

Maximum effect: Parenteral: 1-2 hours

Duration: Oral: 6-8 hours; after repeated doses, duration increases to 22-48 hours

Pharmacokinetics (Adult data unless noted)

Distribution: Crosses the placenta; appears in breast milk

V_d: (Mean ± SD):

Children: 7.1 ± 2.5 L/kg

Adults: 6.1 ± 2.4 L/kg

V_{dss}: Adults: 2-6 L/kg

Protein binding: 85% to 90% (primarily to alpha$_1$-acid glycoprotein)

Metabolism: N-demethylated in the liver to an inactive metabolite

Half-life: May be prolonged with alkaline pH

Children: 19 ± 14 hours (range: 4-62 hours)

Adults: 35 ± 22 hours (range: 9-87 hours)

Elimination: In urine (<10% as unchanged drug); increased renal excretion with urine pH <6; **Note:** Methadone may persist in the liver and other tissues; slow release from tissues may prolong the pharmacologic effect despite low serum concentrations

Dialysis: Hemodialysis, peritoneal dialysis: Not established as effective for increasing the elimination of methadone (or metabolite)

Dosing: Neonatal Note: Doses should be titrated to appropriate effects.

Neonatal abstinence syndrome (opioid withdrawal): Oral, IV: Initial: 0.05-0.2 mg/kg/dose given every 12-24 hours or 0.5 mg/kg/day divided every 8 hours; individualize dose and tapering schedule to control symptoms of withdrawal; usually taper dose by 10% to 20% per week over 1 to 1½ months (AAP, 1998). **Note**: Due to long elimination half-life, tapering is difficult; consider alternate agent.

Dosing: Usual Note: Doses should be titrated to appropriate effects.

Children:

Analgesia: Note: Dosing interval may range from 4-12 hours during initial therapy; decrease in dose or frequency may be required (~2-5 days after initiation of therapy or dosage increase) due to accumulation with repeated doses.

IV: Initial: 0.1 mg/kg/dose every 4 hours for 2-3 doses, then every 6-12 hours as needed; maximum dose: 10 mg/dose

Oral, IM, SubQ: Initial: 0.1 mg/kg/dose every 4 hours for 2-3 doses, then every 6-12 hours as needed or 0.7 mg/kg/24 hours divided every 4-6 hours as needed; maximum dose: 10 mg/dose

Iatrogenic opioid dependency: Oral: Controlled studies have not been conducted; several clinically used dosing regimens have been reported. Methadone dose **must be individualized** and will depend upon patient's previous opioid dose and severity of opioid withdrawal; patients who have received higher doses of opioids will require higher methadone doses.

General guidelines: Initial: 0.05-0.1 mg/kg/dose every 6 hours; increase by 0.05 mg/kg/dose until withdrawal symptoms are controlled; after 24-48 hours, the dosing interval can be lengthened to every 12-24 hours; to taper dose, wean by 0.05 mg/kg/day; if withdrawal symptoms recur, taper at a slower rate

Adults:

Analgesia:

Oral: Initial 5-10 mg; dosing interval may range from 4-12 hours during initial therapy; decrease in dose or frequency may be required (~2-5 days after initiation of therapy or dosage increase) due to accumulation with repeated doses

Manufacturer's recommendations: 2.5-10 mg every 3-4 hours as needed

IV: Manufacturer's recommendations: Opioid-naive patients: Initial: 2.5-10 mg every 8-12 hours; titrate slowly to effect; may also be administered by SubQ or IM injection

Detoxification: Oral: 15-40 mg/day

Maintenance of opioid dependence: Oral: 20-120 mg/day

Dosing adjustment in renal impairment: Children and Adults:

CrCl <10 mL/minute: Administer 50% to 75% of normal dose

Preparation for Administration Oral: Dispersible tablet: Add desired dose to ~120 mL (4 oz) of water, orange juice or other acidic fruit juice and allow to completely dissolve prior administration per the manufacturer; may also be administered in Tang, Kool-Aid, apple juice, and grape Crystal Light (Lauriault 1991)

Administration

Oral: Oral dose for detoxification and maintenance may be administered with juice or water; dispersible tablet should not be chewed or swallowed; completely dissolve before administration; if residue remains in cup after administration rinse with small amount of liquid

Parenteral: May be administered IM, IV or SubQ; rate of IV administration is not defined

Monitoring Parameters Respiratory, cardiovascular, and mental status, pain relief (if used for analgesia), abstinence scoring system (if used for neonatal abstinence syndrome); ECG for monitoring QTc interval prior to and during therapy.

Test Interactions Some quinolones may produce a false-positive urine screening result for opioids using commercially-available immunoassay kits. This has been demonstrated most consistently for levofloxacin and ofloxacin, but other quinolones have shown cross-reactivity in certain assay kits. Confirmation of positive opioid screens by more specific methods should be considered.

Additional Information Methadone accumulates with repeated doses and dosage may need to be adjusted downward after 3-5 days to prevent toxic effects. Some patients may benefit from every 8- to 12-hour dosing interval (pain control).

Methadone 10 mg IM = morphine 10 mg IM

The Center for Substance Abuse and Treatment (CSAT) of the Substance Abuse and Mental Health Services Administration has developed a consensus guideline statement outlining recommendations regarding ECG monitoring in patients being considered for and being treated with methadone regardless of indication. Of note, these recommendations should not supersede clinical judgment or patient preferences and may not apply to patients with terminal, intractable cancer pain. Five recommendations have been developed:

Recommendation 1: Disclosure: Clinicians should inform patients of arrhythmia risk when methadone is prescribed.

Recommendation 2: Clinical History: Clinicians should inquire about any history of structural heart disease, arrhythmia, and syncope.

Recommendation 3: Screening: Clinicians should obtain pretreatment ECG for all patients to measure QTc interval, follow up ECG within 30 days, then annually (monitor more frequently if patient receiving >100 mg/day or if unexplained syncope or seizure occurs while on methadone).

Recommendation 4: Risk Stratification: If before or at anytime during therapy the *QTc >450-499 msecs*: Discuss potential risks and benefits; monitor QTc more frequently. If before or anytime during therapy the *QTc ≥500 msecs*: Consider discontinuation or reducing methadone dose or eliminate factors promoting QTc prolongation (eg, potassium-wasting drugs) or use alternative therapy (eg, buprenorphine).

Recommendation 5: Drug Interactions: Clinicians should be aware of interactions between methadone and other drugs that either prolong the QT interval or reduce methadone elimination.

The panel also concluded that the arrhythmia risk is directly associated with methadone's ability to block the delayed rectifier potassium channel (Ikr) and prolong repolarization. The guideline further states that the use of the Bazett formula is adequate even though it is likely to overcorrect with high heart rates. The patient should remain supine for at least 5 minutes prior to obtaining ECG. In addition, screening for QTc prolongation using automated readings does not require a specialist (eg, cardiologist) and may be performed in a primary care setting. However, in cases when uncertainty exists about whether or not clinically significant QTc prolongation is present, the ECG should be repeated or interpreted by a cardiologist. For more information, Krantz, 2009.

Controlled Substance C-II

Dosage Forms Excipient information presented when available (limited, particularly for generics); consult specific product labeling.

Concentrate, Oral, as hydrochloride:
- Methadone HCl Intensol: 10 mg/mL (30 mL) [unflavored flavor]
- Methadose: 10 mg/mL (1000 mL) [cherry flavor]
- Methadose Sugar-Free: 10 mg/mL (1000 mL) [dye free, sugar free; unflavored flavor]
- Generic: 10 mg/mL (30 mL, 1000 mL)

Solution, Injection, as hydrochloride:
- Generic: 10 mg/mL (20 mL)

Solution, Oral, as hydrochloride:
- Generic: 5 mg/5 mL (500 mL); 10 mg/5 mL (500 mL)

Tablet, Oral, as hydrochloride:
- Dolophine: 5 mg, 10 mg [scored]
- Methadose: 10 mg [scored]
- Generic: 5 mg, 10 mg

Tablet Soluble, Oral, as hydrochloride:
- Methadose: 40 mg [scored]
- Generic: 40 mg

◆ **Methadone HCl Intensol** *see* Methadone *on page 1379*

◆ **Methadone Hydrochloride** *see* Methadone *on page 1379*

◆ **Methadose** *see* Methadone *on page 1379*

◆ **Methadose Sugar-Free** *see* Methadone *on page 1379*

Methamphetamine (meth am FET a meen)

Medication Safety Issues

Sound-alike/look-alike issues:

Desoxyn® may be confused with digoxin

Brand Names: US Desoxyn

Brand Names: Canada Desoxyn

Therapeutic Category Amphetamine; Anorexiant; Central Nervous System Stimulant

Generic Availability (US) Yes

Use Treatment of attention-deficit/hyperactivity disorder (ADHD) (FDA approved in ages ≥6 years and adults); short-term (eg, few weeks) adjunct therapy to treat exogenous obesity refractory to alternative therapy (eg, repeat diets, group programs, and other drugs) (FDA approved in ages ≥12 years and adults)

Medication Guide Available Yes

Pregnancy Risk Factor C

Pregnancy Considerations Adverse effects have been observed in animal reproduction studies. Methamphetamine and amphetamine were detected in newborn tissues following intermittent maternal use of Desoxyn during pregnancy (Garriott, 1973). The majority of human data is based on illicit amphetamine/methamphetamine exposure and not from therapeutic maternal use (Golub, 2005). Use of amphetamines during pregnancy may lead to an increased risk of premature birth and low birth weight; newborns may experience symptoms of withdrawal. Behavioral problems may also occur later in childhood (LaGasse, 2012).

Breast-Feeding Considerations Methamphetamine is excreted in breast milk. The majority of human data is based on illicit amphetamine/methamphetamine exposure and not from therapeutic maternal use (Golub, 2005). Amphetamines may decrease milk production. Increased irritability, agitation, and crying have been reported in nursing infants (ACOG, 2011). Due to the potential for serious adverse reactions in the nursing infant, breast-feeding is not recommended by the manufacturer.

Contraindications

During or within 14 days following MAO inhibitors; glaucoma; advanced arteriosclerosis; symptomatic cardiovascular disease; moderate to severe hypertension; hyperthyroidism; hypersensitivity or idiosyncrasy to sympathomimetic amines; agitated state; patients with a history of drug abuse

Documentation of allergenic cross-reactivity for amphetamines is limited. However, because of similarities in chemical structure and/or pharmacologic actions, the possibility of cross-sensitivity cannot be ruled out with certainty.

Warnings/Precautions CNS stimulant use has been associated with serious cardiovascular events including sudden death in patients with preexisting structural cardiac abnormalities or other serious heart problems (sudden death in children and adolescents; sudden death, stroke and MI in adults). These products should be avoided in the patients with known serious structural cardiac abnormalities, cardiomyopathy, serious heart rhythm abnormalities, or other serious cardiac problems that could increase the risk of sudden death that these conditions alone carry. Patients should be carefully evaluated for cardiac disease prior to initiation of therapy. Patients who develop angina, unexplained syncope, or other symptoms of cardiac disease during therapy should be evaluated immediately. Use with caution in patients with hypertension and other cardiovascular conditions (heart failure, recent MI, ventricular arrhythmia) that might be exacerbated by increases in blood pressure or heart rate. Use is contraindicated in patients with moderate-to-severe hypertension. Amphetamines may impair the ability to engage in potentially hazardous activities; patients must be cautioned about performing tasks which require mental alertness (eg, operating machinery or driving). Stimulants are associated with peripheral vasculopathy, including Raynaud's phenomenon; signs/symptoms are usually mild and intermittent, and generally improve with dose reduction or discontinuation. Digital ulceration and/or soft tissue breakdown have been observed rarely; monitor for digital changes during therapy and seek further evaluation (eg, rheumatology) if necessary. Difficulty in accommodation and blurred vision has been reported with the use of stimulants.

Use with caution in patients with psychiatric disorders, diabetes, or seizure disorders. May exacerbate symptoms of behavior and thought disorder in psychotic patients; new onset psychosis or mania may occur with stimulant use. Patients should be screened for bipolar disorder prior to treatment; consider discontinuation if such symptoms (eg, delusional thinking, hallucinations, or mania) occur. May be associated with aggressive behavior or hostility (causal relationship not established); monitor for development or worsening of these behaviors. May exacerbate motor and phonic tics and Tourette's syndrome. **[U.S. Boxed Warning]: Potential for drug dependency and abuse exists.** Use is contraindicated in patients with history of drug abuse. Prescriptions should be written for the smallest quantity consistent with good patient care to minimize possibility of overdose. Recommended to be used as part of a comprehensive treatment program for attention deficit disorders. Aggression and hostility has been reported with use of medications for ADHD treatment; no evidence suggests that stimulants cause aggressive behavior, but patient should be monitored for the onset or exacerbation of these behaviors. **[U.S. Boxed Warning]: Use in weight reduction programs only when alternative therapy has been ineffective.** Avoid prolonged treatment durations due to potential for drug dependence. Abrupt discontinuation following high doses or for prolonged periods may result in symptoms for withdrawal. Discontinue if satisfactory weight loss has not occurred within the first 4 weeks of treatment, or if tolerance develops.

Therapy is not appropriate for the treatment of fatigue in normal patients. Use caution in the elderly due to the risk for causing dependence, hypertension, angina, and myocardial infarction. Use of stimulants in pediatric patients has been associated with suppression of growth; monitor growth rate during treatment.

Warnings: Additional Pediatric Considerations Serious cardiovascular events, including sudden death, may occur in patients with preexisting structural cardiac abnormalities or other serious heart problems. Sudden death has been reported in children and adolescents; sudden death, stroke, and MI have been reported in adults. Avoid the use of amphetamines in patients with known serious structural cardiac abnormalities, cardiomyopathy, serious heart rhythm abnormalities, coronary artery disease, or other serious cardiac problems that could place patients at an increased risk to the sympathomimetic effects of amphetamines. Patients should be carefully evaluated for cardiac disease prior to initiation of therapy. The American Heart Association recommends that all children diagnosed with ADHD who may be candidates for medication, such as methamphetamine, should have a thorough cardiovascular assessment prior to initiation of therapy. This assessment should include a combination of medical history, family history, and physical examination focusing on cardiovascular disease risk factors. An ECG is not mandatory but should be considered. If a child displays symptoms of cardiovascular disease, including chest pain, dyspnea, or fainting, parents should seek immediate medical care for the child. In a recent retrospective study on the possible association between stimulant medication use and sudden death in children, 564 previously healthy children who died suddenly in motor vehicle accidents were compared to a group of 564 previously healthy children who died suddenly. Two of the 564 (0.4%) children in motor vehicle accidents were taking stimulant medications compared to 10 of 564 (1.8%) children who died suddenly. While the authors of this study conclude there may be an association between stimulant use and sudden death in children, there were a number of limitations to the study and the FDA cannot conclude this information impacts the overall risk: benefit profile of these medications (Gould, 2009). In a large retrospective cohort study involving 1,200,438 children and young adults (aged 2 to 24 years), none of the currently available stimulant medications or atomoxetine were shown to increase the risk of serious cardiovascular events (ie, acute MI, sudden cardiac death, or stroke) in current (adjusted hazard ratio: 0.75; 95% CI: 0.31 to 1.85) or former (adjusted hazard ratio: 1.03; 95% CI: 0.57 to 1.89) users compared to nonusers (Cooper, 2011).

Stimulant medications may increase blood pressure (average increase: 2 to 4 mm Hg) and heart rate (average increase: 3 to 6 bpm); some patients may experience greater increases; use stimulant medications with caution in patients with hypertension and other cardiovascular conditions that may be exacerbated by increases in blood pressure or heart rate.

Adverse Reactions

Cardiovascular: Hypertension, increased blood pressure, palpitations, tachycardia

Central nervous system: Dizziness, drug dependence (prolonged use), dysphoria, euphoria, exacerbation of tics (motor, phonic, and Tourette's syndrome), headache, insomnia, overstimulation, psychotic symptoms, restlessness

Dermatologic: Urticaria

Endocrine & metabolic: Change in libido, growth suppression (children)

Gastrointestinal: Constipation, diarrhea, gastrointestinal distress, unpleasant taste, xerostomia

Genitourinary: Frequent erections, impotence, prolonged erection

Neuromuscular & skeletal: Rhabdomyolysis, tremor

Drug Interactions

Metabolism/Transport Effects Substrate of CYP2D6 (major); **Note:** Assignment of Major/Minor substrate status based on clinically relevant drug interaction potential.

Avoid Concomitant Use

Avoid concomitant use of Methamphetamine with any of the following: Iobenguane I 123; MAO Inhibitors

Increased Effect/Toxicity

Methamphetamine may increase the levels/effects of: Analgesics (Opioid); Sympathomimetics

The levels/effects of Methamphetamine may be increased by: Abiraterone Acetate; Alkalinizing Agents; Antacids; AtoMOXetine; Cannabinoid-Containing Products; Carbonic Anhydrase Inhibitors; Cobicistat; CYP2D6 Inhibitors (Moderate); CYP2D6 Inhibitors (Strong); Darunavir; Linezolid; MAO Inhibitors; Panobinostat; Peginterferon Alfa-2b; Tedizolid; Tricyclic Antidepressants

Decreased Effect

Methamphetamine may decrease the levels/effects of: Antihistamines; Ethosuximide; Iobenguane I 123; Ioflupane I 123; PHENobarbital; Phenytoin

The levels/effects of Methamphetamine may be decreased by: Ammonium Chloride; Antipsychotic Agents; Ascorbic Acid; Gastrointestinal Acidifying Agents; Lithium; Methenamine; Multivitamins/Fluoride (with ADE); Multivitamins/Minerals (with ADEK, Folate, Iron); Multivitamins/Minerals (with AE, No Iron); Peginterferon Alfa-2b; Urinary Acidifying Agents

Food Interactions Amphetamine serum levels may be altered if taken with acidic food, juices, or vitamin C. Management: Administer 30 minutes before a meal.

Storage/Stability Store below 30°C (86°F).

Mechanism of Action A sympathomimetic amine related to ephedrine and amphetamine with CNS stimulant activity; causes release of catecholamines (primarily dopamine and other catecholamines) from their storage sites in the presynaptic nerve terminals. Inhibits reuptake and metabolism of catecholamines through inhibition of monoamine transporters and oxidase.

Pharmacokinetics (Adult data unless noted)

Absorption: Rapid from GI tract

Metabolism: Hepatic via aromatic hydroxylation, N-dealkylation and deamination to several metabolites

Half-life: 4-5 hours

Elimination: Urine primarily (dependent on urine pH; alkaline urine increases the half-life); 62% of dose eliminated in urine within first 24 hours with ~33% as unchanged drug and remainder as metabolites

Dosing: Usual

Children and Adolescents:

Attention-deficit/hyperactivity disorder: Note: Use lowest effective individualized dose; administer first dose in early morning: Children ≥6 years and Adolescents: Oral: Initial: 5 mg once or twice daily; may increase by 5 mg increments weekly until optimum response is achieved; usual effective dose: 20-25 mg/day; dose may be divided twice daily

Exogenous obesity: Children and Adolescents ≥12 years: Oral: 5 mg administered 30 minutes before each meal; treatment duration should not exceed a few weeks

Adults:

Attention-deficit/hyperactivity disorder: Oral: Initial: 5 mg once or twice daily, may increase by 5 mg increments weekly until optimum response is achieved, usually 20-25 mg/day

Exogenous obesity: Oral: Initial: 5 mg administered 30 minutes before each meal; treatment duration should not exceed a few weeks

Administration Avoid late evening doses due to resultant insomnia.

Monitoring Parameters Evaluate patients for cardiac disease prior to initiation of therapy with thorough medical history, family history, and physical exam; consider ECG; perform ECG and echocardiogram if findings suggest cardiac disease; promptly conduct cardiac evaluation in patients who develop chest pain, unexplained syncope, or any other symptom of cardiac disease during treatment. Monitor CNS activity; blood pressure and heart rate (baseline, following dose increases, and periodically during treatment); sleep, appetite, abnormal movements, height, body weight (BMI), growth rate in children. Patients should be re-evaluated at appropriate intervals to assess continued need for the medication. Observe for signs/symptoms of aggression, hostility, or depression. Monitor for visual disturbances.

Test Interactions Amphetamines may elevate plasma corticosteroid levels; may interfere with urinary steroid determinations.

Additional Information Treatment with methamphetamine for ADHD should include "drug holidays" or periodic discontinuation in order to assess the patient's requirements, decrease tolerance, and limit suppression of linear growth and weight. Medications used to treat ADHD should be part of a total treatment program that may include other components such as psychological, educational, and social measures.

Controlled Substance C-II

Dosage Forms Excipient information presented when available (limited, particularly for generics); consult specific product labeling.

Tablet, Oral, as hydrochloride:

Desoxyn: 5 mg [contains sodium aminobenzoate]

Generic: 5 mg

◆ **Methamphetamine Hydrochloride** *see* Methamphetamine *on page 1383*

Methenamine (meth EN a meen)

Medication Safety Issues

Sound-alike/look-alike issues:

Hiprex® may be confused with Mirapex®

Methenamine may be confused with mesalamine, methazolamide, methionine

Urex may be confused with Eurax®, Serax

International issues:

Urex: Brand name for methenamine [U.S. (discontinued)], but also the brand name for furosemide [Australia, China, Turkey]

Urex [U.S. (discontinued)] may be confused with Eurax brand name for crotamitin [U.S., Canada, and multiple international markets]

Brand Names: US Hiprex; Urex

Brand Names: Canada Dehydral®; Hiprex®; Mandelamine®; Urasal®

Therapeutic Category Antibiotic, Miscellaneous

Generic Availability (US) Yes

Use Prophylaxis or suppression of recurrent urinary tract infections

Pregnancy Risk Factor C (methenamine mandelate)

Pregnancy Considerations Methenamine hippurate did not cause adverse fetal effects in animals; animal reproduction studies have not been conducted with methenamine mandelate. Methenamine crosses the placenta and distributes to amniotic fluid (Allgén, 1979). An increased risk of adverse fetal effects has not been observed in available studies (Furness, 1975; Gordon, 1972; Heinonen, 1977). Methenamine use has been shown to interfere with urine estriol concentrations if measured via acid hydrolysis. Use of enzyme hydrolysis prevents this lab interference.

Breast-Feeding Considerations Small amounts of methenamine are excreted into human milk (Allgén, 1979).

Contraindications Hypersensitivity to methenamine or any component of the formulation; severe dehydration, renal insufficiency, severe hepatic insufficiency; concurrent treatment with sulfonamides

Warnings/Precautions Methenamine should not be used to treat infections outside of the lower urinary tract. Use with caution in patients with hepatic disease (contraindicated with severe impairment), gout, and the elderly; doses of 8 g/day for 3 to 4 weeks may cause bladder irritation. Use care to maintain an acid pH of the urine, especially when treating infections due to urea splitting organisms (eg, *Proteus* and strains of *Pseudomonas*); reversible increases in LFTs have occurred during therapy especially in patients with hepatic dysfunction. Hiprex contains tartrazine dye.

Adverse Reactions

Dermatologic: Pruritus, rash

Gastrointestinal: Dyspepsia, nausea, vomiting

Hepatic: ALT increased (reversible; rare), AST increased (reversible; rare)

Note: Large doses (higher than recommended) have resulted in bladder irritation, frequent/painful micturition, albuminuria, and hematuria.

Drug Interactions

Metabolism/Transport Effects None known.

Avoid Concomitant Use

Avoid concomitant use of Methenamine with any of the following: BCG; BCG (Intravesical); Sulfonamide Derivatives

Increased Effect/Toxicity

Methenamine may increase the levels/effects of: ChlorproPAMIDE; Sulfonamide Derivatives

Decreased Effect

Methenamine may decrease the levels/effects of: Alpha-/Beta-Agonists (Indirect-Acting); Amphetamines; BCG; BCG (Intravesical); BCG Vaccine (Immunization); Mecamylamine; Sodium Picosulfate; Typhoid Vaccine

The levels/effects of Methenamine may be decreased by: Antacids; Carbonic Anhydrase Inhibitors

Food Interactions Foods/diets which alkalinize urine (pH >5.5) decrease therapeutic effect of methenamine.

Storage/Stability Store at room temperature of 15°C to 30°C (59°F to 86°F). Protect from light.

Mechanism of Action Methenamine is hydrolyzed to formaldehyde and ammonia in acidic urine; formaldehyde has nonspecific bactericidal action. Other components, hippuric acid or mandelic acid, aid in maintaining urine acidity and may aid in suppressing bacteria.

Pharmacokinetics (Adult data unless noted)

Absorption: Readily from the GI tract; 10% to 30% of the drug will be hydrolyzed by gastric juices unless it is protected by an enteric coating

Distribution: Distributes into breast milk; crosses the placenta

Metabolism: ~10% to 25% in the liver

Half-life: 3-6 hours

Elimination: Excretion occurs via glomerular filtration and tubular secretion with ~70% to 90% of dose excreted unchanged in urine within 24 hours

Dosing: Usual Oral:

Children >2 years to 12 years: Mandelate: 50-75 mg/kg/day divided every 6-8 hours; maximum dose: 4 g/day

Children 6-12 years: Hippurate: 0.5-1 g twice daily

Children >12 years and Adults:

Hippurate: 1 g twice daily

Mandelate: 1 g 4 times/day after meals and at bedtime

Administration Oral: Administer with food to minimize GI upset; shake suspension well before use; patient should drink plenty of fluids to ensure adequate urine flow; administer with cranberry juice, ascorbic acid, or ammonium chloride to acidify urine; avoid intake of alkalinizing agents (sodium bicarbonate, antacids)

Monitoring Parameters Urinary pH, urinalysis, urine cultures, periodic liver function tests in patients receiving hippurate salt

Test Interactions Increased urinary catecholamines, 17-hydroxycorticosteroid and vanillylmandelic acid (VMA) levels; decreased urinary 5-hydroxyindoleacetic acid (5HIAA) and estriol levels

Additional Information Should not be used to treat infections outside of the lower urinary tract (ie, pyelonephritis)

Dosage Forms Excipient information presented when available (limited, particularly for generics); consult specific product labeling.

Tablet, Oral, as hippurate:

Hiprex: 1 g [scored; contains tartrazine (fd&c yellow #5)]

Urex: 1 g [scored]

Generic: 1 g

Tablet, Oral, as mandelate:

Generic: 0.5 g, 1 g

◆ **Methenamine Hippurate** *see* Methenamine *on page 1385*

◆ **Methenamine Mandelate** *see* Methenamine *on page 1385*

Methimazole (meth IM a zole)

Medication Safety Issues

Sound-alike/look-alike issues:

Methimazole may be confused with metolazone

Brand Names: US Tapazole

Brand Names: Canada Dom-Methimazole; PHL-Methimazole; Tapazole

Therapeutic Category Antithyroid Agent

Generic Availability (US) Yes

Use Treatment of hyperthyroidism, including amelioration of hyperthyroid symptoms, prior to thyroidectomy or radioactive iodine therapy [FDA approved in pediatric patients (age not specified) and adults]

Pregnancy Risk Factor D

Pregnancy Considerations Methimazole has been found to readily cross the placenta. Congenital anomalies including esophageal atresia, choanal atresia, aplasia cutis, and dysmorphic facies, have been observed in neonates born to mothers taking methimazole during pregnancy (Stangaro-Green, 2011). Nonteratogenic adverse events, including fetal and neonatal hypothyroidism, have been observed following maternal methimazole use. The transfer of thyroid-stimulating immunoglobulins can stimulate the fetal thyroid *in utero* and transiently after delivery and may increase the risk of fetal or neonatal hyperthyroidism (De Groot, 2012; Stangaro-Green, 2011).

Uncontrolled maternal hyperthyroidism may result in adverse neonatal outcomes (eg, prematurity, low birth weight, infants born small for gestational age) and adverse maternal outcomes (eg, pre-eclampsia, congestive heart failure) (ACOG, 2002; Stangaro-Green, 2011). To prevent adverse fetal and maternal events, normal maternal thyroid function should be maintained prior to conception and throughout pregnancy. Antithyroid treatment is recommended for the control of hyperthyroidism during pregnancy. Due to an increased risk of congenital anomalies with methimazole, propylthiouracil is preferred during the first trimester of pregnancy and methimazole is preferred during the second and third trimesters of pregnancy (ACOG, 2002; De Groot, 2012; Stangaro-Green, 2011). If drug therapy is changed, maternal thyroid function should be monitored after 2 weeks and then every 2 to 4 weeks (De Groot, 2012).

The severity of hyperthyroidism may fluctuate throughout pregnancy and may result in decreased dose requirements or discontinuation of methimazole 2 to 3 weeks prior to delivery.

Breast-Feeding Considerations Methimazole is excreted into human breast milk. The thyroid function and intellectual development of breast-fed infants are not affected by exposure to maternal methimazole during breast-feeding. The American Thyroid Association considers doses of methimazole <30 mg/day to be safe during breast-feeding. Methimazole should be administered after nursing and in divided doses (Stagnaro-Green, 2011).

Contraindications Hypersensitivity to methimazole or any component of the formulation

Warnings/Precautions May cause significant bone marrow depression; the most severe manifestation is agranulocytosis. Aplastic anemia, thrombocytopenia, and leukopenia may also occur. and with concomitant use of other drugs known to cause myelosuppression (particularly agranulocytosis). Monitor patients closely; discontinue if significant bone marrow suppression occurs, particularly agranulocytosis or aplastic anemia.

May cause hypoprothrombinemia and bleeding. Monitoring is recommended, especially before surgical procedures. Antithyroid agents have been associated with rare but severe dermatologic reactions. Discontinue in the presence of exfoliative dermatitis. Hepatotoxicity (including acute liver failure) may occur. Symptoms suggestive of hepatic dysfunction (eg, anorexia, pruritus, right upper quadrant pain) should prompt evaluation. Discontinue in the presence of hepatitis and clinically significant hepatic abnormality, including transaminase >3 times upper limit of normal. May cause hypothyroidism; routinely monitor TSH and free T_4 levels, adjust dose to maintain euthyroid state. ANCA-positive vasculitis may develop during therapy discontinue use in the presence of vasculitis use. Discontinue in the presence of unexplained fever. A lupus-like syndrome may occur. Potentially significant drug-drug interactions may exist, requiring dose or frequency adjustment, additional monitoring, and/or selection of alternative therapy.

Adverse Reactions

Cardiovascular: ANCA-positive vasculitis, edema, leukocytoclastic vasculitis, periarteritis

Central nervous system: Drowsiness, fever, headache, neuritis, vertigo

Dermatologic: Alopecia, exfoliative dermatitis, pruritus, skin pigmentation, skin rash, urticaria

Endocrine & metabolic: Goiter, hypoglycemic coma

Gastrointestinal: Constipation, epigastric distress, loss of taste perception, nausea, salivary gland swelling, vomiting, weight gain

Hematologic: Agranulocytosis, aplastic anemia, granulocytopenia, hypoprothrombinemia, leukopenia, thrombocytopenia

Hepatic: Hepatic necrosis, hepatitis, jaundice

Neuromuscular & skeletal: Arthralgia, myalgia, paresthesia

Renal: Nephritis

Miscellaneous: Insulin autoimmune syndrome, lymphadenopathy, SLE-like syndrome

Drug Interactions

Metabolism/Transport Effects Inhibits CYP1A2 (weak), CYP2A6 (weak), CYP2B6 (weak), CYP2C19 (weak), CYP2C9 (weak), CYP2D6 (weak), CYP2E1 (weak)

Avoid Concomitant Use

Avoid concomitant use of Methimazole with any of the following: BCG (Intravesical); CloZAPine; Dipyrone; Sodium Iodide I131

Increased Effect/Toxicity

Methimazole may increase the levels/effects of: ARIPiprazole; Cardiac Glycosides; CloZAPine; Theophylline Derivatives; TiZANidine

The levels/effects of Methimazole may be increased by: Dipyrone

Decreased Effect

Methimazole may decrease the levels/effects of: BCG (Intravesical); PrednisoLONE (Systemic); Sodium Iodide I131; Vitamin K Antagonists

Storage/Stability Store at 15°C to 30°C (59°F to 86°F).

Mechanism of Action Inhibits the synthesis of thyroid hormones by blocking the oxidation of iodine in the thyroid gland; blocks synthesis of thyroxine and triiodothyronine (T_3); does not inactivate circulating T_4 and T_3

Pharmacodynamics

Onset of action: 12-18 hours

Duration: 36-72 hours (Clark, 2006)

Pharmacokinetics (Adult data unless noted)

Absorption: Almost complete (Clark, 2006)

Distribution: Concentrated in thyroid gland

Bioavailability: ~93% (Clark, 2006)

Metabolism: Hepatic

Half-life: 4-6 hours (Clark, 2006)

Time to peak serum concentration: 1-2 hours (Clark, 2006)

Elimination: Urine

Dosing: Neonatal Congenital Hyperthyroidism: Oral: Initial: 0.25-1 mg/kg/day in 2-3 divided doses; once patient euthyroid, reduce dose (usually by ≥50%) to maintain euthyroid state

Dosing: Usual

Infants, Children, and Adolescent:

Hyperthyroidism: Oral:

Manufacturer's labeling: Initial: 0.4 mg/kg/**day** in 3 divided doses (approximately every 8 hours); maintenance: 0.2 mg/kg/**day** in 3 divided doses

Alternate dosing: Initial: 0.25-1 mg/kg/**day** in 1-3 divided doses; consider doses on low-end of range for younger children; once patient euthyroid, reduce dose (usually by ≥50%) to maintain euthyroid state

Graves' disease (Bahn, 2011): Oral: **Note**: In severe cases, higher doses may be required (50% to 100% higher); once patient euthyroid, reduce dose by ≥50% to maintain euthyroid; duration of therapy usually 1-2 years

Weight-based dosing: Initial: 0.2-0.5 mg/kg/dose once daily (range: 0.1-1 mg/kg/dose)

Fixed dosing (using 1/4, 1/2, or whole tablets):

Infants: 1.25 mg/day

Children 1-5 years: 2.5-5 mg/day

Children 5-10 years: 5-10 mg/day

Children 10-18 years: 10-20 mg/day

Adults

Hyperthyroidism: Oral: Initial: 15 mg/day in 3 divided doses (approximately every 8 hours) for mild hyperthyroidism; 30-40 mg/day in moderately severe hyperthyroidism; 60 mg/day in severe hyperthyroidism; maintenance: 5-15 mg/day (may be given as a single daily dose in many cases)

Adjust dosage as required to achieve and maintain serum T_3, T_4, and TSH levels in the normal range. An elevated T_3 may be the sole indicator of inadequate treatment. An elevated TSH indicates excessive antithyroid treatment.

Graves' disease: Oral: Initial: 10-20 mg once daily to restore euthyroidism; maintenance: 5-10 mg once daily for a total of 12-18 months, then tapered or discontinued if TSH is normal at that time (Bahn, 2011)

Iodine-induced thyrotoxicosis: Oral: 20-40 mg/day given either once or twice daily (Bahn, 2011)

Thyrotoxic crisis: Oral: **Note:** Recommendations vary; use in combination with other specific agents. Dosages of 20-25 mg every 6 hours have been used; once stable, dosing frequency may be reduced to once or twice daily (Nayak, 2006). The American Thyroid Association and the American Association of Clinical Endocrinologists recommend 60-80 mg/day (Bahn, 2011). Rectal administration has also been described (Nabil, 1982).

Thyrotoxicosis (type I amiodarone-induced): Oral: 40 mg once daily to restore euthyroidism (generally 3-6 months). **Note:** If high doses continue to be required, dividing the dose may be more effective (Bahn, 2011).

Dosage adjustment in renal impairment: No adjustment necessary

Administration Oral: Administer consistently in relation to meals every day

Monitoring Parameters Signs of hyper- or hypothyroidism, CBC with differential, liver function (baseline and as needed); serum thyroxine, free thyroxine index, prothrombin time

Dosage Forms Excipient information presented when available (limited, particularly for generics); consult specific product labeling.

Tablet, Oral:

Tapazole: 5 mg, 10 mg [scored]

Generic: 5 mg, 10 mg

Extemporaneous Preparations Suppositories can be made from methimazole tablets; dissolve 1200 mg methimazole in 12 mL of water and add to 52 mL cocoa butter containing 2 drops of Span 80. Stir the resulting mixture to form a water-oil emulsion and pour into 2.6 mL suppository molds to cool.

Nabil N, Miner DJ, and Amatruda JM, "Methimazole: An Alternative Route of Administration," *J Clin Endo Metab*, 1982, 54(1):180-1.

Methocarbamol (meth oh KAR ba mole)

Medication Safety Issues

Sound-alike/look-alike issues:

Methocarbamol may be confused with mephobarbital

Robaxin may be confused with ribavirin, Skelaxin

BEERS Criteria medication:

This drug may be potentially inappropriate for use in geriatric patients (Quality of evidence - moderate; Strength of recommendation - strong).

International issues:

Robaxin [U.S., Canada, Great Britain, Greece, Spain] may be confused with Rubex brand name for ascorbic acid [Ireland]; doxorubicin [Brazil]

Brand Names: US Robaxin; Robaxin-750

Brand Names: Canada Robaxin®

Therapeutic Category Skeletal Muscle Relaxant, Non-paralytic

Generic Availability (US) Yes

Use Adjunctive treatment of muscle spasm associated with acute painful musculoskeletal conditions (eg, tetanus) (FDA approved in ages ≥16 years and adults)

Pregnancy Risk Factor C

Pregnancy Considerations Animal reproduction studies have not been conducted. The manufacturer notes that fetal and congenital abnormalities have been rarely reported following *in utero* exposure. Use during pregnancy only if clearly needed.

Breast-Feeding Considerations It is not known if methocarbamol is excreted in breast milk. The manufacturer recommends that caution be exercised when administering methocarbamol to nursing women.

Contraindications Hypersensitivity to methocarbamol or any component of the formulation; renal impairment (injection formulation)

Warnings/Precautions May cause CNS depression, which may impair physical or mental abilities; patients must be cautioned about performing tasks which require mental alertness (eg, operating machinery or driving). Effects may be potentiated when used with other sedative drugs or ethanol. Plasma protein binding and clearance are decreased and the half-life is increased in patients with hepatic impairment. Muscle relaxants are poorly tolerated by the elderly due to potent anticholinergic effects, sedation, and risk of fracture. Efficacy is questionable at dosages tolerated by elderly patients; avoid use (Beers Criteria).

Injection: Contraindicated in renal impairment. Contains polyethylene glycol. Rate of injection should not exceed 3 mL/minute; solution is hypertonic; avoid extravasation. Use with caution in patients with a history of seizures. Use caution with hepatic impairment. Vial stopper contains latex. Recommended only for the treatment of tetanus in pediatric patients.

Adverse Reactions

Cardiovascular: Bradycardia, flushing, hypotension, syncope

Central nervous system: Amnesia, confusion, coordination impaired (mild), dizziness, drowsiness, fever, headache, insomnia, lightheadedness, sedation, seizures, vertigo

Dermatologic: Angioneurotic edema, pruritus, rash, urticaria

Gastrointestinal: Dyspepsia, metallic taste, nausea, vomiting

Hematologic: Leukopenia

Hepatic: Jaundice

Local: Pain at injection site, thrombophlebitis

Ocular: Blurred vision, conjunctivitis, diplopia, nystagmus

Respiratory: Nasal congestion

Miscellaneous: Hypersensitivity reactions including anaphylaxis

Drug Interactions

Metabolism/Transport Effects None known.

Avoid Concomitant Use

Avoid concomitant use of Methocarbamol with any of the following: Azelastine (Nasal); Orphenadrine; Paraldehyde; Thalidomide

Increased Effect/Toxicity

Methocarbamol may increase the levels/effects of: Alcohol (Ethyl); Azelastine (Nasal); Buprenorphine; CNS Depressants; Hydrocodone; Methotrimeprazine; Metyrosine; Mirtazapine; Orphenadrine; Paraldehyde; Pramipexole; ROPINIRole; Rotigotine; Selective Serotonin Reuptake Inhibitors; Suvorexant; Thalidomide; Zolpidem

The levels/effects of Methocarbamol may be increased by: Brimonidine (Topical); Cannabis; Doxylamine; Dronabinol; Droperidol; Eperisone; HydrOXYzine; Kava Kava; Magnesium Sulfate; Methotrimeprazine; Nabilone; Perampanel; Rufinamide; Sodium Oxybate; Tapentadol; Tetrahydrocannabinol

Decreased Effect

Methocarbamol may decrease the levels/effects of: Pyridostigmine

Storage/Stability

Solution for injection: Prior to dilution, store at controlled room temperature of 20°C to 25°C (68°F to 77°F); excursions permitted to 15°C to 30°C (59°F to 86°F).

Tablet: Store at controlled room temperature of 20°C to 25°C (68°F to 77°F).

Mechanism of Action Causes skeletal muscle relaxation by general CNS depression

Pharmacodynamics Onset of action: 30 minutes

Pharmacokinetics (Adult data unless noted) Oral:

Protein binding: 46% to 50%

Metabolism: Extensive in the liver via dealkylation and hydroxylation

Half-life: 1-2 hours

Time to peak serum concentration: Within ~1-2 hours

Elimination: Clearance: Adults: 0.2-0.8 L/hour/kg

Dosing: Usual

Tetanus: IV:

Children (recommended **only** for use in tetanus): 15 mg/kg/dose or 500 mg/m^2/dose, may repeat every 6 hours if needed; maximum dose: 1.8 g/m^2/day for 3 days only

Adults: 1-2 g by direct IV injection, which may be followed by an additional 1-2 g by infusion (maximum dose: 3 g total); followed by 1-2 g every 6 hours until NG tube or oral therapy possible; total daily dose of up to 24 g may be needed; injection should not be used for more than 3 consecutive days

Muscle spasm:

Oral: Adolescents ≥16 years and Adults: 1.5 g 4 times/day for 2-3 days (up to 8 g/day may be used for severe conditions); decrease dose to 4-4.5 g/day as 1 g 4 times/day or 750 mg every 4 hours or 1.5 g 3 times/day

IM, IV: Adults: Initial: 1 g; may repeat every 8 hours if oral administration not possible; maximum dose: 3 g/day for 3 consecutive days (except when treating tetanus); may be reinstituted after 2 drug-free days

Dosing adjustment in renal impairment: Clearance is reduced by as much as 40% in patients with renal failure on hemodialysis; avoid use or reduce dosage and monitor closely; do not administer parenteral formulation to patients with renal dysfunction

Dosing adjustment in hepatic impairment: Specific dosing guidelines are not available; clearance may be reduced by as much as 70% in cirrhotic patients

Preparation for Administration Parenteral: IV: May further dilute in D_5W or NS to a final concentration of 4 mg/mL

Administration

Parenteral:

IV: May be directly injected undiluted at a maximum rate of >3 mL/minute; may also be further diluted and infused more slowly; patient should be in the recumbent position during and for 10 to 15 minutes after IV administration. Monitor closely for extravasation

IM: Adults: Maximum of 5 mL can be administered into each gluteal region; not recommended for SubQ administration

Oral: Tablet: May be crushed and mixed with food or liquid if needed.

Monitoring Parameters Monitor closely for extravasation (IV administration).

Test Interactions May cause color interference in certain screening tests for 5-HIAA using nitrosonaphthol reagent and in screening tests for urinary VMA using the Gitlow method.

Dosage Forms Excipient information presented when available (limited, particularly for generics); consult specific product labeling.

Solution, Injection:

Robaxin: 1000 mg/10 mL (10 mL) [contains polyethylene glycol 300]

Solution, Injection [preservative free]:

Generic: 1000 mg/10 mL (10 mL)

Tablet, Oral:

Robaxin: 500 mg [scored; contains fd&c yellow #6 (sunset yellow), saccharin sodium]

Robaxin-750: 750 mg [contains fd&c yellow #10 (quinoline yellow), fd&c yellow #6 (sunset yellow), saccharin sodium]

Generic: 500 mg, 750 mg

Methohexital (meth oh HEKS i tal)

Medication Safety Issues

Sound-alike/look-alike issues:

Brevital may be confused with Brevibloc

High alert medication:

The Institute for Safe Medication Practices (ISMP) includes this medication among its list of drugs which have a heightened risk of causing significant patient harm when used in error.

Related Information

Preprocedure Sedatives in Children *on page 2444*

Brand Names: US Brevital Sodium

Brand Names: Canada Brevital

Therapeutic Category Barbiturate; General Anesthetic; Sedative

Generic Availability (US) No

Use Induction of anesthesia prior to the use of other general anesthetic agents (IM, rectal: FDA approved in ages >1 month; IV: FDA approved in adults); adjunct to subpotent inhalational anesthetic agents for short surgical procedures (IM, rectal: FDA approved in ages >1 month; IV: FDA approved in adults); anesthesia for short surgical, diagnostic, or therapeutic procedures associated with minimal painful stimuli (IM, rectal: FDA approved in ages >1 month; IV: FDA approved in adults); anesthesia for use with other parenteral agents, usually opioid analgesics, to supplement subpotent inhalational anesthetic agents for longer surgical procedures (FDA approved in adults); induction of hypnotic state (FDA approved in adults)

Pregnancy Risk Factor B

Pregnancy Considerations Animal studies have not shown fetal or maternal harm. There are no adequate and well-controlled studies in pregnant women. Methohexital crosses the placenta. Use only if potential benefit outweighs risk to fetus.

Breast-Feeding Considerations Methohexital is minimally excreted in breast milk and levels decline rapidly after administration. Interruption of breast-feeding is unnecessary.

Contraindications Hypersensitivity to barbiturates, methohexital, or any component of the formulation; porphyria (latent or manifest); patients in whom general anesthesia is contraindicated

Warnings/Precautions Use with caution in patients with liver impairment, renal impairment, cardiovascular disease (including heart failure), severe anemia, extreme obesity, or seizure disorder, the elderly and children. May cause hypotension; use with caution in hemodynamically unstable patients (hypotension or shock) or severe hypertension. May cause respiratory depression; use with caution in patients with pulmonary disease. Use with caution in patients with asthma and chronic obstructive pulmonary disease. Use with extreme caution in patients with ongoing status asthmaticus; hiccups, coughing, laryngospasm, and muscle twitching have occurred impairing ventilation.

Postmarketing studies have indicated that the use of hypnotic/sedative agents for sleep has been associated with hypersensitivity reactions including anaphylaxis as well as angioedema. Effects with other sedative drugs or ethanol may be potentiated. Repeated dosing or continuous infusions may cause cumulative effects. Ensure patient has intravenous access; extravasation or intra-arterial injection causes necrosis. **[U.S. Boxed Warning]: Should only be administered in hospitals or ambulatory care settings with continuous monitoring of respiratory function; resuscitative drugs, age- and size-appropriate and intubation equipment and trained personnel experienced in handling their use should be readily available. For deeply sedated patients, a healthcare provider other than the individual performing the procedure should be present to continuously monitor the patient.**

Adverse Reactions

Cardiovascular: Cardiorespiratory arrest, circulatory depression, hypotension, peripheral vascular collapse, tachycardia

Central nervous system: Anxiety, emergence delirium, headache, restlessness, seizure

Dermatologic: Erythema, pruritus, urticaria

Gastrointestinal: Abdominal pain, nausea, salivation, vomiting

Hepatic: Transaminases increased

Local: Injection site pain, nerve injury adjacent to injection site, thrombophlebitis

Neuromuscular & skeletal: Involuntary muscle movement, radial nerve palsy, rigidity, tremor, twitching

Respiratory: Apnea, bronchospasm, cough, dyspnea, hiccups, laryngospasm, respiratory depression, rhinitis

Miscellaneous: Anaphylaxis (rare)

Drug Interactions

Metabolism/Transport Effects None known.

Avoid Concomitant Use

Avoid concomitant use of Methohexital with any of the following: Azelastine (Nasal); Mianserin; Orphenadrine; Paraldehyde; Somatostatin Acetate; Thalidomide; Ulipristal

Increased Effect/Toxicity

Methohexital may increase the levels/effects of: Alcohol (Ethyl); Azelastine (Nasal); Buprenorphine; CNS Depressants; Hydrocodone; Hypotensive Agents; Meperidine; Methotrimeprazine; Metyrosine; Mirtazapine; Orphenadrine; Paraldehyde; Pramipexole; ROPINIRole; Rotigotine; Selective Serotonin Reuptake Inhibitors; Suvorexant; Thalidomide; Thiazide Diuretics; Zolpidem

The levels/effects of Methohexital may be increased by: Brimonidine (Topical); Cannabis; Chloramphenicol; Doxylamine; Dronabinol; Droperidol; Felbamate; HydrOXYzine; Kava Kava; Magnesium Sulfate; Methotrimeprazine; Mianserin; Nabilone; Perampanel; Primidone; Rufinamide; Sodium Oxybate; Somatostatin Acetate; Tapentadol; Tetrahydrocannabinol; Valproic Acid and Derivatives

Decreased Effect

Methohexital may decrease the levels/effects of: Acetaminophen; Beta-Blockers; Calcium Channel Blockers; Chloramphenicol; Contraceptives (Estrogens); Contraceptives (Progestins); CycloSPORINE (Systemic); Doxycycline; Etoposide; Etoposide Phosphate; Felbamate; LamoTRIgine; Mianserin; Teniposide; Theophylline Derivatives; Tricyclic Antidepressants; Ulipristal; Valproic Acid and Derivatives; Vitamin K Antagonists

The levels/effects of Methohexital may be decreased by: Mianserin; Multivitamins/Minerals (with ADEK, Folate, Iron); Pyridoxine; Rifamycin Derivatives

Storage/Stability Store at 20°C to 25°C (68°F to 77°F). Reconstituted solutions are chemically stable at room temperature for 24 hours; 0.2% (2 mg/mL) solutions in D_5W or NS are stable at room temperature for 24 hours.

Mechanism of Action Ultra short-acting IV barbiturate anesthetic

Pharmacodynamics

Onset of action:
- IM (pediatric patients): 2-10 minutes
- IV: 1 minute
- Rectal (pediatric patients): 5-15 minutes

Duration:
- IM: 1-1.5 hours
- IV: 7-10 minutes
- Rectal: 1-1.5 hours

Pharmacokinetics (Adult data unless noted)

Metabolism: In the liver via demethylation and oxidation

Bioavailability: Rectal: 17%

Elimination: Through the kidney via glomerular filtration

Dosing: Usual Doses must be titrated to effect

Manufacturer's recommendations: Infants ≥1 month and Children:
- IM: Induction: 6.6-10 mg/kg of a 5% solution
- Rectal: Induction: Usual: 25 mg/kg of a 1% solution

Alternative pediatric dosing:

Children:
- IM: Preoperative: 5-10 mg/kg/dose of a 5% solution
- IV:
  - Induction: 1-2 mg/kg/dose of a 1% solution (Björkman, 1987)
  - Procedural sedation: Initial: 0.5 mg/kg of a 1% solution given immediately prior to procedure; titrate dose to achieve level of sedation as needed, in increments of 0.5 mg/kg to a maximum dose of 2 mg/kg; **Note:** In the prospective phase of a study, 20 children (mean age: 26 months) undergoing emergency CT scans required a mean dose of 1 ± 0.5 mg/kg/dose with a mean total dose of 14 ± 7.5 mg/kg (Sedik, 2001).
- Rectal: Preoperative, anesthesia induction, or preprocedural: Usual: 25 mg/kg/dose; range: 20-35 mg/kg/dose; maximum dose: 500 mg/dose; give as 10% (100 mg/mL) aqueous solution 5-15 minutes prior to procedure (Bjorkman, 1987; Pomeranz, 2000)

Adults: IV:
- Induction: Range: 1-1.5 mg/kg or 50-120 mg/dose
- Maintenance: Intermittent IV bolus injection: 20-40 mg (2-4 mL of a 1% solution) every 4-7 minutes

Preparation for Administration Do not dilute with solutions containing bacteriostatic agents. Solutions should be freshly prepared and used promptly.

Parenteral:

IV:
- Intermittent IV: Prepare a 1% (10 mg/mL) solution:
  - 200 mg vial: Dilute with 20 mL with SWFI (preferred), D_5W, or NS
  - 500 mg vial: Dilute with 50 mL with SWFI (preferred), D_5W, or NS
  - 2.5 g vial: Dilute with 15 mL of SWFI (preferred), D_5W, or NS; solution will be yellow in color; then add to 235 mL of original diluent for a total volume of 250 mL; final solution must be clear and colorless or should not be used.
- Continuous infusion: Prepare a 0.2% (2 mg/mL) solution: 500 mg vial: Dilute with 15 mL D_5W or NS, then add to 235 mL of original diluent for a total volume of 250 mL

IM: Prepare a 5% (50 mg/mL) solution:
- 200 mg vial: Dilute with 4 mL of SWFI (preferred) or NS
- 500 mg vial: Dilute with 10 mL of SWFI (preferred) or NS
- 2.5 g vial: Dilute with 50 mL of SWFI (preferred) or NS

Rectal:
- For a 1% (10 mg/mL) solution:
  - 200 mg vial: Dilute with 20 mL with SWFI (preferred), D_5W, or NS
  - 500 mg vial: Dilute with 50 mL with SWFI (preferred), D_5W, or NS
  - 2.5 g vial: Dilute with 15 mL of SWFI (preferred), D_5W, or NS, solution will be yellow in color; then add to 235 mL of original diluent for a total volume of 250 mL; final solution must be clear and colorless or should not be used.
- For a 10% (100 mg/mL) solution (Pomeranz 2000):
  - 500 mg vial: Dilute with 5 mL of SWFI
  - 2.5 g vial: Dilute with 25 mL of SWFI

Administration

Parenteral:
- IM: Use 5% solution (50 mg/mL)
- IV:
  - Bolus: For induction, infuse a 1% solution (10 mg/mL) at a rate of ~1 mL/5 seconds or ~2 mg/second.
  - Continuous IV infusion: Adults: Use a 0.2% solution (2 mg/mL)

Rectal: Use a 1% solution (10 mg/mL); a 10% solution (100 mg/mL) has also been given rectally (Bjorkman 1987; Pomeranz 2000)

Monitoring Parameters Blood pressure, heart rate, respiratory rate, oxygen saturation, pulse oximetry

Additional Information Does not possess analgesic properties; Brevital® has FDA-approved labeling for IV use in adults, and for rectal and IM use only in pediatric patients >1 month of age; 100 pediatric patients (3 months to 5 years of age) received rectal methohexital (25 mg/kg) for sedation prior to computed tomography (CT) scan; sedation was adequate in 95% of patients; mean time for full sedation = 8.2 ± 3.9 minutes; mean duration of action = 79.3 ± 30.9 minutes; 10% of patients had transient side effects (Pomeranz, 2000)

Controlled Substance C-IV

Dosage Forms Excipient information presented when available (limited, particularly for generics); consult specific product labeling. [DSC] = Discontinued product

Solution Reconstituted, Injection, as sodium:

Brevital Sodium: 200 mg (1 ea [DSC]); 500 mg (1 ea); 2.5 g (1 ea)

◆ **Methohexital Sodium** *see* Methohexital *on page* 1389

Methotrexate (meth oh TREKS ate)

Medication Safety Issues

Sound-alike/look-alike issues:

Methotrexate may be confused with mercaptopurine, methylPREDNISolone sodium succinate, metolazone, metroNIDAZOLE, mitoXANtrone, PRALAtrexate

High alert medication:

The Institute for Safe Medication Practices (ISMP) includes this medication among its list of drugs which have a heightened risk of causing significant patient harm when used in error.

Administration issues:

Errors have occurred (resulting in death) when methotrexate was administered as "daily" dose instead of "weekly" dose recommended for some indications. The ISMP recommends hospitals use a weekly dosage regimen default for oral methotrexate orders, with a hard stop override requiring verification of appropriate oncology indication; manual systems should require verification of an oncology indication prior to dispensing oral methotrexate for daily administration. Pharmacists should provide patient education for patients discharged on weekly oral methotrexate (ISMP, 2014).

Intrathecal medication safety: The American Society of Clinical Oncology (ASCO)/Oncology Nursing Society (ONS) chemotherapy administration safety standards (Jacobson, 2009) encourage the following safety measures for intrathecal chemotherapy:

- Intrathecal medication should not be prepared during the preparation of any other agents
- After preparation, keep in an isolated location or container clearly marked with a label identifying as "intrathecal" use only
- Delivery to the patient should only be with other medications also intended for administration into the central nervous system

Other safety concerns:

MTX is an error-prone abbreviation (mistaken as mitoxantrone or multivitamin)

International issues:

Trexall [U.S.] may be confused with Trexol brand name for tramadol [Mexico]; Truxal brand name for chlorprothixene [multiple international markets]

Related Information

Prevention of Chemotherapy-Induced Nausea and Vomiting in Children *on page 2368*

Safe Handling of Hazardous Drugs *on page 2455*

Brand Names: US Otrexup; Rasuvo; Rheumatrex; Trexall

Brand Names: Canada Apo-Methotrexate; JAMP-Methotrexate; Methotrexate Injection USP; Methotrexate Injection, BP; Methotrexate Sodium Injection; Metoject; ratio-Methotrexate Sodium

Therapeutic Category Antineoplastic Agent, Antimetabolite; Antirheumatic, Disease Modifying

Generic Availability (US) May be product dependent

Use Treatment of trophoblastic neoplasms (gestational choriocarcinoma, chorioadenoma destruens, and hydatidiform mole), acute lymphocytic leukemia, osteosarcoma, breast cancer, head and neck cancer (epidermoid), cutaneous T-Cell lymphoma (advanced mycosis fungoides), lung cancer (squamous cell and small cell) [oral, parenteral: FDA approved in pediatric patients (age not specified) and adults]; treatment of meningeal leukemia [parenteral: FDA approved in pediatric patients (age not specified) and adults]; treatment of active polyarticular juvenile idiopathic arthritis (JIA) in patients who have failed to respond to other agents [oral, parenteral (Otrexup): FDA approved in ages 2-16 years]; treatment of psoriasis (severe, recalcitrant, disabling) and severe, active rheumatoid arthritis [oral, parenteral (Otrexup): FDA approved in adults]. Has also been used for the treatment and maintenance of remission in Crohn's disease, dermatomyositis, uveitis, scleroderma, ectopic pregnancy, central nervous system tumors (including nonleukemic meningeal cancers), acute promyelocytic leukemia (maintenance treatment), soft tissue sarcoma (desmoid tumors)

Pregnancy Risk Factor X (psoriasis, rheumatoid arthritis)

Pregnancy Considerations **[U.S. Boxed Warning]: Methotrexate may cause fetal death and/or congenital abnormalities.** Studies in animals and pregnant women have shown evidence of fetal abnormalities; therefore, the manufacturer classifies methotrexate as pregnancy category X (for psoriasis or RA). A pattern of congenital malformations associated with maternal methotrexate use is referred to as the aminopterin/methotrexate syndrome. Features of the syndrome include CNS, skeletal, and cardiac abnormalities. Low birth weight and developmental delay have also been reported. The use of methotrexate may impair fertility and cause menstrual irregularities or oligospermia during treatment and following therapy. Methotrexate is approved for the treatment of trophoblastic neoplasms (gestational choriocarcinoma, chorioadenoma destruens, and hydatidiform mole) and has been used for the medical management of ectopic pregnancy and the medical management of abortion. **[U.S. Boxed Warning]: Use is contraindicated for the treatment of psoriasis or RA in pregnant women.** Pregnancy should be excluded prior to therapy in women of childbearing potential. Use for the treatment of neoplastic diseases only when the potential benefit to the mother outweighs the possible risk to the fetus. Pregnancy should be avoided for ≥3 months following treatment in male patients and ≥1 ovulatory cycle in female patients. A registry is available for pregnant women exposed to autoimmune medications including methotrexate. For additional information contact the Organization of Teratology Information Specialists, OTIS Autoimmune Diseases Study, at 877-311-8972.

Breast-Feeding Considerations Low amounts of methotrexate are excreted into breast milk. Due to the potential for serious adverse reactions in a breast-feeding infant, use is contraindicated in nursing mothers.

Contraindications Known hypersensitivity to methotrexate or any component of the formulation; breast-feeding

Additional contraindications for patients with psoriasis or rheumatoid arthritis: Pregnancy, alcoholism, alcoholic liver disease or other chronic liver disease, immunodeficiency syndrome (overt or laboratory evidence); preexisting blood dyscrasias (eg, bone marrow hypoplasia, leukopenia, thrombocytopenia, significant anemia)

Warnings/Precautions Hazardous agent - use appropriate precautions for handling and disposal (NIOSH 2014 [group 1]).

[U.S. Boxed Warning]: Methotrexate has been associated with acute (elevated transaminases) and potentially fatal chronic (fibrosis, cirrhosis) hepatotoxicity. Risk is related to cumulative dose (≥1.5 g) and prolonged exposure. Monitor closely (with liver function tests, including serum albumin) for liver toxicities. Liver enzyme elevations may be noted, but may not be predictive of hepatic disease in long term treatment for psoriasis (but generally is predictive in rheumatoid arthritis [RA] treatment). With long-term use, liver biopsy may show histologic changes, fibrosis, or cirrhosis; periodic liver biopsy is recommended with long-term use for psoriasis patients with risk factors for hepatotoxicity and for persistent abnormal liver function tests in psoriasis patients without risk factors for hepatotoxicity and in RA patients; discontinue methotrexate with moderate-to-severe change in liver biopsy. Risk factors for hepatotoxicity include history of above moderate ethanol consumption, persistent abnormal liver chemistries, history of chronic liver disease (including hepatitis B or C), family history of inheritable liver disease, diabetes, obesity, hyperlipidemia, lack of folate supplementation during methotrexate therapy, cumulative methotrexate dose exceeding 1.5 g, continuous daily methotrexate dosing and history of significant exposure to hepatotoxic drugs. Use caution with preexisting liver impairment; may require dosage reduction. Use caution when used with other hepatotoxic agents (azathioprine, retinoids, sulfasalazine). **[U.S. Boxed Warning]: Methotrexate elimination is reduced in patients with ascites and pleural effusions;** resulting in prolonged half-life and toxicity; may require dose reduction or discontinuation. Monitor closely for toxicity.

[U.S. Boxed Warning]: May cause renal damage leading to acute renal failure, especially with high-dose

methotrexate; monitor renal function and methotrexate levels closely, maintain adequate hydration and urinary alkalinization. Use caution in osteosarcoma patients treated with high-dose methotrexate in combination with nephrotoxic chemotherapy (eg, cisplatin). **[U.S. Boxed Warning]: Methotrexate elimination is reduced in patients with renal impairment;** may require dose reduction or discontinuation; monitor closely for toxicity. **[U.S. Boxed Warning]: Tumor lysis syndrome may occur in patients with high tumor burden;** use appropriate prevention and treatment.

[U.S. Boxed Warning]: May cause potentially life-threatening pneumonitis (acute or chronic); may require treatment interruption; may be irreversible. Pulmonary symptoms may occur at any time during therapy and at any dosage; monitor closely for pulmonary symptoms, particularly dry, nonproductive cough. Other potential symptoms include fever, dyspnea, hypoxemia, or pulmonary infiltrate. **[U.S. Boxed Warning]: Methotrexate elimination is reduced in patients with pleural effusions;** may require dose reduction or discontinuation. Monitor closely for toxicity.

[U.S. Boxed Warning]: Bone marrow suppression may occur (sometimes fatal); aplastic anemia has been reported; anemia, pancytopenia, leukopenia, neutropenia, and/or thrombocytopenia may occur. Use caution in patients with preexisting bone marrow suppression. Discontinue treatment (immediately) in RA or psoriasis if a significant decrease in hematologic components is noted. **[U.S. Boxed Warning]: Use of low-dose methotrexate has been associated with the development of malignant lymphomas;** may regress upon treatment discontinuation; treat lymphoma appropriately if regression is not induced by cessation of methotrexate. Discontinue methotrexate if lymphoma does not regress. Other secondary tumors have been reported.

[U.S. Boxed Warning]: Gastrointestinal toxicity may occur; diarrhea and ulcerative stomatitis may require treatment interruption; hemorrhagic enteritis or intestinal perforation (with fatality) may occur. Use with caution in patients with peptic ulcer disease, ulcerative colitis. In children, doses ≥12 g/m^2 (IV) are associated with a high emetic potential; doses ≥250 mg/m^2 (IV) in adults and children are associated with moderate emetic potential (Dupuis, 2011). Antiemetics may be recommended to prevent nausea and vomiting.

May cause neurotoxicity including seizures (usually in pediatric ALL patients receiving intermediate-dose (1 g/m^2 methotrexate), leukoencephalopathy (usually in patients who have received cranial irradiation) and stroke-like encephalopathy (usually with high-dose regimens). Chemical arachnoiditis (headache, back pain, nuchal rigidity, fever) and myelopathy may result from intrathecal administration. Chronic leukoencephalopathy has been reported with high-dose and with intrathecal methotrexate; may be progressive and fatal. May cause dizziness and fatigue; may affect the ability to drive or operate heavy machinery.

[U.S. Boxed Warning]: Any dose level, route of administration, or duration of therapy may cause severe and potentially fatal dermatologic reactions, including toxic epidermal necrolysis, Stevens-Johnson syndrome, exfoliative dermatitis, skin necrosis, and erythema multiforme. Recovery has been reported with treatment discontinuation. Radiation dermatitis and sunburn may be precipitated by methotrexate administration. Psoriatic lesions may be worsened by concomitant exposure to ultraviolet radiation.

Potentially significant drug-drug interactions may exist, requiring dose or frequency adjustment, additional monitoring, and/or selection of alternative therapy. **[U.S. Boxed Warning]: Concomitant administration with NSAIDs may cause severe bone marrow suppression, aplastic anemia, and GI toxicity.** Do not administer NSAIDs prior to or during high-dose methotrexate therapy; may increase and prolong serum methotrexate levels. Doses used for psoriasis may still lead to unexpected toxicities; use caution when administering NSAIDs or salicylates with lower doses of methotrexate for RA. Methotrexate may increase the levels and effects of mercaptopurine; may require dosage adjustments. Vitamins containing folate may decrease response to systemic methotrexate; folate deficiency may increase methotrexate toxicity. Concomitant use of proton pump inhibitors with methotrexate (primarily high-dose methotrexate) may elevate and prolong serum methotrexate and metabolite (hydroxymethotrexate) levels; may lead to toxicities; use with caution. Immunization may be ineffective during methotrexate treatment. Immunization with live vaccines is not recommended; cases of disseminated vaccinia infections due to live vaccines have been reported. **[U.S. Boxed Warning]: Concomitant methotrexate administration with radiotherapy may increase the risk of soft tissue necrosis and osteonecrosis.**

[U.S. Boxed Warnings]: Should be administered under the supervision of a physician experienced in the use of antimetabolite therapy; serious and fatal toxicities have occurred at all dose levels. Immune suppression may lead to potentially fatal opportunistic infections, including *Pneumocystis jirovecii* pneumonia (PCP). Use methotrexate with extreme caution in patients with an active infection (contraindicated in patients with immunodeficiency syndrome). **[U.S. Boxed Warnings]: For rheumatoid arthritis and psoriasis, immunosuppressive therapy should only be used when disease is active, severe, recalcitrant, and disabling; and where less toxic, traditional therapy is ineffective. Methotrexate formulations and/or diluents containing preservatives should not be used for intrathecal or high-dose methotrexate therapy. May cause fetal death or congenital abnormalities; do not use for psoriasis or RA treatment in pregnant women.** May cause impairment of fertility, oligospermia, and menstrual dysfunction. Toxicity from methotrexate or any immunosuppressive is increased in the elderly. Methotrexate injection may contain benzyl alcohol and should not be used in neonates. Errors have occurred (some resulting in death) when methotrexate was administered as a "daily" dose instead of a "weekly" dose intended for some indications. The ISMP Targeted Medication Safety Best Practices for Hospitals recommends hospitals use a weekly dosage regimen default for oral methotrexate orders, with a hard stop override requiring verification of appropriate oncology indication; manual systems should require verification of an oncology indication prior to dispensing oral methotrexate for daily administration. Pharmacists should provide patient education for patients discharged on weekly oral methotrexate; education should include written leaflets that contain clear instructions about the weekly dosing schedule and explain the danger of taking extra doses (ISMP, 2014).

When used for intrathecal administration, should not be prepared during the preparation of any other agents; after preparation, store intrathecal medications in an isolated location or container clearly marked with a label identifying as "intrathecal" use only; delivery of intrathecal medications to the patient should only be with other medications intended for administration into the central nervous system (Jacobson, 2009).

Benzyl alcohol and derivatives: Some dosage forms may contain benzyl alcohol; large amounts of benzyl alcohol (≥99 mg/kg/day) have been associated with a potentially fatal toxicity ("gasping syndrome") in neonates; the "gasping syndrome" consists of metabolic acidosis, respiratory distress, gasping respirations, CNS dysfunction (including convulsions, intracranial hemorrhage), hypotension, and cardiovascular collapse (AAP, 1997; CDC, 1982); some data suggests that benzoate displaces bilirubin from protein binding sites (Ahlfors, 2001); avoid or use dosage forms containing benzyl alcohol with caution in neonates. See manufacturer's labeling.

Adverse Reactions Note: Adverse reactions vary by route and dosage.

Cardiovascular: Arterial thrombosis, cerebral thrombosis, chest pain, deep vein thrombosis, hypotension, pericardial effusion, pericarditis, plaque erosion (psoriasis), pulmonary embolism, retinal thrombosis, thrombophlebitis, vasculitis

Central nervous system: Abnormal cranial sensation, brain disease, chemical arachnoiditis (intrathecal; acute), chills, cognitive dysfunction (has been reported at low dosage), dizziness, drowsiness, fatigue, headache (pJIA), leukoencephalopathy (intravenous administration after craniospinal irradiation or repeated high-dose therapy; may be chronic), malaise, mood changes (has been reported at low dosage), neurological signs and symptoms (at high dosages; including confusion, hemiparesis, transient blindness, seizures, and coma), severe neurotoxicity (reported with unexpectedly increased frequency among pediatric patients with acute lymphoblastic leukemia who were treated with intermediate-dose intravenous methotrexate), speech disturbance

Dermatologic: Acne vulgaris, alopecia, burning sensation of skin (psoriasis), dermal ulcer, dermatitis (rheumatoid arthritis), diaphoresis, ecchymoses, erythema multiforme, erythematous rash, exfoliative dermatitis, furunculosis, hyperpigmentation, hypopigmentation, pruritus (rheumatoid arthritis), skin abnormalities related to radiation recall, skin necrosis, skin photosensitivity, skin rash, Stevens-Johnson syndrome, telangiectasia, toxic epidermal necrolysis, urticaria

Endocrine & metabolic: Decreased libido, decreased serum albumin, diabetes mellitus, gynecomastia, menstrual disease

Gastrointestinal: Abdominal distress, anorexia, aphthous stomatitis, diarrhea, enteritis, gastrointestinal hemorrhage, gingivitis, hematemesis, intestinal perforation, melena, nausea and vomiting, stomatitis

Genitourinary: Azotemia, cystitis, defective oogenesis, defective spermatogenesis, dysuria, hematuria, impotence, infertility, oligospermia, pancreatitis, proteinuria, severe renal disease, vaginal discharge

Hematologic & oncologic: Agranulocytosis, anemia, aplastic anemia, bone marrow depression (nadir: 7-10 days), decreased hematocrit, eosinophilia, gastric ulcer, hypogammaglobulinemia, leukopenia (WBC $<3000/mm^3$), lymphadenopathy, lymphoma, lymphoproliferative disorder, neutropenia, non-Hodgkin's lymphoma (in patients receiving low-dose oral methotrexate), pancytopenia (rheumatoid arthritis), thrombocytopenia (rheumatoid arthritis; platelet count $<100,000/mm^3$), tumor lysis syndrome

Hepatic: Cirrhosis (chronic therapy), hepatic failure, hepatic fibrosis (chronic therapy), hepatitis (acute), hepatotoxicity, increased liver enzymes

Hypersensitivity: Anaphylactoid reaction

Infection: Cryptococcosis, cytomegalovirus disease (including cytomegaloviral pneumonia, sepsis, nocardiosis), herpes simplex infection, herpes zoster, histoplasmosis, infection, pneumonia due to *pneumocystis jiroveci*, vaccinia (disseminated; following smallpox immunization)

Neuromuscular & skeletal: Arthralgia, myalgia, myelopathy (subacute), osteonecrosis (with radiotherapy), osteoporosis, stress fracture

Ophthalmic: Blurred vision, conjunctivitis, eye pain, visual disturbance

Otic: Tinnitus

Renal: Renal failure

Respiratory: Chronic obstructive pulmonary disease, cough, epistaxis, interstitial pneumonitis (rheumatoid arthritis), pharyngitis, pneumonia, pulmonary alveolitis, pulmonary disease, pulmonary fibrosis, respiratory failure, upper respiratory tract infection

Miscellaneous: Fever, nodule, tissue necrosis

Drug Interactions

Metabolism/Transport Effects Substrate of OAT3, P-glycoprotein, SLCO1B1

Avoid Concomitant Use

Avoid concomitant use of Methotrexate with any of the following: Acitretin; BCG; BCG (Intravesical); CloZAPine; Dipyrone; Foscarnet; Natalizumab; Pimecrolimus; Tacrolimus (Topical)

Increased Effect/Toxicity

Methotrexate may increase the levels/effects of: CloZAPine; CycloSPORINE (Systemic); Dipyrone; Leflunomide; Loop Diuretics; Natalizumab; Tegafur; Theophylline Derivatives; Tofacitinib; Vaccines (Live)

The levels/effects of Methotrexate may be increased by: Acitretin; Alitretinoin (Systemic); Ciprofloxacin (Systemic); CycloSPORINE (Systemic); Denosumab; Dexketoprofen; Dipyrone; Eltrombopag; Foscarnet; Fosphenytoin-Phenytoin; Loop Diuretics; Mipomersen; Nonsteroidal Anti-Inflammatory Agents; Penicillins; P-glycoprotein/ABCB1 Inhibitors; Pimecrolimus; Probenecid; Proton Pump Inhibitors; Roflumilast; Salicylates; SulfaSALAzine; Sulfonamide Derivatives; Tacrolimus (Topical); Teriflunomide; Trastuzumab; Trimethoprim

Decreased Effect

Methotrexate may decrease the levels/effects of: BCG; BCG (Intravesical); Coccidioides immitis Skin Test; Fosphenytoin-Phenytoin; Loop Diuretics; Sapropterin; Sipuleucel-T; Vaccines (Inactivated); Vaccines (Live)

The levels/effects of Methotrexate may be decreased by: Bile Acid Sequestrants; Echinacea; P-glycoprotein/ABCB1 Inducers

Food Interactions Methotrexate peak serum levels may be decreased if taken with food. Milk-rich foods may decrease methotrexate absorption. Management: Administer without regard to food.

Storage/Stability

Tablets: Store between 20°C and 25°C (68°F and 77°F); excursions are permitted between 15°C and 30°C (59°F and 86°F). Protect from light.

Injection: Store intact vials and autoinjectors between 20°C and 25°C (68°F and 77°F); excursions may be permitted between 15°C and 30°C (59°F and 86°F). Protect from light.

IV: Solution diluted in D_5W or NS is stable for 24 hours at room temperature (21°C to 25°C).

Intrathecal: Intrathecal dilutions are preservative free and should be used as soon as possible after preparation. After preparation, store intrathecal medications (until use) in an isolated location or container clearly marked with a label identifying as "intrathecal" use only.

Mechanism of Action Methotrexate is a folate antimetabolite that inhibits DNA synthesis, repair, and cellular replication. Methotrexate irreversibly binds to and inhibits dihydrofolate reductase, inhibiting the formation of reduced folates, and thymidylate synthetase, resulting in inhibition of purine and thymidylic acid synthesis, thus interfering with DNA synthesis, repair, and cellular replication. Methotrexate is cell cycle specific for the S phase of the cycle. Actively proliferative tissues are more susceptible to the effects of methotrexate.

The MOA in the treatment of rheumatoid arthritis is unknown, but may affect immune function. In psoriasis, methotrexate is thought to target rapidly proliferating epithelial cells in the skin.

In Crohn disease, it may have immune modulator and anti-inflammatory activity.

Pharmacodynamics Onset of action: Antirheumatic: 3-6 weeks; additional improvement may continue longer than 12 weeks

Pharmacokinetics (Adult data unless noted)

Absorption:

Oral: Pediatric and adult patients: Highly variable; dose-dependent; decreased absorption at higher doses (pediatric patients: >40 mg/m^2; adult patients: >80 mg/m^2); possibly due to saturation effect

IM: Complete

Distribution: Penetrates slowly into 3rd space fluids (eg, pleural effusions, ascites), exits slowly from these compartments (slower than from plasma); sustained concentrations retained in kidney and liver

V_d: IV: ~0.18 L/kg (initial); 0.4-0.8 L/kg (steady state)

Protein binding: ~50 %

Metabolism: Partially metabolized by intestinal flora (after oral administration) to DAMPA by carboxypeptidase; hepatic aldehyde oxidase converts methotrexate to 7-hydroxy methotrexate; polyglutamates are produced intracellularly and are just as potent as methotrexate; their production is dose- and duration-dependent and they are slowly eliminated by the cell once formed. Polyglutamated forms can be converted back to methotrexate.

Bioavailability: Oral: In general, bioavailability is dose dependent and decreases as the dose increases

Pediatric patients: Highly variable: 23% to 95%

Adults: Low doses (≤30 mg/m^2): 60%

Half-life (terminal):

Pediatric patients:

ALL: 0.7-5.8 hours (dose range: 6.3-30 mg/m^2)

JIA: 0.9-2.3 hours (dose range: 3.75-26.2 mg/m^2)

Adults: Low dose: 3-10 hours; high dose: 8-15 hours

Time to peak serum concentration:

Oral:

Pediatric patients: 0.67-4 hours (reported for a 15 mg/m^2 dose)

Adults: 1-2 hours

IM: Pediatric and adult patients: 30-60 minutes

Elimination: Dose and route dependent; IV: Urine (80% to 90% as unchanged drug; 5% to 7% as 7-hydroxy methotrexate); feces (<10%)

Dosing: Usual Note: Methotrexate doses between 100-500 mg/m^2 **may require** leucovorin calcium rescue. Methotrexate doses >500 mg/m^2 **require** leucovorin calcium rescue.

Infants, Children, and Adolescents: **Note:** Dosing may be presented as mg/m^2 or mg/kg; verify dosage unit for calculations; extra precautions should be taken. Frequency of dosing is indication specific (generally weekly or daily); patient harm may occur if administered incorrectly; extra precautions should be taken to verify appropriate frequency.

Acute lymphoblastic leukemia (ALL): Note: Intrathecal therapy is also administered (refer to specific reference for intrathecal dosing used within protocol):

Consolidation/intensification phases (as part of a combination regimen): IV: 1000 mg/m^2 infuse over 24 hours in week 1 of intensification and 20 mg/m^2 IM (use 50% dose reduction if on same day as intrathecal methotrexate) on day 1 of week 2 of intensification phase; Intensification repeats every 2 weeks for a total of 12 courses (Mahoney, 2000) **or** 5000 mg/m^2 IV over 24 hours days 8, 22, 36, and 50 of consolidation phase (Schrappe, 2000) with leucovorin rescue

Interim maintenance (as part of a combination regimen, (Seibel, 2008):

IV: 100 mg/m^2 (escalate dose by 50 mg/m^2 each dose) on days 0, 10, 20, 30, and 40 of increased intensity interim maintenance phase

Oral: 15 mg/m^2 on days 0, 7, 14, 21, 28, and 35 of interim maintenance phase

Maintenance (as part of a combination regimen):

I.M: 20 mg/m^2 weekly on day 1 of weeks 25 to 130 (Mahoney, 2000)

Oral: 20 mg/m^2 on days 7, 14, 21, 28, 35, 42, 49, 56, 63, 70, and 77 (Seibel, 2008)

ALL, T-cell (Asselin, 2011): Children and Adolescents: **Note:** Triple intrathecal therapy is also administered (refer to specific reference for intrathecal dosing used within protocol):

Induction (weeks 1-6; as part of a combination regimen): IV:

Low dose: 40 mg/m^2 on day 2

High dose: 500 mg/m^2 over 30 minutes followed by 4500 mg/m^2 over 23.5 hours (to complete a total dose of 5000 mg/m^2 over 24 hours) on day 22 (with leucovorin rescue)

Consolidation (weeks 7-33; combination chemotherapy): IV: High dose: 500 mg/m^2/dose over 30 minutes followed by 4500 mg/m^2/dose over 23.5 hours (to complete a total dose of 5000 mg/m^2 over 24 hours) (with leucovorin rescue) in weeks 7, 10, and 13

Continuation (weeks 34-108; combination chemotherapy): IV, IM: 30 mg/m^2 weekly until 2 years after documented complete remission

ALL, CNS prophylaxis triple intrathecal therapy: Children <10 years: Intrathecal: Age-based dosing (in combination with cytarabine and hydrocortisone): Days of administration vary based on risk status and protocol; refer to institutional protocols or reference for details (Matloub, 2006):

<2 years: 8 mg

2 to <3 years: 10 mg

3 to ≤8 years: 12 mg

>8 years: 15 mg

Crohn's disease: Limited data available: Children and Adolescents: Oral, SubQ: **Note:** Should be used in patients intolerant or unresponsive to purine analog therapy (eg, azathioprine, mercaptopurine); use in combination with folic acid supplementation

BSA-directed dosing: 15 mg/m^2 once weekly; maximum dose: 25 mg (Mack, 1998; Rufo, 2012; Sandhu, 2010; Turner, 2007)

Fixed-dosing (Kliegman, 2011; Mack, 1998; Turner, 2007; Weiss, 2009)

20-29 kg: 10 mg once weekly

30-39 kg: 15 mg once weekly

40-49 kg: 20 mg once weekly

≥ 50 kg: 25 mg once weekly

Dermatomyositis: Limited data available: Children and Adolescents: Oral, SubQ (preferred): Initial: 15 mg/m^2 **or** 1 mg/kg (whichever is less) once weekly; maximum dose: 40 mg; used in combination with corticosteroids (Huber, 2010; Ramanan, 2005)

Graft-versus-host disease, acute (aGVHD) prophylaxis: Limited data available: Children and Adolescents: IV: 15 mg/m^2/dose on day 1 and 10 mg/m^2/dose on days 3 and 6 after allogeneic transplant (in combination with cyclosporine and prednisone) (Chao, 1993; Chao, 2000; Ross, 1999) or 15 mg/m^2/dose on day 1 and 10 mg/m^2/dose on days 3, 6, and 11 after allogeneic transplant (in combination with cyclosporine) (Chao, 2000)

Juvenile idiopathic arthritis (JIA); polyarticular:

BSA-directed dosing: Children and Adolescents 2-16 years: Oral, IM, SubQ: Initial: 10 mg/m^2 once weekly, adjust gradually up to 20-30 mg/m^2 once weekly;

usual maximum dose: 25 mg; to reduce GI side effects, consider parenteral administration (IM, SubQ) of higher doses (20-30 mg/m^2)

Weight-directed dosing: Children and Adolescents: Oral, SubQ: Initial: 0.5 mg/kg once weekly; maximum initial dose: 15 mg; if symptoms worsen or unchanged after 4 weeks, may increase to SubQ: 1 mg/kg; maximum dose: 30 mg; (Dewitt, 2012)

Meningeal leukemia, prophylaxis or treatment: Intrathecal: 6-12 mg/dose (based on age) every 2-7 days; continue for 1 dose beyond CSF cell count normalization. **Note:** Optimal intrathecal chemotherapy dosing should be based on age rather than on body surface area (BSA); CSF volume correlates with age and not to BSA (Bleyer, 1983; Kerr, 2001):

<1 year: 6 mg/dose
1 year: 8 mg/dose
2 years: 10 mg/dose
≥3 years: 12 mg/dose

Osteosarcoma: Limited data available: IV: MAP regimen (High-dose methotrexate): 12 **g**/m^2 (maximum dose: 20 **g**) over 4 hours (followed by leucovorin rescue) for 4 doses during induction (before surgery) at weeks 3, 4, 8, and 9, and for 8 doses during maintenance (after surgery) at weeks 15, 16, 20, 21, 25, 26, 30, and 31 (in combination with doxorubicin and cisplatin) (Meyers, 2005); other combinations, intervals, and doses (8-14 **g**/m^2/dose) have been described (with leucovorin rescue), refer to specific reference for details (Bacci, 2000; Bacci, 2003; Goorin, 2003; Le Deley, 2007; Meyers, 1992; Weiner, 1986; Winkler, 1988)

Psoriasis, severe; recalcitrant to topical therapy: Limited data available: Children and Adolescents: Oral, SubQ: Usual reported range: 0.2-0.4 mg/kg once weekly; reported treatment duration is highly variable: 6-178 weeks (Dadlani, 2005; deJager, 2010)

Scleroderma, localized (juvenile): Limited data available: Oral, SubQ (preferred): 1 mg/kg once weekly; maximum dose: 25 mg; alone or in combinations with corticosteroids; duration of therapy: 12 months (Li, 2012)

Uveitis, recalcitrant: Limited data available: Children and Adolescents:

BSA-directed dosing: Oral, SubQ: Most frequently reported: 15 mg/m^2 once weekly, usual range: 10-25 mg/m^2 (Foeldvari, 2005; Simonini, 2013); the SubQ route may be preferred for patients with GI symptoms, poor bioavailability or doses >15 mg/m^2 (Simonini, 2010)

Weight-directed dosing: SubQ: 0.5-1 mg/kg once weekly; maximum dose: 25 mg (Weiss, 1998)

Adults: **Note:** For oncologic uses in obese patients, utilize patient's actual body weight (full weight) for calculation of body surface area- or weight-based dosing, particularly when the intent of therapy is curative; manage regimen-related toxicities in the same manner as for nonobese patients; if a dose reduction is utilized due to toxicity, consider resumption of full weight-based dosing with subsequent cycles, especially if cause of toxicity (eg, hepatic or renal impairment) is resolved (Griggs, 2012).

Acute lymphoblastic leukemia (ALL):

Meningeal leukemia prophylaxis or treatment: Intrathecal: Manufacturer's labeling: 12 mg (maximum 15 mg/dose) every 2-7 days; continue for 1 dose beyond CSF cell count normalization. **Note:** Optimal intrathecal chemotherapy dosing should be based on age rather than on body surface area (BSA); CSF volume correlates with age and not to BSA (Bleyer, 1983; Kerr, 2001).

CALGB 8811 regimen (Larson, 1995; combination therapy):

Early intensification: Intrathecal: 15 mg day 1 of early intensification phase, repeat in 4 weeks

CNS prophylaxis/interim maintenance phase:

Intrathecal: 15 mg day 1, 8, 15, 22, and 29

Oral: 20 mg/m^2 days 36, 43, 50, 57, and 64

Prolonged maintenance: Oral: 20 mg/m^2 days 1, 8, 15, and 22 every 4 weeks for 24 months from diagnosis

Dose-intensive regimen (Kantarjian, 2000; combination therapy): IV: 200 mg/m^2 over 2 hours, followed by 800 mg/m^2 over 24 hours beginning day 1 (followed by leucovorin rescue) of even numbered cycles (in combination with cytarabine; alternates with Hyper-CVAD)

CNS prophylaxis: Intrathecal: 12 mg on day 2 of each cycle; duration depends on risk

Maintenance: IV: 10 mg/m^2/day for 5 days every month for 2 years (in combination with prednisone, vincristine, and mercaptopurine)

Breast cancer: IV: CMF regimen: 40 mg/m^2 days 1 and 8 every 4 weeks (in combination with cyclophosphamide and fluorouracil) for 6-12 cycles (Bonadonna, 1995; Levine, 1998)

Choriocarcinoma, chorioadenoma, gestational trophoblastic diseases: 15-30 mg oral or IM daily for a 5 day course; may repeat for 3-5 courses (manufacturer's labeling) **or** 100 mg/m^2 IV over 30 minutes followed by 200 mg/m^2 IV over 12 hours (with leucovorin 24 hours after the start of methotrexate), administer a second course if hCG levels plateau for 3 consecutive weeks (Garrett, 2002)

Head and neck cancer, advanced: IV: 40 mg/m^2 once weekly until disease progression or unacceptable toxicity (Forastiere, 1992; Guardiola, 2004; Stewart, 2009)

Lymphoma, non-Hodgkin: IV:

CODOX-M/IVAC regimen (Mead, 2008): Cycles 1 and 3 of CODOX-M (CODOX-M alternates with IVAC): Adults ≤65 years: IV: 300 mg/m^2 over 1 hour (on day 10) followed by 2700 mg/m^2 over 23 hours (with leucovorin rescue)

Hyper-CVAD alternating with high-dose methotrexate/cytarabine regimen: IV: 1000 mg/m^2 over 24 hours on day 1 during even courses (2, 4, 6, and 8) of 21-day treatment cycles (Thomas, 2006) or 200 mg/m^2 bolus day 1 followed by 800 mg/m^2 over 24 hours during even courses (2, 4, 6, and 8) of 21-day treatment cycles (Khouri, 1998) with leucovorin rescue

Ectopic pregnancy: Limited data available: IM:

Single-dose regimen: Methotrexate 50 mg/m^2 on day 1; Measure serum hCG levels on days 4 and 7; if needed, repeat dose on day 7 (Barnhart, 2009)

Two-dose regimen: Methotrexate 50 mg/m^2 on day 1; Measure serum hCG levels on day 4 and administer a second dose of methotrexate 50 mg/m^2; Measure serum hCG levels on day 7 and if needed, administer a third dose of 50 mg/m^2 (Barnhart, 2009)

Multidose regimen: Methotrexate 1 mg/kg on day 1; measure serum hCG on day 2; methotrexate 1 mg/kg on day 3;alternate days of therapy with leucovorin (ie, day 2 and day 4); measure serum hCG on day 4; continue up to a total of 4 courses based on hCG concentrations (Barnhart, 2009)

Mycosis fungoides (cutaneous T-cell lymphoma): IM, Oral: 5-50 mg once weekly or 15-37.5 mg twice weekly for early stages (manufacturer's labeling) **or** 25 mg orally once weekly, may increase to 50 mg once weekly (Zackheim, 2003)

Osteosarcoma: Adults ≤30 years: IV: MAP regimen: 12 **g**/m^2 (maximum dose: 20 **g**) over 4 hours (followed by leucovorin rescue) for 4 doses during induction (before surgery) at weeks 3, 4, 8, and 9, and for 8 doses during maintenance (after surgery) at weeks 15, 16, 20, 21, 25, 26, 30, and 31 (in combination with doxorubicin and cisplatin) (Meyers, 2005); other combinations, intervals, age ranges, and doses (8-14 **g**/m²/dose) have been described (with leucovorin rescue), refer to specific reference for details (Bacci, 2000; Bacci, 2003; Goorin, 2003; Le Deley, 2007; Meyers, 1992; Weiner, 1986; Winkler, 1988)

Psoriasis: Note: Some experts recommend concomitant daily folic acid (except the day of methotrexate) to reduce hematologic, gastrointestinal, and hepatic adverse events related to methotrexate.

Oral: 2.5-5 mg/dose every 12 hours for 3 doses given weekly **or**

Oral, IM, SubQ: 10-25 mg/dose given once weekly; titrate to lowest effective dose

Note: An initial test dose of 2.5-5 mg is recommended in patients with risk factors for hematologic toxicity or renal impairment (Kalb, 2009).

Rheumatoid arthritis: Note: Some experts recommend concomitant daily folic acid (except the day of methotrexate) to reduce hematologic, gastrointestinal, and hepatic adverse events related to methotrexate.

Oral (manufacturer's labeling): 7.5 mg once weekly or 2.5 mg every 12 hours for 3 doses per week (dosage exceeding 20 mg per week may cause a higher incidence and severity of adverse events); *alternatively,* 10-15 mg once weekly, increased by 5 mg every 2-4 weeks to a maximum of 20-30 mg once weekly has been recommended by some experts (Visser, 2009)

IM, SubQ: 10-25 mg once weekly (dosage varies, similar to oral) or 15 mg once weekly (Braun, 2008)

Dosing adjustment for toxicity: All patients:

Nonhematologic toxicity: Diarrhea, stomatitis, or vomiting which may lead to dehydration: Discontinue until recovery

Hematologic toxicity:

Psoriasis, arthritis (JIA, RA): Significant blood count decrease: Discontinue immediately.

Oncologic uses: Profound granulocytopenia and fever: Evaluate immediately; consider broad-spectrum parenteral antimicrobial coverage

Dosing adjustment in renal impairment: There are no dosage adjustments provided in the manufacturer's labeling. The following adjustments have been recommended:

Infants, Children, and Adolescents (Aronoff, 2007):

CrCl >50 mL/minute/1.73 m²: No adjustment necessary

CrCl 10-50 mL/minute/1.73 m²: Administer 50% of dose

CrCl <10 mL/minute/1.73 m²: Administer 30% of dose

Hemodialysis: Administer 30% of dose

Peritoneal dialysis (PD): Administer 30% of dose

Continuous renal replacement therapy (CRRT): Administer 50% of dose

Adults:

Aronoff, 2007:

CrCl >50 mL/minute/1.73 m²: No adjustment necessary

CrCl 10-50 mL/minute: Administer 50% of dose

CrCl <10 mL/minute: Avoid use

Hemodialysis: Administer 50% of dose

Continuous renal replacement therapy (CRRT): Administer 50% of dose

Kintzel, 1995:

CrCl 46-60 mL/minute: Administer 65% of normal dose

CrCl 31-45 mL/minute: Administer 50% of normal dose

CrCl <30 mL/minute: Avoid use

Hemodialysis patients with cancer (Janus, 2010): Administer 25% of dose after hemodialysis; monitor closely for toxicity

High-dose methotrexate, dose-intensive regimen for ALL (200 mg/m² over 2 hours, followed by 800 mg/m² over 24 hours with leucovorin rescue (Kantarjian, 2000):

Serum creatinine <1.5 mg/dL: No dosage adjustment necessary

Serum creatinine 1.5-2 mg/dL: Administer 75% of dose

Serum creatinine >2 mg/dL: Administer 50% of dose

Dosing adjustment in hepatic impairment: All patients: There are no dosage adjustment provided in the manufacturer's labeling; use with caution in patients with impaired hepatic function or pre-existing hepatic dysfunction. The following adjustments have been recommended (Floyd, 2006):

Bilirubin 3.1-5 mg/dL **or** transaminases >3 times ULN: Administer 75% of dose

Bilirubin >5 mg/dL: Avoid use

Preparation for Administration Hazardous agent; use appropriate precautions for handling and disposal (NIOSH 2014 [group 1]).

Parenteral: **Use preservative-free preparations for intrathecal or high-dose methotrexate administration.**

IV:

Powder for injection: Reconstitute 1 g vial with 19.4 mL of sterile preservative free D_5W or NS to a concentration of 50 mg/mL; further dilute in D_5W or NS; for high doses, dilution of reconstituted solution in D_5W is recommended by the manufacturer; maximum concentration: 25 mg/mL (Gahart 2014)

Solution for injection (25 mg/mL): May further dilute in D_5W or NS

Intrathecal: Prepare intrathecal solutions with preservative-free NS to a final volume of up to 12 mL (volume generally based on institution or practitioner preference). Intrathecal methotrexate concentrations may be institution specific or based on practitioner preference, generally ranging from a final concentration of 1 mg/mL (per prescribing information; Grossman 1993; Lin 2008) up to ~2 to 4 mg/mL (de Lemos 2009; Glantz 1999). For triple intrathecal therapy (methotrexate 12 mg/hydrocortisone 24 mg/cytarabine 36 mg), preparation to final volume of 12 mL is reported (Lin 2008). Intrathecal medications should **NOT** be prepared during the preparation of any other agents.

Administration Hazardous agent; use appropriate precautions for handling and disposal (NIOSH 2014 [group 1]).

Oral: Often preferred when low doses are being administered; administer on an empty stomach.

Parenteral:

IM: May be administered at concentration ≤25 mg/mL; autoinjectors should not be used for IM administration.

IV:

IV push: May be administered as slow IV push at a concentration ≤25 mg/mL; some have suggested a rate of ≤10 mg/minute (Gahart 2014)

Bolus IV infusion, or 24-hour continuous infusion: Route and rate of administration depend upon indication and/or protocol; refer to specific references. For high-dose infusion, preservative-free formulation must be used **[U.S. Boxed Warning]**. Specific dosing schemes vary, but high dose should be followed by leucovorin calcium to prevent toxicity.

SubQ: May be administered SubQ (dependent upon indication and product).

Otrexup and Rasuvo are for once weekly subcutaneous use in the abdomen or thigh; do not inject within 2 inches of the navel or in areas where the skin is tender, bruised, red, scaly, hard or has scars or stretch marks. Patient may self-administer after appropriate training on preparation and administration and with appropriate follow-up monitoring. All schedules should be continually tailored to the individual patient. An initial test dose may be given prior to the regular dosing schedule to detect any extreme sensitivity to adverse effects.

Intrathecal: May be administered intrathecally; must use preservative-free formulation for intrathecal administration.

Monitoring Parameters Laboratory tests should be performed on day 5 or day 6 of the weekly methotrexate cycle (eg, psoriasis, RA, JIA) to detect the leukopenia nadir and to avoid elevated LFTs 1-2 days after taking dose.

Indication-specific recommendations: **Note:** Additional recommendations may vary based upon patient age and specific protocols (refer to specific references); for all pediatric patients receiving long-term therapy (ie, chronic disease), growth parameters should also be monitored.

Psoriasis: CBC with differential and platelets (baseline, 7-14 days after initiating therapy or dosage increase, every 2-4 weeks for first few months, then every 1-3 months); BUN and serum creatinine (baseline and every 2-3 months); consider PPD for latent TB screening (baseline); LFTs (baseline, monthly for first 6 months, then every 1-2 months); chest x-ray (baseline if underlying lung disease); pulmonary function test (if methotrexate-induced lung disease suspected)

Liver biopsy:

Patients **with** risk factors for hepatotoxicity: Baseline or after 2-6 months of therapy and with each 1-1.5 g cumulative dose interval in adults

Patients **without** risk factors for hepatotoxicity: If persistent elevations in 5 of 9 AST levels during a 12-month period, or decline of serum albumin below the normal range with normal nutritional status. In adults, consider biopsy after cumulative dose of 3.5-4 g and after each additional 1.5 g.

Juvenile idiopathic arthritis: Children and Adolescents: PPD screening (baseline and annually); CBC with differential and platelets, C-reactive protein, ESR, ferritin, and LDH [baseline, at follow-up visits (1-2 weeks, 1, 2, 6, and 9 months] and with any treatment change (DeWitt, 2012). Also based on adult recommendations in RA, consider serum creatinine and LFTs (baseline then every 2-4 weeks for initial 3 months of therapy, then every 8-12 weeks for 3-6 months of therapy and then every 12 weeks after 6 months of therapy) and liver biopsy: Baseline (if persistent abnormal baseline LFTs, history of alcoholism, or chronic hepatitis B or C) or during treatment if persistent LFT elevations (6 of 12 tests abnormal over 1 year or 5 of 9 results when LFTs performed at 6-week intervals)

Rheumatoid arthritis:

CBC with differential and platelets, serum creatinine and LFTs (baseline, then every 2-4 weeks for initial 3 months of therapy, then every 8-12 weeks for 3-6 months of therapy and then every 12 weeks after 6 months of therapy); chest x-ray (baseline); pulmonary function test (if methotrexate-induced lung disease suspected); hepatitis B or C testing (baseline)

Liver biopsy: Baseline (if persistent abnormal baseline LFTs, history of alcoholism, or chronic hepatitis B or C) or during treatment if persistent LFT elevations (6 of 12 tests abnormal over 1 year or 5 of 9 results when LFTs performed at 6-week intervals)

Cancer: Baseline and frequently during treatment: CBC with differential and platelets, serum creatinine, BUN, LFTs; chest x-ray (baseline); serum methotrexate concentrations and urine pH (with high-dose therapy); pulmonary function test (if methotrexate-induced lung disease suspected)

Crohn's disease:

Children and Adolescents: In pediatric trials, frequency of monitoring varied with study protocol and duration; may vary based on clinical status and concurrent medication; consider the following: CBC with differential and platelets, LFTs, C-reactive protein, and ESR (baseline, then every 2-4 weeks during initial 8-12 weeks of therapy, then every 4-12 weeks while on therapy); chest x-ray and PFTs (annually) (Mack, 1998; Sandhu, 2010, Turner, 2007; Weiss 2009). Also, based on adult recommendations for Crohn's disease, consider serum creatinine (baseline, then every 2-4 weeks for initial 3 months of therapy, then every 8-12 weeks for 3-6 months of therapy and then every 12 weeks after 6 months of therapy), hepatitis B or C testing (baseline) and liver biopsy: Baseline (if persistent abnormal baseline LFTs, history of alcoholism, or chronic hepatitis B or C) or during treatment if persistent LFT elevations (6 of 12 tests abnormal over 1 year or 5 of 9 results when LFTs performed at 6-week intervals).

Adults: CBC with differential and platelets, serum creatinine and LFTs (baseline then every 2-4 weeks for initial 3 months of therapy, then every 8-12 weeks for 3-6 months of therapy and then every 12 weeks after 6 months of therapy); chest x-ray (baseline); pulmonary function test (if methotrexate-induced lung disease suspected); hepatitis B or C testing (baseline) and liver biopsy: Baseline (if persistent abnormal baseline LFTs, history of alcoholism, or chronic hepatitis B or C) or during treatment if persistent LFT elevations (6 of 12 tests abnormal over 1 year or 5 of 9 results when LFTs performed at 6-week intervals)

Ectopic pregnancy: Prior to therapy, measure serum hCG, CBC with differential, liver function tests, serum creatinine. Serum hCG concentrations should decrease between treatment days 4 and 7. If hCG decreases by >15%, additional courses are not needed; however, continue to measure hCG weekly until no longer detectable. If <15% decrease is observed, repeat dose per regimen (Barnhart, 2009).

Reference Range

Therapeutic levels: Variable; toxic concentration: Variable; therapeutic range is dependent upon therapeutic approach

High-dose regimens produce drug levels that are between 0.1-1 micromole/L 24-72 hours after drug infusion.

Toxic: Low-dose therapy: >0.2 micromole/L; high-dose therapy: >1 micromole/L

Dosage Forms Excipient information presented when available (limited, particularly for generics); consult specific product labeling. [DSC] = Discontinued product

Solution, Injection:

Generic: 25 mg/mL (2 mL, 10 mL)

Solution, Injection [preservative free]:

Generic: 25 mg/mL (2 mL, 4 mL, 8 mL, 10 mL, 40 mL); 50 mg/2 mL (2 mL); 100 mg/4 mL (4 mL); 200 mg/8 mL (8 mL [DSC]); 250 mg/10 mL (10 mL); 1 g/40 mL (40 mL)

Solution Auto-injector, Subcutaneous [preservative free]:

Otrexup: 10 mg/0.4 mL (0.4 mL); 15 mg/0.4 mL (0.4 mL); 20 mg/0.4 mL (0.4 mL); 25 mg/0.4 mL (0.4 mL)

Rasuvo: 7.5 mg/0.15 mL (0.15 mL); 10 mg/0.2 mL (0.2 mL); 12.5 mg/0.25 mL (0.25 mL); 15 mg/0.3 mL (0.3 mL); 17.5 mg/0.35 mL (0.35 mL); 20 mg/0.4 mL (0.4 mL); 22.5 mg/0.45 mL (0.45 mL); 25 mg/0.5 mL (0.5 mL); 27.5 mg/0.55 mL (0.55 mL); 30 mg/0.6 mL (0.6 mL)

Solution Reconstituted, Injection [preservative free]:

Generic: 1 g (1 ea)

Tablet, Oral:

Rheumatrex: 2.5 mg [scored]

Trexall: 5 mg, 7.5 mg, 10 mg, 15 mg [scored]

Generic: 2.5 mg

◆ **Methotrexate Injection, BP (Can)** *see* Methotrexate *on page 1390*

- ◆ **Methotrexate Injection USP (Can)** *see* Methotrexate *on page 1390*
- ◆ **Methotrexate Sodium** *see* Methotrexate *on page 1390*
- ◆ **Methotrexate Sodium Injection (Can)** *see* Methotrexate *on page 1390*
- ◆ **Methotrexatum** *see* Methotrexate *on page 1390*

Methsuximide (meth SUKS i mide)

Medication Safety Issues

Sound-alike/look-alike issues:

Methsuximide may be confused with ethosuximide

Brand Names: US Celontin

Brand Names: Canada Celontin®

Therapeutic Category Anticonvulsant, Succinimide

Generic Availability (US) No

Use Control of refractory absence (petit mal) seizures (FDA approved in children and adults); useful adjunct in refractory, partial complex (psychomotor) seizures

Medication Guide Available Yes

Pregnancy Considerations Patients exposed to methsuximide during pregnancy are encouraged to enroll themselves into the NAAED Pregnancy Registry by calling 1-888-233-2334. Additional information is available at www.aedpregnancyregistry.org.

Contraindications History of hypersensitivity to succinimides

Warnings/Precautions Antiepileptics are associated with an increased risk of suicidal behavior/thoughts with use (regardless of indication); patients should be monitored for signs/symptoms of depression, suicidal tendencies, and other unusual behavior changes during therapy and instructed to inform their healthcare provider immediately if symptoms occur. Use with caution in patients with hepatic or renal disease. Abrupt withdrawal of the drug may precipitate absence status. Methsuximide may increase tonic-clonic seizures when used alone in patients with mixed seizure disorders. Methsuximide must be used in combination with other anticonvulsants in patients with both absence and tonic-clonic seizures. May cause CNS depression, which may impair physical or mental abilities; patients must be cautioned about performing tasks which require mental alertness (eg, operating machinery or driving). Effects with other sedative drugs or ethanol may be potentiated. Consider evaluation of blood counts in patients with signs/symptoms of infection. Succinimides have been associated with severe blood dyscrasias and cases of systemic lupus erythematosus.

Adverse Reactions

Cardiovascular: Hyperemia

Central nervous system: Aggressiveness, ataxia, confusion, depression, dizziness, drowsiness, hallucinations (auditory), headache, hypochondriacal behavior, insomnia, irritability, mental instability, mental slowness, nervousness, psychosis, suicidal behavior

Dermatologic: Pruritus, rash, Stevens-Johnson syndrome, urticaria

Gastrointestinal: Abdominal pain, anorexia, constipation, diarrhea, epigastric pain, nausea, vomiting, weight loss

Genitourinary: Hematuria (microscopic), proteinuria

Hematologic: Eosinophilia, leukopenia, monocytosis, pancytopenia

Ocular: Blurred vision, periorbital edema, photophobia

Miscellaneous: Hiccups, systemic lupus erythematosus

Drug Interactions

Metabolism/Transport Effects Substrate of CYP2C19 (major); **Note:** Assignment of Major/Minor substrate status based on clinically relevant drug interaction potential; **Inhibits** CYP2C19 (weak)

Avoid Concomitant Use

Avoid concomitant use of Methsuximide with any of the following: Azelastine (Nasal); Orphenadrine; Paraldehyde; Thalidomide

Increased Effect/Toxicity

Methsuximide may increase the levels/effects of: Alcohol (Ethyl); Azelastine (Nasal); Buprenorphine; CNS Depressants; Hydrocodone; Methotrimeprazine; Metyrosine; Mirtazapine; Orphenadrine; Paraldehyde; Pramipexole; ROPINIRole; Rotigotine; Selective Serotonin Reuptake Inhibitors; Suvorexant; Thalidomide; Zolpidem

The levels/effects of Methsuximide may be increased by: Brimonidine (Topical); Cannabis; CYP2C19 Inhibitors (Moderate); CYP2C19 Inhibitors (Strong); Doxylamine; Dronabinol; Droperidol; HydrOXYzine; Kava Kava; Luliconazole; Magnesium Sulfate; Methotrimeprazine; Nabilone; Perampanel; Rufinamide; Sodium Oxybate; Tapentadol; Tetrahydrocannabinol

Decreased Effect

The levels/effects of Methsuximide may be decreased by: CYP2C19 Inducers (Strong); Dabrafenib; Mefloquine; Mianserin; Orlistat

Storage/Stability Store at 25°C (77°F); excursions permitted to 15°C to 30°C (59°F to 86°F); protect from excessive heat 40°C (104°F). Protect from light and moisture. **Note:** Methsuximide has a relatively low melting temperature (124°F); do not store in conditions that promote high temperatures (eg, in a closed vehicle).

Mechanism of Action Increases the seizure threshold and suppresses paroxysmal spike-and-wave pattern in absence seizures; depresses nerve transmission in the motor cortex

Pharmacokinetics (Adult data unless noted)

Metabolism: Rapidly demethylated in the liver to N-desmethylmethsuximide (active metabolite)

Half-life: 2-4 hours

- N-desmethylmethsuximide:
  - Children: 26 hours
  - Adults: 28-80 hours

Time to peak serum concentration: Within 1-3 hours

Elimination: <1% in urine as unchanged drug

Dosing: Usual Oral:

Children: Initial: 10-15 mg/kg/day in 3-4 divided doses; increase weekly up to maximum of 30 mg/kg/day; mean dose required:

- <30 kg: 20 mg/kg/day
- >30 kg: 14 mg/kg/day

Adults: 300 mg/day for the first week; may increase by 300 mg/day at weekly intervals up to 1.2 g in 2-4 divided doses/day

Administration Oral: Administer with food

Monitoring Parameters CBC with differential, liver enzymes, urinalysis; measure trough serum levels for efficacy and 3-hour postdose concentrations for toxicity; signs and symptoms of suicidality (eg, anxiety, depression, behavior changes)

Reference Range Measure N-desmethylmethsuximide concentrations:

Therapeutic: 10-40 mcg/mL (SI: 53-212 micromoles/L)

Toxic: >40 mcg/mL (SI: >212 micromoles/L)

Dosage Forms Excipient information presented when available (limited, particularly for generics); consult specific product labeling.

Capsule, Oral:

Celontin: 300 mg

- ◆ **Methylacetoxyprogesterone** *see* MedroxyPROGESTERone *on page 1339*

Methyldopa (meth il DOE pa)

Medication Safety Issues

Sound-alike/look-alike issues:

Methyldopa may be confused with L-dopa, levodopa

BEERS Criteria medication:

This drug may be potentially inappropriate for use in geriatric patients (Quality of evidence - low; Strength of recommendation - strong).

International issues:

Aldomet [Multiple international markets] may be confused with Aldactone brand name for spironolactone [U.S., Canada, multiple international markets]

Brand Names: Canada Methyldopa; Novo-Medopa

Therapeutic Category Alpha-Adrenergic Inhibitors, Central; Antihypertensive Agent

Generic Availability (US) Yes

Use Management of moderate to severe hypertension

Pregnancy Risk Factor B/C (injectable)

Pregnancy Considerations Adverse events have not been observed in animal reproduction studies. Methyldopa crosses the placenta and appears in cord blood. Available data show use during pregnancy does not cause fetal harm and improves fetal outcomes. Untreated chronic maternal hypertension is associated with adverse events in the fetus, infant, and mother. If treatment for chronic hypertension during pregnancy is needed, methyldopa is one of the preferred agents. If an injectable agent is needed for the urgent control of acute hypertension in pregnancy, other agents are preferred (ACOG, 2013).

Breast-Feeding Considerations Methyldopa is excreted into breast milk in concentrations <1% of the weight-adjusted maternal dose (Jones, 1978; White, 1985). The manufacturer recommends that caution be exercised when administering methyldopa to nursing women.

Contraindications Hypersensitivity to methyldopa or any component of the formulation; active hepatic disease; liver disorders previously associated with use of methyldopa; concurrent use of MAO inhibitors

Warnings/Precautions Rare cases of reversible granulocytopenia and thrombocytopenia have been reported. May rarely produce hemolytic anemia; positive Coombs' test occurs in 10% to 20% of patients (perform CBC periodically). If Coombs'-positive hemolytic anemia occurs during therapy, discontinue use and do not reinitiate; Coombs' test may not revert back to normal for weeks to months following discontinuation. Sedation (usually transient) may occur during initial therapy or whenever the dose is increased. May rarely produce liver disorders including fatal hepatic necrosis; use with caution in patients with previous liver disease or dysfunction. Periodically monitor liver function during the first 6-12 weeks of therapy or when unexplained fever occurs; discontinue use if fever, abnormal liver function tests, or jaundice is present. Patients with severe bilateral cerebrovascular disease have exhibited involuntary choreoathetotic movements (rare); discontinue use if these symptoms develop. Patients with impaired renal function may respond to smaller doses. Active metabolites of methyldopa accumulate in patients with renal impairment. Tolerance may occur usually between the second and third month of therapy; adding a diuretic or increasing the dosage of methyldopa frequently restores blood pressure control. May produce clinical edema; discontinue if edema worsens or signs of heart failure arise. Mild edema may be controlled with the concomitant use of diuretic therapy. Patients on methyldopa may need less anesthetic agents (Miller, 1968; Miller, 2010). May be inappropriate in the elderly due to a risk of bradycardia and depression (Beers Criteria); use with caution in the elderly; may experience syncope (avoid by giving smaller doses); not considered a drug of choice in this age group. Often considered the drug of choice for treatment of hypertension in pregnancy. Do not use injectable if bisulfite allergy.

Adverse Reactions

Cardiovascular: Angina pectoris aggravation, bradycardia, carotid sinus hypersensitivity prolonged, heart failure, myocarditis, orthostatic hypotension, paradoxical pressor response (IV use), pericarditis, peripheral edema, symptoms of cerebrovascular insufficiency, vasculitis

Central nervous system: Bell's palsy, dizziness, drug fever, headache, lightheadedness, mental acuity decreased, mental depression, nightmares, parkinsonism, sedation

Dermatologic: Rash, toxic epidermal necrolysis

Endocrine & metabolic: Amenorrhea, breast enlargement, gynecomastia, hyperprolactinemia, lactation, libido decreased

Gastrointestinal: Abdominal distension, colitis, constipation, diarrhea, flatulence, nausea, pancreatitis, sialadenitis, sore or "black" tongue, vomiting, weight gain, xerostomia

Genitourinary: Impotence

Hematologic: Bone marrow suppression, eosinophilia, granulocytopenia, hemolytic anemia; positive tests for ANA, LE cells, rheumatoid factor, Coombs test (positive); leukopenia, thrombocytopenia

Hepatic: Abnormal LFTs, liver disorders (hepatitis), jaundice

Neuromuscular & skeletal: Arthralgia, choreoathetosis, myalgia, paresthesias, weakness

Renal: BUN increased

Respiratory: Nasal congestion

Miscellaneous: SLE-like syndrome

Drug Interactions

Metabolism/Transport Effects Substrate of COMT

Avoid Concomitant Use

Avoid concomitant use of Methyldopa with any of the following: Ceritinib; Iobenguane I 123; MAO Inhibitors

Increased Effect/Toxicity

Methyldopa may increase the levels/effects of: Amifostine; Antihypertensives; Beta-Blockers; Bradycardia-Causing Agents; Ceritinib; DULoxetine; Hypotensive Agents; Ivabradine; Lacosamide; Levodopa; Lithium; Obinutuzumab; RisperiDONE; RiTUXimab

The levels/effects of Methyldopa may be increased by: Alfuzosin; Barbiturates; Beta-Blockers; Bretylium; Brimonidine (Topical); COMT Inhibitors; Diazoxide; Herbs (Hypotensive Properties); MAO Inhibitors; Nicorandil; Pentoxifylline; Phosphodiesterase 5 Inhibitors; Prostacyclin Analogues; Ruxolitinib; Tofacitinib

Decreased Effect

Methyldopa may decrease the levels/effects of: Iobenguane I 123

The levels/effects of Methyldopa may be decreased by: Herbs (Hypertensive Properties); Iron Salts; Methylphenidate; Mirtazapine; Multivitamins/Minerals (with ADEK, Folate, Iron); Serotonin/Norepinephrine Reuptake Inhibitors; Tricyclic Antidepressants; Yohimbine

Storage/Stability

Injection: Store at controlled room temperature 20°C to 25°C (68°F to 77°F); excursions permitted to 15°C to 30°C (59°F to 86°F). Injectable dosage form is most stable at acid to neutral pH. Stability of parenteral admixture at room temperature (25°C) is 24 hours. Parenteral admixture is stable at room temperature for up to 125 hours (Newton, 1981).

Tablets: Store at controlled room temperature 20°C to 25°C (68°F to 77°F).

Mechanism of Action Stimulation of central alpha-adrenergic receptors by a false neurotransmitter (alpha-methylnorepinephrine) that results in a decreased sympathetic outflow to the heart, kidneys, and peripheral vasculature

Pharmacodynamics Hypotensive effects:
Maximum effect: Oral, IV: Single-dose: Within 3-6 hours; multiple-dose: 2-3 days
Duration:
Oral: Single-dose: 12-24 hours; multiple-dose: 1-2 days
IV: 10-16 hours

Pharmacokinetics (Adult data unless noted)
Absorption: Oral: ~50%
Distribution: Crosses placenta; appears in breast milk
Protein binding: <15%
Metabolism: In the intestine and the liver
Half-life: Elimination:
Neonates: 10-20 hours
Adults: 1-3 hours
Elimination: ~70% of systemic dose eliminated in urine as drug and metabolites
Dialysis: Slightly dialyzable (5% to 20%)

Dosing: Usual
Children:
Oral: Initial: 10 mg/kg/day in 2-4 divided doses; increase every 2 days as needed to maximum dose of 65 mg/kg/day; do not exceed 3 g/day
IV: Initial: 2-4 mg/kg/dose; if response is not seen within 4-6 hours, may increase to 5-10 mg/kg/dose; administer doses every 6-8 hours; maximum daily dose: 65 mg/kg or 3 g, whichever is less
Adults:
Oral: Initial: 250 mg 2-3 times/day; increase every 2 days as needed; usual dose 500 mg to 2 g daily in 2-4 divided doses; maximum dose: 3 g/day; usual dosage range (JNC 7): 250-1000 mg/day in 2 divided doses
IV: 250-1000 mg every 6-8 hours; maximum dose: 4 g/day

Dosing interval in renal impairment: Children and Adults:
CrCl >50 mL/minute: Administer normal dose every 8 hours
CrCl 10-50 mL/minute: Administer normal dose every 8-12 hours
CrCl <10 mL/minute: Administer normal dose every 12-24 hours

Preparation for Administration Parenteral: IV: Dilute in D_5W to a final concentration ≤10 mg/mL

Administration
Oral: May be administered without regard to food; administer new dosage increases in the evening to minimize sedation
Parenteral: IV: Infuse over 30 to 60 minutes

Monitoring Parameters Blood pressure, CBC with differential, hemoglobin, hematocrit, Coombs' test [direct], liver enzymes

Test Interactions Methyldopa interferes with the following laboratory tests: urinary uric acid, serum creatinine (alkaline picrate method), AST (colorimetric method), and urinary catecholamines (falsely high levels)

Additional Information Most effective if used with diuretic; titrate dose to optimal blood pressure control with minimal side effects

Dosage Forms Excipient information presented when available (limited, particularly for generics); consult specific product labeling.
Solution, Intravenous, as hydrochloride:
Generic: 250 mg/5 mL (5 mL)
Tablet, Oral:
Generic: 250 mg, 500 mg

Extemporaneous Preparations A 50 mg/mL oral suspension may be made with tablets and either unpreserved Simple Syrup, N.F. or a 1:1 mixture of simple syrup (containing 0.5% citric acid) and hydrochloric acid 0.2 N. Crush ten 250 mg tablets in a glass mortar and reduce to a fine powder. To make formulation with unpreserved simple syrup, add small portions of vehicle and mix to a uniform paste; mix while adding the vehicle in incremental proportions to **almost** 50 mL; transfer to a calibrated bottle; rinse the mortar and pestle several times with vehicle, and add quantity of vehicle sufficient to make 50 mL. To make formulation with the second vehicle, mix powdered tablets with 25 mL of hydrochloric acid 0.2 N (0.73% w/v); dilute this mixture to 50 mL with simple syrup containing 0.5% citric acid by the method described above. Label "shake well" and "protect from light." Stable for 14 days when stored in glass prescription bottles in the dark at room temperature or refrigerated.

Newton DW, Rogers AG, Becker CH, et al, "Extemporaneous Preparation of Methyldopa in Two Syrup Vehicles," *Am J Hosp Pharm*, 1975, 32(8):817-21.

◆ **Methyldopate Hydrochloride** *see* Methyldopa *on page 1399*

Methylene Blue (METH i leen bloo)

Medication Safety Issues
Sound-alike/look-alike issues:
Methylene Blue may be confused with VisionBlue
Other safety concerns:
Due to the potential for dosing errors between mg and mL of methylene blue, prescribing and dosing should only be expressed in terms of mg of methylene blue (and not as mL)
Due to potential toxicity (hemolytic anemia), do not use methylene blue to color enteral feedings to detect aspiration.

Related Information
Serotonin Syndrome *on page 2447*

Therapeutic Category Antidote, Cyanide; Antidote, Drug-induced Methemoglobinemia

Generic Availability (US) Yes

Use Antidote for drug-induced methemoglobinemia (FDA approved in pediatric patients [age not specified] and adults); has also been used for the following: Treatment/prevention of ifosfamide-induced encephalopathy; topically, in conjunction with polychromatic light to photoinactivate viruses such as herpes simplex; alone or in combination with vitamin C for the management of chronic urolithiasis

Pregnancy Risk Factor X

Pregnancy Considerations Use during amniocentesis has shown evidence of fetal abnormalities (atresia of the ileum and jejunum, ileal occlusions); has been used orally without similar adverse events; (Bailey 2003). In addition, hemolytic anemia, methemoglobinemia, and phototoxicity have been reported in neonates following in utero exposure (Burnakis 1995; Porat 1996; Vincer 1987). Based on studies in nonpregnant women, potential exposure to the fetus may be less when methylene blue is used for lymphatic mapping in breast cancer (Pruthi 2011).

Use is contraindicated in women who are or may become pregnant. In general, medications used as antidotes should take into consideration the health and prognosis of the mother (Bailey 2003).

Contraindications Pregnancy; women who are or may become pregnant; intraspinal injection and SubQ injection; hypersensitivity to any component of the formulation.

Warnings/Precautions Inject slowly over a period of several minutes to prevent high local concentration from producing additional methemoglobin. Do not inject SubQ or intrathecally; use with caution in patients with G6PD deficiency. At high doses or in patients with G6PD-deficiency and infants, methylene blue may catalyze the oxidation of ferrous iron in hemoglobin to ferric iron causing paradoxical methemoglobinemia and hemolysis; monitor methemoglobin concentrations regularly during administration. Use with caution in patients with severe renal impairment. Potentially significant drug-drug interactions may exist, requiring dose or frequency adjustment, additional monitoring, and/or selection of alternative therapy. Methylene blue should not be added to enteral feeding products (Durfee 2006; Wessel 2005); safety and efficacy have not been established. Vesicant: If administering as a continuous infusion, ensure proper needle or catheter placement prior to and during infusion; avoid extravasation. Infuse via central line if possible; monitor IV site closely (Dumbarton, 2012).

Adverse Reactions

Cardiovascular: Angina, arrhythmia, hypertension, precordial pain

Central nervous system: Dizziness, headache, fever, mental confusion

Dermatologic: Staining of skin

Gastrointestinal: Abdominal pain, diarrhea, fecal discoloration (blue-green), nausea, vomiting

Genitourinary: Bladder irritation, discoloration of urine (blue-green)

Hematologic: Anemia, paradoxical methemoglobinemia (high doses), transient reduction in oxygen saturation as read by pulse oximetry

Respiratory: Dyspnea

Miscellaneous: Diaphoresis

Postmarketing and/or case reports: Serotonin syndrome

Drug Interactions

Metabolism/Transport Effects Inhibits Monoamine Oxidase

Avoid Concomitant Use

Avoid concomitant use of Methylene Blue with any of the following: Aclidinium; Alcohol (Ethyl); Alpha-/Beta-Agonists (Indirect-Acting); Alpha1-Agonists; Amphetamines; Anilidopiperidine Opioids; Apraclonidine; AtoMOXetine; Atropine (Ophthalmic); Bezafibrate; Buprenorphine; BuPROPion; BusPIRone; CarBAMazepine; Cyclobenzaprine; Cyproheptadine; Dapoxetine; Dexmethylphenidate; Dextromethorphan; Diethylpropion; Eluxadoline; Glucagon; Hydrocodone; HYDROmorphone; Ipratropium (Oral Inhalation); Isometheptene; Levonordefrin; Linezolid; MAO Inhibitors; Maprotiline; Meperidine; Mequitazine; Methyldopa; Methylphenidate; Mianserin; Mirtazapine; Morphine (Liposomal); Morphine (Systemic); Nefazodone; Oxymorphone; Pholcodine; Pizotifen; Potassium Chloride; Selective Serotonin Reuptake Inhibitors; Serotonin 5-HT1D Receptor Agonists; Serotonin/Norepinephrine Reuptake Inhibitors; Tapentadol; Tetrabenazine; Tetrahydrozoline (Nasal); Tiotropium; TraZODone; Tricyclic Antidepressants; Tryptophan; Umeclidinium

Increased Effect/Toxicity

Methylene Blue may increase the levels/effects of: AbobotulinumtoxinA; Alpha-/Beta-Agonists (Indirect-Acting); Alpha1-Agonists; Amphetamines; Analgesics (Opioid); Anticholinergic Agents; Antihypertensives; Antipsychotic Agents; Apraclonidine; AtoMOXetine; Atropine (Ophthalmic); Beta2-Agonists; Betahistine; Bezafibrate; Blood Glucose Lowering Agents; Brimonidine (Ophthalmic); Brimonidine (Topical); BuPROPion; Cannabinoid-Containing Products; Cyproheptadine; Dexmethylphenidate; Dextromethorphan; Diethylpropion; Domperidone; Doxapram; Doxylamine; Eluxadoline; EPINEPHrine (Nasal); Epinephrine (Racemic); EPINEPHrine (Systemic, Oral Inhalation); Glucagon; Hydrocodone; HYDROmorphone; Isometheptene; Levonordefrin; Linezolid; Lithium; Meperidine; Mequitazine; Methadone; Methyldopa; Methylphenidate; Metoclopramide; Mianserin; Mirabegron; Morphine (Liposomal); Morphine (Systemic); Norepinephrine; OnabotulinumtoxinA; Orthostatic Hypotension Producing Agents; OxyCODONE; Pizotifen; Potassium Chloride; Reserpine; RimabotulinumtoxinB; Serotonin 5-HT1D Receptor Agonists; Serotonin Modulators; Tetrahydrozoline (Nasal); Thiazide Diuretics; Tiotropium; Topiramate

The levels/effects of Methylene Blue may be increased by: Aclidinium; Alcohol (Ethyl); Altretamine; Anilidopiperidine Opioids; Antiemetics (5HT3 Antagonists); Antipsychotic Agents; Buprenorphine; BusPIRone; CarBAMazepine; COMT Inhibitors; Cyclobenzaprine; Dapoxetine; Ipratropium (Oral Inhalation); Levodopa; MAO Inhibitors; Maprotiline; Mirtazapine; Nefazodone; Oxymorphone; Pholcodine; Pramlintide; Selective Serotonin Reuptake Inhibitors; Serotonin/Norepinephrine Reuptake Inhibitors; Tapentadol; Tetrabenazine; TraMADol; TraZODone; Tricyclic Antidepressants; Tryptophan; Umeclidinium

Decreased Effect

Methylene Blue may decrease the levels/effects of: Acetylcholinesterase Inhibitors; Domperidone; Itopride; Metoclopramide; Secretin

The levels/effects of Methylene Blue may be decreased by: Acetylcholinesterase Inhibitors; Cyproheptadine; Domperidone

Storage/Stability Store at 20°C to 25°C (68°F to 77°F); excursions permitted to 15°C to 30°C (59°F to 86°F).

Mechanism of Action Weak germicide in low concentrations, hastens the conversion of methemoglobin to hemoglobin; has opposite effect at high concentrations by converting ferrous ion of reduced hemoglobin to ferric ion to form methemoglobin; in cyanide toxicity, it combines with cyanide to form cyanmethemoglobin preventing the interference of cyanide with the cytochrome system

In the treatment of vasoplegia syndrome, methylene blue may be able to restore vascular tone by a direct inhibitory effect on endothelial nitric oxide synthase (eNOS), and probably inducible NOS (iNOS), by oxidation of enzyme-bound ferrous iron. Methylene blue also blocks the formation of cyclic guanosine monophosphate (cGMP) by inhibiting the guanylate cyclase enzyme through binding to iron in the heme complex and subsequently reducing vasorelaxation (Lenglet 2011).

Pharmacodynamics Onset of action: Reduction of methemoglobin: IV: 30 to 60 minutes

Pharmacokinetics (Adult data unless noted)

Absorption: Well-absorbed from GI tract

Bioavailability, oral: 50% to 100%

Time to peak effect: 30 minutes

Metabolism: Peripheral reduction to leukomethylene blue

Elimination: In bile, feces, and urine as leukomethylene blue

Dosing: Neonatal Note: Systemic doses as low as 2 mg/kg have been associated with hemolytic anemia and skin desquamation (Clifton, 2003).

Methemoglobinemia: I.O., IV: 1 mg/kg (Clifton, 2003); a lower range of 0.3 to 1 mg/kg has been recommended for preterm neonates based on a prospective screening study (n=13, GA: 25 to 30 weeks) (Hjelt, 1995)

Shock (vasodilatory) with hypotension unresponsive to fluid resuscitation, exogenous catecholamines and corticosteroids: Limited data available; IV: 1 mg/kg/dose; dosing based on a case series of five neonates (preterm: n=4, GA: 23 to 30 weeks; term: n=1, GA: 40 weeks) with presumed septic shock (Driscoll, 1996)

Dosing: Usual

Pediatric: **Methemoglobinemia:** Infants, Children, and Adolescents: I.O., IV: 1 to 2 mg/kg; may be repeated every 30 to 60 minutes if necessary (Herman, 1999; Kliegman, 2011)

Adult:

Methemoglobinemia: IV: 1 to 2 mg/kg or 25 to 50 mg/m^2; may be repeated after 1 hour if necessary

Ifosfamide-induced encephalopathy: IV: **Note:** Treatment may not be necessary; encephalopathy may improve spontaneously (Patel, 2006, Pelgrims, 2000):

Prevention: 50 mg every 6 to 8 hours

Treatment: 50 mg as a single dose or every 4 to 8 hours until symptoms resolve

Dosing adjustment in renal impairment: There are no dosage adjustments provided in the manufacturer's labeling; however, use with caution in patients with severe renal impairment.

Dosing adjustment in hepatic impairment: There are no dosage adjustments provided in the manufacturer's labeling.

Preparation for Administration Parenteral: For ifosfamide-induced encephalopathy treatment, may be further diluted in 50 mL of NS or D_5W (Patel 2006)

Administration Parenteral: Administer undiluted by direct IV injection over 5 to 10 minutes. When used for the treatment of ifosfamide-induced encephalopathy, may be administered either undiluted as a slow IV push over at least 5 minutes or further diluted and infused over at least 5 minutes (Patel 2006); may be administered intraosseously. **Do not inject intrathecally or subcutaneously.**

Vesicant/Extravasation Risk Vesicant

Monitoring Parameters Arterial blood gases; cardiac monitoring (patients with preexisting pulmonary and/or cardiac disease); CBC; methemoglobin levels (co-oximetry yields a direct and accurate measure of methemoglobin levels); pulse oximeter (will not provide accurate measurement of oxygenation when methemoglobin levels are >35% or following methylene blue administration); renal function; signs and symptoms of methemoglobinemia such as pallor, cyanosis, nausea, muscle weakness, dizziness, confusion, agitation, dyspnea, and tachycardia; transcutaneous O_2 saturation

Reference Range

Methemoglobin levels: **Note:** The level of methemoglobin is expressed as a percent of total hemoglobin affected.

10% to 25%: Cyanosis

35% to 40%: Fatigue, dizziness, dyspnea, headache, tachycardia

60%: Lethargy, stupor

>70%: Death (adults)

Additional Information Has been used topically (compounded 0.1% solutions) in conjunction with polychromatic light to photoinactivate viruses such as herpes simplex; has been used alone or in combination with vitamin C for the management of chronic urolithiasis; skin stains may be removed using a hypochlorite solution

Dosage Forms Excipient information presented when available (limited, particularly for generics); consult specific product labeling.

Solution, Injection:

Generic: 1% (1 mL, 10 mL)

◆ **Methylin** *see* Methylphenidate *on page 1402*

◆ **Methylmorphine** *see* Codeine *on page 525*

Methylphenidate (meth il FEN i date)

Medication Safety Issues

Sound-alike/look-alike issues:

Metadate CD may be confused with Metadate ER

Metadate ER may be confused with methadone

Methylphenidate may be confused with methadone

Ritalin may be confused with Rifadin

Ritalin LA may be confused with Ritalin-SR

Related Information

Oral Medications That Should Not Be Crushed or Altered *on page 2476*

Patient Information for Disposal of Unused Medications *on page 2453*

Brand Names: US Aptensio XR; Concerta; Daytrana; Metadate CD; Metadate ER; Methylin; Quillivant XR; Ritalin; Ritalin LA; Ritalin SR [DSC]

Brand Names: Canada Apo-Methylphenidate; Apo-Methylphenidate SR; Biphentin; Concerta; PHL-Methylphenidate; PMS-Methylphenidate; ratio-Methylphenidate; Ritalin; Ritalin SR; Sandoz-Methylphenidate SR; Teva-Methylphenidate ER-C

Therapeutic Category Central Nervous System Stimulant

Generic Availability (US) May be product dependent

Use

Oral:

Concerta®: Treatment of attention-deficit/hyperactivity disorder (ADHD) (FDA approved in ages 6-65 years)

Ritalin LA®, Quillivant™ XR: Treatment of ADHD (FDA approved in ages 6-12 years)

Metadate CD®: Treatment of ADHD (FDA approved in ages 6-15 years)

Metadate® ER, Methylin®, Ritalin®, Ritalin SR®: Treatment of ADHD, treatment of narcolepsy (All indications: FDA approved in ages ≥6 years and adults)

Topical Patch: Daytrana®: Treatment of ADHD (FDA approved in ages 6-17 years)

Medication Guide Available Yes

Pregnancy Risk Factor C

Pregnancy Considerations Adverse events have been observed in animal reproduction studies. Information related to the use of methylphenidate in pregnant women with attention-deficit/hyperactivity disorder (Bolea-Akmanac, 2013; Dideriksen, 2013) or narcolepsy (Maurovich-Horvat, 2013; Thorpy, 2013) is limited.

Breast-Feeding Considerations Methylphenidate excretion in breast milk has been noted in case reports. In both cases, the authors calculated the relative infant dose to be ≤0.2% of the weight adjusted maternal dose. Adverse events were not noted in either infant, however, both were older (6 months of age and 11 months of age) and exposure was limited (Hackett, 2006; Spigset, 2007). The manufacturer recommends that caution be used if administered to a nursing woman.

Contraindications

US labeling: Hypersensitivity to methylphenidate or any component of the formulation; use during or within 14 days following MAO inhibitor therapy; marked anxiety, tension, and agitation (excluding Aptensio XR and Quillivant XR); glaucoma (excluding Aptensio XR and Quillivant XR); family history or diagnosis of Tourette syndrome or tics (excluding Aptensio XR and Quillivant XR)

Additional contraindications: Metadate CD and Metadate ER: Severe hypertension, heart failure, arrhythmia, hyperthyroidism, recent MI or angina; concomitant use of halogenated anesthetics

Canadian labeling: Hypersensitivity to methylphenidate or any component of the formulation; marked anxiety, tension, and agitation; glaucoma; use during or within 14 days following MAO inhibitor therapy; family history or diagnosis of Tourette's syndrome or tics, thyrotoxicosis, advanced arteriosclerosis, symptomatic cardiovascular disease, or moderate-to-severe hypertension

Additional contraindications: Ritalin and Ritalin SR: Pheochromocytoma

Warnings/Precautions CNS stimulant use has been associated with serious cardiovascular events (eg, sudden death in children and adolescents; sudden death, stroke, and MI in adults) in patients with pre-existing structural cardiac abnormalities or other serious heart problems.

These products should be avoided in patients with known serious structural cardiac abnormalities, cardiomyopathy, serious heart rhythm abnormalities, or other serious cardiac problems that could further increase their risk of sudden death. Patients should be carefully evaluated for cardiac disease prior to initiation of therapy. Use of stimulants can cause an increase in blood pressure (average 2 to 4 mm Hg) and increases in heart rate (average 3 to 6 bpm), although some patients may have larger than average increases. Use caution with hypertension, hyperthyroidism, or other cardiovascular conditions that might be exacerbated by increases in blood pressure or heart rate. Some products are contraindicated in patients with heart failure, arrhythmias, severe hypertension, hyperthyroidism, angina, or recent MI. Stimulants are associated with peripheral vasculopathy, including Raynaud's phenomenon; signs/symptoms are usually mild and intermittent, and generally improve with dose reduction or discontinuation. Digital ulceration and/or soft tissue breakdown have been observed rarely; monitor for digital changes during therapy and seek further evaluation (eg, rheumatology) if necessary. Prolonged and painful erections (priapism), sometimes requiring surgical intervention, have been reported (rarely) with methylphenidate and atomoxetine use in pediatric and adult patients. Priapism has been reported to develop after some time on the drug, often subsequent to an increase in dose but also during a period of drug withdrawal (drug holidays or discontinuation). Patients with certain hematological dyscrasias (eg, sickle cell disease), malignancies, perineal trauma, or concomitant use of alcohol, illicit drugs, or other medications associated with priapism may be at increased risk. Patients who develop abnormally sustained or frequent and painful erections should discontinue therapy and seek immediate medical attention. An emergent urological consultation should be obtained in severe cases. Priapism has been associated with different dosage forms and products; it is not known if rechallenge with a different formulation will risk recurrence. Avoidance of stimulants and atomoxetine may be preferred in patients with severe cases that were slow to resolve and/or required detumescence (Eiland, 2014).

Has demonstrated value as part of a comprehensive treatment program for ADHD. Use with caution in patients with bipolar disorder (may induce mixed/manic episode). May exacerbate symptoms of behavior and thought disorder in psychotic patients; new-onset psychosis or mania may occur with stimulant use. Patients should be screened for bipolar disorder prior to treatment; consider discontinuation if such symptoms (eg, delusional thinking, hallucinations, mania) occur. May be associated with aggressive behavior or hostility (causal relationship not established); monitor for development or worsening of these behaviors. Use caution with seizure disorders (may reduce seizure threshold). Use caution in patients with history of ethanol or drug abuse. May exacerbate symptoms of behavior and thought disorder in psychotic patients. **[US Boxed Warning]: Potential for drug dependency exists - avoid abrupt discontinuation in patients who have received for prolonged periods.** Visual disturbances have been reported (rare). Not labeled for use in children <6 years of age. Use of stimulants has been associated with suppression of growth in children; monitor growth rate during treatment. Hypersensitivity reactions, such as angioedema and anaphylactic reactions have been reported.

Concerta should not be used in patients with esophageal motility disorders or pre-existing severe gastrointestinal narrowing (small bowel disease, short gut syndrome, history of peritonitis, cystic fibrosis, chronic intestinal pseudo-obstruction, Meckel's diverticulum). Concomitant use of Metadate CD and Metadate ER with halogenated anesthetics is contraindicated; may cause sudden elevations in blood pressure; if surgery is planned, do not administer Metadate CD or Metadate ER on the day of surgery. Transdermal system may cause allergic contact sensitization, characterized by intense local reactions (edema, papules) that may spread beyond the patch site; sensitization may subsequently manifest systemically with other routes of methylphenidate administration; monitor closely. Avoid exposure of application site to any direct external heat sources (eg, hair dryers, heating pads, electric blankets); may increase the rate and extent of absorption and risk of overdose. Efficacy of transdermal methylphenidate therapy for >7 weeks has not been established. Potentially significant drug-drug interactions may exist, requiring dose or frequency adjustment, additional monitoring, and/or selection of alternative therapy. Biphentin [Canadian product] controlled release capsules are not interchangeable with other controlled release formulations. Some dosage forms may contain lactose or sucrose; use with caution in patients intolerant to either component (some manufacturer labels recommend avoiding use in such patients).

Benzyl alcohol and derivatives: Some dosage forms may contain sodium benzoate/benzoic acid; benzoic acid (benzoate) is a metabolite of benzyl alcohol; large amounts of benzyl alcohol (≥99 mg/kg/day) have been associated with a potentially fatal toxicity ("gasping syndrome") in neonates; the "gasping syndrome" consists of metabolic acidosis, respiratory distress, gasping respirations, CNS dysfunction (including convulsions, intracranial hemorrhage), hypotension, and cardiovascular collapse (AAP, 1997; CDC, 1982); some data suggests that benzoate displaces bilirubin from protein binding sites (Ahlfors, 2001); avoid or use dosage forms containing benzyl alcohol derivative with caution in neonates. See manufacturer's labeling.

Warnings: Additional Pediatric Considerations Serious cardiovascular events, including sudden death, may occur in patients with preexisting structural cardiac abnormalities or other serious heart problems. Sudden death has been reported in children and adolescents; sudden death, stroke, and MI have been reported in adults. Avoid the use of CNS stimulants in patients with known serious structural cardiac abnormalities, cardiomyopathy, serious heart rhythm abnormalities, coronary artery disease, or other serious cardiac problems that could place patients at an increased risk to the sympathomimetic effects of a stimulant drug. Patients should be carefully evaluated for cardiac disease prior to initiation of therapy. If a child displays symptoms of cardiovascular disease, including chest pain, dyspnea, or fainting, parents should seek immediate medical care for the child.

The American Heart Association recommends that all children diagnosed with ADHD who may be candidates for medication, such as methylphenidate, should have a thorough cardiovascular assessment prior to initiation of therapy. This assessment should include a combination of medical history, family history, and physical examination focusing on cardiovascular disease risk factors. An ECG is not mandatory but should be considered. **Note:** ECG abnormalities and four cases of sudden cardiac death have been reported in children receiving clonidine with methylphenidate; reduce dose of methylphenidate by 40% when used concurrently with clonidine; consider ECG monitoring.

In a recent retrospective study on the possible association between stimulant medication use and sudden death in children, 564 previously healthy children who died suddenly in motor vehicle accidents were compared to a group of 564 previously healthy children who died suddenly. Two of the 564 (0.4%) children in motor vehicle accidents were taking stimulant medications compared to 10 of 564 (1.8%) children who died suddenly. While the authors of this study conclude there may be an association between stimulant use and sudden death in children, there were a number of limitations to the study and the FDA cannot conclude this information impacts the overall risk:benefit profile of these medications (Gould, 2009). In a large retrospective cohort study involving 1,200,438 children and young adults (age: 2 to 24 years), none of the currently available stimulant medications or atomoxetine were shown to increase the risk of serious cardiovascular events (ie, acute MI, sudden cardiac death, or stroke) in current (adjusted hazard ratio: 0.75; 95% CI: 0.31 to 1.85) or former (adjusted hazard ratio: 1.03; 95% CI: 0.57 to 1.89) users compared to nonusers. It should be noted that due to the upper limit of the 95% CI, the study could not rule out a doubling of the risk, albeit low (Cooper, 2011).

Stimulant medications may increase blood pressure (average increase 2 to 4 mm Hg) and heart rate (average increase 3 to 6 bpm). Long-term effects in pediatric patients have not been determined. Use of stimulants in children has been associated with growth suppression (monitor growth; treatment interruption may be needed). Appetite suppression may occur; monitor weight during therapy, particularly in children.

Use with caution in preschool-age children; clinical trials have shown children 3 to 5 years of age are more sensitive to methylphenidate adverse effects resulting in a greater discontinuation of therapy compared to school-age children (discontinuation rate from trials: 11% vs <1 %) (Wigal, 2006). The moderate to severe adverse effect profiles in children are age-related; in preschool children, the most commonly reported adverse effects were crabbiness/irritability, emotional outbursts, difficulty falling asleep, repetitive behavior/thoughts, and decreased appetite; in school-age children, they were decreased appetite, delay of sleep onset, headache, and stomach ache (Wigal, 2006).

Adverse Reactions

All dosage forms:

Cardiovascular: Angina pectoris, cardiac arrhythmia, cerebrovascular accident, cerebrovascular occlusion, decreased pulse, heart murmur, hypertension, hypotension, increased pulse, myocardial infarction, necrotizing angiitis, palpitations, Raynaud's phenomenon, tachycardia, vasculitis

Central nervous system: Aggressive behavior, agitation, anxiety, cerebral arteritis, cerebral hemorrhage, confusion, depression, dizziness (more common in adults), drowsiness, emotional lability (more common in children), fatigue, Gilles de la Tourette's syndrome (rare), headache (more common in adults), hypertonia, hypervigilance, irritability, insomnia, lethargy, nervousness, neuroleptic malignant syndrome (NMS) (rare), outbursts of anger, paresthesia, restlessness, tension, toxic psychosis, vertigo, vocal tics (children)

Dermatologic: Alopecia, erythema multiforme, excoriation (children), exfoliative dermatitis, hyperhidrosis, skin rash (children), urticaria

Endocrine & metabolic: Decreased libido, growth suppression, weight loss

Gastrointestinal: Abdominal pain (children & adolescents), anorexia (more common in children & adolescents), bruxism, constipation, decreased appetite (more common in adults), diarrhea, dyspepsia, motion sickness (children), nausea, vomiting, xerostomia

Genitourinary: Dysmenorrhea, erectile dysfunction

Hematologic & oncologic: Anemia, immune thrombocytopenia, leukopenia, pancytopenia, thrombocytopenia

Hepatic: Abnormal hepatic function tests, hepatic coma, increased serum bilirubin, increased serum transaminases

Hypersensitivity: Hypersensitivity reaction

Neuromuscular & skeletal: Arthralgia, dyskinesia, tremor

Ophthalmic: Accommodation disturbance, blurred vision, dry eye syndrome, eye pain (children), mydriasis

Respiratory: Dyspnea, increased cough, pharyngitis, pharyngolaryngeal pain, rhinitis, sinusitis, upper respiratory tract infection

Miscellaneous: Accidental injury, fever (children & adolescents)

Rare but important or life-threatening: Bradycardia, disorientation, extrasystoles, hallucination, increased serum alkaline phosphatase, mania, migraine, obsessive-compulsive disorder, peripheral vascular insufficiency, priapism, seizure, supraventricular tachycardia, ventricular premature contractions

Transdermal system:

Central nervous system: Headache, insomnia, irritability

Gastrointestinal: Decreased appetite, nausea

Infection: Viral infection

Cardiovascular: Tachycardia

Central nervous system: Dizziness (adolescents), emotional lability, vocal tic

Endocrine & metabolic: Weight loss

Gastrointestinal: Abdominal pain, anorexia, vomiting

Local: Application site reaction

Respiratory: Nasal congestion, nasopharyngitis

Rare but important or life-threatening: Allergic contact dermatitis, allergic contact sensitivity, anaphylaxis, angioedema, hallucination, seizure

Drug Interactions

Metabolism/Transport Effects **Inhibits** CYP2D6 (weak)

Avoid Concomitant Use

Avoid concomitant use of Methylphenidate with any of the following: Alcohol (Ethyl); Inhalational Anesthetics; Iobenguane I 123; MAO Inhibitors

Increased Effect/Toxicity

Methylphenidate may increase the levels/effects of: Anti-Parkinson's Agents (Dopamine Agonist); Antipsychotic Agents; ARIPiprazole; CloNIDine; Fosphenytoin; Inhalational Anesthetics; PHENobarbital; Phenytoin; Primidone; Sympathomimetics; Tricyclic Antidepressants; Vitamin K Antagonists

The levels/effects of Methylphenidate may be increased by: Alcohol (Ethyl); Antacids; Antipsychotic Agents; AtoMOXetine; Cannabinoid-Containing Products; H2-Antagonists; MAO Inhibitors; Proton Pump Inhibitors

Decreased Effect

Methylphenidate may decrease the levels/effects of: Antihypertensives; Iobenguane I 123; Ioflupane I 123

Food Interactions

Ethanol: Alcohol consumption increases the rate of methylphenidate release from Metadate CD and Ritalin LA (extended-release capsules), but not from Concerta (extended-release tablet); an *in vitro* study involving Metadate CD and Ritalin LA showed that an alcohol concentration of 40% resulted in 84% and 98% of the methylphenidate being released in the first hour, respectively. Management: Avoid consuming alcohol during therapy.

Food: Food may increase oral absorption of immediate release tablet/solution and chewable tablet. Management: Administer 30-45 minutes before meals.

Storage/Stability

Capsule:

Extended release:

Aptensio XR: Store at 20°C to 25°C (68°F to 77°F). Protect from moisture.

Metadate CD, Ritalin LA: Store at 25°C (77°F); excursions permitted to 15°C to 30°C (59°F to 86°F). Protect from light.

Controlled release (Biphentin [Canadian product]): Store at 15°C to 30°C (59°F to 86°F).

Solution: *Immediate release (Methylin):* Store at 20°C to 25°C (68°F to 77°F).

Suspension: *Extended release (Quillivant XR):* Store at 25°C (77°F); excursions permitted to 15°C to 30°C (59°F to 86°F), before and after reconstitution. Reconstituted bottle must be used within 4 months.

Tablet:

Chewable (Methylin): Store at 20°C to 25°C (68°F to 77°F). Protect from light and moisture.

Extended release:

Metadate ER: Store at 20°C to 25°C (68°F to 77°F); excursions permitted to 15°C to 30°C (59°F to 86°F). Protect from light and moisture.

Concerta: Store at 25°C (77°F); excursions permitted to 15°C to 30°C (59°F to 86°F). Protect from humidity.

Immediate release (Ritalin): Store at 25°C (77°F); excursions permitted to 15°C to 30°C (59°F to 86°F). Protect from light and moisture.

Sustained release (Ritalin-SR): Store at 25°C (77°F); excursions permitted to 15°C to 30°C (59°F to 86°F). Protect from light and moisture.

Transdermal system: *Daytrana:* Store at 25°C (77°F); excursions permitted to 15°C to 30°C (59°F to 86°F). Keep patches stored in protective pouch. Once tray is opened, use patches within 2 months; once an individual patch has been removed from the pouch and the protective liner removed, use immediately. Do not refrigerate or freeze.

Mechanism of Action Mild CNS stimulant; blocks the reuptake of norepinephrine and dopamine into presynaptic neurons; appears to stimulate the cerebral cortex and subcortical structures similar to amphetamines

Pharmacodynamics

Onset of action (AAP, 2011):

Oral:

Immediate release formulations [chewable tablet, oral solution, tablet (Methylin®, Ritalin®)]: 20-60 minutes

Extended release formulations [Capsule (Metadate CD®, Ritalin LA®), tablets (Concerta®)]: 20-60 minutes

Sustained release tablet (Ritalin-SR®): 60-180 minutes

Transdermal (Daytrana®): 60 minutes

Maximum effect: Oral:

Immediate release tablet: Within 2 hours

Sustained release tablet: Within 4-7 hours

Duration of action (AAP, 2011):

Oral:

Immediate release formulations [Chewable tablet, oral solution, immediate release tablet (Methylin®, Ritalin®)]: 3-5 hours

Extended release capsule (Metadate CD®, Ritalin LA®): 6-8 hours

Extended release tablet (Concerta®): 12 hours

Sustained release tablet (Ritalin-SR®): 2-6 hours

Transdermal (Daytrana®): 11-12 hours

Pharmacokinetics (Adult data unless noted) Note: Values reported below based on pediatric patient data or combined pediatric and adult data.

Absorption: Oral:

Immediate release products: Readily absorbed

Transdermal: Rate and extent of absorption is increased when applied to inflamed skin or exposed to heat; transdermal absorption may increase with chronic therapy

Distribution: V_d: d-methylphenidate: 2.65 ± 1.11 L/kg; l-methylphenidate: 1.80 ± 0.91 L/kg

Protein binding: 15%

Metabolism: Hepatic via hydroxylation (de-esterification by carboxylesterase CES1A1) to ritalinic acid (alpha-phenyl-2-piperidine acetic acid), which has little or no pharmacologic activity

Bioavailability:

Immediate release chewable tablets and oral solution: Bioequivalent to immediate release tablets

Extended release suspension (Quillivant™ XR): 95% (relative to immediate release oral solution)

Transdermal patch (Daytrana®): Lower first-pass effect compared to oral administration; thus, much lower doses (on a mg/kg basis) given via the transdermal route may still produce higher AUCs, compared to the oral route

Half-life:

Oral:

Immediate release formulations:

Chewable tablets, oral solution (Methylin®): 3 hours

Tablet (Ritalin®):

Children: 2.5 hours (range: 1.8-5.3 hours)

Adults: 3.5 hours (range: 1.3-7.7 hours)

Extended release formulations:

Capsule:

Metadate CD®: 6.8 hours

Ritalin LA®:

Children: 2.4 hours (range: 1.5-4 hours)

Adults: 3.3 hours (range: 3-4.2 hours)

Tablet (Concerta®): 3.5 hours

Suspension (Quillivant™ XR): Children ≥9 years, Adolescents, and Adults: ~5 hours

Transdermal patch (Daytrana®): Children and Adolescents 6-17 years: 4-5 hours

Time to peak serum concentration:

Oral:

Immediate release formulations:

Chewable tablets, oral solution (Methylin®): 1-2 hours

Tablet (Ritalin®): Children: 1.9 hours (range: 0.3-4.4 hours)

Extended release formulations:

Capsule (Metadate CD®): 1.5 hours

Tablet:

Concerta®: 6-10 hours

Metadate ER®: Children: 4.7 hours (range: 1.3-8.2 hours)

Powder for oral suspension (Quillivant™ XR):

Children (9-12 years): 4 hours

Adolescents (13-15 years): 2 hours

Adults: 4 hours

Sustained release tablets (Ritalin SR®): Children: 4.7 hours (range: 1.3-8.2 hours)

Transdermal patch (Daytrana®): Children 6-17 years: 8-10 hours

Elimination: 90% of dose is eliminated in the urine as metabolites and unchanged drug; main urinary metabolite (ritalinic acid) accounts for 80% of the dose; drug is also excreted in feces via bile

Dosing: Usual Note: Discontinue medication if no improvement is seen after appropriate dosage adjustment over a 1-month period of time:

Children and Adolescents:

Attention-deficit/hyperactivity disorder:

Oral:

Immediate release products (eg, Methylin®, Ritalin®):

Children 3-5 years, moderate to severe dysfunction: Limited data available; AAP considers first-line agent in this patient population if pharmacological treatment deemed necessary (AAP, 2011): Initial: 1.25 mg twice daily; titrate to effect at weekly intervals; usual reported daily range: 3.75-30 mg/day divided into two or three daily doses (Ghuman, 2008; Greenhill, 2006). In the largest trial, a multicenter, randomized, placebo-controlled, crossover study of 165 preschool children (age range: 3-5.5 years), statistically and clinically significant improvements in ADHD scores were reported with doses of 2.5 mg, 5 mg, and 7.5 mg 3 times daily; in some patients [n=7 (4%)], dose titration to 10 mg 3 times daily was necessary; the mean effective total daily dose: 14.2 ± 8.1 mg/**day**. Although ADHD scores were statistically and clinically improved with methylphenidate use, the effect size was smaller with this younger patient population than that seen in school-age children (Greenhill, 2006).

Children ≥6 years and Adolescents: Initial: 0.3 mg/kg/dose or 2.5-5 mg/dose given before breakfast and lunch; increase by 0.1 mg/kg/dose or by 5-10 mg/day at weekly intervals; usual dose: 0.3-1 mg/kg/day or 20-30 mg/**day** in 2-3 divided doses; maximum daily dose dependent upon patient weight: 2 mg/kg/day or if patient weight ≤50 kg: 60 mg/**day**; in patients >50 kg: 100 mg/day (Dopheide, 2009, Pliszka, 2007); some patients may require 3 doses/day (ie, additional dose at 4 PM)

Extended release, sustained release and long acting products:

Metadate® ER, Ritalin-SR®: Children ≥6 years and Adolescents: Sustained release and extended release tablets (duration of action ~8 hours) may be given in place of regular tablets, once the daily dose is titrated using the immediate release products and the titrated 8-hour dosage corresponds to sustained/extended release tablet size; Ritalin SR® may be administered once or twice daily (AAP, 2011). Maximum daily dose is dependent upon patient weight: ≤50 kg: 60 mg/**day**; >50 kg: 100 mg/**day** (Dopheide, 2009; Pliszka, 2007)

Concerta®: Children ≥6 years and Adolescents:

Methylphenidate-naive patients: Initial: 18 mg once daily

Patients currently using immediate release methylphenidate: Initial dose: Dosing based on current regimen and clinical judgment; suggested dosing listed below:

Switching from methylphenidate immediate release 5 mg 2-3 times daily: Concerta® 18 mg once daily

Switching from methylphenidate immediate release 10 mg 2-3 times daily: Concerta® 36 mg once daily

Switching from methylphenidate immediate release 15 mg 2-3 times daily: Concerta® 54 mg once daily

Switching from methylphenidate immediate release 20 mg 2-3 times daily: Concerta® 72 mg once daily

Dosage adjustment: May increase by Concerta® 18 mg/day increments at weekly intervals. **Note:** A dosage strength of 27 mg is available for situations in which a dosage between 18-36 mg is desired.

Maximum daily dose:

Children 6-12 years: 54 mg/day; for patients >50 kg, higher maximum daily doses may be considered (108 mg/day)

Adolescents:

≤50 kg: 72 mg/day; not to exceed ~2 mg/kg/day

>50 kg:108 mg/day (Dopheide, 2009; Pliszka, 2007)

Metadate CD®: Children ≥6 years and Adolescents: Initial: 20 mg once daily; may increase by 10-20 mg/day increments at weekly intervals; maximum daily dose dependent upon patient weight: ≤50 kg: 60 mg/**day**; >50 kg: 100 mg/**day** (Dopheide, 2009; Pliszka, 2007)

Quillivant™ XR: Children 6-12 years: Initial: 20 mg once daily; may increase by 10-20 mg/day increments at weekly intervals; maximum daily dose: 60 mg/**day**

Ritalin LA®: Children ≥6 years and Adolescents:

Methylphenidate-naive patients: Initial: 20 mg once daily; may increase by 10 mg/day increments at weekly intervals; maximum daily dose dependent upon patient weight: ≤50 kg: 60 mg/**day**; >50 kg: 100 mg/**day** (Dopheide, 2009; Pliszka, 2007). **Note:** If a lower initial dose is desired, patients may begin with Ritalin LA® 10 mg once daily. Alternatively, patients may begin therapy with an immediate release product, and switch to Ritalin LA® once immediate release dosage is titrated to 5 mg twice daily (see below)

Patients currently receiving immediate release methylphenidate: Initial dose: Dosing based on current regimen and clinical judgment; use equivalent total daily dose administered once daily.

Patients currently receiving methylphenidate sustained release (SR): The same total daily dose of Ritalin LA® should be used.

Dosage adjustment: May increase Ritalin LA®: by 10 mg/day increments at weekly intervals

Maximum daily dose: Dependent upon patient weight: ≤50 kg: 60 mg/**day**; >50 kg: 100 mg/**day** (Dopheide, 2009; Pliszka, 2007)

Topical: Transdermal patch (Daytrana®): Children and Adolescents 6-17 years: Initial: 10 mg (12.5 cm^2) patch once daily; apply to hip 2 hours before effect is needed and remove 9 hours after application; titrate dose based on response and tolerability; may increase to next transdermal patch dosage size no more frequently than every week. Patch may be removed before 9 hours if a shorter duration of action is required or if late day adverse effects appear. Plasma concentrations usually start to decline when the patch is removed but drug absorption may continue for several hours after patch removal. **Note:** The manufacturer's labeling recommends patients converting from another formulation of methylphenidate to the transdermal patch should be initiated at 10 mg regardless of their previous dose and titrated as needed due to the differences in bioavailability of the transdermal formulation. However, some clinicians have supported higher starting patch doses for patients converting from oral methylphenidate doses of >20 mg/day; for example, the 15 mg (18.75 cm^2) patch has been investigated to have the same effect as 22.5 mg daily of the immediate release preparation, 27 mg daily of the osmotic release preparation (Concerta®), or 20 mg daily of the encapsulated bead preparation (Metadate CD®) (Arnold, 2007).

Narcolepsy: Children ≥6 years and Adolescents: Oral:

Immediate release tablets and oral solution (Methylin®, Ritalin®): Initial: 5 mg twice daily given before breakfast and lunch; increase by 5-10 increments mg/day at weekly intervals; 2-3 times per day; maximum daily dose: 60 mg/**day** (in 2-3 divided doses)

Extended/sustained release tablets (Metadate® ER, Ritalin-SR®): May be given in place of immediate release products (duration of action: ~8 hours), once the immediate release formulation daily dose is titrated and the titrated 8-hour dosage corresponds to sustained or extended release tablet size; maximum daily dose: 60 mg/**day**

Adults:

Attention-deficit/hyperactivity disorder: Oral:

Immediate release (IR) products (tablets, chewable tablets, and solution): Initial: 5 mg twice daily, before breakfast and lunch; increase by 5-10 mg daily at weekly intervals; maximum dose: 60 mg daily (in 2-3 divided doses)

Extended release (ER), sustained release (SR) products (capsules, tablets, and oral suspension):

Concerta®: Adults <65 years:

Patients not currently taking methylphenidate: Initial dose: 18-36 mg once every morning

Patients currently taking methylphenidate: **Note:** Initial dose: Dosing based on current regimen and clinical judgment; suggested dosing listed below:

Switching from methylphenidate 5 mg 2-3 times daily: 18 mg once every morning

Switching from methylphenidate 10 mg 2-3 times daily: 36 mg once every morning

Switching from methylphenidate 15 mg 2-3 times daily: 54 mg once every morning

Switching from methylphenidate 20 mg 2-3 times daily: 72 mg once every morning

Dose adjustment: May increase dose in increments of 18 mg; dose may be adjusted at weekly intervals. A dosage strength of 27 mg is available for situations in which a dosage between 18-36 mg is desired; maximum dose: 72 mg/day

Metadate® ER, Ritalin-SR®: May be given in place of immediate release products, once the daily dose is titrated and the titrated 8-hour dosage corresponds to sustained or extended release tablet size; maximum: 60 mg/day

Metadate CD®, Quillivant™ XR: Initial: 20 mg once daily; may be adjusted in 10-20 mg increments at weekly intervals; maximum: 60 mg/day

Ritalin LA®: Initial: 20 mg once daily (10 mg once daily may be considered for some patients); may be adjusted in 10 mg increments at weekly intervals; maximum: 60 mg/day

Conversion from immediate release or sustained release methylphenidate formulation to Ritalin LA®: Use equivalent total daily dose administered once daily.

Narcolepsy: Oral:

Immediate release tablets and solution (Methylin®, Ritalin®): Initial: 5 mg twice daily before breakfast and lunch; increase by 5-10 mg daily at weekly intervals; 10 mg 2-3 times per day; maximum daily dose: 60 mg/day (in 2-3 divided doses).

Extended/sustained release tablets (Metadate® ER, Ritalin-SR®): May be given in place of immediate release products (duration of action: ~8 hours), once the immediate release formulation daily dose is titrated and the titrated 8-hour dosage corresponds to sustained or extended release tablet size; maximum: 60 mg/day

Dosing adjustment for renal impairment:

Oral: No dosage adjustment provided in manufacturer's labeling (has not been studied); undergoes extensive metabolism to a renally eliminated metabolite with little or no pharmacologic activity.

Transdermal: No dosage adjustment provided in manufacturer's labeling (has not been studied).

Dosing adjustment for hepatic impairment: There are no dosage adjustments provided in manufacturer's labeling (has not been studied).

Preparation for Administration Oral: Extended release: Powder for oral suspension *(Quillivant XR)*: Prior to dispensing, reconstitute with an appropriate amount of water as specified on the bottle. Shake vigorously for at least 10 seconds until suspended.

Administration

Oral: To avoid insomnia, last daily dose should be administered several hours before retiring.

Immediate release formulations:

Tablet (Ritalin), oral solution (Methylin): Administer on an empty stomach ~30 to 45 minutes before meals. Ensure last daily dose is administered before 6 PM if difficulty sleeping occurs.

Chewable tablet (Methylin): Administer on an empty stomach ~30 to 45 minutes before meals with at least 8 ounces of water or other fluid; choking may occur if not enough fluids are taken. Ensure last daily dose is administered before 6 PM if difficulty sleeping occurs.

Extended/sustained release formulations:

Tablets:

Metadate ER: May be taken with or without food. Swallow whole; do not crush, chew, or break tablets.

Ritalin SR: Administer 30 to 45 minutes before a meal. Swallow whole; do not crush, chew, or break tablets.

Concerta: May be administered without regard to food, but must be taken with water, milk, or juice; administer dose once daily in the morning; do not crush, chew, or divide tablets

Capsules:

Metadate CD: Administer dose once daily in the morning, before breakfast, with water, milk, or juice; capsule may be swallowed whole or opened and contents sprinkled on a small amount (one tablespoonful) of applesauce; immediately consume drug/applesauce mixture; do not store for future use; swallow applesauce without chewing; do not crush or chew capsule contents; drink fluids after consuming drug/applesauce mixture to ensure complete swallowing of beads; do not crush, chew, or divide capsules or its contents

Ritalin LA: Administer dose once daily in the morning; may be administered with or without food (but some food may delay absorption); capsule may be swallowed whole or may be opened and contents sprinkled on a small amount (one spoonful) of applesauce. **Note:** Applesauce should not be warm; immediately consume drug/applesauce mixture; do not store for future use; do not crush, chew, or divide capsule or its contents.

Powder for oral suspension (Quillivant XR): Administer in the morning with or without food. Shake bottle ≥10 seconds prior to administration. Use the oral dosing dispenser provided; wash after each use.

Topical: Transdermal (Daytrana): Apply patch immediately after opening pouch and removing protective liner; do not use patch if pouch seal is broken; do not cut patch; do not use patches that are cut or damaged. If difficulty is experienced when separating the patch from the liner or if any medication (sticky substance) remains on the liner after separation, discard that patch and apply a new patch. Apply to clean, dry, healthy skin on the hip; do not apply to oily, damaged, or irritated skin; do not apply to the waistline; do not premedicate the patch site with hydrocortisone or other solutions, creams, ointments, or emollients. Apply at the same time each day, 2 hours before effect is needed. Alternate site of application daily (ie, use alternate hip). Press patch firmly for 30 seconds to ensure proper adherence. Remove patch 9 hours after application. Patch may be removed earlier if a shorter duration of action is required or if late day adverse effects occur.

Avoid exposure of application site to external heat source (eg, hair dryers, electric blankets, heating pads, heated water beds), which may significantly increase the rate and amount of drug absorbed. Exposure of patch to water during swimming, bathing, or showering may affect patch adherence. Do not reapply patch with dressings, tape, or other adhesives. If patch should become dislodged, may replace with new patch (to different site) but total wear time should not exceed 9 hours.

During removal, peel off patch slowly. If needed, patch removal may be helped by applying an oil-based product (ie, mineral oil, olive oil, or petroleum jelly) to the patch edges, gently working it underneath the patch edges. If a patch is not able to be removed, contact a physician or pharmacist. Nonmedical adhesive removers and acetone-based products, such as nail polish remover, should not be used to remove patches or adhesive. If adhesive residue remains on child's skin after patch removal, use an oil-based product and gently rub area to remove adhesive. Avoid touching the sticky side of the patch. Wash hands with soap and water after handling.

Dispose of used patch by folding adhesive side onto itself, and discard in toilet or appropriate lidded container; discard unused patches that are no longer needed in the same manner; protective pouch and liner should be discarded in an appropriate lidded container. **Note:** Used patches contain residual drug; keep all transdermal patches out of the reach of children.

Monitoring Parameters Evaluate patients for cardiac disease prior to initiation of therapy with thorough medical history, family history, and physical exam; consider ECG; perform ECG and echocardiogram if findings suggest cardiac disease; promptly conduct cardiac evaluation in patients who develop chest pain, unexplained syncope, or any other symptom of cardiac disease during treatment. Monitor CBC with differential, platelet count, liver enzymes, blood pressure, heart rate, height, weight, appetite, abnormal movements, growth in children. Patients should be re-evaluated at appropriate intervals to assess continued need of the medication. Observe for signs/symptoms of aggression or hostility, depression, delusional thinking, hallucinations, or mania. Monitor for visual disturbances. Monitor for signs of misuse, abuse, and addiction.

Transdermal system: Also monitor the application site for local adverse reactions and allergic contact sensitization.

Test Interactions May interfere with urine detection of amphetamines/methamphetamines (false-positive).

Additional Information Methylphenidate is a racemic mixture of d- and l-enantiomers; the d-enantiomer is more active than the l-enantiomer. Treatment with methylphenidate should include "drug holidays" or periodic discontinuation in order to assess the patient's requirements, decrease tolerance and limit suppression of linear growth and weight. Medications used to treat ADHD should be part of a total treatment program that may include other components such as psychological, educational, and social measures. Concerta®, Metadate CD®, and Ritalin LA® are formulated to deliver methylphenidate in a biphasic release profile; Concerta® is an osmotic controlled release formulation, with an immediate release (within 1 hour) outer coating; once daily Concerta® has been shown to be as effective as immediate release methylphenidate tablets administered 3 times/day (Pelham, 2001). Metadate CD® capsules contain both immediate release beads (30% of the dose) and extended release beads (70% of the dose). Ritalin LA® capsules contain both immediate release beads (50% of the dose) and enteric coated, delayed release beads (50% of the dose). Methylin® and Ritalin-SR® tablets are color and additive free; Methylin® oral solution is colorless. Concerta® tablets may be seen on abdominal x-ray under certain conditions (eg, when digital enhancing techniques are used). Quillivant™ XR powder for oral suspension contains a combination of uncoated and coated ion exchange resin complex and a buffering solution based on the Oral XR + platform (Wigal, 2013). Once reconstituted with water forms an extended release suspension that contains approximately 20% immediate release and 80% extended release methylphenidate.

Daytrana™ Transdermal System consists of an adhesive-based matrix containing active drug which is dispersed in acrylic adhesive that is dispersed in a silicone adhesive. The patch consists of 3 layers: A polyester/ethylene vinyl acetate laminate (outside) film backing, the adhesive layer containing methylphenidate, and a flouropolymer-coated polyester protective liner (which must be removed before application). Long-term use of the transdermal system or Concerta® >7 weeks, Metadate® CD >3 weeks, and Ritalin LA® >2 weeks have not been adequately studied; long-term usefulness should be periodically re-evaluated for the individual patient.

Product Availability Aptensio XR: FDA approved April 2015; anticipated availability is currently unknown. Consult prescribing information for additional information.

Controlled Substance C-II

Dosage Forms Excipient information presented when available (limited, particularly for generics); consult specific product labeling. [DSC] = Discontinued product

Capsule Extended Release, Oral, as hydrochloride:
- Metadate CD: 10 mg, 20 mg, 30 mg [contains fd&c blue #2 (indigotine)]
- Metadate CD: 40 mg
- Metadate CD: 50 mg [contains fd&c blue #2 (indigotine)]
- Metadate CD: 60 mg
- Generic: 10 mg, 20 mg, 30 mg, 40 mg, 50 mg, 60 mg

Capsule Extended Release 24 Hour, Oral, as hydrochloride:
- Aptensio XR: 10 mg [contains brilliant blue fcf (fd&c blue #1)]
- Aptensio XR: 15 mg [contains fd&c red #40, fd&c yellow #10 (quinoline yellow)]
- Aptensio XR: 20 mg [contains fd&c yellow #10 (quinoline yellow)]
- Aptensio XR: 30 mg [contains brilliant blue fcf (fd&c blue #1)]
- Aptensio XR: 40 mg [contains brilliant blue fcf (fd&c blue #1), fd&c red #40]
- Aptensio XR: 50 mg [contains fd&c yellow #10 (quinoline yellow)]
- Aptensio XR: 60 mg
- Ritalin LA: 10 mg, 20 mg, 30 mg, 40 mg, 60 mg
- Generic: 20 mg, 30 mg, 40 mg

Patch, Transdermal:
- Daytrana: 10 mg/9 hr (30 ea); 15 mg/9 hr (30 ea); 20 mg/9 hr (30 ea); 30 mg/9 hr (30 ea)

Solution, Oral, as hydrochloride:
- Methylin: 5 mg/5 mL (500 mL); 10 mg/5 mL (500 mL) [contains polyethylene glycol]
- Generic: 5 mg/5 mL (500 mL); 10 mg/5 mL (500 mL)

Suspension Reconstituted, Oral, as hydrochloride:
- Quillivant XR: 25 mg/5 mL (60 mL, 120 mL, 150 mL, 180 mL) [contains sodium benzoate; banana flavor]

Tablet, Oral, as hydrochloride:
- Ritalin: 5 mg
- Ritalin: 10 mg, 20 mg [scored]
- Generic: 5 mg, 10 mg, 20 mg

Tablet Chewable, Oral, as hydrochloride:
- Methylin: 2.5 mg, 5 mg [contains aspartame; grape flavor]
- Methylin: 10 mg [scored; contains aspartame; grape flavor]
- Generic: 2.5 mg, 5 mg, 10 mg

Tablet Extended Release, Oral, as hydrochloride:
- Concerta: 18 mg, 27 mg, 36 mg, 54 mg
- Metadate ER: 20 mg [DSC]
- Metadate ER: 20 mg [additive free, color free]
- Ritalin SR: 20 mg [DSC]
- Generic: 10 mg, 18 mg, 20 mg, 27 mg, 36 mg, 54 mg

◆ **Methylphenidate Hydrochloride** *see* Methylphenidate *on page 1402*

◆ **Methylphenoxy-Benzene Propanamine** *see* AtoMOXetine *on page 217*

◆ **Methylphenyl Isoxazolyl Penicillin** *see* Oxacillin *on page 1576*

◆ **Methylphytyl Napthoquinone** *see* Phytonadione *on page 1698*

MethylPREDNISolone (meth il pred NIS oh lone)

Medication Safety Issues

Sound-alike/look-alike issues:

MethylPREDNISolone may be confused with medroxyPROGESTERone, methotrexate, methylTESTOSTERone, predniSONE

Depo-Medrol may be confused with Solu-Medrol

Medrol may be confused with Mebaral

Solu-MEDROL may be confused with salmeterol, Solu-CORTEF

International issues:

Medrol [U.S., Canada, and multiple international markets] may be confused with Medral brand name for omeprazole [Mexico]

Related Information

Corticosteroids Systemic Equivalencies *on page 2260*

Brand Names: US A-Methapred; Depo-Medrol; Medrol; Medrol (Pak); Solu-MEDROL

Brand Names: Canada Depo-Medrol; Medrol; Methylprednisolone Acetate; Methylprednisolone Sodium Succinate For Injection; Methylprednisolone Sodium Succinate For Injection USP; Solu-Medrol

Therapeutic Category Adrenal Corticosteroid; Anti-inflammatory Agent; Antiasthmatic; Corticosteroid, Systemic; Glucocorticoid

Generic Availability (US) Yes

Use

Systemic: Tablets, parenteral (IV, IM): Anti-inflammatory or immunosuppressant agent in the treatment of a variety of diseases including those of hematologic, allergic, inflammatory, neoplastic, and autoimmune origin (FDA approved in ages >1 month and adults); has also been used for acute spinal cord injury, *Pneumocystis* pneumonia, and prevention and treatment of graft-versus-host disease following allogeneic bone marrow transplantation

Local: Depot formulations (Depo-Medrol®): [FDA approved in pediatric patients (age not specified) and adults]

Intra-articular (or soft tissue): Acute gouty arthritis, acute/subacute bursitis, acute nonspecific tenosynovitis, epicondylitis, rheumatoid arthritis, synovitis of osteoarthritis

Intralesional (injectable suspension): Alopecia areata; discoid lupus erythematosus; infiltrated, inflammatory lesions associated with granuloma annulare, lichen planus, neurodermatitis, and psoriatic plaques; keloids; necrobiosis lipoidica diabeticorum; possibly helpful in cystic tumors of an aponeurosis or tendon (ganglia)

Pregnancy Risk Factor C

Pregnancy Considerations Adverse events have been observed with corticosteroids in animal reproduction studies. Methylprednisolone crosses the placenta (Anderson, 1981). Some studies have shown an association between first trimester systemic corticosteroid use and oral clefts (Park-Wyllie, 2000; Pradat, 2003). Systemic corticosteroids may also influence fetal growth (decreased birth weight); however, information is conflicting (Lunghi, 2010). Hypoadrenalism may occur in newborns following maternal use of corticosteroids in pregnancy; monitor.

When systemic corticosteroids are needed in pregnancy, it is generally recommended to use the lowest effective dose for the shortest duration of time, avoiding high doses during the first trimester (Leachman, 2006; Lunghi, 2010; Makol, 2011; Østensen, 2009). Inhaled corticosteroids are preferred for the treatment of asthma during pregnancy. Systemic corticosteroids such as methylprednisolone may be used for the treatment of severe persistent asthma if needed; the lowest dose administered on alternate days (if possible) should be used (NAEPP, 2005).

Pregnant women exposed to methylprednisolone for antirejection therapy following a transplant may contact the National Transplantation Pregnancy Registry (NTPR) at 215-955-4820. Women exposed to methylprednisolone during pregnancy for the treatment of an autoimmune disease may contact the OTIS Autoimmune Diseases Study at 877-311-8972.

Breast-Feeding Considerations Corticosteroids are excreted in human milk. The manufacturer notes that when used systemically, maternal use of corticosteroids have the potential to cause adverse events in a nursing infant (eg, growth suppression, interfere with endogenous corticosteroid production) and therefore recommends a decision be made whether to discontinue nursing or to discontinue the drug, taking into account the importance of treatment to the mother. If there is concern about exposure to the infant, some guidelines recommend waiting 4 hours after the maternal dose of an oral systemic corticosteroid before breast-feeding in order to decrease potential exposure to the nursing infant (based on a study using prednisolone) (Bae, 2011; Leachman, 2006; Makol, 2011; Ost, 1985). Other guidelines note that maternal use of systemic corticosteroids is not a contraindication to breast-feeding (NAEPP, 2005).

Contraindications Hypersensitivity to methylprednisolone or any component of the formulation; systemic fungal infection; administration of live virus vaccines; methylprednisolone formulations containing benzyl alcohol preservative are contraindicated in premature infants; IM administration in idiopathic thrombocytopenic purpura; intrathecal administration

Warnings/Precautions Corticosteroids are not approved for epidural injection. Serious neurologic events (eg, spinal cord infarction, paraplegia, quadriplegia, cortical blindness, stroke), some resulting in death, have been reported with epidural injection of corticosteroids, with and without use of fluoroscopy.

Use with caution in patients with thyroid disease, hepatic impairment, renal impairment, cardiovascular disease, diabetes, glaucoma, cataracts, myasthenia gravis, multiple sclerosis, osteoporosis, seizures, or GI diseases (diverticulitis, intestinal anastomoses, peptic ulcer, ulcerative colitis) due to perforation risk. Avoid ethanol may enhance gastric mucosal irritation. Not recommended for the treatment of optic neuritis; may increase frequency of new episodes. Use with caution in patients with a history of ocular herpes simplex; corneal perforation has occurred; do not use in active ocular herpes simplex, Use caution following acute MI (corticosteroids have been associated with myocardial rupture). Cardiomegaly and congestive heart failure have been reported following concurrent use of amphotericin B and hydrocortisone for the management of fungal infections.

Because of the risk of adverse effects, systemic corticosteroids should be used cautiously in the elderly in the smallest possible effective dose for the shortest duration. May affect growth velocity; growth should be routinely monitored in pediatric patients. Withdraw therapy with gradual tapering of dose. Patients may require higher doses when subject to stress (ie, trauma, surgery, severe infection).

May cause hypercorticism or suppression of hypothalamic-pituitary-adrenal (HPA) axis, particularly in younger children or in patients receiving high doses for prolonged periods. HPA axis suppression may lead to adrenal crisis. Withdrawal and discontinuation of a corticosteroid should be done slowly and carefully. Particular care is required when patients are transferred from systemic corticosteroids to inhaled products due to possible adrenal insufficiency or withdrawal from steroids, including an increase in allergic symptoms. Adult patients receiving >20 mg per day of prednisone (or equivalent) may be most susceptible. Fatalities have occurred due to adrenal insufficiency in asthmatic patients during and after transfer from systemic corticosteroids to aerosol steroids; aerosol steroids do not provide the systemic steroid needed to treat patients having trauma, surgery, or infections. Use in septic shock or sepsis syndrome may increase mortality in some populations (eg, patients with elevated serum creatinine, patients who develop secondary infections after use).

Acute myopathy has been reported with high dose corticosteroids, usually in patients with neuromuscular transmission disorders; may involve ocular and/or respiratory muscles; monitor creatine kinase; recovery may be delayed. Corticosteroid use may cause psychiatric disturbances, including depression, euphoria, insomnia, mood swings, and personality changes. Preexisting psychiatric conditions may be exacerbated by corticosteroid use. Prolonged use of corticosteroids may increase the incidence of secondary infection, cause activation of latent infections, mask acute infection (including fungal infections), prolong or exacerbate viral or parasitic infections, or limit response to vaccines. Exposure to chickenpox or measles should be avoided; corticosteroids should not be used to treat ocular herpes simplex. Corticosteroids should not be used for cerebral malaria, fungal infections, or viral hepatitis. Close observation is required in patients with latent tuberculosis and/or TB reactivity; restrict use in active TB (only fulminating or disseminated TB in conjunction with antituberculosis treatment). Amebiasis should be ruled out in any patient with recent travel to tropic climates or unexplained diarrhea prior to initiation of corticosteroids. Use with extreme caution in patients with *Strongyloides* infections; hyperinfection, dissemination and fatalities have occurred. Prolonged treatment with corticosteroids has been associated with the development of Kaposi's sarcoma (case reports); discontinuation may result in clinical improvement.

High-dose corticosteroids should not be used to manage acute head injury. Rare cases of anaphylactoid reactions have been observed in patients receiving corticosteroids. Avoid injection or leakage into the dermis; dermal and/or subdermal skin depression may occur at the site of injection. Avoid deltoid muscle injection; subcutaneous atrophy may occur. Potentially significant drug-drug interactions may exist, requiring dose or frequency adjustment, additional monitoring, and/or selection of alternative therapy.

Benzyl alcohol and derivatives: Methylprednisolone **acetate** I.M. injection (multiple-dose vial) and the diluent for methylprednisolone **sodium succinate** injection may contain benzyl alcohol; large amounts of benzyl alcohol (≥99 mg/kg/day) have been associated with a potentially fatal toxicity ("gasping syndrome") in neonates; the "gasping syndrome" consists of metabolic acidosis, respiratory distress, gasping respirations, CNS dysfunction (including convulsions, intracranial hemorrhage), hypotension, and cardiovascular collapse (AAP, 1997; CDC, 1982); some data suggests that benzoate displaces bilirubin from protein binding sites (Ahlfors, 2001); avoid or use dosage forms containing benzyl alcohol with caution in neonates.

Some dosage forms may contain polysorbate 80 (also known as Tweens). Hypersensitivity reactions, usually a delayed reaction, have been reported following exposure to pharmaceutical products containing polysorbate 80 in certain individuals (Isaksson, 2002; Lucente 2000; Shelley, 1995). Thrombocytopenia, ascites, pulmonary deterioration, and renal and hepatic failure have been reported in premature neonates after receiving parenteral products containing polysorbate 80 (Alade, 1986; CDC, 1984). See manufacturer's labeling.

Warnings: Additional Pediatric Considerations May cause osteoporosis (at any age) or inhibition of bone growth in pediatric patients. Use with caution in patients with osteoporosis. In a population-based study of children risk of fracture was shown to be increased with >4 courses of corticosteroids; underlying clinical condition may also impact bone health and osteoporotic effect of corticosteroids (Leonard, 2007). Increased IOP may occur, especially with prolonged use; in children, increased IOP has been shown to be dose dependent and produce a greater IOP in children <6 years than older children treated with ophthalmic dexamethasone (Lam, 2005). Hypertrophic cardiomyopathy has been reported in premature neonates.

Adverse Reactions

Cardiovascular: Arrhythmias, bradycardia, cardiac arrest, cardiomegaly, circulatory collapse, congestive heart failure, edema, fat embolism, hypertension, hypertrophic cardiomyopathy in premature infants, myocardial rupture (post MI), syncope, tachycardia, thromboembolism, vasculitis

Central nervous system: Delirium, depression, emotional instability, euphoria, hallucinations, headache, intracranial pressure increased, insomnia, malaise, mood swings, nervousness, neuritis, personality changes, psychic disorders, pseudotumor cerebri (usually following discontinuation), seizure, vertigo

Dermatologic: Acne, allergic dermatitis, alopecia, dry scaly skin, ecchymoses, edema, erythema, hirsutism, hyper-/hypopigmentation, hypertrichosis, impaired wound healing, petechiae, rash, skin atrophy, sterile abscess, skin test reaction impaired, striae, urticaria

Endocrine & metabolic: Adrenal suppression, amenorrhea, carbohydrate intolerance increased, Cushing's syndrome, diabetes mellitus, fluid retention, glucose intolerance, growth suppression (children), hyperglycemia, hyperlipidemia, hypokalemia, hypokalemic alkalosis, menstrual irregularities, negative nitrogen balance, pituitary-adrenal axis suppression, protein catabolism, sodium and water retention

Gastrointestinal: Abdominal distention, appetite increased, bowel/bladder dysfunction (after intrathecal administration), gastrointestinal hemorrhage, gastrointestinal perforation, nausea, pancreatitis, peptic ulcer, perforation of the small and large intestine, ulcerative esophagitis, vomiting, weight gain

Hematologic: Leukocytosis (transient)

Hepatic: Hepatomegaly, transaminases increased

Local: Postinjection flare (intra-articular use), thrombophlebitis

Neuromuscular & skeletal: Arthralgia, arthropathy, aseptic necrosis (femoral and humoral heads), fractures, muscle mass loss, muscle weakness, myopathy (particularly in conjunction with neuromuscular disease or neuromuscular-blocking agents), neuropathy, osteoporosis, parasthesia, tendon rupture, vertebral compression fractures, weakness

Ocular: Cataracts, exophthalmoses, glaucoma, intraocular pressure increased

Renal: Glycosuria

Respiratory: Pulmonary edema

Miscellaneous: Abnormal fat disposition, anaphylactoid reaction, anaphylaxis, angioedema, avascular necrosis, diaphoresis, hiccups, hypersensitivity reactions, infections, secondary malignancy

Rare but important or life-threatening: Venous thrombosis (Johannesdottir, 2013)

Drug Interactions

Metabolism/Transport Effects Substrate of CYP3A4 (minor); **Note:** Assignment of Major/Minor substrate status based on clinically relevant drug interaction potential; **Inhibits** CYP2C8 (weak)

Avoid Concomitant Use

Avoid concomitant use of MethylPREDNISolone with any of the following: Aldesleukin; Amodiaquine; BCG; BCG (Intravesical); Indium 111 Capromab Pendetide;

Mifepristone; Natalizumab; Pimecrolimus; Tacrolimus (Topical); Tofacitinib

Increased Effect/Toxicity

MethylPREDNISolone may increase the levels/effects of: Acetylcholinesterase Inhibitors; Amodiaquine; Amphotericin B; Androgens; CycloSPORINE (Systemic); Deferasirox; Leflunomide; Loop Diuretics; Natalizumab; Nicorandil; NSAID (COX-2 Inhibitor); NSAID (Nonselective); Quinolone Antibiotics; Thiazide Diuretics; Tofacitinib; Vaccines (Live); Warfarin

The levels/effects of MethylPREDNISolone may be increased by: Aprepitant; CycloSPORINE (Systemic); CYP3A4 Inhibitors (Strong); Denosumab; Estrogen Derivatives; Fosaprepitant; Indacaterol; Mifepristone; Neuromuscular-Blocking Agents (Nondepolarizing); Pimecrolimus; Roflumilast; Salicylates; Tacrolimus (Topical); Telaprevir; Trastuzumab

Decreased Effect

MethylPREDNISolone may decrease the levels/effects of: Aldesleukin; Antidiabetic Agents; BCG; BCG (Intravesical); Calcitriol (Systemic); Coccidioides immitis Skin Test; Corticorelin; CycloSPORINE (Systemic); Hyaluronidase; Indium 111 Capromab Pendetide; Isoniazid; Salicylates; Sipuleucel-T; Telaprevir; Urea Cycle Disorder Agents; Vaccines (Inactivated); Vaccines (Live)

The levels/effects of MethylPREDNISolone may be decreased by: Antacids; Bile Acid Sequestrants; CYP3A4 Inducers (Strong); Echinacea; Mifepristone; Mitotane

Storage/Stability

Methylprednisolone acetate; tablets: Store at 20°C to 25°C (68°F to 77°F).

Methylprednisolone sodium succinate: Store intact vials at controlled room temperature of 20°C to 25°C (68°F to 77°F). Protect from light. Reconstituted solutions of methylprednisolone sodium succinate should be stored at room temperature of 20°C to 25°C (68°F to 77°F) and used within 48 hours. Stability of parenteral admixture at room temperature (25°C) and at refrigeration temperature (4°C) is 48 hours.

Mechanism of Action In a tissue-specific manner, corticosteroids regulate gene expression subsequent to binding specific intracellular receptors and translocation into the nucleus. Corticosteroids exert a wide array of physiologic effects including modulation of carbohydrate, protein, and lipid metabolism and maintenance of fluid and electrolyte homeostasis. Moreover cardiovascular, immunologic, musculoskeletal, endocrine, and neurologic physiology are influenced by corticosteroids. Decreases inflammation by suppression of migration of polymorphonuclear leukocytes and reversal of increased capillary permeability.

Pharmacodynamics The time of maximum effects and the duration of these effects is dependent upon the route of administration. See table.

Route	Maximum Effect	Duration
Oral	1-2 hours	30-36 hours
IM (acetate)	4-8 days	1-4 weeks
Intra-articular	1 week	1-5 weeks

Pharmacokinetics (Adult data unless noted)

Half-life:

Adolescents: 1.9 + 0.7 hours (n=6; patients 12-20 years of age; Rouster-Stevens, 2008)

Adults: 2.4-3.3 hours (Rohatagi, 1997)

Dosing: Usual Note: Adjust dose depending upon condition being treated and response of patient. The lowest possible dose should be used to control the condition; when dose reduction is possible, the dose should be reduced gradually. In life-threatening situations, parenteral doses larger than the oral dose may be needed. **Only sodium succinate salt may be given IV**

Infants, Children, and Adolescents:

Asthma, exacerbation:

Acute, short-course "burst" (NAEPP, 2007):

Infants and Children <12 years:

Oral: 1-2 mg/kg/day in divided doses once or twice daily for 3-10 days; maximum daily dose: 60 mg/**day**; **Note:** Burst should be continued until symptoms resolve or patient achieves peak expiratory flow 80% of personal best; usually requires 3-10 days of treatment (~5 days on average); longer treatment may be required

IM **(acetate)**: **Note:** This may be given in place of short-course "burst" of oral steroids in patients who are vomiting or if compliance is a problem.

Children ≤4 years: 7.5 mg/kg as a one-time dose; maximum dose: 240 mg

Children 5-11 years: 240 mg as a one-time dose

Children ≥12 years and Adolescents:

Oral: 40-60 mg/day in divided doses once or twice daily for 3-10 days; **Note:** Burst should be continued until symptoms resolve and peak expiratory flow is at least 80% of personal best; usually requires 3-10 days of treatment (~5 days on average); longer treatment may be required

IM **(acetate)**: 240 mg as a one-time dose; **Note:** This may be given in place of short-course "burst" of oral steroids in patients who are vomiting or if compliance is a problem

Hospital/emergency medical care doses:

Infants and Children <12 years: Oral, IV: 1-2 mg/kg/day in 2 divided doses; maximum daily dose: 60 mg/**day**; continue until peak expiratory flow is 70% of predicted or personal best

Children ≥12 years and Adolescents: Oral, IV: 40-80 mg/day in divided doses once or twice daily until peak expiratory flow is 70% of predicted or personal best

Status asthmaticus (previous NAEPP guidelines; still used by some clinicians): Children: IV: Loading dose: 2 mg/kg/dose, then 0.5-1 mg/kg/dose every 6 hours; **Note:** See NAEPP 2007 guidelines for asthma exacerbations (emergency medical care or hospital doses) listed above

Asthma, long-term treatment (maintenance) (NAEPP, 2007):

Infants and Children <12 years: Oral: 0.25-2 mg/kg/day once daily in the morning or every other day as needed for asthma control; maximum daily dose: 60 mg/**day**

Children ≥12 years and Adolescents: Oral: 7.5-60 mg daily once daily in the morning or every other day as needed for asthma control

Anti-inflammatory or immunosuppressive: Oral, IM (acetate or succinate), IV (succinate): 0.5-1.7 mg/kg/day or 5-25 mg/**m**^{2}/day in divided doses every 6-12 hours

"Pulse" therapy: IV (succinate): 15-30 mg/kg/dose once daily for 3 days; maximum dose: 1000 mg

Lupus nephritis: Children and Adolescents: IV (succinate): High-dose "pulse" therapy: 30 mg/kg/dose or 600-1000 mg/**m**^{2}/dose once daily for 3 days; maximum dose: 1000 mg (Adams, 2006; Marks, 2010)

Spinal cord injury, acute: Children and Adolescents: IV (succinate): 30 mg/kg over 15 minutes followed in 45 minutes by a continuous infusion of 5.4 mg/kg/hour for 23 hours; **Note:** Due to insufficient evidence of clinical efficacy (ie, preserving or improving spinal cord function), the routine use of methylprednisolone in the treatment of acute spinal cord injury is no longer recommended. If used in this setting, methylprednisolone should not be initiated >8 hours after the injury; not effective in penetrating trauma (eg, gunshot) (Consortium for Spinal Cord Medicine, 2008).

***Pneumocystis* pneumonia; moderate or severe infection: Note:** Initiate therapy within 72 hours of diagnosis, if possible.

Infants and Children: IV (succinate): 1 mg/kg/dose every 6 hours on days 1-7, then 1 mg/kg/dose twice daily on days 8-9, then 0.5 mg/kg/dose twice daily on days 10 and 11, and 1 mg/kg/dose once daily on days 12-16 (CDC, 2009)

Adolescents: IV (succinate): 30 mg twice daily on days 1-5, then 30 mg once daily on days 6-10, then 15 mg once daily on days 11-21 (CDC, 2009a)

Graft-versus-host disease, acute (GVHD): IV (succinate): 1-2 mg/kg/dose once daily; if using low dose (1 mg/kg) and no improvement after 3 days, increase dose to 2 mg/kg. Continue therapy for 5-7 days; if improvement observed, may taper by 10% of starting dose every 4 days; if no improvement, then considered steroid-refractory GVHD and additional agents should be considered (Carpenter, 2010)

Adults:

Allergic conditions: Oral: Tapered-dosage schedule (eg, dose-pack containing 21 x 4 mg tablets):

Day 1: 24 mg on day 1 administered as 8 mg (2 tablets) before breakfast, 4 mg (1 tablet) after lunch, 4 mg (1 tablet) after supper, and 8 mg (2 tablets) at bedtime **OR** 24 mg (6 tablets) as a single dose or divided into 2 or 3 doses upon initiation (regardless of time of day)

Day 2: 20 mg on day 2 administered as 4 mg (1 tablet) before breakfast, 4 mg (1 tablet) after lunch, 4 mg (1 tablet) after supper, and 8 mg (2 tablets) at bedtime

Day 3: 16 mg on day 3 administered as 4 mg (1 tablet) before breakfast, 4 mg (1 tablet) after lunch, 4 mg (1 tablet) after supper, and 4 mg (1 tablet) at bedtime

Day 4: 12 mg on day 4 administered as 4 mg (1 tablet) before breakfast, 4 mg (1 tablet) after lunch, and 4 mg (1 tablet) at bedtime

Day 5: 8 mg on day 5 administered as 4 mg (1 tablet) before breakfast and 4 mg (1 tablet) at bedtime

Day 6: 4 mg on day 6 administered as 4 mg (1 tablet) before breakfast

Anti-inflammatory or immunosuppressive:

Oral: 2-60 mg/day in 1-4 divided doses to start, followed by gradual reduction in dosage to the lowest possible level consistent with maintaining an adequate clinical response

IM (sodium succinate): 10-80 mg/day once daily

IM (acetate): 10-80 mg every 1-2 weeks

IV (sodium succinate): 10-40 mg over a period of several minutes and repeated IV or IM at intervals depending on clinical response; when high dosages are needed, give 30 mg/kg over a period ≥30 minutes and may be repeated every 4-6 hours for 48 hours

Arthritis: Intra-articular (acetate): Administer every 1-5 weeks

Large joints (eg, knee, ankle): 20-80 mg

Medium joints (eg, elbow, wrist): 10-40 mg

Small joints: 4-10 mg

Asthma exacerbations, including status asthmaticus (emergency medical care or hospital doses): Oral, IV: 40-80 mg/day in 1-2 divided doses until peak expiratory flow is 70% of predicted or personal best (NIH Asthma Guidelines, NAEPP, 2007)

Asthma, severe persistent, long-term control: Oral: 7.5-60 mg/day (or on alternate days) (NIH Asthma Guidelines, NAEPP, 2007)

Dermatitis, acute severe: IM (acetate): 80-120 mg as a single dose

Dermatitis, chronic: IM (acetate): 40-120 mg every 5-10 days

Dermatologic conditions (eg, keloids, lichen planus): Intralesional (acetate): 20-60 mg

Dermatomyositis/polymyositis: IV (sodium succinate) 1000 mg/day for 3-5 days for severe muscle weakness followed by conversion to oral prednisone (Drake, 1996)

Lupus nephritis: High-dose "pulse" therapy: IV (sodium succinate): 500-1000 mg/day for 3 days (Ponticelli, 2010)

***Pneumocystis* pneumonia in AIDS patients:** IV: 30 mg twice daily for 5 days, then 30 mg once daily for 5 days, then 15 mg once daily for 11 days

Dosing adjustment in renal impairment: Slightly dialyzable (5% to 20%); administer dose posthemodialysis

Preparation for Administration

Parenteral: Reconstitute vials with provided diluent or bacteriostatic water (see manufacturer's labeling for details). Act-O-Vial (self-contained powder for injection plus diluent [preservative-free SWFI or bacteriostatic water]) may be reconstituted by pressing the activator to force diluent into the powder compartment. Following gentle agitation, solution may be withdrawn via syringe through a needle inserted into the center of the stopper. Neonates should only receive doses reconstituted with preservative free SWFI.

IV infusion: Dilute reconstituted dose in D_5W, NS or D_5NS; in adults the minimum diluent volume is 50 mL; the standard diluent (Solu-Medrol): 40 mg/50 mL D_5W (0.8 mg/mL); 125 mg/50 mL D_5W (2.5 mg/mL). In pediatric patients, a pulse dose (30 mg/kg up to 1,000 mg) has been added to 100 mL of diluent (D_5W, NS or $D_5{}^1/_2NS$) (maximum concentration: 10 mg/mL) (Akikusa 2007; Miller 1980)

Administration

Oral: Administer after meals or with food or milk; do not administer with grapefruit juice; if prescribed once daily, administer dose in the early morning to mimic the normal diurnal variation of endogenous cortisol

Parenteral:

IM: **Acetate, Succinate:** Avoid injection into the deltoid muscle due to a high incidence of subcutaneous atrophy. Do not inject into areas that have evidence of acute local infection. Discard contents of single-dose vial after use.

IV: **Succinate:** Rate dependent upon dose; typically intermittent infusion is administered over 15-60 minutes. Do not administer moderate or high dose IV push; severe adverse effects, including hypotension, cardiac arrhythmia, and sudden death, have been reported in patients receiving high-dose methylprednisolone IV push over <20 minutes (Barron 1982; Ditzian-Kadanoff 1987; Garin 1986; Liebling 1981; Lucas 1993). **Do not give acetate form IV.**

Low dose (eg, ≤1.8 mg/kg or ≤125 mg/dose): IV push over 3 to 15 minutes; maximum concentration: 125 mg/mL

Moderate dose (eg, ≥2 mg/kg or 250 mg/dose): Administer over 15 to 30 minutes

High dose (eg, ≥15 mg/kg or ≥500 mg/dose): Administer over 30 to 60 minutes; doses ≥1,000 mg: Administer over 60 minutes. **Note:** In some of the adult spinal cord injury trials, bolus doses (30 mg/kg) have been administered over 15 minutes.

Monitoring Parameters Blood pressure, serum glucose, potassium, and calcium and clinical presence of adverse effects. Monitor intraocular pressure (if therapy >6 weeks), linear growth of pediatric patients (with chronic use), assess HPA suppression

Test Interactions Interferes with skin tests

Additional Information Sodium content of 1 g sodium succinate injection: 2.01 mEq; methylprednisolone sodium succinate 53 mg = methylprednisolone base 40 mg

Dosage Forms Excipient information presented when available (limited, particularly for generics); consult specific product labeling.

Solution Reconstituted, Injection, as sodium succinate [strength expressed as base]:

A-Methapred: 40 mg (1 ea); 125 mg (1 ea) [contains benzyl alcohol]

Solu-MEDROL: 500 mg (1 ea); 1000 mg (1 ea)

Solu-MEDROL: 2 g (1 ea) [contains benzyl alcohol]

Generic: 40 mg (1 ea); 125 mg (1 ea); 1000 mg (1 ea)

Solution Reconstituted, Injection, as sodium succinate [strength expressed as base, preservative free]:

Solu-MEDROL: 40 mg (1 ea); 125 mg (1 ea); 500 mg (1 ea); 1000 mg (1 ea)

Suspension, Injection, as acetate:

Depo-Medrol: 20 mg/mL (5 mL); 40 mg/mL (5 mL, 10 mL) [contains benzyl alcohol, polyethylene glycol, polysorbate 80]

Depo-Medrol: 40 mg/mL (1 mL) [contains polyethylene glycol]

Depo-Medrol: 80 mg/mL (1 mL)

Depo-Medrol: 80 mg/mL (5 mL) [contains benzyl alcohol, polyethylene glycol, polysorbate 80]

Depo-Medrol: 80 mg/mL (1 mL) [contains polyethylene glycol]

Generic: 40 mg/mL (1 mL, 5 mL, 10 mL); 80 mg/mL (1 mL, 5 mL)

Tablet, Oral:

Medrol: 2 mg, 4 mg, 8 mg, 16 mg, 32 mg [scored]

Medrol (Pak): 4 mg [scored]

Generic: 4 mg, 8 mg, 16 mg, 32 mg

- ◆ **6-α-Methylprednisolone** *see* MethylPREDNISolone *on page 1409*
- ◆ **Methylprednisolone Acetate** *see* MethylPREDNISolone *on page 1409*
- ◆ **Methylprednisolone Sodium Succinate** *see* MethylPREDNISolone *on page 1409*
- ◆ **Methylprednisolone Sodium Succinate For Injection (Can)** *see* MethylPREDNISolone *on page 1409*
- ◆ **Methylprednisolone Sodium Succinate For Injection USP (Can)** *see* MethylPREDNISolone *on page 1409*
- ◆ **4-Methylpyrazole** *see* Fomepizole *on page 933*
- ◆ **Methylrosaniline Chloride** *see* Gentian Violet *on page 970*
- ◆ **Methylthionine Chloride** *see* Methylene Blue *on page 1400*
- ◆ **Methylthioninium Chloride** *see* Methylene Blue *on page 1400*

Metoclopramide (met oh KLOE pra mide)

Medication Safety Issues

Sound-alike/look-alike issues:

Metoclopramide may be confused with metolazone, metoprolol, metroNIDAZOLE

Reglan may be confused with Megace, Regonol, Renagel, Regitine

BEERS Criteria medication:

This drug may be potentially inappropriate for use in geriatric patients (Quality of evidence - moderate; Strength of recommendation - strong).

Brand Names: US Metozolv ODT; Reglan

Brand Names: Canada Apo-Metoclop; Metoclopramide Hydrochloride Injection; Metoclopramide Omega; Metonia; Nu-Metoclopramide; PMS-Metoclopramide

Therapeutic Category Antiemetic; Gastrointestinal Agent, Prokinetic

Generic Availability (US) Yes

Use

Oral (orally disintegrating tablet [Metizolv ODT], solution, tablet): Symptomatic treatment of gastroesophageal reflux; diabetic gastroparesis (All indications: FDA approved in adults)

Parenteral: Symptomatic treatment of acute and recurrent diabetic gastroparesis; prevention of nausea and vomiting associated with chemotherapy; prevention of postoperative nausea and vomiting (All indications: FDA approved in adults); facilitates intubation of the small intestine (postpyloric placement of enteral feeding tube) (FDA approved in pediatric patients [age not specified] and adults)

Medication Guide Available Yes

Pregnancy Risk Factor B

Pregnancy Considerations Adverse events were not observed in animal reproduction studies. Metoclopramide crosses the placenta and can be detected in cord blood and amniotic fluid (Arvela, 1983; Bylsma-Howell, 1983). Available evidence suggests safe use during pregnancy (Berkovitch, 2002; Matok, 2009; Sørensen, 2000). Metoclopramide may be used for the treatment of nausea and vomiting of pregnancy (ACOG, 2004; Levichek, 2002) and prophylaxis for nausea and vomiting associated with cesarean delivery (ASA, 2007; Mahadevan, 2006; Smith, 2011). Other agents are preferred for gastroesophageal reflux (Mahadevan, 2006).

Breast-Feeding Considerations Metoclopramide is excreted in breast milk. Information is available from studies conducted in mothers nursing preterm infants (n=14; delivered at 23-34 weeks gestation) or term infants (n=18) and taking metoclopramide 10 mg 3 times daily. The median concentration of metoclopramide in breast milk was ~45 ng/mL in the preterm infants and the mean concentration was ~48 ng/mL in the full term infants. The authors of both studies calculated the relative infant dose to be 3% to 5%, based on a therapeutic infant dose of 0.5 mg/kg/day. Metoclopramide was also detected in the serum of one nursing full term infant (Hansen, 2005; Kauppila, 1983). Metoclopramide may increase prolactin concentrations and cause galactorrhea and gynecomastia, but studies which evaluated its use to increase milk production for women who want to nurse have had mixed results. In addition, due to the potential for adverse events, nonpharmacologic measure should be considered prior to the use of medications as galactagogues (ABM, 2011). The manufacturer recommends that caution be used if administered to a nursing woman.

Contraindications

Known sensitivity or intolerance to metoclopramide or any component of the formulation; situations where gastrointestinal (GI) motility may be dangerous, including mechanical GI obstruction, perforation, or hemorrhage; pheochromocytoma; history of seizure disorder (eg, epilepsy), concomitant use with other agents likely to increase extrapyramidal reactions

Canadian labeling: Additional contraindications (not in US labeling): Infants <1 year of age.

Warnings/Precautions [US Boxed Warning]: May cause tardive dyskinesia, a serious movement disorder which is often irreversible; the risk of developing tardive dyskinesia increases with duration of treatment and total cumulative dose. Discontinue metoclopramide in patients who develop signs/symptoms of tardive dyskinesia. There is no known treatment for tardive dyskinesia. In some patients, symptoms lessen or resolve after metoclopramide treatment is stopped. Avoid metoclopramide treatment longer than 12 weeks in all but rare cases in which therapeutic benefit is thought to outweigh the risk of developing tardive dyskinesia. Tardive dyskinesia is characterized by involuntary movements of the face, tongue, or extremities and may be disfiguring. An analysis of utilization patterns showed that ~20% of patients who used metoclopramide took it for longer than 12 weeks. Metoclopramide may mask underlying tardive disease by suppressing or partially suppressing tardive dyskinesia signs (metoclopramide should not be used to control tardive dyskinesia symptoms as the long-term course is unknown). The risk for tardive dyskinesia appears to be increased in the elderly, women, and diabetics, although it is not possible to predict which patients will develop tardive dyskinesia. There is no known effective treatment for established cases of tardive dyskinesia, although in some patients, tardive dyskinesia may remit (partially or completely) within several weeks to months after metoclopramide is withdrawn.

May cause extrapyramidal symptoms (EPS), generally manifested as acute dystonic reactions within the initial 24 to 48 hours of use at the usual adult dose (30 to 40 mg/day). Risk of these reactions is increased at higher doses, and in pediatric patients and adults <30 years of age. Symptoms may include involuntary limb movements, facial grimacing, torticollis, oculogyric crisis, rhythmic tongue protrusion, bulbar type speech, trismus, or dystonic reactions resembling tetanus. May also rarely present as stridor and dyspnea (may be due to laryngospasm). Dystonic symptoms may be managed with IM diphenhydramine or benztropine. Pseudoparkinsonism (eg, bradykinesia, tremor, rigidity, mask-like facies) may also occur (usually within first 6 months of therapy) and is generally reversible within 2 to 3 months following discontinuation. Symptoms of Parkinson disease may be exacerbated by metoclopramide; use with extreme caution (or avoid use) in patients with Parkinson disease.

Metoclopramide has been known to cause sinus arrest (usually with rapid IV administration or higher doses) (Bentsen, 2002; Malkoff 1995). The torsadogenic potential for metoclopramide is considered to be low (Claassen, 2005). Based on case reports, however, metoclopramide may cause QT prolongation and torsades de pointes in certain individuals (eg, heart failure patients with renal impairment); use with caution in these patients (Siddiquie, 2009). There is data in healthy male volunteers to show that metoclopramide actually shortens the QT interval while at the same time increasing QT variance (Ellidokuz, 2003). No human data other than case reports; however, has demonstrated a consistent QT prolonging effect with metoclopramide nor is there any substantiated evidence to show a direct association with the development of torsades de pointes.

Metoclopramide use may be associated (rarely) with neuroleptic malignant syndrome (NMS); may be fatal. Monitor for manifestations of NMS, which include hyperthermia, muscle rigidity, altered consciousness, and autonomic instability (irregular pulse or blood pressure, tachycardia, diaphoresis, and cardiac arrhythmias). Discontinue immediately if signs/symptoms of NMS appear and begin intensive symptomatic management and monitoring. Bromocriptine and dantrolene have been used to manage NMS, although effectiveness have not been established.

Mental depression has occurred (in patients with and without a history of depression), and symptoms range from mild to severe (suicidal ideation and suicide); use in patients with a history of depression only if anticipated benefits outweigh potential risks.

In a study in hypertensive patients, IV metoclopramide was associated with catecholamine release. Use with caution in patients with hypertension. There are reports of hypertensive crises in some patients with undiagnosed pheochromocytoma. Immediately discontinue with any rapid rise in blood pressure that is associated with metoclopramide. Hypertensive crises may be managed with phentolamine. Use with caution in patients who are at risk of fluid overload (HF, cirrhosis); metoclopramide causes a transient increase in serum aldosterone and increases the risk for fluid retention/overload; discontinue if adverse events or signs/symptoms appear.

Patients with NADH-cytochrome b5 reductase deficiency are at increased risk of methemoglobinemia and/or sulfhemoglobinemia. Use with caution in patients with renal impairment; dosage adjustment may be needed. Use with caution following surgical anastomosis/closure; promotility agents may theoretically increase pressure in suture lines.

For patients with diabetic gastroparesis, the usual manifestations of delayed gastric emptying (eg, nausea, vomiting, heartburn, persistent fullness after meals, anorexia) appear to respond to metoclopramide within different time intervals. Significant relief of nausea occurs early and continues to improve over a 3-week period; relief of vomiting and anorexia may precede the relief of abdominal fullness by a week or more. If gastroesophageal reflux symptoms are confined to particular situations, such as following the evening meal, consider use of metoclopramide as a single dose prior to the provocative situation, rather than using the drug throughout the day. Symptoms of postprandial and daytime heartburn respond better to metoclopramide, with less observed effect on nocturnal symptoms. Because there is no documented correlation between symptoms and healing of esophageal lesions, patients with documented lesions should be monitored endoscopically. Healing of esophageal ulcers and erosions has been endoscopically demonstrated at the end of a 12-week trial using a dosage of 15 mg 4 times daily.

Avoid use in older adults (except for diabetic gastroparesis) due to risk of extrapyramidal effects, including tardive dyskinesia; risk is potentially even greater in frail older adults (Beers Criteria). In addition, risk of tardive dyskinesia may be increased in older women. EPS are increased in pediatric patients. In neonates, prolonged clearance of metoclopramide may lead to increased serum concentrations. Neonates may also have decreased levels of NADH-cytochrome b5 reductase which increases the risk of methemoglobinemia. The Canadian labeling contraindicates use in infants <1 year of age and recommends avoiding use in children >1 year unless clearly necessary. Potentially significant drug-drug interactions may exist, requiring dose or frequency adjustment, additional monitoring, and/or selection of alternative therapy. CNS effects may be potentiated when used with other sedative drugs or ethanol. Abrupt discontinuation may (rarely) result in withdrawal symptoms (dizziness, headache, nervousness).

Benzyl alcohol and derivatives: Some dosage forms may contain sodium benzoate/benzoic acid; benzoic acid (benzoate) is a metabolite of benzyl alcohol; large amounts of benzyl alcohol (≥99 mg/kg/day) have been associated with a potentially fatal toxicity ("gasping syndrome") in neonates; the "gasping syndrome" consists of metabolic acidosis, respiratory distress, gasping respirations, CNS dysfunction (including convulsions, intracranial hemorrhage), hypotension, and cardiovascular collapse (AAP, 1997; CDC, 1982); some data suggest that benzoate displaces bilirubin from protein binding sites (Ahlfors, 2001); avoid or use dosage forms containing benzyl alcohol derivative with caution in neonates. See manufacturer's labeling.

Adverse Reactions

Cardiovascular: Atrioventricular block, bradycardia, congestive heart failure, flushing (following high IV doses), hypertension, hypotension, supraventricular tachycardia

Central nervous system: Akathisia, confusion, depression, dizziness, drowsiness (dose related), drug-induced Parkinson's disease, dystonic reaction (dose and age related), fatigue, hallucination (rare), headache, insomnia, lassitude, neuroleptic malignant syndrome (rare),

restlessness, seizure, somnolence, suicidal ideation, tardive dyskinesia
Dermatologic: Skin rash, urticaria
Endocrine & metabolic: Amenorrhea, fluid retention, galactorrhea, gynecomastia, hyperprolactinemia, porphyria
Gastrointestinal: Diarrhea, nausea, vomiting
Genitourinary: Impotence, urinary frequency, urinary incontinence
Hematologic & oncologic: Agranulocytosis, leukopenia, methemoglobinemia, neutropenia, sulfhemoglobinemia
Hepatic: Hepatotoxicity (rare)
Hypersensitivity: Angioedema (rare), hypersensitivity reaction
Neuromuscular & skeletal: Laryngospasm (rare)
Ophthalmic: Visual disturbance
Respiratory: Bronchospasm, laryngeal edema (rare)

Drug Interactions

Metabolism/Transport Effects **Substrate** of CYP1A2 (minor), CYP2D6 (minor); **Note:** Assignment of Major/Minor substrate status based on clinically relevant drug interaction potential; **Inhibits** CYP2D6 (weak)

Avoid Concomitant Use

Avoid concomitant use of Metoclopramide with any of the following: Antipsychotic Agents; Droperidol; Promethazine; Rivastigmine; Tetrabenazine; Trimetazidine

Increased Effect/Toxicity

Metoclopramide may increase the levels/effects of: Antipsychotic Agents; CycloSPORINE (Systemic); Highest Risk QTc-Prolonging Agents; Moderate Risk QTc-Prolonging Agents; Prilocaine; Promethazine; Selective Serotonin Reuptake Inhibitors; Serotonin/Norepinephrine Reuptake Inhibitors; Sodium Nitrite; Tetrabenazine; Tricyclic Antidepressants; Trimetazidine

The levels/effects of Metoclopramide may be increased by: Droperidol; Metyrosine; Mifepristone; Nitric Oxide; Rivastigmine; Serotonin Modulators

Decreased Effect

Metoclopramide may decrease the levels/effects of: Anti-Parkinson's Agents (Dopamine Agonist); Atovaquone; Posaconazole; Quinagolide

The levels/effects of Metoclopramide may be decreased by: Anticholinergic Agents

Storage/Stability

Injection: Store intact vials at 20°C to 25°C (68°F to 77°F); injection is photosensitive and should be protected from light during storage; parenteral admixtures in D_5W, $D_5{}^{1/2}NS$, NS, LR, or Ringer's injection are stable for up to 24 hours after preparation at normal light conditions or up to 48 hours if protected from light. When mixed with NS, can be stored frozen for up to 4 weeks; metoclopramide is degraded when admixed and frozen with D_5W.
Oral solution: Store at 20°C to 25°C (68°F to 77°F). Do not freeze. Dispense in tight, light-resistant container.
Tablet: Store at 20°C to 25°C (68°F to 77°F). Dispense in tight, light-resistant container.
Tablet, orally disintegrating: Store at 20°C to 25°C (68°F to 77°F). Keep in original packaging until just prior to use.

Mechanism of Action Blocks dopamine receptors and (when given in higher doses) also blocks serotonin receptors in chemoreceptor trigger zone of the CNS; enhances the response to acetylcholine of tissue in upper GI tract causing enhanced motility and accelerated gastric emptying without stimulating gastric, biliary, or pancreatic secretions; increases lower esophageal sphincter tone

Pharmacodynamics

Onset of action:
Oral: Within 30-60 minutes
IM: Within 10-15 minutes
IV: Within 1-3 minutes
Duration: Therapeutic effects persist for 1-2 hours, regardless of route administered

Pharmacokinetics (Adult data unless noted)

Absorption: Oral: Rapid
Distribution: V_d:
Neonates, PMA 31 to 40 weeks: 6.94 L/kg (Kearns, 1998)
Infants: 4.4 L/kg
Children: 3 L/kg
Adults: 3.5 L/kg
Protein binding: ~30%
Bioavailability: Oral: 80 ± 15.5%
Half-life: Normal renal function:
Neonates, PMA 31 to 40 weeks: 5.4 hours (Kearns, 1998)
Infants: 4.15 hours (range: 2.23 to 10.3 hours) (Kearns, 1988)
Children: ~4 hours (range: 2 to 12.5 hours); half-life and clearance may be dose-dependent
Adults: 5 to 6 hours
Time to peak serum concentration: Oral:
Neonates, PMA 31 to 40 weeks: 2.45 hours (Kearns, 1998)
Infants: 2.2 hours
Adults: 1 to 2 hours
Elimination: Primarily in the urine (~85%) and feces

Dosing: Neonatal **Gastroesophageal reflux:** Limited data available: Oral, IM, IV: Usual dose: 0.1 mg/kg/dose every 6 hours (Avery, 1994; Kimball, 2001); higher doses of 0.15 mg/kg/dose have been reported in a pharmacokinetic study of 10 preterm neonates (PMA: 31 to 40 weeks) (Kearns, 1998). In a small case series of previous VLBW (n=6; GA: 26 to 35 weeks; birth weight: 790 to 1040 g; mean PNA at treatment: 35 days), a lower dose of 0.033 mg/kg every 8 hours was reported effective in all patients (Sankaran, 1982). Doses >0.15 mg/kg may increase potential for adverse effects due to excessive serum concentrations (Kearns, 1998).

Dosing: Usual

Pediatric:

Postpyloric feeding tube placement (short bowel intubation): IV:
Patient age:
<6 years: 0.1 mg/kg as a single dose
6 to 14 years: 2.5 to 5 mg as a single dose
>14 years: 10 mg as a single dose

Gastroesophageal reflux: Limited data available; efficacy results variable (Vandenplas, 2009): **Note:** NASPGHAN/ESPGHAN guidelines do not recommend metoclopramide for routine treatment of GERD; evaluate risk:benefit prior to use (Vandenplas, 2009): Infants, Children, and Adolescents: Oral: 0.1 to 0.2 mg/kg/dose every 6 to 8 hours; maximum dose: 10 mg (Chicella, 2005; Forbes, 1986; Rode, 1987; Tolia, 1989)

Postoperative nausea and vomiting; prevention: Limited data available; optimal dose not established; efficacy results variable: **Note:** Guidelines discourage use of metoclopramide; considered ineffective (Gan, 2007): Children and Adolescents: I.V: 0.1 to 0.5 mg/kg/dose as a single dose administered after induction or on arrival to PACU; maximum dose: 10 mg/dose (Ferrari, 1992; Furst, 1994; Henzi, 1999; Lin, 1992)

Chemotherapy-induced nausea and vomiting (CINV), prevention: Limited data available; optimal dose not established; efficacy results variable. **Note:** Doses required to prevent CINV are high and should not be used first-line due to increased risk of extrapyramidal symptoms (acute dystonic reactions); concurrent administration of diphenhydramine or benztropine is recommended to prevent drug-induced adverse effects (Dupuis, 2013; Roila, 1998).

POGO Guidelines (Dupuis, 2013): Infants, Children and Adolescents: **Note:** For use in patients in whom

corticosteroids are contraindicated; use in combination with 5-HT_3 receptor antagonists.
Initial dose: IV: 1 mg/kg as a single dose prior to chemotherapy
Subsequent doses: Oral: 0.0375 mg/kg/dose every 6 hours
Alternate dosing: Children and Adolescents: IV: 1 to 2 mg/kg/dose prior to and then every 2 to 4 hours up to every 6 hours following chemotherapy; maximum: 5 doses/day (Roila, 1998; Terrin, 1984); another trial administered 2 mg/kg when chemotherapy was started followed by 2 mg/kg/dose 2, 6, and 12 hours later (Marshall, 1989)

Adult:

Diabetic gastroparesis:
Oral: 10 mg up to 4 times daily 30 minutes before meals and at bedtime for 2 to 8 weeks. Treatment >12 weeks is not recommended.
IM, IV (for severe symptoms): 10 mg over 1 to 2 minutes; 10 days of IV therapy may be necessary before symptoms are controlled to allow transition to oral administration

Chemotherapy-induced emesis prophylaxis: IV: 1 to 2 mg/kg 30 minutes before chemotherapy and repeated every 2 hours for 2 doses, then every 3 hours for 3 doses (manufacturer's labeling); pretreatment with diphenhydramine will decrease risk of extrapyramidal reactions
Alternate dosing: **Note:** Metoclopramide is considered an antiemetic with a low therapeutic index; use is generally reserved for agents with low emetogenic potential or in patients intolerant/refractory to first-line antiemetics.
Low-risk chemotherapy: IV, Oral: 10 to 40 mg prior to chemotherapy dose, then every 4 to 6 hours as needed (NCCN Antiemesis guidelines, v.1.2013)
Breakthrough treatment: IV, Oral: 10 to 40 mg every 4 to 6 hours (NCCN Antiemesis guidelines, v.1.2013)
Delayed-emesis prophylaxis: Oral: 20 to 40 mg (or 0.5 mg/kg/dose) 2 to 4 times daily for 3 to 4 days (in combination with dexamethasone (ASCO guidelines [Kris, 2006])
Refractory or intolerant to antiemetics with a higher therapeutic index (Hesketh, 2008):
IV: 1 to 2 mg/kg/dose before chemotherapy and repeat 2 hours after chemotherapy
Oral: 0.5 mg/kg every 6 hours on days 2 to 4

Gastroesophageal reflux: Oral: 10 to15 mg up to 4 times daily 30 minutes before meals or food and at bedtime; single doses of 20 mg are occasionally needed prior to provoking situations. Treatment >12 weeks is not recommended.

Postoperative nausea and vomiting prophylaxis: IM, IV: 10 to 20 mg near end of surgery. **Note:** Guidelines discourage use of 10 mg metoclopramide as being ineffective (Gan, 2007); comparative study indicates higher dose (20 mg) may be efficacious (Quaynor, 2002).

Postpyloric feeding tube placement, radiological exam: IV: 10 mg as a single dose

Dosing adjustment in renal impairment:
Infants, Children, and Adolescents: The following adjustments have been recommended (Aronoff, 2007). **Note:** Renally adjusted dose recommendations are based on doses of 0.1 to 0.2 mg/kg/dose every 6 to 8 hours.
GFR 30 to 50 mL/minute/1.73 m^2: Administer 75% of dose
GFR 10 to 29 mL/minute/1.73 m^2: Administer 50% of dose
GFR <10 mL/minute/1.73 m^2: Administer 25% of dose
Intermittent hemodialysis: Administer 25% of dose
Peritoneal dialysis (PD): Administer 25% of dose
Continuous renal replacement therapy (CRRT): Administer 75% of dose
Adults:
CrCl <40 mL/minute: Administer 50% of recommended dose
Not dialyzable (0% to 5%); supplemental dose is not necessary

Dosing adjustment in hepatic impairment: There are no dosage adjustments provided in the manufacturer's labeling; however, metoclopramide has been used safely in patients with advanced liver disease with normal renal function.

Preparation for Administration Parenteral: Doses >10 mg should be diluted in 50 mL of compatible solution (preferably NS) prior to administration

Administration
Oral:
Orally disintegrating tablets: Administer on an empty stomach at least 30 minutes prior to food. Do not remove from packaging until time of administration. If tablet breaks or crumbles while handling, discard and remove new tablet. Using dry hands, place tablet on tongue and allow to dissolve. Swallow with saliva.
Oral solution, tablet: Administer 30 minutes before meals and at bedtime
Parenteral:
IM: May be administered IM
IV: **Note:** Rapid IV administration is associated with a transient but intense feeling of anxiety and restlessness, followed by drowsiness
IV push: For doses ≤10 mg may be administered undiluted (5 mg/mL) by direct IV push over 1 to 2 minutes.
Intermittent IV infusion: For higher doses (>10 mg), dilute dose prior to use and administer over at least 15 minutes

Monitoring Parameters Blood pressure and heart rate (when rapid IV administration is used); dystonic reactions, agitation, and confusion

Dosage Forms Excipient information presented when available (limited, particularly for generics); consult specific product labeling.
Solution, Injection:
Generic: 5 mg/mL (2 mL)
Solution, Injection [preservative free]:
Generic: 5 mg/mL (2 mL)
Solution, Oral:
Generic: 5 mg/5 mL (10 mL, 473 mL); 10 mg/10 mL (10 mL)
Tablet, Oral:
Reglan: 5 mg [contains fd&c blue #1 aluminum lake, fd&c yellow #10 aluminum lake]
Reglan: 10 mg [dye free]
Generic: 5 mg, 10 mg
Tablet Dispersible, Oral:
Metozolv ODT: 5 mg
Generic: 5 mg

◆ **Metoclopramide Hydrochloride Injection (Can)** *see* Metoclopramide *on page* 1413

◆ **Metoclopramide Omega (Can)** *see* Metoclopramide *on page* 1413

◆ **Metoject (Can)** *see* Methotrexate *on page* 1390

Metolazone (me TOLE a zone)

Medication Safety Issues
Sound-alike/look-alike issues:
Metolazone may be confused with metaxalone, methadone, methazolamide, methimazole, methotrexate, metoclopramide, metoprolol, minoxidil
Zaroxolyn may be confused with Zarontin

Brand Names: US Zaroxolyn [DSC]

Brand Names: Canada Zaroxolyn

Therapeutic Category Antihypertensive Agent; Diuretic, Miscellaneous

Generic Availability (US) Yes

Use Treatment of hypertension (alone or in combination with other antihypertensive agents); treatment of edema in CHF or renal diseases (including nephrotic syndrome and other states of impaired renal function) (All indications: FDA approved in adults)

Pregnancy Risk Factor B

Pregnancy Considerations Adverse events have not been observed in animal reproduction studies. Metolazone crosses the placenta and appears in cord blood. Hypoglycemia, hypokalemia, hyponatremia, jaundice, and thrombocytopenia are reported as complications to the fetus or newborn following maternal use of thiazide diuretics.

Breast-Feeding Considerations Metolazone is excreted in breast milk. Due to the potential for serious adverse reactions in the nursing infant, the manufacturer recommends a decision be made whether to discontinue nursing or to discontinue the drug, taking into account the importance of treatment to the mother.

Contraindications

Hypersensitivity to metolazone or any component of the formulation; anuria; hepatic coma or precoma.

Documentation of allergenic cross-reactivity for diuretics is limited. However, because of similarities in chemical structure and/or pharmacologic actions, the possibility of cross-sensitivity cannot be ruled out with certainty.

Warnings/Precautions Severe hypokalemia and/or hyponatremia can occur rapidly following initial doses. Hypercalcemia, hypochloremic alkalosis, and/or hypomagnesemia can also occur. Correct hypokalemia before initiating therapy. Sensitivity reactions, including angioedema and bronchospasm, may occur. Orthostatic hypotension may also occur. Ethanol may potentiate orthostatic hypotensive effect of metolazone. Instruct patients to avoid ethanol during therapy. If taken concurrently, monitor for hypotensive effects. Use with caution in severe hepatic dysfunction. Hyperuricemia can occur and gout can be precipitated. Cautious use in patients with prediabetes or diabetes; may see a change in glucose control. Can cause SLE exacerbation or activation. Azotemia and oliguria may occur. Use caution in severe renal impairment. If azotemia and oliguria worsen during treatment in these patients, discontinue therapy. Photosensitization may occur. If given the morning of surgery, metolazone may render the patient volume depleted and blood pressure may be labile during general anesthesia.

Potentially significant drug-drug interactions may exist, requiring dose or frequency adjustment, additional monitoring, and/or selection of alternative therapy. Do not interchange Zaroxolyn with other formulations of metolazone that are not therapeutically equivalent at the same doses (eg, Mykrox, no longer available in the US).

Sulfonamide ("sulfa") allergy: The FDA-approved product labeling for many medications containing a sulfonamide chemical group includes a broad contraindication in patients with a prior allergic reaction to sulfonamides. There is a potential for cross-reactivity between members of a specific class (eg, two antibiotic sulfonamides). However, concerns for cross-reactivity have previously extended to all compounds containing the sulfonamide structure (SO_2NH_2). An expanded understanding of allergic mechanisms indicates cross-reactivity between antibiotic sulfonamides and nonantibiotic sulfonamides may not occur or at the very least this potential is extremely low (Brackett 2004; Johnson 2005; Slatore 2004; Tornero 2004). In particular, mechanisms of cross-reaction due to antibody production (anaphylaxis) are unlikely to occur with nonantibiotic sulfonamides. T-cell-mediated (type IV) reactions (eg, maculopapular rash) are less well understood and it is not possible to completely exclude this potential based on current insights. In cases where prior reactions were severe (Stevens-Johnson syndrome/TEN), some clinicians choose to avoid exposure to these classes.

Adverse Reactions

Cardiovascular: Chest pain/discomfort, necrotizing angiitis, orthostatic hypotension, palpitation, syncope, venous thrombosis, vertigo, volume depletion

Central nervous system: Chills, depression, dizziness, drowsiness, fatigue, headache, lightheadedness, restlessness

Dermatologic: Petechiae, photosensitivity, pruritus, purpura, rash, skin necrosis, Stevens-Johnson syndrome, toxic epidermal necrolysis, urticaria

Endocrine & metabolic: Gout attacks, hypercalcemia, hyperglycemia, hyperuricemia, hypochloremia, hypochloremic alkalosis, hypokalemia, hypomagnesemia, hyponatremia, hypophosphatemia

Gastrointestinal: Abdominal bloating, abdominal pain, anorexia, constipation, diarrhea, epigastric distress, nausea, pancreatitis, vomiting, xerostomia

Genitourinary: Impotence

Hematologic: Agranulocytosis, aplastic/hypoplastic anemia, hemoconcentration, leukopenia, thrombocytopenia

Hepatic: Cholestatic jaundice, hepatitis

Neuromuscular & skeletal: Joint pain, muscle cramps/spasm, neuropathy, paresthesia, weakness

Ocular: Blurred vision (transient)

Renal: BUN increased, glucosuria

Drug Interactions

Metabolism/Transport Effects None known.

Avoid Concomitant Use

Avoid concomitant use of Metolazone with any of the following: Dofetilide; Mecamylamine

Increased Effect/Toxicity

Metolazone may increase the levels/effects of: ACE Inhibitors; Allopurinol; Amifostine; Antihypertensives; Calcium Salts; CarBAMazepine; Cardiac Glycosides; Cyclophosphamide; Diazoxide; Dofetilide; DULoxetine; Hypotensive Agents; Ivabradine; Levodopa; Lithium; Mecamylamine; Multivitamins/Minerals (with ADEK, Folate, Iron); Multivitamins/Minerals (with AE, No Iron); Obinutuzumab; OXcarbazepine; Porfimer; RisperiDONE; RiTUXimab; Sodium Phosphates; Topiramate; Toremifene; Verteporfin; Vitamin D Analogs

The levels/effects of Metolazone may be increased by: Alcohol (Ethyl); Alfuzosin; Analgesics (Opioid); Anticholinergic Agents; Barbiturates; Beta2-Agonists; Brimonidine (Topical); Corticosteroids (Orally Inhaled); Corticosteroids (Systemic); Dexketoprofen; Diazoxide; Herbs (Hypotensive Properties); Licorice; MAO Inhibitors; Multivitamins/Fluoride (with ADE); Nicorandil; Pentoxifylline; Phosphodiesterase 5 Inhibitors; Prostacyclin Analogues; Selective Serotonin Reuptake Inhibitors

Decreased Effect

Metolazone may decrease the levels/effects of: Antidiabetic Agents

The levels/effects of Metolazone may be decreased by: Bile Acid Sequestrants; Herbs (Hypertensive Properties); Methylphenidate; Nonsteroidal Anti-Inflammatory Agents; Yohimbine

Storage/Stability Store at 25°C (77°F); excursions are permitted between 15°C and 30°C (59°F and 86°F). Protect from light.

Mechanism of Action Inhibits sodium reabsorption in the distal tubules causing increased excretion of sodium and water, as well as, potassium and hydrogen ions

Pharmacodynamics
Onset of action: 1 hour
Duration: 12-24 hours

Pharmacokinetics (Adult data unless noted)
Absorption: Incomplete
Protein binding: 90% to 95%
Half-life: 6-20 hours
Elimination: Enterohepatic recycling; 70% to 95% excreted unchanged in urine

Dosing: Usual
Pediatric: **Edema, refractory:** Children and Adolescents: Oral: Usual range: 0.2-0.4 mg/kg/day divided every 12-24 hours in combination with furosemide; the usual maximum dose in adults is 20 mg (Arnold, 1984; Nelson, 1996). According to the manufacturer, a lower dose of 0.05-0.1 mg/kg once daily has also been reported to result in weight loss and increase urine output in some pediatric patients.
Adult:
Edema (renal disease): Oral: Initial: 5-20 mg once daily.
Edema (heart failure): Oral: Initial: 2.5 mg once daily; maximum daily dose: 20 mg (ACCF/AHA [Yancy, 2013]); **Note:** Dosing frequency may be adjusted based on patient-specific diuretic needs (eg, administration every other day or weekly) (HFSA [Lindenfeld, 2010]).
Hypertension: Oral: Initial: 2.5-5 mg once daily; adjust dose as necessary to achieve maximum therapeutic effect

Dosing adjustment in renal impairment: There are no dosage adjustments provided in the manufacturer's labeling; use caution in patients with severe renal impairment, as most of the drug is excreted by the renal route and accumulation may occur.

Doing adjustment in hepatic impairment: There are no dosage adjustments provided in manufacturer's labeling; contraindicated in hepatic coma or precoma.

Administration Oral: Administer with food to decrease GI distress; administer early in day to avoid nocturia

Monitoring Parameters Serum electrolytes, renal function, blood pressure, body weight, fluid balance

Additional Information Metolazone 5 mg is approximately equivalent to hydrochlorothiazide 50 mg

Dosage Forms Excipient information presented when available (limited, particularly for generics); consult specific product labeling. [DSC] = Discontinued product
Tablet, Oral:
Zaroxolyn: 2.5 mg [DSC], 5 mg [DSC]
Generic: 2.5 mg, 5 mg, 10 mg

Extemporaneous Preparations A 1 mg/mL oral suspension may be made by with tablets and one of three different vehicles (cherry syrup diluted 1:4 with simple syrup; a 1:1 mixture of Ora-Sweet and Ora-Plus; or a 1:1 mixture of Ora-Sweet SF and Ora-Plus). Crush twelve 10 mg tablets in a mortar and reduce to a fine powder. Add small portions of the chosen vehicle and mix to a uniform paste; mix while adding the vehicle in incremental proportions to **almost** 120 mL; transfer to a calibrated bottle, rinse mortar with vehicle, and add quantity of vehicle sufficient to make 120 mL. Label "shake well" and "refrigerate". Stable for 60 days.

A 0.25 mg/mL oral suspension may be made with tablets and a 1:1 mixture of methylcellulose 1% and simple syrup. Crush one 2.5 mg tablet in a mortar and reduce to a fine powder. Add small portions of the vehicle and mix to a uniform paste; mix while adding the vehicle in incremental proportions to **almost** 10 mL; transfer to a calibrated bottle, rinse mortar with vehicle, and add quantity of vehicle sufficient to make 10 mL. Label "shake well" and "refrigerate". Stable for 91 days refrigerated (preferred), 28 days at room temperature in plastic, and 14 days at room temperature in glass.

Nahata, MC, Pai VB, and Hipple TF, *Pediatric Drug Formulations*, 5th ed, Cincinnati, OH: Harvey Whitney Books Co, 2004.

◆ **Metonia (Can)** *see* Metoclopramide *on page 1413*
◆ **Metopirone** *see* Metyrapone *on page 1426*

Metoprolol (me toe PROE lole)

Medication Safety Issues
Sound-alike/look-alike issues:
Lopressor may be confused with Lyrica
Metoprolol may be confused with metaproterenol, metoclopramide, metolazone, misoprostol
Metoprolol succinate may be confused with metoprolol tartrate
Toprol-XL may be confused with TEGretol, TEGretol-XR, Topamax
High alert medication:
The Institute for Safe Medication Practices (ISMP) includes this medication among its list of drugs which have a heightened risk of causing significant patient harm when used in error.
Administration issues:
Significant differences exist between oral and IV dosing. Use caution when converting from one route of administration to another.

Related Information
Oral Medications That Should Not Be Crushed or Altered *on page 2476*

Brand Names: US Lopressor; Toprol XL

Brand Names: Canada Apo-Metoprolol; Apo-Metoprolol (Type L); Apo-Metoprolol SR; Ava-Metoprolol; Ava-Metoprolol (Type L); Betaloc; Dom-Metoprolol-B; Dom-Metoprolol-L; JAMP-Metoprolol-L; Lopresor; Lopresor SR; Metoprolol Tartrate Injection, USP; Metoprolol-25; Metoprolol-L; Mylan-Metoprolol (Type L); Nu-Metop; PMS-Metoprolol-B; PMS-Metoprolol-L; Riva-Metoprolol-L; Sandoz-Metoprolol (Type L); Sandoz-Metoprolol SR; Teva-Metoprolol

Therapeutic Category Antianginal Agent; Antiarrhythmic Agent, Class II; Antihypertensive Agent; Antimigraine Agent; Beta-Adrenergic Blocker

Generic Availability (US) Yes

Use
Immediate release tablets and injection: Treatment of hypertension, alone or in combination with other agents (FDA approved in adults), angina pectoris (FDA approved in adults), and hemodynamically-stable acute myocardial infarction (to reduce cardiovascular mortality) (FDA approved in adults)
Extended release tablets: Treatment of hypertension, alone or in combination with other agents (FDA approved in ages ≥6 years and adults); angina pectoris (FDA approved in adults); and patients with heart failure (stable NYHA Class II or III) already receiving ACE inhibitors, diuretics, and/or digoxin (to reduce mortality/hospitalization) (FDA approved in adults)

Metoprolol has also been used for the treatment of ventricular arrhythmias, atrial ectopy; prevention and treatment of atrial fibrillation and atrial flutter; multifocal atrial tachycardia; symptomatic treatment of hypertrophic obstructive cardiomyopathy; essential tremor; and migraine headache prophylaxis

Pregnancy Risk Factor C

Pregnancy Considerations Adverse events were observed in animal studies; therefore, the manufacturer classifies metoprolol as pregnancy category C. Metoprolol crosses the placenta and can be detected in cord blood, amniotic fluid, and the serum of newborn infants. In a cohort study, an increased risk of cardiovascular defects was observed following maternal use of beta-blockers during pregnancy. Intrauterine growth restriction (IUGR), small placentas, as well as fetal/neonatal bradycardia, hypoglycemia, and/or respiratory depression have been observed following *in utero* exposure to beta-blockers as a class. Adequate facilities for monitoring infants at birth should be available. Untreated chronic maternal hypertension and pre-eclampsia are also associated with adverse events in the fetus, infant, and mother. The clearance of metoprolol is increased and serum concentrations and AUC of metoprolol are decreased during pregnancy. Metoprolol has been evaluated for the treatment of hypertension in pregnancy, but other agents may be more appropriate for use.

Breast-Feeding Considerations Small amounts of metoprolol can be detected in breast milk. The manufacturer recommends that caution be exercised when administering metoprolol to nursing women.

Contraindications

Hypersensitivity to metoprolol, any component of the formulation, or other beta-blockers

Note: Additional contraindications are formulation and/or indication specific.

Immediate release tablets/injectable formulation:

Hypertension and angina: Sinus bradycardia; second- and third-degree heart block; cardiogenic shock; overt heart failure; sick sinus syndrome (except in patients with a functioning artificial pacemaker); severe peripheral arterial disease; pheochromocytoma (without alpha blockade)

Myocardial infarction: Severe sinus bradycardia (heart rate <45 beats/minute); significant first-degree heart block (P-R interval ≥0.24 seconds); second- and third-degree heart block; systolic blood pressure <100 mm Hg; moderate-to-severe cardiac failure

Extended release tablet: Severe bradycardia, second- and third degree heart block; cardiogenic shock; decompensated heart failure; sick sinus syndrome (except in patients with a functioning artificial pacemaker)

Warnings/Precautions [U.S. Boxed Warning]: Beta-blocker therapy should not be withdrawn abruptly (particularly in patients with CAD), but gradually tapered over 1-2 weeks to avoid acute tachycardia, hypertension, and/or ischemia. Consider pre-existing conditions such as sick sinus syndrome before initiating. Metoprolol commonly produces mild first-degree heart block (P-R interval >0.2-0.24 sec). May also produce severe first- (P-R interval ≥0.26 sec), second-, or third-degree heart block. Patients with acute MI (especially right ventricular MI) have a high risk of developing heart block of varying degrees. If severe heart block occurs, metoprolol should be discontinued and measures to increase heart rate should be employed. Symptomatic hypotension may occur with use. May precipitate or aggravate symptoms of arterial insufficiency in patients with PVD and Raynaud's disease; use with caution and monitor for progression of arterial obstruction. Potentially significant interactions may exist, requiring dose or frequency adjustment, additional monitoring, and/or selection of alternative therapy. Consult drug interactions database for more detailed information.

In general, beta-blockers should be avoided in patients with bronchospastic disease. Metoprolol, with B_1 selectivity, should be used cautiously in bronchospastic disease with close monitoring. Use cautiously in patients with diabetes because it can mask prominent hypoglycemic symptoms. May mask signs of hyperthyroidism (eg, tachycardia); if hyperthyroidism is suspected, carefully manage and monitor; abrupt withdrawal may exacerbate symptoms of hyperthyroidism or precipitate thyroid storm. Alterations in thyroid function tests may be observed. Use caution with hepatic dysfunction. Use with caution in patients with myasthenia gravis or psychiatric disease (may cause CNS depression). Although perioperative beta-blocker therapy is recommended prior to elective surgery in selected patients, use of high-dose extended release metoprolol in patients naïve to beta-blocker therapy undergoing noncardiac surgery has been associated with bradycardia, hypotension, stroke, and death. Chronic beta-blocker therapy should not be routinely withdrawn prior to major surgery. Use of beta-blockers may unmask cardiac failure in patients without a history of dysfunction. Adequate alpha-blockade is required prior to use of any beta-blocker for patients with untreated pheochromocytoma. May induce or exacerbate psoriasis. Use caution with history of severe anaphylaxis to allergens; patients taking beta-blockers may become more sensitive to repeated allergen challenges. Treatment of anaphylaxis (eg, epinephrine) in patients taking beta-blockers may be ineffective or promote undesirable effects. Bradycardia may be observed more frequently in elderly patients (>65 years of age); dosage reductions may be necessary.

Extended release: Use with caution in patients with compensated heart failure; monitor for a worsening of heart failure.

Adverse Reactions

Cardiovascular: Arterial insufficiency (usually Raynaud type), bradycardia, chest pain, CHF, edema (peripheral), first-degree heart block (P-R interval ≥0.26 sec), hypotension, palpitation, syncope

Central nervous system: Confusion, depression, dizziness, fatigue, hallucination, headache, insomnia, memory loss (short-term), nightmares, sleep disturbances, somnolence, vertigo

Dermatology: Photosensitivity, pruritus, psoriasis exacerbated, rash

Endocrine & metabolic: Diabetes exacerbated, libido decreased, Peyronie's disease

Gastrointestinal: Constipation, diarrhea, flatulence, gastrointestinal pain, heartburn, nausea, vomiting, xerostomia

Hematologic: Claudication

Neuromuscular & skeletal: Musculoskeletal pain

Ocular: Blurred vision, visual disturbances

Otic: Tinnitus

Respiratory: Dyspnea, rhinitis, shortness of breath, wheezing

Miscellaneous: Cold extremities

Rare but important or life-threatening: Agranulocytosis, alkaline phosphatase increased, alopecia (reversible), anxiety, arthralgia, arthritis, cardiogenic shock, diaphoresis increased, dry eyes, gangrene, hepatitis, HDL decreased, impotence, jaundice, lactate dehydrogenase increased, nervousness, paresthesia, retroperitoneal fibrosis, second-degree heart block, taste disturbance, third-degree heart block, thrombocytopenia, transaminases increased, triglycerides increased, urticaria, vomiting, weight gain

Other events reported with beta-blockers: Catatonia, emotional lability, fever, hypersensitivity reactions, laryngospasm, nonthrombocytopenic purpura, respiratory distress, thrombocytopenic purpura

Drug Interactions

Metabolism/Transport Effects Substrate of CYP2C19 (minor), CYP2D6 (major); **Note:** Assignment of Major/Minor substrate status based on clinically relevant drug interaction potential; **Inhibits** CYP2D6 (weak)

Avoid Concomitant Use

Avoid concomitant use of Metoprolol with any of the following: Ceritinib; Floctafenine; Methacholine; Rivastigmine

Increased Effect/Toxicity

Metoprolol may increase the levels/effects of: Alpha-/Beta-Agonists (Direct-Acting); Alpha1-Blockers; Alpha2-Agonists; Amifostine; Antihypertensives; Antipsychotic

Agents (Phenothiazines); ARIPiprazole; Bradycardia-Causing Agents; Bupivacaine; Cardiac Glycosides; Ceritinib; Cholinergic Agonists; Disopyramide; Ergot Derivatives; Fingolimod; Grass Pollen Allergen Extract (5 Grass Extract); Hypotensive Agents; Insulin; Ivabradine; Lacosamide; Levodopa; Lidocaine (Systemic); Lidocaine (Topical); Mepivacaine; Methacholine; Midodrine; Obinutuzumab; RisperiDONE; RiTUXimab; Sulfonylureas

The levels/effects of Metoprolol may be increased by: Abiraterone Acetate; Acetylcholinesterase Inhibitors; Alpha2-Agonists; Aminoquinolines (Antimalarial); Anilidopiperidine Opioids; Antipsychotic Agents (Phenothiazines); Barbiturates; Bretylium; Brimonidine (Topical); Calcium Channel Blockers (Nondihydropyridine); Cobicistat; CYP2D6 Inhibitors; Darunavir; Diazoxide; Dipyridamole; Disopyramide; Dronedarone; Floctafenine; Herbs (Hypotensive Properties); Lercanidipine; MAO Inhibitors; Mirabegron; Nicorandil; NIFEdipine; Panobinostat; Peginterferon Alfa-2b; Pentoxifylline; Phosphodiesterase 5 Inhibitors; Propafenone; Prostacyclin Analogues; Regorafenib; Reserpine; Rivastigmine; Ruxolitinib; Selective Serotonin Reuptake Inhibitors; Tofacitinib

Decreased Effect

Metoprolol may decrease the levels/effects of: Beta2-Agonists; Lercanidipine; Theophylline Derivatives

The levels/effects of Metoprolol may be decreased by: Barbiturates; Herbs (Hypertensive Properties); Methylphenidate; Mirabegron; Nonsteroidal Anti-Inflammatory Agents; Peginterferon Alfa-2b; Rifamycin Derivatives; Yohimbine

Food Interactions Food increases absorption. Metoprolol serum levels may be increased if taken with food. Management: Take immediate release tartrate tablets with food; succinate can be taken with or without food.

Storage/Stability

Injection: Store at 25°C (77°F); excursions permitted to 15°C to 30°C (59°F to 86°F). Protect from light and heat.

Tablet: Store at 25°C (77°F); excursions permitted to 15°C to 30°C (59°F to 86°F). Protect from moisture and heat.

Mechanism of Action Selective inhibitor of $beta_1$-adrenergic receptors; competitively blocks $beta_1$-receptors, with little or no effect on $beta_2$-receptors at doses <100 mg; does not exhibit any membrane stabilizing or intrinsic sympathomimetic activity

Pharmacodynamics

Beta blockade:

Onset of action: Oral: Metoprolol tartrate tablets: Within 1 hour

Maximum effect: IV: 20 minutes

Duration: Dose dependent

Antihypertensive effect:

Onset of action: Oral: Metoprolol tartrate tablets: Within 15 minutes

Maximum effect: Oral (multiple dosing): After 1 week

Duration: Oral: Metoprolol tartrate tablets (single dose): 6 hours; metoprolol succinate (extended release tablets): Up to 24 hours

Pharmacokinetics (Adult data unless noted) Note: The pharmacokinetics of metoprolol in hypertensive children 6-17 years of age were found to be similar to adults.

Absorption: Rapid and complete, with large first-pass effect

Distribution: Crosses the blood brain barrier; CSF concentrations are 78% of plasma concentrations

Protein binding: 12% bound to albumin

Metabolism: Significant first-pass metabolism; extensive metabolism in the liver via isoenzyme CYP2D6

Bioavailability: Oral: ~40% to 50% (Johnsson, 1975)

Half-Life:

Neonates: 5-10 hours

Adults: CYP2D6 poor metabolizers: 7.5 hours; CYP2D6 extensive metabolizers: 2.8 hours

Adults with chronic renal failure: Similar to normal adults

Elimination: 10% of an IV dose and <5% of an oral dose is excreted unchanged in the urine

Dosing: Usual

Oral: Hypertension:

Immediate release tablets: Children and Adolescents 1-17 years: Initial: 1-2 mg/kg/day, administered in divided doses; adjust dose based on patient response; maximum: 6 mg/kg/day (≤200 mg/day) (National High Blood Pressure Education Program Working Group on High Blood Pressure in Children and Adolescents, 2004)

Extended release tablets: Manufacturer's recommendation: Children ≥6 years: Initial: 1 mg/kg once daily (maximum initial dose: 50 mg/day); adjust dose based on patient response (maximum: 2 mg/kg/day or 200 mg/day; higher doses have not been studied)

Adults:

Immediate release tablets: Initial: 100 mg/day in single or divided doses, increase at weekly intervals to desired effect; usual dosage range: 100-450 mg/day; doses >450 mg/day have not been studied; usual dosage range (JNC 7): 50-100 mg/day in 1-2 divided doses

Note: Lower once-daily dosing (especially 100 mg/day) may not control blood pressure for 24 hours; larger or more frequent dosing may be needed. Patients with bronchospastic diseases should receive the lowest possible daily dose; dose should initially be divided into 3 doses per day (to avoid high plasma concentrations).

Extended release tablets: Initial: 25-100 mg/day as a single dose; increase at weekly intervals to desired effect; doses >400 mg/day have not been studied; usual dosage range (JNC 7): 50-100 mg once daily

Oral: Congestive heart failure: Adults: Extended release tablets: Initial: NYHA Class II heart failure: 25 mg once daily; more severe heart failure: 12.5 mg once daily; may double the dose every 2 weeks as tolerated; maximum: 200 mg/day

Administration Oral:

Metoprolol tartrate tablets: Administer with food or immediately after meals

Metoprolol succinate extended release tablets: May be administered without regard to meals; Toprol-XL® tablets are scored and may be divided; do not chew or crush the half or whole tablets; swallow whole. Do not chew, crush, or break generic nonscored extended release tablets; swallow whole.

Monitoring Parameters Blood pressure, heart rate, respirations, circulation in extremities

Dosage Forms Excipient information presented when available (limited, particularly for generics); consult specific product labeling. [DSC] = Discontinued product

Solution, Intravenous, as tartrate:

Lopressor: 1 mg/mL (5 mL [DSC])

Generic: 1 mg/mL (5 mL); 5 mg/5 mL (5 mL)

Tablet, Oral, as tartrate:

Lopressor: 50 mg, 100 mg [scored]

Lopressor: 100 mg [scored; contains fd&c blue #2 aluminum lake]

Generic: 25 mg, 50 mg, 100 mg

Tablet Extended Release 24 Hour, Oral, as succinate:

Toprol XL: 25 mg, 50 mg, 100 mg, 200 mg [scored]

Generic: 25 mg, 50 mg, 100 mg, 200 mg

Extemporaneous Preparations A 10 mg/mL oral suspension may be made with metoprolol tartrate tablets and one of three different vehicles (cherry syrup; a 1:1 mixture of Ora-Sweet® and Ora-Plus®; or a 1:1 mixture of Ora-Sweet® SF and Ora-Plus®). Crush twelve 100 mg tablets in a mortar and reduce to a fine powder. Add 20 mL of the chosen vehicle and mix to a uniform paste; mix while adding the vehicle in incremental proportions to **almost** 120 mL; transfer to a calibrated bottle, rinse mortar with vehicle, and add quantity of vehicle sufficient to make 120 mL. Label "shake well" and "protect from light". Stable for 60 days.

Allen LV Jr and Erickson MA 3rd, "Stability of Labetalol Hydrochloride, Metoprolol Tartrate, Verapamil Hydrochloride, and Spironolactone With Hydrochlorothiazide in Extemporaneously Compounded Oral Liquids," *Am J Health Syst Pharm*, 1996, 53(19):2304-9.

- **Metoprolol-25 (Can)** *see* Metoprolol *on page 1418*
- **Metoprolol-L (Can)** *see* Metoprolol *on page 1418*
- **Metoprolol Succinate** *see* Metoprolol *on page 1418*
- **Metoprolol Tartrate** *see* Metoprolol *on page 1418*
- **Metoprolol Tartrate Injection, USP (Can)** *see* Metoprolol *on page 1418*
- **Metozolv ODT** *see* Metoclopramide *on page 1413*
- **Metro** *see* MetroNIDAZOLE (Systemic) *on page 1421*
- **MetroCream** *see* MetroNIDAZOLE (Topical) *on page 1425*
- **Metrogel** *see* MetroNIDAZOLE (Topical) *on page 1425*
- **MetroGel-Vaginal** *see* MetroNIDAZOLE (Topical) *on page 1425*
- **MetroLotion** *see* MetroNIDAZOLE (Topical) *on page 1425*

MetroNIDAZOLE (Systemic)

(met roe NYE da zole)

Medication Safety Issues

Sound-alike/look-alike issues:

MetroNIDAZOLE may be confused with mebendazole, meropenem, metFORMIN, methotrexate, metoclopramide, miconazole

Related Information

H. pylori Treatment in Pediatric Patients *on page 2358*

Oral Medications That Should Not Be Crushed or Altered *on page 2476*

Brand Names: US Flagyl; Flagyl ER; Metro

Brand Names: Canada Flagyl; Metronidazole Injection USP; Novo-Nidazol; PMS-Metronidazole

Therapeutic Category Amebicide; Antibiotic, Anaerobic; Antiprotozoal

Generic Availability (US) May be product dependent

Use

Oral:

Immediate release formulation: Treatment of susceptible amebiasis (intestinal [dysentery] or liver abscess) (FDA approved in pediatric patients [age not specified] and adults); treatment of susceptible anaerobic bacterial and protozoal infections in the following conditions: Symptomatic and asymptomatic trichomoniasis; skin and skin structure infections, bone and joint infections, CNS infections, endocarditis, gynecological infections, intra-abdominal infections, and respiratory tract (lower) infections; septicemia (FDA approved in adults)

Extended release formulation: Treatment of bacterial vaginosis (FDA approved in nonpregnant, postmenarchal females)

Parenteral: Treatment of susceptible anaerobic bacteria in the following conditions: Skin and skin structure infections, bone and joint infections, CNS infections, endocarditis, gynecological infections, intra-abdominal infections, and respiratory tract (lower) infections; septicemia, surgical prophylaxis (colorectal) (all indications: FDA approved in adults)

Has also been used for treatment of giardiasis, pelvic inflammatory disease, tetanus, *H. pylori* and antibiotic-associated pseudomembranous colitis (AAPC) caused by *C. difficile*, and management of inflammatory bowel disease

Pregnancy Risk Factor B

Pregnancy Considerations Adverse events were not observed in animal reproduction studies. Metronidazole crosses the placenta. Cleft lip with or without cleft palate has been reported following first trimester exposure to metronidazole; however, most studies have not shown an increased risk of congenital anomalies or other adverse events to the fetus following maternal use during pregnancy. Because metronidazole was carcinogenic in some animal species, concern has been raised whether metronidazole should be used during pregnancy. Available studies have not shown an increased risk of infant cancer following metronidazole exposure during pregnancy; however, the ability to detect a signal for this may have been limited. Use of metronidazole during the first trimester of pregnancy is contraindicated by the manufacturer.

Metronidazole pharmacokinetics are similar between pregnant and nonpregnant patients (Amon, 1981; Visser, 1984; Wang, 2011). Bacterial vaginosis has been associated with adverse pregnancy outcomes (including preterm labor); metronidazole is recommended for the treatment of symptomatic bacterial vaginosis in pregnant patients (CDC, 2010). Vaginal trichomoniasis has been also associated with adverse pregnancy outcomes (including preterm labor). Treatment may relieve symptoms and prevent sexual transmission; however, metronidazole use has not resulted in reduced perinatal morbidity and should not be used solely to prevent preterm delivery. Some clinicians consider deferring therapy in asymptomatic women until >37 weeks gestation (CDC, 2010). Metronidazole may also be used for the treatment of giardiasis in pregnant women (some sources recommend second and third trimester administration only) (DHHS, 2013; Gardner, 2001) and symptomatic amebiasis during pregnancy (DHHS, 2013; Li, 1996). The use of other agents is preferred when treatment is needed during pregnancy for *Clostridium difficile* (Surawicz, 2013), *Helicobacter pylori* (Mahadevan, 2006), or Crohn disease (Mottet, 2009). Consult current guidelines for appropriate use in pregnant women.

Breast-Feeding Considerations Metronidazole can be detected in breast milk in concentrations similar to the maternal serum. Infant serum concentrations may be near maternal therapeutic concentrations. Due to the potential for tumorigenicity observed in animal studies, the manufacturer recommends a decision be made whether to discontinue nursing or to discontinue the drug, taking into account the importance of treatment to the mother. Alternately, the mother may pump and discard breast milk for 24 hours after the last dose. Some guidelines note if metronidazole is given, breast-feeding should be withheld for 12 to 24 hours after the dose (CDC, 2010). Use of other agents is preferred in some cases, such as when treating breast-feeding women for Crohn disease (Mottet, 2009) or *Clostridium difficile* infection (Surawicz, 2013).

Contraindications Hypersensitivity to metronidazole, nitroimidazole derivatives, or any component of the formulation; pregnant patients (first trimester) with trichomoniasis; use of disulfiram within the past 2 weeks; use of alcohol or propylene glycol-containing products during therapy or within 3 days of therapy discontinuation

Warnings/Precautions [U.S. Boxed Warning]: Possibly carcinogenic based on animal data. Reserve use for conditions described in Use; unnecessary use should be avoided. Use with caution in patients with severe liver impairment and ESRD due to potential accumulation; reduce dosage in patients with severe liver impairment and consider dosage reduction in patients with severe renal impairment (CrCl <10 mL/minute) who are receiving prolonged therapy. Dose should not specifically be reduced in anuric patients (accumulated metabolites may be rapidly removed by dialysis). Hemodialysis patients may need supplemental dosing. Use with caution in patients with blood dyscrasias (monitor CBC with differential at baseline, during and after treatment) or history of seizures.

Aseptic meningitis (symptoms may occur within hours of a dose); encephalopathy (cerebellar toxicity with ataxia, dizziness, dysarthria and/or CNS lesions); seizures; and peripheral and optic neuropathies have been reported especially with increased doses and chronic treatment; monitor and consider discontinuation of therapy if symptoms occur. Prolonged use may result in fungal or bacterial superinfection, including *C. difficile*-associated diarrhea (CDAD) and pseudomembranous colitis; CDAD has been observed >2 months postantibiotic treatment. Guidelines recommend the use of oral metronidazole for initial treatment of mild to moderate *C. difficile* infection and the use of oral vancomycin for initial treatment of severe *C. difficile* infection (with or without IV metronidazole depending on the presence of complications). May treat recurrent mild to moderate infection once with oral metronidazole; avoid use beyond first reoccurrence (Cohen, 2010, Surawicz, 2013). Candidiasis infection (known or unknown) maybe more prominent during metronidazole treatment, antifungal treatment required.

Abdominal cramps, nausea, vomiting, headaches, and flushing have been reported with oral and injectable metronidazole and concomitant alcohol consumption; avoid alcoholic beverages or products containing propylene glycol during oral and injectable therapy and for at least 3 days after oral therapy. Use with caution in the elderly; dosage adjustment may be required based on renal and/or hepatic function. Do not use extended-release tablets in patients with severe hepatic impairment (Child-Pugh class C) unless benefit outweighs risk. Use injection with caution in patients with heart failure, edema or other sodium retaining states, including corticosteroid treatment. In patients receiving continuous nasogastric secretion aspiration, sufficient metronidazole may be removed in the aspirate to cause a reduction in serum levels. Potentially significant drug-drug interactions may exist, requiring dose or frequency adjustment, additional monitoring, and/or selection of alternative therapy.

Adverse Reactions

Cardiovascular: Flattened T-wave on ECG, flushing, local thrombophlebitis (IV), syncope

Central nervous system: Aseptic meningitis, ataxia, brain disease, confusion, depression, disulfiram-like reaction (with alcohol), dizziness, dysarthria, dyspareunia, headache, insomnia, irritability, metallic taste, peripheral neuropathy, seizure, vertigo

Dermatologic: Erythematous rash, pruritus, Stevens-Johnson syndrome, toxic epidermal necrolysis, urticaria

Gastrointestinal: Abdominal cramps, abdominal pain, anorexia, constipation, diarrhea, epigastric distress, glossitis, hairy tongue, nausea, pancreatitis (rare), proctitis, stomatitis, vomiting, xerostomia

Genitourinary: Cystitis, dark urine (rare), decreased libido, dysmenorrhea, dysuria, genital pruritus, sensation of pelvic pressure, urinary incontinence, urinary tract infection, urine abnormality, vaginal dryness, vaginitis, vulvovaginal candidiasis

Hematologic & oncologic: Leukopenia (reversible), thrombocytopenia (reversible, rare)

Immunologic: Serum sickness-like reaction (joint pains)

Infection: Bacterial infection, candidiasis

Neuromuscular & skeletal: Weakness

Ophthalmic: Optic neuropathy

Renal: Polyuria

Respiratory: Flu-like symptoms, nasal congestion, pharyngitis, rhinitis, sinusitis, upper respiratory tract infection

Miscellaneous: Fever, lesion (central nervous system, reversible)

Drug Interactions

Metabolism/Transport Effects Substrate of CYP2A6 (minor); **Note:** Assignment of Major/Minor substrate status based on clinically relevant drug interaction potential. **Inhibits** CYP2C9 (weak)

Avoid Concomitant Use

Avoid concomitant use of MetroNIDAZOLE (Systemic) with any of the following: Alcohol (Ethyl); BCG; BCG (Intravesical); Carbocisteine; Disulfiram; Mebendazole; Ritonavir

Increased Effect/Toxicity

MetroNIDAZOLE (Systemic) may increase the levels/effects of: Alcohol (Ethyl); Busulfan; Capecitabine; Carbocisteine; Fluorouracil (Systemic); Fosphenytoin; Highest Risk QTc-Prolonging Agents; Lopinavir; Moderate Risk QTc-Prolonging Agents; Phenytoin; Tegafur; Tipranavir; Vitamin K Antagonists

The levels/effects of MetroNIDAZOLE (Systemic) may be increased by: Disulfiram; Mebendazole; Mifepristone; Ritonavir

Decreased Effect

MetroNIDAZOLE (Systemic) may decrease the levels/effects of: BCG; BCG (Intravesical); BCG Vaccine (Immunization); Mycophenolate; Sodium Picosulfate; Typhoid Vaccine

The levels/effects of MetroNIDAZOLE (Systemic) may be decreased by: Fosphenytoin; PHENobarbital; Phenytoin; Primidone

Food Interactions Peak antibiotic serum concentration lowered and delayed, but total drug absorbed not affected.

Storage/Stability

Oral:

Extended release: Store at 25°C (77°F); excursions are permitted between 15°C and 30°C (59°F and 86°F).

Immediate release: Store at 15°C to 25°C (59°F to 77°F). Protect the tablets from light.

Injection: Store at 20°C to 25°C (68°F to 77°F). Protect from light. Avoid excessive heat. Do not refrigerate. Do not remove unit from overwrap until ready for use. Discard unused solution.

Mechanism of Action After diffusing into the organism, interacts with DNA to cause a loss of helical DNA structure and strand breakage resulting in inhibition of protein synthesis and cell death in susceptible organisms

Pharmacokinetics (Adult data unless noted)

Absorption: Oral: Well absorbed

Distribution: Widely distributed into body tissues, fluids (including bile), liver, liver abscesses, bone, pleural fluid, and vaginal secretions; crosses blood-brain barrier; saliva and CSF concentrations similar to those in plasma

Protein binding: <20%

Metabolism: Hepatic (30% to 60%) to several metabolites, including an active hydroxyl metabolite which maintains activity ~30% to 65% of the parent compound (Lamp, 1999)

Half-life:

Neonates <7 days (Jager-Roman, 1982): Within first week of life, more prolonged than with lower GA:

GA 28 to 30 weeks: 75.3 ± 16.9 hours

GA 32 to 35 weeks: 35.4 ± 1.5 hours

GA 36 to 40 weeks: 24.8 ± 1.6 hours

Neonates ≥7 days: ~22.5 hours (Upadhyaya, 1988)

Children and Adolescents: 6 to 10 hours (Lamp, 1999)

Adults: ~8 hours

Hepatic impairment: Prolonged

Time to peak serum concentration: Oral: Immediate release: 1 to 2 hours; extended release: ~5 hours

Elimination: Urine (60% to 80% as unchanged drug and metabolites; ~20% of total as unchanged drug); feces (6% to 15%)

Dosing: Neonatal

General dosing, susceptible infection: Limited data available; dosing regimens variable:

Bradley, 2014: IV, Oral:
- Loading dose: 15 mg/kg
- Maintenance dose:
  - Body weight <1 kg:
    - PNA ≤14 days: 7.5 mg/kg/dose every 12 hours
    - PNA 15 to 28 days:
      - PMA <34 weeks: 7.5 mg/kg/dose every 12 hours
      - PMA 34 to 40 weeks: 7.5 mg/kg/dose every 8 hours
    - PNA >28 days (regardless of PMA): 7.5 mg/kg/dose every 6 hours
  - Body weight 1 to 2 kg:
    - PNA ≤7 days: 7.5 mg/kg/dose every 12 hours
    - PNA 8 to 28 days:
      - PMA <34 weeks: 7.5 mg/kg/dose every 12 hours
      - PMA 34 to 40 weeks: 7.5 mg/kg/dose every 8 hours
    - PNA >28 days (regardless of PMA): 7.5 mg/kg/dose every 6 hours
  - Body weight >2 kg:
    - PNA: ≤7 days: 7.5 mg/kg/dose every 8 hours
    - PNA: ≥8 days: 7.5 mg/kg/dose every 6 hours

Red Book [AAP], 2012: IV, Oral:
- Body weight <1 kg:
  - PNA ≤14 days: 15 mg/kg loading dose, then 7.5 mg/kg/dose every 48 hours
  - PNA 15 to 28 days: 15 mg/kg/dose every 24 hours
- Body weight 1 to 2 kg:
  - PNA ≤7 days: 15 mg/kg loading dose, then 7.5 mg/kg/dose every 24 to 48 hours
  - PNA 8 to 28 days: 15 mg/kg/dose every 24 hours
- Body weight >2 kg:
  - PNA ≤7 days: 15 mg/kg/dose every 24 hours
  - PNA 8 to 28 days: 15 mg/kg/dose every 12 hours

Suyagh, 2011: IV: Limited data available; dosing based on pharmacokinetic analysis and modeling of 32 preterm neonates
- Loading dose: 15 mg/kg
- Maintenance dose:
  - PMA ≤25 weeks: 7.5 mg/kg/dose every 24 hours
  - PMA 26 to 27 weeks: 10 mg/kg/dose every 24 hours
  - PMA 28 to 33 weeks: 7.5 mg/kg/dose every 12 hours
  - PMA 34 to 37 weeks: 10 mg/kg/dose every 12 hours

Surgical prophylaxis (IDSA/ASHP [Bratzler], 2013): Limited data available: IV:
- <1.2 kg: 7.5 mg/kg as a single dose 30 to 60 minutes prior to procedure
- ≥1.2 kg: 15 mg/kg as a single dose 30 to 60 minutes prior to procedure

Dosing: Usual

Pediatric: **Note:** Some clinicians recommend using adjusted body weight in obese children. Dosing weight = IBW + 0.45 (TBW-IBW)

General dosing, susceptible infection (*Red Book* [AAP], 2012): Infants, Children, and Adolescents:
- Oral: 30 to 50 mg/kg/day in divided doses 3 times daily; maximum daily dose: 2250 mg/**day**
- Parenteral: IV: 22.5 to 40 mg/kg/day in divided doses 3 times daily; maximum daily dose: 1500 mg/**day**

Amebiasis: Infants, Children, and Adolescents: Oral: 35 to 50 mg/kg/day in divided doses every 8 hours for 7 to 10 days; maximum single dose: 750 mg (*Red Book* [AAP], 2012)

Appendicitis, perforated (divided dosing): Children and Adolescents: IV: 30 mg/kg/day in divided doses 3 times daily (Emil, 2003)

Appendicitis, perforated (once-daily dosing): Limited data available: Children and Adolescents: IV: 30 mg/kg once daily in combination with ceftriaxone; maximum reported daily dose: 1500 mg/day (Yardeni, 2013); however, other pediatric trials did not report a maximum; in adult patients, a maximum daily dose of 1500 mg/day for once-daily dosing is suggested (Solomokin, 2010); in pediatric patients, once-daily metronidazole in combination with ceftriaxone has been shown to have similar efficacy as triple-combination therapy with ampicillin, clindamycin, and gentamicin (Fraser, 2010; St Peter, 2006; St Peter, 2008)

Balantidiasis: Infants, Children, and Adolescents: Oral: 35 to 50 mg/kg/day in divided doses every 8 hours for 5 days; maximum single dose: 750 mg (*Red Book* [AAP], 2012)

***Clostridium difficile* diarrhea:** Infants, Children, and Adolescents: Oral: 30 mg/kg/day in divided doses 4 times daily for 7 to 14 days; maximum daily dose: 2000 mg/**day** (*Red Book* [AAP], 2012; Schutze, 2013)

Dientamoeba fragilis: Infants, Children, and Adolescents: Oral: 35 to 50 mg/kg/day in divided doses every 8 hours for 10 days; maximum dose: 750 mg/dose (*Red Book* [AAP], 2012)

Giardiasis: Infants, Children, and Adolescents: Oral: 15 mg/kg/day in divided doses every 8 hours for 5 to 7 days; maximum dose: 250 mg/dose (*Red Book* [AAP], 2012)

***Helicobacter pylori* infection:** Children and Adolescents: Oral: 20 mg/kg/day in 2 divided doses for 10 to 14 days in combination with amoxicillin and proton pump inhibitor with or without clarithromycin; maximum daily dose: 1000 mg/**day** (NASPGHAN/ESPGHAN [Koletzkol], 2011)

Inflammatory bowel disease:
- *Crohn disease, perianal disease; induction:* Children and Adolescents: Oral: 7.5 mg/kg/dose 3 times daily for 6 weeks with or without ciprofloxacin; maximum dose: 500 mg/dose (Sandhu, 2010)
- *Ulcerative colitis, pouchitis, persistent:* Children and Adolescents: Oral: 20 to 30 mg/kg/day in divided doses 3 times daily for 14 days with or without ciprofloxacin or oral budesonide; maximum dose: 500 mg/dose (Turner, 2012)

Intra-abdominal infection: Infants, Children, and Adolescents: IV: 30 to 40 mg/kg/day in divided doses 3 times daily as part of combination therapy; maximum dose: 500 mg/dose (IDSA [Solomkin], 2010)

Pelvic inflammatory disease: Adolescents: Oral: 500 mg twice daily for 14 days; give with doxycycline plus a cephalosporin (CDC, 2010; *Red Book* [AAP], 2012)

Surgical prophylaxis: Children and Adolescents: IV: 15 mg/kg as a single dose 30 to 60 minutes prior to procedure; maximum single dose: 500 mg (IDSA/ASHP [Bratzler], 2013)
- *Surgical prophylaxis, colorectal:* Children and Adolescents: Oral: 15 mg/kg every 3 to 4 hours for 3 doses, starting after mechanical bowel preparation the afternoon and evening before the procedure, with or without additional oral antibiotics and with an appropriate IV antibiotic prophylaxis regimen; maximum dose: 1000 mg/dose (IDSA/ASHP [Bratzler], 2013)

Tetanus (*Clostridium tetani* infection): Infants, Children, and Adolescents: IV, Oral:.: 30 mg/kg/day in divided doses 4 times daily for 10 to 14 days; maximum daily dose: 4000 mg/**day** (*Red Book* [AAP], 2012)

Trichomoniasis; prophylaxis after sexual victimization and treatment: Oral:
- Children <45 kg: 15 mg/kg/day in divided doses 3 times daily for 7 days; maximum daily dose: 2000 mg/**day** (*Red Book* [AAP], 2012)
- Children ≥45 kg and Adolescents: 2000 mg as a single dose once (CDC, 2010; Red Book [AAP], 2012)

Vaginosis, bacterial: Oral:
Children <45 kg: 15 mg/kg/day in divided doses every 12 hours for 7 days; maximum daily dose: 1000 mg/**day** (*Red Book* [AAP], 2012)
Children >45 kg and Adolescents: 500 mg twice daily for 7 days (CDC, 2010; *Red Book* [AAP], 2012)

Adult:
Amebiasis: Oral: 500 to 750 mg every 8 hours for 5 to 10 days
Anaerobic infections: IV, Oral: 30 mg/kg/day in divided doses every 6 hours (~500 mg every 6 hours for a 70 kg adult); maximum daily dose 4000 mg/**day**; **Note:** Initial: 1000 mg IV loading dose may be administered
Bacterial vaginosis or vaginitis due to *Gardnerella mobiluncus* (CDC, 2010): Oral:
Regular release: 500 mg twice daily for 7 days
Extended release: 750 mg once daily for 7 days
***Clostridium difficile* diarrhea:** IDSA Guidelines (Cohen, 2010):
Mild to moderate infection: Oral: 500 mg 3 times daily for 10 to 14 days
Severe complicated infection: IV: 500 mg 3 times daily with oral vancomycin (recommended agent) for 10 to 14 days
Note: Due to the emergence of a new strain of *C. difficile*, some clinicians recommend converting to oral vancomycin therapy if the patient does not show a clear clinical response after 2 days of metronidazole therapy.
***Helicobacter pylori* infection**: Oral: 250 to 500 mg with meals and at bedtime (4 times daily) for 10 to 14 days; requires combination therapy with at least one other antibiotic and an acid-suppressing agent (proton pump inhibitor or H_2 blocker) (Chey, 2007)
Intra-abdominal infection, complicated, community-acquired, mild to moderate (in combination with cephalosporin or fluoroquinolone): IV: 500 mg every 8 to 12 hours or 1500 mg every 24 hours for 4 to 7 days (provided source controlled) (Solomkin, 2010)
Surgical prophylaxis (colorectal): IV 15 mg/kg 1 hour prior to surgery; followed by 7.5 mg/kg 6 and 12 hours after initial dose
Trichomoniasis: Oral: 250 mg every 8 hours for 7 days **or** 375 mg twice daily for 7 days **or** 2000 mg as a single dose **or** 1000 mg twice daily for 2 doses (on same day)

Dosing adjustment in renal impairment:
Infants, Children, and Adolescents:
Manufacturer's labeling:
Mild, moderate, or severe impairment: There are no dosage adjustments provided in the manufacturer's labeling; however, decreased renal function does not alter the single-dose pharmacokinetics.
ESRD requiring dialysis: Metronidazole metabolites may accumulate; monitor for adverse events; accumulated metabolites may be rapidly removed by dialysis.
Intermittent hemodialysis (IHD): If administration cannot be separated from hemodialysis, consider supplemental dose following hemodialysis.
Peritoneal dialysis (PD): No dosage adjustment necessary
Alternate dosing: Others have used the following the adjustments (Aronoff, 2007). **Note:** Renally adjusted dose recommendations are based on doses of 15 to 30 mg/kg/**day** divided every 6 to 8 hours.
GFR ≥10 mL/minute/1.73 m^2: No adjustment required
GFR <10 mL/minute/1.73 m^2: 4 mg/kg/dose every 6 hours
Intermittent hemodialysis: Extensively removed by hemodialysis: 4 mg/kg/dose every 6 hours
Peritoneal dialysis (PD): Extensively removed by peritoneal dialysis: 4 mg/kg/dose every 6 hours
Continuous renal replacement therapy (CRRT): No adjustment required

Adults:
Manufacturer's labeling:
Mild, moderate, or severe impairment: There are no dosage adjustments provided in the manufacturer's labeling; however, decreased renal function does not alter the single-dose pharmacokinetics.
ESRD requiring dialysis: Metronidazole metabolites may accumulate; monitor for adverse events; accumulated metabolites may be rapidly removed by dialysis.
Intermittent hemodialysis (IHD): If administration cannot be separated from hemodialysis, consider supplemental dose following hemodialysis.
Peritoneal dialysis (PD): No dosage adjustment necessary
Alternate dosing:
Intermittent hemodialysis (IHD) (administer after hemodialysis on dialysis days): Extensively removed by hemodialysis: 500 mg every 8 to 12 hours. **Note:** Dosing regimen highly dependent on clinical indication (trichomoniasis vs *C. difficile* colitis) (Heintz, 2009). **Note:** Dosing dependent on the assumption of thrice-weekly, complete IHD sessions.
Continuous renal replacement therapy (CRRT) (Heintz, 2009; Trotman, 2005): Drug clearance is highly dependent on the method of renal replacement, filter type, and flow rate. Appropriate dosing requires close monitoring of pharmacologic response, signs of adverse reactions due to drug accumulation, as well as drug concentrations in relation to target trough (if appropriate). The following are general recommendations only (based on dialysate flow/ultrafiltration rates of 1 to 2 L/hour and minimal residual renal function) and should not supersede clinical judgment:
CVVH/CVVHD/CVVHDF: 500 mg every 6 to 12 hours (or per clinical indication; dosage reduction generally not necessary)

Dosing adjustment in hepatic impairment: Infants, Children, Adolescents, and Adults:
Manufacturer labeling:
Mild or moderate impairment (Child-Pugh class A or B): No dosage adjustment necessary; use with caution and monitor for adverse events
Severe impairment (Child-Pugh class C):
Immediate release tablets, injection: Reduce dose by 50%
Immediate release capsules:
Amebiasis: Adults: 375 mg 3 times daily
Trichomoniasis: Adults: 375 mg once daily
Extended release tablets: Use is not recommended.
Alternate dosing: The pharmacokinetics of a single oral 500 mg dose were not altered in patients with cirrhosis; initial dose reduction is therefore not necessary (Daneshmend, 1982). In one study of IV metronidazole, patients with alcoholic liver disease (with or without cirrhosis) demonstrated a prolonged elimination half-life (eg, ~18 hours). The authors recommended the dose be reduced accordingly (clearance was reduced by ~62%) and the frequency may be prolonged (eg, every 12 hours instead of every 6 hours) (Lau, 1987). In another single IV dose study using metronidazole metabolism to predict hepatic function, patients classified as Child-Pugh class C demonstrated a half-life of ~21.5 hours (Muscará, 1995).

Administration

Oral: Administer on an empty stomach
Immediate release: May administer with food if GI upset occurs.

Extended release: Should be taken on an empty stomach (1 hour before or 2 hours after meals); do not split, chew, or crush.

Parenteral: Administer undiluted (5 mg/mL) by slow intermittent infusion over 30 to 60 minutes. Avoid contact of drug solution with equipment containing aluminum.

Monitoring Parameters Monitor CBC with differential at baseline and after prolonged or repeated courses of therapy. Closely monitor patients with severe hepatic impairment or ESRD for adverse reactions. Observe patients carefully if neurologic symptoms occur and consider discontinuation of therapy.

Test Interactions May interfere with AST, ALT, triglycerides, glucose, and LDH testing

Additional Information Sodium content of 500 mg ready-to-use single dose plastic container: 14 mEq

Dosage Forms Considerations Parenteral solution contains 28 mEq of sodium/gram of metronidazole.

Dosage Forms Excipient information presented when available (limited, particularly for generics); consult specific product labeling.

Capsule, Oral:
- Flagyl: 375 mg
- Generic: 375 mg

Solution, Intravenous:
- Metro: 500 mg (100 mL)
- Generic: 500 mg (100 mL)

Solution, Intravenous [preservative free]:
- Generic: 500 mg (100 mL)

Tablet, Oral:
- Flagyl: 250 mg, 500 mg
- Generic: 250 mg, 500 mg

Tablet Extended Release 24 Hour, Oral:
- Flagyl ER: 750 mg

Extemporaneous Preparations A 50 mg/mL oral suspension may be made with tablets and a 1:1 mixture of Ora-Sweet and Ora-Plus. Crush twenty-four 250 mg tablets in a mortar and reduce to a fine powder. Add small portions of the vehicle and mix to a uniform paste; mix while adding the vehicle in incremental portions to **almost** 120 mL; transfer to a calibrated bottle, rinse mortar with vehicle, and add quantity of vehicle sufficient to make 120 mL. Label "shake well". Stable for 60 days at room temperature or refrigerated (Allen, 1996).

MetroNIDAZOLE (Topical) (met roe NYE da zole)

Brand Names: US MetroCream; Metrogel; MetroGel-Vaginal; MetroLotion; Noritate; Nuvessa; Rosadan; Vandazole

Brand Names: Canada MetroCream; Metrogel; MetroLotion; Nidagel; Noritate; Rosasol

Therapeutic Category Antibiotic, Topical

Generic Availability (US) May be product dependent

Use

Topical: Treatment of inflammatory lesions (papules and pustules) of rosacea (FDA approved in adults)

Vaginal gel:
- Metrogel: Treatment of bacterial vaginosis (FDA approved in adults)
- Vandazole: Treatment of bacterial vaginosis (FDA approved in nonpregnant, postmenarchal females)

Pregnancy Risk Factor B

Pregnancy Considerations Adverse events have not been observed in animal reproduction studies. Metronidazole crosses the placenta and rapidly distributes into the fetal circulation rapidly following oral administration. The amount of metronidazole available systemically following topical application is less in comparison to oral doses. Metronidazole 1.3% vaginal gel and Vandazole are not indicated for use in pregnant patients. Oral metronidazole is preferred for the treatment of symptomatic bacterial vaginosis in pregnant patients (consult current guidelines) (CDC, 2010).

Breast-Feeding Considerations Metronidazole is excreted in breast milk following oral administration and can be detected in concentrations similar to the maternal serum. The amount of metronidazole available systemically following topical application is less in comparison to oral doses. According to the manufacturer, the decision to continue or discontinue breast-feeding during therapy should take into account the risk of exposure to the infant and the benefits of treatment to the mother; nursing women may consider pumping and discarding their milk during therapy and 24 hours after therapy.

Contraindications Hypersensitivity to metronidazole, parabens, or other ingredients of the formulation or other nitroimidazole derivatives; use of disulfiram within the past 2 weeks; use of alcohol or propylene glycol during therapy or within 24 hours (Nuvessa only) or 3 days of therapy discontinuation.

Warnings/Precautions Possibly carcinogenic based on animal data. Unnecessary use should be avoided. Prolonged use may result in fungal or bacterial superinfection. Approximately 6% to 10% of women treated with the vaginal gel developed *Candida* vaginitis during or immediately after treatment. Aseptic meningitis, encephalopathy, seizures, and neuropathies have been reported with systemic metronidazole, especially with increased doses and chronic treatment; peripheral neuropathy has also been reported with topical products; monitor and consider discontinuation of therapy if symptoms occur. Use with caution in patients with CNS disease. Discontinue immediately if abnormal neurologic signs develop. Use with caution in patients with blood dyscrasias. Use with caution in patients with severe liver impairment due to potential accumulation. May cause tearing of the eye; avoid contact with the eyes. In the event of accidental contact, wash out immediately. Disulfiram-like reaction to ethanol has been reported with systemic metronidazole and may occur with the vaginal gel; consider avoidance of alcoholic beverages during therapy with vaginal gel. Do not administer the vaginal gel to patients who have taken disulfiram within the past 2 weeks. Patient should avoid vaginal intercourse during vaginal gel treatment.

Benzyl alcohol and derivatives: Some dosage forms may contain benzyl alcohol; large amounts of benzyl alcohol (≥99 mg/kg/day) have been associated with a potentially fatal toxicity ("gasping syndrome") in neonates; the "gasping syndrome" consists of metabolic acidosis, respiratory distress, gasping respirations, CNS dysfunction (including convulsions, intracranial hemorrhage), hypotension, and cardiovascular collapse (AAP, 1997; CDC, 1982); some data suggests that benzoate displaces bilirubin from protein binding sites (Ahlfors, 2001); avoid or use dosage forms containing benzyl alcohol with caution in neonates. See manufacturer's labeling.

Warnings: Additional Pediatric Considerations Some dosage forms may contain propylene glycol; in neonates large amounts of propylene glycol delivered orally, intravenously (eg, >3,000 mg/day), or topically have been associated with potentially fatal toxicities which can include metabolic acidosis, seizures, renal failure, and CNS depression; toxicities have also been reported in children and adults including hyperosmolality, lactic acidosis, seizures, and respiratory depression; use caution (AAP, 1997; Shehab, 2009).

Adverse Reactions

Topical:

Cardiovascular: Hypertension

Central nervous system: Headache

Dermatologic: Acne vulgaris, burning sensation of skin, contact dermatitis, erythema, pruritus, skin irritation, skin rash, xeroderma

Gastrointestinal: Metallic taste, nausea, unusual taste, xerostomia
Local: Hypersensitivity reaction
Neuromuscular & skeletal: Numbness of extremities, peripheral neuropathy, tingling of extremities
Ophthalmic: Eye irritation
Respiratory: Flu-like symptoms

Vaginal:
Central nervous system: Dizziness, headache
Gastrointestinal: Abdominal cramps, decreased appetite, diarrhea, gastrointestinal distress, metallic taste (or unusual taste), nausea and vomiting
Genitourinary: Cervical candidiasis (or vaginitis), dysmenorrhea, pelvic pain, vaginal discharge, vulvovaginal candidiasis, vulvovaginal irritation, vulvovaginal pruritus
Rare, but important or life-threatening: Bloating, dark urine, depression, skin rash, xerostomia

Drug Interactions

Metabolism/Transport Effects None known.

Avoid Concomitant Use

Avoid concomitant use of MetroNIDAZOLE (Topical) with any of the following: BCG; BCG (Intravesical)

Increased Effect/Toxicity

MetroNIDAZOLE (Topical) may increase the levels/effects of: Alcohol (Ethyl); Disulfiram; Lopinavir; Tipranavir

Decreased Effect

MetroNIDAZOLE (Topical) may decrease the levels/effects of: BCG; BCG (Intravesical); BCG Vaccine (Immunization); Sodium Picosulfate

Storage/Stability
Topical cream, gel, lotion: Store at 20°C to 25°C (68°F to 77°F).
Vaginal gel: Store at 15°C to 30°C (59°F to 86°F); do not refrigerate or freeze. Avoid exposure to extreme heat.

Mechanism of Action After diffusing into the organism, interacts with DNA to cause a loss of helical DNA structure and strand breakage resulting in inhibition of protein synthesis and cell death in susceptible organisms

Pharmacokinetics (Adult data unless noted)
Absorption:
Topical: Concentrations achieved systemically after application of the 1 g topical gel and cream are <1% of those obtained after a 250 mg oral dose
Vaginal gel: ~50% of oral dose
Time to peak serum concentration:
Topical gel: 6 to 10 hours
Topical cream: 8 to 12 hours
Vaginal gel: 6 to 12 hours

Dosing: Usual
Infants, Children, and Adolescents:
Bacterial vaginosis: Vaginal gel 0.75%: Adolescents: Intravaginal: One applicatorful (~5 g gel contains ~37.5 mg of metronidazole) intravaginally once daily at bedtime for 5 days (CDC, 2010; *Red Book* [AAP], 2012)
Periorifacial dermatitis: Infants ≥6 months, Children, and Adolescents: Limited data available: Topical: 0.75% gel: Apply thin film once or twice daily (Manders, 1992; Miller, 1994; Nguyen, 2006)
Adults:
Acne rosacea: Topical:
0.75%: Apply and rub a thin film twice daily, morning and evening, to entire affected areas after washing
1%: Apply thin film to affected area once daily after washing
Bacterial vaginosis: Intravaginal: One applicatorful (~5 g gel contains ~37.5 mg of metronidazole) intravaginally once or twice daily for 5 days; apply once in morning and evening if using twice daily; apply at bedtime if using once daily

Administration
Intravaginal: Use only **vaginal gel** intravaginally; fill applicator with medication; insert the applicator high into the vagina and press the plunger to release the medication; clean the applicator with warm soapy water and rinse well. Do not apply to the eye
Topical: Wash affected areas with a mild cleanser; then apply a thin film of drug to the affected area and rub in. Cosmetics may be used after application (wait at least 5 minutes after using lotion). Do not apply to the eye.

Dosage Forms Excipient information presented when available (limited, particularly for generics); consult specific product labeling.
Cream, External:
MetroCream: 0.75% (45 g) [contains benzyl alcohol]
Noritate: 1% (60 g) [contains methylparaben, propylparaben, trolamine (triethanolamine)]
Rosadan: 0.75% (45 g) [contains benzyl alcohol]
Generic: 0.75% (45 g)
Gel, External:
Metrogel: 1% (55 g, 60 g) [contains methylparaben, propylparaben]
Rosadan: 0.75% (45 g) [contains edetate disodium, methylparaben, propylene glycol, propylparaben]
Generic: 0.75% (45 g); 1% (55 g, 60 g)
Gel, Vaginal:
MetroGel-Vaginal: 0.75% (70 g) [contains edetate disodium, methylparaben, propylene glycol, propylparaben]
Nuvessa: 1.3% (5 g) [contains benzyl alcohol, methylparaben, polyethylene glycol, propylene glycol, propylparaben]
Vandazole: 0.75% (70 g) [contains methylparaben, propylparaben]
Generic: 0.75% (70 g)
Kit, External:
Rosadan: 0.75% [contains benzyl alcohol]
Rosadan: 0.75% [contains edetate disodium, methylparaben, propylene glycol, propylparaben]
Lotion, External:
MetroLotion: 0.75% (59 mL) [contains benzyl alcohol]
Generic: 0.75% (59 mL)

◆ **Metronidazole Hydrochloride** *see* MetroNIDAZOLE (Systemic) *on page* 1421

◆ **Metronidazole Hydrochloride** *see* MetroNIDAZOLE (Topical) *on page* 1425

◆ **Metronidazole Injection USP (Can)** *see* MetroNIDAZOLE (Systemic) *on page* 1421

Metyrapone (me TEER a pone)

Medication Safety Issues

Sound-alike/look-alike issues:
Metyrapone may be confused with metyrosine

Brand Names: US Metopirone

Therapeutic Category Diagnostic Agent, Hypothalamic-Pituitary ACTH Function

Generic Availability (US) No

Use Diagnostic agent for testing hypothalamic-pituitary ACTH function [FDA approved in pediatric patients (age not specified) and adults]

Prescribing and Access Restrictions Metopirone® is available from HRA Pharma via special allocation only. Contact the manufacturer for additional information at 855-674-7663.

Pregnancy Risk Factor C

Pregnancy Considerations Animal reproduction studies have not been conducted. Subnormal response may occur in pregnant women and the fetal pituitary may be affected.

Breast-Feeding Considerations The excretion of metyrapone and its active metabolite into breast milk are described in a case report. The mother had been taking metyrapone 250 mg 4 times/day for 9 weeks and was 1 week postpartum when milk samples were obtained. Multiple milk samples taken 1-5 hours after the dose contained average concentrations of metyrapone 11.2 mcg/L and metyrapol 48.5 mcg/L over the dosing interval. The relative infant dose (metyrapone and metyrapol) was calculated to be 0.1% of the weight adjusted maternal dose.

Contraindications Hypersensitivity to metyrapone or any component of the formulation; patient with adrenal cortical insufficiency

Warnings/Precautions May cause CNS depression, which may impair physical or mental abilities; patients must be cautioned about performing tasks which require mental alertness (eg, operating machinery or driving). Response to test may be subnormal in patients with hypo- or hyperthyroidism. Acute adrenal insufficiency may be induced in patients with reduced adrenal secretory capacity.

Adverse Reactions

Cardiovascular: Hypotension

Central nervous system: Dizziness, headache, sedation

Dermatologic: Allergic rash

Gastrointestinal: Abdominal discomfort or pain, nausea, vomiting

Hematologic: Bone marrow suppression (rare), white blood cell count decreased (rare)

Drug Interactions

Metabolism/Transport Effects Inhibits CYP2A6 (weak); **Induces** CYP3A4 (weak)

Avoid Concomitant Use There are no known interactions where it is recommended to avoid concomitant use.

Increased Effect/Toxicity

Metyrapone may increase the levels/effects of: Acetaminophen

Decreased Effect

Metyrapone may decrease the levels/effects of: ARIPiprazole; Hydrocodone; NiMODipine; Saxagliptin

The levels/effects of Metyrapone may be decreased by: Fosphenytoin; Phenytoin

Storage/Stability Do not store above 30°C (86°F); protect from heat. Protect from moisture.

Mechanism of Action Metyrapone inhibits the production of cortisol; blockade can be measured by the urinary increase of the metabolites of cortisol precursors in the urine (17-hyroxycorticosteroids [17-OHCS] and 17-ketogenic steroids [17-KGS]).

Pharmacodynamics Maximum effect: Peak excretion of steroid during the first 24 hours after administration

Pharmacokinetics (Adult data unless noted)

Absorption: Oral: Well absorbed; rapid

Metabolism: Reduced to metyrapol (active metabolite); parent drug and metabolite also undergo glucuronide conjugation

Half-life, elimination:

Metyrapone: 1.9 ± 0.7 hours

Metyrapol (active metabolite): Takes twice as long as metyrapone to be eliminated

Time to peak serum concentration: 1 hour

Elimination: Urine; ~5% as metyrapone (primarily as glucuronide conjugate) and ~38% as metyrapol (primarily as glucuronide conjugate)

Dosing: Usual ACTH function, diagnostic test: Oral:

Single-dose/overnight test: Children and Adults: 30 mg/kg as a single dose (maximum dose: 3000 mg) given at midnight the night before the test

Multiple-dose test:

Children: 15 mg/kg/dose every 4 hours for 6 doses; minimum dose: 250 mg; maximum dose: 750 mg

Adults: 750 mg every 4 hours for 6 doses

Administration Oral: May administer with food or milk to reduce GI irritation

Single-dose/overnight test: Administer dose at midnight with yogurt or milk.

Multiple-dose test: Administer with milk or snack 2 days following ACTH test.

Monitoring Parameters Urinary 17-OHCS; urinary 17-KGS; plasma 11-deoxycortisol

Single-dose/overnight test: Blood samples are taken the following morning (7:30-8:00 am).

Multiple-dose test: Urine is collected for 24 hours following the last day of administration.

Reference Range Normal 24-hour urinary excretion of 17-OHCS: 3-12 mg (increases following ACTH infusion)

Normal response to metyrapone:

Plasma ACTH: 44 pmol/L (200 ng/L)

Plasma 11-desoxycortisol: 0.2 micromoles/L (70 mcg/L)

24 hour urinary excretion of 17-OHCS: 2-4 time increase

24 hour urinary excretion of 17-KGS: 2 time increase

A subnormal response may be indicative of panhypopituitarism or partial hypopituitarism. An excessive response is suggestive of Cushing's syndrome associated with adrenal hyperplasia.

Dosage Forms Excipient information presented when available (limited, particularly for generics); consult specific product labeling.

Capsule, Oral:

Metopirone: 250 mg

◆ **Mevacor** *see* Lovastatin *on page* 1305

◆ **Mevinolin** *see* Lovastatin *on page* 1305

Mexiletine (meks IL e teen)

Brand Names: Canada Novo-Mexiletine

Therapeutic Category Antiarrhythmic Agent, Class I-B

Generic Availability (US) Yes

Use Management of serious ventricular arrhythmias; suppression of premature ventricular contractions; diabetic neuropathy

Pregnancy Risk Factor C

Pregnancy Considerations Adverse events have been observed in some animal reproduction studies. A few case reports have demonstrated safe use of mexiletine in pregnant women (Gregg 1988; Lownes 1987; Timmis 1980).

Breast-Feeding Considerations Mexiletine is excreted in breast milk; concentrations in breast milk are similar to those in the maternal plasma. Breast-feeding is not recommended by the manufacturer.

Contraindications Cardiogenic shock; second- or third-degree AV block (except in patients with a functioning artificial pacemaker)

Warnings/Precautions Initiate therapy in the hospital when used to treat life-threatening arrhythmias. Treatment of patients with asymptomatic ventricular premature contractions should be avoided. Has not been shown to enhance survival in patients with ventricular arrhythmias.

[US Boxed Warning]: In the Cardiac Arrhythmia Suppression Trial (CAST), recent (>6 days but <2 years ago) myocardial infarction patients with asymptomatic, nonlife-threatening ventricular arrhythmias did not benefit and may have been harmed by attempts to suppress the arrhythmia with flecainide or encainide. An increased mortality or nonfatal cardiac arrest rate (7.7%) was seen in the active treatment group compared with patients in the placebo group (3%). The applicability of the CAST results to other populations is unknown. Antiarrhythmic agents should be reserved for patients with life-threatening ventricular arrhythmias. In a double-blind placebo controlled trial in patients with recent MI, the use of mexiletine to reduce premature ventricular contractions demonstrated a numerically greater number of deaths compared to placebo (IMPACT Research Group 1984).

[US Boxed Warning]: Abnormal liver function tests have been reported, some in the first few weeks of therapy. Most of these have been observed in the setting of congestive heart failure or ischemia and their relationship to mexiletine has not been established. Marked elevations of AST (>1000 units/L) and rare instances of severe liver injury, including hepatic necrosis, have also been reported. Carefully monitor patients who develop abnormal LFTs or who have signs/symptoms of liver dysfunction. If persistent or worsening elevation of hepatic enzymes occurs, consider discontinuing therapy.

Use cautiously in patients with first-degree block, preexisting sinus node dysfunction, intraventricular conduction delays; use is contraindicated in patients with second- or third-degree AV block (except in patients with a functioning artificial pacemaker). Use with caution in patients with severe HF. Proarrhythmia may occur with the use of mexiletine especially in those with life-threatening arrhythmias (eg, sustained ventricular tachycardia). Aggravation of arrhythmia may also occur; monitor for proarrhythmic effects and correct electrolyte disturbances, especially hypokalemia or hypomagnesemia, prior to use and throughout therapy (Podrid 1987; Podrid 1999; Velebit 1982). Use with caution in patients with hepatic impairment; may prolong the elimination half-life of mexiletine and increase the risk of adverse effects. Use with caution in patients with seizure disorder. Alterations in urinary pH may change urinary excretion; avoid dietary regimens that may markedly alter urinary pH. Rare marked leukopenia, agranulocytosis, and thrombocytopenia have been reported; often occurs in seriously ill patients receiving other medications that can cause these effects. If significant hematologic changes occur, discontinue therapy. Drug reactions with eosinophilia and systemic symptoms (DRESS) has been reported; discontinue use if suspected. Potentially significant drug-drug interactions may exist, requiring dose or frequency adjustment, additional monitoring, and/or selection of alternative therapy.

Adverse Reactions

Cardiovascular: Angina, chest pain, palpitation, premature ventricular contractions, proarrhythmia

Central nervous system: Confusion, depression, dizziness, headache, incoordination, insomnia, lightheadedness, nervousness

Dermatologic: Rash

Gastrointestinal: Abdominal pain, constipation, diarrhea, GI distress, nausea, vomiting, xerostomia

Neuromuscular & skeletal: Arthralgias, ataxia, numbness of fingers or toes, paresthesia, trembling, tremor, unsteady gait, weakness

Ocular: Blurred vision, nystagmus

Otic: Tinnitus

Respiratory: Dyspnea

Rare but important or life-threatening: Agranulocytosis, alopecia, AV block, cardiogenic shock, CHF, dysphagia, exfoliative dermatitis, hallucinations, hepatic necrosis, hepatitis, hypotension, impotence, leukopenia, myelofibrosis, pancreatitis (rare), psychosis, pulmonary fibrosis, seizure, sinus arrest, SLE syndrome, Stevens-Johnson syndrome, syncope, thrombocytopenia, torsade de pointes, upper GI bleeding, urinary retention, urticaria

Drug Interactions

Metabolism/Transport Effects Substrate of CYP1A2 (major), CYP2D6 (major); **Note:** Assignment of Major/Minor substrate status based on clinically relevant drug interaction potential; **Inhibits** CYP1A2 (weak)

Avoid Concomitant Use There are no known interactions where it is recommended to avoid concomitant use.

Increased Effect/Toxicity

Mexiletine may increase the levels/effects of: Theophylline Derivatives; TiZANidine

The levels/effects of Mexiletine may be increased by: Abiraterone Acetate; Cobicistat; CYP1A2 Inhibitors (Moderate); CYP1A2 Inhibitors (Strong); CYP2D6 Inhibitors (Moderate); CYP2D6 Inhibitors (Strong); Darunavir; Deferasirox; Panobinostat; Peginterferon Alfa-2b; Selective Serotonin Reuptake Inhibitors; Vemurafenib

Decreased Effect

The levels/effects of Mexiletine may be decreased by: Cannabis; CYP1A2 Inducers (Strong); Cyproterone; Etravirine; Fosphenytoin; Peginterferon Alfa-2b; Phenytoin; Teriflunomide

Food Interactions Food may decrease the rate, but not the extent of oral absorption; diets which affect urine pH can increase or decrease excretion of mexiletine. Management: Avoid dietary changes that alter urine pH.

Storage/Stability Store at 20°C to 25°C (68°F to 77°F).

Mechanism of Action Class IB antiarrhythmic, structurally related to lidocaine, which inhibits inward sodium current, decreases rate of rise of phase 0, increases effective refractory period/action potential duration ratio

Pharmacodynamics Onset of action: Oral: 30-120 minutes

Pharmacokinetics (Adult data unless noted)

Distribution: V_d: 5-7 L/kg; found in breast milk in similar concentrations as plasma

Protein-binding: 50% to 70%

Metabolism: Extensive in the liver (some minor active metabolites)

Bioavailability: Oral: 88%

Half-life, adults: 10-14 hours; increase in half-life with hepatic or heart failure

Elimination: 10% to 15% excreted unchanged in urine; urinary acidification increases excretion

Dosing: Usual Oral:

Children: Range: 1.4-5 mg/kg/dose (mean: 3.3 mg/kg/dose) given every 8 hours; start with lower initial dose and increase according to effects and serum concentrations

Adults: Initial: 200 mg every 8 hours (may load with 400 mg if necessary); adjust dose every 2-3 days; usual dose: 200-300 mg every 8 hours; some patients may respond to the same daily dose divided every 12 hours; maximum dose: 1.2 g/day

Dosing adjustment in renal impairment: Children and Adults: CrCl <10 mL/minute: Administer 50% to 75% of normal dose

Dosing adjustment in hepatic disease: Children and Adults: Administer 25% to 30% of normal dose; patients with severe liver disease may require even lower doses, monitor closely

Administration Oral: Administer with food, milk, or antacids to decrease GI upset

Monitoring Parameters Liver enzymes, CBC, ECG, heart rate, serum concentrations

Reference Range

Therapeutic range: 0.5-2 mcg/mL

Potentially toxic: >2 mcg/mL

Test Interactions Abnormal liver function test, positive ANA, thrombocytopenia

Additional Information IV form under investigation

Dosage Forms Excipient information presented when available (limited, particularly for generics); consult specific product labeling.

Capsule, Oral, as hydrochloride:

Generic: 150 mg, 200 mg, 250 mg

Extemporaneous Preparations A 10 mg/mL oral suspension may be with made with capsules and either distilled water or sorbitol USP. Empty the contents of eight 150 mg capsules in a mortar and reduce to a fine powder if necessary. Add small portions of the chosen vehicle and mix to a uniform paste; mix while adding the vehicle in incremental proportions to **almost** 120 mL; transfer to a graduated cylinder, rinse mortar with vehicle, and add quantity of vehicle sufficient to make 120 mL. Label "shake well". Sorbitol suspension is stable in plastic prescription bottles for 2 weeks at room temperature and 4 weeks refrigerated; distilled water suspension is stable in plastic prescription bottles for 7 weeks at room temperature and 13 weeks refrigerated. Extended storage under refrigeration is recommended to minimize microbial contamination.

Nahata MC, Morosco RS, and Hipple TF, "Stability of Mexiletine in Two Extemporaneous Liquid Formulations Stored Under Refrigeration and at Room Temperature," *J Am Pharm Assoc (Wash)*, 2000, 40 (2):257-9.

◆ **Mezavant (Can)** *see* Mesalamine *on page 1368*

◆ **$MgSO_4$ (error-prone abbreviation)** *see* Magnesium Sulfate *on page 1317*

◆ **Miacalcin** *see* Calcitonin *on page 337*

◆ **Mi-Acid Gas Relief [OTC]** *see* Simethicone *on page 1927*

◆ **Micaderm [OTC]** *see* Miconazole (Topical) *on page 1431*

Micafungin (mi ka FUN gin)

Brand Names: US Mycamine

Brand Names: Canada Mycamine

Therapeutic Category Antifungal Agent, Echinocandin; Antifungal Agent, Systemic

Generic Availability (US) No

Use Treatment of patients with esophageal candidiasis; treatment of candidemia, acute disseminated candidiasis, *Candida* peritonitis and abscess; prophylaxis of *Candida* infections in patients undergoing hematopoietic stem cell transplant (All indications: FDA approved in ages ≥4 months and adults); has been used for treatment of invasive *Aspergillosis*; micafungin is ineffective against cryptococcosis, fusariosis, and zygomycosis

Pregnancy Risk Factor C

Pregnancy Considerations Adverse events have been observed in animal reproduction studies. There are no adequate and well-controlled studies in pregnant women. Use only if benefit outweighs risk.

Breast-Feeding Considerations It is not known if micafungin is excreted in breast milk. The manufacturer recommends that caution be exercised when administering micafungin to nursing women.

Contraindications Hypersensitivity to micafungin, other echinocandins, or any component of the formulation

Warnings/Precautions Severe anaphylactic reactions, including shock, have been reported. New-onset or worsening hepatic impairment, including hepatitis and hepatic failure, has been reported. Monitor closely and evaluate appropriateness of continued use in patients who develop abnormal liver function tests during treatment. Hemolytic anemia and hemoglobinuria have been reported. Increased BUN, serum creatinine, renal dysfunction, and/or acute renal failure has been reported; use with caution in patients that develop worsening renal function during treatment; monitor closely.

Adverse Reactions

Cardiovascular: Atrial fibrillation, bradycardia, cardiac arrest, edema, hypertension, hypotension, localized phlebitis, myocardial infarction, pericardial effusion, peripheral edema, tachycardia

Central nervous system: Anxiety, brain disease, convulsions, delirium, dizziness, fatigue, headache, insomnia, intracranial hemorrhage, rigors

Dermatologic: Pruritus (more common in pediatric patients ages 3 days through 16 years), skin rash, urticaria (more common in pediatric patients ages 3 days through 16 years)

Endocrine & metabolic: Hyperglycemia, hyperkalemia, hypernatremia, hypervolemia, hypocalcemia, hypoglycemia, hypokalemia, hypomagnesemia

Gastrointestinal: Abdominal distension, abdominal pain, anorexia, constipation, diarrhea, dyspepsia, mucositis, nausea, vomiting

Genitourinary: Decreased urine output, hematuria

Hematologic & oncologic: Anemia (more common in pediatric patients ages 3 days through 16 years), blood coagulation disorder, febrile neutropenia, neutropenia, pancytopenia, thrombocytopenia, thrombotic thrombocytopenic purpura

Hepatic: Abnormal hepatic function tests (more common in pediatric patients ages 3 days through 16 years), hepatic failure, hepatic injury, hepatomegaly, hyperbilirubinemia (more common in pediatric patients ages 3 days through 16 years), increased serum alkaline phosphatase, increased serum ALT (more common in pediatric patients ages 3 days through 16 years), increased serum AST, jaundice

Hypersensitivity: Anaphylaxis, hypersensivity reaction

Infection: Bacteremia, sepsis

Local: Venous thrombosis at injection site

Neuromuscular & skeletal: Back pain

Renal: Renal failure

Respiratory: Cough, dyspnea, epistaxis

Miscellaneous: Fever (more common in pediatric patients ages 3 days through 16 years), infusion related reaction (more common in pediatric patients ages 3 days through 16 years)

Rare but important or life-threatening: Acidosis, acute renal failure, anaphylactoid reaction, anuria, apnea, cardiac arrhythmia, cyanosis, decreased white blood cell count, deep vein thrombosis, disseminated intravascular coagulation, erythema multiforme, hemoglobinuria, hemolysis, hemolytic anemia, hepatic insufficiency, hepatitis, hiccups, hyponatremia, hypoxia, increased blood urea nitrogen, increased serum creatinine, infection, injection site reaction, oliguria, pneumonia, pulmonary embolism, renal insufficiency, renal tubular necrosis, seizure, shock, skin necrosis, Stevens-Johnson syndrome, thrombophlebitis, tissue necrosis at injection site, toxic epidermal necrolysis, vasodilatation

Drug Interactions

Metabolism/Transport Effects Substrate of CYP3A4 (minor); **Note:** Assignment of Major/Minor substrate status based on clinically relevant drug interaction potential

Avoid Concomitant Use

Avoid concomitant use of Micafungin with any of the following: Saccharomyces boulardii

Increased Effect/Toxicity There are no known significant interactions involving an increase in effect.

Decreased Effect

Micafungin may decrease the levels/effects of: Saccharomyces boulardii

Storage/Stability Store at 25°C (77°F); excursions permitted to 15°C to 30°C (59°F to 86°F). Reconstituted and diluted solutions are stable for 24 hours at room temperature. Protect infusion solution from light (it is not necessary to protect the drip chamber or tubing from light).

Mechanism of Action Concentration-dependent inhibition of 1,3-beta-D-glucan synthase resulting in reduced formation of 1,3-beta-D-glucan, an essential polysaccharide comprising 30% to 60% of *Candida* cell walls (absent in mammalian cells); decreased glucan content leads to osmotic instability and cellular lysis

Pharmacokinetics (Adult data unless noted)

Absorption: Oral: Poor

Distribution: Distributes into lung, liver, and spleen; minimally to CNS and eyes (Caudle, 2012)

Preterm infants (ELBW): Reported data highly variable; possibly dependent on GA/weight, and PNA: V_{dss}:
PNA 0-1 day: 0.76 L/kg (Kawada, 2009)
PNA 4 days: 1.52 L/kg (Smith, 2009)
PNA >3 weeks: 0.43 L/kg (range: 0.28-0.66 L/kg) (Heresi, 2006)
Children 2-8 years: V_{dss}: 0.35 ± 0.18 L/kg (Seibel, 2005)
Children and Adolescents 9-17 years: V_{dss}: 0.28 ± 0.09 L/kg (Seibel, 2005)
Adults: V_d: 0.39 ± 0.11 L/kg
Protein binding:
Neonates: 96.7% (Yanni, 2011)
Adults: >99% to albumin
Metabolism: Hepatic to M-1, catechol form by arylsulfatase; further metabolized to M-2, methoxy form by catechol-O-methyltransferase; hydroxylation to M-5 by CYP3A
Half-life:
Preterm infants:
PNA <1 week: 6.7 hours (Kawada, 2009)
PNA >3 weeks: Mean 8.3 hours (range: 5.6-11 hours) (Heresi, 2006)
Pediatric patients 4 months to 16 years of age:
≤30 kg: 12.5 ± 4.6 hours
>30kg: 13.6 ± 8.8 hours
Healthy Adults: 11-21 hours
Adults receiving bone marrow or peripheral stem-cell transplantation: 10.7-13.5 hours (Carver, 2004)
Elimination: <1% of dose is eliminated unchanged renally (Herbert, 2005); 71% is eliminated in the feces
Clearance:
Preterm infants:
PNA 0-1 day: 1.48 mL/minute/kg (Kawada, 2009)
PNA 4 days: 0.58 mL/minute (Smith, 2009)
PNA >3 weeks: 0.64 mL/minute (Heresi, 2006)
Pediatric patients 4 months to 16 years of age:
≤30 kg: 0.328 mL/minute/kg
>30kg: 0.241 mL/minute/kg
Adults: ~0.3 mL/minute/kg

Dosing: Neonatal

Fungal infections, susceptible: Limited data available; dosing based on several pharmacokinetic studies in preterm infants (Benjamin 2010; Caudle 2012; Heresi 2006; Hope 2010; Smith 2009): IV:
<1,000 g: 10 mg/kg/day once daily; doses as high as 15 mg/kg/day have been used; dosages at the higher end of the dosing range should be considered for treating CNS infections due to poor micafungin CNS penetration (Caudle 2012)
≥1,000 g: 7 to 10 mg/kg/day once daily; HIV-exposed/-positive neonates may require up to 10 to 12 mg/kg/day once daily (DHHS [pediatric] 2013)

Dosing: Usual

Pediatric:
Infants <4 months:
Candidiasis:
Disseminated; treatment: Limited data available: IV:
Non-HIV-exposed/-positive: 2 mg/kg/day once daily; may increase higher doses (4 to 10 mg/kg/day) if no improvement in condition, or persistent positive cultures; reported range: 2 to 10 mg/kg/day [Benjamin 2010; Hope 2010; Myacin prescribing information (European Medicines Agency) 2013; Queiroz-Telles 2008)
HIV-exposed/-positive (critically ill): 5 to 7 mg/kg/day once daily; treatment duration variable, continue treatment for 2 weeks following last positive blood culture
Esophageal, treatment: HIV-exposed/-positive: 5 to 7 mg/kg/day once daily; treatment duration: ≥3 weeks and for at least 2 weeks following symptom resolution (DHHS [pediatric] 2013)

Infants ≥4 months, Children, and Adolescents:
Aspergillosis: IV:
Treatment; invasive disease: Limited data available:
Infants and Children: 1.5 to 3 mg/kg/day once daily; titration to a higher dose may be necessary for lack of clinical response or persistent positive cultures; reported usual maximum dose range: 4 to 8.6 mg/kg/day; in infants, initial doses at the higher end of the dosage range may be necessary due to pharmacokinetic differences (Denning 2006, Emiroglu 2011; Flynn 2006; Kobayashi 2007; Singer 2003)
Adolescents:
HIV-exposed/-positive: 100 to 150 mg once daily (DHHS [adult] 2013)
Non-HIV-exposed/-positive: 1.5 mg/kg/day; increase if clinically indicated; maximum daily dose: 150 mg/**day**; dosing based on a noncomparative study of all ages, an abstract describing a study in pediatric patients 3 months to 16 years and single case report of a 13-year old who received 1.5 mg/kg/day for invasive aspergillosis (Denning 2006; Emiroglu 2011; Flynn 2006; Singer 2003).
Prophylaxis in hematopoietic stem cell transplantation: IV: 1 to 3 mg/kg daily; maximum dose: 50 mg (Kusuki 2009; Tomblyn 2009; van Burik 2004)
Candidiasis:
Treatment:
Acute disseminated infection, peritonitis, and abscesses: IV:
Non-HIV-exposed/-positive: 2 mg/kg once daily; maximum dose: 100 mg
HIV-exposed/-positive (DHHS [pediatric] 2013):
Infants <15 kg: 5 to 7 mg/kg once daily
Children 2 to 8 years and ≤40 kg: 3 to 4 mg/kg once daily
Children ≥9 years and Adolescents:
≤40 kg: 2 to 3 mg/kg once daily
>40 kg: 100 mg once daily
Esophageal candidiasis: IV:
Non-HIV-exposed/-positive:
≤30 kg: 3 mg/kg once daily
>30 kg: 2.5 mg/kg once daily; maximum dose:150 mg
HIV-exposed/-positive (DHHS [adult/pediatric] 2013):
Infants <15 kg: 5 to 7 mg/kg once daily
Children 2 to 8 years and ≤40 kg: 3 to 4 mg/kg once daily
Children ≥9 years
≤40 kg: 2 to 3 mg/kg once daily
>40 kg: 100 mg once daily
Adolescents:
<40 kg: 2 to 3 mg/kg once daily
≥40 kg: 150 mg once daily; treatment duration: 14 to 21 days
Prophylaxis in hematopoietic stem cell transplantation: IV: 1 mg/kg daily; maximum dose: 50 mg; doses as high as 3 mg/kg/day have been used in trials (Kusuki 2009)
Adult:
Candidemia, acute disseminated candidiasis, and *Candida* peritonitis and abscesses: IV: 100 mg daily; mean duration of therapy (from clinical trials): 15 days (range: 10 to 47 days)
Esophageal candidiasis: IV: 150 mg daily; mean duration of therapy (from clinical trials): 15 days (range: 10 to 30 days)
Prophylaxis of *Candida* infection in hematopoietic stem cell transplantation: IV: 50 mg daily

Dosing adjustment in renal impairment: Adults: No adjustment required; not dialyzable, supplemental dosing is not required following hemodialysis.

Dosing adjustment in hepatic impairment: Adults: No adjustment required.

Preparation for Administration Parenteral: IV: Reconstitute with 5 mL of NS (preservative free) or D_5W to each 50 or 100 mg vial resulting in a concentration 10 mg/mL or 20 mg/mL, respectively. To minimize foaming, gently swirl to dissolve; do not shake. Further dilution is dose dependent on patient age:

Pediatric patients: Dilute dose in NS or D_5W to a final concentration of 0.5 to 4 mg/mL

Adults: Dilute dose in 100 mL NS or D_5W

Protect infusion solution from light (it is not necessary to protect the drip chamber or tubing from light).

Administration Parenteral: IV: In pediatric patients, final concentrations >1.5 mg/mL should be administered via a central line to minimize risk of infusion reactions. Prior to administration, flush line with NS. Infuse over 1 hour; more rapid infusions may result in a higher incidence of histamine-mediated reactions. Do not coinfuse with other medications since precipitation may occur.

Monitoring Parameters Periodic liver function tests, renal function tests, CBC with differential

Dosage Forms Excipient information presented when available (limited, particularly for generics); consult specific product labeling.

Solution Reconstituted, Intravenous, as sodium:

Mycamine: 50 mg (1 ea); 100 mg (1 ea)

Solution Reconstituted, Intravenous, as sodium [preservative free]:

Mycamine: 50 mg (1 ea); 100 mg (1 ea)

- **Micafungin Sodium** *see* Micafungin *on page 1429*
- **Micatin [OTC]** *see* Miconazole (Topical) *on page 1431*
- **Micatin® (Can)** *see* Miconazole (Topical) *on page 1431*
- **Miconazole 3** *see* Miconazole (Topical) *on page 1431*
- **Miconazole 3 Combo Pack [OTC]** *see* Miconazole (Topical) *on page 1431*
- **Miconazole 7 [OTC]** *see* Miconazole (Topical) *on page 1431*

Miconazole (Topical) (mi KON a zole)

Medication Safety Issues

Sound-alike/look-alike issues:

Miconazole may be confused with metroNIDAZOLE, Micronase, Micronor®

Lotrimin® may be confused with Lotrisone®, Otrivin®

Micatin® may be confused with Miacalcin®

Brand Names: US Aloe Vesta Antifungal [OTC]; Antifungal [OTC]; Azolen Tincture [OTC]; Baza Antifungal [OTC]; Carrington Antifungal [OTC]; Critic-Aid Clear AF [OTC]; Cruex Prescription Strength [OTC]; DermaFungal [OTC]; Desenex Jock Itch [OTC]; Desenex Spray [OTC]; Desenex [OTC]; Fungoid Tincture [OTC]; Lotrimin AF Deodorant Powder [OTC]; Lotrimin AF Jock Itch Powder [OTC]; Lotrimin AF Powder [OTC]; Lotrimin AF [OTC]; Micaderm [OTC]; Micatin [OTC]; Miconazole 3; Miconazole 3 Combo Pack [OTC]; Miconazole 7 [OTC]; Micro Guard [OTC]; Miranel AF [OTC]; Mitrazol [OTC]; Podactin [OTC]; Remedy Antifungal [OTC]; Remedy Phytoplex Antifungal [OTC]; Secura Antifungal Extra Thick [OTC]; Secura Antifungal [OTC]; Soothe & Cool INZO Antifungal [OTC]; Triple Paste AF [OTC]; Vagistat-3 [OTC]; Zeasorb-AF [OTC]

Brand Names: Canada Dermazole; Micatin®; Micozole; Monistat®; Monistat® 3

Therapeutic Category Antifungal Agent, Topical; Antifungal Agent, Vaginal

Generic Availability (US) May be product dependent

Use Treatment of vulvovaginal candidiasis; topical treatment of superficial fungal infections

Pregnancy Considerations Following vaginal administration, small amounts are absorbed systemically (Stevens, 2002). Adverse fetal events have not been observed (Czeizel, 2004). Vaginal products (7-day therapies) may be considered for the treatment of vulvovaginal candidiasis in pregnant women. This product may weaken latex condoms and diaphragms (CDC, 2010).

Breast-Feeding Considerations It is not known if miconazole is excreted in breast milk. The manufacturer recommends that caution be exercised when administering miconazole to nursing women.

Contraindications Hypersensitivity to miconazole or any component of the formulation

Warnings/Precautions For topical use only; avoid contact with eyes. Discontinue if sensitivity or irritation develop. Petrolatum-based vaginal products may damage rubber or latex condoms or diaphragms. Separate use by 3 days. Consult with healthcare provider prior to self-medication (OTC use) of vaginal products if experiencing vaginal itching/discomfort, lower abdominal pain, back or shoulder pain, chills, nausea, vomiting, foul-smelling discharge, if this is the first vaginal yeast infection, or if exposed to HIV. Contact healthcare provider if symptoms do not begin to improve after 3 days or last longer than 7 days. Topical products are not for self-medication (OTC use) in children <2 years of age; vaginal products are not for OTC use in children <12 years of age.

Benzyl alcohol and derivatives: Some dosage forms may contain benzyl alcohol and/or sodium benzoate/benzoic acid; benzoic acid (benzoate) is a metabolite of benzyl alcohol; large amounts of benzyl alcohol (≥99 mg/kg/day) have been associated with a potentially fatal toxicity ("gasping syndrome") in neonates; the "gasping syndrome" consists of metabolic acidosis, respiratory distress, gasping respirations, CNS dysfunction (including convulsions, intracranial hemorrhage), hypotension, and cardiovascular collapse (AAP, 1997; CDC, 1982); some data suggests that benzoate displaces bilirubin from protein binding sites (Ahlfors, 2001); avoid or use dosage forms containing benzyl alcohol and/or benzyl alcohol derivative with caution in neonates. See manufacturer's labeling.

Fungoid® tincture: Patients with diabetes, circulatory problems, renal or hepatic dysfunction should contact healthcare provider prior to self-medication (OTC use).

Warnings: Additional Pediatric Considerations Some dosage forms may contain propylene glycol; in neonates large amounts of propylene glycol delivered orally, intravenously (eg, >3,000 mg/day), or topically have been associated with potentially fatal toxicities which can include metabolic acidosis, seizures, renal failure, and CNS depression; toxicities have also been reported in children and adults including hyperosmolality, lactic acidosis, seizures, and respiratory depression; use caution (AAP, 1997; Shehab, 2009).

Adverse Reactions

Topical: Allergic contact dermatitis, burning, maceration

Vaginal: Abdominal cramps, burning, irritation, itching

Drug Interactions

Metabolism/Transport Effects None known.

Avoid Concomitant Use

Avoid concomitant use of Miconazole (Topical) with any of the following: Progesterone

Increased Effect/Toxicity

Miconazole (Topical) may increase the levels/effects of: Vitamin K Antagonists

Decreased Effect

Miconazole (Topical) may decrease the levels/effects of: Progesterone

Storage/Stability Store at room temperature.

Mechanism of Action Inhibits biosynthesis of ergosterol, damaging the fungal cell wall membrane, which increases permeability causing leaking of nutrients

Pharmacokinetics (Adult data unless noted)

Absorption: Vaginal: Small amount absorbed systemically

Distribution: Into body tissues, joints, and fluids; poor penetration into sputum, saliva, urine, and CSF

Protein binding: 91% to 93%

Metabolism: In the liver

Half-life: Multiphasic degradation:

Alpha: 40 minutes

Beta: 126 minutes

Terminal: 24 hours

Elimination: ~50% excreted in feces and <1% in urine as unchanged drug

Dosing: Usual

Infants, Children, Adolescents, and Adults: Topical:

Tinea pedis and tinea corporis: Apply twice daily for 4 weeks

Tinea cruris: Apply twice daily for 2 weeks

Adolescents and Adults:

Vaginal: Insert contents of 1 applicator of 2% vaginal cream or 100 mg vaginal suppository at bedtime for 7 days; or 1 applicator of 4% vaginal cream or 200 mg vaginal suppository at bedtime for 3 days; or 1200 mg vaginal suppository one-time dose at bedtime or during the day

Note: Many products are available as a combination pack (contains a suppository for vaginal instillation and external cream which is applied twice daily for up to 7 days to relieve external symptoms)

Administration For external use only.

Topical: Apply sparingly to the cleansed, dry affected area; if intertriginous areas are involved, rub cream gently into the skin

Vaginal: Wash hands before using; gently insert tablet or full applicator of cream high into vagina at bedtime. Wash applicator with soap and water following use. Remain lying down for 30 minutes following administration.

Monitoring Parameters Hematocrit, hemoglobin, serum electrolytes and lipids

Dosage Forms Excipient information presented when available (limited, particularly for generics); consult specific product labeling.

Aerosol, External, as nitrate:

Desenex Spray: 2% (133 g)

Lotrimin AF: 2% (150 g)

Aerosol Powder, External, as nitrate:

Cruex Prescription Strength: 2% (85 g)

Desenex Jock Itch: 2% (113 g)

Desenex Spray: 2% (113 g)

Lotrimin AF Deodorant Powder: 2% (133 g)

Lotrimin AF Jock Itch Powder: 2% (133 g)

Lotrimin AF Powder: 2% (133 g)

Cream, External, as nitrate:

Antifungal: 2% (14 g, 28 g, 42.5 g) [contains benzoic acid]

Antifungal: 2% (113 g, 198 g) [contains cetyl alcohol, methylparaben, propylene glycol, propylparaben]

Baza Antifungal: 2% (4 g, 57 g, 142 g)

Carrington Antifungal: 2% (141 g) [contains disodium edta, methylparaben, propylene glycol, propylparaben]

Micaderm: 2% (30 g)

Micatin: 2% (14 g) [contains benzoic acid]

Micro Guard: 2% (57 g)

Podactin: 2% (28.35 g) [contains benzoic acid]

Remedy Antifungal: 2% (118 mL) [contains methylparaben, propylparaben, trolamine (triethanolamine)]

Secura Antifungal: 2% (57 g) [contains cetearyl alcohol, methylparaben, propylparaben]

Secura Antifungal Extra Thick: 2% (92 g) [contains cetearyl alcohol, methylparaben, propylparaben]

Soothe & Cool INZO Antifungal: 2% (56.7 g, 141.7 g)

Generic: 2% (15 g, 28.4 g, 30 g)

Cream, Vaginal, as nitrate:

Miconazole 7: 2% (45 g) [contains benzoic acid]

Generic: 2% (45 g)

Kit, External, as nitrate:

Fungoid Tincture: 2% [contains benzyl alcohol]

Kit, Vaginal, as nitrate:

Miconazole 3 Combo Pack: Cream, topical: 2% (9 g) and Suppository, vaginal: 200 mg (3s)

Miconazole 3 Combo Pack: Cream, topical: 2% (9 g) and Suppository, vaginal: 200 mg (3s) [contains benzoic acid]

Vagistat-3: Cream, topical: 2% (9 g) and Suppository, vaginal: 200 mg (3s) [contains benzoic acid]

Lotion, External, as nitrate:

Zeasorb-AF: 2% (56 g) [contains alcohol, usp]

Ointment, External, as nitrate:

Aloe Vesta Antifungal: 2% (56 g, 141 g)

Critic-Aid Clear AF: 2% (4 g, 57 g, 142 g)

DermaFungal: 2% (113 g)

Triple Paste AF: 2% (56.7 g) [contains polysorbate 80]

Powder, External, as nitrate:

Desenex: 2% (43 g, 85 g)

Lotrimin AF: 2% (90 g)

Micro Guard: 2% (85 g)

Mitrazol: 2% (30 g)

Remedy Antifungal: 2% (85 g)

Remedy Antifungal: 2% (85 g) [talc free; contains methylparaben]

Remedy Phytoplex Antifungal: 2% (85 g) [paraben free; contains sodium benzoate, soy protein]

Zeasorb-AF: 2% (71 g)

Zeasorb-AF: 2% (71 g) [starch free]

Solution, External, as nitrate:

Azolen Tincture: 2% (29.57 mL) [contains benzyl alcohol, isopropyl alcohol]

Fungoid Tincture: 2% (29.57 mL) [contains benzyl alcohol]

Miranel AF: 2% (28 g) [contains disodium edta, menthol, propylene glycol, sd alcohol 40b]

Suppository, Vaginal, as nitrate:

Miconazole 7: 100 mg (7 ea)

Miconazole 3: 200 mg (3 ea)

Generic: 100 mg (7 ea)

◆ **Miconazole Nitrate** *see* Miconazole (Topical) *on page 1431*

◆ **Micozole (Can)** *see* Miconazole (Topical) *on page 1431*

◆ **MICRhoGAM Ultra-Filtered Plus** *see* Rh_o(D) Immune Globulin *on page 1847*

◆ **Micro Guard [OTC]** *see* Miconazole (Topical) *on page 1431*

◆ **Micro-K** *see* Potassium Chloride *on page 1736*

◆ **Micro-K Extencaps (Can)** *see* Potassium Chloride *on page 1736*

◆ **Micronase** *see* GlyBURIDE *on page 975*

◆ **Micronefrin [OTC] [DSC]** *see* EPINEPHrine (Systemic, Oral Inhalation) *on page 760*

◆ **Micronized Colestipol HCl** *see* Colestipol *on page 531*

◆ **Micronor® (Can)** *see* Norethindrone *on page 1530*

◆ **Microzide** *see* Hydrochlorothiazide *on page 1028*

◆ **Midamor** *see* AMILoride *on page 119*

Midazolam (MID aye zoe lam)

Medication Safety Issues

Sound-alike/look-alike issues:

Versed may be confused with VePesid, Vistaril

High alert medication:

The Institute for Safe Medication Practices (ISMP) includes this medication among its list of drugs which have a heightened risk of causing significant patient harm when used in error.

Related Information

Preprocedure Sedatives in Children *on page 2444*

Brand Names: Canada Midazolam Injection

Therapeutic Category Anticonvulsant, Benzodiazepine; Benzodiazepine; Hypnotic; Sedative

Generic Availability (US) Yes

Use

Oral: Sedation, anxiolysis, amnesia prior to procedures or before induction of anesthesia (FDA approved in ages ≥6 months to <16 years)

Parenteral: Preprocedure sedation, anxiolysis, amnesia for diagnostic or radiographic procedures (FDA approved in infants, children, adolescents, and adults); continuous IV sedation of intubated and mechanically ventilated patients (FDA approved in all ages); has also been used for status epilepticus

Buccal: Has been used for acute treatment of seizures

Intranasal: Has been used for preprocedure sedation, anxiolysis, amnesia for diagnostic or radiographic procedures; acute treatment of seizures

Rectal: Has been used for preprocedure sedation

Pregnancy Risk Factor D

Pregnancy Considerations Adverse events were not observed in animal reproduction studies. Midazolam has been found to cross the human placenta and can be detected in the serum of the umbilical vein and artery, as well as the amniotic fluid. Teratogenic effects have been observed with some benzodiazepines; however, additional studies are needed. The incidence of premature birth and low birth weights may be increased following maternal use of benzodiazepines; hypoglycemia and respiratory problems in the neonate may occur following exposure late in pregnancy. Neonatal withdrawal symptoms may occur within days to weeks after birth and "floppy infant syndrome" (which also includes withdrawal symptoms) have been reported with some benzodiazepines (Bergman, 1992; Iqbal, 2002; Wikner, 2007).

Breast-Feeding Considerations Midazolam and hydroxymidazolam can be detected in breast milk. Based on information from two women, 2-3 months postpartum, the half-life of midazolam in breast milk is ~1 hour. Milk concentrations were below the limit of detection (<5 nmol/L) 4 hours after a single maternal dose of midazolam 15 mg. Drowsiness, lethargy, or weight loss in nursing infants have been observed in case reports following maternal use of some benzodiazepines (Iqbal, 2002; Matheson, 1990). The manufacturer recommends that caution be exercised when administering midazolam to nursing women.

Contraindications Hypersensitivity to midazolam or any component of the formulation; intrathecal or epidural injection of parenteral forms containing preservatives (ie, benzyl alcohol); acute narrow-angle glaucoma; concurrent use of potent inhibitors of CYP3A4 (amprenavir, atazanavir, or ritonavir)

Per respective protease inhibitor manufacturer's labeling: Concurrent use of oral midazolam with amprenavir, atazanavir, darunavir, indinavir, lopinavir-ritonavir, nelfinavir, ritonavir, saquinavir, tipranavir and concurrent use of oral or injectable midazolam with fosamprenavir

Warnings/Precautions **[U.S. Boxed Warning]: May cause severe respiratory depression, respiratory arrest, or apnea. Use with extreme caution, particularly in noncritical care settings.** Appropriate resuscitative equipment and qualified personnel must be available for administration and monitoring. Initial dosing must be cautiously titrated and individualized, particularly in elderly or debilitated patients, patients with hepatic impairment (including alcoholics), or in renal impairment, particularly if other CNS depressants (including opioids) are used concurrently. **[U.S. Boxed Warning]: Initial doses in elderly or debilitated patients should be conservative; as little as 1 mg, but not to exceed 2.5 mg.** Use with caution in patients with respiratory disease or impaired gag reflex. Use during upper airway procedures may increase risk of hypoventilation. Prolonged responses have been noted following extended administration by continuous infusion (possibly due to metabolite accumulation) or in the presence of drugs which inhibit midazolam metabolism.

Causes CNS depression (dose-related) resulting in sedation, dizziness, confusion, or ataxia which may impair physical and mental capabilities. Patients must be cautioned about performing tasks which require mental alertness (eg, operating machinery or driving). A minimum of 1 day should elapse after midazolam administration before attempting these tasks. Use with caution in patients receiving other CNS depressants or psychoactive agents. Effects with other sedative drugs or ethanol may be potentiated. Benzodiazepines have been associated with falls and traumatic injury and should be used with extreme caution in patients who are at risk of these events (especially the elderly).

Use with caution in patients receiving CYP3A4 inhibitors; may result in more intense and prolonged sedation; consider reducing midazolam dose and anticipate potential for prolongation and intensity of effect. The concurrent use of all protease inhibitors is contraindicated with oral midazolam per their respective manufacturer's labeling. The concurrent use of fosamprenavir is contraindicated with both oral and parenteral forms of midazolam.

May cause hypotension - hemodynamic events are more common in pediatric patients or patients with hemodynamic instability. Hypotension and/or respiratory depression may occur more frequently in patients who have received opioid analgesics. Use with caution in obese patients, chronic renal failure, and HF. Does not protect against increases in heart rate or blood pressure during intubation. Should not be used in shock, coma, or acute alcohol intoxication. **[U.S. Boxed Warning]: Do not administer by rapid IV injection in neonates; severe hypotension and seizures have been reported; risk may be increased with concomitant fentanyl use.**

Avoid intra-arterial administration or extravasation of parenteral formulation. Some formulations may contain cherry flavoring.

Midazolam causes anterograde amnesia. Paradoxical reactions, including hyperactive or aggressive behavior have been reported with benzodiazepines, particularly in adolescent/pediatric or psychiatric patients; may consider treatment with flumazenil (Massanari, 1997). Does not have analgesic, antidepressant, or antipsychotic properties.

Benzodiazepines have been associated with dependence and acute withdrawal symptoms on discontinuation or reduction in dose. Acute withdrawal, including seizures, may be precipitated after administration of flumazenil to patients receiving long-term benzodiazepine therapy. Midazolam is a short half-life benzodiazepine and may be of benefit in patients where a rapidly and short-acting agent is desired (acute agitation). Tolerance develops to the sedative and anticonvulsant effects. It does not develop to the anxiolytic effects (Vinkers, 2012).

Benzyl alcohol and derivatives: Some dosage forms may contain benzyl alcohol; large amounts of benzyl alcohol (≥99 mg/kg/day) have been associated with a potentially fatal toxicity ("gasping syndrome") in neonates; the "gasping syndrome" consists of metabolic acidosis, respiratory distress, gasping respirations, CNS dysfunction (including convulsions, intracranial hemorrhage), hypotension, and cardiovascular collapse (AAP, 1997; CDC, 1982); some data suggests that benzoate displaces bilirubin from protein binding sites (Ahlfors, 2001); avoid or use dosage forms containing benzyl alcohol with caution in neonates. See manufacturer's labeling.

Warnings: Additional Pediatric Considerations In neonates, particularly premature neonates, several cases of myoclonus (rhythmic myoclonic jerking) have been reported (~8% incidence).

Adverse Reactions

Cardiovascular: Hypotension

Central nervous system: Drowsiness, headache, oversedation, seizure-like activity

Gastrointestinal: Nausea, vomiting

Local: Pain and local reactions at injection site

Neuromuscular & skeletal: Myoclonic jerks (preterm infants)

Ocular: Nystagmus

Respiratory: Apnea, cough, decreased tidal volume and/or respiratory rate

Miscellaneous: Hiccups, paradoxical reaction, physical and psychological dependence with prolonged use

Rare but important or life-threatening: Agitation, amnesia, bigeminy, bronchospasm, emergence delirium, euphoria, hallucinations, laryngospasm, rash

Drug Interactions

Metabolism/Transport Effects Substrate of CYP2B6 (minor), CYP3A4 (major); **Note:** Assignment of Major/Minor substrate status based on clinically relevant drug interaction potential; **Inhibits** CYP2C8 (weak), CYP2C9 (weak)

Avoid Concomitant Use

Avoid concomitant use of Midazolam with any of the following: Amodiaquine; Azelastine (Nasal); Boceprevir; Cobicistat; Conivaptan; Fusidic Acid (Systemic); Idelalisib; Itraconazole; Ketoconazole (Systemic); Methadone; OLANZapine; Orphenadrine; Paraldehyde; Protease Inhibitors; Sodium Oxybate; Telaprevir; Thalidomide

Increased Effect/Toxicity

Midazolam may increase the levels/effects of: Alcohol (Ethyl); Amodiaquine; Azelastine (Nasal); Buprenorphine; CloZAPine; CNS Depressants; Hydrocodone; Methadone; Methotrimeprazine; Metyrosine; Mirtazapine; Orphenadrine; Paraldehyde; Pramipexole; Propofol; ROPINIRole; Rotigotine; Selective Serotonin Reuptake Inhibitors; Sodium Oxybate; Suvorexant; Thalidomide; Zolpidem

The levels/effects of Midazolam may be increased by: Aprepitant; AtorvaSTATin; Boceprevir; Brimonidine (Topical); Cannabis; Cobicistat; Conivaptan; CYP3A4 Inhibitors (Moderate); CYP3A4 Inhibitors (Strong); Dasatinib; Doxylamine; Dronabinol; Droperidol; Fosaprepitant; Fusidic Acid (Systemic); HydrOXYzine; Idelalisib; Itraconazole; Ivacaftor; Kava Kava; Ketoconazole (Systemic); Luliconazole; Macrolide Antibiotics; Magnesium Sulfate; Methotrimeprazine; Mifepristone; Nabilone; Netupitant; OLANZapine; Palbociclib; Perampanel; Propofol; Protease Inhibitors; Rufinamide; Simeprevir; Stiripentol; Tapentadol; Teduglutide; Telaprevir; Tetrahydrocannabinol

Decreased Effect

The levels/effects of Midazolam may be decreased by: Bosentan; CYP3A4 Inducers (Moderate); CYP3A4 Inducers (Strong); Dabrafenib; Deferasirox; Ginkgo Biloba; Mitotane; Siltuximab; St Johns Wort; Theophylline Derivatives; Tocilizumab; Yohimbine

Food Interactions Grapefruit juice may increase serum concentrations of midazolam. Management: Avoid concurrent use of grapefruit juice with oral midazolam.

Storage/Stability

Oral: Store at 25°C (77°F); excursions permitted to 15°C to 30°C (59°F to 86°F).

Injection: Store at 20°C to 25°C (68°F to 77°F), excursions permitted to 15°C to 30°C (59°F to 86°F). The manufacturer states that midazolam, at a final concentration of 0.5 mg/mL, is stable for up to 24 hours when diluted with D_5W or NS. A final concentration of 1 mg/mL in NS has been documented to be stable for up to 10 days (McMullin, 1995). Admixtures do not require protection from light for short-term storage.

Mechanism of Action Binds to stereospecific benzodiazepine receptors on the postsynaptic GABA neuron at several sites within the central nervous system, including the limbic system, reticular formation. Enhancement of the inhibitory effect of GABA on neuronal excitability results by increased neuronal membrane permeability to chloride ions. This shift in chloride ions results in hyperpolarization (a less excitable state) and stabilization. Benzodiazepine receptors and effects appear to be linked to the GABA-A receptors. Benzodiazepines do not bind to GABA-B receptors.

Pharmacodynamics Sedation:

Onset of action:
- Oral: Children: Within 10-20 minutes
- IM:
  - Children: Within 5 minutes
  - Adults: Within 15 minutes
- IV: Within 1-5 minutes
- Intranasal: Within 5 minutes

Maximum effect:
- IM:
  - Children: 15-30 minutes
  - Adults: 30-60 minutes
- IV: 5-7 minutes
- Intranasal: 10 minutes

Duration:
- IM: Mean: 2 hours, up to 6 hours
- IV: 20-30 minutes
- Intranasal: 30-60 minutes
- **Note:** Full recovery may take more than 24 hours

Pharmacokinetics (Adult data unless noted)

Absorption: Oral, nasal: Rapid

Distribution: V_d:
- Preterm infants (n=24; GA: 26-34 weeks; PNA: 3-11 days): Median: 1.1 L/kg (range: 0.4-4.2 L/kg)
- Infants and Children 6 months to 16 years: 1.24-2.02 L/kg
- Adults: 1-3.1 L/kg
- Increased V_d with CHF and chronic renal failure; widely distributed in body including CSF and brain; crosses placenta; enters fetal circulation; crosses into breast milk

Protein binding: Children >1 year and Adults: 97%; primarily to albumin

Metabolism: Extensive in the liver via cytochrome P450 CYP3A4 enzyme; undergoes hydroxylation and then glucuronide conjugation; primary metabolite (alpha-hydroxy-midazolam) is active and equipotent to midazolam

Bioavailability: Oral: 15% to 45% (syrup: 36%); IM: >90%; intranasal: ~60%; rectal: ~40% to 50%

Half-life, elimination: Increased half-life with cirrhosis, CHF, obesity, elderly, and acute renal failure

Preterm infants (n=24; GA: 26-34 weeks; PNA: 3-11 days): Median: 6.3 hours (range: 2.6-17.7 hours)
Neonates: 4-12 hours; seriously ill neonates: 6.5-12 hours
Children: IV: 2.9-4.5 hours; syrup: 2.2-6.8 hours
Adults: 3 hours (range: 1.8-6.4 hours)

Elimination: 63% to 80% excreted as alpha-hydroxy-midazolam glucuronide in urine; ~2% to 10% in feces, <1% eliminated as unchanged drug in the urine
Clearance:
Preterm infants (n=24; GA: 26-34 weeks; PNA: 3-11 days): Median: 1.8 mL/minute/kg (range: 0.7-6.7 mL/minute/kg)
Neonates <39 weeks GA: 1.17 mL/minute/kg
Neonates >39 weeks GA: 1.84 mL/minute/kg
Seriously ill neonates: 1.2-2 mL/minute/kg
Infants >3 months: 9.1 mL/minute/kg
Children >1 year: 3.2-13.3 mL/minute/kg
Healthy adults: 4.2-9 mL/minute/kg
Adults with acute renal failure: 1.9 mL/minute/kg

Dosing: Neonatal Dosage must be individualized and based on patient's age, underlying diseases, concurrent medications, and desired effect; decrease dose (by ~30%) if opioids or other CNS depressants are administered concomitantly. Patients receiving ECMO may require higher doses due to drug absorption in the ECMO circuit (Mulla 2000). To minimize excipient load, preservative free preparations should be used; alternatively use the more concentrated midazolam injection (eg, 5 mg/mL) and dilute with SWI without preservatives.

Sedation, intermittent dosing or procedural (intubation): IM, IV: 0.05 to 0.1 mg/kg/dose over 5 minutes (Kumar 2010; VanLooy 2008)

Sedation, mechanically ventilated patient: IV: **Note:** Use the lowest effective dose.
Manufacturer's labeling: Continuous IV infusion:
GA ≤32 weeks: Initial: 0.03 mg/kg/**hour** (0.5 **mcg**/kg/minute)
GA >32 weeks: Initial: 0.06 mg/kg/**hour** (1 **mcg**/kg/minute)
Alternative dosing:
Loading dose:
GA <34 weeks: **Note:** Some have recommended against the use of a loading or bolus dose due to associated hypotension; to rapidly achieve sedation, it has been suggested to begin the continuous infusion at a faster rate for the first several hours (Jacqz-Aigrain 1992). Others have successfully used loading doses of 0.2 mg/kg given over 1 hour to prevent hypotension (Anand 1999; Treluyer 2005)
GA ≥34 weeks: 0.2 mg/kg/dose once (Anand 1999; Jacqz-Aigrain 1990; Treluyer 2005)
Continuous IV infusion (Anand 1999; Jacqz-Aigrain 1994; Treluyer 2005):
GA 24 to 26 weeks: Initial: 0.02 to 0.03 mg/kg/**hour** (0.33 to 0.5 **mcg**/kg/minute)
GA 27 to 29 weeks: Initial: 0.03 to 0.04 mg/kg/**hour** (0.5 to 0.67 **mcg**/kg/minute)
GA ≥30 weeks: Initial: 0.03 to 0.06 mg/kg/**hour** (0.5 to 1 **mcg**/kg/minute)

Note: After prolonged therapy, consider a slow wean of therapy to prevent signs and symptoms of withdrawal. The following regimen has been reported: If duration of therapy ≤4 days, wean over at least 2 days beginning with an initial dosage reduction of 30% to 50% followed by 20% to 30% dosage reductions every 6-8 hours; monitor closely for signs and symptoms of withdrawal with each reduction in dose. If duration of therapy is >4 days, decrease infusion rate by 25% to 50% every 12 hours, then convert to an intermittent dose every 4 hours and lastly, every 8 hours (Anand 1999).

Seizures, refractory; status epilepticus: IV: Dosage regimens variable, reported doses are higher than sedative doses: **Note:** Consider omitting loading dose if patient has received an IV dose of a benzodiazepine; begin continuous IV infusion at lower end of range and titrate to lowest effective dose: Loading dose: 0.06 to 0.15 mg/kg/dose followed by a continuous infusion of 0.06 to 0.4 mg/kg/**hour** (1 to 7 **mcg**/kg/minute); maximum reported rate: 1.1 mg/kg/**hour** (18 mcg/kg/minute) (Boylan 2004; Conde 2005; Holmes 1999)

Dosing: Usual Dosage must be individualized and based on patient's age, underlying diseases, concurrent medications, and desired effect; decrease dose (by ~30%) if opioids or other CNS depressants are administered concomitantly; use multiple small doses and titrate to desired sedative effect; allow 3 to 5 minutes between doses to decrease the chance of oversedation.

Pediatric:

Sedation, anxiolysis, and amnesia prior to procedure or before induction of anesthesia:
IM: Infants, Children and Adolescents: Usual: 0.1 to 0.15 mg/kg 30-60 minutes before surgery or procedure; range: 0.05 to 0.15 mg/kg; doses up to 0.5 mg/kg have been used in more anxious patients; maximum total dose: 10 mg
IV:
Infants 1 to 5 months: Limited data available in nonintubated infants; infants <6 months are at higher risk for airway obstruction and hypoventilation; titrate dose with small increments to desired clinical effect; monitor carefully
Infants 6 months to Children 5 years: Initial: 0.05 to 0.1 mg/kg; titrate dose carefully; total dose of 0.6 mg/kg may be required; usual total dose maximum: 6 mg
Children 6 to 12 years: Initial: 0.025 to 0.05 mg/kg; titrate dose carefully; total doses of 0.4 mg/kg may be required; usual total dose maximum: 10 mg
Children 12 to 16 years: Dose as adults; usual total dose maximum: 10 mg
Intranasal: Limited data available: **Note:** Some investigators suggest premedication with intranasal lidocaine to decrease irritation and subsequent agitation (Chiaretti 2011; Lugo 1993):
Infants 1 to 5 months: 0.2 mg/kg (single dose) (Harcke 1995; Mittal 2006)
Infants ≥6 months, Children, and Adolescents: 0.2 to 0.3 mg/kg (maximum single dose: 10 mg); may repeat in 5 to 15 minutes to a maximum of 0.5 mg/kg (maximum total dose: 10 mg) (Acworth 2001; Charetti 2011; Harcke 1995; Lane 2008)
Oral: Infants >6 months, Children, and Adolescents ≤16 years: Single dose: 0.25 to 0.5 mg/kg once, depending on patient status and desired effect, usual: 0.5 mg/kg; maximum dose: 20 mg; **Note:** Younger patients (6 months to <6 years) and those less cooperative may require higher doses (up to 1 mg/kg); use lower initial doses (0.25 mg/kg) in patients with cardiac or respiratory compromise, concomitant CNS depressant, or high-risk surgical patients.
Rectal: Limited data available: Infants >6 months and Children: Usual: 0.25-0.5 mg/kg once (Krauss 2006); doses up to 1 mg/kg have been used in infants and young children (7 months to 5 years of age) but may be associated with a higher incidence of postprocedural agitation (Kanegaye 2003; Tanaka 2000)

Sedation, mechanically ventilated patient: Infants, Children, and Adolescents: IV: Loading dose: 0.05 to 0.2 mg/kg given slow IV over 2 to 3 minutes, then follow with initial continuous IV infusion: 0.06 to 0.12 mg/kg/**hour** (1 to 2 **mcg**/kg/minute); titrate to the desired effect; range: 0.024 to 0.36 mg/kg/**hour** (0.4 to 6 **mcg**/kg/minute)

Seizures, acute treatment: Limited data available:

Buccal: Reserve for patients without IV access (Ashrafi 2010; Kutlu 2003; McIntyre 2005; Mpimbaza 2008; Talukdar 2009):

Weight-based dosing: Infants ≥3 months, Children, and Adolescents: 0.2 to 0.5 mg/kg once; maximum dose: 10 mg

Age-based dosing (McIntyre 2005):

Infants 6 to 11 months: 2.5 mg

Children 1 to 4 years: 5 mg

Children 5 to 9 years: 7.5 mg

Children and Adolescents ≥10 years: 10 mg

IM: Infants, Children, and Adolescents: 0.2 mg/kg/dose; repeat every 10 to 15 minutes; maximum dose: 6 mg (Hegenbarth 2008)

Intranasal (Bhattachyaryya 2006; Fişgin 2000; Fişgin 2002; Holsti 2007; Holsti 2010; Kutlu 2000): Reserve for patients without IV access; divide dose between nares:

Infants 1 to 5 months: 0.2 mg/kg once; maximum dose: 10 mg

Infants and Children ≥6 months: 0.2 mg/kg; one study used 0.3 mg/kg (n=9); maximum dose: 10 mg; may repeat once to a total maximum of 0.4 mg/kg

Seizures, refractory; status epilepticus refractory to standard therapy: Limited data available: IV (Hayashi 2007; Hegenbarth 2008; Igartua 1999; Koul 1997; Koul 2002; Morrison 2006; Morrison 2008; Ozdemir 2005; Rivera 1993; Singh 2002; Yoshikawa 2000):

Loading dose: 0.15 to 0.2 mg/kg; 0.5 mg/kg/dose was used in one high-dose midazolam study (n=17); consider using the lower end of the loading dose range in patients with hemodynamic instability or who have received other agents with hypotensive effects

Continuous IV infusion: Initial rate: 0.06 to 0.12 mg/kg/**hour** (1 to 2 mcg/kg/minute); increase rate every 15 minutes in increments of 0.06 to 0.12 mg/kg/**hour** (1 to 2 mcg/kg/minute) until seizure activity ceases; one high dose study increased by 0.24 mg/kg/**hour** (4 mcg/kg/minute); mean required dosage across a number of studies: 0.11 to 0.84 mg/kg/**hour** (1.87 to 14 mcg/kg/minute); the upper end of this range was used in one study; however, patients were titrated to burst suppression on EEG; maximum reported dose (n=1): 3 mg/kg/**hour** (50 mcg/kg/minute)

Seizures, status epilepticus, prehospital treatment: Limited data available: **Note:** Administered by paramedics when convulsions last >5 minutes or if convulsions are occurring after having intermittent seizures without regaining consciousness for >5 minutes: IM: Children and Adolescents (Silbergleit 2012):

<13 kg: Not studied

13 to 40 kg: 5 mg once

>40 kg: 10 mg once

Adult:

Anesthesia: IV:

Induction:

Unpremedicated patients: 0.3 to 0.35 mg/kg (up to 0.6 mg/kg in resistant cases)

Premedicated patients: 0.15 to 0.35 mg/kg

Maintenance: 0.05 to 0.3 mg/kg as needed, or continuous IV infusion 0.25 to 1.5 mcg/kg/minute

Sedation, preoperative:

IM: 0.07 to 0.08 mg/kg 30 to 60 minutes prior to surgery/procedure; usual dose: 5 mg; **Note:** Reduce dose in patients with COPD, high-risk patients, patients ≥60 years of age, and patients receiving other opioids or CNS depressants.

IV: 0.02 to 0.04 mg/kg; repeat every 5 minutes as needed to desired effect or up to 0.1 to 0.2 mg/kg

Sedation, procedural (moderate): IV: Initial: 0.5 to 2 mg slow IV over at least 2 minutes; slowly titrate to effect by repeating doses every 2 to 3 minutes if needed; usual total dose: 2.5 to 5 mg

Healthy Adults <60 years:

Initial: Some patients respond to doses as low as 1 mg; no more than 2.5 mg should be administered over a period of 2 minutes. Additional doses of midazolam may be administered after a 2-minute waiting period and evaluation of sedation after each dose increment. A total dose >5 mg is generally not needed. If opioids or other CNS depressants are administered concomitantly, the midazolam dose should be reduced by 30%. A reduced dose is required for patients ≥60 years, debilitated, or chronically ill.

Maintenance: 25% of dose used to reach sedative effect

Sedation in mechanically ventilated patients: IV:

Manufacturer's labeling: Initial dose: 0.01 to 0.05 mg/kg (~0.5 to 4 mg); may repeat at 5- to 15-minute intervals until adequate sedation achieved; maintenance infusion: 0.02 to 0.1 mg/kg/**hour**. Titrate to reach desired level of sedation.

Alternative dosing: Initial dose: 0.02 to 0.08 mg/kg (~1 to 5 mg in 70 kg adult); may repeat at 5- to 15-minute intervals until adequate sedation achieved; maintenance infusion: 0.04 to 0.2 mg/kg/**hour**. Titrate to reach desired level of sedation (Jacobi 2002).

Status epilepticus, refractory: Note: Intubation required; adjust dose based on hemodynamics, seizure activity, and EEG. IV: 0.15 to 0.3 mg/kg (usual dose: 5 to 15 mg); may repeat every 10 to 15 minutes as needed **or** 0.2 mg/kg bolus followed by a continuous infusion of 0.05 to 0.6 mg/kg/**hour** (Lowenstein 2005; Meierkord 2010)

Status epilepticus, prehospital treatment: Note: Administered by paramedics when convulsions last >5 minutes or if convulsions are occurring after having intermittent seizures without regaining consciousness for >5 minutes: IM: 10 mg once (Silbergleit 2012)

Usual Infusion Concentrations: Neonatal IV Infusion: 0.1 mg/mL **or** 0.5 mg/mL

Usual Infusion Concentrations: Pediatric IV infusion: 0.5 mg/mL **or** 1 mg/mL

Preparation for Administration

Parenteral:

Intermittent IV: For procedural sedation/anxiolysis/amnesia the 1 mg/mL concentration is recommended per the manufacturer. For neonates, use the preservative-free injection; alternatively, if the preservative-free product is not available, may use the 5 mg/mL injection and dilute to 0.5 mg/mL with SWFI (preservative free) to decrease the amount of benzyl alcohol delivered to the neonate (since both concentrations of midazolam injection contain 1% benzyl alcohol)

Continuous IV infusion: Dilute with NS or D_5W to a final concentration of 0.5 mg/mL per the manufacturer; in patients requiring high doses or fluid restriction higher concentrations up to 5 mg/mL (undiluted) may be necessary (Murray 2014; Phillips 2011). ISMP and Vermont Oxford Network recommend a standard concentration of 0.5 mg/mL for neonates (ISMP 2011).

Administration

Buccal: A buccal formulation is not currently available in the US. Some trials used an injectable solution administered buccally. International studies used a 10 mg/mL commercially available buccal formulation. Administer to the buccal mucosa between the gums and the cheek using an oral syringe; gently massage cheek; dose may be divided to both sides of the mouth.

Intranasal: Administer using a needleless syringe into the nares over 15 to 30 seconds; use the 5 mg/mL injection; 1/2 of the dose may be administered to each nare; **Note:** The 5 mg/mL injection has also been administered as a nasal spray using a graded pump device (Ljungman 2000) or using an atomizer such as the MAD Nasal Drug delivery device (Holsti 2007; Holsti 2010).

Oral: Administer on empty stomach (feeding is usually contraindicated prior to sedation for procedures).

Parenteral: Avoid extravasation; do not administer intra-arterially

IV (bolus, loading doses, intermittent therapy): Administer by slow IV injection at a concentration of 1 to 5 mg/mL over at least 2 to 5 minutes. In adults: For induction of anesthesia, may administer IV push over 20 to 30 seconds per the manufacturer.

Neonates: Rapid administration (<2 minutes) has been reported to cause severe hypotension especially if administered concurrently with fentanyl. For procedural sedation (eg, intubation) or intermittent sedation dosing, administration over at least 2 to 5 minutes has been used, monitor for hypotension (Cloherty 2012). For loading doses, administration over 1 hour have successfully prevented hypotension in neonates (Anand 1999; Treluyer 2005); manufacturer recommends against loading doses in neonates and suggests using a faster continuous infusion rate for the first several hours.

Continuous IV infusion: Administer via an infusion pump.

IM: Administer undiluted deep IM into large muscle, generally into anterior-lateral aspect of thigh (vastus lateralis) in pediatric patients (Lam 2005; Malamed 1989)

Rectal: Clinical trials utilized parenteral midazolam for rectal administration; administer a 1 to 5 mg/mL solution through a small, lubricated catheter or tube inserted rectally; hold buttocks closed for ~5 minutes after administration

Monitoring Parameters Level of sedation, respiratory rate, heart rate, blood pressure, oxygen saturation (ie, pulse oximetry)

Additional Information Sodium content of injection: 0.14 mEq/mL. With continuous IV infusion, midazolam may accumulate in peripheral tissues; use lowest effective infusion rate to reduce accumulation effects. Midazolam is 3 to 4 times as potent as diazepam.

Controlled Substance C-IV

Dosage Forms Excipient information presented when available (limited, particularly for generics); consult specific product labeling.

Solution, Injection:

Generic: 2 mg/2 mL (2 mL); 5 mg/5 mL (5 mL); 10 mg/10 mL (10 mL); 5 mg/mL (1 mL, 2 mL, 5 mL, 10 mL); 10 mg/2 mL (2 mL); 25 mg/5 mL (5 mL); 50 mg/10 mL (10 mL)

Solution, Injection [preservative free]:

Generic: 2 mg/2 mL (2 mL); 5 mg/5 mL (5 mL); 5 mg/mL (1 mL); 10 mg/2 mL (2 mL)

Syrup, Oral:

Generic: 2 mg/mL (118 mL)

- ◆ **Midazolam Hydrochloride** *see* Midazolam *on page 1433*
- ◆ **Midazolam Injection (Can)** *see* Midazolam *on page 1433*
- ◆ **Migergot** *see* Ergotamine and Caffeine *on page 776*
- ◆ **Migranal** *see* Dihydroergotamine *on page 659*
- ◆ **Migranal® (Can)** *see* Dihydroergotamine *on page 659*
- ◆ **Milk of Magnesia** *see* Magnesium Hydroxide *on page 1313*
- ◆ **Milk of Magnesia [OTC]** *see* Magnesium Hydroxide *on page 1313*
- ◆ **Milk of Magnesia Concentrate [OTC]** *see* Magnesium Hydroxide *on page 1313*
- ◆ **Millipred** *see* PrednisoLONE (Systemic) *on page 1755*
- ◆ **Millipred DP** *see* PrednisoLONE (Systemic) *on page 1755*
- ◆ **Millipred DP 12-Day** *see* PrednisoLONE (Systemic) *on page 1755*

Milrinone (MIL ri none)

Medication Safety Issues

Sound-alike/look-alike issues:

Primacor may be confused with Primaxin

High alert medication:

The Institute for Safe Medication Practices (ISMP) includes this medication among its list of drugs which have a heightened risk of causing significant patient harm when used in error.

Brand Names: Canada Milrinone Injection; Milrinone Lactate Injection

Therapeutic Category Phosphodiesterase Enzyme Inhibitor

Generic Availability (US) Yes

Use Short-term treatment of acute decompensated heart failure (FDA approved in adults)

Pregnancy Risk Factor C

Pregnancy Considerations Adverse events have not been observed in animal reproduction studies; however, increased resorption was reported in some studies.

Breast-Feeding Considerations It is not known if milrinone is excreted in breast milk. The manufacturer recommends that caution be exercised when administering milrinone to nursing women.

Contraindications Hypersensitivity to milrinone or any component of the formulation

Warnings/Precautions Monitor closely for hypotension. Avoid in severe obstructive aortic or pulmonic valvular disease. Milrinone may aggravate outflow tract obstruction in hypertrophic cardiomyopathy. Ventricular arrhythmias, including nonsustained ventricular tachycardia and supraventricular arrhythmias, have been reported. Observe closely for arrhythmias in this very high-risk patient population; sudden cardiac death has been observed. Due to the prolonged half-life as compared to other inotropic agents, ventricular or atrial arrhythmias may persist even after discontinuation of milrinone especially in patients with renal dysfunction (Cox 2013; Leier 1998). Ensure that ventricular rate is controlled in atrial fibrillation/flutter before initiating; may increase ventricular response rate. In heart transplant candidates, institute appropriate measures to protect patient against risks of sudden cardiac death (Brozena 2004). Monitor and correct fluid and electrolyte problems to minimize the risk of arrhythmias.

Use with caution in patients with renal impairment; reduction in infusion rate recommended. Hypotension may be prolonged in patients with renal dysfunction (Cox 2013; Leier 1998). According to the ACCF/AHA 2013 heart failure guidelines, long-term use of intravenous inotropic therapy without a specific indication or for reasons other than palliation is potentially harmful (ACCF/AHA [Yancy 2013]).

A facility for immediate treatment of potential cardiac events, including life-threatening ventricular arrhythmias, must be available. Safe and effective use beyond 48 hours (prolonged use) has not been demonstrated. An increased risk of death and hospitalization has been observed with prolonged use in NYHA Class III/IV heart failure patients. Sudden cardiac death has been reported with prolonged use. Continuous electrocardiographic monitoring is recommended.

Adverse Reactions

Cardiovascular: Angina, hypotension, supraventricular arrhythmia, ventricular arrhythmia

Central nervous system: Headache

Rare but important or life-threatening: Anaphylaxis, atrial fibrillation, bronchospasm, hypokalemia, injection site reaction, liver function abnormalities, MI, rash, thrombocytopenia, torsade de pointes, tremor, ventricular fibrillation

Drug Interactions

Metabolism/Transport Effects None known.

Avoid Concomitant Use There are no known interactions where it is recommended to avoid concomitant use.

Increased Effect/Toxicity

Milrinone may increase the levels/effects of: Riociguat

Decreased Effect There are no known significant interactions involving a decrease in effect.

Storage/Stability

Injection: Store at 20°C to 25°C (68°F to 77°F); excursions permitted between 15°C and 30°C (59°F and 86°F); avoid freezing. Stable at 0.2 mg/mL in ½NS, NS, or D_5W for 72 hours at room temperature in normal light.

Premixed infusion: Store at room temperature at 25°C (77°F); brief exposure up to 40°C (104°F) will not adversely affect drug; minimize exposure to heat; avoid excessive heat; protect from freezing.

Mechanism of Action A selective phosphodiesterase inhibitor in cardiac and vascular tissue, resulting in vasodilation and inotropic effects with little chronotropic activity.

Pharmacodynamics Onset of action (improved hemodynamic function): Within 5-15 minutes

Pharmacokinetics (Adult data unless noted)

Distribution: V_d beta:
- Infants (after cardiac surgery): 0.9 ± 0.4 L/kg
- Children (after cardiac surgery): 0.7 ± 0.2 L/kg
- Adults:
  - After cardiac surgery: 0.3 ± 0.1 L/kg
  - CHF (with single injection): 0.38 L/kg
  - CHF (with infusion): 0.45 L/kg

Protein binding: 70%

Half-life:
- Infants (after cardiac surgery): 3.15 ± 2 hours
- Children (after cardiac surgery): 1.86 ± 2 hours
- Adults:
  - After cardiac surgery: 1.69 ± 0.18 hours
  - CHF: 2.3-2.4 hours
- Renal impairment: Prolonged half-life

Elimination: Excreted in the urine as unchanged drug (83%) and glucuronide metabolite (12%)
- Clearance:
  - Infants (after cardiac surgery): 3.8 ± 1 mL/kg/minute
  - Children (after cardiac surgery): 5.9 ± 2 mL/kg/minute
  - Children (with septic shock): 10.6 ± 5.3 mL/kg/minute
  - Adults:
    - After cardiac surgery: 2 ± 0.7 mL/kg/minute
    - CHF: 2.2-2.3 mL/kg/minute
  - Renal impairment: Decreased clearance

Dosing: Neonatal

Hemodynamic support: Limited data available: Full-term neonates: IV: Loading dose: 50 to 75 mcg/kg administered over 15 minutes followed by a continuous infusion of 0.5 mcg/kg/minute; titrate to effect; range: 0.25 to 0.75 mcg/kg/minute has been used by several centers. One report used a loading dose of 50 mcg/kg administered over 15 minutes, followed by a continuous infusion of 0.5 mcg/kg/minute for 30 minutes in 10 neonates (3 to 27 days old, median age: 5 days) with low cardiac output after cardiac surgery; results showed improved hemodynamic parameters and milrinone was well tolerated (Chang 1995)

Prevention of postoperative low cardiac output syndrome (CHD corrective surgery): Limited data available: Full-term neonates: IV: Loading dose: 75 mcg/kg administered over 60 minutes followed by a continuous IV infusion of 0.75 mcg/kg/minute for 35 hours was used in a randomized, placebo-controlled trial of 227 patients (age: 2 days to 6.9 years, median: 3 months) and showed 64% relative risk reduction for development of low cardiac output syndrome compared to placebo; a lower milrinone dose used in the study did not show a statistically significant relative risk reduction compared to placebo for the same endpoint (Hoffman 2003)

Dosing: Usual

Infants and Children: IV: A limited number of studies have used different dosing schemes. Two pharmacokinetic studies propose per kg doses for pediatric patients with septic shock that are greater than those recommended for adults (Lindsay 1998) and in infants and children after cardiac surgery (Ramamoorthy 1998). Further pharmacodynamic studies are needed to define pediatric milrinone guidelines. Several centers are using the following guidelines:

Loading dose: 50 mcg/kg administered over 15 minutes followed by a continuous infusion of 0.5 mcg/kg/minute range: 0.25 to 0.75 mcg/kg/minute; titrate dose to effect

PALS Guidelines 2010: IV, I.O.: Loading dose: 50 mcg/kg administered over 10 to 60 minutes followed by a continuous infusion of 0.25 to 0.75 mcg/kg/minute

Adults: IV: Loading dose: 50 mcg/kg slow IV over 10 minutes, followed by a continuous infusion of 0.5 mcg/kg/minute; range: 0.375 to 0.75 mcg/kg/minute; titrate dose to effect; maximum daily dose: 1.13 mg/kg/day

Dosing adjustment in renal impairment: Adult: Continuous IV infusion:

Manufacturer recommended adjustment:
- CrCl 50 mL/minute/1.73 m^2: Administer 0.43 mcg/kg/minute
- CrCl 40 mL/minute/1.73 m^2: Administer 0.38 mcg/kg/minute
- CrCl 30 mL/minute/1.73 m^2: Administer 0.33 mcg/kg/minute
- CrCl 20 mL/minute/1.73 m^2: Administer 0.28 mcg/kg/minute
- CrCl 10 mL/minute/1.73 m^2: Administer 0.23 mcg/kg/minute
- CrCl 5 mL/minute/1.73 m^2: Administer 0.2 mcg/kg/minute

Alternative Dosing Adjustments in Patients with Renal Impairment[1]

CrCl (mL/min)	Starting dose (mcg/kg/min)		
	0.375	**0.5**	**0.75**
50	0.25	0.375	0.5
40	0.125	0.25	0.375
30	0.0625	0.125	0.25
20	Consider alternative therapy	0.0625	0.125
10	Consider alternative therapy		0.0625
5	Consider alternative therapy		

[1]Based on expert opinion

Usual Infusion Concentrations: Pediatric Note: Premixed solutions available

IV infusion: 200 mcg/mL

Preparation for Administration

Loading dose: Adults: May dilute to 10 to 20 mL for ease of administration

Continuous IV infusion: Dilute with ½NS, NS, or D_5W; usual concentration: ≤200 mcg/mL; 250 mcg/mL in NS has been used (Barton 1996). **Note:** Some pediatric centers use a concentration as high as 800 mcg/mL (Murray 2014; Sinclair-Pingel 2006)

Administration

IV:

Loading dose:

Pediatric patients: Administer undiluted slow IV push over 15 minutes

Adults: Administer slow IV push over 10 minutes; loading dose may be given as undiluted solution or may be further diluted for ease of administration

Continuous IV infusion: Administer via infusion pump or syringe pump

Monitoring Parameters Blood pressure, heart rate, cardiac output, CI, SVR, PVR, CVP, ECG, CBC, platelet count, serum electrolytes (especially potassium and magnesium), liver enzymes, renal function; clinical signs and symptoms of CHF; monitor infusion site carefully (avoid extravasation)

Additional Information Dosing schemes and proposed dosing based on pharmacokinetic data:

Infants and children with septic shock: Twelve patients (9 months to 15 years of age) were administered a loading dose of 50 mcg/kg, followed by a continuous infusion of 0.5 mcg/kg/minute. At 1 hour after the loading dose, if patients did not respond (defined as a ≥20% increase in CI or an improvement in peripheral perfusion), an additional loading dose of 25 mcg/kg was given and the infusion rate was increased to 0.75 mcg/kg/minute. Nine of 12 patients required the additional loading dose and increased rate of infusion (Barton, 1996). A subsequent pharmacokinetic analysis of these patients recommended larger loading doses of 75 mcg/kg and infusion rates of 0.75-1 mcg/kg/minute. However, these doses were based on a one-compartment pharmacokinetic model and are higher then the mean infusion rate of 0.69 mcg/kg/minute used in the study (Lindsay, 1998). Further studies are needed.

Infants and Children after open heart surgery: A prospective, open-label trial compared a lower dose of milrinone (Group A) to a higher dose (Group B). Group A: Eleven patients received a loading dose of 25 mcg/kg given over 5 minutes followed by an infusion of 0.25 mcg/kg/minute; 30 minutes later, a second 25 mcg/kg loading dose was given and the infusion was increased to 0.5 mcg/kg/minute. Group B: 8 patients received a loading dose of 50 mcg/kg given over 10 minutes followed by an infusion of 0.5 mcg/kg/minute; 30 minutes later, a second loading dose of 25 mcg/kg was given and the infusion was increased to 0.75 mcg/kg/minute. Patients in both groups received a third loading dose of 25 mcg/kg if needed. A two-compartment model and NONMEM pharmacokinetic analyses were performed. Based on the NONMEM analysis, the authors propose the following doses: Infants: Loading dose: 104 mcg/kg and continuous infusion of 0.49 mcg/kg/minute; children: loading dose: 67 mcg/kg and continuous infusion of 0.61 mcg/kg/minute (Ramamoorthy, 1998). Further studies are needed before these proposed doses can routinely be used in the pediatric population.

Dosage Forms Excipient information presented when available (limited, particularly for generics); consult specific product labeling.

Solution, Intravenous:

Generic: 200 mcg/mL (100 mL, 200 mL); 10 mg/10 mL (10 mL); 20 mg/20 mL (20 mL); 50 mg/50 mL (50 mL)

Solution, Intravenous [preservative free]:

Generic: 200 mcg/mL (100 mL, 200 mL)

◆ **Milrinone Injection (Can)** *see* Milrinone *on page 1437*

◆ **Milrinone Lactate** *see* Milrinone *on page 1437*

◆ **Milrinone Lactate Injection (Can)** *see* Milrinone *on page 1437*

Mineral Oil (MIN er al oyl)

Medication Safety Issues

BEERS Criteria medication:

This drug may be potentially inappropriate for use in geriatric patients (Quality of evidence - moderate; Strength of recommendation - strong).

Brand Names: US Fleet Oil [OTC]

Therapeutic Category Laxative, Lubricant

Generic Availability (US) Yes

Use

Oral: Treatment of occasional constipation (OTC product: FDA approved in ≥6 years and adults)

Rectal: Treatment of occasional constipation; relief of fecal impaction; removal of barium sulfate residues following barium administration (OTC products: Fleet® Mineral Oil Enema; All indications: FDA approved in ages ≥2 years and adults); has also been used as preparation for bowel studies or surgery

Refer to product-specific information to determine FDA approved ages for additional products

Pregnancy Considerations The use of mineral oil for the treatment of constipation in pregnancy is not recommended (Mahadevan, 2006).

Breast-Feeding Considerations The use of mineral oil for the treatment of constipation is not recommended for nursing women (Mahadevan, 2006).

Contraindications Oral: Children <6 years, pregnancy, bedridden patients, elderly, use longer than 1 week, or difficulty swallowing.

Warnings/Precautions Lipid pneumonitis results from aspiration of mineral oil. Aspiration risk increased in patients in prolonged supine position or conditions which interfere with swallowing or epiglottal function (eg, stroke, Parkinson's disease, Alzheimer's disease, esophageal dysmotility). Due to potential for aspiration and other adverse effects, use in the elderly should be avoided (Beers Criteria).

When used for self-medication (OTC): Healthcare provider should be contacted in case of sudden changes in bowel habits which last over 2 weeks or if abdominal pain, nausea, vomiting, or rectal bleeding occur following use; do not use for >1 week, unless otherwise directed by healthcare provider. Do not use orally in children <6 years of age or rectally in children <2 years of age.

Warnings: Additional Pediatric Considerations Not recommended for use in infants due to increased risk of aspiration (NASPHAGAN, 2006).

Adverse Reactions

Gastrointestinal: Abdominal cramps, diarrhea, nausea, vomiting

Respiratory: Lipid pneumonitis with aspiration

Miscellaneous: Large doses may cause anal leakage causing anal itching, hemorrhoids, irritation, perianal discomfort, soiling of clothes

Drug Interactions

Metabolism/Transport Effects None known.

Avoid Concomitant Use There are no known interactions where it is recommended to avoid concomitant use.

Increased Effect/Toxicity There are no known significant interactions involving an increase in effect.

Decreased Effect

Mineral Oil may decrease the levels/effects of: Multivitamins/Fluoride (with ADE); Multivitamins/Minerals (with ADEK, Folate, Iron); Multivitamins/Minerals (with AE, No Iron); Phytonadione; Vitamin D Analogs

Storage/Stability

Oral plain (nonemulsified) liquid: Protect from sunlight.

Oral suspension (emulsion) (Kondremul®): Store at 15°C to 25°C (59°F to 77°F).

Rectal enema: Store at 20°C to 25°C (68°F to 77°F); protect from sunlight.

Mechanism of Action Eases passage of stool by decreasing water absorption and lubricating the intestine; retards colonic absorption of water

Pharmacodynamics

Onset of action:

Enema: 2 to 15 minutes

Oral: ~6 to 8 hours

Pharmacokinetics (Adult data unless noted)

Absorption: Minimal following oral or rectal administration

Distribution: Into intestinal mucosa, liver, spleen, and mesenteric lymph nodes

Elimination: In feces

Dosing: Usual

Pediatric:

Constipation, occasional:

Oral:

Plain (nonemulsified) liquid:

Children 6 to 11 years: 5 to 15 mL/day in a single daily dose at bedtime or in divided doses; maximum daily dose: 15 mL/**day**

Children ≥12 years and Adolescents: 15 to 45 mL/day in a single daily dose at bedtime or in divided doses; maximum daily dose: 45 mL/**day**

Suspension (emulsion) (Kondremul):

Children 6 to 11 years: 10 to 30 mL/day in a single daily dose or in up to 3 divided doses

Children ≥12 years and Adolescents: 30 to 90 mL/day in a single daily dose or in up to 3 divided doses

Rectal:

Children 2 to 11 years: Administer **one half** the contents of a 4.5 oz bottle as a single dose

Children ≥12 years and Adolescents: Administer the contents of one 4.5 oz bottle as a single dose

Constipation, chronic: Limited data available (Tabbers [NASPGHAN 2014]):

Oral: Children and Adolescents: 1 to 3 mL/kg/day divided in 1 to 2 doses; maximum daily dose: 90 mL/**day**

Rectal:

Children 2 to 11 years: 30 to 60 mL once daily

Children >11 years and Adolescents: 60 to 150 mL once daily

Fecal impaction:

Oral: Slow disimpaction: Children and Adolescents: 3 mL/kg twice daily for 7 days (Pashankar 2005; Wyllie 2011)

Rectal:

Children 2 to 11 years: Administer **one half** the contents of a 4.5 oz bottle as a single dose

Children ≥12 years and Adolescents: Administer the contents of one 4.5 oz bottle as a single dose

Removal of barium sulfate residues following barium administration: Rectal:

Children 2 to 11 years: Administer **one half** the contents of a 4.5 oz bottle as a single dose

Children ≥12 years and Adolescents: Administer the contents of one 4.5 oz bottle as a single dose

Adult:

Constipation:

Oral:

Plain (nonemulsified) liquid: 15 to 45 ml/day in a single daily dose at bedtime or in divided doses; maximum daily dose: 45 mL/**day**

Suspension (emulsion) (Kondremul): 30 to 90 mL/day in a single daily dose or in up to 3 divided doses

Rectal: Administer the contents of one 4.5 oz bottle as a single dose

Fecal impaction or following barium studies: Rectal: Administer the contents of one 4.5 oz bottle as a single dose

Administration

Oral: Mineral oil may be more palatable if refrigerated (NASGHAN, 2006). **Note:** Due to risk of aspiration, do not administer to patient in supine position.

Plain (nonemulsified): Administer on an empty stomach. Take at least 2 hours before or after other medications.

Suspension (emulsion) (Kondremul®): Shake well before use. May be administered alone or mixed with warm or cold water, milk, or cocoa; do not take with meals.

Rectal: Administer with patient lying on left side and knees bent or with patient kneeling and head and chest leaning forward until left side of face is resting comfortably. Remove protective shield and gently insert enema tip into rectum with a slight side-to-side movement with tip pointing toward the navel; have patient bear down. Do not force the enema tip into the rectum as this may cause injury. Squeeze the bottle until correct dose is administered. It is not necessary to empty the bottle completely for a one-bottle dose. Remove enema tip from rectum.

Monitoring Parameters Evacuation of stool; anal leakage indicates dose too high or need for disimpaction

Additional Information Fleets® Mineral Oil Enema: 4.5 ounce enema delivers 118 mL

Dosage Forms Excipient information presented when available (limited, particularly for generics); consult specific product labeling.

Enema, Rectal:

Fleet Oil: (133 mL)

Generic: (135 mL)

Oil, Oral:

Generic: (472 mL, 473 mL, 500 mL, 1000 mL, 4000 mL)

◆ **Minims Cyclopentolate (Can)** *see* Cyclopentolate *on page 549*

◆ **Minims Prednisolone Sodium Phosphate (Can)** *see* PrednisoLONE (Ophthalmic) *on page 1758*

◆ **Minipress** *see* Prazosin *on page 1752*

◆ **Minirin (Can)** *see* Desmopressin *on page 607*

◆ **Minitran** *see* Nitroglycerin *on page 1523*

◆ **Minivelle** *see* Estradiol (Systemic) *on page 795*

◆ **Minocin** *see* Minocycline *on page 1440*

Minocycline (mi noe SYE kleen)

Medication Safety Issues

Sound-alike/look-alike issues:

Dynacin may be confused with Dyazide, Dynapen

Minocin may be confused with Indocin, Lincocin, Minizide, niacin

Related Information

Oral Medications That Should Not Be Crushed or Altered *on page 2476*

Brand Names: US Minocin; Solodyn

Brand Names: Canada Apo-Minocycline; Arestin Microspheres; Dom-Minocycline; Mylan-Minocycline; PHL-Minocycline; PMS-Minocycline; Sandoz-Minocycline; Teva-Minocycline

Therapeutic Category Antibiotic, Tetracycline Derivative

Generic Availability (US) May be product dependent

Use

Minocin injection, immediate release oral tablets, and oral capsules: Treatment of susceptible gram-negative and gram-positive infections involving the respiratory tract, urinary tract, and skin/soft tissue; treatment of anthrax (inhalational, cutaneous, and gastrointestinal); brucellosis; asymptomatic meningococcal carrier state; rickettsial diseases (including Rocky Mountain spotted fever, typhus fever, Q fever); nongonococcal urethritis caused by *Ureaplasma urealyticum* or *C. trachomatis*, and gonorrhea; chlamydial infections (All indications: FDA approved in ages >8 years and adults)

Solodyn extended release tablets: Treatment of inflammatory lesions of non-nodular, moderate to severe acne vulgaris (FDA approved in ages ≥12 years and adults)

Pregnancy Risk Factor D

Pregnancy Considerations Tetracyclines cross the placenta and accumulate in developing teeth and long tubular bones. Rare spontaneous reports of congenital anomalies, including limb reduction, have been reported following maternal minocycline use. Due to limited information, a causal association cannot be established. Tetracyclines may discolor fetal teeth following maternal use during pregnancy; the specific teeth involved and the portion of the tooth affected depends on the timing and duration of exposure relative to tooth calcification. As a class, tetracyclines are generally considered second-line antibiotics in pregnant women and their use should be avoided (Mylonas, 2011). Minocycline should not be used for the treatment of acne in pregnant women, or in males or females attempting to conceive a child.

Breast-Feeding Considerations Minocycline is excreted in breast milk (Brogden, 1975). According to the manufacturer, the decision to continue or discontinue breast-feeding during therapy should take into account the risk of exposure to the infant and the benefits of treatment to the mother. Oral absorption is not affected by dairy products; therefore, oral absorption of minocycline by the breast-feeding infant would not be expected to be diminished by the calcium in the maternal milk. Nondose-related effects could include modification of bowel flora. There have been case reports of black discoloration of breast milk in women taking minocycline (Basler, 1985; Hunt, 1996).

Contraindications

Hypersensitivity to minocycline, other tetracyclines, or any component of the formulation

Documentation of allergenic cross-reactivity for tetracyclines is limited. However, because of similarities in chemical structure and/or pharmacologic actions, the possibility of cross-sensitivity cannot be ruled out with certainty.

Warnings/Precautions May be associated with increases in BUN secondary to antianabolic effects; use caution in patients with renal impairment. Hepatotoxicity has been reported; use caution in patients with hepatic insufficiency or in conjunction with other hepatotoxic drugs. Autoimmune syndromes (eg, lupus-like, hepatitis, and vasculitis) have been reported; discontinue if symptoms occur. CNS effects (lightheadedness, dizziness, vertigo) may occur; patients must be cautioned about performing tasks which require mental alertness (eg, operating machinery or driving); symptoms usually disappear with continued therapy and when the drug is discontinued. Intracranial hypertension (headache, blurred vision, diplopia, vision loss, and/or papilledema) has been associated with use. Women of childbearing age who are overweight or have a history of intracranial hypertension are at greater risk. Concomitant use of isotretinoin (known to cause pseudotumor cerebri) and minocycline should be avoided. Intracranial hypertension typically resolves after discontinuation of treatment; however, permanent visual loss is possible. If visual symptoms develop during treatment, prompt ophthalmologic evaluation is warranted. Intracranial pressure can remain elevated for weeks after drug discontinuation; monitor patients until they stabilize.

May cause photosensitivity; discontinue if skin erythema occurs. Prolonged use may result in fungal or bacterial superinfection, including *C. difficile*-associated diarrhea (CDAD) and pseudomembranous colitis; CDAD has been observed >2 months postantibiotic treatment. May cause tissue hyperpigmentation, tooth enamel hypoplasia, or permanent tooth discoloration; more common with long-term use, but observed with repeated, short courses; use of tetracyclines should be avoided during tooth development (infancy and children <8 years of age) unless other drugs are not likely to be effective or are contraindicated. Do not use during pregnancy. In addition to affecting tooth development, tetracycline use has been associated with retardation of skeletal development and reduced bone growth. Rash, along with eosinophilia, fever, and organ failure (Drug Rash with Eosinophilia and Systemic Symptoms [DRESS] syndrome) has been reported; discontinue treatment immediately if DRESS syndrome is suspected. Potentially significant drug-drug interactions may exist, requiring dose or frequency adjustment, additional monitoring, and/or selection of alternative therapy.

Warnings: Additional Pediatric Considerations Pseudotumor cerebri has been reported rarely in infants and adolescents; use with isotretinoin has been associated with cases of pseudotumor cerebri; avoid concomitant treatment with isotretinoin.

Adverse Reactions

Cardiovascular: Myocarditis, pericarditis, vasculitis

Central nervous system: Bulging fontanel, dizziness, fatigue, headache, hypoesthesia, malaise, mood changes, paresthesia, pseudotumor cerebri, sedation, seizure, vertigo

Dermatologic: Alopecia, angioedema, DRESS syndrome, drowsiness, erythema multiforme, erythema nodosum, erythematous rash, exfoliative dermatitis, maculopapular rash, mucous membrane pigmentation, nail hyperpigmentation, pruritus, skin photosensitivity, skin pigmentation, Stevens-Johnson syndrome, toxic epidermal necrolysis, urticaria

Endocrine & metabolic: Microscopic thyroid discoloration, thyroid dysfunction

Gastrointestinal: Anorexia, diarrhea, dyspepsia, dysphagia, enamel hypoplasia, enterocolitis, esophageal ulceration, esophagitis, glossitis, inflammatory anogenital lesion, mouth discoloration, nausea, oral lesion (inflammatory), pancreatitis, pseudomembranous colitis, stomatitis, tooth discoloration, vomiting, xerostomia

Genitourinary: Balanitis, vulvovaginitis

Hematologic & oncologic: Agranulocytosis, eosinophilia, hemolytic anemia, leukopenia, malignant neoplasm of thyroid, neutropenia, pancytopenia, thrombocytopenia

Hepatic: Autoimmune hepatitis, hepatic failure, hepatitis, hyperbilirubinemia, increased liver enzymes, intrahepatic cholestasis, jaundice

Hypersensitivity: Anaphylaxis, hypersensitivity, serum sickness

Infection: Candidiasis

Local: Injection site reaction (IV administration)

Neuromuscular & skeletal: Arthralgia, arthritis, bone discoloration, joint stiffness, joint swelling, lupus erythematosus, lupus-like syndrome, myalgia

Otic: Hearing loss, tinnitus

Renal: Acute renal failure, increased blood urea nitrogen, interstitial nephritis

Respiratory: Asthma, bronchospasm, cough, dyspnea, pneumonitis, pulmonary infiltrates (with eosinophilia)

Miscellaneous: Fever

Rare but important or life-threatening: Hepatotoxicity (idiosyncratic) (Chalasani, 2014)

Drug Interactions

Metabolism/Transport Effects None known.

Avoid Concomitant Use

Avoid concomitant use of Minocycline with any of the following: BCG; BCG (Intravesical); Mecamylamine; Retinoic Acid Derivatives; Strontium Ranelate

Increased Effect/Toxicity

Minocycline may increase the levels/effects of: Mecamylamine; Mipomersen; Neuromuscular-Blocking Agents; Porfimer; Retinoic Acid Derivatives; Verteporfin; Vitamin K Antagonists

Decreased Effect

Minocycline may decrease the levels/effects of: Atazanavir; BCG; BCG (Intravesical); BCG Vaccine (Immunization); Iron Salts; Penicillins; Sodium Picosulfate; Typhoid Vaccine

The levels/effects of Minocycline may be decreased by: Antacids; Bile Acid Sequestrants; Bismuth Subcitrate; Bismuth Subsalicylate; Calcium Salts; Iron Salts; Lanthanum; Magnesium Salts; Multivitamins/Minerals (with ADEK, Folate, Iron); Multivitamins/Minerals (with AE, No Iron); Quinapril; Strontium Ranelate; Sucralfate; Sucroferric Oxyhydroxide; Zinc Salts

Food Interactions Minocycline serum concentrations are not significantly altered if taken with food or dairy products. Management: Administer without regard to food.

Storage/Stability

Capsule (including pellet-filled), tablet: Store at 20°C to 25°C (68°F to 77°F); protect from heat. Protect from light and moisture.

Extended release tablet: Store at 15°C to 30°C (59°F to 86°F); protect from heat. Protect from light and moisture.

Injection: Store vials at 20°C to 25°C (68°F to 77°F) prior to reconstitution. Reconstituted solution is stable at room temperature for up to 24 hours. Final dilutions should be administered immediately.

Mechanism of Action Inhibits bacterial protein synthesis by binding with the 30S and possibly the 50S ribosomal subunit(s) of susceptible bacteria; cell wall synthesis is not affected

Rheumatoid arthritis: The mechanism of action of minocycline in rheumatoid arthritis is not completely understood. It is thought to have antimicrobial, anti-inflammatory, immunomodulatory, and chondroprotective effects. More specifically, it is thought to be a potent inhibitor of metalloproteinases, which are active in rheumatoid arthritis joint destruction.

Pharmacokinetics (Adult data unless noted)

Absorption: Oral: Well absorbed

Distribution: Widely distributed to most body fluids, bile, and tissues; poor CNS penetration; deposits in fat for extended periods

V_d: 0.14 to 0.7 L/kg (Zhanel 2004)

Protein binding: 55% to 96% (Zhanel 2004)

Metabolism: Hepatic to inactive metabolites

Bioavailability: 90% to 100% (Zhanel 2004)

Half-life: IV: 15 to 23 hours; Oral: 16 hours (range: 11 to 22 hours)

Time to peak serum concentration:

Capsules and pellet filled capsules: 1 to 4 hours

Tablet: 1-3 hours

Extended release tablet: 3.5 to 4 hours

Elimination: Urine (5% to 12% excreted unchanged) (Brogden 1975; Zhanel 2004); feces (20% to 34%) (Brogden 1975)

Dosing: Usual

Pediatric:

General dosing, susceptible infection: Children >8 years and Adolescents:

Oral immediate release: Initial: 4 mg/kg (maximum dose: 200 mg), then 2 mg/kg/dose every 12 hours (maximum dose: 100 mg/dose)

I.V.: Initial: 4 mg/kg (maximum dose: 200 mg), then 2 mg/kg/dose (maximum dose 100 mg/dose) every 12 hours; maximum daily dose: 400 mg/**day**

Acne: Adolescents: Oral immediate release: 100 mg once daily, in some patients may increase to 150-200 mg/day (Goulden, 2003)

Acne, inflammatory, non-nodular, moderate to severe: Children ≥12 years and Adolescents: Oral: Extended release tablet: **Note:** Higher doses do not confer greater efficacy and may be associated with more acute vestibular side effects: ~1 mg/kg/dose once daily for 12 weeks

45 to 49 kg: 45 mg once daily
50 to 59 kg: 55 mg once daily
60 to 71 kg: 65 mg once daily
72 to 84 kg: 80 mg once daily
85 to 96 kg: 90 mg once daily
97 to 110 kg: 105 mg once daily
111 to 125 kg: 115 mg once daily
126 to 136 kg: 135 mg once daily

Cellulitis (purulent) infection due to community acquired MRSA: Children >8 years and Adolescents: Oral: Immediate release: Initial: 4 mg/kg (maximum dose: 200 mg), then 2 mg/kg/dose (maximum dose 100 mg/dose) every 12 hours for 5 to 10 days (IDSA [Liu 2011])

Adult:

General dosing, susceptible infection:

Oral: Immediate release: Initial dose: 200 mg, followed by 100 mg every 12 hours; more frequent dosing intervals may be used (100 to 200 mg initially, followed by 50 mg 4 times daily)

IV: Initial dose: 200 mg, followed by 100 mg every 12 hours; maximum daily dose: 400 mg/**day**

Acne, inflammatory, non-nodular, moderate to severe: Extended release tablet: Oral: **Note:** Higher doses do not confer greater efficacy and may be associated with more acute vestibular side effects ~1 mg/kg/dose once daily for 12 weeks

45 to 49 kg: 45 mg once daily
50 to 59 kg: 55 mg once daily
60 to 71 kg: 65 mg once daily
72 to 84 kg: 80 mg once daily
85 to 96 kg: 90 mg once daily
97 to 110 kg: 105 mg once daily
111 to 125 kg: 115 mg once daily
126 to 136 kg: 135 mg once daily

Asymptomatic meningococcal carrier state: Oral Immediate release: 100 mg every 12 hours for 5 days. **Note:** CDC recommendations do not mention use of minocycline for eradicating nasopharyngeal carriage of meningococcus (*Pink Book* [CDC 2012])

Cellulitis (purulent) infection due to community-acquired MRSA: Oral: Immediate release: Initial 200 mg, then: 100 mg every 12 hours for 5 to 10 days, maximum dose: 100 mg/dose (IDSA [Liu 2011])

Chlamydial or *Ureaplasma urealyticum* infection uncomplicated (urethral, endocervical, or rectal): Oral, IV: 100 mg every 12 hours for at least 7 days

Gonococcal infection, uncomplicated (males): Oral IV:

Without urethritis or anorectal infection: Initial: 200 mg followed by 100 mg every 12 hours for at least 4 days (cultures 2 to 3 days post-therapy)

Urethritis: 100 mg every 12 hours for 5 days

***Mycobacterium marinum* cutaneous infection:** Oral Immediate release: 100 mg every 12 hours for 6 to 8 weeks (**Note:** Optimal dosing has not been established)

Syphilis: Oral immediate release tablet, IV: Initial 200 mg, followed by 100 mg every 12 hours for 10 to 15 days

Dosing adjustment in renal impairment:

CrCl ≥80 mL/minute: Adults: No dosage adjustment necessary

CrCl <80 mL/minute: Adults: Consider decreasing dose or extending interval between doses; maximum daily dose: 200 mg/day

Hemodialysis: Not dialyzable (Brogden 1975)

Dosing adjustment in hepatic impairment: There are no dosage adjustments provided in the manufacturer's labeling; however, hepatotoxicity has been reported. Use with caution.

Preparation for Administration IV: Reconstitute vial with 5 mL of SWFI, and further dilute in NS, D_5W, D_5NS, Ringer's injection, or LR to a final concentration not to exceed 0.4 mg/mL.

Administration

IV: Infuse slowly; avoid rapid administration; the manufacturer's labeling does not provide a recommended administration rate; other tetracyclines are typically infused over 1 to 2 hours; the injectable route should be used only if the oral route is not feasible or adequate; prolonged intravenous therapy may be associated with thrombophlebitis

Oral: Administer with adequate fluid to decrease the risk of esophageal irritation and ulceration. Administer with or without food. Swallow pellet-filled capsule and extended release tablet whole; do not chew, crush, or split. Administer antacids, calcium supplements, iron supplements, magnesium-containing laxatives, and cholestyramine 2 hours before or after minocycline.

Monitoring Parameters CBC, serum BUN, creatinine, liver function tests. Observe for changes in bowel frequency.

Test Interactions May cause interference with fluorescence test for urinary catecholamines (false elevations)

Product Availability Minocin for Injection (reformulated): FDA approved April 2015; availability anticipated in third quarter of 2015. The reformulated injection contains magnesium sulfate (inactive excipient), which allows for a lower diluent volume range (100 mL to 1,000 mL) compared to the existing formulation (500 mL to 1,000 mL). The manufacturer, The Medicines Company, has indicated the existing formulation will be removed from the market when the new formulation is available. Consult the prescribing information for additional information.

Dosage Forms Excipient information presented when available (limited, particularly for generics); consult specific product labeling.

Capsule, Oral:
- Minocin: 50 mg, 75 mg, 100 mg [contains brilliant blue fcf (fd&c blue #1), fd&c yellow #10 (quinoline yellow)]
- Generic: 50 mg, 75 mg, 100 mg

Kit, Combination:
- Minocin: 50 mg, 100 mg [contains brilliant blue fcf (fd&c blue #1), disodium edta, fd&c yellow #10 (quinoline yellow), sodium benzoate]

Solution Reconstituted, Intravenous:
- Minocin: 100 mg (1 ea)

Tablet, Oral:
- Generic: 50 mg, 75 mg, 100 mg

Tablet Extended Release 24 Hour, Oral:
- Solodyn: 55 mg [contains fd&c red #40]
- Solodyn: 65 mg [contains brilliant blue fcf (fd&c blue #1), fd&c blue #2 (indigotine), fd&c yellow #10 (quinoline yellow)]
- Solodyn: 80 mg [contains fd&c blue #2 (indigotine), fd&c red #40, fd&c yellow #6 (sunset yellow)]
- Solodyn: 105 mg [contains brilliant blue fcf (fd&c blue #1)]
- Solodyn: 115 mg [contains brilliant blue fcf (fd&c blue #1), fd&c blue #2 (indigotine), fd&c yellow #10 (quinoline yellow)]
- Generic: 45 mg, 90 mg, 135 mg

◆ **Minocycline Hydrochloride** *see* Minocycline *on page 1440*

Minoxidil (Systemic) (mi NOKS i dil)

Medication Safety Issues

Sound-alike/look-alike issues:

Loniten may be confused with Lipitor

Minoxidil may be confused with metolazone, midodrine, Minipress, Minocin, Monopril, Noxafil

International issues:

Noxidil [Thailand] may be confused with Noxafil brand name for posaconazole [U.S. and multiple international markets]

Brand Names: Canada Loniten

Generic Availability (US) Yes

Use Management of severe hypertension

Pregnancy Risk Factor C

Pregnancy Considerations Adverse events were observed in some animal studies. Neonatal hypertrichosis has been reported following exposure to minoxidil during pregnancy.

Breast-Feeding Considerations Excretion in breast milk has been reported in one case report of a woman receiving 10 mg/day orally. Due to the potential for adverse reactions in the nursing infant, breast-feeding is not recommended by the manufacturer.

Contraindications

Hypersensitivity to minoxidil or any component of the formulation; pheochromocytoma

Canadian labeling: Additional contraindications (not in U.S. labeling): Pulmonary hypertension associated with mitral stenosis; severe hepatic impairment

Warnings/Precautions [US Boxed Warning]: Minoxidil may cause pericarditis and pericardial effusion that may progress to tamponade; patients with renal impairment not on dialysis may be at higher risk. Observe patients closely. If effusion persists, consider discontinuation of minoxidil. **[US Boxed Warning]: May increase oxygen demand and exacerbate angina pectoris;** concomitant use with a beta-blocker (if no contraindication exists may help reduce the effect. Use with caution in patients with pulmonary hypertension, significant renal failure, or HF; use with caution in patients with coronary artery disease or recent myocardial infarction; renal failure or dialysis patients may require smaller doses; usually used with a beta-blocker (to treat minoxidil-induced tachycardia) and a diuretic (for treatment of water retention/edema. Compared to placebo minoxidil increased the frequency of clinical events, including increased need for diuretics, angina, ventricular arrhythmias, worsening heart failure and death (Franciosa, 1984). Use with caution in the elderly; initiate at the low end of the dosage range and monitor closely.

[US Boxed Warning]: Maximum therapeutic doses of a diuretic and two antihypertensives should be used before this drug is ever added. Should be given with a diuretic to minimize fluid gain and a beta-blocker (if no contraindications) to prevent tachycardia and increased myocardial workload. Patients with malignant hypertension and those already receiving guanethidine should be hospitalized with close medical supervision to ensure blood pressure is reducing and to prevent too rapid of a reduction in blood pressure. Rapid control of blood pressure in patients with severe hypertension can lead to syncope, cerebrovascular accidents, MI, and/or ischemia of other special sense organs resulting in decrease or loss of vision or hearing. Patients with compromised circulation or cryoglobulinemia may also suffer ischemic episodes of the affected organs. Potentially significant drug-drug interactions may exist, requiring dose or frequency adjustment, additional monitoring, and/or selection of alternative therapy.

Adverse Reactions

Cardiovascular: Angina pectoris, cardiac failure, ECG changes (T-wave changes), edema (reversible), pericardial effusion (occasionally with tamponade), pericarditis, tachycardia

Dermatologic: Bullous rash (rare), hypertrichosis, skin rash, Stevens-Johnson syndrome (rare), toxic epidermal necrolysis

Endocrine & metabolic: Breast tenderness (rare), sodium retention, water retention, weight gain

Gastrointestinal: Nausea, vomiting

Hematologic & oncologic: Decreased hematocrit (transient, hemodilution), decreased red blood cells (transient, hemodilution), hemoglobin (transient, hemodilution), leukopenia (rare), thrombocytopenia (rare)

Hepatic: Ascites, increased serum alkaline phosphatase

Renal: Increased blood urea nitrogen (transient), increased serum creatinine (transient)

Respiratory: Pulmonary edema (Lee 2011)

Rare by important or life-threatening: Breast tenderness (rare)

Drug Interactions

Metabolism/Transport Effects None known.

Avoid Concomitant Use There are no known interactions where it is recommended to avoid concomitant use.

Increased Effect/Toxicity

Minoxidil (Systemic) may increase the levels/effects of: Amifostine; Antihypertensives; DULoxetine; Hypotensive Agents; Levodopa; Obinutuzumab; RisperiDONE; RiTUXimab

The levels/effects of Minoxidil (Systemic) may be increased by: Alfuzosin; Atazanavir; Barbiturates; Brimonidine (Topical); CycloSPORINE (Systemic); Dapoxetine; Diazoxide; Herbs (Hypotensive Properties); MAO Inhibitors; Nicorandil; Pentoxifylline; Phosphodiesterase 5 Inhibitors; Probenecid; Prostacyclin Analogues; Valproic Acid and Derivatives

Decreased Effect

The levels/effects of Minoxidil (Systemic) may be decreased by: Herbs (Hypertensive Properties); Methylphenidate; Yohimbine

Storage/Stability Store between 20°C and 25°C (68°F and 77°F).

Mechanism of Action Produces vasodilation by directly relaxing arteriolar smooth muscle, with little effect on veins; effects may be mediated by cyclic AMP; stimulation of hair growth is secondary to vasodilation, increased cutaneous blood flow and stimulation of resting hair follicles

Pharmacodynamics Hypotensive effects:

Onset of action: Within 30 minutes

Maximum effect: Within 2-8 hours

Duration: Up to 2-5 days

Pharmacokinetics (Adult data unless noted)

Metabolism: 88% primarily via glucuronidation

Protein-binding: None

Bioavailability: 90%

Half-life, adults: 3.5-4.2 hours

Elimination: 12% excreted unchanged in urine

Dialysis: Dialyzable (50% to 100%)

Dosing: Usual Hypertension:

Children <12 years: Initial: 0.1-0.2 mg/kg once daily; maximum dose: 5 mg/day; increase gradually every 3 days; usual dosage: 0.25-1 mg/kg/day in 1-2 divided doses; maximum dose: 50 mg/day

Children >12 years and Adults: Initial: 5 mg once daily, increase gradually every 3 days; usual dose: 10-40 mg/day in 1-2 divided doses; maximum dose: 100 mg/day; **Note:** Usual dosage range for Adolescents ≥18 years and Adults (JNC 7): 2.5-80 mg/day in 1-2 divided doses

Administration May be administered without regard to food

Monitoring Parameters Fluids and electrolytes, body weight, blood pressure

Additional Information May take 1-6 months for hypertrichosis to totally reverse after oral minoxidil therapy is discontinued

Dosage Forms Excipient information presented when available (limited, particularly for generics); consult specific product labeling.

Tablet, Oral:

Generic: 2.5 mg, 10 mg

◆ **Mint-Amlodipine (Can)** *see* AmLODIPine *on page 133*

◆ **Mint-Atenolol (Can)** *see* Atenolol *on page 215*

◆ **Mint-Celecoxib (Can)** *see* Celecoxib *on page 418*

◆ **Mint-Ciproflox (Can)** *see* Ciprofloxacin (Systemic) *on page 463*

◆ **Mint-Ciprofloxacin (Can)** *see* Ciprofloxacin (Systemic) *on page 463*

◆ **Mint-Citalopram (Can)** *see* Citalopram *on page 476*

◆ **Mint-Ezetimibe (Can)** *see* Ezetimibe *on page 832*

◆ **Mint-Fluoxetine (Can)** *see* FLUoxetine *on page 906*

◆ **Mint-Losartan (Can)** *see* Losartan *on page 1302*

◆ **Mint-Metformin (Can)** *see* MetFORMIN *on page 1375*

◆ **Mint-Montelukast (Can)** *see* Montelukast *on page 1459*

◆ **Mint-Olanzapine ODT (Can)** *see* OLANZapine *on page 1546*

◆ **Mint-Ondansetron (Can)** *see* Ondansetron *on page 1564*

◆ **Mint-Pantoprazole (Can)** *see* Pantoprazole *on page 1618*

◆ **Mint-Pravastatin (Can)** *see* Pravastatin *on page 1749*

◆ **Mint-Risperidone (Can)** *see* RisperiDONE *on page 1866*

◆ **Mint-Rosuvastatin (Can)** *see* Rosuvastatin *on page 1886*

◆ **MINT-Sertraline (Can)** *see* Sertraline *on page 1916*

◆ **Mint-Sildenafil (Can)** *see* Sildenafil *on page 1921*

◆ **Mint-Simvastatin (Can)** *see* Simvastatin *on page 1928*

◆ **Mint-Topiramate (Can)** *see* Topiramate *on page 2085*

◆ **Miochol-E** *see* Acetylcholine *on page 56*

◆ **Miochol®-E (Can)** *see* Acetylcholine *on page 56*

◆ **MiraLax [OTC]** *see* Polyethylene Glycol 3350 *on page 1723*

◆ **Miranel AF [OTC]** *see* Miconazole (Topical) *on page 1431*

Misoprostol (mye soe PROST ole)

Medication Safety Issues

Sound-alike/look-alike issues:

Cytotec may be confused with Cytoxan

Misoprostol may be confused with metoprolol, mifepristone

Related Information

Safe Handling of Hazardous Drugs *on page 2455*

Brand Names: US Cytotec

Brand Names: Canada Novo-Misoprostol; PMS-Misoprostol

Therapeutic Category Gastrointestinal Agent, Gastric Ulcer Treatment; Prostaglandin

Generic Availability (US) Yes

Use Prevention of NSAID-induced gastric ulcers (FDA approved in adults)

Pregnancy Risk Factor X

Pregnancy Considerations Teratogenic effects were not observed in animal reproduction studies. Congenital anomalies following first trimester exposure have been reported, including skull defects, cranial nerve palsies, falcial malformations, and limb defects. Misoprostol may produce uterine contractions; fetal death, uterine perforation, and abortion may occur. **[U.S. Boxed Warning]: Use**

of misoprostol during pregnancy may cause abortion, birth defects, or premature birth. It is not to be used to reduce NSAID-induced ulcers in a woman of child-bearing potential unless she is capable of complying with effective contraceptive measures and is at high risk of developing gastric ulcers and/or their complications. If needed, the patient must have a negative pregnancy test within 2 weeks of starting therapy, she must use effective contraception during treatment, and therapy should begin on the second or third day of next normal menstrual period. Written and verbal warnings concerning the hazards of misoprostol should be provided.

Misoprostol is FDA approved for the medical termination of pregnancy of ≤49 days in conjunction with mifepristone.

Because misoprostol may induce or augment uterine contractions, it has been used off-label as a cervical-ripening agent for induction of labor in women who have not had a prior cesarean delivery or major uterine surgery. Hyperstimulation of the uterus, uterine rupture, or adverse events in the fetus or mother may occur with this use.

Breast-Feeding Considerations Misoprostol acid (the active metabolite of misoprostol) has been detected in breast milk. Concentrations following a single oral dose were 7.6-20.9 pg/mL after 1 hour and decreased to <1 pg/mL by 5 hours. Adverse events have not been reported in nursing infants (FIGO, 2012).

Contraindications Hypersensitivity to prostaglandins; pregnancy (when used to reduce NSAID-induced ulcers)

Warnings/Precautions Hazardous agent; use appropriate precautions for handling and disposal (NIOSH 2014 [group 3]).

[U.S. Boxed Warning]: Due to the abortifacient property of this medication, patients must be warned not to give this drug to others. [U.S. Boxed Warning]: Use of misoprostol during pregnancy may cause abortion, birth defects, or premature birth. It is not to be used to reduce NSAID-induced ulcers in a woman of child-bearing potential unless she is capable of complying with effective contraceptive measures and is at high risk of developing gastric ulcers and/or their complications. If needed, the patient must have a negative pregnancy test within two weeks of starting therapy, she must use effective contraception during treatment and therapy should begin on the second or third day of next normal menstrual period. Women of childbearing potential taking this for reducing the risk of NSAID-induced gastric ulcers should be given oral and written warnings of the potential adverse events if pregnancy occurs during treatment. Adverse events have been reported when used outside of current product labeling (cervical ripening, induction of labor, postpartum hemorrhage). Uterine tachysystole may occur and progress to uterine tetany; uteroplacental blood flow may be impaired and uterine rupture or amniotic fluid embolism may occur. The risk of uterine rupture may be increased with advanced gestational age, grand multiparity, or prior uterine surgery. Uterine activity and fetal status should be monitored in a hospital setting. Misoprostol should not be used in situations where uterotonic drugs are otherwise contraindicated or inappropriate.

When used for ulcers, use only in patients at high risk of complications from gastric ulcers (eg, the elderly or patients with concomitant diseases) or patients at high risk for developing gastric ulcers (eg, those with a history of ulcers) taking NSAIDs. Misoprostol must be taken during the duration of NSAID therapy. It is not effective in preventing duodenal ulcers in patients taking NSAIDs.

Use with caution in patients with cardiovascular disease, renal impairment, and the elderly.

Adverse Reactions

Central nervous system: Headache

Gastrointestinal: Abdominal pain, constipation, diarrhea, dyspepsia, flatulence, nausea, vomiting

Rare but important or life-threatening: Abnormal taste, abnormal vision, alkaline phosphatase increased, alopecia, anaphylaxis, anemia, amylase increase, anxiety, arrhythmia, arterial thrombosis, arthralgia, cardiac enzymes increased, chest pain, chills, confusion, CVA, deafness, depression, diaphoresis, dizziness, drowsiness, dysphagia, dyspnea, dysuria, edema, epistaxis, ESR increased, fatigue, fever, GI bleeding, GI inflammation, gingivitis, glycosuria, gout; gynecological disorders, hematuria, hepatobiliary function abnormal, hyper-/hypotension, impotence, loss of libido, MI, muscle cramps, myalgia, neuropathy, neurosis, nitrogen increased, pallor, phlebitis, polyuria, pulmonary embolism, purpura, rash, reflux, rigors, stiffness, syncope, thirst, thrombocytopenia, tinnitus, uterine rupture, weakness, weight changes

Drug Interactions

Metabolism/Transport Effects None known.

Avoid Concomitant Use

Avoid concomitant use of Misoprostol with any of the following: Carbetocin

Increased Effect/Toxicity

Misoprostol may increase the levels/effects of: Carbetocin; Oxytocin

The levels/effects of Misoprostol may be increased by: Antacids

Decreased Effect There are no known significant interactions involving a decrease in effect.

Food Interactions Misoprostol peak serum concentrations may be decreased if taken with food (not clinically significant).

Storage/Stability Store at or below 25°C (77°F).

Mechanism of Action Misoprostol is a synthetic prostaglandin E_1 analog that replaces the protective prostaglandins consumed with prostaglandin-inhibiting therapies (eg, NSAIDs); has been shown to induce uterine contractions

Pharmacodynamics Inhibition of gastric acid secretion:

Onset of action: 30 minutes

Maximum effect: 60-90 minutes

Duration: 3 hours

Pharmacokinetics (Adult data unless noted)

Absorption: Rapid and extensive

Protein binding (misoprostol acid): 80% to 90%

Metabolism: Extensive "first pass" de-esterification to misoprostol acid (active metabolite)

Bioavailability: 88%

Half-life (metabolite): Terminal: 20-40 minutes

Time to peak serum concentration (active metabolite): Fasting: 14 ± 8 minutes

Elimination: In urine (~80%)

Dosing: Usual Oral: Prevention of NSAID-induced ulcers: Adults: 200 mcg 4 times/day; if not tolerated, may decrease dose to 100 mcg 4 times/day; take for the duration of NSAID therapy

Dosage adjustment in renal impairment: Half-life, maximum plasma concentration, and bioavailability may be increased; however, a correlation has not been observed with degree of dysfunction. Decrease dose if recommended dose is not tolerated

Administration Hazardous agent; use appropriate precautions for handling and disposal (NIOSH 2014 [group 3]).

Oral: Administer after meals and at bedtime

Additional Information Has also been used to improve absorption in cystic fibrosis patients 8-16 years of age at doses of 100 mcg 4 times daily, in conjunction with pancreatic enzyme supplements (limited data available)

Dosage Forms Excipient information presented when available (limited, particularly for generics); consult specific product labeling.

Tablet, Oral:
Cytotec: 100 mcg
Cytotec: 200 mcg [scored]
Generic: 100 mcg, 200 mcg

◆ **Mitigare** *see* Colchicine *on page 528*

Mitotane (MYE toe tane)

Medication Safety Issues

Sound-alike/look-alike issues:

Mitotane may be confused with mitoMYcin, mitoXANtrone

High alert medication:

This medication is in a class the Institute for Safe Medication Practices (ISMP) includes among its list of drug classes which have a heightened risk of causing significant patient harm when used in error.

Related Information

Oral Medications That Should Not Be Crushed or Altered *on page 2476*

Prevention of Chemotherapy-Induced Nausea and Vomiting in Children *on page 2368*

Safe Handling of Hazardous Drugs *on page 2455*

Brand Names: US Lysodren

Brand Names: Canada Lysodren

Therapeutic Category Antineoplastic Agent, Miscellaneous

Generic Availability (US) No

Use Treatment of inoperable adrenocortical carcinoma (both functional and nonfunctional types) (FDA approved in adults)

Pregnancy Risk Factor D

Pregnancy Considerations Animal reproduction studies have not been conducted. May cause fetal harm if administered during pregnancy; adverse outcomes have been reported. Women of reproductive potential should use effective contraception during treatment and after treatment until plasma levels are no longer detected.

Breast-Feeding Considerations Mitotane has been detected in human breast milk. Due to the potential for serious adverse reactions in the nursing infant, breastfeeding should be discontinued until plasma levels are no longer detected.

Contraindications Hypersensitivity to mitotane or any component of the formulation

Warnings/Precautions Hazardous agent - use appropriate precautions for handling and disposal (NIOSH 2014 [group 1]). Patients treated with mitotane may develop adrenal insufficiency; steroid replacement with glucocorticoid, and sometimes mineralocorticoid, is necessary. It has been recommended that steroid replacement therapy be initiated at the start of therapy, rather than waiting for evidence of adrenal insufficiency. **[U.S. Boxed Warning]: Because the primary action of mitotane is through adrenal suppression, discontinue mitotane temporarily with onset of shock or severe trauma; administer appropriate steroid coverage.** Because mitotane can increase the metabolism of exogenous steroids, higher than usual replacement steroid doses may be required. Mitotane increases hormone binding proteins; monitor free cortisol and corticotropin levels for optimal replacement. Surgically remove tumor tissues from metastatic masses prior to initiation of treatment; rapid cytotoxic effect may cause tumor hemorrhage. Long-term (>2 years) use may lead to brain damage or functional impairment; observe patients for neurotoxicity (neurologic and behavior) regularly. Plasma concentrations >20 mcg/mL are associated with an increased incidence of higher-grade neurotoxicity. Neurologic impairment may reverse upon discontinuation. Use caution with hepatic impairment (other than metastatic lesions from adrenal cortex); metabolism may be decreased. Other CNS adverse effects, including lethargy, sedation, and vertigo may occur; patients must be cautioned about performing tasks which require mental alertness (eg, operating machinery or driving). CNS effects may be potentiated when used with other sedative drugs or ethanol. The manufacturer recommends initiating treatment within a hospital environment until a stabilized dose is achieved. Continue treatment as long as clinical benefit (maintenance of clinical status or metastatic lesion growth slowing) is observed. Clinical benefit is usually observed within 3 months at maximum tolerated dose, although 10% of patients may require more than 3 months for benefit. Continuous treatment at the maximum tolerated dose is generally the best approach. Some patients have been treated intermittently, restarting when severe symptoms reappear, although often response is no longer observed after 3 or 4 courses of intermittent treatment. Potentially significant drug-drug interactions may exist, requiring dose or frequency adjustment, additional monitoring, and/or selection of alternative therapy. Prolonged bleeding time may occur; consider bleeding possibility prior to any surgical intervention. **[U.S. Boxed Warnings]: Should be administered under the supervision of an experienced cancer chemotherapy physician.** Mitotane is associated with a moderate emetic potential; antiemetics may be needed to prevent nausea and vomiting.

Warnings: Additional Pediatric Considerations Growth, motor skill, and speech delays were observed during therapy in an infant treated for adenocarcinoma (DeLeon, 2002).

Adverse Reactions The majority of adverse events are dose-dependent.

Central nervous system: Central nervous system depression, confusion, dizziness, drowsiness, headache, lethargy, vertigo

Dermatologic: Skin rash

Gastrointestinal: Anorexia, diarrhea, nausea, vomiting

Neuromuscular & skeletal: Tremor, weakness

Rare but important or life-threatening: Abnormal thyroid function test, adrenocortical insufficiency, albuminuria, anemia, autoimmune hepatitis, blurred vision, brain damage (may be reversible), cataract, decreased protein-bound iodine, diplopia, generalized aches, growth suppression, gynecomastia, hematuria, hemorrhagic cystitis, hepatitis, hypercholesterolemia, hyperpyrexia, hypertension, hypertriglyceridemia, hypogonadism (primary), hypouricemia, increased gamma-glutamyl transferase, increased liver enzymes, increased serum transaminases, increased serum triglycerides, increased sex hormone binding globulin, leukopenia, macular edema, maculopathy, memory impairment, mental deficiency, mucositis, myalgia, neuropathy, neutropenia, orthostatic hypotension, prolonged bleeding time, psychological disturbances (neuro), retinopathy (toxic), thrombocytopenia

Drug Interactions

Metabolism/Transport Effects Induces CYP3A4 (strong)

Avoid Concomitant Use

Avoid concomitant use of Mitotane with any of the following: Abiraterone Acetate; Apixaban; Apremilast; Artemether; Axitinib; Bedaquiline; Boceprevir; Bortezomib; Bosutinib; Cabozantinib; Ceritinib; CloZAPine; Crizotinib; Dasabuvir; Dienogest; Dronedarone; Eliglustat; Enzalutamide; Everolimus; Ibrutinib; Idelalisib; Irinotecan; Isavuconazonium Sulfate; Itraconazole; Ivabradine; Ivacaftor; Lapatinib; Lumefantrine; Lurasidone; Macitentan; Mifepristone; Naloxegol; Netupitant; NIFEdipine; Nilotinib; NiMODipine; Nisoldipine; Olaparib; Ombitasvir; Palbociclib; Panobinostat; Paritaprevir; PAZOPanib; Perampanel; PONATinib; Praziquantel; Ranolazine; Regorafenib; Rivaroxaban; Roflumilast; RomiDEPsin; Simeprevir; SORAfenib; Suvorexant; Tasimelteon; Telaprevir; Ticagrelor; Tofacitinib; Tolvaptan; Toremifene;

Trabectedin; Ulipristal; Vandetanib; Vemurafenib; VinCRIStine (Liposomal); Vorapaxar

Increased Effect/Toxicity

Mitotane may increase the levels/effects of: Clarithromycin; Ifosfamide

The levels/effects of Mitotane may be increased by: Clarithromycin; MAO Inhibitors

Decreased Effect

Mitotane may decrease the levels/effects of: Abiraterone Acetate; Apixaban; Apremilast; ARIPiprazole; Artemether; Axitinib; Bedaquiline; Boceprevir; Bortezomib; Bosutinib; Brentuximab Vedotin; Cabozantinib; Cannabidiol; Cannabis; Ceritinib; Clarithromycin; CloZAPine; Corticosteroids (Systemic); Crizotinib; CYP3A4 Substrates; Dasabuvir; Dasatinib; Dexamethasone (Systemic); Dienogest; DOXOrubicin (Conventional); Dronabinol; Dronedarone; Eliglustat; Enzalutamide; Erlotinib; Everolimus; Exemestane; FentaNYL; Gefitinib; GuanFACINE; Ibrutinib; Idelalisib; Ifosfamide; Imatinib; Irinotecan; Isavuconazonium Sulfate; Itraconazole; Ivabradine; Ivacaftor; Ixabepilone; Lapatinib; Linagliptin; Lumefantrine; Lurasidone; Macitentan; Maraviroc; MethylPREDNISolone; Mifepristone; Naloxegol; Netupitant; NIFEdipine; Nilotinib; NiMODipine; Nisoldipine; Olaparib; Ombitasvir; Palbociclib; Panobinostat; Paritaprevir; PAZOPanib; Perampanel; PONATinib; Praziquantel; Propafenone; QUEtiapine; Ranolazine; Regorafenib; Rivaroxaban; Roflumilast; RomiDEPsin; Saxagliptin; Simeprevir; SORAfenib; SUNItinib; Suvorexant; Tadalafil; Tasimelteon; Telaprevir; Tetrahydrocannabinol; Ticagrelor; Tofacitinib; Tolvaptan; Toremifene; Trabectedin; Ulipristal; Vandetanib; Vemurafenib; Vilazodone; VinCRIStine (Liposomal); Vorapaxar; Vortioxetine; Zaleplon; Zuclopenthixol

The levels/effects of Mitotane may be decreased by: Spironolactone

Storage/Stability Store at 25°C (77°F); excursions are permitted between 15°C and 30°C (59°F and 86°F).

Mechanism of Action Adrenolytic agent which causes adrenal cortical atrophy; affects mitochondria in adrenal cortical cells and decreases production of cortisol; also alters the peripheral metabolism of steroids

Pharmacodynamics Onset of action: Antitumor response: Achieved at serum concentrations ≥14 mcg/mL; Pediatric patients: In experience with treatment of adenocarcinoma reported 1.5-12.5 months to reach 10 mcg/mL with subsequent rapid escalation of serum concentration, clinical response may be observed earlier (Rodriguez-Galindo, 2005; Zancanella, 2006); Adults: Typically within 3 months

Pharmacokinetics (Adult data unless noted)

Absorption: Oral: ~40%

Distribution: Stored mainly in fat tissue but is found in all body tissues

Metabolism: Hepatic and other tissues

Half-life, elimination: 18-159 days; serum concentrations undetectable after 6-9 weeks in majority of patients

Time to peak serum concentration: 3-5 hours

Elimination: Urine (~10%, as metabolites); feces (1% to 17%, as metabolites)

Dosing: Usual

Pediatric: **Adrenocortical carcinoma (stage III or IV):** Limited data available: Children and Adolescents: Oral: Initial: 0.5 to 1 g/day in 3 divided doses, titrate dose to target serum concentration range of 14-20 mcg/mL; initially, monitor serum concentrations every 2 to 4 weeks until serum concentration of 10 mcg/mL is achieved, then monitor every 1 to 2 weeks due to rapid drug accumulation and narrow therapeutic window; once target serum concentration (14 to 20 mcg/mL) is reached, continue to monitor every 1 to 2 weeks and adjust dose to maintain therapeutic range (dosage reduction may be necessary in some cases); has also been used in combination with CED regimen (cisplatin, etoposide, and doxorubicin). An initial target daily dose of 4 g/m^2/day was used in an open-label, prospective study (n=11; age range: 2 to 15 years); however, the reported range to initially achieve a serum concentration of 14 ± 2 mcg/mL was 1.6 to 7.3 g/m^2/day; and then further reductions to 1 to 5.3 g/m^2/day were required to maintain therapeutic concentrations (Zancanella 2006). In an ongoing trial at some centers, a similar target dose of 4 g/m^2/day is being evaluated using a titration schedule: Initial dose: 1 to 2 g/m^2/day in 4 divided doses with weekly titration in 1 to 2 g/m^2/day increments; maximum daily dose: 4 g/m^2/day (NCT00304070 2014); **Note:** In general, optimal treatment for pediatric adrenocortical carcinoma is unknown.

Adult: **Adrenocortical carcinoma:** Oral:

Manufacturer's labeling: Initial: 2 to 6 g daily in 3 to 4 divided doses, then increase incrementally to 9 to 10 g daily in 3 to 4 divided doses (maximum tolerated range: 2 to 16 g daily, usually 9 to 10 g daily; maximum dose studied: 18 to 19 g daily); continue as long as clinical benefit is demonstrated

Alternate dosing: Limited data available: Initial: 1 to 2 g daily; increase by 1 to 2 g daily at 1 to 2 week intervals as tolerated to a maximum of 6 to 10 g daily; usual dose 4 to 5 g daily (Veytsman 2009)

Dosing adjustment for toxicity: Adult:

Severe side effects: Reduce dose until a maximum tolerated dose is achieved

Significant neuropsychiatric adverse effects: Withhold treatment for at least 1 week and restart at a lower dose (Allolio 2006)

Dosing adjustment in renal impairment: Adult: There are no dosage adjustments provided in manufacturer's labeling.

Dosing adjustment in hepatic impairment: Adult: There are no dosage adjustments provided in manufacturer's labeling; however, drug accumulation may occur in patients with liver disease; use with caution.

Preparation for Administration Hazardous agent; use appropriate precautions for handling and disposal (NIOSH 2014 [group 1]). Wear impervious gloves when handling; avoid exposure to crushed or broken tablets if possible.

Oral: In pediatric trials, tablets have been crushed and dissolved in MCT (medium-chain triglyceride) oil (ie, each gram mitotane in 2 mL MCT oil); then solution was mixed with a fat-containing food [eg, milk (white or chocolate) or yogurt] (Zancanella 2006)

Administration Hazardous agent; use appropriate precautions for handling and disposal (NIOSH 2014 [group 1]). Wear impervious gloves when handling; avoid exposure to crushed or broken tablets if possible. **Note:** Mitotane is associated with a moderate emetic potential; antiemetics may be needed to prevent nausea and vomiting.

Oral: Per the manufacturer, do not crush tablets; however, in pediatric trials, tablets have been crushed and dissolved in MCT (medium-chain triglyceride) oil (ie, each gram mitotane in 2 mL MCT oil); then solution was mixed with a fat-containing food [eg, milk (white or chocolate) or yogurt] (Zancanella, 2006)

Monitoring Parameters Adrenal function; neurologic assessments (including behavioral) at regular intervals with chronic (>2 years) use.

Pediatric: Monitor mitotane serum concentrations initially every 2-4 weeks until serum concentration of 10 mcg/mL is achieved, then monitor every 1-2 weeks (even after target concentration of 14-20 mcg/mL is reached) and use conservative dose adjustments due to drug accumulation and narrow therapeutic window (Zancanella, 2006)

Adult: Monitor mitotane serum concentrations (gas chromatography-flame ionization assay) every 4-8 weeks until levels at 10-14 mg/L are attained, then monitor every 3 months; urinary free cortisol levels; TSH and free thyroxine every few months (Veytsman, 2009)

Dosage Forms Excipient information presented when available (limited, particularly for generics); consult specific product labeling.

Tablet, Oral:

Lysodren: 500 mg [scored]

MitoXANtrone (mye toe ZAN trone)

Medication Safety Issues

Sound-alike/look-alike issues:

MitoXANtrone may be confused with methotrexate, mitoMYcin, mitotane, Mutamycin

High alert medication:

This medication is in a class the Institute for Safe Medication Practices (ISMP) includes among its list of drug classes which have a heightened risk of causing significant patient harm when used in error.

Related Information

Management of Drug Extravasations *on page 2298*

Prevention of Chemotherapy-Induced Nausea and Vomiting in Children *on page 2368*

Safe Handling of Hazardous Drugs *on page 2455*

Brand Names: Canada Mitoxantrone Injection; Mitoxantrone Injection USP

Therapeutic Category Antineoplastic Agent, Anthracenedione; Antineoplastic Agent, Antibiotic; Antineoplastic Agent, Topoisomerase II Inhibitor

Generic Availability (US) Yes

Use Treatment of acute nonlymphocytic leukemias (ANLL; includes myelogenous, promyelocytic, monocytic, and erythroid leukemias); advanced hormone-refractory prostate cancer, secondary progressive, or relapsing-remitting multiple sclerosis (MS) (FDA approved in adults); has also been used for Hodgkin's lymphoma, non-Hodgkin's lymphomas (NHL), acute lymphocytic leukemia (ALL), myelodysplastic syndrome, breast cancer, pediatric acute myelogenous leukemia (AML), pediatric acute promyelocytic leukemia (APL); part of a conditioning regimen for autologous hematopoietic stem-cell transplantation (HSCT)

Medication Guide Available Yes

Pregnancy Risk Factor D

Pregnancy Considerations Adverse effects were noted in animal reproduction studies. May cause fetal harm if administered to a pregnant woman. Pregnancy should be avoided while on treatment. Women with multiple sclerosis who are of reproductive potential should have a pregnancy test prior to each dose.

Breast-Feeding Considerations Mitoxantrone is excreted in human milk and significant concentrations (18 ng/mL) have been reported for 28 days after the last administration. Because of the potential for serious adverse reactions in infants from mitoxantrone, breast-feeding should be discontinued before starting treatment.

Contraindications Hypersensitivity to mitoxantrone or any component of the formulation

Canadian labeling: Additional contraindications (not in U.S. labeling): Prior hypersensitivity to anthracyclines; prior substantial anthracycline exposure and abnormal cardiac function prior to initiation of mitoxantrone therapy; presence of severe myelosuppression due to prior chemo- and/or radiotherapy; severe hepatic impairment; intrathecal administration

Warnings/Precautions Hazardous agent - use appropriate precautions for handling and disposal (NIOSH 2014 [group 1]).

[U.S. Boxed Warning]: Usually should not be administered if baseline neutrophil count <1500 cells/mm^3 (except for treatment of ANLL). Monitor blood counts and monitor for infection due to neutropenia. Treatment may lead to severe myelosuppression; unless the expected benefit outweighs the risk, use is generally not recommended in patients with pre-existing myelosuppression from prior chemotherapy.

[U.S. Boxed Warning]: May cause myocardial toxicity and potentially-fatal heart failure (HF); risk increases with cumulative dosing. Effects may occur during therapy or may be delayed (months or years after completion of therapy). Predisposing factors for mitoxantrone-induced cardiotoxicity include prior anthracycline or anthracenedione therapy, prior cardiovascular disease, concomitant use of cardiotoxic drugs, and mediastinal/pericardial irradiation, although may also occur in patients without risk factors. Prior to therapy initiation, evaluate all patients for cardiac-related signs/symptoms, including history, physical exam, and ECG; and evaluate baseline left ventricular ejection fraction (LVEF) with echocardiogram or multigated radionuclide angiography (MUGA) or MRI. Not recommended for use in MS patients when LVEF <50%, or baseline LVEF below the lower limit of normal (LLN). Evaluate for cardiac signs/symptoms (by history, physical exam, and ECG) and evaluate LVEF (using same method as baseline LVEF) in MS patients prior to each dose and if signs/symptoms of HF develop. Use in MS should be limited to a cumulative dose of ≤140 mg/m^2, and discontinued if LVEF falls below LLN or a significant decrease in LVEF is observed; decreases in LVEF and HF have been observed in patients with MS who have received cumulative doses <100 mg/m^2. Patients with MS should undergo annual LVEF evaluation following discontinuation of therapy to monitor for delayed cardiotoxicity.

[U.S. Boxed Warning]: For IV administration only, into a free-flowing IV; may cause severe local tissue damage if extravasation occurs; do not administer subcutaneously, intramuscularly, or intra-arterially. Do not administer intrathecally; may cause serious and permanent neurologic damage. Irritant with vesicant-like properties; extravasation resulting in burning, erythema, pain, swelling and skin discoloration (blue) has been reported; may result in tissue necrosis and require debridement for skin graft. Ensure proper needle or catheter placement prior to and during infusion. Avoid extravasation. May cause urine, saliva, tears, and sweat to turn blue-green for 24 hours postinfusion. Whites of eyes may have blue-green tinge. **[U.S. Boxed Warning]: Treatment with mitoxantrone increases the risk of developing secondary acute myelogenous leukemia (AML) in patients with cancer and in patients with MS;** acute promyelocytic leukemia (APL) has also been observed. Symptoms of acute leukemia include excessive bruising, bleeding and recurrent infections. The risk for secondary leukemia is increased in patients who are heavily pretreated, with higher doses, and with combination chemotherapy.

[U.S. Boxed Warning]: Should be administered under the supervision of a physician experienced in cancer chemotherapy agents. Dosage should be reduced in patients with impaired hepatobiliary function (clearance is reduced). Canadian labeling contraindicates use in severe hepatic impairment. Not for treatment of multiple sclerosis in patients with concurrent hepatic impairment. Not for treatment of primary progressive multiple sclerosis. Rapid lysis of tumor cells may lead to hyperuricemia.

Adverse Reactions

Cardiovascular: Arrhythmia, cardiac function changes, CHF, ECG changes, edema, hypertension, ischemia, LVEF decreased

Central nervous system: Anxiety, chills, depression, fatigue, fever, headache, pain, seizure

Dermatologic: Alopecia, cutaneous mycosis, nail bed changes, petechiae/bruising, skin infection

Endocrine & metabolic: Amenorrhea, hypocalcemia, hyperglycemia, hypokalemia, hyponatremia, menorrhagia, menstrual disorder

Gastrointestinal: Abdominal pain, anorexia, aphthosis, constipation, diarrhea, dyspepsia, GI bleeding, mucositis, nausea, stomatitis, vomiting, weight gain/loss

Genitourinary: Abnormal urine, impotence, sterility, urinary tract infection

Hematologic: Anemia, granulocytopenia, hemoglobin decreased, hemorrhage, leukopenia, lymphopenia, neutropenia, neutropenic fever, secondary acute leukemias (includes AML, APL), thrombocytopenia

Hepatic: Alkaline phosphatase increased, GGT increased, jaundice, transaminases increased

Neuromuscular & skeletal: Arthralgia, back pain, myalgia, weakness

Ocular: Blurred vision, conjunctivitis

Renal: BUN increased, creatinine increased, hematuria, proteinuria, renal failure

Respiratory: Cough, dyspnea, pharyngitis, pneumonia, rhinitis, sinusitis, upper respiratory tract infection

Miscellaneous: Diaphoresis, fungal infection, infection, sepsis (ANLL), systemic infection

Rare but important or life-threatening: Allergic reaction, anaphylactoid reactions, anaphylaxis, chest pain, dehydration; extravasation at injection site (may result in burning, erythema, pain, skin discoloration, swelling, or tissue necrosis); interstitial pneumonitis (with combination chemotherapy), hyperuricemia, hypotension, phlebitis at the infusion site, rash, sclera discoloration (blue), tachycardia, urine discoloration (blue-green), urticaria

Drug Interactions

Metabolism/Transport Effects Substrate of BCRP

Avoid Concomitant Use

Avoid concomitant use of MitoXANtrone with any of the following: BCG; BCG (Intravesical); CloZAPine; Dipyrone; Natalizumab; Pimecrolimus; Tacrolimus (Topical); Tofacitinib; Vaccines (Live)

Increased Effect/Toxicity

MitoXANtrone may increase the levels/effects of: CloZAPine; Leflunomide; Natalizumab; Tofacitinib; Vaccines (Live)

The levels/effects of MitoXANtrone may be increased by: CycloSPORINE (Systemic); Denosumab; Dipyrone; Pimecrolimus; Roflumilast; Tacrolimus (Topical); Teriflunomide; Trastuzumab

Decreased Effect

MitoXANtrone may decrease the levels/effects of: BCG; BCG (Intravesical); Coccidioides immitis Skin Test; Sipuleucel-T; Vaccines (Inactivated); Vaccines (Live)

The levels/effects of MitoXANtrone may be decreased by: Echinacea

Storage/Stability Store intact vials at 15°C to 25°C (59°F to 77°F); do not freeze. Opened vials may be stored at room temperature for 7 days or under refrigeration for up to 14 days. Solutions diluted for administration are stable for 7 days at room temperature or under refrigeration, although the manufacturer recommends immediate use.

Mechanism of Action Related to the anthracyclines, mitoxantrone intercalates into DNA resulting in cross-links and strand breaks; binds to nucleic acids and inhibits DNA and RNA synthesis by template disordering and steric obstruction; replication is decreased by binding to DNA topoisomerase II and seems to inhibit the incorporation of uridine into RNA and thymidine into DNA; active throughout entire cell cycle (cell-cycle nonspecific)

Pharmacokinetics (Adult data unless noted)

Distribution: Distributes into thyroid, liver, pancreas, spleen, heart, bone marrow, and red blood cells; prolonged retention in tissues; excreted in breast milk

V_{dss}: >1000 L/m^2

Protein binding: 78%

Half-life, terminal: 23-215 hours (median: 75 hours); may be prolonged with liver impairment

Elimination: 11% of dose excreted in urine (65% as unchanged drug) and 25% in bile as unchanged drug and metabolites

Dosing: Usual

Pediatric: **Note:** Dosing regimens may vary by dose, cycles, and combination therapy; refer to individual protocols.

Acute lymphocytic leukemia (ALL), relapsed: Children and Adolescents: Induction: 10 mg/m^2/dose once daily for 2 days (in combination with other chemotherapeutic agents) (Parker 2010)

Acute nonlymphocytic leukemias (ANLL):

AML:

Induction:

Infants <1 year:

Weight-based dosing: 0.4 mg/**kg**/dose over 1 hour once daily on days 3 to 6 for a total of 4 doses (in combination with cytarabine and gemtuzumab) (Aplenc 2008)

BSA-based dosing: 9 mg/m^2/dose once daily on days 1, 3, and 5 (in combination with cytarabine and etoposide) (Gibson 2011) **or** 8 mg/m^2/dose once daily for 5 days (in combination with cytarabine) (Perel 2002)

Children <3 years:

Weight-based dosing: 0.4 mg/**kg**/dose over 1 hour once daily on days 3 to 6 for a total of 4 doses (in combination with cytarabine and gemtuzumab) (Aplenc 2008)

BSA-based dosing: 12 mg/m^2/dose once daily for 4 to 5 days (in combination with cytarabine); for incomplete response, may repeat at 12 mg/m^2/dose once daily for 2 days (in combination with cytarabine) (Perel 2002; Wells 2003) **or** 12 mg/m^2/dose once daily on days 1, 3, and 5 (in combination with cytarabine and etoposide) (Gibson 2011)

Children ≥3 years and Adolescents: 12 mg/m^2/dose once daily for 4 to 5 days (in combination with cytarabine); for incomplete response, may repeat at 12 mg/m^2/dose once daily for 2 days (in combination with cytarabine) (Perel 2002; Wells 2003) **or** 12 mg/m^2/dose once daily on days 1, 3, and 5 (in combination with cytarabine and etoposide) (Gibson 2011) **or** 12 mg/m^2/dose over 1 hour once daily on days 3 to 6 for a total of 4 doses (in combination with cytarabine and gemtuzumab) (Aplenc 2008)

Consolidation:

Age-directed dosing (Gibson 2011; Stevens 1998):

Infants <1 year: 7.5 mg/m^2/dose once daily for 5 days

Children and Adolescents 1 to 14 years: 10 mg/m^2/dose once daily for 5 days

BSA-directed dosing (Cooper 2012):

BSA <0.6 m^2: 0.4 mg/**kg**/dose once daily on days 3 to 6 (in combination with cytarabine and gemtuzumab)

BSA ≥0.6 m^2: 12 mg/m^2/dose once daily on days 3 to 6 (in combination with cytarabine and gemtuzumab)

APL: Consolidation: Children ≥2 years and Adolescents: 10 mg/m^2/dose once daily for 5 days (Ortega 2005; Sanz 2004)

Adult:

Acute nonlymphocytic leukemias (ANLL):

AML induction: 12 mg/m^2/dose once daily for 3 days (in combination with cytarabine); for incomplete response, may repeat 7 to 10 days later at 12 mg/m^2/dose once daily for 2 days (Arlin 1990)

AML consolidation (beginning ~6 weeks after initiation of the final induction course): 12 mg/m^2/dose once daily for 2 days (in combination with cytarabine), repeat in 4 weeks (Arlin 1990)

Multiple sclerosis: 12 mg/m^2/dose every 3 months; maximum lifetime cumulative dose: 140 mg/m^2 (discontinue use with LVEF <50% or clinically significant reduction in LVEF)

Prostate cancer (advanced hormone-refractory): 12 to 14 mg/m^2/dose every 3 weeks (in combination with corticosteroids)

Dosing adjustment in hepatic impairment: No dosage adjustment provided in the manufacturer's labeling. Dosage reduction of 50% in patients with serum bilirubin of 1.5-3 mg/dL and dosage reduction of 75% in patients with serum bilirubin >3 mg/dL have been recommended; **Note:** MS patients with hepatic impairment should not receive mitoxantrone.

Dosing adjustment for toxicity:

ANLL patients: Severe or life-threatening nonhematologic toxicity: Withhold treatment until toxicity resolves

MS Patients:

Neutrophils <1500/mm^3: Use is not recommended

Signs/symptoms of HF: Evaluate for cardiac signs/symptoms and LVEF

LVEF <50% or baseline LVEF below the lower limit of normal (LLN): Use is not recommended

Preparation for Administration Hazardous agent; use appropriate precautions for handling and disposal (NIOSH 2014 [group 1]).

Parenteral: Must be diluted prior to administration; volume may vary by protocol; manufacturer recommends diluting in at least 50 mL of NS or D_5W.

Administration Hazardous agent; use appropriate precautions for handling and disposal (NIOSH 2014 [group 1]).

Parenteral: For IV administration only; do not administer by SubQ, IM, intrathecal, or intra-arterial injection. Must be diluted prior to use; may administer by IV bolus over 5 to 15 minutes or IV intermittent infusion over 15 to 60 minutes.

Irritant with vesicant-like properties; ensure proper needle or catheter placement prior to and during infusion; avoid extravasation. If extravasation occurs, stop infusion immediately and disconnect (leave cannula/needle in place); gently aspirate extravasated solution (do **NOT** flush the line); remove needle/cannula; elevate extremity. Initiate antidote (dimethyl sulfate [DMSO] **or** dexrazoxane [Adults]) (see Management of Drug Extravasations for more details). Apply dry cold compresses for 20 minutes 4 times daily for 1 to 2 days (Pérez Fidalgo 2012); withhold cooling beginning 15 minutes before dexrazoxane infusion; continue withholding cooling until 15 minutes after infusion is completed. Topical DMSO should not be administered in combination with dexrazoxane; may lessen dexrazoxane efficacy.

Vesicant/Extravasation Risk Irritant with vesicant-like properties

Monitoring Parameters CBC with differential, platelet count, serum uric acid (for leukemia treatment), liver function tests, women with multiple sclerosis of childbearing potential must have a pregnancy test prior to each dose; injection site for signs of extravasation

Cardiac monitoring: Prior to initiation, evaluate all patients for cardiac-related signs/symptoms, including history, physical exam, and echocardiogram; evaluate baseline and periodic left ventricular ejection fraction (LVEF) with ECG or multigated radionuclide angiography (MUGA) or MRI. In patients with MS, evaluate for cardiac signs/symptoms (by history, physical exam, and ECG) and evaluate LVEF (using same method as baseline LVEF) prior to each dose and if signs/symptoms of HF develop. Patients with MS should undergo annual LVEF evaluation following discontinuation of therapy to monitor for delayed cardiotoxicity.

Additional Information Myelosuppression (leukocyte nadir: 10-14 days; recovery: 21 days); injection contains 0.14 mEq of sodium/mL

Dosage Forms Excipient information presented when available (limited, particularly for generics); consult specific product labeling.

Concentrate, Intravenous:

Generic: 20 mg/10 mL (10 mL); 25 mg/12.5 mL (12.5 mL); 30 mg/15 mL (15 mL)

- ◆ **Mitoxantrone Dihydrochloride** *see* MitoXANtrone *on page* *1448*
- ◆ **Mitoxantrone HCl** *see* MitoXANtrone *on page* *1448*
- ◆ **Mitoxantrone Hydrochloride** *see* MitoXANtrone *on page* *1448*
- ◆ **Mitoxantrone Injection (Can)** *see* MitoXANtrone *on page* *1448*
- ◆ **Mitoxantrone Injection USP (Can)** *see* MitoXANtrone *on page* *1448*
- ◆ **Mitozantrone** *see* MitoXANtrone *on page* *1448*
- ◆ **Mitrazol [OTC]** *see* Miconazole (Topical) *on page* *1431*
- ◆ **MK462** *see* Rizatriptan *on page* *1879*
- ◆ **MK 0517** *see* Fosaprepitant *on page* *939*
- ◆ **MK-0518** *see* Raltegravir *on page* *1833*
- ◆ **MK594** *see* Losartan *on page* *1302*
- ◆ **MK0826** *see* Ertapenem *on page* *777*
- ◆ **MK 869** *see* Aprepitant *on page* *186*
- ◆ **MMF** *see* Mycophenolate *on page* *1473*
- ◆ **MMI** *see* Methimazole *on page* *1386*
- ◆ **MMR** *see* Measles, Mumps, and Rubella Virus Vaccine *on page* *1327*
- ◆ **M-M-R II** *see* Measles, Mumps, and Rubella Virus Vaccine *on page* *1327*
- ◆ **MMRV** *see* Measles, Mumps, Rubella, and Varicella Virus Vaccine *on page* *1330*
- ◆ **Mobic** *see* Meloxicam *on page* *1346*
- ◆ **Mobicox (Can)** *see* Meloxicam *on page* *1346*

Modafinil (moe DAF i nil)

Brand Names: US Provigil

Brand Names: Canada Alertec; Apo-Modafinil; Mar-Modafinil; Teva-Modafinil

Therapeutic Category Central Nervous System Stimulant

Generic Availability (US) Yes

Use To improve wakefulness in patients with excessive daytime sleepiness associated with narcolepsy and shift work sleep disorder (SWSD), as adjunctive therapy for obstructive sleep apnea/hypopnea syndrome (OSAHS) (FDA approved in adults); has also been used for attention-deficit/hyperactivity disorder (ADHD); treatment of fatigue in multiple sclerosis (MS) and other disorders

Medication Guide Available Yes

Pregnancy Risk Factor C

Pregnancy Considerations Adverse events have been observed in some animal reproduction studies. An increased risk of spontaneous abortion and intrauterine growth restriction has been reported with modafinil. Efficacy of steroidal contraceptives (including depot and implantable contraceptives) may be decreased; alternate means of contraception should be considered during therapy and for 1 month after modafinil is discontinued.

Health care providers are encouraged to register pregnant patients exposed to modafinil, or pregnant women may enroll themselves, by calling (866-404-4106).

Breast-Feeding Considerations It is not known if modafinil is excreted in breast milk. The manufacturer recommends that caution be exercised when administering modafinil to nursing women.

Contraindications

Hypersensitivity to modafinil, armodafinil, or any component of the formulation

Canadian labeling: Additional contraindications (not in US labeling): Patients in agitated states or with severe anxiety

Warnings/Precautions The degree of sleepiness should be reassessed frequently; some patients may not return to a normal level of wakefulness. In obstructive sleep apnea, modafinil is indicated as treatment for excessive sleepiness and not for the underlying obstruction. If continuous positive airway pressure (CPAP) is the treatment of choice for a patient, a maximal effort to treat with CPAP for an adequate period of time should be made prior to initiating and during treatment with modafinil for excessive sleepiness. Use with caution in patients with cardiovascular disease; increased blood pressure and heart rate monitoring may be required. Use is not recommended in patients with a history of left ventricular hypertrophy or patients with mitral valve prolapse who have developed mitral valve prolapse syndrome with previous CNS stimulant use. Increased monitoring should be considered in patients with a recent history of myocardial infarction or unstable angina.

Serious and life-threatening rashes, including Stevens-Johnson syndrome, toxic epidermal necrolysis and drug rash with eosinophilia and systemic symptoms (DRESS) have been reported. Although initially reported in children during clinical trials, postmarketing cases have occurred in both children and adults. Most cases have occurred within the first 5 weeks of therapy; however, rare cases have occurred after long-term use (eg, 3 months). No risk factors have been identified to predict occurrence or severity. Patients should be advised to discontinue at first sign of rash (unless the rash is clearly not drug-related). As a result of these serious dermatologic adverse events, approval for the use of modafinil in children for ADHD was denied by the FDA. The serious nature of these dermatologic adverse effects, as well reports of psychiatric events, resulted in the FDA's Pediatric Advisory Committee unanimously recommending that a specific warning against the use of modafinil in children be added to the manufacturer's labeling. Modafinil is not FDA-approved for use in pediatrics for any indication.

Rare cases of multiorgan hypersensitivity reactions (with fatality) in association with modafinil use; lone cases of angioedema and anaphylactoid reactions with armodafinil have been reported (angioedema has been noted in postmarketing reports with modafinil). Signs and symptoms are diverse, reflecting the involvement of specific organs; patients typically present with fever and rash associated with organ-system dysfunction. No risk factors have been identified to predict occurrence or severity of multiorgan hypersensitivity reactions. Patients should be advised to report any signs and symptoms related to these effects; discontinuation of therapy is recommended.

Use with caution in patients with a history of psychosis, depression, or mania. Use may result in emergence of or exacerbation of psychiatric symptoms. Observe for symptoms of aggression, hallucinations, mania, delusions, or suicidal ideation. Consider discontinuing therapy if psychiatric symptoms develop. May impair the ability to engage in potentially hazardous activities; patients must be cautioned about performing tasks which require mental alertness (eg, operating machinery or driving). Use with caution in patients with Tourette syndrome; limited evidence suggests stimulants may exacerbate tics and Tourette syndrome (AACAP [Murphy, 2013]; Pringsheim, 2012; Rossner, 2011). Use caution with renal or hepatic impairment (dosage adjustment in severe hepatic impairment is recommended). Instruct patients to avoid concomitant ethanol consumption.

Warnings: Additional Pediatric Considerations Serious cardiovascular adverse events (including sudden death) in patients (both children and adults) taking usual doses of stimulant medications has been reported. Most of these patients were found to have underlying structural heart disease (eg, hypertrophic obstructive cardiomyopathy). The American Heart Association recommends that all children diagnosed with ADHD who may be candidates for stimulant medication, such as modafinil, should have a thorough cardiovascular assessment prior to initiation of therapy. This assessment should include a combination of thorough medical history, family history, and physical examination. An ECG is not mandatory but should be considered.

Use with caution in patients with Tourette syndrome; stimulants may unmask tics. Children may experience a higher frequency of some adverse effects than adults including the following: Insomnia (29% vs 5%), decreased appetite (16% vs 4%), weight loss, and abdominal pain. The following were reported in controlled, open-label clinical studies in children: Cataplexy increased, hostility, hypnagogic hallucinations, suicidal ideation, and Tourette syndrome.

Adverse Reactions

Cardiovascular: Chest pain, edema, hypertension, palpitation, tachycardia, vasodilation

Central nervous system: Agitation, anxiety (dose related), chills, confusion, depression, dizziness, emotional lability, headache (occurs more frequently in adults; dose related), insomnia, nervousness, somnolence, vertigo

Dermatologic: Rash (includes some severe cases requiring hospitalization)

Gastrointestinal: Abdominal pain (occurs more frequently in children), anorexia, appetite decreased (occurs more frequently in children), constipation, diarrhea, dyspepsia, flatulence, mouth ulceration, nausea, taste perversion, weight loss (occurs more frequently in children), xerostomia

Genitourinary: Abnormal urine, hematuria, pyuria

Hematologic: Eosinophilia

Hepatic: LFTs abnormal

Neuromuscular & skeletal: Back pain, dyskinesia, hyperkinesia, hypertonia, neck rigidity, paresthesia, tremor

Ocular: Abnormal vision, amblyopia, eye pain

Respiratory: Asthma, epistaxis, lung disorder, pharyngitis, rhinitis

Miscellaneous: Diaphoresis, flu-like syndrome, herpes simplex infection, thirst

Postmarketing and/or case reports: Agranulocytosis, anaphylactic reaction, angioedema, DRESS syndrome, erythema multiforme, hypersensitivity syndrome (multiorgan), mania, psychosis, Stevens-Johnson syndrome, toxic epidermal necrolysis

Drug Interactions

Metabolism/Transport Effects Substrate of CYP3A4 (major); **Note:** Assignment of Major/Minor substrate status based on clinically relevant drug interaction potential; **Inhibits** CYP2A6 (weak), CYP2C19 (moderate), CYP2C9 (weak), CYP2E1 (weak); **Induces** CYP1A2 (weak/moderate), CYP2B6 (weak/moderate), CYP3A4 (moderate)

Avoid Concomitant Use

Avoid concomitant use of Modafinil with any of the following: Axitinib; Bedaquiline; Bosutinib; Conivaptan; Enzalutamide; Fusidic Acid (Systemic); Idelalisib; Iobenguane I 123; Nisoldipine; Olaparib; Palbociclib; Simeprevir; Sofosbuvir

Increased Effect/Toxicity

Modafinil may increase the levels/effects of: Cilostazol; Citalopram; Clarithromycin; CYP2C19 Substrates; Ifosfamide; Sympathomimetics

The levels/effects of Modafinil may be increased by: Aprepitant; AtoMOXetine; Cannabinoid-Containing Products; Conivaptan; CYP3A4 Inhibitors (Moderate); CYP3A4 Inhibitors (Strong); Dasatinib; Fosaprepitant; Fusidic Acid (Systemic); Idelalisib; Ivacaftor; Linezolid; Luliconazole; Mifepristone; Netupitant; Stiripentol; Tedizolid

Decreased Effect

Modafinil may decrease the levels/effects of: ARIPiprazole; Axitinib; Bedaquiline; Bosutinib; Clarithromycin; Clopidogrel; Contraceptives (Estrogens); CycloSPORINE (Systemic); CYP3A4 Substrates; Dasabuvir; Enzalutamide; FentaNYL; Hydrocodone; Ibrutinib; Ifosfamide; Iobenguane I 123; NiMODipine; Nisoldipine; Olaparib; Ombitasvir; Palbociclib; Paritaprevir; Saxagliptin; Simeprevir; Sofosbuvir

The levels/effects of Modafinil may be decreased by: Bosentan; CYP3A4 Inducers (Moderate); CYP3A4 Inducers (Strong); Dabrafenib; Deferasirox; Mitotane; Siltuximab; St Johns Wort; Tocilizumab

Food Interactions Food delays absorption, but does not affect bioavailability. Management: Administer without regard to meals.

Storage/Stability

Provigil: Store at 20°C to 25°C (68°F to 77°F).

Alertec (Canadian availability; not available in US): Store at 15°C to 30°C (59°F to 86°F).

Mechanism of Action The exact mechanism of action is unclear, it does not appear to alter the release of dopamine or norepinephrine, it may exert its stimulant effects by decreasing GABA-mediated neurotransmission, although this theory has not yet been fully evaluated; several studies also suggest that an intact central alpha-adrenergic system is required for modafinil's activity; the drug increases high-frequency alpha waves while decreasing both delta and theta wave activity, and these effects are consistent with generalized increases in mental alertness

Pharmacokinetics (Adult data unless noted) Modafinil is a racemic compound (at steady state total exposure to the *l*-isomer is ~3 times that for the *d*-isomer) whose enantiomers have different pharmacokinetics and do not interconvert.

Distribution: V_d: 0.9 L/kg

Protein binding: ~60%, primarily to albumin

Metabolism: Hepatic; multiple pathways including CYP3A4

Half-life: Effective half-life: 15 hours

Time to peak serum concentration: 2-4 hours

Elimination: Urine (as metabolites; <10% as unchanged drug)

Dosing: Usual Oral:

Children: **ADHD: Note:** Reports of serious dermatologic adverse effects and psychiatric events has resulted in the FDA's Pediatric Advisory Committee unanimously recommending that a specific warning against the use of modafinil in children be added to the manufacturer's labeling; use only if first- and second-line treatments have failed and the benefits outweigh the risks

Children <30 kg: 200-340 mg once daily

Children >30 kg: 300-425 mg

Adults:

ADHD: 100-400 mg once daily (Taylor, 2000); **Note:** Randomized, double-blind, placebo-controlled pediatric studies have utilized an 85 mg film-coated tablet (currently not commercially available) to provide these dosages. All studies utilized a titration method but varied the length of titration (3 weeks vs 7-9 days); clinical improvement was noted earlier in the shorter titration period.

Narcolepsy, obstructive sleep apnea/hypopnea syndrome (OSAHS): Adults: Initial: 200 mg as a single daily dose in the morning; **Note:** Doses of up to 400 mg/day, given as a single dose, have been well tolerated, but there is no consistent evidence that this dose confers additional benefit.

Shift work sleep disorder (SWSD): Adults: Initial: 200 mg as a single dose taken ~1 hour prior to start of work shift; **Note:** Doses of up to 400 mg/day, given as a single dose, have been well tolerated, but there is no consistent evidence that this dose confers additional benefit.

Dosing adjustment in renal impairment: Safety and efficacy have not been established in severe renal impairment.

Dosing adjustment in hepatic impairment: Severe hepatic impairment: Dose should be reduced to one-half of that recommended for patients with normal liver function.

Administration Oral: May be administer without regard to food, as a single dose in the morning; administer 1 hour prior to the start of work shift in those patients with SWSD

Monitoring Parameters Monitor CNS activity, blood pressure (if hypertensive patient), heart rate, appetite

Controlled Substance C-IV

Dosage Forms Excipient information presented when available (limited, particularly for generics); consult specific product labeling.

Tablet, Oral:

Provigil: 100 mg

Provigil: 200 mg [scored]

Generic: 100 mg, 200 mg

◆ **Moderiba** *see* Ribavirin *on page 1851*

◆ **Modified Burow's Solution** *see* Aluminum Acetate *on page 110*

◆ **Modified Shohl's Solution** *see* Sodium Citrate and Citric Acid *on page 1942*

◆ **MOM** *see* Magnesium Hydroxide *on page 1313*

Mometasone (Oral Inhalation)

(moe MET a sone)

Related Information

Inhaled Corticosteroids *on page 2261*

Brand Names: US Asmanex 120 Metered Doses; Asmanex 14 Metered Doses; Asmanex 30 Metered Doses; Asmanex 60 Metered Doses; Asmanex 7 Metered Doses; Asmanex HFA

Brand Names: Canada Asmanex Twisthaler

Therapeutic Category Anti-inflammatory Agent; Antiasthmatic; Corticosteroid, Inhalant (Oral); Glucocorticoid

Generic Availability (US) No

Use Maintenance treatment of asthma as prophylactic therapy (FDA approved in ages ≥4 years and adults); **NOT** indicated for the relief of acute bronchospasm. Also used to help reduce or discontinue oral corticosteroid therapy in patients with bronchial asthma.

Pregnancy Risk Factor C

Pregnancy Considerations Adverse events were observed in some animal reproduction studies. Hypoadrenalism may occur in infants born to mothers receiving corticosteroids during pregnancy. Based on available data, an overall increased risk of congenital malformations or a decrease in fetal growth has not been associated with maternal use of inhaled corticosteroids during pregnancy (Bakhireva, 2005; NAEPP, 2005; Namazy, 2004). Uncontrolled asthma is associated with adverse events in pregnancy (increased risk of perinatal mortality, pre-eclampsia, preterm birth, low birth weight infants). Inhaled corticosteroids are recommended for the treatment of asthma during pregnancy (most information available using budesonide) (ACOG, 2008; NAEPP, 2005).

Breast-Feeding Considerations Systemic corticosteroids are excreted in human milk. It is not known if sufficient quantities of mometasone are absorbed following oral inhalation to produce detectable amounts in breast milk; however, oral absorption is limited (<1%). The manufacturer recommends that caution be exercised when administering mometasone to nursing women. The use of inhaled corticosteroids is not considered a contraindication to breast-feeding (NAEPP, 2005).

Contraindications

Hypersensitivity to mometasone or any component of the formulation; hypersensitivity to milk proteins (Asmanex Twisthaler only); primary treatment of status asthmaticus or other acute episodes of asthma where intensive measures are required

Documentation of allergenic cross-reactivity for corticosteroids is limited. However, because of similarities in chemical structure and/or pharmacologic actions, the possibility of cross-sensitivity can not be ruled out with certainty.

Canadian labeling: Additional contraindications (not in U.S. labeling): Untreated systemic fungal, bacterial, viral, or parasitic infections; active or quiet tuberculosis infection of the respiratory tract; ocular herpes simplex

Warnings/Precautions May cause hypercorticism or suppression of hypothalamic-pituitary-adrenal (HPA) axis, particularly in younger children or in patients receiving high doses for prolonged periods. HPA axis suppression may lead to adrenal crisis. Withdrawal and discontinuation of a corticosteroid should be done slowly and carefully. Particular care is required when patients are transferred from systemic corticosteroids to inhaled products due to possible adrenal insufficiency or withdrawal from steroids, including an increase in allergic symptoms. Adult patients receiving >20 mg per day of prednisone (or equivalent) may be most susceptible. Fatalities have occurred due to adrenal insufficiency in asthmatic patients during and after transfer from systemic corticosteroids to aerosol steroids; aerosol steroids do not provide the systemic steroid needed to treat patients having trauma, surgery, or infections. Select surgical patients on long-term, high-dose, inhaled corticosteroid (ICS), should be given stress doses of hydrocortisone intravenously during the surgical period and the dose reduced rapidly within 24 hours after surgery (NAEPP, 2007). When transferring to oral inhaler, previously-suppressed allergic conditions (rhinitis, conjunctivitis, eczema) may be unmasked.

Paradoxical bronchospasm may occur with wheezing after inhalation; if this occurs, stop steroid and treat with a fast-acting bronchodilator. Supplemental steroids (oral or parenteral) may be needed during stress or severe asthma attacks. Not to be used in status asthmaticus or for the relief of acute bronchospasm. Corticosteroid use may cause psychiatric disturbances, including depression, euphoria, insomnia, mood swings, and personality changes. Preexisting psychiatric conditions may be exacerbated by corticosteroid use. Prolonged use of corticosteroids may also increase the incidence of secondary infection, mask acute infection (including fungal infections), prolong or exacerbate viral infections, or limit response to vaccines. Exposure to chickenpox and measles should be avoided; corticosteroids should not be used to treat ocular herpes simplex. Corticosteroids should not be used for cerebral malaria or viral hepatitis. Close observation is required in patients with latent tuberculosis and/or TB reactivity; restrict use in active TB (only in conjunction with antituberculosis treatment). Use with extreme caution in untreated systemic fungal, bacterial, viral, or parasitic infections. Canadian labeling contraindicates use in patients with untreated systemic fungal, bacterial, viral, or parasitic infections, active or quiet tuberculosis infection of the respiratory tract and ocular herpes simplex.

Prolonged treatment with corticosteroids has been associated with the development of Kaposi sarcoma (case reports); if noted, discontinuation of therapy should be considered (Goedert, 2002). Local oropharyngeal *Candida* infections have been reported; if occurs treat appropriately while continuing mometasone therapy. Patients should be instructed to rinse mouth after each use.

Hypersensitivity reactions including, allergic dermatitis, anaphylaxis, angioedema, bronchospasm, flushing, pruritus, and rash, and urticaria have been reported; if these symptoms occur discontinue use. Use with caution in patients with thyroid disease, hepatic impairment, renal impairment, cardiovascular disease, diabetes, glaucoma, cataracts, myasthenia gravis, patients with or who are at risk for osteoporosis, patients at risk for seizures, or GI diseases (diverticulitis, peptic ulcer, ulcerative colitis) due to perforation risk. Use caution following acute MI (corticosteroids have been associated with myocardial rupture). Because of the risk of adverse effects, systemic corticosteroids should be used cautiously in the elderly in the smallest possible effective dose for the shortest duration.

Orally-inhaled corticosteroids may cause a reduction in growth velocity in pediatric patients (~1 centimeter per year [range: 0.3 to 1.8 cm per year] and related to dose and duration of exposure). To minimize the systemic effects of orally-inhaled corticosteroids, each patient should be titrated to the lowest effective dose. Growth should be routinely monitored in pediatric patients. Prior to use, the dose and duration of treatment should be based on the risk versus benefit for each individual patient. In general, use the smallest effective dose for the shortest duration of time to minimize adverse events. A gradual tapering of dose may be required prior to discontinuing therapy. There have been reports of systemic corticosteroid withdrawal symptoms (eg, joint/muscle pain, lassitude, depression) when withdrawing inhalation therapy. Asmanex Twisthaler may contain lactose; very rare anaphylactic reactions have been reported in patients with severe milk protein allergy. Potentially significant interactions may exist, requiring dose or frequency adjustment, additional monitoring, and/or selection of alternative therapy.

Adverse Reactions

Central nervous system: Depression, fatigue, headache, pain

Gastrointestinal: Abdominal pain, anorexia, dyspepsia, gastroenteritis, nausea, oral candidiasis, vomiting

Genitourinary: Dysmenorrhea, urinary tract infection

Hematologic & oncologic: Bruise

Infection: Infection, influenza

Neuromuscular & skeletal: Arthralgia, back pain, musculoskeletal pain, myalgia

Ophthalmic: Increased intraocular pressure

Otic: Otalgia

Respiratory: Allergic rhinitis (more common in adolescents & adults), bronchitis, dry throat, epistaxis, flu-like symptoms, nasal discomfort, nasopharyngitis, pharyngitis, sinus congestion, sinusitis, upper respiratory tract infection, voice disorder

Miscellaneous: Fever

Rare but important or life-threatening: Cataract, exacerbation of asthma, glaucoma, growth suppression, hypersensitivity

Drug Interactions

Metabolism/Transport Effects **Substrate** of CYP3A4 (minor); **Note:** Assignment of Major/Minor substrate status based on clinically relevant drug interaction potential

Avoid Concomitant Use

Avoid concomitant use of Mometasone (Oral Inhalation) with any of the following: Aldesleukin; Loxapine

Increased Effect/Toxicity

Mometasone (Oral Inhalation) may increase the levels/effects of: Amphotericin B; Ceritinib; Deferasirox; Loop Diuretics; Loxapine; Thiazide Diuretics

The levels/effects of Mometasone (Oral Inhalation) may be increased by: CYP3A4 Inhibitors (Strong); Telaprevir

Decreased Effect

Mometasone (Oral Inhalation) may decrease the levels/effects of: Aldesleukin; Corticorelin; Hyaluronidase; Telaprevir

Storage/Stability

Asmanex HFA: Store at 20°C to 25°C (68°F to 77°F); excursions permitted to 15°C to 30°C (59°F to 86°F). Do not puncture. Do not use or store near heat or open flame. Exposure to temperatures above 120°F may cause bursting. Discard when the dose counter reads "0".

Asmanex Twisthaler: Store at 25°C (77°F); excursions permitted to 15°C to 30°C (59°F to 86°F). Discard when oral dose counter reads "00" (or 45 days [U.S. labeling] or 60 days [Canadian labeling] after opening the foil pouch).

Mechanism of Action May depress the formation, release, and activity of endogenous chemical mediators of inflammation (kinins, histamine, liposomal enzymes, prostaglandins). Leukocytes and macrophages may have to be present for the initiation of responses mediated by the above substances. Inhibits the margination and subsequent cell migration to the area of injury, and also reverses the dilatation and increased vessel permeability in the area resulting in decreased access of cells to the sites of injury.

Pharmacodynamics Clinical effects are due to direct local effect, rather than systemic absorption

Maximum effect: 1-2 weeks or more

Duration after discontinuation: Several days or more

Pharmacokinetics (Adult data unless noted)

Absorption: Systemic absorption: Single dose: <1%

Distribution: V_{dss}: Adults: 152 L

Protein binding: 98% to 99%

Metabolism: Extensive in the liver to multiple metabolites; no major metabolites are detectable in the plasma; *in vitro* incubation studies identified one minor metabolite, 6 Beta-hydroxymometasone furoate, formed via cytochrome P450 CYP3A4 pathway

Bioavailability: Single dose: <1%

Half-life: Mean: 5 hours

Elimination: Metabolites are excreted primarily via the bile with a limited amount via urine; after oral inhalation, 74% of the dose was excreted in the feces and 8% in the urine (none as unchanged drug)

Dosing: Usual **Note:** Maximum effects may not be seen until 1-2 weeks or longer; doses should be titrated to the lowest effective dose once asthma is controlled.

Children 4-11 years (regardless of prior therapy): **Note:** Use 110 mcg inhaler: Initial: 1 inhalation (110 mcg) once daily, administered in the evening. Maximum dose: 1 inhalation/day (110 mcg/day)

Children ≥12 years and Adults:

Patients previously treated with bronchodilators only or with inhaled corticosteroids: Initial: 1 inhalation (220 mcg) once daily, administered in the evening; may increase dose after 2 weeks if adequate response not obtained. Maximum dose: 2 inhalations/day (440 mcg/day); may be administered as 1 inhalation twice daily or 2 inhalations once daily in the evening

Patients previously treated with oral corticosteroids: Initial: 2 inhalations (440 mcg) twice daily. Maximum dose: 4 inhalations/day (880 mcg/day)

NIH Asthma Guidelines (NAEPP, 2007) (give in divided doses): **Note:** 220 mcg inhaler delivers 200 mcg mometasone furoate per actuation; NAEPP uses doses based on delivery, while manufacturer recommended doses are based on inhaler amount; Children ≥12 years and Adults:

"Low" dose: 200 mcg/day (200 mcg/puff: 1 puff/day)

"Medium" dose: 400 mcg/day (200 mcg/puff: 2 puffs/day)

"High" dose: >400 mcg/day (200 mcg/puff: >2 puffs/day)

Administration Remove inhaler from foil pouch; write date on cap label. Keep inhaler upright while removing cap, twisting in a counterclockwise direction; lifting the cap loads the device with the medication. Exhale fully prior to bringing the inhaler up to the mouth. Place inhaler in mouth, while holding it in a horizontal position. Close lips around the mouthpiece and inhale quickly and deeply. Remove the inhaler from your mouth and hold your breath for about 10 seconds, if possible. Do not exhale into inhaler. Wipe the mouthpiece dry and replace the cap immediately after each inhalation; rotate fully until click is heard. Rinse mouth with water (without swallowing) after inhalation to decrease chance of oral candidiasis. Avoid contact of the inhaler with any liquids; do not wash; wipe with dry cloth or tissue if needed. Discard the inhaler 45 days after opening foil pouch or when dose counter reads "00."

Monitoring Parameters Monitor growth in pediatric patients. Check mucous membranes for signs of fungal infection. Monitor pulmonary function tests (eg, FEV_1, peak flow).

Additional Information When using mometasone oral inhalation to help reduce or discontinue oral corticosteroid therapy, begin prednisone taper after at least 1 week of mometasone inhalation therapy; do not decrease prednisone faster than 2.5 mg/day on a weekly basis; monitor patients for signs of asthma instability and adrenal insufficiency; decrease mometasone to lowest effective dose after prednisone reduction is complete.

Product Availability Asmanex HFA: FDA approved April 2014; anticipated availability is currently unknown.

Dosage Forms Excipient information presented when available (limited, particularly for generics); consult specific product labeling.

Aerosol, Inhalation, as furoate:

Asmanex HFA: 100 mcg/actuation (13 g); 200 mcg/actuation (13 g)

Aerosol Powder Breath Activated, Inhalation, as furoate:

Asmanex 120 Metered Doses: 220 mcg/INH (1 ea) [contains milk protein]

Asmanex 14 Metered Doses: 220 mcg/INH (1 ea) [contains milk protein]

Asmanex 30 Metered Doses: 110 mcg/INH (1 ea); 220 mcg/INH (1 ea) [contains milk protein]

Asmanex 60 Metered Doses: 220 mcg/INH (1 ea) [contains milk protein]

Asmanex 7 Metered Doses: 110 mcg/INH (1 ea) [contains milk protein]

Mometasone (Nasal) (moe MET a sone)

Brand Names: US Nasonex

Brand Names: Canada Apo-Mometasone; Nasonex

Therapeutic Category Anti-inflammatory Agent; Corticosteroid, Intranasal; Glucocorticoid

Generic Availability (US) No

Use Management of nasal symptoms associated with seasonal and perennial allergic rhinitis (FDA approved in ages ≥2 years and adults); prevention of seasonal allergic rhinitis (FDA approved in ages ≥12 years and adults); treatment of nasal polyps (FDA approved in adults); has also been used for management of nasal airway obstruction associated with adenoidal hypertrophy

Intranasal corticosteroids have also been used as an adjunct to antibiotics in empiric treatment of acute bacterial rhinosinusitis primarily in patients with history of allergic rhinitis (Chow, 2012) and in pediatric patients with mild obstructive sleep apnea syndrome who cannot undergo adenotonsillectomy or who still have symptoms after surgery (Marcus, 2012).

Pregnancy Risk Factor C

Pregnancy Considerations Adverse events were observed in some animal reproduction studies. Hypoadrenalism may occur in newborns following maternal use of corticosteroids in pregnancy; monitor. Intranasal corticosteroids are recommended for the treatment of rhinitis during pregnancy; the lowest effective dose should be used (NAEPP 2005; Wallace 2008).

Breast-Feeding Considerations Systemic corticosteroids are excreted in human milk. It is not known if sufficient quantities of mometasone are absorbed following nasal inhalation to produce detectable amounts in breast milk; however, systemic absorption is low (<1%). The use of inhaled corticosteroids is not considered a contraindication to breast-feeding (NAEPP 2005). The manufacturer recommends caution be used if administered to a nursing woman.

Contraindications Hypersensitivity to mometasone or any component of the formulation

Warnings/Precautions Avoid nasal corticosteroid use in patients with recent nasal septal ulcers, nasal surgery or nasal trauma until healing has occurred. Prolonged use of corticosteroids may also increase the incidence of secondary infection, mask acute infection (including fungal infections), prolong or exacerbate viral infections, or limit response to vaccines. Exposure to chickenpox should be avoided. Use caution or avoid in patients with active or latent tuberculosis or in patients with untreated fungal, bacterial, or systemic viral infections. Do not use in untreated localized infection involving the nasal mucosa; concurrent antimicrobial therapy should be administered if bacterial infection of the sinuses is suspected/confirmed.

Prior to use, the dose and duration of treatment should be based on the risk versus benefit for each individual patient. In general, use the smallest effective dose for the shortest duration of time to minimize adverse events. A gradual tapering of dose may be required prior to discontinuing therapy. When recommended doses are exceeded, or in extremely sensitive individuals may cause hypercorticism or suppression of hypothalamic-pituitary-adrenal (HPA) axis. Reports consistent with hypercorticism are rare. HPA axis suppression may lead to adrenal crisis. Withdrawal and discontinuation of a corticosteroid should be done slowly and carefully. Fatalities have occurred due to adrenal insufficiency in asthmatic patients during and after transfer from systemic corticosteroids to aerosol steroids; aerosol steroids do **not** provide the systemic steroid needed to treat patients having trauma, surgery, or infections. Use with caution in patients with cataracts and/or glaucoma; increased intraocular pressure, open-angle glaucoma, and cataracts have occurred with prolonged use. Consider routine eye exams in chronic users.

Avoid using higher than recommended dosages; suppression of linear growth (ie, reduction of growth velocity), reduced bone mineral density, or hypercorticism (Cushing syndrome) may occur; titrate to lowest effective dose. Reduction in growth velocity may occur when corticosteroids are administered to pediatric patients, even at recommended doses via intranasal route (monitor growth).

Adverse Reactions

Central nervous system: Headache

Gastrointestinal: Diarrhea, dyspepsia, vomiting

Neuromuscular & skeletal: Musculoskeletal pain, myalgia

Ocular: Conjunctivitis

Otic: Otitis media

Respiratory: Asthma, bronchitis, nasal irritation, rhinitis, sinusitis, upper respiratory tract infection, wheezing

Miscellaneous: Flu-like syndrome, viral infection (nasal inhalation)

Rare but important or life-threatening: Anaphylaxis, angioedema, growth suppression, nasal burning, nasal candidiasis, nasal septal perforation, nasal ulcers, oral candidiasis (nasal inhalation), smell disturbance (rare), taste disturbance (rare)

Drug Interactions

Metabolism/Transport Effects Substrate of CYP3A4 (minor); **Note:** Assignment of Major/Minor substrate status based on clinically relevant drug interaction potential

Avoid Concomitant Use There are no known interactions where it is recommended to avoid concomitant use.

Increased Effect/Toxicity

Mometasone (Nasal) may increase the levels/effects of: Ceritinib

Decreased Effect There are no known significant interactions involving a decrease in effect.

Storage/Stability Store at 25°C (77°F); excursions permitted to 15°C to 30°C (59°F to 86°F). Protect from light.

Mechanism of Action May depress the formation, release, and activity of endogenous chemical mediators of inflammation (kinins, histamine, liposomal enzymes, prostaglandins). Leukocytes and macrophages may have to be present for the initiation of responses mediated by the above substances. Inhibits the margination and subsequent cell migration to the area of injury, and also reverses the dilatation and increased vessel permeability in the area resulting in decreased access of cells to the sites of injury.

Pharmacodynamics Clinical effects are due to direct local effect, rather than systemic absorption.

Onset of action: Improvement in allergic rhinitis symptoms may be seen within 11 hours.

Maximum effect: Within 1-2 weeks after starting therapy

Pharmacokinetics (Adult data unless noted) Bioavailability: <1%

Dosing: Usual

Children and Adolescents:

Nasal airway obstruction/adenoidal hypertrophy: Intranasal: Limited data available: Children and Adolescents 3-15 years: Initial 100 mcg once daily delivered as 50 mcg (1 spray) **per nostril** once daily for 6 weeks, followed by the same dose given every 24 hours for the first 2 weeks of each month. Dosing based on two studies: The first was a randomized, placebo-controlled study (n=122; treatment arm: 67; age range; 3-15 years) in which patients received therapy for 6 weeks and 67.2% had a significant decrease in adenoid size compared to the control group (p<0.001) (Cengel, 2005). The second was a 2-stage, placebo-controlled, randomized study (n=60, treatment arm: 30; age range: 3-7 years) which showed that after 40 days of daily mometasone therapy, ~77.7% of patients were considered responders and able to avoid adenoidectomy; those who responded continued therapy every 24 or 48 hours for the first 2 weeks of three subsequent months (Berlucchi, 2007). Long-term analysis of children receiving the daily dose for the first 2 weeks of each month continued to show improvement after a mean followup period of 28 months and the need for surgery remained reduced (Berlucchi, 2008).

Allergic rhinitis: Intranasal:

Treatment:

Children 2-11 years: 100 mcg once daily delivered as 50 mcg (1 spray) **per nostril** once daily

Children ≥12 years and Adolescents: 200 mcg once daily delivered as 100 mcg (2 sprays) **per nostril** once daily

Prevention: Children ≥12 years and Adolescents: 200 mcg once daily delivered as 100 mcg (2 sprays) **per nostril** once daily beginning 2-4 weeks prior to pollen season

Nasal polyps, treatment: Intranasal: Adolescents ≥18 years: 200 mcg twice daily delivered as 100 mcg (2 sprays) **per nostril** twice daily; a lower dose of 200 mcg once daily delivered as 100 mcg (2 sprays) **per nostril** once daily may be effective in some patients

Adults:

Allergic rhinitis: Intranasal:

Treatment: 200 mcg once daily delivered as 100 mcg (2 sprays) **per nostril** once daily

Prevention: 200 mcg once daily delivered as 100 mcg (2 sprays) **per nostril** once daily beginning 2-4 weeks prior to pollen season

Nasal polyps, treatment: Intranasal: 200 mcg twice daily delivered as 100 mcg (2 sprays) **per nostril** twice daily; 200 mcg once daily delivered as 100 mcg (2 sprays) **per nostril** once daily may be effective in some patients

Dosing adjustment in renal impairment: There are no dosage adjustments provided in the manufacturer's labeling.

Dosing adjustment in hepatic impairment: There are no dosage adjustments provided in the manufacturer's labeling. Mometasone concentrations appear to increase with the severity of hepatic impairment; use with caution.

Administration Shake well prior to each use. Before first use, prime by pressing pump 10 times or until a fine spray appears. Repeat priming with 2 sprays or until a fine spray appears if ≥1 week between use. Blow nose to clear nostrils before each use. Insert applicator into nostril, keeping bottle upright, and close off the other nostril. Breathe in through nose. While inhaling, press pump to release spray. Do not spray into eyes or mouth. Discard after labeled number of doses has been used, even if bottle is not completely empty.

After removing nasal spray from container, avoid prolonged exposure of product to direct light; brief exposure to light (with normal use) is acceptable.

Monitoring Parameters Mucous membranes for signs of fungal infection, growth (pediatric patients), signs/symptoms of HPA axis suppression/adrenal insufficiency; ocular changes

Additional Information When used short term as adjunctive therapy in acute bacterial rhinosinusitis (ABRS), intranasal steroids show modest symptomatic improvement and few adverse effects; improvement is primarily due to increased sinus drainage. Use should be considered optional in ABRS; however, intranasal corticosteroids should be routinely prescribed to ABRS patients who have a history of or concurrent allergic rhinitis (Chow, 2012).

Dosage Forms Considerations Nasonex 17 g bottles contain 120 sprays.

Dosage Forms Excipient information presented when available (limited, particularly for generics); consult specific product labeling.

Suspension, Nasal, as furoate:

Nasonex: 50 mcg/actuation (17 g) [contains benzalkonium chloride]

Mometasone (Topical) (moe MET a sone)

Medication Safety Issues

Sound-alike/look-alike issues:

Elocon lotion may be confused with ophthalmic solutions. Manufacturer's labeling emphasizes the product is **NOT** for use in the eyes.

Related Information

Topical Corticosteroids *on page 2262*

Brand Names: US Elocon

Brand Names: Canada Elocom; PMS-Mometasone; ratio-Mometasone; Taro-Mometasone

Therapeutic Category Anti-inflammatory Agent; Corticosteroid, Topical; Glucocorticoid

Generic Availability (US) May be product dependent

Use Relief of the inflammation and pruritus associated with corticosteroid-responsive dermatoses (medium potency topical corticosteroid); **Note:** Due to lack of established safety and efficacy in specific age groups, the cream and ointment are not recommended for use in children <2 years of age and the lotion is not recommended for use in children <12 years of age

Pregnancy Risk Factor C

Pregnancy Considerations Adverse events have been observed in animal reproduction studies. When topical corticosteroids are needed during pregnancy, low to mid potency preparations are preferred; higher potency preparations should be used for the shortest time possible and fetal growth should be monitored (Chi, 2011; Chi, 2013). Topical products are not recommended for extensive use, in large quantities, or for long periods of time in pregnant women (Leachman, 2006).

Breast-Feeding Considerations Corticosteroids are excreted in human milk; information specific to mometasone has not been located. It is not known if systemic absorption following topical administration results in detectable quantities in human milk. The manufacturer notes that when used systemically, maternal use of corticosteroids have the potential to cause adverse events in a nursing infant (eg, growth suppression, interfere with endogenous corticosteroid production), therefore caution should be exercised if administered to nursing women. Do not apply topical corticosteroids to nipples; hypertension was noted in a nursing infant exposed to a topical corticosteroid while nursing (Leachman, 2006).

Contraindications

There are no contraindications listed within the manufacturer's U.S. product labeling.

Canadian labeling: Hypersensitivity to mometasone furoate, other corticosteroids, or any component of the formulation; viral (eg, herpes or varicella) lesions of the skin, fungal or bacterial skin infections, parasitic infections, skin manifestations relating to tuberculosis or syphilis, eruptions following vaccinations, acne vulgaris, rosacea, pruritus without inflammation; ophthalmic use; use with occlusive dressings

Warnings/Precautions Topical corticosteroids may be absorbed percutaneously. Absorption may cause manifestations of Cushing's syndrome, hyperglycemia, or glycosuria. Absorption is increased by the use of occlusive dressings, application to denuded skin, or application to large surface areas. Avoid use of topical preparations with occlusive dressings or on weeping or exudative lesions. May cause hypercorticism or suppression of hypothalamic-pituitary-adrenal (HPA) axis, particularly in younger children or in patients receiving high doses for prolonged periods. HPA axis suppression may lead to adrenal crisis.

Prolonged use may result in fungal or bacterial superinfection; discontinue if dermatological infection persists despite appropriate antimicrobial therapy. Allergic contact dermatitis can occur and is usually diagnosed by failure to heal rather than clinical exacerbation; discontinue use if irritation occurs and treat appropriately.

Because of the risk of adverse effects associated with systemic absorption, topical corticosteroids should be used cautiously in the elderly in the smallest possible effective dose for the shortest duration. Not for treatment of diaper dermatitis. Children may absorb proportionally larger amounts after topical application and may be more prone to systemic effects. HPA axis suppression, intracranial hypertension, and Cushing syndrome have been reported in children receiving topical corticosteroids. Prolonged use may affect growth velocity; growth should be routinely monitored in pediatric patients.

Warnings: Additional Pediatric Considerations The extent of percutaneous absorption is dependent on several factors, including epidermal integrity (intact vs abraded skin), formulation, age of the patient, prolonged duration of use, and the use of occlusive dressings. Percutaneous absorption of topical steroids is increased in neonates (especially preterm neonates), infants, and young children. Infants and small children may be more susceptible to HPA axis suppression, intracranial hypertension, Cushing syndrome, or other systemic toxicities due to larger skin surface area to body mass ratio.

Some dosage forms may contain propylene glycol; in neonates large amounts of propylene glycol delivered orally, intravenously (eg, >3,000 mg/day), or topically have been associated with potentially fatal toxicities which can include metabolic acidosis, seizures, renal failure, and CNS depression; toxicities have also been reported in children and adults including hyperosmolality, lactic acidosis, seizures, and respiratory depression; use caution (AAP, 1997; Shehab, 2009).

Adverse Reactions

Dermatologic: Bacterial skin infection, burning, furunculosis, pruritus, skin atrophy, tingling/stinging

Rare but important or life-threatening: Decreased glucocorticoid concentrations (pediatrics), folliculitis, moniliasis, paresthesia, rosacea, skin depigmentation, skin atrophy

Cataract formation, reduction in growth velocity, and HPA axis suppression have been reported with other corticosteroids.

Drug Interactions

Metabolism/Transport Effects Substrate of CYP3A4 (minor); **Note:** Assignment of Major/Minor substrate status based on clinically relevant drug interaction potential

Avoid Concomitant Use

Avoid concomitant use of Mometasone (Topical) with any of the following: Aldesleukin

Increased Effect/Toxicity

Mometasone (Topical) may increase the levels/effects of: Ceritinib; Deferasirox

The levels/effects of Mometasone (Topical) may be increased by: Telaprevir

Decreased Effect

Mometasone (Topical) may decrease the levels/effects of: Aldesleukin; Corticorelin; Hyaluronidase; Telaprevir

Storage/Stability

Cream: Store at 25°C (77°F); excursions permitted to 15°C to 30°C (59°F to 86°F). Avoid excessive heat.

Lotion, ointment: Store at 25°C (77°F); excursions permitted to 15°C to 30°C (59°F to 86°F).

Mechanism of Action Topical corticosteroids have anti-inflammatory, antipruritic, and vasoconstrictive properties. May depress the formation, release, and activity of endogenous chemical mediators of inflammation (kinins, histamine, liposomal enzymes, prostaglandins) through the induction of phospholipase A_2 inhibitory proteins (lipocortins) and sequential inhibition of the release of arachidonic acid. Mometasone has intermediate range potency.

Pharmacokinetics (Adult data unless noted) Absorption: 0.4% of the applied dose of the cream and 0.7% of the applied dose of the ointment enter the circulation after 8 hours of contact with normal skin (without occlusion); absorption is increased by occlusive dressings or with decreased integrity of skin (eg, inflammation or skin disease)

Dosing: Usual Apply sparingly, do not use occlusive dressings. Discontinue therapy when control is achieved; reassess diagnosis if no improvement is seen in 2 weeks.

Cream, ointment: Children ≥2 years and Adults: Apply a thin film to affected area once daily; do not use in pediatric patients for >3 weeks

Lotion: Children ≥12 years and Adults: Apply a few drops to affected area once daily; massage lightly into skin

Administration Apply sparingly; avoid contact with eyes. Do not apply to face, underarms, or groin, unless directed by physician. Do not wrap or bandage affected area unless directed by physician. Do not use for treatment of diaper dermatitis or in diaper area.

Lotion: Hold nozzle of bottle close to affected area and gently squeeze bottle.

Monitoring Parameters Monitor growth in pediatric patients; assess HPA axis suppression in patients using topical steroids applied to a large surface area or to areas under occlusion.

Additional Information Several studies conducted in children 6-23 months of age with atopic dermatitis demonstrated a high incidence of adrenal suppression when topical mometasone products were applied once daily for ~3 weeks over an average body surface area of about 40%. Of the patients with normal baseline adrenal function, adrenal suppression occurred in 16% of patients using the cream, 27% of patients using the ointment, and 29% of patients using the lotion. Follow-up testing 2-4 weeks after discontinuation of therapy demonstrated suppressed HPA axis function in 1 of 5 patients who used the cream, 3 of 8 patients who used the ointment, and 1 of 8 patients who used the lotion.

Dosage Forms Excipient information presented when available (limited, particularly for generics); consult specific product labeling.

Cream, External, as furoate:
- Elocon: 0.1% (15 g, 45 g, 50 g) [contains soybean lecithin]
- Generic: 0.1% (15 g, 45 g)

Lotion, External, as furoate:
- Elocon: 0.1% (30 mL, 60 mL) [contains isopropyl alcohol, propylene glycol]

Ointment, External, as furoate:
- Elocon: 0.1% (15 g, 45 g) [contains propylene glycol stearate]
- Generic: 0.1% (15 g, 45 g)

Solution, External, as furoate:
- Generic: 0.1% (30 mL, 60 mL)

◆ **Mometasone and Eformoterol** *see* Mometasone and Formoterol *on page 1457*

Mometasone and Formoterol

(moe MET a sone & for MOH te rol)

Brand Names: US Dulera

Brand Names: Canada Zenhale

Therapeutic Category Adrenal Corticosteroid; Adrenergic Agonist Agent; Anti-inflammatory Agent; $Beta_2$-Adrenergic Agonist; Bronchodilator; Corticosteroid, Inhalant (Oral); Glucocorticoid

Generic Availability (US) No

Use Maintenance treatment of asthma (FDA approved in ages ≥12 years and adults); **NOT** indicated for the relief of acute bronchospasm

Medication Guide Available Yes

Pregnancy Risk Factor C

Pregnancy Considerations Animal reproduction studies have not been conducted with this combination. See individual agents.

Breast-Feeding Considerations It is not known if mometasone or formoterol are excreted into breast milk. The manufacturer recommends that caution be used if administering this combination to breast-feeding women. Refer to individual agents.

Contraindications

Hypersensitivity to mometasone, formoterol, or any component of the formulation; status asthmaticus or other acute episodes of asthma.

Canadian labeling: Additional contraindications (not in U.S. labeling): Untreated systemic fungal, bacterial, viral or parasitic infections, active tuberculous infection of the respiratory tract, or ocular herpes simplex.

Documentation of allergenic cross-reactivity for corticosteroids and/or sympathomimetics are limited. However, because of similarities in chemical structure and/or pharmacologic actions, the possibility of cross-sensitivity cannot be ruled out with certainty.

Warnings/Precautions **[U.S. Boxed Warning]: Long-acting beta$_2$-agonists (LABAs), such as formoterol, increase the risk of asthma-related deaths; mometasone and formoterol should only be used in patients not adequately controlled on a long-term asthma control medication (ie, inhaled corticosteroid) or whose disease severity requires initiation of two maintenance therapies.** In a large, randomized, placebo-controlled U.S. clinical trial (SMART, 2006), salmeterol was associated with an increase in asthma-related deaths (when added to usual asthma therapy); risk is considered a class effect among all LABAs. Data are not available to determine if the addition of an inhaled corticosteroid lessens this increased risk of death associated with LABA use. Assess patients at regular intervals once asthma control is maintained on combination therapy to determine if step-down therapy is appropriate (without loss of asthma control), and the patient can be maintained on an inhaled corticosteroid only. LABAs are not appropriate in patients whose asthma is adequately controlled on low- or medium-dose inhaled corticosteroids. **[U.S. Boxed Warning]: LABAs may increase the risk of asthma-related hospitalization in pediatric and adolescent patients.**

Do **not** use for acute bronchospasm. Short-acting beta$_2$-agonist (eg, albuterol) should be used for acute symptoms and symptoms occurring between treatments. Do **not** initiate in patients with significantly worsening or acutely deteriorating asthma. Patients must be instructed to use short-acting beta$_2$-agonist (eg, albuterol) for acute asthmatic symptoms and to seek medical attention in cases where acute symptoms are not relieved or a previous level of response is diminished. The need to increase frequency of use of inhaled short-acting beta$_2$-agonist may indicate deterioration of asthma, and medical evaluation must not be delayed. Therapy should not be used more than twice daily; do not use with other long-acting beta$_2$-agonists

Immediate hypersensitivity reactions (allergic dermatitis, angioedema, bronchospasm, flushing, rash, urticaria) have been reported. Do not exceed recommended dose; serious adverse events, including fatalities, have been associated with excessive use of inhaled sympathomimetics. Rarely, paradoxical bronchospasm may occur with use of inhaled bronchodilating agents; this should be distinguished from inadequate response.

Use with caution in patients with cardiovascular disease (arrhythmia, coronary insufficiency, or hypertension); beta agonists may cause elevation in blood pressure, heart rate and result in CNS stimulation/excitation. Beta$_2$-agonists may also increase risk of arrhythmias and electrocardiogram (ECG) changes, such as flattening of the T wave, prolongation of the QTc interval, and ST segment depression. Beta$_2$-agonists may decrease serum potassium (transient), increase serum glucose and aggravate ketoacidosis.

Use with caution in patients with major risk factors for decreased bone mineral count such as prolonged immobilization, family history of osteoporosis, postmenopausal status, tobacco use, advanced age, poor nutrition, or chronic use of drugs that can reduce bone mass (eg, anticonvulsants or oral corticosteroids); high doses and/or long-term use of inhaled corticosteroids have been associated with decreases in bone mineral density. Local oropharyngeal *Candida* infections have been reported; if this occurs, treat appropriately while continuing mometasone/formoterol therapy. Patients should be instructed to rinse mouth after each use. Potentially significant interactions may exist, requiring dose or frequency adjustment, additional monitoring, and/or selection of alternative therapy. Consult drug interactions database for more detailed information.

Mometasone may cause hypercorticism and/or suppression of hypothalamic-pituitary-adrenal (HPA) axis, particularly in younger children or in patients receiving high doses for prolonged periods. Caution is required when patients are transferred from systemic corticosteroids to products with lower systemic bioavailability (ie, inhalation). May lead to possible adrenal insufficiency or withdrawal symptoms, including an increase in allergic symptoms. Adult patients receiving prolonged therapy ≥20 mg per day of prednisone (or equivalent) may be most susceptible. Aerosol steroids do not provide the systemic steroid needed to treat patients having trauma, surgery, or infections.

Orally-inhaled corticosteroids may cause a reduction in growth velocity in pediatric patients (~1 centimeter per year [range 0.3-1.8 cm per year] and related to dose and duration of exposure). To minimize the systemic effects of orally-inhaled corticosteroids, each patient should be titrated to the lowest effective dose. Growth should be routinely monitored in pediatric patients.

Prolonged use of corticosteroids may also increase the incidence of secondary infection, mask acute infection (including fungal infections), prolong or exacerbate viral infections, or limit response to vaccines. Avoid use if possible in patients with ocular herpes; active or quiescent tuberculosis infections of the respiratory tract; or untreated viral, fungal, or bacterial or parasitic systemic infections. Exposure to chickenpox or measles should be avoided; if the patient is exposed to chickenpox, prophylaxis with varicella zoster immune globulin or pooled intravenous immunoglobulin, may be indicated; if chickenpox develops, treatment with antiviral agents may be considered. If exposure to measles, prophylaxis with pooled intramuscular immunoglobulin may be indicated. Withdraw systemic corticosteroid therapy with gradual tapering of dose. Monitor lung function, beta-agonist use, asthma symptoms, and for signs and symptoms of adrenal insufficiency (fatigue, lassitude, weakness, nausea and vomiting, hypotension) during withdrawal. Monitor patients with hepatic impairment; may lead to accumulation of mometasone in plasma.

Adverse Reactions Also see individual agents.

Central nervous system: Headache

Respiratory: Nasopharyngitis, sinusitis, voice disorder

Rare but important or life-threatening: Anaphylactoid reaction, anaphylaxis, angina pectoris, angioedema, atrial fibrillation, cardiac arrhythmia, exacerbation of asthma, hyperglycemia, hypertension, hypokalemia, hypotension (including severe), increased blood pressure, hypersensitivity reaction, oral candidiasis, prolonged Q-T interval on ECG, tachyarrhythmia, ventricular premature contractions

Drug Interactions

Metabolism/Transport Effects Refer to individual components.

Avoid Concomitant Use

Avoid concomitant use of Mometasone and Formoterol with any of the following: Aldesleukin; Beta-Blockers (Nonselective); Iobenguane I 123; Long-Acting Beta2-Agonists; Loxapine

Increased Effect/Toxicity

Mometasone and Formoterol may increase the levels/effects of: Amphotericin B; Atosiban; Ceritinib; Deferasirox; Highest Risk QTc-Prolonging Agents; Long-Acting Beta2-Agonists; Loop Diuretics; Loxapine; Moderate Risk QTc-Prolonging Agents; Sympathomimetics; Thiazide Diuretics

The levels/effects of Mometasone and Formoterol may be increased by: AtoMOXetine; Caffeine and Caffeine Containing Products; Cannabinoid-Containing Products; CYP3A4 Inhibitors (Strong); Inhalational Anesthetics; Linezolid; MAO Inhibitors; Mifepristone; Tedizolid; Telaprevir; Theophylline Derivatives; Tricyclic Antidepressants

Decreased Effect

Mometasone and Formoterol may decrease the levels/effects of: Aldesleukin; Corticorelin; Hyaluronidase; Iobenguane I 123; Telaprevir

The levels/effects of Mometasone and Formoterol may be decreased by: Beta-Blockers (Beta1 Selective); Beta-Blockers (Nonselective); Betahistine

Storage/Stability Store at 20°C to 25°C (68°F to 77°F); excursions are permitted between 15°C and 30°C (59°F and 86°F); temperatures above 49°C (120°F) may cause bursting. Contents under pressure; do not puncture, incinerate, or store near heat or open flame. Discard inhaler after the labeled number of inhalations have been used (the dose counter will read "0"). The 120-actuation inhaler may be stored in any position; store the 60-actuation inhaler with the mouthpiece down or in a horizontal position after priming.

Mechanism of Action Formoterol relaxes bronchial smooth muscle by selective action on $beta_2$ receptors with little effect on heart rate. Formoterol has a long-acting effect.

Mometasone is a corticosteroid which controls the rate of protein synthesis, depresses the migration of polymorphonuclear leukocytes/fibroblasts, and reverses capillary permeability and lysosomal stabilization at the cellular level to prevent or control inflammation.

Pharmacokinetics (Adult data unless noted) See individual agents.

Dosing: Usual Oral inhalation: **Asthma, maintenance treatment:** Initial dose based on previous corticosteroid dosage.

Children and Adolescents ≥12 years:

Previous medium dose inhaled corticosteroids: Mometasone 100 mcg/formoterol 5 mcg (Dulera® 100 mcg/5 mcg): 2 inhalations twice daily; maximum daily dose: 4 inhalations/day. In patients not adequately controlled on the lower combination dose following 2 weeks of therapy, consider the higher dose combination.

Previous high dose inhaled corticosteroids: Mometasone 200 mcg/formoterol 5 mcg (Dulera® 200 mcg/5 mcg): 2 inhalations twice daily; maximum daily dose: 4 inhalations/day

Adults: Dulera® 100 mcg/5 mcg, Dulera® 200 mcg/5 mcg: 2 inhalations twice daily. Do not exceed 4 inhalations/day. In patients not adequately controlled on the lower combination dose following 2 weeks of therapy, consider the higher dose combination.

Dosing adjustment in hepatic impairment: Mometasone systemic exposure appears to increase with increasing extent of impairment; however, there is no dosage adjustment recommended in the manufacturer labeling.

Administration Prior to first use, inhaler must be primed by releasing 4 test sprays into the air; shake well before each spray. Inhaler must be reprimed if not used for >5 days. Shake well before each use. Rinse mouth after each use. Discard inhaler after the labeled number of inhalations have been used.

Monitoring Parameters Pulmonary function tests, check mucous membranes for signs of fungal infection; monitor growth in pediatric patients; serum glucose and serum potassium

Dosage Forms Excipient information presented when available (limited, particularly for generics); consult specific product labeling.

Aerosol, for oral inhalation:

Dulera: Mometasone furoate 100 mcg and formoterol fumarate dihydrate 5 mcg per inhalation (8.8 g) [60 metered actuations]

Dulera: Mometasone furoate 100 mcg and formoterol fumarate dihydrate 5 mcg per inhalation (13 g) [120 metered actuations]

Dulera: Mometasone furoate 200 mcg and formoterol fumarate dihydrate 5 mcg per inhalation (8.8 g) [60 metered actuations]

Dulera: Mometasone furoate 200 mcg and formoterol fumarate dihydrate 5 mcg per inhalation (13 g) [120 metered actuations]

◆ **Mometasone Furoate** *see* Mometasone (Nasal) *on page* 1454

◆ **Mometasone Furoate** *see* Mometasone (Oral Inhalation) *on page* 1452

◆ **Mometasone Furoate** *see* Mometasone (Topical) *on page* 1456

◆ **Monacolin K** *see* Lovastatin *on page* 1305

◆ **Monicure (Can)** *see* Fluconazole *on page* 881

◆ **Monistat® (Can)** *see* Miconazole (Topical) *on page* 1431

◆ **Monistat® 3 (Can)** *see* Miconazole (Topical) *on page* 1431

◆ **Monoclate-P** *see* Antihemophilic Factor (Human) *on page* 167

◆ **Monodox** *see* Doxycycline *on page* 717

◆ **Mononine** *see* Factor IX (Human) *on page* 838

◆ **Monopril** *see* Fosinopril *on page* 943

Montelukast (mon te LOO kast)

Medication Safety Issues

Sound-alike/look-alike issues:

Singulair may be confused with Oralair, SINEquan

Brand Names: US Singulair

Brand Names: Canada ACH-Montelukast; Apo-Montelukast; Auro-Montelukast; Auro-Montelukast Chewable Tablets; Dom-Montelukast; Dom-Montelukast FC; Jamp-Montelukast; Mar-Montelukast; Mint-Montelukast; Montelukast Sodium Tablets; Mylan-Montelukast; PMS-Montelukast; PMS-Montelukast FC; RAN-Montelukast; Riva-Montelukast FC; Sandoz-Montelukast; Sandoz-Montelukast Granules; Singulair; Teva-Montelukast

Therapeutic Category Antiasthmatic; Leukotriene Receptor Antagonist

Generic Availability (US) Yes

Use Prophylaxis and chronic treatment of asthma (FDA approved in ages ≥12 months and adults); relief of symptoms of seasonal allergic rhinitis (FDA approved in ages ≥2 years and adults) and perennial allergic rhinitis (FDA approved in ages ≥6 months and adults); prevention of exercise-induced bronchoconstriction (FDA approved in ages ≥6 years and adults); has also been used as adjunct therapy for asthma exacerbation

Pregnancy Risk Factor B

Pregnancy Considerations Adverse events have not been observed in animal reproduction studies. Structural defects have been reported in neonates exposed to montelukast *in utero*; however, a specific pattern and relationship to montelukast has not been established. Based on available data, an increased risk of teratogenic effects has not been observed with montelukast use in pregnancy (Bakhireva 2007; Nelsen 2012; Sarkar 2009). Uncontrolled asthma is associated with adverse events on pregnancy (increased risk of perinatal mortality, pre-eclampsia, preterm birth, low birth weight infants). Montelukast may be considered for use in women who had a favorable response prior to becoming pregnant; however, initiating a leukotriene receptor antagonist during pregnancy is an alternative (but not preferred) treatment option for mild persistent asthma (NAEPP 2005).

Breast-Feeding Considerations It is not known if montelukast is excreted into breast milk. The manufacturer recommends that caution be exercised when administering montelukast to nursing women.

Contraindications Hypersensitivity to montelukast or any component of the formulation

Warnings/Precautions Montelukast is not FDA approved for use in the reversal of bronchospasm in acute asthma attacks, including status asthmaticus; some studies, however, support its use as adjunctive therapy (Cylly, 2003; Ferreira, 2001; Harmancik, 2006). Appropriate rescue medication should be available. Montelukast treatment should continue during acute asthma exacerbation. When inhaled or systemic corticosteroid reduction is considered in patients initiating or receiving montelukast, appropriate clinical monitoring and a gradual dose reduction of the steroid are recommended.

Postmarketing reports of behavioral changes (eg, agitation, aggression, anxiety, attention deficit, depression, hallucinations, hostility, insomnia, irritability, restlessness, sleep disturbance, suicide ideation/behavior) have been noted in pediatric, adolescent, and adult patients. In a retrospective analysis performed by Merck, serious behavior-related events were rare (Philip, 2009a); assess patients for behavioral changes. Patients should be instructed to notify the prescriber if behavioral changes occur.

Potentially significant drug-drug interactions may exist, requiring dose or frequency adjustment, additional monitoring, and/or selection of alternative therapy. In rare cases, patients on therapy with montelukast may present with systemic eosinophilia, sometimes presenting with clinical features of vasculitis consistent with Churg-Strauss syndrome, a condition which is often treated with systemic corticosteroid therapy. Healthcare providers should be alert to eosinophilia, vasculitic rash, worsening pulmonary symptoms, cardiac complications, and/or neuropathy presenting in their patients. A causal association between montelukast and these underlying conditions has not been established. Montelukast will not interrupt bronchoconstrictor response to aspirin or other NSAIDs; aspirin sensitive asthmatics should continue to avoid these agents. The chewable tablet contains phenylalanine.

Adverse Reactions

Children ≥15 years and Adults:

Central nervous system: Dizziness, fatigue, fever, headache

Dermatologic: Skin rash

Gastrointestinal: Dyspepsia, gastroenteritis, toothache

Hepatic: Increased serum ALT, increased serum AST

Neuromuscular & skeletal: Weakness

Respiratory: Cough, epistaxis, nasal congestion, sinusitis, upper respiratory tract infection

Children 2 to ≤14 years:

Central nervous system: Fever, headache

Dermatologic: Dermatitis, eczema, skin rash, urticaria

Gastrointestinal: Abdominal pain, dyspepsia, gastroenteritis, nausea

Infection: Influenza, varicella, viral infection

Ophthalmic: Conjunctivitis

Otic: Otalgia, otitis

Respiratory: Laryngitis, pharyngitis, pneumonia, rhinorrhea, sinusitis, upper respiratory tract infection

Children 6 to 23 months:

Respiratory: Cough, otitis media, pharyngitis, rhinitis, tonsillitis, upper respiratory tract infection, wheezing

Rare but important or life-threatening: Churg-Strauss syndrome, depression, disorientation, eosinophilia (systemic), eosinophilic pneumonitis, erythema multiforme, erythema nodosum, hallucination, hepatic eosinophilic infiltration, hepatitis (mixed pattern, hepatocellular, and cholestatic), hypersensitivity, insomnia, memory impairment, pancreatitis, paresthesia, seizure, somnambulism, Stevens-Johnson syndrome, suicidal ideation, suicidal tendencies, thrombocytopenia, toxic epidermal necrolysis, urinary incontinence (children)

Drug Interactions

Metabolism/Transport Effects Substrate of CYP2C8 (minor), CYP2C9 (minor), CYP3A4 (minor); **Note:** Assignment of Major/Minor substrate status based on clinically relevant drug interaction potential; **Inhibits** CYP2C8 (weak), CYP2C9 (weak)

Avoid Concomitant Use

Avoid concomitant use of Montelukast with any of the following: Amodiaquine; Loxapine

Increased Effect/Toxicity

Montelukast may increase the levels/effects of: Amodiaquine; Loxapine

The levels/effects of Montelukast may be increased by: Gemfibrozil

Decreased Effect There are no known significant interactions involving a decrease in effect.

Storage/Stability Store at room temperature of 25°C (77°F); excursions permitted to 15°C to 30°C (59°F to 86°F). Store in original package. Protect from moisture and light. Granules must be used within 15 minutes of opening packet.

Mechanism of Action Selective leukotriene receptor antagonist that inhibits the cysteinyl leukotriene receptor. Cysteinyl leukotrienes and leukotriene receptor occupation have been correlated with the pathophysiology of asthma, including airway edema, smooth muscle contraction, and altered cellular activity associated with the inflammatory process, which contribute to the signs and symptoms of asthma. Cysteinyl leukotrienes are also released from the nasal mucosa following allergen exposure leading to symptoms associated with allergic rhinitis (Jarvis, 2000).

Pharmacokinetics (Adult data unless noted)

Absorption: Rapid

Distribution: V_d: Adults: 8-11 L

Protein binding: >99%

Metabolism: Extensive by cytochrome P450 3A4 and 2C9

Bioavailability: Tablet:

- 5 mg: 63% to 73%
- 10 mg: 64%

Time to peak serum concentration: Tablet:

- 4 mg: 2 hours
- 5 mg: 2-2.5 hours
- 10 mg: 3-4 hours

Elimination: Exclusively via bile; <0.2% excreted in urine

Dosing: Usual
Infants, Children, and Adolescents:
Allergic rhinitis: Oral:
6 months to 5 years: 4 mg once daily
6-14 years: 5 mg once daily
≥15 years: 10 mg once daily
Asthma, chronic treatment and prophylaxis: Oral:
12 months to 5 years: 4 mg once daily
6-14 years: 5 mg once daily
≥15 years: 10 mg once daily
Asthma, exacerbation (acute), adjunct therapy: Limited data available: Oral: Children 2-5 years: 4 mg/dose; in a double-blind, placebo-controlled trial of 52 children with acute asthma exacerbation, a single dose of montelukast (4 mg) with concomitant short-acting beta$_2$-agonist (salbutamol) showed lower respiratory rate and improved pulmonary indices compared to placebo (Harmanci, 2006)
Bronchoconstriction, exercise-induced; prevention: Oral: Administer dose at least 2 hours prior to exercise; additional doses should not be administered within 24 hours. Daily administration to prevent exercise-induced bronchospasm has not been evaluated.
Children and Adolescents 6-14 years: Chewable tablet: 5 mg/dose
Adolescents ≥15 years: Tablet: 10 mg/dose
Adults:
Asthma, allergic seasonal or perennial rhinitis: Oral: 10 mg once daily
Bronchoconstriction, exercise-induced (prevention): Oral: 10 mg at least 2 hours prior to exercise; additional doses should not be administered within 24 hours. Daily administration to prevent exercise-induced bronchoconstriction has not been evaluated.
Dosing adjustment in renal impairment: No adjustment necessary.
Dosing adjustment in hepatic impairment:
Mild to moderate impairment: No dosage adjustment necessary.
Severe impairment: There are no dosage adjustments provided in the manufacturer labeling; has not been studied.

Administration Oral: When treating asthma, administer dose in the evening. Patients with allergic rhinitis may individualize administration time (morning or evening). Patients with both asthma and allergic rhinitis should take their dose in the evening.
Granules: May be administered directly into the mouth or mixed in cold or room temperature soft foods; based on stability studies, only applesauce, mashed carrots, rice, and ice cream should be used; granules are not intended to be dissolved in liquid (other than breast milk or infant formula) and must be administered within 15 minutes of opening the packet; liquids may be taken subsequent to administration.

Monitoring Parameters Pulmonary function tests (FEV-1), improvement in asthma symptoms, behavioral effects

Additional Information Recent studies of montelukast use in acute asthma and RSV bronchiolitis have shown promising results. Pulmonary function tests improved significantly in adult patients receiving a single dose (10 mg) montelukast along with IV prednisolone at the onset of an acute asthma exacerbation (Cylly, 2003). Pediatric patients with RSV positive bronchiolitis receiving daily montelukast demonstrated fewer symptoms when compared with placebo treated controls (Bisgaard, 2003).

Dosage Forms Excipient information presented when available (limited, particularly for generics); consult specific product labeling.
Packet, Oral:
Singulair: 4 mg (30 ea)
Generic: 4 mg (1 ea, 30 ea)
Tablet, Oral:
Singulair: 10 mg
Generic: 10 mg
Tablet Chewable, Oral:
Singulair: 4 mg [contains aspartame]
Singulair: 4 mg [contains aspartame; cherry flavor]
Singulair: 5 mg [contains aspartame]
Singulair: 5 mg [contains aspartame; cherry flavor]
Generic: 4 mg, 5 mg

◆ **Montelukast Sodium** *see* Montelukast *on page 1459*
◆ **Montelukast Sodium Tablets (Can)** *see* Montelukast *on page 1459*
◆ **MoreDophilus® [OTC]** *see Lactobacillus on page 1203*
◆ **Morgidox** *see* Doxycycline *on page 717*
◆ **Moroctocog Alfa** *see* Antihemophilic Factor (Recombinant) *on page 168*

Morphine (Systemic) (MOR feen)

Medication Safety Issues
Sound-alike/look-alike issues:
Morphine may be confused with HYDROmorphone, methadone
Morphine sulfate may be confused with magnesium sulfate
Kadian may be confused with Kapidex [DSC]
MS Contin may be confused with OxyCONTIN
MSO_4 and MS are error-prone abbreviations (mistaken as magnesium sulfate)
AVINza may be confused with Evista, INVanz
Roxanol may be confused with OxyFast, Roxicet, Roxicodone
High alert medication:
The Institute for Safe Medication Practices (ISMP) includes this medication (IV formulation) among its list of drug classes which have a heightened risk of causing significant patient harm when used in error.
Other safety concerns:
Use care when prescribing and/or administering morphine solutions. These products are available in different concentrations. Always prescribe dosage in mg; **not** by volume (mL).
Use caution when selecting a morphine formulation for use in neurologic infusion pumps (eg, Medtronic delivery systems). The product should be appropriately labeled as "preservative-free" and suitable for intraspinal use via continuous infusion. In addition, the product should be formulated in a pH range that is compatible with the device operation specifications.
Significant differences exist between oral and IV dosing. Use caution when converting from one route of administration to another.

Related Information
Opioid Conversion Table *on page 2285*
Oral Medications That Should Not Be Crushed or Altered *on page 2476*
Patient Information for Disposal of Unused Medications *on page 2453*
Preprocedure Sedatives in Children *on page 2444*

Brand Names: US Astramorph; AVINza [DSC]; Duramorph; Infumorph 200; Infumorph 500; Kadian; MS Contin

Brand Names: Canada Doloral; Kadian; M-Eslon; M.O.S. 10; M.O.S. 20; M.O.S. 30; M.O.S.-SR; M.O.S.-Sulfate; Morphine Extra Forte Injection; Morphine Forte Injection; Morphine HP; Morphine LP Epidural; Morphine SR; Morphine-EPD; MS Contin; MS Contin SRT; MS-IR; Novo-Morphine SR; PMS-Morphine Sulfate SR; ratio-Morphine; ratio-Morphine SR; Sandoz-Morphine SR; Statex; Teva-Morphine SR

Therapeutic Category Analgesic, Narcotic

Generic Availability (US) Yes

Use

Oral:

Immediate release formulations (oral solution and tablets): Management of moderate to severe acute and chronic pain (FDA approved in ages ≥18 years and adults); has also been used for treatment of neonatal abstinence syndrome, iatrogenic opioid withdrawal, and palliative care management of dyspnea

Controlled and extended release products (eg, Avinza, Kadian, MS Contin): Management of moderate to severe **chronic** pain when continuous, around-the-clock opioid analgesia is required for an extended amount of time (FDA approved in ages ≥18 years and adults); **Note:** Not intended for use as a PRN analgesic or for treatment of mild pain, acute pain, pain that is not expected to persist for an extended period of time, or for immediate postoperative pain (within 12-24 hours after surgery) unless the patient is already receiving chronic opioid therapy prior to surgery or if postoperative pain is expected to be moderate to severe and persist for an extended period of time

Parenteral:

Intravenous: Management of severe acute pain; preanesthetic sedative [FDA approved in pediatric patients (age not specified) and adults]; has also been used for management of hypercyanotic spells associate with tetralogy of Fallot; and for palliative care management of dyspnea (including nebulization)

Epidural (at the lumbar level): Management of pain unresponsive to nonopioid analgesics (Astramorph/PF, Duramorph: FDA approved in adults); treatment of intractable chronic pain as an epidural infusion via microinfusion device (Infumorph: FDA approved in adults)

Intrathecal (at lumbar level): Management of pain unresponsive to nonopioid analgesics (Astramorph/PF, Duramorph: FDA approved in adults); treatment of intractable chronic pain as a continuous infusion via microinfusion device (Infumorph: FDA approved in adults)

Rectal: Suppositories: Management of severe acute and chronic pain (FDA approved in adults)

Medication Guide Available Yes

Pregnancy Risk Factor C

Pregnancy Considerations Adverse events have been observed in some animal reproduction studies. Morphine crosses the human placenta. The frequency of congenital malformations has not been reported to be greater than expected in children from mothers treated with morphine during pregnancy. However, following *in utero* exposure, infants may exhibit withdrawal, decreased brain volume (reversible), small size, decreased ventilatory response to CO_2, and increased risk of sudden infant death syndrome.

Morphine sulfate injection may be used for the management of pain during labor (ACOG, 2002); however, some manufacturers specifically contraindicate use of the injection during labor when a premature birth is anticipated. When used for pain relief during labor, opioids may temporarily affect the heart rate of the fetus. Morphine injection may also be used to treat pain following delivery (ACOG, 2002).

[U.S. Boxed Warning]: Prolonged maternal use of opioids during pregnancy can cause neonatal withdrawal syndrome in the newborn, which may be life-threatening if not recognized and treated according to protocols developed by neonatology experts. If prolonged opioid therapy is required in a pregnant woman, ensure treatment is available and warn patient of risk to the neonate. If chronic opioid exposure occurs in pregnancy, adverse events in the newborn (including withdrawal) may occur; monitoring of the neonate is recommended. The minimum effective dose should be used if opioids are needed (Chou, 2009). Neonatal abstinence syndrome following opioid exposure may present with autonomic (eg, fever, temperature instability), gastrointestinal (eg, diarrhea, vomiting, poor feeding/weight gain), or neurologic (eg, high-pitched crying, increased muscle tone, irritability, seizure, tremor) symptoms (Dow, 2012; Hudak, 2012).

Long-term opioid use may cause secondary hypogonadism, which may lead to sexual dysfunction or infertility (Brennan, 2013).

Breast-Feeding Considerations Morphine concentrates in breast milk, with a milk to plasma AUC ratio of 2.5:1. Detectable serum levels of morphine can be found in infants following morphine administration to nursing mothers.

Parenteral opioids used during labor have the potential to interfere with a newborn's natural reflex to nurse within the first few hours after birth. Morphine is recommended as an analgesic in nursing women due to the limited amounts found in breast milk and poor oral bioavailability in nursing infants. Nursing infants exposed to large doses of opioids should be monitored for apnea and sedation (Montgomery, 2012).

Treatment of the mother with single doses of morphine is not expected to cause detrimental effects in nursing infants. Breast-feeding following chronic use or in neonates with hepatic or renal dysfunction may lead to higher levels of morphine in the infant and a risk of adverse effects (Spigset, 2000).

The manufacturers of extended release products note that due to the potential for serious adverse reactions in the nursing infant, a decision should be made whether to discontinue nursing or to discontinue the drug, taking into account the importance of treatment to the mother.

Contraindications Note: Some contraindications are product specific. For details, please see detailed product prescribing information.

Hypersensitivity to morphine sulfate or any component of the formulation; severe respiratory depression, acute or severe asthma (in an unmonitored setting or without resuscitative equipment); known or suspected paralytic ileus

Additional contraindication information (based on formulation):

Epidural/intrathecal:

Astramorph/PF, Duramorph: Upper airway obstruction

Astramorph/PF, Duramorph, Infumorph: Usual contraindications related to neuraxial analgesia apply (eg, presence of infection at infusion site, concomitant anticoagulant therapy, uncontrolled bleeding diathesis)

Extended release: GI obstruction

Immediate release tablets/solution: Hypercarbia

Injectable formulation: Heart failure due to chronic lung disease, cardiac arrhythmias; increased intracranial pressure, head injuries, brain tumors; acute alcoholism, deliriums tremens; seizure disorders; use during labor when a premature birth is anticipated

Suppository: Severe CNS depression; cardiac arrhythmias, heart failure due to chronic lung disease; increased intracranial or cerebrospinal pressure, head injuries, brain tumor; acute alcoholism, delirium tremens; seizure disorder; use after biliary tract surgery, suspected surgical abdomen, surgical anastomosis; concurrent use or within 2 weeks of MAO inhibitors

Warnings/Precautions An opioid-containing analgesic regimen should be tailored to each patient's needs and based upon the type of pain being treated (acute versus chronic), the route of administration, degree of tolerance for opioids (naive versus chronic user), age, weight, and medical condition. The optimal analgesic dose varies widely among patients. Doses should be titrated to pain relief/prevention. When used as an epidural injection, monitor for delayed sedation.

All morphine sulfate formulations are capable of causing respiratory depression; risk increased in elderly patients, debilitated patients, and patients with conditions associated with hypoxia or hypercapnia. Monitor for respiratory depression, especially during initiation and titration. Extended-release formulations: **[U.S. Boxed Warning]: May cause serious, life-threatening, or fatal respiratory depression. Monitor closely for respiratory depression, especially during initiation or dose escalation. Instruct patients to swallow extended-release morphine formulations whole (or may sprinkle the contents of the Avinza capsule on applesauce and swallow without chewing); crushing, chewing, or dissolving the extended-release formulations can cause rapid release and absorption of a potentially fatal dose of morphine.** Carbon dioxide retention from opioid-induced respiratory depression can exacerbate the sedating effects of opioids. Use with caution and monitor for respiratory depression in patients with significant chronic obstructive pulmonary disease or cor pulmonale, and patients having a substantially decreased respiratory reserve, hypoxia, hypercarbia, or preexisting respiratory depression, particularly when initiating therapy and titrating with morphine; even therapeutic doses may decrease respiratory drive to the point of apnea. Consider the use of alternative nonopioid analgesics in these patients. Some dosage forms may be contraindicated in patients with severe respiratory disorders. Infants <3 months of age are more susceptible to respiratory depression, use with caution and generally in reduced doses in this age group.

Use caution in morbid obesity, adrenal insufficiency, prostatic hyperplasia, thyroid dysfunction, urinary stricture, renal impairment, or severe hepatic dysfunction and in patients with hypersensitivity reactions to other phenanthrene derivative opioid agonists (codeine, hydrocodone, hydromorphone, levorphanol, oxycodone, oxymorphone). Avoid use in patients with CNS depression or coma as these patients are susceptible to intracranial effects of CO_2 retention. Use with caution in patients with biliary tract dysfunction including acute pancreatitis as may cause constriction of sphincter of Oddi. May obscure diagnosis or clinical course of patients with acute abdominal conditions. May cause constipation which may be problematic in patients with unstable angina and patients post-myocardial infarction. Some preparations contain sulfites which may cause allergic reactions.

May cause CNS depression, which may impair physical or mental abilities; patients must be cautioned about performing tasks which require mental alertness (eg, operating machinery or driving). Potentially significant drug interactions may exist, requiring dose or frequency adjustment, additional monitoring, and/or selection of alternative therapy. Effects may be potentiated when used with other CNS depressants (eg, sedatives, anxiolytics, hypnotics, neuroleptics, other opioids). **[U.S. Boxed Warning]: Patients should not consume alcoholic beverages or medication containing ethanol while taking Avinza or Kadian; ethanol may increase morphine plasma levels resulting in a potentially fatal overdose.**

May cause hypotension; use with caution in patients with hypovolemia, cardiovascular disease (including acute MI), circulatory shock, or drugs which may exaggerate hypotensive effects (including phenothiazines or general anesthetics). May cause orthostatic hypotension and syncope in ambulatory patients. Use with extreme caution in patients with head injury, intracranial lesions, or elevated intracranial pressure; exaggerated elevation of ICP may occur if respiratory drive is depressed and CO_2 retention occurs. Use with caution in patients with seizure disorders, may exacerbate preexisting seizures. Tolerance or drug dependence may result from extended use. Concurrent use of mixed agonist/antagonist analgesics (eg, pentazocine, nalbuphine, butorphanol) or partial agonist (eg, buprenorphine) analgesics may precipitate withdrawal symptoms and/or reduced analgesic efficacy in patients following prolonged therapy with mu opioid agonists. Abrupt discontinuation following prolonged use may also lead to withdrawal symptoms; taper dose gradually when discontinuing.

Use epidural/intrathecal formulations with extreme caution in elderly patients.

Extended-release formulations: **[U.S. Boxed Warning]: Users are exposed to the risks of addiction, abuse, and misuse, potentially leading to overdose and death. Assess each patient's risk prior to prescribing; monitor all patients regularly for development of these behaviors or conditions.** Risk of opioid abuse is increased in patients with a history or family history of alcohol or drug abuse or mental illness. Avinza capsules contain fumaric acid; dangerous quantities of fumaric acid may be ingested when >1600 mg/day is used; serious renal toxicity may occur above the maximum dose. **Extended-release products are not interchangeable;** when determining a generic equivalent or switching from one extended-release product to another, review pharmacokinetic properties. **[U.S. Boxed Warning]: Prolonged maternal use of opioids during pregnancy can cause neonatal withdrawal syndrome in the newborn which may be life-threatening if not recognized and treated according to protocols developed by neonatology experts. If prolonged opioid therapy is required in a pregnant woman, ensure treatment is available and warn patient of risk to the neonate.** Signs and symptoms include irritability, hyperactivity, abnormal sleep pattern, high-pitched cry, tremor, vomiting, diarrhea, and failure to gain weight. Onset, duration, and severity depend on the drug used, duration of use, maternal dose, and rate of drug elimination by the newborn. **[U.S. Boxed Warning]: Accidental ingestion of even one dose, especially in children, can result in a fatal overdose of morphine.**

Highly concentrated oral solutions: **[U.S. Boxed Warning]: Check doses carefully when using highly concentrated oral solutions. The 100 mg/5 mL (20 mg/mL) concentration is indicated for use in opioid-tolerant patients only.**

Injections: Products are designed for administration by specific routes (ie, IV, intrathecal, epidural). Use caution when prescribing, dispensing, or administering to use formulations only by intended route(s).

Astramorph/PF, Duramorph, Infumorph: **[U.S. Boxed Warning]: Due to the risk of severe and/or sustained cardiopulmonary depressant effects, must be administered in a fully equipped room for resuscitation and staffed environment.** Naloxone injection should be immediately available. Patient should remain in this environment for at least 24 hours following the initial dose. **[U.S. Boxed Warning]: Accidental dermal exposure to Astramorph/PF, Duramorph, Infumorph should be rinsed with water. Contaminated clothing should be removed.** For patients receiving Infumorph via microinfusion device, patient may be observed, as appropriate, for the first several days after catheter implantation. Thoracic epidural administration has been shown to dramatically increase the risk of early and late respiratory depression.

[U.S. Boxed Warning]: Improper or erroneous substitution of Infumorph for regular Duramorph is likely to result in serious overdosage, leading to seizures, respiratory depression and possibly a fatal outcome. Infumorph should only be used in microinfusion devices; not for IV, IM, or SubQ administration or for single-dose administration. Monitor closely, especially in the first 24 hours. Inflammatory masses (eg, granulomas), some resulting in severe neurologic impairment have occurred when receiving Infumorph via indwelling intrathecal catheter; monitor carefully for new neurologic signs/symptoms. **[U.S. Boxed Warning]: Intrathecal dosage is usually 1/10 (one-tenth) that of epidural dosage.**

Benzyl alcohol and derivatives: Some dosage forms may contain sodium benzoate/benzoic acid; benzoic acid (benzoate) is a metabolite of benzyl alcohol; large amounts of benzyl alcohol (≥99 mg/kg/day) have been associated with a potentially fatal toxicity ("gasping syndrome") in neonates; the "gasping syndrome" consists of metabolic acidosis, respiratory distress, gasping respirations, CNS dysfunction (including convulsions, intracranial hemorrhage), hypotension, and cardiovascular collapse (AAP, 1997; CDC, 1982); some data suggests that benzoate displaces bilirubin from protein binding sites (Ahlfors, 2001); avoid or use dosage forms containing benzyl alcohol derivative with caution in neonates. See manufacturer's labeling.

Warnings: Additional Pediatric Considerations Prolonged use of any morphine product during pregnancy can result in neonatal opioid withdrawal syndrome, which may be life-threatening if not recognized and treated, and requires management according to protocols developed by neonatology experts.

For postoperative tonsillectomy (with/without adenoidectomy) pain management in pediatric patients, morphine has been shown to have a higher risk of adverse effects compared to other analgesics without additional analgesic benefit; patient-specific risk factors for these adverse events are not fully defined (Biesiade 2014; Jimenez 2012; Kelly 2015; Ragjavendran 2010; Sadhasivam 2012). Data is preliminary and large-scale population-based generalizations and recommendations for practice have not been made. However, racial differences in adverse effects have been observed. A statistically significant higher incidence of adverse effects (pruritus, emesis) was reported in Latino children and adolescents following perioperative morphine administration than the comparative non-Latino Caucasian cohort (Jimenez 2012). In another trial, Caucasian children and adolescents receiving peri/postoperative morphine showed a higher incidence of postoperative pruritis and emesis than African-American patients (Sadhasivam 2012). The observed risk for respiratory depression between racial groups has been variable, with some data showing no racial difference in risk between Latino and non-Latino Caucasians or between Caucasians and African-American patients, while other data shows a higher risk in African-American pediatric patients compared to Caucasians (Biesiada 2014; Jimenez 2012, Sadhasivam 2012). Regardless of race, an overall higher and clinically significant incidence of respiratory depression has been observed in patients with sleep disturbances requiring tonsillectomy procedure (eg, obstructive sleep apnea); a lower initial dose has been suggested in these patients (Ragjavendran 2010). Current guidelines recommend that children and adolescents receive intravenous dexamethasone intraoperatively and effective therapy for postoperative tonsillectomy pain; NSAIDs (except ketorolac) can be used safely (AAO-HNS [Baugh 2011]).

Adverse Reactions Note: Individual patient differences are unpredictable. Reactions may be dose-, formulation-, and/or route-dependent.

Cardiovascular: Atrial fibrillation, bradycardia, chest pain, circulatory depression, edema, flushing, hyper-/hypotension, palpitation, peripheral edema, shock, syncope, tachycardia, vasodilation

Central nervous system: Amnesia, agitation, anxiety, apathy, apprehension, ataxia, chills, coma, confusion, delirium, depression, dizziness, dream abnormalities, drowsiness (tolerance usually develops to drowsiness with regular dosing for 1-2 weeks), dysphonia, euphoria, false sense of well being, fever, hallucination, headache (following epidural or intrathecal use), hypoesthesia, insomnia, lethargy, malaise, nervousness, physical and psychological dependence, restlessness, sedation, seizure, slurred speech, somnolence, vertigo

Dermatologic: Dry skin, pruritus (may be dose related), rash, urticaria

Endocrine & metabolic: Antidiuretic hormone release, gynecomastia, hypogonadism, hypokalemia, hyponatremia, libido decreased

Gastrointestinal: Abdominal distension, anorexia, abdominal pain, biliary colic, constipation (tolerance develops very slowly if at all), diarrhea, dyspepsia, dysphagia, flatulence, gastroenteritis, GERD, GI irritation, nausea (tolerance usually develops to nausea and vomiting with chronic use), paralytic ileus, rectal disorder, taste perversion, vomiting, weight loss, xerostomia

Genitourinary: Urinary retention (may be prolonged, up to 20 hours, following epidural or intrathecal use), bladder spasm, dysuria, ejaculation abnormal, impotence, urination decreased

Hematologic: Anemia (following intrathecal use), hematocrit decreased, leukopenia, thrombocytopenia

Hepatic: Liver function tests increased

Local: Pain at injection site

Neuromuscular & skeletal: Arthralgia, back pain, bone mineral density decreased, bone pain, foot drop, gait abnormalities, myoclonus, paresthesia, rigors, skeletal muscle rigidity, tremor, weakness

Ocular: Amblyopia, conjunctivitis, eye pain, vision problems/disturbance

Renal: Oliguria

Respiratory: Asthma, atelectasis, dyspnea, hiccups, hypercapnia, hypoxia, oxygen saturation decreased,pulmonary edema (noncardiogenic), respiratory depression, rhinitis

Miscellaneous: Diaphoresis, flu-like syndrome, histamine release, infection, thirst, voice alteration, withdrawal syndrome

Rare but important or life-threatening: Amenorrhea, anaphylaxis, apnea, biliary tract spasm, blurred vision, bronchospasm, cardiac arrest, cough reflex decreased, dehydration, diplopia, disorientation, hemorrhagic urticaria, intestinal obstruction, intracranial pressure increased, laryngospasm, menstrual irregularities, miosis, myoclonus, nystagmus, paradoxical CNS stimulation, respiratory arrest, sepsis, urinary tract spasm, thermal dysregulation, toxic psychoses

Drug Interactions

Metabolism/Transport Effects Substrate of CYP2D6 (minor), P-glycoprotein; **Note:** Assignment of Major/Minor substrate status based on clinically relevant drug interaction potential

Avoid Concomitant Use

Avoid concomitant use of Morphine (Systemic) with any of the following: Azelastine (Nasal); Eluxadoline; MAO Inhibitors; Mixed Agonist / Antagonist Opioids; Orphenadrine; Paraldehyde; Thalidomide

Increased Effect/Toxicity

Morphine (Systemic) may increase the levels/effects of: Alcohol (Ethyl); Alvimopan; Azelastine (Nasal); CNS Depressants; Desmopressin; Diuretics; Eluxadoline; Hydrocodone; Methotrimeprazine; Metyrosine; Mirtazapine; Orphenadrine; Paraldehyde; Pramipexole; ROPINIRole; Rotigotine; Selective Serotonin Reuptake Inhibitors; Suvorexant; Thalidomide; Zolpidem

The levels/effects of Morphine (Systemic) may be increased by: Amphetamines; Anticholinergic Agents; Antipsychotic Agents (Phenothiazines); Brimonidine (Topical); Cannabis; Doxylamine; Dronabinol; Droperidol; HydrOXYzine; Kava Kava; Magnesium Sulfate; MAO Inhibitors; Methotrimeprazine; Nabilone; Perampanel; P-glycoprotein/ABCB1 Inhibitors; Rufinamide; Sodium Oxybate; Succinylcholine; Tapentadol; Tetrahydrocannabinol

Decreased Effect

Morphine (Systemic) may decrease the levels/effects of: Clopidogrel; Pegvisomant

The levels/effects of Morphine (Systemic) may be decreased by: Ammonium Chloride; Mixed Agonist / Antagonist Opioids; Naltrexone; P-glycoprotein/ABCB1 Inducers; Rifamycin Derivatives

Food Interactions

Ethanol: Alcoholic beverages or ethanol-containing products may disrupt extended release formulation resulting in rapid release of entire morphine dose. Management: Avoid alcohol. **Do not administer Avinza with alcoholic beverages or ethanol-containing prescription or non-prescription products.**

Food: Administration of oral morphine solution with food may increase bioavailability (ie, a report of 34% increase in morphine AUC when morphine oral solution followed a high-fat meal). The bioavailability of Avinza, MS Contin, or Kadian does not appear to be affected by food. Management: Take consistently with or without meals.

Storage/Stability

Capsule, extended release: Store at 25°C (77°F); excursions permitted to 15°C to 30°C (59°F to 86°F). Protect from light and moisture.

Injection: Store at controlled room temperature of 20°C to 25°C (68°F to 77°F); do not freeze. Protect from light. Degradation depends on pH and presence of oxygen; relatively stable in pH ≤4; darkening of solutions indicate degradation.

Astramorph/PF, Duramorph, Infumorph: Store in carton until use at controlled room temperature of 20°C to 25°C (68°F to 77°F); excursions permitted to 15°C to 30°C (59°F to 86°F); do not freeze; do not heat-sterilize. Contains no preservative or antioxidant. Protect from light.

Oral solution: Store at controlled room temperature of 15°C to 30°C (59°F to 86°F); do not freeze. Protect from moisture.

Suppositories: Store below controlled room temperature 25°C (77°F).

Tablet, extended release: Store at controlled room temperature of 25°C (77°F); excursions permitted to 15°C to 30°C (59°F to 86°F).

Tablet, immediate release: Store at controlled room temperature of 15°C to 30°C (59°F to 86°F). Protect from moisture.

Mechanism of Action Binds to opioid receptors in the CNS, causing inhibition of ascending pain pathways, altering the perception of and response to pain; produces generalized CNS depression

Pharmacodynamics See table.

Dosage Form / Route	Analgesia	
	Peak	Duration
Tablets	1 h	3 to 5 h
Oral solution	1 h	3 to 5 h
Epidural	1 h	12 to 20 h
Extended release tablets	3 to 4 h	8 to 12 h
Suppository	20 to 60 min	3 to 7 h
Subcutaneous injection	50 to 90 min	3 to 5 h
IM injection	30 to 60 min	3 to 5 h
IV injection	20 min	3 to 5 h

Pharmacokinetics (Adult data unless noted)

Absorption: Oral: Variable

Distribution: Distributes to skeletal muscle, liver, kidneys, lungs, intestinal tract, spleen and brain

V_d, apparent:

Pediatric cancer patients (age: 1.7 to 18.7 years): Median: 5.2 L/kg; a significantly higher V_d was observed in children <11 years (median: 7.1 L/kg) versus >11 years (median: 4.7 L/kg) (Hunt 1999)

Adults: 1 to 6 L/kg

Protein binding:

Premature Infants: <20%

Adults: 20% to 35%

Metabolism: Hepatic via glucuronide conjugation to morphine-6-glucuronide (active) and morphine-3-glucuronide (inactive)

Bioavailability: Nebulization: 5.5 ± 3.2% (Masood 1996)

Half-life:

Preterm: 10 to 20 hours

Neonates: 7.6 hours (range: 4.5 to 13.3 hours)

Infants 1 to 3 months: Median: 6.2 hours (range: 5 to 10 hours) (McRorie 1992)

Infants 3 to 6 months: Median: 4.5 hours (range: 3.8 to 7.3 hours) (McRorie 1992)

Infants 6 months to Children 2.5 years: Median: 2.9 hours (range: 1.4 to 7.8 hours) (McRorie 1992)

Preschool Children: 1 to 2 hours

Pediatric patients with sickle cell disease (age: 6 to 19 years): ~1.3 hours (Dampier 1995)

Adults: Immediate release: 2 to 4 hours; Avinza: ~24 hours; Kadian: 11 to 13 hours

Elimination: Excreted unchanged in urine:

Neonates: 3% to 15%

Adults: 2% to 12%

Clearance: **Note:** In pediatric patients, adult values are reached by 6 months to 2.5 years of age (McRorie 1992)

Preterm: 0.5 to 3 mL/minute/kg

Neonates 1 to 7 days: Median: 5.5 mL/minute/kg (range: 3.2 to 8.4 mL/minute/kg) (McRorie 1992)

Neonates 8 to 30 days: Median: 7.4 mL/minute/kg (range: 3.4 to 13.8 mL/minute/kg) (McRorie 1992)

Infants 1 to 3 months: Median: 10.5 mL/minute/kg (range: 9.8 to 20.1 mL/minute/kg) (McRorie 1992)

Infants 3 to 6 months: Median: 13.9 mL/minute/kg (range: 8.3 to 24.1 mL/minute/kg) (McRorie 1992)

Infants 6 months to Children 2.5 years: Median: 21.7 mL/minute/kg (range: 5.8 to 28.6 mL/minute/kg) (McRorie 1992)

Preschool Children: 20 to 40 mL/minute/kg

Pediatric cancer patients (age: 1.7 to 18.7 years): Median: 23.1 mL/minute/kg; a significantly higher clearance was observed in children <11 years (median: 37.4 mL/minute/kg) versus >11 years (median: 21.9 mL/minute/kg) (Hunt 1999)

Pediatric patients with sickle cell disease (age: 6 to 19 years): ~36 mL/minute/kg (range: 6 to 59 mL/minute/kg) (Dampier 1995)

Adults: 20 to 30 mL/minute/kg

Dosing: Neonatal Doses should be titrated to appropriate effect; when changing routes of administration in chronically treated patients, please note that oral doses are approximately one-half as effective as parenteral dose; **Note: Use preservative-free formulation:**

Analgesia:

Oral: Oral solution (2 mg/mL or 4 mg/mL): 0.08 mg/kg/dose every 4 to 6 hours (APA 2012)

IM, IV (preferred), SubQ: Initial: 0.05 to 0.1 mg/kg/dose; usual frequency every 4 to 6 hours, although some neonates may require every 8 hour dosing; titrate carefully to effect; maximum dose: 0.1 mg/kg/dose (Anand 2001; Hegenbarth 2008)

Continuous IV infusion: Initial: 0.01 mg/kg/**hour** (10 **mcg**/kg/**hour**); titrate carefully to effect; maximum: 0.03 mg/kg/**hour** (30 **mcg**/kg/**hour**) (Anand, 2001); some have suggested a lower usual maximum infusion rate of 0.015 to 0.02 mg/kg/**hour** (15 to 20 **mcg**/kg/**hour**) due to decreased elimination, increased CNS sensitivity, and adverse effects; **Note:** Some centers may use slightly higher doses, especially in neonates who develop tolerance.

Endotracheal intubation, nonemergent: IM, IV: 0.05 to 0.1 mg/kg; allow at least 5 minutes for onset of analgesia (Kumar 2010)

Neonatal abstinence syndrome: Limited data available: Oral: Oral solution (2 mg/mL or 4 mg/mL): Initial: 0.04 mg/kg/dose every 3 to 4 hours; increase by 0.04 mg/kg/dose if symptoms are not controlled; maximum dose: 0.2 mg/kg/dose (Hudak 2012); dose and weaning schedule should be individualized based on signs and symptoms of withdrawal and/or withdrawal scores; once withdrawal symptoms are controlled, maintain dose for 48 to 72 hours; then taper dose usually by 10% to 20% every 2 to 7 days (Burgos 2009; Hudak 2012).

Dosing: Usual Doses should be titrated to appropriate effect; when changing routes of administration in chronically treated patients, please note that oral doses are approximately one-half as effective as parenteral dose.

Infants, Children, and Adolescents:

Acute pain, moderate to severe: Note: The use of IM injections is no longer recommended, especially for repeated administration due to painful administration, variable absorption, and lag time to peak effect; other routes are more reliable and less painful (American Pain Society 2008).

Infants ≤6 months, nonventilated: **Note:** Infants <3 months of age are more susceptible to respiratory depression; lower doses are recommended (American Pain Society 2008):

Oral: Oral solution (2 mg/mL or 4 mg/mL): 0.08 to 0.1 mg/kg/dose every 3 to 4 hours (American Pain Society 2008; Berde 2002)

IV or SubQ: 0.025 to 0.03 mg/kg/dose every 2 to 4 hours (American Pain Society 2008; Berde 2002)

Infants >6 months, Children, and Adolescents:

Oral: Immediate release tablets, oral solution (2 mg/mL or 4 mg/mL):

Patient weight <50 kg: 0.2 to 0.5 mg/kg/dose every 3 to 4 hours as needed; some experts have recommended an initial dose of 0.3 mg/kg for severe pain; usual initial maximum dose: 15 to 20 mg (American Pain Society 2008; APA 2012; Berde 2002)

Patient weight ≥50 kg: 15 to 20 mg every 3 to 4 hours as needed (American Pain Society 2008; Berde 2002)

IM, IV, or SubQ; intermittent dosing:

Patient weight <50 kg: Initial: 0.05 mg/kg/dose; usual range: 0.1 to 0.2 mg/kg/dose every 2 to 4 hours as needed; usual maximum dose: Infants: 2 mg/dose; Children 1 to 6 years: 4 mg/dose; Children 7 to 12 years: 8 mg/dose; Adolescents: 10 mg/dose

Patient weight ≥50 kg: Initial: 2 to 5 mg every 2 to 4 hours as needed; higher doses have been recommended (5 to 8 mg every 2 to 4 hours as needed) and may be needed in tolerant patients (Berde 2002; Kliegman 2011)

Continuous IV infusion, SubQ continuous infusion:

Patient weight <50 kg: Initial: 0.01 mg/kg/hour (10 mcg/kg/hour); titrate carefully to effect; dosage range: 0.01 to 0.04 mg/kg/**hour** (10 to 40 **mcg**/kg/**hour**) (APA 2012; Friedrichsdorf 2007; Golianu 2000)

Patient weight ≥50 kg: 1.5 mg/**hour** (Berde 2002)

Conversion from intermittent IV morphine: Administer the patient's total daily IV morphine dose over 24 hours as a continuous infusion; titrate dose to appropriate effect

Epidural: Astramorph/PF, Duramorph: Limited data available: **Note: Must use preservative-free formulation:**

Intermittent: 0.015 to 0.05 mg/kg (15 to 50 **mcg**/kg) (APA 2012; Henneberg 1993); a trial evaluating pain relief in pediatric patients after abdominal surgery (n=76; age: newborn to 13 years; median age: 12 months) administered epidural morphine every 8 hours in combination with bupivacaine during the immediate postop period; most children achieved good pain relief with this regimen (Henneberg 1993). Maximum dose: 0.1 mg/kg (100 **mcg**/kg) or 5 mg/24 hours

Continuous epidural infusion: Infants > 6 months, Children, and Adolescents: 0.001 to 0.005 mg/kg/**hour** (1 to 5 **mcg**/kg/**hour**) (Suresh 2012)

Analgesia for minor procedures/sedation: IV: 0.05 to 0.1 mg/kg/dose; administer 5 minutes before the procedure; maximum dose: 4 mg; may repeat dose in 5 minutes if necessary (Cramton 2012; Zeltzer 1990)

Patient-controlled analgesia (PCA), opioid-naïve: Note: All patients should receive an initial loading dose of an analgesic (to attain adequate control of pain) before starting PCA for maintenance. Adjust doses, lockouts, and limits based on required loading dose, age, state of health, and presence of opioid tolerance. Use lower end of dosing range for opioid-naïve. Assess patient and pain control at regular intervals and adjust settings if needed (American Pain Society 2008): IV:

Children ≥5 years and Adolescents, weighing <50 kg: **Note:** PCA has been used in children as young as 5 years of age; however, clinicians need to assess children 5 to 8 years of age to determine if they are able to use the PCA device correctly (American Pain Society 2008).

Usual concentration: 1 mg/mL

Demand dose: Usual initial: 0.02 mg/kg/dose; usual range: 0.01 to 0.03 mg/kg/dose

Lockout: Usual initial: 5 doses/hour

Lockout interval: Range: 6 to 8 minutes

Usual basal rate: 0 to 0.03 mg/kg/hour

Children and Adolescents, weighing ≥50 kg:

Usual concentration: 1 mg/mL

Demand dose: Usual initial: 1 mg; usual range: 0.5 to 2.5 mg

Lockout interval: Usual initial: 6 minutes; usual range: 5 to 10 minutes

Chronic pain: Note: Patients taking opioids chronically may become tolerant and require doses higher than the usual dosage range to maintain the desired effect. Tolerance can be managed by appropriate dose titration. There is no optimal or maximal dose for morphine in chronic pain. The appropriate dose is one that relieves pain throughout its dosing interval without causing unmanageable side effects. Consider total daily dose, potency, prior opioid use, degree of opioid experience and tolerance, conversion from previous opioid (including opioid formulation), patient's general condition, concurrent medications, and type and severity of pain during prescribing process.

Oral: Extended/controlled release preparations: A patient's morphine requirement should be established using immediate release formulations. Conversion to long-acting products may be considered when chronic, continuous treatment is required. Higher dosages should be reserved for use only in opioid-tolerant patients.

Capsules, extended release (Avinza): Adolescents ≥18 years: Daily dose administered once daily (for best results, administer at same time each day)

Opioid-naive: Initial: 30 mg once daily; adjust in increments ≤30 mg daily every 4 days

Conversion from other oral morphine formulations to Avinza: Total daily morphine dose given as once daily. The first dose of Avinza may be taken with the last dose of the immediate release morphine. Patients who experience breakthrough pain may require dose adjustment or rescue with a small dose of immediate release morphine. Maximum: 1,600 mg daily due to fumaric acid content.

Capsules, extended release (Kadian): Adolescents ≥18 years: **Note:** Not intended for use as an initial opioid in the management of pain; use immediate release formulations before initiation. Total daily oral morphine dose may be either administered once daily or in 2 divided doses daily (every 12 hours). The first dose of Kadian may be taken with the last dose of the immediate release morphine.

Tablets, controlled release (MS Contin): Children and Adolescents: Usually not used as an initial opioid in the management of pain; use immediate release formulations to titrate dose. Total daily morphine dose may be administered in 2 divided doses daily (every 12 hours) or in 3 divided doses daily (every 8 hours).

Weight-directed dosing: 0.3 to 0.6 mg/kg/dose every 12 hours (Berde 1990)

Alternate dosing; fixed dosing (Berde 2002):

Patient weight 20 to <35 kg: 10 to 15 mg every 8 to 12 hours; **Note:** 10 mg strength not available in US

Patient weight 35 to <50 kg: 15 to 30 mg every 8 to 12 hours

Patient weight ≥50 kg: 30 to 45 mg every 8 to 12 hours

Conversion from parenteral morphine or other opioids to controlled/extended release formulations: Substantial interpatient variability exists in relative potency. Therefore, it is safer to underestimate a patient's daily oral morphine requirement and provide breakthrough pain relief with immediate release morphine than to overestimate requirements. Consider the parenteral to oral morphine ratio or other oral or parenteral opioids to oral morphine conversions.

Continuous IV infusion, SubQ continuous infusion: Children and Adolescents: 0.01 to 0.04 mg/kg/**hour** (10 to 40 **mcg**/kg/**hour**) (APA 2012; Friedrichsdorf 2007; Golianu 2000); opioid-tolerate patients may require higher doses; in a small study of terminal pediatric oncology patients (n=8; age range: 3-16 years), the median required dose was 0.04 to 0.07 mg/kg/**hour** (40 to 70 **mcg**/kg/**hour**); range: 0.025 to 2.6 mg/kg/**hour** (Miser 1980); another study evaluating subcutaneous continuous infusion in children with cancer (n=17; age range: 22 months to 22 years) had similar findings; median dose: 0.06 mg/kg/**hour** (60 **mcg**/kg/**hour**); range: 0.025 to 1.79 mg/kg/**hour** (Miser 1983)

Conversion from intermittent IV morphine: Administer the patient's total daily IV morphine dose over 24 hours as a continuous infusion; titrate dose to appropriate effect

Sickle cell disease, acute crisis (NHLBI 2002): IV:

Infants ≥6 months and Children weighing ≤50 kg: Loading dose: 0.1-0.15 mg/kg once (maximum dose: 5 mg), then begin 0.05 mg to 0.1 mg/kg/dose every 2 to 4 hours (maximum dose: 2.5 mg)

Children and Adolescents weighing >50 kg: Loading dose: 5 to 10 mg once, then begin 2.5 to 5 mg dose every 2 to 4 hours

Tetralogy of fallot, hypercyanotic spell (infundibular spasm): Limited data available: IM, IV, SubQ: 0.1 mg/kg has been used to decrease ventilatory drive and systemic venous return (Hegenbarth 2008)

Palliative care, dyspnea management: Limited data available:

Inhalation (nebulization; preservative-free injection): Dose should be individualized and is dependent upon patient's previous or current systemic opioid exposure; doses not intended to provide analgesic activity; current systemic analgesia should be continued: Initial dose: Equivalent to patient's 4-hour systemic morphine requirement (eg, IV or oral dose); titrate to effect (Golianu, 2000); every 4-6 hour administration has been suggested (Cohen 2002). In the only pediatric case report (end-stage CF, age: 10 years, weight: 20 kg), an initial dose of 2.5 mg was used and final dose was 10 mg every 4 to 6 hours (Cohen 2002); from experience in adult patients, an initial dose of 5 mg has been used and reported range 2.5 to 30 mg administered up to every 4 hours (Ferraresi 2005; Shirk 2006)

IV: Initial: 25% of 4-hour intermittent dose; titrate until patient is comfortable (Golianu 2000)

Oral: 0.1 mg/kg/dose every 4 hours as needed

Adults:

Acute pain (moderate to severe):

Oral (immediate release formulations): Opioid-naive: Initial: **Note:** Usual dosage range: 10 to 30 mg every 4 hours as needed. Patients with prior opioid exposure may require higher initial doses.

Solution: 10 to 20 mg every 4 hours as needed

Tablet: 15 to 30 mg every 4 hours as needed

IM, SubQ: **Note:** Repeated SubQ administration causes local tissue irritation, pain, and induration. The use of IM injections is no longer recommended, especially for repeated administration due to painful administration, variable absorption, and lag time to peak effect; other routes are more reliable and less painful (American Pain Society 2008).

Initial: Opioid-naive: 5 to 10 mg every 4 hours as needed; usual dosage range: 5 to 15 mg every 4 hours as needed. Patients with prior opioid exposure may require higher initial doses.

IV: Initial: Opioid-naive: 2.5 to 5 mg/dose every 3 to 4 hours as needed; patients with prior opioid exposure may require higher initial doses

Continuous IV infusion, SubQ continuous infusion: 0.8 to 10 mg/hour; may increase depending on pain relief/adverse effects; usual range up to 80 mg/hour. **Note:** May administer a loading dose (amount administered should depend on severity of pain) prior to initiating the infusion. A continuous (basal) infusion is not recommended in an opioid-naive patient (ISMP 2009).

Rectal: 10 to 20 mg every 3 to 4 hours

Patient-controlled analgesia (PCA): Note: In opioid-naïve patients, consider lower end of dosing range:
Usual concentration: 1 mg/mL
Demand dose: Usual initial: 1 mg; usual range: 0.5 to 2.5 mg
Lockout interval: 5 to 10 minutes

Epidural: Note: Use preservative-free formulation; use lower doses and with extreme caution in debilitated patients. Vigilant monitoring is particularly important in these patients:
Single dose: **Lumbar region:** Astramorph/PF, Duramorph: 30 to 100 **mcg**/kg (optimal range: 2.5 to 3.75 mg; may depend upon patient comorbidities; Bujedo 2012; Sultan 2011)
Continuous infusion (may be combined with bupivacaine): 0.2 to 0.4 mg/hour (Bujedo 2012)
Continuous microinfusion (Infumorph):
Opioid-naive: Initial: 3.5 to 7.5 mg over 24 hours
Opioid-tolerant: Initial: 4.5 to 10 mg over 24 hours, titrate to effect; usual maximum is ~30 mg per 24 hours

Intrathecal: Note: Must use preservative-free formulation; use lower doses and with extreme caution in debilitated patients. Intrathecal dose is usually 1/10 (one-tenth) that of epidural dosage.
Opioid-naive: Single dose: **Lumbar region:** Astramorph/PF, Duramorph: 0.1 to 0.3 mg (may provide adequate relief for up to 24 hours; APS 2008); repeat doses **not** recommended. If pain recurs within 24 hours of administration, use of an alternate route of administration is recommended. **Note:** Although product labeling recommends doses up to 1 mg, an analgesic ceiling exists with doses >0.3 mg and the risk of respiratory depression is higher with doses >0.3 mg (Rathmell 2005).
Continuous microinfusion (Infumorph): **Lumbar region:** After initial in-hospital evaluation of response to single-dose injections (Astramorph/PF, Duramorph) the initial dose of Infumorph is 0.2 to 1 mg over 24 hours
Opioid-tolerant: Continuous microinfusion (Infumorph): **Lumbar region:** Dosage range: 1 to 10 mg over 24 hours, titrate to effect; usual maximum: ~20 mg over 24 hours

Chronic pain: Note: Patients taking opioids chronically may become tolerant and require doses higher than the usual dosage range to maintain the desired effect. Tolerance can be managed by appropriate dose titration. There is no optimal or maximal dose for morphine in chronic pain. The appropriate dose is one that relieves pain throughout its dosing interval without causing unmanageable side effects. Consider total daily dose, potency, prior opioid use, degree of opioid experience and tolerance, conversion from previous opioid (including opioid formulation), patient's general condition, concurrent medications, and type and severity of pain during prescribing process.
Oral (extended release formulations): A patient's morphine requirement should be established using immediate release formulations. Conversion to long-acting products may be considered when chronic, continuous treatment is required. Higher dosages should be reserved for use only in opioid-tolerant patients.
Capsules, extended release (Avinza):
Opioid-naive: Initial: 30 mg once daily; adjust in increments ≤30 mg daily every 4 days administered once daily (for best results, administer at same time each day)
Conversion from other oral morphine formulations to Avinza: Total daily morphine dose given once daily. The first dose of Avinza may be taken with the last dose of the immediate release morphine; maximum dose: 1600 mg daily due to fumaric acid content
Capsules, extended release (Kadian): **Note:** Not intended for use as an initial opioid in the management of pain; use immediate release formulations before initiation. Total daily oral morphine dose may be either administered once daily or in 2 divided doses daily (every 12 hours). The first dose of Kadian may be taken with the last dose of the immediate release morphine.
Tablets, extended release (MS Contin): Daily dose divided and administered every 8 or every 12 hours
Conversion from parenteral morphine or other opioids to extended release formulations: Substantial interpatient variability exists in relative potency. Therefore, it is safer to underestimate a patient's daily oral morphine requirement and provide breakthrough pain relief with immediate release morphine than to overestimate requirements. Consider the parenteral to oral morphine ratio or other oral or parenteral opioids to oral morphine conversions.

Dosing adjustment in renal impairment:
Infants, Children and Adolescents: IV, Oral: Dosage adjustments are not provided in the manufacturer's labeling; however, the following adjustments have been recommended (Aronoff 2007). **Note:** Renally adjusted dose recommendations are based on oral (immediate release) doses of 0.2 to 0.5 mg/kg/dose every 4 to 6 hours and IV doses of 0.05 to 0.2 mg/kg/dose every 2 to 4 hours:
GFR >50 mL/minute/1.73 m^2: No dosage adjustment necessary
GFR 10-50 mL/minute/1.73 m^2: Administer 75% of dose
GFR <10 mL/minute/1.73 m^2: Administer 50% of dose
Intermittent hemodialysis: Administer 50% of dose
Peritoneal dialysis (PD): Administer 50% of dose
Continuous renal replacement therapy (CRRT): Administer 75% of dose; titrate to effect
Adults:
CrCl 10 to 50 mL/minute: Administer 75% of normal dose
CrCl <10 mL/minute: Administer 50% of normal dose
Intermittent HD: No dosage adjustment necessary
Continuous renal replacement therapy (CRRT): Administer 75% of normal dose, titrate

Dosing adjustment in hepatic impairment: There are no dosage adjustments provided in manufacturer's labeling. Pharmacokinetics are unchanged in mild liver disease; substantial extrahepatic metabolism may occur. In cirrhosis, increases in half-life and AUC suggest dosage adjustment required.

Usual Infusion Concentrations: Neonatal IV infusion: 0.1 mg/mL

Usual Infusion Concentrations: Pediatric IV infusion: 0.1 mg/mL, 0.5 mg/mL, **or** 1 mg/mL

Preparation for Administration
Parenteral:
IV push/intermittent infusion: May dilute to a final concentration of 0.5 to 5 mg/mL
Continuous IV infusion: Dilute in D_5W, $D_{10}W$, or NS to a usual final concentration of 0.1 to 1 mg/mL; more concentrated solutions may be used in patients requiring fluid restriction or high doses (Murray 2014; Sinclair-Pingel 2006); concentrations >5 mg/mL are rarely needed (Gahart 2014). ISMP and Vermont Oxford Network recommend a standard concentration of 0.1 mg/mL for neonates (ISMP 2011).
Epidural and intrathecal: **Use only preservative-free injections.** Dilution may be required; determined by the individual patient's dosage requirements and the characteristics of the continuous microinfusion device; filter through ≤5 micron microfilter before injecting into microinfusion device

Inhalation: Limited data available; utilize preservative-free parenteral morphine and dilute with NS to a final volume of 5 mL (Cohen 2002; Ferraresi 2005; Shirk 2006)

Administration

Oral: Administer with food

Immediate release: Oral solution: Available in multiple strengths, including a concentrated oral solution (20 mg/mL). Precautions should be taken to avoid confusion between the different concentrations; prescriptions should have the concentration specified as well as the dose clearly represented as milligram (mg) of morphine, not volume (mL). The enclosed calibrated oral syringe should always be used to administer the concentrated oral solution to ensure the dose is measured and administered accurately. The concentrated oral solution (20 mg/mL) should only be used in opioid-tolerant patients (adults taking ≥60 mg/day of morphine or equivalent for ≥1 week).

Extended/controlled release products: Do not chew, crush, break, or dissolve extended and controlled release products; swallow whole. Avinza and Kadian capsules may be opened and contents sprinkled on a small amount of applesauce and eaten immediately without chewing; rinse mouth with water and swallow to ensure all beads have been ingested; do not chew, crush, or dissolve beads or pellets from capsule as it can result in a rapid release and absorption of a potentially fatal dose of morphine. Kadian capsules may be opened and contents sprinkled into ~10 mL of water, then flushed while swirling through a prewetted 16-French gastrostomy tube fitted with a funnel at the port end; flush with water to transfer all pellets and flush the tube; do not attempt to administer via NG tube. Do not administer Avinza with alcohol.

Parenteral: **Note:** Solutions for injection should be visually inspected for particulate matter and discoloration prior to administration. Do not use if contains a precipitate or is darker in color than pale yellow or discolored in any other way.

IV push: Administer undiluted or diluted solution over 4 to 5 minutes (Gahart 2014); rapid IV administration may increase adverse effects

Intermittent IV infusion: Further dilute and administer over 15 to 30 minutes

Continuous IV infusion: Administer as a continuous infusion via an infusion pump.

Epidural and intrathecal: **Use only preservative-free injections.** Adults: Infumorph was developed for use in continuous microinfusion devices only; it may require dilution before use, as determined by the individual patient's dosage requirements and the characteristics of the continuous microinfusion device; not recommended for single dose IV, IM, or SubQ administration; filter through ≤5 micron microfilter before injecting into microinfusion device

Inhalation: Limited data available; utilize preservative free parenteral morphine and further dilute prior to administration (Cohen 2002; Ferraresi 2005; Shirk 2006)

Monitoring Parameters Respiratory rate; oxygen saturation; mental status; blood pressure; heart rate; pain relief; signs of misuse, abuse, and addiction; level of sedation. **Note:** Resedation may occur following epidural administration. Monitor patients receiving Infumorph closely for ≥24 hours after initiation and as appropriate for the first several days after catheter implantation.

Test Interactions Some quinolones may produce a false-positive urine screening result for opioids using commercially-available immunoassay kits. This has been demonstrated most consistently for levofloxacin and ofloxacin, but other quinolones have shown cross-reactivity in certain assay kits. Confirmation of positive opioid screens by more specific methods should be considered.

Additional Information Equianalgesic doses: Codeine: 120 mg IM = morphine 10 mg IM = single dose oral morphine 60 mg or chronic dosing oral morphine 15 to 25 mg

Avinza capsules contain both immediate release and extended release beads; also contains fumaric acid (as an osmotic agent and local pH modifier); this product is intended for once daily oral administration only; not for PRN or postoperative use. Kadian capsules contain extended release pellets that are polymer-coated; this product is intended for every 12- or 24-hour dosing. Kadian capsules also contain talc; parenteral abuse may result in local tissue necrosis, infection, pulmonary granulomas, endocarditis, and valvular heart injury.

Controlled Substance C-II

Dosage Forms Excipient information presented when available (limited, particularly for generics); consult specific product labeling. [DSC] = Discontinued product

Capsule Extended Release 24 Hour, Oral, as sulfate:

AVINza: 30 mg [DSC] [contains fd&c yellow #10 (quinoline yellow), fumaric acid]

AVINza: 45 mg [DSC] [contains fd&c blue #2 (indigotine)]

AVINza: 60 mg [DSC] [contains fumaric acid]

AVINza: 75 mg [DSC]

AVINza: 90 mg [DSC] [contains fd&c red #40, fumaric acid]

AVINza: 120 mg [DSC] [contains brilliant blue fcf (fd&c blue #1), fumaric acid]

Kadian: 10 mg [contains brilliant blue fcf (fd&c blue #1)]

Kadian: 20 mg [contains fd&c yellow #10 (quinoline yellow)]

Kadian: 30 mg [contains brilliant blue fcf (fd&c blue #1)]

Kadian: 40 mg [contains brilliant blue fcf (fd&c blue #1), fd&c yellow #10 (quinoline yellow)]

Kadian: 50 mg, 60 mg [contains brilliant blue fcf (fd&c blue #1), fd&c red #40]

Kadian: 70 mg [DSC] [contains brilliant blue fcf (fd&c blue #1)]

Kadian: 80 mg [contains brilliant blue fcf (fd&c blue #1), fd&c red #40, fd&c yellow #6 (sunset yellow)]

Kadian: 100 mg [contains brilliant blue fcf (fd&c blue #1), fd&c yellow #10 (quinoline yellow)]

Kadian: 130 mg [DSC] [contains brilliant blue fcf (fd&c blue #1), fd&c red #40, fd&c yellow #6 (sunset yellow)]

Kadian: 150 mg [DSC] [contains brilliant blue fcf (fd&c blue #1), fd&c yellow #10 (quinoline yellow)]

Kadian: 200 mg

Generic: 10 mg, 20 mg, 30 mg, 45 mg, 50 mg, 60 mg, 75 mg, 80 mg, 90 mg, 100 mg, 120 mg

Device, Intramuscular, as sulfate:

Generic: 10 mg/0.7 mL (0.7 mL)

Solution, Injection, as sulfate:

Generic: 2 mg/mL (1 mL); 4 mg/mL (1 mL); 5 mg/mL (1 mL); 8 mg/mL (1 mL); 10 mg/mL (1 mL, 10 mL); 15 mg/mL (1 mL, 20 mL)

Solution, Injection, as sulfate [preservative free]:

Astramorph: 0.5 mg/mL (2 mL); 1 mg/mL (2 mL)

Duramorph: 0.5 mg/mL (10 mL); 1 mg/mL (10 mL)

Infumorph 200: 200 mg/20 mL (10 mg/mL) (20 mL) [antioxidant free]

Infumorph 500: 500 mg/20 mL (25 mg/mL) (20 mL) [antioxidant free]

Generic: 0.5 mg/mL (10 mL); 1 mg/mL (10 mL)

Solution, Intravenous, as sulfate:

Generic: 1 mg/mL (10 mL, 30 mL); 25 mg/mL (4 mL, 10 mL); 50 mg/mL (20 mL, 50 mL)

Solution, Intravenous, as sulfate [preservative free]:

Generic: 1 mg/mL (30 mL); 2 mg/mL (1 mL); 4 mg/mL (1 mL); 150 mg/30 mL (30 mL); 8 mg/mL (1 mL); 10 mg/mL (1 mL); 15 mg/mL (1 mL); 25 mg/mL (10 mL)

Solution, Oral, as sulfate:
Generic: 10 mg/5 mL (5 mL, 15 mL, 100 mL, 500 mL); 20 mg/5 mL (5 mL, 100 mL, 500 mL); 20 mg/mL (15 mL, 30 mL, 120 mL, 240 mL); 100 mg/5 mL (30 mL, 120 mL)
Suppository, Rectal, as sulfate:
Generic: 5 mg (12 ea); 10 mg (12 ea); 20 mg (12 ea); 30 mg (12 ea)
Tablet, Oral, as sulfate:
Generic: 15 mg, 30 mg
Tablet Extended Release, Oral, as sulfate:
MS Contin: 15 mg, 30 mg, 60 mg, 100 mg, 200 mg
Generic: 15 mg, 30 mg, 60 mg, 100 mg, 200 mg

- ◆ **Morphine-EPD (Can)** *see* Morphine (Systemic) *on page 1461*
- ◆ **Morphine Extra Forte Injection (Can)** *see* Morphine (Systemic) *on page 1461*
- ◆ **Morphine Forte Injection (Can)** *see* Morphine (Systemic) *on page 1461*
- ◆ **Morphine HP (Can)** *see* Morphine (Systemic) *on page 1461*
- ◆ **Morphine LP Epidural (Can)** *see* Morphine (Systemic) *on page 1461*
- ◆ **Morphine SR (Can)** *see* Morphine (Systemic) *on page 1461*
- ◆ **M.O.S. 10 (Can)** *see* Morphine (Systemic) *on page 1461*
- ◆ **M.O.S. 20 (Can)** *see* Morphine (Systemic) *on page 1461*
- ◆ **M.O.S. 30 (Can)** *see* Morphine (Systemic) *on page 1461*
- ◆ **M.O.S.-SR (Can)** *see* Morphine (Systemic) *on page 1461*
- ◆ **M.O.S.-Sulfate (Can)** *see* Morphine (Systemic) *on page 1461*
- ◆ **Motion Sickness [OTC]** *see* DimenhyDRINATE *on page 664*
- ◆ **Motion-Time [OTC]** *see* Meclizine *on page 1337*
- ◆ **Motrin [OTC]** *see* Ibuprofen *on page 1064*
- ◆ **Motrin (Can)** *see* Ibuprofen *on page 1064*
- ◆ **Motrin (Children's) (Can)** *see* Ibuprofen *on page 1064*
- ◆ **Motrin IB [OTC]** *see* Ibuprofen *on page 1064*
- ◆ **Motrin IB (Can)** *see* Ibuprofen *on page 1064*
- ◆ **Motrin Infants Drops [OTC]** *see* Ibuprofen *on page 1064*
- ◆ **Motrin Junior Strength [OTC]** *see* Ibuprofen *on page 1064*
- ◆ **MoviPrep** *see* Polyethylene Glycol-Electrolyte Solution *on page 1724*
- ◆ **Moxatag** *see* Amoxicillin *on page 138*
- ◆ **Moxeza** *see* Moxifloxacin (Ophthalmic) *on page 1470*

Moxifloxacin (Ophthalmic) (moxs i FLOKS a sin)

Medication Safety Issues

International issues:

Vigamox [U.S., Canada, and multiple international markets] may be confused with Fisamox brand name for amoxicillin [Australia]

Brand Names: US Moxeza; Vigamox

Brand Names: Canada Vigamox

Therapeutic Category Antibiotic, Fluoroquinolone; Antibiotic, Ophthalmic

Generic Availability (US) No

Use Treatment of bacterial conjunctivitis caused by susceptible organisms (Moxeza: FDA approved in ages ≥4 months and adults; Vigamox: FDA approved in ages ≥1 year and adults)

Pregnancy Risk Factor C

Pregnancy Considerations Adverse events have been observed in some animal reproduction studies. When administered orally or IV, moxifloxacin crosses the placenta (Ozyüncü and Beksac 2010; Ozyüncü and Nemutlu, 2010). The amount of moxifloxacin available systemically following topical application of the ophthalmic drops is significantly less in comparison to oral or IV doses. If ophthalmic agents are needed during pregnancy, the minimum effective dose should be used in combination with punctual occlusion for 3 to 5 minutes after application to decrease potential exposure to the fetus (Samples 1988).

Breast-Feeding Considerations It is not known if moxifloxacin is excreted into breast milk. The manufacturer recommends that caution be exercised when administering moxifloxacin ophthalmic drops to nursing women.

Contraindications

Moxeza ophthalmic solution: There are no contraindications listed in manufacturer's labeling

Vigamox: Hypersensitivity to moxifloxacin, other quinolone antibiotics, or any component of the formulation

Warnings/Precautions For topical ophthalmic use only. Not for subconjunctival injection or for direct introduction into the anterior chamber of the eye. Contact lenses should not be worn during therapy. Severe hypersensitivity reactions, including anaphylaxis, angioedema, and dermatologic reactions, have been reported with systemic use of moxifloxacin. Discontinue use if an allergic reaction occurs. Prolonged use may lead to overgrowth of nonsusceptible organisms, including fungi. If superinfection occurs, discontinue use and institute appropriate alternative therapy.

Adverse Reactions Ocular: Conjunctivitis, dry eye, ocular discomfort, ocular hyperemia, ocular irritation, ocular pain, ocular pruritus, subconjunctival hemorrhage, tearing, visual acuity decreased

Drug Interactions

Metabolism/Transport Effects None known.

Avoid Concomitant Use There are no known interactions where it is recommended to avoid concomitant use.

Increased Effect/Toxicity There are no known significant interactions involving an increase in effect.

Decreased Effect There are no known significant interactions involving a decrease in effect.

Storage/Stability Store at 2°C to 25°C (36°F to 77°F).

Mechanism of Action Moxifloxacin is a DNA gyrase inhibitor, and also inhibits topoisomerase IV. DNA gyrase (topoisomerase II) is an essential bacterial enzyme that maintains the superhelical structure of DNA. DNA gyrase is required for DNA replication and transcription, DNA repair, recombination, and transposition; inhibition is bactericidal.

Pharmacokinetics (Adult data unless noted) Absorption: Minimal systemic absorption; resulting serum concentration was 0.02% of that achieved with oral formulation

Dosing: Usual

Pediatric: **Bacterial conjunctivitis:** Ophthalmic:

Moxeza: Infants ≥4 months, Children, and Adolescents: Instill 1 drop into affected eye(s) 2 times daily for 7 days

Vigamox: Children and Adolescents: Instill 1 drop into affected eye(s) 3 times daily for 7 days

Adult: **Bacterial conjunctivitis:** Ophthalmic:

Moxeza: Instill 1 drop into affected eye(s) 2 times daily for 7 days

Vigamox: Instill 1 drop into affected eye(s) 3 times daily for 7 days

Dosing adjustment in renal impairment: There are no dosage adjustments provided in the manufacturer's labeling; however adjustment unlikely needed due to low systemic absorption.

Dosing adjustment in hepatic impairment: There are no dosage adjustments provided in the manufacturer's labeling; however, adjustment unlikely needed due to low systemic absorption.

Administration For topical ophthalmic use only; not for injection. Avoid touching tip of applicator to eye, finger, or other surfaces. Apply gentle pressure to lacrimal sac during and immediately following instillation (1 minute) or instruct patient to gently close eyelid after administration, to decrease systemic absorption of ophthalmic drops (Urrti 1993; Zimmerman 1982).

Monitoring Parameters Signs of infection

Additional Information Evidence of damage to weight-bearing joints in pediatric populations with ophthalmic administration has not been shown.

Dosage Forms Excipient information presented when available (limited, particularly for generics); consult specific product labeling.

Solution, Ophthalmic:
 Moxeza: 0.5% (3 mL)
 Vigamox: 0.5% (3 mL)

- ◆ **Moxifloxacin Hydrochloride** *see* Moxifloxacin (Ophthalmic) *on page 1470*
- ◆ **4-MP** *see* Fomepizole *on page 933*
- ◆ **MPA** *see* MedroxyPROGESTERone *on page 1339*
- ◆ **MPA** *see* Mycophenolate *on page 1473*
- ◆ **6-MP (error-prone abbreviation)** *see* Mercaptopurine *on page 1363*
- ◆ **MPSV** *see* Meningococcal Polysaccharide Vaccine (Groups A / C / Y and W-135) *on page 1357*
- ◆ **MPSV4** *see* Meningococcal Polysaccharide Vaccine (Groups A / C / Y and W-135) *on page 1357*
- ◆ **MRA** *see* Tocilizumab *on page 2079*
- ◆ **MS Contin** *see* Morphine (Systemic) *on page 1461*
- ◆ **MS Contin SRT (Can)** *see* Morphine (Systemic) *on page 1461*
- ◆ **MS (error-prone abbreviation and should not be used)** *see* Morphine (Systemic) *on page 1461*
- ◆ **M-Sildenafil (Can)** *see* Sildenafil *on page 1921*
- ◆ **MS-IR (Can)** *see* Morphine (Systemic) *on page 1461*
- ◆ **MSO_4 (error-prone abbreviation and should not be used)** *see* Morphine (Systemic) *on page 1461*
- ◆ **MTX (error-prone abbreviation)** *see* Methotrexate *on page 1390*
- ◆ **Mucinex [OTC]** *see* GuaiFENesin *on page 988*
- ◆ **Mucinex Allergy [OTC]** *see* Fexofenadine *on page 874*
- ◆ **Mucinex Chest Congestion Child [OTC]** *see* GuaiFENesin *on page 988*
- ◆ **Mucinex DM [OTC]** *see* Guaifenesin and Dextromethorphan *on page 992*
- ◆ **Mucinex DM Maximum Strength [OTC]** *see* Guaifenesin and Dextromethorphan *on page 992*
- ◆ **Mucinex Fast-Max DM Max [OTC]** *see* Guaifenesin and Dextromethorphan *on page 992*
- ◆ **Mucinex For Kids [OTC]** *see* GuaiFENesin *on page 988*
- ◆ **Mucinex Kid's Cough [OTC]** *see* Guaifenesin and Dextromethorphan *on page 992*
- ◆ **Mucinex Kid's Cough Mini-Melts [OTC]** *see* Guaifenesin and Dextromethorphan *on page 992*
- ◆ **Mucinex Maximum Strength [OTC]** *see* GuaiFENesin *on page 988*
- ◆ **Mucinex Nasal Spray Full Force [OTC]** *see* Oxymetazoline (Nasal) *on page 1599*
- ◆ **Mucinex Nasal Spray Moisture [OTC]** *see* Oxymetazoline (Nasal) *on page 1599*
- ◆ **Mucinex Sinus-Max Full Force [OTC]** *see* Oxymetazoline (Nasal) *on page 1599*
- ◆ **Mucinex Sinus-Max Moist Smart [OTC]** *see* Oxymetazoline (Nasal) *on page 1599*
- ◆ **Mucomyst** *see* Acetylcysteine *on page 57*
- ◆ **Mucomyst® (Can)** *see* Acetylcysteine *on page 57*
- ◆ **Mucosa [OTC]** *see* GuaiFENesin *on page 988*
- ◆ **Mucus-ER [OTC]** *see* GuaiFENesin *on page 988*
- ◆ **Mucus Relief [OTC]** *see* GuaiFENesin *on page 988*
- ◆ **Mucus Relief Childrens [OTC]** *see* GuaiFENesin *on page 988*
- ◆ **Multitrace-4** *see* Trace Elements *on page 2097*
- ◆ **Multitrace-4 Concentrate** *see* Trace Elements *on page 2097*
- ◆ **Multitrace-4 Neonatal** *see* Trace Elements *on page 2097*
- ◆ **Multitrace-4 Pediatric** *see* Trace Elements *on page 2097*
- ◆ **Multitrace-5** *see* Trace Elements *on page 2097*
- ◆ **Multitrace-5 Concentrate** *see* Trace Elements *on page 2097*
- ◆ **Mumps, Measles and Rubella Vaccines** *see* Measles, Mumps, and Rubella Virus Vaccine *on page 1327*
- ◆ **Mumps, Rubella, Varicella, and Measles Vaccine** *see* Measles, Mumps, Rubella, and Varicella Virus Vaccine *on page 1330*

Mupirocin (myoo PEER oh sin)

Medication Safety Issues

Sound-alike/look-alike issues:

Bactroban may be confused with bacitracin, baclofen, Bactrim

Brand Names: US Bactroban; Bactroban Nasal; Centany; Centany AT

Brand Names: Canada Bactroban

Therapeutic Category Antibiotic, Topical

Generic Availability (US) May be product dependent

Use

Intranasal ointment: Eradication of *Staphylococcus aureus* from nasal carriage sites as part of an infection control program to reduce the risk of infection among patients at high risk of MRSA infection during institutional outbreaks (FDA approved in ages ≥12 years and adults)

Topical cream: Topical treatment of secondarily-infected traumatic skin lesions due to susceptible strains of *S. aureus* and *Streptococcus pyogenes* (FDA approved in ages ≥3 months and adults); has also been used for prophylaxis at intravenous catheter exit sites

Topical ointment: Topical treatment of impetigo caused by susceptible strains of *S. aureus* and *S. pyogenes* (FDA approved in ages ≥2 months and adults)

Pregnancy Risk Factor B

Pregnancy Considerations Adverse events have not been observed in animal reproduction studies.

Breast-Feeding Considerations It is not known if mupirocin is excreted in breast milk. The manufacturer recommends that caution be exercised when administering mupirocin to nursing women.

Contraindications Hypersensitivity to mupirocin or any component of the formulation

Warnings/Precautions May be associated with systemic allergic reactions, including anaphylaxis, urticarial, angioedema and generalized rash. If a systemic reaction occurs, discontinue use. Potentially toxic amounts of polyethylene glycol contained in some topical products may be absorbed percutaneously in patients with extensive burns or open wounds; use caution with renal impairment. Prolonged use may result in overgrowth of nonsusceptible organisms or fungal or bacterial superinfection, including

C. difficile-associated diarrhea (CDAD) and pseudomembranous colitis; CDAD has been observed >2 months postantibiotic treatment. Topical ointment is for external use only (not for nasal/ophthalmic/mucosal surface use) and should not be used with intravenous (IV) cannulae or at central IV sites because of the potential to promote fungal infections and antimicrobial resistance. With all dosage forms, contact with eyes should be avoided. In case of accidental contact in or near eyes, rinse well with water. Nasal ointment may cause severe burning and tearing in eyes (resolves within days to weeks after discontinuation) and is available in single-use tubes to decrease risk of contamination. If local irritation occurs, discontinue use. There are insufficient data to establish that nasal ointment use is safe and effective as part of an autoinfection prevention program; should not be used for general prophylaxis of any infection in any patient population; 90% of patients had eradication of nasal colonization within 2 to 4 days after therapy was completed; 30% recolonization within 4 weeks of therapy was reported in one study. Potentially significant interactions may exist, requiring dose or frequency adjustment, additional monitoring, and/or selection of alternative therapy.

Benzyl alcohol and derivatives: Some dosage forms may contain benzyl alcohol; large amounts of benzyl alcohol (≥99 mg/kg/day) have been associated with a potentially fatal toxicity ("gasping syndrome") in neonates; the "gasping syndrome" consists of metabolic acidosis, respiratory distress, gasping respirations, CNS dysfunction (including convulsions, intracranial hemorrhage), hypotension, and cardiovascular collapse (AAP, 1997; CDC, 1982); some data suggests that benzoate displaces bilirubin from protein binding sites (Ahlfors, 2001); avoid or use dosage forms containing benzyl alcohol with caution in neonates. See manufacturer's labeling. Potentially significant interactions may exist, requiring dose or frequency adjustment, additional monitoring, and/or selection of alternative therapy.

Warnings: Additional Pediatric Considerations Some dosage forms may contain propylene glycol; in neonates large amounts of propylene glycol delivered orally, intravenously (eg, >3,000 mg/day), or topically have been associated with potentially fatal toxicities which can include metabolic acidosis, seizures, renal failure, and CNS depression; toxicities have also been reported in children and adults including hyperosmolality, lactic acidosis, seizures, and respiratory depression; use caution (AAP, 1997; Shehab, 2009).

Adverse Reactions

Central nervous system: Headache, localized burning, stinging sensation

Dermatologic: Pruritus, skin rash

Gastrointestinal: Dysgeusia, nausea

Local: Local pain

Respiratory: Cough, respiratory congestion, rhinitis, pharyngitis

Rare but important or life-threatening: Aphthous stomatitis, blepharitis, cellulitis, *Clostridium difficile* associated diarrhea, dermatitis, epistaxis, hypersensitivity reaction, increased wound secretion, xeroderma

Drug Interactions

Metabolism/Transport Effects None known.

Avoid Concomitant Use

Avoid concomitant use of Mupirocin with any of the following: BCG; BCG (Intravesical)

Increased Effect/Toxicity There are no known significant interactions involving an increase in effect.

Decreased Effect

Mupirocin may decrease the levels/effects of: BCG; BCG (Intravesical); BCG Vaccine (Immunization); Sodium Picosulfate; Typhoid Vaccine

Storage/Stability

Intranasal: Store between 20°C and 25°C (68°F and 77°F); excursions are permitted between 15°C and 30°C (59°F and 86°F). Do not refrigerate.

Topical cream: Store at or below 25°C (77°F). Do not freeze.

Topical ointment: Store between 20°C and 25°C (68°F and 77°F).

Mechanism of Action Binds to bacterial isoleucyl transfer-RNA synthetase resulting in the inhibition of protein synthesis

Pharmacokinetics (Adult data unless noted)

Absorption: Following topical administration, penetrates the outer layers of the skin; systemic absorption is minimal through intact skin; following intranasal use in neonates significant systemic absorption reported

Protein binding: >97%

Metabolism: Skin: 3% to monic acid (inactive)

Half-life: 17-36 minutes

Elimination: Momic acid [inactive] is renally excreted

Dosing: Neonatal

Intranasal: **MRSA decolonization:** Intranasal ointment: Apply a small amount to both anterior nares 2-3 times/day for 5-10 days in conjunction with umbilical application of topical ointment (Bertin, 2006; Lally, 2004; Liu, 2011)

Topical:

Mild localized impetigo or MRSA skin infections: Ointment: Apply a small amount 3 times/day for 5-10 days (Liu, 2011)

MRSA decolonization: Ointment: Apply a small amount to umbilicus 2-3 times/day for 5-10 days in conjunction with intranasal application (Bertin, 2006; Lally, 2004)

Dosing: Usual

Intranasal: **Eradication of MRSA colonization:** Intranasal ointment:

Manufacturer recommendations: Children ≥12 years, Adolescents, and Adults: Apply 0.5 g (1/2 of unit-dose tube) twice daily for 5 days

Alternate dosing: Infants, Children, and Adults: Apply a small amount twice daily for 5-10 days (Lui, 2011)

Topical:

Cream: **Minor skin infections or infected lesions:** Infants, Children, and Adults: Apply small amount 3 times/day for 10 days; patients not showing clinical response after 5 days should be re-evaluated.

Ointment: **Minor skin infection, impetigo, infected lesions:** Infants, Children, and Adults: Apply a small amount 3-5 times/day for 5-14 days; patients not showing clinical response after 5 days should be re-evaluated.

Administration

Intranasal: Avoid contact with eyes; apply to anterior nares. Press sides of the nose together and gently massage for 1 minute after application to spread ointment throughout the inside of the nostrils.

Topical cream and ointment: For topical use only; not formulated for use on mucosal surfaces; do not apply into the eye or use intranasally; may cover with gauze dressing. Do not mix with Aquaphor®, coal tar solution, or salicylic acid.

Dosage Forms Excipient information presented when available (limited, particularly for generics); consult specific product labeling.

Cream, External, as calcium [strength expressed as base]:

Bactroban: 2% (15 g, 30 g)

Generic: 2% (15 g, 30 g)

Kit, External:

Centany AT: 2% [contains propylene glycol monostearate]

Ointment, External:
Bactroban: 2% (22 g)
Centany: 2% (30 g) [contains propylene glycol monostearate]
Generic: 2% (22 g)
Ointment, Nasal, as calcium [strength expressed as base]:
Bactroban Nasal: 2% (1 g)

◆ **Mupirocin Calcium** *see* Mupirocin *on page 1471*

◆ **Murine Tears® [OTC]** *see* Artificial Tears *on page 201*

◆ **Muro 128 [OTC]** *see* Sodium Chloride *on page 1938*

◆ **Muse** *see* Alprostadil *on page 103*

◆ **Muse Pellet (Can)** *see* Alprostadil *on page 103*

◆ **Mustargen** *see* Mechlorethamine (Systemic) *on page 1335*

◆ **Mustine** *see* Mechlorethamine (Systemic) *on page 1335*

◆ **Myambutol** *see* Ethambutol *on page 810*

◆ **Mycamine** *see* Micafungin *on page 1429*

◆ **Mycelex** *see* Clotrimazole (Oral) *on page 517*

◆ **Mycobutin** *see* Rifabutin *on page 1857*

◆ **Mycocide Clinical NS [OTC]** *see* Tolnaftate *on page 2083*

Mycophenolate (mye koe FEN oh late)

Medication Safety Issues

High alert medication:

This medication is in a class the Institute for Safe Medication Practices (ISMP) includes among its list of drug classes that have a heightened risk of causing significant patient harm when used in error.

Related Information

Oral Medications That Should Not Be Crushed or Altered *on page 2476*

Safe Handling of Hazardous Drugs *on page 2455*

Brand Names: US CellCept; CellCept Intravenous; Myfortic

Brand Names: Canada Ach-Mycophenolate; Apo-Mycophenolate; CellCept; CellCept I.V.; CO Mycophenolate; JAMP-Mycophenolate; Myfortic; Mylan-Mycophenolate; Novo-Mycophenolate; Sandoz-Mycophenolate Mofetil

Therapeutic Category Immunosuppressant Agent

Generic Availability (US) May be product dependent

Use

Oral: Immunosuppressant agent used in conjunction with other immunosuppressive therapies (eg, cyclosporine and corticosteroids with or without antithymocyte induction) for the prophylaxis of organ rejection in patients receiving allogeneic renal (CellCept: FDA approved in ages ≥3 months and adults; Myfortic: FDA approved in ages ≥5 years who are at least 6 months post-transplant and adults), hepatic, or cardiac transplants (CellCept: FDA approved in adults). Has also been used in nephrotic syndrome; intestine, small bowel, and bone marrow transplant patients; moderate to severe psoriasis; chronic graft-versus-host disease; myasthenia gravis; lupus nephritis; autoimmune lymphoproliferative syndrome juvenile localized scleroderma, uveitis and refractory immune thrombocytopenia (ITP).

Parenteral: Immunosuppressant agent used in conjunction with other immunosuppressive therapies (eg, cyclosporine and corticosteroids with or without antithymocyte induction) for the prophylaxis of organ rejection in patients receiving allogeneic renal, hepatic, or cardiac transplants (CellCept: FDA approved in adults)

Medication Guide Available Yes

Pregnancy Risk Factor D

Pregnancy Considerations **[U.S. Boxed Warning]: Mycophenolate is associated with an increased risk of congenital malformations and first trimester pregnancy loss when used by pregnant women. Females of reproductive potential must be counseled about pregnancy prevention and planning.** Alternative agents should be considered for women planning a pregnancy. Adverse events have been reported in animal reproduction studies. In humans, the following congenital malformations have been reported: external ear abnormalities, cleft lip and palate, anomalies of the distal limbs, heart, esophagus and kidney. Spontaneous abortions have also been noted. Females of reproductive potential (girls who have entered puberty, women with a uterus who have not passed through clinically confirmed menopause) should have a negative pregnancy test with a sensitivity of ≥25 mIU/mL immediately before therapy and the test should be repeated 8-10 days later. Pregnancy tests should be repeated during routine follow-up visits. Acceptable forms of contraception should be used during treatment and for 6 weeks after therapy is discontinued. The effectiveness of hormonal contraceptive agents may be affected by mycophenolate. For women with lupus nephritis taking mycophenolate and who are planning a pregnancy, mycophenolate should be discontinued at least 6 weeks prior to trying to conceive (Hahn, 2012).

Healthcare providers should report female exposures to mycophenolate during pregnancy or within 6 weeks of discontinuing therapy to the Mycophenolate Pregnancy Registry (800-617-8191). The National Transplantation Pregnancy Registry (NTPR, Temple University) is a registry for pregnant women taking immunosuppressants following any solid organ transplant. The NTPR encourages reporting of all immunosuppressant exposures during pregnancy in transplant recipients at 877-955-6877.

Breast-Feeding Considerations It is unknown if mycophenolate is excreted in human milk. Due to potentially serious adverse reactions, the decision to discontinue the drug or discontinue breast-feeding should be considered. Breast-feeding is not recommended during therapy or for 6 weeks after treatment is complete.

Contraindications Hypersensitivity to mycophenolate mofetil, mycophenolic acid, mycophenolate sodium, or any component of the formulation

Cellcept: Intravenous formulation is also contraindicated in patients who are allergic to polysorbate 80

Warnings/Precautions Hazardous agent - use appropriate precautions for handling and disposal (NIOSH 2014 [group 2]).

[U.S. Boxed Warning]: Risk for bacterial, viral, fungal, and protozoal infections, including opportunistic infections, is increased with immunosuppressant therapy; infections may be serious and potentially fatal. Due to the risk of oversuppression of the immune system, which may increase susceptibility to infection, combination immunosuppressant therapy should be used with caution. Polyomavirus associated nephropathy (PVAN), JC virus-associated progressive multifocal leukoencephalopathy (PML), cytomegalovirus (CMV) infections, reactivation of hepatitis B (HBV) or hepatitis C (HCV), have been reported with use. A reduction in immunosuppression should be considered for patients with new or reactivated viral infections; however, in transplant recipients, the risk that reduced immunosuppression presents to the functioning graft should also be considered. PVAN, primarily from activation of BK virus, may lead to the deterioration of renal function and/or renal graft loss. PML, a potentially fatal condition, commonly presents with hemiparesis, apathy, ataxia, cognitive deficiencies, confusion, and hemiparesis. Risk factors for development of PML include treatment with immunosuppressants and immune function impairment; consultation with a neurologist should be considered in any patient with neurological symptoms receiving immunosuppressants. Risk of CMV viremia or disease is increased in transplant recipients CMV seronegative at the time of transplant who receive a graft from a CMV seropositive donor. In patients infected with HBV or HCV, viral reactivation may occur; these patients should be monitored for signs of active HBV or HCV. **[U.S. Boxed Warning]: Risk of development of lymphoma and skin malignancy is increased.** The risk for malignancies is related to intensity/duration of therapy. Patients should be monitored appropriately, instructed to limit exposure to sunlight/UV light to decrease the risk of skin cancer, and given supportive treatment should these conditions occur. Post-transplant lymphoproliferative disorder related to EBV infection has been reported in immunosuppressed organ transplant patients; risk is highest in EBV seronegative patients (including many young children). Neutropenia (including severe neutropenia) may occur, requiring dose reduction or interruption of treatment (risk greater from day 31-180 post-transplant). Use may rarely be associated with gastric or duodenal ulcers, GI bleeding and/or perforation. Use caution in patients with active serious digestive system disease; patients with active peptic ulcers were not included in clinical studies. Use caution in renal impairment as toxicity may be increased; may require dosage adjustment in severe impairment.

[U.S. Boxed Warning]: Mycophenolate is associated with an increased risk of congenital malformations and first trimester pregnancy loss when used by pregnant women. Females of reproductive potential must be counseled about pregnancy prevention and planning. Alternative agents should be considered for women planning a pregnancy. Females of reproductive potential should have a negative pregnancy test with a sensitivity of ≥25 mIU/mL immediately before therapy and the test should be repeated 8-10 days later. Pregnancy tests should be repeated during routine follow-up visits. Acceptable forms of contraception should be used during treatment and for 6 weeks after therapy is discontinued. Females of childbearing potential should have a negative pregnancy test within 1 week prior to beginning therapy. Two reliable forms of contraception should be used beginning 4 weeks prior to, during, and for 6 weeks after therapy. Because mycophenolate mofetil has demonstrated teratogenic effects in rats and rabbits, tablets should not be crushed, and capsules should not be opened or crushed. Avoid inhalation or direct contact with skin or mucous membranes of the powder contained in the capsules and the powder for oral suspension. Caution should be exercised in the handling and preparation of solutions of intravenous mycophenolate. Avoid skin contact with the intravenous solution and reconstituted suspension. If such contact occurs, wash thoroughly with soap and water, rinse eyes with plain water.

Theoretically, use should be avoided in patients with the rare hereditary deficiency of hypoxanthine-guanine phosphoribosyltransferase (such as Lesch-Nyhan or Kelley-Seegmiller syndrome). Intravenous solutions should be given over at least 2 hours; never administer intravenous solution by rapid or bolus injection. Live attenuated vaccines should be avoided during use; vaccinations may be less effective during therapy. **[U.S. Boxed Warning]: Should be administered under the supervision of a physician experienced in immunosuppressive therapy.**

Note: CellCept and Myfortic dosage forms should not be used interchangeably due to differences in absorption. Some dosage forms may contain phenylalanine. Some dosage forms may contain polysorbate 80 (also known as Tweens). Hypersensitivity reactions, usually a delayed reaction, have been reported following exposure to pharmaceutical products containing polysorbate 80 in certain individuals (Isaksson, 2002; Lucente 2000; Shelley, 1995). Thrombocytopenia, ascites, pulmonary deterioration, and renal and hepatic failure have been reported in premature neonates after receiving parenteral products containing polysorbate 80 (Alade, 1986; CDC, 1984). See manufacturer's labeling.

Adverse Reactions Note: In general, lower doses used in renal rejection patients had less adverse effects than higher doses. Rates of adverse effects were similar for each indication, except for those unique to the specific organ involved. The type of adverse effects observed in pediatric patients was similar to those seen in adults, with the exception of abdominal pain, anemia, diarrhea, fever, hypertension, infection, pharyngitis, respiratory tract infection, sepsis, and vomiting; lymphoproliferative disorder was the only type of malignancy observed.

As reported in adults following oral dosing of CellCept alone in renal, cardiac, and hepatic allograft rejection studies:

Cardiovascular: Chest pain, edema, hyper-/hypotension, peripheral edema, tachycardia

Central nervous system: Anxiety, dizziness, fever, headache, insomnia, pain

Dermatologic: Rash

Endocrine & metabolic: Hypercholesterolemia, hyperglycemia, hypocalcemia, hyper-/hypokalemia, hypomagnesemia

Gastrointestinal: Abdominal pain, anorexia, constipation, diarrhea, dyspepsia, nausea, vomiting

Genitourinary: Urinary tract infection

Hematologic: Anemia (including hypochromic), leukocytosis, leukopenia, thrombocytopenia

Hepatic: Ascites, liver function tests abnormal

Neuromuscular & skeletal: Back pain, paresthesia, tremor, weakness

Renal: BUN increased, creatinine increased, kidney function abnormal

Respiratory: Cough, dyspnea, lung disorder, pleural effusion, respiratory tract infection, sinusitis

Miscellaneous: *Candida*, herpes simplex, lactate dehydrogenase increased, sepsis

Use in combination with cyclosporine and corticosteroids:

Cardiovascular: Angina, arrhythmia, arterial thrombosis, atrial fibrillation, atrial flutter, bradycardia, cardiac arrest, cardiac failure, CHF, extrasystole, facial edema, hyper-/hypovolemia, orthostatic hypotension, pallor, palpitation, pericardial effusion, peripheral vascular disorder, supraventricular extrasystoles, supraventricular tachycardia, syncope, thrombosis, vasodilation, vasospasm, venous pressure increased, ventricular extrasystole, ventricular tachycardia

Central nervous system: Agitation, chills with fever, confusion, delirium, depression, emotional lability, hallucinations, hypoesthesia, malaise, nervousness, psychosis, seizure, somnolence, thinking abnormal, vertigo

Dermatologic: Acne, alopecia, bruising, cellulitis, fungal dermatitis, hirsutism, petechia, pruritus, skin carcinoma, skin hypertrophy, skin ulcer, vesiculobullous rash

Endocrine & metabolic: Acidosis, alkalosis, Cushing's syndrome, dehydration, diabetes mellitus, gout, hypercalcemia, hyper-hypophosphatemia, hyperlipemia, hyperuricemia, hypochloremia, hypoglycemia, hyponatremia, hypoproteinemia, hypothyroidism, parathyroid disorder

Gastrointestinal: Abdomen enlarged, dysphagia, esophagitis, flatulence, gastritis, gastroenteritis, gastrointestinal hemorrhage, gastrointestinal moniliasis, gingivitis, gum hyperplasia, ileus, melena, mouth ulceration, oral moniliasis, stomach disorder, stomach ulcer, stomatitis, xerostomia, weight gain/loss

Genitourinary: Impotence, nocturia, pelvic pain, prostatic disorder, scrotal edema, urinary frequency, urinary incontinence, urinary retention, urinary tract disorder

Hematologic: Coagulation disorder, hemorrhage, neutropenia, pancytopenia, polycythemia, prothrombin time increased, thromboplastin time increased

Hepatic: Alkaline phosphatase increased, bilirubinemia, cholangitis, cholestatic jaundice, GGT increased, hepatitis, jaundice, liver damage, transaminases increased

Local: Abscess

Neuromuscular & skeletal: Arthralgia, hypertonia, joint disorder, leg cramps, myalgia, myasthenia, neck pain, neuropathy, osteoporosis

Ocular: Amblyopia, cataract, conjunctivitis, eye hemorrhage, lacrimation disorder, vision abnormal

Otic: Deafness, ear disorder, ear pain, tinnitus

Renal: Albuminuria, creatinine increased, dysuria, hematuria, hydronephrosis, oliguria, pyelonephritis, renal failure, renal tubular necrosis

Respiratory: Apnea, asthma, atelectasis, bronchitis, epistaxis, hemoptysis, hiccup, hyperventilation, hypoxia, respiratory acidosis, pharyngitis, pneumonia, pneumothorax, pulmonary edema, pulmonary hypertension, respiratory moniliasis, rhinitis, sputum increased, voice alteration

Miscellaneous: *Candida* (mucocutaneous), CMV tissue invasive disease, CMV viremia/syndrome, herpes zoster cutaneous disease, cyst, diaphoresis, flu-like syndrome, healing abnormal, hernia, ileus infection, neoplasm, peritonitis, thirst

Rare but important or life-threatening: Atypical mycobacterial infection, BK virus-associated nephropathy, bronchiectasis (Boddana 2011, Rook 2006), colitis, gastrointestinal perforation, hypogammaglobulinemia (Boddana 2011, Keven 2003, Robertson 2009), infectious endocarditis, interstitial lung disorder, intestinal villous atrophy, lymphoma, lymphoproliferative disease, malignancy, meningitis, pancreatitis, progressive multifocal leukoencephalopathy (sometimes fatal), pulmonary fibrosis (fatal), pure red cell aplasia, tuberculosis

Drug Interactions

Metabolism/Transport Effects **Substrate** of OAT3, SLCO1B1, UGT1A10, UGT1A8, UGT1A9, UGT2B7

Avoid Concomitant Use

Avoid concomitant use of Mycophenolate with any of the following: BCG; BCG (Intravesical); Bile Acid Sequestrants; Cholestyramine Resin; Natalizumab; Pimecrolimus; Rifamycin Derivatives; Tacrolimus (Topical); Tofacitinib; Vaccines (Live)

Increased Effect/Toxicity

Mycophenolate may increase the levels/effects of: Acyclovir-Valacyclovir; Ganciclovir-Valganciclovir; Leflunomide; Natalizumab; Tofacitinib; Vaccines (Live)

The levels/effects of Mycophenolate may be increased by: Acyclovir-Valacyclovir; Denosumab; Ganciclovir-Valganciclovir; Isavuconazonium Sulfate; Pimecrolimus; Probenecid; Roflumilast; Tacrolimus (Topical); Teriflunomide; Trastuzumab

Decreased Effect

Mycophenolate may decrease the levels/effects of: BCG; BCG (Intravesical); Coccidioides immitis Skin Test; Contraceptives (Estrogens); Contraceptives (Progestins); Sipuleucel-T; Vaccines (Inactivated); Vaccines (Live)

The levels/effects of Mycophenolate may be decreased by: Antacids; Bile Acid Sequestrants; Cholestyramine Resin; CycloSPORINE (Systemic); Echinacea; Magnesium Salts; MetroNIDAZOLE (Systemic); Penicillins; Proton Pump Inhibitors; Quinolone Antibiotics; Rifamycin Derivatives; Sevelamer

Food Interactions Food decreases C_{max} of MPA by 40% following CellCept administration and 33% following Myfortic use; the extent of absorption is not changed. Management: Take CellCept or Myfortic on an empty stomach to decrease variability; however, Cellcept may be taken with food if necessary in stable renal transplant patients.

Storage/Stability

Capsules: Store at 25°C (77°F); excursions permitted to 15°C to 30°C (59°F to 86°F).

Tablets: Store at 25°C (77°F); excursions permitted to 15°C to 30°C (59°F to 86°F). Protect from moisture and light.

Oral suspension: Store powder for oral suspension at 25°C (77°F); excursions permitted to 15°C to 30°C (59°F to 86°F). Once reconstituted, the oral solution may be stored at room temperature or under refrigeration. Do not freeze. The mixed suspension is stable for 60 days.

Injection: Store intact vials and diluted solutions at 25°C (77°F); excursions permitted to 15°C to 30°C (59°F to 86°F). Begin infusion within 4 hours of reconstitution.

Mechanism of Action MPA exhibits a cytostatic effect on T and B lymphocytes. It is an inhibitor of inosine monophosphate dehydrogenase (IMPDH) which inhibits *de novo* guanosine nucleotide synthesis. T and B lymphocytes are dependent on this pathway for proliferation.

Pharmacokinetics (Adult data unless noted)

Absorption: Rapid and extensive; early post-transplant period mycophenolic acid (MPA) AUC values are lower (~45% to 53%) than later post-transplant period (>3 months) MPA AUC values in both pediatric patients and adults

Distribution: Mean V_d:

Mycophenolate mofetil (CellCept): MPA: Oral: 4 L/kg; IV 3.6 L/kg

Mycophenolate sodium delayed release tablet (Myfortic): MPA: Oral: 54 L (at steady state)

Protein binding: Mycophenolic acid (MPA): >97%; Mycophenolic acid glucuronide (MPAG): 82%

Metabolism: Hepatic and via GI tract; undergoes hydrolysis by esterases to mycophenolic acid (MPA is the active metabolite); MPA is metabolized by glucuronyl transferase to mycophenolic acid glucuronide (MPAG is inactive). MPAG is converted to MPA via enterohepatic recirculation.

Bioavailability:

Mycophenolate mofetil (CellCept): 80.7% to 94%; enterohepatic recirculation contributes to MPA concentration (Staatz, 2007); two 500 mg tablets have been shown to be bioequivalent to four 250 mg capsules or 1000 mg of oral suspension

Mycophenolate sodium delayed release tablet (Myfortic): 72%

Half-life:

Mycophenolate mofetil (CellCept): MPA: Oral: 18 hours; IV: 17 hours

Mycophenolate sodium delayed release tablet (Myfortic): MPA: Oral: 8-16 hours; MPAG: 13-17 hours

Time to peak serum concentration: Oral:

Mycophenolate mofetil (CellCept): 0.5-1 hour

Mycophenolate sodium delayed release tablet (Myfortic): Median: 1.5-2.75 hours

Elimination:

Mycophenolate mofetil (CellCept): MPA: Urine (<1%); feces (6%); MPAG: Urine (87%)

Mycophenolate sodium delayed release tablet (Myfortic): MPA: Urine (3%); feces; MPAG: Urine (>60%)

Dosing: Usual Note: May be used IV for up to 14 days; transition to oral therapy as soon as tolerated. Mycophenolate mofetil (CellCept) tablets, capsules, and suspension should not be interchanged with the delayed release tablet formulation (Myfortic) due to differences in the rate of absorption.

Pediatric:

Renal transplantation:

Mycophenolate mofetil (CellCept): Infants ≥3 months, Children, and Adolescents:

Oral:

Suspension: 600 mg/m²/dose twice daily; maximum daily dose: 2000 mg/**day**

Tablets or capsules:

BSA 1.25 m² to 1.5 m²: 750 mg twice daily

BSA >1.5 m²: 1000 mg twice daily

Mycophenolate sodium delayed release tablets (Myfortic): Children ≥5 years and Adolescents: 400 mg/m²/dose twice daily; maximum daily dose: 1440 mg/**day**

Alternate fixed dosing:

BSA <1.19 m²: Use of this formulation is not recommended

BSA 1.19 to 1.58 m²: 540 mg twice daily

BSA >1.58 m²: 720 mg twice daily

Note: Mycophenolate sodium delayed release 720 mg twice daily was shown to be bioequivalent to mycophenolate mofetil 1000 mg twice daily

Lupus nephritis: Limited data available: Mycophenolate mofetil (CellCept): Children and Adolescents: Oral:

BSA-based dosing:

Induction: 300-600 mg/m²/dose twice daily; maximum daily dose: 3000 mg/**day** (Aragon, 2010; Hobbs, 2010; Marks, 2010; Wong, 2009)

Maintenance: Initial: 300-600 mg/m²/dose twice daily; reported maximum daily dose range: 2000-3000 mg/**day** (Baskin, 2010; Cramer, 2007; Marks, 2010); once disease stabilized and remission maintained may consider dosage reduction.

Fixed dosing: Children ≥5 years and Adolescents: Induction or maintenance: Initial: 250-500 mg twice daily and gradually increased up to 750-1000 mg twice daily; doses based on small retrospective studies (n=52); doses equivalent to 10-12.5 mg/kg/dose twice daily (Appel, 2009; Falcini, 2009; Kazyra, 2010)

Nephrotic syndrome: Limited data available: Mycophenolate mofetil (CellCept): Children and Adolescents: Oral:

Frequently relapsing:

BSA-based dosing: 600 mg/m²/dose twice daily for at least 12 months; maximum daily dose: 2000 mg/**day** (Beck, 2013; Gipson, 2009; KDIGO, 2012)

Weight-based dosing: 12.5-18 mg/kg/dose twice daily; maximum daily dose: 2000 mg/**day** for 1-2 years with a tapering dose of prednisone (Gipson, 2009)

Steroid-dependent (for steroid sparing effect):

BSA-based dosing: 600 mg/m²/dose twice daily for at least 12 months; maximum daily dose: 2000 mg/**day** (Gipson, 2009; KDIGO, 2012)

Weight-based dosing: 12-18 mg/kg/dose twice daily; maximum daily dose: 2000 mg/**day** (Gipson, 2009)

Adult: **Note:** May be used IV for up to 14 days; transition to oral therapy as soon as tolerated.

Renal transplantation:

CellCept: IV, Oral: 1000 mg twice daily. Doses >2000 mg daily are not recommended.

Myfortic: Oral: 720 mg twice daily

Cardiac transplantation: *CellCept:* IV, Oral: 1500 mg twice daily

Hepatic transplantation: *CellCept:*

Oral: 1500 mg twice daily

IV: 1000 mg twice daily

Lupus nephritis: *CellCept:* Oral:

Induction: 1000 mg twice daily for 6 months in combination with a glucocorticoid (Ong, 2005) **or** 2000-3000 mg daily for 6 months in combination with glucocorticoids (Hahn, 2012)

Maintenance: 500-3000 mg daily (Contreras, 2004) **or** 1000 mg twice daily (Dooley, 2011) **or** 1000-2000 mg daily (Hahn, 2012)

Dosing adjustment in renal impairment:

Infants, Children, and Adolescents:

Mycophenolate mofetil (CellCept): Infants ≥3 months, Children, and Adolescents: Patients should be carefully observed; no dose adjustments are needed in renal transplant patients experiencing delayed graft function postoperatively. Avoid doses >1 g twice daily.

Mycophenolate delayed release tablet (Myfortic): Children ≥5 years and Adolescents: No dose adjustments are needed in renal transplant patients experiencing delayed graft function postoperatively; however, monitor carefully for potential concentration dependent adverse events.

Adults:

Renal transplant: GFR <25 mL/minute/1.73 m² outside the immediate post-transplant period:

Mycophenolate mofetil (CellCept): Avoid doses >1 g twice daily; patients should also be carefully observed; no dose adjustments are needed in renal transplant patients experiencing delayed graft function postoperatively

Mycophenolate delayed release tablet (Myfortic): No dose adjustments are needed in renal transplant patients experiencing delayed graft function postoperatively; however, monitor carefully for potential concentration dependent adverse events.

Cardiac or liver transplant: No data available; mycophenolate may be used in cardiac or hepatic transplant patients with severe chronic renal impairment if the potential benefit outweighs the potential risk.

Dosing adjustment in hepatic impairment: Infants ≥3 months, Children, Adolescents, and Adults: No dosage adjustment is recommended for renal patients with severe hepatic parenchymal disease; however, it is not currently known whether dosage adjustments are necessary for hepatic disease with other etiologies.

Dosing adjustment for toxicity (neutropenia): ANC <1.3 x 103/µL or anemia; dosing should be interrupted or the dose reduced

Preparation for Administration Hazardous agent; use appropriate precautions for handling and disposal (NIOSH 2014 [group 2]).

Oral suspension: Should be constituted prior to dispensing to the patient and **not** mixed with any other medication. Add 47 mL of water to the bottle and shake well for ~1 minute. Add another 47 mL of water to the bottle and shake well for an additional minute. Final concentration is 200 mg/mL of mycophenolate mofetil.

IV: Reconstitute each vial with 14 mL of D_5W; further dilute the reconstituted solution with D_5W to a final concentration of 6 mg/mL of mycophenolate mofetil. **Note:** Vial is vacuum-sealed; if a lack of vacuum is noted during preparation, the vial should not be used.

Administration Hazardous agent; use appropriate precautions for handling and disposal (NIOSH 2014 [group 2]).

Oral (capsule, tablet, suspension): Administer on an empty stomach 1 hour before or 2 hours after food to avoid variability in absorption; CellCept may be administered with food in stable renal transplant patients when necessary. Shake suspension well before use; may be administered via a nasogastric tube (minimum: 8 French, 1.7 mm interior diameter); oral suspension should not be mixed with other medications. Delayed release tablets should be swallowed whole; do not crush, chew, or cut. If a dose is missed, administer as soon as it is remembered. If it is close to the next scheduled dose, skip the missed dose and resume at next regularly scheduled time; do not double a dose to make up for a missed dose.

IV: **Do not administer IV push** or by rapid IV bolus injection; administer by slow IV infusion over a period of no less than 2 hours.

Monitoring Parameters Complete blood count (weekly for first month, twice monthly during months 2 and 3, then monthly thereafter through the first year); renal and liver function; signs and symptoms of organ rejection; signs and symptoms of bacterial, fungal, protozoal, new or reactivated viral, or opportunistic infections; neurological symptoms (eg, hemiparesis, confusion, cognitive deficiencies, ataxia) suggestive of PML, pregnancy test (immediately prior to initiation and 8-10 days later in females of childbearing potential, followed by repeat tests during therapy); monitor skin (for lesions suspicious of skin cancer); monitor for signs of lymphoma

Additional Information A direct conversion factor from mycophenolate mofetil to mycophenolic acid (delayed release) is not available. In one study, adults on mycophenolate mofetil 1000 mg twice daily were successfully converted to mycophenolic acid (delayed release) 720 mg twice daily. In the same study, children (n=17) were converted from 440 ± 147 mg/m^2 twice daily to mycophenolic acid (delayed release) 432 ± 51 mg/m^2 twice daily (Massari, 2005).

Dosage Forms Considerations Single dose pharmacokinetic studies in adult renal transplant patients suggest that bioavailability is similar between oral mycophenolate mofetil (1000 mg) and delayed release mycophenolic acid (720 mg) (Arns, 2005). In clinical trials, comparative efficacy and safety profiles have been observed in adult renal transplant patients randomized to either oral mycophenolate mofetil (1000 mg twice daily) or delayed release mycophenolic acid (720 mg twice daily) (Budde, 2004; Salvadori, 2003).

Dosage Forms Excipient information presented when available (limited, particularly for generics); consult specific product labeling.

Capsule, Oral, as mofetil:
- CellCept: 250 mg [contains fd&c blue #2 (indigotine)]
- Generic: 250 mg

Solution Reconstituted, Intravenous, as mofetil hydrochloride:
- CellCept Intravenous: 500 mg (1 ea)

Suspension Reconstituted, Oral, as mofetil:
- CellCept: 200 mg/mL (160 mL) [contains aspartame, methylparaben, soybean lecithin; mixed fruit flavor]
- Generic: 200 mg/mL (160 mL)

Tablet, Oral, as mofetil:
- CellCept: 500 mg [contains fd&c blue #2 aluminum lake]
- Generic: 500 mg

Tablet Delayed Release, Oral, as mycophenolic acid:
- Myfortic: 180 mg [contains fd&c blue #2 (indigotine)]
- Myfortic: 360 mg
- Generic: 180 mg, 360 mg

Extemporaneous Preparations Hazardous agent; use appropriate precautions for handling and disposal (NIOSH 2014 [group 2]).

A 50 mg/mL oral suspension may be made with mycophenolate mofetil capsules, Ora-Plus, and cherry syrup. In a vertical flow hood, empty six 250 mg capsules into a mortar; add 7.5 mL Ora-Plus and mix to a uniform paste. Mix while adding 15 mL of cherry syrup in incremental proportions; transfer to a calibrated bottle, rinse mortar with cherry syrup, and add sufficient quantity of cherry syrup to make 30 mL. Label "shake well". Stable for 210 days at 5°C, for 28 days at 25°C to 37°C, and for 11 days at 45°C.

Venkataramanan R, McCombs JR, Zuckerman S, et al, "Stability of Mycophenolate Mofetil as an Extemporaneous Suspension," *Ann Pharmacother*, 1998, 32(7-8):755-7.

◆ **Mycophenolate Mofetil** *see* Mycophenolate *on page 1473*

◆ **Mycophenolate Sodium** *see* Mycophenolate *on page 1473*

◆ **Mycophenolic Acid** *see* Mycophenolate *on page 1473*

◆ **Mydfrin [DSC]** *see* Phenylephrine (Ophthalmic) *on page 1689*

◆ **Mydfrin (Can)** *see* Phenylephrine (Ophthalmic) *on page 1689*

◆ **Mydral [DSC]** *see* Tropicamide *on page 2132*

◆ **Mydriacyl** *see* Tropicamide *on page 2132*

◆ **Myferon 150 [OTC]** *see* Polysaccharide-Iron Complex *on page 1728*

◆ **Myfortic** *see* Mycophenolate *on page 1473*

◆ **Mylan-Acyclovir (Can)** *see* Acyclovir (Systemic) *on page 61*

◆ **Mylan-Almotriptan (Can)** *see* Almotriptan *on page 98*

◆ **Mylan-Alprazolam (Can)** *see* ALPRAZolam *on page 100*

◆ **Mylan-Amantadine (Can)** *see* Amantadine *on page 112*

◆ **Mylan-Amiodarone (Can)** *see* Amiodarone *on page 125*

◆ **Mylan-Amlodipine (Can)** *see* AmLODIPine *on page 133*

◆ **Mylan-Amoxicillin (Can)** *see* Amoxicillin *on page 138*

◆ **Mylan-Anagrelide (Can)** *see* Anagrelide *on page 163*

◆ **Mylan-Atenolol (Can)** *see* Atenolol *on page 215*

◆ **Mylan-Atomoxetine (Can)** *see* AtoMOXetine *on page 217*

◆ **Mylan-Atorvastatin (Can)** *see* AtorvaSTATin *on page 220*

◆ **Mylan-Azathioprine (Can)** *see* AzaTHIOprine *on page 236*

◆ **Mylan-Azithromycin (Can)** *see* Azithromycin (Systemic) *on page 242*

◆ **Mylan-Baclofen (Can)** *see* Baclofen *on page 254*

◆ **Mylan-Beclo AQ (Can)** *see* Beclomethasone (Nasal) *on page 260*

◆ **Mylan-Bosentan (Can)** *see* Bosentan *on page 294*

◆ **Mylan-Budesonide AQ (Can)** *see* Budesonide (Nasal) *on page 311*

◆ **Mylan-Buprenorphine/Naloxone (Can)** *see* Buprenorphine and Naloxone *on page 322*

◆ **Mylan-Bupropion XL (Can)** *see* BuPROPion *on page 324*

◆ **Mylan-Candesartan (Can)** *see* Candesartan *on page 358*

◆ **Mylan-Captopril (Can)** *see* Captopril *on page 364*

◆ **Mylan-Carbamazepine CR (Can)** *see* CarBAMazepine *on page 367*

◆ **Mylan-Carvedilol (Can)** *see* Carvedilol *on page 380*

◆ **Mylan-Celecoxib (Can)** *see* Celecoxib *on page 418*

◆ **Mylan-Cimetidine (Can)** *see* Cimetidine *on page 461*

◆ **Mylan-Ciprofloxacin (Can)** *see* Ciprofloxacin (Systemic) *on page 463*

◆ **Mylan-Citalopram (Can)** *see* Citalopram *on page 476*

◆ **Mylan-Clarithromycin (Can)** *see* Clarithromycin *on page 482*

◆ **Mylan-Clindamycin (Can)** *see* Clindamycin (Systemic) *on page 487*

◆ **Mylan-Clobetasol (Can)** *see* Clobetasol *on page 498*

◆ **Mylan-Clonazepam (Can)** *see* ClonazePAM *on page 506*

◆ **Mylan-Clopidogrel (Can)** *see* Clopidogrel *on page 513*

◆ **Mylan-Cyclobenzaprine (Can)** *see* Cyclobenzaprine *on page 548*

Nabilone (NA bi lone)

Related Information

Prevention of Chemotherapy-Induced Nausea and Vomiting in Children *on page 2368*

Brand Names: US Cesamet

Brand Names: Canada ACT Nabilone; Cesamet; PMS-Nabilone; RAN™-Nabilone; Teva-Nabilone

Therapeutic Category Antiemetic

Generic Availability (US) No

Use Treatment of refractory nausea and vomiting associated with cancer chemotherapy (FDA approved in age 18 years and adults); has also been used to prevent chemotherapy-induced nausea and vomiting in patients receiving moderate to highly emetogenic chemotherapy in whom corticosteroids are contraindicated

Pregnancy Risk Factor C

Pregnancy Considerations Adverse events have been observed in animal reproduction studies.

Breast-Feeding Considerations Because some cannabinoids are excreted in breast milk, use in breast-feeding is not recommended.

Contraindications Hypersensitivity to nabilone, other cannabinoids, or any component of the formulation

Warnings/Precautions May cause tachycardia and orthostatic hypotension; use caution with cardiovascular disease. May affect CNS function (dizziness, drowsiness, ataxia, depression, hallucinations, and psychosis have been reported); use with caution in the elderly and those with pre-existing CNS depression. May cause additive CNS effects with sedatives, hypnotics, or other psychoactive agents; patients must be cautioned about performing tasks which require mental alertness (eg, operating machinery or driving). Use caution in patients with mania, depression, or schizophrenia; cannabinoid use may reveal symptoms of psychiatric disorders. Careful psychiatric monitoring is recommended; psychiatric adverse reactions may persist for up to 3 days after discontinuing treatment. Has potential for abuse and or dependence, use caution in patients with substance abuse history or potential.

Adverse Reactions

Cardiovascular: Hypotension

Central nervous system: Ataxia, concentration decreased, depersonalization, depression, disorientation, dizziness, drowsiness, dysphoria, euphoria, headache, sedation, sleep disturbance, vertigo

Gastrointestinal: Anorexia, appetite increased, nausea, xerostomia

Neuromuscular & skeletal: Weakness

Ocular: Visual disturbance

Rare but important or life-threatening: Abdominal pain, abnormal dreams, akathisia, allergic reaction, amblyopia, anemia, anhydrosis, anxiety, apathy, aphthous ulcer, arrhythmia, back pain, cerebral vascular accident, chest pain, chills, constipation, cough, diaphoresis, diarrhea, dyspepsia, dyspnea, dystonia, emotional disorder, emotional lability, epistaxis, equilibrium dysfunction, eye irritation, fatigue, fever, flushing, gastritis, hallucinations, hot flashes, hyperactivity, hypertension, infection, insomnia, joint pain, leukopenia, lightheadedness, malaise, memory disturbance, mood swings, mouth irritation, muscle pain, nasal congestion, neck pain, nervousness, neurosis (phobic), numbness, orthostatic hypotension, pain, palpitation, panic disorder, paranoia, paresthesia, perception disturbance, pharyngitis, photophobia, photosensitivity, polyuria, pruritus, psychosis (including toxic), pupil dilation, rash, seizure, sinus headache, speech disorder, stupor, syncope, tachycardia, taste perversion, thirst, thought disorder, tinnitus, tremor, urination decreased/increased, urinary retention, visual field defect, voice change, vomiting, wheezing, withdrawal, xerophthalmia

Drug Interactions

Metabolism/Transport Effects None known.

Avoid Concomitant Use There are no known interactions where it is recommended to avoid concomitant use.

Increased Effect/Toxicity

Nabilone may increase the levels/effects of: Alcohol (Ethyl); CNS Depressants; Sympathomimetics

The levels/effects of Nabilone may be increased by: Anticholinergic Agents; Cocaine

Decreased Effect There are no known significant interactions involving a decrease in effect.

Storage/Stability Store at 25°C (77°F); excursion permitted to 15°C and 30°C (59°F and 86°F).

Mechanism of Action Antiemetic activity may be due to effect on cannabinoid receptors (CB1) within the central nervous system.

Pharmacokinetics (Adult data unless noted)

Absorption: Rapid and complete

Distribution: ~12.5 L/kg

Metabolism: Extensively metabolized to several active metabolites by oxidation and stereospecific enzyme reduction; CYP450 enzymes may also be involved

Half-life: Parent compound: ~2 hours; Metabolites: ~35 hours

Time to peak serum concentration: Within 2 hours

Elimination: Feces (~60%); renal (~24%)

Dosing: Usual

Pediatric: **Chemotherapy-induced nausea and vomiting, prevention:** Limited data available: **Note:** Use in patients receiving moderate to highly emetogenic chemotherapy in whom corticosteroids are contraindicated (Dupuis, 2013): Oral:

Infants, Children, and Adolescents (Chan, 1997; Dupuis, 2013):

<18 kg: 0.5 mg twice daily

18 to 30 kg: 1 mg twice daily

>30 kg: 1 mg 3 times daily

Adult: **Chemotherapy-induced nausea and vomiting, refractory:** Oral: 1 to 2 mg twice daily (maximum daily dose: 6 mg/**day** divided in 3 doses); begin with the lower dose in the range and increase if needed. May administer 2 or 3 times per day during the entire chemotherapy course; continue for up to 48 hours after the last chemotherapy dose. A dose of 1 to 2 mg the night before chemotherapy may also be of benefit.

Dosing adjustment in renal impairment: Adults: There are no dosage adjustments provided in the manufacturer's labeling (has not been studied).

Dosing adjustment in hepatic impairment: Adults: There are no dosage adjustments provided in the manufacturer's labeling (has not been studied).

Administration Oral: Initial dose should be given 1 to 3 hours before chemotherapy; may be given 2 to 3 times daily during the entire chemotherapy course and for up to 48 hours after the last dose of chemotherapy; a dose the night before chemotherapy may be useful. One small study (n=22; ages: 8 months to 17 years) described opening capsules and dividing the powder if necessary to obtain the correct dose (Dalzell, 1986).

Monitoring Parameters Blood pressure, heart rate; signs and symptoms of excessive use, abuse, or misuse

Controlled Substance C-II

Dosage Forms Excipient information presented when available (limited, particularly for generics); consult specific product labeling.

Capsule, Oral:

Cesamet: 1 mg [contains fd&c blue #2 (indigotine)]

◆ **NAC** *see* Acetylcysteine *on page 57*

◆ ***N*-Acetyl-L-cysteine** *see* Acetylcysteine *on page 57*

◆ ***N* Acetylcysteine** *see* Acetylcysteine *on page 57*

◆ **N-acetylgalactosamine-6-sulfatase** *see* Elosulfase Alfa *on page 738*

◆ **N-Acetyl-P-Aminophenol** *see* Acetaminophen *on page 44*

◆ **NaCl** *see* Sodium Chloride *on page 1938*

Nadolol (NAY doe lol)

Medication Safety Issues

Sound-alike/look-alike issues:

Corgard may be confused with Cognex, Coreg

International issues:

Nadolol may be confused with Mandol brand name for cefamandole [Belgium, Netherlands, New Zealand, Russia]

Brand Names: US Corgard

Brand Names: Canada Apo-Nadol; Teva-Nadolol

Therapeutic Category Antianginal Agent; Antiarrhythmic Agent, Class II; Antihypertensive Agent; Antimigraine Agent; Beta-Adrenergic Blocker

Generic Availability (US) Yes

Use Treatment of hypertension, alone or in combination with other agents (FDA approved in adults); treatment of angina pectoris (FDA approved in adults); has also been used for supraventricular tachycardia (SVT), thyrotoxicosis, prophylaxis of migraine headaches

Pregnancy Risk Factor C

Pregnancy Considerations Adverse events were observed in some animal reproduction studies; therefore, the manufacturer classifies nadolol as pregnancy category C. Nadolol crosses the placenta and is measurable in infant serum after birth. In a cohort study, an increased risk of cardiovascular defects was observed following maternal use of beta-blockers during pregnancy. Intrauterine growth restriction (IUGR), small placentas, as well as fetal/neonatal bradycardia, hypoglycemia, and/or respiratory depression have been observed following *in utero* exposure to beta-blockers as a class. Adequate facilities for monitoring infants at birth should be available. Untreated chronic maternal hypertension and pre-eclampsia are also associated with adverse events in the fetus, infant, and mother. Nadolol is indicated for the treatment of hypertension, but due to its long half-life and potential effects to the fetus, other agents may be more appropriate for use during pregnancy.

Breast-Feeding Considerations Nadolol is excreted into breast milk in concentrations higher than the maternal serum. According to the manufacturer, the decision to continue or discontinue breast-feeding during therapy should take into account the risk of exposure to the infant and the benefits of treatment to the mother. The time to peak milk concentration is 6 hours after the oral dose, the half-life of nadolol in breast milk is similar to that in the maternal serum, and nadolol can still be detected in breast milk for several days after the last maternal dose.

Contraindications

U.S. labeling: Hypersensitivity to nadolol or any component of the formulation; bronchial asthma; sinus bradycardia; sinus node dysfunction; heart block greater than first degree (except in patients with a functioning artificial pacemaker); cardiogenic shock; uncompensated cardiac failure

Canadian labeling: Hypersensitivity to nadolol or any component of the formulation; bronchial asthma; sinus bradycardia; sinus node dysfunction; heart block greater than first degree (except in patients with a functioning artificial pacemaker); cardiogenic shock; uncompensated cardiac failure; anesthesia with agents that produce myocardial depression; allergic rhinitis; severe chronic obstructive pulmonary disease (COPD)

Warnings/Precautions Consider pre-existing conditions such as sick sinus syndrome before initiating. Administer only with extreme caution in patients with compensated heart failure, monitor for a worsening of the condition. Efficacy in heart failure has not been established for nadolol. **[U.S. Boxed Warning]: Beta-blocker therapy should not be withdrawn abruptly (particularly in patients with CAD), but gradually tapered to avoid acute tachycardia, hypertension, and/or ischemia.** Beta-blockers without alpha1-adrenergic receptor blocking activity should be avoided in patients with Prinzmetal variant angina (Mayer, 1998). Chronic beta-blocker therapy should not be routinely withdrawn prior to major surgery. In general, patients with bronchospastic disease should not receive beta-blockers. Nadolol, if used at all, should be used cautiously in bronchospastic disease with close monitoring. Use cautiously in diabetics because it can mask prominent hypoglycemic symptoms. May mask signs of hyperthyroidism (eg, tachycardia); if hyperthyroidism is suspected, carefully manage and monitor; abrupt withdrawal may exacerbate symptoms of hyperthyroidism or precipitate thyroid storm. Use cautiously in the renally impaired (dosage adjustments are required). Use with caution in patients with myasthenia gravis, peripheral vascular disease, or psychiatric disease (may cause CNS depression). Bradycardia may be observed more frequently in elderly patients (>65 years of age); dosage reductions may be necessary. Potentially significant drug-drug interactions may exist, requiring dose or frequency adjustment, additional monitoring, and/or selection of alternative therapy. Adequate alpha-blockade is required prior to use of any beta-blocker for patients with untreated pheochromocytoma. May induce or exacerbate psoriasis. Use caution with history of severe anaphylaxis to allergens; patients taking beta-blockers may become more sensitive to repeated challenges. Treatment of anaphylaxis (eg, epinephrine) in patients taking beta-blockers may be ineffective or promote undesirable effects.

Adverse Reactions

Cardiovascular: Atrioventricular block, bradycardia, cardiac conduction disturbance, cardiac failure, cold extremities, edema, hypotension, palpitations, peripheral vascular insufficiency, Raynaud's phenomenon

Central nervous system: Depression, dizziness, drowsiness, fatigue, insomnia, sedation

Rare but important or life-threatening: Anorexia, bloating, bronchospasm, cardiac arrhythmia, confusion (especially in the elderly), cough, decreased libido, diarrhea, dyspepsia, facial edema, hallucination, headache, impotence, nasal congestion, nausea, paresthesia, pruritus, sedation, skin rash, slurred speech, thrombocytopenia, transient alopecia, weight gain, xeroderma, xerophthalmia

Drug Interactions

Metabolism/Transport Effects Substrate of P-glycoprotein

Avoid Concomitant Use

Avoid concomitant use of Nadolol with any of the following: Beta2-Agonists; Ceritinib; Floctafenine; Methacholine; Rivastigmine

Increased Effect/Toxicity

Nadolol may increase the levels/effects of: Alpha-/Beta-Agonists (Direct-Acting); Alpha1-Blockers; Alpha2-Agonists; Amifostine; Antihypertensives; Bradycardia-Causing Agents; Bupivacaine; Cardiac Glycosides; Ceritinib; Cholinergic Agonists; Disopyramide; DULoxetine; Ergot Derivatives; Fingolimod; Grass Pollen Allergen Extract (5 Grass Extract); Hypotensive Agents; Insulin; Ivabradine; Lacosamide; Levodopa; Lidocaine (Systemic); Lidocaine (Topical); Mepivacaine; Methacholine; Midodrine; Obinutuzumab; RisperiDONE; RiTUXimab; Sulfonylureas

The levels/effects of Nadolol may be increased by: Acetylcholinesterase Inhibitors; Alpha2-Agonists; Amiodarone; Anilidopiperidine Opioids; Barbiturates; Bretylium; Brimonidine (Topical); Calcium Channel Blockers (Nondihydropyridine); Diazoxide; Dipyridamole; Disopyramide; Dronedarone; Floctafenine; Herbs (Hypotensive Properties); MAO Inhibitors; Nicorandil; NIFEdipine; Pentoxifylline; P-glycoprotein/ABCB1 Inhibitors; Phosphodiesterase 5 Inhibitors; Prostacyclin Analogues;

Regorafenib; Reserpine; Rivastigmine; Ruxolitinib; Tofacitinib

Decreased Effect

Nadolol may decrease the levels/effects of: Beta2-Agonists; Theophylline Derivatives

The levels/effects of Nadolol may be decreased by: Green Tea; Herbs (Hypertensive Properties); Methylphenidate; Nonsteroidal Anti-Inflammatory Agents; P-glycoprotein/ABCB1 Inducers; Yohimbine

Storage/Stability Store at room temperature; avoid excessive heat. Protect from light.

Mechanism of Action Competitively blocks response to $beta_1$- and $beta_2$-adrenergic stimulation; does not exhibit any membrane stabilizing or intrinsic sympathomimetic activity. Nonselective beta-adrenergic blockers (propranolol, nadolol) reduce portal pressure by producing splanchnic vasoconstriction ($beta_2$ effect) thereby reducing portal blood flow.

Pharmacodynamics Duration: 24 hours

Pharmacokinetics (Adult data unless noted)

Absorption: Oral: 30%

Distribution: V_d: ~2 L/kg

Protein-binding: 30%

Metabolism: Not hepatically metabolized

Half-life, elimination:

Increased half-life with decreased renal function

Infants 3-22 months (n=3): 3.2-4.3 hours (Mehta, 1992b)

Children 10 years (n=1): 15.7 hours (Mehta, 1992b)

Children ~15 years (n=1): 7.3 hours (Mehta, 1992b)

Adults: 20-24 hours; prolonged with renal impairment (up to 45 hours in severe impairment) (Herrera, 1979)

Time to peak serum concentration: 3-4 hours

Elimination: Urine (as unchanged drug)

Dosing: Usual

Infants, Children, and Adolescents:

Migraine, prophylaxis: Children >6 years and Adolescents: Limited data available: Oral: 0.25-1 mg/kg once or twice daily; begin at low end of range and slowly titrate upwards every 1-2 weeks (Linder, 2001)

SVT: Limited data available: Oral: Initial: 0.5-1 mg/kg once daily; increase dose gradually to a maximum of 2.5 mg/kg/day; dosing based on a trial of 26 pediatric patients (age range: 3 months to 15 years) which showed SVT was well controlled with a median dose of 1 mg/kg/day (Mehta, 1992)

Adults:

Angina: Oral: Initial: 40 mg once daily; increase dosage gradually by 40-80 mg increments at 3- to 7-day intervals until optimum clinical response is obtained; usual dose: 40-80 mg daily; maximum daily dose: 240 mg/**day**

Hypertension: Oral: Initial: 40 mg once daily; increase dosage gradually by 40-80 mg increments until optimum blood pressure reduction achieved; usual dosage range (JNC 7): 40-120 mg once daily; doses up to 240-320 mg/day in hypertension may be necessary

Thyrotoxicosis: 40-160 mg once daily (Bahn, 2011)

Dosage adjustment for renal impairment: Adults: Manufacturer's recommendation:

CrCl >50 mL/minute/1.73 m^2: Administer every 24 hours

CrCl 31-50 mL/minute/1.73 m^2: Administer every 24-36 hours

CrCl 10-30 mL/minute/1.73 m^2: Administer every 24-48 hours

CrCl <10 mL/minute/1.73 m^2: Administer every 40-60 hours

Dialysis: Moderately dialyzable (20% to 50%). There are no dosage adjustments for dialysis provided in the manufacturer's labeling; however, the following guidelines have been used by some clinicians (Aronoff, 2007):

ESRD requiring hemodialysis: Administer dose postdialysis.

Peritoneal dialysis: Administer every 40-60 hours.

Dosage adjustment for hepatic impairment: There are no dosage adjustments provided in the manufacturer's labeling

Administration Oral: May administer without regard to meals

Monitoring Parameters Blood pressure, heart rate, fluid intake and output, weight

Dosage Forms Excipient information presented when available (limited, particularly for generics); consult specific product labeling.

Tablet, Oral:

Corgard: 20 mg, 40 mg, 80 mg [scored]

Generic: 20 mg, 40 mg, 80 mg

Nafcillin (naf SIL in)

Related Information

Management of Drug Extravasations *on page* 2298

Brand Names: US Nallpen in Dextrose

Therapeutic Category Antibiotic, Penicillin (Antistaphylococcal)

Generic Availability (US) May be product dependent

Use Treatment of bacterial infections such as osteomyelitis, septicemia, endocarditis, and CNS infections due to susceptible penicillinase-producing strains of *Staphylococcus* [FDA approved in pediatric patients (IM) and adults (IM and IV)]

Pregnancy Risk Factor B

Pregnancy Considerations Adverse events have not been observed in animal reproduction studies. Information specific to nafcillin use in pregnancy is limited. Maternal use of penicillins has generally not resulted in an increased risk of birth defects.

Breast-Feeding Considerations Penicillins are excreted into breast milk. The manufacturer recommends that caution be exercised when administering nafcillin to nursing women. Nondose-related effects could include modification of bowel flora.

Contraindications Hypersensitivity to nafcillin, or any component of the formulation, or penicillins

Warnings/Precautions Serious and occasionally severe or fatal hypersensitivity (anaphylactoid) reactions have been reported in patients on penicillin therapy, especially with a history of beta-lactam hypersensitivity, history of sensitivity to multiple allergens, or previous IgE-mediated reactions (eg, anaphylaxis, angioedema, urticaria). Use with caution in asthmatic patients. Contains sodium; use with caution in patients with heart failure. Vesicant; ensure proper catheter or needle position prior to and during IV infusion; avoid extravasation of IV infusions. Large IV or intraventricular doses have been associated with neurotoxicity. Modification of dosage is necessary in patients with both severe renal and hepatic impairment. Elimination may be decreased in pediatric patients. Prolonged use may result in fungal or bacterial superinfection, including *C. difficile*-associated diarrhea (CDAD) and pseudomembranous colitis; CDAD has been observed >2 months postantibiotic treatment. Potentially significant drug-drug interactions may exist, requiring dose or frequency adjustment, additional monitoring, and/or selection of alternative therapy.

Warnings: Additional Pediatric Considerations In a study of pediatric patients (5 to 19 years) receiving outpatient nafcillin for >3 weeks, significantly less rash was reported in the nafcillin group (10.3%) compared to oxacillin group (31.7%) (Maraqa, 2002).

Adverse Reactions

Central nervous system: Neurotoxicity (high doses)
Gastrointestinal: *C. difficile*-associated diarrhea
Hematologic: Agranulocytosis, bone marrow depression, neutropenia
Local: Inflammation, pain, phlebitis, skin sloughing, swelling, and thrombophlebitis at the injection site; tissue necrosis with sloughing (SubQ extravasation)
Renal: Interstitial nephritis (rare), renal tubular damage (rare)
Miscellaneous: Anaphylaxis, hypersensitivity reactions (immediate and delayed; general incidence of 1% to 10% for penicillins), serum sickness
Rare but important or life-threatening: ALT increased, AST increased, bilirubin increased, cholestatic hepatitis, diarrhea, drug-induced lupus erythematosus, fever, hypokalemia, itching, nausea, rash (including bullous skin eruptions), vomiting

Drug Interactions

Metabolism/Transport Effects **Induces** CYP3A4 (moderate)

Avoid Concomitant Use

Avoid concomitant use of Nafcillin with any of the following: Axitinib; BCG; BCG (Intravesical); Bedaquiline; Bosutinib; Enzalutamide; Nisoldipine; Olaparib; Palbociclib; Probenecid; Simeprevir

Increased Effect/Toxicity

Nafcillin may increase the levels/effects of: Clarithromycin; Ifosfamide; Methotrexate

The levels/effects of Nafcillin may be increased by: Probenecid

Decreased Effect

Nafcillin may decrease the levels/effects of: ARIPiprazole; Axitinib; BCG; BCG (Intravesical); BCG Vaccine (Immunization); Bedaquiline; Bosutinib; Calcium Channel Blockers; Clarithromycin; Contraceptives (Estrogens); CycloSPORINE (Systemic); CYP3A4 Substrates; Dasabuvir; Enzalutamide; FentaNYL; Hydrocodone; Ibrutinib; Ifosfamide; Mycophenolate; Nisoldipine; Olaparib; Ombitasvir; Palbociclib; Paritaprevir; Saxagliptin; Simeprevir; Sodium Picosulfate; Typhoid Vaccine; Vitamin K Antagonists

The levels/effects of Nafcillin may be decreased by: Tetracycline Derivatives

Storage/Stability

Premixed infusions: Store in a freezer at -20°C (-4°F). Thaw at room temperature or under refrigeration only. Thawed bags are stable for 21 days under refrigeration or 72 hours at room temperature. Do not refreeze.
Vials: Reconstituted parenteral solution is stable for 3 days at room temperature and 7 days when refrigerated. For IV infusion in NS or D_5W, solution is stable for 24 hours at room temperature and 7 days when refrigerated.
Solutions for ambulatory IV infusion reservoirs (eg, >24-hour supply) may be subject to inadvertent exposure to temperatures higher than recommended due to heat radiation from patient's skin; lower concentrations of preparation may be needed to prevent precipitation of solution in some circumstances (Chan, 2005).

Mechanism of Action Interferes with bacterial cell wall synthesis during active multiplication, causing cell wall destruction and resultant bactericidal activity against susceptible bacteria; resistant to inactivation by staphylococcal penicillinase

Pharmacokinetics (Adult data unless noted)

Distribution: Distributes into bile, synovial, pleural, ascitic, and pericardial fluids and into bone and liver; CSF penetration is poor unless meninges are inflamed
V_d:
Neonates: 0.24-0.53 L/kg
Children: 0.85-0.91 L/kg
Adults: 0.57-1.55 L/kg
Protein binding: ~90%; primarily albumin
Metabolism: Primarily hepatic; undergoes enterohepatic recirculation
Half-life:
Neonates and Infants <9 weeks:
<3 weeks: 2.2-5.5 hours
4-9 weeks: 1.2-2.3 hours
Infants and Children 1 month to 14 years: 0.75-1.9 hours
Adults: Normal renal and hepatic function: 30-60 minutes
Time to peak serum concentration: IM: Within 30-60 minutes
Elimination: Primarily bile/feces; urine (30% as unchanged drug)
Dialysis: Not dialyzable (0% to 5%)

Dosing: Neonatal

General dosing, susceptible infection (non-CNS): (*Red Book*, 2012): IM, IV:
Body weight <1 kg:
PNA ≤14 days: 25 mg/kg/dose every 12 hours
PNA 15-28 days: 25 mg/kg/dose every 8 hours
Body weight 1-2 kg:
PNA ≤7 days: 25 mg/kg/dose every 12 hours
PNA 8-28 days: 25 mg/kg/dose every 8 hours
Body weight >2 kg:
PNA ≤7 days: 25 mg/kg/dose every 8 hours
PNA 8-28 days: 25 mg/kg/dose every 6 hours
Meningitis: IV (Tunkel, 2004):
PNA 0-7 days: 75 mg/kg/day in divided doses every 8-12 hours for 14-21 days
PNA 8-28 days: 100-150 mg/kg/day in divided doses every 6-8 hours for 14-21 days

Dosing: Usual

Infants, Children, and Adolescents:
General dosing, susceptible infection (*Red Book*, 2012): IM, IV:
Mild to moderate infections: 100-150 mg/kg/day in divided doses every 6 hours; maximum daily dose: 4 g/**day**
Severe infections: 150-200 mg/kg/day in divided doses every 4-6 hours; maximum daily dose: 12 g/**day**
Endocarditis, oxacillin/methicillin-susceptible staphylococci (Baddour, 2005):
Native valve: IV: 200 mg/kg/day in divided doses every 4-6 hours for 6 weeks with gentamicin for the first 3-5 days of therapy
Prosthetic valve: IV: 200 mg/kg/day in divided doses every 4-6 hours for ≥6 weeks with rifampin (same duration as nafcillin) and with gentamicin for the first 2 weeks of therapy
Meningitis: IV: 200 mg/kg/day in divided doses every 6 hours; maximum daily dose: 12 g/**day** (Tunkel, 2004)
Skin and soft tissue infections: IV: 100-150 mg/kg/day in divided doses every 6 hours; maximum daily dose: 12 g/**day** (Stevens, 2005)
Adults:
General dosing, susceptible infections:
IM: 500 mg every 4-6 hours
IV: 500-2000 mg every 4-6 hours
Endocarditis, oxacillin/methicillin-susceptible staphylococci: (Baddour, 2005): IV:
Native valve: 12 g/24 hours in 4-6 divided doses for 6 weeks
Prosthetic valve: 12 g/24 hours in 6 divided dose for ≥6 weeks (use with rifampin for entire course and gentamicin for first 2 weeks)
Joint, prosthetic infections: IV: 1500-2000 mg every 4-6 hours for 4-6 weeks (2-6 weeks if in combination with rifampin), followed by oral antibiotic treatment and suppressive regimens (Osmon, 2013)

Skin and soft tissue infections: (Stevens, 2005): IV:
Methicillin-susceptible *Staphylococcus aureus*: 1000-2000 mg every 4 hours
Necrotizing infection *(Staphylococcus aureus)* of fascia, muscle, skin: 1000-2000 mg every 4 hours

Dosing adjustment in renal impairment: Not necessary unless renal impairment is in the setting of concomitant hepatic impairment; poorly dialyzed; no supplemental dose or dosage adjustment necessary, including patients on intermittent hemodialysis, peritoneal dialysis, or continuous renal replacement therapy (eg, CVVHD)

Dosing adjustment in hepatic impairment: No specific dosage adjustments provided in manufacturer's labeling; however, dosage adjustment may be necessary particularly in the setting of concomitant renal impairment; nafcillin primarily undergoes hepatic metabolism. In patients with both hepatic and renal impairment, monitoring of serum drug concentrations and modification of dosage may be necessary.

Preparation for Administration

Parenteral:

IM: Reconstitute with NS, SWFI or bacteriostatic water for injection; resultant concentration is 250 mg/mL

IV: Reconstitute powder for injection with NS, or SWFI, resultant concentration dependent upon product (see manufacturer's labeling for specific details)

Direct IV injection: Further dilute dose in 15 to 30 mL of NS or SWFI

Intermittent IV infusion: Further dilute in an appropriate fluid, final concentration should not exceed 40 mg/mL (Klaus 1989); in fluid-restricted patients, a higher concentration may be used depending on the diluent (D_5W: 71 mg/mL; NS: 62 mg/mL; SWI: 125 mg/mL) (Robinson 1987)

Administration

Parenteral:

IM: Administer reconstituted solution as deep intragluteal injection; rotate injection sites

IV:

Direct IV injection: Further dilute, and administer over 5 to 10 minutes

Intermittent IV infusion: Infuse over 30 to 60 minutes

Vesicant; ensure proper needle or catheter placement prior to and during IV infusion. Avoid extravasation. If extravasation occurs, stop infusion immediately and disconnect (leave needle/cannula in place); gently aspirate extravasated solution (do **NOT** flush the line); initiate hyaluronidase antidote (see Management of Drug Extravasations for more details); remove needle/cannula; apply dry cold compresses (Hurst 2004); elevate extremity.

Vesicant/Extravasation Risk Vesicant

Monitoring Parameters Baseline and periodic CBC with differential, urinalysis, BUN, serum creatinine, AST, and ALT; initial culture and susceptibility test; observe for signs and symptoms of anaphylaxis during first dose and IV site for extravasation

Test Interactions Positive Coombs' test (direct), false-positive urinary and serum proteins; may inactivate aminoglycosides *in vitro*

Additional Information In adults, 1000 mg given IM is expected to yield a peak serum concentration of 7.71 mcg/mL 30-60 minutes after dose.

Sodium content of 1 g injection: 2.9 mEq

Dosage Forms Excipient information presented when available (limited, particularly for generics); consult specific product labeling.

Solution, Intravenous:

Nallpen in Dextrose: 1 g/50 mL (50 mL); 2 g/100 mL (100 mL)

Solution Reconstituted, Injection:

Generic: 1 g (1 ea); 2 g (1 ea); 10 g (1 ea)

Solution Reconstituted, Injection [preservative free]:

Generic: 1 g (1 ea); 2 g (1 ea); 10 g (1 ea)

Solution Reconstituted, Intravenous:

Generic: 1 g (1 ea); 2 g (1 ea)

◆ **Nafcillin Sodium** *see* Nafcillin *on page 1481*

◆ **Naglazyme** *see* Galsulfase *on page 956*

◆ **$NaHCO_3$** *see* Sodium Bicarbonate *on page 1936*

Nalbuphine (NAL byoo feen)

Medication Safety Issues

Sound-alike/look-alike issues:

Nalbuphine may be confused with naloxone

Nubain may be confused with Navane, Nebcin

High alert medication:

The Institute for Safe Medication Practices (ISMP) includes this medication among its list of drug classes which have a heightened risk of causing significant patient harm when used in error.

Therapeutic Category Analgesic, Narcotic; Opioid Partial Agonist

Generic Availability (US) Yes

Use Relief of moderate to severe pain; supplement to balanced anesthesia [for preoperative and postoperative analgesia, and obstetrical analgesia (during labor and delivery)]; prevention or treatment of opioid-induced pruritus

Pregnancy Risk Factor C

Pregnancy Considerations Adverse events were observed in some animal reproduction studies. Nalbuphine crosses the placenta. Nalbuphine is approved for use in obstetrical analgesia during labor and delivery. When used for pain relief during labor, opioids may temporarily affect the heart rate of the fetus (ACOG, 2002) and severe fetal bradycardia has been reported following use of nalbuphine in labor/delivery. Fetal bradycardia may occur when administered earlier in pregnancy (not documented). Use only if clearly needed, with monitoring to detect and manage possible adverse fetal effects. Naloxone has been reported to reverse bradycardia. Newborn should be monitored for respiratory depression or bradycardia following nalbuphine use in labor.

If chronic opioid exposure occurs in pregnancy, adverse events in the newborn (including withdrawal) may occur; monitoring of the neonate is recommended. The minimum effective dose should be used if opioids are needed (Chou, 2009). Neonatal abstinence syndrome following opioid exposure may present with autonomic (eg, fever, temperature instability), gastrointestinal (eg, diarrhea, vomiting, poor feeding/weight gain), or neurologic (eg, high-pitched crying, increased muscle tone, irritability, seizure, tremor) symptoms (Dow, 2012; Hudak, 2012).

Breast-Feeding Considerations Small amounts (<1% of maternal dose) of nalbuphine are excreted in breast milk. The manufacturer recommends that caution be exercised when administering nalbuphine to nursing women.

Parenteral opioids used during labor have the potential to interfere with a newborns natural reflex to nurse within the first few hours after birth. If nalbuphine is administered to a nursing woman, it is recommended to monitor both the mother and baby for psychotomimetic reactions. Nursing infants exposed to large doses of opioids should also be monitored for apnea and sedation (Montgomery, 2012).

Contraindications Hypersensitivity to nalbuphine or any component of the formulation

Warnings/Precautions Use caution in CNS depression. Sedation and psychomotor impairment are likely, and are additive with other CNS depressants or ethanol. May cause respiratory depression. Ambulatory patients must be cautioned about performing tasks which require mental alertness (eg, operating machinery or driving). Potentially significant drug interactions may exist, requiring dose or frequency adjustment, additional monitoring, and/or selection of alternative therapy. Effects may be potentiated when used with other sedative drugs or ethanol. Use with caution in patients with recent myocardial infarction, biliary tract impairment, pancreatitis, morbid obesity, thyroid dysfunction, head trauma, or increased intracranial pressure. Avoid use in patients with CNS depression or coma as these patients are susceptible to intracranial effects of CO_2 retention. Use caution in patients with prostatic hyperplasia and/or urinary stricture, adrenal insufficiency, decreased hepatic or renal function. Use with caution in patients with pre-existing respiratory compromise (hypoxia and/or hypercapnia), COPD or other obstructive pulmonary disease; critical respiratory depression may occur, even at therapeutic dosages. May cause hypotension; use with caution in patients with hypovolemia, cardiovascular disease (including acute MI), or drugs which may exaggerate hypotensive effects (including phenothiazines or general anesthetics). May obscure diagnosis or clinical course of patients with acute abdominal conditions. May result in tolerance and/or drug dependence with chronic use; use with caution in patients with a history of drug dependence. Abrupt discontinuation following prolonged use may lead to withdrawal symptoms. May precipitate withdrawal symptoms in patients following prolonged therapy with mu opioid agonists.

Use with caution in pregnancy (close neonatal monitoring required when used in labor and delivery). After chronic maternal exposure to opioids, neonatal withdrawal syndrome may occur in the newborn; monitor neonate closely. Signs and symptoms include irritability, hyperactivity and abnormal sleep pattern, high pitched cry, tremor, vomiting, diarrhea and failure to gain weight. Onset, duration and severity depend on the drug used, duration of use, maternal dose, and rate of drug elimination by the newborn. Opioid withdrawal syndrome in the neonate, unlike in adults, may be life-threatening and should be treated according to protocols developed by neonatology experts. Use with caution in the elderly and debilitated patients; may be more sensitive to adverse effects.

Adverse Reactions

Central nervous system: Dizziness, headache, sedation
Dermatologic: Cold and clammy skin
Gastrointestinal: Nausea/vomiting, xerostomia
Rare but important or life-threatening: Abdominal pain, abnormal dreams, agitation, anaphylactoid reaction, anaphylaxis, anxiety, asthma, bitter taste, blurred vision, bradycardia, burning sensation, cardiac arrest, confusion, crying, delusions, depersonalization, depression, derealization, diaphoresis, drowsiness, dyspepsia, dysphoria, euphoria, fever, floating feeling, flushing, hallucination, hostility, hypersensitivity reaction, hypertension, hypogonadism (Brennan, 2013; Debono, 2011), hypotension, injection site reaction (pain, swelling, redness, burning), intestinal cramps, laryngeal edema, loss of consciousness, nervousness, numbness, pruritus, pulmonary edema, respiratory depression, respiratory distress, restlessness, seizure, skin rash, speech disturbance, stridor, tachycardia, tingling sensation, tremor, urinary urgency, urticaria

Drug Interactions

Metabolism/Transport Effects None known.

Avoid Concomitant Use

Avoid concomitant use of Nalbuphine with any of the following: Analgesics (Opioid); Azelastine (Nasal); Eluxadoline; Mixed Agonist / Antagonist Opioids; Orphenadrine; Paraldehyde; Thalidomide

Increased Effect/Toxicity

Nalbuphine may increase the levels/effects of: Alcohol (Ethyl); Alvimopan; Azelastine (Nasal); CNS Depressants; Desmopressin; Diuretics; Eluxadoline; Methotrimeprazine; Metyrosine; Mirtazapine; Orphenadrine; Paraldehyde; Pramipexole; ROPINIRole; Rotigotine; Selective Serotonin Reuptake Inhibitors; Suvorexant; Thalidomide; Zolpidem

The levels/effects of Nalbuphine may be increased by: Amphetamines; Anticholinergic Agents; Antipsychotic Agents (Phenothiazines); Brimonidine (Topical); Cannabis; Doxylamine; Dronabinol; Droperidol; HydrOXYzine; Kava Kava; Magnesium Sulfate; Methotrimeprazine; Nabilone; Perampanel; Rufinamide; Sodium Oxybate; Succinylcholine; Tetrahydrocannabinol

Decreased Effect

Nalbuphine may decrease the levels/effects of: Analgesics (Opioid); Pegvisomant

The levels/effects of Nalbuphine may be decreased by: Ammonium Chloride; Mixed Agonist / Antagonist Opioids; Naltrexone

Storage/Stability Store at 20°C to 25°C (68°F to 77°F). Protect from light.

Mechanism of Action Agonist of kappa opiate receptors and partial antagonist of mu opiate receptors in the CNS, causing inhibition of ascending pain pathways, altering the perception of and response to pain; produces generalized CNS depression

Pharmacodynamics

Onset of action:
- IM, SubQ: Within 15 minutes
- IV: 2-3 minutes

Maximum effect:
- IM: 30 minutes
- IV: 1-3 minutes

Duration: 3-6 hours

Pharmacokinetics (Adult data unless noted)

Distribution: Crosses placenta; distributes into breast milk in small amounts (<1% of dose)
Metabolism: In the liver; extensive first-pass metabolism
Protein binding: ~50%
Half-life, terminal:
- Children 1-8 years: 0.9 hours
- Adults 23-32 years: ~2 hours; range: 3.5-5 hours
- Adults 65-90 years: 2.3 hours

Time to peak serum concentration:
- IM: 30 minutes
- IV: 1-3 minutes

Elimination: Metabolites primarily in feces (via bile) and in urine; 4% to 7% eliminated unchanged in the urine

Dosing: Usual

Children 1-14 years: Premedication: IM, IV, SubQ: 0.2 mg/kg; maximum dose: 20 mg/dose
Children: Analgesia: IM, IV, SubQ: 0.1-0.15 mg/kg every 3-6 hours as needed; maximum single-dose: 20 mg/dose; maximum daily dose: 160 mg/day
Adults:
- Analgesia: IM, IV, SubQ: 10 mg/70 kg every 3-6 hours as needed; maximum single-dose: 20 mg/dose; maximum daily dose: 160 mg/day
- Surgical anesthesia supplement: IV: Induction: 0.3-3 mg/kg administered over 10-15 minutes; maintenance doses of 0.25-0.5 mg/kg may be given as required
- Opioid-induced pruritus: IV: 2.5-5 mg; may repeat dose (Cohen, 1992)

Administration Parenteral: IV: Administer over 5-10 minutes; larger doses should be administered over 10-15 minutes

Monitoring Parameters Relief of pain, respiratory and mental status, blood pressure

Test Interactions May interfere with certain enzymatic methods used to detect opioids, depending on sensitivity and specificity of the test (refer to test manufacturer for details)

Additional Information Analgesic potency: 1 mg nalbuphine ~1 mg morphine

Dosage Forms Excipient information presented when available (limited, particularly for generics); consult specific product labeling.

Solution, Injection, as hydrochloride:

Generic: 10 mg/mL (1 mL, 10 mL); 20 mg/mL (1 mL, 10 mL)

◆ **Nalbuphine Hydrochloride** *see* Nalbuphine *on page 1483*

◆ **Nalcrom (Can)** *see* Cromolyn (Systemic, Oral Inhalation) *on page 541*

◆ **Nallpen** *see* Nafcillin *on page 1481*

◆ **Nallpen in Dextrose** *see* Nafcillin *on page 1481*

◆ ***N*-allylnoroxymorphine Hydrochloride** *see* Naloxone *on page 1485*

Naloxone (nal OKS one)

Medication Safety Issues

Sound-alike/look-alike issues:

Naloxone may be confused with Lanoxin, nalbuphine, naltrexone

Narcan may be confused with Marcaine, Norcuron

International issues:

Narcan [multiple international markets] may be confused with Marcen brand name for ketazolam [Spain]

Brand Names: US Evzio

Brand Names: Canada Naloxone Hydrochloride Injection; Naloxone Hydrochloride Injection USP

Therapeutic Category Antidote for Narcotic Agonists

Generic Availability (US) May be product dependent

Use Complete or partial reversal of opioid drug effects, including respiratory depression induced by natural and synthetic opioids; diagnosis and management of known or suspected acute opioid overdose (FDA approved in all ages); has also been used for the prevention and treatment of opioid-induced pruritus

Pregnancy Risk Factor B/C (product-specific)

Pregnancy Considerations Adverse events were not observed in animal reproduction studies. Naloxone crosses the placenta. Consider the benefit to the mother and the risk to the fetus before administering to a pregnant woman who is known or suspected to be opioid dependent; may precipitate withdrawal in both the mother and fetus. In general, medications used as antidotes should take into consideration the health and prognosis of the mother; antidotes should be administered to pregnant women if there is a clear indication for use and should not be withheld because of fears of teratogenicity (Bailey, 2003). Use caution in pregnant women with mild-to-moderate hypertension during labor; severe hypertension may occur.

Breast-Feeding Considerations It is not known if naloxone is excreted into breast milk, however, systemic absorption following oral administration is low (Smith, 2012) and any exposure of naloxone to a nursing infant would therefore be limited. Since naloxone is used for opioid reversal, the opioid concentrations in the milk of a breast-feeding mother and potential transfer of the opioid to the infant should be considered.

Contraindications Hypersensitivity to naloxone or any component of the formulation

Warnings/Precautions Use with caution in patients with cardiovascular disease or in patients receiving medications with potential adverse cardiovascular effects (eg, hypotension, pulmonary edema, or arrhythmias); pulmonary edema and cardiovascular instability, including ventricular fibrillation, have been reported in association with abrupt reversal when using opioid antagonists. Administration of naloxone causes the release of catecholamines, which may precipitate acute withdrawal or unmask pain in those who regularly take opioids. Symptoms of acute withdrawal in opioid-dependent patients may include pain, hypertension, sweating, agitation, and irritability. In neonates born to mothers with narcotic dependence, opioid withdrawal may be life-threatening and symptoms may include shrill cry, failure to feed, seizures, and hyperactive reflexes. Carefully titrate the dose to reverse hypoventilation; do not fully awaken patient or reverse analgesic effect (postoperative patient). Excessive dosages should be avoided after use of opioids in surgery. Abrupt postoperative reversal may result in nausea, vomiting, sweating, tachycardia, hypertension, seizures, and other cardiovascular events (including pulmonary edema and arrhythmias). Reversal of partial opioid agonists or mixed opioid agonist/antagonists (eg, buprenorphine, pentazocine) may be incomplete and large doses of naloxone may be required. Recurrence of respiratory depression is possible if the opioid involved is long-acting; observe patients until there is no reasonable risk of recurrent respiratory depression.

To prevent overdose deaths, there are initiatives to dispense naloxone for self- or buddy-administration to patients at risk of opioid overdose (eg, recipients of high-dose opioids, suspected or confirmed history of illicit opioid use) and individuals likely to be present in an overdose situation (eg, family members of illicit drug users) (Albert, 2011; Bennett, 2011); Evzio is indicated for emergency treatment. Needleless administration via nebulization and the intranasal route by first responders and bystanders has also been described (Doe-Simkins, 2009; Weber, 2012). Needleless administration provides an alternative route of administration in patients with venous scarring due to illicit drug use (eg, heroin). There is a low incidence of death following naloxone reversal of opioid toxicity in patients who refuse transport to a healthcare facility (Wampler, 2011). Nevertheless, patients who received naloxone in the out-of-hospital setting should seek immediate emergency medical assistance after the first dose due to the likelihood that respiratory and/or central nervous system depression will return.

When the auto-injector (Evzio) is administered to infants <1 year of age, monitor the injection site for residual needle parts and signs of infection.

Adverse Reactions Adverse reactions are related to reversing dependency and precipitating withdrawal. Withdrawal symptoms are the result of sympathetic excess. Adverse events occur secondarily to reversal (withdrawal) of opioid analgesia and sedation.

Cardiovascular: Cardiac arrest, fever, flushing, hypertension, hypotension, tachycardia, ventricular fibrillation ventricular tachycardia

Central nervous system: Agitation, coma, crying (excessive [neonates]), encephalopathy, hallucination, irritability, nervousness, restlessness, seizure (neonates), tremulousness

Gastrointestinal: Abdominal cramps, diarrhea, nausea, vomiting

Local: Injection site reaction

Neuromuscular & skeletal: Ache, hyperreflexia (neonates), paresthesia, piloerection, tremor, weakness

Respiratory: Dyspnea, hypoxia, pulmonary edema, respiratory depression, rhinorrhea, sneezing

Miscellaneous: Diaphoresis, hot flashes, shivering, yawning

Drug Interactions

Metabolism/Transport Effects None known.

Avoid Concomitant Use

Avoid concomitant use of Naloxone with any of the following: Methylnaltrexone; Naloxegol

Increased Effect/Toxicity

Naloxone may increase the levels/effects of: Naloxegol

The levels/effects of Naloxone may be increased by: Methylnaltrexone

Decreased Effect There are no known significant interactions involving a decrease in effect.

Storage/Stability

Solution, injection: Store at 20°C to 25°C (68°F to 77°F). Protect from light. Use IV infusion within 24 hours of preparation.

Solution, auto-injector (Evzio): Store at 15°C to 25°C (59°F to 77°F); excursions are permitted between 4°C and 40°C (39°F and 104°F). Store in the outer case provided.

Mechanism of Action Pure opioid antagonist that competes and displaces opioids at opioid receptor sites

Pharmacodynamics

Onset of action:

E.T., IM, SubQ: Within 2-5 minutes

Inhalation via nebulization: ~5 minutes (Mycyk, 2003)

Intranasal: ~8-13 minutes (Kelley, 2005; Robertson, 2009)

IV: Within 2 minutes

Duration: (20-60 minutes) is shorter than that of most opioids; therefore, repeated doses are usually needed

Pharmacokinetics (Adult data unless noted)

Metabolism: Primarily by glucuronidation in the liver

Half-life:

Neonates: 1.2-3 hours

Adults: 0.5-1.5 hours (mean: ~1 hour)

Elimination: In urine as metabolites

Dosing: Neonatal Note: Not recommended as part of initial resuscitative efforts in the delivery room for neonates with respiratory depression; support ventilation to improve oxygenation and heart rate (Kattwinkel, 2010):

Opioid intoxication (full reversal): (PALS Guidelines, 2010):

IV (preferred), I.O.: **Note:** May be administered IM, SubQ, or E.T., but onset of action may be delayed, especially if patient has poor perfusion; E.T. preferred if IV/I.O. route not available; doses may need to be repeated: 0.1 mg/kg/dose; repeat every 2-3 minutes if needed; may need to repeat doses every 20-60 minutes

E.T.: Optimal endotracheal dose unknown; current expert recommendations are 2-3 times the IV dose

Opioid-induced depression: IV, IM, SubQ: Manufacturer's labeling: Initial: Usual: 0.01 mg/kg/dose; **Note:** This dose is **one-tenth** of the dose used for neonatal opioid intoxication (full reversal); may repeat every 2-3 minutes as needed based on response; may need to repeat every 1-2 hours

Reversal of respiratory depression from therapeutic opioid dosing: PALS Guidelines, 2010: IV: 0.001-0.005 mg/kg/dose; titrate to effect. **Note:** AAP recommends a wider dosage range of 0.001-0.015 mg/kg/dose (Hegenbarth, 2008)

Dosing: Usual

Infants, Children, and Adolescents:

Opioid intoxication (full reversal):

PALS Guidelines, 2010:

IV (preferred), I.O.: **Note:** May be administered IM, SubQ, or E.T., but onset of action may be delayed, especially if patient has poor perfusion; E.T. preferred if IV/I.O. route not available; doses may need to be repeated.

Infants and Children ≤5 years or ≤20 kg: 0.1 mg/kg/dose; repeat every 2-3 minutes if needed; may need to repeat doses every 20-60 minutes

Children >5 years or >20 kg and Adolescents: 2 mg/dose; if no response, repeat every 2-3 minutes; may need to repeat doses every 20-60 minutes

E.T.: Optimal endotracheal dose unknown; current expert recommendations are 2-3 times the IV dose

Manufacturer's labeling: IV (preferred), IM, SubQ: Initial 0.01 mg/kg/dose; if no response, a subsequent dose of 0.1 mg/kg may be given; **Note:** If using IM or SubQ route, dose should be given in divided doses.

Continuous IV infusion: Limited data available: Infants, Children, and Adolescents: 24-40 **mcg**/kg/**hour** has been reported (Gourlay, 1983; Lewis, 1984; Tenenbein, 1984). **Note:** Doses as low as 2.5 **mcg**/kg/**hour** have been reported in adults and a dose of 160 **mcg**/kg/**hour** was reported in one neonate (Tenenbein 1984). If continuous infusion is required, calculate the initial dosage/**hour** based on the effective intermittent dose used and duration of adequate response seen (Tenebein, 1984) **or** use two-thirds (2/3) of the initial effective naloxone bolus given as the hourly infusion (Perry, 1996); titrate dose; **Note:** The infusion should be discontinued by reducing the infusion rate in decrements of 25%; closely monitor the patient (eg pulse oximetry and respiratory rate) after each adjustment and after discontinuation of the infusion for recurrence of opioid-induced respiratory depression (Perry, 1996).

Opioid overdose: 1 mg/mL injection: Intranasal administration: Adolescents ≥13 years: 2 mg (1 mg per nostril); **Note:** Onset of action is slightly delayed compared to IM or IV routes (Barton, 2005, Kelly, 2005).

Reversal of respiratory depression from therapeutic opioid dosing:

PALS Guidelines, 2010: IV: 0.001-0.005 mg/kg/dose, titrate to effect; **Note:** AAP recommends a wider dosage range of 0.001-0.015 mg/kg/dose (Hegenbarth, 2008)

Manufacturer's labeling: IV: Initial: 0.005- 0.01 mg repeat every 2-3 minutes as needed based on response

Opioid-induced pruritus: Limited data available:

Prevention: Children ≥6 years and Adolescents ≤17 years: Continuous IV infusion: 0.25 **mcg**/kg/**hour** was used in a double-blind, prospective, randomized placebo-controlled study (n=20) which showed lower incidence and severity of opioid-induced side effects (ie, pruritus, nausea) without a loss of pain control (Maxwell, 2005).

Treatment: Children ≥3 years and Adolescents: Continuous IV infusion: Initial: 2 **mcg**/kg/**hour**; if pruritus continues, may titrate by 0.5 **mcg**/kg/**hour** every few hours; dosing based on a retrospective study (n=30, age range: 3-20 years) with a reported mean (± SD) dose of 2.3 ± 0.68 **mcg**/kg/**hour**; monitor closely; doses ≥3 **mcg**/kg/**hour** may increase risk for loss of pain control and patients may require an increase in opioid dose (Vrchoticky, 2000).

Adults: **Note:** Available routes of administration include IM, IV (preferred), and SubQ routes; other available routes (off-label) include inhalation via nebulization, intranasal, and intraosseous (I.O.). Endotracheal administration is the least desirable and is supported by only anecdotal evidence (case report) (Neumar, 2010):

Opioid overdose (with standard ACLS protocols):

IV, IM, SubQ: Initial: 0.4-2 mg; may need to repeat doses every 2-3 minutes; after reversal, may need to readminister dose(s) at a later interval (ie, 20-60 minutes) depending on type/duration of opioid. If no response is observed after 10 mg, consider other causes of respiratory depression. **Note:** May be given endotracheally as 2-2.5 times the initial IV dose (ie, 0.8-5 mg) (Neumar, 2010).

Continuous IV infusion: **Note:** For use with exposures to long-acting opioids (eg, methadone), sustained release product, and symptomatic body packers after initial naloxone response. Calculate dosage/hour based on effective intermittent dose used and duration of adequate response seen (Tenenbein, 1984) **or** use two-thirds (2/3) of the initial effective naloxone bolus on an hourly basis (typically 0.25-6.25 mg/hour); one-half (1/2) of the initial bolus dose should be readministered 15 minutes after initiation of the continuous infusion to prevent a drop in naloxone levels; adjust infusion rate as needed to assure adequate ventilation and prevent withdrawal symptoms (Goldfrank, 1986).

Inhalation via nebulization: 2 mg; may repeat. Switch to IV or IM administration when possible (Weber, 2012)

Intranasal administration: 2 mg (1 mg per nostril); may repeat in 5 minutes if respiratory depression persists. **Note:** Onset of action is slightly delayed compared to IM or IV routes (Kelly, 2005; Neumar, 2010; Robertson, 2009).

Reversal of respiratory depression with therapeutic opioid doses: IV, IM, SubQ: Initial: 0.04-0.4 mg; may repeat until desired response achieved. If desired response is not observed after 0.8 mg total, consider other causes of respiratory depression. **Note:** May be given endotracheally (off-label route) as 2-2.5 times the initial IV dose (ie, 0.08-1 mg) (Neumar, 2010).

Continuous IV infusion: **Note:** For use with exposures to long-acting opioids (eg, methadone) or sustained release products. Calculate dosage/hour based on effective intermittent dose used and duration of adequate response seen (Tenenbein, 1984) or use two-thirds (2/3) of the initial effective naloxone bolus on an hourly basis (typically 0.2-0.6 mg/hour); one-half (1/2) of the initial bolus dose should be readministered 15 minutes after initiation of the continuous infusion to prevent a drop in naloxone levels; adjust infusion rate as needed to assure adequate ventilation and prevent withdrawal symptoms (Goldfrank, 1986).

Opioid-dependent patients being treated for cancer pain (NCCN guidelines, v.2.2011): IV: 0.04-0.08 mg (40-80 **mcg**) slow IV push; administer every 30-60 seconds until improvement in symptoms; if no response is observed after total naloxone dose 1 mg, consider other causes of respiratory depression

Postoperative opioid reversal: IV: 0.1-0.2 mg every 2-3 minutes until desired response (adequate ventilation and alertness without significant pain). **Note:** Repeat doses may be needed within 1-2 hour intervals depending on type, dose, and timing of the last dose of opioid administered.

Preparation for Administration

Endotracheal: Dilute to 1 to 2 mL with NS

Inhalation via nebulization: Dilute 2 mg of naloxone with 3 mL of NS (Mycyk 2003; Weber 2012)

Parenteral:

IV push: Dilute naloxone 0.4 mg (1 mL ampul) with 9 mL of NS for a total volume of 10 mL to achieve a concentration of 0.04 mg/mL (APS 2008)

IV infusion: Dilute in NS or D_5W to a final concentration of 4 **mcg**/mL (eg, naloxone 2 mg in 500 mL of fluid)

Administration

Endotracheal: Dilute with NS prior to administration; follow with a flush ≥5 mL of NS and 5 consecutive positive-pressure ventilations

Inhalation via nebulization: Adults: Dilute with NS and administer via nebulizer face mask (Mycyk 2003; Weber 2012)

Intranasal: Adolescents and Adults: Administer total dose equally divided into each nostril using a mucosal atomizer device (MAD) (Kelly 2005; Robertson 2009; Vanden Hoek 2010)

Parenteral:

IV push: Administer over 30 seconds as undiluted preparation. May also be diluted and administer slow IV push (APS 2008)

Continuous IV infusion: Administer as continuous IV infusion

IM, I.O., SubQ: May administer IM, I.O., or SubQ if unable to obtain IV access. **Note:** IM or SubQ administration in hypotensive patients or patients with peripheral vasoconstriction or hypoperfusion may result in erratic or delayed absorption.

Monitoring Parameters Respiratory rate, heart rate, blood pressure, temperature, level of consciousness, ABGs, or pulse oximetry

Additional Information For administration to neonates, it is no longer recommended to use a more dilute concentration (0.02 mg/mL) and product has been discontinued. Use of this concentration results in unacceptably high fluid volumes, especially in small neonates. The 0.4 mg/mL preservative-free preparation should be used and can be accurately dosed with appropriately sized syringes (1 mL).

To prevent overdose deaths, there are initiatives to dispense naloxone for self- or buddy-administration to patients at risk of opioid overdose (eg, recipients of high-dose opioids, suspected or confirmed history of illicit opioid use) and individuals likely to be present in an overdose situation (eg, family members of illicit drug users) (Albert, 2011; Bennett, 2011). Needleless administration via nebulization and the intranasal route by first responders and bystanders has also been described (Doe-Simkins, 2009; Weber, 2012). Needleless administration provides an alternative route of administration in patients with venous scarring due to illicit drug use (eg, heroin). There is a low incidence of death following naloxone reversal of opioid toxicity in patients who refuse transport to a healthcare facility (Wampler, 2011).

Some products contain methyl and propylparabens. Naloxone has been used to increase blood pressure in patients with septic shock; increases in blood pressure may last several hours; however, an increase in patient survival has not been demonstrated and in some studies serious adverse effects (eg, agitation, pulmonary edema, hypotension, cardiac arrhythmias, seizures) have been reported; naloxone is generally not used for septic shock, especially in patients with underlying pain or opioid tolerance; optimal dosage for this indication has not been established; one neonatal study (n=2) reported a positive blood pressure response, but one neonate developed intractable seizures and died.

Dosage Forms Excipient information presented when available (limited, particularly for generics); consult specific product labeling.

Solution, Injection, as hydrochloride:
Generic: 0.4 mg/mL (1 mL, 10 mL)

Solution, Injection, as hydrochloride [preservative free]:
Generic: 1 mg/mL (2 mL)

Solution Auto-injector, Injection, as hydrochloride:
Evzio: 0.4 mg/0.4 mL (0.4 mL)

- **Naloxone and Buprenorphine** *see* Buprenorphine and Naloxone *on page* 322
- **Naloxone Hydrochloride** *see* Naloxone *on page* 1485
- **Naloxone Hydrochloride Dihydrate and Buprenorphine Hydrochloride** *see* Buprenorphine and Naloxone *on page* 322
- **Naloxone Hydrochloride Injection (Can)** *see* Naloxone *on page* 1485
- **Naloxone Hydrochloride Injection USP (Can)** *see* Naloxone *on page* 1485
- **NAPA and NABZ** *see* Sodium Phenylacetate and Sodium Benzoate *on page* 1947

Naphazoline (Nasal) (naf AZ oh leen)

Medication Safety Issues

Other safety concerns:

Accidental ingestion: Serious adverse reactions (eg, coma, bradycardia, respiratory depression, sedation) requiring hospitalization have been reported in children ≤5 years of age who have accidentally ingested even small amounts (eg, 1-2 mL) of imidazoline-derivative (ie, tetrahydrozoline, oxymetazoline, or naphazoline) eye drops or nasal sprays. Store these products out of reach of children at all times. Contact poison control or seek medical attention if accidental ingestion occurs.

Brand Names: US Privine® [OTC] [DSC]

Therapeutic Category Decongestant, Nasal; Nasal Agent, Vasoconstrictor

Use Temporarily relieves nasal congestion associated with rhinitis, sinusitis, hay fever, or the common cold (OTC product: FDA approved in ages ≥12 years and adults). **Note:** Approved ages and uses for generic products may vary; consult labeling for specific information.

Contraindications Hypersensitivity to naphazoline or any component of the formulation

Warnings/Precautions Rebound congestion may occur with extended use. Use with caution in the presence of hypertension, diabetes, hyperthyroidism, heart disease, coronary artery disease, or benign prostatic hyperplasia.

Accidental ingestion by children of over-the-counter (OTC) imidazoline-derivative eye drops and nasal sprays may result in serious harm. Serious adverse reactions (eg, coma, bradycardia, respiratory depression, sedation) requiring hospitalization have been reported in children ≤5 years of age who had ingested even small amounts (eg, 1-2 mL). Contact a poison control center and seek emergency medical care immediately for accidental ingestion (FDA Drug Safety Communication, 2012).

When used for self-medication (OTC): Patients should notify healthcare provider if symptoms last >72 hours or if condition worsens.

Warnings: Additional Pediatric Considerations Safety and efficacy for the use of cough and cold products in pediatric patients <4 years of age is limited; the AAP warns against the use of these products for respiratory illnesses in this age group. Serious adverse effects including death have been reported. Many of these products contain multiple active ingredients, increasing the risk of accidental overdose when used with other products. The FDA notes that there are no approved OTC uses for these products in pediatric patients <2 years of age. Health care providers are reminded to ask caregivers about the use of OTC cough and cold products in order to avoid exposure to multiple medications containing the same ingredient (AAP 2012; FDA 2008).

Adverse Reactions

Local: Transient stinging, nasal mucosa irritation, dryness, rebound congestion

Respiratory: Sneezing

Drug Interactions

Metabolism/Transport Effects None known.

Avoid Concomitant Use

Avoid concomitant use of Naphazoline (Nasal) with any of the following: Ergot Derivatives; Iobenguane I 123; MAO Inhibitors

Increased Effect/Toxicity

Naphazoline (Nasal) may increase the levels/effects of: Sympathomimetics

The levels/effects of Naphazoline (Nasal) may be increased by: AtoMOXetine; Cannabinoid-Containing Products; Ergot Derivatives; Linezolid; MAO Inhibitors; Tedizolid; Tricyclic Antidepressants

Decreased Effect

Naphazoline (Nasal) may decrease the levels/effects of: FentaNYL; Iobenguane I 123

The levels/effects of Naphazoline (Nasal) may be decreased by: Alpha1-Blockers; Tricyclic Antidepressants

Storage/Stability Store at room temperature of 20°C to 25°C (68°F to 77°F); avoid excessive heat or freezing.

Mechanism of Action Stimulates alpha-adrenergic receptors in the arterioles of the conjunctiva and the nasal mucosa to produce vasoconstriction

Pharmacodynamics

Onset of action: Decongestion occurs within 10 minutes

Duration: 2 to 6 hours

Dosing: Usual

Pediatric: **Nasal congestion (decongestant):** Intranasal: Children ≥12 years and Adolescents: 0.05%: Instill 1 to 2 drops or 1 to 2 sprays every 6 hours as needed; therapy should not exceed 3 days

Adult: **Nasal congestion (decongestant):** Intranasal: 0.05%: Instill 1 to 2 drops or 1 to 2 sprays every 6 hours as needed; therapy should not exceed 3 days

Dosing adjustment in renal impairment: There are no dosage adjustments provided in manufacturer's labeling.

Dosing adjustment in hepatic impairment: There are no dosage adjustments provided in manufacturer's labeling.

Administration Spray or drop medication into one nostril while gently occluding the other; then reverse procedure

Dosage Forms Excipient information presented when available (limited, particularly for generics); consult specific product labeling. [DSC] = Discontinued product

Solution, intranasal, as hydrochloride [drops]:

Privine®: 0.05% (25 mL) [contains benzalkonium chloride] [DSC]

Solution, intranasal, as hydrochloride [spray]:

Privine®: 0.05% (20 mL) [contains benzalkonium chloride] [DSC]

Naphazoline (Ophthalmic) (naf AZ oh leen)

Medication Safety Issues

Other safety concerns:

Accidental ingestion: Serious adverse reactions (eg, coma, bradycardia, respiratory depression, sedation) requiring hospitalization have been reported in children ≤5 years of age who have accidentally ingested even small amounts (eg, 1-2 mL) of imidazoline-derivative (ie, tetrahydrozoline, oxymetazoline, or naphazoline) eye drops or nasal sprays. Store these products out of reach of children at all times. Contact poison control or seek medical attention if accidental ingestion occurs.

Brand Names: US Clear Eyes Redness Relief [OTC]; VasoClear [OTC]; VasoClear-A [OTC]

Brand Names: Canada Naphcon Forte®; Vasocon®

Therapeutic Category Adrenergic Agonist Agent, Ophthalmic; Ophthalmic Agent, Vasoconstrictor

Generic Availability (US) Yes

Use Topical ocular vasoconstrictor (to soothe, refresh, moisturize, and relieve redness due to minor eye irritation)

Pregnancy Risk Factor C

Pregnancy Considerations Animal reproduction studies have not been conducted.

Breast-Feeding Considerations It is not known if naphazoline is excreted into breast milk. The manufacturer recommends that caution be used if administering to a nursing woman.

Contraindications Hypersensitivity to naphazoline or any component of the formulation; narrow-angle glaucoma or anatomically narrow angle

Warnings/Precautions Use with caution in the presence of hypertension, diabetes, hyperthyroidism, heart disease, coronary artery disease, or local infection or injury. Avoid concurrent use with MAO inhibitors; may cause hypertensive crisis. Not recommended for use in children <6 years of age; may cause CNS depression, coma and marked reduction in body temperature, especially in infants. Products may contain benzalkonium chloride which may be absorbed by soft contact lenses.

Accidental ingestion by children of over-the-counter (OTC) imidazoline-derivative eye drops and nasal sprays may result in serious harm. Serious adverse reactions (eg, coma, bradycardia, respiratory depression, sedation) requiring hospitalization have been reported in children ≤5 years of age who had ingested even small amounts (eg, 1-2 mL). Contact a poison control center and seek emergency medical care immediately for accidental ingestion (FDA Drug Safety Communication, 2012).

Patients should notify healthcare provider if symptoms last >48 hours (>72 hours if using OTC product) or if condition worsens. Contact prescriber in case of eye pain or if changes in vision occur.

Adverse Reactions Ocular: Blurred vision, discomfort, intraocular pressure increased, irritation, lacrimation, mydriasis, punctuate keratitis, redness

Drug Interactions

Metabolism/Transport Effects None known.

Avoid Concomitant Use

Avoid concomitant use of Naphazoline (Ophthalmic) with any of the following: Ergot Derivatives; Iobenguane I 123; MAO Inhibitors

Increased Effect/Toxicity

Naphazoline (Ophthalmic) may increase the levels/effects of: Sympathomimetics

The levels/effects of Naphazoline (Ophthalmic) may be increased by: AtoMOXetine; Cannabinoid-Containing Products; Ergot Derivatives; Linezolid; MAO Inhibitors; Tedizolid; Tricyclic Antidepressants

Decreased Effect

Naphazoline (Ophthalmic) may decrease the levels/effects of: Iobenguane I 123

The levels/effects of Naphazoline (Ophthalmic) may be decreased by: Alpha1-Blockers; Tricyclic Antidepressants

Storage/Stability Store at controlled room temperature.

Mechanism of Action Stimulates alpha-adrenergic receptors in the arterioles of the conjunctiva and the nasal mucosa to produce vasoconstriction

Dosing: Usual Note: Therapy should generally not exceed 3-4 days; not recommended for use in children <6 years of age due to CNS depression (especially in infants). Children >6 years and Adults (0.01% to 0.1%): Instill 1-2 drops every 3-4 hours

Administration Instill drops into conjunctival sac of affected eye; finger pressure should be applied to lacrimal sac during and for 1-2 minutes after instillation to decrease risk of absorption and systemic reactions; avoid contact of bottle tip with skin or eye

Dosage Forms Excipient information presented when available (limited, particularly for generics); consult specific product labeling.

Solution, Ophthalmic, as hydrochloride:

Clear Eyes Redness Relief: 0.012% (6 mL) [contains benzalkonium chloride]

VasoClear: 0.02% (15 mL)

VasoClear-A: 0.02% (15 mL)

Generic: 0.1% (15 mL)

◆ **Naphazoline Hydrochloride** *see* Naphazoline (Nasal) *on page 1488*

◆ **Naphazoline Hydrochloride** *see* Naphazoline (Ophthalmic) *on page 1488*

◆ **Naphcon Forte® (Can)** *see* Naphazoline (Ophthalmic) *on page 1488*

◆ **Naprelan** *see* Naproxen *on page 1489*

◆ **Naprosyn** *see* Naproxen *on page 1489*

Naproxen (na PROKS en)

Medication Safety Issues

Sound-alike/look-alike issues:

Naproxen may be confused with Natacyn, Nebcin

Anaprox may be confused with Anaspaz, Avapro

Naprelan may be confused with Naprosyn

Naprosyn may be confused with Natacyn, Nebcin

BEERS Criteria medication:

This drug may be potentially inappropriate for use in geriatric patients (Quality of evidence - moderate; Strength of recommendation - strong).

International issues:

Flogen [Mexico] may be confused with Flovent brand name for fluticasone [U.S., Canada]

Flogen [Mexico] may be confused with Floxin brand name for flunarizine [Thailand], norfloxacin [South Africa], ofloxacin [U.S., Canada], and perfloxacin [Philippines]

Related Information

Oral Medications That Should Not Be Crushed or Altered *on page 2476*

Brand Names: US Aleve [OTC]; All Day Pain Relief [OTC]; All Day Relief [OTC]; Anaprox; Anaprox DS; EC-Naprosyn; EnovaRX-Naproxen; Equipto-Naproxen; Flanax Pain Relief [OTC]; Mediproxen [OTC]; Naprelan; Naprosyn; Naproxen Comfort Pac; Naproxen DR; Naproxen Kit

Brand Names: Canada Aleve; Anaprox; Anaprox DS; Apo-Napro-Na; Apo-Napro-Na DS; Apo-Naproxen; Apo-Naproxen EC; Apo-Naproxen SR; Ava-Naproxen EC; Maxidol; Mylan-Naproxen EC; Naprelan; Naprosyn; Naproxen EC; Naproxen Sodium DS; Naproxen-NA; Naproxen-NA DF; Pediapharm Naproxen Suspension; PMS-Naproxen; PMS-Naproxen EC; PRO-Naproxen EC; Teva-Naproxen; Teva-Naproxen EC; Teva-Naproxen Sodium; Teva-Naproxen Sodium DS; Teva-Naproxen SR

Therapeutic Category Analgesic, Non-narcotic; Anti-inflammatory Agent; Antipyretic; Nonsteroidal Anti-inflammatory Drug (NSAID), Oral

Generic Availability (US) May be product dependent

Use Management of inflammatory disease and rheumatoid disorders [including rheumatoid arthritis, juvenile idiopathic arthritis (JIA), osteoarthritis, ankylosing spondylitis]; acute gout; mild to moderate pain; primary dysmenorrhea; fever; tendonitis, bursitis. **Note:** Due to delayed absorption, the delayed-release tablets are **not** recommended for initial treatment of pain

Medication Guide Available Yes

Pregnancy Risk Factor C

Pregnancy Considerations Adverse events were not observed in the initial animal reproduction studies; therefore, the manufacturer classifies naproxen as pregnancy category C. Naproxen crosses the placenta and can be detected in fetal tissue and the serum of newborn infants following *in utero* exposure. NSAID exposure during the first trimester is not strongly associated with congenital malformations; however, cardiovascular anomalies and cleft palate have been observed following NSAID exposure in some studies. The use of a NSAID close to conception may be associated with an increased risk of miscarriage. Nonteratogenic effects have been observed following NSAID administration during the third trimester including: Myocardial degenerative changes, prenatal constriction of the ductus arteriosus, fetal tricuspid regurgitation, failure of the ductus arteriosus to close postnatally; renal dysfunction or failure, oligohydramnios; gastrointestinal bleeding or perforation, increased risk of necrotizing enterocolitis; intracranial bleeding (including intraventricular hemorrhage), platelet dysfunction with resultant bleeding; pulmonary hypertension. Because they may cause premature closure of the ductus arteriosus, use of NSAIDs late in pregnancy should be avoided (use after 31 or 32 weeks gestation is not recommended by some clinicians). The Canadian labeling contraindicates use during the third trimester of pregnancy. The chronic use of NSAIDs in women of reproductive age may be associated with infertility that is reversible upon discontinuation of the medication. A registry is available for pregnant women exposed to autoimmune medications including naproxen. For additional information contact the Organization of Teratology Information Specialists, OTIS Autoimmune Diseases Study, at (877) 311-8972.

Breast-Feeding Considerations Small amounts of naproxen are excreted into breast milk. Naproxen has been detected in the urine of a breast-feeding infant. Breast-feeding is not recommended per the U.S. manufacturer labeling and is contraindicated per the Canadian manufacturer labeling. In a study which included 20 mother-infant pairs, there were two cases of drowsiness and one case of vomiting in the breast-fed infants. Maternal naproxen dose, duration, and relationship to breast-feeding were not provided.

Contraindications

Hypersensitivity to naproxen, aspirin, other NSAIDs, or any component of the formulation; treatment of perioperative pain in the setting of coronary artery bypass graft (CABG) surgery

Canadian labeling: Additional contraindications (not in U.S. labeling): Active peptic ulcers; active GI bleeding; cerebrovascular bleeding or other bleeding disorders; active GI inflammatory disease; severe liver impairment or active liver disease; severe renal impairment (Clcr <30 mL/minute) or deteriorating renal disease; severe uncontrolled heart failure; known hyperkalemia; third trimester of pregnancy; breast-feeding; inflammatory lesions or recent bleeding of the rectum or anus (suppository only); use in patients <16 years of age (suppository only); use in patients <18 years of age (naproxen enteric coated and sustained release tablets and naproxen sodium tablets); use in children <2 years (naproxen tablets and suspension).

Warnings/Precautions [U.S. Boxed Warning]: NSAIDs are associated with an increased risk of adverse cardiovascular thrombotic events, including MI and stroke. Risk may be increased with duration of use or preexisting cardiovascular risk factors or disease. Carefully evaluate individual cardiovascular risk profiles prior to prescribing. May cause new-onset hypertension or worsening of existing hypertension. Monitor blood pressure closely with initiation and during therapy. Use caution with fluid retention. Avoid use in heart failure (ACCF/AHA [Yancy, 2013]). Use the lowest effective dose for the shortest duration of time, consistent with individual patient goals, to reduce risk of cardiovascular or GI adverse events. Alternate therapies should be considered for patients at high risk. Concurrent administration of ibuprofen, and potentially other nonselective NSAIDs, may interfere with aspirin's cardioprotective effect. **[U.S. Boxed Warning]: Use is contraindicated for treatment of perioperative pain in the setting of coronary artery bypass graft (CABG) surgery.** Risk of MI and stroke may be increased with use following CABG surgery.

[U.S. Boxed Warning]: NSAIDs may increase risk of gastrointestinal irritation, inflammation, ulceration, bleeding, and perforation. These events may occur at any time during therapy and without warning. Risk for serious events is greater in elderly patients. Use caution with a history of GI disease (bleeding or ulcers). Canadian labeling contraindicates use with active peptic ulcers, GI bleeding, or inflammatory bowel disease. Use caution with concurrent therapy with aspirin, anticoagulants and/or corticosteroids, smoking, use of alcohol, the elderly or debilitated patients. When used concomitantly with aspirin, a substantial increase in the risk of gastrointestinal complications (eg, ulcer) occurs; concomitant gastroprotective therapy (eg, proton pump inhibitors) is recommended (Bhatt, 2008).

May increase the risk of aseptic meningitis, especially in patients with systemic lupus erythematosus (SLE) and mixed connective tissue disorders. Platelet adhesion and aggregation may be decreased; may prolong bleeding time; patients with coagulation disorders or who are receiving anticoagulants should be monitored closely. Anemia may occur; patients on long-term NSAID therapy should be monitored for anemia. Rarely, NSAID use may cause severe blood dyscrasias (eg, agranulocytosis, aplastic anemia, thrombocytopenia).

NSAID use may compromise existing renal function; dose-dependent decreases in prostaglandin synthesis may result from NSAID use, reducing renal blood flow which may cause renal decompensation. NSAID use may increase the risk for hyperkalemia (Canadian labeling contraindicates use in patients with known hyperkalemia). Patients with impaired renal function, dehydration, heart failure, liver dysfunction, those taking diuretics, and ACE inhibitors, and the elderly are at greater risk of renal toxicity and hyperkalemia. Rehydrate patient before starting therapy; monitor renal function closely. Not recommended for use in patients with advanced renal disease. Canadian labeling contraindicates use in severe renal impairment (Clcr <30 mL/minute) or deteriorating renal disease. Long-term NSAID use may result in renal papillary necrosis.

NSAIDs may cause serious skin adverse events including exfoliative dermatitis, Stevens-Johnson Syndrome (SJS) and toxic epidermal necrolysis (TEN); discontinue use at first sign of skin rash or hypersensitivity. Anaphylactoid reactions may occur, even without prior exposure; patients with "aspirin triad" (bronchial asthma, aspirin intolerance, rhinitis) may be at increased risk. Do not use in patients who experience bronchospasm, asthma, rhinitis, or urticaria with NSAID or aspirin therapy. Use caution in other forms of asthma.

Use with caution in patients with decreased hepatic function. Closely monitor patients with any abnormal LFT. Severe hepatic reactions (eg, fulminant hepatitis, liver failure) have occurred with NSAID use, rarely; discontinue if signs or symptoms of liver disease develop, or if systemic manifestations occur. Canadian labeling contraindicates use in severe impairment or with active liver disease.

NSAIDS may cause drowsiness, dizziness, blurred vision and other neurologic effects which may impair physical or mental abilities; patients must be cautioned about performing tasks which require mental alertness (eg, operating machinery or driving). Discontinue use with blurred or diminished vision and perform ophthalmologic exam. Monitor vision with long-term therapy. Withhold for at least 4-6 half-lives prior to surgical or dental procedures.

Use with caution in the elderly, particularly at higher doses; unbound plasma fraction increased. Dose adjustments may be necessary; avoid chronic use (unless alternative agents ineffective and patient can receive concomitant gastroprotective agent); nonselective oral NSAID use is associated with an increased risk of GI bleeding and peptic ulcer disease in older adults in high risk category (eg, >75 years or age or receiving concomitant oral/parenteral corticosteroids, anticoagulants, or antiplatelet agents) (Beers Criteria).

OTC labeling: Prior to self-medication, patients should contact healthcare provider if they have had recurring stomach pain or upset, ulcers, bleeding problems, asthma, high blood pressure, heart or kidney disease, other serious medical problems, are currently taking a diuretic, anticoagulant, other NSAIDs, or are ≥60 years of age. Recommended dosages and duration should not be exceeded, due to an increased risk of GI bleeding, MI, and stroke. Patients should stop use and consult a healthcare provider if symptoms get worse, newly appear, or continue; if an allergic reaction occurs; if feeling faint, vomit blood or have bloody/black stools; if having difficulty swallowing or heartburn, or if fever lasts for >3 days or pain >10 days. Consuming ≥3 alcoholic beverages/day or taking longer than recommended may increase the risk of GI bleeding. Not for self-medication (OTC use) in children <12 years of age. Canadian labeling contraindicates use of certain dosage forms based on age (refer to Contraindications for specific recommendations).

Warnings: Additional Pediatric Considerations Pseudoporphyria (ie, increased skin fragility and blistering with scarring in sun-exposed skin) has been reported in naproxen-treated children with JIA (reported incidence, 12%); discontinue therapy if this occurs.

Adverse Reactions

Cardiovascular: Edema, palpitations

Central nervous system: Dizziness, drowsiness, headache, vertigo

Dermatologic: Diaphoresis, ecchymoses, pruritus, skin rash

Endocrine & metabolic: Fluid retention, increased thirst

Gastrointestinal: Abdominal pain, constipation, diarrhea, dyspepsia, flatulence, gastrointestinal hemorrhage, gastrointestinal perforation, gastrointestinal ulcer, heartburn, nausea, stomatitis, vomiting

Hematologic & oncologic: Anemia, hemolysis, prolonged bleeding time, purpura

Hepatic: Increased liver enzymes

Ophthalmic: Visual disturbance

Otic: Auditory disturbance, tinnitus

Renal: Renal function abnormality

Respiratory: Dyspnea

Rare but important or life-threatening: Abnormal dreams, agranulocytosis, alopecia, anaphylactoid reaction, anaphylaxis, angioedema, aphthous stomatitis, aseptic meningitis, asthma, blurred vision, cardiac arrhythmia, cardiac failure, cognitive dysfunction, colitis, coma, confusion, conjunctivitis, cystitis, depression, dysuria, eosinophilia, eosinophilic pneumonitis, erythema multiforme, exfoliative dermatitis, fever, glossitis, granulocytopenia, hallucination, hematemesis, hepatic failure, hepatitis, hepatotoxicity (idiosyncratic) (Chalasani, 2014), hyperglycemia, hypertension, hypoglycemia, hypotension, infection, interstitial nephritis, melena, jaundice, leukopenia, lymphadenopathy, menstrual disease, malaise, myalgia, myasthenia, myocardial infarction, oliguria, pancreatitis, pancytopenia, paresthesia, pneumonia, polyuria, proteinuria, rectal hemorrhage, renal failure, renal papillary necrosis, respiratory depression, sepsis, skin photosensitivity, Stevens-Johnson syndrome, tachycardia, seizure, syncope, thrombocytopenia, toxic epidermal necrolysis, vasculitis

Drug Interactions

Metabolism/Transport Effects Substrate of CYP1A2 (minor), CYP2C9 (minor); **Note:** Assignment of Major/Minor substrate status based on clinically relevant drug interaction potential

Avoid Concomitant Use

Avoid concomitant use of Naproxen with any of the following: Dexketoprofen; Floctafenine; Ketorolac (Nasal); Ketorolac (Systemic); Morniflumate; NSAID (COX-2 Inhibitor); Omacetaxine; Urokinase

Increased Effect/Toxicity

Naproxen may increase the levels/effects of: 5-ASA Derivatives; Agents with Antiplatelet Properties; Aliskiren; Aminoglycosides; Anticoagulants; Apixaban; Bisphosphonate Derivatives; Collagenase (Systemic); CycloSPORINE (Systemic); Dabigatran Etexilate; Deferasirox; Deoxycholic Acid; Desmopressin; Digoxin; Drospirenone; Eplerenone; Haloperidol; Ibritumomab; Lithium; Methotrexate; Nonsteroidal Anti-Inflammatory Agents; NSAID (COX-2 Inhibitor); Obinutuzumab; Omacetaxine; PEMEtrexed; Porfimer; Potassium-Sparing Diuretics; PRALAtrexate; Quinolone Antibiotics; Rivaroxaban; Salicylates; Tacrolimus (Systemic); Tenofovir; Thrombolytic Agents; Tositumomab and Iodine I 131 Tositumomab; Urokinase; Vancomycin; Verteporfin; Vitamin K Antagonists

The levels/effects of Naproxen may be increased by: ACE Inhibitors; Angiotensin II Receptor Blockers; Antidepressants (Tricyclic, Tertiary Amine); Corticosteroids (Systemic); CycloSPORINE (Systemic); Dasatinib; Dexketoprofen; Diclofenac (Systemic); Floctafenine; Glucosamine; Herbs (Anticoagulant/Antiplatelet Properties); Ibrutinib; Ketorolac (Nasal); Ketorolac (Systemic); Limaprost; Morniflumate; Multivitamins/Fluoride (with ADE); Multivitamins/Minerals (with ADEK, Folate, Iron); Multivitamins/Minerals (with AE, No Iron); Omega-3 Fatty Acids; Pentosan Polysulfate Sodium; Pentoxifylline; Probenecid; Prostacyclin Analogues; Selective Serotonin Reuptake Inhibitors; Serotonin/Norepinephrine Reuptake Inhibitors; Sodium Phosphates; Tipranavir; Treprostinil; Vitamin E

Decreased Effect

Naproxen may decrease the levels/effects of: ACE Inhibitors; Aliskiren; Angiotensin II Receptor Blockers; Beta-Blockers; Eplerenone; HydrALAZINE; Loop Diuretics; Potassium-Sparing Diuretics; Prostaglandins (Ophthalmic); Salicylates; Selective Serotonin Reuptake Inhibitors; Thiazide Diuretics

The levels/effects of Naproxen may be decreased by: Bile Acid Sequestrants; Salicylates

Food Interactions Naproxen absorption rate/levels may be decreased if taken with food. Management: Administer with food, milk, or antacids to decrease GI adverse effects.

Storage/Stability Store at 15°C to 30°C (59°F to 86°F); suspension should not be exposed to excessive heat (>40°C [104°F]).

Mechanism of Action Reversibly inhibits cyclooxygenase-1 and 2 (COX-1 and 2) enzymes, which results in decreased formation of prostaglandin precursors; has antipyretic, analgesic, and anti-inflammatory properties

Other proposed mechanisms not fully elucidated (and possibly contributing to the anti-inflammatory effect to varying degrees), include inhibiting chemotaxis, altering lymphocyte activity, inhibiting neutrophil aggregation/activation, and decreasing proinflammatory cytokine levels.

Pharmacokinetics (Adult data unless noted)

Absorption: Oral: Almost 100%

Distribution: Crosses the placenta; ~1% distributed into breast milk

V_d: Adults: 0.16 L/kg

Protein binding: >99%

Metabolism: Extensively metabolized in the liver to 6-0-desmethyl naproxen; parent drug and desmethyl metabolite undergo further metabolism to their respective acylglucuronide conjugated metabolites

Bioavailability: 95%

Half-life, elimination: Children: Range: 8-17 hours

Children 8-14 years: 8-10 hours

Adults: 12-17 hours

Time to peak serum concentration:

Tablets, naproxen: 2-4 hours

Tablets, naproxen sodium: 1-2 hours

Tablets, delayed-release (empty stomach): 4-6 hours; range 2-12 hours
Tablets, delayed-release (with food): 12 hours; range: 4-24 hours
Suspension: 1-4 hours
Elimination: 95% excreted in urine (<1% as unchanged drug; <1% as 6-0-desmethyl naproxen; 66% to 92% as their conjugates); ≤3% excreted in feces

Dosing: Usual Note: Dosage expressed as naproxen base; 200 mg naproxen base is equivalent to 220 mg naproxen sodium
Oral:
Children >2 years:
Analgesia: 5-7 mg/kg/dose every 8-12 hours
Inflammatory disease, including JIA: Usual: 10-15 mg/kg/day in 2 divided doses; range: 7-20 mg/kg/day; maximum dose: 1000 mg/day. Manufacturer's recommendation for JIA: 10 mg/kg/day in 2 divided doses
Children >12 and Adults ≤65 years: OTC labeling for pain and fever: 200 mg every 8-12 hours; if needed may take 400 mg for the initial dose; maximum dose: 600 mg/day
Adults:
Rheumatoid arthritis, osteoarthritis, and ankylosing spondylitis: 500-1000 mg/day in 2 divided doses
Acute gout: Initial: 750 mg, followed by 250 mg every 8 hours until attack subsides. **Note:** Delayed release tablet is not recommended due to delayed absorption.
Mild to moderate pain, dysmenorrhea, acute tendonitis, or bursitis: Initial: 500 mg, then 500 mg every 12 hours or 250 mg every 6-8 hours as needed; maximum dose: 1250 mg/day initially, then 1000 mg/day thereafter. **Note:** Delayed release tablet is not recommended for treatment of acute pain, due to delayed absorption.
Dosage adjustment in renal impairment: Moderate to severe and severe renal impairment (CrCl <30 mL/minute): Not recommended for use

Administration Oral: Administer with food, milk, or antacids to decrease GI adverse effects. Shake suspension well before use. Do not chew, crush, or break delayed or controlled release tablet, swallow whole. Separate administration of naproxen and antacids, sucralfate, or cholestyramine by 2 hours.

Monitoring Parameters CBC with differential, platelets, BUN, serum creatinine, liver enzymes, occult blood loss, periodic ophthalmologic exams, hemoglobin, hematocrit, blood pressure

Test Interactions Naproxen may interfere with 5-HIAA urinary assays; due to an interaction with m-dinitrobenzene, naproxen should be discontinued 72 hours before adrenal function testing if the Porter-Silber test is used. May interfere with urine detection of cannabinoids and barbiturates (false-positives).

Additional Information In a multicenter, retrospective chart review, 19 children, 4-14 years of age (mean: 9.1 ± 2.9) with rheumatic fever (but without carditis, chorea, or rashes), were treated solely with naproxen (10-20 mg/kg/day divided in 2 doses) until ESR normalized (between 4-8 weeks); fever and arthritis resolved within a median of 1 day of starting therapy; no patient had side effects, or developed carditis over the following 6 months; comparative studies with aspirin that include patients with mild carditis are needed to confirm these findings (Uziel, 2000)

Due to its effects on platelet function, naproxen should be withheld for at least 4-6 half-lives prior to surgical or dental procedures.

Dosage Forms Considerations
EnovaRX-Naproxen and Equipto-Naproxen creams are compounded from a kit. Refer to manufacturer's package insert for compounding instructions.
Naproxen Comfort Pac is a combination kit containing naproxen tablets and Duraflex Comfort Gel

Dosage Forms Excipient information presented when available (limited, particularly for generics); consult specific product labeling.
Capsule, Oral, as sodium:
Aleve: 220 mg [contains brilliant blue fcf (fd&c blue #1)]
Cream, External:
EnovaRX-Naproxen: 10% (60 g, 120 g) [contains cetyl alcohol]
Equipto-Naproxen: 10% (120 g)
Kit, Combination:
Naproxen Comfort Pac: 500 mg [contains methylparaben, trolamine (triethanolamine)]
Suspension, Oral:
Naprosyn: 125 mg/5 mL (480 mL)
Generic: 125 mg/5 mL (500 mL)
Tablet, Oral:
Naprosyn: 250 mg [scored]
Naprosyn: 375 mg
Naprosyn: 500 mg [scored]
Naproxen Kit: 500 mg [scored]
Generic: 250 mg, 375 mg, 500 mg
Tablet, Oral, as sodium:
Aleve: 220 mg [contains fd&c blue #2 aluminum lake]
All Day Pain Relief: 220 mg [contains fd&c blue #2 aluminum lake]
All Day Pain Relief: 220 mg [gluten free; contains fd&c blue #2 aluminum lake]
All Day Relief: 220 mg
All Day Relief: 220 mg [contains fd&c blue #2 aluminum lake]
Anaprox: 275 mg
Anaprox DS: 550 mg [scored]
Flanax Pain Relief: 220 mg [contains fd&c blue #2 (indigotine)]
Mediproxen: 220 mg
Generic: 220 mg, 275 mg, 550 mg
Tablet Delayed Release, Oral:
EC-Naprosyn: 375 mg, 500 mg
Naproxen DR: 375 mg, 500 mg
Tablet Extended Release 24 Hour, Oral, as sodium [strength expressed as base]:
Naprelan: 375 mg, 500 mg, 750 mg
Generic: 500 mg

- ◆ **Naproxen Comfort Pac** *see* Naproxen *on page* 1489
- ◆ **Naproxen DR** *see* Naproxen *on page* 1489
- ◆ **Naproxen EC (Can)** *see* Naproxen *on page* 1489
- ◆ **Naproxen Kit** *see* Naproxen *on page* 1489
- ◆ **Naproxen-NA (Can)** *see* Naproxen *on page* 1489
- ◆ **Naproxen-NA DF (Can)** *see* Naproxen *on page* 1489
- ◆ **Naproxen Sodium** *see* Naproxen *on page* 1489
- ◆ **Naproxen Sodium DS (Can)** *see* Naproxen *on page* 1489
- ◆ **Naramin [OTC]** *see* DiphenhydrAMINE (Systemic) *on page* 668
- ◆ **Narcan** *see* Naloxone *on page* 1485
- ◆ **Naropin** *see* Ropivacaine *on page* 1883
- ◆ **Nasacort Allergy 24HR [OTC]** *see* Triamcinolone (Nasal) *on page* 2115
- ◆ **Nasacort Allergy 24HR (Can)** *see* Triamcinolone (Nasal) *on page* 2115
- ◆ **Nasacort AQ** *see* Triamcinolone (Nasal) *on page* 2115
- ◆ **NasalCrom [OTC]** *see* Cromolyn (Nasal) *on page* 542
- ◆ **Nasal Decongestant [OTC]** *see* Phenylephrine (Systemic) *on page* 1685
- ◆ **Nasal Decongestant [OTC]** *see* Pseudoephedrine *on page* 1801
- ◆ **Nasal Decongestant PE Max St [OTC]** *see* Phenylephrine (Systemic) *on page* 1685

Nedocromil (ne doe KROE mil)

Brand Names: US Alocril
Brand Names: Canada Alocril®
Therapeutic Category Antiallergic, Ophthalmic
Generic Availability (US) No
Use Treatment of itching associated with allergic conjunctivitis (FDA approved in ages ≥3 years and adults)
Pregnancy Risk Factor B
Pregnancy Considerations There are no well-controlled studies in pregnant women. Animal studies show no evidence of teratogenicity or harm to fetus. Additionally, nedocromil has minimal systemic absorption.
Breast-Feeding Considerations It is not known if nedocromil is excreted in breast milk. The manufacturer recommends that caution be exercised when administering nedocromil to nursing women.
Contraindications Hypersensitivity to nedocromil or any component of the formulation
Warnings/Precautions Ophthalmic solution contains benzalkonium chloride, which may be absorbed by contact lenses; users of contact lenses should not wear them during periods of symptomatic allergic conjunctivitis.
Adverse Reactions
Central nervous system: Headache
Gastrointestinal: Unpleasant taste
Ocular: Burning, conjunctivitis, eye redness, irritation, photophobia, stinging
Respiratory: Asthma, nasal congestion, rhinitis
Drug Interactions
Metabolism/Transport Effects None known.
Avoid Concomitant Use There are no known interactions where it is recommended to avoid concomitant use.
Increased Effect/Toxicity There are no known significant interactions involving an increase in effect.
Decreased Effect There are no known significant interactions involving a decrease in effect.
Storage/Stability Store at 2°C to 25°C (36°F to 77°F).
Mechanism of Action Inhibits the activation of and mediator release from a variety of inflammatory cell types associated with hypersensitivity reactions including eosinophils, neutrophils, macrophages, mast cells, monocytes, and platelets; it inhibits the release of histamine, leukotrienes, and slow-reacting substance of anaphylaxis.
Pharmacokinetics (Adult data unless noted)
Absorption: Systemic: Ophthalmic: <4%
Elimination: Excreted unchanged in urine 70%; feces 30%
Dosing: Usual Ophthalmic: Children ≥3 years and Adults: 1-2 drops in each eye twice daily throughout the period of exposure to allergen
Administration Ophthalmic: Instill drops into conjunctival sac; avoid contact of bottle tip with skin or eye
Dosage Forms Excipient information presented when available (limited, particularly for generics); consult specific product labeling.
Solution, Ophthalmic, as sodium:
Alocril: 2% (5 mL) [contains benzalkonium chloride]

Nefazodone (nef AY zoe done)

Medication Safety Issues
Sound-alike/look-alike issues:
Serzone may be confused with selegiline, SEROquel, sertraline
Related Information
Antidepressant Agents *on page 2257*
Therapeutic Category Antidepressant, Serotonin Reuptake Inhibitor/Antagonist
Generic Availability (US) Yes
Use Treatment of depression (FDA approved in adults) **Note:** Due to the risk of hepatic failure, other antidepressant agents are generally tried first
Medication Guide Available Yes
Pregnancy Risk Factor C
Pregnancy Considerations Adverse effects were observed in some animal reproduction studies. When nefazodone is taken during pregnancy, an increased risk of major malformations has not been observed in the limited number of pregnancies studied (Einarson, 2003; Einarson, 2009). The long-term effects of *in utero* exposure to nefazodone on infant development and behavior are not known.

The ACOG recommends that therapy with antidepressants during pregnancy be individualized; treatment of depression during pregnancy should incorporate the clinical expertise of the mental health clinician, obstetrician, primary healthcare provider, and pediatrician. According to the American Psychiatric Association (APA), the risks of medication treatment should be weighed against other treatment options and untreated depression. Consideration should be given to using agents with safety data in pregnancy. For women who discontinue antidepressant medications during pregnancy and who may be at high risk for postpartum depression, the medications can be restarted following delivery. Treatment algorithms have been developed by the ACOG and the APA for the management of depression in women prior to conception and during pregnancy (ACOG, 2008; APA, 2010; Yonkers, 2009).

Breast-Feeding Considerations Nefazodone and its metabolites are excreted in breast milk. Drowsiness, lethargy, poor feeding, and failure to maintain body temperature have been reported in a premature nursing infant. Adverse events were not observed in two case reports of older infants (Dodd, 2000; Yapp, 2000). The long-term effects on neurobehavior have not been studied. The manufacturer recommends that caution be exercised when administering nefazodone to nursing women.

Contraindications Hypersensitivity to nefazodone, related compounds (phenylpiperazines), or any component of the formulation; liver injury due to previous nefazodone treatment, active liver disease, or elevated serum transaminases; concurrent use or use of MAO inhibitors within previous 14 days; concurrent use with carbamazepine, cisapride, or pimozide; concurrent therapy with triazolam is generally contraindicated (dosage must be reduced by 75% for triazolam; such reductions may not be possible with available dosage forms).

Warnings/Precautions [U.S. Boxed Warning]: Antidepressants increase the risk of suicidal thinking and behavior in children, adolescents, and young adults (18-24 years of age) with major depressive disorder (MDD) and other psychiatric disorders; consider risk prior to prescribing. Short-term studies did not show an increased risk in patients >24 years of age and showed a decreased risk in patients ≥65 years. Closely monitor for clinical worsening, suicidality, or unusual changes in behavior, particularly during the initial 1 to 2 months of therapy or during periods of dosage adjustments (increases or decreases); the patient's family or caregiver should be instructed to closely observe the patient and communicate condition with healthcare provider. A medication guide should be dispensed with each prescription. **Nefazodone is not FDA approved for use in children.**

The possibility of a suicide attempt is inherent in major depression and may persist until remission occurs. Use caution in high-risk patients. Worsening depression and severe abrupt suicidality that are not part of the presenting symptoms may require discontinuation or modification of drug therapy. The patient's family or caregiver should be alerted to monitor patients for the emergence of suicidality and associated behaviors (such as agitation, irritability, hostility, impulsivity, and hypomania) and call healthcare provider.

May precipitate a shift to mania or hypomania in patients with bipolar disorder. Patients presenting with depressive symptoms should be screened for bipolar disorder, including details regarding family history of suicide, bipolar disorder, and depression. Monotherapy in patients with bipolar disorder should be avoided. **Nefazodone is not FDA approved for the treatment of bipolar depression.**

[U.S. Boxed Warning]: Cases of life-threatening hepatic failure have been reported. Discontinue if clinical signs or symptoms (such as increased serum AST or ALT levels greater than 3 times the upper limit of normal) suggest liver failure. The time to liver injury in reported, severe cases ranged from 2 weeks to 6 months; not all cases had a clear prodromal onset of symptoms. **Patients who develop symptoms while on nefazodone should not be considered for re-treatment. Treatment should not ordinarily be initiated in patients with active liver disease or elevated baseline serum transaminases.** May cause CNS depression, which may impair physical or mental abilities; patients must be cautioned about performing tasks that require mental alertness (eg, operating machinery or driving). Bone fractures have been associated with antidepressant treatment. Consider the possibility of a fragility fracture if an antidepressant-treated patient presents with unexplained bone pain, point tenderness, swelling, or bruising (Rabenda, 2013; Rizzoli, 2012). Rare reports of priapism have occurred. The incidence of sexual dysfunction with nefazodone is generally lower than with SSRIs.

The risk of sedation, conduction disturbances, orthostatic hypotension, or anticholinergic effects are very low relative to other antidepressants. Use with caution in patients with a history of cardiovascular disease (including previous MI, stroke, tachycardia, or conduction abnormalities). Use with caution in patients with urinary retention, benign prostatic hyperplasia, narrow-angle glaucoma, xerostomia, visual problems, constipation, or history of bowel obstruction (due to anticholinergic effects). May cause mild pupillary dilation which in susceptible individuals can lead to an episode of narrow-angle glaucoma. Consider evaluating patients who have not had an iridectomy for narrow-angle glaucoma risk factors.

Use caution in patients with a previous seizure disorder or condition predisposing to seizures such as brain damage, alcoholism, or concurrent therapy with other drugs which lower the seizure threshold. Use with caution in patients with renal dysfunction, hepatic dysfunction, and in elderly patients. Potentially significant drug-drug interactions may exist, requiring dose or frequency adjustment, additional monitoring, and/or selection of alternative therapy.

Abrupt discontinuation or interruption of antidepressant therapy has been associated with a discontinuation syndrome. Symptoms arising may vary with antidepressant however commonly include nausea, vomiting, diarrhea, headaches, lightheadedness, dizziness, diminished appetite, sweating, chills, tremors, paresthesias, fatigue, somnolence, and sleep disturbances (eg, vivid dreams, insomnia). Greater risks for developing a discontinuation syndrome have been associated with antidepressants with shorter half-lives, longer durations of treatment, and abrupt discontinuation. For antidepressants of short or intermediate half-lives, symptoms may emerge within 2-5 days after treatment discontinuation and last 7-14 days (APA, 2010; Fava, 2006; Haddad, 2001; Shelton, 2001; Warner, 2006).

Adverse Reactions

Cardiovascular: Bradycardia, hypotension, orthostatic hypotension, peripheral edema, vasodilation

Central nervous system: Abnormal dreams, agitation, ataxia, chills, confusion, dizziness, drowsiness, headache, hypertonia, insomnia, lack of concentration, memory impairment, paresthesia, psychomotor retardation

Dermatologic: Pruritus, skin rash

Endocrine & metabolic: Decreased libido, increased thirst

Gastrointestinal: Constipation, diarrhea, dysgeusia, dyspepsia, gastroenteritis, increased appetite, nausea, vomiting, xerostomia

Genitourinary: Mastalgia, impotence, urinary frequency, urinary retention

Hematologic & oncologic: Decreased hematocrit

Infection: Infection

Neuromuscular & skeletal: Arthralgia, neck stiffness, tremor, weakness

Ophthalmic: Blurred vision, eye pain, visual disturbance, visual field defect

Otic: Tinnitus

Respiratory: Bronchitis, cough, dyspnea, flu-like symptoms, pharyngitis

Miscellaneous: Fever

Rare but important or life-threatening: Abnormal liver function tests, angioedema, angle-closure glaucoma, atrioventricular block, galactorrhea, gynecomastia, hallucination, hepatic failure, hepatic necrosis, hepatitis, hypersensitivity reaction, hyponatremia, impotence, increased serum prolactin, leukopenia, priapism, rhabdomyolysis (with lovastatin/simvastatin), seizure, serotonin syndrome, skin photosensitivity, Stevens-Johnson syndrome, thrombocytopenia

Drug Interactions

Metabolism/Transport Effects **Substrate** of CYP2D6 (major), CYP3A4 (major); **Note:** Assignment of Major/Minor substrate status based on clinically relevant drug interaction potential; **Inhibits** CYP1A2 (weak), CYP2B6 (weak), CYP2C8 (weak), CYP2D6 (weak), CYP3A4 (strong); **Induces** P-glycoprotein

Avoid Concomitant Use

Avoid concomitant use of Nefazodone with any of the following: Ado-Trastuzumab Emtansine; Alfuzosin; Amodiaquine; Apixaban; Astemizole; Avanafil; Axitinib; Barnidipine; Bosutinib; Cabozantinib; CarBAMazepine; Ceritinib; Cisapride; Conivaptan; Crizotinib; Dabigatran Etexilate; Dapoxetine; Domperidone; Dronedarone; Eplerenone; Everolimus; Fusidic Acid (Systemic); Halofantrine; Ibrutinib; Idelalisib; Irinotecan; Isavuconazonium Sulfate; Ivabradine; Lapatinib; Ledipasvir; Lercanidipine; Linezolid; Lomitapide; Lovastatin; Lurasidone; Macitentan; MAO Inhibitors; Methylene Blue; Naloxegol; Nilotinib; NiMODipine; Nisoldipine; Olaparib; Palbociclib; Pimozide; Ranolazine; Red Yeast Rice; Regorafenib; Rivaroxaban; Salmeterol; Silodosin; Simeprevir; Simvastatin; Sofosbuvir; Suvorexant; Tamsulosin; Terfenadine; Ticagrelor; Tolvaptan; Toremifene; Trabectedin; Ulipristal; Vemurafenib; VinCRIStine (Liposomal); Vorapaxar

Increased Effect/Toxicity

Nefazodone may increase the levels/effects of: Ado-Trastuzumab Emtansine; Alfuzosin; Almotriptan; Alosetron; Amodiaquine; Antipsychotic Agents; Antipsychotic Agents (Phenothiazines); Apixaban; ARIPiprazole; Astemizole; Avanafil; Axitinib; Barnidipine; Bedaquiline; Bortezomib; Bosentan; Bosutinib; Brentuximab Vedotin; Brinzolamide; Budesonide (Nasal); Budesonide (Systemic, Oral Inhalation); Budesonide (Topical); Cabazitaxel; Cabozantinib; Cannabis; CarBAMazepine; Ceritinib; Cilostazol; Cisapride; CloZAPine; Colchicine; Conivaptan; Corticosteroids (Orally Inhaled); Corticosteroids (Systemic); Crizotinib; CYP3A4 Substrates; Dapoxetine; Dasatinib; Dienogest; Digoxin; Dofetilide; Domperidone; DOXOrubicin (Conventional); Dronabinol; Dronedarone; Drospirenone; Dutasteride; Eliglustat; Eplerenone; Erlotinib; Etizolam; Everolimus; FentaNYL; Fesoterodine; Fluticasone (Nasal); Fluticasone (Oral Inhalation); GuanFACINE; Halofantrine; Hydrocodone; Ibrutinib; Iloperidone; Imatinib; Imidafenacin; Irinotecan; Isavuconazonium Sulfate; Ivabradine; Ivacaftor; Ixabepilone; Lacosamide; Lapatinib; Lercanidipine; Levobupivacaine; Levomilnacipran; Lomitapide; Lovastatin; Lumefantrine; Lurasidone; Macitentan; Maraviroc; MedroxyPROGESTERone; Methylene Blue; MethylPREDNISolone; Metoclopramide; Mifepristone; Naloxegol; Nilotinib; NiMODipine; Nisoldipine; Olaparib; Ospemifene; Oxybutynin; OxyCODONE; Palbociclib; Panobinostat; Parecoxib; Paricalcitol; PAZOPanib; Pimecrolimus; Pimozide; PONATinib; Pranlukast; PrednisoLONE (Systemic); PredniSONE; Propafenone; QUEtiapine; Ramelteon; Ranolazine; Red Yeast Rice; Regorafenib; Repaglinide; Retapamulin; Rilpivirine; Rivaroxaban; RomiDEPsin; Ruxolitinib; Salmeterol; Saxagliptin; Serotonin Modulators; Sildenafil; Silodosin; Simeprevir; Simvastatin; SORAfenib; Suvorexant; Tacrolimus (Systemic); Tacrolimus (Topical); Tadalafil; Tamsulosin; Tasimelteon; Terfenadine; Tetrahydrocannabinol; Ticagrelor; TiZANidine; Tofacitinib; Tolterodine; Tolvaptan; Toremifene; Trabectedin; Ulipristal; Vardenafil; Vemurafenib; Vilazodone; VinCRIStine (Liposomal); Vorapaxar; Zopiclone; Zuclopenthixol

The levels/effects of Nefazodone may be increased by: Abiraterone Acetate; Antiemetics (5HT3 Antagonists); Antipsychotic Agents; Antipsychotic Agents (Phenothiazines); BusPIRone; Conivaptan; CYP2D6 Inhibitors (Moderate); CYP2D6 Inhibitors (Strong); CYP3A4 Inhibitors (Moderate); CYP3A4 Inhibitors (Strong); Dapoxetine; Fusidic Acid (Systemic); Idelalisib; Linezolid; Luliconazole; MAO Inhibitors; Mifepristone; Netupitant; Panobinostat; Peginterferon Alfa-2b; Protease Inhibitors; Selective Serotonin Reuptake Inhibitors; Stiripentol; Tedizolid

Decreased Effect

Nefazodone may decrease the levels/effects of: Afatinib; Brentuximab Vedotin; Dabigatran Etexilate; DOXOrubicin (Conventional); Ifosfamide; Ledipasvir; Linagliptin; P-glycoprotein/ABCB1 Substrates; Prasugrel; Sofosbuvir; Ticagrelor; VinCRIStine (Liposomal)

The levels/effects of Nefazodone may be decreased by: Bosentan; CarBAMazepine; CYP3A4 Inducers (Moderate); CYP3A4 Inducers (Strong); Dabrafenib; Deferasirox; Mitotane; Peginterferon Alfa-2b; Siltuximab; St Johns Wort; Tocilizumab

Food Interactions Nefazodone absorption may be delayed and bioavailability may be decreased if taken with food. Management: Administering after meals may decrease lightheadedness and postural hypotension, but may also decrease absorption and therefore effectiveness.

Storage/Stability Store at 20°C to 25°C (68°F to 77°F).

Mechanism of Action Inhibits neuronal reuptake of serotonin and norepinephrine; also blocks 5-HT_2 and $alpha_1$ receptors; has no significant affinity for $alpha_2$, beta-adrenergic, 5-HT_{1A}, cholinergic, dopaminergic, or benzodiazepine receptors

Pharmacodynamics Maximum antidepressant effect: Adults: 4-6 weeks

Pharmacokinetics (Adult data unless noted)

Absorption: Oral: Rapid and complete

Distribution: Distributes into CNS; V_d: 0.22-0.87 L/kg

Protein binding: >99%

Metabolism: Hepatic, via N-dealkylation and aliphatic and aromatic hydroxylation, to three active metabolites: A triazoledione metabolite, hydroxynefazodone, and m-chlorophenylpiperazine (mCPP); other metabolites have also been identified but not tested for activity

Bioavailability: Oral: Absolute: 20% (variable); AUC increased by 25% in patients with cirrhosis of the liver

Half-life elimination: **Note:** Active metabolites persist longer in all populations.

Children: 4.1 hours

Adolescents: 3.9 hours

Adults: 2-4 hours

Time to peak serum concentration: **Note:** Prolonged in presence of food

Children and Adolescents: 0.5 -1 hour

Adults: 1 hour

Elimination: Primarily urine, as metabolites (<1% is eliminated as unchanged drug in urine); feces

Dialysis: Not likely to be of benefit

Dosing: Usual Oral: Depression:

Children and Adolescents: **Note:** Not FDA approved. Limited information is available: Based on primary outcome measures, no randomized, placebo-controlled trial has shown nefazodone to be effective for the treatment of depression in pediatric patients (Findling, 2006; Laughren, 2004; Wagner, 2005); one study showed a positive trend toward efficacy (Emslie, 2000); two open-label trials [(n=28; age range: 7-17 years) and (n=10; adolescents)] showed nefazodone improved depressive symptom severity scores in children and adolescents (Findling, 2000; Goodnick, 2000); a small case series (n=7; age range: 9-17 years) showed improvement in depression severity scores in treatment refractory children and adolescents with multiple comorbid conditions (Wilens, 1997). Because efficacy has not been established in controlled clinical trials and due to the risk of hepatotoxicity, nefazodone is seldom prescribed in children and adolescents (Dopheide, 2006). If use is indicated, some experts recommend the following doses: Initial: 50 mg twice daily (100 mg/day) for at least 7 days; then increase to 100 mg twice daily (200 mg/day) for at least 7 days; then titrate at weekly intervals using 50 mg/day increments in children and 100 mg/day increments in adolescents; usual target range: 300-400 mg/day

Adults: Initial: 200 mg/day given in 2 divided doses; titrate in 100-200 mg/day increments at ≥1 week intervals; effective dosage: 300-600 mg/day in 2 divided doses

Administration May be administered with or without food

Monitoring Parameters Blood pressure, mental status, liver enzymes, clinical signs and symptoms of liver failure (discontinue nefazodone if clinical signs or symptoms suggestive of liver failure occur or if serum AST or ALT levels increase to ≥3 times the upper limit of normal; do not reinitiate nefazodone in these patients). Monitor patient periodically for symptom resolution; monitor for worsening depression, suicidality, and associated behaviors (especially at the beginning of therapy or when doses are increased or decreased).

Dosage Forms Excipient information presented when available (limited, particularly for generics); consult specific product labeling.

Tablet, Oral, as hydrochloride:

Generic: 50 mg, 100 mg, 150 mg, 200 mg, 250 mg

◆ **Nefazodone Hydrochloride** *see* Nefazodone *on page 1493*

Nelarabine (nel AY re been)

Medication Safety Issues

Sound-alike/look-alike issues:

Nelarabine may be confused with clofarabine

High alert medication:

This medication is in a class the Institute for Safe Medication Practices (ISMP) includes among its list of drug classes which have a heightened risk of causing significant patient harm when used in error.

Related Information

Prevention of Chemotherapy-Induced Nausea and Vomiting in Children *on page 2368*

Safe Handling of Hazardous Drugs *on page 2455*

Brand Names: US Arranon

Brand Names: Canada Atriance™

Therapeutic Category Antineoplastic Agent, Antimetabolite

Generic Availability (US) No

Use Treatment of relapsed or refractory T-cell acute lymphoblastic leukemia (ALL) and T-cell lymphoblastic lymphoma [FDA approved in pediatrics (age not specified) and adults]

Pregnancy Risk Factor D

Pregnancy Considerations Teratogenic effects were observed in animal reproduction studies. May cause fetal harm if administered during pregnancy. Women of childbearing potential should be advised to use effective contraception and avoid becoming pregnant during therapy.

Breast-Feeding Considerations Due to the potential for serious adverse reactions in the nursing infant, the decision to discontinue breast-feeding or discontinue nelarabine should take into account the benefits of treatment to the mother.

Contraindications There are no contraindications listed within the manufacturer's labeling.

Warnings/Precautions Hazardous agent - use appropriate precautions for handling and disposal (NIOSH 2014 [group 1]). **[U.S. Boxed Warning]: Severe neurotoxicity, including mental status changes, severe somnolence, seizure, and peripheral neuropathy (ranging from numbness to motor weakness or paralysis), has been reported. Observe closely for signs and symptoms of neurotoxicity; discontinue if ≥ grade 2. Adverse effects associated with demyelination or similar to Guillain-Barré syndrome (ascending peripheral neuropathies) have also been reported. Neurologic toxicities may not fully return to baseline after treatment cessation.** Neurologic toxicity is dose-limiting. Risk of neurotoxicity may increase in patients with concurrent or previous intrathecal chemotherapy or history of craniospinal irradiation. Tumor lysis syndrome (TLS) may occur as a consequence of leukemia treatment. May lead to life threatening acute renal failure; adequate hydration and prophylactic allopurinol should be instituted prior to treatment to prevent hyperuricemia and TLS; monitor closely. Bone marrow suppression, including leukopenia, thrombocytopenia, anemia, neutropenia and febrile neutropenia are associated with treatment; monitor blood counts regularly. Avoid administration of live vaccines. Use caution in patients with renal impairment; ara-G clearance may be reduced with renal dysfunction. Use caution with severe hepatic impairment; risk of adverse reactions may be higher with hepatic dysfunction.

Adverse Reactions

Cardiovascular: Chest pain, edema, hypotension, peripheral edema, tachycardia

Central nervous system: Amnesia, aphasia, ataxia, attention disturbance, balance disorder, cerebral hemorrhage, coma, confusion, depressed level of consciousness, depression, dizziness, encephalopathy, fatigue, fever, headache, hemiparesis, hydrocephalus, hypoesthesia, insomnia, intracranial hemorrhage, lethargy, leukoencephalopathy, loss of consciousness, mental impairment, motor dysfunction, nerve paralysis, neuropathic pain, nerve palsy, pain, seizure, paralysis, sciatica, sensory disturbance, sensory loss, somnolence, speech disorder

Dermatologic: Petechiae

Endocrine & metabolic: Dehydration, hyper-/hypoglycemia, hypocalcemia,hypokalemia, hypomagnesemia

Gastrointestinal: Abdominal distension, abdominal pain, anorexia, constipation, diarrhea, nausea, stomatitis, taste perversion, vomiting

Hematologic: Anemia, leukopenia, neutropenia, neutropenic fever

Hepatic: Albumin decreased, AST increased, bilirubin increased, transaminases increased

Neuromuscular & skeletal: Abnormal gait, arthralgia, back pain, dysarthria, hypertonia, hyporeflexia, incoordination, limb pain, muscle weakness, myalgia, noncardiac chest pain, paresthesia, peripheral neuropathy, rigors, tremor, weakness

Ocular: Blurred vision, nystagmus

Renal: Creatinine increased

Respiratory: Cough, dyspnea, epistaxis, pleural effusion, pneumonia, sinus headache, sinusitis, wheezing

Miscellaneous: Infection

Rare but important or life-threatening: Craniospinal demyelination, neuropathy (peripheral) (similar to Guillain-Barré syndrome), opportunistic infection, pneumothorax, progressive multifocal leukoencephalopathy (PML), respiratory arrest, rhabdomyolysis, tumor lysis syndrome

Drug Interactions

Metabolism/Transport Effects None known.

Avoid Concomitant Use

Avoid concomitant use of Nelarabine with any of the following: BCG; BCG (Intravesical); CloZAPine; Dipyrone; Natalizumab; Pentostatin; Pimecrolimus; Tacrolimus (Topical); Tofacitinib; Vaccines (Live)

Increased Effect/Toxicity

Nelarabine may increase the levels/effects of: CloZAPine; Leflunomide; Natalizumab; Tofacitinib; Vaccines (Live)

The levels/effects of Nelarabine may be increased by: Denosumab; Dipyrone; Pimecrolimus; Roflumilast; Tacrolimus (Topical); Trastuzumab

Decreased Effect

Nelarabine may decrease the levels/effects of: BCG; BCG (Intravesical); Coccidioides immitis Skin Test; Sipuleucel-T; Vaccines (Inactivated); Vaccines (Live)

The levels/effects of Nelarabine may be decreased by: Echinacea; Pentostatin

Storage/Stability Store unopened vials at 25°C (77°F); excursions permitted to 15°C to 30°C (59°F to 86°F). Stable in plastic (PVC) or glass containers for up to 8 hours at room temperature.

Mechanism of Action Nelarabine, a prodrug of ara-G, is demethylated by adenosine deaminase to ara-G and then converted to ara-GTP. Ara-GTP is incorporated into the DNA of the leukemic blasts, leading to inhibition of DNA synthesis and inducing apoptosis. Ara-GTP appears to accumulate at higher levels in T-cells, which correlates to clinical response.

Pharmacokinetics (Adult data unless noted)

Distribution:

Nelarabine: V_{ss}: Pediatric patients: 213 ± 358 L/m^2; Adults: 197 ± 216 L/m^2

Ara-G: V_{ss}/F: Pediatric patients: 33 ± 9.3 L/m^2; Adults: 50 ± 24 L/m^2

Protein binding: Nelarabine and ara-G: <25%

Metabolism: Hepatic; demethylated by adenosine deaminase to form ara-G (active); also hydrolyzed to form methylguanine. Both ara-G and methylguanine metabolized to guanine. Guanine is deaminated into xanthine, which is further oxidized to form uric acid, which is then oxidized to form allantoin.

Half-life:

Pediatric patients: Nelarabine: 13 minutes; Ara-G: 2 hours

Adults: Nelarabine: 18 minutes; Ara-G: 3 hours

Time to peak serum concentration: Ara-G: 3-25 hours (of day 1)

Elimination: Urine (nelarabine 5% to 10%, ara-G 20% to 30%)

Clearance: Nelarabine clearance is ~30% higher in pediatric patients (259 ± 409 L/hour/m^2) than in adults (197 ± 189 L/hour/m^2); ara-G clearance in pediatric patients (11.3 ± 4.2 L/hour/m^2) is similar to adults (10.5 ± 4.5 L/hour/m^2)

Dosing: Usual Dosing and frequency may vary by protocol and/or treatment phase; refer to specific protocol.

Infants, Children, and Adolescents: **T-cell acute lymphoblastic leukemia (ALL), T-cell lymphoblastic lymphoma, relapsed/refractory:** IV: 650 mg/m^2/dose on days 1 through 5; repeat cycle every 21 days until transplant, disease progression, or unacceptable toxicity

Adults: **T-cell acute lymphoblastic leukemia (ALL), T-cell lymphoblastic lymphoma:** IV: 1500 mg/m^2/dose on days 1, 3, and 5; repeat cycle every 21 days until transplant, disease progression, or unacceptable toxicity. **Note:** In obese adults; utilize patient's actual body weight (full weight) for calculation of body surface area- or weight-based dosing, particularly when the intent of therapy is curative; manage regimen-related toxicities in the same manner as for nonobese patients; if a dose reduction is utilized due to toxicity, consider resumption of full weight-based dosing with subsequent cycles, especially if cause of toxicity (eg, hepatic or renal impairment) is resolved (Griggs, 2012).

Dosage adjustment for toxicity: All patients:

Neurologic toxicity ≥ grade 2: Discontinue treatment

Hematologic or other (non-neurologic) toxicity: Consider treatment delay

Dosage adjustment in renal impairment: All patients:

CrCl ≥50 mL/minute: No adjustment necessary

CrCl <50 mL/minute: There are no dosage adjustments provided in the manufacturer's labeling (although ARA-G clearance is decreased as renal function declines, data is insufficient for a dosing recommendation); monitor closely.

Dosage adjustment in hepatic impairment: All patients: There are no dosage adjustments provided in the manufacturer's labeling (has not been studied); closely monitor with severe impairment (total bilirubin >3 times ULN).

Preparation for Administration Hazardous agent; use appropriate precautions for handling and disposal (NIOSH 2014 [group 1]).

IV: No further dilution required; the appropriate dose should be added to empty plastic (PVC) bag or glass container.

Administration Hazardous agent; use appropriate precautions for handling and disposal (NIOSH 2014 [group 1]). Adequate IV hydration recommended to prevent tumor lysis syndrome; allopurinol may be used if hyperuricemia is anticipated.

IV: Transfer the appropriate nelarabine dose into an empty polyvinyl chloride (PVC) bag or glass container and administered undiluted.

Pediatric patients: Infuse over 1 hour daily for 5 consecutive days

Adults: Infuse over 2 hours on days 1, 3, and 5

Monitoring Parameters Monitor closely for neurologic toxicity (severe somnolence, seizure, peripheral neuropathy, confusion, ataxia, paresthesia, hypoesthesia, coma, or craniospinal demyelination); signs and symptoms of tumor lysis syndrome; hydration status; CBC with platelet counts, renal and liver function tests

Additional Information Contains 4.5 mg of sodium chloride per mL

Dosage Forms Excipient information presented when available (limited, particularly for generics); consult specific product labeling.

Solution, Intravenous:

Arranon: 5 mg/mL (50 mL)

Nelfinavir (nel FIN a veer)

Medication Safety Issues

Sound-alike/look-alike issues:

Nelfinavir may be confused with nevirapine

Viracept may be confused with Viramune, Viramune XR

High alert medication:

This medication is in a class the Institute for Safe Medication Practices (ISMP) includes among its list of drug classes that have a heightened risk of causing significant patient harm when used in error.

Related Information

Adult and Adolescent HIV *on page 2392*

Pediatric HIV *on page 2380*

Perinatal HIV *on page 2400*

Brand Names: US Viracept

Brand Names: Canada Viracept

Therapeutic Category Antiretroviral Agent; HIV Agents (Anti-HIV Agents); Protease Inhibitor

Generic Availability (US) No

Use Treatment of HIV infection in combination with other antiretroviral agents (FDA approved in ages ≥2 years and adults). **Note:** HIV regimens consisting of **three** antiretroviral agents are strongly recommended.

Pregnancy Risk Factor B

Pregnancy Considerations Adverse events were not observed in animal reproduction studies. Nelfinavir has a minimal to low level of transfer across the human placenta.

A modest increased risk of overall birth defects has been observed following first trimester exposure in humans according to data collected by the antiretroviral pregnancy registry. However, no pattern of defects has been detected. The DHHS Perinatal HIV Guidelines do not recommended nelfinavir for initial therapy in antiretroviral-naive pregnant women due to lower viral suppression when compared to other regimens. A dose of 1250 mg twice daily has been shown to provide adequate plasma concentrations although lower and variable levels may occur late in pregnancy. A small increased risk of preterm birth has been associated with maternal use of protease inhibitor-based combination antiretroviral (ARV) therapy during pregnancy; however, the benefits of use generally outweigh this risk and protease inhibitors (PIs) should not be withheld if otherwise recommended. Hyperglycemia, new onset of diabetes mellitus, or diabetic ketoacidosis have been reported with PIs; it is not clear if pregnancy increases this risk.

Regardless of CD4 count or HIV RNA copy number, all HIV-infected pregnant women should receive a combination antiretroviral ARV drug regimen. A combination of antepartum, intrapartum, and infant ARV prophylaxis is recommended. ARV therapy should be started as soon as possible in women with symptomatic infection. Although earlier initiation may be more effective in reducing the perinatal transmission of HIV, initiation may be delayed until after 12 weeks gestation in women who do not require immediate treatment after careful consideration of maternal conditions (eg, nausea and vomiting) and the potential risks of first trimester fetal exposure for specific agents. A scheduled cesarean delivery at 38 weeks gestation is recommended for all women with HIV RNA >1000 copies/mL or unknown concentrations near delivery in order to decrease transmission. If ARV therapy must be interrupted for <24 hours during the peripartum period, stop then restart all medications simultaneously in order to decrease the chance of developing resistance. Long-term follow-up is recommended for all infants exposed to ARV medications. In couples who want to conceive, the HIV-infected partner should attain maximum viral suppression prior to conception.

Health care providers are encouraged to enroll pregnant women exposed to antiretroviral medications in the Antiretroviral Pregnancy Registry (1-800-258-4263 or www.APRegistry.com). Health care providers caring for HIV-infected women and their infants may contact the National Perinatal HIV Hotline (888-448-8765) for clinical consultation (HHS [perinatal], 2014).

Breast-Feeding Considerations Minimal amounts of nelfinavir are excreted into breast milk and plasma concentrations in the nursing infant were undetectable. Maternal or infant antiretroviral therapy does not completely eliminate the risk of postnatal HIV transmission. In addition, multiclass-resistant virus has been detected in breast-feeding infants despite maternal therapy. Therefore, in the United States, where formula is accessible, affordable, safe, and sustainable, and the risk of infant mortality due to diarrhea and respiratory infections is low, complete avoidance of breast-feeding by HIV-infected women is recommended to decrease potential transmission of HIV (HHS [perinatal], 2014).

Contraindications Hypersensitivity to nelfinavir or any component of the formulation; concurrent therapy with alfuzosin, amiodarone, cisapride, ergot derivatives, lovastatin, midazolam (oral), pimozide, quinidine, rifampin, sildenafil (when used for pulmonary artery hypertension [eg, Revatio]), simvastatin, St John's wort, triazolam

Canadian labeling: Additional contraindications (not in U.S. labeling): Concurrent therapy with midazolam (regardless of dosage form)

Warnings/Precautions Potentially significant drug-drug interactions may exist, requiring dose or frequency adjustment, additional monitoring, and/or selection of alternative therapy.

Use caution with hepatic impairment; use not recommended with moderate-to-severe impairment. Diarrhea occurs frequently with use, particularly in children; a secretory diarrhea mediated via a calcium-dependent process may also occur; calcium carbonate administered at the same time as nelfinavir has been used to treat this adverse effect in adults without affecting plasma concentrations of nelfinavir or its major metabolite. Warn patients that redistribution of body fat can occur. New-onset diabetes mellitus, exacerbation of diabetes, and hyperglycemia have been reported in HIV-infected patients receiving protease inhibitors. Use with caution in patients with hemophilia A or B; increased bleeding during protease inhibitor therapy has been reported. Patients may develop immune reconstitution syndrome resulting in the occurrence of an inflammatory response to an indolent or residual opportunistic infection during initial HIV treatment or activation of autoimmune disorders (eg, Graves disease, polymyositis, Guillain-Barré syndrome) later in therapy; further evaluation and treatment may be required.

Warnings: Additional Pediatric Considerations Lipodystrophy was observed in 28% of children after a median of 49 months of receiving a nelfinavir-containing antiretroviral regimen (Scherpbier, 2006).

May cause diarrhea (children: 39% to 47%; adults: 14% to 20%); a secretory diarrhea mediated via a calcium-dependent process may also occur; calcium carbonate administered at the same time as nelfinavir has been used to treat this adverse effect in adults without affecting plasma concentrations of nelfinavir or its major metabolite.

Adverse Reactions

Dermatologic: Rash

Gastrointestinal: Diarrhea, flatulence, nausea

Hematologic: Lymphocytes decreased, neutrophils decreased

Rare but important or life-threatening: Abdominal pain, acute iritis, alkaline phosphatase increased, allergic reaction, amylase increased, anemia, anorexia, anxiety, arthralgia, arthritis, back pain, bilirubinemia, body fat redistribution/accumulation, cramps, creatine phosphokinase increased, dehydration, depression, dermatitis, diaphoresis, dizziness, dyspepsia, dyspnea, emotional lability, epigastric pain, eye disorder, fever, folliculitis, fungal dermatitis, gastrointestinal bleeding, GGTP increased, headache, hepatitis, hyperkinesia, hyper-/hypoglycemia, hyperlipemia; hypersensitivity reaction (bronchospasm, rash, edema); hyperuricemia, immune reconstitution syndrome, insomnia, jaundice, kidney calculus, lactic dehydrogenase increased, leukopenia, lipoatrophy, lipodystrophy, liver function tests abnormal, maculopapular rash, malaise, metabolic acidosis, migraine, mouth ulceration, myalgia, myasthenia, myopathy, pain, pancreatitis, paresthesia, pharyngitis, pruritus, QTc prolongation, rhinitis, seizure, sexual dysfunction, sinusitis, sleep disorder, somnolence, suicidal ideation, thrombocytopenia, torsade de pointes, transaminases increased, urine abnormality, urticaria, vomiting, weakness

Drug Interactions

Metabolism/Transport Effects Substrate of CYP2C19 (major), CYP2C9 (minor), CYP2D6 (minor), CYP3A4 (major), P-glycoprotein; **Note:** Assignment of Major/Minor substrate status based on clinically relevant drug interaction potential; **Inhibits** CYP1A2 (weak), CYP2B6 (weak), CYP2C19 (weak), CYP2C9 (weak), CYP2D6 (weak), CYP3A4 (strong), P-glycoprotein

Avoid Concomitant Use

Avoid concomitant use of Nelfinavir with any of the following: Ado-Trastuzumab Emtansine; Alfuzosin; Amiodarone; Apixaban; Astemizole; Avanafil; Axitinib; Barnidipine; Bosutinib; Cabozantinib; Ceritinib; Cisapride; Conivaptan; Crizotinib; Dapoxetine; Domperidone; Dronedarone; Eplerenone; Ergot Derivatives; Everolimus; Halofantrine; Ibrutinib; Irinotecan; Isavuconazonium Sulfate; Ivabradine; Lapatinib; Lercanidipine; Lomitapide; Lovastatin; Lurasidone; Macitentan; Midazolam; Naloxegol; Nilotinib; NiMODipine; Nisoldipine; Olaparib; Palbociclib; Pimozide; Proton Pump Inhibitors; QuiNIDine; Ranolazine; Red Yeast Rice; Regorafenib; Rifampin; Rivaroxaban; Salmeterol; Silodosin; Simeprevir; Simvastatin; St Johns Wort; Suvorexant; Tamsulosin; Terfenadine; Ticagrelor; Tipranavir; Tolvaptan; Toremifene; Trabectedin; Triazolam; Ulipristal; Vemurafenib; VinCRIStine (Liposomal); Vorapaxar

Increased Effect/Toxicity

Nelfinavir may increase the levels/effects of: Ado-Trastuzumab Emtansine; Alfuzosin; Almotriptan; Alosetron; ALPRAZolam; Amiodarone; Apixaban; ARIPiprazole; Astemizole; AtorvaSTATin; Avanafil; Axitinib; Azithromycin (Systemic); Barnidipine; Bedaquiline; Bortezomib; Bosentan; Bosutinib; Brentuximab Vedotin; Brinzolamide; Budesonide (Nasal); Budesonide (Systemic, Oral Inhalation); Budesonide (Topical); Cabazitaxel; Cabozantinib; Calcium Channel Blockers (Dihydropyridine); Calcium Channel Blockers (Nondihydropyridine); Cannabis; CarBAMazepine; Ceritinib; Cilostazol; Cisapride; Clarithromycin; Colchicine; Conivaptan; Corticosteroids (Orally Inhaled); Corticosteroids (Systemic); Crizotinib; Cyclophosphamide; CycloSPORINE (Systemic); CYP3A4 Substrates; Dapoxetine; Dasatinib; Digoxin; Domperidone; DOXOrubicin (Conventional); Dronabinol; Dronedarone; Dutasteride; Eliglustat; Enfuvirtide; Eplerenone; Ergot Derivatives; Erlotinib; Etizolam; Everolimus; FentaNYL; Fesoterodine; Fluticasone (Nasal); Fluticasone (Oral Inhalation); GuanFACINE; Halofantrine; Highest Risk QTc-Prolonging Agents; Hydrocodone; Ibrutinib; Idelalisib; Iloperidone; Imatinib; Imidafenacin; Irinotecan; Isavuconazonium Sulfate; Ivabradine; Ivacaftor; Ixabepilone; Lacosamide; Lapatinib; Lercanidipine; Levobupivacaine; Levomilnacipran; Lomitapide; Lovastatin; Lurasidone; Macitentan; Maraviroc; Meperidine; MethylPREDNISolone; Midazolam; Mifepristone; Moderate Risk QTc-Prolonging Agents; Naloxegol; Nefazodone; Nilotinib; NiMODipine; Nintedanib; Nisoldipine; Olaparib; Ospemifene; Oxybutynin; OxyCODONE; Palbociclib; Panobinostat; Parecoxib; Paricalcitol; PAZOPanib; Pimecrolimus; Pimozide; PONATinib; Pranlukast; PrednisoLONE (Systemic); PredniSONE; Propafenone; Protease Inhibitors; QUEtiapine; QuiNIDine; Ramelteon; Ranolazine; Red Yeast Rice; Regorafenib; Repaglinide; Retapamulin; Rifabutin; Rilpivirine; Riociguat; Rivaroxaban; RomiDEPsin; Rosuvastatin; Ruxolitinib; Salmeterol; Saxagliptin; Sildenafil; Silodosin; Simeprevir; Simvastatin; Sirolimus; SORAfenib; Suvorexant; Tacrolimus (Systemic); Tacrolimus (Topical); Tadalafil; Tamsulosin; Tasimelteon; Temsirolimus; Terfenadine; Tetrahydrocannabinol; Ticagrelor; TiZANidine; Tofacitinib; Tolterodine; Tolvaptan; Toremifene; Trabectedin; TraMADol; TraZODone; Triazolam; Tricyclic Antidepressants; Ulipristal; Vardenafil; Vemurafenib; Vilazodone; VinCRIStine (Liposomal); Vorapaxar; Warfarin; Zopiclone; Zuclopenthixol

The levels/effects of Nelfinavir may be increased by: Clarithromycin; CycloSPORINE (Systemic); Delavirdine; Enfuvirtide; Etravirine; Lopinavir; Mifepristone; P-glycoprotein/ABCB1 Inhibitors; Simeprevir; Voriconazole

Decreased Effect

Nelfinavir may decrease the levels/effects of: Abacavir; Antidiabetic Agents; Boceprevir; Clarithromycin; Contraceptives (Estrogens); Contraceptives (Progestins); Delavirdine; Etravirine; Fosphenytoin; Ifosfamide; Lopinavir; Meperidine; Methadone; Phenytoin; Prasugrel; Pravastatin; Ticagrelor; Valproic Acid and Derivatives; Warfarin; Zidovudine

The levels/effects of Nelfinavir may be decreased by: Boceprevir; Bosentan; CarBAMazepine; CYP3A4 Inducers (Moderate); CYP3A4 Inducers (Strong); Dabrafenib; Deferasirox; Fosphenytoin; Garlic; H2-Antagonists; Mitotane; Nevirapine; Phenytoin; Proton Pump Inhibitors; Rifabutin; Rifampin; Siltuximab; St Johns Wort; Tipranavir; Tocilizumab

Food Interactions Nelfinavir taken with food increases plasma concentration time curve (AUC) by two- to threefold. Management: Administer with a meal. Do not administer with acidic food or juice (orange juice, apple juice, or applesauce) since the combination may have a bitter taste.

Storage/Stability Store at room temperature of 15°C to 30°C (59°F to 86°F).

Mechanism of Action Binds to the site of HIV-1 protease activity and inhibits cleavage of viral Gag-Pol polyprotein precursors into individual functional proteins required for infectious HIV. This results in the formation of immature, noninfectious viral particles.

Pharmacokinetics (Adult data unless noted)

Absorption: AUC is two- to threefold higher under fed conditions versus fasting; AUC is highly variable in pediatric patients due to increased clearance, problems with compliance, and inconsistent food intake with dosing

Distribution: V_d: 2 to 7 L/kg

Protein binding: >98%

Metabolism: Hepatic via multiple cytochrome P450 isoforms including CYP3A4 and CYP2C19; one active oxidative metabolite with comparable activity to the parent drug and several minor oxidative metabolites are formed

Bioavailability: 20% to 80%; **Note:** The 625 mg and 250 mg tablet formulations were shown to be bioequivalent in HIV-infected patients receiving multiple doses of 1250 mg twice daily (under fed conditions). In healthy volunteers, the 250 mg and 625 mg tablets were **not** bioequivalent; the AUC for the 625 mg tablets was 34% higher than the 250 mg tablets in fasted adults and 24% higher than the 250 mg tablets under fed conditions.

Half-life: 3.5 to 5 hours

Time to peak serum concentration: 2 to 4 hours

Elimination: 98% to 99% excreted in feces (78% as metabolites and 22% as unchanged nelfinavir); 1% to 2% excreted in urine (primarily as unchanged drug)

Dosing: Neonatal HIV infection, treatment: Not approved for use; a reliable, effective dose has not been established; a high interpatient variability in serum drug concentrations occurs; nelfinavir dosing is problematic in neonates, since the drug is best absorbed when taken with a high-fat meal (DHHS [pediatric] 2014; Hirt 2006).

Dosing: Usual

Pediatric: **HIV infection, treatment:** Use in combination with other antiretroviral agents: Oral:

Infants and Children <2 years: Not approved for use; a reliable, effective dose has not been established; high interpatient variability in serum drug concentrations occurs; nelfinavir dosing is problematic in young infants, since the drug is best absorbed when taken with a high-fat meal (DHHS [pediatric] 2014; Hirt 2006).

Children ≥2 years: **Note:** Pediatric guidelines recommend twice daily dosing (DHHS [pediatric], 2014).

Weight-directed dosing: Oral tablets (250 mg): 45 to 55 mg/kg/dose (maximum: 1250 mg) twice daily **or** 25 to 35 mg/kg/dose (maximum: 750 mg) 3 times daily; daily doses >2500 mg/day have not been studied in children. **Note:** Current guidelines rate nelfinavir as an acceptable protease inhibitor for initial therapy in children ≥2 years only in special circumstances (ie, when preferred and alternative drugs are not available or are not tolerated); due to the high variability of nelfinavir plasma concentrations in children, dosage adjustment utilizing measurement of plasma concentrations and pharmacokinetics may be beneficial (Crommentuyn 2006; DHHS [pediatric] 2014; Fletcher 2008).

Fixed dosing: Oral tablets (250 mg):

- 10 to 12 kg: 500 mg (2 tablets) twice daily **or** 250 mg (1 tablet) three times daily
- 13 to 18 kg: 750 mg (3 tablets) twice daily **or** 500 mg (2 tablets) three times daily
- 19 to 20 kg: 1000 mg (4 tablets) twice daily **or** 500 mg (2 tablets) three times daily
- >20 kg: 1000 to 1250 mg (4 to 5 tablets) twice daily **or** 750 mg (3 tablets) three times daily

Adolescents: 1250 mg/dose twice daily **or** 750 mg three times daily (DHHS [adult, pediatric], 2014). **Note:** Some adolescent patients require doses higher than adults to achieve similar nelfinavir AUCs; consider the use of serum drug concentrations to guide optimal dosing (DHHS [pediatric] 2014).

Adult: **HIV infection, treatment:** Use in combination with other antiretroviral agents: Oral: 1250 mg/dose twice daily **or** 750 mg three times daily. **Note:** The DHHS Perinatal HIV Guidelines do not recommend the three times daily dosing in pregnant women (DHHS [perinatal] 2014).

Dosing adjustment in renal impairment: No adjustment necessary (DHHS [adult] 2014); has not been studied; however, since <2% of the drug is eliminated in the urine, renal impairment should have minimal effect on nelfinavir elimination

Dosing adjustment in hepatic impairment:

Mild hepatic impairment (Child-Pugh Class A): Use with caution; no dosage adjustment is necessary. In adults, nelfinavir AUC and C_{max} were not significantly different compared to subjects with normal hepatic function.

Moderate hepatic impairment (Child-Pugh Class B): Not recommended for use. In adults, nelfinavir AUC was increased by 62% and C_{max} was increased by 22% compared to subjects with normal hepatic function.

Severe hepatic impairment (Child-Pugh Class C): Use not recommended; has not been studied

Administration Administer with food to enhance bioavailability and decrease kinetic variability. Tablets can be readily dissolved in water and consumed or mixed with milk or chocolate milk; consume immediately; rinse glass with water and swallow to make sure total dose is consumed; tablets can also be crushed and administered with pudding. If coadministered with didanosine, nelfinavir should be administered 2 hours before or 1 hour after didanosine.

Monitoring Parameters Note: Monitor CD4 percentage (if <5 years of age) or CD4 count (if ≥5 years of age) at least every 3 to 4 months (DHHS [pediatric], 2014).

Prior to initiation of therapy: Genotypic resistance testing, CD4 and viral load (every 3 to 4 months), CBC with differential, LFTs, BUN, creatinine, electrolytes, glucose, urinalysis (every 6 to 12 months), and assessment of readiness for adherence with medication regimen. At initiation and with any change in treatment regimen: CBC with differential, electrolytes, calcium, phosphate, glucose, LFTs, bilirubin, urinalysis (at initiation), BUN, creatinine, albumin, total protein, lipid panel (at initiation), CD4, and viral load. After 1 to 2 weeks of therapy: Signs of medication toxicity and adherence. After 2 to 4 weeks of therapy: CBC with differential, viral load, signs of medication toxicity, and adherence; then every 3 to 4 months: CBC with differential, electrolytes, glucose, LFTs, bilirubin, BUN, creatinine, CD4, viral load, signs of medication toxicity, and adherence. Every 6 to 12 months: Lipid panel and urinalysis. CD4 monitoring frequency may be decreased to every 6 to 12 months in children who are adherent to therapy if the value is well above the threshold for opportunistic infections, viral suppression is sustained, and the clinical status is stable for more than 2 to 3 years (DHHS [pediatric], 2014). Monitor for growth and development, signs of HIV-specific physical conditions, HIV disease progression, opportunistic infections.

Reference Range Plasma trough concentration: ≥800 ng/mL mL (measurable active (M8) metatbolite) (DHHS [adult, pediatric], 2014)

Dosage Forms Excipient information presented when available (limited, particularly for generics); consult specific product labeling.

Tablet, Oral:

Viracept: 250 mg, 625 mg

◆ **Nembutal** *see* PENTobarbital *on page 1666*

◆ **Nembutal Sodium (Can)** *see* PENTobarbital *on page 1666*

◆ **Neo-Fradin [DSC]** *see* Neomycin *on page 1500*

◆ **Neofrin [DSC]** *see* Phenylephrine (Ophthalmic) *on page 1689*

Neomycin (nee oh MYE sin)

Brand Names: US Neo-Fradin [DSC]

Therapeutic Category Ammonium Detoxicant; Antibiotic, Aminoglycoside; Antibiotic, Topical; Hyperammonemia Agent

Generic Availability (US) Yes

Use Adjunct therapy (with erythromycin) for the suppression of normal bacterial flora of the bowel (eg, preoperative preparation); adjunct therapy for hepatic coma (portal-systemic encephalopathy) by reducing ammonia-forming bacteria in the intestinal tract (All indications: FDA approved in ages ≥18 years and adults)

Pregnancy Risk Factor D

Pregnancy Considerations Aminoglycosides cross the placenta; however, neomycin has limited maternal absorption. Therefore the portion of an orally administered maternal dose available to cross the placenta is very low. Teratogenic effects have not been observed following maternal use of neomycin; however, there are several reports of total irreversible bilateral congenital deafness in children whose mothers received another aminoglycoside (streptomycin) during pregnancy.

Breast-Feeding Considerations It is not known if neomycin is excreted into breast milk; however, limited oral absorption by both the mother and infant would minimize exposure to the nursing infant. Due to the potential for serious adverse reactions in the nursing infant, the manufacturer recommends a decision be made whether to discontinue nursing or to discontinue the drug, taking into account the importance of treatment to the mother.

Contraindications Hypersensitivity to the neomycin or any component of the formulation; intestinal obstruction; patients with inflammatory or ulcerative GI disease. Patients with a history of hypersensitivity or serious toxic reaction to other aminoglycosides may have a cross-sensitivity to neomycin.

Warnings/Precautions [US Boxed Warning]: May cause neurotoxicity, nephrotoxicity, and/or neuromuscular blockade and respiratory paralysis; usual risk factors include pre-existing renal impairment, concomitant neuro-/nephrotoxic medications, advanced age and dehydration. The drug's neurotoxicity symptoms also include numbness, skin tingling, muscle twitching and seizures; can result in respiratory paralysis from neuromuscular blockade, especially when the drug is given soon after anesthesia or muscle relaxants. Use with caution in patients with renal impairment, preexisting hearing impairment, neuromuscular disorders; neomycin is more toxic than other aminoglycosides when given parenterally; **do not administer parenterally; do not use as surgical irrigation** due to significant systemic absorption of the drug. Prolonged use may result in fungal or bacterial superinfection, including *C. difficile*-associated diarrhea (CDAD) and pseudomembranous colitis; CDAD has been observed >2 months postantibiotic treatment. Small amounts of neomycin are absorbed through intact intestinal mucosa; increases in fecal bile acid excretion and reduction of intestinal lactase activity may occur. Oral doses of >12 g/day produce malabsorption of fats, nitrogen, cholesterol, carotene, glucose, xylose, lactose, sodium, calcium, cyanocobalamin and iron. Potentially significant interactions may exist, requiring dose or frequency adjustment, additional monitoring, and/or selection of alternative therapy.

Benzyl alcohol and derivatives: Some dosage forms may contain sodium benzoate/benzoic acid; benzoic acid (benzoate) is a metabolite of benzyl alcohol; large amounts of benzyl alcohol (≥99 mg/kg/day) have been associated with a potentially fatal toxicity ("gasping syndrome") in neonates; the "gasping syndrome" consists of metabolic acidosis, respiratory distress, gasping respirations, CNS dysfunction (including convulsions, intracranial hemorrhage), hypotension, and cardiovascular collapse (AAP, 1997; CDC, 1982); some data suggests that benzoate displaces bilirubin from protein binding sites (Ahlfors, 2001); avoid or use dosage forms containing benzyl alcohol derivative with caution in neonates. See manufacturer's labeling.

Adverse Reactions

Gastrointestinal: Diarrhea, irritation or soreness of the mouth or rectal area, nausea, vomiting

Rare but important or life-threatening: Dyspnea, eosinophilia, nephrotoxicity, neurotoxicity, ototoxicity (auditory), ototoxicity (vestibular)

Drug Interactions

Metabolism/Transport Effects None known.

Avoid Concomitant Use

Avoid concomitant use of Neomycin with any of the following: Bacitracin (Systemic); BCG; BCG (Intravesical); Foscarnet; Mannitol; Mecamylamine

Increased Effect/Toxicity

Neomycin may increase the levels/effects of: AbobotulinumtoxinA; Acarbose; Bacitracin (Systemic); Bisphosphonate Derivatives; CARBOplatin; Colistimethate; CycloSPORINE (Systemic); Mecamylamine; Neuromuscular-Blocking Agents; OnabotulinumtoxinA; RimabotulinumtoxinB; Tenofovir; Vitamin K Antagonists

The levels/effects of Neomycin may be increased by: Amphotericin B; Capreomycin; Cephalosporins (2nd Generation); Cephalosporins (3rd Generation); Cephalosporins (4th Generation); CISplatin; Foscarnet; Loop Diuretics; Mannitol; Nonsteroidal Anti-Inflammatory Agents; Tenofovir; Vancomycin

Decreased Effect

Neomycin may decrease the levels/effects of: BCG; BCG (Intravesical); BCG Vaccine (Immunization); Cardiac Glycosides; Sodium Picosulfate; SORAfenib

The levels/effects of Neomycin may be decreased by: Penicillins

Storage/Stability Store at 20° to 25°C (68°F to 77°F).

Mechanism of Action Interferes with bacterial protein synthesis by binding to 30S ribosomal subunits

Pharmacodynamics

Neomycin is bacteriocidal:

Onset of action: Bacterial growth suppression: Rapid

Duration of action: Bacterial growth suppression: 48-72 hours

Pharmacokinetics (Adult data unless noted)

Absorption: Poor orally (3%) or percutaneously; readily absorbed through denuded or abraded skin and body cavities

Distribution: V_d: 0.36 L/kg

Protein binding: 0% to 30%

Half-life: 2-3 hours (age and renal function dependent)

Time to peak serum concentration: 1-4 hours

Elimination: In urine (30% to 50% of absorbed drug as unchanged drug); 97% of an oral dose eliminated unchanged in feces

Dosing: Neonatal Note: Dosage expressed in terms of **neomycin sulfate**.

Diarrhea: Oral: 50-100 mg/kg/day divided every 6 hours (Marks, 1973; *Red Book*, 2009)

Dosing: Usual Note: Dosage expressed in terms of **neomycin sulfate**.

Infants, Children, and Adolescents:

Cholangitis, prophylaxis recurrent episodes after Kasai Portoenterostomy: Limited data available: Infants and Children ≤3 years: Oral: 25-50 mg/kg/day in 4 divided doses 4 days per week; continue until 2-3 years of age. Dosing based on a prospective, randomized, comparative trial and a small case series of patients ≤2 years of age at time of therapy initiation who had an episode of cholangitis after a Kasai Portoenterostomy (n=10). In the trial, two prophylactic regimens were compared (neomycin vs trimethoprim/sulfamethoxazole) against historic controls; the mean age at time of therapy initiation was 6.1 ± 3.6 months; both neomycin and trimethoprim/sulfamethoxazole decreased cholangitis incidence by ~60% and neomycin increased survival. In the case series, dosing was started at 25 mg/kg/day or 50 mg/kg/day for 5 days just prior to discharge then given 4 days per week (4 days on, 3 days off) (Bu, 2003; Mones, 1994).

Enteric infections: Oral: 50-100 mg/kg/day divided every 6-8 hours; maximum dose: 1000 mg (Bradley, 2012; *Red Book*, 2012); duration of treatment should not exceed 3 weeks due to GI absorption which may result in systemic toxicities

Hepatic encephlopathy: Limited data available: Oral: 50-100 mg/kg/day divided every 6 hours for a maximum of 7 days with or without lactulose (Debray, 2006; Lovejoy, 1975); some centers have used 2.5-7 g/m^2/day divided every 4-6 hours for 5-6 days; maximum daily dose: 12 **g**/day

Preoperative intestinal antisepsis: Children and Adolescents: Oral: 15 mg/kg/dose for 3 doses administered over 10 hours (eg, at 1 PM, 2 PM, and 11 PM) the day before surgery; maximum dose: 1000 mg (Bratzler, 2013); some centers have used 90 mg/kg/day divided every 4 hours for 2-3 days; or 25 mg/kg at 1 PM, 2 PM, and 11 PM on the afternoon and evening preceding surgery; maximum dose: 1000 mg; used as an adjunct to mechanical cleansing of the intestine and in combination with erythromycin base

Adults:

Chronic hepatic insufficiency: Oral: 4000 mg/day for an indefinite period

Hepatic encephalopathy: Oral: 500-2000 mg every 6-8 hours or 4-12 g/day divided every 4-6 hours for 5-6 days

Preoperative intestinal antisepsis: Oral: 1000 mg each hour for 4 doses then 1000 mg every 4 hours for 5 doses; or 1000 mg at 1 PM, 2 PM, and 11 PM with oral erythromycin on day preceding surgery as an adjunct to ▶

mechanical cleansing of the bowel; or 6 **g**/day divided every 4 hours for 2-3 days

Dosage adjustment in renal impairment: Dialyzable; there are no specific dosing adjustments provided in the manufacuturer's labeling; however, renal impairment increases the risk for toxicity and consideration should be given to reducing the dose or discontinuing therapy.

Dosage adjustment in hepatic impairment: There are no dosing adjustments provided in the manufacturer's labeling.

Monitoring Parameters Renal function tests (serum creatinine, BUN, creatinine clearance); urinalysis for increased excretion of protein, decreased specific gravity, casts and cells; serial vestibular and audiometric tests

Reference Range Toxic serum concentrations: ≥1.5 mcg/mL (Marks, 1973)

Additional Information Each 500 mg neomycin sulfate tablet contains 350 mg of neomycin base.

Dosage Forms Excipient information presented when available (limited, particularly for generics); consult specific product labeling. [DSC] = Discontinued product

Solution, Oral, as sulfate:

Neo-Fradin: 25 mg/mL (480 mL [DSC]) [cherry flavor]

Tablet, Oral, as sulfate:

Generic: 500 mg

Neomycin and Polymyxin B

(nee oh MYE sin & pol i MIKS in bee)

Brand Names: US Neosporin® G.U. Irrigant

Brand Names: Canada Neosporin® Irrigating Solution

Therapeutic Category Antibiotic, Topical; Antibiotic, Urinary Irrigation; Genitourinary Irrigant

Generic Availability (US) Yes

Use Short-term use as a continuous irrigant or rinse in the urinary bladder to prevent bacteriuria and gram-negative rod septicemia associated with the use of indwelling catheters

Pregnancy Risk Factor D

Pregnancy Considerations Animal reproduction studies have not been conducted with this combination; however, there are reports of total irreversible bilateral congenital deafness in children whose mothers received streptomycin during pregnancy. See individual agents.

Breast-Feeding Considerations It is not known if neomycin or polymyxin B are excreted into breast milk. See individual agents.

Contraindications Hypersensitivity to neomycin, polymyxin B, or any component of the formulation; pregnancy (GU irrigant)

Adverse Reactions

Dermatologic: Contact dermatitis, erythema, rash, urticaria

Genitourinary: Bladder irritation

Local: Burning

Neuromuscular & skeletal: Neuromuscular blockade

Otic: Ototoxicity

Renal: Nephrotoxicity

Drug Interactions

Metabolism/Transport Effects None known.

Avoid Concomitant Use

Avoid concomitant use of Neomycin and Polymyxin B with any of the following: Bacitracin (Systemic); BCG; BCG (Intravesical); Foscarnet; Mannitol; Mecamylamine

Increased Effect/Toxicity

Neomycin and Polymyxin B may increase the levels/effects of: AbobotulinumtoxinA; Acarbose; Bacitracin (Systemic); Bisphosphonate Derivatives; CARBOplatin; Colistimethate; CycloSPORINE (Systemic); Mecamylamine; Neuromuscular-Blocking Agents; OnabotulinumtoxinA; RimabotulinumtoxinB; Tenofovir; Vitamin K Antagonists

The levels/effects of Neomycin and Polymyxin B may be increased by: Amphotericin B; Capreomycin; Cephalosporins (2nd Generation); Cephalosporins (3rd Generation); Cephalosporins (4th Generation); CISplatin; Foscarnet; Loop Diuretics; Mannitol; Nonsteroidal Anti-Inflammatory Agents; Tenofovir; Vancomycin

Decreased Effect

Neomycin and Polymyxin B may decrease the levels/effects of: BCG; BCG (Intravesical); BCG Vaccine (Immunization); Cardiac Glycosides; Sodium Picosulfate; SORAfenib

The levels/effects of Neomycin and Polymyxin B may be decreased by: Penicillins

Storage/Stability Store irrigation solution in refrigerator. The following stability information has also been reported: May be stored at room temperature for up to 6 months if undiluted (Cohen, 2007). Aseptically prepared dilutions (1 mL/1 L) should be stored in the refrigerator and discarded after 48 hours.

Mechanism of Action See individual agents.

Pharmacokinetics (Adult data unless noted) Absorption: Not absorbed following topical application to intact skin; absorbed through denuded or abraded skin, peritoneum, wounds, or ulcers

Dosing: Usual Children and Adults: Bladder irrigation: 1 mL is added to 1 L of NS with administration rate adjusted to patient's urine output; usually administered via a 3-way catheter (approximately 40 mL/hour); continuous irrigation or rinse of the urinary bladder should not exceed 10 days

Preparation for Administration Bladder irrigant: Concentrated irrigant solution must be diluted in 1 liter NS prior to administration

Administration Bladder irrigant: Do not inject irrigant solution; concentrated irrigant solution must be diluted prior to administration; connect irrigation container to the inflow lumen of a 3-way catheter to permit continuous irrigation of the urinary bladder

Monitoring Parameters Urinalysis, renal function

Additional Information GU irrigant contains methylparaben

Dosage Forms Excipient information presented when available (limited, particularly for generics); consult specific product labeling.

Solution, irrigation: Neomycin 40 mg and polymyxin B sulfate 200,000 units per 1 mL (1 mL, 20 mL)

Neosporin® G.U. Irrigant: Neomycin 40 mg and polymyxin sulfate B 200,000 units per 1 mL (1 mL, 20 mL)

◆ **Neomycin, Bacitracin, and Polymyxin B** *see* Bacitracin, Neomycin, and Polymyxin B *on page 253*

◆ **Neomycin, Bacitracin, Polymyxin B, and Hydrocortisone** *see* Bacitracin, Neomycin, Polymyxin B, and Hydrocortisone *on page 253*

Neomycin, Polymyxin B, and Dexamethasone

(nee oh MYE sin, pol i MIKS in bee, & deks a METH a sone)

Brand Names: US Maxitrol

Brand Names: Canada Dioptrol; Maxitrol

Therapeutic Category Antibiotic, Ophthalmic; Corticosteroid, Ophthalmic

Generic Availability (US) Yes

Use Steroid-responsive inflammatory ocular conditions in which a corticosteroid is indicated and where bacterial infection or a risk of bacterial infection exists

Pregnancy Risk Factor C

Pregnancy Considerations Adverse events have been observed with topical corticosteroids in animal reproduction studies.. If ophthalmic agents are needed during pregnancy, the minimum effective dose should be used in combination with punctual occlusion to decrease potential exposure to the fetus (Samples, 1988). Refer to individual agents.

Breast-Feeding Considerations It is not known if systemic absorption following topical administration results in detectable quantities in human milk. The manufacturer recommends that caution be exercised when administering neomycin/polymyxin B/dexamethasone to nursing women. Refer to individual agents.

Contraindications Hypersensitivity to neomycin, polymyxin B, dexamethasone, or any component of the formulation; viral disease of the cornea and conjunctiva (including epithelial herpes simplex keratitis [dendritic keratitis], vaccinia, varicella); mycobacterial ophthalmic infection; fungal diseases of ocular structures.

Warnings/Precautions Prolonged use of corticosteroids (including ophthalmic preparations) may increase the incidence of secondary ocular infections (including fungal infections). Acute purulent ocular infections may be masked or exacerbated with use. Fungal infection should be suspected in any patient with persistent corneal ulceration who has received corticosteroids. Neomycin may cause cutaneous sensitization. Symptoms of neomycin sensitization include itching, reddening, edema, and failure to heal. Discontinuation of product and avoidance of similar products should be considered.

Never directly introduce (eg, inject) into the anterior chamber. Prolonged use of corticosteroids may result in glaucoma; damage to the optic nerve, defects in visual acuity and fields of vision, corneal and scleral thinning (leading to perforation) and posterior subcapsular cataract formation may occur. Use following cataract surgery may delay healing or increase the incidence of bleb formation. A maximum of 8 g of ointment or 20 mL of suspension should be prescribed initially; reevaluate patients (eg, intraocular pressure and exams using magnification and fluorescein staining, where appropriate) prior to additional refills. Use >10 days should include routine monitoring of intraocular pressure. Inadvertent contamination of multiple-dose ophthalmic solutions has caused bacterial keratitis. May contain benzalkonium chloride, which may be absorbed by soft contact lenses; contact lenses should not be worn during treatment of ophthalmologic infections.

Adverse Reactions See individual agents.

Drug Interactions

Metabolism/Transport Effects None known.

Avoid Concomitant Use There are no known interactions where it is recommended to avoid concomitant use.

Increased Effect/Toxicity

Neomycin, Polymyxin B, and Dexamethasone may increase the levels/effects of: Ceritinib

The levels/effects of Neomycin, Polymyxin B, and Dexamethasone may be increased by: NSAID (Ophthalmic)

Decreased Effect There are no known significant interactions involving a decrease in effect.

Storage/Stability

Ointment: Store between 2°C to 25°C (36°F to 77°F).

Suspension: Store between 8°C to 27°C (46°F to 80°F).

Mechanism of Action See individual agents.

Dosing: Usual Children and Adults: Ophthalmic:

Ointment: Apply a small amount (~1/2") in the affected eye 3-4 times/day or apply at bedtime as an adjunct with drops

Suspension: Instill 1-2 drops into affected eye(s) every 4-6 hours; in severe disease, drops may be used hourly and tapered to discontinuation

Administration Ophthalmic: Shake suspension well before using; instill drop into affected eye; avoid contacting bottle tip with skin or eye; apply finger pressure to lacrimal sac during and for 1-2 minutes after instillation to decrease risk of absorption and systemic effects

Monitoring Parameters Intraocular pressure with use >10 days

Dosage Forms Excipient information presented when available (limited, particularly for generics); consult specific product labeling.

Ointment, ophthalmic: Neomycin 3.5 mg, polymyxin B sulfate 10,000 units, and dexamethasone 0.1% per g (3.5 g)

Maxitrol®: Neomycin 3.5 mg, polymyxin B sulfate 10,000 units, and dexamethasone 0.1% per g (3.5 g)

Suspension, ophthalmic [drops]: Neomycin 3.5 mg, polymyxin B sulfate 10,000 units, and dexamethasone 0.1% per 1 mL (5 mL)

Maxitrol®: Neomycin 3.5 mg, polymyxin B sulfate 10,000 units, and dexamethasone 0.1% per 1 mL (5 mL) [contains benzalkonium chloride]

Neomycin, Polymyxin B, and Hydrocortisone

(nee oh MYE sin, pol i MIKS in bee, & hye droe KOR ti sone)

Brand Names: US Cortisporin; Cortomycin

Brand Names: Canada Cortimyxin; Cortisporin Otic

Therapeutic Category Antibacterial, Otic; Antibiotic, Ophthalmic; Antibiotic, Otic; Antibiotic, Topical; Corticosteroid, Ophthalmic; Corticosteroid, Otic; Corticosteroid, Topical

Generic Availability (US) Yes: Excludes topical cream

Use Steroid-responsive inflammatory condition for which a corticosteroid is indicated and where bacterial infection or a risk of bacterial infection exists (Otic preparations: FDA approved in ages 2-16 years and adults; Topical cream, ophthalmic suspension: FDA approved in adults)

Pregnancy Risk Factor C

Pregnancy Considerations Adverse events have been observed with topical corticosteroids in animal reproduction studies If ophthalmic agents are needed during pregnancy, the minimum effective dose should be used in combination with punctual occlusion to decrease potential exposure to the fetus (Samples, 1988). Refer to individual agents.

Breast-Feeding Considerations It is not known if systemic absorption following topical administration results in detectable quantities in human milk. The manufacturer recommends that caution be exercised when administering neomycin/polymyxin B/hydrocortisone to nursing women. Refer to individual agents.

Contraindications Hypersensitivity to neomycin, polymyxin B, hydrocortisone, or any component of the formulation; not for use in viral infections, fungal diseases, mycobacterial infections

Warnings/Precautions Prolonged use of corticosteroids (including ophthalmic preparations) may increase the incidence of secondary ocular infections (including fungal infections). Acute purulent ocular infections may be masked or exacerbated with use. Fungal infection should be suspected in any patient with persistent corneal ulceration who has received corticosteroids. Systemic absorption of topical corticosteroids may cause hypothalamic-pituitary-adrenal (HPA) axis suppression (reversible) particularly in younger children. HPA axis suppression may lead to adrenal crisis. Risk is increased when used over large surface areas, for prolonged periods, or with occlusive dressings. Neomycin may cause cutaneous sensitization. Symptoms of neomycin sensitization include itching, reddening, edema, and failure to heal. Symptoms of neomycin sensitization include itching, reddening, edema, and failure to heal. Discontinuation of product and avoidance of similar products should be considered. Use with caution in patients with glaucoma. Use with extreme caution in patients with a history of ocular herpes simplex; frequent slit lamp microscopy is recommended. Some products may contain sulfites, which may cause allergic-type reactions in susceptible individuals.

Ophthalmic preparations: Prolonged use of corticosteroids may result in ocular hypertension and/or glaucoma; damage to the optic nerve, defects in visual acuity and fields of vision, corneal and scleral thinning (leading to perforation), and posterior subcapsular cataract formation may occur. Use following cataract surgery may delay healing or increase the incidence of bleb formation.

Otic preparations: Risk of ototoxicity is increased in patients with extended use or tympanic perforation; avoid use with tympanic perforation; limit therapy to 10 days.

Warnings: Additional Pediatric Considerations The extent of percutaneous absorption is dependent on several factors, including epidermal integrity (intact vs abraded skin), formulation, age of the patient, prolonged duration of use, and the use of occlusive dressings. Percutaneous absorption of topical steroids is increased in neonates (especially preterm neonates), infants, and young children. Infants and small children may be more susceptible to HPA axis suppression, intracranial hypertension, Cushing syndrome, or other systemic toxicities due to larger skin surface area to body mass ratio.

Adverse Reactions For additional information, see individual agents.

Ophthalmic ointment:

Dermatologic: Delayed wound healing, rash

Ocular: Cataracts, corneal thinning, glaucoma, irritation, keratitis (bacterial), intraocular pressure increase, optic nerve damage, scleral thinning

Miscellaneous: Hypersensitivity (including anaphylaxis), secondary infection, sensitization to kanamycin, paromomycin, streptomycin, and gentamicin

Otic solution and suspension:

Dermatologic: Acneiform eruptions, allergic contact dermatitis, burning skin, dryness, folliculitis, hypertrichosis, hypopigmentation, irritation, maceration of skin, miliaria, perioral dermatitis, pruritus, skin atrophy, striae

Ophthalmic: Ocular hypertension

Otic: Burning, ototoxicity, stinging

Renal: Nephrotoxicity

Miscellaneous: Hypersensitivity (including anaphylaxis), secondary infection, sensitization to karamycin, paromycin, streptomycin, and gentamicin

Drug Interactions

Metabolism/Transport Effects None known.

Avoid Concomitant Use

Avoid concomitant use of Neomycin, Polymyxin B, and Hydrocortisone with any of the following: Aldesleukin

Increased Effect/Toxicity

Neomycin, Polymyxin B, and Hydrocortisone may increase the levels/effects of: Ceritinib; Deferasirox

The levels/effects of Neomycin, Polymyxin B, and Hydrocortisone may be increased by: NSAID (Ophthalmic); Telaprevir

Decreased Effect

Neomycin, Polymyxin B, and Hydrocortisone may decrease the levels/effects of: Aldesleukin; Corticorelin; Hyaluronidase; Telaprevir

Storage/Stability Store at room temperature.

Mechanism of Action See individual agents.

Dosing: Usual

Otic preparations (solution and suspension):

Children: 3 drops into affected ear 3-4 times/day for up to 10 days

Adults: 4 drops into affected ear 3-4 times/day for up to 10 days

Topical cream: Children and Adults: Apply thin layer to affected area 2-4 times/day for up to 7 days. Therapy should be discontinued when control is achieved or after a week; if no improvement is seen, reassessment of diagnosis may be necessary.

Ophthalmic suspension: Children and Adults: Instill 1-2 drops in the affected eye every 3-4 hours

Administration Shake ophthalmic and otic suspension well before use

Ophthalmic: Avoid contamination of the tip of the eye dropper; apply finger pressure to lacrimal sac during and for 1-2 minutes after instillation to decrease risk of absorption and systemic effects

Otic: Drops can be instilled directly into the affected ear, or a cotton wick may be saturated with suspension and inserted in ear canal. Keep wick moist with suspension every 4 hours; wick should be replaced every 24 hours.

Topical: Apply a thin layer to the cleansed, dry affected area

Monitoring Parameters If ophthalmic suspension is used >10 days or in patients with glaucoma, monitor intraocular pressure (IOP).

Additional Information Otic **suspension** is the preferred otic preparation; otic **suspension** can be used for the treatment of infections of mastoidectomy and fenestration cavities caused by susceptible organisms; otic **solution** is used **only** for superficial infections of the external auditory canal (ie, swimmer's ear)

Dosage Forms Excipient information presented when available (limited, particularly for generics); consult specific product labeling.

Cream, topical

Cortisporin: Neomycin 3.5 mg, polymyxin B 10,000 units, and hydrocortisone acetate 5 mg per g (7.5 g)

Solution, otic: Neomycin 3.5 mg, polymyxin B 10,000 units, and hydrocortisone 10 mg per 1 mL (10 mL)

Cortisporin: Neomycin 3.5 mg, polymyxin B 10,000 units, and hydrocortisone 10 mg per 1 mL (10 mL) [contains potassium metabisulfite]

Cortomycin: Neomycin 3.5 mg, polymyxin B 10,000 units, and hydrocortisone 10 mg per 1 mL (10 mL) [contains potassium metabisulfate]

Suspension, ophthalmic [drops]: Neomycin 3.5 mg, polymyxin B 10,000 units, and hydrocortisone 10 mg per 1 mL (7.5 mL)

Suspension, otic: Neomycin 3.5 mg, polymyxin B 10,000 units, and hydrocortisone 10 mg per 1 mL (10 mL)

Cortomycin: Neomycin 3.5 mg, polymyxin B 10,000 units, and hydrocortisone 10 mg per 1 mL (10 mL) [contains thimerosal]

◆ **Neomycin Sulfate** *see* Neomycin *on page* 1500

◆ **Neonatal Trace Metals** *see* Trace Elements *on page* 2097

◆ **Neo-Polycin™** *see* Bacitracin, Neomycin, and Polymyxin B *on page* 253

◆ **Neo-Polycin HC** *see* Bacitracin, Neomycin, Polymyxin B, and Hydrocortisone *on page* 253

◆ **NeoProfen** *see* Ibuprofen *on page* 1064

◆ **Neoral** *see* CycloSPORINE (Systemic) *on page* 556

◆ **Neosar** *see* Cyclophosphamide *on page* 551

◆ **Neosporin® G.U. Irrigant** *see* Neomycin and Polymyxin B *on page* 1502

◆ **Neosporin® Irrigating Solution (Can)** *see* Neomycin and Polymyxin B *on page* 1502

◆ **Neosporin® Neo To Go® [OTC]** *see* Bacitracin, Neomycin, and Polymyxin B *on page* 253

◆ **Neosporin® Topical [OTC]** *see* Bacitracin, Neomycin, and Polymyxin B *on page* 253

Neostigmine (nee oh STIG meen)

Medication Safety Issues

Sound-alike/look-alike issues:

Bloxiverz may be confused with Vazculep (phenylephrine injection) due to similar packaging

Prostigmin may be confused with physostigmine

Brand Names: US Bloxiverz; Prostigmin

Brand Names: Canada Prostigmin

Therapeutic Category Antidote, Neuromuscular Blocking Agent; Cholinergic Agent; Diagnostic Agent, Myasthenia Gravis

Generic Availability (US) May be product dependent

Use

Oral: Treatment of myasthenia gravis (FDA approved in adults)

Parenteral: Reversal of the effects of nondepolarizing neuromuscular blocking agents after surgery (Bloxiverz; FDA approved in all ages; generic injection: FDA approved in adults); treatment of myasthenia gravis when oral therapy impractical (FDA approved in adults); prevention and treatment of postoperative bladder distention and urinary retention (FDA approved in adults)

Pregnancy Risk Factor C

Pregnancy Considerations Animal reproduction studies have not been conducted; anticholinesterases have caused uterine irritability and induced premature labor with IV use in near-term pregnant women. When used as adjunct to analgesia in labor, adverse events to the fetus and mother are dose- and route-dependent (Habib, 2006). Neostigmine may be used to treat myasthenia gravis in pregnant women; however, if an acetylcholinesterase inhibitor is needed during pregnancy, another agent may be preferred (Norwood, 2013; Silvestri, 2012).

Breast-Feeding Considerations It is not known if neostigmine is excreted into breast milk. The manufacturer recommends caution be used if administered to nursing women. Babies born to women with myasthenia gravis may have feeding difficulties due to transient myasthenia gravis of the newborn (Norwood, 2013).

Contraindications

Hypersensitivity to neostigmine or any component of the formulation; history of reaction to bromides (tablets only); peritonitis or mechanical obstruction of the intestinal or urinary tract

Documentation of allergenic cross-reactivity for cholinesterase inhibitors is limited. However, because of similarities in chemical structure and/or pharmacologic actions, the possibility of cross-sensitivity cannot be ruled out with certainty.

Warnings/Precautions Bradycardia, hypotension, and dysrhythmias may occur, particularly with IV use; cardiovascular complications may also be increased in patients with myasthenia gravis. Use with caution in patients with epilepsy, asthma, bradycardia, hypotension, hyperthyroidism, cardiac arrhythmias, coronary artery disease, recent acute coronary syndrome, vagotonia, or peptic ulcer. Cardiovascular complications may also be increased in patients with myasthenia gravis. When IV neostigmine is administered for the reversal of nondepolarizing neuromuscular-blocking agents, atropine or glycopyrrolate should be administered concurrently or prior to neostigmine to lessen the risk of bradycardia. Adequate facilities should be available for cardiopulmonary resuscitation when testing and adjusting dose for myasthenia gravis. Symptoms of hypersensitivity have included urticaria, angioedema, erythema multiforme, generalized rash, facial swelling, peripheral edema, pyrexia, flushing, hypotension, bronchospasm, bradycardia, and anaphylaxis. Have atropine and epinephrine ready to treat hypersensitivity reactions. Overdosage may result in cholinergic crisis, this must be distinguished from myasthenic crisis. Large doses of IV neostigmine administered for the reversal of nondepolarizing neuromuscular blocking-agents when neuromuscular blockade is minimal can result in neuromuscular dysfunction. Reduce the dose of neostigmine if recovery from neuromuscular blockade is nearly complete.

Infants and small children may be at greater risk of complications from incomplete reversal of neuromuscular blockade due to decreased respiratory drive; observe the effects of an anticholinergic agent (eg, atropine) prior to administration of neostigmine to lessen the probability of bradycardia and hypotension. Use with caution in the elderly and monitor for a longer period in the elderly; may experience slower spontaneous recovery from neuromuscular blocking agents. Use with caution in the elderly and monitor for a longer period in the elderly; may experience slower spontaneous recovery from neuromuscular blocking agents.

Adverse Reactions

Cardiovascular: Arrhythmias (especially bradycardia), AV block, cardiac arrest, flushing, hypotension, nodal rhythm, nonspecific ECG changes, syncope, tachycardia

Central nervous system: Convulsions, dizziness, drowsiness, dysarthria, dysphonia, headache, loss of consciousness

Dermatologic: Skin rash, thrombophlebitis (IV), urticaria

Gastrointestinal: Diarrhea, dysphagia, flatulence, hyperperistalsis, nausea, salivation, stomach cramps, vomiting

Genitourinary: Urinary urgency

Neuromuscular & skeletal: Arthralgias, fasciculations, muscle cramps, spasms, weakness

Ocular: Lacrimation, small pupils

Respiratory: Bronchiolar constriction, bronchospasm, dyspnea, increased bronchial secretions, laryngospasm, respiratory arrest, respiratory depression, respiratory muscle paralysis

Miscellaneous: Allergic reactions, anaphylaxis, diaphoresis increased

Drug Interactions

Metabolism/Transport Effects None known.

Avoid Concomitant Use There are no known interactions where it is recommended to avoid concomitant use.

Increased Effect/Toxicity

Neostigmine may increase the levels/effects of: Beta-Blockers; Cholinergic Agonists; Succinylcholine

The levels/effects of Neostigmine may be increased by: Corticosteroids (Systemic)

Decreased Effect

Neostigmine may decrease the levels/effects of: Anticholinergic Agents; Neuromuscular-Blocking Agents (Nondepolarizing)

The levels/effects of Neostigmine may be decreased by: Anticholinergic Agents; Dipyridamole

Storage/Stability

Injection: Store between 20°C and 25°C (68°F and 77°F); excursions permitted to 15°C to 30°C (59°F to 86°F). Protect from light. Store in carton until time of use.

Tablets: Store at 25°C (77°F); excursions permitted to 15°C to 30°C (59°F to 86°F).

Mechanism of Action Inhibits destruction of acetylcholine by acetylcholinesterase which facilitates transmission of impulses across myoneural junction; direct cholinomimetic effect on skeletal muscle and possible on autonomic ganglion cells and neurons of the CNS

Pharmacodynamics

Onset of action:

Oral: 1 to 2 hours

IM: Within 20 to 30 minutes

Duration: IM: 2.5 to 4 hours

Pharmacokinetics (Adult data unless noted)

Absorption: Oral: Poor (~1% to 2%)

Metabolism: Hepatic

Half-life:
IM: 51 to 90 minutes
IV:
Infants 2 to 10 months: Mean: 39 ± 5 minutes
Children 1 to 6 years: Mean: 48 ± 16 minutes
Adult: 24 to 113 minutes
Oral: 42 to 60 minutes
Elimination: Urine (50% excreted as unchanged drug)

Dosing: Neonatal Reversal of nondepolarizing neuromuscular blockade after surgery: IV: *Bloxiverz:* **Note:** An anticholinergic agent (atropine or glycopyrrolate) should be given prior to or in conjunction with neostigmine; in the presence of bradycardia, administer the anticholinergic prior to neostigmine. Peripheral nerve stimulation delivering train-of-four (TOF) stimulus must also be used to determine time of neostigmine initiation and need for additional doses.
Usual dose: 0.03 to 0.07 mg/kg generally achieves a TOF twitch ratio of 90% within 10 to 20 minutes of administration; maximum total dose: 0.07 mg/kg or 5 mg (whichever is less)
Dose selection guide:
The 0.03 mg/kg dose is recommended for reversal of NMBAs with shorter half-lives (eg, rocuronium); or when the first twitch response to the TOF stimulus is substantially >10% of baseline or when a second twitch is present.
The 0.07 mg/kg dose is recommended for NMBAs with longer half-lives (eg, vecuronium, pancuronium); or when the first twitch response is relatively weak (ie, not substantially >10% of baseline); or rapid recovery is needed.

Dosing: Usual Note: Neostigmine (Prostigmin) tablets have been discontinued in the US for more than 1 year.
Pediatric:
Myasthenia gravis: Limited data available:
Diagnosis: **Note:** Pretreatment with atropine is recommended, and atropine should be available. IV fluids also recommended. Children <2 years: IM: 0.04 mg/kg once; if results equivocal or negative, may be repeated once in 4 hours. Typical dose is 0.5 to 1.5 mg (Kliegman 2011)
Treatment: **Note:** Dosage requirements are variable; dosage should be individualized: Children and Adolescents:
Oral: 0.3 to 2 mg/kg/day in divided doses (Silvestri 2012)
IM, IV, SubQ: 0.01 to 0.04 mg/kg every 2 to 6 hours (Kliegman 2007; Kliegman 2011)
Reversal of nondepolarizing neuromuscular blockade after surgery: Infants, Children, and Adolescents: IV:
Manufacturer labeling: Bloxiverz: **Note:** An anticholinergic agent (atropine or glycopyrrolate) should be given prior to or in conjunction with neostigmine; in the presence of bradycardia, administer the anticholinergic prior to neostigmine. Peripheral nerve stimulation delivering train-of-four (TOF) stimulus must also be used to determine time of neostigmine initiation and need for additional doses.
Usual dose: 0.03 to 0.07 mg/kg generally achieves a TOF twitch ratio of 90% within 10 to 20 minutes of administration; maximum total dose: 0.07 mg/kg or 5 mg (whichever is less)
Dose selection guide:
The 0.03 mg/kg dose is recommended for reversal of NMBAs with shorter half-lives (eg, rocuronium); or when the first twitch response to the TOF stimulus is substantially >10% of baseline or when a second twitch is present.
The 0.07 mg/kg dose is recommended for NMBAs with longer half-lives (eg, vecuronium, pancuronium); or when the first twitch response is relatively weak (ie, not substantially >10% of baseline); or rapid recovery is needed.
Alternate dosing: Generic injectable products: Limited data available (Kliegman 2007; Nelson 1996): Infants and Children: 0.025 to 0.1 mg/kg/dose
Adult:
Myasthenia gravis: Treatment:
Manufacturer's labeling:
Oral: Usual dose: 150 mg administered over a 24-hour period; interval between doses is of paramount importance and therapy is frequently required day and night. Dosage range: 15 to 375 mg daily in divided doses.
IM, SubQ: 0.5 mg; subsequent dosing based on individual patient response
Alternative recommendations (off-label dosing):
Oral: Initial: 15 mg every 8 hours; may increase every 1 to 2 days up to 375 mg daily maximum; interval between doses must be individualized to maximal response
IM, IV, SubQ: 0.5 to 2.5 mg every 1 to 3 hours as needed up to 10 mg/24 hours maximum
Reversal of nondepolarizing neuromuscular blockade after surgery *Bloxiverz:* IV: **Note:** An anticholinergic agent (atropine or glycopyrrolate) should be given prior to or in conjunction with neostigmine; in the presence of bradycardia, administer the anticholinergic prior to neostigmine. Peripheral nerve stimulation delivering train-of-four (TOF) stimulus must also be used to determine time of neostigmine initiation and need for additional doses.
Usual dose: 0.03 to 0.07 mg/kg generally achieves a TOF twitch ratio of 90% within 10 to 20 minutes of administration; maximum total dose: 0.07 mg/kg or 5 mg (whichever is less)
Dose selection guide:
The 0.03 mg/kg dose is recommended for reversal of NMBAs with shorter half-lives (eg, rocuronium); or when the first twitch response to the TOF stimulus is substantially >10% of baseline or when a second twitch is present.
The 0.07 mg/kg dose is recommended for NMBAs with longer half-lives (eg, vecuronium, pancuronium); or when the first twitch response is relatively weak (ie, not substantially >10% of baseline); or rapid recovery is needed.
Generic products: IV: 0.5 to 2 mg; repeat as required. Only in exceptional cases should the total dose exceed 5 mg. **Note:** Administer with atropine 0.6 to 1.2 mg in a separate syringe several minutes before neostigmine.
Postoperative urinary retention: IM, SubQ:
Prevention: 0.25 mg as soon as possible after operation; repeat every 4 to 6 hours for 2 to 3 days
Treatment: 0.5 mg; if urination does not occur within an hour, patient should be catheterized. After the bladder has emptied or patient has voided, continue 0.5 mg every 3 hours for at least 5 doses.
Postoperative bladder distention: IM, SubQ:
Prevention: 0.25 mg as soon as possible after operation; repeat every 4 to 6 hours for 2 to 3 days
Treatment: 0.5 mg as needed

Dosing adjustment in renal impairment: There are no dosage adjustment provided in manufacturer's labeling; however, the following adjustments have been recommended (Aronoff 2007): Adults: Oral:
CrCl >50 mL/minute: No dosage adjustment necessary
CrCl 10 to 50 mL/minute: Administer 50% of normal dose.
CrCl <10 mL/minute: Administer 25% of normal dose.
Hemodialysis: No dosage adjustment necessary
Peritoneal dialysis: No dosage adjustment necessary

Continuous renal replacement therapy (CRRT): Administer 50% of normal dose

Dosing adjustment in hepatic impairment: There are no dosage adjustment provided in the manufacturer's labeling.

Administration

Parenteral: May be administered undiluted by slow IV injection over several minutes; may be administered IM or SubQ

Oral: Divide dosages so patient receives larger doses at times of greatest fatigue; may be administered with or without food

Monitoring Parameters ECG, blood pressure, and heart rate especially with IV use; consult individual institutional policies and procedures; muscle strength

Product Availability Neostigmine (Prostigmin) tablets have been discontinued in the US for more than 1 year.

Dosage Forms Excipient information presented when available (limited, particularly for generics); consult specific product labeling. [DSC] = Discontinued product

Solution, Injection, as methylsulfate:
- Prostigmin: 0.5 mg/mL (1 mL, 10 mL)
- Generic: 0.5 mg/mL (10 mL); 1 mg/mL (10 mL)

Solution, Intravenous, as methylsulfate:
- Bloxiverz: 5 mg/10 mL (10 mL); 10 mg/10 mL (10 mL) [contains phenol]
- Generic: 5 mg/10 mL (10 mL); 10 mg/10 mL (10 mL)

Tablet, Oral, as bromide:
- Prostigmin: 15 mg [DSC] [scored]

◆ **Neostigmine Bromide** *see* Neostigmine *on page* 1505

◆ **Neostigmine Methylsulfate** *see* Neostigmine *on page* 1505

◆ **Neo-Synephrine [OTC]** *see* Phenylephrine (Nasal) *on page* 1688

◆ **Neo-Synephrine® (Can)** *see* Phenylephrine (Nasal) *on page* 1688

◆ **Neo-Synephrine 12 Hour Spray [OTC]** *see* Oxymetazoline (Nasal) *on page* 1599

◆ **Neo-Synephrine Cold & Sinus [OTC]** *see* Phenylephrine (Nasal) *on page* 1688

◆ **Nesacaine** *see* Chloroprocaine *on page* 435

◆ **Nesacaine-MPF** *see* Chloroprocaine *on page* 435

◆ **NESP** *see* Darbepoetin Alfa *on page* 585

◆ **Neuac** *see* Clindamycin and Benzoyl Peroxide *on page* 493

◆ **Neulasta** *see* Pegfilgrastim *on page* 1641

◆ **Neulasta Delivery Kit** *see* Pegfilgrastim *on page* 1641

◆ **Neumega** *see* Oprelvekin *on page* 1570

◆ **Neuotrogena T/Gel Therapeutic Shampoo [OTC] (Can)** *see* Coal Tar *on page* 523

◆ **Neupogen** *see* Filgrastim *on page* 876

◆ **Neuro-K-50 [OTC]** *see* Pyridoxine *on page* 1810

◆ **Neuro-K-250 T.D. [OTC]** *see* Pyridoxine *on page* 1810

◆ **Neuro-K-250 Vitamin B6 [OTC]** *see* Pyridoxine *on page* 1810

◆ **Neuro-K-500 [OTC]** *see* Pyridoxine *on page* 1810

◆ **Neurontin** *see* Gabapentin *on page* 954

◆ **Neut** *see* Sodium Bicarbonate *on page* 1936

◆ **NeutraCare** *see* Fluoride *on page* 899

◆ **NeutraGard Advanced** *see* Fluoride *on page* 899

◆ **Neutra-Phos** *see* Potassium Phosphate and Sodium Phosphate *on page* 1746

◆ **Neutra-Phos®-K [OTC] [DSC]** *see* Potassium Phosphate *on page* 1743

◆ **Neutrogena Clear Pore [OTC]** *see* Benzoyl Peroxide *on page* 270

◆ **Neutrogena Oil-Free Acne Wash [OTC]** *see* Salicylic Acid *on page* 1894

◆ **Neutrogena T/Gel Conditioner [OTC]** *see* Coal Tar *on page* 523

◆ **Neutrogena T/Gel Ex St [OTC]** *see* Coal Tar *on page* 523

◆ **Neuvaxin** *see* Capsaicin *on page* 362

Nevirapine (ne VYE ra peen)

Medication Safety Issues

Sound-alike/look-alike issues:

Nevirapine may be confused with nelfinavir

Viramune, Viramune XR may be confused with Viracept, Viramune (herbal product)

High alert medication:

This medication is in a class the Institute for Safe Medication Practices (ISMP) includes among its list of drug classes that have a heightened risk of causing significant patient harm when used in error.

Related Information

Adult and Adolescent HIV *on page* 2392

Oral Medications That Should Not Be Crushed or Altered *on page* 2476

Pediatric HIV *on page* 2380

Perinatal HIV *on page* 2400

Safe Handling of Hazardous Drugs *on page* 2455

Brand Names: US Viramune; Viramune XR

Brand Names: Canada Auro-Nevirapine; Mylan-Nevirapine; Teva-Nevirapine; Viramune; Viramune XR

Therapeutic Category Antiretroviral Agent; HIV Agents (Anti-HIV Agents); Non-nucleoside Reverse Transcriptase Inhibitor (NNRTI)

Generic Availability (US) Yes

Use Treatment of HIV infection in combination with other antiretroviral agents (Immediate release: FDA approved in ages ≥15 days and adults; Extended release: FDA approved in ages ≥6 years and adults). **Note:** HIV regimens consisting of three antiretroviral agents are strongly recommended. Do not start nevirapine therapy in women with CD4+ counts >250 cells/mm^3 or in men with CD4+ counts >400 cells/mm^3 unless benefit of therapy outweighs the risk. Nevirapine has also been used as chemoprophylaxis in newborns to prevent perinatal HIV transmission.

Medication Guide Available Yes

Pregnancy Risk Factor B

Pregnancy Considerations Teratogenic effects were not observed in animal reproduction studies. Nevirapine has a high level of transfer across the human placenta. No increased risk of overall birth defects has been observed following first trimester exposure according to data collected by the antiretroviral pregnancy registry. Pharmacokinetics are not altered during pregnancy and dose adjustment is not needed. The HHS Perinatal HIV Guidelines consider nevirapine to be an alternative NNRTI for use in antiretroviral-naïve pregnant patients. Nevirapine may be initiated in pregnant women with a CD4$^+$ lymphocyte count <250/mm^3 or continued in women who are virologically suppressed and tolerating therapy once pregnancy is detected (regardless of CD4+ lymphocyte count); however, **do not** initiate therapy in pregnant women with a CD4$^+$ lymphocyte count >250/mm^3 unless the benefit of therapy clearly outweighs the risk. Elevated transaminase concentrations at baseline may increase the risk of toxicity; the monitoring recommendation for transaminase levels is generally the same as in nonpregnant women. Hypersensitivity reactions (including hepatic toxicity and rash) are more common in women on NNRTI.

Regardless of CD4 count or HIV RNA copy number, all HIV-infected pregnant women should receive a combination antiretroviral (ARV) drug regimen. A combination of antepartum, intrapartum, and infant ARV prophylaxis is recommended. ARV therapy should be started as soon as possible in women with symptomatic infection. Although earlier initiation may be more effective in reducing the perinatal transmission of HIV, initiation may be delayed until after 12 weeks gestation in women who do not require immediate treatment after careful consideration of maternal conditions (eg, nausea and vomiting) and the potential risks of first trimester fetal exposure for specific agents. A scheduled cesarean delivery at 38 weeks gestation is recommended for all women with HIV RNA >1000 copies/mL or unknown concentrations near delivery in order to decrease transmission. If ARV therapy must be interrupted for <24 hours during the peripartum period, stop then restart all medications simultaneously in order to decrease the chance of developing resistance. Long-term follow-up is recommended for all infants exposed to ARV medications. In couples who want to conceive, the HIV-infected partner should attain maximum viral suppression prior to conception.

Health care providers are encouraged to enroll pregnant women exposed to antiretroviral medications in the Antiretroviral Pregnancy Registry (1-800-258-4263 or www.APRegistry.com). Health care providers caring for HIV-infected women and their infants may contact the National Perinatal HIV Hotline (888-448-8765) for clinical consultation (HHS [perinatal], 2014).

Breast-Feeding Considerations Nevirapine is excreted into breast milk and measurable in the serum of nursing infants. Maternal or infant antiretroviral therapy does not completely eliminate the risk of postnatal HIV transmission. In addition, multiclass resistant virus has been detected in breast-feeding infants despite maternal therapy. Therefore, in the United States, where formula is accessible, affordable, safe, and sustainable, and the risk of infant mortality due to diarrhea and respiratory infections is low, complete avoidance of breast-feeding by HIV-infected women is recommended to decrease potential transmission of HIV (HHS [perinatal], 2014).

Contraindications Moderate-to-severe hepatic impairment (Child-Pugh class B or C); use in occupational or nonoccupational postexposure prophylaxis (PEP) regimens

Canadian labeling: Additional contraindications (not in U.S. labeling): Clinically significant hypersensitivity to nevirapine or any component of the formulation; therapy rechallenge in patients with prior hypersensitivity reactions, severe rash, rash accompanied by constitutional symptoms, or clinical hepatitis due to nevirapine; severe hepatic dysfunction or AST or ALT >5 times ULN (pretreatment or during prior use of nevirapine); hereditary conditions of galactose intolerance (eg, galactosemia, Lapp lactase deficiency, glucose-galactose malabsorption); concomitant use of herbal products containing St John's wort

Warnings/Precautions Hazardous agent - use appropriate precautions for handling and disposal (NIOSH 2014 [group 2]).

[U.S. Boxed Warning]: Severe hepatotoxic reactions may occur (fulminant and cholestatic hepatitis, hepatic necrosis) and, in some cases, have resulted in hepatic failure and death. The greatest risk of these reactions is within the initial 6 weeks of treatment. Patients with a history of chronic hepatitis (B or C) or increased baseline transaminase levels may be at increased risk of hepatotoxic reactions. Female gender and patients with increased CD4⁺-cell counts may be at substantially greater risk of hepatic events (often associated with rash). Therapy in antiretroviral naive patients should not be started with elevated CD4⁺-cell counts unless the benefit of therapy outweighs the risk of serious hepatotoxicity (adult/postpubertal females: CD4⁺-cell counts >250 cells/mm^3; adult males: CD4⁺-cell counts >400 cells/mm^3). Use with caution in patients with pre-existing dysfunction; monitor closely for drug-induced hepatotoxicity. U.S. labeling contraindicates use in patients with moderate-to-severe impairment (Child-Pugh class B or C). Canadian labeling contraindicates use in severe impairment.

[U.S. Boxed Warning]: Severe life-threatening skin reactions (eg, Stevens-Johnson syndrome, toxic epidermal necrolysis, hypersensitivity reactions with rash and organ dysfunction), including fatal cases, have occurred. The greatest risk of these reactions is within the initial 6 weeks of treatment; intensive monitoring is required during the initial 18 weeks of therapy to detect potentially life-threatening dermatologic and hypersensitivity reactions. If a rash occurs within the first 18 weeks of therapy, immediately check serum transaminases. Risk is greatest in African-Americans, Asian, or Hispanic race/ethnicity or in females (DHHS, 2011). If a severe dermatologic or hypersensitivity reaction occurs, nevirapine should be permanently discontinued; these events may include a severe rash, or a rash associated with fever, blisters, oral lesions, conjunctivitis, facial edema, muscle or joint aches, transaminase increases, general malaise, hepatitis, eosinophilia, granulocytopenia, lymphadenopathy, or renal dysfunction. Use of the 14-day lead-in dosing period is necessary to decrease the incidence of rash events. If nonsevere rash (in absence of transaminase elevations) occurs, do not increase dose until resolution of rash. If rash continues beyond 28 days, consider an alternative regimen. Coadministration of prednisone during the first 6 weeks of therapy increases incidence and severity of rash; concomitant prednisone is not recommended to prevent rash.

May cause redistribution of fat (eg, buffalo hump, peripheral wasting with increased abdominal girth, cushingoid appearance). Patients may develop immune reconstitution syndrome resulting in the occurrence of an inflammatory response to an indolent or residual opportunistic infection during initial HIV treatment or activation of autoimmune disorders (eg, Graves' disease, polymyositis, Guillain-Barré syndrome) later in therapy; further evaluation and treatment may be required. Rhabdomyolysis has been observed in conjunction with skin and/or hepatic adverse events during postmarketing surveillance. Termination of therapy is warranted with evidence of severe skin or liver toxicity.

Use with caution in patients taking strong CYP3A4 inhibitors, moderate or strong CYP3A4 inducers and major CYP3A4 substrates (see Drug Interactions); consider alternative agents that avoid or lessen the potential for CYP-mediated interactions. Concurrent use of St John's wort or efavirenz is not recommended; may decrease the therapeutic efficacy (St John's wort) or increase adverse effects (efavirenz). Canadian labeling contraindicates concurrent use with products containing St John's wort.

Nevirapine-based initial regimens should not be used in children <3 years of age if previously exposed to nevirapine during prevention of maternal-to-child transmission of HIV due to increased risk of resistance and treatment failure. Protease inhibitor-based initial regimens preferred in this population.

Due to rapid emergence of resistance, nevirapine should not be used as monotherapy or the only agent added to a failing regimen for the treatment of HIV. Consider alteration of antiretroviral therapies if disease progression occurs while patients are receiving nevirapine. Use care when timing discontinuation of regimens containing nevirapine;

levels are sustained after levels of other medications decrease, leading to nevirapine resistance. Cross-resistance may be conferred to other non-nucleoside reverse transcriptase inhibitors (HHS [adult], 2014).

Some dosage forms may contain polysorbate 80 (also known as Tweens). Hypersensitivity reactions, usually a delayed reaction, have been reported following exposure to pharmaceutical products containing polysorbate 80 in certain individuals (Isaksson, 2002; Lucente 2000; Shelley, 1995). Thrombocytopenia, ascites, pulmonary deterioration, and renal and hepatic failure have been reported in premature neonates after receiving parenteral products containing polysorbate 80 (Alade, 1986; CDC, 1984). See manufacturer's labeling.

Warnings: Additional Pediatric Considerations The incidence of rash in pediatric patients is 21%. Granulocytopenia may occur; more common in neonates and young infants (2 weeks to <3 months of age) compared to older children and adults; also more common in pediatric patients receiving concomitant zidovudine. Anemia may occur at an incidence of 7.3%; it has been reported more commonly in children in postmarketing reports; however, effects of concomitant medications cannot be separated out. In perinatally HIV-exposed infants, the sensitivity of diagnostic virologic assays, particularly HIV RNA assays, may be affected by infant combination antiretroviral prophylactic therapy. Thus, a negative result of a diagnostic virologic assay should be repeated 2 to 4 weeks after cessation of neonatal combination antiretroviral prophylactic therapy (DHHS [pediatric], 2014).

Adverse Reactions Note: Potentially life-threatening nevirapine-associated adverse effects may present with the following symptoms: Abrupt onset of flu-like symptoms, abdominal pain, jaundice, or fever with or without rash; may progress to hepatic failure with encephalopathy.

Central nervous system: Fatigue, fever, headache

Dermatologic: Rash

Endocrine & metabolic: Cholesterol increased, LDL increased

Gastrointestinal: Abdominal pain, amylase increased, diarrhea, nausea

Hematologic: Neutropenia

Hepatic: ALT increased, AST increased, symptomatic hepatic events (including hepatitis and hepatic failure)

Neuromuscular & skeletal: Arthralgia

Rare but important or life-threatening: Allergic reactions, anaphylaxis, anemia, angioedema, bullous eruptions, conjunctivitis, drug reaction with eosinophilia and systemic symptoms (DRESS), eosinophilia, hypersensitivity syndrome, hypophosphatemia, immune reconstitution syndrome, lymphadenopathy, oral lesions, redistribution/accumulation of body fat, renal dysfunction, rhabdomyolysis, Stevens-Johnson syndrome, toxic epidermal necrolysis, ulcerative stomatitis

Drug Interactions

Metabolism/Transport Effects Substrate of CYP2B6 (minor), CYP2D6 (minor), CYP3A4 (major); **Note:** Assignment of Major/Minor substrate status based on clinically relevant drug interaction potential; **Inhibits** CYP1A2 (weak), CYP2D6 (weak); **Induces** CYP2B6 (strong), CYP3A4 (weak)

Avoid Concomitant Use

Avoid concomitant use of Nevirapine with any of the following: Atazanavir; CarBAMazepine; Dolutegravir; Efavirenz; Elvitegravir; Etravirine; Itraconazole; Ketoconazole (Systemic); Rilpivirine; St Johns Wort

Increased Effect/Toxicity

Nevirapine may increase the levels/effects of: Artesunate; Darunavir; Efavirenz; Etravirine; Rifabutin; Rilpivirine; TiZANidine

The levels/effects of Nevirapine may be increased by: Atazanavir; Darunavir; Efavirenz; Fluconazole; Voriconazole

Decreased Effect

Nevirapine may decrease the levels/effects of: ARIPiprazole; Artemether; Artesunate; Atazanavir; CarBAMazepine; Caspofungin; Contraceptives (Estrogens); Contraceptives (Progestins); CYP2B6 Substrates; Dolutegravir; Efavirenz; Elvitegravir; Etravirine; Fosamprenavir; Hydrocodone; Indinavir; Itraconazole; Ketoconazole (Systemic); Lopinavir; Methadone; Nelfinavir; NiMODipine; Rifabutin; Rilpivirine; Saquinavir; Saxagliptin; Voriconazole

The levels/effects of Nevirapine may be decreased by: Bosentan; CarBAMazepine; CYP3A4 Inducers (Moderate); CYP3A4 Inducers (Strong); Dabrafenib; Deferasirox; Mitotane; Rifabutin; Rifampin; Siltuximab; St Johns Wort; Tocilizumab

Storage/Stability Store at 25°C (77°F); excursion permitted to 15°C to 30°C (59°F to 86°F).

Mechanism of Action As a non-nucleoside reverse transcriptase inhibitor, nevirapine has activity against HIV-1 by binding to reverse transcriptase. It consequently blocks the RNA-dependent and DNA-dependent DNA polymerase activities including HIV-1 replication. It does not require intracellular phosphorylation for antiviral activity.

Pharmacokinetics (Adult data unless noted)

Absorption: Rapid and readily absorbed; Immediate release: >90%

Distribution: V_d: 1.21 L/kg; widely distributed; 45% of the plasma concentration in CSF

Metabolism: Metabolized by cytochrome P450 isozymes from the CYP3A family to hydroxylated metabolites; autoinduction of metabolism occurs in 2-4 weeks with a 1.5-2 times increase in clearance; nevirapine is more rapidly metabolized in pediatric patients than in adults

Protein binding, plasma: 60%

Bioavailability:

Single dose: Immediate release: 93%; Extended release (relative to immediate release): 75%; Oral solution: 91%

Multiple dose: Extended release (relative to immediate release): Fasted conditions: 80%; fed conditions: 94%

Half-life: Adults: Single dose (45 hours); multiple dosing (25-30 hours)

Time to peak serum concentration: Immediate release: 4 hours; Extended release: ~24 hours

Elimination: 81.3% in urine as metabolites, 10.1% in feces; <3% of the total dose is eliminated in urine as parent drug

Clearance: Women have a 13.8% lower clearance compared to men; body size does not totally explain the gender difference

Dosing: Neonatal

HIV infection, treatment: Use in combination with other antiretroviral agents: **Note:** If patient experiences a nonsevere rash (in the absence of transaminase elevations) during the first 14 days of therapy, do not increase dose until rash has resolved. If rash continues beyond 28 days, use an alternative regimen. Discontinue nevirapine if severe rash, rash with constitutional symptoms, or rash with elevated hepatic transaminases occurs. If nevirapine therapy is interrupted for >14 days, restart at the initial recommended dose (ie, once daily for the first 14 days) before increasing to twice daily dosing (DHHS [pediatric], 2014).

PNA ≤14 days: Treatment dose is not defined.

PNA ≥15 days: Oral: Immediate release:

Manufacturer's labeling: Initial: 150 mg/m²/dose (maximum: 200 mg/dose) once daily for the first 14 days of therapy; increase to 150 mg/m²/dose twice daily if no rash or other adverse effects occur; maximum dose: 200 mg/dose every 12 hours

AIDS*Info* pediatric guidelines: Initial: 200 mg/m²/dose (maximum: 200 mg/dose) once daily for the first 14 days of therapy; increase to 200 mg/m²/dose (maximum: 200 mg/dose) twice daily if no rash or other adverse effects occur (DHHS [pediatric], 2014)

Prevention of perinatal HIV transmission: [DHHS (perinatal), 2014]; **Note:** Nevirapine is used in combination with a 6-week course of zidovudine in select situations (eg, infants born to HIV-infected mothers with no antiretroviral therapy prior to labor or during labor or infants born to mothers with only intrapartum antiretroviral therapy); and may be considered in other situations (eg, infants born to mothers with suboptimal viral suppression at delivery or infants born to mothers with known antiretroviral drug-resistant virus).

Newborn: Oral: Immediate release: Administer **three** doses of nevirapine within the first week of life; administer the first dose as soon as possible after birth, but within 48 hours (birth to 48 hours); administer the second dose 48 hours after the first dose; administer the third dose 96 hours after the second dose:

Fixed dose:

Birthweight 1.5 to 2 kg: 8 mg

Birthweight >2 kg: 12 mg

Dosing: Usual

Pediatric: **HIV infection, treatment:** Use in combination with other antiretroviral agents: **Note:** If patient experiences a nonsevere rash (in the absence of transaminase elevations) during the first 14 days of therapy, do not increase dose until rash has resolved. If rash continues beyond 28 days, use an alternative regimen. Discontinue nevirapine if severe rash, rash with constitutional symptoms, or rash with elevated hepatic transaminases occurs. **Note:** If nevirapine therapy is interrupted for >7 days (adults/adolescents) or >14 days (infants/children), restart at the initial recommended dose (ie, once daily for the first 14 days) before increasing to twice daily dosing (DHHS [adult, pediatric], 2014).

Manufacturer's labeling: Oral:

Immediate release: Infants, Children, and Adolescents: Initial: 150 mg/m²/dose (maximum: 200 mg/dose) once daily for the first 14 days of therapy; increase to 150 mg/m²/dose (maximum: 200 mg/dose) twice daily if no rash or other adverse effects occur

Extended release: Children ≥6 years and Adolescents (must be able to swallow tablets whole): **Note:** Maintenance therapy using the extended release tablet must follow a 14-day initial dosing period (lead-in) using the immediate release formulation, unless the patient is already maintained on a nevirapine immediate release regimen. Extended release tablets should not be divided to achieve daily dose.

BSA 0.58 to 0.83 m²: 200 mg once daily

BSA 0.84 to 1.16 m²: 300 mg once daily

BSA ≥1.17 m²: 400 mg once daily

AIDS*Info* guidelines (DHHS [pediatric], 2014): Oral:

Immediate release:

Infants and Children <8 years: Initial (lead-in dosing): 200 mg/m²/dose (maximum: 200 mg/dose) once daily for the first 14 days of therapy; increase to 200 mg/m²/dose (maximum: 200 mg/dose) twice daily if no rash or other adverse effects occur; maximum dose: 200 mg twice daily

Children ≥8 years: Initial (lead-in dosing): 120 to 150 mg/m²/dose (maximum: 200 mg/dose) once daily for the first 14 days of therapy; increase to 120 to 150 mg/m²/dose (maximum: 200 mg/dose) twice daily if no rash or other adverse effects occur

Note: In a growing child, do not decrease the mg dose when the child reaches 8 years; leave the mg dose the same to achieve the appropriate mg/m²/dose as the child grows larger (as long as there are no adverse effects)

Adolescents: Initial: 200 mg/dose once daily for the first 14 days; increase to 200 mg every 12 hours if no rash or other adverse effects occur; if patient able to swallow tablets whole, may convert maintenance dose to the extended release formulation (400 mg once daily)

Extended release: Children >6 years and Adolescents (must be able to swallow tablets whole): For patients already on full-dose nevirapine, may initiate extended release preparation without lead-in dosing as long as viral load is undetectable. If initiating nevirapine therapy, begin with the age-appropriate once daily dose of the *immediate release* formulation for the first 14 days of therapy; at 14 days, if no rash or other adverse effects have occurred, increase dose to the age-appropriate dose administered once daily for the extended release formulation; maximum daily dose: 400 mg/**day**

BSA 0.58 to 0.83 m²: 200 mg once daily

BSA 0.84 to 1.16 m²: 300 mg once daily

BSA ≥1.17 m²: 400 mg once daily

Adult: **HIV infection, treatment:** Use in combination with other antiretroviral agents; **Note:** Therapy in antiretroviral-naive patients should not be initiated in patients with elevated CD4⁺ cell counts unless the benefit of therapy outweighs the risk of serious hepatotoxicity (adult/postpubertal females: CD4⁺ cell counts >250 cells/mm³; adult males: CD4⁺ cell counts >400 cells/mm³).

Initial: Immediate release: Oral: 200 mg once daily for the first 14 days

Maintenance:

Immediate release: Oral: 200 mg twice daily if no rash or other adverse effects occur during initial dosing period

Extended release: Oral: 400 mg once daily; **Note:** Maintenance therapy using the extended release tablet must follow a 14-day initial dosing period (lead-in) using the immediate release formulation, unless the patient is already maintained on a nevirapine immediate release regimen.

Dosing adjustment in renal impairment: Adult:

CrCl ≥20 mL/minute: No dosage adjustment required

CrCl <20 mL/minute: There are no dosage adjustments provided in the manufacturer's labeling; however, the following guidelines have been used by some clinicians: No dosage adjustment required

Hemodialysis: An additional 200 mg dose of immediate release tablet is recommended following dialysis. **Note:** Nevirapine metabolites may accumulate in patients on dialysis (clinical significance is unknown)

Dosing adjustment in hepatic impairment:

Mild impairment (Child-Pugh class A): There are no dosage adjustments provided in manufacturer's labeling; use with caution; monitor for symptoms of drug-induced toxicity (increased trough concentrations have been observed in some patients with hepatic fibrosis or cirrhosis).

Moderate to severe impairment (Child-Pugh class B or C): Use is contraindicated; permanently discontinue if symptomatic hepatic events occur.

Administration Hazardous agent; use appropriate precautions for handling and disposal (NIOSH 2014 [group 2]).

Oral:

Immediate release: May be administered with water, milk, or soda, with or without meals; may be administered with an antacid or didanosine. Shake suspension gently prior to administration; the use of an oral dosing syringe is recommended, especially if the dose is <5 mL; if using a dosing cup, after administration, rinse cup with water and also administer rinse.

Extended release: May be administered with or without food; swallow tablet whole; do not chew, crush, or divide.

Monitoring Parameters Note: Monitor CD4 percentage (if <5 years of age) or CD4 count (if ≥5 years of age) at least every 3 to 4 months (DHHS [pediatric], 2014)

Prior to initiation of therapy: Genotypic resistance testing, CD4 and viral load (every 3 to 4 months), CBC with differential, LFTs, BUN, creatinine, electrolytes, glucose, urinalysis (every 6 to 12 months), and assessment of readiness for adherence with medication regimen. At initiation and with any change in treatment regimen: CBC with differential, electrolytes, calcium, phosphate, glucose, LFTs, bilirubin, urinalysis (at initiation), BUN, creatinine, albumin, total protein, lipid panel (at initiation), CD4, and viral load. After 1 to 2 weeks of therapy: Signs of medication toxicity and adherence. After 2 to 4 weeks of therapy: CBC with differential, viral load, signs of toxicity, and adherence; then every 3 to 4 months: CBC with differential, electrolytes, glucose, LFTs, bilirubin, BUN, creatinine, CD4, viral load, signs of medication toxicity, and adherence. Every 6 to 12 months: Lipid panel and urinalysis. CD4 monitoring frequency may be decreased to every 6 to 12 months in children who are adherent to therapy if the value is well above the threshold for opportunistic infections, viral suppression is sustained, and the clinical status is stable for more than 2 to 3 years (DHHS [pediatric], 2014). Monitor for growth and development, signs of HIV-specific physical conditions, HIV disease progression, opportunistic infections, skin rash, or hypersensitivity.

Obtain liver function tests every 2 weeks for the first 4 weeks of therapy, then monthly for 3 months, and every 3 to 4 months thereafter. Also check liver function tests immediately if patient develops signs or symptoms consistent with hepatitis or hypersensitivity reactions and immediately in all patients who develop a rash within the first 18 weeks of therapy (DHHS [pediatric], 2014).

Reference Range Plasma trough concentration: ≥3000 ng/mL (DHHS [adult, pediatric], 2014)

Dosage Forms Excipient information presented when available (limited, particularly for generics); consult specific product labeling.

Suspension, Oral:
- Viramune: 50 mg/5 mL (240 mL) [contains methylparaben, propylparaben]
- Generic: 50 mg/5 mL (240 mL)

Tablet, Oral:
- Viramune: 200 mg [scored]
- Generic: 200 mg

Tablet Extended Release 24 Hour, Oral:
- Viramune XR: 100 mg, 400 mg
- Generic: 400 mg

- ◆ **Nexafed [OTC]** *see* Pseudoephedrine *on page 1801*
- ◆ **NexIUM** *see* Esomeprazole *on page 792*
- ◆ **Nexium (Can)** *see* Esomeprazole *on page 792*
- ◆ **Nexium 24HR** *see* Esomeprazole *on page 792*
- ◆ **Nexium 24HR [OTC]** *see* Esomeprazole *on page 792*
- ◆ **NexIUM I.V.** *see* Esomeprazole *on page 792*
- ◆ **Nexterone** *see* Amiodarone *on page 125*
- ◆ **NFV** *see* Nelfinavir *on page 1497*
- ◆ **NGX-4010** *see* Capsaicin *on page 362*

Niacin (NYE a sin)

Medication Safety Issues

Sound-alike/look-alike issues:

Niacin may be confused with Minocin, niacinamide, Niaspan

Related Information

Oral Medications That Should Not Be Crushed or Altered *on page 2476*

Brand Names: US Niacin-50 [OTC]; Niacor; Niaspan; Slo-Niacin [OTC]

Brand Names: Canada Niaspan; Niaspan FCT; Niodan

Therapeutic Category Antilipemic Agent; Nutritional Supplement; Vitamin, Water Soluble

Generic Availability (US) Yes

Use Adjunctive treatment of hyperlipidemias (FDA approved in adults); adjunctive treatment of hypertriglyceridemia in patients at risk of pancreatitis (FDA approved in adults); to lower the risk of recurrent MI in patients with hyperlipidemia (FDA approved in adults); in combination with a bile acid sequestrant to slow progression (or promote regression) of atherosclerotic disease in patients with CAD and hyperlipidemia (FDA approved in adults); has also been used in the treatment of pellagra; dietary supplement; **Note:** Niacin may be used in combination with lovastatin, simvastatin, or bile acid sequestrants for treatment of hyperlipidemias in patients who fail monotherapy; combination therapy is not indicated as initial therapy

Pregnancy Risk Factor C

Pregnancy Considerations Animal reproduction studies have not been conducted. Water soluble vitamins cross the placenta. When used as a dietary supplement, niacin requirements may be increased in pregnant women compared to nonpregnant women (IOM, 1998). It is not known if niacin at lipid-lowering doses is harmful to the developing fetus. If a woman becomes pregnant while receiving niacin for primary hypercholesterolemia, niacin should be discontinued. If a woman becomes pregnant while receiving niacin for hypertriglyceridemia, the benefits and risks of continuing niacin should be assessed on an individual basis.

Breast-Feeding Considerations Niacin is excreted in breast milk. When used as a dietary supplement, niacin requirements may be increased in breast-feeding women compared to non-breast-feeding women (IOM, 1998). Due to the potential for serious adverse reactions in the breast-feeding infant, the manufacturer recommends a decision be made whether to discontinue breast-feeding or to discontinue the drug, taking into account the importance of treatment to the mother.

Contraindications Hypersensitivity to niacin, niacinamide, or any component of the formulation; active hepatic disease or significant or unexplained persistent elevations in hepatic transaminases; active peptic ulcer; arterial hemorrhage

Warnings/Precautions Prior to initiation, secondary causes for hypercholesterolemia (eg, poorly controlled diabetes mellitus, hypothyroidism) should be excluded; management with diet and other nonpharmacologic measures (eg, exercise or weight reduction) should be attempted prior to initiation. Use has not been evaluated in Fredrickson type I or III dyslipidemias. Use with caution in patients with unstable angina or in the acute phase of an MI or renal disease. In patients with pre-existing coronary artery disease, the incidence of atrial fibrillation was observed more frequently in those receiving immediate release (crystalline) niacin as compared to placebo (Coronary Drug Project Research Group, 1975). Niacin should not be used if patient experiences new-onset atrial fibrillation during therapy (Stone, 2013). Niacin may increase fasting blood glucose, although clinical data suggest increases are generally modest (<5%) (Guyton, 2007). Use niacin with caution in patients with diabetes. Monitor glucose; adjustment of diet and/or hypoglycemic therapy may be necessary. Niacin should not be used if patient experiences persistent hyperglycemia during therapy (Stone, 2013). Use with caution in patients predisposed to gout; niacin should not be used if patient experiences acute gout during therapy (Stone, 2013).

Use with caution in patients with a past history of hepatic impairment and/or who consume substantial amounts of ethanol; contraindicated with active liver disease or unexplained persistent transaminase elevation. Niacin should not be used if hepatic transaminase elevations >2 to 3 times upper limit of normal occur during therapy (Stone, 2013). Rare cases of rhabdomyolysis have occurred during concomitant use with HMG-CoA reductase inhibitors. With concurrent use or if symptoms suggestive of myopathy occur, monitor creatine phosphokinase (CPK) and potassium; use with caution in patients with renal impairment, inadequately treated hypothyroidism, patients with diabetes or the elderly; risk for myopathy and rhabdomyolysis may be increased. May cause gastrointestinal distress, vomiting, diarrhea, or aggravate peptic ulcer. Gastrointestinal distress may be attenuated with a gradual increase in dose and administration with food. Use is contraindicated in patients with active peptic ulcer disease; use with caution in patients with a past history of peptic ulcer. Niacin should not be used if patient experiences unexplained abdominal pain or gastrointestinal symptoms or unexplained weight loss during therapy (Stone, 2013). Dose-related reductions in platelet count and increases of prothrombin time may occur. Has been associated with small but statistically significant dose-related reductions in phosphorus levels. Monitor phosphorus levels periodically in patients at risk for hypophosphatemia.

Formulations of niacin (immediate release versus extended release) are not interchangeable (bioavailability varies); cases of severe hepatotoxicity, including fulminant hepatic necrosis, have occurred in patients who have substituted niacin products at equivalent doses. Patients should be initiated with low doses (eg, niacin extended release 500 mg at bedtime) with titration to achieve desired response. Flushing and pruritus, common adverse effects of niacin, may be attenuated with a gradual increase in dose, administering with food, avoidance of concurrent ingestion of ethanol or hot liquids, and/or by taking aspirin (adults: 325 mg) (Stone, 2013). May also use other NSAIDs according to the manufacturer. Flushing associated with extended release preparation is significantly reduced (Guyton, 2007). For immediate release preparations, may administer in 2 to 3 divided doses to reduce the frequency and severity. Niacin should not be used if patient experiences persistent severe cutaneous symptoms during therapy (Stone, 2013).

Potentially significant interactions may exist, requiring dose or frequency adjustment, additional monitoring, and/or selection of alternative therapy.

Adverse Reactions

Cardiovascular: Arrhythmias, atrial fibrillation, edema, flushing, hypotension, orthostasis, palpitation, syncope (rare), tachycardia

Central nervous system: Chills, dizziness, headache, insomnia, migraine, nervousness, pain

Dermatologic: Acanthosis nigricans, burning skin, dry skin, hyperpigmentation, maculopapular rash, pruritus, rash, skin discoloration, urticaria

Endocrine & metabolic: Glucose tolerance decreased, gout, phosphorous levels decreased, hyperuricemia

Gastrointestinal: Abdominal pain, amylase increased, diarrhea, dyspepsia, eructation, flatulence, nausea, peptic ulcers, vomiting

Hematologic: Platelet counts decreased

Hepatic: Hepatic necrosis (rare), hepatitis, jaundice, transaminases increased (dose-related), prothrombin time increased, total bilirubin increased

Neuromuscular & skeletal: CPK increased, leg cramps, myalgia, myasthenia, myopathy (with concurrent HMG-CoA reductase inhibitor), paresthesia, rhabdomyolysis (with concurrent HMG-CoA reductase inhibitor; rare), weakness

Ocular: Blurred vision, cystoid macular edema, toxic amblyopia

Respiratory: Cough, dyspnea

Miscellaneous: Diaphoresis, hypersensitivity reactions (rare; includes anaphylaxis, angioedema, laryngismus, vesiculobullous rash), LDH increased

Drug Interactions

Metabolism/Transport Effects None known.

Avoid Concomitant Use There are no known interactions where it is recommended to avoid concomitant use.

Increased Effect/Toxicity

Niacin may increase the levels/effects of: HMG-CoA Reductase Inhibitors

The levels/effects of Niacin may be increased by: Alcohol (Ethyl)

Decreased Effect

Niacin may decrease the levels/effects of: Antidiabetic Agents

The levels/effects of Niacin may be decreased by: Bile Acid Sequestrants

Storage/Stability

Niaspan: Store at 20°C to 25°C (68°F to 77°F).

Niacor: Store at 15°C to 30°C (59°F to 86°F).

Mechanism of Action Niacin (nicotinic acid) is bioconverted to nicotinamide which is further converted to nicotinamide adenine dinucleotide (NAD+) and the hydride equivalent (NADH) which are coenzymes necessary for tissue metabolism, lipid metabolism, and glycogenolysis (Belenky, 2006; Suave, 2008). The mechanism by which niacin (in lipid-lowering doses) affects plasma lipoproteins is not fully understood. It may involve several actions including partial inhibition of release of free fatty acids from adipose tissue, and increased lipoprotein lipase activity, which may increase the rate of chylomicron triglyceride removal from plasma. Ultimately, niacin reduces total cholesterol, apolipoprotein (apo) B, triglycerides, VLDL, LDL, lipoprotein (a), and increases HDL and other important components and subfractions (eg, LPA-I) (Kamanna, 2000)

Pharmacodynamics Vasodilation:

Onset of action: Within 20 minutes

Extended release: Within 1 hour

Duration: 20-60 minutes

Extended release: 8-10 hours

Pharmacokinetics (Adult data unless noted)

Absorption: Oral: Rapid and extensive; ≥60% to 76% of dose is absorbed

Distribution: Crosses into breast milk

Metabolism: Extensive first-pass effect; niacin in smaller doses is converted to niacinamide which is metabolized in the liver; niacin undergoes conjugation with glycine to form nicotinuric acid; nicotinamide, nicotinamide adenine dinucleotide (NAD), and other niacin metabolites are formed via saturable pathways; **Note:** It is not clear whether nicotinamide is formed before or after the synthesis of NAD

Bioavailability: Single dose studies indicate that only certain Niaspan® tablet strengths are interchangeable (ie, two 500 mg tablets are equivalent to one 1000 mg tablet; however, three 500 mg tablets are **not** equivalent to two 750 mg tablets)

Half-life: 45 minutes

Time to peak serum concentration: Immediate release: ~45 minutes; extended release: 4-5 hours

Elimination: In urine, with ~33% as unchanged drug; with larger doses, a greater percentage is excreted unchanged in urine

Dosing: Neonatal Oral: Adequate intake: 2 mg/day

Dosing: Usual Note: Formulations of niacin (immediate release versus extended release) are not interchangeable.

Oral:

Infants, Children, and Adolescents:

Adequate intake:

1-5 months: 2 mg/day

6-11 months: 3 mg/day

Recommended daily allowances:

1-3 years: 6 mg/day

4-8 years: 8 mg/day

9-13 years: 12 mg/day

14-18 years: Female: 14 mg/day; Male: 16 mg/day

≥19 years: Refer to adult dosing

Children and Adolescents:

Hyperlipidemia: Initial: **Note:** Routine use is not recommended due to limited safety and efficacy information: 100-250 mg/day (maximum dose: 10 mg/kg/day) in 3 divided doses with meals; increase weekly by 100 mg/day or increase every 2-3 weeks by 250 mg/day as tolerated; evaluate efficacy and adverse effects with laboratory tests at 20 mg/kg/day or 1000 mg/day (whichever is less); continue to increase if needed and as tolerated; re-evaluate at each 500 mg increment; doses up to 2250 mg/day have been used

Pellagra: 50-100 mg/dose 3 times/day (some experts prefer niacinamide for treatment due to a more favorable side effect profile)

Adults:

Recommended daily allowances (RDA) (National Academy of Sciences, 1998):

≥19 years: Female: 14 mg/day; Male: 16 mg/day

Pregnancy (all ages): 18 mg/day

Lactation (all ages): 17 mg/day

Dietary supplement: 50 mg twice daily or 100 mg once daily. **Note:** Many over-the-counter formulations exist.

Hyperlipidemia:

Immediate release formulation (Niacor®): Initial: 250 mg once daily (with evening meal); increase frequency and/or dose every 4-7 days to desired response or first-level therapeutic dose (1.5-2 g/day in 2-3 divided doses); after 2 months, may increase at 2- to 4-week intervals to 3 g/day in 3 divided doses [maximum dose: 6 g/day (NCEP recommends 4.5 g/day) in 3 divided doses]. Usual daily dose after titration (NCEP, 2002): 1.5-3 g/day; **Note:** Many over-the-counter formulations exist.

Sustained release (or controlled release) formulations: Usual daily dose after titration (NCEP, 2002): 1-2 g/day; **Note:** Several over-the-counter formulations exist.

Extended release formulation (Niaspan®): Initial: 500 mg at bedtime for 4 weeks, then 1 g at bedtime for 4 weeks; adjust dose to response and tolerance; may increase dose every 4 weeks by 500 mg/day to a maximum of 2 g/day. Usual daily dose after titration (NCEP, 2002): 1-2 g once daily

If additional LDL-lowering is necessary with lovastatin or simvastatin: Recommended initial lovastatin or simvastatin dose: 20 mg/day; Maximum lovastatin or simvastatin dose: 40 mg/day; **Note:** Lovastatin prescribing information recommends a maximum dose of 20 mg/day with concurrent use of niacin (>1 g/day).

Pellagra: 50-100 mg 3-4 times/day, maximum dose: 500 mg/day (some experts prefer niacinamide for treatment due to more favorable side effect profile)

Dosage adjustment in renal impairment: Studies have not been performed; use with caution

Dosage adjustment in hepatic impairment: Contraindicated in patients with active liver disease, unexplained liver enzyme elevations, significant or unexplained hepatic dysfunction. Use with caution in patients with history of liver disease or those with suspected liver disease (eg, those who consume large quantities of alcohol).

Administration Oral: Administer with food or milk to decrease GI upset; administer Niaspan® with a low-fat snack (do not administer on an empty stomach). Swallow timed release tablet and capsule whole; do not break, chew, or crush. To minimize flushing, administer dose at bedtime, take aspirin (adults: 325 mg) 30 minutes before niacin, and avoid alcohol, hot drinks, or spicy food around the time of administration. Separate administration of bile acid sequestrants by at least 4-6 hours (bile acid sequestrants may decrease the absorption of niacin).

Monitoring Parameters

2013 ACC/AHA Blood Cholesterol Guideline recommendations (Stone, 2013): Baseline hepatic transaminases, fasting blood glucose or hemoglobin A_{1c}, and uric acid before initiation and repeat during uptitration to maintenance dose and every 6 months thereafter.

Manufacturer recommendations: Blood glucose (in diabetic patients); if on concurrent HMG-CoA reductase inhibitor, may periodically check CPK and serum potassium; liver function tests pretreatment, every 6 to 12 weeks for first year, then periodically (approximately every 6 months), monitor liver function more frequently if history of transaminase elevation with prior use; lipid profile; platelets (if on anticoagulants); PT (if on anticoagulants); uric acid (if predisposed to gout); phosphorus (if predisposed to hypophosphatemia)

Test Interactions False elevations in some fluorometric determinations of plasma or urinary catecholamines; false-positive urine glucose (Benedict's reagent)

Dosage Forms Excipient information presented when available (limited, particularly for generics); consult specific product labeling.

Capsule Extended Release, Oral:

Generic: 250 mg, 500 mg

Capsule Extended Release, Oral [preservative free]:

Generic: 250 mg, 500 mg

Tablet, Oral:

Niacin-50: 50 mg [starch free, sugar free, wheat free]

Niacor: 500 mg [scored]

Generic: 50 mg, 100 mg, 250 mg, 500 mg

Tablet, Oral [preservative free]:

Generic: 50 mg, 100 mg, 500 mg

Tablet Extended Release, Oral:

Niaspan: 500 mg, 750 mg, 1000 mg [contains fd&c yellow #6 aluminum lake]

Slo-Niacin: 250 mg [scored]

Slo-Niacin: 500 mg, 750 mg [scored; contains fd&c red #40]

Generic: 500 mg, 750 mg, 1000 mg

Tablet Extended Release, Oral [preservative free]:

Generic: 250 mg, 500 mg, 1000 mg

◆ **Niacin-50 [OTC]** *see* Niacin *on page* 1511

◆ **Niacor** *see* Niacin *on page* 1511

◆ **Niaspan** *see* Niacin *on page* 1511

◆ **Niaspan FCT (Can)** *see* Niacin *on page* 1511

◆ **Niastase (Can)** *see* Factor VIIa (Recombinant) *on page* 835

◆ **Niastase RT (Can)** *see* Factor VIIa (Recombinant) *on page* 835

NiCARdipine (nye KAR de peen)

Medication Safety Issues

Sound-alike/look-alike issues:

NiCARdipine may be confused with niacinamide, NIFEdipine, niMODipine

Cardene may be confused with Cardizem, Cardura, codeine

Administration issues:

Significant differences exist between oral and IV dosing. Use caution when converting from one route of administration to another.

International issues:

Cardene [U.S., Great Britain, Netherlands] may be confused with Cardem brand name for celiprolol [Spain]; Cardin brand name for simvastatin [Poland]

Related Information

Oral Medications That Should Not Be Crushed or Altered *on page 2476*

Brand Names: US Cardene IV; Cardene SR [DSC]

Therapeutic Category Antianginal Agent; Antihypertensive Agent; Calcium Channel Blocker; Calcium Channel Blocker, Dihydropyridine

Generic Availability (US) May be product dependent

Use

Oral:

Immediate release product: Treatment of chronic stable angina and treatment of hypertension (FDA approved in adults)

Sustained release product: Treatment of hypertension (FDA approved in adults)

Parenteral: Short-term treatment of hypertension when oral treatment is not feasible (FDA approved in adults)

Pregnancy Risk Factor C

Pregnancy Considerations Adverse events were observed in some animal reproduction studies. Nicardipine has been used for the treatment of severe hypertension in pregnancy and preterm labor. Nicardipine crosses the placenta; changes in fetal heart rate, neonatal hypotension and neonatal acidosis have been observed following maternal use (rare; based on limited data). Adverse effects reported in pregnant women are generally similar to those reported in nonpregnant patients; however, pulmonary edema has been observed (Nij, 2010). Untreated chronic maternal hypertension is also associated with adverse events in the fetus, infant, and mother. If treatment for hypertension during pregnancy is needed, other agents are preferred (ACOG, 2013).

Breast-Feeding Considerations Nicardipine is minimally excreted into breast milk. Per the manufacturer, the possibility of infant exposure should be considered. In one study, peak milk concentrations ranged from 1.9-18.8 mcg/mL following oral maternal doses of 40-150 mg/day. The estimated exposure to the breast-feeding infant was calculated to be 0.073% of the weight-adjusted maternal oral dose or 0.14% of the weight-adjusted maternal IV dose. Adverse events were not noted in the infants.

Contraindications Hypersensitivity to nicardipine or any component of the formulation; advanced aortic stenosis

Warnings/Precautions Symptomatic hypotension with or without syncope can rarely occur; blood pressure must be lowered at a rate appropriate for the patient's clinical condition. Close monitoring of blood pressure and heart rate is required. Reflex tachycardia may occur resulting in angina and/or MI in patients with obstructive coronary disease especially in the absence of concurrent beta blockade. The most common side effect is peripheral edema (dose-dependent); occurs within 2-3 weeks of starting therapy. Use with caution in CAD (can cause increase in angina), aortic stenosis (may reduce coronary perfusion resulting in ischemia; use is contraindicated in patients with advanced aortic stenosis), and hypertrophic cardiomyopathy with outflow tract obstruction. The ACCF/AHA heart failure guidelines recommend to avoid use in patients with heart failure due to lack of benefit and/or worse outcomes with calcium channel blockers in general (Yancy, 2013). To minimize infusion site reactions, peripheral infusion sites (for IV therapy) should be changed every 12 hours; use of small peripheral veins should be avoided. Titrate IV dose cautiously in patients with renal or hepatic dysfunction. Use the IV form cautiously in patients with portal hypertension (can cause increase in hepatic pressure gradient). Initiate at the low end of the dosage range in the elderly. Some dosage forms may contain propylene glycol; large amounts are potentially toxic and have been associated hyperosmolality, lactic acidosis, seizures and respiratory depression; use caution (AAP, 1997; Zar, 2007).

Adverse Reactions

Cardiovascular: Chest pain (IV), edema, exacerbation of angina pectoris (dose related), extrasystoles (IV), flushing, hemopericardium (IV), hypertension (IV), hypotension (IV), palpitations, pedal edema (dose related), supraventricular tachycardia (IV), tachycardia

Central nervous system: Dizziness, headache, hypoesthesia, intracranial hemorrhage, pain, somnolence

Dermatologic: Diaphoresis, skin rash

Endocrine & metabolic: Hypokalemia (IV)

Gastrointestinal: Abdominal pain (IV), dyspepsia, nausea, nausea and vomiting (IV), xerostomia

Genitourinary: Hematuria

Local: Injection site reaction (IV), pain at injection site (IV)

Neuromuscular & skeletal: Myalgia, paresthesia, weakness

Rare but important or life-threatening: Abnormal dreams, abnormal hepatic function tests, abnormal vision, angina pectoris, arthralgia, atrial fibrillation (not distinguishable from natural history of atherosclerotic vascular disease), cerebral ischemia (not distinguishable from natural history of atherosclerotic vascular disease), conjunctivitis, deep vein thrombophlebitis, depression, ECG abnormal, gingival hyperplasia, heart block (not distinguishable from natural history of atherosclerotic vascular disease), hot flash, hyperkinesia, hypersensitivity reaction, hypertonia, hypophosphatemia, hypotension (exertional; not distinguishable from natural history of atherosclerotic vascular disease), myocardial infarction (chronic therapy; may be due to disease progression), neck pain, nervousness, oxygen saturation decreased (possible pulmonary shunting), parotitis, pericarditis (not distinguishable from natural history of atherosclerotic vascular disease), peripheral vascular disease, respiratory tract disease, sinus node dysfunction (chronic therapy; may be due to disease progression), sustained tachycardia, thrombocytopenia, tinnitus, tremor, urinary frequency, ventricular extrasystoles, ventricular tachycardia, vertigo

Drug Interactions

Metabolism/Transport Effects Substrate of CYP1A2 (minor), CYP2C9 (minor), CYP2D6 (minor), CYP2E1 (minor), CYP3A4 (major), P-glycoprotein; **Note:** Assignment of Major/Minor substrate status based on clinically relevant drug interaction potential; **Inhibits** CYP2C19 (moderate), CYP2C9 (strong), CYP2D6 (moderate), CYP3A4 (weak), P-glycoprotein

Avoid Concomitant Use

Avoid concomitant use of NiCARdipine with any of the following: Bosutinib; Conivaptan; Fusidic Acid (Systemic); Idelalisib; PAZOPanib; Pimozide; Silodosin; Thioridazine; Topotecan; VinCRIStine (Liposomal)

Increased Effect/Toxicity

NiCARdipine may increase the levels/effects of: Afatinib; Amifostine; Antihypertensives; ARIPiprazole; Atosiban; Bosentan; Bosutinib; Brentuximab Vedotin; Calcium Channel Blockers (Nondihydropyridine); Carvedilol; Cilostazol; Citalopram; Colchicine; CYP2C19 Substrates; CYP2C9 Substrates; CYP2D6 Substrates; Dabigatran Etexilate; Diclofenac (Systemic); DOXOrubicin (Conventional); Dronabinol; DULoxetine; Edoxaban; Eliglustat; Everolimus; Fesoterodine; Fosphenytoin; Highest Risk QTc-Prolonging Agents; Hydrocodone; Hypotensive Agents; Lacosamide; Ledipasvir; Levodopa; Lomitapide;

Magnesium Salts; Metoprolol; Moderate Risk QTc-Prolonging Agents; Naloxegol; Nebivolol; Neuromuscular-Blocking Agents (Nondepolarizing); NiMODipine; Nitroprusside; Obinutuzumab; Ospemifene; Parecoxib; PAZOPanib; P-glycoprotein/ABCB1 Substrates; Phenytoin; Pimozide; Prucalopride; Ramelteon; Rifaximin; RisperiDONE; RiTUXimab; Rivaroxaban; Silodosin; Tacrolimus (Systemic); Tetrahydrocannabinol; Thioridazine; Topotecan; VinCRIStine (Liposomal)

The levels/effects of NiCARdipine may be increased by: Alfuzosin; Alpha1-Blockers; Antifungal Agents (Azole Derivatives, Systemic); Aprepitant; Barbiturates; Brimonidine (Topical); Calcium Channel Blockers (Nondihydropyridine); Cannabis; Conivaptan; CycloSPORINE (Systemic); CYP3A4 Inhibitors (Moderate); CYP3A4 Inhibitors (Strong); Dapoxetine; Dasatinib; Diazoxide; Fluconazole; Fosaprepitant; Fusidic Acid (Systemic); Grapefruit Juice; Herbs (Hypotensive Properties); Idelalisib; Ivacaftor; Luliconazole; Macrolide Antibiotics; Magnesium Salts; MAO Inhibitors; Mifepristone; Netupitant; Nicorandil; Palbociclib; Pentoxifylline; P-glycoprotein/ABCB1 Inhibitors; Phosphodiesterase 5 Inhibitors; Propafenone; Prostacyclin Analogues; Protease Inhibitors; Simeprevir; Stiripentol

Decreased Effect

NiCARdipine may decrease the levels/effects of: Clopidogrel; Codeine; Tamoxifen; TraMADol

The levels/effects of NiCARdipine may be decreased by: Barbiturates; Bosentan; Calcium Salts; CarBAMazepine; CYP3A4 Inducers (Moderate); CYP3A4 Inducers (Strong); Dabrafenib; Deferasirox; Efavirenz; Herbs (Hypertensive Properties); Melatonin; Methylphenidate; Mitotane; Nafcillin; P-glycoprotein/ABCB1 Inducers; Rifamycin Derivatives; Siltuximab; St Johns Wort; Tocilizumab; Yohimbine

Food Interactions Nicardipine average peak concentrations may be decreased if taken with food. Serum concentrations/toxicity of nicardipine may be increased by grapefruit juice. Management: Avoid grapefruit juice.

Storage/Stability

IV:

Premixed bags: Store at controlled room temperature of 20°C to 25°C (68°F to 77°F). Protect from light and excessive heat. Do not freeze.

Vials: Store at controlled room temperature of 20°C to 25°C (68°F to 77°F). Protect from light. Diluted solution (0.1 mg/mL) is stable at room temperature for 24 hours in glass or PVC containers. Stability has also been demonstrated at room temperature at concentrations up to 0.5 mg/mL in PVC containers for 24 hours or in glass containers for up to 7 days (Baaske, 1996).

Oral (Cardene®, Cardene SR®): Store at 15°C to 30°C (59°F to 86°F). Protect from light. Freezing does not affect stability.

Mechanism of Action Inhibits calcium ion from entering the "slow channels" or select voltage-sensitive areas of vascular smooth muscle and myocardium during depolarization, producing a relaxation of coronary vascular smooth muscle and coronary vasodilation; increases myocardial oxygen delivery in patients with vasospastic angina

Pharmacodynamics Antihypertensive effects:

Onset of action:

IV: Within minutes

Oral: 0.5-2 hours

Maximum effect:

Immediate capsules: 1-2 hours

Sustained release capsules (at steady state): Sustained from 2-6 hours postdose

IV continuous infusion: 50% of the maximum effect is seen by 45 minutes

Duration:

Immediate release capsules: <8 hours

Sustained release capsules: 12 hours

IV: ≤8 hours

Continuous infusion: Upon discontinuation, a 50% decrease in effect is seen in ~30 minutes with gradual discontinuing antihypertensive effects for ~50 hours.

Pharmacokinetics (Adult data unless noted) Absorption: Oral: ~100%, but large first-pass effect

Distribution: V_d: Adults: 8.3 L/kg

Protein binding: >95%

Metabolism: Extensive, saturable, first-pass effect; dose-dependent (nonlinear) pharmacokinetics; extensive hepatic metabolism; major pathway is via cytochrome P450 isoenzyme CYP3A4

Bioavailability: Oral: 35%

Half-life: Follows dose-dependent (nonlinear) pharmacokinetics; "apparent" or calculated half-life is dependant upon serum concentrations. Half-life over the first 8 hours after oral dosing is 2-4 hours; terminal half-life (oral): 8.6 hours. After IV infusion, serum concentrations decrease tri-exponentially; alpha half-life: 2.7 minutes; beta half-life: 44.8 minutes; terminal half-life: 14.4 hours (**Note:** Terminal half-life can only be seen after long-term infusions)

Time to peak serum concentration: Oral:

Immediate release capsule: 30-120 minutes (mean: 1 hour)

Sustained release capsule: 1-4 hours

Elimination: Urine (oral: 60% as metabolites; IV: 49% as metabolites; <1% as unchanged drug); feces (oral: 35%; IV: 43%)

Clearance: Decreased in patients with hepatic dysfunction; may be decreased in patients with renal impairment

Dosing: Neonatal Note: Oral and IV doses are **not** equivalent on a mg per mg basis; limited data available.

Hypertension: Continuous IV infusion: Initial: 0.5 mcg/kg/minute was used in one prospective, open-label study of 20 hypertensive neonates (15 preterm; median PNA: 15 days). Doses were titrated according to blood pressure; the mean maximal required dose was 0.74 ± 0.41 mcg/kg/minute (range: 0.5-2 mcg/kg/minute) and occurred at 12 ± 19 hours of nicardipine infusion. The median duration of treatment was 11 days (range: 2-43 days) (Milou, 2000). Similar doses were required in a smaller study of eight preterm infants and in one case report of a neonate who received ECMO therapy (Gouyon, 1997; McBride, 2003).

Dosing: Usual Note: Oral and IV doses are **not** equivalent on a mg per mg basis.

Infants, Children, and Adolescents: **Hypertension:**

Continuous IV infusion: **Note:** Use should be reserved for severe hypertension: Limited data available: Initial: 0.5-1 mcg/kg/minute; titrate dose according to blood pressure; rate of infusion may be increased every 15-30 minutes; usual dose: 1-3 mcg/kg/minute; maximum dose: 4-5 mcg/kg/minute (Flynn, 2000; Flynn, 2001; NHBPEP, 2004). In a retrospective analysis (n=29; mean age: 7.8 years; age range: 2 days to 18 years), the mean effective dose was 1.8 ± 0.3 mcg/kg/minute (range: 0.3-4 mcg/kg/minute); blood pressure was controlled within 2.7 ± 2.1 hours (range: 0.5-9 hours) after starting nicardipine continuous infusion (Flynn, 2001).

Alternate dosing (high dose): Infants and Children: Initial dose: 5 mcg/kg/minute; once blood pressure controlled, decrease to a lower maintenance dose. Mean maintenance doses reported: PICU patients (n=10): 2.4 mcg/kg/minute (range: 1-5 mcg/kg/minute); postop cardiac patients (n=9, age range: 6 days to 9 years; mean age: 3.3 years): 3 mcg/kg/minute (range: 2.1-5.5 mcg/kg/minute) (Tobias, 2001)

Oral: Adolescents: Very limited data available; dose not established: One case report used 20 mg every 8 hours in a 14-year old boy following cardiac transplant (Larsen, 1994). Another case transitioned from a continuous infusion (1-4 mcg/kg/minute) to oral dose of 30 mg every 8 hours in a 14-year old girl with renal disease (Michael, 1998).

Adults:

Angina: Immediate release: Oral: 20 mg 3 times daily; usual range: 60-120 mg/day; increase dose at 3-day intervals

Hypertension: Oral:

Immediate release: Initial: 20 mg 3 times daily; titrate to response; usual: 20-40 mg 3 times daily (allow 3 days between dose increases)

Sustained release: Initial: 30 mg twice daily, titrate up to 60 mg twice daily

Note: The total daily dose of immediate release product may not automatically be equivalent to the daily sustained release dose; use caution in converting.

Acute hypertension: IV: Initial: 5 mg/hour increased by 2.5 mg/hour every 5 minutes (for rapid titration) to every 15 minutes (for gradual titration) up to a maximum of 15 mg/hour; rapidly titrated patients, consider reduction to 3 mg/hour after response is achieved.

Substitution for oral nicardipine therapy (approximate equivalents):

Oral dose of 20 mg every 8 hours = 0.5 mg/hour IV infusion

Oral dose of 30 mg every 8 hours = 1.2 mg/hour IV infusion

Oral dose of 40 mg every 8 hours = 2.2 mg/hour IV infusion

Conversion to oral antihypertensive agent:

Oral antihypertensive other than nicardipine: Initiate at the same time that IV nicardipine is discontinued

Oral nicardipine: Initiate 1 hour prior to IV discontinuation

Dosing adjustment in renal impairment: Adults:

IV: There are no dosage adjustments provided in the manufacturer's labeling; titrate slowly; careful monitoring is warranted and dosing adjustment may be necessary.

Oral: Titrate dose carefully beginning with usual initial dose.

Dosing adjustment in hepatic impairment: Adults:

IV: There are no dosage adjustments provided in the manufacturer's labeling; however, nicardipine is extensively metabolized by the liver. Consider initiating at lower doses and titrating slowly; careful monitoring is warranted and dosing adjustment may be necessary.

Oral:

Immediate release: Initial dose: 20 mg twice daily; titrate dose carefully

Sustained release: There are no dosage adjustments provided in the manufacturer's labeling (has not been studied); however, nicardipine is extensively metabolized by the liver; use with caution; titrate dose slowly; careful monitoring is warranted and dosing adjustment may be necessary.

Usual Infusion Concentrations: Pediatric Note: Premixed solutions available

IV infusion: 100 **mcg**/mL **or** 500 **mcg**/mL

Preparation for Administration IV: Vial: Must be diluted prior to administration; may dilute with D_5W, D_5W with KCl 40 mEq, D_5NS, $D_5\frac{1}{2}NS$, NS, $\frac{1}{2}NS$; manufacturer recommended concentration for infusion: 100 mcg/mL; **Note:** One pediatric study used infusions of 500 mcg/mL in D_5W, NS, or other compatible solution (Flynn 2001).

Administration

Oral: May be administered without regard to meals; avoid concurrent administration with high-fat meals. Swallow sustained release capsule whole; do not crush, break, or chew.

IV: Administer by slow IV continuous infusion through a central line or large peripheral vein; avoid extravasation. Peripheral infusion sites should be changed every 12 hours to minimize venous irritation.

Vial: Must be diluted prior to administration

Premixed solution: No further dilution needed. For single use only, discard any unused portion. Use only if solution is clear; per manufacturer's labeling, do not to admix or run in the same line as other medications.

Monitoring Parameters Blood pressure, heart rate, hepatic and renal function; **Note:** Monitor blood pressure carefully during initiation of therapy and with dosage adjustments.

Immediate release product: Measure blood pressure at peak effects (1-2 hours after the dose) especially during initiation of therapy, and just prior to the next dose (to ensure control of blood pressure throughout dosing interval).

Sustained release product: Measure blood pressure 2-4 hours after the first dose or dosage increase and just prior to the next dose

IV: Monitor infusion site for extravasation; monitor blood pressure continuously during IV administration

Additional Information The sustained release capsule contains a powder component (containing 25% of the dose) and a spherical granule component (containing 75% of the dose). The IV product is buffered to a pH of 3.5.

Dosage Forms Excipient information presented when available (limited, particularly for generics); consult specific product labeling. [DSC] = Discontinued product

Capsule, Oral, as hydrochloride:

Generic: 20 mg, 30 mg

Capsule Extended Release 12 Hour, Oral, as hydrochloride:

Cardene SR: 30 mg [DSC] [contains fd&c red #40]

Cardene SR: 60 mg [DSC] [contains fd&c blue #2 (indigotine)]

Solution, Intravenous, as hydrochloride:

Cardene IV: 20 mg (200 mL); 40 mg (200 mL); 2.5 mg/mL (10 mL [DSC])

Generic: 2.5 mg/mL (10 mL)

◆ **Nicardipine Hydrochloride** *see* NiCARdipine *on page 1513*

◆ **NicAzelDoxy 30 [DSC]** *see* Doxycycline *on page 717*

◆ **NicAzelDoxy 60 [DSC]** *see* Doxycycline *on page 717*

◆ **Nicotinic Acid** *see* Niacin *on page 1511*

◆ **Nidagel (Can)** *see* MetroNIDAZOLE (Topical) *on page 1425*

◆ **Nifediac CC** *see* NIFEdipine *on page 1516*

◆ **Nifedical XL** *see* NIFEdipine *on page 1516*

NIFEdipine (nye FED i peen)

Medication Safety Issues

Sound-alike/look-alike issues:

NIFEdipine may be confused with niCARdipine, niMODipine, nisoldipine

Procardia XL may be confused with Cartia XT

BEERS Criteria medication:

This drug may be potentially inappropriate for use in geriatric patients (Quality of evidence - high; Strength of recommendation - strong).

International issues:

Depin [India] may be confused with Depen brand name for penicillamine [US]; Depon brand name for acetaminophen [Greece]; Dipen brand name for diltiazem [Greece]

Nipin [Italy and Singapore] may be confused with Nipent brand name for pentostatin [US, Canada, and multiple international markets]

Related Information

Oral Medications That Should Not Be Crushed or Altered *on page 2476*

Brand Names: US Adalat CC; Afeditab CR; Nifediac CC; Nifedical XL; Procardia; Procardia XL

Brand Names: Canada Adalat XL; Apo-Nifed PA; Mylan-Nifedipine Extended Release; Nifedipine ER; PMS-Nifedipine; PMS-Nifedipine ER

Therapeutic Category Antianginal Agent; Antihypertensive Agent; Calcium Channel Blocker; Calcium Channel Blocker, Dihydropyridine

Generic Availability (US) Yes

Use

Immediate release: Treatment of chronic stable or vasospastic angina (FDA approved in adults); has also been used for treatment of hypertensive emergency in pediatric patients and high altitude pulmonary edema

Extended release:

Adalat® CC, Afeditab® CR, Nifediac CC®: Treatment of hypertension alone or in combinations with other hypertensive agents (FDA approved in adults)

Procardia XL®, Nifedical XL®: Treatment of chronic stable or vasospastic angina (FDA approved in adults); treatment of hypertension alone or in combination with other antihypertensive agents (FDA approved in adults)

Pregnancy Risk Factor C

Pregnancy Considerations Adverse events were observed in animal reproduction studies. Nifedipine crosses the placenta and small amounts can be detected in the urine of newborn infants (Manninen, 1991; Silberschmidt, 2008). An increase in perinatal asphyxia, cesarean delivery, prematurity, and intrauterine growth retardation have been reported following maternal use. Untreated chronic maternal hypertension is also associated with adverse events in the fetus, infant, and mother. If treatment for chronic hypertension during pregnancy is needed, nifedipine is one of the preferred agents (ACOG, 2013; SOGC [Magee, 2014]). Nifedipine is also recommended for the management of acute onset, severe hypertension (systolic BP ≥160 mm Hg or diastolic BP ≥110 mm Hg) with preeclampsia or eclampsia in pregnant and postpartum women (ACOG, 2015; Magee, 2014).

Nifedipine has also been evaluated for the treatment of preterm labor. Tocolytics may be used for the short-term (48 hour) prolongation of pregnancy to allow for the administration of antenatal steroids and should not be used prior to fetal viability or when the risks of use to the fetus or mother are greater than the risk of preterm birth (ACOG, 2012). Nifedipine is ineffective for maintenance tocolytic therapy (ACOG, 2012; Roos, 2013).

Breast-Feeding Considerations Nifedipine is excreted into breast milk. Reported concentrations are low and similar to those in the maternal serum (Ehrenkranz, 1989; Manninen, 1991; Penny, 1989). Breast-feeding is not recommended by the U.S. manufacturer (Canadian labeling contraindicates use). Nifedipine has been used for the treatment of Raynaud's phenomenon of the nipple in breast-feeding mothers (Barrett, 2013; Wu, 2012).

Contraindications

Hypersensitivity to nifedipine or any component of the formulation; concomitant use with strong CYP3A4 inducers (eg, rifampin); cardiogenic shock

Note: Considered contraindicated in patients with ST-elevation myocardial infarction (STEMI) (ACCF/AHA [O'Gara, 2013]).

Canadian labeling: Additional contraindications (not in U.S. labeling): Severe hypotension; patients with a Kock pouch (ileostomy after proctocolectomy; extended release tablets only); breast-feeding; pregnancy or women of childbearing potential. **Note:** SOGC and ACOG guidelines recommend nifedipine as a preferred agent for maternal hypertension (ACOG, 2013; SOGC [Magee, 2014]).

Warnings/Precautions Symptomatic hypotension with or without syncope can rarely occur; blood pressure must be lowered at a rate appropriate for the patient's clinical condition. **The use of immediate release nifedipine (sublingually or orally) in hypertensive emergencies and urgencies is neither safe nor effective.** Serious adverse events (eg, death, cerebrovascular ischemia, syncope, stroke, acute myocardial infarction, and fetal distress) have been reported. **Immediate release nifedipine should not be used for acute blood pressure reduction.**

Blood pressure lowering should be done at a rate appropriate for the patient's condition. Rapid drops in blood pressure can lead to arterial insufficiency. Increased angina and/or MI have occurred with initiation or dosage titration of dihydropyridine calcium channel blockers; use with caution in patients with obstructive coronary disease especially in the absence of concurrent beta-blockade. In patients with unstable angina/non-STEMI, the use of immediate-release nifedipine is not recommended except with concomitant beta-blockade (ACCF/AHA [Anderson, 2013]). Use with caution before major surgery. Cardiopulmonary bypass, intraoperative blood loss or vasodilating anesthesia may result in severe hypotension and/or increased fluid requirements. Consider withdrawing nifedipine (>36 hours) before surgery if possible.

The most common side effect is peripheral edema; occurs within 2-3 weeks of starting therapy. Reflex tachycardia may occur with use. Use with caution in severe aortic stenosis (especially with concomitant beta-adrenergic blocker), severe left ventricular dysfunction, renal impairment, hypertrophic cardiomyopathy (especially obstructive), concomitant therapy with beta-blockers or digoxin, and edema. The ACCF/AHA heart failure guidelines recommend to avoid use in patients with heart failure due to lack of benefit and/or worse outcomes with calcium channel blockers in general (Yancy, 2013). Use caution in patients with severe hepatic impairment. Clearance of nifedipine is reduced in cirrhotic patients leading to increased systemic exposure; monitor closely for adverse effects/toxicity and consider dose adjustments. Mild and transient elevations in liver function enzymes may be apparent within 8 weeks of therapy initiation. Abrupt withdrawal may cause rebound angina in patients with CAD. In the elderly, immediate release nifedipine should be avoided in due to potential to cause hypotension and risk of precipitating myocardial ischemia (Beers Criteria). Immediate release formulations should not be used to manage primary hypertension, adequate studies to evaluate outcomes have not been conducted. Avoid use of extended release tablets (Procardia XL) in patients with known stricture/narrowing of the GI tract. Adalat CC tablets contain lactose; do not use with galactose intolerance, Lapp lactase deficiency, or glucose-galactose malabsorption syndromes.

Potentially significant drug-drug interactions may exist, requiring dose or frequency adjustment, additional monitoring, and/or selection of alternative therapy.

Adverse Reactions

Cardiovascular: CHF, flushing, palpitation, peripheral edema (dose related), transient hypotension (dose related)

Central nervous system: Chills difficulties in balance, dizziness, fatigue, fever, giddiness, headache, jitteriness, lightheadedness, mood changes, nervousness, shakiness, sleep disturbances

Dermatologic: Dermatitis, pruritus, urticaria

Endocrine & metabolic: Sexual difficulties

Gastrointestinal: Constipation, cramps, diarrhea, flatulence, gingival hyperplasia, heartburn, nausea
Neuromuscular & skeletal: Inflammation, joint stiffness, muscle cramps, tremor, weakness
Ocular: Blurred vision
Respiratory: Chest congestion, cough, dyspnea, nasal congestion, sore throat, wheezing
Miscellaneous: Diaphoresis
Rare but important or life-threatening: Agranulocytosis, allergic hepatitis, alopecia, anemia, angina, angioedema, aplastic anemia, arrhythmia, arthritis with positive ANA, bezoars (Procardia XL®), cerebral ischemia, depression, dysosmia, epistaxis, EPS, erectile dysfunction, erythema multiforme, erythromelalgia, exanthematous pustulosis, exfoliative dermatitis, facial edema, gastroesophageal reflux, gastrointestinal obstruction (Procardia XL®), gastrointestinal ulceration (Procardia XL®), gynecomastia, hematuria, ischemia, leukopenia, lip cancer (Friedman, 2012), memory dysfunction, migraine, myalgia, myoclonus, nocturia, paranoid syndrome, parotitis, periorbital edema, photosensitivity, polyuria, purpura, Stevens-Johnson syndrome, syncope, tachycardia, taste perversion, thrombocytopenia, tinnitus, toxic epidermal necrolysis, transient blindness, ventricular arrhythmia
Reported with use of sublingual short-acting nifedipine: Acute MI, cerebrovascular ischemia, ECG changes, fetal distress, heart block, severe hypotension, sinus arrest, stroke, syncope

Drug Interactions

Metabolism/Transport Effects **Substrate** of CYP2D6 (minor), CYP3A4 (major); **Note:** Assignment of Major/Minor substrate status based on clinically relevant drug interaction potential; **Inhibits** CYP1A2 (weak), CYP2C9 (weak), CYP2D6 (weak)

Avoid Concomitant Use

Avoid concomitant use of NIFEdipine with any of the following: Conivaptan; CYP3A4 Inducers (Strong); Fusidic Acid (Systemic); Grapefruit Juice; Idelalisib; St Johns Wort

Increased Effect/Toxicity

NIFEdipine may increase the levels/effects of: Amifostine; Antihypertensives; ARIPiprazole; Atosiban; Beta-Blockers; Calcium Channel Blockers (Nondihydropyridine); Digoxin; DULoxetine; Hypotensive Agents; Levodopa; Magnesium Salts; Neuromuscular-Blocking Agents (Nondepolarizing); Nitroprusside; Obinutuzumab; QuiNIDine; RisperiDONE; RiTUXimab; Tacrolimus (Systemic); TiZANidine; VinCRIStine; VinCRIStine (Liposomal)

The levels/effects of NIFEdipine may be increased by: Alcohol (Ethyl); Alfuzosin; Alpha1-Blockers; Antifungal Agents (Azole Derivatives, Systemic); Aprepitant; Barbiturates; Brimonidine (Topical); Calcium Channel Blockers (Nondihydropyridine); Cimetidine; Cisapride; Conivaptan; CycloSPORINE (Systemic); CYP3A4 Inhibitors (Moderate); CYP3A4 Inhibitors (Strong); Dapoxetine; Dasatinib; Diazoxide; Fluconazole; FLUoxetine; Fosaprepitant; Fusidic Acid (Systemic); Grapefruit Juice; Herbs (Hypotensive Properties); Idelalisib; Ivacaftor; Luliconazole; Macrolide Antibiotics; Magnesium Salts; MAO Inhibitors; Mifepristone; Netupitant; Nicorandil; Palbociclib; Pentoxifylline; Phosphodiesterase 5 Inhibitors; Prostacyclin Analogues; Protease Inhibitors; QuiNIDine; Simeprevir; Stiripentol

Decreased Effect

NIFEdipine may decrease the levels/effects of: Clopidogrel; QuiNIDine

The levels/effects of NIFEdipine may be decreased by: Barbiturates; Bosentan; Calcium Salts; CYP3A4 Inducers (Moderate); CYP3A4 Inducers (Strong); Dabrafenib; Deferasirox; Efavirenz; Herbs (Hypertensive Properties); Melatonin; Methylphenidate; Nafcillin; Siltuximab; St Johns Wort; Tocilizumab; Yohimbine

Food Interactions Nifedipine serum levels may be decreased if taken with food. Food may decrease the rate but not the extent of absorption of Procardia XL®. Increased nifedipine concentrations resulting in therapeutic and vasodilator side effects, including severe hypotension and myocardial ischemia, may occur if nifedipine is taken by patients ingesting grapefruit. Management: Avoid grapefruit/grapefruit juice.

Storage/Stability

Adalat CC, Afeditab CR, Procardia XL: Store below 30°C (86°F); protect from light and moisture.
Nifediac CC, Nifedical XL: Store at 25°C (77°F); excursions permitted to 15°C to 30°C (59°F to 86°F); protect from light and moisture.
Immediate release capsules (Procardia): Store at 15°C to 25°C (59°F to 77°F); prevent capsules from freezing; protect from light and moisture.

Mechanism of Action Inhibits calcium ion from entering the "slow channels" or select voltage-sensitive areas of vascular smooth muscle and myocardium during depolarization, producing a relaxation of coronary vascular smooth muscle and coronary vasodilation; increases myocardial oxygen delivery in patients with vasospastic angina; also reduces peripheral vascular resistance, producing a reduction in arterial blood pressure.

Pharmacodynamics

Onset of action:
- "Bite and swallow": Within 1-5 minutes
- Oral:
  - Immediate release: Within 20-30 minutes
  - Extended release: 2.5-5 hours

Duration:
- Immediate release: 4-8 hours
- Extended release: 24 hours

Pharmacokinetics (Adult data unless noted)

Protein-binding: 92% to 98% (concentration-dependent); **Note:** Protein-binding may be significantly decreased in patients with renal or hepatic impairment
Metabolism: Hepatic via CYP3A4 to inactive metabolites
Bioavailability: Capsule: 40% to 77%; Extended release: 84% to 89% relative to immediate release capsules; bioavailability increased with significant hepatic disease
Half-life: Adults:
- Normal: Immediate release: 2-5 hours; Extended release: 7 hours
- Cirrhosis: 7 hours

Elimination: Urine (60% to 80% as inactive metabolites); feces

Dosing: Usual

Children and Adolescents: **Note:** Doses are usually titrated upward over 7-14 days; may increase over 3 days if clinically necessary:

Hypertensive urgency: Immediate release: Oral or "bite and swallow" (eg, bite capsule to release liquid contents then swallow): 0.1-0.25 mg/kg/dose; maximum single dose: 10 mg; may repeat if needed every 4-6 hours; monitor carefully; typically reserved for inpatient use; maximum daily dose: 1-2 mg/kg/**day** (Blaszak, 2001; Egger, 2002; Singh, 2012). **Note:** Current pediatric blood pressure guidelines do not recommend use (NHBPEP, 2004).

Hypertension (chronic treatment): Extended release: Oral: Initial: 0.25-0.5 mg/kg/**day** given once daily or divided in 2 doses per **day**; do not exceed initial adult dose (30-60 mg/**day**); titrate dose to effect; maximum dose: 3 mg/kg/**day** up to 120 mg/**day** (NHBPEP, 2004; NHLBI, 2011); some centers use a higher maximum dose: 3 mg/kg/**day** up to 180 mg/day (Flynn, 2000)

High altitude pulmonary edema (Pollard, 2001): Limited data available: Children and Adolescents: **Note:** Reserve treatment with NIFEdipine for unsatisfactory response to oxygen and/or altitude descent: Oral:

Immediate release: 0.5 mg/kg/dose every 8 hours; maximum dose: 20 mg

Extended release (preferred): 1.5 mg/kg/day given once daily or divided in 2 doses per **day**; maximum dose: 40 mg

Adults: **Note:** Dosage adjustments should occur at 7- to 14-day intervals, to allow for adequate assessment of new dose; when switching from immediate release to sustained release formulations, use same total daily dose.

Chronic stable or vasospastic angina: Oral:

Immediate release: Initial: 10 mg 3 times daily; usual dose: 10-20 mg 3 times daily; coronary artery spasm may require up to 20-30 mg 3-4 times daily; single doses >30 mg and total daily doses >120 mg are rarely needed; maximum daily dose: 180 mg/**day**; **Note:** Do not use for acute anginal episodes; may precipitate myocardial infarction.

Extended release: Initial: 30 or 60 mg once daily; maximum: 120-180 mg/day

Hypertension: Oral: Extended release: Initial: 30 or 60 mg once daily; maximum: 90-120 mg/day

High altitude pulmonary edema (Luks, 2010): Oral:

Prevention: Extended release: 30 mg every 12 hours starting the day before ascent and may be discontinued after staying at the same elevation for 5 days or if descent initiated

Treatment: Extended release: 30 mg every 12 hours

Administration Oral:

Immediate release: Administer with or without food. Liquid-filled capsule may be punctured and drug solution administered orally. When nifedipine is administered sublingually, only a small amount is absorbed sublingually; the observed effects are actually due to swallowing of the drug with subsequent rapid oral absorption. When measuring smaller doses from the liquid-filled capsules, completely empty the capsule to determine the concentration (may vary based on strength and by manufacturer) and administer the appropriate volume for the desired dose; the following concentrations are for Procardia®: 10 mg capsule = 10 mg/0.34 mL; 20 mg capsule = 20 mg/0.45 mL

Extended release: Tablets should be swallowed whole; do not crush, break, chew, or divide. Adalat® CC, Afeditab® CR, Nifediac CC®: Administer on an empty stomach (per manufacturer); other extended release products may not have this recommendation; consult product labeling.

Monitoring Parameters CBC, platelets, periodic liver enzymes; blood pressure, heart rate, signs and symptoms of CHF, peripheral edema

Dosage Forms Excipient information presented when available (limited, particularly for generics); consult specific product labeling.

Capsule, Oral:

Procardia: 10 mg

Generic: 10 mg, 20 mg

Tablet Extended Release 24 Hour, Oral:

Adalat CC: 30 mg, 60 mg, 90 mg

Afeditab CR: 30 mg, 60 mg

Nifediac CC: 30 mg, 60 mg

Nifediac CC: 90 mg [contains tartrazine (fd&c yellow #5)]

Nifedical XL: 30 mg, 60 mg

Procardia XL: 30 mg, 60 mg, 90 mg

Generic: 30 mg, 60 mg, 90 mg

Extemporaneous Preparations A 4 mg/mL oral suspension may be made with liquid capsules (**Note:** Concentration inside capsule may vary depending on manufacturer. Procardia: 10 mg capsule contains a concentration of 10 mg/0.34 mL [29.4 mg/mL]). Puncture the top of twelve 10 mg liquid capsules with one needle to create a vent. Insert a second needle attached to a syringe and extract the liquid; transfer to a calibrated bottle and add sufficient quantity of a 1:1 mixture of Ora-Sweet and Ora-Plus to make 30 mL. Label "shake well". Stable 90 days under refrigeration or at room temperature.

Nahata MC, Morosco RS, and Willhite EA, "Stability of Nifedipine in Two Oral Suspensions Stored at Two Temperatures," *J Am Pharm Assoc*, 2002, 42(6):865-7.

- **Nifedipine ER (Can)** *see* NIFEdipine *on page 1516*
- **Nighttime Sleep Aid [OTC]** *see* DiphenhydrAMINE (Systemic) *on page 668*
- **Nimbex** *see* Cisatracurium *on page 472*
- **Niodan (Can)** *see* Niacin *on page 1511*
- **Nipent** *see* Pentostatin *on page 1668*
- **Nipride (Can)** *see* Nitroprusside *on page 1526*
- **Niravam** *see* ALPRAZolam *on page 100*
- **Nitalapram** *see* Citalopram *on page 476*

Nitazoxanide (nye ta ZOX a nide)

Brand Names: US Alinia

Therapeutic Category Antiprotozoal

Generic Availability (US) No

Use Treatment of diarrhea caused by *Giardia lamblia* (FDA approved in ages ≥1 year and adults); treatment of diarrhea caused by *Cryptosporidium parvum* in immunocompetent patients (FDA approved in ages ≥1 year and adults); has also been used for the treatment of amebiasis, dwarf tapeworm infection, fluke infections, and refractory or recurrent *Clostridium difficile*-associated diarrhea

Pregnancy Risk Factor B

Pregnancy Considerations Teratogenic effects were not observed in animal reproduction studies.

Breast-Feeding Considerations It is not known if nitazoxanide is excreted in breast milk. The manufacturer recommends that caution be exercised when administering nitazoxanide to nursing women.

Contraindications Hypersensitivity to nitazoxanide or any component of the formulation

Warnings/Precautions Use caution with renal or hepatic impairment. Safety and efficacy have not been established in patients with HIV infection or immunodeficiency. Oral suspension contains sucrose; use caution in patients with diabetes mellitus.

Benzyl alcohol and derivatives: Some dosage forms may contain sodium benzoate/benzoic acid; benzoic acid (benzoate) is a metabolite of benzyl alcohol; large amounts of benzyl alcohol (≥99 mg/kg/day) have been associated with a potentially fatal toxicity ("gasping syndrome") in neonates; the "gasping syndrome" consists of metabolic acidosis, respiratory distress, gasping respirations, CNS dysfunction (including convulsions, intracranial hemorrhage), hypotension, and cardiovascular collapse (AAP, 1997; CDC, 1982); some data suggests that benzoate displaces bilirubin from protein binding sites (Ahlfors, 2001); avoid or use dosage forms containing benzyl alcohol derivative with caution in neonates. See manufacturer's labeling.

Adverse Reactions

Central nervous system: Headache

Gastrointestinal: Abdominal pain, diarrhea, nausea, vomiting

Rare but important or life-threatening: Allergic reaction, ALT increased, anemia, anorexia, appetite increased, creatinine increased, diaphoresis, dizziness, eye discoloration (pale yellow), fever, flatulence, hypertension, infection, malaise, pruritus, rhinitis, salivary glands enlarged, tachycardia, urine discoloration

Drug Interactions

Metabolism/Transport Effects None known.

Avoid Concomitant Use There are no known interactions where it is recommended to avoid concomitant use.

Increased Effect/Toxicity There are no known significant interactions involving an increase in effect.

Decreased Effect There are no known significant interactions involving a decrease in effect.

Food Interactions Food increases AUC. Management: Take with food.

Storage/Stability

Suspension: Prior to and following reconstitution, store at 25°C (77°F); excursions permitted to 15°C to 30°C (59°F to 86°F). For preparation at time of dispensing, add 48 mL incrementally to 60 mL bottle; shake vigorously. Resulting suspension is 20 mg/mL (100 mg per 5 mL). Following reconstitution, discard unused portion of suspension after 7 days.

Tablet: Store at 25°C (77°F); excursions permitted to 15°C to 30°C (59°F to 86°F).

Mechanism of Action Nitazoxanide is rapidly metabolized to the active metabolite tizoxanide *in vivo*. Activity may be due to interference with the pyruvate:ferredoxin oxidoreductase (PFOR) enzyme-dependent electron transfer reaction which is essential to anaerobic metabolism. *In vitro*, nitazoxanide and tizoxanide inhibit the growth of sporozoites and oocysts of *Cryptosporidium parvum* and trophozoites of *Giardia lamblia*.

Pharmacokinetics (Adult data unless noted) Note: In pediatric patients (1-18 years of age), pharmacokinetic properties similar to adult when dosed equivalently.

Protein binding: Tizoxanide: >99%

Metabolism: Hepatic, to an active metabolite, tizoxanide. Tizoxanide undergoes conjugation to form tizoxanide glucuronide. Nitazoxanide is not detectable in the serum following oral administration.

Bioavailability: Relative bioavailability of the suspension to the tablet is 70%; tablet and suspension are not bioequivalent

Half-life: Tizoxanide: 1-1.6 hours

Time to peak serum concentration: Tizoxanide: 1-4 hours

Elimination: Tizoxanide is excreted in urine (<10%), bile, and feces (60%); tizoxanide glucuronide is excreted in urine and bile

Dosing: Usual Oral:

Cryptosporidium parvum or *Giardia lamblia* treatment of diarrhea (**Note:** May consider increasing duration up to 14 days in HIV-exposed/HIV-infected patients (CDC, 2009):

- Children 1-3 years: 100 mg every 12 hours for 3 days
- Children 4-11 years: 200 mg every 12 hours for 3 days
- Adolescents ≥12 years and Adults: 500 mg every 12 hours for 3 days

Fasciola hepatica (sheep liver fluke) (*Red Book*, 2009):

- Children 1-3 years: 100 mg every 12 hours for 7 days
- Children 4-11years: 200 mg every 12 hours for 7 days
- Adolescents ≥12 years and Adults: 500 mg every 12 hours for 7 days

Hymenolepis nana (dwarf tapeworm) (*Red Book*, 2009):

- Children 1-3 years: 100 mg twice daily for 3 days
- Children 4-11 years: 200 mg twice daily for 3 days
- Adults: 500 mg once or twice daily for 3 days

C. difficile-associated diarrhea: Adults: 500 mg every 12 hours for 7-10 days

Dosage adjustment in renal and/or hepatic impairment: Specific recommendations are not available; use with caution

Preparation for Administration Oral suspension: Prior to dispensing, add 48 mL incrementally to 60 mL bottle; shake vigorously. Resulting suspension is 20 mg/mL (100 mg per 5 mL).

Administration Oral: Minimize gastric irritation by administering with food; shake suspension well prior to administration

Monitoring Parameters Periodic liver function tests, stool frequency

Additional Information The oral suspension contains sucrose 1.48 g/5 mL.

Dosage Forms Excipient information presented when available (limited, particularly for generics); consult specific product labeling.

Suspension Reconstituted, Oral:

Alinia: 100 mg/5 mL (60 mL) [contains fd&c red #40, sodium benzoate; strawberry flavor]

Tablet, Oral:

Alinia: 500 mg [contains fd&c blue #2 aluminum lake, fd&c yellow #10 aluminum lake, fd&c yellow #6 aluminum lake, soybean lecithin]

◆ **Nitetime Sleep-Aid [OTC]** *see* Doxylamine *on page 721*

◆ **Nithiodote** *see* Sodium Nitrite and Sodium Thiosulfate *on page 1945*

Nitisinone (ni TIS i known)

Brand Names: US Orfadin

Therapeutic Category Tyrosinemia Type 1, Treatment Agent

Generic Availability (US) No

Use Adjunct to dietary restriction of tyrosine and phenylalanine in the treatment of hereditary tyrosinemia type 1 (HT-1) (FDA approved in all ages)

Prescribing and Access Restrictions Distributed by Orfadin4U comprehensive patient support program. Information regarding acquisition of product may be obtained by calling 877-473-3179. Additional information can be found at http://www.orfadin.com

Pregnancy Risk Factor C

Pregnancy Considerations Adverse events have been observed in animal reproduction studies.

Breast-Feeding Considerations It is not known if nitisinone is excreted in breast milk. Due to the potential for serious adverse reactions in the nursing infant, the manufacturer recommends a decision be made whether to discontinue nursing or to discontinue the drug, taking into account the importance of treatment to the mother.

Contraindications There are no contraindications listed in the manufacturer's labeling.

Warnings/Precautions Must be used with dietary restriction of tyrosine and phenylalanine; inadequate restriction can result in toxic effects to the eyes (eg, conjunctivitis, corneal ulcers, corneal opacities, eye pain, keratitis, photophobia), skin (eg, hyperkeratotic plaques on the soles and palms), and nervous system (eg, developmental delay, mental retardation). Evaluate plasma tyrosine concentrations in patients who develop signs and symptoms of toxicity; slit-lamp examination of the eyes and immediate measurement of plasma tyrosine concentration are recommended for the development of ocular toxicity. Nutritional consultation is recommended. Leukopenia and/or thrombocytopenia have been reported; may be due to underlying liver disease as opposed to drug-related (McKiernan, 2006). Monitor platelets and WBC regularly during therapy.

Adverse Reactions

Dermatologic: Alopecia, dry skin, exfoliative dermatitis, maculopapular rash, pruritus

Hematologic: Epistaxis, granulocytopenia, leukopenia, porphyria, thrombocytopenia

Hepatic: Hepatic failure, hepatic neoplasm

Ocular: Blepharitis, cataracts, conjunctivitis, corneal opacity, eye pain, keratitis, photophobia

Rare but important or life-threatening: Abdominal pain, amenorrhea, brain tumor, bronchitis, corneal ulceration, cyanosis, dehydration, diarrhea, enanthema, encephalopathy, gastritis, gastroenteritis, gastrointestinal hemorrhage, headache, hepatic dysfunction, hepatomegaly, hyperkinesias, hypoglycemia, infection, liver enzymes increased, melena, nervousness, otitis, pathologic fracture, respiratory insufficiency, seizure, septicemia, somnolence, thirst, tooth discoloration, tyrosine levels increased

Drug Interactions

Metabolism/Transport Effects None known.

Avoid Concomitant Use There are no known interactions where it is recommended to avoid concomitant use.

Increased Effect/Toxicity There are no known significant interactions involving an increase in effect.

Decreased Effect There are no known significant interactions involving a decrease in effect.

Food Interactions Effect of taking with food is unknown. Tyrosine toxicity can occur without proper dietary restriction of tyrosine and phenylalanine. Management: Administer at least 1 hour prior to, or 2 hours after a meal. Dietary restriction of tyrosine and phenylalanine is required.

Storage/Stability Store refrigerated at 2°C to 8°C (36°F to 46°F).

Mechanism of Action In patients with HT-1, tyrosine metabolism is interrupted due to a lack of the enzyme (fumarylacetoacetate hydrolase) needed in the last step of tyrosine degradation. Toxic metabolites of tyrosine accumulate and cause liver and kidney toxicity. Nitisinone competitively inhibits 4-hydroxyphenyl-pyruvate dioxygenase, an enzyme present early in the tyrosine degradation pathway, thereby preventing the build-up of the toxic metabolites.

Pharmacokinetics (Adult data unless noted) Note: Limited pharmacokinetic studies exist in HT-1 patients.

Bioavailability: >90% (animal studies)

Half-life: 54 hours (healthy volunteers)

Time to peak serum concentration: 3 hours (healthy volunteers)

Excretion: Equal amounts in urine and feces (McKiernan, 2006)

Dosing: Usual Oral: HT-1: **Note:** Must be used in conjunction with a diet restricted in tyrosine and phenylalanine.

Infants, Children, and Adults: Initial: 1 mg/kg/day in two divided doses; adjust dose if inadequate response, as defined by continued abnormal biological parameters (erythrocyte PBG-synthase activity, urine 5-ALA, and urine succinylacetone) despite treatment. If the aforementioned parameters are not available, may use urine succinylacetone, liver function tests, alpha-fetoprotein, serum tyrosine, and serum phenylalanine to evaluate response (exceptions may include during initiation of therapy and exacerbations).

Abnormal biological parameters at 1 month: Increase dose to 1.5 mg/kg/day

Abnormal biological parameters at 3 months: Increase to maximum dose of 2 mg/kg/day

Administration Oral: Administer in two divided doses in the morning and evening, at least 1 hour prior to, or 2 hours after a meal. The total daily dose does not need to be split evenly; divide the total dose to limit the total number of capsules administered at each interval. Capsules may be opened and contents suspended in a small quantity of water, formula, or applesauce; use immediately.

Monitoring Parameters

Dietary tyrosine and phenylalanine intake; platelets, WBC, plasma and urine succinylacetone concentrations, serum alpha-fetoprotein, serum phosphate (if renal dysfunction), hepatic

Function (ultrasound, computerized tomography, magnetic resonance imaging)

Ophthalmic exam (Slit-lamp examination prior to initiation of therapy and in patients who develop symptoms of ocular toxicity)

Plasma tyrosine concentrations should be kept <500 µmol/L to avoid toxicity

Reference Range Plasma tyrosine concentration <500 micromoles/L

Dosage Forms Excipient information presented when available (limited, particularly for generics); consult specific product labeling.

Capsule, Oral:

Orfadin: 2 mg, 5 mg, 10 mg

◆ **Nitro-Bid** *see* Nitroglycerin *on page 1523*

◆ **Nitro-Dur** *see* Nitroglycerin *on page 1523*

Nitrofurantoin (nye troe fyoor AN toyn)

Medication Safety Issues

Sound alike/look alike issues:

Macrobid may be confused with microK, Nitro-Bid

Nitrofurantoin may be confused with Neurontin®, nitroglycerin

BEERS Criteria medication:

This drug may be potentially inappropriate for use in geriatric patients (Quality of evidence - moderate; Strength of recommendation - strong).

Brand Names: US Furadantin; Macrobid; Macrodantin

Brand Names: Canada Apo-Nitrofurantoin; Macrobid; Macrodantin; Novo-Furantoin; Teva-Nitrofurantoin

Therapeutic Category Antibiotic, Miscellaneous

Generic Availability (US) Yes

Use Prevention and treatment of urinary tract infections caused by susceptible gram-negative and some gram-positive organisms including *E. coli*, *Klebsiella*, *Enterobacter*, enterococci, *S. saprophyticus*, and *S. aureus*; *Pseudomonas*, *Serratia*, and most species of *Proteus* are generally resistant to nitrofurantoin.

Macrodantin® and Furadantin® (FDA approved in ages ≥1 month)

Macrobid® (FDA approved in ages ≥12 years)

Pregnancy Risk Factor B (contraindicated at term)

Pregnancy Considerations Adverse effects have not been observed in animal reproduction studies. Nitrofurantoin crosses the placenta (Perry, 1967) and maternal serum concentrations may be lower in pregnancy (Philipson, 1979). Current studies evaluating maternal use of nitrofurantoin during pregnancy and the development of birth defects have had mixed results (ACOG, 2011). An increased risk of neonatal jaundice was observed following maternal nitrofurantoin use during the last 30 days of pregnancy (Nordeng, 2013). Nitrofurantoin may be used to treat infections in pregnant women; use during the first trimester should be limited to situations where no alternative therapies are available. Prescriptions should be written when clinically appropriate and for the shortest effective duration for confirmed infections (ACOG, 2011). Nitrofurantoin is contraindicated in pregnant patients at term (38-42 weeks gestation), during labor and delivery, or when the onset of labor is imminent due to the possibility of hemolytic anemia in the neonate. Alternative antibiotics should be considered in pregnant women with G-6-PD deficiency (Nordeng, 2013).

Breast-Feeding Considerations Trace amounts of nitrofurantoin can be detected in breast milk. Due to the potential for serious adverse reactions in the nursing infant, the manufacturer recommends a decision be made whether to discontinue nursing or to discontinue the drug, taking into account the importance of treatment to the mother. The therapeutic use of nitrofurantoin is contraindicated in neonates (<1 month of age) due to the possibility of hemolytic anemia caused by immature erythrocyte enzyme systems. In case reports, diarrhea was reported in two nursing infants and decreased milk volume was reported by one mother (dose, duration, relationship to breast-feeding not provided) (Ito, 1993).

Contraindications

Anuria, oliguria, or significant impairment of renal function (creatinine clearance [CrCl] <60 mL/minute or clinically significant elevated serum creatinine); previous history of cholestatic jaundice or hepatic dysfunction associated with prior nitrofurantoin use; hypersensitivity to drug or any component of the formulation.

Note: The manufacturer's contraindication in patients with CrCl <60 mL/minute has been challenged in the literature; limited data suggest that an alternative creatinine clearance threshold may be considered (Oplinger, 2013).

Because of the possibility of hemolytic anemia caused by immature erythrocyte enzyme systems (glutathione instability), the drug is contraindicated in pregnant patients at term (38 to 42 weeks gestation), during labor and delivery, or when the onset of labor is imminent; also contraindicated in neonates younger than 1 month of age.

Warnings/Precautions Use with caution in patients with G6PD deficiency (increased risk of hemolytic anemia). Urinary nitrofurantoin concentrations are variable in patients with impaired renal function. The manufacturer contraindicates use in CrCl <60 mL/minute; however, limited data suggest clinicians may consider using a lower threshold of CrCl ≥40 mL/minute when treatment is short term (≤1 week) for an uncomplicated UTI (Oplinger, 2013).

Use with caution if prolonged therapy is anticipated due to possible pulmonary toxicity. Acute, subacute, or chronic (usually after 6 months of therapy) pulmonary reactions (possibly fatal) have been observed in patients treated with nitrofurantoin; if these occur, discontinue therapy immediately; monitor closely for malaise, dyspnea, cough, fever, radiologic evidence of diffuse interstitial pneumonitis or fibrosis. Rare, but severe and sometimes fatal hepatic reactions (eg, cholestatic jaundice, hepatitis, hepatic necrosis) have been associated with nitrofurantoin (onset may be insidious); discontinue immediately if hepatitis occurs. Use is contraindicated in patients with a history of nitrofurantoin associated cholestatic jaundice or hepatic dysfunction. Monitor liver function test periodically. Has been associated with peripheral neuropathy (rare); risk may be increased in patients with anemia, renal impairment (CrCl <60 mL/minute), diabetes, vitamin B deficiency, debilitating disease, or electrolyte imbalance; use caution. Potentially significant drug-drug interactions may exist, requiring dose or frequency adjustment, additional monitoring, and/or selection of alternative therapy. Effects may be potentiated when used with other sedative drugs or ethanol. Use in the elderly, particularly females receiving long-term prophylaxis for recurrent UTIs, has been associated with an increased risk of hepatic and pulmonary toxicity, and peripheral neuropathy. In the elderly, avoid use for long-term suppression due to potential for pulmonary toxicity and availability of safer alternative agents (Beers Criteria). Use in the elderly, particularly females receiving long-term prophylaxis for recurrent UTIs, has also been associated with an increased risk of hepatic toxicity and peripheral neuropathy; monitor closely for toxicities during use. Prolonged use may result in fungal or bacterial superinfection, including *C. difficile*-associated diarrhea (CDAD) and pseudomembranous colitis; CDAD has been observed >2 months postantibiotic treatment. Use is contraindicated in children <1 month of age (at increased risk for hemolytic anemia). Not indicated for the treatment of pyelonephritis or perinephric abscesses. Postmarketing cases of optic neuritis have been reported.

Warnings: Additional Pediatric Considerations Nitrofurantoin should not be used to treat UTIs in febrile infants and young children in whom renal involvement is likely; not indicated for the treatment of pyelonephritis or perinephric abscesses.

Adverse Reactions

Cardiovascular: ECG changes (nonspecific ST/T wave changes, bundle branch block)

Central nervous system: Bulging fontanel (infants), chills, confusion, depression, dizziness, drowsiness, headache, malaise, numbness, paresthesia, peripheral neuropathy, pseudotumor cerebri, psychotic reaction, vertigo

Dermatologic: Alopecia, erythema multiforme, exfoliative dermatitis, pruritus, skin rash (eczematous, erythematous, maculopapular), Stevens-Johnson syndrome, urticaria

Endocrine & metabolic: Hyperphosphatemia

Gastrointestinal: Abdominal pain, anorexia, *Clostridium difficile* associated diarrhea, constipation, diarrhea, dyspepsia, flatulence, nausea, pancreatitis, pseudomembranous colitis, sialadenitis, vomiting

Genitourinary: Urine discoloration (brown)

Hematologic & oncologic: Agranulocytosis, aplastic anemia, eosinophilia, glucose-6-phosphate dehydrogenase deficiency anemia, granulocytopenia, hemoglobin decreased, hemolytic anemia, leukopenia, megaloblastic anemia, thrombocytopenia

Hepatic: Cholestatic jaundice, hepatitis, hepatic necrosis, increased serum transaminases

Hypersensitivity: Anaphylaxis, angioedema, hypersensitivity (including acute pulmonary hypersensitivity)

Infection: Superinfection (eg, *Pseudomonas* or *Candida*)

Neuromuscular & skeletal: Arthralgia, lupus-like syndrome, myalgia, weakness

Ophthalmic: Amblyopia, nystagmus, optic neuritis

Respiratory: Acute pulmonary reaction (symptoms include chills, chest pain, cough, dyspnea, fever, and eosinophilia), cough, cyanosis, dyspnea, pneumonitis, pulmonary fibrosis (with long-term use), pulmonary infiltration

Miscellaneous: Fever

Rare but important or life-threatening: Hepatotoxicty (idiosyncratic) (Chalasani, 2014)

Drug Interactions

Metabolism/Transport Effects None known.

Avoid Concomitant Use

Avoid concomitant use of Nitrofurantoin with any of the following: BCG; BCG (Intravesical); Magnesium Trisilicate; Norfloxacin

Increased Effect/Toxicity

Nitrofurantoin may increase the levels/effects of: Eplerenone; Prilocaine; Sodium Nitrite; Spironolactone

The levels/effects of Nitrofurantoin may be increased by: Nitric Oxide; Probenecid

Decreased Effect

Nitrofurantoin may decrease the levels/effects of: BCG; BCG (Intravesical); BCG Vaccine (Immunization); Norfloxacin; Sodium Picosulfate; Typhoid Vaccine

The levels/effects of Nitrofurantoin may be decreased by: Magnesium Trisilicate

Food Interactions Nitrofurantoin serum concentrations may be increased if taken with food. Management: Administer with meals.

Storage/Stability

Capsules: Store at controlled room temperature, 15°C to 30°C (59°F to 86°F). Dispense in a tight container using a child-resistant closure.

Oral suspension: Avoid exposure to strong light, which may darken the drug. It is stable when stored between 20°C and 25°C (68°F and 77°F). Protect from freezing. Dispense in glass amber bottles.

Mechanism of Action Nitrofurantoin is reduced by bacterial flavoproteins to reactive intermediates that inactivate or alter bacterial ribosomal proteins leading to inhibition of protein synthesis, aerobic energy metabolism, DNA, RNA, and cell wall synthesis. Nitrofurantoin is bactericidal in urine at therapeutic doses. The broad-based nature of this mode of action may explain the lack of acquired bacterial resistance to nitrofurantoin, as the necessary multiple and simultaneous mutations of the target macromolecules would likely be lethal to the bacteria.

Pharmacokinetics (Adult data unless noted)

Absorption: Well absorbed from the GI tract; macrocrystalline form is absorbed more slowly due to slower dissolution, but causes less GI distress than formulations containing microcrystals of the drug

Distribution: V_d: 0.8 L/kg; crosses the placenta; appears in breast milk and bile

Protein binding: ~40% to 60%

Metabolism: Partially in the liver

Bioavailability: Presence of food increases bioavailability

Half-life: 20-60 minutes and is prolonged with renal impairment

Elimination: As metabolites and unchanged drug (40%) in the urine and small amounts in the bile; renal excretion is via glomerular filtration and tubular secretion

Dialysis: Dialyzable

Dosing: Usual Oral:

Infants >1 month and Children: 5-7 mg/kg/day divided every 6 hours; maximum dose: 400 mg/day

Macrocrystal/monohydrate: Children >12 years: 100 mg every 12 hours for 7 days

Prophylaxis of UTI: 1-2 mg/kg/day as a single daily dose; maximum dose: 100 mg/day

Adults: 50-100 mg/dose every 6 hours; macrocrystal/monohydrate: 100 mg twice daily for 7 days

Prophylaxis of UTI: 50-100 mg/dose at bedtime

Dosing adjustment in renal impairment: CrCl <60 mL/minute: Avoid use

Administration Oral: Administer with food or milk; do not administer with antacid preparations containing magnesium trisilicate; suspension may be mixed with water, milk, fruit juice, or infant formula. Shake suspension well before use.

Monitoring Parameters Signs of pulmonary reaction; signs of numbness or tingling of the extremities; periodic liver and renal function tests; CBC; urine culture and *in vitro* susceptibility tests. Observe for change in bowel frequency.

Test Interactions False-positive urine glucose (Benedict's and Fehling's methods); no false positives with enzymatic tests

Dosage Forms Excipient information presented when available (limited, particularly for generics); consult specific product labeling.

Capsule, Oral:

Macrobid: 100 mg [contains brilliant blue fcf (fd&c blue #1), fd&c red #40, fd&c yellow #10 (quinoline yellow)]

Macrodantin: 25 mg

Macrodantin: 50 mg, 100 mg [contains fd&c yellow #10 (quinoline yellow), fd&c yellow #6 (sunset yellow)]

Generic: 50 mg, 100 mg

Suspension, Oral:

Furadantin: 25 mg/5 mL (230 mL)

Generic: 25 mg/5 mL (230 mL, 240 mL)

◆ **Nitrogen Mustard** *see* Mechlorethamine (Systemic) *on page 1335*

Nitroglycerin (nye troe GLI ser in)

Medication Safety Issues

Sound-alike/look-alike issues:

Nitroglycerin may be confused with nitrofurantoin, nitroprusside

Nitro-Bid may be confused with Macrobid

Nitroderm may be confused with NicoDerm

Nitrol may be confused with Nizoral

Nitrostat may be confused with Nilstat, nystatin

Other safety concerns:

Transdermal patch may contain conducting metal (eg, aluminum); remove patch prior to MRI.

International issues:

Nitrocor [Italy, Russia, and Venezuela] may be confused with Natrecor brand name for nesiritide [U.S., Canada, and multiple international markets]; Nutracort brand name for hydrocortisone in the [U.S. and multiple international markets]; Nitro-Dur [U.S., Canada, and multiple international markets]

Related Information

Management of Drug Extravasations *on page 2298*

Oral Medications That Should Not Be Crushed or Altered *on page 2476*

Safe Handling of Hazardous Drugs *on page 2455*

Brand Names: US Minitran; Nitro-Bid; Nitro-Dur; Nitro-Time; Nitrolingual; NitroMist; Nitronal; Nitrostat; Rectiv

Brand Names: Canada Minitran; Mylan-Nitro Sublingual Spray; Nitro-Dur; Nitroglycerin Injection, USP; Nitrol; Nitrostat; Rho-Nitro Pump Spray; Transderm-Nitro; Trinipatch

Therapeutic Category Antianginal Agent; Antihypertensive Agent; Nitrate; Vasodilator; Vasodilator, Coronary

Generic Availability (US) May be product dependent

Use Treatment or prevention of angina pectoris (FDA approved in adults)

IV administration: Treatment or prevention of angina pectoris; acute decompensated heart failure (especially when associated with acute myocardial infarction); perioperative hypertension (especially during cardiovascular surgery); induction of intraoperative hypotension (FDA approved in adults)

Intra-anal administration (Rectiv™ ointment): Treatment of moderate to severe pain associated with chronic anal fissure (FDA approved in adults)

Pregnancy Risk Factor B/C (product specific)

Pregnancy Considerations Animal reproduction studies have not been conducted with all products; adverse events were not observed in animal reproduction studies conducted using the ointment. Nitroglycerin crosses the placenta (David, 2000). Concentrations following application of a transdermal patch 0.4 mg/hour were low but detectable in the fetal serum (fetal/maternal ratio: 0.23) (Bustard, 2003). Nitroglycerin may be used in pregnancy when immediate relaxation of the uterus is needed (ACOG, 2006; Axemo, 1998; Chandraharan, 2005). Intravenous nitroglycerin may be used to treat pre-eclampsia with pulmonary edema (ESG, 2011).

Breast-Feeding Considerations It is not known if nitroglycerin is excreted in breast milk. The manufacturer recommends that caution be exercised when administering nitroglycerin to nursing women. Information related to the use of nitroglycerin and breast-feeding is limited (Böttiger, 2010; O'Sullivan, 2011).

Contraindications

Hypersensitivity to organic nitrates or any component of the formulation (includes adhesives for transdermal product); concurrent use with phosphodiesterase-5 (PDE-5) inhibitors (avanafil, sildenafil, tadalafil, or vardenafil); concurrent use with riociguat

Additional contraindications for IV product: Hypersensitivity to corn or corn products (solutions containing dextrose); constrictive pericarditis; pericardial tamponade; restrictive cardiomyopathy

Additional contraindications for sublingual product and rectal ointment: Early myocardial infarction (sublingual product only; see **Note**); increased intracranial pressure; severe anemia

Additional contraindications for translingual product: Increased intracranial pressure; severe anemia; acute circulatory failure or shock (Nitrolingual only)

Canadian labeling: Additional contraindications for transdermal patch (not in US labeling): Acute circulatory failure associated with marked hypotension (shock and states of collapse); orthostatic hypotension; myocardial insufficiency due to obstruction (eg, presence of aortic or mitral stenosis or of constrictive pericarditis); increased intracranial pressure; increased intraocular pressure; severe anemia

Note: According to the 2013 American College of Cardiology Foundation/American Heart Association (ACCF/AHA) guidelines of the management of ST-elevation myocardial infarction (STEMI) and the 2013 ACCF/AHA guidelines for the management of unstable angina/non-ST-elevation myocardial infarction, avoid nitrates in the following conditions: Hypotension (SBP <90 mm Hg or ≥30 mm Hg below baseline), marked bradycardia or tachycardia, and right ventricular infarction. Sublingual nitroglycerin may be used as initial treatment of ongoing chest pain in patients who may have STEMI or UA/NSTEMI (Anderson, 2013; O'Gara, 2013).

Warnings/Precautions Severe hypotension can occur. Use with caution in volume depletion, moderate hypotension, constrictive pericarditis, aortic or mitral stenosis, and extreme caution with inferior wall MI and suspected right ventricular involvement. The Canadian labeling contraindicates use in myocardial insufficiency due to obstruction such as constrictive pericarditis and aortic or mitral stenosis. According to the ACCF/AHA, avoid use in patients with severe hypotension (SBP <90 mm Hg or ≥30 mm Hg below baseline), marked bradycardia or tachycardia, and right ventricular MI (ACCF/AHA [Anderson, 2013]; ACCF/AHA [O'Gara, 2013]). Avoid use in patients with hypertrophic cardiomyopathy (HCM) with outflow tract obstruction; nitrates may reduce preload, exacerbating obstruction and cause hypotension or syncope and/or worsening of heart failure (ACCF/AHA [Gersh, 2011]).

Paradoxical bradycardia and increased angina pectoris can accompany hypotension. Orthostatic hypotension can also occur. Ethanol can accentuate this. Dose-related headaches may occur, especially during initial dosing. Tolerance does develop to nitrates and appropriate dosing is needed to minimize this (drug-free interval). Avoid use of long-acting agents in acute MI or acute HF; cannot easily reverse effects. Nitrates may aggravate angina caused by hypertrophic cardiomyopathy. Nitroglycerin may precipitate or aggravate increased intracranial pressure and subsequently may worsen clinical outcomes in patients with neurologic injury (eg, intracranial hemorrhage, traumatic brain injury). The Canadian labeling contraindicates use with increased intracranial pressure. Nitroglycerin transdermal patches may contain conducting metal (eg, aluminum); remove patch prior to MRI. Some dosage forms may contain propylene glycol; large amounts are potentially toxic and have been associated hyperosmolality, lactic acidosis, seizures and respiratory depression; use caution (AAP, 1997; Zar, 2007). Potentially significant drug-drug interactions may exist, requiring dose or frequency adjustment, additional monitoring, and/or selection of alternative therapy.

Use caution when treating rectal anal fissures with nitroglycerin ointment formulation in patients with suspected or known significant cardiovascular disorders (eg, cardiomyopathies, heart failure, acute MI); intra-anal nitroglycerin administration may decrease systolic blood pressure and decrease arterial vascular resistance.

Warnings: Additional Pediatric Considerations Some dosage forms may contain propylene glycol; in neonates large amounts of propylene glycol delivered orally, intravenously (eg, >3,000 mg/day), or topically have been associated with potentially fatal toxicities which can include metabolic acidosis, seizures, renal failure, and CNS depression; toxicities have also been reported in children and adults including hyperosmolality, lactic acidosis, seizures, and respiratory depression; use caution (AAP, 1997; Shehab, 2009).

Adverse Reactions

Cardiovascular: Bradycardia, flushing, hypotension, orthostatic hypotension, peripheral edema, syncope, tachycardia

Central nervous system: Headache (common), dizziness, lightheadedness

Gastrointestinal: Nausea, vomiting, xerostomia

Neuromuscular & skeletal: Paresthesia, weakness

Respiratory: Dyspnea, pharyngitis, rhinitis

Miscellaneous: Diaphoresis

Rare but important or life-threatening): Allergic reactions, anaphylactoid reaction, application site irritation (patch), blurred vision, cardiovascular collapse, contact dermatitis (ointment, patch), crescendo angina, exfoliative dermatitis, fixed drug eruption (ointment, patch), methemoglobinemia (rare; overdose), pallor, palpitation, rash, rebound hypertension, restlessness, shock, vertigo

Drug Interactions

Metabolism/Transport Effects None known.

Avoid Concomitant Use

Avoid concomitant use of Nitroglycerin with any of the following: Ergot Derivatives; Phosphodiesterase 5 Inhibitors; Riociguat

Increased Effect/Toxicity

Nitroglycerin may increase the levels/effects of: DULoxetine; Ergot Derivatives; Hypotensive Agents; Levodopa; Prilocaine; Riociguat; RisperiDONE; Rosiglitazone; Sodium Nitrite

The levels/effects of Nitroglycerin may be increased by: Alcohol (Ethyl); Alfuzosin; Barbiturates; Dapoxetine; Nicorandil; Nitric Oxide; Phosphodiesterase 5 Inhibitors

Decreased Effect

Nitroglycerin may decrease the levels/effects of: Alteplase; Heparin

The levels/effects of Nitroglycerin may be decreased by: Ergot Derivatives

Storage/Stability

IV solution: Doses should be made in glass bottles, EXCEL® or PAB® containers. Adsorption occurs to soft plastic (eg, PVC). Nitroglycerin diluted in D_5W or NS in glass containers is physically and chemically stable for 48 hours at room temperature and 7 days under refrigeration. In D_5W or NS in EXCEL®/PAB® containers it is physically and chemically stable for 24 hours at room temperature.

Sublingual tablets, slow-release capsules, topical ointment, and rectal ointment: Store at 20°C to 25°C (68°F to 77°F)

Transdermal patch: Store at 15°C to 30°C (59°F to 86°F)

Translingual spray: Store at 25°C (77°F); excursions permitted to 15°C to 30°C (59°F to 86°F). Do not forcefully open or burn container after use. Do not spray toward flames.

Mechanism of Action Nitroglycerin forms free radical nitric oxide. In smooth muscle, nitric oxide activates guanylate cyclase which increases guanosine 3'5' monophosphate (cGMP) leading to dephosphorylation of myosin light chains and smooth muscle relaxation. Produces a vasodilator effect on the peripheral veins and arteries with more prominent effects on the veins. Primarily reduces cardiac oxygen demand by decreasing preload (left ventricular end-diastolic pressure); may modestly reduce afterload; dilates coronary arteries and improves collateral flow to ischemic regions. For use in rectal fissures, intra-anal administration results in decreased sphincter tone and intra-anal pressure.

Pharmacodynamics

Onset of action: Sublingual tablet: 1-3 minutes; Translingual spray: Similar to sublingual tablet; Sustained release: ~60 minutes; Topical: 15-30 minutes; Transdermal: ~30 minutes; IV: Immediate

Peak effect: Sublingual tablet: 5 minutes; Translingual spray: 4-10 minutes; Sustained release: 2.5-4 hours; Topical: ~60 minutes; Transdermal: 120 minutes; IV: Immediate

Duration: Sublingual tablet: At least 25 minutes; Translingual spray: Similar to sublingual tablet; Sustained release: 4-8 hours; Topical: 7 hours; Transdermal: 10-12 hours; IV: 3-5 minutes

Pharmacokinetics (Adult data unless noted)

Distribution: V_d: ~3 L/kg

Protein binding: 60%

Metabolism: Extensive first-pass; metabolized hepatically to glycerol di- and mononitrate metabolites via liver reductase enzyme; subsequent metabolism to glycerol and organic nitrate; nonhepatic metabolism via red blood cells and vascular walls also occurs

Half-life: 1-4 minutes

Elimination: Excretion of inactive metabolites in urine

Dosing: Neonatal Vasodilation; perioperative, congenital heart defect repair: Limited data available: Continuous IV infusion: Initial: 0.25 to 0.5 mcg/kg/minute; titrate by 0.5 to 1 mcg/kg/minute every 3 to 5 minutes as needed; usual dose: 1 to 3 mcg/kg/minute; usual maximum dose: 5 mcg/kg/minute. In one clinical study of 16 pediatric patients <24 months of age (median: 4.4 months, range: 3 days to 23.7 months), a median dose of 1.8 mcg/kg/minute (range: 0.5 to 4 mcg/kg/minute) was reported following cardiac surgery with bypass (Williams 1994); another trial describes a fixed dose of 1 mcg/kg/minute administered to 15 neonates (mean: 8 days of age) after cardiac surgery in conjunction with dopamine (Laitinen 1999)

Dosing: Usual Tolerance to the hemodynamic and antianginal effects can develop within 24 to 48 hours of continuous use.

Infants and Children: Continuous IV infusion: Initial: 0.25 to 0.5 mcg/kg/minute; titrate by 0.5 to 1 mcg/kg/minute every 3 to 5 minutes as needed; usual dose: 1 to 3 mcg/kg/minute; usual maximum dose: 5 mcg/kg/minute; doses up to 20 mcg/kg/minute may be used

Adults:

Anal fissure, chronic: Intra-anal: 0.4% ointment: 1 inch (equals 1.5 mg of nitroglycerin) every 12 hours for up to 3 weeks

Angina/coronary artery disease:

Continuous IV infusion: **Note:** Do **not** dose per kg; adult dose is in units of mcg/minute; Initial: 5 mcg/minute, increase by 5 mcg/minute every 3 to 5 minutes to 20 mcg/minute, then increase as needed by 10 to 20 mcg/minute every 3 to 5 minutes (generally accepted maximum dose: 400 mcg/minute)

Oral: 2.5 to 6.5 mg 3 to 4 times daily (maximum dose: 26 mg)

Patch, transdermal: Initial: 0.2 to 0.4 mg/hour, titrate to 0.4 to 0.8 mg/hour; use a "patch-on" period of 12 to 14 hours per day and a "patch-off" period of 10 to 12 hours per day to minimize tolerance

Sublingual: 0.3 to 0.6 mg every 5 minutes for maximum of 3 doses in 15 minutes; may also use prophylactically 5 to 10 minutes prior to activities which may provoke an attack

Topical: 2% Ointment: Apply 0.5 inch upon rising and 0.5 inch 6 hours later; if necessary, the dose may be doubled to 1 inch and subsequently doubled again to 2 inches if response is inadequate. Doses of 0.5 to 2 inches were used in clinical trials. Recommended maximum: 2 doses/day; include a nitrate-free interval ~10 to 12 hours/day

Translingual: 1 to 2 sprays into mouth onto or under tongue every 3 to 5 minutes for maximum of 3 sprays in 15 minutes; may administer 5 to 10 minutes before activities that may precipitate angina

Usual Infusion Concentrations: Pediatric Note: Premixed solutions available

IV infusion: 100 **mcg**/mL, 200 **mcg**/mL, or 400 **mcg**/mL

Preparation for Administration Parenteral: Continuous IV infusion: Dilute in D_5W or NS to 50 to 100 mcg/mL; maximum concentration not to exceed 400 mcg/mL; prepare in glass bottles, EXCEL or PAB containers (adsorption occurs to soft plastic [eg, PVC]).

Nitronal (glyceryl trinitrate) 1 mg/mL (temporarily available in the US):

To prepare a 100 **mcg**/mL solution: Withdraw 25 mL D_5W from a 250 mL bottle of D_5W and replace volume with 25 mg (25 mL) of Nitronal.

To prepare a 200 **mcg**/mL solution: Withdraw 50 mL D_5W from a 250 mL bottle of D_5W and replace volume with 50 mg (50 mL) of Nitronal.

Administration

Intra-anal ointment: Using a finger covering (eg, plastic wrap, surgical glove, finger cot), place finger beside 1 inch measuring guide on the box and squeeze ointment the length of the measuring line directly onto covered finger. Insert ointment into the anal canal using the covered finger up to first finger joint (do not insert further than the first finger joint) and apply ointment around the side of the anal canal. If intra-anal application is too painful, may apply the ointment to the outside of the anus. Wash hands following application.

Oral:

Capsule (sustained release): Administer with a full glass of water on an empty stomach; swallow whole, do not crush or chew

Sublingual tablet: Place under tongue and allow to dissolve, do not swallow, chew, or crush; do not eat or drink while tablet dissolves

Translingual spray: Do not shake container. Pump must be primed prior to first use by spraying 5 times (Nitrolingual) or 10 times (Nitromist); direct priming sprays into the air, away from patient and others; if pump is unused for 6 weeks, a single priming spray (Nitrolingual) or 2 priming sprays (Nitromist) should be completed. To administer dose, spray onto or under tongue with container as close to mouth as possible; close mouth after administration; do not inhale spray; avoid swallowing immediately after spray; do not expectorate or rinse mouth for 5 to 10 minutes after use

Parenteral: Continuous IV infusion: Administer via infusion pump. Adsorption occurs to soft plastic (eg, PVC); special administration sets intended for nitroglycerin (nonpolyvinyl chloride) must be used

Transdermal patch: Place on hair-free area of skin; rotate patch sites; **Note:** Some products are a membrane-controlled system (eg, Transderm-Nitro); do **not** cut these patches to deliver partial doses; rate of drug delivery, reservoir contents, and adhesion may be affected; if partial dose is needed, surface area of patch can be blocked proportionally using adhesive bandage (Lee 1997 and see specific product labeling)

Monitoring Parameters Blood pressure, heart rate (continuously with IV use)

Test Interactions IV formulation: Due to propylene glycol content, triglyceride assays dependent on glycerol oxidase may be falsely elevated.

Additional Information IV preparations contain alcohol and/or propylene glycol; may need to use nitrate-free interval (10-12 hours/day) to avoid tolerance development; tolerance may possibly be reversed with acetylcysteine; gradually decrease dose in patients receiving NTG for prolonged period to avoid withdrawal reaction; lingual spray contains 20% alcohol, do not spray toward flames

Dosage Forms Excipient information presented when available (limited, particularly for generics); consult specific product labeling.

Aerosol Solution, Translingual:

NitroMist: 400 mcg/spray (4.1 g, 8.5 g) [contains menthol]

Generic: 400 mcg/spray (4.1 g, 8.5 g)

Capsule Extended Release, Oral:

Nitro-Time: 2.5 mg [contains brilliant blue fcf (fd&c blue #1), fd&c red #40, fd&c yellow #10 (quinoline yellow)]

Nitro-Time: 6.5 mg [contains brilliant blue fcf (fd&c blue #1), fd&c yellow #10 (quinoline yellow), fd&c yellow #6 (sunset yellow)]

Nitro-Time: 9 mg [contains fd&c yellow #10 (quinoline yellow), fd&c yellow #6 (sunset yellow)]

Generic: 2.5 mg, 6.5 mg, 9 mg

Ointment, Rectal:

Rectiv: 0.4% (30 g) [contains propylene glycol]

Ointment, Transdermal:

Nitro-Bid: 2% (1 g, 30 g, 60 g)

Patch 24 Hour, Transdermal:

Minitran: 0.1 mg/hr (30 ea); 0.2 mg/hr (30 ea); 0.4 mg/hr (30 ea); 0.6 mg/hr (30 ea)

Nitro-Dur: 0.1 mg/hr (30 ea, 100 ea); 0.2 mg/hr (30 ea, 100 ea); 0.3 mg/hr (30 ea, 100 ea); 0.4 mg/hr (30 ea, 100 ea); 0.6 mg/hr (30 ea, 100 ea); 0.8 mg/hr (30 ea, 100 ea)

Generic: 0.1 mg/hr (30 ea, 4350 ea); 0.2 mg/hr (30 ea, 4350 ea); 0.4 mg/hr (30 ea, 4350 ea); 0.6 mg/hr (30 ea, 4350 ea)

Solution, Intravenous:

Nitronal: 1 mg/mL (25 mL, 50 mL)

Generic: 25 mg (250 mL); 50 mg (250 mL, 500 mL); 100 mg (250 mL); 200 mg (500 mL); 5 mg/mL (10 mL)

Solution, Translingual:

Nitrolingual: 0.4 mg/spray (4.9 g, 12 g) [contains alcohol, usp]

Generic: 0.4 mg/spray (4.9 g, 12 g)

Tablet Sublingual, Sublingual:

Nitrostat: 0.3 mg, 0.4 mg, 0.6 mg

- ◆ **Nitroglycerin Injection, USP (Can)** *see* Nitroglycerin *on page* 1523
- ◆ **Nitroglycerol** *see* Nitroglycerin *on page* 1523
- ◆ **Nitrol (Can)** *see* Nitroglycerin *on page* 1523
- ◆ **Nitrolingual** *see* Nitroglycerin *on page* 1523
- ◆ **NitroMist** *see* Nitroglycerin *on page* 1523
- ◆ **Nitronal** *see* Nitroglycerin *on page* 1523
- ◆ **Nitronal** *see* Nitroglycerin *on page* 1523
- ◆ **Nitropress** *see* Nitroprusside *on page* 1526

Nitroprusside (nye troe PRUS ide)

Medication Safety Issues

Sound-alike/look-alike issues:

Nitroprusside may be confused with nitroglycerin

High alert medication:

The Institute for Safe Medication Practices (ISMP) includes this medication among its list of drugs which have a heightened risk of causing significant patient harm when used in error.

Related Information

Serotonin Syndrome *on page* 2447

Brand Names: US Nitropress

Brand Names: Canada Nipride

Therapeutic Category Antihypertensive Agent; Vasodilator

Generic Availability (US) No

Use Management of hypertensive crises; CHF; used for controlled hypotension during anesthesia

Pregnancy Risk Factor C

Pregnancy Considerations Animal studies have shown that nitroprusside may cross the placental barrier and result in fetal cyanide levels that are dose-related to maternal nitroprusside levels. However, information related to use in pregnancy is limited.

Breast-Feeding Considerations It is not known if nitroprusside is excreted in breast milk. Due to the potential for serious adverse reactions in the nursing infant, a decision should be made whether to discontinue nursing or to discontinue the drug, taking into account the importance of treatment to the mother.

Contraindications Treatment of compensatory hypertension (aortic coarctation, arteriovenous shunting); to produce controlled hypotension during surgery in patients with known inadequate cerebral circulation or in moribund patients requiring emergency surgery; high output heart failure associated with reduced systemic vascular resistance (eg, septic shock); congenital optic atrophy or tobacco amblyopia

Warnings/Precautions **[U.S. Boxed Warning] Excessive hypotension resulting in compromised perfusion of vital organs may occur; continuous blood pressure monitoring by experienced personnel is required. Except when used briefly or at low (<2 mcg/kg/minute) infusion rates, nitroprusside gives rise to large cyanide quantities. Do not use the maximum dose for more than 10 minutes; if blood pressure is not controlled by the maximum rate (ie, 10 mcg/kg/minute) after 10 minutes, discontinue infusion. Monitor for cyanide toxicity via acid-base balance and venous oxygen concentration; however, clinicians should note that these indicators may not always reliably indicate cyanide toxicity.** Patients at risk of cyanide toxicity include those who are malnourished, have hepatic impairment, or those undergoing cardiopulmonary bypass, or therapeutic hypothermia (Rindone, 1992). Discontinue use of nitroprusside if signs and/or symptoms of cyanide toxicity (eg, metabolic acidosis, decreased oxygen saturation, bradycardia, confusion, convulsions) occur. Although not routinely done, sodium thiosulfate has been co-administered with nitroprusside using a 10:1 ratio of sodium thiosulfate to nitroprusside when higher doses of nitroprusside are used (eg, 4-10 mcg/kg/minute) for extended periods of time in order to prevent cyanide toxicity (Varon, 2008; Shulz, 2010); thiocyanate toxicity may still occur with this approach (Rindone, 1992). The use of other agents (eg, clevidipine, labetalol, nicardipine) should be considered if blood pressure is not controlled with nitroprusside. Use the lowest end of the dosage range with renal impairment. Cyanide toxicity may occur in patients with decreased liver function. Thiocyanate toxicity occurs in patients with renal impairment or those on prolonged infusions.

When nitroprusside is used for controlled hypotension during surgery, correct pre-existing anemia and hypovolemia prior to use when possible. Use with extreme caution in patients with elevated intracranial pressure (head trauma, cerebral hemorrhage), myocardial infarction, severe renal impairment, hepatic failure, hypothyroidism. **[U.S. Boxed Warning]: Solution must be further diluted with 5% dextrose in water. Do not administer by direct injection.**

Adverse Reactions

Cardiovascular: Bradycardia, ECG changes, flushing, hypotension (excessive), palpitation, substernal distress, tachycardia

Central nervous system: Apprehension, dizziness, headache, intracranial pressure increased, restlessness

Dermatologic: Rash

Endocrine & metabolic: Metabolic acidosis (secondary to cyanide toxicity), hypothyroidism

Gastrointestinal: Abdominal pain, ileus, nausea, retching, vomiting
Hematologic: Methemoglobinemia, platelet aggregation decreased
Local: Injection site irritation
Neuromuscular & skeletal: Hyperreflexia (secondary to thiocyanate toxicity), muscle twitching
Ocular: Miosis (secondary to thiocyanate toxicity)
Otic: Tinnitus (secondary to thiocyanate toxicity)
Respiratory: Hyperoxemia (secondary to cyanide toxicity)
Miscellaneous: Cyanide toxicity, diaphoresis, thiocyanate toxicity

Drug Interactions

Metabolism/Transport Effects None known.

Avoid Concomitant Use There are no known interactions where it is recommended to avoid concomitant use.

Increased Effect/Toxicity

Nitroprusside may increase the levels/effects of: Amifostine; Antihypertensives; DULoxetine; Hypotensive Agents; Levodopa; Obinutuzumab; Prilocaine; RisperiDONE; RiTUXimab; Sodium Nitrite

The levels/effects of Nitroprusside may be increased by: Alfuzosin; Barbiturates; Brimonidine (Topical); Calcium Channel Blockers; Diazoxide; Herbs (Hypotensive Properties); MAO Inhibitors; Nicorandil; Nitric Oxide; Pentoxifylline; Phosphodiesterase 5 Inhibitors; Prostacyclin Analogues

Decreased Effect

The levels/effects of Nitroprusside may be decreased by: Herbs (Hypertensive Properties); Methylphenidate; Yohimbine

Storage/Stability Store the intact vial at 20°C to 25°C (68°F to 77°F). Protect from light.

Stability of parenteral admixture at room temperature (25°C) and at refrigeration temperature (4°C) is 24 hours.

Mechanism of Action Causes peripheral vasodilation by direct action on venous and arteriolar smooth muscle, thus reducing peripheral resistance; will increase cardiac output by decreasing afterload; reduces aortal and left ventricular impedance

Pharmacodynamics Hypotensive effects:
Onset of action: Within 2 minutes
Duration: 1-10 minutes

Pharmacokinetics (Adult data unless noted)
Metabolism: Converted to cyanide by erythrocyte and tissue sulfhydryl group interactions; cyanide is converted in the liver by the enzyme rhodanase to thiocyanate
Half-life: <10 minutes
Thiocyanate: 2.7-7 days
Elimination: Thiocyanate is excreted in the urine

Dosing: Neonatal Continuous IV infusion: Initial: 0.2 mcg/kg/minute and titrate to effect; doses up to 8 mcg/kg/minute have been reported; however, doses ≥1.8 mcg/kg/minute are associated with increased cyanide concentration in pediatric patients, including neonates (Moffett, 2008); reported duration of therapy was typically <6-7 days. Use in neonates has been described in several retrospective reports and case series; most recent and majority of patient experience is during cardiac surgery requiring cardiopulmonary bypass and postoperatively for afterload reduction (Benitz, 1985; Cachat, 2004; Furck, 2010; Kiran, 2006; Motta, 1995; Williams, 1994); use for 6 days at a maximum dose of 2.5 mcg/kg/minute produced profound lactic acidosis in one neonate (Meyer, 2005)

Dosing: Usual
Infants and Children: Continuous IV infusion: Start 0.3-0.5 mcg/kg/minute, titrate to effect; doses ≥1.8 mcg/kg/minute are associated with increased cyanide concentration in pediatric patients (Moffett, 2008); rarely need >4 mcg/kg/minute; maximum dose: 8-10 mcg/kg/minute
Adults: Continuous IV infusion: Initial: 0.3-0.5 mcg/kg/minute; increase in increments of 0.5 mcg/kg/minute, titrating to the desired hemodynamic effect or the appearance of headache or nausea; usual dose: 3 mcg/kg/minute; rarely need >4 mcg/kg/minute; maximum: 10 mcg/kg/minute. When >500 mcg/kg is administered by prolonged infusion of faster than 2 mcg/kg/minute, cyanide is generated faster than an unaided patient can handle.

Usual Infusion Concentrations: Pediatric IV infusion: 100 **mcg**/mL **or** 200 **mcg**/mL

Preparation for Administration
Parenteral: Must dilute prior to administration; dilute with D_5W (preferred), LR, or NS to a concentration of 50 to 200 mcg/mL; in fluid restricted patients, concentrations up to 1,000 mcg/mL in D_5W have been used (Murray 2014; Pramer 1991). Do not add other medications to nitroprusside solutions.

Use only clear solutions; solutions of nitroprusside exhibit a color described as brownish, brown, brownish-pink, light orange, and straw. Solutions are highly sensitive to light. Exposure to light causes decomposition, resulting in a highly colored solution of orange, dark brown or blue. **A blue color indicates almost complete decomposition.** Do not use discolored solutions (eg, blue, green, red) or solutions in which particulate matter is visible.

Prepared solutions should be wrapped with aluminum foil or other opaque material to protect from light (do as soon as possible).

Administration Parenteral: Not for direct injection; must dilute prior to administration. Administer as continuous IV infusion via infusion pump. Solution should be protected from light, but not necessary to wrap administration set or IV tubing.

Monitoring Parameters Blood pressure, heart rate; monitor for cyanide and thiocyanate toxicity; monitor acid-base status as acidosis can be the earliest sign of cyanide toxicity; monitor thiocyanate levels if requiring prolonged infusion (>3 days) or dose ≥4 mcg/kg/minute or patient has renal dysfunction; monitor cyanide blood levels in patients with decreased hepatic function

Reference Range
Thiocyanate:
Toxic: 35-100 mcg/mL
Fatal: >200 mcg/mL
Cyanide:
Normal <0.2 mcg/mL
Normal (smoker): <0.4 mcg/mL
Toxic: >2 mcg/mL
Potentially lethal: >3 mcg/mL

Additional Information Thiocyanate toxicity includes psychoses, blurred vision, confusion, weakness, tinnitus, seizures; cyanide toxicity includes metabolic acidosis, tachycardia, pink skin, decreased pulse, decreased reflexes, altered consciousness, coma, almond smell on breath, methemoglobinemia, dilated pupils

Dosage Forms Excipient information presented when available (limited, particularly for generics); consult specific product labeling.
Solution, Intravenous, as sodium:
Nitropress: 25 mg/mL (2 mL)

◆ **Nitroprusside Sodium** *see* Nitroprusside *on page* 1526
◆ **Nitrostat** *see* Nitroglycerin *on page* 1523
◆ **Nitro-Time** *see* Nitroglycerin *on page* 1523
◆ **Nix [OTC] (Can)** *see* Permethrin *on page* 1675

Nizatidine (ni ZA ti deen)

Medication Safety Issues

Sound-alike/look-alike issues:

Axid may be confused with Ansaid

International issues:

Tazac [Australia] may be confused with Tazact brand name for piperacillin/tazobactam [India]; Tiazac brand name for diltiazem [U.S., Canada]

Brand Names: US Axid; Axid AR [OTC]

Brand Names: Canada Apo-Nizatidine; Axid; Gen-Nizatidine; Novo-Nizatidine; Nu-Nizatidine; PMS-Nizatidine

Therapeutic Category Gastrointestinal Agent, Gastric or Duodenal Ulcer Treatment; Histamine H_2 Antagonist

Generic Availability (US) May be product dependent

Use Treatment and maintenance therapy of duodenal ulcer; treatment of active benign gastric ulcer; esophagitis; gastroesophageal reflux disease (GERD); adjunctive therapy in the treatment of *Helicobacter pylori*-associated duodenal ulcer

Pregnancy Risk Factor B

Pregnancy Considerations Adverse events have not been observed in animal reproduction studies; therefore, the nizatidine is classified as pregnancy category B. Nizatidine crosses the placenta. An increased risk of congenital malformations or adverse events in the newborn has generally not been observed following maternal use of nizatidine during pregnancy. Histamine H_2 antagonists have been evaluated for the treatment of gastroesophageal reflux disease (GERD), as well as gastric and duodenal ulcers during pregnancy. Although if needed, nizatidine is not the agent of choice. Histamine H_2 antagonists may be used for aspiration prophylaxis prior to cesarean delivery.

Breast-Feeding Considerations Following oral administration of nizatidine, 0.1% of the maternal dose is found in breast milk. The highest milk concentrations appear ~2 hours after a maternal dose. According to the manufacturer, the decision to continue or discontinue breast-feeding during therapy should take into account the risk of exposure to the infant and the benefits of treatment to the mother.

Contraindications Hypersensitivity to nizatidine or any component of the formulation; hypersensitivity to other H_2 antagonists (cross-sensitivity has been observed)

Warnings/Precautions Relief of symptoms does not preclude the presence of a gastric malignancy. Use with caution in patients with liver and renal impairment. Dosage modification required in patients with renal impairment.

Prolonged treatment (≥2 years) may lead to vitamin B_{12} malabsorption and subsequent vitamin B_{12} deficiency. The magnitude of the deficiency is dose-related and the association is stronger in females and those younger in age (<30 years); prevalence is decreased after discontinuation of therapy (Lam, 2013).

Adverse Reactions

Central nervous system: Anxiety, dizziness, fever (reported in children), headache, insomnia, irritability (reported in children), nervousness, somnolence

Dermatologic: Pruritus, rash

Gastrointestinal: Abdominal pain, anorexia, constipation, diarrhea, dry mouth, flatulence, heartburn, nausea, vomiting

Respiratory: Reported in children: Cough, nasal congestion, nasopharyngitis

Rare but important or life-threatening: Alkaline phosphatase increased, ALT increased, anaphylaxis, anemia, AST increased, bronchospasm, confusion, eosinophilia, exfoliative dermatitis, gynecomastia, hepatitis, jaundice, laryngeal edema, serum-sickness like reactions, thrombocytopenia, thrombocytopenic purpura, vasculitis, ventricular tachycardia

Drug Interactions

Metabolism/Transport Effects None known.

Avoid Concomitant Use

Avoid concomitant use of Nizatidine with any of the following: Dasatinib; Delavirdine; PAZOPanib; Risedronate

Increased Effect/Toxicity

Nizatidine may increase the levels/effects of: Dexmethylphenidate; Methylphenidate; Risedronate; Saquinavir; Varenicline

Decreased Effect

Nizatidine may decrease the levels/effects of: Atazanavir; Bosutinib; Cefditoren; Cefpodoxime; Cefuroxime; Dabrafenib; Dasatinib; Delavirdine; Erlotinib; Fosamprenavir; Gefitinib; Indinavir; Iron Salts; Itraconazole; Ketoconazole (Systemic); Ledipasvir; Mesalamine; Multivitamins/Minerals (with ADEK, Folate, Iron); Nelfinavir; Nilotinib; PAZOPanib; Posaconazole; Rilpivirine

Food Interactions Prolonged treatment (≥2 years) may lead to malabsorption of dietary vitamin B_{12} and subsequent vitamin B_{12} deficiency (Lam, 2013).

Storage/Stability

Store at 25°C (77°F); excursions permitted to 15°C to 30°C (59°F to 86°F).

Nizatidine is stable for 48 hours at room temperature when the contents of a capsule are mixed in Gatorade® lemon-lime, Cran-Grape® grape-cranberry drink, V8®, or aluminum- and magnesium hydroxide suspension (approximate concentration 2.5 mg/mL) (Lantz, 1990)

Mechanism of Action Competitive inhibition of histamine at H_2-receptors of the gastric parietal cells resulting in reduced gastric acid secretion, gastric volume and hydrogen ion concentration reduced. In healthy volunteers, nizatidine suppresses gastric acid secretion induced by pentagastrin infusion or food.

Pharmacodynamics Maximum effect: Duodenal ulcer: 4 weeks

Pharmacokinetics (Adult data unless noted)

Distribution: V_d: Adults: 0.8-1.5 L/kg; breast milk: 0.1% excreted into breast milk

Protein binding: 35%

Bioavailability: Oral: 70%

Half-life, elimination: Adults: 1-2 hours; anuric: 3.5-11 hours

Time to peak serum concentration: 0.5-3 hours

Elimination: 60% excreted unchanged in urine

Dosing: Usual Oral:

Infants 6 months to Children 11 years: Limited information available: 5-10 mg/kg/day divided twice daily

GERD, esophagitis: Children ≥12 years and Adults: 150 mg twice daily

Active duodenal and gastric ulcers: Adults: 300 mg once daily at bedtime or 150 mg twice daily

Maintenance of healed duodenal ulcer: Adults: 150 mg once daily

Helicobacter pylori-associated duodenal ulcer (limited information): Adults: 150 mg twice daily for 4 weeks (combined with clarithromycin and bismuth formulation; followed by 300 mg/day)

Dosing adjustment in renal impairment: Adults:

Active treatment:

CrCl 20-50 mL/minute: 150 mg once daily

CrCl <20 mL/minute: 150 mg every other day

Maintenance treatment:

CrCl 20-50 mL/minute: 150 every other day

CrCl <20 mL/minute: 150 mg every 3 days

Administration Oral: May administer with or without food; do not administer or mix with apple juice

Test Interactions False-positive urine protein using Multistix®, gastric acid secretion test, skin tests allergen extracts, serum creatinine and serum transaminase concentrations, urine protein test

Dosage Forms Excipient information presented when available (limited, particularly for generics); consult specific product labeling.

Capsule, Oral:
Axid: 300 mg
Generic: 150 mg, 300 mg

Solution, Oral:
Axid: 15 mg/mL (480 mL) [contains methylparaben, propylparaben, saccharin sodium; bubble-gum flavor]
Generic: 15 mg/mL (473 mL, 480 mL)

Tablet, Oral:
Axid AR: 75 mg

Extemporaneous Preparations A 2.5 mg/mL oral solution may be made with capsules and one of three different vehicles (lemon-lime Gatorade®, Ocean Spray® Cran-Grape® juice or V8® 100% vegetable juice). Empty the contents of one 300 mg capsule in a mortar. Add small portions of the chosen vehicle and mix to a uniform paste; mix while adding the vehicle in incremental proportions to **almost** 120 mL; transfer to a calibrated bottle, rinse mortar with vehicle, and add quantity of vehicle sufficient to make 120 mL. Label "shake well". Stable for 2 days refrigerated.

Nahata MC, Pai VB, and Hipple TF, *Pediatric Drug Formulations*, 5th ed, Cincinnati, OH: Harvey Whitney Books Co, 2004.

- ◆ **Nizoral** *see* Ketoconazole (Systemic) *on page 1188*
- ◆ **Nizoral** *see* Ketoconazole (Topical) *on page 1191*
- ◆ **Nizoral A-D [OTC]** *see* Ketoconazole (Topical) *on page 1191*
- ◆ **N-Methylhydrazine** *see* Procarbazine *on page 1772*
- ◆ **Nocdurna (Can)** *see* Desmopressin *on page 607*
- ◆ **No Doz Maximum Strength [OTC]** *see* Caffeine *on page 335*
- ◆ **Nolvadex** *see* Tamoxifen *on page 2005*
- ◆ **Nolvadex-D (Can)** *see* Tamoxifen *on page 2005*
- ◆ **Non-Aspirin Pain Reliever [OTC]** *see* Acetaminophen *on page 44*
- ◆ **Non-Pseudo Sinus Decongestant [OTC]** *see* Phenylephrine (Systemic) *on page 1685*
- ◆ **Nora-BE** *see* Norethindrone *on page 1530*
- ◆ **Noradrenaline** *see* Norepinephrine *on page 1529*
- ◆ **Noradrenaline Acid Tartrate** *see* Norepinephrine *on page 1529*
- ◆ **Norco** *see* Hydrocodone and Acetaminophen *on page 1032*
- ◆ **Norcuron** *see* Vecuronium *on page 2163*
- ◆ **Norcuron® (Can)** *see* Vecuronium *on page 2163*
- ◆ **Nordeoxyguanosine** *see* Ganciclovir (Ophthalmic) *on page 959*
- ◆ **Nordeoxyguanosine** *see* Ganciclovir (Systemic) *on page 958*
- ◆ **Norditropin FlexPro** *see* Somatropin *on page 1957*
- ◆ **Norditropin Nordiflex (Can)** *see* Somatropin *on page 1957*
- ◆ **Norditropin NordiFlex Pen** *see* Somatropin *on page 1957*
- ◆ **Norditropin Simplexx (Can)** *see* Somatropin *on page 1957*

Norepinephrine (nor ep i NEF rin)

Medication Safety Issues

Sound-alike/look-alike issues:
Levophed® may be confused with levofloxacin

High alert medication:
The Institute for Safe Medication Practices (ISMP) includes this medication among its list of drugs which have a heightened risk of causing significant patient harm when used in error.

Related Information

Emergency Drip Calculations *on page 2229*
Management of Drug Extravasations *on page 2298*
Serotonin Syndrome *on page 2447*

Brand Names: US Levophed

Brand Names: Canada Levophed®

Therapeutic Category Adrenergic Agonist Agent; Alpha-Adrenergic Agonist; Sympathomimetic

Generic Availability (US) Yes

Use Treatment of shock which persists after adequate fluid volume replacement; severe hypotension; cardiogenic shock

Pregnancy Risk Factor C

Pregnancy Considerations Animal reproduction studies have not been conducted. Norepinephrine is an endogenous catecholamine and crosses the placenta (Minzter, 2010; Wang, 1999).

Breast-Feeding Considerations It is not known if norepinephrine is excreted in breast milk. The manufacturer recommends that caution be exercised when administering norepinephrine to nursing women.

Contraindications Hypersensitivity to norepinephrine, bisulfites (contains metabisulfite), or any component of the formulation; hypotension from hypovolemia except as an emergency measure to maintain coronary and cerebral perfusion until volume could be replaced; mesenteric or peripheral vascular thrombosis unless it is a lifesaving procedure; during anesthesia with cyclopropane (not available in U.S.) or halothane (not available in U.S.) anesthesia (risk of ventricular arrhythmias)

Warnings/Precautions Assure adequate circulatory volume to minimize need for vasoconstrictors. Avoid hypertension; monitor blood pressure closely and adjust infusion rate. Use with extreme caution in patients taking MAO-Inhibitors. Vesicant; ensure proper needle or catheter placement prior to and during infusion. Avoid extravasation; infuse into a large vein if possible. Avoid infusion into leg veins. Montior IV site closely. **[U.S. Boxed Warning]: If extravasation occurs, infiltrate the area with diluted phentolamine (5-10 mg in 10-15 mL of saline) with a fine hypodermic needle. Phentolamine should be administered as soon as possible after extravasation is noted to prevent sloughing/necrosis.** Product may contain sodium metabisulfite.

Adverse Reactions

Cardiovascular: Arrhythmias, bradycardia, peripheral (digital) ischemia
Central nervous system: Anxiety, headache (transient)
Local: Skin necrosis (with extravasation)
Respiratory: Dyspnea, respiratory difficulty

Drug Interactions

Metabolism/Transport Effects Substrate of COMT

Avoid Concomitant Use

Avoid concomitant use of Norepinephrine with any of the following: Ergot Derivatives; Inhalational Anesthetics; Iobenguane I 123

Increased Effect/Toxicity

Norepinephrine may increase the levels/effects of: Droxidopa; Sympathomimetics

The levels/effects of Norepinephrine may be increased by: AtoMOXetine; Beta-Blockers; Cannabinoid-Containing Products; COMT Inhibitors; Ergot Derivatives; Hyaluronidase; Inhalational Anesthetics; Linezolid; MAO Inhibitors; Serotonin/Norepinephrine Reuptake Inhibitors; Tedizolid; Tricyclic Antidepressants

Decreased Effect

Norepinephrine may decrease the levels/effects of: Benzylpenicilloyl Polylysine; Iobenguane I 123; Ioflupane I 123

The levels/effects of Norepinephrine may be decreased by: Alpha1-Blockers; Spironolactone

Storage/Stability Readily oxidized. Protect from light. Do not use if brown coloration. Stability of parenteral admixture at room temperature (25°C) is 24 hours.

Mechanism of Action Stimulates $beta_1$-adrenergic receptors and alpha-adrenergic receptors causing increased contractility and heart rate as well as vasoconstriction, thereby increasing systemic blood pressure and coronary blood flow; clinically, alpha effects (vasoconstriction) are greater than beta effects (inotropic and chronotropic effects)

Pharmacodynamics

Onset of action: Very rapid

Duration: Limited duration following IV injection

Pharmacokinetics (Adult data unless noted)

Metabolism: By catechol-o-methyltransferase (COMT) and monoamine oxidase (MAO)

Elimination: In urine (84% to 96% as inactive metabolites)

Dosing: Usual Continuous IV infusion: **Note:** Dose stated in terms of **norepinephrine base**:

Children: Initial: 0.05-0.1 mcg/kg/minute, titrate to desired effect; maximum dose: 1-2 mcg/kg/minute

Adults: Initial: 0.5-1 mcg/minute; titrate to desired response

Usual range: 8-30 mcg/minute as an infusion

ACLS dosage range: 0.5-30 mcg/minute

Usual Infusion Concentrations: Neonatal IV infusion: 10 **mcg**/mL **or** 16 **mcg**/mL

Usual Infusion Concentrations: Pediatric IV infusion: 8 **mcg**/mL **or** 16 **mcg**/mL

Preparation for Administration Continuous IV infusion: Dilute with D_5W, D_5NS, or NS; dilution in NS is not recommended by the manufacturer; however, stability in NS has been demonstrated (Tremblay 2008). Concentrations ranging from 4 to 16 mcg/mL are typically used in clinical practice (Phillips 2011). ISMP and Vermont Oxford Network recommend a standard concentration of 16 mcg/mL for neonates (ISMP 2011).

Administration Continuous IV infusion: Administer as a continuous infusion via an infusion pump. Central line administration is preferred; extravasation may cause severe ischemic necrosis. Do not administer sodium bicarbonate (or any alkaline solution) through an IV line containing norepinephrine; inactivation of norepinephrine may occur.

Rate of infusion (mL/hour) = dose (mcg/kg/minute) x weight (kg) x 60 minutes/hour divided by the concentration (mcg/mL)

Vesicant; ensure proper needle or catheter placement prior to and during infusion; avoid extravasation. If extravasation occurs, stop infusion immediately and disconnect (leave cannula/needle in place); gently aspirate extravasated solution (do **NOT** flush the line); remove needle/cannula; elevate extremity. Initiate phentolamine (or alternative) antidote (see Management of Drug Extravasations for more details). Apply dry warm compresses (Hurst 2004).

Vesicant/Extravasation Risk Vesicant

Monitoring Parameters Blood pressure, heart rate, urine output, peripheral perfusion

Additional Information Treat extravasations with local injections of phentolamine.

Dosage Forms Excipient information presented when available (limited, particularly for generics); consult specific product labeling.

Solution, Intravenous [strength expressed as base]:

Levophed: 1 mg/mL (4 mL) [contains sodium metabisulfite]

Generic: 1 mg/mL (4 mL)

Solution, Intravenous [strength expressed as base, preservative free]:

Generic: 1 mg/mL (4 mL)

◆ **Norepinephrine Bitartrate** *see* Norepinephrine *on page 1529*

Norethindrone (nor ETH in drone)

Medication Safety Issues

Sound-alike/look-alike issues:

Micronor® may be confused with miconazole, Micronase

Related Information

Contraceptive Comparison Table *on page 2309*

Safe Handling of Hazardous Drugs *on page 2455*

Brand Names: US Aygestin; Camila; Deblitane; Errin; Heather; Jencycla; Jolivette; Lyza; Nor-QD; Nora-BE; Norlyroc; Ortho Micronor; Sharobel

Brand Names: Canada Micronor®; Norlutate®

Therapeutic Category Contraceptive, Oral; Contraceptive, Progestin Only; Progestin

Generic Availability (US) Yes

Use Treatment of amenorrhea, abnormal uterine bleeding, endometriosis, oral contraceptive

Pregnancy Risk Factor X

Pregnancy Considerations First trimester exposure may cause genital abnormalities including hypospadias in male infants and mild virilization of external female genitalia. Significant adverse events related to growth and development have not been observed (limited studies). Use is contraindicated during pregnancy. May be started immediately postpartum if not breast-feeding.

Breast-Feeding Considerations Small amounts of progestins are found in breast milk (1% to 6% of maternal serum concentration). Norethindrone can cause changes in milk production in the mother. When used for contraception, may start 3 weeks after delivery in women who are partially breast-feeding, or 6 weeks after delivery in women who are fully breast-feeding.

Contraindications Hypersensitivity to norethindrone or any component of the formulation; history of or current thrombophlebitis or venous thromboembolic disorders (including DVT, PE); hepatic dysfunction or tumor; known or suspected breast carcinoma; undiagnosed vaginal bleeding; pregnancy; missed abortion or as a diagnostic test for pregnancy

Warnings/Precautions Hazardous agent - use appropriate precautions for handling and disposal (NIOSH 2014 [group 2]).

Progestin only contraceptives do not protect against HIV infection or other sexually-transmitted diseases. Irregular menstrual bleeding patterns are common with progestin-only contraceptives; nonpharmacologic causes of abnormal bleeding should be ruled out. Progestin use has been associated with retinal vascular lesions; discontinue pending examination in case of sudden vision loss, complete loss of vision, sudden onset of proptosis, diplopia or migraine. May have adverse effects on glucose tolerance; use caution in women with diabetes. May have adverse effects on lipid metabolism; use caution in women with hyperlipidemias. Use with caution in patients with depression.

Use with caution in patients with diseases which may be exacerbated by fluid retention, including asthma, epilepsy, migraine, cardiac or renal dysfunction. Use caution in patients at increased risk of thromboembolism; includes elective surgery associated with an increased risk of thromboembolism or during periods of prolonged immobilization. The use of combination hormonal contraceptives has been associated with a slight increase in the frequency of breast cancer, however studies are not consistent. Data is insufficient to determine if progestin-only contraceptives also increase this risk. The risk of cardiovascular side effects increases in women using estrogen containing combined hormonal contraceptives and who smoke cigarettes, especially those who are >35 years of age. This risk relative to progestin-only contraceptives has not been established. Extremely rare hepatic adenomas and focal nodular hyperplasia resulting in fatal intra-abdominal hemorrhage have been reported in association with long-term combination oral contraceptive use. Data is insufficient to determine if progestin-only contraceptives also increase this risk. Not for use prior to menarche.

The use of estrogens and/or progestins may change the results of some laboratory tests (eg, coagulation factors, lipids, glucose tolerance, binding proteins). The dose, route, and the specific estrogen/progestin influences these changes. In addition, personal risk factors (eg, cardiovascular disease, smoking, diabetes, age) also contribute to adverse events; use of specific products may be contraindicated in women with certain risk factors.

Adverse Reactions

Cardiovascular: Cerebral embolism, cerebral thrombosis, deep vein thrombosis, edema, pulmonary embolism, retinal thrombosis

Central nervous system: Depression, dizziness, fatigue, headache, insomnia, migraine, emotional lability, nervousness

Dermatologic: Acne vulgaris, alopecia, chloasma, pruritus, skin rash, urticaria

Endocrine & metabolic: Amenorrhea, hirsutism, hypermenorrhea, menstrual disease, weight gain

Gastrointestinal: Abdominal pain, nausea, vomiting

Genitourinary: Breakthrough bleeding, breast hypertrophy, breast tenderness, cervical erosion, change in cervical secretions, decreased lactation, genital discharge, mastalgia, spotting, vaginal hemorrhage

Hypersensitivity: Anaphylaxis, hypersensitivity

Hepatic: Cholestatic jaundice, hepatitis, abnormal hepatic function tests

Neuromuscular & skeletal: Arm pain, leg pain

Ophthalmic: Optic neuritis (with or without vision loss)

Drug Interactions

Metabolism/Transport Effects Substrate of CYP3A4 (major); **Note:** Assignment of Major/Minor substrate status based on clinically relevant drug interaction potential; **Induces** CYP2C19 (weak/moderate)

Avoid Concomitant Use

Avoid concomitant use of Norethindrone with any of the following: Griseofulvin; Tranexamic Acid; Ulipristal

Increased Effect/Toxicity

Norethindrone may increase the levels/effects of: C1 inhibitors; Selegiline; Thalidomide; Tranexamic Acid; Voriconazole

The levels/effects of Norethindrone may be increased by: Atazanavir; Boceprevir; Cobicistat; Herbs (Progestogenic Properties); Lopinavir; Metreleptin; Mifepristone; Tipranavir; Voriconazole

Decreased Effect

Norethindrone may decrease the levels/effects of: Anticoagulants; Antidiabetic Agents; Fosamprenavir; Ulipristal; Vitamin K Antagonists

The levels/effects of Norethindrone may be decreased by: Acitretin; Aprepitant; Artemether; Barbiturates; Bexarotene (Systemic); Bile Acid Sequestrants; Bosentan; CarBAMazepine; CloBAZam; Colesevelam; CYP3A4 Inducers (Moderate); CYP3A4 Inducers (Strong); Dabrafenib; Darunavir; Deferasirox; Efavirenz; Eslicarbazepine; Exenatide; Felbamate; Fosamprenavir; Fosaprepitant; Fosphenytoin; Griseofulvin; LamoTRIgine; Lopinavir; Metreleptin; Mifepristone; Mitotane; Mycophenolate; Nelfinavir; Nevirapine; OXcarbazepine; Perampanel; Phenytoin; Primidone; Prucalopride; Retinoic Acid Derivatives; Rifamycin Derivatives; Rufinamide; Saquinavir; Siltuximab; St Johns Wort; Sugammadex; Telaprevir; Tocilizumab; Topiramate; Ulipristal

Storage/Stability Store at controlled room temperature of 25°C (77°F).

Mechanism of Action Inhibits secretion of pituitary gonadotropin (LH) which prevents follicular maturation and ovulation

Pharmacokinetics (Adult data unless noted)

Absorption: Oral: Rapidly absorbed

Distribution: V_d: 4 L/kg

Protein binding: 61% to albumin and 36% to sex hormone-binding globulin (SHBG)

Metabolism: Hepatic via reduction and conjugation; first-pass effect

Bioavailability: ~65%

Half-life: ~8 hours

Time to peak serum concentration: 1 hour (range: 0.5-2 hours)

Elimination: Urine (>50% as metabolites); feces (20% to 40% as metabolites)

Dosing: Usual Adolescents and Adults: Female: Oral: Not indicated for use before menarche

Amenorrhea and abnormal uterine bleeding: Norethindrone acetate 2.5-10 mg/day for 5-10 days beginning during the latter half of the menstrual cycle

Endometriosis: Norethindrone acetate 5 mg/day for 14 days; increase at increments of 2.5 mg/day every 2 weeks up to 15 mg/day

Contraception: Progesterone only: Norethindrone 0.35 mg every day of the year starting on first day of menstrual period or the day after a miscarriage or abortion. If switching from a combined oral contraceptive, begin the day after finishing the last active combined tablet. If dose is missed, take as soon as remembered. An additional method of contraception should be used for 48 hours if dose is taken >3 hours late.

Administration Hazardous agent; use appropriate precautions for handling and disposal (NIOSH 2014 [group 2]).

Oral: Administer at the same time each day; may administer with food

Dosage Forms Excipient information presented when available (limited, particularly for generics); consult specific product labeling.

Tablet, Oral:

Camila: 0.35 mg

Deblitane: 0.35 mg [contains fd&c blue #2 aluminum lake, fd&c red #40 aluminum lake, fd&c yellow #10 aluminum lake, soybean lecithin]

Errin: 0.35 mg

Heather: 0.35 mg [contains fd&c yellow #10 aluminum lake, fd&c yellow #6 aluminum lake]

Jencycla: 0.35 mg [contains brilliant blue fcf (fd&c blue #1), fd&c yellow #10 (quinoline yellow)]

Jolivette: 0.35 mg

Lyza: 0.35 mg [contains fd&c yellow #10 (quinoline yellow)]

Nor-QD: 0.35 mg

Nora-BE: 0.35 mg

Norlyroc: 0.35 mg

Ortho Micronor: 0.35 mg [contains fd&c yellow #10 (quinoline yellow)]

Sharobel: 0.35 mg [contains fd&c blue #1 aluminum lake, fd&c yellow #6 aluminum lake, soybean lecithin]
Generic: 0.35 mg
Tablet, Oral, as acetate:
Aygestin: 5 mg [scored]
Generic: 5 mg

- ◆ **Norethindrone Acetate** *see* Norethindrone *on page 1530*
- ◆ **Norethisterone** *see* Norethindrone *on page 1530*
- ◆ **Noritate** *see* MetroNIDAZOLE (Topical) *on page 1425*
- ◆ **Norlutate® (Can)** *see* Norethindrone *on page 1530*
- ◆ **Norlyroc** *see* Norethindrone *on page 1530*
- ◆ **Normal Human Serum Albumin** *see* Albumin *on page 79*
- ◆ **Normal Immunoglobulin** *see* Immune Globulin *on page 1089*
- ◆ **Normal Saline** *see* Sodium Chloride *on page 1938*
- ◆ **Normal Serum Albumin (Human)** *see* Albumin *on page 79*
- ◆ **Normodyne (Can)** *see* Labetalol *on page 1197*
- ◆ **Norpace** *see* Disopyramide *on page 689*
- ◆ **Norpace CR** *see* Disopyramide *on page 689*
- ◆ **Norpramin** *see* Desipramine *on page 602*
- ◆ **Nor-QD** *see* Norethindrone *on page 1530*
- ◆ **Nortemp Children's [OTC]** *see* Acetaminophen *on page 44*
- ◆ **North American Antisnake-Bite Serum, FAB (Ovine)** *see Crotalidae* Polyvalent Immune Fab (Ovine) *on page 543*

Nortriptyline (nor TRIP ti leen)

Medication Safety Issues

Sound-alike/look-alike issues:

Aventyl HCl may be confused with Bentyl
Nortriptyline may be confused with amitriptyline, desipramine, Norpramin
Pamelor may be confused with Demerol, Tambocor [DSC]

BEERS Criteria medication:

This drug may be potentially inappropriate for use in geriatric patients (Quality of evidence - high [moderate for SIADH]; Strength of recommendation - strong).

Related Information

Antidepressant Agents *on page 2257*

Brand Names: US Pamelor

Brand Names: Canada Apo-Nortriptyline; Ava-Nortriptyline; Aventyl; Dom-Nortriptyline; Norventyl; Nu-Nortriptyline; PMS-Nortriptyline; Teva-Nortriptyline

Therapeutic Category Antidepressant, Tricyclic (Secondary Amine)

Generic Availability (US) Yes

Use Treatment of depression (FDA approved in adolescents and adults); has also been used in the treatment of attention deficit hyperactivity disorder (ADHD), nocturnal enuresis, and neuropathic pain

Medication Guide Available Yes

Pregnancy Considerations Animal reproduction studies are inconclusive. Nortriptyline and its metabolites cross the human placenta and can be detected in cord blood (Loughhead, 2006). Tricyclic antidepressants may be associated with irritability, jitteriness, and convulsions (rare) in the neonate (Yonkers, 2009).

The ACOG recommends that therapy for depression during pregnancy be individualized; treatment should incorporate the clinical expertise of the mental health clinician, obstetrician, primary healthcare provider, and pediatrician (ACOG, 2008). According to the American Psychiatric Association (APA), the risks of medication treatment should be weighed against other treatment options and untreated depression. For women who discontinue antidepressant medications during pregnancy and who may be at high risk for postpartum depression, the medications can be restarted following delivery (APA, 2010). Treatment algorithms have been developed by the ACOG and the APA for the management of depression in women prior to conception and during pregnancy (Yonkers, 2009).

Breast-Feeding Considerations Nortriptyline is excreted into breast milk and the M/P ratio ranged from 0.87 to 3.71 in one case report (Matheson, 1988). Based on available information, nortriptyline has not been detected in the serum of nursing infants; however, low levels of the active metabolite E-10-hydroxynortriptyline have been detected in the serum of newborns following breast-feeding (Wisner, 1991). Based on information from one mother-infant pair, following maternal use of nortriptyline 125 mg/day, the estimated exposure to the breast-feeding infant would be 0.6% to 3% of the weight-adjusted maternal dose. Adverse events have not been reported in nursing infants. Infants should be monitored for signs of adverse events; routine monitoring of infant serum concentrations is not recommended (Fortinguerra, 2009).

Contraindications Hypersensitivity to nortriptyline and similar chemical class, or any component of the formulation; use in a patient during the acute recovery phase of MI; use of MAO inhibitors intended to treat psychiatric disorders (concurrently or within 14 days of discontinuing either nortriptyline or the MAO inhibitor); initiation of nortriptyline in a patient receiving linezolid or intravenous methylene blue

Warnings/Precautions [U.S. Boxed Warning]: Antidepressants increase the risk of suicidal thinking and behavior in children, adolescents, and young adults (18-24 years of age) with major depressive disorder (MDD) and other psychiatric disorders; consider risk prior to prescribing. Short-term studies did not show an increased risk in patients >24 years of age and showed a decreased risk in patients ≥65 years. Closely monitor for clinical worsening, suicidality, or unusual changes in behavior, particularly during the initial 1-2 months of therapy or during periods of dosage adjustments (increases or decreases); the patient's family or caregiver should be instructed to closely observe the patient and communicate condition with healthcare provider. A medication guide should be dispensed with each prescription. **Nortriptyline is not FDA approved for use in children.**

The possibility of a suicide attempt is inherent in major depression and may persist until remission occurs. Use caution in high-risk patients. Worsening depression and severe abrupt suicidality that are not part of the presenting symptoms may require discontinuation or modification of drug therapy. The patient's family or caregiver should be alerted to monitor patients for the emergence of suicidality and associated behaviors (such as agitation, irritability, hostility, impulsivity, and hypomania) and call healthcare provider.

May worsen psychosis in some patients or precipitate a shift to mania or hypomania in patients with bipolar disorder. Patients presenting with depressive symptoms should be screened for bipolar disorder. Monotherapy in patients with bipolar disorder should be avoided. **Nortriptyline is not FDA approved for the treatment of bipolar depression.**

Potentially life-threatening serotonin syndrome (SS) has occurred with serotonergic agents (eg, SSRIs, SNRIs), particularly when used in combination with other serotonergic agents (eg, triptans, TCAs, fentanyl, lithium, tramadol, buspirone, St John's wort, tryptophan) or agents that impair metabolism of serotonin (eg, MAO inhibitors intended to treat psychiatric disorders, other MAO inhibitors [ie, linezolid and intravenous methylene blue]). Discontinue treatment (and any concomitant serotonergic agent) immediately if signs/symptoms arise. TCAs may rarely cause bone marrow suppression; monitor for any signs of infection and obtain CBC if symptoms (eg, fever, sore throat) evident. The risk of sedation and orthostatic effects are low relative to other antidepressants. However, nortriptyline may result in impaired performance of tasks requiring alertness (eg, operating machinery or driving). The degree of anticholinergic blockade produced by this agent is moderate relative to other cyclic antidepressants, however, caution should still be used in patients with urinary retention, benign prostatic hyperplasia, narrow-angle glaucoma, xerostomia, visual problems, constipation, or history of bowel obstruction. May cause orthostatic hypotension (risk is low relative to other antidepressants) or conduction disturbances. Use with caution in patients with a history of cardiovascular disease (including previous MI, stroke, tachycardia, or conduction abnormalities). The risk conduction abnormalities with this agent is moderate relative to other antidepressants. CNS effects may be potentiated when used with other sedative drugs or ethanol.

Recommended by the manufacturer to discontinue prior to elective surgery; risks exist for drug interactions with anesthesia and for cardiac arrhythmias. However, definitive drug interactions have not been widely reported in the literature and continuation of tricyclic antidepressants is generally recommended as long as precautions are taken to reduce the significance of any adverse events that may occur (Pass, 2004). May alter glucose regulation - use caution in patients with diabetes. Use caution in patients with a previous seizure disorder or condition predisposing to seizures such as brain damage, alcoholism, or concurrent therapy with other drugs which lower the seizure threshold. May increase the risks associated with electroconvulsive therapy. Bone fractures have been associated with antidepressant treatment. Consider the possibility of a fragility fracture if an antidepressant-treated patient presents with unexplained bone pain, point tenderness, swelling, or bruising (Rabenda, 2013; Rizzoli, 2012). Use with caution in patients with hepatic or renal dysfunction.

Use caution in elderly patients; may cause or exacerbate syndrome of inappropriate antidiuretic hormone secretion or hyponatremia; monitor sodium closely with initiation or dosage adjustments in older adults. May be inappropriate in older adults depending on comorbidities (eg, dementia, delirium) or in patients with a history of falls and fractures due to its potent anticholinergic effects (Beers Criteria).

Benzyl alcohol and derivatives: Some dosage forms may contain sodium benzoate/benzoic acid; benzoic acid (benzoate) is a metabolite of benzyl alcohol; large amounts of benzyl alcohol (≥99 mg/kg/day) have been associated with a potentially fatal toxicity ("gasping syndrome") in neonates; the "gasping syndrome" consists of metabolic acidosis, respiratory distress, gasping respirations, CNS dysfunction (including convulsions, intracranial hemorrhage), hypotension, and cardiovascular collapse (AAP, 1997; CDC, 1982); some data suggests that benzoate displaces bilirubin from protein binding sites (Ahlfors, 2001); avoid or use dosage forms containing benzyl alcohol derivative with caution in neonates. See manufacturer's labeling.

Abrupt discontinuation or interruption of antidepressant therapy has been associated with a discontinuation syndrome. Symptoms arising may vary with antidepressant however commonly include nausea, vomiting, diarrhea, headaches, lightheadedness, dizziness, diminished appetite, sweating, chills, tremors, paresthesias, fatigue, somnolence, and sleep disturbances (eg, vivid dreams, insomnia). Greater risks for developing a discontinuation syndrome have been associated with antidepressants with shorter half-lives, longer durations of treatment, and abrupt discontinuation. For antidepressants of short or intermediate half-lives, symptoms may emerge within 2-5 days after treatment discontinuation and last 7-14 days (APA, 2010; Fava, 2006; Haddad, 2001; Shelton, 2001; Warner, 2006).

Adverse Reactions Some reactions listed are based on reports for other agents in this same pharmacologic class and may not be specifically reported for nortriptyline.

Cardiovascular: Cardiac arrhythmia, cerebrovascular accident, edema, flushing, heart block, hypertension, hypotension, myocardial infarction, palpitations, tachycardia

Central nervous system: Agitation, anxiety, ataxia, confusion, delusions, disorientation, dizziness, drowsiness, drug fever, EEG pattern changes, extrapyramidal reaction, fatigue, hallucination, headache, hypomania, insomnia, nightmares, numbness, panic, peripheral neuropathy, psychosis (exacerbation), restlessness, seizure, tingling of extremities, tingling sensation, withdrawal symptoms

Dermatologic: Alopecia, diaphoresis (excessive), pruritus, skin photosensitivity, skin rash, urticaria

Endocrine & metabolic: Decreased libido, decreased serum glucose, galactorrhea, gynecomastia, increased libido, increased serum glucose, SIADH, weight gain, weight loss

Gastrointestinal: Abdominal cramps, anorexia, constipation, diarrhea, epigastric distress, melanoglossia, nausea, paralytic ileus, parotid gland enlargement, stomatitis, sublingual adenitis, unpleasant taste, vomiting, xerostomia

Genitourinary: Breast hypertrophy, impotence, nocturia, testicular swelling, urinary hesitance, urinary retention, urinary tract dilation

Hematologic & oncologic: Agranulocytosis, eosinophilia, petechia, purpura, thrombocytopenia

Hepatic: Abnormal hepatic function tests, cholestatic jaundice

Neuromuscular & skeletal: Tremor, weakness

Ophthalmic: Accommodation disturbance, blurred vision, eye pain, mydriasis

Otic: Tinnitus

Renal: Polyuria

Rare but important or life-threatening: Angle-closure glaucoma, serotonin syndrome, suicidal ideation

Drug Interactions

Metabolism/Transport Effects **Substrate** of CYP1A2 (minor), CYP2C19 (minor), CYP2D6 (major), CYP3A4 (minor); **Note:** Assignment of Major/Minor substrate status based on clinically relevant drug interaction potential; **Inhibits** CYP2D6 (weak), CYP2E1 (weak)

Avoid Concomitant Use

Avoid concomitant use of Nortriptyline with any of the following: Aclidinium; Azelastine (Nasal); Dapoxetine; Eluxadoline; Glucagon; Iobenguane I 123; Ipratropium (Oral Inhalation); Linezolid; MAO Inhibitors; Methylene Blue; Moxonidine; Orphenadrine; Paraldehyde; Potassium Chloride; Thalidomide; Tiotropium; Umeclidinium

Increased Effect/Toxicity

Nortriptyline may increase the levels/effects of: AbobotulinumtoxinA; Alcohol (Ethyl); Alpha-/Beta-Agonists (Direct-Acting); Alpha1-Agonists; Amphetamines; Analgesics (Opioid); Anticholinergic Agents; Antipsychotic Agents; ARIPiprazole; Azelastine (Nasal); Beta2-Agonists; Buprenorphine; Citalopram; CNS Depressants; Desmopressin; Eluxadoline; Escitalopram; Glucagon; Highest Risk QTc-Prolonging Agents; Hydrocodone; Methotrimeprazine; Methylene Blue; Metyrosine; Mirabegron; Moderate Risk QTc-Prolonging Agents; Nicorandil; OnabotulinumtoxinA; Orphenadrine; Paraldehyde; Potassium Chloride; Pramipexole; QuiNIDine;

RimabotulinumtoxinB; ROPINIRole; Rotigotine; Serotonin Modulators; Sodium Phosphates; Sulfonylureas; Suvorexant; Thalidomide; Thiazide Diuretics; Tiotropium; Topiramate; TraMADol; Vitamin K Antagonists; Yohimbine; Zolpidem

The levels/effects of Nortriptyline may be increased by: Abiraterone Acetate; Aclidinium; Altretamine; Antiemetics (5HT3 Antagonists); Antipsychotic Agents; Brimonidine (Topical); BuPROPion; Cannabis; Cimetidine; Cinacalcet; Citalopram; Cobicistat; CYP2D6 Inhibitors (Moderate); CYP2D6 Inhibitors (Strong); Dapoxetine; Darunavir; Dexmethylphenidate; Doxylamine; Dronabinol; Droperidol; DULoxetine; Escitalopram; FLUoxetine; FluvoxaMINE; HydrOXYzine; Ipratropium (Oral Inhalation); Kava Kava; Linezolid; Lithium; Magnesium Sulfate; MAO Inhibitors; Methotrimeprazine; Methylphenidate; Metoclopramide; Metyrosine; Mianserin; Mifepristone; Nabilone; Panobinostat; PARoxetine; Peginterferon Alfa-2b; Perampanel; Pramlintide; Protease Inhibitors; QuiNIDine; Rufinamide; Sertraline; Sodium Oxybate; Tapentadol; Tedizolid; Terbinafine (Systemic); Tetrahydrocannabinol; Thyroid Products; TraMADol; Umeclidinium; Valproic Acid and Derivatives

Decreased Effect

Nortriptyline may decrease the levels/effects of: Acetylcholinesterase Inhibitors; Alpha1-Agonists; Alpha2-Agonists; Alpha2-Agonists (Ophthalmic); Iobenguane I 123; Itopride; Moxonidine; Secretin

The levels/effects of Nortriptyline may be decreased by: Acetylcholinesterase Inhibitors; Barbiturates; CarBAMazepine; Peginterferon Alfa-2b; St Johns Wort

Storage/Stability Store at 20°C to 25°C (68°F to 77°F). Protect from light.

Mechanism of Action Traditionally believed to increase the synaptic concentration of serotonin and/or norepinephrine in the central nervous system by inhibition of their reuptake by the presynaptic neuronal membrane. However, additional receptor effects have been found including desensitization of adenyl cyclase, down regulation of beta-adrenergic receptors, and down regulation of serotonin receptors.

Pharmacodynamics

Onset of action:

Antidepressant effect: Initial: 7 to 21 days; maximum effects may not occur for ≥2 to 3 weeks

ADHD response: 2 to 4 weeks (Wilens, 1993)

Antineuritic effect: Within 24 hours (Rushton, 1989)

Pharmacokinetics (Adult data unless noted)

Absorption: Oral: Rapid; well absorbed

Distribution: V_d: 14 to 22 L/kg

Protein binding: 93% to 95%

Metabolism: Undergoes significant first-pass metabolism; primarily detoxified hepatically via hydroxylation followed by glucuronide conjugation

Half-life:

Children: 18 ± 4 hours

Adults: 28 to 31 hours

Time to peak serum concentration: Oral: 7 to 8.5 hours

Elimination: Urine (as metabolites and small amounts of unchanged drug); feces (small amounts)

Dosing: Usual

Pediatric:

Attention-deficit/hyperactivity disorder (ADHD): Limited data available: **Note:** Should not be used first-line; use should be reserved for cases where other therapies have failed or not tolerated (AACAP [Pliszka], 2007; Dolpheide, 2005; Prince, 2000; Spencer, 1996; Wilens, 1993).

Children ≥6 years and Adolescents: Oral: Initial: 0.5 mg/kg/day; may increase by 0.5 mg/kg/day increments at weekly intervals; maximum daily dose range: 2 to 2.5 mg/kg/**day** up to 100 mg/**day**; in one trial, the daily dose was divided twice daily with a dose administered before school and a dose after dinner; reported mean effective dose: 1.8 mg/kg/day (Prince, 2000).

Enuresis: Limited data available: Children ≥6 years and Adolescents: Oral: **Note:** Due to the risk of serious side effects (eg, arrhythmias, heart block, seizures), TCAs are considered third line treatment for enuresis; may consider use in patients who have failed all other therapies; high relapse rate when discontinued (Deshpande, 2012; Kliegman, 2007). Administer dose 30 minutes before bedtime; usual treatment duration: ≤3 months (Sweetman, 2012).

General dosing: Initial: 10 to 20 mg/day; titrate up to maximum daily dose of 40 mg/**day** (Kliegman, 2007)

Age-directed dosing (Sweetman, 2012):

6 to 7 years (20 to 25 kg): 10 mg

8 to 11 years (25 to 35 kg): 10 to 20 mg

>11 years (35 to 54 kg): 25 to 35 mg

Depression: Oral: **Note:** Controlled clinical trials have not shown tricyclic antidepressants to be superior to placebo for the treatment of depression in children and adolescents; not recommended as first line medication; may be beneficial for patient with comorbid conditions (ADHD, enuresis) (Biramaher, 2007; Dopheide, 2006; Wagner, 2005).

Children 6 to 12 years: Limited data available: 1 to 3 mg/kg/day in 4 divided doses; maximum daily dose: 150 mg/**day** (Kliegman, 2007)

Adolescents: 30 to 50 mg/day in 3 to 4 divided doses or as a single daily dose; maximum daily dose: 150 mg/**day**

Neuropathic pain: Limited data available: Children and Adolescents: Oral: Usual range: 0.05 to 1 mg/kg/dose at bedtime; begin at the lower end of dosing range and titrate every 3 days to effect; the analgesic effects of TCA's are typically observed at a lower dose compared to TCA doses for depression; maximum daily dose: 3 mg/kg/day or 150 mg/**day**, whichever is less (APS, 2008; Kliegman, 2011)

Adult: **Depression:** Oral: 25 mg 3 to 4 times daily or as a single daily dose; maximum daily dose: 150 mg/day

Dosing adjustment for concomitant MAO inhibitor therapy: Adolescents and Adults:

Switching to or from a MAO inhibitor intended to treat psychiatric disorders:

Allow 14 days to elapse between discontinuing an MAO inhibitor intended to treat psychiatric disorders and initiation of nortriptyline.

Allow 14 days to elapse between discontinuing nortriptyline and initiation of an MAO inhibitor intended to treat psychiatric disorders.

Use with other MAO inhibitors (linezolid or IV methylene blue):

Do not initiate nortriptyline in patients receiving linezolid or IV methylene blue; consider other interventions for psychiatric condition.

If urgent treatment with linezolid or IV methylene blue is required in a patient already receiving nortriptyline and potential benefits outweigh potential risks, discontinue nortriptyline promptly and administer linezolid or IV methylene blue. Monitor for serotonin syndrome for 2 weeks or until 24 hours after the last dose of linezolid or IV methylene blue, whichever comes first. May resume nortriptyline 24 hours after the last dose of linezolid or IV methylene blue.

Dosing adjustment for renal impairment: Not dialyzable. There are no dosage adjustments provided in the manufacturer's labeling.

Dosing adjustment in hepatic impairment: Use lower doses and slower titration; individualization of dosage is recommended.

Administration Oral: May administer without regards to food; in pediatric patients, the timing of doses dependent upon use; for nocturnal enuresis and neuropathic pain, doses administered at bedtime; for ADHD, daily doses may be administered once daily in the morning or some have divided doses twice daily with a morning dose and a dose at dinner.

Monitoring Parameters Heart rate, blood pressure, ECG, mental status, weight, liver enzymes, CBC with differential, serum drug concentrations. Monitor patient periodically for symptom resolution; monitor for worsening depression, suicidality, and associated behaviors (especially at the beginning of therapy or when doses are increased or decreased); signs/symptoms of serotonin syndrome.

ADHD: Evaluate patients for cardiac disease prior to initiation of therapy for ADHD with thorough medical history, family history, and physical exam; consider ECG; perform ECG and echocardiogram if findings suggest cardiac disease; promptly conduct cardiac evaluation in patients who develop chest pain, unexplained syncope, or any other symptom of cardiac disease during treatment.

Reference Range Therapeutic: 50-150 ng/mL (SI: 190-570 nmol/L)

Dosage Forms Excipient information presented when available (limited, particularly for generics); consult specific product labeling.

Capsule, Oral:

Pamelor: 10 mg, 25 mg [contains fd&c yellow #10 (quinoline yellow), fd&c yellow #6 (sunset yellow)]

Pamelor: 50 mg

Pamelor: 75 mg [contains fd&c yellow #10 (quinoline yellow), fd&c yellow #6 (sunset yellow)]

Generic: 10 mg, 25 mg, 50 mg, 75 mg

Solution, Oral:

Generic: 10 mg/5 mL (473 mL)

◆ **Nortriptyline Hydrochloride** *see* Nortriptyline *on page 1532*

◆ **Norvasc** *see* AmLODIPine *on page 133*

◆ **Norventyl (Can)** *see* Nortriptyline *on page 1532*

◆ **Norvir** *see* Ritonavir *on page 1871*

◆ **NovaFerrum 50 [OTC]** *see* Polysaccharide-Iron Complex *on page 1728*

◆ **NovaFerrum Pediatric Drops [OTC]** *see* Polysaccharide-Iron Complex *on page 1728*

◆ **Novamoxin (Can)** *see* Amoxicillin *on page 138*

◆ **Novantrone** *see* MitoXANtrone *on page 1448*

◆ **Novarel** *see* Chorionic Gonadotropin (Human) *on page 453*

◆ **Novasen (Can)** *see* Aspirin *on page 206*

◆ **Novel Erythropoiesis-Stimulating Protein** *see* Darbepoetin Alfa *on page 585*

◆ **Novo-Ampicillin (Can)** *see* Ampicillin *on page 156*

◆ **Novo-Atorvastatin (Can)** *see* AtorvaSTATin *on page 220*

◆ **Novo-Azithromycin (Can)** *see* Azithromycin (Systemic) *on page 242*

◆ **Novo-AZT (Can)** *see* Zidovudine *on page 2207*

◆ **Novo-Baclofen (Can)** *see* Baclofen *on page 254*

◆ **Novo-Bupropion SR (Can)** *see* BuPROPion *on page 324*

◆ **Novo-Carvedilol (Can)** *see* Carvedilol *on page 380*

◆ **Novo-Cefaclor (Can)** *see* Cefaclor *on page 386*

◆ **Novo-Chloroquine (Can)** *see* Chloroquine *on page 437*

◆ **Novo-Cholamine (Can)** *see* Cholestyramine Resin *on page 450*

◆ **Novo-Cholamine Light (Can)** *see* Cholestyramine Resin *on page 450*

◆ **Novo-Cimetidine (Can)** *see* Cimetidine *on page 461*

◆ **Novo-Clavamoxin (Can)** *see* Amoxicillin and Clavulanate *on page 141*

◆ **Novo-Clobazam (Can)** *see* CloBAZam *on page 495*

◆ **Novo-Clobetasol (Can)** *see* Clobetasol *on page 498*

◆ **Novo-Clomipramine (Can)** *see* ClomiPRAMINE *on page 502*

◆ **Novo-Clonidine (Can)** *see* CloNIDine *on page 508*

◆ **Novo-Clopate (Can)** *see* Clorazepate *on page 516*

◆ **Novo-Cycloprine (Can)** *see* Cyclobenzaprine *on page 548*

◆ **Novo-Desipramine (Can)** *see* Desipramine *on page 602*

◆ **Novo-Desmopressin (Can)** *see* Desmopressin *on page 607*

◆ **Novo-Dimenate [OTC] (Can)** *see* DimenhyDRINATE *on page 664*

◆ **Novo-Dipam (Can)** *see* Diazepam *on page 635*

◆ **Novo-Divalproex (Can)** *see* Valproic Acid and Derivatives *on page 2143*

◆ **Novo-Docusate Calcium [OTC] (Can)** *see* Docusate *on page 697*

◆ **Novo-Docusate Sodium [OTC] (Can)** *see* Docusate *on page 697*

◆ **Novo-Doxepin (Can)** *see* Doxepin (Systemic) *on page 711*

◆ **Novoeight** *see* Antihemophilic Factor (Recombinant) *on page 168*

◆ **Novo-Ferrogluc (Can)** *see* Ferrous Gluconate *on page 870*

◆ **Novo-Fluconazole (Can)** *see* Fluconazole *on page 881*

◆ **Novo-Fluoxetine (Can)** *see* FLUoxetine *on page 906*

◆ **Novo-Flurprofen (Can)** *see* Flurbiprofen (Systemic) *on page 915*

◆ **Novo-Fluvoxamine (Can)** *see* FluvoxaMINE *on page 928*

◆ **Novo-Furantoin (Can)** *see* Nitrofurantoin *on page 1521*

◆ **Novo-Gesic (Can)** *see* Acetaminophen *on page 44*

◆ **Novo-Hydroxyzin (Can)** *see* HydrOXYzine *on page 1058*

◆ **Novo-Hylazin (Can)** *see* HydrALAZINE *on page 1027*

◆ **Novo-Ipramide (Can)** *see* Ipratropium (Oral Inhalation) *on page 1155*

◆ **Novo-Ketorolac (Can)** *see* Ketorolac (Systemic) *on page 1192*

◆ **Novo-Levobunolol (Can)** *see* Levobunolol *on page 1238*

◆ **Novo-Levofloxacin (Can)** *see* Levofloxacin (Systemic) *on page 1243*

◆ **NovoLIN 70/30** *see* Insulin NPH and Insulin Regular *on page 1141*

◆ **Novolin ge 30/70 (Can)** *see* Insulin NPH and Insulin Regular *on page 1141*

◆ **Novolin ge 40/60 (Can)** *see* Insulin NPH and Insulin Regular *on page 1141*

◆ **Novolin ge 50/50 (Can)** *see* Insulin NPH and Insulin Regular *on page 1141*

◆ **Novolin® ge NPH (Can)** *see* Insulin NPH *on page 1138*

◆ **Novolin ge Toronto (Can)** *see* Insulin Regular *on page 1143*

◆ **NovoLIN N [OTC]** *see* Insulin NPH *on page 1138*

◆ **NovoLIN N ReliOn [OTC]** *see* Insulin NPH *on page 1138*

- ◆ **Nu-Prochlor (Can)** *see* Prochlorperazine *on page 1774*
- ◆ **Nu-Propranolol (Can)** *see* Propranolol *on page 1789*
- ◆ **Nu-Sotalol (Can)** *see* Sotalol *on page 1963*
- ◆ **Nu-Sucralate (Can)** *see* Sucralfate *on page 1978*
- ◆ **Nu-Terazosin (Can)** *see* Terazosin *on page 2020*
- ◆ **Nu-Tetra (Can)** *see* Tetracycline *on page 2035*
- ◆ **Nutracort** *see* Hydrocortisone (Topical) *on page 1041*
- ◆ **Nu-Trazodone (Can)** *see* TraZODone *on page 2105*
- ◆ **Nu-Trazodone D (Can)** *see* TraZODone *on page 2105*
- ◆ **Nutr-E-Sol [OTC]** *see* Vitamin E *on page 2188*
- ◆ **Nutrilipid** *see* Fat Emulsion (Plant Based) *on page 850*
- ◆ **Nutropin [DSC]** *see* Somatropin *on page 1957*
- ◆ **Nutropin AQ NuSpin (Can)** *see* Somatropin *on page 1957*
- ◆ **Nutropin AQ NuSpin 5** *see* Somatropin *on page 1957*
- ◆ **Nutropin AQ NuSpin 10** *see* Somatropin *on page 1957*
- ◆ **Nutropin AQ NuSpin 20** *see* Somatropin *on page 1957*
- ◆ **Nutropin AQ Pen** *see* Somatropin *on page 1957*
- ◆ **Nuvessa** *see* MetroNIDAZOLE (Topical) *on page 1425*
- ◆ **NuZon [DSC]** *see* Hydrocortisone (Topical) *on page 1041*
- ◆ **NVA237** *see* Glycopyrrolate *on page 979*
- ◆ **NVP** *see* Nevirapine *on page 1507*
- ◆ **Nyaderm (Can)** *see* Nystatin (Topical) *on page 1537*
- ◆ **Nyamyc** *see* Nystatin (Topical) *on page 1537*
- ◆ **Nycoff [OTC]** *see* Dextromethorphan *on page 631*

Nystatin (Oral) (nye STAT in)

Medication Safety Issues

Sound-alike/look-alike issues:

Nystatin may be confused with HMG-CoA reductase inhibitors (also known as "statins"; eg, atorvaSTATin, fluvastatin, lovastatin, pitavastatin, pravastatin, rosuvastatin, simvastatin), Nitrostat

Brand Names: US Bio-Statin

Brand Names: Canada PMS-Nystatin

Generic Availability (US) Yes

Use Treatment of susceptible cutaneous, mucocutaneous, and oral cavity fungal infections normally caused by the *Candida* species

Pregnancy Risk Factor C

Pregnancy Considerations Animal reproduction studies have not been conducted. Adverse events in the fetus or newborn have not been reported following maternal use of vaginal nystatin during pregnancy. Absorption following oral use is poor.

Breast-Feeding Considerations Excretion into breast milk is not known; however, absorption following oral use is poor.

Contraindications Hypersensitivity to nystatin or any component of the formulation

Adverse Reactions

Gastrointestinal: Diarrhea, nausea, stomach pain, vomiting

Rare but important or life-threatening: Hypersensitivity reactions

Drug Interactions

Metabolism/Transport Effects None known.

Avoid Concomitant Use

Avoid concomitant use of Nystatin (Oral) with any of the following: Saccharomyces boulardii

Increased Effect/Toxicity There are no known significant interactions involving an increase in effect.

Decreased Effect

Nystatin (Oral) may decrease the levels/effects of: Saccharomyces boulardii

Storage/Stability

Tablet and suspension: Store at controlled room temperature of 15°C to 25°C (59°F to 77°F).

Powder for suspension: Store under refrigeration at 2°C to 8°C (36°F to 46°F).

Mechanism of Action Binds to sterols in fungal cell membrane, changing the cell wall permeability allowing for leakage of cellular contents

Pharmacodynamics Onset of action: Symptomatic relief from candidiasis: Within 24-72 hours

Pharmacokinetics (Adult data unless noted)

Absorption: Poorly absorbed from the GI tract

Elimination: In feces as unchanged drug

Dosing: Neonatal Oral candidiasis:

Prophylaxis: 100,000 units/dose 4 times/day divided as 50,000 units to each side of the mouth (Ganesan, 2009)

Treatment: 100,000-400,000 units/dose 4 times/day; one study of 14 patients (neonates and infants) found higher cure rates using 400,000 unit/dose 4 times/day (Hoppe, 1997)

Dosing: Usual

Oral candidiasis:

Infants: 200,000-400,000 units 4 times/day or 100,000 units to each side of mouth 4 times/day; one study of 14 patients (neonates and infants) found higher cure rates using 400,000 unit/dose 4 times/day (Hoppe, 1997)

Children and Adults: 400,000-600,000 units 4 times/day

Intestinal infections: Adults: Oral: 500,000-1,000,000 units every 8 hours

Administration Shake suspension well before use; suspension should be swished about the mouth and retained in the mouth for as long as possible (several minutes) before swallowing. For neonates and infants, paint nystatin suspension into recesses of the mouth.

Monitoring Parameters KOH smears or cultures should be used to confirm diagnosis of cutaneous or mucocutaneous candidiasis.

Dosage Forms Excipient information presented when available (limited, particularly for generics); consult specific product labeling.

Capsule, Oral [preservative free]:

Bio-Statin: 500,000 units, 1,000,000 units [dye free]

Powder, Oral:

Bio-Statin: (1 ea)

Generic: (1 ea)

Suspension, Mouth/Throat:

Generic: 100,000 units/mL (5 mL, 60 mL, 473 mL, 480 mL)

Tablet, Oral:

Generic: 500,000 units

Nystatin (Topical) (nye STAT in)

Medication Safety Issues

Sound-alike/look-alike issues:

Nystatin may be confused with HMG-CoA reductase inhibitors (also known as "statins"; eg, atorvaSTATin, fluvastatin, lovastatin, pitavastatin, pravastatin, rosuvastatin, simvastatin), Nitrostat

Brand Names: US Nyamyc; Nystop; Pedi-Dri [DSC]; Pediaderm AF Complete

Brand Names: Canada Nyaderm; Ratio-Nystatin

Therapeutic Category Antifungal Agent, Topical; Antifungal Agent, Vaginal

Generic Availability (US) May be product dependent

Use Treatment of cutaneous and mucocutaneous fungal infections caused by susceptible *Candida* species (FDA approved in all ages)

Pregnancy Risk Factor C

Pregnancy Considerations Animal reproduction studies have not been conducted. Absorption following oral use is poor and nystatin is not absorbed following application to mucous membranes or intact skin.

Breast-Feeding Considerations It is not known if nystatin is excreted in breast milk; however, absorption following oral use is poor and nystatin is not absorbed following application to mucous membranes or intact skin. The manufacturer recommends that caution be exercised when administering nystatin to nursing women.

Contraindications Hypersensitivity to nystatin or any component of the formulation

Warnings/Precautions For topical use only; not for systemic, oral, intravaginal, or ophthalmic use. Hypersensitivity reactions may occur; immediately discontinue if signs of a hypersensitivity reaction occurs. Discontinue use if irritation occurs.

Warnings: Additional Pediatric Considerations Some dosage forms may contain propylene glycol; in neonates large amounts of propylene glycol delivered orally, intravenously (eg, >3,000 mg/day), or topically have been associated with potentially fatal toxicities which can include metabolic acidosis, seizures, renal failure, and CNS depression; toxicities have also been reported in children and adults including hyperosmolality, lactic acidosis, seizures, and respiratory depression; use caution (AAP, 1997; Shehab, 2009).

Adverse Reactions

Dermatologic: Contact dermatitis, Stevens-Johnson syndrome

Rare but important or life-threatening: Hypersensitivity reactions

Drug Interactions

Metabolism/Transport Effects None known.

Avoid Concomitant Use

Avoid concomitant use of Nystatin (Topical) with any of the following: Progesterone

Increased Effect/Toxicity There are no known significant interactions involving an increase in effect.

Decreased Effect

Nystatin (Topical) may decrease the levels/effects of: Progesterone

Storage/Stability

Cream, ointment: Store at room temperature.

Topical powder: Store between 15°C to 30°C (59°F to 86°F). Avoid excessive heat (40°C [104°F]).

Mechanism of Action Binds to sterols in fungal cell membrane, changing the cell wall permeability allowing for leakage of cellular contents

Pharmacodynamics Onset of action: Symptomatic relief from candidiasis: Within 24 to 72 hours

Pharmacokinetics (Adult data unless noted) Absorption: Not absorbed through mucous membranes or intact skin

Dosing: Neonatal

Diaper dermatitis, candidal: Topical: Ointment, cream: Apply to affected area 2 to 4 times daily; most studies have used 4 times daily dosing (Hoppe 1997)

Mucocutaneous candidal infection:

Manufacturer's labeling:

Cream; ointment: Topical: Apply to affected area twice daily

Powder: Topical: Apply to affected area 2 to 3 times daily

Alternate dosing: Limited data available: Cream, ointment, powder: Topical: Apply to affected area 2 to 4 times daily (Bradley 2015)

Dosing: Usual

Pediatric:

Diaper dermatitis, candidal: Limited data available: Infants: Ointment, cream: Topical: Apply 2 to 4 times daily to affected area; most studies have used 4 times daily dosing (Hoppe, 1997; Munz 1982)

Mucocutaneous candidal infections: Infants, Children, and Adolescents:

Manufacturer's labeling:

Cream/ointment: Topical: Apply to affected area twice daily

Powder: Topical: Apply to affected area 2 to 3 times daily

Alternate dosing: Limited data available: Cream, ointment, powder: Topical: Apply to affected area 2 to 4 times daily (Bradley 2015)

Adult: **Mucocutaneous infections:**

Cream/ointment: Topical: Apply to affected area twice daily

Powder: Topical: Apply to affected area 2 to 3 times daily

Dosing adjustment in renal impairment: There are no dosage adjustments provided in the manufacturer's labeling; however, dosage adjustment unlikely due to low systemic absorption.

Dosing adjustment in hepatic impairment: There are no dosage adjustments provided in the manufacturer's labeling; however, dosage adjustment unlikely due to low systemic absorption.

Administration

Cream or ointment: Gently massage formulation into the skin.

Powder: Dust in shoes, in stockings, and on feet for treatment of candidal infection of the feet; also used on very moist lesions

Monitoring Parameters KOH smears or cultures should be used to confirm diagnosis of cutaneous or mucocutaneous candidiasis.

Dosage Forms Excipient information presented when available (limited, particularly for generics); consult specific product labeling. [DSC] = Discontinued product

Cream, External:

Generic: 100,000 units/g (15 g, 30 g)

Kit, External:

Pediaderm AF Complete: 100,000 units/g [contains methylparaben, propylene glycol, propylparaben]

Ointment, External:

Generic: 100,000 units/g (15 g, 30 g)

Powder, External:

Nyamyc: 100,000 units/g (15 g, 30 g, 60 g)

Nystop: 100,000 units/g (15 g, 30 g, 60 g)

Pedi-Dri: 100,000 units/g (56.7 g [DSC])

Generic: 100,000 units/g (15 g, 30 g, 60 g)

◆ **Nystop** *see* Nystatin (Topical) *on page 1537*

◆ **Nytol [OTC]** *see* DiphenhydrAMINE (Systemic) *on page 668*

◆ **Nytol (Can)** *see* DiphenhydrAMINE (Systemic) *on page 668*

◆ **Nytol Extra Strength (Can)** *see* DiphenhydrAMINE (Systemic) *on page 668*

◆ **Nytol Maximum Strength [OTC]** *see* DiphenhydrAMINE (Systemic) *on page 668*

◆ **OC8 [OTC]** *see* Benzoyl Peroxide *on page 270*

◆ **OCBZ** *see* OXcarbazepine *on page 1584*

◆ **Occlusal-HP (Can)** *see* Salicylic Acid *on page 1894*

◆ **Ocean Complete Sinus Rinse [OTC]** *see* Sodium Chloride *on page 1938*

◆ **Ocean for Kids [OTC]** *see* Sodium Chloride *on page 1938*

◆ **Oceanic Selenium [OTC]** *see* Selenium *on page 1912*

◆ **Ocean Nasal Spray [OTC]** *see* Sodium Chloride *on page 1938*

◆ **Ocean Ultra Saline Mist [OTC]** *see* Sodium Chloride *on page 1938*

- ◆ **Ocphyl (Can)** *see* Octreotide *on page 1539*
- ◆ **Octacog Alfa** *see* Antihemophilic Factor (Recombinant) *on page 168*
- ◆ **Octagam** *see* Immune Globulin *on page 1089*
- ◆ **Octagam 10%** *see* Immune Globulin *on page 1089*
- ◆ **Octostim (Can)** *see* Desmopressin *on page 607*

Octreotide (ok TREE oh tide)

Medication Safety Issues

Sound-alike/look-alike issues:

Octreotide may be confused with pasireotide

SandoSTATIN may be confused with SandIMMUNE, SandoSTATIN LAR, sargramostim, simvastatin

Brand Names: US SandoSTATIN; SandoSTATIN LAR Depot

Brand Names: Canada Ocphyl; Octreotide Acetate Omega; Octreotide Injection; Sandostatin; Sandostatin LAR

Therapeutic Category Antidiarrheal; Antidote; Antihemorrhagics; Antisecretory Agent; Somatostatin Analog

Generic Availability (US) May be product dependent

Use Control of symptoms, including secretory diarrhea in patients with metastatic carcinoid or vasoactive intestinal peptide-secreting tumors (VIPomas) (FDA approved in adults); treatment of acromegaly (FDA approved in adults). Other uses include control of bleeding of esophageal varices, Cushing's syndrome, insulinomas, glucagonoma, small bowel fistulas, postgastrectomy dumping syndrome, chemotherapy-induced diarrhea, graft-versus-host disease (GVHD)-associated diarrhea, Zollinger-Ellison syndrome, persistent hyperinsulinemic hypoglycemia of infancy (nesidioblastosis), postoperative chylothorax, second-line treatment for thymic malignancies; islet cell tumors; treatment of malignant bowel obstruction; treatment of sulfonylurea overdosage (nondepot formulation); hypothalamic obesity

Pregnancy Risk Factor B

Pregnancy Considerations Adverse effects were not observed in animal reproduction studies. Octreotide crosses the placenta and can be detected in the newborn at delivery (Caron, 1995; Fassnacht, 2001; Maffei, 2010); data concerning use in pregnancy is limited. In case reports of acromegalic women who received normal doses of octreotide during pregnancy, no congenital malformations were reported. Because normalization of IGF-1 and GH may restore fertility in women with acromegaly, women of childbearing potential should use adequate contraception during treatment. Long-acting formulations should be discontinued 2 to 3 months prior to a planned pregnancy when possible; however, octreotide therapy may be resumed in pregnant women with worsening symptoms if needed (Katznelson, 2011).

Breast-Feeding Considerations Octreotide is excreted in breast milk. In a case report, a woman was taking octreotide SubQ in doses up to 2400 mcg/day prior to and throughout pregnancy. Octreotide was measurable in the colostrum in concentrations similar to those in the maternal serum (Maffei, 2010); however, oral absorption of octreotide is considered to be poor (Battershill, 1989). The manufacturer recommends that caution be exercised when administering octreotide to nursing women.

Contraindications Hypersensitivity to octreotide or any component of the formulation

Warnings/Precautions May impair gallbladder function; monitor patients for cholelithiasis. The incidence of gallbladder stone or biliary sludge increases with a duration of therapy of ≥12 months. In patients with neuroendocrine tumors, the NCCN guidelines (v.1.2011) recommend considering prophylactic cholecystectomy in patients undergoing abdominal surgery if octreotide treatment is planned. Use with caution in patients with renal and/or hepatic impairment; dosage adjustment may be required in patients receiving dialysis and in patients with established cirrhosis. Somatostatin analogs may affect glucose regulation. In type I diabetes, severe hypoglycemia may occur; in type II diabetes or patients without diabetes, hyperglycemia may occur. Insulin and other hypoglycemic medication requirements may change. Octreotide may worsen hypoglycemia in patients with insulinomas; use with caution. Do not use depot formulation for the treatment of sulfonylurea-induced hypoglycemia. Bradycardia, conduction abnormalities, and arrhythmia have been observed in acromegalic and carcinoid syndrome patients; use caution with CHF or concomitant medications that alter heart rate or rhythm. Cardiovascular medication requirements may change. Octreotide may enhance the adverse/toxic effects of other QTc-prolonging agents. May alter absorption of dietary fats; monitor for pancreatitis. May reduce excessive fluid loss in patients with conditions that cause such loss; monitor for elevations in zinc levels in such patients that are maintained on total parenteral nutrition (TPN). Chronic treatment has been associated with abnormal Schillings test; monitor vitamin B_{12} levels. Suppresses secretion of TSH; monitor for hypothyroidism.

Postmarketing cases of serious and fatal events, including hypoxia and necrotizing enterocolitis, have been reported with octreotide use in children (usually with serious underlying conditions), particularly in children <2 years of age. In studies with octreotide depot, the incidence of cholelithiasis in children is higher than the reported incidences for adults and efficacy was not demonstrated. Therapy may restore fertility; females of childbearing potential should use adequate contraception. Dosage adjustment may be necessary in the elderly; significant increases in elimination half-life have been observed in older adults. Vehicle used in depot injection (polylactide-co-glycolide microspheres) has rarely been associated with retinal artery occlusion in patients with abnormal arteriovenous anastomosis.

Warnings: Additional Pediatric Considerations The incidence of gallbladder stone or increase in sludge is ~33% in children with a duration of therapy ≥12 months.

Adverse Reactions Adverse reactions vary by route of administration or dosage form.

Cardiovascular: Angina, arrhythmia, cardiac failure, chest pain (non-depot formulations), conduction abnormalities, edema, flushing, hematoma, hypertension, palpitation, peripheral edema, phlebitis, sinus bradycardia

Central nervous system: Abnormal gait, amnesia, anxiety, confusion, depression, dizziness, dysphonia, fatigue, fever, hallucinations, headache, hypoesthesia, insomnia, malaise, nervousness, neuralgia, neuropathy, pain, somnolence, tremor, vertigo

Dermatologic: Acne, alopecia, bruising, cellulitis, pruritus, rash (depot formulation)

Endocrine & metabolic: Breast pain, cachexia, goiter (non-depot formulations), gout, hyper-/hypoglycemia, hypokalemia, hypoproteinemia, hypothyroidism (non-depot formulations), impotence

Gastrointestinal: Abdominal pain, anorexia, biliary duct dilatation, biliary sludge (length of therapy dependent), cholelithiasis (length of therapy dependent), colitis, constipation, cramping, dehydration, diarrhea, diverticulitis, dyspepsia, dysphagia, fat malabsorption, feces discoloration, flatulence, gastritis, gastroenteritis, gingivitis, glossitis, loose stools, melena, nausea, steatorrhea, stomatitis, taste perversion, tenesmus, vomiting, xerostomia

Genitourinary: Incontinence, pollakiuria (non-depot formulations), urinary tract infection

Hematologic: Anemia (more common with depot formulations)

Local: Injection site hematoma/pain (dose and formulation related)
Neuromuscular & skeletal: Arthralgia, arthropathy, back pain, hyperkinesia, hypertonia, joint pain, myalgia, neuropathy, paresthesia, rigors, tremor, weakness
Ocular: Blurred vision, visual disturbance
Otic: Earache, tinnitus
Renal: Albuminuria, renal abscess, renal calculus
Respiratory: Bronchitis, cough, dyspnea (non-depot formulations), epistaxis, pharyngitis, rhinitis, sinusitis, upper respiratory infection
Miscellaneous: Allergy, antibodies to octreotide, bacterial infection, cold symptoms, diaphoresis, flu symptoms, moniliasis
Rare but important or life-threatening: Amenorrhea, anaphylactic shock, anaphylactoid reactions, aneurysm, aphasia, appendicitis, arthritis, ascending cholangitis, ascites, atrial fibrillation, basal cell carcinoma, Bell's palsy, biliary obstruction, breast carcinoma, cardiac arrest, cerebral vascular disorder, CHF, cholecystitis, cholestatic hepatitis, CK increased, deafness, diabetes insipidus, diabetes mellitus, fatty liver, galactorrhea, gallbladder polyp, GI bleeding, GI hemorrhage, GI ulcer, glaucoma, gynecomastia, hematuria, hepatitis, hypoadrenalism, hypoxia (children), intestinal obstruction, intracranial hemorrhage, intraocular pressure increased, ischemia, joint effusion, malignant hyperpyrexia, MI, migraine, necrotizing enterocolitis (neonates), nephrolithiasis, neuritis, oligomenorrhea, orthostatic hypotension, pancreatitis, pancytopenia, paresis, pituitary apoplexy, pleural effusion, pneumonia, pneumothorax, polymenorrhea, pulmonary embolism, pulmonary hypertension, pulmonary nodule, Raynaud's syndrome, renal failure, renal insufficiency, retinal vein thrombosis, seizures, status asthmaticus, suicide attempt, syncope, tachycardia, thrombocytopenia, thrombophlebitis, thrombosis, weight loss

Drug Interactions

Metabolism/Transport Effects None known.

Avoid Concomitant Use

Avoid concomitant use of Octreotide with any of the following: Ceritinib

Increased Effect/Toxicity

Octreotide may increase the levels/effects of: Bradycardia-Causing Agents; Bromocriptine; Ceritinib; Codeine; Highest Risk QTc-Prolonging Agents; Hypoglycemia-Associated Agents; Ivabradine; Lacosamide; Moderate Risk QTc-Prolonging Agents; Pegvisomant

The levels/effects of Octreotide may be increased by: Androgens; Antidiabetic Agents; Bretylium; Herbs (Hypoglycemic Properties); MAO Inhibitors; Mifepristone; Pegvisomant; Quinolone Antibiotics; Ruxolitinib; Salicylates; Selective Serotonin Reuptake Inhibitors; Tofacitinib

Decreased Effect

Octreotide may decrease the levels/effects of: Antidiabetic Agents; CycloSPORINE (Systemic)

The levels/effects of Octreotide may be decreased by: Quinolone Antibiotics

Food Interactions Octreotide may alter absorption of dietary fats. Management: Administer injections between meals to decrease GI effects.

Storage/Stability

Solution: Octreotide is a clear solution and should be stored at refrigerated temperatures between 2°C and 8°C (36°F and 46°F). Protect from light. May be stored at room temperature of 20°C to 30°C (68°F and 86°F) for up to 14 days when protected from light. Stable as a parenteral admixture in NS or D_5W for 24 hours. Discard multidose vials within 14 days after initial entry.

Suspension: Prior to dilution, store at refrigerated temperatures between 2°C and 8°C (36°F and 46°F). Protect from light. Additionally, the manufacturer reports that octreotide suspension may be stored at room temperature of 20°C to 25°C (68°F and 77°F) for up to 10 days when protected from light (data on file [Novartis, 2011]). Depot drug product kit may be at room temperature for 30 to 60 minutes prior to use. Use suspension immediately after preparation.

Mechanism of Action Mimics natural somatostatin by inhibiting serotonin release, and the secretion of gastrin, VIP, insulin, glucagon, secretin, motilin, and pancreatic polypeptide. Decreases growth hormone and IGF-1 in acromegaly. Octreotide provides more potent inhibition of growth hormone, glucagon, and insulin as compared to endogenous somatostatin. Also suppresses LH response to GnRH, secretion of thyroid-stimulating hormone and decreases splanchnic blood flow.

Pharmacodynamics Duration (immediate release formulation): SubQ: 6-12 hours

Pharmacokinetics (Adult data unless noted)

Absorption: SubQ: Rapid; IM (depot formulation): Released slowly (via microsphere degradation in the muscle)
Bioavailability: SubQ: 100%; IM: 60% to 63% of SubQ dose
Distribution: V_d:
Adults: 13.6 L
Adults with acromegaly: 21.6 ± 8.5 L
Protein binding: 65% primarily to lipoprotein (41% in acromegaly)
Metabolism: Extensive by the liver
Half-life: 1.7-1.9 hours; up to 3.7 hours with cirrhosis; up to 3.4 hours with fatty liver disease; up to 3.1 hours in renal impairment
Time to peak serum concentration: SubQ: 0.4 hours (0.7 hours acromegaly); IM: 1 hour
Elimination: 32% excreted unchanged in urine
Clearance:
Adults: 10 L/hour
Adults with acromegaly: 18 L/hour
Note: When using Sandostatin LAR® Depot formulation, steady-state levels are achieved after 3 injections (3 months of therapy)

Dosing: Neonatal

Chylothorax: Continuous IV infusion: 0.3-10 mcg/kg/**hour** titrated to response (median: 2.8 mcg/kg/**hour**) has been described in case reports; treatment duration is usually 1-3 weeks but may vary with the clinical response (Das, 2010; Roehr, 2006)

Persistent hyperinsulinemic hypoglycemia of infancy (Stanley, 1997):
Continuous IV infusion: Initial: 0.08-0.4 mcg/kg/**hour**; titrate dosage depending upon patient response; maximum dose: 1.67 mcg/kg/**hour**
SubQ: Initial: 2-10 mcg/kg/day divided 3-4 times daily; titrate dosage depending upon patient response; maximum daily dose: 40 mcg/kg/day

Dosing: Usual Dosage should be individualized according to the patient's response

Sandostatin®:

Infants and Children (data limited to small studies and case reports): **Note:** The following are effective dosing ranges for specific therapies: IV, SubQ:
Diarrhea:
Continuous IV infusion: Initial: 1 mcg/kg bolus dose, followed by a continuous infusion of 1 mcg/kg/**hour** has been used successfully in several cases of severe diarrhea secondary to graft vs host disease
IV, SubQ: Doses of 1-10 mcg/kg/dose every 12 hours have been used in children beginning at the low end of the range and increasing based upon the clinical response

Chylothorax:

Continuous IV infusion: 0.3-10 mcg/kg/**hour** titrated to response (median: 2.8 mcg/kg/**hour**) has been described in case reports; treatment duration is usually 1-3 weeks but may vary with the clinical response (Roehr, 2006)

SubQ: 40 mcg/kg/day; case reports of effective dosage range from 2-68 mcg/kg/day (Chan, 2006; Roehr, 2006)

Esophageal varices/GI bleed: 1-2 mcg/kg initial IV bolus followed by 1-2 mcg/kg/**hour** continuous infusion; titrate infusion rate to response; taper dose by 50% every 12 hours when no active bleeding occurs for 24 hours; may discontinue when dose is 25% of initial dose (Eroglu, 2004)

Hypothalamic obesity (from cranial insult): SubQ: 5 mcg/kg/day divided into 3 daily doses; dose may be increased bimonthly at 5 mcg/kg/day increments to a maximum of 15 mcg/kg/day divided into 3 daily doses (Lustig, 2003)

Persistent hyperinsulinemic hypoglycemia of infancy: SubQ: 2-10 mcg/kg/day divided 3-4 times daily; titrate dosage depending upon patient response; maximum daily dose: 40 mcg/kg/day (Stanley, 1997)

Treatment of sulfonylurea overdose: **Note:** SubQ is the preferred route of administration; repeat dosing, dose escalation, or initiation of a continuous infusion may be required in patients who experience recurrent hypoglycemia. Duration of treatment may exceed 24 hours. Optimal care decisions should be made based upon patient-specific details; SubQ: 1-1.5 mcg/kg/dose; repeat in 6-12 hours as needed based upon blood glucose concentrations

Adults:

Acromegaly:

SubQ, IV: Initial: 50 mcg 3 times/day; titrate to achieve growth hormone levels <5 ng/mL or IGF-I (somatomedin C) levels <1.9 units/mL in males and <2.2 units/mL in females. Usual effective dose is 100-200 mcg 3 times/day; range: 300-1500 mcg/day. **Note:** Should be withdrawn yearly for a 4-week interval (8 weeks for depot injection) in patients who have received irradiation. Resume if levels increase and signs/symptoms recur.

IM depot injection: Patients must be stabilized on subcutaneous octreotide for at least 2 weeks before switching to the long-acting depot. Upon switch: 20 mg IM intragluteally every 4 weeks for 3 months, then the dose may be modified based upon response.

Dosage adjustment: After 3 months of depot injections, the dosage may be continued or modified as follows:

GH ≤1 ng/mL, IGF-1 normal, and symptoms controlled: Reduce octreotide LAR® to 10 mg IM every 4 weeks

GH ≤2.5 ng/mL, IGF-1 normal, and symptoms controlled: Maintain octreotide LAR® at 20 mg IM every 4 weeks

GH >2.5 ng/mL, IGF-1 elevated, and/or symptoms uncontrolled: Increase octreotide LAR® to 30 mg IM every 4 weeks

Note: Patients not adequately controlled at a dose of 30 mg may increase dose to 40 mg every 4 weeks. Dosages >40 mg are not recommended.

Carcinoid tumors:

SubQ, IV: Initial 2 weeks: 100-600 mcg/day in 2-4 divided doses; usual range: 50-750 mcg/day (some patients may require up to 1500 mcg/day)

IM depot injection: Patients must be stabilized on subcutaneous octreotide for at least 2 weeks before switching to the long-acting depot. Upon switch: 20 mg IM intragluteally every 4 weeks for 2 months, then the dose may be modified based upon response

Note: Patients should continue to receive their SubQ injections for the first 2 weeks at the same dose in order to maintain therapeutic levels (some patients may require 3-4 weeks of continued SubQ injections). Patients who experience periodic exacerbations of symptoms may require temporary SubQ injections in addition to depot injections (at their previous SubQ dosing regimen) until symptoms have resolved.

Dosage adjustment: See dosing adjustment for VIPomas.

VIPomas:

SubQ, IV: Initial 2 weeks: 200-300 mcg/day in 2-4 divided doses; titrate dose based on response/tolerance; range: 150-750 mcg/day (doses >450 mcg/day are rarely required)

IM depot injection: Patients must be stabilized on subcutaneous octreotide for at least 2 weeks before switching to the long-acting depot. Upon switch: 20 mg IM intragluteally every 4 weeks for 2 months, then the dose may be modified based upon response.

Note: Patients receiving depot injection should continue to receive their SubQ injections for the first 2 weeks at the same dose in order to maintain therapeutic levels (some patients may require 3-4 weeks of continued SubQ injections). Patients who experience periodic exacerbations of symptoms may require temporary SubQ injections in addition to depot injections (at their previous SubQ dosing regimen) until symptoms have resolved.

Dosage adjustment: After 2 months of depot injections, the dosage may be continued or modified as follows:

Increase to 30 mg IM every 4 weeks if symptoms are inadequately controlled

Decrease to 10 mg IM every 4 weeks, for a trial period, if initially responsive to 20 mg dose

Dosage >30 mg is not recommended

Dosage adjustment in renal impairment: Clearance is decreased by 50% in patients with severe renal failure requiring dialysis; consider dosage modification in these patients as follows:

- Nondialysis-dependent renal impairment: No dosage adjustment required
- Dialysis-dependent renal impairment: Depot injection: Initial dose: IM: 10 mg every 4 weeks; titrate based upon response (clearance is reduced by ~50%

Dosage adjustment in hepatic impairment: Patients with established cirrhosis of the liver: Depot injection: Initial dose: IM: 10 mg every 4 weeks; titrate based upon response

Preparation for Administration

Parenteral:

IV infusion: Dilute Sandostatin injection in 50 to 200 mL NS or D_5W

IM: Sandostatin LAR: Allow Sandostatin LAR Depot vial and provided diluent-filled syringe to reach room temperature slowly (approximately 30 to 60 minutes). Reconstitute with provided diluent; see detailed mixing instructions included with the product. Administer immediately after preparation.

Administration Parenteral: Only Sandostatin injection may be administered IV and SubQ; Sandostatin LAR Depot may only be administered IM

SubQ: Use the concentration with smallest volume to deliver dose to reduce injection site pain; rotate injection site; may bring to room temperature prior to injection

IV infusion: Dilute Sandostatin injection and infuse over 15 to 30 minutes or over 24 hours as a continuous infusion; in emergency situations, may be administered undiluted by direct IV push over 3 minutes; allow solution to come to room temperature before administration

IM: Administer into gluteal area only; avoid deltoid injections due to significant pain and discomfort at injection site

Monitoring Parameters Baseline and periodic ultrasound evaluations for cholelithiasis, blood sugar, baseline and periodic thyroid function tests, fluid and electrolyte balance, fecal fat, and serum carotene determinations; for carcinoid, monitor urinary 5-hydroxyindole acetic acid (5-HIAA), plasma serotonin, plasma substance P; for VIPoma, monitor VIP; vitamin B_{12} levels (chronic therapy); for acromegaly: growth hormone levels, IGF-I (somatomedin C), glycemic control, and antidiabetic regimen (patients with diabetes mellitus)

Reference Range Vasoactive intestinal peptide (VIP): <75 ng/L; levels vary considerably between laboratories; growth hormone level: <5 ng/mL; IGF-I (somatomedin C): males: <1.9 units/mL, females: <2.2 units/mL

Dosage Forms Excipient information presented when available (limited, particularly for generics); consult specific product labeling.

Kit, Intramuscular:

SandoSTATIN LAR Depot: 10 mg, 20 mg, 30 mg

Solution, Injection:

SandoSTATIN: 50 mcg/mL (1 mL); 100 mcg/mL (1 mL)

SandoSTATIN: 200 mcg/mL (5 mL) [contains phenol]

SandoSTATIN: 500 mcg/mL (1 mL)

SandoSTATIN: 1000 mcg/mL (5 mL) [contains phenol]

Generic: 50 mcg/mL (1 mL); 100 mcg/mL (1 mL); 200 mcg/mL (5 mL); 1000 mcg/5 mL (5 mL); 500 mcg/mL (1 mL); 1000 mcg/mL (5 mL)

Solution, Injection [preservative free]:

Generic: 100 mcg/mL (1 mL); 500 mcg/mL (1 mL)

- ◆ **Octreotide Acetate** *see* Octreotide *on page 1539*
- ◆ **Octreotide Acetate Omega (Can)** *see* Octreotide *on page 1539*
- ◆ **Octreotide Injection (Can)** *see* Octreotide *on page 1539*
- ◆ **Ocudox [DSC]** *see* Doxycycline *on page 717*
- ◆ **Ocufen** *see* Flurbiprofen (Ophthalmic) *on page 916*
- ◆ **Ocuflox** *see* Ofloxacin (Ophthalmic) *on page 1544*
- ◆ **Ocuflox® (Can)** *see* Ofloxacin (Ophthalmic) *on page 1544*

Ocular Lubricant (OK yoo lar LOO bri kant)

Brand Names: US Akwa Tears® [OTC]; Refresh® Lacri-Lube® [OTC]; Tears Renewed® [OTC]

Therapeutic Category Lubricant, Ocular; Ophthalmic Agent, Miscellaneous

Use Ocular lubricant

Contraindications Known hypersensitivity to any of the components

Mechanism of Action Forms an occlusive film on the surface of the eye to lubricate and protect the eye from drying

Dosing: Neonatal Note: Neonatal data are unavailable. Dose extrapolated from older patients. Ophthalmic: Apply 1/4" of ointment to the inside of the lower lid as needed.

Dosing: Usual Infants, Children, Adolescents, and Adults: Ophthalmic: Apply 1/4" of ointment to the inside of the lower lid as needed.

Administration Ophthalmic: Do not use with contact lenses; to avoid contamination, do not touch tip of container to any surface

Additional Information Contains petrolatum, mineral oil, chlorobutanol and lanolin alcohols

Dosage Forms Excipient information presented when available (limited, particularly for generics); consult specific product labeling. [DSC] = Discontinued product

Ointment, ophthalmic: (1 g [DSC], 3.5 g [DSC])

Akwa Tears®: 3.5 g (3.5 g)

Ointment, ophthalmic [preservative free]:

Tears Renewed®: 3.5 g (3.5 g)

- ◆ **Odans Liquor Carbonis Detergens [OTC] (Can)** *see* Coal Tar *on page 523*
- ◆ **Oesclim (Can)** *see* Estradiol (Systemic) *on page 795*
- ◆ **Ofirmev** *see* Acetaminophen *on page 44*

Ofloxacin (Systemic) (oh FLOKS a sin)

Brand Names: Canada Apo-Oflox; Novo-Ofloxacin

Therapeutic Category Antibiotic, Quinolone

Generic Availability (US) Yes

Use Treatment of acute bacterial exacerbations of chronic bronchitis, community-acquired pneumonia, uncomplicated skin and skin structure infections, urethral and cervical gonorrhea (acute, uncomplicated), urethritis and cervicitis (nongonococcal), pelvic inflammatory disease, uncomplicated cystitis, complicated urinary tract infections, and prostatitis caused by susceptible organisms including *S. pneumoniae*, *S. aureus*, *S. pyrogenes*, *C. koseri*, *E. aerogenes*, E. *coli*, *H. influenzae*, *K. pneumoniae*, *N. gonorrhoeae*, *P. mirabilis*, *C. trachomatis*, and *P. aeruginosa*

Medication Guide Available Yes

Pregnancy Risk Factor C

Pregnancy Considerations Adverse events have been observed in some animal reproduction studies. Ofloxacin crosses the placenta and produces measurable concentrations in the amniotic fluid. Serum concentrations of ofloxacin may be lower during pregnancy than in non-pregnant patients (Giamarellou 1989). Based on available data, an increased risk of teratogenic effects has not been observed following ofloxacin use during pregnancy (Padberg 2014).

Breast-Feeding Considerations Ofloxacin is excreted in breast milk. Due to the potential for serious adverse reactions in the nursing infant, the manufacturer recommends a decision be made whether to discontinue nursing or to discontinue the drug, taking into account the importance of treatment to the mother.

Contraindications Hypersensitivity to ofloxacin or other members of the quinolone group, such as oxolinic acid, cinoxacin, norfloxacin, and ciprofloxacin; hypersensitivity to any component of the formulation

Warnings/Precautions [U.S. Boxed Warning]: There have been reports of tendon inflammation and/or rupture with quinolone antibiotics; risk may be increased with concurrent corticosteroids, organ transplant recipients, and in patients >60 years of age. Rupture of the Achilles tendon sometimes requiring surgical repair has been reported most frequently; but other tendon sites (eg, rotator cuff, biceps) have also been reported. Strenuous physical activity, rheumatoid arthritis, and renal impairment may be an independent risk factor for tendonitis. Discontinue at first sign of tendon inflammation or pain. May occur even after discontinuation of therapy. Use with caution in patients with rheumatoid arthritis; may increase risk of tendon rupture. CNS effects may occur (tremor, restlessness, confusion, and very rarely hallucinations, increased intracranial pressure [including pseudotumor cerebri] or seizures). Use with caution in patients with known or suspected CNS disorder. Potential for seizures, although very rare, may be increased with concomitant NSAID therapy. Use with caution in individuals at risk of seizures. Use with caution in patients with renal or hepatic impairment. Peripheral neuropathy has been reported (rare); may occur soon after initiation of therapy and may be irreversible; discontinue if symptoms of sensory or sensorimotor neuropathy occur.

Fluoroquinolones have been associated with the development of serious, and sometimes fatal, hypoglycemia, most often in elderly diabetics, but also in patients without diabetes. This occurred most frequently with gatifloxacin (no longer available systemically) but may occur at a lower frequency with other quinolones.

Rare cases of torsade de pointes have been reported in patients receiving ofloxacin and other quinolones. Risk may be minimized by avoiding use in patients with known prolongation of the QT interval, bradycardia, hypokalemia, hypomagnesemia, cardiomyopathy, or in those receiving concurrent therapy with Class Ia or Class III antiarrhythmics.

Severe hypersensitivity reactions, including anaphylaxis, have occurred with quinolone therapy. Reactions may present as typical allergic symptoms after a single dose, or may manifest as severe idiosyncratic dermatologic, vascular, pulmonary, renal, hepatic, and/or hematologic events, usually after multiple doses. Prompt discontinuation of drug should occur if skin rash or other symptoms arise. Prolonged use may result in fungal or bacterial superinfection, including *C. difficile*-associated diarrhea (CDAD) and pseudomembranous colitis; CDAD has been observed >2 months postantibiotic treatment. **[U.S. Boxed Warning]: Quinolones may exacerbate myasthenia gravis; avoid use (rare, potentially life-threatening weakness of respiratory muscles may occur).** Avoid excessive sunlight and take precautions to limit exposure (eg, loose fitting clothing, sunscreen); may cause moderate-to-severe phototoxicity reactions. Discontinue use if photosensitivity occurs. Since ofloxacin is ineffective in the treatment of syphilis and may mask symptoms, all patients should be tested for syphilis at the time of gonorrheal diagnosis and 3 months later. Hemolytic reactions may (rarely) occur with quinolone use in patients with latent or actual G6PD deficiency.

Adverse Reactions

Cardiovascular: Chest pain

Central nervous system: dizziness, fatigue, headache, insomnia, nervousness, pyrexia, sleep disorders, somnolence

Dermatologic: Pruritus, rash

Gastrointestinal: Abdominal cramps, abnormal taste, appetite decreased, constipation, diarrhea, flatulence, GI distress, nausea, vomiting, xerostomia

Genitourinary: External genital pruritus in women, vaginitis

Ocular: Visual disturbances

Respiratory: Pharyngitis

Miscellaneous: Trunk pain

Rare but important or life-threatening: Anaphylaxis reactions, anxiety, blurred vision, chills, cognitive change, cough, depression, dream abnormality, ecchymosis, edema, erythema nodosum, euphoria, extremity pain, hallucinations, hearing acuity decreased, hepatic dysfunction, hepatic failure (some fatal), hepatitis, hepatotoxicity (idiosyncratic) (Chalasani, 2014), hyper-/hypoglycemia, hypertension, interstitial nephritis, intracranial pressure increased, lightheadedness, malaise, myasthenia gravis exacerbation, palpitation, paresthesia, peripheral neuropathy, photophobia, photosensitivity, pneumonitis, pseudotumor cerebri, psychotic reactions, rhabdomyolysis, seizure, Stevens-Johnson syndrome, syncope, tendonitis and tendon rupture, thirst, tinnitus, torsade de pointes, Tourette's syndrome, toxic epidermal necrolysis, vasculitis, vasodilation, vertigo, weakness, weight loss

Drug Interactions

Metabolism/Transport Effects Inhibits CYP1A2 (strong)

Avoid Concomitant Use

Avoid concomitant use of Ofloxacin (Systemic) with any of the following: Agomelatine; BCG; BCG (Intravesical); DULoxetine; Highest Risk QTc-Prolonging Agents; Ivabradine; Mifepristone; Pomalidomide; Strontium Ranelate; Tasimelteon; TiZANidine

Increased Effect/Toxicity

Ofloxacin (Systemic) may increase the levels/effects of: Agomelatine; Bendamustine; Blood Glucose Lowering Agents; CloZAPine; CYP1A2 Substrates; DULoxetine; Highest Risk QTc-Prolonging Agents; Moderate Risk QTc-Prolonging Agents; Pentoxifylline; Pirfenidone; Pomalidomide; Porfimer; Rasagiline; Tasimelteon; Theophylline Derivatives; TiZANidine; Varenicline; Verteporfin; Vitamin K Antagonists

The levels/effects of Ofloxacin (Systemic) may be increased by: Corticosteroids (Systemic); Ivabradine; Mifepristone; Nonsteroidal Anti-Inflammatory Agents; Probenecid; QTc-Prolonging Agents (Indeterminate Risk and Risk Modifying)

Decreased Effect

Ofloxacin (Systemic) may decrease the levels/effects of: BCG; BCG (Intravesical); BCG Vaccine (Immunization); Blood Glucose Lowering Agents; Didanosine; Mycophenolate; Sodium Picosulfate; Typhoid Vaccine

The levels/effects of Ofloxacin (Systemic) may be decreased by: Antacids; Calcium Salts; Didanosine; Iron Salts; Lanthanum; Magnesium Salts; Multivitamins/Minerals (with ADEK, Folate, Iron); Multivitamins/Minerals (with AE, No Iron); Quinapril; Sevelamer; Strontium Ranelate; Sucralfate; Zinc Salts

Food Interactions Ofloxacin average peak serum concentrations may be decreased by 20% if taken with food. Management: Do not administer within 2 hours of food or any antacids which contain zinc, magnesium, or aluminum.

Storage/Stability Store at 25°C (77°F); excursions permitted to 15°C to 30°C (59°F to 86°F).

Mechanism of Action Ofloxacin is a DNA gyrase inhibitor. DNA gyrase is an essential bacterial enzyme that maintains the superhelical structure of DNA. DNA gyrase is required for DNA replication and transcription, DNA repair, recombination, and transposition; bactericidal

Pharmacokinetics (Adult data unless noted)

Absorption: Well-absorbed

Distribution: Widely distributed into body tissues and fluids, including blister fluid, cervix, lung, ovary, prostatic tissue, skin, and sputum; crosses the placenta; excreted into breast milk

V_d: 2.4-3.5 L/kg

Protein binding: 20% to 32%

Bioavailability: 98%

Half-life, biphasic: 4-7.4 hours and 20-25 hours; prolonged with renal impairment

Time to peak, serum concentration: 1-2 hours

Elimination: 68% to 90% is excreted unchanged in urine; 4% to 8% excreted in feces; <10% is metabolized

Dosing: Usual

Children: Oral: **Note:** Limited information regarding ofloxacin use in pediatric patients is currently available in the literature; some centers recommend doses of 15 mg/kg/day divided every 12 hours.

Adults:

Cervicitis/urethritis: Oral:

Nongonococcal: 300 mg every 12 hours for 7 days

Gonococcal (acute, uncomplicated): 400 mg as a single dose; **Note:** As of April 2007, the CDC no longer recommends the use of fluoroquinolones for the treatment of uncomplicated gonococcal disease.

Chronic bronchitis (acute exacerbation), community-acquired pneumonia, skin and skin structure infections (uncomplicated): Oral: 400 mg every 12 hours for 10 days

Pelvic inflammatory disease (acute): Oral: 400 mg every 12 hours for 10 to 14 days; **Note:** The CDC recommends use only if standard cephalosporin therapy is not feasible and community prevalence of quinolone-resistant gonococcal organisms is low. Culture sensitivity must be confirmed.

Prostatitis: Oral:

Acute: 400 mg for 1 dose, then 300 mg twice daily for 10 days

Chronic: 200 mg every 12 hours for 6 weeks

UTI: Oral:

Uncomplicated: 200 mg every 12 hours for 3 to 7 days

Complicated: 200 mg every 12 hours for 10 days

Dosing adjustment in renal impairment: Adults: Oral: After a normal initial dose, adjust as follows:

CrCl 20 to 50 mL/minute: Administer usual dose every 24 hours

CrCl <20 mL/minute: Administer half the usual dose every 24 hours

Dosing adjustment in hepatic impairment: Adults: Severe impairment: Maximum dose: 400 mg/day

Administration May administer ofloxacin tablets with or without food; avoid antacids, vitamins with iron or minerals, sucralfate, or didanosine; use within 2 hours of administration; drink plenty of fluids to maintain proper hydration and urine output

Monitoring Parameters Patients receiving concurrent ofloxacin and theophylline should have serum levels of theophylline monitored; monitor INR in patients receiving warfarin; monitor blood glucose in patients receiving antidiabetic agents; monitor renal, hepatic, hematopoietic function, and electrolytes periodically; number and type of stools/day for diarrhea

Test Interactions Some quinolones may produce a false-positive urine screening result for opioids using commercially-available immunoassay kits. This has been demonstrated most consistently for levofloxacin and ofloxacin, but other quinolones have shown cross-reactivity in certain assay kits. Confirmation of positive opioid screens by more specific methods should be considered.

Dosage Forms Excipient information presented when available (limited, particularly for generics); consult specific product labeling. [DSC] = Discontinued product

Tablet, Oral:

Generic: 200 mg [DSC], 300 mg, 400 mg

Ofloxacin (Ophthalmic) (oh FLOKS a sin)

Medication Safety Issues

Sound-alike/look-alike issues:

Ocuflox may be confused with Occlusal-HP, Ocufen

Brand Names: US Ocuflox

Brand Names: Canada Ocuflox®

Therapeutic Category Antibiotic, Ophthalmic; Antibiotic, Quinolone

Generic Availability (US) Yes

Use Treatment of bacterial keratitis due to susceptible organisms including *P. aeruginosa*, *Propionibacterium acnes*, *S. marcescens*, *S. aureus*, *S. epidermidis*, and *S. pneumoniae*; treatment of severe bacterial conjunctivitis due to susceptible organisms, including *Enterobacter cloacae*, *H. influenzae*, *P. mirabilis*, *P. aeruginosa*, *S. aureus*, *S. epidermidis*, or *S. pneumoniae*

Pregnancy Risk Factor C

Pregnancy Considerations Adverse events have been observed in some animal reproduction studies. When administered orally, ofloxacin crosses the placenta (Giamarellou 1989). The amount of ofloxacin available systemically following topical application of the ophthalmic drops is significantly less in comparison to oral doses. If ophthalmic agents are needed during pregnancy, the minimum effective dose should be used in combination with punctual occlusion for 3 to 5 minutes after application to decrease potential exposure to the fetus (Samples 1988).

Breast-Feeding Considerations When administered orally, ofloxacin enters breast milk. It is not known if ofloxacin is excreted into breast milk following ophthalmic application. Due to the potential for serious adverse reactions in the nursing infant, the manufacturer recommends a decision be made whether to discontinue nursing or to discontinue the drug, taking into account the importance of treatment to the mother.

Contraindications Hypersensitivity to ofloxacin or other members of the quinolone group, such as oxolinic acid, cinoxacin, norfloxacin, and ciprofloxacin; hypersensitivity to any component of the formulation

Warnings/Precautions Not for subconjunctival injection or for introduction into the ocular anterior chamber. Severe hypersensitivity reactions, including anaphylaxis, have occurred with quinolone therapy (primarily with systemic use). The spectrum of these reactions can vary widely; reactions may present as typical allergic symptoms (eg, itching, urticaria, rash, edema) after a single dose or may manifest as severe idiosyncratic dermatologic (eg, Stevens-Johnson, toxic epidermal necrolysis), vascular (eg, vasculitis), pulmonary (eg, pneumonitis), renal (eg, nephritis), hepatic (eg, hepatic failure, necrosis), and/or hematologic (eg, anemia, cytopenias) events, usually after multiple doses. Prompt discontinuation of drug should occur if skin rash or other symptoms arise. Prolonged use may result in fungal or bacterial superinfection. If superinfection is suspected, institute appropriate alternative therapy. There have been reports of tendon inflammation and/or rupture with systemic quinolone antibiotics. Exposure following ophthalmic administration is substantially lower than with systemic therapy. Discontinue at first sign of tendon inflammation or pain. Safety and efficacy have not been established in children <1 year of age.

Adverse Reactions

Central nervous system: Dizziness

Dermatologic: Stevens-Johnson syndrome (rare), toxic epidermal necrolysis (rare)

Gastrointestinal: Nausea

Ocular: Blurred vision, burning, chemical conjunctivitis/keratitis, discomfort, dryness, edema, eye pain, foreign body sensation, itching, photophobia, redness, stinging, tearing

Drug Interactions

Metabolism/Transport Effects None known.

Avoid Concomitant Use There are no known interactions where it is recommended to avoid concomitant use.

Increased Effect/Toxicity There are no known significant interactions involving an increase in effect.

Decreased Effect There are no known significant interactions involving a decrease in effect.

Storage/Stability Store 15°C to 25°C (59°F to 77°F).

Mechanism of Action Ofloxacin is a DNA gyrase inhibitor. DNA gyrase is an essential bacterial enzyme that maintains the superhelical structure of DNA. DNA gyrase is required for DNA replication and transcription, DNA repair, recombination, and transposition; bactericidal

Pharmacokinetics (Adult data unless noted) Absorption: Ocular: Minimal absorption unless inflammation or epithelial defect is present

Dosing: Usual Children >1 year and Adults:

Conjunctivitis: Instill 1-2 drops in affected eye(s) every 2-4 hours while awake for the first 2 days, then 4 times/day for an additional 5 days

Corneal ulcer: Instill 1-2 drops in affected eye(s) every 30 minutes while awake and every 4-6 hours at night for the first 2 days; then starting day 3, instill 1-2 drops every hour while awake for 4-6 additional days; thereafter, 1-2 drops 4 times/day until clinical cure is achieved

Administration Not for subconjunctival or direct injection into the anterior chamber of the eye. Apply gentle pressure to lacrimal sac during and immediately following instillation

(1 minute) or instruct patient to gently close eyelid after administration, to decrease systemic absorption of ophthalmic drops; avoid contact of bottle tip with skin or eye. Remove contact lenses prior to administration (ophthalmic solution contains benzalkonium chloride which may adsorb to soft contact lenses); lenses may be inserted 15 minutes after administration.

Monitoring Parameters Slit-lamp biomicroscopy and fluorescein staining may be necessary

Dosage Forms Excipient information presented when available (limited, particularly for generics); consult specific product labeling.

Solution, Ophthalmic:

Ocuflox: 0.3% (5 mL) [contains benzalkonium chloride]

Generic: 0.3% (5 mL, 10 mL)

Ofloxacin (Otic) (oh FLOKS a sin)

Medication Safety Issues

Sound-alike/look-alike issues:

Floxin may be confused with Flexeril®

International issues:

Floxin: Brand name for ofloxacin [U.S., Canada], but also the brand name for flunarizine [Thailand], norfloxacin [South Africa], and perfloxacin [Philippines]

Floxin [U.S., Canada] may be confused with Flexin brand name for diclofenac [Argentina], cyclobenzaprine [Chile], and orphenadrine [Israel]; Flogen brand name for naproxen [Mexico]

Therapeutic Category Antibiotic, Otic; Antibiotic, Quinolone

Generic Availability (US) Yes

Use Treatment of acute otitis externa (FDA approved in ages 6 months and adults); treatment of acute otitis media in patients with tympanostomy tubes (FDA approved in ages ≥1 to 12 years); treatment of chronic suppurative otitis media with perforation of the tympanic membrane (FDA approved in ages ≥12 years and adults)

Pregnancy Risk Factor C

Pregnancy Considerations Adverse events have been observed in some animal reproduction studies. When administered orally, ofloxacin crosses the placenta (Giamarellou 1989). The amount of ofloxacin available systemically following topical application of the otic drops is significantly less in comparison to oral doses.

Breast-Feeding Considerations When administered orally, ofloxacin enters breast milk. It is not known if ofloxacin can be detected in breast milk following otic administration. Due to the potential for serious adverse reactions in the nursing infant, the manufacturer recommends a decision be made whether to discontinue nursing or to discontinue the drug, taking into account the importance of treatment to the mother.

Contraindications Hypersensitivity to ofloxacin or other members of the quinolone group, such as oxolinic acid, cinoxacin, norfloxacin, and ciprofloxacin; hypersensitivity to any component of the formulation

Warnings/Precautions Not for injection or for ophthalmic use. Severe hypersensitivity reactions, including anaphylaxis, have occurred with quinolone therapy (primarily with systemic use). The spectrum of these reactions can vary widely; reactions may present as typical allergic symptoms (eg, itching, urticaria, rash, edema) after a single dose or may manifest as severe idiosyncratic dermatologic (eg, Stevens-Johnson, toxic epidermal necrolysis), vascular (eg, vasculitis), pulmonary (eg, pneumonitis), renal (eg, nephritis), hepatic (eg, hepatic failure or necrosis), and/or hematologic (eg, anemia, cytopenias) events, usually after multiple doses. Prompt discontinuation of drug should occur if skin rash or other symptoms arise. Prolonged use may result in fungal or bacterial superinfection. If superinfection is suspected, institute appropriate alternative therapy. There have been reports of tendon inflammation and/or rupture with systemic quinolone antibiotics. Exposure following otic administration is substantially lower than with systemic therapy. Discontinue at first sign of tendon inflammation or pain. Safety and efficacy have not been established in children <6 months of age (otitis externa with intact tympanic membranes, < 1 year of age (acute otitis media with tympanostomy tubes), or <12 years of age (chronic suppurative otitis media with perforated tympanic membranes).

Adverse Reactions

Central nervous system: Dizziness, vertigo

Dermatologic: Pruritus, rash

Gastrointestinal: Taste perversion

Local: Application site reaction

Neuromuscular & skeletal: Paresthesia

Rare but important or life-threatening: Diarrhea, fever, headache, hearing loss transient, hypertension, nausea, otorrhagia, tinnitus, transient neuropsychiatric disturbances, tremor, vomiting, xerostomia

Drug Interactions

Metabolism/Transport Effects None known.

Avoid Concomitant Use There are no known interactions where it is recommended to avoid concomitant use.

Increased Effect/Toxicity There are no known significant interactions involving an increase in effect.

Decreased Effect There are no known significant interactions involving a decrease in effect.

Storage/Stability

Solution: Store at 25°C (77°F); excursions permitted to 15°C to 30°C (59°F to 86°F).

Otic Singles™: Store at 25°C (77°F); excursions permitted to 15°C to 30°C (59°F to 86°F). Protect from light.

Mechanism of Action Ofloxacin is a DNA gyrase inhibitor. DNA gyrase is an essential bacterial enzyme that maintains the superhelical structure of DNA. DNA gyrase is required for DNA replication and transcription, DNA repair, recombination, and transposition; bactericidal

Pharmacokinetics (Adult data unless noted) Absorption: Minimal absorption unless tympanic membrane is perforated

Dosing: Usual

Pediatric:

Otitis media, acute (with tympanostomy tubes): Children: Otic: Instill 5 drops (0.25 mL) into the affected ear(s) twice daily for 10 days

Otitis media, chronic suppurative (with perforated tympanic membranes): Children ≥12 years and Adolescents: Otic: Instill 10 drops (0.5 mL) into the affected ear(s) twice daily for 14 days

Otitis externa, acute:

Infants ≥6 months and Children: Otic: Instill 5 drops (0.25 mL) into the affected ear(s) once daily for 7 days

Adolescents: Otic: Instill 10 drops (0.5 mL) into the affected ear(s) once daily for 7 days

Adult:

Otitis media, chronic suppurative (with perforated tympanic membranes): Otic: Instill 10 drops (0.5 mL) into affected ear(s) twice daily for 14 days

Otitis externa, acute: Otic: Instill 10 drops (0.5 mL) into affected ear(s) once daily for 7 days

Dosing adjustment in renal impairment: Infants ≥6 months, Children, Adolescents, and Adults: There are no dosing adjustments provided in the manufacturer's labeling.

Dosing adjustment in hepatic impairment: Infants ≥6 months, Children, Adolescents, and Adults: There are no dosing adjustments provided in the manufacturer's labeling.

Administration Not for ophthalmic use or injection. Gently clean any discharge that can be easily removed from the outer ear. Warm otic solution by holding bottle in hand for 1 to 2 minutes prior to instillation. The tip of the bottle should not touch the fingers, ear, or any surface. Patient should lie on side with affected ear upward. For middle ear infections, gently press the tragus 4 times in a pumping motion to allow the drops to pass through the hole or tube in the eardrum and into the middle ear. For otitis externa infection, pull the outer ear upward and backward to allow the ear drops to flow down into the ear canal. Patient should remain on his/her side for at least 5 minutes. If necessary, repeat procedure for the other ear.

Monitoring Parameters Presence of otorrhea, cultures

Dosage Forms Excipient information presented when available (limited, particularly for generics); consult specific product labeling.

Solution, Otic:

Generic: 0.3% (5 mL, 10 mL)

◆ **17OHPC** *see* Hydroxyprogesterone Caproate *on page 1054*

◆ **9-OH-risperidone** *see* Paliperidone *on page 1604*

OLANZapine (oh LAN za peen)

Medication Safety Issues

Sound-alike/look-alike issues:

OLANZapine may be confused with olsalazine, QUEtiapine

ZyPREXA may be confused with CeleXA, Reprexain, Zestril, ZyrTEC

ZyPREXA Zydis may be confused with Zelapar, zolpidem

ZyPREXA Relprevv may be confused with ZyPREXA IntraMuscular

BEERS Criteria medication:

This drug may be potentially inappropriate for use in geriatric patients (Quality of evidence - moderate; Strength of recommendation - strong).

Brand Names: US ZyPREXA; ZyPREXA Relprevv; ZyPREXA Zydis

Brand Names: Canada Abbott-Olanzapine ODT; Accel-Olanzapine; ACT Olanzapine; ACT Olanzapine ODT; Apo-Olanzapine; Apo-Olanzapine ODT; JAMP-Olanzapine ODT; Mar-Olanzapine; Mar-Olanzapine ODT; Mint-Olanzapine ODT; Mylan-Olanzapine; Mylan-Olanzapine ODT; Olanzapine for injection; Olanzapine ODT; PHL-Olanzapine; PHL-Olanzapine ODT; PMS-Olanzapine; PMS-Olanzapine ODT; RAN-Olanzapine; RAN-Olanzapine ODT; Riva-Olanzapine; Riva-Olanzapine ODT; Sandoz-Olanzapine; Sandoz-Olanzapine ODT; Teva-Olanzapine; Teva-Olanzapine OD; Zyprexa; Zyprexa Intramuscular; Zyprexa Zydis

Therapeutic Category Second Generation (Atypical) Antipsychotic

Generic Availability (US) May be product dependent

Use

Oral: Treatment of schizophrenia (FDA approved in ages ≥13 years and adults); acute and maintenance treatment of manic or mixed episodes of bipolar I disorder (FDA approved in ages ≥13 years and adults); adjunctive therapy (to lithium or valproate) for treatment of manic or mixed episodes of bipolar I disorder (FDA approved in adults); in combination with fluoxetine for treatment-resistant depression or depressive episodes associated with bipolar I disorder (FDA approved in adults). Has also been used for anorexia nervosa, autism spectrum disorders, Tourette syndrome, and tic disorders. Therapy should only be initiated in pediatric patients after a thorough diagnostic evaluation and an assessment of potential long-term risks; adolescent patients experience a higher incidence of weight gain, and greater increases in total cholesterol, triglycerides, LDL, prolactin, and hepatic transaminase concentrations than adult patients; other agents with fewer risks may be preferred as first-line treatment.

Parenteral:

IM extended release (Zyprexa® Relprevv™): Treatment of schizophrenia (FDA approved in adults)

IM short-acting (Zyprexa® IntraMuscular): Treatment of acute agitation associated with schizophrenia and bipolar I mania (FDA approved in adults)

Prescribing and Access Restrictions As a requirement of the REMS program, only prescribers, healthcare facilities, and pharmacies registered with the Zyprexa Relprevv Patient Care Program are able to prescribe, distribute, or dispense Zyprexa Relprevv for patients who are enrolled in and meet all conditions of the program. Zyprexa Relprevv must be administered at a registered healthcare facility. Prescribers will need to be recertified every 3 years. Contact the Zyprexa Relprevv Patient Care Program at 1-877-772-9390.

Medication Guide Available Yes

Pregnancy Risk Factor C

Pregnancy Considerations Adverse events were observed in animal reproduction studies. Olanzapine crosses the placenta and can be detected in cord blood at birth (Newport 2007). Information related to olanzapine use in pregnancy is limited (Goldstein 2000). Antipsychotic use during the third trimester of pregnancy has a risk for abnormal muscle movements (extrapyramidal symptoms [EPS]) and/or withdrawal symptoms in newborns following delivery. Symptoms in the newborn may include agitation, feeding disorder, hypertonia, hypotonia, respiratory distress, somnolence, and tremor; these effects may be self-limiting or require hospitalization. Olanzapine may cause hyperprolactinemia, which may decrease reproductive function in both males and females.

The ACOG recommends that therapy during pregnancy be individualized; treatment with psychiatric medications during pregnancy should incorporate the clinical expertise of the mental health clinician, obstetrician, primary healthcare provider, and pediatrician. Safety data related to atypical antipsychotics during pregnancy is limited and routine use is not recommended. However, if a woman is inadvertently exposed to an atypical antipsychotic while pregnant, continuing therapy may be preferable to switching to a typical antipsychotic that the fetus has not yet been exposed to; consider risk:benefit (ACOG 2008). Evaluate risk factors for gestational diabetes and weight gain if considering use of olanzapine in a pregnant woman (NICE 2007).

Healthcare providers are encouraged to enroll women 18 to 45 years of age exposed to olanzapine during pregnancy in the Atypical Antipsychotics Pregnancy Registry (1-866-961-2388 or http://www.womensmentalhealth.org/pregnancyregistry).

Breast-Feeding Considerations Olanzapine is excreted into breast milk. At steady-state concentrations, it is estimated that a breast-fed infant may be exposed to ~2% of the maternal dose. In one study, the median time to peak milk concentration was ~5 hours after the maternal dose and serum concentrations in the nursing infants were low (<5 ng/mL; n=5) (Gardiner 2003). An increased risk of adverse events in nursing infants has not been reported (Gardiner 2003; Gilad 2011). Breast-feeding is not recommended by the manufacturer.

Contraindications There are no contraindications listed in the manufacturer's labeling.

Canadian labeling: Hypersensitivity to olanzapine or any component of the formulation

Warnings/Precautions [US Boxed Warning]: Elderly patients with dementia-related psychosis treated with antipsychotics are at an increased risk of death

compared with placebo. Most deaths appeared to be either cardiovascular (eg, heart failure, sudden death) or infectious (eg, pneumonia) in nature. In addition, an increased incidence of cerebrovascular effects (eg, transient ischemic attack, stroke) has been reported in studies of placebo-controlled trials of olanzapine in elderly patients with dementia-related psychosis. Use with caution in dementia with Lewy bodies; antipsychotics may worsen dementia symptoms and patients with dementia with Lewy bodies are more sensitive to the extrapyramidal side effects (APA, [Rabins 2007]). Olanzapine is not approved for the treatment of dementia-related psychosis.

May cause CNS depression, which impair physical and mental abilities; patients must be cautioned about performing tasks that require mental alertness (eg, operating machinery, driving). May be moderate to highly sedating in comparison with other antipsychotics (APA [Lehman 2004]); dose-related effects have been observed. Use caution in patients with cardiac disease. Use with caution in Parkinson disease, predisposition to seizures, or severe hepatic or renal disease. Life-threatening arrhythmias have occurred with therapeutic doses of some neuroleptics. May induce orthostatic hypotension; use caution with history of cardiovascular disease, hemodynamic instability, prior myocardial infarction, or ischemic heart disease. Dose-related increases in cholesterol and triglycerides have been noted. Use with caution in patients with preexisting abnormal lipid profile. Esophageal dysmotility and aspiration have been associated with antipsychotic use; use with caution in patients at risk of aspiration pneumonia. May cause dose-related increases in prolactin levels; clinical significance of hyperprolactinemia in patients with breast cancer or other prolactin-dependent tumors is unknown. Clinical manifestations of increased prolactin levels included menstrual-, sexual- and breast-related events. Significant dose-related weight gain (>7% of baseline weight) may occur; monitor waist circumference and BMI. Impaired core body temperature regulation may occur; caution with strenuous exercise, heat exposure, dehydration, and concomitant medication possessing anticholinergic effects.

Leukopenia, neutropenia, and agranulocytosis (sometimes fatal) have been reported in clinical trials and postmarketing reports with antipsychotic use; presence of risk factors (eg, preexisting low WBC or history of drug-induced leuko-/neutropenia) should prompt periodic blood count assessment. Discontinue therapy at first signs of blood dyscrasias or if absolute neutrophil count <1,000/mm^3.

May cause anticholinergic effects; use with caution in patients with decreased gastrointestinal motility, urinary retention, BPH, xerostomia, or narrow-angle glaucoma. Relative to other neuroleptics, olanzapine has a moderate potency of cholinergic blockade. May cause extrapyramidal symptoms (EPS), although risk of these reactions is lower relative to other neuroleptics. Risk of dystonia (and probably other EPS) may be greater with increased doses, use of conventional antipsychotics, males, and younger patients. May be associated with neuroleptic malignant syndrome (NMS). May cause extreme and life-threatening hyperglycemia; use with caution in patients with diabetes or other disorders of glucose regulation; monitor. Olanzapine levels may be lower in patients who smoke. Smokers may require a daily dose 30% higher than nonsmokers in order to obtain an equivalent olanzapine concentration (Tsuda 2014); however, the manufacturer does not routinely recommend dosage adjustments.

Use in adolescent patients ≥13 years of age may result in increased weight gain and sedation, as well as greater increases in LDL cholesterol, total cholesterol, triglycerides, prolactin, and liver transaminase levels when compared with adults. Adolescent patients should be maintained on the lowest dose necessary. Use in elderly patients with dementia is associated with an increased risk of mortality and cerebrovascular accidents; avoid antipsychotic use for behavioral problems associated with dementia unless alternative nonpharmacologic therapies have failed and patient may harm self or others. In addition, use may cause or exacerbate syndrome of inappropriate antidiuretic hormone secretion or hyponatremia; monitor sodium closely with initiation or dosage adjustments in older adults. May also be inappropriate in older adults depending on comorbidities (eg, dementia, delirium) due to its potent anticholinergic effects (Beers Criteria).

The possibility of a suicide attempt is inherent in psychotic illness or bipolar disorder; use caution in high-risk patients during initiation of therapy. Prescriptions should be written for the smallest quantity consistent with good patient care.

Some dosage forms may contain polysorbate 80 (also known as Tweens). Hypersensitivity reactions, usually a delayed reaction, have been reported following exposure to pharmaceutical products containing polysorbate 80 in certain individuals (Isaksson 2002; Lucente 2000; Shelley 1995). Thrombocytopenia, ascites, pulmonary deterioration, and renal and hepatic failure have been reported in premature neonates after receiving parenteral products containing polysorbate 80 (Alade 1986; CDC 1984). See manufacturer's labeling.

There are two Zyprexa formulations for intramuscular injection: Zyprexa Relprevv is an extended-release formulation and Zyprexa Intramuscular is short-acting:

Extended-release IM injection (Zyprexa Relprevv): **[US Boxed Warning]: Sedation (including coma) and delirium (including agitation, anxiety, confusion, disorientation) have been observed following use of *Zyprexa Relprevv*.** Administer at a registered health care facility where patients should be continuously monitored (≥3 hours) for symptoms of olanzapine overdose; symptom development highest in first hour but may occur within or after 3 hours; risk of syndrome is cumulative with each injection; recovery expected by 72 hours. Upon determining alert status, patient should be escorted to their destination and not drive or operate heavy machinery for the remainder of the day.

Two unexplained deaths in patients who received *Zyprexa Relprevv* have been reported. The patients died 3 to 4 days after receiving an appropriate dose of the drug. Both patients were found to have high blood concentrations of olanzapine postmortem. It is unclear if these deaths were the result of postinjection delirium sedation syndrome (PDSS) (FDA Safety Communication 2013).

Zyprexa Relprevv is only available under a restricted distribution program. Only prescribers, health care facilities, and pharmacies registered with the program are able to prescribe, distribute, or dispense *Zyprexa Relprevv* for patients who are enrolled in and meet all conditions of the program.

Short-acting IM injection (Zyprexa IntraMuscular): Patients should remain recumbent if drowsy/dizzy until hypotension, bradycardia, and/or hypoventilation have been ruled out. Concurrent use of IM/IV benzodiazepines is not recommended (fatalities have been reported, though causality not determined).

Warnings: Additional Pediatric Considerations Pediatric psychiatric disorders are frequently serious mental disorders which present with variable symptoms that do not always match adult diagnostic criteria. Conduct a thorough diagnostic evaluation and carefully consider risks of psychotropic medication before initiation in pediatric patients. Medication therapy for pediatric patients with bipolar disorder and schizophrenia is indicated as part of a total treatment program that frequently includes educational, psychological, and social interventions.

A higher incidence of hyperprolactinemia has been observed in adolescent patients treated with olanzapine than adults (47% vs 30%), high concentrations of prolactin may reduce pituitary gonadotropin secretion; galactorrhea, amenorrhea, gynecomastia, impotence, decreased bone density may occur. Use with caution in children and adolescents as adverse effects due to elevated serum prolactin concentrations have been observed; long-term effects on growth or sexual maturation have not been evaluated. In adolescent patients, increases in fasting total cholesterol, LDL cholesterol, and triglycerides were generally greater than in adult patients; measure fasting serum lipids at the beginning of therapy and periodically during therapy in these patients. Compared to adult patients, adolescent patients had both greater magnitude of weight gain and proportion of patients who had clinically significant weight gain (incidence: 29% to 40% vs 6%). With long-term olanzapine exposure (≥24 weeks), 89% of adolescents gained at least 7% of their baseline body weight, 55% gained at least 15% of their baseline body weight, and 29% gained at least 25% of their baseline body weight; discontinuation due to weight gain occurred in 2.2%. Monitor growth (including weight, height, BMI, and waist circumference) in pediatric and adolescent patients receiving olanzapine; compare weight gain to standard growth curves. **Note:** A prospective, nonrandomized, cohort study followed 338 antipsychotic naive pediatric patients (age: 4 to 19 years) for a median of 10.8 weeks (range: 10.5 to 11.2 weeks) and showed that olanzapine was associated with greater increases in weight, fat mass, BMI, and waist circumference than other atypical antipsychotics evaluated (ie, quetiapine, risperidone, and aripiprazole). The following significant mean increases in weight in kg (and % change from baseline) were reported: Olanzapine: 8.5 kg (15.2%), quetiapine: 6.1 kg (10.4%), risperidone: 5.3 kg (10.4%), and aripiprazole: 4.4 kg (8.1%) compared to the control cohort: 0.2 kg (0.65%). Also, compared to the other atypical antipsychotics evaluated, olanzapine showed higher increases in metabolic indices (eg, serum glucose, total cholesterol and LDL-C). Biannual monitoring of cardiometabolic indices after the first 3 months of therapy is suggested (Correll, 2009).

Olanzapine is moderate to highly sedating; a higher frequency of sedation-related adverse events (defined as hypersomnia, lethargy, sedation, and somnolence) have been observed in adolescents compared to adults.

Adverse Reactions

Oral: Unless otherwise noted, adverse events are reported for placebo-controlled trials in adult patients on monotherapy:

Cardiovascular: Chest pain, hypertension, orthostatic hypotension, peripheral edema, tachycardia

Central nervous system: Drowsiness (dose dependent), extrapyramidal reaction (dose dependent; more common in adults), akathisia, parkinsonian-like syndrome (includes akinesia, cogwheel rigidity, extrapyramidal syndrome, hypertonia, hypokinesia, maked facies, and tremor), dizziness (more common in adults), headache, fatigue (dose dependent), insomnia, personality disorder, abnormal gait, hypertonia, restlessness, falling, articulation impairment

Endocrine & metabolic: Increased serum prolactin (more common in adolescents), weight gain (more common in adolescents), increased gamma-glutamyl transferase, menstrual disease (including amenorrhea, hypomenorrhea, delayed menstruation, oligomenorrhea), breast changes (including discharge, enlargement, galactorrhea, gynecomastia, lactation disorder)

Gastrointestinal: Increased appetite (more common in adolescents), xerostomia (dose dependent; more common in adults), dyspepsia (more common in adults), constipation, abdominal pain (adolescents), vomiting, diarrhea (adolescents)

Genitourinary: urinary incontinence, sexual disorder (less common in adolescents; anorgasmia, delayed ejaculation, erectile dysfunction, changes in libido, abnormal orgasm, sexual dysfunction), urinary tract infection

Hematologic & oncologic: Bruise

Hepatic: Increased serum AST, decreased serum bilirubin, increased serum ALT, increased liver enzymes

Neuromuscular & skeletal: Weakness (dose dependent), tremor (dose dependent), limb pain, arthralgia (more common in adults), back pain, muscle rigidity (adolescents), dyskinesia

Ophthalmic: Amblyopia

Respiratory: Rhinitis, cough, nasopharyngitis, pharyngitis, epistaxis, respiratory tract infection, sinusitis

Miscellaneous: Accidental injury, fever

Rare but important or life-threatening: Accommodation disturbance, agranulocytosis, alopecia, anaphylactoid reaction, angioedema, ataxia, cerebrovascular accident, coma, confusion, diabetes mellitus, diabetic ketoacidosis, diabetic coma, hepatic injury (cholestatic or mixed), hepatitis, hypercholesterolemia, hyperglycemia, hyperlipidemia, hypertriglyceridemia, hypoproteinemia, intestinal obstruction, jaundice, ketosis, leukocytosis (eosinophilia), leukopenia, liver steatosis, myopathy, neuroleptic malignant syndrome, neutropenia, osteoporosis, pancreatitis, priapism, pruritus, pulmonary embolism, rhabdomyolysis, seizure, skin rash, suicidal tendencies, syncope, tardive dyskinesia, thrombocytopenia, tongue edema, transient ischemic attacks, urticaria, venous thrombosis, withdrawal syndrome

Injection: Unless otherwise noted, adverse events are reported for placebo-controlled trials in adult patients on extended release IM injection (Zyprexa Relprevv). Also refer to adverse reactions noted with oral therapy.

Cardiovascular: Hypertension, hypotension, prolonged Q-T interval on ECG, orthostatic hypotension

Central nervous system: Drowsiness, akathisia, dizziness, fatigue, extrapyramidal reaction, abnormality in thinking, auditory hallucination, parkinsonian-like syndrome, restlessness, pain, abnormal dreams, procedural pain, sleep disorder, dysarthria, headache, sedation

Dermatologic: Acne vulgaris

Endocrine & metabolic: Weight gain

Gastrointestinal: Diarrhea, vomiting, xerostomia, increased appetite, nausea (more common in long-acting IM formula), tooth infection, toothache, abdominal pain, flatulence

Genitourinary: Vaginal discharge

Hepatic: Increased liver enzymes

Infection: Viral infection

Local: Pain at injection site

Neuromuscular & skeletal: Arthralgia, back pain, muscle spasm, stiffness, tremor (more common in long-acting IM formula)

Otic: Otalgia

Respiratory: Cough, nasal congestion, nasopharyngitis, upper respiratory tract infection, pharyngolaryngeal pain, sneezing

Miscellaneous: Fever

Rare but important or life-threatening: Delirium, increased creatine phosphokinase (short-acting solution for IM injection), postinjection delirium/sedation syndrome, syncope (short-acting solution for IM injection)

Drug Interactions

Metabolism/Transport Effects Substrate of CYP1A2 (major), CYP2D6 (minor); **Note:** Assignment of Major/Minor substrate status based on clinically relevant drug interaction potential; **Inhibits** CYP1A2 (weak), CYP2C19 (weak), CYP2C9 (weak), CYP2D6 (weak)

Avoid Concomitant Use

Avoid concomitant use of OLANZapine with any of the following: Aclidinium; Amisulpride; Azelastine (Nasal); Benzodiazepines; Eluxadoline; Glucagon; Ipratropium (Oral Inhalation); Metoclopramide; Orphenadrine; Paraldehyde; Potassium Chloride; Sulpiride; Thalidomide; Tiotropium; Umeclidinium

Increased Effect/Toxicity

OLANZapine may increase the levels/effects of: AbobotulinumtoxinA; Alcohol (Ethyl); Amisulpride; Analgesics (Opioid); Anticholinergic Agents; ARIPiprazole; Azelastine (Nasal); Benzodiazepines; Buprenorphine; CNS Depressants; Eluxadoline; Glucagon; Highest Risk QTc-Prolonging Agents; Hydrocodone; Mequitazine; Methotrimeprazine; Methylphenidate; Metyrosine; Mirabegron; Mirtazapine; Moderate Risk QTc-Prolonging Agents; OnabotulinumtoxinA; Orphenadrine; Paraldehyde; Potassium Chloride; RimabotulinumtoxinB; Selective Serotonin Reuptake Inhibitors; Serotonin Modulators; Sulpiride; Suvorexant; Thalidomide; Thiazide Diuretics; Tiotropium; TiZANidine; Topiramate; Zolpidem

The levels/effects of OLANZapine may be increased by: Abiraterone Acetate; Acetylcholinesterase Inhibitors (Central); Aclidinium; Brimonidine (Topical); Cannabis; CYP1A2 Inhibitors (Moderate); CYP1A2 Inhibitors (Strong); Deferasirox; Doxylamine; Dronabinol; Droperidol; FluvoxaMINE; HydrOXYzine; Ipratropium (Oral Inhalation); Kava Kava; LamoTRIgine; Lithium; Magnesium Sulfate; Methotrimeprazine; Methylphenidate; Metoclopramide; Metyrosine; Mianserin; Mifepristone; Nabilone; Peginterferon Alfa-2b; Perampanel; Pramlintide; Rufinamide; Serotonin Modulators; Sodium Oxybate; Tapentadol; Tetrahydrocannabinol; Umeclidinium; Vemurafenib

Decreased Effect

OLANZapine may decrease the levels/effects of: Acetylcholinesterase Inhibitors; Amphetamines; Antidiabetic Agents; Anti-Parkinson's Agents (Dopamine Agonist); Itopride; Quinagolide; Secretin

The levels/effects of OLANZapine may be decreased by: Acetylcholinesterase Inhibitors; Cannabis; CYP1A2 Inducers (Strong); Cyproterone; Lithium; Ritonavir; Teriflunomide; Valproic Acid and Derivatives

Storage/Stability

Injection, extended-release: Store at controlled room temperature, not to exceed 30°C (86°F).

Injection, short-acting: Store at 20°C to 25°C (68°F to 77°F); excursions permitted to 15°C to 30°C (59°F to 86°F); do not freeze. Protect from light.

Tablet and orally disintegrating tablet: Store at 20°C to 25°C (68°F to 77°F); excursions permitted to 15°C to 30°C (59°F to 86°F). Protect from light and moisture.

Mechanism of Action Olanzapine is a second generation thienobenzodiazepine antipsychotic which displays potent antagonism of serotonin 5-HT_{2A} and 5-HT_{2C}, dopamine D_{1-4}, histamine H_1, and alpha$_1$-adrenergic receptors. Olanzapine shows moderate antagonism of 5-HT_3 and muscarinic M_{1-5} receptors, and weak binding to GABA-A, BZD, and beta-adrenergic receptors. Although the precise mechanism of action in schizophrenia and bipolar disorder is not known, the efficacy of olanzapine is thought to be mediated through combined antagonism of dopamine and serotonin type 2 receptor sites.

Pharmacodynamics Onset of action: Within 1-2 weeks for control of aggression, agitation, insomnia; 3-6 weeks for control of mania and positive psychotic symptoms. Adequate trial: Typically 6 weeks at maximum tolerated doses

Pharmacokinetics (Adult data unless noted)

Absorption:
- IM (short-acting): Rapidly absorbed
- Oral: Well absorbed; not affected by food; tablets and orally disintegrating tablets are bioequivalent

Distribution: Extensive throughout body; V_d: 1000 L

Protein binding: 93% primarily to albumin and alpha$_1$-glycoprotein

Metabolism: Highly metabolized via direct glucuronidation and cytochrome P450 mediated oxidation (CYP1A2, CYP2D6); 40% removed via first pass metabolism

Half-life:
- Oral and IM (short-acting):
  - Pediatric patients (10-18 years; n=8): 37.2 ± 5.1 hours (Grothe, 2000)
  - Adults: 30 hours [21-54 hours (5th to 95th percentile)]
- IM (extended release): 30 days (effective half-life)

Time to peak serum concentration: Maximum plasma concentrations after IM (short-acting product) administration are 5 times higher than maximum plasma concentrations produced by an oral dose.
- IM (short-acting): 15-45 minutes
- IM (extended release): ~7 days
- Oral:
  - Pediatric patients (10-18 years; n=8): 4.7 ± 3.7 hours (Grothe, 2000)
  - Adults: ~6 hours

Elimination: Urine (57%; 7% as unchanged drug); feces (30%)
- Clearance: Oral:
  - Pediatric patients (10-18 years; n=8): Apparent: 9.6 ± 2.4 L/hour (Grothe, 2000)
  - Adult: Apparent: 25 L/hour [12-47 L/hour (5th to 95th percentile)]; 40% increase in olanzapine clearance in smokers; 30% decrease in females

Dialysis: Not removed by dialysis

Dosing: Usual

Oral:

Children and Adolescents:

Bipolar I disorder (acute manic or mixed episodes):

Children 4 to <6 years: Limited data available: Initial: 1.25 mg once daily; increase at weekly intervals according to response and tolerability to target dose: 10 mg/day. Dosing based on an open-label trial in 15 children (mean age: 5 ± 0.8 years; mean weight: 20.8 kg; mean required dose: 6.3 ± 2.3 mg/day) that showed significant improvement in manic symptoms (Biederman, 2005)

Children 6-12 years: Limited data available: Initial: 2.5 mg once daily; increase dose in 2.5 or 5 mg increments at weekly intervals to target dose of 10 mg once daily; maximum dose: 20 mg/day (Frazier, 2001; Kowatch, 2006; Wozniak, 2009)

Adolescents: Initial: 2.5-5 mg once daily; increase dose in 2.5 or 5 mg increments at weekly intervals to target dose of 10 mg once daily; maximum dose: 20 mg/day. In adolescent flexible-dosing (2.5-20 mg/day) clinical trials, the mean modal dose was 10.7 mg/day (mean dose: 8.9 mg/day) (Kowatch, 2006; Tohen, 2007)

Schizophrenia: Children ≥8 years (Limited data available) and Adolescents: Initial: 2.5-5 mg once daily; increase dose in 2.5 or 5 mg increments at weekly intervals to target dose of 10 mg once daily; maximum dose: 20 mg/day. **Note:** Doses up to 30 mg/day were used in one study of adolescents who were treatment refractory; however, some patients did not tolerate doses > 20 mg/day (Kumra, 2008); safety and efficacy of doses >20 mg/day have not been fully evaluated. In adolescent flexible-dosing (2.5-20 mg/day) clinical trials, the mean modal dose was 12.5 mg/day (mean dose: 11.1 mg/day). Dosing in children is based on two double-blind comparison studies which included both children and adolescents [n=35, age: 8-19 years with seven children; n=13, age: 7-16 years (mean age: 12.8 + 2.4 years)] (Shaw, 2006; Sikich, 2008).

Anorexia nervosa: Children ≥9 years and Adolescents: Limited data available: 1.25-2.5 mg once daily has been shown in one small trial and several case reports to improve BMI and other disease-related symptoms (eg, eating attitudes, anxiety); another case series used initial doses of 2.5 mg once daily and final doses of 5 mg to 10 mg once daily; reported range: 1.25-12.5 mg/day; however, it has been suggested that higher doses (>2.5 mg once daily) may not be associated with greater efficacy (Boachie, 2003; Dunican, 2007; Legerro, 2010; Mehler, 2001; Mehler-Wex, 2007).

Tourette syndrome, tic disorder: Children ≥7 years and Adolescents: Limited data available:

Patient weight ≤40 kg: Initial: 2.5 mg every other day for 3 days, increase to 2.5 mg every day for remainder of week; increase to 5 mg/day by second week if needed; then increase in 5 mg increments at weekly intervals as tolerated; maximum dose: 20 mg/day

Patient weight >40 kg: Initial: 2.5 mg every day for 3 days; increase to 5 mg every day for remainder of week if needed, then increase in 5 mg increments at weekly intervals as tolerated; maximum dose: 20 mg/day

An open-label study of 10 pediatric patients (7-13 years of age) reported significant reductions in tic severity [Yale Global Tic Severity Scale (YGTSS)] from baseline at a mean final dose of 14.5 mg/day after 8 weeks of treatment (Stephens, 2004). An open-label trial of 12 children and adolescents (7-14 years of age) reported a significant reduction (30%) in total tic severity (YGTSS) at a final mean dose of 11.3 mg/day (range: 2.5-20 mg/day) (McCracken, 2008)

Adults:

Acute mania associated with bipolar disorder:

Monotherapy: Initial: 10-15 mg once daily; increase by 5 mg/day at intervals of not less than 24 hours. Maintenance: 5-20 mg/day; recommended maximum dose: 20 mg/day

Combination therapy (with lithium or valproate): Initial: 10 mg once daily; dosing range: 5-20 mg/day

Schizophrenia: Initial: 5-10 mg once daily (increase to 10 mg once daily within 5-7 days); thereafter, adjust by 5 mg/day at 1-week intervals, up to a recommended maximum of 20 mg/day. Maintenance: 10-20 mg once daily. Doses of 30-50 mg/day have been used; however, doses >10 mg/day have not demonstrated better efficacy, and safety and efficacy of doses >20 mg/day have not been evaluated.

IM (short-acting): **Agitation** (acute, associated with bipolar disorder or schizophrenia):

Pediatric patients: Limited data available: Children: 5 mg; Adolescents: 10 mg. Dosing based on a retrospective report of IM olanzapine use in an inpatient psychiatric setting which included 50 pediatric patients [children (n=15; mean age: 11 years); adolescents (n=35; mean age: 15 years)] and evaluated 163 doses administered; results showed a 90.2% response rate (Khan, 2006)

Adults: Initial dose: 10 mg (a lower dose of 5-7.5 mg may be considered when clinical factors warrant); additional doses (up to 10 mg) may be considered; however, 2-4 hours should be allowed between doses to evaluate response (maximum total daily dose: 30 mg)

IM (extended release): Adults:

Schizophrenia: Note: Establish tolerance to oral olanzapine prior to changing to extended release IM injection. It may take up to 3 months to re-establish steady-state when switching from oral olanzapine to long-acting IM injection. Maximum dose: 300 mg/2 weeks or 405 mg/4 weeks

Patients established on oral olanzapine 10 mg/day: Initial dose: 210 mg every 2 weeks for 4 doses or 405 mg every 4 weeks for 2 doses; Maintenance dose: 150 mg every 2 weeks or 300 mg every 4 weeks

Patients established on oral olanzapine 15 mg/day: Initial dose: 300 mg every 2 weeks for 4 doses; Maintenance dose: 210 mg every 2 weeks or 405 mg every 4 weeks

Patients established on oral olanzapine 20 mg/day: Initial and maintenance dose: 300 mg every 2 weeks

Patients who are debilitated, predisposed to hypotensive reactions, exhibit multiple factors that may result in slower metabolism, or may be more sensitive to olanzapine: Initial dose: 150 mg every 4 weeks; increase dose with caution and only if clinically needed

Dosage adjustment in renal impairment: No dosage adjustment required.

Dosage adjustment in hepatic impairment: Use with caution. Dosage adjustment may be necessary; however no specific recommendations exist. Monitor closely.

Preparation for Administration

Parenteral:

IM (short acting): Reconstitute 10 mg vial with 2.1 mL SWFI; resulting solution is ~5 mg/mL; should have a clear and yellow appearance. Use immediately (within 1 hour) following reconstitution. Discard any unused portion. Do not mix diazepam, lorazepam, or haloperidol in the same syringe.

IM (extended release): Dilute as directed with provided diluent to final concentration of 150 mg/mL. Shake vigorously to mix; will form yellow, opaque suspension. Following reconstitution, suspension may be stored at room temperature and used within 24 hours. If foam develops, let vial stand to allow foam to dissipate. If suspended drug is not used right away, agitate vial again vigorously to resuspend drug prior to withdrawal from vial. Use immediately once suspension is in syringe. Suspension may be irritating to skin; wear gloves during reconstitution; flush skin with water if drug comes into contact with skin. Do not mix diazepam, lorazepam, or haloperidol in the same syringe.

Administration

Oral:

Tablet: May be administered with or without food.

Orally disintegrating tablet: Remove from foil blister by peeling back foil (do not push tablet through the foil); place tablet in mouth immediately upon removal; tablet dissolves rapidly in saliva and may be swallowed with or without liquid. May be administered with or without food/meals.

Parenteral:

IM (short-acting): For IM administration only; do not administer IV or subcutaneously; inject slowly, deep into muscle mass. If dizziness and/or drowsiness are noted patient should remain recumbent until examination indicates postural hypotension and/or bradycardia are not a problem.

IM (extended release): Adults: For deep IM gluteal administration only; do not administer injection intravenously. After needle insertion into muscle, aspirate to verify that no blood appears; inject slowly, deep into muscle. Do not massage injection site. Use diluent, syringes, and needles provided in convenience kit obtain a new kit if aspiration of blood occurs.

Monitoring Parameters Vital signs; CBC with differential fasting lipid profile, and fasting blood glucose/Hgb A_{1c} (prior to treatment, at 3 months, then annually or as symptoms warrant); periodic assessment of hepatic transaminases; weight, BMI, waist circumference; personal/family history of diabetes or obesity; orthostatic blood pressure; mental status, abnormal involuntary movement scale (AIMS), extrapyramidal symptoms (EPS). Weight should be assessed prior to treatment, at 4 weeks, 8 weeks, 12 weeks, and then at quarterly intervals. Consider switching to a different antipsychotic agent for a weight gain ≥5% of the initial weight. Monitor patient periodically for symptom resolution. Following IM administration, if dizziness and/or drowsiness are noted, patient should remain recumbent until resolved. Extended release IM injection (Zyprexa® Relprevv™): Monitor patients continuously for 3 hours after injection for symptoms of post-injection sedation syndrome and olanzapine overdose; once patient is alert, escort patient to their destination; patient should not drive or operate heavy machinery for the remainder of the day.

Additional Information Long-term usefulness of olanzapine should be periodically re-evaluated in patients receiving the drug for extended periods of time.

Additional detailed olanzapine dosing information for Children and Adolescents: Oral:

Autism spectrum disorders: Note: Limited information exists in the literature; dose not established; efficacy results have been variable; further studies are needed. A double-blind, placebo-controlled study (n=11, 6-14 years of age, study duration: 8 weeks) reported a response in only 3 of 6 treatment arm patients using an initial dose of: 2.5 mg every other day (patient weight: <40 kg) or 2.5 mg every day (patient weight: ≥40 kg); dose increased at weekly intervals in 2.5-5 mg increments as tolerated (maximum dose allowed: 20 mg/day); final dosage range: 7.5-12.5 mg/day; mean: 10 mg/day (Hollander, 2006). An open-label, 6-week, comparative study with haloperidol in 12 children (4.8-11.8 years of age) used a similar dosing regimen and reported responses in 5 of 6 patients in the olanzapine treatment arm; final dosage range: 5-10 mg/day (mean: 7.9 ± 2.5 mg/day) (Malone, 2001). However, an open-label, 12-week study in 25 pediatric patients (6-16 years) reported a response in only three patients, final dosage range: 2.5-20 mg/day (mean: 10.7 mg/day) (Kemner, 2002).

Dosage Forms Excipient information presented when available (limited, particularly for generics); consult specific product labeling.

Solution Reconstituted, Intramuscular:
- ZyPREXA: 10 mg (1 ea) [contains tartaric acid]
- Generic: 10 mg (1 ea)

Suspension Reconstituted, Intramuscular:
- ZyPREXA Relprevv: 210 mg (1 ea); 300 mg (1 ea); 405 mg (1 ea) [contains polysorbate 80]

Tablet, Oral:
- ZyPREXA: 2.5 mg, 5 mg, 7.5 mg, 10 mg
- ZyPREXA: 15 mg [contains fd&c blue #2 aluminum lake]
- ZyPREXA: 20 mg
- Generic: 2.5 mg, 5 mg, 7.5 mg, 10 mg, 15 mg, 20 mg

Tablet Dispersible, Oral:
- ZyPREXA Zydis: 5 mg, 10 mg, 15 mg, 20 mg [contains aspartame, methylparaben sodium, propylparaben sodium]
- Generic: 5 mg, 10 mg, 15 mg, 20 mg

- ◆ **Olanzapine for injection (Can)** *see* OLANZapine *on page 1546*
- ◆ **Olanzapine ODT (Can)** *see* OLANZapine *on page 1546*
- ◆ **Olanzapine Pamoate** *see* OLANZapine *on page 1546*
- ◆ **Oleovitamin A** *see* Vitamin A *on page 2186*
- ◆ **Oleptro** *see* TraZODone *on page 2105*
- ◆ **Olestyr (Can)** *see* Cholestyramine Resin *on page 450*
- ◆ **Oleum Ricini** *see* Castor Oil *on page 385*
- ◆ **Olex (Can)** *see* Omeprazole *on page 1555*

Olmesartan (ole me SAR tan)

Medication Safety Issues

Sound-alike/look-alike issues:

Benicar may be confused with Mevacor

Brand Names: US Benicar

Brand Names: Canada Olmetec

Therapeutic Category Angiotensin II Receptor Blocker; Antihypertensive Agent

Generic Availability (US) No

Use Treatment of hypertension alone or in combination with other antihypertensive agents (FDA approved in ages 6-16 years and adults)

Pregnancy Risk Factor D

Pregnancy Considerations [U.S. Boxed Warning]: Drugs that act on the renin-angiotensin system can cause injury and death to the developing fetus. Discontinue as soon as possible once pregnancy is detected. The use of drugs which act on the renin-angiotensin system are associated with oligohydramnios. Oligohydramnios, due to decreased fetal renal function, may lead to fetal lung hypoplasia and skeletal malformations. Use is also associated with anuria, hypotension, renal failure, skull hypoplasia, and death in the fetus/neonate. The exposed fetus should be monitored for fetal growth, amniotic fluid volume, and organ formation. Infants exposed *in utero* should be monitored for hyperkalemia, hypotension, and oliguria (exchange transfusions or dialysis may be needed). These adverse events are generally associated with maternal use in the second and third trimesters.

Untreated chronic maternal hypertension is also associated with adverse events in the fetus, infant, and mother. The use of angiotensin II receptor blockers is not recommended to treat chronic uncomplicated hypertension in pregnant women and should generally be avoided in women of reproductive potential (ACOG, 2013).

Breast-Feeding Considerations It is not known if olmesartan is excreted into breast milk. Due to the potential for serious adverse reactions in the nursing infant, the manufacturer recommends a decision be made whether to discontinue nursing or to discontinue the drug, taking into account the importance of treatment to the mother.

Contraindications Concomitant use with aliskiren in patients with diabetes mellitus

Canadian labeling: Additional contraindications (not in U.S. labeling): Hypersensitivity to olmesartan or any component of the formulation; concomitant use with aliskiren in patients with moderate to severe renal impairment (GFR <60 mL/minute/1.73 m^2)

Documentation of allergenic cross-reactivity for angiotensin II receptor blockers is limited. However, because of similarities in chemical structure and/or pharmacologic actions, the possibility of cross-sensitivity cannot be ruled out with certainty.

Warnings/Precautions [U.S. Boxed Warning]: Drugs that act on the renin-angiotensin system can cause injury and death to the developing fetus. Discontinue as soon as possible once pregnancy is detected. May cause hyperkalemia; avoid potassium supplementation unless specifically required by healthcare provider. Avoid use or use a smaller dose in patients who are volume depleted; correct depletion first. May be associated with deterioration of renal function and/or increases in serum creatinine, particularly in patients with low renal blood flow (eg, renal artery stenosis, heart failure) whose glomerular filtration rate (GFR) is dependent on efferent arteriolar vasoconstriction by angiotensin II. Use with caution in unstented unilateral/bilateral renal artery stenosis. When unstented bilateral renal artery stenosis is present, use is generally avoided due to the elevated risk of deterioration in renal function unless possible benefits outweigh risks. Use with caution with pre-existing renal insufficiency; significant aortic/mitral stenosis. Potentially significant drug-drug interactions may exist, requiring dose or frequency adjustment, additional monitoring, and/or selection of alternative therapy. In surgical patients on chronic angiotensin receptor blocker (ARB) therapy, intraoperative hypotension may occur with induction and maintenance of general anesthesia.

Symptoms of sprue-like enteropathy (ie, severe, chronic diarrhea with significant weight loss) has been reported; may develop months to years after treatment initiation with villous atrophy commonly found on intestinal biopsy. Once other etiologies have been excluded, discontinue treatment and consider other antihypertensive treatment. Clinical and histologic improvement was noted after treatment was discontinued in a case series of 22 patients (Ianiro, 2014; Rubio-Tapia, 2012).

Angioedema has been reported rarely with some angiotensin II receptor antagonists (ARBs) and may occur at any time during treatment (especially following first dose). It may involve the head and neck (potentially compromising airway) or the intestine (presenting with abdominal pain). Patients with idiopathic or hereditary angioedema or previous angioedema associated with ACE-inhibitor therapy may be at an increased risk. Prolonged frequent monitoring may be required, especially if tongue, glottis, or larynx are involved, as they are associated with airway obstruction. Patients with a history of airway surgery may have a higher risk of airway obstruction. Discontinue therapy immediately if angioedema occurs. Aggressive early management is critical. Intramuscular (IM) administration of epinephrine may be necessary. Do not readminister to patients who have had angioedema with ARBs.

Olmesartan has not been shown to be effective for hypertension in children younger than 6 years. Children younger than 1 year must not receive olmesartan for hypertension. The renin-angiotensin-aldosterone system plays a critical role in kidney development. Administering drugs that act directly on the renin-angiotensin-aldosterone system can have effects on the development of immature kidneys and alter normal renal development.

Adverse Reactions

Central nervous system: Dizziness, headache

Endocrine & metabolic: Hyperglycemia, hypertriglyceridemia

Gastrointestinal: Diarrhea

Neuromuscular & skeletal: Back pain, CPK increased

Renal: Hematuria

Respiratory: Bronchitis, pharyngitis, rhinitis, sinusitis

Miscellaneous: Flu-like syndrome

Rare but important or life-threatening: Acute renal failure, alopecia, anaphylaxis, angioedema, arthritis, gastroenteritis, hypercholesterolemia, hyperkalemia, hyperlipidemia, hyperuricemia, liver enzymes increased, peripheral edema, rhabdomyolysis, serum creatinine increased, sprue-like symptoms, tachycardia

Drug Interactions

Metabolism/Transport Effects Substrate of SLCO1B1

Avoid Concomitant Use There are no known interactions where it is recommended to avoid concomitant use.

Increased Effect/Toxicity

Olmesartan may increase the levels/effects of: ACE Inhibitors; Amifostine; Antihypertensives; Ciprofloxacin (Systemic); CycloSPORINE (Systemic); Drospirenone; DULoxetine; Hypotensive Agents; Levodopa; Lithium; Nonsteroidal Anti-Inflammatory Agents; Obinutuzumab; Potassium-Sparing Diuretics; RisperiDONE; RiTUXimab; Sodium Phosphates

The levels/effects of Olmesartan may be increased by: Alfuzosin; Aliskiren; Barbiturates; Brimonidine (Topical); Canagliflozin; Dapoxetine; Diazoxide; Eltrombopag; Eplerenone; Heparin; Heparin (Low Molecular Weight); Herbs (Hypotensive Properties); MAO Inhibitors; Nicorandil; Pentoxifylline; Phosphodiesterase 5 Inhibitors; Potassium Salts; Prostacyclin Analogues; Teriflunomide; Tolvaptan; Trimethoprim

Decreased Effect

The levels/effects of Olmesartan may be decreased by: Colesevelam; Herbs (Hypertensive Properties); Methylphenidate; Nonsteroidal Anti-Inflammatory Agents; Yohimbine

Storage/Stability Store at 20°C to 25°C (68°F to 77°F).

Mechanism of Action As a selective and competitive nonpeptide angiotensin II receptor antagonist, olmesartan blocks the vasoconstrictor and aldosterone-secreting effects of angiotensin II; olmesartan interacts reversibly at the AT1 and AT2 receptors of many tissues and has slow dissociation kinetics; its affinity for the AT1 receptor is 12,500 times greater than the AT2 receptor. Angiotensin II receptor antagonists may induce a more complete inhibition of the renin-angiotensin system than ACE inhibitors, they do not affect the response to bradykinin, and are less likely to be associated with nonrenin-angiotensin effects (eg, cough and angioedema). Olmesartan increases urinary flow rate and, in addition to being natriuretic and kaliuretic, increases excretion of chloride, magnesium, uric acid, calcium, and phosphate.

Pharmacokinetics (Adult data unless noted)

Distribution: V_d: ~17 L

Protein binding: 99%

Metabolism: Olmesartan medoxomil is hydrolyzed during absorption from the GI tract to active olmesartan. Virtually no further metabolism occurs

Bioavailability: ~26%

Half-life elimination: Terminal: ~13 hours

Time to peak serum concentration: 1-2 hours

Elimination: All as unchanged drug: Feces (50% to 65%); urine (35% to 50%)

Clearance: 1.3 L/hour; similar data reported in pediatric patients (1-16 years) when adjusted by body weight

Dialysis: Effects of hemodialysis have not been studied

Dosing: Usual Note: Consider lower starting dose in patients with possible depletion of intravascular volume (eg, patients receiving diuretics).

Children and Adolescents: **Hypertension:** Oral:

Children 1-5 years and ≥5 kg: Limited data available: Initial: 0.3 mg/kg/dose once daily; if initial response inadequate after 2 weeks, dose may be increased to 0.6 mg/kg/dose once daily. Dosing was evaluated in a double-blind, placebo-controlled study of 59 patients and some efficacy was demonstrated; however, results were not statistically significant (NCT00151775, 2010).

Children and Adolescents 6-16 years:

20 to <35 kg: 10 mg once daily; if initial response inadequate after 2 weeks, dose may be increased (maximum: 20 mg/day)

≥35 kg: 20 mg once daily; if initial response inadequate after 2 weeks, dose may be increased (maximum: 40 mg/day)

Adolescents >16 years: Initial: 20 mg once daily; if initial response is inadequate, may be increased to 40 mg once daily after 2 weeks. May administer with other antihypertensive agents if blood pressure inadequately controlled with olmesartan.

Adults: **Hypertension:** Oral: Initial: 20 mg once daily; if initial response is inadequate, may be increased to 40 mg once daily after 2 weeks. May administer with other antihypertensive agents if blood pressure inadequately controlled with olmesartan.

Dosing adjustment in renal impairment: No specific guidelines for dosage adjustment; patients undergoing hemodialysis have not been studied. **Note:** In patients with severe renal impairment (CrCl <20 mL/minute), the AUC was tripled after repeated dosing.

Dosing adjustment in hepatic impairment: No initial dosage adjustment necessary. **Note:** In patients with moderate hepatic impairment, an increase in AUC of ~60% was observed.

Administration May be administered with or without food.

Monitoring Parameters Blood pressure, serum creatinine, serum potassium

Additional Information The antihypertensive effects of olmesartan are smaller in black patients (usually a low-renin patient population); this effect of race is also seen with ACE inhibitors, beta-blockers, and other angiotensin receptor blockers. A pediatric study of olmesartan in patients 6-16 years of age found numerically smaller reductions in blood pressure in black patients compared to a racially-mixed cohort (Hazan, 2010).

Dosage Forms Excipient information presented when available (limited, particularly for generics); consult specific product labeling.

Tablet, Oral, as medoxomil:

Benicar: 5 mg, 20 mg, 40 mg

Extemporaneous Preparations A 2 mg/mL oral suspension may be made with olmesartan tablets. Combine 50 mL purified water and twenty 20 mg tablets in an 8-ounce amber bottle and allow to stand for ≥5 minutes. Shake well for ≥1 minute, then allow to stand for ≥1 minute. Repeat shaking and standing process four additional times. Add 100 mL Ora-Sweet® and 50 mL Ora-Plus® to the suspension and shake well for ≥1 minute. Label "shake well" and "refrigerate". Stable for 28 days refrigerated.

Benicar® prescribing information, Daiichi Sankyo, Inc, Parsippany, NJ, 2010.

- **Olmesartan Medoxomil** *see* Olmesartan *on page 1551*
- **Olmetec (Can)** *see* Olmesartan *on page 1551*

Olsalazine (ole SAL a zeen)

Medication Safety Issues

Sound-alike/look-alike issues:

Olsalazine may be confused with OLANZapine

Dipentum® may be confused with Dilantin®

Brand Names: US Dipentum

Brand Names: Canada Dipentum®

Therapeutic Category 5-Aminosalicylic Acid Derivative; Anti-inflammatory Agent

Generic Availability (US) No

Use Maintenance of remission of ulcerative colitis in patients intolerant to sulfasalazine (FDA approved in adults)

Pregnancy Risk Factor C

Pregnancy Considerations Animal studies have demonstrated fetal developmental toxicities. There are no well-controlled studies in pregnant women. Use during pregnancy only if clearly necessary.

Breast-Feeding Considerations The active metabolite, 5-aminosalicylic acid may pass into breast milk. Diarrhea has been reported in breast-fed infants whose mothers took olsalazine.

Contraindications Hypersensitivity to olsalazine, salicylates, or any component of the formulation

Warnings/Precautions Diarrhea is a common adverse effect of olsalazine. May exacerbate symptoms of colitis. Use with caution in patients with renal or hepatic impairment. Use with caution in elderly patients. Use with caution in patients with severe allergies or asthma.

Adverse Reactions

Central nervous system: Depression, dizziness, vertigo

Dermatologic: Pruritus, rash

Gastrointestinal: Abdominal pain/cramps, bloating, diarrhea (dose related), nausea, stomatitis, vomiting

Neuromuscular & skeletal: Arthralgia

Respiratory: Upper respiratory infection

Rare but important or life-threatening: Alkaline phosphatase increased, Alopecia, ALT increased, anemia, angioedema, aplastic anemia, AST increased, bilirubin increased, blood in stool, blurred vision, bronchospasm, cholestatic hepatitis, cholestatic jaundice, chest pain, chills, cirrhosis, dehydration, dry eyes, dyspnea, dysuria, eosinophilia, epigastric discomfort, erythema, erythema nodosum, fever, flare of symptoms, flatulence, GGT increased, heart block (second degree), hematuria, hemolytic anemia, hepatitis, hepatic failure, hepatic necrosis, hot flashes, hypertension, impotence, insomnia, interstitial nephritis, interstitial pneumonia, irritability, jaundice, Kawasaki-like syndrome, LDH increased, leukopenia, lymphopenia, menorrhagia, mood swings, muscle cramps, myalgia, myocarditis, nephrotic syndrome, neutropenia, orthostatic hypotension, palpitation, pancreatitis, pancytopenia, paresthesia, pericarditis, peripheral edema, peripheral neuropathy, photosensitivity, proteinuria, rectal bleeding, rectal discomfort, reticulocytosis, rigors, tachycardia, thrombocytopenia, tinnitus, tremor, urinary frequency, watery eyes, xerostomia

Drug Interactions

Metabolism/Transport Effects None known.

Avoid Concomitant Use There are no known interactions where it is recommended to avoid concomitant use.

Increased Effect/Toxicity

Olsalazine may increase the levels/effects of: Heparin; Heparin (Low Molecular Weight); Thiopurine Analogs; Varicella Virus-Containing Vaccines

The levels/effects of Olsalazine may be increased by: Nonsteroidal Anti-Inflammatory Agents

Decreased Effect

Olsalazine may decrease the levels/effects of: Cardiac Glycosides

Storage/Stability Store at 20°C to 25°C (77°F); excursions permitted to 15°C to 30°C (59°F to 86°F).

Mechanism of Action Mesalamine (5-aminosalicylic acid) is the active component of olsalazine; the specific mechanism of action of mesalamine is unknown; however, it is thought that it modulates local chemical mediators of the inflammatory response, especially leukotrienes, and is also postulated to be a free radical scavenger or an inhibitor of tumor necrosis factor (TNF); action appears topical rather than systemic.

Pharmacokinetics (Adult data unless noted)

Absorption: <3%; very little intact olsalazine is systemically absorbed

Protein binding: >99%

Metabolism: Mostly by colonic bacteria to the active drug, 5-aminosalicylic acid

Bioavailability: 2.4%

Half-life, elimination: 54 minutes (in serum)

Elimination: Primarily in feces; <1% eliminated in urine

Dosing: Usual Adults: Oral: 1 g/day in 2 divided doses

Administration Oral: Administer with food in evenly divided doses

Dosage Forms Excipient information presented when available (limited, particularly for generics); consult specific product labeling.

Capsule, Oral, as sodium:

Dipentum: 250 mg

- **Olsalazine Sodium** *see* Olsalazine *on page 1553*
- **Olux** *see* Clobetasol *on page 498*
- **Olux-E** *see* Clobetasol *on page 498*

Omalizumab (oh mah lye ZOO mab)

Medication Safety Issues

Sound-alike/look-alike issues:

Omalizumab may be confused with obinutuzumab, ofatumumab

Brand Names: US Xolair

Brand Names: Canada Xolair

Therapeutic Category Monoclonal Antibody, Anti-Asthmatic

Generic Availability (US) No

Use Treatment of moderate to severe, persistent allergic asthma not adequately controlled with inhaled corticosteroids

Medication Guide Available Yes

Pregnancy Risk Factor B

Pregnancy Considerations Adverse events have not been observed in animal reproduction studies. IgG molecules are known to cross the placenta. A registry has been established to monitor outcomes of women exposed to omalizumab during pregnancy or within 8 weeks prior to pregnancy (http://www.xolairpregnancyregistry.com or 866-496-5247).

Breast-Feeding Considerations It is not known if omalizumab is excreted in breast milk; however, IgG is excreted in human milk and excretion of omalizumab is expected. The manufacturer recommends that caution be exercised when administering omalizumab to breast-feeding women.

Contraindications Severe hypersensitivity reaction to omalizumab or any component of the formulation

Warnings/Precautions [U.S. Boxed Warning]: Anaphylaxis, including delayed-onset anaphylaxis, has been reported following administration; anaphylaxis may present as bronchospasm, hypotension, syncope, urticaria, and/or angioedema of the throat or tongue. Anaphylaxis has occurred after the first dose and in some cases >1 year after initiation of regular treatment. Due to the risk, patients should be observed closely for an appropriate time period after administration and should receive treatment only under direct medical supervision. Healthcare providers should be prepared to administer appropriate therapy for managing potentially life-threatening anaphylaxis. Patients should be instructed on identifying signs/symptoms of anaphylaxis and to seek immediate care if they arise. In postmarketing reports, anaphylaxis usually occurred with the first or second dose and with a time to onset of ≤60 minutes; however, reactions have been reported with subsequent doses (after 39 doses) and with a time to onset of up to 4 days after administration. Discontinue therapy following any severe reaction.

In rare cases, patients may present with systemic eosinophilia, sometimes presenting with clinical features of vasculitis consistent with Churg-Strauss syndrome, a condition which is often treated with systemic corticosteroid therapy. Healthcare providers should be alert to eosinophilia, vasculitic rash, worsening pulmonary symptoms, cardiac complications, and/or neuropathy presenting in their patients. A causal association between omalizumab and these underlying conditions has not been established. Reports of a constellation of symptoms including fever, arthritis or arthralgia, rash, and lymphadenopathy have been reported with postmarketing use (symptoms resemble those seen in patients experiencing serum sickness, although circulating immune complexes or a skin biopsy consistent with a Type III hypersensitivity reaction were not seen with these cases). Onset of symptoms generally occurred 1-5 days following the first or subsequent doses. Discontinue therapy in any patient reporting this constellation of signs/symptoms. Malignant neoplasms have been reported rarely with use in short-term studies; impact of long-term use is not known. Use caution with and monitor patients at high risk for parasitic (helminth) infections (risk of infection may be increased).

Therapy has not been shown to alleviate acute asthma exacerbations; do not use to treat acute bronchospasm or status asthmaticus. Do not use to treat forms of urticaria other than chronic idiopathic urticaria. Dosing for allergic asthma is based on body weight and pretreatment total IgE serum levels. IgE levels remain elevated up to 1 year following treatment; therefore, levels taken during treatment or for up to 1 year following treatment cannot and should not be used as a dosage guide. Dosing in chronic idiopathic urticaria is not dependent on serum IgE (free or total) level or body weight. Gradually taper systemic or inhaled corticosteroid therapy; do not discontinue corticosteroids abruptly following initiation of omalizumab therapy. The combined use of omalizumab and corticosteroids in patients with chronic idiopathic urticaria has not been evaluated. Potentially significant drug-drug interactions may exist, requiring dose or frequency adjustment, additional monitoring, and/or selection of alternative therapy.

Adverse Reactions

Asthma:

Cardiovascular: Myocardial infarction, pulmonary embolism, unstable angina pectoris, venous thrombosis

Central nervous system: Dizziness, fatigue, pain

Dermatologic: Dermatitis, pruritus

Local: Injection site reaction (includes bruising, redness, warmth, burning, stinging, itching, hive formation, pain, indurations, mass, and inflammation; most reactions occurred within 1 hour, lasted <8 days, and decreased in frequency with additional dosing)

Neuromuscular & skeletal: Arm pain, arthralgia, bone fracture, leg pain

Otic: Otalgia

Rare but important or life-threatening: Alopecia, anaphylaxis, antibody development, arthritis, lymphadenopathy, malignant neoplasm, syncope, thrombocytopenia

Chronic idiopathic urticaria:

Cardiovascular: Peripheral edema

Central nervous system: Anxiety, headache, migraine

Dermatologic: Alopecia

Gastrointestinal: Toothache

Genitourinary: Urinary tract infection

Infection: Fungal infection

Local: Injection site reaction

Neuromuscular & skeletal: Arthralgia, limb pain, musculoskeletal pain, myalgia

Respiratory: Asthma, cough, nasopharyngitis, oropharyngeal pain, sinus headache, sinusitis, upper respiratory tract infection, viral upper respiratory tract infection

Miscellaneous: Fever

All indications: Rare but important or life-threatening: Alopecia, anaphylaxis, antibody development, arthritis, chest tightness, Churg-Strauss syndrome, lymphadenopathy, malignant neoplasm, pulmonary hypertension, syncope, thrombocytopenia, transient ischemic attacks

Drug Interactions

Metabolism/Transport Effects None known.

Avoid Concomitant Use

Avoid concomitant use of Omalizumab with any of the following: Belimumab; Loxapine

Increased Effect/Toxicity

Omalizumab may increase the levels/effects of: Belimumab; Loxapine

Decreased Effect There are no known significant interactions involving a decrease in effect.

Storage/Stability Prior to reconstitution, store under refrigeration at 2°C to 8°C (36°F to 46°F); product may be shipped at room temperature. Following reconstitution, protect from direct sunlight. May be stored for up to 8 hours if refrigerated or 4 hours if stored at room temperature.

Mechanism of Action

Asthma: Omalizumab is an IgG monoclonal antibody (recombinant DNA derived) which inhibits IgE binding to the high-affinity IgE receptor on mast cells and basophils. By decreasing bound IgE, the activation and release of mediators in the allergic response (early and late phase) is limited. Serum free IgE levels and the number of high affinity IgE receptors are decreased. Long-term treatment in patients with allergic asthma showed a decrease in asthma exacerbations and corticosteroid usage.

Chronic idiopathic urticaria: Omalizumab binds to IgE and lowers free IgE levels. Subsequently, IgE receptors (FcεRI) on cells down-regulate. The mechanism by which these effects of omalizumab result in an improvement of chronic idiopathic urticaria symptoms is unknown.

Pharmacodynamics Response to therapy: ~12-16 weeks (87% of patients had measurable response in 12 weeks)

Pharmacokinetics (Adult data unless noted)

Absorption: Slow after SubQ administration

Distribution: V_d: 78 ± 32 mL/kg

Metabolism: Hepatic: IgG degradation by reticuloendothelial system and endothelial cells

Bioavailability: Absolute: 62%

Half-life: Adults: 1-4 weeks

Time to peak serum concentration: 7-8 days

Excretion: Primarily via hepatic degradation; intact IgG may be secreted in bile

Clearance: 2.4 ± 1.1 mL/kg/day

Dosing: Usual Dosage and frequency of administration are dependent upon the serum total IgE level and body weight. Measure total IgE level prior to beginning treatment. Total IgE levels are elevated during treatment and remain elevated for up to one year after the discontinuation of treatment. Remeasurement of IgE levels during omalizumab treatment should not be used as a guide to dosage.

Asthma: Children ≥12 years, Adolescents, and Adults: SubQ: 0.016 mg/kg/unit of IgE every 4 weeks.

Manufacturer's labeling:

- IgE ≥30-100 units/mL:
  - 30-90 kg: 150 mg every 4 weeks
  - >90-150 kg: 300 mg every 4 weeks
- IgE >100-200 units/mL:
  - 30-90 kg: 300 mg every 4 weeks
  - >90-150 kg: 225 mg every 2 weeks
- IgE >200-300 units/mL:
  - 30-60 kg: 300 mg every 4 weeks
  - >60-90 kg: 225 mg every 2 weeks
  - >90-150 kg: 300 mg every 2 weeks
- IgE >300-400 units/mL:
  - 30-70 kg: 225 mg every 2 weeks
  - >70-90 kg: 300 mg every 2 weeks
  - >90 kg: Do not use*
- IgE >400-500 units/mL:
  - 30-70 kg: 300 mg every 2 weeks
  - >70-90 kg: 375 mg every 2 weeks
  - >90 kg: Do not use*
- IgE >500-600 units/mL:
  - 30-60 kg: 300 mg every 2 weeks
  - >60-70 kg: 375 mg every 2 weeks
  - >70 kg: Do not use*
- IgE >600-700 units/mL:
  - 30-60 kg: 375 mg every 2 weeks
  - >60 kg: Do not use*

*Dosage has not been studied and approved for this weight and IgE level

Preparation for Administration SubQ: Reconstitute using SWFI only; add SWFI 1.4 mL to upright vial using a 1-inch, 18-gauge needle on a 3 mL syringe and swirl gently for ~1 minute to evenly wet the powder; do not shake. Then gently swirl the upright vial for 5 to 10 seconds approximately every 5 minutes until dissolved; generally takes 15 to 20 minutes to dissolve completely. If it takes >20 minutes to dissolve completely, continue to swirl the upright vial for 5 to 10 seconds every 5 minutes until no gel-like particles are visible in the solution; do not use if contents are not completely dissolved after 40 minutes. Resulting solution is 150 mg/1.2 mL. Invert the vial for 15 seconds so the solution drains toward the stopper. Remove all of the solution by inserting a new 3 mL syringe with a 1-inch, 18-gauge needle into the inverted vial. Replace the 18-gauge needle with a 25-gauge needle for subcutaneous injection, and expel any air, bubbles, or excess solution to obtain the 1.2 mL dose.

Administration SubQ: Doses >150 mg should be divided into more than one injection site. Due to viscosity, injection may take 5 to 10 seconds to administer. Administer only under direct medical supervision and observe patient for a minimum of 2 hours following administration of any dose given.

Monitoring Parameters Baseline total serum IgE, pulmonary function tests, anaphylactic/hypersensitivity reactions

Test Interactions Total IgE levels are elevated for up to 1 year following treatment. Total serum IgE may be retested after interruption of therapy for 1 year or more.

Additional Information Omalizumab was used successfully in a double-blind, randomized, placebo-controlled study of 334 children between the ages of 6-12 years; omalizumab dosage was based on body weight and initial serum total IgE. Patients received omalizumab at either 2- or 4-week intervals with a dosage equal to 0.016 mg/kg/IgE (units/mL) per 4 weeks. 55% of patients were able to discontinue corticosteroid use (Milgrom, 2003). A registry has been established to monitor outcomes of women exposed to omalizumab during pregnancy or within 8 weeks prior to pregnancy (866-496-5247).

Dosage Forms Excipient information presented when available (limited, particularly for generics); consult specific product labeling.

Solution Reconstituted, Subcutaneous [preservative free]:
Xolair: 150 mg (1 ea)

Omeprazole (oh MEP ra zole)

Medication Safety Issues

Sound-alike/look-alike issues:

Omeprazole may be confused with aripiprazole, esomeprazole, fomepizole

PriLOSEC may be confused with Plendil, Prevacid, predniSONE, prilocaine, Prinivil, Pristiq, Proventil, PROzac

International issues:

Losec [multiple international markets] may be confused with Lasix brand name for furosemide [U.S., Canada, and multiple international markets]

Medral [Mexico] may be confused with Medrol brand name for methylprednisolone [U.S., Canada, and multiple international markets]

Norpramin: Brand name for omeprazole [Spain], but also the brand name for desipramine [U.S., Canada] and enalapril/hydrochlorothiazide [Portugal]

Protonix: Brand name for omeprazole [Phillipines] but also the brand name for pantoprazole [U.S.]

Related Information

H. pylori Treatment in Pediatric Patients *on page 2358*

Oral Medications That Should Not Be Crushed or Altered *on page 2476*

Brand Names: US First-Omeprazole; Omeprazole+Syrspend SF Alka; PriLOSEC; PriLOSEC OTC [OTC]

Brand Names: Canada Apo-Omeprazole; Auro-Omeprazole; Ava-Omeprazole; Dom-Omeprazole DR; JAMP-Omeprazole DR; Losec; Mylan-Omeprazole; Olex; PMS-Omeprazole; PMS-Omeprazole DR; Q-Omeprazole; RAN-Omeprazole; ratio-Omeprazole; Riva-Omeprazole DR; Sandoz-Omeprazole; Teva-Omeprazole

Therapeutic Category Gastric Acid Secretion Inhibitor; Gastrointestinal Agent, Gastric or Duodenal Ulcer Treatment; Proton Pump Inhibitor

Generic Availability (US) May be product dependent

Use Short-term treatment (4-8 weeks) and maintenance of healing of severe erosive esophagitis (FDA approved in ages ≥1 year and adults); treatment of symptomatic gastroesophageal reflux disease (GERD) (FDA approved in ages ≥1 year and adults); short-term treatment (4-8 weeks)

of active duodenal ulcers and active benign gastric ulcers (FDA approved in adults); adjunctive treatment of duodenal ulcers associated with *Helicobacter pylori* (FDA approved in adults); treatment of pathological hypersecretory conditions (FDA approved in adults); relief of frequent heartburn (OTC products; FDA approved in adults)

Medication Guide Available Yes

Pregnancy Risk Factor C

Pregnancy Considerations Adverse events have been observed in some animal reproduction studies. An increased risk of hypospadias was reported following maternal use of proton pump inhibitors (PPIs) during pregnancy (Anderka, 2012), but this was based on a small number of exposures and the same association was not found in another study (Erichsen, 2012). Most available studies have not shown an increased risk of major birth defects following maternal use of omeprazole during pregnancy (Diav-Citrin, 2005; Källén, 2001; Lalkin, 1998; Matok, 2012; Pasternak, 2010). When treating GERD in pregnancy, PPIs may be used when clinically indicated (Katz, 2013).

Breast-Feeding Considerations Omeprazole is excreted in breast milk. Milk concentrations of omeprazole were studied in a breast-feeding woman at 3 weeks postpartum. The mother had taken omeprazole 20 mg daily starting her 29th week of gestation and continued after delivery. Following administration of omeprazole 20 mg, peak concentrations in the maternal serum occurred 240 minutes after the dose and peak concentrations in the breast milk were 180 minutes after the dose. The concentrations of omeprazole detected in the breast milk were <7% of the highest maternal serum concentration (Marshall, 1998).The manufacturer recommends caution be used if administered to a nursing woman. The acidic content of the nursing infants' stomach may potentially inactivate any ingested omeprazole (Marshall, 1998).

Contraindications Hypersensitivity (eg, anaphylaxis, anaphylactic shock, angioedema, bronchospasm, acute interstitial nephritis, urticaria) to omeprazole, other substituted benzimidazole proton pump inhibitors, or any component of the formulation

Warnings/Precautions Use of proton pump inhibitors (PPIs) may increase the risk of gastrointestinal infections (eg, *Salmonella, Campylobacter*). Relief of symptoms does not preclude the presence of a gastric malignancy. Atrophic gastritis (by biopsy) has been noted with long-term omeprazole therapy. In long-term (2-year) studies in rats, omeprazole produced a dose-related increase in gastric carcinoid tumors. While available endoscopic evaluations and histologic examinations of biopsy specimens from human stomachs have not detected a risk from short-term exposure to omeprazole, further human data on the effect of sustained hypochlorhydria and hypergastrinemia are needed to rule out the possibility of an increased risk for the development of tumors in humans receiving long-term therapy. Use of PPIs may increase risk of *Clostridium difficile*-associated diarrhea (CDAD), especially in hospitalized patients; consider CDAD diagnosis in patients with persistent diarrhea that does not improve. Use the lowest dose and shortest duration of PPI therapy appropriate for the condition being treated.

PPIs may diminish the therapeutic effect of clopidogrel, thought to be due to reduced formation of the active metabolite of clopidogrel. The manufacturer of clopidogrel recommends either avoidance both omeprazole (even when scheduled 12 hours apart) and esomeprazole or use of a PPI with comparatively less effect on the active metabolite of clopidogrel (eg, pantoprazole). In contrast to these warnings, others have recommended the continued use of PPIs, regardless of the degree of inhibition, in patients with a history of GI bleeding or multiple risk factors for GI bleeding who are also receiving clopidogrel since no evidence has established clinically meaningful differences in outcome; however, a clinically significant interaction cannot be excluded in those who are poor metabolizers of clopidogrel (Abraham, 2010; Levine, 2011). Potentially significant interactions may exist, requiring dose or frequency adjustment, additional monitoring, and/or selection of alternative therapy.

Increased incidence of osteoporosis-related bone fractures of the hip, spine, or wrist may occur with PPI therapy. Patients on high-dose (multiple daily doses) or long-term (≥1 year) therapy should be monitored. Use the lowest effective dose for the shortest duration of time, use vitamin D and calcium supplementation, and follow appropriate guidelines to reduce risk of fractures in patients at risk. Acute interstitial nephritis has been observed in patients taking PPIs; may occur at any time during therapy and is generally due to an idiopathic hypersensitivity reaction. Discontinue if acute interstitial nephritis develops.

Hypomagnesemia, reported rarely, usually with prolonged PPI use of >3 months (most cases >1 year of therapy) may be symptomatic or asymptomatic; severe cases may cause tetany, seizures, and cardiac arrhythmias. Consider obtaining serum magnesium concentrations prior to beginning long-term therapy, especially if taking concomitant digoxin, diuretics, or other drugs known to cause hypomagnesemia; and periodically thereafter. Hypomagnesemia may be corrected by magnesium supplementation, although discontinuation of omeprazole may be necessary; magnesium levels typically return to normal within 1 week of stopping. Serum chromogranin A levels may be increased if assessed while patient on omeprazole; may lead to diagnostic errors related to neuroendocrine tumors.

Prolonged treatment (≥2 years) may lead to vitamin B_{12} malabsorption and subsequent vitamin B_{12} deficiency. The magnitude of the deficiency is dose-related and the association is stronger in females and those younger in age (<30 years); prevalence is decreased after discontinuation of therapy (Lam, 2013).

Decreased *H. pylori* eradication rates have been observed with short-term (≤7 days) combination therapy. The American College of Gastroenterology recommends 10 to 14 days of therapy (triple or quadruple) for eradication of *H. pylori* (Chey, 2007). Bioavailability may be increased in Asian populations and patients with hepatic dysfunction; consider dosage reductions, especially for maintenance healing of erosive esophagitis. Bioavailability may be increased in the elderly. When used for self-medication (OTC), do not use for >14 days.

Benzyl alcohol and derivatives: Some dosage forms may contain benzyl alcohol; large amounts of benzyl alcohol (≥99 mg/kg/day) have been associated with a potentially fatal toxicity ("gasping syndrome") in neonates; the "gasping syndrome" consists of metabolic acidosis, respiratory distress, gasping respirations, CNS dysfunction (including convulsions, intracranial hemorrhage), hypotension, and cardiovascular collapse (AAP, 1997; CDC, 1982); some data suggests that benzoate displaces bilirubin from protein binding sites (Ahlfors, 2001); avoid or use dosage forms containing benzyl alcohol with caution in neonates. See manufacturer's labeling.

Adverse Reactions

Central nervous system: Dizziness, headache

Dermatologic: Skin rash

Gastrointestinal: Abdominal pain, acid regurgitation, constipation, diarrhea, flatulence, nausea, vomiting

Neuromuscular & skeletal: Back pain, weakness

Respiratory: Cough, upper respiratory infection

Rare but important or life-threatening: Abdominal swelling, abnormal dreams, aggression, agranulocytosis, allergic reactions, alopecia, anaphylaxis, anemia, angina pectoris, angioedema, anorexia, apathy, arthralgia, atrophic gastritis, benign gastric polyps, blurred vision, bone fracture, bradycardia, bronchospasm, chest pain, cholestatic hepatitis, *Clostridium difficile*-associated diarrhea (CDAD), confusion, depression, dermatitis, diplopia, drowsiness, epistaxis, erythema multiforme, esophageal candidiasis, fecal discoloration, gastroduodenal carcinoids, glycosuria, gynecomastia, hallucinations, hematuria, hemolytic anemia, hepatic disease (hepatocellular, cholestatic, mixed), hepatic encephalopathy, hepatic failure, hepatic necrosis, hepatitis, hepatocellular hepatitis, hepatotoxicity (idiosyncratic) (Chalasani, 2014), hyperhidrosis, hypersensitivity, hypertension, hypocalcemia, hypoglycemia, hypokalemia, hypomagnesemia, hyponatremia, increased gamma glutamyl transferase, increased serum alkaline phosphatase, increased serum bilirubin, increased serum creatinine, increased serum transaminases, insomnia, interstitial nephritis, irritable bowel syndrome, jaundice, leg pain, leukocytosis, leukopenia, malaise, microscopic colitis, microscopic pyuria, mucosal atrophy (tongue), muscle cramps, myalgia, myasthenia, nervousness, neutropenia, ocular irritation, optic atrophy, optic neuritis, optic neuropathy (anterior ischemic), osteoporosis-related fracture, pain, palpitation, pancreatitis, pancytopenia, paresthesia, peripheral edema, petechiae, photophobia, pneumonia, proteinuria, pruritus, psychiatric disturbance, purpura, sleep disturbance, sore throat, Stevens-Johnson syndrome, stomatitis, tachycardia, testicular pain, thrombocytopenia, toxic epidermal necrolysis, tremor, urinary tract infection, urticaria, weight gain, xeroderma, xerophthalmia, xerostomia

Drug Interactions

Metabolism/Transport Effects **Substrate** of CYP2A6 (minor), CYP2C19 (major), CYP2C9 (minor), CYP2D6 (minor), CYP3A4 (minor); **Note:** Assignment of Major/Minor substrate status based on clinically relevant drug interaction potential; **Inhibits** CYP1A2 (weak), CYP2C19 (moderate), CYP2C9 (moderate), CYP2D6 (weak); **Induces** CYP1A2 (weak/moderate)

Avoid Concomitant Use

Avoid concomitant use of Omeprazole with any of the following: Clopidogrel; Dasatinib; Delavirdine; Erlotinib; Nelfinavir; PAZOPanib; Rifampin; Rilpivirine; Risedronate; St Johns Wort

Increased Effect/Toxicity

Omeprazole may increase the levels/effects of: Amphetamine; ARIPiprazole; Bosentan; Cannabis; Carvedilol; Cilostazol; Citalopram; CloZAPine; CycloSPORINE (Systemic); CYP2C19 Substrates; CYP2C9 Substrates; Dexmethylphenidate; Dextroamphetamine; Dronabinol; Escitalopram; Fosphenytoin; Methotrexate; Methylphenidate; Phenytoin; Raltegravir; Risedronate; Saquinavir; Tacrolimus (Systemic); Tetrahydrocannabinol; TiZANidine; Vitamin K Antagonists; Voriconazole

The levels/effects of Omeprazole may be increased by: Fluconazole; Ketoconazole (Systemic); Voriconazole

Decreased Effect

Omeprazole may decrease the levels/effects of: Atazanavir; Bisphosphonate Derivatives; Bosutinib; Cefditoren; Clopidogrel; CloZAPine; Dabigatran Etexilate; Dabrafenib; Dasatinib; Delavirdine; Erlotinib; Gefitinib; Indinavir; Iron Salts; Itraconazole; Ketoconazole (Systemic); Ledipasvir; Mesalamine; Multivitamins/Minerals (with ADEK, Folate, Iron); Mycophenolate; Nelfinavir; Nilotinib; PAZOPanib; Posaconazole; Rilpivirine; Riociguat; Risedronate

The levels/effects of Omeprazole may be decreased by: CYP2C19 Inducers (Strong); Dabrafenib; Fosphenytoin; Phenytoin; Rifampin; St Johns Wort; Tipranavir

Food Interactions Prolonged treatment (≥2 years) may lead to malabsorption of dietary vitamin B_{12} and subsequent vitamin B_{12} deficiency (Lam, 2013).

Storage/Stability

Capsules, tablets: Store at 15°C to 30°C (59°F to 86°F). Protect from light and moisture.

Granules for oral suspension: Store at 25°C (77°F); excursions permitted to 15°C to 30°C (59°F to 86°F).

Powder for suspension (compounding kit): Prior to compounding, store at 15°C to 30°C (59°F to 86°F). Once compounded, the product is stable for 30 days under refrigeration [2°C to 8°C (36°F to 46°F)]; protect from light; protect from freezing.

OTC capsules: Store at 20°C to 25°C (68°F to 77°F); protect from moisture.

Mechanism of Action Proton pump inhibitor; suppresses gastric basal and stimulated acid secretion by inhibiting the parietal cell H+/K+ ATP pump

Pharmacodynamics

Onset of action: 1 hour

Maximum effect: 2 hours

Duration: 72 hours; 50% of maximum effect at 24 hours; after stopping treatment, secretory activity gradually returns over 3-5 days

Maximum secretory inhibition: 4 days

Pharmacokinetics (Adult data unless noted)

Absorption: Rapid

Protein binding: 95%

Metabolism: Hepatic via CYP2C19 primarily and to a lesser extent via 3A4 to hydroxy, desmethyl, and sulfone metabolites (all inactive); saturable first pass effect

Bioavailability: 30% to 40%; improves slightly with repeated administration; hepatic dysfunction: ~100%; in Asians, the AUC increased up to fourfold compared to Caucasians

Half-life: 0.5-1 hour; chronic hepatic disease: 3 hours

Time to peak serum concentration: 0.5-3.5 hours

Elimination: Urine (~77% as metabolites; very small amount as unchanged drug); feces

Clearance: 500-600 mL/minute; chronic hepatic disease: 70 mL/minute

Note: Half-life and AUC were significantly reduced for omeprazole suspension when compared with an equivalent dose via the commercially available capsule in 7 adults (Song, 2001).

Dosing: Neonatal **GERD:** Oral: 0.7 mg/kg/dose once daily reduced the percentage of time gastric and esophageal pH <4, as well as the number of reflux episodes in 10 infants (mean PMA: 36.1 weeks; range: 34 to 40 weeks) in a double-blind, placebo-controlled trial (Omari 2007); higher doses of 1 to 1.5 mg/kg/day have been reported (Gibbons 2005)

Dosing: Usual

Infants, Children, and Adolescents:

Erosive esophagitis: Oral: Children ≥1 year and Adolescents:
- 5 kg to <10 kg: 5 mg once daily
- 10 kg to <20 kg: 10 mg once daily
- ≥20 kg: 20 mg once daily

GERD: Oral:

Infants: 0.7 mg/kg/dose once daily reduced the percentage of time gastric and esophageal pH <4, as well as the number of reflux episodes in 10 infants [mean PMA: 36.1 weeks, (34-40 weeks)] in a double-blind, placebo-controlled trial (Omari, 2007); higher doses of 1-1.5 mg/kg/day have been reported (Gibbons, 2005)

Children ≥1 year and Adolescents:

Manufacturer labeling:
- 5 kg to <10 kg: 5 mg once daily
- 10 kg to <20 kg: 10 mg once daily
- ≥20 kg: 20 mg once daily

Alternate dosing: Infants, Children, and Adolescents: 0.7-3.3 mg/kg/day; maximum daily dose: 20 mg/**day**; the dose most frequently reported to provide healing of esophagitis and relief of GERD symptoms is 1 mg/kg/day (Lightdale, 2013; Zimmerman, 2001).

In critically ill children to maintain gastric pH >5, administration every 6-8 hours may be necessary (1.5-2 mg/kg/day) (Kaufman, 2002)

***Helicobacter pylori* eradication:** Oral: Children and Adolescents: **Note:** Usual duration of therapy is 7-14 days; use in combination with antimicrobials (eg, clarithromycin, metronidazole, amoxicillin).

Weight-based: 1-2 mg/kg/day divided into 2 doses; maximum single dose: 20 mg (Gold, 2000; Koletzko, 2011)

Fixed-dosing (Gottrand, 2001):

15-30 kg: 10 mg twice daily

>30 kg: 20 mg twice daily

Adults:

Active duodenal ulcer: Oral: 20 mg once daily for 4-8 weeks

Gastric ulcers: Oral: 40 mg once daily for 4-8 weeks

GERD, symptomatic: Oral: 20 mg once daily for up to 4 weeks

Erosive esophagitis: Oral: 20 mg once daily for 4-8 weeks

***Helicobacter pylori* eradication:** Oral: Dose varies with regimen: 20 mg twice daily for 10 days (in combination with clarithromycin and amoxicillin) or 40 mg once daily for 14 days (in combination with clarithromycin)

Note: Presence of ulcer at the time of therapy initiation may necessitate an additional 14-18 days of omeprazole 20 mg daily (monotherapy) after completion of combination therapy

Pathological hypersecretory conditions: Oral: Initial: 60 mg once daily; doses up to 120 mg 3 times daily have been administered; administer daily doses >80 mg in divided doses

Frequent heartburn (OTC labeling): Oral: 20 mg once daily for 14 days; treatment may be repeated after 4 months if needed

Dosing adjustment in renal impairment: Children, Adolescents, and Adults: No dosage adjustments are recommended

Dosing adjustment in hepatic impairment: Children, Adolescents, and Adults: There are no dosage adjustments provided in the manufacturer's labeling. However, based on increased bioavailability, dosage adjustment should be considered, especially for maintenance healing of erosive esophagitis. Specific guidelines are not available.

Preparation for Administration

Oral suspension:

Oral: Mix the contents of the 2.5 mg packet into 5 mL of water or the contents of the 10 mg packet into 15 mL of water; stir; the suspension should be left to thicken for 2 to 3 minutes prior to administration.

Nasogastric tube: Add 5 mL of water into a catheter-tipped syringe, and then add the contents of a 2.5 mg packet **or** 15 mL water for the 10 mg packet; shake; the suspension should be left to thicken for 2 to 3 minutes prior to administration.

Administration

Oral: Should be taken before meals; best if taken 30 minutes before a meal (Lightdale 2013); may be administered with antacids

Capsule: Should be swallowed whole; do not chew or crush. Delayed release capsule may be opened and contents added to 1 tablespoon of applesauce; use immediately after adding to applesauce; do not chew. Follow with a cool glass of water. Applesauce should not be heated.

Oral suspension: Empty the contents of the 2.5 mg packet or 10 mg packet into 5 mL or 15 mL of water, respectively; stir, the suspension should be left to thicken for 2 to 3 minutes and administered within 30 minutes. If any material remains after administration, add more water, stir, and administer immediately.

Tablet: Should be swallowed whole; do not crush or chew.

Nasogastric tube administration:

Capsule: The manufacturer of Prilosec does not give recommendations for extemporaneous preparation of omeprazole capsules for NG/OG administration. Consider using the packets for oral suspension. If packets are unavailable, methods of preparation of capsules for NG/OG administration have been described (Balaban 1997; Phillips 1996). An extemporaneously prepared suspension with extended stability may also be used (DiGiacinto 2000; Quercia 1997; Sharma 1999).

Oral suspension: Add 5 mL of water to a catheter-tipped syringe and then add the contents of a 2.5 mg packet (or 15 mL of water for the 10 mg packet), shake the suspension well and leave to thicken for 2 to 3 minutes. Administer within 30 minutes of reconstitution. Use an NG or gastric tube that is a French size 6 or larger; refill syringe with an equal amount of water, shake, and flush remaining contents through NG or gastric tube.

Test Interactions Omeprazole may falsely elevate serum chromogranin A (CgA) levels. The increased CgA level may cause false-positive results in the diagnosis of a neuroendocrine tumor. Temporarily stop omeprazole ≥14 days prior to assessing CgA level; repeat level if initially elevated; use the same laboratory for all testing of CgA levels.

Dosage Forms Excipient information presented when available (limited, particularly for generics); consult specific product labeling.

Capsule Delayed Release, Oral:

PriLOSEC: 10 mg, 20 mg, 40 mg

Generic: 10 mg, 20 mg, 40 mg, 20 mg

Packet, Oral:

PriLOSEC: 2.5 mg (30 ea); 10 mg (30 ea)

Suspension, Oral:

First-Omeprazole: 2 mg/mL (90 mL, 150 mL, 300 mL [contains benzyl alcohol, fd&c red #40, saccharin sodium; strawberry flavor]

Omeprazole+Syrspend SF Alka: 2 mg/mL (100 mL [cherry flavor]

Tablet Delayed Release, Oral:

PriLOSEC OTC: 20 mg

Generic: 20 mg

Extemporaneous Preparations Note: More palatable omeprazole (2 mg/mL) suspensions are commercially available as compounding kits (First-Omeprazole, Omeprazole+Syrspend SF Alka Cherry Kit).

A 2 mg/mL oral omeprazole solution (Simplified Omeprazole Solution) may be made with five omeprazole 20 mg delayed release capsules and 50 mL sodium bicarbonate 8.4%. Empty capsules into beaker. Add sodium bicarbonate solution. Gently stir (about 15 minutes) until a white suspension forms. Transfer to amber-colored syringe or bottle. Stable for 14 days at room temperature or for 30 days refrigerated.

DiGiacinto JL, Olsen KM, Bergman KL, et al, "Stability of Suspension Formulations of Lansoprazole and Omeprazole Stored in Amber Colored Plastic Oral Syringes," *Ann Pharmacother*, 2000, 34(5):600-5.

Quercia R, Fan C, Liu X, et al, "Stability of Omeprazole in an Extemporaneously Prepared Oral Liquid," *Am J Health Syst Pharm*, 1997, 54(16):1833-6.

Sharma V, "Comparison of 24-hour Intragastric pH Using Four Liquid Formulations of Lansoprazole and Omeprazole," *Am J Health Syst Pharm*, 1999, 56(23 Suppl 4):18-21.

Omeprazole and Sodium Bicarbonate

(oh MEP ra zole & SOW dee um bye KAR bun ate)

Medication Safety Issues

Sound-alike/look-alike issues:

Zegerid may be confused with Zestril

Related Information

Oral Medications That Should Not Be Crushed or Altered *on page 2476*

Brand Names: US Zegerid; Zegerid OTC [OTC]

Therapeutic Category Proton Pump Inhibitor; Substituted Benzimidazole

Generic Availability (US) Yes: Capsule

Use Short-term (4-8 weeks) treatment of active duodenal ulcer disease or active benign gastric ulcer; treatment of symptomatic gastroesophageal reflux disease (GERD) treatment and maintenance healing of erosive esophagitis (Capsule, oral suspension: FDA approved in adults); reduction of risk of upper gastrointestinal bleeding in critically ill patients (Oral suspension: FDA approved in adults); relief of frequent (≥2 days/week), uncomplicated heartburn (OTC products: FDA approved in adults)

Medication Guide Available Yes

Pregnancy Risk Factor C

Pregnancy Considerations Adverse events have been observed in animal reproduction studies with omeprazole. Refer to individual agents.

Breast-Feeding Considerations Omeprazole is excreted in breast milk. Due to the potential for serious adverse reactions in the nursing infant, the manufacturer recommends a decision be made whether to discontinue nursing or to discontinue the drug, taking into account the importance of treatment to the mother. Refer to individual agents.

Contraindications Hypersensitivity (eg, anaphylaxis, anaphylactic shock, angioedema, bronchospasm, acute interstitial nephritis, urticaria) to omeprazole, other substituted benzimidazole proton pump inhibitors, or any component of the formulation

Warnings/Precautions See individual agents.

Adverse Reactions

Cardiovascular: Atrial fibrillation, bradycardia, edema, hyper-/hypotension, supraventricular tachycardia, tachycardia, ventricular tachycardia

Central nervous system: Agitation, hyperpyrexia, pyrexia

Dermatological: Decubitus ulcer, rash

Endocrine & metabolic: Fluid overload, hyper-/hypoglycemia, hyper-/hypokalemia, hyper-/hyponatremia, hypocalcemia, hypomagnesemia, hypophosphatemia

Gastrointestinal: Constipation, diarrhea, hypomotility

Genitourinary: Urinary tract infection

Hematological: Anemia, anemia increased, thrombocytopenia

Hepatic: LFTs increased

Respiratory: ARDS, cough, nosocomial pneumonia, pneumothorax, respiratory failure

Miscellaneous: Candidal infection, oral candidiasis, sepsis

Rare but important or life-threatening (adverse event occurrence may vary based on formulation): Agranulocytosis, allergic reactions, alopecia, anaphylaxis, angina, angioedema, anorexia, atrophic gastritis, benign gastric polyps, bronchospasm, *Clostridium difficile*-associated diarrhea (CDAD), creatinine increased, depression, erythema multiforme, esophageal candidiasis, fracture, glycosuria, gynecomastia, hallucinations, hematuria, hemifacial dysesthesia, hemolytic anemia, hepatic encephalopathy, hepatic failure, hepatic necrosis, hepatotoxicity (idiosyncratic) (Chalasani, 2014), hypersensitivity, interstitial nephritis, leukocytosis, leukopenia, liver disease (hepatocellular, cholestatic, mixed), metabolic alkalosis, microscopic pyuria, microscopic colitis, mucosal atrophy (tongue), neutropenia, optic neuritis, optic neuropathy, osteoporosis-related fracture, pancreatitis, pancytopenia, photosensitivity, pneumonia (CAP), proteinuria, psychiatric disturbance, purpura, seizure, Stevens-Johnson syndrome, taste perversion, tinnitus, toxic epidermal necrolysis, vertigo, xerostomia

Drug Interactions

Metabolism/Transport Effects Refer to individual components.

Avoid Concomitant Use

Avoid concomitant use of Omeprazole and Sodium Bicarbonate with any of the following: Clopidogrel; Dasatinib; Delavirdine; Erlotinib; Nelfinavir; PAZOPanib; Rifampin; Rilpivirine; Risedronate; St Johns Wort

Increased Effect/Toxicity

Omeprazole and Sodium Bicarbonate may increase the levels/effects of: Alpha-/Beta-Agonists (Indirect-Acting); Amphetamines; ARIPiprazole; Bosentan; Calcium Polystyrene Sulfonate; Cannabis; Carvedilol; Cilostazol; Citalopram; CloZAPine; CycloSPORINE (Systemic); CYP2C19 Substrates; CYP2C9 Substrates; Dexmethylphenidate; Dronabinol; Escitalopram; Flecainide; Fosphenytoin; Mecamylamine; Memantine; Methotrexate; Methylphenidate; Phenytoin; QuiNIDine; QuiNINE; Raltegravir; Risedronate; Saquinavir; Tacrolimus (Systemic); Tetrahydrocannabinol; TiZANidine; Vitamin K Antagonists; Voriconazole

The levels/effects of Omeprazole and Sodium Bicarbonate may be increased by: AcetaZOLAMIDE; Fluconazole; Ketoconazole (Systemic); Voriconazole

Decreased Effect

Omeprazole and Sodium Bicarbonate may decrease the levels/effects of: Antipsychotic Agents (Phenothiazines); Atazanavir; Bisacodyl; Bismuth Subcitrate; Bisphosphonate Derivatives; Bosutinib; Captopril; Cefditoren; Cefpodoxime; Cefuroxime; Chloroquine; Clopidogrel; CloZAPine; Corticosteroids (Oral); Dabigatran Etexilate; Dabrafenib; Dasatinib; Delavirdine; Elvitegravir; Erlotinib; Flecainide; Fosinopril; Gabapentin; Gefitinib; HMG-CoA Reductase Inhibitors; Hyoscyamine; Indinavir; Iron Salts; Isoniazid; Itraconazole; Ketoconazole (Systemic); Ledipasvir; Lithium; Mesalamine; Methenamine; Multivitamins/Minerals (with ADEK, Folate, Iron); Mycophenolate; Nelfinavir; Nilotinib; PAZOPanib; PenicillAMINE; Phosphate Supplements; Posaconazole; Potassium Acid Phosphate; Rilpivirine; Riociguat; Risedronate; Sotalol; Sulpiride; Tetracycline Derivatives; Trientine

The levels/effects of Omeprazole and Sodium Bicarbonate may be decreased by: CYP2C19 Inducers (Strong); Dabrafenib; Fosphenytoin; Phenytoin; Rifampin; St Johns Wort; Tipranavir

Food Interactions See individual agents.

Storage/Stability

Capsules, powder for oral suspension: Store at 25°C (77°F); excursions permitted to 15°C to 30°C (59°F to 86°F). Protect from light.

OTC capsules: Store at 20°C to 25°C (68°F to 77°F).

Mechanism of Action Suppresses gastric basal and stimulated acid secretion by inhibiting the parietal cell H+/K+ ATP pump

Pharmacodynamics

Onset of action: 1 hour

Maximum effect: 2 hours

Duration: 72 hours; 50% of maximum effect at 24 hours

Maximum secretory inhibition: 4 days

Pharmacokinetics (Adult data unless noted)

Absorption: Rapid

Protein binding: 95%

Metabolism: Hepatic via CYP2C19 primarily and to a lesser extent via 3A4 to hydroxy, desmethyl, and sulfone metabolites (all inactive); saturable first pass effect

Bioavailability: 30% to 40%; improves slightly with repeated administration; hepatic dysfunction: ~100%; increased in Asian patients; AUC increased up to fourfold compared to Caucasians

Half-life: ~1 hour (range: 0.4-3.2 hours); chronic hepatic disease: 3 hours

Time to peak serum concentration: ~30 minutes

Elimination: Urine (77% as metabolites, very small amount as unchanged drug); feces

Clearance: 500-600 mL/minute; chronic hepatic disease: 70 mL/minute

Dosing: Usual Note: Dosage listed is for omeprazole component; both strengths of Zegerid® capsule and powder for oral suspension have identical sodium bicarbonate content. Do not substitute two 20 mg capsules/packets for one 40 mg dose.

Children and Adolescents: **Note:** Recognizing that this formulation has not received FDA approval for use in children despite an approved dosage for omeprazole in children and considering that omeprazole has been used safely in children as an extemporaneous formulation with sodium bicarbonate, the following dosage is recommended:

Erosive esophagitis: Oral:

5 kg to <10 kg: 5 mg once daily

10 kg to <20 kg: 10 mg once daily

≥20 kg: 20 mg once daily

GERD, symptomatic: Oral:

5 kg to <10 kg: 5 mg once daily

10 kg to ≤20 kg: 10 mg once daily

>20 kg: 20 mg once daily

Alternate dosing: Infants, Children, and Adolescents: 0.7-3.3 mg/kg/day (Lightdale, 2013); maximum daily dose: 20 mg/day; 1 mg/kg/day is the dose reported most often to provide healing of esophagitis and relief of GERD symptoms (Zimmerman, 2001). To maintain gastric pH >5 in critically ill children, administration every 6-8 hours may be necessary (1.5-2 mg/kg/day) (Kaufman, 2002).

Adults:

Active duodenal ulcer: Oral: 20 mg once daily for 4-8 weeks

Erosive esophagitis: Oral: 20 mg once daily for 4-8 weeks; maintenance of healing: 20 mg once daily for up to 12 months total therapy (including treatment period of 4-8 weeks)

Gastric ulcers: Oral: 40 mg once daily for 4-8 weeks

GERD, symptomatic: Oral: 20 mg once daily for up to 4 weeks

Heartburn (OTC labeling): Oral: 20 mg once daily for 14 days. Do not take for >14 days or more often than every 4 months, unless instructed by healthcare provider.

Risk reduction of upper GI bleeding in critically ill patients (Zegerid® powder for oral suspension): Oral:

Loading dose: Day 1: 40 mg every 6-8 hours for two doses

Maintenance dose: 40 mg daily for up to 14 days; therapy >14 days has not been evaluated

Dosing adjustment in renal impairment: Adults: No dosage adjustments are recommended

Dosing adjustment in hepatic impairment: Adults: There are no dosage adjustments provided in the manufacturer's labeling; however, based on increased bioavailability, a dosage adjustment should be considered, especially for maintenance of healing of erosive esophagitis. Specific guidelines are not available.

Preparation for Administration

Powder for oral suspension: **Note:** Both strengths of Zegerid powder for oral suspension have identical sodium bicarbonate content, respectively. Do not substitute two 20 mg packets for one 40 mg dose.

Oral: Mix 1 packet with 15 to 30 mL of water; stir well and administer immediately. Do not mix with other liquids or food; only water.

Nasogastric/orogastric tube: Mix well 1 packet with 20 mL of water and administer immediately; do not mix with other liquids or food; only water.

Administration Note: Both strengths of capsule and Zegerid powder for oral suspension have identical sodium bicarbonate content, respectively. Do not substitute two 20 mg capsules/packets for one 40 mg dose.

Capsule: Should be swallowed whole with water (do not use other liquids); do not chew or crush. Capsules should **not** be opened, sprinkled on food, or administered via NG. Best if taken at least 1 hour before breakfast.

Powder for oral suspension:

Oral: Administer 1 hour before a meal. Mix with 15 to 30 mL of water; stir well and drink immediately. Rinse cup with water and drink. Do not mix with other liquids or food; only water.

Nasogastric/orogastric tube: Mix well with 20 mL of water and administer immediately; flush tube with an additional 20 mL of water. Suspend enteral feeding for 3 hours before and 1 hour after administering. Do not mix with other liquids or food; only water.

Test Interactions Omeprazole may falsely elevate serum chromogranin A (CgA) levels. The increased CgA level may cause false-positive results in the diagnosis of a neuroendocrine tumor. Temporarily stop omeprazole ≥14 days prior to assessing CgA level; repeat test if CgA level is initially elevated; use the same laboratory for all testing of CgA levels.

Additional Information Each capsule of omeprazole-sodium bicarbonate contains 1100 mg (13 mEq) of sodium bicarbonate; total Na content is 304 mg and 303 mg for the prescription and OTC product, respectively. Each packet of omeprazole-sodium bicarbonate powder for oral suspension contains 1680 mg (20 mEq) of sodium bicarbonate; total Na content is 460 mg.

Dosage Forms Excipient information presented when available (limited, particularly for generics); consult specific product labeling.

Capsule, oral: Omeprazole 20 mg [immediate release] and sodium bicarbonate 1100 mg; omeprazole 40 mg [immediate release] and sodium bicarbonate 1100 mg

Zegerid: Omeprazole 20 mg [immediate release] and sodium bicarbonate 1100 mg [contains sodium 304 mg (13 mEq) per capsule]

Zegerid: Omeprazole 40 mg [immediate release] and sodium bicarbonate 1100 mg [contains sodium 304 mg (13 mEq) per capsule]

Zegerid OTC: Omeprazole 20 mg [immediate release] and sodium bicarbonate 1100 mg [contains sodium 303 mg (13 mEq) per capsule]

Powder for suspension, oral:

Zegerid: Omeprazole 20 mg and sodium bicarbonate 1680 mg per packet (30s) [contains sodium 460 mg (20 mEq) per packet]

Zegerid: Omeprazole 40 mg and sodium bicarbonate 1680 mg per packet (30s) [contains sodium 460 mg (20 mEq) per packet]

Extemporaneous Preparations A 2 mg/mL oral suspension may be made with omeprazole-sodium bicarbonate powder and water. Pour the contents of six 20 mg omeprazole-sodium bicarbonate packets into a glass mortar. Add 30 mL water to the powder and mix to a uniform paste mix while adding water in incremental proportions to **almost** 60 mL; transfer to a 60 mL bottle, rinse mortar with water, and add sufficient quantity of water to make 60 mL. Label "shake well" and "refrigerate". Stable for 45 days refrigerated.

Johnson CE, Cober MP, and Ludwig JL, "Stability of Partial Doses of Omeprazole-Sodium Bicarbonate Oral Suspension," *Ann Pharmacother*, 2007, 41(12):1954-61.

- **Omeprazole Magnesium** *see* Omeprazole *on page 1555*
- **Omeprazole+Syrspend SF Alka** *see* Omeprazole *on page 1555*
- **Omnaris** *see* Ciclesonide (Nasal) *on page 454*

◆ **Omnaris HFA (Can)** *see* Ciclesonide (Nasal) *on page 454*

◆ **Omnicef** *see* Cefdinir *on page 390*

◆ **Omni Gel [OTC]** *see* Fluoride *on page 899*

◆ **Omnipred** *see* PrednisoLONE (Ophthalmic) *on page 1758*

◆ **Omnitrope** *see* Somatropin *on page 1957*

OnabotulinumtoxinA

(oh nuh BOT yoo lin num TOKS in aye)

Medication Safety Issues

Other safety concerns:

Botulinum products are not interchangeable; potency differences may exist between the products.

Brand Names: US Botox; Botox Cosmetic

Brand Names: Canada Botox; Botox Cosmetic

Therapeutic Category Muscle Contracture, Treatment; Ophthalmic Agent, Toxin

Generic Availability (US) No

Use Treatment of strabismus and blepharospasm associated with dystonia (including benign essential blepharospasm or VII nerve disorders) (FDA approved in ages >12 years and adults); treatment of dynamic muscle contracture in pediatric cerebral palsy patients (orphan drug); treatment of cervical dystonia (FDA approved in ages >16 and adults); treatment of severe primary axillary hyperhidrosis (not adequately controlled with topical treatments) (FDA approved in adults); temporary improvement in the appearance of lines and wrinkles of the face (moderate to severe glabellar lines associated with corrugator and/or procerus muscle activity) in adult patients ≤65 years of age; focal spasticity, specifically upper limb spasticity (FDA approved in adults); prophylaxis of chronic migraine headache (≥15 days/month with ≥4 hours/day headache duration) (FDA approved in adults). Other uses include treatment of sialorrhea, palmar hyperhidrosis, esophageal achalasia, chronic anal fissure.

Medication Guide Available Yes

Pregnancy Risk Factor C

Pregnancy Considerations Adverse events were observed in some animal reproduction studies.

Breast-Feeding Considerations It is not known if onabotulinumtoxinA is excreted in breast milk. The manufacturer recommends that caution be exercised when administering onabotulinumtoxinA to nursing women.

Contraindications Hypersensitivity to botulinum toxin, or any component of the formulation; infection at the proposed injection site(s); intradetrusor injection in patients with overactive bladder or detrusor overactivity with a neurologic condition who have a urinary tract infection; intradetrusor injection in patients with urinary retention and in patients with post-void residual (PVR) urine volume >200 mL who are not routinely performing clean intermittent self-catheterization

Warnings/Precautions [US Boxed Warning]: Distant spread of botulinum toxin beyond the site of injection has been reported; dysphagia and breathing difficulties have occurred and may be life threatening; other symptoms reported include blurred vision, diplopia, dysarthria, dysphonia, generalized muscle weakness, ptosis, and urinary incontinence which may develop within hours or weeks following injection. The risk is likely greatest in children treated for the unapproved use of spasticity. Systemic effects have occurred following use in approved and unapproved uses, including low doses. Immediate medical attention required if respiratory, speech, or swallowing difficulties appear. Higher doses or more frequent administration may result in neutralizing antibody formation and loss of efficacy. Use caution in patients with bleeding disorders and/or receiving anticoagulation therapy. May impair ability to drive and/or operate machinery; if loss of strength, muscle weakness, or impaired vision occurs, patients should avoid driving or engaging in other hazardous activities.

Product contains albumin and may carry a remote risk of virus transmission. Use caution if there is inflammation or excessive weakness or atrophy at the proposed injection site(s); use is contraindicated if infection is present at injection site. Serious events (including fatalities) have been observed with direct injection into the esophagus, stomach, salivary glands and oro-lingual-pharyngeal region. Use caution when administering in close proximity to the lungs (especially the apices); pneumothorax has been reported following administration near the thorax. Have appropriate support in case of anaphylactic reaction. Use with caution in patients with neuromuscular diseases (such as myasthenia gravis or Lambert-Eaton syndrome), neuropathic disorders (such as amyotrophic lateral sclerosis), patients taking aminoglycosides, neuromuscular-blocking agents, or other drugs that interfere with neuromuscular transmission and patients with preexisting cardiovascular disease (rare reports of arrhythmia and MI). Long-term effects of chronic therapy are unknown. Botulinum products (abobotulinumtoxinA, onabotulinumtoxinA, rimabotulinumtoxinB) are not interchangeable; potency units are specific to each preparation and cannot be compared or converted to any other botulinum product. Serious and/or immediate hypersensitivity reactions (eg, anaphylaxis, serum sickness, urticaria, soft tissue edema, and dyspnea) have occurred. If a reaction occurs, discontinue and institute immediate treatment.

Cervical dystonia: Dysphagia is common. It may be severe requiring alternative feeding methods and may persist anywhere from 2 weeks up to 5 months after administration. Risk factors include smaller neck muscle mass, bilateral injections into the sternocleidomastoid muscle, or injections into the levator scapulae. Use extreme caution in patients with preexisting respiratory disease; may weaken accessory muscles that are necessary for these patients to maintain adequate ventilation. Risk of aspiration resulting from severe dysphagia is increased in patients with decreased respiratory function.

Bladder dysfunction (overactive bladder or detrusor overactivity associated with a neurologic condition): Rule out acute urinary tract infection (UTI) prior to treatment; appropriate prophylactic antimicrobial therapy is required prior to, during, and following treatment. Discontinue antiplatelet therapy at least 3 days prior to administration. An increased incidence of urinary retention and need for catheterization has been observed in patients receiving therapy for bladder dysfunction; due to the risk of urinary retention, treatment should only be used in patients able and willing to initiate post-treatment catheterization, if required. Therapy in patients with overactive bladder increases the incidence of urinary tract infections; clinical trials for overactive bladder excluded patients with >2 UTIs in the previous 6 months and those taking chronic antibiotics for prophylaxis of recurrent UTIs. Consider risks vs. benefits when contemplating use in these patients or patients experiencing recurrent UTIs during treatment. Patients with diabetes had an increased incidence of urinary retention and urinary tract infection. Patients experiencing difficulty in voiding should be instructed to consult their healthcare provider. Autonomic dysreflexia has been observed with therapy in patients with detrusor overactivity associated with a neurologic condition; acts as stimuli to trigger an exaggerated sympathetic and parasympathetic response. Clinical presentation often includes headache, a marked increase in blood pressure, and diaphoresis;

prompt treatment may be required in patients presenting with severe symptoms (eg, hypertensive crisis).

Episodic migraines: Safety and efficacy have not been established in patients with 14 or fewer headaches per month.

Ocular disease: Blepharospasm: Reduced blinking from injection of the orbicularis muscle can lead to corneal exposure and ulceration. Strabismus: Retrobulbar hemorrhages may occur from needle penetration into orbit. Spatial disorientation, double vision, or past-pointing may occur if one or more extraocular muscles are paralyzed. Covering the affected eye may help. Careful testing of corneal sensation, avoidance of lower lid injections, and treatment of epithelial defects are necessary. Use with caution in angle closure glaucoma.

Primary axillary hyperhidrosis: Evaluate for secondary causes prior to treatment (eg, hyperthyroidism). Safety and efficacy for treatment of hyperhidrosis in other areas of the body have not been established.

Temporary reduction in glabellar lines: Do not use more frequently than every 3 months (Canadian labeling states not to use more frequently than every 2 months). Patients with marked facial asymmetry, ptosis, excessive dermatochalasis, deep dermal scarring, thick sebaceous skin, or the inability to substantially lessen glabellar lines by physically spreading them apart were excluded from clinical trials. Use with caution in patients with surgical alterations to the facial anatomy. Reduced blinking from injection of the orbicularis muscle can lead to corneal exposure and ulceration. Spatial disorientation, double vision, or past pointing may occur if one or more extraocular muscles are paralyzed.

Warnings: Additional Pediatric Considerations The U.S. Food and Drug Administration (FDA) and Health Canada have issued respective communications to health care professionals alerting them of serious adverse events (including fatalities) in association with the use of onabotulinumtoxinA (Botox, Botox Cosmetic) and rimabotulinumtoxinB (Myobloc). Events reported are suggestive of botulism, indicating systemic spread of the botulinum toxin beyond the site of injection. Reactions were observed in both adult and pediatric patients treated for a variety of conditions with varying doses; however, the most serious outcomes, including respiratory failure and death, were associated with the use in children for cerebral palsy limb spasticity. The FDA has evaluated postmarketing cases and now reports that systemic and potentially fatal toxicity may result from local injection of the botulinum toxins in the treatment of other underlying conditions, such as cerebral palsy associated with limb spasticity. Monitor patients closely for signs/symptoms of systemic toxic effects (possibly occurring 1 day to several weeks after treatment) and instruct patients to seek immediate medical attention with worsening symptoms or dysphagia, dyspnea, muscle weakness, or difficulty speaking.

Adverse Reactions Adverse effects usually occur in 1 week and may last up to several months.

Bladder dysfunction:

Central nervous system: Abnormal gait, falling, myasthenia

Gastrointestinal: Constipation

Genitourinary: Bacteriuria, dysuria, hematuria, increased post-void residual urine volume (not requiring catheterization), urinary retention, urinary tract infection

Neuromuscular & skeletal: Muscle spasm

Cervical dystonia:

Central nervous system: Dizziness, drowsiness, headache, hypertonia, numbness, speech disturbance

Gastrointestinal: Dysphagia, nausea, xerostomia

Immunologic: Antibody development

Local: Injection site reaction, soreness

Neuromuscular & skeletal: Back pain, neck pain, stiffness, weakness

Ophthalmic: Blepharoptosis, diplopia

Respiratory: Cough, dyspnea, flu-like symptoms, rhiniti upper respiratory tract infection

Miscellaneous: Fever

Chronic migraines:

Cardiovascular: Hypertension

Central nervous system: Exacerbation of migraine headache, headache, facial paresis

Local: Pain at injection site

Neuromuscular & skeletal: Myasthenia, muscle spasm musculoskeletal pain, myalgia, neck pain, stiffness

Ophthalmic: Blepharoptosis

Respiratory: Bronchitis

Upper Limb Spasticity:

Central nervous system: Fatigue

Gastrointestinal: Nausea

Neuromuscular & skeletal: Limb pain, myasthenia

Respiratory: Bronchitis

Other indications (blepharospasm, primary axillar hyperhidrosis, strabismus):

Central nervous system: Anxiety, dizziness, headache facial pain, facial paresis, pain

Dermatologic: Diaphoresis (nonaxillary), pruritus skin rash

Gastrointestinal: Nausea

Immunologic: Antibody development

Infection: Infection

Local: Injection site reaction: Hemorrhage, pair soreness

Neuromuscular & skeletal: back pain, neck pair weakness

Ophthalmic: Blepharoptosis (strabismus more common diplopia, dry eye syndrome, ectropion, entropion, ey irritation (includes dry eye, lagophthalmos, photophc bia), eyelid edema, keratitis, lacrimation, superfici punctate keratitis, vertical deviation of eyes (stra bismus)

Respiratory: Flu-like symptoms, pharyngitis

Miscellaneous: Fever

Rare but important or life-threatening: *Any indicatio* Abdominal distension, acute angle-closure glaucoma alopecia, amyotrophy, anaphylaxis, anorexia, anteric segment ischemia, antibody development (neutralizing aspiration pneumonia, asthma, brachial plexopathy, ca diac arrhythmia, cardiac insufficiency, ciliary ganglio damage, circulatory shock, colitis, corneal perforatio corneal ulceration, denervation, diarrhea, ectropior entropion, erythema, erythema multiforme, exacerbatio of myasthenia gravis, eye pain, focal facial paralysis glaucoma, hearing loss, herpes zoster, hyperreflexi hypersensitivity reaction, hypoacusis, lymphadenopath madarosis, myalgia, myocardial infarction, ocular edema paresthesia, peripheral edema, peripheral neuropathy pneumonia, psoriasiform eruption, radiculopath reduced blinking, respiratory depression, respiratory fai ure, retinal vein occlusion, retrobulbar hemorrhage, seiz ure, serum sickness, syncope, trismus, urinar incontinence, vertigo with nystagmus, visual disturbar ces, vitreous hemorrhage, voice disorder

Drug Interactions

Metabolism/Transport Effects None known.

Avoid Concomitant Use There are no known interac tions where it is recommended to avoid concomitant use

Increased Effect/Toxicity

OnabotulinumtoxinA may increase the levels/effects o AbobotulinumtoxinA; RimabotulinumtoxinB

The levels/effects of OnabotulinumtoxinA may b increased by: Aminoglycosides; Anticholinergic Agents Neuromuscular-Blocking Agents

Decreased Effect There are no known significant interactions involving a decrease in effect.

Storage/Stability Store unopened vials under refrigeration at 2°C to 8°C (36°F to 46°F) for up to 36 months (Botox 100 unit vial) or up to 24 months (Botox 200 unit vial), or until the expiration date on the vial (Botox Cosmetic). After reconstitution, store in refrigerator at 2°C to 8°C (36°F to 46°F) and use within 24 hours (does not contain a preservative).

Botox 100-unit vial: The following stability information has also been reported: May be stored at room temperature for up to 5 days (Cohen, 2007).

Mechanism of Action OnabotulinumtoxinA (previously known as botulinum toxin type A) is a neurotoxin produced by *Clostridium botulinum*, spore-forming anaerobic bacillus, which appears to affect only the presynaptic membrane of the neuromuscular junction in humans, where it prevents calcium-dependent release of acetylcholine and produces a state of denervation. Muscle inactivation persists until new fibrils grow from the nerve and form junction plates on new areas of the muscle-cell walls. Intradetrusor injection affects efferent pathways of detrusor activity by inhibiting release of acetylcholine. Intradermal injection results in temporary sweat gland denervation, reducing local sweating.

Pharmacodynamics

Strabismus:
- Onset of action: 1-2 days after injection
- Duration of paralysis: 2-6 weeks

Blepharospasm:
- Onset of action: 3 days after injection
- Maximum effect: 1-2 weeks
- Duration of paralysis: 3 months

Spasticity associated with cerebral palsy
- Onset of action: Several days
- Duration of paralysis: 3-8 months

Reduction in axillary sweat production:
- Duration of effect: 201 days (mean)

Dosing: Usual IM:

Strabismus:

Children 2 months to 12 years:
- Horizontal or vertical deviations <20 prism diopters: 1.25 units into any one muscle
- Horizontal or vertical deviations 20-50 prism diopters: 1-2.5 units into any one muscle
- Persistent VI nerve palsy of ≥1 month duration: 1-1.25 units into the medial rectus muscle

Children ≥12 years and Adults:
- Horizontal or vertical deviations <20 prism diopters: 1.25-2.5 units into any one muscle
- Horizontal or vertical deviations 20-50 prism diopters: 2.5-5 units into any one muscle
- Persistent VI nerve palsy of ≥1 month duration: 1.25-2.5 units into the medial rectus muscle

Note: Re-examine patient 7-14 days after each injection to assess effects; dosage may be increased up to twofold of the previously administered dose; do not exceed 25 units as a single injection for any one muscle

Spasticity associated with cerebral palsy: Children >18 months to Adolescents: Small muscle: 1-2 units/kg; large muscle: 3-6 units/kg; maximum dose per injection site: 50 units; maximum dose for any one visit: 12 units/kg, up to 400 units; no more than 400 units should be administered during a 3-month period

Blepharospasm: Adults: Initial: 1.25-2.5 units injected into the medial and lateral pretarsal orbicularis oculi of the upper lid and into the lateral pretarsal orbicularis oculi of the lower lid; dose may be increased up to 2.5-5 units at repeat treatment sessions; do not exceed 5 units per injection or cumulative dose of 200 units in a 30-day period

Cervical dystonia: Adults: Initial and sequential doses should be individualized related to the patient's head and neck position, localization of pain, muscle hypertrophy, and patient response; mean dosage used in research trials: 236 units (range: 198-300 units) (maximum: ≤50 units/site) divided among affected muscles; limit total dose into sternocleidomastoid muscles to ≤100 units to decrease the occurrence of dysphagia

Severe primary axillary hyperhidrosis: Adults: Intradermal: 50 units per axilla injected in 0.1-0.2 mL aliquots

Reduction of glabellar lines: Adults ≤65 years: IM: An effective dose is determined by gross observation of the patient's ability to activate the superficial muscles injected. The location, size and use of muscles may vary markedly among individuals. Inject 0.1 mL dose into each of five sites, two in each corrugator muscle and one in the procerus muscle (total dose 0.5 mL).

Chronic migraine: Adults: IM: Administer 5 units/0.1 mL per site. Recommended total dose is 155 units once every 12 weeks. Each 155-unit dose should be equally divided and administered bilaterally, into 31 total sites as described below (refer to prescribing information for specific diagrams of recommended injection sites):
- Corrugator: 5 units to each side (2 sites)
- Procerus: 5 units (1 site only)
- Frontalis: 10 units to each side (divided into 2 sites/side)
- Temporalis: 20 units to each side (divided into 4 sites/side)
- Occipitalis: 15 units to each side (divided into 3 sites/side)
- Cervical paraspinal: 10 units to each side (divided into 2 sites/side)
- Trapezius: 15 units to each side (divided into 3 sites/side)

Spasticity (focal): Adults: IM: Individualize dose based on patient size, extent, and location of muscle involvement, degree of spasticity, local muscle weakness, and response to prior treatment. In clinical trials, total doses up to 360 units were administered as separate injections typically divided among selected muscles; may repeat therapy at ≥3 months with appropriate dosage based upon the clinical condition of patient at time of retreatment.

Suggested guidelines for the treatment of upper limb spasticity. The lowest recommended starting dose should be used and ≤50 units/site should be administered. **Note:** Dose listed is total dose administered as individual or separate intramuscular injection(s):
- Biceps brachii: 100-200 units (up to 4 sites)
- Flexor digitorum profundus: 30-50 units (1 site)
- Flexor digitorum sublimes: 30-50 units (1 site)
- Flexor carpi radialis: 12.5-50 units (1 site)
- Flexor carpi ulnaris: 12.5-50 units (1 site)

Preparation for Administration

Parenteral: Reconstitute with sterile, preservative free NS:

Note: Dilution information (excludes recommendations for preparing the solution for use in detrusor overactivity associated with a neurologic condition):

Botox 100-unit vial: Reconstitute vials with 1 mL of diluent to obtain concentration of 10 units per 0.1 mL; 2 mL of diluent to obtain concentration of 5 units per 0.1 mL; 4 mL of diluent to obtain concentration of 2.5 units per 0.1 mL; 8 mL of diluent to obtain concentration of 1.25 units per 0.1 mL; 10 mL of diluent to obtain concentration of 1 unit per 0.1 mL. Gently mix by rotating vial; discard vial if vacuum does not pull diluent into the vial.

Botox 200-unit vial: Reconstitute vials with 1 mL of diluent to obtain concentration of 20 units per 0.1 mL; 2 mL of diluent to obtain concentration of 10 units per 0.1 mL; 4 mL of diluent to obtain concentration of 5 units per 0.1 mL; 8 mL of diluent to obtain concentration of 2.5 units per 0.1 mL; 10 mL of diluent to obtain concentration of 2 units per 0.1 mL. Gently mix by rotating vial; discard vial if vacuum does not pull diluent into the vial.

Botox Cosmetic: Reconstitute 50-unit vial with 1.25 mL of diluent or 100-unit vial with 2.5 mL of diluent to obtain concentration of 4 units per 0.1 mL (20 units per 0.5 mL for glabellar lines and 24 units per 0.6 mL for lateral canthal lines). Reconstitute vial using an appropriate sized needle and syringe by inserting needle into vial at a 45° angle and allowing vacuum to pull diluent into vial (do not use if vacuum has been lost); mix gently.

Detrusor overactivity associated with a neurologic condition: Dilution recommendations:

Botox 100-unit vial: Reconstitute two 100 unit vials, each with 6 mL of preservative free NS; mix gently. Withdraw 4 mL from each vial into each of two 10 mL syringes; withdraw remaining 2 mL from each vial into the third 10 mL syringe for a total of 4 mL in each of the three 10 mL syringes. To complete dilution, add 6 mL of preservative-free NS into each of the three 10 mL syringes and mix gently; each of the 10 mL syringes will contain 10 mL (~6.7 units/mL) for a total of 200 units.

Botox 200-unit vial: Reconstitute with 6 mL of preservative free NS; mix gently. Withdraw 2 mL from the vial into each of three 10 mL syringes. To complete dilution, add 8 mL of preservative free NS into each of the three 10 mL syringes and mix gently; each of the 10 mL syringes will contain 10 mL (~6.7 units/mL) for a total of 200 units.

Administration

Parenteral: **Note:** For IM or intradermal administration only by individuals understanding the relevant neuromuscular and orbital anatomy and any alterations to the anatomy due to prior surgical procedures and standard electromyographic techniques. Local site reactions may be minimized by careful injection into the target muscle, using a minimal volume, and slowing the rate of injection.

IM: **Note:** Dilution concentration is dependent on indication; see product labeling for details.

Blepharospasm: Administer IM using a 27- or 30-gauge needle without electromyography guidance. Avoid injecting near the levator palpebrae superioris (may decrease ptosis); avoid medial lower lid injections (may decrease diplopia). Apply pressure at the injection site to prevent ecchymosis in the soft eyelid tissues.

Cervical dystonia: Administer IM using 25-, 27-, or 30-gauge needle for superficial muscles and a longer 22-gauge needle for deeper musculature; electromyography may help localize the involved muscles.

Chronic migraines: Adults: Administer IM using a 0.5-inch, 30-gauge needle to administer 5 units/0.1 mL to each of the 31 sites in the head/neck muscle areas; a 1-inch needle may be needed in the neck region for patients with thick neck muscles. All muscles except the procerus muscle (single injection only) should be injected bilaterally with half the number of injections administered on the left side and the other half administered on the right side.

Spasticity (focal): Administer IM using a 25-, 27-, or 30-gauge needle for superficial muscles and a longer 22-gauge needle for deeper musculature; electromyography or nerve stimulation may help localize the involved muscles.

Strabismus injections: Administer IM into extraocular muscles utilizing the electrical activity recorded from the tip of the injections needle as a guide to placement within the target muscle. Local anesthetic and ocular decongestant should be given before injection. Injection without surgical exposure or EMG guidance should not be attempted. Health care providers should be familiar with EMG technique. To prepare the eye for injection, it is recommended that several drops of a local anesthetic and an ocular decongestant be given several minutes prior to injection. The volume of injection should be 0.05 to 0.15 mL per muscle. Many patients will require additional doses because of inadequate response to initial dose.

Reduction of glabellar lines (Botox Cosmetic): Adults: Administer IM using a 30- to 33-gauge needle. Inject into each of 5 sites (2 injections in each corrugator muscle and 1 injection in the procerus muscle). Ensure injected volume/dose is accurate and where feasible keep to a minimum. Avoid injection near the levator palpebrae superioris. Lateral corrugator injections should be at least 1 cm above the bony supraorbital ridge. Do not inject toxin closer than 1 cm above the central eyebrow.

Reduction of lateral canthal lines (Botox Cosmetic): Adults: Administer IM using a 30- to 33-gauge needle and give injections with the needle bevel tip up and oriented away from the eye. Inject into 3 sites per side (6 total injection points) in the lateral orbicularis oculi muscle. The first injection should be approximately 1.5 to 2.0 cm temporal to the lateral canthus and just temporal to the orbital rim. If the lines are above and below the lateral canthus, administer the next 2 injections above and below the first injection point. Inject at a similar distance from the orbital rim at a position approximately 30° from the first injection. If the lines in the lateral canthal region are primarily below the lateral canthus, inject the next 2 injections below the first injection at a similar distance from the orbital rim.

Intradermal: **Primary axillary hyperhidrosis:** Adults: Administer intradermally using a 30-gauge needle. Inject each dose intradermally to a depth of ~2 mm and at a 45° angle with the bevel side up to minimize leakage and to ensure the injections remain intradermal. If injection sites are marked in ink, do not inject directly into areas marked in ink to avoid permanent tattoo effect. Prior to administration, injection area should be defined by standard staining techniques such as Minor's Iodine-Starch Test.

Monitoring Parameters Monitor patients closely for signs/symptoms of systemic toxic effects (possibly occurring 1 day to several weeks after treatment)

Cervical dystonia: Toronto Western Spasmodic Torticollis Rating Scale (TWSTRS) which evaluates severity, disability, and pain

Cerebral palsy: Modified Ashworth Scale, Tardieu Scale, Gross Motor Function Measure; treatment goals include improved gait and balance, facilitation of patient care, increased comfort with therapy, improved tolerance of bracing, and prevention of musculoskeletal complications

Dosage Forms Excipient information presented when available (limited, particularly for generics); consult specific product labeling.

Solution Reconstituted, Injection:

Botox: 100 units (1 ea)

Solution Reconstituted, Injection [preservative free]:

Botox: 200 units (1 ea)

Solution Reconstituted, Intramuscular:

Botox Cosmetic: 100 units (1 ea) [contains albumin human]

Solution Reconstituted, Intramuscular [preservative free]:

Botox Cosmetic: 50 units (1 ea) [contains albumin human]

◆ **Oncaspar** *see* Pegaspargase *on page 1639*

◆ **Oncovin** *see* VinCRIStine *on page 2179*

Ondansetron (on DAN se tron)

Medication Safety Issues

Sound-alike/look-alike issues:

Ondansetron may be confused with dolasetron, granisetron, palonosetron

Zofran may be confused with Zantac, Zosyn

Related Information

Prevention of Chemotherapy-Induced Nausea and Vomiting in Children *on page 2368*

Serotonin Syndrome *on page 2447*

Brand Names: US Zofran; Zofran ODT; Zuplenz

Brand Names: Canada Apo-Ondansetron; Ava-Ondansetron; CO Ondansetron; Dom-Ondansetron; JAMP-Ondansetron; Mar-Ondansetron; Mint-Ondansetron; Mylan-Ondansetron; Ondansetron Injection; Ondansetron Injection USP; Ondansetron-Odan; Ondansetron-Omega; Ondissolve ODF; PHL-Ondansetron; PMS-Ondansetron; RAN-Ondansetron; ratio-Ondansetron; Riva-Ondansetron; Sandoz-Ondansetron; Septa-Ondansetron; Teva-Ondansetron; Zofran; Zofran ODT

Therapeutic Category 5-HT_3 Receptor Antagonist; Antiemetic

Generic Availability (US) May be product dependent

Use

Oral:

Orally disintegrating tablets, oral solution, oral tablets: Prevention of nausea and vomiting associated with moderately emetogenic cancer chemotherapy (FDA approved in ages ≥4 years and adults); prevention of nausea and vomiting associated with highly emetogenic cancer chemotherapy (including cisplatin) (FDA approved in ages ≥4 years and adults); prevention of nausea and vomiting associated with radiotherapy (FDA approved in adults); prevention of postoperative nausea and vomiting (FDA approved in adults); has also been used in the treatment of hyperemesis gravidarum

Soluble Film (Zuplenz): Prevention of nausea and vomiting associated with moderately emetogenic cancer chemotherapy (FDA approved in ages ≥4 years and adults); prevention of nausea and vomiting associated with highly emetogenic cancer chemotherapy or radiotherapy (FDA approved in adults); prevention of postoperative nausea and vomiting (PONV) (FDA approved in adults)

Parenteral: Prevention of nausea and vomiting associated emetogenic cancer chemotherapy [including high-dose cisplatin (highly emetogenic)] (FDA approved in ages ≥6 months and adults); prevention of postoperative nausea and vomiting (FDA approved in ages ≥1 month and adults); has also been used in the treatment of acute gastroenteritis, cyclic vomiting syndrome, and hyperemesis gravidarum

Pregnancy Risk Factor B

Pregnancy Considerations Teratogenic effects were not observed in animal reproduction studies. Ondansetron readily crosses the human placenta in the first trimester of pregnancy and can be detected in fetal tissue (Siu, 2006). The use of ondansetron for the treatment of nausea and vomiting of pregnancy (NVP) has been evaluated. Although a significant increase in birth defects has not been described in case reports and some studies (Ferreira, 2012; Pasternak, 2013), other studies have shown a possible association with ondansetron exposure and adverse fetal events (Anderka, 2012; Einarson, 2004). Additional studies are needed to determine safety to the fetus, particularly during the first trimester. Based on available data, use is generally reserved for severe NVP (hyperemesis gravidarum) or when conventional treatments are not effective (ACOG, 2004; Koren, 2012; Levicheck, 2002; Tan, 2011). Because a dose-dependent QT-interval prolongation occurs with use, the manufacturer recommends ECG monitoring in patients with electrolyte abnormalities (which can be associated with some cases of NVP; Koren, 2012). An international consensus panel recommends that 5-HT_3 antagonists (including ondansetron) should not be withheld in pregnant patients receiving chemotherapy for the treatment of gynecologic cancers, when chemotherapy is given according to general recommendations for chemotherapy use during pregnancy (Amant, 2010).

Breast-Feeding Considerations It is not known if ondansetron is excreted into breast milk. The U.S. manufacturer labeling recommends caution be used if administered to nursing women. The Canadian labeling recommends avoiding nursing during ondansetron treatment.

Contraindications Hypersensitivity to ondansetron or any component of the formulation; concomitant use of apomorphine

Warnings/Precautions Antiemetics are most effective when used prophylactically (Roila, 2010). If emesis occurs despite optimal antiemetic prophylaxis, reevaluate emetic risk, disease, concurrent morbidities and medications to assure antiemetic regimen is optimized (Basch, 2011). Does not stimulate gastric or intestinal peristalsis; may mask progressive ileus and/or gastric distension. Use with caution in patients allergic to other 5-HT_3 receptor antagonists; cross-reactivity has been reported.

Dose-dependent QT interval prolongation occurs with ondansetron use. Cases of torsade de pointes have also been reported to the manufacturer. Selective 5-HT_3 antagonists, including ondansetron, have been associated with a number of dose-dependent increases in ECG intervals (eg, PR, QRS duration, QT/QTc, JT), usually occurring 1 to 2 hours after IV administration. Single doses >16 mg ondansetron IV are no longer recommended due to the potential for an increased risk of QT prolongation. In most patients, these changes are not clinically relevant; however, when used in conjunction with other agents that prolong these intervals or in those at risk for QT prolongation, arrhythmia may occur. When used with agents that prolong the QT interval (eg, Class I and III antiarrhythmics) or in patients with cardiovascular disease, clinically relevant QT interval prolongation may occur resulting in torsade de pointes. Avoid ondansetron use in patients with congenital long QT syndrome. Use caution and monitor ECG in patients with other risk factors for QT prolongation (eg, medications known to prolong QT interval, electrolyte abnormalities [hypokalemia or hypomagnesemia], heart failure, bradyarrhythmias, and cumulative high-dose anthracycline therapy). IV formulations of 5-HT_3 antagonists have more association with ECG interval changes, compared to oral formulations. Dose limitations are recommended for patients with severe hepatic impairment (Child-Pugh class C); use with caution in mild-moderate hepatic impairment; clearance is decreased and half-life increased in hepatic impairment.

Serotonin syndrome has been reported with 5-HT_3 receptor antagonists, predominantly when used in combination with other serotonergic agents (eg, SSRIs, SNRIs, MAOIs, mirtazapine, fentanyl, lithium, tramadol, and/or methylene blue). Some of the cases have been fatal. The majority of serotonin syndrome reports due to 5-HT_3 receptor antagonist have occurred in a postanesthesia setting or in an infusion center. Serotonin syndrome has also been reported following overdose of ondansetron. Monitor patients for signs of serotonin syndrome, including mental status changes (eg, agitation, hallucinations, delirium, coma); autonomic instability (eg, tachycardia, labile blood pressure, diaphoresis, dizziness, flushing, hyperthermia); neuromuscular changes (eg, tremor, rigidity, myoclonus, hyperreflexia, incoordination); gastrointestinal symptoms (eg, nausea, vomiting, diarrhea); and/or seizures. If serotonin syndrome occurs, discontinue 5-HT_3 receptor antagonist treatment and begin supportive management. Potentially significant drug-drug interactions may exist, requiring dose or frequency adjustment, additional monitoring, and/or selection of alternative therapy. Orally disintegrating tablets contain phenylalanine.

Benzyl alcohol and derivatives: Some dosage forms may contain sodium benzoate/benzoic acid; benzoic acid (benzoate) is a metabolite of benzyl alcohol; large amounts of benzyl alcohol (≥99 mg/kg/day) have been associated with a potentially fatal toxicity ("gasping syndrome") in neonates; the "gasping syndrome" consists of metabolic acidosis, respiratory distress, gasping respirations, CNS dysfunction (including convulsions, intracranial hemorrhage), hypotension, and cardiovascular collapse (AAP, 1997; CDC, 1982); some data suggests that benzoate displaces bilirubin from protein binding sites (Ahlfors, 2001); avoid or use dosage forms containing benzyl alcohol derivative with caution in neonates. See manufacturer's labeling.

Adverse Reactions

Central nervous system: Agitation (oral), anxiety (oral), dizziness, drowsiness (IV), fatigue (oral), headache (more common in oral), malaise (oral), paresthesia (IV), sedation (IV), sensation of cold (IV)

Dermatologic: Pruritus, skin rash

Gastrointestinal: Constipation, diarrhea (more common in oral)

Genitourinary: Gynecologic disease (oral), urinary retention (oral)

Hepatic: Increased serum ALT (>2 times ULN; transient), increased serum AST (>2 times ULN; transient)

Local: Injection site reaction (IV, includes burning sensation at injection site, erythema at injection site, injection site pain)

Respiratory: Hypoxia (oral)

Miscellaneous: Fever

Rare but important or life-threatening: Abdominal pain, accommodation disturbance, atrial fibrillation, cardiorespiratory arrest (IV), depression of ST segment on ECG, dyspnea, extrapyramidal reaction (IV), flushing, hepatic failure (when used with other hepatotoxic medications), hiccups, hypersensitivity reaction, hypokalemia, hypotension, laryngospasm (IV), liver enzyme disorder, mucosal tissue reaction, myocardial infarction, neuroleptic malignant syndrome, positive lymphocyte transformation test, prolonged Q-T interval on ECG (dose dependent), second-degree atrioventricular block, serotonin syndrome, shock (IV), Stevens-Johnson syndrome, supraventricular tachycardia, syncope, tachycardia, tonic-clonic seizures, torsades de pointes, transient blindness (lasted ≤48 hours), transient blurred vision (following infusion), vascular occlusive events, ventricular premature contractions, ventricular tachycardia, weakness

Drug Interactions

Metabolism/Transport Effects Substrate of CYP1A2 (minor), CYP2C9 (minor), CYP2D6 (minor), CYP2E1 (minor), CYP3A4 (major), P-glycoprotein; **Note:** Assignment of Major/Minor substrate status based on clinically relevant drug interaction potential; **Inhibits** CYP1A2 (weak), CYP2C9 (weak), CYP2D6 (weak)

Avoid Concomitant Use

Avoid concomitant use of Ondansetron with any of the following: Apomorphine; Highest Risk QTc-Prolonging Agents; Ivabradine; Mifepristone

Increased Effect/Toxicity

Ondansetron may increase the levels/effects of: Apomorphine; ARIPiprazole; Highest Risk QTc-Prolonging Agents; Moderate Risk QTc-Prolonging Agents; Panobinostat; Serotonin Modulators; TiZANidine

The levels/effects of Ondansetron may be increased by: Ivabradine; Mifepristone; P-glycoprotein/ABCB1 Inhibitors; QTc-Prolonging Agents (Indeterminate Risk and Risk Modifying)

Decreased Effect

Ondansetron may decrease the levels/effects of: Tapentadol; TraMADol

The levels/effects of Ondansetron may be decreased by: Bosentan; CYP3A4 Inducers (Moderate); CYP3A4 Inducers (Strong); Dabrafenib; Deferasirox; Mitotane; P-glycoprotein/ABCB1 Inducers; Siltuximab; St Johns Wort; Tocilizumab

Food Interactions Tablet: Food slightly increases the extent of absorption. Management: Administer without regard to meals.

Storage/Stability

Oral soluble film: Store between 20°C and 25°C (68°F and 77°F). Store pouches in cartons; keep film in individual pouch until ready to use.

Oral solution: Store between 15°C and 30°C (59°F and 86°F). Protect from light.

Tablet: Store between 2°C and 30°C (36°F and 86°F).

Vial: Store between 2°C and 30°C (36°F and 86°F). Protect from light. Stable when mixed in D_5W or NS for 48 hours at room temperature.

Premixed bag in D_5W: Store at 20°C to 25°C (68°F to 77°F), excursions permitted from 15°C to 30°C (59°F to 86°F); may refrigerate; avoid freezing and excessive heat; protect from light.

Mechanism of Action Selective 5-HT_3-receptor antagonist, blocking serotonin, both peripherally on vagal nerve terminals and centrally in the chemoreceptor trigger zone

Pharmacokinetics (Adult data unless noted)

Absorption: Oral: 100%; nonlinear absorption occurs with increasing oral doses; Zofran ODT tablets are bioequivalent to Zofran tablets; absorption does not occur via oral mucosa

Distribution: V_d:
- Infants and Children: Surgical patients:
  - 1 to 4 months: 3.5 L/kg
  - 5 to 24 months: 2.3 L/kg
  - 3 to 12 years: 1.65 L/kg
- Children and Adolescents: Cancer patients: 4 to 18 years: 1.9 L/kg
- Adults: 1.9 L/kg

Protein binding, plasma: 70% to 76%

Metabolism: Some first-pass metabolism; primarily by hydroxylation, followed by glucuronidation and sulfate conjugation; CYP1A2, CYP2D6, and CYP3A4 substrate; some demethylation occurs

Bioavailability: Oral: 50% to 70% due to some first-pass metabolism; in cancer patients (adults) 85% to 87% bioavailability possibly related to changes in metabolism

Half-life:
- Pediatric:
  - Cancer patients: Children and Adolescents: 4 to 18 years: 2.8 hours
  - Surgical patients:
    - Infants 1 to 4 months: 6.7 hours
    - Infants and Children 5 months to 12 years: 2.9 hours
- Adult: 3.5 to 5.5 hours
  - Mild to moderate hepatic impairment (Child-Pugh A-B): 12 hours
  - Severe hepatic impairment (Child-Pugh C): 20 hours

Elimination: In urine and feces; <5% of the parent drug is recovered unchanged in urine
- Pediatric:
  - Cancer patients: Children and Adolescents 4 to 18 years: 0.599 L/kg/hour
  - Surgical patients: Infants and Children:
    - 1 to 4 months: 0.401 L/kg/hour
    - 5 to 24 months: 0.581 L/kg/hour
    - 3 to 12 years: 0.439 L/kg/hour
- Adult (normal):
  - 19 to 40 years: 0.381 L/kg/hour
  - 61 to 74 years: 0.319 L/kg/hour
  - >75 years: 0.262 L/kg/hour

Dosing: Usual

Pediatric:

Chemotherapy-induced nausea and vomiting, prevention: IV: Infants (Limited data available in infants <6 months), Children, and Adolescents:

Manufacturer's labeling:

IV: Infants ≥6 months, Children, and Adolescents: *Moderately to highly emetogenic antineoplastic therapy:* 0.15 mg/kg/dose; maximum dose: 16 mg/dose; administer first dose 30 minutes before the start chemotherapy with subsequent doses administered 4 and 8 hours after the first dose for 3 doses total

Oral: *Highly and moderately emetogenic antineoplastic therapy:*

Children 4 to 11 years: 4 mg beginning 30 minutes before chemotherapy; repeat 4 and 8 hours after initial dose, then 4 mg every 8 hours for 1 to 2 days after chemotherapy completed

Children and Adolescents ≥12 years: 8 mg beginning 30 minutes before chemotherapy; repeat dose 8 hours after initial dose, then 8 mg every 12 hours for 1 to 2 days after chemotherapy completed

Alternate dosing:

Weight-directed dosing: Infants, Children, and Adolescents:

Highly emetogenic antineoplastic therapy: IV, Oral: 0.15 mg/kg/dose; maximum dose: 16 mg/dose; administer first dose before the start chemotherapy and then every 8 hours (Dupuis, 2013); a once-daily single dose of 0.3 mg/kg or 0.45 mg/kg (maximum dose: 16 mg) dependent upon emetogenic potential of chemotherapy has also been reported (Holdsworth, 2006)

Moderately emetogenic antineoplastic therapy: IV, Oral: 0.15 mg/kg/dose; maximum dose: 8 mg/dose; administer first dose before the start of chemotherapy with subsequent doses every 12 hours (Dupuis, 2013)

Low emetogenic antineoplastic therapy: IV, Oral: 0.3 mg/kg/dose once; maximum dose: 16 mg/dose; administered 30 minutes before the start of chemotherapy (Dupuis, 2013)

BSA-directed dosing:

Highly emetogenic antineoplastic therapy: Infants, Children, and Adolescents: IV, Oral: 5 mg/m^2/dose; maximum dose: 16 mg/dose; administer first dose before the start chemotherapy with subsequent doses administered every 8 hours (Dupuis, 2013)

Moderately emetogenic antineoplastic therapy: Infants, Children, and Adolescents: IV, Oral: 5 mg/m^2/dose; maximum dose: 8 mg/dose; administer first before the start of chemotherapy with subsequent doses every 12 hours (Dupuis, 2013)

Low emetogenic antineoplastic therapy: Infants, Children, and Adolescents: IV, Oral: 10 mg/m^2/dose once; maximum dose: 16 mg/dose; administered before the start of chemotherapy (Dupuis, 2013)

Cyclic vomiting syndrome (CVS); treatment of acute attack Limited data available; dosing based on case reports and clinical experience: Children >2 years and Adolescents:

Low dose: IV: 0.15 mg/kg every 4 hours as needed for up to 3 doses; maximum dose: 16 mg/dose (Fleisher, 1995)

High dose: IV: 0.3 to 0.4 mg/kg/dose every 4 to 6 hours; maximum dose: 16 mg/dose (Li, 2008); per manufacturer labeling, should not exceed 3 doses in a 24-hour period

Gastroenteritis, acute; treatment: Note: Routine use of ondansetron is not recommended in most cases of acute gastroenteritis (AAP, 2004; CDC, 2003)

IV: Infants and Children ≥1 month: 0.15 or 0.3 mg/kg/dose once; maximum dose: 16 mg/dose (DeCamp, 2008)

Oral: Infants and Children 6 months to 10 years, ≥8 kg (Freedman, 2006):

8 to 15 kg: 2 mg/dose once

>15 to 30 kg: 4 mg/dose once

>30 kg: 8 mg/dose once

Postoperative nausea and vomiting; prevention: IV: Administer immediately before or following induction of anesthesia, or postoperatively if the patient is symptomatic:

Infants and Children 1 month to 12 years and ≤40 kg: 0.1 mg/kg/dose; maximum dose: 4 mg/dose

Children >40 kg and Adolescents: 4 mg/dose

Note: Repeat doses given in response to inadequate control of nausea/vomiting from preoperative doses are generally ineffective.

Radiation-induced nausea and vomiting, prevention: Limited data available: Oral:

Weight-directed dosing: Infants ≥ 5 months, Children, and Adolescents: 0.2 mg/kg/dose (maximum dose: 8 mg/dose) administered every 8 hours throughout total body irradiation (TBI) prior to HSCT (n = 68; mean age: 6.7 years; range: 5 months to 20 years); doses were generally rounded to 4 mg/dose in children 4 to11 years and 8 mg/dose in children ≥12 years and adolescents (Applegate, 1998)

Alternate weight-based dosing: Children and Adolescents: 0.15 mg/kg/dose administered 3 to 4 times daily throughout TBI (n = 33; mean age: 9 years; range: 13 months to 16 years) (Farah, 1998)

Fixed dose: **Note:** Derived from rounding weight based (0.2 mg/kg/dose) doses (Applegate, 1998)

Children 4 to 11 years: 4 mg every 8 hours throughout total body irradiation (TBI) prior to HSCT

Children ≥12 years and Adolescents: 8 mg every 8 hours throughout total body irradiation (TBI) prior to HSCT

Alternate fixed-dosing: Children ≥9 years and Adolescents: 8 mg every 12 hours on days of TBI prior to bone marrow transplantation (age range: 9 to 67 years; median age range: 39 to 49 years). **Note:** Administered in combination with dexamethasone (Bredeson, 2002).

Adult:

Chemotherapy-induced nausea and vomiting, prevention:

IV: 0.15 mg/kg/dose (maximum dose: 16 mg) over 15 minutes for 3 doses, beginning 30 minutes prior to chemotherapy, followed by subsequent doses 4 and 8 hours after the first dose

Oral:

Highly emetogenic chemotherapy: 24 mg given as three 8 mg tablets 30 minutes prior to the start of single-day chemotherapy

Moderately emetogenic chemotherapy: 8 mg beginning 30 minutes before chemotherapy; repeat dose 8 hours after initial dose, then 8 mg every 12 hours for 1 to 2 days after chemotherapy completed

Postoperative nausea and vomiting (PONV), prevention: Note: The manufacturer recommends administration immediately before induction of anesthesia; however, this has been shown not to be as effective as administration at the end of surgery (Sun, 1997). Repeat doses given in response to inadequate control of nausea/vomiting from preoperative doses are generally ineffective.

IM, IV: 4 mg as a single dose administered ~30 minutes before the end of anesthesia or as treatment if vomiting occurs after surgery (Gan, 2007).

Oral: 16 mg administered 1 hour prior to induction of anesthesia

Radiation-induced nausea and vomiting, prevention:
Total body irradiation: Oral: 8 mg administered 1 to 2 hours before each daily fraction of radiotherapy
Single high-dose fraction radiotherapy to abdomen: Oral: 8 mg administered 1 to 2 hours before irradiation, then 8 mg every 8 hours after first dose for 1 to 2 days after completion of radiotherapy
Daily fractionated radiotherapy to abdomen: Oral: 8 mg administered 1 to 2 hours before irradiation, then 8 mg 8 hours after first dose for each day of radiotherapy
Hyperemesis gravidum, treatment:
IV: 8 mg administered over 15 minutes every 12 hours (ACOG, 2004)
Oral: 8 mg every 12 hours (Levichek, 2002)
Dosing adjustment in renal impairment: No dosage adjustments are recommended (there is no experience for oral ondansetron beyond day 1).
Dosing adjustment in hepatic impairment: Adults:
Mild to moderate impairment: No dosage adjustment necessary.
Severe impairment (Child-Pugh C):
IV: Day 1: Maximum dose: 8 mg (there is no experience beyond day 1)
Oral: Maximum daily dose: 8 mg/day

Preparation for Administration
Parenteral: IVPB infusion:
Prevention of chemotherapy-induced nausea and vomiting: Dilute to a maximum concentration of 1 mg/mL
Cyclic vomiting syndrome: Dilute in 50 to100 mL of D_5W (Fleischer 1995)

Administration
Oral (all dosage forms): May administer without regard to meals. Administer 30 minutes prior to chemotherapy and 1 to 2 hours prior to radiotherapy.
Orally disintegrating tablet (Zofran ODT): Do not remove from blister until needed. Peel backing off the blister; do not push tablet through foil backing. Using dry hands, place tablet on tongue and allow to dissolve; swallow with saliva
Soluble film (Zuplenz): Do not remove from pouch until immediately before use. Using dry hands, place film on top of tongue and allow to dissolve (4 to 20 seconds). Swallow with or without liquid. If using more than one film, allow each film to dissolve completely before administering the next film.
Parenteral:
IV:
IVPB infusion:
Prevention of chemotherapy-induced nausea and vomiting: Infuse over 15 minutes
Cyclic vomiting syndrome: Infuse over 15 to 30 minutes (Fleischer 1995)
IV push: May be administered undiluted IV over 2 to 5 minutes for prevention of PONV
IM: Administer as undiluted injection; use only in adults

Monitoring Parameters Closely monitor patients <4 months of age; baseline ECG (if applicable); serum electrolytes (K/Mg); emesis episodes

Dosage Forms Excipient information presented when available (limited, particularly for generics); consult specific product labeling.
Film, Oral:
Zuplenz: 4 mg (1 ea, 10 ea); 8 mg (1 ea, 10 ea)
Solution, Injection:
Zofran: 40 mg/20 mL (20 mL) [contains methylparaben, propylparaben]
Generic: 4 mg/2 mL (2 mL); 40 mg/20 mL (20 mL)
Solution, Injection [preservative free]:
Generic: 4 mg/2 mL (2 mL)
Solution, Oral:
Zofran: 4 mg/5 mL (50 mL) [strawberry flavor]
Generic: 4 mg/5 mL (50 mL)
Tablet, Oral:
Zofran: 4 mg, 8 mg
Generic: 4 mg, 8 mg, 24 mg
Tablet Dispersible, Oral:
Zofran ODT: 4 mg, 8 mg [contains aspartame, methylparaben sodium, propylparaben sodium; strawberry flavor]
Generic: 4 mg, 8 mg

Extemporaneous Preparations Note: Commercial oral solution is available (0.8 mg/mL)

If commercial oral solution is unavailable, a 0.8 mg/mL syrup may be made with ondansetron tablets, Ora-Plus® (Paddock), and any of the the following syrups: Cherry syrup USP, Syrpalta® (HUMCO), Ora-Sweet® (Paddock), or Ora-Sweet® Sugar-Free (Paddock). Crush ten 8 mg tablets in a mortar and reduce to a fine powder (flaking of the tablet coating occurs). Add 50 mL Ora-Plus® in 5 mL increments, mixing thoroughly; mix while adding the chosen syrup in incremental proportions to **almost** 100 mL; transfer to a calibrated bottle, rinse mortar with syrup, and add sufficient quantity of syrup to make 100 mL. Label "shake well" and "refrigerate". Stable for 42 days refrigerated (Trissel, 1996).

Rectal suppositories: Calibrate a suppository mold for the base being used. Determine the displacement factor (DF) for ondansetron for the base being used (Fattibase® = 1.1; Polybase® = 0.6). Weigh the ondansetron tablet(s). Divide the tablet weight by the DF; this result is the weight of base displaced by the drug. Subtract the weight of base displaced from the calculated weight of base required for each suppository. Grind the ondansetron tablets in a mortar and reduce to a fine powder. Weigh out the appropriate weight of suppository base. Melt the base over a water bath (<55°C). Add the ondansetron powder to the suppository base and mix well. Pour the mixture into the suppository mold and cool. Stable for at least 30 days refrigerated (Tenjarla, 1998).

Tenjarla SN, Ward ES, and Fox JL, "Ondansetron Suppositories: Extemporaneous Preparation, Drug Release, Stability and Flux Through Rabbit Rectal Membrane," *Int J Pharm Compound*, 1998, 2(1):83-8.
Trissel LA, *Trissel's Stability of Compounded Formulations*, Washington, DC: American Pharmaceutical Association, 1996.

◆ **Ondansetron Hydrochloride** *see* Ondansetron *on page 1564*
◆ **Ondansetron Injection (Can)** *see* Ondansetron *on page 1564*
◆ **Ondansetron Injection USP (Can)** *see* Ondansetron *on page 1564*
◆ **Ondansetron-Odan (Can)** *see* Ondansetron *on page 1564*
◆ **Ondansetron-Omega (Can)** *see* Ondansetron *on page 1564*
◆ **Ondissolve ODF (Can)** *see* Ondansetron *on page 1564*
◆ **One Step Callus Remover [OTC]** *see* Salicylic Acid *on page 1894*
◆ **Onexton** *see* Clindamycin and Benzoyl Peroxide *on page 493*
◆ **Onfi** *see* CloBAZam *on page 495*
◆ **Onmel** *see* Itraconazole *on page 1176*
◆ **Onsolis [DSC]** *see* FentaNYL *on page 857*
◆ **Onxyl** *see* PACLitaxel (Conventional) *on page 1602*
◆ **OPC-14597** *see* ARIPiprazole *on page 193*
◆ **o,p'-DDD** *see* Mitotane *on page 1446*
◆ **Ophtho-Dipivefrin™ (Can)** *see* Dipivefrin *on page 687*
◆ **Opium and Belladonna** *see* Belladonna and Opium *on page 264*

Opium Tincture (OH pee um TING chur)

Medication Safety Issues

Sound-alike/look-alike issues:

Opium tincture may be confused with camphorated tincture of opium (paregoric)

High alert medication:

The Institute for Safe Medication Practices (ISMP) includes this medication among its list of drugs which have a heightened risk of causing significant patient harm when used in error.

Administration issues:

Use care when prescribing opium tincture; opium tincture is 25 times more concentrated than paregoric; each undiluted mL of opium tincture contains the equivalent of morphine 10 mg/mL.

If opium tincture is used in neonates (off-label), a 25-fold dilution should be prepared (final concentration: 0.4 mg/mL morphine). Of note, paregoric (which contains the equivalent of morphine 0.4 mg/mL) is **not** recommended for use in neonates due to the high alcohol content (~45%) and the presence of other additives; as an alternative to the use of diluted opium tincture or paregoric, ISMP recommends using a diluted preservative free injectable morphine solution orally.

Although historically opium tincture is dosed as mL/kg, the preferred dosing units are **mg**/kg (Levine, 2001). ISMP suggests hospitals evaluate the need for this product at their institution.

Other safety concerns:

DTO is an error-prone abbreviation and should never be used as an abbreviation for opium tincture (also known as *Deodorized* Tincture of Opium) due to potential for being mistaken as *Diluted* Tincture of Opium

Therapeutic Category Analgesic, Narcotic; Antidiarrheal

Generic Availability (US) Yes

Use Treatment of diarrhea in adults; has also been used for the treatment of neonatal abstinence syndrome (opioid withdrawal) using **a 25-fold dilution with water** (final concentration 0.4 mg/mL morphine)

Pregnancy Risk Factor C

Pregnancy Considerations Animal reproduction studies have not been conducted. Opium tincture contains morphine; refer to the Morphine (Systemic) monograph for additional information. In addition, this preparation contains large amounts of alcohol (19%).

Breast-Feeding Considerations Opium tincture contains morphine, which is excreted into breast milk; refer to the Morphine (Systemic) monograph for additional information. In addition, this preparation contains large amounts of alcohol (19%). The manufacturer recommends that caution be used if administered to a nursing woman.

Contraindications

Use in children; diarrhea caused by poisoning until the toxic material is eliminated from the GI tract

Documentation of allergenic cross-reactivity for opioids is limited. However, because of similarities in chemical structure and/or pharmacologic actions, the possibility of cross-sensitivity cannot be ruled out with certainty.

Warnings/Precautions May cause CNS depression, which may impair physical or mental abilities; patients must be cautioned about performing tasks which require mental alertness (eg, operating machinery or driving). Use with caution in patients with morbid obesity, adrenal insufficiency, hepatic impairment, biliary tract impairment, pancreatitis, head trauma, GI hemorrhage, thyroid dysfunction, prostatic hyperplasia/urinary stricture, respiratory disease, or a history of drug abuse. Avoid use in patients with CNS depression or coma as these patients are susceptible to intracranial effects of CO_2 retention. May cause hypotension; use with caution in patients with hypovolemia, cardiovascular disease (including acute MI), or with drugs which may exaggerate hypotensive effects (including phenothiazines or general anesthetics). May obscure diagnosis or clinical course of patients with acute abdominal conditions. Concurrent use of agonist/antagonist analgesics may precipitate withdrawal symptoms and/or reduced analgesic efficacy in patients following prolonged therapy with mu opioid agonists. Abrupt discontinuation following prolonged use may also lead to withdrawal symptoms. Use with caution in the elderly and debilitated patients; may be more sensitive to adverse effects. Potentially significant interactions may exist, requiring dose or frequency adjustment, additional monitoring, and/or selection of alternative therapy.

Do not confuse opium tincture with paregoric; opium tincture is 25 times more potent than paregoric; opium shares the toxic potential of opioid agonists, usual precautions of opioid agonist therapy should be observed; abrupt discontinuation after prolonged use may result in withdrawal symptoms. Infants <3 months of age are more susceptible to respiratory depression; if used (off-label), diluted doses are recommended and use with caution. Contraindicated for use in children according to the manufacturer. Opium tincture is not routinely used as a source of morphine to treat neonatal abstinence syndrome in infants exposed to chronic opioids *in utero*. If used, then dilution is necessary. In addition, use for this purpose may increase the risk of drug error and morphine overdose in the infant (AAP, 1998; Dow, 2012; Hudack, 2012).

Adverse Reactions

Cardiovascular: Bradycardia, hypotension, palpitations, peripheral vasodilation

Central nervous system: Central nervous system depression, depression, dizziness, drowsiness, drug dependence, headache, increased intracranial pressure, insomnia, malaise, restlessness

Gastrointestinal: Anorexia, biliary tract spasm, constipation, nausea, stomach cramps, vomiting

Genitourinary: Decreased urine output, genitourinary tract spasm

Hypersensitivity: Histamine release

Neuromuscular & skeletal: Weakness

Ophthalmic: Miosis

Respiratory: Respiratory depression

Rare but important or life-threatening: Hypogonadism (Brennan, 2013; Debono, 2011)

Drug Interactions

Metabolism/Transport Effects None known.

Avoid Concomitant Use

Avoid concomitant use of Opium Tincture with any of the following: Azelastine (Nasal); Eluxadoline; Mixed Agonist / Antagonist Opioids; Orphenadrine; Paraldehyde; Thalidomide

Increased Effect/Toxicity

Opium Tincture may increase the levels/effects of: Alcohol (Ethyl); Alvimopan; Azelastine (Nasal); CNS Depressants; Desmopressin; Diuretics; Eluxadoline; Hydrocodone; Methotrimeprazine; Metyrosine; Mirtazapine; Orphenadrine; Paraldehyde; Pramipexole; ROPINIRole; Rotigotine; Selective Serotonin Reuptake Inhibitors; Suvorexant; Thalidomide; Zolpidem

The levels/effects of Opium Tincture may be increased by: Amphetamines; Anticholinergic Agents; Antipsychotic Agents (Phenothiazines); Brimonidine (Topical); Cannabis; Doxylamine; Dronabinol; Droperidol; HydrOXYzine; Kava Kava; Magnesium Sulfate; Methotrimeprazine; Nabilone; Perampanel; Rufinamide; Sodium Oxybate; Succinylcholine; Tapentadol; Tetrahydrocannabinol

Decreased Effect

Opium Tincture may decrease the levels/effects of: Pegvisomant

The levels/effects of Opium Tincture may be decreased by: Ammonium Chloride; Mixed Agonist / Antagonist Opioids; Naltrexone

Storage/Stability Store at 68°F to 77°F (20°C to 25°C). Protect from light.

Mechanism of Action Contains many opioid alkaloids including morphine; its mechanism for gastric motility inhibition is primarily due to this morphine content; it results in a decrease in digestive secretions, an increase in GI muscle tone, and therefore a reduction in GI propulsion

Pharmacodynamics Duration: 4-5 hours

Pharmacokinetics (Adult data unless noted)

Absorption: Variable from GI tract

Metabolism: In the liver

Elimination: In urine and bile

Dosing: Neonatal Oral: **Note:** The following doses are expressed in **mg/kg** or **mg** dosing units of morphine.

Full-term neonates: Neonatal abstinence syndrome (opioid withdrawal): **Use a 25-fold dilution of opium tincture** (final concentration: 0.4 mg/mL morphine)

Initial: Give 0.04 **mg/kg**/dose of a 0.4 mg/mL solution with feedings every 3-4 hours; increase as needed by 0.04 **mg/kg**/dose of a 0.4 mg/mL solution every 3-4 hours until withdrawal symptoms are controlled

Usual dose: 0.08-0.2 **mg**/dose given every 3-4 hours; it is rare to exceed 0.28 **mg**/dose; stabilize withdrawal symptoms for 3-5 days, then gradually decrease the dosage (keeping the same dosage interval) over a 2- to 4-week period

Dosing: Usual Oral: **Note:** The following doses are expressed in **mg/kg** or **mg** dosing units of morphine.

Adults: Diarrhea: Usual: 6 **mg** of undiluted opium tincture (10 mg/mL morphine) every 6 hours

Preparation for Administration Note: Each undiluted mL of opium tincture contains the equivalent of morphine 10 mg/mL.

Oral: Neonatal abstinence syndrome (opioid withdrawal): Must be diluted prior to administration, use a 25-fold dilution of opium tincture; final concentration: 0.4 mg/mL of morphine

Administration Oral: May administer with food to decrease GI upset; for neonatal abstinence syndrome (opioid withdrawal), use a 25-fold dilution of opium tincture (final concentration 0.4 mg/mL morphine)

Monitoring Parameters Respiratory rate, blood pressure, heart rate, resolution of diarrhea, mental status; if using a 25-fold dilution to treat neonatal abstinence syndrome, monitor for resolution of withdrawal symptoms (such as irritability, high-pitched cry, stuffy nose, rhinorrhea, vomiting, poor feeding, diarrhea, sneezing, yawning etc), and signs of overtreatment (such as bradycardia, lethargy, hypotonia, irregular respirations, respiratory depression etc). An abstinence scoring system (eg, Finnegan abstinence scoring system) can be used to more objectively assess neonatal opioid withdrawal symptoms and the need for dosage adjustment.

Test Interactions Increased aminotransferase [ALT/AST] (S)

Additional Information Opium tincture contains 10 mg/mL morphine; for treatment of neonatal abstinence syndrome, a 25-fold dilution of opium tincture (final concentration: 0.4 mg/mL morphine) is preferred over paregoric; the 25-fold dilution of opium tincture contains the same morphine concentration as paregoric, but without the high amount of alcohol or additives of paregoric

Controlled Substance C-II

Dosage Forms Excipient information presented when available (limited, particularly for generics); consult specific product labeling.

Tincture, Oral:

Generic: 10 mg/mL (1%) (118 mL, 473 mL)

◆ **Opium Tincture, Deodorized** *see* Opium Tincture *on page 1569*

Oprelvekin (oh PREL ve kin)

Medication Safety Issues

Sound-alike/look-alike issues:

Oprelvekin may be confused with aldesleukin, Proleukin

Neumega may be confused with Neulasta, Neupogen

Brand Names: US Neumega

Therapeutic Category Biological Response Modulator; Thrombopoietic Growth Factor

Generic Availability (US) No

Use Prevention of severe thrombocytopenia and the reduction of the need for platelet transfusions following myelosuppressive chemotherapy in adult patients with nonmyeloid malignancies who are at high risk of severe thrombocytopenia (FDA approved in adults)

Pregnancy Risk Factor C

Pregnancy Considerations Adverse events have been observed in animal reproduction studies

Breast-Feeding Considerations It is not known if oprelvekin is excreted in breast milk. Due to the potential for serious adverse reactions in breast-feeding infants, the manufacturer recommends a decision be made to discontinue breast-feeding or the drug, taking into account the importance of treatment to the mother.

Contraindications Hypersensitivity to oprelvekin or any component of the formulation

Warnings/Precautions [US Boxed Warning]: Allergic or hypersensitivity reactions, including anaphylaxis, have been reported. Permanently discontinue in any patient developing an allergic or hypersensitivity reaction. Reaction may occur with the first or with subsequent doses. Allergic reactions included facial/tongue/larynx edema, dyspnea, wheezing, chest pain, hypotension (including shock), rash, urticaria, flushing, fever, loss of consciousness, mental status changes, and/or dysarthria.

Arrhythmias, pulmonary edema, and cardiac arrest have been reported; use in patients with a history of atrial arrhythmia only if the potential benefit exceeds possible risks. Stroke has been reported in patients who develop atrial fibrillation/flutter while receiving oprelvekin. Ventricular arrhythmia has also been reported, occurring within 2 to 7 days of treatment initiation. May cause serious fluid retention, which may result in peripheral edema, dyspnea, pulmonary edema, capillary leak syndrome, atrial arrhythmias, and exacerbation of preexisting pleural effusion. Serious fluid retention (sometimes fatal) has been reported. Use with caution in patients with clinically evident heart failure or who may be susceptible to developing heart failure, patients receiving aggressive hydration, patients with a history of heart failure who are well compensated and receiving appropriate medical therapy, and patients who may develop fluid retention as a result of associated medical conditions or whose medical condition may be exacerbated by fluid retention. Monitor fluid and electrolyte status; preexisting fluid collections, including pericardial effusions or ascites, should also be monitored. Dilutional anemia may occur due to increased plasma volume; presenting as moderate decreases in hemoglobin concentration, hematocrit, and red blood cells without a decrease in red blood cell mass; effect generally appears within 3 to 5 days of initiation of therapy and resolves over approximately 1 week following oprelvekin discontinuation.

Papilledema has occurred, usually following repeated cycles. The incidence of papilledema occurred more frequently in children. Use with caution in patients with preexisting papilledema or with CNS tumors; may worsen or develop during treatment. Patients experiencing oprelvekin-related papilledema may be at risk for visual acuity changes and/or visual field defects ranging from blurred vision to blindness. Use with caution in patients with renal impairment (oprelvekin is renally eliminated); dosage adjustment required in severe renal impairment.

Begin 6 to 24 hours following completion of chemotherapy; safety and efficacy of oprelvekin administered immediately before or during cytotoxic chemotherapy or initiated at the time of expected nadir has not been established. Not indicated following myeloablative chemotherapy; increased toxicities (hypotension, tachycardia, edema, and conjunctival bleeding) were reported and efficacy was not demonstrated. A higher incidence of adverse events (fluid retention/overload, facial/pulmonary edema, capillary leak syndrome) has also been reported when used following bone marrow transplantation. Efficacy has not been evaluated with chemotherapy regimens >5 days' duration or with regimens associated with delayed myelosuppression (eg, nitrosoureas, mitomycin). Safety and efficacy have not been established with chronic administration.

Warnings: Additional Pediatric Considerations Reported adverse events that occurred more frequently in children than adults include tachycardia (84%), conjunctival injection (57%), cardiomegaly (21%), and periosteal changes (11%). Papilledema (dose-limiting) also reported more frequently in children than adults (16% vs 2%).

Adverse Reactions

Cardiovascular: Atrial arrhythmia, cardiomegaly, edema, palpitation, syncope, tachycardia, vasodilation

Central nervous system: Dizziness, fatigue, fever, headache, insomnia, neutropenic fever

Dermatologic: Rash

Endocrine & metabolic: Fluid retention

Gastrointestinal: Diarrhea, mucositis, nausea/vomiting, oral moniliasis, weight gain

Hematologic: Anemia (dilutional)

Neuromuscular & skeletal: Arthralgia, periostitis, weakness

Ocular: Conjunctival injection/redness/swelling, papilledema

Respiratory: Cough, dyspnea, rhinitis, pharyngitis, pleural effusion

Rare but important or life-threatening: Allergic reaction, amblyopia, anaphylaxis/anaphylactoid reactions, blindness, blurred vision, capillary leak syndrome, cardiac arrest, chest pain, dehydration, dysarthria, exfoliative dermatitis, eye hemorrhage, facial edema, fibrinogen increased, fluid overload, HF, hypoalbuminemia, hypocalcemia, hypokalemia, hypotension, injection site reactions (dermatitis, pain, discoloration), loss of consciousness, mental status changes, optic neuropathy, paresthesia, pericardial effusion, peripheral edema, pneumonia, pulmonary edema, renal failure, shock, skin discoloration, stroke, urticaria, ventricular arrhythmia, visual acuity changes, visual field defect, von Willebrand factor concentration increased, wheezing

Drug Interactions

Metabolism/Transport Effects None known.

Avoid Concomitant Use There are no known interactions where it is recommended to avoid concomitant use.

Increased Effect/Toxicity There are no known significant interactions involving an increase in effect.

Decreased Effect There are no known significant interactions involving a decrease in effect.

Storage/Stability Store intact vials (and prefilled diluent syringe) refrigerated between 2°C and 8°C (36°F and 46°F); do not freeze. Protect from light. Store reconstituted solution in the vial at either 2°C to 8°C (36°F to 46°F) or room temperature of ≤25°C (77°F); use within 3 hours of reconstitution. Do not freeze or shake reconstituted solution.

Mechanism of Action Oprelvekin is a thrombopoietic growth factor that stimulates megakaryocytopoiesis and thrombopoiesis, resulting in proliferation of megakaryocyte progenitors and megakaryocyte maturation, thereby increasing platelet production.

Pharmacodynamics

Onset of action: 5-9 days

Maximum effect: 14-19 days

Duration: Up to 7 days after discontinuation

Pharmacokinetics (Adult data unless noted)

Distribution: V_d: Adults: 112-152 mL/kg

Bioavailability: >80%

Metabolism: Uncertain

Half-life: Terminal: 6.9-8.1 hours

Time to peak serum concentration: 3.2 ± 2.4 hours

Elimination: Urine (primarily as metabolites)

Clearance: Adults: 2.2-2.7 mL/min/kg; clearance decreases with age and is about 1.2-1.6 times faster in children than in adults

Dosing: Usual SubQ: **Note:** First dose should not be administered until 6-24 hours after the end of chemotherapy. Discontinue the drug at least 48 hours before beginning the next cycle of chemotherapy.

Children: 25-50 mcg/kg once daily for 27 days was shown to be efficacious with decreased toxicities as compared to higher doses in one study with 47 pediatric patients (Cairo, 2005); dosing should continue until postnadir platelet count ≥50,000/mm^3

Note: The manufacturer states that, until efficacy/toxicity parameters are established, the use of oprelvekin in pediatric patients (particularly those <12 years of age) should be restricted to use in controlled clinical trials.

Adults: 50 mcg/kg once daily for 10-21 days (until postnadir platelet count ≥50,000/mm^3)

Dosage adjustment in renal failure: Adults: CrCl <30 mL/minute: 25 mcg/kg once daily for 10-21 days (until postnadir platelet count ≥50,000/mm^3)

Preparation for Administration SubQ: Reconstitute with 1 mL preservative free SWFI, resulting in a final concentration of 5 mg/mL; direct diluent down side of vial, swirl gently, do not shake.

Administration SubQ: Administer subcutaneously in either the abdomen, thigh, hip, or upper arm (if not self-injected).

Monitoring Parameters Monitor electrolytes and fluid balance during therapy; obtain a CBC at regular intervals during therapy; monitor platelet counts until adequate recovery has occurred; renal function (at baseline)

Dosage Forms Excipient information presented when available (limited, particularly for generics); consult specific product labeling.

Solution Reconstituted, Subcutaneous [preservative free]:
Neumega: 5 mg (1 ea)

- ◆ **Opticrom® (Can)** *see* Cromolyn (Ophthalmic) *on page 543*
- ◆ **Optimyxin® (Can)** *see* Bacitracin and Polymyxin B *on page 252*
- ◆ **Optivar [DSC]** *see* Azelastine (Ophthalmic) *on page 241*
- ◆ **Oracea** *see* Doxycycline *on page 717*
- ◆ **Oracit®** *see* Sodium Citrate and Citric Acid *on page 1942*
- ◆ **Oracort (Can)** *see* Triamcinolone (Topical) *on page 2117*
- ◆ **Ora-film [OTC]** *see* Benzocaine *on page 268*
- ◆ **Oralair** *see* Grass Pollen Allergen Extract (5 Grass Extract) *on page 984*
- ◆ **Oralone** *see* Triamcinolone (Topical) *on page 2117*
- ◆ **Oral Pain Relief Max St [OTC] [DSC]** *see* Benzocaine *on page 268*
- ◆ **Orap** *see* Pimozide *on page 1704*
- ◆ **Orap® (Can)** *see* Pimozide *on page 1704*
- ◆ **Orapred [DSC]** *see* PrednisoLONE (Systemic) *on page 1755*

- ◆ **Orapred ODT** *see* PrednisoLONE (Systemic) *on page 1755*
- ◆ **Oraqix** *see* Lidocaine and Prilocaine *on page 1263*
- ◆ **OraVerse (Can)** *see* Phentolamine *on page 1684*
- ◆ **Orazinc [OTC]** *see* Zinc Sulfate *on page 2214*
- ◆ **Orciprenaline Sulfate** *see* Metaproterenol *on page 1374*
- ◆ **Orencia** *see* Abatacept *on page 41*
- ◆ **Orfadin** *see* Nitisinone *on page 1520*
- ◆ **ORG 9426** *see* Rocuronium *on page 1881*
- ◆ **Organ-I NR [OTC]** *see* GuaiFENesin *on page 988*
- ◆ **ORG NC 45** *see* Vecuronium *on page 2163*
- ◆ **ORO-Clense (Can)** *see* Chlorhexidine Gluconate *on page 434*
- ◆ **Ortho-CS 250** *see* Ascorbic Acid *on page 202*
- ◆ **Ortho Micronor** *see* Norethindrone *on page 1530*
- ◆ **Ortho,para-DDD** *see* Mitotane *on page 1446*
- ◆ **OrthoWash** *see* Fluoride *on page 899*
- ◆ **Oscal** *see* Calcium Carbonate *on page 343*
- ◆ **Os-Cal [OTC] [DSC]** *see* Calcium Carbonate *on page 343*
- ◆ **Os-Cal (Can)** *see* Calcium Carbonate *on page 343*
- ◆ **Oscimin** *see* Hyoscyamine *on page 1061*
- ◆ **Oscimin SR** *see* Hyoscyamine *on page 1061*
- ◆ **Oscion Cleanser** *see* Benzoyl Peroxide *on page 270*

Oseltamivir (oh sel TAM i vir)

Medication Safety Issues

Sound-alike/look-alike issues:

Tamiflu may be confused with Tambocor, Thera-Flu

Other safety concerns:

Oseltamivir (Tamiflu) oral suspension is available in a 6 mg/mL concentration and is packaged with an oral syringe calibrated in **milliliters** up to a total of 10 mL. **Instructions to the patient should be provided based on these units of measure (ie, mL). When providing oseltamivir suspension for children <1 year of age, use a lower calibrated (ie, <10 mL) oral syringe to ensure accurate dosing.**

When commercially-prepared oseltamivir oral suspension is not available, an extemporaneously prepared suspension may be compounded to provide a 6 mg/mL concentration.

Brand Names: US Tamiflu

Brand Names: Canada Tamiflu

Therapeutic Category Antiviral Agent, Oral; Neuraminidase Inhibitor

Generic Availability (US) No

Use Treatment of influenza infection in patients who have been symptomatic for no more than 2 days (FDA approved in ages ≥2 weeks and adults); prophylaxis of influenza exposures (FDA approved in ages ≥1 year and adults)

Has also been used for prophylaxis of influenza in ages <1 year and treatment of patients symptomatic for >2 days with severe illness (CDC, 2010)

The Advisory Committee on Immunization Practices (ACIP) recommends that antiviral **treatment** be considered for the following (see specific antiviral product monograph for appropriate patient selection):

- Persons with severe, complicated or progressive illness
- Hospitalized persons
- Persons at higher risk for influenza complications
  - Children <2 years of age (highest risk in children <6 months of age)
  - Adults ≥65 years of age
  - Persons with chronic disorders of the pulmonary (including asthma) or cardiovascular systems (except hypertension)
  - Persons with chronic metabolic diseases (including diabetes mellitus), hepatic disease, renal dysfunction, hematologic disorders (including sickle cell disease), or immunosuppression (including immunosuppression caused by medications or HIV)
  - Persons with neurologic/neuromuscular conditions (including conditions such as spinal cord injuries, seizure disorders, cerebral palsy, stroke, mental retardation, moderate to severe developmental delay, or muscular dystrophy) which may compromise respiratory function, the handling of respiratory secretions, or that can increase the risk of aspiration
  - Pregnant or postpartum women (≤2 weeks after delivery)
  - Persons <19 years of age on long-term aspirin therapy
  - American Indians and Alaskan Natives
  - Persons who are morbidly obese (BMI ≥40)
  - Residents of nursing homes or other chronic care facilities
- Use may also be considered for previously healthy, non-high-risk outpatients with confirmed or suspected influenza based on clinical judgment when treatment can be started within 48 hours of illness onset.

The ACIP recommends that **prophylaxis** be considered for the following (**Note**: Postexposure chemoprophylaxis is generally only recommended when it can be started within 48 hours of most recent exposure) (see specific antiviral product monograph for appropriate patient selection):

- Postexposure prophylaxis may be considered for family or close contacts of suspected or confirmed cases, who are at higher risk of influenza complications, and who have not been vaccinated against the circulating strain at the time of the exposure or if exposure occurred within 2 weeks of vaccination.
- Postexposure prophylaxis may be considered for unvaccinated healthcare workers who had occupational exposure without protective equipment.
- Pre-exposure prophylaxis should only be used for persons at very high risk of influenza complications and who cannot be otherwise protected at times of high risk for exposure.
- Prophylaxis should also be administered to all eligible residents of institutions that house patients at high risk when needed to control outbreaks.

The ACIP recommends that treatment and prophylaxis be given to children <1 year of age when indicated.

Tamiflu® oral suspension: 75 mg dose delivers 2 g sorbitol

Hospitalized patients with severe 2009 H1N1 influenza infection may require longer (eg, ≥10 days) treatment courses. Some experts also recommend empirically doubling the treatment dose. Doubling the dose in adult outpatients was not associated with increased adverse events. As no double dose studies have been published in children, use caution. Initiate as early as possible in any hospitalized patient with suspected/confirmed influenza [interim recommendations (CDC, 2010)].

The absence of symptoms does not rule out viral influenza infection and clinical judgment should guide the decision for therapy. Treatment should not be delayed while waiting for the results of diagnostic tests. Treatment should be considered for high-risk patients with symptoms despite a negative rapid influenza test when the illness cannot be contributed to another cause. Use of oseltamivir is not a substitute for vaccination (when available); susceptibility to influenza infection returns once therapy is discontinued.

Pregnancy Risk Factor C

Pregnancy Considerations Adverse events were observed in some animal reproduction studies. Oseltamivir phosphate and its active metabolite oseltamivir carboxylate cross the placenta (Meijer, 2012). An increased risk of adverse neonatal or maternal outcomes has generally not been observed following maternal use of oseltamivir during pregnancy (CDC, 60[1], 2011; CDC, March 13, 2014).

Untreated influenza infection is associated with an increased risk of adverse events to the fetus and an increased risk of complications or death to the mother. Neuraminidase inhibitors are currently recommended for the treatment or prophylaxis of influenza in pregnant women and women up to 2 weeks postpartum (CDC 60 [1], 2011; CDC March 13, 2014; January 2015).

Breast-Feeding Considerations Low concentrations of oseltamivir and oseltamivir carboxylate (OC) have been detected in breast milk; levels are unlikely to lead to toxicity in a breast-fed infant. The manufacturer recommends that caution be used if administered to a nursing woman.

Influenza may cause serious illness in postpartum women and prompt evaluation for febrile respiratory illnesses is recommended (Louie, 2011).

Contraindications Hypersensitivity to oseltamivir or any component of the formulation

Warnings/Precautions Oseltamivir is not a substitute for the influenza virus vaccine. It has not been shown to prevent primary or concomitant bacterial infections that may occur with influenza virus. Use caution with renal impairment; dosage adjustment is required. Safety and efficacy for use in patients with chronic cardiac and/or kidney disease, severe hepatic impairment, or for treatment or prophylaxis in immunocompromised patients have not been established. Rare but severe hypersensitivity reactions, including anaphylaxis and severe dermatologic reactions (eg, Stevens-Johnson syndrome, erythema multiforme), have been associated with use. Discontinue use immediately if hypersensitivity occurs or is suspected and treat appropriately. Rare occurrences of neuropsychiatric events (including confusion, delirium, hallucinations, and/or self-injury) have been reported from postmarketing surveillance (primarily in pediatric patients); direct causation is difficult to establish (influenza infection may also be associated with behavioral and neurologic changes). Monitor closely for signs of any unusual behavior.

Antiviral treatment should begin within 48 hours of symptom onset. However, the CDC recommends that treatment may still be beneficial and should be started in hospitalized patients with severe, complicated or progressive illness if >48 hours. Treatment should not be delayed while awaiting results of laboratory tests for influenza. Nonhospitalized persons who are not at high risk for developing severe or complicated illness and who have a mild disease are not likely to benefit if treatment is started >48 hours after symptom onset. Nonhospitalized persons who are already beginning to recover do not need treatment. Oral suspension contains sorbitol (delivers ~2 g sorbitol per 75 mg dose) which is greater than the maximum daily limit for some patients; may cause diarrhea and dyspepsia; use with caution in patients with hereditary fructose intolerance. The Canadian labeling does not approve of use (treatment or prophylaxis) in infants <1 year of age.

Benzyl alcohol and derivatives: Some dosage forms may contain sodium benzoate/benzoic acid; benzoic acid (benzoate) is a metabolite of benzyl alcohol; large amounts of benzyl alcohol (≥99 mg/kg/day) have been associated with a potentially fatal toxicity ("gasping syndrome") in neonates; the "gasping syndrome" consists of metabolic acidosis, respiratory distress, gasping respirations, CNS dysfunction (including convulsions, intracranial hemorrhage), hypotension, and cardiovascular collapse (AAP, 1997; CDC, 1982); some data suggests that benzoate displaces bilirubin from protein binding sites (Ahlfors, 2001); avoid or use dosage forms containing benzyl alcohol derivative with caution in neonates. See manufacturer's labeling.

Adverse Reactions

Gastrointestinal: Abdominal pain, diarrhea, nausea, vomiting

Ocular: Conjunctivitis

Respiratory: Epistaxis

Rare but important or life-threatening: Allergy, anaphylactic/anaphylactoid reaction, angina, arrhythmia, confusion, erythema multiforme, fracture, gastrointestinal bleeding, hemorrhagic colitis, hepatitis, liver function tests abnormal, neuropsychiatric events, pseudomembranous colitis, pyrexia, seizure, Stevens-Johnson syndrome, swelling of face or tongue, toxic epidermal necrolysis

Drug Interactions

Metabolism/Transport Effects None known.

Avoid Concomitant Use There are no known interactions where it is recommended to avoid concomitant use.

Increased Effect/Toxicity

The levels/effects of Oseltamivir may be increased by: Probenecid

Decreased Effect

Oseltamivir may decrease the levels/effects of: Influenza Virus Vaccine (Live/Attenuated)

Storage/Stability

Capsules: Store at 25°C (77°F); excursions permitted to 15°C to 30°C (59°F to 86°F).

Oral suspension: Store powder for suspension at 25°C (77°F); excursions permitted to 15°C to 30°C (59°F to 86°F). Once reconstituted, store suspension under refrigeration at 2°C to 8°C (36°F to 46°F) or at room temperature; do not freeze. Use within 10 days of preparation if stored at room temperature or within 17 days of preparation if stored under refrigeration.

Mechanism of Action Oseltamivir, a prodrug, is hydrolyzed to the active form, oseltamivir carboxylate (OC). OC inhibits influenza virus neuraminidase, an enzyme known to cleave the budding viral progeny from its cellular envelope attachment point (neuraminic acid) just prior to release.

Pharmacodynamics Reduction in the median time to improvement: 1.3 days

Pharmacokinetics (Adult data unless noted)

Absorption: Well absorbed from the GI tract

Distribution: Adults: V_{dss}: 23 to 26 L; may be significantly increased in patients receiving ECMO (Lemaitre 2012; Mulla 2013)

Protein binding: 3% (oseltamivir carboxylate); 42% (oseltamivir phosphate)

Metabolism: Prodrug oseltamivir phosphate is metabolized by hepatic esterases to oseltamivir carboxylate (active); neither oseltamivir phosphate or oseltamivir carboxylate are a substrate, inducer, or inhibitor of cytochrome P450 isoenzymes

Half-life:

Oseltamivir phosphate: 1 to 3 hours

Oseltamivir carboxylate: 6 to 10 hours

Elimination: >99% of oseltamivir carboxylate is eliminated by renal excretion via glomerular filtration and tubular secretion

Dosing: Neonatal Influenza, treatment: Note: Treatment should ideally begin within 48 hours; however, initiation after 48 hours may decrease mortality or duration of illness.

Premature neonates: Limited data available: GA: 24 to 37 weeks: Oral: 1 mg/kg/dose twice daily; duration not determined. This dose is expected to produce serum concentrations similar to treatment doses in infants and young children based on retrospective pharmacokinetic trial of 20 neonates (Acosta 2010; Bradley 2011; CDC 2011).

Full-term neonates (Bautista 2010; Bradley 2011; CDC 2011; WHO 2010):
PNA 0 to 13 days: Limited data available: Oral: 3 mg/kg/dose once daily for 5 days
PNA 14 to 28 days: Oral: 3 mg/kg/dose twice daily for 5 days

Dosing: Usual

Pediatric:

Influenza, treatment: Note: Treatment should ideally begin within 48 hours; however, initiation after 48 hours may decrease mortality or duration of illness. Hospitalized patients may require longer (eg, ≥10 days) treatment courses. Initiate as early as possible in any hospitalized patient with suspected/confirmed influenza (CDC, 2011).

Infants:

Weight-based dosing (preferred):

CDC Recommendations (independent of HIV status) (CDC 2012; DHHS [pediatric] 2013): Manufacturer's labeling: Oral: 3 mg/kg/dose twice daily for 5 days

IDSA/PIDS Recommendations (Bradley 2011): Oral:
1 to 8 months: 3 mg/kg/dose twice daily
9 to 11 months: 3.5 mg/kg/dose twice daily

*Fixed dosing (use **only** if weight not available)* (AAP 2010): Limited data available: Oral:
<3 months: 12 mg twice daily for 5 days
3 to 5 months: 20 mg twice daily for 5 days
6 to 11 months: 25 mg twice daily for 5 days

Children 12 to 23 months:

CDC Recommendations (independent of HIV status) (CDC 2012; DHHS [pediatric] 2013): Oral:
≤15 kg: 30 mg twice daily for 5 days
>15 to 23 kg: 45 mg twice daily for 5 days
>23 kg: See dosage recommendations below for children ≥2 years

IDSA/PIDS Recommendations (Bradley 2011): Oral: 3.5 mg/kg/dose twice daily; weight-dependent maximum dose: Weight ≤15 kg: 30 mg; Weight >15 to 23 kg: 45 mg

Children ≥2-12 years and Adolescents (independent of HIV status): **Note:** Manufacturer's labeling consistent with current CDC and IDSA/PIDS recommendations (Bradley 2011; CDC 2012; DHHS [pediatric] 2013): Oral:
≤15 kg: 30 mg twice daily for 5 days
>15 to 23 kg: 45 mg twice daily for 5 days
>23 to 40 kg: 60 mg twice daily for 5 days
>40 kg: 75 mg twice daily for 5 days

Influenza, prophylaxis: Note: Initiate treatment within 48 hours of contact with an infected individual. Duration of prophylaxis dependent upon type of exposure or outbreak (eg, household exposure vs hospital outbreak); see below for further details.

Infants: Limited data available

Weight-directed dosing (preferred):

CDC Recommendation (independent of HIV status) (CDC 2012; DHHS [pediatric] 2013): Oral:
<3 months: Not recommended unless clinically critical
3 to 11 months: 3 mg/kg/dose once daily

IDSA/PIDS Recommendations (Bradley 2011): Oral:
3 to 8 months: 3 mg/kg/dose once daily
9 to 11 months: 3.5 mg/kg/dose once daily

*Fixed dosing (use **only** if weight not available)* (AAP 2010): Oral:
<3 months: Not recommended unless clinically critical
3 to 5 months: 20 mg once daily
6 to 11 months: 25 mg once daily

Children 12 to 23 months:

CDC Recommendations (independent of HIV status) (CDC 2012; DHHS [pediatric] 2013): Oral:
≤15 kg: 30 mg once daily
>15 to 23 kg: 45 mg dose once daily
>23 kg: See dosage recommendations below for weight.

IDSA/PIDS Recommendations (Bradley 2011): Oral: 3.5 mg/kg/dose once daily; weight-dependent maximum dose: Weight: ≤15 kg: 30 mg; Weight >15 to 23 kg: 45 mg

Children: 2 to 12 years and Adolescents (independent of HIV status): **Note:** Manufacturer's labeling consistent with current CDC and IDSA/PIDS recommendations (Bradley 2011; CDC 2012; DHHS [pediatric] 2013): Oral:
≤15 kg: 30 mg once daily
>15 kg to ≤23 kg: 45 mg once daily
>23 kg to ≤40 kg: 60 mg once daily
>40 kg: 75 mg once daily

Prophylaxis duration:

Individual/household exposure:
Manufacturer labeling: 10 days
Alternate recommendations:
Non-HIV-exposed/-positive: 7 days (CDC 2012)
HIV-exposed/-positive: 10 days for household exposure; 7 days for other exposures (DHHS [pediatric] 2013)

Community/institutional outbreak:
Manufacturer recommendation: May be used for up to 6 weeks
Alternate recommendations: Continue for ≥2 weeks and until ~7 days after identification of illness onset in the last patient (CDC 2012) or until influenza activity in community subsides or immunity obtained from immunization (Bradley 2011). During community outbreaks, duration of protection lasts for length of dosing period; safety and efficacy have been demonstrated for use up to 6 weeks in immunocompetent patients and safety has been demonstrated for use up to 12 weeks in patients who are immunocompromised.

Adult:

Influenza, prophylaxis: Oral: 75 mg once daily; initiate prophylaxis within 48 hours of contact with an infected individual; duration of prophylaxis: 10 days (manufacturer recommendation) or alternatively 7 days (CDC, 2012). During community outbreaks, duration of protection lasts for length of dosing period; safety and efficacy have been demonstrated for use up to 6 weeks in immunocompetent patients and safety has been demonstrated for use up to 12 weeks in patients who are immunocompromised.

Prophylaxis (institutional outbreak; CDC 2012): Continue for ≥2 weeks and until ~7 days after identification of illness onset in the last patient

Influenza, treatment: Oral: 75 mg twice daily initiated within 48 hours of onset of symptoms; duration of treatment: 5 days. However, optimal duration is uncertain for severe or complicated influenza. Consider longer duration (eg, >5 days) of therapy in severely ill patients who remain severely ill after 5 days of therapy.

Note: Data suggest that increased doses (>150 mg daily) in critically ill patients is not necessary since blood concentrations of oseltamivir were comparable or higher compared to ambulatory patients given similar dosing regimens (Ariano 2010; CDC [Influenza Antiviral Medications] 2014). Initiate as early as possible in any hospitalized patient with suspected/confirmed influenza regardless of the time of presentation from symptom onset (even if >48 hours) (CDC [Influenza Antiviral Medications] 2014); may be administered via naso- or orogastric tube in mechanically ventilated patients (Taylor 2008).

Dosing adjustment in renal impairment:

Children >1 year: **Treatment** (Schreuder 2010): Limited data available:

Intermittent hemodialysis (IHD) (CrCl ≤10 mL/minute): Fixed dosing:

≤15 kg: 7.5 mg after each hemodialysis session

>15 kg to ≤23 kg: 10 mg after each hemodialysis session

>23 kg to ≤40 kg: 15 mg after each hemodialysis session

>40 kg: 30 mg after each hemodialysis session

Adults:

Treatment:

CrCl >60 mL/minute: No dosage adjustment necessary.

CrCl >30 to 60 mL/minute: 30 mg twice daily for 5 days

CrCl >10 to 30 mL/minute: 30 mg once daily for 5 days

End-stage renal disease (ESRD) not undergoing dialysis: Use is not recommended (has not been studied).

Intermittent hemodialysis (IHD) (CrCl ≤10 mL/minute):

Manufacturer labeling: 30 mg after every hemodialysis session for 5 days. **Note:** Assumes three hemodialysis sessions in the 5-day period. Treatment may be initiated immediately if influenza symptoms develop during the 48 hours between hemodialysis sessions; however, the posthemodialysis dose should still be administered independently of the time of the initial dose administration.

Alternate recommendations (AMMI Canada [Aoki 2012]):

Low-flux hemodialysis: 30 mg after each dialysis session for 5 days

High-flux hemodialysis: 75 mg after each dialysis session for 5 days

CAPD: 30 mg for one dose to provide a 5-day duration. Administer immediately after a dialysis exchange

Continuous renal replacement therapy (CRRT) (high-flux): Limited data available: 30 mg once daily for 5 days or 75 mg every 48 hours to provide a 5-day duration (AMMI Canada [Aoki, 2012]; Ariano, 2010)

Continuous veno-venous hemodialysis (CVVHD): **Note:** Limited data available; optimal dosing has not been established: 150 mg twice daily administered via nasogastric or postpyloric feeding tube for suspected or confirmed H1N1 influenza demonstrated supratherapeutic oseltamivir carboxylate concentrations at effluent rates of 3,300 ± 919 mL/hour; the authors determined that the manufacturer recommended dosage of 75 mg once daily for patients with CrCl 10 to 30 mL/minute will likely achieve concentrations necessary to inhibit viral neuraminidase activity at these effluent rates; however, doses greater than 75 mg once daily may be required when using higher effluent rates (Eyler, 2012).

CVVHD and concurrent use of ECMO: Lower oseltamivir carboxylate concentrations (~981 ng/mL) were observed as compared to those with the use of CVVHD alone (~2,760 ng/mL) when patients were administered 150 mg twice daily for suspected or confirmed H1N1 influenza (n=4; Eyler 2012).

Prophylaxis:

CrCl >60 mL/minute: No dosage adjustment necessary.

CrCl >30 to 60 mL/minute: 30 mg once daily

CrCl >10 to 30 mL/minute: 30 mg every other day

ESRD not undergoing dialysis: Use is not recommended (has not been studied).

Intermittent hemodialysis (IHD) (CrCl ≤10 mL/minute): 30 mg once after alternate hemodialysis sessions for the recommended prophylaxis duration. **Note:** An initial dose may be administered prior to the start of dialysis.

CAPD: 30 mg once weekly for the recommended prophylaxis duration. Administer immediately after a dialysis exchange.

Continuous renal replacement therapy (CRRT) (high-flux): No data (AMMI Canada [Aoki 2012])

Dosing adjustment in hepatic impairment:

Mild to moderate impairment (Child-Pugh score ≤9): No dosage adjustment necessary.

Severe impairment: There are no dosage adjustments provided in manufacturer's labeling (has not been studied).

Preparation for Administration Oral suspension: Reconstitute with 55 mL of water to a final concentration of 6 mg/mL (to make 60 mL total suspension).

Administration

Oral: May administer with or without food; may decrease stomach upset if administered with food

Capsules: May be opened and mixed with sweetened liquid [eg, chocolate syrup, corn syrup, caramel topping, or light brown sugar (dissolved in water)]. May be administered via naso- or orogastric tube in mechanically ventilated patients; for a 150 mg dose (in adults), dissolve powder from two 75 mg capsules in 20 mL of sterile water and inject down the NG/OG tube; follow with a 10 mL sterile water flush (Taylor 2008)

Oral suspension: Shake suspension well before use; measure dose in calibrated oral syringe; the manufacturer provided oral syringe should not be used to measure the dose for infants (<1 year of age); a smaller total volume syringe (ie, <10 mL) should be used to accurately measure dose

Monitoring Parameters Renal function, serum glucose in patients with diabetes mellitus; signs or symptoms of unusual behavior, including attempts at self-injury, confusion, and/or delirium

Critically ill patients: Repeat rRT-PCR or viral culture may help to determine ongoing viral replication

Dosage Forms Excipient information presented when available (limited, particularly for generics); consult specific product labeling.

Capsule, Oral, as phosphate:

Tamiflu: 30 mg, 45 mg, 75 mg

Suspension Reconstituted, Oral, as base:

Tamiflu: 6 mg/mL (60 mL) [contains saccharin sodium, sodium benzoate; tutti-frutti flavor]

Extemporaneous Preparations

If the commercially prepared oral suspension is not available, the manufacturer provides the following compounding information to prepare a **6 mg/mL** suspension in emergency situations.

1. Place the specified amount of water into a polyethyleneterephthalate (PET) or glass bottle.
2. Carefully separate the capsule body and cap and pour the contents of the required number of 75 mg capsules into the PET or glass bottle.
3. Gently swirl the suspension to ensure adequate wetting of the powder for at least 2 minutes.
4. Slowly add the specified amount of vehicle to the bottle.
5. Close the bottle using a child-resistant cap and shake well for 30 seconds to completely dissolve the active drug.
6. Label "Shake Well Before Use."

Stable for 35 days at 2°C to 8°C (36°F to 46°F) or 5 days at 25° C (77°F). The Canadian labeling suggests that preparations made with water containing preservative (ie, 0.05% sodium benzoate) are stable for 49 days at 2°C to 8°C (36°F to 46°F) and 10 days at 25°C (77°F). Shake gently prior to use. Do **not** dispense with dosing device provided with commercially-available product.

Preparation of Oseltamivir 6 mg/mL Suspension

Body Weight	Total Volume per Patient[1]	# of 75 mg Capsules[2]	Required Volume of Water	Required Volume of Vehicle[2,3]	Treatment Dose (wt based)[4]	Prophylactic Dose (wt based)[4]
≤15 kg	75 mL	6	5 mL	69 mL	5 mL (30 mg) twice daily for 5 days	5 mL (30 mg) once daily for 10 days
16 to 23 kg	100 mL	8	7 mL	91 mL	7.5 mL (45 mg) twice daily for 5 days	7.5 mL (45 mg) once daily for 10 days
24 to 40 kg	125 mL	10	8 mL	115 mL	10 mL (60 mg) twice daily for 5 days	10 mL (60 mg) once daily for 10 days
≥41 kg	150 mL	12	10 mL	137 mL	12.5 mL (75 mg) twice daily for 5 days	12.5 mL (75 mg) once daily for 10 days

[1]Entire course of therapy.

[2]Based on total volume per patient.

[3]Acceptable vehicles are cherry syrup (Humco®), Ora-Sweet® SF, or simple syrup.

[4]Using 6 mg/mL suspension.

Canadian labeling:

Preparation of Oseltamivir 6 mg/mL Suspension

(using water with preservative (ie, 0.05% sodium benzoate)

Body Weight	Total Volume per Patient[1]	# of 75 mg Capsules[2]	Required Volume of Water (with preservative)	Treatment Dose (wt based)[2,3]	Prophylactic Dose (wt based)[2,3]
≤15 kg	75 mL	6	74 mL	5 mL (30 mg) twice daily for 5 days	5 mL (30 mg) once daily for 10 days
16 to 23 kg	100 mL	8	98 mL	7.5 mL (45 mg) twice daily for 5 days	7.5 mL (45 mg) once daily for 10 days
24 to 40 kg	125 mL	10	123 mL	10 mL (60 mg) twice daily for 5 days	10 mL (60 mg) once daily for 10 days
≥41 kg	150 mL	12	147 mL	12.5 mL (75 mg) twice daily for 5 days	12.5 mL (75 mg) once daily for 10 days

[1]Entire course of therapy.

[2]Using 6 mg/mL suspension.

[3]Measured dose should be mixed with an equal amount of sweetened liquid (eg, chocolate syrup, cherry syrup) to mask bitter taste.

- ◆ **Osmitrol** *see* Mannitol *on page* 1321
- ◆ **Osmitrol® (Can)** *see* Mannitol *on page* 1321
- ◆ **OsmoPrep** *see* Sodium Phosphates *on page* 1949
- ◆ **Osteocit® (Can)** *see* Calcium Citrate *on page* 348
- ◆ **OTFC (Oral Transmucosal Fentanyl Citrate)** *see* FentaNYL *on page* 857
- ◆ **Otrexup** *see* Methotrexate *on page* 1390
- ◆ **Ovace Plus** *see* Sulfacetamide (Topical) *on page* 1982
- ◆ **Ovace Plus Wash** *see* Sulfacetamide (Topical) *on page* 1982
- ◆ **Ovace Wash** *see* Sulfacetamide (Topical) *on page* 1982
- ◆ **Ovide** *see* Malathion *on page* 1321
- ◆ **Ovol (Can)** *see* Simethicone *on page* 1927

Oxacillin (oks a SIL in)

Brand Names: US Bactocill in Dextrose

Therapeutic Category Antibiotic, Penicillin (Antistaphylococcal)

Generic Availability (US) May be product dependent

Use Treatment of bacterial infections, such as osteomyelitis, septicemia, endocarditis, and CNS infections, due to susceptible penicillinase-producing strains of *Staphylococcus* (FDA approved in all ages)

Pregnancy Risk Factor B

Pregnancy Considerations Adverse events have not been observed in animal reproduction studies. Oxacillin is distributed into the amniotic fluid and is detected in cord blood. Maternal use of penicillins has generally not resulted in an increased risk of adverse fetal effects.

Breast-Feeding Considerations Oxacillin is excreted in breast milk. The manufacturer recommends that caution be exercised when administering oxacillin to nursing women. Nondose-related effects could include modification of bowel flora.

Contraindications Hypersensitivity (eg, anaphylaxis) to oxacillin, any penicillin or any component of the formulation.

Warnings/Precautions Serious and occasionally fatal hypersensitivity (anaphylactic) reactions have been reported in patients on penicillin therapy, especially with a history of beta-lactam hypersensitivity, history of sensitivity to multiple allergens, or previous IgE-mediated reactions (eg, anaphylaxis, angioedema, urticaria). Use with caution in patients with histories of significant allergies and/or asthma. Acute hepatitis and reversible elevations of serum transaminases have been reported, sometimes accompanied by rash and leukopenia; onset after 2 to 3 weeks of therapy; monitor periodically throughout therapy (Dahlgren 1997; Faden 2009; Maraqa 2002). May contain a significant amount of sodium; consult product specific labeling for amount. The elderly population may respond with a blunted natriuresis to salt loading. This may be clinically important in diseases such as congestive heart failure. Use with caution in neonates (elimination of oxacillin is slow) and patients with renal impairment; dosage adjustment recommended. Prolonged use may result in fungal or bacterial superinfection, including *C. difficile*-associated diarrhea (CDAD) and pseudomembranous colitis; CDAD has been observed >2 months postantibiotic treatment. Potentially significant interactions may exist, requiring dose or frequency adjustment, additional monitoring, and/or selection of alternative therapy.

Warnings: Additional Pediatric Considerations In neonates, elimination rate is decreased due to immature renal function; dosage adjustment is needed; hematuria and azotemia have occurred in neonates and infants receiving high-dose oxacillin. In a study of pediatric patients (5 to 19 years) receiving outpatient oxacillin, significantly less rash was reported in the nafcillin group (10.3%) compared to the oxacillin group (31.7%) (Maraqa, 2002).

Adverse Reactions

Central nervous system: Fever
Dermatologic: Rash
Gastrointestinal: Diarrhea, nausea, vomiting
Hematologic: Agranulocytosis, eosinophilia, leukopenia, neutropenia, thrombocytopenia
Hepatic: Hepatotoxicity, AST increased
Renal: Acute interstitial nephritis, hematuria
Miscellaneous: Serum sickness-like reactions

Drug Interactions

Metabolism/Transport Effects None known.

Avoid Concomitant Use

Avoid concomitant use of Oxacillin with any of the following: BCG; BCG (Intravesical); Probenecid

Increased Effect/Toxicity

Oxacillin may increase the levels/effects of: Methotrexate; Vitamin K Antagonists

The levels/effects of Oxacillin may be increased by: Probenecid

Decreased Effect

Oxacillin may decrease the levels/effects of: BCG; BCG (Intravesical); BCG Vaccine (Immunization); Mycophenolate; Sodium Picosulfate; Typhoid Vaccine

The levels/effects of Oxacillin may be decreased by: Tetracycline Derivatives

Storage/Stability

Premixed infusions: Store in a freezer at -20°C (4°F). Thaw at room temperature or under refrigeration only. Thawed bags are stable for 21 days under refrigeration or 48 hours at room temperature. Do not refreeze.

Vials: Store intact vials at 20°C to 25°C (68°F to 77°F); refer to manufacturer's labeling for specific storage instructions after dilution (varies by concentration and diluent).

Mechanism of Action Inhibits bacterial cell wall synthesis by binding to one or more of the penicillin-binding proteins (PBPs); which in turn inhibits the final transpeptidation step of peptidoglycan synthesis in bacterial cell walls, thus inhibiting cell wall biosynthesis. Bacteria eventually lyse due to ongoing activity of cell wall autolytic enzymes (autolysins and murein hydrolases) while cell wall assembly is arrested.

Pharmacokinetics (Adult data unless noted)

Distribution: Distributes into bile, pleural, and amniotic fluids; insignificant concentrations in CNS and aqueous humor
Protein binding: ~94%; primarily albumin
Metabolism: Hepatic to inactive metabolites
Half-life:
- Neonates (PNA: 8 to 15 days): 1.6 hours
- Infants and Children ≤2 years: 0.9 to 1.8 hours
- Adults: 20 to 60 minutes

Time to peak serum concentration:
- IM: Within 30 to 60 minutes
- IV: Within 5 minutes

Elimination: Urine and feces/bile (unchanged drug)

Dosing: Neonatal

General dosing, susceptible infection (nonmeningitis): IM, IV:
- Manufacturer labeling: Premature Infants and Neonates: 25 mg/kg/day
- Alternate dosing (*Red Book* [AAP 2012]):
  - Body weight <1 kg:
    - PNA ≤14 days: 25 mg/kg/dose every 12 hours
    - PNA 15 to 28 days: 25 mg/kg/dose every 8 hours
  - Body weight 1 to 2 kg:
    - PNA ≤7 days: 25 mg/kg/dose every 12 hours
    - PNA 8 to 28 days: 25 mg/kg/dose every 8 hours
  - Body weight >2 kg:
    - PNA ≤7 days: 25 mg/kg/dose every 8 hours
    - PNA 8 to 28 days: 25 mg/kg/dose every 6 hours

Meningitis: IV (Tunkel 2004):
- PNA 0 to 7 days: 75 mg/kg/day in divided doses every 8 to 12 hours
- PNA 8 to 28 days: 150 to 200 mg/kg/day in divided doses every 6 to 8 hours

Dosing: Usual

Pediatric:

General dosing, susceptible infection: Infants, Children, and Adolescents:
- Mild to moderate infections: IM, IV:
  - Manufacturer's labeling:
    - Infants and Children <40 kg: 50 mg/kg/day in divided doses every 6 hours
    - Children ≥40 kg and Adolescents: 250 to 500 mg every 4 to 6 hours
  - Alternate dosing: 100 to 150 mg/kg/day in divided doses every 6 hours; maximum daily dose: 4000 mg/**day** (*Red Book* [AAP 2012])
- Severe infections: IM, IV:
  - Manufacturer's labeling:
    - Infants and Children <40 kg: 100 mg/kg/day in divided doses every 4 to 6 hours; maximum daily dose: 4,000 mg/**day**
    - Children ≥40 kg and Adolescents: 1,000 mg every 4 to 6 hours; maximum daily dose: 4,000 mg/**day**
  - Alternate dosing: 150 to 200 mg/kg/day in divided doses every 4 to 6 hours; maximum daily dose: 12 g/**day**; however, recent manufacturer labeling suggests a maximum daily dose of 6 g/**day** in adults when treating severe infection (*Red Book* [AAP 2012])

Endocarditis, oxacillin/methicillin-susceptible staphylococci (Baddour 2005): Infants, Children, and Adolescents: IV:
Native valve: 200 mg/kg/day in divided doses every 4 to 6 hours for 6 weeks with gentamicin for the first 3 to 5 days of therapy
Prosthetic valve: 200 mg/kg/day in divided doses every 4 to 6 hours for ≥6 weeks with rifampin (same duration as oxacillin) and with gentamicin for the first 2 weeks of therapy
Meningitis: Infants, Children, and Adolescents: IV: 200 mg/kg/day in divided doses every 6 hours; maximum daily dose: 12 g/**day** (Tunkel 2004)
Pneumonia, community-acquired (CAP) moderate to severe infection, *S. aureus* (methicillin-susceptible): Infants ≥3 months, Children, and Adolescents: IV: 150 to 200 mg/kg/day divided every 6 to 8 hours (Bradley 2011),
Skin and soft tissue infections: IV: 100 to 150 mg/kg/day in divided doses every 6 hours; maximum daily dose: 12 g/**day** (Stevens 2005)
Adult:
General dosing, susceptible infection:
Mild to moderate infections: IM, IV: 250 to 500 mg every 4 to 6 hours
Severe infections: IM, IV: 1,000 mg every 4 to 6 hours
Dosing adjustment in renal impairment: Not dialyzable (0% to 5%). There are no dosage adjustments provided in the manufacturer's labeling.
Dosing adjustment in hepatic impairment: There are no dosage adjustments provided in the manufacturer's labeling.

Preparation for Administration
Parenteral:
IM: Reconstitute according to vial size; resulting concentration will be oxacillin 167 mg/1 mL
1-gram vial: Add 5.7 mL SWFI; shake well
2-gram vial: Add 11.5 mL SWFI; shake well
IV: Reconstitute according to vial size; resulting concentration will be oxacillin 100 mg/mL
1-gram vial: Add 10 mL SWFI or NS; shake well
2-gram vial: Add 20 mL SWFI or NS; shake well
10-gram vial: Add 93 mL SWFI or NS; shake well; requires further dilution prior to administration
Direct IV injection: No further dilution needed if prepared from 1 g or 2 g vial; maximum concentration: 100 mg/mL
Intermittent IV infusion: Further dilute in a compatible solution to a concentration ≤40 mg/mL; some ambulatory centers limit the concentration to 20 mg/mL for peripheral administration in home care patients (Dahlgren 1997). In fluid restricted patients, a concentration of ~106 mg/mL using SWFI results in a maximum recommended osmolality for peripheral infusion (Robinson 1987).

Administration Parenteral:
IM: Administer by deep IM injection into a large muscle mass (eg, gluteus maximus); avoid sciatic nerve injury
IV:
Direct IV injection: Administer over 10 minutes at a concentration of 100 mg/mL
Intermittent IV infusion: Administer over 15 to 30 minutes (Klaus 1989); extending the infusion over 60 minutes has been used for peripheral administration by some ambulatory centers to decrease the risk of phlebitis in homecare patients (Dahlgren 1997)

Monitoring Parameters Periodic CBC with differential, urinalysis, BUN, serum creatinine, AST and ALT; number and type of stools/day for diarrhea; observe IV site for extravasation

Test Interactions May interfere with urinary glucose tests using cupric sulfate (Benedict's solution, Clinitest®); may inactivate aminoglycosides *in vitro*; false-positive urinary and serum proteins

Additional Information May contain a significant amount of sodium; consult product specific labeling for amount.

Dosage Forms Excipient information presented when available (limited, particularly for generics); consult specific product labeling.
Solution, Intravenous:
Bactocill in Dextrose: 1 g/50 mL (50 mL); 2 g/50 mL (50 mL)
Solution Reconstituted, Injection:
Generic: 1 g (1 ea); 2 g (1 ea); 10 g (1 ea)
Solution Reconstituted, Injection [preservative free]:
Generic: 1 g (1 ea); 2 g (1 ea); 10 g (1 ea)

◆ **Oxacillin Sodium** *see* Oxacillin *on page 1576*
◆ **Oxalatoplatin** *see* Oxaliplatin *on page 1578*
◆ **Oxalatoplatinum** *see* Oxaliplatin *on page 1578*

Oxaliplatin (ox AL i pla tin)

Medication Safety Issues
Sound-alike/look-alike issues:
Oxaliplatin may be confused with Aloxi, carboplatin, cisplatin
High alert medication:
This medication is in a class the Institute for Safe Medication Practices (ISMP) includes among its list of drug classes which have a heightened risk of causing significant patient harm when used in error.

Related Information
Management of Drug Extravasations *on page 2298*
Prevention of Chemotherapy-Induced Nausea and Vomiting in Children *on page 2368*
Safe Handling of Hazardous Drugs *on page 2455*

Brand Names: US Eloxatin
Brand Names: Canada Eloxatin
Therapeutic Category Antineoplastic Agent, Alkylating Agent
Generic Availability (US) Yes
Use Treatment of stage III colon cancer (adjuvant) and advanced colorectal carcinoma (FDA approved in adults); has also been used in the treatment of relapsed/refractory childhood solid tumors including CNS and non-CNS tumors
Pregnancy Risk Factor D
Pregnancy Considerations Adverse events were observed in animal reproduction studies at one-tenth the equivalent human dose. Women of childbearing potential should be advised to avoid pregnancy and use effective contraception during treatment.

Canadian labeling: Use in pregnant women is contraindicated in the Canadian labeling. Males should be advised not to father children during and for up to 6 months following therapy. May cause permanent infertility in males. Prior to initiating therapy, advise males desiring to father children, to seek counseling on sperm storage.

Breast-Feeding Considerations It is not known if oxaliplatin is excreted in breast milk. Due to the potential for serious adverse reactions in the nursing infant, the decision to discontinue breast-feeding or to discontinue oxaliplatin should take into account the benefits of treatment to the mother.

Contraindications
Hypersensitivity to oxaliplatin, other platinum-containing compounds, or any component of the formulation
Canadian labeling: Additional contraindications (not in US labeling): Pregnancy, breast-feeding; severe renal impairment (CrCl <30 mL/minute)

Warnings/Precautions Hazardous agent - use appropriate precautions for handling and disposal (NIOSH 2014

[group 1]). **[US Boxed Warning]: Anaphylactic/anaphylactoid reactions have been reported with oxaliplatin (may occur within minutes of administration); symptoms may be managed with epinephrine, corticosteroids, antihistamines,** and discontinuation; oxygen and bronchodilators have also been used (Kim, 2009). Grade 3 or 4 hypersensitivity has been observed. Allergic reactions are similar to reactions reported with other platinum analogs, and may occur with any cycle. Reactions typically occur after multiple cycles; in retrospective reviews, reaction occurred at a median of 7 to 9 cycles, with an onset of 5 to 70 minutes (Kim, 2009; Polyzos, 2009). Symptoms may include bronchospasm (rare), erythema, hypotension (rare), pruritus, rash, and/or urticaria; previously-untreated patients have also experienced flushing, diaphoresis, diarrhea, shortness of breath, chest pain, hypotension, syncope, and disorientation. According to the manufacturer, rechallenge is contraindicated (deaths due to anaphylaxis have been associated with platinum derivatives). In patients rechallenged after mild hypersensitivity, reaction recurred at a higher level of severity; for patients with severe hypersensitivity, rechallenge (with 2 to 3 days of antihistamine and corticosteroid premedication, and prolongation of infusion time) allowed for 2 to 4 additional oxaliplatin cycles; however, rechallenge was not feasible in nearly two-thirds of patients due to the severity of the initial reaction (Polyzos, 2009).

Two different types of peripheral sensory neuropathy may occur: First, an acute (within hours to 1 to 2 days), reversible (resolves within 14 days), with primarily peripheral symptoms that are often exacerbated by cold (may include pharyngolaryngeal dysesthesia); commonly recur with subsequent doses; avoid mucositis prophylaxis with ice chips, exposure to cold temperatures, or consumption of cold food/beverages during or within hours after oxaliplatin infusion. Cold-triggered neuropathy may last up to 7 days after oxaliplatin administration (Grothey, 2011). Secondly, a more persistent (>14 days) presentation that often interferes with daily activities (eg, writing, buttoning, swallowing), these symptoms may improve in some patients upon discontinuing treatment. In a retrospective evaluation of patients treated with oxaliplatin for colorectal cancer, the incidence of peripheral sensory neuropathy was similar between diabetic and nondiabetic patients (Ramanathan, 2010). Several retrospective studies (as well as a small, underpowered randomized trial) have suggested calcium and magnesium infusions before and after oxaliplatin administration may reduce incidence of cumulative sensory neuropathy; however, a recent abstract of an ongoing randomized, placebo-controlled, double-blind study in patients with colorectal cancer suggests there is no benefit of calcium and magnesium in preventing sensory neuropathy or in decreasing oxaliplatin discontinuation rates (Loprinzi, 2013).

Oxaliplatin is associated with a moderate emetic potential; antiemetics are recommended to prevent nausea and vomiting (Basch, 2011; Dupuis, 2011; Roila, 2010). Cases of reversible posterior leukoencephalopathy syndrome (RPLS) have been reported. Signs/symptoms include headache, mental status changes, seizure, blurred vision, blindness and/or other vision changes; may be associated with hypertension; diagnosis is confirmed with brain imaging. May cause pulmonary fibrosis; withhold treatment for unexplained pulmonary symptoms (eg, crackles, dyspnea, nonproductive cough, pulmonary infiltrates) until interstitial lung disease or pulmonary fibrosis are excluded. Hepatotoxicity (including rare cases of hepatitis and hepatic failure) has been reported. Liver biopsy has revealed peliosis, nodular regenerative hyperplasia, sinusoidal alterations, perisinusoidal fibrosis, and veno-occlusive lesions; the presence of hepatic vascular disorders (including veno-occlusive disease) should be considered, especially in individuals developing portal hypertension or who present with increased liver function tests. Use caution with renal dysfunction; increased toxicity may occur; reduce initial dose in severe impairment. The Canadian labeling contraindicates use in severe renal impairment (CrCl <30 mL/minute). Potentially significant drug-drug interactions may exist, requiring dose or frequency adjustment, additional monitoring, and/or selection of alternative therapy. Elderly patients are more sensitive to some adverse events including diarrhea, dehydration, hypokalemia, leukopenia, fatigue and syncope. Oxaliplatin is an irritant with vesicant-like properties; ensure proper needle or catheter placement prior to and during infusion; avoid extravasation.

Adverse Reactions

Cardiovascular: Chest pain, edema, flushing, peripheral edema, thromboembolism

Central nervous system: Dizziness, fatigue, fever, headache, insomnia, pain, peripheral neuropathy (may be dose limiting), rigors

Dermatologic: Alopecia, palmar-plantar erythrodysesthesia, skin rash

Endocrine & metabolic: Dehydration, hypokalemia

Gastrointestinal: Abdominal pain, anorexia, constipation, diarrhea, hiccups, palmar-plantar erythrodysesthesia, dyspepsia, dysphagia, flatulence, gastroesophageal reflux, mucositis, nausea, stomatitis, vomiting

Genitourinary: Dysuria

Hematologic & oncologic: Anemia, leukopenia, neutropenia, thrombocytopenia

Hepatic: Increased serum ALT, increased serum AST, increased serum bilirubin

Hypersensitivity: Hypersensitivity reaction (includes urticaria, pruritus, facial flushing, shortness of breath, bronchospasm, diaphoresis, hypotension, syncope)

Local: Injection site reaction (redness/swelling/pain)

Neuromuscular & skeletal: Arthralgia, back pain

Ocular: Abnormal lacrimation

Renal: Increased serum creatinine

Respiratory: Cough, dyspnea, epistaxis, pharyngitis, pharyngolaryngeal dysesthesia, rhinitis, upper respiratory tract infection

Miscellaneous: Fever

Rare but important or life-threatening (reported with mono- and combination therapy): Abnormal gait, acute renal failure, anaphylaxis, anaphylactic shock, anaphylactoid reaction, angioedema, aphonia, ataxia, blepharoptosis, cerebral hemorrhage, colitis, cranial nerve palsy, decreased deep tendon reflex, deafness, decreased visual acuity, diplopia, dysarthria, eosinophilic pneumonitis, fasciculations, febrile neutropenia,hematuria, hemolysis, hemolytic anemia (immuno-allergic), hemolytic-uremic syndrome, hemorrhage, hepatic failure, hepatic sinusoidal obstruction syndrome (SOS; veno-occlusive disease), hepatitis, hepatotoxicity, hypertension, hypomagnesemia, hypoxia, idiopathic noncirrhotic portal hypertension (nodular regenerative hyperplasia), increased INR, increased serum alkaline phosphatase, infusion related reaction (extravasation [including necrosis]), interstitial nephritis (acute), interstitial pulmonary disease, intestinal obstruction, laryngospasm, Lhermittes' sign, metabolic acidosis, muscle spasm, myoclonus, neutropenic enterocolitis, neutropenic infection (sepsis), optic neuritis, pancreatitis, prolonged prothrombin time, purpura, rectal hemorrhage, renal tubular necrosis, reversible posterior leukoencephalopathy syndrome (RPLS), rhabdomyolysis, seizure, sepsis, temporary vision loss, thrombocytopenia (immuno-allergic), trigeminal neuralgia, visual field loss, voice disorder

Drug Interactions

Metabolism/Transport Effects Substrate of OCT2

Avoid Concomitant Use

Avoid concomitant use of Oxaliplatin with any of the following: BCG; BCG (Intravesical); CloZAPine; Dipyrone; Natalizumab; Pimecrolimus; Tacrolimus (Topical); Tofacitinib; Vaccines (Live)

Increased Effect/Toxicity

Oxaliplatin may increase the levels/effects of: CloZAPine; Leflunomide; Natalizumab; Taxane Derivatives; Tofacitinib; Topotecan; Vaccines (Live)

The levels/effects of Oxaliplatin may be increased by: BuPROPion; Denosumab; Dipyrone; Pimecrolimus; Roflumilast; Tacrolimus (Topical); Trastuzumab

Decreased Effect

Oxaliplatin may decrease the levels/effects of: BCG; BCG (Intravesical); Coccidioides immitis Skin Test; Fosphenytoin-Phenytoin; Sipuleucel-T; Vaccines (Inactivated); Vaccines (Live)

The levels/effects of Oxaliplatin may be decreased by: Echinacea

Storage/Stability Store intact vials at room temperature of 25°C (77°F); excursions permitted to 15°C to 30°C (59°F to 86°F); do not freeze. Protect concentrated solution from light (store in original outer carton). According to the manufacturer, solutions diluted for infusion are stable up to 6 hours at room temperature of 20°C to 25°C (68°F to 77°F) or up to 24 hours under refrigeration at 2°C to 8°C (36°F to 46°F). Oxaliplatin solution diluted with D_5W to a final concentration of 0.7 mg/mL (polyolefin container) has been shown to retain >90% of the original concentration for up to 30 days when stored at room temperature or refrigerated; artificial light did not affect the concentration (Andre, 2007). As this study did not examine sterility, refrigeration would be preferred to limit microbial growth. Solutions diluted for infusion do not require protection from light.

Mechanism of Action Oxaliplatin, a platinum derivative, is an alkylating agent. Following intracellular hydrolysis, the platinum compound binds to DNA forming cross-links which inhibit DNA replication and transcription, resulting in cell death. Cytotoxicity is cell-cycle nonspecific.

Pharmacokinetics (Adult data unless noted)

Distribution: V_d: 440 L

Protein binding: >90%

Metabolism: Nonenzymatic biotransformation (rapid and extensive), forms active and inactive derivatives

Half-life:

- Children: Oxaliplatin ultrafilterable platinum (terminal): Median: 293 hours; range: 187-662 hours (Beaty, 2010)
- Adults: Oxaliplatin ultrafilterable platinum:
  - Distribution:
    - Alpha phase: 0.4 hours
    - Beta phase: 16.8 hours
  - Terminal: 391 hours

Elimination: Urine (~54%); feces (~2%)

Dosing: Usual Refer to individual protocols; details concerning dosing in combination regimens should also be consulted.

Children and Adolescents: **Refractory or relapsed solid tumors:** Limited data available; efficacy results highly variable; has shown limited activity in pediatric patients (primarily some delayed tumor progression reported) and an acceptable safety profile; should not be used first-line; reserved for refractory cases. IV:

85 mg/m^2 or 100 mg/m^2 on day 1 of a 14 day cycle in combination with gemcitabine or fluorouracil/leucovorin (Georger, 2011; Macy, 2013); **or** 105 or 130 mg/m^2 on day 1 of a 21 day cycle in combination with doxorubicin or etoposide (respectively) (MacGregor, 2009; Mascarenhas, 2013).

Adults:

Advanced colorectal cancer: IV: 85 mg/m^2 every 2 weeks until disease progression or unacceptable toxicity; administer in combination with fluorouracil/leucovorin calcium

Stage III colon cancer (adjuvant): IV: 85 mg/m^2 every 2 weeks for 12 cycles; administer in combination with fluorouracil/leucovorin calcium

Dosing adjustment for obesity: Adults: ASCO Guidelines for appropriate chemotherapy dosing in obese adults with cancer: Utilize patient's actual body weight (full weight) for calculation of body surface area- or weight-based dosing, particularly when the intent of therapy is curative; manage regimen-related toxicities in the same manner as for nonobese patients; if a dose reduction is utilized due to toxicity, consider resumption of full weight-based dosing with subsequent cycles, especially if cause of toxicity (eg, hepatic or renal impairment) is resolved (Griggs, 2012).

Dosing adjustments for toxicity: Adults:

Acute toxicities: Longer infusion time (6 hours) may mitigate acute toxicities (eg, pharyngolaryngeal dysesthesia)

Neurosensory events:

Persistent (>7 days) grade 2 neurosensory events:

- Adjuvant treatment of stage III colon cancer: Reduce dose to 75 mg/m^2
- Advanced colorectal cancer: Reduce dose to 65 mg/m^2

Consider withholding oxaliplatin for grade 2 neuropathy lasting >7 days despite dose reduction.

Persistent (>7 days) grade 3 neurosensory events: Consider discontinuing oxaliplatin.

Gastrointestinal toxicity (grade 3/4):

Adjuvant treatment of stage III colon cancer: Delay next dose until recovery from toxicity, then reduce dose to 75 mg/m^2

Advanced colorectal cancer: Delay next dose until recovery from toxicity, then reduce dose to 65 mg/m^2

Hematologic toxicity (grade 4 neutropenia or grade 3/4 thrombocytopenia):

Adjuvant treatment of stage III colon cancer: Delay next dose until neutrophils recover to ≥1500/mm^3 and platelets recover to ≥75,000/mm^3, then reduce dose to 75 mg/m^2.

Advanced colorectal cancer: Delay next dose until neutrophils recover to ≥1500/mm^3 and platelets recover to ≥75,000/mm^3, then reduce dose to 65 mg/m^2.

Pulmonary toxicity (unexplained respiratory symptoms, including nonproductive cough, dyspnea, crackles, pulmonary infiltrates): Discontinue until interstitial lung disease or pulmonary fibrosis have been excluded.

Dosing adjustment in renal impairment: Adults:

Mild to moderate impairment: No dosage adjustment required

Severe impairment: Reduce dose to 65 mg/m^2

Dosing adjustment in hepatic impairment: Adults: There are no dosage adjustments provided in the manufacturer's labeling; however, some have suggested that dosage adjustment is not necessary (Doroshow, 2003; Synold, 2007)

Preparation for Administration Hazardous agent; use appropriate precautions for handling and disposal (NIOSH 2014 [group 1]).

Do not prepare using a chloride-containing solution such as NaCl due to rapid conversion to monochloroplatinum, dichloroplatinum, and diaquoplatinum; all highly reactive in sodium chloride (Takimoto 2007). Do not use needles or administration sets containing aluminum during preparation.

Aqueous solution: Dilution with D_5W (250 or 500 mL) is required prior to administration.

Lyophilized powder: Use only SWFI or D_5W to reconstitute powder. To obtain final concentration of 5 mg/mL add 10 mL of diluent to 50 mg vial or 20 mL diluent to 100 mg vial. Gently swirl vial to dissolve powder. Dilution with D_5W (250 or 500 mL) is required prior to administration. Discard unused portion of vial.

Administration Hazardous agent; use appropriate precautions for handling and disposal (NIOSH 2014 [group 1]). Oxaliplatin is associated with moderate emetic potential and preventative antiemetics recommended (Basch 2011; Dupuis 2011; Roila 2010).

IV: Administer as IV infusion over 2 to 6 hours. Flush infusion line with D_5W prior to administration of any concomitant medication. Do **not** use IV administration sets containing aluminum. When used in combination with a fluoropyrimidine (eg, 5-FU), infuse oxaliplatin first.

Irritant with vesicant-like properties; ensure proper needle or catheter placement prior to and during infusion. Avoid extravasation; monitor IV site for redness, swelling, or pain. If extravasation occurs, stop infusion immediately and disconnect (leave cannula/needle in place); gently aspirate extravasated solution (do **NOT** flush the line); remove needle/cannula; elevate extremity. Information conflicts regarding use of warm or cold compresses. Cold compresses could potentially precipitate or exacerbate peripheral neuropathy (de Lemos 2005).

Vesicant/Extravasation Risk Irritant with vesicant-like properties

Cold compress may cause local vasoconstriction and reduce cellular injury; however, may cause or exacerbate peripheral neuropathy; warm compresses may increase local drug removal, although may also increase cellular uptake and injury (de Lemos, 2005).

Monitoring Parameters CBC with differential, hemoglobin, platelet count, blood chemistries (including serum creatinine, ALT, AST, and bilirubin) prior to each cycle; INR and prothrombin time (in patients on oral anticoagulant therapy); signs of neuropathy, hypersensitivity reaction, respiratory effects, and/or RPLS.

Dosage Forms Excipient information presented when available (limited, particularly for generics); consult specific product labeling.

Solution, Intravenous [preservative free]:
- Eloxatin: 50 mg/10 mL (10 mL); 100 mg/20 mL (20 mL); 200 mg/40 mL (40 mL)
- Generic: 50 mg/10 mL (10 mL); 100 mg/20 mL (20 mL)

Solution Reconstituted, Intravenous [preservative free]:
- Generic: 50 mg (1 ea); 100 mg (1 ea)

◆ **Oxandrin** *see* Oxandrolone *on page* *1581*

Oxandrolone (oks AN droe lone)

Brand Names: US Oxandrin

Therapeutic Category Anabolic Steroid; Androgen

Generic Availability (US) Yes

Use Adjunctive therapy to promote weight gain after weight loss following extensive surgery, chronic infections, or severe trauma, and in some patients who, without definite pathophysiologic reasons, fail to gain or to maintain normal weight; to offset protein catabolism with prolonged corticosteroid administration and for the relief of bone pain associated with osteoporosis (All indications: FDA approved in children and adults); has also been used in the management of Turner syndrome in girls, constitutional delay of growth and puberty (CDGP), and for postoperative burn management to increase lean muscle mass and promote wound healing.

Pregnancy Risk Factor X

Pregnancy Considerations Use is contraindicated in women who are or may become pregnant; masculinization of the fetus has been reported.

Breast-Feeding Considerations It is not known if oxandrolone is excreted in breast milk. Due to the potential for serious adverse reactions in the nursing infant, breast-feeding is not recommended.

Contraindications Nephrosis; carcinoma of breast (women with hypercalcemia or men) or prostate; hypercalcemia; pregnancy

Warnings/Precautions **[U.S. Boxed Warning]: Anabolic steroids may cause peliosis hepatis or liver cell tumors which may not be apparent until liver failure or intra-abdominal hemorrhage develops.** Discontinue in case of cholestatic hepatitis with jaundice or abnormal liver function tests. Use caution with concomitant warfarin therapy; warfarin dose may need significantly decreased. **[U.S. Boxed Warning]: May cause blood lipid changes with increased risk of arteriosclerosis.** Use with caution in elderly patients, they may be at greater risk for prostatic hyperplasia, prostate cancer, fluid retention, and transaminase elevations. Use with caution in patients with cardiac, renal, or hepatic disease; COPD; diabetes; migraine; or epilepsy. Use with caution in patients with breast cancer; may cause hypercalcemia by stimulating osteolysis. May cause mild virilization in females; monitor for signs of virilization (deepening of the voice, hirsutism, acne, clitoromegaly). Discontinue with evidence of mild virilization in female patients; early discontinuation may prevent irreversible virilization. May accelerate bone maturation without producing compensatory gain in linear growth in children; effect may continue for 6 months after the drug is stopped; in prepubertal children perform radiographic examination of the left hand and wrist every 6 months to determine the rate of bone maturation and to assess the effect of treatment on the epiphyseal centers. Anabolic steroids have not been shown to improve athletic ability.

Adverse Reactions

Cardiovascular: Edema

Central nervous system: Depression, excitation, insomnia

Dermatologic: Acne (females and prepubertal males)
- Also reported in females: Hirsutism, male-pattern baldness

Endocrine & metabolic: Electrolyte imbalances, glucose intolerance, gonadotropin secretion inhibited, gynecomastia, HDL decreased, LDL increased, libido changes
- Also reported in females: Clitoral enlargement, menstrual irregularities

Genitourinary:
- Prepubertal males: Erections increased or persistent, penile enlargement
- Postpubertal males: Bladder irritation, epididymitis, impotence, oligospermia, priapism (chronic), testicular atrophy, testicular function

Hematologic: Prothrombin time increased, suppression of clotting factors

Hepatic: Alkaline phosphatase increased, ALT increased, AST increased, bilirubin increased, cholestatic jaundice, hepatic necrosis (rare), hepatocellular neoplasms, peliosis hepatis (with long-term therapy)

Neuromuscular & skeletal: CPK increased, premature closure of epiphyses (in children)

Renal: Creatinine excretion increased

Miscellaneous: Bromsulfophthalein retention, habituation, voice alteration (deepening, in females)

Rare but important or life-threatening: Hepatotoxicity (idiosyncratic) (Chalasani, 2014)

Drug Interactions

Metabolism/Transport Effects None known.

Avoid Concomitant Use There are no known interactions where it is recommended to avoid concomitant use.

Increased Effect/Toxicity

Oxandrolone may increase the levels/effects of: Blood Glucose Lowering Agents; C1 inhibitors; CycloSPORINE (Systemic); Vitamin K Antagonists

The levels/effects of Oxandrolone may be increased by: Corticosteroids (Systemic)

Decreased Effect There are no known significant interactions involving a decrease in effect.

Storage/Stability Store at 20°C to 25°C (68°F to 77°F).

Mechanism of Action Synthetic testosterone derivative with similar androgenic and anabolic actions

Pharmacokinetics (Adult data unless noted)

Absorption: Oral: Well absorbed (Orr, 2004)

Protein binding: 95% (Orr, 2004)

Half-life elimination: 10-13 hours

Time to peak serum concentration: ~1 hour (Orr, 2004)

Elimination: Urine (28% as unchanged drug) (Orr, 2004)

Dosing: Usual

Pediatric:

Weight gain, adjunct: Children and Adolescents: Oral: Total daily dose: ≤0.1 mg/kg; may be repeated intermittently as needed; in adult patients, the daily dose is divided 2-4 times daily; typical duration of therapy: 2-4 weeks

Burn management, severe; to increase lean muscle mass and promote wound healing: Limited data available: Children and Adolescents: Oral: 0.1 mg/kg/dose twice daily for up to 12 months has been shown to increase lean body mass, bone mineral density, and muscle strength; shortened length of ICU stay and improved donor site wound healing were also observed (Hart, 2001; Jeschke, 2007; Murphy, 2004; Porro, 2012; Pzkora, 2005). Benefits have been shown to persist for up to 5 years post burn (Porro, 2012; Przkora, 2005).

Constitutional delay of growth and puberty (CDGP) (males): Limited data available: Children and Adolescents 9-16 years: Oral: 1.25-2.5 mg once daily in the evening; usual duration: 3-12 months although longer (~5 years) has been reported (Albanese, 1994; Buyukgebiz, 1990; Papadimitriou, 1991; Schroor, 1995; Stanhope, 1985; Stanhope, 1988; Tse, 1990)

Turner Syndrome (females): Limited data available: Children and Adolescents ≥8 years: Oral: Reported range: 0.03-0.06 mg/kg/day at bedtime in combination with growth hormone and/or estrogen; maximum single dose: 2.5 mg; due to risks of dose-related virilization, doses ≥0.05 mg/kg/day should generally be avoided. Typically, therapy initiated at 8-9 years of age and continued until goal height attained or further growth is unlikely (bone age ≥14 years and growth velocity <2 cm/year) [Bareille, 1997; NIH (Bondy), 2007, Freriks, 2013; Gault, 2011; Haeusler, 1995; Menke, 2010, Nilsson, 1996).

Adult: **Weight gain, adjunct:** Oral: 2.5-20 mg/day in 2-4 divided based on individual response; a course of therapy of 2-4 weeks is usually adequate. This may be repeated intermittently as needed.

Dosing adjustment in renal impairment: There are no dosage adjustments provided in the manufacturer's labeling. Caution is recommended because of the propensity of oxandrolone to cause edema and water retention.

Dosing adjustment in hepatic impairment: There are no dosage adjustments provided in the manufacturer's labeling.

Monitoring Parameters Liver function tests, lipid profile, hemoglobin/hematocrit; INR/PT in patients on anticoagulant therapy

Children: Radiographs of left wrist every 6 months to assess bone maturation

Females: Signs of virilization (deepening voice, hirsutism, acne, clitoromegaly); urine and serum calcium in women with breast cancer

Test Interactions May suppress factors II, V, VII, and X; may increase PT; may decrease thyroxine-binding globulin and radioactive iodine uptake

Controlled Substance C-III

Dosage Forms Excipient information presented when available (limited, particularly for generics); consult specific product labeling.

Tablet, Oral:

Oxandrin: 2.5 mg [scored]

Oxandrin: 10 mg

Generic: 2.5 mg, 10 mg

Extemporaneous Preparations A 1 mg/mL oral suspension may be made with tablets and either a 1:1 mixture of Ora-Sweet® and Ora-Plus®, or a 1:1 mixture of Ora-Sweet® SF and Ora-Plus®. Crush twenty-four 2.5 mg tablets in a mortar to a fine powder. Add small portions of chosen vehicle and mix to a uniform paste; mix while adding the vehicle in incremental proportions to **almost** 60 mL; transfer to a calibrated bottle, rinse mortar with vehicle, and add quantity of vehicle sufficient to make 60 mL. Thoroughly mix the suspension by shaking. Label "shake well" and "protect from light". Stable for 90 days at room temperature (Johnson, 2011).

Johnson CE, Cober MP, Hawkins KA, et al, "Stability of Extemporaneously Prepared Oxandrolone Oral Suspensions," *Am J Health-Syst Pharm*, 2011, 68(6):519-21.

Oxaprozin (oks a PROE zin)

Medication Safety Issues

Sound-alike/look-alike issues:

Oxaprozin may be confused with oxazepam, OXcarbazepine

BEERS Criteria medication:

This drug may be potentially inappropriate for use in geriatric patients (Quality of evidence - moderate; Strength of recommendation - strong).

Brand Names: US Daypro

Brand Names: Canada Apo-Oxaprozin

Therapeutic Category Analgesic, Non-narcotic; Anti-inflammatory Agent; Nonsteroidal Anti-inflammatory Drug (NSAID), Oral

Generic Availability (US) Yes

Use Symptomatic relief of the signs and symptoms of osteoarthritis; adult and juvenile idiopathic arthritis(JIA)

Medication Guide Available Yes

Pregnancy Risk Factor C

Pregnancy Considerations Adverse events were not observed in the initial animal reproduction studies; therefore, the manufacturer classifies oxaprozin as pregnancy category C. NSAID exposure during the first trimester is not strongly associated with congenital malformations; however, cardiovascular anomalies and cleft palate have been observed following NSAID exposure in some studies. The use of an NSAID close to conception may be associated with an increased risk of miscarriage. Nonteratogenic effects have been observed following NSAID administration during the third trimester including myocardial degenerative changes, prenatal constriction of the ductus arteriosus, fetal tricuspid regurgitation, failure of the ductus arteriosus to close postnatally; renal dysfunction or failure, oligohydramnios; gastrointestinal bleeding or perforation, increased risk of necrotizing enterocolitis; intracranial bleeding (including intraventricular hemorrhage), platelet dysfunction with resultant bleeding; pulmonary hypertension. Because they may cause premature closure of the ductus arteriosus, use of NSAIDs late in pregnancy should be avoided (use after 31 or 32 weeks gestation is not recommended by some clinicians). The chronic use of NSAIDs in women of reproductive age may be associated with infertility that is reversible upon discontinuation of the medication. A registry is available for pregnant women exposed to autoimmune medications including oxaprozin. For additional information, contact the Organization of Teratology Information Specialists, OTIS Autoimmune Diseases Study, at 877-311-8972.

Breast-Feeding Considerations The amount of oxaprozin found in breast milk is not known; however, distribution into breast milk would be expected. Breast-feeding is not recommended by the manufacturer.

Contraindications Hypersensitivity to oxaprozin, aspirin, other NSAIDs, or any component of the formulation; perioperative pain in the setting of coronary artery bypass graft (CABG) surgery

Warnings/Precautions **[U.S. Boxed Warning]: NSAIDs are associated with an increased risk of adverse cardiovascular thrombotic events, including MI and stroke.** Risk may be increased with duration of use or pre-existing cardiovascular risk factors or disease. Carefully evaluate individual cardiovascular risk profiles prior to prescribing. May cause new onset hypertension or worsening of existing hypertension. Use caution with fluid retention. Avoid use in heart failure (ACCF/AHA [Yancy, 2013]). Concurrent administration of ibuprofen, and potentially other nonselective NSAIDs, may interfere with aspirin' s cardioprotective effect. **[U.S. Boxed Warning]: Use is contraindicated for treatment of perioperative pain in the setting of coronary artery bypass graft (CABG) surgery.** Risk of MI and stroke may be increased with use following CABG surgery.

Platelet adhesion and aggregation may be decreased; may prolong bleeding time; patients with coagulation disorders or who are receiving anticoagulants should be monitored closely. Anemia may occur; patients on long-term NSAID therapy should be monitored for anemia. Rarely, NSAID use may cause severe blood dyscrasias (eg, agranulocytosis, aplastic anemia, thrombocytopenia).

NSAID use may compromise existing renal function; dose-dependent decreases in prostaglandin synthesis may result from NSAID use, reducing renal blood flow which may cause renal decompensation. NSAID use may increase the risk for hyperkalemia. Patients with impaired renal function, dehydration, heart failure, liver dysfunction, those taking diuretics, and ACE inhibitors, and the elderly are at greater risk of renal toxicity and hyperkalemia. In the elderly, may be inappropriate for long-term use due to potential for GI bleeding, hypertension, heart failure, and renal failure (Beers Criteria). Rehydrate patient before starting therapy; monitor renal function closely. Not recommended for use in patients with advanced renal disease. Long-term NSAID use may result in renal papillary necrosis.

[U.S. Boxed Warning]: NSAIDs may increase risk of gastrointestinal irritation, inflammation, ulceration, bleeding, and perforation. These events may occur at any time during therapy and without warning. Use caution with a history of GI disease (bleeding or ulcers); concurrent therapy with aspirin, anticoagulants, and/or corticosteroids; smoking; use of alcohol; and the elderly or debilitated patients. When used concomitantly with aspirin, a substantial increase in the risk of gastrointestinal complications (eg, ulcer) occurs; concomitant gastroprotective therapy (eg, proton pump inhibitors) is recommended (Bhatt, 2008).

Use the lowest effective dose for the shortest duration of time, consistent with individual patient goals, to reduce risk of cardiovascular or GI adverse events. Alternate therapies should be considered for patients at high risk.

NSAIDs may cause serious skin adverse events including exfoliative dermatitis, Stevens-Johnson syndrome (SJS), and toxic epidermal necrolysis (TEN); discontinue use at first sign of skin rash or hypersensitivity. Anaphylactoid reactions may occur, even without prior exposure; patients with "aspirin triad" (bronchial asthma, aspirin intolerance, rhinitis) may be at increased risk. Do not use in patients who experience bronchospasm, asthma, rhinitis, or urticaria with NSAID or aspirin therapy. Use caution in other forms of asthma.

Use with caution in patients with decreased hepatic function. Closely monitor patients with any abnormal LFT. Severe hepatic reactions (eg, fulminant hepatitis, liver failure) have occurred with NSAID use, rarely; discontinue if signs or symptoms of liver disease develop, or if systemic manifestations occur.

NSAIDS may cause drowsiness, dizziness, blurred vision and other neurologic effects which may impair physical or mental abilities; patients must be cautioned about performing tasks which require mental alertness (eg, operating machinery or driving). Discontinue use with blurred or diminished vision and perform ophthalmologic exam. Monitor vision with long-term therapy.

In the elderly, avoid chronic use (unless alternative agents ineffective and patient can receive concomitant gastroprotective agent); nonselective oral NSAID use is associated with an increased risk of GI bleeding and peptic ulcer disease in older adults in high risk category (eg, >75 years or age or receiving concomitant oral/parenteral corticosteroids, anticoagulants, or antiplatelet agents) (Beers Criteria).

Withhold for at least 4-6 half-lives prior to surgical or dental procedures. May cause mild photosensitivity reactions.

Adverse Reactions

Cardiovascular: Edema

Central nervous system: Confusion, depression, dizziness, headache, sedation, sleep disturbance, somnolence

Dermatologic: Pruritus, rash

Gastrointestinal: Abdominal distress, abdominal pain, anorexia, constipation, diarrhea, dyspepsia, flatulence, gastrointestinal ulcer, gross bleeding with perforation, heartburn, nausea, vomiting

Hematologic: Anemia, bleeding time increased

Hepatic: Liver enzymes increased

Otic: Tinnitus

Renal: Dysuria, renal function abnormal, urinary frequency

Rare but important or life-threatening (effects reported with oxaprozin or other NSAIDs): Acute interstitial nephritis, acute renal failure, agranulocytosis, alopecia, anaphylaxis, angioedema, anxiety, aplastic anemia, appetite changes, arrhythmia, asthma, blurred vision, bruising, coma, conjunctivitis, cystitis, death, diaphoresis, dream abnormalities, drowsiness, dyspnea, eosinophilia, eructation, erythema multiforme, esophagitis, exfoliative dermatitis, fever, gastritis, GI bleeding, glossitis, hallucinations, hearing decreased, heart failure, hematemesis, hematuria, hemolytic anemia, hemorrhoidal bleeding, hepatitis, hepatitis, hepatotoxicity (idiosyncratic) (Chalasani, 2014), hyperglycemia, hypersensitivity reaction, hyper-/hypotension, infection, insomnia, jaundice, leukopenia, liver failure, liver function abnormalities, lymphadenopathy, malaise, melena, meningitis, menstrual flow increased/decreased, myocardial infarction, nephrotic syndrome, nervousness, oliguria, palpitation, pancreatitis, pancytopenia, paresthesia, peptic ulcer, photosensitivity, pneumonia, polyuria, proteinuria, pseudoporphyria, pulmonary infection, purpura, rectal bleeding, renal insufficiency, respiratory depression, seizures, sepsis, serum sickness, sinusitis, Stevens-Johnson syndrome, stomatitis, syncope, tachycardia, taste alteration, thrombocytopenia, toxic epidermal necrolysis, tremor, upper respiratory tract infection, urticaria, vasculitis, vertigo, weakness, weight changes, xerostomia

Drug Interactions

Metabolism/Transport Effects None known.

Avoid Concomitant Use

Avoid concomitant use of Oxaprozin with any of the following: Dexketoprofen; Floctafenine; Ketorolac

(Nasal); Ketorolac (Systemic); Morniflumate; NSAID (COX-2 Inhibitor); Omacetaxine; Urokinase

Increased Effect/Toxicity

Oxaprozin may increase the levels/effects of: 5-ASA Derivatives; Agents with Antiplatelet Properties; Aliskiren; Aminoglycosides; Anticoagulants; Apixaban; Bisphosphonate Derivatives; Collagenase (Systemic); CycloSPORINE (Systemic); Dabigatran Etexilate; Deferasirox; Deoxycholic Acid; Desmopressin; Digoxin; Drospirenone; Eplerenone; Haloperidol; Ibritumomab; Lithium; Methotrexate; Nonsteroidal Anti-Inflammatory Agents; NSAID (COX-2 Inhibitor); Obinutuzumab; Omacetaxine; PEMEtrexed; Porfimer; Potassium-Sparing Diuretics; PRALAtrexate; Quinolone Antibiotics; Rivaroxaban; Salicylates; Tacrolimus (Systemic); Tenofovir; Thrombolytic Agents; Tositumomab and Iodine I 131 Tositumomab; Urokinase; Vancomycin; Verteporfin; Vitamin K Antagonists

The levels/effects of Oxaprozin may be increased by: ACE Inhibitors; Angiotensin II Receptor Blockers; Antidepressants (Tricyclic, Tertiary Amine); Corticosteroids (Systemic); CycloSPORINE (Systemic); Dasatinib; Dexketoprofen; Diclofenac (Systemic); Floctafenine; Glucosamine; Herbs (Anticoagulant/Antiplatelet Properties); Ibrutinib; Ketorolac (Nasal); Ketorolac (Systemic); Limaprost; Morniflumate; Multivitamins/Fluoride (with ADE); Multivitamins/Minerals (with ADEK, Folate, Iron); Multivitamins/Minerals (with AE, No Iron); Omega-3 Fatty Acids; Pentosan Polysulfate Sodium; Pentoxifylline; Probenecid; Prostacyclin Analogues; Selective Serotonin Reuptake Inhibitors; Serotonin/Norepinephrine Reuptake Inhibitors; Sodium Phosphates; Tipranavir; Treprostinil; Vitamin E

Decreased Effect

Oxaprozin may decrease the levels/effects of: ACE Inhibitors; Aliskiren; Angiotensin II Receptor Blockers; Beta-Blockers; Eplerenone; HydrALAZINE; Loop Diuretics; Potassium-Sparing Diuretics; Prostaglandins (Ophthalmic); Salicylates; Selective Serotonin Reuptake Inhibitors; Thiazide Diuretics

The levels/effects of Oxaprozin may be decreased by: Bile Acid Sequestrants; Salicylates

Storage/Stability Store at 25°C (77°F); excursions permitted to 15°C to 30°C (59°F to 86°C). Protect from light; keep bottle tightly closed.

Mechanism of Action Reversibly inhibits cyclooxygenase-1 and 2 (COX-1 and 2) enzymes, which results in decreased formation of prostaglandin precursors; has antipyretic, analgesic, and anti-inflammatory properties.

Other proposed mechanisms not fully elucidated (and possibly contributing to the anti-inflammatory effect to varying degrees) include inhibiting chemotaxis, altering lymphocyte activity, inhibiting neutrophil aggregation/activation, and decreasing proinflammatory cytokine levels.

Pharmacodynamics Maximum effect: Due to its long half-life, several days of treatment are required for oxaprozin to reach its full effect

Pharmacokinetics (Adult data unless noted)

Absorption: Oral: 95%

Distribution: Distributes into synovial tissues at twice the concentration of plasma and 3 times the concentration of synovial fluid; expected to distribute into breast milk (exact amount not known)

V_d (apparent): Adults: 11-17 L per 70 kg

Protein binding: 99%, primarily to albumin; protein binding is saturable (nonlinear protein binding)

Metabolism: Hepatic via microsomal oxidation (65%) and conjugation with glucuronic acid (35%); major conjugated metabolites are ester and ether glucuronide (inactive); small amounts of an active phenolic metabolite is produced (<5%) but has limited contribution to overall activity

Half-life: Adults: 41-55 hours

Time to peak serum concentration: 2.4-3.1 hours

Elimination: Excreted in the urine (5% as unchanged drug, 65% as metabolites) and feces (35% as metabolites)

Clearance: After adjusting for body weight, no clinically important age-related differences in apparent clearance of unbound drug were identified between adult and pediatric patients ≥6 years of age

Dialysis: Not significantly removed by hemodialysis or CAPD due to high protein binding

Dosing: Usual Note: Use lowest effective dose; dose may be divided if patient does not tolerate once daily dosing; Oral:

Children 6-16 years: JIA: Dose according to body weight. **Note:** Doses greater than 1200 mg have not been evaluated:

22-31 kg: 600 mg once daily

32-54 kg: 900 mg once daily

≥55 kg: 1200 mg once daily

Adults: Osteoarthritis or Rheumatoid arthritis: Usual: 1200 mg once daily; titrate to lowest effective dose; patients with low body weight should start with 600 mg daily; a one-time loading dose of 1200 mg to 1800 mg or 26 mg/kg (whichever is lower) may be given if needed; maximum daily dose: 1800 mg or 26 mg/kg (whichever is lower) in divided doses

Note: Chronic administration of doses >1200 mg/day should be reserved for adult patients >50 kg with severe disease, low risk for peptic ulcer disease, and normal hepatic and renal function; ensure that patient tolerates lower doses before advancing to larger dose

Dosing adjustment in renal impairment: Severe renal impairment or patients on dialysis: Initial: 600 mg once daily; may increase dose if needed to 1200 mg once daily with close monitoring

Dosing adjustment in hepatic impairment: Use with caution in patients with severe hepatic dysfunction (dosage reduction is not required in patients with well compensated cirrhosis)

Administration May be administered without regard to food; administer with food or milk to decrease GI distress

Monitoring Parameters CBC, occult blood loss, liver enzymes, renal function tests; blood pressure, signs and symptoms of GI bleeding

Test Interactions False-positive urine immunoassay screening tests for benzodiazepines have been reported and may occur several days after discontinuing oxaprozin.

Additional Information An open-label study of oxaprozin (10-20 mg/kg/dose once daily) in 59 JIA patients [3-16 years of age (mean age: 9 years)], reported adverse events in 58% of patients; GI symptoms occurred at a higher incidence than historically reported in adults; 9 of 30 patients (30%) who continued therapy for a total of 19-48 weeks, developed a vesicular rash on sun-exposed areas of skin; 5 of these 9 patients with rash discontinued the drug (Bass, 1985).

Dosage Forms Excipient information presented when available (limited, particularly for generics); consult specific product labeling.

Tablet, Oral:

Daypro: 600 mg [scored]

Generic: 600 mg

◆ **Oxaydo** *see* OxyCODONE *on page* 1590

OXcarbazepine (ox car BAZ e peen)

Medication Safety Issues

Sound-alike/look-alike issues:

OXcarbazepine may be confused with carBAMazepine, oxaprozin, oxazepam

Trileptal may be confused with TriLipix

Related Information

Oral Medications That Should Not Be Crushed or Altered *on page 2476*

Safe Handling of Hazardous Drugs *on page 2455*

Brand Names: US Oxtellar XR; Trileptal

Brand Names: Canada Jamp-Oxcarbazepine; Trileptal

Therapeutic Category Anticonvulsant, Miscellaneous

Generic Availability (US) May be product dependent

Use Oral:

Immediate release; suspension, tablet (Trileptal®): Treatment of partial seizures (FDA approved as monotherapy in ages ≥4 years and adults; FDA approved as adjunctive therapy in ages ≥2 years and adults)

Extended release; tablet (Oxtellar XR™): Adjunctive therapy for treatment of partial seizures (FDA approved in ages ≥6 years and adults)

Medication Guide Available Yes

Pregnancy Risk Factor C

Pregnancy Considerations Adverse events have been observed in animal reproduction studies; therefore, the manufacturer classifies oxcarbazepine as pregnancy category C. Oxcarbazepine, the active metabolite MHD and the inactive metabolite DHD, crosses the placenta and can be detected in the newborn. An increased risk in the overall rate of major congenital malformations has not been observed following maternal use of oxcarbazepine. Available studies have not been large enough to determine if there is an increased risk of specific defects. In general, the risk of teratogenic effects is higher with AED polytherapy than monotherapy. Plasma concentrations of MHD gradually decrease due to physiologic changes which occur during pregnancy; patients should be monitored during pregnancy and postpartum. Oxcarbazepine may decrease plasma concentrations of hormonal contraceptives.

Patients exposed to oxcarbazepine during pregnancy are encouraged to enroll themselves into the NAAED Pregnancy Registry by calling 1-888-233-2334. Additional information is available at www.aedpregnancyregistry.org.

Breast-Feeding Considerations Oxcarbazepine and the active 10-hydroxy metabolite (MHD) are found in breast milk (small amounts). According to the manufacturer, the decision to continue or discontinue breast-feeding during therapy should take into account the risk of exposure to the infant and the benefits of treatment to the mother.

Contraindications Hypersensitivity to oxcarbazepine or any component of the formulation

Warnings/Precautions Hazardous agent - use appropriate precautions for handling and disposal (NIOSH 2014 [group 2]).

Antiepileptics are associated with an increased risk of suicidal behavior/thoughts with use (regardless of indication); patients should be monitored for signs/symptoms of depression, suicidal tendencies, and other unusual behavior changes during therapy and instructed to inform their healthcare provider immediately if symptoms occur.

Clinically-significant hyponatremia (serum sodium <125 mmol/L) may develop during oxcarbazepine use. Rare cases of anaphylaxis and angioedema have been reported, even after initial dosing; permanently discontinue should symptoms occur. Use caution in patients with previous hypersensitivity to carbamazepine (cross-sensitivity occurs in 25% to 30% of patients). Potentially serious, sometimes fatal, dermatologic reactions (eg, Stevens-Johnson, toxic epidermal necrolysis) and drug reaction with eosinophilia and systemic symptoms (DRESS) also known as multiorgan hypersensitivity reactions have been reported in adults and children; monitor for signs and symptoms of skin reactions and possible disparate manifestations associated with lymphatic, hepatic, renal, cardiovascular, and/or hematologic organ systems; discontinuation and conversion to alternate therapy may be required. Considering screening patients of Asian descent for the variant human leukocyte antigen (HLA) allele B*1502 prior to initiating therapy. This genetic variant has been associated with a significantly increased risk of developing Stevens-Johnson syndrome and/or toxic epidermal necrolysis in patients receiving carbamazepine. Structural similarity of oxcarbazepine to carbamazepine, available clinical evidence, and data from nonclinical studies showing a direct interaction of oxcarbazepine with the HLA-B*1502 protein suggest patients receiving oxcarbazepine may be at a similar risk. Consider avoiding use of oxcarbazepine in patients with a positive result. Screening is not recommending in low-risk populations or in current oxcarbazepine patients (risk usually during first few months of therapy). Clinical trials excluded patients with significant cardiovascular disease or ECG abnormalities; Canadian labeling recommends using caution with cardiac conduction abnormalities or concomitant drugs that depress atrioventricular (AV) conduction and to avoid use in patients with AV block. Monitor body weight/fluid retention in patients with HF; evaluate serum sodium with worsening cardiac function or fluid retention.

Hepatitis and hepatic failure have been reported rarely (Hsu 2010; Trileptal Canadian product monograph 2013). Promptly evaluate any symptoms of hepatic dysfunction (eg, anorexia, nausea/vomiting, right upper quadrant pain, pruritus) and discontinue therapy immediately if significant abnormalities are confirmed. Agranulocytosis, leukopenia, and pancytopenia have been reported rarely. Discontinuation and conversion to alternate therapy may be required. Long term use has been associated with decreased bone mineral density, osteopenia, osteoporosis, and fractures.

As with all antiepileptic drugs, oxcarbazepine should be withdrawn gradually to minimize the potential of increased seizure frequency. Use of oxcarbazepine has been associated with CNS-related adverse events, most significant of these were cognitive symptoms including psychomotor slowing, difficulty with concentration, speech or language problems, somnolence or fatigue, and coordination abnormalities, including ataxia and gait disturbances. Single-dose studies show that half-life of the primary active metabolite is prolonged 3- to 4-fold and AUC is doubled in patients with CrCl <30 mL/minute; dose adjustment required in these patients. Potentially significant drug-drug interactions may exist, requiring dose or frequency adjustment, additional monitoring, and/or selection of alternative therapy. Oral suspension contains sorbitol; Canadian labeling recommends avoiding use in patients with fructose intolerance

Warnings: Additional Pediatric Considerations Usual onset of hyponatremia (ie, serum sodium <125 mEq/L) is within first 3 months of therapy with immediate release formulation, but has been reported in patients >1 year after initiation; reported incidence: Immediate release: 2.5%; extended release: 1.2%.

CNS adverse effects may occur, including somnolence (children: ~35%), fatigue, coordination abnormalities [ataxia and gait disturbances (children: 23%)], and cognitive symptoms [eg, difficulty concentrating, speech or language problems, and psychomotor slowing (5.8%)]; these effects may be more common when oxcarbazepine is used as add-on therapy versus monotherapy.

Trileptal and Oxtellar XR are not bioequivalent and not interchangeable on a mg-per-mg basis; systemic absorption and resulting serum concentrations are lower with once daily Oxtellar XR compared to twice daily Trileptal when administered at the same total daily dose; higher doses of Oxtellar XR may be necessary.

Some dosage forms may contain propylene glycol; in neonates large amounts of propylene glycol delivered orally, intravenously (eg, >3,000 mg/day), or topically have been associated with potentially fatal toxicities which can include metabolic acidosis, seizures, renal failure, and CNS depression; toxicities have also been reported in children and adults including hyperosmolality, lactic acidosis, seizures, and respiratory depression; use caution (AAP, 1997; Shehab, 2009).

Adverse Reactions

Cardiovascular: Bradycardia, cardiac failure, flushing, hypertension, hypotension, lower extremity edema, orthostatic hypotension, palpitations, syncope, tachycardia

Central nervous system: Abnormal gait, abnormal electroencephalogram, abnormality in thinking, aggressive behavior, agitation, amnesia, anxiety, apathy, aphasia, ataxia, aura, cerebral hemorrhage, confusion, convulsions, delirium, delusion, depression, dizziness, drowsiness, dysmetria, dystonia, emotional lability, equilibrium disturbance, euphoria extrapyramidal reaction, falling, fatigue, feeling abnormal, headache, hemiplegia, hyperkinesia, hyperreflexia, hypertonia, hypokinesia, hyporeflexia, hypotonia, hysteria, impaired consciousness, insomnia, intoxicated feeling, lack of concentration, malaise, manic behavior, migraine, myasthenia, nervousness, neuralgia, nightmares, oculogyric crisis, panic disorder, paralysis, personality disorder, precordial pain, psychosis, rigors, seizure (aggravated), speech disorder, stupor, vertigo, voice disorder

Dermatologic: Acne vulgaris, alopecia, contact dermatitis, diaphoresis, eczema, erythematosus rash, facial rash, folliculitis, genital pruritus, maculopapular rash, miliaria, psoriasis, skin photosensitivity, skin rash, urticaria, vitiligo

Endocrine & metabolic: Change in libido, decreased serum sodium (<135 mEq/L), hyponatremia, hot flash, hyperglycemia, hypermenorrhea, hypocalcemia, hypoglycemia, hypokalemia, increased gamma-glutamyl transferase, intermenstrual bleeding, weight gain, weight loss

Gastrointestinal: Aphthous stomatitis, biliary colic, bloody stools, cholelithiasis, colitis, constipation, diarrhea, duodenal ulcer, dysgeusia,dyspepsia, dysphagia, enteritis, eructation, esophagitis, flatulence, gastric ulcer, gastritis, gingival hemorrhage, gingival hyperplasia, hematemesis, hemorrhoids, hiccups, increased appetite, retching, sialadenitis, stomatitis, upper abdominal pain, xerostomia

Gastrointestinal: Abdominal pain, nausea, vomiting

Genitourinary: Dysuria, hematuria, leukorrhea, priapism, urinary frequency, urinary tract pain

Hematologic & oncologic: Bruise, purpura, rectal hemorrhage, thrombocytopenia

Hepatic: Increased liver enzymes

Hypersensitivity: Angioedema, hypersensitivity reaction

Neuromuscular & skeletal: Back pain, muscle spasm right hypochondrium pain, sprain, systemic lupus erythematosus, tetany, tremor, weakness

Ophthalmic: Accommodation disturbance, blepharoptosis, blurred vision, cataract, conjunctival hemorrhage, diplopia, hemianopia, mydriasis, nystagmus, ocular edema, photophobia, scotoma, visual disturbance, xerophthalmia

Otic: Otitis externa, tinnitus

Renal: Nephrolithiasis, polyuria, renal pain

Respiratory: asthma, dyspnea, epistaxis, laryngismus, nasopharyngitis, pleurisy, pneumonia, pulmonary infection, rhinitis, sinusitis, upper respiratory tract infection

Miscellaneous: Fever

Rare but important or life-threatening: Abnormal thyroid function test (decreased total T_4 and/or free T_4), acute generalized exanthematous pustulosis, agranulocytosis, anaphylaxis, aplastic anemia, bone fracture (long-term therapy), decreased bone mineral density (long-term therapy), DRESS syndrome, erythema multiforme, folate deficiency, hepatic failure, hepatitis (Hsu, 2010), hypersensitivity reaction, hypothyroidism, increased serum amylase, increased serum lipase, leukopenia, multiorgan hypersensitivity (eosinophilia, arthralgia, rash, fever, lymphadenopathy), osteopenia (long-term therapy), osteoporosis (long-term therapy), pancreatitis, pancytopenia, Stevens-Johnson syndrome, suicidal ideation, suicidal tendencies, toxic epidermal necrolysis

Drug Interactions

Metabolism/Transport Effects **Induces** CYP3A4 (weak)

Avoid Concomitant Use

Avoid concomitant use of OXcarbazepine with any of the following: Dolutegravir; Eslicarbazepine; Ledipasvir; Rilpivirine; Selegiline; Sofosbuvir; Ulipristal

Increased Effect/Toxicity

OXcarbazepine may increase the levels/effects of: Fosphenytoin-Phenytoin; PHENobarbital; Selegiline

The levels/effects of OXcarbazepine may be increased by: Alcohol (Ethyl); Eslicarbazepine; Perampanel; Thiazide Diuretics

Decreased Effect

OXcarbazepine may decrease the levels/effects of: ARIPiprazole; Cobicistat; Contraceptives (Estrogens); Contraceptives (Progestins); Dolutegravir; Elvitegravir; Hydrocodone; Ledipasvir; NiMODipine; Perampanel; Rilpivirine; Saxagliptin; Sofosbuvir; Ulipristal

The levels/effects of OXcarbazepine may be decreased by: CarBAMazepine; Fosphenytoin-Phenytoin; Mefloquine; Mianserin; Orlistat; PHENobarbital; Valproic Acid and Derivatives

Storage/Stability Store tablets and suspension at 25°C (77°F); excursions permitted to 15°C to 30°C (59°F to 86°F). Store suspension in the original container; use within 7 weeks of first opening container.

Mechanism of Action Pharmacological activity results from both oxcarbazepine and its monohydroxy metabolite (MHD). Precise mechanism of anticonvulsant effect has not been defined. Oxcarbazepine and MHD block voltage-sensitive sodium channels, stabilizing hyperexcited neuronal membranes, inhibiting repetitive firing, and decreasing the propagation of synaptic impulses. These actions are believed to prevent the spread of seizures. Oxcarbazepine and MHD also increase potassium conductance and modulate the activity of high-voltage activated calcium channels.

Pharmacokinetics (Adult data unless noted)

Absorption: Complete

Distribution: MHD: V_d (apparent): 49 L

Protein binding: Oxcarbazepine: 67%; MHD: 40%, primarily to albumin; parent drug and metabolite do not bind to alpha-1 acid glycoprotein

Metabolism: Oxcarbazepine is extensively metabolized in the liver to its active 10-monohydroxy metabolite (MHD); MHD undergoes further metabolism via glucuronide conjugation; 4% of dose is oxidized to the 10,11-dihydroxy metabolite (DHD) (inactive); 70% of serum concentration appears as MHD, 2% as unchanged oxcarbazepine, and the rest as minor metabolites; **Note:** Unlike carbamazepine, autoinduction of metabolism has not been observed and biotransformation of oxcarbazepine does not result in an epoxide metabolite

Bioavailability: Immediate release tablets and suspension have similar bioavailability (based on MDH serum concentrations). Extended release tablets and immediate release products are **not** bioequivalent.

Half-life:

Children (Rey, 2004):

2-5 years: MHD: Single dose: Mean range: 4.8-6.7 hours

6-12 years: MHD: Single dose: Mean range: 7.2-9.3 hours
Adults:
Immediate release: Oxcarbazepine: 2 hours; MHD: 9 hours
Extended release: Oxcarbazepine: 7-11 hours; MHD: 9-11 hours
Adults with renal impairment (CrCl <30 mL/minute): MHD: 19 hours
Time to peak serum concentration:
Children 2-12 years: Immediate release: Oxcarbazepine: 1 hour; MHD: 3-4 hours (Rey, 2004)
Adults:
Immediate release: MHD: Tablets: Median: 4.5 hours (range: 3-13 hours); Suspension: Median 6 hours
Extended release: MHD: 7 hours
Elimination: Urine (>95% of dose is excreted in the urine with <1% as unchanged parent drug), 27% as unchanged MHD, 49% as MHD glucuronides, 3% as DHD (inactive), and 13% as conjugate of oxcarbazepine and MHD); feces (<4%)
Clearance (per body weight):
Children 2 to <4 years: Increased by ~80% compared to adults
Children 4-12 years: Increased by ~40% compared to adults
Children ≥13 years: Values approach adult clearance

Dosing: Usual Note: Immediate release preparations (oral suspension and tablets) are interchangeable on a mg per mg basis; immediate release and extended release preparations are **not** bioequivalent and not interchangeable on a mg per mg basis.
Children and Adolescents:
Partial seizures, monotherapy: Oral: Immediate release (Trileptal®): Children and Adolescents 4-16 years:
Initiation of monotherapy:
Initial: 8-10 mg/kg/day in 2 divided doses; increase dose every third day by 5 mg/kg/day to achieve the recommended monotherapy maintenance dose by weight, as follows:
Maintenance dose:
20 to <25 kg: 600-900 mg/day in 2 divided doses
25 to <35 kg: 900-1200 mg/day in 2 divided doses
35 to <45 kg: 900-1500 mg/day in 2 divided doses
45 to <50 kg: 1200-1500 mg/day in 2 divided doses
50 to <60 kg: 1200-1800 mg/day in 2 divided doses
60 to <70 kg: 1200-2100 mg/day in 2 divided doses
≥70 kg: 1500-2100 mg/day in 2 divided doses
Conversion to monotherapy: Initial: 8-10 mg/kg/day in 2 divided doses, with a simultaneous initial reduction of the dose of concomitant antiepileptic drugs (AEDs); withdraw concomitant AEDs completely over 3-6 weeks, while increasing oxcarbazepine dose as needed by no more than 10 mg/kg/day at approximately weekly intervals; increase oxcarbazepine dose to achieve the recommended monotherapy maintenance dose.
Partial seizures, adjunctive therapy: Oral:
Immediate release (Trileptal®):
Children 2 to <4 years: Initial: 8-10 mg/kg/day in 2 divided doses (usual maximum initial daily dose: 600 mg/day); patients <20 kg may require a higher initial dose of 16-20 mg/kg/day in 2 divided doses; increase dose slowly over 2-4 weeks; maximum daily dose: 60 mg/kg/day
Children and Adolescents 4-16 years:
Initial: 8-10 mg/kg/day in 2 divided doses (usual maximum initial daily dose: 600 mg/day); increase dose slowly over 2 weeks to the target maintenance dose by weight, as follows:
Maintenance dose:
20-29 kg: 900 mg/day in 2 divided doses
29.1-39 kg: 1200 mg/day in 2 divided doses
>39 kg: 1800 mg/day in 2 divided doses
Note: Use of these pediatric target maintenance doses in one clinical trial resulted in doses ranging from 6-51 mg/kg/day (median dose: 31 mg/kg/day) in pediatric patients 4-16 years of age (Glauser, 2000). In children 2-4 years of age, 50% of patients were titrated to a final dose of at least 55 mg/kg/day with target dose of 60 mg/kg/day. Due to a higher drug clearance, children 2 to <4 years of age may require up to twice the dose per body weight compared to adults; children 4 to ≤12 years of age may require a 50% higher dose per body weight compared to adults.
Extended release (Oxtellar XR™): Children and Adolescents 6-17 years:
Initial: 8-10 mg/kg/day once daily; maximum initial daily dose: 600 mg/day during the first week of therapy; increase dose at weekly intervals in 8-10 mg/kg/day increments (maximum dosage incremental increase: 600 mg) to the target maintenance dose by weight, as follows:
Maintenance dose:
20-29 kg: 900 mg once daily
29.1-39 kg: 1200 mg once daily
>39 kg: 1800 mg once daily
Conversion from immediate release (Trileptal®) to extended release (Oxtellar XR™): Higher doses of Oxtellar XR™ may be necessary; on a mg per mg basis dosage forms are not bioequivalent.
Adults:
Partial seizures; adjunctive therapy (epilepsy): Oral:
Immediate release (Trileptal®): Initial: 600 mg daily in 2 divided doses; dose may be increased by as much as 600 mg/day increments at weekly intervals; recommended daily dose: 1200 mg daily in 2 divided doses. Although daily doses >1200 mg daily were somewhat more efficacious, most patients were unable to tolerate 2400 mg daily (due to CNS effects).
Extended release (Oxtellar XR™): Initial: 600 mg once daily; dosage may be increased by 600 mg/day increments at weekly intervals. Recommended daily dose is 1200-2400 mg once daily. Although daily doses >1200 mg daily were somewhat more efficacious, most patients were unable to tolerate 2400 mg daily (due to CNS effects).
Conversion to monotherapy, partial seizures (epilepsy): Patients receiving concomitant antiepileptic drugs (AEDs): Oral: Immediate release (Trileptal®): Initial: 600 mg daily in 2 divided doses while simultaneously reducing the dose of concomitant AEDs. Withdraw concomitant AEDs completely over 3-6 weeks, while increasing the oxcarbazepine dose in increments of 600 mg daily at weekly intervals, reaching the maximum oxcarbazepine dose (2400 mg daily in 2 divided doses) in about 2-4 weeks (lower doses have been effective in patients in whom monotherapy has been initiated).
Partial seizures; monotherapy (epilepsy): Patients not receiving prior AEDs: Oral: Immediate release (Trileptal®): Initial: 600 mg daily in 2 divided doses. Increase dose by 300 mg daily every third day to a dose of 1200 mg daily. Higher dosages (2400 mg daily) have been shown to be effective in patients converted to monotherapy from other AEDs.
Conversion from immediate release (Trileptal®) to extended release (Oxtellar XR™): Higher doses of Oxtellar XR™ may be necessary.

Dosing adjustment with concomitant antiepileptic drugs (AEDs): Adults: Concomitant use with enzyme-inducing antiepileptic drugs (eg, carbamazepine, phenobarbital, phenytoin): Extended release (Oxtellar XR™): Consider initiating dose at 900 mg once daily.

Dosing adjustment in renal impairment: Children, Adolescents, and Adults:

Severe impairment (CrCl <30 mL/minute): Immediate release (Trileptal®), Extended release (Oxtellar XR™): Therapy should be initiated at lower starting dose [eg, one-half the usual starting dose (adults: 300 mg daily)] and increased slowly to achieve desired clinical response (eg, adults: Increase in 300-450 mg daily increments at weekly intervals).

ESRD (on dialysis): Immediate release formulations should be used instead of extended release formulation.

Dosing adjustment in hepatic impairment: Children, Adolescents, and Adults:

Mild to moderate impairment: Immediate release (Trileptal®), Extended release (Oxtellar XR™): No dosage adjustments are recommended.

Severe impairment:

Immediate release (Trileptal®): Use caution (not studied).

Extended release (Oxtellar XR™): Not recommended (not studied).

Administration Hazardous agent; use appropriate precautions for handling and disposal (NIOSH 2014 [group 2]).

Oral:

Immediate release: May be taken without regard to meals

Suspension: Prior to using for the first time, firmly insert the manufacturer supplied plastic adapter into the neck of the bottle; cover the adapter with child-resistant cap when not in use; shake suspension well (for at least 10 seconds) before use; use manufacturer supplied oral syringe to withdraw appropriate dose; dose may be administered directly from syringe or mixed in a small amount of water immediately prior to use; after use, rinse oral syringe with warm water and allow to dry thoroughly; discard any unused portion 7 weeks after first opening bottle

Extended release: Administer on an empty stomach at least 1 hour before or 2 hours after food. Swallow whole; do not cut, crush, or chew the tablets.

Monitoring Parameters Seizure frequency, duration and severity; symptoms of CNS depression (dizziness, headache, somnolence); consider monitoring serum sodium (particularly during first three months of therapy) especially in patients who receive other drugs that may cause hyponatremia and in patients with symptoms of hyponatremia; signs and symptoms of suicidality (eg, anxiety, depression, behavior changes); hypersensitivity reactions; periodic thyroid function tests (particularly pediatric patients); CBC

Reference Range The metabolite of oxcarbazepine, 10-monohydroxy metabolite (MHD), is considered the active entity primarily responsible for the therapeutic effects. A clear correlation between MHD plasma concentrations and therapeutic response has not been demonstrated. A number of studies which included pediatric patients down to 1 year of age have suggested optimal MHD concentrations for efficacy may range from 2 to 55 mcg/mL and some experts suggest a target range of 8 to 35 mcg/mL based on clinical experience; however, a high degree of variability has been observed and within the pediatric population, the influence of pharmacokinetic differences in younger pediatric patients (faster MHD clearance) on therapeutic range have not been defined. Therapeutic drug monitoring of MHD is not routinely warranted; however, it may be beneficial in optimizing seizure control in the following situations: Extremes of age, pregnancy, to investigate the correlation between drug concentrations and toxicity especially with concurrent disease states such as renal impairment, to identify potential drug interactions, to assess reasons for therapeutic failure, or to rule out noncompliance (Bring 2008; May 2003).

Test Interactions Thyroid function tests; may depress serum T_4 without affecting T_3 levels or TSH

Additional Information Oxcarbazepine is a keto analogue of carbamazepine; symptoms of overdose may include CNS depression (somnolence, ataxia, obtundation)

Dosage Forms Excipient information presented when available (limited, particularly for generics); consult specific product labeling.

Suspension, Oral:

Trileptal: 300 mg/5 mL (250 mL) [contains alcohol, usp, methyl hydroxybenzoate, propyl hydroxybenzoate, propylene glycol, saccharin sodium; lemon flavor]

Generic: 300 mg/5 mL (250 mL)

Tablet, Oral:

Trileptal: 150 mg, 300 mg, 600 mg [scored]

Generic: 150 mg, 300 mg, 600 mg

Tablet Extended Release 24 Hour, Oral:

Oxtellar XR: 150 mg, 300 mg, 600 mg

- ◆ **Oxecta** *see* OxyCODONE *on page* *1590*
- ◆ **Oxecta [DSC]** *see* OxyCODONE *on page* *1590*
- ◆ **Oxeze Turbuhaler (Can)** *see* Formoterol *on page* *934*
- ◆ **Oxpentifylline** *see* Pentoxifylline *on page* *1670*
- ◆ **Oxtellar XR** *see* OXcarbazepine *on page* *1584*
- ◆ **Oxybutyn (Can)** *see* Oxybutynin *on page* *1588*

Oxybutynin (oks i BYOO ti nin)

Medication Safety Issues

Sound-alike/look-alike issues:

Oxybutynin may be confused with OxyCONTIN

Ditropan may be confused with Detrol, diazepam, Diprivan, dithranol

BEERS Criteria medication:

This drug may be potentially inappropriate for use in geriatric patients (Quality of evidence - varies based on comorbidity; Strength of recommendation - varies based on comorbidity)

Other safety concerns:

Transdermal patch may contain conducting metal (eg, aluminum); remove patch prior to MRI.

Related Information

Oral Medications That Should Not Be Crushed or Altered *on page 2476*

Brand Names: US Ditropan XL; Gelnique; Oxytrol; Oxytrol For Women [OTC]

Brand Names: Canada Apo-Oxybutynin; Ditropan XL; Dom-Oxybutynin; Gelnique; Mylan-Oxybutynin; Novo-Oxybutynin; Nu-Oxybutyn; Oxybutyn; Oxybutynine; Oxytrol; PHL-Oxybutynin; PMS-Oxybutynin; Riva-Oxybutynin; Uromax

Therapeutic Category Antispasmodic Agent, Urinary

Generic Availability (US) May be product dependent

Use Relief of bladder spasms associated with voiding in patients with uninhibited and reflex neurogenic bladder; treatment of overactive bladder with symptoms of urge urinary incontinence, urgency, and frequency (FDA approved in ages >5 and adults); symptoms of detrus or overactivity associated with a neurological condition (XL product FDA approved in ages >6 years)

Pregnancy Risk Factor B

Pregnancy Considerations Adverse events were not observed in animal reproduction studies.

Breast-Feeding Considerations It is not known if oxybutynin is excreted into breast milk. The manufacturer recommends that caution be used if administered to a nursing woman. Suppression of lactation has been reported.

Contraindications Hypersensitivity to oxybutynin or any component of the formulation; patients with or at risk for uncontrolled narrow-angle glaucoma, urinary retention, gastric retention or conditions with severely decreased GI motility

OTC labeling: When used for self-medication, do not use if you have pain or burning when urinating, blood in urine, unexplained lower back or side pain, cloudy or foul-smelling urine; in males; age <18 years; only experience accidental urine loss when cough, sneeze, or laugh; diagnosis of urinary or gastric retention; glaucoma; hypersensitivity to oxybutynin.

Warnings/Precautions May cause hypersensitivity reactions, including anaphylaxis and angioedema. Cases of angioedema involving the face, lips, tongue, and/or larynx have been reported with oral oxybutynin; some cases have occurred after a single dose. Discontinue immediately if tongue, hypopharynx, or larynx is involved; promptly initiate appropriate management. Use with caution in patients with bladder outflow obstruction (may increase the risk of urinary retention), Parkinson disease (may aggravate symptoms of disease), treated angle-closure glaucoma (use is contraindicated in uncontrolled narrow-angle glaucoma), hyperthyroidism, coronary artery disease, heart failure, hypertension, cardiac arrhythmias, hepatic or renal impairment, prostatic hyperplasia (may cause urinary retention), hiatal hernia, myasthenia gravis, dementia, automonic neuropathy (may aggravate symptoms of decreased GI motility). Use with caution in patients with decreased GI motility or gastrointestinal obstructive disorders (eg, ulcerative colitis, intestinal atony, pyloric stenosis); may increase the risk of gastric retention. In patients with ulcerative colitis, use may decrease gastric motility to the point of increasing the risk of paralytic ileus or toxic megacolon. Use with caution in patients with gastroesophageal reflux or with medications that may exacerbate esophagitis (eg, bisphosphonates). May increase the risk of heat prostration. Anticholinergics may cause agitation, confusion, drowsiness, dizziness, hallucinations, headache, and/or blurred vision, which may impair physical or mental abilities; patients must be cautioned about performing tasks which require mental alertness (eg, operating machinery or driving). Dose reduction or discontinuation should be considered if CNS effects occur.

Potentially significant drug-drug interactions may exist, requiring dose or frequency adjustment, additional monitoring, and/or selection of alternative therapy. This medication is associated with potent anticholinergic properties which may be inappropriate in older adults depending on comorbidities (eg, dementia, delirium) (Beers Criteria).

The extended release formulation consists of drug within a nondeformable matrix; following drug release/absorption, the matrix/shell is expelled in the stool. The use of nondeformable products in patients with known stricture/narrowing of the GI tract has been associated with symptoms of obstruction. Transdermal patch may contain conducting metal (eg, aluminum); remove patch prior to MRI. When using the topical gel, cover treatment area with clothing after gel has dried to minimize transferring medication to others. Discontinue gel if skin irritation occurs. Gel contains ethanol; do not expose to open flame or smoking until gel has dried.

When used for self-medication (OTC), other causes of frequent urination (UTI, diabetes, early pregnancy, other serious conditions) may need to be considered prior to use. Patients should contact a health care provider if symptoms do not improve within 2 weeks of initial use or for new or worsening symptoms.

Warnings: Additional Pediatric Considerations Some dosage forms may contain propylene glycol; in neonates large amounts of propylene glycol delivered orally, intravenously (eg, >3,000 mg/day), or topically have been associated with potentially fatal toxicities which can include metabolic acidosis, seizures, renal failure, and CNS depression; toxicities have also been reported in children and adults including hyperosmolality, lactic acidosis, seizures, and respiratory depression; use caution (AAP, 1997; Shehab, 2009).

Adverse Reactions

Oral:

Cardiovascular: Cardiac arrhythmia (sinus), decreased blood pressure, chest pain, edema, flushing, hypertension, palpitations, peripheral edema

Central nervous system: Confusion, depression, dizziness, drowsiness, fatigue, headache, insomnia, nervousness, pain

Dermatologic: Pruritus, xeroderma

Endocrine & metabolic: Fluid retention, hyperglycemia

Gastrointestinal: Abdominal pain, constipation, diarrhea, dry throat, dyspepsia, dysphagia, eructation, flatulence, gastroesophageal reflux disease, nausea, unpleasant taste, vomiting, xerostomia

Genitourinary: Cystitis, dysuria, pollakiuria, urinary hesitancy, urinary retention, urinary tract infection

Infection: Fungal infection

Neuromuscular & skeletal: Arthralgia, back pain, flank pain, limb pain, weakness

Ophthalmic: Blurred vision, eye irritation, keratoconjunctivitis sicca, xerophthalmia

Respiratory: Asthma, bronchitis, cough, dry nose, dry throat, hoarseness, nasal congestion, nasal dryness, nasopharyngitis, pharyngolaryngeal pain, sinus congestion, upper respiratory tract infection

Miscellaneous: Increased thirst

Rare but important or life-threatening: Anaphylaxis, anorexia, cycloplegia, decreased gastrointestinal motility, glaucoma, hallucination, hypersensitivity reaction, impotence, suppressed lactation, memory impairment, mydriasis, psychotic reaction, prolonged Q-T interval on ECG, seizure, tachycardia

Topical gel:

Central nervous system: Dizziness, fatigue, headache

Dermatologic: Pruritus

Gastrointestinal: Constipation, gastroenteritis, xerostomia

Genitourinary: Urinary tract infection

Local: Application site reaction (includes anesthesia, dermatitis, erythema, irritation, pain, papules, pruritus, rash)

Ophthalmic: Blurred vision, conjunctivitis, xerophthalmia

Respiratory: Nasopharyngitis, upper respiratory tract infection

Transdermal:

Gastrointestinal: Constipation, diarrhea, xerostomia

Genitourinary: Dysuria

Local: Erythema, localized vesiculation, macular eruption, pruritus, skin rash

Ophthalmic: Visual disturbance

Rare but important or life-threatening: Dizziness, drowsiness

Drug Interactions

Metabolism/Transport Effects Substrate of CYP3A4 (minor); **Note:** Assignment of Major/Minor substrate status based on clinically relevant drug interaction potential; **Inhibits** CYP2C8 (weak), CYP2D6 (weak)

Avoid Concomitant Use

Avoid concomitant use of Oxybutynin with any of the following: Aclidinium; Amodiaquine; Eluxadoline; Glucagon; Ipratropium (Oral Inhalation); Potassium Chloride; Tiotropium; Umeclidinium

Increased Effect/Toxicity

Oxybutynin may increase the levels/effects of: AbobotulinumtoxinA; Amodiaquine; Analgesics (Opioid); Anticholinergic Agents; ARIPiprazole; Cannabinoid-Containing Products; Eluxadoline; Glucagon; Mirabegron;

OnabotulinumtoxinA; Potassium Chloride; RimabotulinumtoxinB; Thiazide Diuretics; Tiotropium; Topiramate

The levels/effects of Oxybutynin may be increased by: Aclidinium; Alcohol (Ethyl); CYP3A4 Inhibitors (Strong); Ipratropium (Oral Inhalation); Mianserin; Pramlintide; Umeclidinium

Decreased Effect

Oxybutynin may decrease the levels/effects of: Acetylcholinesterase Inhibitors; Itopride; Metoclopramide; Secretin

The levels/effects of Oxybutynin may be decreased by: Acetylcholinesterase Inhibitors

Storage/Stability

Immediate release tablet and syrup: Store at 20°C to 25°C (68°F to 77°F). Protect from light.

Extended release tablet: Store at 25°C (77°F); excursions permitted to 15°C to 30°C (59°F to 86°F). Protect from moisture and humidity.

Topical gel (pump or sachets): Store at 25°C (77°F); excursions permitted to 15°C to 30°C (59°F to 86°F). Protect from moisture and humidity. Keep gel away from open flame. Do not store sachets outside the sealed pouch; apply immediately after removal from the protective pouch. Discard used sachets such that accidental application or ingestion by children, pets, or others is avoided.

Transdermal patch: Store at 20°C to 25°C (68°F to 77°F). Protect from moisture and humidity. Do not store outside the sealed pouch; apply immediately after removal from the protective pouch. Discard used patches such that accidental application or ingestion by children, pets, or others is avoided.

Mechanism of Action Direct antispasmodic effect on smooth muscle, also inhibits the action of acetylcholine on smooth muscle (exhibits 1/5 the anticholinergic activity of atropine, but has 4-10 times the antispasmodic activity); does not block effects at skeletal muscle or at autonomic ganglia; increases bladder capacity, decreases uninhibited contractions, and delays desire to void, therefore, decreases urgency and frequency

Pharmacodynamics

Immediate release formulation:
- Onset of action: Oral: Within 30-60 minutes
- Maximum effect: 3-6 hours
- Duration: 6-10 hours

Extended release formulation: Maximum effects: 3 days

Transdermal formulation: Duration: 96 hours

Pharmacokinetics (Adult data unless noted)

Absorption: Oral: Rapid and well absorbed

Distribution: V_d: Adults: 193 L

Metabolism: Hepatic via cytochrome isozyme CYP3A4 found mostly in liver and gut wall; extensive first pass effect (not with IV or transdermal use); metabolized in the liver to active and inactive metabolites

Bioavailability: Oral: Immediate release: 6% (range: 1.6% to 10.9%)

Half-life: Adults: 2-3 hours

Time to peak serum concentration:
- Immediate release: Within 60 minutes
- Extended release: 4-6 hours
- Transdermal: 24-48 hours

Elimination: <0.1% excreted unchanged in urine

Dosing: Usual

Children: Oral:

Immediate release:
- 1-5 years: 0.2 mg/kg/dose 2-3 times/day
- >5 years: 5 mg twice daily, up to 5 mg 3 times/day

Extended release: ≥6 years: 5 mg once daily; increase as tolerated in 5 mg increments to a maximum of 20 mg/day

Adults:

Oral: 5 mg 2-3 times/day up to 5 mg 4 times/day maximum **or** extended release tablet (Ditropan® XL) 5-10 mg once daily; increase in 5 mg increments to a maximum of 30 mg/day

Topical gel: Apply contents of one sachet (100 mg/g) once daily

Transdermal: 3.9 mg/day system applied twice weekly (every 3-4 days)

Note: Should be discontinued periodically to determine whether the patient can manage without the drug and to minimize tolerance to the drug

Administration

Oral: May be administered with or without food; swallow extended release tablets whole; do not chew or crush.

Topical gel: For topical use only. Apply to clean, dry, intact skin on abdomen, thighs, or upper arms/shoulders. Rotate site; do not apply to same site on consecutive days. Wash hands after use. Cover treated area with clothing after gel has dried to prevent transfer of medication to others. Do not bathe, shower, or swim until 1 hour after gel applied.

Transdermal: Apply to dry intact skin on the abdomen, hip, or buttock. Rotate site of application with each administration and avoid application to the same site within 7 days

Test Interactions May suppress the wheal and flare reactions to skin test antigens.

Dosage Forms Excipient information presented when available (limited, particularly for generics); consult specific product labeling.

Gel, Transdermal:
- Gelnique: 3% (92 g) [contains propylene glycol]

Gel, Transdermal, as chloride:
- Gelnique: 10% (1 g) [contains alcohol, usp]

Patch Twice Weekly, Transdermal:
- Oxytrol: 3.9 mg/24 hr (1 ea, 2 ea, 4 ea, 8 ea)
- Oxytrol For Women: 3.9 mg/24 hr (8 ea); 3.9 mg/24hr (4 ea)

Syrup, Oral, as chloride:
- Generic: 5 mg/5 mL (473 mL)

Tablet, Oral, as chloride:
- Generic: 5 mg

Tablet Extended Release 24 Hour, Oral, as chloride:
- Ditropan XL: 5 mg, 10 mg, 15 mg [contains polysorbate 80]
- Generic: 5 mg, 10 mg, 15 mg

◆ **Oxybutynin Chloride** *see* Oxybutynin *on page 1588*

◆ **Oxybutynine (Can)** *see* Oxybutynin *on page 1588*

◆ **Oxycodan® (Can)** *see* Oxycodone and Aspirin *on page 1597*

OxyCODONE (oks i KOE done)

Medication Safety Issues

Sound-alike/look-alike issues:

OxyCODONE may be confused with HYDROcodone, OxyCONTIN, oxymorphone

OxyCONTIN may be confused with MS Contin, oxybutynin

OxyFast may be confused with Roxanol

Roxicodone may be confused with Roxanol

High alert medication:

The Institute for Safe Medication Practices (ISMP) includes this medication among its list of drug classes which have a heightened risk of causing significant patient harm when used in error.

Related Information

Opioid Conversion Table *on page 2285*

Oral Medications That Should Not Be Crushed or Altered *on page 2476*

Patient Information for Disposal of Unused Medications *on page 2453*

Brand Names: US Oxecta [DSC]; OxyCONTIN; Roxicodone

Brand Names: Canada ACT Oxycodone CR; Apo-Oxycodone CR; Oxy.IR; OxyNEO; PMS-Oxycodone; PMS-Oxycodone CR; Supeudol

Therapeutic Category Analgesic, Narcotic

Generic Availability (US) May be product dependent

Use

Immediate release formulations (capsules, oral solution, and tablets): Management of moderate to severe pain (FDA approved in ages ≥18 years and adults)

Controlled release tablets (OxyContin®): For around-the-clock management of moderate to severe pain when an analgesic is needed for an extended period of time (FDA approved in ages ≥18 years and adults); immediate post-operative pain management in patients who received OxyContin® prior to surgery or if moderate to severe persistent pain is anticipated (FDA approved in ages ≥18 years and adults) **Note:** Not intended for use as a PRN analgesic or for treatment of mild pain, pain that is not expected to persist for an extended period of time, or for immediate postoperative pain (within 12-24 hours after surgery)

Prescribing and Access Restrictions As a requirement of the REMS program, healthcare providers who prescribe OxyContin need to receive training on the proper use and potential risks of OxyContin. For training, please refer to http://www.oxycontinrems.com. Prescribers will need retraining every 2 years or following any significant changes to the OxyContin REMS program.

Medication Guide Available Yes

Pregnancy Risk Factor B/C (manufacturer specific)

Pregnancy Considerations Adverse events were observed in some animal reproduction studies. Opioids cross the placenta. Oxycodone should not be used immediately prior to or during labor.

[U.S. Boxed Warning]: Prolonged maternal use of opioids during pregnancy can cause neonatal withdrawal syndrome in the newborn which may be life-threatening if not recognized and treated according to protocols developed by neonatology experts. If prolonged opioid therapy is required in a pregnant woman, ensure treatment is available and warn patient of risk to the neonate. If chronic opioid exposure occurs in pregnancy, adverse events in the newborn (including withdrawal) may occur; monitoring of the neonate is recommended. The minimum effective dose should be used if opioids are needed (Chou, 2009). Neonatal abstinence syndrome following opioid exposure may present with autonomic (eg, fever, temperature instability), gastrointestinal (eg, diarrhea, vomiting, poor feeding/weight gain), or neurologic (eg, high-pitched crying, increased muscle tone, irritability, seizure, tremor) symptoms (Dow, 2012; Hudak, 2012).

Long-term opioid use may cause secondary hypogonadism, which may lead to sexual dysfunction or infertility (Brennan, 2013).

Breast-Feeding Considerations Oxycodone is excreted into breast milk. Breast-feeding is not recommended by the manufacturer. Sedation and/or respiratory depression may occur in the infant; symptoms of opioid withdrawal may occur following the cessation of breast-feeding. Nursing infants exposed to large doses of opioids should be monitored for apnea and sedation. Use caution in a woman who may be an ultrarapid metabolizer; oxycodone is a substrate for CYP2D6 and their nursing infants may be at higher risk for adverse events (Montgomery, 2012).

Contraindications Hypersensitivity to oxycodone or any component of the formulation; significant respiratory depression; hypercarbia; acute or severe bronchial asthma; paralytic ileus (known or suspected); GI obstruction

Warnings/Precautions May cause CNS depression, which may impair physical or mental abilities; patients must be cautioned about performing tasks which require mental alertness (eg, operating machinery or driving). Potentially significant drug interactions may exist, requiring dose or frequency adjustment, additional monitoring, and/or selection of alternative therapy. Effects may be potentiated when used with other CNS depressants (eg, sedatives, anxiolytics, hypnotics, neuroleptics, other opioids). Use with caution in patients with hypersensitivity reactions to other phenanthrene derivative opioid agonists (morphine, hydrocodone, hydromorphone, levorphanol, oxymorphone). Use with caution in pancreatitis or biliary tract disease, acute alcoholism (including delirium tremens), morbid obesity, adrenocortical insufficiency, history of seizure disorders, hypothyroidism (including myxedema), prostatic hyperplasia, urethral stricture, and toxic psychosis. Use with caution and monitor for respiratory depression in patients with significant chronic obstructive pulmonary disease or cor pulmonale, and patients having a substantially decreased respiratory reserve, hypoxia, hypercarbia, or preexisting respiratory depression, particularly when initiating therapy and titrating with oxycodone; even therapeutic doses may decrease respiratory drive to the point of apnea. Consider the use of alternative non-opioid analgesics in these patients. May obscure diagnosis or clinical course of patients with acute abdominal conditions. Avoid use in patients with CNS depression/coma as these patients are susceptible to intracranial effects of CO_2 retention.

Use with caution in the elderly, debilitated, or cachectic patients, and hepatic or renal dysfunction. Hemodynamic effects (hypotension, orthostasis) may be exaggerated in patients with hypovolemia, concurrent vasodilating drugs, or in patients with head injury. Monitor for symptoms of hypotension following initiation or dose titration. Respiratory depressant effects and capacity to elevate CSF pressure may be exaggerated in presence of head injury, other intracranial lesion, or pre-existing intracranial pressure. May cause constipation which may be problematic in patients with unstable angina and patients post-myocardial infarction. Concurrent use of mixed agonist/antagonist analgesics (eg, pentazocine, nalbuphine, butorphanol) or partial agonist (eg, buprenorphine) analgesics may precipitate withdrawal symptoms and/or reduced analgesic efficacy in patients following prolonged therapy with mu opioid agonists. Taper dose gradually when discontinuing. Potentially significant interactions may exist, requiring dose or frequency adjustment, additional monitoring, and/or selection of alternative therapy.

Extended release tablets: Therapy should only be prescribed by healthcare professionals familiar with the use of potent opioids for chronic pain. **[U.S. Boxed Warning]: May cause serious, life-threatening, or fatal respiratory depression. Monitor closely for respiratory depression, especially during initiation or dose escalation. Patients should swallow tablets whole; crushing, chewing, or dissolving can cause rapid release and a potentially fatal dose.** Carbon dioxide retention from opioid-induced respiratory depression can exacerbate the sedating effects of opioids. **[U.S. Boxed Warning]: Use with all CYP3A4 inhibitors may result in increased effects and potentially fatal respiratory depression. In addition, discontinuation of a concomitant CYP 3A4 inducer may result in increased oxycodone**

concentrations. Monitor patients receiving any CYP 3A4 inhibitor or inducer. Tablets may be difficult to swallow and could become lodged in throat; patients with swallowing difficulties may be at increased risk. Cases of intestinal obstruction or diverticulitis exacerbation have also been reported, including cases requiring medical intervention to remove the tablet; patients with an underlying GI disease (eg, esophageal cancer, colon cancer) may be at increased risk. **[U.S. Boxed Warning]: Users are exposed to the risks of addiction, abuse, and misuse, potentially leading to overdose and death. Assess each patient's risk prior to prescribing; monitor all patients regularly for development of these behaviors or conditions.** Risk of opioid abuse is increased in patients with a history or family history of alcohol or drug abuse or mental illness. **[U.S. Boxed Warning]: Accidental ingestion of even one dose, especially in children, can result in a fatal overdose of oxycodone. [U.S. Boxed Warning]: Prolonged maternal use of opioids during pregnancy can cause neonatal withdrawal syndrome in the newborn which may be life-threatening if not recognized and treated according to protocols developed by neonatology experts. If prolonged opioid therapy is required in a pregnant woman, ensure treatment is available and warn patient of risk to the neonate.** Signs and symptoms include irritability, hyperactivity and abnormal sleep pattern, high pitched cry, tremor, vomiting, diarrhea and failure to gain weight. Onset, duration and severity depend on the drug used, duration of use, maternal dose, and rate of drug elimination by the newborn.

Oral solutions: **[U.S. Boxed Warning]: Highly concentrated oral solution (20 mg/mL) should only be used in opioid tolerant patients (taking ≥30 mg/day of oxycodone or equivalent for ≥1 week). [U.S. Boxed Warning]: Orders for oxycodone oral solutions (20 mg/mL or 5 mg/5 mL) should be clearly written to include the intended dose (in mg vs mL) and the intended product concentration to be dispensed to avoid potential dosing errors. Products should be stored out of reach of children; seek immediate medical care in the event of accidental ingestion.**

Benzyl alcohol and derivatives: Some dosage forms may contain sodium benzoate/benzoic acid; benzoic acid (benzoate) is a metabolite of benzyl alcohol; large amounts of benzyl alcohol (≥99 mg/kg/day) have been associated with a potentially fatal toxicity ("gasping syndrome") in neonates; the "gasping syndrome" consists of metabolic acidosis, respiratory distress, gasping respirations, CNS dysfunction (including convulsions, intracranial hemorrhage), hypotension, and cardiovascular collapse (AAP, 1997; CDC, 1982); some data suggests that benzoate displaces bilirubin from protein binding sites (Ahlfors, 2001); avoid or use dosage forms containing benzyl alcohol derivative with caution in neonates. See manufacturer's labeling.

Adverse Reactions

Cardiovascular: Orthostatic hypotension

Central nervous system: Abnormal dreams, abnormality in thinking, anxiety, chills, confusion, dizziness, drowsiness, dysphoria, euphoria, headache, insomnia, nervousness, twitching

Dermatologic: Diaphoresis, pruritus, skin rash

Gastrointestinal: Abdominal pain, anorexia, constipation, diarrhea, dyspepsie, gastritis, hiccups, nausea, xerostomia, vomiting

Miscellaneous: Fever

Neuromuscular & skeletal: Weakness

Respiratory: Dyspnea

Rare but important or life-threatening: Abnormal stools (tablet in stool [some controlled release dosage forms]), agitation, amnesia, anaphylactoid reaction, anaphylaxis, chest pain, dehydration, depression, depression of ST segment on ECG, diverticulitis (exacerbation), dysphagia (or other swallowing difficulties due to properties of controlled release tablets), dysuria, edema (including facial and peripheral), emotional lability, eructation, hallucination, hematuria, histamine release, hyperalgesia, hyperkinesia, hypoesthesia, hypogonadism (Brennan, 2013; Debono, 2011), hyponatremia, hypotonia, increased intracranial pressure, intestinal obstruction, malaise, paresthesia, seizure, SIADH, speech disturbance, stomatitis, stupor, syncope, tremor, urinary retention, vertigo, withdrawal syndrome

Drug Interactions

Metabolism/Transport Effects Substrate of CYP2D6 (minor), CYP3A4 (major); **Note:** Assignment of Major/Minor substrate status based on clinically relevant drug interaction potential

Avoid Concomitant Use

Avoid concomitant use of OxyCODONE with any of the following: Azelastine (Nasal); Conivaptan; Eluxadoline; Fusidic Acid (Systemic); Idelalisib; Mixed Agonist / Antagonist Opioids; Orphenadrine; Paraldehyde; Thalidomide

Increased Effect/Toxicity

OxyCODONE may increase the levels/effects of: Alcohol (Ethyl); Alvimopan; Azelastine (Nasal); CNS Depressants; Desmopressin; Diuretics; Eluxadoline; Hydrocodone; Methotrimeprazine; Metyrosine; Mirtazapine; Orphenadrine; Paraldehyde; Pramipexole; ROPINIRole; Rotigotine; Selective Serotonin Reuptake Inhibitors; Suvorexant; Thalidomide; Zolpidem

The levels/effects of OxyCODONE may be increased by: Amphetamines; Anticholinergic Agents; Antipsychotic Agents (Phenothiazines); Brimonidine (Topical); Cannabis; Conivaptan; CYP3A4 Inhibitors (Moderate); CYP3A4 Inhibitors (Strong); Dasatinib; Doxylamine; Dronabinol; Droperidol; Fusidic Acid (Systemic); HydrOXYzine; Idelalisib; Ivacaftor; Kava Kava; Luliconazole; Magnesium Sulfate; MAO Inhibitors; Methotrimeprazine; Mifepristone; Nabilone; Palbociclib; Perampanel; Rufinamide; Simeprevir; Sodium Oxybate; Stiripentol; Succinylcholine; Tapentadol; Tetrahydrocannabinol; Voriconazole

Decreased Effect

OxyCODONE may decrease the levels/effects of: Pegvisomant

The levels/effects of OxyCODONE may be decreased by: Ammonium Chloride; Bosentan; CYP3A4 Inducers (Moderate); CYP3A4 Inducers (Strong); Dabrafenib; Deferasirox; Mitotane; Mixed Agonist / Antagonist Opioids; Naltrexone; Rifampin; Siltuximab; St Johns Wort; Tocilizumab

Storage/Stability Store at 25°C (77°F); excursions permitted between 15°C to 30°C (59°F to 86°F). Protect from light.

Mechanism of Action Binds to opiate receptors in the CNS, causing inhibition of ascending pain pathways, altering the perception of and response to pain; produces generalized CNS depression

Pharmacodynamics Duration of action: Analgesia:

Immediate release: 4-5 hours

Controlled release (OxyContin): 12 hours

Pharmacokinetics (Adult data unless noted)

Distribution: Distributes into skeletal muscle, liver, intestinal tract, lungs, spleen, and brain; V_{dss}:

Children 2-10 years: 2.1 L/kg (range: 1.2-3.7 L/kg)

Adults: 2.6 L/kg

Protein binding: 38% to 45%

Metabolism: In the liver primarily to noroxycodone (via demethylation) and oxymorphone (via CYP2D6); noroxycodone is the major circulating metabolite, but has much weaker activity than oxycodone; oxymorphone is active, but present in low concentrations; <15% of the dose is metabolized to oxymorphone via CYP2D6; drug and metabolites undergo glucuronide conjugation

Bioavailability: 60% to 87%

Half-life, apparent:

Immediate release: 3.2 hours

Controlled release (OxyContin): 4.5 hours

Half-life, elimination:

Children 2-10 years: 1.8 hours (range: 1.2-3 hours)

Adults: 3.7 hours

Adults with renal dysfunction (CrCl <60 mL/minute): Half-life increases by 1 hour, but peak oxycodone concentrations increase by 50% and AUC increases by 60%

Adults with mild to moderate hepatic dysfunction: Half-life increases by 2.3 hours, peak oxycodone concentrations increase by 50%, and AUC increases by 95%

Elimination: In the urine as unchanged drug (≤19%) and metabolites: Conjugated oxycodone (≤50%), conjugated oxymorphone (≤14%), noroxycodone, and conjugated noroxycodone

Dosing: Usual Note: Doses should be titrated to appropriate effect:

Infants, Children, and Adolescents:

Analgesic, moderate to severe: Oral: Immediate release:

Infants ≤6 months: Limited data available: Initial dose: 0.025-0.05 mg/kg/dose every 4-6 hours as needed (Berde, 2002)

Infants >6 months, Children, and Adolescents:

Patient weight <50 kg: Initial dose: 0.1-0.2 mg/kg/dose every 4-6 hours as needed; for severe pain some experts have recommended an initial dose of 0.2 mg/kg; usual maximum dose range: 5-10 mg (American Pain Society, 2008; APA, 2012; Berde, 2002)

Patient weight ≥50 kg: Initial dose: 5-10 mg every 4-6 hours as needed; for severe pain an initial dose of 10 mg may be used; usual maximum dose: 20 mg/dose (American Pain Society, 2008; Berde, 2002)

Adolescents ≥18 years and Adults: **Analgesic, moderate to severe:** Oral:

Immediate release: Initial: 5-15 mg every 4-6 hours as needed; dosing range: 5-20 mg/dose (American Pain Society, 2008). For severe chronic pain, administer on a regularly scheduled basis, every 4-6 hours, at the lowest dose that will achieve adequate analgesia.

Controlled release (OxyContin): **Note:** Only opioid-tolerant patients should receive the 60 mg and 80 mg strengths, a single dose >40 mg, or a total dose of >80 mg/day.

Opioid-naïve: 10 mg every 12 hours

Concurrent CNS depressants: Reduce usual initial oxycodone dose by one-third (1/3) to one-half (1/2)

Conversion from transdermal fentanyl: For each 25 mcg/hour transdermal dose, substitute 10 mg controlled release oxycodone every 12 hours; should be initiated 18 hours after the removal of the transdermal fentanyl patch

Currently on opioids: Use standard conversion chart to convert daily opioid dose to oxycodone equivalent. Initiate controlled release oxycodone with one-half (1/2) the estimated oxycodone daily dose (mg/day) and provide rescue medication in the form of immediate release oxycodone. Divide the initial controlled release oxycodone daily dose in 2 (for twice-daily dosing, usually every 12 hours) and round down to nearest dosage form.

Dose adjustment: Doses may be adjusted by changing the total daily dose (not by changing the dosing interval). Doses may be adjusted every 1-2 days and may be increased by 25% to 50%. Dose should be gradually tapered when no longer required in order to prevent withdrawal.

Dosing adjustment in renal impairment:

Children and Adolescents: Dosage adjustments are not provided in the manufacturer's labeling; however, the following adjustments have been recommended (Aronoff, 2007):

GFR 10-50 mL/minute/1.73 m^2: Administer 75% of dose

GFR <10 mL/minute/1.73 m^2: Administer 50% of dose

Hemodialysis: Administer 50% of dose posthemodialysis

Peritoneal dialysis: Administer 50% of dose

Adults: CrCl <60 mL/minute: Initiate doses conservatively and carefully titrate dose to appropriate effect

Dosing adjustment in hepatic impairment: Adults:

Immediate release: Reduced initial doses may be necessary (use a conservative approach to initial dosing); adjust dose based on clinical situation.

Controlled release products: Initial: One-third (1/3) to one-half (1/2) of the usual starting dose; carefully titrate dose to appropriate effect

Administration May administer with food to decrease GI upset

Immediate release (capsule, oral solution, tablets):

Oral solution: Available in two strengths; 1 mg/mL and a concentrated oral solution (20 mg/mL). Precautions should be taken to avoid confusion between the different concentrations; prescriptions should have the concentration specified as well as the dose clearly represented as milligram (mg) of oxycodone, not volume (mL). The enclosed calibrated oral syringe should always be used to administer the concentrated oral solution to ensure the dose is measured and administered accurately. The concentrated oral solution (20 mg/mL) should only be used in opioid-tolerant patients (taking ≥30 mg/day of oxycodone or equivalent for ≥1 week).

Tablet (Oxecta): Swallow whole with adequate water to ensure complete swallowing immediately after placing in the mouth; the formulation uses technology designed to discourage common methods of tampering to prevent misuse/abuse. The tablet should not be wet prior to placing in the mouth. Do not crush, chew, or dissolve nor administer via feeding tubes (eg, gastric, NG) due to potential for obstruction.

Controlled release tablet (OxyContin): Swallow whole; do not moisten, dissolve, cut, crush, chew, or break as this would result in rapid release of oxycodone and absorption of a potentially fatal dose of drug. Administer one at a time and follow each with water immediately after placing in the mouth. For oral use only, do not administer rectally; increased risk of adverse events due to better rectal absorption.

Monitoring Parameters Pain relief, respiratory rate, mental status, blood pressure; signs of misuse, abuse, and addiction

Test Interactions Some quinolones may produce a false-positive urine screening result for opioids using commercially-available immunoassay kits. This has been demonstrated most consistently for levofloxacin and ofloxacin, but other quinolones have shown cross-reactivity in certain assay kits. Confirmation of positive opioid screens by more specific methods should be considered.

Additional Information OxyContin tablets deliver medication over 12 hours; release is pH independent. Equianalgesic doses: oral oxycodone 30 mg = morphine 10 mg IM = single oral dose morphine 60 mg **or** chronic dosing oral morphine 30 mg

Oxecta utilizes Acura Pharmaceutical's Aversion technology which may help discourage misuse and abuse potential. Reduced abuse potential of Oxecta compared to other immediate release oxycodone tablet formulations has not been proven; the FDA is requiring Pfizer to complete a post approval epidemiological study to determine whether the formulation actually results in a decrease of misuse/abuse. In one clinical trial in non-dependent recreational opioid users, the "drug-liking" responses and safety of crushed Oxecta tablets were compared to crushed immediate-release oxycodone tablets following the self-administered intranasal use. A small difference in "drug-liking" scores was observed, with lower scores reported in the crushed Oxecta group. In regards to safety, there was an increased incidence of nasopharyngeal and facial adverse events in the Oxecta group. In addition, there was decreased ability in the Oxecta group to completely administer the two crushed Oxecta tablets intranasally within a set time period. However, whether these differences translate into a significant clinical difference is unknown. Of note, pharmacokinetic studies showed that Oxecta is bioequivalent with oxycodone immediate release tablets with no differences in T_{max} and half-life when administered in the fasted state.

Product Availability

Oxaydo: FDA approved immediate-release oxycodone product formulated to discourage abuse via snorting; availability anticipated in the third quarter of 2015.

Oxaydo is indicated for the management of acute and chronic moderate to severe pain where the use of an opioid analgesic is appropriate. Oxaydo is formerly known as Oxecta (Pfizer).

Controlled Substance C-II

Dosage Forms Excipient information presented when available (limited, particularly for generics); consult specific product labeling. [DSC] = Discontinued product

Capsule, Oral, as hydrochloride:
- Generic: 5 mg

Concentrate, Oral, as hydrochloride:
- Generic: 100 mg/5 mL (15 mL, 30 mL)

Solution, Oral, as hydrochloride:
- Generic: 5 mg/5 mL (5 mL, 15 mL, 500 mL)

Tablet, Oral, as hydrochloride:
- Roxicodone: 5 mg [scored]
- Roxicodone: 15 mg [scored; contains fd&c blue #2 (indigotine), fd&c yellow #10 (quinoline yellow)]
- Roxicodone: 30 mg [scored]
- Generic: 5 mg, 10 mg, 15 mg, 20 mg, 30 mg

Tablet Abuse-Deterrent, Oral, as hydrochloride:
- Oxecta: 5 mg [DSC], 7.5 mg [DSC]

Tablet ER 12 Hour Abuse-Deterrent, Oral, as hydrochloride:
- OxyCONTIN: 10 mg, 15 mg, 20 mg, 30 mg, 40 mg, 60 mg
- OxyCONTIN: 80 mg [contains fd&c blue #2 aluminum lake]
- Generic: 10 mg, 20 mg, 40 mg, 80 mg

Oxycodone and Acetaminophen

(oks i KOE done & a seet a MIN oh fen)

Medication Safety Issues

Sound-alike/look-alike issues:

Oxycodone and Acetaminophen may be confused with Hydrocodone and Acetaminophen

Endocet may be confused with Indocid

Percocet may be confused with Fioricet, Percodan, Procet-30

Roxicet may be confused with Roxanol

High alert medication:

The Institute for Safe Medication Practices (ISMP) includes this medication among its list of drug classes which have a heightened risk of causing significant patient harm when used in error.

Other safety concerns:

Duplicate therapy issues: This product contains acetaminophen, which may be a component of other combination products. Do not exceed the maximum recommended daily dose of acetaminophen.

Brand Names: US Endocet; Percocet; Primlev; Roxicet; Xartemis XR; Xolox [DSC]

Brand Names: Canada Apo-Oxycodone/Acet; Endocet; Percocet; Percocet-Demi; PMS-Oxycodone-Acetaminophen; Ratio-Oxycocet; Rivacocet; Sandoz-Oxycodone/Acetaminophen

Therapeutic Category Analgesic, Narcotic

Generic Availability (US) Yes: Excludes solution

Use Relief of moderate to moderately severe pain (FDA approved in adults)

Medication Guide Available Yes

Pregnancy Risk Factor C

Pregnancy Considerations Animal reproduction studies have not been conducted with this combination. Refer to individual monographs for additional information.

[U.S. Boxed Warning]: Prolonged use of oxycodone/acetaminophen during pregnancy can result in neonatal opioid withdrawal syndrome, which may be life-threatening if not recognized and requires management according to protocols developed by neonatology experts. If opioid use is required for a prolonged period in a pregnant woman, advise the patient of the risk of neonatal opioid withdrawal syndrome.

Breast-Feeding Considerations Oxycodone and acetaminophen are both excreted into breast milk. Somnolence and lethargy have been reported in nursing infants following maternal use of this combination. Breast-feeding is not recommended by the manufacturer. Refer to individual monographs for additional information.

Contraindications

Hypersensitivity to oxycodone, acetaminophen, or any component of the formulation; severe respiratory depression (in absence of resuscitative equipment or ventilatory support); bronchial asthma (acute or severe) or hypercarbia; paralytic ileus (suspected or known)

Documentation of allergenic cross-reactivity for opioids is limited. However, because of similarities in chemical structure and/or pharmacologic actions, the possibility of cross-sensitivity cannot be ruled out with certainty.

Warnings/Precautions Hypersensitivity and anaphylactic reactions have been reported with acetaminophen use; discontinue immediately if symptoms of allergic or hypersensitivity reactions occur. Serious and potentially fatal skin reactions, including acute generalized exanthematous pustulosis (AGEP), Stevens-Johnson syndrome (SJS), and toxic epidermal necrolysis (TEN), have occurred rarely with acetaminophen use; discontinue therapy at the first appearance of skin rash. Use with caution in patients with hypersensitivity reactions to other phenanthrene-derivative opioid agonists (morphine, codeine, hydrocodone, hydromorphone, levorphanol, oxymorphone); liver or renal insufficiency; thyroid dysfunction; adrenal insufficiency, including Addison's disease; seizure disorder; toxic psychosis; morbid obesity; biliary tract impairment; acute pancreatitis; prostatic hyperplasia; or urethral stricture. Use with caution in patients with known G6PD deficiency. May obscure diagnosis or clinical course of patients with acute abdominal conditions. Avoid use in patients with CNS depression or coma as these patients are susceptible to intracranial effects of CO_2 retention. Some preparations contain sulfites which may cause allergic reactions. May be habit-forming. Causes sedation; caution must be used in performing tasks which require alertness (eg, operating machinery or driving). May cause hypotension; use with caution in patients with hypovolemia, cardiovascular disease (including acute MI), or drugs which may exaggerate hypotensive effects (including phenothiazines or general anesthetics). May produce orthostatic hypotension in ambulatory patients. Use with caution to patients in circulatory shock. Opioids decrease bowel motility; monitor for decrease bowel motility in postop patients receiving opioids. Concurrent use of agonist/antagonist analgesics may precipitate withdrawal symptoms and/or reduced analgesic efficacy in patients following prolonged therapy with mu opioid agonists. Abrupt discontinuation following prolonged use may also lead to withdrawal symptoms.

Use with caution in patients with pre-existing respiratory compromise (hypoxia and/or hypercapnia), cor pulmonale, COPD or other obstructive pulmonary disease, and kyphoscoliosis or other skeletal disorder which may alter respiratory function; critical respiratory depression may occur, even at therapeutic dosages. Use with caution in patients with head injury, intracranial lesions, or increased intracranial pressure. Risk of respiratory depression is increased in elderly and debilitated patients. Oxycodone clearance may also be slightly reduced in the elderly; use with caution and consider dosage adjustments. Use with caution in patients with alcoholic liver disease; consuming ≥3 alcoholic drinks/day may increase the risk of liver damage. Limit acetaminophen dose from all sources (prescription and OTC) to <4 g/day in adults. Do not use oxycodone/acetaminophen concomitantly with other acetaminophen-containing products. Oxycodone may cause constipation which may be problematic in patients with unstable angina and patients post- myocardial infarction.

Potentially significant drug-drug interactions may exist, requiring dose or frequency adjustment, additional monitoring, and/or selection of alternative therapy.

[U.S. Boxed Warning]: Prolonged use of oxycodone/acetaminophen during pregnancy can cause neonatal withdrawal syndrome in the newborn which may be life-threatening if not recognized and treated according to protocols developed by neonatology experts. If prolonged opioid therapy is required in a pregnant woman, ensure treatment is available and warn of risk to the neonate. Signs and symptoms include irritability, hyperactivity and abnormal sleep pattern, high pitched cry, tremor, vomiting, diarrhea and failure to gain weight. Onset, duration and severity depend on the drug used, duration of use, maternal dose, and rate of drug elimination by the newborn.

[U.S. Boxed Warning]: Oxycodone/acetaminophen ER exposes patients and other users to the risks of opioid addiction, abuse, and misuse, which can lead to overdose and death. Assess each patient's risk prior to prescribing oxycodone/acetaminophen ER, and monitor all patients regularly for the development of these behaviors or conditions. Use with caution in patients with a history of drug abuse or acute alcoholism; potential for drug dependency exists. Tolerance, psychological and physical dependence may occur with prolonged use. Abuse or misuse of XR tablets by crushing, chewing, snorting, or injecting the dissolved product will result in the uncontrolled delivery of the oxycodone and can result in overdose and death

[U.S. Boxed Warning]: Serious, life-threatening, or fatal respiratory depression may occur with use of opioids. Monitor for respiratory depression, especially during initiation of therapy or following a dose increase. [U.S. Boxed Warning]: Serious, life-threatening, or fatal respiratory depression may occur with use of oxycodone/acetaminophen ER. Monitor for respiratory depression, especially during initiation of therapy or following a dose increase. To reduce the risk of respiratory depression, proper dosing and titration is essential. Overestimating the oxycodone/acetaminophen ER dose when converting patients from another opioid product can result in fatal overdose with the first dose.

[U.S. Boxed Warning]: Acetaminophen may cause severe hepatotoxicity, potentially requiring liver transplant or resulting in death; hepatotoxicity is usually associated with excessive acetaminophen intake (>4 g/day) in adults. Risk is increased with alcohol use, pre-existing liver disease, and intake of more than one source of acetaminophen-containing medications. Chronic daily dosing in adults has also resulted in liver damage in some patients.

[U.S. Boxed Warning]: Accidental ingestion of oxycodone/acetaminophen ER, especially in children, can result in a fatal overdose of oxycodone. Do not to presoak, lick or otherwise wet ER tablets prior to placing in the mouth; take one tablet at a time with enough water to ensure complete swallowing. Do not break, chew, crush, cut, dissolve or split the ER tablets; breaking, chewing, crushing, cutting, dissolving or splitting will result in uncontrolled delivery of oxycodone and can lead to overdose or death. Oxycodone/acetaminophen ER is not interchangeable with other oxycodone/acetaminophen products because of differing pharmacokinetic profiles that affect the frequency of administration. Do not abruptly stop ER tablets in patients who may be physically dependent; gradually decrease dose by 50% every 2 to 4 days to prevent signs and symptoms of withdrawal. Due to characteristics of the ER formulation that cause the tablets to swell and become sticky when wet, consider use of an alternative analgesic in patients who have difficulty swallowing and patients at risk for underlying GI disorders resulting in a small GI lumen.

Benzyl alcohol and derivatives: Some dosage forms may contain sodium benzoate/benzoic acid; benzoic acid (benzoate) is a metabolite of benzyl alcohol; large amounts of benzyl alcohol (≥99 mg/kg/day) have been associated with a potentially fatal toxicity ("gasping syndrome") in neonates; the "gasping syndrome" consists of metabolic acidosis, respiratory distress, gasping respirations, CNS dysfunction (including convulsions, intracranial hemorrhage), hypotension, and cardiovascular collapse (AAP, 1997; CDC, 1982); some data suggests that benzoate displaces bilirubin from protein binding sites (Ahlfors, 2001); avoid or use dosage forms containing benzyl alcohol derivative with caution in neonates. See manufacturer's labeling.

Adverse Reactions Also see individual agents.

Cardiovascular: Circulatory depression, hypotension, peripheral edema, shock

Central nervous system: Dizziness, drowsiness, dysphoria, fatigue, headache, insomnia

Dermatologic: Erythema, erythematous dermatitis, excoriation, pruritus, skin blister, skin rash

Endocrine & metabolic: Hot flash

Gastrointestinal: Constipation, diarrhea, dyspepsia, nausea, vomiting, xerostomia

Genitourinary: Dysuria

Hematologic & oncologic: Hemolytic anemia, neutropenia, pancytopenia, thrombocytopenia

Hepatic: Increased liver enzymes

Respiratory: Apnea, cough, respiratory arrest, respiratory depression

Rare but important or life-threatening: Abdominal pain, acidosis, agitation, alkalosis, altered mental status, anxiety, arthralgia, aspiration, asthma, bradycardia, cardiac arrhythmia, cerebral edema, chest discomfort, chills, cognitive dysfunction, confusion, decreased appetite, dehydration, depression, dermatitis, diaphoresis, disorientation, dysphoria, drug abuse, drug dependence, drug overdose (accidental and nonaccidental), dysgeusia, dyspnea, ecchymoses, emotional lability, esophageal spasm, euphoria, eye redness, falling, fever, flushing, hallucination, hearing loss, hepatic failure, hepatitis, hepatotoxicity, hiccups, hyperglycemia, hyperhidrosis, hyperkalemia, hypersensitivity, hypersensitivity reaction, hypertension, hypoesthesia, hypoglycemia, hypothermia, hypoventilation, impaired consciousness, increased blood pressure, increased gamma-glutamyl transferase, increased lactate dehydrogenase, increased serum alanine aminotransferase, increased serum aspartate aminotransferase, increased serum bilirubin, interstitial nephritis, intestinal obstruction, jitteriness, laryngeal edema, lethargy, malaise, memory impairment, metabolic acidosis, migraine, miosis, musculoskeletal chest pain, musculoskeletal stiffness, myalgia, myoclonus, noncardiac chest pain, obstructive sleep apnea hypopnea syndrome, oropharyngeal pain, orthostatic hypotension, palpitations, pancreatitis, paresthesia, proteinuria, pulmonary edema, renal failure, renal insufficiency, renal papillary necrosis, respiratory alkalosis, reduced urine flow, respiratory depression, rhabdomyolysis, sedation, seizure, sleep disorder, stupor, suicide, tachycardia, tachypnea, tinnitus, tremor, urinary retention, visual disturbance, weakness, withdrawal syndrome

Drug Interactions

Metabolism/Transport Effects Refer to individual components.

Avoid Concomitant Use

Avoid concomitant use of Oxycodone and Acetaminophen with any of the following: Azelastine (Nasal); Conivaptan; Eluxadoline; Fusidic Acid (Systemic); Idelalisib; Mixed Agonist / Antagonist Opioids; Orphenadrine; Paraldehyde; Thalidomide

Increased Effect/Toxicity

Oxycodone and Acetaminophen may increase the levels/effects of: Alvimopan; Azelastine (Nasal); Busulfan; CNS Depressants; Dasatinib; Desmopressin; Diuretics; Eluxadoline; Hydrocodone; Methotrimeprazine; Metyrosine; Mipomersen; Mirtazapine; Orphenadrine; Paraldehyde; Phenylephrine (Systemic); Pramipexole; Prilocaine; ROPINIRole; Rotigotine; Selective Serotonin Reuptake Inhibitors; Sodium Nitrite; SORAfenib; Suvorexant; Thalidomide; Vitamin K Antagonists; Zolpidem

The levels/effects of Oxycodone and Acetaminophen may be increased by: Alcohol (Ethyl); Amphetamines; Anticholinergic Agents; Antipsychotic Agents (Phenothiazines); Brimonidine (Topical); Cannabis; Conivaptan; CYP3A4 Inhibitors (Moderate); CYP3A4 Inhibitors (Strong); Dasatinib; Doxylamine; Dronabinol; Droperidol; Fusidic Acid (Systemic); HydrOXYzine; Idelalisib; Isoniazid; Ivacaftor; Kava Kava; Luliconazole; Magnesium Sulfate; MAO Inhibitors; Methotrimeprazine; Metyrapone; Mifepristone; Nabilone; Nitric Oxide; Palbociclib; Perampanel; Probenecid; Rufinamide; Simeprevir; Sodium Oxybate; SORAfenib; Stiripentol; Succinylcholine; Tapentadol; Tetrahydrocannabinol; Voriconazole

Decreased Effect

Oxycodone and Acetaminophen may decrease the levels/effects of: Pegvisomant

The levels/effects of Oxycodone and Acetaminophen may be decreased by: Ammonium Chloride; Barbiturates; Bosentan; Cholestyramine Resin; CYP3A4 Inducers (Moderate); CYP3A4 Inducers (Strong); Dabrafenib; Deferasirox; Mitotane; Mixed Agonist / Antagonist Opioids; Naltrexone; Rifampin; Siltuximab; St Johns Wort; Tocilizumab

Storage/Stability

Extended-release: Store at 25°C (77°F); excursions permitted between 15°C and 30°C (59°F and 86°F).

Immediate-release: Store at 20°C to 25°C (68°F to 77°F). Protect from moisture.

Mechanism of Action

Oxycodone, as with other opioid analgesics, blocks pain perception in the cerebral cortex by binding to specific receptor molecules (opiate receptors) within the neuronal membranes of synapses. This binding results in a decreased synaptic chemical transmission throughout the CNS thus inhibiting the flow of pain sensations into the higher centers. Mu and kappa are the two subtypes of the opiate receptor to which oxycodone binds to cause analgesia.

Acetaminophen inhibits the synthesis of prostaglandins in the CNS and peripherally blocks pain impulse generation; produces antipyresis from inhibition of hypothalamic heat-regulating center.

Pharmacodynamics

Onset of action: Within 10 to 15 minutes

Maximum effect: Within 1 hour

Duration: 3 to 6 hours

Pharmacokinetics (Adult data unless noted) See individual agents.

Dosing: Usual

Children and Adolescents: **Note:** Doses based on total oxycodone content; titrate dose to appropriate analgesic effects; maximum daily acetaminophen dose: 75 mg/kg/**day** not to exceed 4000 mg/**day**; do **not** exceed 5 doses in 24 hours

Analgesic, moderate: Oral: 0.1 to 0.2 mg/kg/dose; doses typically given every 4 to 6 hours as needed; manufacturer's labeling recommends every 6 hours; maximum initial oxycodone dose: 5 mg/dose (American Pain Society, 2008)

Analgesic, severe: Initial dose: Oral: 0.2 mg/kg/dose; doses typically given every 4 to 6 hours as needed; manufacturer's labeling recommends every 6 hours; maximum initial oxycodone dose: 10 mg (American Pain Society, 2008)

Adults: **Analgesic:** Initial dose is based on oxycodone content; however, the maximum daily dose is based on the acetaminophen content. Doses should be given every 4 to 6 hours as needed and titrated to appropriate analgesic effects.

Manufacturer's labeling: Moderate to moderately severe pain: Initial dose, based on oxycodone content: Oral: 2.5 to 10 mg every 6 hours as needed. Titrate according to pain severity and individual response. Do not exceed acetaminophen 4 **g**/day.

Alternate recommendations (American Pain Society, 2008):

Moderate pain: Initial dose, based on oxycodone content: Oral: 5 mg; doses typically given every 4 to 6 hours as needed; manufacturer's labeling recommends every 6 hours as needed. Do not exceed acetaminophen 4 **g**/day

Severe pain: Initial dose, based on oxycodone content: Oral: 10 to 20 mg; doses typically given every 4 to 6 hours as needed; manufacturer's labeling recommends every 6 hours as needed. Do not exceed acetaminophen 4 **g**/day

Administration Oral: May administer with food or milk to decrease GI upset

Monitoring Parameters Pain relief, respiratory rate, mental status, blood pressure; signs of misuse, abuse, and addiction

Test Interactions See individual agents.

Controlled Substance C-II

Dosage Forms Excipient information presented when available (limited, particularly for generics); consult specific product labeling. [DSC] = Discontinued product

Capsule, Oral: 5/500: Oxycodone hydrochloride 5 mg and acetaminophen 500 mg [DSC]

Solution, Oral:

Roxicet: Oxycodone hydrochloride 5 mg and acetaminophen 325 mg per 5 mL (5 mL, 500 mL) [contains ethanol <0.5%; mint flavor]

Tablet, Oral: 2.5/325: Oxycodone hydrochloride 2.5 mg and acetaminophen 325 mg; 5/325: Oxycodone hydrochloride 5 mg and acetaminophen 325 mg; 7.5/325: Oxycodone hydrochloride 7.5 mg and acetaminophen 325 mg; 7.5/500: Oxycodone hydrochloride 7.5 mg and acetaminophen 500 mg [DSC]; 10/325: Oxycodone hydrochloride 10 mg and acetaminophen 325 mg;

10/650: Oxycodone hydrochloride 10 mg and acetaminophen 650 mg [DSC]
Endocet 2.5/325: Oxycodone hydrochloride 2.5 mg and acetaminophen 325 mg
Endocet 5/325 [scored]: Oxycodone hydrochloride 5 mg and acetaminophen 325 mg
Endocet 7.5/325: Oxycodone hydrochloride 7.5 mg and acetaminophen 325 mg
Endocet 7.5/500: Oxycodone hydrochloride 7.5 mg and acetaminophen 500 mg [DSC]
Endocet 10/325: Oxycodone hydrochloride 10 mg and acetaminophen 325 mg
Endocet 10/650: Oxycodone hydrochloride 10 mg and acetaminophen 650 mg [DSC]
Magnacet 5/400: Oxycodone hydrochloride 5 mg and acetaminophen 400 mg [DSC]
Magnacet 7.5/400: Oxycodone hydrochloride 7.5 mg and acetaminophen 400 mg [DSC]
Magnacet 10/400: Oxycodone hydrochloride 10 mg and acetaminophen 400 mg [DSC]
Percocet 2.5/325: Oxycodone hydrochloride 2.5 mg and acetaminophen 325 mg
Percocet 5/325 [scored]: Oxycodone hydrochloride 5 mg and acetaminophen 325 mg
Percocet 7.5/325: Oxycodone hydrochloride 7.5 mg and acetaminophen 325 mg
Percocet 7.5/500: Oxycodone hydrochloride 7.5 mg and acetaminophen 500 mg [DSC]
Percocet 10/325: Oxycodone hydrochloride 10 mg and acetaminophen 325 mg
Percocet 10/650: Oxycodone hydrochloride 10 mg and acetaminophen 650 mg [DSC]
Primlev 5/300: Oxycodone hydrochloride 5 mg and acetaminophen 300 mg
Primlev 7.5/300: Oxycodone hydrochloride 7.5 mg and acetaminophen 300 mg
Primlev 10/300: Oxycodone hydrochloride 10 mg and acetaminophen 300 mg
Roxicet 5/325 [scored]: Oxycodone hydrochloride 5 mg and acetaminophen 325 mg

Tablet, Extended Release, Oral:
Xartemis XR: Oxycodone hydrochloride 7.5 mg and acetaminophen 325 mg

Oxycodone and Aspirin (oks i KOE done & AS pir in)

Medication Safety Issues

Sound-alike/look-alike issues:
Percodan® may be confused with Decadron, Percocet®, Percogesic®, Periactin

High alert medication:
The Institute for Safe Medication Practices (ISMP) includes this medication among its list of drug classes which have a heightened risk of causing significant patient harm when used in error.

Brand Names: US Endodan®; Percodan®

Brand Names: Canada Endodan®; Oxycodan®; Percodan®

Therapeutic Category Analgesic, Narcotic

Generic Availability (US) Yes

Use Relief of moderate to moderately severe pain (FDA approved in adults)

Pregnancy Risk Factor B (oxycodone); D (aspirin)

Pregnancy Considerations See individual agents.

Breast-Feeding Considerations See individual agents.

Contraindications Hypersensitivity to oxycodone, salicylates, other NSAIDs, or any component of the formulation; patients with the syndrome of asthma, rhinitis, and nasal polyps; inherited or acquired bleeding disorders (including factor VII and factor IX deficiency); do not use in children and teenagers in the presence of viral infections (chickenpox or flu symptoms), with or without fever, due to a potential association with Reye's syndrome; significant respiratory depression; hypercarbia; known or suspected paralytic ileus; acute or severe bronchial asthma

Warnings/Precautions Use with caution in patients with hypersensitivity reactions to other phenanthrene-derivative opioid agonists (morphine, hydrocodone, hydromorphone, levorphanol, oxycodone, oxymorphone), respiratory diseases including asthma, emphysema, or COPD. Use with caution in pancreatitis or biliary tract disease, acute alcoholism (including delirium tremens), adrenocortical insufficiency, kyphoscoliosis (or other skeletal disorder which may alter respiratory function), hypothyroidism (including myxedema), seizure disorder, morbid obesity, prostatic hyperplasia, urethral stricture, and toxic psychosis. Avoid use in patients with CNS depression or coma as these patients are susceptible to intracranial effects of CO_2 retention. May obscure diagnosis or clinical course of patients with acute abdominal conditions.

Causes sedation; caution must be used in performing tasks which require alertness (eg, operating machinery or driving). Effects may be potentiated when used with other sedative drugs or ethanol. Use with caution in elderly or debilitated patients. Use with caution in patients with renal and/or hepatic impairment; avoid use of aspirin-containing products in patients with severe hepatic or renal dysfunction. Hemodynamic effects (hypotension, orthostasis) may be exaggerated in patients with dehydration, hypovolemia, concurrent vasodilating drugs, or in patients with head injury. Respiratory depressant effects and capacity to elevate CSF pressure may be exaggerated in presence of head injury, other intracranial lesion, or pre-existing elevation of intracranial pressure. Tolerance or drug dependence may result from extended use. Healthcare provider should be alert to problems of abuse, misuse, and diversion. Taper dose gradually to avoid withdrawal symptoms in physically-dependent patients.

Prolonged use of oxycodone/aspirin during pregnancy can cause neonatal withdrawal syndrome in the newborn which may be life-threatening if not recognized and treated according to protocols developed by neonatology experts. If prolonged opioid therapy is required in a pregnant woman, ensure treatment is available and warn of risk to the neonate. Signs and symptoms include irritability, hyperactivity and abnormal sleep pattern, high pitched cry, tremor, vomiting, diarrhea and failure to gain weight. Onset, duration and severity depend on the drug used, duration of use, maternal dose, and rate of drug elimination by the newborn.

Use with caution in patients with platelet and bleeding disorders, erosive gastritis, or peptic ulcer disease. Heavy ethanol use (>3 drinks/day) can increase bleeding risks. Discontinue use if tinnitus or impaired hearing occurs. Patients with sensitivity to tartrazine dyes, nasal polyps, and asthma may have an increased risk of salicylate sensitivity. Surgical patients should avoid ASA if possible, for 1-2 weeks prior to surgery, to reduce the risk of excessive bleeding.

Adverse Reactions Note: Also see individual agents

Cardiovascular: Circulatory depression, hypotension, shock
Central nervous system: Dizziness, drowsiness, dysphoria, euphoria, sedation
Dermatologic: Pruritus
Gastrointestinal: Constipation, nausea, vomiting
Respiratory: Apnea, respiratory arrest, respiratory depression
Rare but important or life-threatening: Agitation, anaphylactoid reaction, anaphylaxis, angioedema, asthma, bradycardia, bronchospasm, bruise, cerebral edema, coma, confusion, diaphoresis, disseminated intravascular coagulation, drug dependence, duodenal ulcer, dyspnea,

fever, gastric ulcer, gastrointestinal hemorrhage, hallucination, hearing loss, hemorrhage, hepatitis, hepatotoxicity, hyperglycemia, hyperkalemia, hypersensitivity reaction, hypoglycemia, hypogonadism (Brennan, 2013; Debono, 2011), hypothermia, interstitial nephritis, intestinal obstruction, intestinal perforation, laryngeal edema, leukopenia, metabolic acidosis, palpitations, pancreatitis, paresthesia, prolonged prothrombin time, proteinuria, pulmonary edema, purpura, renal failure, renal papillary necrosis, respiratory alkalosis, Reye's syndrome, rhabdomyolysis, seizure, skin rash, tachycardia, thrombocytopenia, tinnitus, urinary retention, visual disturbance

Drug Interactions

Metabolism/Transport Effects Refer to individual components.

Avoid Concomitant Use

Avoid concomitant use of Oxycodone and Aspirin with any of the following: Azelastine (Nasal); Conivaptan; Dexketoprofen; Eluxadoline; Floctafenine; Fusidic Acid (Systemic); Idelalisib; Influenza Virus Vaccine (Live/Attenuated); Ketorolac (Nasal); Ketorolac (Systemic); Mixed Agonist / Antagonist Opioids; Omacetaxine; Orphenadrine; Paraldehyde; Thalidomide; Urokinase

Increased Effect/Toxicity

Oxycodone and Aspirin may increase the levels/effects of: Agents with Antiplatelet Properties; Alcohol (Ethyl); Alendronate; Alvimopan; Anticoagulants; Apixaban; Azelastine (Nasal); Blood Glucose Lowering Agents; Carbonic Anhydrase Inhibitors; Carisoprodol; CNS Depressants; Collagenase (Systemic); Corticosteroids (Systemic); Dabigatran Etexilate; Deoxycholic Acid; Desmopressin; Dexketoprofen; Diuretics; Eluxadoline; Heparin; Hydrocodone; Ibritumomab; Methotrexate; Methotrimeprazine; Metyrosine; Mirtazapine; Nicorandil; NSAID (COX-2 Inhibitor); Obinutuzumab; Omacetaxine; Orphenadrine; Paraldehyde; PRALAtrexate; Pramipexole; Rivaroxaban; ROPINIRole; Rotigotine; Salicylates; Suvorexant; Thalidomide; Thrombolytic Agents; Ticagrelor; Tositumomab and Iodine I 131 Tositumomab; Urokinase; Valproic Acid and Derivatives; Varicella Virus-Containing Vaccines; Vitamin K Antagonists; Zolpidem

The levels/effects of Oxycodone and Aspirin may be increased by: Agents with Antiplatelet Properties; Ammonium Chloride; Amphetamines; Anticholinergic Agents; Antidepressants (Tricyclic, Tertiary Amine); Antipsychotic Agents (Phenothiazines); Brimonidine (Topical); Cannabis; Conivaptan; CYP3A4 Inhibitors (Moderate); CYP3A4 Inhibitors (Strong); Dasatinib; Doxylamine; Dronabinol; Droperidol; Floctafenine; Fusidic Acid (Systemic); Ginkgo Biloba; Glucosamine; Herbs (Anticoagulant/Antiplatelet Properties); HydrOXYzine; Ibrutinib; Idelalisib; Influenza Virus Vaccine (Live/Attenuated); Ivacaftor; Kava Kava; Ketorolac (Nasal); Ketorolac (Systemic); Limaprost; Loop Diuretics; Luliconazole; Magnesium Sulfate; MAO Inhibitors; Methotrimeprazine; Mifepristone; Multivitamins/Fluoride (with ADE); Multivitamins/Minerals (with ADEK, Folate, Iron); Multivitamins/Minerals (with AE, No Iron); Nabilone; NSAID (Nonselective); Omega-3 Fatty Acids; Palbociclib; Pentosan Polysulfate Sodium; Pentoxifylline; Perampanel; Potassium Acid Phosphate; Prostacyclin Analogues; Rufinamide; Selective Serotonin Reuptake Inhibitors; Serotonin/Norepinephrine Reuptake Inhibitors; Simeprevir; Sodium Oxybate; Stiripentol; Succinylcholine; Tapentadol; Tetrahydrocannabinol; Tipranavir; Treprostinil; Vitamin E; Voriconazole

Decreased Effect

Oxycodone and Aspirin may decrease the levels/effects of: ACE Inhibitors; Carisoprodol; Dexketoprofen; Hyaluronidase; Loop Diuretics; Multivitamins/Fluoride (with ADE); Multivitamins/Minerals (with ADEK, Folate, Iron); Multivitamins/Minerals (with AE, No Iron); NSAID (Nonselective); Pegvisomant; Probenecid; Ticagrelor; Tiludronate

The levels/effects of Oxycodone and Aspirin may be decreased by: Ammonium Chloride; Bosentan; Corticosteroids (Systemic); CYP3A4 Inducers (Moderate); CYP3A4 Inducers (Strong); Dabrafenib; Deferasirox; Dexketoprofen; Floctafenine; Ketorolac (Nasal); Ketorolac (Systemic); Mitotane; Mixed Agonist / Antagonist Opioids; Naltrexone; NSAID (Nonselective); Rifampin; Siltuximab; St Johns Wort; Tocilizumab

Storage/Stability Store at 25°C (77°F); excursions permitted to 15°C to 30°C (59°F to 86°F).

Mechanism of Action

Oxycodone, as with other opioid analgesics, blocks pain perception in the cerebral cortex by binding to specific receptor molecules (opiate receptors) within the neuronal membranes of synapses. This binding results in a decreased synaptic chemical transmission throughout the CNS, thus inhibiting the flow of pain sensations into the higher centers. Mu and kappa are the two subtypes of the opiate receptor to which oxycodone binds to cause analgesia.

Aspirin inhibits prostaglandin synthesis by decreasing the activity of the enzyme, cyclooxygenase, which results in decreased formation of prostaglandin precursors, acts on the hypothalamic heat-regulating center to reduce fever, blocks thromboxane synthetase action which prevents formation of the platelet-aggregating substance thromboxane A_2

Pharmacokinetics (Adult data unless noted) See individual agents.

Dosing: Usual Oral:

Children and Adolescents: **Note:** Dosed based on total oxycodone content; titrate dose to appropriate analgesic effects; maximum daily aspirin dose: 4 g/day

Analgesic, moderate: 0.1-0.2 mg/kg/dose every 4-6 hours as needed; maximum oxycodone dose: 5 mg/dose (American Pain Society, 2008)

Analgesic, severe: Initial dose: 0.2 mg/kg/dose every 4-6 hours as needed (American Pain Society, 2008)

Adults: 1 tablet every 6 hours as needed for pain; maximum aspirin dose should not exceed 4 g/**day**

Dosing adjustment in renal impairment:

Children and Adolescents: **Note:** No dosing recommendations are available for the combination product. The following guidelines have been used by some clinicians:

GFR 10-50 mL/minute/1.73m^2: Administer 75% of dose (Aronoff, 2007); **Note:** Based on the oxycodone component only

GFR <10 mL/minute/1.73m^2: No data available; avoid use due to aspirin component

Adults: CrCl <10 mL/minute: Adults: Avoid use due to aspirin component

Dosing adjustment in hepatic impairment: Adults: The FDA-approved labeling does not contain dosing adjustment guidelines; use with caution; if severe impairment, avoid use of aspirin

Administration May administer with food or milk to decrease GI upset

Monitoring Parameters Pain relief, respiratory rate, mental status, blood pressure; signs of misuse, abuse, and addiction

Test Interactions May cross-react with urine tests for cocaine or marijuana.

Additional Information One generic tablet contains ~5 mg oxycodone as combined salt

Controlled Substance C-II

Dosage Forms Excipient information presented when available (limited, particularly for generics); consult specific product labeling.

Tablet: Oxycodone hydrochloride 4.8355 mg and aspirin 325 mg

Endodan®, Percodan®: Oxycodone hydrochloride 4.8355 mg and aspirin 325 mg

- **Oxycodone Hydrochloride** *see* OxyCODONE *on page 1590*
- **OxyCONTIN** *see* OxyCODONE *on page 1590*
- **Oxyderm™ (Can)** *see* Benzoyl Peroxide *on page 270*
- **Oxy.IR (Can)** *see* OxyCODONE *on page 1590*

Oxymetazoline (Nasal) (oks i met AZ oh leen)

Medication Safety Issues

Sound-alike/look-alike issues:

Oxymetazoline may be confused with oxymetholone
Afrin may be confused with aspirin
Afrin (oxymetazoline) may be confused with Afrin (saline)
Neo-Synephrine (oxymetazoline) may be confused with Neo-Synephrine (phenylephrine, nasal)

Other safety concerns:

Accidental ingestion: Serious adverse reactions (eg, coma, bradycardia, respiratory depression, sedation) requiring hospitalization have been reported in children ≤5 years of age who have accidentally ingested even small amounts (eg, 1-2 mL) of imidazoline-derivative (ie, tetrahydrozoline, oxymetazoline, or naphazoline) eye drops or nasal sprays. Store these products out of reach of children at all times. Contact poison control or seek medical attention if accidental ingestion occurs.

Brand Names: US 12 Hour Nasal Relief Spray [OTC]; 12 Hour Nasal Spray [OTC]; Afrin 12 Hour [OTC]; Afrin Extra Moisturizing [OTC]; Afrin Menthol Spray [OTC]; Afrin Nasal Spray [OTC]; Afrin NoDrip Original [OTC]; Afrin NoDrip Sinus [OTC]; Afrin Sinus [OTC]; Dristan Spray [OTC]; Long Lasting Nasal Spray [OTC]; Mucinex Nasal Spray Full Force [OTC]; Mucinex Nasal Spray Moisture [OTC]; Mucinex Sinus-Max Full Force [OTC]; Mucinex Sinus-Max Moist Smart [OTC]; Nasal Decongestant Spray [OTC]; Nasal Spray 12 Hour [OTC]; Nasal Spray Extra Moisturizing [OTC]; Neo-Synephrine 12 Hour Spray [OTC]; NRS Nasal Relief [OTC]; Sinus Nasal Spray [OTC]

Brand Names: Canada Claritin Allergic Decongestant; Dristan Long Lasting Nasal; Drixoral Nasal

Therapeutic Category Decongestant, Nasal; Nasal Agent, Vasoconstrictor; Vasoconstrictor, Nasal

Generic Availability (US) Yes

Use Symptomatic relief of nasal mucosal congestion associated with acute or chronic rhinitis, the common cold, sinusitis, hay fever, or other allergies (OTC product: FDA approved in ages ≥6 years and adults). **Note:** Approved ages and uses for generic products may vary; consult labeling for specific information.

Pregnancy Considerations Adverse fetal or neonatal effects have not been observed following normal maternal doses of oxymetazoline during the third trimester of pregnancy. Adverse events have been noted in case reports following large doses or extended use. Decongestants are not the preferred agents for the treatment of rhinitis during pregnancy. Short-term (<3 days) use of intranasal oxymetazoline may be beneficial to some patients although its safety during pregnancy has not been studied.

Contraindications Hypersensitivity to oxymetazoline or any component of the formulation

Warnings/Precautions Rebound congestion may occur with extended use. Use with caution in the presence of hypertension, diabetes, hyperthyroidism, heart disease, coronary artery disease, or benign prostatic hyperplasia.

Accidental ingestion by children of over-the-counter (OTC) imidazoline-derivative eye drops and nasal sprays may result in serious harm. Serious adverse reactions (eg, coma, bradycardia, respiratory depression, sedation) requiring hospitalization have been reported in children ≤5 years of age who had ingested even small amounts (eg, 1-2 mL). Contact a poison control center and seek emergency medical care immediately for accidental ingestion (FDA Drug Safety Communication, 2012).

Benzyl alcohol and derivatives: Some dosage forms may contain benzyl alcohol; large amounts of benzyl alcohol (≥99 mg/kg/day) have been associated with a potentially fatal toxicity ("gasping syndrome") in neonates; the "gasping syndrome" consists of metabolic acidosis, respiratory distress, gasping respirations, CNS dysfunction (including convulsions, intracranial hemorrhage), hypotension, and cardiovascular collapse (AAP, 1997; CDC, 1982); some data suggests that benzoate displaces bilirubin from protein binding sites (Ahlfors, 2001); avoid or use dosage forms containing benzyl alcohol with caution in neonates. See manufacturer's labeling.

Warnings: Additional Pediatric Considerations Safety and efficacy for the use of cough and cold products in pediatric patients <4 years of age is limited; the AAP warns against the use of these products for respiratory illnesses in this age group. Serious adverse effects including death have been reported. Many of these products contain multiple active ingredients, increasing the risk of accidental overdose when used with other products. The FDA notes that there are no approved OTC uses for these products in pediatric patients <2 years of age. Health care providers are reminded to ask caregivers about the use of OTC cough and cold products in order to avoid exposure to multiple medications containing the same ingredient (AAP 2012; FDA 2008).

Some dosage forms may contain propylene glycol; in neonates large amounts of propylene glycol delivered orally, intravenously (eg, >3,000 mg/day), or topically have been associated with potentially fatal toxicities which can include metabolic acidosis, seizures, renal failure, and CNS depression; toxicities have also been reported in children and adults including hyperosmolality, lactic acidosis, seizures, and respiratory depression; use caution (AAP 1997; Shehab 2009).

Adverse Reactions Respiratory: Dryness of the nasal mucosa, nasal irritation (temporary), rebound congestion (chronic use), sneezing

Drug Interactions

Metabolism/Transport Effects None known.

Avoid Concomitant Use

Avoid concomitant use of Oxymetazoline (Nasal) with any of the following: Ergot Derivatives; Iobenguane I 123; MAO Inhibitors

Increased Effect/Toxicity

Oxymetazoline (Nasal) may increase the levels/effects of: Sympathomimetics

The levels/effects of Oxymetazoline (Nasal) may be increased by: AtoMOXetine; Cannabinoid-Containing Products; Ergot Derivatives; Linezolid; MAO Inhibitors; Tedizolid; Tricyclic Antidepressants

Decreased Effect

Oxymetazoline (Nasal) may decrease the levels/effects of: FentaNYL; Iobenguane I 123

The levels/effects of Oxymetazoline (Nasal) may be decreased by: Alpha1-Blockers; Tricyclic Antidepressants

Storage/Stability Store at room temperature.

Mechanism of Action Stimulates alpha-adrenergic receptors in the arterioles of the nasal mucosa to produce vasoconstriction

Pharmacodynamics

Onset of action: Within seconds
Duration: 5 to 6 hours

Dosing: Usual

Pediatric: **Note:** Intranasal not recommended for use in children <6 years of age (especially in infants) due to CNS depression.

Nasal congestion: Children ≥6 years and Adolescents: 0.05%: Intranasal: Instill 2 to 3 sprays into each nostril twice daily; therapy should not exceed 3 days

Adult:

Nasal congestion: Intranasal: 0.05%: Instill 2 to 3 sprays into each nostril twice daily; therapy should not exceed 3 days

Dosing adjustment in renal impairment: There are no dosage adjustments provided in manufacturer's labeling.

Dosing adjustment in hepatic impairment: There are no dosage adjustments provided in manufacturer's labeling.

Administration Spray or apply drops into each nostril while gently occluding the other

Dosage Forms Excipient information presented when available (limited, particularly for generics); consult specific product labeling.

Solution, Nasal, as hydrochloride:

12 Hour Nasal Relief Spray: 0.05% (15 mL, 30 mL)

12 Hour Nasal Spray: 0.05% (30 mL) [contains benzalkonium chloride]

12 Hour Nasal Spray: 0.05% (30 mL) [contains benzalkonium chloride, benzyl alcohol, edetate disodium, polyethylene glycol]

Afrin 12 Hour: 0.05% (30 mL) [contains benzalkonium chloride, disodium edta, polyethylene glycol, propylene glycol]

Afrin Extra Moisturizing: 0.05% (30 mL)

Afrin Menthol Spray: 0.05% (15 mL)

Afrin Nasal Spray: 0.05% (15 mL)

Afrin Nasal Spray: 0.05% (15 mL, 20 mL, 30 mL) [contains benzalkonium chloride, disodium edta]

Afrin NoDrip Original: 0.05% (15 mL) [contains benzalkonium chloride]

Afrin NoDrip Sinus: 0.05% (15 mL) [contains benzalkonium chloride, menthol]

Afrin Sinus: 0.05% (15 mL)

Dristan Spray: 0.05% (15 mL) [contains benzalkonium chloride, disodium edta]

Long Lasting Nasal Spray: 0.05% (30 mL) [contains benzalkonium chloride]

Mucinex Nasal Spray Full Force: 0.05% (22 mL) [contains benzalkonium chloride, disodium edta, menthol, polysorbate 80]

Mucinex Nasal Spray Moisture: 0.05% (22 mL) [contains benzalkonium chloride, edetate disodium, propylene glycol]

Mucinex Sinus-Max Full Force: 0.05% (22 mL) [contains benzalkonium chloride, disodium edta, menthol, polysorbate 80, propylene glycol]

Mucinex Sinus-Max Moist Smart: 0.05% (22 mL) [contains benzalkonium chloride, disodium edta, propylene glycol]

Nasal Decongestant Spray: 0.05% (15 mL, 30 mL) [contains benzalkonium chloride]

Nasal Decongestant Spray: 0.05% (15 mL, 30 mL) [contains benzalkonium chloride, edetate disodium, polyethylene glycol, propylene glycol]

Nasal Spray 12 Hour: 0.05% (30 mL) [contains benzalkonium chloride, benzyl alcohol, edetate disodium, polyethylene glycol, propylene glycol]

Nasal Spray Extra Moisturizing: 0.05% (30 mL) [contains benzalkonium chloride, benzyl alcohol, edetate disodium, polyethylene glycol, propylene glycol]

Neo-Synephrine 12 Hour Spray: 0.05% (15 mL)

NRS Nasal Relief: 0.05% (15 mL) [contains benzalkonium chloride, benzyl alcohol, disodium edta, propylene glycol]

Sinus Nasal Spray: 0.05% (30 mL) [contains benzalkonium chloride, edetate disodium, menthol, polysorbate 80, propylene glycol]

Generic: 0.05% (30 mL)

Oxymetazoline (Ophthalmic)

(oks i met AZ oh leen)

Medication Safety Issues

Sound-alike/look-alike issues:

Oxymetazoline may be confused with oxymetholone

Visine® may be confused with Visken®

Other safety concerns:

Accidental ingestion: Serious adverse reactions (eg, coma, bradycardia, respiratory depression, sedation) requiring hospitalization have been reported in children ≤5 years of age who have accidentally ingested even small amounts (eg, 1-2 mL) of imidazoline-derivative (ie, tetrahydrozoline, oxymetazoline, or naphazoline) eye drops or nasal sprays. Store these products out of reach of children at all times. Contact poison control or seek medical attention if accidental ingestion occurs.

Brand Names: US Visine-LR [OTC]

Therapeutic Category Adrenergic Agonist Agent, Ophthalmic; Vasoconstrictor, Ophthalmic

Generic Availability (US) No

Use Relief of redness of eye due to minor eye irritations

Contraindications Hypersensitivity to oxymetazoline or any component of the formulation

Warnings/Precautions Use caution in patients with glaucoma; may exacerbate condition. Accidental ingestion by children of over-the-counter (OTC) imidazoline-derivative eye drops and nasal sprays may result in serious harm. Serious adverse reactions (eg, coma, bradycardia, respiratory depression, sedation) requiring hospitalization have been reported in children ≤5 years of age who had ingested even small amounts (eg, 1-2 mL). Contact a poison control center and seek emergency medical care immediately for accidental ingestion (FDA Drug Safety Communication, 2012).

Adverse Reactions Local: Transient burning, stinging

Drug Interactions

Metabolism/Transport Effects None known.

Avoid Concomitant Use There are no known interactions where it is recommended to avoid concomitant use.

Increased Effect/Toxicity There are no known significant interactions involving an increase in effect.

Decreased Effect There are no known significant interactions involving a decrease in effect.

Storage/Stability Store at controlled room temperature of 15°C to 25°C (59°F to 77°F).

Dosing: Usual Children ≥6 years and Adults: Instill 1-2 drops into the affected eye(s) 2-4 times/day (≥6 hours apart)

Administration Instill drops into conjunctival sac of affected eye(s); avoid contact of bottle tip with skin or eye; finger pressure should be applied to lacrimal sac during and for 1-2 minutes after instillation to decrease the risk of absorption and systemic reactions

Dosage Forms Excipient information presented when available (limited, particularly for generics); consult specific product labeling.

Solution, Ophthalmic, as hydrochloride:

Visine-LR: 0.025% (15 mL) [contains benzalkonium chloride]

◆ **Oxymetazoline Hydrochloride** *see* Oxymetazoline (Nasal) *on page* 1599

◆ **Oxymetazoline Hydrochloride** *see* Oxymetazoline (Ophthalmic) *on page* 1600

Oxymetholone (oks i METH oh lone)

Medication Safety Issues

Sound-alike/look-alike issues:

Oxymetholone may be confused with oxymetazoline, oxymorphone

Brand Names: US Anadrol-50

Therapeutic Category Anabolic Steroid; Androgen

Generic Availability (US) No

Use Treatment of anemias caused by deficient red cell production (FDA approved in children and adults)

Pregnancy Risk Factor X

Pregnancy Considerations Oligospermia or amenorrhea may occur resulting in an impairment of fertility. Use is contraindicated in women who are or may become pregnant.

Breast-Feeding Considerations It is not known if oxymetholone is excreted in breast milk. Breast-feeding is not recommended by the manufacturer.

Contraindications Hypersensitivity to oxymetholone or any component of the formulation; breast cancer in men; breast cancer in women with hypercalcemia; prostate cancer; severe hepatic dysfunction; nephrosis or nephrotic phase of nephritis; pregnancy or use in women who may become pregnant

Warnings/Precautions [U.S. Boxed Warnings]: Androgenic anabolic steroid treatment may cause peliosis hepatis, which occurs when splenic or hepatic tissue is replaced by cysts (blood-filled); may only cause minimal hepatic dysfunction although has been associated with hepatic failure. Androgenic liver cell tumors, which may be benign, although malignant tumors have also been reported; generally regress when anabolic steroid treatment is withdrawn. Both conditions (peliosis and tumors) may not be apparent until liver failure or intra-abdominal hemorrhage develops. Androgen use (low doses) has also been associated with cholestatic hepatitis and jaundice; may be associated with hepatomegaly and right upper-quadrant pain; jaundice is typically reversible upon discontinuation (continuing treatment has been associated with coma and death); monitor liver function periodically. **[U.S. Boxed Warning]: Anabolic steroids may cause changes in blood lipids (decreased high density lipoproteins and sometimes increased low density lipoproteins), increasing the risk of arteriosclerosis and coronary artery disease.**

Monitor diabetic patients carefully (insulin or oral hypoglycemic needs may be altered). Anabolic steroids may suppress clotting factors II, V, VII, and X; prothrombin time may be increased. Use with caution in elderly men; they may be at greater risk for prostate hyperplasia and cancer. Use caution with cardiac or renal disease; may develop edema. In women with breast cancer, may cause hypercalcemia by stimulating osteolysis. Discontinue with evidence of mild virilization in women. May accelerate bone maturation without producing compensatory gain in linear growth in children; effect may continue for 6 months after treatment discontinuation; in prepubertal children perform radiographic examination of the hand and wrist every 6 months to determine the rate of bone maturation and to assess the effect of treatment on the epiphyseal centers. Oxymetholone should not replace other anemia treatment supportive measures such as transfusion, correction of iron, folic acid, vitamin B_{12} or pyridoxine deficiency, antibacterial therapy, and the appropriate use of corticosteroids.

Warnings: Additional Pediatric Considerations In children, androgens are not recommended for management of anemia associated with chronic kidney disease and should not be used (KDIGO, 2006).

Oxymetholone may cause virilization in females; monitor for signs of virilization (eg, deepening of voice, hirsutism, acne, and clitoromegaly); discontinue use if evidence of mild virilization; discontinuation may prevent irreversible virilization.

Adverse Reactions

Cardiovascular: Coronary artery disease, peripheral edema

Central nervous system: Chills, excitation, insomnia

Dermatologic: Acne, hirsutism (women), hyperpigmentation, male-pattern baldness (postpubertal males, women)

Endocrine & metabolic: Amenorrhea, clitoromegaly, glucose tolerance decreased, gynecomastia, HDL-cholesterol decreased, hypercalcemia, hyperchloremia, hyperkalemia, hypernatremia, hyperphosphatemia, LDL-cholesterol increased, libido increased/decreased, menstrual irregularities, virilism (women)

Gastrointestinal: Diarrhea, nausea, vomiting

Genitourinary: Bladder irritability, epididymitis, impotence, oligospermia, penile enlargement, penile erections increased (prepubertal males), priapism, prostate cancer, prostatic hyperplasia (elderly males), seminal volume decreased, testicular atrophy, testicular dysfunction

Hematologic: Bleeding, INR increased, iron-deficiency anemia, leukemia, prothrombin time increased, clotting factors (II, V, VII, X) suppressed

Hepatic: Alkaline phosphatase increased, bilirubin increased, cholestatic hepatitis, cholestatic jaundice, hepatic failure, hepatic necrosis, hepatocellular carcinoma, liver cell tumors, peliosis hepatis, transaminases increased

Neuromuscular & skeletal: Creatine phosphokinase increased, premature closure of epiphysis (children)

Renal: Creatinine increased

Respiratory: Hoarseness (women)

Miscellaneous: Voice deepening (women)

Rare but important or life-threatening: Hepatotoxicity (idiosyncratic) (Chalasani, 2014)

Drug Interactions

Metabolism/Transport Effects None known.

Avoid Concomitant Use There are no known interactions where it is recommended to avoid concomitant use.

Increased Effect/Toxicity

Oxymetholone may increase the levels/effects of: Blood Glucose Lowering Agents; C1 inhibitors; CycloSPORINE (Systemic); Vitamin K Antagonists

The levels/effects of Oxymetholone may be increased by: Corticosteroids (Systemic)

Decreased Effect There are no known significant interactions involving a decrease in effect.

Storage/Stability Store at room temperature 20°C to 25°C (68°F to 77°F); excursions permitted to 15°C to 30°C (59°F to 86°F). Protect from light.

Mechanism of Action Enhances production of erythropoietin in patients with anemias which are due to bone marrow failure; stimulates erythropoiesis in anemias due to deficient red cell production

Pharmacodynamics Onset of action: Response is not often immediate; a minimum trial of 3 to 6 months is recommended

Dosing: Usual Note: The National Kidney Foundation does not recommend the use of androgens as an adjuvant to ESA treatment in anemic patients with chronic kidney disease (KDOQI, 2006).

Pediatric: **Anemia; treatment (erythropoietic effect [eg, aplastic or Fanconi anemias]):** Children and Adolescents: Oral: 1 to 5 mg/kg/day once daily; usual effective dose: 1 to 2 mg/kg/day; some have suggested higher dosing initially (2 to 5 mg/kg/day) and then tapering to lowest effective dose (Carmitta, 1979; Lanzkowsky, 2010); response often is not immediate; give for a minimum trial of 3 to 6 months

Adult: **Erythropoietic effects:** Oral: 1 to 5 mg/kg/day once daily; usual effective dose: 1 to 2 mg/kg/day; response often is not immediate; give for a minimum trial of 3 to 6 months

Dosing adjustment in renal impairment: Children, Adolescents, and Adults: There are no dosage adjustments provided in manufacturer's labeling. Use with caution due to risk of edema in patients with renal impairment; use is contraindicated in patients with nephrosis or patients in the nephrotic phase of nephritis.

Dosing adjustment in hepatic impairment: Children, Adolescents, and Adults:

Mild to moderate hepatic impairment: There are no dosage adjustments provided in manufacturer's labeling. Use with caution in patients with liver dysfunction because of its hepatotoxic potential.

Severe hepatic impairment: Use is contraindicated

Monitoring Parameters Liver function tests, lipid profile, serum glucose (monitor patients with diabetes), hemoglobin/hematocrit, iron studies; INR/PT in patients on anticoagulant therapy

Children: Radiographs of left wrist every 6 months to assess bone maturation

Females: Signs of virilization (deepening voice, hirsutism, acne, clitoromegaly); urine and serum calcium in women with breast cancer

Test Interactions Decreased thyroxine-binding globulin, T_4; increased resin uptake of T_3 and T_4

Controlled Substance C-III

Dosage Forms Excipient information presented when available (limited, particularly for generics); consult specific product labeling.

Tablet, Oral:

Anadrol-50: 50 mg [scored]

- ◆ **OxyNEO (Can)** *see* OxyCODONE *on page* 1590
- ◆ **Oxytrol** *see* Oxybutynin *on page* 1588
- ◆ **Oxytrol For Women [OTC]** *see* Oxybutynin *on page* 1588
- ◆ **Oysco 500 [OTC]** *see* Calcium Carbonate *on page* 343
- ◆ **Ozurdex** *see* Dexamethasone (Ophthalmic) *on page* 614
- ◆ **P-071** *see* Cetirizine *on page* 423
- ◆ **Pacerone** *see* Amiodarone *on page* 125

PACLitaxel (Conventional)

(pac li TAKS el con VEN sha nal)

Medication Safety Issues

Sound-alike/look-alike issues:

PACLitaxel may be confused with cabazitaxel, DOCEtaxel, PARoxetine, Paxil

PACLitaxel (conventional) may be confused with PACLitaxel (protein-bound)

Taxol may be confused with Abraxane, Paxil, Taxotere

High alert medication:

This medication is in a class the Institute for Safe Medication Practices (ISMP) includes among its list of drug classes which have a heightened risk of causing significant patient harm when used in error.

Related Information

Management of Drug Extravasations *on page* 2298

Prevention of Chemotherapy-Induced Nausea and Vomiting in Children *on page* 2368

Safe Handling of Hazardous Drugs *on page* 2455

Brand Names: Canada Apo-Paclitaxel; Paclitaxel for Injection; Paclitaxel Injection USP

Therapeutic Category Antineoplastic Agent, Antimicrotubular; Antineoplastic Agent, Taxane Derivative

Generic Availability (US) Yes

Use Treatment of breast cancer, advanced ovarian cancer, non-small cell lung cancer, and second-line treatment of AIDS-related Kaposi's sarcoma (FDA approved in adults); has also been used in head and neck cancer, bladder cancer, cervical cancer, small cell lung cancer, and unknown primary adenocarcinomas

Pregnancy Risk Factor D

Pregnancy Considerations Adverse events (embryotoxicity, fetal toxicity, and maternal toxicity) have been observed in animal reproduction studies at doses less than the recommended human dose. An *ex vivo* human placenta perfusion model illustrated that paclitaxel crossed the placenta at term. Placental transfer was low and affected by the presence of albumin; higher albumin concentrations resulted in lower paclitaxel placental transfer (Berveiller, 2012). Some pharmacokinetic properties of paclitaxel may be altered in pregnant women (van Hasselt, 2014). Women of childbearing potential should be advised to avoid becoming pregnant. A pregnancy registry is available for all cancers diagnosed during pregnancy at Cooper Health (877-635-4499).

Breast-Feeding Considerations Paclitaxel is excreted in breast milk (case report). The mother (3 months postpartum) was treated with paclitaxel 30 mg/m^2 (56.1 mg) and carboplatin once weekly for papillary thyroid cancer. Milk samples were obtained 4-316 hours after the infusion given at the sixth and final week of therapy. The average paclitaxel milk concentration over the testing interval was 0.78 mg/L. Although maternal serum concentrations were not noted in the report, the relative infant dose to a nursing infant was calculated to be ~17% of the maternal dose. Paclitaxel continued to be detected in breast milk when sampled at 172 hours after the dose and was below the limit of detection when sampled at 316 hours after the infusion (Griffin, 2012). Due to the potential for serious adverse reactions in a nursing infant, breast-feeding is not recommended.

Contraindications Hypersensitivity to paclitaxel, Cremophor EL (polyoxyethylated castor oil), or any component of the formulation; treatment of solid tumors in patients with baseline neutrophil counts <1,500/mm^3; treatment of Kaposi sarcoma in patients with baseline neutrophil counts <1,000/mm^3.

Warnings/Precautions Hazardous agent - use appropriate precautions for handling and disposal (NIOSH 2014 [group 1]). **[U.S. Boxed Warning]: Anaphylaxis and severe hypersensitivity reactions (dyspnea requiring bronchodilators, hypotension requiring treatment, angioedema, and/or generalized urticaria) have occurred in 2% to 4% of patients in clinical studies; premedicate with corticosteroids, diphenhydramine, and H_2 antagonists prior to infusion. Some reactions have been fatal despite premedication. If severe hypersensitivity occurs, stop infusion and do not rechallenge.** Minor hypersensitivity reactions (flushing, skin reactions, dyspnea, hypotension, or tachycardia) do not require interruption of treatment. Infusion-related hypotension, bradycardia, and/or hypertension may occur; frequent monitoring of vital signs is recommended, especially during the first hour of the infusion. Conventional paclitaxel formulations contain polyoxyethylated castor oil (Cremophor El) which is associated with hypersensitivity reactions. Formulations also contain dehydrated alcohol which may cause adverse CNS effects.

[U.S. Boxed Warning]: Bone marrow suppression (primarily neutropenia; may be severe or result in infection) may occur. Monitor blood counts frequently. Do not administer if baseline neutrophil count is <1,500/mm^3 (for solid tumors) or <1,000/mm^3 (for patients with AIDS-related Kaposi sarcoma). Bone marrow suppression (usually neutropenia) is dose-dependent and is the dose-limiting toxicity; neutrophil nadir is usually at a median of 11 days. Subsequent cycles should not be administered until neutrophils are >1,500/mm^3 (for solid tumors) and 1,000/mm^3 (for Kaposi sarcoma); platelets should recover to 100,000/mm^3. Reduce future doses by 20% for severe neutropenia (<500/mm^3 for 7 days or more) and consider the use of supportive therapy, including growth factor treatment.

Use extreme caution with hepatic dysfunction (myelotoxicity may be worsened in patients with total bilirubin >2 times ULN); dose reductions are recommended. Peripheral neuropathy may commonly occur; patients with preexisting neuropathies from prior chemotherapy or coexisting conditions (eg, diabetes mellitus) may be at a higher risk; reduce dose by 20% for severe neuropathy. Rare but severe conduction abnormalities have been reported; conduct continuous cardiac monitoring during subsequent infusions for these patients. Elderly patients have an increased risk of toxicity (neutropenia, neuropathy, and cardiovascular events); use with caution. Intraperitoneal administration of paclitaxel is associated with a higher incidence of chemotherapy-related toxicity (Armstrong, 2006).

Paclitaxel is an irritant with vesicant-like properties; ensure proper needle or catheter placement prior to and during infusion; avoid extravasation. Injection site reactions are generally mild (skin discoloration, tenderness, erythema, or swelling) and occur more commonly with an extended infusion duration (eg, 24 hours); injection site reactions may be delayed (7 to 10 days). More severe reactions (phlebitis, cellulitis, skin exfoliation, necrosis, fibrosis, and induration) have also been reported. Recall skin reactions may occur despite administering through a different IV site. **[U.S. Boxed Warning]: Should be administered under the supervision of an experienced cancer chemotherapy physician; administer in a facility sufficient to appropriately diagnose and manage complications.** Potentially significant drug-drug interactions may exist, requiring dose or frequency adjustment, additional monitoring, and/or selection of alternative therapy.

Warnings: Additional Pediatric Considerations CNS toxicity has been reported in pediatric patients receiving high doses of paclitaxel (350 to 420 mg/m^2 as a 3-hour infusion) possibly due to the ethanol contained in the formulation.

Adverse Reactions Myelosuppression is dose related, schedule related, and infusion-rate dependent (increased incidences with higher doses, more frequent doses, and longer infusion times) and, in general, rapidly reversible upon discontinuation.

Cardiovascular: Bradycardia, ECG abnormal, edema, flushing, hyper-/hypotension, rhythm abnormalities, syncope, tachycardia, venous thrombosis

Dermatologic: Alopecia, nail changes, rash

Gastrointestinal: Abdominal pain (with intraperitoneal paclitaxel), diarrhea, mucositis, nausea/vomiting, stomatitis

Hematologic: Anemia, bleeding, febrile neutropenia, leukopenia; neutropenia (onset 8-10 days, median nadir 11 days, recovery 15-21 days); thrombocytopenia

Hepatic: Alkaline phosphatase increased, AST increased, bilirubin increased

Local: Injection site reaction (erythema, tenderness, skin discoloration, swelling)

Neuromuscular & skeletal: Arthralgia/myalgia, peripheral neuropathy, weakness

Renal: Creatinine increased (observed in KS patients only)

Miscellaneous: Hypersensitivity reaction, infection

Rare but important or life-threatening: Anaphylaxis, arrhythmia, ataxia, atrial fibrillation, AV block, back pain, cardiac conduction abnormalities, cellulitis, CHF, chills, conjunctivitis, dehydration, enterocolitis, extravasation recall, hepatic encephalopathy, hepatic necrosis, induration, intestinal obstruction, intestinal perforation, interstitial pneumonia, ischemic colitis, lacrimation increased, maculopapular rash, malaise, MI, myocardial ischemia, necrotic changes and ulceration following extravasation, neuroencephalopathy, neutropenic enterocolitis, neutropenic typhlitis, ototoxicity (tinnitus and hearing loss), pancreatitis, paralytic ileus, phlebitis, pneumonitis, pruritus, pulmonary embolism, pulmonary fibrosis, radiation recall, radiation pneumonitis, renal insufficiency, seizure, skin exfoliation, skin fibrosis, skin necrosis, Stevens-Johnson syndrome, supraventricular tachycardia, toxic epidermal necrolysis, ventricular tachycardia (asymptomatic), visual disturbances (scintillating scotomata)

Drug Interactions

Metabolism/Transport Effects Substrate of CYP2C8 (major), CYP3A4 (major), P-glycoprotein; **Note:** Assignment of Major/Minor substrate status based on clinically relevant drug interaction potential; **Induces** CYP3A4 (weak)

Avoid Concomitant Use

Avoid concomitant use of PACLitaxel (Conventional) with any of the following: Atazanavir; BCG; BCG (Intravesical); CloZAPine; Conivaptan; Dipyrone; Fusidic Acid (Systemic); Idelalisib; Natalizumab; Pimecrolimus; SORAfenib; Tacrolimus (Topical); Tofacitinib; Vaccines (Live)

Increased Effect/Toxicity

PACLitaxel (Conventional) may increase the levels/effects of: Antineoplastic Agents (Anthracycline, Systemic); Bexarotene (Systemic); CloZAPine; DOXOrubicin (Conventional); Leflunomide; Natalizumab; Tofacitinib; Trastuzumab; Vaccines (Live); Vinorelbine

The levels/effects of PACLitaxel (Conventional) may be increased by: Abiraterone Acetate; Aprepitant; Atazanavir; Conivaptan; CYP2C8 Inhibitors (Moderate); CYP2C8 Inhibitors (Strong); CYP3A4 Inhibitors (Moderate); CYP3A4 Inhibitors (Strong); Dasatinib; Deferasirox; Denosumab; Dipyrone; Fosaprepitant; Fusidic Acid (Systemic); Idelalisib; Ivacaftor; Luliconazole; Mifepristone; Netupitant; Palbociclib; P-glycoprotein/ABCB1 Inhibitors; Pimecrolimus; Platinum Derivatives; Roflumilast; Simeprevir; SORAfenib; Stiripentol; Tacrolimus (Topical)

Decreased Effect

PACLitaxel (Conventional) may decrease the levels/effects of: ARIPiprazole; BCG; BCG (Intravesical); Coccidioides immitis Skin Test; Hydrocodone; NiMODipine; Saxagliptin; Sipuleucel-T; Vaccines (Inactivated); Vaccines (Live)

The levels/effects of PACLitaxel (Conventional) may be decreased by: Bexarotene (Systemic); Bosentan; CYP2C8 Inducers (Strong); CYP3A4 Inducers (Moderate); CYP3A4 Inducers (Strong); Dabrafenib; Deferasirox; Echinacea; Mitotane; P-glycoprotein/ABCB1 Inducers; Siltuximab; St Johns Wort; Tocilizumab; Trastuzumab

Storage/Stability Store intact vials at room temperature of 20°C to 25°C (68°F to 77°F). Protect from light. Solutions diluted for infusion in D_5W and NS are stable for up to 27 hours at ambient temperature (~25°C).

Paclitaxel should be dispensed in either glass or non-PVC containers (eg, Excel/PAB). Use **nonpolyvinyl** (non-PVC) tubing (eg, polyethylene) to minimize leaching. Formulated in a vehicle known as Cremophor EL (polyoxyethylated castor oil). Cremophor EL has been found to leach the plasticizer DEHP from polyvinyl chloride infusion bags or administration sets. Contact of the undiluted concentrate with plasticized polyvinyl chloride (PVC) equipment or devices is not recommended.

Mechanism of Action Paclitaxel promotes microtubule assembly by enhancing the action of tubulin dimers, stabilizing existing microtubules, and inhibiting their disassembly, interfering with the late G_2 mitotic phase, and inhibiting cell replication. In addition, the drug can distort mitotic spindles, resulting in the breakage of chromosomes. Paclitaxel may also suppress cell proliferation and modulate immune response.

Pharmacokinetics (Adult data unless noted)

Distribution: Biphasic with initial rapid distribution to the peripheral compartment; later phase is a slow efflux of paclitaxel from the peripheral compartment

V_d: 227-688 L/m^2

Protein binding: 89% to 98%

Metabolism: Cytochrome P450 hepatic isoenzymes metabolize paclitaxel to 6 alpha-hydroxypaclitaxel

Half-life (varies with dose and infusion duration):

Children: 4.6-17 hours

Adults: 1.5-8.4 hours

Elimination: Urinary recovery of unchanged drug: 1.3% to 12.6%

Dialysis: No significant drug removal by hemodialysis

Dosing: Usual IV infusion (refer to individual protocols):

Children:

Treatment for refractory leukemia is still undergoing investigation: 250-360 mg/m^2/dose infused over 24 hours every 14 days

Recurrent Wilms' tumor: 250-350 mg/m^2/dose infused over 24 hours every 3 weeks

Adults:

Ovarian carcinoma: 135-175 mg/m^2/dose infused over 1-24 hours every 3 weeks

Metastatic breast cancer: 175 mg/m^2/dose infused over 3 hours every 3 weeks (protocols have used dosages ranging between 135-250 mg/m^2/dose over 1-24 hours every 3 weeks)

Kaposi's sarcoma: 135 mg/m^2/dose infused over 3 hours every 3 weeks, or 100 mg/m^2/dose infused over 3 hours every 2 weeks

Dosage adjustment in renal impairment: None

Dosage adjustment in hepatic impairment:

Total bilirubin ≤1.5 mg/dL and AST >2x normal limits: Total dose <135 mg/m^2

Total bilirubin 1.6-3.0 mg/dL: Total dose ≤75 mg/m^2

Total bilirubin ≥3.1 mg/dL: Total dose ≤50 mg/m^2

Preparation for Administration Hazardous agent; use appropriate precautions for handling and disposal (NIOSH 2014 [group 1]).

Parenteral: IV: Dilute for infusion in D_5W, D_5LR, D_5NS, or NS to a concentration of 0.3 to 1.2 mg/mL. To minimize patient exposure to the plasticizer diethylhexylphthalate (DEHP) prepare paclitaxel infusions in a non-PVC container (glass or polyethylene). Chemotherapy dispensing devices (eg, Chemo Dispensing Pin) should not be used to withdraw paclitaxel from the vial; closed system transfer devices may not be compatible with undiluted paclitaxel.

Administration Hazardous agent; use appropriate precautions for handling and disposal (NIOSH 2014 [group 1]).

Parenteral: IV: Infuse over 3 or 24 hours (depending on indication/protocol); some protocols use a 1-hour infusion. Infuse through a 0.22-micron in-line filter and polyethylene-lined (non-PVC) administration set. When administered as a part of a combination chemotherapy regimen, sequence of administration may vary by regimen; refer to specific protocol for sequence recommendation. Patients should be premedicated with a corticosteroid, diphenhydramine and an H_2-receptor antagonist prior to paclitaxel administration.

Irritant with vesicant-like properties; avoid extravasation. Ensure proper needle or catheter position prior to administration. If extravasation occurs, stop infusion immediately and disconnect (leave cannula/needle in place); gently aspirate extravasated solution (do **NOT** flush the line); remove needle/cannula; initiate antidote (hyaluronidase) (see Management of Drug Extravasations for more details); remove needle/cannula; elevate extremity. Information conflicts regarding the use of warm or cold compresses (Pérez Fidalgo 2012; Polovich 2009).

Vesicant/Extravasation Risk Irritant with vesicant-like properties

Monitoring Parameters CBC with differential, platelet count, vital signs, ECG, liver function test; observe IV injection site for extravasation

Dosage Forms Considerations Paclitaxel injection contains Cremophor EL

Dosage Forms Excipient information presented when available (limited, particularly for generics); consult specific product labeling.

Concentrate, Intravenous:

Generic: 100 mg/16.7 mL (16.7 mL); 30 mg/5 mL (5 mL); 150 mg/25 mL (25 mL); 300 mg/50 mL (50 mL)

Concentrate, Intravenous [preservative free]:

Generic: 100 mg/16.7 mL (16.7 mL); 30 mg/5 mL (5 mL); 300 mg/50 mL (50 mL)

◆ **Paclitaxel for Injection (Can)** *see* PACLitaxel (Conventional) *on page* 1602

◆ **Paclitaxel Injection USP (Can)** *see* PACLitaxel (Conventional) *on page* 1602

◆ **Pain Eze [OTC]** *see* Acetaminophen *on page* 44

◆ **Pain & Fever Children's [OTC]** *see* Acetaminophen *on page* 44

◆ **Palafer® (Can)** *see* Ferrous Fumarate *on page* 869

◆ **Palgic [DSC]** *see* Carbinoxamine *on page* 372

Paliperidone (pal ee PER i done)

Medication Safety Issues

Sound-alike/look-alike issues:

Invega may be confused with Intuniv

BEERS Criteria medication:

This drug may be potentially inappropriate for use in geriatric patients (Quality of evidence - moderate; Strength of recommendation - strong).

Related Information

Oral Medications That Should Not Be Crushed or Altered *on page* 2476

Brand Names: US Invega; Invega Sustenna; Invega Trinza

Brand Names: Canada Invega; Invega Sustenna

Therapeutic Category Antipsychotic Agent, Benzisoxazole; Second Generation (Atypical) Antipsychotic

Generic Availability (US) No

Use

Oral: Treatment of schizophrenia (FDA approved in ages ≥12 years and adults); treatment of schizoaffective disorder as monotherapy or adjunctive therapy to mood stabilizers and/or antidepressants (FDA approved in adults); has also been used for treatment of irritability associated with autistic disorder

Parenteral: Treatment of schizophrenia (acute and maintenance) (FDA approved in adults)

Pregnancy Risk Factor C

Pregnancy Considerations Adverse events have not been observed in animal reproduction studies. Antipsychotic use during the third trimester of pregnancy has a risk for extrapyramidal symptoms (EPS) and/or withdrawal symptoms in newborns following delivery. Symptoms in the newborn may include agitation, feeding disorder, hypertonia, hypotonia, respiratory distress, somnolence, and tremor. These effects may be self-limiting and allow recovery within hours or days with no specific treatment, or they may be severe requiring prolonged hospitalization.

Paliperidone may cause hyperprolactinemia, which may decrease reproductive function in both males and females.

Paliperidone is the active metabolite of risperidone; refer to Risperidone monograph for additional information.

The ACOG recommends that therapy during pregnancy be individualized; treatment with psychiatric medications during pregnancy should incorporate the clinical expertise of the mental health clinician, obstetrician, primary healthcare provider, and pediatrician. Safety data related to atypical antipsychotics during pregnancy is limited and routine use is not recommended. However, if a woman is inadvertently exposed to an atypical antipsychotic while pregnant, continuing therapy may be preferable to switching to a typical antipsychotic that the fetus has not yet been exposed to; consider risk:benefit (ACOG, 2008).

Healthcare providers are encouraged to enroll women 18 to 45 years of age exposed to paliperidone during pregnancy in the Atypical Antipsychotics Pregnancy Registry (1-866-961-2388 or http://www.womensmentalhealth.org/pregnancyregistry).

Breast-Feeding Considerations Paliperidone is excreted in breast milk. According to the manufacturer, the decision to continue or discontinue breast-feeding during therapy should take into account the risk of exposure to the infant and the benefits of treatment to the mother.

Contraindications Hypersensitivity to paliperidone, risperidone, or any component of the formulation

Warnings/Precautions [U.S. Boxed Warning]: Elderly patients with dementia-related psychosis treated with antipsychotics are at an increased risk of death compared to placebo. Most deaths appeared to be either cardiovascular (eg, heart failure, sudden death) or infectious (eg, pneumonia) in nature. In addition, an increased incidence of cerebrovascular adverse effects (eg, transient ischemic attack, cerebrovascular accidents) has been reported in studies of placebo-controlled trials of risperidone (paliperidone is the primary active metabolite of risperidone) in elderly patients with dementia-related psychosis. Paliperidone is not approved for the treatment of dementia-related psychosis. In addition, patients with Lewy body dementia (LBD) may be more sensitive to CNS-related and extrapyramidal effects.

May cause CNS depression, which may impair physical or mental abilities; patients must be cautioned about performing tasks that require mental alertness (eg, operating machinery or driving). Use with caution in mild renal dysfunction; dose reduction recommended. Not recommended in patients with moderate to severe impairment. Esophageal dysmotility and aspiration have been associated with antipsychotic use; use with caution in patients at risk of aspiration pneumonia (eg, Alzheimer disease).

Leukopenia, neutropenia, and agranulocytosis (sometimes fatal) have been reported in clinical trials and postmarketing reports with antipsychotic use; presence of risk factors (eg, preexisting low WBC or history of drug-induced leuko-/neutropenia) should prompt periodic blood count assessment. Discontinue therapy at first signs of blood dyscrasias or if absolute neutrophil count <1,000/mm^3.

Paliperidone is associated with increased prolactin levels; clinical significance of hyperprolactinemia in patients with breast cancer or other prolactin-dependent tumors is unknown. May alter temperature regulation. May mask toxicity of other drugs or conditions (eg, intestinal obstruction, Reye's syndrome, brain tumor) due to antiemetic effects. Priapism has been reported rarely with use. Hypersensitivity reactions, including anaphylactic reactions and angioedema, have been reported.

May cause orthostasis and syncope; use with caution in patients with known cardiovascular disease (heart failure, history of myocardial infarction or ischemia, conduction abnormalities), cerebrovascular disease, or conditions that predispose the patient to hypotension (dehydration, hypovolemia, and treatment with antihypertensive medications). May alter cardiac conduction; life-threatening arrhythmias have occurred with therapeutic doses of neuroleptics. Avoid use in combination with QTc-prolonging drugs. Avoid use in patients with congenital long QT syndrome and in patients with history of cardiac arrhythmia.

May cause extrapyramidal symptoms (EPS), including pseudoparkinsonism, acute dystonic reactions, akathisia, and tardive dyskinesia (risk of these reactions is low relative to other neuroleptics, and is dose dependent). Risk of dystonia (and probably other EPS) may be greater with increased doses, use of conventional antipsychotics, males, and younger patients. Risk of neuroleptic malignant syndrome (NMS) may be increased in patients with Parkinson disease or Lewy body dementia; monitor for symptoms of confusion, obtundation, postural instability and extrapyramidal symptoms. May cause hyperglycemia; in some cases may be extreme and associated with ketoacidosis, hyperosmolar coma, or death. All patients should be monitored for symptoms of hyperglycemia (eg, polydipsia, polyuria, polyphagia, weakness). Use with caution in patients with diabetes (or risk factors) or other disorders of glucose regulation; monitor for worsening of glucose control. Patients with risk factors for diabetes (eg, obesity or family history) should have a baseline fasting blood sugar (FBS) and periodically during treatment. Significant weight gain has been observed with antipsychotic therapy; incidence varies with product. Monitor waist circumference and BMI. May cause lipid abnormalities (LDL and triglycerides increased; HDL decreased). Few case reports describe intraoperative floppy iris syndrome (IFIS) in patients receiving risperidone and undergoing cataract surgery (Ford, 2011). IFIS has not been reported with paliperidone but caution is advised since it is the active metabolite of risperidone. Prior to cataract surgery, evaluate for prior or current paliperidone or risperidone use. The benefits or risks of interrupting paliperidone or risperidone prior to surgery have not been established; clinicians are advised to proceed with surgery cautiously.

The possibility of a suicide attempt is inherent in psychotic illness or bipolar disorder; use caution in high-risk patients during initiation of therapy. Prescriptions should be written for the smallest quantity consistent with good patient care.

Use in elderly patients with dementia is associated with an increased risk of mortality and cerebrovascular accidents; avoid antipsychotic use for behavioral problems associated with dementia unless alternative nonpharmacologic therapies have failed and patient may harm self or others. Paliperidone is not approved for the treatment of dementia-related psychosis. In addition, use may cause or exacerbate syndrome of inappropriate antidiuretic hormone secretion or hyponatremia; monitor sodium closely with initiation or dosage adjustments in older adults (Beers Criteria).

The tablet formulation consists of drug within a nonabsorbable shell that is expelled and may be visible in the stool. Use is not recommended in patients with preexisting severe gastrointestinal narrowing disorders. Patients with upper GI tract alterations in transit time may have increased or decreased bioavailability of paliperidone. Do not use in patients unable to swallow the tablet whole.

Warnings: Additional Pediatric Considerations Risk of dystonia is increased with the use of high potency and higher doses of conventional antipsychotics and in males and younger patients; occurring in up to 18% of children. Use with caution in children and adolescents; adverse effects due to elevated prolactin levels have been observed; long-term effects on growth or sexual maturation have not been evaluated.

Paliperidone may cause a higher than normal weight gain in children and adolescents; monitor growth (including weight, height, BMI, and waist circumference) in pediatric patients receiving paliperidone; in adolescent trials, ≤19% of patients experienced a weight gain of ≥7%; monitor weight and compare to standard growth curves.

Paliperidone may cause increases in metabolic indices (eg, serum cholesterol, triglycerides). Biannual monitoring of cardiometabolic indices after the first 3 months of therapy is suggested for atypical antipsychotics (Correll, 2009).

Adolescents may experience a higher frequency of certain adverse effects than adults, particularly akathisia (4% to 17% vs 1% to 10%; dose dependent), somnolence (9% to 26% vs 1% to 12%), and vomiting (≤11% vs 2% to 5%). Adolescents may experience some adverse effects not reported in adults, including amenorrhea, blurred vision, galactorrhea, gynecomastia, and tongue swelling.

Adverse Reactions Unless otherwise noted, frequency of adverse effects is reported for the oral/IM formulation in adults.

Cardiovascular: Bundle branch block, orthostatic hypotension (dose dependent), tachycardia (adolescents and adults)

Central nervous system: Agitation, akathisia (adolescents and adults; dose dependent), anxiety (adolescents and adults), dizziness (adolescents and adults), drowsiness (more common in adolescents; dose dependent), dysarthria (dose dependent), dystonia (adolescents and adults; dose dependent), extrapyramidal reaction (more common in adolescents; dose dependent), fatigue (adolescents and adults), headache (adolescents and adults), lethargy (adolescents and adults), parkinsonian-like syndrome (adolescents and adults; dose dependent), sleep disorder

Endocrine & metabolic: Abnormal triglycerides (adolescents and adults), altered serum glucose (adolescents and adults), amenorrhea (adolescents and adults), blood cholesterol abnormal (adolescents and adults), galactorrhea (adolescents and adults), gynecomastia (adolescents and adults), weight gain (adolescents and adults; dose dependent)

Gastrointestinal: Abdominal pain, constipation, diarrhea, dyspepsia, increased appetite, nausea, sialorrhea (adolescents and adults; dose dependent), swollen tongue (adolescents and adults), toothache, vomiting (adolescents and adults), xerostomia (adolescents and adults)

Hematologic & oncologic: Change in HDL (adolescents and adults), change in LDL (adolescents and adults)

Local: IM formulation: Injection site reaction

Neuromuscular & skeletal: Back pain, dyskinesia (adolescents and adults), hyperkinesia (adolescents and adults; dose dependent), limb pain, myalgia (dose dependent), tongue paralysis (adolescents), tremor (adolescents and adults), weakness (adolescents and adults)

Ophthalmic: Blurred vision (adolescents and adults)

Respiratory: cough (dose dependent), nasopharyngitis (adolescents and adults; dose dependent), rhinitis (dose dependent), upper respiratory tract infection

Rare but important or life-threatening: Agranulocytosis, alopecia, anaphylaxis, antiemetic effect, aspiration pneumonia, atrial fibrillation, cerebrovascular accident, deep vein thrombosis, diabetes mellitus, diabetic ketoacidosis, edema, epistaxis, erectile dysfunction, first degree atrioventricular block, hyperprolactinemia, hypertension, hypertonia, hypothermia, increased serum ALT, increased serum AST, insomnia, intestinal obstruction, intraoperative floppy iris syndrome, ischemia, jaundice, mania, neuroleptic malignant syndrome, orthostatic dizziness, pancreatitis, postural orthostatic tachycardia, priapism, psychomotor agitation, pulmonary embolism, retrograde ejaculation, seizure, SIADH, sleep apnea, suicidal ideation, syncope, tardive dyskinesia, thrombocytopenia, thrombotic thrombocytopenic purpura, trismus, urinary incontinence, urinary retention, venous thromboembolism

Drug Interactions

Metabolism/Transport Effects **Substrate** of P-glycoprotein

Avoid Concomitant Use

Avoid concomitant use of Paliperidone with any of the following: Amisulpride; Azelastine (Nasal); Highest Risk QTc-Prolonging Agents; Ivabradine; Metoclopramide; Mifepristone; Moderate Risk QTc-Prolonging Agents; Orphenadrine; Paraldehyde; Sulpiride; Thalidomide

Increased Effect/Toxicity

Paliperidone may increase the levels/effects of: Alcohol (Ethyl); Amisulpride; Azelastine (Nasal); Buprenorphine; CNS Depressants; Highest Risk QTc-Prolonging Agents; Hydrocodone; Methotrimeprazine; Methylphenidate; Metyrosine; Orphenadrine; Paraldehyde; Selective Serotonin Reuptake Inhibitors; Serotonin Modulators; Sulpiride; Suvorexant; Thalidomide; Zolpidem

The levels/effects of Paliperidone may be increased by: Acetylcholinesterase Inhibitors (Central); Brimonidine (Topical); Cannabis; Doxylamine; Dronabinol; Itraconazole; Ivabradine; Kava Kava; Magnesium Sulfate; Methotrimeprazine; Methylphenidate; Metoclopramide; Metyrosine; Mifepristone; Moderate Risk QTc-Prolonging Agents; Nabilone; Perampanel; P-glycoprotein/ABCB1 Inhibitors; QTc-Prolonging Agents (Indeterminate Risk and Risk Modifying); RisperiDONE; Rufinamide; Serotonin Modulators; Sodium Oxybate; Tapentadol; Tetrahydrocannabinol; Valproic Acid and Derivatives

Decreased Effect

Paliperidone may decrease the levels/effects of: Amphetamines; Antidiabetic Agents; Anti-Parkinson's Agents (Dopamine Agonist); Quinagolide

The levels/effects of Paliperidone may be decreased by: CarBAMazepine; Inducers of CYP3A4 and P-glycoprotein; P-glycoprotein/ABCB1 Inducers

Storage/Stability

Oral, Monthly IM: Store at ≤25°C (77°F); excursions permitted to 15°C to 30°C (59°F to 86°F). Protect tablets from moisture.

3-month IM: Store at 20°C to 25°C (68°F to 77°F); excursions permitted to 15°C to 30°C (59°F to 86°F).

Mechanism of Action Paliperidone is considered a benzisoxazole atypical antipsychotic as it is the primary active metabolite of risperidone. As with other atypical antipsychotics, its therapeutic efficacy is believed to result from mixed central serotonergic and dopaminergic antagonism. The addition of serotonin antagonism to dopamine antagonism (classic neuroleptic mechanism) is thought to improve negative symptoms of psychoses and reduce the incidence of extrapyramidal side effects. Similar to risperidone, paliperidone demonstrates high affinity to α_1, D_2, H_1, and 5-HT_{2C} receptors, and low affinity for muscarinic and 5-HT_{1A} receptors. In contrast to risperidone, paliperidone displays nearly 10-fold lower affinity for α_2 and 5-HT_{2A} receptors, and nearly three- to fivefold less affinity for 5-HT_{1A} and 5-HT_{1D}, respectively.

Pharmacokinetics (Adult data unless noted) Note: Pharmacokinetic parameters in adolescent patients weighing >51 kg were similar to adults; an increased drug exposure (23%) was observed in adolescent patient weighing <51 kg compared to adults and was not considered clinically significant.

Absorption: IM: Slow release (begins on day 1 and continues up to 126 days)

Distribution, apparent V_d: 391-487 L

Protein binding: 74%

Metabolism: Hepatic via CYP2D6 and 3A4 (limited role in elimination); minor metabolism (<10% each) via dealkylation, hydroxylation, dehydrogenation, and benzisoxazole scission

Bioavailability: Oral: 28%

Half-life:

Oral: 23 hours; prolonged with renal impairment (CrCl <80 mL/minute): 24-51 hours

IM (single dose): Range: 25-49 days

Time to peak serum concentration: Oral: ~24 hours; IM: 13 days

Elimination: Urine (80%; 59% as unchanged drug); feces (11%)

Dosing: Usual

Children and Adolescents:

Schizophrenia: Children ≥12 and Adolescents: Oral: 3 mg once daily; titration not necessary; if after clinical assessment a dosage increase is required, may increase dose in 3 mg/day increments at least every 5 days; maximum daily dose is weight dependent: <51 kg: 6 mg/**day**; ≥51 kg: 12 mg/**day**; **Note:** During adolescent clinical trials, higher doses were not associated with greater efficacy, but increased risk of adverse effects.

Irritability associated with autistic disorder: Limited data available: Children ≥12 years and Adolescents: Oral: Initial: 3 mg once daily; titrate on a weekly basis in 3 mg/day increments until clinical response or intolerance; maximum daily dose: 12 mg/**day**. Dosing based on an open-label trial of 25 patients (mean age: 15.3 years; age range: 12-21 years); therapeutic response was reported in 84% of patients at a mean final dose: 7.1 mg/day (Stigler, 2012)

Adults:

Schizoaffective disorder, schizophrenia: Oral: Usual: 6 mg once daily in the morning; titration not required, though some may benefit from higher or lower doses. If dose exceeding 6 mg/day, increases of 3 mg/day are recommended no more frequently than every 4 days in schizoaffective disorder or every 5 days in schizophrenia, up to a maximum of 12 mg/day. Some patients may require only 3 mg/day.

Schizophrenia: IM: **Note:** Prior to initiation of I.M therapy, tolerability should be established with oral paliperidone or oral risperidone. Previous oral antipsychotics can be discontinued at the time of initiation of IM therapy. **Dosing based on paliperidone palmitate.**

Initiation of therapy:

Initial: 234 mg on treatment day 1 followed by 156 mg 1 week later. The second dose may be administered 2 days before or after the weekly timepoint.

Maintenance: Following the 1-week initiation regimen, begin a maintenance dose of 117 mg every month. Some patients may benefit from higher or lower monthly maintenance doses (monthly maintenance dosage range: 39-234 mg). The monthly maintenance dose may be administered 7 days before or after the monthly timepoint.

Conversion from oral paliperidone to I.M paliperidone: Initiate IM therapy as described using the 1-week initiation regimen. Patients previously stabilized on oral doses can expect similar steady state exposure during maintenance treatment with IM therapy using the following conversion:

Oral extended release dose of 12 mg, then IM maintenance dose of 234 mg

Oral extended release dose of 6 mg, then IM maintenance dose of 117 mg

Oral extended release dose of 3 mg, then IM maintenance dose of 39-78 mg

Switching from other long acting injectable antipsychotics to IM paliperidone: Initiate IM paliperidone in the place of the next scheduled injection and continue at monthly intervals. The 1-week initiation regimen is not required in these patients.

Dosage adjustments: Adjustments may be made monthly (full effect from adjustments may not be seen for several months)

Missed doses:

If <6 weeks has elapsed since the last monthly injection: Administer the missed dose as soon as possible and continue therapy at monthly intervals.

If >6 weeks and ≤6 months has elapsed since the last monthly injection:

If the maintenance dose was <234 mg: Administer the same dose the patient was previously stabilized on as soon as possible, followed by a second equivalent dose 1 week later, then resume maintenance dose at monthly intervals

If the maintenance dose was 234 mg: Administer a 156 mg dose as soon as possible, followed by a second dose of 156 mg 1 week later, then resume maintenance dose at monthly intervals.

If >6 months has elapsed since last monthly maintenance injection: Therapy must be reinitiated following dosing recommendations for initiation of therapy.

Dosing adjustment in renal impairment:

Children ≥12 years and Adolescents: There are no dosing adjustments provided in manufacturer's labeling.

Adults:

Oral:

CrCl 50-79 mL/minute: Initial: 3 mg once daily; maximum dose: 6 mg once daily

CrCl 10-49 mL/minute: Initial: 1.5 mg once daily; maximum dose: 3 mg once daily

CrCl <10 mL/minute: Use not recommended; not studied in this population

IM:

CrCl 50-79 mL/minute: Initiation of therapy: 156 mg on treatment day 1, followed by 117 mg 1 week later, followed by a maintenance dose of 78 mg every month

CrCl <50 mL/minute: Use not recommended

Dosing adjustment hepatic impairment: Oral, IM: No adjustment necessary for mild to moderate (Child-Pugh class A or B) impairment. Not studied in severe impairment.

Administration

Oral: Administer in the morning without regard to meals; swallow extended release tablets whole with liquids; do not crush, chew, or divide.

IM (Invega® Sustenna™): Shake prefilled syringe for at least 10 seconds to ensure a homogenous suspension; administer IM as a single injection (do not divide doses) injection should be slow and deep into the muscle. When initiating therapy, the deltoid muscle should be used for the first two doses to rapidly attain therapeutic concentrations (see manufacturer labeling for specific needle length/gauge). Monthly maintenance doses can be administered in either the deltoid muscle or upper, outer quadrant of gluteal muscle; may alternate injection sites. Do not administer IV or subQ; avoid inadvertent injection into vasculature.

Monitoring Parameters Blood pressure (including orthostatic) and heart rate, particularly during dosage titration; mental status, abnormal involuntary movement scale (AIMS), extrapyramidal symptoms; growth, BMI, waist circumference, and weight (in adults, weight should be assessed prior to treatment, at 4 weeks, 8 weeks, 12 weeks, and then at quarterly intervals; consider titrating to a different antipsychotic agent for a weight gain ≥5% of the initial weight); CBC with differential; liver enzymes in children (especially obese children or those who are rapidly gaining weight while receiving therapy); lipid profile; fasting blood glucose/Hgb A_{1c} (prior to treatment, at 3 months, then annually); prolactin serum concentrations

Additional Information Long-term usefulness of paliperidone should be periodically re-evaluated in patients receiving the drug for extended periods of time. Invega® is an extended release tablet based on the OROS® osmotic delivery system. Water from the GI tract enters through a semipermeable membrane coating the tablet, solubilizing the drug into a gelatinous form which, through hydrophilic expansion, is then expelled through laser-drilled holes in the coating.

Dosage Forms Excipient information presented when available (limited, particularly for generics); consult specific product labeling.

Suspension, Intramuscular, as palmitate:

Invega Sustenna: 39 mg/0.25 mL (0.25 mL); 78 mg/0.5 mL (0.5 mL); 117 mg/0.75 mL (0.75 mL); 156 mg/mL (1 mL); 234 mg/1.5 mL (1.5 mL) [contains polyethylene glycol]

Invega Trinza: 410 mg/1.315 mL (1.315 mL); 273 mg/0.875 mL (0.875 mL); 546 mg/1.75 mL (1.75 mL); 819 mg/2.625 mL (2.625 mL) [contains polyethylene glycol]

Tablet Extended Release 24 Hour, Oral:

Invega: 1.5 mg, 3 mg, 6 mg, 9 mg

◆ **Paliperidone Palmitate** *see* Paliperidone *on page* 1604

Palivizumab (pah li VIZ u mab)

Medication Safety Issues

Sound-alike/look-alike issues:

Synagis may be confused with Synalgos-DC, Synflorix, Synvisc

Brand Names: US Synagis

Brand Names: Canada Synagis

Therapeutic Category Monoclonal Antibody

Generic Availability (US) No

Use Prevention of serious lower respiratory tract disease caused by respiratory syncytial virus (RSV) in infants and children at high risk for RSV disease including patients with bronchopulmonary disease, a gestational age ≤35 weeks, or hemodynamically significant congenital heart disease (FDA approved ≤24 months of age); has also been used for IV treatment of active RSV infections in patients at high-risk for severe disease.

The American Academy of Pediatrics (AAP, 2014) recommends RSV prophylaxis with palivizumab during RSV season for:

- Infants born at ≤28 weeks 6 days gestational age and <12 months at the start of RSV season
- Infants <12 months of age with chronic lung disease (CLD) of prematurity
- Infants <12 months of age with hemodynamically significant congenital heart disease (CHD)
- Infants and children <24 months of age with CLD necessitating medical therapy (eg, supplemental oxygen, bronchodilator, diuretic, or chronic steroid therapy) within 6 months prior to the beginning of RSV season

AAP also suggests that palivizumab prophylaxis may be considered in the following circumstances:

- Infants <12 months of age with congenital airway abnormality or neuromuscular disorder that decreases the ability to manage airway secretions
- Infants <12 months of age with cystic fibrosis with clinical evidence of CLD and/or nutritional compromise
- Children <24 months with cystic fibrosis with severe lung disease (previous hospitalization for pulmonary exacerbation in the first year of life or abnormalities on chest radiography or chest computed tomography that persist when stable) or weight for length less than the 10th percentile.
- Infants and children <24 months profoundly immunocompromised
- Infants and children <24 months undergoing cardiac transplantation during RSV season

Pregnancy Risk Factor C

Pregnancy Considerations Not for adult use; reproduction studies have not been conducted

Contraindications Significant prior hypersensitivity reaction to palivizumab or any component of the formulation

Warnings/Precautions Very rare cases of anaphylaxis, some fatal, have been observed following palivizumab. Rare cases of severe acute hypersensitivity reactions have also been reported. Use with caution after mild hypersensitivity reaction; permanently discontinue for severe hypersensitivity reaction. Safety and efficacy of palivizumab have not been demonstrated in the treatment of established RSV disease. Palivizumab is not recommended for the prevention of health care-associated RSV disease (AAP, 2014). Use with caution in patients with thrombocytopenia or any coagulation disorder; bleeding/hematoma may occur from IM administration.

Adverse Reactions

Central nervous system: Fever

Dermatologic: Rash

Miscellaneous: Antibody formation

Rare but important or life-threatening: Anaphylaxis (very rare - includes angioedema, dyspnea, hypotonia, pruritus, respiratory failure, unresponsiveness, urticaria); hypersensitivity reactions, injection site reactions, thrombocytopenia

Drug Interactions

Metabolism/Transport Effects None known.

Avoid Concomitant Use

Avoid concomitant use of Palivizumab with any of the following: Belimumab

Increased Effect/Toxicity

Palivizumab may increase the levels/effects of: Belimumab

Decreased Effect There are no known significant interactions involving a decrease in effect.

Storage/Stability Store between 2°C and 8°C (36°F and 46°F) in original container; do not freeze. Extended storage information may be available; contact product manufacturer to obtain current recommendations.

Mechanism of Action Exhibits neutralizing and fusion-inhibitory activity against RSV; these activities inhibit RSV replication in laboratory and clinical studies

Pharmacodynamics Protective trough concentrations (≥40 mcg/mL) are achieved following the second dose.

Pharmacokinetics (Adult data unless noted)

Bioavailability: 70%

Half-life: Infants and Children <24 months: 20 days

Time to achieve adequate serum antibody titers: 48 hours

Dosing: Neonatal

RSV, prevention: IM: 15 mg/kg once monthly throughout RSV season; **Note:** AAP recommends a maximum of 5 doses per season; hospitalized neonates who qualify for prophylaxis during RSV season should receive the first palivizumab dose 48 to 72 hours before discharge or promptly after discharge.

Cardiopulmonary bypass patients: IM: Administer a 15 mg/kg dose as soon as possible after cardiopulmonary bypass procedure or at the conclusion of extracorporeal membrane oxygenation, even if <1 month from previous dose. A 58% decrease in palivizumab serum concentrations has been noted after cardiopulmonary bypass (AAP, 2014).

Dosing: Usual Pediatric:

RSV, prevention: Infants and Children <24 months: IM: 15 mg/kg once monthly throughout RSV season; first dose administered prior to commencement of RSV season; **Note:** AAP recommends a maximum 5 doses per season; if hospitalization occurs for breakthrough RSV infection, monthly prophylaxis should be discontinued for the remainder of that season (AAP, 2014).

Cardiopulmonary bypass patients: Administer a 15 mg/kg dose as soon as possible after cardiopulmonary bypass procedure or at the conclusion of extracorporeal membrane oxygenation, even if <1 month from previous dose. A 58% decrease in palivizumab serum concentrations has been noted after cardiopulmonary bypass (AAP, 2014).

RSV, treatment in patients at high-risk for severe disease: Limited data available: Infants, Children, and Adolescents: IV: 15 mg/kg as a single dose; in most patients, used in combination with ribavirin therapy; in two patients with disease progression, a single repeat dose at 3 to 5 days after the initial dose was reported (Chávez-Bueno, 2007). Dosing based on experience in 85 patients the majority of which are pediatric patients and mostly ≤2 years of age. Reported efficacy results variable, an initial double-blind, placebo-controlled trial (n=17 treatment group; all patients ≤2 years) showed statistically significant decreases in RSV tracheal aspirate concentrations vs placebo (Malley, 1998); in another double-blind, placebo-controlled trial (n=22 treatment group; all patients ≤2 years) a decrease in the days of RSV hospitalization, days of supplemental oxygen, and lower respiratory infection scores were reported relative to placebo (Sáez-Llorens, 2004); in an underpowered, observational study of hematopoietic stem cell patients (n=15; age range: 2 to 60 years) a decrease viral shedding and increased 30 day-survival vs ribavirin monotherapy (83.3% vs ~55%) was reported (Boeckh, 2001).

Dosing adjustment in renal impairment: Infants and Children <24 months: There are no dosage adjustments provided in the manufacturer's labeling.

Dosing adjustment in hepatic impairment: Infants and Children <24 months: There are no dosage adjustments provided in the manufacturer's labeling.

Administration

IM: Administer undiluted solution IM, preferably in the anterolateral aspect of the thigh; gluteal muscle should not be used routinely as an injection site because of the risk of damage to the sciatic nerve; injection volume over 1 mL should be given as a divided dose. Do **not** dilute product; do not shake or vigorously agitate the vial.

IV: In clinical trials in pediatric patients ≤2 years, palivizumab has been administered IVP over 2 to 5 minutes or IV infusion through a 0.2 micron filter at a rate not to exceed 1 to 2 mL/minute at a final concentration of 10 to 20 mg/mL (Boeckh 2001; Sáez-Llorens 2004; Subramanian 1998).

Monitoring Parameters Observe for anaphylactic or severe allergic reactions

Test Interactions May interfere (false negatives) with immunological-based RSV diagnostic tests (antigen detection) and viral culture assays; rely on reverse-transcriptase-polymerase chain reaction-based assays and clinical findings.

Additional Information Antipalivizumab antibodies may develop after the fourth injection in some patients (~1%). This has not been associated with any risk of adverse events or altered serum concentrations.

Dosage Forms Excipient information presented when available (limited, particularly for generics); consult specific product labeling.

Solution, Intramuscular [preservative free]:

Synagis: 50 mg/0.5 mL (0.5 mL); 100 mg/mL (1 mL) [contains glycine, histidine]

Palonosetron (pal oh NOE se tron)

Medication Safety Issues

Sound-alike/look-alike issues:

Aloxi may be confused with Eloxatin, oxaliplatin

Palonosetron may be confused with dolasetron, granisetron, ondansetron

Brand Names: US Aloxi

Therapeutic Category 5-HT_3 Receptor Antagonist; Antiemetic

Generic Availability (US) No

Use Prevention of acute and delayed chemotherapy-induced nausea and vomiting associated with initial and repeat courses of emetogenic chemotherapy (including highly emetogenic) (FDA approved in ages ≥1 month and adults); prevention of postoperative nausea and vomiting (PONV) for up to 24 hours following surgery (FDA approved in adults)

Pregnancy Risk Factor B

Pregnancy Considerations Adverse events have not been observed in animal reproduction studies. Use during pregnancy only if clearly needed.

Breast-Feeding Considerations It is not known if palonosetron is excreted in breast milk. Due to the potential for adverse reactions in the nursing infant, the manufacturer recommends a decision be made whether to discontinue nursing or to discontinue palonosetron, taking into account the importance of treatment to the mother.

Contraindications Hypersensitivity to palonosetron or any component of the formulation

Warnings/Precautions Hypersensitivity (including anaphylaxis) has been reported in patients with or without known hypersensitivity to other 5-HT_3 receptor antagonists. Serotonin syndrome has been reported with 5-HT_3 receptor antagonists, predominantly when used in combination with other serotonergic agents (eg, SSRIs, SNRIs, MAOIs, mirtazapine, fentanyl, lithium, tramadol, and/or methylene blue). Some of the cases have been fatal. The majority of serotonin syndrome reports due to 5-HT_3 receptor antagonists have occurred in a post-anesthesia setting or in an infusion center. Serotonin syndrome has also been reported following overdose of another 5-HT_3 receptor antagonist. Monitor patients for signs of serotonin syndrome, including mental status changes (eg, agitation, hallucinations, delirium, coma); autonomic instability (eg, tachycardia, labile blood pressure, diaphoresis, dizziness, flushing, hyperthermia); neuromuscular changes (eg, tremor, rigidity, myoclonus, hyperreflexia, incoordination); gastrointestinal symptoms (eg, nausea, vomiting, diarrhea); and/or seizures. If serotonin syndrome occurs, discontinue 5-HT_3 receptor antagonist treatment and begin supportive management.

Although other selective 5-HT_3 receptor antagonists have been associated with dose-dependent increases in ECG intervals (eg, PR, QRS duration, QT/QTc, JT), palonosetron has not been shown to significantly affect the QT/QTc interval (Gonullu, 2012; Morganroth, 2008). Reduction in heart rate may occur with the 5-HT_3 antagonists, including palonosetron (Gonullu, 2012). Antiemetics are most effective when used prophylactically (Roila, 2010). Potentially significant drug-drug interactions may exist, requiring dose or frequency adjustment, additional monitoring, and/or selection of alternative therapy. If emesis occurs despite optimal antiemetic prophylaxis, re-evaluate emetic risk, disease, concurrent morbidities and medications to assure antiemetic regimen is optimized (Basch, 2011). For postoperative nausea and vomiting (PONV), may use for low expectation of PONV if it is essential to avoid nausea and vomiting in the postoperative period; use is not recommended if there is little expectation of nausea and vomiting.

Adverse Reactions Adverse events reported for adults unless otherwise noted.

Cardiovascular: Bradycardia (chemotherapy-associated), prolonged Q-T interval on ECG (more common in PONV), sinus bradycardia (PONV), tachycardia (may be nonsustained), hypotension

Central nervous system: Anxiety (chemotherapy-associated), dizziness (infants, children, adolescents, and adults), headache (chemotherapy-associated; more common in adults)

Dermatologic: Pruritus (PONV)

Endocrine & metabolic: Hyperkalemia (chemotherapy-associated)

Gastrointestinal: Constipation (chemotherapy-associated), diarrhea, flatulence

Genitourinary: Urinary retention

Hepatic: Increased serum ALT (may be transient), increased serum AST (may be transient)

Neuromuscular & skeletal: Weakness (chemotherapy-associated)

Rare but important or life-threatening: Amblyopia, anasarca, anemia, anorexia, arthralgia, chills, decreased appetite, decreased blood pressure, decreased gastrointestinal motility, decreased platelet count, dermatological disease (infants, children, and adolescents), distended vein, drowsiness, dyskinesia (infants, children, and adolescents), dyspepsia, epistaxis, erythema, euphoria, extrasystoles, eye irritation, flattened T wave on ECG, flu-like symptoms, hiccups, hot flash, hyperglycemia, hypersensitivity (very rare), hypertension, hypokalemia, hypoventilation, increased bilirubin (transient), increased liver enzymes, infusion site pain (infants, children, and adolescents), injection site reaction (very rare; includes burning sensation at injection site, discomfort at injection site, induration at injection site, pain at injection site), insomnia, ischemic heart disease, limb pain, metabolic acidosis, motion sickness, paresthesia, serotonin syndrome, sialorrhea, sinus arrhythmia, sinus tachycardia, supraventricular extrasystole, tinnitus, vein discoloration, ventricular premature contractions

Drug Interactions

Metabolism/Transport Effects Substrate of CYP1A2 (minor), CYP2D6 (minor), CYP3A4 (minor); **Note:** Assignment of Major/Minor substrate status based on clinically relevant drug interaction potential

Avoid Concomitant Use

Avoid concomitant use of Palonosetron with any of the following: Apomorphine

Increased Effect/Toxicity

Palonosetron may increase the levels/effects of: Apomorphine; Serotonin Modulators

Decreased Effect

Palonosetron may decrease the levels/effects of: Tapentadol; TraMADol

Storage/Stability Store intact vials at 20°C to 25°C (68°F to 77°F); excursions permitted to 15°C to 30°C (59°F to 86°F). Do not freeze. Protect from light. Solutions of 5 mcg/mL and 30 mcg/mL in NS, D_5W, $D_5{}^1/_2NS$, and D_5LR injection are stable for 48 hours at room temperature and 14 days under refrigeration (Trissel, 2004a).

Mechanism of Action Selective 5-HT_3 receptor antagonist, blocking serotonin, both on vagal nerve terminals in the periphery and centrally in the chemoreceptor trigger zone

Pharmacokinetics (Adult data unless noted)

Distribution: V_{dss}:

Pediatric patients 1 month to 17 years: Mean range: 5.3 to 6.3 L/kg

Adults: 8.3 ± 2.5 L/kg

Protein binding: ~62%

Metabolism: ~50% metabolized via CYP enzymes (and likely other pathways) to relatively inactive metabolites (N-oxide-palonosetron and 6-S-hydroxy-palonosetron); CYP1A2, 2D6, and 3A4 contribute to its metabolism

Half-life:

Pediatric patients 1 month to 17 years: Median: 29.5 hours (range: 20 to 30 hours)

Adults: ~40 hours

Elimination: Urine (80%; 40% as unchanged drug)

Clearance:

Infants and children <2 years: 0.31 L/hour/kg

Children 2 to <12 years: Mean range: 0.19 to 0.23 L/hour/kg

Children ≥12 years, Adolescents, and Adults: 0.160 L/hour/kg

Dosing: Usual

Pediatric: **Note:** Dosing presented in both mcg and mg; use extra caution to verify correct units

Chemotherapy-induced nausea and vomiting; prevention: IV:

Manufacturer's labeling:

Infants, Children, and Adolescents <17 years: 20 **mcg**/kg as a single dose; maximum dose: 1500 **mcg**/dose (1.5 mg/dose); beginning ~30 minutes prior to the start of chemotherapy

Adolescents ≥17 years: 0.25 mg as a single dose administered ~30 minutes before chemotherapy

Alternate dosing: Fixed dosing: Limited data available: Children and Adolescents 2 to 15 years: 0.25 mg single dose beginning ~30 minutes prior to the start of chemotherapy; dosing based on a randomized comparison trial with ondansetron which evaluated 100 chemotherapy courses in each arm and showed a statistically significant reduction in emetic events on days 0 to 3 in the palonosetron group and clinically significant reduction in emetic events on days 4 to 7 (up to 6 emetic events in the ondansetron group vs none with palonosetron) (Sepúlveda-Vildósola, 2008)

Postoperative nausea and vomiting (PONV); prevention: IV:

Infants, Children, and Adolescents < 17 years: Limited data available; efficacy results variable: 1 **mcg**/kg as a single dose; maximum dose: 75 **mcg**/dose (0.075 mg/dose) immediately prior to anesthesia induction; dosing based on a double-blind randomized comparative trial with ondansetron which showed complete response in 78.2% of the palonsetron group and 82.7% of the ondansetron; however, palonsetron efficacy data did not meet noninferiority margin; safety analysis showed no unexpected adverse effects, similar data as adult patients.

Adolescents ≥17 years: Limited data available in 17 years of age: 0.075 mg immediately prior to anesthesia induction

Adult:

Chemotherapy-induced nausea and vomiting; prevention: IV: 0.25 mg as a single dose administered ~30 minutes prior to the start of chemotherapy

Postoperative nausea and vomiting; prevention (PONV): IV: 0.075 mg immediately prior to anesthesia induction

Dosing adjustment in renal impairment: Infants, Children, Adolescents, and Adults: No adjustment is necessary

Dosing adjustment in hepatic impairment: Infants, Children, Adolescents, and Adults: No adjustment is necessary

Preparation for Administration Parenteral: Prevention of chemotherapy-induced nausea and vomiting: May further dilute in NS, D_5W, $D_5{}^1/_2NS$, or $D_5{}^1/_2LR$ injection to 5 mcg/mL or 30 mcg/mL has been shown to be stable (Trissel 2004a)

Administration Parenteral: Flush IV line with NS prior to and following administration

Prevention of chemotherapy-induced nausea and vomiting:

Infants, Children, and Adolescents: May administer IV undiluted or further dilute (Trissel 2004a) and infuse over 15 minutes, beginning ~30 minutes prior to the start of chemotherapy

Adolescents ≥17 years and Adults: Administer IV undiluted, infuse over 30 seconds, beginning ~30 minutes prior to the start of chemotherapy

Prevention of postoperative nausea and vomiting: May administer IV undiluted and infuse over 10 seconds immediately prior to anesthesia induction

Monitoring Parameters Hypersensitivity reactions; emesis episodes; HR

Dosage Forms Excipient information presented when available (limited, particularly for generics); consult specific product labeling.

Solution, Intravenous:

Aloxi: 0.25 mg/5 mL (5 mL) [contains edetate disodium]

- **Palonosetron Hydrochloride** *see* Palonosetron *on page 1609*
- **2-PAM** *see* Pralidoxime *on page 1747*
- **Pamelor** *see* Nortriptyline *on page 1532*

Pamidronate (pa mi DROE nate)

Medication Safety Issues

Sound-alike/look-alike issues:

Aredia may be confused with Adriamycin

Pamidronate may be confused with papaverine

Related Information

Safe Handling of Hazardous Drugs *on page 2455*

Brand Names: Canada Aredia; Pamidronate Disodium; Pamidronate Disodium Omega; PMS-Pamidronate

Therapeutic Category Antidote, Hypercalcemia; Bisphosphonate Derivative

Generic Availability (US) Yes

Use Treatment of moderate or severe hypercalcemia associated with malignancy with or without bone metastases (in conjunction with adequate hydration); treatment of osteolytic bone lesions associated with multiple myeloma or metastatic breast cancer; treatment of moderate to severe Paget's disease of bone (All indications: FDA approved in adults); has also been used in the treatment of osteogenesis imperfecta and osteopenia in cerebral palsy patients

Pregnancy Risk Factor D

Pregnancy Considerations Adverse events were observed in animal reproduction studies. It is not known if bisphosphonates cross the placenta, but fetal exposure is expected (Djokanovic, 2008; Stathopoulos, 2011). Bisphosphonates are incorporated into the bone matrix and gradually released over time. The amount available in the systemic circulation varies by dose and duration of therapy. Theoretically, there may be a risk of fetal harm when pregnancy follows the completion of therapy; however, available data have not shown that exposure to bisphosphonates during pregnancy significantly increases the risk of adverse fetal events (Djokanovic, 2008; Levy, 2009; Stathopoulos, 2011). Until additional data is available, most sources recommend discontinuing bisphosphonate therapy in women of reproductive potential as early as possible prior to a planned pregnancy; use in premenopausal women should be reserved for special circumstances when rapid bone loss is occurring (Bhalla, 2010; Pereira, 2012; Stathopoulos, 2011). Because hypocalcemia has been described following *in utero* bisphosphonate exposure, exposed infants should be monitored for hypocalcemia after birth (Djokanovic, 2008; Stathopoulos, 2011).

Breast-Feeding Considerations It is not known if pamidronate is excreted in breast milk. Pamidronate was not detected in the milk of a nursing woman receiving pamidronate 30 mg IV monthly (therapy started ~6 months postpartum). Following the first infusion, milk was pumped and collected for 0-24 hours and 25-48 hours, and each day pooled for analysis. Pamidronate readings were below the limit of quantification (<0.4 micromole/L). During therapy, breast milk was pumped and discarded for the first 48 hours following each infusion prior to resuming nursing. The infant was breast-fed >80% of the time; adverse events were not observed in the nursing infant (Simonoski, 2000). Monitoring the serum calcium concentrations of nursing infants is recommended (Stathopoulos, 2011). Due to the potential for serious adverse reactions in the nursing infant, the manufacturer recommends a decision be made whether to discontinue nursing or to discontinue the drug, taking into account the importance of treatment to the mother.

Contraindications Hypersensitivity to pamidronate, other bisphosphonates, or any component of the formulation

Warnings/Precautions Hazardous agent - use appropriate precautions for handling and disposal (meets NIOSH 2014 criteria). Osteonecrosis of the jaw (ONJ) has been reported in patients receiving bisphosphonates. Risk factors include invasive dental procedures (eg, tooth extraction, dental implants, boney surgery); a diagnosis of cancer, with concomitant chemotherapy, radiotherapy, or corticosteroids; poor oral hygiene, ill-fitting dentures; and comorbid disorders (anemia, coagulopathy, infection, preexisting dental disease). Most reported cases occurred after IV bisphosphonate therapy; however, cases have been reported following oral therapy. A dental exam and preventive dentistry should be performed prior to placing patients with risk factors on chronic bisphosphonate therapy. There is no evidence that discontinuing therapy reduces the risk of developing ONJ (Assael, 2009). The benefit/risk must be assessed by the treating physician and/or dentist/surgeon prior to any invasive dental procedure. Patients developing ONJ while on bisphosphonates should receive care by an oral surgeon.

Atypical femur fractures (after minimal or no trauma) have been reported. The fractures include subtrochanteric femur (bone just below the hip joint) and diaphyseal femur (long segment of the thigh bone). Some patients experience prodromal pain weeks or months before the fracture occurs. It is unclear if bisphosphonate therapy is the cause for these fractures. Patients receiving long-term (>3 to 5 years) bisphosphonate therapy may be at an increased risk. Consider discontinuing pamidronate in patients with a suspected femoral shaft fracture. Patients who present with thigh or groin pain in the absence of trauma should be evaluated. Infrequently, severe (and occasionally debilitating) musculoskeletal (bone, joint, and/or muscle) pain have been reported during bisphosphonate treatment. The onset of pain ranged from a single day to several months. Consider discontinuing therapy in patients who experience severe symptoms; symptoms usually resolve upon discontinuation. Some patients experienced recurrence when rechallenged with same drug or another bisphosphonate; avoid use in patients with a history of these symptoms in association with bisphosphonate therapy.

Initial or single doses have been associated with renal deterioration, progressing to renal failure and dialysis. Withhold pamidronate treatment (until renal function returns to baseline) in patients with evidence of renal deterioration. Glomerulosclerosis (focal segmental) with or without nephrotic syndrome has also been reported. Longer infusion times (>2 hours) may reduce the risk for renal toxicity, especially in patients with preexisting renal insufficiency. Single pamidronate doses should not exceed 90 mg. Patients with serum creatinine >3 mg/dL were not studied in clinical trials; limited data are available in patients with CrCl <30 mL/minute. Evaluate serum creatinine prior to each treatment. For the treatment of bone metastases, use is not recommended in patients with severe renal impairment; for renal impairment in indications other than bone metastases, use clinical judgment to determine if benefits outweigh potential risks.

Use has been associated with asymptomatic electrolyte abnormalities (including hypophosphatemia, hypokalemia, hypomagnesemia, and hypocalcemia). Rare cases of symptomatic hypocalcemia, including tetany have been reported. Patients with a history of thyroid surgery may have relative hypoparathyroidism; predisposing them to pamidronate-related hypocalcemia. Patients with preexisting anemia, leukopenia, or thrombocytopenia should be closely monitored during the first 2 weeks of treatment.

Hypercalcemia of malignancy (HCM): Adequate hydration is required during treatment (urine output ~2 L/day); avoid overhydration, especially in patients with heart failure.

Multiple myeloma: Patients with Bence-Jones proteinuria and dehydration should be adequately hydrated prior to therapy. The American Society of Clinical Oncology (ASCO) has also published guidelines on bisphosphonates use for prevention and treatment of bone disease in multiple myeloma (Kyle, 2007). Bisphosphonate (pamidronate or zoledronic acid) use is recommended in multiple myeloma patients with lytic bone destruction or compression spine fracture from osteopenia. Bisphosphonates may also be considered in patients with pain secondary to osteolytic disease, adjunct therapy to stabilize fractures or impending fractures, and for multiple myeloma patients with osteopenia but no radiographic evidence of lytic bone disease. Bisphosphonates are not recommended in patients with solitary plasmacytoma, smoldering (asymptomatic) or indolent myeloma, or monoclonal gammopathy of undetermined significance. The guidelines recommend monthly treatment for a period of 2 years. At that time, consider discontinuing in responsive and stable patients, and reinitiate if a new-onset skeletal-related event occurs. The ASCO guidelines are in alignment with the prescribing information for dosing, renal dose adjustments, infusion times, prevention and management of osteonecrosis of the jaw, and monitoring of laboratory parameter recommendations. According to the guidelines, in patients with extensive bone disease with existing severe renal disease (a serum creatinine >3 mg/dL or CrCl <30 mL/minute) pamidronate at a dose of 90 mg over 4 to 6 hours should be used (unless preexisting renal disease in which case a reduced initial dose should be considered). Monitor for albuminuria every 3 to 6 months; in patients with unexplained albuminuria >500 mg/24 hours, withhold the dose until level returns to baseline, then recheck every 3 to 4 weeks. Pamidronate may be reinitiated at a dose not to exceed 90 mg every 4 weeks with a longer infusion time of at least 4 hours.

Breast cancer (metastatic): The American Society of Clinical Oncology (ASCO) updated guidelines on the role of bone-modifying agents (BMAs) in the prevention and treatment of skeletal-related events for metastatic breast cancer patients (Van Poznak, 2011). The guidelines recommend initiating a BMA (denosumab, pamidronate, zoledronic acid) in patients with metastatic breast cancer to the bone. There is currently no literature indicating the superiority of one particular BMA. Optimal duration is not yet defined; however, the guidelines recommend continuing therapy until substantial decline in patient's performance status. The ASCO guidelines are in alignment with prescribing information for dosing, renal dose adjustments, infusion times, prevention and management of osteonecrosis of the jaw, and monitoring of laboratory parameter recommendations. BMAs are not the first-line therapy for pain. BMAs are to be used as adjunctive therapy for cancer-related bone pain associated with bone metastasis, demonstrating a modest pain control benefit. BMAs should be used in conjunction with agents such as NSAIDS, opioid and nonopioid analgesics, corticosteroids, radiation/surgery, and interventional procedures.

Warnings: Additional Pediatric Considerations Maintain adequate hydration with therapy (pediatric patients: 2 to 3 L/m^2 [Kerdudo, 2005]) and urinary output during treatment; use with caution with other potentially nephrotoxic drugs.

Bisphosphonate therapy may not be appropriate for patients with mild osteogenesis imperfect; risk:benefit has not been established. Potential adverse effects in growing children include infusion reactions and effects on bone growth. Influenza-like reactions are common after the first dose occurring at 12 to 36 hours after the infusion and may include fever, rash, and vomiting; treatment with standard antipyretic therapy is usually adequate and symptoms do not generally recur after later doses. Increased height has been reported and theoretical effects of diminishing bone remodeling in a growing child may result in bone malformation or delayed recovery after fractures (Rauch, 2004).

Adverse Reactions

Cardiovascular: Atrial fibrillation, atrial flutter, cardiac failure, edema, hypertension, syncope, tachycardia

Central nervous system: Drowsiness, fatigue, headache, insomnia, psychosis, seizure

Endocrine & metabolic: Hypocalcemia, hypokalemia, hypomagnesemia, hypophosphatemia, hypothyroidism

Gastrointestinal: Abdominal pain, anorexia, constipation, diarrhea, dyspepsia, gastrointestinal hemorrhage, nausea, stomatitis, vomiting

Genitourinary: Uremia, urinary tract infection

Hematologic & oncologic: Anemia, granulocytopenia, leukopenia, metastases, neutropenia, thrombocytopenia

Infection: Candidiasis

Local: Infusion site reaction (includes induration, pain, redness, and swelling)

Neuromuscular & skeletal: Arthralgia, back pain, myalgia, ostealgia, osteonecrosis of the jaw, weakness

Renal: Increased serum creatinine

Respiratory: Cough, dyspnea, pleural effusion, rales, rhinitis, sinusitis, upper respiratory tract infection

Miscellaneous: Fever

Rare but important or life-threatening: Acute renal failure, anaphylactic shock, angioedema, cardiac failure, confusion, episcleritis, focal segmental glomerulosclerosis (including collapsing variant), hallucination (visual), hematuria, herpes virus infection (reactivation), hyperkalemia, hypernatremia, hypersensitivity reaction, hypervolemia, hypotension, inflammation at injection site, injection site phlebitis, iridocyclitis, iritis, left heart failure, lymphocytopenia, nephrotic syndrome, osteonecrosis (other than jaw), renal failure, renal insufficiency, scleritis, uveitis, xanthopsia

Drug Interactions

Metabolism/Transport Effects None known.

Avoid Concomitant Use There are no known interactions where it is recommended to avoid concomitant use.

Increased Effect/Toxicity

Pamidronate may increase the levels/effects of: Deferasirox

The levels/effects of Pamidronate may be increased by: Aminoglycosides; Nonsteroidal Anti-Inflammatory Agents; Systemic Angiogenesis Inhibitors; Thalidomide

Decreased Effect

The levels/effects of Pamidronate may be decreased by: Proton Pump Inhibitors

Storage/Stability

Powder for reconstitution: Store at 20°C to 25°C (68°F to 77°F). The reconstituted solution is stable for 24 hours stored under refrigeration at 2°C to 8°C (36°F to 46°F). The diluted solution for infusion is stable at room temperature for up to 24 hours.

Solution for injection: Store at 20°C to 25°C (68°F to 77°F). The diluted solution for infusion is stable at room temperature for up to 24 hours.

Mechanism of Action Nitrogen-containing bisphosphonate; inhibits bone resorption and decreases mineralization by disrupting osteoclast activity (Gralow, 2009; Rogers, 2011)

Pharmacodynamics

Onset of action:

Hypercalcemia of malignancy: Reduction of albumin-corrected serum calcium: Children: ~48 hours (Kerdudo, 2005); Adults: ≤24 hours

Paget's disease: ~1 month for ≥50% decrease in serum alkaline phosphatase

Maximum effect: Hypercalcemia of malignancy: ≤7 days

Duration: Hypercalcemia of malignancy: 7-14 days; Paget's disease: 1-372 days

Pharmacokinetics (Adult data unless noted)

Absorption: Poorly from the GI tract

Metabolism: Not metabolized

Half-life, elimination: 28 ± 7 hours

Elimination: Biphasic: Urine (30% to 62% as unchanged drug; lower in patients with renal dysfunction) within 120 hours

Dosing: Neonatal Osteogenesis imperfecta: Limited data available: Full-term neonates, PNA ≥14 days: IV: Initial: 0.25 mg/kg once on day 1, then 0.5 mg/kg/dose daily days 2 and 3 of the first cycle, then 0.5 mg/kg/dose once daily for 3 days for subsequent cycles; cycles are repeated every 2 months for a total yearly dose of 9 mg/kg (Rauch 2003; Zietlin 2003)

Dosing: Usual Note: Due to increased risk of nephrotoxicity, single doses should not exceed 90 mg.

Pediatric:

Hypercalcemia: Limited data available: Children and Adolescents: Dosing based on several case reports and retrospective studies for treatment of hypercalcemia due to malignancy and/or immobility. Administer as a single infusion. Retreatment may be necessary if serum calcium does not return to normal or does not remain normal after initial treatment; reported interval for multiple doses is ≥24 hours.

Initial treatment: IV: 0.5 to 1 mg/kg; maximum dose: 90 mg (Kerdudo 2005; Kutluk 1999; Lteif 1998; Young 1998)

Severe, life-threatening: IV: 1.5 to 2 mg/kg; maximum dose: 90 mg; in one case report, a higher dose of 4 mg/kg was used to treat a serum calcium concentration of 18.9 mg/dL associated with bone metastases in a 4-year old child with non-Hodgkin lymphoma (Kerdudo 2005; Kutluk 1997; Kutluk 1999)

Osteogenesis imperfecta: Limited data available: **Note:** Reported dosing regimens variable (ie, weight-directed vs BSA-directed); duration of treatment has not been established; however, the most benefit has been shown to occur in the first 2 to 4 years of treatment (Rauch 2006).

Weight-directed dosing (Rauch 2003; Zietlin 2003):

Infants and Children <2 years: IV: Initial: 0.25 mg/kg once on day 1, then 0.5 mg/kg/dose daily days 2 and 3 of the first cycle, then 0.5 mg/kg/dose once daily for 3 days for subsequent cycles; cycles are repeated every 2 months for a total yearly dose of 9 mg/kg

Children 2 to 3 years: IV: Initial: 0.38 mg/kg once on day 1, then 0.75 mg/kg/dose daily days 2 and 3 of the first cycle, then 0.75 mg/kg/dose once daily for 3 days for subsequent cycles; cycles are repeated every 3 months for a total yearly dose of 9 mg/kg

Children >3 years and Adolescents: IV: Initial: 0.5 mg/kg once on day 1, then 1 mg/kg/dose daily days 2 and 3 of the first cycle, then 1 mg/kg/dose once daily for 3 days for subsequent cycles; cycles are repeated every 4 months for a total yearly dose of 9 mg/kg

BSA-directed dosing: Infants, Children, and Adolescents: IV: Initial: 10 mg/**m²**/dose once a month for 3 months, then increase to 20 mg/**m²**/dose once a month for 3 months, then increase to 30 mg/**m²**/dose once a month for subsequent doses; maximum dose: 40 mg/**m²**/dose was used in six patients after 1-2 years due to skeletal pain and less bone mineral gain; improvements in mobility and vertebral height was noted in patients who received this regimen for 3 to 6 years (n=11, median age at initiation of therapy: 3.6 months, range: 3 to 13 months) (Astrom 2007); another study used the same dosing in 14 prepubescent patients with mild disease (Heino 2011)

Osteopenia associated with cerebral palsy (nonambulatory): Limited data available; dosing regimens variable: Children and Adolescents: IV: Initial: 1 mg/kg/dose daily for 3 days; administer every 3 to 4 months; minimum dose: 15 mg; maximum dose: 35 mg. Dosing based on two trials; the first included 14 pediatric patients (age range: 6 to 16 years, treatment group: n=7), and reported an increase in bone mineral density; therapy was used in combination with calcium and vitamin D supplementation (Henderson 2002). In the other trial (n=25, age range: 3 to 19 years), a decreased incidence of fractures was noted after 1 year of therapy (Bachrach 2010). A lower dose was used in a trial of 23 pediatric patients (age range: 4 to 17 years); the initial dose was 0.37 mg/kg on day 1, followed by 0.75 mg/kg on day 2, then 0.75 mg/kg/dose once daily for 2 days was used for subsequent cycles; cycles were repeated every 4 months for 1 year; maximum single dose: 45 mg (Plotkin 2006).

Adult:

Hypercalcemia of malignancy: IV:

Moderate cancer-related hypercalcemia (corrected serum calcium 12 to 13.5 mg/dL): 60-90 mg as a single dose over 2 to 24 hours

Severe cancer-related hypercalcemia (corrected serum calcium >13.5 mg/dL): 90 mg as a single dose over 2 to 24 hours

Retreatment in patients who show an initial complete or partial response (allow at least 7 days to elapse prior to retreatment): May retreat at the same dose if serum calcium does not return to normal or does not remain normal after initial treatment

Multiple myeloma, osteolytic bone lesions: IV: 90 mg over 4 hours once monthly

Breast cancer, osteolytic bone metastases: IV: 90 mg over 2 hours every 3 to 4 weeks

Paget's disease, moderate to severe: IV: 30 mg over 4 hours daily for 3 consecutive days (total dose = 90 mg); may retreat at initial dose if clinically indicated

Dosing adjustment in renal impairment: Adults:

Baseline: Patients with serum creatinine >3 mg/dL were excluded from clinical trials; there are only limited pharmacokinetic data in patients with CrCl <30 mL/minute

Manufacturer's recommendations:

Treatment of bone metastases: Use is not recommended in patients with severe renal impairment.

Renal impairment in indications other than bone metastases: Use clinical judgment to determine if benefit outweighs risks.

The following recommendations have been used by some clinicians:

Multiple myeloma: American Society of Clinical Oncology (ASCO) guidelines (Kyle 2007):

Severe renal impairment (serum creatinine >3 mg/dL **or** CrCl <30 mL/minute) and extensive bone disease: 90 mg over 4 to 6 hours; however, a reduced initial dose should be considered if renal impairment was preexisting.

Albuminuria >500 mg/24 hours (unexplained): Withhold dose until returns to baseline, then recheck every 3 to 4 weeks; consider reinitiating at a dose not to exceed 90 mg every 4 weeks and with a longer infusion time of at least 4 hours

During therapy: In patients with bone metastases, treatment should be withheld for deterioration in renal function (increase of serum creatinine ≥0.5 mg/dL in patients with normal baseline or ≥1 mg/dL in patients with abnormal baseline). Resumption of therapy may be considered when serum creatinine returns to within 10% of baseline.

Dosing adjustment in hepatic impairment: Adults:

Mild to moderate impairment (Child-Pugh class A or B): No adjustment recommended.

Severe hepatic impairment (Child-Pugh class C): There are no dosage adjustments provided in manufacturer's labeling; not studied.

Preparation for Administration Hazardous agent; use appropriate precautions for handling and disposal (meets NIOSH, 2014 criteria).

Powder for injection: Reconstitute by adding 10 mL of SWFI to each vial of lyophilized powder, the resulting solution will be 30 mg/10 mL or 90 mg/10 mL; further dilute solution for injection or reconstituted solution with D_5W, $^1/_2$NS, or NS to a final concentration of 0.06 to 0.36 mg/mL; final concentration is determined by dose and condition being treated; refer to manufacturer's labeling for specific information for adult patients. In pediatric osteogenesis imperfecta trials, for neonates, infants and children <3 years, the dose was diluted in NS to a final concentration of ≤0.1 mg/mL; in children ≥3 years and adolescents, doses were added to 250 mL or 500 mL of NS (final concentration not specified) (Glorieaux 1998; Plotkin 2000).

Administration Hazardous agent; use appropriate precautions for handling and disposal (meets NIOSH, 2014 criteria).

Infusion rate varies by indication; longer infusion times (>2 hours) may reduce the risk for renal toxicity, especially in patients with preexisting renal insufficiency. In adults, the manufacturer recommends infusing over 2 to 24 hours for hypercalcemia of malignancy, over 2 hours for osteolytic bone lesions with metastatic breast cancer, and over 4 hours for Paget's disease and for osteolytic bone lesions with multiple myeloma. In pediatric trials, infusion times were 4 hours for osteogenesis imperfecta, 3 to 4 hours for osteopenia from immobility, and 4 to 6 hours for hypercalcemia; a 24-hour infusion has also been used (Henderson 2002; Kerdudo 2005; Kutluk 1997; Lteif 1998; Rauch 2003; Young 1998).

Monitoring Parameters Monitor serum creatinine prior to each dose; monitor serum calcium, phosphate, potassium, and magnesium; monitor for hypocalcemia for at least 2 weeks after therapy; patients with pre-existing anemia, leukopenia, or thrombocytopenia should have hemoglobin, hematocrit, and CBC with differential monitored closely, particularly in the first 2 weeks following treatment; dental exam and preventative dentistry prior to therapy for patients at risk for osteonecrosis

Additional indication-specific monitoring:

Multiple myeloma: Urine albumin every 3-6 months

Osteogenesis imperfecta: In pediatric trials, motor milestones, ambulation assessment, total body length, sitting height, and arm span were recorded every 6 months. Bone density was measured every 6 months. Conventional x-rays were obtained once yearly (Heino, 2011). Urinary excretion of calcium, alkaline phosphatase, and other bone-related chemistries were also monitored.

Osteopenia associated with cerebral palsy: In pediatric trials, bone mineral density, number and location of fractures, conventional x-rays, serum vitamin D concentrations, alkaline phosphatase, and other bone related chemistries were monitored (Bachrach, 2010; Henderson, 2002; Plotkin, 2006)

Paget's disease: Monitor serum alkaline phosphatase and urinary hydroxyproline excretion

Test Interactions Bisphosphonates may interfere with diagnostic imaging agents such as technetium-99m-diphosphonate in bone scans.

Dosage Forms Excipient information presented when available (limited, particularly for generics); consult specific product labeling.

Solution, Intravenous, as disodium:

Generic: 30 mg/10 mL (10 mL); 90 mg/10 mL (10 mL)

Solution, Intravenous, as disodium [preservative free]:

Generic: 30 mg/10 mL (10 mL); 6 mg/mL (10 mL); 90 mg/10 mL (10 mL)

Solution Reconstituted, Intravenous, as disodium:

Generic: 30 mg (1 ea); 90 mg (1 ea)

◆ **Pamidronate Disodium** *see* Pamidronate *on page 1611*

◆ **Pamidronate Disodium Omega (Can)** *see* Pamidronate *on page 1611*

◆ **Pamix [OTC]** *see* Pyrantel Pamoate *on page 1806*

◆ **Pamprin Ibuprofen Formula (Can)** *see* Ibuprofen *on page 1064*

◆ **Pancrease MT (Can)** *see* Pancrelipase *on page 1614*

◆ **Pancreatic Enzymes** *see* Pancrelipase *on page 1614*

◆ **Pancreaze** *see* Pancrelipase *on page 1614*

Pancrelipase (pan kre LYE pase)

Medication Safety Issues

Sound-alike/look-alike issues:

Pancrelipase may be confused with pancreatin

Related Information

Oral Medications That Should Not Be Crushed or Altered *on page 2476*

Brand Names: US Creon; Pancreaze; Pancrelipase (Lip-Prot-Amyl); Pertzye; Ultresa; Viokace; Zenpep

Brand Names: Canada Cotazym; Creon; Pancrease MT; Ultrase; Ultrase MT; Viokase

Therapeutic Category Enzyme, Pancreatic; Pancreatic Enzyme

Generic Availability (US) No

Use

Creon: Treatment of exocrine pancreatic insufficiency due to cystic fibrosis, chronic pancreatitis, pancreatectomy, or other conditions (FDA approved in infants, children, adolescents, and adults)

Pancrelipase, Pancreaze, Zenpep: Treatment of exocrine pancreatic insufficiency due to cystic fibrosis or other conditions (FDA approved in infants, children, adolescents, and adults)

Pertzye: Treatment of exocrine pancreatic insufficiency due to cystic fibrosis or other conditions (FDA approved in ages >12 months and weighing ≥8 kg and adults)

Ultresa: Treatment of exocrine pancreatic insufficiency due to cystic fibrosis or other conditions (FDA approved in ages >12 months and weighing ≥14 kg and adults)

Viokace: Treatment of exocrine pancreatic insufficiency due to chronic pancreatitis or pancreatectomy in combination with a proton pump inhibitor (FDA approved in adults)

Medication Guide Available Yes

Pregnancy Risk Factor C

Pregnancy Considerations Animal reproduction studies have not been conducted. Nutrition should be optimized in pregnancy; in cystic fibrosis patients with malabsorption, pancreatic enzyme replacement is not considered to cause a risk to the pregnancy.

Breast-Feeding Considerations It is not known if pancrelipase is excreted in breast milk. The manufacturer recommends that caution be exercised when administering pancrelipase to nursing women.

Contraindications There are no contraindications listed in the manufacturer's labeling.

Warnings/Precautions Hypersensitivity reactions (eg anaphylaxis, asthma, hives, pruritus) have rarely been observed. Use with caution in patients hypersensitive to pork proteins, taking into consideration the patient's overall clinical needs. Fibrosing colonopathy advancing to colonic strictures have been reported (rarely) with doses of lipase >6,000 units/kg/meal usually over long periods of time and most commonly in children <12 years of age. Patients taking doses of lipase >6,000 units/kg/meal should be examined and the dose decreased. Doses of lipase >2,500 units/kg/meal, lipase >10,000 units/kg/day, or lipase >4,000 units/g fat daily should be used with caution and only with documentation of 3-day fecal fat measures. Crushing or chewing the contents of the capsules or tablets, or mixing the capsule contents with foods outside of product labeling, may cause early release of the enzymes, causing irritation of the oral mucosa and/or loss of enzyme activity. Pancrelipase should not be mixed in foods with pH >4.5. When mixing the contents of capsules with food, the mixture should be swallowed immediately and followed with water or juice to ensure complete ingestion. Use caution in patients with gout, hyperuricemia, or renal impairment; porcine-derived products contain purines which may increase uric acid concentrations. Use Viokace tablets with caution in patients with lactose intolerance; tablets contain lactose. Products are derived from porcine pancreatic glands. Transmission of porcine viruses is theoretically a risk; however, testing and/or inactivation or removal of certain viruses, reduces the risk. There have been no cases of transmission of an infectious illness reported. Available brand products are **not** interchangeable.

Adverse Reactions The following adverse reactions were reported in a short-term safety studies; actual frequency varies with different products; adverse events, particularly gastrointestinal events, were often greater with placebo:

Cardiovascular: Peripheral edema

Central nervous system: Dizziness, headache

Dermatologic: Rash

Endocrine & metabolic: Diabetes mellitus exacerbation, hyper-/hypoglycemia

Gastrointestinal: Abdominal pain, anal itching, biliary tract stones, diarrhea, dyspepsia, early satiety, feces abnormal, flatulence, upper abdominal pain, vomiting, weight loss

Hematologic: Anemia

Hepatic: Ascites, hydrocholecystis

Neuromuscular & skeletal: Neck pain

Otic: Ear pain

Renal: Renal cyst

Respiratory: Beta-hemolytic streptococcal infection, cough, epistaxis, nasopharyngitis, pharyngolaryngeal pain

Miscellaneous: Lymphadenopathy, viral infection

Rare but important or life-threatening (reported with various formulations of pancrelipase): Allergic reactions (severe), anaphylaxis, asthma, carcinoma recurrence, constipation, distal intestinal obstruction syndrome (DIOS), duodenitis, fibrosing colonopathy, gastritis, hives, hyperuricemia, muscle spasm, myalgia, nausea, neutropenia (transient), pruritus, transaminases increased (asymptomatic), urticaria, vision blurred

Drug Interactions

Metabolism/Transport Effects None known.

Avoid Concomitant Use There are no known interactions where it is recommended to avoid concomitant use.

Increased Effect/Toxicity There are no known significant interactions involving an increase in effect.

Decreased Effect

Pancrelipase may decrease the levels/effects of: Iron Salts; Multivitamins/Minerals (with ADEK, Folate, Iron)

Food Interactions Delayed release capsules: Enteric coated contents of delayed release capsules opened and sprinkled on alkaline foods may result in early release of pancrelipase followed by enzyme inactivation by gastric acid in the stomach after swallowing. Management: Avoid placing contents of opened capsules on alkaline food (using soft acidic foods with a pH of ≤4.5 is recommended for patients who cannot swallow capsules).

Storage/Stability

Avoid heat. Protect from moisture. After opening, keep the container tightly closed between uses to protect from moisture.

Creon: Store at room temperature up to 25°C (77°F); excursions are permitted between 25°C and 40°C (77°F and 104°F) for ≤30 days. Discard if moisture conditions are >70%. Bottles of 3,000 USP units of lipase must be stored and dispensed in the original container.

Pancreaze: Store at ≤25°C (77°F). Store in the original container.

Pancrelipase: Store at 20°C to 25°C (68°F to 77°F); brief excursions are permitted between 15°C and 40°C (59°F and 104°F).

Pertzye: Store at 20°C to 25°C (68°F to 77°F); excursions are permitted between 15°C and 40°C (59°F and 104°F). Store in the original container.

Ultresa: Store at 20°C to 25°C (68°F to 77°F). Store in the original container.

Viokace: Store at 20°C to 25°C (68°F to 77°F); brief excursions are permitted up to 40°C (104°F) for up to 24 hours.

Zenpep:

Original glass container: Store at 20°C to 25°C (68°F to 77°F); excursions are permitted between 15°C and 40°C (59°F and 104°F).

Repackaged HDPE container: Store at ≤30°C (86°F) for up to 6 months; excursions are permitted between 15°C and 40°C (59°F and 104°F) for ≤30 days.

Mechanism of Action Pancrelipase is a natural product harvested from the porcine pancreatic glands. It contains a combination of lipase, amylase, and protease. Products are formulated to dissolve in the more basic pH of the duodenum so that they may act locally to break down fats, protein, and starch.

Pharmacokinetics (Adult data unless noted)

Absorption: Not significantly absorbed, acts locally in the GI tract

Elimination: In feces

Dosing: Neonatal Pancreatic insufficiency: Limited data available: Oral: Lipase 2000-5000 units per feeding of formula, breast milk, or per breast-feeding. Adjust dose based on clinical symptoms and stool fat content up to 2500 units/kg/feeding. Allow several days between dose adjustments. Maximum daily dose: Lipase 10,000 units/kg/**day** (Borowitz, 2009). **Note:** A review of data from the CF Foundation Patient Registry suggests that the maximum daily dose of lipase may be insufficient in young infants with CF; however, the optimal dose is not established (Borowitz, 2013).

Dosing: Usual Note: Adjust dose based on body weight, clinical symptoms, and stool fat content. Allow several days between dose adjustments. Total daily dose reflects ~3 meals/day and 2-3 snacks/day, with half the mealtime dose given with a snack. Doses of lipase >2500 units/kg/meal should be used with caution and only with documentation of 3-day fecal fat measures. Doses of lipase >6000 units/kg/meal are associated with colonic stricture and should be decreased.

Infants, Children, and Adolescents: **Pancreatic insufficiency:**

Oral:

Infants: Lipase 2000-5000 units per feeding of formula, breast milk, or per breast-feeding. Maximum daily dose: Lipase 10,000 units/kg/**day** up to 2500 units/kg/feeding (Borowitz, 2009). **Note:** A review of data from the CF Foundation Patient Registry suggests that the maximum daily dose may be insufficient in young infants with CF; however, the optimal dose is not established (Borowitz, 2013).

Children 1 to <2 years: Dosage requirements may fluctuate as diet transitions to more solid foods. Initial dose: Lipase 1000 units/kg/meal. Dosage range: Lipase 1000-2500 units/kg/meal. Maximum daily dose: Lipase 10,000 units/kg/**day** or lipase 4000 units/g of fat/day. Higher dosing similar to infant dosing (Lipase: 2000-5000 units per feeding of formula, breast milk, or per breast-feeding) may be necessary in some patients (Borowitz, 2009).

Children 2 to <4 years: Initial dose: Lipase 1000 units/kg/meal. Dosage range: Lipase 1000-2500 units/kg/meal. Maximum daily dose: Lipase 10,000 units/kg/**day** or lipase 4000 units/g of fat/day.

≥4 years: Initial dose: Lipase 500 units/kg/meal. Dosage range: Lipase 500-2500 units/kg/meal. Maximum daily dose: Lipase 10,000 units/kg/**day** or lipase 4000 units per g of fat/day.

Enteral tube feedings: Limited data available: **Note:** With low-fat or elemental enteral formulas, pancreatic enzyme supplementation may not be necessary (Ferrie, 2011).

Continuous enteral feeding: Lipase 1000 units/g of fat provided by the daily amount of feeds administered in divided doses every 2-3 hours (Ferrie, 2011)

Overnight enteral feeding: Administer premeal dose at beginning of feeding; additional dose may be given if midway through or at the end of a feeding (Borowitz, 2002). Some centers recommend using 1000 units/g of fat provided by the overnight feed administered in 2 divided doses with the first dose as 50% of requirement or enough to cover 3 hours of feeds and the additional dose given if patient awakens at night or at the end of a feeding (Ferrie, 2011).

Adults:

Pancreatic insufficiency due to conditions such as cystic fibrosis: Oral: Initial: Lipase 500 units/kg/meal. Dosage range: Lipase 500-2500 units/kg/meal. Maximum single dose: Lipase ≤2500 units/kg/**meal**; maximum daily dose: Lipase ≤10,000 units/kg/**day** or lipase <4000 units/g of fat daily

Pancreatic insufficiency due to chronic pancreatitis or pancreatectomy: Oral:

Creon: Lipase 72,000 units/meal while consuming ≥100 g of fat per day; alternatively, lower initial doses of lipase 500 units/kg/meal with individualized dosage titrations have also been used.

Viokace (administer in combination with a proton pump inhibitor): Initial: Lipase 500 units/kg/meal. Dosage range: Lipase 500-2500 units/kg/meal. Maximum single dose: Lipase ≤2500 units/kg/**meal**; maximum daily dose: Lipase ≤10,000 units/kg/**day** or lipase <4000 units/g of fat daily.

Administration Administer with meals or snacks and swallow capsules or tablets whole with a generous amount of liquid, water, or juice. Do not crush or chew; retention in the mouth before swallowing may cause mucosal irritation and stomatitis.

Oral:

Capsules: If necessary, capsules may also be opened and contents added to a small amount of an acidic food (pH ≤4.5), such as applesauce. The food should be at room temperature and swallowed immediately after mixing. The contents of the capsule should not be crushed or chewed. Follow with water or juice to ensure complete ingestion and that no medication remains in the mouth. Creon capsules contain enteric coated spheres which are 0.71-1.6 mm in diameter. Pancreaze capsules contain enteric coated microtablets which are ~2 mm in diameter. Zenpep capsules contain enteric coated beads which are 1.8-2.5 mm in diameter.

Infants <1 year: Avoid mixing with breast milk or infant formula. Open capsule and place the contents directly into the mouth or mix with a small amount of acidic soft food (pH ≤4.5) such as applesauce, or other commercially prepared baby food (pears or bananas) at room temperature. Administer immediately after mixing (or within 15 minutes of mixing using Pancreaze). Follow with infant formula or breast milk to ensure complete ingestion and that no medication remains in the mouth.

Tablets: Tablets are not enteric coated and should be taken with a proton pump inhibitor.

Gastrostomy tube (GT): Capsules: An *in vitro* study demonstrated that Creon delayed release capsules sprinkled on a small amount of baby food (pH<4.5; applesauce or bananas manufacturered by both Gerber and Beech-Nut) may be administered through the following G-tubes without significant loss of lipase activity: Kimberly-Clark MIC Bolus® size 18 Fr, Kimberly-Clark MIC-KEY size 16 Fr, Bard® Tri-Funnel size 18 Fr, and Bard® Button size 18 Fr (Shlieout, 2011). Some centers use sodium bicarbonate to dissolve the beads before administering into GT; may cause increase in serum bicarbonate, monitor closely (Ferrie, 2011; Nicolo, 2013).

Monitoring Parameters Stool fat content, abdominal symptoms, nutritional intake, weight, growth, stool character, serum bicarbonate if using bicarbonate for GT administration.

Additional Information Concomitant administration with an H_2-receptor antagonist or proton pump inhibitor has been used to decrease acid inactivation of enzyme activity; concomitant antacid administration may decrease effectiveness of enzymes.

Product Availability Ultresa (Lipase 4,000 USP units, protease 8,000 USP units, and amylase 8,000 USP units) capsules: FDA approved October 2014; availability anticipated in mid-2015. Consult prescribing information for additional information.

Dosage Forms Excipient information presented when available (limited, particularly for generics); consult specific product labeling.

Capsule, delayed release, bicarbonate buffered enteric coated microspheres, oral [porcine derived]:

Pertzye: Lipase 8,000 USP units, protease 28,750 USP units, and amylase 30,250 USP units

Pertzye: Lipase 16,000 USP units, protease 57,500 USP units, and amylase 60,500 USP units

Capsule, delayed release, enteric coated beads, oral [porcine derived]:

Pancrelipase (Lip-Prot-Amyl): Lipase 5000 USP units, protease 17,000 USP units, amylase 27,000 USP units

Zenpep: Lipase 3000 USP units, protease 10,000 USP units, and amylase 16,000 USP units

Zenpep: Lipase 5000 USP units, protease 17,000 USP units, and amylase 27,000 USP units
Zenpep: Lipase 10,000 USP units, protease 34,000 USP units, and amylase 55,000 USP units
Zenpep: Lipase 15,000 USP units, protease 51,000 USP units, and amylase 82,000 USP units
Zenpep: Lipase 20,000 USP units, protease 68,000 USP units, and amylase 109,000 USP units
Zenpep: Lipase 25,000 USP units, protease 85,000 USP units, and amylase 136,000 USP units
Zenpep: Lipase 40,000 USP units, protease 136,000 USP units, and amylase 218,000 USP units

Capsule, delayed release, enteric coated microspheres, oral [porcine derived]:
Creon: Lipase 3000 USP units, protease 9500 USP units, and amylase 15,000 USP units
Creon: Lipase 6000 USP units, protease 19,000 USP units, and amylase 30,000 USP units
Creon: Lipase 12,000 USP units, protease 38,000 USP units, and amylase 60,000 USP units
Creon: Lipase 24,000 USP units, protease 76,000 USP units, and amylase 120,000 USP units
Creon: Lipase 36,000 USP units, protease 114,000 USP units, and amylase 180,000 USP units

Capsule, delayed release, enteric coated microtablets, oral [porcine derived]:
Pancreaze: Lipase 4200 USP units, protease 10,000 USP units, and amylase 17,500 USP units
Pancreaze: Lipase 10,500 USP units, protease 25,000 USP units, and amylase 43,750 USP units
Pancreaze: Lipase 16,800 USP units, protease 40,000 USP units, and amylase 70,000 USP units
Pancreaze: Lipase 21,000 USP units, protease 37,000 USP units, and amylase 61,000 USP units

Capsule, delayed release, enteric coated minitablets, oral [porcine derived]:
Ultresa: Lipase 13,800 USP units, protease 27,600 USP units, and amylase 27,600 USP units
Ultresa: Lipase 20,700 USP units, protease 41,400 USP units, and amylase 41,400 USP units
Ultresa: Lipase 23,000 USP units, protease 46,000 USP units, and amylase 46,000 USP units

Tablet, oral [porcine derived]:
Viokace: Lipase 10,440 USP units, protease 39,150 USP units, and amylase 39,150 USP units
Viokace: Lipase 20,880 USP units, protease 78,300 USP units, and amylase 78,300 USP units

◆ **Pancrelipase (Lip-Prot-Amyl)** *see* Pancrelipase *on page 1614*

Pancuronium (pan kyoo ROE nee um)

Medication Safety Issues

High alert medication:

The Institute for Safe Medication Practices (ISMP) includes this medication among its list of drugs which have a heightened risk of causing significant patient harm when used in error.

Other safety concerns:

United States Pharmacopeia (USP) 2006: The Interdisciplinary Safe Medication Use Expert Committee of the USP has recommended the following:

- Hospitals, clinics, and other practice sites should institute special safeguards in the storage, labeling, and use of these agents and should include these safeguards in staff orientation and competency training.
- Healthcare professionals should be on high alert (especially vigilant) whenever a neuromuscular-blocking agent (NMBA) is stocked, ordered, prepared, or administered.

Brand Names: Canada Pancuronium Bromide®

Therapeutic Category Neuromuscular Blocker Agent, Nondepolarizing; Skeletal Muscle Relaxant, Paralytic

Generic Availability (US) Yes

Use Adjunct to anesthesia, to facilitate endotracheal intubation and provide skeletal muscle relaxation during surgery or mechanical ventilation (FDA approved in all ages)

Pregnancy Risk Factor C

Pregnancy Considerations Animal reproduction studies have not been conducted. Small amounts of pancuronium cross the placenta (Daily, 1984). May be used short-term in cesarean section; reduced doses recommended in patients also receiving magnesium sulfate due to enhanced effects.

Contraindications Hypersensitivity to pancuronium, bromide, or any component of the formulation

Warnings/Precautions Ventilation must be supported during neuromuscular blockade. Elimination half-life is doubled due to reduced clearance of pancuronium and recovery is prolonged; use with caution in patients with renal and/or hepatic impairment (adjust dose appropriately); certain clinical conditions may result in potentiation or antagonism of neuromuscular blockade:

Antagonism: Respiratory alkalosis, hypercalcemia, demyelinating lesions, peripheral neuropathies, denervation, and muscle trauma

Potentiation: Electrolyte abnormalities (eg, severe hypocalcemia, severe hypokalemia, hypermagnesemia), neuromuscular diseases, metabolic acidosis, metabolic alkalosis, respiratory acidosis, Eaton-Lambert syndrome and myasthenia gravis

Resistance may occur in burn patients (≥20% of total body surface area), usually several days after the injury, and may persist for several months after wound healing. Resistance may occur in patients who are immobilized. Cross-sensitivity with other neuromuscular-blocking agents may occur; use extreme caution in patients with previous anaphylactic reactions. Use caution in the elderly. **[US Boxed Warning]: Should be administered by adequately trained individuals familiar with its use.**

Benzyl alcohol and derivatives: Some dosage forms may contain benzyl alcohol; large amounts of benzyl alcohol (≥99 mg/kg/day) have been associated with a potentially fatal toxicity ("gasping syndrome") in neonates; the "gasping syndrome" consists of metabolic acidosis, respiratory distress, gasping respirations, CNS dysfunction (including convulsions, intracranial hemorrhage), hypotension, and cardiovascular collapse (AAP, 1997; CDC, 1982); some data suggests that benzoate displaces bilirubin from protein binding sites (Ahlfors, 2001); avoid or use dosage forms containing benzyl alcohol with caution in neonates. See manufacturer's labeling.

Adverse Reactions

Cardiovascular: Circulatory collapse, edema, elevated blood pressure and cardiac output, elevation in pulse rate, skin flushing, tachycardia

Dermatologic: Burning sensation along the vein, erythema, itching, rash

Gastrointestinal: Excessive salivation

Neuromuscular & skeletal: Profound muscle weakness

Respiratory: Bronchospasm, wheezing

Miscellaneous: Hypersensitivity reaction

Postmarketing and/or case reports: Acute quadriplegic myopathy syndrome (prolonged use), anaphylactoid reactions, anaphylaxis, myositis ossificans (prolonged use)

Drug Interactions

Metabolism/Transport Effects None known.

Avoid Concomitant Use

Avoid concomitant use of Pancuronium with any of the following: QuiNINE

Increased Effect/Toxicity

Pancuronium may increase the levels/effects of: Cardiac Glycosides; Corticosteroids (Systemic); OnabotulinumtoxinA; RimabotulinumtoxinB

The levels/effects of Pancuronium may be increased by: AbobotulinumtoxinA; Aminoglycosides; Calcium Channel Blockers; Capreomycin; Clindamycin (Topical); Colistimethate; CycloSPORINE (Systemic); Fosphenytoin-Phenytoin; Inhalational Anesthetics; Ketorolac (Nasal); Ketorolac (Systemic); Lincosamide Antibiotics; Lithium; Loop Diuretics; Magnesium Salts; Polymyxin B; Procainamide; QuiNIDine; QuiNINE; Spironolactone; Tetracycline Derivatives; Theophylline Derivatives; Vancomycin

Decreased Effect

The levels/effects of Pancuronium may be decreased by: Acetylcholinesterase Inhibitors; Fosphenytoin-Phenytoin; Loop Diuretics; Theophylline Derivatives

Storage/Stability Refrigerate; however, stable for up to 6 months at room temperature.

Mechanism of Action Blocks neural transmission at the myoneural junction by binding with cholinergic receptor sites

Pharmacodynamics

Onset of action (Martin, 1999):
- Infants: 2-5 minutes
- Children: 2-4 minutes
- Adults: 3-5 minutes

Duration: Dose-dependent
- Children: 24 minutes (Martin, 1999)
- Adults: 22 minutes (Martin, 1999)

Pharmacokinetics (Adult data unless noted)

Distribution: V_d: 0.24-0.28 L/kg

Protein binding: 87%

Metabolism: Hepatic: 30% to 40%; active metabolite 3-hydroxypancuronium (1/2 the activity of parent drug)

Half-life: 89-161 minutes

Elimination: Urine (40%); bile (11%)
- Clearance: ~1-2 mL/kg/minute

Dosing: Neonatal Paralysis/skeletal muscle relaxation: IV: 0.05-0.1 mg/kg/dose (Kumar, 2010); may repeat dose every 30-60 minutes as needed or as continuous IV infusion of 0.02-0.04 mg/kg/**hour** or 0.4-0.6 **mcg**/kg/minute

Dosing: Usual Paralysis/skeletal muscle relaxation: IV:

Infants: 0.1 mg/kg/dose every 30-60 minutes as needed or as continuous IV infusion of 0.02-0.04 mg/kg/**hour** or 0.4-0.6 **mcg**/kg/minute

Children: 0.15 mg/kg/dose every 30-60 minutes as needed or as continuous IV infusion 0.03-0.1 mg/kg/**hour** or 0.5-1.7 **mcg**/kg/minute

Adolescents and Adults: 0.15 mg/kg/dose every 30-60 minutes as needed or as a continuous IV infusion 0.02-0.04 mg/kg/**hour** or 0.4-0.6 **mcg**/kg/minute

Dosing adjustment in renal impairment:
- CrCl 10-50 mL/minute: Administer 50% of normal dose
- CrCl <10 mL/minute: Do not use

Preparation for Administration Parenteral: Continuous I.V. infusion: Dilute in D_5NS, D_5W, LR, or NS; final concentrations of 0.01 to 1 mg/mL have been used by some centers (Murray 2014; Sinclair-Pingel 2006). Product formulations may contain benzyl alcohol; in neonates, consider using the 2 mg/mL product for preparation to decrease amount of benzyl alcohol delivered.

Administration

Parenteral:
- IV push: Administer undiluted by rapid IV injection
- Continuous IV Infusion: Further dilute in an appropriate fluid and administer via an infusion pump

Monitoring Parameters Heart rate, blood pressure, assisted ventilation status, peripheral nerve stimulator measuring twitch response

Additional Information Patients with hepatic and biliar disease have a larger V_d which may result in a higher tota initial dose and possibly a slower onset of effect; th duration of neuromuscular blocking effects may be pro longed in patients with hepatic, biliary, or renal dysfunctio

Dosage Forms Excipient information presented whe available (limited, particularly for generics); consult specifi product labeling.

Solution, Intravenous, as bromide:
- Generic: 1 mg/mL (10 mL); 2 mg/mL (2 mL, 5 mL)

- ◆ **Pancuronium Bromide** *see* Pancuronium *on page 161*
- ◆ **Pancuronium Bromide® (Can)** *see* Pancuronium *on page 1617*
- ◆ **Pandel** *see* Hydrocortisone (Topical) *on page 1041*
- ◆ **Panglobulin** *see* Immune Globulin *on page 1089*
- ◆ **PanOxyl [OTC]** *see* Benzoyl Peroxide *on page 270*
- ◆ **PanOxyl® (Can)** *see* Benzoyl Peroxide *on page 270*
- ◆ **PanOxyl-4 Creamy Wash [OTC]** *see* Benzoyl Peroxide *on page 270*
- ◆ **PanOxyl-8 Creamy Wash [OTC]** *see* Benzoyl Peroxide *on page 270*
- ◆ **PanOxyl Wash [OTC]** *see* Benzoyl Peroxide *on page 270*
- ◆ **Panto I.V. (Can)** *see* Pantoprazole *on page 1618*
- ◆ **Pantoloc (Can)** *see* Pantoprazole *on page 1618*

Pantoprazole (pan TOE pra zole)

Medication Safety Issues

Sound-alike/look-alike issues:
- Pantoprazole may be confused with ARIPiprazole
- Protonix may be confused with Lotronex, Lovenox, prot amine

Administration issues:
- Vials containing Protonix IV for injection are not recom mended for use with spiked IV system adaptors. Nurse and pharmacists have reported breakage of the glas vials during attempts to connect spiked IV syster adaptors, which may potentially result in injury to health care professionals.

International issues:
- Protonix [US] may be confused with Pretanix brand nam for indapamide [Hungary]
- Protonix: Brand name for pantoprazole [US] but also th brand name for omeprazole [Phillipines]

Related Information

Oral Medications That Should Not Be Crushed or Altere *on page 2476*

Brand Names: US Protonix

Brand Names: Canada Abbott-Pantoprazole; ACT Pan toprazole; Apo-Pantoprazole; Ava-Pantoprazole; Dom Pantoprazole; JAMP-Pantoprazole; Mint-Pantoprazole Mylan-Pantoprazole; Panto I.V.; Pantoloc; Pantoprazol for Injection; Pantoprazole Sodium for Injection; PMS Pantoprazole; Q-Pantoprazole; RAN-Pantoprazole; ratio Pantoprazole; Riva-Pantoprazole; Sandoz-Pantoprazole Tecta; Teva-Pantoprazole

Therapeutic Category Gastric Acid Secretion Inhibitor Gastrointestinal Agent, Gastric or Duodenal Ulcer Treat ment; Proton Pump Inhibitor

Generic Availability (US) May be product dependent

Use

Oral: Short-term treatment (up to 8 weeks) of erosiv esophagitis associated with gastroesophageal reflux dis ease (GERD) (FDA approved in ages ≥5 years an adults); maintenance of healing of erosive esophagiti (FDA approved in adults); treatment of pathologica hypersecretory conditions, including Zollinger-Elliso syndrome (FDA approved in adults); has also been use as adjunctive therapy of duodenal ulcers associated with *Helicobacter pylori*

IV: Short-term treatment (7-10 days) of patients with GERD with a history of erosive esophagitis (FDA approved in adults); treatment of pathological hypersecretory conditions, including Zollinger-Ellison syndrome (FDA approved in adults); has also been used as an alternative to oral therapy in patients who are unable to continue taking oral pantoprazole

Medication Guide Available Yes

Pregnancy Risk Factor B

Pregnancy Considerations Adverse events have not been observed in animal reproduction studies. Most available studies have not shown an increased risk of major birth defects following maternal use of proton pump inhibitors during pregnancy (Diav-Citrin, 2005; Erichsen, 2012; Matok, 2012; Pasternak, 2010). When treating GERD in pregnancy, PPIs may be used when clinically indicated (Katz, 2013).

Breast-Feeding Considerations Pantoprazole is excreted in breast milk. The excretion of pantoprazole into breast milk was studied in a nursing woman, 10 months postpartum. Following a single dose of pantoprazole 40 mg, maternal milk and serum samples were obtained over 24 hours. Peak concentrations appeared in both the plasma and milk 2 hours after the dose. Pantoprazole concentrations in breast milk were below the limits of detection during most of the study period. Based on this single dose study, the authors calculated the expected exposure to a nursing infant to be 0.14% of the weight-adjusted maternal dose (Plante, 2004). Due to the potential for serious adverse reactions in the nursing infant, the manufacturer recommends a decision be made whether to discontinue nursing or to discontinue the drug, taking into account the importance of treatment to the mother; however, the acidic content of the nursing infants' stomach may potentially inactivate any ingested pantoprazole (Plante, 2004).

Contraindications Hypersensitivity (eg, anaphylaxis, anaphylactic shock, angioedema, bronchospasm, acute interstitial nephritis, urticaria) to pantoprazole, other substituted benzimidazole proton pump inhibitors, or any component of the formulation

Warnings/Precautions Use of proton pump inhibitors (PPIs) may increase the risk of gastrointestinal infections (eg, *Salmonella, Campylobacter*). Relief of symptoms does not preclude the presence of a gastric malignancy. Long-term pantoprazole therapy (especially in patients who were *H. pylori* positive) has caused biopsy-proven atrophic gastritis. Benign and malignant neoplasia has been observed in long-term rodent studies; while not reported in humans, the relevance of these findings in regards to tumorigenicity in humans is not known. Use of PPIs may increase risk of *Clostridium difficile*-associated diarrhea (CDAD), especially in hospitalized patients; consider CDAD diagnosis in patients with persistent diarrhea that does not improve. Use the lowest dose and shortest duration of PPI therapy appropriate for the condition being treated. Prolonged treatment (≥2 years) may lead to vitamin B_{12} malabsorption and subsequent vitamin B_{12} deficiency. The magnitude of the deficiency is dose-related and the association is stronger in females and those younger in age (<30 years); prevalence is decreased after discontinuation of therapy (Lam, 2013).

Intravenous preparation contains edetate sodium (EDTA); use caution in patients who are at risk for zinc deficiency if other EDTA-containing solutions are coadministered. Some dosage forms may contain polysorbate 80 (also known as Tweens). Hypersensitivity reactions, usually a delayed reaction, have been reported following exposure to pharmaceutical products containing polysorbate 80 in certain individuals (Isaksson, 2002; Lucente 2000; Shelley, 1995). Thrombocytopenia, ascites, pulmonary deterioration, and renal and hepatic failure have been reported in premature neonates after receiving parenteral products containing polysorbate 80 (Alade, 1986; CDC, 1984). See manufacturer's labeling. Decreased *H. pylori* eradication rates have been observed with short-term (≤7 days) combination therapy. The American College of Gastroenterology recommends 10-14 days of therapy (triple or quadruple) for eradication of *H. pylori* (Chey, 2007).

PPIs may diminish the therapeutic effect of clopidogrel, thought to be due to reduced formation of the active metabolite of clopidogrel. The manufacturer of clopidogrel recommends either avoidance of both omeprazole (even when scheduled 12 hours apart) and esomeprazole or use of a PPI with comparatively less effect on the active metabolite of clopidogrel. Of the PPIs, pantoprazole has the lowest degree of CYP2C19 inhibition *in vitro* (Li, 2004) and has been shown to have less effect on conversion of clopidogrel to its active metabolite compared to omeprazole (Angiolillo, 2011). In contrast to these warnings, others have recommended the continued use of PPIs, regardless of the degree of inhibition, in patients with a history of GI bleeding or multiple risk factors for GI bleeding who are also receiving clopidogrel since no evidence has established clinically meaningful differences in outcome; however, a clinically-significant interaction cannot be excluded in those who are poor metabolizers of clopidogrel (Abraham, 2010; Levine, 2011). Potentially significant drug-drug interactions may exist, requiring dose or frequency adjustment, additional monitoring, and/or selection of alternative therapy.

Increased incidence of osteoporosis-related bone fractures of the hip, spine, or wrist may occur with PPI therapy. Patients on high-dose or long-term therapy (≥1 year) should be monitored. Use the lowest effective dose for the shortest duration of time, use vitamin D and calcium supplementation, and follow appropriate guidelines to reduce risk of fractures in patients at risk. Acute interstitial nephritis has been observed in patients taking PPIs; may occur at any time during therapy and is generally due to an idiopathic hypersensitivity reaction. Discontinue if acute interstitial nephritis develops. Thrombophlebitis and hypersensitivity reactions including anaphylaxis, Stevens-Johnson syndrome, and toxic epidermal necrolysis have been reported with IV administration.

Hypomagnesemia, reported rarely, usually with prolonged PPI use of >3 months (most cases >1 year of therapy); may be symptomatic or asymptomatic; severe cases may cause tetany, seizures, and cardiac arrhythmias. Consider obtaining serum magnesium concentrations prior to beginning long-term therapy, especially if taking concomitant digoxin, diuretics, or other drugs known to cause hypomagnesemia; and periodically thereafter. Hypomagnesemia may be corrected by magnesium supplementation, although discontinuation of pantoprazole may be necessary; magnesium levels typically return to normal within 2 weeks of stopping.

Some dosage forms may contain polysorbate 80 (also known as Tweens). Hypersensitivity reactions, usually a delayed reaction, have been reported following exposure to pharmaceutical products containing polysorbate 80 in certain individuals (Isaksson, 2002; Lucente 2000; Shelley, 1995). Thrombocytopenia, ascites, pulmonary deterioration, and renal and hepatic failure have been reported in premature neonates after receiving parenteral products containing polysorbate 80 (Alade, 1986; CDC, 1984). See manufacturer's labeling.

Adverse Reactions

Cardiovascular: Edema, facial edema

Central nervous system: Depression, dizziness, headache, vertigo

Dermatologic: Pruritus, skin photosensitivity, skin rash (more common in children), urticaria
Endocrine & metabolic: Increased serum triglycerides
Gastrointestinal: Abdominal pain, constipation, diarrhea, flatulence, nausea, vomiting, xerostomia
Hematologic & oncologic: Leukopenia, thrombocytopenia
Hepatic: Abnormal hepatic function tests, hepatitis
Hypersensitivity: Hypersensitivity reaction
Local: Inflammation at injection site
Neuromuscular & skeletal: Arthralgia, increased creatine phosphokinase, myalgia
Ophthalmic: Blurred vision
Respiratory: Upper respiratory tract infection
Miscellaneous: Fever (more common in children)
Rare but important or life-threatening: Ageusia, agranulocytosis, albuminuria, anaphylaxis (including anaphylactic shock), anemia, angioedema, angina pectoris, aphthous stomatitis, atrial fibrillation, atrial flutter, atrophic gastritis, biliary colic, bone fracture, bursitis, candidiasis (gastrointestinal), cardiac arrhythmia, cardiac failure, cataract, cholecystitis, cholelithiasis, *Clostridium difficile*-associate diarrhea, colitis, contact dermatitis, cystitis, deafness, dehydration, diabetes mellitus, diplopia, duodenitis, dysmenorrhea, dysphagia, dysuria, ecchymoses, ECG abnormality, eosinophilia, epididymitis, epistaxis, erythema multiforme, exacerbation of asthma, extraocular palsy, fungal dermatitis, gastric ulcer, gastrointestinal carcinoma, gastrointestinal hemorrhage, gingivitis, glaucoma, glossitis, glycosuria, goiter, gout, hallucination, hematemesis, hematuria, hemorrhage, hepatic failure, hepatotoxicity (idiosyncratic) (Chalasani, 2014), hernia, hyperbilirubinemia, hyperesthesia, hypertension, hyperkinesia, hyperuricemia, hypokinesia, hypomagnesemia, hyponatremia, hypotension, impotence, increased gamma-glutamyl transferase, increased serum alkaline phosphatase, increased serum creatinine, interstitial nephritis, ischemic heart disease, jaundice, leukocytosis, lichenoid dermatitis, maculopapular rash, mastalgia, melena, myocardial infarction, neoplasm, nephrolithiasis, neuralgia, neuritis, optic neuropathy (including anterior ischemic), oral mucosa ulcer, ostealgia, palpitations, pancreatitis, pancytopenia, paresthesia, periodontitis, pneumonia, pyelonephritis, rectal hemorrhage, renal pain, retinal vascular disease, rhabdomyolysis, scrotal edema, seizure, Stevens-Johnson syndrome, stomatitis, syncope, tachycardia, tenosynovitis, thrombosis, tinnitus, tongue discoloration, toxic epidermal necrolysis, urethritis, visual disturbance

Drug Interactions

Metabolism/Transport Effects Substrate of CYP2C19 (major), CYP2D6 (minor), CYP3A4 (minor); **Note:** Assignment of Major/Minor substrate status based on clinically relevant drug interaction potential; **Inhibits** BCRP, CYP2C19 (weak); **Induces** CYP1A2 (weak/moderate)

Avoid Concomitant Use

Avoid concomitant use of Pantoprazole with any of the following: Dasatinib; Delavirdine; Erlotinib; Nelfinavir; PAZOPanib; Rilpivirine; Risedronate

Increased Effect/Toxicity

Pantoprazole may increase the levels/effects of: Amphetamine; Dexmethylphenidate; Dextroamphetamine; Methotrexate; Methylphenidate; PAZOPanib; Raltegravir; Risedronate; Saquinavir; Topotecan; Voriconazole

The levels/effects of Pantoprazole may be increased by: Fluconazole; Ketoconazole (Systemic); Voriconazole

Decreased Effect

Pantoprazole may decrease the levels/effects of: Atazanavir; Bisphosphonate Derivatives; Bosutinib; Cefditoren; Clopidogrel; Dabigatran Etexilate; Dabrafenib; Dasatinib; Delavirdine; Erlotinib; Gefitinib; Indinavir; Iron Salts; Itraconazole; Ketoconazole (Systemic); Ledipasvir; Mesalamine; Multivitamins/Minerals (with ADEK, Folate, Iron); Mycophenolate; Nelfinavir; Nilotinib; PAZOPanib; Posaconazole; Rilpivirine; Riociguat; Risedronate

The levels/effects of Pantoprazole may be decreased by: CYP2C19 Inducers (Strong); Dabrafenib; Tipranavir

Food Interactions Prolonged treatment (≥2 years) may lead to malabsorption of dietary vitamin B_{12} and subsequent vitamin B_{12} deficiency (Lam, 2013).

Storage/Stability

Oral: Store tablet and oral suspension at 20°C to 25°C (68°F to 77°F); excursions permitted to 15°C to 30°C (59°F to 86°F).

IV: Prior to reconstitution, store at 20°C to 25°C (68°F to 77°F); excursions permitted to 15°C to 30°C (59°F to 86°F). Do not freeze. Protect from light prior to reconstitution; upon reconstitution, protection from light is not required. Per manufacturer's labeling, reconstituted solution is stable at room temperature for 6 hours; further diluted (admixed) solution should be stored at room temperature and used within 24 hours from the time of initial reconstitution. However, studies have shown that reconstituted solution (4 mg/mL) in polypropylene syringes is stable up to 96 hours at room temperature (Johnson, 2005). Upon further dilution, the admixed solution should be used within 96 hours from the time of initial reconstitution. The preparation should be stored at 3°C to 5°C (37°F to 41°F) if it is stored beyond 48 hours to minimize discoloration.

Mechanism of Action Suppresses gastric acid secretion by inhibiting the parietal cell H^+/K^+ ATP pump

Pharmacodynamics Acid secretion:

Onset of action:
- Oral: 2.5 hours
- IV: 15-30 minutes

Maximum effect: IV: 2 hours
Duration: Oral, IV: 24 hours

Pharmacokinetics (Adult data unless noted)

Absorption: Rapid, well-absorbed
Distribution: V_d:
- Children and Adolescents (Kearns, 2008):
  - IV: 2-16 years: 0.22 ± 0.14 L/kg
  - Oral: 5-16 years: 0.24 ± 0.09 L/kg
- Adults: 11-23.6 L

Protein binding: 98%
Metabolism: Extensively hepatic; CYP2C19 (demethylation), CYP3A4; no evidence that metabolites have pharmacologic activity
Bioavailability: ~77%
Half-life:
- Neonates (PMA: 37-44 weeks): ~3 hours (Ward, 2010)
- Children and Adolescents (Kearns, 2008):
  - IV: 2-16 years: 1.22 ± 0.68 hours
  - Oral: 5-16 years: 1.27 ± 1.29 hours
- Adults: 1 hour; prolonged half-life (3.5-10 hours) in slow metabolizers (CYP2C19 deficiency)

Time to peak serum concentration:
- Children and Adolescents (Kearns, 2008):
  - IV: 2-16 years: 0.34 ± 0.12 hours
  - Oral: 5-16 years: 2.54 ± 0.72 hours
- Adults: Oral: 2.5 hours

Elimination: Urine (71% as metabolites); feces (18%); pantoprazole clearance increased with weight and age (Peterson, 2009)

Dosing: Neonatal GERD, symptomatic: Limited data available: Preterm (PMA <44 weeks and weighing ≥1.5 kg) and Term Neonates: Oral: 2.5 mg (~1.2 mg/kg/dose) once daily administered 30 minutes prior to first feeding of the day was evaluated in a pharmacokinetic trial in 21 neonatal patients (preterm: 19; term: 2; mean GA: 28 weeks; range: 23-41 weeks); this dose produced slightly higher systemic exposure than adolescents and adults receiving 40 mg, but there was no evidence of accumulation with repeated administration noted; although there was a significant increase in gastric pH and the amount of time the pH >4, there was no significant difference in reflux episodes. A lower dose of 1.25 mg (0.6 mg/kg/dose) was also evaluated (n=19); however, this dose did not provide statistically significant improvements in pH-metry parameters (Kierkus, 2011; Ward, 2010).

Dosing: Usual Note: Parenteral therapy should be discontinued as soon as the patient tolerates oral therapy.

Pediatric:

GERD, symptomatic: Limited data available:

Infants and Children <5 years: Oral: 1.2 mg/kg/day once daily for 4 weeks was shown to reduce GERD symptoms but was not significantly different from placebo (n=128; age range: 1 to 11 months) (Winter 2010); a pharmacokinetic trial showed this dose produced similar serum concentrations as adults receiving 40 mg in infants 1 to 11 months (mean age: 6.3 months) and slightly lower concentrations in children 1 to <6 years (mean age: 3.2 years) (Tammara 2011)

Children 5 to 11 years: Oral: 20 or 40 mg once daily have been shown to reduce severity and frequency of symptoms within 1 week based on the GERD Assessment of Symptoms in Pediatric Patients Questionnaire (n=53, age range: 5 to 11 years); results also showed that while a lower dose of 10 mg improved symptoms, it took longer (3 weeks) for results (Tolia 2006); a pharmacokinetic trial in patients 6 to 11 years old (n=24) showed that 40 mg once daily produced similar systemic exposure as adults receiving 40 mg; however, the authors suggested that 20 mg once daily may be appropriate for small children (Ward 2011)

Children and Adolescents 12 to 16 years: Oral: 20 or 40 mg once daily was shown to reduce symptoms in patients with confirmed or clinically suspected diagnosis of GERD (n=136) based on the GERD Assessment of Symptoms in Pediatric Patients Questionnaire (Tsou 2011); a pharmacokinetic trial showed that a 40 mg dose produced similar systemic exposure as adults receiving 40 mg; however, suggested that 20 mg once daily may be appropriate for smaller adolescents (<40 kg) (Ward 2011)

Erosive esophagitis associated with GERD:

Children 1 to 5 years: Limited data available: Oral: 0.3, 0.6, or 1.2 mg/kg/day once daily for 8 weeks was used in a dose-finding study of 60 patients with histologic or erosive esophagitis. High-dose treatment (1.2 mg/kg/day) was administered as a fixed dose of either: 15 mg for 1-year-olds **or** 20 mg for 2- to 5-year-olds. Patients with erosive esophagitis (n=4) received either 0.6 or 1.2 mg/kg/day. All patients had symptomatic improvement and patients with erosive esophagitis were healed by week 8; no dose response relationship was demonstrated (Baker 2010)

Children ≥5 years and Adolescents: Oral:

≥15 to <40 kg: 20 mg once daily for up to 8 weeks

≥40 kg: 40 mg once daily for up to 8 weeks

Gastric acid suppression; oral therapy not appropriate or tolerated: Limited data available; dosing regimens variable: Infants, Children, and Adolescents: IV: Dosing based on pharmacokinetic data from 39 pediatric patients (age range: 10 days to 16 years) which has shown doses within this range produce similar AUC as adult patients with comparable dosing; efficacy was not evaluated in either trial (Kearns 2008; Petersen 2009).

Weight-based dosing: Children ≥2 years and Adolescents: IV: 0.8 or 1.6 mg/kg once daily; maximum single dose: 80 mg; dosing from a single dose pharmacokinetic study in 18 patients (age range: 2 to 14 years) (Kearns 2008). In the BSA-based dosing trial (Petersen 2009), the final median dose when standardized to weight was 1.1 mg/kg/day (range: 0.5 to 4.6 mg/kg/day). (**Note:** The 4.6 mg/kg/day dose was a prescription error; however, the patient experienced no adverse consequences due to high dose). Additionally, some clinicians have used 1 to 2 mg/kg/day in single or divided doses. **Note:** In a very small trial (n=8), a median dose of 1.1 mg/kg (0.9 to 2.5 mg/kg) produced similar AUC values as adults, but only produced a definable response (gastric pH >4) in one patient; in the remaining seven patients the mean percentage of time with intragastric pH ≥4 was 7.4 % (Petersen 2005); the pharmacodynamic profile needs further defined (Petersen 2009)

Body surface area (BSA)-based dosing: Infants, Children, and Adolescents: IV: 40 mg/1.73 m^2/day; if inadequate response (eg, continued symptoms or target gastric pH not achieved) may titrate up to a maximum dose of 80 mg/1.73 m^2/day; dosing based on multidose pharmacokinetic analysis; in the final analysis, the median reported dose was 41.8 mg/1.73 m^2/day (range: 19.9-140.6 mg/1.73 m^2/day) (**Note:** The 140.6 mg/1.73 m^2/day dose was a prescription error; however, the patient experienced no adverse consequences due to high dose) (Petersen 2009).

Adult:

Erosive esophagitis associated with GERD:

Oral:

Treatment: 40 mg once daily for up to 8 weeks; an additional 8 weeks may be used in patients who have not healed after an 8-week course

Maintenance of healing: 40 mg once daily

IV: 40 mg once daily for 7 to 10 days

Hypersecretory conditions (including Zollinger-Ellison syndrome):

Oral: Initial: 40 mg twice daily; adjust dose based on patient response; doses up to 240 mg daily have been administered

IV: Initial: 80 mg every 12 hours; adjust dosage to maintain acid output; 160-240 mg daily in divided doses has been used for a limited period (up to 7 days)

Dosing adjustment in renal impairment: Adults: No dosage adjustment needed

Hemodialysis: Not appreciably removed by hemodialysis

Dosing adjustment in hepatic impairment: Adults: No dosage adjustment for doses up to 40 mg/day. Doses higher than 40 mg/day have not been studied in patients with hepatic impairment.

Preparation for Administration

IV:

IV push: Reconstitute powder for injection with 10 mL NS; final concentration: 4 mg/mL

Intermittent IV infusion: After reconstitution, further dilute in NS, D_5W, or LR to a final concentration of 0.4 to 0.8 mg/mL

Administration

Parenteral: IV: Not for IM or SubQ use. Flush IV line with NS, D_5W, or LR before and after administration.

IV push: Administer over 2 minutes at a concentration of 4 mg/mL

Intermittent IV infusion: Using a 0.4 to 0.8 mg/mL solution, infuse over 15 minutes at a rate not to exceed 7 mL/minute

Oral:

Tablet: Should be swallowed whole; do not chew or crush. May be taken without regard to meals; however, best if taken 30 minutes before a meal (Lightdale 2013); may be administered with antacids.

Delayed release oral suspension: Should only be administered in apple juice or applesauce and administered 30 minutes before a meal. Do not administer in water, other liquids, or foods. Per manufacturer's labeling, do not divide the 40 mg delayed release oral suspension packet to create a 20 mg dosage for pediatric patients who are unable to take the tablet formulation.

Oral administration in apple juice: Empty intact granules into 5 mL of apple juice, stir for 5 seconds, and swallow immediately. Rinse container once or twice with apple juice and swallow immediately.

Oral administration in applesauce: Sprinkle intact granules on 1 teaspoonful of applesauce; swallow within 10 minutes of preparation.

Nasogastric tube administration: Separate the plunger from the barrel of a 60 mL catheter tip syringe and connect to a ≥16 French nasogastric tube. Holding the syringe attached to the tubing as high as possible, empty granules into barrel of syringe, add 10 mL of apple juice, and gently tap/shake the barrel of the syringe to help empty the syringe. Add an additional 10 mL of apple juice and gently tap/shake the barrel to help rinse. Repeat rinse with at least 2 to 10 mL aliquots of apple juice. No granules should remain in the syringe.

Oral administration in syringe: In neonatal trials, fixed dosage packets of 2.5 mg pantoprazole were mixed with grape flavoring and 2.5 mL of water and administered immediately (Ward 2010).

Test Interactions False-positive urine screening tests for tetrahydrocannabinol (THC) have been noted in patients receiving proton pump inhibitors, including pantoprazole.

Dosage Forms Excipient information presented when available (limited, particularly for generics); consult specific product labeling. [DSC] = Discontinued product

Packet, Oral:
- Protonix: 40 mg (1 ea, 30 ea) [contains polysorbate 80]

Solution Reconstituted, Intravenous:
- Protonix: 40 mg (1 ea) [contains edetate disodium]
- Generic: 40 mg (1 ea [DSC])

Tablet Delayed Release, Oral:
- Protonix: 20 mg, 40 mg
- Generic: 20 mg, 40 mg

Extemporaneous Preparations A 2 mg/mL pantoprazole oral suspension may be made with pantoprazole tablets, sterile water, and sodium bicarbonate powder. Remove the Protonix® imprint from twenty 40 mg tablets with a paper towel dampened with ethanol (improves the look of product). Let tablets air dry. Crush the tablets in a mortar and reduce to a fine powder. Transfer to a 600 mL beaker, and add 340 mL sterile water. Place beaker on a magnetic stirrer. Add 16.8 g of sodium bicarbonate powder and stir for about 20 minutes until the tablet remnants have disintegrated. While stirring, add another 16.8 g of sodium bicarbonate powder and stir for about 5 minutes until powder has dissolved. Add enough sterile water for irrigation to bring the final volume to 400 mL. Mix well. Transfer to amber-colored bottle. Label "shake well" and "refrigerate". Stable for 62 days refrigerated.

Dentinger PJ, Swenson CF, and Anaizi NH, "Stability of Pantoprazole in an Extemporaneously Compounded Oral Liquid," *Am J Health Syst Pharm*, 2002, 59(10):953-6.

◆ **Pantoprazole for Injection (Can)** *see* Pantoprazole *on page 1618*

◆ **Pantoprazole Magnesium** *see* Pantoprazole *on page 1618*

◆ **Pantoprazole Sodium** *see* Pantoprazole *on page 1618*

◆ **Pantoprazole Sodium for Injection (Can)** *see* Pantoprazole *on page 1618*

Papaverine (pa PAV er een)

Medication Safety Issues

Sound-alike/look-alike issues:

Papaverine may be confused with pamidronate

Therapeutic Category Antimigraine Agent; Vasodilator

Generic Availability (US) Yes

Use Various vascular spasms associated with smooth muscle spasms as in myocardial infarction, angina, peripheral and pulmonary embolism, peripheral vascular disease; cerebral angiospastic states; visceral spasms (ureteral, biliary, and GI colic) (FDA approved in adults); has also been used for peripheral arterial catheter patency. **Note:** Labeled uses have fallen out of favor; safer and more effective alternatives are available.

Pregnancy Risk Factor C

Pregnancy Considerations Teratogenic effects have not been observed in animal reproduction studies.

Breast-Feeding Considerations It is not known if papaverine is excreted in breast milk. The manufacturer recommends that caution be exercised when administering papaverine to nursing women.

Contraindications Patients with complete AV block

Warnings/Precautions Use with caution in patients with glaucoma. Administer IV cautiously since apnea and arrhythmias may result. May, in large doses, depress cardiac conduction (eg, AV node) leading to arrhythmias. May cause hepatic hypersensitivity; discontinue use if GI symptoms, jaundice, eosinophilia, or abnormal LFTs occur. Not indicated for treatment of impotence by intracorporeal injection; persistent priapism may occur.

Warnings: Additional Pediatric Considerations Administer IV slowly and with caution since arrhythmias and apnea may occur with rapid IV use. Avoid use in neonates due to the increased risk of drug-induced cerebral vasodilation and possibility of an intracranial bleed.

Adverse Reactions

Cardiovascular: Arrhythmias (with rapid IV use), flushing, mild hypertension, tachycardia

Central nervous system: Headache, malaise, sedation, vertigo

Dermatologic: Rash

Gastrointestinal: Abdominal distress, anorexia, constipation, diarrhea, nausea

Hepatic: Cirrhosis, hepatic hypersensitivity, hepatitis (rare)

Respiratory: Apnea (with rapid IV use)

Miscellaneous: Diaphoresis

Drug Interactions

Metabolism/Transport Effects None known.

Avoid Concomitant Use There are no known interactions where it is recommended to avoid concomitant use.

Increased Effect/Toxicity

Papaverine may increase the levels/effects of: DULoxetine; Hypotensive Agents; Levodopa; RisperiDONE

The levels/effects of Papaverine may be increased by: Barbiturates; Nicorandil

Decreased Effect

Papaverine may decrease the levels/effects of: Levodopa

Storage/Stability Store at 20°C to 25°C (68°F to 77°F); excursions permitted to 15°C to 30°C (59°F to 86°F). Protect from light.

Mechanism of Action Smooth muscle spasmolytic producing a generalized smooth muscle relaxation including vasodilatation, gastrointestinal sphincter relaxation, bronchiolar muscle relaxation, and potentially a depressed myocardium (with large doses); muscle relaxation may occur due to inhibition or cyclic nucleotide phosphodiesterase, increasing cyclic AMP; muscle relaxation is unrelated to nerve innervation; papaverine increases cerebral blood flow in normal subjects; oxygen uptake is unaltered

Pharmacodynamics Onset of action: Oral: Rapid

Pharmacokinetics (Adult data unless noted)

Protein binding: 90%

Metabolism: Rapid in the liver

Bioavailability: Oral: ~54%

Half-life: 30-120 minutes

Elimination: Primarily as metabolites in urine

Dosing: Neonatal Peripheral arterial catheter patency: Limited data available: Full-term neonates: Add 30 mg preservative-free papaverine to an admixture of 250 mL NS or 1/2NS with heparin 1 unit/mL; infuse via peripheral arterial catheter at ≤1 mL/hour (see Heparin monograph). A double-blind, placebo-controlled trial of 141 neonates (median GA: 27 weeks; median birth weight: 910 to 952 g) demonstrated prolonged functionality of peripherally inserted arterial catheters (Griffin 2005). **Note:** Due to the risk of IVH, the use of papaverine in preterm neonates <3 weeks of age is not recommended (Griffin 2005).

Dosing: Usual

Pediatric:

Peripheral arterial catheter patency: Limited data available: Infants, Children, and Adolescents: Add 30 mg papaverine to an admixture of 250 mL NS or 1/2NS with heparin 1 unit/mL (Heulitt 1993; Kliegman 2007); infuse via peripheral arterial catheter; some centers report infusions at ≤1 mL/hour

Adult: **Note:** Labeled uses have fallen out of favor; safer and more effective alternatives are available. The manufacturer's labeling recommends the following dosing:

Arterial spasm: IM, IV: 30 to 120 mg; may repeat dose every 3 hours; if cardiac extrasystole occurs during use, may administer 2 doses 10 minutes apart

Preparation for Administration Parenteral: IV infusion: Peripheral arterial catheter patency: Add 30 mg papaverine to an admixture of 250 mL NS or 1/2NS with heparin 1 unit/mL

Administration

Parenteral: IV infusion: Neonates, Infants, Children, and Adolescents: Administer through designated peripheral arterial catheter at prescribed rate, usually ≤1 mL/hour

IV injection: Adults: Rapid IV administration may result in arrhythmias and fatal apnea; administer undiluted slow IV over 1 to 2 minutes

IM: Adults: Administer undiluted

Monitoring Parameters Liver enzymes; intraocular pressure in glaucoma patients

Additional Information Evidence of therapeutic value of systemic use for relief of peripheral and cerebral ischemia related to arterial spasm is lacking

Further studies are needed to determine the benefit of adding papaverine (60 mg/500 mL) to arterial catheter infusions containing NS or 1/2NS and heparin 1 unit/mL. One investigation showed a lower risk of arterial catheter failure and longer duration of arterial catheter function in patients 7 months to 5.5 years of age who received papaverine in their arterial catheter solutions; these results should be verified by additional studies before the addition of papaverine to arterial catheter solutions can be recommended.

Dosage Forms Excipient information presented when available (limited, particularly for generics); consult specific product labeling.

Solution, Injection, as hydrochloride:

Generic: 30 mg/mL (2 mL, 10 mL)

◆ **Papaverine Hydrochloride** *see* Papaverine *on page 1622*

Papillomavirus (9-Valent) Vaccine (Human, Recombinant)

(pap ih LO ma VYE rus nine VAY lent vak SEEN YU man ree KOM be nant)

Medication Safety Issues

Sound-alike/look-alike issues:

Papillomavirus vaccine 9-valent (Gardasil 9) may be confused with Papillomavirus vaccine types 6, 11, 16, 18 (Gardasil)

Brand Names: US Gardasil 9

Therapeutic Category Vaccine; Vaccine, Inactivated (Viral)

Generic Availability (US) No

Use

Prevention of the following: Cervical, vulvar, vaginal, and anal cancer caused by HPV types 16, 18, 31, 33, 45, 52, and 58; genital warts caused by HPV types 6 and 11; cervical adenocarcinoma in situ; and vulvar, vaginal, cervical, or anal intraepithelial neoplasia caused by HPV types 6, 11, 16, 18, 31, 33, 45, 52, and 58 (FDA approved in females ages 9 to 26 years)

Prevention of the following: genital warts caused by HPV types 6 and 11; anal cancer caused by HPV types 16, 18, 31, 33, 45, 52, and 58; and anal intraepithelial neoplasia caused by HPV types 6, 11, 16, 18, 31, 33, 45, 52, and 58 (FDA approved in males ages 9 to 15 years)

The Advisory Committee on Immunization Practices (ACIP) recommends routine vaccination for females and males 11 to 12 years of age; can be administered as young as 9 years; catch-up vaccination is recommended for females 13 to 26 years of age and males 13 to 21 years of age. Vaccination for males 22 through 26 years of age is recommended if immunocompromised (including HIV) and for men who have sex with men and may be considered for any other male in this age group (CDC/ACIP [Petrosky 2015]).

Pregnancy Risk Factor B

Pregnancy Considerations Adverse events were not observed in animal reproduction studies. In clinical trials, women who were found to be pregnant before the completion of the 3-dose regimen were instructed to defer any remaining dose until pregnancy resolution. In pregnancies detected within 30 days of vaccination, no cases of congenital abnormalities were noted. Pregnancies with onset beyond 30 days of vaccination had a rate of congenital anomalies consistent with the general population. Administration of the vaccine in pregnancy is not recommended. Until additional information is available, the vaccine series (or completion of the series) should be delayed until pregnancy is completed. Pregnancy testing is not required prior to administration of the vaccine (CDC/ACIP [Petrosky 2015]).

A registry has been established for women exposed to the Gardasil 9 HPV vaccine during pregnancy (1-800-986-8999).

Breast-Feeding Considerations It is not known if this vaccine is excreted into breast milk. The manufacturer recommends that caution be exercised when administering papilloma virus vaccine to nursing women.

Contraindications Hypersensitivity, including severe allergic reactions to yeast (a vaccine component), or a previous dose of this vaccine or human papillomavirus vaccine (recombinant) for types 6, 11, 16, 18

Warnings/Precautions Immediate treatment (including epinephrine 1:1,000) for anaphylactoid and/or hypersensitivity reactions should be available during vaccine use (NCIRD/ACIP 2011). There is no evidence that individuals already infected with HPV will be protected; those already infected with 1 or more HPV types were protected from disease caused by the remaining HPV types. Not for the treatment of active disease; will not protect against diseases not caused by human papillomavirus (HPV) vaccine types contained in the vaccine. Does not eliminate the necessity for recommended cervical or anal cancer screenings. The decision to administer or delay vaccination because of current or recent febrile illness depends on the severity of symptoms and the etiology of the disease. Consider deferring administration in patients with moderate or severe acute illness (with or without fever); vaccination should not be delayed for patients with mild acute illness (with or without fever) (NCIRD/ACIP 2011).

Vaccination may not result in effective immunity in all patients. Response depends upon multiple factors (eg, type of vaccine, age of patient) and may be improved by administering the vaccine at the recommended dose, route, and interval. Vaccines may not be effective if administered during periods of altered immune competence (NCIRD/ACIP 2011). Use with caution in severely immunocompromised patients (eg, patients receiving chemo/radiation therapy or other immunosuppressive therapy [including high dose corticosteroids]); may have a reduced response to vaccination. In general, household and close contacts of persons with altered immunocompetence may receive all age-appropriate vaccines (IDSA [Rubin 2014]; NCIRD/ACIP 2011); inactivated vaccines should be administered ≥2 weeks prior to planned immunosuppression when feasible (IDSA [Rubin 2014]).

Use with caution in patients with a history of bleeding disorders (including thrombocytopenia) and/or patients on anticoagulant therapy; bleeding/hematoma may occur from IM administration; if the patient receives antihemophilia or other similar therapy, IM injection can be scheduled shortly after such therapy is administered (NCIRD/ACIP 2011). The entire 3-dose regimen should be completed for maximum efficacy. Safety and immunogenicity of Gardasil 9 were assessed in individuals who previously completed a 3-dose vaccination series with Gardasil (quadrivalent). Studies using a mixed regimen of HPV vaccines to assess interchangeability were not performed. Per the ACIP, if the provider does not have available or does not know the HPV product used previously, any gender appropriate product can be used to complete the series (CDC/ACIP [Petrovsky 2015]).

Syncope has been reported with use of injectable vaccines and may result in serious secondary injury (eg skull fracture, cerebral hemorrhage); typically reported in adolescents and young adults and within 15 minutes after vaccination. Procedures should be in place to avoid injuries from falling and to restore cerebral perfusion if syncope occurs (NCIRD/ACIP 2011). Product may contain yeast. In order to maximize vaccination rates, the ACIP recommends simultaneous administration of all age-appropriate vaccines (live or inactivated) for which a person is eligible at a single clinic visit, unless contraindications exist. The ACIP prefers each dose of a specific vaccine in a series come from the same manufacturer when possible (NCIRD/ACIP 2011).

Adverse Reactions To report **suspected adverse reactions**, contact Merck Sharp & Dohme Corp., a subsidiary of Merck & Co., Inc., at (877) 888-4231 or VAERS at (800) 822-7967 or http://www.vaers.hhs.gov.

Cardiovascular: Syncope

Central nervous system: Dizziness, fatigue, headache

Gastrointestinal: Diarrhea, nausea, upper abdominal pain

Immunologic: Autoimmune disease

Local: bleeding at injection site, bruising at injection site, erythema at injection site (erythema increases with successive doses), hematoma at injection site, induration at injection site, itching at injection site, injection site nodule, injection site reaction, pain at injection site, swelling at injection site (swelling increased with successive doses and/or concomitant vaccines)

Neuromuscular & skeletal: Myalgia

Respiratory: Oropharyngeal pain

Miscellaneous: Fever

Rare but important or life-threatening: Anaphylactoid reaction, hypersomnia, postural orthostatic tachycardia, status asthmaticus, tonsillitis

Drug Interactions

Metabolism/Transport Effects None known.

Avoid Concomitant Use There are no known interactions where it is recommended to avoid concomitant use.

Increased Effect/Toxicity There are no known significant interactions involving an increase in effect.

Decreased Effect

The levels/effects of Papillomavirus (9-Valent) Vaccine (Human, Recombinant) may be decreased by: Belimumab; Fingolimod; Immunosuppressants

Storage/Stability Store refrigerated at 2°C to 8°C (36°F to 46°F). Do not freeze. Protect from light.

Administer as soon as possible after being removed from refrigeration. HPV 9-valent vaccine can be administered provided total (cumulative multiple excursion) time out of refrigeration (at temperatures between 8°C and 25°C) does not exceed 72 hours. Cumulative multiple excursions between 0°C and 2°C are also permitted as long as the total time between 0°C and 2°C does not exceed 72 hours. These are not, however, recommendations for storage.

Mechanism of Action Contains inactive human papillomavirus (HPV) proteins (types 6 L1,11 L1, 16 L1, 18 L1, 31 L1, 33 L1, 45 L1, 52 L1, and 58 L1) which produce neutralizing antibodies to prevent cervical, vulvar, vaginal, and anal cancers, cervical adenocarcinoma, cervical, vaginal, vulvar, and anal neoplasia, and genital warts caused by HPV. Efficacy of HPV 9-valent vaccine against anogenital diseases related to the vaccine HPV types in humans is thought to be mediated by humoral immune responses induced by the vaccine, although the exact mechanism of protection is unknown.

Dosing: Usual

Pediatric: **Immunization: Note:** If the HPV product previously administered is not known or not available, any available HPV vaccine product may be used to continue or complete the series for females for protection against HPV 16 and 18; the 9-valent HPV or 4-valent HPV may be used to continue or complete the series for males (CDC/ACIP [Petrosky 2015]).

CDC/ACIP recommended immunization schedule: Children ≥9 years and Adolescents: IM: 0.5 mL per dose for a total of 3 doses administered as follows: Initial dose followed by a second dose at 1 to 2 months after initial and a third dose at 6 months after the initial.

Administer first dose at age 11 to 12 years although series may be initiated as early as 9 years of age. Minimum interval between first and second doses is 4 weeks; the minimum interval between the second and third dose is 12 weeks; the minimum interval between first and third doses is 24 weeks. (CDC/ACIP [Petrosky 2015]).

Manufacturer's labeling:

Females: Children and Adolescents 9 to 15 years: IM 0.5 mL per dose for a total of 3 doses; administer the second and third doses at 2 and 6 months after initial dose

Males: Children and Adolescents 9 to 15 years: IM: 0.5 mL per dose for a total of 3 doses; administer the second and third doses at 2 and 6 months after initial dose

Adult: **Immunization:**

Manufacturer's labeling: Females ≤26 years: IM: 0.5 mL per dose for a total of 3 doses; administer the second and third doses at 2 and 6 months after initial dose

CDC/ACIP recommended immunization schedule: Begin series in females ≤26 years or males ≤21 years if not previously vaccinated or completed the 3-dose series (typically administer first dose at age 11 to 12 years). Vaccination for males 22 through 26 years of age is recommended if immunocompromised (including HIV) and for men who have sex with men and may be considered for any other male in this age group. Administer the second and third doses at 1 to 2 months and 6 months after the first dose. Second and third doses may be given after age 26 years to complete a previously initiated series. (CDC/ACIP [Petrosky 2015].

Dosing adjustment in renal impairment: There are no dosage adjustments provided in the manufacturer's labeling.

Dosing adjustment in hepatic impairment: There are no dosage adjustments provided in the manufacturer's labeling.

Administration Shake suspension well before use. Do not use if discolored or if contains particulate matter, or if syringe is cracked. Inject the entire dose IM into the deltoid region of the upper arm or higher anterolateral thigh area. To prevent syncope related injuries, adolescents and adults should be vaccinated while seated or lying down (NCIRD/ACIP 2011). US law requires that the date of administration, the vaccine manufacturer, lot number of vaccine, and the administering person's name, title, and address be entered into the patient's permanent medical record.

For patients at risk of hemorrhage following intramuscular injection, the vaccine should be administered intramuscularly if, in the opinion of the physician familiar with the patient's bleeding risk, the vaccine can be administered by this route with reasonable safety. If the patient receives antihemophilia or other similar therapy, intramuscular vaccination can be scheduled shortly after such therapy is administered. A fine needle (23 gauge or smaller) can be used for the vaccination and firm pressure applied to the site (without rubbing) for at least 2 minutes. The patient should be instructed concerning the risk of hematoma from the injection. Patients on anticoagulant therapy should be considered to have the same bleeding risks and treated as those with clotting factor disorders (NCIRD/ACIP 2011).

Monitoring Parameters Screening for HPV is not required prior to vaccination. Monitor for syncope for 15 minutes following administration (NCIRD/ACIP 2011). If seizure-like activity associated with syncope occurs, maintain patient in supine or Trendelenburg position to reestablish adequate cerebral perfusion. Continue recommended anal cancer screening.

Females: Gynecologic screening exam, papillomavirus test; screening for cervical cancer should continue per current guidelines following vaccination

Additional Information Ideally, administration of vaccine should occur prior to potential HPV exposure. Benefits of vaccine decrease once infected with ≥1 of the HPV vaccine types, although patients are protected from precancerous cervical lesions and external genital lesions caused by other HPV vaccine types.

Comparison of HPV vaccines: Cervarix, Gardasil, and Gardasil 9 are all vaccines formulated to protect against infection with the human papillomavirus. All are inactive vaccines which contain proteins HPV16 L1 and HPV 18 L1, the cause of >70% of invasive cervical cancer. The vaccines differ in that Gardasil also contains HPV 6 L1 and HPV 11 L1 proteins which protect against 75% to 90% of genital warts. Gardasil 9 adds HPV 31 L1, HPV 33 L1, HPV 45 L1, HPV 52 L1, and HPV 58 L1. The vaccines also differ in their preparation and adjuvants used. The viral proteins in Cervarix are prepared using *Trichoplusia ni* (insect cells) which are adsorbed on to an aluminum salt which is also combined with a monophosphoryl lipid. The viral proteins in Gardasil and Gardasil 9 are prepared using *Saccharomyces cerevisiae* (baker's yeast) which are then adsorbed to an aluminum salt. Results from a short term study (measurements obtained 1 month following the third vaccination in the series) have shown that the immune response to HPV 16 and HPV 18 may be greater with Cervarix than with Gardasil; although the clinical significance of this difference is not known, local adverse events may occur more frequently with Cervarix. Both vaccines were effective and results from long term studies are pending (Einstein 2009).

Dosage Forms Excipient information presented when available (limited, particularly for generics); consult specific product labeling.

Suspension, Intramuscular [preservative free]:
- Gardasil 9: (0.5 mL) [contains polysorbate 80, yeast extract]

Suspension Prefilled Syringe, Intramuscular [preservative free]:
- Gardasil 9: (0.5 mL) [contains polysorbate 80, yeast extract]

Papillomavirus (Types 6, 11, 16, 18) Vaccine (Human, Recombinant)

(pap ih LO ma VYE rus typs six e LEV en SIX teen AYE teen vak SEEN YU man ree KOM be nant)

Medication Safety Issues

Sound-alike/look-alike issues:

Papillomavirus vaccine types 6, 11, 16, 18 (Gardasil) may be confused with Papillomavirus vaccine types 16, 18 (Cervarix)

Papillomavirus vaccine types 6, 11, 16, 18 (Gardasil) may be confused with Papillomavirus vaccine 9-valent (Gardasil 9)

Related Information

Centers for Disease Control and Prevention (CDC) and Other Links *on page 2424*

Immunization Administration Recommendations *on page 2411*

Immunization Schedules *on page 2416*

Brand Names: US Gardasil

Brand Names: Canada Gardasil

Therapeutic Category Vaccine; Vaccine, Inactivated Virus

Generic Availability (US) No

Use

Prevention of cervical, vulvar, vaginal, and anal cancer caused by HPV types 16 and 18; genital warts caused by HPV types 6 and 11; cervical adenocarcinoma *in situ*; and vulvar, vaginal, cervical, or anal intraepithelial neoplasia caused by HPV types 6, 11, 16, 18 (FDA approved in females ages 9 to 26 years)

Prevention of genital warts caused by HPV types 6 and 11; anal cancer caused by HPV types 16 and 18; and anal intraepithelial neoplasia caused by HPV types 6, 11, 16, and 18 (FDA approved in males ages 9 to 26 years)

The Advisory Committee on Immunization Practices (ACIP) recommends routine vaccination for females and males 11 to 12 years of age; can be administered as young as 9 years; catch-up vaccination is recommended for females 13 to 26 years of age and males 13 to 21 years of age. Vaccination for males 22 through 26 years of age is recommended if immunocompromised (including HIV) and for men who have sex with men and may be considered for any other male in this age group (CDC/ACIP [Markowitz 2014]; CDC/ACIP [Strikas 2015]).

Medication Guide Available Yes

Pregnancy Risk Factor B

Pregnancy Considerations Teratogenic effects were not observed in animal reproduction studies. In clinical trials, women who were found to be pregnant before the completion of the 3-dose regimen were instructed to defer any remaining dose until pregnancy resolution. Pregnancies detected within 30 days of vaccination had a higher rate of congenital anomalies (pyloric stenosis, congenital megacolon, congenital hydronephrosis, hip dysplasia, club foot) than the placebo group. Pregnancies with onset beyond 30 days of vaccination had a rate of congenital anomalies consistent with the general population. Overall, the types of teratogenic events were the same as those generally observed for this age group. Administration of the vaccine in pregnancy is not recommended; until additional information is available, the vaccine series (or completion of the series) should be delayed until pregnancy is completed. Pregnancy testing is not required prior to administration of the vaccine (CDC/ACIP [Petrosky 2015]).

A registry has been established for women exposed to the HPV vaccine during pregnancy (1-877-888-4231).

Breast-Feeding Considerations It is not known if this vaccine is excreted into breast milk. Infants had a higher incidence of acute respiratory illness when breast-fed by mothers within 30 days postvaccination. The manufacturer recommends that caution be exercised when administering papilloma virus vaccine to nursing women. Lactating women may receive vaccine (CDC/ACIP [Markowitz 2014]).

Contraindications Hypersensitivity, including severe allergic reactions to yeast (a vaccine component), or a previous dose of the vaccine

Warnings/Precautions Immediate treatment (including epinephrine 1:1,000) for anaphylactoid and/or hypersensitivity reactions should be available during vaccine use (NCIRD/ACIP 2011). There is no evidence that individuals already infected with HPV will be protected; those already infected with 1 or more HPV types were protected from disease in the remaining HPV types. Not for the treatment of active disease; will not protect against diseases not caused by human papillomavirus (HPV) vaccine types 6, 11, 16, and 18. The decision to administer or delay vaccination because of current or recent febrile illness depends on the severity of symptoms and the etiology of the disease. Consider deferring administration in patients with moderate or severe acute illness (with or without fever); vaccination should not be delayed for patients with mild acute illness (with or without fever) (CDC/ACIP [Markowitz 2014]; NCIRD/ACIP 2011). Vaccination may not result in effective immunity in all patients. Response depends upon multiple factors (eg, type of vaccine, age of patient) and may be improved by administering the vaccine at the recommended dose, route, and interval. Vaccines may not be effective if administered during periods of altered immune competence (NCIRD/ACIP 2011). May be administered to those who are immunosuppressed (CDC/ACIP [Markowitz 2014]). Use with caution in severely immunocompromised patients (eg, patients receiving chemo/radiation therapy or other immunosuppressive therapy [including high dose corticosteroids]); may have a reduced response to vaccination (CDC/ACIP [Markowitz 2014]; NCIRD/ACIP 2011). In general, household and close contacts of persons with altered immunocompetence may receive all age-appropriate vaccines (IDSA [Rubin 2014]; NCIRD/ACIP 2011); inactivated vaccines should be administered ≥2 weeks prior to planned immunosuppression when feasible (IDSA [Rubin 2014]). Use with caution in patients with a history of bleeding disorders (including thrombocytopenia) and/or patients on anticoagulant therapy; bleeding/hematoma may occur from IM administration; if the patient receives antihemophilia or other similar therapy, IM injection can be scheduled shortly after such therapy is administered (NCIRD/ACIP 2011). The entire 3-dose regimen should be completed for maximum efficacy. Not recommended for use during pregnancy. Syncope has been reported with use of injectable vaccines and may result in serious secondary injury (eg, skull fracture, cerebral hemorrhage); typically reported in adolescents and young adults and within 15 minutes after vaccination. Procedures should be in place to avoid injuries from falling and to restore cerebral perfusion if syncope occurs (NCIRD/ACIP 2011). Product may contain yeast.

Some dosage forms may contain polysorbate 80 (also known as Tweens). Hypersensitivity reactions, usually a delayed reaction, have been reported following exposure to pharmaceutical products containing polysorbate 80 in certain individuals (Isaksson 2002; Lucente 2000; Shelle 1995). Thrombocytopenia, ascites, pulmonary deterioration, and renal and hepatic failure have been reported in premature neonates after receiving parenteral products containing polysorbate 80 (Alade, 1986; CDC, 1984). See manufacturer's labeling.

In order to maximize vaccination rates, the ACIP recommends simultaneous administration (ie, >1 vaccine on the same day at different anatomic sites) of all age-appropriate vaccines (live or inactivated) for which a person is eligible at a single clinic visit, unless contraindications exist. Use of this vaccine for specific medical and/or other indications (eg, immunocompromising conditions, hepatic or kidney disease, diabetes) is also addressed in the ACIP Adult Recommended Immunization Schedule (CDC/ACIP [Ki 2015]). Specific recommendations for use of this vaccine in immunocompromised patients with asplenia, cancer, HIV infection, cerebrospinal fluid leaks, cochlear implants, hematopoietic stem cell transplant (prior to or after), sickle cell disease, solid organ transplant (prior to or after), or those receiving immunosuppressive therapy for chronic conditions are available from the IDSA (IDSA [Rubin 2014]).

Adverse Reactions All serious adverse reactions must be reported to the U.S. Department of Health and Human Services (DHHS) Vaccine Adverse Event Reporting System (VAERS) 1-800-822-7967 or online at https://vaers.hhs.gov/esub/index. In Canada, adverse reactions may be reported to local provincial/territorial health agencies or to the Vaccine Safety Section at Public Health Agency of Canada (1-866-844-0018).

Central nervous system: Dizziness, fever, headache, insomnia, malaise

Local: Injection site: Bruising, erythema, hematoma, pain, pruritus, swelling

Gastrointestinal: Diarrhea, nausea, toothache, vomiting

Neuromuscular & skeletal: Arthralgia, myalgia

Respiratory: Cough, nasal congestion, pharyngolaryngeal pain

Rare but important or life-threatening: Acute disseminated encephalomyelitis, alopecia areata, anaphylactic/anaphylactoid reaction, appendicitis, arrhythmia, arthritis, asthma, autoimmune hemolytic anemia and other autoimmune diseases, bronchospasm, cellulitis, cerebrovascular accident, chills, DVT, fatigue, gastroenteritis, Guillain-Barré syndrome, hypersensitivity reaction, hyper-/hypothyroidism, injection site joint movement impairment, ITP, JIA, lymphadenopathy, motor neuron disease, pancreatitis, paralysis, pelvic inflammatory disease, pulmonary embolus, RA, renal failure (acute), seizure, sepsis, syncope (may result in falls with injury or be associated with tonic-clonic movements), transverse myelitis, urticaria, weakness

Drug Interactions

Metabolism/Transport Effects None known.

Avoid Concomitant Use There are no known interactions where it is recommended to avoid concomitant use.

Increased Effect/Toxicity There are no known significant interactions involving an increase in effect.

Decreased Effect

The levels/effects of Papillomavirus (Types 6, 11, 16, 18) Vaccine (Human, Recombinant) may be decreased by: Belimumab; Fingolimod; Immunosuppressants

Storage/Stability Store refrigerated at 2°C to 8°C (36°F to 46°F). Do not freeze. Protect from light. Administer as soon as possible after removing it from refrigeration; can be out of refrigeration (at temperatures at or below 25°C [77°F]) for a total time of not more than 72 hours.

Mechanism of Action Contains inactive human papillomavirus (HPV) proteins HPV 6 L1, HPV 11 L1, HPV 16 L1

and HPV 18 L1 which produce neutralizing antibodies to prevent cervical cancer, cervical adenocarcinoma, cervical, vaginal and vulvar neoplasia, and genital warts caused by HPV. The vaccine has not been shown to provide cross-protective efficacy to HPV types not contained in the vaccine. Immunogenicity has been measured by the percentage of persons who became seropositive for antibodies contained in the vaccine; the minimum anti-HPV antibody concentration needed to protect against disease has not been determined. The population benefit to vaccination is influenced by the prevalence of HPV within the geographic area and subject characteristics (eg, lifetime sexual partners).

Efficacy: Vaccination with HPV4 reduced the incidence of CIN 2/3 and AIS by 98% to 100% in several randomized clinical trials. Efficacy against vulvar or vaginal intraepithelial neoplasia grades 2/3 was 100%. Against HPV 6- and 11-related genital warts, HPV4 vaccination reduced incidence in women by 99% in several clinical trials. In men and boys, HPV4 vaccination reduced the incidence of the following end points: external genital warts, 89% penile intraepithelial neoplasia of any severity, 100%; anal intraepithelial neoplasia (AIN) of any severity, 78%. (CDC/ACIP [Markowitz 2014])

Pharmacodynamics

Onset of action: Peak seroconversion was observed 1 month following the last dose of vaccine

Duration: Not well defined; at least 5 years

Dosing: Usual

Pediatric:

Primary immunization:

CDC (ACIP) recommended immunization schedule: Children ≥9 years and Adolescents: IM: 0.5 mL per dose for a total of 3 doses administered as follows: Initial dose followed by a second dose at 1 to 2 months after initial and third doses at 6 months after the initial.

Administer first dose at age 11 to 12 years although series may be initiated as early as 9 years of age. Minimum interval between first and second doses is 4 weeks; the minimum interval between the second and third dose is 12 weeks (16 weeks preferred); the minimum interval between first and third doses is 24 weeks. If the dose is given in an interval shorter than recommended, the dose should be repeated. The HPV vaccine series should be completed with the same product whenever possible (CDC/ACIP [Markowitz, 2014]; CDC/ACIP [Strikas 2015]).

Manufacturer's labeling: Children ≥9 years and Adolescents: IM: 0.5 mL per dose for a total of 3 doses; administer the second and third doses at 2 and 6 months after initial dose

Catch-up immunization: CDC (ACIP) recommendations (Strikas 2015): **Note:** Do not restart the series. If doses have been given, begin the below schedule at the applicable dose number. IM: 0.5 mL per dose for a total of 3 doses in females ages 13 to 26 years or males 13 through 18 years who were not previously vaccinated, administered as follows:

First dose given on the elected date

Second dose given at least 4 weeks after the first dose

Third dose given at 16 weeks after the second dose (minimum interval: 12 weeks) and at least 24 weeks after the first dose

Adult: **Immunization:**

CDC (ACIP) recommended immunization schedule: IM: 0.5 mL per dose for a total of 3 doses administered as follows: Initial dose followed by a second and third dose at 1 to 2 months and 6 months after the first dose. Begin series in females ≤26 years or males ≤21 years if not previously vaccinated or have not completed the 3-dose series (typically administer first dose at age 11 to 12 years). Vaccination for males 22 through 26 years of age is recommended if immunocompromised (including HIV) and for men who have sex with men and may be considered for any other male in this age group. Administer the second and third doses at 1 to 2 months and 6 months after the first dose. Minimum interval between first and second doses is 4 weeks; the minimum interval between the second and third dose is 12 weeks (16 weeks preferred); the minimum interval between first and third doses is 24 weeks. Inadequate doses or doses received following a shorter than recommended dosing interval should be repeated. Second and third doses may be given after age 26 years to complete a previously initiated series. The HPV vaccine series should be completed with the same product whenever possible (CDC/ACIP [Kim 2015]; CDC/ACIP [Markowitz, 2014]).

Manufacturer's labeling: Adults ≤26 years: IM: 0.5 mL per dose for a total of 3 doses; administer the second and third doses at 2 and 6 months after initial dose

Dosage adjustment in renal impairment: There are no dosage adjustments provided in the manufacturer's labeling.

Dosage adjustment in hepatic impairment: There are no dosage adjustments provided in the manufacturer's labeling.

Administration IM: Shake suspension well prior to use; do not use suspension if it is discolored or contains particulate matter; do not dilute or mix with other vaccines. Administer IM into the deltoid region of the upper arm or in the higher anterolateral area of the thigh; **not for IV, intradermal, or SubQ administration**. To prevent syncope related injuries, adolescents and adults should be vaccinated while seated or lying down (NCIRD/ACIP 2011). U.S. law requires that the date of administration, the vaccine manufacturer, lot number of vaccine, and the administering person's name, title and address be entered into the patient's permanent medical record.

For patients at risk of hemorrhage following intramuscular injection, the vaccine should be administered intramuscularly if, in the opinion of the physician familiar with the patient's bleeding risk, the vaccine can be administered by this route with reasonable safety. If the patient receives antihemophilia or other similar therapy, intramuscular vaccination can be scheduled shortly after such therapy is administered. A fine needle (23 gauge or smaller) can be used for the vaccination and firm pressure applied to the site (without rubbing) for at least 2 minutes. The patient should be instructed concerning the risk of hematoma from the injection. Patients on anticoagulant therapy should be considered to have the same bleeding risks and treated as those with clotting factor disorders (NCIRD/ACIP 2011).

Monitoring Parameters Screening for HPV is not required prior to vaccination. Observe for syncope for 15 minutes following administration (NCIRD/ACIP 2011). If seizure-like activity associated with syncope occurs, maintain patient in supine or Trendelenburg position to reestablish adequate cerebral perfusion.

Females: Gynecologic screening exam, papillomavirus test; screening for cervical cancer should continue per current guidelines following vaccination

Additional Information Comparison of HPV vaccines: Cervarix and Gardasil are both vaccines formulated to protect against infection with the human papillomavirus. Both are inactive vaccines which contain proteins HPV16 L1 and HPV 18 L1, the cause of >70% of invasive cervical cancer. The vaccines differ in that Gardasil also contains HPV 6 L1 and HPV 11 L1 proteins which protect against 75% to 90% of genital warts. The vaccines also differ in their preparation and adjuvants used. The viral proteins in Cervarix are prepared using *Trichoplusia ni* (insect cells) which are adsorbed onto an aluminum salt which is also combined with a monophosphoryl lipid. The viral proteins in Gardasil are prepared using *S. cerevisiae* (baker's yeast) which are then adsorbed onto an aluminum salt. Results from a short-term study (measurements obtained 1 month following the third vaccination in the series) have shown that the immune response to HPV 16 and HPV 18 may be greater with Cervarix; although the clinical significance of this difference is not known, local adverse events may also occur more frequently with this preparation. Both vaccines were effective and results from long-term studies are pending (Einstein, 2009).

Dosage Forms Excipient information presented when available (limited, particularly for generics); consult specific product labeling.

Injection, suspension [preservative free]:

Gardasil: HPV 6 L1 protein 20 mcg, HPV 11 L1 protein 40 mcg, HPV 16 L1 protein 40 mcg, and HPV 18 L1 protein 20 mcg per 0.5 mL (0.5 mL) [contains aluminum, polysorbate 80; manufactured using *S. cerevisiae* (baker's yeast)]

Papillomavirus (Types 16, 18) Vaccine (Human, Recombinant)

(pap ih LO ma VYE rus typs SIX teen AYE teen vak SEEN YU man ree KOM be nant)

Medication Safety Issues

Sound-alike/look-alike issues:

Papillomavirus vaccine types 16, 18 (Cervarix) may be confused with Papillomavirus vaccine types 6, 11, 16, 18 (Gardasil)

Cervarix may be confused with Cerebyx, CeleBREX

Related Information

Centers for Disease Control and Prevention (CDC) and Other Links *on page 2424*

Immunization Administration Recommendations *on page 2411*

Immunization Schedules *on page 2416*

Brand Names: US Cervarix

Brand Names: Canada Cervarix

Therapeutic Category Vaccine; Vaccine, Inactivated (Viral)

Generic Availability (US) No

Use

Prevention of cervical cancer and cervical intraepithelial neoplasia with or without cervical adenocarcinoma in situ caused by Human Papillomavirus (HPV) types 16 and 18 (FDA approved in girls ≥9 years and women ≤25 years of age)

The Advisory Committee on Immunization Practices (ACIP) recommends routine vaccination for females 11 to 12 years of age; may be started at 9 years of age; catch-up vaccination is recommended for females 13 to 26 years of age (CDC/ACIP [Markowitz 2014]; CDC/ACIP [Strikas 2015])

Medication Guide Available Yes

Pregnancy Risk Factor B

Pregnancy Considerations Adverse events were not observed in animal reproduction studies. In clinical trials, pregnancy testing was conducted prior to each vaccine administration and vaccination was discontinued if the woman was found to be pregnant; women were also instructed to avoid pregnancy for 2 months after receiving the vaccine. Pregnancies with vaccination within 1 month of their last menstrual period (LMP) had a higher rate of spontaneous abortions. The association between vaccination and spontaneous abortion occurring between gestation weeks 1 to 19 was evaluated in a postmarketing study. Women who were vaccinated within 1 month of their LMP were compared to women vaccinated 18 months prior to and 120 days after their LMP. The rate of spontaneous abortion was not statistically significant (HR 1.26, 95% CI 0.77 to 2.09). Based on available registry data, the rate of major birth defects is within the reported background rates (CDC/ACIP [Markowitz, 2014]).

Administration of the vaccine in pregnancy is not recommended; until additional information is available, the vaccine series (or completion of the series) should be delayed until pregnancy is completed. Pregnancy testing is not required prior to administration of the vaccine (CDC/ACIP [Petrosky, 2015]).

Breast-Feeding Considerations It is not known if this vaccine is excreted into breast milk. The manufacturer recommends that caution be exercised when administering papilloma virus vaccine to nursing women. Breast-feeding women may receive vaccine (CDC/ACIP [Markowitz, 2014]). Inactivated vaccines do not affect the safety of breast-feeding for the mother or the infant. Breast-feeding infants should be vaccinated according to the recommended schedules (NCIRD/ACIP, 2011).

Contraindications Severe hypersensitivity (eg, anaphylaxis) to papillomavirus recombinant vaccine or any component of the formulation

Warnings/Precautions Immediate treatment (including epinephrine 1:1000) for anaphylactoid and/or hypersensitivity reactions should be available during vaccine use (NCIRD/ACIP, 2011). The decision to administer or delay vaccination because of current or recent febrile illness depends on the severity of symptoms and the etiology of the disease. Consider deferring administration in patients with moderate or severe acute illness (with or without fever); vaccination should not be delayed for patients with mild acute illness (with or without fever) (NCIRD/ACIP, 2011). Vaccination may not result in effective immunity in all patients. Response depends upon multiple factors (eg type of vaccine, age of patient) and may be improved by administering the vaccine at the recommended dose, route, and interval. Vaccines may not be effective if administered during periods of altered immune competence (NCIRD/ACIP, 2011). Use with caution in patients with a history of bleeding disorders (including thrombocytopenia) and/or patients on anticoagulant therapy; bleeding/hematoma may occur from IM administration; if the patient receives antihemophilia or other similar therapy, IM injection can be scheduled shortly after such therapy is administered (NCIRD/ACIP, 2011). There is no evidence that individuals already exposed to or infected with HPV will be protected; those already infected with 1 or more HPV types were protected from disease in the remaining HPV types. Will not provide therapeutic benefit for active HPV disease or abnormal Pap test; will not protect against diseases not caused by HPV vaccine types 16 and 18. Use with caution in severely immunocompromised patients (eg, patients receiving chemo/radiation therapy or other immunosuppressive therapy [including high-dose corticosteroids]); may have a reduced response to vaccination. In general, household and close contacts of persons with altered immunocompetence may receive all age appropriate vaccines (IDSA [Rubin 2014]; NCIRD/ACIP, 2011); inactivated vaccines should be administered ≥2 weeks prior to planned immunosuppression when feasible (IDSA [Rubin, 2014]). Syncope has been reported with use of injectable vaccines and may result in serious secondary injury (e.g. skull fracture, cerebral hemorrhage); typically reported in adolescents and young adults and within 15 minutes after vaccination. Procedures should be in place to avoid injuries from falling and to restore cerebral perfusion if syncope occurs (NCIRD/ACIP, 2011).

Packaging may contain natural rubber/natural latex. Safety and efficacy have not been established in males. In order to maximize vaccination rates, the ACIP recommends simultaneous administration (ie, >1 vaccine on the same day at different anatomic sites) of all age-appropriate vaccines (live or inactivated) for which a person is eligible at a single clinic visit, unless contraindications exist. The

ACIP prefers each dose of a specific vaccine in a series come from the same manufacturer when possible (NCIRD/ACIP, 2011). Use of this vaccine for specific medical and/or other indications (eg, immunocompromising conditions, hepatic or kidney disease, diabetes) is also addressed in the ACIP Adult Recommended Immunization Schedule (CDC/ACIP [Kim, 2015]). Specific recommendations for use of this vaccine in immunocompromised patients with asplenia, cancer, HIV infection, cerebrospinal fluid leaks, cochlear implants, hematopoietic stem cell transplant (prior to or after), sickle cell disease, solid organ transplant (prior to or after), or those receiving immunosuppressive therapy for chronic conditions are available from the IDSA (Rubin, 2014).

Adverse Reactions **All serious adverse reactions must be reported to the U.S. Department of Health and Human Services (DHHS) Vaccine Adverse Event Reporting System (VAERS) 1-800-822-7967 or online at https://vaers.hhs.gov/esub/index.** In Canada, adverse reactions may be reported to local provincial/territorial health agencies or to the Vaccine Safety Section at Public Health Agency of Canada (1-866-844-0018).

Central nervous system: Fatigue

Dermatologic: Urticaria

Local: Injection site reactions: Pain, pruritus, redness, swelling

Neuromuscular & skeletal: Arthralgia, myalgia

Respiratory: Nasopharyngitis, pharyngitis, pharyngolaryngeal pain, upper respiratory tract infection

Miscellaneous: Chlamydia infection, influenza, vaginal infection

Rare but important or life-threatening: Allergic reactions, anaphylactic/anaphylactoid reactions, angioedema, erythema multiforme, lymphadenopathy, syncope (may be associated with tonic-clonic movements), vasovagal response

Drug Interactions

Metabolism/Transport Effects None known.

Avoid Concomitant Use There are no known interactions where it is recommended to avoid concomitant use.

Increased Effect/Toxicity There are no known significant interactions involving an increase in effect.

Decreased Effect

The levels/effects of Papillomavirus (Types 16, 18) Vaccine (Human, Recombinant) may be decreased by: Belimumab; Fingolimod; Immunosuppressants

Storage/Stability

U.S. labeling: Store under refrigeration at 2°C to 8°C (36°F to 46°F); do not freeze; discard if frozen. May develop a fine, white deposit with a clear, colorless supernatant during storage (not a sign of deterioration).

Canadian labeling: Store under refrigeration at 2°C to 8°C (36°F to 46°F); do not freeze; discard if frozen. Vaccine can be administered if stored between 8°C and 25°C (46°F to 77°F) for up to 3 days or stored between 25°C and 37°C (77°F to 98.6°F) for up to 1 day. Discard vaccine if exposed to temperatures >37°C (98.6°F). Protect from light.

Mechanism of Action Contains inactive human papillomavirus (HPV) proteins HPV 16 L1, and HPV 18 L1 which produce neutralizing antibodies to prevent cervical cancer, cervical adenocarcinoma, and cervical neoplasia cause by HPV.

Efficacy: Moderate- to high-grade cervical intraepithelial neoplasia (CIN 2/3) and adenocarcinoma in situ (AIS) are the immediate and necessary precursors of squamous cell carcinoma and adenocarcinoma of the cervix, respectively. Vaccination with HPV2 reduced the incidence of CIN 2/3 and AIS by 87% to 98% in several randomized clinical trials (CDC/ACIP [Markowitz, 2014]).

Pharmacodynamics

Onset of action: Peak seroconversion was observed 1 month following the last dose of vaccine

Duration: Not well defined; >5 years

Dosing: Usual

Pediatric:

Primary immunization:

CDC (ACIP) recommendations: Female only: Children ≥9 years and Adolescents: IM: 0.5 mL per dose for a total of 3 doses administered as follows: Initial dose followed by a second dose at 1 to 2 months after initial and third dose at 6 months after the initial dose. Administer first dose to females at age 11 to 12 years although series may be initiated as early as 9 years of age. Minimum interval between the first and second dose is 4 weeks; minimum interval between the second and third dose of vaccine is 12 weeks (16 weeks preferred); minimum interval between first and third dose is 24 weeks. If the dose is given in an interval shorter than recommended, the dose should be repeated. The HPV vaccine series should be completed with the same product whenever possible (CDC/ACIP [Markowitz 2014]; CDC/ACIP [Strikas 2015]).

Manufacturer's labeling: Females: Children ≥9 years and Adolescents: IM: 0.5 mL per dose for a total of 3 doses. Administer the second and third doses at 1 and 6 months after initial dose.

Catch-up immunization: CDC (ACIP) recommendations (Strikas 2015): **Note:** Do not restart the series. If doses have been given, begin the below schedule at the applicable dose number. IM: 0.5 mL per dose for a total of 3 doses in females ages 13 to 18 years who are incompletely vaccinated or were not previously vaccinated, administered as follows:

First dose given on the elected date

Second dose given at least 4 weeks after the first dose

Third dose given at 16 weeks after the second dose (minimum interval: 12 weeks) and at least 24 weeks after the first dose

Adult: **Immunization:**

CDC (ACIP) recommendations: Begin series in females ≤26 years if not previously vaccinated or who have not completed the 3 dose series (typically administer first dose at age 11 to 12 years). If a female reaches 27 years of age before the vaccination series is complete, the remaining doses can be administered after age 26 years. Administer the second and third doses at 1 to 2 months and 6 months after the first dose. Minimum interval between first and second doses is 4 weeks; the minimum interval between the second and third dose is 12 weeks (16 weeks preferred); the minimum interval between first and third doses is 24 weeks. Inadequate doses or doses received following a shorter than recommended dosing interval should be repeated. The HPV vaccine series should be completed with the same product whenever possible (CDC/ACIP [Kim 2015]; CDC/ACIP [Markowitz 2014]).

Manufacturer's labeling: Females ≤25 years: IM: 0.5 mL per dose for a total of 3 doses. Administer the second and third doses at 1 and 6 months after initial dose.

Dosing adjustment in renal impairment: There are no dosage adjustments provided in the manufacturer's labeling.

Dosing adjustment in hepatic impairment: There are no dosage adjustments provided in the manufacturer's labeling.

Administration IM: Shake suspension well prior to use; do not use suspension if it is discolored or contains particulate matter; should be a homogenous, turbid, white suspension. Do not dilute or mix with other vaccines. Administer IM into the deltoid region of the upper arm; **not for IV, intradermal, or SubQ administration**. To prevent syncope related injuries, adolescents and adults should be vaccinated while seated or lying down (NCIRD/ACIP 2011). US law requires that the date of administration, the vaccine manufacturer, lot number of vaccine, and the administering person's name, title and address be entered into the patient's permanent medical record.

For patients at risk of hemorrhage following intramuscular injection, the vaccine should be administered intramuscularly if, in the opinion of the physician familiar with the patient's bleeding risk, the vaccine can be administered by this route with reasonable safety. If the patient receives antihemophilia or other similar therapy, intramuscular vaccination can be scheduled shortly after such therapy is administered. A fine needle (23 gauge or smaller) should be used for the vaccination and firm pressure on the site (without rubbing) for at least 2 minutes. The patient should be instructed concerning the risk of hematoma from the injection. Patients on anticoagulant therapy should be considered to have the same bleeding risks and treated as those with clotting factor disorders (NCIRD/ACIP 2011).

Monitoring Parameters Gynecologic screening exam, papillomavirus test as per current guidelines; screening for HPV is not required prior to vaccination and screening for cervical cancer should continue as recommended following vaccination (NCIRD/ACIP 2011). Observe for syncope for 15 minutes following administration. If seizure-like activity associated with syncope occurs, maintain patient in supine or Trendelenburg position to reestablish adequate cerebral perfusion.

Additional Information Comparison of HPV vaccines: Cervarix and Gardasil are both vaccines formulated to protect against infection with the human papillomavirus. Both are inactive vaccines which contain proteins HPV16 L1 and HPV 18 L1, the cause of >70% of invasive cervical cancer. The vaccines differ in that Gardasil also contains HPV 6 L1 and HPV 11 L1 proteins which protect against 75% to 90% of genital warts. The vaccines also differ in their preparation and adjuvants used. The viral proteins in Cervarix are prepared using *Trichoplusia ni* (insect cells) which are adsorbed onto an aluminum salt which is also combined with a monophosphoryl lipid. The viral proteins in Gardasil are prepared using *S. cerevisiae* (baker's yeast) which are then adsorbed onto an aluminum salt. Results from a short-term study (measurements obtained 1 month following the third vaccination in the series) have shown that the immune response to HPV 16 and HPV 18 may be greater with Cervarix; although the clinical significance of these differences is not known, local adverse events may also occur more frequently with this preparation. Both vaccines are effective and results from long-term studies are pending (Einstein 2009).

Dosage Forms Excipient information presented when available (limited, particularly for generics); consult specific product labeling.

Injection, suspension [preservative free]:

Cervarix: HPV 16 L1 protein 20 mcg and HPV 18 L1 protein 20 mcg per 0.5 mL (0.5 mL) [contains aluminum, natural rubber/natural latex in prefilled syringe; manufactured using *Trichoplusia ni* (insect cells)]

◆ **Papillomavirus Vaccine, Recombinant** *see* Papillomavirus (Types 6, 11, 16, 18) Vaccine (Human, Recombinant) *on page 1625*

◆ **Papillomavirus Vaccine, Recombinant** *see* Papillomavirus (Types 16, 18) Vaccine (Human, Recombinant) *on page 1628*

◆ **Paracetamol** *see* Acetaminophen *on page 44*

◆ **Parafon Forte DSC** *see* Chlorzoxazone *on page 447*

◆ **Paraplatin** *see* CARBOplatin *on page 374*

◆ **Parcaine [DSC]** *see* Proparacaine *on page 1785*

Paregoric (par e GOR ik)

Medication Safety Issues

Sound-alike/look-alike issues:

Camphorated tincture of opium is an error-prone synonym (mistaken as opium tincture)

Paregoric may be confused with Percogesic

High alert medication:

The Institute for Safe Medication Practices (ISMP) includes this medication among its list of drug classes which have a heightened risk of causing significant patient harm when used in error.

Administration issues:

Use care when prescribing opium products; paregoric contains the equivalent of morphine 0.4 mg/mL; opium tincture contains the equivalent of morphine 10 mg/mL and is 25 times more potent than paregoric.

Therapeutic Category Analgesic, Narcotic; Antidiarrheal

Generic Availability (US) Yes

Use Treatment of diarrhea (FDA approved in pediatric patients [age not specified] and adults); has also been used in management of neonatal abstinence syndrome (neonatal opioid withdrawal)

Pregnancy Risk Factor C

Pregnancy Considerations Animal reproduction studies have not been conducted. Paregoric contains morphine; refer to the Morphine (Systemic) monograph for additional information. In addition, this preparation contains large amounts of alcohol (47%).

Breast-Feeding Considerations Paregoric contains morphine, which is excreted into breast milk; refer to the Morphine (Systemic) monograph for additional information. In addition, this preparation contains large amounts of alcohol (47%). The manufacturer recommends that caution be used if administered to a nursing woman.

Contraindications

Hypersensitivity to morphine or any component of the formulation; diarrhea caused by poisoning until the toxic material is eliminated from the GI tract; convulsive states (eg, status epilepticus, tetanus, strychnine poisoning).

Documentation of allergenic cross-reactivity for opioids is limited. However, because of similarities in chemical structure and/or pharmacologic actions, the possibility of cross-sensitivity cannot be ruled out with certainty.

Warnings/Precautions May cause CNS depression, which may impair physical or mental abilities; patients must be cautioned about performing tasks which require mental alertness (eg, operating machinery or driving). May cause hypotension; use with caution in patients with hypovolemia, cardiovascular disease (including acute MI), or drugs which may exaggerate hypotensive effects (including phenothiazines or general anesthetics). Use with caution in patients with atrial flutter or other supraventricular tachycardias, respiratory compromise, severe hepatic or severe renal dysfunction, adrenal insufficiency, morbid obesity, severe prostatic hyperplasia, urinary stricture, head trauma, thyroid dysfunction, seizure disorder, or history of drug abuse or acute alcoholism. Avoid use in patients with CNS depression or coma as these patients are susceptible to intracranial effects of CO_2 retention. Use with caution in patients with biliary tract dysfunction including acute pancreatitis; use may cause constriction of sphincter of Oddi. May obscure diagnosis or clinical course of patients with acute abdominal conditions. Opium shares the toxic potential of opioid agonists, and usual precautions of opioid agonist therapy should be observed; tolerance or drug dependence may result from extended use. Concurrent use of agonist/antagonist analgesics may precipitate withdrawal symptoms and/or reduced analgesic efficacy in patients following prolonged therapy with mu opioid agonists. Abrupt discontinuation following prolonged use may also lead to withdrawal symptoms.

Additives in paregoric (eg, alcohol, benzoic acid, noscapine, and papaverine) may be harmful to neonates. Paregoric is no longer recommended as a source of morphine to treat neonatal abstinence syndrome in infants exposed to chronic opioids *in utero* (Dow, 2012; Hudack, 2012). Infants <3 months of age are more susceptible to respiratory depression; use with caution and generally in reduced doses in this age group. Use with caution in the elderly and debilitated patients; may be more sensitive to adverse effects. Do not confuse paregoric with opium tincture which is 25 times **more** potent. Contains ≤47% alcohol. Potentially significant interactions may exist, requiring dose or frequency adjustment, additional monitoring, and/or selection of alternative therapy.

Benzyl alcohol and derivatives: Some dosage forms may contain sodium benzoate/benzoic acid; benzoic acid (benzoate) is a metabolite of benzyl alcohol; large amounts of benzyl alcohol (≥99 mg/kg/day) have been associated with a potentially fatal toxicity ("gasping syndrome") in neonates; the "gasping syndrome" consists of metabolic acidosis, respiratory distress, gasping respirations, CNS dysfunction (including convulsions, intracranial hemorrhage), hypotension, and cardiovascular collapse (AAP, 1997; CDC, 1982); some data suggests that benzoate displaces bilirubin from protein binding sites (Ahlfors, 2001); avoid or use dosage forms containing benzyl alcohol derivative with caution in neonates. See manufacturer's labeling.

Warnings: Additional Pediatric Considerations Do not confuse paregoric with opium tincture which is 25 times more potent. Each 5 mL of paregoric contains 2 mg morphine equivalent, 0.02 mL anise oil, 20 mg benzoic acid, 20 mg camphor, 0.2 mL glycerin, and alcohol; final alcohol content 45%; paregoric also contains papaverine and noscapine; the excipients and additives in paregoric may be harmful to neonates; thus, paregoric is no longer recommended for treatment of neonatal absence syndrome (Dow 2012; Hudak 2012).

Adverse Reactions

Cardiovascular: Hypotension, peripheral vasodilation

Central nervous system: Central nervous system depression, depression, dizziness, drowsiness, drug dependence (physical and psychological), dysphoria, euphoria, headache, increased intracranial pressure, insomnia, malaise, restlessness, sedation

Dermatologic: Pruritus

Gastrointestinal: Anorexia, biliary tract spasm, constipation, nausea, stomach cramps, vomiting

Genitourinary: Decreased urine output, ureteral spasm

Hepatic: Increased liver enzymes

Hypersensitivity: Histamine release

Neuromuscular & skeletal: Weakness

Ophthalmic: Miosis

Respiratory: Respiratory depression

Rare but important or life-threatening: Hypogonadism (Brennan, 2013; Debono, 2011)

Drug Interactions

Metabolism/Transport Effects None known.

Avoid Concomitant Use

Avoid concomitant use of Paregoric with any of the following: Azelastine (Nasal); Eluxadoline; Mixed Agonist / Antagonist Opioids; Orphenadrine; Paraldehyde; Thalidomide

Increased Effect/Toxicity

Paregoric may increase the levels/effects of: Alcohol (Ethyl); Alvimopan; Azelastine (Nasal); CNS Depressants; Desmopressin; Diuretics; Eluxadoline; Hydrocodone; Methotrimeprazine; Metyrosine; Mirtazapine; Orphenadrine; Paraldehyde; Pramipexole; ROPINIRole; Rotigotine; Selective Serotonin Reuptake Inhibitors; Suvorexant; Thalidomide; Zolpidem

The levels/effects of Paregoric may be increased by: Amphetamines; Anticholinergic Agents; Antipsychotic Agents (Phenothiazines); Brimonidine (Topical); Cannabis; Doxylamine; Dronabinol; Droperidol; HydrOXYzine; Kava Kava; Magnesium Sulfate; Methotrimeprazine; Nabilone; Perampanel; Rufinamide; Sodium Oxybate; Succinylcholine; Tapentadol; Tetrahydrocannabinol

Decreased Effect

Paregoric may decrease the levels/effects of: Pegvisomant

The levels/effects of Paregoric may be decreased by: Ammonium Chloride; Mixed Agonist / Antagonist Opioids; Naltrexone

Storage/Stability Store at 15°C to 30°C (59°F to 86°F). Protect from light; avoid excessive heat. A sediment may deposit if exposed to low temperatures.

Mechanism of Action Increases smooth muscle tone in GI tract, decreases motility and peristalsis, diminishes digestive secretions

Pharmacokinetics (Adult data unless noted)

Metabolism: Hepatic

Elimination: In urine, primarily as morphine glucuronide conjugates and as parent compound (morphine, codeine, papaverine, etc)

Dosing: Neonatal Note: Paregoric oral liquid contains morphine 2 mg per 5 mL (0.4 mg/mL)

Neonatal abstinence syndrome: Note: Due to potential adverse effects from the excipients and additives, paregoric is no longer recommended for treatment of neonatal abstinence syndrome (Dow 2012; Hudak 2012). Full-term neonates: Oral: Initial: 0.1 mL/kg or 2 drops/kg with feedings every 3 to 4 hours; may increase dosage by 0.1 mL/kg or 2 drops/kg every 3 to 4 hours until withdrawal symptoms are controlled; it is rare to exceed 0.7 mL/dose. Stabilize withdrawal symptoms for 3 to 5 days, then gradually decrease the dosage (keeping the same dosing interval) over a 2- to 4-week period (AAP 1998; Kraus 2009; Levy 1993).

Dosing: Usual Note: Paregoric oral liquid contains morphine 2 mg per 5 mL (0.4 mg/mL)

Pediatric: **Diarrhea:** Children and Adolescents: Oral: 0.25 to 0.5 mL/kg 1 to 4 times/day; maximum dose: 10 mL/dose

Adult: **Diarrhea:** Oral: 5 to 10 mL 1 to 4 times daily

Dosing adjustment in renal impairment: There are no dosing adjustments provided in the manufacturer's labeling.

Dosing adjustment in hepatic impairment: There are no dosing adjustments provided in the manufacturer's labeling.

Administration Oral: Shake well before use.

Monitoring Parameters Respiratory rate, blood pressure, heart rate, level of sedation

Neonatal abstinence syndrome (opioid withdrawal; **Note:** Paregoric is no longer recommended): Monitor for resolution of withdrawal symptoms (such as irritability, high-pitched cry, stuffy nose, rhinorrhea, vomiting, poor feeding, diarrhea, sneezing, yawning, etc) and signs of over treatment (such as bradycardia, lethargy, hypotonia, irregular respirations, respiratory depression, etc); an abstinence scoring system (eg, Finnegan abstinence scoring system) can be used to more objectively assess neonatal opioid withdrawal symptoms and the need for dosage adjustment

Controlled Substance C-III

Dosage Forms Excipient information presented when available (limited, particularly for generics); consult specific product labeling.

Tincture, Oral:

Generic: 2 mg/5 mL (473 mL)

Paricalcitol (pah ri KAL si tole)

Medication Safety Issues

Sound alike/look alike issues:

Paricalcitol may be confused with calcitriol

Zemplar may be confused with zaleplon, Zelapar, zolpidem, ZyPREXA Zydis

Brand Names: US Zemplar

Brand Names: Canada Zemplar

Therapeutic Category Vitamin D Analog; Vitamin, Fat Soluble

Generic Availability (US) Yes

Use

IV: Prevention and treatment of secondary hyperparathyroidism associated with stage 5 chronic kidney disease (CKD) (FDA approved in children ≥5 years and adults)

Oral: Prevention and treatment of secondary hyperparathyroidism associated with stages 3 and 4 chronic kidney disease (CKD) and stage 5 CKD patients on hemodialysis or peritoneal dialysis (FDA approved in adults)

Pregnancy Risk Factor C

Pregnancy Considerations Adverse events were observed in some animal reproduction studies.

Breast-Feeding Considerations It is not known if paricalcitol is excreted in breast milk. Due to the potential for serious adverse reactions in the nursing infant, a decision should be made whether to discontinue nursing or to discontinue the drug, taking into account the importance of treatment to the mother.

Contraindications Hypersensitivity to paricalcitol or any component of the formulation; patients with evidence of vitamin D toxicity; hypercalcemia

Warnings/Precautions Excessive administration may lead to over suppression of PTH, hypercalcemia, hypercalciuria, hyperphosphatemia and adynamic bone disease. Acute hypercalcemia may increase risk of cardiac arrhythmias and seizures; use caution with cardiac glycosides as digitalis toxicity may be increased. Chronic hypercalcemia may lead to generalized vascular and other soft-tissue calcification. Phosphate and vitamin D (and its derivatives) should be withheld during therapy to avoid hypercalcemia. Risk of hypercalcemia may be increased by concomitant use of calcium-containing supplements and/or medications that increase serum calcium (eg, thiazide diuretics). Avoid regular administration of aluminum-containing preparations (eg, antacids, phosphate binders) to prevent aluminum overload and bone toxicity. Dialysate concentration of aluminum should be maintained at <10 mcg/L.

Warnings: Additional Pediatric Considerations Some dosage forms may contain propylene glycol; in neonates large amounts of propylene glycol delivered orally, intravenously (eg, >3,000 mg/day), or topically have been associated with potentially fatal toxicities which can include metabolic acidosis, seizures, renal failure, and CNS depression; toxicities have also been reported in children and adults including hyperosmolality, lactic acidosis, seizures, and respiratory depression; use caution (AAP, 1997; Shehab, 2009).

Adverse Reactions

Cardiovascular: Chest pain, edema, hypertension, hypotension, palpitations, peripheral edema, syncope

Central nervous system: Anxiety, chills, depression, dizziness, fatigue, headache, insomnia, malaise, pain, vertigo

Dermatologic: Dermal ulcer, ecchymoses, skin rash

Endocrine & metabolic: Dehydration, hypervolemia, hypoglycemia

Gastrointestinal: Abdominal pain, constipation, diarrhea, dyspepsia, gastrointestinal hemorrhage, nausea, peritonitis, vomiting, xerostomia

Genitourinary: Uremia, urinary tract infection

Hypersensitivity: Hypersensitivity reaction

Infection: Infection (bacterial, fungal, viral), influenza, sepsis

Neuromuscular & skeletal: Arthralgia, arthritis, back pain, leg cramps, muscle spasm, weakness

Respiratory: Bronchitis, cough, nasopharyngitis, oropharyngeal pain, pneumonia, rhinitis, sinusitis

Miscellaneous: Fever

Rare but important or life-threatening:Abnormal gait, abnormal hepatic function tests, anemia, angioedema (including laryngeal edema), atrial flutter, burning sensation of skin, cardiac arrest, cardiac arrhythmia, cerebrovascular accident, confusion, conjunctivitis, delirium, dysphagia, erectile dysfunction, extravasation reactions, gastritis, gastroesophageal reflux disease, glaucoma, hirsutism, hypercalciuria, hypercalcemia, hyperparathyroidism, hyperkalemia, hyperphosphatemia, hypocalcemia, hypoparathyroidism, increased serum creatinine, ischemic bowel disease, lymphadenopathy, malignant neoplasm of breast, myalgia, myoclonus, night sweats, ocular hyperemia, orthopnea, paresthesia, prolonged bleeding time, pruritus, pulmonary edema, rectal hemorrhage, upper respiratory tract infection, urticaria, vaginal infection, weight loss, wheezing

Drug Interactions

Metabolism/Transport Effects Substrate of CYP3A4 (minor); **Note:** Assignment of Major/Minor substrate status based on clinically relevant drug interaction potential

Avoid Concomitant Use

Avoid concomitant use of Paricalcitol with any of the following: Aluminum Hydroxide; Multivitamins/Fluoride (with ADE); Multivitamins/Minerals (with ADEK, Folate, Iron); Sucralfate; Vitamin D Analogs

Increased Effect/Toxicity

Paricalcitol may increase the levels/effects of: Aluminum Hydroxide; Cardiac Glycosides; Digoxin; Sucralfate; Vitamin D Analogs

The levels/effects of Paricalcitol may be increased by: Calcium Salts; CYP3A4 Inhibitors (Strong); Danazol; Multivitamins/Fluoride (with ADE); Multivitamins/Minerals (with ADEK, Folate, Iron); Thiazide Diuretics

Decreased Effect

The levels/effects of Paricalcitol may be decreased by: Bile Acid Sequestrants; Mineral Oil; Orlistat

Storage/Stability Store at 25°C (77°F); excursions permitted between 15°C to 30°C (59°F to 86°F).

Mechanism of Action Decreased renal conversion of vitamin D to its primary active metabolite (1,25-hydroxyvitamin D) in chronic renal failure leads to reduced activation of vitamin D receptor (VDR), which subsequently removes inhibitory suppression of parathyroid hormone (PTH) release; increased serum PTH (secondary hyperparathyroidism) reduces calcium excretion and enhances bone resorption. Paricalcitol is a synthetic vitamin D analog which binds to and activates the VDR in kidney, parathyroid gland, intestine and bone, thus reducing PTH levels and improving calcium and phosphate homeostasis.

Pharmacokinetics (Adult data unless noted)

Distribution: V_d:

Healthy subjects: Oral: 34 L; IV: 24 L

Stage 3 and 4 CKD: Oral: 44-46 L

Stage 5 CKD: Oral: 38-49 L; IV: 31-35 L

Protein binding: >99%

Metabolism: Hydroxylation and glucuronidation via hepatic and nonhepatic enzymes, including CYP24, CYP3A4, UGT1A4; forms metabolites (at least one active)

Bioavailability: Oral: 72% to 86% in healthy subjects

Time to peak serum concentration: Oral: 3 hours

Half-life: Adults:

Healthy subjects: Oral: 4-6 hours; IV: 5-7 hours

Stage 3 and 4 CKD: Oral: 14-20 hours

Stage 5 CKD: Oral: 14-20 hours; IV: 14-15 hours

Elimination: Healthy subjects: Feces (Oral: 70%; IV: 63%); urine (Oral: 18%, IV: 19%); 51% to 59% as metabolites

Dosing: Usual In stage 3-5 CKD maintain Ca x P <55 mg^2/dL^2 (adults and children >12 years) or <65 mg^2/dL^2 (children <12 years), reduce or interrupt dosing if recommended Ca x P is exceeded or hypercalcemia is observed (K/DOQI Clinical Practice Guidelines, 2005).

Secondary hyperparathyroidism associated with chronic renal failure (stage 5 CKD): Children ≥5 years (limited small studies) and Adults: IV: 0.04-0.1 mcg/kg no more frequently than every other day; dose may be increased by 2-4 mcg every 2-4 weeks (0.04-0.1 mcg/kg for children); doses as high as 0.24 mcg/kg (16.8 mcg) have been administered safely; children may require higher weight-based doses; 0.2 ± 0.7 mcg/kg/dose (Seeherunvong, 2006); the dose of paricalcitol should be adjusted based on serum intact parathyroid hormone (iPTH) levels, as follows:

Same or increasing iPTH level: Increase paricalcitol dose

iPTH level decreased by <30%: Increase paricalcitol dose

iPTH level decreased by >30% and <60%: Maintain paricalcitol dose

iPTH level decrease by >60%: Decrease paricalcitol dose

iPTH level 1.5-3 times upper limit of normal: Maintain paricalcitol dose

Adults: Oral: Initial dose, in mcg, based on baseline iPTH level divided by 80. Administer 3 times weekly; no more frequently than every other day. **Note:** To reduce the risk of hypercalcemia initiate only after baseline serum calcium has been adjusted to ≤9.5 mg/dL.

Dose titration: Titration dose (mcg) = most recent iPTH level (pg/ml) divided by 80

Note: In situations where monitoring of iPTH, calcium, and phosphorus occurs less frequently than once per week, a more modest initial and dose titration rate may be warranted: Modest titration dose (mcg) = Most recent iPTH level (pg/mL) divided by 100

Dosage adjustment for hypercalcemia or elevated Ca x P: Decrease calculated dose by 2-4 mcg. If further adjustment is required, dose should be reduced or interrupted until these parameters are normalized. If applicable, phosphate binder dosing may also be adjusted or withheld, or switch to a noncalcium-based phosphate binder

Secondary hyperparathyroidism associated with stage 3 and 4 CKD: Adults: Oral: Initial dose based on baseline serum iPTH:

iPTH ≤500 pg/mL: 1 mcg/day or 2 mcg 3 times/week*

iPTH >500 pg/mL: 2 mcg/day or 4 mcg 3 times/week*

*Do not administer 3 times/week regimen more frequently than every other day

Dosage adjustment based on iPTH level relative to baseline, adjust dose at 2-4 week intervals:

iPTH same or increased: Increase paricalcitol dose by 1 mcg/day or 2 mcg 3 times/week

iPTH decreased by <30%: Increase paricalcitol dose by 1 mcg/day or 2 mcg 3 times/week

iPTH decreased by ≥30% and ≤60%: Maintain paricalcitol dose

iPTH decreased by >60%: Decrease paricalcitol dose by 1 mcg/day* or 2 mcg 3 times/week

iPTH <60 pg/mL: Decrease paricalcitol dose by 1 mcg/day* or 2 mcg 3 times/week

*If patient is taking the lowest dose on an every other day regimen, but further dose reduction is needed, decrease dose to 1 mcg 3 times/week. If further dose reduction is required, withhold drug as needed and restart at a lower dose. If applicable, calcium-phosphate binder dosing may also be adjusted or withheld, or switch to noncalcium-based binder.

Dosage adjustment in hepatic impairment: Adjustment not needed for mild-to-moderate impairment. Paricalcitol has not been evaluated in severe hepatic impairment.

Administration

Oral: May be administered with or without food. With the 3 times/week dosing schedule, doses should not be given more frequently than every other day.

Parenteral: Administer undiluted as an IV bolus dose at anytime during dialysis. Doses should not be administered more often than every other day.

Monitoring Parameters Signs and symptoms of vitamin D intoxication

Serum calcium and phosphorus (closely monitor levels during dosage titration and after initiation of a strong CYP3A4 inhibitor):

IV: Twice weekly during initial phase, then at least monthly once dose established

Oral: At least every 2 weeks for 3 months or following dose adjustment, then monthly for 3 months, then every 3 months

Calcium phosphorus product (Ca x P): Maintain Ca x P <55 mg^2/dL^2 (adults and children >12 years) or <65 mg^2/dL^2 (children <12 years) in stage 3-5 CKD

Serum or plasma intact parathyroid hormone (iPTH): At least every 2 weeks for 3 months or following dose adjustment, then monthly for 3 months, then as per K/DOQI Guidelines below

Per Kidney Disease Outcome Quality Initiative Practice Guidelines - Children (K/DOQI, 2005):

Stage 3 CKD: iPTH every 6 months

Stage 4 CKD: iPTH every 3 months

Stage 5 CKD: iPTH every 3 months

Per Kidney Disease Outcome Quality Initiative Practice Guidelines - Adults (K/DOQI, 2003):

Stage 3 CKD: iPTH every 12 months

Stage 4 CKD: iPTH every 3 months

Stage 5 CKD: iPTH every 3 months

Reference Range Chronic kidney disease (CKD) is defined either as kidney damage or GFR <60 mL/minute/1.73 m^2 for ≥3 months); stages of CKD are described below:

CKD Stage 1: Kidney damage with normal or increased GFR; GFR ≥90 mL/minute/1.73 m^2

CKD Stage 2: Kidney damage with mild decrease in GFR; GFR 60-89 mL/minute/1.73 m^2

CKD Stage 3: Moderate decrease in GFR; GFR 30-59 mL/minute/1.73 m^2

CKD Stage 4: Severe decrease in GFR; GFR 15-29 mL/minute/1.73 m^2

CKD Stage 5: Kidney failure; GFR <15 mL/minute/1.73 m^2 or dialysis

Target range for iPTH:

Stage 2 CKD: Children: 35-70 pg/mL (3.85-7.7 pmol/L)

Children and Adults:

Stage 3 CKD: Children and Adults: 35-70 pg/mL (3.85-7.7 pmol/L)

Stage 4 CKD: Children and Adults: 70-110 pg/mL (7.7-12.1 pmol/L)

Stage 5 CKD:

Children: 200-300 pg/mL (22-33 pmol/L)

Adults: 150-300 pg/mL (16.5-33 pmol/L)

Serum phosphorous:

Stages 1-4 CKD: Children: At or above the age-appropriate lower limits and no higher than age-appropriate upper limits

Stage 3 and 4 CKD: Adults: ≥2.7 to <4.6 mg/dL (≥0.87 to <1.49 mmol/L)

Stage 5 CKD:

Children 1-12 years: 4-6 mg/dL (1.29-1.94 mmol/L)

Children >12 years and Adults: 3.5-5.5 mg/dL (1.13-1.78 mmol/L)

Test Interactions In predialysis patients, paricalcitol may increase serum creatinine and therefore decrease the estimated GFR (eGFR).

Dosage Forms Excipient information presented when available (limited, particularly for generics); consult specific product labeling.

Capsule, Oral:

Zemplar: 1 mcg, 2 mcg, 4 mcg [contains alcohol, usp]

Generic: 1 mcg, 2 mcg, 4 mcg

Solution, Intravenous:

Zemplar: 2 mcg/mL (1 mL); 5 mcg/mL (1 mL, 2 mL) [contains alcohol, usp, propylene glycol]

Generic: 2 mcg/mL (1 mL); 5 mcg/mL (1 mL, 2 mL)

- ◆ **Pariet (Can)** *see* RABEprazole *on page 1828*
- ◆ **Paripazole** *see* RABEprazole *on page 1828*
- ◆ **Parlodel** *see* Bromocriptine *on page 303*
- ◆ **Paroex** *see* Chlorhexidine Gluconate *on page 434*

Paromomycin (par oh moe MYE sin)

Brand Names: Canada Humatin

Therapeutic Category Amebicide

Generic Availability (US) Yes

Use Treatment of acute and chronic intestinal amebiasis due to susceptible *Entamoeba histolytica* (not effective in the treatment of extraintestinal amebiasis) (FDA approved in pediatric patients [age not specified] and adults); adjunctive management of hepatic coma (FDA approved in adults); has also been used for the treatment of cryptosporidial diarrhea

Pregnancy Considerations Paromomycin is poorly absorbed when given orally. Information related to the use of paromomycin in pregnancy is limited (Kreutner, 1981). Use may be considered for the treatment of giardiasis throughout pregnancy (Gardner, 2001) or cryptosporidiosis after the first trimester (DHHS, 2013) in pregnant women.

Breast-Feeding Considerations Paromomycin is poorly absorbed when given orally. Available information suggests that paromomycin may be used in nursing women when renal function is normal in both the mother and infant (Davidson, 2009).

Contraindications Hypersensitivity to paromomycin or any component of the formulation; intestinal obstruction

Warnings/Precautions Use with caution in patients with impaired renal function or ulcerative bowel lesions (may lead to renal toxicity due to inadvertent absorption). Prolonged use may result in fungal or bacterial superinfection, including *C. difficile*-associated diarrhea (CDAD) and pseudomembranous colitis; CDAD has been observed >2 months postantibiotic treatment. Use in the absence of proven (or strongly suspected) susceptible infection is unlikely to provide benefit and may increase the risk for drug-resistance.

Adverse Reactions

Gastrointestinal: Abdominal cramps, diarrhea, heartburn, nausea, vomiting

Rare but important or life-threatening: Enterocolitis (secondary), eosinophilia, ototoxicity, pruritus, rash, steatorrhea

Drug Interactions

Metabolism/Transport Effects None known.

Avoid Concomitant Use There are no known interactions where it is recommended to avoid concomitant use.

Increased Effect/Toxicity There are no known significant interactions involving an increase in effect.

Decreased Effect There are no known significant interactions involving a decrease in effect.

Storage/Stability Store at 20°C to 25°C (68°F to 77°F). Protect from moisture.

Mechanism of Action Acts directly on ameba; has antibacterial activity against normal and pathogenic organisms in the GI tract; interferes with bacterial protein synthesis by binding to 30S ribosomal subunits

Pharmacokinetics (Adult data unless noted)

Absorption: Poor from the GI tract

Elimination: Excreted unchanged in feces

Dosing: Usual

Pediatric:

Intestinal amebiasis *(Entamoeba histolytica)*: Infants, Children, and Adolescents: Oral: 25 to 35 mg/kg/day divided every 8 hours for 5 to 10 days; usual duration 7 days (*Red Book* [AAP 2015])

Cryptosporidial diarrhea: Limited data available: Adolescents with HIV: Oral: 500 mg 4 times daily for 14 to 21 days in combination with optimized ART (DHHS [adult] 2015)

***Dientamoeba fragilis* infection:** Limited data available: Infants, Children, and Adolescents: Oral: 25 to 35 mg/kg/day divided every 8 hours for 7 days (*Red Book* [AAP 2015]; Vandenberg 2007)

Adult:

Hepatic coma: Oral: 4,000 mg/day in divided doses for 5 to 6 days

Intestinal amebiasis *(Entamoeba histolytica)*: Oral: 25 to 35 mg/kg/day divided every 8 hours for 5 to 10 days

Dosing adjustment in renal impairment: There are no dosage adjustments provided in the manufacturer's labeling; however, dosage adjustment is unlikely needed due to low systemic absorption.

Dosing adjustment in hepatic impairment: There are no dosage adjustments provided in the manufacturer's labeling; however dosage adjustment is unlikely needed due to low systemic absorption.

Administration Oral: Administer with meals

Dosage Forms Excipient information presented when available (limited, particularly for generics); consult specific product labeling.

Capsule, Oral:

Generic: 250 mg

- ◆ **Paromomycin Sulfate** *see* Paromomycin *on page 1634*

PARoxetine (pa ROKS e teen)

Medication Safety Issues

Sound-alike/look-alike issues:

PARoxetine may be confused with FLUoxetine, PACLitaxel, piroxicam, pyridoxine, vortioxetine

Paxil may be confused with Doxil, PACLitaxel, Plavix, PROzac, Taxol

Pexeva may be confused with Lexiva

BEERS Criteria medication:

This drug may be potentially inappropriate for use in geriatric patients with a history of falls or fractures (Quality of evidence - high [moderate for SIADH]; Strength of recommendation - strong).

Related Information

Antidepressant Agents *on page 2257*

Oral Medications That Should Not Be Crushed or Altered *on page 2476*

Safe Handling of Hazardous Drugs *on page 2455*

Brand Names: US Brisdelle; Paxil; Paxil CR; Pexeva

Brand Names: Canada Apo-Paroxetine; Auro-Paroxetine; CO Paroxetine; Dom-Paroxetine; JAMP-Paroxetine; Mylan-Paroxetine; Novo-Paroxetine; Paxil; Paxil CR; PHL-Paroxetine; PMS-Paroxetine; Q-Paroxetine; ratio-Paroxetine; Riva-Paroxetine; Sandoz-Paroxetine; Teva-Paroxetine

Therapeutic Category Antidepressant, Selective Serotonin Reuptake Inhibitor (SSRI)

Generic Availability (US) May be product dependent

Use

Brisdelle: Treatment of moderate to severe vasomotor symptoms associated with menopause (FDA approved in adults)

Paxil: Treatment of major depressive disorder (MDD), panic disorder (with or without agoraphobia), obsessive-compulsive disorder (OCD), social anxiety disorder (social phobia), generalized anxiety disorder (GAD), and post-traumatic stress disorder (PTSD) (All indications: FDA approved in adults); has also been used for self-injurious behavior

Paxil CR: Treatment of major depressive disorder (MDD), panic disorder (with or without agoraphobia), social anxiety disorder (social phobia), and premenstrual dysphoric disorder (PMDD) (FDA approved in adults)

Pexeva: Treatment of major depressive disorder (MDD), obsessive-compulsive disorder (OCD), panic disorder (with or without agoraphobia), and generalized anxiety disorder (GAD) (FDA approved in adults)

Medication Guide Available Yes

Pregnancy Risk Factor D//X (product specific)

Pregnancy Considerations Studies in pregnant women have demonstrated a risk to the fetus. Paroxetine crosses the placenta. An increased risk of teratogenic effects, including cardiovascular defects, may be associated with maternal use of paroxetine or other SSRIs; however, available information is conflicting. Nonteratogenic effects in the newborn following SSRI/SNRI exposure late in the third trimester include respiratory distress, cyanosis, apnea, seizures, temperature instability, feeding difficulty, vomiting, hypoglycemia, hypo- or hypertonia, hyperreflexia, jitteriness, irritability, constant crying, and tremor. Symptoms may be due to the toxicity of the SSRIs/SNRIs or a discontinuation syndrome and may be consistent with serotonin syndrome associated with SSRI treatment. Persistent pulmonary hypertension of the newborn (PPHN) has also been reported with SSRI exposure. The long-term effects of *in utero* SSRI exposure on infant development and behavior are not known.

Due to pregnancy-induced physiologic changes, some pharmacokinetic parameters of paroxetine may be altered. The maternal CYP2D6 genotype also influences paroxetine plasma concentrations during pregnancy.

The manufacturer suggests discontinuing paroxetine or switching to another antidepressant unless the benefits of therapy justify continuing treatment during pregnancy; consider other treatment options for women who are planning to become pregnant. The ACOG recommends that therapy with SSRIs or SNRIs during pregnancy be individualized; treatment of depression during pregnancy should incorporate the clinical expertise of the mental health clinician, obstetrician, primary healthcare provider, and pediatrician. The ACOG also recommends that therapy with paroxetine be avoided during pregnancy if possible and that fetuses exposed in early pregnancy be assessed with a fetal echocardiography. According to the American Psychiatric Association (APA), the risks of medication treatment should be weighed against other treatment options and untreated depression. The use of paroxetine is not recommended as first line therapy during pregnancy. For women who discontinue antidepressant medications during pregnancy and who may be at high risk for postpartum depression, the medications can be restarted following delivery. Treatment algorithms have been developed by the ACOG and the APA for the management of depression in women prior to conception and during pregnancy. Menopausal vasomotor symptoms do not occur during pregnancy; therefore, the use of paroxetine for the treatment of menopausal vasomotor symptoms is contraindicated in pregnant women.

Breast-Feeding Considerations Paroxetine is excreted in breast milk and concentrations in the hindmilk are higher than in foremilk. Paroxetine has not been detected in the serum of nursing infants. Adverse reactions have been reported in nursing infants exposed to some SSRIs. The manufacturer recommends that caution be exercised when administering paroxetine to nursing women. Maternal use of an SSRI during pregnancy may cause delayed milk secretion. The American Academy of Breastfeeding Medicine suggests that paroxetine may be considered for the treatment of postpartum depression in appropriately selected women who are nursing. Mothers should be monitored for changes in symptoms and infants should be monitored for growth. The long-term effects on development and behavior have not been studied.

Contraindications Concurrent use with or within 14 days of MAOIs intended to treat psychiatric disorders; initiation in patients being treated with linezolid or methylene blue IV; concomitant use with pimozide or thioridazine; hypersensitivity to paroxetine or any of its inactive ingredients; pregnancy (Brisdelle only).

Warnings/Precautions Hazardous agent - use appropriate precautions for handling and disposal (NIOSH 2014 [group 3]). **[U.S. Boxed Warning]: Antidepressants increase the risk of suicidal thinking and behavior in children, adolescents, and young adults (18 to 24 years of age) with major depressive disorder (MDD) and other psychiatric disorders;** consider risk prior to prescribing. Short-term studies did not show an increased risk in patients >24 years of age and showed a decreased risk in patients ≥65 years. Closely monitor patients for clinical worsening, suicidality, or unusual changes in behavior, particularly during the initial 1 to 2 months of therapy or during periods of dosage adjustments (increases or decreases); the patient's family or caregiver should be instructed to closely observe the patient and communicate condition with healthcare provider. A medication guide concerning the use of antidepressants should be dispensed with each prescription. **Paroxetine is not FDA approved for use in children.**

The possibility of a suicide attempt is inherent in major depression and may persist until remission occurs. Use caution in high-risk patients. Worsening depression and severe abrupt suicidality that are not part of the presenting symptoms may require discontinuation or modification of drug therapy. The patient's family or caregiver should be alerted to monitor patients for the emergence of suicidality and associated behaviors (such as agitation, irritability, hostility, impulsivity, and hypomania) and call health care provider.

May worsen psychosis in some patients or precipitate a shift to mania or hypomania in patients with bipolar disorder. Patients presenting with depressive symptoms should be screened for bipolar disorder. Monotherapy in patients with bipolar disorder should be avoided. **Paroxetine is not FDA approved for the treatment of bipolar depression.**

Potentially life-threatening serotonin syndrome (SS) has occurred with serotonergic agents (eg, SSRIs, SNRIs), particularly when used in combination with other serotonergic agents (eg, triptans, TCAs, fentanyl, lithium, tramadol, buspirone, St John's wort, tryptophan) or agents that impair metabolism of serotonin (eg, MAO inhibitors intended to treat psychiatric disorders, other MAO inhibitors [ie, linezolid and intravenous methylene blue]). Discontinue treatment (and any concomitant serotonergic agent) immediately if signs/symptoms arise.

Paroxetine may increase the risks associated with electroconvulsive therapy. Has a low potential to impair cognitive or motor performance - use caution when operating hazardous machinery or driving. Symptoms of agitation and/or restlessness may occur during initial few weeks of therapy. Low potential for sedation or anticholinergic effects relative to cyclic antidepressants. Bone fractures have been associated with SSRI treatment. Consider the possibility of a fragility fracture if an SSRI-treated patient presents with unexplained bone pain, point tenderness, swelling, or bruising.

Use caution in elderly patients; may be potentially inappropriate in patients with a history of falls or fractures, and may cause or exacerbate syndrome of inappropriate antidiuretic hormone secretion or hyponatremia; monitor sodium closely with initiation or dosage adjustments in older adults. Medication associated with potent anticholinergic properties which may be inappropriate in older adults depending on comorbidities (eg, dementia, delirium) (Beers Criteria).

Use caution in patients with a previous seizure disorder or condition predisposing to seizures such as brain damage or alcoholism. Use with caution in patients with hepatic dysfunction. May cause SIADH; volume depletion and/or diuretics may increase risk. Potentially significant drug-drug interactions may exist, requiring dose or frequency adjustment, additional monitoring, and/or selection of alternative therapy. Use with caution in patients with renal insufficiency or other concurrent illness (due to limited experience); dose reduction recommended with severe renal impairment. May cause or exacerbate sexual dysfunction. May cause mild pupillary dilation, which can lead to an episode of narrow-angle glaucoma in susceptible individuals. Consider evaluating patients who have not had an iridectomy for narrow-angle glaucoma risk factors. Avoid use in the first trimester of pregnancy. Menopausal vasomotor symptoms do not occur during pregnancy; therefore, the use of paroxetine for the treatment of menopausal vasomotor symptoms is contraindicated in pregnant women.

Brisdelle contains a lower dose than what is required for the treatment of psychiatric conditions. Patients who require paroxetine for the treatment of psychiatric conditions should discontinue Brisdelle and begin treatment with a paroxetine-containing medication which provides an adequate dosage.

Abrupt discontinuation or interruption of antidepressant therapy has been associated with a discontinuation syndrome. Symptoms arising may vary with antidepressant however commonly include nausea, vomiting, diarrhea, headaches, lightheadedness, dizziness, diminished appetite, sweating, chills, tremors, paresthesias, fatigue, somnolence, and sleep disturbances (eg, vivid dreams, insomnia). Greater risks for developing a discontinuation syndrome have been associated with antidepressants with shorter half-lives, longer durations of treatment, and abrupt discontinuation. For antidepressants of short or intermediate half-lives, symptoms may emerge within 2 to 5 days after treatment discontinuation and last 7 to 14 days (APA, 2010; Fava, 2006; Haddod, 2001; Shelton, 2001; Warner, 2006).

Some dosage forms may contain polysorbate 80 (also known as Tweens). Hypersensitivity reactions, usually a delayed reaction, have been reported following exposure to pharmaceutical products containing polysorbate 80 in certain individuals (Isaksson, 2002; Lucente 2000; Shelley, 1995). Thrombocytopenia, ascites, pulmonary deterioration, and renal and hepatic failure have been reported in premature neonates after receiving parenteral products containing polysorbate 80 (Alade, 1986; CDC, 1984). See manufacturer's labeling.

Warnings: Additional Pediatric Considerations The FDA recommends that paroxetine not be used in pediatric patients for the treatment of depression. Three well-controlled trials in pediatric patients with depression have failed to show therapeutic superiority over placebo; in addition, an increased risk for suicidal behavior was observed in patients receiving paroxetine when compared to other SSRIs (Dopheide, 2006). SSRI-associated behavioral activation (ie, restlessness, hyperkinesis, hyperactivity, agitation) is two- to threefold more prevalent in children compared to adolescents; it is more prevalent in adolescents compared to adults. Somnolence (including sedation and drowsiness) is more common in adults compared to children and adolescents (Safer, 2006).

An SSRI discontinuation syndrome similar to that described in adults has been reported in six children (Diler, 2002). May cause abnormal bleeding (eg, ecchymosis, purpura, upper GI bleeding); use with caution in patients with impaired platelet aggregation and with concurrent use of aspirin, NSAIDs, or other drugs that affect coagulation. A recent report describes five children (age: 8 to 15 years) who developed epistaxis (n=4) or bruising (n=1) while receiving SSRI therapy (sertraline) (Lake, 2000). SSRI-associated vomiting is two- to threefold more prevalent in children compared to adolescents and is more prevalent in adolescents compared to adults (Safer, 2006).

Some dosage forms may contain propylene glycol; in neonates large amounts of propylene glycol delivered orally, intravenously (eg, >3,000 mg/day), or topically have been associated with potentially fatal toxicities which can include metabolic acidosis, seizures, renal failure, and CNS depression; toxicities have also been reported in children and adults including hyperosmolality, lactic acidosis, seizures, and respiratory depression; use caution (AAP, 1997; Shehab, 2009).

Adverse Reactions

Cardiovascular: Chest pain, hypertension, palpitations, tachycardia, vasodilatation

Central nervous system: Abnormal dreams, agitation, amnesia, anxiety, chills, confusion, depersonalization, dizziness, drowsiness, emotional lability, fatigue, headache, insomnia, lack of concentration, myasthenia, myoclonus, nervousness, paresthesia, vertigo, yawning

Dermatologic: Diaphoresis, pruritus, skin rash

Endocrine & metabolic: Decreased libido, dysmenorrhea, orgasm disturbance, weight gain

Gastrointestinal: Abdominal pain, constipation, decreased appetite, diarrhea, dysgeusia, dyspepsia, flatulence, increased appetite, nausea, vomiting, xerostomia

Genitourinary: Ejaculatory disorder, female genital tract disease, impotence, male genital disease, urinary frequency, urinary tract infection

Infection: Infection

Neuromuscular & skeletal: Arthralgia, back pain, myalgia, myopathy, tremor, weakness

Ophthalmic: Blurred vision, visual disturbance

Otic: Tinnitus

Respiratory: Dyspnea, pharyngitis, rhinitis, sinusitis

Rare but important or life-threatening: Abnormal hepatic function tests, acute angle-closure glaucoma, acute renal failure, adrenergic syndrome, agranulocytosis, akathisia, akinesia, anaphylactoid reaction, anaphylaxis, anemia (various), angina pectoris, angioedema, aphasia, aphthous stomatitis, aplastic anemia, asthma, atrial arrhythmia, atrial fibrillation, bilirubinemia, bloody diarrhea, bone marrow aplasia, bradycardia, bronchitis, bulimia nervosa, bundle branch block, cardiac failure, cataract, cellulitis, cerebral ischemia, cerebrovascular accident, change in platelet count, cholelithiasis, colitis, deafness, dehydration, delirium, depression, diabetes mellitus, disorientation, drug dependence, dyskinesia, dysphagia, dystonia, eclampsia, electrolyte disturbance, emphysema, esophageal achalasia, exfoliative dermatitis, extrapyramidal reaction, fecal impaction, fungal skin infection, gastroenteritis, glaucoma, goiter, Guillain-Barre syndrome, hallucination, hematemesis, hematologic abnormality, hematologic disease, hematoma, hemoptysis, hemorrhage, hemorrhagic pancreatitis, hepatic failure, hepatic necrosis, hepatitis, hepatotoxicity, homicidal ideation, hypercholesteremia, hypergammaglobulinemia, hyperglycemia, hyperhidrosis, hypersensitivity reaction, hyperthyroidism, hypoglycemia, hyponatremia, hypotension, hypothyroidism, immune thrombocytopenia, increased blood urea nitrogen, increased creatine phosphokinase, increased lactate dehydrogenase, increased serum alkaline phosphatase, intestinal obstruction, ischemic heart disease, jaundice, ketosis, low cardiac output, lymphadenopathy, meningitis, migraine, mydriasis, myelitis, myocardial infarction, neuroleptic malignant syndrome, neuropathy, osteoarthritis, osteoporosis, pancreatitis, pancytopenia, paralytic ileus, peptic ulcer, peritonitis, phlebitis, pneumonia, prolonged bleeding time, pulmonary edema, pulmonary embolism, pulmonary fibrosis, pulmonary hypertension, restlessness, seizure, sepsis, serotonin syndrome, spermatozoa disorder (activity altered, DNA fragmentation [abnormal] increased), status epilepticus, Stevens-Johnson syndrome, suicidal ideation, suicidal tendencies, syncope, tetany, thrombophlebitis, thrombosis, torsades de pointes, toxic epidermal necrolysis, uncontrolled diabetes mellitus, vasculitis, ventricular arrhythmia, ventricular fibrillation, ventricular tachycardia, withdrawal syndrome (including increased dreaming/nightmares, muscle cramps/spasms/twitching, headache, nervousness/anxiety, fatigue/tiredness, restless feeling in legs, and trouble sleeping/insomnia)

Drug Interactions

Metabolism/Transport Effects **Substrate** of CYP2D6 (major); **Note:** Assignment of Major/Minor substrate status based on clinically relevant drug interaction potential; **Inhibits** CYP1A2 (weak), CYP2B6 (moderate), CYP2C19 (weak), CYP2C9 (weak), CYP2D6 (strong)

Avoid Concomitant Use

Avoid concomitant use of PARoxetine with any of the following: Dapoxetine; Dosulepin; Iobenguane I 123; Linezolid; MAO Inhibitors; Mequitazine; Methylene Blue; Pimozide; Tamoxifen; Thioridazine; Tryptophan; Urokinase

Increased Effect/Toxicity

PARoxetine may increase the levels/effects of: Agents with Antiplatelet Properties; Anticoagulants; Antidepressants (Serotonin Reuptake Inhibitor/Antagonist); Antipsychotic Agents; Apixaban; ARIPiprazole; Asenapine; Aspirin; AtoMOXetine; Beta-Blockers; Blood Glucose Lowering Agents; BusPIRone; CarBAMazepine; CloZAPine; Collagenase (Systemic); CYP2B6 Substrates; CYP2D6 Substrates; Dabigatran Etexilate; Deoxycholic Acid; Desmopressin; Dextromethorphan; Dosulepin; DOXOrubicin (Conventional); DULoxetine; Eliglustat; Fesoterodine; Galantamine; Highest Risk QTc-Prolonging Agents; Ibritumomab; Iloperidone; Mequitazine; Methadone; Methylene Blue; Metoprolol; Mexiletine; Moderate Risk QTc-Prolonging Agents; Nebivolol; NSAID (COX-2 Inhibitor); NSAID (Nonselective); Obinutuzumab; Pimozide; Propafenone; Rivaroxaban; Salicylates; Serotonin Modulators; Tamsulosin; Tetrabenazine; Thiazide Diuretics; Thioridazine; Thrombolytic Agents; TiZANidine; Tositumomab and Iodine I 131 Tositumomab; TraMADol; Tricyclic Antidepressants; Urokinase; Vitamin K Antagonists; Vortioxetine

The levels/effects of PARoxetine may be increased by: Abiraterone Acetate; Alcohol (Ethyl); Analgesics (Opioid); Antiemetics (5HT3 Antagonists); Antipsychotic Agents; ARIPiprazole; Asenapine; BuPROPion; BusPIRone; Cimetidine; CNS Depressants; Cobicistat; CYP2D6 Inhibitors (Moderate); CYP2D6 Inhibitors (Strong); Dapoxetine; Dasatinib; DULoxetine; Glucosamine; Herbs (Anticoagulant/Antiplatelet Properties); Ibrutinib; Limaprost; Linezolid; Lithium; MAO Inhibitors; Metoclopramide; Metyrosine; Mifepristone; Multivitamins/Fluoride (with ADE); Multivitamins/Minerals (with ADEK, Folate, Iron); Multivitamins/Minerals (with AE, No Iron); Omega-3 Fatty Acids; Panobinostat; Peginterferon Alfa-2b; Pentosan Polysulfate Sodium; Pentoxifylline; Pravastatin; Prostacyclin Analogues; Tedizolid; TraMADol; Tryptophan; Vitamin E

Decreased Effect

PARoxetine may decrease the levels/effects of: Aprepitant; Codeine; Fosaprepitant; Hydrocodone; Iloperidone; Iobenguane I 123; Ioflupane I 123; Tamoxifen; Thyroid Products

The levels/effects of PARoxetine may be decreased by: Aprepitant; CarBAMazepine; Cyproheptadine; Darunavir; Fosamprenavir; Fosaprepitant; NSAID (COX-2 Inhibitor); NSAID (Nonselective); Peginterferon Alfa-2b

Food Interactions Peak concentration is increased, but bioavailability is not significantly altered by food. Management: Administer without regard to meals.

Storage/Stability

Capsules: Store between 20°C and 25°C (68°F and 77°F); excursions permitted between 15°C and 30°C (59°F and 86°F). Protect from light and humidity.

Tablets: Store immediate-release tablets between 15°C and 30°C (59°F and 86°F) and controlled-release tablets at or below 25°C (77°F).

Suspension: Store at or below 25°C (77°F).

Mechanism of Action Paroxetine is a selective serotonin reuptake inhibitor, chemically unrelated to tricyclic, tetracyclic, or other antidepressants; presumably, the inhibition of serotonin reuptake from brain synapse stimulated serotonin activity in the brain

Pharmacodynamics

Onset of action: Antidepressant effects: The onset of action is within a week; however, individual response varies greatly and full response may not be seen until 8-12 weeks after initiation of treatment.

Antiobsessional and antipanic effects: Up to several weeks

Pharmacokinetics (Adult data unless noted)

Absorption: Oral: Well absorbed

Distribution: V_d: Mean: 8.7 L/kg; range: 3-28 L/kg

Protein binding: 93% to 95%

Metabolism: Extensive by cytochrome P450 enzymes via oxidation and methylation followed by glucuronide and sulfate conjugation; nonlinear kinetics may be seen with higher doses and longer duration of therapy due to saturation of P450 2D6 (CYP2D6), an enzyme partially responsible for metabolism. **Note:** Paroxetine pharmacokinetics have not been studied in patients deficient in CYP2D6 (ie, poor metabolizers)

Bioavailability: Immediate release tablet and oral suspension have equal bioavailability

Half-life:

- Paxil: 21 hours
- Paxil CR: 15-20 hours
- Pexeva: 33.2 hours

Time to peak serum concentration:

- Immediate release capsule: Brisdelle: Median: 6 hours (range: 3-8 hours)
- Immediate release tablet:
  - Hydrochloride (Paxil): Mean: 5.2 hours
  - Mesylate (Pexeva): Mean: 8.1 hours
- Controlled release tablet: 6-10 hours

Elimination: Urine (64%; 2% as unchanged drug); feces (36% primarily via bile, <1% as unchanged drug)

Dosing: Usual Note: For maintenance therapy, use lowest effective dose and periodically reassess need for continued treatment

Pediatric:

Obsessive-compulsive disorder (OCD): Limited data available: Children and Adolescents 7 to 17 years: Oral: Initial: 10 mg once daily; titrate every 7 to 14 days in

10 mg/day increments; maximum daily dose: 60 mg/**day**. Dosing based on two trials. The first was a 12-week open-label trial of paroxetine in 20 outpatients 8 to 17 years of age that demonstrated the potential clinical usefulness in pediatric OCD (Rosenberg 1999). The second trial demonstrated efficacy of paroxetine in a 10-week, randomized, double-blind, placebo-controlled trial conducted in 207 pediatric patients (aged 7 to 17 years) with OCD; the overall mean dose was 20.3 mg/day for children and 26.8 mg/day for adolescents (Geller 2004).

Social anxiety disorder: Children and Adolescents 8 to 17 years: Oral: Initial: 10 mg once daily; titrate at intervals of at least 7 days in 10 mg/day increments; maximum daily dose: 50 mg/**day**. Dosing based on a 16-week multicenter, randomized, double-blind, placebo-controlled trial that reported the efficacy of paroxetine in pediatric patients (aged 8 to 17 years) with social anxiety disorder; 163 patients were randomized to receive paroxetine; the overall mean dose was 21.7 mg/day for children and 26.1 mg/day for adolescents (Wagner 2004).

Adult:

Major depressive disorder (MDD): Oral:

Paxil, Pexeva: Initial: 20 mg once daily, preferably in the morning; increase if needed by 10 mg/day increments at intervals of at least 1 week; maximum daily dose: 50 mg/**day**

Paxil CR: Initial: 25 mg once daily; increase if needed by 12.5 mg/day increments at intervals of at least 1 week; maximum daily dose: 62.5 mg/**day**

Generalized anxiety disorder (GAD): Paxil, Pexeva: Oral: Initial: 20 mg once daily, preferably in the morning; if dose is increased, adjust in increments of 10 mg/day at 1-week intervals; doses of 20-50 mg/day were used in clinical trials; however, no greater benefit was seen with doses >20 mg.

Obsessive compulsive disorder (OCD): Paxil, Pexeva: Oral: Initial: 20 mg once daily, preferably in the morning; increase if needed by 10 mg/day increments at intervals of at least 1 week; recommended dose: 40 mg/day; range: 20 to 60 mg/day; maximum daily dose: 60 mg/**day**

Panic disorder: Oral:

Paxil, Pexeva: Initial: 10 mg once daily, preferably in the morning; increase if needed by 10 mg/day increments at intervals of at least 1 week; recommended dose: 40 mg/day; range: 10 to 60 mg/day; maximum daily dose: 60 mg/**day**

Paxil CR: Initial: 12.5 mg once daily, preferably in the morning; increase if needed by 12.5 mg/day increments at intervals of at least 1 week; maximum daily dose: 75 mg/**day**

Post-traumatic stress disorder (PTSD): Paxil: Oral: Initial: 20 mg once daily, preferably in the morning; increase if needed by 10 mg/day increments at intervals of at least 1 week; range: 20 to 50 mg/day. Limited data suggest doses of 40 mg/day were not more efficacious than 20 mg/day.

Premenstrual dysphoric disorder: Paxil CR: Oral: Initial: 12.5 mg once daily in the morning; may be increased to 25 mg/day; dosing changes should occur at intervals of at least 1 week; may be given daily throughout the menstrual cycle **or** limited to the luteal phase

Social anxiety disorder: Oral:

Paxil: Initial: 20 mg once daily, preferably in the morning; recommended dose: 20 mg/day; range: 20 to 60 mg/day; doses >20 mg may not have additional benefit

Paxil CR: Initial: 12.5 mg once daily, preferably in the morning; may be increased by 12.5 mg/day increments at intervals of at least 1 week; maximum daily dose: 37.5 mg/**day**

Vasomotor symptoms of menopause: Brisdelle: Oral: 7.5 mg once daily at bedtime.

Discontinuation of therapy: Upon discontinuation of antidepressant therapy, gradually taper the dose to minimize the incidence of withdrawal symptoms and allow for the detection of reemerging symptoms. Evidence supporting ideal taper rates is limited. APA and NICE guidelines suggest tapering therapy over at least several weeks with consideration to the half-life of the antidepressant; antidepressants with a shorter half-life may need to be tapered more conservatively. In addition, for long-term treated patients, WFSBP guidelines recommend tapering over 4-6 months. If intolerable withdrawal symptoms occur following a dose reduction, consider resuming the previously prescribed dose and/or decrease dose at a more gradual rate (APA 2010; Bauer 2002; Haddod 2001; NCCMH 2010; Schatzberg 2006; Shelton 2001; Warner 2006).

MAO inhibitor recommendations:

Switching to or from an MAO inhibitor intended to treat psychiatric disorders:

Allow 14 days to elapse between discontinuing an MAO inhibitor intended to treat psychiatric disorders and initiation of paroxetine.

Allow 14 days to elapse between discontinuing paroxetine and initiation of an MAO inhibitor intended to treat psychiatric disorders.

Use with other MAO inhibitors (linezolid or IV methylene blue):

Do not initiate paroxetine in patients receiving linezolid or IV methylene blue; consider other interventions for psychiatric condition.

If urgent treatment with linezolid or IV methylene blue is required in a patient already receiving paroxetine and potential benefits outweigh potential risks, discontinue paroxetine promptly and administer linezolid or IV methylene blue. Monitor for serotonin syndrome for 2 weeks or until 24 hours after the last dose of linezolid or IV methylene blue, whichever comes first. May resume paroxetine 24 hours after the last dose of linezolid or IV methylene blue.

Dosing adjustment in renal impairment: Adults:

Brisdelle: No dosage adjustments necessary

Paxil, Paxil CR, Pexeva:

CrCl >60 mL/minute: No dosage adjustment necessary

CrCl 30 to 60 mL/minute: Plasma concentration is 2 times that seen in normal function. There are no dosage adjustments provided in manufacturer's labeling.

Severe impairment (CrCl <30 mL/minute): Mean plasma concentration is ~4 times that seen in normal function.

Paxil, Pexeva: Initial: 10 mg/day; increase if needed by 10 mg/day increments at intervals of at least 1 week; maximum dose: 40 mg/day

Paxil CR: Initial: 12.5 mg/day; increase if needed by 12.5 mg/day increments at intervals of at least 1 week; maximum dose: 50 mg/day

Dosing adjustment in hepatic impairment: Adults:

Brisdelle: No dosage adjustments necessary.

Paxil, Paxil CR, Pexeva:

Mild to moderate impairment: There are no dosage adjustments provided in manufacturer's labeling.

Severe impairment:

Paxil, Pexeva: Initial: 10 mg/day; increase if needed by 10 mg/day increments at intervals of at least 1 week; maximum dose: 40 mg/day

Paxil CR: Initial: 12.5 mg/day; increase if needed by 12.5 mg/day increments at intervals of at least 1 week; maximum dose: 50 mg/day

Administration Hazardous agent; use appropriate precautions for handling and disposal (NIOSH 2014 [group 3]). May be administered without regard to meals; administration with food may decrease GI side effects; shake suspension well before use. Paxil, Paxil CR, and Pexeva should preferentially be administered in the morning; whereas Brisdelle is recommended to be administered at bedtime. Do not chew or crush immediate or controlled release tablet, swallow whole

Monitoring Parameters Blood pressure, heart rate, liver and renal function. Monitor patient periodically for symptom resolution; monitor for worsening depression, suicidality, and associated behaviors (especially at the beginning of therapy or when doses are increased or decreased); signs and symptoms of serotonin syndrome; akathisia

Additional Information Paroxetine is more potent and more selective than other SSRIs (eg, fluoxetine, fluvoxamine, sertraline, and clomipramine) in the inhibition of serotonin reuptake. If used for an extended period of time, long-term usefulness of paroxetine should be periodically re-evaluated for an individual patient. Paxil CR® tablets contain a degradable polymeric matrix (that controls the dissolution rate over ~4-5 hours) and an entering coating (that delays drug release until tablets leave the stomach).

Dosage Forms Excipient information presented when available (limited, particularly for generics); consult specific product labeling.

Capsule, Oral, as mesylate [strength expressed as base]:
- Brisdelle: 7.5 mg [contains fd&c red #40, fd&c yellow #6 (sunset yellow)]

Suspension, Oral, as hydrochloride [strength expressed as base]:
- Paxil: 10 mg/5 mL (250 mL) [contains fd&c yellow #6 aluminum lake, methylparaben, propylene glycol, propylparaben, saccharin sodium; orange flavor]

Tablet, Oral, as hydrochloride [strength expressed as base]:
- Paxil: 10 mg, 20 mg [scored]
- Paxil: 30 mg, 40 mg
- Generic: 10 mg, 20 mg, 30 mg, 40 mg

Tablet, Oral, as mesylate [strength expressed as base]:
- Pexeva: 10 mg
- Pexeva: 20 mg [scored]
- Pexeva: 30 mg, 40 mg

Tablet Extended Release 24 Hour, Oral, as hydrochloride [strength expressed as base]:
- Paxil CR: 12.5 mg [contains fd&c yellow #10 aluminum lake, fd&c yellow #6 aluminum lake]
- Paxil CR: 25 mg
- Paxil CR: 37.5 mg [contains fd&c blue #2 aluminum lake]
- Generic: 12.5 mg, 25 mg, 37.5 mg

- ◆ **Paroxetine Hydrochloride** *see* PARoxetine *on page 1634*
- ◆ **Paroxetine Mesylate** *see* PARoxetine *on page 1634*
- ◆ **Parvolex® (Can)** *see* Acetylcysteine *on page 57*
- ◆ **Pat-Rabeprazole (Can)** *see* RABEprazole *on page 1828*
- ◆ **Pavabid** *see* Papaverine *on page 1622*
- ◆ **Pavulon [DSC]** *see* Pancuronium *on page 1617*
- ◆ **Paxil** *see* PARoxetine *on page 1634*
- ◆ **Paxil CR** *see* PARoxetine *on page 1634*
- ◆ **PCA (error-prone abbreviation)** *see* Procainamide *on page 1769*
- ◆ **PCB** *see* Procarbazine *on page 1772*
- ◆ **PCC (Caution: Confusion-prone synonym)** *see* Factor IX Complex (Human) [(Factors II, IX, X)] *on page 836*
- ◆ **PCE** *see* Erythromycin (Systemic) *on page 779*
- ◆ **PCEC** *see* Rabies Vaccine *on page 1832*
- ◆ **PC-Tar [OTC]** *see* Coal Tar *on page 523*
- ◆ **PCV13** *see* Pneumococcal Conjugate Vaccine (13-Valent) *on page 1715*
- ◆ **PCZ** *see* Procarbazine *on page 1772*
- ◆ **PDP-Isoniazid (Can)** *see* Isoniazid *on page 1168*
- ◆ **PediaCare Childrens Allergy [OTC]** *see* DiphenhydrAMINE (Systemic) *on page 668*
- ◆ **PediaCare Childrens Long-Act [OTC]** *see* Dextromethorphan *on page 631*
- ◆ **Pediacel (Can)** *see* Diphtheria and Tetanus Toxoids, Acellular Pertussis, Poliovirus and *Haemophilus* b Conjugate Vaccine *on page 679*
- ◆ **Pediaderm AF Complete** *see* Nystatin (Topical) *on page 1537*
- ◆ **Pediaderm HC** *see* Hydrocortisone (Topical) *on page 1041*
- ◆ **Pediaderm TA** *see* Triamcinolone (Topical) *on page 2117*
- ◆ **Pedia-Lax [OTC]** *see* Docusate *on page 697*
- ◆ **Pedia-Lax [OTC]** *see* Glycerin *on page 978*
- ◆ **Pedia-Lax [OTC]** *see* Magnesium Hydroxide *on page 1313*
- ◆ **Pediapharm Naproxen Suspension (Can)** *see* Naproxen *on page 1489*
- ◆ **Pediapred** *see* PrednisoLONE (Systemic) *on page 1755*
- ◆ **Pediarix** *see* Diphtheria, Tetanus Toxoids, Acellular Pertussis, Hepatitis B (Recombinant), and Poliovirus (Inactivated) Vaccine *on page 685*
- ◆ **Pediatex TD [DSC]** *see* Triprolidine and Pseudoephedrine *on page 2129*
- ◆ **Pediatric Digoxin CSD (Can)** *see* Digoxin *on page 652*
- ◆ **Pediatrix (Can)** *see* Acetaminophen *on page 44*
- ◆ **Pediazole® (Can)** *see* Erythromycin and Sulfisoxazole *on page 784*
- ◆ **Pedi-Boro [OTC]** *see* Aluminum Acetate *on page 110*
- ◆ **Pedi-Dri [DSC]** *see* Nystatin (Topical) *on page 1537*
- ◆ **Pedipirox-4 Nail [DSC]** *see* Ciclopirox *on page 458*
- ◆ **Peditrace** *see* Trace Elements *on page 2097*
- ◆ **PedvaxHIB** *see* *Haemophilus* b Conjugate Vaccine *on page 998*
- ◆ **PEG** *see* Polyethylene Glycol 3350 *on page 1723*
- ◆ **PEG-L-asparaginase** *see* Pegaspargase *on page 1639*
- ◆ **Peg 3350 (Can)** *see* Polyethylene Glycol 3350 *on page 1723*
- ◆ **Pegalax (Can)** *see* Polyethylene Glycol 3350 *on page 1723*
- ◆ **PEG-ASP** *see* Pegaspargase *on page 1639*
- ◆ **PEG-asparaginase** *see* Pegaspargase *on page 1639*

Pegaspargase (peg AS par jase)

Medication Safety Issues

Sound-alike/look-alike issues:

Oncaspar may be confused with Elspar

Pegaspargase may be confused with asparaginase (*E. coli*), asparaginase (*Erwinia*), peginesatide

High alert medication:

This medication is in a class the Institute for Safe Medication Practices (ISMP) includes among its list of drug classes that have a heightened risk of causing significant patient harm when used in error.

Related Information

Prevention of Chemotherapy-Induced Nausea and Vomiting in Children *on page 2368*

Brand Names: US Oncaspar

Therapeutic Category Antineoplastic Agent, Enzyme; Antineoplastic Agent, Miscellaneous

Generic Availability (US) No

Use First-line treatment of newly diagnosed acute lymphoblastic leukemia (ALL) as part of a multiple chemotherapeutic drug regimen (FDA approved in ages ≥1 year and adults); induction treatment of acute lymphoblastic leukemia in combination with other chemotherapeutic agents in patients who have developed hypersensitivity to native forms of L-asparaginase derived from *E. coli* and/or *Erwinia chrysanthemia* (FDA approved in ages ≥1 year and adults); has been used for the treatment of lymphoma and acute myelogenous leukemia (AML)

Pregnancy Risk Factor C

Pregnancy Considerations Animal reproduction studies have not been conducted with pegaspargase.

Breast-Feeding Considerations It is not known if pegaspargase is excreted in breast milk. Due to the potential for serious adverse reactions in the nursing infant, the manufacturer recommends a decision be made whether to discontinue nursing or to discontinue the drug, taking into account the importance of treatment to the mother.

Contraindications History of serious allergic reactions to pegaspargase; history of any of the following with prior L-asparaginase treatment: serious thrombosis, pancreatitis, and/or serious hemorrhagic events

Warnings/Precautions Anaphylaxis and serious allergic reactions (eg, bronchospasm, hypotension, laryngeal edema, local erythema or swelling, systemic rash, urticaria) may occur; discontinue in patients with serious allergic reaction. The risk of serious allergic reactions is increased in patients with a history of hypersensitivity reactions to other L-asparaginase products. Observe patients for 1 hour after administration; equipment and immediate treatment for hypersensitivity reactions should be available during administration.

Serious thrombotic events, including sagittal sinus thrombosis may occur; discontinue with serious thrombotic event. Anticoagulation prophylaxis during therapy may be considered in some patients (Farge, 2013). Pancreatitis may occur; promptly evaluate patients with abdominal pain. The manufacturer recommends discontinuing pegaspargase if pancreatitis occurs during treatment. May consider continuing therapy for asymptomatic chemical pancreatitis (amylase or lipase >3 times ULN) or only radiologic abnormalities; monitor closely for rising amylase and/or lipase levels (Stock, 2011). Discontinue permanently for clinical pancreatitis (eg, vomiting, severe abdominal pain) with amylase/lipase elevation >3 times ULN for >3 days and/or development of a pancreatic pseudocyst. Avoid alcohol use (Stock, 2011). May cause glucose intolerance; irreversible in some cases; use with caution in patients with hyperglycemia, or diabetes. Increased prothrombin time, increased partial thromboplastin time, and hypofibrinogenemia may occur. Severe or symptomatic coagulopathy may require treatment with fresh-frozen plasma; use with caution in patients with underlying coagulopathy or previous hematologic complications from asparaginase. Monitor coagulation parameters at baseline and periodically during and after therapy. Altered liver function tests (eg, increased AST, ALT, alkaline phosphatase, bilirubin [direct and indirect], and decreased serum albumin, plasma fibrinogen) may occur with therapy. Use with caution in patients with pre-existing hepatic impairment. Monitor liver function tests at baseline and periodically during treatment. Potentially significant drug-drug interactions may exist, requiring dose or frequency adjustment, additional monitoring, and/or selection of alternative therapy. Do not interchange pegaspargase for asparaginase (*E. coli*) or asparaginase (*Erwinia*); ensure the proper asparaginase formulation, route of administration, and dose prior to administration.

Adverse Reactions

Cardiovascular: Thrombosis

Central nervous system: Cerebral thrombosis (or hemorrhage of the brain)

Endocrine & metabolic: Hyperglycemia (some patients required insulin therapy)

Gastrointestinal: Pancreatitis (includes 3 deaths)

Hematologic: Blood coagulation disorder (includes increased prothrombin time or partial thromboplastin time or decreased serum fibrogen)

Hepatic: Abnormal hepatic function tests, hyperbilirubinemia, increased serum transaminases (ALT, AST)

Hypersensitivity: Hypersensitivity reaction (includes anaphylaxis, bronchospasm, erythema, hives, hypotension, laryngeal edema, skin rash, swelling, urticaria; relapsed ALL with no prior asparaginase hypersensitivity, relapsed ALL with prior asparaginase hypersensitivity)

Hepatic:

Immunologic: Hypersensitivity to L-asparaginase

Rare but important or life-threatening: Abdominal pain, anemia, arthralgia, bronchospasm, chest pain, coagulation time increased, colitis, confusion, constipation, deep vein thrombosis, disseminated intravascular coagulation, dizziness, dyspnea, emotional lability, endocarditis, facial edema, gastrointestinal pain, headache, hemorrhagic cystitis, hepatic failure, hyperuricemia, hypoglycemia, increased thirst, lip edema, liver steatosis, myalgia, night sweats, ostealgia, pancytopenia, paresthesia, purpura, renal failure, sagittal sinus thrombosis, seizure, septic shock, superficial venous thrombosis

Drug Interactions

Metabolism/Transport Effects None known.

Avoid Concomitant Use

Avoid concomitant use of Pegaspargase with any of the following: BCG; BCG (Intravesical); Natalizumab; Pimecrolimus; Tacrolimus (Topical); Tofacitinib; Vaccines (Live)

Increased Effect/Toxicity

Pegaspargase may increase the levels/effects of: Leflunomide; Natalizumab; Tofacitinib; Vaccines (Live)

The levels/effects of Pegaspargase may be increased by: Denosumab; Pimecrolimus; Roflumilast; Tacrolimus (Topical); Trastuzumab

Decreased Effect

Pegaspargase may decrease the levels/effects of: BCG; BCG (Intravesical); Coccidioides immitis Skin Test; Sipuleucel-T; Vaccines (Inactivated); Vaccines (Live)

The levels/effects of Pegaspargase may be decreased by: Echinacea; Pegloticase

Storage/Stability Store intact vials at 2°C to 8°C (36°F to 46°F); do not freeze. Do not shake; protect from light. Discard vial if previously frozen, stored at room temperature for >48 hours, excessively shaken/agitated, or if cloudy, discolored, or if precipitate is present. If not used immediately, solutions for infusion should be protected from light, refrigerated at 2°C to 8°C (36°F to 46°F) and used within 48 hours (including administration time).

Mechanism of Action Pegaspargase is a modified version of L-asparaginase, conjugated with polyethylene glycol. In leukemic cells, asparaginase hydrolyzes L-asparagine to ammonia and L-aspartic acid, leading to depletion of asparagine. Leukemia cells, especially lymphoblasts, require exogenous asparagine; normal cells can synthesize asparagine. Asparagine depletion in leukemic cells leads to inhibition of protein synthesis and apoptosis. Asparaginase is cycle-specific for the G_1 phase of the cell cycle.

Pharmacodynamics

Onset of action: Asparagine depletion: IM: Within 4 days

Duration: Asparagine depletion:
IM: ~21 days
IV: 2-4 weeks (in asparaginase-naïve adults)

Pharmacokinetics (Adult data unless noted)
Absorption: Not absorbed from the GI tract; therefore, requires parenteral administration; IM: Slow
Distribution:
Apparent V_d: Plasma volume:
IM: Children: 1.5 L/m^2
IV: Adults (asparaginase-naïve): 2.4 L/m^2
Half-life:
IM: Children: 5.8 days; Adults: 5.5-6 days; 3.2 ± 1.8 days in patients who previously had a hypersensitivity reaction to native L-asparaginase
IV: Adults (asparaginase-naïve): 7 days
Time to peak serum concentration: IM: 3-4 days
Elimination: Clearance is unaffected by age, renal function, or hepatic function; not detected in urine

Dosing: Usual (Refer to individual protocols): Children >1 year, Adolescents and Adults: IM, IV: 2,500 units/m^2/dose ≥ every 14 days (as part of a combination chemotherapy regimen)

Preparation for Administration IV: Dilute in 100 mL NS or D_5W

Administration
IM: Limit the volume at a single injection site to 2 mL; for IM administration, if the volume to be administered is >2 mL, use multiple injection sites
IV: Administer dose as an IV infusion over a period of 1 to 2 hours through a running IV infusion line. Use of a 0.2 micron filter may result in some loss of potency.

Monitoring Parameters Vital signs during administration, CBC with differential, platelet count, urinalysis, serum amylase, liver enzymes, bilirubin, prothrombin time, renal function tests, urine glucose, blood glucose, uric acid, fibrinogen levels. Observe patients for 1 hour after administration for signs of anaphylaxis and serious allergic reactions.

Dosage Forms Excipient information presented when available (limited, particularly for generics); consult specific product labeling.
Solution, Injection [preservative free]:
Oncaspar: 750 units/mL (5 mL)

◆ **Pegasys** *see* Peginterferon Alfa-2a *on page 1642*

◆ **Pegasys ProClick** *see* Peginterferon Alfa-2a *on page 1642*

Pegfilgrastim (peg fil GRA stim)

Medication Safety Issues
Sound-alike/look-alike issues:
Neulasta may be confused with Lunesta, Neumega, Neupogen, Nuedexta

Brand Names: US Neulasta; Neulasta Delivery Kit

Brand Names: Canada Neulasta

Therapeutic Category Colony Stimulating Factor; Hematopoietic Agent

Generic Availability (US) No

Use Reduction of the duration of neutropenia and the associated risk of infection in patients with nonmyeloid malignancies receiving myelosuppressive chemotherapeutic regimens associated with a significant incidence of febrile neutropenia

Pregnancy Risk Factor C

Pregnancy Considerations Adverse events were observed in some animal reproduction studies.

Women who are exposed to Neulasta during pregnancy are encouraged to enroll in the Amgen Pregnancy Surveillance Program (800-772-6436).

Breast-Feeding Considerations It is not known if pegfilgrastim is excreted in breast milk. The manufacturer recommends that caution be exercised when administering pegfilgrastim to nursing women.

Contraindications Hypersensitivity (serious allergic reaction) to pegfilgrastim, filgrastim, or any component of the formulation

Warnings/Precautions Do not use pegfilgrastim in the period 14 days before to 24 hours after administration of cytotoxic chemotherapy because of the potential sensitivity of rapidly dividing myeloid cells to cytotoxic chemotherapy. Safety and efficacy have not been established with dose-dense chemotherapy regimens (Smith 2006). Not indicated for peripheral blood progenitor cell (PBPC) mobilization for hematopoietic stem cell transplantation.

Serious allergic reactions (including anaphylaxis) may occur, usually with the initial dose; may recur within days after discontinuation of initial antiallergic treatment. Permanently discontinue for severe reactions. Do not administer in patients with a history of serious allergic reaction to pegfilgrastim or filgrastim. Acute respiratory distress syndrome (ARDS) has been reported with use; evaluate patients with pulmonary symptoms such as fever, pulmonary infiltrates, or respiratory distress for ARDS. Discontinue pegfilgrastim if ARDS occurs. Rare cases of splenic rupture have been reported (some fatal); patients must be instructed to report left upper abdominal pain or shoulder pain. May precipitate sickle cell crises in patients with sickle cell disorders (severe and sometimes fatal sickle cell crises have occurred with filgrastim). The granulocyte-colony stimulating factor (G-CSF) receptor through which pegfilgrastim (and filgrastim) work has been located on tumor cell lines. May potentially act as a growth factor for any tumor type, including myeloid malignancies and myelodysplasia (pegfilgrastim is not approved for myeloid malignancies). Capillary leak syndrome (CLS), characterized by hypotension, hypoalbuminemia, edema, and hemoconcentration, may occur in patients receiving human granulocyte colony-stimulating factors (G-CSF). If CLS develops, monitor closely and manage symptomatically (may require intensive care). CLS may be life-threatening if treatment is delayed.

The On-body injector contains an acrylic adhesive; may result in a significant reaction in patients who react to acrylic adhesives. A health care provider must fill the On-body injector prior to applying to the patient's skin. The On-body delivery system may be applied on the same day as chemotherapy administration as long as pegfilgrastim is delivered no less than 24 hours after chemotherapy is administered. The prefilled syringe provided in the On-body kit contains overfill to compensate for loss during delivery; do not use for manual subcutaneous injection (will result in higher than recommended dose). Do not use prefilled syringe intended for manual injection to fill the On-body injector; may result in lower than intended dose. The On-body injector is only for use with pegfilgrastim; do not use to deliver other medications. Do not expose the On-body injector to oxygen-rich environments (eg, hyperbaric chambers), MRI, x-ray (including airport x-ray), CT scan, or ultrasound (may damage injector system). Keep the On-body injector at least 4 inches away from electrical equipment, including cell phones, cordless phones, microwaves, and other common appliances (injector may not work properly).

The 6 mg fixed dose should not be used in infants, children, and adolescents weighing <45 kg (Smith 2006). The packaging (needle cover) contains latex.

Adverse Reactions
Neuromuscular & Skeletal: Limb pain, ostealgia
Rare but important or life-threatening: Acute respiratory distress syndrome (ARDS), anaphylaxis, antibody ▶

development, capillary leak syndrome, chest pain, erythema, fever, flushing, hypersensitivity angiitis, hypertonia, increased serum alkaline phosphatase, increased uric acid, injection site reactions, leukocytosis, musculoskeletal pain, periorbital edema, peripheral edema, polyarthralgia, polymyalgia rheumatic, severe sickle cell crisis, splenic rupture, spelenomegaly, Sweet's syndrome, urticaria, weakness

Drug Interactions

Metabolism/Transport Effects None known.

Avoid Concomitant Use There are no known interactions where it is recommended to avoid concomitant use.

Increased Effect/Toxicity There are no known significant interactions involving an increase in effect.

Decreased Effect

The levels/effects of Pegfilgrastim may be decreased by: Pegloticase

Storage/Stability Store under refrigeration at 2°C to 8°C (36°F to 46°F); do not freeze. If syringe for manual injection is inadvertently frozen, allow to thaw in refrigerator; discard if frozen more than one time. Protect from light. Do not shake. Allow to reach room temperature prior to injection. Prefilled syringe for manual injection may be kept at room temperature for up to 48 hours. The On-body injector kit should not be held at room temperature for longer than 12 hours prior to use (discard if stored at room temperature for >12 hours).

Mechanism of Action Stimulates the production, maturation, and activation of neutrophils, pegfilgrastim activates neutrophils to increase both their migration and cytotoxicity. Pegfilgrastim has a prolonged duration of effect relative to filgrastim and a reduced renal clearance.

Pharmacokinetics (Adult data unless noted)

Half-life: Adults: 15-80 hours; Children (100 mcg/kg dose): ~20-30 hours (range: Up to 68 hours)

Elimination: Primarily through binding to neutrophils

Dosing: Usual SubQ: **Note:** Do not administer in the period between 14 days before and 24 hours after administration of cytotoxic chemotherapy. According to the NCCN guidelines, efficacy has been demonstrated with every 2-week chemotherapy regimens; however, benefit has not been demonstrated with regimens under a 2-week duration (Myeloid Growth Factor Guidelines, v.1, 2009)

Children (limited studies in children): 100 mcg/kg (maximum dose: 6 mg) once per chemotherapy cycle, beginning 24-72 hours after completion of chemotherapy

Adolescents >45 kg and Adults: 6 mg once per chemotherapy cycle, beginning 24-72 hours after completion of chemotherapy

Dosage adjustment in renal impairment: No adjustment necessary

Administration Parenteral: SubQ: Administer undiluted solution; do not shake

Monitoring Parameters Temperature, CBC with differential and platelet count

Evaluate for left upper abdominal pain, shoulder tip pain, or splenomegaly. Monitor for sickle cell crisis (in patients with sickle cell anemia).

Test Interactions May interfere with bone imaging studies; increased hematopoietic activity of the bone marrow may appear as transient positive bone imaging changes

Dosage Forms Excipient information presented when available (limited, particularly for generics); consult specific product labeling.

Solution, Subcutaneous [preservative free]:

Neulasta: 6 mg/0.6 mL (0.6 mL)

Neulasta Delivery Kit: 6 mg/0.6 mL (0.6 mL)

◆ **PEG-IFN Alfa-2a** *see* Peginterferon Alfa-2a *on page 1642*

◆ **PEG-IFN Alfa-2b** *see* Peginterferon Alfa-2b *on page 1646*

Peginterferon Alfa-2a

(peg in ter FEER on AL fa too aye)

Related Information

Prevention of Chemotherapy-Induced Nausea and Vomiting in Children *on page 2368*

Brand Names: US Pegasys; Pegasys ProClick

Brand Names: Canada Pegasys

Therapeutic Category Interferon

Generic Availability (US) No

Use

Chronic hepatitis C: Treatment of chronic hepatitis C virus (HCV) infection in patients with compensated liver disease and who have not been previously treated with interferon alfa alone or in combination with ribavirin (monotherapy with peginterferon alfa-2a is not recommended for treatment of chronic hepatitis C infection unless a patient has a contraindication to or significant intolerance of ribavirin) (FDA approved in ages ≥5 years and adults); treatment of chronic hepatitis C virus (HCV) infection in patients with histological evidence of cirrhosis (Child-Pugh class A) and compensated liver disease (FDA approved in adults); treatment of patients coinfected with HCV and clinically stable HIV disease (CD_4 count >100 cells/mm^3) (FDA approved in adults)

Combination with ribavirin is indicated in patients with HCV genotypes other than 1, pediatric patients (5-17 years), or patients with HCV genotype 1 where use of an HCV NS3/4A protease inhibitor is not warranted based on tolerability, contraindications, or other clinical factors.

Combination with ribavirin and an HCV NS3/4A protease inhibitor is indicated in adults with HCV genotype 1.

Chronic hepatitis B: Treatment with hepatitis B e antigen (HBeAg)-positive and HBeAG-negative chronic hepatitis B virus (HBV) infection who have compensated liver disease and evidence of viral replication and liver inflammation (FDA approved in adults)

Medication Guide Available Yes

Pregnancy Risk Factor C / X in combination with ribavirin

Pregnancy Considerations Reproduction studies with pegylated interferon alfa have not been conducted. Animal studies with nonpegylated interferon alfa-2b have demonstrated abortifacient effects. Disruption of the normal menstrual cycle was also observed in animal studies; therefore, the manufacturer recommends that reliable contraception is used in women of childbearing potential. Alfa interferon is endogenous to normal amniotic fluid (Lebon, 1982). *In vitro* administration studies have reported that when administered to the mother, it does not cross the placenta (Waysbort, 1993). Case reports of use in pregnant women are limited. The DHHS Perinatal HIV Guidelines do not recommend that peginterferon-alfa be used during pregnancy (DHHS [perinatal], 2012). **Combination therapy with ribavirin may cause birth defects and/or fetal mortality; avoid pregnancy in females and female partners of male patients.** Combination therapy with ribavirin is contraindicated in pregnancy (refer to Ribavirin monograph). Female patients of childbearing potential and male patients with female partners of childbearing potential must use 2 forms of contraception along with monthly pregnancy tests during therapy and for 6 months after therapy has been discontinued.

A pregnancy registry has been established for women inadvertently exposed to ribavirin while pregnant (800-593-2214).

Breast-Feeding Considerations Breast milk samples obtained from a lactating mother prior to and after administration of interferon alfa-2b showed that interferon alfa is present in breast milk and administration of the medication did not significantly affect endogenous levels (Kumar,

2000). Breast-feeding is not linked to the spread of hepatitis C virus (ACOG, 2007); however, if nipples are cracked or bleeding, breast-feeding is not recommended (CDC, 2010). Due to the potential for serious adverse reactions in the nursing infant, the manufacturer recommends a decision be made whether to discontinue nursing or to discontinue the drug. Mothers coinfected with HIV are discouraged from breast-feeding to decrease potential transmission of HIV (DHHS [perinatal], 2012).

Contraindications

Hypersensitivity reactions (eg, urticaria, angioedema, bronchoconstriction, anaphylaxis, Stevens-Johnson syndrome) to peginterferon alfa-2a, other alfa interferons, or any component of the formulation; autoimmune hepatitis; hepatic decompensation in cirrhotic patients (Child-Pugh score >6, class B and C) before treatment; hepatic decompensation with Child-Pugh score ≥6 in cirrhotic CHC coinfected with HIV before treatment; neonates and infants (due to benzyl alcohol component)

Combination therapy with peginterferon alfa-2a and ribavirin is also contraindicated in pregnancy; men whose female partners are pregnant

Documentation of allergenic cross-reactivity for interferons is limited. However, because of similarities in chemical structure and/or pharmacologic actions, the possibility of cross-sensitivity cannot be ruled out with certainty

Warnings/Precautions [US Boxed Warning]: May cause or exacerbate life-threatening neuropsychiatric disorders; monitor closely; discontinue treatment with worsening or persistently severe signs/symptoms of neuropsychiatric disorders. In most cases these effects were reversible following discontinuation, but not all cases. Neuropsychiatric adverse effects include depression, suicidal ideation, suicide attempt, homicidal ideation, drug overdose, and relapse of drug addiction, and may occur in patients with or without a prior history of psychiatric disorder. Avoid use in severe psychiatric disorders; use with extreme caution in patients with a history of depression. May cause CNS depression, which may impair physical or mental abilities; patients must be cautioned about performing tasks that require mental alertness (eg, operating machinery or driving).

[US Boxed Warning]: May cause or exacerbate autoimmune disorders; monitor closely; discontinue treatment in patients with worsening or persistently severe signs/symptoms of autoimmune disease. In most cases these effects were reversible following discontinuation, but not all cases. Thyroiditis, idiopathic thrombocytopenic purpura, immune thrombocytopenia (ITP), rheumatoid arthritis, interstitial nephritis, systemic lupus erythematosus, myositis, hepatitis, and psoriasis have been reported with interferon therapy; use with caution in patients with autoimmune disorders.

[US Boxed Warning]: May cause or aggravate infectious disorders; monitor closely; discontinue treatment in patients with worsening or persistently severe signs/symptoms of infectious disorders. In most cases these effects were reversible following discontinuation, but not all cases. Serious and severe infections (bacterial, viral, and fungal), some fatal, have been reported with treatment. Interferon therapy is commonly associated with flu-like symptoms, including fever; however, rule out other causes/infection with persistent or high fever.

[US Boxed Warning]: May cause or aggravate ischemic disorders and hemorrhagic cerebrovascular events; monitor closely. Discontinue treatment in patients with worsening or persistent ischemia. In most cases these effects were reversible following discontinuation, but not all cases. Has been reported in patients without risk factors for stroke.

Causes bone marrow suppression, including potentially severe cytopenias; alfa interferons may (rarely) cause aplastic anemia. Ribavirin may potentiate these effects. When used in combination with ribavirin, use caution with baseline neutrophil count <1,500/mm^3, platelet count <90,000/mm^3, or hemoglobin <10 g/dL. Discontinue therapy (at least temporarily) if ANC <500/mm^3 or platelet count <25,000/mm^3. Severe neutropenia and thrombocytopenia may occur with a greater incidence in HIV coinfected patients than monoinfected patients. Obtain CBC before treatment and monitor routinely during therapy.

Hepatic decompensation and death have been associated with the use of alpha interferons including Pegasys®, in cirrhotic chronic hepatitis C patients; patients coinfected with HIV and receiving highly active antiretroviral therapy have shown an increased risk. Monitor hepatic function closely during use; discontinue if decompensation occurs (Child-Pugh score >6) in monoinfected patients and (Child-Pugh score ≥6, class B and C) in patients coinfected with HIV. In hepatitis B patients, flares (transient and potentially severe increases in serum ALT) may occur during or after treatment; more frequent monitoring of LFTs and a dose reduction are recommended. Discontinue immediately if ALT elevation continues despite dose reduction or if increased bilirubin or hepatic decompensation occur. Instruct patients to avoid alcohol; may increase hepatic effects.

Gastrointestinal hemorrhage, ulcerative and hemorrhagic/ischemic colitis (may be fatal) have been observed with interferon alfa treatment; may be severe and/or life-threatening; discontinue if symptoms of colitis (eg, abdominal pain, bloody diarrhea, and/or fever) develop. Colitis generally resolves within 1 to 3 weeks of discontinuation. Withhold treatment for suspected pancreatitis; discontinue therapy for confirmed pancreatitis.

Use with caution in patients with diabetes mellitus; hyper- or hypoglycemia have been reported which may require adjustments in medications. Use with caution in patients with preexisting thyroid disease; thyroid disorders (hyper- or hypothyroidism) or exacerbations have been reported. Use with caution in patients with prior cardiovascular disease; hypertension, supraventricular arrhythmias, chest pain, and MI have been observed with treatment. Patients with a history of significant or unstable cardiac disease should not receive combination treatment with ribavirin.

Severe acute hypersensitivity reactions (eg, urticaria, angioedema, bronchoconstriction, anaphylaxis) have been reported; prompt discontinuation and management is recommended. Serious cutaneous reactions, including vesiculobullous eruptions, Stevens-Johnson syndrome, and exfoliative dermatitis, have been reported with use, with or without ribavirin therapy; discontinue with signs or symptoms of severe skin reactions.

Decreased or loss of vision and retinopathy, including macular edema, optic neuritis, papilledema, retinal hemorrhages, retinal detachment (serous), cotton wool spots, and retinal artery or vein thrombosis may occur or be aggravated during treatment; if any ocular symptoms occur during use, a complete eye exam should be performed promptly. Prior to use, all patients should have a visual exam and patients with pre-existing disorders (eg, diabetic or hypertensive retinopathy) should have exams periodically during therapy. Discontinue if new or worsening ophthalmologic disorders occur.

May cause or aggravate dyspnea, pulmonary infiltrates, pneumonia, bronchiolitis obliterans, interstitial pneumonitis, pulmonary hypertension, and sarcoidosis, which may result in potentially fatal respiratory failure; may recur upon rechallenge with interferons. Monitor closely. Discontinue with unexplained pulmonary infiltrates or evidence of impaired pulmonary function. Use with caution in patients with pulmonary dysfunction or a history of pulmonary disease.

Use with caution in patients with renal dysfunction (CrCl <30 mL/minute); monitor for signs/symptoms of toxicity (dosage adjustment required if toxicity occurs).

Safety and efficacy have not been established in patients who have been coinfected with HBV **and** HCV or HIV, have been coinfected with HCV **and** HBV or HIV with a CD4$^+$ cell count <100 cells/mm^3, or been treated for >48 weeks.

Potentially significant drug-drug interactions may exist, requiring dose or frequency adjustment, additional monitoring, and/or selection of alternative therapy. **Due to differences in dosage, patients should not change brands of interferon without the concurrence of their health care provider.**

Growth velocity (height and weight) was decreased in children on combination treatment with ribavirin, during the length of treatment. In clinical studies, decreases were noted in weight and height for age z-scores and normative growth curve percentiles. Following treatment, rebound growth and weight gain occurred in most patients; however, a small percentage did not. For most children, posttreatment recovery in growth at 2 years posttreatment was maintained to 6 years posttreatment. Growth should be closely monitored in children during therapy and posttreatment until growth catch-up has occurred. Use with caution in the elderly; certain adverse effects (eg, neuropsychiatric, cardiac, flu-like reactions) may be more severe.

Benzyl alcohol and derivatives: Some dosage forms may contain benzyl alcohol; large amounts of benzyl alcohol (≥99 mg/kg/day) have been associated with a potentially fatal toxicity ("gasping syndrome") in neonates; the "gasping syndrome" consists of metabolic acidosis, respiratory distress, gasping respirations, CNS dysfunction (including convulsions, intracranial hemorrhage), hypotension, and cardiovascular collapse (AAP, 1997; CDC, 1982); some data suggests that benzoate displaces bilirubin from protein binding sites (Ahlfors, 2001); avoid or use dosage forms containing benzyl alcohol with caution in neonates. See manufacturer's labeling.

Polysorbate 80: Some dosage forms may contain polysorbate 80 (also known as Tweens). Hypersensitivity reactions, usually a delayed reaction, have been reported following exposure to pharmaceutical products containing polysorbate 80 in certain individuals (Isaksson, 2002; Lucente 2000; Shelley, 1995). Thrombocytopenia, ascites, pulmonary deterioration, and renal and hepatic failure have been reported in premature neonates after receiving parenteral products containing polysorbate 80 (Alade, 1986; CDC, 1984). See manufacturer's labeling.

Warnings: Additional Pediatric Considerations Inhibition of growth velocity in pediatric patients may occur; in clinical trials, growth suppression of ≥15 percentiles on the normal growth curve was reported for weight in 43% of pediatric patients and for height in 25% of patients after 48 weeks of therapy. At the two-year follow-up after treatment, most children had returned to their baseline growth curve percentile; monitor growth at baseline and during therapy.

Adverse Reactions

Central nervous system: Anxiety, depression, dizziness, fatigue, headache, insomnia, irritability, lack of concentration, memory impairment, mood changes, nervousness, pain, rigors

Dermatologic: Alopecia, dermatitis, diaphoresis, eczema, pruritus, skin rash, xeroderma

Endocrine & metabolic: Growth suppression (children, percentile decrease [≥15 percentiles], height, and weight), hyperthyroidism, hypothyroidism, weight loss

Gastrointestinal: Abdominal pain, anorexia, diarrhea, nausea, vomiting, xerostomia

Hematologic & oncologic: neutropenia, anemia, lymphocytopenia, thrombocytopenia

Hepatic: Hepatic decompensation (in CHC/HIV), increased serum ALT

Infection: Bacterial infection

Local: Injection site reaction

Neuromuscular & skeletal: Arthralgia, back pain, myalgia, weakness

Ophthalmic: Blurred vision

Respiratory: Cough, dyspnea

Miscellaneous: Fever (more common in hepatitis B)

Rare but important or life-threatening: Aggressive behavior, angina pectoris, aplastic anemia, arrhythmia, auditory impairment, autoimmune disorders, bipolar mood disorder, bronchiolitis obliterans, cerebral hemorrhage, cholangitis, colitis, coma, corneal ulcer, dehydration, diabetes mellitus, dyspepsia, dyspnea on exertion, endocarditis, erythema multiforme major, exacerbation of hepatitis B, exfoliative dermatitis, gastrointestinal hemorrhage, graft rejection (hepatic, renal), hallucination, hearing loss, hematocrit decreased, hemoglobin decreased, hepatic insufficiency, hyperglycemia, hyperpigmentation, hypersensitivity reaction, hypertension, hypoglycemia, increased serum triglycerides, influenza, interstitial pneumonitis, macular edema, mania, myocardial infarction, myositis, optic neuritis, pancreatitis, papilledema, peptic ulcer, peripheral neuropathy, pneumonia, psychosis, pulmonary embolism, pulmonary infiltrates, pure red cell aplasia, retinal cotton-wool spot, retinal detachment, retinal hemorrhage, retinal thrombosis (in artery or vein), retinopathy, rheumatoid arthritis, sarcoidosis, seizures, Stevens-Johnson syndrome, suicidal ideation, supraventricular cardiac arrhythmia, systemic lupus erythematosus, thrombotic thrombocytopenic purpura, vesiculobullous reaction, vision loss

Drug Interactions

Metabolism/Transport Effects Inhibits CYP1A2 (weak)

Avoid Concomitant Use

Avoid concomitant use of Peginterferon Alfa-2a with any of the following: BCG (Intravesical); CloZAPine; Dipyrone; Telbivudine

Increased Effect/Toxicity

Peginterferon Alfa-2a may increase the levels/effects of: Aldesleukin; CloZAPine; Methadone; Ribavirin; Telbivudine; Theophylline Derivatives; TiZANidine; Zidovudine

The levels/effects of Peginterferon Alfa-2a may be increased by: Dipyrone

Decreased Effect

Peginterferon Alfa-2a may decrease the levels/effects of: BCG (Intravesical)

The levels/effects of Peginterferon Alfa-2a may be decreased by: Pegloticase

Storage/Stability Store in refrigerator at 2°C to 8°C (36°F to 46°F). Do not leave out of the refrigerator for more than 24 hours. Do not freeze or shake. Protect from light. Discard any unused portion. The following stability information has also been reported:

Intact vial: May be stored at room temperature for up to 14 days (Cohen, 2007).

Prefilled syringe: May be stored at room temperature for up to 6 days (Cohen, 2007).

Mechanism of Action Alpha interferons are a family of proteins, produced by nucleated cells that have antiviral, antiproliferative, and immune-regulating activity. There are 16 known subtypes of alpha interferons. Interferons interact with cells through high affinity cell surface receptors. Following activation, multiple effects can be detected including induction of gene transcription. Interferons inhibit cellular growth, alter the state of cellular differentiation, interfere with oncogene expression, alter cell surface antigen expression, increase phagocytic activity of macrophages, and augment cytotoxicity of lymphocytes for target cells.

Pharmacokinetics (Adult data unless noted)

Half-life elimination: Terminal: 50-160 hours; increased with renal dysfunction

Time to peak serum concentration: 72-96 hours

Dosing: Usual

Children ≥5 years and Adolescents: **Chronic hepatitis C virus (HCV) infection:** SubQ: 104 mcg/m^2 once weekly; maximum dose: 180 mcg; in combination with ribavirin (Copegus) (Schwartz, 2011); **Note:** Dosing presented is mathematically equivalent to weekly dosing presented in manufacturer's labeling: 180 mcg/1.73 m^2 x Body Surface Area (BSA); adolescents who reach their 18th birthday during treatment should remain on the pediatric regimen

Duration of therapy (based on genotype):

Genotype 1, 4, 5, 6: 48 weeks

Genotype 2, 3: 24 weeks

Adults:

Chronic hepatitis B: SubQ: 180 mcg once weekly for 48 weeks

Chronic hepatitis C virus (HCV) infection (monoinfection or coinfection with HIV): SubQ: 180 mcg once weekly for 48 weeks as monotherapy or in combination with ribavirin (Copegus®)

Duration of therapy: Monoinfection (based on genotype):

Genotypes 1, 4: 48 weeks

Genotypes 2, 3: 24 weeks

Genotypes 5, 6: No dosing recommendations provided; data insufficient

Duration of therapy: Coinfection with HIV: 48 weeks

Note: American Association for the Study of Liver Diseases (AASLD) guidelines recommendation: Adults with chronic HCV infection (Ghany, 2009): Treatment of choice: Ribavirin plus **peginterferon**; clinical condition and ability of patient to tolerate therapy should be evaluated to determine length and/or likely benefit of therapy. Recommended treatment duration (AASLD guidelines): Genotypes 1,4: 48 weeks; Genotypes 2,3: 24 weeks; Coinfection with HIV: 48 weeks

Dosing adjustment for renal impairment:

Children and Adolescents: There are no dosage adjustment provided in manufacturer's labeling; has not been studied.

Adults:

CrCl ≥30 mL/minute: No adjustment required

CrCl <30 mL/minute: Reduce dose to 135 mcg weekly; monitor for interferon toxicity

End-stage renal disease (ESRD) requiring hemodialysis: 135 mcg weekly; monitor for interferon toxicity

Dosing adjustment for hepatic impairment:

Children ≥5 years and Adolescents: *Chronic Hepatitis C:*

ALT ≥5 but <10 x ULN: Decrease interferon dose to 78 mcg/m^2 once weekly. Monitor weekly; further modify dose if needed until ALT stabilizes or decreases (Schwartz, 2011). **Note:** Dosing presented is mathematically equivalent to adjusted weekly dose in manufacturer's labeling: 135 mcg/1.73 m^2 x Body Surface Area (BSA)

ALT ≥10 x ULN (persistent): Discontinue interferon

Adults:

Chronic hepatitis C (HCV): ALT progressively rising above baseline: Decrease dose to 135 mcg weekly **and** monitor LFTs more frequently. If ALT continues to rise despite dose reduction or ALT increase is accompanied by increased bilirubin or hepatic decompensation, discontinue therapy immediately. Therapy may resume after ALT flare subsides.

Chronic hepatitis B (HBV):

ALT >5 x ULN: Consider decreasing dose to 135 mcg weekly or temporarily discontinuing (may resume after ALT flare subsides) **and** monitor LFTs more frequently. If ALT continues to rise despite dose reduction or ALT increase is accompanied by increased bilirubin or hepatic decompensation, discontinue therapy immediately.

ALT >10 x ULN: Consider discontinuing

Dosing adjustment for toxicity: Note: Pediatric dosing adjustments shown below correspond to the following doses in manufacturer's labeling: 78 mcg/m^2 = 135 mcg/1.73 m^2; 52 mcg/m^2 = 90 mcg/1.73 m^2; and 26 mcg/m^2 = 45 mcg/1.73 m^2 (Schwartz, 2011).

For moderate to severe adverse reactions:

Children ≥5 years and Adolescents: Decrease to 78 mcg/m^2 once weekly for initial dose reduction; further dose reductions to 52 mcg/m^2 once weekly and then 26 mcg/m^2 once weekly may be necessary in some cases if reaction persists or recurs. Up to three dosing adjustments for toxicity may be made before discontinuation is considered.

Adults: HCV, HBV infection: For moderate to severe adverse reactions: Decrease to 135 mcg/week for initial dose reduction; further dose reductions to 90 mcg/week may be necessary in some cases if reaction persists or recurs

Depression (severity based upon DSM-IV criteria):

Mild depression: Children ≥5 years, Adolescents, and Adults: No dosage adjustment required; evaluate once weekly by visit/phone call. If depression remains stable, continue weekly visits. If depression improves, resume normal visit schedule.

Moderate depression:

Children ≥5 years and Adolescents: Initially decrease interferon dose to 78 mcg/m^2 once weekly and based upon response of adverse effect further dose modifications may be necessary in stepwise approach; next decrease to 52 mcg/m^2 once weekly and then 26 mcg/m^2 once weekly; evaluate once weekly with an office visit at least every other week. If symptoms improve and remain stable for 4 weeks, resume normal visit schedule; may continue reduced dosing or return to normal dose. If depression remains stable, consider psychiatric evaluation and continue reduced dosing. If symptoms worsen, considered further dosage reduction; discontinue therapy if no improvement after three dosage reductions.

Adults: Decrease interferon dose to 135 mcg once weekly (or to 90 mcg once weekly); evaluate once weekly with an office visit at least every other week. If depression remains stable, consider psychiatric evaluation and continue with reduced dosing. If symptoms improve and remain stable for 4 weeks, resume normal visit schedule; continue reduced dosing or return to normal dose.

Severe depression: Children ≥5 years, Adolescents, and Adults: Discontinue interferon permanently. Obtain immediate psychiatric consultation. Discontinue ribavirin.

Based on hematological parameters: **Note:** Management dependent upon weeks of therapy.

Children ≥5 years and Adolescents:

Neutropenia:

ANC 750-999/mm^3:

Week 1-2: Decrease dose to 78 mcg/m^2 once weekly

Weeks 3-48: No modification

ANC 500-749/mm^3:

Week 1-2: Hold dose until ANC >750/mm^3 then resume therapy at 78 mcg/m^2 once weekly. Assess WBC weekly for 3 weeks to verify ANC >750/mm^3.

Weeks 3-48: Decrease dose to 78 mcg/m^2 once weekly
ANC 250-499/mm^3:
Week 1-2: Hold dose until ANC >750/mm^3 then resume dose at 52 mcg/m^2 once weekly
Weeks 3-48: Hold dose until ANC >750/mm^3 then resume dose at 78 mcg/m^2 once weekly
ANC <250/mm^3 or febrile neutropenia: Discontinue treatment.
Thrombocytopenia: Platelet count <50,000/mm^3: Decrease dose to 52 mcg/m^2 once weekly
Adults:
Neutropenia:
ANC <750/mm^3: 135 mcg once weekly
ANC <500/mm^3: Suspend therapy until >1000/mm^3, then restart at 90 mcg once weekly; monitor ANC
Thrombocytopenia:
Platelet count <50,000/mm^3: 90 mcg once weekly
Platelet count <25,000/mm^3: Discontinue therapy

Administration SubQ: Do not shake vial, prefilled syringe, or autoinjector. Allow syringe, autoinjector, or vial to reach room temperature before use; wait for condensation on the outside of the syringe or autoinjector to disappear before use. The vial may be warmed by gently rolling in the palms of the hand for ~1 minute. Allow the autoinjector to come to room temperature on its own for ~20 minutes; do not warm autoinjector any other way. Do not use if solution contains particulate matter or is discolored.

Administer in the abdomen or thigh. Rotate injection site. Discard unused solution. Administration should be done on the same day and at approximately the same time each week.

Monitoring Parameters
The following were used during clinical trials:
Children ≥5 years and Adolescents: Hematologic and biochemical assessments were made at weeks 1, 3, 5, and 8, and then every 4 weeks thereafter; TSH measured every 12 weeks; growth parameters (height, weight, percentiles on growth curve) (Schwarz, 2011)
Adults: CBC (including hemoglobin, WBC, and platelets) and chemistries (including liver function tests and uric acid) measured at weeks 1, 2, 4, 6, and 8, and then every 4-6 weeks (more frequently if abnormal); TSH measured every 12 weeks
Additionally, the following baseline values were used as entrance criteria in adults:
Platelet count ≥90,000/mm^3 (as low as 75,000/mm^3 in patients with cirrhosis or 70,000/mm^3 in patients with HCV coinfected with HIV)
ANC ≥1500/mm^3
Serum creatinine <1.5 times ULN
TSH and T_4 within normal limits or adequately controlled
$CD4^+$ cell count ≥200 cells/mm^3 or $CD4^+$ cell count ≥100 cells/mm^3, but <200 cells/mm^3 and HIV-1 RNA <5000 copies/mL in HCV patients coinfected with HIV
Hemoglobin ≥12 g/dL for women and ≥13 g/dL for men in HCV monoinfected patients
Hemoglobin ≥11 g/dL for women and ≥12 g/dL for men in HCV patients coinfected with HIV
Also in adults, serum HCV RNA levels (pretreatment, 12- and 24 weeks after therapy initiation, 24 weeks after completion of therapy). **Note:** Discontinuation of therapy may be considered after 12 weeks in patients with HCV (genotype 1) who fail to achieve an early virologic response (defined as ≥2-log decrease in HCV RNA compared to pretreatment) or after 24 weeks with detectable HCV RNA (Ghany, 2009).
Prior to treatment, pregnancy screening should occur for women of childbearing age who are receiving treatment or who have male partners who are receiving treatment. In combination therapy with ribavirin, pregnancy tests should continue monthly up to 6 months after discontinuation of therapy. Evaluate for depression and other psychiatric symptoms before and during therapy; baseline eye examination and periodically in patients with baseline disorders; baseline echocardiogram in patients with cardiac disease.

Dosage Forms Excipient information presented when available (limited, particularly for generics); consult specific product labeling.
Kit, Subcutaneous [preservative free]:
Pegasys: 180 mcg/0.5 mL [contains benzyl alcohol]
Solution, Subcutaneous [preservative free]:
Pegasys: 180 mcg/mL (1 mL) [contains benzyl alcohol]
Pegasys: 180 mcg/0.5 mL (0.5 mL) [contains benzyl alcohol, polysorbate 80]
Pegasys ProClick: 135 mcg/0.5 mL (0.5 mL) [contains benzyl alcohol, polysorbate 80]
Pegasys ProClick: 180 mcg/0.5 mL (0.5 mL) [contains benzyl alcohol]

Peginterferon Alfa-2b
(peg in ter FEER on AL fa too bee)

Medication Safety Issues
Sound-alike/look-alike issues:
Peginterferon alfa-2b may be confused with interferon alfa-2a, interferon alfa-2b, interferon alfa-n3, peginterferon alfa-2a, peginterferon beta-1a
PegIntron may be confused with Intron A, Pegasys
International issues:
Peginterferon alfa-2b may be confused with interferon alpha multi-subtype which is available in international markets

Related Information
Prevention of Chemotherapy-Induced Nausea and Vomiting in Children *on page* 2368

Brand Names: US Peg-Intron; Peg-Intron Redipen; Peg-Intron Redipen Pak 4; PegIntron; Sylatron

Brand Names: Canada PegIntron

Therapeutic Category Antineoplastic Agent, Biologic Response Modulator; Biological Response Modulator; Immunomodulator, Systemic; Interferon

Generic Availability (US) No

Use
PegIntron®: Treatment of chronic hepatitis C (in combination with ribavirin) in patients who have compensated liver disease (FDA approved in ages ≥3 years and adults); treatment of chronic hepatitis C (as monotherapy) in patients with compensated liver disease who have never received alfa interferons (FDA approved in adults); has also be used for treatment of chronic hepatitis C with HIV coinfection and chronic hepatitis B with HIV coinfection
Sylatron™: Adjuvant treatment of melanoma (with microscopic or gross nodal involvement within 84 days of definitive surgical resection, including lymphadenectomy) (FDA approved in ages ≥18 years and adults)

Medication Guide Available Yes

Pregnancy Risk Factor C / X in combination with ribavirin

Pregnancy Considerations Reproduction studies with pegylated interferon alfa have not been conducted. Animal reproduction studies with nonpegylated interferon alfa-2b have demonstrated abortifacient effects. Disruption of the normal menstrual cycle was also observed in animal studies; therefore, the manufacturer recommends that reliable contraception is used in women of childbearing potential. Alfa interferon is endogenous to normal amniotic fluid (Lebon, 1982). *In vitro* administration studies have reported that when administered to the mother, it does not cross the placenta (Waysbort, 1993). Case reports of use in pregnant women are limited. The DHHS Perinatal HIV Guidelines do not recommend that peginterferon alfa be used during pregnancy (DHHS [perinatal], 2012). **[U.S.**

Boxed Warning]: Combination therapy with ribavirin may cause birth defects and/or fetal mortality; avoid pregnancy in females and female partners of male patients; combination therapy with ribavirin is contraindicated in pregnancy. Two forms of contraception should be used along with monthly pregnancy tests during combination therapy and for 6 months after therapy has been discontinued.

A pregnancy registry has been established for women inadvertently exposed to ribavirin while pregnant (800-593-2214).

Breast-Feeding Considerations Breast milk samples obtained from a lactating mother prior to and after administration of interferon alfa-2b showed that interferon alfa is present in breast milk and administration of the medication did not significantly affect endogenous levels (Kumar, 2000). Breast-feeding is not linked to the spread of hepatitis C virus (ACOG, 2007); however, if nipples are cracked or bleeding, breast-feeding is not recommended (CDC, 2010). Mothers coinfected with HIV are discouraged from breast-feeding to decrease potential transmission of HIV (DHHS [perinatal], 2012).

Contraindications

Hypersensitivity (including urticaria, angioedema, bronchoconstriction, anaphylaxis, Stevens Johnson syndrome and toxic epidermal necrolysis) to peginterferon alfa-2b, interferon alfa-2b, other alfa interferons, or any component of the formulation; autoimmune hepatitis; decompensated liver disease (Child-Pugh score >6, classes B and C)

Documentation of allergenic cross-reactivity for interferons is limited. However, because of similarities in chemical structure and/or pharmacologic actions, the possibility of cross-sensitivity cannot be ruled out with certainty

Combination therapy with peginterferon alfa-2b and ribavirin is also contraindicated in pregnancy, women who may become pregnant, males with pregnant partners; hemoglobinopathies (eg, thalassemia major, sickle-cell anemia); renal dysfunction (CrCl <50 mL/minute)

Warnings/Precautions [U.S. Boxed Warnings]: May cause or aggravate severe depression or other neuropsychiatric adverse events (including suicide and suicidal ideation) in patients with and without a history of psychiatric disorder; monitor closely with clinical evaluations (periodic); discontinue treatment with worsening or persistently severe signs/symptoms of neuropsychiatric disorders (eg, depression, encephalopathy, psychosis). Many cases resolve upon discontinuation, although some cases may persist. May cause or aggravate fatal or life-threatening autoimmune disorders, infectious disorders, ischemic disorders; monitor closely with clinical evaluations (periodic); discontinue treatment in patients with worsening or persistently severe signs/symptoms of infectious disorders; may resolve with discontinuation. May also cause hemorrhagic cerebrovascular events.

Neuropsychiatric disorders: Neuropsychiatric effects may occur in patients with and without a history of psychiatric disorder; addiction relapse, aggression, depression, homicidal ideation and suicidal behavior/ideation have been observed with peginterferon alfa-2b; bipolar disorder, encephalopathy, hallucinations, mania, and psychosis have been observed with other alfa interferons. Onset may be delayed (up to 6 months after discontinuation). Higher doses may be associated with the development of encephalopathy (higher risk in elderly patients). Use with caution in patients with a history of psychiatric disorders, including depression or substance abuse history. New or exacerbated neuropsychiatric or substance abuse disorders are best managed with early intervention. Drug screening and periodic health evaluation (including monitoring of psychiatric symptoms) is recommended if initiating treatment in patients with coexisting psychiatric condition or substance abuse disorders. Monitor all patients for evidence of depression and other psychiatric symptoms; patients being treated for melanoma should be monitored for depression and psychiatric symptoms every 3 weeks during the first 8 weeks of treatment and every 6 months thereafter; permanently discontinue treatment if psychiatric symptoms persist, worsen or if suicidal behavior develops. Patients should continue to be monitored for 6 months after completion of therapy.

Bone marrow suppression: Causes bone marrow suppression, including potentially severe cytopenias; alfa interferons may (rarely) cause aplastic anemia. Use with caution in patients who are chronically immunosuppressed, with low peripheral blood counts or myelosuppression, including concurrent use of myelosuppressive therapy. Dosage modification may be necessary for hematologic toxicity. Combination therapy with ribavirin may potentiate the neutropenic effects of alfa interferons. When used in combination with ribavirin, an increased incidence of anemia was observed when using ribavirin weight-based dosing, as compared to flat-dose ribavirin.

Hepatic disease: Use is contraindicated in patients with hepatic decompensation or autoimmune hepatitis. Discontinue treatment immediately with hepatic decompensation (Child Pugh score >6) or evidence of severe hepatic injury. Patients with chronic hepatitis C (CHC) with cirrhosis receiving peginterferon alfa-2b are at risk for hepatic decompensation. CHC patients coinfected with human immunodeficiency virus (HIV) are at increased risk for hepatic decompensation when receiving highly active antiretroviral therapy (HAART); monitor closely. A transient increase in ALT (2-5 times above baseline) which is not associated with deterioration of liver function may occur with peginterferon alfa-2b use (for the treatment of chronic hepatitis C); therapy generally may continue with monitoring. Instruct patients to avoid alcohol; may increase hepatic effects.

Gastrointestinal disorders: Pancreatitis (including fatal cases) has been observed with alfa interferon therapy; discontinue therapy if known or suspected pancreatitis develops. Ulcerative or hemorrhagic/ischemic colitis has been observed with alfa interferons (within 12 weeks of initiation); withhold treatment for suspected pancreatitis; discontinue therapy for known pancreatitis. Ulcerative or hemorrhagic/ischemic colitis has been observed with alfa interferons; discontinue therapy if signs of colitis (abdominal pain, bloody diarrhea, fever) develop; symptoms typically resolve within 1-3 weeks.

Autoimmune disorders: Thyroiditis, thrombotic thrombocytopenic purpura, immune thrombocytopenia (ITP), rheumatoid arthritis, interstitial nephritis, systemic lupus erythematosus, and psoriasis have been reported with therapy; use with caution in patients with autoimmune disorders.

Cardiovascular disease: Use with caution in patients with cardiovascular disease or a history of cardiovascular disease; hypotension, arrhythmia, bundle branch block, tachycardia, cardiomyopathy, angina pectoris and MI have been observed with treatment. Patients with pre-existing cardiac abnormalities should have baseline ECGs prior to combination treatment with ribavirin; closely monitor patients with a history of MI or arrhythmia. Patients with a history of significant or unstable cardiac disease should not receive combination treatment with ribavirin. Discontinue treatment (permanently) for new-onset ventricular arrhythmia or cardiovascular decompensation.

Endocrine disorders: Diabetes mellitus (including new-onset type I diabetes), hyperglycemia, and thyroid disorders have been reported; discontinue peginterferon alfa-2b if cannot be effectively managed with medication. Use caution in patients with a history of diabetes mellitus, particularly if prone to DKA. Use with caution in patients with thyroid disorders; may cause or aggravate hyper- or hypothyroidism.

Pulmonary disease: May cause or aggravate dyspnea, pulmonary infiltrates, pneumonia, bronchiolitis obliterans, interstitial pneumonitis, pulmonary hypertension, and sarcoidosis which may result in respiratory failure; may recur upon rechallenge with treatment; monitor closely. Use with caution in patients with existing pulmonary disease (eg, chronic obstructive pulmonary disease). Withhold combination therapy with ribavirin for development of pulmonary infiltrate or pulmonary function impairment.

Ophthalmic disorders: Ophthalmologic disorders (including decreased visual acuity, blindness, macular edema, retinal hemorrhages, optic neuritis, papilledema, cotton wool spots, retinal detachment [serous], and retinal artery or vein thrombosis) have occurred with peginterferon alfa-2b and/or with other alfa interferons. Prior to start of therapy, ophthalmic exams are recommended for all patients; patients with diabetic or hypertensive retinopathy should have periodic ophthalmic exams during treatment; a complete eye exam should be done promptly in patients who develop ocular symptoms. Permanently discontinue treatment with new or worsening ophthalmic disorder.

[U.S. Boxed Warning]: Combination treatment with ribavirin may cause birth defects and/or fetal mortality (avoid pregnancy in females and female partners of male patients); hemolytic anemia (which may worsen cardiac disease), genotoxicity, mutagenicity, and may possibly be carcinogenic. Potentially significant drug-drug interactions may exist, requiring dose or frequency adjustment, additional monitoring, and/or selection of alternative therapy. Peripheral neuropathy has been reported with alpha interferons when used in combination with telbivudine. Interferon therapy is commonly associated with flu-like symptoms, including fever; rule out other causes/infection with persistent or high fever. Acute hypersensitivity reactions (eg, urticaria, angioedema, bronchoconstriction, anaphylaxis) and cutaneous reactions (eg, Stevens-Johnson syndrome, toxic epidermal necrolysis) have been reported (rarely) with alfa interferons; prompt discontinuation is recommended; transient rashes do not require interruption of therapy. Hypertriglyceridemia has been reported (may result in pancreatitis); periodically monitor and manage with appropriate treatment; consider discontinuing peginterferon if persistent and severe (triglycerides >1000 mg/dL), particularly if combined with symptoms of pancreatitis. Interferons are commonly associated with flu-like symptoms. Use with caution in patients with debilitating conditions. Use with caution in patients with renal impairment (CrCl <50 mL/minute); monitor closely for signs of interferon toxicity. For the treatment of chronic hepatitis C, dosage adjustments are recommended with monotherapy in patients with moderate-to-severe impairment; do not use combination therapy with ribavirin in adult patients renal dysfunction (CrCl <50 mL/minute); discontinue if serum creatinine >2 mg/dL in children. Dosage adjustment is also recommended when used for the treatment of melanoma. Serum creatinine increases have been reported in patients with renal insufficiency. Use with caution in the elderly; the potential adverse effects (eg, neuropsychiatric events, cardiac events, systemic effects) may be more pronounced. Encephalopathy has also been observed in primarily elderly patients treated with higher doses of peginterferon alfa-2b. For the treatment of hepatitis, elderly patients generally do not respond to interferon treatment as well as younger patients. When used in combination with ribavirin, closely monitor adults >50 years of age for the development of anemia. Dental/periodontal disorders have been reported with combination therapy; dry mouth may affect teeth and mucous membranes; instruct patients to brush teeth twice daily; encourage regular dental exams; rinse mouth thoroughly after vomiting.

Combination therapy with ribavirin is preferred over monotherapy for the treatment of chronic hepatitis C. Safety and efficacy have not been established in patients who have received organ transplants or are coinfected with HIV or hepatitis B. Patients with significant bridging fibrosis or cirrhosis, genotype 1 infection or who have not responded to prior therapy, including previous pegylated interferon treatment are less likely to benefit from combination therapy with peginterferon alfa-2b and ribavirin. Growth velocity (height and weight) was decreased in children on combination treatment with ribavirin during the length of treatment. Severely inhibited growth velocity has been noted. Long-term follow-up data indicate that combination therapy may inhibit growth, resulting in reduced adult height in some patients. Growth should be closely monitored in pediatric patients during therapy and posttreatment. **[U.S. Boxed Warning]: Combination therapy with ribavirin is contraindicated in pregnancy.** Due to differences in dosage, patients should not change brands of interferon. Some dosage forms may contain polysorbate 80 (also known as Tweens). Hypersensitivity reactions, usually a delayed reaction, have been reported following exposure to pharmaceutical products containing polysorbate 80 in certain individuals (Isaksson, 2002; Lucente 2000; Shelley, 1995). Thrombocytopenia, ascites, pulmonary deterioration, and renal and hepatic failure have been reported in premature neonates after receiving parenteral products containing polysorbate 80 (Alade, 1986; CDC, 1984). See manufacturer's labeling.

Warnings: Additional Pediatric Considerations Suicidal ideation or attempts may occur more frequently in pediatric patients as compared to adults (2.4% vs 1%, respectively).

Severe inhibition of growth velocity, <3rd percentile and affecting height and weight, was reported in 70% of pediatric patients during clinical trials on combination therapy; monitor closely; dosage adjustment may be required. After therapy, 20% continued to have severely inhibited growth; however, in majority of patients, growth velocity rates increased such that by 6 months post-treatment, weight gain stabilized to 53rd percentile (similar to predicted based on average baseline weight: 57th percentile) and height gain stabilized to 44th percentile (less than predicted based on average baseline height: 51st percentile).

A higher incidence of some adverse effects has been reported in children compared to adults, including fever (80% vs 46%) and vomiting (27% vs 14%).

Adverse Reactions

Cardiovascular: Bundle branch block, chest pain, flushing, myocardial infarction, supraventricular arrhythmia, ventricular tachycardia

Central nervous system: Agitation, anxiety, chills, depression (may be severe), dizziness, emotional liability, fatigue, fever, headache, impaired concentration, insomnia, irritability, malaise, nervousness, olfactory nerve disorder, suicidal behavior (ideation/attempt/suicide)

Dermatologic: Alopecia, dry skin, pruritus, rash

Endocrine & metabolic: Hyper-/hypothyroidism, menstrual disorder

Gastrointestinal: Abdominal pain, anorexia, constipation, diarrhea, dyspepsia, nausea, taste perversion, vomiting, weight loss, xerostomia

Hematologic: Anemia (in combination with ribavirin), neutropenia, thrombocytopenia

Hepatic: Alkaline phosphatase increased, ALT/AST increased, GGT increased, hepatomegaly
Local: Injection site inflammation/reaction, injection site pain
Neuromuscular & skeletal: Arthralgia, musculoskeletal pain, myalgia, paresthesia, rigors, weakness
Ocular: Blurred vision, conjunctivitis
Renal: Proteinuria
Respiratory: Cough, dyspnea, pharyngitis, rhinitis, sinusitis
Miscellaneous: Binding antibodies (melanoma patients), diaphoresis, neutralizing antibodies, viral infection
Rare but important or life-threatening: Addiction (drug) relapse, anaphylaxis, angina, angioedema, aphthous stomatitis, aplastic anemia, arrhythmia, autoimmune thrombocytopenia (with or without purpura), bacterial infection, bipolar disorders, blindness, bronchiolitis obliterans, cardiac arrest, cardiomyopathy, cellulitis, colitis, cotton wool spots, cytopenia, diabetes mellitus, diabetic ketoacidosis, drug overdose, emphysema, encephalopathy, erythema multiforme, fungal infection, gastroenteritis, gout, hallucinations, hearing impairment/loss, hemorrhagic colitis, homicidal ideation, hyperglycemia, hyper-/hypotension, hypersensitivity reactions, hypertriglyceridemia, injection site necrosis, interstitial nephritis, interstitial pneumonitis, ischemic colitis, leukopenia, loss of consciousness, lupus-like syndrome, macular edema, mania, memory loss, migraine, myositis, nerve palsy (facial/oculomotor), optic neuritis, palpitation, pancreatitis, papilledema, pericardial effusion, peripheral neuropathy, phototoxicity, pleural effusion, pneumonia, psoriasis, psychosis, pulmonary hypertension, pulmonary infiltrates, pure red cell aplasia, renal failure, renal insufficiency, retinal artery or vein thrombosis, retinal detachment (serous), retinal hemorrhage, retinal ischemia, retinopathy, rhabdomyolysis, rheumatoid arthritis, sarcoidosis, seizure, sepsis, serum creatinine increased, Stevens-Johnson syndrome, stroke, systemic lupus erythematosus, tachycardia, thrombotic thrombocytopenic purpura, thyroiditis, toxic epidermal necrolysis, transient ischemic attack, ulcerative colitis, vasculitis, vision decrease/loss, Vogt-Koyanagi-Harada syndrome

Drug Interactions

Metabolism/Transport Effects **Inhibits** CYP1A2 (weak), CYP2D6 (weak)

Avoid Concomitant Use

Avoid concomitant use of Peginterferon Alfa-2b with any of the following: BCG (Intravesical); CloZAPine; Dipyrone; Telbivudine

Increased Effect/Toxicity

Peginterferon Alfa-2b may increase the levels/effects of: Aldesleukin; ARIPiprazole; CloZAPine; CYP1A2 Substrates; CYP2D6 Substrates; Methadone; Ribavirin; Telbivudine; TiZANidine; Zidovudine

The levels/effects of Peginterferon Alfa-2b may be increased by: Dipyrone

Decreased Effect

Peginterferon Alfa-2b may decrease the levels/effects of: BCG (Intravesical); CYP2D6 Substrates; FLUoxetine

The levels/effects of Peginterferon Alfa-2b may be decreased by: Pegloticase

Storage/Stability Prior to reconstitution, store Redipen at 2°C to 8°C (36°F to 46°F). Store intact vials at 25°C (77°F); excursions permitted to 15°C to 30°C (59°F to 86°F). Do not freeze. Once reconstituted each product should be used immediately or may be stored for ≤24 hours at 2°C to 8°C (36°F to 46°F); do not freeze. Do not shake. Keep away from heat. Products do not contain preservative (single use; do not reuse).

Mechanism of Action Alpha interferons are a family of proteins, produced by nucleated cells, that have antiviral, antiproliferative, and immune-regulating activity. There are 16 known subtypes of alpha interferons. Interferons interact with cells through high affinity cell surface receptors. Following activation, multiple effects can be detected including induction of gene transcription. Inhibits cellular growth, alters the state of cellular differentiation, interferes with oncogene expression, alters cell surface antigen expression, increases phagocytic activity of macrophages, and augments cytotoxicity of lymphocytes for target cells.

Pharmacokinetics (Adult data unless noted) Note: Peginterferon alfa-2b has a prolonged duration of effect relative to interferon alfa-2b and a reduced renal clearance (sevenfold lower). Data in children similar to adult values.
Bioavailability: Increases with chronic dosing
Half-life elimination: Chronic hepatitis C: ~40 hours (range: 22-60 hours)
Time to peak serum concentration: 15-44 hours
Elimination: Urine (30%); clearance reduced in renal impairment by 17% in moderate dysfunction, 44% in severe dysfunction

Dosing: Usual Note: Due to differences in dosage, patients should not change brands of interferon alfa therapy.

Children and Adolescents:

Chronic hepatitis B virus (HBV) infection (HIV-exposed/-positive): Adolescents: PegIntron: SubQ: 1.5 mcg/kg once weekly for 48 weeks (DHHS [adult], 2013)

Chronic hepatitis C virus (HCV) infection:

Non-HIV-exposed/-infected:

Manufacturer's labeling: Children ≥3 years and Adolescents: PegIntron: SubQ: 60 mcg/m^2 once weekly (in combination with ribavirin). Treatment duration: 48 weeks (genotype 1); 24 weeks (genotypes 2 and 3). Consider discontinuation of combination therapy in patients with HCV (genotype 1) at 12 weeks if a 2 log decrease in HCV-RNA has not been achieved or if HCV-RNA is still detectable at 24 weeks. **Note:** Adolescents who reach their 18th birthday during treatment should remain on the pediatric regimen.

Alternate dosing: American Association for the Study of Liver Diseases (AASLD) recommendations: Children ≥2 years and Adolescents: PegIntron: SubQ: 60 mcg/m^2 once weekly (in combination with oral ribavirin) for 48 weeks (all genotypes) (Ghany, 2009)

HIV-exposed/-positive (coinfection):

Children ≥3 years: PegIntron: SubQ: 60 mcg/m^2 once weekly (in combination with ribavirin). Treatment duration: 48 weeks, regardless of genotype (DHHS [pediatric], 2013)

Adolescents: PegIntron: SubQ: 1.5 mcg/kg once weekly (in combination with ribavirin). Treatment duration: 48 weeks, regardless of genotype (DHHS [adult], 2013)

Adults:

Melanoma: Sylatron: SubQ: 6 mcg/kg/week for 8 doses, followed by 3 mcg/kg/week for up to 5 years. **Note:** Premedicate with acetaminophen (500-1000 mg orally) 30 minutes prior to the first dose and as needed for subsequent doses thereafter.

Chronic hepatitis C: PegIntron: Sub Q: Administer dose once weekly. **Note:** Discontinue in patients with HCV (genotype 1) after 12 weeks if HCV RNA does not decrease by at least 2 log (compared to pretreatment) or if detectable HCV RNA present at 24 weeks. Discontinuation is also recommended in patients who previously failed therapy (regardless of genotype) if detectable HCV RNA present at 12 or 24 weeks.

Monotherapy: Duration of treatment is 1 year; Initial dose (based on average dose of 1 mcg/kg/week):
≤45 kg: 40 mcg once weekly
46-56 kg: 50 mcg once weekly
57-72 kg: 64 mcg once weekly
73-88 kg: 80 mcg once weekly
89-106 kg: 96 mcg once weekly

107-136 kg: 120 mcg once weekly
137-160 kg: 150 mcg once weekly
Combination therapy with ribavirin: Treatment duration is 48 weeks for genotype 1, 24 weeks for genotypes 2 and 3, or 48 weeks for patients who previously failed therapy (regardless of genotype). Initial dose (based on an average dose of 1.5 mcg/kg/week):
<40 kg: 50 mcg once weekly
40-50 kg: 64 mcg once weekly
51-60 kg: 80 mcg once weekly
61-75 kg: 96 mcg once weekly
76-85 kg: 120 mcg once weekly
86-105 kg: 150 mcg once weekly
>105 kg: 1.5 mcg/kg once weekly
Note: American Association for the Study of Liver Diseases (AASLD) recommendation: Adults with chronic HCV infection: Treatment of choice: Ribavirin plus **peginterferon**; clinical condition and ability of patient to tolerate therapy should be evaluated to determine length and/or likely benefit of therapy. Recommended treatment duration (AASLD guidelines; Ghany, 2009): Genotypes 1,4: 48 weeks; Genotypes 2,3: 24 weeks; Coinfection with HIV: 48 weeks

Dosing adjustment in renal impairment: Chronic hepatitis C:
Children and Adolescents: *Combination therapy with ribavirin:* Serum creatinine >2 mg/dL: Discontinue treatment
Adults:
Monotherapy:
CrCl 30-50 mL/minute: Reduce dose by 25%
CrCl 10-29 mL/minute: Reduce dose by 50%
Hemodialysis: Reduce dose by 50%
Discontinue use if renal function declines during treatment.
Combination therapy with ribavirin: CrCl <50 mL/minute: Combination therapy with ribavirin is not recommended.

Dosing adjustment hepatic impairment:
Decompensated liver disease or autoimmune hepatitis: Use is contraindicated.
Hepatic decompensation or severe hepatic injury during treatment (Child-Pugh class B or C): Discontinue immediately

Dosing adjustment for toxicity:
***Chronic hepatitis C:* Dosage adjustment for depression (severity based upon DSM-IV criteria):**
Mild depression: Children, Adolescents, and Adults: No dosage adjustment required; evaluate once weekly by visit/phone call. If depression remains stable, continue weekly visits. If depression improves, resume normal visit schedule. For worsening depression, see "Moderate depression" below.
Moderate depression: Evaluate once weekly with an office visit at least every other week. If depression remains stable, consider psychiatric evaluation and continue with reduced dosing. If symptoms improve and remain stable for 4 weeks, resume normal visit schedule; continue reduced dosing or return to normal dose. For worsening depression or development of severe depression, discontinue therapy permanently and obtain immediate psychiatric consultation. Utilize followup psychiatric therapy as needed.
Children and Adolescents: Decrease to 40 mcg/m^2 once weekly, may further decrease to 20 mcg/m^2 once weekly if needed
Adults:
Monotherapy: Refer to adult weight-based dosage reduction with monotherapy for depression below
Combination therapy: Refer to adult weight-based dosage reduction with combination therapy for depression below
Severe depression: Children, Adolescent, and Adults: Discontinue peginterferon alfa-2b and ribavirin permanently. Obtain immediate psychiatric consultation.

***Chronic hepatitis C:* Dosage adjustment in hematologic toxicity:**
Children and Adolescents:
Hemoglobin decrease >2 g/dL in any 4-week period in patients *with stable cardiac disease:* Reduce peginterferon alfa-2b dose by 50%; monitor and evaluate weekly. If after 4 weeks of dose reduction the hemoglobin remains <12 g/dL: Permanently discontinue both peginterferon alfa-2b and ribavirin.
Hemoglobin 8.5 to <10 g/dL in patients *without history of cardiac disease*: No dosage adjustment for peginterferon alfa-2b. Decrease ribavirin dose.
WBC 1000 to <1500/mm^3, neutrophils 500 to <750/mm^3, or platelets 50,000 to <70,000/mm^3: Reduce peginterferon alfa-2b dose to 40 mcg/m^2 once weekly; may further reduce to 20 mcg/m^2 once weekly
Hemoglobin <8.5 g/dL, WBC <1000/mm^3, neutrophils <500/mm^3, or platelets <50,000/mm^3: Permanently discontinue peginterferon alfa-2b and ribavirin
Adults:
Hemoglobin decrease ≥2 g/dL in any 4-week period and stable cardiac disease: Decrease peginterferon alfa-2b dose by 50%; decrease ribavirin dose. If after 4 weeks of dose reduction hemoglobin <12 g/dL: Permanently discontinue both peginterferon alfa-2b and ribavirin.
Hemoglobin 8.5 to <10 g/dL and no history of cardiac disease: No dosage adjustment necessary for peginterferon alfa-2b. Decrease ribavirin dose; may further reduce ribavirin dose if needed
WBC 1000 to <1500/mm^3, neutrophils 500 to <750/mm^3, or platelets <25,000 to <50,000/mm^3:
Peginterferon alfa-2b monotherapy: Refer to adult weight-based dosage reduction with combination therapy for hematologic toxicity below.
Peginterferon alfa-2b combination therapy: Refer to adult weight-based dosage reduction monotherapy for hematologic toxicity below.
Hemoglobin <8.5 g/dL, WBC <1000/mm^3, neutrophils <500/mm^3, or platelets <25,000/mm^3: Permanently discontinue peginterferon alfa-2b and ribavirin.

***Chronic hepatitis C:* Adult weight-based dosage reduction for depression or hematologic toxicity:**
Adults:
Peginterferon alfa-2b monotherapy: Reduce to average weekly dose of 0.5 mcg/kg as follows:
≤45 kg: 20 mcg once weekly
46-56 kg: 25 mcg once weekly
57-72 kg: 30 mcg once weekly
73-88 kg: 40 mcg once weekly
89-106 kg: 50 mcg once weekly
107-136 kg: 64 mcg once weekly
≥137 kg: 80 mcg once weekly
Peginterferon alfa-2b combination therapy: Initially reduce to average weekly dose of 1 mcg/kg; may further reduce to average weekly dose 0.5 mcg/kg if needed as follows:
<40 kg: 35 mcg once weekly; may further reduce to 20 mcg once weekly if needed
40-50 kg: 45 mcg once weekly; may further reduce to 25 mcg once weekly if needed
51-60 kg: 50 mcg once weekly; may further reduce to 30 mcg once weekly if needed
61-75 kg: 64 mcg once weekly; may further reduce to 35 mcg once weekly if needed
76-85 kg: 80 mcg once weekly; may further reduce to 45 mcg once weekly if needed
86-104 kg: 96 mcg once weekly; may further reduce to 50 mcg once weekly if needed

105-125 kg: 108 mcg once weekly; may further reduce to 64 mcg once weekly if needed

>125 kg: 135 mcg once weekly; may further reduce to 72 mcg once weekly if needed

Melanoma: Adults:

Discontinue for any of the following: Persistent or worsening severe neuropsychiatric disorders (depression, psychosis, encephalopathy), grade 4 nonhematologic toxicity, new or worsening retinopathy, new-onset ventricular arrhythmia or cardiovascular decompensation, evidence of hepatic injury (severe) or hepatic decompensation, development of hyper- or hypothyroidism or diabetes that cannot be effectively managed with medication, or inability to tolerate a dose of 1 mcg/kg/week

Temporarily withhold for any of the following: ANC <500/mm³, platelets <50,000/mm³, ECOG performance status (PS) ≥2, nonhematologic toxicity ≥ grade 3

May reinitiate at a reduced dose once ANC ≥500/mm³, platelets ≥50,000/mm³, ECOG PS at 0-1, and nonhematologic toxicity completely resolved or improved to grade 1.

Reduced dose schedule, Weeks 1-8:

First dose reduction (if prior dose 6 mcg/kg/week): 3 mcg/kg/week

Second dose reduction (if prior dose 3 mcg/kg/week): 2 mcg/kg/week

Third dose reduction (if prior dose 2 mcg/kg/week): 1 mcg/kg/week

Discontinue permanently if unable to tolerate 1 mcg/kg/week

Reduced dose schedule, Weeks 9-260:

First dose reduction (if prior dose 3 mcg/kg/week): 2 mcg/kg/week

Second dose reduction (if prior dose 2 mcg/kg/week): 1 mcg/kg/week

Discontinue permanently if unable to tolerate 1 mcg/kg/week

Preparation for Administration

PegIntron:

Redipen: Hold cartridge upright and press the two halves together until there is a "click". Gently invert to mix; do not shake; do not reuse (single use).

Vial: Add 0.7 mL SWFI (supplied single-use diluent) to the vial. Gently swirl. Do not re-enter vial after dose removed. Discard unused reconstituted portion; do not reuse.

Sylatron (vial): Add 0.7 mL SWFI and swirl gently (do not withdraw more than 0.5 mL), resulting in the following concentrations:

296 mcg vial: 40 mcg/0.1 mL

444 mcg vial: 60 mcg/0.1 mL

888 mcg vial: 120 mcg/0.1 mL

Administration SubQ: Rotate injection site; thigh, outer surface of upper arm, and abdomen are preferred injection sites; do not inject near navel or waistline; patients who are thin should only use thigh or upper arm. Do not inject into bruised, infected, irritated, red, or scarred skin. The weekly dose may be administered at bedtime to reduce flu-like symptoms. Administration volume depends on the patient's weight and peginterferon concentration used.

Monitoring Parameters CBC with differential and platelets; serum chemistries, liver function tests, renal function, triglycerides. Clinical studies (for combination therapy) tested as follows: CBC (including hemoglobin, WBC, and platelets) and chemistries (including liver function tests and uric acid) measured at weeks 2, 4, 8, and 12, and then every 6 weeks; TSH measured every 12 weeks during treatment. ECG at baseline for patients with preexisting cardiac abnormalities (for combination therapy with ribavirin)

Hepatitis C:

Serum HCV RNA levels (pretreatment, 12 and 24 weeks after therapy initiation, 24 weeks after completion of therapy). **Note:** Discontinuation of therapy may be considered after 12 weeks in patients with HCV (genotype 1) who fail to achieve an early virologic response (EVR) (defined as ≥2-log decrease in HCV RNA compared to pretreatment) or after 24 weeks with detectable HCV RNA. Treat patients with HCV (genotypes 2,3) for 24 weeks (if tolerated) and then evaluate HCV RNA levels (Ghany, 2009).

Evaluate for depression and other psychiatric symptoms before and after initiation of therapy; patients being treated for melanoma should be monitored for depression and psychiatric symptoms every 3 weeks during the first eight weeks of treatment and every 6 months thereafter; baseline ophthalmic eye examination; periodic ophthalmic exam in patients with diabetic or hypertensive retinopathy; baseline ECG in patients with cardiac disease; serum glucose or Hb A1c (for patients with diabetes mellitus). In combination therapy with ribavirin, pregnancy tests (for women of childbearing age who are receiving treatment or who have male partners who are receiving treatment), continue monthly up to 6 months after discontinuation of therapy.

Dosage Forms Excipient information presented when available (limited, particularly for generics); consult specific product labeling. [DSC] = Discontinued product

Kit, Subcutaneous:

Sylatron: 4 x 200 mcg, 4 x 300 mcg, 4 x 600 mcg [DSC] [contains polysorbate 80]

Kit, Subcutaneous [preservative free]:

Peg-Intron: 50 mcg/0.5 mL, 80 mcg/0.5 mL, 120 mcg/0.5 mL, 150 mcg/0.5 mL

Peg-Intron Redipen: 50 mcg/0.5 mL, 80 mcg/0.5 mL, 120 mcg/0.5 mL, 150 mcg/0.5 mL

Peg-Intron Redipen Pak 4: 50 mcg/0.5 mL, 80 mcg/0.5 mL [DSC], 120 mcg/0.5 mL, 150 mcg/0.5 mL

PegIntron: 50 mcg/0.5 mL, 80 mcg/0.5 mL, 120 mcg/0.5 mL, 150 mcg/0.5 mL [contains polysorbate 80]

Sylatron: 200 mcg, 300 mcg, 600 mcg [contains polysorbate 80]

- ◆ **Peg-Intron** *see* Peginterferon Alfa-2b *on page 1646*
- ◆ **PegIntron (Can)** *see* Peginterferon Alfa-2b *on page 1646*
- ◆ **Peg-Intron Redipen** *see* Peginterferon Alfa-2b *on page 1646*
- ◆ **Peg-Intron Redipen Pak 4** *see* Peginterferon Alfa-2b *on page 1646*
- ◆ **PEGLA** *see* Pegaspargase *on page 1639*
- ◆ **PegLyte (Can)** *see* Polyethylene Glycol-Electrolyte Solution *on page 1724*
- ◆ **Pegylated G-CSF** *see* Pegfilgrastim *on page 1641*
- ◆ **Pegylated Interferon Alfa-2a** *see* Peginterferon Alfa-2a *on page 1642*
- ◆ **Pegylated Interferon Alfa-2b** *see* Peginterferon Alfa-2b *on page 1646*
- ◆ **PEGyLAX** *see* Polyethylene Glycol 3350 *on page 1723*

Penciclovir (pen SYE kloe veer)

Medication Safety Issues

Sound-alike/look-alike issues:

Denavir may be confused with indinavir

Brand Names: US Denavir

Therapeutic Category Antiviral Agent, Topical

Generic Availability (US) No

Use Topical treatment of recurrent herpes labialis (cold sores, fever blisters) (FDA approved in ages ≥12 years and adults)

Pregnancy Risk Factor B

Pregnancy Considerations Adverse events have not been observed in animal reproduction studies following intravenous administration.

Breast-Feeding Considerations According to the manufacturer, the decision to continue or discontinue breast-feeding during therapy should take into account the risk of exposure to the infant and the benefits of treatment to the mother.

Contraindications Hypersensitivity to the penciclovir or any component of the formulation

Warnings/Precautions Penciclovir should only be used on herpes labialis on the lips and face; because no data are available, application to mucous membranes is not recommended. Avoid application in or near eyes since it may cause irritation. The effect of penciclovir has not been established in immunocompromised patients.

Warnings: Additional Pediatric Considerations Some dosage forms may contain propylene glycol; in neonates large amounts of propylene glycol delivered orally, intravenously (eg, >3,000 mg/day), or topically have been associated with potentially fatal toxicities which can include metabolic acidosis, seizures, renal failure, and CNS depression; toxicities have also been reported in children and adults including hyperosmolality, lactic acidosis, seizures, and respiratory depression; use caution (AAP, 1997; Shehab, 2009).

Adverse Reactions

Central nervous system: Headache

Dermatologic: Mild erythema

Local: Application site reaction

Rare but important or life-threatening: Erythematous rash, local anesthesia, local edema, oropharyngeal edema, pain, paresthesia, parosmia, pruritus, skin discoloration, urticaria

Drug Interactions

Metabolism/Transport Effects None known.

Avoid Concomitant Use There are no known interactions where it is recommended to avoid concomitant use.

Increased Effect/Toxicity There are no known significant interactions involving an increase in effect.

Decreased Effect There are no known significant interactions involving a decrease in effect.

Storage/Stability Store at controlled room temperature of 20°C to 25°C (68°F to 77°F).

Mechanism of Action In cells infected with HSV-1 or HSV-2, viral thymidine kinase phosphorylates penciclovir to a monophosphate form which, in turn, is converted to penciclovir triphosphate by cellular kinases. Penciclovir triphosphate inhibits HSV polymerase competitively with deoxyguanosine triphosphate. Consequently, herpes viral DNA synthesis and, therefore, replication are selectively inhibited

Pharmacodynamics

Resolution of pain: Adults: 3.5 days (Spruance, 1997)

Cutaneous healing: Adults: 4.8 days (Spruance, 1997)

Pharmacokinetics (Adult data unless noted) Absorption: Topical: Negligible

Dosing: Usual Topical: Children ≥12 years, Adolescents, and Adults: Apply every 2 hours during waking hours for 4 days; start at the first sign or symptom of cold sore (eg, tingling, redness, itching, swelling)

Administration Topical: Apply only to herpes labialis on the lips and face. Apply sufficient amount to cover lesions and gently rub into the affected area. Avoid application in or near eyes since it may cause irritation.

Monitoring Parameters Resolution of pain and healing of cold sore lesion

Additional Information Penciclovir is the active metabolite of the prodrug famciclovir.

Dosage Forms Excipient information presented when available (limited, particularly for generics); consult specific product labeling. [DSC] = Discontinued product

Cream, External:

Denavir: 1% (1.5 g [DSC], 5 g) [contains cetostearyl alcohol, propylene glycol]

PenicillAMINE (pen i SIL a meen)

Medication Safety Issues

Sound-alike/look-alike issues:

Penicillamine may be confused with penicillin

International issues:

Depen [U.S.] may be confused with Depin brand name for nifedipine [India]; Depon brand name for acetaminophen [Greece]; Dipen brand name for diltiazem [Greece]

Pemine [Italy] may be confused with Pamine brand name for methscopolamine [U.S., Canada]

Brand Names: US Cuprimine; Depen Titratabs

Brand Names: Canada Cuprimine®

Therapeutic Category Antidote, Copper Toxicity; Antidote, Lead Toxicity; Chelating Agent, Oral

Generic Availability (US) No

Use Treatment of Wilson's disease, cystinuria, adjunct in the treatment of severe rheumatoid arthritis (FDA approved in adults); has also been used for lead poisoning, primary biliary cirrhosis (as adjunctive therapy following initial treatment with calcium EDTA or BAL); has also been used in lead poisoning

Pregnancy Risk Factor D

Pregnancy Considerations Birth defects, including congenital cutix laxa and associated defects, have been reported in infants following penicillamine exposure during pregnancy. Use for the treatment of rheumatoid arthritis during pregnancy is contraindicated. Use for the treatment of cystinuria only if the possible benefits to the mother outweigh the potential risks to the fetus. Continued treatment of Wilson's disease during pregnancy protects the mother against relapse. Discontinuation has detrimental maternal and fetal effects. Daily dosage should be limited to 750 mg. For planned cesarean section, reduce dose to 250 mg/day for the last 6 weeks of pregnancy, and continue at this dosage until wound healing is complete.

Breast-Feeding Considerations It is not known if penicillamine is excreted in breast milk. Use while breast-feeding is contraindicated by the manufacturer.

Contraindications Renal insufficiency (in patients with rheumatoid arthritis); patients with previous penicillamine-related aplastic anemia or agranulocytosis; breast-feeding; pregnancy (in patients with rheumatoid arthritis)

Canadian labeling: Additional contraindications (not in U.S. labeling): Hypersensitivity to penicillamine or any component of the formulation; use in patients with chronic lead poisoning who have radiographic evidence of lead-containing substances in the GI tract; pregnancy (in patients with chronic lead poisoning); concomitant use with gold therapy, antimalarial or cytotoxic drugs, oxyphenbutazone or phenylbutazone

Warnings/Precautions Approximately 33% of patients will experience an allergic reaction; toxicity may be dose related; use caution in the elderly. Once instituted for Wilson's disease or cystinuria, continue treatment on a daily basis; interruptions of even a few days have been followed by hypersensitivity with reinstitution of therapy. Rash may occur early (more commonly) or late in therapy; early-onset rash typically resolves within days of discontinuation of therapy and does not recur upon rechallenge with reduced dose; discontinue therapy for late-onset rash (eg, after >6 months) and do not rechallenge; rash typically recurs with rechallenge. Drug fever sometimes in conjunction with macular cutaneous eruptions may be observed usually 2-3 weeks after therapy initiation. Discontinue use in patients with rheumatoid arthritis, Wilson's disease or cystinuria who develop a marked febrile response. Consider alternative therapy for patients with rheumatoid arthritis due to high incidence of fever reoccurrence with penicillamine rechallenge. May resume therapy at a reduced dose in Wilson's disease or cystinuria upon resolution of fever. Discontinue therapy for skin reactions accompanied by lymphadenopathy, fever, arthralgia, or other allergic reactions. Patients with a penicillin allergy may theoretically have cross-sensitivity to penicillamine; however, the possibility has been eliminated now that penicillamine is produced synthetically and no longer contains trace amounts of penicillin.

[U.S. Boxed Warning]: Patients should be warned to report promptly any symptoms suggesting toxicity (fever, sore throat, chills, bruising, or bleeding); penicillamine has been associated with fatalities due to agranulocytosis, aplastic anemia, and thrombocytopenia. Use caution with other hematopoietic-depressant drugs (eg, gold, immunosuppressants, antimalarials, phenylbutazone; Canadian labeling contraindicates concomitant use with these agents). Discontinue therapy for WBC <3500/mm^3. Withhold therapy at least temporarily for platelet counts <100,000/mm^3 or a progressive fall in WBC or platelets in 3 successive determinations, even though values may remain within the normal range. Proteinuria or hematuria may develop; monitor for membranous glomerulopathy which can lead to nephrotic syndrome. In rheumatoid arthritis patients, discontinue if gross hematuria or persistent microscopic hematuria develop and discontinue therapy or reduce dose for proteinuria that is either >1 g/day or progressively increasing. Dose reduction may lead to resolution of proteinuria.

[U.S. Boxed Warning]: Should be administered under the close supervision of a physician familiar with the toxicity and dosage considerations. Monitor liver function tests periodically due to rare reports of intrahepatic cholestasis or toxic hepatitis. Has been associated with myasthenic syndrome which in some cases progressed to myasthenia gravis. Resolution of symptoms has been observed in most cases following discontinuation of therapy. Bronchiolitis obliterans has been reported rarely with use. Pemphigus may occur early or late in therapy; discontinue use with suspicion of pemphigus. Lupus erythematosus-like syndrome may be observed in some patients; Taste alteration may occur (rare in Wilson's disease); usually self-limited with continued therapy, however may last ≥2 months and result in total loss of taste. Oral ulceration (eg, stomatitis) may occur; typically recurs on rechallenge, but often resolves with dose reduction. Other dose-related lesions (eg, glossitis, gingivostomatitis) have been observed with use and may require therapy discontinuation. Pyridoxine supplementation (25-50 mg/day) is recommended in Wilson's disease (Roberts, 2008) or 25 mg/day in cystinuria or in rheumatoid arthritis patients with impaired nutrition.

Penicillamine increases the amount of soluble collagen; may increase skin friability, particularly at sites subject to pressure or trauma (eg, knees, elbows shoulders). Purpuric areas with localized bleeding (if skin is broken) or vesicles with dark blood may be observed. Effects are considered localized and do not necessitate discontinuation of therapy; may not recur with dose reduction. Dose reduction may be considered prior to surgical procedures. May resume normal recommended dosing postoperatively once wound healing is complete.

Lead poisoning: Investigate, identify, and remove sources of lead exposure and confirm lead-containing substances are absent from the GI tract prior to initiating therapy. Do not permit patients to re-enter the contaminated environment until lead abatement has been completed. Penicillamine is considered to be a third-line agent for the treatment of lead poisoning in children due to the overall toxicity associated with its use (AAP, 2005; Chandran, 2010); penicillamine should only be used when unacceptable reactions have occurred with edetate CALCIUM disodium and succimer. Primary care providers should consult experts in the chemotherapy of lead toxicity before using chelation drug therapy.

Adverse Reactions

Cardiovascular: Vasculitis

Central nervous system: Anxiety, agitation, fever, Guillain-Barré syndrome, hyperpyrexia, psychiatric disturbances, worsening neurologic symptoms

Dermatologic: Alopecia, cheilosis, dermatomyositis, drug eruptions, exfoliative dermatitis, lichen planus, pemphigus, pruritus, rash (early and late), skin friability increased, toxic epidermal necrolysis, urticaria, wrinkling (excessive), yellow nail syndrome

Endocrine & metabolic: Hypoglycemia, thyroiditis

Gastrointestinal: Anorexia, diarrhea, epigastric pain, gingivostomatitis, glossitis, nausea, oral ulcerations, pancreatitis, peptic ulcer reactivation, taste alteration, vomiting

Hematologic: Agranulocytosis, aplastic anemia, eosinophilia, hemolytic anemia, leukocytosis, leukopenia, monocytosis, red cell aplasia, sideroblastic anemia, thrombocytopenia, thrombotic thrombocytopenia purpura, thrombocytosis

Hepatic: Alkaline phosphatase increased, hepatic failure, intrahepatic cholestasis, toxic hepatitis

Local: Thrombophlebitis, white papules at venipuncture and surgical sites

Neuromuscular & skeletal: Arthralgia, dystonia, myasthenia gravis, muscle weakness, neuropathies, polyarthralgia (migratory, often with objective synovitis), polymyositis

Ocular: Diplopia, extraocular muscle weakness, optic neuritis, ptosis, visual disturbances

Otic: Tinnitus

Renal: Goodpasture's syndrome, hematuria, nephrotic syndrome, proteinuria, renal failure, renal vasculitis

Respiratory: Asthma, interstitial pneumonitis, pulmonary fibrosis, obliterative bronchiolitis

Miscellaneous: Allergic alveolitis, anetoderma, elastosis perforans serpiginosa, lupus-like syndrome, lactic dehydrogenase increased, lymphadenopathy, mammary hyperplasia, positive ANA test

Drug Interactions

Metabolism/Transport Effects None known.

Avoid Concomitant Use There are no known interactions where it is recommended to avoid concomitant use.

Increased Effect/Toxicity

The levels/effects of PenicillAMINE may be increased by: Multivitamins/Minerals (with ADEK, Folate, Iron)

Decreased Effect

PenicillAMINE may decrease the levels/effects of: Digoxin

The levels/effects of PenicillAMINE may be decreased by: Antacids; Iron Salts; Polaprezinc

Food Interactions Penicillamine serum levels may be decreased if taken with food. Management: Administer on an empty stomach 1 hour before or 2 hours after meals and at least 1 hour apart from other drugs, milk, antacids, and zinc- or iron-containing products. Certain disease states require further diet adjustment.

Storage/Stability Store in tight, well-closed containers.

Mechanism of Action Chelates with lead, copper, mercury and other heavy metals to form stable, soluble complexes that are excreted in urine; depresses circulating IgM rheumatoid factor, depresses T-cell but not B-cell activity; combines with cystine to form a compound which is more soluble, thus cystine calculi are prevented

Pharmacodynamics Onset of action:

Rheumatoid arthritis: 2-3 months

Wilson's disease: 1-3 months

Pharmacokinetics (Adult data unless noted)

Absorption: 40% to 70%

Protein binding: 80%

Metabolism: In the liver

Half-life: 1.7-7 hours

Time to peak serum concentration: Within 1-3 hours

Elimination: Primarily (30% to 60%) in urine as unchanged drug

Dosing: Usual Oral:

Rheumatoid arthritis: **Note:** The optimal duration of therapy has not been determined; in patients experiencing a remission for ≥6 months, the daily dosage may be decreased in a stepwise fashion in 3-month intervals:

Children: Initial: 3 mg/kg/day (≤250 mg/day) for 3 months, then 6 mg/kg/day (≤500 mg/day) in 2 divided doses for 3 months to a maximum of 10 mg/kg/day (≤1-1.5 g/day) in 3-4 divided doses

Adults: 125-250 mg/day, may increase dose by 125-250 mg/day; if therapy still ineffective after 2-3 months of treatment and no signs of adverse effects, increases of 250 mg/day at 2-3 month intervals up to a maximum daily dose of 1.5 g may be done; doses >500 mg/day should be given in divided doses

Wilson's disease: **Note:** Dose that results in an initial 24-hour urinary copper excretion >2 mg/day should be continued for ~3 months; maintenance dose defined by amount resulting in <10 mcg serum free copper/dL.

Children: AASLD guidelines: 20 mg/kg/day in 2-3 divided doses, round off to the nearest 250 mg dose; reduce dose by 25% when clinically stable; administer with a pyridoxine supplement (25-50 mg/day)

Adults: 750-1500 mg/day in divided doses; maximum dose: 2000 mg/day; administer with a pyridoxine supplement (25-50 mg/day)

Note: In pregnant patients, limit daily dose to 1 g; if a cesarean section is planned, limit daily dose to 250 mg during the last 6 weeks before delivery and postoperatively until the wound has healed.

AASLD guidelines recommend to increase tolerability, therapy may be initiated at 250-500 mg/day and then titrated upward by 250 mg every 4-7 days; usual maintenance dose: 750-1000 mg/day in 2 divided doses; maximum: 1000-1500 mg/day in 2-4 divided doses; reduce dose by 25% when clinically stable (Roberts, 2008)

Cystinuria (doses titrated to maintain urinary cystine excretion at <100-200 mg/day in patients without a history of stones and <100 mg/day in patients who have had stone formation and/or pain):

Children: 30 mg/kg/day in 4 divided doses; maximum dose: 4 g/day

Adults: Initial: 2 g/day divided every 6 hours (range: 1-4 g/day)

Lead poisoning (treatment duration varies from 4-12 weeks depending upon the pretreatment blood lead level; goal of therapy is to reduce the total body content so that the blood lead level does not rebound to unacceptable levels post-treatment):

Children: 20-30 mg/kg/day in 3-4 divided doses; initiating treatment at 25% of this dose and gradually increasing to the full dose over 2-3 weeks may minimize adverse reactions; maximum dose: 1.5 g/day; a reduced dosage of 15 mg/kg/day in 2 divided doses has been shown to be effective in the treatment of mild to moderate lead poisoning (blood lead concentration 20-40 mcg/dL) with a reduction in adverse effects (Shannon, 2000)

Adults: 1-1.5 g/day in 3-4 divided doses; initiating treatment at 25% of this dose and gradually increasing to the full dose over 2-3 weeks may minimize adverse reactions

Primary biliary cirrhosis: Adults: 250 mg/day to start, increase by 250 mg every 2 weeks up to a maintenance dose of 1 g/day, as 250 mg 4 times/day

Dosing adjustment in renal impairment: CrCl <50 mL/minute: Avoid use

Administration Oral: Administer on an empty stomach 1 hour before or 2 hours after meals, milk, or other medications; patients unable to swallow capsules may mix contents of capsule with fruit juice or chilled pureed fruit; patients with cystinuria should drink copious amounts of water

Monitoring Parameters Urinalysis, CBC with differential, hemoglobin, and platelet count are recommended twice weekly for the first month then every 2 weeks for 6 months and monthly thereafter; in addition, monitor the patient's skin, lymph nodes, and body temperature; liver function tests are recommended every 6 months; weekly measurements of urinary and blood concentrations of the intoxicating metal are indicated; quantitative 24-hour urine protein at 1- to 2-week intervals initially (first 2-3 months); annual x-ray for renal stones (when used for cystinuria)

Wilson's disease: Periodic ophthalmic exam; 24-hour urinary copper excretion; copper excretion is highest initially after treatment and may exceed 1000 mcg/day; chronic treatment should produce urinary copper excretion of 200-500 mcg/day on treatment; values <200 mcg/day may be due to either noncompliance or overtreatment which may be differentiated by measuring nonceruloplamin bound copper (high in noncompliance and low in overtreatment)

Reference Range Wilson's disease: Adequate treatment: "Free" (unbound) serum copper <10 mcg/dL (Free serum copper = Total copper - ceruloplasmin copper); 24-hour urinary copper excretion 200-500 mcg (3-8 micromoles)/day

Additional Information The racemic mixture interferes with pyridoxine action and is no longer used; however, supplemental pyridoxine is still recommended.

Dosage Forms Excipient information presented when available (limited, particularly for generics); consult specific product labeling.

Capsule, Oral:

Cuprimine: 250 mg [contains fd&c yellow #10 (quinoline yellow)]

Tablet, Oral:

Depen Titratabs: 250 mg [scored]

Extemporaneous Preparations A 50 mg/mL oral suspension may be made with capsules. Mix the contents of sixty 250 mg capsules with 3 g carboxymethylcellulose, 150 g sucrose, 300 mg citric acid, and parabens (methylparaben 120 mg, propylparaben 12 mg). Add quantity of propylene glycol sufficient to make 100 mL, then add quantity of purified water sufficient to make 300 mL. Cherry flavor may be added. Label "shake well" and "refrigerate". Stable for 30 days refrigerated.

DeCastro FJ, Jaeger RQ, and Rolfe UT, "An Extemporaneously Prepared Penicillamine Suspension Used to Treat Lead Intoxication," *Hosp Pharm*, 1977, 2:446-8.

Penicillin G Benzathine

(pen i SIL in jee BENZ a theen)

Medication Safety Issues

Sound-alike/look-alike issues:

Penicillin may be confused with penicillamine

Bicillin may be confused with Wycillin

Administration issues:

Penicillin G benzathine may only be administered by deep intramuscular injection; intravenous administration of penicillin G benzathine has been associated with cardiopulmonary arrest and death.

Other safety concerns:

Bicillin C-R (penicillin G benzathine and penicillin G procaine) may be confused with Bicillin L-A (penicillin G benzathine). Penicillin G benzathine is the only product currently approved for the treatment of syphilis. Administration of penicillin G benzathine and penicillin G procaine combination instead of Bicillin L-A may result in inadequate treatment response.

Brand Names: US Bicillin L-A

Brand Names: Canada Bicillin L-A

Therapeutic Category Antibiotic, Penicillin

Generic Availability (US) No

Use Active against many gram-positive organisms and some spirochetes; treatment of syphilis; used only for the treatment of mild-to-moderate infections (ie, *Streptococcus* pharyngitis) caused by organisms susceptible to low concentrations of penicillin G, or for prophylaxis of infections caused by these organisms, such as rheumatic fever disease and acute glomerulonephritis (FDA approved in all ages)

Pregnancy Risk Factor B

Pregnancy Considerations Adverse events have not been observed in animal reproduction studies. Penicillin crosses the placenta and distributes into amniotic fluid. Maternal use of penicillins has generally not resulted in an increased risk of adverse fetal effects. Penicillin G is the drug of choice for treatment of syphilis during pregnancy.

Breast-Feeding Considerations Penicillins are excreted in breast milk. The manufacturer recommends that caution be exercised when administering penicillin to nursing women. Nondose-related effects could include modification of bowel flora and allergic sensitization.

Contraindications Hypersensitivity to penicillin(s) or any component of the formulation

Warnings/Precautions Use with caution in patients with impaired renal function, seizure disorder, or history of hypersensitivity to other beta-lactams. Serious anaphylactic reactions require immediate emergency treatment with epinephrine, oxygen, intravenous steroids and airway management (including intubation) as indicated. CDC and AAP do not currently recommend the use of penicillin G benzathine to treat congenital syphilis or neurosyphilis due to reported treatment failures and lack of published clinical data on its efficacy. Use only for infections susceptible to the low and very prolonged serum concentrations of benzathine penicillin G. Prolonged use may result in fungal or bacterial superinfection, including *C. difficile*-associated diarrhea (CDAD) and pseudomembranous colitis; CDAD has been observed >2 months postantibiotic treatment. **[U.S. Boxed Warning]: Not for intravenous use; cardiopulmonary arrest and death have occurred from inadvertent IV administration;** administer by deep IM injection only; injection into or near an artery or nerve could result in severe neurovascular damage or permanent neurological damage. Quadriceps femoris fibrosis and atrophy have been reported after repeated IM injections of penicillin preparations into the anterolateral thigh. Extended duration of therapy or use associated with high serum concentrations may be associated with an increased risk for some adverse reactions.

Warnings: Additional Pediatric Considerations Injection into or near a nerve may result in permanent neurovascular and neurological damage, gangrene requiring amputation of proximal portions of extremities, necrosis, and sloughing at the injection site. These effects have most often occurred in infants and small children. Avoid repeated IM injections into the anterolateral thigh in neonates and infants since quadriceps femoris fibrosis and atrophy may occur.

Adverse Reactions

Cardiovascular: Cardiac arrest, cerebral vascular accident, cyanosis, gangrene, hypotension, pallor, palpitations, syncope, tachycardia, vasodilation, vasospasm, vasovagal reaction

Central nervous system: Anxiety, coma, confusion, dizziness, euphoria, fatigue, headache, nervousness, pain, seizure, somnolence

In addition, a syndrome of CNS symptoms has been reported which includes: Severe agitation with confusion, hallucinations (auditory and visual), and fear of death (Hoigne's syndrome); other symptoms include cyanosis, dizziness, palpitations, psychosis, seizures, tachycardia, taste disturbance, tinnitus

Gastrointestinal: Bloody stool, intestinal necrosis, nausea, vomiting

Genitourinary: Impotence, priapism

Hepatic: AST increased

Local: Injection site reactions: Abscess, atrophy, bruising, cellulitis, edema, hemorrhage, inflammation, lump, necrosis, pain, skin ulcer

Neuromuscular & skeletal: Arthritis exacerbation, joint disorder, neurovascular damage, numbness, periostitis, rhabdomyolysis, transverse myelitis, tremor, weakness

Ocular: Blindness, blurred vision

Renal: BUN increased, creatinine increased, hematuria, myoglobinuria, neurogenic bladder, proteinuria, renal failure

Miscellaneous: Diaphoresis, hypersensitivity reactions, Jarisch-Herxheimer reaction, lymphadenopathy, mottling, warmth

Drug Interactions

Metabolism/Transport Effects Substrate of OAT3

Avoid Concomitant Use

Avoid concomitant use of Penicillin G Benzathine with any of the following: BCG; BCG (Intravesical); Probenecid

Increased Effect/Toxicity

Penicillin G Benzathine may increase the levels/effects of: Methotrexate; Vitamin K Antagonists

The levels/effects of Penicillin G Benzathine may be increased by: Probenecid; Teriflunomide

Decreased Effect

Penicillin G Benzathine may decrease the levels/effects of: BCG; BCG (Intravesical); BCG Vaccine (Immunization); Mycophenolate; Sodium Picosulfate; Typhoid Vaccine

The levels/effects of Penicillin G Benzathine may be decreased by: Tetracycline Derivatives

Storage/Stability Store at 2°C to 8°C (36°F to 46°F); do not freeze. The following stability information has also been reported: May be stored at 25°C (77°F) for 7 days (Cohen, 2007).

Mechanism of Action Interferes with bacterial cell wall synthesis during active multiplication, causing cell wall death and resultant bactericidal activity against susceptible bacteria

Pharmacokinetics (Adult data unless noted)

Absorption: IM: Slow

Distribution: Minimal concentrations attained in CSF with inflamed or uninflamed meninges; highest levels in the kidneys; lesser amounts in liver, skin, intestine; excreted in breast milk

Protein binding: ~60%

Time to peak serum concentration: Within 12-24 hours; serum levels are usually detectable for 1-4 weeks depending on the dose; larger doses result in more sustained levels rather than higher levels

Elimination: Excreted by renal tubular excretion; penicillin G is detected in urine for up to 12 weeks after a single IM injection; renal clearance is delayed in neonates, young infants, and patients with impaired renal function

Dosing: Neonatal Syphilis, congenital: IM: 50,000 units/kg as a single dose (*Red Book*, 2012)

Dosing: Usual

Infants, Children, and Adolescents:

Group A streptococcal upper respiratory infection (Gerber, 2009): IM:

Rheumatic fever, primary prevention:

≤27 kg: 600,000 units as a single dose

>27 kg: 1.2 million units as a single dose

Rheumatic fever, secondary prevention: **Note:** Duration of secondary rheumatic fever prophylaxis varies: Rheumatic fever with carditis and residual heart disease: 10 years or until 40 years of age (whichever is longer), sometimes lifelong prophylaxis; rheumatic fever with carditis but no residual heart disease: 10 years or until 21 years of age (whichever is longer); rheumatic fever without carditis: 5 years or until 21 years of age (whichever is longer)

≤27 kg: 600,000 units every 3-4 weeks

>27 kg: 1.2 million units every 3-4 weeks

Syphilis: (CDC, 2010; *Red Book*, 2012): IM

Primary, Secondary, or Early Latent (<1 year duration): 50,000 units/kg once; maximum dose: 2.4 million units

Late Latent or Latent with unknown duration: 50,000 units/kg once weekly for 3 doses; maximum dose: 2.4 million units

Adults:

Group A streptococcal upper respiratory infection: IM: 1.2 million units as a single dose

Rheumatic fever, secondary prevention: IM: 600,000 units twice monthly or 1.2 million units every 4 weeks

Syphilis: (CDC, 2010): IM:

Primary, Secondary, or Early Latent (<1 year duration): 2.4 million units as a single dose

Late Latent or Latent with unknown duration: 2.4 million units once weekly for 3 doses

Neurosyphilis: Not indicated as single-drug therapy, but may be given once weekly for 3 weeks following IV treatment; refer to Penicillin G (Parenteral/Aqueous) monograph for dosing

Administration Administer undiluted as deep IM injection in the upper outer quadrant of the buttock (adolescents and adults) or into the midlateral aspect of the thigh (neonates, infants, and children); do **not** give IV, intra-arterially or SubQ; **inadvertent IV administration has resulted in thrombosis, severe neurovascular damage, cardiac arrest, and death**

Monitoring Parameters CBC, urinalysis, culture, renal function tests, stool frequency

Test Interactions Positive Coombs' [direct], false-positive urinary and/or serum proteins; false-positive or negative urinary glucose using Clinitest®

Additional Information Use a penicillin G benzathine/penicillin G procaine combination (ie, Bicillin® C-R) to achieve early peak levels in acute infections. Do not administer Bicillin® C-R to treat patients infected with syphilis since this may result in inadequate treatment.

Dosage Forms Excipient information presented when available (limited, particularly for generics); consult specific product labeling.

Suspension, Intramuscular:

Bicillin L-A: 600,000 units/mL (1 mL); 1,200,000 units/2 mL (2 mL); 2,400,000 units/4 mL (4 mL) [contains methylparaben, propylparaben]

Penicillin G (Parenteral/Aqueous)

(pen i SIL in jee, pa REN ter al, AYE kwee us)

Medication Safety Issues

Sound-alike/look-alike issues:

Penicillin may be confused with penicillamine

Brand Names: US Pfizerpen-G

Brand Names: Canada Crystapen

Therapeutic Category Antibiotic, Penicillin

Generic Availability (US) Yes

Use Treatment of sepsis, meningitis, pericarditis, endocarditis, pneumonia, and other infections due to susceptible gram-positive organisms (except *Staphylococcus aureus*), some gram-negative organisms such as *Neisseria gonorrhoeae*, or *N. meningitidis* and some anaerobes and spirochetes (FDA approved in all ages)

Pregnancy Risk Factor B

Pregnancy Considerations Adverse events have not been observed in animal reproduction studies. Penicillin crosses the placenta and distributes into amniotic fluid. Maternal use of penicillins has generally not resulted in an increased risk of adverse fetal effects. Penicillin G is the drug of choice for treatment of syphilis during pregnancy and penicillin G (parenteral/aqueous) is the drug of choice for the prevention of early-onset Group B Streptococcal (GBS) disease in newborns (consult current guidelines).

Breast-Feeding Considerations Very small amounts of penicillin G transfer into breast milk. Peak milk concentrations occur at approximately 1 hour after an IM dose and are higher if multiple doses are given. The manufacturer recommends that caution be exercised when administering penicillin to nursing women. Nondose-related effects could include modification of bowel flora and allergic sensitization.

Contraindications Hypersensitivity to penicillin or any component of the formulation

Warnings/Precautions Avoid intra-arterial administration or injection into or near major peripheral nerves or blood vessels since such injections may cause severe and/or permanent neurovascular damage; use with caution in patients with renal impairment (dosage reduction required), concomitant renal and hepatic impairment (further dosage adjustment may be required), pre-existing seizure disorders, or with a history of hypersensitivity to cephalosporins. Prolonged use may result in fungal or bacterial superinfection, including *C. difficile*-associated diarrhea (CDAD) and pseudomembranous colitis; CDAD has been observed >2 months postantibiotic treatment. Serious and occasionally severe or fatal hypersensitivity (anaphylactoid) reactions have been reported in patients on penicillin therapy, especially with a history of beta-lactam hypersensitivity, history of sensitivity to multiple allergens, or previous IgE-mediated reactions (eg, anaphylaxis, angioedema, urticaria). Use with caution in asthmatic patients. Extended duration of therapy or use associated with high serum concentrations may be associated with an increased risk for some adverse reactions. Neonates may have decreased renal clearance of penicillin and require frequent dosage adjustments depending on age. Product contains sodium and potassium; high doses of IV therapy may alter serum levels.

Adverse Reactions

Cardiovascular: Localized phlebitis, local thrombophlebitis

Central nervous system: Coma (high doses), hyperreflexia (high doses), myoclonus (high doses), seizure (high doses)

Dermatologic: Contact dermatitis, skin rash

Endocrine & metabolic: Electrolyte disturbance (high doses)

Gastrointestinal: Pseudomembranous colitis

Hematologic & oncologic: Neutropenia, positive direct Coombs test (rare, high doses)

Hypersensitivity: Anaphylaxis, hypersensitivity reaction (immediate and delayed), serum sickness
Immunologic: Jarisch-Herxheimer reaction
Local: Injection site reaction
Renal: Acute interstitial nephritis (high doses), renal tubular disease (high doses)

Drug Interactions

Metabolism/Transport Effects **Substrate** of OAT3

Avoid Concomitant Use

Avoid concomitant use of Penicillin G (Parenteral/Aqueous) with any of the following: BCG; BCG (Intravesical); Probenecid

Increased Effect/Toxicity

Penicillin G (Parenteral/Aqueous) may increase the levels/effects of: Methotrexate; Vitamin K Antagonists

The levels/effects of Penicillin G (Parenteral/Aqueous) may be increased by: Probenecid; Teriflunomide

Decreased Effect

Penicillin G (Parenteral/Aqueous) may decrease the levels/effects of: BCG; BCG (Intravesical); BCG Vaccine (Immunization); Mycophenolate; Sodium Picosulfate; Typhoid Vaccine

The levels/effects of Penicillin G (Parenteral/Aqueous) may be decreased by: Tetracycline Derivatives

Storage/Stability

Penicillin G potassium powder for injection should be stored below 86°F (30°C). Following reconstitution, solution may be stored for up to 7 days under refrigeration. Premixed bags for infusion should be stored in the freezer (-20°C or -4°F); frozen bags may be thawed at room temperature or in refrigerator. Once thawed, solution is stable for 14 days if stored in refrigerator or for 24 hours when stored at room temperature. Do not refreeze once thawed.

Penicillin G sodium powder for injection should be stored at controlled room temperature. Reconstituted solution may be stored under refrigeration for up to 3 days.

Mechanism of Action Interferes with bacterial cell wall synthesis during active multiplication, causing cell wall death and resultant bactericidal activity against susceptible bacteria

Pharmacokinetics (Adult data unless noted)

Distribution: Penetration across the blood-brain barrier is poor with uninflamed meninges
Protein binding: 65%
Metabolism: Hepatic (10% to 30%) to penicilloic acid
Half-life:
- Neonates:
  - <6 days: 3.2-3.4 hours
  - 7-13 days: 1.2-2.2 hours
  - >14 days: 0.9-1.9 hours
- Infants and Children: 0.5-1.2 hours
- Adults: 0.5-0.75 hours with normal renal function

Time to peak serum concentration: IM: Within 30 minutes
Elimination: Renal (58% to 85% unchanged drug and metabolites); mainly by tubular secretion and bile
Dialysis: Moderately dialyzable (20% to 50%)

Dosing: Neonatal

General dosing, susceptible infection (non-CNS) (*Red Book*, 2012): IM, IV:
- Body weight <1 kg:
  - PNA ≤14 days: 25,000-50,000 units/kg/**dose** every 12 hours
  - PNA 15-28 days: 25,000-50,000 units/kg/**dose** every 8 hours
- Body weight ≥1 kg:
  - PNA ≤7 days: 25,000-50,000 units/kg/**dose** every 12 hours
  - PNA 8-28 days: 25,000-50,000 units/kg/**dose** every 8 hours

Meningitis: IV:
- Group B streptococcus (*Red Book*, 2012):
  - PNA 0-7 days: 250,000-450,000 units/kg/day in divided doses every 8 hours
  - PNA 8-28 days: 450,000-500,000 units/kg/day in divided doses every 6 hours
- Other susceptible organisms (Tunkel, 2004):
  - PNA 0-7 days: 50,000 units/kg/day in divided doses every 8-12 hours
  - PNA 8-28 days: 200,000 units/kg/day in divided doses every 6-8 hours

Syphilis, congenital (CDC, 2010): IV:
- PNA 0-7 days: 50,000 units/kg/**dose** every 12 hours for 10 days
- PNA 8-28 days: 50,000 units/kg/**dose** every 8 hours for 10 days

Dosing: Usual

Infants, Children, and Adolescents:

General dosing, susceptible infection (*Red Book*, 2012): IM, IV:
- Mild to moderate infection: 100,000-150,000 units/kg/day in divided doses every 6 hours maximum daily dose: 8 million units/day
- Severe infections: 200,000-300,000 units/kg/day in divided doses every 4 hours; maximum daily dose: 24 million units/day

Anthrax, community-acquired: IV: 100,000-150,000 units/kg/day in divided doses every 4-6 hours (Stevens, 2005)

Arthritis, gonococcal: IM, IV:
- Weight <45 kg: 100,000 units/kg/day divided every 6 hours for 7-10 days
- Weight ≥45 kg: 2.5 million units every 6 hours for 7-10 days

Clostridial myonecrosis (gas gangrene): IV: 250,000-400,000 units/kg/day in divided doses every 4-6 hours with or without clindamycin (*Red Book*, 2012)

Diphtheria: IM, IV: 150,000-250,000 units/kg/day in divided doses every 6 hours for 7-10 days. AAP suggests a duration of 14 days (*Red Book*, 2012)

Endocarditis, bacterial, treatment (Baddour, 2005): IV:
- Enterococcal endocarditis (native or prosthetic valve): 300,000 units/kg/day in divided doses every 4-6 hours with gentamicin for 4-6 weeks
- Viridans group streptococci and *Streptococcus bovis* (highly penicillin susceptible):
  - Native valve: 200,000 units/kg/day in divided doses every 4-6 hours for 4 weeks or 2 weeks if given with gentamicin
  - Prosthetic valve: 300,000 units/kg/day in divided doses every 4-6 hours for 6 weeks with 2-6 weeks of gentamicin
- Viridans group streptococci and *Streptococcus bovis* (relatively resistant):
  - Native valve: 300,000 units/kg/day in divided doses every 4-6 hours for 4 weeks with 2 weeks of gentamicin
  - Prosthetic valve: 300,000 units/kg/day in divided doses every 4-6 hours for 6 weeks with 2-6 weeks of gentamicin

Lyme disease: IV: 200,000-400,000 units/kg/day in divided doses every 4 hours; maximum daily dose: 24 million units/day (Halperin, 2007; Wormser, 2006)

Meningitis: Note: Dosing varies based on organism being treated. IV:
- Group B streptococcus: Infants: 450,000-500,000 units/kg/day divided every 6 hours (*Red Book*, 2012)
- *S. pneumonia:* 250,000-400,000 units/kg/day divided every 4-6 hours (*Red Book*, 2012)
- Other susceptible organisms: 300,000 units/kg/day divided every 4-6 hours; maximum daily dose: 24 million units/day (Tunkel, 2004)

Meningococcal disease: IV: 300,000 units/kg/day in divided doses every 4-6 hours; maximum daily dose: 12 million units/day (*Red Book*, 2012)

Pneumonia, community-acquired (CAP): IV: Infants and Children >3 months:

Empiric treatment or *S. pneumoniae* (moderate to severe; MICs to penicillin ≤2.0 mcg/mL): 200,000-250,000 units/kg/day divided every 4-6 hours (Bradley, 2011)

Alternate dosing (AAP recommendation): 250,000-400,000 units/kg/day divided every 4-6 hours (*Red Book*, 2012)

Group A *Streptococcus* (moderate to severe): 100,000-250,000 units/kg/day divided every 4-6 hours (Bradley, 2011)

Rat-bite fever/Haverhill fever: IV: 150,000-250,000 units/kg/day in divided doses every 4 hours for 4 weeks; maximum daily dose: 20 million units/day (*Red Book*, 2012)

Syphilis: IV:

Congenital: Infants ≥1 month: 200,000-300,000 units/kg/day in divided doses every 4-6 hours for 10 days (CDC, 2009)

Neurosyphilis:

Non-HIV-exposed/-positive: 200,000-300,000 units/kg/day in divided doses every 4-6 hours for 10-14 days; maximum dose: 24 million units/day (*Red Book*, 2012)

HIV-exposed/-positive: 200,000-300,000 units/kg/day divided every 6 hours for 10-14 days; maximum dose: 24 million units/day (CDC, 2009)

Tetanus: IV: 100,000 units/kg/day in divided doses every 4-6 hours for 10-14 days; maximum daily dose: 12 million units/day (*Red Book*, 2012)

Adults:

***Actinomyces* species:** IV: 10-20 million units/day in divided doses every 4-6 hours for 4-6 weeks

Clostridium perfringens: IV: 24 million units/day in divided doses every 4-6 hours with clindamycin

Corynebacterium diptheriae: IV: 2-3 million units/day in divided doses every 4-6 hours for 10-12 days

Erysipelas: IV: 1-2 million units every 4-6 hours

Erysipelothrix: IV: 2-4 million units every 4 hours

Fascial space infections: IV: 2-4 million units every 4-6 hours with metronidazole

Leptospirosis: IV: 1.5 million units every 6 hours for 7 days

Listeria: IV: 15-20 million units/day in divided doses every 4-6 hours for 2 weeks (meningitis) or 4 weeks (endocarditis)

Lyme disease (meningitis): IV: 20 million units/day in divided doses

Neurosyphilis: IV: 18-24 million units/day in divided doses every 4 hours (or by continuous infusion) for 10-14 days (CDC, 2010)

Prosthetic joint infection: IV:

Enterococcus spp (penicillin-susceptible), streptococci (beta-hemolytic): 20-24 million units daily continuous infusion every 24 hours or in divided doses every 4 hours for 4-6 weeks (Osmon, 2013); **Note:** For penicillin-susceptible *Enterococcus* spp, consider addition of aminoglycoside.

Propionibacterium acnes: 20 million units daily continuous infusion every 24 hours or in divided doses every 4 hours for 4-6 weeks (Osmon, 2013)

Streptococcus sp.:

Brain abscess: IV: 18-24 million units/day in divided doses every 4 hours with metronidazole

Endocarditis or osteomyelitis: IV: 3-4 million units every 4 hours for at least 4 weeks

Group B streptococcus (neonatal prophylaxis) IV: 5 million units once then 2.5 to 3.0 million units every 4 hours until delivery (CDC, 2010)

Skin and soft tissue: IV: 3-4 million units every 4 hours for 10 days

Toxic shock: IV: 24 million units/day in divided doses with clindamycin

Streptococcal pneumonia: IV: 2-3 million units every 4 hours

Whipple's disease: IV: 2 million units every 4 hours for 2 weeks, followed by oral trimethoprim/sulfamethoxazole or doxycycline for 1 year

Relapse or CNS involvement: 4 million units every 4 hours for 4 weeks

Dosing adjustment in renal impairment:

Manufacturer's labeling: Infants, Children, Adolescents, and Adults: IM, IV:

Uremic patients with CrCl >10 mL/minute: Administer a normal dose followed by 50% of the normal dose every 4-5 hours

CrCl <10 mL/minute: Administer a normal dose followed by 50% of the normal dose every 8-10 hours

Alternate recommendation: Adults:

GFR >50 mL/minute: No dosage adjustments are necessary (Aronoff, 2007)

GFR 10-50 mL/minute: Administer 75% of the normal dose (Aronoff, 2007)

GFR <10 mL/minute: Administer 20% to 50% of the normal dose (Aronoff, 2007)

Intermittent hemodialysis (IHD) (administer after hemodialysis on dialysis days) (Heintz, 2009): Administer a normal dose followed by either 25% to 50% of normal dose every 4-6 hours **or** 50% to 100% of normal dose every 8-12 hours. *For mild to moderate infections,* administer 0.5-1 million units every 4-6 hours **or** 1-2 million units every 8-12 hours. *For neurosyphilis, endocarditis, or serious infections,* administer up to 2 million units every 4-6 hours; administer after dialysis on dialysis days **or** supplement with 500,000 units after dialysis. **Note:** Dosing dependent on the assumption of 3 times weekly, complete IHD sessions.

Continuous renal replacement therapy (CRRT) (Heintz, 2009; Trotman, 2005): Drug clearance is highly dependent on the method of renal replacement, filter type, and flow rate. Appropriate dosing requires close monitoring of pharmacologic response, signs of adverse reactions due to drug accumulation, as well as drug concentrations in relation to target trough (if appropriate). The following are general recommendations only (based on dialysate flow/ultrafiltration rates of 1-2 L/hour and minimal residual renal function) and should not supersede clinical judgment:

CVVH: Loading dose of 4 million units, followed by 2 million units every 4-6 hours

CVVHD: Loading dose of 4 million units, followed by 2-3 million units every 4-6 hours

CVVHDF: Loading dose of 4 million units, followed by 2-4 million units every 4-6 hours

Dosing adjustment in hepatic impairment: There are no dosage adjustments provided in the manufacturer's labeling.

Preparation for Administration

IM: 5 million unit vial: Solutions containing ≤100,000 units/mL may be used with minimal discomfort

IV:

Intermittent IV infusion: 5 million unit vial: Reconstitute powder for injection with SWFI, NS or D_5W to a resultant concentration of 500,000 to 1,000,000 units/mL (see manufacturer's labeling for specific details). Further dilute in an appropriate fluid to usual final concentration range of 50,000 to 100,000 units/mL prior to infusion. In fluid-restricted patients, ~150,000 units/mL in SWFI results in a maximum recommended osmolality for peripheral infusion (Robinson 1987). In neonates a concentration of 25,000 units/mL has been used (Prober 1990).

Continuous IV infusion: 20 million unit vial: Add 11.5 mL for a resultant concentration of 1,000,000 units/mL. Determine the volume of an appropriate fluid and rate of its administration (the potassium content of the dose should be considered when determining the infusion rate) required by the patient in a 24-hour period. Add the appropriate daily dosage of penicillin to this fluid. For example, if the daily dose is 10 million units and 2 L of fluid/day is required, add 5 million units to 1 L and adjust the rate of flow so the liter will be infused over 12 hours (83 mL/hour). Repeat steps (5 million units/L at 83 mL/hour) for the remaining 12 hours.

Administration

Parenteral:

IM: Administer IM by deep injection in the upper outer quadrant of the buttock. Administer injection around-the-clock to promote less variation in peak and trough levels.

IV: Usually administered by intermittent infusion. In some centers, large doses may be administered by continuous IV infusion. The potassium or sodium content of the dose should be considered when determining the infusion rate.

Intermittent IV: Infuse over 15 to 30 minutes

Continuous IV infusion: Daily dose may be administered as a continuous infusion over 24 hours, or smaller increments (eg, 24 hour dose divided into two 12-hour infusions)

Monitoring Parameters Periodic serum electrolytes, renal and hematologic function tests, cardiac and hematologic function tests during prolonged/high-dose therapy; observe for signs and symptoms of anaphylaxis during first dose

Test Interactions False-positive or negative urinary glucose determination using Clinitest®; positive Coombs' [direct]; false-positive urinary and/or serum proteins

Additional Information

Penicillin G potassium: 1.7 mEq of potassium and 0.3 mEq of sodium per 1 million units of penicillin G

Penicillin G sodium: 2 mEq of sodium per 1 million units of penicillin G

Dosage Forms Excipient information presented when available (limited, particularly for generics); consult specific product labeling.

Solution, Intravenous, as potassium:

Generic: 20,000 units/mL (50 mL); 40,000 units/mL (50 mL); 60,000 units/mL (50 mL)

Solution Reconstituted, Injection, as potassium:

Pfizerpen-G: 5,000,000 units (1 ea); 20,000,000 units (1 ea)

Pfizerpen-G: 5,000,000 units (1 ea); 20,000,000 units (1 ea) [pyrogen free]

Generic: 5,000,000 units (1 ea); 20,000,000 units (1 ea)

Solution Reconstituted, Injection, as potassium [preservative free]:

Generic: 20,000,000 units (1 ea)

Solution Reconstituted, Injection, as sodium:

Generic: 5,000,000 units (1 ea)

◆ **Penicillin G Potassium** *see* Penicillin G (Parenteral/Aqueous) *on page 1656*

Penicillin G Procaine (pen i SIL in jee PROE kane)

Medication Safety Issues

Sound-alike/look-alike issues:

Penicillin G procaine may be confused with penicillin V potassium

Wycillin may be confused with Bicillin

Brand Names: Canada Pfizerpen-AS®; Wycillin®

Therapeutic Category Antibiotic, Penicillin

Generic Availability (US) Yes

Use Moderately severe infections due to *Treponema pallidum* and other penicillin G-sensitive microorganisms that are susceptible to low but prolonged serum penicillin concentrations

Pregnancy Risk Factor B

Pregnancy Considerations Adverse events have not been observed in animal reproduction studies. Penicillin crosses the placenta and distributes into amniotic fluid. Maternal use of penicillins has generally not resulted in an increased risk of adverse fetal effects.

Breast-Feeding Considerations Penicillins are excreted in breast milk. The manufacturer recommends that caution be used when administering penicillin to nursing women. Nondose-related effects could include modification of bowel flora and allergic sensitization.

Contraindications Hypersensitivity to any penicillin or any component of the formulation.

Warnings/Precautions May need to modify dosage in patients with severe renal impairment or seizure disorders; avoid IV, intravascular, or intra-arterial administration of penicillin G procaine since severe and/or permanent neurovascular damage may occur. Serious and occasionally severe or fatal hypersensitivity (anaphylactic) reactions have been reported in patients on penicillin therapy, especially with a history of beta-lactam hypersensitivity, and/or sensitivity to multiple allergens. If an allergic reaction occurs, discontinue therapy and institute appropriate supportive measures. If there is a history of hypersensitivity to procaine, test with 0.1 mL of 1% or 2% procaine solution. If erythema, wheal, flare, or eruption occurs, patient may be sensitive to procaine; do not use penicillin G procaine in these patients. Treat sensitivity with supportive measures, including antihistamines. Immediate toxic reactions (eg, anxiety, confusion, agitation, depression, weakness, seizures, hallucinations, combativeness and expressed "fear of impending death") have been reported. Mental disturbance reactions are more common in patients receiving a large single dose (eg 4.8 million units). Reactions are transient and last 15 to 30 minutes (eg, transverse myelitis with permanent paralysis, gangrene requiring digit or proximal extremity amputation, necrosis and sloughing at and surrounding the injection site) may occur. These reactions have occurred following injection into the deltoid, thigh or buttock areas. Other serious complications of suspected intravascular administration (eg, immediate distal and proximal pallor, mottling or cyanosis of the extremity around the injection site followed by bleb formation or severe edema requiring anterior and/or posterior compartment fasciotomy in the lower extremity) occur most often in infants and small children. If any evidence of blood supply compromise is noted, consult appropriate specialists promptly. Quadriceps femoris fibrosis and atrophy have been reported following repeated IM injections of penicillins into the anterolateral thigh. Extended duration of therapy or use associated with high serum concentrations may be associated with an increased risk for some adverse reactions. Prolonged use may result in fungal or bacterial superinfection, including *C. difficile*-associated diarrhea (CDAD) and pseudomembranous colitis; CDAD has been observed >2 months postantibiotic treatment. Do not use for the treatment of gonorrhea. Penicillin G procaine is not the same preparation as penicillin G benzathine-penicillin G procaine (eg, *Bicillin C-R*). Dispensing errors have occurred. Potentially significant drug-drug interactions may exist, requiring dose or frequency adjustment, additional monitoring, and/or selection of alternative therapy.

Warnings: Additional Pediatric Considerations Avoid repeated IM injections into the anterolateral thigh in neonates and infants since quadriceps femoris fibrosis and atrophy may occur.

Adverse Reactions

Cardiovascular: Conduction disturbances, myocardial depression, vasodilation

Central nervous system: CNS stimulation, confusion, drowsiness, myoclonus, seizure

Hematologic: Hemolytic anemia, neutropenia, positive Coombs' reaction

Local: Pain at injection site, sterile abscess at injection site, thrombophlebitis

Renal: Interstitial nephritis

Miscellaneous: Hypersensitivity reactions, Jarisch-Herxheimer reaction, pseudoanaphylactic reactions, serum sickness

Drug Interactions

Metabolism/Transport Effects Substrate of OAT3

Avoid Concomitant Use

Avoid concomitant use of Penicillin G Procaine with any of the following: BCG; BCG (Intravesical); Probenecid

Increased Effect/Toxicity

Penicillin G Procaine may increase the levels/effects of: Methotrexate; Vitamin K Antagonists

The levels/effects of Penicillin G Procaine may be increased by: Probenecid; Teriflunomide

Decreased Effect

Penicillin G Procaine may decrease the levels/effects of: BCG; BCG (Intravesical); BCG Vaccine (Immunization); Mycophenolate; Sodium Picosulfate; Typhoid Vaccine

The levels/effects of Penicillin G Procaine may be decreased by: Tetracycline Derivatives

Storage/Stability Store at 2°C to 8°C (36°F to 46°F). Keep from freezing.

Mechanism of Action Inhibits bacterial cell wall synthesis by binding to one or more of the penicillin-binding proteins (PBPs); which in turn inhibits the final transpeptidation step of peptidoglycan synthesis in bacterial cell walls, thus inhibiting cell wall biosynthesis. Bacteria eventually lyse due to ongoing activity of cell wall autolytic enzymes (autolysins and murein hydrolases) while cell wall assembly is arrested.

Pharmacokinetics (Adult data unless noted)

Absorption: IM: Slow

Distribution: Penetration across the blood-brain barrier is poor, despite inflamed meninges; appears in breast milk

Time to peak serum concentration: Within 1-4 hours and can persist within the therapeutic range for 15-24 hours

Elimination: Renal clearance is delayed in neonates, young infants, and patients with impaired renal function

Dialysis: Moderately dialyzable (20% to 50%)

Dosing: Neonatal Note: Use in this age group should be avoided since sterile abscesses and procaine toxicity occur more frequently with neonates than older patients

Congenital syphilis: IM: Patient weight >1200 g: 50,000 units/kg/day once daily for 10 days; if more than 1 day of therapy is missed, the entire course should be restarted

Dosing: Usual

Infants and Children: IM: 25,000-50,000 units/kg/day in divided doses every 12-24 hours; not to exceed 4.8 million units/24 hours

Congenital syphilis: IM: 50,000 units/kg/day once daily for 10 days; if more than 1 day of therapy is missed, the entire course should be restarted

Adults: IM: 0.6-4.8 million units/day in divided doses every 12-24 hours

When used in conjunction with an aminoglycoside for the treatment of endocarditis caused by susceptible *S. viridans*: IM: 1.2 million units every 6 hours for 2-4 weeks

Neurosyphilis: IM: 2.4 million units once daily for 10 days with probenecid 500 mg every 6 hours

Administration Parenteral: **Do not give IV, intra-arterially, or SubQ**; procaine suspension for deep IM injection only; inadvertent IV administration has resulted in neurovascular damage; in infants and children it is preferable to administer IM into the midlateral muscles of the thigh; in adults, administer into the gluteus maximus or into the midlateral muscles of the thigh

Monitoring Parameters Periodic renal and hematologic function tests with prolonged therapy

Test Interactions Positive Coombs' [direct], false-positive urinary and/or serum proteins

Dosage Forms Excipient information presented when available (limited, particularly for generics); consult specific product labeling.

Suspension, Intramuscular:

Generic: 600,000 units/mL (1 mL, 2 mL)

◆ **Penicillin G Sodium** *see* Penicillin G (Parenteral/Aqueous) *on page 1656*

Penicillin V Potassium

(pen i SIL in vee poe TASS ee um)

Medication Safety Issues

Sound-alike/look-alike issues:

Penicillin V procaine may be confused with penicillin G potassium

Brand Names: Canada Apo-Pen VK; Novo-Pen-VK; Nu-Pen-VK

Therapeutic Category Antibiotic, Penicillin

Generic Availability (US) Yes

Use Treatment of mild to moderately severe susceptible bacterial infections involving the upper respiratory tract, skin, and soft tissues; prophylaxis of rheumatic fever (all indications: FDA approved in ages ≥12 years and adults); has also been used for prophylaxis of invasive pneumococcal infections in high-risk patients, treatment of community-acquired cutaneous anthrax, and treatment of community-acquired pneumonia caused by group A streptococcus

Pregnancy Considerations Penicillin crosses the placenta and distributes into amniotic fluid. Maternal use of penicillins has generally not resulted in an increased risk of adverse fetal effects. Due to pregnancy-induced physiologic changes, some pharmacokinetic parameters of penicillin V may be altered in the second and third trimester. Higher doses or increased dosing frequency may be required.

Breast-Feeding Considerations Penicillin V is excreted into breast milk (low concentrations) and may be detected in the urine of some breast-feeding infants. Loose stools and rash have been reported in nursing infants.

Contraindications Hypersensitivity to penicillin or any component of the formulation

Warnings/Precautions Use with caution in patients with severe renal impairment or history of seizures. Serious and occasionally severe or fatal hypersensitivity (anaphylactoid) reactions have been reported in patients on penicillin therapy, especially with a history of beta-lactam hypersensitivity, history of sensitivity to multiple allergens, or previous IgE-mediated reactions (eg, anaphylaxis, angioedema, urticaria). Use with caution in asthmatic patients. Extended duration of therapy or use associated with high serum concentrations may be associated with an increased risk for some adverse reactions. Prolonged use may result in fungal or bacterial superinfection, including *C. difficile*-associated diarrhea (CDAD) and pseudomembranous colitis; CDAD has been observed >2 months postantibiotic treatment.

Benzyl alcohol and derivatives: Some dosage forms may contain sodium benzoate/benzoic acid; benzoic acid (benzoate) is a metabolite of benzyl alcohol; large amounts of benzyl alcohol (≥99 mg/kg/day) have been associated with a potentially fatal toxicity ("gasping syndrome") in neonates; the "gasping syndrome" consists of metabolic acidosis, respiratory distress, gasping respirations, CNS dysfunction (including convulsions, intracranial hemorrhage), hypotension, and cardiovascular collapse (AAP, 1997; CDC, 1982); some data suggests that benzoate displaces bilirubin from protein binding sites (Ahlfors 2001); avoid or use dosage forms containing benzyl alcohol derivative with caution in neonates. See manufacturer's labeling.

Adverse Reactions

Gastrointestinal: Melanoglossia, mild diarrhea, nausea, oral candidiasis, vomiting

Rare but important or life-threatening: Acute interstitial nephritis, convulsions, exfoliative dermatitis, hemolytic anemia, hypersensitivity reaction, positive Coombs' reaction, serum-sickness like reactions

Drug Interactions

Metabolism/Transport Effects None known.

Avoid Concomitant Use

Avoid concomitant use of Penicillin V Potassium with any of the following: BCG; BCG (Intravesical); Probenecid

Increased Effect/Toxicity

Penicillin V Potassium may increase the levels/effects of: Methotrexate; Vitamin K Antagonists

The levels/effects of Penicillin V Potassium may be increased by: Probenecid

Decreased Effect

Penicillin V Potassium may decrease the levels/effects of: BCG; BCG (Intravesical); BCG Vaccine (Immunization); Mycophenolate; Sodium Picosulfate; Typhoid Vaccine

The levels/effects of Penicillin V Potassium may be decreased by: Tetracycline Derivatives

Food Interactions Food decreases drug absorption rate; decreases drug serum concentration. Management: Take on an empty stomach 1 hour before or 2 hours after meals around-the-clock to promote less variation in peak and trough serum levels.

Storage/Stability Refrigerate suspension after reconstitution; discard after 14 days.

Mechanism of Action Inhibits bacterial cell wall synthesis by binding to one or more of the penicillin-binding proteins (PBPs); which in turn inhibits the final transpeptidation step of peptidoglycan synthesis in bacterial cell walls, thus inhibiting cell wall biosynthesis. Bacteria eventually lyse due to ongoing activity of cell wall autolytic enzymes (autolysins and murein hydrolases) while cell wall assembly is arrested.

Pharmacokinetics (Adult data unless noted)

Absorption: Oral: 60% to 73% from the GI tract

Distribution: Widely distributed to kidneys, liver, skin, tonsils, and into synovial, pleural, and pericardial fluids

Protein binding: 80%

Metabolism: 10% to 30%

Half-life: 30 minutes; prolonged in patients with renal impairment

Time to peak serum concentration: Within 30-60 minutes

Elimination: Penicillin V and its metabolites are excreted in urine mainly by tubular secretion

Dosing: Usual

Infants, Children, and Adolescents:

General dosing, susceptible infections: Oral:

Infants and Children <12 years: Mild to moderate infection: 25-50 mg/kg/day in divided doses every 6-8 hours; maximum daily dose: 2000 mg/**day** (*Red Book*, 2012)

Children ≥12 years and Adolescents:

Manufacturer's labeling (fixed dosing): 125-500 mg every 6-8 hours

Alternate dosing (weight-based): Mild to moderate infection: 25-50 mg/kg/day in divided doses every 6-8 hours; maximum daily dose: 2000 mg/**day** (*Red Book*, 2012)

Anthrax (cutaneous), community-acquired: Oral: Infants, Children, and Adolescents: 25-50 mg/kg/day in divided doses 2 **or** 4 times daily; maximum single dose: 500 mg (Stevens, 2005)

Fusospirochetosis (Vincent infection), mild to moderately severe infections: Oral: Children ≥12 years and Adolescents: 250-500 mg every 6-8 hours

Tonsillopharyngitis; Group A streptococcal infection, treatment and primary prevention of rheumatic fever: Oral:

Acute treatment (Gerber, 2009; Shulman, 2012; WHO, 2004):

Children ≤27 kg: 250 mg 2-3 times daily for 10 days

Children >27 kg and Adolescents: 500 mg 2-3 times daily for 10 days; in adolescents, 250 mg 4 times daily has also been suggested

Chronic carrier treatment (Group A *streptococci*): 50 mg/kg/day in 4 divided doses for 10 days in combination with oral rifampin; maximum daily dose: 2000 mg/**day** (Shulman, 2012)

Recurrent rheumatic fever, prophylaxis: Children and Adolescents: 250 mg twice daily (Gerber, 2009)

Pneumococcal infection prophylaxis for anatomic or functional asplenia [eg, sickle cell disease (SCD)] (AAP, 2000; AAP, 2002; Kavanagh, 2011; NHLBI, 2002): Oral: Infants and Children:

Before 2 months of age (or as soon as SCD diagnosed or asplenia occurs) to 3 years of age: 125 mg twice daily

>3 years: 250 mg twice daily; the decision to discontinue penicillin prophylaxis after 5 years of age in children who have not experienced invasive pneumococcal infection and have received recommended pneumococcal immunizations is patient and clinician dependent; **Note:** Some clinicians recommend in patients <5 years, a lower dose of 125 mg twice daily (*Red Book*, 2012)

Pneumonia, community-acquired; Group A *Streptococcus*, mild infection or step-down therapy: Oral: Infants ≥3 months, Children, and Adolescents: 50-75 mg/kg/day in 3-4 divided doses (Bradley, 2011); maximum daily dose: 2000 mg/**day**

Adults:

Anthrax (cutaneous), community-acquired: Oral: 250-500 mg 4 times daily for 5-9 days (Stevens, 2005)

Fusospirochetosis (Vincent infection): Oral: 250-500 mg 3-4 times daily

Pharyngitis (streptococcal): Oral:

Acute treatment, group A streptococci (IDSA guidelines): 250 mg 4 times daily or 500 mg twice daily for 10 days (Shulman, 2012)

Chronic carrier treatment, group A streptococcal (IDSA guidelines): 500 mg 4 times daily for 10 days in combination with oral rifampin (Shulman, 2012)

Prophylaxis of recurrent rheumatic fever infections: Oral: 250 mg twice daily

Dosing adjustment in renal impairment: Children ≥12 years, Adolescents, and Adults: There are no dosage adjustments provided in manufacturer's labeling. Use with caution; excretion is prolonged in patients with renal impairment.

Dosing adjustment in hepatic impairment: Children ≥12 years, Adolescents, and Adults: There are no dosage adjustments provided in the manufacturer's labeling.

Preparation for Administration Oral: Reconstitute powder for oral solution with appropriate amount of water as specified on the bottle. Shake vigorously until suspended.

Administration Oral: Administer with water on an empty stomach 1 hour before or 2 hours after meals; may be administered with food to decrease GI upset

Monitoring Parameters With prolonged therapy, monitor renal and hematologic function periodically; observe for change in bowel frequency; monitor for signs of anaphylaxis during first dose

Test Interactions False-positive or negative urinary glucose determination using Clinitest®; positive Coombs' [direct]; false-positive urinary and/or serum proteins

Additional Information 0.7 mEq of potassium/250 mg penicillin V; 250 mg = 400,000 units of penicillin

Dosage Forms Excipient information presented when available (limited, particularly for generics); consult specific product labeling.

Solution Reconstituted, Oral:

Generic: 125 mg/5 mL (100 mL, 200 mL); 250 mg/5 mL (100 mL, 200 mL)

Tablet, Oral:

Generic: 250 mg, 500 mg

- ◆ **Penicilloyl-polylysine** *see* Benzylpenicilloyl Polylysine *on page 274*
- ◆ **Penlac** *see* Ciclopirox *on page 458*
- ◆ **Pentacel** *see* Diphtheria and Tetanus Toxoids, Acellular Pertussis, Poliovirus and *Haemophilus* b Conjugate Vaccine *on page 679*
- ◆ **Pentahydrate** *see* Sodium Thiosulfate *on page 1955*
- ◆ **Pentam** *see* Pentamidine *on page 1662*

Pentamidine (pen TAM i deen)

Brand Names: US Nebupent; Pentam

Therapeutic Category Antibiotic, Miscellaneous; Antifungal Agent; Antiprotozoal

Generic Availability (US) No

Use

Aerosol: Prevention of pneumonia caused by *Pneumocystis jirovecii* (formerly *carinii*) (PCP) (FDA approved in ages ≥17 years and adults)

Parenteral: Treatment of pneumonia caused by *Pneumocystis jirovecii* (formerly *carinii*) (PCP) (FDA approved in ages >4 months and adults). **Note:** The CDC recommends pentamidine for patients who cannot tolerate or who fail to respond to sulfamethoxazole and trimethoprim; has also been used in the treatment of African trypanosomiasis, cutaneous leishmaniasis, and amebic meningoencephalitis.

Pregnancy Risk Factor C

Pregnancy Considerations Animal reproduction studies were not conducted by the manufacturer. Pentamidine crosses the human placenta (Fortunato, 1989). Information related to fetal outcomes following maternal use of pentamidine is limited. If administered via the aerosolized route, maternal serum concentrations are lower, minimizing the exposure to the fetus (Gates, 1993; Nanda, 1992; Sperling, 1992). Concern regarding occupational exposure of pregnant health care workers has been discussed in the literature. Pregnant health care workers should avoid aerosolized exposure if possible (Conover, 1988; Ito, 1994; Smaldone, 1991). Pentamidine may be used in pregnant women as an alternative agent for the prophylaxis or treatment of PCP if the patient is unable to take preferred medications (DHHS [OI], 2013).

Breast-Feeding Considerations It is not known if pentamidine is excreted in human milk. Due to the potential for serious adverse reactions in the nursing infant, the manufacturer recommends a decision be made whether to discontinue nursing or to discontinue the drug, taking into account the importance of treatment to the mother.

In the United States, where formula is accessible, affordable, safe, and sustainable, and the risk of infant mortality due to diarrhea and respiratory infections is low, complete avoidance of breast-feeding by HIV-infected women is recommended to decrease potential transmission of HIV (DHHS [perinatal], 2014).

Contraindications Hypersensitivity to pentamidine isethionate or any component of the formulation

Warnings/Precautions Severe hypotension (some fatalities) has been observed (even after a single dose); may occur with either IV or IM administration, although more common with rapid IV administration; monitor blood pressure during (and after) infusion. May cause QT prolongation and subsequent torsade de pointes; avoid use in patients with diagnosed or suspected congenital long QT syndrome. Use with caution in patients with pre-existing cardiovascular disease; hyper-/hypotension and arrhythmia, including ventricular tachycardia (eg, torsade de pointes) have been reported.

Use with caution in patients with diabetes mellitus or hypocalcemia; hyper-/hypoglycemia and pancreatic islet cell necrosis with hyperinsulinemia has been reported. Symptoms may occur months after therapy; monitor blood glucose daily on therapy and periodically thereafter. Use with caution in patients with a history of pancreatic disease or elevated amylase/lipase levels; acute pancreatitis (with fatality) has been reported. Discontinue if signs/symptoms of acute pancreatitis occur. Concurrent use with other bone marrow suppressants may increase the risk for myelotoxicity; use with caution in patients with current evidence and/or prior history of hematologic disorders; anemia, leukopenia and/or thrombocytopenia have been reported. Use with caution in patients with hepatic or renal disease. Concurrent use with other nephrotoxic drugs may increase the risk for nephrotoxicity. Avoid concurrent use with other drugs known to prolong QTc interval. Stevens-Johnson syndrome has been reported with use. Intravenous pentamidine is an irritant with vesicant-like properties. Ensure proper needle or catheter placement prior to and during infusion; avoid extravasation. Ulceration, tissue necrosis, and/or sloughing have been reported with extravasation.

Aerosolized pentamidine may induce bronchospasm or cough, especially in patients with a smoking or asthma history (an inhaled bronchodilator prior to pentamidine may ameliorate symptoms). Use appropriate precautions to minimize exposure to healthcare personnel; refer to individual institutional policy. Acute PCP may develop despite aerosolized pentamidine prophylaxis. Although rare, extrapulmonary PCP disease may occur and has been associated with aerosolized pentamidine.

Adverse Reactions

Aerosol:

Central nervous system: Dizziness/lightheadedness, fatigue, fever, headache

Gastrointestinal: Appetite decreased, nausea, oral candida, taste alteration

Hematologic: Anemia

Respiratory: Bronchitis, chest pain, cough, dyspnea, pharyngitis, sinusitis, upper respiratory tract infection, wheezing

Miscellaneous: Herpes infection, infection, influenza, night sweats

Injection:

Cardiovascular: Hypotension

Central nervous system: Confusion/hallucinations

Dermatologic: Rash

Endocrine & metabolic: Hypoglycemia

Gastrointestinal: Nausea/anorexia, taste alteration

Hematologic: Anemia, leukopenia, thrombocytopenia

Hepatic: Liver function tests increased

Local: Local reactions at IM injection site (includes sterile abscess, necrosis, pain, induration)

Renal: Azotemia, BUN increased, creatinine increased, renal function impaired

Miscellaneous: Herpes infection, infection, influenza, night sweats

Aerosol or injection: Rare but important or life-threatening: Abdominal pain, allergic reaction, anaphylaxis, anxiety, arthralgia, asthma, blepharitis, blurred vision, bronchitis, bronchospasm, cardiac arrhythmia, central venous line related sepsis, cerebrovascular accident, chest tightness, chills, clotting time prolonged, CMV infection, colitis, confusion, congestion (chest, nasal), conjunctivitis, cough, cryptococcal meningitis, cyanosis, defibrination, depression, dermatitis, desquamation, diabetes mellitus, diabetic ketoacidosis, diarrhea, dizziness, drowsiness, dyspepsia, dyspnea, emotional lability, eosinophilia, erythema, esophagitis, extrapulmonary pneumocystosis, extravasation (tissue ulceration, necrosis, and/or sloughing), facial edema, flank pain, gait unsteady, gagging, gingivitis, headache, hearing loss, hematochezia, hematuria, hemoptysis, hepatic dysfunction, hepatitis, hepatomegaly, histoplasmosis, hyperglycemia, hyperkalemia, hypersalivation, hypertension, hyperventilation, hypesthesia, hypocalcemia, hypomagnesemia, incontinence, insomnia, laryngitis, laryngospasm, leg edema, melena, memory loss, nephritis, nervousness, neuralgia, neuropathy, neutropenia, night sweats, palpitation, pancreatitis, pancytopenia, paranoia, paresthesia, peripheral neuropathy, phlebitis, pleuritis, pneumonitis (eosinophilic or interstitial), pneumothorax, pruritus, rales, renal dysfunction, renal failure, rhinitis, seizure, splenomegaly, Stevens-Johnson syndrome, ST segment abnormal, syncope, syndrome of inappropriate antidiuretic hormone (SIADH), tachycardia, tachypnea, temperature abnormal, torsade de pointes, tremor, vasodilation, vasculitis, ventricular tachycardia, vertigo, vomiting, urticaria, xerostomia

Drug Interactions

Metabolism/Transport Effects Substrate of CYP2C19 (major); **Note:** Assignment of Major/Minor substrate status based on clinically relevant drug interaction potential; **Inhibits** CYP2C19 (weak), CYP2C9 (weak), CYP2D6 (weak)

Avoid Concomitant Use

Avoid concomitant use of Pentamidine with any of the following: BCG; BCG (Intravesical); Highest Risk QTc-Prolonging Agents; Ivabradine; Mifepristone

Increased Effect/Toxicity

Pentamidine may increase the levels/effects of: ARIPiprazole; Foscarnet; Highest Risk QTc-Prolonging Agents; Hypoglycemia-Associated Agents; Mequitazine; Moderate Risk QTc-Prolonging Agents

The levels/effects of Pentamidine may be increased by: Androgens; Antidiabetic Agents; CYP2C19 Inhibitors (Moderate); CYP2C19 Inhibitors (Strong); Herbs (Hypoglycemic Properties); Ivabradine; Luliconazole; MAO Inhibitors; Mifepristone; Pegvisomant; QTc-Prolonging Agents (Indeterminate Risk and Risk Modifying); Quinolone Antibiotics; Salicylates; Selective Serotonin Reuptake Inhibitors

Decreased Effect

Pentamidine may decrease the levels/effects of: Antidiabetic Agents; BCG; BCG (Intravesical); BCG Vaccine (Immunization); Sodium Picosulfate; Typhoid Vaccine

The levels/effects of Pentamidine may be decreased by: CYP2C19 Inducers (Strong); Dabrafenib; Quinolone Antibiotics

Storage/Stability Store intact vials at 20°C to 25°C (68°F to 77°F); protect from light. Do not use sodium chloride for initial reconstitution (sodium chloride will cause precipitation).

Aerosol: The manufacturer recommends the use of freshly prepared solutions for inhalation; however, may be stored for up to 48 hours in the vial at room temperature if protected from light.

Injection: Reconstituted solution is stable for 48 hours in the vial at room temperature and protected from light. Solutions for injection (1-2.5 mg/mL) in D_5W are stable for at least 24 hours at room temperature. Store at room temperature to avoid crystallization.

Mechanism of Action Interferes with microbial RNA/DNA, phospholipids and protein synthesis, through inhibition of oxidative phosphorylation and/or interference with incorporation of nucleotides and nucleic acids into RNA and DNA

Pharmacokinetics (Adult data unless noted)

Absorption: IM: Well absorbed; Aerosol: Limited systemic absorption

Distribution: Binds to tissues and plasma protein; high concentrations are found in the liver, kidney, adrenals, spleen, lungs and pancreas; poor penetration into CNS; following oral inhalation, high concentrations are found in bronchoalveolar fluid; V_{dss}: IV: 821 ± 535 L; IM: 2724 ± 1066 L

Half-life: IV: 5-8 hours; IM: 7-11 hours; half-life may be prolonged in patients with severe renal impairment

Elimination: IV: ≤12% in urine as unchanged drug

Dialysis: Not appreciably removed by hemodialysis or peritoneal dialysis

Dosing: Usual

Infants, Children, and Adolescents:

***Pneumocystis jirovecii* (PCP), prophylaxis (primary and secondary):** Limited data available: **Note:** For patients intolerant to sulfamethoxazole and trimethoprim.

HIV-exposed/-positive: Children ≥5 years and Adolescents: Inhalation: 300 mg once monthly via Respirgard® II nebulizer (DHHS [adult and pediatric], 2013)

Oncology patients: Children ≥2 years and Adolescents: IV: 4 mg/kg/dose once a month (Kim, 2008; Prasad, 2007)

PCP, treatment (moderate-severe disease): Note: For patients who cannot tolerate or who fail to respond to 5-7 days of sulfamethoxazole and trimethoprim.

Manufacturer's labeling: Infants ≥5 months, Children, and Adolescents: IM, IV: 4 mg/kg/dose once daily for 14-21 days

HIV-exposed/-positive:

Infants and Children: IV: 4 mg/kg/dose once daily; if clinical improvement after 7-10 days of therapy, may change to an oral regimen to complete a 21-day course (DHHS [pediatric], 2013)

Adolescents: IV: 4 mg/kg/dose once daily for 21 days; some experts recommend a dose reduction to 3 mg/kg/dose for toxicity (DHHS [adult], 2013)

Non-HIV-exposed/-positive: IV: 3-4 mg/kg/dose once daily for 21 days (*Red Book*, 2012)

Trypanosomiasis; treatment (non-CNS disease): IM: 4 mg/kg/dose once daily for 7 days (*Red Book*, 2012)

Cutaneous leishmaniasis; treatment: IM, IV: 2-3 mg/kg/dose once daily or every 2 days for 4-7 doses (*Red Book*, 2012)

Adults:

***Pneumocystis jirovecii* (PCP), prophylaxis (primary and secondary):** Inhalation: 300 mg/dose every 4 weeks via Respirgard® II nebulizer

PCP, treatment (moderate-severe disease):

Manufacturer's labeling: IM, IV: 4 mg/kg/dose once daily for 14-21 days

CDC recommendation: IV: 3-4 mg/kg/dose once daily for 21 days

AIDS*Info* guidelines (HIV-infected/-exposed): IV: 4 mg/kg/dose once daily; some experts recommend a dose reduction to 3 mg/kg/dose for toxicity (DHHS [adult], 2013)

Dosing adjustment in renal impairment: The FDA-approved labeling recommends that caution should be used in patients with renal impairment; however, no specific dosage adjustment guidelines are provided. The following guidelines have been used by some clinicians (Aronoff, 2007):

Infants, Children, and Adolescents: IV:

GFR >30 mL/minute/1.73 m^2: No adjustment required

GFR 10-30 mL/minute/1.73 m^2: Administer 4 mg/kg/dose every 36 hours

GFR <10 mL/minute/1.73 m^2 and peritoneal dialysis: Administer 4 mg/kg/dose every 48 hours

Hemodialysis: Administer 4 mg/kg/dose every 48 hours, after dialysis on dialysis days

Peritoneal dialysis: 4 mg/kg/dose every 48 hours

Continuous renal replacement therapy: No adjustment required

Adults: IV:

CrCl ≥10 mL/minute: No adjustment required

CrCl <10 mL/minute: Administer 4 mg/kg/dose every 24-36 hours

Hemodialysis: Administer 4 mg/kg/dose every 48 hours and 750 mg after each dialysis

Peritoneal dialysis: 4 mg/kg/dose every 48 hours

Continuous renal replacement therapy: No adjustment required

Preparation for Administration Do not use sodium chloride for initial reconstitution (sodium chloride will cause precipitation).

Oral inhalation: Reconstitute powder for nebulization with 6 mL SWFI. Do not mix with other nebulizer solutions.

Parenteral:

IM: Reconstitute with 3 mL SWFI to a final concentration of 100 mg/mL

IV: Reconstitute with 3 to 5 mL SWFI or D_5W; the manufacturer recommends further dilution in D_5W; however, stability with further dilution in NS has also been documented. The final concentration for administration should not exceed 6 mg/mL.

Administration

Oral inhalation: Safe and effective administration via nebulization in children is dependent on patients wearing an appropriately sized pediatric face mask. Deliver via Respirgard II nebulizer until nebulizer is emptied (30 to 45 minutes). Use appropriate precautions to minimize exposure to health care personnel; refer to individual institutional policy. The manufacturer recommends the use of freshly prepared solutions for inhalation. Do not mix with other nebulizer solutions.

Parenteral:

IM: Administer deep IM

IV: Administer by slow IV infusion over a period of at least 60 to 120 minutes; rapid IV administration can cause severe hypotension.

Irritant with vesicant-like properties; ensure proper needle or catheter placement prior to and during infusion. Avoid extravasation. If extravasation occurs, stop infusion immediately and disconnect (leave cannula/needle in place); gently aspirate extravasated solution (do **NOT** flush the line); remove needle/cannula; elevate extremity. Apply dry warm compresses (Reynolds 2014).

Vesicant/Extravasation Risk Irritant with vesicant-like properties

Monitoring Parameters Liver function tests, renal function tests (daily), blood glucose (daily), serum potassium and calcium, CBC with differential and platelet count, ECG, blood pressure

Dosage Forms Excipient information presented when available (limited, particularly for generics); consult specific product labeling.

Solution Reconstituted, Inhalation, as isethionate:

Nebupent: 300 mg (1 ea)

Solution Reconstituted, Injection, as isethionate:

Pentam: 300 mg (1 ea)

◆ **Pentamidine Isethionate** *see* Pentamidine *on page 1662*

◆ **Pentamycetin® (Can)** *see* Chloramphenicol *on page 432*

◆ **Pentasa** *see* Mesalamine *on page 1368*

◆ **Pentasodium Colistin Methanesulfonate** *see* Colistimethate *on page 532*

◆ **Pentavalent Human-Bovine Reassortant Rotavirus Vaccine (PRV)** *see* Rotavirus Vaccine *on page 1889*

Pentazocine (pen TAZ oh seen)

Medication Safety Issues

Sound-alike/look-alike issues:

Talwin may be confused with Targin

High alert medication:

The Institute for Safe Medication Practices (ISMP) includes this medication among its list of drug classes which have a heightened risk of causing significant patient harm when used in error.

BEERS Criteria medication:

This drug may be potentially inappropriate for use in geriatric patients (Quality of evidence - low; Strength of recommendation - strong).

Related Information

Opioid Conversion Table *on page 2285*

Brand Names: US Talwin

Brand Names: Canada Talwin

Therapeutic Category Analgesic, Narcotic; Opioid Partial Agonist; Sedative

Generic Availability (US) No

Use Relief of moderate to severe pain (FDA approved in adults); a sedative prior to surgery (FDA approved in ages ≥1 year and adults); supplement to surgical anesthesia (FDA approved in adults)

Pregnancy Risk Factor C

Pregnancy Considerations Adverse events were not found in animal reproduction studies. Pentazocine is approved for pain relief during labor. When used for pain relief during labor, opioids may temporarily affect the heart rate of the fetus (ACOG, 2002).

If chronic opioid exposure occurs in pregnancy, adverse events in the newborn (including withdrawal) may occur; monitoring of the neonate is recommended. The minimum effective dose should be used if opioids are needed (Chou, 2009). Neonatal abstinence syndrome following opioid exposure may present with autonomic (eg, fever, temperature instability), gastrointestinal (eg, diarrhea, vomiting, poor feeding/weight gain), or neurologic (eg, high-pitched crying, increased muscle tone, irritability, seizure, tremor) symptoms (Dow, 2012; Hudak, 2012). Neonatal abstinence syndrome has been reported following prolonged use of pentazocine during pregnancy.

Breast-Feeding Considerations It is not known if pentazocine is excreted into breast milk. Parenteral opioids used during labor have the potential to interfere with a newborn's natural reflex to nurse within the first few hours after birth. If pentazocine is administered to a nursing woman, it is recommended to monitor both the mother and baby for psychotomimetic reactions. Nursing infants exposed to large doses of opioids should be monitored for apnea and sedation (Montgomery, 2012).

Contraindications Hypersensitivity to pentazocine or any component of the formulation

Warnings/Precautions May increase systemic and pulmonary arterial pressure and systemic vascular resistance; use with caution in patients who may not tolerate these alterations in hemodynamics (eg, heart failure). May cause CNS depression, which may impair physical or mental abilities; patients must be cautioned about performing tasks which require mental alertness (eg, operating machinery or driving). Potentially significant drug interactions may exist, requiring dose or frequency adjustment, additional monitoring, and/or selection of alternative therapy. Effects may be potentiated when used with other sedative drugs or ethanol. Avoid use in patients with CNS depression or coma as these patients are susceptible to intracranial effects of CO_2 retention. Use with caution in seizure-prone patients, acute myocardial infarction, biliary tract impairment, pancreatitis, thyroid dysfunction, prostatic hyperplasia/urinary stricture, patients with respiratory, adrenal insufficiency, morbid obesity, renal and hepatic dysfunction, head trauma, increased intracranial pressure, and patients with a history of prior opioid dependence or abuse; pentazocine may precipitate opioid withdrawal symptoms in patients who have been receiving opioids regularly; injection contains sulfites which may cause allergic reaction; tolerance or drug dependence may result from extended use. May cause hypotension; use with caution in patients with hypovolemia, cardiovascular disease (including acute MI), or drugs which may exaggerate hypotensive effects (including phenothiazines or general anesthetics). May obscure diagnosis or clinical course of patients with acute abdominal conditions. Abrupt discontinuation may result in withdrawal symptoms; taper dose to decrease risk of withdrawal symptoms. After chronic maternal exposure to opioids, neonatal withdrawal syndrome may occur in the newborn; monitor neonate closely. Signs and symptoms include irritability, hyperactivity and abnormal sleep pattern, high pitched cry, tremor, vomiting, diarrhea and failure to gain weight. Onset, duration and severity depend on the drug used, duration of use, maternal dose, and rate of drug elimination by the newborn. Opioid withdrawal syndrome in the neonate, unlike in adults, may be life-threatening and should be treated according to protocols developed by neonatology experts. Severe sclerosis has occurred at the injection-site following multiple injections; rotate sites of injection. Use with caution in the elderly and debilitated patients; may be more sensitive to adverse effects.

Avoid use in the elderly due to increased risk of CNS effects (confusion and hallucinations) compared to other opioids; safer alternative agents preferred (Beers Criteria). If used, use lower initial doses.

Adverse Reactions

Cardiovascular: Circulatory depression, facial edema, flushing, hypertension, hypotension, increased peripheral vascular resistance, shock, syncope, tachycardia

Central nervous system: Central nervous system depression, chills, confusion, disorientation, dizziness, drowsiness, drug dependence (physical and psychological), euphoria, excitement, hallucination, headache, insomnia, irritability, malaise, nightmares, paresthesia, sedation

Dermatologic: Dermatitis, diaphoresis, erythema multiforme, pruritus, skin rash, Stevens-Johnson syndrome, toxic epidermal necrolysis, urticaria

Gastrointestinal: Abdominal distress, anorexia, constipation, diarrhea, dysgeusia, nausea, vomiting, xerostomia

Genitourinary: Urinary retention

Hematologic & oncologic: Agranulocytosis (rare), decreased white blood cell count, eosinophilia

Hypersensitivity: Anaphylaxis

Local: Injection site reaction (tissue damage and irritation)

Neuromuscular & skeletal: Tremor, weakness

Ophthalmic: Blurred vision, diplopia, miosis, nystagmus

Otic: Tinnitus

Respiratory: Dyspnea, respiratory depression (rare)

Rare but important or life-threatening: Hypogonadism (Brennan, 2013; Debono, 2011)

Drug Interactions

Metabolism/Transport Effects None known.

Avoid Concomitant Use

Avoid concomitant use of Pentazocine with any of the following: Analgesics (Opioid); Azelastine (Nasal); Eluxadoline; Orphenadrine; Paraldehyde; Thalidomide

Increased Effect/Toxicity

Pentazocine may increase the levels/effects of: Alcohol (Ethyl); Alvimopan; Azelastine (Nasal); CNS Depressants; Desmopressin; Diuretics; Eluxadoline; Methotrimeprazine; Metyrosine; Mirtazapine; Orphenadrine; Paraldehyde; Pramipexole; ROPINIRole; Rotigotine; Selective Serotonin Reuptake Inhibitors; Suvorexant; Thalidomide; Zolpidem

The levels/effects of Pentazocine may be increased by: Amphetamines; Anticholinergic Agents; Antipsychotic Agents (Phenothiazines); Brimonidine (Topical); Cannabis; Doxylamine; Dronabinol; Droperidol; HydrOXYzine; Kava Kava; Magnesium Sulfate; Methotrimeprazine; Nabilone; Perampanel; Rufinamide; Sodium Oxybate; Succinylcholine; Tetrahydrocannabinol

Decreased Effect

Pentazocine may decrease the levels/effects of: Analgesics (Opioid); Pegvisomant

The levels/effects of Pentazocine may be decreased by: Ammonium Chloride; Naltrexone

Storage/Stability Store at 20°C to 25°C (68°F to 77°F).

Mechanism of Action Agonist of kappa opiate receptors and partial agonist of mu opiate receptors in the CNS, causing inhibition of ascending pain pathways, altering the perception of and response to pain; produces analgesia, respiratory depression and sedation similar to opioids

Pharmacodynamics

Onset of action:
- IM, SubQ: Within 15-30 minutes
- IV: Within 2-3 minutes

Duration: Parenteral: 2-3 hours

Pharmacokinetics (Adult data unless noted)

Distribution: Children 4-8 years (mean ± SD): V_{dss}: 4 ± 1.2 L/kg (Hanunen, 1993)

Protein binding: 60%

Metabolism: In the liver via oxidative and glucuronide conjugation pathways

Half-life: Increased half-life with decreased hepatic function
- Neonates: 8-12 hours (estimated; Osifo, 2008)
- Children 4-8 years (mean ± SD): 3 ± 1.5 hours (Hanunen, 1993)
- Adults: 2-3 hours

Elimination: Small amounts excreted unchanged in urine

Dosing: Neonatal Not recommended for use; safety, efficacy, and dose are not established.

Dosing: Usual

Infants and Children: Limited information available

Preoperative sedation: Manufacturer recommendations:

Infants <1 year: Safety, efficacy, and dose not established

Children 1-16 years: IM: 0.5 mg/kg as a single dose

Note: In 300 children (1-14 years) IM doses ranging from approximately 0.45-1.5 mg/kg in children <27 kg to 0.65-1.9 mg/kg in children >27 kg were used preoperatively (Rita, 1970)

Postoperative pain: IM: Doses of 15 mg for children 5-8 years of age and 30 mg for children 9-14 years of age have been used (n=30) (Waterworth, 1974)

Intraoperative analgesia: IV: Titrating doses of 0.5 mg/kg every 30-45 minutes as needed have been given in 50 children 5-9 years of age; total dose required: 1-1.5 mg/kg (Ray, 1994)

Adults:
Analgesia (excluding labor pain):
IM, SubQ: 30-60 mg every 3-4 hours; do **not** exceed 60 mg/dose; maximum: 360 mg/day
IV: 30 mg every 3-4 hours; do **not** exceed 30 mg/dose; maximum: 360 mg/day
Labor pain:
IM: 30 mg once
IV: 20 mg every 2-3 hours as needed; maximum total dose: 60 mg

Dosing adjustment in renal impairment: Children and Adults:
CrCl 10-50 mL/minute: Administer 75% of normal dose
CrCl <10 mL/minute: Administer 50% of normal dose

Administration SubQ route not advised due to tissue damage; rotate injection site for IM, SubQ use; avoid intra-arterial injection

Monitoring Parameters Respiratory and cardiovascular status; level of pain relief and sedation; blood pressure

Additional Information Use only in patients who are not tolerant to or physically dependent upon opioids

A retrospective study assessed the use of pentazocine 0.5 mg/kg every 8 hours in neonates undergoing surgery; pentazocine use was associated with life-threatening morbidity and unacceptable high mortality due to persistent respiratory depression; the authors of the study recommend the use of alternative neonatal analgesics (Osifo, 2008).

Controlled Substance C-IV

Dosage Forms Excipient information presented when available (limited, particularly for generics); consult specific product labeling.
Solution, Injection:
Talwin: 30 mg/mL (1 mL)
Talwin: 30 mg/mL (10 mL) [contains methylparaben, sodium bisulfite]

◆ **Pentazocine Lactate** *see* Pentazocine *on page 1664*

PENTobarbital (pen toe BAR bi tal)

Medication Safety Issues
Sound-alike/look-alike issues:
PENTobarbital may be confused with PHENobarbital
Nembutal may be confused with Myambutol
BEERS Criteria medication:
This drug may be potentially inappropriate for use in geriatric patients (Quality of evidence - high; Strength of recommendation - strong).

Related Information
Preprocedure Sedatives in Children *on page 2444*

Brand Names: US Nembutal

Brand Names: Canada Nembutal Sodium

Therapeutic Category Anticonvulsant, Barbiturate; Barbiturate; General Anesthetic; Hypnotic; Sedative

Generic Availability (US) No

Use Sedation, preanesthetic, short-term treatment of insomnia, and emergency treatment of acute convulsive episodes associated with certain conditions such as status epilepticus, eclampsia, tetanus, cholera, meningitis, and toxic reactions to local anesthetics or strychnine [FDA approved in pediatric patients (age not specified) and adults]; has also been used for procedural sedation (parenteral, oral, and rectal), treatment of increased intracranial pressure, and sedation for the mechanically ventilated ICU patient

Pregnancy Risk Factor D

Pregnancy Considerations Barbiturates can be detected in the placenta, fetal liver and fetal brain. Fetal and maternal blood concentrations may be similar following parenteral administration. An increased incidence of fetal abnormalities may occur following maternal use. When used during the third trimester of pregnancy, withdrawal symptoms may occur in the neonate including seizures and hyperirritability; symptoms may be delayed up to 14 days. Use during labor does not impair uterine activity; however, respiratory depression may occur in the newborn; resuscitation equipment should be available, especially for premature infants.

Breast-Feeding Considerations Small amounts of barbiturates are found in breast milk.

Contraindications Hypersensitivity to barbiturates or any component of the formulation; porphyria

Warnings/Precautions May cause hypotension particularly when administered intravenously; use with caution in hemodynamically unstable patients (hypotension or shock). High doses used to induce pentobarbital coma cause hypotension requiring vasopressor therapy. May cause respiratory depression particularly when administered intravenously; use with caution in patients with respiratory disease. Intubation is typically required prior to treatment for status epilepticus or traumatic brain injury. Anticonvulsants should not be discontinued abruptly because of the possibility of increasing seizure frequency; therapy should be withdrawn gradually to minimize the potential of increased seizure frequency, unless safety concerns require a more rapid withdrawal. Do not administer to patients in acute pain; may heighten/worsen sense of pain.

Use with caution in patients with hepatic or renal impairment; reduce dose as appropriate. Do not use in patients with premonitory signs of hepatic coma. Use with caution in patients with a history of drug abuse; potential for drug dependency exists. Tolerance, psychological and physical dependence may occur with prolonged use. Use with caution in patients with depression or suicidal tendencies. Avoid use in the elderly due to risk of overdose with low dosages, tolerance to sleep effects, and increased risk of physical dependence (Beers Criteria). May cause CNS depression, which may impair physical or mental abilities; patients must be cautioned about performing tasks which require mental alertness (eg, operating machinery or driving). Effects with other sedative drugs or ethanol may be potentiated.

Solution for injection is highly alkaline and extravasation may cause local tissue damage. Intravenous solution may contain propylene glycol (PG). One case report has described a patient who developed lactic acidosis possibly secondary to PG accumulation following a continuous infusion of pentobarbital (Miller, 2008). Consider monitoring for signs of PG toxicity (eg, lactic acidosis, acute renal failure, osmol gap) in patients who require a continuous infusion of pentobarbital.

Warnings: Additional Pediatric Considerations Some dosage forms may contain propylene glycol; in neonates large amounts of propylene glycol delivered orally, intravenously (eg, >3,000 mg/day), or topically have been associated with potentially fatal toxicities which can include metabolic acidosis, seizures, renal failure, and CNS depression; toxicities have also been reported in children and adults including hyperosmolality, lactic acidosis, seizures, and respiratory depression; use caution (AAP, 1997; Shehab, 2009).

Adverse Reactions
Cardiovascular: Bradycardia, hypotension, syncope
Central nervous system: Abnormal thinking, agitation, anxiety, ataxia, CNS excitation, confusion, depression, dizziness, drowsiness, fever, hallucinations, headache, hyperkinesia, insomnia, nervousness, nightmares, psychiatric disturbances, somnolence
Dermatologic: Angioedema, exfoliative dermatitis, rash
Gastrointestinal: Constipation, nausea, vomiting
Hematologic: Megaloblastic anemia
Hepatic: Hepatotoxicity

Local: Injection site reactions

Respiratory: Apnea (especially with rapid IV use), hypoventilation, laryngospasm, respiratory depression

Miscellaneous: Gangrene with inadvertent intra-arterial injection, hypersensitivity reactions

Drug Interactions

Metabolism/Transport Effects Induces CYP2A6 (strong)

Avoid Concomitant Use

Avoid concomitant use of PENTobarbital with any of the following: Azelastine (Nasal); Mianserin; Orphenadrine; Paraldehyde; Somatostatin Acetate; Thalidomide; Ulipristal

Increased Effect/Toxicity

PENTobarbital may increase the levels/effects of: Alcohol (Ethyl); Azelastine (Nasal); Buprenorphine; CNS Depressants; Hydrocodone; Hypotensive Agents; Meperidine; Methotrimeprazine; Metyrosine; Mirtazapine; Orphenadrine; Paraldehyde; Pramipexole; ROPINIRole; Rotigotine; Selective Serotonin Reuptake Inhibitors; Suvorexant; Thalidomide; Thiazide Diuretics; Zolpidem

The levels/effects of PENTobarbital may be increased by: Brimonidine (Topical); Cannabis; Chloramphenicol; Doxylamine; Dronabinol; Droperidol; Felbamate; HydrOXYzine; Kava Kava; Magnesium Sulfate; Methotrimeprazine; Mianserin; Nabilone; Perampanel; Primidone; Rufinamide; Sodium Oxybate; Somatostatin Acetate; Tapentadol; Tetrahydrocannabinol; Valproic Acid and Derivatives

Decreased Effect

PENTobarbital may decrease the levels/effects of: Acetaminophen; Beta-Blockers; Calcium Channel Blockers; Chloramphenicol; Contraceptives (Estrogens); Contraceptives (Progestins); CycloSPORINE (Systemic); CYP2A6 Substrates; Doxycycline; Etoposide; Etoposide Phosphate; Felbamate; Griseofulvin; LamoTRIgine; Mianserin; Teniposide; Theophylline Derivatives; Tricyclic Antidepressants; Ulipristal; Valproic Acid and Derivatives; Vitamin K Antagonists

The levels/effects of PENTobarbital may be decreased by: Mefloquine; Mianserin; Multivitamins/Minerals (with ADEK, Folate, Iron); Pyridoxine; Rifamycin Derivatives

Storage/Stability Store at controlled room temperature of 20°C to 25°C (68°F to 77°F); brief excursions of 15°C to 30°C (59°F to 86°F) permitted. Protect from freezing and avoid excessive heat. When mixed with an acidic solution, precipitate may form. Use only clear solution.

Mechanism of Action Barbiturate with sedative, hypnotic, and anticonvulsant properties. Barbiturates depress the sensory cortex, decrease motor activity, alter cerebellar function, and produce drowsiness, sedation, and hypnosis. In high doses, barbiturates exhibit anticonvulsant activity; barbiturates produce dose-dependent respiratory depression; reduce brain metabolism and cerebral blood flow in order to decrease intracranial pressure

Pharmacodynamics Note: Values below are for sedation in pediatric and adult patients.

Onset of action (Krauss, 2006):

IM: Within 10-15 minutes

IV: Almost immediate, within 3-5 minutes

Oral, Rectal: 15-60 minutes

Duration (Krauss, 2006):

IM: 1-2 hours

IV: 15-45 minutes

Oral, Rectal: 1-4 hours

Pharmacokinetics (Adult data unless noted)

Distribution: V_d:

Children: 0.8 L/kg (Schiable, 1982)

Adults: 1 L/kg (Ehrnebo, 1974)

Protein binding: 45% to 70%

Metabolism: Extensive in the liver via hydroxylation and glucuronidation (Wermeling, 1985)

Half-life, terminal:

Children: 26 ± 16 hours (Schaible, 1982)

Adults (healthy): 22 hours (15-50 hours, dose-dependent) (Ehrnebo, 1974)

Elimination: <1% excreted unchanged in urine

Dosing: Usual Note: Adjust dose based on patient's age, weight, and medical condition.

Infants, Children, and Adolescents: **Note:** Consider the potential for delayed metabolism or elimination in infants <6 months of age (Krauss, 2006).

Hypnotic: Children: IM: 2-6 mg/kg; maximum dose: 100 mg/dose

Preoperative sedation: Infants and Children:

IM: 2-6 mg/kg; maximum dose: 100 mg/dose

IV: 1-3 mg/kg to a maximum of 100 mg to desired effect

Procedural (moderate) sedation:

Infants: Oral: 4 mg/kg, if needed supplemental 2-4 mg/kg every 30 minutes; maximum total dose: 8 mg/kg (Mason, 2004)

Infants and Children:

IM: 2-6 mg/kg; maximum dose: 100 mg

IV: Initial 1-2 mg/kg; additional doses of 1-2 mg/kg every 3-5 minutes to desired effect; usual effective total dose: 1-6 mg/kg (maximum: 100 mg/dose) (Krauss, 2006; Mason, 2004). **Note:** Patients receiving concurrent barbiturate therapy may require higher total mg/kg doses (up to 9 mg/kg) (Mason, 2004).

Children: Oral, Rectal: (Krauss, 2006):

<4 years: 3-6 mg/kg; maximum dose: 100 mg

≥4 years: 1.5-3 mg/kg; maximum dose: 100 mg

Adolescents: IV: 100 mg prior to procedure

Reduction of elevated ICP: IV: **Note:** Intubation is required; adjust dose based on hemodynamics, ICP, cerebral perfusion pressure, and EEG.

Low dose: Children and Adolescents: 5 mg/kg every 4-6 hours (Mazzola, 2002)

High-dose pentobarbital coma: Children and Adolescents: Loading dose: 10 mg/kg over 30 minutes, then 5 mg/kg every hour for 3 hours; initial maintenance infusion: 1 mg/kg/**hour**; adjust to maintain burst suppression on EEG; maintenance dose range: 1-2 mg/kg/**hour** (Adelson, 2003; Rangel-Castillo, 2008)

Sedation of mechanically ventilated ICU patient (who failed standard therapy): IV: Infants, Children, and Adolescents: Loading dose: 1 mg/kg followed by 1 mg/kg/**hour** infusion. Additional boluses at a dose equal to hourly rate may be given every 2 hours as needed. If ≥4-6 boluses are administered within 24 hours, then increase maintenance rate by 1 mg/kg/**hour**; reported required range: 1-6 mg/kg/**hour** (median: 2 mg/kg/**hour**). Tapering of dose and/or conversion to oral phenobarbital has been reported for therapy ≥5 days (Tobias, 1995; Tobias, 2000; Tobias 2000a). **Note:** Higher rates of adverse effects were observed in a small report that used higher loading and initial maintenance doses (Yanay, 2004).

Status epilepticus refractory to standard therapy: Note: Intubation is required; adjust dose based on hemodynamics, seizure activity, and EEG.

IV: Infants, Children, and Adolescents: Loading dose: 5 mg/kg; maintenance infusion: Initial: 1 mg/kg/**hour**, may increase up to 3 mg/kg/**hour** (usual range: 1-3 mg/kg/**hour**); maintain burst suppression on EEG for 12-48 hours (no seizure activity), tapering pentobarbital rate by 0.5 mg/kg every 12 hours has been reported (Abend, 2008; Holmes, 1999; Kim, 2001)

High-dose pentobarbital coma: IV: Infants and Children: Loading dose: 10-15 mg/kg given slowly over 1-2 hours; monitor blood pressure and respiratory rate. Maintenance infusion: Initial: 1 mg/kg/**hour**; may increase up to 5 mg/kg/**hour** (usual range: 0.5-3 mg/kg/**hour**); maintain burst suppression on EEG (Holmes, 1999). **Note:** Loading doses of 20-35 mg/kg (given over 1-2 hours) have been utilized in pediatric patients for pentobarbital coma, but these higher loading doses often cause hypotension requiring vasopressor therapy.

Adults:

Hypnotic/sedative:

IM: 150-200 mg

IV: Initial: 100 mg; decrease dose for elderly or debilitated patients. If needed, may administer additional increments after at least 1 minute, up to a total dose of 200-500 mg

Refractory status epilepticus: IV: **Note:** Intubation required; adjust dose based on hemodynamics, seizure activity, and EEG (Abou Khaled 2008; Millikan, 2009; Mirski, 2008; Yaffe, 1993). Various regimens available:

Loading dose: 10-15 mg/kg (5-10 mg/kg in patients with pre-existing hypotension) administer slowly over 1 hour; initial maintenance infusion: 0.5-1 mg/kg/hour; adjust to maintain burst suppression pattern on EEG; maintenance dose range: 0.5-5 mg/kg/hour (Yaffe, 1993). **Note:** Patients may require infusion rates up to 10 mg/kg/hour (Abou Khaled, 2008; Mirski, 2008).

Loading dose: 5 mg/kg (up to 25-50 mg/minute); repeat 5 mg/kg boluses until seizures stop; maintenance dose: 1 mg/kg/hour (range: 0.5-10 mg/kg/hour) (Abou Khaled, 2008)

When increasing maintenance infusion rate during active seizure activity, some experts suggest administration of an additional 5 mg/kg bolus, given the long half-life of pentobarbital.

Preparation for Administration Parenteral: Continuous IV infusion: May dilute in D_5W, $D_{10}W$, NS, 1/2NS, LR, Ringer's injection, D_5LR, and dextrose/saline combinations to a concentration <50 mg/mL; in clinical practice concentrations have been reported as 4, 8, and 25 mg/mL (Murray 2014; Wermeling 1987).

Administration

Parenteral:

IM: May be administered by deep IM; inject into a large muscle. No more than 5 mL should be injected at any one site because of possible tissue irritation.

IV:

Intermittent IV injection: Administer undiluted (50 mg/mL) by slow IV injection; infuse over 10 to 30 minutes not to exceed >50 mg/minute; rapid IV injection may cause respiratory depression, apnea, laryngospasm, bronchospasm, and hypotension; loading doses have been infused over 30 to 180 minutes in head injury patients to decrease the risk of hypotension (Schaible 1982; Wermeling 1987)

Continuous IV infusion: Administer at a concentration ≤50 mg/mL via infusion pump. Solution highly alkaline (pH=9.5); care should be taken to avoid extravasation; consider administration using large bore vein (not hand or wrist) or via a running IV line at port farthest from patient's vein.

Oral: Parenteral solution may be mixed with cherry syrup prior to administration to improve palatability (Chung 2000; Mason 2004).

Monitoring Parameters Vital signs, respiratory status (including pulse oximetry for moderate sedation), cardiovascular status, CNS status. Monitor EEG when using pentobarbital to treat status epilepticus or to reduce ICP. Monitor ICP and cerebral perfusion pressure (CPP) (CPP = MAP - ICP) when using pentobarbital coma to reduce ICP. Consider monitoring for signs of propylene glycol toxicity (eg, lactic acidosis, acute renal failure, osmolal gap) in patients who require a continuous infusion of pentobarbital. Periodically monitor renal, hepatic, and hematopoietic function with prolonged therapy.

Reference Range Therapeutic:

Hypnotic: 1-5 mcg/mL (SI: 4-22 micromoles/L)

Coma: 20-50 mcg/mL (SI: 88-221 micromoles/L)

Toxic: >10 mcg/mL (SI: >44 µmol/L)

Additional Information Tolerance to hypnotic effect can occur; taper dose to prevent withdrawal; in pediatric patients, a total cumulative pentobarbital dose ≥25 mg/kg or duration ≥5-7 days have been reported to have a higher probability of withdrawal. To prevent withdrawal in susceptible pediatric patients, the following dosing approach transitioning to PHENobarbital has been described: Discontinue PENTobarbital infusion, administer half of the PHENobarbital IV loading dose (see table) over 1 hour followed 6 hours later by the remaining half of PHENObarbital loading dose IV (over 1 hour). Begin maintenance PHENobarbital dose 6 hours after loading dose completed; the maintenance PHENobarbital dose should be 1/3 of the initial loading dose IV given every 12 hours. Once patient is stabilized, may switch to oral therapy and begin tapering 10% to 20% weekly (Tobias, 2000; Tobias, 2000a). **Note:** This conversion method is based on preliminary data and further studies are needed to confirm the efficacy of this regimen.

PENTobarbital Infusion Rate (mg/kg/hour)	PHENobarbital IV Loading Dose (mg/kg)
1-2	8
2-3	15
3-4	20

Controlled Substance C-II

Dosage Forms Excipient information presented when available (limited, particularly for generics); consult specific product labeling.

Solution, Injection, as sodium:

Nembutal: 50 mg/mL (20 mL, 50 mL) [latex free; contains alcohol, usp, propylene glycol]

◆ **Pentobarbital Sodium** *see* PENTobarbital *on page 1666*

Pentostatin (pen toe STAT in)

Medication Safety Issues

Sound-alike/look-alike issues:

Pentostatin may be confused with pentamidine, pentosan

High alert medication:

This medication is in a class the Institute for Safe Medication Practices (ISMP) includes among its list of drug classes which have a heightened risk of causing significant patient harm when used in error.

International issues:

Nipent [U.S., Canada, and multiple international markets] may be confused with Nipin brand name for nifedipine [Italy, Singapore]

Related Information

Prevention of Chemotherapy-Induced Nausea and Vomiting in Children *on page 2368*

Safe Handling of Hazardous Drugs *on page 2455*

Brand Names: US Nipent

Brand Names: Canada Nipent

Therapeutic Category Antineoplastic Agent, Antimetabolite; Antineoplastic Agent, Antimetabolite (Purine Analog); Antineoplastic Agent, Antimetabolite (Purine Antagonist)

Generic Availability (US) No

Use Treatment (as a single-agent) of untreated and interferon-refractory hairy cell leukemia in patients with active disease (clinically significant anemia, neutropenia, thrombocytopenia, or disease-related symptoms) (FDA approved in adults); has also been used for treatment of cutaneous T-cell lymphoma, chronic lymphocytic leukemia (CLL), and acute and chronic graft-versus-host disease (GVHD)

Pregnancy Risk Factor D

Pregnancy Considerations Adverse events were observed in animal reproduction studies. Women of child-bearing potential should be advised to avoid becoming pregnant during treatment.

Breast-Feeding Considerations It is not known if pentostatin is excreted in breast milk. Due to the potential for serious adverse reactions in nursing the infant, a decision should be made to discontinue pentostatin or to discontinue breast feeding, taking into account the importance of treatment to the mother.

Contraindications Hypersensitivity to pentostatin or any component of the formulation

Warnings/Precautions Hazardous agent; use appropriate precautions for handling and disposal (NIOSH 2014 [group 1]). **[U.S. Boxed Warnings]: Severe renal, liver, pulmonary, and CNS toxicities have occurred with doses higher than recommended; do not exceed the recommended dose.** May cause elevations (usually reversible) in liver function tests. Withhold treatment or discontinue for CNS toxicity. Serum creatinine elevations occurring at recommended doses are usually minor and reversible. Withhold treatment for elevated serum creatinine and determine creatinine clearance. May require dosage adjustment or therapy discontinuation. Use with caution in patients with renal dysfunction (CrCl <60 mL/minute); the terminal half-life is prolonged; may require dosage adjustment.

Myelosuppression may occur, primarily early in treatment (first few courses). Neutropenia may worsen during initial courses for the treatment of hairy cell leukemia. If severe neutropenia persists beyond early cycles, evaluate for disease status. Monitor blood counts during treatment (more frequently in the initial cycles). In patients who present with infections prior to treatment, infections should be resolved, if possible, prior to initiation of treatment; preexisting infections may worsen with pentostatin treatment. Treatment should be temporarily withheld for active infections during therapy. Use in patients with infections only if the potential benefit justifies the potential risk.

Severe rashes may occur and worsen with therapy continuation; may require treatment interruption or discontinuation. Potentially significant drug-drug interactions may exist, requiring dose or frequency adjustment, additional monitoring, and/or selection of alternative therapy. **[U.S. Boxed Warnings]: Do not administer concurrently with fludarabine; concomitant use has resulted in serious or fatal pulmonary toxicity.** Fatal pulmonary edema and hypotension have been reported in patients treated with pentostatin in combination with carmustine, etoposide, or high-dose cyclophosphamide as part of a myeloablative regimen for bone marrow transplant. **[U.S. Boxed Warning]: Should be administered under the supervision of an experienced cancer chemotherapy physician.**

Adverse Reactions

Cardiovascular: Angina, arrhythmia, AV block, bradycardia, cardiac arrest, chest pain, deep thrombophlebitis, facial edema, heart failure, hypertension, hypotension, pericardial effusion, peripheral edema, sinus arrest, syncope, tachycardia, vasculitis, ventricular extrasystoles

Central nervous system: Abnormal dreams/thinking, amnesia, anxiety, ataxia, chills, CNS toxicity, confusion, depression, dizziness, emotional lability, encephalitis, fatigue, fever, hallucination, headache, hostility, insomnia, meningism, nervousness, neuritis, neurosis, pain, seizure, somnolence, vertigo

Dermatologic: Abscess, acne, alopecia, cellulitis, dry skin, eczema, furunculosis, petechial rash, photosensitivity, pruritus, rash, skin disorder, urticaria

Endocrine & metabolic: Amenorrhea, gout, hypercalcemia, hyponatremia, libido decreased/loss

Gastrointestinal: Abdominal pain, anorexia, constipation, diarrhea, dyspepsia, dysphagia, flatulence, gingivitis, glossitis, ileus, nausea/vomiting, oral moniliasis, stomatitis, taste perversion

Genitourinary: Impotence, urinary tract infection

Hematologic: Acute leukemia, agranulocytosis, anemia, aplastic anemia, hemolytic anemia, hemorrhage, leukopenia, myelosuppression, thrombocytopenia

Hepatic: Transaminases increased

Local: Phlebitis

Neuromuscular & skeletal: Arthralgia, arthritis, dysarthria, hyperkinesia, myalgia, neuralgia, neuropathy, osteomyelitis, paralysis, paresthesia, twitching, weakness

Ocular: Amblyopia, conjunctivitis, eyes nonreactive, lacrimation disorder, photophobia, retinopathy, vision abnormal, watery eyes, xerophthalmia

Otic: Deafness, earache, labyrinthitis, tinnitus

Renal: Creatinine increased, nephropathy, renal failure, renal insufficiency, renal function abnormal, renal stone

Respiratory: Asthma, bronchitis, bronchospasm, cough, dyspnea, laryngeal edema, pharyngitis, pneumonia, pulmonary embolus, rhinitis, sinusitis, upper respiratory infection

Miscellaneous: Allergic reaction, bacterial infection, diaphoresis, flu-like syndrome, herpes simplex, herpes zoster, infection, sepsis, viral infection

Rare but important or life-threatening: Dysuria, fungal infection (skin), hematuria, lethargy, pulmonary edema, pulmonary toxicity (fatal; in combination with fludarabine), uveitis/vision loss

Drug Interactions

Metabolism/Transport Effects None known.

Avoid Concomitant Use

Avoid concomitant use of Pentostatin with any of the following: BCG; BCG (Intravesical); CloZAPine; Dipyrone; Fludarabine; Natalizumab; Nelarabine; Pegademase Bovine; Pimecrolimus; Tacrolimus (Topical); Tofacitinib; Vaccines (Live)

Increased Effect/Toxicity

Pentostatin may increase the levels/effects of: CloZAPine; Cyclophosphamide; Fludarabine; Leflunomide; Natalizumab; Tofacitinib; Vaccines (Live)

The levels/effects of Pentostatin may be increased by: Denosumab; Dipyrone; Fludarabine; Pimecrolimus; Roflumilast; Tacrolimus (Topical); Trastuzumab

Decreased Effect

Pentostatin may decrease the levels/effects of: BCG; BCG (Intravesical); Coccidioides immitis Skin Test; Nelarabine; Pegademase Bovine; Sipuleucel-T; Vaccines (Inactivated); Vaccines (Live)

The levels/effects of Pentostatin may be decreased by: Echinacea; Pegademase Bovine

Storage/Stability Store intact vials under refrigeration at 2°C to 8°C (36°F to 46°F). Reconstituted vials and solutions diluted for infusion (in D_5W or NS) may be stored at room temperature for 8 hours.

Mechanism of Action Pentostatin is a purine antimetabolite that inhibits adenosine deaminase, preventing the deamination of adenosine to inosine. Accumulation of deoxyadenosine (dAdo) and deoxyadenosine 5'-triphosphate (dATP) results in a reduction of purine metabolism which blocks DNA synthesis and leads to cell death.

Pharmacokinetics (Adult data unless noted)

Distribution: IV: V_d: Adults: 36.1 L (20.1 L/m^2); rapidly to body tissues

Protein binding: ~4%

Half-life elimination: Adults:
Distribution half-life: 11 to 85 minutes
Terminal half-life: 3 to 7 hours; renal impairment (CrCl <50 mL/minute): 4 to 18 hours
Elimination: Urine (~50% to 96%) within 24 hours (30% to 90% as unchanged drug)
Clearance: Adults: 68 mL/minute/m^2 (mean)

Dosing: Usual

Pediatric: **Chronic graft-versus-host disease (GVHD), steroid-refractory:** Limited data available: Infant, Children, and Adolescents: IV: Initial: 4 mg/m^2 once every 2 weeks; after 6 months of therapy, discontinue for sustained objective response, or continue same dose every 2 to 4 weeks for up to 12 months if still improving (Jacobsohn 2007; Jacobsohn 2009) **or** 4 mg/m^2 once every 2 weeks for 3 months (Wolff 2011)

Adult: **Note**: Utilize patient's actual body weight (full weight) for calculation of body surface area- or weight-based dosing, particularly when the intent of therapy is curative; manage regimen-related toxicities in the same manner as for nonobese patients; if a dose reduction is utilized due to toxicity, consider resumption of full weight-based dosing with subsequent cycles, especially if cause of toxicity (eg, hepatic or renal impairment) is resolved (Griggs 2012). Utilize actual body weight (full weight) for calculation of body surface area in pentostatin dosing for hematopoietic stem cell transplant conditioning regimens in adults (Bubalo 2014).

Hairy cell leukemia: IV: 4 mg/m^2 every 2 weeks. **Note:** The optimal duration has not been determined; in the absence of unacceptable toxicity, may continue until complete response is achieved or until 2 doses after complete response. Discontinue after 6 months if partial or complete response is not achieved.

Acute graft-versus-host disease (GVHD), steroid-refractory: IV:
Initial therapy: 1.5 mg/m^2 days 1 to 3 and days 15 to 17 (in combination with corticosteroids) (Alousi 2009)
Steroid-refractory disease: 1.5 mg/m^2 daily for 3 days; may repeat after 2 weeks if needed (Bolanos-Meade 2005)

Chronic graft-versus-host disease (GVHD), steroid-refractory: IV: 4 mg/m^2 once every 2 weeks; discontinue after 6 months for sustained objective response or continue every 2 to 4 weeks for up to 12 months if still improving (Jacobsohn 2007; Jacobsohn 2009), **or** 4 mg/m^2 once every 2 weeks for 3 months (Wolff 2011)

Dosing adjustment in renal impairment: There are no dosage adjustments provided in the manufacturer's labeling; although not adequately studied, two adult patients with CrCl 50 to 60 mL/minute achieved responses when treated with 2 mg/m^2/dose. For renal toxicity during treatment, withhold for elevated serum creatinine and determine creatinine clearance. The following adjustments have also been recommended (some are indication specific):

Infants, Children, and Adolescents: **GVHD treatment** (Jacobsohn 2009; Wolff 2011):
CrCl 30 to 50 mL/minute/1.73 m^2: Reduce dose by 50%
CrCl <30 mL/minute/1.73 m^2: Withhold dose

Adults:
Kintzel 1995:
CrCl 46 to 60 mL/minute: Administer 70% of dose
CrCl 31 to 45 mL/minute: Administer 60% of dose
CrCl <30 mL/minute: Consider use of alternative drug
Lathia 2002:
CrCl ≥60 mL/minute: Administer 4 mg/m^2/dose
CrCl 40 to 59 mL/minute: Administer 3 mg/m^2/dose
CrCl 20 to 39 mL/minute: Administer 2 mg/m^2/dose
Alousi 2009; Jacobsohn 2009; Poi 2013 (for GVHD treatment):
CrCl 30 to 50 mL/minute/1.73 m^2: Reduce dose by 50%
CrCl <30 mL/minute/1.73 m^2: Withhold dose

Dosing adjustment in hepatic impairment: There are no dosage adjustments provided in the manufacturer's labeling.

Dosing adjustment for toxicity:

Infants, Children, and Adolescents (Jacobsohn 2007; Jacobsohn 2009; Wolff 2011):
ANC 500 to 1,000/mm^3: Reduce dose by 25%
ANC <500/mm^3, platelets <20,000/mm^3, or neutropenic fever: Reduce dose by 50%
Infection, severe: Interrupt treatment until infection is controlled

Adults:
ANC <200/mm^3 (with baseline ANC >500/mm^3): Temporarily interrupt treatment until ANC returns to predose levels.
CNS toxicity: Withhold treatment or discontinue.
Infection, active: Interrupt treatment until infection is controlled.
Rash: Severe rashes may require treatment interruption or discontinuation.
Other severe adverse reactions: Withhold treatment or discontinue.

Preparation for Administration Hazardous agent; use appropriate precautions for handling and disposal (NIOSH 2014 [group 1]).

IV: Reconstitute with 5 mL SWFI to a concentration of 2 mg/mL

IV infusion: Further dilute in NS or D_5W; to achieve compatibility in PVC containing infusion bags and sets a target concentration of 0.18 to 0.33 mg/mL should be used; in adults, doses are diluted in 25 to 50 mL fluid.

Administration Hazardous agent; use appropriate precautions for handling and disposal (NIOSH 2014 [group 1]). At concentrations of 0.18 to 0.33 mg/mL, pentostatin is compatible with PVC containing infusion bags and infusion sets.

IV: **Note:** Hydration with fluids prior to pentostatin dose is necessary; in adults, 500 to 1,000 mL fluid prior to dose and 500 mL after dose is recommended per the manufacturer; in one pediatric study 5 mL/kg fluid boluses were given prior to and after the infusion (Jacobsohn 2009).
Infants, Children, and Adolescents: After further dilution, administer as IV infusion over 20 to 30 minutes (Jacobsohn 2007; Jacobsohn 2009)
Adults: Administer as an IV bolus (2 mg/mL) or as an infusion over 20 to 30 minutes (after further dilution).

Monitoring Parameters CBC with differential and platelet count (prior to each dose; more frequently during initial cycles), peripheral blood smears (periodically for hairy cells and to assess treatment response), liver function, serum uric acid, renal function (serum creatinine and/or creatinine clearance at baseline, and serum creatinine prior to each dose), bone marrow evaluation, signs/symptoms of pulmonary and CNS toxicity

Dosage Forms Excipient information presented when available (limited, particularly for generics); consult specific product labeling.

Solution Reconstituted, Intravenous:
Nipent: 10 mg (1 ea)

Pentoxifylline (pen toks IF i lin)

Medication Safety Issues

Sound-alike/look-alike issues:
Pentoxifylline may be confused with tamoxifen
TRENtal may be confused with Bentyl, TEGretol, Trandate

Related Information

Oral Medications That Should Not Be Crushed or Altered *on page 2476*

Brand Names: US TRENtal [DSC]

Brand Names: Canada Pentoxifylline SR

Therapeutic Category Blood Viscosity Reducer Agent

Generic Availability (US) Yes

Use Symptomatic management of peripheral vascular disease, mainly intermittent claudication (FDA approved in adults)

Has also been studied for use in AIDS patients with increased tumor necrosis factor, cerebrovascular accidents, cerebrovascular diseases, new onset type I diabetes mellitus, diabetic atherosclerosis, diabetic neuropathy, diabetic nephropathy, gangrene, cutaneous polyarteritis nodosa, hemodialysis shunt thrombosis, cerebral malaria, septic shock, sepsis in premature neonates, sickle cell syndromes, vasculitis, Kawasaki disease, Raynaud's syndrome, cystic fibrosis, bone marrow transplant-related toxicities (ie, graft-versus-host disease, veno-occlusive disease, and interstitial pneumonitis), and persistent pulmonary hypertension of the newborn

Pregnancy Risk Factor C

Pregnancy Considerations Adverse events have been observed in animal reproduction studies. Information related to use in pregnant women has not been located. Pentoxifylline may be used to test sperm viability when evaluating nonfertile males (ASRM, 2012). It has also been evaluated for the treatment of infertility due to endometriosis, but use for this purpose is not currently recommended (Lu, 2012).

Breast-Feeding Considerations Pentoxifylline and its metabolites are excreted into breast milk. Five nursing women (~6 weeks postpartum) were given a single dose of pentoxifylline 400 mg and maternal milk and serum samples were measured 2 and 4 hours later. The mean M/P ratio of pentoxifylline was 0.87 at 4 hours; actual milk concentrations ranged from below the limit of detection to 67.4 ng/mL. Three metabolites were also measured in breast milk, with mean M/P ratios ranging from 0.54-1.13 at 4 hours (Witter, 1985). Due to the potential for serious adverse reactions in the nursing infant, the manufacturer recommends a decision be made whether to discontinue nursing or to discontinue the drug, taking into account the importance of treatment to the mother.

Contraindications Patients previously exhibiting intolerance to pentoxifylline, xanthines (eg, caffeine, theophylline), or any component of the formulation; recent cerebral and/or retinal hemorrhage

Canadian labeling: Additional contraindications (not in U.S. labeling): Acute MI, severe coronary artery disease when myocardial stimulation might prove harmful, peptic ulcers (current or recent)

Warnings/Precautions Discontinue at first sign of anaphylaxis or anaphylactoid reaction. Use with caution in patients with mild to moderate hepatic impairment; the bioavailability of pentoxifylline and metabolite I is increased. Has not been studied in patients with severe hepatic disease. Use with caution in patients with renal impairment; bioavailability of active metabolite V may be increased. Use with caution in the elderly due to the potential for cardiac, hepatic, or renal impairment.

Adverse Reactions

Gastrointestinal: Nausea, vomiting

Rare but important or life-threatening: Anaphylactic shock, anaphylactoid reaction, anaphylaxis, angioedema, angina, anorexia, aplastic anemia, arrhythmia, aseptic meningitis, blurred vision, chest pain, cholecystitis, conjunctivitis, depression, fibrinogen decreased (serum), hallucinations, hepatitis, hypotension, leukemia, leukopenia, liver enzymes increased, pancytopenia, scotoma, seizure, tachycardia, thrombocytopenia

Drug Interactions

Metabolism/Transport Effects Inhibits CYP1A2 (weak)

Avoid Concomitant Use

Avoid concomitant use of Pentoxifylline with any of the following: Ketorolac (Nasal); Ketorolac (Systemic)

Increased Effect/Toxicity

Pentoxifylline may increase the levels/effects of: Agents with Antiplatelet Properties; Antihypertensives; Heparin; Heparin (Low Molecular Weight); Theophylline Derivatives; TiZANidine; Vitamin K Antagonists

The levels/effects of Pentoxifylline may be increased by: Cimetidine; CYP1A2 Inhibitors (Strong); Ketorolac (Nasal); Ketorolac (Systemic)

Decreased Effect There are no known significant interactions involving a decrease in effect.

Food Interactions Food may decrease rate but not extent of absorption. Pentoxifylline peak serum levels may be decreased if taken with food.

Storage/Stability Store between 20°C to 25°C (68°F to 77°F); protect from light.

Mechanism of Action Pentoxifylline increases blood flow to the affected microcirculation. Although the precise mechanism of action is not well-defined, blood viscosity is lowered, erythrocyte flexibility is increased, leukocyte deformability is increased, and neutrophil adhesion and activation are decreased. Overall, tissue oxygenation is significantly increased.

Pharmacodynamics Onset of action: 2-4 weeks with multiple doses

Pharmacokinetics (Adult data unless noted)

Absorption: Oral: Well absorbed

Distribution: Pentoxifylline and metabolites distribute into breast milk

Metabolism: Undergoes first-pass in the liver, dose-related (nonlinear) pharmacokinetics; 2 active metabolites (M-I and M-V); **Note:** Plasma concentrations of M-1 and M-V are 5 and 8 times greater, respectively, than pentoxifylline

Half-life, apparent:

Parent drug: 24-48 minutes

Metabolites: 60-96 minutes

Time to peak serum concentration: Within 2-4 hours

Elimination: Metabolites excreted in urine; 0% eliminated unchanged in the urine: 50% to 80% eliminated as M-V metabolite in the urine; 20% as other metabolites

Dosing: Usual Oral:

Children: Minimal information available; one investigation (Furukawa, 1994) found a lower incidence of coronary artery lesions in 22 children (mean age: 2 years) treated for acute Kawasaki disease with versus without pentoxifylline 20 mg/kg/day (given in 3 divided doses); all patients received aspirin and IV gamma globulin therapy; a lower dose (10 mg/kg/day) was not effective; higher doses have been used investigationally for the treatment of cystic fibrosis (Aronoff, 1994)

Adults: 400 mg 3 times/day with meals; decrease to 400 mg twice daily if CNS or GI side effects occur. **Note:** Although clinical benefit may be seen within 2-4 weeks, treatment should be continued for at least 8 weeks.

Dosing adjustment in renal impairment: Use with caution; monitor for enhanced therapeutic and toxic effects; **Note:** Pentoxifylline is not eliminated unchanged in the urine; however, the pharmacologically active metabolite (M-V) is; M-V may accumulate in patients with renal impairment and add to pharmacologic and toxic effects.

Adults: Dosage adjustments not listed by manufacturer; adjust dose based on degree of renal impairment (Aronoff, 2007)

CrCl >50 mL/minute: 400 mg every 8-12 hours

CrCl 10-50 mL/minute: 400 mg every 12-24 hours

CrCl <10 mL/minute: 400 mg every 24 hours; **Note:** Further dosage reduction may be required; Paap (1996) suggests a further reduction to 200 mg once daily but current products (extended or controlled release; unscored) may require adaptation to 400 mg once every other day

Administration Oral: Administer with food or antacids to decrease GI upset. Do not crush, break, or chew extended or controlled release tablet, swallow whole.

Test Interactions Concomitant administration increases theophylline levels

Dosage Forms Excipient information presented when available (limited, particularly for generics); consult specific product labeling. [DSC] = Discontinued product

Tablet Extended Release, Oral:

TRENtal: 400 mg [DSC] [contains benzyl alcohol]

Generic: 400 mg

Extemporaneous Preparations A 20 mg/mL oral suspension may be made using tablets. Crush ten 400 mg tablets and reduce to a fine powder. Add a small amount of purified water and mix to a uniform paste; mix while adding purified water to **almost** 200 mL; transfer to a calibrated bottle, rinse mortar with vehicle, and add quantity of vehicle sufficient to make 200 mL. Label "shake well" and "refrigerate". Stable 91 days.

Nahata MC, Pai VB, and Hipple TF, *Pediatric Drug Formulations*, 5th ed, Cincinnati, OH: Harvey Whitney Books Co, 2004.

- **Pentoxifylline SR (Can)** *see* Pentoxifylline *on page 1670*
- **Pentrax Gold [OTC]** *see* Coal Tar *on page 523*
- **Pentrax Gold Shampoo [OTC] (Can)** *see* Coal Tar *on page 523*
- **Pentrax Tar Shampoo [OTC] (Can)** *see* Coal Tar *on page 523*
- **Pen VK** *see* Penicillin V Potassium *on page 1660*
- **Pepcid** *see* Famotidine *on page 847*
- **Pepcid AC (Can)** *see* Famotidine *on page 847*
- **Pepcid Complete (Can)** *see* Famotidine *on page 847*
- **Peptic guard (Can)** *see* Famotidine *on page 847*
- **Peptic Relief [OTC]** *see* Bismuth Subsalicylate *on page 290*
- **Pepto-Bismol [OTC]** *see* Bismuth Subsalicylate *on page 290*
- **Pepto-Bismol To-Go [OTC]** *see* Bismuth Subsalicylate *on page 290*

Peramivir (pe RA mi veer)

Brand Names: US Rapivab

Therapeutic Category Antiviral Agent; Neuraminidase Inhibitor

Generic Availability (US) No

Use Treatment of acute, uncomplicated influenza in patients who have been symptomatic ≤2 days (FDA approved in ages ≥18 years and adults). **Note:** Efficacy has not been established for patients with serious influenza requiring hospitalization; efficacy is based on clinical trials in which influenza A was the predominant virus; a limited number of subjects with influenza B have been studied.

Pregnancy Risk Factor C

Pregnancy Considerations Adverse events were observed in some animal reproduction studies. Information related to the use of peramivir in pregnancy is limited (Hernandez 2011; Sorbello 2012). Based on information from one case, the pharmacokinetics of peramivir may be changed with pregnancy (Clay 2011).

Untreated influenza infection is associated with an increased risk of adverse events to the fetus and an increased risk of complications or death to the mother (CDC 62[07], 2013). Neuraminidase inhibitors are currently recommended for the treatment or prophylaxis of influenza in pregnant women and women up to 2 weeks postpartum (CDC 60[1], 2011; CDC March 13, 2014; CDC January 2015).

Breast-Feeding Considerations It is not known if peramivir is excreted into breast milk. According to the manufacturer, the decision to breast-feed during therapy should take into account the risk of exposure to the infant and the benefits of treatment to the mother. Influenza may cause serious illness in postpartum women and prompt evaluation for febrile respiratory illnesses is recommended (Louie 2011).

Contraindications There are no contraindications listed in the manufacturer's labeling.

Warnings/Precautions Rare serious skin reactions (eg, erythema multiforme, Stevens-Johnson syndrome)) have been reported. If skin reactions are suspected or occur, institute appropriate supportive treatment. Serious hypersensitivity reactions (eg, anaphylaxis, urticaria, angioedema) have been reported with other neuraminidase inhibitors. Although these reactions have not yet been observed with peramivir, discontinue infusion immediately and treat reaction if hypersensitivity is suspected. Rare occurrences of neuropsychiatric events (including abnormal behavior, delirium, and hallucinations), including fatalities, have been reported, primarily among pediatric patients. Onset is often abrupt and subsequent resolution is rapid. These events may occur in patients with encephalitis, encephalopathy, or in uncomplicated influenza. Closely monitor for signs of abnormal behavior. Emergence of resistance substitutions or other factors (eg, viral virulence) could decrease drug effectiveness. Consider available information on influenza drug susceptibility patterns/treatment effects when using; efficacy in patients with serious influenza requiring hospitalization has not been established. Has not been shown to prevent secondary serious bacterial infections occurring during influenza course; if bacterial infections occur, treat with antibiotics as appropriate. Elimination is primarily renal; dosage adjustment is required in renal impairment. Potentially significant drug-drug interactions may exist, requiring dose or frequency adjustment, additional monitoring, and/or selection of alternative therapy.

Warnings: Additional Pediatric Considerations In pediatric trials, most frequently reported adverse effects included diarrhea and abnormal behavior (Komeda 2014).

Adverse Reactions

Cardiovascular: Hypertension

Central nervous system: Insomnia

Endocrine: Increased serum glucose

Gastrointestinal: Constipation, diarrhea

Hematologic and oncologic: Neutropenia

Hepatic: Increased serum ALT, increased serum AST

Neuromuscular & skeletal: Increased creatine phosphokinase

Rare but important or life-threatening: Abnormal behavior, delirium, erythema multiforme, exfoliative dermatitis, hallucination, skin rash, Stevens-Johnson syndrome

Drug Interactions

Metabolism/Transport Effects None known.

Avoid Concomitant Use There are no known interactions where it is recommended to avoid concomitant use.

Increased Effect/Toxicity There are no known significant interactions involving an increase in effect.

Decreased Effect

Peramivir may decrease the levels/effects of: Influenza Virus Vaccine (Live/Attenuated)

Storage/Stability Store intact vials at 20°C to 25°C (68°F to 77°F); excursions are permitted between 15°C and 30°C (59°F and 86°F).

Mechanism of Action Peramivir, a cyclopentane analogue, selectively inhibits the influenza virus neuraminidase enzyme, preventing the release of viral particles from infected cells.

Pharmacokinetics (Adult data unless noted)

Bioavailability: Oral: Low (investigational agent) (Hata, 2014)

Distribution: V_d central: 12.6 L

Protein binding: <30%

Half-life elimination: ~20 hours (normal renal function)

Elimination: Urine: 90% (primarily unchanged)

Dosing: Neonatal Influenza, treatment: Very limited data available describing use in neonates diagnosed with influenza A; dosing based on recommendations and experience from H1N1 epidemic 2009-10 (Hata 2014; Louis 2013). Full term neonate: IV: 6 mg/kg once daily for 5 to 10 days (FDA 2009; Hata 2014); **Note:** Treatment duration >10 days may be permitted in certain situations, such as critical illness (eg, respiratory failure or intensive care unit admission), continued viral shedding, or unresolved clinical influenza illness.

Dosing adjustment in renal impairment: Dosage must be adjusted in patients with a CrCl <50 mL/minute. **Note:** Dosage adjustments based on Schwartz formula (FDA 2009).

CrCl ≥50 mL/minute/1.73 m^2: No adjustment necessary

CrCl 31 to 49 mL/minute/1.73 m^2: 1.5 mg/kg once daily for 5 to 10 days

CrCl 10 to 30 mL/minute/1.73 m^2: 1 mg/kg once daily for 5 to 10 days

CrCl <10 mL/minute/1.73 m^2 (**not** on intermittent HD or CRRT): 1 mg/kg on day 1, followed by 0.15 mg/kg once daily for 5 to 10 days

CrCl <10 mL/minute/1.73 m^2 (**on** intermittent HD): 1 mg/kg on day 1, followed by 1 mg/kg given 2 hours after each HD session **on dialysis days only**

Dosing: Usual

Pediatric: **Influenza, treatment:** Limited data available; optimal dosing not established; use in pediatric patients diagnosed with influenza A; dosing based on recommendations and experience from H1N1 epidemic 2009-10 (FDA 2009; Hata 2014; Louis 2013; Randolph 2011) and postmarketing data from Japan with unclassified virus subtypes (Komeda, 2014). **Note:** Treatment duration >10 days may be permitted in certain situations, such as critical illness (eg, respiratory failure or intensive care unit admission), continued viral shedding, or unresolved clinical influenza illness. Infants, Children, and Adolescents: IV:

29 to 30 days of life: 6 mg/kg once daily for 5 to 10 days (FDA 2009; Hata 2014); doses up to 10 mg/kg once daily have been used (Komeda 2014)

31 to 90 days of life: 8 mg/kg once daily for 5 to 10 days (FDA 2009; Hata 2014); others have used 10 mg/kg once daily (Komeda 2014)

91 to 180 days of life: 10 mg/kg once daily for 5 to 10 days (FDA 2009; Hata 2014; Komeda 2014)

181 days of life through 5 years: 12 mg/kg once daily for 5 to 10 days (FDA 2009; Hata 2014); others have used 10 mg/kg once daily (Komeda 2014); maximum daily dose: 600 mg/**day**

6 to 17 years: 10 mg/kg once daily for 5 to 10 days (FDA 2009; Hata, 2014; Kometa 2014); maximum daily dose: 600 mg/**day**

≥18 years: 600 mg once daily for 5 to 10 days (Hata 2014)

Adult: 600 mg as a single dose

Dosing adjustment in renal impairment: Dosage must be adjusted in patients with a CrCl <50 mL/minute. **Note:** Dosage adjustments based on Schwartz formula (children) and Cockroft and Gault equation (adults).

Infants, Children, and Adolescents <18 years: Limited data available: Dosing adjustment based on recommendations from H1N1 epidemic 2009-10 (FDA 2009):

CrCl ≥ 50 mL/minute/1.73 m^2: No adjustment necessary

CrCl 31 to 49 mL/minute/1.73 m^2:

29 to 30 days of life: 1.5 mg/kg once daily for 5 to 10 days

31 to 90 days of life: 2 mg/kg once daily for 5 to 10 days

91 to 180 days of life: 2.5 mg/kg once daily for 5 to 10 days

181 days of life through 5 years: 3 mg/kg once daily for 5 to 10 days; maximum dose: 150 mg/dose

6 to 17 years: 2.5 mg/kg once daily for 5 to 10 days; maximum dose: 150 mg/dose

CrCl 10 to 30 mL/minute/1.73 m^2:

29 to 30 days of life: 1 mg/kg once daily for 5 to 10 days

31 to 90 days of life: 1.3 mg/kg once daily for 5 to 10 days

91 to 180 days of life: 1.6 mg/kg once daily for 5 to 10 days

181 days of life through 5 years: 1.9 mg/kg once daily for 5 to 10 days; maximum dose: 100 mg/dose

6 to 17 years: 1.6 mg/kg once daily for 5 to 10 days; maximum dose: 100 mg/dose

CrCl <10 mL/minute/1.73 m^2 (**not** on intermittent HD or CRRT):

29 to 30 days of life: 1 mg/kg on day 1, followed by 0.15 mg/kg once daily for 5 to 10 days

31 to 90 days of life: 1.3 mg/kg on day 1, followed by 0.2 mg/kg once daily for 5 to 10 days

91 to 180 days of life: 1.6 mg/kg on day 1, followed by 0.25 mg/kg once daily for 5 to 10 days

181 days of life through 5 years: 1.9 mg/kg on day 1 (maximum dose day 1: 100 mg), followed by 0.3 mg/kg once daily for 5 to 10 days; maximum dose: 15 mg/dose

6 to 17 years: 1.6 mg/kg on day 1 (maximum dose day 1: 100 mg), followed by 0.25 mg/kg once daily for 5 to 10 days; maximum dose: 15 mg/dose

CrCl <10 mL/minute/1.73 m^2 (**on** intermittent HD):

29 to 30 days of life: 1 mg/kg on day 1, followed by 1 mg/kg given 2 hours after each HD session **on dialysis days only**

31 to 90 days of life: 1.3 mg/kg on day 1, followed by 1.3 mg/kg given 2 hours after each HD session **on dialysis days only**

91 to 180 days of life: 1.6 mg/kg on day 1, followed by 1.6 mg/kg given 2 hours after each HD session **on dialysis days only**

181 days of life through 5 years: 1.9 mg/kg on day 1, followed by 1.9 mg/kg given 2 hours after each HD session **on dialysis days only**; maximum dose: 100 mg/dose

6 to 17 years: 1.6 mg/kg on day 1, followed by 1.6 mg/kg given 2 hours after each HD session **on dialysis days only**; maximum dose: 100 mg/dose

Continuous renal replacement therapy (CRRT): Limited data exist. Estimate total clearance by calculating CLCRRT depending on CRRT modality used (eg, CVVHD, SCUF), plus any residual renal function, and adjust dosage according to CrCl recommendation.

Adolescents ≥18 years and Adults:

CrCl ≥50 mL/minute: No adjustment necessary

CrCl 30 to 49 mL/minute: 200 mg once daily

CrCl 10 to 29 mL/minute: 100 mg once daily

Hemodialysis: 100 mg as a single dose administered after dialysis

Dosing adjustment in hepatic impairment: There are no dosage adjustments provided in the manufacturer's labeling (has not been studied); however, not significantly metabolized hepatically.

Preparation for Administration Parenteral: Dilute peramivir dose in NS, ½NS, D_5W, or LR to a final concentration ≤6 mg/mL; maximum total volume: 100 mL

Administration Parenteral: IV: For IV use only, do not administer intramuscularly. Administer diluted dose intravenously over 15 to 30 minutes; in pediatric patients, an infusion time of ≥15 minutes has been used (Komeda 2014)

Monitoring Parameters CBC with differential and a renal function (prior to initiation and during therapy); vital signs (daily at minimum); development of diarrhea; signs or symptoms of unusual behavior (including attempts at self-injury, confusion, and/or delirium)

Dosage Forms Excipient information presented when available (limited, particularly for generics); consult specific product labeling.

Solution, Intravenous [preservative free]:

Rapivab: 200 mg/20 mL (20 mL)

Perampanel (per AM pa nel)

Brand Names: US Fycompa

Therapeutic Category AMPA Glutamate Receptor Antagonist; Anticonvulsant, Miscellaneous

Generic Availability (US) No

Use Adjunctive therapy in the treatment of partial-onset seizures with or without secondarily generalized seizures (FDA approved in ages ≥12 years and adults)

Medication Guide Available Yes

Pregnancy Risk Factor C

Pregnancy Considerations Adverse events have been observed in animal reproduction studies at doses equivalent to the human dose (based on BSA). Contraceptives containing levonorgestrel may be less effective; additional nonhormonal forms of contraception are recommended during perampanel therapy.

Patients exposed to perampanel during pregnancy are encouraged to enroll in the North American Antiepileptic Drug (NAAED) Pregnancy Registry by calling 1-888-233-2334. Additional information is available at www.aedpregnancyregistry.org.

Breast-Feeding Considerations It is not known if perampanel is excreted in breast milk. The manufacturer recommends that caution be exercised when administering perampanel to nursing women.

Contraindications There are no contraindications listed in manufacturer's labeling.

Warnings/Precautions [US Boxed Warning]: Dose-related serious and/or life-threatening neuropsychiatric events (including aggression, anger, homicidal ideation and threats, hostility, and irritability) have been reported most often occurring in first 6 weeks of therapy in patients with or without prior psychiatric history, prior aggressive behavior, or concomitant use of medications associated with hostility and aggression; monitor patients closely especially during dosage adjustments and when receiving higher doses. Adjust dose or immediately discontinue use if severe or worsening symptoms occur; permanently discontinue for persistent severe or worsening psychiatric symptoms or behaviors. Inform patients and caregivers to contact their healthcare provider immediately if they experience any atypical behavioral and/or mood changes while taking perampanel or after discontinuing perampanel. Pooled analysis of trials involving various antiepileptics (regardless of indication) showed an increased risk of suicidal thoughts/behavior (incidence rate: 0.43% treated patients compared to 0.24% of patients receiving placebo); risk observed as early as 1 week after initiation and continued through duration of trials (most trials ≤24 weeks). Monitor all patients for notable changes in behavior that might indicate suicidal thoughts or depression; notify healthcare provider immediately if symptoms occur. Dizziness, fatigue (including lethargy and weakness), gait disturbances (including abnormal coordination, ataxia, and balance disorder), and somnolence may occur during therapy; patients should be cautioned about performing tasks which require alertness (eg, operating machinery or driving). Concomitant use with CNS depressant (including alcohol) may increase the risk of CNS depression. Use caution if a CNS depressant must be used concurrently with perampanel. Not recommended for use in patients with severe hepatic impairment, severe renal impairment, or on hemodialysis; dosage adjustment recommended for mild-to-moderate hepatic impairment and consider slower titration in patients with moderate renal impairment. Use with extreme caution in patients who are at risk of falls (including head injuries and bone fracture); perampanel has been associated with falls and traumatic injury. Anticonvulsants should not be discontinued abruptly because of the possibility of increasing seizure frequency; therapy should be withdrawn gradually (≥1 week) to minimize the potential of increased seizure frequency, unless safety concerns require a more rapid withdrawal. Use caution in elderly due to increased risk of dizziness, gait or coordination disturbances, somnolence, fatigue-related events, and falls; proceed slowly with dosing titration in patients ≥65 years of age. Potentially significant drug-drug interactions may exist, requiring dose or frequency adjustment, additional monitoring, and/or selection of alternative therapy.

Adverse Reactions

Cardiovascular: Peripheral edema

Central nervous system: Aggression, anger, anxiety, ataxia, balance impaired, confusion, coordination impaired, dizziness, euphoria, fatigue, gait disturbance, headache, hypersomnia, hypoesthesia, irritability, memory impaired, mood changes, somnolence, vertigo

Dermatologic: Bruising, skin laceration

Endocrine & metabolic: Hyponatremia

Gastrointestinal: Constipation, nausea, vomiting, weight gain

Neuromuscular & skeletal: Arthralgia, back pain, dysarthria, falling, limb injury, limb pain, musculoskeletal pain, myalgia, paresthesia, weakness

Ocular: Blurred vision, diplopia

Respiratory: Cough, oropharyngeal pain, upper respiratory tract infection

Miscellaneous: Head injury

Drug Interactions

Metabolism/Transport Effects Substrate of CYP1A2 (minor), CYP2B6 (minor), CYP3A4 (major); **Note:** Assignment of Major/Minor substrate status based on clinically relevant drug interaction potential; **Induces** CYP3A4 (weak)

Avoid Concomitant Use

Avoid concomitant use of Perampanel with any of the following: Alcohol (Ethyl); Azelastine (Nasal); CYP3A4 Inducers (Strong); Orphenadrine; Paraldehyde; St Johns Wort; Thalidomide

Increased Effect/Toxicity

Perampanel may increase the levels/effects of: Alcohol (Ethyl); Azelastine (Nasal); Buprenorphine; CNS Depressants; Hydrocodone; Methotrimeprazine; Metyrosine; Orphenadrine; OXcarbazepine; Paraldehyde; Pramipexole; ROPINIRole; Rotigotine; Selective Serotonin Reuptake Inhibitors; Suvorexant; Thalidomide; Zolpidem

The levels/effects of Perampanel may be increased by: Brimonidine (Topical); Cannabis; Dronabinol; Droperidol; Kava Kava; Magnesium Sulfate; Methotrimeprazine; Nabilone; Rufinamide; Sodium Oxybate; Tapentadol; Tetrahydrocannabinol

Decreased Effect

Perampanel may decrease the levels/effects of: ARIPiprazole; Contraceptives (Progestins); NiMODipine; Saxagliptin

The levels/effects of Perampanel may be decreased by: Bosentan; CarBAMazepine; CYP3A4 Inducers (Moderate); CYP3A4 Inducers (Strong); Dabrafenib; Deferasirox; Fosphenytoin; Mefloquine; Orlistat; OXcarbazepine; Phenytoin; Siltuximab; St Johns Wort; Tocilizumab

Storage/Stability Store at 20°C to 25°C (68°F to 77°F); excursions permitted between 15°C to 30°C (59°F to 86°F).

Mechanism of Action The exact mechanism by which perampanel exerts antiseizure activity is not definitively known; it is a noncompetitive antagonist of the ionotropic alpha-amino-3-hydroxy-5-methyl-4-isoxazolepropionic acid (AMPA) glutamate receptor on postsynaptic neurons. Glutamate is a primary excitatory neurotransmitter in the central nervous center causing many neurological disorders from neuronal over excitation.

Pharmacokinetics (Adult data unless noted) Note: Pharmacokinetic data are similar in pediatric patients ≥12 years as adults.

Absorption: Rapid and complete

Protein binding: 95% to 96%; primarily albumin and alpha$_1$-acid glycoprotein

Metabolism: Extensive via primary oxidation mediated by CYP3A4 and/or CYP3A5 and sequential glucuronidation

Half-life elimination: 105 hours

Time to peak: Median range: 0.5 to 2.5 hours, delayed when given with food

Excretion: Feces (48%); urine (22%)

Dosing: Usual Note: Dosing should be individualized based upon response and tolerability.

Pediatric: **Partial seizures (adjunct):** Children ≥12 years and Adolescents: Oral:

Patients **not** receiving enzyme-inducing AED regimens: Initial: 2 mg once daily at bedtime; may increase daily dose by 2 mg increments at no more frequent than weekly intervals; recommended dose: 8 to 12 mg once daily at bedtime. Although 12 mg doses showed somewhat greater efficacy (reduction in seizure rate) than 8 mg doses, the 12 mg dose was associated with substantially higher adverse effects

Patients receiving enzyme-inducing AED regimens (eg, phenytoin, carbamazepine, oxcarbazepine): Initial: 4 mg once daily at bedtime; may increase daily dose by 2 mg increments at weekly intervals; recommended dose: 8 to 12 mg once daily at bedtime. (French, 2012; Krauss, 2012). Although 12 mg doses showed somewhat greater efficacy (reduction in seizure rate) than 8 mg doses, the 12 mg dose was associated with substantially higher adverse effects.

Adult: **Partial seizures (adjunct):** Oral:

Patients **not** receiving enzyme-inducing AED regimens: Initial: 2 mg once daily at bedtime; may increase daily dose by 2 mg at weekly intervals based on response and tolerability. Recommended dose: 8 to 12 mg once daily at bedtime

Patients receiving enzyme-inducing AED regimens (eg, phenytoin, carbamazepine, oxcarbazepine): Initial: 4 mg once daily at bedtime; may increase daily dose by 2 mg at weekly intervals based on response and tolerability; recommended dose: 8 to 12 mg once daily at bedtime

Dosing adjustment in renal impairment: Children ≥12 years, Adolescents, and Adults:

CrCl ≥50 mL/minute: No dosage adjustment necessary.

CrCl 30 to 49 mL/minute: No dosage adjustment necessary; monitor closely and consider slower titration based on response and tolerability.

CrCl <30 mL/minute: Use not recommended (has not been studied).

Hemodialysis: Use not recommended (has not been studied).

Dosing adjustment in hepatic impairment: Children ≥12 years, Adolescents, and Adults:

Mild impairment (Child-Pugh class A): Initial: 2 mg once daily; may increase daily dose by 2 mg every 2 weeks based on response and tolerability. Maximum daily dose: 6 mg/**day**

Moderate impairment (Child-Pugh class B): Initial: 2 mg once daily; may increase daily dose by 2 mg after 2 weeks based on response and tolerability. Maximum daily dose: 4 mg/**day**

Severe impairment (Child-Pugh class C): Use not recommended (has not been studied).

Administration Oral: Administer at bedtime. May be administered without regard to meals.

Monitoring Parameters Seizure frequency/duration; mental status/suicidality (eg, suicidal thoughts, depression, behavioral changes); weight

Controlled Substance C-III

Dosage Forms Excipient information presented when available (limited, particularly for generics); consult specific product labeling.

Tablet, Oral:

Fycompa: 2 mg, 4 mg, 6 mg, 8 mg

Fycompa: 10 mg, 12 mg [contains fd&c blue #2 aluminum lake]

- ◆ **Percocet** *see* Oxycodone and Acetaminophen *on page 1594*
- ◆ **Percocet-Demi (Can)** *see* Oxycodone and Acetaminophen *on page 1594*
- ◆ **Percodan®** *see* Oxycodone and Aspirin *on page 1597*
- ◆ **Perdiem Overnight Relief [OTC]** *see* Senna *on page 1914*
- ◆ **Perforomist** *see* Formoterol *on page 934*
- ◆ **Periactin** *see* Cyproheptadine *on page 562*
- ◆ **Perichlor (Can)** *see* Chlorhexidine Gluconate *on page 434*
- ◆ **Peri-Colace [OTC]** *see* Docusate and Senna *on page 698*
- ◆ **Peridex** *see* Chlorhexidine Gluconate *on page 434*
- ◆ **Peridex Oral Rinse (Can)** *see* Chlorhexidine Gluconate *on page 434*
- ◆ **Periogard** *see* Chlorhexidine Gluconate *on page 434*
- ◆ **PerioMed** *see* Fluoride *on page 899*
- ◆ **Periostat (Can)** *see* Doxycycline *on page 717*

Permethrin (per METH rin)

Brand Names: US Acticin; Elimite

Brand Names: Canada Kwellada-P [OTC]; Nix [OTC]

Therapeutic Category Antiparasitic Agent, Topical; Pediculocide; Scabicidal Agent

Generic Availability (US) Yes

Use Single application treatment of infestation with *Pediculus humanus capitis* (head louse) and its nits; treatment of *Sarcoptes scabiei* (scabies) (FDA approved in ages ≥2 months and adults)

Pregnancy Risk Factor B

Pregnancy Considerations Adverse effects have not been observed in oral animal reproduction studies. The amount of permethrin available systemically following topical application is ≤2%. The CDC considers the use of permethrin or pyrethrins with piperonyl butoxide the drugs of choice for the treatment of pubic lice during pregnancy (CDC, 2010).

Breast-Feeding Considerations It is not known if permethrin is excreted in breast milk. Because many drugs are excreted in human milk and because of the evidence for tumorigenic potential of permethrin in animal studies, consideration should be given to discontinuing nursing temporarily or withholding the drug while the mother is nursing.

Contraindications Hypersensitivity to pyrethyroid, pyrethrin, chrysanthemums, or any component of the formulation

OTC labeling (Lotion): When used for self-medication, do not use on infants <2 months of age; near the eyes; inside the nose, ear, mouth, or vagina. Consult physician for use in eyebrows or eyelashes.

Warnings/Precautions Treatment may temporarily exacerbate the symptoms of itching, redness, swelling; for external use only

Adverse Reactions

Dermatologic: Erythema, pruritus, rash of scalp

Local: Burning, numbness, scalp discomfort, stinging, or tingling; edema

Drug Interactions

Metabolism/Transport Effects None known.

Avoid Concomitant Use There are no known interactions where it is recommended to avoid concomitant use.

Increased Effect/Toxicity There are no known significant interactions involving an increase in effect.

Decreased Effect There are no known significant interactions involving a decrease in effect.

Mechanism of Action Inhibits sodium ion influx through nerve cell membrane channels in parasites resulting in delayed repolarization and thus paralysis and death of the pest

Pharmacokinetics (Adult data unless noted)

Absorption: Topical: Minimal (<2%)

Metabolism: By ester hydrolysis to inactive metabolites

Dosing: Neonatal Topical: Full-term neonates: Scabies: A single application of permethrin 5% cream was shown to be safe and effective in a full-term neonate (PNA: 21 days) when applied from scalp to toes for 6 hours before rinsing with soap and water (Quarterman, 1994).

Dosing: Usual Topical: Infants and Children ≥2 months and Adults:

Head lice: After hair has been washed with shampoo, rinsed with water and towel dried, apply a sufficient volume of creme rinse to saturate the hair and scalp; also apply behind the ears and at the base of the neck; leave on hair for 10 minutes before rinsing off with water; remove remaining nits. May repeat in 1 week if lice or nits still present; in areas of head lice resistance to 1% permethrin, 5% permethrin has been applied to clean, dry hair and left on overnight (8-14 hours) under a shower cap.

Scabies: Apply cream from head to toe; leave on for 8-14 hours before washing off with water; for infants, also apply on the hairline, neck, scalp, temple, and forehead; may reapply in 1 week if live mites appear.

Administration Topical: Avoid contact with eyes during application; shake creme rinse well before using. Apply cream in the evening and leave on overnight to maximize exposure of the mites to the drug.

Additional Information Topical cream formulation contains formaldehyde which is a contact allergen

Dosage Forms Excipient information presented when available (limited, particularly for generics); consult specific product labeling.

Cream, External:

Acticin: 5% (60 g)

Elimite: 5% (60 g) [contains formaldehyde solution]

Generic: 5% (60 g)

Lotion, External:

Generic: 1% (59 mL)

◆ **Pernox Lemon [OTC]** *see* Sulfur and Salicylic Acid *on page 1992*

◆ **Pernox Regular [OTC]** *see* Sulfur and Salicylic Acid *on page 1992*

◆ **Peroxide** *see* Hydrogen Peroxide *on page 1044*

Perphenazine (per FEN a zeen)

Medication Safety Issues

Sound-alike/look-alike issues:

Trilafon may be confused with Tri-Levlen®

BEERS Criteria medication:

This drug may be potentially inappropriate for use in geriatric patients (Quality of evidence - moderate; Strength of recommendation - strong).

Brand Names: Canada Apo-Perphenazine®

Therapeutic Category Antiemetic; Antipsychotic Agent, Typical, Phenothiazine; First Generation (Typical) Antipsychotic; Phenothiazine Derivative

Generic Availability (US) Yes

Use Treatment of schizophrenia (FDA approved in ages ≥12 years and adults); severe nausea and vomiting (FDA approved in adults); other psychotic disorders (eg, schizoaffective disorder), psychotic depression

Pregnancy Considerations Jaundice or hyper- or hyporeflexia have been reported in newborn infants following maternal use of phenothiazines. Antipsychotic use during the third trimester of pregnancy has a risk for abnormal muscle movements (extrapyramidal symptoms [EPS]) and withdrawal symptoms in newborns following delivery. Symptoms in the newborn may include agitation, feeding disorder, hypertonia, hypotonia, respiratory distress, somnolence, and tremor; these effects may be self-limiting or require hospitalization.

Breast-Feeding Considerations Based on information from two mother-infant pairs, following maternal use of perphenazine 16-24 mg/day, the estimated exposure to the breast-feeding infant would be 0.1% to 0.2% of the weight-adjusted maternal dose. Adverse events have not been reported in nursing infants (information from four cases). Infants should be monitored for signs of adverse events; routine monitoring of infant serum concentrations is not recommended.

Contraindications Hypersensitivity to perphenazine or any component of the formulation (cross-reactivity between phenothiazines may occur); severe CNS depression (comatose or patients receiving large doses of CNS depressants); subcortical brain damage (with or without hypothalamic damage); bone marrow suppression; blood dyscrasias; liver damage

Warnings/Precautions [U.S. Boxed Warning]: Elderly patients with dementia-related psychosis treated with antipsychotics are at an increased risk of death compared to placebo. Most deaths appeared to be either cardiovascular (eg, heart failure, sudden death) or infectious (eg, pneumonia) in nature. Perphenazine is not approved for the treatment of dementia-related psychosis.

Leukopenia, neutropenia, and agranulocytosis (sometimes fatal) have been reported in clinical trials and postmarketing reports with antipsychotic use; presence of risk factors (eg, preexisting low WBC or history of drug-induced leuko-/neutropenia) should prompt periodic blood count assessment. Discontinue therapy at first signs of blood dyscrasias or if absolute neutrophil count <1000/mm^3.

May cause hypotension. May be sedating, use with caution in disorders where CNS depression is a feature. Use with caution in depressed patients. Use with caution in Parkinson's disease. Caution in patients with hemodynamic instability; predisposition to seizures; severe cardiac, renal, or respiratory disease. Monitor hepatic and renal function during use; contraindicated in patients with liver damage. Esophageal dysmotility and aspiration have been associated with antipsychotic use; use with caution in patients at risk of pneumonia (eg, Alzheimer's disease). Use associated with increased prolactin levels; clinical significance of hyperprolactinemia in patients with breast cancer or other prolactin-dependent tumors is unknown. May alter temperature regulation or mask toxicity of other drugs due to antiemetic effects. May alter cardiac conduction; life-threatening arrhythmias have occurred with therapeutic doses of phenothiazines. May cause orthostatic hypotension; use with caution in patients at risk of this effect or those who would tolerate transient hypotensive episodes (cerebrovascular disease, cardiovascular disease, or other medications which may predispose).

Phenothiazines may cause anticholinergic effects (confusion, agitation, constipation, xerostomia, blurred vision, urinary retention); therefore, they should be used with caution in patients with decreased gastrointestinal motility, urinary retention, BPH, xerostomia, visual problems, or narrow-angle glaucoma (screening is recommended). Relative to other neuroleptics, perphenazine has a low potency of cholinergic blockade. Use with caution in patients with reduced functional alleles of CYP2D6. Poor metabolizers may have higher plasma concentrations at usual doses, increasing risk for adverse reactions.

May cause extrapyramidal symptoms, including pseudoparkinsonism, acute dystonic reactions, akathisia, and tardive dyskinesia. Risk of dystonia (and possibly other EPS) may be greater with increased doses, use of conventional antipsychotics, males, and younger patients. Risk of tardive dyskinesia and potential for irreversibility may be increased in elderly patients (particularly women), prolonged therapy, and higher total cumulative dose. May be associated with neuroleptic malignant syndrome (NMS). May cause pigmentary retinopathy, and lenticular and corneal deposits, particularly with prolonged therapy. May cause photosensitization. Use with caution in the elderly.

Use in elderly patients with dementia is associated with an increased risk of mortality and cerebrovascular accidents; avoid antipsychotic use for behavioral problems associated with dementia unless alternative nonpharmacologic therapies have failed and patient may harm self or others. In addition, use may cause or exacerbate syndrome of inappropriate antidiuretic hormone secretion or hyponatremia; monitor sodium closely with initiation or dosage adjustments in older adults. May also be inappropriate in older adults depending on comorbidities (eg, dementia, delirium) due to its potent anticholinergic effects (Beers Criteria). Potential for an increased risk of adverse events (eg, sedation, orthostatic hypotension, anticholinergic effects) and an increased risk for developing tardive dyskinesia, particularly in elderly women.

Adverse Reactions

Cardiovascular: Bradycardia, cardiac arrest, ECG changes, hyper-/hypotension, orthostatic hypotension, pallor, peripheral edema, sudden death, tachycardia

Central nervous system: Bizarre dreams, catatonic-like states, cerebral edema, dizziness, drowsiness, extrapyramidal symptoms (pseudoparkinsonism, akathisia, dystonias, tardive dyskinesia), faintness, headache, hyperactivity, hyperpyrexia, impairment of temperature regulation, insomnia, lethargy, neuroleptic malignant syndrome (NMS), nocturnal confusion, paradoxical excitement, paranoid reactions, restlessness, seizure

Dermatologic: Discoloration of skin (blue-gray), photosensitivity

Endocrine & metabolic: Amenorrhea, breast enlargement, hyper-/hypoglycemia, galactorrhea, lactation, libido changes, gynecomastia, menstrual irregularity, parotid swelling (rare), SIADH

Gastrointestinal: Adynamic ileus, anorexia, appetite increased, constipation, diarrhea, fecal impaction, obstipation, nausea, salivation, vomiting, weight gain, xerostomia

Genitourinary: Bladder paralysis, ejaculatory disturbances, incontinence, polyuria, urinary retention

Hematologic: Agranulocytosis, eosinophilia, hemolytic anemia, leukopenia, pancytopenia, thrombocytopenic purpura

Hepatic: Hepatotoxicity, jaundice

Neuromuscular & skeletal: Muscle weakness

Ocular: Blurred vision, cornea and lens changes, epithelial keratopathies, glaucoma, mydriasis, myosis, photophobia, pigmentary retinopathy

Renal: Glycosuria

Respiratory: Nasal congestion

Miscellaneous: Allergic reactions, diaphoresis, systemic lupus erythematosus-like syndrome

Drug Interactions

Metabolism/Transport Effects Substrate of CYP1A2 (minor), CYP2C19 (minor), CYP2C9 (minor), CYP2D6 (major), CYP3A4 (minor); **Note:** Assignment of Major/Minor substrate status based on clinically relevant drug interaction potential; **Inhibits** CYP1A2 (weak), CYP2D6 (weak)

Avoid Concomitant Use

Avoid concomitant use of Perphenazine with any of the following: Aclidinium; Amisulpride; Azelastine (Nasal); Eluxadoline; Glucagon; Ipratropium (Oral Inhalation); Metoclopramide; Orphenadrine; Paraldehyde; Potassium Chloride; Sulpiride; Thalidomide; Tiotropium; Umeclidinium

Increased Effect/Toxicity

Perphenazine may increase the levels/effects of: AbobotulinumtoxinA; Alcohol (Ethyl); Amisulpride; Analgesics (Opioid); Anticholinergic Agents; Antidepressants (Serotonin Reuptake Inhibitor/Antagonist); ARIPiprazole; Azelastine (Nasal); Beta-Blockers; Buprenorphine; CNS Depressants; Eluxadoline; Glucagon; Hydrocodone; Mequitazine; Methotrimeprazine; Methylphenidate; Metyrosine; Mirabegron; Mirtazapine; OnabotulinumtoxinA; Orphenadrine; Paraldehyde; Porfimer; Potassium Chloride; RimabotulinumtoxinB; Selective Serotonin Reuptake Inhibitors; Serotonin Modulators; Sulpiride; Suvorexant; Thalidomide; Thiazide Diuretics; Thiopental; Tiotropium; TiZANidine; Topiramate; Verteporfin; Zolpidem

The levels/effects of Perphenazine may be increased by: Abiraterone Acetate; Acetylcholinesterase Inhibitors (Central); Aclidinium; Antidepressants (Serotonin Reuptake Inhibitor/Antagonist); Antimalarial Agents; Beta-Blockers; Brimonidine (Topical); Cannabis; Cobicistat; CYP2D6 Inhibitors (Moderate); CYP2D6 Inhibitors (Strong); Darunavir; Doxylamine; Dronabinol; Droperidol; HydrOXYzine; Ipratropium (Oral Inhalation); Kava Kava; Lithium; Magnesium Sulfate; Methotrimeprazine; Methylphenidate; Metoclopramide; Metyrosine; Mianserin; Nabilone; Panobinostat; Peginterferon Alfa-2b; Perampanel; Pramlintide; Rufinamide; Serotonin Modulators; Sodium Oxybate; Tapentadol; Tetrabenazine; Tetrahydrocannabinol; Umeclidinium

Decreased Effect

Perphenazine may decrease the levels/effects of: Acetylcholinesterase Inhibitors; Amphetamines; Anti-Parkinson's Agents (Dopamine Agonist); Itopride; Quinagolide; Secretin

The levels/effects of Perphenazine may be decreased by: Acetylcholinesterase Inhibitors; Antacids; Anti-Parkinson's Agents (Dopamine Agonist); Lithium; Peginterferon Alfa-2b

Storage/Stability Store at controlled room temperature of 20°C to 25°C (68°F to 77°F). Protect from light.

Mechanism of Action Perphenazine is a piperazine phenothiazine antipsychotic which blocks postsynaptic mesolimbic dopaminergic receptors in the brain; exhibits alpha-adrenergic blocking effect and depresses the release of hypothalamic and hypophyseal hormones

Pharmacodynamics

Onset of action: 2-4 weeks for control of psychotic symptoms (hallucinations, disorganized thinking or behavior, delusions)

Adequate trial: 6 weeks at moderate to high dose based on tolerability

Duration: Variable

Pharmacokinetics (Adult data unless noted)

Absorption: Well absorbed

Distribution: Crosses placenta

Metabolism: Extensively hepatic to metabolites via sulfoxidation, hydroxylation, dealkylation, and glucuronidation; **Note:** Metabolism is subject to genetic polymorphism; CYP2D6 poor metabolizers will have higher plasma concentrations of perphenazine compared with normal or extensive metabolizers.

Half-life: Perphenazine: 9-12 hours; 7-hydroxyperphenazine: 9.9-18.8 hours

Time to peak serum concentration: Perphenazine: 1-3 hours; 7-hydroxyperphenazine: 2-4 hours

Elimination: Urine and feces, primarily as metabolites

Dialysis: Not dialyzable (0% to 5%)

Dosing: Usual Oral: **Note:** Dosage should be individualized; use lowest effective dose and shortest effective duration; periodically reassess the need for continued treatment

Children: **Note:** Safety and efficacy have not been established in children <12 years of age; use in this age group is not recommended by manufacturer. Some centers use the following doses:

Schizophrenia/psychoses:

<1 year: Dosage not established

1-6 years: 4-6 mg/day in divided doses

6-12 years: 6 mg/day in divided doses

\>12 years: 4-16 mg 2-4 times/day

Postoperative vomiting: Dosage not established; use not recommended. Previous studies used an IV dose of 70 mcg/kg (maximum: 5 mg/dose) in children 2-12 years of age to decrease postoperative vomiting; perphenazine was shown to be more effective than placebo (Splinter, 1997), more effective than dexamethasone (Splinter, 1997a), and similar in efficacy to ondansetron (Splinter, 1998). However, IV granisetron was shown to be more effective than IV perphenazine (Fujii, 1999). Only one study has assessed oral perphenazine; doses of 70 mcg/kg were administered 1 hour prior to surgery to 100 children, 4-10 years of age, to reduce postoperative vomiting; oral granisetron was more effective than oral perphenazine (Fujii, 1999a).

Adults:

Schizophrenia/psychoses: 4-16 mg 2-4 times/day; maximum: 64 mg/day (exceptions occur; indication specific)

Nausea/vomiting: 8-16 mg/day in divided doses; maximum: 24 mg/day

Dosing adjustment in hepatic impairment: Specific guidelines are not available; consider dosage reduction in patients with liver disease

Administration May be administered without regard to meals; do not administer within 2 hours of antacids

Monitoring Parameters Vital signs; periodic eye exam, CBC with differential, liver enzyme tests; renal function in patients with long-term use; fasting blood glucose/Hgb A_{1c}; BMI; therapeutic response (mental status, mood, affect, gait), and adverse reactions at beginning of therapy and periodically with long-term use [eg, excess sedation, extrapyramidal symptoms, tardive dyskinesia, CNS changes, abnormal involuntary movement scale (AIMS)]

Reference Range 2-6 nmol/L

Additional Information Long-term usefulness of perphenazine should be periodically re-evaluated in patients receiving the drug for extended periods; consideration should be given whether to decrease the maintenanc dose or discontinue drug therapy

Dosage Forms Excipient information presented whe available (limited, particularly for generics); consult specifi product labeling.

Tablet, Oral:

Generic: 2 mg, 4 mg, 8 mg, 16 mg

- **Persantine** *see* Dipyridamole *on page 688*
- **Persantine® (Can)** *see* Dipyridamole *on page 688*
- **Pertussis, Acellular (Adsorbed)** *see* Diphtheria anc Tetanus Toxoids, Acellular Pertussis, Poliovirus and *Hae mophilus* b Conjugate Vaccine *on page 679*
- **Pertzye** *see* Pancrelipase *on page 1614*
- **Pethidine Hydrochloride** *see* Meperidine *on page 135*
- **Petrolatum White and Mineral Oil Ophthalmic Oint ment** *see* Ocular Lubricant *on page 1542*
- **Pexeva** *see* PARoxetine *on page 1634*
- **PFA** *see* Foscarnet *on page 941*
- **Pfizerpen-AS® (Can)** *see* Penicillin G Procaine *on page 1659*
- **Pfizerpen-G** *see* Penicillin G (Parenteral/Aqueous) *on page 1656*
- **PGE$_1$** *see* Alprostadil *on page 103*
- **PGI$_2$** *see* Epoprostenol *on page 769*
- **PGX** *see* Epoprostenol *on page 769*
- **Pharbechlor [OTC]** *see* Chlorpheniramine *on page 44*
- **Pharbedryl** *see* DiphenhydrAMINE (Systemic) *on page 668*
- **Pharbetol [OTC]** *see* Acetaminophen *on page 44*
- **Pharbetol Extra Strength [OTC]** *see* Acetaminophen *on page 44*
- **Pharmabase Barrier [OTC]** *see* Zinc Oxide *on page 2214*
- **Phazyme [OTC]** *see* Simethicone *on page 1927*
- **Phazyme (Can)** *see* Simethicone *on page 1927*
- **Phazyme Maximum Strength [OTC]** *see* Simethicone *on page 1927*
- **Phazyme Ultra Strength [OTC]** *see* Simethicone *on page 1927*
- **Pheburane (Can)** *see* Sodium Phenylbutyrate *on page 1948*
- **Phenadoz** *see* Promethazine *on page 1777*

Phenazopyridine (fen az oh PEER i deen)

Medication Safety Issues

Sound-alike/look-alike issues:

Phenazopyridine may be confused with phenoxybenz amine

Pyridium may be confused with Dyrenium, Perdiem pyridoxine, pyrithione

Brand Names: US Azo-Gesic [OTC]; Baridium [OTC] Pyridium; Urinary Pain Relief [OTC]

Therapeutic Category Analgesic, Urinary; Local Anes thetic, Urinary

Generic Availability (US) Yes

Use Symptomatic relief of urinary burning, itching, fre quency and urgency in association with urinary trac infection, or following urologic procedures

Pregnancy Risk Factor B

Pregnancy Considerations Adverse events have no been observed in animal reproduction studies. Phenazo pyridine crosses the placenta and can be detected i amniotic fluid (Meyer, 1991).

Breast-Feeding Considerations It is not known if phenazopyridine is excreted into breast milk.

Contraindications Hypersensitivity to phenazopyridine or any component of the formulation; kidney or liver disease; patients with a CrCl <50 mL/minute

Warnings/Precautions Does not treat urinary infection, acts only as an analgesic; drug should be discontinued if skin or sclera develop a yellow color; use with caution in patients with renal impairment. Use of this agent in the elderly is limited since accumulation of phenazopyridine can occur in patients with renal insufficiency. Use is contraindicated in patients with a CrCl <50 mL/minute.

Adverse Reactions

Central nervous system: Dizziness, headache

Gastrointestinal: Stomach cramps

Rare but important or life-threatening: Acute renal failure, hemolytic anemia, hepatitis, methemoglobinemia

Drug Interactions

Metabolism/Transport Effects None known.

Avoid Concomitant Use There are no known interactions where it is recommended to avoid concomitant use.

Increased Effect/Toxicity

Phenazopyridine may increase the levels/effects of: Prilocaine; Sodium Nitrite

The levels/effects of Phenazopyridine may be increased by: Nitric Oxide

Decreased Effect There are no known significant interactions involving a decrease in effect.

Mechanism of Action An azo dye which exerts local anesthetic or analgesic action on urinary tract mucosa through an unknown mechanism

Pharmacokinetics (Adult data unless noted)

Metabolism: In the liver and other tissues

Elimination: In urine (where it exerts its action); renal excretion (as unchanged drug) is rapid and accounts for 65% of the drug's elimination

Dosing: Usual Oral:

Children: 12 mg/kg/day in 3 divided doses for 2 days if used concomitantly with an antibacterial agent for UTI

Adults: 95-200 mg 3-4 times/day for 2 days if used concomitantly with an antibacterial agent for UTI

Dosing interval in renal impairment:

CrCl 50-80 mL/minute: Administer every 8-16 hours

CrCl <50 mL/minute: Avoid use

Administration Oral: Administer with food to decrease GI distress

Test Interactions Phenazopyridine may cause delayed reactions with glucose oxidase reagents (Clinistix®, Tes-Tape®); occasional false-positive tests occur with Tes-Tape®; cupric sulfate tests (Clinitest®) are not affected; interference may also occur with urine ketone tests (Acetest®, Ketostix®) and urinary protein tests; tests for urinary steroids and porphyrins may also occur

Dosage Forms Excipient information presented when available (limited, particularly for generics); consult specific product labeling.

Tablet, Oral, as hydrochloride:

Azo-Gesic: 95 mg

Baridium: 97.2 mg

Pyridium: 100 mg, 200 mg

Urinary Pain Relief: 95 mg

Generic: 95 mg, 100 mg, 200 mg

◆ **Phenazopyridine Hydrochloride** *see* Phenazopyridine *on page 1678*

◆ **Phenergan** *see* Promethazine *on page 1777*

PHENobarbital (fee noe BAR bi tal)

Medication Safety Issues

Sound-alike/look-alike issues:

PHENobarbital may be confused with PENTobarbital, Phenergan, phenytoin

BEERS Criteria medication:

This drug may be potentially inappropriate for use in geriatric patients (Quality of evidence - high; Strength of recommendation - strong).

Brand Names: Canada PMS-Phenobarbital

Therapeutic Category Anticonvulsant, Barbiturate; Barbiturate; Hypnotic; Sedative

Generic Availability (US) Yes

Use

Oral: Management of generalized tonic-clonic and partial seizures [FDA approved in pediatric patients (age not specified) and adults]; sedation (tablets: FDA approved in children and adults; elixir, oral solution: FDA approved in adults); insomnia (hypnotic) (FDA approved in adults)

Parenteral: Treatment of generalized tonic-clonic seizures including status epilepticus and cortical focal seizures (FDA approved in adults); sedation (FDA approved in adults)

Phenobarbital has also been used in neonatal and febrile seizures (treatment and prevention); prevention and treatment of neonatal hyperbilirubinemia; hyperbilirubinemia associated with chronic cholestasis; management of sedative/hypnotic withdrawal; management of neonatal abstinence syndrome

Pregnancy Risk Factor B/D (manufacturer dependent)

Pregnancy Considerations Barbiturates can be detected in the placenta, fetal liver, and fetal brain. Fetal and maternal blood concentrations may be similar following parenteral administration. An increased incidence of fetal abnormalities may occur following maternal use. The use of folic acid throughout pregnancy and vitamin K during the last month of pregnancy is recommended; epilepsy itself, number of medications, genetic factors, or a combination of these probably influence the teratogenicity of anticonvulsant therapy. When used during the third trimester of pregnancy, withdrawal symptoms may occur in the neonate, including seizures and hyperirritability; symptoms of withdrawal may be delayed in the neonate up to 14 days after birth. Use during labor does not impair uterine activity; however, respiratory depression may occur in the newborn; resuscitation equipment should be available, especially for premature infants.

Breast-Feeding Considerations Phenobarbital is excreted into breast milk. Infantile spasms and other withdrawal symptoms have been reported following the abrupt discontinuation of breast-feeding.

Contraindications Hypersensitivity to barbiturates or any component of the formulation; marked hepatic impairment; dyspnea or airway obstruction; porphyria (manifest and latent); intra-arterial administration, subcutaneous administration (not recommended); use in patients with a history of sedative/hypnotic addiction; nephritic patients (large doses)

Warnings/Precautions Potential for drug dependency exists, abrupt cessation may precipitate withdrawal, including status epilepticus in epileptic patients. Do not administer to patients in acute pain. Use caution in debilitated, renal or hepatic dysfunction, and pediatric patients. May cause paradoxical responses, including agitation and hyperactivity, particularly in acute pain and pediatric patients. Avoid use in the elderly due to risk of overdose with low dosages, tolerance to sleep effects, and increased risk of physical dependence (Beers Criteria). Use with caution in patients with depression or suicidal tendencies, or in patients with a history of drug abuse. Tolerance, psychological and physical dependence may occur with prolonged use. May cause CNS depression, which may impair physical or mental abilities. Effects with other sedative drugs or ethanol may be potentiated. May cause respiratory depression or hypotension, particularly when administered intravenously. Use with caution in hemodynamically unstable patients (hypovolemic shock, CHF) or patients with respiratory disease. Due to its long half-life and risk of dependence, phenobarbital is not recommended as a sedative in the elderly. Phenobarbital has been associated with cognitive deficits in children receiving chronic therapy for febrile seizures. Use with caution in patients with hypoadrenalism. Intra-arterial administration may cause reactions ranging from transient pain to gangrene and is contraindicated. Subcutaneous administration may cause tissue irritation (eg, redness, tenderness, necrosis) and is not recommended. Some dosage forms may contain propylene glycol; large amounts are potentially toxic and have been associated hyperosmolality, lactic acidosis, seizures and respiratory depression; use caution (AAP 1997; Zar 2007).

Warnings: Additional Pediatric Considerations Rapid IV administration may cause respiratory depression, apnea, laryngospasm, or hypotension; use with caution in hemodynamically unstable patients (hypotension or shock). Phenobarbital may cause CNS depression and effects with other sedative drugs may be potentiated; when treating status epilepticus, additional respiratory support may be required particularly when maximizing loading dose or if concurrent sedative therapy (Hegenbarth, 2008).

Pediatric patients may be at increased risk for vitamin D deficiency; with chronic therapy; phenobarbital may cause catabolism of vitamin D; the daily vitamin D requirement may be increased in these patients (≥400 units/day); vitamin D status should be periodically monitored with laboratory data (Misra, 2008; Wagner, 2008). A retrospective study demonstrated that enzyme-inducing antiepileptic drugs (AEDs) (carbamazepine, phenobarbital, and phenytoin) increased systemic clearance of antileukemic drugs (teniposide and methotrexate) and were associated with a worse event-free survival, CNS relapse, and hematologic relapse (ie, lower efficacy), in B-lineage ALL children receiving chemotherapy; the authors recommend using nonenzyme-inducing AEDs in patients receiving chemotherapy for ALL (Relling, 2000).

Adverse Reactions

Cardiovascular: Bradycardia, hypotension, syncope

Central nervous system: Agitation, anxiety, ataxia, CNS excitation or depression, confusion, dizziness drowsiness, hallucinations, "hangover" effect, headache, hyperkinesia, impaired judgment, insomnia, lethargy, nervousness, nightmares, somnolence

Dermatologic: Exfoliative dermatitis, rash, Stevens-Johnson syndrome

Gastrointestinal: Constipation, nausea, vomiting

Hematologic: Agranulocytosis, megaloblastic anemia, thrombocytopenia

Local: Pain at injection site, thrombophlebitis with IV use

Renal: Oliguria

Respiratory: Apnea (especially with rapid IV use), hypoventilation, laryngospasm, respiratory depression

Miscellaneous: Gangrene with inadvertent intra-arterial injection

Drug Interactions

Metabolism/Transport Effects Substrate of CYP2C19 (major), CYP2C9 (minor), CYP2E1 (minor); **Note:** Assignment of Major/Minor substrate status based on clinically relevant drug interaction potential; **Induces** CYP1A2 (strong), CYP2A6 (strong), CYP2B6 (strong), CYP2C8 (strong), CYP2C9 (strong), CYP3A4 (strong), P-glycoprotein

Avoid Concomitant Use

Avoid concomitant use of PHENobarbital with any of the following: Abiraterone Acetate; Apixaban; Apremilast; Artemether; Axitinib; Azelastine (Nasal); Bedaquiline; Boceprevir; Bortezomib; Bosutinib; Cabozantinib; Ceritinib; CloZAPine; Crizotinib; Dabigatran Etexilate; Dasabuvir; Dienogest; Dolutegravir; Dronedarone; Eliglustat; Enzalutamide; Etravirine; Everolimus; Ibrutinib; Idelalisib; Irinotecan; Isavuconazonium Sulfate; Itraconazole; Ivabradine; Ivacaftor; Lapatinib; Ledipasvir; Lumefantrine; Lurasidone; Macitentan; Mianserin; Mifepristone; Naloxegol; Netupitant; NIFEdipine; Nilotinib; NiMODipine; Nintedanib; Nisoldipine; Olaparib; Ombitasvir; Orphenadrine; Palbociclib; Panobinostat; Paraldehyde; Paritaprevir; PAZOPanib; Perampanel; Pirfenidone; PONATinib; Praziquantel; Ranolazine; Regorafenib; Rilpivirine; Rivaroxaban; Roflumilast; RomiDEPsin; Simeprevir; Sofosbuvir; Somatostatin Acetate; SORAfenib; Stiripentol; Suvorexant; Tasimelteon; Telaprevir; Thalidomide; Ticagrelor; Tofacitinib; Tolvaptan; Toremifene; Trabectedin; Ulipristal; Vandetanib; Vemurafenib; VinCRIStine (Liposomal); Vorapaxar; Voriconazole

Increased Effect/Toxicity

PHENobarbital may increase the levels/effects of: Alcohol (Ethyl); Azelastine (Nasal); Buprenorphine; Clarithromycin; CNS Depressants; Hydrocodone; Hypotensive Agents; Meperidine; Methotrimeprazine; Metyrosine; Orphenadrine; Paraldehyde; Pramipexole; Prilocaine; QuiNIDine; Rotigotine; Selective Serotonin Reuptake Inhibitors; Sodium Nitrite; Thalidomide; Thiazide Diuretics; Zolpidem

The levels/effects of PHENobarbital may be increased by: Brimonidine (Topical); Cannabis; Chloramphenicol; Clarithromycin; Cosyntropin; CYP2C19 Inhibitors (Moderate); CYP2C19 Inhibitors (Strong); Dexmethylphenidate; Doxylamine; Dronabinol; Droperidol; Felbamate; Fosphenytoin; HydrOXYzine; Kava Kava; Luliconazole; Magnesium Sulfate; Methotrimeprazine; Methylphenidate; Mianserin; Nabilone; Nitric Oxide; OXcarbazepine; Phenytoin; Primidone; QuiNINE; Rufinamide; Sodium Oxybate; Somatostatin Acetate; Tapentadol; Tetrahydrocannabinol; Valproic Acid and Derivatives

Decreased Effect

PHENobarbital may decrease the levels/effects of: Abiraterone Acetate; Acetaminophen; Afatinib; Albendazole; Apixaban; Apremilast; ARIPiprazole; Artemether; Axitinib; Bazedoxifene; Bedaquiline; Bendamustine; Beta-Blockers; Boceprevir; Bortezomib; Bosutinib; Brentuximab Vedotin; Cabozantinib; Calcium Channel Blockers; Canagliflozin; Cannabidiol; Cannabis; Ceritinib; Chloramphenicol; Clarithromycin; CloZAPine; Cobicistat; Contraceptives (Estrogens); Contraceptives (Progestins); Corticosteroids (Systemic); Crizotinib; CycloSPORINE (Systemic); CYP1A2 Substrates; CYP2A6 Substrates; CYP2B6 Substrates; CYP2C8 Substrates; CYP2C9 Substrates; CYP3A4 Substrates; Dabigatran Etexilate; Dasabuvir; Dasatinib; Deferasirox; Dexamethasone (Systemic); Diclofenac (Systemic); Dienogest; Disopyramide; Dolutegravir; DOXOrubicin (Conventional); Doxycycline; Dronabinol; Dronedarone; Eliglustat; Elvitegravir; Enzalutamide; Erlotinib; Eslicarbazepine; Etoposide; Etravirine; Everolimus; Exemestane; Felbamate; FentaNYL; Fosphenytoin; Gefitinib; Griseofulvin; GuanFACINE; Hydrocortisone (Systemic); Ibrutinib; Idelalisib; Imatinib; Irinotecan; Isavuconazonium Sulfate; Itraconazole; Ivabradine; Ivacaftor; Ixabepilone; Lacosamide; LamoTRIgine; Lapatinib; Ledipasvir; Linagliptin; Lopinavir; Lumefantrine; Lurasidone; Macitentan; Maraviroc; Methadone; MethylPREDNISolone; MetroNIDAZOLE (Systemic); Mianserin; Mifepristone; Naloxegol; Netupitant; NIFEdipine; Nilotinib; NiMODipine; Nintedanib; Nisoldipine; Olaparib; Ombitasvir; OXcarbazepine;

Palbociclib; Paliperidone; Panobinostat; Paritaprevir; PAZOPanib; Perampanel; P-glycoprotein/ABCB1 Substrates; Phenytoin; Pirfenidone; PONATinib; Praziquantel; PrednisoLONE (Systemic); PredniSONE; Propafenone; QUEtiapine; QuiNIDine; QuiNINE; Ranolazine; Regorafenib; Rilpivirine; Rivaroxaban; Roflumilast; RomiDEPsin; Rufinamide; Saxagliptin; Simeprevir; Sofosbuvir; SORAfenib; Stiripentol; SUNItinib; Suvorexant; Tadalafil; Tasimelteon; Telaprevir; Teniposide; Tetrahydrocannabinol; Ticagrelor; Tipranavir; Tofacitinib; Tolvaptan; Toremifene; Trabectedin; Treprostinil; Tricyclic Antidepressants; Ulipristal; Valproic Acid and Derivatives; Vandetanib; Vemurafenib; Vilazodone; VinCRIStine (Liposomal); Vitamin K Antagonists; Vorapaxar; Voriconazole; Vortioxetine; Zaleplon; Zonisamide; Zuclopenthixol

The levels/effects of PHENobarbital may be decreased by: Amphetamines; Cholestyramine Resin; CYP2C19 Inducers (Strong); Dabrafenib; Darunavir; Folic Acid; Leucovorin Calcium-Levoleucovorin; Levomefolate; Mefloquine; Methylfolate; Mianserin; Multivitamins/Minerals (with ADEK, Folate, Iron); Orlistat; Pyridoxine; Rifamycin Derivatives; Tipranavir

Food Interactions May cause decrease in vitamin D and calcium.

Storage/Stability

Elixir: Protect from light.

Injection: Protect from light. Not stable in aqueous solutions; use only clear solutions. Do not add to acidic solutions; precipitation may occur.

Mechanism of Action Long-acting barbiturate with sedative, hypnotic, and anticonvulsant properties. Barbiturates depress the sensory cortex, decrease motor activity, alter cerebellar function, and produce drowsiness, sedation, and hypnosis. In high doses, barbiturates exhibit anticonvulsant activity; barbiturates produce dose-dependent respiratory depression.

Pharmacodynamics Hypnosis:

Onset of action:

- Oral: Within 20-60 minutes
- IV: Within 5 minutes

Maximum effect: IV: Within 30 minutes

Duration:

- Oral: 6-10 hours
- IV: 4-10 hours

Pharmacokinetics (Adult data unless noted)

Absorption: Oral: 70% to 90%

Distribution: V_d:

- Neonates: 0.8-1 L/kg
- Infants: 0.7-0.8 L/kg
- Children: 0.6-0.7 L/kg

Protein binding: 35% to 50%, decreased protein binding in neonates

Metabolism: In the liver via hydroxylation and glucuronide conjugation

Half-life:

- Neonates: 45-500 hours
- Infants: 20-133 hours
- Children: 37-73 hours
- Adults: 53-140 hours

Time to peak serum concentration: Oral: Within 1-6 hours

Elimination: 20% to 50% excreted unchanged in urine; clearance can be increased with alkalinization of urine or with oral multiple-dose activated charcoal

Dialysis: Moderately dialyzable (20% to 50%)

Dosing: Neonatal

Status epilepticus; neonatal seizures: Limited data available: IV: Initial: 15-20 mg/kg as a single dose; may repeat doses of 5-10 mg/kg every 15-20 minutes as needed (maximum total dose: 40 mg/kg) (Cloherty, 2012; Gilman, 1989; Lockman, 1979; Painter, 1978; Painter, 1981). **Note:** Additional respiratory support may be required, especially when maximizing loading dose (Hegenbarth, 2008).

Seizures, maintenance therapy: Oral, IV: 3-4 mg/kg/day given once daily; maintenance dose usually starts 12-24 hours after loading dose; assess serum concentrations; increase to 5 mg/kg/day if needed (usually by second week of therapy) (Bourgeois, 1995; Cloherty, 2012; Kleigman, 2011)

Neonatal abstinence syndrome (AAP, 1998; Burgos, 2009; Hudak, 2012): Limited data available:

Loading dose (optional): IV, Oral: 16 mg/kg

- IV: Administer as a single dose; follow with maintenance dose 12-24 hours after loading dose
- Oral: Administer divided into 2 doses and administered every 4-6 hours; follow with maintenance dose 12-24 hours after loading dose

Maintenance dose: Oral, IV: Initial: 5 mg/kg/day divided every 12 hours; adjust dose according to abstinence scores and serum concentrations; usual required dose: 2-8 mg/kg/day. After patient is stabilized, decrease phenobarbital dose 20% every other day or such that drug concentration decreases by 10% to 20% per day (AAP, 1998; Burgos, 2009; Finnegan, 1979).

Neuroprotectant following anoxic injury (with or without cooling): Limited data available: IV: 40 mg/kg once; if introducing therapeutic hypothermia, administer prior to cooling (Hall, 1998; Meyn, 2010).

Dosing: Usual

Pediatric:

Status epilepticus: Infants, Children, and Adolescents: IV: Initial: 15-20 mg/kg; maximum dose: 1000 mg; may repeat once after 10-15 minutes if needed; maximum total dose: 40 mg/kg; repeat doses administered sooner than 10-15 minutes may not allow adequate time for peak CNS concentrations to be achieved and may lead to CNS depression (Brophy, 2012; Hegenbarth, 2008). **Note:** Additional respiratory support may be required particularly when maximizing loading dose or if concurrent sedative therapy.

Seizures, maintenance therapy: Note: Maintenance dose usually starts 12 hours after loading dose:

Manufacturer's labeling: Infants, Children, and Adolescents: Oral: 3-6 mg/kg/day

Alternate dosing: Limited data available (Geurinni, 2006; Kliegman, 2011):

Initial: Oral, IV:

- Infants and Children ≤5 years: 3-5 mg/kg/day in 1-2 divided doses
- Children >5 years: 2-3 mg/kg/day in 1-2 divided doses
- Adolescents: 1-3 mg/kg/day in 1-2 divided doses (Nelson, 1996)

Usual dosing range: **Note:** Dosage should be individualized based upon clinical response and serum concentration; once daily doses usually administered at bedtime in children and adolescents. Some centers have used:

- Infants: 5-6 mg/kg/day in 1-2 divided doses
- Children:
  - 1-5 years: 6-8 mg/kg/day in 1-2 divided doses
  - 5-12 years: 4-6 mg/kg/day in 1-2 divided doses
- Adolescents: 1-3 mg/kg/day in 1-2 divided doses

Sedation: Note: Newer, shorter-acting agents may be preferable.

Manufacturer's labeling: Children and Adolescents: Oral: 2 mg/kg/**dose** 3 times daily; maximum dose: 40 mg

Alternate dosing: Limited data available: Infants and Children: IM, Oral: 2-3 mg/kg/day in divided doses every 8-12 hours (Nelson, 1996)

Insomnia (hypnotic): Limited data available; shorter-acting agents may be preferable: Infants and Children: IM, Oral: 2-3 mg/kg/**dose**; may repeat dose as needed after 12-24 hours (Nelson, 1996); some centers have used: IM, IV: 3-5 mg/kg at bedtime

Hyperbilirubinemia: Limited data available: Infants and Children: Oral: Usual range: 3-8 mg/kg/day in 2-3 divided doses; doses up to 10 mg/kg/day in divided doses have been used in case reports (Cies, 2007; Nelson, 1996); for the treatment of hyperbilirubinemia in Crigler-Najjar Syndrome, a dose of 5 mg/kg/day has been used to reduce serum bilirubin concentrations (Kliegman, 2011); not recommended for management of biliary cirrohisis due to sedation and other adverse effects (Lindor-AASLD, 2009)

Sedative/hypnotic withdrawal; prevention; conversion of PENTobarbital to PHENobarbital (PENTobarbital infusion, a total cumulative PENTobarbital dose ≥25 mg/kg or duration ≥5-7 days): Limited data available: Infants, Children, and Adolescents: The following approach transitioning from PENTobarbital to PHENobarbital has been described: Discontinue PENTobarbital infusion, administer half of the PHENobarbital IV loading dose (see table) over 1 hour followed 6 hours later by the remaining half of PHENobarbital loading dose IV (over 1 hour). Begin IV maintenance PHENobarbital dose 6 hours after loading dose completed; the maintenance PHENobarbital dose should be 1/3of the initial loading dose and given every 12 hours. Once patient is stabilized, may switch to oral therapy and begin tapering 10% to 20% weekly (Tobias, 2000; Tobias, 2000a). **Note:** This conversion method is based on preliminary data in mechanically ventilated patients. Closely monitor respiratory status and evaluate patient for withdrawal symptoms.

PENTobarbital Infusion Rate (mg/kg/hour)	PHENobarbital IV Loading Dose (mg/kg)
1-2	8
2-3	15
3-4	20

Adult:

Sedation: Oral, IM: 30-120 mg/day in 2-3 divided doses

Preoperative sedation: IM: 100-200 mg 1-1.5 hours before procedure

Anticonvulsant/status epilepticus:

Loading dose: IV: 10-20 mg/kg (maximum rate: ≤60 mg/minute in patients ≥60 kg); may repeat dose in 20-minute intervals as needed; maximum total dose: 30 mg/kg

Maintenance dose: Oral, IV: 1-3 mg/kg/day in divided doses or 50-100 mg 2-3 times/day

Dosing adjustment in renal impairment: No specific dosage adjustment provided in manufacturer's labeling; reduced doses are recommended. The following guidelines have been used by some clinicians (Aronoff, 2007):

Infants, Children, and Adolescents: **Note:** Renally adjusted dose recommendations are based on doses of 3-7 mg/kg/day every 12-24 hours

GFR ≥10 mL/minute/1.73 m^2: No adjustment necessary

GFR <10 mL/minute/1.73 m^2: Decrease normal dose by 50% and administer every 24 hours

Intermittent hemodialysis [moderately dialyzable (20% to 50%)]: Supplemental dose may be needed during and after dialysis depending on individual seizure threshold

Peritoneal dialysis (PD): 40% to 50% removed; amount varies depending on number of cycles

Continuous renal replacement therapy (CRRT): Monitor serum concentrations; a case report suggests that clearance and volume of distribution increased with CVVH; more frequent and higher dosing may be necessary in some cases (Pasko, 2004)

Adults:

CrCl ≥10 mL/minute: No dosage adjustment necessary

CrCl <10 mL/minute: Administer every 12-16 hours.

Hemodialysis [moderately dialyzable (20% to 50%)]: Administer dose before dialysis and 50% of dose after dialysis.

Peritoneal dialysis: Administer 50% of normal dose.

CRRT: Administer normal dose and monitor levels.

Dosing adjustment in hepatic impairment: No specific dosage adjustment provided in manufacturer's labeling; reduced doses are recommended. Phenobarbital exposure is increased with hepatic impairment; use with caution.

Administration

Oral: Administer elixir or solution with water, milk, or juice

Parenteral: Do not inject IV faster than 1 mg/kg/minute with a maximum of 30 mg/minute for infants and children and 60 mg/minute for adults ≥60 kg. Neonatal studies that used a loading dose of 40 mg/kg for perinatal asphyxia infused the dose over 60 minutes (Hall, 1998). Do not administer intra-arterially. Avoid extravasation. SubQ administration is not recommended. For IM administration, inject deep into muscle; do not exceed 5 mL per injection site (adults) due to potential for tissue irritation.

Monitoring Parameters CNS status, seizure activity, liver enzymes, CBC with differential, renal function, serum concentrations; signs and symptoms of suicidality (eg, anxiety, depression, behavior changes). With IV use: Respiratory rate, heart rate, blood pressure, IV site (stop injection if patient complains of pain in the limb). For treatment of hyperbilirubinemia: Monitor bilirubin (total and direct)

Reference Range

Therapeutic:

Infants, Children, and Adolescents: 15-40 mcg/mL (SI: 65-172 micromole/L)

Adults: 20-40 mcg/mL (SI: 86-172 micromole/L)

Toxic: >40 mcg/mL (SI: >172 micromole/L)

Toxic concentration: Slowness, ataxia, nystagmus: 35-80 mcg/mL (SI: 150-344 micromole/L)

Coma with reflexes: 65-117 mcg/mL (SI: 279-502 micromole/L)

Coma without reflexes: >100 mcg/mL (SI: >430 micromole/L)

Test Interactions Assay interference of LDH

Controlled Substance C-IV

Dosage Forms Excipient information presented when available (limited, particularly for generics); consult specific product labeling.

Elixir, Oral:

Generic: 20 mg/5 mL (473 mL)

Solution, Oral:

Generic: 20 mg/5 mL (473 mL)

Solution, Injection, as sodium:

Generic: 65 mg/mL (1 mL); 130 mg/mL (1 mL)

Tablet, Oral:

Generic: 15 mg, 16.2 mg, 30 mg, 32.4 mg, 60 mg, 64.8 mg, 97.2 mg, 100 mg

Extemporaneous Preparations An alcohol-free 10 mg/mL phenobarbital oral suspension may be made from tablets and one of two different vehicles (a 1:1 mixture of Ora-Plus® and Ora-Sweet® or a 1:1 mixture of Ora-Plus® and Ora-Sweet® SF). Crush ten phenobarbital 60 mg tablets in a glass mortar and reduce to a fine powder. Mix 30 mL of Ora-Plus® and 30 mL of either Ora-Sweet® or Ora-Sweet® SF; stir vigorously. Add 15 mL of the vehicle to the powder and mix to a uniform paste. Transfer the mixture to a 2 ounce amber plastic prescription bottle. Rinse mortar and pestle with 15 mL of the vehicle; transfer to bottle. Repeat, then add quantity of vehicle sufficient to make 60 mL. Label "shake well." May mix dose with chocolate syrup (1:1 volume) immediately before administration to mask the bitter aftertaste. Stable for 115 days when stored in amber plastic prescription bottles at room temperature.

Cober M and Johnson CE, "Stability of an Extemporaneously Prepared Alcohol-Free Phenobarbital Suspension," *Am J Health Syst Pharm*, 2007, 64(6):644-6.

◆ **Phenobarbital, Hyoscyamine, Atropine, and Scopolamine** *see* Hyoscyamine, Atropine, Scopolamine, and Phenobarbital *on page 1062*

◆ **Phenobarbital Sodium** *see* PHENobarbital *on page 1679*

◆ **Phenobarbitone** *see* PHENobarbital *on page 1679*

◆ **Phenoptin** *see* Sapropterin *on page 1900*

Phenoxybenzamine (fen oks ee BEN za meen)

Medication Safety Issues

Sound-alike/look-alike issues:

Phenoxybenzamine may be confused with phenazopyridine

Related Information

Oral Medications That Should Not Be Crushed or Altered *on page 2476*

Safe Handling of Hazardous Drugs *on page 2455*

Brand Names: US Dibenzyline

Therapeutic Category Alpha-Adrenergic Blocking Agent, Oral; Antihypertensive Agent; Vasodilator

Generic Availability (US) No

Use Symptomatic management of hypertension and sweating in patients with pheochromocytoma

Pregnancy Risk Factor C

Pregnancy Considerations Adequate animal reproduction studies have not been conducted. It is not known whether phenoxybenzamine can cause fetal harm when administered to a pregnant woman or can affect reproduction capacity.

Breast-Feeding Considerations It is not known if phenoxybenzamine is excreted in breast milk. Due to the potential for serious adverse reactions in the nursing infant, a decision should be made whether to discontinue nursing or to discontinue the drug, taking into account the importance of treatment to the mother.

Contraindications Hypersensitivity to phenoxybenzamine or any component of the formulation; conditions in which a fall in blood pressure would be undesirable (eg, shock)

Warnings/Precautions Hazardous agent - use appropriate precautions for handling and disposal (NIOSH 2014 [group 2]).

Use with caution in patients with renal impairment. Can exacerbate symptoms of respiratory tract infections; use caution. Use with caution in patients with obstructive cerebral or coronary atherosclerosis, since a marked reduction in blood pressure may induce ischemic symptoms. An exaggerated hypotensive response and tachycardia may occur when administered concurrently with compounds that stimulate both alpha- and beta-adrenergic receptors or in the setting of pheochromocytoma. Discontinue if symptoms of severe hypotension or angina occur. Hypotensive effect may last for a few days after discontinuation. Use with caution in the elderly; may be at higher risk of adverse effects. Not recommended for long-term use due to case reports of cancer in humans.

Benzyl alcohol and derivatives: Some dosage forms may contain benzyl alcohol; large amounts of benzyl alcohol (≥99 mg/kg/day) have been associated with a potentially fatal toxicity ("gasping syndrome") in neonates; the "gasping syndrome" consists of metabolic acidosis, respiratory distress, gasping respirations, CNS dysfunction (including convulsions, intracranial hemorrhage), hypotension, and cardiovascular collapse (AAP, 1997; CDC, 1982); some data suggests that benzoate displaces bilirubin from protein binding sites (Ahlfors, 2001); avoid or use dosage forms containing benzyl alcohol with caution in neonates. See manufacturer's labeling.

Adverse Reactions

Cardiovascular: Orthostatic hypotension, tachycardia

Central nervous system: Drowsiness, fatigue

Gastrointestinal: GI irritation

Genitourinary: Inhibition of ejaculation

Ocular: Miosis

Respiratory: Nasal congestion

Drug Interactions

Metabolism/Transport Effects None known.

Avoid Concomitant Use

Avoid concomitant use of Phenoxybenzamine with any of the following: Alpha1-Blockers

Increased Effect/Toxicity

Phenoxybenzamine may increase the levels/effects of: Alpha1-Blockers; Amifostine; Antihypertensives; Calcium Channel Blockers; Obinutuzumab; RiTUXimab

The levels/effects of Phenoxybenzamine may be increased by: Beta-Blockers; Brimonidine (Topical); Dapoxetine; Diazoxide; Herbs (Hypotensive Properties); MAO Inhibitors; Pentoxifylline; Phosphodiesterase 5 Inhibitors; Prostacyclin Analogues

Decreased Effect

Phenoxybenzamine may decrease the levels/effects of: Alpha-/Beta-Agonists; Alpha1-Agonists

The levels/effects of Phenoxybenzamine may be decreased by: Herbs (Hypertensive Properties); Methylphenidate; Yohimbine

Storage/Stability Store at controlled room temperature of 25°C (77°F).

Mechanism of Action Produces long-lasting noncompetitive alpha-adrenergic blockade of postganglionic synapses in exocrine glands and smooth muscle; relaxes urethra and increases opening of the bladder

Pharmacodynamics Oral:

Onset of action: Within 2 hours

Maximum effect: Within 4-6 hours

Duration: Effects can continue for up to 4 days

Pharmacokinetics (Adult data unless noted)

Absorption: Oral: ~20% to 30%

Distribution: Distributes to and may accumulate in adipose tissues

Half-life: Adults: 24 hours

Elimination: Primarily in urine and bile

Dosing: Usual Oral:

Children: Initial: 0.2 mg/kg once daily; maximum dose: 10 mg/dose; increase every 4 days by 0.2 mg/kg/day increments; usual maintenance dose: 0.4-1.2 mg/kg/day every 6-8 hours; maximum doses of up to 2-4 mg/kg/day have been recommended

Adults: Initial: 10 mg twice daily; increase dose every other day to usual dose of 10-40 mg every 8-12 hours; higher doses may be needed

Administration Hazardous agent; use appropriate precautions for handling and disposal (NIOSH 2014 [group 2]).

Oral: May administer with milk to decrease GI upset

Monitoring Parameters Blood pressure, orthostasis, heart rate

Dosage Forms Excipient information presented when available (limited, particularly for generics); consult specific product labeling.

Capsule, Oral, as hydrochloride:

Dibenzyline: 10 mg [contains fd&c yellow #6 (sunset yellow)]

Extemporaneous Preparations Hazardous agent; use appropriate precautions for handling and disposal (NIOSH 2014 [group 2]).

A 2 mg/mL oral suspension may be made with capsules, propylene glycol 1%, and citric acid 0.15% in distilled water. Prepare the vehicle by dissolving 150 mg citric acid in a minimal amount of distilled water. Add 1 mL propylene glycol and mix well; add quantity of distilled water sufficient to make 100 mL (only a small portion of this vehicle will be used to make the final product). Grind the contents of two phenoxybenzamine 10 mg capsules in a mortar and reduce to a fine powder. Add a small portion of the vehicle and mix to a uniform paste; transfer to a graduated cylinder, rinse mortar with vehicle, and add quantity of prepared vehicle sufficient to make 10 mL. Transfer to an amber glass prescription bottle with tight-fitting cap; label "shake well" and "refrigerate". Stable for 7 days when stored in amber glass prescription bottles and refrigerated.

A stock solution of 10 mg/mL in propylene glycol was stable for 30 days refrigerated. When this stock solution was diluted 1:4 (v/v) with syrup (66.7% sucrose) to 2 mg/mL, the preparation was stable for 1 hour refrigerated. **Note:** Although the stock solution is stable for 30 days, it must be diluted before administration to decrease the amount of propylene glycol delivered to the patient.

Lim LY, Tan LL, Chan EW, et al, "Stability of Phenoxybenzamine Hydrochloride in Various Vehicles," *Am J Health Syst Pharm*, 1997, 54(18):2073-8.

◆ **Phenoxybenzamine Hydrochloride** *see* Phenoxybenzamine *on page 1683*

◆ **Phenoxymethyl Penicillin** *see* Penicillin V Potassium *on page 1660*

Phentolamine (fen TOLE a meen)

Medication Safety Issues

Sound-alike/look-alike issues:

Phentolamine may be confused with phentermine, Ventolin

Regitine may be confused with Reglan

Related Information

Management of Drug Extravasations *on page 2298*

Brand Names: Canada OraVerse; Rogitine

Therapeutic Category Alpha-Adrenergic Blocking Agent, Parenteral; Antidote, Extravasation; Antihypertensive Agent; Diagnostic Agent, Pheochromocytoma; Vasodilator

Generic Availability (US) Yes

Use Diagnosis of pheochromocytoma; treatment of hypertension associated with pheochromocytoma or other causes of excess sympathomimetic amines; local treatment and prevention of dermal necrosis after extravasation of drugs with alpha-adrenergic effects (dobutamine, dopamine, epinephrine, metaraminol, norepinephrine, phenylephrine)

Pregnancy Risk Factor C

Pregnancy Considerations Adverse events were observed in some oral animal reproduction studies. Diagnosing and treating pheochromocytoma is critical for favorable maternal and fetal outcomes (Schenker, 1971; Schenker, 1982).

Breast-Feeding Considerations It is not known if phentolamine is excreted in breast milk. Due to the potential for serious adverse reaction in the nursing infant, the decision to discontinue phentolamine or discontinue breast-feeding during treatment should take in account the benefits of treatment to the mother.

Contraindications

Hypersensitivity to phentolamine, any component of the formulation, or related compounds; MI (or history of MI), coronary insufficiency, angina, or other evidence suggestive of coronary artery disease

Canadian labeling: Additional contraindications (not in US labeling): Hypotension

OraVerse:

US labeling: There are no contraindications listed in the manufacturer's labeling.

Canadian labeling: Hypersensitivity to phentolamine or any component of the formulation.

Warnings/Precautions MI, cerebrovascular spasm, and cerebrovascular occlusion have been reported following administration, usually associated with hypotensive episodes. Tachycardia and cardiac arrhythmias may occur. Discontinue if symptoms of angina occur or worsen. The use of phentolamine as a blocking agent in the screening of patients with hypertension has predominantly been replaced with urinary/biochemical assays; phentolamine use should be reserved for situations where additional confirmation is necessary and after risks associated with use have been considered. Use with caution in patients with gastritis or peptic ulcer disease. Use with caution in patients with renal impairment; primarily eliminated by the kidneys. Potentially significant drug-drug interactions may exist, requiring dose or frequency adjustment, additional monitoring, and/or selection of alternative therapy.

Adverse Reactions

Cardiovascular: Bradycardia (OraVerse), cerebrovascular occlusion, hypertension (OraVerse), hypotension, myocardial infarction, tachycardia (OraVerse)

Central nervous system: Cerebrovascular spasm, headache (OraVerse), mouth pain (OraVerse), paresthesia (OraVerse; mild, transient)

Dermatologic: Facial swelling (OraVerse), pruritus (OraVerse)

Gastrointestinal: Diarrhea (OraVerse), nausea, upper abdominal pain (OraVerse), vomiting (OraVerse)

Local: Pain at injection site (OraVerse)

Rare but important or life-threatening: Cardiac arrhythmia, orthostatic hypotension

Drug Interactions

Metabolism/Transport Effects None known.

Avoid Concomitant Use

Avoid concomitant use of Phentolamine with any of the following: Alpha1-Blockers

Increased Effect/Toxicity

Phentolamine may increase the levels/effects of: Alpha1-Blockers; Amifostine; Antihypertensives; Calcium Channel Blockers; Obinutuzumab; RiTUXimab

The levels/effects of Phentolamine may be increased by: Beta-Blockers; Brimonidine (Topical); Dapoxetine; Diazoxide; Herbs (Hypotensive Properties); MAO Inhibitors; Pentoxifylline; Phosphodiesterase 5 Inhibitors; Prostacyclin Analogues

Decreased Effect

Phentolamine may decrease the levels/effects of: Alpha-/Beta-Agonists; Alpha1-Agonists

The levels/effects of Phentolamine may be decreased by: Herbs (Hypertensive Properties); Methylphenidate; Yohimbine

Storage/Stability

Powder for injection: Store intact vials at room temperature of 15°C to 30°C (59°F to 86°F). Reconstituted solution should be used immediately after preparation (per manufacturer).

Solution for injection (OraVerse): Store at 20°C to 25°C (68°F to 77°F); brief excursions permitted between 15°C to 30°C (59°F to 86°F). Protect from heat and light. Do not freeze.

Mechanism of Action Competitively blocks alpha-adrenergic receptors (nonselective) to produce brief antagonism of circulating epinephrine and norepinephrine to reduce hypertension caused by alpha effects of these catecholamines and minimizes tissue injury due to extravasation of these and other sympathomimetic vasoconstrictors (eg, dopamine, phenylephrine); also has a positive inotropic and chronotropic effect on the heart thought to be due to presynaptic alpha-2 receptor blockade which results in release of presynaptic norepinephrine (Hoffman, 1980)

OraVerse: Causes vasodilation and increased blood flow in injection area via alpha-adrenergic blockade to accelerate reversal of soft tissue anesthesia

Pharmacodynamics

Onset of action:
 IM: Within 15-20 minutes
 IV: Immediate
Maximum effect:
 IM: Within 20 minutes
 IV: Within 2 minutes
Duration:
 IM: 30-45 minutes
 IV: Within 15-30 minutes

Pharmacokinetics (Adult data unless noted)

Metabolism: In the liver
Half-life: Adults: 19 minutes
Elimination: 10% to 13% excreted in urine as unchanged drug

Dosing: Neonatal Note: Phentolamine mesylate (5 mg) injection is no longer available in the US. Treatment of alpha-adrenergic agonist drug extravasation: SubQ: **Note:** Total dose required depends on the size of extravasation; dose may be repeated if required. Infiltrate area of extravasation with a small amount (eg, 1 mL given in 0.1-0.2 mL aliquots) of a 0.25-0.5 mg/mL solution (made by diluting 2.5-5 mg in 10 mL of preservative free NS) within 12 hours of extravasation; in general, do not exceed 2.5 mg total; monitor blood pressure, especially when dose exceeds the recommended IM/IV dose of 0.1 mg/kg

Dosing: Usual Note: Phentolamine mesylate (5 mg) injection is no longer available in the US.

Treatment of alpha-adrenergic agonist drug extravasation: SubQ: **Note:** Total dose required depends on the size of extravasation; dose may be repeated if required: Infants, Children, and Adults: Infiltrate area of extravasation with a small amount (eg, 1 mL given in 0.2 mL aliquots) of a 0.5-1 mg/mL solution (made by diluting 5-10 mg in 10 mL of NS) within 12 hours of extravasation; in general, do not exceed 0.1-0.2 mg/kg or 5 mg total; **Note:** Doses of <5 mg total are usually effective; one **adult** case using a total dose of 50 mg (given over 1 hour in 0.5 ml aliquots of a 1 mg/mL solution) for a large extravasation has been reported (Cooper, 1989).

Diagnosis of pheochromocytoma: IM, IV:
 Children: 0.05-0.1 mg/kg/dose, maximum single dose: 5 mg
 Adults: 5 mg

Hypertension (prior to surgery for pheochromocytoma): IM, IV:
 Children: 0.05-0.1 mg/kg/dose given 1-2 hours before pheochromocytomectomy; repeat as needed to control blood pressure; maximum single dose: 5 mg
 Adults: 5 mg given 1-2 hours before pheochromocytomectomy; repeat as needed to control blood pressure

Hypertensive crisis due to MAO inhibitor/sympathomimetic amine interaction: IM, IV: Adults: 5-20 mg

Preparation for Administration Parenteral: Powder for injection: Reconstitute 5 mg vial with 1 mL SWFI. For treatment of extravasation, further dilute 5 to 10 mg in 10 mL of NS (manufacturer's recommendation) or in 10 to 15 mL of saline (Peberdy 2010).

Administration Parenteral: Treatment of extravasation: Infiltrate area of extravasation with multiple small injections of a diluted solution; use 27- or 30-gauge needles and change needle between each skin entry to prevent bacterial contamination and minimize pain; do not inject a volume such that swelling of the extremity or digit with resultant compartment syndrome occurs

Monitoring Parameters Blood pressure, heart rate, orthostasis; treatment of extravasation: site of extravasation, skin color, local perfusion

Additional Information When drugs with alpha-adrenergic effects extravasate, they cause local vasoconstriction which causes blanching of the skin and a pale, cold, hard appearance; SubQ phentolamine blocks the alpha-adrenergic receptors and reverses the vasoconstriction; the extravasation area should "pink up" and return to normal skin color following SubQ administration of phentolamine. Dobutamine primarily stimulates beta$_1$-adrenergic receptors, but does possess alpha (and beta$_2$) adrenergic effects; the alpha-adrenergic effects (vasoconstriction) may be seen when dobutamine extravasates (since high concentrations of dobutamine would be present locally); although infrequent, cases of dermal necrosis from dobutamine extravasation have been reported; thus, phentolamine may help prevent dermal necrosis following dobutamine extravasations (Hoff, 1979; MacCara, 1983). Injection contains mannitol 25 mg/vial

Product Availability Phentolamine mesylate (5 mg) injection is no longer available in the US.

Dosage Forms Excipient information presented when available (limited, particularly for generics); consult specific product labeling. [DSC] = Discontinued product
Solution, Injection, as mesylate:
 Generic: 5 mg/mL (1 mL)
Solution Reconstituted, Injection, as mesylate:
 Generic: 5 mg (1 ea [DSC])

◆ **Phentolamine Mesylate** *see* Phentolamine *on page 1684*

◆ **Phenylalanine Mustard** *see* Melphalan *on page 1348*

◆ **Phenylazo Diamino Pyridine Hydrochloride** *see* Phenazopyridine *on page 1678*

Phenylephrine (Systemic) (fen il EF rin)

Medication Safety Issues

Sound-alike/look-alike issues:
 Sudafed PE may be confused with Sudafed
 Vazculep may be confused with Bloxiverz (neostigmine) due to similar packaging

High alert medication:
 The Institute for Safe Medication Practices (ISMP) includes this medication among its list of drugs which have a heightened risk of causing significant patient harm when used in error.

Related Information

Management of Drug Extravasations *on page 2298*
Serotonin Syndrome *on page 2447*

Brand Names: US Little Colds Decongestant [OTC]; Medi-Phenyl [OTC]; Nasal Decongestant PE Max St [OTC]; Nasal Decongestant [OTC]; Non-Pseudo Sinus Decongestant [OTC]; Sudafed PE Childrens [OTC]; Sudafed PE Maximum Strength [OTC]; Sudogest PE [OTC]; Vazculep

Therapeutic Category Adrenergic Agonist Agent; Alpha-Adrenergic Agonist; Sympathomimetic

Generic Availability (US) May be product dependent

Use

Parenteral: Treatment of hypotension and vascular failure in shock; supraventricular tachycardia; as a vasoconstrictor in regional analgesia (All indications: FDA approved adults); treatment of hypotension during spinal anesthesia (FDA approved in pediatric patients [age not specified] and adults)

Oral: Temporary relief of nasal congestion due to the common cold, hay fever, or other upper respiratory allergies (OTC products: FDA approved in ages ≥4 years and adults; consult specific product formulation for appropriate age group

Pregnancy Risk Factor C

Pregnancy Considerations Animal reproduction studies have not been conducted; therefore, the manufacturer classifies phenylephrine as pregnancy category C. Phenylephrine crosses the placenta at term. Maternal use of phenylephrine during the first trimester of pregnancy is not strongly associated with an increased risk of fetal malformations; maternal dose and duration of therapy were not reported in available publications. Phenylephrine is available over-the-counter (OTC) for the symptomatic relief of nasal congestion. Decongestants are not the preferred agents for the treatment of rhinitis during pregnancy. Oral phenylephrine should be avoided during the first trimester of pregnancy; short-term use (<3 days) of intranasal phenylephrine may be beneficial to some patients although its safety during pregnancy has not been studied. Phenylephrine injection is used at delivery for the prevention and/or treatment of maternal hypotension associated with spinal anesthesia in women undergoing cesarean section. Phenylephrine may be associated with a more favorable fetal acid base status than ephedrine; however, overall fetal outcomes appear to be similar. Nausea or vomiting may be less with phenylephrine than ephedrine but is also dependent upon blood pressure control. Phenylephrine may be preferred in the absence of maternal bradycardia.

Breast-Feeding Considerations It is not known if phenylephrine is excreted into breast milk. The manufacturer recommends that caution be exercised when administering phenylephrine to nursing women.

Contraindications Hypersensitivity to phenylephrine or any component of the formulation

Injection: Severe hypertension; ventricular tachycardia

Vazculep: There are no contraindications listed in the manufacturer's labeling.

OTC labeling (Oral): When used for self-medication: Use with or within 14 days of MAO inhibitor therapy

Warnings/Precautions Some products contain sulfites which may cause allergic reactions in susceptible individuals. Use with extreme caution in patients taking MAO inhibitors. Use with caution in patients with hyperthyroidism.

Intravenous: Phenylephrine may cause severe bradycardia (likely baroreflex mediated) and reduced cardiac output due to an increase in cardiac afterload especially in patients with preexisting cardiac dysfunction (Goertz 1993; Yamazaki 1982). May also precipitate angina in patients with severe coronary artery disease and increase pulmonary arterial pressure. Use with caution in patients with preexisting bradycardia, partial heart block, myocardial disease, or severe coronary artery disease. Avoid or use with extreme caution in patients with heart failure or cardiogenic shock; increased systemic vascular resistance may significantly reduce cardiac output. Avoid use in patients with hypertension (contraindicated in severe hypertension); monitor blood pressure closely and adjust infusion rate. Assure adequate circulatory volume to minimize need for vasoconstrictors. Vesicant; ensure proper needle or catheter placement prior to and during infusion; avoid extravasation. **[U.S. Boxed Warning]: Should be administered by adequately trained individuals familiar with its use.** Acidosis may reduce the efficacy of phenylephrine; correct acidosis prior to or during use of phenylephrine. Patients with autonomic dysfunction (eg, spinal cord injury) may exhibit an exaggerated increase in blood pressure response to phenylephrine.

Oral: When used for self-medication (OTC), use caution with asthma, bowel obstruction/narrowing, hyperthyroidism, diabetes mellitus, cardiovascular disease, ischemic heart disease, hypertension, increased intraocular pressure, prostatic hyperplasia or in the elderly. Notify healthcare provider if symptoms do not improve within 7 days or are accompanied by fever. Discontinue and contact health care provider if nervousness, dizziness, or sleeplessness occur.

Benzyl alcohol and derivatives: Some dosage forms may contain sodium benzoate/benzoic acid; benzoic acid (benzoate) is a metabolite of benzyl alcohol; large amounts of benzyl alcohol (≥99 mg/kg/day) have been associated with a potentially fatal toxicity ("gasping syndrome") in neonates; the "gasping syndrome" consists of metabolic acidosis, respiratory distress, gasping respirations, CNS dysfunction (including convulsions, intracranial hemorrhage), hypotension, and cardiovascular collapse (AAP 1997; CDC 1982); some data suggests that benzoate displaces bilirubin from protein binding sites (Ahlfors 2001); avoid or use dosage forms containing benzyl alcohol derivative with caution in neonates. See manufacturer's labeling.

Warnings: Additional Pediatric Considerations Safety and efficacy for the use of cough and cold products in pediatric patients <4 years of age is limited; the AAP warns against the use of these products for respiratory illnesses in this age group. Serious adverse effects including death have been reported. Many of these products contain multiple active ingredients, increasing the risk of accidental overdose when used with other products. The FDA notes that there are no approved OTC uses for these products in pediatric patients <2 years of age. Health care providers are reminded to ask caregivers about the use of OTC cough and cold products in order to avoid exposure to multiple medications containing the same ingredient (AAP 2012; FDA 2008).

Adverse Reactions

Injection:

Cardiovascular: Cardiac arrhythmia (rare), exacerbation of angina, hypertension, hypertensive crisis, ischemia, localized blanching, low cardiac output, peripheral vasoconstriction (severe), reflex bradycardia, visceral vasoconstriction (severe), worsening of heart failure

Central nervous system: Anxiety, dizziness, excitability, headache, insomnia, nervousness, paresthesia, precordial pain (or discomfort), restlessness

Dermatologic: Pallor, piloerection, pruritus

Endocrine & metabolic: Metabolic acidosis

Gastrointestinal: Epigastric pain, gastric irritation, nausea, vomiting

Genitourinary: Decreased renal blood flow, decreased urine output

Hypersensitivity: Hypersensitivity reaction (including skin rash, urticaria, leukopenia, agranulocytosis, thrombocytopenia)

Local: Extravasation which may lead to necrosis and sloughing of surrounding tissue

Neuromuscular & skeletal: Neck pain, tremor, weakness

Ophthalmic: Blurred vision

Respiratory: Dyspnea, exacerbation of pulmonary arterial hypertension, respiratory distress

Oral: Central nervous system: Anxiety, dizziness, excitability, headache, insomnia, nervousness, restlessness

Drug Interactions

Metabolism/Transport Effects None known.

Avoid Concomitant Use

Avoid concomitant use of Phenylephrine (Systemic) with any of the following: Ergot Derivatives; Hyaluronidase; Iobenguane I 123; MAO Inhibitors

Increased Effect/Toxicity

Phenylephrine (Systemic) may increase the levels/effects of: Sympathomimetics

The levels/effects of Phenylephrine (Systemic) may be increased by: Acetaminophen; AtoMOXetine; Cannabinoid-Containing Products; Ergot Derivatives; Hyaluronidase; Linezolid; MAO Inhibitors; Tedizolid; Tricyclic Antidepressants

Decreased Effect

Phenylephrine (Systemic) may decrease the levels/effects of: Benzylpenicilloyl Polylysine; FentaNYL; Iobenguane I 123; Ioflupane I 123

The levels/effects of Phenylephrine (Systemic) may be decreased by: Alpha1-Blockers; Tricyclic Antidepressants

Storage/Stability

Solution for injection: Store vials at controlled room temperature of 15°C to 25°C (59°F to 77°F). Protect from light. Do not use solution if brown or contains a precipitate.

Oral: Store at controlled room temperature of 15°C to 25°C (59°F to 77°F). Protect from light.

Mechanism of Action Potent, direct-acting alpha-adrenergic agonist with virtually no beta-adrenergic activity; produces systemic arterial vasoconstriction. Such increases in systemic vascular resistance result in dose dependent increases in systolic and diastolic blood pressure and reductions in heart rate and cardiac output especially in patients with heart failure.

Pharmacodynamics

Onset of action:

Blood pressure increase/vasoconstriction:

IM, SubQ: Within 10-15 minutes

IV: Immediate

Nasal decongestant: Oral: 15-30 minutes (Kollar, 2007)

Duration: Blood pressure increase/vasoconstriction:

IM: 1 to 2 hours

IV: 15 to 20 minutes

SubQ: 50 minutes

Nasal decongestant: Oral: 2 to 4 hours

Pharmacokinetics (Adult data unless noted)

Absorption: Oral: Rapid and complete (Kanfer, 1993)

Distribution: V_d initial: 26-61 L; V_{dss} 184-543 L (mean: 340 L) (Hengstmann, 1982)

Metabolism: Hepatic via oxidative deamination (oral: 24%; IV: 50%); undergoes sulfation [oral (mostly within gut wall): 46%; IV: 8%] and some glucuronidation; forms inactive metabolites (Kanfer, 1993)

Bioavailability: Oral: ≤38% (Hengstmann, 1982; Kanfer, 1993)

Half-life: Alpha phase: ~5 minutes: terminal phase: 2-3 hours (Hengstmann, 1982; Kanfer, 1993)

Time to peak serum concentration: Oral: 0.75-2 hours (Kanfer, 1993)

Elimination: Urine (mostly as inactive metabolites)

Dosing: Neonatal Hypotension, low cardiac output: Continuous IV infusion: Usual initial range: 0.1 to 0.5 mcg/kg/minute; titrate to desired response (Wessel, 2001); in cases of shock or intraoperative hypotension, doses up to 2 mcg/kg/minute have been reported (Kliegman, 2011; Shaddy, 1989) and for management of infundibular spasm (Tet Spell), even higher doses up to 5 mcg/kg/minute may be required (AAP, 1998; Shaddy, 1989)

Dosing: Usual

Pediatric: **Note:** Dosing presented in both mg (oral) and mcg (parenteral); use caution when ordering and dispensing.

Nasal congestion: Oral:

Children 4 to 5 years: 2.5 mg every 4 hours; maximum daily dose: 15 mg in 24 hours

Children 6 to 11 years: 5 mg every 4 hours; maximum daily dose: 30 mg in 24 hours

Children ≥12 years and Adolescents: 10 mg every 4 hours; maximum daily dose: 60 mg in 24 hours

Hypotension, low cardiac output: Infants, Children, and Adolescents:

IM, SubQ: 100 mcg/kg/dose every 1 to 2 hours as needed; maximum dose: 5000 mcg

IV bolus: 5 to 20 mcg/kg/dose every 10 to 15 minutes as needed (AAP, 1998; Shaddy, 1989); initial dose should not exceed 500 mcg; maximum dose: 1000 mcg

Continuous IV infusion: Usual initial dose: 0.1 to 0.5 mcg/kg/minute; titrate to desired response (Di Gennaro, 2010; Stewart, 2002; Wessel, 2001); in cases of shock or intraoperative hypotension, doses up to 2 mcg/kg/minute have been reported (Di Gennaro, 2010; Kliegman, 2011; Shaddy, 1989; Stewart, 2002) and for management of infundibular spasm (Tet Spell), even higher doses up to 5 mcg/kg/minute may be required (AAP, 1998; Shaddy, 1989)

Hypotension during spinal anesthesia: IM, SubQ: Infants, Children, and Adolescents: 44 to 88 mcg/kg/dose; maximum dose: 500 mcg

Adult:

Hypotension/shock:

IV bolus: 100 to 500 mcg/dose every 10 to 15 minutes as needed (initial dose should not exceed 500 mcg)

IV infusion: 100 to 180 mcg/minute, **or alternatively**, 0.5 mcg/kg/minute; titrate to desired response. Dosing ranges between 0.4 to 9.1 mcg/kg/minute have been reported (Gregory, 1991)

Nasal congestion: Oral: OTC labeling: 10 mg every 4 hours as needed for ≤7 days; maximum total dose: 60 mg in 24 hours

Paroxysmal supraventricular tachycardia: Note: Not recommended for routine use in treatment of supraventricular tachycardias: IV: 250 to 500 mcg over 20 to 30 seconds

Usual Infusion Concentrations: Pediatric IV infusion: 20 **mcg**/mL, 40 **mcg**/mL, or 60 **mcg**/mL

Preparation for Administration

Parenteral:

IV bolus: May dilute with SWFI, NS, or D5W to a concentration of 1 mg/mL; may also prepare a 100 mcg/mL (0.1 mg/mL) solution for bolus administration.

Stability in syringes (Kiser 2007): Concentration of 0.1 mg/mL in NS (polypropylene syringes) is stable for at least 30 days at -20°C (-4°F), 3°C to 5°C (37°F to 41°F), or 23°C to 25°C (73.4°F to 77°F).

IV infusion: May dilute in NS or D_5W; in pediatric patients, the usual concentration range is from 20 to 60 mcg/mL (Klaus 1989; Murray 2014; Sinclair-Pingel 2006); in some cases, higher concentrations of 100 mcg/mL and 120 mcg/mL may be used in pediatric patients (Klaus 1989; Sinclair-Pingel 2006); 200 mcg/mL prepared in NS has been used in adults).

Administration

Oral: OTC products: Administer without regard to food

Parenteral:

IV bolus: Dilute and administer dose over 20 to 30 seconds (Klaus, 1989)

Continuous IV infusion: After further dilution in an appropriate fluid, administer via an infusion pump; central line administration is preferred; administration into an umbilical arterial catheter is **not** recommended.

Vesicant; ensure proper needle or catheter placement prior to and during infusion; avoid extravasation. If extravasation occurs, stop infusion immediately and disconnect (leave cannula/needle in place); gently aspirate extravasated solution (do **not** flush the line); remove needle/cannula; elevate extremity. Initiate phentolamine (or alternative antidote). (See Management of Drug Extravasations on page 2298 for more details.) Apply dry warm compresses (Hurs, 2004).

Vesicant/Extravasation Risk Vesicant

Monitoring Parameters Heart rate, blood pressure, central venous pressure, arterial blood gases (hypotension/shock treatment)

Product Availability

Vazculep (10 mg/mL injection): FDA approved July 2014; anticipated availability is currently unknown.

Vazculep is indicated for the treatment of clinically important hypotension resulting primarily from vasodilation in the setting of anesthesia.

Dosage Forms Excipient information presented when available (limited, particularly for generics); consult specific product labeling.

Liquid, Oral, as hydrochloride:

Little Colds Decongestant: 2.5 mg/mL (30 mL) [alcohol free, dye free, saccharin free; contains sodium benzoate; grape flavor]

Solution, Injection, as hydrochloride:

Generic: 10 mg/mL (1 mL, 5 mL, 10 mL)

Solution, Intravenous, as hydrochloride:

Vazculep: 10 mg/mL (1 mL, 5 mL, 10 mL) [contains sodium metabisulfite]

Solution, Oral, as hydrochloride:

Sudafed PE Childrens: 2.5 mg/5 mL (118 mL) [alcohol free, sugar free; contains edetate disodium, fd&c red #40, sodium benzoate; berry flavor]

Tablet, Oral, as hydrochloride:

Medi-Phenyl: 5 mg

Nasal Decongestant: 10 mg [contains fd&c blue #2 (indigotine), fd&c red #40, fd&c yellow #6 aluminum lake]

Nasal Decongestant PE Max St: 10 mg [pseudoephedrine free; contains fd&c red #40 aluminum lake]

Non-Pseudo Sinus Decongestant: 10 mg [contains fd&c red #40 aluminum lake, fd&c yellow #6 aluminum lake]

Sudafed PE Maximum Strength: 10 mg [contains fd&c red #40 aluminum lake, fd&c yellow #10 aluminum lake, fd&c yellow #6 aluminum lake]

Sudafed PE Maximum Strength: 10 mg [contains fd&c red #40 aluminum lake, fd&c yellow #6 aluminum lake]

Sudafed PE Maximum Strength: 10 mg [pseudoephedrine free; contains fd&c red #40 aluminum lake, fd&c yellow #10 aluminum lake, fd&c yellow #6 aluminum lake]

Sudogest PE: 10 mg [contains fd&c red #40]

Phenylephrine (Nasal) (fen il EF rin)

Medication Safety Issues

Sound-alike/look-alike issues:

Neo-Synephrine (phenylephrine, nasal) may be confused with Neo-Synephrine (oxymetazoline)

Brand Names: US 4-Way Fast Acting [OTC]; 4-Way Menthol [OTC]; Afrin Childrens [OTC]; Nasal Four [OTC]; Neo-Synephrine Cold & Sinus [OTC]; Neo-Synephrine [OTC]; Rhinall [OTC]

Brand Names: Canada Neo-Synephrine®

Therapeutic Category Adrenergic Agonist Agent; Alpha-Adrenergic Agonist; Nasal Agent, Vasoconstrictor; Sympathomimetic

Generic Availability (US) Yes

Use Symptomatic relief of nasal and nasopharyngeal mucosal congestion (OTC products: FDA approved in adults; refer to product specific information regarding FDA approval in pediatric patients)

Pregnancy Considerations When administered intravenously, phenylephrine crosses the placenta. Refer to the Phenylephrine (Systemic) monograph for details. Decongestants are not the preferred agents for the treatment of rhinitis during pregnancy. Short-term use (<3 days) of intranasal phenylephrine may be beneficial to some patients, although its safety during pregnancy has not been studied.

Breast-Feeding Considerations It is not known if phenylephrine is excreted into breast milk.

Contraindications Hypersensitivity to phenylephrine or any component of the formulation; hypertension; ventricular tachycardia

Warnings/Precautions Use caution in patients with hyperthyroidism, diabetes mellitus, cardiovascular disease, ischemic heart disease, increased intraocular pressure, prostatic hyperplasia, or in the elderly. Rebound congestion may occur when nasal products are discontinued after chronic use. When used for self-medication (OTC), notify healthcare provider if symptoms do not improve within 3 days.

Warnings: Additional Pediatric Considerations Safety and efficacy for the use of cough and cold products in pediatric patients <4 years of age is limited; the AAP warns against the use of these products for respiratory illnesses in this age group. Serious adverse effects, including death, have been reported. Many of these products contain multiple active ingredients, increasing the risk of accidental overdose when used with other products. The FDA notes that there are no approved OTC uses for these products in pediatric patients <2 years of age. Health care providers are reminded to ask caregivers about the use of OTC cough and cold products in order to avoid exposure to multiple medications containing the same ingredient (AAP 2012; FDA 2008).

Adverse Reactions Nasal: Burning, nasal discharge, sneezing, stinging

Drug Interactions

Metabolism/Transport Effects None known.

Avoid Concomitant Use

Avoid concomitant use of Phenylephrine (Nasal) with any of the following: Ergot Derivatives; Iobenguane I 123; MAO Inhibitors

Increased Effect/Toxicity

Phenylephrine (Nasal) may increase the levels/effects of: Sympathomimetics

The levels/effects of Phenylephrine (Nasal) may be increased by: AtoMOXetine; Cannabinoid-Containing Products; Ergot Derivatives; Linezolid; MAO Inhibitors; Tedizolid; Tricyclic Antidepressants

Decreased Effect

Phenylephrine (Nasal) may decrease the levels/effects of: FentaNYL; Iobenguane I 123

The levels/effects of Phenylephrine (Nasal) may be decreased by: Alpha1-Blockers; Tricyclic Antidepressants

Storage/Stability Store at room temperature; protect from light.

Mechanism of Action Potent, direct-acting alpha-adrenergic agonist with virtually no beta-adrenergic activity; produces local vasoconstriction resulting in nasal decongestion.

Pharmacodynamics

Onset of action: Intranasal: ≤2 minutes (Chua, 1989)

Duration of action: Intranasal: 2.5-4 hours (dose dependent) (Chua, 1989)

Dosing: Usual

Pediatric: **Nasal congestion: Note:** Therapy should not exceed 3 days:

Infants and Children <2 years: Limited data available: 0.5% solution: Intranasal: Instill 0.1 mL in each nostril as a single dose (Ralston 2008; Turner 1996). In a double-blind, placebo-controlled trial in 20 infants (mean age: 4 months) with bronchiolitis results showed, improved respiratory scores and oxygen saturation; however statistical significance was not reached (Ralston 2008). In another randomized, double-blind, placebo-controlled trial, 23 pediatric patients (age range: 6 to 18 months) with the common cold showed improvement in nasal obstruction which was not considered significant; no effect on middle ear pressures was observed (Turner 1996).

Children ≥2 years:

2 to <6 years: 0.125% solution: Intranasal: Instill 1 drop in each nostril every 2-4 hours as needed. **Note:** Consult product specific information for further details.

Little Noses Decongestant: Instill 2 to 3 drops in each nostril every 4 hours as needed

6 to 12 years: 0.25% solution: Intranasal: Instill 1 to 3 sprays in each nostril every 4 hours as needed

Children >12 years and Adolescents: 0.25% to 1% solutions: Intranasal: Instill 1 to 3 drops or sprays every 4 hours as needed

Adults: **Nasal congestion:** 0.25% to 1% solution: Intranasal: Instill 2 to 3 sprays or 2 to 3 drops in each nostril every 4 hours as needed for ≤3 days

Dosing adjustment in renal impairment: There are no dosage adjustments provided in manufacturer's labeling.

Dosing adjustment in hepatic impairment: There are no dosage adjustments provided in manufacturer's labeling.

Administration Spray or apply drops into each nostril while gently occluding the other.

Dosage Forms Excipient information presented when available (limited, particularly for generics); consult specific product labeling.

Solution, Nasal, as hydrochloride:

4-Way Fast Acting: 1% (14.8 mL, 29.6 mL) [contains benzalkonium chloride]

4-Way Menthol: 1% (14.8 mL, 29.6 mL) [contains benzalkonium chloride, menthol, polysorbate 80]

Afrin Childrens: 0.25% (15 mL)

Nasal Four: 1% (29.6 mL) [contains benzalkonium chloride]

Neo-Synephrine: 0.25% (15 mL); 0.5% (15 mL); 1% (15 mL) [contains benzalkonium chloride]

Neo-Synephrine Cold & Sinus: 0.25% (15 mL); 0.5% (15 mL); 1% (15 mL) [contains benzalkonium chloride]

Rhinall: 0.25% (30 mL, 40 mL)

Phenylephrine (Ophthalmic) (fen il EF rin)

Medication Safety Issues

Sound-alike/look-alike issues:

Mydfrin may be confused with Midrin

Brand Names: US Altafrin; Mydfrin [DSC]; Neofrin [DSC]

Brand Names: Canada Dionephrine; Mydfrin

Therapeutic Category Adrenergic Agonist Agent; Adrenergic Agonist Agent, Ophthalmic; Alpha-Adrenergic Agonist; Ophthalmic Agent, Mydriatic; Sympathomimetic

Generic Availability (US) Yes

Use As a mydriatic in ophthalmic procedures and treatment of wide-angle glaucoma; OTC use as symptomatic relief of eye irritation

Pregnancy Risk Factor C

Pregnancy Considerations Animal reproduction studies have not been conducted; therefore, the manufacturer classifies phenylephrine ophthalmic as pregnancy category C. When administered intravenously, phenylephrine crosses the placenta (refer to the Phenylephrine (Systemic) monograph for details). The amount of phenylephrine available systemically following ophthalmic application is generally less in comparison to oral or IV doses.

Breast-Feeding Considerations It is not known if phenylephrine is excreted into breast milk. The manufacturer recommends that caution be exercised when administering phenylephrine to nursing women.

Contraindications

2.5% solution: There are no contraindications listed in the manufacturer's labeling.

10% solution: Hypertension; thyrotoxicosis; infants younger than 1 year

Documentation of allergenic cross-reactivity for ophthalmic decongestants is limited. However, because of similarities in chemical structure and/or pharmacologic actions, the possibility of cross-sensitivity cannot be ruled out with certainty.

Warnings/Precautions For ophthalmic use only; not for injection. Some products contain sulfites which may cause allergic reactions in susceptible individuals. Although rare, ventricular arrhythmias and myocardial infarction (including fatalities) have been reported with use of the 10% solution. Patients with preexisting cardiovascular disease may be at increased risk; consider use of 2.5% solution in these patients. Significant blood pressure elevation has been reported with the 10% solution; risk is less with 2.5% solution. Use caution when using 10% solution in children <5 years of age, patients with hyperthyroidism or patients with cardiovascular disease. Carefully monitor post-treatment blood pressure in patients with endocrine or cardiac diseases, or any patient who develops symptoms during treatment. Rebound miosis has been reported 1 day after treatment; reinstallation of the drug produced a lesser mydriatic effect. The 10% should NOT be used in infants <1 year of age (2.5% solution should be used). Use caution when using 10% solution in children <5 years of age. Potentially significant interactions may exist, requiring dose or frequency adjustment, additional monitoring, and/or selection of alternative therapy.

Adverse Reactions Systemic effects are rare at normal dosages.

Cardiovascular: Arrhythmia (rare), hypertension (rare), myocardial infarction (rare), subarachnoid hemorrhage (rare), syncope (rare)

Ocular: Burning, irritation, vision changes, rebound miosis, floaters (transient)

Drug Interactions

Metabolism/Transport Effects None known.

Avoid Concomitant Use

Avoid concomitant use of Phenylephrine (Ophthalmic) with any of the following: Ergot Derivatives; Iobenguane I 123; MAO Inhibitors

Increased Effect/Toxicity

Phenylephrine (Ophthalmic) may increase the levels/effects of: Sympathomimetics

The levels/effects of Phenylephrine (Ophthalmic) may be increased by: AtoMOXetine; Cannabinoid-Containing Products; Ergot Derivatives; Linezolid; MAO Inhibitors; Tedizolid; Tricyclic Antidepressants

Decreased Effect

Phenylephrine (Ophthalmic) may decrease the levels/effects of: Iobenguane I 123

The levels/effects of Phenylephrine (Ophthalmic) may be decreased by: Alpha1-Blockers; Tricyclic Antidepressants

Storage/Stability Ophthalmic solution: 2.5% and 10%: Refer to product labeling. Some products are labeled to store at room temperature; others should be stored under refrigeration at 2°C to 8°C (36°F to 46°F). Do not use solution if brown or contains a precipitate.

Mechanism of Action Potent, direct-acting alpha-adrenergic agonist with virtually no beta-adrenergic activity; produces local vasoconstriction

Pharmacodynamics

Onset of action: Mydriasis: 15-30 minutes

Duration: Mydriasis 2.5% solution: 1-3 hours

Pharmacokinetics (Adult data unless noted)

Absorption: Minimal systemic absorption (Kumar, 1986)

Time to peak serum concentration: ≤20 minutes (Kumar, 1986)

Dosing: Neonatal Ophthalmic procedures: Use combination products containing 1% phenylephrine (see specific monographs for details). In neonates, 2.5% phenylephrine has been shown to cause significant increases in blood pressure compared to 1% preparations (Chew, 2005).

Dosing: Usual

Ophthalmic procedures:

Infants <1 year: Instill 1 drop of 2.5% 15-30 minutes before procedures

Children and Adults: Instill 1 drop of 2.5% or 10% solution, may repeat in 10-60 minutes as needed

Ophthalmic irritation (OTC formulation for relief of eye redness): Adults: Instill 1-2 drops 0.12% solution into affected eye, up to 4 times/day; do not use for >72 hours

Administration Instill drops into conjunctival sac of affected eye(s); avoid contact of bottle tip with skin or eye; finger pressure should be applied to the lacrimal sac during and for 1-2 minutes after instillation to decrease risk of absorption and systemic reactions

Dosage Forms Excipient information presented when available (limited, particularly for generics); consult specific product labeling. [DSC] = Discontinued product

Solution, Ophthalmic, as hydrochloride:

Altafrin: 2.5% (15 mL); 10% (5 mL) [contains benzalkonium chloride]

Mydfrin: 2.5% (3 mL [DSC], 5 mL [DSC]) [contains benzalkonium chloride, edetate disodium]

Neofrin: 2.5% (15 mL [DSC]) [contains benzalkonium chloride, edetate disodium, sodium bisulfite]

Neofrin: 10% (5 mL [DSC]) [contains benzalkonium chloride]

Generic: 2.5% (2 mL, 3 mL, 5 mL, 15 mL); 10% (5 mL)

Solution, Ophthalmic, as hydrochloride [preservative free]:

Generic: 2.5% (1 ea)

Phenylephrine (Topical) (fen il EF rin)

Brand Names: US Anu-Med [OTC]; GRX Hemorrhoidal [OTC]; Hem-Prep [OTC]; Hemorrhoidal [OTC]; Preparation H [OTC]; Rectacaine [OTC]

Therapeutic Category Adrenergic Agonist Agent; Alpha-Adrenergic Agonist; Hemorrhoidal Treatment Agent; Sympathomimetic

Generic Availability (US) Yes

Use Symptomatic relief of hemorrhoidal symptoms

Pregnancy Considerations When administered intravenously, phenylephrine crosses the placenta. Refer to the Phenylephrine (Systemic) monograph for details. There is limited information available supporting the use of topical agents for the treatment of hemorrhoids. Products containing phenylephrine should be used with caution in pregnant women, especially patients with hypertension or diabetes.

Breast-Feeding Considerations It is not known if phenylephrine is excreted into breast milk.

Contraindications Hypersensitivity to phenylephrine or any component of the formulation; hypertension; ventricular tachycardia

Warnings/Precautions Use with caution in patients with hyperthyroidism, diabetes mellitus, cardiovascular disease, ischemic heart disease, increased intraocular pressure, prostatic hyperplasia, or in the elderly. Notify healthcare provider if symptoms do not improve within 7 days or if bleeding occurs.

Adverse Reactions Rare systemic effects may occur.

Drug Interactions

Metabolism/Transport Effects None known.

Avoid Concomitant Use

Avoid concomitant use of Phenylephrine (Topical) with any of the following: Ergot Derivatives; Iobenguane I 123; MAO Inhibitors

Increased Effect/Toxicity

Phenylephrine (Topical) may increase the levels/effects of: Sympathomimetics

The levels/effects of Phenylephrine (Topical) may be increased by: AtoMOXetine; Cannabinoid-Containing Products; Ergot Derivatives; Linezolid; MAO Inhibitors; Tedizolid; Tricyclic Antidepressants

Decreased Effect

Phenylephrine (Topical) may decrease the levels/effects of: Iobenguane I 123

The levels/effects of Phenylephrine (Topical) may be decreased by: Alpha1-Blockers; Tricyclic Antidepressants

Mechanism of Action Potent, direct-acting alpha-adrenergic agonist with virtually no beta-adrenergic activity; produces local vasoconstriction.

Dosing: Usual Treatment of hemorrhoidal symptoms: Children ≥12 years and Adults: Apply to rectal area or by applicator into rectum up to 4 times/day

Administration Apply to clean and dry rectal area at night, in the morning, or after each bowel movement; when using applicator, remove protective cover from applicator and attach to tube. Lubricate applicator well, then gently insert into rectum. Thoroughly cleanse applicator after each use and replace protective cover.

Dosage Forms Excipient information presented when available (limited, particularly for generics); consult specific product labeling.

Ointment, Rectal, as hydrochloride:

GRX Hemorrhoidal: 0.25% (43 g) [contains benzoic acid, methylparaben, propylparaben]

Hemorrhoidal: 0.25% (57 g) [contains benzoic acid, methylparaben, propylparaben]

Preparation H: 0.25% (28 g, 57 g)

Rectacaine: 0.25% (30 g)

Suppository, Rectal, as hydrochloride:

Anu-Med: 0.25% (12 ea)

Hem-Prep: 0.25% (24 ea)

Hemorrhoidal: 0.25% (24 ea); 0.25% (12 ea) [contains methylparaben, propylparaben]

Preparation H: 0.25% (12 ea, 24 ea, 48 ea)

Preparation H: 0.25 % (48 ea) [contains methylparaben, propylparaben]

Rectacaine: 0.25% (12 ea)

◆ **Phenylephrine and Cyclopentolate** *see* Cyclopentolate and Phenylephrine *on page* 550

◆ **Phenylephrine and Promethazine** *see* Promethazine and Phenylephrine *on page* 1781

◆ **Phenylephrine Hydrochloride** *see* Phenylephrine (Nasal) *on page* 1688

◆ **Phenylephrine Hydrochloride** *see* Phenylephrine (Ophthalmic) *on page* 1689

◆ **Phenylephrine Hydrochloride** *see* Phenylephrine (Systemic) *on page* 1685

◆ **Phenylephrine Hydrochloride** *see* Phenylephrine (Topical) *on page* 1690

◆ **Phenylephrine, Promethazine, and Codeine** *see* Promethazine, Phenylephrine, and Codeine *on page* 1782

◆ **Phenylethylmalonylurea** *see* PHENobarbital *on page* 1679

◆ **Phenytek** *see* Phenytoin *on page* 1690

Phenytoin (FEN i toyn)

Medication Safety Issues

Sound-alike/look-alike issues:

Phenytoin may be confused with phenelzine, phentermine, PHENobarbital

Dilantin may be confused with Dilaudid, diltiazem, Dipentum

International issues:

Dilantin [US, Canada, and multiple international markets] may be confused with Dolantine brand name for pethidine [Belgium]

Related Information

Management of Drug Extravasations *on page 2298*

Oral Medications That Should Not Be Crushed or Altered *on page 2476*

Safe Handling of Hazardous Drugs *on page 2455*

Brand Names: US Dilantin; Dilantin Infatabs; Phenytek; Phenytoin Infatabs

Brand Names: Canada Dilantin; Novo-Phenytoin; Taro-Phenytoin; Tremytoine Inj

Therapeutic Category Antiarrhythmic Agent, Class I-B; Anticonvulsant, Hydantoin

Generic Availability (US) Yes

Use

Oral: Management of generalized tonic-clonic (grand mal) and complex partial seizures and the prevention of seizures following head trauma/neurosurgery [FDA approved in pediatric patients (age not specified) and adults]. Has also been used for simple partial seizures; ventricular arrhythmias, including those associated with digitalis intoxication, prolonged QT interval, and surgical repair of congenital heart diseases in children

Parenteral: Management of status epilepticus of the grand mal type and prevention and treatment of seizures occurring during neurosurgery [FDA approved in neonatal and pediatric patients (age not specified) and adults]

Medication Guide Available Yes

Pregnancy Risk Factor D

Pregnancy Considerations Phenytoin crosses the placenta (Harden and Pennell, 2009). An increased risk of congenital malformations and adverse outcomes may occur following *in utero* phenytoin exposure. Reported malformations include orofacial clefts, cardiac defects, dysmorphic facial features, nail/digit hypoplasia, growth abnormalities including microcephaly, and mental deficiency. Isolated cases of malignancies (including neuroblastoma) and coagulation defects in the neonate (may be life threatening) following delivery have also been reported. Maternal use of phenytoin should be avoided when possible to decrease the risk of cleft palate and poor cognitive outcomes. Polytherapy may also increase the risk of congenital malformations; monotherapy is recommended (Harden and Meader, 2009). The maternal use of folic acid throughout pregnancy is recommended to reduce the risk of major congenital malformations (Harden and Pennell, 2009).

Total plasma concentrations of phenytoin are decreased in the mother during pregnancy; unbound plasma (free) concentrations are also decreased and plasma clearance is increased. Due to pregnancy-induced physiologic changes, women who are pregnant may require dose adjustments of phenytoin in order to maintain clinical response; monitoring during pregnancy should be considered (Harden and Pennell, 2009). For women with epilepsy who are planning a pregnancy in advance, baseline serum concentrations should be measured once or twice prior to pregnancy during a period when seizure control is optimal. Monitoring can then be continued once each trimester during pregnancy and postpartum; more frequent monitoring may be needed in some patients. Monitoring of unbound plasma concentrations is recommended (Patsalos, 2008). In women taking phenytoin who are trying to avoid pregnancy, potentially significant interactions may exist with hormone-containing contraceptives; consult drug interactions database for more detailed information.

Patients exposed to phenytoin during pregnancy are encouraged to enroll themselves into the North American Antiepileptic Drug (NAAED) Pregnancy Registry by calling 1-888-233-2334. Additional information is available at https:\\aedpregnancyregistry.org.

Breast-Feeding Considerations Phenytoin is excreted in breast milk; however, the amount to which the infant is exposed is considered small. The manufacturers of phenytoin do not recommend breast-feeding during therapy.

Contraindications Hypersensitivity to phenytoin, other hydantoins, or any component of the formulation; concurrent use of delavirdine (due to loss of virologic response and possible resistance to delavirdine or other non-nucleoside reverse transcriptase inhibitors [NNRTIs])

IV: Sinus bradycardia, sinoatrial block, second- and third-degree heart block, Adams-Stokes syndrome

Warnings/Precautions Hazardous agent - use appropriate precautions for handling and disposal (NIOSH 2014 [group 2]).

Antiepileptics are associated with an increased risk of suicidal behavior/thoughts with use (regardless of indication); patients should be monitored for signs/symptoms of depression, suicidal tendencies, and other unusual behavior changes during therapy and instructed to inform their healthcare provider immediately if symptoms occur.

[US Boxed Warning]: Phenytoin must be administered slowly. Intravenous administration should not exceed 50 mg/minute in adult patients. In pediatric patients, intravenous administration rate should not exceed 1-3 mg/kg/minute or 50 mg/minute whichever is slower. Hypotension and severe cardiac arrhythmias (eg, heart block, ventricular tachycardia, ventricular fibrillation) may occur with rapid administration; adverse cardiac events have been reported at or below the recommended infusion rate. Cardiac monitoring is necessary during and after administration of intravenous phenytoin; reduction in rate of administration or discontinuation of infusion may be necessary. For nonemergency use, intravenous phenytoin should be administered more slowly; the use of oral phenytoin should be used whenever possible. Vesicant (intravenous administration); ensure proper catheter or needle position prior to and during infusion; avoid extravasation; IV form may cause soft tissue irritation and inflammation, and skin necrosis at IV site; avoid IV administration in small veins. The "purple glove syndrome" (ie, discoloration with edema and pain of distal limb) may occur following peripheral IV administration of phenytoin; may or may not be associated with drug extravasation; symptoms may resolve spontaneously; however, skin necrosis and limb ischemia may occur; interventions such as fasciotomies, skin grafts, and amputation (rare) may be required. May increase frequency of petit mal seizures; use with caution in patients with porphyria; discontinue if rash or lymphadenopathy occurs; a spectrum of hematologic effects have been reported with use (eg, agranulocytosis, neutropenia, leukopenia, thrombocytopenia, pancytopenia, and anemias); use with caution in patients with hepatic dysfunction, hypothyroidism, or underlying cardiac disease; IV use is contraindicated in patients with sinus bradycardia, sinoatrial block, or second- and third-degree heart block; use with caution in elderly or debilitated patients, or in any condition associated with low serum albumin levels, which will increase the free fraction of phenytoin in the serum and, therefore, the pharmacologic response. Sedation, confusional states, or cerebellar dysfunction (loss of motor coordination) may occur at higher total serum concentrations, or at lower total serum concentrations when the free fraction of phenytoin is increased. Effects with other sedative drugs or ethanol may be potentiated. Abrupt withdrawal may precipitate status epilepticus. Severe reactions, including toxic epidermal necrolysis and Stevens-Johnson syndromes, although rarely reported, have resulted in fatalities; drug should be discontinued if there are any signs of rash and evaluate for signs and symptoms of drug reaction with eosinophilia and systemic symptoms (DRESS). Preliminary data suggests that patients testing positive for the human leukocyte antigen (HLA) allele HLA-B*1502 have an increased risk of developing Stevens-Johnson syndrome (SJS) and/or toxic epidermal necrolysis (TEN). The risk appears to be highest in the early months of therapy initiation. The presence of this genetic variant exists in up to 15% of people of Asian descent in China, Thailand, Malaysia, Indonesia, Taiwan, and the Philippines, and may vary from <1% in Japanese and Koreans, to 2% to 4% of South Asians and Indians; this variant is virtually absent in those of Caucasian, African-American, Hispanic, or European ancestry; consider avoiding phenytoin use in patients HLA-B*1502 allele positive if other therapeutic options available. Carbamazepine, another antiepileptic with a chemical structure similar to phenytoin, includes in the manufacturer labeling a recommendation to screen patients of Asian descent for the HLA-B*1502 allele prior to initiating therapy; this is not a current recommendation in the phenytoin manufacturer labeling. Chronic use of phenytoin has been associated with decreased bone mineral density (osteopenia, osteoporosis, and osteomalacia) and bone fractures. Chronic use may result in decreased vitamin D concentrations due to hepatic enzyme induction and may lead to hypocalcemia and hypophosphatemia; monitor as appropriate and consider implementing vitamin D and calcium supplementation.

Benzyl alcohol and derivatives: Some dosage forms may contain sodium benzoate/benzoic acid; benzoic acid (benzoate) is a metabolite of benzyl alcohol; large amounts of benzyl alcohol (≥99 mg/kg/day) have been associated with a potentially fatal toxicity ("gasping syndrome") in neonates; the "gasping syndrome" consists of metabolic acidosis, respiratory distress, gasping respirations, CNS dysfunction (including convulsions, intracranial hemorrhage), hypotension, and cardiovascular collapse (AAP, 1997; CDC, 1982); some data suggests that benzoate displaces bilirubin from protein binding sites (Ahlfors, 2001); avoid or use dosage forms containing benzyl alcohol derivative with caution in neonates. See manufacturer's labeling.

Propylene glycol: Some dosage forms may contain propylene glycol; large amounts are potentially toxic and have been associated hyperosmolality, lactic acidosis, seizures and respiratory depression; use caution (AAP, 1997; Zar, 2007).

Warnings: Additional Pediatric Considerations In neonates, the FDA labeled maximum IV administration rate is 1 to 3 mg/kg/minute; **Note:** Most clinicians use a lower maximum rate of infusion in neonates: 0.5 to 1 mg/kg/minute; in infants and children: 1 to 3 mg/kg/minute.

Chronic use of phenytoin has been associated with decreased bone mineral density (osteopenia, osteoporosis, and osteomalacia) and bone fractures. Pediatric patients may be at increased risk for vitamin D deficiency; with chronic therapy, phenytoin may cause catabolism of vitamin D; the daily vitamin D requirement may be increased in these patients (≥400 units/day); vitamin D status should be periodically monitored with laboratory data (Misra, 2008; Wagner, 2008). May cause gingival overgrowth or hyperplasia; reported incidence up to 60%; some data suggest development is associated with higher doses and serum concentrations; folic acid supplementation (0.5 mg/day in pediatric patients ≥6 years) may help to prevent or decrease gingival overgrowth; patients should be counseled regarding the importance of proper dental hygiene (Arya, 2011).

Adverse Reactions Frequency not defined.

Cardiovascular: Atrial conduction depression (IV administration), bradycardia (IV administration), cardiac arrhythmia (IV administration), circulatory shock (IV administration), hypotension (IV administration), periarteritis nodosa, ventricular conduction depression (IV adminsitration), ventricular fibrillation (IV administration)

Central nervous system: Ataxia, confusion, dizziness, drowsiness, headache, insomnia, mood changes, nervousness, paresthesia, peripheral neuropathy (associated with chronic treatment), slurred speech, twitching, vertigo

Dermatologic: Bullous dermatitis, exfoliative dermatitis, hypertrichosis, morbilliform rash (most common), scarlatiniform rash, skin or other tissue necrosis (IV administration), skin rash, toxic epidermal necrolysis

Endocrine & metabolic: Hyperglycemia, vitamin D deficiency (associated with chronic treatment)

Gastrointestinal: Constipation, dysgeusia (metallic taste), gingival hyperplasia, nausea, enlargement of facial features (lips), vomiting

Genitourinary: Peyronie's disease

Hematologic & oncologic: Agranulocytosis, granulocytopenia, Hodgkin lymphoma, immunoglobulin abnormality, leukopenia, lymphadenopathy, macrocytosis, malignant lymphoma, megaloblastic anemia, pancytopenia, pseudolymphoma, purpuric dermatitis, thrombocytopenia

Hepatic: Acute hepatic failure, hepatic injury, hepatitis, toxic hepatitis

Hypersensitivity: Anaphylaxis

Immunologic: DRESS syndrome

Local: Injection site reaction ("purple glove syndrome", edema, discoloration, and pain distal to injection site), local inflammation (IV administration), local irritation (IV administration), localized tenderness (IV administration), local tissue necrosis (IV administration)

Neuromuscular & skeletal: Coarsening of facial features, osteomalacia, systemic lupus erythematosus, tremor

Ophthalmic: Nystagmus

Miscellaneous: Fever, tissue sloughing (IV administration)

Rare but important or life-threatening: Dyskinesia, hepatotoxicity (idiosyncratic) (Chalasani 2014)

Drug Interactions

Metabolism/Transport Effects Substrate of CYP2C19 (major), CYP2C9 (major), CYP3A4 (minor); **Note:** Assignment of Major/Minor substrate status based on clinically relevant drug interaction potential; **Induces** CYP2B6 (strong), CYP2C19 (strong), CYP2C8 (strong), CYP2C9 (strong), CYP3A4 (strong), P-glycoprotein

Avoid Concomitant Use

Avoid concomitant use of Phenytoin with any of the following: Abiraterone Acetate; Apixaban; Apremilast; Artemether; Axitinib; Azelastine (Nasal); Bedaquiline; Boceprevir; Bortezomib; Bosutinib; Cabozantinib; Ceritinib; CloZAPine; Crizotinib; Dabigatran Etexilate; Dasabuvir; Delavirdine; Dienogest; Dolutegravir; Dronedarone; Eliglustat; Enzalutamide; Etravirine; Everolimus; Ibrutinib; Idelalisib; Irinotecan; Isavuconazonium Sulfate; Itraconazole; Ivabradine; Ivacaftor; Lapatinib; Ledipasvir; Lumefantrine; Lurasidone; Macitentan; Mifepristone; Naloxegol; Netupitant; NIFEdipine; Nilotinib; NiMODipine; Nintedanib; Nisoldipine; Olaparib; Ombitasvir; Orphenadrine; Palbociclib; Panobinostat; Paraldehyde; Paritaprevir; PAZOPanib; PONATinib; Praziquantel; Ranolazine; Regorafenib; Rilpivirine; Rivaroxaban; Roflumilast; RomiDEPsin; Simeprevir; Sofosbuvir; SORAfenib; Stiripentol; Suvorexant; Tasimelteon; Telaprevir; Thalidomide; Ticagrelor; Tofacitinib; Tolvaptan; Toremifene; Trabectedin; Ulipristal; Vandetanib; Vemurafenib; VinCRIStine (Liposomal); Vorapaxar

Increased Effect/Toxicity

Phenytoin may increase the levels/effects of: Azelastine (Nasal); Buprenorphine; Clarithromycin; CNS Depressants; Fosamprenavir; Hydrocodone; Lithium; Methotrexate; Methotrimeprazine; Metyrosine; Neuromuscular-Blocking Agents (Nondepolarizing); Orphenadrine; Paraldehyde; PHENobarbital; Pramipexole; Prilocaine; ROPINIRole; Rotigotine; Selective Serotonin Reuptake

Inhibitors; Sodium Nitrite; Thalidomide; Vitamin K Antagonists; Zolpidem

The levels/effects of Phenytoin may be increased by: Alcohol (Ethyl); Amiodarone; Antifungal Agents (Azole Derivatives, Systemic); Benzodiazepines; Brimonidine (Topical); Calcium Channel Blockers; Cannabis; Capecitabine; CarBAMazepine; Carbonic Anhydrase Inhibitors; CeFAZolin; Chlorpheniramine; Cimetidine; Clarithromycin; Cosyntropin; CYP2C19 Inhibitors (Moderate); CYP2C19 Inhibitors (Strong); CYP2C9 Inhibitors (Moderate); CYP2C9 Inhibitors (Strong); Delavirdine; Dexamethasone (Systemic); Dexketoprofen; Dexmethylphenidate; Disulfiram; Doxylamine; Dronabinol; Droperidol; Efavirenz; Eslicarbazepine; Ethosuximide; Felbamate; Floxuridine; Fluconazole; Fluorouracil (Systemic); Fluorouracil (Topical); FLUoxetine; FluvoxaMINE; Halothane; HydrOXYzine; Isoniazid; Kava Kava; Luliconazole; Magnesium Sulfate; Methotrimeprazine; Methylphenidate; MetroNIDAZOLE (Systemic); Miconazole (Oral); Nabilone; Nitric Oxide; Omeprazole; OXcarbazepine; Rufinamide; Sertraline; Sodium Oxybate; Sulfamethoxazole; Tacrolimus (Systemic); Tapentadol; Tegafur; Telaprevir; Tetrahydrocannabinol; Ticlopidine; Topiramate; TraZODone; Trimethoprim; Vitamin K Antagonists

Decreased Effect

Phenytoin may decrease the levels/effects of: Abiraterone Acetate; Acetaminophen; Afatinib; Albendazole; Amiodarone; Antifungal Agents (Azole Derivatives, Systemic); Apixaban; Apremilast; ARIPiprazole; Artemether; Axitinib; Bazedoxifene; Bedaquiline; Boceprevir; Bortezomib; Bosutinib; Brentuximab Vedotin; Busulfan; Cabozantinib; Canagliflozin; Cannabidiol; Cannabis; CarBAMazepine; Caspofungin; Ceritinib; Clarithromycin; CloZAPine; Cobicistat; Contraceptives (Estrogens); Contraceptives (Progestins); Corticosteroids (Systemic); Crizotinib; CycloSPORINE (Systemic); CYP2B6 Substrates; CYP2C19 Substrates; CYP2C8 Substrates; CYP2C9 Substrates; CYP3A4 Substrates; Dabigatran Etexilate; Dasabuvir; Dasatinib; Deferasirox; Delavirdine; Dexamethasone (Systemic); Diclofenac (Systemic); Dienogest; Disopyramide; Dolutegravir; DOXOrubicin (Conventional); Doxycycline; Dronabinol; Dronedarone; Efavirenz; Eliglustat; Elvitegravir; Enzalutamide; Erlotinib; Eslicarbazepine; Ethosuximide; Etoposide; Etoposide Phosphate; Etravirine; Everolimus; Exemestane; Ezogabine; Felbamate; FentaNYL; Flunarizine; Gefitinib; GuanFACINE; HMG-CoA Reductase Inhibitors; Hydrocortisone (Systemic); Ibrutinib; Idelalisib; Imatinib; Irinotecan; Isavuconazonium Sulfate; Itraconazole; Ivabradine; Ivacaftor; Ixabepilone; Lacosamide; LamoTRIgine; Lapatinib; Ledipasvir; Levodopa; Linagliptin; Loop Diuretics; Lopinavir; Lumefantrine; Lurasidone; Macitentan; Maraviroc; Mebendazole; Meperidine; Methadone; MethylPREDNISolone; MetroNIDAZOLE (Systemic); Metyrapone; Mexiletine; Mianserin; Mifepristone; Naloxegol; Nelfinavir; Netupitant; Neuromuscular-Blocking Agents (Nondepolarizing); NIFEdipine; Nilotinib; NiMODipine; Nintedanib; Nisoldipine; Olaparib; Ombitasvir; Omeprazole; OXcarbazepine; Palbociclib; Paliperidone; Panobinostat; Paritaprevir; PAZOPanib; Perampanel; P-glycoprotein/ABCB1 Substrates; PONATinib; Praziquantel; PrednisoLONE (Systemic); PredniSONE; Primidone; Propafenone; QUEtiapine; QuiNIDine; QuiNINE; Ranolazine; Regorafenib; Rilpivirine; Ritonavir; Rivaroxaban; Roflumilast; RomiDEPsin; Rufinamide; Saxagliptin; Sertraline; Simeprevir; Sirolimus; Sofosbuvir; SORAfenib; SUNItinib; Suvorexant; Tacrolimus (Systemic); Tadalafil; Tasimelteon; Telaprevir; Temsirolimus; Teniposide; Tetrahydrocannabinol; Theophylline Derivatives; Thyroid Products; Ticagrelor; Tipranavir; Tofacitinib; Tolvaptan; Topiramate; Topotecan; Toremifene; Trabectedin; TraZODone; Treprostinil; Trimethoprim; Ulipristal; Valproic Acid and Derivatives; Vandetanib; Vemurafenib; Vilazodone; VinCRIStine; VinCRIStine (Liposomal); Vorapaxar; Vortioxetine; Zaleplon; Zonisamide; Zuclopenthixol

The levels/effects of Phenytoin may be decreased by: Alcohol (Ethyl); Amphetamines; Bleomycin; CarBAMazepine; Ciprofloxacin (Systemic); Colesevelam; CYP2C9 Inducers (Strong); Dabrafenib; Darunavir; Dexamethasone (Systemic); Diazoxide; Enzalutamide; Folic Acid; Fosamprenavir; Leucovorin Calcium-Levoleucovorin; Levomefolate; Lopinavir; Mefloquine; Methotrexate; Methylfolate; Mianserin; Multivitamins/Minerals (with ADEK, Folate, Iron); Nelfinavir; Orlistat; PHENobarbital; Platinum Derivatives; Pyridoxine; Rifampin; Ritonavir; Stiripentol; Theophylline Derivatives; Tipranavir; Valproic Acid and Derivatives; Vigabatrin; VinCRIStine

Food Interactions

Ethanol:

Acute use: Ethanol inhibits metabolism of phenytoin and may also increase CNS depression. Management: Monitor patients. Caution patients about effects.

Chronic use: Ethanol stimulates metabolism of phenytoin. Management: Monitor patients.

Food: Phenytoin serum concentrations may be altered if taken with food. If taken with enteral nutrition, phenytoin serum concentrations may be decreased. Tube feedings decrease bioavailability. Phenytoin may decrease calcium, folic acid, and vitamin D levels. Supplementing folic acid may lower the seizure threshold. Management: Hold tube feedings 1-2 hours before and 1-2 hours after phenytoin administration. Do not supplement folic acid. Consider vitamin D supplementation. Take preferably on an empty stomach.

Storage/Stability

Capsule, tablet: Store at 20°C to 25°C (68°F to 77°F). Protect capsules from light. Protect capsules and tablets from moisture.

Oral suspension: Store at room temperature of 20°C to 25°C (68°F to 77°F); do not freeze. Protect from light.

Solution for injection: Store at room temperature of 15°C to 30°C (59°F to 86°F). Use only clear solutions free of precipitate and haziness; slightly yellow solutions may be used. Precipitation may occur if solution is refrigerated and may dissolve at room temperature.

Mechanism of Action Stabilizes neuronal membranes and decreases seizure activity by increasing efflux or decreasing influx of sodium ions across cell membranes in the motor cortex during generation of nerve impulses; prolongs effective refractory period and suppresses ventricular pacemaker automaticity, shortens action potential in the heart

Pharmacokinetics (Adult data unless noted)

Absorption: Oral: Slow, variable; dependent on product formulation; decreased in neonates

Distribution: V_d:

- Neonates:
  - Premature: 1-1.2 L/kg
  - Full-term: 0.8-0.9 L/kg
- Infants: 0.7-0.8 L/kg
- Children: 0.7 L/kg
- Adults: 0.6-0.7 L/kg

Protein binding: Adults: 90% to 95%; Neonates: Decreased protein binding and increased free fraction of phenytoin (up to 20%); Infants: Decreased protein binding and increased free fraction of phenytoin (up to 15%); also increased free fraction in patients with hyperbilirubinemia, hypoalbuminemia, renal dysfunction, or uremia

Metabolism: Follows dose-dependent (Michaelis-Menten) pharmacokinetics; "apparent" or calculated half-life is dependent upon serum concentration, therefore, metabolism is best described in terms of K_m and V_{max}; V_{max} is increased in infants >6 months and children compared to adults; major metabolite (via oxidation) HPPA undergoes enterohepatic recycling and elimination in urine as glucuronides

Bioavailability: Formulation dependent

Half-life, elimination (apparent): 7-42 hours; newborns (PNA <7 days): Apparent half-life greatly prolonged (clearance decreased) and then rapidly accelerates to infant levels by 5 weeks of life; **Note:** Elimination is not first-order and follows Michaelis-Menten pharmacokinetics; half-life increases with increasing phenytoin concentrations

Time to peak serum concentration: Oral: Dependent upon formulation

Extended release capsule: Within 4-12 hours

Immediate release preparation: Within 2-3 hours

Elimination: <5% excreted unchanged in urine; increased clearance and decreased serum concentrations with febrile illness; highly variable clearance, dependent upon intrinsic hepatic function and dose administered

Dosing: Neonatal Note: Dosage should be individualized based upon clinical response and serum concentrations. Phenytoin base (eg, oral suspension, chewable tablets) contains ~8% more drug than phenytoin sodium (~92 mg base is equivalent to 100 mg phenytoin sodium). Dosage adjustments and closer serum monitoring may be necessary when switching dosage forms.

Status epilepticus; neonatal seizures:

Manufacturer labeling: IV: 15 to 20 mg/kg in a single or divided dose; then begin maintenance therapy usually 12 hours after dose

Alternate dosing: AAP recommendation: IV: 10 mg/kg in a single dose; then begin maintenance therapy usually 12 hours after dose. **Note:** Phenobarbital is the preferred treatment for treatment of neonatal seizures. Fosphenytoin is preferred over phenytoin if available due to lower risk of cardiac adverse effects (Hegenbarth 2008).

Seizures; maintenance therapy: IV, Oral: Initial: 5 mg/kg/day in 2 divided doses; usual range: 4 to 8 mg/kg/day in 2 divided doses; some patients may require dosing every 8 hours

Dosing: Usual Note: Dosage should be individualized based upon clinical response and serum concentrations; maintenance therapy dosage adjustments are typically not made more frequently than every 7 days. Phenytoin base (eg, oral suspension, chewable tablets) contains ~8% more drug than phenytoin sodium (~92 mg base is equivalent to 100 mg phenytoin sodium). Dosage adjustments and closer serum monitoring may be necessary when switching dosage forms.

Pediatric:

Status epilepticus: Infants, Children, and Adolescents:

Manufacturer labeling: Loading dose: IV: 15 to 20 mg/kg in a single or divided dose; then begin maintenance therapy usually 12 hours after dose

Alternate dosing: AAP, NCS recommendations: Loading dose: IV: 20 mg/kg in a single or divided doses; maximum dose: 1000 mg; then begin maintenance therapy usually 12 hours after dose (Brophy 2012; Hegenbarth 2008). An additional load of 5 to 10 mg/kg if status epilepticus is not resolved has been used; however, some experts recommend trying another agent once a total loading dose of 20 mg/kg has been given (Brophy 2012).

Seizures: Infants, Children, and Adolescents:

Loading dose (if not previously on phenytoin): IV, Oral: 15 to 20 mg/kg; if currently on phenytoin, reloading dose should be based upon serum concentrations and recent dosing history; an oral loading dose should be divided into 3 doses and administered every 2-4 hours to decrease GI adverse effects and to ensure complete oral absorption

Maintenance therapy: IV, Oral: Initial: 5 mg/kg/day in divided doses (based upon dosage form, see below); usual range: 4 to 8 mg/kg/day; maximum daily dose: 300 mg/**day**. Some experts suggest higher maintenance doses (8 to 10 mg/kg/day) may be necessary in infants and young children (Guerrini 2006). Dosing should be based upon ideal body weight (IBW).

Usual dosing range (Bauer 1983; Chiba 1980; Suzuki 1994):

6 months to 3 years: 8 to 10 mg/kg/day

4 to 6 years: 7.5 to 9 mg/kg/day

7 to 9 years: 7 to 8 mg/kg/day

10 to 16 years: 6 to 7 mg/kg/day

Dosing interval (product specific):

Immediate release preparations (including injection, suspension, and chewable tablets): Divide daily dose into 2 to 3 doses per day

Extended release preparations: In most pediatric patients, usually dosed every 12 hours; however, in adolescent patients with sufficiently long half-life, may be dosed every 24 hours

Seizure prophylaxis, traumatic brain injury: Limited data available; efficacy results variable: Infants, Children, and Adolescents: IV: Initial: 18 mg/kg over 20 minutes; followed by 6 mg/kg/day divided every 8 hours for 48 hours was used in a double-blind, placebo-controlled trial of 102 pediatric patients (n=46 treatment group; median age: 6.4 years) and showed no significance difference in seizure frequency between groups; however, the trial was stopped early due to a very low seizure frequency among both study groups (Young 2004). In a retrospective trial, reduced seizure frequency with prophylactic phenytoin use was described (Lewis 1993). **Note:** Current guidelines suggest that prophylactic phenytoin may be considered to reduce the incidence of early post-traumatic seizures in pediatric patients with severe traumatic brain injuries but it does not reduce the risk of long-term seizures or improve neurologic outcome (Kochanek 2012).

Adult: **Note:** Phenytoin base (eg, oral suspension, chewable tablets) contains ~8% more drug than phenytoin sodium (~92 mg base is equivalent to 100 mg phenytoin sodium). Dosage adjustments and closer serum monitoring may be necessary when switching dosage forms.

Status epilepticus: IV: Loading dose: Manufacturer recommends 10 to 15 mg/kg; however, 15 to 20 mg/kg at a maximum rate of 50 mg/minute is generally recommended (Kälviäinen 2007; Lowenstein 2005); initial maintenance dose: IV, Oral: 100 mg every 6 to 8 hours

Anticonvulsant: Oral: Loading dose: 15 to 20 mg/kg; consider prior phenytoin serum concentrations and/or recent dosing history if available; administer oral loading dose in 3 divided doses given every 2 to 4 hours to decrease GI adverse effects and to ensure complete oral absorption; initial maintenance dose: 300 mg/day in 3 divided doses; may also administer in 1 to 2 divided doses using extended release formulation; adjust dosage based on individual requirements; usual maintenance dose range: 300 to 600 mg/day

Dosing adjustment in renal impairment: Phenytoin serum concentrations may be difficult to interpret in renal failure. Monitoring of free (unbound) concentrations or adjustment to allow interpretation is recommended.

Dosing adjustment in hepatic impairment: Safe in usual doses in mild liver disease; clearance may be substantially reduced in cirrhosis and plasma concentration monitoring with dose adjustment advisable. Free phenytoin concentrations should be monitored closely.

Preparation for Administration Hazardous agent; use appropriate precautions for handling and disposal (NIOSH 2014 [group 2]).

Parenteral: IV: May be further diluted in NS to a final concentration ≥5 mg/mL; infusion must be completed within 4 hours after preparation. Do not refrigerate.

Administration Hazardous agent; use appropriate precautions for handling and disposal (NIOSH 2014 [group 2]).

Oral:

Extended release capsules: May be administered without regard to meals

Suspension: Shake well prior to use; measure and administer dose using a calibrated oral dosing syringe (or other accurate dose-measuring device). Absorption is impaired when phenytoin suspension is given concurrently to patients who are receiving continuous nasogastric feedings. A method to resolve this interaction is to divide the daily dose of phenytoin and withhold the administration of nutritional supplements for 1-2 hours before and after each phenytoin dose.

Parenteral: **Note:** Fosphenytoin may be considered for loading in patients who are in status epilepticus, hemodynamically unstable, or develop hypotension/bradycardia with IV administration of phenytoin.

IV: Phenytoin may be administered IV directly into a large vein through a large gauge needle or IV catheter; however, it is preferred that phenytoin be administered via infusion pump either undiluted or diluted in NS to prevent exceeding the maximum infusion rate (monitor closely for extravasation during infusion). An in-line 0.22 to 0.55 micron filter is recommended for IVPB solutions due to the potential for precipitation of the solution.

Neonates: Administer slowly, usual maximum recommended rate: 0.5 to 1 mg/kg/minute (Hegenbarth 2008). **Note:** The manufacturer recommends a maximum rate: 1 to 3 mg/kg/minute; however, a lower maximum rate of infusion of 1 mg/kg/minute has been recommended (Hanhan 2001; Hegenbarth 2008)

Infants, Children, Adolescents, and Adults: Administer slowly, maximum recommended rate: 1 to 3 mg/kg/minute or maximum rate: 50 mg/minute, whichever is slower

Following IV administration, NS should be injected through the same needle or IV catheter to prevent irritation. Avoid IM use due to erratic absorption, pain on injection, and precipitation of drug at injection site.

Vesicant; ensure proper needle or catheter placement prior to and during IV infusion. Avoid extravasation. If extravasation occurs, stop infusion immediately and disconnect (leave needle/cannula in place); gently aspirate extravasated solution (do NOT flush the line); remove needle/cannula; elevate extremity. There is conflicting information regarding an antidote; some sources recommend not to use an antidote (Montgomery, 1999), while other sources recommend hyaluronidase (see Management of Drug Extravasations for more details).

Vesicant/Extravasation Risk Vesicant

Monitoring Parameters CBC with differential, liver function, suicidality (eg, suicidal thoughts, depression, behavioral changes), bone growth or BMD

Serum phenytoin concentrations: If available, free phenytoin concentrations should be obtained in patients with hyperbilirubinemia, renal impairment, uremia, or hypoalbuminemia; in adult patients, if free phenytoin concentrations are unavailable, the adjusted total concentration may be determined based upon equations. Trough serum concentrations are generally recommended for routine monitoring. To ensure therapeutic concentration is attained, peak serum concentrations may be measured 1 hour after the end of an IV infusion (particularly after a loading dose).

Additional monitoring with IV use: Continuous cardiac monitoring (rate, rhythm, blood pressure) and clinical observation during administration is recommended; blood pressure and pulse should be monitored every 15 minutes for 1 hour after administration with nonemergency use (Meek, 1999); emergency use may require more frequent monitoring and for a longer time after administration; infusion site reactions

Reference Range

Timing of serum samples: Because phenytoin is slowly absorbed, peak serum concentrations may occur 4-8 hours after ingestion of an oral dose. The apparent serum half-life varies with the dosage and the drug follows Michaelis-Menten kinetics. In adults, the average apparent half-life is about 24 hours; in pediatric patients, the apparent half-life is age-dependent (longer in neonates). Steady-state concentrations are reached in 5-10 days.

Toxicity is measured clinically, and some patients may require levels outside the suggested therapeutic range.

Therapeutic range:

Total phenytoin:

Neonates: 8-15 mcg/mL

Pediatric patients ≥1 month and Adults: 10-20 mcg/mL

Concentrations of 5-10 mcg/mL may be therapeutic for some patients, but concentrations <5 mcg/mL are not likely to be effective

50% of adult patients show decreased frequency of seizures at concentrations >10 mcg/mL

86% of adult patients show decreased frequency of seizures at concentrations >15 mcg/mL

Add another anticonvulsant if satisfactory therapeutic response is not achieved with a phenytoin concentration of 20 mcg/mL

Free phenytoin: 1-2.5 mcg/mL

Total phenytoin:

Toxic: >30 mcg/mL (SI: >119 micromole/L)

Lethal: >100 mcg/mL (SI: >400 micromole/L)

When to draw serum concentrations: This is dependent on the disease state being treated and the clinical condition of the patient.

Key points:

Slow absorption of extended capsules and prolonged apparent half-life minimize fluctuations between peak and trough concentrations, thus timing of sampling is not crucial.

Trough concentrations are generally recommended for routine monitoring (capsules, oral suspension, chewable tablets, and intermittent IV dosing). Daily levels are not necessary and may result in incorrect dosage adjustments. If it is determined essential to monitor free phenytoin concentrations, concomitant monitoring of total phenytoin concentrations is not necessary and expensive.

After a loading dose: If rapid therapeutic serum concentrations are needed, initial concentrations may be drawn after 1 hour (after end of IV loading dose) or within 24 hours (after last oral loading dose) to aid in determining maintenance dose or need to reload.

Early assessment of serum concentrations: Draw within 2-3 days of therapy initiation to ensure that the patient's metabolism is not remarkably different from that which would be predicted by average literature-derived pharmacokinetic parameters; early serum concentrations should be used cautiously in design of new dosing regimens.

Second concentration: Draw within 6-7 days with subsequent doses of phenytoin adjusted accordingly.

If plasma concentrations have not changed over a 3- to 5-day period, monitoring interval may be increased to once weekly in the acute clinical setting. In stable patients requiring long-term therapy, generally monitor levels at 3- to 12-month intervals.

Adjustment of serum concentration: See tables.

Note: Although it is ideal to obtain free phenytoin concentrations to assess serum concentrations in patients with hypoalbuminemia or renal failure (CrCl ≤10 mL/minute), it may not always be possible. If free phenytoin concentrations are unavailable, the following equations may be utilized in adult patients.

Adjustment of Serum Concentration in Adults With Low Serum Albumin

Measured Total Phenytoin Concentration (mcg/mL)	Adult Patient's Serum Albumin (g/dL)			
	3.5	3	2.5	2
	Adjusted Total Phenytoin Concentration (mcg/mL)[1]			
[1]Adjusted concentration = measured total concentration divided by [(0.2 x albumin) + 0.1].				
5	6	7	8	10
10	13	14	17	20
15	19	21	25	30

Adjustment of Serum Concentration in Adults With Renal Failure (CrCl ≤10 mL/min)

Measured Total Phenytoin Concentration (mcg/mL)	Adult Patient's Serum Albumin (g/dL)				
	4	3.5	3	2.5	2
	Adjusted Total Phenytoin Concentration (mcg/mL)[1]				
[1]Adjusted concentration = measured total concentration divided by [(0.1 x albumin) + 0.1].					
5	10	11	13	14	17
10	20	22	25	29	33
15	30	33	38	43	50

Dosage Forms Considerations The capsule dosage form represents *Extended Phenytoin Sodium Capsules,* USP, a designation differentiating the drug from *Prompt Phenytoin Sodium Capsules,* USP (no longer available) as the extended form was characterized by a slow and extended rate of absorption when the two were compared.

Dosage Forms Excipient information presented when available (limited, particularly for generics); consult specific product labeling.

Capsule, Oral, as sodium:
- Dilantin: 30 mg [contains fd&c yellow #10 (quinoline yellow)]
- Dilantin: 100 mg
- Phenytek: 200 mg, 300 mg [contains brilliant blue fcf (fd&c blue #1), fd&c blue #1 aluminum lake, fd&c blue #2 aluminum lake, fd&c red #40 aluminum lake, fd&c yellow #10 aluminum lake]
- Generic: 100 mg, 200 mg, 300 mg

Solution, Injection, as sodium:
- Generic: 50 mg/mL (2 mL, 5 mL)

Suspension, Oral:
- Dilantin: 125 mg/5 mL (237 mL) [orange-vanilla flavor]
- Generic: 125 mg/5 mL (4 mL, 237 mL)

Tablet Chewable, Oral:
- Dilantin Infatabs: 50 mg [scored]
- Phenytoin Infatabs: 50 mg [scored; contains fd&c yellow #10 aluminum lake, fd&c yellow #6 aluminum lake, saccharin sodium]
- Generic: 50 mg

◆ **Phenytoin Infatabs** *see* Phenytoin *on page 1690*
◆ **Phenytoin Sodium** *see* Phenytoin *on page 1690*
◆ **Phenytoin Sodium, Extended** *see* Phenytoin *on page 1690*
◆ **Phenytoin Sodium, Prompt** *see* Phenytoin *on page 1690*
◆ **Phisohex [DSC]** *see* Hexachlorophene *on page 1021*
◆ **pHisoHex (Can)** *see* Hexachlorophene *on page 1021*
◆ **PHL-Amantadine (Can)** *see* Amantadine *on page 112*
◆ **PHL-Amiodarone (Can)** *see* Amiodarone *on page 125*
◆ **PHL-Amlodipine (Can)** *see* AmLODIPine *on page 133*
◆ **PHL-Amoxicillin (Can)** *see* Amoxicillin *on page 138*
◆ **PHL-Azithromycin (Can)** *see* Azithromycin (Systemic) *on page 242*
◆ **PHL-Baclofen (Can)** *see* Baclofen *on page 254*
◆ **PHL-Bethanechol (Can)** *see* Bethanechol *on page 284*
◆ **PHL-Ciprofloxacin (Can)** *see* Ciprofloxacin (Systemic) *on page 463*
◆ **PHL-Citalopram (Can)** *see* Citalopram *on page 476*
◆ **PHL-Clonazepam (Can)** *see* ClonazePAM *on page 506*
◆ **PHL-Clonazepam-R (Can)** *see* ClonazePAM *on page 506*
◆ **PHL-Cyclobenzaprine (Can)** *see* Cyclobenzaprine *on page 548*
◆ **PHL-Dexamethasone (Can)** *see* Dexamethasone (Systemic) *on page 610*
◆ **PHL-Divalproex (Can)** *see* Valproic Acid and Derivatives *on page 2143*
◆ **PHL-Docusate Sodium [OTC] (Can)** *see* Docusate *on page 697*
◆ **PHL-Doxycycline (Can)** *see* Doxycycline *on page 717*
◆ **PHL-Fluconazole (Can)** *see* Fluconazole *on page 881*
◆ **PHL-Fluoxetine (Can)** *see* FLUoxetine *on page 906*
◆ **PHL-Fluvoxamine (Can)** *see* FluvoxaMINE *on page 928*
◆ **PHL-Gabapentin (Can)** *see* Gabapentin *on page 954*
◆ **PHL-Levetiracetam (Can)** *see* LevETIRAcetam *on page 1234*
◆ **PHL-Lorazepam (Can)** *see* LORazepam *on page 1299*
◆ **PHL-Lovastatin (Can)** *see* Lovastatin *on page 1305*
◆ **PHL-Meloxicam (Can)** *see* Meloxicam *on page 1346*
◆ **PHL-Metformin (Can)** *see* MetFORMIN *on page 1375*
◆ **PHL-Methimazole (Can)** *see* Methimazole *on page 1386*
◆ **PHL-Methylphenidate (Can)** *see* Methylphenidate *on page 1402*
◆ **PHL-Minocycline (Can)** *see* Minocycline *on page 1440*
◆ **PHL-Olanzapine (Can)** *see* OLANZapine *on page 1546*
◆ **PHL-Olanzapine ODT (Can)** *see* OLANZapine *on page 1546*
◆ **PHL-Ondansetron (Can)** *see* Ondansetron *on page 1564*
◆ **PHL-Oxybutynin (Can)** *see* Oxybutynin *on page 1588*
◆ **PHL-Paroxetine (Can)** *see* PARoxetine *on page 1634*
◆ **PHL-Pravastatin (Can)** *see* Pravastatin *on page 1749*
◆ **PHL-Quetiapine (Can)** *see* QUEtiapine *on page 1815*
◆ **PHL-Ranitidine (Can)** *see* Ranitidine *on page 1836*
◆ **PHL-Risperidone (Can)** *see* RisperiDONE *on page 1866*
◆ **PHL-Salbutamol (Can)** *see* Albuterol *on page 81*
◆ **PHL-Sertraline (Can)** *see* Sertraline *on page 1916*
◆ **PHL-Simvastatin (Can)** *see* Simvastatin *on page 1928*
◆ **PHL-Sotalol (Can)** *see* Sotalol *on page 1963*
◆ **PHL-Sumatriptan (Can)** *see* SUMAtriptan *on page 1995*
◆ **PHL-Terazosin (Can)** *see* Terazosin *on page 2020*

- ◆ **PHL-Terbinafine (Can)** *see* Terbinafine (Systemic) *on page 2021*
- ◆ **PHL-Topiramate (Can)** *see* Topiramate *on page 2085*
- ◆ **PHL-Trazodone (Can)** *see* TraZODone *on page 2105*
- ◆ **PHL-Ursodiol C (Can)** *see* Ursodiol *on page 2136*
- ◆ **PHL-Valacyclovir (Can)** *see* ValACYclovir *on page 2138*
- ◆ **PHL-Valproic Acid (Can)** *see* Valproic Acid and Derivatives *on page 2143*
- ◆ **PHL-Valproic Acid E.C. (Can)** *see* Valproic Acid and Derivatives *on page 2143*
- ◆ **PHL-Verapamil SR (Can)** *see* Verapamil *on page 2170*
- ◆ **Phos-Flur** *see* Fluoride *on page 899*
- ◆ **Phos-Flur Rinse [OTC]** *see* Fluoride *on page 899*
- ◆ **PhosLo** *see* Calcium Acetate *on page 341*
- ◆ **PhosLo® (Can)** *see* Calcium Acetate *on page 341*
- ◆ **Phoslyra** *see* Calcium Acetate *on page 341*
- ◆ **Phos-NaK** *see* Potassium Phosphate and Sodium Phosphate *on page 1746*
- ◆ **Phospha 250 Neutral** *see* Potassium Phosphate and Sodium Phosphate *on page 1746*
- ◆ **Phosphate, Potassium** *see* Potassium Phosphate *on page 1743*
- ◆ **Phosphates, Sodium** *see* Sodium Phosphates *on page 1949*
- ◆ **Phosphonoformate** *see* Foscarnet *on page 941*
- ◆ **Phosphonoformic Acid** *see* Foscarnet *on page 941*
- ◆ ***p*-Hydroxyampicillin** *see* Amoxicillin *on page 138*
- ◆ **Phylloquinone** *see* Phytonadione *on page 1698*
- ◆ **Physicians EZ Use B-12** *see* Cyanocobalamin *on page 545*
- ◆ **Physicians EZ Use Flu** *see* Influenza Virus Vaccine (Inactivated) *on page 1108*

Physostigmine (fye zoe STIG meen)

Medication Safety Issues

Sound-alike/look-alike issues:

Physostigmine may be confused with Prostigmin®, pyridostigmine

Related Information

Safe Handling of Hazardous Drugs *on page 2455*

Therapeutic Category Antidote, Anticholinergic Agent; Cholinergic Agent; Cholinergic Agent, Ophthalmic

Generic Availability (US) Yes

Use Reverse toxic, life-threatening delirium caused by atropine, diphenhydramine, dimenhydrinate, *Atropa belladonna* (deadly nightshade), or jimson weed (*Datura* spp)

Pregnancy Considerations In general, medications used as antidotes should take into consideration the health and prognosis of the mother; antidotes should be administered to pregnant women if there is a clear indication for use and should not be withheld because of fears of teratogenicity (Bailey, 2003).

Breast-Feeding Considerations It is not known if physostigmine is excreted in breast milk. According to the manufacturer, the decision to continue or discontinue breast-feeding during therapy should take into account the risk of exposure to the infant and the benefits of treatment to the mother.

Contraindications Gastrointestinal or genitourinary obstruction; asthma; gangrene; diabetes; cardiovascular disease; any vagotonic state; coadministration of choline esters and depolarizing neuromuscular-blocking agents (eg, succinylcholine)

Warnings/Precautions Hazardous agent - use appropriate precautions for handling and disposal (EPA, P-listed). Patient must have a normal QRS interval, as measured by ECG, in order to receive; use caution in poisoning with agents known to prolong intraventricular conduction (Howland, 2011). Discontinue if symptoms of excessive cholinergic activity occur (eg, salivation, urinary incontinence, defecation, vomiting); overdosage may result in cholinergic crisis, which must be distinguished from myasthenic crisis. If excessive diaphoresis or nausea occurs, reduce subsequent doses. Due to the possibility of hypersensitivity or overdose/cholinergic crisis, atropine should be readily available. When administering by IV injection, administer no faster than 1 mg/minute in adults or 0.5 mg/minute in children to prevent bradycardia, respiratory distress, and seizures from too rapid administration. Although the use of continuous infusions of physostigmine have been described in the literature (Eyer, 2008; Hail, 2013), experts do not recommend the routine use of continuous infusions. It is preferable to titrate physostigmine to patient needs through the use of intermittent administration; intermittent administration will minimize the risk of cholinergic toxicity, which can be associated with considerable morbidity. Asystole and seizures have been reported when physostigmine was administered to TCA poisoned patients. Physostigmine is not recommended in patients with known or suspected TCA intoxication. Products may contain sodium metabisulfite which may cause allergic reactions in some individuals. Hazardous agent; use appropriate precautions for handling and disposal (EPA, P-listed).

Benzyl alcohol and derivatives: Some dosage forms may contain benzyl alcohol; large amounts of benzyl alcohol (≥99 mg/kg/day) have been associated with a potentially fatal toxicity ("gasping syndrome") in neonates; the "gasping syndrome" consists of metabolic acidosis, respiratory distress, gasping respirations, CNS dysfunction (including convulsions, intracranial hemorrhage), hypotension, and cardiovascular collapse (AAP, 1997; CDC, 1982); some data suggests that benzoate displaces bilirubin from protein binding sites (Ahlfors, 2001); avoid or use dosage forms containing benzyl alcohol with caution in neonates. See manufacturer's labeling.

Adverse Reactions

Cardiovascular: Asystole, bradycardia, palpitation

Central nervous system: Hallucinations, nervousness, restlessness, seizure

Gastrointestinal: Defecation, diarrhea, nausea, salivation, stomach pain, vomiting

Genitourinary: Urinary frequency

Neuromuscular & skeletal: Twitching

Ocular: Lacrimation, miosis

Respiratory: Bronchospasm, dyspnea, pulmonary edema, respiratory distress, respiratory paralysis

Miscellaneous: Diaphoresis, hypersensitivity

Drug Interactions

Metabolism/Transport Effects None known.

Avoid Concomitant Use There are no known interactions where it is recommended to avoid concomitant use.

Increased Effect/Toxicity

Physostigmine may increase the levels/effects of: Beta-Blockers; Cholinergic Agonists; Succinylcholine

The levels/effects of Physostigmine may be increased by: Corticosteroids (Systemic)

Decreased Effect

Physostigmine may decrease the levels/effects of: Anticholinergic Agents; Neuromuscular-Blocking Agents (Nondepolarizing)

The levels/effects of Physostigmine may be decreased by: Anticholinergic Agents; Dipyridamole

Storage/Stability Store at 20°C to 25°C (68°F to 77°F).

Mechanism of Action Physostigmine is a carbamate which inhibits the enzyme acetylcholinesterase and prolongs the central and peripheral effects of acetylcholine

Pharmacodynamics Parenteral:
Onset of action: Within 3-8 minutes
Duration: 30 minutes to 1 hour

Pharmacokinetics (Adult data unless noted)
Distribution: Widely distributed throughout the body; crosses into the CNS
Half-life: 1-2 hours
Elimination: Via hydrolysis by cholinesterases

Dosing: Usual
Reversal of toxic anticholinergic effects: **Note:** Administer slowly over 5 minutes to prevent respiratory distress and seizures. Continuous infusions of physostigmine should never be used.
Children: Reserve for life-threatening situations only: IV: 0.01-0.03 mg/kg/dose; may repeat after 15-20 minutes to a maximum total dose of 2 mg
Adults: IM, IV, SubQ: 0.5-2 mg initially, repeat every 20 minutes until response or adverse effect occurs; repeat 1-4 mg every 30-60 minutes as life-threatening symptoms recur
Preanesthetic reversal: Children and Adults:
IM, IV: Give twice the dose, on a weight basis, of the anticholinergic drug (atropine, scopolamine)

Administration Hazardous agent; use appropriate precautions for handling and disposal (EPA, P-listed).
Parenteral:
IM: May administer as undiluted solution
IV: Infuse undiluted solution slowly; maximum rate: Pediatric patients: 0.5 mg/minute; adults: 1 mg/minute. Too rapid administration can cause bradycardia and hypersalivation leading to respiratory distress and seizures.

Monitoring Parameters Heart rate, respiratory rate, ECG

Test Interactions Increased aminotransferase [ALT/AST] (S), increased amylase (S)

Dosage Forms Excipient information presented when available (limited, particularly for generics); consult specific product labeling.
Solution, Injection, as salicylate:
Generic: 1 mg/mL (2 mL)

- **Physostigmine Salicylate** *see* Physostigmine *on page 1697*
- **Physostigmine Sulfate** *see* Physostigmine *on page 1697*
- **Phytomenadione** *see* Phytonadione *on page 1698*

Phytonadione (fye toe na DYE one)

Medication Safety Issues
Sound-alike/look-alike issues:
Mephyton may be confused with melphalan, methadone

Brand Names: US Mephyton®

Brand Names: Canada AquaMEPHYTON®; Konakion; Mephyton®

Therapeutic Category Nutritional Supplement; Vitamin, Fat Soluble

Generic Availability (US) Yes

Use
Injection: Prophylaxis and treatment of hemorrhagic disease of the newborn (FDA approved in newborns); prevention and treatment of hypoprothrombinemia caused by vitamin K deficiency, vitamin K antagonist (VKA)-induced (eg, warfarin-induced), other drug-induced vitamin K deficiency, altered activity, or altered metabolism (FDA approved in adults); hypoprothrombinemia caused by malabsorption or inability to synthesize vitamin K (FDA approved in adults)
Oral: Prevention and treatment of hypoprothrombinemia caused by vitamin K deficiency, vitamin K antagonist (VKA)-induced (eg, warfarin-induced), other drug-induced vitamin K deficiency, altered activity, or altered metabolism; hypoprothrombinemia caused by malabsorption or inability to synthesize vitamin K (FDA approved in adults)

Pregnancy Risk Factor C

Pregnancy Considerations Animal reproduction studies have not been conducted. Phytonadione crosses the placenta in limited concentrations (Kazzi, 1990). The dietary requirements of vitamin K are the same in pregnant and nonpregnant women (IOM, 2000). In general, medications used as antidotes should take into consideration the health and prognosis of the mother; antidotes should be administered to pregnant women if there is a clear indication for use and should not be withheld because of fears of teratogenicity (Bailey, 2003).

Breast-Feeding Considerations Small amounts of dietary vitamin K can be detected in breast milk and the dietary requirements of vitamin K are the same in nursing and non-nursing women (IOM, 2000). Information following the use of phytonadione has not been located. The manufacturer recommends caution be used if phytonadione is administered to a nursing woman.

Contraindications Hypersensitivity to phytonadione or any component of the formulation

Warnings/Precautions [U.S. Boxed Warning]: Severe reactions resembling hypersensitivity reactions (eg, anaphylaxis) have occurred rarely during or immediately after IV administration (even with proper dilution and rate of administration); some patients had no previous exposure to phytonadione. Anaphylactoid reactions typically occurred when patients received large IV doses administered rapidly with formulations containing polyethoxylated castor oil; proper dosing, dilution, and administration will minimize risk (Ageno, 2012; Riegert-Johnson, 2002). Limit IV administration to situations where an alternative route of administration is not feasible and the benefit of therapy outweighs the risk of hypersensitivity reactions. Allergic reactions have also occurred with IM and SubQ injections, albeit less frequently. In obstructive jaundice or with biliary fistulas concurrent administration of bile salts is necessary. Manufacturers recommend the SubQ route over other parenteral routes. SubQ is less predictable when compared to the oral route. The American College of Chest Physicians recommends the IV route in patients with major bleeding secondary to warfarin. The IV route should be restricted to emergency situations where oral phytonadione cannot be used. Efficacy is delayed regardless of route of administration; patient management may require other treatments in the interim. In patients receiving a therapeutic vitamin K antagonist (VKA) (eg, warfarin), administer a dose of phytonadione that will quickly lower the INR into a safe range without causing resistance to warfarin. High phytonadione doses may lead to warfarin resistance for at least one week. Patients with LAAR-induced coagulopathy require much larger doses and longer treatment durations (up to months) after exposure compared to that needed to reverse VKA-induced coagulopathy. Use with caution in neonates, especially premature infants; severe hemolytic anemia, jaundice, and hyperbilirubinemia have been reported with larger than recommended doses (10 to 20 mg). In liver disease, if initial doses do not reverse coagulopathy then higher doses are unlikely to have any effect. Ineffective in hereditary hypoprothrombinemia.

Benzyl alcohol and derivatives: Some dosage forms may contain benzyl alcohol; large amounts of benzyl alcohol (≥99 mg/kg/day) have been associated with a potentially fatal toxicity ("gasping syndrome") in neonates; the "gasping syndrome" consists of metabolic acidosis, respiratory distress, gasping respirations, CNS dysfunction (including convulsions, intracranial hemorrhage), hypotension, and cardiovascular collapse (AAP, 1997; CDC, 1982); some data suggests that benzoate displaces bilirubin from protein binding sites (Ahlfors, 2001); avoid or use dosage forms containing benzyl alcohol with caution in neonates. See manufacturer's labeling.

The parenteral product may contain aluminum; toxic aluminum concentrations may be seen with high doses, prolonged use, or renal dysfunction. Premature neonates are at higher risk due to immature renal function and aluminum intake from other parenteral sources. Parenteral aluminum exposure of >4 to 5 mcg/kg/day is associated with CNS and bone toxicity; tissue loading may occur at lower doses (Federal Register, 2002). See manufacturer's labeling.

Some dosage forms may contain polysorbate 80 (also known as Tweens). Hypersensitivity reactions, usually a delayed reaction, have been reported following exposure to pharmaceutical products containing polysorbate 80 in certain individuals (Isaksson, 2002; Lucente 2000; Shelley, 1995). Thrombocytopenia, ascites, pulmonary deterioration, and renal and hepatic failure have been reported in premature neonates after receiving parenteral products containing polysorbate 80 (Alade, 1986; CDC, 1984). See manufacturer's labeling.

Some dosage forms contain Cremophor EL which has been associated with anaphylactoid reactions; use these formulations with caution.

Adverse Reactions

Cardiovascular: Cyanosis, flushing, hyper-/hypotension
Central nervous system: Dizziness
Dermatologic: Erythematous skin eruptions, pruritus, scleroderma-like lesions
Endocrine & metabolic: Hyperbilirubinemia (newborn; greater than recommended doses)
Gastrointestinal: Abnormal taste
Local: Injection site reactions
Respiratory: Dyspnea
Miscellaneous: Diaphoresis, hypersensitivity reactions, nonimmunologic anaphylaxis (formerly known as anaphylactoid reaction), sweating

Drug Interactions

Metabolism/Transport Effects None known.

Avoid Concomitant Use There are no known interactions where it is recommended to avoid concomitant use.

Increased Effect/Toxicity There are no known significant interactions involving an increase in effect.

Decreased Effect

Phytonadione may decrease the levels/effects of: Vitamin K Antagonists

The levels/effects of Phytonadione may be decreased by: Mineral Oil; Orlistat

Storage/Stability

Injection: Store at 15°C to 30°C (59°F to 86°F). Protect from light. **Note:** Store Hospira product at 20°C to 25°C (68°F to 77°F).
Oral: Store tablets at 15°C to 30°C (59°F to 86°F). Protect from light.

Mechanism of Action Promotes liver synthesis of clotting factors (II, VII, IX, X); however, the exact mechanism as to this stimulation is unknown. Menadiol is a water soluble form of vitamin K; phytonadione has a more rapid and prolonged effect than menadione; menadiol sodium diphosphate (K_4) is half as potent as menadione (K_3).

Pharmacodynamics

Onset of action: Blood coagulation factors increase: Oral: Within 6 to 12 hours; Parenteral: Within 1 to 2 hours
Maximum effect: Normalization prothrombin time (INR): Oral: 24 to 48 hours; Parenteral: 12 to 14 hours

Pharmacokinetics (Adult data unless noted)

Absorption: Oral: From the intestines in the presence of bile; SubQ: Variable; IM: Readily absorbed
Metabolism: Rapidly in the liver
Elimination: In bile and urine as metabolites

Dosing: Neonatal Note: Dosing presented in **mcg** and mg; verify dosing units.

Adequate intake (Vanek 2012): Oral:
Preterm neonates: 8 to 10 **mcg**/kg/day
Term neonates: 2 **mcg**/day

Parenteral nutrition, maintenance requirement (Vanek 2012): IV:
Preterm neonate: 10 **mcg**/kg/day
Term neonates: 200 **mcg**/day

Vitamin K deficiency bleeding (formerly known as hemorrhagic disease of the newborn):

Prophylaxis: IM: **Note:** Administer within 1 hour of birth
AAP recommendations (AAP 2003; AAP 2009, AAP 2013):
Preterm neonate: Optimal dose not established (AAP 2003)
Birth weight <1,000 g: 0.3 to 0.5 mg/kg
Birth weight ≥1,000 g: 0.5 to 1 mg
Term neonate: 0.5 to 1 mg
Alternate dosing: GA <32 weeks: 0.2 mg; may repeat dose for prolonged prothrombin time or clinical signs of bleeding (Clarke 2006)
Treatment: SubQ, IM: 1 to 2 mg/day

Dosing: Usual Note: SubQ route is preferred; IV and IM routes should be restricted for situations when the SubQ route is not feasible. Dosing presented in **mcg** and mg; verify dosing units.

Pediatric:

Adequate intake (IOM 2001; Vanek 2013):
1 to 6 months: 2 **mcg**/day
7 to 12 months: 2.5 **mcg**/day
1 to 3 years: 30 **mcg**/day
4 to 8 years: 55 **mcg**/day
9 to 13 years: 60 **mcg**/day
14 to 18 years: 75 **mcg**/day

Vitamin K deficiency, prevention, and supplementation (Disease-specific): Limited data available:

Biliary atresia (Shneider 2012): **Note:** Dose and route are determined by INR value: Infants 1 to 6 months:
INR >1.2 to 1.5: 2.5 mg once daily orally
INR >1.5 to 1.8: Initial: 2 to 5 mg IM once followed by 2.5 mg once daily orally
INR >1.8: Initial: 2 to 5 mg IM once followed by 5 mg once daily orally

Cholestasis: Infants, Children, and Adolescents: Oral:: 2.4 to 15 mg/day (Sathe 2010)

Cystic fibrosis: Infants, Children, and Adolescents: Oral: 0.3 to 0.5 mg/day (Borowitz 2002; Sathe 2010)

Liver disease: Infants, Children, and Adolescents: Oral: 2.5 to 5 mg/day (Nightingale 2009; Sathe 2010)

Reversal of Vitamin K antagonists (eg, warfarin): Limited data available: Infants, Children, and Adolescents:

Weight-based dosing (preferred): *Chest* recommendations: IV: 0.03 mg/kg/dose is recommended for excessively prolonged INR (usually INR >8; no evidence of bleeding) due to vitamin K-antagonist (eg, warfarin): if significant bleeding, consider use of fresh frozen plasma, prothrombin complex concentrates, or recombinant factor VIIa (Bolton-Maggs 2002; Monagle 2012)

Alternate dosing: Fixed dosing: **Note:** Smaller pediatric patients should receive doses on the low end of dosing range; excessive dosages may cause warfarin-resistance (Bolton-Maggs 2002; Michelson 1998)
No bleeding, rapid reversal needed, patient will require further oral anticoagulant therapy: SubQ, IV: 0.5 to 2 mg
No bleeding, rapid reversal needed, patient will not require further oral anticoagulant therapy: SubQ, IV: 2 to 5 mg

Significant bleeding, not life-threatening: SubQ, IV: 0.5 to 2 mg

Significant bleeding, life-threatening: SubQ, IV: 5 mg

Parenteral nutrition, maintenance requirement Limited data available (Vanek 2012): IV: **Note:** Patients receiving warfarin may not require TPN supplementation of phytonadione.

Infants: 10 **mcg**/kg/day

Children and Adolescents: 200 **mcg**/day

Adult:

Adequate intake (IOM 2001):

Male: 120 **mcg**/day

Female: 90 **mcg**/day

Pregnant, ≤18 years of age: 75 **mcg**/day

Pregnant, ≥19 years of age: 90 **mcg**/day

Breast-feeding, ≤18 years of age: 75 **mcg**/day

Breast-feeding, ≥19 years of age: 90 **mcg**/day

Vitamin K deficiency due to drugs (other than coumarin derivatives) or factors limiting absorption or synthesis: Oral, SubQ, IM, IV: Initial: 2.5 to 25 mg (rarely up to 50 mg)

Vitamin K deficiency (supratherapeutic INR) secondary to VKAs (eg, warfarin):

If INR above therapeutic range to <4.5 (no evidence of bleeding): Lower or hold next VKA dose and monitor frequently; when INR approaches desired range, resume VKA dosing with a lower dose (Patriquin 2011)

If INR 4.5 to 10 (no evidence of bleeding): The 2012 *Chest* guidelines recommend against routine phytonadione (ie, vitamin K) administration in this setting (Guyatt 2012). Previously, the 2008 ACCP guidelines recommended if no risk factors for bleeding exist, to omit next 1 or 2 VKA doses, monitor INR more frequently, and resume with an appropriately adjusted VKA dose when INR in desired range; may consider administering vitamin K orally 1 to 2.5 mg if other risk factors for bleeding exist (Hirsh 2008). Others have recommended consideration of vitamin K 1 mg orally or 0.5 mg IV (Patriquin 2011).

If INR >10 (no evidence of bleeding): The 2012 ACCP guidelines recommend administration of oral vitamin K (dose not specified) in this setting (Guyatt 2012). Previously, the 2008 ACCP guidelines recommended to hold warfarin, administer vitamin K orally 2.5 to 5 mg, expect INR to be reduced within 24 to 48 hours, monitor INR more frequently and give additional vitamin K at an appropriate dose if necessary; resume warfarin at an appropriately adjusted dose when INR is in desired range (Hirsh 2008). Others have recommended consideration of vitamin K 2 to 2.5 mg orally or 0.5 to 1 mg IV (Patriquin 2011).

If minor bleeding at any INR elevation: Hold warfarin, may administer vitamin K orally 2.5 to 5 mg, monitor INR more frequently, may repeat dose after 24 hours if INR correction incomplete; resume warfarin at an appropriately adjusted dose when INR is in desired range (Patriquin 2011)

If major bleeding at any INR elevation: The 2012 ACCP guidelines recommend administration of four-factor prothrombin complex concentrate (PCC) and IV vitamin K 5 to 10 mg in this setting (Guyatt 2012); however, in the US, the available PCCs (Bebulin VH and Profilnine SD) are **three**-factor PCCs and do not contain adequate levels of factor VII. Four-factor PCCs include Beriplex P/N, Cofact, Konyne, or Octaplex all of which are **not** available in the US. Previously, the 2008 ACCP guidelines recommended to hold warfarin, administer vitamin K 10 mg by slow IV infusion and supplement with PCC depending on the urgency of the situation; IV vitamin K may be repeated every 12 hours (Hirsh 2008).

Note: Use of high doses of vitamin K (eg, 10 to 15 mg) may cause warfarin resistance for ≥1 week. During this period of resistance, heparin or low molecular-weight heparin (LMWH) may be given until INR responds (Ansell 2008).

Preprocedural/surgical INR normalization in patients receiving warfarin (routine use): Oral: 1 to 2.5 mg once administered on the day before surgery; recheck INR on day of procedure/surgery (Douketis 2012). Others have recommended the use of vitamin K 1 mg orally for mild INR elevations (ie, INR 3.0 to 4.5) (Patriquin 2011).

Preparation for Administration Parenteral: IV: Dilute phytonadione injection in preservative-free NS, D_5W, or D_5NS. To reduce the incidence of anaphylactoid reaction upon IV administration dilution of dose is recommended; in adults, dilute dose in a minimum of 50 mL of compatible solution (Ageno 2012).

Administration

Oral: May be administered with or without food. The parenteral formulation may also be used for small oral doses (eg, 1 mg) or situations in which tablets cannot be swallowed (Crowther,2000; O'Connor 1986).

Parenteral: **Note:** Limit IV administration to situations where an alternative route of administration is not feasible and the benefit of therapy outweighs the risk of hypersensitivity reactions; proper dosing, dilution, and administration will minimize risk (Ageno 2012; Riegert-Johnson 2002). Allergic reactions have also occurred with IM and SubQ injections, albeit less frequently.

SubQ: Administer undiluted; preferred route of administration

IM: Administer undiluted; for use in neonatal patients, verify appropriate concentration (1 mg/0.5 mL)

IV: After dilution, infuse slowly. In pediatric patients, IV doses have been infused over 15 to 30 minutes (Kliegman 2007; Michelson 1998); in adults, administration using an infusion pump over at least 20 minutes has been suggested (Ageno 2012); maximum rate of infusion: 1 mg/minute

Monitoring Parameters PT, INR

Dosage Forms Considerations Injectable products may contain benzyl alcohol, polysorbate 80, propylene glycol, or castor derivatives.

Dosage Forms Excipient information presented when available (limited, particularly for generics); consult specific product labeling.

Injection, aqueous colloidal: 1 mg/0.5 mL (0.5 mL); 10 mg/mL (1 mL)

Injection, aqueous colloidal [preservative free]: 1 mg/0.5 mL (0.5 mL)

Tablet, oral: 100 mcg

Mephyton®: 5 mg [scored]

Extemporaneous Preparations A 1 mg/mL oral suspension may be made with tablets. Crush six 5 mg tablets in a mortar and reduce to a fine powder. Add 5 mL each of water and methylcellulose 1% and mix to a uniform paste. Mix while adding sorbitol in incremental proportions to **almost** 30 mL; transfer to a calibrated bottle, rinse mortar with sorbitol, and add quantity of sorbitol sufficient to make 30 mL. Label "shake well" and "refrigerate". Stable for 3 days.

Nahata MC and Hipple TF, *Pediatric Drug Formulations*, 3rd ed, Cincinnati, OH: Harvey Whitney Books Co, 1997.

Note: The parenteral formulation may also be used for small oral doses (eg, 1 mg) or situations in which tablets cannot be swallowed (Crowther, 2000; O'Connor, 1986).

◆ **PIC 200 [OTC]** *see* Polysaccharide-Iron Complex *on page 1728*

Pilocarpine (Systemic) (pye loe KAR peen)

Medication Safety Issues

Sound-alike/look-alike issues:

Salagen may be confused with selegiline

Brand Names: US Salagen

Brand Names: Canada Salagen®

Therapeutic Category Cholinergic Agent

Generic Availability (US) Yes

Use Symptomatic treatment of xerostomia caused by salivary gland hypofunction resulting from radiotherapy for cancer of the head and neck; and in Sjögren's syndrome

Pregnancy Risk Factor C

Pregnancy Considerations Adverse events were observed in some animal reproduction studies.

Breast-Feeding Considerations It is not known if pilocarpidine systemic is excreted in breast milk. Due to the potential for serious adverse reactions in the nursing infant, a decision should be made whether to discontinue nursing or to discontinue the drug, taking into account the importance of treatment to the mother.

Contraindications Hypersensitivity to pilocarpine or any component of the formulation; uncontrolled asthma; angle-closure glaucoma, severe hepatic impairment

Warnings/Precautions Use caution with cardiovascular disease; patients may have difficulty compensating for transient changes in hemodynamics or rhythm induced by pilocarpine. Use caution with controlled asthma, chronic bronchitis, or COPD; may increase airway resistance, bronchial smooth muscle tone, and bronchial secretions. Use caution with cholelithiasis, biliary tract disease, and nephrolithiasis; adjust dose with moderate hepatic impairment.

Adverse Reactions

Cardiovascular: Edema, facial edema, flushing, hypertension, palpitation, tachycardia

Central nervous system: Chills, dizziness, fever, headache, pain, somnolence

Dermatologic: Pruritus, rash

Gastrointestinal: Diarrhea, dyspepsia, constipation, flatulence, glossitis, increased salivation, nausea, stomatitis, taste perversion, vomiting

Genitourinary: Urinary frequency, urinary incontinence, vaginitis

Neuromuscular & skeletal: Myalgias, tremor, weakness

Ocular: Abnormal vision, amblyopia, blurred vision, conjunctivitis lacrimation

Otic: Tinnitus

Respiratory: Dysphagia, epistaxis, increased cough, rhinitis, sinusitis

Miscellaneous: Allergic reaction, diaphoresis, voice alteration

Rare but important or life-threatening: Abnormal dreams, alopecia, angina pectoris, anorexia, anxiety, arrhythmia, body odor, bone disorder, cholelithiasis, colitis, confusion, dry eyes, dry mouth, ECG abnormality, myasthenia, photosensitivity reaction, nervousness, pancreatitis, paresthesia, salivary gland enlargement, sputum increased, taste loss, tongue disorder, urinary impairment, urinary urgency, yawning

Drug Interactions

Metabolism/Transport Effects Inhibits CYP2A6 (weak), CYP2E1 (weak)

Avoid Concomitant Use There are no known interactions where it is recommended to avoid concomitant use.

Increased Effect/Toxicity

The levels/effects of Pilocarpine (Systemic) may be increased by: Acetylcholinesterase Inhibitors; Beta-Blockers

Decreased Effect There are no known significant interactions involving a decrease in effect.

Food Interactions Fat decreases the rate of absorption, maximum concentration and increases the time it takes to reach maximum concentration. Management: Avoid administering with a high-fat meal.

Storage/Stability Store at controlled room temperature of 15°C to 30°C (59°F to 86°F).

Pharmacodynamics Increased salivary flow

Onset of action: 20 minutes

Maximum effect: 1 hour

Duration: 3-5 hours

Pharmacokinetics (Adult data unless noted)

Half-life, elimination: 0.76-1.35 hours

Mild to moderate hepatic impairment: 2.1 hours

Elimination: Urine

Dosing: Usual

Xerostomia: Adults: Oral:

Following head and neck cancer: 5 mg 3 times/day, titration up to 10 mg 3 times/day may be considered for patients who have not responded adequately; not to exceed 10 mg/dose

Sjögren's syndrome: 5 mg 4 times/day

Dosage adjustment in hepatic impairment: Adults: Oral: Patients with moderate impairment: 5 mg 2 times/day regardless of indication; avoid use in severe hepatic impairment

Administration May be administered with or without food; avoid administration with high-fat meal

Monitoring Parameters Salivation (xerostomia treatment)

Dosage Forms Excipient information presented when available (limited, particularly for generics); consult specific product labeling.

Tablet, Oral, as hydrochloride:

Salagen: 5 mg

Salagen: 7.5 mg [contains fd&c blue #2 aluminum lake]

Generic: 5 mg, 7.5 mg

Pilocarpine (Ophthalmic) (pye loe KAR peen)

Medication Safety Issues

Sound-alike/look-alike issues:

Isopto® Carpine may be confused with Isopto® Carbachol

Brand Names: US Isopto Carpine; Pilopine HS

Brand Names: Canada Diocarpine; Isopto® Carpine; Pilopine HS®

Therapeutic Category Cholinergic Agent; Cholinergic Agent, Ophthalmic; Ophthalmic Agent, Miotic

Generic Availability (US) May be product dependent

Use Management of chronic simple glaucoma, chronic and acute angle-closure glaucoma; counter effects of cycloplegics

Pregnancy Risk Factor C

Pregnancy Considerations Animal reproduction studies have not been conducted.

Breast-Feeding Considerations It is not known if pilocarpine (ophthalmic) is excreted in breast milk. The manufacturer recommends that caution be exercised when administering pilocarpine (ophthalmic) to nursing women.

Contraindications Hypersensitivity to pilocarpine or any component of the formulation; acute inflammatory disease of the anterior chamber of the eye

Warnings/Precautions May cause decreased visual acuity, especially at night or with reduced lighting.

Adverse Reactions

Cardiovascular: Hypertension, tachycardia

Dermatologic: Diaphoresis

Gastrointestinal: Diarrhea, nausea, salivation, vomiting

Ocular: Burning, ciliary spasm, conjunctival vascular congestion, corneal granularity, lacrimation, lens opacity, myopia, retinal detachment, supraorbital or temporal headache, visual acuity decreased

Respiratory: Bronchial spasm, pulmonary edema

Drug Interactions

Metabolism/Transport Effects Inhibits CYP2A6 (weak), CYP2E1 (weak)

Avoid Concomitant Use There are no known interactions where it is recommended to avoid concomitant use.

Increased Effect/Toxicity

The levels/effects of Pilocarpine (Ophthalmic) may be increased by: Acetylcholinesterase Inhibitors; Beta-Blockers

Decreased Effect There are no known significant interactions involving a decrease in effect.

Storage/Stability

Gel: Store at room temperature of 2°C to 27°C (36°F to 80°F); do not freeze. Avoid excessive heat.

Solution: Store at controlled room temperature of 15°C to 30°C (59°F to 86°F).

Isopto® Carpine solution: Store at 8°C to 27°C (46°F to 80°F).

Mechanism of Action Directly stimulates cholinergic receptors in the eye causing miosis (by contraction of the iris sphincter), loss of accommodation (by constriction of ciliary muscle), and lowering of intraocular pressure (with decreased resistance to aqueous humor outflow)

Pharmacodynamics

Ophthalmic solution instillation: Miosis:

Onset of action: Within 10-30 minutes

Duration: 4-8 hours

Intraocular pressure reduction:

Onset of action: 1 hour

Duration: 4-12 hours

Dosing: Usual Children and Adults:

Gel: 0.5" (1.3 cm) ribbon applied to lower conjunctival sac once daily at bedtime; adjust dosage as required to control elevated intraocular pressure

Solution: Instill 1-2 drops up to 6 times/day; adjust the concentration and frequency as required to control elevated intraocular pressure

To counteract the mydriatic effects of sympathomimetic agents: Instill 1 drop of a 1% solution in the affected eye

Administration

Gel: Instill gel into affected eye(s); close the eye for 1-2 minutes and instruct patient to roll the eyeball in all directions; avoid contact of bottle tip with eye or skin

Solution: Shake well before use; instill into affected eye(s); apply finger pressure to lacrimal sac during and for 1-2 minutes after instillation to decrease drainage into the nose and throat and minimize possible systemic absorption

Monitoring Parameters Intraocular pressure, funduscopic exam, visual field testing

Dosage Forms Excipient information presented when available (limited, particularly for generics); consult specific product labeling.

Gel, Ophthalmic, as hydrochloride:

Pilopine HS: 4% (4 g) [contains benzalkonium chloride, edetate disodium]

Solution, Ophthalmic, as hydrochloride:

Isopto Carpine: 1% (15 mL); 2% (15 mL); 4% (15 mL)

Generic: 1% (15 mL); 2% (15 mL); 4% (15 mL)

◆ **Pilocarpine Hydrochloride** *see* Pilocarpine (Ophthalmic) *on page 1701*

◆ **Pilocarpine Hydrochloride** *see* Pilocarpine (Systemic) *on page 1701*

◆ **Pilopine HS** *see* Pilocarpine (Ophthalmic) *on page 1701*

◆ **Pilopine HS® (Can)** *see* Pilocarpine (Ophthalmic) *on page 1701*

Pimecrolimus (pim e KROE li mus)

Medication Safety Issues

Sound-alike/look-alike issues:

Pimecrolimus may be confused with tacrolimus

High alert medication:

This medication is in a class the Institute for Safe Medication Practices (ISMP) includes among its list of drug classes that have a heightened risk of causing significant patient harm when used in error.

Related Information

Safe Handling of Hazardous Drugs *on page 2455*

Brand Names: US Elidel

Brand Names: Canada Elidel

Therapeutic Category Immunomodulating Agent, Topical

Generic Availability (US) No

Use Second-line agent for short-term and intermittent treatment of mild to moderate atopic dermatitis in nonimmunocompromised patients unresponsive to, or intolerant of other treatments

Medication Guide Available Yes

Pregnancy Risk Factor C

Pregnancy Considerations Adverse events were not observed in animal reproduction studies following topical application.

Breast-Feeding Considerations It is not known if pimecrolimus is excreted in breast milk. Due to the potential for serious adverse reactions in the nursing infant, the manufacturer recommends a decision be made whether to discontinue nursing or to discontinue the drug, taking into account the importance of treatment to the mother.

Contraindications Hypersensitivity to pimecrolimus or any component of the formulation

Warnings/Precautions Hazardous agent; use appropriate precautions for handling and disposal (meets NIOSH 2014 criteria). **[U.S. Boxed Warning]: Topical calcineurin inhibitors (including pimecrolimus) have been associated with rare cases of lymphoma and skin malignancy.** Avoid use on malignant or premalignant skin conditions (eg, cutaneous T-cell lymphoma). **[U.S. Boxed Warning]: Continuous long-term use of calcineurin inhibitors (including pimecrolimus) should be avoided and application of cream should be limited to areas of involvement with atopic dermatitis. Safety of intermittent use for >1 year has not been established.** Diagnosis should be reconfirmed if sign/symptoms do not improve within 6 weeks of treatment.

May cause local symptoms (eg, burning, pruritus, soreness, stinging) during first few days of treatment; usually self-resolving as atopic dermatitis lesions heal. Should not be used in immunocompromised patients, including patients on concomitant systemic immunosuppressive therapy. Patients with atopic dermatitis are predisposed to skin infections; therapy has been associated with an increased risk of developing eczema herpeticum, varicella zoster, and herpes simplex. Do not apply to areas of active bacterial or viral infection; local infections at the treatment site should be resolved prior to therapy. Skin papilloma (warts) have been observed with use; discontinue use if there is worsening of skin papillomas or they do not respond to conventional treatment. Pimecrolimus may be associated with development of lymphadenopathy; possible infectious causes should be investigated. Discontinue use in patients with unknown cause of lymphadenopathy or acute infectious mononucleosis. Not recommended for use in patients with skin disease which may increase the potential for systemic absorption (eg, Netherton's syndrome). Avoid artificial or natural sunlight exposure, even when pimecrolimus is not on the skin. Safety not established in patients with generalized erythroderma. **[U.S. Boxed Warning]: The use of pimecrolimus in children**

<2 years of age is not recommended, particularly since the effect on immune system development is unknown.

Benzyl alcohol and derivatives: Some dosage forms may contain benzyl alcohol; large amounts of benzyl alcohol (≥99 mg/kg/day) have been associated with a potentially fatal toxicity ("gasping syndrome") in neonates; the "gasping syndrome" consists of metabolic acidosis, respiratory distress, gasping respirations, CNS dysfunction (including convulsions, intracranial hemorrhage), hypotension, and cardiovascular collapse (AAP, 1997; CDC, 1982); some data suggests that benzoate displaces bilirubin from protein binding sites (Ahlfors, 2001); avoid or use dosage forms containing benzyl alcohol with caution in neonates. See manufacturer's labeling.

Warnings: Additional Pediatric Considerations Some dosage forms may contain propylene glycol; in neonates large amounts of propylene glycol delivered orally, intravenously (eg, >3,000 mg/day), or topically have been associated with potentially fatal toxicities which can include metabolic acidosis, seizures, renal failure, and CNS depression; toxicities have also been reported in children and adults including hyperosmolality, lactic acidosis, seizures, and respiratory depression; use caution (AAP, 1997; Shehab, 2009).

Adverse Reactions

Central nervous system: Fever (more common in children and adolescents), headache (more common in children and adolescents)

Dermatologic: Acne vulgaris, folliculitis (more common in adults), herpes simplex dermatitis, impetigo, molluscum contagiosum (children and adolescents), skin infection, urticaria, warts (children and adolescents)

Gastrointestinal: Abdominal pain, constipation (children and adolescents), diarrhea (more common in children and adolescents), gastroenteritis (more common in children and adolescents), nausea, toothache, vomiting

Genitourinary: Dysmenorrhea

Hypersensitivity: Hypersensitivity

Infection: Bacterial infection, herpes simplex infection, influenza, staphylococcal infection, varicella, viral infection (children and adolescents)

Local: Application site reaction (more common in adults), local burning (more common in adults; tends to resolve/improve as lesions resolve), local irritation (more common in adults), localized erythema, local pruritus

Neuromuscular & skeletal: Arthralgia, back pain

Ocular: Conjunctivitis, eye infection

Otic: Otic infection, otitis media

Respiratory: Asthma, asthma aggravated (children and adolescents), bronchitis (more common in children and adolescents), cough (more common in children and adolescents), dyspnea, epistaxis, flu-like symptoms, nasal congestion, nasopharyngitis (more common in infants, children, and adolescents), pharyngitis (more common in children and adolescents), pneumonia, rhinitis, rhinorrhea (children and adolescents), sinusitis, sore throat, streptococcal pharyngitis (children and adolescents), tonsillitis (more common in children and adolescents), upper respiratory tract infection (more common in children and adolescents), viral upper respiratory tract infection, wheezing (children and adolescents)

Miscellaneous: Laceration (children and adolescents)

Rare but important or life-threatening: Anaphylaxis, angioedema, eczema (herpeticum), lymphadenopathy, malignant neoplasm (basal cell carcinoma, squamous cell carcinoma, malignant melanoma, malignant lymphoma), skin discoloration

Drug Interactions

Metabolism/Transport Effects Substrate of CYP3A4 (minor); **Note:** Assignment of Major/Minor substrate status based on clinically relevant drug interaction potential

Avoid Concomitant Use

Avoid concomitant use of Pimecrolimus with any of the following: Immunosuppressants

Increased Effect/Toxicity

Pimecrolimus may increase the levels/effects of: Immunosuppressants

The levels/effects of Pimecrolimus may be increased by: CYP3A4 Inhibitors (Moderate); CYP3A4 Inhibitors (Strong)

Decreased Effect There are no known significant interactions involving a decrease in effect.

Storage/Stability Store at 25°C (77°F); excursions permitted to 15°C to 30°C (59°F to 86°F); do not freeze.

Mechanism of Action Penetrates inflamed epidermis to inhibit T cell activation by blocking transcription of proinflammatory cytokine genes such as interleukin-2, interferon gamma (Th1-type), interleukin-4, and interleukin-10 (Th2-type). Pimecrolimus binds to the intracellular protein FKBP-12, inhibiting calcineurin, which blocks cytokine transcription and inhibits T-cell activation. Prevents release of inflammatory cytokines and mediators from mast cells *in vitro* after stimulation by antigen/IgE.

Pharmacodynamics Onset of action: Time to significant improvement: 8 days

Pharmacokinetics (Adult data unless noted)

Absorption: Topical: Low systemic absorption; blood concentration of pimecrolimus was routinely <2 ng/mL with treatment of atopic dermatitis in adult patients (13% to 62% BSA involvement); blood concentration of pimecrolimus was <3 ng/mL in 26 pediatric patients 2-14 years of age with atopic dermatitis (20% to 69% BSA involvement). Detectable blood levels were observed in a higher proportion of children as compared to adults and may be due to the larger surface area to body mass ratio seen in pediatric patients.

Protein binding: 99.5%, primarily to various lipoproteins

Metabolism: In the liver by the cytochrome P450 3A4 system

Half-life: Terminal: 30-40 hours

Time to peak serum concentration: Topical: 2-6 hours

Elimination: 80% in the feces as metabolites

Dosing: Usual Children ≥2 years of age and Adults: Topical: Apply twice daily; use smallest amount of cream needed to control symptoms; continue therapy for as long as symptoms persist; re-evaluate patient at 6 weeks. **Note:** Pimecrolimus is not approved for use in children <2 years of age since the drug's long-term effect on the developing immune system is unknown. Detectable blood levels were observed in a higher proportion of children as compared to adults and may be due to the larger surface area to body mass ratio seen in pediatric patients. Children <2 years of age treated with pimecrolimus had a higher rate of upper respiratory infections than those treated with placebo.

Preparation for Administration Hazardous agent; use appropriate precautions for handling and disposal (meets NIOSH, 2014 criteria).

Administration Hazardous agent; use appropriate precautions for handling and disposal (meets NIOSH, 2014 criteria).

Topical: Avoid contact with eyes, nose, mouth, and cut, scraped, or infected skin areas. Wash hands with soap and water prior to and after cream application. If applying cream after a bath or shower, make sure skin is dry. Apply thin layer of cream by gently rubbing it in over affected skin surfaces which may include head and neck areas. The use of occlusive dressings is not recommended.

Monitoring Parameters Check skin for signs of worsening condition (increase in pruritus, erythema, excoriation, and lichenification)

Dosage Forms Excipient information presented when available (limited, particularly for generics); consult specific product labeling.

Cream, External:

Elidel: 1% (30 g, 60 g, 100 g) [contains benzyl alcohol, cetyl alcohol, propylene glycol]

Pimozide (PI moe zide)

Medication Safety Issues

BEERS Criteria medication:

This drug may be potentially inappropriate for use in geriatric patients (Quality of evidence - moderate; Strength of recommendation - strong).

Brand Names: US Orap

Brand Names: Canada Apo-Pimozide®; Orap®; PMS-Pimozide

Therapeutic Category First Generation (Typical) Antipsychotic

Generic Availability (US) No

Use Suppression of severe motor and phonic (vocal) tics in patients with Tourette's disorder who have failed to respond satisfactorily to standard treatment and whose daily life function and/or development is severely compromised by the presence of motor and phonic tics (FDA approved in ages ≥2 years and adults)

Note: A trial of standard treatment is currently recommended before a trial of pimozide because of pimozide's potential cardiac toxicity (Scahill, 2006).

Pregnancy Risk Factor C

Pregnancy Considerations Adverse events were observed in some animal reproduction studies. Antipsychotic use during the third trimester of pregnancy has a risk for abnormal muscle movements (extrapyramidal symptoms [EPS]) and withdrawal symptoms in newborns following delivery. Symptoms in the newborn may include agitation, feeding disorder, hypertonia, hypotonia, respiratory distress, somnolence, and tremor; these effects may be self-limiting or require hospitalization.

Breast-Feeding Considerations It is not known if pimozide is excreted in breast milk. Due to the potential for serious adverse reactions in the nursing infant, a decision should be made whether to discontinue nursing or to discontinue the drug, taking into account the importance of treatment to the mother.

Contraindications Hypersensitivity to pimozide or any component of the formulation; severe toxic CNS depression; coma; history of cardiac arrhythmias; congenital long QT syndrome; concurrent use with QTc-prolonging agents; hypokalemia or hypomagnesemia; concurrent use of drugs that are inhibitors of CYP3A4, including concurrent use of the azole antifungals itraconazole and ketoconazole, macrolide antibiotics (eg, clarithromycin or erythromycin [**Note:** The manufacturer lists azithromycin, dirithromycin, and troleandomycin in its list of contraindicated macrolides; however, azithromycin does not inhibit CYP3A4, but may interact with pimozide on the basis of QTc prolongation]), protease inhibitors (ie, atazanavir, indinavir, nelfinavir, ritonavir, saquinavir), citalopram, escitalopram, nefazodone, sertraline, and other less potent inhibitors of CYP3A4 (eg, fluvoxamine, zileuton); concurrent use with strong CYP2D6 inhibitors (eg, paroxetine); concurrent use with medications that may cause motor or phonic tics (eg, amphetamines, methylphenidate, pemoline) until it is determined if medications or Tourette's is causing tics; treatment of simple tics or tics other than Tourette's

Warnings/Precautions May alter cardiac conduction; life-threatening arrhythmias have occurred with therapeutic doses of antipsychotics. Contraindicated in patients with underlying QT prolongation, in those taking medicines that prolong the QT interval, or cause polymorphic ventricular tachycardia; monitor ECG closely for dose-related QT effects. Sudden unexplained deaths have occurred in patients taking high doses (~1 mg/kg).

Leukopenia, neutropenia, and agranulocytosis (sometimes fatal) have been reported in clinical trials and postmarketing reports with antipsychotic use; presence of risk factors (eg, pre-existing low WBC or history of drug-induced leuko-/neutropenia) should prompt periodic blood count assessment. Discontinue therapy at first signs of blood dyscrasias or if absolute neutrophil count <1000/mm^3.

Antipsychotic use has been associated with esophageal dysmotility and aspiration; use with caution in patients at risk of pneumonia (ie, Alzheimer's disease). May cause extrapyramidal symptoms, including pseudoparkinsonism, acute dystonic reactions, akathisia, and tardive dyskinesia. Risk of dystonia (and possibly other EPS) may be greater with increased doses, use of conventional antipsychotics, males, and younger patients. Risk of tardive dyskinesia and potential for irreversibility may be increased in elderly patients (particularly women), prolonged therapy, and higher total cumulative dose. Use may be associated with NMS; monitor for mental status changes, fever, muscle rigidity, and/or autonomic instability; may also be associated with increased CPK, myogloburia, and acute renal failure. Discontinue use; may recur upon rechallenge. May be associated with pigmentary retinopathy. Impaired core body temperature regulation may occur; caution with strenuous exercise, heat exposure, dehydration, and concomitant medication possessing anticholinergic effects.

May be sedating, use with caution in disorders where CNS depression is a feature; patients must be cautioned about performing tasks which require mental alertness (eg, operating machinery or driving). Effects may be potentiated when used with other sedative drugs or ethanol. May cause anticholinergic effects (constipation, xerostomia, blurred vision, urinary retention); use with caution in patients with decreased gastrointestinal motility, paralytic ileus, urinary retention, BPH, xerostomia, or visual problems. Relative to neuroleptics, pimozide has a moderate potency of cholinergic blockade. Antipsychotics are associated with increased prolactin levels; clinical significance of hyperprolactinemia in patients with breast cancer or other prolactin-dependent tumors is unknown.

Use with caution in patients with severe cardiovascular disease, narrow-angle glaucoma, hepatic impairment, Parkinson's disease, renal impairment, or seizure disorder. Use with caution in the elderly and in CYP2D6 poor metabolizers (dose adjustment required).

Use in patients with dementia is associated with an increased risk of mortality and cerebrovascular accidents; avoid antipsychotic use for behavioral problems associated with dementia unless alternative nonpharmacologic therapies have failed and patient may harm self or others. In addition, use may cause or exacerbate syndrome of inappropriate antidiuretic hormone secretion or hyponatremia; monitor sodium closely with initiation or dosage adjustments in older adults. May also be inappropriate in older adults depending on comorbidities (eg, dementia, delirium) due to its potent anticholinergic effects (Beers Criteria). Increased risk for developing tardive dyskinesia, particularly elderly women.

Warnings: Additional Pediatric Considerations Pimozide may have a tumorigenic potential; a dose related increase in pituitary tumors was observed in studies of mice; full significance in humans is unknown; however, this finding should be considered when deciding to use pimozide chronically in a young patient. Limited information exists about the use of pimozide in children <12 years of age.

Adverse Reactions

Cardiovascular: Abnormal ECG

Central nervous system: Akathisia, akinesia, behavior changes, depression, dreams abnormal, drowsiness, headache, hyperkinesias, insomnia, nervousness, sedation, somnolence
Dermatologic: Rash
Gastrointestinal: Appetite increased, constipation, diarrhea, dysphagia, salivation increased, taste disturbance, thirst, xerostomia
Genitourinary: Impotence
Neuromuscular & skeletal: Handwriting change, muscle tightness, myalgia, rigidity, stooped posture, torticollis, tremor, weakness
Ocular: Accommodation decreased, photophobia, visual disturbance
Rare but important or life-threatening (some reported for other than Tourette's disorder): Anorexia, blurred vision, cataracts, chest pain, diaphoresis, dizziness, excitement; extrapyramidal symptoms (dystonia, pseudoparkinsonism, tardive dyskinesia); GI distress, gingival hyperplasia (case report), hemolytic anemia, hyper-/hypotension, hyponatremia, libido decreased, nausea, neuroleptic malignant syndrome, orthostatic hypotension, nocturia, palpitation, periorbital edema, polyuria, QTc prolongation, seizure, skin irritation, syncope, tachycardia, ventricular arrhythmia, vomiting, weight gain/loss

Drug Interactions

Metabolism/Transport Effects Substrate of CYP1A2 (major), CYP2D6 (major), CYP3A4 (major); **Note:** Assignment of Major/Minor substrate status based on clinically relevant drug interaction potential; **Inhibits** CYP2C19 (weak), CYP2D6 (weak), CYP2E1 (weak)

Avoid Concomitant Use

Avoid concomitant use of Pimozide with any of the following: Aclidinium; Amisulpride; Antifungal Agents (Azole Derivatives, Systemic); Aprepitant; Azelastine (Nasal); Boceprevir; Conivaptan; Crizotinib; CYP2D6 Inhibitors (Strong); CYP3A4 Inhibitors (Moderate); CYP3A4 Inhibitors (Strong); CYP3A4 Inhibitors (Weak); Eluxadoline; Enzalutamide; FLUoxetine; Fosaprepitant; Fusidic Acid (Systemic); Glucagon; Grapefruit Juice; Highest Risk QTc-Prolonging Agents; Idelalisib; Ipratropium (Oral Inhalation); Ivabradine; Macrolide Antibiotics; Metoclopramide; Mifepristone; Moderate Risk QTc-Prolonging Agents; Nefazodone; Orphenadrine; Paraldehyde; Potassium Chloride; Protease Inhibitors; Selective Serotonin Reuptake Inhibitors; Sulpiride; Telaprevir; Thalidomide; Tiotropium; Umeclidinium; Zileuton

Increased Effect/Toxicity

Pimozide may increase the levels/effects of: AbobotulinumtoxinA; Alcohol (Ethyl); Amisulpride; Analgesics (Opioid); Anticholinergic Agents; Azelastine (Nasal); Buprenorphine; CNS Depressants; Eluxadoline; Glucagon; Highest Risk QTc-Prolonging Agents; Hydrocodone; Methylphenidate; Metyrosine; OnabotulinumtoxinA; Orphenadrine; Paraldehyde; Potassium Chloride; RimabotulinumtoxinB; Serotonin Modulators; Sulpiride; Suvorexant; Thalidomide; Thiazide Diuretics; Tiotropium; Topiramate; Zolpidem

The levels/effects of Pimozide may be increased by: Abiraterone Acetate; Acetylcholinesterase Inhibitors (Central); Aclidinium; Antifungal Agents (Azole Derivatives, Systemic); Aprepitant; Boceprevir; Brimonidine (Topical); Cannabis; Conivaptan; Crizotinib; CYP1A2 Inhibitors (Moderate); CYP1A2 Inhibitors (Strong); CYP2D6 Inhibitors (Moderate); CYP2D6 Inhibitors (Strong); CYP3A4 Inhibitors (Moderate); CYP3A4 Inhibitors (Strong); CYP3A4 Inhibitors (Weak); Deferasirox; Doxylamine; Dronabinol; FLUoxetine; Fosaprepitant; Fusidic Acid (Systemic); Grapefruit Juice; Idelalisib; Ipratropium (Oral Inhalation); Ivabradine; Kava Kava; Luliconazole; Macrolide Antibiotics; Magnesium Sulfate; Methylphenidate; Metoclopramide; Metyrosine; Mifepristone; Moderate Risk QTc-Prolonging Agents; Nabilone; Nefazodone; Peginterferon Alfa-2b; Perampanel; Pramlintide; Protease Inhibitors; QTc-Prolonging Agents (Indeterminate Risk and Risk Modifying); Rufinamide; Selective Serotonin Reuptake Inhibitors; Serotonin Modulators; Simeprevir; Sodium Oxybate; Tapentadol; Telaprevir; Tetrahydrocannabinol; Umeclidinium; Zileuton

Decreased Effect

Pimozide may decrease the levels/effects of: Acetylcholinesterase Inhibitors; Amphetamines; Anti-Parkinson's Agents (Dopamine Agonist); Itopride; Quinagolide; Secretin

The levels/effects of Pimozide may be decreased by: Acetylcholinesterase Inhibitors; Anti-Parkinson's Agents (Dopamine Agonist); Bosentan; Cannabis; CYP1A2 Inducers (Strong); CYP3A4 Inducers (Moderate); CYP3A4 Inducers (Strong); Cyproterone; Dabrafenib; Deferasirox; Enzalutamide; Mitotane; Peginterferon Alfa-2b; Siltuximab; St Johns Wort; Teriflunomide; Tocilizumab

Food Interactions Pimozide serum concentration may be increased when taken with grapefruit juice due to CYP3A4 inhibition. Management: Avoid concurrent use with grapefruit juice.

Storage/Stability Store at 25°C (77°F); excursion permitted to 15°C to 30°C (59°F to 86°F).

Mechanism of Action Pimozide, a diphenylbutylperidine conventional antipsychotic, is a potent centrally-acting dopamine-receptor antagonist resulting in its characteristic neuroleptic effects

Pharmacodynamics Onset of action: Within one week
Maximum effect: 4-6 weeks
Duration: Variable

Pharmacokinetics (Adult data unless noted)

Absorption: Oral: >50%
Protein binding: 99%
Metabolism: Hepatic via N-dealkylation primarily by CYP3A4, but with contributions by CYP1A2 and CYP2D6; significant first-pass effect
Half-life:
Tourette's disorder (Sallee, 1987):
Children 6-13 years (n=4): Mean ± SD: 66 ± 49 hours
Adults 23-39 years (n=7): Mean ± SD: 111 ± 57 hours
Schizophrenia: Adults: Mean: 55 hours
Time to peak serum concentration: 6-8 hours; range: 4-12 hours
Elimination: Urine

Dosing: Usual Note: Slow titration is recommended to improve tolerability; use lowest effective dose. An ECG should be performed baseline and periodically thereafter, especially during dosage adjustment.

Children and Adolescents: **Tourette's disorder:** Oral: Manufacturer's labeling: Children ≥2 years and Adolescents: Initial: 0.05 mg/kg/dose (maximum dose: 1 mg) once daily, preferably at bedtime; may increase dose every third day if needed; maximum daily dose: 0.2 mg/kg/**day** not to exceed 10 mg/**day**; in pediatric trials of children ≥7 years old, reported mean effective dose: 2.4-3.4 mg/day (range: 1-6 mg) (Gilbert, 2004; Sallee, 1997). **Note:** If therapy requires exceeding dose of 0.05 mg/kg/**day**, CYP2D6 geno-/phenotyping should be performed; CYP2D6 poor metabolizers should be dose titrated in ≥14-day increments and should not receive doses in excess of 0.05 mg/kg/**day**.

Adults: **Tourette's disorder:** Oral: Initial: 1-2 mg/day in divided doses, then increase dose as needed every other day; maximum daily dose: 10 mg/**day** or 0.2 mg/kg/**day** (whichever is less). **Note:** If therapy requires exceeding dose of 4 mg/day, CYP2D6 geno-/phenotyping should be performed; CYP2D6 poor metabolizers should be dose titrated in ≥14-day increments and should not receive doses in excess of 4 mg/**day**.

Dosing adjustment in renal impairment: Children ≥2 years, Adolescents, and Adults: There are no dosage adjustments provided in the manufacturer's labeling; use with caution.

Dosing adjustment in hepatic impairment: Children ≥ 2 years, Adolescents, and Adults: There are no dosage adjustments provided in the manufacturer's labeling; use with caution.

Dosing adjustment for toxicity: Children ≥ 2 years, Adolescents, and Adults:

ECG changes:

Children: QTc prolongation >0.47 seconds or >25% above baseline: Decrease dose.

Adults: QTc prolongation >0.52 seconds or >25% above baseline: Decrease dose.

Neuroleptic malignant syndrome: Discontinue; monitor carefully if therapy is reinitiated.

Tardive dyskinesia signs/symptoms: Consider discontinuing.

Administration May be administered without regard to meals.

Monitoring Parameters ECG should be performed at baseline and periodically thereafter, especially during dosage adjustment; vital signs; serum potassium; magnesium, sodium; renal and hepatic function; height, weight, BMI; mental status, abnormal involuntary movement scale (AIMS), extrapyramidal symptoms (EPS) screening; CBC with differential (patients with a history of low WBC or drug-induced leukopenia or neutropenia)

Test Interactions Increased prolactin (S)

Dosage Forms Excipient information presented when available (limited, particularly for generics); consult specific product labeling.

Tablet, Oral:

Orap: 1 mg, 2 mg [scored]

- **Pin-X [OTC]** *see* Pyrantel Pamoate *on page* *1806*
- **Pink Bismuth** *see* Bismuth Subsalicylate *on page* *290*
- **Pink Bismuth [OTC]** *see* Bismuth Subsalicylate *on page* *290*
- **Pinnacaine Otic** *see* Benzocaine *on page* *268*

Piperacillin and Tazobactam

(pi PER a sil in & ta zoe BAK tam)

Medication Safety Issues

Sound-alike/look-alike issues:

Zosyn may be confused with Zofran, Zyvox

International issues:

Tazact [India] may be confused with Tazac brand name for nizatidine [Australia]; Tiazac brand name for diltiazem [U.S., Canada]

Brand Names: US Zosyn

Brand Names: Canada AJ-PIP/TAZ; Piperacillin and Tazobactam for Injection; Tazocin

Therapeutic Category Antibiotic, Beta-lactam and Beta-lactamase Inhibitor Combination; Antibiotic, Penicillin (Antipseudomonal)

Generic Availability (US) Yes: Excludes infusion

Use Treatment of moderate to severe infections caused by susceptible organisms (FDA approved in ages ≥2 months and adults); including sepsis, postpartum endometritis or pelvic inflammatory disease, intra-abdominal infections, uncomplicated or complicated infections involving skin and skin structures, moderate severity community-acquired pneumonia, and moderate to severe nosocomial pneumonia. Tazobactam expands activity of piperacillin to include beta-lactamase producing strains of *S. aureus*, *H. influenzae*, *B. fragilis*, *Klebsiella*, *E. coli*, and *Acinetobacter*. When piperacillin and tazobactam is used to treat nosocomial pneumonia caused by *P. aeruginosa*, combination therapy with an aminoglycoside is recommended.

Pregnancy Risk Factor B

Pregnancy Considerations Adverse events have not been observed in animal reproduction studies. Piperacillin and tazobactam both cross the placenta and are found in the fetal serum, placenta, amniotic fluid, and fetal urine. When used during pregnancy, the clearance and volume of distribution of piperacillin/tazobactam are increased; half-life and AUC are decreased (Bourget, 1998). Piperacillin/tazobactam is approved for the treatment of postpartum gynecologic infections, including endometritis or pelvic inflammatory disease, caused by susceptible organisms.

Breast-Feeding Considerations Low concentrations of piperacillin are excreted in breast milk; information for tazobactam is not available. The manufacturer recommends that caution be used when administering piperacillin/tazobactam to nursing women. Nondose-related effects could include modification of bowel flora.

Contraindications Hypersensitivity to penicillins, cephalosporins, beta-lactamase inhibitors, or any component of the formulation

Warnings/Precautions Serious and occasionally severe or fatal hypersensitivity (anaphylactic/anaphylactoid) reactions have been reported in patients on penicillin therapy, especially with a history of beta-lactam hypersensitivity, history of sensitivity to multiple allergens, or previous IgE-mediated reactions (eg, anaphylaxis, angioedema, urticaria). Serious skin reactions, including toxic epidermal necrolysis (TEN) and Stevens-Johnson syndrome (SJS), have been reported. If a skin rash develops, monitor closely. Discontinue if lesions progress.

Bleeding disorders have been observed, particularly in patients with renal impairment; discontinue if thrombocytopenia or bleeding occurs. Leukopenia/neutropenia may occur; appears to be reversible and most frequently associated with prolonged administration. Assess hematologic parameters periodically, especially with prolonged (≥21 days) use.

Assess electrolytes periodically in patients with low potassium reserves, especially those receiving cytotoxic therapy or diuretics. Due to sodium load and to the adverse effects of high serum concentrations of penicillins, dosage modification is required in patients with impaired or underdeveloped renal function; use with caution in patients with seizures or in patients with history of beta-lactam allergy; associated with an increased incidence of rash and fever in cystic fibrosis patients. Use may result in fungal or bacterial superinfection, including *C. difficile*-associated diarrhea (CDAD) and pseudomembranous colitis; CDAD has been observed >2 months postantibiotic treatment.

Potentially significant drug-drug interactions may exist, requiring dose or frequency adjustment, additional monitoring, and/or selection of alternative therapy.

Adverse Reactions

Cardiovascular: Chest pain, edema, hypertension, phlebitis

Central nervous system: Agitation, anxiety, dizziness, headache, insomnia, pain

Dermatologic: Pruritus, skin rash

Gastrointestinal: Abdominal pain, change in stool, constipation, diarrhea, dyspepsia, nausea, oral candidiasis, vomiting

Hepatic: Increased serum AST

Local: Local irritation

Infection: Abscess, candidiasis, infection, sepsis

Respiratory: Dyspnea, pharyngitis, rhinitis

Miscellaneous: Fever

Rare but important or life-threatening: Agranulocytosis, anaphylactoid reaction, anaphylaxis, anemia, aphthous stomatitis, atrial fibrillation, bradycardia, cardiac arrest, cardiac arrhythmia, cardiac failure, change in platelet count, cholestatic jaundice, circulatory arrest, *Clostridium difficile* associated diarrhea, confusion, convulsions, decreased hematocrit, decreased hemoglobin, decreased serum albumin, depression, dysgeusia, dysuria, electrolyte disturbance, eosinophilia, epistaxis, erythema multiforme, gastritis, genital pruritus, hallucination, hematuria, hemolytic anemia, hemorrhage, hepatitis, hiccups, hyperglycemia, hypersensitivity reaction, hypoglycemia, increased blood glucose, increased blood urea nitrogen, increased gamma-glutamyl transferase, increased serum alkaline phosphatase, increased serum ALT, increased serum AST, increased serum bilirubin, increased serum creatinine, increased thirst, inflammation, interstitial nephritis, intestinal obstruction, leukopenia, leukorrhea, melena, mesenteric embolism, myalgia, myocardial infarction, neutropenia, oliguria, pancytopenia, photophobia, positive direct Coombs test, prolonged partial thromboplastin time, prolonged prothrombin time, pulmonary edema, pulmonary embolism, purpura, renal failure, rigors, Stevens-Johnson syndrome, supraventricular tachycardia, syncope, thrombocythemia, thrombocytopenia, thrombophlebitis, toxic epidermal necrolysis, urinary incontinence, urinary retention, vaginitis, ventricular fibrillation, ventricular tachycardia

Drug Interactions

Metabolism/Transport Effects None known.

Avoid Concomitant Use

Avoid concomitant use of Piperacillin and Tazobactam with any of the following: BCG; BCG (Intravesical); Probenecid

Increased Effect/Toxicity

Piperacillin and Tazobactam may increase the levels/effects of: Flucloxacillin [Floxacillin]; Methotrexate; Vancomycin; Vecuronium; Vitamin K Antagonists

The levels/effects of Piperacillin and Tazobactam may be increased by: Probenecid

Decreased Effect

Piperacillin and Tazobactam may decrease the levels/effects of: Aminoglycosides; BCG; BCG (Intravesical); BCG Vaccine (Immunization); Mycophenolate; Sodium Picosulfate; Typhoid Vaccine

The levels/effects of Piperacillin and Tazobactam may be decreased by: Tetracycline Derivatives

Storage/Stability

Vials: Store at 20°C to 25°C (68°F to 77°F) prior to reconstitution. Use single-dose or bulk vials immediately after reconstitution. Discard any unused portion after 24 hours if stored at 20°C to 25°C (68°F to 77°F) or after 48 hours if stored refrigerated (2°C to 8°C [36°F to 46°F]). Do not freeze vials after reconstitution. Stability in IV bags has been demonstrated for up to 24 hours at room temperature and up to 1 week at refrigerated temperature. Stability in an ambulatory IV infusion pump has been demonstrated for a period of 12 hours at room temperature.

Galaxy containers: Store at or below -20°C (-4°F). The thawed solution is stable for 14 days under refrigeration (2°C to 8°C [36°F to 46°F]) or 24 hours at 20°C to 25°C (68°F to 77°F). Do not refreeze.

Mechanism of Action Piperacillin inhibits bacterial cell wall synthesis by binding to one or more of the penicillin-binding proteins (PBPs); which in turn inhibits the final transpeptidation step of peptidoglycan synthesis in bacterial cell walls, thus inhibiting cell wall biosynthesis. Bacteria eventually lyse due to ongoing activity of cell wall autolytic enzymes (autolysins and murein hydrolases) while cell wall assembly is arrested. Piperacillin exhibits time-dependent killing. Tazobactam inhibits many beta-lactamases, including staphylococcal penicillinase and Richmond-Sykes types 2, 3, 4, and 5, including extended spectrum enzymes; it has only limited activity against class 1 beta-lactamases other than class 1C types.

Pharmacokinetics (Adult data unless noted) Both AUC and peak concentrations are dose proportional

Distribution: Widely distributed into tissues and body fluids including lungs, intestinal mucosa, female reproductive tissues, interstitial fluid, gallbladder, and bile; penetration into CSF is poor when meninges are uninflamed

- V_d: Children and Adults: 0.243 L/kg

Protein binding:

- Piperacillin: ~26% to 33%
- Tazobactam: 31% to 32%

Metabolism:

- Piperacillin: 6% to 9% to desethyl metabolite (weak activity)
- Tazobactam: ~22% to inactive metabolite

Bioavailability: IM:

- Piperacillin: 71%
- Tazobactam: 84%

Half-life (Pediatric data: Reed 1994):

- Piperacillin:
  - Infants 2 to 5 months: 1.4 hours
  - Children 6 to 23 months: 0.9 hour
  - Children 2 to 12 years: 0.7 hour
  - Adults: 0.7 to 1.2 hours
- Metabolite: 1 to 1.5 hours
- Tazobactam:
  - Infants 2 to 5 months: 1.6 hours
  - Children 6 to 23 months: 1 hour
  - Children 2 to 12 years: 0.8-0.9 hour
  - Adults: 0.7 to 0.9 hour

Elimination: Piperacillin and tazobactam are both eliminated by renal tubular secretion and glomerular filtration. Piperacillin, tazobactam, and desethylpiperacillin are also secreted into bile.

- Piperacillin: 50% to 70% eliminated unchanged in urine
- Tazobactam: Found in urine at 24 hours, with 20% as the inactive metabolite and 80% as unchanged drug
- Clearance: Children 9 months to 12 years: 5.64 mL/minute/kg

Dosing: Neonatal Note: Zosyn (piperacillin and tazobactam) is a combination product; each 3.375 g vial contains 3 g piperacillin sodium and 0.375 g tazobactam sodium in an 8:1 ratio. Dosage recommendations are based on the **piperacillin** component.

General dosing, susceptible infection:

Weight-directed dosing (*Red Book*, 2012): IV:

- Body weight <1 kg:
  - PNA ≤14 days: 100 mg piperacillin/kg/dose every 12 hours
  - PNA 15 to 28 days: 100 mg piperacillin/kg/dose every 8 hours
- Body weight ≥1 kg:
  - PNA ≤7 days: 100 mg piperacillin/kg/dose every 12 hours
  - PNA 8 to 28 days: 100 mg piperacillin/kg/dose every 8 hours

Age-directed dosing: **Note:** Limited data available, positive efficacy results, dosage regimens variable, dosing partially extrapolated from piperacillin data (Kacet 1992)

- GA <36 weeks:
  - PNA 0 to 7 days: 75 mg piperacillin/kg/dose every 12 hours
  - PNA 8 to 28 days: 75 mg piperacillin/kg/dose every 8 hours
  - Meningitis: PNA 0 to 7 days: 200 mg piperacillin/kg/dose every 12 hours was used in two neonates (GA: 31, 35 weeks) (Placzek 1983)
- GA ≥36 weeks:
  - PNA 0 to 7 days: 75 mg piperacillin/kg/dose every 8 hours
  - PNA 8 to 28 days: 75 mg piperacillin/kg/dose every 6 hours

Dosing: Usual

Pediatric: **Note:** Zosyn (piperacillin and tazobactam) is a combination product; each 3.375 g vial contains 3 g piperacillin sodium and 0.375 g tazobactam sodium in an 8:1 ratio. Dosage recommendations are based on the **piperacillin** component. **Note:** Some centers divide doses every 6 hours for enhanced pharmacodynamic profile. Unless otherwise specified, dosing presented is based on traditional infusion method (IV infusion over 30 minutes). Dosing is presented in mg/kg/dose and mg/kg/day; use precaution.

General dosing, susceptible infection (*Red Book* [AAP] 2012): IV: Severe infection:

Infants <2 months: 100 mg piperacillin/kg/dose every 6 hours (Bradley 2014)

Infants 2 to 9 months: 80 mg piperacillin/kg/dose every 8 hours

Infants >9 months, Children, and Adolescents: 100 mg piperacillin/kg/dose every 8 hours; maximum daily dose: 16 g piperacillin/**day**

Appendicitis and/or peritonitis: IV:

Infants 2 to 9 months: 80 mg of piperacillin/kg/dose every 8 hours

Infants >9 months and Children weighing ≤40 kg: 100 mg piperacillin/kg/dose every 8 hours; maximum dose: 3,000 mg piperacillin/dose

Children weighing >40 kg and Adolescents: 3,000 mg piperacillin every 6 hours; maximum daily dose: 16 g piperacillin/**day**

Cystic fibrosis, pseudomonal lung infection: Infants, Children, and Adolescents: **Note:** Multiple dosing approaches have been evaluated; optimal dose may vary based on disease severity, susceptibility patterns (eg, MIC), or patient tolerability:

Standard dosing range: IV: 240 to 400 mg piperacillin/kg/**day** divided every 8 hours (Kliegman 2011); others have used 350 to 400 mg/kg/**day** divided every 4 hours in early piperacillin trials (Zobell 2013)

High-dose: Limited data available: IV: 450 mg piperacillin/kg/**day** every 4 to 6 hours or 600 mg piperacillin/kg/**day** divided every 4 hours has been described from early studies of piperacillin alone; usual maximum daily dose: 18 to 24 g piperacillin/**day**. **Note:** Piperacillin doses >600 mg/kg/day or an extended duration of therapy (>14 days) have been associated with dose-related adverse effects including serum sickness, immune-mediated hemolytic anemia and bone marrow suppression (Zobell 2013).

Intra-abdominal infection, complicated: Infants, Children, and Adolescents: IV: 200 to 300 mg piperacillin/kg/day divided every 6 to 8 hours; maximum daily dose: 12 g piperacillin/**day** (Solomkin 2010)

Surgical antimicrobial prophylaxis (Bratzler, 2013): IV:

Infants 2 to 9 months: 80 mg piperacillin/kg 30 to 60 minutes prior to procedure; may repeat in 2 hours

Infants >9 months, Children, and Adolescents weighing ≤40 kg: 100 mg piperacillin/kg 30 to 60 minutes prior to procedure; may repeat in 2 hours. Maximum dose: 3,000 mg piperacillin/dose

Adolescents weighing >40 kg: 3000 mg piperacillin 30 to 60 minutes prior to procedure; may repeat in 2 hours

Extended-infusion method: Limited data available: Children and Adolescents: IV: 100 mg piperacillin/kg/dose infused over 4 hours 3 times daily. Dosing based on a prospective, observational study (n=332) in a single children's hospital comparing the extended interval method to traditional dosing (Nichols 2012).

Adult: **Note:** Dosing expressed as total dose of combination product (piperacillin/tazobactam); dosing presented is based on traditional infusion method (IV infusion over 30 minutes) unless otherwise specified as the extended infusion method (IV infusion over 4 hours)

General dosing, susceptible infection: IV: 3.375 **g** (3,000 mg piperacillin/375 mg tazobactam) every 6 hours or 4.5 g (4,000 mg piperacillin/500 mg tazobactam) every 6 to 8 hours; maximum: 16 g piperacillin/day

Diverticulitis, intra-abdominal abscess, peritonitis: IV: 3.375 **g** every 6 hours; **Note:** Some clinicians use 4.5 **g** every 8 hours for empiric coverage since the % time>MIC is similar between the regimens for most pathogens; however, this regimen is **not** recommended for nosocomial pneumonia or *Pseudomonas* coverage.

Pneumonia, nosocomial: IV: 4.5 **g** every 6 hours for 7 to 14 days (when used empirically, combination with an aminoglycoside or antipseudomonal fluoroquinolone is recommended; consider discontinuation of additional agent if *P. aeruginosa* is not isolated)

Skin and soft tissue infection: IV: 3.375 **g** every 6 to 8 hours for 7 to 14 days. **Notes:** When used for necrotizing infection of skin, fascia, or muscle, combination with clindamycin and ciprofloxacin is recommended (Stevens 2005); for severe diabetic foot infections, recommended treatment duration is up to 4 weeks depending on severity of infection and response to therapy (Lipsky, 2012).

Dosing adjustment in renal impairment:

Infants, Children, and Adolescents: There are no dosage adjustments provided in the manufacturer's labeling; however, the following have been used by some clinicians (Aronoff 2007): **Note:** Dosage recommendations are based on the piperacillin component. Dosing based on a usual dose of 200 to 300 mg piperacillin kg/day in divided doses every 6 hours.

GFR >50 mL/minute/1.73 m^2: No adjustment required

GFR 30 to 50 mL/minute/1.73 m^2: 35 to 50 mg piperacillin/kg/dose every 6 hours

GFR <30 mL/minute/1.73 m^2: 35 to 50 mg piperacillin/kg/dose every 8 hours

Intermittent hemodialysis (IHD): Hemodialysis removes 30% to 40% of a piperacillin/tazobactam dose: 50 to 75 mg piperacillin/kg/dose every 12 hours

Peritoneal dialysis (PD): Peritoneal dialysis removes 21% of tazobactam and 6% of piperacillin: 50 to 75 mg piperacillin/kg/dose every 12 hours

Continuous renal replacement therapy (CRRT): 35 to 50 mg piperacillin kg/dose every 8 hours

Adults: **Note:** Dosing expressed as total dose of combination product (piperacillin/tazobactam).

Traditional infusion method (ie, IV infusion over 30 minutes): Manufacturer's labeling:

Nosocomial pneumonia:

CrCl >40 mL/minute: No adjustment needed

CrCl 20 to 40 mL/minute: 3.375 **g** every 6 hours

CrCl <20 mL/minute: 2.25 **g** every 6 hours

Hemodialysis: 2.25 **g** every 8 hours with an additional dose of 0.75 **g** after each dialysis

CAPD: Adults: 2.25 **g** every 8 hours

All other indications:

CrCl >40 mL/minute: No adjustment needed

CrCl 20 to 40 mL/minute: 2.25 **g** every 6 hours

CrCl <20 mL/minute: 2.25 **g** every 8 hours

Hemodialysis: Hemodialysis removes 30% to 40% of a piperacillin/tazobactam dose: 2.25 **g** every 12 hours with an additional dose of 0.75 **g** after each dialysis

CAPD: Peritoneal dialysis removes 21% of tazobactam and 6% of piperacillin: 2.25 **g** every 12 hours

Dosing adjustment in hepatic impairment: No dosing adjustment required

Preparation for Administration

Parenteral:

Reconstitution:

Single-dose vials: Reconstitute with 5 mL of diluent (NS, D_5W, or SWFI) per 1,000 mg of piperacillin to yield a concentration of piperacillin 200 mg/mL and tazobactam 25 mg/mL

Pharmacy bulk vial: Reconstitute with 152 mL of diluent (NS, D_5W or SWFI) to yield a concentration of piperacillin 200 mg/mL and tazobactam 25 mg/mL

Intermittent IV infusion: Further dilute dose in a volume of 50 to 150 mL for a usual final concentration of piperacillin 20 to 80 mg/mL; dilution of doses in volumes as low 25 or 37.5 mL have been used in ambulatory infusion pumps

Administration

Parenteral:

Intermittent IV infusion: Administer over 30 minutes

Extended IV infusion: Administration over 3 to 4 hours has been reported in pediatric and adult patients (Kim 2007; Nichols 2012; Shea 2009).

Some penicillins (eg, carbenicillin, ticarcillin, and piperacillin) have been shown to inactivate aminoglycosides *in vitro*. This has been observed to a greater extent with tobramycin and gentamicin, while amikacin has shown greater stability against inactivation. Concurrent use of these agents may pose a risk of reduced antibacterial efficacy *in vivo*, particularly in the setting of profound renal impairment. However, definitive clinical evidence is lacking. If combination penicillin/aminoglycoside therapy is desired in a patient with renal dysfunction, separation of doses (if feasible), and routine monitoring of aminoglycoside levels, CBC, and clinical response should be considered. **Note:** Reformulated Zosyn containing EDTA has been shown to be compatible *in vitro* for Y-site infusion with amikacin and gentamicin diluted in NS or D_5W (applies **only** to specific concentrations and varies by product; consult manufacturer's labeling). Reformulated Zosyn containing EDTA is **not** compatible with tobramycin.

Monitoring Parameters Serum electrolytes, bleeding time especially in patients with renal impairment; periodic tests of renal, hepatic, and hematologic function; observe for changes in bowel frequency, CBC with differential; monitor for signs of anaphylaxis during first dose

Test Interactions Positive Coombs' [direct] test; false positive reaction for urine glucose using copper-reduction method (Clinitest); may result in false positive results with the Platelia *Aspergillus* enzyme immunoassay (EIA)

Some penicillin derivatives may accelerate the degradation of aminoglycosides *in vitro*, leading to a potential underestimation of aminoglycoside serum concentration. **Note:** Reformulated Zosyn containing EDTA has been shown to be compatible *in vitro* for Y-site infusion with amikacin and gentamicin diluted in NS or D_5W (applies **only** to specific concentrations and varies by product; consult manufacturer's labeling). Reformulated Zosyn containing EDTA is **not** compatible with tobramycin.

Additional Information Some penicillins (eg, carbenicillin, ticarcillin, and piperacillin) have been shown to inactivate aminoglycosides *in vitro*. This has been observed to a greater extent with tobramycin and gentamicin, while amikacin has shown greater stability against inactivation. Concurrent use of these agents may pose a risk of reduced antibacterial efficacy *in vivo*, particularly in the setting of profound renal impairment. However, definitive clinical evidence is lacking. If combination penicillin/aminoglycoside therapy is desired in a patient with renal dysfunction, separation of doses (if feasible), and routine monitoring of aminoglycoside levels, CBC, and clinical response should be considered. **Note:** Reformulated Zosyn® containing EDTA has been shown to be compatible *in vitro* for Y-site infusion with amikacin and gentamicin diluted in NS or D_5W (applies only to specific concentrations and varies by product; consult manufacturer's labeling). Reformulated Zosyn® containing EDTA is not compatible with tobramycin.

Dosage Forms Excipient information presented when available (limited, particularly for generics); consult specific product labeling.

Note: 8:1 ratio of piperacillin sodium/tazobactam sodium

Infusion [premixed iso-osmotic solution]:

Zosyn: 2.25 g: Piperacillin 2 g and tazobactam 0.25 g (50 mL) [contains edetate disodium, sodium 128 mg (5.58 mEq)]

Zosyn: 3.375 g: Piperacillin 3 g and tazobactam 0.375 g (50 mL) [contains edetate disodium, sodium 192 mg (8.38 mEq)]

Zosyn: 4.5 g: Piperacillin 4 g and tazobactam 0.5 g (100 mL) [contains edetate disodium, sodium 256 mg (11.17 mEq)]

Injection, powder for reconstitution: 2.25 g: Piperacillin 2 g and tazobactam 0.25 g; 3.375 g: Piperacillin 3 g and tazobactam 0.375 g; 4.5 g: Piperacillin 4 g and tazobactam 0.5 g; 40.5 g: Piperacillin 36 g and tazobactam 4.5 g

Zosyn: 2.25 g: Piperacillin 2 g and tazobactam 0.25 g [contains edetate disodium, sodium 128 mg (5.58 mEq)]

Zosyn: 3.375 g: Piperacillin 3 g and tazobactam 0.375 g [contains edetate disodium, sodium 192 mg (8.38 mEq)]

Zosyn: 4.5 g: Piperacillin 4 g and tazobactam 0.5 g [contains edetate disodium, sodium 256 mg (11.17 mEq)]

Zosyn: 40.5 g: Piperacillin 36 g and tazobactam 4.5 g [contains edetate disodium, sodium 2304 mg (100.4 mEq); bulk pharmacy vial]

◆ **Piperacillin and Tazobactam for Injection (Can)** *see* Piperacillin and Tazobactam *on page 1706*

◆ **Piperacillin and Tazobactam Sodium** *see* Piperacillin and Tazobactam *on page 1706*

◆ **Piperacillin Sodium and Tazobactam Sodium** *see* Piperacillin and Tazobactam *on page 1706*

Pirbuterol (peer BYOO ter ole)

Brand Names: US Maxair Autohaler [DSC]

Therapeutic Category Adrenergic Agonist Agent; Antiasthmatic; $Beta_2$-Adrenergic Agonist; Bronchodilator; Sympathomimetic

Generic Availability (US) No

Use Prevention and treatment of bronchospasm in patients with reversible airway obstruction due to asthma or COPD

Pregnancy Risk Factor C

Pregnancy Considerations Adverse events have been observed in some animal reproduction studies. Beta-agonists may interfere with uterine contractility if administered during labor.

Uncontrolled asthma is associated with adverse events on pregnancy (increased risk of perinatal mortality, preeclampsia, preterm birth, low birth weight infants). Other $beta_2$-receptor agonists are preferred for the treatment of asthma during pregnancy (NAEPP, 2005).

Breast-Feeding Considerations It is not known if pirbuterol is excreted into breast milk. The manufacturer recommends that pirbuterol be used in breast-feeding women only if the potential benefit to the mother outweighs the possible risk to the infant. The use of $beta_2$-receptor agonists are not considered a contraindication to breastfeeding (NAEPP, 2005).

Contraindications Hypersensitivity to pirbuterol or any component of the formulation

Warnings/Precautions Optimize anti-inflammatory treatment before initiating maintenance treatment with pirbuterol. Do not use as a component of chronic therapy without an anti-inflammatory agent. Only the mildest form of asthma (Step 1 and/or exercise-induced) would not require concurrent use based upon asthma guidelines. Patient must be instructed to seek medical attention in cases where acute symptoms are not relieved or a previous level of response is diminished. The need to increase frequency of use may indicate deterioration of asthma, and treatment must not be delayed.

Use caution in patients with cardiovascular disease (arrhythmia or hypertension or CHF), convulsive disorders, diabetes, glaucoma, hyperthyroidism, or hypokalemia. Beta-agonists may cause elevation in blood pressure, heart rate, and result in CNS stimulation/excitation. $Beta_2$-agonists may increase risk of arrhythmia, increase serum glucose, or decrease serum potassium.

Do not exceed recommended dose; serious adverse events including fatalities, have been associated with excessive use of inhaled sympathomimetics. Rarely, paradoxical bronchospasm may occur with use of inhaled bronchodilating agents (may occur more frequently with the first use of a new canister); this should be distinguished from inadequate response. All patients should utilize a spacer device when using a metered-dose inhaler.

Adverse Reactions

Cardiovascular: Palpitations, tachycardia

Central nervous system: Dizziness, headache, nervousness, tremor

Endocrine & metabolic: Decreased serum potassium, increased serum glucose

Gastrointestinal: Nausea

Rare but important or life-threatening: Chest pain, confusion, depression, hypotension, insomnia, numbness of extremities, pruritus, skin rash, sore throat, syncope

Drug Interactions

Metabolism/Transport Effects None known.

Avoid Concomitant Use

Avoid concomitant use of Pirbuterol with any of the following: Beta-Blockers (Nonselective); Iobenguane I 123; Loxapine

Increased Effect/Toxicity

Pirbuterol may increase the levels/effects of: Atosiban; Loop Diuretics; Loxapine; Sympathomimetics; Thiazide Diuretics

The levels/effects of Pirbuterol may be increased by: AtoMOXetine; Cannabinoid-Containing Products; Linezolid; MAO Inhibitors; Tedizolid; Tricyclic Antidepressants

Decreased Effect

Pirbuterol may decrease the levels/effects of: Iobenguane I 123

The levels/effects of Pirbuterol may be decreased by: Beta-Blockers (Beta1 Selective); Beta-Blockers (Nonselective); Betahistine

Storage/Stability Store between 15°C and 30°C (59°F and 86°F).

Mechanism of Action Pirbuterol is a $beta_2$-adrenergic agonist with a similar structure to albuterol, specifically a pyridine ring has been substituted for the benzene ring in albuterol. The increased $beta_2$ selectivity of pirbuterol results from the substitution of a tertiary butyl group on the nitrogen of the side chain, which additionally imparts resistance of pirbuterol to degradation by monoamine oxidase and provides a lengthened duration of action in comparison to the less selective beta-agonist agents.

Pharmacodynamics

Onset of action: 5 minutes

Maximum effect: 30-60 minutes

Duration: 5 hours

Pharmacokinetics (Adult data unless noted)

Metabolism: Liver (by sulfate conjugation)

Half-life: 2 hours

Elimination: 51% excreted in the urine as pirbuterol plus its sulfate conjugate

Dosing: Usual Oral inhalation:

Acute asthma exacerbation (NIH guidelines):

Children: 4-8 inhalations every 20 minutes for 3 doses then every 1-4 hours

Children >12 years and Adults: 4-8 inhalations every 20 minutes for up to 4 hours then every 1-4 hours

Maintenance therapy (nonacute) (NIH guidelines): Children and Adults: 2 inhalations 3-4 times/day

Administration Oral inhalation: Shake well before administration; "prime" (test spray) inhaler prior to first use and if it has not been used for 48 hours; use spacer for children <8 years of age (Maxair™ Inhaler only); Maxair™ Autohaler™ is breath activated; after sealing lips around mouthpiece, inhale deeply with steady, moderate force; inhalation triggers the release "puff" of medication; do not stop inhalation when puff occurs, but continue to take a deep, full breath; hold breath for 10 seconds, then exhale slowly

Monitoring Parameters Serum potassium, heart rate, pulmonary function tests, respiratory rate; arterial or capillary blood gases (if patient's condition warrants)

Product Availability Maxair Autohaler has been discontinued in the US for more than 1 year.

Dosage Forms Considerations

Maxair Autohaler 14 g canisters contain 400 inhalations.

Maxair Autohaler contains chlorofluorocarbons

Dosage Forms Excipient information presented when available (limited, particularly for generics); consult specific product labeling. [DSC] = Discontinued product

Aerosol Breath Activated, Inhalation, as acetate:

Maxair Autohaler: 200 mcg/INH (14 g [DSC])

◆ **Pirbuterol Acetate** *see* Pirbuterol *on page 1709*

Piroxicam (peer OKS i kam)

Medication Safety Issues

Sound-alike/look-alike issues:

Feldene may be confused with FLUoxetine

Piroxicam may be confused with PARoxetine

BEERS Criteria medication:

This drug may be potentially inappropriate for use in geriatric patients (Quality of evidence - moderate; Strength of recommendation - strong).

International issues:

Flogene [Brazil] may be confused with Flogen brand name for naproxen [Mexico]; Florone brand name for diflorasone [Germany, Greece]; Flovent brand name for fluticasone [U.S., Canada]

Related Information

Oral Medications That Should Not Be Crushed or Altered *on page 2476*

Brand Names: US Feldene

Brand Names: Canada Apo-Piroxicam; Dom-Piroxicam; Novo-Pirocam; PMS-Piroxicam

Therapeutic Category Analgesic, Non-narcotic; Anti-inflammatory Agent; Nonsteroidal Anti-inflammatory Drug (NSAID), Oral

Generic Availability (US) Yes

Use Management of rheumatoid arthritis and osteoarthritis (FDA approved in adults); has also been used to treat juvenile idiopathic arthritis

Medication Guide Available Yes

Pregnancy Risk Factor C (first and second trimester)/D (third trimester)

Pregnancy Considerations Adverse events were observed in some animal reproduction studies. NSAID exposure during the first trimester is not strongly associated with congenital malformations; however, cardiovascular anomalies and cleft palate have been observed following NSAID exposure in some studies (Ericson, 2001; Källén, 2003; Ofori, 2006). The use of a NSAID close to conception may be associated with an increased risk of miscarriage (Li, 2003; Nielsen, 2001; Nielsen, 2004). Nonteratogenic effects have been observed following NSAID administration during the third trimester including: Myocardial degenerative changes, prenatal constriction of the ductus arteriosus, fetal tricuspid regurgitation, failure of the ductus arteriosus to close postnatally; renal dysfunction or failure, oligohydramnios; gastrointestinal bleeding or perforation, increased risk of necrotizing enterocolitis; intracranial bleeding (including intraventricular hemorrhage), platelet dysfunction with resultant bleeding; pulmonary hypertension (Van den Veyver, 1993). Because they may cause premature closure of the ductus arteriosus, use of NSAIDs late in pregnancy should be avoided (use after 31 or 32 weeks gestation is not recommended by some clinicians) (Moise, 1993; Van den Veyver, 1993; Vermillion, 1997; Vermillion, 1998). The chronic use of NSAIDs in women of reproductive age may be associated with infertility that is reversible upon discontinuation of the medication (Smith, 1996).

Breast-Feeding Considerations Piroxicam is excreted into breast milk at ~1% to 3% of the maternal concentration. The manufacturer recommends that caution be used if administered to a nursing woman.

Contraindications Treatment of perioperative pain in the setting of coronary artery bypass graft (CABG) surgery; hypersensitivity to piroxicam or to any component of the formulation; patients who have experienced asthma, urticaria, or allergic-type reactions after taking aspirin or other NSAIDs.

Canadian labeling: Additional contraindications (not in U.S. labeling): Recent or recurrent history of GI bleeding; active GI inflammatory disease; inflammatory bowel disease; cerebrovascular bleeding or other bleeding disorders; severe liver impairment or active liver disease; severe renal impairment (CrCl <30 mL/minute) or deteriorating renal disease; known hyperkalemia; children and adolescents <16 years of age; use in the third trimester of pregnancy; breast-feeding, severe uncontrolled heart failure; inflammatory lesions or recent bleeding of the rectum or anus (suppository only)

Warnings/Precautions **[U.S. Boxed Warning]: NSAIDs are associated with an increased risk of adverse cardiovascular thrombotic events, including MI and stroke.** Risk may be increased with duration of use or pre-existing cardiovascular risk factors or disease. Carefully evaluate individual cardiovascular risk profiles prior to prescribing. May cause new-onset hypertension or worsening of existing hypertension. Use caution with fluid retention. Avoid use in heart failure (ACCF/AHA [Yancy, 2013]). Use is contraindicated in severe heart failure. Concurrent administration of ibuprofen, and potentially other nonselective NSAIDs, may interfere with aspirin's cardioprotective effect. **[U.S. Boxed Warning]: Use is contraindicated for treatment of perioperative pain in the setting of coronary artery bypass graft (CABG) surgery.** Risk of MI and stroke may be increased with use following CABG surgery.

Platelet adhesion and aggregation may be decreased; may prolong bleeding time; patients with coagulation disorders or who are receiving anticoagulants should be monitored closely. Anemia may occur; patients on long-term NSAID therapy should be monitored for anemia. Rarely, NSAID use may cause severe blood dyscrasias (eg, agranulocytosis, aplastic anemia, thrombocytopenia).

NSAID use may compromise existing renal function; dose-dependent decreases in prostaglandin synthesis may result from NSAID use, reducing renal blood flow which may cause renal decompensation. NSAID use may increase the risk for hyperkalemia. Patients with impaired renal function, dehydration, heart failure, liver dysfunction, those taking diuretics, and ACE inhibitors, and the elderly are at greater risk of renal toxicity and hyperkalemia. Rehydrate patient before starting therapy; monitor renal function closely. Use is contraindicated in severe renal failure (Canadian labeling also contraindicates use in patients with deteriorating renal disease or known hyperkalemia). Long-term NSAID use may result in renal papillary necrosis.

[U.S. Boxed Warning]: NSAIDs may increase risk of gastrointestinal irritation, inflammation, ulceration, bleeding, and perforation. These events may occur at any time during therapy and without warning. Use caution with a history of GI disease (bleeding or ulcers), concurrent therapy with aspirin, anticoagulants and/or corticosteroids, smoking, use of alcohol, the elderly or debilitated patients. When used concomitantly with aspirin, a substantial increase in the risk of gastrointestinal complications (eg, ulcer) occurs; concomitant gastroprotective therapy (eg, proton pump inhibitors) is recommended (Bhatt, 2008).

Use the lowest effective dose for the shortest duration of time, consistent with individual patient goals, to reduce risk of cardiovascular or GI adverse events. Alternate therapies should be considered for patients at high risk.

Rupture of ovarian follicles may be delayed or prevented resulting in reversible infertility; some studies have also shown a reversible delay in ovulation. Discontinuation of treatment should be considered in women who have difficulty conceiving or who are undergoing infertility treatment.

NSAIDs may cause serious skin adverse events including exfoliative dermatitis, Stevens-Johnson syndrome (SJS) and toxic epidermal necrolysis (TEN); discontinue use at first sign of skin rash or hypersensitivity. Anaphylactoid reactions may occur, even without prior exposure; patients with "aspirin triad" (bronchial asthma, aspirin intolerance, rhinitis) may be at increased risk. Do not use in patients who experience bronchospasm, asthma, rhinitis, or urticaria with NSAID or aspirin therapy. Use caution with other forms of asthma. A serum sickness-like reaction can rarely occur; watch for arthralgias, pruritus, fever, fatigue, and rash.

Use with caution in patients with decreased hepatic function (contraindicated in severe hepatic impairment). Closely monitor patients with any abnormal LFT. Severe hepatic reactions (eg, fulminant hepatitis, liver failure) have occurred with NSAID use, rarely; discontinue if signs or symptoms of liver disease develop, or if systemic manifestations occur. Use with caution in poor CYP2C9 metabolizers as hepatic metabolism may be reduced resulting in elevated serum concentrations.

NSAIDS may cause drowsiness, dizziness, blurred vision and other neurologic effects which may impair physical or mental abilities; patients must be cautioned about performing tasks which require mental alertness (eg, operating machinery or driving). Discontinue use with blurred or diminished vision and perform ophthalmologic exam. Monitor vision with long-term therapy.

In the elderly, avoid chronic use (unless alternative agents ineffective and patient can receive concomitant gastroprotective agent); nonselective oral NSAID use is associated with an increased risk of GI bleeding and peptic ulcer disease in older adults in high risk category (eg, >75 years or age or receiving concomitant oral/parenteral corticosteroids, anticoagulants, or antiplatelet agents) (Beers Criteria).

Withhold for at least 4 to 6 half-lives prior to surgical or dental procedures. Potentially significant interactions may exist, requiring dose or frequency adjustment, additional monitoring, and/or selection of alternative therapy.

Adverse Reactions

Cardiovascular: Edema

Central nervous system: Dizziness, headache

Dermatologic: Pruritus, skin rash

Gastrointestinal: Abdominal pain, anorexia, constipation, diarrhea, dyspepsia, flatulence, gastrointestinal hemorrhage, gastrointestinal perforation, heartburn, nausea, ulcer (gastric, duodenal), vomiting

Hematologic & oncologic: Anemia, prolonged bleeding time

Hepatic: Increased liver enzymes

Otic: Tinnitus

Renal: Renal function abnormality

Rare but important or life-threatening: Agranulocytosis, anaphylactoid reactions, anaphylaxis, aplastic anemia, aseptic meningitis, bone marrow depression, cardiac arrhythmia, cardiac failure, cystitis, erythema multiforme, exacerbation of angina pectoris, gastritis, glomerulonephritis, hallucination, hearing loss, hemolytic anemia, hepatic failure, hepatitis, hepatotoxicity (idiosyncratic) (Chalasani 2014), hyperkalemia, hypertension, hypoglycemia, interstitial nephritis, leukopenia, myocardial infarction, nephrotic syndrome, pancreatitis, pancytopenia, reduced fertility (female), renal failure, Stevens-Johnson syndrome, tachycardia, thrombocytopenia, toxic epidermal necrolysis

Drug Interactions

Metabolism/Transport Effects **Substrate** of CYP2C9 (major); **Note:** Assignment of Major/Minor substrate status based on clinically relevant drug interaction potential; **Inhibits** CYP2C9 (weak)

Avoid Concomitant Use

Avoid concomitant use of Piroxicam with any of the following: Dexketoprofen; Floctafenine; Ketorolac (Nasal); Ketorolac (Systemic); Morniflumate; NSAID (COX-2 Inhibitor); Omacetaxine; Urokinase

Increased Effect/Toxicity

Piroxicam may increase the levels/effects of: 5-ASA Derivatives; Agents with Antiplatelet Properties; Aliskiren; Aminoglycosides; Anticoagulants; Apixaban; Bisphosphonate Derivatives; Collagenase (Systemic); CycloSPORINE (Systemic); Dabigatran Etexilate; Deferasirox; Deoxycholic Acid; Desmopressin; Digoxin; Drospirenone; Eplerenone; Haloperidol; Ibritumomab; Lithium; Methotrexate; Nonsteroidal Anti-Inflammatory Agents; NSAID (COX-2 Inhibitor); Obinutuzumab; Omacetaxine; PEMEtrexed; Porfimer; Potassium-Sparing Diuretics; PRALAtrexate; Quinolone Antibiotics; Rivaroxaban; Salicylates; Tacrolimus (Systemic); Tenofovir; Thrombolytic Agents; Tositumomab and Iodine I 131 Tositumomab; Urokinase; Vancomycin; Verteporfin; Vitamin K Antagonists

The levels/effects of Piroxicam may be increased by: ACE Inhibitors; Angiotensin II Receptor Blockers; Antidepressants (Tricyclic, Tertiary Amine); Ceritinib; Corticosteroids (Systemic); CycloSPORINE (Systemic); CYP2C9 Inhibitors (Moderate); CYP2C9 Inhibitors (Strong); Dasatinib; Dexketoprofen; Diclofenac (Systemic); Floctafenine; Glucosamine; Herbs (Anticoagulant/Antiplatelet Properties); Ibrutinib; Ketorolac (Nasal); Ketorolac (Systemic); Limaprost; Mifepristone; Morniflumate; Multivitamins/Fluoride (with ADE); Multivitamins/Minerals (with ADEK, Folate, Iron); Multivitamins/Minerals (with AE, No Iron); Omega-3 Fatty Acids; Pentosan Polysulfate Sodium; Pentoxifylline; Probenecid; Prostacyclin Analogues; Selective Serotonin Reuptake Inhibitors; Serotonin/Norepinephrine Reuptake Inhibitors; Sodium Phosphates; Tipranavir; Treprostinil; Vitamin E

Decreased Effect

Piroxicam may decrease the levels/effects of: ACE Inhibitors; Aliskiren; Angiotensin II Receptor Blockers; Beta-Blockers; Eplerenone; HydrALAZINE; Loop Diuretics; Potassium-Sparing Diuretics; Prostaglandins (Ophthalmic); Salicylates; Selective Serotonin Reuptake Inhibitors; Thiazide Diuretics

The levels/effects of Piroxicam may be decreased by: Bile Acid Sequestrants; CYP2C9 Inducers (Strong); Dabrafenib; Salicylates

Food Interactions Onset of effect may be delayed if piroxicam is taken with food. Management: May administer with food or milk to decrease GI upset.

Storage/Stability

Capsule: Store below 30°C (86°F)

Suppository [Canadian product]: Store at 15°C to 25°C (59°F to 77°F)

Mechanism of Action Reversibly inhibits cyclooxygenase-1 and 2 (COX-1 and 2) enzymes, which results in decreased formation of prostaglandin precursors; has antipyretic, analgesic, and anti-inflammatory properties

Other proposed mechanisms not fully elucidated (and possibly contributing to the anti-inflammatory effect to varying degrees), include inhibiting chemotaxis, altering lymphocyte activity, inhibiting neutrophil aggregation/activation, and decreasing proinflammatory cytokine levels.

Pharmacodynamics Analgesia:

Onset of action: Oral: Within 1 hour

Maximum effect: 3-5 hours

Pharmacokinetics (Adult data unless noted)

Absorption: Oral: Well absorbed

Distribution:

V_d:

Children and Adolescents 7-16 years: 0.16 L/kg (range: 0.12-0.25 L/kg) (Mäkelä, 1991)

Adults: 0.14 L/kg

Protein binding: 99%

Metabolism: Hepatic predominantly via CYP2C9; metabolites are inactive

Half-life:

Children and Adolescents 7-16 years: 32.6 hours (range: 22-40 hours)(Mäkelä, 1991)

Adults: 50 hours

Time to peak: 3-5 hours

Elimination: Excreted as metabolites and unchanged drug (~5% to 10%) in the urine; small amount excreted in feces

Dosing: Usual

Children and Adolescents: **Juvenile idiopathic arthritis (JIA):** Oral: 0.2-0.4 mg/kg/**day** once daily; maximum daily dose: 15 mg/day (American Pain Society, 2008); **Note:** 15 mg strength not available in U.S.

Adults: **Osteoarthritis, rheumatoid arthritis:** Oral: 10-20 mg/day in 1-2 divided doses; maximum daily dose: 20 mg/**day**

Dosing adjustment in renal impairment: Adults:

Mild to moderate impairment: There are no dosage adjustments provided in manufacturer's labeling.

Severe impairment: Use is not recommended (has not been studied); if therapy must be initiated, close monitoring is recommended.

Dosing adjustment in hepatic impairment: Adults: There are no specific dosage adjustments provided in manufacturer's labeling; however, a dosage reduction is recommended.

Administration May administer with food or milk to decrease GI upset

Monitoring Parameters Occult blood loss, CBC, BUN, serum creatinine, liver enzymes; periodic ophthalmologic exams with chronic use

Test Interactions Increased bleeding time

Dosage Forms Excipient information presented when available (limited, particularly for generics); consult specific product labeling.

Capsule, Oral:
Feldene: 10 mg, 20 mg
Generic: 10 mg, 20 mg

◆ **p-Isobutylhydratropic Acid** *see* Ibuprofen *on page 1064*

◆ **Pitressin Synthetic [DSC]** *see* Vasopressin *on page 2161*

◆ **Pitrex (Can)** *see* Tolnaftate *on page 2083*

◆ **Pix Carbonis** *see* Coal Tar *on page 523*

◆ **Plantago Seed** *see* Psyllium *on page 1804*

◆ **Plantain Seed** *see* Psyllium *on page 1804*

◆ **Plaquenil** *see* Hydroxychloroquine *on page 1052*

◆ **Plasbumin-5** *see* Albumin *on page 79*

◆ **Plasbumin-25** *see* Albumin *on page 79*

◆ **Platinol** *see* CISplatin *on page 473*

◆ **Platinol-AQ** *see* CISplatin *on page 473*

◆ **Plavix** *see* Clopidogrel *on page 513*

◆ **Plendil** *see* Felodipine *on page 855*

◆ **Pliaglis** *see* Lidocaine and Tetracaine *on page 1266*

◆ **PMPA** *see* Tenofovir *on page 2017*

◆ **PMS-Acetaminophen with Codeine Elixir (Can)** *see* Acetaminophen and Codeine *on page 50*

◆ **PMS-Adenosine (Can)** *see* Adenosine *on page 73*

◆ **PMS-Amantadine (Can)** *see* Amantadine *on page 112*

◆ **PMS-Amiodarone (Can)** *see* Amiodarone *on page 125*

◆ **PMS-Amitriptyline (Can)** *see* Amitriptyline *on page 131*

◆ **PMS-Amlodipine (Can)** *see* AmLODIPine *on page 133*

◆ **PMS-Amoxicillin (Can)** *see* Amoxicillin *on page 138*

◆ **PMS-Anagrelide (Can)** *see* Anagrelide *on page 163*

◆ **PMS-Atenolol (Can)** *see* Atenolol *on page 215*

◆ **PMS-Atomoxetine (Can)** *see* AtoMOXetine *on page 217*

◆ **PMS-Atorvastatin (Can)** *see* AtorvaSTATin *on page 220*

◆ **PMS-Azithromycin (Can)** *see* Azithromycin (Systemic) *on page 242*

◆ **PMS-Baclofen (Can)** *see* Baclofen *on page 254*

◆ **PMS-Benztropine (Can)** *see* Benztropine *on page 272*

◆ **PMS-Bethanechol (Can)** *see* Bethanechol *on page 284*

◆ **PMS-Bisacodyl [OTC] (Can)** *see* Bisacodyl *on page 289*

◆ **PMS-Bosentan (Can)** *see* Bosentan *on page 294*

◆ **PMS-Brimonidine Tartrate (Can)** *see* Brimonidine (Ophthalmic) *on page 301*

◆ **PMS-Bromocriptine (Can)** *see* Bromocriptine *on page 303*

◆ **PMS-Bupropion SR (Can)** *see* BuPROPion *on page 324*

◆ **PMS-Buspirone (Can)** *see* BusPIRone *on page 328*

◆ **PMS-Candesartan (Can)** *see* Candesartan *on page 358*

◆ **PMS-Captopril (Can)** *see* Captopril *on page 364*

◆ **PMS-Carbamazepine (Can)** *see* CarBAMazepine *on page 367*

◆ **PMS-Carvedilol (Can)** *see* Carvedilol *on page 380*

◆ **PMS-Cefaclor (Can)** *see* Cefaclor *on page 386*

◆ **PMS-Celecoxib (Can)** *see* Celecoxib *on page 418*

◆ **PMS-Cephalexin (Can)** *see* Cephalexin *on page 422*

◆ **PMS-Cetirizine (Can)** *see* Cetirizine *on page 423*

◆ **PMS-Chloral Hydrate (Can)** *see* Chloral Hydrate *on page 429*

◆ **PMS-Cholestyramine (Can)** *see* Cholestyramine Resin *on page 450*

◆ **PMS-Ciclopirox (Can)** *see* Ciclopirox *on page 458*

◆ **PMS-Cimetidine (Can)** *see* Cimetidine *on page 461*

◆ **PMS-Ciprofloxacin (Can)** *see* Ciprofloxacin (Systemic) *on page 463*

◆ **PMS-Ciprofloxacin XL (Can)** *see* Ciprofloxacin (Systemic) *on page 463*

◆ **PMS-Citalopram (Can)** *see* Citalopram *on page 476*

◆ **PMS-Clarithromycin (Can)** *see* Clarithromycin *on page 482*

◆ **PMS-Clindamycin (Can)** *see* Clindamycin (Systemic) *on page 487*

◆ **PMS-Clobazam (Can)** *see* CloBAZam *on page 495*

◆ **PMS-Clobetasol (Can)** *see* Clobetasol *on page 498*

◆ **PMS-Clonazepam (Can)** *see* ClonazePAM *on page 506*

◆ **PMS-Clonazepam-R (Can)** *see* ClonazePAM *on page 506*

◆ **PMS-Clopidogrel (Can)** *see* Clopidogrel *on page 513*

◆ **PMS-Codeine (Can)** *see* Codeine *on page 525*

◆ **PMS-Colchicine (Can)** *see* Colchicine *on page 528*

◆ **PMS-Conjugated Estrogens C.S.D. (Can)** *see* Estrogens (Conjugated/Equine, Systemic) *on page 801*

◆ **PMS-Cyclobenzaprine (Can)** *see* Cyclobenzaprine *on page 548*

◆ **PMS-Cyclopentolate (Can)** *see* Cyclopentolate *on page 549*

◆ **PMS-Cyproheptadine (Can)** *see* Cyproheptadine *on page 562*

◆ **PMS-Deferoxamine (Can)** *see* Deferoxamine *on page 598*

◆ **PMS-Desipramine (Can)** *see* Desipramine *on page 602*

◆ **PMS-Desmopressin (Can)** *see* Desmopressin *on page 607*

◆ **PMS-Dexamethasone (Can)** *see* Dexamethasone (Systemic) *on page 610*

◆ **PMS-Diazepam (Can)** *see* Diazepam *on page 635*

◆ **PMS-Dicitrate (Can)** *see* Sodium Citrate and Citric Acid *on page 1942*

◆ **PMS-Diclofenac (Can)** *see* Diclofenac (Systemic) *on page 641*

◆ **PMS-Diclofenac K (Can)** *see* Diclofenac (Systemic) *on page 641*

◆ **PMS-Diclofenac-SR (Can)** *see* Diclofenac (Systemic) *on page 641*

◆ **PMS-Digoxin (Can)** *see* Digoxin *on page 652*

◆ **PMS-Diltiazem CD (Can)** *see* Diltiazem *on page 661*

◆ **PMS-Dimenhydrinate [OTC] (Can)** *see* DimenhyDRINATE *on page 664*

◆ **PMS-Diphenhydramine (Can)** *see* DiphenhydrAMINE (Systemic) *on page 668*

◆ **PMS-Dipivefrin (Can)** *see* Dipivefrin *on page 687*

◆ **PMS-Divalproex (Can)** *see* Valproic Acid and Derivatives *on page 2143*

◆ **PMS-Docusate Calcium [OTC] (Can)** *see* Docusate *on page 697*

◆ **PMS-Docusate Sodium [OTC] (Can)** *see* Docusate *on page 697*

◆ **PMS-Doxazosin (Can)** *see* Doxazosin *on page 709*

◆ **PMS-Doxycycline (Can)** *see* Doxycycline *on page 717*

◆ **PMS-Enalapril (Can)** *see* Enalapril *on page 744*

◆ **PMS-Entecavir (Can)** *see* Entecavir *on page 756*

◆ **PMS-Erythromycin (Can)** *see* Erythromycin (Ophthalmic) *on page 782*

◆ **PMS-Escitalopram (Can)** *see* Escitalopram *on page 786*

- ◆ **PMS-Esomeprazole DR (Can)** *see* Esomeprazole *on page 792*
- ◆ **PMS-Ezetimibe (Can)** *see* Ezetimibe *on page 832*
- ◆ **PMS-Famciclovir (Can)** *see* Famciclovir *on page 846*
- ◆ **PMS-Fentanyl MTX (Can)** *see* FentaNYL *on page 857*
- ◆ **PMS-Fluconazole (Can)** *see* Fluconazole *on page 881*
- ◆ **PMS-Fluorometholone (Can)** *see* Fluorometholone *on page 903*
- ◆ **PMS-Fluoxetine (Can)** *see* FLUoxetine *on page 906*
- ◆ **PMS-Flurazepam (Can)** *see* Flurazepam *on page 913*
- ◆ **PMS-Fluvoxamine (Can)** *see* FluvoxaMINE *on page 928*
- ◆ **PMS-Fosinopril (Can)** *see* Fosinopril *on page 943*
- ◆ **PMS-Furosemide (Can)** *see* Furosemide *on page 951*
- ◆ **PMS-Gabapentin (Can)** *see* Gabapentin *on page 954*
- ◆ **PMS-Gentamicin (Can)** *see* Gentamicin (Ophthalmic) *on page 968*
- ◆ **PMS-Gentamicin (Can)** *see* Gentamicin (Topical) *on page 969*
- ◆ **PMS-Glyburide (Can)** *see* GlyBURIDE *on page 975*
- ◆ **PMS-Haloperidol (Can)** *see* Haloperidol *on page 1002*
- ◆ **PMS-Haloperidol LA (Can)** *see* Haloperidol *on page 1002*
- ◆ **PMS-Hydrochlorothiazide (Can)** *see* Hydrochlorothiazide *on page 1028*
- ◆ **PMS-Hydromorphone (Can)** *see* HYDROmorphone *on page 1044*
- ◆ **PMS-Hydroxyzine (Can)** *see* HydrOXYzine *on page 1058*
- ◆ **PMS-Ibuprofen (Can)** *see* Ibuprofen *on page 1064*
- ◆ **PMS Imipramine (Can)** *see* Imipramine *on page 1086*
- ◆ **PMS-Ipratropium (Can)** *see* Ipratropium (Oral Inhalation) *on page 1155*
- ◆ **PMS-Irbesartan (Can)** *see* Irbesartan *on page 1158*
- ◆ **PMS-Lactulose (Can)** *see* Lactulose *on page 1204*
- ◆ **PMS-Lamotrigine (Can)** *see* LamoTRIgine *on page 1211*
- ◆ **PMS-Lansoprazole (Can)** *see* Lansoprazole *on page 1219*
- ◆ **PMS-Letrozole (Can)** *see* Letrozole *on page 1224*
- ◆ **PMS-Levetiracetam (Can)** *see* LevETIRAcetam *on page 1234*
- ◆ **PMS-Levobunolol (Can)** *see* Levobunolol *on page 1238*
- ◆ **PMS-Levofloxacin (Can)** *see* Levofloxacin (Systemic) *on page 1243*
- ◆ **PMS-Lisinopril (Can)** *see* Lisinopril *on page 1280*
- ◆ **PMS-Lithium Carbonate (Can)** *see* Lithium *on page 1284*
- ◆ **PMS-Lithium Citrate (Can)** *see* Lithium *on page 1284*
- ◆ **PMS-Loperamine (Can)** *see* Loperamide *on page 1288*
- ◆ **PMS-Lorazepam (Can)** *see* LORazepam *on page 1299*
- ◆ **PMS-Losartan (Can)** *see* Losartan *on page 1302*
- ◆ **PMS-Lovastatin (Can)** *see* Lovastatin *on page 1305*
- ◆ **PMS-Medroxyprogesterone (Can)** *see* MedroxyPROGESTERone *on page 1339*
- ◆ **PMS-Meloxicam (Can)** *see* Meloxicam *on page 1346*
- ◆ **PMS-Metformin (Can)** *see* MetFORMIN *on page 1375*
- ◆ **PMS-Methylphenidate (Can)** *see* Methylphenidate *on page 1402*
- ◆ **PMS-Metoclopramide (Can)** *see* Metoclopramide *on page 1413*
- ◆ **PMS-Metoprolol-L (Can)** *see* Metoprolol *on page 1418*
- ◆ **PMS-Metoprolol-B (Can)** *see* Metoprolol *on page 1418*
- ◆ **PMS-Metronidazole (Can)** *see* MetroNIDAZOLE (Systemic) *on page 1421*
- ◆ **PMS-Minocycline (Can)** *see* Minocycline *on page 1440*
- ◆ **PMS-Misoprostol (Can)** *see* Misoprostol *on page 1444*
- ◆ **PMS-Mometasone (Can)** *see* Mometasone (Topical) *on page 1456*
- ◆ **PMS-Montelukast (Can)** *see* Montelukast *on page 1459*
- ◆ **PMS-Montelukast FC (Can)** *see* Montelukast *on page 1459*
- ◆ **PMS-Morphine Sulfate SR (Can)** *see* Morphine (Systemic) *on page 1461*
- ◆ **PMS-Nabilone (Can)** *see* Nabilone *on page 1478*
- ◆ **PMS-Naproxen (Can)** *see* Naproxen *on page 1489*
- ◆ **PMS-Naproxen EC (Can)** *see* Naproxen *on page 1489*
- ◆ **PMS-Nifedipine (Can)** *see* NIFEdipine *on page 1516*
- ◆ **PMS-Nifedipine ER (Can)** *see* NIFEdipine *on page 1516*
- ◆ **PMS-Nizatidine (Can)** *see* Nizatidine *on page 1528*
- ◆ **PMS-Nortriptyline (Can)** *see* Nortriptyline *on page 1532*
- ◆ **PMS-Nystatin (Can)** *see* Nystatin (Oral) *on page 1537*
- ◆ **PMS-Olanzapine (Can)** *see* OLANZapine *on page 1546*
- ◆ **PMS-Olanzapine ODT (Can)** *see* OLANZapine *on page 1546*
- ◆ **PMS-Omeprazole (Can)** *see* Omeprazole *on page 1555*
- ◆ **PMS-Omeprazole DR (Can)** *see* Omeprazole *on page 1555*
- ◆ **PMS-Ondansetron (Can)** *see* Ondansetron *on page 1564*
- ◆ **PMS-Oxybutynin (Can)** *see* Oxybutynin *on page 1588*
- ◆ **PMS-Oxycodone (Can)** *see* OxyCODONE *on page 1590*
- ◆ **PMS-Oxycodone-Acetaminophen (Can)** *see* Oxycodone and Acetaminophen *on page 1594*
- ◆ **PMS-Oxycodone CR (Can)** *see* OxyCODONE *on page 1590*
- ◆ **PMS-Pamidronate (Can)** *see* Pamidronate *on page 1611*
- ◆ **PMS-Pantoprazole (Can)** *see* Pantoprazole *on page 1618*
- ◆ **PMS-Paroxetine (Can)** *see* PARoxetine *on page 1634*
- ◆ **PMS-Phenobarbital (Can)** *see* PHENobarbital *on page 1679*
- ◆ **PMS-Pimozide (Can)** *see* Pimozide *on page 1704*
- ◆ **PMS-Piroxicam (Can)** *see* Piroxicam *on page 1710*
- ◆ **PMS-Polytrimethoprim (Can)** *see* Trimethoprim and Polymyxin B *on page 2128*
- ◆ **PMS-Pravastatin (Can)** *see* Pravastatin *on page 1749*
- ◆ **PMS-Prednisolone Sodium Phosphate Forte (Can)** *see* PrednisoLONE (Ophthalmic) *on page 1758*
- ◆ **PMS-Prochlorperazine (Can)** *see* Prochlorperazine *on page 1774*
- ◆ **PMS-Promethazine (Can)** *see* Promethazine *on page 1777*
- ◆ **PMS-Propofol (Can)** *see* Propofol *on page 1786*
- ◆ **PMS-Propranolol (Can)** *see* Propranolol *on page 1789*
- ◆ **PMS-Pseudoephedrine (Can)** *see* Pseudoephedrine *on page 1801*
- ◆ **PMS-Quetiapine (Can)** *see* QUEtiapine *on page 1815*
- ◆ **PMS-Quinapril (Can)** *see* Quinapril *on page 1820*
- ◆ **PMS-Rabeprazole EC (Can)** *see* RABEprazole *on page 1828*

- ◆ **PMS-Ranitidine (Can)** *see* Ranitidine *on page 1836*
- ◆ **PMS-Risperidone (Can)** *see* RisperiDONE *on page 1866*
- ◆ **PMS-Risperidone ODT (Can)** *see* RisperiDONE *on page 1866*
- ◆ **PMS-Rizatriptan RDT (Can)** *see* Rizatriptan *on page 1879*
- ◆ **PMS-Rosuvastatin (Can)** *see* Rosuvastatin *on page 1886*
- ◆ **PMS-Salbutamol (Can)** *see* Albuterol *on page 81*
- ◆ **PMS-Sertraline (Can)** *see* Sertraline *on page 1916*
- ◆ **PMS-Sildenafil (Can)** *see* Sildenafil *on page 1921*
- ◆ **PMS-Simvastatin (Can)** *see* Simvastatin *on page 1928*
- ◆ **PMS-Sodium Cromoglycate (Can)** *see* Cromolyn (Systemic, Oral Inhalation) *on page 541*
- ◆ **PMS-Sodium Polystyrene Sulfonate (Can)** *see* Sodium Polystyrene Sulfonate *on page 1953*
- ◆ **PMS-Sotalol (Can)** *see* Sotalol *on page 1963*
- ◆ **PMS-Sucralate (Can)** *see* Sucralfate *on page 1978*
- ◆ **PMS-Sulfacetamide (Can)** *see* Sulfacetamide (Ophthalmic) *on page 1981*
- ◆ **PMS-Sulfasalazine (Can)** *see* SulfaSALAzine *on page 1990*
- ◆ **PMS-Sumatriptan (Can)** *see* SUMAtriptan *on page 1995*
- ◆ **PMS-Tamoxifen (Can)** *see* Tamoxifen *on page 2005*
- ◆ **PMS-Terazosin (Can)** *see* Terazosin *on page 2020*
- ◆ **PMS-Terbinafine (Can)** *see* Terbinafine (Systemic) *on page 2021*
- ◆ **PMS-Testosterone (Can)** *see* Testosterone *on page 2025*
- ◆ **PMS-Theophylline (Can)** *see* Theophylline *on page 2044*
- ◆ **PMS-Timolol (Can)** *see* Timolol (Ophthalmic) *on page 2067*
- ◆ **PMS-Tobramycin (Can)** *see* Tobramycin (Ophthalmic) *on page 2078*
- ◆ **PMS-Topiramate (Can)** *see* Topiramate *on page 2085*
- ◆ **PMS-Trazodone (Can)** *see* TraZODone *on page 2105*
- ◆ **PMS-Trihexyphenidyl (Can)** *see* Trihexyphenidyl *on page 2124*
- ◆ **PMS-Ursodiol C (Can)** *see* Ursodiol *on page 2136*
- ◆ **PMS-Valacyclovir (Can)** *see* ValACYclovir *on page 2138*
- ◆ **PMS-Valproic Acid (Can)** *see* Valproic Acid and Derivatives *on page 2143*
- ◆ **PMS-Valproic Acid E.C. (Can)** *see* Valproic Acid and Derivatives *on page 2143*
- ◆ **PMS-Valsartan (Can)** *see* Valsartan *on page 2149*
- ◆ **PMS-Vancomycin (Can)** *see* Vancomycin *on page 2151*
- ◆ **PMS-Venlafaxine XR (Can)** *see* Venlafaxine *on page 2166*
- ◆ **PMS-Verapamil SR (Can)** *see* Verapamil *on page 2170*
- ◆ **Pneumo 23 (Can)** *see* Pneumococcal Polysaccharide Vaccine (23-Valent) *on page 1718*
- ◆ **Pneumococcal 13-Valent Conjugate Vaccine** *see* Pneumococcal Conjugate Vaccine (13-Valent) *on page 1715*

Pneumococcal Conjugate Vaccine (13-Valent)

(noo moe KOK al KON ju gate vak SEEN, thur TEEN vay lent)

Medication Safety Issues

Sound-alike/look-alike issues:

Pneumococcal 13-Valent Conjugate Vaccine (Prevnar 13) may be confused with Pneumococcal 7-Valent Conjugate Vaccine (Prevnar) or with Pneumococcal 23-Valent Polysaccharide Vaccine (Pneumovax 23)

Related Information

Centers for Disease Control and Prevention (CDC) and Other Links *on page 2424*

Immunization Administration Recommendations *on page 2411*

Immunization Schedules *on page 2416*

Brand Names: US Prevnar 13

Brand Names: Canada Prevnar 13

Therapeutic Category Vaccine; Vaccine, Inactivated (Bacterial)

Generic Availability (US) No

Use

Immunization against *Streptococcus pneumoniae* infection caused by serotypes 1, 3, 4, 5, 6A, 6B, 7F, 9V, 14, 18C, 19A, 19F, and 23F (FDA approved in ages 6 weeks to 17 years and adults ≥50 years). Prevention of otitis media in infants and children caused by *Streptococcus pneumoniae* serotypes 4, 6B, 9V, 14, 18C, 19F, and 23F (FDA approved in ages 6 weeks to 5 years)

The Advisory Committee on Immunization Practices (ACIP) recommends routine vaccination for the following (CDC/ACIP [Nuorti 2010]):

- All infants and children age 2 to 59 months
- Children 60 to 71 months with underlying medical conditions including:
  - Immunocompetent children with chronic heart disease (particularly cyanotic congenital heart disease and heart failure), chronic lung disease (including asthma if treated with high dose corticosteroids), diabetes, cerebrospinal fluid leaks, or cochlear implants
  - Children with functional or anatomic asplenia, including sickle cell disease or other hemoglobinopathies, congenital or acquired asplenia, or splenic dysfunction
  - Children with immunocompromising conditions, including congenital immunodeficiency (includes B or T cell deficiency, compliment deficiencies and phagocytic disorders; excludes chronic granulomatous disease), HIV infection, chronic renal failure, nephrotic syndrome, leukemia, lymphoma, Hodgkin disease, generalized malignancies, solid organ transplant, or other diseases requiring immunosuppressive drugs (including long-term systemic corticosteroids and radiation therapy)
- Children who received ≥1 dose of 7-valent pneumococcal vaccine (PCV7): **Note:** Routine use is not recommended for healthy children ≥5 years

Children ≥6 years, Adolescents, and Adults with the following immunocompromising conditions (CDC/ACIP, 61[40], 2012; CDC/ACIP, 62[25], 2013):

- Immunocompetent persons with cerebrospinal fluid leaks or cochlear implants
- Persons with functional or anatomic asplenia, including sickle cell disease or other hemoglobinopathies, or congenital or acquired asplenia
- Persons with immunocompromising conditions including congenital or acquired immunodeficiency (includes B or T cell deficiency, compliment deficiencies and phagocytic disorders; excludes chronic granulomatous disease), HIV infection, chronic renal failure, nephrotic syndrome, leukemia, lymphoma, Hodgkin disease,

generalized malignancies, solid organ transplant, multiple myeloma, or other diseases requiring immunosuppressive drugs (including long-term systemic corticosteroids and radiation therapy)

Medication Guide Available Yes

Pregnancy Risk Factor B

Pregnancy Considerations Animal reproduction studies have not shown adverse fetal effects. Inactivated vaccines have not been shown to cause increased risks to the fetus (NCIRD/ACIP 2011).

Breast-Feeding Considerations It is not known if this vaccine is excreted into breast milk. The manufacturer recommends that caution be exercised when administering this vaccine to nursing women. Inactivated vaccines do not affect the safety of breast-feeding for the mother or the infant. Breast-feeding infants should be vaccinated according to the recommended schedules (NCIRD/ACIP 2011).

Contraindications Severe allergic reaction (eg, anaphylaxis) to pneumococcal vaccine, any component of the formulation, or any diphtheria toxoid-containing vaccine

Warnings/Precautions Immediate treatment (including epinephrine 1:1000) for anaphylactoid and/or hypersensitivity reactions should be available during vaccine use (NCIRD/ACIP 2011). Use with caution in patients with bleeding disorders (including thrombocytopenia) and patients on anticoagulant therapy; bleeding/hematoma may occur from IM administration; if the patient receives antihemophilia or other similar therapy, IM injection can be scheduled shortly after such therapy is administered (NCIRD/ACIP 2011).. Use with caution in severely immunocompromised patients (eg, patients receiving chemo/radiation therapy or other immunosuppressive therapy including high-dose corticosteroids); may have a reduced response to vaccination. In general, household and close contacts of persons with altered immunocompetence may receive all age appropriate vaccines (IDSA [Rubin 2014]; NCIRD/ACIP 2011). Syncope has been reported with use of injectable vaccines and may result in serious secondary injury (e.g. skull fracture, cerebral hemorrhage); typically reported in adolescents and young adults and within 15 minutes after vaccination.Procedures should be in place to avoid injuries from falling and to restore cerebral perfusion if syncope occurs (NCIRD/ACIP 2011).

The decision to administer or delay vaccination because of current or recent febrile illness depends on the severity of symptoms and the etiology of the disease. Consider deferring administration in patients with moderate or severe acute illness (with or without fever); vaccination should not be delayed for patients with mild acute illness (with or without fever) (NCIRD/ACIP 2011).

Receipt of PPSV23 within 1 year prior to pneumococcal conjugate vaccine (PCV13) diminishes response to PCV13 when compared to response in PPSV23 naïve individuals. In order to maximize vaccination rates, the ACIP recommends simultaneous administration (ie, >1 vaccine on the same day at different anatomic sites) of all age-appropriate vaccines (live or inactivated) for which a person is eligible at a single clinic visit, unless contraindications exist (NCIRD/ACIP 2011). Vaccination may not result in effective immunity in all patients. Response depends upon multiple factors (eg, type of vaccine, age of patient) and may be improved by administering the vaccine at the recommended dose, route, and interval. Vaccines may not be effective if administered during periods of altered immune competence (NCIRD/ACIP 2011).

Use of pneumococcal conjugate vaccine does not replace use of the 23-valent pneumococcal polysaccharide vaccine in children ≥24 months of age with chronic illness, asplenia, sickle cell disease or are immunocompromised or have HIV infection (CDC/ACIP [Nuorti 2010]); inactivated vaccines should be administered ≥2 weeks prior to planned immunosuppression when feasible (IDSA [Rubin 2014]). Antibody responses were lower in older adults >65 years of age compared to adults 50 to 59 years of age and lower in preterm infants (<37 weeks gestational age) compared to term infants (≥37 weeks gestational age). Apnea has been reported following IM vaccine administration in premature infants; consider clinical status implications. Not to be used to treat pneumococcal infections or to provide immunity against diphtheria. Use of this vaccine for specific medical and/or other indications (eg, immunocompromising conditions, hepatic or kidney disease, diabetes) is also addressed in the ACIP Recommended Adult Immunization Schedule (CDC/ACIP [Kim 2015]). Specific recommendations for use of this vaccine in immunocompromised patients with asplenia, cancer, HIV infection, cerebrospinal fluid leaks, cochlear implants, hematopoietic stem cell transplant (prior to or after), sickle cell disease, solid organ transplant (prior to or after), or those receiving immunosuppressive therapy for chronic conditions are available from the IDSA (Rubin 2014).

Antipyretics have not been shown to prevent febrile seizures; antipyretics may be used to treat fever or discomfort following vaccination (NCIRD/ACIP 2011). One study reported that routine prophylactic administration of acetaminophen to prevent fever prior to vaccination decreased the immune response of some vaccines; the clinical significance of this reduction in immune response has not been established (Prymula 2009).

Some dosage forms may contain polysorbate 80 (also known as Tweens). Hypersensitivity reactions, usually a delayed reaction, have been reported following exposure to pharmaceutical products containing polysorbate 80 in certain individuals (Isaksson 2002; Lucente 2000; Shelley 1995). Thrombocytopenia, ascites, pulmonary deterioration, and renal and hepatic failure have been reported in premature neonates after receiving parenteral products containing polysorbate 80 (Alade 1986; CDC 1984). See manufacturer's labeling.

Warnings: Additional Pediatric Considerations Febrile seizures have been reported; CDC reports indicate that young children appear to be at increased risk of febrile seizures when given the pneumococcal conjugate vaccine (PCV13) at the same time as the inactivated influenza virus vaccine (TIV); the risk appears to be greatest from ages 12 to 23 months. Because febrile seizures are typically benign and occur in 2% to 5% of all young children, the ACIP does not recommend a delay in administration of either vaccine or altering the vaccine schedule in any manner due to the potential risk of infection.

Adverse Reactions All serious adverse reactions must be reported to the U.S. Department of Health and Human Services (DHHS) Vaccine Adverse Event Reporting System (VAERS) 1-800-822-7967 or online at https://vaers.hhs.gov/esub/index.

Central nervous system: Chills, drowsiness, fatigue, fever, headache, insomnia, irritability

Dermatologic: Hives, rash

Gastrointestinal: Appetite decreased, diarrhea, vomiting

Local: Erythema, limitation of arm motion, pain, swelling, tenderness

Neuromuscular & skeletal: Arthralgia, myalgia

Rare but important or life-threatening: Abnormal crying, erythema multiforme, febrile seizures, hypersensitivity reaction (bronchospasm, dyspnea, facial edema), seizure, urticaria, urticaria-like rash

Adverse reactions observed with PCV7 which may also be seen with PCV-13: Anaphylactic reaction, angioneurotic edema, apnea, breath holding, edema, hypotonic hyporesponsive episode, injection site reaction (dermatitis, pruritus), lymphadenopathy (localized), shock

Drug Interactions

Metabolism/Transport Effects None known.

Avoid Concomitant Use There are no known interactions where it is recommended to avoid concomitant use.

Increased Effect/Toxicity There are no known significant interactions involving an increase in effect.

Decreased Effect

Pneumococcal Conjugate Vaccine (13-Valent) may decrease the levels/effects of: Influenza Virus Vaccine (Inactivated)

The levels/effects of Pneumococcal Conjugate Vaccine (13-Valent) may be decreased by: Belimumab; Fingolimod; Immunosuppressants; Influenza Virus Vaccine (Inactivated)

Storage/Stability Store under refrigeration at 2°C to 8°C (36°F to 46°F); do not freeze; discard if frozen. **Note:** The Canadian labeling suggests that the vaccine is stable at temperatures up to 25°C (77°F) for 4 days.

Mechanism of Action Promotes active immunization against invasive disease caused by *S. pneumoniae* capsular serotypes 1, 3, 4, 5, 6A, 6B, 7F, 9V, 14, 18C, 19A, 19F, and 23F, all which are individually conjugated to CRM197 protein

Dosing: Usual

Pediatric:

Primary immunization; all patients: Note: Preterm infants should be vaccinated according to their chronological age from birth.

Infants and Children 6 weeks to 15 months: IM: 0.5 mL per dose for a total of 4 doses given as follows: the first dose may be given as young as 6 weeks of age, but is typically given at 8 weeks (2 months of age); the 3 remaining doses are usually given at 4, 6, and 12 to 15 months of age. The recommended dosing interval is 4 to 8 weeks. The minimum interval between doses in infants <1 year of age is 4 weeks. The minimum interval between the third and fourth dose is 8 weeks.

Catch-up immunization, healthy patients: CDC (ACIP) recommendations (Strikas 2015): Infants and Children 4 months to 6 years: **Note:** Do not restart the series. If doses have been given (PCV7 or PCV13), begin the below schedule at the applicable dose number. IM: 0.5 mL per dose for a total of 1 to 4 doses administered as follows:

First dose given on the elected date.

Second dose given at least 4 weeks after the first dose (if first dose at age <12 months) **or** at least 8 weeks after the first dose (if first dose at ≥12 months of age). This dose is not needed in healthy patients if the first dose was given at ≥24 months of age.

Third dose given at least 4 weeks after the second dose (if age <12 months) or at least 8 weeks after the first dose if: previous dose between 7 to 11 months of age (wait until at least 12 months of age) or age ≥12 months and at least 1 dose given before age 12 months. This dose is not needed in healthy patients if the previous dose was given at ≥24 months of age.

Fourth dose given at least 8 weeks after the third dose. This dose is only needed for children 12 to 59 months of age who received 3 doses before age 12 months.

High-risk conditions; catch-up or revaccination:

Infants ≥4 months and Children <24 months: For catch-up immunization, refer to Catch-up immunization, healthy patients dosing.

Children 2 through 5 years [CDC/ACIP [Nuorti 2010]):

Pneumococcal vaccine-naïve (no previous PCV13): IM: 0.5 mL for a total of 2 doses at least 8 weeks apart

Previously vaccinated with PCV7 and/or PCV13:

Previously received <3 doses of PCV (PCV7 and/or PCV13): IM: 0.5 mL dose for a total of 2 doses at least 8 weeks apart and at least 8 weeks after the most recent dose,

Previously received three doses of PCV (PCV7 and/ or PCV13): IM: 0.5 mL as a single dose ≥8 weeks after most recent dose.

Previously received 4 doses of PCV7 or other age-appropriate complete PCV7 series: IM: 0.5 mL as a single dose ≥8 weeks after most recent dose

Children and Adolescents 6 to 18 years (CDC/ACIP 62 [25] 2013):

Pneumococcal vaccine-naïve (no previous PCV13 or PPSV23 vaccine): IM: 0.5 mL as a single dose

Previously vaccinated with PPSV23 vaccine: If PCV13 has never been administered, give PCV13 vaccine: IM: 0.5 mL as a single dose ≥8 weeks after the last dose of PPSV23 vaccine. The PCV13 vaccine should be administered even if child has previously received PCV7.

Adult: **Immunization:**

Adults 19 to <65 years with specified underlying medical conditions: IM: 0.5 mL as a single dose

Note: Which vaccines are indicated (pneumococcal conjugate vaccine [PCV 13] and/or pneumococcal polysaccharide vaccine [PPSV23]) is dependent on previous pneumococcal vaccination history; some medical conditions do not require PCV13 [see guidelines for details] (CDC/ACIP [Kim 2015]):

Pneumococcal vaccine-naive or vaccination status unknown: Administer PCV13 followed by PPSV23 at least 8 weeks later

Previously received PPSV23 but not PCV 13: Administer PCV13 ≥1 year after the PPSV23 dose

Previously received PCV 13 but not PPSV23: No additional PCV 13 doses are needed

Revaccination: Administration of additional doses is not recommended for adults (CDC/ACIP [Kim 2015]).

Adults ≥65 years: IM: 0.5 mL as a single dose

Note: All patients should receive both pneumococcal conjugate vaccine (PCV 13) and pneumococcal polysaccharide vaccine (PPSV23) (CDC/ACIP [Tomczyk 2014]):

Pneumococcal vaccine-naive or vaccination status unknown: Administer PCV13 followed by PPSV23 6 to 12 months later (minimum interval of 8 weeks)

Previously received PPSV23 (at age ≥65 years) but not PCV 13: Administer PCV13 ≥1 year after the last dose of PPSV23

Previously received PPSV23 (at age <65 years) but not PCV13: Administer PCV13 ≥1 year after the last dose of PPSV23; administer PPSV23 6 to 12 months later (and at least 5 years after the last PPSV23 dose)

Dosing adjustment in renal impairment: There are no dosage adjustments provided in the manufacturer's labeling.

Dosing adjustment in hepatic impairment: There are no dosage adjustments provided in the manufacturer's labeling.

Administration IM: Shake vial well before withdrawing the dose; administer IM into midlateral aspect of the thigh in infants and small children; administer in the deltoid area to older children and adults; not for IV or SubQ administration. To prevent syncope-related injuries, adolescents and adults should be vaccinated while seated or lying down (NCIRD/ACIP 2011). US law requires that the date of administration; the vaccine manufacturer; lot number of vaccine; and the administering person's name, title, and address be entered into the patient's permanent medical record.

For patients at risk of hemorrhage following intramuscular injection, the vaccine should be administered intramuscularly if, in the opinion of the physician familiar with the patient's bleeding risk, the vaccine can be administered by this route with reasonable safety. If the patient receives antihemophilia or other similar therapy, intramuscular vaccination can be scheduled shortly after such therapy is administered. A fine needle (23 gauge or smaller) can be used for the vaccination and firm pressure applied to the site (without rubbing) for at least 2 minutes. The patient should be instructed concerning the risk of hematoma from the injection. Patients on anticoagulant therapy should be considered to have the same bleeding risks and treated as those with clotting factor disorders (NCIRD/ACIP 2011).

Monitoring Parameters Observe for syncope for 15 minutes following administration (NCIRD/ACIP 2011). If seizure-like activity associated with syncope occurs, maintain patient in supine or Trendelenburg position to reestablish adequate cerebral perfusion.

Additional Information Pneumococcal 13-valent conjugate vaccine (PCV13; Prevnar 13) is the successor to the previously-marketed pneumococcal 7-valent conjugate vaccine (PCV7; Prevnar). Prevnar 13 contains an additional six serotypes of *Streptococcus pneumoniae*, compared to the seven serotypes provided in the original Prevnar formulation.

Dosage Forms Excipient information presented when available (limited, particularly for generics); consult specific product labeling.

Injection, suspension:

Prevnar 13: 2 mcg of each capsular saccharide for serotypes 1, 3, 4, 5, 6A, 7F, 9V, 14, 18C, 19A, 19F, and 23F, and 4 mcg of serotype 6B [bound to diphtheria CRM_{197} protein ~34 mcg] per 0.5 mL (0.5 mL) [contains aluminum, polysorbate 80, and yeast]

Pneumococcal Polysaccharide Vaccine (23-Valent)

(noo moe KOK al pol i SAK a ride vak SEEN, TWEN tee three VAY lent)

Medication Safety Issues

Sound-alike/look-alike issues:

Pneumococcal 23-Valent Polysaccharide Vaccine (Pneumovax 23) may be confused with Pneumococcal 7-Valent Conjugate Vaccine (Prevnar) or with Pneumococcal 13-Valent Conjugate Vaccine (Prevnar 13)

Related Information

Centers for Disease Control and Prevention (CDC) and Other Links *on page 2424*

Immunization Administration Recommendations *on page 2411*

Immunization Schedules *on page 2416*

Brand Names: US Pneumovax 23

Brand Names: Canada Pneumo 23; Pneumovax 23

Therapeutic Category Vaccine; Vaccine, Inactivated Bacteria

Generic Availability (US) No

Use To provide immunization against pneumococcal disease caused by serotypes included in the vaccine (FDA approved in ages ≥2 years and adults).

The Advisory Committee on Immunization Practices (ACIP) recommends routine vaccination for patients with the following underlying medical conditions (CDC/ACI, 59 [34], 2010; CDC/ACIP 61[40], 2012; CDC/ACIP [Nuorti 2010]; CDC/ACIP [Tomczyk 2014]):

- Immunocompromised children ≥2 years, adolescents, and adults ≤64 years with congenital or acquired immunodeficiency (includes B or T cell deficiency, compliment deficiencies and phagocytic disorders; excludes chronic granulomatous disease), HIV infection, chronic renal failure, nephrotic syndrome, leukemia, lymphoma, Hodgkin disease, generalized malignancies, solid organ transplant, multiple myeloma, or other diseases requiring immunosuppressive drugs (including long-term systemic corticosteroids and radiation therapy)
- Children ≥2 years, adolescents, and adults 19 to 64 years with functional or anatomic asplenia, including sickle cell disease or other hemoglobinopathies, congenital or acquired asplenia, splenic dysfunction, or splenectomy
- Immunocompetent children ≥2 years and adolescents with chronic heart disease (particularly cyanotic congenital heart disease and heart failure), chronic lung disease (including asthma if treated with high dose corticosteroids), diabetes, cerebrospinal fluid leaks, or cochlear implants
- Immunocompetent adults 19 to 64 years with chronic heart disease (including heart failure and cardiomyopathies; excluding hypertension), chronic lung disease (including COPD, emphysema, and asthma), diabetes, cerebrospinal fluid leaks, cochlear implants, alcoholism, chronic liver disease, cirrhosis, and cigarette smokers
- All adults ≥65 years

Medication Guide Available Yes

Pregnancy Risk Factor C

Pregnancy Considerations Animal reproduction studies have not been conducted. Vaccination should be considered in pregnant women at high risk for infection. Inactivated vaccines have not been shown to cause increased risks to the fetus (NCIRD/ACIP 2011).

Breast-Feeding Considerations It is not known if the components of this vaccine are excreted into breast milk. The manufacturer recommends that caution be used if administered to nursing women. Inactivated vaccines do not affect the safety of breast-feeding for the mother or the infant. Breast-feeding infants should be vaccinated according to the recommended schedules (NCIRD/ACIP 2011).

Contraindications Severe allergic reaction (eg, anaphylactic/anaphylactoid reaction) to pneumococcal vaccine or any component of the formulation

Warnings/Precautions Use caution in patients with severely compromised cardiovascular function or pulmonary disease where a systemic reaction may pose a significant risk. May cause relapse in patients with stable idiopathic thrombocytopenia purpura. Immediate treatment (including epinephrine 1:1000) must be immediately available during vaccine use (NCIRD/ACIP 2011). Syncope has been reported with use of injectable vaccines and may result in serious secondary injury (eg, skull fracture, cerebral hemorrhage); typically reported in adolescents and young adults and within 15 minutes after vaccination. Procedures should be in place to avoid injuries from falling and to restore cerebral perfusion if syncope occurs (NCIRD/ACIP 2011). Use with caution in patients with bleeding disorders (including thrombocytopenia) and patients on anticoagulant therapy; bleeding/hematoma may occur from IM administration; if the patient receives antihemophilia or other similar therapy, IM injection can be scheduled shortly after such therapy is administered (NCIRD/ACIP 2011).

Patients who will be receiving immunosuppressive therapy (including Hodgkin's disease, cancer chemotherapy, or transplantation) should be vaccinated at least 2 weeks prior to the initiation of therapy. Immune responses may be impaired for several months following intensive immunosuppressive therapy (up to 2 years in Hodgkin disease patients). Vaccination may not result in effective immunity in all patients. Response depends upon multiple factors (eg, type of vaccine, age of patient) and may be improved by administering the vaccine at the recommended dose, route, and interval. Vaccines may not be effective if administered during periods of altered immune competence (NCIRD/ACIP 2011). Patients who will undergo splenectomy or who will undergo cochlear implant placement should also be vaccinated at least 2 weeks prior to surgery, if possible (IDSA [Rubin 2014]). In general, household and close contacts of persons with altered immunocompetence may receive all age appropriate vaccines (IDSA [Rubin 2014]; NCIRD/ACIP 2011). Patients with HIV should be vaccinated as soon as possible (following confirmation of the diagnosis) (CDC/ACIP, 61[40] 2012). In general, inactivated vaccines should be administered ≥2 weeks prior to planned immunosuppression when feasible (IDSA [Rubin 2014]). The decision to administer or delay vaccination because of current or recent febrile illness depends on the severity of symptoms and the etiology of the disease. Consider deferring administration in patients with moderate or severe acute illness (with or without fever); vaccination should not be delayed for patients with mild acute illness (with or without fever) (NCIRD/ACIP 2011).

Pneumococcal vaccine may not be effective in patients with chronic CSF leaks due to congenital lesions, skull fractures, or neurosurgical procedures. Vaccination does not replace the need for antibiotic prophylaxis against pneumococcal infection when otherwise required.

In order to maximize vaccination rates, the ACIP recommends simultaneous administration (ie, >1 vaccine on the same day at different anatomic sites) of all age-appropriate vaccines (live or inactivated) for which a person is eligible at a single clinic visit, unless contraindications exist. If a person has not received any pneumococcal vaccine or if pneumococcal vaccination status is unknown, PPSV23 should be administered as indicated. Pneumococcal vaccine is not approved for use in children <2 years of age. Children in this age group do not develop an effective immune response to the capsular types contained in this polysaccharide vaccine. Postmarketing reports of adverse effects in the elderly, especially those with comorbidities, have been significant enough to require hospitalization. Use of this vaccine for specific medical and/or other indications (eg, immunocompromising conditions, hepatic or kidney disease, diabetes) is also addressed in the ACIP Recommended Adult Immunization Schedule (CDC/ACIP [Kim 2015]). Specific recommendations for use of this vaccine in immunocompromised patients with asplenia, cancer, HIV infection, cerebrospinal fluid leaks, cochlear implants, hematopoietic stem cell transplant (prior to or after), sickle cell disease, solid organ transplant (prior to or after), or those receiving immunosuppressive therapy for chronic conditions are available from the IDSA (Rubin 2014).

Antipyretics have not been shown to prevent febrile seizures; antipyretics may be used to treat fever or discomfort following vaccination (NCIRD/ACIP 2011). One study reported that routine prophylactic administration of acetaminophen to prevent fever prior to vaccination decreased the immune response of some vaccines; the clinical significance of this reduction in immune response has not been established (Prymula 2009).

Warnings: Additional Pediatric Considerations Not recommended for use in infants and children <2 years of age.

Adverse Reactions All serious adverse reactions must be reported to the U.S. Department of Health and Human Services (DHHS) Vaccine Adverse Event Reporting System (VAERS) 1-800-822-7967 or online at https://vaers.hhs.gov/esub/index. In Canada, adverse reactions may be reported to local provincial/territorial health agencies or to the Vaccine Safety Section at Public Health Agency of Canada (1-866-844-0018).

Central nervous system: Chills, Guillain-Barré syndrome, fever ≤102°F*, fever >102°F, headache, malaise, pain, radiculoneuropathy, seizure (febrile)

Dermatologic: Angioneurotic edema, cellulitis, rash, urticaria

Gastrointestinal: Nausea, vomiting

Hematologic: Hemolytic anemia (in patients with other hematologic disorders), leukocytosis, thrombocytopenia (in patients with stabilized ITP)

Local: Injection site reaction* (erythema, induration, swelling, soreness, warmth); peripheral edema in injected extremity

Neuromuscular & skeletal: Arthralgia, arthritis, limb mobility decreased, myalgia, paresthesia, weakness

Miscellaneous: Anaphylactoid reaction, C-reactive protein increased, lymphadenitis, lymphadenopathy, serum sickness

*Reactions most commonly reported in clinical trials.

Drug Interactions

Metabolism/Transport Effects None known.

Avoid Concomitant Use There are no known interactions where it is recommended to avoid concomitant use.

Increased Effect/Toxicity There are no known significant interactions involving an increase in effect.

Decreased Effect

Pneumococcal Polysaccharide Vaccine (23-Valent) may decrease the levels/effects of: Zoster Vaccine

The levels/effects of Pneumococcal Polysaccharide Vaccine (23-Valent) may be decreased by: Belimumab; Fingolimod; Immunosuppressants

Storage/Stability Store at 2°C to 8°C (36°F to 46°F).

Mechanism of Action

Pneumococcal polysaccharide polyvalent is an inactive bacterial vaccine that induces active immunization to the serotypes contained in the vaccine. Although there are more than 80 known pneumococcal capsular types, pneumococcal disease is mainly caused by only a few types of pneumococci. Pneumococcal vaccine polyvalent contains capsular polysaccharides of 23 pneumococcal types of *Streptococcal pneumoniae* which represent at least 85% to 90% of pneumococcal disease isolates in the United States. The 23 capsular pneumococcal vaccine contains purified capsular polysaccharides of pneumococcal types 1, 2, 3, 4, 5, 6B, 7F, 8, 9N, 9V, 10A, 11A, 12F, 14, 15B, 17F, 18C, 19F, 19A, 20, 22F, 23F, and 33F.

Efficacy: In adults, PPSV23 demonstrated 50% to 80% efficacy in preventing invasive pneumococcal disease due to relevant serotypes of *S. pneumoniae* (CDC/ACIP 59[34] 2010).

Dosing: Usual

Pediatric:

Primary immunization: Children ≥2 years and Adolescents with specified underlying medical conditions: IM, SubQ: 0.5 mL as a single dose; immunization with pneumococcal conjugate vaccine (PCV13) should be completed prior to pneumococcal polysaccharide vaccine (PPSV23) as recommended. The minimum interval between the last dose of PCV13 and PPSV23 is 8 weeks (AAP, 2010; CDC/ACIP [Nuorti 2010]).

Revaccination: Children ≥2 and Adolescents with functional or anatomic asplenia, those who are immunocompromised, and others with high-risk medical conditions [see guidelines for specific details]: One revaccination dose ≥5 years after the first dose of PPSV23. Revaccination of immunocompetent individuals is generally not recommended (CDC/ACIP [Strikas 2015]).

Adult:

Primary immunization:

Adults 19 to <65 years with specified underlying medical conditions: IM, SubQ: 0.5 mL as a single dose

Note: Some medical conditions do not require PCV13 [see guidelines for details] (CDC/ACIP [Kim 2015]):

Pneumococcal vaccine-naive or vaccination status unknown: Administer PCV13 followed by PPSV23 at least 8 weeks later

Previously received PPSV23 but not PCV13: No additional PPSV23 doses needed for primary vaccination; administer PCV13 ≥ 1 year after the last PPSV23 dose was received.

Previously received PCV13 but not PPSV23: Administer PPSV23 at least 8 weeks after PCV13

Adults ≥65 years: IM, SubQ: 0.5 mL as a single dose

Note: All patients should receive both PCV13 and PPSV23 [see guidelines for specific details] (CDC/ACIP [Tomczyk 2014]):

Revaccination: Adults 19 to 64 years of age with chronic renal failure or nephrotic syndrome, functional, or anatomic asplenia or who are immunocompromised: One revaccination dose ≥5 years after first dose of PPSV23 (CDC/ACIP, 59[34], 2010) and ≥8 weeks after PCV13 (CDC/ACIP, 61[40], 2012)

Dosing adjustment in renal impairment: There are no dosage adjustments provided in the manufacturer's labeling.

Dosing adjustment in hepatic impairment: There are no dosage adjustments provided in the manufacturer's labeling.

Administration Administer SubQ or IM either the anterolateral aspect of the thigh or the deltoid muscle; not for IV or intradermal administration. To prevent syncope-related injuries, adolescents and adults should be vaccinated while seated or lying down (NCIRD/ACIP 2011). US law requires that the date of administration; the vaccine manufacturer; lot number of vaccine; and the administering person's name, title, and address be entered into the patient's permanent medical record.

For patients at risk of hemorrhage following intramuscular injection, the vaccine should be administered intramuscularly if, in the opinion of the physician familiar with the patient's bleeding risk, the vaccine can be administered by this route with reasonable safety. If the patient receives antihemophilia or other similar therapy, intramuscular vaccination can be scheduled shortly after such therapy is administered. A fine needle (23 gauge or smaller) can be used for the vaccination and firm pressure applied to the site (without rubbing) for at least 2 minutes. The patient should be instructed concerning the risk of hematoma from the injection. Patients on anticoagulant therapy should be considered to have the same bleeding risks and treated as those with clotting factor disorders (NCIRD/ACIP 2011).

Monitoring Parameters Observe for syncope for 15 minutes following administration (NCIRD/ACIP 2011). If seizure-like activity associated with syncope occurs, maintain patient in supine or Trendelenburg position to reestablish adequate cerebral perfusion.

Dosage Forms Excipient information presented when available (limited, particularly for generics); consult specific product labeling.

Injection, solution:

Pneumovax 23: 25 mcg each of 23 capsular polysaccharide isolates/0.5 mL (0.5 mL, 2.5 mL)

◆ **Pneumococcal Polysaccharide Vaccine (Polyvalent)** *see* Pneumococcal Polysaccharide Vaccine (23-Valent) *on page* 1718

◆ **Pneumovax 23** *see* Pneumococcal Polysaccharide Vaccine (23-Valent) *on page* 1718

◆ **PNU-140690E** *see* Tipranavir *on page* 2070

◆ **Podactin [OTC]** *see* Miconazole (Topical) *on page* 1431

◆ **Podactin [OTC]** *see* Tolnaftate *on page* 2083

◆ **Podocon** *see* Podophyllum Resin *on page* 1720

◆ **Podofilm® (Can)** *see* Podophyllum Resin *on page* 1720

◆ **Podophyllin** *see* Podophyllum Resin *on page* 1720

Podophyllum Resin (po DOF fil um REZ in)

Brand Names: US Podocon

Brand Names: Canada Podofilm®

Therapeutic Category Keratolytic Agent

Generic Availability (US) Yes

Use Topical treatment of benign growths including external genital and perianal warts (condylomata acuminata), papillomas, fibroids

Pregnancy Considerations Reports in pregnant women have shown evidence of fetal abnormalities, fetal death, and stillbirth; use is contraindicated in women who are or may become pregnant

Breast-Feeding Considerations It is not known of podophyllum resin is excreted into breast milk. Use in nursing women is contraindicated by the manufacturer.

Contraindications Not to be used on bleeding warts, birthmarks, moles, or warts with hair growth; not to be used by patients with diabetes or poor circulation; concurrent use of steroids; pregnancy; breast-feeding

Warnings/Precautions Use of large amounts of drug should be avoided. For external use only; avoid contact with the eyes as it can cause severe corneal damage; do not apply to moles, birthmarks, or unusual warts; do not use if wart or surrounding tissue is inflamed/irritated. To be applied by a physician only.

Adverse Reactions

Central nervous system: Coma, fever, polyneuritis

Gastrointestinal: Paralytic ileus

Hematologic: Leukopenia, thrombocytopenia

Neuromuscular & skeletal: Paresthesia

Miscellaneous: Death

Drug Interactions

Metabolism/Transport Effects None known.

Avoid Concomitant Use There are no known interactions where it is recommended to avoid concomitant use.

Increased Effect/Toxicity There are no known significant interactions involving an increase in effect.

Decreased Effect There are no known significant interactions involving a decrease in effect.

Storage/Stability Store at controlled room temperature of 20°C to 25°C (68°F to 77°F). Protect from light.

Mechanism of Action Directly affects epithelial cell metabolism by arresting mitosis through binding to a protein subunit of spindle microtubules (tubulin)

Dosing: Usual Children and Adults: Topical: 10% to 25% solution in compound benzoin tincture; use 1 drop at a time allowing drying between drops until area is covered; total volume should be limited to <0.5 mL to an area <10 cm^2 for genital or perianal warts or <2 cm^2 for vaginal warts per treatment session; therapy may be repeated once weekly for up to 4 applications for the treatment of genital or perianal warts; use 10% solution when applied to or near mucous membranes

Verrucae: 25% solution is applied directly to the wart; remove drug from area of application within 6 hours

Administration Topical: Clean and dry affected area prior to application. Use applicator provided with product. When applying for the first time leave on for only 30-40 minutes to determine patient sensitivity. After first use may leave on 1-4 hours depending on severity of lesion; systemic absorption may occur with prolonged contact. Do not treat large areas or many warts at one time. Remove drug with alcohol or soap and water once treatment time has elapsed.

Dosage Forms Excipient information presented when available (limited, particularly for generics); consult specific product labeling.

Solution, External:

Podocon: 25% (15 mL)

◆ **Polio Vaccine** *see* Poliovirus Vaccine (Inactivated) *on page* 1721

◆ **Poliovirus, Inactivated (IPV)** *see* Diphtheria and Tetanus Toxoids, Acellular Pertussis, and Poliovirus Vaccine *on page 677*

◆ **Poliovirus, Inactivated (IPV)** *see* Diphtheria and Tetanus Toxoids, Acellular Pertussis, Poliovirus and *Haemophilus* b Conjugate Vaccine *on page 679*

Poliovirus Vaccine (Inactivated)

(POE lee oh VYE rus vak SEEN, in ak ti VAY ted)

Medication Safety Issues

Administration issues:

Poliovirus vaccine (inactivated) may be confused with tuberculin products. Medication errors have occurred when poliovirus vaccine (IPV) has been inadvertently administered instead of tuberculin skin tests (PPD). These products are refrigerated and often stored in close proximity to each other.

Related Information

Centers for Disease Control and Prevention (CDC) and Other Links *on page 2424*

Immunization Administration Recommendations *on page 2411*

Immunization Schedules *on page 2416*

Brand Names: US IPOL

Brand Names: Canada Imovax Polio

Therapeutic Category Vaccine; Vaccine, Inactivated Virus

Generic Availability (US) No

Use Provide active immunity to poliovirus (FDA approved in ages ≥6 weeks and adults)

The Advisory Committee on Immunization Practices (ACIP) recommends routine vaccination for the following:

- All infants and children (first dose given at 2 months of age) (CDC/ACIP 58[30] 2009)

Routine immunization of adults in the United States is generally not recommended. Adults with previous wild poliovirus disease, who have never been immunized, or those who are incompletely immunized may receive inactivated poliovirus vaccine if they fall into one of the following categories (CDC/ACIP [Prevots 2000]):

- Travelers to regions or countries where poliomyelitis is endemic or epidemic
- Health care workers in close contact with patients who may be excreting poliovirus
- Laboratory workers handling specimens that may contain poliovirus
- Members of communities or specific population groups with diseases caused by wild poliovirus
- Incompletely vaccinated or unvaccinated adults in a household or with other close contact with children receiving oral poliovirus (may be at increased risk of vaccine associated paralytic poliomyelitis)

Medication Guide Available Yes

Pregnancy Risk Factor C

Pregnancy Considerations Animal reproduction studies have not been conducted. Although adverse effects of IPV have not been documented in pregnant women or their fetuses, vaccination of pregnant women should be avoided on theoretical grounds. Pregnant women at increased risk for infection and requiring immediate protection against polio may be administered the vaccine.

Breast-Feeding Considerations Inactivated virus vaccines do not affect the safety of breast-feeding for the mother or the infant. Breast-feeding infants should be vaccinated according to the recommended schedules (NCIRD/ACIP, 2011).

Contraindications Hypersensitivity to any component of the vaccine

Warnings/Precautions Patients with prior clinical poliomyelitis, incomplete immunization with oral poliovirus vaccine (OPV), HIV infection, severe combined immunodeficiency, hypogammaglobulinemia, agammaglobulinemia, or altered immunity (due to corticosteroids, alkylating agents, antimetabolites or radiation) may receive inactivated poliovirus vaccine (IPV). In general, household and close contacts of persons with altered immunocompetence may receive all age appropriate vaccines (IDSA [Rubin, 2014]; NCIRD/ACIP, 2011); inactivated vaccines should be administered ≥2 weeks prior to planned immunosuppression when feasible (IDSA [Rubin, 2014]). Immune response may be decreased in patients receiving immune globulin. The decision to administer or delay vaccination because of current or recent febrile illness depends on the severity of symptoms and the etiology of the disease. Consider deferring administration in patients with moderate or severe acute illness (with or without fever); vaccination should not be delayed for patients with mild acute illness (with or without fever) (NCIRD/ACIP, 2011).

Vaccination may not result in effective immunity in all patients. Response depends upon multiple factors (eg, type of vaccine, age of patient) and may be improved by administering the vaccine at the recommended dose, route, and interval. Vaccines may not be effective if administered during periods of altered immune competence (NCIRD/ACIP, 2011). Immediate treatment (including epinephrine 1:1,000) for anaphylactoid and/or hypersensitivity reactions should be available during vaccine use (NCIRD/ACIP, 2011). In order to maximize vaccination rates, the ACIP recommends simultaneous administration of all age-appropriate vaccines (live or inactivated) for which a person is eligible at a single clinic visit, unless contraindications exist. The use of combination vaccines is generally preferred over separate injections, taking into consideration provider assessment, patient preference, and adverse events. When using combination vaccines, the minimum age for administration is the oldest minimum age for any individual component; the minimum interval between dosing is the greatest minimum interval between any individual components. The ACIP prefers each dose of a specific vaccine in a series come from the same manufacturer when possible (NCIRD/ACIP, 2011). Syncope has been reported with use of injectable vaccines and may result in serious secondary injury (eg, skull fracture, cerebral hemorrhage); typically reported in adolescents and young adults and within 15 minutes after vaccination. Procedures should be in place to avoid injuries from falling and to restore cerebral perfusion if syncope occurs (NCIRD/ACIP, 2011).

The injection contains 2-phenoxyethanol, calf serum protein, formaldehyde, neomycin, streptomycin, and polymyxin B. Use of the minimum age and minimum intervals during the first 6 months of life should only be done when the vaccine recipient is at risk for imminent exposure to circulating poliovirus (shorter intervals and earlier start dates may lead to lower seroconversion). Specific recommendations for use of this vaccine in immunocompromised patients with asplenia, cancer, HIV infection, cerebrospinal fluid leaks, cochlear implants, hematopoietic stem cell transplant (prior to or after), sickle cell disease, solid organ transplant (prior to or after), or those receiving immunosuppressive therapy for chronic conditions as well as contacts of immunocompromised patients are available from the IDSA (Rubin, 2014).

Antipyretics have not been shown to prevent febrile seizures; antipyretics may be used to treat fever or discomfort following vaccination (NCIRD/ACIP, 2011). One study reported that routine prophylactic administration of acetaminophen to prevent fever prior to vaccination decreased the immune response of some vaccines; the clinical significance of this reduction in immune response has not been established (Prymula, 2009). Apnea has occurred following intramuscular vaccine administration in premature infants; consider clinical status implications. In general, preterm infants should be vaccinated at the same chronological age as full-term infants (NCIRD/ACIP, 2011).

Adverse Reactions All serious adverse reactions must be reported to the U.S. Department of Health and Human Services (DHHS) Vaccine Adverse Event Reporting System (VAERS) 1-800-822-7967 or online at https://vaers.hhs.gov/esub/index. In Canada, adverse reactions may be reported to local provincial/territorial health agencies or to the Vaccine Safety Section at Public Health Agency of Canada (1-866-844-0018).

Central nervous system: Fever (>39°C), irritability (most common in infants 2 months of age), tiredness
Gastrointestinal: Anorexia
Local: Injection site: Swelling, tenderness
Gastrointestinal: Vomiting
Local: Injection site: Erythema
Miscellaneous: Persistent crying
Rare but important or life-threatening: Allergic reaction, anaphylactic shock, anaphylaxis, febrile seizures, hypersensitivity reactions, lymphadenopathy, seizures; Guillain-Barré syndrome has been temporally related to another inactivated poliovirus vaccine

Drug Interactions

Metabolism/Transport Effects None known.

Avoid Concomitant Use There are no known interactions where it is recommended to avoid concomitant use.

Increased Effect/Toxicity There are no known significant interactions involving an increase in effect.

Decreased Effect

The levels/effects of Poliovirus Vaccine (Inactivated) may be decreased by: Belimumab; Fingolimod; Immunosuppressants

Storage/Stability Store under refrigeration 2°C to 8°C (35°F to 46°F); do not freeze. Protect from light

Mechanism of Action As an inactivated virus vaccine, poliovirus vaccine induces active immunity against poliovirus types 1, 2, and 3 infection

Dosing: Usual

Pediatric: **Note:** Use of the minimum age and minimum intervals (4 weeks) during the first 6 months of life should only be done when the vaccine recipient is at risk for imminent exposure to circulating poliovirus (shorter intervals and earlier start dates may lead to lower seroconversion).

Primary immunization: Infants and Children 6 weeks to 47 months: IM, SubQ: 0.5 mL per dose for a total of 3 doses administered as follows: 2 months, 4 months, and 6 to 18 months of age

Booster immunization: Children 4 to 6 years: IM, SubQ: 0.5 mL as a single dose; administered at least 6 months from the previous dose

Catch-up immunization (CDC/ACIP [Strikas 2015]): Infants, Children, and Adolescents 4 months to 18 years: **Note:** Do not restart the series if doses have been given (OPV or IPV). Begin the below schedule at the applicable dose number. IM, SubQ: 0.5 mL per dose for a total of 1 to 4 doses administered as follows:

First dose given on the elected date
Second dose given at least 4 weeks after the first dose
Third dose given at least 4 weeks after the second dose
Fourth dose given at least 6 months after the third dose and at age ≥4 years; fourth dose not needed if the third dose was given at least 6 months after second dose and at ≥4 years of age

Note: If 4 or more doses were administered before age of 4 years, an additional dose should be given at age 4 to 6 years, at least 6 months after the previous dose.

Adult: **Note:** Not routinely recommended unless at increased risk of exposure.

Immunization:

Poliovirus vaccine-naïve (no previous IPV or OPV vaccine): IM, SubQ: Administer 0.5 mL per dose for a total of 3 doses given as follows: Two 0.5 mL doses administered at 1- to 2-month intervals, followed by a third dose 6 to 12 months later. If <3 months, but at least 2 months are available before protection is needed, 3 doses may be administered at least 1 month apart. If administration must be completed within 1 to 2 months, give 2 doses at least 1 month apart. If <1 month is available, give 1 dose.

Previously vaccinated with at least at least 1 previous dose of OPV, <3 doses of IPV, or a combination of OPV and IPV equaling <3 doses: IM, SubQ: Administer at least one 0.5 mL dose of IPV. Additional doses to complete the series may be given if time permits.

Immunization for increased risk of exposure (completely vaccinated): I.M, SubQ: 0.5 mL as a single dose

Dosing adjustment in renal impairment: There are no dosage adjustments provided in the manufacturer's labeling.

Dosing adjustment in hepatic impairment: There are no dosage adjustments provided in the manufacturer's labeling.

Administration Administer IM or SubQ into midlateral aspect of the thigh in infants and small children; administer in the deltoid area to older children and adults; not for IV administration. To prevent syncope related injuries, adolescents and adults should be vaccinated while seated or lying down (NCIRD/ACIP 2011). US law requires that the date of administration, the vaccine manufacturer, lot number of vaccine, and the administering person's name, title, and address be entered into the patient's permanent medical record.

For patients at risk of hemorrhage following intramuscular injection, the vaccine should be administered intramuscularly if, in the opinion of the physician familiar with the patient's bleeding risk, the vaccine can be administered by this route with reasonable safety. If the patient receives antihemophilia or other similar therapy, intramuscular vaccination can be scheduled shortly after such therapy is administered. A fine needle (23 gauge or smaller) should be used for the vaccination and firm pressure on the site (without rubbing) for at least 2 minutes. The patient should be instructed concerning the risk of hematoma from the injection. Patients on anticoagulant therapy should be considered to have the same bleeding risks and treated as those with clotting factor disorders (NCIRD/ACIP 2011).

Monitoring Parameters Observe for syncope for 15 minutes following administration (NCIRD/ACIP 2011). If seizure-like activity associated with syncope occurs, maintain patient in supine or Trendelenburg position to reestablish adequate cerebral perfusion.

Test Interactions May temporarily suppress tuberculin skin test sensitivity (4-6 weeks)

Additional Information Oral polio vaccine (OPV) is no longer distributed in the United States; OPV is the vaccine of choice for global eradication in areas with continued or recent circulation of wild-type poliovirus, most developing countries where the higher cost of IPV prohibits its use or where inadequate sanitation necessitates an optimal barrier to wild-type virus circulation (*Red Book* [AAP], 2012)

Dosage Forms Excipient information presented when available (limited, particularly for generics); consult specific product labeling.

Injection, suspension:

IPOL: Type 1 poliovirus 40 D-antigen units, type 2 poliovirus 8 D-antigen units, and type 3 poliovirus 32 D-antigen units per 0.5 mL (0.5 mL, 5 mL) [contains 2-phenoxyethanol, formaldehyde, calf serum protein, neomycin (may have trace amounts), streptomycin (may have trace amounts), and polymyxin B (may have trace amounts)]

- **Polocaine** *see* Mepivacaine *on page 1362*
- **Polocaine® (Can)** *see* Mepivacaine *on page 1362*
- **Polocaine-MPF** *see* Mepivacaine *on page 1362*
- **Polycin™** *see* Bacitracin and Polymyxin B *on page 252*
- **Polycitra** *see* Citric Acid, Sodium Citrate, and Potassium Citrate *on page 479*
- **Polycitra K** *see* Potassium Citrate and Citric Acid *on page 1738*
- **Polyethylene Glycol-L-asparaginase** *see* Pegaspargase *on page 1639*

Polyethylene Glycol 3350

(pol i ETH i leen GLY kol 3350)

Medication Safety Issues

Sound-alike/look-alike issues:

MiraLax may be confused with Mirapex

Polyethylene glycol 3350 may be confused with polyethylene glycol electrolyte solution

International issues:

MiraLax may be confused with Murelax brand name for oxazepam [Australia]

Polyethylene glycol 3350 may be confused with polyethylene glycol 4000 [international markets]

Brand Names: US GaviLAX [OTC]; GlycoLax [OTC]; HealthyLax [OTC]; MiraLax [OTC]; PEGyLAX

Brand Names: Canada Peg 3350; Pegalax; Relaxa

Therapeutic Category Laxative, Osmotic

Generic Availability (US) Yes

Use Treatment of occasional constipation (OTC product: FDA approved in ages ≥17 years and adults)

Pregnancy Considerations Polyethylene glycol (PEG) has minimal systemic absorption and would be unlikely to cause fetal malformations. However, until additional information is available, use to treat constipation in pregnancy should be avoided unless other preferred methods are inadequate (Mahadevan, 2006). Use as a bowel preparation prior to colonoscopy in pregnant women may be considered (Wexner, 2006).

Contraindications

Hypersensitivity to polyethylene glycol or any component of the formulation

Canadian labeling: Relaxa: Additional contraindications (not in U.S. labeling): Known or suspected bowel obstruction; use in children <18 years of age unless advised by a physician

Warnings/Precautions Evaluate patients with symptoms of bowel obstruction (nausea, vomiting, abdominal pain, or distension) prior to use; avoid use in patients with known or suspected bowel obstruction. Use with caution in patients with renal impairment. Do not use for longer than 1 week; 2-4 days may be required to produce bowel movement. Prolonged, frequent, or excessive use may lead to electrolyte imbalance. When using for self medication, patients should consult healthcare provider prior to use if they have nausea, vomiting, or abdominal pain, irritable bowel syndrome, kidney disease, or a sudden change in bowel habits for >2 weeks. Patients should be instructed to discontinue use and consult healthcare provider if they have diarrhea, rectal bleeding, if abdominal pain, bloating, cramping, or nausea gets worse, or if need to use for >1 week.

Warnings: Additional Pediatric Considerations The effects of long-term use or large doses of polyethylene glycol in children are unknown. The FDA has received reports of metabolic acidosis (with and without anion gap) and neuropsychiatric events in children taking polyethylene glycol; however, direct causality with the drug has not been established. Neuropsychiatric adverse events reported may include seizures, tremors, tics, headache, anxiety, lethargy, sedation, aggression, rages, obsessive-compulsive behaviors (including repetitive chewing and sucking), paranoia and mood swings. Studies are underway to define the metabolic processes and pathways polyethylene glycol (and any metabolites) in pediatric patients and to determine gastrointestinal absorption properties if any (FDA 2013). As of 2014, the FDA decided no action was necessary based upon available data (FDA 2014). Monitor pediatric patients closely for signs of metabolic acidosis or neuropsychiatric changes.

Adverse Reactions

Dermatologic: Urticaria

Gastrointestinal: Abdominal bloating, cramping, diarrhea, flatulence, nausea

Rare but important or life-threatening: Anaphylactic shock (observed with PEG 6000)

Drug Interactions

Metabolism/Transport Effects None known.

Avoid Concomitant Use There are no known interactions where it is recommended to avoid concomitant use.

Increased Effect/Toxicity There are no known significant interactions involving an increase in effect.

Decreased Effect

Polyethylene Glycol 3350 may decrease the levels/effects of: Digoxin

Storage/Stability Store at room temperature before reconstitution.

Mechanism of Action An osmotic agent, polyethylene glycol 3350 causes water retention in the stool; increases stool frequency.

Pharmacodynamics Onset of action: Produces bowel movement in 1 to 3 days

Pharmacokinetics (Adult data unless noted)

Absorption: Minimal; <0.28% (Pelham 2008)

Elimination: Feces (93%); urine (0.2%) (Pelham 2008)

Dosing: Usual

Pediatric:

Bowel preparation: Limited data available: Children >2 years and Adolescents: Oral: 1.5 g/kg/day for 4 days; maximum daily dose: 100 g/**day** (Pashankar 2004)

Constipation: Limited data available: Infants, Children, and Adolescents: Oral: 0.2 to 0.8 g/kg/day (NASPGHAN [Tabbers] 2014); higher initial dose of 1 g/kg have been suggested (Loening-Buck 2004; Pashankar 2001); maximum daily dose: 17 g/day. **Note:** Dosage should be individualized to achieved desired effect, infants and young children may require higher doses than school aged children (Loening-Buck 2004; Pashankar 2001)

Fecal impaction, slow disimpaction: Limited data available: Children and Adolescents: Oral: 1 to 1.5 g/kg daily for 3 to 6 consecutive days (NASPGHAN [Tabbers] 2014; Youssef 2002); maximum daily dose: 100 g/**day** (Youssef 2002); following disimpaction maintenance dose of 0.4 g/kg daily should be continued for ≥ 2 months (NASPGHAN [Tabbers] 2014)

Adult:

Bowel preparation: Oral: Mix 17 g of powder (~1 heaping tablespoon) in 8 ounces of clear liquid and administer the entire mixture every 10 minutes until 2 liters are consumed (start within 6 hours after administering 20 mg bisacodyl delayed release tablets) (Wexner 2006)

Constipation, occasional: Oral: 17 g of powder (~1 heaping tablespoon) dissolved in 4 to 8 ounces of beverage, once daily; do not use for >1 week unless directed by healthcare provider

Administration Oral:

Bowel preparation for colonoscopy: Stir powder in 8 ounces of clear liquid until dissolved and drink. Oral medications should not be administered within 1 hour of start of therapy.

Constipation: Stir powder in 4 to 8 ounces of water, juice, soda, coffee or tea until dissolved and administer.

Monitoring Parameters Stool frequency

Dosage Forms Excipient information presented when available (limited, particularly for generics); consult specific product labeling.

Packet, Oral:
- HealthyLax: (1 ea, 14 ea)
- MiraLax: (1 ea, 10 ea, 12 ea, 24 ea)
- Generic: (1 ea, 14 ea, 30 ea, 100 ea)

Powder, Oral:
- GaviLAX: (238 g, 510 g)
- GlycoLax: (119 g, 255 g, 527 g)
- MiraLax: (1 ea, 119 g, 238 g, 510 g)
- PEGyLAX: (527 g)
- Generic: 17 g/dose (119 g, 238 g, 510 g); (119 g, 238 g, 250 g, 255 g, 500 g, 510 g, 527 g, 850 g)

Polyethylene Glycol-Electrolyte Solution

(pol i ETH i leen GLY kol ee LEK troe lite soe LOO shun)

Medication Safety Issues

Sound-alike/look-alike issues:

GoLYTELY may be confused with NuLYTELY

TriLyte may be confused with TriLipix

International issues:

Polyethylene glycol 3350 may be confused with polyethylene glycol 4000 [international markets]

Brand Names: US Colyte; GaviLyte-C; GaviLyte-G; GaviLyte-N; GoLYTELY; MoviPrep; NuLYTELY; TriLyte

Brand Names: Canada Colyte; Klean-Prep; PegLyte

Therapeutic Category Laxative, Bowel Evacuant; Laxative, Osmotic

Generic Availability (US) Yes

Use Bowel cleansing prior to GI procedure (GaviLyte-N, NuLYTELY, Trilyte: FDA approved in ages ≥6 months and adults; MoviPrep: FDA approved in ages ≥18 and adults; Colyte, GaviLyte-C, GaviLyte-G: FDA approved in adults); has also been used for whole bowel irrigation after toxic ingestions and for treatment of fecal impaction

Medication Guide Available Yes

Pregnancy Risk Factor C

Pregnancy Considerations Animal reproduction studies have not been conducted. Information related to the use of polyethylene glycol-electrolyte solution in pregnancy is limited (Neri, 2004). Colonoscopy in pregnant women is generally reserved for strong indications or life-threatening emergencies; until additional safety data for polyethylene glycol-electrolyte solution is available, other agents may be preferred for this purpose (Siddiqui, 2006; Wexner, 2006).

Breast-Feeding Considerations It is not known if polyethylene glycol-electrolyte solution is excreted into breast milk. Significant changes in the mother's fluid or electrolyte balance would not be expected with most products.

Contraindications Hypersensitivity to polyethylene glycol or any component of the formulation; ileus, gastrointestinal obstruction, gastric retention, bowel perforation, toxic colitis, toxic megacolon

Warnings/Precautions Evaluate patients with symptoms of bowel obstruction or perforation (nausea, vomiting, abdominal pain or distension) prior to use; if a patient develops severe bloating, distention or abdominal pain during administration, slow the rate of administration or temporarily discontinue use until the symptoms subside. Correct electrolyte abnormalities in patients prior to use. No additional ingredients or flavors (other than the flavor packets provided) should be added to the polyethylene glycol-electrolyte solution.

Fluid and electrolyte disturbances can lead to arrhythmias, seizures, and renal impairment. Advise patients to maintain adequate hydration before, during, and after treatment. If patient becomes dehydrated or experiences significant vomiting after treatment, consider post-colonoscopy lab tests (electrolytes, creatinine, and BUN). Serious arrhythmias have been reported (rarely) with the use of ionic osmotic laxative products. Use with caution in patients who may be at risk of cardiac arrhythmias (eg, patients with a history of prolonged QT, uncontrolled arrhythmias, recent MI, unstable angina, CHF, or cardiomyopathy). Consider pre-dose and post-colonoscopy ECGs in these patients. Generalized tonic-clonic seizures and/or loss of consciousness have occurred rarely in patients with no prior history of seizures. Seizures resolved with the correction of fluid and electrolyte abnormalities. Use with caution in patients with a history of seizures or who are at an increased risk of seizures (eg concomitant administration of medications that lower the seizures threshold, patients withdrawing from alcohol or benzodiazepines) and in patients with known or suspected hyponatremia or low serum osmolality.

Cases of ischemic colitis have been reported; concomitant use of stimulant laxatives may increase the risk and is not recommended. The potential for mucosal aphthous ulcerations as a result of the bowel preparation should be considered, especially when evaluating colonoscopy results in patients with known or suspected inflammatory bowel disease. Use with caution in patients with severe ulcerative colitis. Use with caution in patients with renal impairment and/or in patients taking medications that may adversely affect renal function (eg, diuretics, NSAIDs, ACE inhibitors, ARBs). Patients with impaired renal function should be instructed to remain adequately hydrated; consider pre-dose and post-colonoscopy lab tests (electrolytes, creatinine, BUN) in these patients. Observe unconscious or semiconscious patients with impaired gag reflex or those who are otherwise prone to regurgitation or aspiration during administration; use with caution.

MoviPrep: Use with caution in patients with G6PD deficiency (especially patients with an active infection, history of hemolysis, or taking concomitant medications known to precipitate hemolytic reactions) due to the presence of sodium ascorbate and ascorbic acid in the formulation. Contains phenylalanine.

Use in patients <2 years of age may result in hypoglycemia, dehydration, and hypokalemia; use with caution and monitor closely. Use with caution in patients >60 years of age; serious adverse events have been reported (eg, asystole, esophageal perforation, chest infiltration following vomiting and aspiration, Mallory-Weiss tear with GI bleeding, pulmonary edema with sudden dyspnea).

Warnings: Additional Pediatric Considerations

The effects of long-term use or large doses of polyethylene glycol in children are unknown. The FDA has received reports of metabolic acidosis (with and without anion gap) and neuropsychiatric events in children taking polyethylene glycol products; however, direct causality with the drug has not been established. Neuropsychiatric adverse events reported may include seizures, tremors, tics, headache, anxiety, lethargy, sedation, aggression, rages, obsessive-compulsive behaviors (including repetitive chewing and sucking), paranoia, and mood swings. Studies are underway to define the metabolic processes and pathways of polyethylene glycol (and any metabolites) in pediatric patients and to determine gastrointestinal absorption properties if any (FDA 2013). As of 2014, the FDA decided no action was necessary based upon available data (FDA 2014). Monitor pediatric patients closely for signs of metabolic acidosis or neuropsychiatric changes.

Adverse Reactions

Central nervous system: Dizziness, headache, malaise, rigors, sleep disorder

Endocrine & metabolic: Increased thirst

Gastrointestinal: Abdominal distention, abdominal pain, anorectal pain, bloating, dyspepsia, hunger, nausea, vomiting

Rare but important or life-threatening: Anaphylaxis, angioedema, aspiration, asystole (older adults >60 years), chest tightness, esophageal perforation (older adults >60 years), hypersensitivity reaction, ischemic colitis, Mallory-Weiss syndrome (older adults >60 years), pulmonary edema (older adults >60 years), rhinorrhea, seizure, shock, tightness in chest and throat, upper gastrointestinal hemorrhage (older adults >60 years), urticaria

Drug Interactions

Metabolism/Transport Effects None known.

Avoid Concomitant Use There are no known interactions where it is recommended to avoid concomitant use.

Increased Effect/Toxicity There are no known significant interactions involving an increase in effect.

Decreased Effect There are no known significant interactions involving a decrease in effect.

Storage/Stability

CoLyte, GaviLyte-C, GaviLyte-G, GaviLyte-N, GoLYTELY, NuLYTELY, TriLyte: Prior to reconstitution, store at 25°C (77°F); excursions permitted to 15°C to 30°C (59°F to 86°F). Refrigerate reconstituted solution. Use within 48 hours of preparation; discard any unused portion.

MoviPrep: Prior to reconstitution, store at 20°C to 25°C (68°F to 77°F); excursions permitted to 15°C to 30°C (59°F to 86°F). Refrigerate reconstituted solution in an upright position. Use within 24 hours of preparation; discard any unused portion.

Mechanism of Action Induces catharsis by strong electrolyte and osmotic effects

Pharmacodynamics Onset of action: Bowel cleansing: Within 1-2 hours

Dosing: Usual

Pediatric:

Bowel cleansing (to prevent excessive fluid and electrolyte changes, use only products containing supplemental electrolytes for bowel cleansing): Patient should fast at least 2 hours (preferably 3 to 4 hours) prior to ingestion:

Infants ≥6 months, Children, and Adolescents: Oral, nasogastric: GaviLyte-N, NuLYTELY, and TriLyte: 25 mL/kg/hour until rectal effluent is clear (usually in ~4 hours). One study used 40 mL/kg/hour intermittently by mouth or continuously by nasogastric drip in patients ≥18 months (Sondheimer 1991). Although not FDA approved for pediatric patients, other preparations have been used in pediatric studies: Colyte, GoLYTELY (Sondheimer 1991; Tuggle 1987).

Fecal impaction; slow disimpaction: Limited data available: Children> 2 years and Adolescents: Oral, Nasogastric: 20 mL/kg/hour up to a maximum dose of 1 L/hour for 4 hours per day for 2 days was evaluated in a study comparing polyethylene glycol with electrolytes lavage (n=19, mean age: 6.44 ± 2.36 years) to mineral oil (n=17, mean age: 6.88 ± 3.26 years) (Tolia 1993)

Toxic ingestion (AACT 2004): Nasogastric:

Infants ≥9 months and Children <6 years: 500 mL/hour until rectal effluent is clear

Children ≥6 years: 1,000 mL/hour until rectal effluent is clear

Adolescents: 1,500 to 2,000 mL/hour until rectal effluent is clear

Note: Continue treatment at least until the rectal effluent is clear; treatment duration may be extended based on corroborative evidence of continued presence of poisons in the GI tract as determined by radiographic means or the presence of the poison in the effluent.

Adult: **Bowel cleansing:**

CoLyte, GaviLyte-C, GaviLyte-G, GaviLyte-N, GoLYTELY, NuLYTELY, TriLyte:

Oral: 240 mL (8 oz) every 10 minutes until 4 L are consumed or the rectal effluent is clear; rapid drinking of each portion is preferred to drinking small amounts continuously

Nasogastric: 20 to 30 mL/minute until 4 L are administered or the rectal effluent is clear

MoviPrep: Oral: Administer 2 L total with an additional 1 L of clear fluid prior to colonoscopy as follows:

Split dose (2-day regimen) (preferred method):

Dose 1: Evening before colonoscopy (10 to 12 hours before dose 2): 240 mL (8 oz) every 15 minutes until 1 L (entire contents of container) is consumed. Then fill container with 480 mL (16 oz) of clear liquid and consume prior to going to bed.

Dose 2: On the morning of the colonoscopy (beginning at least 3.5 hours prior to procedure): 240 mL (8 oz) every 15 minutes until 1 L (entire contents of container) is consumed. Then fill container with 480 mL (16 oz) of clear liquid and consume at least 2 hours before the procedure.

Evening only dose (1-day regimen) (alternate method):

Dose 1: Evening before colonoscopy (at least 3.5 hours before bedtime): 240 mL (8 oz) every 15 minutes until 1 L (entire contents of container) is consumed

Dose 2: ~90 minutes after starting dose 1: 240 mL (8 oz) every 15 minutes until 1 L (entire contents of container) is consumed. Then fill container with 1 L (32 oz) of clear liquid and consume all of the liquid prior to going to bed.

Dosing adjustment in renal impairment: There are no dosage adjustments provided in manufacturer's labeling (not studied). Use with caution due to risks of fluid and electrolyte abnormalities.

Dosing adjustment in hepatic impairment: There are no dosage adjustments provided in manufacturer's labeling (not studied).

Preparation for Administration

CoLyte, GaviLyte-C, GaviLyte-G, GaviLyte-N, GoLYTELY, NuLYTELY, TriLyte: If using a flavor packet provided, add the flavor packet contents to the existing powder in the provided container and shake well prior to adding water. Add lukewarm water (may use tap water) up to the 4 L water mark; shake vigorously several times to ensure dissolution of the powder. No additional ingredients or flavors should be added to the solution (other than the flavor packets provided).

MoviPrep: Mix the contents of pouch A and pouch B (one each) in container provided. Add lukewarm water to fill line (~1 L); mix the solution until dissolved. No additional ingredients or flavors should be added to the solution.

Administration Oral: For bowel cleansing, no solid foods for 2 to 4 hours prior to initiation of therapy; rapid drinking is preferred to drinking small amounts continuously; chilled solution often more palatable, but not recommended for infants; refrigerate reconstituted solution when not in use; do not add ingredients as flavorings before use; discard any unused portion. The solution may be administered via nasogastric tube for bowel cleansing or whole bowel irrigation in patients who are unwilling or unable to drink the solution.

Monitoring Parameters Electrolytes, BUN, serum glucose, urine osmolality; children <2 years of age should be monitored for hypoglycemia, dehydration, hypokalemia

Additional Information Concentrations for reconstituted solutions:

When prepared as recommended by the manufacturer, the solutions will contain:

CoLyte, GaviLyte-C: When dissolved in sufficient water to make 4,000 mL, the final solution contains PEG-3350 60 g/L, sodium 125 mEq/L, sulfate 80 mEql/L, chloride 35 mEql/L, bicarbonate 20 mEq/L, and potassium 10 mEq/L

GaviLyte-G, GoLYTELY: When dissolved in sufficient water to make 4,000 mL, the final solution contains PEG-3350 59 g/L, sodium 125 mEq/L, sulfate 40 mEq/L, chloride 35 mEq/L, bicarbonate 20 mEq/L, and potassium 10 mEq/L

GaviLyte-N, NuLYTELY, TriLyte: When dissolved in sufficient water to make 4,000 mL, the final solution contains PEG-3350 105 g/L, sodium 65 mEq/L, chloride 53 mEq/L, bicarbonate 17 mEq/L, and potassium 5 mEq/L

Dosage Forms Excipient information presented when available (limited, particularly for generics); consult specific product labeling.

Powder, for solution, oral: PEG 3350 240 g, sodium sulfate 22.72 g, sodium bicarbonate 6.72 g, sodium chloride 5.84 g, and potassium chloride 2.98 g (4000 mL); PEG 3350 236 g, sodium sulfate 22.74 g, sodium bicarbonate 6.74 g, sodium chloride 5.86 g, and potassium chloride 2.97 g (4000 mL); PEG 3350 240 g, sodium bicarbonate 5.72 g, sodium chloride 11.2 g, and potassium chloride 1.48 g (4000 mL); PEG 3350 420 g, sodium bicarbonate 5.72 g, sodium chloride 11.2 g, and potassium chloride 1.48 g (4000 mL)

Colyte: PEG 3350 227.1 g, sodium sulfate 21.5 g, sodium bicarbonate 6.36 g, sodium chloride 5.53 g, and potassium chloride 2.82 g (3785 mL) [supplied with cherry, lemon lime, and orange flavor packs]

Colyte: PEG 3350 240 g, sodium sulfate 22.72 g, sodium bicarbonate 6.72 g, sodium chloride 5.84 g, and potassium chloride 2.98 g (4000 mL) [supplied with cherry, citrus berry, lemon lime, orange, and pineapple flavor packs]

GaviLyte-C: PEG 3350 240 g, sodium sulfate 22.72 g, sodium bicarbonate 6.72 g, sodium chloride 5.84 g, and potassium chloride 2.98 g (4000 mL) [supplied with lemon flavor packet]

GaviLyte-G: PEG 3350 236 g, sodium sulfate 22.74 g, sodium bicarbonate 6.74 g, sodium chloride 5.86 g, and potassium chloride 2.97 g (4000 mL) [supplied with lemon flavor packet]

GaviLyte-N: PEG 3350 420 g, sodium bicarbonate 5.72 g, sodium chloride 11.2 g, and potassium chloride 1.48 g (4000 mL) [supplied with lemon flavor packet]

GoLYTELY: PEG 3350 227.1 g, sodium sulfate 21.5 g, sodium bicarbonate 6.36 g, sodium chloride 5.53 g, and potassium chloride 2.82 g per packet (1s) [regular flavor; makes 1 gallon of solution after mixing]

GoLYTELY: PEG 3350 236 g, sodium sulfate 22.74 g, sodium bicarbonate 6.74 g, sodium chloride 5.86 g, and potassium chloride 2.97 g (4000 mL) [regular and pineapple flavor]

MoviPrep: Pouch A: PEG 3350 100g, sodium sulfate 7.5 g, sodium chloride 2.69 g, potassium chloride 1.02 g; Pouch B: Ascorbic acid 4.7 g, sodium ascorbate 5.9 g (1000 mL) [contains phenylalanine 131 mg/treatment; lemon flavor; packaged with 2 of Pouch A and 2 of Pouch B in carton and a disposable reconstitution container]

NuLYTELY: PEG 3350 420 g, sodium bicarbonate 5.72 g, sodium chloride 11.2 g, and potassium chloride 1.48 g (4000 mL) [supplied with cherry, lemon-lime, orange, and pineapple flavor packs]

TriLyte: PEG 3350 420 g, sodium bicarbonate 5.72 g, sodium chloride 11.2 g, and potassium chloride 1.48 g (4000 mL) [supplied with cherry, citrus berry, lemon lime, orange, and pineapple flavor packs]

- ◆ **Polyethylene Glycol Interferon Alfa-2b** *see* Peginterferon Alfa-2b *on page 1646*
- ◆ **Poly-Iron 150 [OTC]** *see* Polysaccharide-Iron Complex *on page 1728*

Polymyxin B (pol i MIKS in bee)

Medication Safety Issues

High alert medication:

The Institute for Safe Medication Practices (ISMP) includes this medication (intrathecal administration) among its list of drug classes which have a heightened risk of causing significant patient harm when used in error.

Therapeutic Category Antibiotic, Miscellaneous; Antibiotic, Ophthalmic; Antibiotic, Urinary Irrigation

Generic Availability (US) Yes

Use

Parenteral: **Note:** Parenteral use of polymyxin B has mainly been replaced by less toxic antibiotics. Due to increased toxicity risks, systemic use of polymyxin B should be limited to life-threatening, multidrug resistant infections where less toxic alternatives are not effective or not tolerated.

IM, IV: Treatment of acute systemic infections (excluding meningitis) caused by susceptible strains of *Pseudomonas aeruginosa* (FDA approved in all ages); treatment of serious acute infection caused by other susceptible gram negative organisms when other less potentially toxic agents are ineffective or contraindicated (FDA approved in all ages); solution for injection has also been used topically for wound irrigation

Intrathecal: Treatment of meningeal infection caused by susceptible strains of *Pseudomonas aeruginosa* or *Haemophilus influenza* (FDA approved in infants, children, adolescents, and adults); has also been administered intraventricularly for the treatment of CSF shunt infection/ventriculitis

Topical: Ophthalmic (topical or subconjunctival injection): Treatment of acute ophthalmic infections caused by susceptible strains of *Pseudomonas aeruginosa* (FDA approved in all ages); treatment of serious acute infection caused by other susceptible gram negative organisms when other less potentially toxic agents are ineffective or contraindicated (FDA approved in all ages)

Pregnancy Considerations [U.S. Boxed Warning]: Safety in pregnant women has not been established. Animal reproduction studies are lacking. A teratogenic potential has not been identified for polymyxin b, but very limited data is available (Heinonen, 1977; Kazy, 2005). Based on the relative toxicity compared to other antibiotics, systemic use in pregnancy is not recommended (Knothe, 1985). Due to poor tissue diffusion, topical use would be expected to have only minimal risk to the mother or fetus (Leachman, 2006).

Breast-Feeding Considerations It is not known if polymyxin b is excreted in human milk. If present in breast milk, polymyxin b is not absorbed well from a normal gastrointestinal tract. Nondose-related effects could include modification of the bowel flora.

Contraindications Hypersensitivity to polymyxin B or any component of the formulation; concurrent use of neuromuscular blockers

Warnings/Precautions [U.S. Boxed Warning]: May cause neurotoxicity, nephrotoxicity, and/or neuromuscular blockade and respiratory paralysis; usual risk factors include pre-existing renal impairment, concomitant neuro-/nephrotoxic medications, advanced age and dehydration. Use with caution in patients with impaired renal function (modify dosage); polymyxin B-induced nephrotoxicity may be manifested by albuminuria, cellular casts, and azotemia. Discontinue therapy with decreasing urinary output and increasing BUN; neurotoxic reactions are usually associated with high serum levels, often in patients with renal dysfunction. Avoid concurrent or sequential use of other nephrotoxic and neurotoxic drugs (eg, aminoglycosides). The drug's neurotoxicity can result in respiratory paralysis from neuromuscular blockade, especially when the drug is given soon after anesthesia or muscle relaxants. Polymyxin B sulfate is most toxic when given parenterally; avoid parenteral use whenever possible. Prolonged use may result in fungal or bacterial superinfection, including *C. difficile*-associated diarrhea (CDAD) and pseudomembranous colitis; CDAD has been observed >2 months postantibiotic treatment. **[U.S. Boxed Warnings]: Safety in pregnant women not established; intramuscular/intrathecal administration only to hospitalized patients.** May cause severe pain at IM injection site or thrombophlebitis at IV infusion site.

Warnings: Additional Pediatric Considerations IM use is not routinely recommended in infants and children due to severe pain at injection site.

Adverse Reactions

Cardiovascular: Facial flushing

Central nervous system: Neurotoxicity (irritability, drowsiness, ataxia, perioral paresthesia, numbness of the extremities, and blurred vision); dizziness, drug fever, meningeal irritation with intrathecal administration

Dermatologic: Urticarial rash

Endocrine & metabolic: Hypocalcemia, hyponatremia, hypokalemia, hypochloremia

Local: Pain at injection site

Neuromuscular & skeletal: Neuromuscular blockade, weakness

Renal: Nephrotoxicity

Respiratory: Respiratory arrest

Miscellaneous: Anaphylactoid reaction

Drug Interactions

Metabolism/Transport Effects None known.

Avoid Concomitant Use

Avoid concomitant use of Polymyxin B with any of the following: Bacitracin (Systemic); BCG; BCG (Intravesical); Mecamylamine

Increased Effect/Toxicity

Polymyxin B may increase the levels/effects of: Bacitracin (Systemic); Colistimethate; Mecamylamine; Neuromuscular-Blocking Agents

The levels/effects of Polymyxin B may be increased by: Capreomycin

Decreased Effect

Polymyxin B may decrease the levels/effects of: BCG; BCG (Intravesical); BCG Vaccine (Immunization); Sodium Picosulfate

Storage/Stability Prior to reconstitution, store at room temperature of 15°C to 30°C (59°F to 86°F) and protect from light. After reconstitution, store under refrigeration at 2°C to 8°C (36°F to 46°F). Discard any unused solution after 72 hours.

Mechanism of Action Binds to phospholipids, alters permeability, and damages the bacterial cytoplasmic membrane permitting leakage of intracellular constituents

Pharmacokinetics (Adult data unless noted)

Absorption: Well absorbed from the peritoneum; minimal absorption (<10%) from the GI tract (except in neonates), mucous membranes, or intact skin. Clinically insignificant amounts are absorbed following irrigation of an intact urinary bladder; systemic absorption may occur from a denuded bladder. Small amounts are systemically absorbed following ophthalmic instillation.

Distribution: Tissue diffusion is poor; critically ill patients: Central V_d: ~0.09 L/kg; peripheral V_d: 0.33 L/kg (Sandri, 2013); does not cross blood brain barrier into CSF or into the eye (Hoeprich, 1970)

Protein binding: ~56%; critically ill patients: 79% to 92% (Zavascki, 2008)

Half-life: 6 hours, increased with reduced renal function (Evans, 1999)

Time to peak serum concentration: IM: Within 2 hours (Hoeprich, 1970)

Elimination: Urine (<1% as unchanged drug within first 12 hours; as therapy continues up to 60% as unchanged drug in the urine [Evans, 1999]); in critically ill adults: Urine (median: 4% [range: 0.98% to 17.4%] as unchanged drug) (Sandri, 2013)

Dosing: Neonatal Note: Due to toxicity risks, systemic use of polymyxin B should be limited to life-threatening multidrug resistant infection where less toxic alternatives are not effective or not tolerated.

Severe, life-threatening, multidrug resistant infection (excluding meningitis):

IM: 25,000 to 40,000 units/kg/day divided every 6 hours; in premature neonates or newborns, doses as high as 45,000 units/kg/day have been used for *Pseudomonas aeruginosa* sepsis with limited clinical experience; **Note:** Routine IM administration not recommended due to severe pain at injection site.

IV: 15,000 to 40,000 units/kg/day divided every 12 hours

Dosing: Usual Note: Due to increased toxicity risks, the systemic use of polymyxin B should be limited to life-threatening, multidrug resistant infection where less toxic alternatives are not effective or not tolerated. Multiple routes of administration available for use (eg, IV, IM, intrathecal, ophthalmic) and dosing is different based upon route; use extra precaution to verify dose and route of administration.

Pediatric: **Note:** Dosing may be presented as units or mg; 10,000 units = 1 mg, use extra caution with prescribing and/or dispensing.

Severe, life-threatening, multidrug resistant infection (excluding meningitis): Note: Total daily dose should not exceed 2,000,000 units/**day**

Infants:

IM: 25,000 to 40,000 units/kg/day divided every 4 to 6 hours; **Note:** Routine IM administration not recommended due to severe pain at injection site.

IV: 15,000 to 40,000 units/kg/day divided every 12 hours

Children and Adolescents:

IM: 25,000 to 30,000 units/kg/day divided every 4 to 6 hours; **Note:** Routine IM administration not recommended due to severe pain at injection site.

IV:

Manufacturer's labeling: 15,000 to 25,000 units/kg/day divided every 12 hours

Alternate dosing: Children ≥ 2 years and Adolescents: Very limited data available: Dosing based on previous recommendations (Hoeprich, 1970) and extrapolations from adult pharmacokinetic modeling (Sandri, 2013) which assumes that dosing for pediatric patients ≥2 years and adults is the same (per current manufacturer's labeling); some centers have used the following:

Loading dose: 25,000 units/kg

Maintenance dose: 25,000 to 30,000 units/kg/day divided every 12 hours; consider higher doses for organisms with higher MIC

Meningitis; *Pseudomonas aeruginosa* or *Haemophilus influenzae:*

Infants and Children <2 years: Intrathecal: 20,000 units once daily for 3 to 4 days **or** 25,000 units once every other day; continue 25,000 units once every other day for at least 2 weeks after cultures of the CSF are negative

Children ≥2 years and Adolescents: Intrathecal: 50,000 units daily for 3 to 4 days, then every other day for at least 2 weeks after cultures of CSF are negative

CNS infection (VP-shunt infection, ventriculitis): Limited data available: Children and Adolescents: Intraventricular/intrathecal: 2 to 5 mg/day; lower doses should be used in smaller patients (Hoeprich, 1970; Tunkel, 2004)

Ocular infection; *Pseudomonas aeruginosa:* Infants, Children, and Adolescents: Ophthalmic:

Topical: 0.1% to 0.25% solution (prepared from parenteral injection): 1 to 3 drops every hour, then increasing the interval as response indicates

Subconjunctival injection: Up to 100,000 units/day not to exceed 25,000 units/**kg**/day

Note: Combined total therapy (systemic and ophthalmic instillation) should not exceed 25,000 units/kg/**day**

Adult:

Ocular infections: Ophthalmic: A concentration of 0.1% to 0.25% is administered as 1 to 3 drops every hour, then increasing the interval as response indicates to 1 to 3 drops 4 to 6 times daily.

Systemic infections:

IM: 25,000 to 30,000 units/kg/day divided every 4 to 6 hours

IV: 15,000 to 25,000 units/kg/day divided every 12 hours

Intrathecal: 50,000 units daily for 3 to 4 days, then every other day for at least 2 weeks

Note: Total daily dose should not exceed 2,000,000 units.

Topical irrigation or topical solution: 500,000 units/L of normal saline; maximum daily dose should not exceed 2,000,000 units

Dosing adjustment in renal impairment: Note: Some adult data suggest that renal adjustment may not be necessary since total body clearance of polymyxin B is not altered in the setting of renal impairment and nonrenal pathways are primarily responsible for elimination (Sandri, 2013; Zavascki, 2008). These authors suggest that renal dosage adjustment recommendations should await further data from larger clinical trials.

Manufacturer's labeling: Infants, Children, Adolescents, and Adults: For individuals with renal impairment, the manufacturer's labeling recommends a dosage reduction so that the dose does not exceed 15,000 units/kg/day

Alternate dosing: Infants, Children, Adolescents, and Adults: The following adjustments have been used by some clinicians (modified from Hoeprich, 1970): IV, IM:

Loading dose (first day of therapy): CrCl <80 mL/minute: 25,000 units/kg in 2 equally divided doses every 12 hours

Subsequent dosage:

CrCl 30 to 80 mL/minute: 10,000 to 15,000 units/kg every 24 hours

CrCl <30 mL/minute: 10,000 to 15,000 units/kg every 2 to 3 days

Anuric patients: 10,000 units/kg every 5 to 7 days

Hemodialysis: Adult: IM: 250,000 units every 24 hours; no supplemental dose necessary (Cunha, 1988)

Peritoneal dialysis: Adult: IM: 250,000 units every 24 hours; no supplemental dose necessary (Cunha, 1988)

Dosing adjustment in hepatic impairment: There are no dosage adjustments provided in manufacturer's labeling

Preparation for Administration Note: Polymyxin B 10,000 units = 1 mg

Parenteral:

IM: Dissolve 500,000 units in 2 mL NS, SWFI, or 1% procaine HCl to a final concentration of 250,000 units/mL

IV infusion: Dissolve 500,000 units in 300 to 500 mL D_5W to a final concentration of 1,000 to 1,667 units/mL

Intrathecal: Dissolve 500,000 units in 10 mL NS (preservative free); final concentration: 50,000 units/mL

Topical: Ophthalmic: Dissolve 500,000 units in 20 to 50 mL SWFI or NS; final concentration: 10,000 to 25,000 units/mL (0.1 to 0.25%)

Administration

Parenteral: Due to increased toxicity risks, the systemic use of polymyxin B should be avoided when possible.

IM: Not recommended for routine use in infants and children because of the severe pain associated with injection; should only be administered to hospitalized patients. Administer IM injections deep into the upper outer quadrant of the gluteal muscles

IV: Infuse drug slowly, most data reports over 60 to 120 minutes (Teng 2008; Zavascki 2008) or by continuous infusion (per manufacturer's labeling)

Intrathecal: May be administered intrathecally; only administer intrathecally to hospitalized patients.

Topical: Ophthalmic: May be administered as a subconjunctival injection or as topical ophthalmic drops

Monitoring Parameters Neurologic symptoms and signs of superinfection; renal function (baseline and frequently during therapy; decreasing urine output and increasing BUN may require discontinuance of therapy); observe for changes in bowel frequency

Dosage Forms Excipient information presented when available (limited, particularly for generics); consult specific product labeling.

Solution Reconstituted, Injection:

Generic: 500,000 units (1 ea)

Solution Reconstituted, Injection [preservative free]:

Generic: 500,000 units (1 ea)

◆ **Polymyxin B and Bacitracin** *see* Bacitracin and Polymyxin B *on page* 252

◆ **Polymyxin B and Neomycin** *see* Neomycin and Polymyxin B *on page* 1502

◆ **Polymyxin B and Trimethoprim** *see* Trimethoprim and Polymyxin B *on page* 2128

◆ **Polymyxin B, Bacitracin, and Neomycin** *see* Bacitracin, Neomycin, and Polymyxin B *on page* 253

◆ **Polymyxin B, Bacitracin, Neomycin, and Hydrocortisone** *see* Bacitracin, Neomycin, Polymyxin B, and Hydrocortisone *on page* 253

◆ **Polymyxin B, Neomycin, and Dexamethasone** *see* Neomycin, Polymyxin B, and Dexamethasone *on page* 1502

◆ **Polymyxin B, Neomycin, and Hydrocortisone** *see* Neomycin, Polymyxin B, and Hydrocortisone *on page* 1503

◆ **Polymyxin B Sulfate** *see* Polymyxin B *on page* 1726

◆ **Polymyxin E** *see* Colistimethate *on page* 532

Polysaccharide-Iron Complex

(pol i SAK a ride-EYE ern KOM pleks)

Brand Names: US EZFE 200 [OTC]; Ferrex 150 [OTC]; Ferric x-150 [OTC]; FerUS [OTC] [DSC]; iFerex 150 [OTC]; Myferon 150 [OTC]; NovaFerrum 50 [OTC]; NovaFerrum Pediatric Drops [OTC]; Nu-Iron [OTC]; PIC 200 [OTC]; Poly-Iron 150 [OTC]

Therapeutic Category Iron Salt

Generic Availability (US) May be product dependent

Use Prevention and treatment of iron deficiency anemias (OTC: FDA approved in adults); has also been used as supplemental therapy for patients receiving epoetin alfa

Pregnancy Considerations It is recommended that pregnant women meet the dietary requirements of iron with diet and/or supplements in order to prevent adverse events associated with iron deficiency anemia in pregnancy. Treatment of iron deficiency anemia in pregnant women is the same as in nonpregnant women and in most cases, oral iron preparations may be used. Except in severe cases of maternal anemia, the fetus achieves normal iron stores regardless of maternal concentrations.

Breast-Feeding Considerations Iron is normally found in breast milk. Breast milk or iron fortified formulas generally provide enough iron to meet the recommended dietary requirements of infants. The amount of iron in breast milk is generally not influenced by maternal iron status.

Contraindications Known hypersensitivity to polysaccharide-iron complex or any component of the formulations; hemochromatosis; hemosiderosis

Documentation of allergenic cross-reactivity for other iron-containing products is limited. However, because of similarities in chemical structure and/or pharmacologic actions, the possibility of cross-sensitivity cannot be ruled out with certainty.

Warnings/Precautions **Accidental overdose of iron-containing products is a leading cause of fatal poisoning in children under 6 years of age. Keep this product out of the reach of children. In case of accidental overdose call the poison control center immediately.** Investigate type of anemia and potential underlying causes (eg, recurrent blood loss) prior to initiating iron supplementation. Some formulations may contain tartrazine, which is associated with allergic-type reactions. Although rare, hypersensitivity is more frequently seen in individuals with aspirin allergy. Potentially significant drug-drug interactions may exist, requiring dose or frequency adjustment, additional monitoring, and/or selection of alternative therapy. May interfere with absorption of antibiotics.

Warnings: Additional Pediatric Considerations Consider all iron sources when evaluating the dose of iron, including combination products, infant formulas, and liquid nutritional supplements.

Adverse Reactions

Gastrointestinal: Constipation, dark stools, diarrhea, epigastric pain, GI irritation, heartburn, nausea, stomach cramping, vomiting

Genitourinary: Discolored urine

Miscellaneous: Staining of teeth

Rare but important or life-threatening: Contact irritation

Drug Interactions

Metabolism/Transport Effects None known.

Avoid Concomitant Use

Avoid concomitant use of Polysaccharide-Iron Complex with any of the following: Dimercaprol

Increased Effect/Toxicity

The levels/effects of Polysaccharide-Iron Complex may be increased by: Dimercaprol

Decreased Effect

Polysaccharide-Iron Complex may decrease the levels/effects of: Alpha-Lipoic Acid; Bisphosphonate Derivatives; Cefdinir; Deferiprone; Dolutegravir; Eltrombopag; Levodopa; Levothyroxine; Methyldopa; PenicillAMINE; Phosphate Supplements; Quinolone Antibiotics; Tetracycline Derivatives; Trientine

The levels/effects of Polysaccharide-Iron Complex may be decreased by: Alpha-Lipoic Acid; Antacids; H2-Antagonists; Pancrelipase; Proton Pump Inhibitors; Tetracycline Derivatives; Trientine

Storage/Stability Store between 15°C and 30°C (59°F and 86°F).

Pharmacodynamics

Onset of action: Hematologic response: Red blood cells form within 3-10 days; similar onset as parenteral iron salts

Maximum effect: Peak reticulocytosis occurs in 5-10 days, and hemoglobin values increase within 2-4 weeks

Pharmacokinetics (Adult data unless noted)

Absorption: Oral: Iron is absorbed in the duodenum and upper jejunum; in persons with normal iron stores 10% of an oral dose is absorbed; this is increased to 20% to 30% in persons with inadequate iron stores; food and achlorhydria will decrease absorption

Protein binding: To transferrin

Elimination: Excreted in the urine, sweat, sloughing of intestinal mucosa, and by menses

Dosing: Usual

Infants, Children, and Adolescents: **Note:** Dosages are expressed in terms of **elemental** iron.

Recommended daily allowance (RDA): Oral:

4-8 years: 10 mg/day

9-13 years: 8 mg/day

14-18 years: Males: 11 mg/day; Females: 15 mg/day;

Iron deficiency: Oral: Children ≥6 years: 50-100 mg/day; may be given in divided doses

Adults:

Recommended daily allowance (RDA): Oral:

19-50 years: Males: 8 mg/day; Females: 18 mg/day; Pregnant females: 27 mg/day; Lactating females: 9 mg/day

≥50 years: 8 mg/day

Iron deficiency: Oral: 150-300 mg/day

Administration Administer with water or juice between meals for maximum absorption; may administer with food if GI upset occurs; do not administer with milk or milk products.

Monitoring Parameters Serum iron, total iron binding capacity, reticulocyte count, hemoglobin, ferritin

Reference Range

Serum iron: 22-184 mcg/dL

Total iron binding capacity:

Infants: 100-400 mcg/dL

Children and Adults: 250-400 mcg/dL

Additional Information 100% elemental iron. When treating iron deficiency anemias, treat for 3-4 months after hemoglobin/hematocrit return to normal in order to replenish total body stores.

Dosage Forms Excipient information presented when available (limited, particularly for generics); consult specific product labeling. [DSC] = Discontinued product

Capsule, Oral:

EZFE 200: 200 mg [non-toxic; contains brilliant blue fcf (fd&c blue #1), fd&c red #40, fd&c yellow #10 (quinoline yellow)]

Ferrex 150: 150 mg [contains fd&c blue #1 aluminum lake, fd&c red #40 aluminum lake, fd&c yellow #5 aluminum lake]

Ferric x-150: 150 mg [contains brilliant blue fcf (fd&c blue #1), fd&c red #40, tartrazine (fd&c yellow #5)]

FerUS: 150 mg [DSC]

iFerex 150: 150 mg [contains brilliant blue fcf (fd&c blue #1), fd&c red #40, fd&c yellow #10 (quinoline yellow)]

Myferon 150: 150 mg

NovaFerrum 50: 50 mg

Nu-Iron: 150 mg [contains brilliant blue fcf (fd&c blue #1), fd&c red #40]

PIC 200: 200 mg

Poly-Iron 150: 150 mg

Liquid, Oral:

NovaFerrum Pediatric Drops: 15 mg/mL (120 mL) [alcohol free, dye free, gluten free, lactose free, sodium free, sugar free; contains sodium benzoate; raspberry-grape flavor]

◆ **Polysporin® [OTC]** *see* Bacitracin and Polymyxin B *on page 252*

◆ **Polytar [OTC]** *see* Coal Tar *on page 523*

◆ **Polytrim®** *see* Trimethoprim and Polymyxin B *on page 2128*

◆ **Polytrim™ (Can)** *see* Trimethoprim and Polymyxin B *on page 2128*

◆ **Polyvinyl Alcohol** *see* Artificial Tears *on page 201*

◆ **Pontocaine (Can)** *see* Tetracaine (Systemic) *on page 2034*

◆ **Pontocaine (Can)** *see* Tetracaine (Topical) *on page 2035*

Poractant Alfa (por AKT ant AL fa)

Brand Names: US Curosurf

Brand Names: Canada Curosurf

Therapeutic Category Lung Surfactant

Generic Availability (US) No

Use Treatment of respiratory distress syndrome (RDS) in premature infants

Pregnancy Considerations This drug is not indicated for use in adults.

Breast-Feeding Considerations This drug is not indicated for use in adults.

Contraindications There are no contraindications listed in the manufacturer's labeling.

Warnings/Precautions For intratracheal administration only. Rapidly affects oxygenation and lung compliance; restrict use to a highly-supervised clinical setting with immediate availability of clinicians experienced in intubation and ventilatory management of premature infants. Transient episodes of bradycardia, decreased oxygen saturation, hypotension, or endotracheal tube blockage may occur. Discontinue dosing procedure and initiate measures to alleviate the condition; may reinstitute after the patient is stable. Pulmonary hemorrhage is a known complication of premature birth and very low birth-weight; has been reported in both clinical trials and postmarketing reports in infants who have received poractant. Produces rapid improvements in lung oxygenation and compliance; may require frequent adjustments to oxygen delivery and ventilator settings.

Adverse Reactions All reported adverse reactions occurred in premature neonates as safety and efficacy has not been established in full term neonates and older pediatric patients with respiratory failure.

Cardiovascular: Bradycardia, hypotension, patent ductus arteriosus

Hematologic & oncologic: Oxygen desaturation

Miscellaneous: Obstruction of endotracheal tube

Rare but important or life-threatening: Pulmonary hemorrhage

Drug Interactions

Metabolism/Transport Effects None known.

Avoid Concomitant Use

Avoid concomitant use of Poractant Alfa with any of the following: Ceritinib

Increased Effect/Toxicity

Poractant Alfa may increase the levels/effects of: Bradycardia-Causing Agents; Ceritinib; Ivabradine; Lacosamide

The levels/effects of Poractant Alfa may be increased by: Bretylium; Ruxolitinib; Tofacitinib

Decreased Effect There are no known significant interactions involving a decrease in effect.

Storage/Stability Store under refrigeration at defined temperature of 2°C to 8°C (36°F to 46°F). Unopened, unused vials that have been warmed to room temperature can be returned to refrigerator storage within 24 hours for future use. Do not warm and then refrigerate more than once. Vials are for single use only. Protect from light. Do not shake.

Mechanism of Action Endogenous pulmonary surfactant reduces surface tension at the air-liquid interface of the alveoli during ventilation and stabilizes the alveoli against collapse at resting transpulmonary pressures. A deficiency of pulmonary surfactant in preterm infants results in respiratory distress syndrome characterized by poor lung expansion, inadequate gas exchange, and atelectasis. Poractant alfa compensates for the surfactant deficiency and restores surface activity to the infant's lungs. It reduces mortality and pneumothoraces associated with RDS.

Dosing: Neonatal Endotracheal: Initial: 2.5 mL/kg/dose (200 mg/kg/dose); may repeat 1.25 mL/kg/dose (100 mg/kg/dose) at 12-hour intervals for up to 2 additional doses; maximum total dose: 5 mL/kg

Administration Intratracheal: For intratracheal administration only; suction infant prior to administration; inspect solution to verify complete mixing of the suspension; do not shake; gently turn vial upside-down to obtain uniform suspension; administer intratracheally by instillation through a 5-French end-hole catheter inserted into the infant's endotracheal tube; each dose should be administered as two aliquots, with each aliquot administered into one of the two main bronchi by positioning the infant with either the right or left side dependent; alternatively, it may be administered through a secondary lumen of a dual lumen endotracheal tube as a single dose administered over 1 minute without interrupting mechanical ventilation

Monitoring Parameters Continuous heart rate and transcutaneous O_2 saturation should be monitored during administration; frequent ABG sampling is necessary to prevent postdosing hyperoxia and hypocarbia

Dosage Forms Excipient information presented when available (limited, particularly for generics); consult specific product labeling.

Suspension, Inhalation [preservative free]:

Curosurf: 80 mg/mL (1.5 mL, 3 mL) [contains sodium chloride]

◆ **Porcine Lung Surfactant** *see* Poractant Alfa *on page 1730*

Posaconazole (poe sa KON a zole)

Medication Safety Issues

Sound-alike/look-alike issues:

Noxafil may be confused with minoxidil

Posaconazole may be confused with itraconazole

International issues:

Noxafil [US and multiple international markets] may be confused with Noxidil brand name for minoxidil [Thailand]

Related Information

Oral Medications That Should Not Be Crushed or Altered *on page 2476*

Brand Names: US Noxafil

Brand Names: Canada Posanol

Therapeutic Category Antifungal Agent, Systemic; Antifungal Agent, Triazole

Generic Availability (US) No

Use Prophylaxis of invasive *Aspergillus* and *Candida* infections in high-risk, severely immunocompromised patients (eg, hematopoietic stem cell transplant [HSCT] recipients with graft-versus-host disease or those with hematologic malignancies with prolonged neutropenia secondary to chemotherapy) (Oral suspension and delayed release tablets: FDA approved in ages ≥13 years and adults; Parenteral: FDA approved in ages ≥18 years and adults); treatment of oropharyngeal candidiasis (including patients refractory to itraconazole and/or fluconazole) (Oral suspension: FDA approved in ages ≥13 years and adults); has also been used for treatment of serious invasive fungal infections in patients intolerant of, or refractory to, conventional antifungal therapy

Pregnancy Risk Factor C

Pregnancy Considerations Adverse events have been observed in animal reproduction studies.

Breast-Feeding Considerations It is not known if posaconazole is excreted in breast milk. Due to the potential for serious adverse reactions in the nursing infant, the manufacturer recommends a decision be made to discontinue nursing or the drug, taking into account the importance of treatment to the mother.

Contraindications

Coadministration with sirolimus, ergot alkaloids (eg, ergotamine, dihydroergotamine), HMG-CoA reductase inhibitors that are primarily metabolized through CYP3A4 (eg, atorvastatin, lovastatin, simvastatin), or CYP3A4 substrates that prolong the QT interval (eg, pimozide, quinidine); hypersensitivity to posaconazole, other azole antifungal agents, or any component of the formulation.

Canadian labeling: Additional contraindications (not in US labeling): Coadministration with terfenadine, astemizole, or cisapride (each drug is no longer marketed in Canada).

Warnings/Precautions The delayed-release tablet and oral suspension are not to be used interchangeably due to dosing differences for each formulation. Hepatic dysfunction has occurred, ranging from mild/moderate increases of ALT, AST, alkaline phosphatase, total bilirubin, and/or clinical hepatitis to severe reactions (cholestasis, hepatic failure including death). Consider discontinuation of therapy in patients who develop clinical evidence of liver disease that may be secondary to posaconazole. Elevations in liver function tests have been generally reversible after posaconazole has been discontinued; some cases resolved without drug interruption. More severe reactions have been observed in patients with underlying serious medical conditions (eg, hematologic malignancy) and primarily with suspension total daily doses of 800 mg. Monitor liver function tests at baseline and periodically during therapy. If increases occur, monitor for severe hepatic injury development. Use caution in patients with an increased risk of arrhythmia (long QT syndrome, concurrent QTc-prolonging drugs, drugs metabolized through CYP3A4, hypokalemia). Correct electrolyte abnormalities (eg, potassium, magnesium, and calcium) before initiating therapy. Potentially significant drug-drug interactions may exist, requiring dose or frequency adjustment, additional monitoring, and/or selection of alternative therapy.

US labeling contraindicates use in patients with hypersensitivity to other azole antifungal agents; Canadian labeling does not contraindicate use, but recommends using caution in hypersensitivity with other azole antifungal agents; cross-reaction may occur, but has not been established. Consider alternative therapy or closely monitor for breakthrough fungal infections in patients receiving drugs that decrease absorption or increase the metabolism of posaconazole or in any patient unable to eat or tolerate an oral liquid nutritional supplement. Do not give IV formulation as an intravenous bolus injection. Avoid/limit use of IV formulation in patients with eGFR <50 mL/minute/1.73 m^2; injection contains excipient cyclodextrin (sulfobutyl ether beta-cyclodextrin [SBECD]), which may accumulate; consider using oral posaconazole in these patients unless benefit of injection outweighs the risk. Evaluate renal function (particularly serum creatinine) at baseline and periodically during therapy. If increases occur, consider oral therapy. Monitor for breakthrough fungal infections. Patients weighing >120 kg may have lower plasma drug exposure; monitor closely for breakthrough fungal infections. Oral suspension contains glucose; patients with rare glucose-galactose malabsorption may require alternative agents.

Benzyl alcohol and derivatives: Some dosage forms may contain sodium benzoate/benzoic acid; benzoic acid (benzoate) is a metabolite of benzyl alcohol; large amounts of benzyl alcohol (≥99 mg/kg/day) have been associated with a potentially fatal toxicity ("gasping syndrome") in neonates; the "gasping syndrome" consists of metabolic acidosis, respiratory distress, gasping respirations, CNS dysfunction (including convulsions, intracranial hemorrhage), hypotension, and cardiovascular collapse (AAP 1997; CDC 1982); some data suggests that benzoate displaces bilirubin from protein binding sites (Ahlfors 2001); avoid or use dosage forms containing benzyl alcohol derivative with caution in neonates. See manufacturer's labeling.

Polysorbate 80: Some dosage forms may contain polysorbate 80 (also known as Tweens). Hypersensitivity reactions, usually a delayed reaction, have been reported following exposure to pharmaceutical products containing polysorbate 80 in certain individuals (Isaksson 2002; Lucente 2000; Shelley 1995). Thrombocytopenia, ascites, pulmonary deterioration, and renal and hepatic failure have been reported in premature neonates after receiving parenteral products containing polysorbate 80 (Alade 1986; CDC 1984). See manufacturer's labeling.

Adverse Reactions Note: Unless otherwise specified, adverse reactions are identified with oral formulations and reflect data from use in comparator trials with multiple concomitant conditions and medications; some adverse reactions may be due to underlying condition(s). Systemic includes oral and intravenous routes.

Cardiovascular: Edema, hypertension (systemic), hypotension, peripheral edema (systemic), pulmonary embolism, tachycardia, thrombophlebitis (intravenous via peripheral venous catheter), torsades de pointes

Central nervous system: Anxiety, chills (systemic), dizziness, fatigue (systemic), headache (systemic), insomnia, lower extremity edema, pain, paresthesia, rigors

Dermatologic: Diaphoresis, pruritus, skin rash (systemic)

Endocrine & metabolic: Adrenocortical insufficiency, dehydration, hyperglycemia, hypocalcemia, hypokalemia (systemic), hypomagnesemia (systemic), weight loss

Gastrointestinal: Abdominal pain (systemic), anorexia, constipation (systemic), decreased appetite (systemic), diarrhea (systemic), dyspepsia, mucositis, nausea (systemic), oral candidiasis, stomatitis, upper abdominal pain (systemic), vomiting (systemic)

Genitourinary: Vaginal hemorrhage

Hematologic & oncologic: Anemia (systemic), febrile neutropenia, hemolytic-uremic syndrome, neutropenia, petechia (systemic), thrombocytopenia (systemic), thrombotic thrombocytopenic purpura

Hepatic: Hepatic failure, hepatitis, hepatomegaly, hyperbilirubinemia, increased liver enzymes, increased serum alkaline phosphatase, increased serum ALT, increased serum AST, jaundice

Hypersensitivity: Hypersensitivity reaction

Infection: Bacteremia, cytomegalovirus disease, herpes simplex infection

Neuromuscular & skeletal: Arthralgia, back pain, musculoskeletal pain, weakness

Renal: Acute renal failure

Respiratory: Cough (systemic), dyspnea (systemic), epistaxis (systemic), pharyngitis, pneumonia, upper respiratory tract infection

Miscellaneous: Fever (systemic)

Rare but important or life-threatening: Atrial fibrillation, cholestasis, hypersensitivity, prolonged Q-T interval on ECG, reduced ejection fraction, syncope

Drug Interactions

Metabolism/Transport Effects **Inhibits** CYP3A4 (strong)

Avoid Concomitant Use

Avoid concomitant use of Posaconazole with any of the following: Ado-Trastuzumab Emtansine; Alfuzosin; Apixaban; Astemizole; AtorvaSTATin; Avanafil; Axitinib; Barnidipine; Bosutinib; Cabozantinib; Ceritinib; Cisapride; Conivaptan; Crizotinib; Dapoxetine; Dihydroergotamine; Dofetilide; Domperidone; Dronedarone; Efavirenz;

Eletriptan; Eplerenone; Ergoloid Mesylates; Ergonovine; Ergotamine; Everolimus; Halofantrine; Ibrutinib; Irinotecan; Isavuconazonium Sulfate; Ivabradine; Lapatinib; Lercanidipine; Lomitapide; Lovastatin; Lurasidone; Macitentan; Methadone; Methylergonovine; Naloxegol; Nilotinib; NiMODipine; Nisoldipine; Olaparib; Palbociclib; Pimozide; QuiNIDine; Ranolazine; Red Yeast Rice; Regorafenib; Rivaroxaban; Saccharomyces boulardii; Salmeterol; Silodosin; Simeprevir; Simvastatin; Sirolimus; Suvorexant; Tamsulosin; Terfenadine; Ticagrelor; Tolvaptan; Toremifene; Trabectedin; Ulipristal; Vemurafenib; VinCRIStine (Liposomal); Vorapaxar

Increased Effect/Toxicity

Posaconazole may increase the levels/effects of: Ado-Trastuzumab Emtansine; Alfuzosin; Almotriptan; Alosetron; Antineoplastic Agents (Vinca Alkaloids); Apixaban; ARIPiprazole; Astemizole; Atazanavir; AtorvaSTATin; Avanafil; Axitinib; Barnidipine; Bedaquiline; Boceprevir; Bortezomib; Bosentan; Bosutinib; Brentuximab Vedotin; Brinzolamide; Budesonide (Nasal); Budesonide (Systemic, Oral Inhalation); Budesonide (Topical); BusPIRone; Busulfan; Cabazitaxel; Cabozantinib; Calcium Channel Blockers; Cannabis; Ceritinib; Cilostazol; Cisapride; Colchicine; Conivaptan; Corticosteroids (Orally Inhaled); Corticosteroids (Systemic); Crizotinib; CycloSPORINE (Systemic); CYP3A4 Substrates; Dapoxetine; Dasatinib; Dienogest; Digoxin; Dihydroergotamine; DOCEtaxel; Dofetilide; Domperidone; DOXOrubicin (Conventional); Dronabinol; Dronedarone; Drospirenone; Dutasteride; Eletriptan; Eliglustat; Enzalutamide; Eplerenone; Ergoloid Mesylates; Ergonovine; Ergotamine; Erlotinib; Etizolam; Etravirine; Everolimus; FentaNYL; Fesoterodine; Fluticasone (Nasal); Fluticasone (Oral Inhalation); Fosamprenavir; Fosphenytoin; GlipiZIDE; GuanFACINE; Halofantrine; Highest Risk QTc-Prolonging Agents; Hydrocodone; Ibrutinib; Idelalisib; Iloperidone; Imatinib; Imidafenacin; Irinotecan; Isavuconazonium Sulfate; Ivabradine; Ivacaftor; Ixabepilone; Lacosamide; Lapatinib; Lercanidipine; Levobupivacaine; Levomilnacipran; Lomitapide; Losartan; Lovastatin; Lurasidone; Macitentan; Maraviroc; MedroxyPROGESTERone; Methadone; Methylergonovine; MethylPREDNISolone; Mifepristone; Moderate Risk QTc-Prolonging Agents; Naloxegol; Nilotinib; NiMODipine; Nisoldipine; Olaparib; Ospemifene; Oxybutynin; OxyCODONE; Palbociclib; Panobinostat; Parecoxib; Paricalcitol; PAZOPanib; Phenytoin; Pimecrolimus; Pimozide; PONATinib; Pranlukast; PrednisoLONE (Systemic); PredniSONE; Propafenone; QUEtiapine; QuiNIDine; Ramelteon; Ranolazine; Red Yeast Rice; Regorafenib; Repaglinide; Retapamulin; Rifamycin Derivatives; Rilpivirine; Ritonavir; Rivaroxaban; RomiDEPsin; Ruxolitinib; Salmeterol; Saxagliptin; Sildenafil; Silodosin; Simeprevir; Simvastatin; Sirolimus; Solifenacin; SORAfenib; SUNItinib; Suvorexant; Tacrolimus (Systemic); Tacrolimus (Topical); Tadalafil; Tamsulosin; Tasimelteon; Telaprevir; Temsirolimus; Terfenadine; Tetrahydrocannabinol; Ticagrelor; Tofacitinib; Tolterodine; Tolvaptan; Toremifene; Trabectedin; TraMADol; Ulipristal; Vardenafil; Vemurafenib; Vilazodone; VinCRIStine (Liposomal); Vitamin K Antagonists; Vorapaxar; Zolpidem; Zopiclone; Zuclopenthixol

The levels/effects of Posaconazole may be increased by: Boceprevir; Etravirine; Mifepristone; Telaprevir

Decreased Effect

Posaconazole may decrease the levels/effects of: Amphotericin B; Ifosfamide; Prasugrel; Saccharomyces boulardii; Ticagrelor

The levels/effects of Posaconazole may be decreased by: Didanosine; Efavirenz; Etravirine; Fosamprenavir; Fosphenytoin; H2-Antagonists; Metoclopramide; Phenytoin; Proton Pump Inhibitors; Rifamycin Derivatives; Sucralfate

Food Interactions Bioavailability increased ~3 times when posaconazole suspension was administered with a nonfat meal or an oral liquid nutritional supplement; increased ~4 times when administered with a high-fat meal. Following administration of posaconazole delayed-release tablets, the AUC increased 51% when given with a high-fat meal compared with a fasted state. Management: Suspension must be administered with or within 20 minutes of a full meal or an oral liquid nutritional supplement, or may be administered with an acidic carbonated beverage (eg, ginger ale). Take tablet with food. Consider alternative antifungal therapy in patients with inadequate oral intake or severe diarrhea/vomiting.

Storage/Stability

Suspension: Store at 25°C (77°F); excursions are permitted between 15°C and 30°C (59°F and 86°F). Do not freeze.

Tablets: Store between 20°C and 25°C (68°F and 77°F); excursions are permitted between 15°C and 30°C (59°F and 86°F).

Injection: Store at 2°C to 8°C (36°F to 46°F).

Mechanism of Action Interferes with fungal cytochrome P450 (latosterol-14α-demethylase) activity, decreasing ergosterol synthesis (principal sterol in fungal cell membrane) and inhibiting fungal cell membrane formation.

Pharmacokinetics (Adult data unless noted)

Absorption: Coadministration with food and/or liquid nutritional supplements increases absorption; fasting states do not provide sufficient absorption to ensure adequate plasma concentrations

Distribution: V_d: Oral: 287 L; IV: ~261 L

Protein binding: >98%, predominantly bound to albumin

Metabolism: Not significantly metabolized; ~15% to 17% undergoes non-CYP-mediated metabolism, primarily via hepatic glucuronidation into metabolites

Bioavailability: Oral: Suspension and delayed release tablets are not bioequivalent; higher plasma exposure observed with delayed release tablets

Suspension: Dependent upon gastric pH environment (decreased with higher pH or increased motility) and fed-conditions (increased in high-fat environment)

Delayed release tablets: Dependent upon fed condition: Fasted conditions: 54%; higher under high-fat fed conditions (51% increase in AUC)

Half-life:

Oral: Suspension: 35 hours (range: 20 to 66 hours); delayed release tablets: 26 to 31 hours

IV: ~27 hours

Time to peak serum concentration: Oral: Suspension: 3 to 5 hours; delayed release tablets: 4 to 5 hours

Elimination: Feces 71% (66% as unchanged drug); urine 13% (<0.2% as unchanged drug)

Dosing: Usual Note: Verify correct dosage form; the delayed release tablet and oral suspension are **not** interchangeable.

Pediatric:

Antifungal prophylaxis, HSCT recipients: Limited data available:

Infants ≥8 months and Children <12 years: Oral suspension: 4 mg/kg/dose 3 times daily; begin 2-4 days prior to discharge and continue until either day 100 post-HSCT or until CD_3 T cells reach 200/mm^3 and CD_4 cells reach 100/mm^3 whichever is longer. Dosing based on experience in 60 pediatric patients (median age: 6 years; age range: 0.7-11.5 years); pharmacokinetic analysis showed 12 mg/kg/day (4 mg/kg 3 times daily) produced morning serum trough concentration similar to effective adult values. The other evaluated regimen of 10 mg/kg/day (5 mg/kg twice daily) produced morning trough levels that were approximately 3 times lower than the thrice daily regimen and was subsequently removed from the protocol. Overall, no patients developed invasive mycosis (probable or proven), the median duration of therapy was 127 days (range: 12-188 days), and no severe adverse effects were observed (Döring, 2012).

Adolescents ≥13 years: Oral suspension: 200 mg 3 times daily beginning with GVHD diagnosis, continue until GVHD resolves (Science, 2014)

Antifungal prophylaxis, acute myeloid leukemia (AML) or myelodysplastic syndrome (MDS): Limited data available: Adolescents ≥13 years: Oral suspension: 200 mg 3 times daily during chemotherapy associated neutropenia (Science, 2014). **Note:** Consider in centers with high incidence of mold infections or if fluconazole not available.

Aspergillosis, invasive; prophylaxis:

Oral: Adolescents ≥13 years:

Oral delayed release tablets (preferred): Initial: 300 mg twice daily for 1 day; maintenance dose: 300 mg once daily starting on Day 2; duration is based on recovery from neutropenia or immunosuppression. Missed doses: Take as soon as remembered. If it is <12 hours until the next dose, skip the missed dose and return to the regular schedule. Do not double doses.

Oral suspension: 200 mg 3 times daily; duration of therapy is based on recovery from neutropenia or immunosuppression. Missed doses: Take as soon as remembered. If it is <12 hours until the next dose, skip the missed dose and return to the regular schedule. Do not double doses.

IV: Adolescents ≥18 years: Loading dose: 300 mg twice a day on day 1; maintenance dose: 300 mg once daily on day 2 and thereafter. Duration is based on recovery from neutropenia or immunosuppression.

Candidiasis:

Esophageal infection; azole -refractory (HIV-exposed/-positive): Treatment: Adolescent: Oral suspension: 400 mg twice daily for 28 days; **Note:** If patient has frequent or severe recurrences may continue for suppressive therapy; consider discontinuing when CD_4 >200/mm^3 (DHHS [adult], 2014)

Invasive infections:

Prophylaxis: Adolescents ≥13 years:

Oral delayed release tablets (preferred): Initial: 300 mg twice daily for 1 day; maintenance dose: 300 mg once daily. Duration is based on recovery from neutropenia or immunosuppression. Missed doses: Take as soon as remembered. If it is <12 hours until the next dose, skip the missed dose and return to the regular schedule. Do not double doses.

Oral suspension: 200 mg 3 times daily; duration of therapy is based on recovery from neutropenia or immunosuppression. Missed doses: Take as soon as remembered. If it is <12 hours until the next dose, skip the missed dose and return to the regular schedule. Do not double doses.

Treatment (refractory infection): Limited data available: Children ≥8 years and Adolescents: Oral suspension: 800 mg/day administered as either 200 mg 4 times daily **or** 400 mg twice daily; this regimen produced similar plasma concentrations in both children (n=12; age range: 8-17 years; weight: 24-76 kg) and adults (Krishna, 2007)

Oropharyngeal infection:

Non-HIV-exposed/-positive: Adolescents ≥13 years:

Treatment: Oral suspension: Initial: 100 mg twice daily on day 1; maintenance: 100 mg once daily for 13 days

Treatment (refractory infection): Oral suspension: 400 mg twice daily; duration of therapy is based on underlying disease and clinical response

HIV-exposed/-positive: Treatment: Adolescents: Oral suspension: Initial: 400 mg twice daily on day 1; maintenance: 400 mg once daily for 28 days (DHHS [adult], 2014)

Adult:

Aspergillosis, invasive; prophylaxis:

Oral delayed release tablets (preferred): Initial: 300 mg twice daily for 1 day; maintenance dose: 300 mg once daily starting on Day 2. Duration is based on recovery from neutropenia or immunosuppression; initiate posaconazole in patients with acute myelogenous leukemia (AML) or myelodysplastic syndromes (MDS) several days before the anticipated onset of neutropenia (eg, at the time of chemotherapy initiation) and discontinue once neutropenia is resolved (Cornely 2007; NCCN 2009). Missed doses: Take as soon as remembered. If it is <12 hours until the next dose, skip the missed dose and return to the regular schedule. Do not double doses.

Oral suspension: 200 mg 3 times daily; duration of therapy is based on recovery from neutropenia or immunosuppression. Initiate posaconazole in patients with acute myelogenous leukemia (AML) or myelodysplastic syndromes (MDS) several days before the anticipated onset of neutropenia (eg, at the time of chemotherapy initiation) and discontinue once neutropenia is resolved (Cornely 2007; NCCN 2009).

IV: Loading dose: 300 mg twice a day on day 1; maintenance dose: 300 mg once daily on day 2 and thereafter. Duration is based on recovery from neutropenia or immunosuppression.

Candidal infections:

Prophylaxis:

Oral delayed release tablets (preferred): Initial: 300 mg twice daily for 1 day; maintenance dose: 300 mg once daily starting on Day 2; duration of therapy is based on recovery from neutropenia or immunosuppression. Missed doses: Take as soon as remembered. If it is <12 hours until the next dose, skip the missed dose and return to the regular schedule. Do not double doses.

Oral suspension: 200 mg 3 times daily; duration of therapy is based on recovery from neutropenia or immunosuppression

IV: Loading dose: 300 mg twice a day on day 1; maintenance dose: 300 mg once daily on day 2 and thereafter. Duration is based on recovery from neutropenia or immunosuppression.

Treatment:

Oropharyngeal infection: Oral suspension: Initial: 100 mg twice daily for 1 day; maintenance: 100 mg once daily starting on Day 2 for 13 days

Refractory oropharyngeal infection: Oral suspension: 400 mg twice daily; duration of therapy is based on underlying disease and clinical response

Dosing adjustment in renal impairment:

Adolescents ≥13 years and Adults: Delayed-release tablets and oral suspension:

eGFR ≥20 mL/minute/1.73 m^2: No dosage adjustment necessary.

eGFR <20 mL/minute/1.73 m^2: No dosage adjustment necessary; however, monitor for breakthrough fungal infections due to variability in posaconazole exposure.

Adolescents ≥18 years and Adults: IV:

eGFR ≥50 mL/minute/1.73 m^2: No dosage adjustment recommended.

eGFR <50 mL/minute/1.73m^2: Avoid use unless risk/benefit has been assessed; the intravenous vehicle may accumulate. Monitor serum creatinine levels; if increases occur, consider oral therapy.

Dosing adjustment in hepatic impairment: Adolescents ≥13 years and Adults: Mild to severe insufficiency (Child-Pugh class A, B, or C): No dosage adjustment necessary.

Note: If patient shows clinical signs and symptoms of liver disease due to posaconazole, consider discontinuing therapy. Hepatic impairment studies were only conducted with oral suspension; however, recommendations also apply to patients receiving injection or delayed release tablets.

Preparation for Administration IV: Equilibrate the refrigerated vial to room temperature. Contents of vial should be withdrawn and admixed with 150 mL D_5W or NS. The admixed solution may be colorless to yellow. Color variations in this range do not affect potency. Admixture should be used immediately; if not used immediately, may be stored for up to 24 hours refrigerated at 2°C to 8°C (36°F to 46°F).

Administration

IV: Infuse over 90 minutes via a central venous line. Do not administer IV push or bolus. Must be infused through an in-line filter (0.22-micron polyethersulfone [PES] or polyvinylidene difluoride [PVDF]). Infusion through a peripheral line should only be used as a one-time infusion over 30 minutes in a patient who will be receiving a central venous line for subsequent doses, or to bridge a period during which a central venous line is to be replaced or is in use for another infusion. **Note:** In clinical trials, multiple peripheral infusions given through the same vein resulted in infusion-site reactions.

Oral: **Note:** The delayed release tablet and oral suspension are not to be used interchangeably due to dosing differences for each formulation.

Suspension: Shake well before use. Administer during or within 20 minutes following a full meal, liquid nutritional supplement, or an acidic carbonated beverage (eg, ginger ale). In patients able to swallow, administer oral suspension using dosing spoon provided by the manufacturer; spoon should be rinsed clean with water after each use and before storage. **Note:** Nasogastric administration results in decreased absorption; monitor for breakthrough infection if this route is used.

Tablets (delayed release): Swallow tablets whole; do not divide, crush, or chew. Administer with food. If a dose is missed, take as soon as remembered. If it is <12 hours until the next dose, skip the missed does and return to the regular schedule. Do not double doses.

Consider alternative antifungal therapy in patients with inadequate oral intake or severe diarrhea/vomiting; if alternative therapy is not an option, closely monitoring for breakthrough fungal infections. Adequate posaconazole absorption from GI tract and subsequent plasma concentrations are dependent on food for efficacy. Lower average plasma concentrations have been associated with an increased risk of treatment failure.

Monitoring Parameters Hepatic function tests and bilirubin prior to initiation and periodically during therapy, serum electrolytes (eg, calcium, potassium and magnesium), serum creatinine, renal function, especially in patients on IV therapy if eGFR <50 mL/minute/1.73 m^2, ECG; breakthrough fungal infections, oral intake

Dosage Forms Excipient information presented when available (limited, particularly for generics); consult specific product labeling.

Solution, Intravenous:

Noxafil: 300 mg/16.7 mL (16.7 mL) [contains edetate disodium]

Suspension, Oral:

Noxafil: 40 mg/mL (105 mL) [contains polysorbate 80, sodium benzoate; cherry flavor]

Tablet Delayed Release, Oral:

Noxafil: 100 mg

◆ **Posanol (Can)** *see* Posaconazole *on page 1730*

Potassium Acetate (poe TASS ee um AS e tate)

Medication Safety Issues

Sound-alike/look-alike issues:

Potassium acetate may be confused with sodium acetate

Other safety concerns:

Consider special storage requirements for intravenous potassium salts; IV potassium salts have been administered IVP in error, leading to fatal outcomes.

Related Information

Management of Drug Extravasations *on page 2298*

Therapeutic Category Electrolyte Supplement, Parenteral

Generic Availability (US) Yes

Use Treatment and prevention of hypokalemia when it is necessary to avoid chloride or acid/base status requires an additional source of bicarbonate

Pregnancy Risk Factor C

Pregnancy Considerations Animal reproduction studies have not been conducted. Potassium requirements are the same in pregnant and nonpregnant women. Adverse events have not been observed following use of potassium supplements in healthy women with normal pregnancies. Use caution in pregnant women with other medical conditions (eg, pre-eclampsia; may be more likely to develop hyperkalemia) (IOM, 2004).

Breast-Feeding Considerations Potassium is excreted into breast milk (IOM, 2004).

Contraindications Severe renal impairment or adrenal insufficiency; hyperkalemia

Warnings/Precautions Close monitoring of serum potassium concentrations is needed to avoid hyperkalemia. Use with caution in patients with renal impairment (contraindicated in severe renal insufficiency), cardiac disease, acid/base disorders, or potassium-altering conditions/disorders. Use with caution in digitalized patients or patients receiving concomitant medications or therapies that increase potassium (eg, ACEIs, potassium-sparing diuretics, potassium containing salt substitutes). Do **NOT** administer undiluted or IV push; inappropriate parenteral administration may be fatal. Always administer potassium further diluted; refer to appropriate dilution and administration rate recommendations. Vesicant/irritant (at concentrations >0.1 mEq/mL); ensure proper catheter or needle position prior to and during infusion; avoid extravasation. Pain and phlebitis may occur during parenteral infusion requiring a decrease in infusion rate or potassium concentration. The parenteral product may contain aluminum; toxic aluminum concentrations may be seen with high doses, prolonged use, or renal dysfunction. Premature neonates are at higher risk due to immature renal function and aluminum intake from other parenteral sources. Parenteral aluminum exposure of >4 to 5 mcg/kg/day is associated with CNS and bone toxicity; tissue loading may occur at lower doses (Federal Register, 2002). See manufacturer's labeling.

Adverse Reactions

Cardiovascular: Arrhythmias, EEG abnormalities, heart block, hypotension

Central nervous system: Confusion, listlessness

Neuromuscular & skeletal: Paralysis, paresthesia, weakness

Local: Local tissue necrosis with extravasation

Drug Interactions

Metabolism/Transport Effects None known.

Avoid Concomitant Use There are no known interactions where it is recommended to avoid concomitant use.

Increased Effect/Toxicity

Potassium Acetate may increase the levels/effects of: ACE Inhibitors; Aliskiren; Angiotensin II Receptor Blockers; Potassium-Sparing Diuretics

The levels/effects of Potassium Acetate may be increased by: Eplerenone; Heparin; Heparin (Low Molecular Weight); Nicorandil

Decreased Effect There are no known significant interactions involving a decrease in effect.

Storage/Stability Store at room temperature; do not freeze.

Mechanism of Action Potassium is the major cation of intracellular fluid and is essential for the conduction of nerve impulses in heart, brain, and skeletal muscle; contraction of cardiac, skeletal and smooth muscles; maintenance of normal renal function, acid-base balance, carbohydrate metabolism, and gastric secretion

Pharmacokinetics (Adult data unless noted)

Distribution: Enters cells via active transport from extracellular fluid

Elimination: Primarily urine; skin and feces (small amounts); most intestinal potassium reabsorbed

Dosing: Neonatal IV doses should be incorporated into the patient's maintenance IV fluids; intermittent IV potassium administration should be reserved for severe depletion situations; continuous ECG monitoring should be used for intermittent doses >0.5 mEq/kg/**hour**. **Note:** Doses listed as mEq of **potassium**.

Normal daily requirement: IV: 2-6 mEq/kg/day

Treatment of hypokalemia: Intermittent IV infusion (must be diluted prior to administration): 0.5-1 mEq/kg/dose, infuse at 0.3-0.5 mEq/kg/**hour** (maximum dose/rate: 1 mEq/kg/**hour**); then repeated as needed based on frequently obtained lab values; severe depletion or ongoing losses may require >200% of normal daily limit needs

Dosing: Usual IV doses should be incorporated into the patient's maintenance IV fluids; intermittent IV potassium administration should be reserved for severe depletion situations; continuous ECG monitoring should be used for intermittent doses >0.5 mEq/kg/**hour**. **Note:** Doses listed as mEq of **potassium**.

Normal daily requirement: IV:
- Infants: 2-6 mEq/kg/day
- Children: 2-3 mEq/kg/day
- Adults: 40-80 mEq/day

Treatment of hypokalemia:

Infants and Children:

Intermittent IV infusion (must be diluted prior to administration): 0.5-1 mEq/kg/dose (maximum dose: 40 mEq), infuse at 0.3-0.5 mEq/kg/**hour** (maximum dose/rate: 1 mEq/kg/**hour**); then repeated as needed based on frequently obtained lab values; severe depletion or ongoing losses may require >200% of normal daily limit needs

Adults:

Intermittent IV infusion: 5-10 mEq/hour (continuous cardiac monitor recommended for rates >5 mEq/hour), not to exceed 40 mEq/hour; usual adult maximum per 24 hours: 400 mEq

Potassium dosage/rate of infusion guidelines:

Serum potassium ≥2.5 mEq/L (and <desired): 10 mEq with additional doses if needed; maximum infusion rate: 10 mEq/hour; maximum 24-hour dose: 200 mEq

Serum potassium <2.5 mEq/L: Up to 40 mEq with additional doses based upon frequent lab monitoring; maximum infusion rate: 40 mEq/hour; maximum 24-hour dose: 400 mEq; deficits at a plasma level of 2 mEq/L may be as high as 400-800 mEq of potassium

Preparation for Administration

Parenteral: Potassium must be diluted prior to parenteral administration. The concentration of infusion may be dependent on patient condition and specific institution policy. The maximum concentrations should be reserved for specific clinical situations (eg, fluid restricted).

Pediatric: Specific pediatric data limited and based on recommendations in adult patients and reported clinical experience for some pediatric centers (Corkins 2010; Hamill 1990; Klaus 1989; Kraft 2005; Kruse 1990; Lafraniere 2006; Murray 2014; Schaber 1985).

For peripheral administration, further dilution to a concentration ≤80 mEq/L (0.08 mEq/mL) for continuous infusion has been used; usual reported concentration is 40 to 60 mEq/L (0.04 to 0.06 mEq/mL).

For central line infusion, a maximum concentration up to 200 mEq/L (0.2 mEq/mL) has been used for infusions; usual reported concentration is 120 to 150 mEq/L (0.12 to 0.15 mEq/L); for potassium replacement (intermittent), higher concentration of 400 mEq/L (0.4 mEq/mL) has been used.

Adult: Some clinicians recommend that the maximum concentration for peripheral infusion is 10 mEq/100 mL and 20 to 40 mEq/100 mL for central infusions.

Administration

Parenteral: Potassium must be diluted prior to parenteral administration. Do not administer IV push. In general, the dose, concentration of infusion, and rate of administration may be dependent on patient condition and specific institution policy.

Infusion rates (including all sources):

Pediatric: Non-critical care settings: Usual range: 0.2 to 0.5 mEq/kg/hour up to 10 mEq to 20 mEq/hour have been used. Critical care settings/situations: Higher rates may be used; maximum rate: 1 mEq/kg/hour up to 40 mEq/hour; continuous cardiac monitoring recommended for rates >0.5 mEq/kg/hour (Fuhrman 2011; Hamill 1991; Klaus 1989; Kliegman 2011; Kruse 1990; Lafraniere 2006; Schaber 1985)

Adult: Some clinicians recommend that the maximum concentration for peripheral infusion is 10 mEq/100 mL and maximum rate of administration for peripheral infusion is 10 mEq/hour (Kraft 2005). ECG monitoring is recommended for peripheral or central infusions >10 mEq/hour in adults (Kraft 2005). Concentration and rate of infusion may be greater with central line administration. Concentration of 20 to 40 mEq/100 mL at a maximum rate of 40 mEq/hour via central line have been safely administered (Hamill 1991; Kruse 1990).

Vesicant/irritant (at concentrations >0.1 mEq/mL); ensure proper needle or catheter placement prior to and during IV infusion. Avoid extravasation. If extravasation occurs, stop infusion immediately and disconnect (leave needle/cannula in place); gently aspirate extravasated solution (do **NOT** flush the line); initiate hyaluronidase antidote (see Management of Drug Extravasations for more details); remove needle/cannula; apply dry cold compresses (Hurst, 2004); elevate extremity.

Vesicant/Extravasation Risk Vesicant/irritant (at concentrations >0.1 mEq/mL)

Monitoring Parameters Serum potassium, glucose, chloride, pH, urine output (if indicated), cardiac monitor [if intermittent IV infusion or potassium IV infusion rates >0.5 mEq/kg/hour or 5 mEq/hour (adults)]

Additional Information 1 mEq of acetate is equivalent to the alkalinizing effect of 1 mEq of bicarbonate. Hypokalemia is highly arrhythmogenic, particularly in the setting of ischemia or digitalis toxicity. ECG evidence of hypokalemia includes flattening of the T wave. As the T wave shrinks, U waves may appear. There is no prolongation of the QT interval. Hyperkalemia may present as tall peaked symmetrical T waves. S-T elevation may present in severe hyperkalemia. QRS complex progressively widens with eventual apparent sine waves on the ECG. Hyperkalemia will also induce cardiac slowing and AV conduction abnormalities.

Dosage Forms Excipient information presented when available (limited, particularly for generics); consult specific product labeling.

Solution, Intravenous:

Generic: 2 mEq/mL (20 mL, 50 mL, 100 mL); 4 mEq/mL (50 mL)

Potassium Chloride (poe TASS ee um KLOR ide)

Medication Safety Issues

Sound-alike/look-alike issues:

Kaon-Cl-10 may be confused with kaolin

KCl may be confused with HCl

Klor-Con may be confused with Klaron

microK may be confused with Macrobid, Micronase

High alert medication:

The Institute for Safe Medication Practices (ISMP) includes this medication (IV formulation) among its list of drugs which have a heightened risk of causing significant patient harm when used in error.

Other safety concerns:

Per JCAHO recommendations, concentrated electrolyte solutions should not be available in patient care areas.

Consider special storage requirements for intravenous potassium salts; IV potassium salts have been administered IVP in error, leading to fatal outcomes.

Related Information

Management of Drug Extravasations *on page 2298*

Oral Medications That Should Not Be Crushed or Altered *on page 2476*

Brand Names: US K-Sol; K-Tab; K-Vescent; Klor-Con; Klor-Con 10; Klor-Con M10; Klor-Con M15; Klor-Con M20; Micro-K

Brand Names: Canada Apo-K; K-10; K-Dur; Micro-K Extencaps; Roychlor; Slo-Pot; Slow-K

Therapeutic Category Electrolyte Supplement, Oral; Electrolyte Supplement, Parenteral

Generic Availability (US) Yes

Use Treatment or prevention of hypokalemia

Pregnancy Risk Factor C

Pregnancy Considerations Reproduction studies have not been conducted. Potassium requirements are the same in pregnant and nonpregnant women. Adverse events have not been observed following use of potassium supplements in healthy women with normal pregnancies. Use caution in pregnant women with other medical conditions (eg, pre-eclampsia; may be more likely to develop hyperkalemia) (IOM, 2004). Potassium supplementation (that does not cause maternal hyperkalemia) would not be expected to cause adverse fetal events.

Breast-Feeding Considerations Potassium is excreted into breast milk (IOM, 2004). The normal content of potassium in human milk is ~13 mEq/L. Supplementation (that does not cause maternal hyperkalemia) would not be expected to affect normal concentrations.

Contraindications Hypersensitivity to any component of the formulation; hyperkalemia. In addition, solid oral dosage forms are contraindicated in patients in whom there is a structural, pathological, and/or pharmacologic cause for delay or arrest in passage through the GI tract.

Warnings/Precautions Close monitoring of serum potassium concentrations is needed to avoid hyperkalemia. Use with caution in patients with renal impairment, cardiac disease, acid/base disorders, or potassium-altering conditions/disorders. Use with caution in digitalized patients or patients receiving concomitant medications or therapies that increase potassium (eg, ACEI, potassium-sparing diuretics, potassium containing salt substitutes). Do **NOT** administer undiluted or IV push; inappropriate parenteral administration may be fatal. Always administer potassium further diluted; refer to appropriate dilution and administration rate recommendations. Vesicant/irritant (at concentrations >0.1 mEq/mL); ensure proper catheter or needle position prior to and during infusion; avoid extravasation. Pain and phlebitis may occur during parenteral infusion requiring a decrease in infusion rate or potassium concentration. Avoid administering potassium diluted in dextrose solutions during initial therapy; potential for transient decreases in serum potassium due to intracellular shift of potassium from dextrose-stimulated insulin release. May cause GI upset (eg, nausea, vomiting, diarrhea, abdominal pain, discomfort) and lead to GI ulceration, bleeding, perforation, and/or obstruction. Oral liquid preparations (not solid) should be used in patients with esophageal compression or delayed gastric emptying.

Adverse Reactions

Dermatologic: Rash

Endocrine & metabolic: Hyperkalemia

Gastrointestinal: Abdominal pain/discomfort, diarrhea, flatulence, GI bleeding (oral), GI obstruction (oral), GI perforation (oral), nausea, vomiting

Drug Interactions

Metabolism/Transport Effects None known.

Avoid Concomitant Use

Avoid concomitant use of Potassium Chloride with any of the following: Anticholinergic Agents; Glycopyrrolate

Increased Effect/Toxicity

Potassium Chloride may increase the levels/effects of: ACE Inhibitors; Aliskiren; Angiotensin II Receptor Blockers; Potassium-Sparing Diuretics

The levels/effects of Potassium Chloride may be increased by: Anticholinergic Agents; Eplerenone; Glycopyrrolate; Heparin; Heparin (Low Molecular Weight); Nicorandil

Decreased Effect There are no known significant interactions involving a decrease in effect.

Storage/Stability

Capsule: MicroK®: Store between 20°C to 25°C (68°F to 77°F).

Powder for oral solution: Klor-Con®: Store at room temperature of 15°C to 30°C (59°F to 86°F).

Solution for injection: Store at room temperature; do not freeze. Use only clear solutions. Use admixtures within 24 hours.

Tablet: K-Tab®: Store below 30°C (86°F).

Mechanism of Action Potassium is the major cation of intracellular fluid and is essential for the conduction of nerve impulses in heart, brain, and skeletal muscle; contraction of cardiac, skeletal and smooth muscles; maintenance of normal renal function, acid-base balance, carbohydrate metabolism, and gastric secretion

Pharmacokinetics (Adult data unless noted)

Absorption: Well absorbed from upper GI tract; enters cells via active transport from extracellular fluid

Distribution: Enters cells via active transport from extracellular fluid

Elimination: Primarily urine; skin and feces (small amounts); most intestinal potassium reabsorbed

Dosing: Neonatal Note: IV doses should be incorporated into the patient's maintenance IV fluids; intermittent IV potassium administration should be reserved for severe depletion situations; continuous ECG monitoring should be used for intermittent doses >0.5 mEq/kg/**hour**. Doses listed as mEq of **potassium**.

Normal daily requirements: Oral, IV: 2-6 mEq/kg/day

Prevention of hypokalemia during diuretic therapy: 1-2 mEq/kg/day in 1-2 divided doses

Treatment of hypokalemia: **Note:** High variability exists in dosing/infusion rate recommendations; therapy should be guided by patient condition and specific institutional guidelines.

Oral: 2-5 mEq/kg/day in divided doses; not to exceed 1-2 mEq/kg as a single dose; if deficits are severe or ongoing losses are great, IV route should be considered preferred route of administration

Intermittent IV infusion (must be diluted prior to administration): 0.5-1 mEq/kg/dose, infuse at 0.3-0.5 mEq/kg/**hour** (maximum dose/rate: 1 mEq/kg/**hour**); then repeated as needed based on frequently obtained lab values; severe depletion or ongoing losses may require >200% of normal daily limit needs

Dosing: Usual Note: IV doses should be incorporated into the patient's maintenance IV fluids; intermittent IV potassium administration should be reserved for severe depletion situations; continuous ECG monitoring should be used for intermittent doses >0.5 mEq/kg/**hour**. Doses listed as mEq of **potassium**. When using microencapsulated or wax matrix formulations, use no more than 20 mEq as a single dose.

Normal daily requirements: Oral, IV:

Infants: 2-6 mEq/kg/day

Children: 2-3 mEq/kg/day

Adults: 40-80 mEq/day

Prevention of hypokalemia during diuretic therapy: Oral:

Infants and Children: 1-2 mEq/kg/day in 1-2 divided doses

Adults: 20-40 mEq/day in 1-2 divided doses

Treatment of hypokalemia: **Note:** High variability exists in dosing/infusion rate recommendations; therapy should be guided by patient condition and specific institutional guidelines.

Infants and Children:

Oral: 2-5 mEq/kg/day in divided doses; not to exceed 1-2 mEq/kg as a single dose; if deficits are severe or ongoing losses are great, IV route should be considered preferred route of administration

Intermittent IV infusion (must be diluted prior to administration): 0.5-1 mEq/kg/dose (maximum dose: 40 mEq) to infuse at 0.3-0.5 mEq/kg/hour (maximum dose/rate: 1 mEq/kg/hour); then repeated as needed based on frequently obtained lab values; severe depletion or ongoing losses may require >200% of normal daily limit needs

Adults:

Intermittent IV infusion: 5-10 mEq/hour (continuous cardiac monitor recommended for rates >5 mEq/hour), not to exceed 40 mEq/hour; usual adult maximum per 24 hours: 400 mEq

Potassium dosage/rate of infusion guidelines:

Serum potassium ≥2.5 mEq/L (and <desired): 10 mEq with additional doses if needed; maximum infusion rate: 10 mEq/hour; maximum 24-hour dose: 200 mEq

Serum potassium <2.5 mEq/L: Up to 40 mEq, with additional doses based upon frequent lab monitoring; maximum infusion rate: 40 mEq/hour; maximum 24-hour dose: 400 mEq; deficits at a plasma level of 2 mEq/L may be as high as 400-800 mEq of potassium

Oral:

Asymptomatic, mild hypokalemia: Usual dosage range: 40-100 mEq/day divided in 2-5 doses; generally recommended to limit doses to 20-25 mEq/dose to avoid GI discomfort

Mild to moderate hypokalemia: Some clinicians may administer up to 120-240 mEq/day divided in 3-4 doses; limit doses to 40-60 mEq/dose. If deficits are severe or ongoing losses are great, IV route should be considered.

Preparation for Administration

Oral:

Oral solution: Available in two concentrations: 20 mEq/15 mL (1.33 mEq/mL) and 40 mEq/15 mL (2.67 mEq/mL); verify product formulation for dosage calculations. To avoid gastrointestinal irritation, the manufacturer recommends diluting 15 mL of KCl oral solution (either strength) in at least 6 ounces of water or juice. In postcardiac surgery pediatric patients (including neonates and infants), oral KCl solution was administered at a concentration of 2.67 mEq/mL followed by an equivalent volume of sterile water as a flush (Moffett 2011).

Powder:

Klor-Con: Dissolve one 20 mEq packet in 4 ounces of water or other beverage

Klor-Con/25: Dissolve one 25 mEq packet in 5 ounces of water or other beverage

Tablet (Klor-Con M): May dissolve whole tablet in approximately 4 ounces of water; allow approximately 2 minutes to dissolve, stir well, and drink immediately.

Parenteral: Potassium must be diluted prior to parenteral administration. The concentration of infusion may be dependent on patient condition and specific institution policy. The maximum concentrations should be reserved for specific clinical situations (eg, fluid-restricted).

Pediatric: Specific pediatric data limited and based on recommendations in adult patients and reported clinical experience for some pediatric centers (Corkins 2010; Hamill 1990; Klaus 1989; Kraft 2005; Kruse 1990; Lafraniere 2006; Murray 2014; Schaber 1985).

For peripheral administration, further dilution to a concentration ≤80 mEq/L (0.08 mEq/mL) for continuous infusion has been used; usual reported concentration is 40 to 60 mEq/L (0.04 to 0.06 mEq/mL).

For central line infusion, a maximum concentration up to 200 mEq/L (0.2 mEq/mL) has been used for infusions; usual reported concentration is 120 to 150 mEq/L (0.12 to 0.15 mEq/L); for potassium replacement (intermittent), higher concentration of 400 mEq/L (0.4 mEq/mL) has been used.

Adult: Some clinicians recommend that the maximum concentration for peripheral infusion is 10 mEq/100 mL and 20 to 40 mEq/100 mL for central infusions.

Administration

Oral: **Note:** Should be taken with meals and a full glass of water or other liquid to minimize the risk of GI irritation. Prescribing information for the various oral preparations recommend that no more than 20 mEq or 25 mEq should be given as single dose.

Capsule: MicroK: Swallow whole, do not chew; may also be opened and contents sprinkled on a spoonful of applesauce or pudding and swallowed immediately without chewing

Oral solution: Do not administer full strength; must be diluted prior to administration

Powder (Klor-Con): Dissolve in water or juice

Tablets, Sustained release and wax matrix:

K-Tab, Kaon-Cl-10, Klor-Con: Swallow whole, do not crush or chew; administer with food

Klor-Con M: Tablet may be broken in half and each half swallowed separately; the whole tablet may also be dissolved in water

Parenteral: Potassium must be diluted prior to parenteral administration. Do not administer IV push. In general, the dose, concentration of infusion and rate of administration may be dependent on patient condition and specific institution policy.

Infusion rates (including all sources):

Pediatric: Noncritical care settings: Usual range: 0.2 to 0.5 mEq/kg/hour up to 10 mEq to 20 mEq/hour have been used. Critical care settings/situations: Higher rates may be used; maximum rate: 1 mEq/kg/hour up to 40 mEq/hour; continuous cardiac monitoring recommended for rates >0.5 mEq/kg/hour (Fuhrman 2011; Hamill 1991; Klaus 1989; Kliegman 2011; Kruse 1990; Lafraniere 2006; Schaber 1985)

Adult: Some clinicians recommend that the maximum concentration for peripheral infusion is 10 mEq/100 mL and maximum rate of administration for peripheral infusion is 10 mEq/hour (Kraft 2005). ECG monitoring is recommended for peripheral or central infusions >10 mEq/hour in adults (Kraft 2005). Concentrations and rates of infusion may be greater with central line administration. Concentrations of 20 to 40 mEq/100 mL at a maximum rate of 40 mEq/hour via central line have been safely administered (Hamill 1991; Kruse 1990).

Vesicant/irritant (at concentrations >0.1 mEq/mL); ensure proper needle or catheter placement prior to and during IV infusion. Avoid extravasation. If extravasation occurs, stop infusion immediately and disconnect (leave needle/cannula in place); gently aspirate extravasated solution (do NOT flush the line); initiate hyaluronidase antidote (see Management of Drug Extravasations for more details); remove needle/cannula; apply dry cold compresses (Hurst 2004); elevate extremity.

Vesicant/Extravasation Risk Vesicant/irritant (at concentrations >0.1 mEq/mL)

Monitoring Parameters Serum potassium, glucose, chloride, pH, urine output (if indicated), cardiac monitor [if intermittent IV infusion or potassium IV infusion rates >0.5 mEq/kg/hour or >10 mEq/hour (adults)]

Additional Information Hypokalemia is highly arrhythmogenic, particularly in the setting of ischemia or digitalis toxicity. ECG evidence of hypokalemia includes flattening of the T wave. As the T wave shrinks, U waves may appear. There is no prolongation of the QT interval. Hyperkalemia may present as tall peaked symmetrical T waves. S-T elevation may present in severe hyperkalemia. QRS complex progressively widens with eventual apparent sine waves on the ECG. Hyperkalemia will also induce cardiac slowing and AV conduction abnormalities.

Dosage Forms Considerations 750 mg potassium chloride = elemental potassium 390 mg = potassium 10 mEq = potassium 10 mmol

Dosage Forms Excipient information presented when available (limited, particularly for generics); consult specific product labeling.

Capsule Extended Release, Oral:
- Micro-K: 8 mEq, 10 mEq
- Generic: 8 mEq, 10 mEq

Liquid, Oral:
- Generic: 20 mEq/15 mL (10%) (473 mL); 40 mEq/15 mL (20%) (473 mL)

Packet, Oral:
- K-Vescent: 20 mEq (100 ea)
- Klor-Con: 20 mEq (1 ea, 30 ea, 100 ea); 25 mEq (30 ea, 100 ea) [sugar free; contains fd&c yellow #6 (sunset yellow); fruit flavor]
- Generic: 20 mEq (1 ea, 30 ea, 100 ea)

Solution, Intravenous:
- Generic: 5 mEq (250 mL); 10 mEq (500 mL, 1000 mL); 20 mEq (1000 mL); 30 mEq (1000 mL); 40 mEq (1000 mL); 0.4 mEq/mL (50 mL); 10 mEq/100 mL (100 mL); 10 mEq/50 mL (50 mL); 20 mEq/100 mL (100 mL); 20 mEq/50 mL (50 mL); 40 mEq/100 mL (100 mL); 2 mEq/mL (5 mL, 10 mL, 15 mL, 20 mL, 30 mL, 250 mL); 20 mEq/L (1000 mL); 40 mEq/L (1000 mL)

Solution, Oral:
- K-Sol: 20 mEq/15 mL (10%) (473 mL) [alcohol free, dye free, sugar free; contains methylparaben, propylene glycol, propylparaben, saccharin sodium]
- K-Sol: 40 mEq/15 mL (20%) (473 mL) [alcohol free, sugar free; contains fd&c red #40, saccharin sodium, sodium benzoate]
- Generic: 20 mEq/15 mL (10%) (15 mL, 30 mL, 473 mL)

Tablet Extended Release, Oral:
- K-Tab: 8 mEq, 10 mEq [contains fd&c yellow #10 (quinoline yellow)]
- K-Tab: 20 mEq
- Klor-Con: 8 mEq [contains fd&c blue #1 aluminum lake, fd&c blue #2 aluminum lake]
- Klor-Con 10: 10 mEq [contains fd&c yellow #10 aluminum lake, fd&c yellow #6 aluminum lake]
- Klor-Con M10: 10 mEq
- Klor-Con M15: 15 mEq [scored]
- Klor-Con M20: 20 mEq [scored]
- Generic: 8 mEq, 10 mEq, 20 mEq

Potassium Citrate and Citric Acid

(poe TASS ee um SIT rate & SI trik AS id)

Medication Safety Issues

Sound-alike/look-alike issues:

Polycitra may be confused with Bicitra

Brand Names: US Cytra-K; Virtrate-K

Therapeutic Category Alkalinizing Agent, Oral

Generic Availability (US) Yes

Use As long-term therapy to alkalinize the urine for control and/or dissolution of uric acid and cystine calculi of the urinary tract [FDA approved in pediatric patients (age not specified) and adults]; treatment of chronic metabolic acidosis secondary to chronic renal insufficiency or syndrome of renal tubular acidosis when use of sodium salt is undesirable [FDA approved in pediatric patients (age not specified) and adults]

Contraindications Severe renal insufficiency, oliguria, or azotemia; potassium-restricted diet; untreated Addison's disease; adynamia episodica hereditaria; acute dehydration; heat cramps; anuria; severe myocardial damage; hyperkalemia from any cause

Warnings/Precautions Use caution in patients with acid/base disorders, cardiovascular disease, potassium-altering conditions/disorders, or renal impairment. Citrate is converted to bicarbonate in the liver; this conversion may be blocked in patients who are severely ill, in shock, or in hepatic failure. Use with caution in patients receiving concomitant medications or therapies that increase potassium (eg, ACEI, potassium-sparing diuretics, potassium containing salt substitutes). Close monitoring of serum potassium concentrations is needed to avoid hyperkalemia. May cause GI upset (eg, nausea, vomiting, diarrhea, abdominal pain, discomfort) and lead to GI ulceration, bleeding, perforation and/or obstruction.

Benzyl alcohol and derivatives: Some dosage forms may contain sodium benzoate/benzoic acid; benzoic acid (benzoate) is a metabolite of benzyl alcohol; large amounts of benzyl alcohol (≥99 mg/kg/day) have been associated with a potentially fatal toxicity ("gasping syndrome") in neonates; the "gasping syndrome" consists of metabolic acidosis, respiratory distress, gasping respirations, CNS dysfunction (including convulsions, intracranial hemorrhage), hypotension, and cardiovascular collapse (AAP, 1997; CDC, 1982); some data suggests that benzoate displaces bilirubin from protein binding sites (Ahlfors, 2001); avoid or use dosage forms containing benzyl alcohol derivative with caution in neonates. See manufacturer's labeling.

Propylene glycol: Some dosage forms may contain propylene glycol; large amounts are potentially toxic and have been associated hyperosmolality, lactic acidosis, seizures and respiratory depression; use caution (AAP, 1997; Zar, 2007).

Warnings: Additional Pediatric Considerations Some dosage forms may contain propylene glycol; in neonates large amounts of propylene glycol delivered orally, intravenously (eg, >3,000 mg/day), or topically have been associated with potentially fatal toxicities which can include metabolic acidosis, seizures, renal failure, and CNS depression; toxicities have also been reported in children and adults including hyperosmolality, lactic acidosis, seizures, and respiratory depression; use caution (AAP, 1997; Shehab, 2009).

Drug Interactions

Metabolism/Transport Effects None known.

Avoid Concomitant Use There are no known interactions where it is recommended to avoid concomitant use.

Increased Effect/Toxicity

Potassium Citrate and Citric Acid may increase the levels/effects of: ACE Inhibitors; Aliskiren; Aluminum Hydroxide; Angiotensin II Receptor Blockers; Potassium-Sparing Diuretics

The levels/effects of Potassium Citrate and Citric Acid may be increased by: Eplerenone; Heparin; Heparin (Low Molecular Weight); Nicorandil

Decreased Effect There are no known significant interactions involving a decrease in effect.

Storage/Stability Store at controlled room temperature. Protect from excessive heat or freezing. Diluted formulations may be refrigerated to improve palatability.

Pharmacokinetics (Adult data unless noted)

Metabolism: ≥95% via hepatic oxidation to bicarbonate; may be impaired in patients with hepatic failure, in shock, or who are severely ill

Elimination: <5% unchanged in the urine

Dosing: Neonatal Oral: **Note:** 1 mL of oral solution contains 2 mEq of bicarbonate and 2 mEq of potassium; 1 packet of crystals contains 30 mEq of bicarbonate and 30 mEq of potassium: 2 to 3 mEq bicarbonate/kg/**day** (1 to 1.5 mL/kg/**day**) in 3 to 4 divided doses

Dosing: Usual Oral: **Note:** 1 mL of oral solution contains 2 mEq of bicarbonate and 2 mEq of potassium; 1 packet of crystals contains 30 mEq of bicarbonate and 30 mEq of potassium.

Manufacturer's recommendation: Pediatric patients: 5 to 15 mL (10 to 30 mEq bicarbonate) per dose after meals and at bedtime

Alternative recommendation: Dosing per mEq of bicarbonate:

Infants and Children: 2 to 3 mEq bicarbonate/kg/**day** (1 to 1.5 mL/kg/**day**) in 3 to 4 divided doses

Adults:

Powder: One packet (30 mEq bicarbonate) dissolved in 6 oz water after meals and at bedtime

Solution: 15 to 30 mL (30 to 60 mEq bicarbonate) per dose after meals and at bedtime

Note: When using to alkalinize the urine, 10 to 15 mL doses given 4 times/day typically maintain urinary pH 6.5 to 7.4; doses 15 to 20 mL 4 times/day usually maintain urinary pH at 7.0 to 7.6

Preparation for Administration

Oral:

Powder: Dilute contents of each packet with at least 6 ounces of cool water or juice.

Solution: Dilute each dose with water; pediatric patients dilute with 4 oz (1/2 glass) and adults with 8 oz (full glass)

Administration Oral: Dose should be diluted prior to administration to minimize injury due to high concentration of potassium; administer after meals and at bedtime to prevent saline laxative effect; may follow dose with additional water if necessary; dose may be chilled to improve palatability.

Dosage Forms Excipient information presented when available (limited, particularly for generics); consult specific product labeling. [DSC] = Discontinued product

Powder for solution, oral:

Cytra-K: Potassium citrate monohydrate 3300 mg and citric acid monohydrate 1002 mg per packet (100s) [sugar free; fruit-punch flavor; each packet contains potassium 30 mEq equivalent to bicarbonate 30 mEq]

Solution, oral:

Cytra-K: Potassium citrate monohydrate 1100 mg and citric acid monohydrate 334 mg per 5 mL (480 mL) [ethanol free, sugar free; contains propylene glycol; cherry flavor; contains potassium 2 mEq/mL equivalent to bicarbonate 2 mEq /mL]

Virtrate-K: Potassium citrate monohydrate 1100 mg and citric acid monohydrate 334 mg per 5 mL (480 mL) [contains propylene glycol; cherry flavor; contains potassium 2 mEq/mL equivalent to bicarbonate 2 mEq /mL]

Generic: Potassium citrate monohydrate 1100 mg and citric acid monohydrate 334 mg per 5 mL (473 mL)

◆ **Potassium Citrate, Citric Acid, and Sodium Citrate** *see* Citric Acid, Sodium Citrate, and Potassium Citrate *on page 479*

Potassium Gluconate

(poe TASS ee um GLOO coe nate)

Brand Names: US K-99 [OTC]

Therapeutic Category Electrolyte Supplement, Oral

Generic Availability (US) Yes

Use Treatment or prevention of hypokalemia

Pregnancy Considerations Potassium requirements are the same in pregnant and non-pregnant women. Adverse events have not been observed following use of potassium supplements in healthy women with normal pregnancies. Use caution in pregnant women with other medical conditions (eg, pre-eclampsia; may be more likely to develop hyperkalemia) (IOM, 2004).

Breast-Feeding Considerations Potassium is excreted into breast milk (IOM, 2004).

Contraindications Hyperkalemia

Warnings/Precautions Use caution in patients with acid/base disorders, cardiovascular disease, potassium-altering conditions/disorders, or renal impairment. Use with caution in patients receiving concomitant medications or therapies that increase potassium (eg, ACEI, potassium-sparing diuretics, potassium containing salt substitutes). Close monitoring of serum potassium concentrations is needed to avoid hyperkalemia. May cause GI upset (eg, nausea, vomiting, diarrhea, abdominal pain, discomfort) and lead to GI ulceration, bleeding, perforation and/or obstruction. Oral liquid preparations (not solid) should be used in patients with esophageal compression or delayed gastric emptying.

Drug Interactions

Metabolism/Transport Effects None known.

Avoid Concomitant Use There are no known interactions where it is recommended to avoid concomitant use.

Increased Effect/Toxicity

Potassium Gluconate may increase the levels/effects of: ACE Inhibitors; Aliskiren; Angiotensin II Receptor Blockers; Potassium-Sparing Diuretics

The levels/effects of Potassium Gluconate may be increased by: Eplerenone; Heparin; Heparin (Low Molecular Weight); Nicorandil

Decreased Effect There are no known significant interactions involving a decrease in effect.

Storage/Stability Store at room temperature.

Mechanism of Action Potassium is the major cation of intracellular fluid and is essential for the conduction of nerve impulses in heart, brain, and skeletal muscle; contraction of cardiac, skeletal and smooth muscles; maintenance of normal renal function, acid-base balance, carbohydrate metabolism, and gastric secretion

Pharmacokinetics (Adult data unless noted)

Absorption: Well absorbed from upper GI tract

Distribution: Enters cells via active transport from extracellular fluid

Elimination: Primarily urine; skin and feces (small amounts); most intestinal potassium reabsorbed

Dosing: Usual Oral: **Note:** Doses listed as mEq of potassium (approximately 4.3 mEq potassium/g potassium gluconate; 1 mEq potassium is equivalent to 39 mg elemental potassium)

Normal daily requirement:

Children: 2-3 mEq/kg/day

Adults: 40-80 mEq/day

Prevention of hypokalemia during diuretic therapy:

Children: 1-2 mEq/kg/day in 1-2 divided doses

Adults: 20-40 mEq/day in 1-2 divided doses

Treatment of hypokalemia:

Children: 2-5 mEq/kg/day in divided doses; not to exceed 1-2 mEq/kg as a single dose; if deficits are severe or ongoing losses are great, IV route should be considered preferred route of administration

Adults: 40-100 mEq/day in 2-4 divided doses

Administration Oral: Sustained release and wax matrix tablets should be swallowed whole, do not crush or chew; administer with food

Monitoring Parameters Serum potassium, chloride, glucose, pH, urine output (if indicated)

Test Interactions Decreased ammonia (B)

Additional Information 9.4 g potassium gluconate is approximately equal to 40 mEq potassium (4.3 mEq potassium/g potassium gluconate). Hypokalemia is highly arrhythmogenic, particularly in the setting of ischemia or digitalis toxicity. ECG evidence of hypokalemia includes flattening of the T wave. As the T wave shrinks, U waves may appear. There is no prolongation of the QT interval. Hyperkalemia may present as tall peaked symmetrical T waves. S-T elevation may present in severe hyperkalemia. QRS complex progressively widens with eventual apparent sine waves on the ECG. Hyperkalemia will also induce cardiac slowing and AV conduction abnormalities.

Dosage Forms Considerations 1 g potassium gluconate = elemental potassium 167 mg = potassium 4.3 mEq = potassium 4.3 mmol

Dosage Forms Excipient information presented when available (limited, particularly for generics); consult specific product labeling.

Capsule, Oral [preservative free]:

K-99: 595 mg [dye free, sugar free, yeast free]

Tablet, Oral:

Generic: 2 mEq, 2.5 mEq

Tablet, Oral [strength expressed as base]:

Generic: 80 mg

Potassium Iodide (poe TASS ee um EYE oh dide)

Medication Safety Issues

Sound-alike/look-alike issues:

Potassium iodide products, including saturated solution of potassium iodide (SSKI®) may be confused with potassium iodide and iodine (Strong Iodide Solution or Lugol's solution)

Other safety concerns:

Dosage volume: Dosing errors have been reported during the prescribing, dispensing, and administration of potassium iodide-containing solutions (eg, Lugol's, SSKI). Errors have occurred when **mL** doses were administered, when only **drops** were indicated for the dose. Carefully review dosage and administration information; appropriate oral dosage is most commonly expressed as drops to provide doses less than 1 mL. Dispensing unit doses is also highly recommended; pharmacists should never dispense quantities that could be lethal if consumed as a single dose. (ISMP, 2011).

Brand Names: US SSKI; ThyroShield [OTC]

Therapeutic Category Antithyroid Agent; Expectorant

Generic Availability (US) No

Use Expectorant for the symptomatic treatment of chronic pulmonary diseases complicated by mucous (SSKI: FDA approved in adults); block thyroidal uptake of radioactive isotopes of iodine in a nuclear radiation emergency (Iosat, ThyroSafe, ThyroShield: FDA approved in all ages); has also been used to reduce thyroid vascularity prior to thyroidectomy and management of thyrotoxic crisis; lymphocutaneous and cutaneous sporotrichosis; to block thyroidal uptake of radioactive isotopes of iodine after therapeutic or diagnostic exposure to radioactive iodine

Pregnancy Risk Factor D

Pregnancy Considerations Iodide crosses the placenta (may cause hypothyroidism and goiter in fetus/newborn). Use as an expectorant during pregnancy is contraindicated by the AAP. Use for protection against thyroid cancer secondary to radioactive iodine exposure is considered acceptable based upon risk:benefit, keeping in mind the dose and duration. In general, medications used as antidotes should take into consideration the health and prognosis of the mother; antidotes should be administered to pregnant women if there is a clear indication for use and should not be withheld because of fears of teratogenicity (Bailey, 2003). Pregnant women should take as instructed by public officials and contact their physician. Repeat dosing should be avoided if possible. Refer to Iodine monograph for additional information.

Breast-Feeding Considerations Potassium iodide is excreted in breast milk. May cause skin rash in nursing infant. Nursing mothers should take as instructed by public officials and contact their physician. Refer to Iodine monograph for additional information.

Contraindications Hypersensitivity to iodide, iodine, or any component of the formulation; dermatitis herpetiformis; hypocomplementemic vasculitis, nodular thyroid condition with heart disease

Warnings/Precautions Prolonged use can lead to hypothyroidism; iodide may cause underactive or overactive thyroid; thyroid enlargement may also occur; use with caution in patients with a history of hyperthyroidism; use is contraindicated in patients with nodular thyroid condition (goiter) with heart disease. Iodism or chronic iodide poisoning may occur with high doses or prolonged treatment; symptoms include burning of mouth/throat, sore teeth/gums, severe headache, metallic taste, eye irritation/eye lid swelling, increased salivation, acneform skin lesions, and (rarely) severe skin lesions; withhold potassium iodide treatment and manage with supportive care.

May cause acne flare-ups, can cause dermatitis; use with caution in patients with a history of renal impairment, Addison's disease, cardiac disease, myotonia congenita, tuberculosis, and/or acute bronchitis. Iodide hypersensitivity may occur, manifesting as angioedema, cutaneous/mucosal hemorrhage, and serum sickness-like symptoms (fever, arthralgia, lymph node enlargement, and eosinophilia). Potentially significant drug-drug interactions may exist, requiring dose or frequency adjustment, additional monitoring, and/or selection of alternative therapy. For thyroid gland protection (radiopharmaceutical use), potassium iodide must be administered prior to receiving radiopharmaceuticals that require thyroid gland protection. For nuclear radiation emergency, take only when instructed by public health officials; do not take more or more often than instructed; follow other emergency measures recommended by officials. In a nuclear radiation emergency, infants and children are more likely to experience thyroid damage. Neonates <1 month are at higher risk for hypothyroidism with potassium iodide use; evaluate thyroid function if repeat dosing is required in this patient population.

Warnings: Additional Pediatric Considerations Use with caution in patients with cystic fibrosis; may have exaggerated susceptibility to goitrogenic effects.

Some dosage forms may contain propylene glycol; in neonates large amounts of propylene glycol delivered orally, intravenously (eg, >3,000 mg/day), or topically have been associated with potentially fatal toxicities which can include metabolic acidosis, seizures, renal failure, and CNS depression; toxicities have also been reported in children and adults including hyperosmolality, lactic acidosis, seizures, and respiratory depression; use caution (AAP, 1997; Shehab, 2009).

Adverse Reactions

Cardiovascular: Cardiac arrhythmia

Central nervous system: Confusion, fatigue, fever, numbness, tingling sensation

Dermatologic: Skin rash, urticaria

Endocrine & metabolic: Goiter, hyperthyroidism (prolonged use), hypothyroidism (prolonged use), myxedema

Gastrointestinal: Diarrhea, enlargement of salivary glands, gastric distress, gastrointestinal hemorrhage, metallic taste, nausea, stomach pain, vomiting

Hematologic & oncologic: Lymphedema, thyroid adenoma

Hypersensitivity: Hypersensitivity reaction (angioedema, cutaneous and mucosal hemorrhage, serum sickness-like symptoms)

Neuromuscular & skeletal: Weakness

Respiratory: Dyspnea, wheezing

Miscellaneous: Iodine poisoning (with prolonged treatment/high doses)

Drug Interactions

Metabolism/Transport Effects None known.

Avoid Concomitant Use

Avoid concomitant use of Potassium Iodide with any of the following: Sodium Iodide I131

Increased Effect/Toxicity

Potassium Iodide may increase the levels/effects of: ACE Inhibitors; Aliskiren; Angiotensin II Receptor Blockers; Cardiac Glycosides; Lithium; Potassium-Sparing Diuretics; Theophylline Derivatives

The levels/effects of Potassium Iodide may be increased by: Eplerenone; Heparin; Heparin (Low Molecular Weight); Nicorandil

Decreased Effect

Potassium Iodide may decrease the levels/effects of: Sodium Iodide I131; Vitamin K Antagonists

Storage/Stability Store at room temperature of 25°C (77°F); excursions permitted to 15°C to 30°C (59°F to 86°F). Protect from light. Keep tightly closed.

SSKI®: If exposed to cold, crystallization may occur. Warm and shake to redissolve. If solution becomes brown/yellow, it should be discarded.

iOSAT™, Thyrosafe®: Keep dry and keep intact in foil.

Mechanism of Action Reduces viscosity of mucus by increasing respiratory tract secretions; inhibits secretion of thyroid hormone, fosters colloid accumulation in thyroid follicles. Following radioactive iodine exposure, potassium iodide blocks the uptake of radioactive iodine by the thyroid, reducing the risk of thyroid cancer.

Pharmacodynamics

Antithyroid effects:

Onset of action: 24 to 48 hours

Maximum effect: 10 to 15 days after continuous therapy

Duration: May persist up to 6 weeks

Radioactive iodine exposure: Duration: 24 hours

Dosing: Neonatal

Thyroid block following nuclear radiation emergency: Iosat, ThyroSafe, ThyroShield: Oral: 16.25 mg once daily; **Note:** Continue treatment until the risk of exposure has passed and/or until other measures (evacuation, sheltering, control of the food and milk supply) have been successfully implemented

Thyroid gland protection during radiopharmaceutical use: ThyroShield: Oral: 16 mg once on the day before radiopharmaceutical use (Olivier, 2003)

Dosing: Usual

Pediatric:

Sporotrichosis, cutaneous: Limited data available: Children and Adolescents: SSKI: Oral: Initial: 50 mg (1 drop **or** 0.05 mL) 3 times daily; increase as tolerated to ≤50 mg/kg/dose (≤1 drop/**kg**/dose **or** ≤0.05 mL/**kg**/dose) 3 times daily; Maximum dose: 2500 mg/dose (50 drops/dose or 2.5 mL/dose); continued at the maximum tolerated dosage for several weeks after lesions have resolved (Kauffman, 2007; *Red Book* [AAP], 2012)

Thyroid block following nuclear radiation emergency: Iosat, ThyroSafe, ThyroShield: Oral: **Note:** Continue treatment until the risk of exposure has passed and/or until other measures (evacuation, sheltering, control of the food and milk supply) have been successfully implemented.

Infants and Children ≤3 years: 32.5 mg once daily

Children >3 to 12 years: 65 mg once daily

Adolescents:

Weight <68 kg: 65 mg once daily

Weight ≥68 kg: 130 mg once daily

Thyroid gland protection during radiopharmaceutical use: Limited data available; **Note:** Begin at 1 to 48 hours prior to exposure; continue potassium iodide after radiopharmaceutical administration until risk of exposure has diminished (treatment duration and time of initiation is dependent on the radiopharmaceutical; consult specific protocol: Iostat, ThyroSafe, ThyroShield: Oral:

Age-directed dosing (Olivier, 2003):

Infants and Children <3 years: 32 mg once daily

Children and Adolescents 3 to 13 years: 65 mg once daily

Adolescents >13 years: 130 mg once daily

Weight-directed dosing (Giammarile, 2008):

<5 kg: 16 mg once daily

5 to <15 kg: 32 mg once daily

15 to <50 kg: 65 mg once daily

≥50 kg: 130 mg once daily

Thyroidectomy, preoperative preparation: Children and Adolescents: SSKI: Oral: 150 to 350 mg (3 to 7 drops or 0.15 to 0.35 mL) 3 times daily; administer for 10 days before surgery; if not euthyroid prior to surgery, consider concurrent beta-blockade (eg, propranolol) in the immediate preoperative period to reduce the risk of thyroid storm (Bahn, 2011)

Thyrotoxic crisis/thyroid storm: (Eyal, 2008): **Note:** Administer at least 1 hour after antithyroid drug (eg, methimazole) administration:

Infants: SSKI: Oral: 100 mg (2 drops **or** 0.1 mL) 4 times daily

Children and Adolescents: SSKI: Oral: 250 mg (5 drops **or** 0.25 mL) 2 to 4 times daily

Adult:

Expectorant: SSKI: Oral: 300 to 600 mg (0.3 to 0.6 mL) 3 to 4 times daily

Thyroidectomy, preparation: Oral: 50 to 100 mg (1 to 2 drops **or** 0.05 to 0.1 mL SSKI) 3 times daily; administer for 10 days before surgery; if not euthyroid prior to surgery, consider concurrent beta-blockade (eg, propranolol) in the immediate preoperative period to reduce the risk of thyroid storm (Bahn, 2011)

Sporotrichosis (cutaneous, lymphocutaneous): SSKI: Oral: Initial: 250 mg (5 drops **or** 0.25 mL) 3 times daily; increase to 2,000 to 2,500 mg (40 to 50 drops **or** 2 to 2.5 mL) 3 times daily as tolerated until 2 to 4 weeks after lesions have resolved (usual duration: 3 to 6 months) (Kauffman, 2007)

Thyroid gland protection during radiopharmaceutical use: Oral: Tablet: 130 mg once daily **or** Solution (SSKI): 200 mg (4 drops **or** 0.2 mL) 3 times daily (Bexxar prescribing information, 2012). **Note:** Begin at 1 to 48 hours prior to exposure. Continue potassium iodide after radiopharmaceutical administration until risk of exposure has diminished (treatment duration and time of initiation is dependent on the radiopharmaceutical, consult specific protocol).

Thyrotoxic crisis/thyroid storm: SSKI: Oral: **Note:** Administer at least 1 to 2 hours after antithyroid drug administration: 250 mg (5 drops **or** 0.25 mL) every 6 hours (Bahn, 2011)

Thyroid block following nuclear radiation emergency: Iosat, ThyroSafe, ThyroShield: Includes pregnant/lactating women: Oral: 130 mg once daily, continue for 10 to 14 days or as directed by public officials (until risk of exposure has passed or other measures are implemented).

Dosing adjustment in renal impairment: Infants, Children, Adolescents, and Adults: There are no dosage adjustments provided in the manufacturer's labeling.

Dosing adjustment in hepatic impairment: Infants, Children, Adolescents, and Adults: There are no dosage adjustments provided in the manufacturer's labeling.

Preparation for Administration

Oral: To make potassium iodide (KI) mixture from tablet:

Iosat: Grind one 130 mg tablet into a fine powder; add 20 mL of water and mix until powder is dissolved. Take mixture and add to 20 mL of low fat milk (white or chocolate), orange juice, soda (flat), raspberry syrup, or infant formula. This results in a concentration of 16.25 mg/5 mL. KI liquid may be kept for 7 days in the refrigerator. Discard unused portion.

Thyrosafe: Grind one 65 mg tablet into a fine powder; add 20 mL of water and mix until powder is dissolved. Take mixture and add to 20 mL of low fat milk (white or chocolate), orange juice, soda (flat), raspberry syrup, or infant formula. This results in a concentration of 8.125 mg/5 mL

Administration Oral:

SSKI: Dilute with a large quantity of water, fruit juice, milk, or broth; take with food or milk to decrease gastric irritation.

Iosat, Thyrosafe, Thyroshield: Take as soon as possible after instructed to do so by public officials. Take every 24 hours; do not take more than 1 dose in 24 hours. Tablets may be crushed and mixed with water, low fat milk (white or chocolate), orange juice, soda (flat), raspberry syrup, or infant formula.

Monitoring Parameters Thyroid function tests; sign/symptoms of hyperthyroidism; thyroid function should be monitored in pregnant or breast-feeding women, neonates, and young infants if repeat doses are required following radioactive iodine exposure

Test Interactions Iodide may alter thyroid function tests.

Additional Information SSKI 10 drops = potassium iodide 500 mg

Dosage Forms Excipient information presented when available (limited, particularly for generics); consult specific product labeling.

Solution, Oral:

SSKI: 1 g/mL (30 mL, 237 mL)

ThyroShield: 65 mg/mL (30 mL) [contains brilliant blue fcf (fd&c blue #1), fd&c red #40, methylparaben, propylene glycol, propylparaben, saccharin sodium; black raspberry flavor]

Extemporaneous Preparations A 16.25 mg/5 mL oral solution may be made with tablets. Crush one 130 mg tablet and reduce to a fine powder. Add 20 mL of water and mix until powder is dissolved. Add an additional 20 mL of low-fat milk (white or chocolate), orange juice, flat soda, raspberry syrup, or infant formula. Stable for 7 days under refrigeration.

To prepare an 8.125 mg/5 mL oral solution, crush one 65 mg tablet and reduce to a fine powder. Add 20 mL of water and mix until powder is dissolved. Add an additional 20 mL of low-fat milk (white or chocolate), orange juice, flat soda, raspberry syrup, or infant formula. Stable for 7 days under refrigeration.

Potassium Iodide and Iodine

(poe TASS ee um EYE oh dide & EYE oh dine)

Medication Safety Issues

Sound-alike/look-alike issues:

Potassium iodide and iodine (Strong Iodide Solution or Lugol's solution) may be confused with potassium iodide products, including saturated solution of potassium iodide (SSKI®)

Other safety concerns:

Dosage volume: Dosing errors have been reported during the prescribing, dispensing, and administration of potassium iodide-containing solutions (eg, Lugol's, SSKI). Errors have occurred when **mL** doses were administered, when only **drops** were indicated for the dose. Carefully review dosage and administration information; appropriate oral dosage is most commonly expressed as drops to provide doses less than 1 mL. Dispensing unit doses is also highly recommended; pharmacists should never dispense quantities that could be lethal if consumed as a single dose. (ISMP, 2011).

Therapeutic Category Antibacterial, Topical; Antithyroid Agent

Generic Availability (US) Yes

Use

Oral solution: Reduce thyroid vascularity prior to thyroidectomy and management of thyrotoxic crisis (FDA approved in adults); has also been used to block thyroidal uptake of radioactive isotopes of iodine in a radiation emergency or after therapeutic/diagnostic use of radioactive iodine

Topical solution: Provide topical antisepsis (FDA approved in adults)

Pregnancy Risk Factor D (potassium iodide)

Pregnancy Considerations Iodide crosses the placenta (may cause hypothyroidism and goiter in fetus/newborn). Use for protection against thyroid cancer secondary to radioactive iodine exposure is considered acceptable based upon risk:benefit, keeping in mind the dose and duration. Repeat dosing should be avoided if possible. Refer to Iodine for additional information.

Breast-Feeding Considerations Skin rash in the nursing infant has been reported with maternal intake of potassium iodide. Refer to Iodine monograph for additional information.

Contraindications Hypersensitivity to iodine or any component of the formulation; iodine-induced goiter; dermatitis herpetiformis; hypocomplementemic vasculitis; nodular thyroid disease with heart disease

Warnings/Precautions Prolonged use can lead to hypothyroidism; can cause acne flare-ups and/or dermatitis; use with caution in patients with a history of renal impairment, hyperthyroidism, Addison's disease, cardiac disease, myotonia congenita, tuberculosis, acute bronchitis. Potentially significant interactions may exist, requiring dose or frequency adjustment, additional monitoring, and/or selection of alternative therapy. Potassium iodide and iodine solution must be administered prior to receiving radiopharmaceuticals that require thyroid gland protection.

Adverse Reactions

Cardiovascular: Irregular heart beat

Central nervous system: Confusion, tiredness, fever

Dermatologic: Skin rash

Endocrine & metabolic: Goiter, salivary gland swelling/tenderness, thyroid adenoma, swelling of neck/throat, myxedema, lymph node swelling, hyper-/hypothyroidism

Gastrointestinal: Diarrhea, gastrointestinal bleeding, metallic taste, nausea, stomach pain, stomach upset, vomiting

Neuromuscular & skeletal: Numbness, tingling, weakness, joint pain

Miscellaneous: Chronic iodine poisoning (with prolonged treatment/high doses); iodism, hypersensitivity reactions (angioedema, cutaneous and mucosal hemorrhage, serum sickness-like symptoms)

Drug Interactions

Metabolism/Transport Effects None known.

Avoid Concomitant Use

Avoid concomitant use of Potassium Iodide and Iodine with any of the following: Sodium Iodide I131

Increased Effect/Toxicity

Potassium Iodide and Iodine may increase the levels/effects of: ACE Inhibitors; Aliskiren; Angiotensin II Receptor Blockers; Cardiac Glycosides; Lithium; Potassium-Sparing Diuretics; Theophylline Derivatives

The levels/effects of Potassium Iodide and Iodine may be increased by: Eplerenone; Heparin; Heparin (Low Molecular Weight); Nicorandil

Decreased Effect

Potassium Iodide and Iodine may decrease the levels/effects of: Sodium Iodide I131; Vitamin K Antagonists

Storage/Stability Store at room temperature of 15°C to 30°C (59°F to 86°F). Protect from light and keep container tightly closed.

Mechanism of Action In hyperthyroidism, iodine temporarily inhibits thyroid hormone synthesis and secretion into the circulation; use also decreases thyroid gland size and vascularity. Serum T_4 and T_3 concentrations can be reduced for several weeks with use but effect will not be maintained.

Following radioactive iodine exposure, potassium iodide blocks uptake of radioiodine by the thyroid, reducing the risk of thyroid cancer.

Pharmacodynamics Antithyroid effects:

Onset of action: 24-48 hours

Maximum effect: 10-15 days after continuous therapy

Duration: May persist up to 6 weeks

Dosing: Neonatal Graves' disease: Oral: Lugol's solution: 1 drop/dose 3 times daily

Dosing: Usual

Children:

Thyroidectomy, preoperative preparation: Oral: Lugol's solution: 3-5 drops (0.1-0.3 mL)/dose 3 times daily; administer for 10 days before surgery

Thyrotoxic crisis: Oral: Lugol's solution: 4-8 drops/dose 3 times daily, begin therapy preferably 2 hours following the initial dose of either propylthiouracil or methimazole

Adults:

Thyroidectomy, preoperative preparation: Oral: Lugol's solution: 5-7 drops (0.25-0.35 mL)/dose 3 times daily; administer for 10 days before surgery; if not euthyroid prior to surgery, consider concurrent beta-blockade (eg, propranolol) in the immediate preoperative period to reduce the risk of thyroid storm (Bahn, 2011)

Thyrotoxic crisis: Oral: Lugol's solution: 4-8 drops/dose every 6-8 hours; begin administration ≥1 hour following the initial dose of either propylthiouracil or methimazole (Nayak, 2006)

Administration

Oral: Dilute with a large quantity of water, fruit juice, or milk or administer after meals with food or milk

Topical: For external use only; apply to area requiring antiseptic

Monitoring Parameters Thyroid function tests, signs/symptoms of hyperthyroidism; thyroid function should be monitored in pregnant women, neonates, and young infants if repeat doses are required following radioactive iodine exposure

Test Interactions Iodide may alter thyroid function tests.

Dosage Forms Excipient information presented when available (limited, particularly for generics); consult specific product labeling.

Solution, oral: Potassium iodide 100 mg/mL and iodine 50 mg/mL (473 mL)

Solution, topical: Potassium iodide 100 mg/mL and iodine 50 mg/mL (8 mL)

Potassium Phosphate (poe TASS ee um FOS fate)

Medication Safety Issues

Sound-alike/look-alike issues:

Neutra-Phos-K [DSC] may be confused with K-Phos Neutral

High alert medication:

The Institute for Safe Medication Practices (ISMP) includes this medication (IV formulation) among its list of drugs which have a heightened risk of causing significant patient harm when used in error.

Other safety concerns:

Per JCAHO recommendations, concentrated electrolyte solutions should not be available in patient care areas.

Consider special storage requirements for intravenous potassium salts; IV potassium salts have been administered IVP in error, leading to fatal outcomes.

Safe Prescribing: Because inorganic phosphate exists as monobasic and dibasic anions, with the mixture of valences dependent on pH, ordering by mEq amounts is unreliable and may lead to large dosing errors. In addition, IV phosphate is available in the sodium and potassium salt; therefore, the content of these cations must be considered when ordering phosphate. The most reliable method of ordering IV phosphate is by millimoles, then specifying the potassium or sodium salt. For example, an order for 15 mmol of phosphate as potassium phosphate in one liter of normal saline.

Related Information

Management of Drug Extravasations *on page 2298*

Brand Names: US Neutra-Phos®-K [OTC] [DSC]

Therapeutic Category Electrolyte Supplement, Parenteral; Phosphate Salt; Potassium Salt

Generic Availability (US) Yes: Injection

Use Treatment and prevention of hypophosphatemia; source of phosphate in large volume IV fluids (All indications: FDA approved in all ages)

Pregnancy Risk Factor C

Pregnancy Considerations Reproduction studies have not been conducted. Phosphorus requirements are the same in pregnant and nonpregnant women (IOM, 1997). Although this product is not used for potassium supplementation, adverse events have not been observed following use of potassium supplements in healthy women with normal pregnancies. Use caution in pregnant women with other medical conditions (eg, pre-eclampsia; may be more likely to develop hyperkalemia) (IOM, 2004).

Breast-Feeding Considerations Phosphorus, sodium, and potassium are normal constituents of human milk.

Contraindications Hyperphosphatemia, hyperkalemia, hypocalcemia

Warnings/Precautions Close monitoring of serum potassium concentrations is needed to avoid hyperkalemia. Use with caution in patients with renal insufficiency, cardiac disease, metabolic alkalosis. Use with caution in digitalized patients and patients receiving concomitant potassium-altering therapies. Parenteral potassium may cause pain and phlebitis, requiring a decrease in infusion rate or potassium concentration. Vesicant/irritant (may depend on concentration); ensure proper catheter or needle position prior to and during infusion; avoid extravasation. The parenteral product may contain aluminum; toxic aluminum concentrations may be seen with high doses, prolonged use, or renal dysfunction. Premature neonates are at higher risk due to immature renal function and aluminum intake from other parenteral sources. Parenteral aluminum exposure of >4 to 5 mcg/kg/day is associated with CNS and bone toxicity; tissue loading may occur at lower doses (Federal Register, 2002). See manufacturer's labeling.

Adverse Reactions

Cardiovascular: Arrhythmia, bradycardia, chest pain, ECG changes, edema, heart block, hypotension

Central nervous system: Listlessness, mental confusion, tetany (with large doses of phosphate)

Endocrine & metabolic: Hyperkalemia

Gastrointestinal: Diarrhea, nausea, stomach pain, vomiting

Genitourinary: Urine output decreased

Local: Phlebitis

Neuromuscular & skeletal: Paralysis, paresthesia, weakness

Renal: Acute renal failure

Respiratory: Dyspnea

Drug Interactions

Metabolism/Transport Effects None known.

Avoid Concomitant Use There are no known interactions where it is recommended to avoid concomitant use.

Increased Effect/Toxicity

Potassium Phosphate may increase the levels/effects of: ACE Inhibitors; Aliskiren; Angiotensin II Receptor Blockers; Potassium-Sparing Diuretics

The levels/effects of Potassium Phosphate may be increased by: Eplerenone; Heparin; Heparin (Low Molecular Weight); Nicorandil

Decreased Effect

The levels/effects of Potassium Phosphate may be decreased by: Antacids; Calcium Salts; Iron Salts; Magnesium Salts; Multivitamins/Minerals (with ADEK, Folate, Iron); Sucralfate

Food Interactions Avoid administering with oxalate (berries, nuts, chocolate, beans, celery, tomato) or phytate-containing foods (bran, whole wheat).

Storage/Stability Store intact vials at 20°C to 25°C (68°F to 77°F); excursions permitted between 15°C and 30°C (59°F and 86°F).

Mechanism of Action

Phosphorus in the form of organic and inorganic phosphate has a variety of important biochemical functions in the body and is involved in many significant metabolic and enzymatic reactions in almost all organs and tissues. It exerts a modifying influence on the steady state of calcium levels, a buffering effect on acid-base equilibrium and a primary role in the renal excretion of hydrogen ion.

Potassium is the major cation of intracellular fluid and is essential for the conduction of nerve impulses in heart, brain, and skeletal muscle; contraction of cardiac, skeletal and smooth muscles; maintenance of normal renal function, acid-base balance, carbohydrate metabolism, and gastric secretion.

Pharmacokinetics (Adult data unless noted) Elimination: Excreted in the urine with over 80% to 90% of dose reabsorbed by the kidney

Dosing: Neonatal Note: If phosphate repletion is required and a phosphate product is not available at your institution, consider the use of sodium glycerophosphate pentahydrate (Glycophos) as a suitable substitute. Concentration and dosing are different from FDA approved products; use caution when switching between products. Refer to Sodium Glycerophosphate Pentahydrate monograph.

Caution: With orders for IV phosphate, there is considerable confusion associated with the use of millimoles (mmol) versus milliequivalents (mEq) to express the phosphate requirement. The most reliable method of ordering IV phosphate is by millimoles, then specifying the potassium or sodium salt. Intravenous doses listed as mmol of phosphate. **Note:** Consider the contribution of potassium when determining the appropriate phosphate replacement.

Phosphorus Estimated Average Requirement (EAR): Oral: 3.2 mmol/day (adequate intake)

Parenteral nutrition, maintenance requirement: IV: 1-2 mmol/kg/day (Mirtallo, 2004)

Dosing: Usual Note: If phosphate repletion is required and a phosphate product is not available at your institution, consider the use of sodium glycerophosphate pentahydrate (Glycophos) as a suitable substitute. Concentration and dosing are different from FDA approved products; use caution when switching between products. Refer to Sodium Glycerophosphate Pentahydrate monograph.

Caution: With orders for IV phosphate, there is considerable confusion associated with the use of millimoles (mmol) versus milliequivalents (mEq) to express the phosphate requirement. The most reliable method of ordering IV phosphate is by millimoles, then specifying the potassium or sodium salt. Intravenous doses listed as mmol of phosphate. **Note:** Consider the contribution of potassium when determining the appropriate phosphate replacement.

Infants, Children, and Adolescents:

Phosphorus - Recommended Daily Allowance (RDA) and Estimated Average Requirement (EAR):

1-6 months:
- EAR: 3.2 mmol/day (adequate intake)

7-12 months:
- EAR: 8.9 mmol/day (adequate intake)

1-3 years:
- RDA: 14.8 mmol/day
- EAR: 12.3 mmol/day

4-8 years:
- RDA: 16.1 mmol/day
- EAR: 13.1 mmol/day

9-18 years:
- RDA: 40.3 mmol/day
- EAR: 34 mmol/day

19-30 years:
- RDA: 22.6 mmol/day
- EAR: 18.7 mmol/day

Hypophosphatemia, acute: Hypophosphatemia does not necessarily equate with phosphate depletion. Hypophosphatemia may occur in the presence of low, normal, or high total body phosphate and conversely, phosphate depletion may exist with normal, low, or elevated levels of serum phosphate (Gaasbeek, 2005). It is difficult to provide concrete guidelines for the treatment of severe hypophosphatemia because the extent of total body deficits and response to therapy are difficult to predict. Aggressive doses of phosphate may result in a transient serum elevation followed by redistribution into intracellular compartments or bone tissue. Intermittent IV infusion should be reserved for severe depletion situations; requires continuous cardiac monitoring. Guidelines differ based on degree of illness, need/use of TPN, and severity of hypophosphatemia. If hyperkalemia exists, consider phosphate replacement strategy without potassium (eg, sodium phosphates). Various regimens for replacement of phosphate in adults have been studied. The regimens below have only been studied in adult patients, however, many institutions have used them in children safely and successfully. Obese patients and/or severe renal impairment were excluded from phosphate supplement trials. **Note:** 1 mmol phosphate = 31 mg phosphorus; 1 mg phosphorus = 0.032 mmol phosphate

IV doses may be incorporated into the patient's maintenance IV fluids; intermittent IV infusion should be reserved for severe depletion situations. **Note:** Doses listed as mmol of **phosphate**

Children and Adolescents: **Note:** There are no prospective studies of parenteral phosphate replacement in children. The following weight-based guidelines for adult dosing may be cautiously employed in pediatric patients. Guidelines differ based on degree of illness, use of TPN, and severity of hypophosphatemia.

General replacement guidelines (Lentz, 1978): **Note:** The initial dose may be increased by 25% to 50% if the patient is symptomatic secondary to hypophosphatemia and lowered by 25% to 50% if the patient is hypercalcemic.

Low dose: 0.08 mmol/kg over 6 hours; use if losses are recent and uncomplicated

Intermediate dose: 0.16-0.24 mmol/kg over 4-6 hours; use if serum phosphorus level 0.5-1 mg/dL (0.16-0.32 mmol/L)

High dose: 0.36 mmol/kg over 6 hours; use if serum phosphorus <0.5 mg/dL (<0.16 mmol/L)

Patients receiving TPN (Clark, 1995):

Low dose: 0.16 mmol/kg over 4-6 hours; use if serum phosphorus level 2.3-3 mg/dL (0.73- 0.96 mmol/L)

Intermediate dose: 0.32 mmol/kg over 4-6 hours; use if serum phosphorus level 1.6-2.2 mg/dL (0.51-0.72 mmol/L)

High dose: 0.64 mmol/kg over 8-12 hours; use if serum phosphorus <1.5 mg/dL (< 0.5 mmol/L)

Critically ill adult trauma patients receiving TPN (Brown, 2006):

Low dose: 0.32 mmol/kg over 4-6 hours; use if serum phosphorus level 2.3-3 mg/dL (0.73-0.96 mmol/L)

Intermediate dose: 0.64 mmol/kg over 4-6 hours; use if serum phosphorus level 1.6-2.2 mg/dL (0.51-0.72 mmol/L)

High dose: 1 mmol/kg over 8-12 hours; use if serum phosphorus <1.5 mg/dL (<0.5 mmol/L)

Alternative method in critically ill patients (Kingston, 1985):

Low dose: 0.25 mmol/kg over 4 hours; use if serum phosphorus level 0.5-1 mg/dL (0.16-0.32 mmol/L)

Moderate dose: 0.5 mmol/kg over 4 hours; use if serum phosphorus level <0.5 mg/dL (<0.16 mmol/L)

Parenteral nutrition, maintenance requirement (Mirtallo, 2004): IV:

Infants and Children ≤50 kg: 0.5-2 mmol/kg/day

Children >50 kg and Adolescents: 10-40 mmol/day

Adults: IV:

Hypophosphatemia, acute treatment: Repletion of severe hypophosphatemia should be done IV because large doses of oral phosphate may cause diarrhea and intestinal absorption may be unreliable. Reserve intermittent IV infusion for severe depletion situations; may require continuous cardiac monitoring depending on potassium administration rate. If potassium >4.0 mEq/L consider phosphate replacement strategy without potassium (eg, sodium phosphates). Guidelines differ based on degree of illness, need/use of parenteral nutrition, and severity of hypophosphatemia. Patients with severe renal impairment were excluded from phosphate supplement trials. **Note:** 1 mmol phosphate = 31 mg phosphorus; 1 mg phosphorus = 0.032 mmol phosphate

General replacement guidelines (Lentz, 1978):

Low dose, if serum phosphate losses are recent and uncomplicated: 0.08 mmol/kg over 6 hours

Intermediate dose, if serum phosphorus level 0.5-1 mg/dL (0.16-0.32 mmol/L): 0.16-0.24 mmol/kg over 4-6 hours

Note: The initial dose may be increased by 25% to 50% if the patient is symptomatic secondary to hypophosphatemia and lowered by 25% to 50% if the patient is hypercalcemic.

Critically ill adult patients receiving concurrent enteral/parenteral nutrition (Brown, 2006; Clark, 2006): **Note:** Round doses to the nearest 7.5 mmol for ease of preparation. If administering with phosphate-containing parenteral nutrition, do not exceed 15 mmol/L within parenteral nutrition.

Low dose, serum phosphorus level 2.3-3 mg/dL (0.74-0.96 mmol/L): 0.16-0.32 mmol/kg over 4-6 hours

Intermediate dose, serum phosphorus level 1.6-2.2 mg/dL (0.51-0.71 mmol/L): 0.32-0.64 mmol/kg over 4-6 hours

High dose, serum phosphorus <1.5 mg/dL (<0.5 mmol/L): 0.64-1 mmol/kg over 8-12 hours

Obesity: May use adjusted body weight for patients weighing >130% of ideal body weight (and BMI<40 kg/m^2) by using [IBW + 0.25 (ABW-IBW)].

Parenteral nutrition: IV: 10-15 mmol/1000 kcal (Hicks, 2001) **or** 20-40 mmol/24 hours (Mirtallo, 2004)

Preparation for Administration

Parenteral: Observe the vial for the presence of translucent visible particles. Do not use vial if particles are present. Injection must be diluted in appropriate IV solution and volume prior to administration. **Note:** Due to the potential presence of particulates, American Regent, Inc recommends the use of a 5 micron filter when preparing IV potassium phosphate-containing solutions (Important Drug Administration Information, American Regent 2011); a similar recommendation has not been noted by other manufacturers.

Intermittent IV infusion: In general, the dose, concentration of infusion, and rate of administration may be dependent on patient condition and specific institution policy. Intermittent infusion doses of potassium phosphate for adults are typically prepared in 100 to 250 mL of NS or D_5W (usual phosphate concentration range: 0.15 to 0.6 mmol/mL) (Charron 2003; Rosen 1995).

Pediatric suggested maximum concentrations used by some centers (with consideration for maximum potassium concentration):

Central line administration: 12 mmoL potassium phosphate/100 mL (~18 mEq potassium/100 mL)

Peripheral line administration: 5 mmol potassium phosphate/100 mL (~7.5 mEq potassium /100 mL)

Adult suggested maximum concentrations:

Central line administration: 26.8 mmoL potassium phosphate/100 mL (40 mEq potassium/100 mL)

Peripheral line administration: 6.7 mmoL potassium phosphate/100 mL (10 mEq potassium/100 mL)

Administration

Parenteral: **Note:** In general, the dose, concentration of infusion, and rate of administration may be dependent on patient condition and specific institution policy. Must consider administration precautions for both phosphate and potassium when prescribing. Due to the potential presence of translucent visible particles, American Regent, Inc recommends the use of a 0.22-micron in-line filter for IV administration (1.2-micron filter if admixture contains lipids) (Important Drug Administration Information, American Regent 2011); a similar recommendation has not been noted by other manufacturers.

Intermittent IV infusion: Must be diluted prior to administration and infused slowly to avoid potassium and/or phosphate toxicity; in pediatric patients, suggested maximum concentrations used by some centers: Peripheral line: 0.05 mmol/mL; Central line: 0.12 mmol/mL (maximum concentrations were determined with consideration for maximum potassium concentrations). Infusion of dose over 4 to 6 hours for mild/moderate hypophosphatemia or 8 to 12 hours for severe hypophosphatemia has been recommended (Brown 2006; Clark 1995; Lentz 1978); for adult patients with severe symptomatic hypophosphatemia (ie, <1.5 mg/dL), may administer at rates up to 15 mmol phosphate/hour (this rate will deliver potassium at 22.5 mEq/hour) (Charron, 2003; Rosen, 1995). Verify infusion time does not exceed acceptable potassium infusion rates: Usual pediatric infusion rates for potassium (including all sources): 0.3 to 0.5 mEq/kg/hour; maximum rate: 1 mEq/kg/hour up to 40 mEq/hour; ECG monitoring is recommended for potassium infusions >0.5 mEq/kg/hour in pediatric patients or >10 mEq/hour in adults. Do not infuse with calcium-containing IV fluids.

Parenteral nutrition solution: Calcium-phosphate stability in parenteral nutrition solutions is dependent upon the pH of the solution, temperature, and relative concentration of each ion. The pH of the solution is primarily dependent upon the amino acid concentration. The higher the percentage amino acids the lower the pH, the more soluble the calcium and phosphate. Individual commercially available amino acid solutions vary significantly with respect to pH lowering potential and subsequent calcium phosphate compatibility; consult product specific labeling for additional information.

Vesicant/Extravasation Risk Vesicant/irritant (may depend on concentration)

Monitoring Parameters Serum potassium, calcium, and phosphorus concentrations; renal function; in pediatric patients after IV phosphate repletion, repeat serum phosphorus concentration should be checked 2 hours later (ASPEN Pediatric Nutrition Support Core Curriculum, 2010; cardiac monitor (if intermittent infusion or potassium infusion rates >0.5 mEq/kg/hour in children or >10 mEq/hour in adults)

Reference Range Note: There is a diurnal variation with the nadir at 1100, plateau at 1600, and peak in the early evening (Gaasbeek, 2005); 1 mmol/L phosphate = 3.1 mg/dL phosphorus

Newborn 0-5 days: 4.8-8.2 mg/dL

1-3 years: 3.8-6.5 mg/dL

4-11 years: 3.7-5.6 mg/dL

12-15 years: 2.9-5.4 mg/dL

16-19 years: 2.7-4.7 mg/dL

Additional Information Cow's milk is a good source of phosphate with 1 mg elemental (0.032 mmol) elemental phosphate per mL.

Dosage Forms Considerations

Potassium 4.4 mEq is equivalent to potassium 170 mg

Phosphorous 3 mmol is equivalent to phosphorus 93 mg

Dosage Forms Excipient information presented when available (limited, particularly for generics); consult specific product labeling.

Injection, solution: Potassium 4.4 mEq and phosphorus 3 mmol per mL (5 mL, 15 mL, 50 mL) [equivalent to potassium 170 mg and elemental phosphorus 93 mg per mL]

Potassium Phosphate and Sodium Phosphate

(poe TASS ee um FOS fate & SOW dee um FOS fate)

Medication Safety Issues

Sound-alike/look-alike issues:

K-Phos Neutral may be confused with Neutra-Phos-K [DSC]

Brand Names: US K-Phos Neutral; K-Phos No. 2; Phos-NaK; Phospha 250 Neutral; Virt-Phos 250 Neutral

Therapeutic Category Electrolyte Supplement, Oral; Phosphate Salt; Potassium Salt; Sodium Salt

Generic Availability (US) Yes

Use Treatment and prevention of hypophosphatemia (FDA approved in ages ≥4 years and adults); urinary acidification (FDA approved in adults)

Pregnancy Risk Factor C

Pregnancy Considerations Animal reproduction studies have not been conducted.

Breast-Feeding Considerations It is not known if the combination product is excreted in breast milk. The manufacturer recommends that caution be exercised when administering potassium phosphate and sodium phosphate to nursing women. Refer to individual agents.

Contraindications Hyperphosphatemia, infected phosphate stones, patients with severely impaired renal function

Warnings/Precautions Use with caution in patients with severe adrenal insufficiency (eg, Addison disease), peripheral or pulmonary edema, renal impairment or chronic renal disease (contraindicated in severe renal impairment), cardiac disease (including heart failure [especially patients receiving digoxin] and hypertension), myotonia congenita, hypoparathyroidism, rickets (may increase the risk of extraskeletal calcification), acute dehydration, acute pancreatitis, extensive tissue breakdown (eg, severe burns), pregnant patients with preeclampsia, cirrhosis or severe hepatic impairment, and hypernatremia. Patients with renal calculi may pass preformed stones when phosphate therapy is initiated. Close monitoring of serum potassium concentrations is needed to avoid hyperkalemia; severe hyperkalemia may lead to muscle weakness/paralysis and cardiac conduction abnormalities (eg, heart block, ventricular arrhythmias, asystole). Use with caution in patients receiving concomitant medications or therapies that increase potassium (eg, ACEI, potassium-sparing diuretics, potassium-containing salt substitutes).

Adverse Reactions

Cardiovascular: Bradycardia, cardiac arrhythmia, chest pain, edema, lower extremity edema, tachycardia

Central nervous system: Confusion, dizziness, fatigue, headache, paresthesia, seizure, tetany (with large doses of phosphate)

Endocrine & metabolic: Alkalosis, hyperkalemia, weight gain

Gastrointestinal: Diarrhea, flatulence, nausea, sore throat, stomach pain, vomiting

Genitourinary: Decreased urine output

Neuromuscular & skeletal: Arthralgia, limb pain, muscle cramps, ostealgia, paralysis, weakness

Renal: Acute renal failure

Respiratory: Dyspnea

Miscellaneous: Increased thirst

Drug Interactions

Metabolism/Transport Effects None known.

Avoid Concomitant Use There are no known interactions where it is recommended to avoid concomitant use

Increased Effect/Toxicity

Potassium Phosphate and Sodium Phosphate may increase the levels/effects of: ACE Inhibitors; Aliskiren

Angiotensin II Receptor Blockers; Potassium-Sparing Diuretics

The levels/effects of Potassium Phosphate and Sodium Phosphate may be increased by: Eplerenone; Heparin; Heparin (Low Molecular Weight); Nicorandil

Decreased Effect

The levels/effects of Potassium Phosphate and Sodium Phosphate may be decreased by: Antacids; Calcium Salts; Iron Salts; Magnesium Salts; Multivitamins/Minerals (with ADEK, Folate, Iron); Sucralfate

Storage/Stability Tablets: Store at 20°C to 25°C (68°F to 77°F).

Pharmacodynamics Onset of action (catharsis): Oral: 3-6 hours

Pharmacokinetics (Adult data unless noted)

Absorption: Oral: 1% to 20%

Elimination: Oral forms excreted in feces

Dosing: Neonatal Note: Consider the contribution of potassium when determining the appropriate phosphate replacement. **Phosphorus Estimated Average Requirement (EAR)**: Oral: 3.2 mmol/day (adequate intake)

Dosing: Usual Note: Consider the contribution of sodium and potassium cations when determining appropriate phosphate replacement.

Phosphorus-Recommended Daily Allowance (RDA) and Estimated Average Requirement (EAR):

1-6 months:
- EAR: 3.2 mmol/day (adequate intake)

7-12 months:
- EAR: 8.9 mmol/day (adequate intake)

1-3 years:
- RDA: 14.8 mmol/day
- EAR: 12.3 mmol/day

4-8 years:
- RDA: 16.1 mmol/day
- EAR: 13.1 mmol/day

9-18 years:
- RDA: 40.3 mmol/day
- EAR: 34 mmol/day

19-30 years:
- RDA: 22.6 mmol/day
- EAR: 18.7 mmol/day

Maintenance: Oral:

Children: 2-3 mmol/kg/day in divided doses

Adults: 50-150 mmol/day in divided doses

Supplementation:

K-Phos® Neutral, Phospha 250™ Neutral:
- Children >4 years and Adolescents: 1 tablet 4 times/day
- Adults: 1-2 tablets 4 times/day

Phos-NaK:
- Children 4-8 years: 1 packet 2 times/day
- Children ≥9 years, Adolescents, and Adults: 1 packet 4 times/day

Urinary acidification: Oral: **Note:** Packets are **not** an appropriate substitution for this indication due to the higher potassium content.

Adults: K-Phos® No. 2: 1 tablet 4 times/day; may administer 1 tablet every 2 hours (maximum: 8 tablets/24 hours) when urine is difficult to acidify

Preparation for Administration Oral powder: Phos-NaK: Contents of 1 packet should be diluted in 75 mL water or juice; stir well and use promptly.

Administration

Oral:

Tablets: Administer with a full glass of water; administration with food may reduce the risk of diarrhea

Oral powder: Phos-NaK: Must be diluted in water or juice prior to administration; following dilution solution may be chilled to increase palatability

Monitoring Parameters Serum potassium, sodium, calcium, phosphorus, renal function, reflexes

Reference Range Note: There is a diurnal variation with the nadir at 1100, plateau at 1600, and peak in the early evening (Gaasbeek, 2005); 1 mmol/L phosphate = 3.1 mg/dL phosphorus

Newborns: 4.2-9 mg/dL phosphorus (1.36-2.91 mmol/L phosphate)

6 weeks to 18 months: 3.8-6.7 mg/dL phosphorus (1.23-2.16 mmol/L phosphate)

18 months to 3 years: 2.9-5.9 mg/dL phosphorus (0.94-1.91 mmol/L phosphate)

3-15 years: 3.6-5.6 mg/dL phosphorus (1.16-1.81 mmol/L phosphate)

>15 years: 2.5-5 mg/dL phosphorus (0.81-1.62 mmol/L phosphate)

Hypophosphatemia:
- Moderate: 1-2 mg/dL phosphorus (0.32-0.65 mmol/L phosphate)
- Severe: <1 mg/dL phosphorus (<0.32 mmol/L phosphate)

Additional Information Each mmol of phosphate contains 31 mg elemental phosphorus; 1 mmol/L phosphate = 3.1 mg/dL phosphorus; cow's milk is a good source of phosphate with 1 mg elemental (0.032 mmol) phosphate per mL

Dosage Forms Excipient information presented when available (limited, particularly for generics); consult specific product labeling.

Powder for solution, oral:

Phos-NaK: Dibasic potassium phosphate, monobasic potassium phosphate, dibasic sodium phosphate, and monobasic sodium phosphate per packet (100s) [sugar free; equivalent to elemental phosphorus 250 mg (8 mmol), sodium 160 mg (6.9 mEq), and potassium 280 mg (7.1 mEq) per packet; fruit flavor]

Tablet, oral:

K-Phos Neutral: Monobasic potassium phosphate 155 mg, dibasic sodium phosphate 852 mg, and monobasic sodium phosphate 130 mg [equivalent to elemental phosphorus 250 mg (8 mmol), sodium 298 mg (13 mEq), and potassium 45 mg (1.1 mEq)]

K-Phos No. 2: Potassium acid phosphate 305 mg and sodium acid phosphate 700 mg [equivalent to elemental phosphorus 250 mg (8 mmol), sodium 134 mg (5.8 mEq), and potassium 88 mg (2.3 mEq)]

Phospha 250 Neutral: Monobasic potassium phosphate 155 mg, dibasic sodium phosphate 852 mg, and monobasic sodium phosphate 130 mg [equivalent to elemental phosphorus 250 mg (8 mmol), sodium 298 mg (13 mEq), and potassium 45 mg (1.1 mEq)]

Virt-Phos 250 Neutral: Monobasic potassium phosphate 155 mg, dibasic sodium phosphate 852 mg, and monobasic sodium phosphate 130 mg [equivalent to elemental phosphorus 250 mg (8 mmol), sodium 298 mg (13 mEq), and potassium 45 mg (1.1 mEq)]

◆ **PPL** *see* Benzylpenicilloyl Polylysine *on page* 274

◆ **PPSV** *see* Pneumococcal Polysaccharide Vaccine (23-Valent) *on page* 1718

◆ **PPSV23** *see* Pneumococcal Polysaccharide Vaccine (23-Valent) *on page* 1718

◆ **PPV23** *see* Pneumococcal Polysaccharide Vaccine (23-Valent) *on page* 1718

Pralidoxime (pra li DOKS eem)

Medication Safety Issues

Sound-alike/look-alike issues:

Pralidoxime may be confused with pramoxine, pyridoxine

Protopam® may be confused with protamine

Brand Names: US Protopam Chloride

Therapeutic Category Antidote, Anticholinesterase; Antidote, Organophosphate Poisoning

Generic Availability (US) May be product dependent

Use Treatment of muscle weakness and/or respiratory depression secondary to poisoning due to organophosphate anticholinesterase pesticides and chemicals (eg, nerve agents) [FDA approved in pediatric patients (age not specified) and adults]; control of overdose of anticholinesterase medications used to treat myasthenia gravis (ambenonium, neostigmine, pyridostigmine) [FDA approved in pediatric patients (age not specified) and adults]

Pregnancy Risk Factor C

Pregnancy Considerations Animal reproduction studies have not been conducted. A case report did not show evidence of adverse events after pralidoxime administration during the second trimester (Kamha, 2005). In general, medications used as antidotes should take into consideration the health and prognosis of the mother; antidotes should be administered to pregnant women if there is a clear indication for use and should not be withheld because of fears of teratogenicity (Bailey, 2003).

Breast-Feeding Considerations It is not known if pralidoxime is excreted in breast milk. The manufacturer recommends that caution be exercised when administering pralidoxime to nursing women.

Contraindications There are no absolute contraindications listed within the manufacturer's labeling. **Note:** According to the manufacturer, relative contraindications include hypersensitivity to pralidoxime or any component of the formulation and other situations where the risk of administration clearly outweighs possible benefit.

Warnings/Precautions Pralidoxime is not indicated for the treatment of poisoning due to phosphorus, inorganic phosphates, organophosphates without anticholinesterase activity, or carbamate pesticides (acetylcholinesterase is weakly, but not permanently, affected by carbamates). Use with caution in patients with myasthenia gravis (may precipitate a myasthenic crisis); dosage modification required in patients with impaired renal function. Clinical symptoms that are consistent with suspected organophosphate poisoning (eg, organophosphate anticholinesterase pesticides and nerve agents) should be treated with the antidote immediately; administration should not be delayed for confirmatory laboratory tests. Treatment should include proper evacuation and decontamination procedures as indicated; medical personnel should protect themselves from inadvertent contamination. Antidote administration is intended only for initial management; definitive and more intensive medical care is required following administration. Individuals should not rely solely on antidote for treatment; the concomitant use of atropine will be necessary and other supportive measures (eg, artificial respiration) may still be required.

Warnings: Additional Pediatric Considerations Rapid IV infusion may be associated with temporary worsening of cholinergic manifestations (eg, tachycardia, laryngospasm, muscle rigidity, cardiac arrest) in adults; in children, muscle fasciculations, apnea, and convulsions have also been reported.

Adverse Reactions

Cardiovascular: Cardiac arrest, hypertension, tachycardia

Central nervous system: Dizziness, drowsiness, headache, paralysis, seizure

Dermatologic: Skin rash

Gastrointestinal: Nausea

Hepatic: Increased serum ALT (transient), increased serum AST (transient)

Local: Pain at injection site (IM)

Neuromuscular & skeletal: Fasciculations, increased creatine phosphokinase, laryngospasm, muscle rigidity, weakness

Ophthalmic: Accommodation disturbance, blurred vision, diplopia

Renal: Renal insufficiency

Respiratory: Apnea, hyperventilation

Drug Interactions

Metabolism/Transport Effects None known.

Avoid Concomitant Use There are no known interactions where it is recommended to avoid concomitant use.

Increased Effect/Toxicity There are no known significant interactions involving an increase in effect.

Decreased Effect There are no known significant interactions involving a decrease in effect.

Storage/Stability Store at 20°C to 25°C (68°F to 77°F); excursions permitted to 15°C to 30°C (59°F to 86°F).

Mechanism of Action Reactivates cholinesterase that had been inactivated by phosphorylation due to exposure to organophosphate pesticides and cholinesterase-inhibiting nerve agents (eg, terrorism and chemical warfare agents such as sarin) by displacing the enzyme from its receptor sites; removes the phosphoryl group from the active site of the inactivated enzyme

Pharmacokinetics (Adult data unless noted)

Distribution: V_{dss}: 0.6-2.7 L/kg; severely poisoned pediatric patients (n=11; age: 0.8-18 years): ~9 L/kg (range: 1.7-13.8 L/kg) (Schexnayder, 1998); may increase with increasing severity of organophosphate intoxication

Protein binding: None

Metabolism: Hepatic

Half-life: Apparent: 74-77 minutes; pediatric patients (n=11; age: 0.8-18 years): 2.4-5 hours

Time to peak serum concentration: IM: 35 minutes

Elimination: Urine (~80% as metabolites and unchanged drug)

Dosing: Usual Note: Use in conjunction with atropine; atropine effects should be established before pralidoxime is administered.

Organophosphate poisoning: Note: IV administration is preferable; if IV route not feasible, may be given IM or SubQ

IV:

Infants, Children, and Adolescents ≤16 years: Loading dose: 20-50 mg/kg (maximum: 2000 mg/dose); Maintenance infusion: 10-20 mg/kg/**hour**; alternatively, a repeat bolus of 20-50 mg/kg (maximum: 2000 mg/dose) may be administered after 1 hour if muscle weakness is not relieved and repeated every 10-12 hours thereafter, as needed if muscle weakness persists

Adolescents >16 years and Adults: Loading dose 1000-2000 mg; Maintenance: Repeat bolus of 1000-2000 mg after 1 hour and repeated every 10-12 hours thereafter, as needed

IM:

Infants, Children, and Adolescents <40 kg:

Mild symptoms: 15 mg/kg/dose; repeat as needed for persistent mild symptoms every 15 minutes to a maximum total dose of 45 mg/kg; may administer doses in rapid succession if severe symptoms develop

Severe symptoms: 15 mg/kg/dose; repeat twice in rapid succession to deliver a total dose of 45 mg/kg

Persistent symptoms: May repeat the entire series (45 mg/kg in 3 divided doses) beginning ~1 hour after administration of the last injection

Children and Adolescents ≥40 kg and Adults:

Mild symptoms: 600 mg; repeat as needed for persistent mild symptoms every 15 minutes to a maximum total dose of 1800 mg; may administer doses in rapid succession if severe symptoms develop

Severe symptoms: 600 mg; repeat twice in rapid succession to deliver a total dose of 1800 mg

Persistent symptoms: May repeat the entire series (1800 mg in 3 divided doses) beginning ~1 hour after administration of the last injection

Anticholinesterase poisoning (eg, neostigmine, pyridostigmine): Adults: IV: 1000-2000 mg; followed by increments of 250 mg every 5 minutes as needed

Dosage adjustment in renal impairment: Pediatric patients (age not specified) and Adults: Dose should be reduced; no specific recommendations are provided by the manufacturer

Preparation for Administration Parenteral: Powder for solution:

IM: Reconstitute 1,000 mg vial with 3.3 mL SWFI to a final concentration of ~300 mg/mL; discard any unused portion of vial.

IV: Reconstitute 1,000 mg vial with 20 mL SWFI to make a concentration of 50 mg/mL; further dilute with NS to a final concentration range of 10 to 20 mg/mL. In fluid-restricted patients or situations where a more rapid administration is required, may use reconstituted solution (50 mg/mL) without further diution. Discard any unused portion of vial.

Administration Parenteral:

IM: Use a 300 mg/mL solution; either autoinjector or reconstituted powder for injection may be used; in infants and children, administer intramuscularly in the anterolateral aspect of the thigh

IV:

Loading dose: Infuse over 15 to 30 minutes; if maximally concentrated solution (50 mg/mL) may be administered over ≥5 minutes not to exceed 200 mg/minute

Maintenance dose (intermittent infusion): Infuse over 15 to 30 minutes a rate not to exceed 200 mg/minute

Monitoring Parameters Heart rate, respiratory rate, muscle fasciculations and strength, pulse oximetry, blood pressure and cardiac monitoring with IV administration

Additional Information Most effective when given as soon as possible after exposure, typically within 36 hours after termination of exposure to poison.

Dosage Forms Excipient information presented when available (limited, particularly for generics); consult specific product labeling.

Solution Auto-injector, Intramuscular, as chloride:
Generic: 600 mg/2 mL (2 mL)

Solution Reconstituted, Intravenous, as chloride:
Protopam Chloride: 1 g (1 ea)

◆ **Pralidoxime Chloride** *see* Pralidoxime *on page 1747*

◆ **Pravachol** *see* Pravastatin *on page 1749*

Pravastatin (prav a STAT in)

Medication Safety Issues

Sound-alike/look-alike issues:

Pravachol may be confused with atorvaSTATin, Prevacid, Prinivil, propranolol

Pravastatin may be confused with nystatin, pitavastatin, prasugrel

Brand Names: US Pravachol

Brand Names: Canada ACT Pravastatin; Apo-Pravastatin; Dom-Pravastatin; JAMP-Pravastatin; Mint-Pravastatin; Mylan-Pravastatin; PHL-Pravastatin; PMS-Pravastatin; Pravachol; RAN-Pravastatin; Riva-Pravastatin; Sandoz-Pravastatin; Teva-Pravastatin

Therapeutic Category Antilipemic Agent; HMG-CoA Reductase Inhibitor

Generic Availability (US) Yes

Use Adjunct to dietary therapy in patients with heterozygous familial hypercholesterolemia (HFH) hypercholesterolemia if LDL-C remains ≥190 mg/dL or if ≥160 mg/dL with family history of premature cardiovascular (CVD) or presence of ≥2 cardiovascular risk [FDA approved in children ≥8 years of age and adolescents]. Adjunct to dietary therapy to decrease elevated serum total and low density lipoprotein cholesterol (LDL-C), apolipoprotein B (apo-B), and triglyceride levels, and to increase high density lipoprotein cholesterol (HDL-C) in patients with primary hypercholesterolemia (heterozygous, familial, and nonfamilial) and mixed dyslipidemia (Fredrickson types IIa and IIb) (FDA approved in adults); adjunct to dietary therapy in patients with isolated hypertriglyceridemia (Fredrickson type IV) (FDA approved in adults); treatment of primary dysbetalipoproteinemia (Fredrickson Type III) who do not respond adequately to diet (FDA approved in adults); primary and secondary prevention of cardiovascular disease in high risk patients (FDA approved in adults)

Primary prevention of cardiovascular disease in high-risk patients (FDA approved in adults); risk factors include: Age ≥55 years, smoking, hypertension, low HDL-C, or family history of early coronary heart disease; secondary prevention of cardiovascular disease to reduce the risk of MI, stroke, revascularization procedures, and angina in patients with evidence of coronary heart disease.

Pregnancy Risk Factor X

Pregnancy Considerations Adverse events were observed in some animal reproduction studies. Pravastatin was found to cross the placenta in an *ex vivo* study using term human placentas (Nanovskaya, 2013). There are reports of congenital anomalies following maternal use of HMG-CoA reductase Inhibitors in pregnancy; however, maternal disease, differences in specific agents used, and the low rates of exposure limit the interpretation of the available data (Godfrey, 2012; Lecarpentier, 2012). Cholesterol biosynthesis may be important in fetal development; serum cholesterol and triglycerides increase normally during pregnancy. The discontinuation of lipid lowering medications temporarily during pregnancy is not expected to have significant impact on the long term outcomes of primary hypercholesterolemia treatment.

Use of pravastatin is contraindicated in pregnancy. HMG-CoA reductase Inhibitors should be discontinued prior to pregnancy (ADA, 2013). If treatment of dyslipidemias is needed in pregnant women or in women of reproductive age, other agents are preferred (Berglund, 2012; Stone, 2013). The manufacturer recommends administration to women of childbearing potential only when conception is highly unlikely and patients have been informed of potential hazards.

Breast-Feeding Considerations A small amount of pravastatin is excreted into breast milk. Data is available from eight lactating females administered pravastatin 20 mg twice daily for 2.5 days. After the fifth dose, maximum maternal serum concentrations were ~40 ng/mL (pravastatin) and ~26 ng/mL (metabolite) and maximum milk concentrations were ~3.9 ng/mL (pravastatin) and ~2.1 ng/mL (metabolite). Maximum milk concentrations were detected ~3 hours after the dose (Pan, 1988). Due to the potential for serious adverse reactions in a nursing infant, use while breast-feeding is contraindicated by the manufacturer.

Contraindications Hypersensitivity to pravastatin or any component of the formulation; active liver disease; unexplained persistent elevations of serum transaminases; pregnancy; breast-feeding

Warnings/Precautions Secondary causes of hyperlipidemia should be ruled out prior to therapy. Liver function must be monitored by periodic laboratory assessment. Rhabdomyolysis with acute renal failure has occurred. Risk may be increased with concurrent use of other drugs which may cause rhabdomyolysis (including colchicine, gemfibrozil, fibric acid derivatives, or niacin at doses ≥1 g/day). Discontinue in any patient in which CPK levels are markedly elevated (>10 times ULN) or if myopathy is suspected/diagnosed. Immune-mediated necrotizing myopathy (IMNM), an autoimmune-mediated myopathy, has been reported (rarely) with HMG-CoA reductase inhibitor therapy. IMNM presents as proximal muscle weakness with elevated CPK levels, which persists despite discontinuation of HMG-CoA reductase inhibitor therapy; additionally, muscle biopsy may show necrotizing myopathy with limited inflammation; immunosuppressive therapy (eg, corticosteroids, azathioprine) may be used for treatment. The manufacturer recommends temporary discontinuation for elective major surgery, acute medical or surgical conditions, or in any patient experiencing an acute or serious condition predisposing to renal failure (eg, sepsis, hypotension, trauma, uncontrolled seizures). Based on current research and clinical guidelines (Fleisher, 2009), HMG-CoA reductase inhibitors should be continued in the perioperative period. Postoperative discontinuation of statin therapy is associated with an increased risk of cardiac morbidity and mortality. Use with caution in patients with advanced age, these patients are predisposed to myopathy. Use caution in patients with previous liver disease or heavy ethanol use. If serious hepatotoxicity with clinical symptoms and/or hyperbilirubinemia or jaundice occurs during treatment, interrupt therapy. If an alternate etiology is not identified, do not restart pravastatin. Liver enzyme tests should be obtained at baseline and as clinically indicated; routine periodic monitoring of liver enzymes is not necessary. Increases in HbA_{1c} and fasting blood glucose have been reported with HMG-CoA reductase inhibitors; however, the benefits of statin therapy far outweigh the risk of dysglycemia. Treatment in patients <8 years of age is not recommended.

Adverse Reactions

Cardiovascular: Chest pain

Central nervous system: Dizziness, fatigue, headache

Dermatologic: Rash

Gastrointestinal: Diarrhea, heartburn, nausea, vomiting

Hepatic: Transaminases increased

Neuromuscular & skeletal: Myalgia

Respiratory: Cough

Miscellaneous: Influenza

Rare but important or life-threatening: Allergy, amnesia (reversible), anaphylaxis, angioedema, cholestatic jaundice, cirrhosis, cognitive impairment (reversible), confusion (reversible), cranial nerve dysfunction, dermatomyositis, erythema multiforme, ESR increase, fulminant hepatic necrosis, gynecomastia, hemolytic anemia, hepatitis, hepatoma, lens opacity, libido change, lupus erythematosus-like syndrome, memory disturbance (reversible), memory impairment (reversible), muscle weakness, myopathy, neuropathy, pancreatitis, paresthesia, peripheral nerve palsy, polymyalgia rheumatica, positive ANA, purpura, rhabdomyolysis, Stevens-Johnson syndrome, taste disturbance, tremor, vasculitis, vertigo

Additional class-related events or case reports (not necessarily reported with pravastatin therapy): Angioedema, blood glucose increased, cataracts, depression, diabetes mellitus (new onset), dyspnea, eosinophilia, erectile dysfunction, facial paresis, glycosylated hemoglobin ($Hb\ A_{1c}$) increased, hypersensitivity reaction, immune-mediated necrotizing myopathy (IMNM), impaired extraocular muscle movement, impotence, interstitial lung disease, leukopenia, malaise, memory loss, ophthalmoplegia, paresthesia, peripheral neuropathy, photosensitivity, psychic disturbance, skin discoloration, thrombocytopenia, thyroid dysfunction, toxic epidermal necrolysis, transaminases increased, vomiting

Drug Interactions

Metabolism/Transport Effects **Substrate** of CYP3A4 (minor), P-glycoprotein, SLCO1B1; **Note:** Assignment of Major/Minor substrate status based on clinically relevant drug interaction potential; **Inhibits** CYP2C9 (weak), CYP2D6 (weak)

Avoid Concomitant Use

Avoid concomitant use of Pravastatin with any of the following: Fusidic Acid (Systemic); Gemfibrozil; Red Yeast Rice

Increased Effect/Toxicity

Pravastatin may increase the levels/effects of: ARIPiprazole; CycloSPORINE (Systemic); DAPTOmycin; PARoxetine; PAZOPanib; Trabectedin; Vitamin K Antagonists

The levels/effects of Pravastatin may be increased by: Acipimox; Bezafibrate; Boceprevir; Ciprofibrate; Clarithromycin; Colchicine; CycloSPORINE (Systemic); Darunavir; Eltrombopag; Erythromycin (Systemic); Fenofibrate and Derivatives; Fusidic Acid (Systemic); Gemfibrozil; Itraconazole; Niacin; Niacinamide; Paritaprevir; Raltegravir; Red Yeast Rice; Simeprevir; Telaprevir; Telithromycin; Teriflunomide

Decreased Effect

Pravastatin may decrease the levels/effects of: Lanthanum

The levels/effects of Pravastatin may be decreased by: Antacids; Bile Acid Sequestrants; Efavirenz; Fosphenytoin; Nelfinavir; Phenytoin; Rifamycin Derivatives; Saquinavir

Storage/Stability Store at 25°C (77°F); excursions permitted to 15°C to 30°C (59°F to 86°F). Protect from moisture and light.

Mechanism of Action Pravastatin is a competitive inhibitor of 3-hydroxy-3-methylglutaryl coenzyme A (HMG-CoA) reductase, which is the rate-limiting enzyme involved in *de novo* cholesterol synthesis. In addition to the ability of HMG-CoA reductase inhibitors to decrease levels of high-sensitivity C-reactive protein (hsCRP), they also possess pleiotropic properties including improved endothelial function, reduced inflammation at the site of the coronary plaque, inhibition of platelet aggregation, and anticoagulant effects (de Denus, 2002; Ray, 2005).

Pharmacodynamics

Onset of action: 2 weeks

Maximum effect: After 4 weeks

LDL-reduction: 40 mg/day: 34% (for each doubling of this dose, LDL-C is lowered by ~6%)

Pharmacokinetics (Adult data unless noted)

Absorption: Oral: 34%; Rapidly absorbed

Distribution: V_d: 0.46 L/kg

Protein binding: 50%

Metabolism: Hepatic to multiple metabolites; primary metabolite is 3α-hydroxy-iso-pravastatin (2.5% to 10% activity of parent drug); extensive first-pass metabolism

Bioavailability: Absolute: 17%

Half-life:

Children and Adolescents (4.9-15.6 years): 1.6 hours range: 0.85-4.2 hours (Hedman, 2003)

Adults: 77 hours (including all metabolites); pravastatin: 2.3 hours; 3α-hydroxy-iso-pravastatin: ~1.5 hours (Gustavson, 2005)

Time to peak serum concentration: 1-1.5 hours

Elimination: ~20% excreted in urine unchanged and 70% in feces

Dosing: Usual Dosage should be individualized according to the baseline LDL-C level, the recommended goal of therapy, and patient response; adjustments should be made at intervals of 4 weeks

Children and Adolescents: Oral: **Hyperlipidemia or heterozygous familial and nonfamilial hypercholesterolemia: Note:** Begin treatment if after adequate trial of diet the following are present: LDL-C ≥190 mg/dL or LDL-C remains ≥160 mg/dL and positive family history of premature cardiovascular disease or meets NCEP classification. (NHLBI 2011). Therapy may be considered for children 8-9 years of age meeting the above criteria or for children with diabetes mellitus and LDL-C ≥130 mg/dL (Daniels, 2008).

Children and Adolescents 8-13 years: 20 mg once daily; doses >20 mg have not been studied

Adolescents 14-18 years: 40 mg once daily; doses >40 mg have not been studied

Adults: **Hyperlipidemias, primary prevention of coronary events, secondary prevention of cardiovascular events:** Oral: Initial: 40 mg once daily; titrate dosage to response (usual range: 10-80 mg) (maximum daily dose: 80 mg/**day**)

Dosing adjustment in renal impairment: Adults: Significant impairment: Initiate dosage at 10 mg once daily

Dosing adjustment in hepatic impairment: There are no dosage adjustments provided in the manufacturer labeling; contraindicated in active liver disease or in patients with unexplained persistent elevations of serum transaminases.

Dosing adjustment for pravastatin with concomitant medications: Adults:

Clarithromycin: Maximum daily dose: 40 mg/**day**

Cyclosporine: Initial: 10 mg pravastatin daily at bedtime; titrate with caution (maximum daily dose: 20 mg/**day**)

Administration Oral: May be taken without regard to meals or time of day. Give at least 1 hour before or 4 hours after bile acid resins.

Monitoring Parameters

Pediatric patients: Baseline: ALT, AST, and creatine phosphokinase levels (CPK); fasting lipid panel (FLP) and repeat ALT and AST should be checked after 4 weeks of therapy; if no myopathy symptoms or laboratory abnormalities, then monitor FLP, ALT, and AST every 3 to 4 months during the first year and then every 6 months thereafter (NHLBI, 2011).

Adults:

2013 ACC/AHA Blood Cholesterol Guideline recommendations (Stone, 2013):

Lipid panel (total cholesterol, HDL, LDL, triglycerides): Baseline lipid panel; fasting lipid profile within 4 to 12 weeks after initiation or dose adjustment and every 3 to 12 months (as clinically indicated) thereafter. If 2 consecutive LDL levels are <40 mg/dL, consider decreasing the dose.

Hepatic transaminase levels: Baseline measurement of hepatic transaminase levels (ie, ALT); measure hepatic function if symptoms suggest hepatotoxicity (eg, unusual fatigue or weakness, loss of appetite, abdominal pain, dark-colored urine or yellowing of skin or sclera) during therapy.

CPK: CPK should not be routinely measured. Baseline CPK measurement is reasonable for some individuals (eg, family history of statin intolerance or muscle disease, clinical presentation, concomitant drug therapy that may increase risk of myopathy). May measure CPK in any patient with symptoms suggestive of myopathy (pain, tenderness, stiffness, cramping, weakness, or generalized fatigue).

Evaluate for new-onset diabetes mellitus during therapy; if diabetes develops, continue statin therapy and encourage adherence to a heart-healthy diet, physical activity, a healthy body weight, and tobacco cessation.

If patient develops a confusional state or memory impairment, may evaluate patient for nonstatin causes (eg, exposure to other drugs), systemic and neuropsychiatric causes, and the possibility of adverse effects associated with statin therapy.

Manufacturer recommendations: Liver enzyme tests at baseline and repeated when clinically indicated. **Upon initiation or titration, lipid panel should be analyzed at intervals of 4 weeks or more.**

Dosage Forms Excipient information presented when available (limited, particularly for generics); consult specific product labeling.

Tablet, Oral, as sodium:

Pravachol: 20 mg, 40 mg, 80 mg

Generic: 10 mg, 20 mg, 40 mg, 80 mg

◆ **Pravastatin Sodium** *see* Pravastatin *on page 1749*

◆ **Praxis ASA EC 81 Mg Daily Dose (Can)** *see* Aspirin *on page 206*

Praziquantel (pray zi KWON tel)

Related Information

Oral Medications That Should Not Be Crushed or Altered *on page 2476*

Brand Names: US Biltricide

Brand Names: Canada Biltricide

Therapeutic Category Anthelmintic

Generic Availability (US) No

Use Treatment of all stages of schistosomiasis caused by *Schistosoma* species pathogenic to humans; treatment of clonorchiasis, opisthorchiasis (FDA approved in ages ≥4 years and adults); has also been used in the treatment of cysticercosis and many intestinal tapeworm and trematode infections

Pregnancy Risk Factor B

Pregnancy Considerations Adverse effects have not been observed in animal reproduction studies. Use in pregnant women only if clearly needed.

Breast-Feeding Considerations Appears in breast milk at a concentration of ¼ that of maternal serum. Women should be advised to not breast-feed on the day of treatment and for 72 hours after treatment.

Contraindications Hypersensitivity to praziquantel or any component of the formulation; ocular cysticercosis; concomitant administration with strong cytochrome P450 (CYP450) inducers, such as rifampin

Warnings/Precautions Use caution in patients with cardiac abnormalities or patients with moderate-to-severe hepatic disease; reduced liver drug metabolism may result in higher and longer lasting plasma concentrations of unmetabolized praziquantel. It is recommended to hospitalize patients with cerebral cysticercosis for the duration of treatment. Use not recommended in patients with a history of seizures or signs of central nervous system involvement (eg, subcutaneous nodules suggestive of cysticercosis); may exacerbate condition. Praziquantel may not be effective against migrating shistosomulae; observational data indicate that praziquantel treatment in the acute phase of the infection may not prevent progression from asymptomatic to acute shistosomiasis, or from asymptomatic/acute disease to chronic disease. In addition, use in patients with shistosomiasis may be associated with clinical deterioration such as paradoxical reactions or serum sickness Jarisch-Herxheimer like reactions, which is a sudden inflammatory immune response likely caused by the release of shistosomal antigens. Such reactions typically occur during the acute disease phase, and may lead to life-threatening events such as respiratory failure, encephalopathy, and/or cerebral vasculitis. Potentially significant drug-drug interactions may exist, requiring dose or frequency adjustment, additional monitoring, and/or selection of alternative therapy. Therapeutic levels of praziquantel may not be achieved with concurrent administration of strong inducers of cytochrome P450 (eg, rifampin); concurrent use is contraindicated. Patients should be instructed to not drive or operate machinery on the day of treatment and the day after treatment.

Adverse Reactions May be more serious in patients with a heavy worm burden.

Central nervous system: Dizziness, headache, malaise

Dermatologic: Urticaria

Gastrointestinal: Abdominal distress, nausea

Miscellaneous: Fever

Rare but important or life-threatening: Abdominal pain, anorexia, atrioventricular block, bloody diarrhea, bradycardia, cardiac arrhythmia, ectopic beats, eosinophilia, hypersensitivity, hypersensitivity reaction, myalgia, paradoxical reaction (in schistosomiasis), polyserositis, pruritus, seizure, serum sickness (in schistosomiasis; Jarisch-Herxheimer-like reaction), ventricular fibrillation,vomiting

Drug Interactions

Metabolism/Transport Effects **Substrate** of CYP3A4 (major); **Note:** Assignment of Major/Minor substrate status based on clinically relevant drug interaction potential; **Inhibits** CYP2D6 (weak)

Avoid Concomitant Use

Avoid concomitant use of Praziquantel with any of the following: Conivaptan; CYP3A4 Inducers (Strong); Fusidic Acid (Systemic); Idelalisib

Increased Effect/Toxicity

Praziquantel may increase the levels/effects of: ARIPiprazole

The levels/effects of Praziquantel may be increased by: Aprepitant; Cimetidine; Conivaptan; CYP3A4 Inhibitors (Moderate); CYP3A4 Inhibitors (Strong); Dasatinib; Fosaprepitant; Fusidic Acid (Systemic); Idelalisib; Ivacaftor; Ketoconazole (Systemic); Luliconazole; Mifepristone; Netupitant; Palbociclib; Simeprevir; Stiripentol

Decreased Effect

The levels/effects of Praziquantel may be decreased by: Aminoquinolines (Antimalarial); Bosentan; CYP3A4 Inducers (Moderate); CYP3A4 Inducers (Strong); Dabrafenib; Deferasirox; Siltuximab; St Johns Wort; Tocilizumab

Storage/Stability Store below 30°C (86°F).

Mechanism of Action Increases the cell permeability to calcium in schistosomes, causing strong contractions and paralysis of worm musculature leading to detachment of suckers from the blood vessel walls and to dislodgment

Pharmacokinetics (Adult data unless noted)

Absorption: Oral: ~80%

Distribution: CSF concentration is 14% to 20% of plasma concentration

Protein binding: ~80%

Metabolism: Extensive first-pass effect; metabolized by the liver to hydroxylated and conjugated metabolites

Half-life: 0.8-1.5 hours

Metabolites: 4.5 hours

Time to peak serum concentration: Within 1-3 hours

Elimination: Praziquantel and metabolites excreted mainly in urine 80% (>99% as metabolites)

Dosing: Usual Oral:

Children and Adolescents:

Flukes:

Clonorchiasis [*Clonorchis sinesis* (Chinese liver fluke)]; Opisthorchiasis [Opisthorchis viverrini (Southeast Asian liver fluke)]:

Manufacturer's labeling: Children ≥4 years and Adolescents: 25 mg/kg/dose 3 times daily (at 4- to 6-hour intervals) for 1 day

Alternative dosing (*Red Book*, 2009): 25 mg/kg/dose 3 times daily for 2 days

Fasciolopsis buski, Heterophyes heterophyes, Metagonimus yokogawi (intestinal flukes); *Metorchis conjunctus* (North American liver fluke): 25 mg/kg/dose 3 times daily for 1 day (*Red Book*, 2009)

Nanophyetus salmincola: 20 mg/kg/dose 3 times daily for 1 day (*Red Book*, 2009)

Paragonimus westermani (lung fluke): 25 mg/kg/dose 3 times daily for 2 days (*Red Book*, 2009)

Schistosomiasis:

Manufacturer's labeling: Children >4 years and Adolescents: 20 mg/kg/dose 3 times daily (at 4- to 6-hour intervals) for 1 day

Alternative dosing (*Red Book*, 2009): **Note:** Praziquantel does not kill developing worms; therapy started within 1-2 months of exposure should be repeated in 1-2 months.

S. mansoni, S. haematobium: 20 mg/kg/dose twice daily for 1 day

S. japonicum, S. mekongi: 20 mg/kg/dose 3 times daily for 1 day

Tapeworms (*Red Book*, 2009):

Cysticercosis [*Taenia solium* (pork tapeworm)]; tissue (larvae) stage: 33.3 mg/kg/dose 3 times daily for 1 day followed by 16.7 mg/kg/dose 3 times daily for 29 days; **Note:** May be used in conjunction with antiseizure medication and/or corticosteroids.

Diphyllobothrium latum (fish), *Taenia saginata* (beef), *Taenia solium* (pork), *Dipylidium caninum* (dog); intestinal (adult) stage: 5-10 mg/kg as a single dose

Hymenolepis nana (dwarf tapeworm): 25 mg/kg as a single dose

Adults:

Schistosomiasis: 20 mg/kg/dose 3 times daily (at 4- to 6-hour intervals) for 1 day

Clonorchiasis/opisthorchiasis: 25 mg/kg/dose 3 times daily (at 4- to 6-hour intervals) for 1 day

Dosage adjustment in renal impairment: No dosage adjustments are recommended

Dosage adjustments in hepatic impairment: Moderate to severe impairment (Child-Pugh classes B and C): Use caution; decreased metabolism may lead to higher and prolonged serum concentrations; there are no dosage adjustments provided in the manufacturer's labeling.

Administration Oral: Administer tablets with water during meals; tablets can be halved or quartered; do not chew tablets due to bitter taste

Dosage Forms Excipient information presented when available (limited, particularly for generics); consult specific product labeling.

Tablet, Oral:

Biltricide: 600 mg [scored]

Prazosin (PRAZ oh sin)

Medication Safety Issues

Sound-alike/look-alike issues:

Prazosin may be confused with predniSONE

BEERS Criteria medication:

This drug may be potentially inappropriate for use in geriatric patients (Quality of evidence - moderate; Strength of recommendation - strong).

Brand Names: US Minipress

Brand Names: Canada Apo-Prazo; Minipress; Teva-Prazosin

Therapeutic Category Alpha-Adrenergic Blocking Agent, Oral; Antihypertensive Agent; Vasodilator

Generic Availability (US) Yes

Use Treatment of hypertension alone or in combination with diuretics or beta-blockers (FDA approved in adults); has also been used in the management of the sympathetic stimulatory cardiovascular effects of scorpion envenomation usually due to non-*Centruroides* species stings (typically found outside North America)

Pregnancy Risk Factor C

Pregnancy Considerations Adverse events were observed in some animal reproduction studies. Prazosin crosses the placenta and its pharmacokinetics may be slightly altered during pregnancy (Bourget 1995; Rubin 1983). Limited use in pregnant women has not demonstrated any fetal abnormalities or adverse effects (Dommisse 1983).

Untreated chronic maternal hypertension is associated with adverse events in the fetus, infant, and mother. It treatment for hypertension during pregnancy is needed, other agents are generally preferred (ACOG 2013).

Breast-Feeding Considerations Small amounts of prazosin are excreted in breast milk. The manufacturer recommends that caution be exercised when administering prazosin to nursing women.

Contraindications Known sensitivity to quinazolines, prazosin, or any component of the formulation

Warnings/Precautions May cause significant orthostatic hypotension and syncope with sudden loss of consciousness, especially within 30 to 90 minutes of the first dose; anticipate a similar effect if therapy is interrupted for a few days, if dosage is rapidly increased, or if another antihypertensive drug (particularly vasodilators or a beta-blocker) or a phosphodiesterase 5 (PDE 5) inhibitor is introduced. Severe tachycardia (120 to 160 beats/minute) has occasionally been reported prior to a syncopal episode. Intraoperative floppy iris syndrome has been observed during cataract surgery in some patients treated with $alpha_1$-blockers; modification to surgical technique may be necessary. Patients should be cautioned about alcohol use and performing hazardous tasks when starting new therapy or adjusting dosage upward. Discontinue if symptoms of angina occur or worsen. Should rule out prostatic carcinoma before beginning therapy. In the elderly, avoid use as an antihypertensive due to high risk of orthostatic hypotension; alternative agents are preferred due to a more favorable risk/benefit profile (Beers Criteria). Priapism and prolonged erections have been reported; seek immediate medical assistance for erections lasting longer than 4 hours. May cause CNS depression, which may impair physical or mental abilities; patients must be cautioned about performing tasks that require mental alertness (eg, operating machinery or driving). Potentially significant drug-drug interactions may exist, requiring dose or frequency adjustment, additional monitoring, and/or selection of alternative therapy.

Adverse Reactions

Cardiovascular: Edema, orthostatic hypotension, palpitation, syncope

Central nervous system: Depression, dizziness, drowsiness, headache, nervousness, vertigo

Dermatologic: Rash

Endocrine & metabolic: Decreased energy

Gastrointestinal: Constipation, diarrhea, nausea, vomiting, xerostomia

Genitourinary: Urinary frequency

Neuromuscular & skeletal: Weakness

Ocular: Blurred vision, reddened sclera

Respiratory: Dyspnea, epistaxis, nasal congestion

Rare but important or life-threatening: Abdominal discomfort, allergic reaction, alopecia, angina, arthralgia, bradycardia, cataplexy, cataracts (both development and disappearance have been reported), diaphoresis, enuresis, eye pain, fever, flushing, gynecomastia, hallucinations, impotence, insomnia, leukopenia, lichen planus, liver function abnormalities, malaise, MI, narcolepsy (worsened), pain, pancreatitis, paresthesia, pigmentary mottling and serous retinopathy, positive ANA titer, priapism, pruritus, systemic lupus erythematosus, tachycardia, tinnitus, urticaria, vasculitis

Reported in association with other $alpha_1$-blockers: Intraoperative floppy iris syndrome (with cataract surgery)

Drug Interactions

Metabolism/Transport Effects None known.

Avoid Concomitant Use

Avoid concomitant use of Prazosin with any of the following: Alpha1-Blockers

Increased Effect/Toxicity

Prazosin may increase the levels/effects of: Alpha1-Blockers; Amifostine; Antihypertensives; Calcium Channel Blockers; DULoxetine; Hypotensive Agents; Levodopa; Obinutuzumab; RisperiDONE; RiTUXimab

The levels/effects of Prazosin may be increased by: Barbiturates; Beta-Blockers; Brimonidine (Topical); Dapoxetine; Diazoxide; Herbs (Hypotensive Properties); MAO Inhibitors; Nicorandil; Pentoxifylline; Phosphodiesterase 5 Inhibitors; Prostacyclin Analogues

Decreased Effect

Prazosin may decrease the levels/effects of: Alpha-/Beta-Agonists; Alpha1-Agonists

The levels/effects of Prazosin may be decreased by: Herbs (Hypertensive Properties); Methylphenidate; Yohimbine

Food Interactions Food has variable effects on absorption. Management: Administer without regard to food.

Storage/Stability

Store at 20°C to 25°C (68°F to 77°F). Protect from moisture and light.

Extended-release tablet [Canadian product]: Store between 15°C and 30°C (59°F and 86°F). Protect from moisture.

Mechanism of Action Competitively inhibits postsynaptic alpha-adrenergic receptors which results in vasodilation of veins and arterioles and a decrease in total peripheral resistance and blood pressure

Pharmacodynamics

Onset of action: Antihypertensive: Within 2 hours

Maximum effect: Antihypertensive: 2-4 hours

Duration: 10-24 hours

Pharmacokinetics (Adult data unless noted)

Distribution: V_d: 0.5 L/kg

Protein-binding: 92% to 97%

Metabolism: Extensive in the liver, metabolites may be active

Bioavailability: 43% to 82%

Time to peak serum concentration: ~3 hours

Half-life: 2-3 hours, prolonged with CHF

Elimination: Feces; urine (6% to 10% renally as unchanged drug)

Dosing: Usual

Infants, Children, and Adolescents:

Hypertension: Children and Adolescents: Limited data available: Oral: Initial: 0.05-0.1 mg/kg/**day** in divided doses every 8 hours; may titrate up to 0.5 mg/kg/**day** in divided doses 3 times daily; maximum daily dose: 20 mg/**day** (NHBPEP, 2004; NHLBI, 2011)

Scorpion envenomation: Limited data available:

Weight-directed: Infants ≥4 months, Children, and Adolescents: Oral: 0.03 mg/kg/dose; second dose has been administered at 3 or 6 hours after initial dose; subsequent doses every 6 hours; therapy has been continued for 48 hours or until extremities are warm and dry (Bosnak, 2009; Gupta, 2010)

Fixed dosing: Infants >6 months, Children, and Adolescents: Oral: 0.25 mg every 3 hours until extremities are warm and dry (Bawaskar, 2010)

Adults: **Hypertension:** Oral: Initial: 1 mg/dose 2-3 times/day; usual maintenance dose: 2-20 mg/day in divided doses 2-3 times/day (JNC 7); maximum daily dose: 20 mg

Administration Oral: Administer without regard to meals at the same time each day.

Monitoring Parameters Blood pressure (standing and sitting or supine)

Test Interactions Increased urinary VMA 17%, norepinephrine metabolite 42%; therefore, false positives may occur in screening for pheochromocytoma. If elevated VMA is found, discontinue prazosin and retest after one month.

Dosage Forms Excipient information presented when available (limited, particularly for generics); consult specific product labeling.

Capsule, Oral:
Minipress: 1 mg, 2 mg, 5 mg
Generic: 1 mg, 2 mg, 5 mg

- **Prazosin Hydrochloride** *see* Prazosin *on page 1752*
- **PR Benzoyl Peroxide Wash** *see* Benzoyl Peroxide *on page 270*
- **Precedex** *see* Dexmedetomidine *on page 617*
- **Precose** *see* Acarbose *on page 43*
- **Predator [OTC]** *see* Lidocaine (Topical) *on page 1258*
- **Pred Forte** *see* PrednisoLONE (Ophthalmic) *on page 1758*
- **Pred-G** *see* Prednisolone and Gentamicin *on page 1759*
- **Pred Mild** *see* PrednisoLONE (Ophthalmic) *on page 1758*

Prednicarbate (pred ni KAR bate)

Medication Safety Issues

Sound-alike/look-alike issues:

Dermatop may be confused with Dimetapp

Related Information

Topical Corticosteroids *on page 2262*

Brand Names: US Dermatop

Brand Names: Canada Dermatop

Therapeutic Category Adrenal Corticosteroid; Anti-inflammatory Agent; Corticosteroid, Topical; Glucocorticoid

Generic Availability (US) Yes

Use

Cream: Relief of the inflammatory and pruritic manifestations of corticosteroid-responsive dermatoses (medium potency topical corticosteroid) (FDA approved in ages ≥1 year and adults) **Note:** In pediatric patients, safety and efficacy ≥3 weeks has not been established)

Ointment: Relief of the inflammatory and pruritic manifestations of corticosteroid-responsive dermatoses (medium-potency topical corticosteroid) (FDA approved in ages ≥10 years and adults)

Pregnancy Risk Factor C

Pregnancy Considerations Adverse events have been observed in animal reproduction studies. Topical corticosteroids are not recommended for extensive use, in large quantities, or for long periods of time in pregnant women (Koutroulis, 2011; Leachman, 2006).

Breast-Feeding Considerations Systemic corticosteroids are excreted in human milk. It is not known if sufficient quantities of prednicarbate are absorbed following topical administration to produce detectable amounts in breast milk. Do not apply topical corticosteroids to nipples; hypertension was noted in a nursing infant exposed to a topical corticosteroid while nursing (Leachman, 2006). The manufacturer recommends that caution be exercised when administering prednicarbate to nursing women.

Contraindications

Hypersensitivity to prednicarbate or any component of the formulation

Documentation of allergenic cross-reactivity for corticosteroids is limited. However, because of similarities in chemical structure and/or pharmacologic actions, the possibility of cross-sensitivity cannot be ruled out with certainty.

Warnings/Precautions For topical use only; do not use intravaginally. Avoid contact with eyes, face, underarms, or groin area. Do not use occlusive dressings; discontinue use if irritation occurs. Topical corticosteroids may be absorbed percutaneously. Absorption of topical corticosteroids may cause manifestations of Cushing syndrome, hyperglycemia, or glycosuria. Absorption is increased by the use of occlusive dressings, application to denuded skin, or application to large surface areas. May cause hypercorticism or suppression of hypothalamic-pituitary-adrenal (HPA) axis, particularly in younger children or in patients receiving high doses for prolonged periods. HPA axis suppression may lead to adrenal crisis. Prolonged use of corticosteroids may result in fungal or bacterial superinfection; discontinue if dermatological infection persists despite appropriate antimicrobial therapy. Allergic contact dermatitis can occur and it is usually diagnosed by failure to heal rather than clinical exacerbation. Prolonged treatment with corticosteroids has been associated with the development of Kaposi sarcoma (case reports); if noted, discontinuation of therapy should be considered (Goedert 2002). Children may absorb proportionally larger amounts after topical application and may be more prone to systemic effects. HPA axis suppression, intracranial hypertension, and Cushing's syndrome have been reported in children receiving topical corticosteroids. Prolonged use may affect growth velocity; growth should be routinely monitored in pediatric patients. Do not use for diaper dermatitis. Avoid contact with latex-containing products; may damage or reduce effectiveness of latex condoms or diaphragms. If contact occurs, throw away latex product. Do not use prednicarbate intravaginally.

Warnings: Additional Pediatric Considerations The extent of percutaneous absorption is dependent on several factors, including epidermal integrity (intact vs abraded skin), formulation, age of the patient, prolonged duration of use, and the use of occlusive dressings. Percutaneous absorption of topical steroids is increased in neonates (especially preterm neonates), infants, and young children. Infants and small children may be more susceptible to HPA axis suppression, intracranial hypertension, Cushing syndrome, or other systemic toxicities due to larger skin surface area to body mass ratio.

Adverse Reactions

Dermatologic: Mild telangiectasia, shininess, skin atrophy, thinness

Rare but important or life-threatening: Acneiform eruptions, allergic contact dermatitis, burning, edema, folliculitis, hypopigmentation, miliaria, paresthesia, perioral dermatitis, pruritus, rash, secondary infection, striae, urticaria

Drug Interactions

Metabolism/Transport Effects None known.

Avoid Concomitant Use

Avoid concomitant use of Prednicarbate with any of the following: Aldesleukin

Increased Effect/Toxicity

Prednicarbate may increase the levels/effects of: Ceritinib; Deferasirox

The levels/effects of Prednicarbate may be increased by: Telaprevir

Decreased Effect

Prednicarbate may decrease the levels/effects of: Aldesleukin; Corticorelin; Hyaluronidase; Telaprevir

Storage/Stability

Cream: Store at 5°C to 25°C (41°F to 77°F).

Ointment: Store at 15°C to 30°C (59°F to 86°F).

Mechanism of Action Topical corticosteroids have anti-inflammatory, antipruritic, and vasoconstrictive properties. May depress the formation, release, and activity of endogenous chemical mediators of inflammation (kinins, histamine, liposomal enzymes, prostaglandins) through the induction of phospholipase A_2 inhibitory proteins (lipocortins) and sequential inhibition of the release of arachidonic acid. Prednicarbate has intermediate range potency.

Pharmacokinetics (Adult data unless noted) Absorption: Topical corticosteroids are absorbed percutaneously. The extent is dependent on several factors, including epidermal integrity (intact vs abraded skin), formulation, age of the patient, and the use of occlusive dressings. Percutaneous absorption of topical steroids is increased in neonates (especially preterm neonates), infants, and young children.

Dosing: Usual Topical: **Note:** Therapy should be discontinued once control is achieved; if no improvement is seen within 2 weeks, reassessment of diagnosis may be necessary.

Cream: Children ≥1 year and Adults: Apply a thin film to affected area twice daily

Ointment: Children ≥10 year and Adults: Apply a thin film to affected area twice daily

Administration Apply a thin film to clean, dry skin and rub in gently. For external use only. Do not use on diaper area, face, groin area, underarm, or open wounds. Do not cover with occlusive dressings.

Monitoring Parameters Growth in pediatric patients; assess HPA axis suppression (eg, ACTH stimulation test, morning plasma cortisol test, urinary free cortisol test)

Dosage Forms Excipient information presented when available (limited, particularly for generics); consult specific product labeling.

Cream, External:

Dermatop: 0.1% (60 g) [contains cetostearyl alcohol, edetate disodium]

Generic: 0.1% (15 g, 60 g)

Ointment, External:

Dermatop: 0.1% (60 g) [contains propylene glycol]

Generic: 0.1% (15 g, 60 g)

PrednisoLONE (Systemic) (pred NISS oh lone)

Medication Safety Issues

Sound-alike/look-alike issues:

PrednisoLONE may be confused with predniSONE

Pediapred may be confused with Pediazole

Prelone may be confused with PROzac

Related Information

Corticosteroids Systemic Equivalencies *on page 2260*

Brand Names: US Flo-Pred; Millipred; Millipred DP; Millipred DP 12-Day; Orapred ODT; Orapred [DSC]; Pediapred; Prelone; Veripred 20

Brand Names: Canada Hydeltra T.B.A.; Novo-Prednisolone; Pediapred

Therapeutic Category Adrenal Corticosteroid; Anti-inflammatory Agent; Antiasthmatic; Corticosteroid, Systemic; Glucocorticoid

Generic Availability (US) May be product dependent

Use Treatment of endocrine disorders, rheumatic disorders, collagen diseases, dermatologic diseases, allergic states, respiratory diseases, hematologic disorders, neoplastic diseases, edematous states, and GI diseases

Pregnancy Risk Factor C/D (manufacturer specific)

Pregnancy Considerations Adverse events have been observed with corticosteroids in animal reproduction studies. Prednisolone crosses the placenta; prior to reaching the fetus, prednisolone is converted by placental enzymes to prednisone. As a result, the amount of prednisolone reaching the fetus is ~8-10 times lower than the maternal serum concentration (healthy women at term; similar results observed with preterm pregnancies complicated by HELLP syndrome) (Beitins 1972; van Runnard Heimel 2005). Some studies have shown an association between first trimester systemic corticosteroid use and oral clefts (Park-Wyllie 2000; Pradat 2003). Systemic corticosteroids may also influence fetal growth (decreased birth weight); however, information is conflicting (Lunghi 2010). Hypoadrenalism may occur in newborns following maternal use of corticosteroids in pregnancy; monitor.

When systemic corticosteroids are needed in pregnancy, it is generally recommended to use the lowest effective dose for the shortest duration of time, avoiding high doses during the first trimester (Leachman 2006; Lunghi 2010; Makol 2011; Østensen 2009). Inhaled corticosteroids are preferred for the treatment of asthma during pregnancy. Oral corticosteroids, such as prednisolone, may be used for the treatment of severe persistent asthma if needed; the lowest dose administered on alternate days (if possible) should be used (NAEPP 2005). Prednisolone may be used to treat women during pregnancy who require therapy for congenital adrenal hyperplasia (Speiser 2010). Topical agents are preferred for managing atopic dermatitis in pregnancy; for severe symptomatic or recalcitrant atopic dermatitis, a short course of prednisolone may be used during the third trimester (Koutroulis 2011).

Women exposed to prednisolone during pregnancy for the treatment of an autoimmune disease may contact the OTIS Autoimmune Diseases Study at 877-311-8972.

Breast-Feeding Considerations Prednisolone is excreted into breast milk. In one study (n=6), milk concentrations were 5% to 25% of the maternal serum concentration with peak concentrations occurring ~1 hour after the maternal dose. The milk/plasma ratio was found to be 0.2 with doses ≥30 mg/day and 0.1 with doses <30 mg/day. Following a maternal dose of prednisolone 80 mg/day, it was calculated that a breast-feeding infant would ingest <0.1% of the maternal dose (Ost 1985). One manufacturer notes that when used systemically, maternal use of corticosteroids have the potential to cause adverse events in a nursing infant (eg, growth suppression, interfere with endogenous corticosteroid production) and therefore caution should be used when administered to nursing women. In order to decrease potential exposure to a nursing infant, one manufacturer recommends administering the dose after nursing, at the time of day with the longest interval between feeds. Other sources recommend waiting 4 hours after the maternal dose before breast-feeding (Bae 2012; Leachman 2006; Makol 2011; Ost 1985). Other guidelines note that maternal use of systemic corticosteroids is not a contraindication to breast-feeding (NAEPP 2005).

Contraindications Hypersensitivity to prednisolone or any component of the formulation; acute superficial herpes simplex keratitis; live or attenuated virus vaccines (with immunosuppressive doses of corticosteroids); systemic fungal infections; varicella

Warnings/Precautions May cause hypercorticism or suppression of hypothalamic-pituitary-adrenal (HPA) axis, particularly in younger children or in patients receiving high doses for prolonged periods. HPA axis suppression may lead to adrenal crisis. Withdrawal and discontinuation of a corticosteroid should be done slowly and carefully. Particular care is required when patients are transferred from systemic corticosteroids to inhaled products due to possible adrenal insufficiency or withdrawal from steroids, including an increase in allergic symptoms. Patients receiving >20 mg per day of prednisone (or equivalent) may be most susceptible. Fatalities have occurred due to adrenal insufficiency in asthmatic patients during and after transfer from systemic corticosteroids to aerosol steroids; aerosol steroids do **not** provide the systemic steroid needed to treat patients having trauma, surgery, or infections.

Acute myopathy has been reported with high dose corticosteroids, usually in patients with neuromuscular transmission disorders; may involve ocular and/or respiratory muscles; monitor creatine kinase; recovery may be delayed. Corticosteroid use may cause psychiatric disturbances, including depression, euphoria, insomnia, mood swings, and personality changes. Pre-existing psychiatric conditions may be exacerbated by corticosteroid use. Prolonged use of corticosteroids may also increase the incidence of secondary infection, mask acute infection (including fungal infections), prolong or exacerbate viral infections, or limit response to vaccines. Exposure to chickenpox should be avoided; corticosteroids should not be used to treat ocular herpes simplex. Corticosteroids should not be used for cerebral malaria or viral hepatitis. Close observation is required in patients with latent tuberculosis and/or TB reactivity; restrict use in active TB (only in conjunction with antituberculosis treatment). Prolonged use of corticosteroids may result in glaucoma; cataract formation may occur. Prolonged treatment with corticosteroids has been associated with the development of Kaposi's sarcoma (case reports); if noted, discontinuation of therapy should be considered.

Use with caution in patients with thyroid disease, hepatic impairment, renal impairment, cardiovascular disease, diabetes, glaucoma, cataracts, myasthenia gravis, patients at risk for osteoporosis, patients at risk for seizures, or GI diseases (diverticulitis, peptic ulcer, ulcerative colitis) due to perforation risk. Avoid ethanol may enhance gastric mucosal irritation. Use caution following acute MI (corticosteroids have been associated with myocardial rupture). Because of the risk of adverse effects, systemic corticosteroids should be used cautiously in the elderly in the smallest possible effective dose for the shortest duration. Withdraw therapy with gradual tapering of dose. May affect growth velocity; growth should be routinely monitored in pediatric patients. Potentially significant drug-drug interactions may exist, requiring dose or frequency adjustment, additional monitoring, and/or selection of alternative therapy.

Benzyl alcohol and derivatives: Some dosage forms may contain sodium benzoate/benzoic acid; benzoic acid (benzoate) is a metabolite of benzyl alcohol; large amounts of benzyl alcohol (≥99 mg/kg/day) have been associated with a potentially fatal toxicity ("gasping syndrome") in neonates; the "gasping syndrome" consists of metabolic acidosis, respiratory distress, gasping respirations, CNS dysfunction (including convulsions, intracranial hemorrhage), hypotension, and cardiovascular collapse (AAP 1997; CDC 1982); some data suggests that benzoate displaces bilirubin from protein binding sites (Ahlfors 2001); avoid or use dosage forms containing benzyl alcohol derivative with caution in neonates. See manufacturer's labeling.

Propylene glycol: Some dosage forms may contain propylene glycol; large amounts are potentially toxic and have been associated hyperosmolality, lactic acidosis, seizures, and respiratory depression; use caution (AAP 1997; Zar 2007).

Warnings: Additional Pediatric Considerations May cause osteoporosis (at any age) or inhibition of bone growth in pediatric patients. Use with caution in patients with osteoporosis. In a population-based study of children, risk of fracture was shown to be increased with >4 courses of corticosteroids; underlying clinical condition may also impact bone health and osteoporotic effect of corticosteroids (Leonard, 2007). Increased IOP may occur, especially with prolonged use; in children, increased IOP has been shown to be dose dependent and produce a greater IOP in children <6 years than older children treated with ophthalmic dexamethasone (Lam, 2005). Corticosteroids have been associated with myocardial rupture; hypertrophic cardiomyopathy has been reported in premature neonates.

Some dosage forms may contain propylene glycol; in neonates large amounts of propylene glycol delivered orally, intravenously (eg, >3,000 mg/day), or topically have been associated with potentially fatal toxicities which can include metabolic acidosis, seizures, renal failure, and CNS depression; toxicities have also been reported in children and adults including hyperosmolality, lactic acidosis, seizures, and respiratory depression; use caution (AAP, 1997; Shehab, 2009).

Adverse Reactions

Cardiovascular: Cardiomyopathy, CHF, edema, facial edema, hypertension

Central nervous system: Headache, insomnia, malaise, nervousness, pseudotumor cerebri, psychic disorders, seizure, vertigo

Dermatologic: Bruising, facial erythema, hirsutism, petechiae, skin test reaction suppression, thin fragile skin, urticaria

Endocrine & metabolic: Carbohydrate tolerance decreased, Cushing's syndrome, diabetes mellitus, growth suppression, hyperglycemia, hypernatremia, hypokalemia, hypokalemic alkalosis, menstrual irregularities, negative nitrogen balance, pituitary adrenal axis suppression

Gastrointestinal: Abdominal distention, increased appetite, indigestion, nausea, pancreatitis, peptic ulcer, ulcerative esophagitis, weight gain

Hepatic: LFTs increased (usually reversible)

Neuromuscular & skeletal: Arthralgia, aseptic necrosis (humeral/femoral heads), fractures, muscle mass decreased, muscle weakness, osteoporosis, steroid myopathy, tendon rupture, weakness

Ocular: Cataracts, exophthalmus, eyelid edema, glaucoma, intraocular pressure increased, irritation

Respiratory: Epistaxis

Miscellaneous: Diaphoresis increased, impaired wound healing

Rare but important or life-threatening: Venous thrombosis (Johannesdottir, 2013)

Drug Interactions

Metabolism/Transport Effects Substrate of CYP3A4 (minor); **Note:** Assignment of Major/Minor substrate status based on clinically relevant drug interaction potentia

Avoid Concomitant Use

Avoid concomitant use of PrednisoLONE (Systemic) with any of the following: Aldesleukin; BCG; BCG (Intravesical); Indium 111 Capromab Pendetide; Mifepristone; Natalizumab; Pimecrolimus; Tacrolimus (Topical); Tofacitinib

Increased Effect/Toxicity

PrednisoLONE (Systemic) may increase the levels/effects of: Acetylcholinesterase Inhibitors; Amphotericin B; Androgens; Ceritinib; CycloSPORINE (Systemic); Deferasirox; Leflunomide; Loop Diuretics; Natalizumab; Nicorandil; NSAID (COX-2 Inhibitor); NSAID (Nonselective); Quinolone Antibiotics; Thiazide Diuretics; Tofacitinib; Vaccines (Live); Warfarin

The levels/effects of PrednisoLONE (Systemic) may be increased by: Aprepitant; Boceprevir; CycloSPORINE (Systemic); CYP3A4 Inhibitors (Strong); Denosumab; Estrogen Derivatives; Fosaprepitant; Indacaterol; Mifepristone; Neuromuscular-Blocking Agents (Nondepolarizing); Pimecrolimus; Ritonavir; Roflumilast; Salicylates; Tacrolimus (Topical); Telaprevir; Trastuzumab

Decreased Effect

PrednisoLONE (Systemic) may decrease the levels/effects of: Aldesleukin; Antidiabetic Agents; BCG; BCG (Intravesical); Calcitriol (Systemic); Coccidioides immitis Skin Test; Corticorelin; CycloSPORINE (Systemic); Hyaluronidase; Indium 111 Capromab Pendetide; Isoniazid; Salicylates; Sipuleucel-T; Telaprevir; Urea Cycle Disorder Agents; Vaccines (Inactivated); Vaccines (Live)

The levels/effects of PrednisoLONE (Systemic) may be decreased by: Antacids; Bile Acid Sequestrants; Carbimazole; CYP3A4 Inducers (Strong); Echinacea; Methimazole; Mifepristone; Mitotane

Storage/Stability

Flo-Pred: Store at 20°C to 25°C (68°F to 77°F). Flo-Pred™ should be dispensed in the original container (to avoid loss of formulation during transfer).

Millipred: Store at 20°C to 25°C (68°F to 77°F).

Orapred ODT: Store at 20°C to 25°C (68°F to 77°F) in blister pack. Protect from moisture.

Orapred, Veripred 20: 2°C to 8°C (36°F to 46°F).

Pediapred: 4°C to 25°C (39°F to 77°F); may be refrigerated.

Mechanism of Action Decreases inflammation by suppression of migration of polymorphonuclear leukocytes and reversal of increased capillary permeability; suppresses the immune system by reducing activity and volume of the lymphatic system

Pharmacokinetics (Adult data unless noted)

Absorption: Well-absorbed

Protein binding: 70% to 90% (concentration dependent)

Metabolism: Primarily in the liver, but also metabolized in most tissues, to inactive compounds

Half-life, serum: 2-4 hours

Elimination: In urine, principally as glucuronide and sulfate-conjugated metabolites

Dosing: Neonatal Bronchopulmonary dysplasia, treatment: See Dosing: Usual for dosing in infants

Dosing: Usual Dose depends upon condition being treated and response of patient; dosage for infants and children should be based on disease severity and patient response, rather than by rigid adherence to dosage guidelines by age, weight, or body surface area. Consider alternate day therapy for long-term therapy. Discontinuation of long-term therapy requires gradual withdrawal by tapering the dose.

Pediatric:

Bronchopulmonary dysplasia, treatment: Infants: Oral: 2 mg/kg/day divided twice daily for 5 days, followed by 1 mg/kg/day once daily for 3 days, followed by 1 mg/kg/dose every other day for 3 doses was used in 131 former premature neonates (postmenstrual age: ≥36 weeks) with BPD; results showed weaning of supplemental oxygen was facilitated in patients with capillary pCO_2 <48.5 mm Hg and pulmonary acuity score <0.5 (Bhandari 2006)

Asthma: NIH Asthma Guidelines (NAEPP 2007):

Infants and Children <12 years: Oral:

Asthma exacerbations (emergency care or hospital doses): 1 to 2 mg/kg/day in 2 divided doses (maximum: 60 mg/day) until peak expiratory flow is 70% of predicted or personal best

Short-course "burst" (acute asthma): 1 to 2 mg/kg/day in divided doses 1 to 2 times/day for 3 to 10 days; maximum dose: 60 mg/day; **Note:** Burst should be continued until symptoms resolve or patient achieves peak expiratory flow 80% of personal best; usually requires 3 to 10 days of treatment (~5 days on average); longer treatment may be required

Long-term treatment: 0.25 to 2 mg/kg/day given as a single dose in the morning or every other day as needed for asthma control; maximum dose: 60 mg/day

Children ≥12 years and Adolescents: Oral:

Asthma exacerbations (emergency care or hospital doses): 40 to 80 mg/day in divided doses 1 to 2 times/day until peak expiratory flow is 70% of predicted or personal best

Short-course "burst" (acute asthma): 40 to 60 mg/day in divided doses 1 to 2 times/day for 3 to 10 days; **Note:** Burst should be continued until symptoms resolve and peak expiratory flow is at least 80% of personal best; usually requires 3 to 10 days of treatment (~5 days on average); longer treatment may be required

Long-term treatment: 7.5 to 60 mg daily given as a single dose in the morning or every other day as needed for asthma control

Anti-inflammatory or immunosuppressive dose: Infants, Children, and Adolescents: Oral: 0.1 to 2 mg/kg/day in divided doses 1 to 4 times/day

Nephrotic syndrome; steroid-sensitive (SSNS): Children and Adolescents: **Note:** Obese patients should be dosed based on ideal body weight: Oral:

Initial episode: 2 mg/kg/day or 60 mg/m²/day once daily, maximum daily dose: 60 mg/**day** for 4 to 6 weeks; then adjust to an alternate-day schedule of 1.5 mg/kg/dose or 40 mg/m²/dose on alternate days as a single dose, maximum dose: 40 mg/dose (Gipson 2009; KDIGO 2012; KDOQI 2013); duration of therapy based on patient response.

Relapse: 2 mg/kg/day or 60 mg/m²/day once daily, maximum daily dose: 60 mg/**day**; continue until complete remission for at least 3 days; then adjust to an alternate-day schedule of 1.5 mg/kg/dose or 40 mg/m²/dose on alternate days as a single dose, maximum dose: 40 mg/dose, recommended duration of alternate day dosing is variable: may continue for at least 4 weeks then taper. Longer duration of treatment may be necessary in patients who relapse frequently, some patients may require up to 3 months of treatment (Gipson 2009; KDIGO 2012; KDOQI 2013).

Maintenance therapy for frequently relapsing SSNS: Taper previous dose down to lowest effective dose which maintains remission using an alternate day schedule; usual effective range: 0.1 to 0.5 mg/kg/dose on alternating days; other patients may require doses up to 0.7 mg/kg/dose every other day (KDIGO 2012, KDOQI 2013)

Adult:

Usual dose (range): Oral: 5 to 60 mg daily

Rheumatoid arthritis: Oral: Initial: 5 to 7.5 mg daily, adjust dose as necessary

Multiple sclerosis: Oral: 200 mg daily for 1 week followed by 80 mg every other day for 1 month

Administration Administer after meals or with food or milk to decrease GI upset.

Flo-Pred™: Administer using the provided calibrated syringe (supplied by manufacturer) to accurately measure the dose. Syringe should be washed prior to next use.

Orapred ODT®: Do not cut, split, or break tablets; do not use partial tablets. Remove tablet from blister pack immediately prior to use. May swallow tablet whole or allow to dissolve on tongue.

Monitoring Parameters Blood pressure, weight, electrolytes, serum glucose; IOP (use >6 weeks); bone mineral density (long-term use); children's height and growth

Test Interactions Response to skin tests

Dosage Forms Considerations

Orapred oral solution contains fructose.

Orapred ODT dispersible tablets contain sucrose.

Prelone oral syrup contains sucrose.

Dosage Forms Excipient information presented when available (limited, particularly for generics); consult specific product labeling. [DSC] = Discontinued product

Solution, Oral, as base:

Generic: 15 mg/5 mL (240 mL, 480 mL)

Solution, Oral, as sodium phosphate [strength expressed as base]:

Millipred: 10 mg/5 mL (237 mL) [alcohol free, dye free; contains edetate disodium, methylparaben, saccharin sodium; grape flavor]

Orapred: 15 mg/5 mL (20 mL [DSC], 237 mL [DSC]) [dye free; contains alcohol, usp, sodium benzoate; grape flavor]

Pediapred: 5 mg/5 mL (120 mL) [alcohol free, dye free, sugar free; contains edetate disodium, methylparaben; raspberry flavor]

Veripred 20: 20 mg/5 mL (237 mL) [alcohol free, dye free; contains edetate disodium, methylparaben, saccharin sodium; grape flavor]

Generic: 15 mg/5 mL (237 mL); 25 mg/5 mL (237 mL); 5 mg/5 mL (120 mL)
Suspension, Oral, as acetate [strength expressed as base]:
Flo-Pred: 15 mg/5 mL (30 mL) [contains butylparaben, disodium edta, propylene glycol; cherry flavor]
Syrup, Oral, as base:
Prelone: 15 mg/5 mL (240 mL) [contains alcohol, usp, benzoic acid, brilliant blue fcf (fd&c blue #1), fd&c red #40, propylene glycol, saccharin sodium; cherry flavor]
Generic: 15 mg/5 mL (240 mL, 480 mL)
Tablet, Oral, as base:
Millipred: 5 mg [scored; contains fd&c yellow #10 (quinoline yellow), fd&c yellow #6 (sunset yellow), sodium benzoate]
Millipred DP: 5 mg [scored; contains fd&c yellow #10 (quinoline yellow), fd&c yellow #6 (sunset yellow), sodium benzoate]
Millipred DP 12-Day: 5 mg [scored; contains fd&c yellow #10 (quinoline yellow), fd&c yellow #6 (sunset yellow), sodium benzoate]
Tablet Dispersible, Oral, as sodium phosphate [strength expressed as base]:
Orapred ODT: 10 mg, 15 mg, 30 mg [grape flavor]
Generic: 10 mg, 15 mg, 30 mg

PrednisoLONE (Ophthalmic) (pred NISS oh lone)

Medication Safety Issues
Sound-alike/look-alike issues:
PrednisoLONE may be confused with predniSONE
Brand Names: US Omnipred; Pred Forte; Pred Mild
Brand Names: Canada Minims Prednisolone Sodium Phosphate; PMS-Prednisolone Sodium Phosphate Forte; Pred Forte; Pred Mild; Ratio-Prednisolone; Sandoz Prednisolone
Therapeutic Category Anti-inflammatory Agent, Ophthalmic; Corticosteroid, Ophthalmic
Generic Availability (US) Yes
Use Treatment of inflammatory conditions of the palpebral and bulbar conjunctiva, cornea, and anterior segment of the globe; corneal injury from chemical, radiation, thermal burns, or foreign body penetration (All indications: FDA approved in adults)
Pregnancy Risk Factor C
Pregnancy Considerations Ophthalmic prednisolone was shown to be teratogenic in animal studies. When administered systemically, prednisolone crosses the placenta. The amount of prednisolone available systemically following topical application of the ophthalmic drops is unknown; refer to the PrednisoLONE (Systemic) monograph for additional information.
Breast-Feeding Considerations The amount of prednisolone available systemically following topical application of the ophthalmic drops is unknown. Due to the potential for serious adverse reactions in the nursing infant, the manufacturer recommends a decision be made whether to discontinue nursing or to discontinue the drug, taking into account the importance of treatment to the mother. When administered systemically, prednisolone is excreted in breast milk. Refer to the PrednisoLONE (Systemic) monograph for additional information.
Contraindications Hypersensitivity to prednisolone, any component of the formulation, or other corticosteroids; acute untreated purulent ocular infections; viral diseases of the cornea and conjunctiva (eg, epithelial herpes simplex keratitis (dendritic keratitis), vaccinia, varicella); mycobacterial or fungal infections of the eye; use after uncomplicated removal of a superficial corneal foreign body (prednisolone sodium phosphate solution only)
Warnings/Precautions Prolonged use of corticosteroids may result in posterior subcapsular cataract formation. Use following cataract surgery may delay healing or increase the incidence of bleb formation. Prolonged use of corticosteroids may result in elevated intraocular pressure (IOP) and/or glaucoma; damage to the optic nerve; and defects in visual acuity and fields of vision. Use with caution in patients with glaucoma; monitor IOP in any patient receiving treatment for ≥10 days.

Prolonged use of corticosteroids may increase the incidence of secondary infection, mask acute infection (including fungal infections), or prolong or exacerbate viral infections. Corticosteroids should not be used to treat ocular herpes simplex. Fungal infection should be suspected in any patient with persistent corneal ulceration who has received corticosteroids. Various ophthalmic disorders, as well as prolonged use of corticosteroids, may result in corneal and scleral thinning. Continued use in a patient with thinning may result in rupture.

Not effective in Sjogren's keratoconjunctivitis or mustard gas keratitis. Some products may contain sodium bisulfite, which may cause allergic reactions in susceptible individuals. In chronic conditions, withdraw therapy with gradual tapering of dose. Some dosage forms may contain polysorbate 80 (also known as Tweens). Hypersensitivity reactions, usually a delayed reaction, have been reported following exposure to pharmaceutical products containing polysorbate 80 in certain individuals (Isåksson, 2002; Lucente 2000; Shelley, 1995). Thrombocytopenia, ascites, pulmonary deterioration, and renal and hepatic failure have been reported in premature neonates after receiving parenteral products containing polysorbate 80 (Alade, 1986; CDC, 1984). See manufacturer's labeling.
Warnings: Additional Pediatric Considerations Increased IOP may occur especially with prolonged use; in children, increased IOP has been shown to be dose dependent and produce a greater IOP in children <6 years than older children (Lam, 2005).
Adverse Reactions Ocular: Conjunctival hyperemia, conjunctivitis, corneal ulcers, delayed wound healing, glaucoma, intraocular pressure increased, keratitis, loss of accommodation, optic nerve damage, mydriasis, posterior subcapsular cataract formation, ptosis, secondary ocular infection
Drug Interactions
Metabolism/Transport Effects Substrate of CYP3A4 (minor); **Note:** Assignment of Major/Minor substrate status based on clinically relevant drug interaction potential
Avoid Concomitant Use There are no known interactions where it is recommended to avoid concomitant use.
Increased Effect/Toxicity
PrednisoLONE (Ophthalmic) may increase the levels/effects of: Ceritinib

The levels/effects of PrednisoLONE (Ophthalmic) may be increased by: NSAID (Ophthalmic)
Decreased Effect There are no known significant interactions involving a decrease in effect.
Storage/Stability
Omnipred: Store at 8°C to 24°C (46°F to 75°F).
Pred Forte: Store up to 25°C (77°F). Protect from freezing.
Pred Mild: Store at 15°C to 30°C (59°F to 86°F). Protect from freezing.
Prednisolone sodium phosphate (solution): Store at 15°C to 25°C (59°F to 77°F). Protect from light.
Mechanism of Action Reduces inflammation by inhibiting edema, leukocyte migration, fibrin deposition, capillary proliferation and dilation, collagen deposition and scar formation.
Dosing: Usual
Pediatric: **Ophthalmic inflammation, treatment:** Limited data available: Children and Adolescents: Prednisolone acetate 1% (suspension): Instill 1 to 2 drops into conjunctival sac 3 to 6 times daily. If signs and symptoms fail

to improve after 2 days, re-evaluate. Initiate with more frequent dosing, and decrease as clinically indicated. If signs and symptoms fail to improve after 2 days, re-evaluate (Wilson, 2009).

Adult: **Ophthalmic inflammation, treatment:**

Prednisolone acetate 1% (suspension):

Omnipred: Instill 2 drops into conjunctival sac 4 times daily. If signs and symptoms fail to improve after 2 days, re-evaluate.

Pred Forte: Instill 1 to 2 drops into conjunctival sac 2 to 4 times daily. During the initial 24 to 48 hours, the dosing frequency may be increased if necessary. If signs and symptoms fail to improve after 2 days, re-evaluate.

Prednisolone sodium phosphate 1% (solution): Instill 1 to 2 drops into conjunctival sac every hour during the day and every 2 hours at night until favorable response is obtained, then use 1 drop every 4 hours; later further reduction to 1 drop 3 to 4 times daily may be adequate

Dosing adjustment in renal impairment: There are no dosage adjustments provided in manufacturer's labeling.

Dosing adjustment in hepatic impairment: There are no dosage adjustments provided in manufacturer's labeling.

Administration Not for injection into eye; for topical use only. Shake suspension well before use; instill drops into affected eye(s); avoid contact of container tip with skin or eye; apply finger pressure to lacrimal sac during and for 1-2 minutes after instillation to decrease risk of absorption and systemic effects

Dosage Forms Excipient information presented when available (limited, particularly for generics); consult specific product labeling.

Solution, Ophthalmic, as sodium phosphate:

Generic: 1% (10 mL)

Suspension, Ophthalmic, as acetate:

Omnipred: 1% (5 mL, 10 mL) [contains benzalkonium chloride, edetate disodium, polysorbate 80]

Pred Forte: 1% (1 mL, 5 mL, 10 mL, 15 mL) [contains benzalkonium chloride, edetate disodium, polysorbate 80, sodium bisulfite]

Pred Mild: 0.12% (5 mL, 10 mL)

Generic: 1% (5 mL, 10 mL, 15 mL)

◆ **Prednisolone Acetate, Ophthalmic** *see* PrednisoLONE (Ophthalmic) *on page 1758*

Prednisolone and Gentamicin

(pred NIS oh lone & jen ta MYE sin)

Brand Names: US Pred-G

Therapeutic Category Antibiotic, Ophthalmic; Corticosteroid, Ophthalmic

Generic Availability (US) No

Use Treatment of steroid responsive inflammatory conditions and superficial ocular infections due to strains of microorganisms susceptible to gentamicin such as *Staphylococcus*, *E. coli*, *H. influenzae*, *Klebsiella*, *Neisseria*, *Pseudomonas*, *Proteus*, and *Serratia* species

Pregnancy Risk Factor C

Pregnancy Considerations Animal reproduction studies have not been conducted with this combination. See individual agents.

Breast-Feeding Considerations It is not known whether topical administration of corticosteroids could result in sufficient systemic absorption to produce detectable quantities in human milk. The amount of gentamicin available systemically following application of the ophthalmic drops is below the limit of detection (<0.5 mcg/mL). Due to the potential for serious adverse reactions in the nursing infant, the manufacturer recommends a decision be made whether to discontinue nursing or to discontinue the drug, taking into account the importance of treatment to the mother. See individual agents.

Contraindications Hypersensitivity to gentamicin, prednisolone, other corticosteroids, or any component of the formulation; viral disease of the cornea and conjunctiva (including epithelial herpes simplex keratitis [dendritic keratitis], vaccinia, varicella); mycobacterial or fungal infection of the eye

Warnings/Precautions For ophthalmic use only. Do not inject subconjunctivally or introduce into the anterior chamber of the eye. Steroids may mask infection or enhance existing ocular infection (including herpes simplex); prolonged use may result in secondary bacterial or fungal superinfection due to immunosuppression. Ocular irritation and punctate keratitis have occurred. Prolonged use of corticosteroids may result in glaucoma; damage to the optic nerve, defects in visual acuity and fields of vision, corneal and scleral thinning leading to perforation, and posterior subcapsular cataract formation may occur. Use following cataract surgery may delay healing or increase the incidence of bleb formation.

A maximum of 20 mL of suspension or a maximum of 8 g of ointment should be prescribed initially; patients should be re-evaluated (eg, intraocular pressure and exams using magnification and fluorescein staining, where appropriate) prior to additional refills. Use >10 days should include routine monitoring of intraocular pressure. Some products contain benzalkonium chloride which may be absorbed by soft contact lenses; contact lenses should not be worn during treatment of ophthalmologic infections.

Use with caution in patients with glaucoma and/or ophthalmic herpes simplex; frequent monitoring is advised. Ocular steroids are indicated in inflammatory conditions of the palpebral and bulbar conjunctiva, cornea, and anterior segment of the globe; also indicated in chronic anterior uveitis and corneal injury from chemical, radiation, or thermal burns or penetration of foreign bodies.

Adverse Reactions

Dermatologic: Delayed wound healing

Local: Discomfort, irritation

Ocular: Glaucoma, intraocular pressure increased, optic nerve damage (infrequent), posterior subcapsular cataract formation, superficial punctate keratitis

Miscellaneous: Secondary infection

Drug Interactions

Metabolism/Transport Effects Refer to individual components.

Avoid Concomitant Use There are no known interactions where it is recommended to avoid concomitant use.

Increased Effect/Toxicity

Prednisolone and Gentamicin may increase the levels/effects of: Ceritinib

The levels/effects of Prednisolone and Gentamicin may be increased by: NSAID (Ophthalmic)

Decreased Effect There are no known significant interactions involving a decrease in effect.

Storage/Stability

Ointment: Store at 15°C to 25°C (59°F to 77°F).

Suspension: Store at 15°C to 25°C (59°F to 77°F). Avoid excessive heat (≥40°C [104°F]). Do not freeze.

Mechanism of Action

Gentamicin: Interferes with bacterial protein synthesis by binding to 30S and 50S ribosomal subunits resulting in a defective bacterial cell membrane

Prednisolone: Reduces inflammation by inhibiting edema, leukocyte migration, fibrin deposition, capillary proliferation and dilation, collagen deposition and scar formation.

Dosing: Usual Children and Adults: Ophthalmic: Instill 1 drop 2-4 times/day; during the initial 24-48 hours, the dosing frequency may be increased if necessary, up to 1 drop every hour; or small amount (1/2" ribbon) of ointment can be applied into the conjunctival sac 1-3 times/day

Administration Suspension: Shake well before using; instill drop into affected eye; avoid contacting bottle tip with skin or eye; apply finger pressure to lacrimal sac during and for 1-2 minutes after instillation to decrease risk of absorption and systemic effects

Monitoring Parameters With use >10 days, monitor intraocular pressure

Dosage Forms Excipient information presented when available (limited, particularly for generics); consult specific product labeling. [DSC] = Discontinued product

Ointment, ophthalmic:

Pred-G: Prednisolone acetate 0.6% and gentamicin sulfate 0.3% (3.5 g)

Suspension, ophthalmic:

Pred-G: Prednisolone acetate 1% and gentamicin sulfate 0.3% (5 mL) [contains benzalkonium chloride]

◆ **Prednisolone Sodium Phosphate** *see* PrednisoLONE (Systemic) *on page 1755*

◆ **Prednisolone Sodium Phosphate, Ophthalmic** *see* PrednisoLONE (Ophthalmic) *on page 1758*

PredniSONE (PRED ni sone)

Medication Safety Issues

Sound-alike/look-alike issues:

PredniSONE may be confused with methylPREDNISolone, Pramosone, prazosin, prednisoLONE, PriLOSEC, primidone, promethazine

Related Information

Corticosteroids Systemic Equivalencies *on page 2260*

Brand Names: US PredniSONE Intensol; Rayos

Brand Names: Canada Apo-Prednisone; Novo-Prednisone; Winpred

Therapeutic Category Adrenal Corticosteroid; Anti-inflammatory Agent; Antiasthmatic; Corticosteroid, Systemic; Glucocorticoid

Generic Availability (US) May be product dependent

Use Anti-inflammatory or immunosuppressant agent in the treatment of a variety of diseases, including those of allergic, hematologic, dermatologic, gastrointestinal, inflammatory, ophthalmic, neoplastic, rheumatic, autoimmune, nervous system, renal, and respiratory origin (Immediate release: FDA approved in infants, children, adolescents, and adults; delayed release [Rayos]: FDA approved in pediatric patients [age not specified] and adults); primary or secondary adrenocorticoid deficiency (not first-line) (Immediate release: FDA approved in infants, children, adolescents, and adults; delayed release [Rayos]: FDA approved in pediatric patients [age not specified] and adults); solid organ rejection (acute/chronic) (delayed release [Rayos]: FDA approved in pediatric patients [age not specified] and adults); has also been used for treatment of Bell palsy, autoimmune hepatitis, and *Pneumocystis jirovecii* pneumonia

Pregnancy Risk Factor C/D (product specific)

Pregnancy Considerations Adverse events have been observed with corticosteroids in animal reproduction studies. Prednisone and its metabolite, prednisolone, cross the human placenta. In the mother, prednisone is converted to the active metabolite prednisolone by the liver. Prior to reaching the fetus, prednisolone is converted by placental enzymes back to prednisone. As a result, the level of prednisone remaining in the maternal serum and reaching the fetus are similar; however, the amount of prednisolone reaching the fetus is ~8-10 times lower than the maternal serum concentration (healthy women at term) (Beitins, 1972). Some studies have shown an association between first trimester systemic corticosteroid use and oral clefts (Park-Wyllie, 2000; Pradat, 2003). Systemic corticosteroids may also influence fetal growth (decreased birth weight); however, information is conflicting (Lunghi, 2010). Hypoadrenalism may occur in newborns following maternal use of corticosteroids in pregnancy; monitor.

When systemic corticosteroids are needed in pregnancy, it is generally recommended to use the lowest effective dose for the shortest duration of time, avoiding high doses during the first trimester (Leachman, 2006; Lunghi, 2010; Makol, 2011; Østensen, 2009). Inhaled corticosteroids are preferred for the treatment of asthma during pregnancy. Oral corticosteroids, such as prednisone, may be used for the treatment of severe persistent asthma if needed; the lowest dose administered on alternate days (if possible) should be used (NAEPP, 2005). Prednisone may be used to treat lupus nephritis in pregnant women who have active nephritis or substantial extrarenal disease activity (Hahn, 2012).

Pregnant women exposed to prednisone for antirejection therapy following a transplant may contact the National Transplantation Pregnancy Registry (NTPR) at 215-955-4820. Women exposed to prednisone during pregnancy for the treatment of an autoimmune disease (eg, rheumatoid arthritis) may contact the OTIS Autoimmune Diseases Study at 877-311-8972.

Breast-Feeding Considerations Prednisone and its metabolite, prednisolone, are found in low concentrations in breast milk. Following a maternal dose of 10 mg (n=1), milk concentrations were measured ~2 hours after the maternal dose (prednisone 0.0016 mcg/mL; prednisolone 0.0267 mcg/mL) (Katz, 1975). In a study which included six mother/infant pairs, adverse events were not observed in nursing infants (maternal prednisone dose not provided) (Ito, 1993).

The manufacturer notes that when used systemically, maternal use of corticosteroids have the potential to cause adverse events in a nursing infant (eg, growth suppression, interfere with endogenous corticosteroid production) and therefore, a decision should be made whether to discontinue nursing or to discontinue the drug, taking into account the importance of treatment to the mother. If there is concern about exposure to the infant, some guidelines recommend waiting 4 hours after the maternal dose of an oral systemic corticosteroid before breast-feeding in order to decrease potential exposure to the nursing infant (based on a study using prednisolone) (Bae, 2011; Leachman, 2006; Makol, 2011; Ost, 1985). Other guidelines note that maternal use of prednisone is not a contraindication to breast-feeding (NAEPP, 2005).

Contraindications Hypersensitivity to any component of the formulation; systemic fungal infections; administration of live or live attenuated vaccines with immunosuppressive doses of prednisone

Warnings/Precautions May cause hypercorticism or suppression of hypothalamic-pituitary-adrenal (HPA) axis, particularly in younger children or in patients receiving high doses for prolonged periods. HPA axis suppression may lead to adrenal crisis. Withdrawal and discontinuation of a corticosteroid should be done slowly and carefully. Particular care is required when patients are transferred from systemic corticosteroids to inhaled products due to possible adrenal insufficiency or withdrawal from steroids, including an increase in allergic symptoms. Patients receiving >20 mg per day of prednisone (or equivalent) may be most susceptible. Fatalities have occurred due to adrenal insufficiency in asthmatic patients during and after transfer from systemic corticosteroids to aerosol steroids; aerosol steroids do **not** provide the systemic steroid needed to treat patients having trauma, surgery, or infections.

Acute myopathy has been reported with high dose corticosteroids, usually in patients with neuromuscular transmission disorders; may involve ocular and/or respiratory muscles; monitor creatine kinase; recovery may be delayed. Prolonged use of corticosteroids may increase the incidence of secondary infection, mask acute infection (including fungal infections), prolong or exacerbate viral infections, or limit response to vaccines. Exposure to chickenpox should be avoided. Corticosteroids should not be used to treat ocular herpes simplex or cerebral malaria. Close observation is required in patients with latent tuberculosis and/or TB reactivity; restrict use in active TB (only in conjunction with antituberculosis treatment). Prolonged treatment with corticosteroids has been associated with the development of Kaposi's sarcoma (case reports); if noted, discontinuation of therapy should be considered. Prolonged use may cause posterior subcapsular cataracts, glaucoma (with possible nerve damage) and may increase the risk for ocular infections. Corticosteroid use may cause psychiatric disturbances, including depression, euphoria, insomnia, mood swings, and personality changes. Pre-existing psychiatric conditions may be exacerbated by corticosteroid use.

Use with caution in patients with HF, diabetes, GI diseases (diverticulitis, peptic ulcer, ulcerative colitis; due to risk of perforation), hepatic impairment, myasthenia gravis, MI, patients with or who are at risk for osteoporosis, seizure disorders or thyroid disease. Avoid ethanol may enhance gastric mucosal irritation. May affect growth velocity; growth should be routinely monitored in pediatric patients.

Prior to use, the dose and duration of treatment should be based on the risk versus benefit for each individual patient. In general, use the smallest effective dose for the shortest duration of time to minimize adverse events. A gradual tapering of dose may be required prior to discontinuing therapy. Potentially significant drug-drug interactions may exist, requiring dose or frequency adjustment, additional monitoring, and/or selection of alternative therapy.

Benzyl alcohol and derivatives: Some dosage forms may contain sodium benzoate/benzoic acid; benzoic acid (benzoate) is a metabolite of benzyl alcohol; large amounts of benzyl alcohol (≥99 mg/kg/day) have been associated with a potentially fatal toxicity ("gasping syndrome") in neonates; the "gasping syndrome" consists of metabolic acidosis, respiratory distress, gasping respirations, CNS dysfunction (including convulsions, intracranial hemorrhage), hypotension, and cardiovascular collapse (AAP, 1997; CDC, 1982); some data suggests that benzoate displaces bilirubin from protein binding sites (Ahlfors, 2001); avoid or use dosage forms containing benzyl alcohol derivative with caution in neonates. See manufacturer's labeling.

Propylene glycol: Some dosage forms may contain propylene glycol; large amounts are potentially toxic and have been associated hyperosmolality, lactic acidosis, seizures, and respiratory depression; use caution (AAP, 1997; Zar, 2007).

Warnings: Additional Pediatric Considerations May cause osteoporosis (at any age) or inhibition of bone growth in pediatric patients. Use with caution in patients with osteoporosis. In a population-based study of children, risk of fracture was shown to be increased with >4 courses of corticosteroids; underlying clinical condition may also impact bone health and osteoporotic effect of corticosteroids (Leonard 2007). Increased IOP may occur, especially with prolonged use; in children, increased IOP has been shown to be dose dependent and produce a greater IOP in children <6 years than older children treated with ophthalmic dexamethasone (Lam 2005). Corticosteroids have been associated with myocardial rupture; hypertrophic cardiomyopathy has been reported in premature neonates.

Adverse Reactions

Cardiovascular: Congestive heart failure (in susceptible patients), hypertension

Central nervous system: Emotional instability, headache, intracranial pressure increased (with papilledema), psychic derangements (including euphoria, insomnia, mood swings, personality changes, severe depression), seizure, vertigo

Dermatologic: Bruising, facial erythema, petechiae, thin fragile skin, urticaria, wound healing impaired

Endocrine & metabolic: Adrenocortical and pituitary unresponsiveness (in times of stress), carbohydrate intolerance, Cushing's syndrome, diabetes mellitus, fluid retention, growth suppression (in children), hypokalemic alkalosis, hypothyroidism enhanced, menstrual irregularities, negative nitrogen balance due to protein catabolism, potassium loss, sodium retention

Gastrointestinal: Abdominal distension, pancreatitis, peptic ulcer (with possible perforation and hemorrhage), ulcerative esophagitis

Hepatic: ALT increased, AST increased, alkaline phosphatase increased

Neuromuscular & skeletal: Aseptic necrosis of femoral and humeral heads, muscle mass loss, muscle weakness, osteoporosis, pathologic fracture of long bones, steroid myopathy, tendon rupture (particularly Achilles tendon), vertebral compression fractures

Ocular: Exophthalmos, glaucoma, intraocular pressure increased, posterior subcapsular cataracts

Miscellaneous: Allergic reactions, anaphylactic reactions, diaphoresis, hypersensitivity reactions, infections, Kaposi's sarcoma

Rare but important or life-threatening: Venous thrombosis (Johannesdottir, 2013)

Drug Interactions

Metabolism/Transport Effects **Substrate** of CYP3A4 (minor); **Note:** Assignment of Major/Minor substrate status based on clinically relevant drug interaction potential; **Induces** CYP2C19 (weak/moderate), CYP3A4 (weak)

Avoid Concomitant Use

Avoid concomitant use of PredniSONE with any of the following: Aldesleukin; BCG; BCG (Intravesical); Indium 111 Capromab Pendetide; Mifepristone; Natalizumab; Pimecrolimus; Tacrolimus (Topical); Tofacitinib

Increased Effect/Toxicity

PredniSONE may increase the levels/effects of: Acetylcholinesterase Inhibitors; Amphotericin B; Androgens; Ceritinib; CycloSPORINE (Systemic); Deferasirox; Leflunomide; Loop Diuretics; Natalizumab; Nicorandil; NSAID (COX-2 Inhibitor); NSAID (Nonselective); Quinolone Antibiotics; Thiazide Diuretics; Tofacitinib; Vaccines (Live); Warfarin

The levels/effects of PredniSONE may be increased by: Aprepitant; Boceprevir; CycloSPORINE (Systemic); CYP3A4 Inhibitors (Strong); Denosumab; Estrogen Derivatives; Fluconazole; Fosaprepitant; Indacaterol; Mifepristone; Neuromuscular-Blocking Agents (Nondepolarizing); Pimecrolimus; Ritonavir; Roflumilast; Salicylates; Tacrolimus (Topical); Telaprevir; Trastuzumab

Decreased Effect

PredniSONE may decrease the levels/effects of: Aldesleukin; Antidiabetic Agents; ARIPiprazole; BCG; BCG (Intravesical); Calcitriol (Systemic); Coccidioides immitis Skin Test; Corticorelin; CycloSPORINE (Systemic); Hyaluronidase; Hydrocodone; Indium 111 Capromab Pendetide; Isoniazid; NiMODipine; Salicylates; Saxagliptin; Sipuleucel-T; Telaprevir; Urea Cycle Disorder Agents; Vaccines (Inactivated); Vaccines (Live)

The levels/effects of PredniSONE may be decreased by: Antacids; Bile Acid Sequestrants; CYP3A4 Inducers (Strong); Echinacea; Mifepristone; Mitotane; Somatropin; Tesamorelin

Mechanism of Action Decreases inflammation by suppression of migration of polymorphonuclear leukocytes and reversal of increased capillary permeability;

suppresses the immune system by reducing activity and volume of the lymphatic system; suppresses adrenal function at high doses. Antitumor effects may be related to inhibition of glucose transport, phosphorylation, or induction of cell death in immature lymphocytes. Antiemetic effects are thought to occur due to blockade of cerebral innervation of the emetic center via inhibition of prostaglandin synthesis.

Pharmacokinetics (Adult data unless noted)

Absorption: 50% to 90% (may be altered in irritable bowel syndrome or hyperthyroidism)

Protein binding (concentration dependent): 65% to 91%

Metabolism: Hepatically converted from prednisone (inactive) to prednisolone (active); may be impaired with hepatic dysfunction

Half-life elimination: ~3.5 hours

Time to peak serum concentration: Oral:

Immediate release tablet: 2 hours

Delayed release tablet (Rayos): 6 to 6.5 hours

Elimination: Urine (small portion)

Dosing: Usual

Pediatric: **Note:** All pediatric dosing based on immediate release products. Dose depends upon condition being treated and response of patient; dosage for infants and children should be based on disease severity and patient response rather than by rigid adherence to dosage guidelines by age, weight, or body surface area. Consider alternate day therapy for long-term therapy. Discontinuation of long-term therapy requires gradual withdrawal by tapering the dose.

General dosing; anti-inflammatory or immunosuppressive: Infants, Children, and Adolescents: Oral 0.05 to 2 mg/kg/day divided every 6 to 24 hours (Bertsias 2012; Kliegman 2007)

Asthma, acute exacerbation:

NAEPP 2007:

Infants and Children <12 years: Oral:

Emergency care or hospital doses: 1 to 2 mg/kg/day in 2 divided doses; maximum daily dose: 60 mg/**day**; continue until peak expiratory flow is 70% of predicted or personal best

Short-course "burst" (Outpatient): 1 to 2 mg/kg/day in divided doses 1 to 2 times daily for 3 to 10 days; maximum daily dose: 60 mg/**day**; **Note:** Burst should be continued until symptoms resolve or patient achieves peak expiratory flow 80% of personal best; usually requires 3 to 10 days of treatment (~5 days on average); longer treatment may be required

Children ≥12 years and Adolescents: Oral:

Emergency care or hospital doses: 40 to 80 mg/day in divided doses 1 to 2 times daily until peak expiratory flow is 70% of predicted or personal best

Short-course "burst" (Outpatient): 40 to 60 mg/day in divided doses 1 to 2 times daily for 3 to 10 days; **Note:** Burst should be continued until symptoms resolve and peak expiratory flow is at least 80% of personal best; usually requires 3 to 10 days of treatment (~5 days on average); longer treatment may be required

GINA 2014:

Infants and Children <12 years: Oral: 1 to 2 mg/kg/day for 3 to 5 days

Maximum daily dose age-dependent:

Infants and Children <2 years: 20 mg/**day**

Children 2 to 5 years: 30 mg/**day**

Children 6 to 11 years: 40 mg/**day**

Children ≥12 years and Adolescents: Oral: 1 mg/kg/day for 5 to 7 days; maximum daily dose 50 mg/**day**

Asthma, maintenance therapy (nonacute) (NAEPP 2007):

Infants and Children <12 year: Oral: 0.25 to 2 mg/kg/day administered as a single dose in the morning or every other day as needed for asthma control; maximum daily dose: 60 mg/**day**

Children ≥12 years and Adolescents: Oral: 7.5 to 60 mg daily administered as a single dose in the morning or every other day as needed for asthma control

Autoimmune hepatitis (monotherapy or in combination with azathioprine): Limited data available: Infants, Children, and Adolescents: Oral: Initial: 1 to 2 mg/kg/day for 2 weeks; maximum daily dose: 60 mg/**day**; taper upon response over 6 to 8 weeks to a dose of 0.1 to 0.2 mg/kg/day or 2.5 to 5 mg daily; an alternate day schedule to decrease risk of adverse effect has been used; however, a higher incidence of relapse has been observed in some cases and use is not suggested (AASLD [Manns 2010]; Della Corte 2012).

Bell palsy: Limited data available:

Infants, Children, and Adolescents <16 years: Oral: 1 mg/kg/day for 1 week, then taper over 1 week; ideally start within the 72 hours of onset of symptoms; maximum daily dose: 60 mg/**day** (Kliegman 2011)

Adolescents ≥16 years: Oral: 60 mg daily for 5 days, followed by a 5-day taper. Treatment should begin within 72 hours of onset of symptoms (OHNS [Baugh 2013]).

Congenital adrenal hyperplasia: Note: Individualize dose by monitoring growth, hormone levels, and bone age; mineralocorticoid (eg, fludrocortisone) and sodium supplement may be required in salt losers (AAP 2000; Endocrine Society [Speiser] 2010):

Infants, Children, and Adolescents (actively growing): Not recommended because impedes statural growth more so than shorter-acting systemic glucocorticoid (ie, hydrocortisone) (Endocrine Society [Speiser] 2010)

Adolescents (fully grown): Oral: 5 to 7.5 mg daily in divided doses 2 times daily (Endocrine Society [Speiser] 2010)

Crohn disease: Children and Adolescents: Oral: 1 to 2 mg/kg/day; maximum daily dose: 60 mg/**day**; continue for 2 to 4 weeks until remission, then gradually taper (Kliegman 2011; Rufo 2012; Sandhu 2010)

Dermatomyositis, moderately severe; initial treatment: Limited data available: Children and Adolescents: Oral: Initial: 2 mg/kg/day divided once or twice daily; maximum daily dose: 60 mg/**day**; continue for 4 weeks then if adequate patient response, begin taper; most recommend an initial 20% reduction in dose with subsequent wean based upon response; use in combination with other immunosuppressants (eg, methotrexate) (CARRA [Huber 2010])

Immune thrombocytopenia (ITP): Infants, Children, and Adolescents: Oral: 1 to 2 mg/kg/day; titrate dose according to platelet count; when and if able, a rapid taper is recommended; a maximum duration of therapy of 14 days has been suggested; others have used a higher dose with shorter course of 4 mg/kg/day for 3 to 4 days (Neunert 2011; Provan 2010)

Juvenile idiopathic arthritis: Infants ≥ 6 months, Children and Adolescents: Oral: Initial: 1 mg/kg/day administered once daily (maximum daily dose: 60 mg/**day**); may be used in combination with methylprednisolone pulse therapy; evaluate initial response at 1 to 2 weeks and then at 1 month of therapy; if patient improves then taper prednisone, if unchanged then continue current prednisone therapy and if worsened then increase dose to 2 mg/kg/day (maximum daily dose: 100 mg/day). After 1 month, if improvement, begin taper; if condition worsens or unchanged then increase or continue prednisone dose at 2 mg/kg/day (maximum daily dose: 100 mg/day) and/or may add or repeat methylprednisolone pulse therapy. After 3 months of glucocorticoid therapy, if improvement (prednisone dose <50% starting dose), continue taper and reassess monthly; if patient remains unchanged (prednisone dose >50% of starting dose) or worsened, additional therapy should be considered (CARRA [Dewitt 2012])

Lupus nephritis: Children and Adolescents: Oral: Initial therapy:

With concurrent methylprednisolone pulse therapy: Prednisone: 0.5 to 1.5 mg/kg/day; maximum daily dose: 60 mg/**day**, taper usually over 6 months to a dose ≤10 mg/day according to clinical response; use in combination with cyclophosphamide or mycophenolate (Bertsias 2012; KDIGO 2012; KDOQI 2013; Mina 2012)

Without concurrent methylprednisolone pulse therapy: Prednisone: 2 mg/kg/day for 6 weeks, maximum daily dose variable: for weeks 1 to 4: maximum daily dose: 80 mg/**day** and for weeks 5 and 6: 60 mg/**day**; taper over 6 months; use in combination with cyclophosphamide or mycophenolate (Mina 2012)

Malignancy (antineoplastic): Note: Used for various types of malignancy and neoplasm; see specific protocols for details concerning dosing in combination regimens.

Hodgkin lymphoma (BEACOPP regimen): Children and Adolescents: Oral: 40 mg/m^2/day in 2 divided doses on days 0 to 13; in combination with bleomycin, etoposide, doxorubicin, cyclophosphamide, vincristine, and procarbazine (Kelly 2002; Kelly 2011)

Nephrotic syndrome; steroid-sensitive (SSNS): Children and Adolescents: **Note:** Obese patients should be dosed based on ideal body weight: Oral:

Initial episode: 2 mg/kg/day or 60 mg/m^2/day once daily, maximum daily dose: 60 mg/**day** for 4 to 6 weeks; then adjust to an alternate-day schedule of 1.5 mg/kg/dose or 40 mg/m^2/dose on alternate days as a single dose, maximum dose: 40 mg/dose (Gipson 2009; KDIGO 2012; KDOQI 2013); duration of therapy based on patient response.

Relapse: 2 mg/kg/day or 60 mg/m^2/day once daily, maximum daily dose: 60 mg/**day** continue until complete remission for at least 3 days; then adjust to an alternate-day schedule of 1.5 mg/kg/dose or 40 mg/m^2/dose on alternate days as a single dose, maximum dose: 40 mg/dose, recommended duration of alternate day dosing is variable: may continue for at least 4 weeks then taper. Longer duration of treatment may be necessary in patients who relapse frequently, some patients may require up to 3 months of treatment (Gipson 2009; KDIGO 2012; KDOQI 2013).

Maintenance therapy for frequently relapsing SSNS: Taper previous dose down to lowest effective dose which maintains remission using an alternate day schedule; usual effective range: 0.1 to 0.5 mg/kg/dose on alternating days; other patients may require doses up to 0.7 mg/kg/dose every other day (KDIGO 2012, KDOQI 2013)

Physiologic replacement: Children and Adolescents: Oral: 2 to 2.5 mg/m^2/day (Ahmet 2011; Gupta 2008). **Note:** Hydrocortisone is generally preferred in growing children and adolescents due to its lower growth suppressant effects compared to prednisone (Gupta 2008).

***Pneumocystis jirovecii* pneumonia (PCP), treatment; HIV-exposed/-positive: Note:** Begin as soon as possible after diagnosis and within 72 hours of PCP therapy initiation.

Infants and Children: Oral: 1 mg/kg/dose twice daily on days 1 to 5, then 0.5 to 1 mg/kg/dose twice daily on days 6 to 10, then 0.5 mg/kg/dose once daily for days 11 to 21 (DHHS [pediatric] 2013)

Adolescents: Oral: 40 mg twice daily on days 1 to 5, followed by 40 mg once daily on days 6 to 10, followed by 20 mg once daily on days 11 to 21 or until antimicrobial regimen is completed (DHHS [adult] 2014).

Ulcerative colitis: Children and Adolescents: Oral: 1 to 2 mg/kg/day administered in the morning; maximum daily dose: 60 mg/**day**; if no response after 7 to 14 days optimal dosing and compliance should be assessed (Kliegman 2011; Rufo 2012; Turner 2012)

Adult:

General dosing range: Oral: Initial: 5 to 60 mg daily: **Note:** Dose depends upon condition being treated and response of patient. Consider alternate day therapy for long-term therapy. Discontinuation of long-term therapy requires gradual withdrawal by tapering the dose.

Prednisone taper (other regimens also available):

- Day 1: 30 mg/day divided as 10 mg before breakfast, 5 mg at lunch, 5 mg at dinner, 10 mg at bedtime
- Day 2: 5 mg at breakfast, 5 mg at lunch, 5 mg at dinner, 10 mg at bedtime
- Day 3: 5 mg 4 times daily (with meals and at bedtime)
- Day 4: 5 mg 3 times daily (breakfast, lunch, bedtime)
- Day 5: 5 mg 2 times daily (breakfast, bedtime)
- Day 6: 5 mg before breakfast

Acute asthma (NAEPP 2007): Oral: 40 to 60 mg per day for 3 to 10 days; administer as single or 2 divided doses

Acute gout (ACR guidelines [Khanna 2012]): Oral: Initial: ≥0.5 mg/kg for 5 to 10 days

Antineoplastic: Oral: Usual range: 10 mg daily to 100 mg/m^2/day (depending on indication). **Note:** Details concerning dosing in combination regimens should also be consulted.

Dermatomyositis/polymyositis: Oral: 1 mg/kg daily (range: 0.5 to 1.5 mg/kg/day), often in conjunction with steroid-sparing therapies; depending on response/tolerance, consider slow tapering after 2 to 8 weeks depending on response; taper regimens vary widely, but often involve 5 to 10 mg decrements per week and may require 6 to 12 months to reach a low once-daily or every-other-day dose to prevent disease flare (Briemberg 2003; Hengstman 2009; Iorizzo 2008; Wiendl 2008)

Immune thrombocytopenia (ITP) (American Society of Hematology 1997): Oral: 1 to 2 mg/kg/day

Lupus nephritis, induction (Hahn 2012): Oral:

Class III-IV lupus nephritis: 0.5 to 1 mg/kg/day (after glucocorticoid pulse) tapered after a few weeks to lowest effective dose, in combination with an immunosuppressive agent

Class V lupus nephritis: 0.5 mg/kg/day for 6 months in combination mycophenolate mofetil; if not improved after 6 months, use 0.5 to 1 mg/kg/day (after a glucocorticoid pulse) for an additional 6 months in combination with cyclophosphamide

Rheumatoid arthritis (American College of Rheumatology 2002): Oral: ≤10 mg daily

Dosing adjustment in renal impairment: There are no dosage adjustments provided in the manufacturer's labeling; use with caution.

Dosing adjustment in hepatic impairment: There are no dosage adjustments provided in the manufacturer's labeling. Prednisone is inactive and must be metabolized by the liver to prednisolone. This conversion may be impaired in patients with liver disease; however, prednisolone levels are observed to be higher in patients with severe liver failure than in normal patients. Therefore, compensation for the inadequate conversion of prednisone to prednisolone occurs.

Administration Oral: Administer after meals or with food or milk to decrease GI upset. Delayed release tablet (Rayos) should be swallowed whole; do not crush, divide, or chew.

Monitoring Parameters Blood pressure; weight; serum glucose; electrolytes; growth in pediatric patients; presence of infection, bone mineral density; assess HPA axis suppression (eg, ACTH stimulation test, morning plasma cortisol test, urinary free cortisol test); Hgb, occult blood loss. Monitor IOP with therapy >6 weeks.

Test Interactions Decreased response to skin tests

Dosage Forms Excipient information presented when available (limited, particularly for generics); consult specific product labeling.

Concentrate, Oral:

PredniSONE Intensol: 5 mg/mL (30 mL) [contains alcohol, usp; unflavored flavor]

Solution, Oral:

Generic: 5 mg/5 mL (5 mL, 120 mL, 500 mL)

Tablet, Oral:

Generic: 1 mg, 2.5 mg, 5 mg, 10 mg, 20 mg, 50 mg

Tablet Delayed Release, Oral:

Rayos: 1 mg, 2 mg, 5 mg

- ◆ **PredniSONE Intensol** *see* PredniSONE *on page* *1760*
- ◆ **Pregnyl** *see* Chorionic Gonadotropin (Human) *on page* *453*
- ◆ **Pregnyl® (Can)** *see* Chorionic Gonadotropin (Human) *on page* *453*
- ◆ **Prelone** *see* PrednisoLONE (Systemic) *on page* *1755*
- ◆ **Premarin** *see* Estrogens (Conjugated/Equine, Systemic) *on page* *801*
- ◆ **Premarin** *see* Estrogens (Conjugated/Equine, Topical) *on page* *803*
- ◆ **Premarin® (Can)** *see* Estrogens (Conjugated/Equine, Systemic) *on page* *801*
- ◆ **Premarin® (Can)** *see* Estrogens (Conjugated/Equine, Topical) *on page* *803*
- ◆ **Premium Activated Charcoal [OTC] (Can)** *see* Charcoal, Activated *on page* *425*
- ◆ **Premium Lidocaine** *see* Lidocaine (Topical) *on page* *1258*
- ◆ **Preparation H [OTC]** *see* Phenylephrine (Topical) *on page* *1690*
- ◆ **Preparation H Hydrocortisone [OTC]** *see* Hydrocortisone (Topical) *on page* *1041*
- ◆ **Pre-Pen** *see* Benzylpenicilloyl Polylysine *on page* *274*
- ◆ **Pressyn (Can)** *see* Vasopressin *on page* *2161*
- ◆ **Pressyn AR (Can)** *see* Vasopressin *on page* *2161*
- ◆ **Pretz [OTC]** *see* Sodium Chloride *on page* *1938*
- ◆ **Pretz Irrigation [OTC]** *see* Sodium Chloride *on page* *1938*
- ◆ **Prevacare [OTC]** *see* Alcohol (Ethyl) *on page* *86*
- ◆ **Prevacid** *see* Lansoprazole *on page* *1219*
- ◆ **Prevacid 24HR [OTC]** *see* Lansoprazole *on page* *1219*
- ◆ **Prevacid FasTab (Can)** *see* Lansoprazole *on page* *1219*
- ◆ **Prevacid SoluTab** *see* Lansoprazole *on page* *1219*
- ◆ **Prevalite** *see* Cholestyramine Resin *on page* *450*
- ◆ **Prevex B (Can)** *see* Betamethasone (Topical) *on page* *280*
- ◆ **Prevex® HC (Can)** *see* Hydrocortisone (Topical) *on page* *1041*
- ◆ **PreviDent** *see* Fluoride *on page* *899*
- ◆ **PreviDent 5000 Booster** *see* Fluoride *on page* *899*
- ◆ **PreviDent 5000 Booster Plus** *see* Fluoride *on page* *899*
- ◆ **PreviDent 5000 Dry Mouth** *see* Fluoride *on page* *899*
- ◆ **PreviDent 5000 Plus** *see* Fluoride *on page* *899*
- ◆ **Prevnar 13** *see* Pneumococcal Conjugate Vaccine (13-Valent) *on page* *1715*
- ◆ **Prezista** *see* Darunavir *on page* *588*
- ◆ **Prilocaine and Lidocaine** *see* Lidocaine and Prilocaine *on page* *1263*
- ◆ **PriLOSEC** *see* Omeprazole *on page* *1555*
- ◆ **PriLOSEC OTC [OTC]** *see* Omeprazole *on page* *1555*
- ◆ **Primaclone** *see* Primidone *on page* *1766*

Primaquine (PRIM a kween)

Medication Safety Issues

Sound-alike/look-alike issues:

Primaquine may be confused with primidone

Therapeutic Category Antimalarial Agent

Generic Availability (US) Yes

Use For the radical cure (prevention of relapse) of vivax malaria (*P. vivax*) [FDA approved in adults]; has also been used for prevention relapse of *P. ovale*, prevention of malaria (primarily *P. vivax*), malaria postexposure prophylaxis, and treatment of *Pneumocystis jirovecii* (PCP) pneumonia

Pregnancy Considerations Animal reproduction studies have not been conducted. Primaquine use is not recommended in pregnant women (CDC 2013). Consult current CDC guidelines for the treatment of malaria during pregnancy.

Breast-Feeding Considerations It is not known if primaquine is excreted in breast milk. If therapy is needed, the mother and infant should be tested for G6PD deficiency; primaquine may be used in breast-feeding mothers and infants with normal G6PD levels and concentrations (CDC 2012).

Contraindications

Use in acutely ill patients who have a tendency to develop granulocytopenia (eg, rheumatoid arthritis, SLE); concurrent use with other medications causing hemolytic anemia or myeloid bone marrow suppression; concurrent use with or recent use of quinacrine

Canadian labeling: Additional contraindications (not in US labeling): Hypersensitivity to primaquine or any component of the formulation

Documentation of allergenic cross-reactivity for aminoquinolines is limited. However, because of similarities in chemical structure and/or pharmacologic actions, the possibility of cross-sensitivity cannot be ruled out with certainty.

Warnings/Precautions Use with caution in patients with G6PD deficiency (hemolytic anemia may occur), NADH methemoglobin reductase deficiency (methemoglobinemia may occur); do not exceed recommended dosage and duration. Moderate to severe hemolytic reactions may occur in individuals with G6PD deficiency and personal or familial history of favism. Geographic regions with a high prevalence of G6PD deficiency (eg, Africa, southern Europe, Mediterranean region, Middle East, southeast Asia, Oceania) are associated with a higher incidence of hemolytic anemia. Promptly discontinue with signs of hemolytic anemia (darkening of urine, marked fall in hemoglobin or erythrocyte count). The CDC recommends screening for G6PD deficiency prior to therapy initiation (CDC 2013). Anemia, methemoglobinemia, and leukopenia have been associated with primaquine use; monitor during treatment. Immediately discontinue if marked darkening of the urine or sudden decrease in hemoglobin concentration or leukocyte count occurs.

May cause QT prolongation; monitor ECG in patients with cardiac disease, long QT syndrome, a history of ventricular arrhythmias, uncorrected hypokalemia and/or hypomagnesemia, or bradycardia (<50 beats per minute), and during concomitant administration with QT interval prolonging agents. Some dosage forms may contain polysorbate 80 (also known as Tweens). Hypersensitivity reactions, usually a delayed reaction, have been reported following exposure to pharmaceutical products containing polysorbate 80 in certain individuals (Isaksson 2002; Lucente

2000; Shelley 1995). Thrombocytopenia, ascites, pulmonary deterioration, and renal and hepatic failure have been reported in premature neonates after receiving parenteral products containing polysorbate 80 (Alade 1986; CDC 1984). See manufacturer's labeling. Potentially significant drug-drug interactions may exist, requiring dose or frequency adjustment, additional monitoring, and/or selection of alternative therapy.

Adverse Reactions

Cardiovascular: Cardiac arrhythmias, prolonged Q-T interval on ECG

Gastrointestinal: Abdominal cramps, epigastric distress, nausea, vomiting

Hematologic & oncologic: Anemia, hemolytic anemia (in patients with G6PD deficiency), leukopenia, methemoglobinemia (in NADH-methemoglobin reductase-deficient individuals)

Ophthalmic: Accommodation disturbance

Drug Interactions

Metabolism/Transport Effects **Substrate** of CYP2D6 (major), CYP3A4 (major); **Note:** Assignment of Major/Minor substrate status based on clinically relevant drug interaction potential; **Inhibits** CYP1A2 (strong), CYP2D6 (weak); **Induces** CYP1A2 (weak/moderate)

Avoid Concomitant Use

Avoid concomitant use of Primaquine with any of the following: Agomelatine; Artemether; DULoxetine; Highest Risk QTc-Prolonging Agents; Ivabradine; Lumefantrine; Mefloquine; Mifepristone; Pomalidomide; Tasimelteon; TiZANidine

Increased Effect/Toxicity

Primaquine may increase the levels/effects of: Agomelatine; Antipsychotic Agents (Phenothiazines); ARIPiprazole; Bendamustine; Beta-Blockers; Cardiac Glycosides; CloZAPine; CYP1A2 Substrates; Dapsone (Systemic); Dapsone (Topical); DULoxetine; Highest Risk QTc-Prolonging Agents; Lumefantrine; Mefloquine; Moderate Risk QTc-Prolonging Agents; Pentoxifylline; Pirfenidone; Pomalidomide; Prilocaine; Rasagiline; Sodium Nitrite; Tasimelteon; TiZANidine

The levels/effects of Primaquine may be increased by: Abiraterone Acetate; Artemether; Cobicistat; CYP2D6 Inhibitors (Moderate); CYP2D6 Inhibitors (Strong); Dapsone (Systemic); Darunavir; Ivabradine; Mefloquine; Mifepristone; Nitric Oxide; Panobinostat; Peginterferon Alfa-2b; QTc-Prolonging Agents (Indeterminate Risk and Risk Modifying)

Decreased Effect

Primaquine may decrease the levels/effects of: Anthelmintics

The levels/effects of Primaquine may be decreased by: Bosentan; CYP3A4 Inducers (Moderate); CYP3A4 Inducers (Strong); Dabrafenib; Deferasirox; Mitotane; Peginterferon Alfa-2b; Siltuximab; St Johns Wort; Tocilizumab

Storage/Stability Store at 25°C (77°F); excursions permitted to 15°C to 30°C (59°F to 86°F). Protect from light.

Mechanism of Action Primaquine is an antiprotozoal agent active against exoerythrocytic stages of *Plasmodium ovale* and *P. vivax*, also active against the primary exoerythrocytic stages of *P. falciparum* and gametocytes of *Plasmodia*; disrupts mitochondria and binds to DNA

Pharmacokinetics (Adult data unless noted)

Absorption: Oral: Well absorbed

Metabolism: Hepatic metabolism to carboxyprimaquine, an active metabolite via CYP1A2

Half-life: 7 hours; reported range: 3.7-9.6 hours

Time to peak serum concentration: Within 3 hours

Elimination: Small amount of unchanged drug excreted in urine

Dosing: Usual Oral: **Note:** Dosage expressed as mg of **base** (15 mg base = 26.3 mg primaquine phosphate):

Pediatric:

Malaria: Oral:

Treatment or relapse prevention of *P. vivax* malaria: Infants, Children, and Adolescents: 0.5 mg base/kg once daily for 14 days; maximum single dose: 30 mg base (CDC, 2013)

Treatment of uncomplicated malaria (*P. vivax* and *P. ovale*): Infants, Children, and Adolescents: 0.5 mg base/kg once daily for 14 days with chloroquine or hydroxychloroquine; maximum single dose: 30 mg base (CDC, 2013)

Prevention of malaria (primarily *P. vivax*):

Non-HIV-exposed/-positive: Infants, Children and Adolescents: 0.5 mg base/kg once daily; maximum single dose: 30 mg base; initiate 1 to 2 days prior to travel and continue once daily while in the area with malaria risk, and for 7 days after departure from malaria-endemic area (CDC, 2014)

HIV-exposed/-positive:

Primary prophylaxis: Infants and Children: 0.6 mg base/kg once daily; maximum single dose: 30 mg base; initiate 1 day prior to travel and continue once daily while in the area with malaria risk, and for 3 to 7 days after departure from malaria-endemic area (DHHS [pediatric], 2013)

Secondary prophylaxis and antirelapse therapy: Infants, Children, and Adolescents: 0.5 mg base/kg once daily for 14 days after departure from malaria-endemic area; maximum single dose: 30 mg base (CDC, 2014)

***Pneumocystis jirovecii* pneumonia (PCP) (HIV-exposed/-positive) treatment:** Oral:

Infants and Children: 0.3 mg base/kg once daily for 21 days in combination with clindamycin; maximum single dose: 30 mg base (DHHS [pediatric], 2013)

Adolescents: 30 mg base once daily for 21 days in combination with clindamycin (DHHS [adult], 2013)

Adult:

Malaria: Oral:

Treatment or prevention of relapse of *P. vivax* malaria: 30 mg base once daily for 14 days

Treatment of uncomplicated *P. vivax* and *P. ovale* malaria: 30 mg base once daily for 14 days with chloroquine or hydroxychloroquine; alternative regimen (for mild G-6-PD deficiency or as an alternative to daily regimen): 45 mg base once weekly for 8 weeks (use only after consultation with an infectious disease/tropical medicine expert) (CDC, 2011)

Chemoprophylaxis: 30 mg base once daily; start 1 to 2 days prior to travel and continue once daily while in the area with malaria risk, and for 7 days after departure from malaria-endemic area (CDC, 2012)

Presumptive antirelapse therapy for *P. vivax* and *P. ovale* malaria: 30 mg base once daily for 14 days after departure from malaria-endemic area (CDC, 2012)

***Pneumocystis jirovecii* pneumonia (PCP); treatment:** Oral: 30 mg base once daily for 21 days (in combination with clindamycin) (DHHS [adult], 2013)

Administration Oral: Administer with meals to decrease adverse GI effects; drug has a bitter taste

Monitoring Parameters Periodic CBC, visual color check of urine, hemoglobin, glucose; if hemolysis is suspected, monitor CBC, haptoglobin, peripheral smear, urinalysis dipstick for occult blood; G-6-PD deficiency screening (prior to initiating treatment; CDC recommendation)

Dosage Forms Excipient information presented when available (limited, particularly for generics); consult specific product labeling.

Tablet, Oral, as phosphate:

Generic: 26.3 mg

Extemporaneous Preparations A 6 mg base/5 mL oral suspension may be made using tablets. Crush ten 15 mg base tablets and reduce to a fine powder. In small amounts, add a total of 10 mL Carboxymethylcellulose 1.5% and mix to a uniform paste; mix while adding Simple Syrup, NF to **almost** 125 mL; transfer to a calibrated bottle, rinse mortar with vehicle, and add quantity of vehicle sufficient to make 125 mL. Label "shake well" and "refrigerate". Stable 7 days.

Nahata MC, Pai VB, and Hipple TF, *Pediatric Drug Formulations*, 5th ed, Cincinnati, OH: Harvey Whitney Books Co, 2004.

- ◆ **Primaquine Phosphate** *see* Primaquine *on page 1764*
- ◆ **Primaxin (Can)** *see* Imipenem and Cilastatin *on page 1083*
- ◆ **Primaxin I.M. [DSC]** *see* Imipenem and Cilastatin *on page 1083*
- ◆ **Primaxin® I.V.** *see* Imipenem and Cilastatin *on page 1083*

Primidone (PRI mi done)

Medication Safety Issues

Sound-alike/look-alike issues:

Primidone may be confused with predniSONE, primaquine, pyridoxine

Brand Names: US Mysoline

Brand Names: Canada Apo-Primidone®

Therapeutic Category Anticonvulsant, Barbiturate; Barbiturate

Generic Availability (US) Yes

Use Management of generalized tonic-clonic (grand mal), complex partial and simple partial (focal) seizures

Medication Guide Available Yes

Pregnancy Considerations Primidone and its metabolites (PEMA, phenobarbital, and p-hydroxyphenobarbital) cross the placenta; neonatal serum concentrations at birth are similar to those in the mother. Withdrawal symptoms may occur in the neonate and may be delayed due to the long half-life of primidone and its metabolites. Use may be associated with birth defects and adverse events; the use of folic acid throughout pregnancy and vitamin K during the last month of pregnancy is recommended. Epilepsy itself, number of medications, genetic factors, or a combination of these probably influence the teratogenicity of anticonvulsant therapy.

Patients exposed to primidone during pregnancy are encouraged to enroll themselves into the NAAED Pregnancy Registry by calling 1-888-233-2334. Additional information is available at www.aedpregnancyregistry.org.

Breast-Feeding Considerations Primidone and its metabolites (PEMA, phenobarbital, and p-hydroxyphenobarbital) are found in breast milk (variable concentrations). The manufacturer recommends discontinuing breast-feeding if undue drowsiness and somnolence occur in the newborn.

Contraindications Hypersensitivity to phenobarbital; porphyria

Warnings/Precautions Antiepileptics are associated with an increased risk of suicidal behavior/thoughts with use (regardless of indication); patients should be monitored for signs/symptoms of depression, suicidal tendencies, and other unusual behavior changes during therapy and instructed to inform their healthcare provider immediately if symptoms occur.

Use with caution in patients with renal or hepatic impairment, pulmonary insufficiency; abrupt withdrawal may precipitate status epilepticus. Potential for drug dependency exists. Do not administer to patients in acute pain. Use caution in elderly, debilitated, or pediatric patients - may cause paradoxical responses. May cause CNS depression, which may impair physical or mental abilities. Patients must cautioned about performing tasks which require mental alertness (eg, operating machinery or driving). Effects with other sedative drugs or ethanol may be potentiated. Use with caution in patients with depression or suicidal tendencies, or in patients with a history of drug abuse. Tolerance or psychological and physical dependence may occur with prolonged use. Primidone's active metabolite, phenobarbital, has been associated with cognitive deficits in children receiving chronic therapy for febrile seizures. Use with caution in patients with hypoadrenalism.

Benzyl alcohol and derivatives: Some dosage forms may contain sodium benzoate/benzoic acid; benzoic acid (benzoate) is a metabolite of benzyl alcohol; large amounts of benzyl alcohol (≥99 mg/kg/day) have been associated with a potentially fatal toxicity ("gasping syndrome") in neonates; the "gasping syndrome" consists of metabolic acidosis, respiratory distress, gasping respirations, CNS dysfunction (including convulsions, intracranial hemorrhage), hypotension, and cardiovascular collapse (AAP, 1997; CDC, 1982); some data suggests that benzoate displaces bilirubin from protein binding sites (Ahlfors, 2001); avoid or use dosage forms containing benzyl alcohol derivative with caution in neonates. See manufacturer's labeling.

Adverse Reactions

Central nervous system: Ataxia, drowsiness, emotional disturbances, fatigue, hyperirritability, suicidal ideation, vertigo

Dermatologic: Morbilliform skin eruptions

Gastrointestinal: Anorexia, nausea, vomiting

Genitourinary: Impotence

Hematologic: Agranulocytosis, granulocytopenia, megaloblastic anemia (idiosyncratic), red cell aplasia/hypoplasia

Ocular: Diplopia, nystagmus

Drug Interactions

Metabolism/Transport Effects **Induces** CYP1A2 (strong), CYP2B6 (strong), CYP2C8 (strong), CYP2C9 (strong), CYP3A4 (strong), P-glycoprotein

Avoid Concomitant Use

Avoid concomitant use of Primidone with any of the following: Abiraterone Acetate; Apixaban; Apremilast; Artemether; Axitinib; Azelastine (Nasal); Bedaquiline; Boceprevir; Bortezomib; Bosutinib; Cabozantinib; Ceritinib; CloZAPine; Crizotinib; Dabigatran Etexilate; Dasabuvir; Dienogest; Dolutegravir; Dronedarone; Eliglustat; Enzalutamide; Etravirine; Everolimus; Ibrutinib; Idelalisib; Irinotecan; Isavuconazonium Sulfate; Itraconazole; Ivabradine; Ivacaftor; Lapatinib; Ledipasvir; Lumefantrine; Lurasidone; Macitentan; Mifepristone; Naloxegol; Netupitant; NIFEdipine; Nilotinib; NiMODipine; Nintedanib; Nisoldipine; Olaparib; Ombitasvir; Orphenadrine; Palbociclib; Panobinostat; Paraldehyde; Paritaprevir; PAZOPanib; Perampanel; Pirfenidone; PONATinib; Praziquantel; Ranolazine; Regorafenib; Rilpivirine; Rivaroxaban; Roflumilast; RomiDEPsin; Simeprevir; Sofosbuvir; SORAfenib; Suvorexant; Tasimelteon; Telaprevir; Thalidomide; Ticagrelor; Tofacitinib; Tolvaptan; Toremifene; Trabectedin; Ulipristal; Vandetanib; Vemurafenib; VinCRIStine (Liposomal); Vorapaxar

Increased Effect/Toxicity

Primidone may increase the levels/effects of: Alcohol (Ethyl); Azelastine (Nasal); Barbiturates; Buprenorphine; Clarithromycin; CNS Depressants; Hydrocodone; Methotrimeprazine; Metyrosine; Orphenadrine; Paraldehyde; Pramipexole; Rotigotine; Selective Serotonin Reuptake Inhibitors; Thalidomide; Valproic Acid and Derivatives; Zolpidem

The levels/effects of Primidone may be increased by: Brimonidine (Topical); Cannabis; Carbonic Anhydrase Inhibitors; Clarithromycin; Cosyntropin;

Dexmethylphenidate; Doxylamine; Dronabinol; Droperidol; Felbamate; HydrOXYzine; Kava Kava; Magnesium Sulfate; Methotrimeprazine; Methylphenidate; Nabilone; Sodium Oxybate; Tapentadol; Tetrahydrocannabinol; Valproic Acid and Derivatives

Decreased Effect

Primidone may decrease the levels/effects of: Abiraterone Acetate; Afatinib; Apixaban; Apremilast; ARIPiprazole; Artemether; Axitinib; Bazedoxifene; Bedaquiline; Bendamustine; Boceprevir; Bortezomib; Bosutinib; Brentuximab Vedotin; Cabozantinib; Canagliflozin; Cannabidiol; Cannabis; Ceritinib; Clarithromycin; CloZAPine; Cobicistat; Contraceptives (Progestins); Corticosteroids (Systemic); Crizotinib; CYP1A2 Substrates; CYP2B6 Substrates; CYP2C8 Substrates; CYP2C9 Substrates; CYP3A4 Substrates; Dabigatran Etexilate; Dasabuvir; Dasatinib; Dexamethasone (Systemic); Diclofenac (Systemic); Dienogest; Dolutegravir; DOXOrubicin (Conventional); Dronabinol; Dronedarone; Eliglustat; Enzalutamide; Erlotinib; Eslicarbazepine; Etravirine; Everolimus; Exemestane; Felbamate; FentaNYL; Gefitinib; GuanFACINE; Hydrocortisone (Systemic); Ibrutinib; Idelalisib; Imatinib; Irinotecan; Isavuconazonium Sulfate; Itraconazole; Ivabradine; Ivacaftor; Ixabepilone; LamoTRIgine; Lapatinib; Ledipasvir; Linagliptin; Lumefantrine; Lurasidone; Macitentan; Maraviroc; Methadone; MethylPREDNISolone; MetroNIDAZOLE (Systemic); Mifepristone; Naloxegol; Netupitant; NIFEdipine; Nilotinib; NiMODipine; Nintedanib; Nisoldipine; Olaparib; Ombitasvir; Palbociclib; Paliperidone; Panobinostat; Paritaprevir; PAZOPanib; Perampanel; P-glycoprotein/ABCB1 Substrates; Pirfenidone; PONATinib; Praziquantel; PrednisoLONE (Systemic); PredniSONE; Propafenone; QUEtiapine; QuiNIDine; Ranolazine; Regorafenib; Rilpivirine; Rivaroxaban; Roflumilast; RomiDEPsin; Rufinamide; Saxagliptin; Simeprevir; Sofosbuvir; SORAfenib; SUNItinib; Suvorexant; Tadalafil; Tasimelteon; Telaprevir; Tetrahydrocannabinol; Ticagrelor; Tofacitinib; Tolvaptan; Toremifene; Trabectedin; Treprostinil; Ulipristal; Vandetanib; Vemurafenib; Vilazodone; VinCRIStine (Liposomal); Vorapaxar; Vortioxetine; Zaleplon; Zuclopenthixol

The levels/effects of Primidone may be decreased by: Carbonic Anhydrase Inhibitors; Folic Acid; Fosphenytoin; Leucovorin Calcium-Levoleucovorin; Levomefolate; Mefloquine; Methylfolate; Orlistat; Phenytoin

Food Interactions Protein-deficient diets increase duration of action of primidone.

Storage/Stability Store at 20°C to 25°C (68°F to 77°F).

Mechanism of Action Decreases neuron excitability, raises seizure threshold similar to phenobarbital; primidone has two active metabolites, phenobarbital and phenylethylmalonamide (PEMA); PEMA may enhance the activity of phenobarbital

Pharmacokinetics (Adult data unless noted)

Distribution: V_d: Adults: 2-3 L/kg

Protein-binding: 99%

Metabolism: In the liver to phenobarbital (active) and phenylethylmalonamide (PEMA)

Bioavailability: 60% to 80%

Half-life:

- Primidone: 10-12 hours
- PEMA: 16 hours
- Phenobarbital: 52-118 hours (age-dependent)

Time to peak serum concentration: Oral: Within 4 hours

Elimination: Urinary excretion of both active metabolites and unchanged primidone (15% to 25%)

Dosing: Neonatal Oral: Seizure disorder: 12-20 mg/kg/day in 2-4 divided doses; start with lower dosage and titrate upward

Dosing: Usual Oral: Seizure disorder:

Children <8 years: Initial: 50-125 mg/day given at bedtime; increase by 50-125 mg/day increments every 3-7 days; usual dose: 10-25 mg/kg/day in 3-4 divided doses

Children ≥8 years and Adults: Initial: 125-250 mg/day at bedtime; increase by 125-250 mg/day every 3-7 days; usual dose: 750-1500 mg/day in 3-4 divided doses with maximum dosage of 2 g/day

Administration Oral: Administer with food to decrease GI upset

Monitoring Parameters Serum primidone and phenobarbital concentrations; CBC with differential; neurological status, seizure frequency, duration, severity; signs and symptoms of suicidality (eg, anxiety, depression, behavior changes)

Reference Range Monitor both primidone and phenobarbital concentrations.

Primidone:

- Therapeutic: 5-12 mcg/mL (SI: 23-55 micromoles/L)
- Toxic effects rarely present with levels <10 mcg/mL (SI: 46 micromoles/L) if phenobarbital concentrations are low
- Toxic: >15 mcg/mL (SI: >69 micromoles/L)

Phenobarbital:

- Therapeutic: 15-40 mcg/mL (SI: 65-172 micromoles/L)
- Potentially toxic: >40 mcg/mL (SI: >172 micromoles/L)
- Coma: >50 mcg/mL (SI: >215 micromoles/L)
- Potentially lethal: >80 mcg/mL (SI: >344 micromoles/L)

Additional Information Mysoline® suspension was discontinued in February 2001

Dosage Forms Excipient information presented when available (limited, particularly for generics); consult specific product labeling.

Tablet, Oral:

- Mysoline: 50 mg, 250 mg [scored]
- Generic: 50 mg, 250 mg

- ◆ **Primlev** *see* Oxycodone and Acetaminophen *on page 1594*
- ◆ **Primsol** *see* Trimethoprim *on page 2126*
- ◆ **Prinivil** *see* Lisinopril *on page 1280*
- ◆ **Priorix (Can)** *see* Measles, Mumps, and Rubella Virus Vaccine *on page 1327*
- ◆ **Priorix-Tetra (Can)** *see* Measles, Mumps, Rubella, and Varicella Virus Vaccine *on page 1330*
- ◆ **Priva-Celecoxib (Can)** *see* Celecoxib *on page 418*
- ◆ **Priva-Escitalopram (Can)** *see* Escitalopram *on page 786*
- ◆ **Priva-Ezetimibe (Can)** *see* Ezetimibe *on page 832*
- ◆ **Privigen** *see* Immune Globulin *on page 1089*
- ◆ **Privine® [OTC] [DSC]** *see* Naphazoline (Nasal) *on page 1488*
- ◆ **Pro-AAS EC-80 (Can)** *see* Aspirin *on page 206*
- ◆ **ProAir HFA** *see* Albuterol *on page 81*
- ◆ **ProAir RespiClick** *see* Albuterol *on page 81*
- ◆ **ProAir RespiClick** *see* Albuterol *on page 81*
- ◆ **PRO-Amiodarone (Can)** *see* Amiodarone *on page 125*
- ◆ **Pro-Amox-250 (Can)** *see* Amoxicillin *on page 138*
- ◆ **Pro-Amox-500 (Can)** *see* Amoxicillin *on page 138*
- ◆ **PRO-Azithromycine (Can)** *see* Azithromycin (Systemic) *on page 242*

Probenecid (proe BEN e sid)

Medication Safety Issues

Sound-alike/look-alike issues:

Probenecid may be confused with Procanbid

Brand Names: Canada Benuryl

Therapeutic Category Adjuvant Therapy, Penicillin Level Prolongation; Antigout Agent; Uric Acid Lowering Agent; Uricosuric Agent

Generic Availability (US) Yes

Use Adjuvant to therapy with penicillins to prolong serum concentrations (FDA approved in ages ≥2 years and adults); treatment of hyperuricemia associated with gout and gouty arthritis (FDA approved in adults); has also been used with cephalosporin therapy to prolong serum concentrations and to prevent nephrotoxicity associated with cidofovir therapy

Pregnancy Considerations Probenecid crosses the placenta. Based on available data, an increased risk of adverse fetal events have not been reported (Gutman, 2012).

Contraindications Hypersensitivity to probenecid or any component of the formulation; small- or large-dose aspirin therapy; blood dyscrasias; uric acid kidney stones; children <2 years of age; initiation during an acute gout attack

Warnings/Precautions Use with caution in patients with peptic ulcer. Salicylates may diminish the therapeutic effect of probenecid. This effect may be more pronounced with high, chronic doses, however, the manufacturer recommends the use of an alternative analgesic even in place of small doses of aspirin. Use of probenecid with penicillin in patients with renal insufficiency is not recommended. Probenecid monotherapy may not be effective in patients with a creatinine clearance <30 mL/minute. The American College of Rheumatology guidelines for the treatment of hyperuricemia do **not** recommend probenecid as first-line or an alternative first-line therapy in patients with a creatinine clearance <50 mL/minute (ACR guidelines [Khanna, 2012]). Probenecid may increase the serum concentration of methotrexate. Avoid concomitant use of probenecid and methotrexate if possible. If used together, consider lower methotrexate doses and monitor for methotrexate toxicity. May cause exacerbation of acute gouty attack. If hypersensitivity reaction or anaphylaxis occurs, discontinue medication. Use caution in patients with G6PD deficiency; may increase risk for hemolytic anemia.

Adverse Reactions

Cardiovascular: Flushing

Central nervous system: Dizziness, fever, headache

Dermatologic: Alopecia, dermatitis, pruritus, rash

Gastrointestinal: Anorexia, dyspepsia, gastroesophageal reflux, nausea, sore gums, vomiting

Genitourinary: Hematuria, polyuria

Hematologic: Anemia, aplastic anemia, hemolytic anemia (in G6PD deficiency), leukopenia

Hepatic: Hepatic necrosis

Neuromuscular & skeletal: Costovertebral pain, gouty arthritis (acute)

Renal: Nephrotic syndrome, renal colic

Miscellaneous: Anaphylaxis, hypersensitivity

Drug Interactions

Metabolism/Transport Effects Inhibits CYP2C19 (weak), UGT1A6

Avoid Concomitant Use

Avoid concomitant use of Probenecid with any of the following: Avibactam; Doripenem; Ketorolac (Nasal); Ketorolac (Systemic); Meropenem; Pegloticase; Penicillins

Increased Effect/Toxicity

Probenecid may increase the levels/effects of: Acetaminophen; Avibactam; Cefotaxime; Cephalosporins; Dapsone (Systemic); Deferiprone; Dexketoprofen; Doripenem; Ertapenem; Ganciclovir-Valganciclovir; Gemifloxacin; Imipenem; Ketoprofen; Ketorolac (Nasal); Ketorolac (Systemic); Loop Diuretics; LORazepam; Meropenem; Methotrexate; Minoxidil (Systemic); Mycophenolate; Nitrofurantoin; Nonsteroidal Anti-Inflammatory Agents; Oseltamivir; Pegloticase; Penicillins; PRALAtrexate; Quinolone Antibiotics; Sodium Benzoate; Sodium Phenylacetate; Sulfonylureas; Theophylline Derivatives; Urea Cycle Disorder Agents; Zidovudine

Decreased Effect

Probenecid may decrease the levels/effects of: Loop Diuretics

The levels/effects of Probenecid may be decreased by: Salicylates

Storage/Stability Store at 20°C to 25°C (68°F to 77°F). Protect from light.

Mechanism of Action Competitively inhibits the reabsorption of uric acid at the proximal convoluted tubule, thereby promoting its excretion and reducing serum uric acid levels; increases plasma levels of weak organic acids (penicillins, cephalosporins, or other beta-lactam antibiotics) by competitively inhibiting their renal tubular secretion

Pharmacodynamics

Maximum effect:

Penicillin concentrations: After 2 hours

Uric acid renal clearance: 30 minutes

Pharmacokinetics (Adult data unless noted)

Absorption: Rapid and complete from GI tract

Protein binding: 85% to 95%

Metabolism: Hepatic

Half-life: 6-12 hours

Time to peak serum concentration: Within 2-4 hours

Dosing: Usual

Infants, Children, and Adolescents:

Prolongation of penicillin serum levels: Children ≥2 years and Adolescents: **Note:** Dosing per manufacturer; some indication-specific dosing may vary.

Patient weight ≤50 kg: Oral: Initial: 25 mg/kg/dose or 700 mg/**m²**/dose as a single dose; maintenance: 40 mg/kg/**day** or 1200 mg /**m²/day** in 4 divided doses; maximum dose: 500 mg

Patient weight >50 kg: Oral: 500 mg 4 times daily

Gonorrhea, uncomplicated infections of cervix, urethra, and rectum: Adolescents >45 kg: Oral: 1000 mg as a single dose with cefoxitin (CDC, 2010)

Pelvic inflammatory disease: Adolescents >50 kg: Oral: 1000 mg as a single dose with cefoxitin in combination with doxycycline with/without metronidazole (CDC, 2010)

Neurosyphilis: Adolescents >50 kg: Oral: 500 mg 4 times daily with procaine penicillin for 10-14 days (CDC, 2010)

Prevention of cidofovir nephrotoxicity: Infants, Children, and Adolescents: Limited data available; various regimens have been reported (Anderson, 2008; Bhadri, 2009; Cesaro, 2005; Doan, 2007; Williams, 2009): Oral:

Weight-directed dosing: 25-40 mg/kg/dose (maximum dose: 2000 mg) administered 3 hours before cidofovir infusion and 10-20 mg/kg/dose (maximum dose: 1000 mg) at 2-3 hours and 8-9 hours after cidofovir infusion

Body surface area (BSA)-directed dosing: 1000-2000 mg/**m²**/dose administered 3 hours prior to cidofovir, followed by 500-1250 mg/**m²**/dose 1-2 hours and 8 hours after completion

Adults:

Gonorrhea, uncomplicated infections of cervix, urethra, and rectum: Oral: 1000 mg as a single dose with cefoxitin (CDC, 2010)

Hyperuricemia with gout: Oral: Initial: 250 mg twice daily for 1 week; may increase to 500 mg twice daily; if needed, may increase in 500 mg increments every 4 weeks; maximum daily dose: 2000 mg/**day**. If serum uric acid levels are within normal limits and gout attacks have been absent for 6 months, daily dosage may be reduced by 500 mg increments every 6 months.

Prolongation of penicillin serum levels: Oral: 500 mg 4 times daily; **Note:** Dosing per manufacturer, some indication-specific dosing may vary.

Dosing adjustment in renal impairment: Children ≥2 years, Adolescents, and Adults: CrCl <30 mL/minute: Avoid use

Dosing adjustment in hepatic impairment: There are no dosage adjustments provided in manufacturer's labeling.

Administration Oral: Administer with food or antacids to minimize GI effects

Monitoring Parameters Uric acid, renal function, CBC

Test Interactions False-positive glucosuria with Clinitest®, a falsely high determination of theophylline has occurred and the renal excretion of phenolsulfonphthalein 17-ketosteroids and bromsulfophthalein (BSP) may be inhibited

Dosage Forms Excipient information presented when available (limited, particularly for generics); consult specific product labeling.

Tablet, Oral:

Generic: 500 mg

Procainamide (pro KANE a mide)

Medication Safety Issues

Sound-alike/look-alike issues:

Procanbid may be confused with probenecid, Procan SR

Pronestyl may be confused with Ponstel

High alert medication:

The Institute for Safe Medication Practices (ISMP) includes this medication among its list of drugs which have a heightened risk of causing significant patient harm when used in error.

BEERS Criteria medication:

This drug may be potentially inappropriate for use in geriatric patients (Quality of evidence - high; Strength of recommendation - strong).

Administration issues:

Procainamide hydrochloride is available in 10 mL vials of 100 mg/mL and in 2 mL vials with 500 mg/mL. Note that **BOTH** vials contain 1 gram of drug; confusing the strengths can lead to massive overdoses or underdoses.

Other safety concerns:

PCA is an error-prone abbreviation (mistaken as patient controlled analgesia)

Related Information

Adult ACLS Algorithms *on page 2236*

Pediatric ALS (PALS) Algorithms *on page 2233*

Brand Names: Canada Apo-Procainamide; Procainamide Hydrochloride Injection, USP; Procan SR

Therapeutic Category Antiarrhythmic Agent, Class I-A

Generic Availability (US) Yes

Use Treatment of life-threatening ventricular arrhythmias (FDA approved in adults); has also been used for treatment of paroxysmal supraventricular tachycardia (PSVT) and symptomatic premature ventricular contractions; and to prevent recurrence of ventricular tachycardia

PALS guidelines: Tachycardia with pulses and poor perfusion (probable SVT [unresponsive to vagal maneuvers and adenosine and/or synchronized cardioversion]; probable VT [unresponsive to synchronized cardioversion or adenosine])

ACLS guidelines: Treatment of the following arrhythmias in patients with preserved left ventricular function: Stable monomorphic VT; pre-excited atrial fibrillation; stable wide complex regular tachycardia (likely VT)

Pregnancy Risk Factor C

Pregnancy Considerations Animal reproduction studies have not been conducted. Procainamide crosses the placenta; procainamide and its active metabolite (N-acetyl procainamide) can be detected in the cord blood and neonatal serum.

Breast-Feeding Considerations Procainamide and its metabolite are found in breast milk and concentrations may be higher than in the maternal serum. In a case report, procainamide was used throughout pregnancy with a dose of 2 g/day prior to delivery. After birth (39 weeks gestation) milk and maternal serum concentrations were obtained over 15 hours of a dosing interval. Mean maternal serum concentrations were procainamide 1.1 mcg/mL and N-acetyl procainamide 1.6 mcg/mL. Mean milk concentrations were procainamide 5.4 mcg/mL and N-acetyl procainamide 3.5 mcg/mL. Due to the potential for adverse events in the nursing infant, breast-feeding is not recommended by the manufacturer.

Contraindications Hypersensitivity to procainamide, procaine, other ester-type local anesthetics, or any component of the formulation; complete heart block; second-degree AV block or various types of hemiblock (without a functional artificial pacemaker); SLE; torsade de pointes

Warnings/Precautions Monitor and adjust dose to prevent QTc prolongation. Watch for proarrhythmic effects. Avoid use in patients with QT prolongation (ACLS, 2010). May precipitate or exacerbate HF due to negative inotropic actions; use with caution or avoid (ACLS, 2010) in patients with HF. Correct electrolyte disturbances, especially hypokalemia or hypomagnesemia, prior to use and throughout therapy. Reduce dosage in renal impairment. May increase ventricular response rate in patients with atrial fibrillation or flutter; control AV conduction before initiating. Correct hypokalemia before initiating therapy; hypokalemia may worsen toxicity. Reduce dose if first-degree heart block occurs. Use caution with concurrent use of other antiarrhythmics; may exacerbate or increase the risk of conduction disturbances. Avoid concurrent use with other drugs known to prolong QTc interval. Avoid use in myasthenia gravis (may worsen condition).

Use caution and dose cautiously in older adults; renal clearance of procainamide/NAPA declines in patients ≥50 years of age (independent of creatinine clearance reductions) and in the presence of concomitant renal impairment. In the treatment of atrial fibrillation, avoid antiarrhythmics as first-line treatment. In older adults, data suggests rate control may provide more benefits than risks compared to rhythm control for most patients (Beers Criteria).

The injectable product contains sodium metabisulfite which may cause allergic-type reactions, including anaphylactic symptoms and life-threatening asthmatic episodes in susceptible people; this is seen more frequently in asthmatics. **Note:** Canadian injectable product does not contain sodium metabisulfite.

[U.S. Boxed Warning]: Potentially fatal blood dyscrasias (eg, agranulocytosis) have occurred with therapeutic doses; weekly monitoring is recommended during the first 3 months of therapy and periodically thereafter. Discontinue procainamide if this occurs.

[U.S. Boxed Warning]: Long-term administration leads to the development of a positive antinuclear antibody (ANA) test in 50% of patients which may result in a drug-induced lupus erythematosus-like syndrome (in 20% to 30% of patients); discontinue procainamide with rising ANA titers or with SLE symptoms and choose an alternative agent.

[U.S. Boxed Warning] In the Cardiac Arrhythmia Suppression Trial (CAST), recent (>6 days but <2 years ago) myocardial infarction patients with asymptomatic, non-life-threatening ventricular arrhythmias did not benefit and may have been harmed by attempts to suppress the arrhythmia with flecainide or

encainide. An increased mortality or nonfatal cardiac arrest rate (7.7%) was seen in the active treatment group compared with patients in the placebo group (3%). The applicability of the CAST results to other populations is unknown. Procainamide should be reserved for patients with life-threatening ventricular arrhythmias.

Adverse Reactions

Cardiovascular: Hypotension

Dermatologic: Rash

Gastrointestinal: Diarrhea, nausea, taste disorder, vomiting

Rare but important or life-threatening: Agranulocytosis, alkaline phosphatase increased, angioedema, anorexia, aplastic anemia, arrhythmia exacerbated, arthralgia, asystole, bone marrow suppression, cerebellar ataxia, confusion, demyelinating polyradiculoneuropathy, disorientation, dizziness, drug fever, fever, first degree heart block, flushing, granulomatous hepatitis, hallucinations, hemolytic anemia, hepatic failure, hyperbilirubinemia, hypoplastic anemia, intrahepatic cholestasis, leukopenia, lightheadedness, maculopapular rash, mania, mental depression, myasthenia gravis worsened, myocardial contractility depressed, myocarditis, myopathy, neuromuscular blockade, neutropenia, pancreatitis, pancytopenia, paradoxical increase in ventricular rate in atrial fibrillation/flutter, peripheral/polyneuropathy, pleural effusion, positive Coombs' test, proarrhythmia, pseudo-obstruction, psychosis, pulmonary embolism, QTc-interval prolongation, pruritus, rash, respiratory failure due to myopathy, second-degree heart block, tachycardia, thrombocytopenia, torsade de pointes, transaminases increased, urticaria, vasculitis, ventricular fibrillation, weakness

Drug Interactions

Metabolism/Transport Effects Substrate of CYP2D6 (major), OCT2; **Note:** Assignment of Major/Minor substrate status based on clinically relevant drug interaction potential

Avoid Concomitant Use

Avoid concomitant use of Procainamide with any of the following: Amiodarone; Fingolimod; Highest Risk QTc-Prolonging Agents; Ivabradine; Mifepristone; Moderate Risk QTc-Prolonging Agents; Propafenone

Increased Effect/Toxicity

Procainamide may increase the levels/effects of: Highest Risk QTc-Prolonging Agents; Neuromuscular-Blocking Agents

The levels/effects of Procainamide may be increased by: Abiraterone Acetate; Amiodarone; Cimetidine; Cobicistat; CYP2D6 Inhibitors (Moderate); CYP2D6 Inhibitors (Strong); Darunavir; Fingolimod; Ivabradine; LamoTRIgine; Lurasidone; Mifepristone; Moderate Risk QTc-Prolonging Agents; Peginterferon Alfa-2b; Propafenone; QTc-Prolonging Agents (Indeterminate Risk and Risk Modifying); Ranitidine; Trimethoprim

Decreased Effect

The levels/effects of Procainamide may be decreased by: Peginterferon Alfa-2b

Food Interactions Acute ethanol administration reduces procainamide serum concentrations. Management: Avoid ethanol.

Storage/Stability Store at 20°C to 25°C (68°F to 77°F). The solution is initially colorless but may turn slightly yellow on standing. Injection of air into the vial causes solution to darken. Discard solutions darker than light amber. Color formation may occur upon refrigeration. When admixed in NS or D_5W to a final concentration of 2 to 4 mg/mL, solution is stable at room temperature for 24 hours and for 7 days under refrigeration.

Mechanism of Action Decreases myocardial excitability and conduction velocity and may depress myocardial contractility, by increasing the electrical stimulation threshold of ventricle, His-Purkinje system and through direct cardiac effects

Pharmacodynamics Onset of action: IM 10-30 minutes

Pharmacokinetics (Adult data unless noted)

Distribution: V_d (decreased with CHF or shock):
- Children: 2.2 L/kg
- Adults: 2 L/kg

Protein binding: 15% to 20%

Metabolism: By acetylation in the liver to produce N-acetyl procainamide (NAPA) (active metabolite)

Half-life:
- Procainamide (dependent upon hepatic acetylator phenotype, cardiac function, and renal function):
  - Children: 1.7 hours
  - Adults with normal renal function: 2.5-4.7 hours
- NAPA (dependent upon renal function):
  - Children: 6 hours
  - Adults with normal renal function: 6-8 hours

Time to peak serum concentration: IM: 15-60 minutes

Elimination: Urinary excretion (25% as NAPA)

Dosing: Neonatal Note: Dose must be individualized and titrated to patient's response; monitor serum concentrations.

Supraventricular tachycardia: Limited data available: IV: Loading dose: 7 to 10 mg/kg infused over 60 minutes followed by a continuous IV infusion of 20 to 80 **mcg**/kg/minute; a retrospective study of 20 neonates (GA: ≥25 weeks) reported a mean loading dose of 9.6 ± 1.5 mg/kg and a mean continuous infusion rate of 37.56 ± 13.52 **mcg**/kg/minute; **Note:** Procainamide serum concentrations were supratherapeutic in five neonates studied; four of the five were <36 weeks GA and all five had CrCl < 30 mL/minute/1.73m^2; these results indicate that doses may need to be decreased in preterm neonates and in those with renal impairment (Moffett, 2006)

Dosing: Usual Note: Dose must be individualized and titrated to patient's response; monitor serum concentrations.

Pediatric: **Antiarrhythmic:** Limited data available:

IM: Children and Adolescents: 20 to 30 mg/kg/day divided every 4 to 6 hours; maximum daily dose: 4000 mg/**day** (Nelson, 1996)

IV, I.O.: Infants, Children, and Adolescents:

Loading dose: 10 to 15 mg/kg over 30 to 60 minutes; in adults, maximum dose range: 1000 to 1500 mg (Hegenbarth, 2008; Kliegman, 2011)

Maintenance: Continuous IV infusion: 20 to 80 **mcg**/kg/minute; maximum daily dose: 2000 mg/24 hours (Kliegman, 2011)

Stable wide-complex tachycardia of unknown origin (atrial or ventricular) or SVT (PALS [Kleinman, 2010]): Infants, Children, and Adolescents: **Note:** Avoid or use extreme caution when administering procainamide with other drugs that prolong QT interval (eg, amiodarone); consider consulting with cardiology expert

IV, I.O.: Loading dose: 15 mg/kg infused over 30-60 minutes; monitor ECG and blood pressure; stop the infusion if hypotension occurs or QRS complex widens by >50% of baseline

Adult: **Antiarrhythmic:**

IM: 50 mg/kg/day divided every 3 to 6 hours **or** 0.5 to 1 g every 4 to 8 hours (Koch-Weser, 1971)

IV: Loading dose: 15 to 18 mg/kg administered as slow infusion over 25 to 30 minutes **or** 100 mg/dose at a rate not to exceed 50 mg/minute repeated every 5 minutes as needed to a total dose of 1000 mg

Hemodynamically stable monomorphic VT or pre-excited atrial fibrillation (ACLS [Neumar, 2010]):

Loading dose: Infuse 20 to 50 mg/minute **or** 100 mg every 5 minutes until arrhythmia controlled, hypotension occurs, QRS complex widens by 50% of its original width, or total of 17 mg/kg is given. Follow with a continuous infusion of 1 to 4 mg/minute. **Note:** Not recommended for use in ongoing ventricular fibrillation (VF) or pulseless ventricular tachycardia (VT) due to prolonged administration time and uncertain efficacy.

Maintenance dose: 1 to 4 mg/minute by continuous IV infusion. Maintenance infusions should be reduced by one-third in patients with moderate renal or cardiac impairment and by two-thirds in patients with severe renal or cardiac impairment.

Dosing adjustment in renal impairment:

Infants, Children, and Adolescents: There are no specific recommendations provided in the manufacturer's labeling; dose must be individualized and titrated to patient's response; monitor serum concentrations; some have suggested the following (Aronoff, 2007): **Note:** Renally adjusted dose recommendations are based on a dose of loading dose of 15 mg/kg total.

GFR <10 mL/minute/1.73 m^2:

Loading dose: Reduce dose to 12 mg/kg

Maintenance infusion: Start at lower end of continuous infusion range of 20 to 80 **mcg**/kg/minute

Adults: IV:

Loading dose: Reduce dose to 12 mg/kg in severe renal impairment

Maintenance infusion: Reduce dose by one-third in patients with mild renal impairment. Reduce dose by two-thirds in patients with severe renal impairment.

Dialysis: All patients:

Procainamide: Moderately hemodialyzable (20% to 50%): Monitor procainamide/N-acetylprocainamide (NAPA) levels; supplementation may be necessary

NAPA: Not dialyzable (0% to 5%)

Procainamide/NAPA: Not peritoneal dialyzable (0% to 5%)

Procainamide/NAPA: Replace by blood level during continuous arteriovenous or venovenous hemofiltration

Dosing adjustment in hepatic impairment: Adults:

Manufacturer's labeling: Manufacturer recommends reduction in frequency of administration; specific frequency reduction not described; however, close monitoring of procainamide and NAPA concentrations and clinical effectiveness recommended.

Alternate dosing (Bauer, 2008):

Oral (not available in the U.S.):

Child-Pugh score 8–10: Reduce initial daily dose by 25%. Monitor procainamide/NAPA concentrations closely.

Child-Pugh score >10: Reduce initial daily dose by 50%. Monitor procainamide/NAPA concentrations closely.

IV:

Child-Pugh score 8–10: Reduce continuous infusion dose by 25%. Monitor procainamide/NAPA concentrations closely.

Child-Pugh score >10: Reduce continuous infusion dose by 50%. Monitor procainamide/NAPA concentrations closely.

Preparation for Administration

IV:

Loading dose: Dilute loading dose to a maximum concentration of 20 mg/mL per the manufacturer; concentrations as high as 30 mg/mL have been used in adult studies (Halpern 1980)

Continuous IV infusion: Dilute to a usual final concentration of 2 to 4 mg/mL in D_5W per the manufacturer; in adult patients, concentrations as high as 8 mg/mL have been shown to be stable (Raymond 1988) and utilized by some institutions.

Administration

IM: Not for emergent situations; may be administered undiluted

IV:

Pediatric: **Note:** Infusion rate should be decreased if QT interval becomes prolonged or patient develops heart block; discontinue the infusion if patient develops hypotension or QRS interval widens to >50% of baseline; severe hypotension can occur with rapid IV administration (Hegenbarth 2008; PALS [Kleinman 2010])

Loading dose:

Neonates: Administer over 60 minutes (Moffett 2006)

Infants and Children: Administer over 30 to 60 minutes (Hegenberth 2008; PALS [Kleinman 2010])

Adolescents: Administer at usual infusion rate: 20 to 50 mg/minute not to exceed 50 mg/minute (ACLS [Neumar 2010]; Hegenberth 2008; PALS [Kleinman 2010])

Adult: Usual rate of infusion: 20 to 50 mg/minute; do not administer faster than 50 mg/minute (ACLS [Neumar 2010]); severe hypotension can occur with rapid IV administration.

Continuous IV infusion: Administer via an infusion pump

Rate of infusion (mL/hour) = dose (mcg/kg/minute) x weight (kg) x 60 minutes/hour divided by the concentration

Monitoring Parameters ECG, blood pressure; CBC with differential and platelet counts at weekly intervals for the first 3 months of treatment, periodically thereafter, or if signs of infection, bruising or bleeding occur; antinuclear antibody test (ANA); renal function; serum drug concentrations (procainamide and NAPA) especially in patients with hepatic impairment, renal failure, or those receiving higher maintenance doses (eg, adults: >3 mg/minute) for >24 hours

Reference Range Timing of serum samples: Draw 6 to 12 hours after start of IV infusion; half-life is 2.5 to 5 hours in adults

Therapeutic: Optimal ranges must be ascertained for individual patients, with ECG monitoring

Procainamide: 4 to 10 mcg/mL (SI: 15 to 37 micromoles/L)

Sum of procainamide and N-acetyl procainamide: 10 to 30 mcg/mL (SI: <110 micromoles/L)

Toxic (procainamide): >10-12 mcg/mL (SI: >37-44 micromoles/L)

Test Interactions In the presence of propranolol or supra-pharmacologic concentrations of lidocaine or meprobamate, tests which depend on fluorescence to measure procainamide/NAPA concentrations may be affected.

Dosage Forms Excipient information presented when available (limited, particularly for generics); consult specific product labeling.

Solution, Injection, as hydrochloride:

Generic: 100 mg/mL (10 mL); 500 mg/mL (2 mL)

- **Procainamide Hydrochloride** *see* Procainamide *on page 1769*
- **Procainamide Hydrochloride Injection, USP (Can)** *see* Procainamide *on page 1769*
- **Procaine Amide Hydrochloride** *see* Procainamide *on page 1769*
- **Procaine Benzylpenicillin** *see* Penicillin G Procaine *on page 1659*
- **Procaine Penicillin G** *see* Penicillin G Procaine *on page 1659*
- **Procanbid** *see* Procainamide *on page 1769*
- **Procan SR (Can)** *see* Procainamide *on page 1769*

Procarbazine (proe KAR ba zeen)

Medication Safety Issues

Sound-alike/look-alike issues:

Procarbazine may be confused with dacarbazine

International issues:

Matulane [U.S., Canada] may be confused with Materna brand name for vitamin with minerals [multiple international markets]

High alert medication:

This medication is in a class the Institute for Safe Medication Practices (ISMP) includes among its list of drug classes which have a heightened risk of causing significant patient harm when used in error.

Related Information

Oral Medications That Should Not Be Crushed or Altered *on page 2476*

Prevention of Chemotherapy-Induced Nausea and Vomiting in Children *on page 2368*

Safe Handling of Hazardous Drugs *on page 2455*

Brand Names: US Matulane

Brand Names: Canada Matulane; Natulan

Therapeutic Category Antineoplastic Agent, Miscellaneous

Generic Availability (US) No

Use Treatment of Hodgkin lymphoma [FDA approved in pediatrics (age not specified) and adults]

Pregnancy Risk Factor D

Pregnancy Considerations Adverse events were observed in animal reproduction studies. There are case reports of fetal malformations in the offspring of pregnant women exposed to procarbazine as part of a combination chemotherapy regimen. Women of reproductive potential should avoid becoming pregnant during treatment.

Breast-Feeding Considerations It is not known if procarbazine is excreted in breast milk. Due to the potential for serious adverse reactions in the nursing infant, nursing is not recommended during treatment with procarbazine.

Contraindications Hypersensitivity to procarbazine or any component of the formulation; inadequate bone marrow reserve

Warnings/Precautions Hazardous agent - use appropriate precautions for handling and disposal (NIOSH 2014 [group 1]). Hematologic toxicity (leukopenia and thrombocytopenia) may occur 2-8 weeks after treatment initiation. Allow ≥1 month interval between radiation therapy or myelosuppressive chemotherapy and initiation of procarbazine treatment. Withhold treatment for leukopenia (WBC $<4000/mm^3$) or thrombocytopenia (platelets $<100,000/mm^3$). Monitor for infections due to neutropenia. May cause hemolysis and/or presence of Heinz inclusion bodies in erythrocytes. Procarbazine is associated with a high emetic potential; antiemetics are recommended to prevent nausea and vomiting (Dupuis, 2011; Roila, 2010). May cause diarrhea and stomatitis; withhold treatment for diarrhea or stomatitis. Withhold treatment for CNS toxicity, hemorrhage, or hypersensitivity. Azoospermia and infertility have been reported with procarbazine when used in combination with other chemotherapy agents. Possibly carcinogenic; acute myeloid leukemia and lung cancer have been reported following use.

Use with caution in patients with hepatic or renal impairment. Potentially significant drug-drug interactions may exist, requiring dose or frequency adjustment, additional monitoring, and/or selection of alternative therapy. Possesses MAO inhibitor activity and has potential for severe drug and food interactions; follow MAOI diet (avoid tyramine-containing foods). Avoid ethanol consumption, may cause disulfiram-like reaction. **[U.S. Boxed Warning]: Should be administered under the supervision of an experienced cancer chemotherapy physician.**

Warnings: Additional Pediatric Considerations In pediatric patients, undue toxicity characterized as tremors, coma, and convulsions have been reported rarely; monitor closely with use.

Adverse Reactions

Cardiovascular: Edema, flushing, hypotension, syncope, tachycardia

Central nervous system: Apprehension, ataxia, chills, coma, confusion, depression, dizziness, drowsiness, falling, fatigue, hallucination, headache, hyporeflexia, insomnia, lethargy, nervousness, neuropathy, nightmares, pain, paresthesia, seizure, slurred speech, unsteadiness

Dermatologic: Alopecia, dermatitis, diaphoresis, hyperpigmentation, pruritus, skin rash, urticaria

Endocrine & metabolic: Gynecomastia (in prepubertal and early pubertal males)

Gastrointestinal: Abdominal pain, anorexia, constipation, diarrhea, dysphagia, hematemesis, melena, nausea and vomiting (increasing the dose in a stepwise fashion over several days may minimize), stomatitis, xerostomia

Genitourinary: Azoospermia (reported with combination chemotherapy), hematuria, nocturia, reduced fertility

Hematologic & oncologic: Anemia, bone marrow depression, eosinophilia, hemolysis (in patients with G6PD deficiency), hemolytic anemia, malignant neoplasm (secondary; nonlymphoid; reported with combination therapy), pancytopenia, petechia, purpura, thrombocytopenia

Hepatic: Hepatic insufficiency, jaundice

Hypersensitivity: Hypersensitivity reaction

Infection: Herpes virus infection, increased susceptibility to infection

Neuromuscular & skeletal: Arthralgia, foot-drop, myalgia, tremor, weakness

Ophthalmic: Accommodation disturbance, diplopia, nystagmus, papilledema, photophobia, retinal hemorrhage

Otic: Hearing loss

Renal: Polyuria

Respiratory: Cough, epistaxis, hemoptysis, hoarseness, pleural effusion, pneumonitis, pulmonary toxicity

Miscellaneous: Fever

Drug Interactions

Metabolism/Transport Effects Inhibits Monoamine Oxidase

Avoid Concomitant Use

Avoid concomitant use of Procarbazine with any of the following: Alpha-/Beta-Agonists (Indirect-Acting); Alpha1-Agonists; Amphetamines; Anilidopiperidine Opioids; Antidepressants (Serotonin Reuptake Inhibitor/Antagonist); Apraclonidine; AtoMOXetine; Atropine (Ophthalmic); BCG; BCG (Intravesical); Bezafibrate; Buprenorphine; BuPROPion; BusPIRone; CarBAMazepine; CloZAPine; Cyclobenzaprine; Cyproheptadine; Dapoxetine; Dexmethylphenidate; Dextromethorphan; Diethylpropion; Dipyrone; Hydrocodone; HYDROmorphone; Isometheptene; Levonordefrin; Linezolid; Maprotiline; Meperidine; Mequitazine; Methyldopa; Methylene Blue; Methylphenidate; Mianserin; Mirtazapine; Morphine (Liposomal); Morphine (Systemic); Natalizumab; Oxymorphone; Pholcodine; Pimecrolimus; Pizotifen; Selective Serotonin Reuptake Inhibitors; Serotonin 5-HT1D Receptor Agonists; Serotonin/Norepinephrine Reuptake Inhibitors; Tacrolimus (Topical); Tapentadol; Tetrabenazine; Tetrahydrozoline (Nasal); Tofacitinib; Tricyclic Antidepressants; Tryptophan; Vaccines (Live)

Increased Effect/Toxicity

Procarbazine may increase the levels/effects of: Alpha-/Beta-Agonists (Indirect-Acting); Alpha1-Agonists; Amphetamines; Antidepressants (Serotonin Reuptake Inhibitor/Antagonist); Antihypertensives; Antipsychotic Agents; Apraclonidine; AtoMOXetine; Atropine (Ophthalmic); Beta2-Agonists; Betahistine; Bezafibrate; Blood Glucose Lowering Agents; Brimonidine (Ophthalmic);

Brimonidine (Topical); BuPROPion; Carbocisteine; CloZAPine; Cyproheptadine; Dexmethylphenidate; Dextromethorphan; Diethylpropion; Domperidone; Doxapram; Doxylamine; EPINEPHrine (Nasal); Epinephrine (Racemic); EPINEPHrine (Systemic, Oral Inhalation); Hydrocodone; HYDROmorphone; Isometheptene; Leflunomide; Levonordefrin; Linezolid; Lithium; Meperidine; Mequitazine; Methadone; Methyldopa; Methylene Blue; Methylphenidate; Metoclopramide; Mianserin; Mirtazapine; Morphine (Liposomal); Morphine (Systemic); Natalizumab; Norepinephrine; Orthostatic Hypotension Producing Agents; OxyCODONE; Pizotifen; Reserpine; Selective Serotonin Reuptake Inhibitors; Serotonin 5-HT1D Receptor Agonists; Serotonin Modulators; Serotonin/Norepinephrine Reuptake Inhibitors; Tetrahydrozoline (Nasal); Tofacitinib; Tricyclic Antidepressants; Vaccines (Live)

The levels/effects of Procarbazine may be increased by: Altretamine; Anilidopiperidine Opioids; Antiemetics (5HT3 Antagonists); Antipsychotic Agents; Buprenorphine; BusPIRone; CarBAMazepine; COMT Inhibitors; Cyclobenzaprine; Dapoxetine; Denosumab; Dipyrone; Levodopa; MAO Inhibitors; Maprotiline; Oxymorphone; Pholcodine; Pimecrolimus; Roflumilast; Tacrolimus (Topical); Tapentadol; Tedizolid; Tetrabenazine; TraMADol; Trastuzumab; Tryptophan

Decreased Effect

Procarbazine may decrease the levels/effects of: BCG; BCG (Intravesical); Coccidioides immitis Skin Test; Domperidone; Sipuleucel-T; Vaccines (Inactivated); Vaccines (Live)

The levels/effects of Procarbazine may be decreased by: Cyproheptadine; Domperidone; Echinacea

Food Interactions

Ethanol: Ethanol may cause a disulfiram reaction. Management: Avoid ethanol.

Food: Concurrent ingestion of foods rich in tyramine, dopamine, tyrosine, phenylalanine, tryptophan, or caffeine may cause sudden and severe high blood pressure (hypertensive crisis or serotonin syndrome). Management: Avoid tyramine-containing foods (aged or matured cheese, air-dried or cured meats including sausages and salamis; fava or broad bean pods, tap/draft beers, Marmite concentrate, sauerkraut, soy sauce, and other soybean condiments). Food's freshness is also an important concern; improperly stored or spoiled food can create an environment in which tyramine concentrations may increase. Avoid foods containing dopamine, tyrosine, phenylalanine, tryptophan, or caffeine.

Storage/Stability Protect from light.

Mechanism of Action Inhibits DNA, RNA, and protein synthesis by inhibiting transmethylation of methionine into transfer RNA; may also damage DNA directly through alkylation.

Pharmacokinetics (Adult data unless noted)

Absorption: Oral: Well absorbed

Distribution: Crosses the blood-brain barrier and distributes into CSF, liver, kidney, intestine, and skin

Metabolism: In the liver; first-pass conversion to cytotoxic metabolites

Half-life: 10 minutes

Time to peak serum concentration: Within 1 hour

Elimination: In urine (<5% as unchanged drug) and 70% as metabolites

Dosing: Usual Note: Refer to individual protocols for specific dosage and interval information. Procarbazine is associated with a high emetic potential; antiemetics are recommended to prevent nausea and vomiting. The manufacturer suggests that an estimated lean body mass be used in obese patients and patients with rapid weight gain due to edema, ascites, or abnormal fluid retention.

Pediatric: **Hodgkin lymphoma:** Oral:

MOPP regimen: **Note:** While procarbazine is approved as part of the MOPP regimen, the MOPP regimen is generally no longer used due to improved toxicity profiles with other combination regimens used in the treatment of Hodgkin lymphoma (Kelly, 2012). Manufacturer's labeling: Infants, Children, and Adolescents: 50-100 mg/m²/day once daily for 14 days of a 28-day cycle (Longo, 1986).

BEACOPP regimen: Limited data available: Children and Adolescents: 100 mg/m² days 0-6 of a 21-day treatment cycle (in combination with bleomycin, etoposide, doxorubicin, cyclophosphamide, vincristine, and prednisone) for 4 cycles (Kelly, 2011)

Adult: **Hodgkin lymphoma:** Oral:

MOPP regimen: While procarbazine is approved as part of the MOPP regimen, the MOPP regimen is generally no longer used due to improved toxicity profiles with other combination regimens used in the treatment of Hodgkin lymphoma.

BEACOPP, standard or escalated regimen: Limited data available: 100 mg/m² days 1-7 every 21 days (in combination with bleomycin, etoposide, doxorubicin, cyclophosphamide, vincristine, and prednisone) for 8 cycles (Diehl, 2003)

Dosing adjustment in renal impairment: All patients: There are no dosage adjustments provided in manufacturer's labeling; use with caution; may result in increased toxicity. However, because predominantly inactive metabolites are excreted via the kidneys, dosage adjustment is not necessary (Kintzel, 1995).

Dosing adjustment in hepatic impairment: All patients: There are no dosage adjustments provided in manufacturer's labeling; use with caution; may result in increased toxicity. The following adjustments have been reported in literature:

Floyd, 2006:

Transaminases 1.6-6 times ULN: Administer 75% of dose

Transaminases >6 times ULN: Use clinical judgment

Serum bilirubin >5 mg/dL or transaminases >3 times ULN: Avoid use

King, 2001: Adults: Serum bilirubin >5 mg/dL or transaminases >180 units/L: Avoid use

Administration Hazardous agent; use appropriate precautions for handling and disposal (NIOSH 2014 [group 1]).

Oral: Total daily dose may be administered as a single daily dose or in divided doses throughout the day to minimize GI toxicity. Procarbazine is associated with a high emetic potential; antiemetics are recommended to prevent nausea and vomiting.

Monitoring Parameters CBC with differential, platelet and reticulocyte count (at least every 3-4 days); also urinalysis (weekly), liver function test (prior to therapy and weekly), renal function test (prior to therapy and weekly), alkaline phosphatase (weekly). Monitor for infections, CNS toxicity, and gastrointestinal toxicities.

Dosage Forms Excipient information presented when available (limited, particularly for generics); consult specific product labeling.

Capsule, Oral, as hydrochloride:

Matulane: 50 mg

Extemporaneous Preparations Hazardous agent: Use appropriate precautions for handling and disposal (NIOSH 2014 [group 1]).

A 10 mg/mL oral suspension may be prepared using capsules, glycerin, and strawberry syrup. Empty the contents of ten 50 mg capsules into a mortar. Add 2 mL glycerin and mix to a thick uniform paste. Add 10 mL strawberry syrup in incremental proportions; mix until uniform. Transfer the mixture to an amber glass bottle and rinse mortar with small amounts of strawberry syrup; add rinses to the bottle in sufficient quantity to make 50 mL. Label "shake well" and "protect from light". Stable for 7 days at room temperature.

Matulane® data on file, Sigma Tau Pharmaceuticals, Inc.

- **Procarbazine Hydrochloride** *see* Procarbazine *on page 1772*
- **Procardia** *see* NIFEdipine *on page 1516*
- **Procardia XL** *see* NIFEdipine *on page 1516*
- **PRO-Cefadroxil (Can)** *see* Cefadroxil *on page 387*
- **PRO-Cefuroxime (Can)** *see* Cefuroxime *on page 414*
- **ProCentra** *see* Dextroamphetamine *on page 625*
- **Procet-30 (Can)** *see* Acetaminophen and Codeine *on page 50*

Prochlorperazine (proe klor PER a zeen)

Medication Safety Issues

Sound-alike/look-alike issues:

Prochlorperazine may be confused with chlorproMAZINE

Compazine may be confused with Copaxone, Coumadin

BEERS Criteria medication:

This drug may be potentially inappropriate for use in geriatric patients (Quality of evidence - varies based on comorbidity; Strength of recommendation - varies based on comorbidity)

Other safety concerns:

CPZ (occasional abbreviation for Compazine) is an error-prone abbreviation (mistaken as chlorpromazine)

Brand Names: US Compazine; Compro

Brand Names: Canada Apo-Prochlorperazine; Nu-Prochlor; PMS-Prochlorperazine; Sandoz-Prochlorperazine

Therapeutic Category Antiemetic; Antipsychotic Agent, Typical, Phenothiazine; First Generation (Typical) Antipsychotic; Phenothiazine Derivative

Generic Availability (US) Yes

Use

Oral: Management of nonsurgical nausea and vomiting [FDA approved in ages ≥2 years (and at least 9 kg) and adults]; management of surgery-related nausea and vomiting (FDA approved in adults); treatment of acute and chronic psychosis [FDA approved in ages ≥2 years (and at least 9 kg) and adults]; has also been used for treatment of intractable migraine headaches

Parenteral: Management of severe nonsurgical nausea and vomiting [FDA approved in ages ≥2 years (and at least 9 kg) and adults]; treatment of schizophrenia [FDA approved in ages ≥2 years (and at least 9 kg) and adults]

Rectal: Management of severe nausea and vomiting (FDA approved in adults)

Pregnancy Considerations Jaundice or hyper- or hyporeflexia have been reported in newborn infants following maternal use of phenothiazines. Antipsychotic use during the third trimester of pregnancy has a risk for abnormal muscle movements (extrapyramidal symptoms [EPS]) and withdrawal symptoms in newborns following delivery. Symptoms in the newborn may include agitation, feeding disorder, hypertonia, hypotonia, respiratory distress, somnolence, and tremor; these effects may be self-limiting or require hospitalization. Use may interfere with pregnancy tests, causing false positive results. Prochlorperazine has been used for the treatment of nausea and vomiting associated with pregnancy (Levicheck 2002; Mahadevan 2006); however, other agents may be preferred (ACOG 2004).

Breast-Feeding Considerations Other phenothiazines are excreted in human milk; excretion of prochlorperazine is not known.

Contraindications

Hypersensitivity to prochlorperazine or any component of the formulation (cross-reactivity between phenothiazines may occur); coma or presence of large amounts of CNS depressants (eg, alcohol, opioids, barbiturates); postoperative management of nausea/vomiting following pediatric surgery; use in infants and children <2 years or <9 kg; pediatric conditions for which dosage has not been established

Documentation of allergenic cross-reactivity for phenothiazines is limited. However, because of similarities in chemical structure and/or pharmacologic actions, the possibility of cross-sensitivity cannot be ruled out with certainty.

Canadian labeling: Additional contraindications (not in US labeling): Presence of circulatory collapse; severe cardiovascular disorders; altered state of consciousness; concomitant use of high dose hypnotics; severe depression; presence of blood dyscrasias, hepatic or renal impairment, or pheochromocytoma; suspected or established subcortical brain damage with or without hypothalamic damage

Warnings/Precautions [US Boxed Warning]: Elderly patients with dementia-related psychosis treated with antipsychotics are at an increased risk of death (compared to placebo). This was based on analyses of 17 placebo-controlled trials (duration ~10 weeks), predominantly in patients taking atypical antipsychotics which revealed a risk of death in drug-treated patients between 1.6 and 1.7 times the risk of death in placebo-treated patients. Over the course of a typical 10-week controlled trial, the rate of death in drug-treated patients was ~4.5% compared with ~2.6% in the placebo group. Although the causes of death varied, most deaths appeared to be either cardiovascular (eg, heart failure, sudden death) or infectious (eg, pneumonia) in nature. Observational studies suggest that, similar to atypical antipsychotic drugs, treatment with conventional antipsychotic drugs may increase mortality, although the extent to which increased mortality may be attributed to the antipsychotic drug as opposed to some characteristic(s) of the patients is not clear. Prochlorperazine is not approved for the treatment of dementia-related psychosis.

Prochlorperazine may cause extrapyramidal symptoms (EPS), including pseudoparkinsonism, acute dystonic reactions, akathisia, and tardive dyskinesia. Risk of dystonia (and possibly other EPS) may be greater with increased doses, use of conventional antipsychotics, males, and younger patients. Risk of tardive dyskinesia and potential for irreversibility often associated with total cumulative dose and therapy duration and may also be increased in elderly patients (particularly elderly women); antipsychotics may also mask signs/symptoms of tardive dyskinesia. Consider therapy discontinuation with signs/symptoms of tardive dyskinesia. Antipsychotic use has been associated with esophageal dysmotility and aspiration; use with caution in patients at risk of pneumonia (ie, Alzheimer's disease).

May be sedating and impair physical or mental abilities; use with caution in disorders where CNS depression is a feature. Use with caution in Parkinson's disease; hemodynamic instability; predisposition to seizures; subcortical brain damage; and in severe cardiac, hepatic, or renal disease. Canadian labeling contraindicates use in patients with severe cardiac disease, hepatic or renal impairment, subcortical brain damage, and circulatory collapse. May alter temperature regulation, obscure intestinal obstruction or brain tumor or mask toxicity of other drugs. May alter cardiac conduction. Hypotension may occur following administration, particularly when parenteral form is used or in high dosages. May cause orthostatic hypotension; use with caution in patients at risk of this effect or in those who would not tolerate transient hypotensive episodes (cerebrovascular disease, cardiovascular disease, hypovolemia, or concurrent medication use which may predispose to hypotension/bradycardia).

Leukopenia, neutropenia, and agranulocytosis (sometimes fatal) have been reported in clinical trials and postmarketing reports with antipsychotic use; presence of risk factors (eg, preexisting low WBC or history of drug-induced leuko-/neutropenia) should prompt periodic blood count assessment. Discontinue therapy at first signs of blood dyscrasias or if absolute neutrophil count <1000/mm^3.

Due to its potent anticholinergic effects, may be inappropriate in older adults depending on comorbidities (eg, dementia, delirium) (Beers Criteria). Use with caution in patients with decreased gastrointestinal motility, urinary retention, BPH, xerostomia, visual problems, or narrow-angle glaucoma (screening is recommended). Use caution with exposure to heat. May cause pigmentary retinopathy, and lenticular and corneal deposits, particularly with prolonged therapy. Use associated with increased prolactin levels; clinical significance of hyperprolactinemia in patients with breast cancer or other prolactin-dependent tumors is unknown. Avoid use in patients with signs/symptoms suggestive of Reye's syndrome. Children with acute illness or dehydration are more susceptible to neuromuscular reactions; use cautiously. May be associated with neuroleptic malignant syndrome (NMS). Some dosage forms may contain sodium sulfite.

Benzyl alcohol and derivatives: Some dosage forms may contain benzyl alcohol; large amounts of benzyl alcohol (≥99 mg/kg/day) have been associated with a potentially fatal toxicity ("gasping syndrome") in neonates; the "gasping syndrome" consists of metabolic acidosis, respiratory distress, gasping respirations, CNS dysfunction (including convulsions, intracranial hemorrhage), hypotension, and cardiovascular collapse (AAP 1997; CDC 1982); some data suggests that benzoate displaces bilirubin from protein binding sites (Ahlfors 2001); avoid or use dosage forms containing benzyl alcohol with caution in neonates. See manufacturer's labeling. Potentially significant drug-drug interactions may exist, requiring dose or frequency adjustment, additional monitoring, and/or selection of alternative therapy.

Warnings: Additional Pediatric Considerations High incidence of extrapyramidal reactions especially in children reported, reserve use in children <5 years of age to those who are unresponsive to other antiemetics. Incidence of extrapyramidal reactions is increased with acute illnesses such as chicken pox, measles, CNS infections, gastroenteritis, and dehydration, Extrapyramidal reactions may also be confused with CNS signs of Reye syndrome or other encephalopathies; avoid use in these clinical conditions.

Adverse Reactions Reported with prochlorperazine or other phenothiazines.

Cardiovascular: Cardiac arrest, cerebral edema, hypotension, peripheral edema, Q-wave distortions, sudden death, T-wave distortions

Central nervous system: Agitation, altered cerebrospinal fluid proteins, catatonia, coma, cough reflex suppressed, dizziness, drowsiness, fever (mild [IM]), headache, hyperpyrexia, impairment of temperature regulation, insomnia, neuroleptic malignant syndrome (NMS), oculogyric crisis, opisthotonos, restlessness, seizure, somnolence, tremulousness

Dermatologic: Angioedema, contact dermatitis, epithelial keratopathy, erythema, eczema, exfoliative dermatitis, itching, photosensitivity, skin pigmentation, urticaria

Endocrine & metabolic: Amenorrhea, galactorrhea, gynecomastia, glucosuria, hyper-/hypoglycemia, lactation, libido (changes in), menstrual irregularity

Gastrointestinal: Appetite increased, atonic colon, constipation, ileus, nausea, obstipation, vomiting, weight gain, xerostomia

Genitourinary: Ejaculating dysfunction, ejaculatory disturbances, impotence, priapism, urinary retention

Hematologic: Agranulocytosis, aplastic anemia, eosinophilia, hemolytic anemia, leukopenia, pancytopenia, thrombocytopenic purpura

Hepatic: Biliary stasis, cholestatic jaundice, hepatotoxicity

Neuromuscular & skeletal: Dystonias (torticollis, carpopedal spasm, trismus, protrusion of tongue); extrapyramidal symptoms (pseudoparkinsonism, akathisia, dystonias, tardive dyskinesia, hyperreflexia); SLE-like syndrome, tremor

Ocular: Blurred vision, lenticular/corneal deposits, miosis, mydriasis, pigmentary retinopathy

Respiratory: Asthma, laryngeal edema, nasal congestion

Miscellaneous: Allergic reactions, asphyxia, diaphoresis

Drug Interactions

Metabolism/Transport Effects None known.

Avoid Concomitant Use

Avoid concomitant use of Prochlorperazine with any of the following: Aclidinium; Amisulpride; Azelastine (Nasal); Dofetilide; Eluxadoline; Glucagon; Ipratropium (Oral Inhalation); Metoclopramide; Orphenadrine; Paraldehyde; Potassium Chloride; Sulpiride; Thalidomide; Tiotropium; Umeclidinium

Increased Effect/Toxicity

Prochlorperazine may increase the levels/effects of: AbobotulinumtoxinA; Alcohol (Ethyl); Amisulpride; Analgesics (Opioid); Anticholinergic Agents; Antidepressants (Serotonin Reuptake Inhibitor/Antagonist); Azelastine (Nasal); Beta-Blockers; Buprenorphine; CNS Depressants; Dofetilide; Eluxadoline; Glucagon; Hydrocodone; Mequitazine; Methotrimeprazine; Methylphenidate; Metyrosine; Mirabegron; Mirtazapine; OnabotulinumtoxinA; Orphenadrine; Paraldehyde; Porfimer; Potassium Chloride; RimabotulinumtoxinB; Selective Serotonin Reuptake Inhibitors; Serotonin Modulators; Sulpiride; Suvorexant; Thalidomide; Thiazide Diuretics; Thiopental; Tiotropium; Topiramate; Verteporfin; Zolpidem

The levels/effects of Prochlorperazine may be increased by: Acetylcholinesterase Inhibitors (Central); Aclidinium; Antidepressants (Serotonin Reuptake Inhibitor/Antagonist); Antimalarial Agents; Beta-Blockers; Brimonidine (Topical); Cannabis; Deferoxamine; Doxylamine; Dronabinol; Droperidol; HydrOXYzine; Ipratropium (Oral Inhalation); Kava Kava; Lithium; Magnesium Sulfate; Methotrimeprazine; Methylphenidate; Metoclopramide; Metyrosine; Mianserin; Nabilone; Perampanel; Pramlintide; Rufinamide; Serotonin Modulators; Sodium Oxybate; Tapentadol; Tetrabenazine; Tetrahydrocannabinol; Umeclidinium

Decreased Effect

Prochlorperazine may decrease the levels/effects of: Acetylcholinesterase Inhibitors; Amphetamines; Anti-Parkinson's Agents (Dopamine Agonist); Itopride; Quinagolide; Secretin

The levels/effects of Prochlorperazine may be decreased by: Acetylcholinesterase Inhibitors; Antacids; Anti-Parkinson's Agents (Dopamine Agonist); Lithium

Storage/Stability

Injection:

Edisylate: Store at 20°C to 25°C (68°F to 77°F); do not freeze. Protect from light. Clear or slightly yellow solutions may be used.

Mesylate (Canadian availability; not available in US): Store at 15°C to 30°C (59°F to 86°F). Protect from light. Do not use if solution is discolored or hazy.

IV infusion: Injection may be diluted in 50 to 100 mL NS or D_5W.

Suppository: Store at 20°C to 25°C (68°F to 77°F). Do not remove from wrapper until ready to use.

Tablet: Store at 20°C to 25°C (68°F to 77°F). Protect from light.

Mechanism of Action Prochlorperazine is a piperazine phenothiazine antipsychotic which blocks postsynaptic mesolimbic dopaminergic D_1 and D_2 receptors in the brain, including the chemoreceptor trigger zone; exhibits a strong alpha-adrenergic and anticholinergic blocking effect and depresses the release of hypothalamic and hypophyseal hormones; believed to depress the reticular activating system, thus affecting basal metabolism, body temperature, wakefulness, vasomotor tone and emesis

Pharmacodynamics

Onset of action:

Oral: 30-40 minutes

IM: Within 10-20 minutes

Rectal: Within 60 minutes

Duration:

IM: 3-4 hours

Rectal, oral immediate release: 3-4 hours

Dosing: Usual

Children and Adolescents: **Note:** Use lowest possible dose in pediatric patients to decrease incidence of extrapyramidal reactions

Antiemetic: Children ≥2 years and weight ≥9 kg and Adolescents:

Oral:

9-13 kg: 2.5 mg every 12-24 hours as needed; maximum daily dose: 7.5 mg/**day**

>13-18 kg: 2.5 mg every 8-12 hours as needed; maximum daily dose: 10 mg/**day**

>18-39 kg: 2.5 mg every 8 hours **or** 5 mg every 12 hours as needed; maximum daily dose: 15 mg/**day**

>39 kg: 5-10 mg every 6-8 hours; usual maximum daily dose: 40 mg/**day**

Parenteral (as edisylate): Administer based upon patient response, typically every 8-12 hours; convert to oral therapy as soon as possible.

Manufacturer's labeling: IM: 0.13 mg/kg/dose; maximum single dose: 10 mg

Alternate dosing: IM, IV: 0.1-0.15 mg/kg/dose; maximum single dose: 10 mg

Migraine, intractable: Limited data available: Children ≥8 years and Adolescents: IV (as edisylate): 0.1-0.15 mg/kg as a single dose has been studied in 20 children between the ages of 8-17 years combined with IV hydration (Kabbouche, 2001)

Psychoses; schizophrenia: Children 2-12 years and ≥9 kg:

Oral: 2.5 mg every 8-12 hours; initial maximum daily dose: 10 mg/day on first day; may increase dosage as needed; maximum daily dose: Children 2-5 years: 20 mg/**day**; Children 6-12 years: 25 mg/**day**

IM (as edisylate): 0.13 mg/kg/dose, control usually obtained with single dose; change to oral as soon as possible

Adults:

Antiemetic:

Oral (tablet): 5-10 mg 3-4 times/**day**; usual maximum: 40 mg/day; larger doses may rarely be required

IM (as edisylate): 5-10 mg every 3-4 hours; usual maximum: 40 mg/**day**

IV (as edisylate): 2.5-10 mg; maximum: 10 mg/dose or 40 mg/**day**; may repeat dose every 3-4 hours as needed

Rectal: 25 mg twice daily

Surgical nausea/vomiting: Note: Should not exceed 40 mg/**day**:

IM (as edisylate): 5-10 mg 1-2 hours before induction or to control symptoms during or after surgery; may repeat once if necessary

IV (as edisylate): 5-10 mg 15-30 minutes before induction or to control symptoms during or after surgery; may repeat once if necessary

Antipsychotic:

Oral: 5-10 mg 3-4 times/day; titrate dose slowly every 2-3 days; doses up to 150 mg/**day** may be required in some patients for treatment of severe disturbances

IM (as edisylate): Initial: 10-20 mg; if necessary repeat initial dose every 1-4 hours to gain control; more than 3-4 doses are rarely needed. If parenteral administration is still required, give 10-20 mg every 4-6 hours; change to oral as soon as possible.

Nonpsychotic anxiety: Oral (tablet): Usual dose: 15-20 mg/**day** in divided doses; do not give doses >20 mg/**day** or for longer than 12 weeks

Administration

Oral: Administer with food or water

Parenteral: IM is preferred; avoid IV administration; if necessary, may be administered by direct IV injection at a maximum rate of 5 mg/minute; do not administer by SubQ route (tissue damage may occur)

Monitoring Parameters CBC with differential and periodic ophthalmic exams (if chronically used)

Test Interactions False-positives for phenylketonuria, pregnancy

Additional Information Previously recommended rectal dosages in pediatric patients were similar to the oral formulation dosages; however, an appropriate dosage form for rectal administration to pediatric patients is no longer available in the U.S.

Dosage Forms Excipient information presented when available (limited, particularly for generics); consult specific product labeling.

Solution, Injection, as edisylate [strength expressed as base]:

Generic: 5 mg/mL (2 mL, 10 mL)

Suppository, Rectal:

Compazine: 25 mg (12 ea)

Compro: 25 mg (12 ea)

Generic: 25 mg (12 ea, 1000 ea)

Tablet, Oral, as maleate [strength expressed as base]:

Compazine: 5 mg, 10 mg

Generic: 5 mg, 10 mg

◆ **Prochlorperazine Edisylate** *see* Prochlorperazine *on page 1774*

◆ **Prochlorperazine Maleate** *see* Prochlorperazine *on page 1774*

◆ **Prochlorperazine Mesylate** *see* Prochlorperazine *on page 1774*

◆ **PRO-Ciprofloxacin (Can)** *see* Ciprofloxacin (Systemic) *on page 463*

◆ **PRO-Clonazepam (Can)** *see* ClonazePAM *on page 506*

◆ **Procrit** *see* Epoetin Alfa *on page 765*

◆ **Proctocort** *see* Hydrocortisone (Topical) *on page 1041*

◆ **Procto-Pak** *see* Hydrocortisone (Topical) *on page 1041*

◆ **Proctosol HC** *see* Hydrocortisone (Topical) *on page 1041*

◆ **Proctozone-HC** *see* Hydrocortisone (Topical) *on page 1041*

◆ **Procysbi™** *see* Cysteamine (Systemic) *on page 564*

◆ **Procysbi** *see* Cysteamine (Systemic) *on page 564*

◆ **Procytox (Can)** *see* Cyclophosphamide *on page 551*

◆ **PRO-Dexamethasone (Can)** *see* Dexamethasone (Systemic) *on page 610*

◆ **PRO-Diclo-Rapide (Can)** *see* Diclofenac (Systemic) *on page 641*

◆ **PRO-Enalapril (Can)** *see* Enalapril *on page 744*

- ◆ **Profilnine SD** *see* Factor IX Complex (Human) [(Factors II, IX, X)] *on page 836*
- ◆ **PRO-Fluconazole (Can)** *see* Fluconazole *on page 881*
- ◆ **PRO-Fluoxetine (Can)** *see* FLUoxetine *on page 906*
- ◆ **PRO-Gabapentin (Can)** *see* Gabapentin *on page 954*
- ◆ **PRO-Glyburide (Can)** *see* GlyBURIDE *on page 975*
- ◆ **Proglycem** *see* Diazoxide *on page 639*
- ◆ **Proglycem® (Can)** *see* Diazoxide *on page 639*
- ◆ **Prograf** *see* Tacrolimus (Systemic) *on page 1999*
- ◆ **Proguanil and Atovaquone** *see* Atovaquone and Proguanil *on page 224*
- ◆ **Proguanil Hydrochloride and Atovaquone** *see* Atovaquone and Proguanil *on page 224*
- ◆ **PRO-Hydroxyquine (Can)** *see* Hydroxychloroquine *on page 1052*
- ◆ **Pro-Indo (Can)** *see* Indomethacin *on page 1101*
- ◆ **Prokine** *see* Sargramostim *on page 1905*
- ◆ **Proleukin** *see* Aldesleukin *on page 89*
- ◆ **PRO-Levetiracetam (Can)** *see* LevETIRAcetam *on page 1234*
- ◆ **PRO-Lisinopril (Can)** *see* Lisinopril *on page 1280*
- ◆ **PRO-Lorazepam (Can)** *see* LORazepam *on page 1299*
- ◆ **PRO-Lovastatin (Can)** *see* Lovastatin *on page 1305*
- ◆ **PRO-Metformin (Can)** *see* MetFORMIN *on page 1375*

Promethazine (proe METH a zeen)

Medication Safety Issues

Sound-alike/look-alike issues:

Promethazine may be confused with chlorproMAZINE, predniSONE

Phenergan may be confused with PHENobarbital, Phrenilin, Theragran

High alert medication:

The Institute for Safe Medication Practices (ISMP) includes this medication (IV formulation) among its list of drugs which have a heightened risk of causing significant patient harm when used in error.

BEERS Criteria medication:

This drug may be potentially inappropriate for use in geriatric patients (Quality of evidence - high; Strength of recommendation - strong).

Administration issues:

To prevent or minimize tissue damage during IV administration, the Institute for Safe Medication Practices (ISMP) has the following recommendations:

- Limit concentration available to the 25 mg/mL product
- Consider limiting initial doses to 6.25 to 12.5 mg
- Further dilute the 25 mg/mL strength into 10 to 20 mL NS
- Administer through a large bore vein (not hand or wrist)
- Administer via running IV line at port farthest from patient's vein
- Consider administering over 10 to 15 minutes
- Instruct patients to report immediately signs of pain or burning

International issues:

Sominex: Brand name for promethazine in Great Britain, but also is a brand name for diphenhydrAMINE in the US

Related Information

Management of Drug Extravasations *on page 2298*

Brand Names: US Phenadoz; Phenergan; Promethegan

Brand Names: Canada Bioniche Promethazine; Histantil; Phenergan; PMS-Promethazine

Therapeutic Category Antiemetic; Phenothiazine Derivative; Sedative

Generic Availability (US) Yes

Use Symptomatic treatment of various allergic conditions and motion sickness, sedative, antiemetic; adjunct to postoperative analgesia and anesthesia (FDA approved in ages ≥2 years and adults)

Pregnancy Risk Factor C

Pregnancy Considerations Teratogenic effects were not observed in animal reproduction studies. Promethazine crosses the placenta. Maternal promethazine use has generally not resulted in an increased risk of birth defects. Platelet aggregation may be inhibited in newborns following maternal use of promethazine within 2 weeks of delivery. Promethazine is used for the treatment of nausea and vomiting of pregnancy (refer to current guidelines). Promethazine is also indicated for use during labor for obstetric sedation and may be used alone or as an adjunct to opioid analgesics.

Breast-Feeding Considerations It is not known if promethazine is excreted in breast milk. According to the manufacturer, the decision to continue or discontinue breast-feeding during therapy should take into account the risk of exposure to the infant and the benefits of treatment to the mother. Antihistamines may decrease maternal serum prolactin concentrations when administered prior to the establishment of nursing.

Contraindications Hypersensitivity to promethazine or any component of the formulation (cross-reactivity between phenothiazines may occur); coma; treatment of lower respiratory tract symptoms, including asthma; children <2 years of age; intra-arterial or subcutaneous administration

Warnings/Precautions **[US Boxed Warning]: Respiratory fatalities have been reported in children <2 years of age. Contraindicated in children <2 years of age. In children ≥2 years, use the lowest possible dose; other drugs with respiratory depressant effects should be avoided.**

[US Boxed Warning]: Promethazine injection can cause severe tissue injury (including gangrene) regardless of the route of administration. Tissue irritation and damage may result from perivascular extravasation, unintentional intra-arterial administration, and intraneuronal or perineuronal infiltration. In addition to gangrene, adverse events reported include tissue necrosis, abscesses, burning, pain, erythema, edema, paralysis, severe spasm of distal vessels, phlebitis, thrombophlebitis, venous thrombosis, sensory loss, paralysis, and palsies. Surgical intervention including fasciotomy, skin graft, and/or amputation have been necessary in some cases. The preferred route of administration is by deep intramuscular (IM) injection. Subcutaneous administration is contraindicated. Discontinue intravenous injection immediately with onset of pain and evaluate for arterial injection or perivascular extravasation. Although there is no proven successful management of unintentional intra-arterial injection or perivascular extravasation, sympathetic block and heparinization have been used in the acute management of unintentional intra-arterial injection based on results from animal studies. Vesicant; for IV administration (**not** the preferred route of administration), ensure proper needle or catheter placement prior to and during administration; avoid extravasation.

May be sedating; use with caution in disorders where CNS depression is a feature. May impair physical or mental abilities; patients must be cautioned about performing tasks which require mental alertness. Use with caution in hemodynamic instability; bone marrow suppression;

subcortical brain damage; and in severe cardiac or respiratory disease. Use with caution in patients with hepatic impairment; cholestatic jaundice has been reported with use. Avoid use in pediatric patients with signs and symptoms of hepatic disease (extrapyramidal symptoms caused by promethazine may be confused with CNS signs of hepatic disease). Avoid use in Reye's syndrome. May lower seizure threshold; use caution in persons with seizure disorders or in persons using opioids or local anesthetics which may also affect seizure threshold. May alter temperature regulation or mask toxicity of other drugs due to antiemetic effects. May alter cardiac conduction (life-threatening arrhythmias have occurred with therapeutic doses of phenothiazines). May cause orthostatic hypotension; use with caution in patients at risk of hypotension or where transient hypotensive episodes would be poorly tolerated (cardiovascular disease or cerebrovascular disease).

Phenothiazines may cause anticholinergic effects; therefore, they should be used with caution in patients with decreased gastrointestinal motility, GI or GU obstruction, urinary retention, BPH, xerostomia, or visual problems. Conditions which also may be exacerbated by cholinergic blockade include narrow-angle glaucoma (screening is recommended) and worsening of myasthenia gravis. Use with caution in Parkinson's disease. May cause extrapyramidal symptoms, including pseudoparkinsonism, acute dystonic reactions, akathisia, and tardive dyskinesia. May be associated with neuroleptic malignant syndrome (NMS). May cause photosensitivity. In the elderly, avoid use of this potent anticholinergic agent due to increased risk of confusion, dry mouth, constipation, and other anticholinergic effects; clearance decreases in patients of advanced age (Beers Criteria). Injection may contain sodium metabisulfite.

Warnings: Additional Pediatric Considerations Children with dehydration are at increased risk for development of dystonic reactions from promethazine.

Adverse Reactions

Cardiovascular: Bradycardia, hyper-/hypotension, nonspecific QT changes, orthostatic hypotension, tachycardia,

Central nervous system: Agitation akathisia, catatonic states, confusion, delirium, disorientation, dizziness, drowsiness, dystonias, euphoria, excitation, extrapyramidal symptoms, faintness, fatigue, hallucinations, hysteria, insomnia, lassitude, pseudoparkinsonism, tardive dyskinesia, nervousness, neuroleptic malignant syndrome, nightmares, sedation, seizure, somnolence

Dermatologic: Angioneurotic edema, dermatitis, photosensitivity, skin pigmentation (slate gray), urticaria

Endocrine & metabolic: Amenorrhea, breast engorgement, gynecomastia, hyperglycemia, lactation

Gastrointestinal: Constipation, nausea, vomiting, xerostomia

Genitourinary: Ejaculatory disorder, impotence, urinary retention

Hematologic: Agranulocytosis, leukopenia, thrombocytopenia, thrombocytopenic purpura

Hepatic: Jaundice

Local: Abscess, distal vessel spasm, gangrene, injection site reactions (burning, edema, erythema, pain), palsies, paralysis, phlebitis, sensory loss, thrombophlebitis, tissue necrosis, venous thrombosis

Neuromuscular & skeletal: Incoordination, tremor

Ocular: Blurred vision, corneal and lenticular changes, diplopia, epithelial keratopathy, pigmentary retinopathy

Otic: Tinnitus

Respiratory: Apnea, asthma, nasal congestion, respiratory depression

Drug Interactions

Metabolism/Transport Effects Substrate of CYP2B6 (major), CYP2D6 (major); **Note:** Assignment of Major/Minor substrate status based on clinically relevant drug interaction potential; **Inhibits** CYP2D6 (weak)

Avoid Concomitant Use

Avoid concomitant use of Promethazine with any of the following: Aclidinium; Azelastine (Nasal); Dapoxetine; Eluxadoline; Glucagon; Ipratropium (Oral Inhalation); Metoclopramide; Orphenadrine; Paraldehyde; Potassium Chloride; Thalidomide; Tiotropium; Umeclidinium

Increased Effect/Toxicity

Promethazine may increase the levels/effects of: AbobotulinumtoxinA; Alcohol (Ethyl); Analgesics (Opioid); Anticholinergic Agents; Antipsychotic Agents; ARIPiprazole; Azelastine (Nasal); Buprenorphine; CNS Depressants; Eluxadoline; Glucagon; Highest Risk QTc-Prolonging Agents; Hydrocodone; Methotrimeprazine; Mirabegron; Moderate Risk QTc-Prolonging Agents; OnabotulinumtoxinA; Orphenadrine; Paraldehyde; Potassium Chloride; Pramipexole; RimabotulinumtoxinB; ROPINIRole; Rotigotine; Serotonin Modulators; Suvorexant; Thalidomide; Thiazide Diuretics; Tiotropium; Topiramate; Zolpidem

The levels/effects of Promethazine may be increased by: Abiraterone Acetate; Aclidinium; Antiemetics (5HT3 Antagonists); Antipsychotic Agents; Brimonidine (Topical); Cannabis; Cobicistat; CYP2B6 Inhibitors (Moderate); CYP2D6 Inhibitors (Moderate); CYP2D6 Inhibitors (Strong); Dapoxetine; Darunavir; Doxylamine; Dronabinol; Droperidol; HydrOXYzine; Ipratropium (Oral Inhalation); Kava Kava; Magnesium Sulfate; MAO Inhibitors; Methotrimeprazine; Metoclopramide; Metyrosine; Mianserin; Mifepristone; Nabilone; Panobinostat; Peginterferon Alfa-2b; Perampanel; Pramlintide; Quazepam; Rufinamide; Sodium Oxybate; Tapentadol; Tedizolid; Tetrahydrocannabinol; Umeclidinium

Decreased Effect

Promethazine may decrease the levels/effects of: Acetylcholinesterase Inhibitors; EPINEPHrine (Nasal); Epinephrine (Racemic); EPINEPHrine (Systemic, Oral Inhalation); Itopride; Secretin

The levels/effects of Promethazine may be decreased by: Acetylcholinesterase Inhibitors; CYP2B6 Inducers (Strong); Dabrafenib; Peginterferon Alfa-2b

Storage/Stability

Injection: Prior to dilution, store at 20°C to 25°C (68°F to 77°F). Protect from light. Solutions in NS or D_5W are stable for 24 hours at room temperature.

Oral solution: Store at 15°C to 25°C (59°F to 77°F). Protect from light.

Suppositories: Store refrigerated at 2°C to 8°C (36°F to 46°F).

Tablets: Store at 20°C to 25°C (68°F to 77°F). Protect from light.

Mechanism of Action Phenothiazine derivative; blocks postsynaptic mesolimbic dopaminergic receptors in the brain; exhibits a strong alpha-adrenergic blocking effect and depresses the release of hypothalamic and hypophyseal hormones; competes with histamine for the H_1-receptor; muscarinic-blocking effect may be responsible for antiemetic activity; reduces stimuli to the brainstem reticular system

Pharmacodynamics

Onset of action:

Oral, IM: Within 20 minutes

IV: 5 minutes

Duration: Usually 4 to 6 hours (up to 12 hours)

Pharmacokinetics (Adult data unless noted)

Absorption: Oral: Rapid and complete; large first pass effect limits systemic bioavailability (Sharma, 2003)

Distribution: V_d:13.4 ± 3.6 L/kg (Brunton, 2011)

Protein binding: 93% (Brunton, 2011)
Bioavailability: Oral: ~25% (Sharma, 2003); rectal: 21.7% to 23.4% (Brunton, 2011)
Half-life:
Parenteral: IM: ~10 hours; IV: 9 to 16 hours
Oral (syrup); Rectal (suppository): 16 to 19 hours (range: 4 to 34 hours) (Strenkoski-Nix, 2000)
Time to peak serum concentrations (Brunton, 2011):
Oral (syrup): 2.8 ± 1.4 hours
Rectal: 8.2 ± 3.4 hours
Metabolism: Hepatic; hydroxylation via CYP2D6 and N-demethylation via CYP2B6; significant first-pass effect (Sharma, 2003)
Elimination: Principally as inactive metabolites in the urine and in the feces

Dosing: Usual
Pediatric: **Note:** Use with extreme caution utilizing the lowest most effective dose:
Allergic conditions: Children ≥2 years and Adolescents: Oral: 0.1 mg/kg/dose (maximum dose: 12.5 mg/dose) every 6 hours during the day and 0.5 mg/kg/dose (maximum dose: 25 mg/dose) at bedtime as needed
Antiemetic: Children ≥2 years and Adolescents: Oral, IM, IV, rectal: 0.25 to 1 mg/kg every 4 to 6 hours as needed; maximum dose: 25 mg/dose
Motion sickness: Children ≥2 years and Adolescents: Oral, rectal: 0.5 mg/kg 30 minutes to 1 hour before departure, then every 12 hours as needed; maximum dose: 25 mg/dose
Pre/postoperative analgesia/hypnotic adjunct: Children ≥2 years and Adolescents: IM, IV: 1.1 mg/kg once in combination with an analgesic or hypnotic (at reduced dosage) and with an atropine-like agent (at appropriate dosage). **Note:** Promethazine dosage should not exceed 12.5 to 25 mg (ie, half of suggested adult dosage).
Sedation: Oral, IM, IV, rectal: 0.5 to 1 mg/kg/dose every 6 hours as needed; maximum dose: 25 mg/dose
Adult:
Allergic conditions (including allergic reactions to blood or plasma):
Oral, rectal: 25 mg at bedtime **or** 12.5 mg before meals and at bedtime (range: 6.25 to 12.5 mg 3 times daily)
IM, IV: 25 mg, may repeat in 2 hours when necessary; switch to oral route as soon as feasible
Antiemetic: Oral, IM, IV, rectal: 12.5 to 25 mg every 4 to 6 hours as needed
Motion sickness: Oral, rectal: 25 mg 30 to 60 minutes before departure, then every 12 hours as needed
Obstetrics (labor) as adjunct to analgesia: IM, IV: Early labor: 50 mg; established labor: 25 to 75 mg in combination with analgesic at reduced dosage; may repeat every 4 hours for up to 2 additional doses (maximum: 100 mg/day while in labor)
Pre/postoperative analgesia/hypnotic adjunct: IM, IV: 25 to 50 mg in combination with analgesic or hypnotic (at reduced dosage)
Sedation: Oral, IM, IV, rectal: 25 to 50 mg/dose
Dosing adjustment in renal impairment: Children ≥ 2 years, Adolescents, and Adults: There are no dosage adjustments provided in manufacturer's labeling.
Dosing adjustment in hepatic impairment:
Children ≥2 years and Adolescents: The manufacturer recommends to avoid use in pediatric patients with signs and symptoms of hepatic disease (extrapyramidal symptoms may be confused with CNS signs of hepatic disease).
Adults: There are no dosage adjustments provided in manufacturer's labeling; use with caution (cholestatic jaundice has been reported with use).

Preparation for Administration Parenteral: IV: Although IV administration should be avoided, promethazine has been administered IV in select patients. Solution for injection may be administered at a maximum concentration of 25 mg/mL; however, to minimize phlebitis further dilution is recommended. Some have suggested further diluting the 25 mg/mL with 10 to 20 mL NS (ISMP 2006).

Administration
Oral: Administer with food, water, or milk to decrease GI distress
Parenteral: Not for SubQ administration; promethazine is a chemical irritant which may produce necrosis.
IM: Preferred route of administration; administer as a deep IM injection
IV: IV use should be avoided when possible since severe tissue damage has occurred with IV administration; in selected patients, promethazine has been diluted and infused at a maximum rate of 25 mg/minute. To minimize phlebitis, consider administering over 10 to 15 minutes, limiting initial dose to 1/4 or 1/2 the usual dose (eg, in adults 6.25 to 12.5 mg), further diluting the 25 mg/mL strength in 10 to 20 mL NS, and administering through a large bore vein (not hand or wrist) or via a running IV line at port farthest from patient's vein (ISMP 2006).
Vesicant; ensure proper needle or catheter placement prior to and during infusion; avoid extravasation. Discontinue immediately if burning or pain occurs with administration; evaluate for inadvertent arterial injection or extravasation. If extravasation occurs, stop infusion immediately and disconnect (leave cannula/needle in place); gently aspirate extravasated solution (do **NOT** flush the line); remove needle/cannula; elevate extremity. Apply dry cold compresses (Hurst 2004).

Vesicant/Extravasation Risk Vesicant

Monitoring Parameters Relief of symptoms, mental status; monitor for signs and symptoms of tissue injury (burning or pain at injection site, phlebitis, edema) with IV administration

Test Interactions May interfere with urine detection of amphetamine/methamphetamine (false-positive); alters the flare response in intradermal allergen tests; hCG-based pregnancy tests may result in false-negatives or false-positives

Additional Information Although promethazine has been used in combination with meperidine and chlorpromazine as a premedication (lytic cocktail), this combination may have a higher rate of adverse effects compared to alternative sedative/analgesics

Dosage Forms Excipient information presented when available (limited, particularly for generics); consult specific product labeling.
Solution, Injection, as hydrochloride:
Phenergan: 50 mg/mL (1 mL) [contains edetate disodium, phenol, sodium metabisulfite]
Phenergan: 25 mg/mL (1 mL) [pyrogen free; contains edetate disodium, phenol, sodium metabisulfite]
Generic: 25 mg/mL (1 mL); 50 mg/mL (1 mL)
Solution, Oral, as hydrochloride:
Generic: 6.25 mg/5 mL (118 mL, 473 mL)
Suppository, Rectal, as hydrochloride:
Phenadoz: 12.5 mg (12 ea); 25 mg (12 ea)
Phenergan: 12.5 mg (12 ea); 25 mg (12 ea); 50 mg (12 ea)
Promethegan: 12.5 mg (12 ea); 25 mg (12 ea, 1000 ea); 50 mg (12 ea)
Generic: 12.5 mg (1 ea, 12 ea); 25 mg (1 ea, 12 ea); 50 mg (12 ea)
Syrup, Oral, as hydrochloride:
Generic: 6.25 mg/5 mL (118 mL, 473 mL)
Tablet, Oral, as hydrochloride:
Generic: 12.5 mg, 25 mg, 50 mg

Promethazine and Codeine

(proe METH a zeen & KOE deen)

Medication Safety Issues

High alert medication:

The Institute for Safe Medication Practices (ISMP) includes this medication among its list of drug classes which have a heightened risk of causing significant patient harm when used in error.

Therapeutic Category Antitussive; Cough Preparation; Phenothiazine Derivative

Generic Availability (US) Yes

Use Temporary relief of coughs and upper respiratory symptoms associated with allergy or the common cold (FDA approved in ages ≥6 years and adults)

Pregnancy Risk Factor C

Pregnancy Considerations Reproduction studies have not been conducted with this combination. See individual agents.

Breast-Feeding Considerations See individual agents.

Contraindications Hypersensitivity to promethazine or other phenothiazines, codeine, or any component of the formulation; children <6 years of age; postoperative pain management in children who have undergone tonsillectomy and/or adenoidectomy; coma; treatment of lower respiratory tract symptoms, including asthma

Warnings/Precautions [US Boxed Warning]: Promethazine and codeine combination use is contraindicated in children <6 years of age; respiratory depression, including fatalities, is associated with concomitant administration of promethazine and other respiratory depressants in children. Fatalities associated with respiratory depression have also been reported with promethazine use in children <2 years of age. Avoid use in children who may have Reyes syndrome or hepatic disease as adverse reactions caused by promethazine may be confused with signs of primary disease. Due to the incidence of serious side effects and fatalities associated with codeine use in children, Health Canada does not recommend codeine use in any child <12 years of age. Use caution in atopic children. **[US Boxed Warning]: Respiratory depression and death have occurred in children who received codeine following tonsillectomy and/or adenoidectomy and were found to have evidence of being ultra-rapid metabolizers of codeine due to a CYP2D6 polymorphism.** Deaths have also occurred in nursing infants after being exposed to high concentrations of morphine because the mothers were ultra-rapid metabolizers. Use of codeine is contraindicated in the postoperative pain management of children who have undergone tonsillectomy and/or adenoidectomy.

Use the lowest effective dose for the shortest period of time. Dose should not be increased if cough does not respond; re-evaluate within 5 days for possible underlying pathology. Codeine is not recommended for cough control in patients with a productive cough or chronic respiratory disease. May be sedating; use with caution in disorders where CNS depression is a feature. May impair physical or mental abilities; patients must be cautioned about performing tasks which require mental alertness (eg, operating machinery or driving). May cause orthostatic hypotension; use with caution in patients at risk of hypotension or where transient hypotensive episodes would be poorly tolerated (cardiovascular disease or cerebrovascular disease).

Codeine should be used with caution in patients with hypersensitivity reactions to other phenanthrene-derivative opioid agonists (eg, morphine, hydrocodone, hydromorphone, levorphanol, oxycodone, oxymorphone). Avoid use in patients with head injury or increased intracranial pressure; exaggerated elevation of intracranial pressure may occur. May obscure diagnosis or clinical course of patients with acute abdominal conditions. Use caution in patients with seizure disorder, respiratory disease, severe biliary tract impairment, pancreatitis, renal impairment, thyroid disease, adrenal insufficiency, prostatic hypertrophy, the elderly and debilitated. Use with caution in patients with hepatic impairment; cholestatic jaundice has been reported with promethazine use. Avoid use in pediatric patients with signs and symptoms of hepatic disease (extrapyramidal symptoms caused by promethazine may be confused with CNS signs of hepatic disease). Use caution in patients with two or more copies of the variant CYP2D6*2 allele; may have extensive conversion to morphine and thus increased opioid-mediated effects. Avoid the use of codeine in these patients; consider alternative analgesics such as morphine or a nonopioid agent (Crews, 2012). The occurrence of this phenotype is seen in 0.5% to 1% of Chinese and Japanese, 0.5% to 1% of Hispanics, 1% to 10% of Caucasians, 3% of African-Americans, and 16% to 28% of North Africans, Ethiopians, and Arabs.

Use promethazine with caution in Parkinson's disease; hemodynamic instability; bone marrow suppression; subcortical brain damage; pyloroduodenal obstruction; and in severe cardiac, hepatic or respiratory disease. Avoid use in Reye's syndrome. May lower seizure threshold; use caution in persons with seizure disorders or in persons using opioids or local anesthetics which may also affect seizure threshold. May alter temperature regulation or mask toxicity of other drugs due to antiemetic effects. May alter cardiac conduction (life-threatening arrhythmias have occurred with therapeutic doses of phenothiazines). Use with caution in patients with bone marrow depression; leukopenia and agranulocytosis have been reported.

Phenothiazines may cause anticholinergic effects (constipation, xerostomia, blurred vision, urinary retention); therefore, they should be used with caution in patients with decreased gastrointestinal motility, urinary retention, BPH, xerostomia, or visual problems. Conditions which also may be exacerbated by cholinergic blockade include narrow-angle glaucoma (screening is recommended) and worsening of myasthenia gravis. May cause extrapyramidal symptoms, including pseudoparkinsonism, acute dystonic reactions, akathisia, and tardive dyskinesia. May be associated with neuroleptic malignant syndrome (NMS). Potentially significant drug interactions may exist, requiring dose or frequency adjustment, additional monitoring, and/or selection of alternative therapy.

After chronic maternal exposure to opioids, neonatal withdrawal syndrome may occur in the newborn; monitor neonate closely. Signs and symptoms include irritability, hyperactivity and abnormal sleep pattern, high pitched cry, tremor, vomiting, diarrhea and failure to gain weight. Onset, duration and severity depend on the drug used, duration of use, maternal dose, and rate of drug elimination by the newborn. Opioid withdrawal syndrome in the neonate, unlike in adults, may be life-threatening and should be treated according to protocols developed by neonatology experts.

Warnings: Additional Pediatric Considerations Safety and efficacy for the use of cough and cold products in pediatric patients <4 years of age is limited; the AAP warns against the use of these products for respiratory illnesses in this age group. Serious adverse effects including death have been reported. Many of these products contain multiple active ingredients, increasing the risk of accidental overdose when used with other products. (AAP 2012; FDA 2008). In July 2015, the FDA announced that it would be further evaluating the risk of serious adverse effects of codeine-containing products to treat cough and colds in pediatric patients <18 years including slowed or difficulty breathing. In April 2015, the European Medicines

Agency (EMA) stated that codeine-containing medicines should not be used in children <12 years, and use is not recommended in pediatric patients 12 to 18 years who have breathing problems including asthma or other chronic breathing problems (FDA 2015)

Children with dehydration are at increased risk for development of dystonic reactions from promethazine.

Adverse Reactions Also see individual agents.

Rare but important or life-threatening: Hypogonadism (Brennan, 2013; Debono, 2011)

Drug Interactions

Metabolism/Transport Effects Refer to individual components.

Avoid Concomitant Use

Avoid concomitant use of Promethazine and Codeine with any of the following: Aclidinium; Azelastine (Nasal); Dapoxetine; Eluxadoline; Glucagon; Ipratropium (Oral Inhalation); Metoclopramide; Mixed Agonist / Antagonist Opioids; Orphenadrine; Paraldehyde; Potassium Chloride; Thalidomide; Tiotropium; Umeclidinium

Increased Effect/Toxicity

Promethazine and Codeine may increase the levels/effects of: AbobotulinumtoxinA; Alcohol (Ethyl); Alvimopan; Analgesics (Opioid); Anticholinergic Agents; Antipsychotic Agents; ARIPiprazole; Azelastine (Nasal); CNS Depressants; Desmopressin; Diuretics; Eluxadoline; Glucagon; Highest Risk QTc-Prolonging Agents; Hydrocodone; Methotrimeprazine; Mirabegron; Moderate Risk QTc-Prolonging Agents; OnabotulinumtoxinA; Orphenadrine; Paraldehyde; Potassium Chloride; Pramipexole; RimabotulinumtoxinB; ROPINIRole; Rotigotine; Serotonin Modulators; Suvorexant; Thalidomide; Thiazide Diuretics; Tiotropium; Topiramate; Zolpidem

The levels/effects of Promethazine and Codeine may be increased by: Abiraterone Acetate; Aclidinium; Amphetamines; Anticholinergic Agents; Antiemetics (5HT3 Antagonists); Antipsychotic Agents; Antipsychotic Agents (Phenothiazines); Brimonidine (Topical); Cannabis; Cobicistat; CYP2B6 Inhibitors (Moderate); Dapoxetine; Darunavir; Doxylamine; Dronabinol; Droperidol; HydrOXYzine; Ipratropium (Oral Inhalation); Kava Kava; Magnesium Sulfate; MAO Inhibitors; Methotrimeprazine; Metoclopramide; Metyrosine; Mianserin; Mifepristone; Nabilone; Panobinostat; Peginterferon Alfa-2b; Perampanel; Pramlintide; Quazepam; Rufinamide; Sodium Oxybate; Somatostatin Analogs; Succinylcholine; Tapentadol; Tedizolid; Tetrahydrocannabinol; Umeclidinium

Decreased Effect

Promethazine and Codeine may decrease the levels/effects of: Acetylcholinesterase Inhibitors; EPINEPHrine (Nasal); Epinephrine (Racemic); EPINEPHrine (Systemic, Oral Inhalation); Itopride; Pegvisomant; Secretin

The levels/effects of Promethazine and Codeine may be decreased by: Acetylcholinesterase Inhibitors; Ammonium Chloride; CYP2B6 Inducers (Strong); CYP2D6 Inhibitors (Moderate); CYP2D6 Inhibitors (Strong); Dabrafenib; Mixed Agonist / Antagonist Opioids; Naltrexone; Peginterferon Alfa-2b

Storage/Stability Store at controlled room temperature of 20°C to 25°C (68°F to 77°F). Protect from light.

Dosing: Usual Note: Dosage expressed as mL based on product formulation: Promethazine 6.25 mg and codeine 10 mg per 5 mL.

Children and Adolescents: **Antitussive (nonproductive cough):** Oral:

Children 6-11 years: 2.5-5 mL every 4-6 hours as needed; maximum total dose: 30 mL/24 hours

Children ≥12 years and Adolescents: 5 mL every 4-6 hours as needed; maximum total dose: 30 mL/24 hours

Adults: **Upper respiratory symptoms:** Oral: 5 mL every 4-6 hours as needed; maximum total dose: 30 mL/24 hours

Dosing adjustment in renal impairment: Children ≥6 years, Adolescents, and Adults: There are no specific dosage adjustments provided in the manufacturer's labeling; use with caution; consider decreasing dose.

Dosing adjustment in hepatic impairment:

Children ≥6 years and Adolescents: Avoid use in pediatric patients with signs and symptoms of hepatic disease (extrapyramidal symptoms caused by promethazine may be confused with CNS signs of hepatic disease).

Adults: There are no specific dosage adjustments provided in the manufacturer's labeling; use with caution; consider decreasing dose. Cholestatic jaundice has been reported with promethazine use and codeine clearance may be reduced.

Administration Oral: Administer with food or water to decrease GI upset. Administer with accurate measuring device; do not use household teaspoon (overdosage may occur).

Test Interactions

Codeine: Amylase and lipase plasma levels may by unreliable for 24 hours after codeine administration.

Promethazine: Pregnancy tests (hCG-based) may result in false-negatives or false-positives; increased serum glucose may be seen with glucose tolerance tests; may suppress the wheal and flare reactions to skin test antigens

Controlled Substance C-V

Dosage Forms Excipient information presented when available (limited, particularly for generics); consult specific product labeling.

Syrup, oral: Promethazine hydrochloride 6.25 mg and codeine phosphate 10 mg per 5 mL (5 mL, 118 mL, 473 mL)

Promethazine and Phenylephrine

(proe METH a zeen & fen il EF rin)

Related Information

Phenylephrine (Systemic) *on page 1685*

Promethazine *on page 1777*

Brand Names: US Promethazine VC

Therapeutic Category Antihistamine/Decongestant Combination

Generic Availability (US) Yes

Use Temporary relief of upper respiratory symptoms associated with allergy or the common cold (FDA approved in ages ≥2 years and adults)

Pregnancy Risk Factor C

Pregnancy Considerations Reproduction studies have not been conducted with this combination. Refer to individual monographs.

Contraindications Hypersensitivity to promethazine, phenylephrine, or any component of the formulation (cross-reactivity between phenothiazines may occur;) treatment of lower respiratory tract symptoms, including asthma; hypertension; ventricular tachycardia; peripheral vascular insufficiency; use with or within 14 days of MAO inhibitor therapy

Warnings/Precautions See individual agents.

Warnings: Additional Pediatric Considerations Children with dehydration are at increased risk for development of dystonic reactions from promethazine.

Safety and efficacy for the use of cough and cold products in pediatric patients <4 years of age is limited; the AAP warns against the use of these products for respiratory illnesses in this age group. Serious adverse effects including death have been reported. Many of these products contain multiple active ingredients, increasing the risk of accidental overdose when used with other products. Health care providers are reminded to ask caregivers about the use of OTC cough and cold products in order to avoid exposure to multiple medications containing the same ingredient (AAP 2012; FDA 2008).

Some dosage forms may contain propylene glycol; in neonates large amounts of propylene glycol delivered orally, intravenously (eg, >3,000 mg/day), or topically have been associated with potentially fatal toxicities which can include metabolic acidosis, seizures, renal failure, and CNS depression; toxicities have also been reported in children and adults including hyperosmolality, lactic acidosis, seizures, and respiratory depression; use caution (AAP 1997; Shehab 2009).

Adverse Reactions See individual agents.

Drug Interactions

Metabolism/Transport Effects Refer to individual components.

Avoid Concomitant Use

Avoid concomitant use of Promethazine and Phenylephrine with any of the following: Aclidinium; Azelastine (Nasal); Dapoxetine; Eluxadoline; Ergot Derivatives; Glucagon; Hyaluronidase; Iobenguane I 123; Ipratropium (Oral Inhalation); MAO Inhibitors; Metoclopramide; Orphenadrine; Paraldehyde; Potassium Chloride; Thalidomide; Tiotropium; Umeclidinium

Increased Effect/Toxicity

Promethazine and Phenylephrine may increase the levels/effects of: AbobotulinumtoxinA; Alcohol (Ethyl); Analgesics (Opioid); Anticholinergic Agents; Antipsychotic Agents; ARIPiprazole; Azelastine (Nasal); Buprenorphine; CNS Depressants; Eluxadoline; Glucagon; Highest Risk QTc-Prolonging Agents; Hydrocodone; Methotrimeprazine; Mirabegron; Moderate Risk QTc-Prolonging Agents; OnabotulinumtoxinA; Orphenadrine; Paraldehyde; Potassium Chloride; Pramipexole; RimabotulinumtoxinB; ROPINIRole; Rotigotine; Serotonin Modulators; Suvorexant; Sympathomimetics; Thalidomide; Thiazide Diuretics; Tiotropium; Topiramate; Zolpidem

The levels/effects of Promethazine and Phenylephrine may be increased by: Abiraterone Acetate; Acetaminophen; Aclidinium; Antiemetics (5HT3 Antagonists); Antipsychotic Agents; AtoMOXetine; Brimonidine (Topical); Cannabis; Cobicistat; CYP2B6 Inhibitors (Moderate); CYP2D6 Inhibitors (Moderate); CYP2D6 Inhibitors (Strong); Dapoxetine; Darunavir; Doxylamine; Dronabinol; Droperidol; Ergot Derivatives; Hyaluronidase; HydrOXYzine; Ipratropium (Oral Inhalation); Kava Kava; Linezolid; Magnesium Sulfate; MAO Inhibitors; Methotrimeprazine; Metoclopramide; Metyrosine; Mianserin; Mifepristone; Nabilone; Panobinostat; Peginterferon Alfa-2b; Perampanel; Pramlintide; Quazepam; Rufinamide; Sodium Oxybate; Tapentadol; Tedizolid; Tetrahydrocannabinol; Umeclidinium

Decreased Effect

Promethazine and Phenylephrine may decrease the levels/effects of: Acetylcholinesterase Inhibitors; Benzylpenicilloyl Polylysine; EPINEPHrine (Nasal); Epinephrine (Racemic); EPINEPHrine (Systemic, Oral Inhalation); Iobenguane I 123; Ioflupane I 123; Itopride; Secretin

The levels/effects of Promethazine and Phenylephrine may be decreased by: Acetylcholinesterase Inhibitors; Alpha1-Blockers; CYP2B6 Inducers (Strong); Dabrafenib; Peginterferon Alfa-2b

Dosing: Usual Note: Dosage expressed as mL based on product formulation: Promethazine 6.25 mg and phenylephrine 5 mg per 5 mL

Pediatric: **Upper respiratory symptoms: Note:** Promethazine with phenylephrine is contraindicated for use in infants or children <2 years old.

Children 2 to <6 years: Oral: 1.25 to 2.5 mL every 4 to 6 hours; not to exceed 15 mL in 24 hours

Children 6 to <12 years: Oral: 2.5 to 5 mL every 4 to 6 hours; not to exceed 30 mL in 24 hours

Children ≥12 years and Adolescents: Oral: 5 mL every 4 to 6 hours; not to exceed 30 mL in 24 hours

Adult: **Upper respiratory symptoms:** Oral: 5 mL every 4 to 6 hours; not to exceed 30 mL in 24 hours

Dosing adjustment in renal impairment: There are no dosage adjustments provided in manufacturer's labeling.

Dosing adjustment in hepatic impairment:

Children ≥2 years and Adolescents: The manufacturer recommends to avoid use in pediatric patients with signs and symptoms of hepatic disease (extrapyramidal symptoms caused by promethazine may be confused with CNS signs of hepatic disease).

Adults: There are no dosage adjustments provided in manufacturer's labeling; use with caution (cholestatic jaundice has been reported with use.

Administration Oral: Administer with food, water, or milk to decrease GI distress

Test Interactions May suppress the wheal and flare reactions to skin test antigens; false negative and positive reactions with pregnancy tests relying on immunological reactions between hCG and anti-hCG

Dosage Forms Excipient information presented when available (limited, particularly for generics); consult specific product labeling.

Syrup, oral:

Promethazine VC: Promethazine hydrochloride 6.25 mg and phenylephrine hydrochloride 5 mg per 5 mL (118 mL, 473 mL) [contains ethanol 7%, menthol, propylene glycol, sodium benzoate; apricot-peach flavor]

◆ **Promethazine Hydrochloride** *see* Promethazine *on page 1777*

Promethazine, Phenylephrine, and Codeine (proe METH a zeen, fen il EF rin, & KOE deen)

Brand Names: US Promethazine VC/Codeine

Therapeutic Category Antihistamine/Decongestant Combination; Antitussive; Cough Preparation

Generic Availability (US) Yes

Use Temporary relief of coughs and upper respiratory symptoms including nasal congestion (FDA approved in ages ≥6 years and adults)

Pregnancy Risk Factor C

Pregnancy Considerations Reproduction studies have not been conducted with this combination. See individual agents.

Breast-Feeding Considerations Codeine enters breast milk; excretion of promethazine and phenylephrine is unknown. See individual agents.

Contraindications Hypersensitivity to promethazine or other phenothiazines, phenylephrine, codeine, or any component of the formulation; children <6 years of age; coma; treatment of lower respiratory tract symptoms, including asthma; hypertension; peripheral vascular insufficiency; use with or within 14 days of MAO inhibitor therapy; postoperative pain management in children who have undergone tonsillectomy and/or adenoidectomy

Warnings/Precautions [U.S. Boxed Warning]: Promethazine, codeine, and phenylephrine combination use is contraindicated in children <6 years of age; respiratory depression, including fatalities, is associated with concomitant administration of promethazine and other respiratory depressants in children. Fatalities associated with respiratory depression have also been reported with promethazine use in children <2 years of age. Avoid use in children who may have Reye syndrome or hepatic disease as adverse reactions caused by promethazine may be confused with signs of primary disease. Use with caution in atopic children. **[U.S. Boxed Warning]: Respiratory depression and death have occurred in children who received codeine following tonsillectomy and/or adenoidectomy and were found to have evidence of being ultra-rapid metabolizers of codeine due to a CYP2D6 polymorphism.** Deaths have also occurred in nursing infants after being exposed to high concentrations of morphine because the mothers were ultra-rapid metabolizers. Use of codeine is contraindicated in the postoperative pain management of children who have undergone tonsillectomy and/or adenoidectomy.

After chronic maternal exposure to opioids, neonatal withdrawal syndrome may occur in the newborn; monitor neonate closely. Signs and symptoms include irritability, hyperactivity and abnormal sleep pattern, high pitched cry, tremor, vomiting, diarrhea and failure to gain weight. Onset, duration and severity depend on the drug used, duration of use, maternal dose, and rate of drug elimination by the newborn. Opioid withdrawal syndrome in the neonate, unlike in adults, may be life-threatening and should be treated according to protocols developed by neonatology experts.

Use the lowest effective dose for the shortest period of time. Dose should not be increased if cough does not respond; reevaluate within 5 days for possible underlying pathology. Codeine is not recommended for cough control in patients with a productive cough or chronic respiratory disease. May be sedating; use with caution in disorders where CNS depression is a feature. May impair physical or mental abilities; patients must be cautioned about performing tasks which require mental alertness (eg, operating machinery or driving). Effects may be potentiated when used with other sedative drugs or ethanol. May cause orthostatic hypotension; use with caution in patients at risk of hypotension or where transient hypotensive episodes would be poorly tolerated (cardiovascular disease or cerebrovascular disease).

Codeine should be used with caution in patients with hypersensitivity reactions to other phenanthrene-derivative opioid agonists (morphine, hydrocodone, hydromorphone, levorphanol, oxycodone, oxymorphone). Avoid use in patients with head injury or increased intracranial pressure; exaggerated elevation of intracranial pressure may occur. May obscure diagnosis or clinical course of patients with acute abdominal conditions. Use caution in patients with seizure disorder, respiratory disease, biliary tract impairment, pancreatitis, renal impairment, thyroid disease, adrenal insufficiency, prostatic hypertrophy, the elderly and debilitated. Use with caution in patients with hepatic impairment; cholestatic jaundice has been reported with promethazine use. Avoid use in pediatric patients with signs and symptoms of hepatic disease (extrapyramidal symptoms caused by promethazine may be confused with CNS signs of hepatic disease). Use codeine with caution in patients with two or more copies of the variant CYP2D6*2 allele; may have extensive conversion to morphine and thus increased opioid-mediated effects. Avoid the use of codeine in these patients; consider alternative analgesics such as morphine or a non-opioid agent (Crews, 2012). The occurrence of this phenotype is seen in 0.5% to 1% of Chinese and Japanese, 0.5% to 1% of Hispanics, 1% to 10% of Caucasians, 3% of African-Americans, and 16% to 28% of North Africans, Ethiopians, and Arabs.

Use promethazine with caution in Parkinson's disease; hemodynamic instability; bone marrow suppression; subcortical brain damage; pyloroduodenal obstruction; and in severe cardiac, hepatic or respiratory disease. Avoid use in Reye's syndrome. May lower seizure threshold; use caution in persons with seizure disorders or in persons using opioids or local anesthetics which may also affect seizure threshold. May alter temperature regulation or mask toxicity of other drugs due to antiemetic effects. Potentially significant drug interactions may exist, requiring dose or frequency adjustment, additional monitoring, and/or selection of alternative therapy. Effects may be potentiated when used with other sedative drugs or ethanol. May alter cardiac conduction (life-threatening arrhythmias have occurred with therapeutic doses of phenothiazines). Use with caution in patients with bone marrow depression; leukopenia and agranulocytosis have been reported.

Phenothiazines may cause anticholinergic effects (constipation, xerostomia, blurred vision, urinary retention); therefore, they should be used with caution in patients with decreased gastrointestinal motility, urinary retention, BPH, xerostomia, or visual problems. Conditions which also may be exacerbated by cholinergic blockade include narrow-angle glaucoma (screening is recommended) and worsening of myasthenia gravis. May cause extrapyramidal symptoms, including pseudoparkinsonism, acute dystonic reactions, akathisia, and tardive dyskinesia. May be associated with neuroleptic malignant syndrome (NMS).

Phenylephrine should be used with caution in patients with hyperthyroidism, diabetes mellitus, cardiovascular disease, ischemic heart disease, increased intraocular pressure, prostatic hyperplasia or in the elderly.

Warnings: Additional Pediatric Considerations Children with dehydration are at increased risk for development of dystonic reactions from promethazine.

Safety and efficacy for the use of cough and cold products in pediatric patients <4 years of age is limited; the AAP warns against the use of these products for respiratory illnesses in this age group. Serious adverse effects including death have been reported. Many of these products contain multiple active ingredients, increasing the risk of accidental overdose when used with other products. Health care providers are reminded to ask caregivers about the use of OTC cough and cold products in order to avoid exposure to multiple medications containing the same ingredient (AAP 2012; FDA 2008). In July 2015, the FDA announced that it would be further evaluating the risk of serious adverse effects of codeine-containing products to treat cough and colds in pediatric patients <18 years including slowed or difficulty breathing. In April 2015, the European Medicines Agency (EMA) stated that codeine-containing medicines should not be used in children <12 years, and use is not recommended in pediatric patients 12 to 18 years who have breathing problems including asthma or other chronic breathing problems (FDA 2015).

Some dosage forms may contain propylene glycol; in neonates large amounts of propylene glycol delivered orally, intravenously (eg, >3,000 mg/day), or topically have been associated with potentially fatal toxicities which can include metabolic acidosis, seizures, renal failure, and CNS depression; toxicities have also been reported in children and adults including hyperosmolality, lactic acidosis, seizures, and respiratory depression; use caution (AAP, 1997; Shehab, 2009).

Adverse Reactions Also see individual agents.Rare but important or life-threatening: Hypogonadism (Brennan, 2013; Debono, 2011)

Drug Interactions

Metabolism/Transport Effects Refer to individual components.

Avoid Concomitant Use

Avoid concomitant use of Promethazine, Phenylephrine, and Codeine with any of the following: Aclidinium; Azelastine (Nasal); Dapoxetine; Eluxadoline; Ergot Derivatives; Glucagon; Hyaluronidase; Iobenguane I 123; Ipratropium (Oral Inhalation); MAO Inhibitors; Metoclopramide; Mixed Agonist / Antagonist Opioids;

Orphenadrine; Paraldehyde; Potassium Chloride; Thalidomide; Tiotropium; Umeclidinium

Increased Effect/Toxicity

Promethazine, Phenylephrine, and Codeine may increase the levels/effects of: AbobotulinumtoxinA; Alcohol (Ethyl); Alvimopan; Analgesics (Opioid); Anticholinergic Agents; Antipsychotic Agents; ARIPiprazole; Azelastine (Nasal); CNS Depressants; Desmopressin; Diuretics; Eluxadoline; Glucagon; Highest Risk QTc-Prolonging Agents; Hydrocodone; Methotrimeprazine; Mirabegron; Moderate Risk QTc-Prolonging Agents; OnabotulinumtoxinA; Orphenadrine; Paraldehyde; Potassium Chloride; Pramipexole; RimabotulinumtoxinB; ROPINIRole; Rotigotine; Serotonin Modulators; Suvorexant; Sympathomimetics; Thalidomide; Thiazide Diuretics; Tiotropium; Topiramate; Zolpidem

The levels/effects of Promethazine, Phenylephrine, and Codeine may be increased by: Abiraterone Acetate; Acetaminophen; Aclidinium; Amphetamines; Anticholinergic Agents; Antiemetics (5HT3 Antagonists); Antipsychotic Agents; Antipsychotic Agents (Phenothiazines); AtoMOXetine; Brimonidine (Topical); Cannabis; Cobicistat; CYP2B6 Inhibitors (Moderate); Dapoxetine; Darunavir; Doxylamine; Dronabinol; Droperidol; Ergot Derivatives; Hyaluronidase; HydrOXYzine; Ipratropium (Oral Inhalation); Kava Kava; Linezolid; Magnesium Sulfate; MAO Inhibitors; Methotrimeprazine; Metoclopramide; Metyrosine; Mianserin; Mifepristone; Nabilone; Panobinostat; Peginterferon Alfa-2b; Perampanel; Pramlintide; Quazepam; Rufinamide; Sodium Oxybate; Somatostatin Analogs; Succinylcholine; Tapentadol; Tedizolid; Tetrahydrocannabinol; Umeclidinium

Decreased Effect

Promethazine, Phenylephrine, and Codeine may decrease the levels/effects of: Acetylcholinesterase Inhibitors; Benzylpenicilloyl Polylysine; EPINEPHrine (Nasal); Epinephrine (Racemic); EPINEPHrine (Systemic, Oral Inhalation); Iobenguane I 123; Ioflupane I 123; Itopride; Pegvisomant; Secretin

The levels/effects of Promethazine, Phenylephrine, and Codeine may be decreased by: Acetylcholinesterase Inhibitors; Alpha1-Blockers; Ammonium Chloride; CYP2B6 Inducers (Strong); CYP2D6 Inhibitors (Moderate); CYP2D6 Inhibitors (Strong); Dabrafenib; Mixed Agonist / Antagonist Opioids; Naltrexone; Peginterferon Alfa-2b

Storage/Stability Store at controlled room temperature of 20°C to 25°C (68°F to 77°F). Protect from light.

Dosing: Usual Note: Dosage expressed as mL based on product formulation: Promethazine 6.25 mg, phenylephrine 5 mg, and codeine 10 mg per 5 mL

Pediatric: **Antitussive (nonproductive cough) and upper respiratory symptoms:** Oral:

Children 6 to 11 years: 2.5 to 5 mL every 4 to 6 hours as needed; maximum daily dose: 30 mL/24 hours

Children ≥12 years and Adolescents: 5 mL every 4 to 6 hours as needed; maximum daily dose: 30 mL/24 hours

Adult: **Cough and upper respiratory symptoms:** Oral: 5 mL every 4 to 6 hours as needed; maximum daily dose: 30 mL/24 hours

Dosing adjustment in renal impairment: There are no specific dosage adjustments provided in the manufacturer's labeling; use with caution; consider decreasing dose.

Dosing adjustment in hepatic impairment:

Children ≥6 years and Adolescents: Avoid use in pediatric patients with signs and symptoms of hepatic disease (extrapyramidal symptoms caused by promethazine may be confused with CNS signs of hepatic disease).

Adults: There are no specific dosage adjustments provided in the manufacturer's labeling; use with caution; consider decreasing dose. Cholestatic jaundice has been reported with promethazine use and codeine clearance may be reduced.

Administration Oral: Administer with food or water to decrease GI upset. Administer with an accurate measuring device; do not use a household teaspoon (overdosage may occur).

Test Interactions

Codeine: Amylase and lipase plasma levels may by unreliable for 24 hours after codeine administration.

Promethazine: Pregnancy tests (hCG-based) may result in false-negatives or false-positives; increased serum glucose may be seen with glucose tolerance tests.

Controlled Substance C-V

Dosage Forms Excipient information presented when available (limited, particularly for generics); consult specific product labeling.

Syrup, Oral:

Promethazine VC/Codeine: Promethazine hydrochloride 6.25 mg, phenylephrine hydrochloride 5 mg, and codeine phosphate 10 mg per 5 mL (120 mL, 480 mL) [contains alcohol, fd&c yellow #6 (sunset yellow),methylparaben,propylene glycol,propylparaben,saccharin sodium, sodium benzoate]

Generic: Promethazine hydrochloride 6.25 mg, phenylephrine hydrochloride 5 mg, and codeine phosphate 10 mg per 5 mL (120 mL, 480 mL)

- ◆ **Promethazine VC** *see* Promethazine and Phenylephrine *on page* 1781
- ◆ **Promethazine VC/Codeine** *see* Promethazine, Phenylephrine, and Codeine *on page* 1782
- ◆ **Promethegan** *see* Promethazine *on page* 1777
- ◆ **Promolaxin [OTC]** *see* Docusate *on page* 697
- ◆ **PRO-Naproxen EC (Can)** *see* Naproxen *on page* 1489
- ◆ **Pronestyl** *see* Procainamide *on page* 1769
- ◆ **Pronutrients Vitamin D3 [OTC]** *see* Cholecalciferol *on page* 448

Propantheline (proe PAN the leen)

Medication Safety Issues

BEERS Criteria medication:

This drug may be potentially inappropriate for use in geriatric patients (Quality of evidence - moderate; Strength of recommendation - strong).

Therapeutic Category Anticholinergic Agent; Antispasmodic Agent, Gastrointestinal; Antispasmodic Agent, Urinary

Generic Availability (US) Yes

Use Adjunctive treatment of peptic ulcer, irritable bowel syndrome, pancreatitis, ureteral and urinary bladder spasm; to reduce duodenal motility during diagnostic radiologic procedures

Pregnancy Risk Factor C

Pregnancy Considerations Animal reproduction studies have not been conducted.

Breast-Feeding Considerations It is not known if propantheline is excreted in breast milk. The manufacturer recommends that caution be exercised when administering propantheline to nursing women.

Contraindications Severe ulcerative colitis, toxic megacolon, obstructive disease of the GI or urinary tract; glaucoma; myasthenia gravis; unstable cardiovascular adjustment in acute hemorrhage; intestinal atony of elderly or debilitated patients

Warnings/Precautions May cause drowsiness and/or blurred vision, which may impair physical or mental abilities; patients must be cautioned about performing tasks which require mental alertness (eg, operating machinery or driving). Use with caution in patients with hyperthyroidism, hiatal hernia with reflux esophagitis, autonomic neuropathy, hepatic, cardiac, or renal disease, hypertension, GI infections, or other endocrine diseases. Avoid use in the elderly due to potent anticholinergic adverse effects and uncertain effectiveness (Beers Criteria). Heat prostration may occur in the presence of increased environmental temperature; use caution in hot weather and/or exercise. Diarrhea may be a sign of incomplete intestinal obstruction, treatment should be discontinued if this occurs.

Warnings: Additional Pediatric Considerations Infants, patients with Down syndrome, and children with spastic paralysis or brain damage may be hypersensitive to antimuscarinic effects.

Adverse Reactions

Cardiovascular: Palpitation, tachycardia

Central nervous system: Confusion, dizziness, drowsiness, headache, insomnia, nervousness

Endocrine & metabolic: Suppression of lactation

Gastrointestinal: Bloated feeling, constipation, loss of taste, nausea, vomiting, xerostomia

Genitourinary: Impotence, urinary hesitancy, urinary retention

Neuromuscular & skeletal: Weakness

Ocular: Blurred vision, cycloplegia, mydriasis, ocular tension increased

Miscellaneous: Allergic reactions, anaphylaxis, diaphoresis decreased

Drug Interactions

Metabolism/Transport Effects None known.

Avoid Concomitant Use

Avoid concomitant use of Propantheline with any of the following: Aclidinium; Eluxadoline; Glucagon; Ipratropium (Oral Inhalation); Potassium Chloride; Tiotropium; Umeclidinium

Increased Effect/Toxicity

Propantheline may increase the levels/effects of: AbobotulinumtoxinA; Analgesics (Opioid); Anticholinergic Agents; Cannabinoid-Containing Products; Eluxadoline; Glucagon; Mirabegron; OnabotulinumtoxinA; Potassium Chloride; RimabotulinumtoxinB; Thiazide Diuretics; Tiotropium; Topiramate

The levels/effects of Propantheline may be increased by: Aclidinium; Ipratropium (Oral Inhalation); MAO Inhibitors; Mianserin; Pramlintide; Umeclidinium

Decreased Effect

Propantheline may decrease the levels/effects of: Acetylcholinesterase Inhibitors; Itopride; Metoclopramide; Secretin

The levels/effects of Propantheline may be decreased by: Acetylcholinesterase Inhibitors

Storage/Stability Store at 20°C to 25°C (68°F to 77°F).

Mechanism of Action Competitively blocks the action of acetylcholine at postganglionic parasympathetic receptor sites

Pharmacodynamics

Onset of action: Within 30-45 minutes

Duration: 4-6 hours

Pharmacokinetics (Adult data unless noted)

Metabolism: In the liver and GI tract

Elimination: In urine, bile, and other body fluids

Dosing: Usual Oral:

Antisecretory:

Children: 1-2 mg/kg/day in 3-4 divided doses

Adults: 15 mg 3 times/day before meals or food and 30 mg at bedtime; for mild manifestations: 7.5 mg 3 times/day

Antispasmodic:

Children: 2-3 mg/kg/day in divided doses every 4-6 hours and at bedtime

Adults: 15 mg 3 times/day before meals or food and 30 mg at bedtime

Administration Oral: Administer 30 minutes before meals and at bedtime

Dosage Forms Excipient information presented when available (limited, particularly for generics); consult specific product labeling.

Tablet, Oral, as bromide:

Generic: 15 mg

◆ **Propantheline Bromide** *see* Propantheline *on page 1784*

Proparacaine (proe PAR a kane)

Brand Names: US Alcaine; Parcaine [DSC]

Brand Names: Canada Alcaine®; Diocaine®

Therapeutic Category Local Anesthetic, Ophthalmic

Generic Availability (US) Yes

Use Local anesthesia for tonometry, gonioscopy; suture removal from cornea; removal of corneal foreign body; cataract extraction, glaucoma surgery; short operative procedure involving the cornea and conjunctiva

Pregnancy Risk Factor C

Pregnancy Considerations Animal reproduction studies have not been conducted.

Breast-Feeding Considerations It is not known if proparacaine is excreted in breast milk. The manufacturer recommends that caution be exercised when administering proparacaine to nursing women.

Contraindications Hypersensitivity to proparacaine or any component of the formulation

Warnings/Precautions For topical ophthalmic use only; prolonged use may result in permanent corneal opacification and visual loss and is not recommended.

Adverse Reactions

Dermatologic: Allergic contact dermatitis

Hypersensitivity: Hypersensitivity reaction (corneal; characterized by acute, intense, and diffuse epithelial keratitis; gray, ground glass appearance; exfoliation of skin; corneal filaments; and can include iritis with descemetitis)

Ophthalmic: Burning sensation of eyes, conjunctival hemorrhage, conjunctival hyperemia, corneal erosion, cycloplegia, eye redness, mydriasis, stinging of eyes

Drug Interactions

Metabolism/Transport Effects None known.

Avoid Concomitant Use There are no known interactions where it is recommended to avoid concomitant use.

Increased Effect/Toxicity There are no known significant interactions involving an increase in effect.

Decreased Effect There are no known significant interactions involving a decrease in effect.

Storage/Stability Store under refrigeration at 2°C to 8°C (36°F to 46°F). Protect from light. The following stability information has also been reported for Alcaine®: May be stored at room temperature for up to 30 days (Cohen, 2007).

Mechanism of Action Prevents initiation and transmission of impulse at the nerve cell membrane by decreasing ion permeability through stabilizing

Pharmacodynamics

Onset of action: Within 20 seconds of instillation

Duration: 15-20 minutes

Dosing: Neonatal Ophthalmic: Instill 2 drops of 0.5% solution 30 seconds prior to procedure; a crossover study in 22 premature neonates (GA: <30 weeks) undergoing examination for retinopathy of prematurity showed decreased pain scores compared to placebo (Marsh, 2005)

Dosing: Usual Children and Adults:

Ophthalmic surgery: Instill 1 drop of 0.5% solution in eye every 5-10 minutes for 5-7 doses

Tonometry, gonioscopy, suture removal: Instill 1-2 drops of 0.5% solution in eye just prior to procedure

Administration Ophthalmic: Instill drops into affected eye(s); avoid contact of bottle tip with skin or eye

Dosage Forms Excipient information presented when available (limited, particularly for generics); consult specific product labeling. [DSC] = Discontinued product

Solution, Ophthalmic, as hydrochloride:

Alcaine: 0.5% (15 mL)

Parcaine: 0.5% (15 mL [DSC])

Generic: 0.5% (15 mL)

◆ **Proparacaine Hydrochloride** *see* Proparacaine *on page 1785*

◆ **Propine® (Can)** *see* Dipivefrin *on page 687*

Propofol (PROE po fole)

Medication Safety Issues

Sound-alike/look-alike issues:

Diprivan may be confused with Diflucan, Ditropan

Propofol may be confused with fospropofol

Propofol may be confused with bupivacaine (liposomal) due to similar white, milky appearance.

High alert medication:

The Institute for Safe Medication Practices (ISMP) includes this medication among its list of drugs which have a heightened risk of causing significant patient harm when used in error.

Administration issues:

Propofol may be confused with bupivacaine liposome injectable suspension (Exparel) in operating rooms and other surgical areas due to their similar white, milky appearance especially when prepared in syringes. Bupivacaine liposome injectable suspension (Exparel) is intended only for administration via infiltration into the surgical site (and **not** for systemic use). Confusion with propofol may lead to accidental intravenous administration of Exparel instead of the intended propofol. Therefore, to avoid potential confusion ISMP recommends that all vials be separated when stocked in common areas and all prepared syringes be labeled.

Brand Names: US Diprivan; Fresenius Propoven

Brand Names: Canada Diprivan; PMS-Propofol; Propofol Injection

Therapeutic Category General Anesthetic

Generic Availability (US) Yes

Use Induction of general anesthesia (FDA approved in ages ≥3 years and adults); maintenance of general anesthesia (FDA approved in ages ≥2 months and adults); initiation and maintenance of monitored anesthesia care sedation (FDA approved in adults); sedation of intubated, mechanically ventilated ICU patients (FDA approved in adults); combined sedation and regional anesthesia (FDA approved in adults)

Note: Consult local regulations and individual institutional policies and procedures.

Pregnancy Risk Factor B

Pregnancy Considerations Propofol crosses the placenta and may be associated with neonatal CNS and respiratory depression. Propofol is not recommended by the manufacturer for obstetrics, including cesarean section deliveries.

Breast-Feeding Considerations Propofol is excreted in breast milk. Breast-feeding is not recommended by the manufacturer. A green discoloration to the breast milk was noted in a woman following administration of propofol during surgery for removal of an ectopic pregnancy. Although other medications were also administered, propofol was detected in the milk and assumed to be the cause; resolution of this effect occurred within 48 hours after surgery (Birkholz, 2009).

Contraindications Hypersensitivity to propofol or any component of the formulation; hypersensitivity to eggs, egg products, soybeans, or soy products; when general anesthesia or sedation is contraindicated

Note: Fresenius Propoven is also contraindicated in patients who are hypersensitive to peanuts. In July 2012, the FDA initiated temporary importation of Fresenius Propoven 1% (propofol) injection into the U.S. market to address a propofol shortage.

Warnings/Precautions May rarely cause hypersensitivity, anaphylaxis, anaphylactoid reactions, angioedema, bronchospasm, and erythema; medications for the treatment of hypersensitivity reactions should be available for immediate use. Use with caution in patients with history of hypersensitivity/anaphylactic reaction to peanuts; a low risk of crossreactivity between soy and peanuts may exist. Use is contraindicated in patients who are hypersensitive to eggs, egg products, soybeans, or soy products. The major cardiovascular effect of propofol is hypotension especially if patient is hypovolemic or if bolus dosing is used; use with caution in patients who are hemodynamically unstable, hypovolemic, or have abnormally low vascular tone (eg, sepsis). Use requires careful patient monitoring, should only be used by experienced personnel who are not actively engaged in the procedure or surgery. If used in a nonintubated and/or non–mechanically ventilated patient, qualified personnel and appropriate equipment for rapid institution of respiratory and/or cardiovascular support must be immediately available. Use to induce moderate (conscious) sedation in patients warrants monitoring equivalent to that seen with deep anesthesia. Consult local regulations and individual institutional policies and procedures.

Use a lower induction dose, a slower maintenance rate of administration, and avoid rapidly administered boluses in the elderly, debilitated, or ASA-PS (American Society of Anesthesiologists - Physical Status) 3/4 patients to reduce the incidence of unwanted cardiorespiratory depressive events. Use caution in patients with severe cardiac disease (ejection fraction <50%) or respiratory disease; may have more profound adverse cardiovascular responses to propofol. Use caution in patients with a history of epilepsy or seizures; seizure may occur during recovery phase. Use caution in patients with increased intracranial pressure or impaired cerebral circulation; substantial decreases in mean arterial pressure and subsequent decreases in cerebral perfusion pressure may occur; consider continuous infusion or administer as a slow bolus. In most cases, propofol does not significantly affect the QT interval (Staikou, 2014). However, prolongation of the QT interval, usually within normal limits, has occurred in case reports and small prospective studies and may be dose dependent (Hume-Smith, 2008; Kim, 2008; McConachie, 1989; Saarnivaara, 1990; Saarnivaara, 1993; Sakabe, 2002). Shortening of the QT interval has also occurred (Erdil, 2009; Tanskanen, 2002).

Propofol-related infusion syndrome (PRIS) is a serious side effect with a high mortality rate (up to 33%) characterized by dysrhythmia (eg, bradycardia or tachycardia), heart failure, hyperkalemia, lipemia, metabolic acidosis, and/or rhabdomyolysis or myoglobinuria with subsequent renal failure. Risk factors include poor oxygen delivery, sepsis, serious cerebral injury, and the administration of high doses of propofol (usually doses >83 mcg/kg/minute or >5 mg/kg/hour for >48 hours), but has also been reported following large dose, short term infusions during surgical anesthesia. PRIS has also been reported with lower-dose infusions (Chukwuemeka, 2006; Merz, 2006). The onset of the syndrome is rapid, occurring within 4 days of initiation. Alternate sedative therapy should be considered for patients with escalating doses of vasopressors or inotropes, when cardiac failure occurs during high-dose propofol infusion, when metabolic acidosis is observed, or in whom lengthy and/or high-dose sedation is needed (Barr, 2013; Corbett, 2008).

Because propofol is formulated within a 10% fat emulsion, hypertriglyceridemia is an expected side effect. Patients who develop hypertriglyceridemia (eg, >500 mg/dL) are at risk of developing pancreatitis. An alternative sedative agent should be employed if significant hypertriglyceridemia occurs. Use with caution in patients with preexisting pancreatitis; use of propofol may exacerbate this condition. Use caution in patients with preexisting hyperlipidemia as evidenced by increased serum triglyceride levels or serum turbidity. Transient local pain may occur during IV injection; perioperative myoclonia has occurred. Propofol should only be used in pregnancy if clearly needed. Not recommended for use in obstetrics, including cesarean section deliveries. Safety and efficacy in pediatric intensive care unit patients have not been established. Concurrent use of fentanyl and propofol in pediatric patients may result in bradycardia.

Concomitant use with opioids may lead to increased sedative or anesthetic effects of propofol, more pronounced decreases in systolic, diastolic, and mean arterial pressures and cardiac output; lower doses of propofol may be needed. In addition, fentanyl may cause serious bradycardia when used with propofol in pediatric patients. Alfentanil use with propofol has precipitated seizure activity in patients without any history of epilepsy. Discontinue opioids and paralytic agents prior to weaning. Avoid abrupt discontinuation prior to weaning or daily wake up assessments. Abrupt discontinuation can result in rapid awakening, anxiety, agitation, and resistance to mechanical ventilation; wean the infusion rate so the patient awakens slowly. Propofol lacks analgesic properties; pain management requires specific use of analgesic agents, at effective dosages, propofol must be titrated separately from the analgesic agent.

Propofol vials and prefilled syringes have the potential to support the growth of various microorganisms despite product additives intended to suppress microbial growth. To limit the potential for contamination, recommendations in product labeling for handling and administering propofol should be strictly adhered to. Some formulations may contain edetate disodium which may lead to decreased zinc levels in patients with prolonged therapy (>5 days) or a predisposition to zinc deficiency (eg, burns, diarrhea, or sepsis). A holiday from propofol infusion should take place after 5 days of therapy to allow for evaluation and necessary replacement of zinc. Some formulations may contain sulfites.

Benzyl alcohol and derivatives: Some dosage forms may contain benzyl alcohol; large amounts of benzyl alcohol (≥99 mg/kg/day) have been associated with a potentially fatal toxicity ("gasping syndrome") in neonates; the "gasping syndrome" consists of metabolic acidosis, respiratory distress, gasping respirations, CNS dysfunction (including convulsions, intracranial hemorrhage), hypotension, and cardiovascular collapse (AAP, 1997; CDC, 1982); some data suggests that benzoate displaces bilirubin from protein binding sites (Ahlfors, 2001); avoid or use dosage forms containing benzyl alcohol with caution in neonates. See manufacturer's labeling.

Warnings: Additional Pediatric Considerations Metabolic acidosis with fatal cardiac failure has occurred in several infants and children (4 weeks to 11 years of age) who received propofol infusions at average rates of infusion of 4.5 to 10 mg/kg/hour for 66 to 115 hours (maximum rates of infusion: 6.2 to 11.5 mg/kg/hour) (Bray, 1995; Parke, 1992; Strickland, 1995). Anecdotal reports of serious adverse events, including death, have been reported in pediatric patients with upper respiratory tract infections receiving propofol for ICU sedation. Not recommended for ICU sedation of pediatric patients; an increased number of deaths was observed in a multicenter clinical trial of pediatric ICU patients who received propofol (9% mortality) versus patients who received other sedative agents (4% mortality); although causality was not established, propofol is not indicated for sedation in PICU patients until further studies can document its safety in this population.

Adverse Reactions

Cardiovascular: Arrhythmia, bradycardia, cardiac output decreased, hyper-/hypotension, tachycardia

Central nervous system: Movement

Dermatologic: Pruritus, rash

Endocrine & metabolic: Hypertriglyceridemia

Local: Injection site burning, stinging, or pain

Respiratory: Apnea, respiratory acidosis during weaning

Rare but important or life-threatening: Agitation, amblyopia, anaphylaxis, anaphylactoid reaction, anticholinergic syndrome, asystole, atrial arrhythmia, bigeminy, cardiac arrest, chills, cough, dizziness, delirium, discoloration (green [urine, hair, or nailbeds]), extremity pain, fever, flushing, hemorrhage, hypersalivation, hypertonia, hypomagnesemia, hypoxia, infusion site reactions (including pain, swelling, blisters and/or tissue necrosis following accidental extravasation); laryngospasm, leukocytosis, lung function decreased, myalgia, myoclonia (rarely including convulsions and opisthotonos), nausea, pancreatitis, paresthesia, phlebitis, postoperative unconsciousness with or without increase in muscle tone, premature atrial contractions, premature ventricular contractions, pulmonary edema, propofol-related infusion syndrome, rhabdomyolysis, somnolence, syncope, thrombosis, urine cloudy, vision abnormality, wheezing

Drug Interactions

Metabolism/Transport Effects Substrate of CYP1A2 (minor), CYP2A6 (minor), CYP2B6 (major), CYP2C19 (minor), CYP2C9 (minor), CYP2D6 (minor), CYP2E1 (minor), CYP3A4 (minor); **Note:** Assignment of Major/Minor substrate status based on clinically relevant drug interaction potential; **Inhibits** CYP1A2 (weak), CYP2C9 (weak), CYP2D6 (weak), CYP2E1 (weak), CYP3A4 (weak)

Avoid Concomitant Use

Avoid concomitant use of Propofol with any of the following: Azelastine (Nasal); Orphenadrine; Paraldehyde; Pimozide; Thalidomide

Increased Effect/Toxicity

Propofol may increase the levels/effects of: Alcohol (Ethyl); ARIPiprazole; Azelastine (Nasal); Buprenorphine; CNS Depressants; Highest Risk QTc-Prolonging Agents; Hydrocodone; Lomitapide; Methotrimeprazine; Metyrosine; Midazolam; Mirtazapine; Moderate Risk QTc-Prolonging Agents; NiMODipine; Orphenadrine; Paraldehyde; Pimozide; Pramipexole; ROPINIRole; Ropivacaine; Rotigotine; Selective Serotonin Reuptake Inhibitors; Suvorexant; Thalidomide; TiZANidine; Zolpidem

The levels/effects of Propofol may be increased by: Alfentanil; Brimonidine (Topical); Cannabis; CYP2B6 Inhibitors (Moderate); Doxylamine; Dronabinol; Droperidol; HydrOXYzine; Kava Kava; Magnesium Sulfate; Methotrimeprazine; Midazolam; Mifepristone; Nabilone; Perampanel; Quazepam; Rifampin; Rufinamide; Sodium Oxybate; Tapentadol; Tetrahydrocannabinol

Decreased Effect There are no known significant interactions involving a decrease in effect.

Food Interactions Edetate disodium, an ingredient of propofol emulsion, may lead to decreased zinc levels in patients on prolonged therapy (>5 days) or those predisposed to deficiency (burns, diarrhea, and/or major sepsis). Management: Zinc replacement therapy may be needed.

Storage/Stability Store between 4°C to 22°C (40°F to 72°F); refrigeration is not required. Do not freeze. If transferred to a syringe or other container prior to administration, use within 6 hours. If used directly from vial/prefilled syringe, use within 12 hours. If diluted in 5% dextrose stable for 8 hours at room temperature. Shake well before use. Do not use if there is evidence of separation of phases of emulsion.

Mechanism of Action Propofol is a short-acting, lipophilic intravenous general anesthetic. The drug is unrelated to any of the currently used barbiturate, opioid, benzodiazepine, arylcyclohexylamine, or imidazole intravenous anesthetic agents. Propofol causes global CNS depression, presumably through agonism of $GABA_A$ receptors and perhaps reduced glutamatergic activity through NMDA receptor blockade.

Pharmacodynamics

Onset of anesthesia: Within 30 seconds after bolus infusion

Duration: ~3-10 minutes depending on the dose, rate and duration of administration; with prolonged use (eg, 10 days ICU sedation), propofol accumulates in tissues and redistributes into plasma when the drug is discontinued, so that the time to awakening (duration of action) is increased; however, if dose is titrated on a daily basis, so that the minimum effective dose is utilized, time to awakening may be within 10-15 minutes even after prolonged use

Pharmacokinetics (Adult data unless noted)

Distribution: Large volume of distribution; highly lipophilic

V_d (apparent): Children 4-12 years: 5-10 L/kg

V_{dss}:

Adults: 170-350 L

Adults (10-day infusion): 60 L/kg

Protein binding: 97% to 99%

Metabolism: Hepatic via glucuronide and sulfate conjugation

Half-life (three-compartment model):

Alpha: 2-8 minutes

Beta (second distribution): ~40 minutes

Terminal: ~200 minutes; range: 300-700 minutes

Terminal (after 10-day infusion): 1-3 days

Elimination: Urine (~88% as metabolites, 40% as glucuronide metabolite); feces (<2%)

Dosing: Usual Consult local regulations and individual institutional policies and procedures. Dosage must be individualized based on total body weight and titrated to the desired clinical effect; wait at least 3-5 minutes between dosage adjustments to clinically assess drug effects; smaller doses are required when used with opioids; the following are general dosing guidelines (see "Abbreviations, Acronyms, and Symbols" section in front section for explanation of ASA-PS classes). **Note:** Increase dose in patients with chronic alcoholism (Fassoulaki, 1993); decrease dose with acutely intoxicated (alcoholic) patients.

Pediatric: **General anesthesia:**

Induction of general anesthesia: Children and Adolescents (healthy) 3 to 16 years, ASA-PS 1 or 2: IV: 2.5 to 3.5 mg/kg over 20 to 30 seconds; use a lower dose for ASA-PS 3 or 4

Maintenance of general anesthesia: Infants, Children, and Adolescents (healthy) ≥2 months to ≤16 years, ASA-PS 1 or 2: IV infusion: General range: 125 to 300 mcg/kg/minute (7.5 to 18 mg/kg/**hour**); Initial dose immediately following induction: 200 to 300 mcg/kg/minute; then decrease dose after 30 minutes if clinical signs of light anesthesia are absent; usual infusion rate after initial 30 minutes: 125 to 150 mcg/kg/minute (7.5 to 9 mg/kg/**hour**); infants and children ≤5 years may require higher infusion rates compared to older children.

Adult:

General anesthesia:

Induction of general anesthesia:

Healthy adults, ASA-PS 1 or 2, <55 years: IV: 2 to 2.5 mg/kg (~40 mg every 10 seconds until onset of induction)

Debilitated, ASA-PS 3 or 4: IV: 1 to 1.5 mg/kg (~20 mg every 10 seconds until onset of induction)

Maintenance of general anesthesia:

Healthy adults, ASA-PS 1 or 2, <55 years:

IV infusion: Initial: 100 to 200 mcg/kg/minute (or 6 to 12 mg/kg/**hour**) for 10 to 15 minutes; usual maintenance infusion rate: 50 to 100 mcg/kg/minute (or 3 to 6 mg/kg/**hour**) to optimize recovery time

IV intermittent bolus: 25 to 50 mg increments as needed

Debilitated, ASA-PS 3 or 4: IV Infusion: 50 to 100 mcg/kg/minute (or 3 to 6 mg/kg/hour)

Monitored anesthesia care sedation:

Healthy adults, ASA-PS 1 or 2, <55 years: Slow IV infusion: 100 to 150 mcg/kg/minute (or 6 to 9 mg/kg/**hour**) for 3 to 5 minutes **or** slow injection: 0.5 mg/kg over 3 to 5 minutes followed by IV infusion of 25 to 75 mcg/kg/minute (or 1.5 to 4.5 mg/kg/**hour**) **or** incremental bolus doses: 10 mg or 20 mg

Debilitated or ASA-PS 3 or 4 patients: Use 80% of healthy adult dose

ICU sedation in intubated mechanically-ventilated patients: Avoid rapid bolus injection; individualize dose and titrate to response. Continuous IV infusion: Initial: 5 mcg/kg/minute (or 0.3 mg/kg/**hour**); increase by 5 to 10 mcg/kg/minute (or 0.3 to 0.6 mg/kg/**hour**) every 5 to 10 minutes until desired sedation level is achieved; usual maintenance: 5 to 50 mcg/kg/minute (or 0.3 to 3 mg/kg/**hour**); reduce dose after adequate sedation established and adjust to response (eg, evaluate frequently to use minimum dose for sedation). Daily interruption with retitration or a light target level of sedation is recommended to minimize prolonged sedative effects (Barr, 2013).

Debilitated or ASA-PS 3 or 4 patients: Use 80% of healthy adult dose; reduce dose after adequate sedation established and adjust to response (eg, evaluate frequently to use minimum dose for sedation). Daily interruption with retitration or a light target level of sedation is recommended to minimize prolonged sedative effects (Barr, 2013).

Dosing adjustment in renal impairment: No dosage adjustment necessary.

Dosing adjustment in hepatic impairment: No dosage adjustment necessary.

Preparation for Administration Parenteral: IV: May be further diluted in D_5W to a concentration of ≥2 mg/mL; diluted emulsion is more stable in glass (stability in plastic: 95% potency after 2 hours). To reduce pain associated with administration, may add lidocaine to propofol immediately before administration in a quantity not to exceed 20 mg lidocaine per 200 mg propofol. Strict aseptic technique must be maintained in handling. Prepare drug for single-patient use only. Shake emulsion well before use.

Administration Note: Consult local regulations and individual institutional policies and procedures.

Parenteral: IV: Shake emulsion well before use. May be administered undiluted or may be further diluted with D_5W. Do not administer via filter with <5-micron pore size. Do not administer through the same IV catheter with blood or plasma. Tubing and any unused portions of propofol vials should be discarded after 12 hours.

To reduce pain associated with injection, use larger veins of forearm or antecubital fossa; lidocaine IV (1 mL of a 1% solution) may also be used prior to administration or lidocaine may be added to propofol immediately before administration.

Induction: Administer pediatric induction doses over 20 to 30 seconds; may be administered more rapidly in adults

Maintenance: Administer at a concentration of 2 to 10 mg/mL at prescribed rate

Monitoring Parameters Cardiac monitor, blood pressure, oxygen saturation (during monitored anesthesia care sedation), arterial blood gas (with prolonged infusions). With prolonged infusions (eg, ICU sedation), monitor for metabolic acidosis, hyperkalemia, rhabdomyolysis or elevated CPK, hepatomegaly, and progression of cardiac and renal failure.

ICU sedation: Adult: Assess and adjust sedation according to scoring system (Richmond Agitation-Sedation Scale [RASS] or Sedation-Agitation Scale [SAS]) (Barr, 2013); assess CNS function daily. Serum triglyceride levels should be obtained prior to initiation of therapy and every 3 to 7 days thereafter, especially if receiving for >48 hours with doses exceeding 50 mcg/kg/minute (Devlin, 2005); use intravenous port opposite propofol infusion or temporarily suspend infusion and flush port prior to blood draw.

Diprivan: Monitor zinc levels in patients predisposed to deficiency (burns, diarrhea, major sepsis) or after 5 days of treatment.

Additional Information Propofol injection contains ~0.1 g of fat/mL (1.1 kcal/mL)

Acute febrile reactions: In June 2007, the FDA alerted clinicians of several reports of chills, fever, and body aches occurring in clusters of patients after administration of propofol for sedation in gastrointestinal suites. These reports were received from several facilities and involved multiple vials and lots. Symptoms appeared 6 to 18 hours following propofol therapy and persisted for ≤3 days. There is no evidence that any patient had sepsis or that the vials were contaminated. The FDA has tested multiple propofol vials and lots used in these patients and presently have found no evidence of bacterial contamination. Regardless, propofol vials and prefilled syringes have the potential to support the growth of various microorganisms despite product additives intended to suppress microbial growth. To limit the potential for contamination, the FDA is reminding healthcare professionals to strictly adhere to recommendations in product labeling for handling and administering propofol. Clinicians should also be vigilant for signs and symptoms of acute febrile reactions and evaluate patients for bacteremia. The FDA is continuing to work with the Centers for Disease Control and Prevention to investigate factors contributing to these occurrences. Additional information is available at http://www.fda.gov/Drugs/DrugSafety/PostmarketDrugSafetyInformationforPatientsandProviders/ucm109357.htm.

Dosage Forms Excipient information presented when available (limited, particularly for generics); consult specific product labeling.

Emulsion, Intravenous:

Diprivan: 10 mg/mL (10 mL, 20 mL, 50 mL, 100 mL) [contains edetate disodium, egg phospholipids (egg lecithin), glycerin, soybean oil]

Generic: 10 mg/mL (20 mL, 50 mL, 100 mL)

Emulsion, Intravenous [preservative free]:

Fresenius Propoven: 10 mg/mL (20 mL, 50 mL, 100 mL) [contains egg phosphatides, soybean oil]

Generic: 10 mg/mL (20 mL, 50 mL, 100 mL)

◆ **Propofol Injection (Can)** *see* Propofol *on page 1786*

Propranolol (proe PRAN oh lole)

Medication Safety Issues

Sound-alike/look-alike issues:

Propranolol may be confused with prasugrel, Pravachol, Propulsid

Inderal may be confused with Adderall, Enduron, Imdur, Imuran, Inderide, Isordil, Toradol

High alert medication:

The Institute for Safe Medication Practices (ISMP) includes this medication among its list of drugs which have a heightened risk of causing significant patient harm when used in error.

Administration issues:

Significant differences exist between oral and IV dosing. Use caution when converting from one route of administration to another.

International issues:

Deralin [Australia, Israel] may be confused with Deptran brand name for doxepin [Australia]

Inderal [Canada and multiple international markets], Inderal LA [U.S.], and Inderal XL [U.S.] may be confused with Indiaral brand name for loperamide [France] or Indamol brand name for indapamide [Italy]

Related Information

Oral Medications That Should Not Be Crushed or Altered *on page 2476*

Serotonin Syndrome *on page 2447*

Brand Names: US Hemangeol; Inderal LA; Inderal XL; InnoPran XL

Brand Names: Canada Apo-Propranolol; Dom-Propranolol; Inderal; Inderal LA; Novo-Pranol; Nu-Propranolol; PMS-Propranolol; Propranolol Hydrochloride Injection, USP; Teva-Propranolol

Therapeutic Category Antianginal Agent; Antiarrhythmic Agent, Class II; Antihypertensive Agent; Antimigraine Agent; Beta-Adrenergic Blocker

Generic Availability (US) Yes

Use

Oral:

Immediate release products (oral solutions, tablets):

Hemangeol: Treatment of proliferating infantile hemangioma requiring systemic therapy (FDA approved in infants ≥5 weeks weighing ≥2 kg)

Other immediate release products: Management of hypertension alone or in combination with other agents, angina pectoris, symptomatic treatment of hypertrophic subaortic stenosis, migraine headache prophylaxis, pheochromocytoma, essential tremor, atrial fibrillation, reduction of mortality post-MI (all indications FDA approved in adults); has also been used for tetralogy of Fallot cyanotic spells; short-term adjunctive therapy of thyrotoxicosis

Extended release capsules (Inderal XL, InnoPran XL): Management of hypertension alone or in combination with other agents (FDA approved in adults)

Long acting capsules (Inderal LA): Management of hypertension alone or in combination with other agents, angina pectoris, symptomatic treatment of hypertrophic subaortic stenosis, migraine headache prophylaxis (all indications: FDA approved in adults)

IV: Supraventricular arrhythmias (such as atrial fibrillation and flutter, AV nodal re-entrant tachycardias), ventricular tachycardias (catecholamine-induced arrhythmias, digoxin toxicity) (all indications FDA approved in adults); has also been used for tetralogy of Fallot cyanotic spells; short-term adjunction therapy of thyrotoxicosis

Prescribing and Access Restrictions Prescriptions for Hemangeol may be obtained via the Hemangeol Patient Access program. Visit http://www.hemangeol.com/hcp/hemangeol-direct/ or call 855-618-4950 for ordering information.

Pregnancy Risk Factor C

Pregnancy Considerations Adverse events have been observed in some animal reproduction studies; therefore, the manufacturer classifies propranolol as pregnancy category C. Propranolol crosses the placenta and is measurable in the newborn serum following maternal use during pregnancy. In a cohort study, an increased risk of cardiovascular defects was observed following maternal use of beta-blockers during pregnancy. Intrauterine growth restriction (IUGR), small placentas, as well as fetal/neonatal bradycardia, hypoglycemia, and/or respiratory depression have been observed following *in utero* exposure to beta-blockers as a class. Adequate facilities for monitoring infants at birth should be available. Untreated chronic maternal hypertension and pre-eclampsia are also associated with adverse events in the fetus, infant, and mother. The peak maternal serum concentrations of propranolol and the active metabolite 4-hydroxypropranolol do not change during pregnancy; peak serum concentrations of naphthoxylactic acid are lower in the third trimester when compared to postpartum. Propranolol is recommended for use in the management of thyrotoxicosis in pregnancy. Propranolol has been evaluated for the treatment of hypertension in pregnancy, but other agents may be more appropriate for use. Propranolol has also been used in the management of hypertrophic obstructive cardiomyopathy in pregnancy and has been studied for use as an adjunctive agent in the management of dysfunctional labor (dystocia).

Breast-Feeding Considerations Propranolol is excreted into breast milk with peak concentrations occurring ~2-3 hours after an oral dose. The inactive metabolites of propranolol have also been detected in breast milk. The manufacturer recommends that caution be exercised when administering propranolol to nursing women. Due to immature hepatic metabolism in newborns, breast-feeding infants should be monitored for adverse events.

Contraindications

Hypersensitivity to propranolol, beta-blockers, or any component of the formulation; uncompensated congestive heart failure (unless the failure is due to tachyarrhythmias being treated with propranolol), cardiogenic shock; severe sinus bradycardia, sick sinus syndrome, or heart block greater than first-degree (except in patients with a functioning artificial pacemaker); bronchial asthma

Hemangeol (additional contraindications): Premature infants with corrected age <5 weeks; infants weighing <2 kg; heart rate <80 bpm; blood pressure <50/30 mm Hg; pheochromocytoma; history of bronchospasm

Warnings/Precautions Consider preexisting conditions such as sick sinus syndrome before initiating. Administer cautiously in compensated heart failure and monitor for a worsening of the condition (efficacy of propranolol in HF has not been demonstrated). **[U.S. Boxed Warning]: Beta-blocker therapy should not be withdrawn abruptly (particularly in patients with CAD), but gradually tapered to avoid acute tachycardia, hypertension, and/or ischemia.** Beta-blockers without alpha1-adrenergic receptor blocking activity should be avoided in patients with Prinzmetal variant angina (Mayer, 1998). Chronic beta-blocker therapy should not be routinely withdrawn prior to major surgery. May precipitate or aggravate symptoms of arterial insufficiency in patients with PVD and Raynaud's disease; use with caution and monitor for progression of arterial obstruction. Bradycardia may be observed more frequently in elderly patients (>65 years of age); dosage reductions may be necessary. Potentially significant drug-drug interactions may exist, requiring dose or frequency adjustment, additional monitoring, and/or selection of alternative therapy. Cigarette smoking may decrease plasma levels of propranolol by increasing metabolism. Patients should be advised to avoid smoking. Use cautiously in patients with diabetes because it can mask prominent hypoglycemic symptoms. May mask signs of hyperthyroidism (eg, tachycardia); if hyperthyroidism is suspected, carefully manage and monitor; abrupt withdrawal may exacerbate symptoms of hyperthyroidism or precipitate thyroid storm. May alter thyroid-function tests. Use with caution in myasthenia gravis or psychiatric disease (may cause CNS depression). Use cautiously in renal and hepatic dysfunction; dosage adjustment may be required in hepatic impairment. In general, patients with bronchospastic disease should not receive beta-blockers; if used at all, should be used cautiously with close monitoring. Adequate alpha-blockade is required prior to use of any beta-blocker for patients with untreated pheochromocytoma. May induce or exacerbate psoriasis. Use caution with history of severe anaphylaxis to allergens; patients taking beta-blockers may become more sensitive to repeated challenges. Treatment of anaphylaxis (eg, epinephrine) in patients taking beta-blockers may be ineffective or promote undesirable effects.

Considerations when treating infantile hemangioma: Bradycardia and/or hypotension may occur or be worsened; monitor heart rate and blood pressure after propranolol initiation or increase in dose; discontinue treatment if severe (<80 bpm) or symptomatic bradycardia or hypotension (systolic blood pressure <50 mm Hg) occurs. Infants with large facial infantile hemangioma should be investigated for potential arteriopathy associated with PHACE syndrome prior to propranolol therapy; decreases in blood pressure caused by propranolol may increase risk of stroke in PHACE syndrome patients with cerebrovascular anomalies. May potentiate hypoglycemia and/or mask signs and symptoms. Withhold the dose in infants or children who are not feeding regularly or who are vomiting; discontinue therapy and seek immediate treatment if hypoglycemia occurs. May cause bronchospasm. Interrupt therapy in infants or children with lower respiratory tract infection associated with dyspnea or wheezing.

Adverse Reactions

Cardiovascular: Angina pectoris, atrioventricular conduction disturbance, bradycardia, cardiogenic shock, cold extremities, congestive heart failure, hypotension, ineffective myocardial contractions, syncope

Central nervous system: Agitation, amnesia, carpal tunnel syndrome, catatonia, cognitive dysfunction, confusion, dizziness, drowsiness, fatigue, hypersomnia, irritability, lethargy, nightmares, paresthesia, psychosis, sleep disorder, vertigo

Dermatologic: Changes in nails, contact dermatitis, dermal ulcer, eczematous rash, erosive lichen planus, hyperkeratosis, pruritus, skin rash

Endocrine & metabolic: Hyperglycemia, hyperkalemia, hyperlipidemia, hypoglycemia

Gastrointestinal: Abdominal pain, anorexia, constipation, decreased appetite, diarrhea, stomach discomfort

Genitourinary: Oliguria, proteinuria

Hematologic & oncologic: Immune thrombocytopenia, thrombocytopenia

Hepatic: Increased serum alkaline phosphatase, increased serum transaminases

Neuromuscular & skeletal: Arthropathy, oculomucocutaneous syndrome, polyarthritis

Ophthalmic: Conjunctival hyperemia, decreased visual acuity, mydriasis

Renal: Increased blood urea nitrogen, interstitial nephritis (rare)

Respiratory: Bronchiolitis (infants; associated with cough, fever, diarrhea, and vomiting), bronchitis (infants; associated with cough, fever, diarrhea, and vomiting), bronchospasm, dyspnea, pulmonary edema, wheezing

Miscellaneous: Ulcer

Rare but important or life-threatening: Agranulocytosis, alopecia, arterial insufficiency, arterial mesenteric thrombosis, decreased heart rate (infants), decreased serum glucose (infants), depression, emotional lability, epigastric distress, erythema multiforme, fever combined with generalized ache, sore throat, laryngospasm, and respiratory distress), hallucination, hypersensitivity reaction (including anaphylaxis, anaphylactoid reaction), impotence, insomnia, ischemic colitis, lupus-like syndrome, myotonia, myopathy, nonthrombocytopenic purpura, peripheral arterial disease (exacerbation), Peyronie's disease, pharyngitis, psoriasiform eruption, purpura, Raynaud's phenomenon, second degree atrioventricular block (infants; in a patient with an underlying conduction disorder), slightly clouded sensorium, Stevens-Johnson syndrome, systemic lupus erythematosus, temporary amnesia, tingling of extremities (hands), toxic epidermal necrolysis, urticaria, visual disturbance, weakness, xerophthalmia

Drug Interactions

Metabolism/Transport Effects Substrate of CYP1A2 (major), CYP2C19 (minor), CYP2D6 (major), CYP3A4 (minor); **Note:** Assignment of Major/Minor substrate status based on clinically relevant drug interaction potential; **Inhibits** CYP1A2 (weak), CYP2D6 (weak), P-glycoprotein

Avoid Concomitant Use

Avoid concomitant use of Propranolol with any of the following: Beta2-Agonists; Bosutinib; Ceritinib; Floctafenine; Methacholine; PAZOPanib; Rivastigmine; Silodosin; Topotecan; VinCRIStine (Liposomal)

Increased Effect/Toxicity

Propranolol may increase the levels/effects of: Afatinib; Alpha-/Beta-Agonists (Direct-Acting); Alpha1-Blockers; Alpha2-Agonists; Amifostine; Antihypertensives; Antipsychotic Agents (Phenothiazines); ARIPiprazole; Bosutinib; Bradycardia-Causing Agents; Brentuximab Vedotin; Bupivacaine; Cardiac Glycosides; Ceritinib; Cholinergic Agonists; Colchicine; Dabigatran Etexilate; Disopyramide; DOXOrubicin (Conventional); DULoxetine; Edoxaban; Ergot Derivatives; Everolimus; Fingolimod; Grass Pollen Allergen Extract (5 Grass Extract); Hypotensive Agents; Insulin; Ivabradine; Lacosamide; Ledipasvir; Levodopa; Lidocaine (Systemic); Lidocaine (Topical); Mepivacaine; Methacholine; Midodrine; Naloxegol; Obinutuzumab; PAZOPanib; P-glycoprotein/ABCB1 Substrates; Prucalopride; Rifaximin; RisperiDONE; RiTUXimab; Rivaroxaban; Rizatriptan; Silodosin; Sulfonylureas; TiZANidine; Topotecan; VinCRIStine (Liposomal); ZOLMitriptan

The levels/effects of Propranolol may be increased by: Abiraterone Acetate; Acetylcholinesterase Inhibitors; Alcohol (Ethyl); Alpha2-Agonists; Aminoquinolines (Antimalarial); Amiodarone; Anilidopiperidine Opioids; Antipsychotic Agents (Phenothiazines); Barbiturates; Bretylium; Brimonidine (Topical); Calcium Channel Blockers (Nondihydropyridine); Cobicistat; CYP1A2 Inhibitors (Moderate); CYP1A2 Inhibitors (Strong); CYP2D6 Inhibitors (Moderate); CYP2D6 Inhibitors (Strong); Darunavir; Deferasirox; Diazoxide; Dipyridamole; Disopyramide; Dronedarone; Floctafenine; FluvoxaMINE; Herbs (Hypotensive Properties); Lacidipine; MAO Inhibitors; Nicorandil; NIFEdipine; Panobinostat; Peginterferon Alfa-2b; Pentoxifylline; Phosphodiesterase 5 Inhibitors; Propafenone; Prostacyclin Analogues; QuiNIDine; Regorafenib; Reserpine; Rivastigmine; Ruxolitinib; Selective Serotonin Reuptake Inhibitors; Tofacitinib; Vemurafenib; Zileuton

Decreased Effect

Propranolol may decrease the levels/effects of: Beta2-Agonists; Lacidipine; Theophylline Derivatives

The levels/effects of Propranolol may be decreased by: Alcohol (Ethyl); Barbiturates; Bile Acid Sequestrants; Cannabis; CYP1A2 Inducers (Strong); Cyproterone; Herbs (Hypertensive Properties); Methylphenidate; Nonsteroidal Anti-Inflammatory Agents; Peginterferon Alfa-2b; Rifamycin Derivatives; Teriflunomide; Yohimbine

Food Interactions

Ethanol: Ethanol may increase or decrease plasma levels of propranolol. Reports are variable and have shown both enhanced as well as inhibited hepatic metabolism (of propranolol). Management: Caution advised with consumption of ethanol and monitor for heart rate and/or blood pressure changes.

Food: Propranolol serum levels may be increased if taken with food. Protein-rich foods may increase bioavailability; a change in diet from high carbohydrate/low protein to low carbohydrate/high protein may result in increased oral clearance. Management: Tablets (immediate release) should be taken on an empty stomach. Capsules (extended release) may be taken with or without food, but be consistent with regard to food.

Storage/Stability

Injection: Store at 20°C to 25°C (68°F to 77°F); protect from freezing or excessive heat. Once diluted, propranolol is stable for 24 hours at room temperature in D_5W or NS. Protect from light. Solution has a maximum stability at pH of 3 and decomposes rapidly in alkaline pH.

Capsule, tablet, oral solution: Store at controlled room temperature; protect from freezing or excessive heat. Protect from light and moisture. Dispense Hemangeol in original container; discard 2 months after first opening.

Mechanism of Action Nonselective beta-adrenergic blocker (class II antiarrhythmic); competitively blocks response to $beta_1$- and $beta_2$-adrenergic stimulation which results in decreases in heart rate, myocardial contractility, blood pressure, and myocardial oxygen demand. Nonselective beta-adrenergic blockers (propranolol, nadolol) reduce portal pressure by producing splanchnic vasoconstriction ($beta_2$ effect) thereby reducing portal blood flow.

Pharmacodynamics Beta blockade: Oral:

Onset of action: Immediate release: Within 1 to 2 hours

Duration: Immediate release: 6 to 12 hours; Extended release: ~24 to 27 hours

Maximum effect: Hypertension: A few days to several weeks

Pharmacokinetics (Adult data unless noted)

Absorption: Oral: Rapid and complete

Distribution: V_d: 4 L/kg; crosses the blood-brain barrier

Protein-binding: $Alpha_1$-acid glycoprotein and albumin; **Note:** The S-isomer of propranolol preferentially binds to $alpha_1$-acid glycoprotein and the R-isomer preferentially binds to albumin

Newborns: 60% to 68%

Adults: 90%

Metabolism: Extensive first-pass effect, hepatically metabolized to active and inactive compounds; the 3 main metabolic pathways include: Aromatic hydroxylation (primarily 4-hydroxylation), N-dealkylation followed by further side-chain oxidation and direct glucuronidation; the 4 primary metabolites include: Propranolol glucuronide, naphthyloxylactic acid, and sulfate and glucuronic acid conjugates of 4-hydroxy propranolol; **Note:** Aromatic hydroxylation is catalyzed primarily by isoenzyme CYP2D6; side chain oxidation is mainly via CYP1A2, but also CYP2D6; 4-hydroxypropranolol possesses beta-adrenergic receptor blocking activity and is a weak inhibitor of CYP2D6.

Bioavailability: Oral: ~25%; oral bioavailability may be increased in Down syndrome children; protein-rich foods increase bioavailability of immediate release formulations by ~50%

Half-life, elimination:

Neonates: Possible increased half-life

Infants 35 to 150 days: Median 3.5 hours

Children: 3.9 to 6.4 hours

Adults: Immediate release: 3 to 6 hours; Extended release formulations: 8 to 10 hours

Time to peak serum concentration: Oral:

Infants: Immediate release: ≤2 hours

Adults:

Immediate release: 1 to 4 hours

Extended release capsule (Inderal XL, InnoPran XL): 12 to 14 hours

Long acting capsule (Inderal LA): 6 hours

Elimination: Metabolites are excreted primarily in urine (96% to 99%); <1% excreted in urine as unchanged drug

Dosing: Neonatal Note: Dosage should be individualized based on patient response.

Hypertension, tachyarrhythmias: Limited data available:

Oral: Immediate release formulations: Initial: 0.25 mg/kg/dose every 6 to 8 hours; increase slowly as needed to maximum daily dose of 5 mg/kg/**day** (Rasoulpour, 1992)

IV: Initial: 0.01 mg/kg slow IV push over 10 minutes; may repeat every 6 to 8 hours as needed; increase slowly to maximum dose of 0.15 mg/kg/dose every 6 to 8 hours (Rasoulpour, 1992)

Thyrotoxicosis: Limited data available: Oral: Immediate release formulations: 0.5 to 2 mg/kg/day in divided doses every 6 to 12 hours (Kliegman, 2011; Léger, 2013; Smith, 2001); occasionally higher doses may be required

Dosing: Usual Note: Dosage should be individualized based on patient response.

Pediatric:

Essential tremor: Limited data available: Children and Adolescents: Oral: Immediate release formulations: Initial: 0.5 to 1 mg/kg/day in 3 divided doses; maximum daily dose: 4 mg/kg/**day** (Ferrara, 2009)

Hemangioma, infantile; proliferating: Oral:

Manufacturer's labeling (Hemangeol): Infants ≥5 weeks weighing at least 2 kg: **Note:** Therapy should be initiated at age 5 weeks to 5 months: Initial dose: 0.6 mg/kg/**dose** twice daily for 1 week then beginning with week 2, increase dose to 1.1 mg/kg/**dose** twice daily and then for week 3 begin maintenance dose of 1.7 mg/kg/**dose** twice daily; doses should be separated by at least 9 hours; continue maintenance dose for 6 months; readjust dose for patient growth. May repeat course if hemangiomas recur.

Alternate dosing: Infants and Children <5 years: Limited data available: Oral: Immediate release formulations: Initial: 0.5 to 1 mg/kg/day in 2 or 3 divided doses, titrate gradually (most trials titrated dose every 2 or 3 days, up to 1 week) to maintenance dose; usual daily maintenance dose: 2 mg/kg/day; some patients may require 3 mg/kg/day. Optimal duration not defined; mean/median duration in clinical studies ranged from 6 to 12 months(Fuchsmann, 2011; Gan, 2013; Georgountzou, 2012; Hermans, 2013; Hogeling, 2011; Price, 2011; Sans, 2009).

Hypertension: Children and Adolescents 1 to 17 years: Oral: Immediate release formulations: Initial: 1 to 2 mg/kg/day divided in 2 to 3 doses/day; titrate dose to effect; maximum dose: 4 mg/kg/day up to 640 mg/day; sustained release formulation may be dosed once daily (NHBPEP, 2004; NHLBI, 2011). Others have suggested a higher maximum daily dose of 16 mg/kg/**day**; 640 mg/**day** (Kavay 2010; Park, 2008)

Migraine headache; prophylaxis: Limited data available; efficacy results variable; optimal dose not established: Oral: Immediate release formulations:

Weight-directed dosing: Children ≥3 years and Adolescents: Reported range: 0.5 to 3 mg/kg/day in 2 to 3 divided doses; some trials initiated therapy at the low end of the range and titrated upward to response; doses as low as 0.5 to 1 mg/kg/day may be effective; doses up to 4 mg/kg/day have been used; maximum daily dose: 120 mg/**day** (AAN [Lewis, 2004]; AAP [Drolet, 2011]; Ashrafi, 2005; Bonfert, 2013; Eidlitz-Markus, 2012; El-Chammas, 2013; Lanteri-Minet, 2014)

Fixed dose: Children ≥7 years and Adolescents: Initial: 10 mg daily; increase at weekly intervals in 10 mg increments; usual dose range: 10 to 20 mg 3 times daily (Kliegman, 2011); doses as high as 120 mg daily have been used (AAN [Lewis, 2004])

Tachyarrhythmias: Limited data available: Infants, Children, and Adolescents:

Oral: Immediate release formulations: Initial: 0.5 to 1 mg/kg/day in divided doses every 6 to 8 hours; titrate dosage upward every 3 to 5 days; usual daily dose: 2 to 4 mg/kg/day; higher doses may be needed; maximum daily dose: 16 mg/kg/**day** or 60 mg/**day** (Kliegman, 2011; Park, 2008)

IV: 0.01 to 0.15 mg/kg slow IV over 10 minutes; may repeat every 6 to 8 hours as needed; maximum dose is age-dependent: Infants: 1 mg/dose; children and adolescents: 3 mg/dose (Nelson, 1996; Park, 2008)

Tetralogy spells:

Oral: Palliative therapy: Infants and Children: 0.5 to 1 mg/kg/dose every 6 hours (Kliegman, 2011). Others have used the following: Initial: 0.25 mg/kg/dose every 6 hours (1 mg/kg/day); if ineffective within first week of therapy, may increase by 1 mg/kg/day every 24 hours to maximum of 5 mg/kg/day; if patient becomes refractory may increase slowly to a maximum of 10 to 15 mg/kg/day but must carefully monitor heart rate, heart size, and cardiac contractility; average dose: 2.3 mg/kg/day; range: 0.8 to 5 mg/kg/day (Garson, 1981).

IV: Infants and Children: 0.15 to 0.25 mg/kg/dose infused over 10 minutes; maximum initial dose: 1 mg; may repeat dose once (AAP [Hegenbarth, 2008]); alternatively, initiate lower doses of 0.015 to 0.02 mg/kg/dose and titrate to effect, up to 0.1 to 0.2 mg/kg/dose (Anderson, 2009)

Thyrotoxicosis; thyroid storm (Kliegman, 2011):

Infants and Children: Oral: Immediate release formulations: 0.5 to 2 mg/kg/day divided every 8 hours; maximum dose: 40 mg/dose

Adolescents:

Oral: 20 to 40 mg every 4 to 6 hours

IV: 1 mg slow IV push over 10 minutes; **Note:** May need to repeat dose; interval in adolescents not defined. Adult doses are repeated every 3 hours (Gardner, 2011).

Adult:

Essential tremor: Oral: 40 mg twice daily initially; maintenance doses: Usually 120 to 320 mg/day

Hypertension:

Initial: Oral: Immediate release: 40 mg twice daily; increase dosage every 3 to 7 days; usual dose: 120 to 240 mg divided in 2 to 3 doses daily; maximum daily dose: 640 mg; usual dosage range (ASH/ISH [Weber, 2014]): 40 to 160 mg twice daily

Extended release formulations:

Inderal LA: Initial: 80 mg once daily; usual maintenance: 120 to 160 mg once daily; maximum daily dose: 640 mg/**day**

Inderal XL, InnoPran XL: Initial: 80 mg once daily at bedtime; if initial response is inadequate, may be increased at 2 to 3 week intervals to a maximum daily dose of 120 mg/**day**

Hypertrophic subaortic stenosis: Oral: Immediate release: 20 to 40 mg 3 to 4 times daily

Inderal LA: 80 to 160 mg once daily

Migraine headache prophylaxis: Oral: Immediate release: Initial: 80 mg/day divided every 6 to 8 hours; increase by 20 to 40 mg/dose every 3 to 4 weeks to a maximum of 160 to 240 mg/day given in divided doses every 6 to 8 hours; if satisfactory response not achieved within 6 weeks of starting therapy, drug should be withdrawn gradually over several weeks

Inderal LA: Initial: 80 mg once daily; effective dose range: 160 to 240 mg once daily

Pheochromocytoma: Oral: 30 to 60 mg/day in divided doses

Post-MI mortality reduction: Oral: 180 to 240 mg/day in 3 to 4 divided doses

Stable angina: Oral: Immediate release: 80 to 320 mg/day in doses divided 2 to 4 times/day

Inderal LA: Initial: 80 mg once daily; maximum dose: 320 mg once daily

Tachyarrhythmias:

Oral: 10 to 30 mg/dose every 6 to 8 hours or a usual maintenance dose of 10 to 40 mg 3 or 4 times daily for rate control in patients with atrial fibrillation (AHA/ACC/HRS [January, 2014]).

IV: 1 to 3 mg/dose slow IVP; repeat every 2 to 5 minutes up to a total of 5 mg; titrate initial dose to desired response. **Note:** Once response achieved or maximum dose administered, additional doses should not be given for at least 4 hours.

or

0.5 to 1 mg over 1 minute; may repeat, if necessary, up to a total maximum dose of 0.1 mg/kg (ACLS guidelines [Neumar, 2010])

or

1 mg over 1 minute; may be repeated every 2 minutes up to 3 doses for rate control in patients with atrial fibrillation (AHA/ACC/HRS [January, 2014])

Dosing adjustment in renal impairment: Not dialyzable (0% to 5%). There are no dosage adjustments provided in the manufacturer's labeling; however, renal impairment increases systemic exposure to propranolol. Use with caution. Some clinicians suggest dosage adjustment is not necessary (Aronoff, 2007).

Dosing adjustment in hepatic impairment: There are no dosage adjustments provided in the manufacturer's labeling; however, hepatic impairment increases systemic exposure to propranolol. Use with caution.

Administration

Oral:

Immediate release tablets: Take on an empty stomach

Extended release capsules: Administer consistently either with food or on an empty stomach; do not chew or crush sustained or extended release capsules, swallow whole

Oral solution: Mix concentrated oral solution with water, fruit juice, liquid, or semisolid food before administration.

Hemangeol oral solution: Infants: Administer during or after a feeding to minimize the risk for hypoglycemia; skip the dose if the patient is not eating or is vomiting. Administer doses at least 9 hours apart. Do not shake before use. Administer Hemangeol directly into the child's mouth using the supplied oral dosing syringe; if needed, may be diluted with a small quantity of milk or fruit juice and administered in a baby's bottle.

Parenteral: **Note:** IV dose is much smaller than oral dose. When administered acutely for cardiac treatment, monitor ECG and blood pressure; consult individual institutional policies and procedures.

IV push (rapid injection): May be administered undiluted by IV push at a rate not to exceed 1 mg/minute

Slow IV injection/infusion: May be administered undiluted by slow IV over 10 minutes in children (AAP [Hegenbarth 2008]); in adults, infused over 30 minutes

Monitoring Parameters Monitor ECG, blood pressure, heart rate with IV administration; heart rate and blood pressure with oral administration

Infantile hemangioma: Monitor heart rate and blood pressure for 2 hours after initiation of therapy or dose increases.

Reference Range Therapeutic: 50 to 100 ng/mL (SI: 190 to 390 nmol/L) at end of dosing interval

Dosage Forms Excipient information presented when available (limited, particularly for generics); consult specific product labeling.

Capsule Extended Release 24 Hour, Oral, as hydrochloride:

Inderal LA: 60 mg, 80 mg, 120 mg, 160 mg [contains brilliant blue fcf (fd&c blue #1)]

Inderal XL: 80 mg, 120 mg

InnoPran XL: 80 mg, 120 mg

Generic: 60 mg, 80 mg, 120 mg, 160 mg

Solution, Intravenous, as hydrochloride:

Generic: 1 mg/mL (1 mL)

Solution, Oral, as hydrochloride:

Hemangeol: 4.28 mg/mL (120 mL) [alcohol free, paraben free, sugar free; contains saccharin sodium]

Generic: 20 mg/5 mL (500 mL); 40 mg/5 mL (500 mL)

Tablet, Oral, as hydrochloride:

Generic: 10 mg, 20 mg, 40 mg, 60 mg, 80 mg

◆ **Propranolol Hydrochloride** *see* Propranolol *on page 1789*

◆ **Propranolol Hydrochloride Injection, USP (Can)** *see* Propranolol *on page 1789*

◆ **Proprinal® Cold and Sinus [OTC]** *see* Pseudoephedrine and Ibuprofen *on page 1803*

◆ **Propulsid®** *see* Cisapride *on page 470*

◆ **Propylene Glycol Diacetate, Acetic Acid, and Hydrocortisone** *see* Acetic Acid, Propylene Glycol Diacetate, and Hydrocortisone *on page 56*

◆ **2-Propylpentanoic Acid** *see* Valproic Acid and Derivatives *on page 2143*

Propylthiouracil (proe pil thye oh YOOR a sil)

Medication Safety Issues

Sound-alike/look-alike issues:

Propylthiouracil may be confused with Purinethol [DSC]

PTU is an error-prone abbreviation (mistaken as mercaptopurine [Purinethol; 6-MP])

High alert medication:

The Institute for Safe Medication Practices (ISMP) includes this medication among its list of drugs that have a heightened risk of causing significant patient harm when used in error.

Related Information

Safe Handling of Hazardous Drugs *on page 2455*

Brand Names: Canada Propyl-Thyracil

Therapeutic Category Antithyroid Agent

Generic Availability (US) Yes

Use Adjunctive therapy in patients intolerant of methimazole to ameliorate hyperthyroidism symptoms in preparation for surgical treatment or radioactive iodine therapy (FDA approved in adults); treatment of hyperthyroidism in patients with Graves' disease or toxic multinodular goiter intolerant of methimazole and not candidates for surgical/radiotherapy (FDA approved in adults); has also been used for treatment of neonatal hyperthyroidism (including infants born to mothers with Graves' disease)

Medication Guide Available Yes

Pregnancy Risk Factor D

Pregnancy Considerations Propylthiouracil has been found to readily cross the placenta. Teratogenic effects have not been observed; however, nonteratogenic adverse effects, including fetal and neonatal hypothyroidism, goiter, and hyperthyroidism, have been reported following maternal propylthiouracil use. The transfer of thyroid-stimulating immunoglobulins can stimulate the fetal thyroid in utero and transiently after delivery and may increase the risk of fetal or neonatal hyperthyroidism (De Groot 2012; Peleg 2002).

Antithyroid treatment is recommended for the control of hyperthyroidism during pregnancy (Casey 2006; De Groot 2012). Uncontrolled maternal hyperthyroidism may result in adverse neonatal outcomes (eg, prematurity, low birth weight) and adverse maternal outcomes (eg, preeclampsia, congestive heart failure, stillbirth, and abortion). To prevent adverse fetal and maternal events, normal maternal thyroid function should be maintained prior to conception and throughout pregnancy (De Groot 2012).

[US Boxed Warning]: Because of the risk of fetal abnormalities associated with methimazole, propylthiouracil may be the treatment of choice when an antithyroid drug is indicated during or just prior to the first trimester of pregnancy. Due to an increased risk of liver toxicity, use of methimazole may be preferred during the second and third trimesters. If drug therapy is changed, maternal thyroid function should be monitored after 2 weeks and then every 2 to 4 weeks (De Groot 2012). Propylthiouracil, along with other medications, is used for the treatment of thyroid storm in pregnant women (ACOG 2015).

The pharmacokinetics of propylthiouracil are not significantly changed during pregnancy; however, the severity of hyperthyroidism may fluctuate throughout pregnancy (DeGroot 2012; Sitar 1979; Sitar 1982). Doses of propylthiouracil may be decreased as pregnancy progresses and discontinued weeks to months prior to delivery.

Breast-Feeding Considerations Propylthiouracil is excreted in human breast milk; however, the infant dose is considered low and unlikely to affect infant thyroid hormones. The American Thyroid Association considers doses <300 mg/day to be safe during breast-feeding (Stagnaro-Green 2011).

Contraindications

Hypersensitivity to propylthiouracil or any component of the formulation

Canadian labeling: Additional contraindications (not in US labeling): Breast-feeding

Warnings/Precautions Hazardous agent - use appropriate precautions for handling and disposal (NIOSH 2014 [group 2]).

[US Boxed Warning]: Severe liver injury and acute liver failure (sometimes fatal) have been reported and have included cases requiring liver transplantation in adult and pediatric patients, including pregnant women. Reserve propylthiouracil for patients who cannot tolerate methimazole and in whom radioactive iodine therapy or surgery are not appropriate treatments for the management of hyperthyroidism. Routine liver function test monitoring may not reduce risk due to unpredictable and rapid onset. Patients should be counseled to recognize and report symptoms suggestive of hepatic dysfunction (eg, anorexia, pruritus, right upper quadrant pain), especially in first 6 months of treatment, which should prompt immediate discontinuation.

[US Boxed Warning]: Due to the risk of fetal abnormalities associated with methimazole, propylthiouracil may be the treatment of choice when an antithyroid drug is indicated during or just prior to the first trimester of pregnancy.

May cause significant bone marrow depression; the most severe manifestation is agranulocytosis (usually occurs within first 3 months of therapy). Aplastic anemia, thrombocytopenia, and leukopenia may also occur. Use with caution in patients receiving other drugs known to cause myelosuppression (particularly agranulocytosis); discontinue if significant bone marrow suppression occurs, particularly agranulocytosis or aplastic anemia.

A lupus-like syndrome (including splenomegaly and vasculitis) may occur. Interstitial pneumonitis has been reported; discontinue if this reaction occurs. Has been associated with nephritis and glomerulonephritis, sometimes leading to acute renal failure. ANCA-positive vasculitis or leukocytoclastic vasculitis may occur; discontinue in patients who develop vasculitis during therapy. May cause hypoprothrombinemia and bleeding. Monitoring is recommended, especially before surgical procedures. May cause hypothyroidism; routinely monitor TSH and free T_4 levels, adjust dose to maintain euthyroid state. Dermatologic toxicity may occur; discontinue in the presence of exfoliative dermatitis.

Potentially significant interactions may exist, requiring dose or frequency adjustment, additional monitoring, and/or selection of alternative therapy.

Warnings: Additional Pediatric Considerations In pediatric patients, severe liver injury including hepatic failure requiring transplantation or resulting in death have been reported with propylthiouracil (most cases with doses ≥300 mg, but has also been reported with the lower 50 mg dose). Routine liver function test monitoring may not reduce risk due to unpredictable and rapid onset. Use is not recommended and should be limited to patients who have developed minor toxic reactions to methimazole and who are not candidates for surgery or radioactive iodine treatment. If use necessary, patients and parents should be informed of risks and propylthiouracil therapy limited to a short course with close patient monitoring (baseline CBC, liver profile including LFTs, bilirubin and alkaline phosphatase recommended). Discontinue use, contact prescriber, and obtain CBC (WBC) and LFTs (transaminases) if any of the following occur: Tiredness, nausea, anorexia, fever, pharyngitis, malaise, pruritis, rash, jaundice, light-colored stool or dark urine, joint pain, right upper quadrant pain, abdominal bloating (Bahn [ATA/AACE 2011]).

Adverse Reactions

Cardiovascular: Edema, periarteritis, vasculitis (ANCA-positive, cutaneous, leukocytoclastic)

Central nervous system: Drowsiness, drug fever, headache, neuritis, paresthesia, vertigo

Dermatologic: Alopecia, dermal ulcer, erythema nodosum, exfoliative dermatitis, pruritus, skin pigmentation, skin rash, Stevens-Johnson syndrome, toxic epidermal necrolysis, urticaria

Gastrointestinal: Ageusia, dysgeusia, nausea, salivary gland disease, stomach pain, vomiting

Hematologic & oncologic: Agranulocytosis, aplastic anemia, granulocytopenia, hemorrhage, hypoprothrombinemia, leukopenia, lymphadenopathy, splenomegaly, thrombocytopenia

Hepatic: Acute hepatic failure, hepatitis, hepatotoxicity (idiosyncratic) (Chalasani 2014), jaundice

Neuromuscular & skeletal: Arthralgia, lupus-like syndrome, myalgia

Renal: Acute renal failure, glomerulonephritis, nephritis

Respiratory: Interstitial pneumonitis, pulmonary alveolar hemorrhage

Miscellaneous: Fever

Drug Interactions

Metabolism/Transport Effects None known.

Avoid Concomitant Use

Avoid concomitant use of Propylthiouracil with any of the following: BCG (Intravesical); CloZAPine; Dipyrone; Sodium Iodide I131

Increased Effect/Toxicity

Propylthiouracil may increase the levels/effects of: Cardiac Glycosides; CloZAPine; Theophylline Derivatives

The levels/effects of Propylthiouracil may be increased by: Dipyrone

Decreased Effect

Propylthiouracil may decrease the levels/effects of: BCG (Intravesical); Sodium Iodide I131; Vitamin K Antagonists

Storage/Stability Store at 15°C to 30°C (59°F to 86°F).

Mechanism of Action Inhibits the synthesis of thyroid hormones by blocking the conversion of thyroxine to triiodothyronine in peripheral tissues (does not inactivate existing thyroxine and triiodothyronine stores in circulating blood and the thyroid and does not interfere with replacement thyroid hormones.

Pharmacodynamics For significant therapeutic effects 24-36 hours are required; remission of hyperthyroidism usually does not occur before 4 months of continued therapy

Pharmacokinetics (Adult data unless noted)

Protein binding: 75% to 80%

Metabolism: Hepatic

Bioavailability: 80% to 95%

Half-life: 1.5-5 hours

End-stage renal disease: 8.5 hours

Time to peak serum concentration: Oral: Within 1 hour; persists for 2-3 hours

Elimination: 35% excreted in urine

Dosing: Neonatal Note: Severe liver toxicity reported in pediatric patients; monitor closely.

Hyperthyroidism (including born to mothers with Graves' disease): Limited data available: Oral: 5 to 10 mg/kg/day in divided doses every 8 hours; begin with low dose and adjust dosage every few days to maintain total T_3, free T_4, and TSH in normal range; usual duration of therapy 2 to 3 months (Cloherty, 2012). Elevated T_3 may be sole indicator of inadequate treatment and elevated TSH indicates excessive antithyroid treatment.

Dosing: Usual Note: Adjust dosage to maintain T_3, T_4, and TSH in normal range; elevated T_3 may be sole indicator of inadequate treatment. Elevated TSH indicates excessive antithyroid treatment.

Pediatric: **Note:** Due to reports of severe liver toxicity, propylthiouracil is not recommended for use in pediatric patients and dosing is no longer FDA-approved for pediatric patients; use should be limited to patients who have developed minor toxic reactions to methimazole and who are not candidates for surgery or radioactive iodine treatment. If used, limit duration to short course of therapy. Discontinue therapy if transaminases reach 2 to 3 times ULN and fail to resolve within a week of repeat testing (Bahn [ATA/AACE 2011]).

Hyperthyroidism: Oral:

Children: ≥6 years and Adolescents: Limited data available [Propyl-Thyracil Prescribing Information (Canada)]:

Initial: 150 mg/m^2/day

6 to 10 years: 50 to 150 mg/day divided every 8 hours

≥10 years: 150 to 300 mg/day divided every 8 hours

Maintenance (once euthyroid): Dose should be individualized based on patient response: Usual dose: 50 mg twice daily

Adult: **Hyperthydroidism:** Oral: Initial: 300 mg daily in 3 equally divided doses (~8-hour intervals); 400 mg daily in patients with severe hyperthyroidism and/or very large goiters; an occasional patient will require 600 to 900 mg daily; usual maintenance: 100 to 150 mg daily in 3 equally divided doses

Dosing adjustment in renal impairment: There are no dosage adjustments provided in the US manufacturer's labeling.

Administration Hazardous agent; use appropriate precautions for handling and disposal (NIOSH 2014 [group 2]).

Oral: Administer same time in relation to meals each day, either always with meals or always between meals

Monitoring Parameters CBC with differential, liver function tests, platelets, thyroid function tests (TSH, T_3, T_4), prothrombin time, INR

Reference Range

Thyroid Function Tests

Lab Parameters	Age	Normal Range
T_4 (thyroxine) serum concentration	1-7 days	10.1-20.9 mcg/dL
	8-14 days	9.8-16.6 mcg/dL
	1 month to 1 year	5.5-16.0 mcg/dL
	>1 year	4.0-12.0 mcg/dL
Free thyroxine index (FTI)	1-3 days	9.3-26.6
	1-4 weeks	7.6-20.8
	1-4 months	7.4-17.9
	4-12 months	5.1-14.5
	1-6 years	5.7-13.3
	>6 years	4.8-14.0
T_3 serum concentration	Newborns	100-470 ng/dL
	1-5 years	100-260 ng/dL
	5-10 years	90-240 ng/dL
	10 years to Adult	70-210 ng/dL
T_3 uptake		35%-45%
TSH serum concentration	Cord	3-22 micro international units/mL
	1-3 days	<40 micro international units/mL
	3-7 days	<25 micro international units/mL
	>7 days	0-10 micro international units/mL

Dosage Forms Excipient information presented when available (limited, particularly for generics); consult specific product labeling.

Tablet, Oral:

Generic: 50 mg

Extemporaneous Preparations Hazardous agent; use appropriate precautions for handling and disposal (NIOSH 2014 [group 2]). When manipulating tablets, NIOSH recommends double gloving, a protective gown, and preparation in a controlled device; if not prepared in a controlled device, respiratory and eye protection as well as ventilated engineering controls are recommended (NIOSH 2014).

A 5 mg/mL oral suspension may be made with tablets and a 1:1 mixture of Ora-Plus and Ora-Sweet. Crush twenty 50 mg propylthiouracil tablets in a mortar and reduce to a fine powder. Add small portions of vehicle and mix to a uniform paste; mix while adding vehicle in incremental proportions to **almost** 200 mL; transfer to a calibrated bottle, rinse mortar with vehicle, and add quantity of vehicle sufficient to make 200 mL. Label "shake well" and "refrigerate". Stable for 91 days refrigerated (preferred) and 70 days at room temperature.

Nahata MC, Pai VB, and Hipple TF, *Pediatric Drug Formulations*, 5th ed, Cincinnati, OH: Harvey Whitney Books Co, 2004.

- **Propyl-Thyracil (Can)** *see* Propylthiouracil *on page 1793*
- **2-Propylvaleric Acid** *see* Valproic Acid and Derivatives *on page 2143*
- **ProQuad** *see* Measles, Mumps, Rubella, and Varicella Virus Vaccine *on page 1330*
- **PRO-Quetiapine (Can)** *see* QUEtiapine *on page 1815*

◆ **PRO-Rabeprazole (Can)** *see* RABEprazole *on page 1828*
◆ **PRO-Risperidone (Can)** *see* RisperiDONE *on page 1866*
◆ **PRO-Sotalol (Can)** *see* Sotalol *on page 1963*
◆ **Prostacyclin** *see* Epoprostenol *on page 769*
◆ **Prostaglandin E_1** *see* Alprostadil *on page 103*
◆ **Prostigmin** *see* Neostigmine *on page 1505*
◆ **Prostin VR** *see* Alprostadil *on page 103*

Protamine (PROE ta meen)

Medication Safety Issues

Sound-alike/look-alike issues:

Protamine may be confused with ProAmatine, Protonix, Protopam

Therapeutic Category Antidote, Heparin

Generic Availability (US) Yes

Use Treatment of heparin overdosage; neutralize heparin during surgery or dialysis procedures

Pregnancy Risk Factor C

Pregnancy Considerations Animal reproduction studies have not been conducted. In general, medications used as antidotes should take into consideration the health and prognosis of the mother; antidotes should be administered to pregnant women if there is a clear indication for use and should not be withheld because of fears of teratogenicity (Bailey, 2003). Protamine sulfate may be used during delivery to reduce the risk of bleeding following maternal use of heparin or low molecular weight heparin (LMWH) (Bates, 2012).

Breast-Feeding Considerations It is not known if protamine is excreted in breast milk. The manufacturer recommends that caution be exercised when administering protamine to nursing women.

Contraindications Hypersensitivity to protamine or any component of the formulation

Warnings/Precautions May not be totally effective in some patients following cardiac surgery despite adequate doses. May cause hypersensitivity reaction in patients (have epinephrine 1:1000 and resuscitation equipment available). **[U.S. Boxed Warning]: Hypotension, cardiovascular collapse, noncardiogenic pulmonary edema, pulmonary vasoconstriction, and pulmonary hypertension may occur. Risk factors for such events include: use of high doses or overdose, repeated doses, previous protamine administration (including protamine-containing drugs), fish allergy, vasectomy, severe left ventricular dysfunction, abnormal preoperative pulmonary hemodynamics.** Too rapid administration can cause severe hypotensive and anaphylactoid-like reactions. Heparin rebound associated with anticoagulation and bleeding has been reported to occur occasionally; symptoms typically occur 8-9 hours after protamine administration, but may occur as long as 18 hours later.

Adverse Reactions

Cardiovascular: Bradycardia, flushing, hypotension, sudden fall in blood pressure

Central nervous system: Lassitude

Gastrointestinal: Nausea, vomiting

Hematologic: Hemorrhage

Respiratory: Dyspnea, pulmonary hypertension

Miscellaneous: Hypersensitivity reactions

Drug Interactions

Metabolism/Transport Effects None known.

Avoid Concomitant Use There are no known interactions where it is recommended to avoid concomitant use.

Increased Effect/Toxicity There are no known significant interactions involving an increase in effect.

Decreased Effect There are no known significant interactions involving a decrease in effect.

Storage/Stability Refrigerate; do not freeze. Stable for at least 2 weeks at room temperature. Preservative-free formulation does not require refrigeration.

Mechanism of Action Combines with strongly acidic heparin to form a stable complex (salt) neutralizing the anticoagulant activity of both drugs

Pharmacodynamics Onset of action: Heparin neutralization occurs within 5 minutes following IV injection

Pharmacokinetics (Adult data unless noted) Elimination: Unknown

Dosing: Neonatal Note: Limited data in neonates. Doses are extrapolated from adult information.

IV: Protamine dosage is determined by the most recent dosage of heparin or low molecular weight heparin (LMWH); 1 mg of protamine sulfate neutralizes 90 USP units of heparin (lung), 115 USP units of heparin (intestinal), and 1 mg of enoxaparin; maximum dose: 50 mg

Heparin overdosage: Since blood heparin concentrations decrease rapidly **after** heparin administration, adjust the protamine dosage depending upon the duration of time since heparin administration as follows (see table):

Time Since Last Heparin Dose (min)	Dose of Protamine (mg) to Neutralize 100 units of Heparin
<30	1
30-60	0.5-0.75
60-120	0.375-0.5
>120	0.25-0.375

LMWH overdosage: If most recent LMWH dose has been administered within the last 4 hours, use 1 mg protamine per 1 mg (100 units) LMWH; a second dose of 0.5 mg protamine per 1 mg (100 units) LMWH may be given if APTT remains prolonged 2-4 hours after the first dose; one report described dividing the total protamine dose and administering to a target Anti-Xa level to avoid potential protamine toxicity (Wiernikowski, 2007)

Dosing: Usual IV: Infants, Children and Adults: Protamine dosage is determined by the most recent dosage of heparin or low molecular weight heparin (LMWH); 1 mg of protamine neutralizes 90 USP units of heparin (lung), 115 USP units of heparin (intestinal), and 1 mg (100 units) LMWH; maximum dose: 50 mg

Heparin overdosage: Since blood heparin concentrations decrease rapidly **after** heparin administration, adjust the protamine dosage depending upon the duration of time since heparin administration as follows (see table):

Time Since Last Heparin Dose (min)	Dose of Protamine (mg) to Neutralize 100 units of Heparin
<30	1
30-60	0.5-0.75
60-120	0.375-0.5
>120	0.25-0.375

If heparin is administered by deep SubQ injection, use 1-1.5 mg protamine per 100 units heparin; this may be done by administering a portion of the dose (eg, 25-50 mg) slowly IV followed by the remaining portion as a continuous infusion over 8-16 hours (the expected absorption time of the SubQ heparin dose)

LMWH overdosage: If most recent LMWH dose has been administered within the last 4 hours, use 1 mg protamine per 1 mg (100 units) LMWH; a second dose of 0.5 mg protamine per 1 mg (100 units) LMWH may be given if APTT remains prolonged 2-4 hours after the first dose

Administration Parenteral: Inject without further dilution over 10 minutes not to exceed 5 mg/minute; maximum of 50 mg in any 10-minute period

Monitoring Parameters Coagulation tests, APTT or ACT, cardiac monitor, and blood pressure monitor required during administration

Dosage Forms Excipient information presented when available (limited, particularly for generics); consult specific product labeling.

Solution, Intravenous, as sulfate:

Generic: 10 mg/mL (5 mL, 25 mL)

Solution, Intravenous, as sulfate [preservative free]:

Generic: 10 mg/mL (5 mL, 25 mL)

- ◆ **Protamine Sulfate** *see* Protamine *on page 1796*
- ◆ **Protease, Lipase, and Amylase** *see* Pancrelipase *on page 1614*
- ◆ **Protection Plus [OTC]** *see* Alcohol (Ethyl) *on page 86*
- ◆ **Protein C** *see* Protein C Concentrate (Human) *on page 1797*

Protein C Concentrate (Human)

(PROE teen cee KON suhn trate HYU man)

Medication Safety Issues

Sound-alike/look-alike issues:

Ceprotin may be confused with aprotinin, Cipro®

Protein C concentrate (human) may be confused with activated protein C (human, recombinant) which refers to drotrecogin alfa

Brand Names: US Ceprotin

Therapeutic Category Anticoagulant; Blood Product Derivative; Enzyme

Generic Availability (US) No

Use Replacement therapy for severe congenital protein C deficiency for the prevention and/or treatment of venous thromboembolism and purpura fulminans (FDA approved in neonatal, pediatric, and adult patients). Has also been used in patients with purpura fulminans secondary to meningococcemia.

Pregnancy Risk Factor C

Pregnancy Considerations Reproductive studies have not been performed. It is unknown if administration during pregnancy will result in fetal harm.

Breast-Feeding Considerations Use in nursing mothers has not been studied.

Contraindications Hypersensitivity to protein C or any component of the formulation

Warnings/Precautions Formulation may contain small amounts of mouse protein and/or heparin. Hypersensitivity reactions may occur. Discontinue use in the presence of allergy related symptoms. Use of products derived from human plasma carries the potential risk for the transmission of infectious agents including viruses. Consideration should be given for patients to receive appropriate vaccinations during therapy. Concomitant use with other anticoagulants may increase risk of bleeding. Small amounts of heparin within formulation may induce thrombocytopenia. Use with caution in patients with renal impairment or in whom sodium overload is a concern.

Adverse Reactions As with all drugs which may affect hemostasis, bleeding may be associated with protein C administration. Hemorrhage may occur at virtually any site. Risk is dependent on multiple variables, including the concurrent use of multiple agents that alter hemostasis and patient susceptibility.

Central nervous system: Lightheadedness

Hematologic: Bleeding

Miscellaneous: Hypersensitivity reactions (itching and rash)

Postmarketing and/or case reports: Fever, hemothorax, hypotension, hyperhidrosis, restlessness

Drug Interactions

Metabolism/Transport Effects None known.

Avoid Concomitant Use

Avoid concomitant use of Protein C Concentrate (Human) with any of the following: Apixaban; Dabigatran Etexilate; Edoxaban; Omacetaxine; Rivaroxaban; Urokinase; Vorapaxar

Increased Effect/Toxicity

Protein C Concentrate (Human) may increase the levels/effects of: Anticoagulants; Collagenase (Systemic); Deferasirox; Deoxycholic Acid; Ibritumomab; Nintedanib; Obinutuzumab; Omacetaxine; Rivaroxaban; Tositumomab and Iodine I 131 Tositumomab

The levels/effects of Protein C Concentrate (Human) may be increased by: Agents with Antiplatelet Properties; Apixaban; Dabigatran Etexilate; Dasatinib; Edoxaban; Herbs (Anticoagulant/Antiplatelet Properties); Ibrutinib; Limaprost; Nonsteroidal Anti-Inflammatory Agents; Omega-3 Fatty Acids; Pentosan Polysulfate Sodium; Prostacyclin Analogues; Salicylates; Sugammadex; Thrombolytic Agents; Tibolone; Tipranavir; Urokinase; Vitamin E; Vorapaxar

Decreased Effect

The levels/effects of Protein C Concentrate (Human) may be decreased by: Estrogen Derivatives; Progestins

Storage/Stability Store under refrigeration at 2°C to 8°C (36°F to 46°F); do not freeze. Protect from light. Administer within 3 hours of reconstitution and discard any unused portion.

Mechanism of Action Converted to activated protein C (APC). APC is a serine protease which inactivates factors Va and VIIIa, limiting thrombotic formation. *In vitro* data also suggest inhibition of plasminogen activator inhibitor-1 (PAF-1) resulting in profibrinolytic activity, inhibition of macrophage production of tumor necrosis factor, blocking of leukocyte adhesion, and limitation of thrombin-induced inflammatory responses.

Pharmacodynamics Onset of action: 30 minutes

Pharmacokinetics (Adult data unless noted) Note: Limited data suggests that infants and very young children may have a faster clearance, lower AUC and maximum serum concentration, larger volume of distribution, and shorter half-life than older subjects.

Distribution: V_d: Median: 0.074L/kg (range: 0.044-0.165 L/kg)

Metabolism: Activated protein C (APC) inactivated by plasma protease inhibitors

Half-life elimination: Median: 9.8 hours (range: 4.9-14.7 hours)

Time to peak, serum concentration: Median: 0.5 hours (range: 0.17-1.33 hours)

Dosing: Neonatal Note: Patient variables (including age, clinical condition, and plasma levels of protein C) will influence dosing and duration of therapy. Individualize dosing based on protein C activity and patient's pharmacokinetic profile.

Severe congenital protein C deficiency: IV:

Acute episode/short-term prophylaxis:

Initial dose: 100-120 units/kg/dose (for determination of recovery and half-life); followed by subsequent 3 doses: 60-80 units/kg/dose every 6 hours adjusted to maintain peak protein C activity of 100%

Maintenance dose: 45-60 units/kg/dose every 6 or 12 hours adjusted to maintain recommended maintenance trough protein C activity levels >25%

Long-term prophylaxis: Maintenance dose: 45-60 units/kg/dose every 12 hours (recommended maintenance trough protein C activity levels >25%)

Note: Maintain target peak protein C activity of 100% during acute episodes and short-term prophylaxis. Maintain trough levels of protein C activity >25%.

Higher peak levels of protein C may be necessary in prophylactic therapy of patients at increased risk for thrombosis (eg, infection, trauma, surgical intervention).

Purpura fulminans secondary to meningococcemia: Limited data available. IV: A retrospective review of 94 pediatric patients (0-18 years including eight newborns) reported a median dose of 100 units/kg/day divided every 4-6 hours was used in the majority of patients (78 of the 94 patients); the other dosing in the remaining patients was an initial bolus with the remainder of daily dose administered as a continuous IV infusion (dosing specifics were not provided); median treatment duration of 33 hours (range: 1-645 hours); daily dose range: 28-375 units/kg/day (Veldman, 2010).

Dosing: Usual Note: Patient variables (including age, clinical condition, and plasma levels of protein C) will influence dosing and duration of therapy. Individualize dosing based on protein C activity and patient's pharmacokinetic profile.

Severe congenital protein C deficiency: IV: Infants, Children, Adolescents, and Adults:

Acute episode/short-term prophylaxis:

Initial dose: 100-120 units/kg/dose (for determination of recovery and half-life) followed by subsequent 3 doses: 60-80 units/kg/dose every 6 hours adjusted to maintain peak protein C activity of 100%

Maintenance dose: 45-60 units/kg/dose every 6 or 12 hours adjusted to maintain recommended maintenance trough protein C activity levels >25%

Long-term prophylaxis: Maintenance dose: 45-60 units/kg/dose every 12 hours (recommended maintenance trough protein C activity levels >25%)

Note: Maintain target peak protein C activity of 100% during acute episodes and short-term prophylaxis. Maintain trough levels of protein C activity >25%. Higher peak levels of protein C may be necessary in prophylactic therapy of patients at increased risk for thrombosis (eg, infection, trauma, surgical intervention).

Purpura fulminans secondary to meningococcemia: Limited data available: Infants >1month, Children, and Adolescents: IV: 100-150 units/kg/dose every 6 hours for 72 hours then 50-150 units/kg/dose every 12 hours until target symptom/sign resolution or treatment duration reaches 7 days. This protocol was used in a Phase II, double-blind, placebo-controlled, dose-finding study of 40 pediatric patients [median age: 2.3 years (range: 2.4 months-16.1 years)] (de Kleinjn, 2003). A retrospective review of 94 pediatric patients (newborn to 18 years) reported a median dose of 100 units/kg/day divided every 4-6 hours or as an initial bolus with the remainder of daily dose administered as a continuous IV infusion (dosing specifics were not provided); median treatment duration of 2 days (range: 1-24 days); daily dose range: 28-375 units/kg/day (Veldman, 2010). An open-label, prospective study of 36 patients (3 months to 76 years) reported an initial dose of 100 units/kg followed by a continuous IV infusion with an initial rate of 10 units/kg/hour adjusted daily to maintain plasma protein C concentration 80-120 units/mL (White, 2000).

Preparation for Administration Parenteral: Allow ceprotin and sterile water vial to warm to room temperature prior to reconstitution. Using provided transfer set, reconstitute vial with appropriate volume of SWFI for final concentration of ~100 units/mL (ie, 500 units vial with 5 mL and 1,000 units vial with 10 mL). Gently swirl vial after adding the diluent until powder is completely dissolved; discard vial if vacuum does not pull diluent into the vial. Use provided filter needle to withdraw solution from vial; remove filter needle prior to administration.

Administration Parenteral: Administer by IV injection; infusion must be completed within 3 hours of solution preparation.

Neonates, Infants, and Children <10 kg: Rate should not exceed 0.2 mL/kg/minute

Children ≥10 kg, Adolescents, and Adults: Rate should not exceed 2 mL/minute

Monitoring Parameters Protein C activity (chromogenic assay) prior to and during therapy (if acute thrombotic event, check protein C activity immediately before next injection); signs and symptoms of bleeding; hemoglobin/hematocrit, PT/INR, platelet count

Reference Range Maintain target peak protein C activity of 100% during acute episodes and short-term prophylaxis. Maintain trough levels of protein C activity >25%. Higher peak levels of protein C may be necessary in prophylactic therapy of patients at increased risk for thrombosis (eg, infection, trauma, surgical intervention).

Additional Information Conversion to vitamin K antagonist therapy may cause a transient hypercoagulable state during therapy initiation due to shorter half-life of protein C than other vitamin K-dependent clotting factors. For patients requiring conversion to oral vitamin K antagonists, it is recommended to continue protein C therapy during oral anticoagulant initiation until anticoagulation stabilized. It is also advised to begin with a low dose of oral anticoagulant instead of a loading dose.

Prescribers should register their patients to assist in the collection and assessment of protein C concentration deficiency, treatment, safety, and outcomes of subjects. More information may be found at the following website: http://clinicaltrials.gov/ct2/show/NCT01127529.

Dosage Forms Excipient information presented when available (limited, particularly for generics); consult specific product labeling.

Solution Reconstituted, Intravenous [preservative free]:

Ceprotin: 500 units (1 ea); 1000 units (1 ea) [contains albumin human, heparin, mouse protein (murine) (hamster)]

◆ **Prothrombin Complex Concentrate (Caution: Confusion-prone synonym)** *see* Factor IX Complex (Human) [(Factors II, IX, X)] *on page 836*

◆ **Protonix** *see* Pantoprazole *on page 1618*

◆ **Protopam Chloride** *see* Pralidoxime *on page 1747*

◆ **Protopic** *see* Tacrolimus (Topical) *on page 2004*

◆ **Protopic® (Can)** *see* Tacrolimus (Topical) *on page 2004*

◆ **PRO-Topiramate (Can)** *see* Topiramate *on page 2085*

◆ **Protrin DF (Can)** *see* Sulfamethoxazole and Trimethoprim *on page 1986*

Protriptyline (proe TRIP ti leen)

Medication Safety Issues

Sound-alike/look-alike issues:

Vivactil® may be confused with Vyvanse®

BEERS Criteria medication:

This drug may be potentially inappropriate for use in geriatric patients (Quality of evidence - high [moderate for SIADH]; Strength of recommendation - strong).

Related Information

Antidepressant Agents *on page 2257*

Brand Names: US Vivactil [DSC]

Therapeutic Category Antidepressant, Tricyclic (Secondary Amine)

Generic Availability (US) Yes

Use Treatment of depression (FDA approved in adults)

Medication Guide Available Yes

Pregnancy Considerations Adverse events have not been observed in animal reproduction studies. Tricyclic antidepressants may be associated with irritability, jitteriness, and convulsions (rare) in the neonate (Yonkers, 2009).

The ACOG recommends that therapy for depression during pregnancy be individualized; treatment should incorporate the clinical expertise of the mental health clinician, obstetrician, primary healthcare provider, and pediatrician (ACOG, 2008). According to the American Psychiatric Association (APA), the risks of medication treatment should be weighed against other treatment options and untreated depression. For women who discontinue antidepressant medications during pregnancy and who may be at high risk for postpartum depression, the medications can be restarted following delivery (APA, 2010). Treatment algorithms have been developed by the ACOG and the APA for the management of depression in women prior to conception and during pregnancy (Yonkers, 2009).

Breast-Feeding Considerations It is not known if protriptyline is excreted in breast milk. According to the manufacturer, the decision to continue or discontinue breast-feeding during therapy should take into account the risk of exposure to the infant and the benefits of treatment to the mother.

Contraindications

Hypersensitivity to protriptyline or any component of the formulation; use of MAOIs (concurrently or within 14 days of stopping an MAOI or protriptyline); use of cisapride; use in a patient during the acute recovery phase of MI

Documentation of allergenic cross-reactivity for tricyclic antidepressants is limited. However, because of similarities in chemical structure and/or pharmacologic actions, the possibility of cross-sensitivity cannot be ruled out with certainty.

Warnings/Precautions [U.S. Boxed Warning]: Antidepressants increase the risk of suicidal thinking and behavior in children, adolescents, and young adults (18-24 years of age) with major depressive disorder (MDD) and other psychiatric disorders; consider risk prior to prescribing. Short-term studies did not show an increased risk in patients >24 years of age and showed a decreased risk in patients ≥65 years. Closely monitor for clinical worsening, suicidality, or unusual changes in behavior, particularly during the initial 1 to 2 months of therapy or during periods of dosage adjustments (increases or decreases); the patient's family or caregiver should be instructed to closely observe the patient and communicate condition with healthcare provider. A medication guide should be dispensed with each prescription. **Protriptyline is FDA approved for the treatment of depression in adolescents.**

The possibility of a suicide attempt is inherent in major depression and may persist until remission occurs. Use caution in high-risk patients. Worsening depression and severe abrupt suicidality that are not part of the presenting symptoms may require discontinuation or modification of drug therapy. The patient's family or caregiver should be alerted to monitor patients for the emergence of suicidality and associated behaviors (such as agitation, irritability, hostility, impulsivity, and hypomania) and call healthcare provider.

May precipitate a shift to mania or hypomania in patients with bipolar disorder. Patients presenting with depressive symptoms should be screened for bipolar disorder, including details regarding family history of suicide, bipolar disorder, and depression. Monotherapy in patients with bipolar disorder should be avoided. **Protriptyline is not FDA approved for the treatment of bipolar depression.**

TCAs may rarely cause bone marrow suppression; monitor for any signs of infection and obtain CBC if symptoms (eg, fever, sore throat) evident. May cause CNS depression, which may impair physical or mental abilities; patients must be cautioned about performing tasks that require mental alertness (eg, operating machinery or driving). Recommended by the manufacturer to discontinue prior to elective surgery; risks exist for drug interactions with anesthesia and for cardiac arrhythmias. However, definitive drug interactions have not been widely reported in the literature and continuation of tricyclic antidepressants is generally recommended as long as precautions are taken to reduce the significance of any adverse events that may occur (Pass, 2004). May alter glucose regulation - use with caution in patients with diabetes (APA, 2010).

May cause orthostatic hypotension or conduction abnormalities (risks are moderate relative to other antidepressants). Use with caution in patients with a history of cardiovascular disease (including previous MI, stroke, tachycardia, or conduction abnormalities). The degree of anticholinergic blockade produced by this agent is high relative to other cyclic antidepressants; however, caution should still be used in patients with urinary retention, benign prostatic hyperplasia, narrow-angle glaucoma, xerostomia, visual problems, constipation, or history of bowel obstruction (APA, 2010; Bauer, 2013).

Hyperpyrexia has been observed with TCAs in combination with anticholinergics and/or neuroleptics, particularly during hot weather. Use caution in patients with a previous seizure disorder or condition predisposing to seizures such as brain damage, alcoholism, or concurrent therapy with other drugs which lower the seizure threshold. May increase the risks associated with electroconvulsive therapy. Bone fractures have been associated with antidepressant treatment. Consider the possibility of a fragility fracture if an antidepressant-treated patient presents with unexplained bone pain, point tenderness, swelling, or bruising (Rabenda, 2013; Rizzoli, 2012). Use with caution in patients with hepatic or renal dysfunction.

May cause mild pupillary dilation which in susceptible individuals can lead to an episode of narrow-angle glaucoma. Consider evaluating patients who have not had an iridectomy for narrow-angle glaucoma risk factors. Use caution in elderly patients; may cause or exacerbate syndrome of inappropriate antidiuretic hormone secretion or hyponatremia; monitor sodium closely with initiation or dosage adjustments in older adults. May be inappropriate in older adults depending on comorbidities (eg, dementia, delirium) or in patients with a history of falls and fractures due to its potent anticholinergic effects (Beers Criteria).

Abrupt discontinuation or interruption of antidepressant therapy has been associated with a discontinuation syndrome. Symptoms arising may vary with antidepressant however commonly include nausea, vomiting, diarrhea, headaches, lightheadedness, dizziness, diminished appetite, sweating, chills, tremors, paresthesias, fatigue, somnolence, and sleep disturbances (eg, vivid dreams, insomnia). Greater risks for developing a discontinuation syndrome have been associated with antidepressants with shorter half-lives, longer durations of treatment, and abrupt discontinuation. For antidepressants of short or intermediate half-lives, symptoms may emerge within 2-5 days after treatment discontinuation and last 7-14 days (APA, 2010; Fava, 2006; Haddad, 2001; Shelton, 2001; Warner, 2006).

Adverse Reactions Some reactions listed are based on reports for other agents in this same pharmacologic class and may not be specifically reported for protriptyline.

Cardiovascular: Cardiac arrhythmia, cerebrovascular accident, edema, flushing, heart block, hypertension, hypotension, myocardial infarction, orthostatic hypotension, palpitations, tachycardia

Central nervous system: Agitation, anxiety, ataxia, confusion, delusions, disorientation, dizziness, drowsiness, drug fever, EEG pattern changes, extrapyramidal reaction, fatigue, hallucination, headache, hyperpyrexia, hypomania, insomnia, nightmares, numbness, panic, peripheral neuropathy, psychosis (exacerbation), restlessness, seizure, tingling of extremities, tingling sensation, withdrawal syndrome

Dermatologic: Alopecia, diaphoresis (excessive), pruritus, skin photosensitivity, skin rash, urticaria

Endocrine & metabolic: Decreased libido, decreased serum glucose, galactorrhea, gynecomastia, increased libido, increased serum glucose, SIADH, weight gain, weight loss

Gastrointestinal: Abdominal cramps, anorexia, constipation, diarrhea, epigastric distress, melanoglossia, nausea, paralytic ileus, parotid gland enlargement, stomatitis, sublingual adenitis, unpleasant taste, vomiting, xerostomia

Genitourinary: Breast hypertrophy, impotence, nocturia, testicular swelling, urinary hesitancy, urinary retention, urinary tract dilation

Hematologic & oncologic: Agranulocytosis, eosinophilia, leukopenia, petechia, purpura, thrombocytopenia

Hepatic: Abnormal hepatic function tests, cholestatic jaundice

Neuromuscular & skeletal: Tremor, weakness

Ophthalmic: Accommodation disturbance, blurred vision, eye pain, increased intraocular pressure

Otic: Tinnitus

Renal: Polyuria

Rare but important or life-threatening: Angle-closure glaucoma, suicidal ideation

Drug Interactions

Metabolism/Transport Effects Substrate of CYP2D6 (major); **Note:** Assignment of Major/Minor substrate status based on clinically relevant drug interaction potential

Avoid Concomitant Use

Avoid concomitant use of Protriptyline with any of the following: Aclidinium; Azelastine (Nasal); Cisapride; Dapoxetine; Eluxadoline; Glucagon; Iobenguane I 123; Ipratropium (Oral Inhalation); Linezolid; MAO Inhibitors; Methylene Blue; Moxonidine; Orphenadrine; Paraldehyde; Potassium Chloride; Thalidomide; Tiotropium; Umeclidinium

Increased Effect/Toxicity

Protriptyline may increase the levels/effects of: AbobotulinumtoxinA; Alcohol (Ethyl); Alpha-/Beta-Agonists (Direct-Acting); Alpha1-Agonists; Amphetamines; Analgesics (Opioid); Anticholinergic Agents; Antipsychotic Agents; Azelastine (Nasal); Beta2-Agonists; Buprenorphine; Cisapride; Citalopram; CNS Depressants; Desmopressin; Eluxadoline; Escitalopram; Glucagon; Highest Risk QTc-Prolonging Agents; Hydrocodone; Methotrimeprazine; Methylene Blue; Metyrosine; Mirabegron; Moderate Risk QTc-Prolonging Agents; Nicorandil; OnabotulinumtoxinA; Orphenadrine; Paraldehyde; Potassium Chloride; Pramipexole; QuiNIDine; RimabotulinumtoxinB; ROPINIRole; Rotigotine; Serotonin Modulators; Sodium Phosphates; Sulfonylureas; Suvorexant; Thalidomide; Thiazide Diuretics; Tiotropium; Topiramate; TraMADol; Vitamin K Antagonists; Yohimbine; Zolpidem

The levels/effects of Protriptyline may be increased by: Abiraterone Acetate; Aclidinium; Altretamine; Antiemetics (5HT3 Antagonists); Antipsychotic Agents; Brimonidine (Topical); Cannabis; Cimetidine; Cinacalcet; Citalopram; Cobicistat; CYP2D6 Inhibitors (Moderate); CYP2D6 Inhibitors (Strong); Dapoxetine; Darunavir; Dexmethylphenidate; Doxylamine; Dronabinol; Droperidol; DULoxetine; Escitalopram; FLUoxetine; FluvoxaMINE; HydrOXYzine; Ipratropium (Oral Inhalation); Kava Kava; Linezolid; Lithium; Magnesium Sulfate; MAO Inhibitors; Methotrimeprazine; Methylphenidate; Metoclopramide; Metyrosine; Mianserin; Mifepristone; Nabilone; Panobinostat; PARoxetine; Peginterferon Alfa-2b; Perampanel; Pramlintide; Protease Inhibitors; QuiNIDine; Rufinamide; Sertraline; Sodium Oxybate; Tapentadol; Tedizolid; Terbinafine (Systemic); Tetrahydrocannabinol; Thyroid Products; TraMADol; Umeclidinium; Valproic Acid and Derivatives

Decreased Effect

Protriptyline may decrease the levels/effects of: Acetylcholinesterase Inhibitors; Alpha1-Agonists; Alpha2-Agonists; Alpha2-Agonists (Ophthalmic); Iobenguane I 123; Itopride; Moxonidine; Secretin

The levels/effects of Protriptyline may be decreased by: Acetylcholinesterase Inhibitors; Barbiturates; CarBAMazepine; Peginterferon Alfa-2b; St Johns Wort

Storage/Stability Store at 20°C to 25°C (68°F to 77°F).

Mechanism of Action Increases the synaptic concentration of serotonin and/or norepinephrine in the central nervous system by inhibition of their reuptake by the presynaptic neuronal membrane

Pharmacodynamics

Onset of action: 1-2 weeks

Maximum effect: 4-12 weeks

Duration: 1-2 days

Pharmacokinetics (Adult data unless noted)

Protein binding: 92%

Metabolism: Extensively hepatic via N-oxidation, hydroxylation, and glucuronidation; first-pass effect (10% to 25%)

Half-life: 54-92 hours (average: 74 hours)

Time to peak serum concentration: 24-30 hours

Elimination: Urine

Dosing: Usual Oral:

Children: **Note:** Safe and effective use in children has not been established; controlled clinical trials have not shown tricyclic antidepressants to be superior to placebo for the treatment of depression in children and adolescents (Dopheide, 2006; Wagner, 2005).

Adolescents: Manufacturer labeling: Initial: 5 mg/dose given 2-3 times/day; may increase in 2 weeks as tolerated; slow titration is recommended in order to facilitate monitoring for adverse effects such as behavioral activation; usual dose: 15-20 mg/day in divided doses

Adults: Initial: 10 mg/dose given twice daily; may increase every week as tolerated to a goal of 30-60 mg/day in 3-4 divided doses

Administration Oral: May administer with food to decrease GI upset; do not administer with grapefruit juice.

Monitoring Parameters Heart rate, blood pressure, mental status, weight. Monitor patient periodically for symptom resolution; monitor for worsening depression, suicidality, and associated behaviors (especially at the beginning of therapy or when doses are increased or decreased).

Reference Range Therapeutic: 70-250 ng/mL (SI: 266-950 nmol/L); Toxic: >500 ng/mL (SI: >1900 nmol/L)

Dosage Forms Excipient information presented when available (limited, particularly for generics); consult specific product labeling. [DSC] = Discontinued product

Tablet, Oral, as hydrochloride:

Vivactil: 5 mg [DSC] [contains fd&c red #40, fd&c yellow #6 (sunset yellow)]

Vivactil: 10 mg [DSC] [contains fd&c yellow #10 (quinoline yellow)]

Generic: 5 mg, 10 mg

◆ **Protriptyline Hydrochloride** *see* Protriptyline *on page 1798*

◆ **Protylol (Can)** *see* Dicyclomine *on page 645*

◆ **PRO-Valacyclovir (Can)** *see* ValACYclovir *on page 2138*

◆ **Proventil HFA** *see* Albuterol *on page 81*

◆ **Provera** *see* MedroxyPROGESTERone *on page 1339*

◆ **Provera-Pak (Can)** *see* MedroxyPROGESTERone *on page 1339*

◆ **PRO-Verapamil SR (Can)** *see* Verapamil *on page 2170*

◆ **Provigil** *see* Modafinil *on page 1450*

- ◆ **Provil [OTC]** *see* Ibuprofen *on page 1064*
- ◆ **Proxymetacaine** *see* Proparacaine *on page 1785*
- ◆ **PROzac** *see* FLUoxetine *on page 906*
- ◆ **Prozac (Can)** *see* FLUoxetine *on page 906*
- ◆ **PROzac Weekly** *see* FLUoxetine *on page 906*
- ◆ **Prozena** *see* Lidocaine (Topical) *on page 1258*
- ◆ **PRP-OMP (PedvaxHIB)** *see Haemophilus* b Conjugate Vaccine *on page 998*
- ◆ **PRP-T (ActHIB)** *see Haemophilus* b Conjugate Vaccine *on page 998*
- ◆ **PRP-T (Hiberix)** *see Haemophilus* b Conjugate Vaccine *on page 998*
- ◆ **Prymaccone** *see* Primaquine *on page 1764*
- ◆ **P & S [OTC]** *see* Salicylic Acid *on page 1894*
- ◆ **23PS** *see* Pneumococcal Polysaccharide Vaccine (23-Valent) *on page 1718*

Pseudoephedrine (soo doe e FED rin)

Medication Safety Issues

Sound-alike/look-alike issues:

Sudafed may be confused with sotalol, Sudafed PE, Sufenta

Sudafed 12 Hour may be confused with Sudafed 12 Hour Pressure + Pain

Related Information

Oral Medications That Should Not Be Crushed or Altered *on page 2476*

Brand Names: US Childrens Silfedrine [OTC]; Decongestant 12Hour Max St [OTC]; ElixSure Congestion [OTC]; Genaphed [OTC]; Nasal Decongestant [OTC]; Nexafed [OTC]; Psudatabs [OTC]; Shopko Nasal Decongestant Max [OTC]; Shopko Nasal Decongestant [OTC]; Simply Stuffy [OTC]; Sudafed 12 Hour [OTC]; Sudafed 24 Hour [OTC]; Sudafed Childrens [OTC]; Sudafed [OTC]; Sudanyl [OTC]; SudoGest 12 Hour [OTC]; SudoGest [OTC]; Suphedrine [OTC]; Zephrex-D [OTC]

Brand Names: Canada Balminil Decongestant; Benylin® D for Infants; Contac® Cold 12 Hour Relief Non Drowsy; Drixoral® ND; Eltor®; PMS-Pseudoephedrine; Pseudofrin; Robidrine®; Sudafed® Decongestant

Therapeutic Category Adrenergic Agonist Agent; Decongestant; Sympathomimetic

Generic Availability (US) May be product dependent

Use Temporary symptomatic relief of nasal congestion due to common cold, upper respiratory allergies, and sinusitis; also promotes nasal or sinus drainage (immediate release formulations: FDA approved in ages >4 years and adults; extended release formulations: FDA approved in ages >12 years and adults). **Note:** Approved ages and uses for generic products may vary; consult labeling for specific information.

Pregnancy Considerations Use of pseudoephedrine during the first trimester may be associated with a possible risk of gastroschisis, small intestinal atresia, and hemifacial microsomia due to pseudoephedrine's vasoconstrictive effects; additional studies are needed to define the magnitude of risk. Single doses of pseudoephedrine were not found to adversely affect the fetus during the third trimester of pregnancy (limited data); however, fetal tachycardia was noted in a case report following maternal use of an extended release product for multiple days. Decongestants are not the preferred agents for the treatment of rhinitis during pregnancy. Oral pseudoephedrine should be avoided during the first trimester.

Breast-Feeding Considerations Pseudoephedrine is excreted into breast milk in concentrations that are ~4% of the weight adjusted maternal dose. The time to maximum milk concentration is ~1-2 hours after the maternal dose. Irritability has been reported in nursing infants (limited data; dose, duration, relationship to breast-feeding not provided). Milk production may be decreased in some women.

Contraindications Hypersensitivity to pseudoephedrine or any component of the formulation; with or within 14 days of MAO inhibitor therapy

Warnings/Precautions Use with caution in the elderly; may be more sensitive to adverse effects; administer with caution to patients with hypertension, hyperthyroidism, diabetes mellitus, cardiovascular disease, ischemic heart disease, increased intraocular pressure, prostatic hyperplasia, seizure disorders, or renal impairment. When used for self-medication (OTC), notify healthcare provider if symptoms do not improve within 7 days or are accompanied by fever. Discontinue and contact healthcare provider if nervousness, dizziness, or sleeplessness occur. Some products may contain sodium. Not for OTC use in children <4 years of age.

Benzyl alcohol and derivatives: Some dosage forms may contain sodium benzoate/benzoic acid; benzoic acid (benzoate) is a metabolite of benzyl alcohol; large amounts of benzyl alcohol (≥99 mg/kg/day) have been associated with a potentially fatal toxicity ("gasping syndrome") in neonates; the "gasping syndrome" consists of metabolic acidosis, respiratory distress, gasping respirations, CNS dysfunction (including convulsions, intracranial hemorrhage), hypotension, and cardiovascular collapse (AAP, 1997; CDC, 1982); some data suggests that benzoate displaces bilirubin from protein binding sites (Ahlfors, 2001); avoid or use dosage forms containing benzyl alcohol derivative with caution in neonates. See manufacturer's labeling.

Warnings: Additional Pediatric Considerations Safety and efficacy for the use of cough and cold products in pediatric patients <4 years of age is limited; the AAP warns against the use of these products for respiratory illnesses in this age group. Serious adverse effects including death have been reported (in some cases, high blood concentrations of pseudoephedrine were found). Many of these products contain multiple active ingredients, increasing the risk of accidental overdose when used with other products. The FDA notes that there are no approved OTC uses for these products in pediatric patients <2 years of age. Health care providers are reminded to ask caregivers about the use of OTC cough and cold products in order to avoid exposure to multiple medications containing the same ingredient (AAP 2012; FDA 2008).

Some dosage forms may contain propylene glycol; in neonates large amounts of propylene glycol delivered orally, intravenously (eg, >3,000 mg/day), or topically have been associated with potentially fatal toxicities which can include metabolic acidosis, seizures, renal failure, and CNS depression; toxicities have also been reported in children and adults including hyperosmolality, lactic acidosis, seizures, and respiratory depression; use caution (AAP 1997; Shehab 2009).

Adverse Reactions

Cardiovascular: Arrhythmia, cardiovascular collapse with hypotension, hypertension, palpitation, tachycardia

Central nervous system: Chills, confusion, coordination impaired, dizziness, drowsiness, excitability, fatigue, hallucination, headache, insomnia, nervousness, neuritis, restlessness, seizure, transient stimulation, vertigo

Dermatologic: Photosensitivity, rash, urticaria

Gastrointestinal: Anorexia, constipation, diarrhea, dry throat, ischemic colitis, nausea, vomiting, xerostomia

Genitourinary: Difficult urination, dysuria, polyuria, urinary retention

Hematologic: Agranulocytosis, hemolytic anemia, thrombocytopenia

Neuromuscular & skeletal: Tremor, weakness

Ocular: Blurred vision, diplopia
Otic: Tinnitus
Respiratory: Chest/throat tightness, dry nose, dyspnea, nasal congestion, thickening of bronchial secretions, wheezing
Miscellaneous: Anaphylaxis, diaphoresis

Drug Interactions

Metabolism/Transport Effects None known.

Avoid Concomitant Use

Avoid concomitant use of Pseudoephedrine with any of the following: Ergot Derivatives; Iobenguane I 123; MAO Inhibitors

Increased Effect/Toxicity

Pseudoephedrine may increase the levels/effects of: Sympathomimetics

The levels/effects of Pseudoephedrine may be increased by: Alkalinizing Agents; AtoMOXetine; Cannabinoid-Containing Products; Carbonic Anhydrase Inhibitors; Ergot Derivatives; Linezolid; MAO Inhibitors; Serotonin/Norepinephrine Reuptake Inhibitors; Tedizolid

Decreased Effect

Pseudoephedrine may decrease the levels/effects of: Benzylpenicilloyl Polylysine; FentaNYL; Iobenguane I 123

The levels/effects of Pseudoephedrine may be decreased by: Alpha1-Blockers; Spironolactone; Urinary Acidifying Agents

Food Interactions Onset of effect may be delayed if pseudoephedrine is taken with food. Management: Administer without regard to food.

Mechanism of Action Directly stimulates alpha-adrenergic receptors of respiratory mucosa causing vasoconstriction; directly stimulates beta-adrenergic receptors causing bronchial relaxation, increased heart rate and contractility

Pharmacodynamics

Onset of action: Decongestant: Oral: 30 minutes (Chua 1989)
Maximum effect: Decongestant: Oral: ~1 to 2 hours (Chua 1989)
Duration: Immediate release tablet: 3 to 8 hours (Chua 1989)

Pharmacokinetics (Adult data unless noted)

Absorption: Rapid (Simons 1996)
Distribution: V_d:
Children: ~2.5 L/kg (Simons 1996)
Adults: 2.64 to 3.51 L/kg (Kanfer 1993)
Metabolism: Undergoes n-demethylation to norpseudoephedrine (active) (Chua 1989; Kanfer 1993); hepatic (<1%) (Kanfer 1993)
Half-life elimination: Varies by urine pH and flow rate; alkaline urine decreases renal elimination of pseudoephedrine (Kanfer 1993)
Children: ~3 hours (urine pH ~6.5) (Simons 1996)
Adults: 9 to 16 hours (pH 8); 3-6 hours (pH 5) (Chua 1989)
Time to peak serum concentration:
Children: Immediate release tablet: ~2 hours (Simons 1996)
Adults: Immediate release tablet: 1 to 3 hours (dose-dependent) (Kanfer 1993)
Elimination: Urine (43% to 96% as unchanged drug, 1% to 6% as active norpseudoephedrine); dependent on urine pH and flow rate; alkaline urine decreases renal elimination of pseudoephedrine (Kanfer 1993)

Dosing: Usual

Pediatric: **Nasal congestion (decongestant):** Oral:
Children <4 years: Limited data available: Immediate release: 1 mg/kg/dose every 6 hours; maximum dose: 15 mg/dose (Gentile 2000)
Children 4 to <6 years: Immediate release:
Manufacturer's labeling: 15 mg every 4 to 6 hours; maximum daily dose: 60 mg/**24 hours**
Alternate dosing: 1 mg/kg/dose every 6 hours; maximum dose: 15 mg/dose (Gentile 2000)
Children 6 to <12 years: Immediate release: 30 mg every 4 to 6 hours; maximum daily dose: 120 mg/**24 hours**
Children ≥12 years and Adolescents:
Immediate release: 60 mg every 4 to 6 hours; maximum daily dose: 240 mg/day
Extended release: 120 mg every 12 hours **or** 240 mg once daily; maximum daily dose: 240 mg/**24 hours**
Adult: **Nasal congestion (decongestant):** General dosing guidelines: Oral:
Immediate release: 60 mg every 4 to 6 hours; maximum daily dose: 240 mg/**24 hours**
Extended release: 120 mg every 12 hours **or** 240 mg every 24 hours; maximum daily dose: 240 mg/**24 hours**
Dosing adjustment in renal impairment: There are no dosage adjustments provided in manufacturer's labeling.
Dosing adjustment in hepatic impairment: There are no dosage adjustments provided in manufacturer's labeling.

Administration Oral: Administer with water or milk to decrease GI distress; swallow timed release tablets or capsules whole, do not chew or crush; Sudafed 24 Hour tablet may not completely dissolve and appear in stool

Test Interactions Interferes with urine detection of amphetamine (false-positive)

Additional Information Because ephedrine and pseudoephedrine have been used to synthesize methamphetamine, the DEA has placed them in the category of "Schedule Listed Products"; restrictions are in place to reduce the potential for misuse (diversion) and abuse (eg, storage requirements, additional documentation of sale); the DEA limit for a single transaction to a single individual for drug products containing ephedrine or pseudoephedrine is 3.6 g/24 hours, 9 g/30 days, or if mail-order transaction 7.5 g/30 days.

Dosage Forms Excipient information presented when available (limited, particularly for generics); consult specific product labeling.

Gel, Oral, as hydrochloride:
ElixSure Congestion: 15 mg/5 mL (120 mL) [alcohol free; contains brilliant blue fcf (fd&c blue #1), carbomer 934p, propylene glycol, propylparaben; grape bubblegum flavor]
Liquid, Oral, as hydrochloride:
Childrens Silfedrine: 15 mg/5 mL (118 mL, 237 mL) [grape flavor]
Nasal Decongestant: 30 mg/5 mL (118 mL) [contains fd&c red #40, methylparaben, saccharin sodium, sodium benzoate; raspberry flavor]
Sudafed Childrens: 15 mg/5 mL (118 mL) [alcohol free, sugar free; contains brilliant blue fcf (fd&c blue #1), edetate disodium, fd&c red #40, menthol, polyethylene glycol, saccharin sodium, sodium benzoate; grape flavor]
Syrup, Oral, as hydrochloride:
Nasal Decongestant: 30 mg/5 mL (473 mL) [contains fd&c red #40, methylparaben, saccharin sodium, sodium benzoate; raspberry flavor]
Tablet, Oral, as hydrochloride:
Genaphed: 30 mg
Nasal Decongestant: 30 mg [contains fd&c red #40 aluminum lake, fd&c yellow #6 aluminum lake]
Nasal Decongestant: 30 mg [contains fd&c red #40 aluminum lake, polysorbate 80]
Psudatabs: 30 mg [contains fd&c red #40, fd&c yellow #10 (quinoline yellow), fd&c yellow #6 (sunset yellow)]
Shopko Nasal Decongestant Max: 30 mg [contains fd&c red #40 aluminum lake]
Simply Stuffy: 30 mg
Sudafed: 30 mg

Sudafed: 30 mg [contains fd&c red #40 aluminum lake, fd&c yellow #10 aluminum lake, fd&c yellow #6 aluminum lake]
Sudanyl: 30 mg
SudoGest: 30 mg [contains fd&c red #40 aluminum lake, fd&c yellow #10 aluminum lake, fd&c yellow #6 aluminum lake]
SudoGest: 30 mg [contains fd&c red #40 aluminum lake, fd&c yellow #6 aluminum lake]
SudoGest: 60 mg [scored]
Suphedrine: 30 mg
Generic: 30 mg, 60 mg
Tablet Abuse-Deterrent, Oral, as hydrochloride:
Nexafed: 30 mg
Zephrex-D: 30 mg
Tablet Extended Release 12 Hour, Oral, as hydrochloride:
Decongestant 12Hour Max St: 120 mg [contains polysorbate 80]
Shopko Nasal Decongestant: 120 mg
Sudafed 12 Hour: 120 mg
Sudafed 12 Hour: 120 mg [contains fd&c blue #1 aluminum lake]
SudoGest 12 Hour: 120 mg
Generic: 120 mg
Tablet Extended Release 24 Hour, Oral, as hydrochloride:
Sudafed 24 Hour: 240 mg

◆ **Pseudoephedrine and Brompheniramine** *see* Brompheniramine and Pseudoephedrine *on page 305*

Pseudoephedrine and Ibuprofen

(soo doe e FED rin & eye byoo PROE fen)

Brand Names: US Advil® Cold & Sinus [OTC]; Proprinal® Cold and Sinus [OTC]

Brand Names: Canada Advil® Cold & Sinus; Advil® Cold & Sinus Daytime; Children's Advil® Cold; Sudafed® Sinus Advance

Therapeutic Category Decongestant/Analgesic

Generic Availability (US) Yes: Caplet

Use Temporary relief of cold, sinus, and flu symptoms (including nasal congestion, headache, sore throat, minor body aches and pains, and fever) (OTC product: FDA approved in ages ≥4 years and adults). **Note:** Approved ages and uses for generic products may vary; consult labeling for specific information.

Pregnancy Considerations Refer to individual agents.

Breast-Feeding Considerations Refer to individual agents.

Contraindications

Hypersensitivity to ibuprofen, pseudoephedrine, or any component of the formulation; hypersensitivity to aspirin or other NSAIDs; use with or within 2 weeks of discontinuing MAO inhibitor; immediately prior to or after coronary bypass graft (CABG)

OTC labeling: Do not use in children <12 years of age.

Warnings/Precautions NSAIDs are associated with an increased risk of adverse cardiovascular events, including MI, stroke, and new-onset or worsening of pre-existing hypertension. Use caution with fluid retention. Avoid use in heart failure. NSAIDs may increase risk of gastrointestinal irritation, inflammation, ulceration, bleeding, and perforation. When used concomitantly with ≤325 mg of aspirin, a substantial increase in the risk of gastrointestinal complications (eg, ulcer) occurs; concomitant gastroprotective therapy (eg, proton pump inhibitors) is recommended (Bhatt, 2008). Even in patients without prior exposure to NSAIDs anaphylactoid reactions may occur; patients with "aspirin triad" (bronchial asthma, aspirin intolerance, rhinitis) may be at increased risk. Do not use in patients who experience bronchospasm, asthma, rhinitis, or urticaria with NSAID or aspirin therapy. NSAIDs may cause serious skin adverse events including exfoliative dermatitis, Stevens-Johnson syndrome (SJS), and toxic epidermal necrolysis (TEN); discontinue at the first sign of skin rash or hypersensitivity. May increase the risk of aseptic meningitis. Platelet adhesion and aggregation may be decreased. Anemia may occur; patients on long-term NSAID therapy should be monitored for anemia. Use is contraindicated when used immediately prior to or after coronary artery bypass graft (CABG) surgery. Risk of MI and stroke may be increased with use following CABG surgery.

Use caution with heart disease, high blood pressure, thyroid disease, diabetes, enlarged prostate, hepatic impairment, renal impairment, asthma, the elderly or GI disease (bleeding or ulcers). Use caution in patients consuming ≥3 alcoholic beverages per day; may increase risk of stomach bleeding.

Benzyl alcohol and derivatives: Some dosage forms may contain sodium benzoate/benzoic acid; benzoic acid (benzoate) is a metabolite of benzyl alcohol; large amounts of benzyl alcohol (≥99 mg/kg/day) have been associated with a potentially fatal toxicity ("gasping syndrome") in neonates; the "gasping syndrome" consists of metabolic acidosis, respiratory distress, gasping respirations, CNS dysfunction (including convulsions, intracranial hemorrhage), hypotension, and cardiovascular collapse (AAP, 1997; CDC, 1982); some data suggests that benzoate displaces bilirubin from protein binding sites (Ahlfors, 2001); avoid or use dosage forms containing benzyl alcohol derivative with caution in neonates. See manufacturer's labeling.

Prior to self-medication, patients should contact healthcare provider if they have had recurring stomach pain or upset, ulcers, bleeding problems, asthma, high blood pressure, heart or kidney disease, thyroid disease, diabetes, enlarged prostate, other serious medical problems, are currently taking a diuretic, aspirin, anticoagulant, or are ≥60 years of age. Recommended dosages should not be exceeded, due to an increased risk of GI bleeding. Stop use and consult a healthcare provider if symptoms get worse, newly appear, or continue; if an allergic reaction occurs; if nervousness, dizziness, or sleeplessness occurs; or if fever lasts for >3 days, congestion lasts for >7 days, or pain >10 days. Consuming ≥3 alcoholic beverages/day or taking longer than recommended may increase the risk of GI bleeding. Not for self medication (OTC use) use in children <12 years of age.

Warnings: Additional Pediatric Considerations Safety and efficacy for the use of cough and cold products in pediatric patients <4 years of age is limited; the AAP warns against the use of these products for respiratory illnesses in this age group. Serious adverse effects including death have been reported (in some cases, high blood concentrations of pseudoephedrine were found). Many of these products contain multiple active ingredients, increasing the risk of accidental overdose when used with other products. The FDA notes that there are no approved OTC uses for these products in pediatric patients <2 years of age. Health care providers are reminded to ask caregivers about the use of OTC cough and cold products in order to avoid exposure to multiple medications containing the same ingredient (AAP 2012; FDA 2008).

Adverse Reactions See individual agents.

Drug Interactions

Metabolism/Transport Effects Refer to individual components.

Avoid Concomitant Use

Avoid concomitant use of Pseudoephedrine and Ibuprofen with any of the following: Dexketoprofen; Ergot Derivatives; Floctafenine; Iobenguane I 123; Ketorolac

(Nasal); Ketorolac (Systemic); MAO Inhibitors; Morniflumate; NSAID (COX-2 Inhibitor); Omacetaxine; Urokinase

Increased Effect/Toxicity

Pseudoephedrine and Ibuprofen may increase the levels/effects of: 5-ASA Derivatives; Agents with Antiplatelet Properties; Aliskiren; Aminoglycosides; Anticoagulants; Apixaban; Bisphosphonate Derivatives; Collagenase (Systemic); CycloSPORINE (Systemic); Dabigatran Etexilate; Deferasirox; Deoxycholic Acid; Desmopressin; Digoxin; Drospirenone; Eplerenone; Haloperidol; Ibritumomab; Lithium; Methotrexate; Nonsteroidal Anti-Inflammatory Agents; NSAID (COX-2 Inhibitor); Obinutuzumab; Omacetaxine; PEMEtrexed; Porfimer; Potassium-Sparing Diuretics; PRALAtrexate; Quinolone Antibiotics; Rivaroxaban; Salicylates; Sympathomimetics; Tacrolimus (Systemic); Tenofovir; Thrombolytic Agents; Tositumomab and Iodine I 131 Tositumomab; Urokinase; Vancomycin; Verteporfin; Vitamin K Antagonists

The levels/effects of Pseudoephedrine and Ibuprofen may be increased by: ACE Inhibitors; Alkalinizing Agents; Angiotensin II Receptor Blockers; Antidepressants (Tricyclic, Tertiary Amine); AtoMOXetine; Cannabinoid-Containing Products; Carbonic Anhydrase Inhibitors; Corticosteroids (Systemic); CycloSPORINE (Systemic); Dasatinib; Dexketoprofen; Diclofenac (Systemic); Ergot Derivatives; Floctafenine; Glucosamine; Herbs (Anticoagulant/Antiplatelet Properties); Ibrutinib; Ketorolac (Nasal); Ketorolac (Systemic); Limaprost; Linezolid; MAO Inhibitors; Morniflumate; Multivitamins/Fluoride (with ADE); Multivitamins/Minerals (with ADEK, Folate, Iron); Multivitamins/Minerals (with AE, No Iron); Omega-3 Fatty Acids; Pentosan Polysulfate Sodium; Pentoxifylline; Probenecid; Prostacyclin Analogues; Selective Serotonin Reuptake Inhibitors; Serotonin/Norepinephrine Reuptake Inhibitors; Sodium Phosphates; Tedizolid; Tipranavir; Treprostinil; Vitamin E; Voriconazole

Decreased Effect

Pseudoephedrine and Ibuprofen may decrease the levels/effects of: ACE Inhibitors; Aliskiren; Angiotensin II Receptor Blockers; Benzylpenicilloyl Polylysine; Beta-Blockers; Eplerenone; FentaNYL; HydrALAZINE; Imatinib; Iobenguane I 123; Loop Diuretics; Potassium-Sparing Diuretics; Prostaglandins (Ophthalmic); Salicylates; Selective Serotonin Reuptake Inhibitors; Thiazide Diuretics

The levels/effects of Pseudoephedrine and Ibuprofen may be decreased by: Alpha1-Blockers; Bile Acid Sequestrants; Salicylates; Spironolactone; Urinary Acidifying Agents

Food Interactions See individual agents.

Storage/Stability Store at 20°C to 25°C (68°F to 77°F); avoid excessive heat.

Pharmacodynamics See individual monographs for Pseudoephedrine and Ibuprofen.

Pharmacokinetics (Adult data unless noted) See individual monographs for Pseudoephedrine and Ibuprofen.

Dosing: Usual

Pediatric: **Analgesic/decongestant:** Oral:

Oral suspension (Ibuprofen 100 mg and pseudoephedrine 15 mg per 5 mL):

Children 4 to 5 years: 5 mL every 6 hours; maximum daily dose: 4 doses/**24 hours**

Children 6 to 11 years: 10 mL every 6 hours; maximum daily dose: 4 doses/**24 hours**

Oral capsule/caplet (ibuprofen 200 mg and pseudoephedrine 30 mg per dose): Children ≥12 years and Adolescents: One dose every 4 to 6 hours as needed; may increase to 2 doses if necessary; maximum daily dose: 6 doses/**24 hours**

Adult: **Analgesic/decongestant:** Oral: Ibuprofen 200 mg and pseudoephedrine 30 mg per dose: One dose every 4 to 6 hours as needed; may increase to 2 doses if necessary; maximum daily dose: 6 doses/**24 hours. Note:** Contact health care provider if symptoms have not improved within 7 days when treating cold symptoms.

Administration Oral: Administer with food

Test Interactions See individual agents.

Dosage Forms Excipient information presented when available (limited, particularly for generics); consult specific product labeling.

Caplet:

Advil® Cold & Sinus, Proprinal® Cold and Sinus: Pseudoephedrine hydrochloride 30 mg and ibuprofen 200 mg

Capsule, liquid filled:

Advil® Cold & Sinus: Pseudoephedrine hydrochloride 30 mg and ibuprofen 200 mg [solubilized ibuprofen as free acid and potassium salt; contains potassium 20 mg/capsule and coconut oil]

- ◆ **Pseudoephedrine and Loratadine** *see* Loratadine and Pseudoephedrine *on page* *1298*
- ◆ **Pseudoephedrine and Triprolidine** *see* Triprolidine and Pseudoephedrine *on page* *2129*
- ◆ **Pseudoephedrine Hydrochloride** *see* Pseudoephedrine *on page* *1801*
- ◆ **Pseudoephedrine Sulfate** *see* Pseudoephedrine *on page* *1801*
- ◆ **Pseudofrin (Can)** *see* Pseudoephedrine *on page* *1801*
- ◆ **Pseudomonic Acid A** *see* Mupirocin *on page* *1471*
- ◆ **Psoriasin [OTC]** *see* Coal Tar *on page* *523*
- ◆ **Psoriasin [OTC]** *see* Salicylic Acid *on page* *1894*
- ◆ **Psudatabs [OTC]** *see* Pseudoephedrine *on page* *1801*

Psyllium (SIL i yum)

Medication Safety Issues

Sound-alike/look-alike issues:

Fiberall® may be confused with Feverall®

Brand Names: US Dietary Fiber Laxative [OTC]; Evac [OTC]; Fiber Therapy [OTC]; Geri-Mucil [OTC]; Konsyl [OTC]; Konsyl-D [OTC]; Metamucil MultiHealth Fiber [OTC]; Natural Fiber Therapy [OTC]; Natural Psyllium Seed [OTC]; Natural Vegetable Fiber [OTC]; Reguloid [OTC]; Sorbulax [OTC]

Brand Names: Canada Metamucil®

Therapeutic Category Laxative, Bulk-Producing

Generic Availability (US) May be product dependent

Use Dietary fiber supplement (OTC: All products: FDA approved in adults; refer to product specific information regarding FDA approval in pediatric patients, most products FDA approved in ages ≥12 years); treatment of occasional constipation (OTC: All products: FDA approved in adults; refer to product specific information regarding FDA approval in pediatric patients, most products FDA approved in ages ≥6 years); has also been used for adjunctive treatment with dietary management for hyperlipidemia (eg, LDL, total cholesterol, or triglycerides) and treatment of chronic constipation; management of irritable bowel syndrome. **Note:** Although approved for treatment of occasional constipation in pediatric patients and improved bowel movement frequency, current guidelines do not recommend for treatment of functional constipation (NASPGHAN/ESPGHAN [Tabbers 2014]).

Pregnancy Considerations Psyllium is not absorbed systemically. When administered with adequate fluids use is considered safe for the treatment of occasional constipation during pregnancy (Wald, 2003).

Contraindications Hypersensitivity to psyllium or any component of the formulation; fecal impaction; GI obstruction

Warnings/Precautions Use with caution in patients with esophageal strictures, ulcers, stenosis, intestinal adhesions, or difficulty swallowing. Use with caution in the elderly; may have insufficient fluid intake which may predispose them to fecal impaction and bowel obstruction. Products must be taken with at least 8 ounces of fluid in order to prevent choking. Hypersensitivity reactions have been reported with ingestion or inhalation of psyllium in susceptible individuals. To reduce the risk of CHD, the soluble fiber from psyllium should be used in conjunction with a diet low in saturated fat and cholesterol. Some products may contain calcium, potassium, sodium, soy lecithin, or phenylalanine.

When used for self-medication (OTC), do not use in the presence of abdominal pain, nausea, or vomiting. Notify healthcare provider in case of sudden changes of bowel habits which last >2 weeks or in case of rectal bleeding. Not for self-treatment of constipation lasting >1 week

Adverse Reactions

Gastrointestinal: Abdominal cramps, constipation, diarrhea, esophageal or bowel obstruction

Respiratory: Bronchospasm

Miscellaneous: Anaphylaxis upon inhalation in susceptible individuals, rhinoconjunctivitis

Drug Interactions

Metabolism/Transport Effects None known.

Avoid Concomitant Use There are no known interactions where it is recommended to avoid concomitant use.

Increased Effect/Toxicity There are no known significant interactions involving an increase in effect.

Decreased Effect There are no known significant interactions involving a decrease in effect.

Storage/Stability Store at room temperature; protect from moisture (consult product labeling for specific information).

Mechanism of Action Psyllium is a soluble fiber. It absorbs water in the intestine to form a viscous liquid which promotes peristalsis and reduces transit time.

Pharmacodynamics Onset of action: 12-72 hours

Pharmacokinetics (Adult data unless noted) Absorption: Oral: Generally not absorbed; small amounts of grain extract present in the preparation have been reportedly absorbed following colonic hydrolysis

Dosing: Usual

Pediatric:

Adequate intake for total fiber: Oral: **Note:** The definition of "fiber" varies; however, the soluble fiber in psyllium is only one type of fiber which makes up the daily recommended intake of total fiber; contribution from other food sources should also be considered when assessing intake. Reported requirements variable:

AAP/NHLBI recommendation (NHLBI 2011): Minimum intake: Children 2 to 10 years: Daily dietary intake (g/day) = Age (years) + 5 g

IOM recommendation:

Children 1 to 3 years: 19 g/day

Children 4 to 8 years: 25 g/day

Children and Adolescents 9 to 13 years: Male: 31 g/day; Female: 26 g/day

Adolescents: 14 to 18 years: Male: 38 g/day; Female: 26 g/day

Bowel movement regularity: Oral: **Note:** General dosing guidelines (Federal Register 1985); consult specific product labeling.

Children 6 to <12 years: 1.25 to 15 g/day in 1 to 3 divided doses

Children ≥12 years and Adolescents: 2.5 to 30 g/day in 1 to 3 divided doses

Hypercholesterolemia; adjunct treatment with dietary management (NHLBI 2011): Oral:

Children 2 to <12 years: 6 g/day in 1 to 3 divided doses

Children ≥12 years and Adolescents: 12 g/day in 1 to 3 divided doses

Adults:

Adequate intake for total fiber: Oral: **Note:** The definition of "fiber" varies; however, the soluble fiber in psyllium is only one type of fiber which makes up the daily recommended intake of total fiber.

Adults 19 to 50 years: Male: 38 g/day; Female: 25 g/day

Adults ≥51 years: Male: 30 g/day; Female: 21 g/day

Pregnancy: 28 g/day

Lactation: 29 g/day

Constipation: Oral: Psyllium: 2.5 to 30 g per day in divided doses

Reduce risk of coronary heart disease: Oral: Soluble fiber ≥7 g (psyllium seed husk ≥10.2 g) per day (DHHS 1998)

Administration Oral: Granules and powder must be mixed in an 8 ounce glass of water or juice; drink an 8 ounce glass of liquid with each dose of wafers or capsules; capsules should be swallowed one at a time. When more than one dose is required, divide throughout the day. Separate dose by at least 2 hours from other drug therapies. Inhalation of psyllium dust may cause sensitivity to psyllium (eg, runny nose, watery eyes, wheezing).

Monitoring Parameters Dependent upon use, may include stool output and frequency; serum lipids, weight

Dosage Forms Considerations Psyllium hydrophilic mucilloid 3.4 g is equivalent to 2 g Soluble fiber

Dosage Forms Excipient information presented when available (limited, particularly for generics); consult specific product labeling. [DSC] = Discontinued product

Capsule, Oral:

Konsyl: 520 mg [gluten free, sugar free]

Reguloid: 0.52 g [contains fd&c yellow #6 aluminum lake]

Packet, Oral:

Konsyl: 28.3% (1 ea) [gluten free, kosher certified; contains fd&c yellow #10 (quinoline yellow), fd&c yellow #6 (sunset yellow)]

Konsyl: 28.3% (30 ea) [gluten free, kosher certified; contains fd&c yellow #10 (quinoline yellow), fd&c yellow #6 (sunset yellow); orange flavor]

Konsyl: 60.3% (1 ea, 30 ea) [gluten free, kosher certified, sugar free; contains aspartame, fd&c yellow #6 (sunset yellow); orange flavor]

Konsyl: 100% (1 ea, 30 ea, 100 ea) [gluten free, kosher certified, sugar free; bland flavor]

Metamucil MultiHealth Fiber: 58.12% (1 ea, 30 ea, 44 ea) [gluten free, sugar free; contains aspartame, fd&c yellow #6 (sunset yellow)]

Powder, Oral:

Dietary Fiber Laxative: 28.3% (283 g, 300 g, 425 g, 660 g) [contains fd&c yellow #6 (sunset yellow)]

Fiber Therapy: 58.6% (283 g) [sugar free; contains aspartame, fd&c yellow #6 (sunset yellow)]

Geri-Mucil: 68% (368 g)

Geri-Mucil: 68% (368 g) [contains fd&c yellow #6 aluminum lake]

Geri-Mucil: 68% (284 g) [sugar free]

Geri-Mucil: 68% (283 g) [sugar free; contains aspartame, fd&c yellow #6 aluminum lake]

Konsyl: 28.3% (538 g) [gluten free, kosher certified; contains fd&c yellow #10 (quinoline yellow), fd&c yellow #6 (sunset yellow); orange flavor]

Konsyl: 30.9% (397 g) [gluten free, kosher certified; contains fd&c yellow #6 (sunset yellow); orange flavor]

Konsyl: 60.3% (450 g) [gluten free, kosher certified, sugar free; contains aspartame, fd&c yellow #6 (sunset yellow); orange flavor]

Konsyl: 71.67% (300 g) [gluten free, kosher certified, sugar free; bland flavor]
Konsyl: 100% (300 g, 450 g) [gluten free, kosher certified, sugar free]
Konsyl: 100% (300 g, 450 g) [gluten free, kosher certified, sugar free; bland flavor]
Konsyl: 60.3% (283 g) [sugar free; contains aspartame, fd&c yellow #6 (sunset yellow); orange flavor]
Konsyl-D: 52.3% (397 g, 500 g [DSC]) [flavor free; sweet flavor]
Metamucil MultiHealth Fiber: 58.6% (425 g) [gluten free, sugar free; contains aspartame, brilliant blue fcf (fd&c blue #1), fd&c red #40]
Metamucil MultiHealth Fiber: 63% (660 g) [gluten free, sugar free]
Natural Fiber Therapy: 30.9% (368 g, 539 g); 48.57% (368 g, 538 g)
Natural Psyllium Seed: 100% (480 g) [animal products free, gelatin free, gluten free, kosher certified, lactose free, no artificial color(s), no artificial flavor(s), starch free, sugar free, yeast free]
Natural Vegetable Fiber: 48.57% (368 g)
Reguloid: 48.57% (369 g, 540 g)
Reguloid: 28.3% (369 g, 540 g) [contains fd&c yellow #6 (sunset yellow), fd&c yellow #6 aluminum lake; orange flavor]
Reguloid: 58.6% (284 g, 426 g) [sugar free; natural flavor]
Reguloid: 58.6% (284 g, 426 g) [sugar free; contains aspartame, fd&c yellow #6 (sunset yellow), fd&c yellow #6 aluminum lake]
Sorbulax: 100% (420 g)

Powder, Oral [preservative free]:
Evac: (480 g) [dye free]

- ◆ **Psyllium Husk** *see* Psyllium *on page 1804*
- ◆ **Psyllium Hydrophilic Mucilloid** *see* Psyllium *on page 1804*
- ◆ **Pteroylglutamic Acid** *see* Folic Acid *on page 931*
- ◆ **PTG** *see* Teniposide *on page 2015*
- ◆ **PTU (error-prone abbreviation)** *see* Propylthiouracil *on page 1793*
- ◆ **Pulmicort** *see* Budesonide (Systemic, Oral Inhalation) *on page 307*
- ◆ **Pulmicort Flexhaler** *see* Budesonide (Systemic, Oral Inhalation) *on page 307*
- ◆ **Pulmicort Turbuhaler (Can)** *see* Budesonide (Systemic, Oral Inhalation) *on page 307*
- ◆ **Pulmophylline (Can)** *see* Theophylline *on page 2044*
- ◆ **PulmoSal** *see* Sodium Chloride *on page 1938*
- ◆ **Pulmozyme** *see* Dornase Alfa *on page 705*
- ◆ **Puralube [OTC]** *see* Artificial Tears *on page 201*
- ◆ **Purell [OTC]** *see* Alcohol (Ethyl) *on page 86*
- ◆ **Purell 2 in 1 [OTC]** *see* Alcohol (Ethyl) *on page 86*
- ◆ **Purell Lasting Care [OTC]** *see* Alcohol (Ethyl) *on page 86*
- ◆ **Purell Moisture Therapy [OTC]** *see* Alcohol (Ethyl) *on page 86*
- ◆ **Purell with Aloe [OTC]** *see* Alcohol (Ethyl) *on page 86*
- ◆ **Purified Chick Embryo Cell** *see* Rabies Vaccine *on page 1832*
- ◆ **Purinethol** *see* Mercaptopurine *on page 1363*
- ◆ **Purinethol [DSC]** *see* Mercaptopurine *on page 1363*
- ◆ **Purixan** *see* Mercaptopurine *on page 1363*

Pyrantel Pamoate (pi RAN tel PAM oh ate)

Brand Names: US Pamix [OTC]; Pin-X [OTC]; Reeses Pinworm Medicine [OTC]

Brand Names: Canada Combantrin

Therapeutic Category Anthelmintic

Generic Availability (US) May be product dependent

Use Treatment of pinworm (*Enterobius vermicularis*) infestation (OTC products: FDA approved in ages ≥2 years weighing at least 11 kg and adults); has also been used for the treatment of hookworm (*Ancylostoma duodenale* and *Necator americanus*) infestations, trichostrongyliasis and moniliformis infections

Pregnancy Considerations Pyrantel pamoate has minimal systemic absorption. Systemic absorption would be required in order for pyrantel pamoate to cross the placenta and reach the fetus.

Contraindications Hypersensitivity to pyrantel or any component of the formulation

Warnings/Precautions Use with caution in patients with hepatic impairment. Since pinworm infections are easily spread to others, treat all family members in close contact with the patient. When used for self-medication, patients should be instructed to contact health care provider if symptoms or pinworm infection persists after treatment or if any worms other than pinworms are present before or after treatment. Patients should not repeat dose unless directed to by their health care provider.

Benzyl alcohol and derivatives: Some dosage forms may contain sodium benzoate/benzoic acid; benzoic acid (benzoate) is a metabolite of benzyl alcohol; large amounts of benzyl alcohol (≥99 mg/kg/day) have been associated with a potentially fatal toxicity ("gasping syndrome") in neonates; the "gasping syndrome" consists of metabolic acidosis, respiratory distress, gasping respirations, CNS dysfunction (including convulsions, intracranial hemorrhage), hypotension, and cardiovascular collapse (AAP, 1997; CDC, 1982); some data suggests that benzoate displaces bilirubin from protein binding sites (Ahlfors, 2001); avoid or use dosage forms containing benzyl alcohol derivative with caution in neonates. See manufacturer's labeling.

Warnings: Additional Pediatric Considerations Some dosage forms may contain propylene glycol; in neonates large amounts of propylene glycol delivered orally, intravenously (eg, >3,000 mg/day), or topically have been associated with potentially fatal toxicities which can include metabolic acidosis, seizures, renal failure, and CNS depression; toxicities have also been reported in children and adults including hyperosmolality, lactic acidosis, seizures, and respiratory depression; use caution (AAP, 1997; Shehab, 2009).

Adverse Reactions

Central nervous system: Dizziness, headache

Gastrointestinal: Abdominal cramps, diarrhea, nausea, vomiting

Drug Interactions

Metabolism/Transport Effects Substrate of CYP2D6 (minor); **Note:** Assignment of Major/Minor substrate status based on clinically relevant drug interaction potential

Avoid Concomitant Use There are no known interactions where it is recommended to avoid concomitant use.

Increased Effect/Toxicity There are no known significant interactions involving an increase in effect.

Decreased Effect

The levels/effects of Pyrantel Pamoate may be decreased by: Aminoquinolines (Antimalarial)

Storage/Stability Store at 15°C to 30°C (59°F to 86°F).

Mechanism of Action Causes the release of acetylcholine and inhibits cholinesterase; acts as a depolarizing neuromuscular blocker, paralyzing the helminths

Pharmacokinetics (Adult data unless noted)

Absorption: Oral: Poor

Metabolism: Undergoes partial hepatic metabolism

Time to peak serum concentration: Within 1-3 hours

Elimination: In feces (50% as unchanged drug) and urine (7% as unchanged drug and metabolites)

Dosing: Usual

Pediatric: **Note:** Dose is expressed as pyrantel base.

***Enterobius vermicularis* (pinworm):**

Manufacturer's labeling: Children ≥2 years and Adolescents: Oral:

Weight-directed dosing: 11 mg/kg administered as a single dose; maximum dose: 1,000 mg/dose

Fixed-dosing (weight band):

11 to 16 kg: 125 mg
17 to 28 kg: 250 mg
29 to 39 kg: 375 mg
40 to 50 kg: 500 mg
51 to 62 kg: 625 mg
63 to 73 kg: 750 mg
74 to 84 kg: 875 mg
>84 kg: 1,000 mg

Alternate dosing: Limited data available: Children and Adolescents: Oral: 11 mg/kg/dose every 2 weeks for 2 doses; maximum dose: 1,000 mg/dose (*Red Book* [AAP], 2012)

***Ancylostoma duodenale* (hookworm), *Necator americanus* (hookworm):** Limited data available: Children and Adolescents: Oral: 11 mg/kg once daily for 3 days; maximum dose: 1,000 mg/dose (*Red Book* [AAP], 2012)

Moniliformis: Limited data available: Children and Adolescents: Oral: 11 mg/kg/dose every 2 weeks for 3 doses(*Red Book* [AAP], 2012)

Trichostrongylus: Limited data available: Children and Adolescents: Oral: 11 mg/kg administered as a single dose; maximum dose: 1,000 mg/dose (*Red Book* [AAP], 2012)

Adult: **Note:** Dose is expressed as pyrantel base; not preferred therapy since newer treatments are available.

***Enterobius vermicularis* (pinworm):** Oral: 11 mg/kg administered as a single dose; maximum dose: 1,000 mg/dose

Dosing adjustment in renal impairment: Children, Adolescents, and Adults: There are no dosage adjustments provided in the manufacturer's labeling.

Dosing adjustment in hepatic impairment: Children, Adolescents, and Adults: There are no dosage adjustments provided in the manufacturer's labeling; use with caution.

Administration Oral: May be taken alone or mixed with milk or fruit juice. May be administered without regard to meals. The use of a laxative is not required prior to, during, or after use.

Suspension: Shake well before use.

Tablet: Chewable tablet must be chewed thoroughly before swallowing.

Monitoring Parameters Stool for presence of eggs, worms, and occult blood

Dosage Forms Excipient information presented when available (limited, particularly for generics); consult specific product labeling.

Suspension, Oral [strength expressed as base]:

Pamix: 50 mg/mL (30 mL, 60 mL, 240 mL)

Pin-X: 50 mg/mL (30 mL, 60 mL) [sugar free; contains methylparaben, propylene glycol, propylparaben, saccharin sodium, sodium benzoate; caramel flavor]

Reeses Pinworm Medicine: 50 mg/mL (30 mL) [contains saccharin sodium, sodium benzoate]

Tablet, Oral [strength expressed as base]:

Reeses Pinworm Medicine: 62.5 mg [scored]

Tablet Chewable, Oral [strength expressed as base]:

Pin-X: 250 mg [scored; contains aspartame, fd&c yellow #6 aluminum lake; orange flavor]

Pyrazinamide (peer a ZIN a mide)

Brand Names: Canada Tebrazid™

Therapeutic Category Antitubercular Agent

Generic Availability (US) Yes

Use Adjunctive treatment of *Mycobacterium* tuberculosis infection in combination with other antituberculosis agents (FDA approved in children and adults); especially useful in disseminated and meningeal tuberculosis; CDC currently recommends a 3 or 4 multidrug regimen which includes pyrazinamide, rifampin, INH, and at times ethambutol or streptomycin for the treatment of tuberculosis

Pregnancy Risk Factor C

Pregnancy Considerations Teratogenic effects have not been observed in animal reproduction studies. Due to the risk of tuberculosis to the fetus, treatment is recommended when the probability of maternal disease is moderate to high. Although not recommended as the initial treatment regimen, the use of pyrazinamide during pregnancy is recommended by The World Health Organization (Blumberg, 2003).

Breast-Feeding Considerations Low concentrations of pyrazinamide have been detected in breast milk; concentrations are less than maternal plasma concentration (Holdiness, 1984). The amount of drug in breast milk is considered insufficient for the treatment of tuberculosis in breast-fed infants.

Contraindications Hypersensitivity to pyrazinamide or any component of the formulation; acute gout; severe hepatic damage

Warnings/Precautions Use with caution in patients with a history of alcoholism, renal failure, chronic gout, diabetes mellitus, or porphyria. Dose-related hepatotoxicity ranging from transient ALT/AST elevations to jaundice, hepatitis and/or liver atrophy (rare) has occurred. Use with caution in patients receiving concurrent medications associated with hepatotoxicity (particularly with rifampin). The 2-month rifampin-pyrazinamide regimen for the treatment of latent tuberculosis infection (LTBI) has been associated with severe and fatal liver injuries; incidence increased with pyrazinamide doses >30 mg/kg/day. The Infectious Diseases Society of America and Centers for Disease Control and Prevention recommend that the 2-month rifampin-pyrazinamide regimen should not generally be used in patients with LTBI.

Adverse Reactions

Central nervous system: Malaise

Gastrointestinal: Anorexia, nausea, vomiting

Neuromuscular & skeletal: Arthralgia, myalgia

Rare but important or life-threatening: Acne, angioedema (rare), anticoagulant effect, dysuria, fever, gout, hepatotoxicity, interstitial nephritis, itching, photosensitivity, porphyria, rash, sideroblastic anemia, thrombocytopenia, urticaria

Drug Interactions

Metabolism/Transport Effects None known.

Avoid Concomitant Use There are no known interactions where it is recommended to avoid concomitant use.

Increased Effect/Toxicity

Pyrazinamide may increase the levels/effects of: CycloSPORINE (Systemic); Rifampin

Decreased Effect There are no known significant interactions involving a decrease in effect.

Storage/Stability Store at controlled room temperature of 15°C to 30°C (59°F to 86°F).

Mechanism of Action Converted to pyrazinoic acid in susceptible strains of *Mycobacterium* which lowers the pH of the environment; exact mechanism of action has not been elucidated

Pharmacokinetics (Adult data unless noted)

Absorption: Oral: Well absorbed

Distribution: Widely distributed into body tissues and fluids including the liver, lung, and CSF

Protein binding: 50%

Metabolism: In the liver

Half-life: 9-10 hours, prolonged with reduced renal or hepatic function

Time to peak serum concentration: Within 2 hours

Elimination: In urine (4% as unchanged drug)

Dosing: Usual Oral: Tuberculosis, treatment: **Note:** Used as part of a multidrug regimen. Treatment regimens consist of an initial 2-month phase, followed by a continuation phase of 4 or 7 additional months; frequency of dosing may differ depending on phase of therapy.

Infants, Children < 40 kg, and Adolescents ≤14 years and <40 kg:

Non-HIV patients (CDC, 2003):

Daily therapy: 15-30 mg/kg/dose (maximum: 2 g/dose) once daily

Directly observed therapy (DOT): 50 mg/kg/dose (maximum: 2 g/dose) twice weekly

HIV-exposed/infected patients: (CDC, 2009): Daily therapy: 20-40 mg/kg/dose once daily (maximum: 2 g/day) (CDC, 2009)

Adults: Suggested dosing based on lean body weight (Blumberg, 2003):

Daily therapy:

40-55 kg: 1000 mg

56-75 kg: 1500 mg

76-90 kg: 2000 mg (maximum dose regardless of weight)

Twice weekly directly observed therapy (DOT):

40-55 kg: 2000 mg

56-75 kg: 3000 mg

76-90 kg: 4000 mg (maximum dose regardless of weight)

3 times/week DOT:

40-55 kg: 1500 mg

56-75 kg: 2500 mg

76-90 kg: 3000 mg (maximum dose regardless of weight)

Monitoring Parameters Periodic liver function tests, serum uric acid

Test Interactions Reacts with Acetest® and Ketostix® to produce pinkish-brown color

Dosage Forms Excipient information presented when available (limited, particularly for generics); consult specific product labeling.

Tablet, Oral:

Generic: 500 mg

Extemporaneous Preparations A 100 mg/mL oral suspension may be made with tablets. Crush two-hundred pyrazinamide 500 mg tablets and mix with a suspension containing 500 mL methylcellulose 1% and 500 mL simple syrup. Add to this a suspension containing one-hundred forty crushed pyrazinamide tablets in 350 mL methylcellulose 1% and 350 mL simple syrup to make 1.7 L suspension. Label "shake well" and "refrigerate". Stable for 60 days refrigerated (preferred) and 45 days at room temperature.

Nahata MC, Morosco RS, and Peritre SP, "Stability of Pyrazinamide in Two Suspensions," *Am J Health Syst Pharm*, 1995, 52(14):1558-60.

◆ **Pyrazinoic Acid Amide** *see* Pyrazinamide *on page 1807*

◆ **Pyri 500 [OTC]** *see* Pyridoxine *on page 1810*

◆ **2-Pyridine Aldoxime Methochloride** *see* Pralidoxime *on page 1747*

◆ **Pyridium** *see* Phenazopyridine *on page 1678*

Pyridostigmine (peer id oh STIG meen)

Medication Safety Issues

Sound-alike/look-alike issues:

Pyridostigmine may be confused with physostigmine

Regonol may be confused with Reglan, Renagel

Related Information

Oral Medications That Should Not Be Crushed or Altered *on page 2476*

Brand Names: US Mestinon; Regonol

Brand Names: Canada Mestinon; Mestinon-SR

Therapeutic Category Antidote, Neuromuscular Blocking Agent; Cholinergic Agent

Generic Availability (US) May be product dependent

Use

Oral: Mestinon®: Treatment of myasthenia gravis (FDA approved in adults); has also been used for treatment of vincristine induced neurotoxicity, congenital myasthenic syndrome, and pretreatment for Soman nerve gas exposure (military use only)

Parenteral: Regonol®: Reversal agent for effects of nondepolarizing neuromuscular blocking agents (FDA approved in adults); has also been used for treatment of myasthenia gravis

Pregnancy Risk Factor B/C (manufacturer dependent)

Pregnancy Considerations Adverse events were not observed in animal reproduction studies. Pyridostigmine may cross the placenta (Buckley, 1968). Use of pyridostigmine may be continued during pregnancy for the treatment of myasthenia gravis (Skie, 2010; Norwood, 2013) and its use should be continued during labor (Norwood, 2013). Transient neonatal myasthenia gravis may occur in 10% to 20% of neonates due to placental transfer of maternal antibodies (Skie, 2010; Varner, 2013).

In general, medications used as antidotes should take into consideration the health and prognosis of the mother; antidotes should be administered to pregnant women if there is a clear indication for use and should not be withheld because of fears of teratogenicity (Bailey, 2003).

Breast-Feeding Considerations Pyridostigmine is excreted in breast milk (Hardell, 1992). The manufacturer recommends that caution be exercised when administering pyridostigmine to nursing women.

Information is available from two mothers using pyridostigmine for myasthenia gravis throughout pregnancy and postpartum. Maternal doses ranged from 180 mg to 300 mg/day. Milk concentrations averaged ≤0.1% of the weight adjusted maternal dose (n=2); infant plasma concentrations were less than the limit of quantification (<2 ng/mL; n=1) (Hardell, 1992). Disease exacerbations may occur in nursing women with poorly controlled myasthenia gravis due to fatigue associated with breast-feeding. Babies born to women with myasthenia gravis may have feeding difficulties due to transient myasthenia gravis of the newborn (Norwood, 2013). Nursing infants should be monitored for fatigue associated with transient neonatal myasthenia gravis (Varner, 2013), however current guidelines note that nursing is not contraindicated in women taking pyridostigmine for myasthenia gravis (Norwood, 2013).

Contraindications Hypersensitivity to pyridostigmine, anticholinesterase agents, or any component of the formulation; mechanical intestinal or urinary obstruction

Documentation of allergenic cross-reactivity for anticholinergic muscle stimulants is limited. However, because of similarities in chemical structure and/or pharmacologic actions, the possibility of cross-sensitivity cannot be ruled out with certainty.

Warnings/Precautions Symptoms of excess cholinergic activity may occur (eg, salivation, sweating, urinary incontinence). Overdosage may result in cholinergic crisis (eg, muscle weakness), which must be distinguished from myasthenic crisis; discontinue immediately in the presence of cholinergic crisis. Hypersensitivity reactions may occur; have atropine and epinephrine ready to treat hypersensitivity reactions. Inadequate reversal induced by nondepolarizing muscle relaxants is possible; manage with manual or mechanical ventilation until recovery is adequate (additional doses not recommended). Failure to produce prompt (within 30 minutes) reversal of neuromuscular blockade may occur in the presence of extreme debilitation, carcinomatosis, or with concomitant use of certain broad-spectrum antibiotics, or anesthetic agents and other drugs which enhance neuromuscular blockade or cause respiratory depression.

Use with caution in patients with bradycardia or other cardiac arrhythmias, glaucoma, renal impairment, asthma, bronchospastic disease, COPD, or bromide sensitivity. Potentially significant interactions may exist, requiring dose or frequency adjustment, additional monitoring, and/or selection of alternative therapy.

Injection not indicated for use in neonates; may contain benzyl alcohol which has been associated with "gasping syndrome" in neonates. Injection must be administered by trained personnel; use of peripheral nerve stimulation to monitor neuromuscular function recovery and continuous patient observation until recovery of normal respiration is recommended. To counteract anticholinergic effects, use of glycopyrrolate or atropine sulfate simultaneously with or prior to administration is recommended. Adequate facilities should be available for cardiopulmonary resuscitation when testing and adjusting dose for myasthenia gravis.

Military use: Only for pretreatment for exposure to Soman; discontinue pyridostigmine at the first sign of Soman exposure (do not administer pyridostigmine after Soman exposure); atropine and pralidoxime must be administered after Soman exposure (pyridostigmine pretreatment offers no benefit against Soman unless atropine and pralidoxime are administered once symptoms of poisoning appear). Use in conjunction with protective garments, including gas mask, hood and overgarments.

Warnings: Additional Pediatric Considerations Neonates of myasthenic mothers may have transient difficulties in swallowing, sucking, and breathing; use of pyridostigmine may be of benefit; use edrophonium test to assess neonate with these symptoms.

Adverse Reactions

Cardiovascular: Arrhythmias (especially bradycardia), AV block, cardiac arrest, decreased carbon monoxide, flushing, hypotension, nodal rhythm, nonspecific ECG changes, syncope, tachycardia

Central nervous system: Convulsions, dizziness, drowsiness, dysphonia, headache, loss of consciousness

Dermatologic: Skin rash, thrombophlebitis (IV), urticaria

Gastrointestinal: Abdominal pain, diarrhea, dysphagia, flatulence, hyperperistalsis, nausea, salivation, stomach cramps, vomiting

Genitourinary: Urinary urgency

Neuromuscular & skeletal: Arthralgia, dysarthria, fasciculations, muscle cramps, myalgia, spasms, weakness

Ocular: Amblyopia, lacrimation, small pupils

Respiratory: Bronchial secretions increased, bronchiolar constriction, bronchospasm, dyspnea, laryngospasm, respiratory arrest, respiratory depression, respiratory muscle paralysis

Miscellaneous: Allergic reactions, anaphylaxis, diaphoresis increased

Drug Interactions

Metabolism/Transport Effects None known.

Avoid Concomitant Use There are no known interactions where it is recommended to avoid concomitant use.

Increased Effect/Toxicity

Pyridostigmine may increase the levels/effects of: Beta-Blockers; Cholinergic Agonists; Succinylcholine

The levels/effects of Pyridostigmine may be increased by: Corticosteroids (Systemic)

Decreased Effect

Pyridostigmine may decrease the levels/effects of: Anticholinergic Agents; Neuromuscular-Blocking Agents (Nondepolarizing)

The levels/effects of Pyridostigmine may be decreased by: Anticholinergic Agents; Dipyridamole; Methocarbamol

Storage/Stability

Store at 25°C (77°F); excursions permitted to 15°C to 30°C (59°F to 86°F); protect from light.

Military use: Store between 2°C and 8°C (36°F to 46°F); protect from light. Discard 3 months after issue. Do not dispense after removal from the refrigerator for more than a total of 3 months.

Mechanism of Action Inhibits destruction of acetylcholine by acetylcholinesterase which facilitates transmission of impulses across myoneural junction

Pharmacodynamics

Recovery from vincristine neurotoxicity: Onset of action: 1-2 weeks (Akbayram, 2010)

Myasthenia gravis:

Onset of action:

Oral: Within 30 minutes (Maggi, 2011)

IM: 15-30 minutes

IV: Within 2-5 minutes

Duration:

Oral: 3-4 hours (Maggi, 2011)

IM, IV: 2-3 hours

Pharmacokinetics (Adult data unless noted)

Absorption: Oral: Very poor

Distribution: V_d: 0.53-1.76 L/kg (Aquilonius, 1986)

Protein Binding: None (Aquilonius, 1986)

Metabolism: Hepatic and at tissue site by cholinesterases

Bioavailability: Oral: 10% to 20% (Aquilonius, 1986)

Half-life: 1-2 hours; renal failure: ~6 hours (Aquilonius, 1986)

Time to peak serum concentration: Oral: 1-2 hours (Aquilonius, 1986)

Elimination: Urine (80% to 90% as unchanged drug) (Aquilonius, 1986)

Dosing: Neonatal Myasthenic syndrome; congenital: Limited data available: Oral: 1 mg/kg/dose every 4 hours; maximum daily dose: 7 mg/kg/**day** divided in 5-6 doses (Lorenzoni, 2012)

Dosing: Usual

Pediatric: **Note:** All pediatric dosing recommendations based on immediate release product formulations. Dosage should be individualized based on patient response.

Myasthenic syndromes, congenital: Limited data available: Infants, Children, and Adolescents: Oral: 1 mg/kg/dose every 4 hours; usual range: 4 to 5 mg/kg/day in 4 to 6 divided doses; maximum daily dose: 7 mg/kg/**day** divided in 5-6 doses (Kleigman, 2011; Lorenzoni, 2012)

Myasthenia gravis, autoimmune (juvenile): Limited data available: Infants, Children, and Adolescents: **Note:** Dosage should be adjusted such that larger doses administered prior to time of greatest fatigue.

Oral: 1 mg/kg/dose every 4-6 hours; maximum daily dose: 7 mg/kg/**day** divided in 5-6 doses; usual daily dose: 600 mg/**day**; doses as high as 1500 mg/**day** have been used (Andrews, 1998; Maggi, 2011)

IM, IV: 0.05-0.15 mg/kg/dose; maximum dose: 10 mg (Kleigman, 2007)

Reversal of nondepolarizing neuromuscular blocker: Limited data available: Infants, Children, and Adolescents: IM, IV: 0.1-0.25 mg/kg/dose (Kleigman, 2007).

Note: Give atropine or glycopyrrolate immediately prior to minimize side effects.

Vincristine-induced neurotoxicity: Limited data available: Children ≥2 years and Adolescents: Oral: 3 mg/kg/day divided in 2 doses, given with pyridoxine for 3 weeks; dosing based on a case series of four children (age: 2-13 years) receiving vincristine for treatment of ALL (Akbayram, 2010) and a 2-year old receiving vincristine for a cervical synovial sarcoma (Muller, 2004)

Adults:

Myasthenia gravis:

Oral:

Immediate release: Highly individualized dosing ranges: 60-1500 mg/day, usually 600 mg/day divided into 5-6 doses, spaced to provide maximum relief

Sustained release formulation: Highly individualized dosing ranges: 180-540 mg once or twice daily (doses separated by at least 6 hours); **Note:** Most clinicians reserve sustained release dosage form for bedtime dose only.

IM or slow IV push: To supplement oral dosage pre- and postoperatively during labor and postpartum, during myasthenic crisis, or when oral therapy is impractical: ~1/30th of oral dose; observe patient closely for cholinergic reactions

IV infusion: To supplement oral dosage pre- and postoperatively, during labor and postpartum, during myasthenic crisis, or when oral therapy is impractical: Initial: 2 mg/hour with gradual titration in increments of 0.5-1 mg/hour, up to a maximum rate of 4 mg/hour

Reversal of nondepolarizing neuromuscular blocker: IV: 0.1-0.25 mg/kg/dose; 10-20 mg is usually sufficient (full recovery usually occurs ≤15 minutes, but ≥30 minutes may be required)

Soman nerve gas exposure; pretreatment (military use): Oral: 30 mg every 8 hours beginning several hours before exposure; discontinue at first sign of nerve agent exposure, then begin atropine and pralidoxime

Dosage adjustment in renal impairment: There are no dosage adjustments are provided in the manufacturer's labeling; however, lower doses may be required due to prolonged elimination; dosage titration should be based on drug effects.

Dosage adjustment in hepatic impairment: There are no dosage adjustments are provided in the manufacturer's labeling.

Administration

Oral: Swallow sustained release tablets whole, do not chew or crush

Parenteral: May administer IM or as a direct IV slowly over 2-4 minutes; patients receiving large parenteral doses should be pretreated with atropine

Monitoring Parameters Muscle strength, heart rate, respiration; vital capacity; observe for cholinergic reactions, particularly when administered IV

Dosage Forms Excipient information presented when available (limited, particularly for generics); consult specific product labeling.

Solution, Intravenous, as bromide:

Regonol: 10 mg/2 mL (2 mL) [contains benzyl alcohol]

Syrup, Oral, as bromide:

Mestinon: 60 mg/5 mL (473 mL) [contains alcohol, usp, brilliant blue fcf (fd&c blue #1), fd&c red #40, sodium benzoate; raspberry flavor]

Tablet, Oral, as bromide:

Mestinon: 60 mg [scored]

Generic: 60 mg

Tablet Extended Release, Oral, as bromide:

Mestinon: 180 mg [scored]

Generic: 180 mg

◆ **Pyridostigmine Bromide** *see* Pyridostigmine *on page 1808*

Pyridoxine (peer i DOKS een)

Medication Safety Issues

Sound-alike/look-alike issues:

Pyridoxine may be confused with paroxetine, pralidoxime, Pyridium

International issues:

Doxal [Brazil] may be confused with Doxil brand name for DOXOrubicin [U.S.]

Doxal: Brand name for pyridoxine/thiamine combination [Brazil], but also the brand name for doxepin [Finland]

Brand Names: US Neuro-K-250 T.D. [OTC]; Neuro-K-250 Vitamin B6 [OTC]; Neuro-K-50 [OTC]; Neuro-K-500 [OTC]; Pyri 500 [OTC]

Therapeutic Category Antidote, Cycloserine Toxicity; Antidote, Hydrazine Toxicity; Antidote, Mushroom Toxicity; Drug-induced Neuritis, Treatment Agent; Nutritional Supplement; Vitamin, Water Soluble

Generic Availability (US) May be product dependent

Use Prevention and treatment of vitamin B_6 deficiency; treatment of drug-induced deficiency (eg, isoniazid or oral contraceptives); treatment of inborn errors of metabolism (eg, B_6-dependent seizures or anemia); injection may be used when oral route not feasible (All indications: FDA approved in adults); has also been used for the treatment of pyridoxine-dependent seizures and treatment of acute intoxication of isoniazid, cycloserine, hydrazine, and mushroom (genus *Gyromitra*)

Pregnancy Risk Factor A

Pregnancy Considerations Water soluble vitamins cross the placenta. Maternal pyridoxine plasma concentrations may decrease as pregnancy progresses and requirements may be increased in pregnant women (IOM, 1998). Pyridoxine is used to treat nausea and vomiting of pregnancy (Neibyl, 2010). In general, medications used as antidotes should take into consideration the health and prognosis of the mother; antidotes should be administered to pregnant women if there is a clear indication for use and should not be withheld because of fears of teratogenicity (Bailey, 2003).

Breast-Feeding Considerations Pyridoxine is found in breast milk and concentrations vary by maternal intake. Pyridoxine requirements are increased in nursing women compared to non-nursing women (IOM, 1998). Possible inhibition of lactation at doses >600 mg/day when taken immediately postpartum (Foukas, 1973).

Contraindications Hypersensitivity to pyridoxine or any component of the formulation

Warnings/Precautions Severe, permanent peripheral neuropathies have been reported; neurotoxicity is more common with long-term administration of large doses (>2 g/day). Dependence and withdrawal may occur with doses >200 mg/day. Single vitamin deficiency is rare; evaluate for other deficiencies. The parenteral product may contain aluminum; toxic aluminum concentrations may be seen with high doses, prolonged use, or renal dysfunction. Premature neonates are at higher risk due to immature renal function and aluminum intake from other parenteral sources. Parenteral aluminum exposure of >4 to 5 mcg/kg/day is associated with CNS and bone toxicity; tissue loading may occur at lower doses (Federal Register, 2002). See manufacturer's labeling.

Pharmacy supply of emergency antidotes: Guidelines suggest that at least 8-24 g be stocked. This is enough to treat 1 patient weighing 100 kg for an initial 8- to 24-hour period. In areas where tuberculosis is common, hospitals should consider stocking 24 g. This is enough to treat 1 patient for 24 hours (Dart, 2009).

Adverse Reactions

Central nervous system: Headache, seizure (following very large IV doses), somnolence
Endocrine & metabolic: Acidosis, folic acid decreased
Gastrointestinal: Nausea
Hepatic: AST increased
Neuromuscular & skeletal: Neuropathy, paresthesia
Miscellaneous: Allergic reactions

Drug Interactions

Metabolism/Transport Effects None known.

Avoid Concomitant Use There are no known interactions where it is recommended to avoid concomitant use.

Increased Effect/Toxicity There are no known significant interactions involving an increase in effect.

Decreased Effect

Pyridoxine may decrease the levels/effects of: Altretamine; Barbiturates; Fosphenytoin; Levodopa; Phenytoin

Storage/Stability Injection: Store at 20°C to 25°C (68°F to 77°F). Protect from light.

Mechanism of Action Precursor to pyridoxal, which functions in the metabolism of proteins, carbohydrates, and fats; pyridoxal also aids in the release of liver and muscle-stored glycogen and in the synthesis of GABA (within the central nervous system) and heme

Pharmacokinetics (Adult data unless noted)

Absorption: Readily from the GI tract; primarily in jejunum
Metabolism: Hepatic to pyridoxal phosphate and pyridoxamine phosphate
Half-life, biologic: 15-20 days
Elimination: Urine (as metabolites)

Dosing: Neonatal

Adequate intake (AI): Oral: 0.1 mg/day (0.01 mg/kg/day)

Pyridoxine-dependent seizures: Oral, IM, IV:
Initial: IV preferred: 50 to 100 mg (Rajesh, 2003)
Maintenance: Oral preferred: Usual: 50 to 100 mg/day; range: 10 to 200 mg (Rajesh, 2003); an observational study in UK described a usual dose of 30 mg/kg/day (Baxter, 1999)

Dosing: Usual

Pediatric:

Adequate intake (AI): Oral: Infants:
1 to <6 months: 0.1 mg (0.01 mg/kg)
6 to 12 months: 0.3 mg (0.03 mg/kg)

Recommended daily allowance (RDA): Oral:
1 to 3 years: 0.5 mg
4 to 8 years: 0.6 mg
9 to 13 years: 1 mg
14 to 18 years:
Male: 1.3 mg
Female: 1.2 mg

Dietary deficiency; treatment: Oral, IM, IV:
Children: 5 to 25 mg/day for 3 weeks, then 2.5 to 5 mg/day in multivitamin product
Adolescents: 10 to 20 mg/day for 3 weeks, then 2 to 5 mg/day (usual dosage found in multivitamin products)

Pyridoxine-dependent seizures, treatment: Oral, IM, IV: Infants and Children:
Initial: IV preferred: 50 to 100 mg (Rajesh, 2003)
Maintenance: Oral preferred: Usual: 50 to 100 mg/day; range: 10 to 200 mg (Rajesh, 2003); an observational study in UK described a usual dose of 30 mg/kg/day (Baxter, 1999)

Drug-induced deficiency/toxicity (cycloserine, isoniazid, penicillamine); chronic use: Oral, IM, IV:
Isoniazid/Cycloserine:
Prevention: **Note:** Recommended for patients at risk: Exclusively breast-fed infants, meat- and milk-deficient diet, nutritional deficiency, pregnant adolescents (*Red Book*, 2012).
Non-HIV-exposed/-positive:
Infants and Children: 1 mg/kg/day; usual range: 10 to 50 mg/day (*Red Book* [AAP], 2012)
Adolescents: 30 mg/day
HIV-exposed/-positive:
Infants and Children: 1 to 2 mg/kg once daily; maximum daily dose: 50 mg/day (DHHS [pediatric], 2013)
Adolescents: 25 mg/day (DHHS [adult], 2013)
Treatment:
Infants and Children: Optimal dose not established, higher doses than prophylaxis are necessary for treatment of neuritis (ataxia), some clinicians have suggested the following: 100 mg/day; higher doses (ie, 200mg/day) may be necessary to alleviate signs/symptoms
Adolescents: Initial: 100 mg/day for 3 weeks followed by 30 mg/day
Penicillamine (in Wilson Disease patients): Limited data available: Children and Adolescents: 25 to 50 mg/day (Roberts, 2008)

Acute isoniazid ingestion:
Treatment of isoniazid-induced seizures and/or coma: IV: Children and Adolescents:
Acute ingestion of known amount: Initial: A total dose of pyridoxine equal to the amount of isoniazid ingested (maximum dose: 70 mg/kg up to 5 g); administer at a rate of 0.5 to 1 g/minute until seizures stop or the maximum initial dose has been administered; may repeat every 5 to 10 minutes as needed to control persistent seizure activity and/or CNS toxicity. If seizures stop prior to the administration of the calculated initial dose, infuse the remaining pyridoxine over 4 to 6 hours (Howland, 2006; Morrow, 2006).
Acute ingestion of unknown amount: Initial: 70 mg/kg (maximum dose: 5 g); administer at a rate of 0.5 to 1 g/minute; may repeat every 5 to 10 minutes as needed to control persistent seizure activity and/or CNS toxicity (Howland, 2006; Morrow, 2006; Santucci, 1999)
Prevention of isoniazid-induced seizures and/or coma: IV: Children: Asymptomatic patients who present within 2 hours of ingesting a potentially toxic amount of isoniazid should receive a prophylactic dose of pyridoxine (Boyer, 2006). Dosing recommendations are the same as for the treatment of symptomatic patients.

Acute intoxication: Children and Adolescents: Mushroom ingestion (genus *Gyromitra*): IV: 25 mg/kg/dose; repeat as necessary to a maximum total dose of 15 to 20 g (Lheureaux, 2005)

Adult:

Recommended daily allowance: Oral:
19 to 50 years: 1.3 mg
>50 years:
Female: 1.5 mg
Male: 1.7 mg
Pregnancy: 1.9 mg
Lactation: 2 mg

Dietary deficiency: Oral, IM, IV: Adults: 10 to 20 mg/day for 3 weeks, then 2-5 mg/day (usual dosage found in multivitamin products). Doses up to 600 mg/day may be needed with pyridoxine dependency syndrome.

Drug-induced neuritis (eg, isoniazid): Oral, IM, IV: Prophylaxis: HIV-exposed/-positive: 25 mg/day; 50 mg/day if pregnant (DHHS [adult], 2013)

Treatment of isoniazid-induced seizures and/or coma following acute ingestion: IV:
Acute ingestion of known amount: Initial: A total dose of pyridoxine equal to the amount of isoniazid ingested (maximum dose: 5000 mg); administer at a rate of 500 to 1000 mg/minute until seizures stop or the maximum

initial dose has been administered; may repeat every 5 to 10 minutes as needed to control persistent seizure activity and/or CNS toxicity. If seizures stop prior to the administration of the calculated initial dose, infuse the remaining pyridoxine over 4 to 6 hours (Howland, 2006; Morrow, 2006).

Acute ingestion of unknown amount: Initial: 5000 mg; administer at a rate of 500 to 1000 mg/minute; may repeat every 5 to 10 minutes as needed to control persistent seizure activity and/or CNS toxicity (Howland, 2006; Morrow, 2006)

Prevention of isoniazid-induced seizures and/or coma following acute ingestion: IV: Asymptomatic patients who present within 2 hours of ingesting a potentially toxic amount of isoniazid should receive a prophylactic dose of pyridoxine (Boyer, 2006). Dosing recommendations are the same as for the treatment of symptomatic patients.

Acute intoxication: Mushroom ingestion (genus *Gyromitra*): IV: 25 mg/kg/dose; repeat as necessary to a maximum total dose of 15 to 20 g (Lheureaux, 2005)

Administration

Oral: Administer without regard to meals

Parenteral: May be administered IM or slow IV; seizures have been precipitated following large IV doses

Isoniazid toxicity: Initial doses should be administered at a rate of 500-1000 mg/minute. If the parenteral formulation is not available, anecdotal reports suggest that pyridoxine tablets may be crushed and made into a slurry and given at the same dose orally or via nasogastric (NG) tube (Boyer, 2006) or an extemporaneous compounded solution may be used. Oral administration is not recommended for acutely poisoned patients with seizure activity.

Monitoring Parameters When administering large IV doses, monitor respiratory rate, heart rate, and blood pressure

For treatment of isoniazid, hydrazine, or gyromitrin-containing mushroom toxicity: Anion gap, arterial blood gases, electrolytes, neurological exam, seizure activity

Reference Range 30-80 ng/mL

Test Interactions False positive urobilinogen spot test using Ehrlich's reagent

Dosage Forms Excipient information presented when available (limited, particularly for generics); consult specific product labeling.

Capsule, Oral, as hydrochloride:
- Neuro-K-250 T.D.: 250 mg [corn free, rye free, starch free, sugar free, wheat free]

Solution, Injection, as hydrochloride:
- Generic: 100 mg/mL (1 mL)

Tablet, Oral, as hydrochloride:
- Neuro-K-50: 50 mg
- Neuro-K-500: 500 mg
- Neuro-K-250 Vitamin B6: 250 mg
- Pyri 500: 500 mg
- Generic: 25 mg, 50 mg, 100 mg, 250 mg

Tablet, Oral, as hydrochloride [preservative free]:
- Generic: 25 mg, 50 mg, 100 mg

Tablet Extended Release, Oral, as hydrochloride:
- Generic: 200 mg

Extemporaneous Preparations A 1 mg/mL oral solution may be made using pyridoxine injection. Withdraw 100 mg (1 mL of a 100 mg/mL injection) from a vial with a needle and syringe; add to 99 mL simple syrup in an amber bottle. Label "refrigerate". Stable for 30 days refrigerated.

Nahata MC, Pai VB, and Hipple TF, *Pediatric Drug Formulations*, 5th ed, Cincinnati, OH: Harvey Whitney Books Co, 2004.

◆ **Pyridoxine Hydrochloride** *see* Pyridoxine *on page 1810*

Pyrimethamine (peer i METH a meen)

Medication Safety Issues

Sound-alike/look-alike issues:

Daraprim may be confused with Dantrium, Daranide

Brand Names: US Daraprim

Brand Names: Canada Daraprim [DSC]

Therapeutic Category Antimalarial Agent

Generic Availability (US) No

Use Used in combination with sulfadiazine for treatment of toxoplasmosis [FDA approved in pediatric patients (age not specified) and adults]; chemoprophylaxis and treatment of malaria [FDA approved in pediatric patients (age not specified) and adults]; has also been used in combination with dapsone as primary or secondary prophylaxis for *Pneumocystis jirovecii* in HIV-infected patients. **Note:** Although an FDA labeled indication, the use of pyrimethamine for chemoprophylaxis or treatment of malaria is not routinely recommended due to severe adverse reactions and reports of resistance (CDC, 2013).

Pregnancy Risk Factor C

Pregnancy Considerations Adverse events have been observed in animal reproduction studies. If administered during pregnancy (ie, for toxoplasmosis), supplementation of folate is strongly recommended. Pregnancy should be avoided during therapy.

Breast-Feeding Considerations Pyrimethamine enters breast milk and may result in significant systemic concentrations in breast-fed infants. The effect of concurrent therapy with sulfonamide or dapsone (frequently used with pyrimethamine as combination treatment) must be considered.

Contraindications Hypersensitivity to pyrimethamine or any component of the formulation; megaloblastic anemia secondary to folate deficiency

Warnings/Precautions Administer leucovorin calcium to prevent hematologic complications due to pyrimethamine-induced folic acid deficiency-state; continue leucovorin during therapy and for 1 week after therapy is discontinued (to account for the long half-life of pyrimethamine) (DHHS [pediatric], 2013). Megaloblastic anemia, leukopenia, thrombocytopenia, and pancytopenia have been reported; most commonly with high doses. Monitor CBC and platelets twice weekly in patients receiving high-dose therapy (eg, when used for toxoplasmosis treatment). Use with caution in patients with impaired renal or hepatic function or with possible G6PD deficiency. Use caution in patients with seizure disorders or possible folate deficiency (eg, malabsorption syndrome, pregnancy, alcoholism). Potentially significant interactions may exist, requiring dose or frequency adjustment, additional monitoring, and/or selection of alternative therapy.

Adverse Reactions

Cardiovascular: Arrhythmias (large doses)

Dermatologic: Erythema multiforme, rash, Stevens-Johnson syndrome, toxic epidermal necrolysis

Gastrointestinal: Anorexia, atrophic glossitis, vomiting

Hematologic: Leukopenia, megaloblastic anemia, pancytopenia, pulmonary eosinophilia, thrombocytopenia

Genitourinary: Hematuria

Miscellaneous: Anaphylaxis

Drug Interactions

Metabolism/Transport Effects Inhibits CYP2C9 (moderate)

Avoid Concomitant Use

Avoid concomitant use of Pyrimethamine with any of the following: Artemether; Lumefantrine

Increased Effect/Toxicity

Pyrimethamine may increase the levels/effects of: Antipsychotic Agents (Phenothiazines); Bosentan; Cannabis; Carvedilol; CYP2C9 Substrates; Dapsone (Systemic)

Dapsone (Topical); Dronabinol; Lumefantrine; Tetrahydrocannabinol

The levels/effects of Pyrimethamine may be increased by: Artemether; Dapsone (Systemic)

Decreased Effect

The levels/effects of Pyrimethamine may be decreased by: Methylfolate

Storage/Stability Store at 15°C to 25°C (59°F to 77°F). Protect from light.

Mechanism of Action Inhibits parasitic dihydrofolate reductase, resulting in inhibition of vital tetrahydrofolic acid synthesis

Pharmacokinetics (Adult data unless noted)

Absorption: Oral: Well absorbed

Distribution: V_d: Adults: 2.9 L/kg; distributed to the kidneys, lung, liver, and spleen

Protein binding: 80% to 87%

Half-life: 96 hours

Time to peak serum concentration: Within 2 to 6 hours

Elimination: Pyrimethamine and metabolites are excreted in urine

Dosing: Neonatal Congenital toxoplasmosis (independent of HIV status); treatment: Oral: Initial: 2 mg/kg/day once daily for 2 days, then 1 mg/kg/day once daily given with sulfadiazine for 2 to 6 months; then 1 mg/kg/day 3 times/week (eg, MWF) with sulfadiazine; total treatment duration: 12 months; oral leucovorin should be administered throughout the entire course to prevent hematologic toxicity (DHHS [pediatric], 2013; McAuley, 2008)

Dosing: Usual

Pediatric:

Isosporiasis *(Isospora belli)*, HIV-exposed/-positive:

Oral:

Treatment:

Infants and Children: 1 mg/kg once daily in combination with leucovorin for 14 days; maximum daily dose: 75 mg/day (DHHS [pediatric], 2013)

Adolescents: 50 to 75 mg once daily in combination with leucovorin (DHHS [adult], 2013)

Chronic maintenance:

Infants and Children: 1 mg/kg once daily in combination with leucovorin; maximum daily dose: 25 mg/day (DHHS [pediatric], 2013)

Adolescents: 25 mg once daily in combination with leucovorin (DHHS [adult], 2013)

Toxoplasmosis: Oral:

Treatment:

Congenital toxoplasmosis (independent of HIV status): Infants: Initial: 2 mg/kg/dose once daily for 2 days, then 1 mg/kg/day once daily given with sulfadiazine for 2 to 6 months; then 1 mg/kg/day 3 times/week (eg, MWF) with sulfadiazine; oral leucovorin should be administered throughout entire course to prevent hematologic toxicity (total treatment duration: 12 months) (DHHS [pediatric], 2013; McAuley, 2008)

Acquired infection:

HIV-exposed/-positive:

Infants and Children: 2 mg/kg (maximum dose: 50 mg) once daily for 3 days followed by 1 mg/kg (maximum dose: 25 mg) once daily in combination with sulfadiazine or clindamycin and leucovorin; continue for at least 6 weeks; consider longer duration if clinical or radiologic disease is extensive or incomplete response; follow with chronic suppressive therapy (DHHS [pediatric], 2013)

Adolescents: Encephalitis: 200 mg once as a single dose, followed by weight-based daily dosing: For weight <60 kg: 50 mg or for weight ≥60 kg: 75 mg once daily, typically used in combination with sulfadiazine and leucovorin; other combination regimens include clindamycin, atovaquone, or azithromycin and leucovorin; continue for at least 6 weeks; consider longer duration if clinical or radiologic disease is extensive or incomplete response (DHHS [adult], 2013)

Non-HIV-exposed/-positive (*Red Book* [AAP, 2012]):

Note: Use in combination with sulfadiazine or clindamycin; oral leucovorin should be administered to prevent hematologic toxicity. Continue therapy until 1 to 2 weeks after the resolution of symptoms.

Children: 2 mg/kg (maximum dose: 50 mg) once daily for 2 days, followed by 1 mg/kg/day (maximum dose: 25 mg) once daily for 3 to 6 weeks

Adolescents: 200 mg once as a single dose; then 50 to 75 mg once daily for 3 to 6 weeks

Prophylaxis:

First episode of *Toxoplasma gondii:*

HIV-exposed/-positive (CDC, 2009):

Infants and Children (DHHS [pediatric], 2013):

In combination with dapsone: 1 mg/kg/day once daily (maximum dose: 25 mg) with dapsone plus oral leucovorin

In combination with atovaquone: Infants and Children 4 to 24 months: 1 mg/kg or 15 mg/m^2 once daily (maximum dose: 25 mg) with atovaquone plus oral leucovorin

Adolescents (DHHS [adult], 2013):

In combination with dapsone: 50 mg or 75 mg once **weekly** plus oral leucovorin

In combination with atovaquone: 25 mg once **daily** plus leucovorin

Hematopoietic cell transplantation recipients (Tomblyn, 2009):

Infants and Children: 1 mg/kg/day of pyrimethamine once daily (maximum single dose: 75 mg) with clindamycin and leucovorin. Start after engraftment and administer as long as the patient remains on immunosuppressive therapy.

Adolescents: 25 to 75 mg once daily with clindamycin and leucovorin. Start after engraftment and administer as long as the patient remains on immunosuppressive therapy.

Recurrence of *Toxoplasma gondii* (secondary prophylaxis; suppressive therapy): HIV-exposed/-positive:

Infants and Children: 1 mg/kg or 15 mg/m^2 once daily (maximum dose: 25 mg) with sulfadiazine, clindamycin, or atovaquone, plus oral leucovorin (DHHS [pediatric], 2013)

Adolescents (DHHS [adult], 2013):

In combinations with sulfadiazine or clindamycin: 25 to 50 mg once daily plus leucovorin

In combination with atovaquone: 25 mg once daily plus leucovorin

Malaria: Oral: **Note:** Current CDC recommendations for malaria prophylaxis or treatment do not include the use of pyrimethamine; resistance to pyrimethamine is prevalent worldwide. (CDC, 2013); however, pyrimethamine is still discussed in the World Health Organization (WHO) treatment guidelines (WHO, 2010; WHO, 2011).

Chemoprophylaxis: Begin prophylaxis before entering endemic area:

Infants and Children <4 years: 6.25 mg once weekly

Children 4 to 10 years: 12.5 mg once weekly

Children >10 years and Adolescents: 25 mg once weekly

Treatment (non-*falciparum* malaria; use in conjunction with a sulfonamide [eg, sulfadoxine]):

Children 4 to 10 years: 25 mg daily for 2 days; following clinical cure, administer a once-weekly chemoprophylaxis regimen for ≥10 weeks. **Note:** Pyrimethamine monotherapy is generally not recommended.

Children >10 years and Adolescents: 25 mg daily for 2 days; following clinical cure, administer a once-weekly chemoprophylaxis regimen for ≥10 weeks. **Note:** Pyrimethamine monotherapy is **not** recommended; if circumstances arise where it must be used alone in semi-immune patients, give 50 mg daily for 2 days; then (following clinical cure) administer a once-weekly chemoprophylaxis regimen for ≥10 weeks.

***Pneumocystis jirovecii* pneumonia (PCP) (HIV-exposed/-positive)** (DHHS [adult], 2013): Oral: Adolescents: Primary prophylaxis or chronic maintenance (secondary prophylaxis):

In combination with dapsone and leucovorin: 50 to 75 mg once **weekly** with dapsone and leucovorin

In combination with atovaquone and leucovorin: 25 mg once **daily**with atovaquone and leucovorin

Adult:

Isosporiasis (*Isospora belli* infection) in HIV-positive/-exposed patients (DHHS [adult], 2013): Oral:

Treatment: 50 to 75 mg once daily in combination with leucovorin

Chronic maintenance (secondary prophylaxis): 25 mg once daily in combination with leucovorin

Malaria chemoprophylaxis: Oral: **Note:** Current CDC recommendations for malaria prophylaxis do not include the use of pyrimethamine; resistance to pyrimethamine is prevalent worldwide.

Manufacturer's labeling: 25 mg once weekly

Malaria treatment (non-*falciparum* malaria; use in conjunction with a sulfonamide [eg, sulfadoxine]): Oral: **Note:** Current CDC recommendations for malaria treatment do not include the use of pyrimethamine; resistance to pyrimethamine is prevalent worldwide.

Manufacturer's labeling: 25 mg daily for 2 days; following clinical cure, administer a once-weekly chemoprophylaxis regimen for ≥10 weeks. **Note:** Pyrimethamine use alone is **not** recommended; if circumstances arise where it must be used alone in semi-immune patients, give 50 mg daily for 2 days; then (following clinical cure) administer a once-weekly chemoprophylaxis regimen for ≥10 weeks.

Toxoplasmosis in HIV-positive/-exposed patients: (DHHS [adult], 2013): Oral:

Prophylaxis for first episode of *Toxoplasma gondii*: 50 mg or 75 mg once weekly with dapsone, plus oral leucovorin **or** 25 mg once daily with atovaquone plus leucovorin

Prophylaxis to prevent recurrence of *Toxoplasma gondii*: 25 to 50 mg once daily in combination with sulfadiazine plus oral leucovorin **or** 25 to 50 mg once daily with clindamycin in combination with oral leucovorin **or** 25 mg once daily with atovaquone in combination with leucovorin

Treatment of *Toxoplasma gondii* encephalitis: 200 mg as a single dose, followed by 50 mg (<60 kg patients) or 75 mg (≥60 kg patients) daily, plus sulfadiazine and leucovorin **or** 200 mg as a single dose, followed by 50 mg (<60 kg patients) or 75 mg (≥60 kg patients) daily, with clindamycin, atovaquone, or azithromycin in combination with oral leucovorin; continue treatment for at least 6 weeks; longer if clinical or radiologic disease is extensive or response is incomplete at 6 weeks.

Dosing adjustment in renal impairment: There are no dosage adjustments provided in the manufacturer's labeling.

Dosing adjustment in hepatic impairment: There are no dosage adjustments provided in the manufacturer's labeling.

Administration Oral: Administer with meals to minimize vomiting

Monitoring Parameters CBC, including platelet counts twice weekly with high-dose therapy (eg, when used for toxoplasmosis treatment; frequency not defined for lower doses); liver and renal function

Dosage Forms Excipient information presented when available (limited, particularly for generics); consult specific product labeling.

Tablet, Oral:

Daraprim: 25 mg [scored]

Extemporaneous Preparations A 2 mg/mL oral suspension may be made with tablets and a 1:1 mixture of Simple Syrup, NF and methylcellulose 1%. Crush forty 25 mg tablets in a mortar and reduce to a fine powder. Add small portions of vehicle and mix to a uniform paste; mix while adding vehicle in incremental proportions to **almost** 500 mL; transfer to a calibrated bottle, rinse mortar with vehicle, and add quantity of vehicle sufficient to make 500 mL. Label "shake well" and "refrigerate". Stable for 91 days.

Nahata MC, Pai VB, and Hipple TF, *Pediatric Drug Formulations*, 5th ed, Cincinnati, OH: Harvey Whitney Books Co, 2004.

◆ **Q-Amlodipine (Can)** *see* AmLODIPine *on page* 133

◆ **Q-Citalopram (Can)** *see* Citalopram *on page* 476

◆ **Q-Cyclobenzaprine (Can)** *see* Cyclobenzaprine *on page* 548

◆ **Q-Dryl [OTC]** *see* DiphenhydrAMINE (Systemic) *on page* 668

◆ **Q-Fluoxetine (Can)** *see* FLUoxetine *on page* 906

◆ **Q-Lansoprazole (Can)** *see* Lansoprazole *on page* 1219

◆ **QlearQuil 24 Hour Relief [OTC]** *see* Loratadine *on page* 1296

◆ **Q-Metformin (Can)** *see* MetFORMIN *on page* 1375

◆ **Qnasl** *see* Beclomethasone (Nasal) *on page* 260

◆ **Qnasl Childrens** *see* Beclomethasone (Nasal) *on page* 260

◆ **Q-Omeprazole (Can)** *see* Omeprazole *on page* 1555

◆ **Q-Pantoprazole (Can)** *see* Pantoprazole *on page* 1618

◆ **Q-Pap [OTC]** *see* Acetaminophen *on page* 44

◆ **Q-Pap Children's [OTC]** *see* Acetaminophen *on page* 44

◆ **Q-Pap Extra Strength [OTC]** *see* Acetaminophen *on page* 44

◆ **Q-Pap Infant's [OTC]** *see* Acetaminophen *on page* 44

◆ **Q-Paroxetine (Can)** *see* PARoxetine *on page* 1634

◆ **Qroxin** *see* Capsaicin *on page* 362

◆ **Q-Sertraline (Can)** *see* Sertraline *on page* 1916

◆ **Q-Simvastatin (Can)** *see* Simvastatin *on page* 1928

◆ **Q-Tapp Cold & Allergy [OTC]** *see* Brompheniramine and Pseudoephedrine *on page* 305

◆ **Q-Terbinafine (Can)** *see* Terbinafine (Systemic) *on page* 2021

◆ **Q-Topiramate (Can)** *see* Topiramate *on page* 2085

◆ **Q-Tussin [OTC]** *see* GuaiFENesin *on page* 988

◆ **Q-Tussin DM [OTC]** *see* Guaifenesin and Dextromethorphan *on page* 992

◆ **Quadracel** *see* Diphtheria and Tetanus Toxoids, Acellular Pertussis, and Poliovirus Vaccine *on page* 677

- ◆ **Quadrivalent Human Papillomavirus Vaccine** *see* Papillomavirus (Types 6, 11, 16, 18) Vaccine (Human, Recombinant) *on page 1625*
- ◆ **Qualaquin** *see* QuiNINE *on page 1825*
- ◆ **Qudexy XR** *see* Topiramate *on page 2085*
- ◆ **Quelicin** *see* Succinylcholine *on page 1976*
- ◆ **Quelicin® (Can)** *see* Succinylcholine *on page 1976*
- ◆ **Quelicin-1000** *see* Succinylcholine *on page 1976*
- ◆ **Quenalin [OTC]** *see* DiphenhydrAMINE (Systemic) *on page 668*
- ◆ **Questran** *see* Cholestyramine Resin *on page 450*
- ◆ **Questran Light** *see* Cholestyramine Resin *on page 450*
- ◆ **Questran Light Sugar Free (Can)** *see* Cholestyramine Resin *on page 450*

QUEtiapine (kwe TYE a peen)

Medication Safety Issues

Sound-alike/look-alike issues:

QUEtiapine may be confused with OLANZapine

SEROquel may be confused with Desyrel, SEROquel XR, Serzone, SINEquan

BEERS Criteria medication:

This drug may be potentially inappropriate for use in geriatric patients (Quality of evidence - moderate; Strength of recommendation - strong).

Related Information

Oral Medications That Should Not Be Crushed or Altered *on page 2476*

Brand Names: US SEROquel; SEROquel XR

Brand Names: Canada Abbott-Quetiapine; ACT-Quetiapine; Apo-Quetiapine; Auro-Quetiapine; Dom-Quetiapine; JAMP-Quetiapine; Mar-Quetiapine; Mylan-Quetiapine; PHL-Quetiapine; PMS-Quetiapine; PRO-Quetiapine; Quetiapine XR; RAN-Quetiapine; Riva-Quetiapine; Sandoz-Quetiapine; Sandoz-Quetiapine XRT; Seroquel; Seroquel XR; Teva-Quetiapine; Teva-Quetiapine XR

Therapeutic Category Second Generation (Atypical) Antipsychotic

Generic Availability (US) May be product dependent

Use

Immediate release (Seroquel®): Acute treatment (adjunct and monotherapy) of manic episodes associated with bipolar I disorder (FDA approved in ages ≥10 years and adults); treatment of schizophrenia (FDA approved in ages ≥13 years and adults); acute treatment of depressive episodes associated with bipolar disorder (FDA approved in adults); adjunct therapy for maintenance in bipolar I disorder (FDA approved in adults); has also been used for autism

Extended release (Seroquel XR®): Acute treatment (adjunct and monotherapy) of manic or mixed episodes associated with bipolar I disorder (FDA approved in ages ≥10 years and adults); treatment of schizophrenia (FDA approved in ages ≥13 years and adults); acute treatment of depressive episodes associated with bipolar disorder (FDA approved in adults); adjunct maintenance therapy of bipolar I disorder (FDA approved in adults); adjunct treatment of major depressive disorder (FDA approved in adults)

Medication Guide Available Yes

Pregnancy Risk Factor C

Pregnancy Considerations Adverse events were observed in animal reproduction studies. Quetiapine crosses the placenta and can be detected in cord blood (Newport 2007). Congenital malformations have not been observed in humans (based on limited data). Antipsychotic use during the third trimester of pregnancy has a risk for abnormal muscle movements (extrapyramidal symptoms [EPS]) and/or withdrawal symptoms in newborns following delivery. Symptoms in the newborn may include agitation, feeding disorder, hypertonia, hypotonia, respiratory distress, somnolence, and tremor; these effects may be self-limiting or require hospitalization. Quetiapine may cause hyperprolactinemia, which may decrease reproductive function in both males and females.

Treatment algorithms have been developed by the ACOG and the APA for the management of depression in women prior to conception and during pregnancy (Yonkers 2009). The ACOG recommends that therapy during pregnancy be individualized; treatment with psychiatric medications during pregnancy should incorporate the clinical expertise of the mental health clinician, obstetrician, primary healthcare provider, and pediatrician. Safety data related to atypical antipsychotics during pregnancy is limited and routine use is not recommended. However, if a woman is inadvertently exposed to an atypical antipsychotic while pregnant, continuing therapy may be preferable to switching to a typical antipsychotic that the fetus has not yet been exposed to; consider risk:benefit (ACOG 2008).

Healthcare providers are encouraged to enroll women 18-45 years of age exposed to quetiapine during pregnancy in the Atypical Antipsychotics Pregnancy Registry (1-866-961-2388 or http://www.womensmentalhealth.org/pregnancyregistry).

Breast-Feeding Considerations Quetiapine is excreted into breast milk. Based on information from 8 mother-infant pairs, concentrations of quetiapine in breast milk have been reported from undetectable to 170 mcg/L. The estimated exposure to the breast-feeding infant would be up to 0.1 mg/kg/day (relative infant dose up to 0.43% based on a weight adjusted maternal dose of 400 mg/day). Due to the potential for serious adverse reactions in the nursing infant, the manufacturer recommends a decision be made whether to discontinue nursing or to discontinue the drug, taking into account the importance of treatment to the mother.

Contraindications Hypersensitivity to quetiapine or any component of the formulation

Warnings/Precautions [US Boxed Warning]: Antidepressants increase the risk of suicidal thinking and behavior in children, adolescents, and young adults (18-24 years of age) with major depressive disorder (MDD) and other psychiatric disorders; consider risk prior to prescribing. Short-term studies did not show an increased risk in patients >24 years of age and showed a decreased risk in patients ≥65 years. Closely monitor all patients for clinical worsening, suicidality, or unusual changes in behavior; particularly during the initial 1-2 months of therapy or during periods of dosage adjustments (increased or decreases); the patient's family or caregiver should be instructed to closely observe the patient and communicate condition with healthcare provider. A medication guide concerning the use of antidepressants should be dispensed with each prescription. **Quetiapine is not approved in the U.S. for use in children <10 years of age.**

May precipitate a shift to mania or hypomania in patients with bipolar disorder. Patients presenting with depressive symptoms should be screened for bipolar disorder; the screening should include a detailed psychiatric history covering a family history of suicide, bipolar disorder, and depression. Quetiapine is approved in the US for the treatment of bipolar depression. Pharmacologic treatment for pediatric bipolar I disorder or schizophrenia should be initiated only after thorough diagnostic evaluation and a careful consideration of potential risks vs benefits. If a pharmacologic agent is initiated, it should be a component of a total treatment program including psychological, educational and social interventions. Increased blood pressure (including hypertensive crisis) has been reported in children and adolescents; monitor blood pressure at baseline and periodically during use.

Leukopenia, neutropenia, and agranulocytosis (sometimes fatal) have been reported with antipsychotic use; presence of risk factors (eg, pre-existing low WBC or history of drug-induced leuko-/neutropenia) should prompt periodic blood count assessment. Discontinue therapy at first signs of blood dyscrasias or if absolute neutrophil count <1000/mm^3.

May cause orthostatic hypotension; use with caution in patients at risk of this effect or in those who would not tolerate transient hypotensive episodes (cerebrovascular disease, cardiovascular disease, dehydration, hypovolemia, or concurrent medication use which may predispose to hypotension/bradycardia) especially during the initial dose titration period. Use has been associated with QT prolongation; postmarketing reports have occurred in patients with concomitant illness, quetiapine overdose, or who were receiving concomitant therapy known to increase QT interval or cause electrolyte imbalance. Avoid use in patients at increased risk of torsade de pointes/ sudden death (eg, hypokalemia, hypomagnesemia, history of cardiac arrhythmias, congenital prolongation of QT interval, concomitant medications with QTc interval-prolonging properties). Use with caution in patients at increased risk of QT prolongation (eg, cardiovascular disease, heart failure, cardiac hypertrophy, elderly, family history of QT prolongation). May cause hyperglycemia; in some cases may be extreme and associated with ketoacidosis, hyperosmolar coma, or death. All patients should be monitored for symptoms of hyperglycemia (eg, polydipsia, polyuria, polyphagia, weakness) and undergo a fasting blood glucose test if symptoms develop during treatment. Patients with risk factors for diabetes (eg, obesity or family history) should have a baseline fasting blood sugar (FBS) and periodically during treatment. Use with caution in patients with pre-existing abnormal lipid profile. Significant weight gain has been observed with antipsychotic therapy; incidence varies with product. Monitor waist circumference and BMI.

[US Boxed Warning]: Elderly patients with dementia-related psychosis treated with antipsychotics are at an increased risk of death compared to placebo. Most deaths appeared to be either cardiovascular (eg, heart failure, sudden death) or infectious (eg, pneumonia) in nature. Use with caution in dementia with Lewy bodies; antipsychotics may worsen dementia symptoms and patients with dementia with Lewy bodies are more sensitive to the extrapyramidal side effects (APA, [Rabins 2007]). Quetiapine is not approved for the treatment of dementia-related psychosis. Avoid antipsychotic use for behavioral problems associated with dementia unless alternative nonpharmacologic therapies have failed and patient may harm self or others. In addition, use may cause or exacerbate syndrome of inappropriate antidiuretic hormone secretion or hyponatremia; monitor sodium closely with initiation or dosage adjustments in older adults (Beers Criteria).

May cause dose-related decreases in thyroid levels, including cases requiring thyroid replacement therapy. Measure both TSH and free T_4, along with clinical assessment, at baseline and follow-up to determine thyroid status; measurement of TSH alone may not be accurate (exact mechanism of quetiapine's effect on the thyroid axis is unknown). Due to anticholinergic effects, use with caution in patients with decreased gastrointestinal motility, urinary retention, BPH, xerostomia, visual problems, and narrow-angle glaucoma. Relative to other antipsychotics, quetiapine has a moderate potency of cholinergic blockade. May cause extrapyramidal symptoms (EPS) and/or tardive dyskinesia. Risk of dystonia (and probably other EPS) may be greater with increased doses, use of conventional antipsychotics, males, and younger patients. Impaired core body temperature regulation may occur; caution with strenuous exercise, heat exposure, dehydration, and concomitant medication possessing anticholinergic effects. Use may be associated with neuroleptic malignant syndrome (NMS); monitor for mental status changes, fever, muscle rigidity and/or autonomic instability. Rare cases have been reported with quetiapine. Esophageal dysmotility and aspiration have been associated with antipsychotic use; use with caution in patients at risk of aspiration pneumonia (eg, Alzheimer disease). Development of cataracts has been observed in animal studies; lens changes have been observed in humans during long-term treatment. Lens examination, such as a slit-lamp exam, on initiation of therapy and every 6 months thereafter is recommended by manufacturer. Use caution with Parkinson disease, history of seizures, and renal impairment. Use caution with hepatic impairment; may cause elevations of liver enzymes. May cause CNS depression, which may impair physical or mental abilities; patients must be cautioned about performing tasks that require mental alertness (eg, operating machinery or driving). Anaphylactic reactions have been reported with use. May increase prolactin levels; clinical significance of hyperprolactinemia in patients with breast cancer or other prolactin-dependent tumors is unknown. Potentially significant drug-drug interactions may exist, requiring dose or frequency adjustment, additional monitoring, and/or selection of alternative therapy. May cause withdrawal symptoms (rare) with abrupt cessation; gradually taper dose during discontinuation.

Warnings: Additional Pediatric Considerations Significant weight gain has been observed with antipsychotic therapy; incidence varies with specific drug. Monitor growth (including weight, height, BMI, and waist circumference) in pediatric patients receiving quetiapine; compare weight gain to standard growth curves. The SATIETY (Second-Generation Antipsychotic Treatment Indications, Effectiveness and Tolerability in Youth) study showed children and adolescents aged 4 to 19 years taking second-generation antipsychotics for the first time experienced significant weight gain, increase in BMI from baseline, and an increase in waist circumference with aripiprazole, olanzapine, quetiapine, and risperidone compared to untreated patients. Average weight gain after a median of 10.8 weeks was 8.5 kg with olanzapine, 6.1 kg with quetiapine, 5.3 kg with risperidone, and 4.4 kg with aripiprazole compared to 0.2 kg in untreated group. A significant increase in total cholesterol, triglycerides, and nonhigh density lipoprotein was seen with quetiapine and olanzapine. Biannual monitoring of cardiometabolic indices after the first 3 months of therapy is suggested (Correll 2009). Increases in cholesterol and triglycerides have been noted; in pediatric trials (ages: 10 to 17 years), total cholesterol increased to a clinically significant level (≥200 mg/dL) in 10% to 12% of patients, and triglycerides (≥150 mg/dL) in 17% to 22% of patients. Use with caution in patients with preexisting abnormal lipid profile; monitor lipid profile. Hyperglycemia has been reported with atypical antipsychotics, which may be severe and include potentially fatal ketoacidosis or hyperosmolar coma. In pediatric (ages 10 to 17 years) clinical trials of quetiapine, slight increases in fasting glucose levels were reported (mean change: 3.62 mg/dL); however, no pediatric patients with baseline fasting glucose <126 mg/dL developed treatment-emergent hyperglycemia (≥126 mg/dL). Quetiapine increases prolactin concentrations; in pediatric clinical trials (ages: 10 to 17 years), development of clinically significant prolactin levels occurred in 13.4% of male patients and 8.7% of females; high concentrations of prolactin may reduce pituitary gonadotropin secretion, galactorrhea, amenorrhea, gynecomastia, impotence decreased bone density may occur. Use with caution in children and adolescents; adverse effects due to increased prolactin concentrations have been observed; long-term effects on growth or sexual maturation have not been evaluated.

In children and adolescents, increases in blood pressure (including hypertensive crisis) have been reported. In pediatric clinical trials (ages: 10 to 17 years), an increase in SBP (≥20 mm Hg) and DBP (≥10 mm Hg) was observed more frequently with quetiapine than placebo (SBP: 15.2% vs 5.5%; DBP: 40.6% vs 24.5%). Monitor blood pressure at baseline and periodically during therapy with quetiapine.

Pediatric psychiatric disorders are frequently serious mental disorders which present with variable symptoms that do not always match adult diagnostic criteria. Conduct a thorough diagnostic evaluation and carefully consider risks of psychotropic medication before initiation in pediatric patients. Medication therapy for pediatric patients with bipolar disorder and schizophrenia is indicated as part of a total treatment program that frequently includes educational, psychological, and social interventions.

Adverse Reactions Actual frequency may be dependent upon dose and/or indication.

Cardiovascular: Hypertension (diastolic; children and adolescents), hypertension (systolic; children and adolescents), hypotension, increased heart rate, orthostatic hypotension (more common in adults), palpitations, peripheral edema, syncope, tachycardia

Central nervous system: Abnormal dreams, abnormality in thinking, aggressive behavior (children and adolescents), agitation, akathisia, anxiety, ataxia, confusion, decreased mental acuity, depression, disorientation, disturbance in attention, dizziness, drowsiness, drug-induced Parkinson's disease, dysarthria, dystonic reaction, extrapyramidal reaction, falling, fatigue, headache, hypersomnia, hypertonia, hypoesthesia, irritability, lack of concentration, lethargy, migraine, pain, paresthesia, restless leg syndrome, restlessness, twitching, vertigo

Dermatologic: Acne vulgaris (children and adolescents), diaphoresis, pallor (children and adolescents), skin rash

Endocrine & metabolic: Decreased HDL cholesterol (≤40 mg/dL), decreased libido, hyperglycemia (≥200 mg/dL post glucose challenge or fasting glucose ≥126 mg/dL), hyperprolactinemia, hypothyroidism, increased LDL cholesterol (≥160 mg/dL), increased serum triglycerides (≥200 mg/dL), increased thirst (children and adolescents), total cholesterol increased (≥240 mg/dL), weight gain (dose related)

Gastrointestinal: Abdominal pain, anorexia, constipation, decreased appetite, dyspepsia (dose related), dysphagia, flatulence, gastroenteritis, gastroesophageal reflux disease, increased appetite, nausea, periodontal abscess (adolescents), toothache, vomiting, xerostomia (more common in adults)

Genitourinary: Pollakiuria, urinary tract infection

Hematologic & oncologic: Leukopenia, neutropenia

Hepatic: Increased serum transaminases

Hypersensitivity: Seasonal allergy

Neuromuscular & skeletal: Arthralgia, back pain, dyskinesia, limb pain, muscle rigidity, muscle spasm, myalgia, neck pain, stiffness (children and adolescents), tremor, weakness

Ophthalmic: Amblyopia, blurred vision

Otic: Otalgia

Respiratory: Cough, dyspnea, epistaxis (adolescents), influenza, nasal congestion, pharyngitis, rhinitis, sinus congestion, sinus headache, sinusitis, upper respiratory tract infection

Miscellaneous: Fever

Rare but important or life-threatening: Abnormality of blepharitis, abnormal T waves on ECG, accommodation, acute hepatic failure, acute renal failure, agranulocytosis, alcohol intolerance, amenorrhea, amnesia, anemia, angina pectoris, apathy, aphasia, arthritis, atrial fibrillation, atrioventricular block, bone pain, bruxism, buccoglossal syndrome, bundle branch block, cardiac failure, cardiomyopathy, cataract, catatonic reaction, cerebrovascular accident, choreoathetosis, cyanosis, cystitis, deafness, deep vein thrombophlebitis, dehydration, delirium, delusions, depersonalization, diabetes mellitus, dysmenorrhea, dysuria, ecchymosis, eosinophilia, facial edema, first degree atrioventricular block, flattened T wave on ECG, galactorrhea, glossitis, hemiplegia, hemolysis, hepatic injury (cholestatic or mixed), hepatitis (with or without jaundice), hyperkinesia, hyperlipemia, hypersensitivity, hyperthyroidism, hyperventilation, hypochromic anemia, hypoglycemia, increased creatinine phosphokinase, increased gamma-glutamyl transferase, increased libido, increased QRS duration, increased salivation, increased serum alkaline phosphatase, increased ST segment on ECG, intestinal obstruction, irregular pulse, leukocytosis, leukorrhea, liver steatosis, lymphadenopathy, malaise, manic reaction, melena, myasthenia, myocarditis, myoclonus, neuralgia, neuroleptic malignant syndrome, orchitis, pancreatitis, paranoid reaction, pathological fracture, pelvic pain, pneumonia, priapism, prolonged Q-T interval on ECG, pruritus, psoriasis, psychosis, rectal hemorrhage, rhabdomyolysis, seborrhea, seizure, SIADH, stomatitis, ST segment changes on ECG, stupor, subdural hematoma, suicidal ideation, tardive dyskinesia, thrombocytopenia, thrombophlebitis, tongue edema, uterine hemorrhage, vaginal hemorrhage, vaginitis, vasodilatation, vulvovaginal moniliasis, vulvovaginitis, widened QRS complex on ECG

Drug Interactions

Metabolism/Transport Effects Substrate of CYP2D6 (minor), CYP3A4 (major); **Note:** Assignment of Major/Minor substrate status based on clinically relevant drug interaction potential

Avoid Concomitant Use

Avoid concomitant use of QUEtiapine with any of the following: Aclidinium; Amisulpride; Azelastine (Nasal); Conivaptan; Eluxadoline; Fusidic Acid (Systemic); Glucagon; Highest Risk QTc-Prolonging Agents; Idelalisib; Ipratropium (Oral Inhalation); Ivabradine; Methadone; Metoclopramide; Mifepristone; Moderate Risk QTc-Prolonging Agents; Orphenadrine; Paraldehyde; Potassium Chloride; Sulpiride; Thalidomide; Tiotropium; Umeclidinium

Increased Effect/Toxicity

QUEtiapine may increase the levels/effects of: AbobotulinumtoxinA; Alcohol (Ethyl); Amisulpride; Analgesics (Opioid); Anticholinergic Agents; Azelastine (Nasal); Buprenorphine; CarBAMazepine; CNS Depressants; DULoxetine; Eluxadoline; Glucagon; Highest Risk QTc-Prolonging Agents; Hydrocodone; Hypotensive Agents; Methadone; Methotrimeprazine; Methylphenidate; Metyrosine; OnabotulinumtoxinA; Orphenadrine; Paraldehyde; Potassium Chloride; RimabotulinumtoxinB; Selective Serotonin Reuptake Inhibitors; Serotonin Modulators; St Johns Wort; Sulpiride; Suvorexant; Thalidomide; Thiazide Diuretics; Tiotropium; Topiramate; Zolpidem

The levels/effects of QUEtiapine may be increased by: Acetylcholinesterase Inhibitors (Central); Aclidinium; Aprepitant; Barbiturates; Brimonidine (Topical); Cannabis; Conivaptan; CYP3A4 Inhibitors (Moderate); CYP3A4 Inhibitors (Strong); Doxylamine; Dronabinol; Fosaprepitant; Fusidic Acid (Systemic); Idelalisib; Ipratropium (Oral Inhalation); Ivabradine; Ivacaftor; Kava Kava; Luliconazole; Magnesium Sulfate; Methadone; Methotrimeprazine; Methylphenidate; Metoclopramide; Metyrosine; Mifepristone; Moderate Risk QTc-Prolonging Agents; Nabilone; Netupitant; Nicorandil; Palbociclib; Perampanel; Pramlintide; QTc-Prolonging Agents (Indeterminate

Risk and Risk Modifying); Rufinamide; Serotonin Modulators; Simeprevir; Sodium Oxybate; Stiripentol; Tapentadol; Tetrahydrocannabinol; Umeclidinium

Decreased Effect

QUEtiapine may decrease the levels/effects of: Acetylcholinesterase Inhibitors; Amphetamines; Antidiabetic Agents; Anti-Parkinson's Agents (Dopamine Agonist); Itopride; Quinagolide; Secretin

The levels/effects of QUEtiapine may be decreased by: Acetylcholinesterase Inhibitors; Bosentan; CarBAMazepine; CYP3A4 Inducers (Moderate); CYP3A4 Inducers (Strong); Dabrafenib; Deferasirox; Mitotane; Siltuximab; St Johns Wort; Tocilizumab

Food Interactions In healthy volunteers, administration of quetiapine (immediate release) with food resulted in an increase in the peak serum concentration and AUC by 25% and 15%, respectively, compared to the fasting state. Administration of the extended release formulation with a high-fat meal (~800-1000 calories) resulted in an increase in peak serum concentration by 44% to 52% and AUC by 20% to 22% for the 50 mg and 300 mg tablets; administration with a light meal (≤300 calories) had no significant effect on the C_{max} or AUC. Management: Administer without food or with a light meal (≤300 calories).

Storage/Stability Store at 25°C (77°F); excursions permitted between 15°C and 30°C (59°F and 86°F).

Mechanism of Action Quetiapine is a dibenzothiazepine atypical antipsychotic. It has been proposed that this drug's antipsychotic activity is mediated through a combination of dopamine type 2 (D_2) and serotonin type 2 ($5\text{-}HT_2$) antagonism. It is an antagonist at multiple neurotransmitter receptors in the brain: Serotonin $5\text{-}HT_{1A}$ and $5\text{-}HT_2$, dopamine D_1 and D_2, histamine H_1, and adrenergic $alpha_1$- and $alpha_2$-receptors; but appears to have no appreciable affinity at cholinergic muscarinic and benzodiazepine receptors. Norquetiapine, an active metabolite, differs from its parent molecule by exhibiting high affinity for muscarinic M1 receptors.

Antagonism at receptors other than dopamine and $5\text{-}HT_2$ with similar receptor affinities may explain some of the other effects of quetiapine. The drug's antagonism of histamine H_1-receptors may explain the somnolence observed. The drug's antagonism of adrenergic $alpha_1$-receptors may explain the orthostatic hypotension observed.

Pharmacokinetics (Adult data unless noted)

Absorption: Rapidly absorbed following oral administration; parent compound AUC and C_{max} were 41% and 39% lower, respectively, in pediatric patients (10-17 years) compared to adults when adjusted for weight, but pharmacokinetics of active metabolite were similar to adult values after adjusting for weight.

Distribution: V_d: 10 ± 4 L/kg

Protein binding, plasma: 83%

Metabolism: Primarily hepatic; via CYP3A4; forms the metabolite N-desalkyl quetiapine (active) and two inactive metabolites [sulfoxide metabolite (major metabolite) and parent acid metabolite]

Bioavailability: 100% (relative to oral solution)

Half-life elimination:

- Children and Adolescents (ages 12-17): Quetiapine: 5.3 hours (McConville, 2000)
- Adults: Quetiapine: ~6 hours; Extended release: ~7 hours

Time to peak serum concentration:

- Children and Adolescents ages 12-17: Immediate release: 0.5-3 hours (McConville, 2000)
- Adults: Immediate release: 1.5 hours; Extended release: 6 hours

Elimination: Urine (73% as metabolites, <1% of total dose as unchanged drug); feces (20%)

Dosing: Usual Note: Patients who have interrupted therapy for >1 week should generally be restarted at the initial dosing and retitrated; patients who have interrupted therapy for <1 week can generally be reinitiated on their previous dose.

Children and Adolescents:

Bipolar disorder, mania or mixed episodes: Children and Adolescents ≥10 years: Oral:

Immediate release tablet: Initial: 25 mg twice daily on day 1; increase to 50 mg twice daily on day 2, then 100 mg twice daily on day 3, then 150 mg twice daily on day 4, then continue at the target dose of 200 mg twice daily beginning on day 5. May increase further based on clinical response and tolerability at increments ≤100 mg/day up to 300 mg twice daily; however, no additional benefit was seen with 300 mg twice daily vs 200 mg twice daily. Usual dosage range: 200-300 mg twice daily; maximum daily dose: 600 mg/**day**. Total daily doses may also be divided into 3 doses per day. Continue therapy at lowest dose needed to maintain remission; periodically assess maintenance treatment needs

Extended release: Initial: 50 mg once daily on day 1; increase to 100 mg once daily on day 2, then increase in 100 mg/day increments each day until a target dose of 400 mg once daily is reached on day 5. Usual dosage range: 400-600 mg once daily; maximum daily dose: 600 mg/**day**; continue therapy at lowest dose needed to maintain remission; periodically assess maintenance treatment needs

Switching from immediate release to extended release: May convert patients from immediate release to extended release tablets at the equivalent total daily dose and administer once daily; individual dosage adjustments may be necessary.

Schizophrenia: Adolescents: Oral:

Immediate release tablet: Initial: 25 mg twice daily on day 1; increase to 50 mg twice daily on day 2, 100 mg twice daily on day 3, then 150 mg twice daily on day 4, then continue at a target dose of 200 mg twice daily beginning on day 5. May increase further based on clinical response and tolerability at increments ≤100 mg/day up to 400 mg twice daily; however, no additional benefit was seen with 400 mg twice daily vs 200 mg twice daily. Usual dosage range: 200-400 mg twice daily; maximum daily dose: 800 mg/**day**. Total daily doses may also be divided into 3 doses per day. Periodically assess maintenance treatment needs.

Extended release: Initial: 50 mg once daily on day 1; increase to 100 mg once daily on day 2, then increase in 100 mg/day increments each day until a target dose of 400 mg once daily is reached on day 5. Usual dosage range: 400-800 mg once daily; maximum daily dose: 800 mg/**day**. Periodically assess maintenance treatment needs.

Switching from immediate release to extended release: May convert patients from immediate release to extended release tablets at the equivalent total daily dose and administer once daily; individual dosage adjustments may be necessary.

Adults:

Bipolar disorder: Oral:

Depression:

Immediate release tablet: Initial: 50 mg once daily at bedtime the first day; increase to 100 mg once daily at bedtime on day 2, then increase by 100 mg/day increments each day until a target dose of 300 mg once daily at bedtime is reached by day 4. Further increases up to 600 mg once daily by day 8 have been evaluated in clinical trials, but no additional antidepressant efficacy was noted. Maximum daily dose: 300 mg/**day**

Extended release tablet: Initial: 50 mg once daily the first day; increase to 100 mg once daily on day 2, then increase by 100 mg/day increments each day until a target dose of 300 mg once daily is reached by day 4. Maximum daily dose: 300 mg/**day**

Switching from immediate release to extended release: May convert patients from immediate release to extended release tablets at the equivalent total daily dose and administer once daily; individual dosage adjustments may be necessary.

Mania:

Immediate release tablet: Initial: 50 mg twice daily on day 1, increase dose in increments of 100 mg/day each day to 200 mg twice daily on day 4; may increase at increments ≤200 mg/day to 400 mg twice daily by day 6. Usual dosage range: 200-400 mg twice daily. Maximum daily dose: 800 mg/**day**

Extended release tablet: Initial: 300 mg once daily on day 1; increase to 600 mg once daily on day 2 and adjust dose to 400-800 mg once daily on day 3, depending on response and tolerance. Maximum daily dose: 800 mg/**day**

Switching from immediate release to extended release: May convert patients from immediate release to extended release tablets at the equivalent total daily dose and administer once daily; individual dosage adjustments may be necessary.

Maintenance therapy:

Immediate release tablet (twice daily dosing) or extended release tablet (once daily dosing): 400-800 mg/day with lithium or divalproex; **Note:** In the maintenance phase, patients generally continue on the same dose on which they were stabilized. Maximum daily dose: 800 mg/**day**. Average time of stabilization was 15 weeks in clinical trials. During maintenance treatment, periodically reassess need for continued therapy and the appropriate dose. Patients who have discontinued therapy for >1 week should generally be retitrated following reinitiation of therapy; patients who have discontinued therapy for <1 week can generally be reinitiated at their previous dose.

Major depressive disorder (adjunct to antidepressants): Oral: Extended release tablet: Initial: 50 mg once daily on days 1 and 2; may be increased to 150 mg once daily on day 3. Usual dosage range: 150-300 mg once daily. Maximum daily dose: 300 mg/**day**

Schizophrenia/psychoses: Oral:

Immediate release tablet: Initial: 25 mg twice daily; followed by increases in the total daily dose on the second and third day in increments of 25-50 mg divided 2-3 doses daily, if tolerated, to a target dose of 300-400 mg/day in 2-3 divided doses by day 4. Make further adjustments of 50-100 mg/day as needed at intervals of at least 2 days. Usual maintenance range: 150-750 mg/day. Maximum daily dose: 750 mg/**day**

Extended release tablet: Initial: 300 mg once daily; increase in increments of up to 300 mg/day (in intervals ≥1 day). Usual maintenance range: 400-800 mg once daily. Maximum daily dose: 800 mg/**day**

Switching from immediate release to extended release: May convert patients from immediate release to extended release tablets at the equivalent total daily dose and administer once daily; individual dosage adjustments may be necessary.

Note: During maintenance treatment, periodically reassess the need for continued therapy and the appropriate dose.

Dosage adjustment for concomitant therapy: Children ≥10 years, Adolescents, and Adults:

Concomitant use with a strong CYP3A4 inhibitor (eg, ketoconazole, itraconazole, indinavir, ritonavir, nefazodone): Immediate release or extended release: Decrease quetiapine to one-sixth of the original dose; when strong CYP3A4 inhibitor is discontinued, increase quetiapine dose by sixfold.

Concomitant use with a strong CYP3A4 inducer (eg, phenytoin, carbamazepine, rifampin, St. John's wort): Immediate release or extended release: Increase quetiapine up to fivefold of the original dose when combined with chronic treatment (>7-14 days) of a strong CYP3A4 inducer; titrate based on clinical response and tolerance; when the strong CYP3A4 inducer is discontinued, decrease quetiapine to the original dose within 7-14 days.

Dosing adjustment in renal impairment: No adjustment required

Dosing adjustment in hepatic impairment: Lower clearance in hepatic impairment (30% lower); higher plasma levels expected; dosage adjustment may be needed. Adults:

Immediate release tablet: Initial: 25 mg daily; increase dose by 25-50 mg daily increments to effective dose, based on clinical response and tolerability. If initiated with immediate-release formulation, patient may transition to extended-release formulation (at equivalent total daily dose) when effective dose has been reached.

Extended release tablet: Initial: 50 mg once daily; increase dose by 50 mg daily increments to effective dose, based on clinical response and tolerability.

Administration

Oral:

Immediate release tablet: May be administered with or without food.

Extended release tablet: Administer without food or with a light meal (≤300 calories), preferably in the evening. Swallow tablet whole; do not break, crush, or chew.

Nasogastric/enteral tube: Immediate release tablet: Adults: Hold tube feeds for 30 minutes before administration; flush with 25 mL of sterile water. Crush dose, mix in 10 mL water and administer via NG/enteral tube; follow with a 50 mL flush of sterile water. Restart tube feedings after drug administration (Devlin, 2010).

Monitoring Parameters Vital signs, including for children and adolescents, BP at baseline and periodically; CBC with differential; fasting lipid profile and fasting blood glucose/Hb A_{1c} (prior to treatment, at 3 months, then annually); weight, growth, BMI, and waist circumference (especially in children), personal/family history of diabetes, blood pressure, mental status, abnormal involuntary movement scale (AIMS), extrapyramidal symptoms (EPS). In adults, weight should be assessed prior to treatment, at 4 weeks, 8 weeks, 12 weeks, and then at quarterly intervals; consider titrating to a different antipsychotic agent for a weight gain ≥5% of the initial weight. Monitor patient periodically for symptom resolution; monitor for worsening depression, suicidality, and associated behaviors (especially at the beginning of therapy or when doses are increased or decreased). Patients should have eyes checked for cataracts every 6 months while on this medication.

Measure both TSH and free T4, along with clinical assessment, at baseline and follow-up to determine thyroid status; measurement of TSH alone may not be accurate; the exact mechanism of the effect of quetiapine on the thyroid axis is unknown.

Test Interactions May interfere with urine detection of methadone (false-positives); may cause false-positive serum TCA screen

Dosage Forms Excipient information presented when available (limited, particularly for generics); consult specific product labeling.

Tablet, Oral:

SEROquel: 25 mg, 50 mg, 100 mg, 200 mg, 300 mg, 400 mg

Generic: 25 mg, 50 mg, 100 mg, 200 mg, 300 mg, 400 mg

Tablet Extended Release 24 Hour, Oral:

SEROquel XR: 50 mg, 150 mg, 200 mg, 300 mg, 400 mg

◆ **Quetiapine Fumarate** *see* QUEtiapine *on page 1815*

◆ **Quetiapine XR (Can)** *see* QUEtiapine *on page 1815*

◆ **Quillivant XR** *see* Methylphenidate *on page 1402*

◆ **Quinalbarbitone Sodium** *see* Secobarbital *on page 1910*

Quinapril (KWIN a pril)

Medication Safety Issues

Sound-alike/look-alike issues:

Accupril may be confused with Accolate, Accutane, AcipHex, Monopril

International issues:

Accupril [U.S., Canada] may be confused with Acepril which is a brand name for captopril [Great Britain]; enalapril [Hungary, Switzerland]; lisinopril [Malaysia]

Brand Names: US Accupril

Brand Names: Canada Accupril; Apo-Quinapril; GD-Quinapril; PMS-Quinapril

Therapeutic Category Angiotensin-Converting Enzyme (ACE) Inhibitor; Antihypertensive Agent

Generic Availability (US) Yes

Use Treatment of hypertension alone or in combination with thiazide diuretics (FDA approved in adults); management of heart failure as adjunctive therapy in combination with conventional therapy (eg, diuretics, digitalis) (FDA approved in adults)

Pregnancy Risk Factor D

Pregnancy Considerations [U.S. Boxed Warning]: Drugs that act on the renin-angiotensin system can cause injury and death to the developing fetus. Discontinue as soon as possible once pregnancy is detected. Quinapril crosses the placenta; teratogenic effects may occur following maternal use during pregnancy. Drugs that act on the renin-angiotensin system are associated with oligohydramnios. Oligohydramnios, due to decreased fetal renal function, may lead to fetal lung hypoplasia and skeletal malformations. Their use in pregnancy is also associated with anuria, hypotension, renal failure, skull hypoplasia, and death in the fetus/neonate. Chronic maternal hypertension itself is also associated with adverse events in the fetus/infant. ACE inhibitors are not recommended during pregnancy to treat maternal hypertension or heart failure. Use of an ACE inhibitor should also be avoided in any woman of reproductive age. Women who are planning a pregnancy should be considered for other medication options if an ACE inhibitor is currently prescribed or the ACE inhibitor should be discontinued as soon as possible once pregnancy is detected. The exposed fetus should be monitored for fetal growth, amniotic fluid volume, and organ formation. Infants exposed to an ACE inhibitor *in utero* should be monitored for hyperkalemia, hypotension, and oliguria (exchange transfusions or dialysis may be needed). These adverse events are generally associated with maternal use in the second and third trimesters.

Untreated chronic maternal hypertension is also associated with adverse events in the fetus, infant, and mother. The use of ACE inhibitors is not recommended to treat chronic uncomplicated hypertension in pregnant women and should generally be avoided in women of reproductive potential (ACOG, 2013).

Breast-Feeding Considerations Quinapril is excreted in breast milk. The manufacturer recommends that caution be exercised when administering quinapril to nursing women. The Canadian labeling contraindicates use in nursing women.

Contraindications

Hypersensitivity to quinapril or any component of the formulation; angioedema related to previous treatment with an ACE inhibitor; concomitant use with aliskiren in patients with diabetes mellitus.

Documentation of allergenic cross-reactivity for ACE inhibitors is limited. However, because of similarities in chemical structure and/or pharmacologic actions, the possibility of cross-sensitivity cannot be ruled out with certainty.

Canadian labeling: Additional contraindications (not in U.S. labeling): Women who are pregnant, intend to become pregnant, or of childbearing potential and not using adequate contraception; breast-feeding; concomitant use with aliskiren, angiotensin receptor blockers (ARBs) or other ACE inhibitors in patients with moderate-to-severe renal impairment (GFR <60 mL/minute/1.73 m^2); hyperkalemia (>5 mmol/L), or congestive heart failure who are hypotensive; concomitant use with angiotensin receptor blockers (ARBs) or other ACE inhibitors in diabetic patients with end organ damage; hereditary problems of galactose intolerance, glucose-galactose malabsorption or Lapp lactase deficiency

Warnings/Precautions Anaphylactic reactions may occur rarely with ACE inhibitors. At any time during treatment (especially following first dose) angioedema may occur rarely with ACE inhibitors; it may involve the head and neck (potentially compromising airway) or the intestine (presenting with abdominal pain). African-Americans and patients with idiopathic or hereditary angioedema may be at an increased risk. Prolonged frequent monitoring may be required especially if tongue, glottis, or larynx are involved as they are associated with airway obstruction. Patients with a history of airway surgery may have a higher risk of airway obstruction. Aggressive early and appropriate management is critical. Use in patients with previous angioedema associated with ACE inhibitor therapy is contraindicated. Severe anaphylactoid reactions may be seen during hemodialysis (eg, CVVHD) with high-flux dialysis membranes (eg, AN69), and rarely, during low density lipoprotein apheresis with dextran sulfate cellulose. Rare cases of anaphylactoid reactions have been reported in patients undergoing sensitization treatment with hymenoptera (bee, wasp) venom while receiving ACE inhibitors. Formulation may contain lactose.

Symptomatic hypotension with or without syncope can occur with ACE inhibitors (usually with the first several doses); effects are most often observed in volume-depleted patients; close monitoring of patient is required especially with initial dosing and dosing increases; blood pressure must be lowered at a rate appropriate for the patient's clinical condition. Initiation of therapy in patients with ischemic heart disease or cerebrovascular disease warrants close observation due to the potential consequences posed by falling blood pressure (eg, MI, stroke). Use with caution in hypertrophic cardiomyopathy with outflow tract obstruction and severe aortic stenosis. In patients on chronic ACE inhibitor therapy, intraoperative hypotension may occur with induction and maintenance of general anesthesia; use with caution before, during, or immediately after major surgery. Cardiopulmonary bypass, intraoperative blood loss, or vasodilating anesthesia increases endogenous renin release. Use of ACE inhibitors perioperatively will blunt angiotensin II formation and may result in hypotension. However, discontinuation of therapy prior to surgery is controversial. If continued preoperatively, avoidance of hypotensive agents during surgery is prudent (Hillis, 2011). **[U.S. Boxed Warning]: Drugs that act on the renin-angiotensin system can cause injury and death to the developing fetus. Discontinue as soon as possible once pregnancy is detected.**

Hyperkalemia may occur with ACE inhibitors; risk factors include renal dysfunction, diabetes mellitus, concomitant use of potassium-sparing diuretics, potassium supplements, and/or potassium-containing salts. Use cautiously, if at all, with these agents and monitor potassium closely. Cough may occur with ACE inhibitors. Other causes of cough should be considered (eg, pulmonary congestion in patients with heart failure) and excluded prior to discontinuation.

May be associated with deterioration of renal function and/ or increases in serum creatinine, particularly in patients with low renal blood flow (eg, renal artery stenosis, heart failure) whose glomerular filtration rate (GFR) is dependent on efferent arteriolar vasoconstriction by angiotensin II; deterioration may result in oliguria, acute renal failure, and progressive azotemia. Small increases in serum creatinine may occur following initiation; consider discontinuation only in patients with progressive and/or significant deterioration in renal function. Use with caution in patients with unstented unilateral/bilateral renal artery stenosis. When unstented bilateral renal artery stenosis is present, use is generally avoided due to the elevated risk of deterioration in renal function unless possible benefits outweigh risks. Potentially significant drug-drug interactions may exist, requiring dose or frequency adjustment, additional monitoring, and/or selection of alternative therapy.

Rare toxicities associated with ACE inhibitors include cholestatic jaundice (which may progress to fulminant hepatic necrosis), agranulocytosis, neutropenia, or leukopenia with myeloid hypoplasia. Patients with collagen vascular diseases (especially with concomitant renal impairment) or renal impairment alone may be at increased risk for hematologic toxicity; periodically monitor CBC with differential in these patients.

Warnings: Additional Pediatric Considerations In pediatric patients, an isolated dry hacking cough lasting >3 weeks was reported in seven of 42 pediatric patients (17%) receiving ACE inhibitors (von Vigier, 2000); a review of pediatric randomized-controlled ACE inhibitor trials reported a lower incidence of 3.2% (Baker-Smith, 2010). Other causes of cough should be considered (eg, pulmonary congestion in patients with heart failure) and excluded prior to discontinuation.

Adverse Reactions

Cardiovascular: Chest pain, first-dose hypotension, hypotension

Central nervous system: Dizziness, fatigue, headache

Dermatologic: Rash

Endocrine & metabolic: Hyperkalemia

Gastrointestinal: Diarrhea, nausea, vomiting

Neuromuscular & skeletal: Back pain, myalgia

Renal: BUN/serum creatinine increased, worsening of renal function (in patients with bilateral renal artery stenosis or hypovolemia)

Respiratory: Cough, dyspnea, upper respiratory symptoms,

Rare but important or life-threatening: Acute renal failure, agranulocytosis, alopecia, amblyopia, anaphylactoid reaction, angina, angioedema, arrhythmia, cerebrovascular accident, depression, dermatopolymyositis, eosinophilic pneumonitis, exfoliative dermatitis, gastrointestinal hemorrhage, heart failure, hemolytic anemia, hepatitis, hyperkalemia, hypertensive crisis, impotence, insomnia, MI, orthostatic hypotension, pancreatitis, pemphigus, photosensitivity, shock, stroke, syncope, thrombocytopenia, viral infection, visual hallucinations (Doane, 2013)

A syndrome which may include arthralgia, elevated ESR, eosinophilia and positive ANA, fever, interstitial nephritis, myalgia, rash, and vasculitis has been reported with ACE inhibitors. In addition, hepatic necrosis, neutropenia, pancreatitis, and/or agranulocytosis (particularly in patients with collagen-vascular disease or renal impairment) have been associated with many ACE inhibitors.

Drug Interactions

Metabolism/Transport Effects None known.

Avoid Concomitant Use There are no known interactions where it is recommended to avoid concomitant use.

Increased Effect/Toxicity

Quinapril may increase the levels/effects of: Allopurinol; Amifostine; Antihypertensives; AzaTHIOprine; Drospirenone; DULoxetine; Ferric Gluconate; Gold Sodium Thiomalate; Grass Pollen Allergen Extract (5 Grass Extract); Hypotensive Agents; Iron Dextran Complex; Levodopa; Lithium; Nonsteroidal Anti-Inflammatory Agents; Obinutuzumab; Pregabalin; RisperiDONE; RiTUXimab; Sodium Phosphates

The levels/effects of Quinapril may be increased by: Alfuzosin; Aliskiren; Angiotensin II Receptor Blockers; Barbiturates; Brimonidine (Topical); Canagliflozin; Dapoxetine; Diazoxide; DPP-IV Inhibitors; Eplerenone; Everolimus; Heparin; Heparin (Low Molecular Weight); Herbs (Hypotensive Properties); Loop Diuretics; MAO Inhibitors; Nicorandil; Pentoxifylline; Phosphodiesterase 5 Inhibitors; Potassium Salts; Potassium-Sparing Diuretics; Prostacyclin Analogues; Sirolimus; Temsirolimus; Thiazide Diuretics; TiZANidine; Tolvaptan; Trimethoprim

Decreased Effect

Quinapril may decrease the levels/effects of: Quinolone Antibiotics; Tetracycline Derivatives

The levels/effects of Quinapril may be decreased by: Aprotinin; Herbs (Hypertensive Properties); Icatibant; Lanthanum; Methylphenidate; Nonsteroidal Anti-Inflammatory Agents; Salicylates; Yohimbine

Storage/Stability Store at 15°C to 30°C (59°F to 86°F). Protect from light.

Mechanism of Action Competitive inhibitor of angiotensin-converting enzyme (ACE); prevents conversion of angiotensin I to angiotensin II, a potent vasoconstrictor; results in lower levels of angiotensin II which causes an increase in plasma renin activity and a reduction in aldosterone secretion; a CNS mechanism may also be involved in hypotensive effect as angiotensin II increases adrenergic outflow from CNS; vasoactive kallikreins may be decreased in conversion to active hormones by ACE inhibitors, thus reducing blood pressure

Pharmacodynamics

Onset of action: Antihypertensive: 1 hour

Maximum effect: Antihypertensive: 2-4 hours postdose

Duration: 24 hours (chronic dosing)

Pharmacokinetics (Adult data unless noted)

Absorption: Quinapril: ≥60%

Distribution:

- Infants and Children <6 years: 0.7 L/kg (range: 0.27-1.48 L/kg) (Blumer, 2003)
- Adults: 1.5 L/kg (Aronoff, 2007)

Protein binding: Quinapril: 97%; Quinaprilat: 97%

Metabolism: Rapidly hydrolyzed to quinaprilat, the active metabolite (~38% of an oral dose)

Half-life:
Infants and Children <7 years: Quinaprilat: 2.3 hours (Blumer, 2003)
Adults: Quinaprilat: 3 hours; increases as CrCl decreases
Time to peak serum concentration:
Infants and Children <7 years: 1.7 hours (range: 1-4 hours) (Blumer, 2003)
Adults: Quinaprilat: ~2 hours
Elimination: Urine (50% to 60% primarily as quinaprilat)

Dosing: Usual
Children and Adolescents: **Hypertension:** Limited data available: Oral: Initial: 5-10 mg once daily; may titrate every 2 weeks; maximum daily dose: 80 mg/day; for younger patients or those who are small for age, begin at lower end of range. A pharmacokinetic analyses of a 0.2 mg/kg single-dose in 24 pediatric patients <7 years of age, reported similar serum concentrations to those in adults who received a single 10 mg dose (Blumer, 2003; NHLBI, 2011)
Adults:
Heart failure: Oral: Initial: 5 mg once or twice daily, titrated at weekly intervals to 20-40 mg daily in 2 divided doses; target dose (heart failure): 20 mg twice daily (ACC/AHA 2009 Heart Failure Guidelines)
Hypertension: Oral: Initial: 10-20 mg once daily, adjust according to blood pressure response at peak and trough blood levels; initial dose may be reduced to 5 mg in patients receiving diuretic therapy if the diuretic is continued.
Usual dose range (JNC 7): 10-40 mg once daily
Dosing adjustment in renal impairment: Adults: Lower initial doses should be used; after initial dose (if tolerated), administer initial dose twice daily; may be increased at weekly intervals to optimal response:
Heart failure: Oral: Initial:
CrCl >30 mL/minute: Administer 5 mg/day
CrCl 10-30 mL/minute: Administer 2.5 mg/day
CrCl <10 mL/minute: No recommendations; insufficient data available
Hypertension: Oral: Initial:
CrCl >60 mL/minute: Administer 10 mg/day
CrCl 30-60 mL/minute: Administer 5 mg/day
CrCl 10-30 mL/minute: Administer 2.5 mg/day
CrCl <10 mL/minute: No recommendations; insufficient data available
Dosing adjustment in hepatic impairment: Adults: In patients with alcoholic cirrhosis, hydrolysis of quinapril to quinaprilat is impaired; however, the subsequent elimination of quinaprilat is unaltered.

Administration Oral: May be administered without regard to food

Monitoring Parameters Blood pressure, BUN, serum creatinine, renal function, urine dipstick for protein, serum potassium, WBC with differential, especially during first 3 months of therapy for patients with renal impairment and/or collagen vascular disease; monitor for angioedema and anaphylactoid reactions; hypovolemia and postural hypotension when beginning therapy, adjusting dosage, and on a regular basis throughout

Dosage Forms Excipient information presented when available (limited, particularly for generics); consult specific product labeling.
Tablet, Oral:
Accupril: 5 mg [scored; contains magnesium carbonate]
Accupril: 10 mg, 20 mg, 40 mg [contains magnesium carbonate]
Generic: 5 mg, 10 mg, 20 mg, 40 mg

Extemporaneous Preparations A 1 mg/mL quinapril oral suspension may be made with tablets, K-Phos® Neutral (equivalent to 250 mg elemental phosphorus, 13 mEq sodium, and 1.1 mEq potassium per tablet), Bicitra®, and Ora-Sweet SF™. Place ten quinapril 20 mg tablets in an amber plastic prescription bottle (eg, 240 mL). In a separate container, prepare a buffer solution by crushing one K-Phos® Neutral tablet and dissolving it in 100 mL sterile water for irrigation. Add 30 mL of the prepared K-Phos® buffer solution to the quinapril tablets. Shake for at least 2 minutes, then remove cap and allow the concentrate to stand for 15 minutes, then shake the concentrate again for an additional minute. Add 30 mL of Bicitra® and shake for 2 minutes. Add quantity sufficient of Ora-Sweet SF® (~140 mL) to make 200 mL and shake the suspension. Store in amber plastic prescription bottles; label "shake well" and "refrigerate." Stable for 28 days refrigerated (Freed, 2005).

Freed A, Silbering SB, Kolodsick KJ, et al, "The Development and Stability Assessment of Extemporaneous Pediatric Formulations of Accupril," *Int J Pharm*, 2005, 304(1-2):135-44.

◆ **Quinapril Hydrochloride** *see* Quinapril *on page 1820*
◆ **Quinate (Can)** *see* QuiNIDine *on page 1822*

QuiNIDine (KWIN i deen)

Medication Safety Issues
Sound-alike/look-alike issues:
QuiNIDine may be confused with cloNIDine, quiNINE
High alert medication:
The Institute for Safe Medication Practices (ISMP) includes this medication (IV formulation) among its list of drug classes which have a heightened risk of causing significant patient harm when used in error.
BEERS Criteria medication:
This drug may be potentially inappropriate for use in geriatric patients (Quality of evidence - high; Strength of recommendation - strong).

Related Information
Oral Medications That Should Not Be Crushed or Altered *on page 2476*

Brand Names: Canada Apo-Quinidine; BioQuin Durules; Novo-Quinidin; Quinate

Therapeutic Category Antiarrhythmic Agent, Class I-A; Antimalarial Agent

Generic Availability (US) Yes

Use
Quinidine **sulfate**: Treatment of life-threatening *Plasmodium falciparum* malaria [Oral: Immediate release: FDA approved in pediatric patients (age not specified) and adults]; conversion of atrial fibrillation and/or flutter; prophylaxis after cardioversion of atrial fibrillation and/or flutter to maintain normal sinus rhythm; suppression of serious recurrent ventricular arrhythmias (eg, life-threatening ventricular tachycardia) (Oral: Immediate/extended release: FDA approved in adults); has also been used to prevent reoccurrence of paroxysmal supraventricular tachycardia, paroxysmal A-V junctional rhythm, paroxysmal ventricular tachycardia, paroxysmal atrial fibrillation, and atrial or ventricular premature contractions
Quinidine **gluconate**: Treatment of life-threatening *Plasmodium falciparum* malaria [Parenteral: FDA approved in pediatric patients (age not specified) and adults]; conversion of atrial fibrillation and/or flutter; prophylaxis after cardioversion of atrial fibrillation and/or flutter to maintain normal sinus rhythm; suppression of serious recurrent ventricular arrhythmias (eg, life-threatening ventricular tachycardia) (Parenteral, Oral: Extended release: FDA approved in adults); has also been used to prevent reoccurrence of paroxysmal supraventricular tachycardia, paroxysmal A-V junctional rhythm, paroxysmal ventricular tachycardia, paroxysmal atrial fibrillation, and atrial or ventricular premature contractions; **Note:** The use of IV quinidine gluconate for these indications has been replaced by more effective/safer antiarrhythmic agents (eg, amiodarone and procainamide).

Pregnancy Risk Factor C

Pregnancy Considerations Animal reproduction studies have not been conducted. Quinidine crosses the placenta and can be detected in the amniotic fluid, cord blood, and neonatal serum. Quinidine is indicated for use in the treatment of severe malaria infection in pregnant women (CDC, 2011; Smereck, 2011) and has also been used to treat arrhythmias in pregnancy when other agents are ineffective (European Society of Cardiology, 2003).

Breast-Feeding Considerations Quinidine can be detected in breast milk at concentrations slightly lower than those in the maternal serum. The manufacturer recommends avoiding use in nursing women.

Contraindications Hypersensitivity to quinidine or any component of the formulation; thrombocytopenia; thrombocytopenic purpura; myasthenia gravis; heart block greater than first degree; idioventricular conduction delays (except in patients with a functioning artificial pacemaker); those adversely affected by anticholinergic activity; concurrent use of quinolone antibiotics which prolong QT interval, cisapride, amprenavir, or ritonavir

Warnings/Precautions Watch for proarrhythmic effects; may cause QT prolongation and subsequent torsade de pointes. Monitor and adjust dose to prevent QTc prolongation. Avoid use in patients with diagnosed or suspected congenital long QT syndrome. Correct hypokalemia before initiating therapy. Hypokalemia may worsen toxicity. **[U.S. Boxed Warning]: Antiarrhythmic drugs have not been shown to enhance survival in non-life-threatening ventricular arrhythmias and may increase mortality; the risk is greatest with structural heart disease. Quinidine may increase mortality in treatment of atrial fibrillation/flutter.** May precipitate or exacerbate HF. Reduce dosage in hepatic impairment. Use may cause digoxin-induced toxicity (adjust digoxin's dose). Use caution with concurrent use of other antiarrhythmics. Hypersensitivity reactions can occur. Can unmask sick sinus syndrome (causes bradycardia); use with caution in patients with heart block. In the treatment of atrial fibrillation in the elderly, avoid antiarrhythmics as first-line treatment. In older adults, data suggests rate control may provide more benefits than risks compared to rhythm control for most patients (Beers Criteria).

Has been associated with severe hepatotoxic reactions, including granulomatous hepatitis. Hemolysis may occur in patients with G6PD (glucose-6-phosphate dehydrogenase) deficiency. Different salt products are not interchangeable.

Adverse Reactions

Cardiovascular: Angina, new or worsened arrhythmia (proarrhythmic effect), hypotension, palpitation, QTc prolongation (modest prolongation is common, however, excessive prolongation is rare and indicates toxicity), syncope

Central nervous system: Fatigue, headache, incoordination, lightheadedness, nervousness, sleep disturbance, syncope, tremor

Dermatologic: Rash

Gastrointestinal: Anorexia, bitter taste, diarrhea, nausea, stomach cramping, upper GI distress, vomiting

Neuromuscular & skeletal: Weakness

Ocular: Blurred vision

Otic: Tinnitus

Respiratory: Wheezing

Rare but important or life-threatening: Abnormal pigmentation, acute psychotic reactions, agranulocytosis, angioedema, arthralgia, bronchospasm, cerebral hypoperfusion (possibly resulting in ataxia, apprehension, and seizure), cholestasis, confusion, CPK increased, delirium, depression, drug-induced lupus-like syndrome, eczematous dermatitis, esophagitis, exacerbated bradycardia (in sick sinus syndrome), exfoliative rash, fever, flushing, granulomatous hepatitis, hallucinations, hearing impaired, heart block, hemolytic anemia, hepatotoxic reaction (rare), lichen planus, livedo reticularis, lymphadenopathy, melanin pigmentation of the hard palate, myalgia, mydriasis, nephropathy, optic neuritis, pancytopenia, paradoxical increase in ventricular rate during atrial fibrillation/flutter, photosensitivity, pneumonitis, pruritus, psoriaform rash, QTc prolongation (excessive), respiratory depression, sicca syndrome, tachycardia, thrombocytopenia, thrombocytopenic purpura, torsade de pointes, urticaria, uveitis, vascular collapse, vasculitis, ventricular fibrillation, ventricular tachycardia, vertigo, visual field loss

Note: Cinchonism, a syndrome which may include tinnitus, high-frequency hearing loss, deafness, vertigo, blurred vision, diplopia, photophobia, headache, confusion, and delirium has been associated with quinidine use. Usually associated with chronic toxicity, this syndrome has also been described after brief exposure to a moderate dose in sensitive patients. Vomiting and diarrhea may also occur as isolated reactions to therapeutic quinidine levels.

Drug Interactions

Metabolism/Transport Effects **Substrate** of CYP2C9 (minor), CYP2E1 (minor), CYP3A4 (major), P-glycoprotein; **Note:** Assignment of Major/Minor substrate status based on clinically relevant drug interaction potential; **Inhibits** CYP2C9 (weak), CYP2D6 (strong), CYP3A4 (weak), P-glycoprotein

Avoid Concomitant Use

Avoid concomitant use of QuiNIDine with any of the following: Amiodarone; Antifungal Agents (Azole Derivatives, Systemic); Bosutinib; Conivaptan; Crizotinib; Enzalutamide; Fingolimod; Fusidic Acid (Systemic); Haloperidol; Highest Risk QTc-Prolonging Agents; Idelalisib; Ivabradine; Lopinavir; Macrolide Antibiotics; Mefloquine; Mequitazine; Mifepristone; Moderate Risk QTc-Prolonging Agents; Nelfinavir; PAZOPanib; Pimozide; Propafenone; Ritonavir; Saquinavir; Silodosin; Tamoxifen; Thioridazine; Tipranavir; Topotecan; VinCRIStine (Liposomal)

Increased Effect/Toxicity

QuiNIDine may increase the levels/effects of: Afatinib; ARIPiprazole; AtoMOXetine; Bosutinib; Brentuximab Vedotin; Calcium Channel Blockers (Dihydropyridine); Cardiac Glycosides; Colchicine; CYP2D6 Substrates; Dabigatran Etexilate; Dalfampridine; Dextromethorphan; DOXOrubicin (Conventional); Edoxaban; Everolimus; Fesoterodine; FluvoxaMINE; Haloperidol; Highest Risk QTc-Prolonging Agents; Ledipasvir; Lomitapide; Mefloquine; Mequitazine; Metoprolol; Naloxegol; Nebivolol; Neuromuscular-Blocking Agents; NiMODipine; PAZOPanib; P-glycoprotein/ABCB1 Substrates; Pimozide; Propafenone; Propranolol; Prucalopride; Rifaximin; Rivaroxaban; Silodosin; Tamsulosin; Thioridazine; Topotecan; TraMADol; Tricyclic Antidepressants; Verapamil; VinCRIStine (Liposomal); Vitamin K Antagonists; Vortioxetine

The levels/effects of QuiNIDine may be increased by: Amiodarone; Antacids; Antifungal Agents (Azole Derivatives, Systemic); Aprepitant; Atazanavir; Boceprevir; Calcium Channel Blockers (Dihydropyridine); Carbonic Anhydrase Inhibitors; Cimetidine; Cobicistat; Conivaptan; Crizotinib; CYP3A4 Inhibitors (Moderate); CYP3A4 Inhibitors (Strong); Darunavir; Diltiazem; Fingolimod; FluvoxaMINE; Fosamprenavir; Fosaprepitant; Fosphenytoin; Fusidic Acid (Systemic); Haloperidol; Idelalisib; Indinavir; Ivabradine; Ivacaftor; Lopinavir; Luliconazole; Lurasidone; Macrolide Antibiotics; Mifepristone; Moderate Risk QTc-Prolonging Agents; Nelfinavir; Netupitant; Palbociclib; P-glycoprotein/ABCB1 Inhibitors; PHENobarbital; QTc-Prolonging Agents (Indeterminate Risk and Risk Modifying); Reserpine; Ritonavir; Saquinavir; Simeprevir; Stiripentol; Telaprevir; Tipranavir; Tricyclic Antidepressants; Verapamil

Decreased Effect

QuiNIDine may decrease the levels/effects of: Codeine; Dihydrocodeine; Hydrocodone; Tamoxifen; TraMADol

The levels/effects of QuiNIDine may be decreased by: Bosentan; Calcium Channel Blockers (Dihydropyridine); CYP3A4 Inducers (Moderate); CYP3A4 Inducers (Strong); Dabrafenib; Deferasirox; Enzalutamide; Etravirine; Fosphenytoin; Kaolin; Mitotane; P-glycoprotein/ABCB1 Inducers; PHENobarbital; Phenytoin; Potassium-Sparing Diuretics; Primidone; Rifamycin Derivatives; Siltuximab; St Johns Wort; Sucralfate; Tocilizumab

Food Interactions Changes in dietary salt intake may alter the rate and extent of quinidine absorption. Quinidine serum levels may be increased if taken with food. Food has a variable effect on absorption of sustained release formulation. The rate of absorption of quinidine may be decreased following the ingestion of grapefruit juice. Excessive intake of fruit juice or vitamin C may decrease urine pH and result in increased clearance of quinidine with decreased serum concentration. Alkaline foods may result in increased quinidine serum concentrations. Management: Avoid changes in dietary salt intake. Grapefruit juice should be avoided. Take around-the-clock to avoid variation in serum levels and with food or milk to avoid GI irritation.

Storage/Stability

Solution for injection: Store at room temperature of 25°C (77°F).

Tablets: Store at controlled room temperature of 20°C to 25°C (68°F to 77°F). Protect from light.

Mechanism of Action Class Ia antiarrhythmic agent; depresses phase O of the action potential; decreases myocardial excitability and conduction velocity, and myocardial contractility by decreasing sodium influx during depolarization and potassium efflux in repolarization; also reduces calcium transport across cell membrane

Pharmacokinetics (Adult data unless noted)

Distribution: V_d: Adults: 2-3.5 L/kg, decreased V_d with CHF, malaria; increased V_d with cirrhosis

Protein-binding: Binds mainly to alpha$_1$-acid glycoprotein and to a lesser extent albumin; protein-binding changes may occur in periods of stress due to increased alpha$_1$-acid glycoprotein concentrations (eg, acute myocardial infarction) or in certain disease states due to decreased alpha$_1$-acid glycoprotein concentrations (eg, cirrhosis, hyperthyroidism, malnutrition)

Newborns: 60% to 70%

Adults: 80% to 90%

Metabolism: Extensively hepatic (50% to 90%) to inactive compounds

Bioavailability: Sulfate: ~70% with wide variability between patients (45% to 100%); Gluconate: 70% to 80%

Time to peak serum concentration: Oral: Sulfate: Immediate release: 2 hours; Extended release: 6 hours; Gluconate: Extended release: 3-5 hours

Half-life, plasma (increased half-life with cirrhosis and CHF):

Children: 2.5-6.7 hours

Adults: 6-8 hours

Elimination: Urine (15% to 25% as unchanged drug)

Dialysis: Slightly dialyzable (5% to 20%) by hemodialysis; not removed by peritoneal dialysis

Dosing: Usual Note: Quinidine is available in gluconate and sulfate salt formulations which are not interchangeable on a mg per mg basis, due to differences in the amount of quinidine base supplied.

Pediatric:

Malaria, treatment (severe, life-threatening): Infants, Children, and Adolescents: IV: **Quinidine gluconate:** 10 mg/kg infused over 60-120 minutes, followed by 0.02 mg/kg/minute continuous infusion for ≥24 hours; alternatively, may administer 24 mg/kg loading dose over 4 hours, followed by 12 mg/kg over 4 hours every 8 hours (beginning 8 hours after loading dose). Change to oral quinine once parasite density is <1% and patient can receive oral medication to complete treatment course; total duration of treatment (quinidine/quinine): 3 days in Africa or South America; 7 days in Southeast Asia; use in combination with doxycycline, tetracycline, or clindamycin; omit quinidine loading dose if patient received >40 mg/kg of quinine in preceding 48 hours or mefloquine within preceding 12 hours (CDC, 2009). **Note:** Close monitoring, including telemetry, is **required**; if severe cardiac adverse effects occur, infusion rate may need to be decreased or drug temporarily discontinued.

Arrhythmias: Children and Adolescents: Limited data available:

Oral: Quinidine **sulfate**; immediate release: Usual: 30 mg/kg/day or 900 mg/m^2/day in 5 daily doses or 6 mg/kg every 4-6 hours; range: 15-60 mg/kg/day in 4-5 divided doses; usual maximum dose: 600 mg; maximum daily dose: 3000-4000 mg/**day**

IV: Quinidine **gluconate**: 2-10 mg/kg/dose every 3-6 hours as needed (IV route **not** recommended)

Adults:

Malaria: IV: Quinidine **gluconate**: 10 mg/kg infused over 60-120 minutes, followed by 0.02 mg/kg/minute continuous infusion for ≥24 hours; alternatively, may administer 24 mg/kg loading dose over 4 hours, followed by 12 mg/kg over 4 hours every 8 hours (beginning 8 hours after loading dose). Change to oral quinine once parasite density is <1% and patient can receive oral medication to complete treatment course; total duration of treatment (quinidine/quinine): 3 days in Africa or South America; 7 days in Southeast Asia; use in combination with doxycycline, tetracycline, or clindamycin; omit quinidine loading dose if patient received >40 mg/kg of quinine in preceding 48 hours or mefloquine within preceding 12 hours (CDC, 2009). **Note:** Close monitoring, including telemetry, is required; if severe cardiac adverse effects occur, infusion rate may need to be decreased or drug temporarily discontinued.

Arrythmias: Oral:

Immediate release formulations: Quinidine **sulfate**: Initial: 200-400 mg/dose every 6 hours; the dose may be increased cautiously to desired effect; maximum daily dose range: 3000-4000 mg/**day**

Extended release formulations:

Quinidine **sulfate**: Initial: 300 mg every 8-12 hours; the dose may be increased cautiously to desired effect

Quinidine **gluconate**: Initial: 324 mg every 8-12 hours; the dose may be increased cautiously to desired effect

Dosing adjustment in renal impairment: The FDA-approved labeling recommends that caution should be used in patients with renal impairment; however, no specific dosage adjustment guidelines are available. The following guidelines have been used by some clinicians (Aronoff, 2007): Oral: Adults:

CrCl ≥10 mL/minute: No adjustment required.

CrCl <10 mL/minute: Administer 75% of normal dose.

Hemodialysis: Administer dose following hemodialysis session.

Peritoneal dialysis: Supplemental dose is not necessary.

CRRT: No dosage adjustment required; monitor serum concentrations.

Dosing adjustment in hepatic impairment: Use caution; hepatic impairment decreases clearance; dosage adjustments are not provided in the manufacturers' labeling although toxicity may occur if the dose is not appropriately adjusted; larger loading dose may be indicated

Preparation for Administration Parenteral: Quinidine gluconate: IV: Dilute with D_5W to a maximum concentration of 16 mg/mL

Administration

Oral: Administer with water on an empty stomach, but may administer with food or milk to decrease GI upset; best to administer in a consistent manner with regards to meals and around-the-clock to promote less variation in peak and trough serum concentrations; swallow extended release tablets whole, do not chew or crush; some preparations of quinidine **gluconate** extended release tablets may be split in half to facilitate dosage titration; tablets are not scored.

Parenteral: Quinidine gluconate: **Note:** Length of IV tubing should be minimized (quinidine may be significantly adsorbed to polyvinyl chloride tubing)

Malaria: IV: Infusion duration of loading and subsequent dosing determined by regimen used, refer to Dosing: Usual for specific details.

Arrhythmia: Intermittent IV infusion: After dilution, infuse slowly using an infusion pump; maximum rate: 0.25 mg/kg/minute; monitor ECG along with closely monitoring patient for possible hypersensitivity or idiosyncratic reactions. **Note:** The use of IV quinidine gluconate for these indications has been replaced by more effective/safer antiarrhythmic agents

Monitoring Parameters CBC with differential, platelet count, liver and renal function tests. Serum concentrations should be routinely performed during long-term administration. Continuously monitor blood pressure and ECG (for widening QRS complex and lengthening of QTc interval) and periodically monitor blood glucose for hypoglycemia with IV use.

Reference Range Optimal therapeutic level is method dependent

Therapeutic: 2-5 mcg/mL (SI: 6.2-15.4 micromole/L).

Patient-dependent therapeutic response occurs at levels of 3-6 mcg/mL (SI: 9.2-18.5 micromole/L).

Additional Information Quinidine **gluconate**: 267 mg = quinidine **sulfate**: 200 mg

Formation of a concretion of tablets or bezoar in the stomach has been reported following tablet ingestion by a 16-month old infant; diagnostic or therapeutic endoscopy may be required in patients with massive overdose and prolonged elevated serum quinidine concentrations

Dosage Forms Excipient information presented when available (limited, particularly for generics); consult specific product labeling.

Solution, Injection, as gluconate:
Generic: 80 mg/mL (10 mL)

Tablet, Oral, as sulfate:
Generic: 200 mg, 300 mg

Tablet Extended Release, Oral, as gluconate:
Generic: 324 mg

Tablet Extended Release, Oral, as sulfate:
Generic: 300 mg

Extemporaneous Preparations A 10 mg/mL oral liquid preparation may be made with tablets and one of three different vehicles (cherry syrup, a 1:1 mixture of Ora-Sweet® and Ora-Plus®, or a 1:1 mixture of Ora-Sweet® SF and Ora-Plus®). Crush six 200 mg tablets in a mortar and reduce to a fine powder. Add 15 mL of the chosen vehicle and mix to a uniform paste; mix while adding vehicle in incremental proportions to **almost** 120 mL; transfer to a calibrated bottle, rinse mortar with vehicle, and add quantity of vehicle sufficient to make 120 mL. Label "shake well" and "protect from light". Stable for 60 days when stored in amber plastic prescription bottles in the dark at room temperature or refrigerated.

Allen LV and Erickson MA, "Stability of Bethanechol Chloride, Pyrazinamide, Quinidine Sulfate, Rifampin, and Tetracycline in Extemporaneously Compounded Oral Liquids," *Am J Health Syst Pharm*, 1998, 55(17):1804-9.

- ◆ **Quinidine Gluconate** *see* QuiNIDine *on page* 1822
- ◆ **Quinidine Polygalacturonate** *see* QuiNIDine *on page* 1822
- ◆ **Quinidine Sulfate** *see* QuiNIDine *on page* 1822

QuiNINE (KWYE nine)

Medication Safety Issues

Sound-alike/look-alike issues:

QuiNINE may be confused with quiNIDine

Brand Names: US Qualaquin

Brand Names: Canada Apo-Quinine®; Novo-Quinine; Quinine-Odan

Therapeutic Category Antimalarial Agent; Skeletal Muscle Relaxant, Miscellaneous

Generic Availability (US) Yes

Use Treatment of chloroquine-resistant, uncomplicated *P. falciparum* malaria infection (inactive against sporozoites, pre-erythrocytic or exoerythrocytic forms of plasmodia) in conjunction with other antimalarial agents [FDA approved in pediatrics (age not specified) and adults]; has also been used for the treatment of uncomplicated chloroquine-resistant *P. vivax* malaria (in conjunction with other antimalarial agents); treatment of *Babesia microti* infection in conjunction with clindamycin

Medication Guide Available Yes

Pregnancy Risk Factor C

Pregnancy Considerations Teratogenic effects have been reported in some animal studies. Quinine crosses the human placenta. Cord plasma to maternal plasma quinine ratios have been reported as 0.18-0.46 and should not be considered therapeutic to the infant. Teratogenic effects, optic nerve hypoplasia, and deafness have been reported in the infant following maternal use of very high doses; however, therapeutic doses used for malaria are generally considered safe. Quinine may also cause significant hypoglycemia when used during pregnancy. Malaria infection in pregnant women may be more severe than in nonpregnant women. Because *P. falciparum* malaria can cause maternal death and fetal loss, pregnant women traveling to malaria-endemic areas must use personal protection against mosquito bites. Quinine may be used for the treatment of malaria in pregnant women; consult current CDC guidelines. Pregnant women should be advised not to travel to areas of *P. falciparum* resistance to chloroquine.

Breast-Feeding Considerations Based on limited data, it is estimated that nursing infants would receive <0.4% of the maternal dose from breast-feeding.

Contraindications Hypersensitivity to quinine or any component of the formulation; hypersensitivity to mefloquine or quinidine (cross sensitivity reported); history of potential hypersensitivity reactions (including black water fever, thrombotic thrombocytopenia purpura [TTP], hemolytic uremic syndrome [HUS], or thrombocytopenia) associated with prior quinine use; prolonged QT interval; myasthenia gravis; optic neuritis; G6PD deficiency

Warnings/Precautions **[U.S. Boxed Warning]: Quinine is not recommended for the prevention/treatment of nocturnal leg cramps due to the potential for severe and/or life-threatening side effects (eg, cardiac arrhythmias, thrombocytopenia, HUS/TTP, severe hypersensitivity reactions).** These risks, as well as the absence of clinical effectiveness, do not justify its use in the unapproved/off-label prevention and/or treatment of leg cramps.

Quinine may cause QT-interval prolongation, with maximum increase corresponding to maximum plasma concentration. Fatal torsade de pointes and ventricular fibrillation has been reported. Use contraindicated in patients with QT prolongation. Concurrent use of Class IA (eg, quinidine, procainamide) or Class III (eg, amiodarone, dofetilide, sotalol) antiarrhythmic agents or with other drugs known to prolong the QT interval is not recommended. Quinine may also cause concentration-dependent prolongation of the PR and QRS intervals. Risk of prolonged PR and/or QRS intervals is higher in patients with underlying structural heart disease, myocardial ischemia, preexisting conduction system abnormalities, elderly patients with sick sinus syndrome, patients with atrial fibrillation with slow ventricular response and concomitant use of drugs known to prolong the PR interval (eg, verapamil) or QRS interval (eg, flecainide or quinidine). Use caution with clinical conditions which may further prolong the QT interval or cause cardiac arrhythmias. Use caution with atrial fibrillation or flutter (paradoxical increase in heart rate may occur), or renal impairment. Use with caution with mild-to-moderate hepatic impairment; avoid use with severe hepatic impairment. Potentially significant drug-drug interactions may exist, requiring dose or frequency adjustment, additional monitoring, and/or selection of alternative therapy.

Severe hypersensitivity reactions (eg, Stevens-Johnson syndrome, anaphylactic shock) have occurred; discontinue following any signs of sensitivity. Other events (including acute interstitial nephritis, neutropenia, and granulomatous hepatitis) may also be attributed to hypersensitivity reactions. Immune-mediated thrombocytopenia, including life-threatening cases and hemolytic uremic syndrome/thrombotic thrombocytopenic purpura (HUS/TTP), has occurred with use. Chronic renal failure associated with TTP has also been reported. Thrombocytopenia generally resolves within a week upon discontinuation. Re-exposure may result in increased severity of thrombocytopenia and faster onset.

Use may cause significant hypoglycemia due to quinine-induced insulin release. Use with caution in patients with hepatic impairment. Use with caution in patients with renal impairment; dosage adjustment recommended. Quinine should not be used for the prevention of malaria or in the treatment of complicated or severe *P. falciparum* malaria (oral antimalarial agents are not appropriate for initial therapy of severe malaria).

Adverse Reactions

Cardiovascular: Atrial fibrillation, atrioventricular block, bradycardia, cardiac arrest, chest pain, hypotension, irregular rhythm, nodal escape beats, orthostatic hypotension, palpitation, QT prolongation, syncope, tachycardia, torsade de pointes, unifocal premature ventricular contractions, U waves, vasodilation, ventricular fibrillation, ventricular tachycardia

Central nervous system: Aphasia, ataxia, chills, coma, confusion, disorientation, dizziness, dystonic reaction, fever, flushing, headache, mental status altered, restlessness, seizure, suicide, vertigo

Dermatologic: Acral necrosis, allergic contact dermatitis, bullous dermatitis, bruising, cutaneous rash (urticaria, papular, scarlatinal), cutaneous vasculitis, exfoliative dermatitis, erythema multiforme, petechiae, photosensitivity, pruritus, Stevens-Johnson syndrome, toxic epidermal necrolysis

Endocrine & metabolic: Hypoglycemia

Gastrointestinal: Abdominal pain, anorexia, diarrhea, esophagitis, gastric irritation, nausea, vomiting

Hematologic: Agranulocytosis, aplastic anemia, coagulopathy, disseminated intravascular coagulation, hemolytic anemia, hemolytic uremic syndrome, hemorrhage, hypoprothrombinemia, immune thrombocytopenia (ITP), leukopenia, neutropenia, pancytopenia, thrombocytopenia, thrombotic thrombocytopenic purpura

Hepatic: Granulomatous hepatitis, hepatitis, jaundice, liver function test abnormalities

Neuromuscular & skeletal: Myalgia, tremor, weakness

Ocular: Blindness, blurred vision (with or without scotomata), color vision disturbance, diminished visual fields, diplopia, night blindness, optic neuritis, photophobia, pupillary dilation, vision loss (sudden)

Otic: Deafness, hearing impaired, tinnitus

Renal: Acute interstitial nephritis, hemoglobinuria, renal failure, renal impairment

Respiratory: Asthma, dyspnea, pulmonary edema

Miscellaneous: Black water fever, diaphoresis, hypersensitivity reaction, lupus anticoagulant, lupus-like syndrome

Drug Interactions

Metabolism/Transport Effects Substrate of CYP1A2 (minor), CYP2C19 (minor), CYP3A4 (major), P-glycoprotein; **Note:** Assignment of Major/Minor substrate status based on clinically relevant drug interaction potential; **Inhibits** CYP2C8 (moderate), CYP2C9 (moderate), CYP2D6 (moderate), P-glycoprotein

Avoid Concomitant Use

Avoid concomitant use of QuiNINE with any of the following: Amodiaquine; Antacids; Artemether; Bosutinib; Conivaptan; Fusidic Acid (Systemic); Halofantrine; Highest Risk QTc-Prolonging Agents; Idelalisib; Ivabradine; Lopinavir; Lumefantrine; Macrolide Antibiotics; Mefloquine; Mifepristone; Moderate Risk QTc-Prolonging Agents; Neuromuscular-Blocking Agents; PAZOPanib; Rifampin; Ritonavir; Silodosin; Thioridazine; Topotecan; VinCRIStine (Liposomal)

Increased Effect/Toxicity

QuiNINE may increase the levels/effects of: Afatinib; Amodiaquine; Antihypertensives; Antipsychotic Agents (Phenothiazines); Bosentan; Bosutinib; Brentuximab Vedotin; Cannabis; CarBAMazepine; Carvedilol; Colchicine; CYP2C8 Substrates; CYP2C9 Substrates; CYP2D6 Substrates; Dabigatran Etexilate; Dapsone (Systemic); Dapsone (Topical); Digoxin; DOXOrubicin (Conventional); Dronabinol; Edoxaban; Everolimus; Fesoterodine; Halofantrine; Herbs (Hypotensive Properties); Highest Risk QTc-Prolonging Agents; HMG-CoA Reductase Inhibitors; Hypoglycemia-Associated Agents; Ledipasvir; Lumefantrine; Mefloquine; Metoprolol; Naloxegol; Nebivolol; Neuromuscular-Blocking Agents; PAZOPanib; P-glycoprotein/ABCB1 Substrates; PHENobarbital; Prilocaine; Prucalopride; Rifaximin; Ritonavir; Rivaroxaban; Silodosin; Sodium Nitrite; Tetrahydrocannabinol; Theophylline Derivatives; Thioridazine; Topotecan; VinCRIStine (Liposomal); Vitamin K Antagonists

The levels/effects of QuiNINE may be increased by: Alkalinizing Agents; Androgens; Antidiabetic Agents; Aprepitant; Artemether; Cimetidine; Conivaptan; CYP3A4 Inhibitors (Moderate); CYP3A4 Inhibitors (Strong); Dapsone (Systemic); Fosaprepitant; Fusidic Acid (Systemic); Herbs (Hypoglycemic Properties); Idelalisib; Ivabradine; Ivacaftor; Luliconazole; Macrolide Antibiotics; MAO Inhibitors; Mefloquine; Mifepristone; Moderate Risk QTc-Prolonging Agents; Netupitant; Nitric Oxide; Palbociclib; Pegvisomant; P-glycoprotein/ABCB1 Inhibitors; QTc-Prolonging Agents (Indeterminate Risk and Risk Modifying); Quinolone Antibiotics; Ritonavir; Salicylates; Selective Serotonin Reuptake Inhibitors; Simeprevir; Stiripentol; Tetracycline

Decreased Effect

QuiNINE may decrease the levels/effects of: Codeine; Tamoxifen; TraMADol

The levels/effects of QuiNINE may be decreased by: Antacids; Bosentan; CarBAMazepine; CYP3A4 Inducers (Moderate); CYP3A4 Inducers (Strong); Dabrafenib; Deferasirox; Fosphenytoin; Lopinavir; Mitotane; P-glycoprotein/ABCB1 Inducers; PHENobarbital; Phenytoin; Quinolone Antibiotics; Rifampin; Ritonavir; Siltuximab; St Johns Wort; Tocilizumab

Storage/Stability Store at 20°C to 25°C (68°F to 77°F).

Mechanism of Action Depresses oxygen uptake and carbohydrate metabolism; intercalates into DNA, disrupting the parasite's replication and transcription; cardiovascular effects similar to quinidine

Pharmacokinetics (Adult data unless noted)

Absorption: Oral: Readily absorbed, mainly from the upper small intestine

Distribution: Widely distributed to body tissues and fluids including small amounts into bile and CSF (2% to 7% of plasma concentration); crosses the placenta; excreted into breast milk

V_d (children): 0.8 L/kg

V_d (adults): 1.9 L/kg

Protein binding: 70% to 90%

Metabolism: Primarily in the liver via hydroxylation pathways

Half-life:

Children: 6-12 hours

Adults: 8-14 hours

Time to peak serum concentration: Within 2-4 hours

Elimination: In bile and saliva with ~20% excreted unchanged in urine; renal excretion is twofold in the presence of acidic urine

Dialysis: Not effectively removed by peritoneal dialysis; removed by hemodialysis

Dosing: Usual Oral: **Note:** Actual duration of quinine treatment for malaria may be dependent upon the geographic region or pathogen. Dosage expressed in terms of the **salt**; 1 capsule Qualaquin® = 324 mg of quinine sulfate = 269 mg of base.

Children:

Treatment of uncomplicated chloroquine-resistant *P. falciparum* malaria: CDC guidelines: 30 mg/kg/day in divided doses every 8 hours for 3-7 days depending on region (maximum dose: 1944 mg/day).Tetracycline, doxycycline, or clindamycin (consider risk versus benefit of using tetracycline or doxycycline in children <8 years of age) should also be given.

Treatment of uncomplicated chloroquine-resistant *P. vivax* malaria: CDC guidelines: 30 mg/kg/day in divided doses every 8 hours for 3-7 days depending on region (maximum dose: 1944 mg/day). Tetracycline or doxycycline (consider risk versus benefit of using tetracycline or doxycycline in children <8 years of age) **plus** primaquine should also be given.

Babesiosis: 30 mg/kg/day, divided every 8 hours for 7-10 days with clindamycin; maximum dose: 648 mg/dose

Adults:

Treatment of uncomplicated chloroquine-resistant *P. falciparum* malaria: CDC guidelines: 648 mg every 8 hours for 3-7 days. Tetracycline, doxycycline, or clindamycin should also be given.

Treatment of uncomplicated chloroquine-resistant *P. vivax* malaria: CDC guidelines: 648 mg every 8 hours for 3-7 days. Tetracycline or doxycycline **plus** primaquine should also be given.

Babesiosis: 648 mg every 8 hours for 7-10 days with clindamycin

Dosing adjustment in renal impairment: Adult:

CrCl 10-50 mL/minute: Administer every 8-12 hours

CrCl <10 mL/minute: Administer every 24 hours

Severe chronic renal failure not on dialysis: Initial dose: 648 mg followed by 324 mg every 12 hours

Administration Oral: Do not crush capsule to avoid bitter taste

Monitoring Parameters CBC with platelet count, liver function tests, blood glucose, ophthalmologic examination

Test Interactions May interfere with urine detection of opioids (false-positive); positive Coombs' [direct]; false elevation of urinary steroids (when assayed by Zimmerman method) and catecholamines; qualitative and quantitative urine dipstick protein assays

Additional Information Parenteral form of quinine (dihydrochloride) is no longer available from the CDC; quinidine gluconate should be used instead; the FDA has banned over-the-counter (OTC) drug products containing quinine sold for treatment and/or prevention of malaria, as well as, products labeled for treatment or prevention of nocturnal leg cramps

Dosage Forms Excipient information presented when available (limited, particularly for generics); consult specific product labeling.

Capsule, Oral, as sulfate:

Qualaquin: 324 mg

Generic: 324 mg

◆ **Quinine-Odan (Can)** *see* QuiNINE *on page 1825*

◆ **Quinine Sulfate** *see* QuiNINE *on page 1825*

Quinupristin and Dalfopristin

(kwi NYOO pris tin & dal FOE pris tin)

Brand Names: US Synercid®

Brand Names: Canada Synercid®

Therapeutic Category Antibiotic, Streptogramin

Generic Availability (US) No

Use Treatment of complicated skin and skin structure infections caused by *Staphylococcus aureus* (methicillin-susceptible) or *Streptococcus pyogenes* (FDA approved in ages ≥12 years and adults); has also been used for salvage therapy for invasive MRSA infections in cases of vancomycin treatment failure

Pregnancy Risk Factor B

Pregnancy Considerations Because adverse effects were not observed in animal reproduction studies, quinupristin/dalfopristin is classified pregnancy category B. There are no adequate and well-controlled studies of quinupristin/dalfopristin in pregnant women.

Breast-Feeding Considerations It is not known if quinupristin/dalfopristin is excreted in human milk. The manufacturer recommends caution if administering quinupristin/dalfopristin to a nursing woman. The increased molecular weight of quinupristin/dalfopristin may minimize excretion into human milk. Nondose-related effects could include modification of bowel flora.

Contraindications Hypersensitivity to quinupristin, dalfopristin, pristinamycin, or virginiamycin, or any component of the formulation

Warnings/Precautions Use with caution in patients with hepatic or renal dysfunction. May cause pain and phlebitis when infused through a peripheral line (not relieved by hydrocortisone or diphenhydramine). Prolonged use may result in fungal or bacterial superinfection, including *C. difficile*-associated diarrhea (CDAD) and pseudomembranous colitis; CDAD has been observed >2 months post-antibiotic treatment. May cause arthralgias, myalgias, and hyperbilirubinemia. May inhibit the metabolism of many drugs metabolized by CYP3A4. Concurrent therapy with cisapride (which may prolong QTc interval and lead to arrhythmias) should be avoided.

Adverse Reactions

Central nervous system: Headache, pain

Dermatologic: Pruritus, rash

Endocrine & metabolic: Hyperglycemia

Gastrointestinal: Diarrhea, nausea, vomiting

Hematologic: Anemia

Hepatic: Hyperbilirubinemia, increased GGT, increased LDH

Local: Inflammation at infusion site, infusion site reaction, local edema, local pain, thrombophlebitis

Neuromuscular & skeletal: Arthralgia, CPK increased, myalgia

Rare but important or life-threatening: Allergic reaction, anaphylactoid reaction, angina, apnea, arrhythmia, cardiac arrest, coagulation disorder, dysautonomia, dyspnea, encephalopathy, gout, hematuria, hemolytic anemia, hepatitis, hyperkalemia, hypotension, maculopapular rash, mesenteric artery occlusion, myasthenia, neuropathy, pancreatitis, pancytopenia, paraplegia, paresthesia, pericarditis, pleural effusion, pseudomembranous colitis, respiratory distress, seizure, shock, stomatitis, syncope, thrombocytopenia, urticaria

Drug Interactions

Metabolism/Transport Effects Refer to individual components.

Avoid Concomitant Use

Avoid concomitant use of Quinupristin and Dalfopristin with any of the following: Pimozide

Increased Effect/Toxicity

Quinupristin and Dalfopristin may increase the levels/effects of: ARIPiprazole; CycloSPORINE (Systemic); Dofetilide; Hydrocodone; Lomitapide; NiMODipine; Pimozide

Decreased Effect There are no known significant interactions involving a decrease in effect.

Storage/Stability Store unopened vials under refrigeration at 2°C to 8°C (36°F to 46°F). Stability of the diluted solution prior to the infusion is established as 5 hours at room temperature or 54 hours if refrigerated at 2°C to 8°C (36°F to 46°F). The following stability information has also been reported: May be stored at room temperature for up to 7 days (Cohen, 2007).

Mechanism of Action Quinupristin/dalfopristin inhibits bacterial protein synthesis by binding to different sites on the 50S bacterial ribosomal subunit thereby inhibiting protein synthesis

Pharmacokinetics (Adult data unless noted)

Distribution: V_d: Quinupristin: 0.45 L/kg; Dalfopristin: 0.24 L/kg

Metabolism: Quinupristin is conjugated with glutathione and cysteine to active metabolites; dalfopristin is hydrolyzed to an active metabolite

Half-life:

Quinupristin: 0.85 hour

Dalfopristin: 0.7 hour

Elimination: Feces (75% to 77% as unchanged drug and metabolites); urine (15% to 19%)

Dosing: Usual Dosage is expressed in terms of combined "mg" of quinupristin plus dalfopristin:

Infants, Children, and Adolescents: Limited data in infants and children <12 years:

General dosing, susceptible infection (*Red Book*, 2012): IV: Severe infection: 15-22.5 mg/kg/day in divided doses every 8-12 hours

Enterococcus faecium, vancomycin resistant (VREF): Limited data available: IV: 7.5 mg/kg/dose every 8 hours; dosing based on an Emergency-Use Program [n=127, mean age: 7.3 years (range: 1.2 months to 17 years)] (Loeffler, 2002) and a case series (n=8, range: 17 months to 18 years) (Gray, 2000)

MRSA, vancomycin failure salvage therapy: IV: 7.5 mg/kg/dose every 8 hours (Liu, 2011; Loeffler, 2002)

Skin and skin structure infection; complicated, treatment: IV: 7.5 mg/kg/dose every 12 hours for at least 7 days

VP-shunt infection, ventriculitis: Limited data available: Intraventricular/intrathecal **(use a preservative-free preparation)**: Usual dose: 1-2 mg/**day**; reported range: 1-5 mg; administered with concurrent IV quinupristin/dalfopristin therapy (Nachman, 1995; Tunkel, 2004; Tush, 1998)

Adults:

Bacteremia, MRSA (persistent, vancomycin failure): IV: 7.5 mg/kg every 8 hours (Liu, 2011)

Skin and skin structure infection; complicated, treatment: IV: 7.5 mg/kg/dose every 12 hours for at least 7 days

Dosing adjustment in renal impairment: No dosage adjustment is required for use in patients with renal impairment or patients undergoing peritoneal dialysis. Not removed by peritoneal dialysis or hemodialysis

Dosing adjustment in hepatic impairment: There are no dosage adjustments provided in the manufacturer labeling; not studied; pharmacokinetic data suggest adjustment may be necessary.

Preparation for Administration Parenteral: Reconstitute vial by slowly adding 5 mL D_5W or SWFI to make a 100 mg/mL solution; gently swirl the vial contents without shaking to minimize foam formation; further dilute the reconstituted solution with D_5W to a final maximum concentration for administration via peripheral line of 2 mg/mL; maximum concentration for administration via a central line is 5 mg/mL; if an injection site reaction occurs, the dose can be further diluted to a final concentration of <1 mg/mL. Do not freeze solution.

Administration Parenteral: Administer infusion over 60 minutes (toxicity may be increased with shorter infusion); prior to and following administration, the infusion line should be flushed with D_5W to minimize venous irritation; **DO NOT FLUSH** with saline or heparin solutions due to incompatibility. If severe venous irritation occurs following peripheral administration, quinupristin/dalfopristin may be further diluted, infusion site changed, or infused by a peripherally inserted central catheter (PICC) or a central venous catheter.

Monitoring Parameters CBC, liver function test; monitor infusion site closely; number and type of stools/day for diarrhea

Dosage Forms Excipient information presented when available (limited, particularly for generics); consult specific product labeling.

Injection, powder for reconstitution:

Synercid®: 500 mg: Quinupristin 150 mg and dalfopristin 350 mg

◆ **Qutenza** *see* Capsaicin *on page 362*

◆ **Qvar** *see* Beclomethasone (Oral Inhalation) *on page 262*

◆ **QVAR (Can)** *see* Beclomethasone (Oral Inhalation) *on page 262*

◆ **R-1569** *see* Tocilizumab *on page 2079*

◆ **RabAvert** *see* Rabies Vaccine *on page 1832*

RABEprazole (ra BEP ra zole)

Medication Safety Issues

Sound-alike/look-alike issues:

AcipHex may be confused with Acephen, Accupril, Aricept, pHisoHex

RABEprazole may be confused with ARIPiprazole, donepezil, lansoprazole, omeprazole, raloxifene

Related Information

Oral Medications That Should Not Be Crushed or Altered *on page 2476*

Brand Names: US Aciphex; AcipHex Sprinkle

Brand Names: Canada Apo-Rabeprazole; Pariet; Pat-Rabeprazole; PMS-Rabeprazole EC; PRO-Rabeprazole; Rabeprazole EC; RAN-Rabeprazole; Riva-Rabeprazole EC; Sandoz-Rabeprazole; Teva-Rabeprazole EC

Therapeutic Category Gastric Acid Secretion Inhibitor; Gastrointestinal Agent, Gastric or Duodenal Ulcer Treatment; Proton Pump Inhibitor

Generic Availability (US) May be product dependent

Use Treatment of symptomatic gastroesophageal reflux disease (GERD) (FDA approved in ages ≥1 year and adults); short-term treatment (4-8 weeks) and maintenance of erosive or ulcerative GERD (FDA approved in adults); short-term treatment (4 weeks) of duodenal ulcers (FDA approved in adults); long-term treatment of pathological hypersecretory conditions (eg, Zollinger-Ellison syndrome) (FDA approved in adults); in combination with clarithromycin and amoxicillin, adjunctive treatment of duodenal ulcers associated with *Helicobacter pylori* (FDA approved in adults)

Medication Guide Available Yes

Pregnancy Risk Factor C

Pregnancy Considerations Adverse events have not been observed in animal reproduction studies. Available studies have not shown an increased risk of major birth defects following maternal use of proton pump inhibitors during pregnancy; however, information specific to rabeprazole is limited (Pasternak, 2010); most information available for omeprazole. When treating GERD in pregnancy, PPIs may be used when clinically indicated (Katz, 2013).

Breast-Feeding Considerations It is not known if rabeprazole is excreted in breast milk. The manufacturer recommends that caution be exercised when administering rabeprazole to nursing women.

Contraindications Hypersensitivity (eg, anaphylaxis, anaphylactic shock, angioedema, bronchospasm, acute interstitial nephritis, urticaria) to rabeprazole, other substituted benzimidazole proton pump inhibitors, or any component of the formulation

Warnings/Precautions Use of proton pump inhibitors (PPIs) may increase the risk of gastrointestinal infections (eg, *Salmonella, Campylobacter*). Use caution in severe hepatic impairment. Relief of symptoms with rabeprazole does not preclude the presence of a gastric malignancy. Use of PPIs may increase risk of *Clostridium difficile*-associated diarrhea (CDAD), especially in hospitalized patients; consider CDAD diagnosis in patients with persistent diarrhea that does not improve. Use the lowest dose and shortest duration of PPI therapy appropriate for the condition being treated. Decreased *H. pylori* eradication rates have been observed with short-term (≤7 days) combination therapy. The American College of Gastroenterology recommends 10 to 14 days of therapy (triple or quadruple) for eradication of *H. pylori* (Chey, 2007).

PPIs may diminish the therapeutic effect of clopidogrel, thought to be due to reduced formation of the active metabolite of clopidogrel. The manufacturer of clopidogrel recommends either avoidance of both omeprazole (even when scheduled 12 hours apart) and esomeprazole or use of a PPI with comparatively less effect on the active metabolite of clopidogrel. Avoidance of rabeprazole appears prudent due to potent *in vitro* CYP2C19 inhibition (Li, 2004) and lack of sufficient comparative *in vivo* studies with other PPIs. In contrast to these warnings, others have recommended the continued use of PPIs, regardless of the degree of inhibition, in patients with a history of GI bleeding or multiple risk factors for GI bleeding who are also receiving clopidogrel since no evidence has established clinically meaningful differences in outcome; however, a clinically-significant interaction cannot be excluded in those who are poor metabolizers of clopidogrel (Abraham, 2010; Levine, 2011). Potentially significant drug-drug interactions may exist, requiring dose or frequency adjustment, additional monitoring, and/or selection of alternative therapy.

Increased incidence of osteoporosis-related bone fractures of the hip, spine, or wrist may occur with PPI therapy. Patients on high-dose (multiple daily doses) or long-term therapy (≥1 year) should be monitored. Acute interstitial nephritis has been observed in patients taking PPIs; may occur at any time during therapy and is generally due to an idiopathic hypersensitivity reaction. Discontinue if acute interstitial nephritis develops. Use the lowest effective dose for the shortest duration of time, use vitamin D and calcium supplementation, and follow appropriate guidelines to reduce risk of fractures in patients at risk.

Hypomagnesemia, reported rarely, usually with prolonged PPI use of >3 months (most cases >1 year of therapy); may be symptomatic or asymptomatic; severe cases may cause tetany, seizures, and cardiac arrhythmias. Consider obtaining serum magnesium concentrations prior to beginning long-term therapy, especially if taking concomitant digoxin, diuretics, or other drugs known to cause hypomagnesemia; and periodically thereafter. Hypomagnesemia may be corrected by magnesium supplementation, although discontinuation of rabeprazole may be necessary; magnesium levels typically return to normal within 1 week of stopping.

Prolonged treatment (≥2 years) may lead to vitamin B_{12} malabsorption and subsequent vitamin B_{12} deficiency. The magnitude of the deficiency is dose-related and the association is stronger in females and those younger in age (<30 years); prevalence is decreased after discontinuation of therapy (Lam, 2013).

Adverse Reactions

Cardiovascular: Peripheral edema

Central nervous system: Dizziness, headache, pain

Gastrointestinal: Abdominal pain, constipation, diarrhea, flatulence, nausea, vomiting, xerostomia

Hepatic: Hepatic encephalopathy, hepatitis, increased liver enzymes

Infection: Increased susceptibility to infection

Neuromuscular & skeletal: Arthralgia, myalgia

Respiratory: Pharyngitis

Rare but important or life-threatening:Agranulocytosis, albuminuria, alopecia, amblyopia, anaphylaxis, anemia, angioedema, bone fracture, bullous rash, cholecystitis, cholelithiasis, *Clostridium difficile* associated diarrhea (CDAD), colitis, coma, delirium, disorientation, erythema multiforme, gynecomastia, hematuria, hemolytic anemia, hepatotoxicity (idiosyncratic) (Chalasani, 2014), hyperammonemia, hypersensitivity reaction, hypertension, hypokalemia, hypomagnesemia, hyponatremia, increased thyroid stimulating hormone level, interstitial nephritis, jaundice, leukocytosis, leukopenia, melena, migraine, neutropenia, osteoporosis, palpitation, pancreatitis, pancytopenia, pathological fracture due to osteoporosis, pneumonia, rhabdomyolysis, sinus bradycardia, Stevens-Johnson syndrome, thrombocytopenia, toxic epidermal necrolysis

Drug Interactions

Metabolism/Transport Effects **Substrate** of CYP2C19 (major), CYP3A4 (major); **Note:** Assignment of Major/Minor substrate status based on clinically relevant drug interaction potential; **Inhibits** CYP2C19 (weak), CYP2C8 (moderate), CYP2D6 (weak)

Avoid Concomitant Use

Avoid concomitant use of RABEprazole with any of the following: Amodiaquine; Dasatinib; Delavirdine; Erlotinib; Nelfinavir; PAZOPanib; Rilpivirine; Risedronate

Increased Effect/Toxicity

RABEprazole may increase the levels/effects of: Amodiaquine; Amphetamine; ARIPiprazole; CYP2C8 Substrates; Dexmethylphenidate; Dextroamphetamine; Methotrexate; Methylphenidate; Raltegravir; Risedronate; Saquinavir; Tacrolimus (Systemic); Voriconazole

The levels/effects of RABEprazole may be increased by: Fluconazole; Ketoconazole (Systemic); Voriconazole

Decreased Effect

RABEprazole may decrease the levels/effects of: Atazanavir; Bisphosphonate Derivatives; Bosutinib; Cefditoren; Clopidogrel; Dabigatran Etexilate; Dabrafenib; Dasatinib; Delavirdine; Erlotinib; Gefitinib; Indinavir; Iron Salts; Itraconazole; Ketoconazole (Systemic); Ledipasvir; Mesalamine; Multivitamins/Minerals (with ADEK, Folate, Iron); Mycophenolate; Nelfinavir; Nilotinib; PAZOPanib; Posaconazole; Rilpivirine; Riociguat; Risedronate

The levels/effects of RABEprazole may be decreased by: Bosentan; CYP2C19 Inducers (Strong); CYP3A4 Inducers (Moderate); CYP3A4 Inducers (Strong); Dabrafenib; Deferasirox; Mitotane; Siltuximab; St Johns Wort; Tipranavir; Tocilizumab

Food Interactions Prolonged treatment (≥2 years) may lead to malabsorption of dietary vitamin B_{12} and subsequent vitamin B_{12} deficiency (Lam, 2013).

Storage/Stability Store at 25°C (77°F); excursions are permitted between 15°C and 30°C (59°F and 86°F). Protect from moisture.

Mechanism of Action Potent proton pump inhibitor; suppresses gastric acid secretion by inhibiting the parietal cell H+/K+ ATP pump

Pharmacodynamics

Onset of action: 1 hour

Duration: 24 hours

Pharmacokinetics (Adult data unless noted)

Protein binding: 96.3%

Metabolism: Extensive hepatic metabolism via cytochrome isoenzymes CYP3A and CYP2C19 to inactive metabolites; CYP2C19 exhibits a known genetic polymorphism due to its deficiency in some subpopulations (3% to 5% of Caucasians and 17% to 20% of Asians) which results in slower metabolism

Bioavailability: Tablet: 52%

Half-life:

Adolescents: ~0.55-1 hour (James, 2007)

Adults: 1-2 hours

Time to peak serum concentration:

Adolescents: Tablet: 3.3-4.1 hours (James, 2007)

Adults: Capsule: 1-6.5 hours; Tablet: 2-5 hours

Excretion: 90% in urine

Dosing: Usual

Children and Adolescents:

GERD, symptomatic: Oral:

Children 1-11 years:

<15 kg: 5 mg once daily for ≤12 weeks; if inadequate response may increase to 10 mg once daily

≥15 kg: 10 mg once daily for ≤12 weeks

Children ≥12 years and Adolescents: 20 mg once daily for up to 8 weeks

Adults:

GERD, erosive/ulcerative: Oral: Treatment: 20 mg once daily for 4-8 weeks; if inadequate response, may repeat up to an additional 8 weeks; maintenance: 20 mg once daily

GERD, symptomatic: Oral: Treatment: 20 mg once daily for 4 weeks; if inadequate response, may repeat for an additional 4 weeks

Duodenal ulcer: Oral: 20 mg once daily for ≤4 weeks; additional therapy may be required for some patients

***Helicobacter pylori* eradication:** Oral: 20 mg twice daily administered for 7 days (in combination with clarithromycin and amoxicillin)

Hypersecretory conditions (eg, Zollinger-Ellison Syndrome): Oral: 60 mg once daily; dose may need to be adjusted as necessary. Doses as high as 100 mg once daily and 60 mg twice daily have been used and continued as long as necessary (up to 1 year in some patients).

Dosing adjustment in renal impairment: Children ≥1 year, Adolescents, and Adults: No dosage adjustments are recommended

Dosing adjustment in hepatic impairment: Children ≥1 year, Adolescents, and Adults:

Mild to moderate: No dosage adjustments are recommended

Severe impairment: There are no dosage adjustments provided in the manufacturer's labeling (has not been studied). Use with caution; elimination may be decreased.

Administration

Oral: May administer with an antacid.

Capsules: Administer 30 minutes before a meal. Open capsule and sprinkle contents on a small amount of soft food (eg, applesauce, fruit- or vegetable-based baby food, yogurt) or empty contents into a small amount of liquid (eg, infant formula, apple juice, pediatric electrolyte solution); food or liquid should be at or below room temperature. Do not chew or crush granules; administer whole dose within 15 minutes of preparation; do not store for future use.

Tablets: May be administered without regard to food; best if taken 30 minutes before a meal when treating GERD (Lightdale, 2013). Tablets should be swallowed whole, do not chew, crush, or split.

Monitoring Parameters Magnesium levels in patients on long-term treatment or those taking digoxin, diuretics, or other drugs that cause hypomagnesemia; susceptibility testing recommended in patients who fail *H. pylori* eradication regimen.

Dosage Forms Excipient information presented when available (limited, particularly for generics); consult specific product labeling.

Capsule Sprinkle, Oral, as sodium:

AcipHex Sprinkle: 5 mg [contains fd&c blue #2 aluminum lake]

AcipHex Sprinkle: 10 mg [contains fd&c yellow #6 (sunset yellow)]

Tablet Delayed Release, Oral, as sodium:

Aciphex: 20 mg

Generic: 20 mg

◆ **Rabeprazole EC (Can)** *see* RABEprazole *on page 1828*

Rabies Immune Globulin (Human)

(RAY beez i MYUN GLOB yoo lin, HYU man)

Medication Safety Issues

International issues:

Bayrab [Philippines, Turkey] may be confused with Bayhep-B which is a brand name for hepatitis B immune globulin [Philippines, Turkey]; Bayrho-D which is brand name for Rh_oD immune globulin [Israel, Turkey]

Related Information

Centers for Disease Control and Prevention (CDC) and Other Links *on page 2424*

Immunization Administration Recommendations *on page 2411*

Immunization Schedules *on page 2416*

Brand Names: US HyperRAB S/D; Imogam Rabies-HT

Brand Names: Canada HyperRAB S/D; Imogam Rabies Pasteurized

Therapeutic Category Immune Globulin

Generic Availability (US) No

Use Part of postexposure prophylaxis of persons with suspected rabies exposure. Provides passive immunity until active immunity with rabies vaccine is established (FDA approved in all patients). Not for use in persons with a history of preexposure vaccination or postexposure prophylaxis with human diploid cell vaccine (HDCV), purified chick embryo cell vaccine, or rabies vaccine adsorbed, or previous vaccination with any other rabies vaccine and documentation of antibody response. Each exposure to possible rabies infection should be individually evaluated.

Factors to consider include: Species of biting animal, circumstances of biting incident (provoked vs unprovoked bite), type of exposure to rabies infection (bite vs nonbite), vaccination status of biting animal, and presence of rabies in the region. See product information for additional details.

Pregnancy Risk Factor C

Pregnancy Considerations Animal reproduction studies have not been conducted. Pregnancy is not a contraindication to postexposure prophylaxis. Pre-exposure prophylaxis may be indicated during pregnancy if the risk for exposure to rabies is significant.

Breast-Feeding Considerations Immunoglobulins are excreted in breast milk. The manufacturer recommends that caution be exercised when administering Imogam Rabies-HT immune globulin to nursing women.

Contraindications

Imogam Rabies-HT: Should not be administered in repeated doses once vaccine treatment has been initiated.

HyperRAB SD: There are no contraindications listed in the manufacturer's labeling.

Documentation of allergenic cross-reactivity for immune globulins is limited. However, because of similarities in chemical structure and/or pharmacologic actions, the possibility of cross-sensitivity cannot be ruled out with certainty.

Warnings/Precautions Hypersensitivity and anaphylactic reactions can occur; immediate treatment (including epinephrine 1:1000) should be available. Use with caution in patients with isolated immunoglobulin A deficiency or a history of systemic hypersensitivity to human immunoglobulins. Use with caution in patients with a history of bleeding disorders (including thrombocytopenia) and/or patients on anticoagulant therapy; bleeding/hematoma may occur from IM administration. Product of human plasma; may potentially contain infectious agents which could transmit disease. Screening of donors, as well as testing and/or inactivation or removal of certain viruses, reduces the risk. Infections thought to be transmitted by this product should be reported to the manufacturer. Administration is a medical urgency (not emergency); however, do not delay decision to treat. Not for intravenous administration. A single dose is recommended; repeating the dose may interfere with maximum active immunity expected from the vaccine. Repeated doses of Imogam Rabies-HT after vaccine treatment has been initiated are contraindicated. after vaccine treatment has been initiated. Live vaccines (eg, measles vaccine) should be given ≥3 months after rabies immune globulin; antibodies may interfere with the immune response to the live vaccine.

Adverse Reactions

Central nervous system: Fever (mild), headache, malaise

Dermatologic: Angioneurotic edema, rash

Local: Injection site: Pain, stiffness, soreness, tenderness

Renal: Nephrotic syndrome

Miscellaneous: Anaphylaxis

Drug Interactions

Metabolism/Transport Effects None known.

Avoid Concomitant Use There are no known interactions where it is recommended to avoid concomitant use.

Increased Effect/Toxicity There are no known significant interactions involving an increase in effect.

Decreased Effect

Rabies Immune Globulin (Human) may decrease the levels/effects of: Vaccines (Live)

Storage/Stability Store between 2°C to 8°C (36°F to 46°F); do not freeze. Discard unused portion immediately and any product exposed to freezing. The following stability information has also been reported for HyperRAB S/D: May be exposed to room temperature for a cumulative 7 days (Cohen, 2007).

Mechanism of Action Rabies immune globulin is a solution of globulins dried from the plasma or serum of selected adult human donors who have been immunized with rabies vaccine and have developed high titers of rabies antibody. It generally contains 10% to 18% of protein of which not less than 80% is monomeric immunoglobulin G.

Pharmacokinetics (Adult data unless noted) Half-life: 21 days (CDC [Manning], 2008)

Dosing: Neonatal

Postexposure prophylaxis (ACIP Recommendation): Local wound infiltration: 20 units/kg single dose administered as soon as possible after exposure. If anatomically feasible, the full rabies immune globulin (RIG) dose should be infiltrated around and into the wound(s); any remaining volume should be administered IM at a site distant from the vaccine administration site. If rabies vaccine was initiated without rabies immune globulin, rabies immune globulin may be administered through the seventh day after the first vaccine dose. Administration of RIG is not recommended after the seventh day postvaccine since an antibody response to the vaccine is expected during this time period (CDC, 2010).

Dosing: Usual Note: Not recommended for use in persons with a history of preexposure vaccination or postexposure prophylaxis with human diploid cell vaccine (HDCV), purified chick embryo cell vaccine, rabies vaccine adsorbed, or previous vaccination with any other rabies vaccine and documentation of antibody response.

Pediatric: **Postexposure prophylaxis:** Local wound infiltration: Infants, Children, and Adolescents: 20 units/kg single dose administered as soon as possible after exposure; do not exceed recommended dose since passive antibody can interfere with response to rabies vaccine. If anatomically feasible, the full rabies immune globulin (RIG) dose should be infiltrated around and into the wound(s); any remaining volume should be administered IM at a site distant from the vaccine administration site. If rabies vaccine was initiated without rabies immune globulin, rabies immune globulin may be administered through the seventh day after the first vaccine dose. Administration of RIG is not recommended after the seventh day postvaccine since an antibody response to the vaccine is expected during this time period (CDC 59 [RR2], 2010).

Adult: **Postexposure prophylaxis:** Local wound infiltration: 20 units/kg single dose administered as soon as possible after exposure; do not exceed recommended dose since passive antibody can interfere with response to rabies vaccine. If anatomically feasible, the full rabies immune globulin (RIG) dose should be infiltrated around and into the wound(s); any remaining volume should be administered IM at a site distant from the vaccine administration site. If rabies vaccine was initiated without rabies immune globulin, rabies immune globulin may be administered through the seventh day after the first vaccine dose. Administration of RIG is not recommended after the seventh day postvaccine since an antibody response to the vaccine is expected during this time period.

Dosing adjustment in renal impairment: There are no dosage adjustments provided in manufacturer's labeling.

Dosing adjustment in hepatic impairment: There are no dosage adjustments provided in manufacturer's labeling.

Administration Do **not** administer IV Do not administer rabies vaccine in the same syringe or at same administration site as RIG.

Wound infiltration: Thoroughly cleanse wound(s) with soap and water; use povidone-iodine solution to irrigate the wound(s); infiltrate with RIG in the area around and into the wound(s); any remaining dose should be administered IM If RIG dose volume is insufficient for wound(s) infiltration, dilute RIG two- to threefold in NS to an adequate volume to insure that all wound areas receive infiltrate (*Red Book*, 2012).

IM: Inject into the deltoid muscle of the upper arm or lateral thigh muscle at a site distant from rabies vaccine administration. The gluteal area should be avoided to reduce the risk of sciatic nerve damage. Infants and children with small muscle mass may require multiple IM sites for dose delivery.

Monitoring Parameters Serum rabies antibody titer (if rabies immune globulin is inadvertently administered after the eighth day from the first rabies vaccine dose).

Dosage Forms Excipient information presented when available (limited, particularly for generics); consult specific product labeling.

Injectable, Intramuscular:
 Imogam Rabies-HT: 150 units/mL (2 mL, 10 mL)

Injectable, Intramuscular [preservative free]:
 HyperRAB S/D: 150 units/mL (2 mL, 10 mL)

Rabies Vaccine (RAY beez vak SEEN)

Related Information

Centers for Disease Control and Prevention (CDC) and Other Links *on page 2424*

Immunization Administration Recommendations *on page 2411*

Immunization Schedules *on page 2416*

Brand Names: US Imovax Rabies; RabAvert

Brand Names: Canada Imovax Rabies; RabAvert

Therapeutic Category Vaccine; Vaccine, Inactivated Virus

Generic Availability (US) No

Use

Pre-exposure immunization: To provide protection against rabies virus to persons with unrecognized exposure or to those in areas where postexposure treatment would be delayed (FDA approved in all ages). Vaccinate persons with greater than usual risk due to occupation or avocation, including veterinarians, rangers, animal handlers, certain laboratory workers, and persons living in or visiting countries for longer than 1 month where rabies is a constant threat. **Note:** Routine pre-exposure prophylaxis for the general U.S. population or routine travelers to areas where rabies is not enzootic is not recommended

Postexposure prophylaxis: To provide protection against rabies virus. If a bite from a carrier animal is unprovoked or if the animal is not captured and rabies is present in that species and area, administer rabies immune globulin (RIG) and the vaccine as indicated (FDA approved in all ages)

Medication Guide Available Yes

Pregnancy Risk Factor C

Pregnancy Considerations Animal reproduction studies have not been conducted. Pregnancy is not a contraindication to postexposure prophylaxis. Pre-exposure prophylaxis during pregnancy may also be considered if risk of rabies is great.

Breast-Feeding Considerations Breast-feeding mothers may be vaccinated. Inactivated virus vaccines do not affect the safety of breast-feeding for the mother or the infant. Breast-feeding infants should be vaccinated according to the recommended schedules (CDC, 2011)

Contraindications

Pre-exposure prophylaxis: Hypersensitivity to rabies vaccine or any component of the formulation

Postexposure prophylaxis: There are no contraindications listed within the FDA-approved manufacturer's labeling.

Warnings/Precautions Rabies vaccine should not be used in persons with a confirmed diagnosis of rabies; use after the onset of symptoms may be detrimental. Postexposure vaccination may begin regardless of the length of time from documented or likely exposure, as long as clinical signs of rabies are not present. Immediate treatment (including epinephrine 1:1000) for anaphylactoid and/or hypersensitivity reactions should be available during vaccine use. Once postexposure prophylaxis has begun, administration should generally not be interrupted or discontinued due to local or mild adverse events. Continuation of vaccination following severe systemic reactions should consider the persons risk of developing rabies. Report serious reactions to the State Health Department or the manufacturer/distributor. An immune complex reaction is possible 2-21 days following booster doses of HDCV. Symptoms may include arthralgia, arthritis, angioedema, fever, generalized urticaria, malaise, nausea, and vomiting. Syncope has been reported with use of injectable vaccines and may be accompanied by transient visual disturbances, weakness, or tonic-clonic movements. Procedures should be in place to avoid injuries from falling and to restore cerebral perfusion if syncope occurs. Vaccination may not result in effective immunity in all patients. Response depends upon multiple factors (eg, type of vaccine, age of patient) and may be improved by administering the vaccine at the recommended dose, route, and interval. Vaccines may not be effective if administered during periods of altered immune competence (CDC, 2011). Use with caution in severely immunocompromised patients (eg, patients receiving chemo/radiation therapy or other immunosuppressive therapy [including high-dose corticosteroids]); may have a reduced response to vaccination. Withhold nonessential immunosuppressive agents during postexposure prophylaxis; if possible postpone pre-exposure prophylaxis until the immunocompromising condition is resolved. Persons with altered immunocompetence should receive the five-dose postexposure vaccine regimen. In general, household and close contacts of persons with altered immunocompetence may receive all age appropriate vaccines. Products may contain albumin and therefore carry a remote risk of transmitting Creutzfeldt-Jakob or other viral diseases. Imovax® Rabies contains neomycin. RabAvert® contains amphotericin B, bovine gelatin, chicken protein, chlortetracycline, and neomycin. For I. M. administration only.

Warnings: Additional Pediatric Considerations Antipyretics have not been shown to prevent febrile seizures; antipyretics may be used to treat fever or discomfort following vaccination (CDC, 2011). One study reported that routine prophylactic administration of acetaminophen to prevent fever prior to vaccination decreased the immune response of some vaccines; the clinical significance of this reduction in immune response has not been established (Prymula, 2009).

Adverse Reactions All serious adverse reactions must be reported to the U.S. Department of Health and Human Services (DHHS) Vaccine Adverse Event Reporting System (VAERS) 1-800-822-7967 or online at https://vaers.hhs.gov/esub/index. In Canada, adverse reactions may be reported to local provincial/territorial health agencies or to the Vaccine Safety Section at Public Health Agency of Canada (1-866-844-0018).

Cardiovascular: Circulatory reactions, edema, palpitation

Central nervous system: Chills, dizziness, encephalitis, fatigue, fever >38°C (100°F), Guillain-Barré syndrome, headache, malaise, meningitis, multiple sclerosis, myelitis, neuroparalysis, seizures, vertigo

Dermatologic: Pruritus, urticaria, urticaria pigmentosa

Endocrine & metabolic: Hot flashes

Gastrointestinal: Diarrhea, vomiting

Local: Hematoma, limb swelling (extensive)

Neuromuscular & skeletal: Arthralgia, limb pain, monoarthritis, neuropathy, paralysis (transient), paresthesias (transient), weakness

Ocular: Retrobulbar neuritis, visual disturbances

Respiratory: Bronchospasm, dyspnea, wheezing

Miscellaneous: Allergic reactions, anaphylaxis, hypersensitivity reactions, serum sickness, swollen lymph nodes

Drug Interactions

Metabolism/Transport Effects None known.

Avoid Concomitant Use There are no known interactions where it is recommended to avoid concomitant use.

Increased Effect/Toxicity There are no known significant interactions involving an increase in effect.

Decreased Effect

The levels/effects of Rabies Vaccine may be decreased by: Belimumab; Chloroquine; Fingolimod; Immunosuppressants

Storage/Stability Prior to reconstitution, store under refrigeration at 2°C to 8°C (36°F to 46°F); do not freeze. Protect from light.

Mechanism of Action Rabies vaccine is an inactivated virus vaccine which promotes immunity by inducing an active immune response. The production of specific antibodies requires about 7-10 days to develop. Rabies immune globulin or antirabies serum, equine (ARS) is given in conjunction with rabies vaccine to provide immune protection until an antibody response can occur.

Pharmacodynamics

Onset of action: IM: Rabies antibody: ~7-10 days

Peak effect: ~30-60 days

Duration: ≥1 year

Dosing: Neonatal Postexposure prophylaxis: All postexposure treatment should begin with immediate cleansing of the wound with soap and water (for ~15 minutes); immunization should begin as soon as possible after exposure.

ACIP Recommendations: IM: 1 mL/dose for 4 doses, on days 0, 3, 7, and 14; **Note:** Immunocompromised patients should receive a fifth dose on day 28. Administer rabies immune globulin (RIG) 20 units/kg body weight around and into the wound(s) if anatomically feasible; administer any remaining volume of the RIG dose IM at a distant anatomical site (CDC, 2010).

Dosing: Usual Infants, Children, Adolescents, and Adults: IM:

Pre-exposure prophylaxis: 1 mL/dose for 3 doses, on days 0, 7, and 21 or 28. Frequency of booster doses dependent upon rabies exposure risk and may include using antibody titers drawn every 6 months to 2 years to determine booster dose need. **Note:** Prolonging the interval between doses does not interfere with immunity achieved after the concluding dose of the basic series.

Postexposure prophylaxis: All postexposure treatment should begin with immediate cleansing of the wound with soap and water (for ~15 minutes); immunization should begin as soon as possible after exposure.

Persons not previously immunized (ACIP Recommendation): 1 mL/dose for 4 doses, on days 0, 3, 7, and 14; **Note:** Immunocompromised patients should receive a fifth dose on day 28. Administer rabies immune globulin (RIG) 20 units/kg body weight around and into the wound(s) if anatomically feasible; administer any remaining volume of the RIG dose IM at a distant anatomical site (CDC, 2010).

Persons who have previously received vaccine (either previous postexposure prophylaxis or pre-exposure series of vaccination) or have a previously documented rabies antibody titer considered adequate: 1 mL/dose on days 0 and 3; do not administer RIG

Preparation for Administration

IM: Reconstitute with entire contents of provided diluent; slowly inject diluent into the vaccine vial; gently swirl to dissolve to avoid foaming. Use immediately after reconstitution.

Imovax: Suspension will appear pink to red.

RabAvert: Suspension will appear clear to slightly opaque.

Administration IM: **Not for IV or SubQ administration;** reconstitute immediately before administration; administer injections in the deltoid muscle, not the gluteal; for infants and small children the outer aspect of the thigh may be used. Do not administer in same syringe as RIG. Adolescents and adults should be vaccinated while seated or lying down.

Monitoring Parameters Serum rabies antibody titers are not routinely recommended in postexposure patients unless the patient was immunocompromised; to determine the need for repeat booster treatment, titers may be measured every 6 months to 2 years in persons at high risk for exposure. Observe for syncope for 15 minutes following administration. If seizure-like activity associated with syncope occurs, maintain patient in supine or Trendelenburg position to reestablish adequate cerebral perfusion.

Additional Information In order to maximize vaccination rates, the ACIP recommends simultaneous administration (ie, >1 vaccine on the same day at different anatomic sites) of all age-appropriate vaccines (live or inactivated) for which a person is eligible at a single visit, unless contraindications exist. If available, the use of combination vaccines is generally preferred over separate injections, taking into consideration provider assessment, patient preference, and potential adverse events. If separate vaccines being used, evaluate product information regarding same syringe compatibility of vaccines. Separate needles and syringes should be used for each injection. The ACIP prefers each dose of specific vaccine in a series come from the same manufacturer if possible. (CDC, 2011)

For additional information, please refer to the following website: http://www.cdc.gov/vaccines/vpd-vac/.

Dosage Forms Excipient information presented when available (limited, particularly for generics); consult specific product labeling.

Injectable, Intramuscular [preservative free]:

Imovax Rabies: 2.5 units/mL (1 ea) [contains albumin human, neomycin sulfate]

Suspension Reconstituted, Intramuscular:

RabAvert: 2.5 units (1 ea) [contains albumin human, chicken protein, edetate disodium, gelatin (bovine), neomycin]

- **Racemic Epinephrine** *see* EPINEPHrine (Systemic, Oral Inhalation) *on page 760*
- **Racepinephrine** *see* EPINEPHrine (Systemic, Oral Inhalation) *on page 760*
- **RAD001** *see* Everolimus *on page 825*
- **rAHF** *see* Antihemophilic Factor (Recombinant) *on page 168*
- **RAL** *see* Raltegravir *on page 1833*
- **R-albuterol** *see* Levalbuterol *on page 1233*
- **Ralivia (Can)** *see* TraMADol *on page 2098*

Raltegravir (ral TEG ra vir)

Medication Safety Issues

High alert medication:

This medication is in a class the Institute for Safe Medication Practices (ISMP) includes among its list of drug classes that have a heightened risk of causing significant patient harm when used in error.

Related Information

Adult and Adolescent HIV *on page 2392*

Pediatric HIV *on page 2380*

Perinatal HIV *on page 2400*

Brand Names: US Isentress

Brand Names: Canada Isentress

Therapeutic Category Antiretroviral, Integrase Inhibitor (Anti-HIV); Antiviral Agent; HIV Agents (Anti-HIV Agents); Integrase Inhibitor

Generic Availability (US) No

Use Treatment of HIV-1 infection in combination with other antiretroviral agents (FDA approved in ages ≥4 weeks weighing ≥3 kg and adults). **Note:** HIV regimens consisting of **three** antiretroviral agents are strongly recommended.

Pregnancy Risk Factor C

Pregnancy Considerations Adverse events were observed in some animal reproduction studies. Raltegravir has high transfer across the human placenta and can be detected in neonatal serum after delivery. Standard doses appear to be appropriate in pregnant women. The DHHS Perinatal HIV Guidelines consider raltegravir to be an alternative for use in antiretroviral-naïve pregnant patients when drug interactions with protease inhibitors are a concern. Because of its ability to rapidly suppress viral load, some experts have suggested using raltegravir in late pregnancy in women who have high viral loads; however, this use is not routinely recommended at this time. Reversible elevation of liver enzymes occurred in a patient who initiated raltegravir late in pregnancy; monitor liver enzymes if used during pregnancy.

Regardless of CD4 count or HIV RNA copy number, all HIV-infected pregnant women should receive a combination antiretroviral (ARV) drug regimen. A combination of antepartum, intrapartum, and infant ARV prophylaxis is recommended. ARV therapy should be started as soon as possible in women with symptomatic infection. Although earlier initiation may be more effective in reducing the perinatal transmission of HIV, initiation may be delayed until after 12 weeks gestation in women who do not require immediate treatment after careful consideration of maternal conditions (eg nausea and vomiting) and the potential risks of first trimester fetal exposure for specific agents. A scheduled cesarean delivery at 38 weeks gestation is recommended for all women with HIV RNA >1000 copies/mL or unknown concentrations near delivery in order to decrease transmission. If ARV therapy must be interrupted for <24 hours during the peripartum period, stop then restart all medications simultaneously in order to decrease the chance of developing resistance. Long-term follow-up is recommended for all infants exposed to ARV medications. In couples who want to conceive, the HIV-infected partner should attain maximum viral suppression prior to conception.

Health care providers are encouraged to enroll pregnant women exposed to antiretroviral medications in the Antiretroviral Pregnancy Registry (1-800-258-4263 or www.-APRegistry.com). Health care providers caring for HIV-infected women and their infants may contact the National Perinatal HIV Hotline (888-448-8765) for clinical consultation (HHS [perinatal], 2014).

Breast-Feeding Considerations It is not known if raltegravir is excreted into breast milk. Maternal or infant antiretroviral therapy does not completely eliminate the risk of postnatal HIV transmission. In addition, multiclass-resistant virus has been detected in breast-feeding infants despite maternal therapy. Therefore, in the United States, where formula is accessible, affordable, safe, and sustainable, and the risk of infant mortality due to diarrhea and respiratory infections is low, complete avoidance of breast-feeding by HIV-infected women is recommended to decrease potential transmission of HIV (HHS [perinatal], 2014).

Contraindications

There are no contraindications listed in the manufacturer's labeling.

Canadian labeling: Hypersensitivity to raltegravir or any other component of the formulation

Warnings/Precautions Patients may develop immune reconstitution syndrome resulting in the occurrence of an inflammatory response to an indolent or residual opportunistic infection during initial HIV treatment or activation of autoimmune disorders (eg, Graves' disease, polymyositis, Guillain-Barré syndrome) later in therapy; further evaluation and treatment may be required. Severe, life-threatening or fatal cases of Stevens-Johnson syndrome and toxic epidermal necrolysis have been reported. Hypersensitivity reactions (rash [may occur with fever, fatigue, malaise, conjunctivitis, or other constitutional symptoms], organ dysfunction and/or hepatic failure) have also been reported. Discontinue immediately if a severe skin reaction or hypersensitivity symptoms develop. Monitor liver transaminases and start supportive therapy. Myopathy and rhabdomyolysis have been reported; use caution in patients with risk factors for CK elevations and/or skeletal muscle abnormalities. Potentially significant drug-drug interactions may exist, requiring dose or frequency adjustment, additional monitoring, and/or selection of alternative therapy. Avoid use as a boosted PI replacement in antiretroviral experienced patients with documented resistance to nucleoside reverse transcriptase inhibitors. Chewable tablet contains phenylalanine. Raltegravir film-coated tablets and chewable tablets or oral suspension are not bioequivalent and are not substitutable on a mg/mg basis.

Adverse Reactions

Central nervous system: Dizziness, fatigue, headache, insomnia

Endocrine & metabolic: Increased serum glucose

Gastrointestinal: Increased serum amylase, increased serum lipase, nausea

Hematologic: Abnormal absolute neutrophil count, thrombocytopenia

Hepatic: Hyperbilirubinemia, increased serum alkaline phosphatase, increased serum ALT (incidence higher with hepatitis B and/or C coinfection), increased serum AST (incidence higher with hepatitis B and/or C coinfection)

Neuromuscular & skeletal: Increased creatine phosphokinase

Rare but important or life-threatening: Anemia, cerebellar ataxia, depression (particularly in subjects with a preexisting history of psychiatric illness), drug rash with eosinophilia and systemic symptoms (DRESS; Perry, 2013), gastritis, hepatic failure, hepatitis, hypersensitivity, myopathy, nephrolithiasis, psychomotor agitation (children; grade 3), renal failure, rhabdomyolysis, Stevens-Johnson syndrome, suicidal ideation, toxic epidermal necrolysis

Drug Interactions

Metabolism/Transport Effects Substrate of UGT1A1

Avoid Concomitant Use

Avoid concomitant use of Raltegravir with any of the following: Aluminum Hydroxide; Magnesium Salts

Increased Effect/Toxicity

Raltegravir may increase the levels/effects of: Fibric Acid Derivatives; HMG-CoA Reductase Inhibitors; Zidovudine

The levels/effects of Raltegravir may be increased by: Proton Pump Inhibitors; Rifapentine

Decreased Effect

Raltegravir may decrease the levels/effects of: Fosamprenavir

The levels/effects of Raltegravir may be decreased by: Aluminum Hydroxide; Fosamprenavir; Magnesium Salts; Rifabutin; Rifampin; Rifapentine; Tipranavir

Food Interactions Variable absorption depending upon meal type (low- vs high-fat meal) and dosage form. Management: Raltegravir was administered without regard to meals in clinical trials.

Storage/Stability

Store at 20°C to 25°C (68°F to 77°F); excursions are permitted between 15°C and 30°C (59°F and 86°F).

Chewable tablets: Store in the original package; keep desiccant in the bottle to protect from moisture.

Oral suspension: Store in the original container; do not open foil packet until ready for reconstitution and use.

Mechanism of Action Incorporation of viral DNA into the host cell's genome is required to produce a self-replicating provirus and propagation of infectious virion particles. The viral cDNA strand produced by reverse transcriptase is subsequently processed and inserted into the human genome by the enzyme HIV-1 integrase (encoded by the pol gene of HIV). Raltegravir inhibits the catalytic activity of integrase, thus preventing integration of the proviral gene into human DNA.

Pharmacokinetics (Adult data unless noted)

Protein binding: ~83%

Metabolism: Primarily hepatic glucuronidation mediated by UGT1A1

Bioavailability: Film-coated tablet: Not established; Chewable tablet: Higher oral bioavailability compared to film-coated tablet; dosage forms are not interchangeable.

Half-life elimination: ~9 hours

Time to peak, serum concentration: Film-coated tablet: ~3 hours

Elimination: Feces (~51% as unchanged drug); urine (~32%; 9% as unchanged drug)

Dosing: Usual Note: Chewable tablets and oral suspension are not bioequivalent with film-coated tablets; dosing is not interchangeable.

Pediatric: **HIV infection, treatment:** Oral: **Note:** Use in combination with other antiretroviral agents.

Oral suspension (20 mg/mL): Infants and Children weighing 3 to <20 kg:

Weight-directed dosing: 6 mg/kg/dose twice daily; maximum dose: 100 mg/dose

Fixed-dosing:

3 to <4 kg: 20 mg (1 mL) twice daily
4 to <6 kg: 30 mg (1.5 mL) twice daily
6 to <8 kg: 40 mg (2 mL) twice daily
8 to <11 kg: 60 mg (3 mL) twice daily
11 to <14 kg: 80 mg (4 mL) twice daily
14 to <20 kg: 100 mg (5 mL) twice daily

Chewable tablets: Children weighing ≥11 kg:

Weight-directed dosing: 6 mg/kg/dose twice daily; maximum dose: 300 mg/dose

Fixed-dosing:

11 to <14 kg: 75 mg (3 x 25 mg tablet) twice daily
14 to <20 kg: 100 mg (1 x 100 mg tablet) twice daily
20 to <28 kg: 150 mg (1.5 x 100 mg tablet) twice daily
28 to <40 kg: 200 mg (2 x 100 mg tablet) twice daily
≥40 kg: 300 mg (3 x 100 mg tablet) twice daily

Film-coated tablets: Children and Adolescents weighing ≥25 kg: 400 mg twice daily

Adult: **HIV infection, treatment:** Oral: **Note:** Use in combination with other antiretroviral agents: Film-coated tablet: 400 mg twice daily

Dosing adjustment for concomitant therapy: Adults: Concomitant rifampin therapy: Raltegravir dose: Film-coated tablet: 800 mg twice daily

Dosing adjustment in renal impairment: Infants, Children, Adolescents, and Adults: No dosage adjustment required

Dosing adjustment in hepatic impairment: Infants, Children, Adolescents, and Adults:

Mild to moderate hepatic impairment: No dosage adjustment required

Severe impairment: No data available

Preparation for Administration Oral suspension: Open foil packet of drug (100 mg). Measure 5 mL water in provided mixing cup. Pour packet contents into 5 mL water, close lid, and swirl for 30 to 60 seconds; do not turn the mixing cup upside down; resulting concentration: 20 mg/mL. Once mixed, measure recommended suspension dose with an oral syringe. Discard any remaining suspension in the trash.

Administration Oral: May be administered without regard to meals.

Chewable tablets: May be chewed or swallowed whole; 100 mg chewable tablet can be broken in half.

Film-coated tablets: Must be swallowed whole.

Oral suspension: Administer dose (at a concentration of 20 mg/mL) within 30 minutes of mixing with water.

Monitoring Parameters Note: Monitor CD4 percentage (if <5 years of age) or CD4 count (if ≥5 years of age) at least every 3 to 4 months (DHHS [pediatric], 2014).

Prior to initiation of therapy: Genotypic resistance testing, CD4 and viral load (every 3 to 4 months), CBC with differential, LFTs, BUN, creatinine, electrolytes, glucose, urinalysis (every 6 to 12 months), and assessment of readiness for adherence with medication regimen. At initiation and with any change in treatment regimen: CBC with differential, electrolytes, calcium, phosphate, glucose, LFTs, bilirubin, urinalysis (at initiation), BUN, creatinine, albumin, total protein, lipid panel (at initiation), CD4, and viral load. After 1 to 2 weeks of therapy: Signs of medication toxicity and adherence. After 2 to 4 weeks of therapy: CBC with differential, viral load, signs of medication toxicity, and adherence; then every 3 to 4 months: CBC with differential, electrolytes, glucose, LFTs, bilirubin, BUN, creatinine, CD4, viral load, signs of medication toxicity, and adherence. Every 6 to 12 months: Lipid panel and urinalysis. CD4 monitoring frequency may be decreased to every 6 to 12 months in children who are adherent to therapy if the value is well above the threshold for opportunistic infections, viral suppression is sustained, and the clinical status is stable for more than 2 to 3 years (DHHS [pediatric], 2014). Monitor for growth and development, signs of HIV-specific physical conditions, HIV disease progression, opportunistic infections.

Reference Range Trough concentration (Limited data available; range utilized in trials): Median 72 ng/mL (Range: 29 to 118 ng/mL) (DHHS [adult, pediatric], 2014)

Dosage Forms Excipient information presented when available (limited, particularly for generics); consult specific product labeling.

Packet, Oral:

Isentress: 100 mg (60 ea) [contains polyethylene glycol; banana flavor]

Tablet, Oral:

Isentress: 400 mg [contains polyethylene glycol]

Tablet Chewable, Oral:

Isentress: 25 mg [contains aspartame, saccharin sodium; orange banana flavor]

Isentress: 100 mg [scored; contains aspartame, saccharin sodium; orange banana flavor]

- ◆ **RAN-Amlodipine (Can)** *see* AmLODIPine *on page 133*
- ◆ **RAN-Atenolol (Can)** *see* Atenolol *on page 215*
- ◆ **RAN-Atorvastatin (Can)** *see* AtorvaSTATin *on page 220*
- ◆ **Ran-Candesartan (Can)** *see* Candesartan *on page 358*
- ◆ **RAN-Carvedilol (Can)** *see* Carvedilol *on page 380*
- ◆ **RAN-Cefprozil (Can)** *see* Cefprozil *on page 405*
- ◆ **RAN-Celecoxib (Can)** *see* Celecoxib *on page 418*
- ◆ **RAN-Ciproflox (Can)** *see* Ciprofloxacin (Systemic) *on page 463*
- ◆ **RAN-Citalo (Can)** *see* Citalopram *on page 476*
- ◆ **RAN-Clarithromycin (Can)** *see* Clarithromycin *on page 482*
- ◆ **RAN-Clopidogrel (Can)** *see* Clopidogrel *on page 513*
- ◆ **RAN-Enalapril (Can)** *see* Enalapril *on page 744*
- ◆ **RAN-Escitalopram (Can)** *see* Escitalopram *on page 786*
- ◆ **RAN-Ezetimibe (Can)** *see* Ezetimibe *on page 832*
- ◆ **RAN-Fentanyl Matrix Patch (Can)** *see* FentaNYL *on page 857*
- ◆ **RAN-Fosinopril (Can)** *see* Fosinopril *on page 943*
- ◆ **RAN-Gabapentin (Can)** *see* Gabapentin *on page 954*
- ◆ **RAN-Imipenem-Cilastatin (Can)** *see* Imipenem and Cilastatin *on page 1083*

◆ **RAN-Irbesartan (Can)** *see* Irbesartan *on page 1158*

Ranitidine (ra NI ti deen)

Medication Safety Issues

Sound-alike/look-alike issues:

Ranitidine may be confused with amantadine, rimantadine

Zantac may be confused with Xanax, Zarontin, Zofran, ZyrTEC

Brand Names: US Acid Reducer Maximum Strength [OTC] [DSC]; Acid Reducer [OTC]; Deprizine FusePaq; GoodSense Acid Reducer [OTC]; Ranitidine Acid Reducer [OTC]; Zantac; Zantac 150 Maximum Strength [OTC]; Zantac 75 [OTC]

Brand Names: Canada Acid Reducer; ACT Ranitidine; Apo-Ranitidine; Dom-Ranitidine; Myl-Ranitidine; Mylan-Ranitidine; PHL-Ranitidine; PMS-Ranitidine; RAN-Ranitidine; Ranitidine Injection, USP; ratio-Ranitidine; Riva-Ranitidine; Sandoz-Ranitidine; ScheinPharm Ranitidine; Teva-Ranitidine; Zantac; Zantac 75; Zantac Maximum Strength Non-Prescription

Therapeutic Category Gastrointestinal Agent, Gastric or Duodenal Ulcer Treatment; Histamine H_2 Antagonist

Generic Availability (US) May be product dependent

Use

Oral: Short-term and maintenance treatment of duodenal ulcers and benign gastric ulcers, treatment of gastroesophageal reflux disease (GERD) and treatment of erosive esophagitis (All indications: FDA approved in ages ≥1 month and adults); treatment of pathologic hypersecretory conditions and maintenance of erosive esophagitis (FDA approved in adults)

Relief of heartburn associated with acid indigestion and sour stomach (OTC product: FDA approved in ages ≥12 years and adults)

Injection: Treatment of intractable duodenal ulcers (FDA approved in ages ≥1 month and adults); treatment of pathologic hypersecretory conditions in hospitalized patients (FDA approved in adults); alternative to oral ranitidine in patients unable to take oral medication (FDA approved in ages ≥1 month and adults)

Has also been used for stress ulcer prophylaxis, upper GI bleeding and as adjunct treatment for anaphylaxis

Pregnancy Risk Factor B

Pregnancy Considerations Adverse events were not observed in animal studies; therefore, ranitidine is classified as pregnancy category B. Ranitidine crosses the placenta. An increased risk of congenital malformations or adverse events in the newborn has generally not been observed following maternal use of ranitidine during pregnancy. Histamine H_2 antagonists have been evaluated for the treatment of gastroesophageal reflux disease (GERD) as well as gastric and duodenal ulcers during pregnancy. If needed, ranitidine is the agent of choice. Histamine H_2 antagonists may be used for aspiration prophylaxis prior to cesarean delivery.

Breast-Feeding Considerations Ranitidine is excreted into breast milk. The manufacturer recommends that caution be exercised when administering ranitidine to nursing women. Peak milk concentrations of ranitidine occur ~5.5 hours after the dose (case report).

Contraindications Hypersensitivity to ranitidine or any component of the formulation

Warnings/Precautions Ranitidine has been associated with confusional states (rare). Use with caution in patients with hepatic impairment; use with caution in renal impairment, dosage modification required. Avoid use in patients with history of acute porphyria (may precipitate attacks). Prolonged treatment (≥2 years) may lead to vitamin B_{12} malabsorption and subsequent vitamin B_{12} deficiency. The magnitude of the deficiency is dose-related and the association is stronger in females and those younger in age (<30 years); prevalence is decreased after discontinuation of therapy (Lam, 2013). Symptoms of GI distress may be associated with a variety of conditions; symptomatic response to H_2 antagonists does not rule out the potential for significant pathology (eg, malignancy).

Warnings: Additional Pediatric Considerations Use of gastric acid inhibitors, including proton pump inhibitors and H_2 blockers, has been associated with an increased risk for development of acute gastroenteritis and community-acquired pneumonia in pediatric patients (Canani, 2006). A large epidemiological study has suggested an increased risk for developing pneumonia in patients receiving H_2 receptor antagonists; however, a causal relationship with ranitidine has not been demonstrated. A cohort analysis including over 11,000 neonates reported an association of H_2 blocker use and an increased incidence of NEC in VLBW neonates (Guillet, 2006). An approximate sixfold increase in mortality, NEC, and infection (ie, sepsis, pneumonia, UTI) was reported in patients receiving ranitidine in a cohort analysis of 274 VLBW neonates (Terrin, 2011).

Adverse Reactions

Cardiovascular: Asystole, atrioventricular block, bradycardia (with rapid IV administration), premature ventricular beats, tachycardia, vasculitis

Central nervous system: Agitation, dizziness, depression, hallucinations, headache, insomnia, malaise, mental confusion, somnolence, vertigo

Dermatologic: Alopecia, erythema multiforme, rash

Endocrine & metabolic: Prolactin levels increased

Gastrointestinal: Abdominal discomfort/pain, constipation, diarrhea, nausea, necrotizing enterocolitis (VLBW neonates; Guillet, 2006), pancreatitis, vomiting

Hematologic: Acquired immune hemolytic anemia, acute porphyritic attack, agranulocytosis, aplastic anemia, granulocytopenia, leukopenia, pancytopenia, thrombocytopenia

Hepatic: Cholestatic hepatitis, hepatic failure, hepatitis, jaundice

Local: Transient pain, burning or itching at the injection site

Neuromuscular & skeletal: Arthralgia, involuntary motor disturbance, myalgia

Ocular: Blurred vision

Renal: Acute interstitial nephritis, serum creatinine increased

Respiratory: Pneumonia (causal relationship not established)

Miscellaneous: Anaphylaxis, angioneurotic edema, hypersensitivity reactions (eg, bronchospasm, fever, eosinophilia)

Drug Interactions

Metabolism/Transport Effects Substrate of CYP1A2 (minor), CYP2C19 (minor), CYP2D6 (minor), OCT2, P-glycoprotein; **Note:** Assignment of Major/Minor substrate status based on clinically relevant drug interaction potential; **Inhibits** CYP1A2 (weak), CYP2D6 (weak)

Avoid Concomitant Use

Avoid concomitant use of Ranitidine with any of the following: Dasatinib; Delavirdine; PAZOPanib; Risedronate

Increased Effect/Toxicity

Ranitidine may increase the levels/effects of: ARIPiprazole; Dexmethylphenidate; Methylphenidate; Procainamide; Risedronate; Saquinavir; Sulfonylureas; TiZANidine; Varenicline; Warfarin

The levels/effects of Ranitidine may be increased by: BuPROPion; P-glycoprotein/ABCB1 Inhibitors

Decreased Effect

Ranitidine may decrease the levels/effects of: Atazanavir; Bosutinib; Cefditoren; Cefpodoxime; Cefuroxime; Dabrafenib; Dasatinib; Delavirdine; Erlotinib; Fosamprenavir; Gefitinib; Indinavir; Iron Salts; Itraconazole;

Ketoconazole (Systemic); Ledipasvir; Mesalamine; Multivitamins/Minerals (with ADEK, Folate, Iron); Nelfinavir; Nilotinib; PAZOPanib; Posaconazole; Prasugrel; Rilpivirine

The levels/effects of Ranitidine may be decreased by: P-glycoprotein/ABCB1 Inducers

Food Interactions Prolonged treatment (≥2 years) may lead to malabsorption of dietary vitamin B_{12} and subsequent vitamin B_{12} deficiency (Lam, 2013).

Storage/Stability

Injection: Vials: Store between 4°C to 25°C (39°F to 77°F); excursion permitted to 30°C (86°F). Protect from light. Solution is a clear, colorless to yellow solution; slight darkening does not affect potency. Vials mixed with NS or D_5W are stable for 48 hours at room temperature.

Syrup: Store between 4°C to 25°C (39°F to 77°F). Protect from light.

Tablets: Store in dry place, between 15°C to 30°C (59°F to 86°F). Protect from light.

Mechanism of Action Competitive inhibition of histamine at H_2-receptors of the gastric parietal cells, which inhibits gastric acid secretion, gastric volume, and hydrogen ion concentration are reduced. Does not affect pepsin secretion, pentagastrin-stimulated intrinsic factor secretion, or serum gastrin.

Pharmacokinetics (Adult data unless noted)

Absorption: Oral: 50%

Distribution: Minimally penetrates the blood-brain barrier

V_d:

Infants, Children, and Adolescents: IV, Oral: 1 to 2.3 L/kg

Adults: 1.4 L/kg

Protein binding: 15%

Metabolism: Hepatic to N-oxide, S-oxide, and N-desmethyl metabolites

Bioavailability:

Oral: ~50%

IM: 90% to 100%

Half-life:

Neonates (receiving ECMO): IV: 6.6 hours

Infants, Children, and Adolescents: IV: 1.7 to 2.4 hours

Adults:

Oral: Normal renal function: 2.5 to 3 hours

IV: Normal renal function: 2 to 2.5 hours; CrCl 25 to 35 mL/minute: 4.8 hours

Time to peak serum concentration:

Oral: 2 to 3 hours

IM: ≤15 minutes

Elimination: Urine (as unchanged drug): Oral: 30%, IV: 70% (IV); feces (as metabolites)

Dosing: Neonatal Note: Consider judicial use in neonatal population due to an association of H_2 blocker use and an increased incidence of NEC in VLBW neonates (Guillet, 2006) and a reported approximate sixfold increase in mortality, NEC, and infection (ie, sepsis, pneumonia, UTI) in VLBW neonates receiving ranitidine (Terrin, 2011).

Gastroesophageal reflux: Limited data available: Corrected age <44 weeks: Oral: 2 mg/kg/dose every 8 hours (Birch, 2009; Sutphen, 1989, Wheatley, 2012)

GI bleed or stress ulcer; prophylaxis: Limited data available; dosing regimens variable: IV:

Intermittent IV:

GA <37 weeks: 0.5 mg/kg/dose every 12 hours (ASHP, 1999; Kuusela, 1998); others have used 1.5 to 3 mg/kg/**day** divided every 12 hours

GA ≥37 weeks: 1.5 to 2 mg/kg/**day** in divided doses every 8 hours (Crill, 1999); others have recommended higher dosing at 1.5 mg/kg/dose every 8 hours (Kuusela, 1998)

ECMO: 2 mg/kg/dose every 12 to 24 hours

Continuous IV infusion: **Note:** Reported ranges are similar to the total daily dose with intermittent IV dosing. Loading dose: 1.5 mg/kg/dose, followed by usual range of 0.04 to 0.08 mg/kg/hour infusion (1-2 mg/kg/**day**); reported range of 0.031 to 0.125 mg/kg/hour (0.75 to 3 mg/kg/**day**); in a trial of premature neonates on concurrent dexamethasone, an infusion rate of 0.0625 mg/kg/hour was shown to maintain neonatal gastric pH >4; higher rates of 0.125 mg/kg/hour have been used without additional clinical benefit (Crill, 1999; Kelly, 1993)

ECMO: Term neonates: Loading dose: 2 mg/kg/dose over 10 minutes followed by 0.083 mg/kg/hour infusion (2 mg/kg/**day**), begin infusion 24 hours after loading dose; rate of infusion was increased by 0.042 mg/kg/hour (1 mg/kg/**day**) if gastric pH fell to <4 (Wells, 1998)

Dosing: Usual

Pediatric:

Duodenal or gastric ulcer:

Oral:

Treatment:

Infants, Children, and Adolescents ≤16 years: 4 to 8 mg/kg/day divided twice daily; maximum daily dose: 300 mg/**day**

Adolescents >16 years:

Duodenal ulcer: 150 mg twice daily **or** 300 mg once daily after the evening meal or at bedtime

Gastric ulcer: 150 mg twice daily

Maintenance:

Infants, Children, and Adolescents ≤16 years: 2 to 4 mg/kg/day once daily; maximum daily dose: 150 mg/day

Adolescents >16 years: 150 mg once daily at bedtime

IM: Adolescents >16 years: 50 mg every 6 to 8 hours

IV:

Infants, Children, and Adolescents ≤16 years: 2 to 4 mg/kg/day divided every 6 to 8 hours; maximum dose: 50 mg/dose

Adolescents >16 years: 50 mg every 6 to 8 hours

Erosive esophagitis:

Infants, Children, and Adolescents ≤16 years: Oral: 5 to 10 mg/kg/day divided twice daily; maximum dose: 150 mg/dose

Adolescents >16 years: Oral

Treatment: 150 mg 4 times daily

Maintenance: 150 mg twice daily

GI bleed or stress ulcer; prophylaxis: Limited data available; dosing regimens variable: IV:

Intermittent infusion:

Infants: 2 to 6 mg/kg/day divided every 8 hours (ASHP, 1999; Crill, 1999)

Children and Adolescents: 3 to 6 mg/kg/day divided every 6 hours; maximum daily dose: 300 mg/**day** (ASHP, 1999; Crill, 1999)

Continuous infusion: Infants, Children, and Adolescents: Initial: 0.15 to 0.5 mg/kg/dose for 1 dose, followed by infusion of 0.08 to 0.2 mg/kg/hour (2 to 5 mg/kg/day) (Kleigman, 2007; Lugo, 2001; Osteyee, 1994)

GERD: Oral:

Infants, Children, and Adolescents ≤16 years: 5 to 10 mg/kg/day divided twice daily; maximum daily dose: 300 mg/**day**

Adolescents >16 years: 150 mg twice daily

Heartburn: OTC labeling: **Note: Do not use for more than 14 days.**

Prevention: Children ≥12 years and Adolescents: Oral: 75 to 150 mg 30 to 60 minutes before eating food or drinking beverages which cause heartburn; maximum daily dose: 2 doses/day

Relief of symptoms: Children ≥12 years and Adolescents: Oral: 75 to 150 mg twice daily; maximum daily dose: 2 doses/day

Patients not able to take oral medication:
Infants, Children, and Adolescents <16 years: IV: 2 to 4 mg/kg/day divided every 6 to 8 hours; maximum dose: 50 mg/dose
Adolescents ≥ 16 years:
IM, IV: 50 mg every 6 to 8 hours
Continuous IV infusion: 6.25 mg/hour

Pathological hypersecretory conditions (eg, Zollinger-Ellison): Adolescents >16 years:
Oral: 150 mg twice daily; adjust dose or frequency as clinically indicated; doses of up to 6 g/day have been used
Continuous IV infusion: Initial: 1 mg/kg/hour; measure gastric acid output at 4 hours, if >10 mEq/hour or if patient is symptomatic, increase dose in increments of 0.5 mg/kg/hour; doses of up to 2.5 mg/kg/hour (or 220 mg/hour) have been used

Anaphylaxis, adjunct therapy: Infants, Children, and Adolescents: IV: 1 mg/kg/dose; maximum dose: 50 mg/dose; **Note:** Should not be used as monotherapy or as first line therapy (AAAAI/ACAAI [Lieberman, 2010]; Canadian Paediatric Society [Cheng, 2011])

Adult:

Duodenal ulcer; treatment: Oral: 150 mg twice daily or 300 mg once daily after the evening meal or at bedtime; maintenance: 150 mg once daily at bedtime

Pathological hypersecretory conditions:
Oral: 150 mg twice daily; adjust dose or frequency as clinically indicated; doses of up to 6 **g**/day have been used
IV: Continuous infusion for Zollinger-Ellison: Initial: 1 mg/kg/hour; measure gastric acid output at 4 hours, if >10 mEq/hour or if patient is symptomatic, increase dose in increments of 0.5 mg/kg/hour; doses of up to 2.5 mg/kg/hour (or 220 mg/hour) have been used

Gastric ulcer, benign: Oral: 150 mg twice daily; maintenance: 150 mg once daily at bedtime

GERD: Oral: 150 mg twice daily

Erosive esophagitis; treatment: Oral: 150 mg 4 times daily; maintenance: 150 mg twice daily

Heartburn, prevention or relief [OTC labeling]: Oral:
Prevention: 75 mg to 150 mg 30 to 60 minutes before eating food or drinking beverages which cause heartburn; maximum in 24 hours; do not use for more than 14 days
Relief of symptoms: 75 mg to 150 mg twice daily; do not use for more than 14 days

Patients not able to take oral medication:
IM: 50 mg every 6 to 8 hours
IV: Intermittent bolus or infusion: 50 mg every 6 to 8 hours
Continuous IV infusion: 6.25 mg/hour

Dosing adjustment in renal impairment:
Infants, Children, and Adolescents(Aronoff, 2007):
Oral: Based on a usual dose of 2-6 mg/kg/day divided every 8-12 hours
GFR >50 mL/minute/1.73 m^2: No adjustment required
GFR 30-50 mL/minute/1.73 m^2: 2 mg/kg/dose every 12 hours
GFR 10-29 mL/minute/1.73 m^2: 1 mg/kg/dose every 12 hours
GFR <10 mL/minute/1.73 m^2: 1 mg/kg/dose every 24 hours
Hemodialysis: 1 mg/kg/dose every 24 hours
Peritoneal dialysis: 1 mg/kg/dose every 24 hours
Continuous renal replacement therapy: 2 mg/kg/dose every 12 hours
Parenteral (IV): Based on a usual dose of 2-4 mg/kg/day divided every 6-24 hours
GFR >50 mL/minute/1.73 m^2: No adjustment required
GFR 30-50 mL/minute/1.73 m^2: 1 mg/kg/dose every 12 hours
GFR 10-29 mL/minute/1.73 m^2: 0.5 mg/kg/dose every 12 hours
GFR <10 mL/minute/1.73 m^2: 0.5 mg/kg/dose every 24 hours
Hemodialysis: 0.5 mg/kg/dose every 24 hours
Peritoneal dialysis: 0.5 mg/kg/dose every 24 hours
Continuous renal replacement therapy: 1 mg/kg/dose every 12 hours
Adults:
CrCl ≥50 mL/minute: No dosage adjustment necessary
CrCl <50 mL/minute:
Oral: 150 mg every 24 hours; adjust dose cautiously if needed
IV: 50 mg every 18-24 hours; adjust dose cautiously if needed
Hemodialysis: Adjust dose schedule to administer dose at the end of dialysis

Dosing adjustment in hepatic impairment: There are no dosage adjustments provided in the manufacturer's labeling; however dosage adjustment unlikely necessary due to minimal hepatic metabolism.

Usual Infusion Concentrations: Pediatric Note: Premixed solutions available
IV infusion: 0.5 mg/mL

Preparation for Administration
Parenteral: Solution may be further diluted with NS or D_5W.
Intermittent IV infusion: Dilute to maximum concentration of 0.5 mg/mL
IV push: Dilute to maximum concentration of 2.5 mg/mL
Continuous IV infusion: Dilute to a concentration of ≤0.6 mg/mL; concentrations up to 2.5 mg/mL have been used when treating Zollinger-Ellison syndrome

Administration
Oral: Administer with meals and/or at bedtime
Parenteral:
IV: Must be diluted prior to administration; may be administered IV push, intermittent IV infusion, or continuous IV infusion
Intermittent IV infusion: Preferred over IV push to decrease risk of bradycardia; infuse over 15 to 20 minutes
IV push: Manufacturer recommends administering over a period of at least 5 minutes, not to exceed 10 mg/minute (4 mL/minute)
Continuous IV infusion: Administer at ordered rate; titration may be necessary for some conditions.
IM: Administer undiluted

Monitoring Parameters AST, ALT, serum creatinine, occult blood with GI bleeding, signs/symptoms of peptic ulcer disease; when used to prevent stress-related GI bleeding, measure the intragastric pH and try to maintain pH >4; when used for Zollinger-Ellison syndrome, monitor gastric acid secretion (goal: <10 mEq/hour)

Test Interactions False-positive urine protein using Multistix®; gastric acid secretion test; skin test allergen extracts. May also interfere with urine detection of amphetamine/methamphetamine (false-positive).

Dosage Forms Considerations Deprizine FusePaq is a compounding kit for the preparation of an oral suspension. Refer to manufacturer's labeling for compounding instructions.

Dosage Forms Excipient information presented when available (limited, particularly for generics); consult specific product labeling. [DSC] = Discontinued product
Capsule, Oral:
Generic: 150 mg, 300 mg
Solution, Injection:
Zantac: 50 mg/2 mL (2 mL); 150 mg/6 mL (6 mL); 1000 mg/40 mL (40 mL) [contains phenol]
Generic: 50 mg/2 mL (2 mL); 150 mg/6 mL (6 mL); 1000 mg/40 mL (40 mL)

Suspension Reconstituted, Oral:
Deprizine FusePaq: 22.4 mg/mL (250 mL) [contains sodium benzoate]
Syrup, Oral:
Zantac: 15 mg/mL (480 mL [DSC]) [contains alcohol, usp, butylparaben, propylparaben, saccharin sodium; peppermint flavor]
Generic: 15 mg/mL (10 mL, 473 mL, 474 mL, 480 mL); 75 mg/5 mL (473 mL, 480 mL); 150 mg/10 mL (10 mL)
Tablet, Oral:
Acid Reducer: 75 mg, 150 mg
Acid Reducer: 150 mg [sodium free, sugar free]
Acid Reducer: 75 mg [DSC] [sugar free]
Acid Reducer Maximum Strength: 150 mg [DSC] [sugar free; contains fd&c yellow #6 (sunset yellow)]
GoodSense Acid Reducer: 75 mg [gluten free]
Ranitidine Acid Reducer: 75 mg
Zantac 75: 75 mg
Zantac: 150 mg, 300 mg
Zantac 150 Maximum Strength: 150 mg
Zantac 150 Maximum Strength: 150 mg [sodium free, sugar free; contains brilliant blue fcf (fd&c blue #1); mint flavor]
Generic: 75 mg, 150 mg, 300 mg

- **Ranitidine Acid Reducer [OTC]** *see* Ranitidine *on page 1836*
- **Ranitidine Hydrochloride** *see* Ranitidine *on page 1836*
- **Ranitidine Injection, USP (Can)** *see* Ranitidine *on page 1836*
- **RAN-Lansoprazole (Can)** *see* Lansoprazole *on page 1219*
- **RAN-Letrozole (Can)** *see* Letrozole *on page 1224*
- **RAN-Levetiracetam (Can)** *see* LevETIRAcetam *on page 1234*
- **RAN-Lisinopril (Can)** *see* Lisinopril *on page 1280*
- **RAN-Losartan (Can)** *see* Losartan *on page 1302*
- **RAN-Metformin (Can)** *see* MetFORMIN *on page 1375*
- **RAN-Montelukast (Can)** *see* Montelukast *on page 1459*
- **RAN™-Nabilone (Can)** *see* Nabilone *on page 1478*
- **RAN-Olanzapine (Can)** *see* OLANZapine *on page 1546*
- **RAN-Olanzapine ODT (Can)** *see* OLANZapine *on page 1546*
- **RAN-Omeprazole (Can)** *see* Omeprazole *on page 1555*
- **RAN-Ondansetron (Can)** *see* Ondansetron *on page 1564*
- **RAN-Pantoprazole (Can)** *see* Pantoprazole *on page 1618*
- **RAN-Pravastatin (Can)** *see* Pravastatin *on page 1749*
- **RAN-Quetiapine (Can)** *see* QUEtiapine *on page 1815*
- **RAN-Rabeprazole (Can)** *see* RABEprazole *on page 1828*
- **RAN-Ranitidine (Can)** *see* Ranitidine *on page 1836*
- **RAN-Risperidone (Can)** *see* RisperiDONE *on page 1866*
- **RAN-Rosuvastatin (Can)** *see* Rosuvastatin *on page 1886*
- **Ran-Sertraline (Can)** *see* Sertraline *on page 1916*
- **RAN-Sildenafil (Can)** *see* Sildenafil *on page 1921*
- **RAN-Simvastatin (Can)** *see* Simvastatin *on page 1928*
- **RAN-Topiramate (Can)** *see* Topiramate *on page 2085*
- **Ran-Valsartan (Can)** *see* Valsartan *on page 2149*
- **Ran-Venlafaxine XR (Can)** *see* Venlafaxine *on page 2166*
- **Rapamune** *see* Sirolimus *on page 1931*
- **Rapamycin** *see* Sirolimus *on page 1931*
- **Rapivab** *see* Peramivir *on page 1672*

Rasburicase (ras BYOOR i kayse)

Brand Names: US Elitek
Brand Names: Canada Fasturtec
Therapeutic Category Enzyme; Uric Acid Lowering Agent
Generic Availability (US) No
Use Initial management of plasma uric acid levels in patients with leukemia, lymphoma, and solid tumor malignancies who are receiving anticancer therapy expected to result in tumor lysis and subsequent elevation of plasma uric acid (FDA approved in ages ≥1 month and adults)
Pregnancy Risk Factor C
Pregnancy Considerations Adverse effects were observed in animal reproduction studies. Use during pregnancy only if the benefit to the mother outweighs the potential risk to the fetus.
Breast-Feeding Considerations It is not known if rasburicase is excreted in breast milk. Due to the potential for serious adverse reactions in the nursing infant, a decision should be made to discontinue breast-feeding or the drug, taking into account the benefits of treatment to the mother. The Canadian labeling does not recommend use in breast-feeding women.
Contraindications History of anaphylaxis or severe hypersensitivity to rasburicase or any component of the formulation; history of hemolytic reaction or methemoglobinemia associated with rasburicase; glucose-6-phosphatase dehydrogenase (G6PD) deficiency
Warnings/Precautions **[US Boxed Warning]: Severe hypersensitivity reactions (including anaphylaxis) have been reported; immediately and permanently discontinue in patients developing serious hypersensitivity reaction;** reactions may occur at any time during treatment, including the initial dose. Signs and symptoms of hypersensitivity may include bronchospasm, chest pain/tightness, dyspnea, hypotension, hypoxia, shock, or urticaria. The safety and efficacy of more than one course of administration has not been established. **[US Boxed Warning]: Due to the risk for hemolysis (<1%), rasburicase is contraindicated in patients with G6PD deficiency; discontinue immediately and permanently in any patient developing hemolysis. Patients at higher risk for G6PD deficiency (eg, African or Mediterranean descent) should be screened prior to therapy;** severe hemolytic reactions occurred within 2 to 4 days of rasburicase initiation. **[US Boxed Warning]: Methemoglobinemia has been reported (<1%). Discontinue immediately and permanently in any patient developing methemoglobinemia;** initiate appropriate treatment (eg, transfusion, methylene blue) if methemoglobinemia occurs.

[US Boxed Warning]: Enzymatic degradation of uric acid in blood samples will occur if left at room temperature, which may interfere with serum uric acid measurements; specific guidelines for the collection of plasma uric acid samples must be followed, including collection in prechilled tubes with heparin anticoagulant, immediate ice water bath immersion and assay within 4 hours. Patients at risk for tumor lysis syndrome should receive appropriate IV hydration as part of uric acid management; however, alkalinization (with sodium bicarbonate) concurrently with rasburicase is not recommended (Coiffier 2008). Rasburicase is immunogenic and can elicit an antibody response; efficacy may be reduced with subsequent courses of therapy.
Warnings: Additional Pediatric Considerations Data suggest that children <2 years of age may experience a

higher frequency of adverse effects than adults, particularly vomiting (75% vs 55%), diarrhea (63% vs 20%), fever (50% vs 38%), and rash (38% vs 10%).

Adverse Reactions

Cardiovascular: Fluid overload, ischemic coronary disease, peripheral edema, supraventricular arrhythmia

Central nervous system: Anxiety, fever, headache,

Dermatologic: Rash

Endocrine & metabolic: Hyper-/hypophosphatemia

Gastrointestinal: Abdominal/gastrointestinal infection, abdominal pain, constipation, diarrhea, mucositis, nausea, vomiting

Hematologic: Neutropenia, neutropenia with fever

Hepatic: ALT increased, hyperbilirubinemia

Respiratory: Pharyngolaryngeal pain, pulmonary hemorrhage, respiratory distress/failure

Miscellaneous: Antibody formation, hypersensitivity, sepsis

Rare but important or life-threatening: Acute renal failure, anaphylaxis, arrhythmia, cardiac arrest, cardiac failure, cellulitis, cerebrovascular disorder, chest pain, cyanosis, dehydration, hemolysis, hemorrhage, hot flashes, ileus, infection, intestinal obstruction, liver enzymes increased, methemoglobinemia, MI, pancytopenia, paresthesia, pneumonia, pulmonary edema, pulmonary hypertension, retinal hemorrhage, rigors, seizure, thrombosis, thrombophlebitis

Drug Interactions

Metabolism/Transport Effects None known.

Avoid Concomitant Use There are no known interactions where it is recommended to avoid concomitant use.

Increased Effect/Toxicity There are no known significant interactions involving an increase in effect.

Decreased Effect There are no known significant interactions involving a decrease in effect.

Storage/Stability The lyophilized drug product and the diluent for reconstitution should be stored at 2°C to 8°C (36°F to 46°F); do not freeze. Protect from light. Reconstituted solution and solution diluted for infusion may be stored for up to 24 hours at 2°C to 8°C (36°F to 46°F). Discard unused product.

Mechanism of Action Rasburicase is a recombinant urate-oxidase enzyme, which converts uric acid to allantoin (an inactive and soluble metabolite of uric acid); it does not inhibit the formation of uric acid.

Pharmacodynamics Onset: Uric acid levels decrease within 4 hours of initial administration

Pharmacokinetics (Adult data unless noted)

Distribution: V_d: Children: 110-127 mL/kg

Half-life: Children: 18 hours

Dosing: Usual

Infants, Children, and Adolescents: **Hyperuricemia associated with malignancy:** IV:

Multiple-dosing:

Manufacturer's labeling (Elitek): 0.2 mg/kg/dose once daily for up to 5 days. **Note:** Limited data suggest that a single prechemotherapy dose (versus multiple-day administration) may be sufficiently efficacious. Monitoring electrolytes, hydration status, and uric acid concentrations are necessary to identify the need for additional doses. Other clinical manifestations of tumor lysis syndrome (eg, hyperphosphatemia, hypocalcemia, and hyperkalemia) may occur.

Alternate dosing (Coiffier, 2008): Limited data available: 0.05-0.2 mg/kg once daily for 1-7 days (average of 2-3 days) with the duration of treatment dependent on plasma uric acid levels and clinical judgment (patients with significant tumor burden may require an increase to twice daily); the following dose levels are recommended based on risk of tumor lysis syndrome (TLS):

High risk and baseline uric acid level >7.5 mg/dL: 0.2 mg/kg once daily (duration is based on plasma uric acid levels)

Intermediate risk and baseline uric acid level <7.5 mg/dL: 0.15 mg/kg once daily (duration is based on plasma uric acid levels); may consider managing initially with a single dose

Low risk and baseline uric acid level <7.5 mg/dL: 0.1 mg/kg once daily (duration is based on clinical judgment); a dose of 0.05 mg/kg was used (with good results) in one trial

Single-dose: Limited data available: 0.15 mg/kg; additional doses may be needed based on serum uric acid levels (Liu, 2005)

Adults: **Hyperuricemia associated with malignancy:** IV:

Manufacturer's labeling: 0.2 mg/kg once daily for up to 5 days (manufacturer recommended dose) **or**

Alternate dosing (Coiffier, 2008): 0.05-0.2 mg/kg once daily for 1-7 days (average: 2-3 days) with the duration of treatment dependent on plasma uric acid levels and clinical judgment (patients with significant tumor burden may require an increase to twice daily); the following dose levels are recommended based on risk of tumor lysis syndrome (TLS):

High risk: 0.2 mg/kg once daily (duration is based on plasma uric acid levels)

Intermediate risk: 0.15 mg/kg once daily (duration is based on plasma uric acid levels)

Low risk: 0.1 mg/kg once daily (duration is based on clinical judgment); a dose of 0.05 mg/kg was used effectively in one trial

Dosing adjustment in renal impairment: There is no dosage adjustment provided in manufacturer's labeling.

Dosing adjustment in hepatic impairment: There is no dosage adjustment provided in manufacturer's labeling.

Preparation for Administration IV: Reconstitute vials with provided diluent (use 1 mL diluent for the 1.5 mg vial and 5 mL diluent for the 7.5 mg vial). Mix by gently swirling; do **not** shake or vortex. Discard if discolored or containing particulate matter. Total dose should be further diluted in NS to a final volume of 50 mL.

Administration IV: Infuse over 30 minutes; do **not** administer as a bolus infusion. Do not filter or mix with other medications. If not possible to administer through a separate line, IV line should be flushed with at least 15 mL NS prior to and following rasburicase infusion. The optimal timing of rasburicase administration (with respect to chemotherapy administration) is not specified in the manufacturer's labeling. In some studies, chemotherapy was administered 4 to 24 hours after the first rasburicase dose (Cortes 2010; Kikuchi 2009; Vadhan-Raj 2012); however, rasburicase generally may be administered irrespective of chemotherapy timing.

Monitoring Parameters Plasma uric acid levels (4 hours after rasburicase administration, then every 6-8 hours until TLS resolution), CBC, G6PD deficiency screening (in patients at high risk for deficiency); monitor for hypersensitivity

Test Interactions Specific handling procedures must be followed to prevent the degradation of uric acid in plasma samples. Blood must be collected in prechilled tubes containing heparin anticoagulant. Samples must then be **immediately** immersed and maintained in an ice water bath. Prepare samples by centrifugation in a precooled centrifuge (4°C). Samples must be analyzed within 4 hours of collection.

Dosage Forms Excipient information presented when available (limited, particularly for generics); consult specific product labeling.

Solution Reconstituted, Intravenous:

Elitek: 1.5 mg (1 ea); 7.5 mg (1 ea)

◆ **Rasuvo** *see* Methotrexate *on page* 1390

◆ **rATG** *see* Antithymocyte Globulin (Rabbit) *on page* 180

◆ **ratio-Aclavulanate (Can)** *see* Amoxicillin and Clavulanate *on page* 141

◆ **ratio-Acyclovir (Can)** *see* Acyclovir (Systemic) *on page 61*
◆ **ratio-Amlodipine (Can)** *see* AmLODIPine *on page 133*
◆ **ratio-Atenolol (Can)** *see* Atenolol *on page 215*
◆ **ratio-Atorvastatin (Can)** *see* AtorvaSTATin *on page 220*
◆ **ratio-Baclofen (Can)** *see* Baclofen *on page 254*
◆ **ratio-Bisacodyl [OTC] (Can)** *see* Bisacodyl *on page 289*
◆ **ratio-Brimonidine (Can)** *see* Brimonidine (Ophthalmic) *on page 301*
◆ **ratio-Bupropion SR (Can)** *see* BuPROPion *on page 324*
◆ **ratio-Carvedilol (Can)** *see* Carvedilol *on page 380*
◆ **ratio-Cefuroxime (Can)** *see* Cefuroxime *on page 414*
◆ **ratio-Ciprofloxacin (Can)** *see* Ciprofloxacin (Systemic) *on page 463*
◆ **ratio-Clobetasol (Can)** *see* Clobetasol *on page 498*
◆ **ratio-Clonazepam (Can)** *see* ClonazePAM *on page 506*
◆ **ratio-Codeine (Can)** *see* Codeine *on page 525*
◆ **ratio-Cyclobenzaprine (Can)** *see* Cyclobenzaprine *on page 548*
◆ **ratio-Dexamethasone (Can)** *see* Dexamethasone (Systemic) *on page 610*
◆ **ratio-Diltiazem CD (Can)** *see* Diltiazem *on page 661*
◆ **ratio-Docusate Sodium [OTC] (Can)** *see* Docusate *on page 697*
◆ **ratio-Ectosone (Can)** *see* Betamethasone (Topical) *on page 280*
◆ **ratio-Emtec-30 (Can)** *see* Acetaminophen and Codeine *on page 50*
◆ **ratio-Fluoxetine (Can)** *see* FLUoxetine *on page 906*
◆ **ratio-Fluticasone (Can)** *see* Fluticasone (Nasal) *on page 917*
◆ **ratio-Fluvoxamine (Can)** *see* FluvoxaMINE *on page 928*
◆ **ratio-Gabapentin (Can)** *see* Gabapentin *on page 954*
◆ **ratio-Gentamicin (Can)** *see* Gentamicin (Topical) *on page 969*
◆ **ratio-Glyburide (Can)** *see* GlyBURIDE *on page 975*
◆ **ratio-Indomethacin (Can)** *see* Indomethacin *on page 1101*
◆ **ratio-Ipra-Sal (Can)** *see* Albuterol *on page 81*
◆ **ratio-Ipratropium UDV (Can)** *see* Ipratropium (Oral Inhalation) *on page 1155*
◆ **ratio-Irbesartan (Can)** *see* Irbesartan *on page 1158*
◆ **ratio-Ketorolac (Can)** *see* Ketorolac (Ophthalmic) *on page 1195*
◆ **Ratio-Lactulose (Can)** *see* Lactulose *on page 1204*
◆ **ratio-Lamotrigine (Can)** *see* LamoTRIgine *on page 1211*
◆ **ratio-Lenoltec (Can)** *see* Acetaminophen and Codeine *on page 50*
◆ **Ratio-Levobunolol (Can)** *see* Levobunolol *on page 1238*
◆ **ratio-Meloxicam (Can)** *see* Meloxicam *on page 1346*
◆ **ratio-Metformin (Can)** *see* MetFORMIN *on page 1375*
◆ **ratio-Methotrexate Sodium (Can)** *see* Methotrexate *on page 1390*
◆ **ratio-Methylphenidate (Can)** *see* Methylphenidate *on page 1402*
◆ **ratio-Mometasone (Can)** *see* Mometasone (Topical) *on page 1456*
◆ **ratio-Morphine (Can)** *see* Morphine (Systemic) *on page 1461*
◆ **ratio-Morphine SR (Can)** *see* Morphine (Systemic) *on page 1461*
◆ **Ratio-Nystatin (Can)** *see* Nystatin (Topical) *on page 1537*
◆ **ratio-Omeprazole (Can)** *see* Omeprazole *on page 1555*
◆ **ratio-Ondansetron (Can)** *see* Ondansetron *on page 1564*
◆ **ratio-Orciprenaline® (Can)** *see* Metaproterenol *on page 1374*
◆ **Ratio-Oxycocet (Can)** *see* Oxycodone and Acetaminophen *on page 1594*
◆ **ratio-Pantoprazole (Can)** *see* Pantoprazole *on page 1618*
◆ **ratio-Paroxetine (Can)** *see* PARoxetine *on page 1634*
◆ **Ratio-Prednisolone (Can)** *see* PrednisoLONE (Ophthalmic) *on page 1758*
◆ **ratio-Ranitidine (Can)** *see* Ranitidine *on page 1836*
◆ **ratio-Risperidone (Can)** *see* RisperiDONE *on page 1866*
◆ **ratio-Salbutamol (Can)** *see* Albuterol *on page 81*
◆ **ratio-Sertraline (Can)** *see* Sertraline *on page 1916*
◆ **ratio-Sildenafil R (Can)** *see* Sildenafil *on page 1921*
◆ **ratio-Sotalol (Can)** *see* Sotalol *on page 1963*
◆ **ratio-Tamsulosin (Can)** *see* Tamsulosin *on page 2008*
◆ **ratio-Terazosin (Can)** *see* Terazosin *on page 2020*
◆ **ratio-Theo-Bronc (Can)** *see* Theophylline *on page 2044*
◆ **Ratio-Topilene (Can)** *see* Betamethasone (Topical) *on page 280*
◆ **Ratio-Topisone (Can)** *see* Betamethasone (Topical) *on page 280*
◆ **ratio-Trazodone (Can)** *see* TraZODone *on page 2105*
◆ **ratio-Valproic (Can)** *see* Valproic Acid and Derivatives *on page 2143*

Raxibacumab (rax i BAK ue mab)

Therapeutic Category Antidote; Monoclonal Antibody

Generic Availability (US) No

Use Treatment of inhalational anthrax following exposure to *Bacillus anthracis* in combination with appropriate antimicrobial therapy; prophylaxis of inhalational anthrax when alternative therapies are unavailable or not appropriate (All indications: FDA approved in all ages)

Prescribing and Access Restrictions Raxibacumab is not available for general public use. All supplies are currently owned by the federal government for inclusion in the Strategic National Stockpile and for use by the U.S. military.

Pregnancy Risk Factor B

Pregnancy Considerations Adverse events were not observed in animal reproduction studies. In general, medications used as antidotes should take into consideration the health and prognosis of the mother; antidotes should be administered to pregnant women if there is a clear indication for use and should not be withheld because of fears of teratogenicity (Bailey, 2003).

Breast-Feeding Considerations In general, an increase in maternal immunoglobulins is not observed in infants following nursing. The potential effects of raxibacumab on a nursing infant are not known.

Contraindications There are no contraindications listed in the manufacturer's labeling.

Warnings/Precautions Raxibacumab is not an antimicrobial agent; use should always be in combination with appropriate antimicrobial therapy. Raxibacumab does not cross the blood brain barrier and is not appropriate for the prevention or treatment of meningitis due to anthrax infection. The efficacy of raxibacumab in humans is presumptive and based solely on efficacy studies in animals.

Infusion-related reactions (eg, rash, urticaria, pruritus) have been reported. Premedication with diphenhydramine is recommended to reduce the risk. The administration rate is slowed over the first 20 minutes to monitor for adverse reactions; slow or interrupt infusion if adverse reactions (including infusion-related reactions) occur.

Some dosage forms may contain polysorbate 80 (also known as Tweens). Hypersensitivity reactions, usually a delayed reaction, have been reported following exposure to pharmaceutical products containing polysorbate 80 in certain individuals (Isaksson, 2002; Lucente 2000; Shelley, 1995). Thrombocytopenia, ascites, pulmonary deterioration, and renal and hepatic failure have been reported in premature neonates after receiving parenteral products containing polysorbate 80 (Alade, 1986; CDC, 1984). See manufacturer's labeling.

Adverse Reactions

Central nervous system: Pain, somnolence

Dermatologic: Pruritus

Local: Infusion-related rash

Rare but important or life-threatening: Amylase increased, anemia, back pain, creatinine phosphokinase increased, fatigue, flushing, hypertension, insomnia, leukopenia, lymphadenopathy, muscle spasm, pain (infusion site), palpitations, peripheral edema, prothrombin time increased, somnolence, syncope (vasovagal), vertigo

Drug Interactions

Metabolism/Transport Effects None known.

Avoid Concomitant Use

Avoid concomitant use of Raxibacumab with any of the following: Belimumab

Increased Effect/Toxicity

Raxibacumab may increase the levels/effects of: Belimumab

Decreased Effect There are no known significant interactions involving a decrease in effect.

Storage/Stability Unused vials should be stored at 2°C to 8°C (36°F to 46°F); do not freeze. Protect from light. Diluted solutions are stable for 8 hours at room temperature.

Mechanism of Action Raxibacumab is a recombinant human IgG1 lambda monoclonal antibody which binds and neutralizes free protective antigen (PA) component of *Bacillus anthracis* toxin; as a result, PA-mediated delivery of lethal toxin and edema toxin via the anthrax toxin receptor (ATR) into host cells of anthrax-infected individuals is inhibited.

Pharmacokinetics (Adult data unless noted)

Distribution: V_d: 0.07 L/kg (Migone, 2009)

Half-life elimination: Terminal: 20.44 ± 6.46 (Migone, 2009)

Elimination: Nonrenal

Dosing: Neonatal Note: Administer diphenhydramine (oral or IV depending on the proximity to start of raxibacumab infusion) ≤1 hour prior to administration of raxibacumab to reduce the risk of infusion reactions. Must be administered in combination with antimicrobial therapy.

Anthrax, prophylaxis or treatment: IV: 80 mg/kg as a single dose

Dosing: Usual Note: Administer diphenhydramine (oral or IV depending on the proximity to start of raxibacumab infusion) ≤1 hour prior to administration of raxibacumab to reduce the risk of infusion reactions. Must be administered in combination with antimicrobial therapy.

Pediatric: **Anthrax, prophylaxis or treatment:** Infants, Children, and Adolescents: IV:

≤15 kg: 80 mg/kg as a single dose

>15 kg to 50 kg: 60 mg/kg as a single dose

>50 kg: 40 mg/kg as a single dose

Adult: **Anthrax, prophylaxis or treatment:** IV: 40 mg/kg as a single dose

Dosing adjustment in renal impairment: There are no dosage adjustments provided in manufacturer's labeling; however, dosage adjustment unlikely as clearance is nonrenal.

Dosing adjustment in hepatic impairment: There are no dosage adjustment provided in manufacturer's labeling (has not been studied).

Preparation for Administration IV: Single-use vial (50 mg/mL solution) requires dilution prior to administration; each vial delivers 1,700 mg of raxibacumab (34 mL). Diluent based on weight: In patients <11 kg dilute with either ½NS or NS; in patients ≥11 kg, dilute with NS; final volume based on weight. May be prepared for administration in a syringe or infusion bag depending on volume required for administration. Gently mix solution; do not shake.

Body weight: ≤1 kg: Dilute to a final volume of 7 mL

Body weight 1.1 to 2 kg: Dilute to a final volume of 15 mL

Body weight 2.1 to 3 kg: Dilute to a final volume of 20 mL

Body weight 3.1 to 4.9 kg: Dilute to a final volume of 25 mL

Body weight 5 to 10 kg: Dilute to a final volume of 50 mL

Body weight 11 to 30 kg: Dilute to a final volume of 100 mL

Body weight ≥31 kg: Dilute to a final volume of 250 mL

Administration IV: Must be diluted prior to administration. Premedicate with diphenhydramine ≤1 hour prior to raxibacumab infusion. Administer entire dose over 2 hours and 15 minutes; administration rate should be slower over the first 20 minutes to monitor for adverse reactions; slow or interrupt infusion if adverse reactions (including infusion-related reactions) occur. Administer as follows:

Body weight: ≤1 kg: Infuse at 0.5 mL/hour for 20 minutes; increase rate to 3.5 mL/hour for the remaining infusion

Body weight 1.1 to 2 kg: Infuse at 1 mL/hour for 20 minutes; increase rate to 7 mL/hour for the remaining infusion

Body weight 2.1 to 3 kg: Infuse at 1.2 mL/hour for 20 minutes; increase rate to 10 mL/hour for the remaining infusion

Body weight 3.1 to 4.9 kg: Infuse at 1.5 mL/hour for 20 minutes; increase rate to 12 mL/hour for the remaining infusion

Body weight 5 to 10 kg: Infuse at 3 mL/hour for 20 minutes; increase rate to 25 mL/hour for the remaining infusion

Body weight 11 to 30 kg: Infuse at 6 mL/hour for 20 minutes; increase rate to 50 mL/hour for the remaining infusion

Body weight ≥31 kg: Infuse at 15 mL/hour for 20 minutes; increase rate to 125 mL/hour for the remaining infusion

Monitoring Parameters Infusion-related adverse effects (eg, rash, urticaria, pruritus)

Dosage Forms Excipient information presented when available (limited, particularly for generics); consult specific product labeling.

Injection, solution: 50 mg/mL (34 mL) [contains polysorbate 80, sucrose 10 mg/mL]

◆ **Rayos** *see* PredniSONE *on page* 1760

◆ **6R-BH4** *see* Sapropterin *on page* 1900

◆ **Reactine (Can)** *see* Cetirizine *on page* 423

◆ **Rebetol** *see* Ribavirin *on page* 1851

◆ **Recombinant α-L-Iduronidase (Glycosaminoglycan α-L-Iduronohydrolase)** *see* Laronidase *on page* 1222

◆ **Recombinant Granulocyte-Macrophage Colony Stimulating Factor** *see* Sargramostim *on page* 1905

◆ **Recombinant Human Deoxyribonuclease** *see* Dornase Alfa *on page* 705

◆ **Recombinant Human Insulin-Like Growth Factor-1** *see* Mecasermin *on page* 1334

Remifentanil (rem i FEN ta nil)

Medication Safety Issues

Sound-alike/look-alike issues:

Remifentanil may be confused with alfentanil

High alert medication:

The Institute for Safe Medication Practices (ISMP) includes this medication among its list of drug classes which have a heightened risk of causing significant patient harm when used in error.

Brand Names: US Ultiva

Brand Names: Canada Ultiva®

Therapeutic Category Analgesic, Narcotic; General Anesthetic

Generic Availability (US) No

Use Analgesic for use during the induction of general anesthesia (FDA approved in adults); maintenance of general anesthesia (FDA approved in ages 0-2 months, 1-12 years, and adults); continued analgesia into the immediate postoperative period (FDA approved in adults); as the analgesic component of monitored anesthesia (FDA approved in adults); has also been used as adjunct for analgesia during endotracheal intubation, for total intravenous anesthesia (TIVA), and for continuous analgesia/sedation in critically ill mechanically ventilated patients.

Pregnancy Risk Factor C

Pregnancy Considerations Adverse events were not observed in animal reproduction studies. Remifentanil has been shown to cross the placenta; fetal and maternal concentrations may be similar.

Breast-Feeding Considerations It is not known if remifentanil is excreted into breast milk. The manufacturer recommends that caution be used if administered to a nursing woman. Remifentanil has a limited duration of action; use may be appropriate for breast-feeding women undergoing short procedures (Montgomery, 2012).

Contraindications Not for intrathecal or epidural administration, due to the presence of glycine in the formulation; hypersensitivity to remifentanil, fentanyl, or fentanyl analogs, or any component of the formulation

Warnings/Precautions Remifentanil is not recommended as the sole agent for induction of anesthesia, because the loss of consciousness cannot be assured. Due to the high incidence of apnea, hypotension, respiratory depression, tachycardia and muscle rigidity remifentanil should only be administered by individuals specifically trained in the use of anesthetic agents and should not be used in diagnostic or therapeutic procedures outside the monitored anesthesia setting; resuscitative and intubation equipment should be readily available. May cause hypotension; use with caution in patients with hypovolemia, cardiovascular disease (including acute MI), or drugs which may exaggerate hypotensive effects (including phenothiazines or general anesthetics). Shares the toxic potentials of opioid agonists, and precautions of opioid agonist therapy should be observed. In patients <55 years of age, intraoperative awareness has been reported when used with propofol rates of ≤75 mcg/kg/minute.

Rapid IV infusion (single dose >1 mcg/kg over 30-60 seconds and infusion rates >0.1 mcg/kg/minute) should only be used during maintenance of general anesthesia; may result in skeletal muscle and chest wall rigidity, impaired ventilation, or respiratory distress/arrest; nondepolarizing skeletal muscle relaxant may be required. Chest wall rigidity may resolve by decreasing the infusion rate or temporarily stopping the infusion. Inadequate clearing of IV tubing following remifentanil administration could result in chest wall rigidity, respiratory depression, and apnea when another fluid is administered through the same line. Interruption of an infusion will result in offset of effects within 5-10 minutes; the discontinuation of remifentanil infusion should be preceded by the establishment of adequate postoperative analgesia orders, especially for patients in whom postoperative pain is anticipated. Use caution in the morbidly obese. Use with caution in patients with a history of drug abuse or acute alcoholism; potential for drug dependency exists. Tolerance, psychological and physical dependence may occur with prolonged use.

Adverse Reactions

Cardiovascular: Bradycardia (dose dependent), flushing, hypertension (dose dependent), hypotension, tachycardia (dose dependent)

Central nervous system: Agitation, chills, dizziness, fever, headache, postoperative pain

Dermatologic: Pruritus

Gastrointestinal: Nausea, vomiting

Local: Pain at injection site

Neuromuscular & skeletal: Muscle rigidity

Respiratory: Apnea, hypoxia, respiratory depression

Miscellaneous: Diaphoresis, shivering, warm sensation

Rare but important or life-threatening: Abdominal discomfort, amnesia, anaphylaxis, anxiety, arrhythmias, awareness under anesthesia without pain, bronchitis, bronchospasm, chest pain, confusion, constipation, cough, CPK increased, diarrhea, disorientation, dysphagia, dysphoria, dyspnea, dysuria, ECG changes, electrolyte disorders, erythema, gastroesophageal reflux, hallucinations, heart block, heartburn, hiccups, hyperglycemia, ileus, incontinence, involuntary movement, laryngospasm, leukocytosis, liver dysfunction, lymphopenia, nasal congestion, nightmares, nystagmus, oliguria, paresthesia, pharyngitis, pleural effusion, prolonged emergence from anesthesia, pulmonary edema, rales, rapid awakening from anesthesia, rash, rhinorrhea, rhonchi, seizure, sleep disturbance, stridor, syncope, temperature regulation impaired, thrombocytopenia, tremors, twitching, urine retention, urticaria, xerostomia

Drug Interactions

Metabolism/Transport Effects None known.

Avoid Concomitant Use

Avoid concomitant use of Remifentanil with any of the following: Azelastine (Nasal); Eluxadoline; MAO Inhibitors; Mixed Agonist / Antagonist Opioids; Orphenadrine; Paraldehyde; Thalidomide

Increased Effect/Toxicity

Remifentanil may increase the levels/effects of: Alcohol (Ethyl); Alvimopan; Azelastine (Nasal); Beta-Blockers; Calcium Channel Blockers (Nondihydropyridine); CNS Depressants; Desmopressin; Diuretics; Eluxadoline; Hydrocodone; MAO Inhibitors; Methotrimeprazine; Metyrosine; Mirtazapine; Orphenadrine; Paraldehyde; Pramipexole; ROPINIRole; Rotigotine; Selective Serotonin Reuptake Inhibitors; Suvorexant; Thalidomide; Zolpidem

The levels/effects of Remifentanil may be increased by: Amphetamines; Anticholinergic Agents; Antipsychotic Agents (Phenothiazines); Brimonidine (Topical); Cannabis; Doxylamine; Dronabinol; Droperidol; HydrOXYzine; Kava Kava; Magnesium Sulfate; Methotrimeprazine; Nabilone; Perampanel; Rufinamide; Sodium Oxybate; Succinylcholine; Tapentadol; Tetrahydrocannabinol

Decreased Effect

Remifentanil may decrease the levels/effects of: Pegvisomant

The levels/effects of Remifentanil may be decreased by: Ammonium Chloride; Mixed Agonist / Antagonist Opioids; Naltrexone

Storage/Stability Prior to reconstitution, store at 2°C to 25°C (36°F to 77°F). Stable for 24 hours at room temperature after reconstitution and further dilution to concentrations of 20-250 mcg/mL (4 hours if diluted with LR).

Mechanism of Action Binds with stereospecific mu-opioid receptors at many sites within the CNS, increases pain threshold, alters pain reception, inhibits ascending pain pathways

Pharmacodynamics

Analgesia:

- Onset of action: 1-3 minutes
- Maximum effect: 3-5 minutes
- Duration: 3-10 minutes (Scott, 2005)

Pharmacokinetics (Adult data unless noted) Note: In pediatric patients (neonates through adolescents), pharmacokinetic data showed variable age-related changes with distribution (ie, highest V_d associated with lowest age) and clearance (ie, fastest clearance in the youngest patients); however, no age-related changes with half-life (Ross, 2001).

Distribution:

- Pediatric patients (Ross, 2001): V_{dss}:
  - Neonates ≤2 months: 453 ± 145 mL/kg
  - Infants and Children >2 months to <2 years: 308 ± 89 mL/kg
  - Children 2-6 years: 240 mL/kg ± 131 mL/kg
  - Children 7-12 years: 249 mL/kg ± 91 mL/kg
  - Adolescents 13 to <16 years: 223 ± 31 mL/kg
  - Adolescents 16-18 years: 243 ± 109 mL/kg
- Adults: V_d: Initial: 100 mL/kg; V_{dss}: 350 mL/kg

Protein binding: ~70% (primarily $alpha_1$ acid glycoprotein)

Metabolism: Rapid via blood and tissue esterases; not metabolized by plasma cholinesterase (pseudocholinesterase) and is not appreciably metabolized by the liver

Half-life (dose dependent):

- Pediatric patients (Ross, 2001): Effective:
  - Neonates ≤2 months: 5.4 minutes (range: 3-8 minutes)
  - Infants and Children >2 months to <2 years: 3.4 minutes (range: 2-6 minutes)
  - Children 2-6 years: 3.6 minutes (range: 1-6 minutes)
  - Children 7-12 years: 5.3 minutes (range: 3-7 minutes)
  - Adolescents: 13 to <16 years: 3.7 minutes (range: 2-5 minutes)
  - Adolescents 16-18 years: 5.7 minutes (range: 5-6 minutes)
- Adults: Terminal: 10-20 minutes; effective: 3-10 minutes

Time to peak serum concentration: Intranasal: Children ≤7 years: ~3.5 minutes (Verghese, 2008)

Elimination: Clearance:

- Pediatric patients (Ross, 2001):
  - Neonates ≤2 months of age: 90.5 ± 36.8 mL/minute/kg
  - Infants and Children >2 months to <2 years: 92.1 ± 25.8 mL/minute/kg
  - Children 2-6 years: 76.0 ± 22.4 mL/minute/kg
  - Children 7-12 years: 59.7 ± 22.5 mL/minute/kg
  - Adolescents 13 to <16 years: 57.2 ± 21.2 mL/minute/kg
  - Adolescents 16-18 years: 46.5 ± 2.1 mL/minute/kg
- Adults: ~40 mL/minute/kg

Dosing: Neonatal

Anesthesia, maintenance of anesthesia with nitrous oxide (70%): Continuous IV infusion: 0.4 mcg/kg/minute (range: 0.4-1 mcg/kg/minute); supplemental bolus dose of 1 mcg/kg may be administered; smaller bolus dose may be required with potent inhalation agents, potent neuraxial anesthesia, significant comorbidities, significant fluid shifts, or without atropine pretreatment. Clearance in neonates is highly variable; dose should be carefully titrated.

Analgesia/sedation in mechanically ventilated patients: Limited data available, dosage not established: Continuous IV infusion:

Preterm infants: Initial: 0.075 mcg/kg/minute, titrate to effect; dosing based on a trial in 48 preterm infants requiring mechanical ventilation (GA: Mean: 28.5 weeks, range: 25-33 weeks; PNA: 1-17 days); in a large majority of the patients (73%), dose escalation from the initial dose was required within the first 6 hours of therapy; mean effective dose: 0.11 ± 0.05 mcg/kg/minute, maximum reported dose: 0.94 mcg/kg/minute.

No cardiovascular or respiratory adverse effects were observed (Giannantonio, 2009).

Term infants: Initial: 0.15 mcg/kg/minute, titrate to effect; dosing based on a randomized, double-blind, comparative study of neonates and young infants (n=23; GA: ≥36 weeks; PNA: <60 days) requiring mechanical ventilation who were given a combination of either midazolam/remifentanil (n=11) or midazolam/fentanyl (n=12); mean remifentanil effective dose: 0.23 mcg/kg/minute; maximum reported dose: 0.5 mcg/kg/minute; efficacy data and adverse effect profile were similar to fentanyl (Welzing, 2012)

Endotracheal intubation, nonemergent: Limited data available: IV: 1-3 mcg/kg/dose; may repeat dose in 2-3 minutes if needed (Choong, 2010; Kumar, 2010; Silva, 2008)

Dosing: Usual

Infants, Children, and Adolescents: **Note:** Continuous IV infusion: Dose should be based on ideal body weight (IBW) in obese patients (>30% over IBW).

Analgesia (postoperative); mechanically ventilated patient: Limited data available: Children and Adolescents 3-16 years: Continuous IV infusion: 0.1 mcg/kg/minute with or without adjunctive medication, titrate to effect; dosing based on a randomized, double-blind comparative trial of remifentanil versus fentanyl in 22 postoperative orthopedic spinal surgery patients requiring mechanical ventilation (remifentanil group, n=11; age: Mean:13 years, range: 3-16 years); similar efficacy and adverse effect profile were reported with both treatment groups (Akinci, 2005)

Analgesia/sedation in mechanically ventilated patients: Limited data available: Infants ≤2 months: Continuous IV infusion: Initial: 0.15 mcg/kg/minute, titrate to effect; dosing based on a randomized, double-blind, comparative study of neonates and young infants (n=23; GA: ≥36 weeks; PNA: <60 days) requiring mechanical ventilation who were given a combination of either midazolam/remifentanil (n=11) or midazolam/fentanyl (n=12); mean remifentanil effective dose: 0.23 mcg/kg/minute; maximum reported dose: 0.5 mcg/kg/minute; efficacy data and adverse effect profile were similar to fentanyl (Welzing, 2012)

Anesthesia, maintenance of anesthesia: Continuous IV infusion:

Infants 1-2 months: Maintenance of anesthesia with nitrous oxide (70%): 0.4 mcg/kg/minute (range: 0.4-1 mcg/kg/minute); supplemental bolus dose of 1 mcg/kg may be administered, smaller bolus dose may be required with potent inhalation agents, potent neuraxial anesthesia, significant comorbidities, significant fluid shifts, or without atropine pretreatment

Infants ≥3 months, Children, and Adolescents: Limited data available: Maintenance of anesthesia with halothane, sevoflurane, or isoflurane: 0.25 mcg/kg/minute (range: 0.05-1.3 mcg/kg/minute); supplemental bolus dose of 1 mcg/kg may be administered every 2-5 minutes. Consider increasing concomitant anesthetics with infusion rate >1 mcg/kg/minute. Infusion rate can be titrated upward in increments up to 50% or titrated downward in decrements of 25% to 50%. May titrate every 2-5 minutes.

Anesthesia, total intravenous (TIVA); with or without propofol induction: Limited data available: IV: Loading dose (may omit if propofol induction used): 0.5 mcg/kg/minute for 3 minutes (total dose: 1.5 mcg/kg) or 1 mcg/kg over 1 minute; followed by an initial maintenance dose: 0.05-1 mcg/kg/minute; titrate in 0.05 mcg/kg/minute increments every 3 minutes to effect; usual effective range: 0.2-0.5 mcg/kg/minute; has been used in combination with propofol (bolus and/or infusion) (Malherbe, 2010a; Malherbe, 2010b; Mani, 2010; Shen, 2012)

Endotracheal intubation for elective procedures: Limited data available:

IV: Usual range: 1-3 mcg/kg/dose, doses as high as 4 mcg/kg have been used. Dosing based on multiple trials in patients undergoing elective procedures requiring intubation who were not receiving neuromuscular blockers and remifentanil administered in combination with other induction agents such as propofol, ketamine, or sevoflurane. (Begec, 2009; Blair, 2004; Hume-Smith, 2010; Klemola, 2000; Morgan, 2007; Park, 2009)

Intranasal (using parenteral 100 mcg/mL formulation): Children ≤7 years: 4 mcg/kg/dose; administer half of the total dose in each nostril; wait 2-3 minutes before attempting intubation. Dosing based on a double-blind, randomized, controlled trial (n=188), remifentanil was administered after sevoflurane induction and overall, was found more effective than saline placebo at both endpoints of 2 minutes and 3 minutes post-dose. Results also showed that within the remifentanil treatment groups, good or excellent intubation conditions were reported more often at 3 minutes post-dose than at 2 minutes (91.7% vs 68.2%) (Verghese, 2008).

Procedural sedation: Limited data available, dosage not established: IV: 0.5 mcg/kg with propofol has been used to induce analgesia and adjunct sedation prior to esophagogastroduodenoscopy (n=22; age range: 2-12 years) and short hemato-oncologic invasive procedures (n=30, age range: 2-18 years) (Hirsh, 2010; Ince, 2013). A higher dose of 3 mcg/kg was used in already sedated (sevoflurane) infants and young children who required apnea for CT or MRI imaging (n=12, age range: 6-16 months) (Joshi, 2009). In a dose-finding trial, continuous IV infusion of remifentanil at 0.2 mcg/kg/minute has been shown more effective than a lower 0.1 mcg/kg/minute in 60 children 2-12 years undergoing diagnostic cardiac catheterization; pretreatment with oral midazolam and local groin anesthetic also utilized (Kaynar, 2011).

Adults:

Induction of anesthesia: 0.5-1 mcg/kg/minute; if endotracheal intubation is to occur in <8 minutes, an initial dose of 1 mcg/kg may be given over 30-60 seconds; in coronary bypass surgery: 1 mcg/kg/minute

Maintenance of anesthesia: Note: Supplemental bolus dose of 1 mcg/kg may be administered every 2-5 minutes. Consider increasing concomitant anesthetics with infusion rate >1 mcg/kg/minute. Infusion rate can be titrated upward in increments of 25% to 100% or downward in decrements of 25% to 50%. May titrate every 2-5 minutes.

With nitrous oxide (66%): 0.4 mcg/kg/minute (range: 0.1-2 mcg/kg/minute)

With isoflurane: 0.25 mcg/kg/minute (range: 0.05-2 mcg/kg/minute)

With propofol: 0.25 mcg/kg/minute (range: 0.05-2 mcg/kg/minute)

Coronary bypass surgery: 1 mcg/kg/minute (range: 0.125-4 mcg/kg/minute); supplemental dose: 0.5-1 mcg/kg

Continuation as an analgesic in immediate postoperative period: 0.1 mcg/kg/minute (range: 0.025-0.2 mcg/kg/minute). Infusion rate may be adjusted every 5 minutes in increments of 0.025 mcg/kg/minute. Bolus doses are not recommended. Infusion rates >0.2 mcg/kg/minute are associated with respiratory depression.

Coronary bypass surgery, continuation as an analgesic into the ICU: 1 mcg/kg/minute (range: 0.05-1 mcg/kg/minute)

Analgesic component of monitored anesthesia care:
Note: Supplemental oxygen is recommended:
Single IV dose given 90 seconds prior to local anesthetic:
Remifentanil alone: 1 mcg/kg over 30-60 seconds
With midazolam: 0.5 mcg/kg over 30-60 seconds
Continuous infusion beginning 5 minutes prior to local anesthetic:
Remifentanil alone: 0.1 mcg/kg/minute
With midazolam: 0.05 mcg/kg/minute
Continuous infusion given after local anesthetic:
Remifentanil alone: 0.05 mcg/kg/minute (range: 0.025-0.2 mcg/kg/minute)
With midazolam: 0.025 mcg/kg/minute (range: 0.025-0.2 mcg/kg/minute)
Note: Following local or anesthetic block, infusion rate should be decreased to 0.05 mcg/kg/minute; rate adjustments of 0.025 mcg/kg/minute may be done at 5-minute intervals

Dosing adjustment in renal impairment: Removed by hemodialysis (30%). There are no dosage adjustments provided in the manufacturer's labeling; however, remifentanil pharmacokinetics are unchanged in patients with end stage renal disease.

Dosing adjustment in hepatic impairment: There are no dosage adjustments provided in the manufacturer's labeling; however, remifentanil pharmacokinetics are unchanged in patients with severe hepatic impairment.

Preparation for Administration IV: Prepare solution by adding 1 mL of diluent per 1 mg of remifentanil. Shake well. Further dilute to a final concentration of 20, 25, 50, or 250 mcg/mL.

Administration IV: An infusion pump should be used to administer continuous infusions. During the maintenance of general anesthesia, IV boluses ≤1 mcg/kg may be administered over 30 to 60 seconds; for doses >1 mcg/kg, administer over >60 seconds (to reduce the potential to develop skeletal muscle and chest wall rigidity). Injections should be given into IV tubing close to the venous cannula; tubing should be cleared after treatment to prevent residual effects when other fluids are administered through the same IV line.

Monitoring Parameters Respiratory and cardiovascular status, blood pressure, heart rate

Controlled Substance C-II

Dosage Forms Excipient information presented when available (limited, particularly for generics); consult specific product labeling.
Solution Reconstituted, Intravenous [preservative free]:
Ultiva: 1 mg (1 ea); 2 mg (1 ea); 5 mg (1 ea)

- ◆ **Remsima (Can)** *see* InFLIXimab *on page 1104*
- ◆ **Renagel** *see* Sevelamer *on page 1920*
- ◆ **Renova** *see* Tretinoin (Topical) *on page 2111*
- ◆ **Renova Pump** *see* Tretinoin (Topical) *on page 2111*
- ◆ **Renovo** *see* Capsaicin *on page 362*
- ◆ **Renvela** *see* Sevelamer *on page 1920*
- ◆ **Repository Corticotropin** *see* Corticotropin *on page 536*
- ◆ **Resectisol** *see* Mannitol *on page 1321*
- ◆ **Restasis** *see* CycloSPORINE (Ophthalmic) *on page 561*
- ◆ **Restasis® (Can)** *see* CycloSPORINE (Ophthalmic) *on page 561*

Retapamulin (re te PAM ue lin)

Brand Names: US Altabax

Therapeutic Category Antibiotic, Pleuromutilin; Antibiotic, Topical

Generic Availability (US) No

Use Treatment of impetigo caused by susceptible strains of *S. pyrogenes* or methicillin-susceptible *S. aureus* (FDA approved in ages ≥9 months and adults)

Pregnancy Risk Factor B

Pregnancy Considerations Adverse events have not been observed in animal reproduction studies.

Breast-Feeding Considerations It is not known if retapamulin is excreted in breast milk. The manufacturer recommends that caution be exercised when administering retapamulin to nursing women.

Contraindications There are no contraindications listed in the manufacturer's labeling.

Warnings/Precautions For external use only; not for intranasal, intravaginal, ophthalmic, oral, or mucosal application. Prolonged use may result in fungal or bacterial superinfection, including *C. difficile*-associated diarrhea (CDAD) and pseudomembranous colitis; CDAD has been observed >2 months postantibiotic treatment. Concomitant use with other topical products to the same treatment area has not been evaluated. If sensitization or severe local skin irritation occurs, wipe ointment off and discontinue use.

Adverse Reactions
Central nervous system: Headache
Dermatologic: Eczema (infants, children, and adolescents)
Gastrointestinal: Diarrhea, nausea
Local: Application site irritation (adults), application site pruritus (infants, children, and adolescents)
Respiratory: Nasopharyngitis
Rare but important or life-threatening: Contact dermatitis, creatine phosphokinase increased, epistaxis, hypersensitivity

Drug Interactions

Metabolism/Transport Effects Substrate of CYP3A4 (minor); **Note:** Assignment of Major/Minor substrate status based on clinically relevant drug interaction potential

Avoid Concomitant Use There are no known interactions where it is recommended to avoid concomitant use.

Increased Effect/Toxicity
The levels/effects of Retapamulin may be increased by: CYP3A4 Inhibitors (Strong)

Decreased Effect There are no known significant interactions involving a decrease in effect.

Storage/Stability Store at 25°C (77°F); excursions permitted between 15°C and 30°C (59°F and 86°F).

Mechanism of Action Primarily bacteriostatic; inhibits normal bacterial protein biosynthesis by binding at a unique site (protein L3) on the ribosomal 50S subunit; prevents formation of active 50S ribosomal subunits by inhibiting peptidyl transfer and blocking P-site interactions at this site

Pharmacokinetics (Adult data unless noted)
Absorption: Topical: Increased when applied to abraded skin; age dependent; absorption highest in younger patients
Infants and Children 2 to 24 months: Overall, in trials, 46% of subjects 2 to 24 months of age had measurable serum concentration compared to 7% of those ≥2 years. Within the 2 to 24 month age group, the aggregate of infants 2 to 9 months had a higher proportion of patients with measurable serum concentration than those aged 9 to 24 months (69% vs 32%)
Children ≥ 2 years, Adolescents, and Adults: Low; increased when applied to abraded skin
Protein binding: 94%
Metabolism: Hepatic via CYP 3A4; extensively metabolized by mono-oxygenation and di-oxygenation to multiple metabolites

Dosing: Usual
Pediatric: **Impetigo: Note:** Total treatment area should not exceed 2% of total body surface area or 100 cm^2 total body surface area, whichever is less.

Infants 1 to <9 months: Limited data available: Topical: Apply to lesions twice daily for 5 days (Stevens, 2014); **Note:** In trials, infants 2 to 9 months of age had higher systemic exposure than older pediatric patients, monitor closely for systemic effects.

Infants ≥9 months, Children, and Adolescents: Topical: Apply to affected area (lesions) twice daily for 5 days

Adult: **Impetigo:** Topical: Apply to affected area twice daily for 5 days. Total treatment area should not exceed 100 cm^2 total body surface area.

Dosing adjustment in renal impairment: There are no dosage adjustments provided in manufacturer's labeling

Dosing adjustment in hepatic impairment: There are no dosage adjustments provided in manufacturer's labeling

Administration Topical: May cover treatment area with sterile bandage or gauze dressing if needed to prevent accidental transfer of ointment into eyes, mouth, or other areas. Concomitant use with other topical products to the same treatment area has not been evaluated.

Dosage Forms Excipient information presented when available (limited, particularly for generics); consult specific product labeling.

Ointment, External:

Altabax: 1% (15 g, 30 g)

- **Retin-A** *see* Tretinoin (Topical) *on page 2111*
- **Retin-A Micro** *see* Tretinoin (Topical) *on page 2111*
- **Retin-A Micro Pump** *see* Tretinoin (Topical) *on page 2111*
- **Retinoic Acid** *see* Tretinoin (Topical) *on page 2111*
- **Retinova (Can)** *see* Tretinoin (Topical) *on page 2111*
- **Retisert** *see* Fluocinolone (Ophthalmic) *on page 895*
- **Retrovir** *see* Zidovudine *on page 2207*
- **Retrovir (AZT) (Can)** *see* Zidovudine *on page 2207*
- **Revatio** *see* Sildenafil *on page 1921*
- **Revonto** *see* Dantrolene *on page 576*
- **Reyataz** *see* Atazanavir *on page 210*
- **rFVIIa** *see* Factor VIIa (Recombinant) *on page 835*
- **R-Gene 10** *see* Arginine *on page 190*
- **rhASB** *see* Galsulfase *on page 956*
- **rhDNase** *see* Dornase Alfa *on page 705*
- **Rheumatrex** *see* Methotrexate *on page 1390*
- **rhGAA** *see* Alglucosidase Alfa *on page 94*
- **r-h α-GAL** *see* Agalsidase Beta *on page 76*
- **RhIG** *see* $Rh_o(D)$ Immune Globulin *on page 1847*
- **rhIGF-1 (Mecasermin [Increlex®])** *see* Mecasermin *on page 1334*
- **rhIL-11** *see* Oprelvekin *on page 1570*
- **Rhinalar® (Can)** *see* Flunisolide (Nasal) *on page 894*
- **Rhinall [OTC]** *see* Phenylephrine (Nasal) *on page 1688*
- **Rhinaris [OTC]** *see* Sodium Chloride *on page 1938*
- **Rhinaris-CS Anti-Allergic Nasal Mist (Can)** *see* Cromolyn (Nasal) *on page 542*
- **Rhinocort Allergy OTC** *see* Budesonide (Nasal) *on page 311*
- **Rhinocort Aqua** *see* Budesonide (Nasal) *on page 311*
- **Rhinocort Turbuhaler (Can)** *see* Budesonide (Nasal) *on page 311*
- **Rho(D) Immune Globulin (Human)** *see* $Rh_o(D)$ Immune Globulin *on page 1847*

$Rh_o(D)$ Immune Globulin

(ar aych oh (dee) i MYUN GLOB yoo lin)

Medication Safety Issues

International issues:

Bayrho-D [Israel, Turkey] may be confused with Bayhep-B which is a brand name for hepatitis B immune globulin [Philippines, Turkey]; Bayrab which is brand name for rabies immune globulin [Philippines, Turkey]

Brand Names: US HyperRHO S/D; MICRhoGAM Ultra-Filtered Plus; RhoGAM Ultra-Filtered Plus; Rhophylac; WinRho SDF

Brand Names: Canada WinRho SDF

Therapeutic Category Immune Globulin

Generic Availability (US) No

Use

Suppression of Rh isoimmunization: Use in the following situations when an $Rh_o(D)$-negative individual is exposed to $Rh_o(D)$-positive blood: During delivery of an $Rh_o(D)$-positive infant; abortion; amniocentesis; chorionic villus sampling; ruptured tubal pregnancy; abdominal trauma; transplacental hemorrhage. Used when the mother is $Rh_o(D)$ negative, the father of the child is either $Rh_o(D)$ positive or $Rh_o(D)$ unknown, the baby is either $Rh_o(D)$ positive or $Rh_o(D)$ unknown (FDA approved in pregnant women)

Transfusion: Suppression of Rh isoimmunization in $Rh_o(D)$-negative individuals transfused with $Rh_o(D)$ antigen-positive RBCs or blood components containing $Rh_o(D)$ antigen-positive RBCs (FDA approved in adults)

Treatment of immune thrombocytopenia (ITP): Used intravenously in the following nonsplenectomized $Rh_o(D)$ positive individuals: Acute ITP (WinRho SDF: FDA approved in children), chronic ITP (Rhophylac: FDA approved in adults; WinRho SDF: FDA approved in children and adults), ITP secondary to HIV infection (WinRho SDF: FDA approved in ages <16 years and adults)

Pregnancy Risk Factor C

Pregnancy Considerations Animal reproduction studies have not been conducted.

$Rh_o(D)$ immune globulin (RhIG) is administered to pregnant women to prevent alloimmunization of $Rh_o(D)$ negative mothers who may potentially have a fetus who is $Rh_o(D)$ positive. Administration of the immune globulin prevents the mother from developing antibodies to the D antigen and the development of hemolytic anemia in the newborn. Current guidelines recommend administration of RhIG to pregnant women who are $Rh_o(D)$ negative and who are not already $Rh_o(D)$ alloimmunized at ~28 weeks gestation (unless the father is known to be $Rh_o(D)$ negative), within 72 hours of delivery of an $Rh_o(D)$ positive infant, after a first trimester pregnancy loss, or after invasive procedures such as amniocentesis, chorionic villus sampling (CVS), or fetal blood sampling (ACOG, 1999). Available evidence suggests that $Rh_o(D)$ immune globulin administration during pregnancy does not harm the fetus or affect future pregnancies.

In pregnant women who require treatment for ITP, other agents are preferred. RhIG for this indication in pregnancy is limited to case reports and small studies (Neunert, 2011).

Breast-Feeding Considerations Adverse events in the nursing infant have not been observed when administered to women for the suppression of Rh isoimmunization. The manufacturer recommends that caution be used if administered to nursing women. The purified immune globulin in these products is obtained from human donors; the $Rh_o(D)$ antibodies are endogenous to human plasma.

Contraindications

HyperRHO S/D Full Dose, HyperRHO S/D Mini Dose: There are no contraindications listed in the manufacturer's labeling.

MICRhoGAM Ultra-Filtered Plus, RhoGAM Ultra-Filtered Plus: Use in Rh-positive individuals.

Rhophylac: Anaphylactic or severe systemic reaction to a previous dose of human immune globulin; use in IgA-deficient patients with antibodies to IgA and a history of hypersensitivity.

WinRho SDF: Anaphylactic or severe systemic reaction to a previous dose of human immune globulin; use in IgA-deficient patients with antibodies to IgA and a history of hypersensitivity; autoimmune hemolytic anemia; preexisting hemolysis or at high risk for hemolysis; suppression of $Rh_o(D)$ isoimmunization in infants.

WinRho SDF Canadian labeling: Additional contraindications (not in US labeling): All uses: Use in IgA-deficient patients; hypersensitivity to $Rh_o(D)$ immune globulin or any component of the formulation.

Rh Immunization prophylaxis: Use in $Rh_o(D)$-positive women; $Rh_o(D)$ negative women who are Rh immunized.

Immune thrombocytopenia (ITP): $Rh_o(D)$-negative patients; splenectomized patients; ITP secondary to other conditions including leukemia, lymphoma, or active viral infections with EBV or HCV; elderly patients with underlying cardiac, renal, or hepatic comorbidities that would predispose them to acute hemolytic reactions (AHR) complications; autoimmune hemolytic anemia (Evan syndrome); systemic lupus erythematosus (SLE); antiphospholipid antibody syndrome.

Documentation of allergenic cross-reactivity for immune globulins is limited. However, because of similarities in chemical structure and/or pharmacologic actions, the possibility of cross-sensitivity cannot be ruled out with certainty.

Warnings/Precautions Rhophylac, WinRho SDF: **[U.S. Boxed Warning]: May cause fatal intravascular hemolysis (IVH) in patients treated with intravenous (IV) $Rh_o(D)$ immune globulin for immune thrombocytopenia (ITP). IVH may result in clinically compromising anemia and multiorgan system failure, including acute respiratory distress syndrome. Acute renal insufficiency, renal failure, severe anemia, and disseminated intravascular coagulation (DIC) have also been reported. Patients should be closely monitored for at least 8 hours after administration.** ITP patients should be advised of the signs and symptoms of IVH (eg, back pain, shaking, chills, fever, discolored urine) and instructed to report them immediately. Previous administration of IV $Rh_o(D)$ immune globulin does not preclude the possibility of IVH.

Immediate treatment (including epinephrine 1:1000) for anaphylactoid and/or hypersensitivity reactions should be available during use. Some products are specifically contraindicated in patients with a previous anaphylactic or severe systemic reaction to an immune globulin. Use with caution in patients with IgA deficiency, may contain trace amounts of IgA; patients who are IgA deficient may have the potential for developing IgA antibodies, anaphylactic reactions may occur.

Acute renal dysfunction/failure, osmotic nephropathy, and death may occur with IGIV products. Use with caution and administer at the minimum infusion rate possible in patients at risk for renal disease (eg, diabetes mellitus, >65 years of age, volume depletion, sepsis, paraproteinemia, concomitant use of nephrotoxic medications); ensure adequate hydration prior to administration in these patients. Thrombotic events have been reported with administration of intravenous immune globulins (IVIG); use with caution in patients with a history of atherosclerosis or cardiovascular and/or thrombotic risk factors or patients with known/suspected hyperviscosity. Consider a baseline assessment of blood viscosity in patients at risk for hyperviscosity. Administer at the minimum practical infusion rate. Monitor for adverse pulmonary events including transfusion-related acute lung injury (TRALI); noncardiogenic pulmonary edema has been reported with IVIG use. TRALI is characterized by severe respiratory distress, pulmonary edema, hypoxemia, and fever in the presence of normal left ventricular function and usually occurs within 1 to 6 hours after infusion; may be managed with oxygen and respiratory support.

Use with caution in patients with thrombocytopenia or coagulation disorders; bleeding/hematoma may occur from IM administration. Use with caution in patients with renal impairment or those at risk for renal disease (eg, diabetes mellitus, advanced age [>65 years], volume depletion, sepsis, paraproteinemia, concomitant use of nephrotoxic medications). In patients at risk of renal dysfunction, ensure adequate hydration prior to administration; administer at the minimum practical infusion rate. Product of human plasma; may potentially contain infectious agents which could transmit disease. Screening of donors, as well as testing and/or inactivation or removal of certain viruses, reduces the risk. Infections thought to be transmitted by this product should be reported to the manufacturer.

Some products may contain maltose, which may result in falsely elevated blood glucose readings. Some dosage forms may contain polysorbate 80 (also known as Tweens). Hypersensitivity reactions, usually a delayed reaction, have been reported following exposure to pharmaceutical products containing polysorbate 80 in certain individuals (Isaksson, 2002; Lucente 2000; Shelley, 1995). Thrombocytopenia, ascites, pulmonary deterioration, and renal and hepatic failure have been reported in premature neonates after receiving parenteral products containing polysorbate 80 (Alade, 1986; CDC, 1984). See manufacturer's labeling.

Immune globulin deficiency syndromes: Not for replacement therapy in immune globulin deficiency syndromes.

ITP: Appropriate use: Safety and efficacy of WinRho not established in $Rh_o(D)$ negative, non-ITP thrombocytopenia, or splenectomized patients; safety and efficacy of Rhophylac not established in patients with preexisting anemia. Dose adjustment may be required with decreased hemoglobin. Do not administer IM or SubQ; administer dose I.V. only. Although $Rh_o(D)$ immune globulin is not the preferred pharmacologic agent for the management of ITP, a single dose may be used in nonsplenectomized children who are $Rh_o(D)$ positive and require treatment, or in adults when corticosteroids are contraindicated (Neunert, 2011).

$Rh_o(D)$ suppression: For use in the mother; do not administer to the neonate. If $Rh_o(D)$ antibodies are already present in the mother, use of the $Rh_o(D)$ immune globulin is not beneficial. In addition, if the father is known to be $Rh_o(D)$ negative, administration of the immune globulin is not needed. When treatment is indicated, administration should be within the time frame recommended. However, there may still be benefit if therapy is given as late as 28 days postpartum. The longer treatment is delayed, the less protection will be provided (ACOG, 1999).

Adverse Reactions

Cardiovascular: Hyper-/hypotension, pallor, vasodilation

Central nervous system: Chills, dizziness, fever, headache, malaise, somnolence

Dermatologic: Pruritus, rash

Gastrointestinal: Abdominal pain, diarrhea, nausea, vomiting

Hematologic: Haptoglobin decreased, hemoglobin decreased (patients with ITP), intravascular hemolysis (patients with ITP)

Hepatic: Bilirubin increased, LDH increased

Local: Injection site reaction: Discomfort, induration, mild pain, redness, swelling

Neuromuscular & skeletal: Arthralgia, back pain, hyperkinesia, myalgia, weakness

Renal: Acute renal insufficiency

Miscellaneous: Anaphylaxis, diaphoresis, infusion-related reactions, positive anti-C antibody test (transient), shivering

Postmarketing and/or case reports: Anemia (clinically-compromising), anuria, ARDS, cardiac arrest, cardiac failure, chest pain, chromaturia, DIC, edema, erythema, fatigue, hematuria, hemoglobinemia, hemoglobinuria (transient in patients with ITP), hyperhidrosis, hypersensitivity, injection site irritation, jaundice, myocardial infarction, muscle spasm, nausea, pain in extremities, renal failure, renal impairment, tachycardia, transfusion-related acute lung injury

Drug Interactions

Metabolism/Transport Effects None known.

Avoid Concomitant Use There are no known interactions where it is recommended to avoid concomitant use.

Increased Effect/Toxicity There are no known significant interactions involving an increase in effect.

Decreased Effect

Rho(D) Immune Globulin may decrease the levels/effects of: Vaccines (Live)

Storage/Stability

Store at 2°C to 8°C (35°F to 46°F); do not freeze.

Rhophylac: Protect from light.

Mechanism of Action

Rh suppression: Not completely characterized; prevents isoimmunization by suppressing the immune response and antibody formation by $Rh_o(D)$-negative individuals to $Rh_o(D)$-positive red blood cells. When administered within 72 hours of a full term delivery, the incidence of Rh isoimmunization decreases from 12% to 13% to 1% to 2%. The rate further decreases to <1% with administration at both 28 weeks' gestation and postpartum.

ITP: Not completely characterized; $Rh_o(D)$ immune globulin is thought to form anti-D-coated red blood cell complexes which bind to macrophage Fc receptors within the reticuloendothelial system (RES); blocks or saturates the RES ability to clear antibody-coated cells, including platelets. Thus, platelets are spared from destruction.

Pharmacodynamics

Onset of action:

- Rh isoimmunization: IV: 8 hours
- ITP: IV: 1-2 days

Maximum effect: ITP: 7-14 days

Duration:

- ITP (single dose): IV: 30 days
- Passive anti-$Rh_o(D)$ antibodies (after 120 mcg dose): IV: 6 weeks

Pharmacokinetics (Adult data unless noted)

Distribution: Appears in breast milk, however, not absorbed by the nursing infant

Half-life, elimination:

- IM: 18-30 days
- IV: 16-24 days

Time to peak serum concentration:

- IM: 5-10 days
- IV: 2 hours

Dosing: Usual

Infants, Children, and Adolescents: **ITP:**

Manufacturer's labeling: WinRho SDF: IV: Children and Adolescents <16 years:

Initial:

- Hemoglobin <10 g/dL: 25-40 mcg/kg as single dose or divided into 2 doses given on separate days
- Hemoglobin ≥10 g/dL: 50 mcg/kg as single dose or divided into 2 doses given on separate days

Maintenance: **Note:** Usage dependent upon clinical response, platelet count, hemoglobin, red blood cell counts, and reticulocyte levels; platelet counts >50,000/mm^3 rarely require treatment

Response to initial dose: 25-60 mcg/kg as single dose

Nonresponse to initial therapy:

- Hemoglobin <8 g/dL: Alternative therapy should be used
- Hemoglobin 8-10 g/dL: 25-40 mcg/kg as single dose
- Hemoglobin >10 g/dL: 50-60 mcg/kg as single dose

Alternate dosing: IV: **Note:** Recommended as first-line in Rh-positive, nonsplenectomized pediatric patients (Neunert, 2011; Provan, 2010)

First-line; initial treatment or chronic: 50-75 mcg/kg (Provan, 2010)

Serious or life-threatening bleeding: 75 mcg/kg in combination with platelet infusion(s) and corticosteroids (Provan, 2010)

Adults:

ITP:

Rhophylac: IV: 50 mcg/kg

WinRho SDF: IV:

Initial: 50 mcg/kg as a single injection, or can be given as a divided dose on separate days. If hemoglobin is <10 g/dL: Dose should be reduced to 25-40 mcg/kg

Subsequent dosing: 25-60 mcg/kg can be used if required to increase platelet count

Maintenance dosing if patient **did respond** to initial dosing: 25-60 mcg/kg based on platelet count and hemoglobin concentration

Maintenance dosing if patient **did not respond** to initial dosing:

- Hemoglobin <8 g/dL: Alternative treatment should be used
- Hemoglobin 8-10 g/dL: Redose between 25-40 mcg/kg
- Hemoglobin >10 g/dL: Redose between 50-60 mcg/kg

$Rh_o(D)$ suppression: Note: One "full dose" (300 mcg) provides enough antibody to prevent Rh sensitization if the volume of RBC entering the circulation is ≤15 mL. When >15 mL is suspected, a fetal red cell count should be performed to determine the appropriate dose.

Pregnancy:

Antepartum prophylaxis: In general, single dose is given at 28 weeks. If given early in pregnancy, administer every 12 weeks to ensure adequate levels of passively acquired anti-Rh.

- HyperRHO S/D Full Dose, RhoGAM: IM: 300 mcg
- Rhophylac, WinRho SDF: IM, IV: 300 mcg

Postpartum: In general, dose is administered as soon as possible after delivery, preferably within 72 hours. Can be given up to 28 days following delivery

- HyperRHO S/D Full Dose, RhoGAM: IM: 300 mcg
- Rhophylac: IM, IV: 300 mcg
- WinRho SDF: IM, IV: 120 mcg

Threatened abortion, any time during pregnancy (with continuation of pregnancy):

- HyperRHO S/D Full Dose, RhoGAM: IM: 300 mcg; administer as soon as possible
- Rhophylac, WinRho SDF: IM, IV: 300 mcg; administer as soon as possible

Abortion, miscarriage, termination of ectopic pregnancy:

RhoGAM: IM: ≥13 weeks gestation: 300 mcg

HyperRHO S/D Mini Dose, MICRhoGAM: IM: <13 weeks gestation: 50 mcg
Rhophylac: IM, IV: 300 mcg
WinRho SDF: IM, IV: After 34 weeks gestation: 120 mcg; administer immediately or within 72 hours

Amniocentesis, chorionic villus sampling:
HyperRHO S/D Full Dose, RhoGAM: IM: At 15-18 weeks gestation or during the 3rd trimester: 300 mcg. If dose is given between 13-18 weeks, repeat at 26-28 weeks and within 72 hours of delivery.
Rhophylac: IM, IV: 300 mcg
WinRho SDF: IM, IV:
Before 34 weeks gestation: 300 mcg; administer immediately, repeat dose every 12 weeks during pregnancy
After 34 weeks gestation: 120 mcg, administered immediately or within 72 hours

Excessive fetomaternal hemorrhage (>15 mL): Rhophylac: IM, IV: 300 mcg within 72 hours plus 20 mcg/mL fetal RBCs in excess of 15 mL if excess transplacental bleeding is quantified or 300 mcg/dose if bleeding cannot be quantified

Abdominal trauma, manipulation:
HyperRHO S/D Full Dose, RhoGAM: IM: 2nd or 3rd trimester: 300 mcg. If dose is given between 13-18 weeks, repeat at 26-28 weeks and within 72 hours of delivery.
Rhophylac: IM, IV: 300 mcg within 72 hours
WinRho SDF: IM, IV: After 34 weeks gestation: 120 mcg; administer immediately or within 72 hours

Transfusion:
HyperRHO S/D Full Dose, RhoGAM: IM: Multiply the volume of Rh positive whole blood administered by the hematocrit of the donor unit to equal the volume of RBCs transfused. The volume of RBCs is then divided by 15 mL, providing the number of 300 mcg doses (vials/syringes) to administer. If the dose calculated results in a fraction, round up to the next higher whole 300 mcg dose (vial/syringe).
WinRho SDF: Administer within 72 hours after exposure of incompatible blood transfusions or massive fetal hemorrhage.
IV: Calculate dose as follows; administer 600 mcg every 8 hours until the total dose is administered:
Exposure to Rh_o(D) positive whole blood: 9 mcg/mL blood
Exposure to Rh_o(D) positive red blood cells: 18 mcg/mL cells
IM: Calculate dose as follows; administer 1200 mcg every 12 hours until the total dose is administered:
Exposure to Rh_o(D) positive whole blood: 12 mcg/mL blood
Exposure to Rh_o(D) positive red blood cells: 24 mcg/mL cells
Rhophylac: IM, IV: 20 mcg per 2 mL transfused blood or 1 mL erythrocyte concentrate

Preparation for Administration Parenteral: WinRho SDF: IV: May dilute in NS prior to IV administration; do not dilute with D_5W.

Administration
Parenteral: Bring products to room temperature prior to administration. When used for the prevention of rhesus (Rh) isoimmunization in an Rh-incompatible pregnancy, the dose is administered to the mother, not the neonate. WinRho SDF and Rhophylac are the only immune globulin products available that can be administered both IM and IV; however, for the treatment of ITP, it must be administered IV.
IM: HyperRHO S/D Full Dose, HyperRHO S/D Mini Dose, MICRhoGAM Ultra-Filtered Plus and RhoGAM Ultra-Filtered Plus, Rhophylac, WinRho SDF: Administer into the deltoid muscle of upper arm or the anterolateral aspect of the upper thigh; the gluteal region is not recommended for routine administration due to the potential risk of sciatic nerve injury; if gluteal area is used, administer only in the upper, outer quadrant. The total volume can be given in divided doses at different sites at one time
IV: Product and rate depends on indication
Prevention of Rh isoimmunization: WinRho SDF: Infuse at 2 mL per 5 to 15 seconds
ITP:
WinRho SDF: Infuse over 3 to 5 minutes; may be further diluted if desired when used for ITP treatment
Rhophylac: Infuse at 2 mL per 15 to 60 seconds

Monitoring Parameters Signs and symptoms of intravascular hemolysis (IVH), anemia, renal insufficiency, back pain, shaking, chills, discolored urine, or hematuria; observe patient for side effects for 8 hours following administration
Patients with suspected IVH: CBC, haptoglobin, plasma hemoglobin, urine dipstick, BUN, serum creatinine, liver function tests, DIC-specific tests [D-dimer, fibrin degradation products (FDP) or fibrin split products (FSP)] for differential diagnosis. In patients at increased risk of developing acute renal failure, periodically monitor renal function and urine output. Clinical response may be determined by monitoring platelets, red blood cell (RBC) counts, hemoglobin, and reticulocyte levels.
ITP: Check blood type, CBC, reticulocyte count, DAT before initiating treatment with WinRho SDF; check urine dipstick before initiating treatment with WinRho SDF or Rhophylac and repeat urine dipstick at 2 and 4 hours after administration and prior to end of the 8-hour monitoring period.

Test Interactions Some infants born to women given Rh_o(D) antepartum have a weakly positive Coombs' test at birth. Fetal-maternal hemorrhage may cause false blood-typing result in the mother; when there is any doubt to the patients' Rh type, Rh_o(D) immune globulin should be administered. WinRho SDF liquid contains maltose; may result in falsely elevated blood glucose levels with dehydrogenase pyrroloquinolinequinone or glucose-dye-oxidoreductase testing methods. WinRho SDF contains trace amounts of anti-A, B, C and E; may alter Coombs' tests following administration.

Additional Information 1 mcg = 5 units

Treatment of ITP in Rh-positive patients with an intact spleen appears to be about as effective as IVIG.

HyperRho S/D and RhoGAM, which are prepared using cold ethanol fraction and ultrafiltration, must be administered intramuscularly because trace amounts of IgA and other plasma proteins in the product could cause anaphylaxis if they were given intravenously. Rhophylac and WinRho SDF are prepared by ion-exchange chromatography isolation and are purer, allowing them to be given intramuscularly or intravenously.

Dosage Forms Excipient information presented when available (limited, particularly for generics); consult specific product labeling. [DSC] = Discontinued product
Solution, Injection:
WinRho SDF: 2500 units/2.2 mL (2.2 mL); 5000 units/4.4 mL (4.4 mL); 1500 units/1.3 mL (1.3 mL); 15,000 units/13 mL (13 mL)
Solution, Injection [preservative free]:
WinRho SDF: 2500 units/2.2 mL (2.2 mL); 5000 units/4.4 mL (4.4 mL); 1500 units/1.3 mL (1.3 mL); 15,000 units/13 mL (13 mL) [contains polysorbate 80]
Solution Prefilled Syringe, Injection [preservative free]:
Rhophylac: 1500 units/2 mL (2 mL)
Solution Prefilled Syringe, Intramuscular:
HyperRHO S/D: 250 units (1 ea [DSC])

Solution Prefilled Syringe, Intramuscular [preservative free]:
HyperRHO S/D: 250 units (1 ea); 1500 units (1 ea) [latex free]
MICRhoGAM Ultra-Filtered Plus: 250 units (1 ea) [latex free, thimerosal free; contains polysorbate 80]
RhoGAM Ultra-Filtered Plus: 1500 units (1 ea) [latex free, thimerosal free; contains polysorbate 80]

- ◆ **RhoGAM Ultra-Filtered Plus** *see* Rh_o(D) Immune Globulin *on page 1847*
- ◆ **RhoIGIV** *see* Rh_o(D) Immune Globulin *on page 1847*
- ◆ **RhoIVIM** *see* Rh_o(D) Immune Globulin *on page 1847*
- ◆ **Rho®-Loperamide (Can)** *see* Loperamide *on page 1288*
- ◆ **Rho-Nitro Pump Spray (Can)** *see* Nitroglycerin *on page 1523*
- ◆ **Rhophylac** *see* Rh_o(D) Immune Globulin *on page 1847*
- ◆ **Rhoxal-loperamide (Can)** *see* Loperamide *on page 1288*
- ◆ **Rhoxal-sotalol (Can)** *see* Sotalol *on page 1963*
- ◆ ***r*HuEPO** *see* Epoetin Alfa *on page 765*
- ◆ **rhuGM-CSF** *see* Sargramostim *on page 1905*
- ◆ **rhuMAb-E25** *see* Omalizumab *on page 1553*
- ◆ **rhuMAb-VEGF** *see* Bevacizumab *on page 285*
- ◆ **Riax** *see* Benzoyl Peroxide *on page 270*
- ◆ **Ribasphere** *see* Ribavirin *on page 1851*
- ◆ **Ribasphere RibaPak** *see* Ribavirin *on page 1851*

Ribavirin (rye ba VYE rin)

Medication Safety Issues

Sound-alike/look-alike issues:

Ribavirin may be confused with riboflavin, rifampin, Robaxin

Related Information

Safe Handling of Hazardous Drugs *on page 2455*

Brand Names: US Copegus; Moderiba; Rebetol; Ribasphere; Ribasphere RibaPak; Virazole

Brand Names: Canada Ibavyr; Virazole

Therapeutic Category Antiviral Agent, Inhalation Therapy; Antiviral Agent, Oral

Generic Availability (US) Yes: Capsule, tablet

Use

Inhalation: Treatment of hospitalized patients with severe RSV infections (FDA approved in infants and young children); especially indicated for treatment of severe lower respiratory tract RSV infections in patients with an underlying compromising condition (prematurity, cardiopulmonary disease, or immunosuppression). **Note:** Due to potential toxic effects to exposed health care workers and variable efficacy results in clinical trials, the AAP recommends against routine use of ribavirin to treat RSV; use should be reserved for patients with documented, potentially life-threatening disease (AAP, 2006; *Red Book* [AAP], 2012); has also been used in other viral infections including influenza A and B and adenovirus.

Oral:

Capsule and solution (Rebetol, Ribasphere): Treatment of chronic hepatitis C (in combination with interferon alfa-2b [pegylated or nonpegylated]) in patients with compensated liver disease (FDA approved in ages ≥3 years and adults). Patients likely to fail retreatment after a prior failed course include previous nonresponders, those who received previous pegylated interferon treatment, patients who have significant bridging fibrosis or cirrhosis, and those with genotype 1 infection.

Tablets: Treatment of chronic hepatitis C [in combination with peginterferon alfa-2a] in previously untreated patients with compensated liver disease (Copegus: FDA approved in ages ≥5 years and adults; Moderiba, Ribasphere: FDA approved in ages ≥18 years and adults); treatment of chronic hepatitis C in patients coinfected with HIV (All tablets: FDA approved in adults).

Medication Guide Available Yes

Pregnancy Risk Factor X

Pregnancy Considerations [US Boxed Warning]: Significant teratogenic and/or embryocidal effects have been observed in all animal studies. Use is contraindicated in pregnant women or male partners of pregnant women. Avoid pregnancy in female patients and female partners of male patients during therapy by using two effective forms of contraception; continue contraceptive measures for at least 6 months after completion of therapy. A negative pregnancy test is required immediately before initiation, monthly during therapy, and for 6 months after treatment is discontinued. If patient or female partner becomes pregnant during treatment, she should be counseled about potential risks of exposure. The manufacturer recommends that pregnant health care workers take precautions to limit exposure to ribavirin aerosol; potential occupational exposure may be greatest if administration is via oxygen tent or hood, and lower if administered via mechanical ventilation.

Health care providers and patients are encouraged to enroll women exposed to ribavirin during pregnancy or within 6 months after treatment in the Ribavirin Pregnancy Registry (800-593-2214).

Breast-Feeding Considerations It is not known if ribavirin is excreted in breast milk. Due to the potential for serious adverse reactions in the nursing infant, the manufacturer recommends that a decision be made whether to discontinue nursing or to discontinue the drug, taking into account the importance of treatment to the mother.

Contraindications

Inhalation: Hypersensitivity to ribavirin or any component of the formulation; women who are pregnant or may become pregnant

Oral formulations: Hypersensitivity to ribavirin or any component of the formulation; women who are pregnant or may become pregnant; males whose female partners are pregnant; patients with hemoglobinopathies (eg, thalassemia major, sickle cell anemia); concomitant use with didanosine

Ribasphere capsules and Rebetol capsules/solution: Additional contraindications: Patients with a CrCl <50 mL/minute

Oral combination therapy with alfa interferons: Autoimmune hepatitis, hepatic decompensation (Child-Pugh score >6; class B and C) in cirrhotic chronic hepatitis C monoinfected patients prior to treatment, hepatic decompensation (Child-Pugh score ≥6) in cirrhotic chronic hepatitis C patients coinfected with HIV prior to treatment. Also refer to individual monographs for Interferon Alfa-2b (Intron A), Peginterferon Alfa-2b, and Peginterferon Alfa-2a (Pegasys) for additional contraindication information.

Warnings/Precautions Hazardous agent - use appropriate precautions for handling and disposal (NIOSH 2014 [group 3]).

Oral: Safety and efficacy have not been established in patients who have received organ transplants, or been coinfected with hepatitis B or HIV (ribavirin tablets may be used in adult HIV-coinfected patients unless CD4+ cell count is ≤100 cells/microliter and HIV-1 RNA <5000 cells/mm^3). Hemoglobin at initiation must be ≥12 g/dL (women) or ≥13 g/dL (men) in CHC monoinfected patients and ≥11 g/dL (women) or ≥12 g/dL (men) in CHC and HIV coinfected patients. Oral ribavirin should not be used for adenovirus, RSV, influenza or parainfluenza infections; ribavirin inhalation is approved for severe RSV infection ▶

in children. Severe psychiatric events have occurred including depression and suicidal/homicidal ideation during combination therapy. Avoid use in patients with a psychiatric history; discontinue if severe psychiatric symptoms occur. Acute hypersensitivity reactions (eg, anaphylaxis, angioedema, bronchoconstriction, and urticaria) have been observed with ribavirin and alfa interferon combination therapy. Severe cutaneous reactions, including Stevens-Johnson syndrome and exfoliative dermatitis have been reported (rarely) with ribavirin and alfa interferon combination therapy; discontinue with signs or symptoms of severe skin reactions. Use with caution in patients with renal impairment; dosage adjustment or discontinuation may be required. Elderly patients are more susceptible to adverse effects; use caution.

[US Boxed Warning]: Monotherapy not effective for chronic hepatitis C infection.

[US Boxed Warning]: Hemolytic anemia is the primary clinical toxicity of oral therapy; anemia associated with ribavirin may worsen underlying cardiac disease and lead to fatal and nonfatal myocardial infarctions. Avoid use in patients with significant/unstable cardiac disease. Anemia usually occurs within 1 to 2 weeks of therapy initiation; observed in ~10% to 13% of patients when alfa interferons were combined with ribavirin. Assess cardiac function before initiation of therapy. If patient has underlying cardiac disease, assess electrocardiogram prior to and periodically during treatment. If any deterioration in cardiovascular status occurs, discontinue therapy. Use caution in patients with baseline risk of severe anemia. Assess hemoglobin and hematocrit at baseline and, at minimum, weeks 2 and 4 of therapy since initial drop may be significant. Patients with renal dysfunction and/or those >50 years of age should be carefully assessed for development of anemia. Pancytopenia and bone marrow suppression have been reported with the combination of ribavirin, interferon, and azathioprine. Use caution in pulmonary disease; pulmonary symptoms have been associated with administration. Discontinue therapy if evidence of hepatic decompensation is observed. Use caution in patients with sarcoidosis (exacerbation reported). Dental and periodontal disorders have been reported with ribavirin and interferon therapy; patients should be instructed to brush teeth twice daily and have regular dental exams. Serious ophthalmologic disorders have occurred with combination therapy. All patients require an eye exam at baseline; those with preexisting ophthalmologic disorders (eg, diabetic or hypertensive retinopathy) require periodic follow up. Delay in weight and height increases have been noted in children treated with combination therapy for CHC. In clinical studies, decreases were noted in weight and height for age z-scores and normative growth curve percentiles. Following treatment, rebound growth and weight gain occurred in most patients; however, a small percentage did not. Long-term data indicate that combination therapy may inhibit growth resulting in reduced adult height. Growth should be closely monitored in pediatric patients during therapy and post-treatment for growth catch-up.

Inhalation: **[US Boxed Warning]: Use with caution in patients requiring assisted ventilation because precipitation of the drug in the respiratory equipment may interfere with safe and effective patient ventilation; sudden deterioration of respiratory function has been observed;** monitor carefully in patients with COPD and asthma for deterioration of respiratory function. Ribavirin is potentially mutagenic, tumor-promoting, and gonadotoxic. Although anemia has not been reported with inhalation therapy, consider monitoring for anemia 1 to 2 weeks post-treatment. Hazardous agent - use appropriate precautions for handling and disposal.

[US Boxed Warning]: Sudden respiratory deterioration has been observed during the initiation of aerosolized ribavirin in infants; carefully monitor during treatment. If deterioration of respiratory function occurs, stop treatment; reinstitute with extreme caution, continuous monitoring, and consider concomitant administration of bronchodilators.

[US Boxed Warning]: Significant teratogenic and/or embryocidal effects have been observed in all animal studies. Use is contraindicated in pregnant women or male partners of pregnant women. Avoid pregnancy in female patients and female partners of male patients during therapy by using two effective forms of contraception; continue contraceptive measures for at least 6 months after completion of therapy. The manufacturer recommends that pregnant health care workers take precautions to limit exposure to ribavirin aerosol.

Benzyl alcohol and derivatives: Some dosage forms may contain sodium benzoate/benzoic acid; benzoic acid (benzoate) is a metabolite of benzyl alcohol; large amounts of benzyl alcohol (≥99 mg/kg/day) have been associated with a potentially fatal toxicity ("gasping syndrome") in neonates; the "gasping syndrome" consists of metabolic acidosis, respiratory distress, gasping respirations, CNS dysfunction (including convulsions, intracranial hemorrhage), hypotension, and cardiovascular collapse (AAP, 1997; CDC, 1982); some data suggests that benzoate displaces bilirubin from protein binding sites (Ahlfors, 2001); avoid or use dosage forms containing benzyl alcohol derivative with caution in neonates. See manufacturer's labeling.

Warnings: Additional Pediatric Considerations Sudden respiratory deterioration has been observed during the initiation of aerosolized ribavirin in infants; carefully monitor infants. If deterioration of respiratory function occurs, stop treatment; reinstitute with extreme caution, continuous monitoring, and consider concomitant administration of bronchodilators.

Pediatric patients treated with ribavirin in combination with alfa interferon lag behind in height and weight gains compared to normative population growth curves for the duration of treatment. Severe inhibition of growth velocity (<3rd percentile) was reported in 70% of pediatric patients during clinical trials. After therapy, 20% continued to have severely inhibited growth; however, in the majority of patients, growth velocity rates increased such that by 6 months post-treatment, weight gain stabilized to 53rd percentile (similar to predicted based on average baseline weight: 57th percentile) and height gain stabilized to 44th percentile (less than predicted based on average baseline height: 51st percentile). Post-treatment, rebound growth occurred in most patients; however, long-term data indicate that combination therapy may result in reduced adult height in some patients. Growth should be closely monitored in pediatric patients during therapy and post-treatment for growth catch-up.

Some dosage forms may contain propylene glycol; in neonates large amounts of propylene glycol delivered orally, intravenously (eg, >3,000 mg/day), or topically have been associated with potentially fatal toxicities which can include metabolic acidosis, seizures, renal failure, and CNS depression; toxicities have also been reported in children and adults including hyperosmolality, lactic acidosis, seizures, and respiratory depression; use caution (AAP, 1997; Shehab, 2009).

Adverse Reactions

Inhalation:

Cardiovascular: Cardiac arrest, digitalis toxicity, hypotension

Central nervous system: Fatigue, headache, insomnia

Gastrointestinal: Nausea, anorexia

Hematologic: Anemia
Ocular: Conjunctivitis
Respiratory: Apnea, mild bronchospasm, worsening of respiratory function

Oral (all adverse reactions are documented while receiving combination therapy with alfa interferons; as reported in adults unless noted; most common pediatric adverse reactions were similar to adults):
Cardiovascular: Chest pain, flushing
Central nervous system: Agitation, anxiety, depression, dizziness, emotional lability, fatigue (children and adults), fever, headache, insomnia (children and adults), impaired concentration, irritability, malaise, memory impairment, mood alteration, nervousness, pain, suicidal ideation
Dermatologic: Alopecia (children and adults), dermatitis, dry skin, eczema, pruritus (children and adults), rash
Endocrine & metabolic: Growth suppression (pediatric), hyperuricemia, hypothyroidism, menstrual disorder
Gastrointestinal: Abdominal pain, anorexia, constipation, diarrhea, dyspepsia, nausea (children and adults), RUQ pain, taste perversion, vomiting, weight loss, xerostomia
Hematologic: Anemia, hemoglobin decreased, hemolytic anemia, leukopenia, lymphopenia, neutropenia, thrombocytopenia
Hepatic: Bilirubin increased, hepatic decompensation, hepatomegaly, transaminases increased
Local: Inflammation at injection site, injection site reaction
Neuromuscular & skeletal: Arthralgia, back pain, decreased linear skeletal growth (including lagging weight gain), musculoskeletal pain (children and adults), myalgia (children and adults), rigors, weakness
Ocular: Blurred vision, conjunctivitis
Respiratory: Cough, dyspnea (including exertional), pharyngitis, rhinitis, sinusitis, upper respiratory tract infection (children)
Miscellaneous: Bacterial infection, diaphoresis, flu-like syndrome (children and adults), fungal infection, viral infection

Rare but important or life-threatening: Aggression, angina, aplastic anemia, arrhythmia; autoimmune disorders (systemic lupus erythematosus, rheumatoid arthritis, sarcoidosis); bone marrow suppression, cerebral hemorrhage, cholangitis, colitis, coma, corneal ulcer, dehydration, diabetes mellitus, drug abuse relapse/overdose, exfoliative dermatitis, fatty liver, hearing impairment/loss, gastrointestinal bleeding, gout, hallucination, hepatic dysfunction, hyper-/hypothyroidism, hypersensitivity (including anaphylaxis, angioedema, bronchoconstriction, and urticaria), macular edema, myositis, optic neuritis, papilledema, pancreatitis, peptic ulcer, peripheral neuropathy, pneumonitis, psychosis, psychotic disorder, pulmonary dysfunction, pulmonary embolism, pulmonary infiltrates, pure red cell aplasia, retinal artery/vein thrombosis, retinal detachment, retinal hemorrhage, retinopathy, sarcoidosis exacerbation; skin reactions (erythema multiforme, exfoliative dermatitis, urticaria, vesiculobullous eruptions); Stevens-Johnson syndrome, suicide, thrombotic thrombocytopenic purpura, thyroid function test abnormalities; transplant rejection (kidney, liver); vision loss

Note: Incidence of headache, fever, suicidal ideation, and vomiting are higher in children.

Drug Interactions

Metabolism/Transport Effects None known.

Avoid Concomitant Use

Avoid concomitant use of Ribavirin with any of the following: Didanosine

Increased Effect/Toxicity

Ribavirin may increase the levels/effects of: AzaTHIOprine; Didanosine; Reverse Transcriptase Inhibitors (Nucleoside)

The levels/effects of Ribavirin may be increased by: Interferons (Alfa); Zidovudine

Decreased Effect

Ribavirin may decrease the levels/effects of: Influenza Virus Vaccine (Live/Attenuated)

Food Interactions Oral: High-fat meal increases the AUC and C_{max}. Management: Capsule (in combination with peginterferon alfa-2b) and tablet should be administered with food. Other dosage forms and combinations should be taken consistently in regards to food.

Storage/Stability

Inhalation: Store vials in a dry place at 15°C to 30°C (59°F to 86°F). Reconstituted solution is stable for 24 hours at room temperature.
Oral: Store at 25°C (77°F); excursions permitted between 15°C and 30°C (59°F and 86°F). Solution may also be refrigerated at 2°C to 8°C (36°F to 46°F).

Mechanism of Action Inhibits replication of RNA and DNA viruses; inhibits influenza virus RNA polymerase activity and inhibits the initiation and elongation of RNA fragments resulting in inhibition of viral protein synthesis

Pharmacokinetics (Adult data unless noted)

Absorption: Inhalation: Systemically absorbed from the respiratory tract following nasal and oral inhalation; absorption is dependent upon respiratory factors and method of drug delivery; maximal absorption occurs with the use of the aerosol generator via an endotracheal tube
Distribution:
Inhalation: Highest concentrations are found in the respiratory tract and erythrocytes
Oral: Single dose (capsule): V_d: 2825 L; distribution significantly prolonged in the erythrocyte (16 to 40 days), which can be used as a marker for intracellular metabolism
Protein binding: Oral: None
Metabolism: Occurs intracellularly and may be necessary for drug action; metabolized hepatically to deribosylated ribavirin (active metabolite)
Bioavailability: Oral: 64%
Half-life:
Respiratory tract secretions: Infants and Children 6 weeks to 7 years: ~2 hours (Englund, 1990)
Plasma:
Infants and Children: Inhalation: 9.5 hours
Adults: Oral:
Capsule, single dose: 24 hours in healthy adults, 44 hours with chronic hepatitis C infection (increases to ~298 hours at steady state)
Tablet, single dose: ~120 to 170 hours
Time to peak serum concentration:
Aerosol inhalation: At the end of the inhalation period
Oral capsule, multiple doses:
Children and Adolescents 3 to 16 years: ~2 hours
Adults: 3 hours
Tablet: 2 hours
Elimination: Inhalation: Urine (40% as unchanged drug and metabolites); oral capsule: Urine (61%), feces (12%)

Dosing: Usual

Pediatric:
RSV infection: Note: Due to potential toxic effects of exposed healthcare workers and variable efficacy results in trials, the AAP recommends against routine use of ribavirin to treat RSV; use should be reserved for patients with documented, potentially life-threatening disease (AAP, 2006; *Red Book* [AAP], 2012).
Infants and Children: Aerosol inhalation: Use with Viratek small particle aerosol generator (SPAG-2). **Note:** Dose actually delivered to the patient will depend on patient's minute ventilation.
Continuous aerosolization: 6 **g** administered over 12 to 18 hours/day for 3 to 7 days
Intermittent aerosolization: 2,000 mg over 2 hours 3 times daily in **nonmechanically ventilated** patients

for 3 to 7 days has been used to permit easier accessibility for patient care and limit environmental exposure of healthcare worker. Due to apparent increased potential for crystallization of the high-dose 60 mg/mL solution around areas of turbulent flow such as bends in tubing or connector pieces, use of high-dose therapy in individuals with an endotracheal tube in place is not recommended (Englund, 1994).

Chronic hepatitis C monoinfection: Note: Children who start treatment prior to age 18 years should continue on pediatric dosing regimen through therapy completion. Recommended therapy duration (manufacturer labeling): Genotypes 2, 3: 24 weeks; all other genotypes: 48 weeks. Consider discontinuation of combination therapy in patients with HCV (genotype 1) at 12 weeks if a 2 log decrease in HCV-RNA has not been achieved or if HCV-RNA is still detectable at 24 weeks.

Capsule or oral solution (Rebetol, Ribasphere) in combination with pegylated or nonpegylated interferon alfa-2b: **Note:** Oral solution should be used in children <47 kg or those unable to swallow capsules.

Manufacturer's labeling: Children ≥3 years and Adolescents: Oral:

<47 kg: 15 mg/kg/day in 2 divided doses as oral solution

47 to 59 kg: 400 mg twice daily

60 to 73 kg: 400 mg in the morning; 600 mg in the evening

>73 kg: 600 mg twice daily

Alternate dosing:

AAP recommendations: Children ≥3 years and Adolescents: Oral: **Note:** Use in combination with interferon alfa-2b (*Red Book*, [AAP] 2012):

<25 kg: 15 mg/kg/day in 2 divided doses as oral solution

25 to 36 kg: 200 mg twice daily

>36 to 49 kg: 200 mg in the morning; 400 mg in the evening

>49 to 61 kg: 400 mg twice daily

>61 to 75 kg: 400 mg in the morning; 600 mg in the evening

>75 kg: 600 mg twice daily

AASLD recommendations (Ghany, 2009): Children ≥2 years and Adolescents: Oral: 15 mg/kg/day in 2 divided doses in combination with weekly peginterferon alfa-2b for 48 weeks

NASPGHAN recommendations (Mack, 2012): Children ≥3 years and Adolescents: Oral: 15 mg/kg/day in 2 divided doses in combination with weekly peginterferon alfa-2a **or** 2b; duration is either 24 weeks (genotypes 2 or 3) or 48 weeks (genotypes 1 or 4)

Tablets (Copegus) in combination with peginterferon alfa-2a: Children ≥5 years and Adolescents: Oral: **Note:** Assess child's ability to swallow tablet.

23 to 33 kg: 200 mg twice daily

34 to 46 kg: 200 mg in the morning; 400 mg in the evening

47 to 59 kg: 400 mg twice daily

60 to 74 kg: 400 mg in the morning; 600 mg in the evening

≥75 kg: 600 mg twice daily

Chronic hepatitis C coinfection with HIV:

Children ≥3 years (DHHS [pediatric], 2013): Oral: **Note:** Use in combination with peginterferon alfa-2a **or** 2b; recommended therapy duration: 48 weeks, regardless of genotype

Weight-based dosing: 15 mg/kg/day in 2 divided doses

Fixed dosing:

25 to 36 kg: 200 mg twice daily

>36 to 49 kg: 200 mg in morning; 400 mg in evening

>49 to 61 kg: 400 mg twice daily

>61 to 75 kg: 400 mg in the morning; 600 mg in the evening

>75 kg: 600 mg twice daily

Adolescents (DHHS [adult], 2013): Oral:

Genotype 1: Use in combination with peginterferon alfa-2a **or** 2b ± boceprevir **or** telaprevir (based on antiretroviral therapy)

<75 kg: 400 mg in the morning, 600 mg in the evening for 48 weeks

≥75 kg: 600 mg twice daily 48 weeks

Genotype, all others: 400 mg twice daily in combination with peginterferon alfa-2a **or** 2b for 48 weeks

Adult:

Chronic hepatitis C monoinfection (in combination with peginterferon alfa-2b): Oral capsule, oral solution (Rebetol, Ribasphere): **Note:** Recommended therapy duration [manufacturer labeling]: Genotype 1: 48 weeks; genotypes 2, 3: 24 weeks; recommended therapy duration for patients who previously failed therapy: 48 weeks (regardless of genotype)

<66 kg: 400 mg in the morning and evening

66 to 80 kg: 400 mg in the morning, 600 mg in the evening

81 to 105 kg: 600 mg in the morning, 600 mg in the evening

>105 kg: 600 mg in the morning, 800 mg in the evening

Chronic hepatitis C monoinfection (in combination with interferon alfa-2b): Oral capsule (Rebetol, Ribasphere): **Note:** Individualized therapy duration [manufacturer labeling] 24 to 48 weeks:

≤75 kg: 400 mg in the morning; 600 mg in the evening

>75 kg: 600 mg twice daily

Chronic hepatitis C monoinfection (in combination with peginterferon alfa-2a): Oral tablet (Copegus, Moderiba, Ribasphere):

Genotype 1, 4:

<75 kg: 1000 mg daily in 2 divided doses for 48 weeks

≥75 kg: 1200 mg daily in 2 divided doses for 48 weeks

Genotype 2, 3: 800 mg daily in 2 divided doses for 24 weeks

Chronic hepatitis C coinfection with HIV (in combination with peginterferon alfa-2a): Oral tablet (Copegus, Moderiba, Ribasphere): 800 mg daily in 2 divided doses for 48 weeks (regardless of genotype)

Dosing adjustment in renal impairment: Chronic hepatitis C infection: Oral:

Capsules/solution (Rebetol, Ribasphere):

Children ≥3 years and Adolescents: Serum creatinine >2 mg/dL: Permanently discontinue treatment

Children ≥3 years, Adolescents and Adults:

CrCl ≥50 mL/minute: No dosage adjustments are recommended.

CrCl <50 mL/minute: Use is contraindicated

Tablets:

Moderiba, Ribasphere: Adults:

CrCl ≥50 mL/minute: No dosage adjustments are recommended.

CrCl <50 mL/minute: Use is contraindicated

Copegus: Adults:

CrCl >50 mL/minute: No dosage adjustments are recommended.

CrCl 30 to 50 mL/minute: Alternate 200 mg and 400 mg every other day

CrCl <30 mL/minute: 200 mg once daily

ESRD requiring hemodialysis: 200 mg once daily

Note: The dose of Copegus should not be further modified in patients with renal impairment. If severe adverse reactions or laboratory abnormalities develop it should be discontinued, if appropriate, until the adverse reactions resolve or decrease in severity. If abnormalities persist after restarting, therapy should be discontinued.

Dosing adjustment in hepatic impairment: Chronic hepatitis C infection: Hepatic decompensation (Child-Pugh class B and C): Children, Adolescents, and Adults: Use is contraindicated

Dosing adjustment for toxicity: Oral:

Notes:

Children and Adolescents: Once a laboratory abnormality or clinical adverse event has resolved, the ribavirin dose may be increased, based on clinical judgment, to its original assigned dose. Initiate restart at 50% of the full dose.

Adults: Once ribavirin has been withheld due to clinical adverse event or laboratory abnormality, an attempt can be made to restart ribavirin, in divided doses, at 600 mg daily, with a further ribavirin increase to 800 mg daily. Increasing the ribavirin dose to its original assigned dose (1000 or 1200 mg daily) is not recommended.

Patient **without** cardiac history:

Hemoglobin 8.5 to <10 g/dL:

Capsules, oral solution:

Children ≥3 years and Adolescents: Decrease ribavirin dose to 12 mg/kg/day; may further reduce to 8 mg/kg/day

Adult:

First reduction:

≤105 kg: Decrease by 200 mg daily

>105 kg: Decrease by 400 mg daily

Second reduction: Decrease by an additional 200 mg daily (not weight-based)

Tablets:

Children ≥5 years: Copegus:

23 to 33 kg: Decrease dose to 200 mg daily (in the morning)

34 to 59 kg: Decrease dose to 400 mg/day (200 mg twice daily)

≥60 kg: Decrease dose to 600 mg/day (200 mg in the morning and 400 mg in the evening)

Adults: Decrease dose to 600 mg/day (200 mg in the morning, 400 mg in the evening)

Hemoglobin <8.5 g/dL: Children, Adolescents and Adults: Oral capsules, solution, tablets: Permanently discontinue ribavirin

WBC <1000 mm^3, neutrophils <500 mm^3: Children, Adolescents, and Adults: Oral capsules, solution: Permanently discontinue treatment.

Platelets <50 x 10^9/L: Children and Adolescents: Oral capsules, solution: Permanently discontinue treatment.

Platelets <25 x 10^9/L: Adults: Oral capsules, solution: Permanently discontinue treatment.

Patient **with** cardiac history:

Hemoglobin decrease ≥2 g/dL in any 4-week period of treatment:

Capsules, oral solution: Children ≥3 years, Adolescents, and Adults: Decrease by 200 mg daily (regardless of the patient's initial dose); monitor and evaluate weekly

Tablets:

Children ≥5 years and Adolescents: Copegus:

23 to 33 kg: Decrease dose to 200 mg daily (in the morning)

34 to 59 kg: Decrease dose to 400 mg/day (200 mg twice daily)

≥60 kg: Decrease to 600 mg/day (200 mg in the morning, 400 mg in the evening)

Adults: Decrease dose to 600 mg/day (200 mg in the morning, 400 mg in the evening)

Hemoglobin <12 g/dL after 4 weeks of reduced dose: Children ≥ 3 years, Adolescents, and Adults: Capsules, oral solution, tablets: Permanently discontinue ribavirin

Hemoglobin <8.5 g/dL: Children, Adolescents, and Adults: Oral capsules, solution, tablets: Permanently discontinue ribavirin

WBC <1000 mm^3, neutrophils <500 mm^3: Children, Adolescents, and Adults: Oral capsules, solution: Permanently discontinue treatment

Platelets <50 x 10^9/L: Children and Adolescents: Oral capsules, solution: Permanently discontinue treatment

Platelets <25 x 10^9/L: Adults: Oral capsules, solution: Permanently discontinue treatment

Preparation for Administration Hazardous agent; use appropriate precautions for handling and disposal (NIOSH 2014 [group 3]).

Inhalation:

Continuous aerosolization: Per the manufacturer, reconstitute 6 g vial with at least 75 mL of preservative free sterile water for injection or inhalation; shake vial well to mix. Transfer vial contents to the clean, sterile 500 mL SPAG-2 reservoir and further dilute to a final volume of 300 mL with preservative free sterile water for injection or inhalation; final concentration: 20 mg/mL. Alternatively, sterile NS has been used for dilution rather than sterile water to achieve a near isotonic solution (Meert 1994)

Intermittent aerosolization: Reconstitute 6 g vial with 100 mL of preservative free sterile water; final concentration: 60 mg/mL (Englund 1994).

Administration Hazardous agent; use appropriate precautions for handling and disposal (NIOSH 2014 [group 3]).

Inhalation: Ribavirin should be administered in well-ventilated rooms (at least 6 air changes/hour)

Mechanically ventilated patients: Ribavirin can potentially be deposited in the ventilator delivery system depending on temperature, humidity, and electrostatic forces; this deposition can lead to malfunction or obstruction of the expiratory valve, resulting in inadvertently high positive end-expiratory pressures. The use of one-way valves in the inspiratory lines, use of a breathing circuit filter in the expiratory line, and frequent monitoring and filter replacement have been effective in preventing these problems. Solutions in SPAG-2 unit should be discarded at least every 24 hours and when the liquid level is low before adding newly reconstituted solution. Should not be mixed with other aerosolized medication.

Oral: Administer concurrently with interferon alfa injection (pegylated or nonpegylated).

Capsule: Administer with food; capsule should not be opened, crushed, chewed, or broken.

Oral solution: Administer with food; use in patients <47 kg or those who cannot swallow capsules.

Tablet: Administer with food

Monitoring Parameters

Inhalation: Respiratory function, hemoglobin, reticulocyte count, CBC, I & O

Oral: Laboratory tests recommended for all patients prior to therapy and then periodically during treatment: Hemoglobin, hematocrit, CBC with differential, platelet count, liver function tests, TSH, HCV-RNA, ophthalmic exam pretreatment (all patients) and periodically for those with preexisting ophthalmologic disorders. Pregnancy screening (prior to therapy and monthly until 6 months after therapy discontinuation if woman of childbearing age), ECG (if preexisting cardiac abnormalities) and regular dental exams are also recommended. Monitor for depression, suicidal ideation and other psychiatric symptoms before and during therapy. In pediatric patients, growth velocity and weight should also be monitored during and periodically after treatment discontinuation. The following schedule has been recommended for pediatric patients (NASPGHAN [Mack], 2012):

CBC with differential, ANC, LFTs, glucose: Check on weeks 0, 1, 2, 4, 8, 12 and every 4 to 8 weeks thereafter

TSH/total T4: Check on weeks 0, 12, 24, 36, 48

HCV RNA: Check on weeks 0, 24, 48, 72
Prothrombin time, Urinalysis: Check at week 0; repeat if clinically indicated
In adults, hematologic tests should be at treatment weeks 2 and 4, biochemical tests at week 4, TSH at week 12, and pregnancy tests monthly during and for 6 months after treatment discontinuation.
Baseline values used in adult clinical trials in combination with alfa interferons:
Platelet count ≥90,000/mm^3 (75,000/mm^3 for cirrhosis or 70,000/mm^3 for coinfection with HIV)
ANC ≥1500/mm^3
Hemoglobin ≥12 g/dL for women and ≥13 g/dL for men (11 g/dL for HIV coinfected women and 12 g/dL for HIV coinfected men)
TSH and T_4 within normal limits or adequately controlled
CD4$^+$ cell count ≥200 cells/microL or CD4$^+$ cell count 100-200 cells/microL and HIV-1 RNA <5000 copies/mL for coinfection with HIV
Serum HCV RNA levels (pretreatment, 12- and 24 weeks after therapy initiation, 24 weeks after completion of therapy). **Note:** Discontinuation of therapy may be considered after 12 weeks in patients with HCV (genotype 1) who fail to achieve an early virologic response (EVR) (defined as ≥2-log decrease in HCV RNA compared to pretreatment) or after 24 weeks with detectable HCV RNA. Treat patients with HCV (genotypes 2, 3) for 24 weeks (if tolerated) and then evaluate HCV RNA levels (AASLD [Ghany], 2009).

Additional Information
Response definitions (NASPGHAN [Mack], 2012):
Rapid virological response (RVR): Absence of detectable HCV RNA (<50 units/mL) after 4 weeks of treatment
Early viral response (EVR): ≥2-log decrease in HCV RNA after 12 weeks of treatment
End of treatment response (ETR): Absence of detectable HCV RNA (<50 units/mL) at end of the recommended treatment period
Sustained virologic response (SVR): Absence of HCV RNA (<50 units/mL) in the serum 6 months following completion of full treatment course

Dosage Forms Excipient information presented when available (limited, particularly for generics); consult specific product labeling.
Capsule, Oral:
Rebetol: 200 mg
Ribasphere: 200 mg
Generic: 200 mg
Powder for solution, for nebulization:
Virazole: 6 g [reconstituted product contains ribavirin 20 mg/mL]
Solution, Oral:
Rebetol: 40 mg/mL (100 mL) [contains propylene glycol, sodium benzoate; bubblegum flavor]
Tablet, Oral:
Copegus: 200 mg
Moderiba: 200 mg
Ribasphere: 200 mg, 400 mg, 600 mg
Generic: 200 mg
Tablet, Oral [dose-pack]:
Moderiba 600 Dose Pack: 200 mg & 400 mg (56s)
Moderiba 800 Dose Pack: 400 mg (56s)
Moderiba 1000 Dose Pack: 400 mg & 600 mg (56s)
Moderiba 1200 Dose Pack: 600 mg (56s)
Ribasphere RibaPak 600: 200 mg AM dose, 400 mg PM dose (14s, 56s)
Ribasphere RibaPak 800: 400 mg AM dose, 400 mg PM dose (14s, 56s)
Ribasphere RibaPak 1000: 600 mg AM dose, 400 mg PM dose (14s, 56s)
Ribasphere RibaPak 1200: 600 mg AM dose, 600 mg PM dose (14s, 56s)

Riboflavin (RYE boe flay vin)

Medication Safety Issues
Sound-alike/look-alike issues:
Riboflavin may be confused with ribavirin

Brand Names: US B-2-400 [OTC]

Therapeutic Category Nutritional Supplement; Vitamin, Water Soluble

Generic Availability (US) Yes

Use Prevention of riboflavin deficiency and treatment of ariboflavinosis; microcytic anemia associated with glutathione reductase deficiency

Pregnancy Considerations Water-soluble vitamins cross the placenta. Riboflavin requirements may be increased in pregnant women compared to nonpregnant women (IOM, 1998).

Breast-Feeding Considerations Riboflavin is found in breast milk. Concentrations may be influenced by supplements or maternal deficiency. Riboflavin requirements may be increased in nursing women compared to non-nursing women (IOM, 1998).

Warnings/Precautions Riboflavin deficiency often occurs in the presence of other B vitamin deficiencies.

Adverse Reactions Genitourinary: Discoloration of urine (yellow-orange)

Drug Interactions
Metabolism/Transport Effects None known.
Avoid Concomitant Use There are no known interactions where it is recommended to avoid concomitant use.
Increased Effect/Toxicity There are no known significant interactions involving an increase in effect.
Decreased Effect There are no known significant interactions involving a decrease in effect.

Storage/Stability Protect from light.

Mechanism of Action Component of flavoprotein enzymes that work together, which are necessary for normal tissue respiration; also needed for activation of pyridoxine and conversion of tryptophan to niacin

Pharmacokinetics (Adult data unless noted)
Absorption: Readily via GI tract; GI absorption is decreased in patients with hepatitis, cirrhosis, or biliary obstruction
Metabolism: Metabolic fate unknown
Half-life, biologic: 66-84 minutes
Elimination: 9% eliminated unchanged in urine

Dosing: Neonatal Oral: Adequate intake: 0.3 mg/day (0.04 mg/kg/day)

Dosing: Usual Oral:
Riboflavin deficiency:
Children: 3-10 mg/day in divided doses
Adults: 5-30 mg/day in divided doses
Adequate intake: Infants:
1 to <6 months: 0.3 mg (0.04 mg/kg)
6-12 months: 0.4 mg (0.04 mg/kg)
Recommended daily allowance (RDA): Children and Adults:
1-3 years: 0.5 mg
4-8 years: 0.6 mg
9-13 years: 0.9 mg
14-18 years:
Male: 1.3 mg
Female: 1 mg
19-70 years:
Male: 1.3 mg
Female: 1.1 mg
Microcytic anemia associated with glutathione reductase deficiency: Adults: 10 mg daily for 10 days

Administration Oral: Administer with food

Monitoring Parameters CBC and reticulocyte counts (if anemic when treating deficiency)

Test Interactions Large doses may interfere with urinalysis based on spectrometry; may cause false elevations in fluorometric determinations of catecholamines and urobilinogen

Dosage Forms Excipient information presented when available (limited, particularly for generics); consult specific product labeling.

Capsule, Oral:
B-2-400: 400 mg
Generic: 50 mg

Tablet, Oral:
Generic: 25 mg, 50 mg, 100 mg

Tablet, Oral [preservative free]:
Generic: 100 mg

◆ **Ridaura** *see* Auranofin *on page 231*

◆ **Ridaura® (Can)** *see* Auranofin *on page 231*

Rifabutin (rif a BYOO tin)

Medication Safety Issues

Sound-alike/look-alike issues:
Rifabutin may be confused with rifampin

Brand Names: US Mycobutin

Brand Names: Canada Mycobutin

Therapeutic Category Antibiotic, Miscellaneous; Antitubercular Agent

Generic Availability (US) Yes

Use Prevention of disseminated *Mycobacterium avium* complex (MAC) in patients with advanced HIV infection (FDA approved in adults); has also been utilized in multiple drug regimens for treatment of MAC; alternative to rifampin as prophylaxis for latent tuberculosis infection (LTBI) or part of multidrug regimen for treatment active tuberculosis infection; alternative as agent for prophylaxis of *Mycobacterium avium* complex in children >6 years; add-on therapy for severe *Mycobacterium avium* complex infection

Pregnancy Risk Factor B

Pregnancy Considerations Adverse events were seen in some animal reproduction studies.

Breast-Feeding Considerations In the United States, where formula is accessible, affordable, safe, and sustainable, and the risk of infant mortality due to diarrhea and respiratory infections is low, complete avoidance of breast-feeding by HIV-infected women is recommended to decrease potential transmission of HIV (DHHS [perinatal], 2011).

Contraindications Hypersensitivity to rifabutin, any other rifamycins, or any component of the formulation

Warnings/Precautions Rifabutin must not be administered for MAC prophylaxis to patients with active tuberculosis since its use may lead to the development of tuberculosis that is resistant to both rifabutin and rifampin. Caution that active TB in the HIV-positive patient may present atypically (ie, negative PPD or extrapulmonary manifestations). Uveitis may occur; carefully monitor patients when used in combination with macrolides or azole antifungals. If uveitis is suspected, refer patient to an ophthalmologist and consider temporarily discontinuing treatment. May be associated with neutropenia and/or thrombocytopenia (rarely); consider blood monitoring and discontinue permanently if signs of thrombocytopenia (eg, petechial rash) (DHHS, 2014). Use with caution in patients with renal impairment; dosage reduction recommended in severe renal impairment (CrCl <30 mL/minute). Use with caution in patients with liver impairment; discontinue in patients with AST >3 x ULN (symptomatic) or ≥5 x ULN (regardless of symptoms) or if significant bilirubin and/or alkaline phosphatase elevations occur (DHHS, 2014). Prolonged use may result in fungal or bacterial superinfection, including *C. difficile*-associated diarrhea (CDAD) and pseudomembranous colitis; CDAD has been observed >2 months postantibiotic treatment. May cause brown/orange discoloration of urine, feces, saliva, sweat, tears, and skin. Remove soft contact lenses during therapy since permanent staining may occur. Potentially significant drug-drug interactions may exist, requiring dose or frequency adjustment, additional monitoring, and/or selection of alternative therapy.

Adverse Reactions

Dermatologic: Skin rash

Genitourinary: Discoloration of urine

Hematologic & oncologic: Leukopenia, neutropenia, thrombocytopenia

Gastrointestinal: abdominal pain, dysgeusia, dyspepsia, eructation, flatulence, nausea, vomiting

Neuromuscular & skeletal: Myalgia

Miscellaneous: Fever

Rare but important or life-threatening: Aphasia, arthralgia, chest pain, confusion, dyspnea, flu-like syndrome, hepatitis, hemolysis, myositis, parasthesia, seizures, skin discoloration, T-wave abnormalities, uveitis

Drug Interactions

Metabolism/Transport Effects Substrate of CYP1A2 (minor), CYP3A4 (major); **Note:** Assignment of Major/Minor substrate status based on clinically relevant drug interaction potential; **Induces** CYP3A4 (strong)

Avoid Concomitant Use

Avoid concomitant use of Rifabutin with any of the following: Abiraterone Acetate; Apixaban; Apremilast; Artemether; Atovaquone; Axitinib; BCG; BCG (Intravesical); Bedaquiline; Boceprevir; Bortezomib; Bosutinib; Cabozantinib; Ceritinib; CloZAPine; Crizotinib; Dasabuvir; Delavirdine; Dienogest; Dronedarone; Eliglustat; Elvitegravir; Enzalutamide; Everolimus; Ibrutinib; Idelalisib; Irinotecan; Isavuconazonium Sulfate; Itraconazole; Ivabradine; Ivacaftor; Lapatinib; Ledipasvir; Lumefantrine; Lurasidone; Macitentan; Mifepristone; Mycophenolate; Naloxegol; Netupitant; NIFEdipine; Nilotinib; NiMODipine; Nisoldipine; Olaparib; Ombitasvir; Palbociclib; Panobinostat; Paritaprevir; PAZOPanib; Perampanel; PONATinib; Praziquantel; Ranolazine; Regorafenib; Rivaroxaban; Roflumilast; RomiDEPsin; Simeprevir; Sofosbuvir; SORAfenib; Suvorexant; Tasimelteon; Telaprevir; Ticagrelor; Tofacitinib; Tolvaptan; Toremifene; Trabectedin; Ulipristal; Vandetanib; Vemurafenib; VinCRIStine (Liposomal); Vorapaxar; Voriconazole

Increased Effect/Toxicity

Rifabutin may increase the levels/effects of: Clarithromycin; Clopidogrel; Darunavir; Fosamprenavir; Ifosfamide; Isoniazid; Lopinavir; Pitavastatin

The levels/effects of Rifabutin may be increased by: Antifungal Agents (Azole Derivatives, Systemic); Atazanavir; Boceprevir; Clarithromycin; Darunavir; Delavirdine; Fosamprenavir; Indinavir; Lopinavir; Macrolide Antibiotics; Nelfinavir; Nevirapine; Ritonavir; Saquinavir; Telaprevir; Tipranavir; Voriconazole

Decreased Effect

Rifabutin may decrease the levels/effects of: Abiraterone Acetate; Alfentanil; Antiemetics (5HT3 Antagonists); Antifungal Agents (Azole Derivatives, Systemic); Apixaban; Apremilast; ARIPiprazole; Artemether; Atovaquone; Axitinib; Barbiturates; BCG; BCG (Intravesical); BCG Vaccine (Immunization); Bedaquiline; Boceprevir; Bortezomib; Bosutinib; Brentuximab Vedotin; BusPIRone; Cabozantinib; Calcium Channel Blockers; Cannabidiol; Cannabis; Ceritinib; Clarithromycin; CloZAPine; Contraceptives (Estrogens); Contraceptives (Progestins); Corticosteroids (Systemic); Crizotinib; CycloSPORINE (Systemic); CYP3A4 Substrates; Dapsone (Systemic); Dasabuvir; Dasatinib; Delavirdine; Dexamethasone (Systemic); Dienogest; DOXOrubicin (Conventional); Dronabinol; Dronedarone; Efavirenz; Eliglustat; Elvitegravir; Enzalutamide; Erlotinib; Etravirine; Everolimus;

Exemestane; FentaNYL; Gefitinib; GuanFACINE; HMG-CoA Reductase Inhibitors; Hydrocodone; Hydrocortisone (Systemic); Ibrutinib; Idelalisib; Ifosfamide; Imatinib; Indinavir; Irinotecan; Isavuconazonium Sulfate; Itraconazole; Ivabradine; Ivacaftor; Ixabepilone; Lapatinib; Ledipasvir; Linagliptin; Lumefantrine; Lurasidone; Macitentan; Maraviroc; MethylPREDNISolone; Mifepristone; Morphine (Systemic); Mycophenolate; Naloxegol; Nelfinavir; Netupitant; Nevirapine; NIFEdipine; Nilotinib; NiMODipine; Nisoldipine; Olaparib; Ombitasvir; Palbociclib; Panobinostat; Paritaprevir; PAZOPanib; Perampanel; PONATinib; Praziquantel; PrednisoLONE (Systemic); PredniSONE; Propafenone; QUEtiapine; QuiNIDine; Raltegravir; Ramelteon; Ranolazine; Regorafenib; Rilpivirine; Rivaroxaban; Roflumilast; RomiDEPsin; Saquinavir; Saxagliptin; Simeprevir; Sodium Picosulfate; Sofosbuvir; SORAfenib; SUNItinib; Suvorexant; Tacrolimus (Systemic); Tadalafil; Tamoxifen; Tasimelteon; Telaprevir; Temsirolimus; Tetrahydrocannabinol; Ticagrelor; Tofacitinib; Tolvaptan; Toremifene; Trabectedin; Typhoid Vaccine; Ulipristal; Vandetanib; Vemurafenib; Vilazodone; VinCRIStine (Liposomal); Vitamin K Antagonists; Vorapaxar; Voriconazole; Vortioxetine; Zaleplon; Zolpidem; Zuclopenthixol

The levels/effects of Rifabutin may be decreased by: Bosentan; CYP3A4 Inducers (Moderate); CYP3A4 Inducers (Strong); Dabrafenib; Deferasirox; Efavirenz; Mitotane; Nevirapine; Siltuximab; St Johns Wort; Tocilizumab

Food Interactions High-fat meal may decrease the rate but not the extent of absorption. Management: May administer with meals.

Storage/Stability Store at 25°C (77°F); excursions permitted to 15°C to 30°C (59°F to 86°F).

Mechanism of Action Inhibits DNA-dependent RNA polymerase at the beta subunit which prevents chain initiation

Pharmacokinetics (Adult data unless noted)

Absorption: Oral: Readily absorbed

Distribution: To body tissues including the lungs, liver, spleen, eyes, and kidneys

V_d: Adults: 9.3 ± 1.5 L/kg

Protein binding: 85%

Metabolism: Hepatically to 5 metabolites; predominantly 25-O-desacetyl-rifabutin (antimicrobial activity equivalent to parent drug; serum AUC 10% of parent drug) and 31-hydroxy-rifabutin (serum AUC 7% of parent drug)

Bioavailability: 20% in HIV patients

Half-life, terminal: 45 hours (range: 16-69 hours)

Time to peak serum concentration: 2-4 hours

Elimination: Renal and biliary clearance of unchanged drug is 10%; 30% excreted in feces; 53% excreted in urine

Dosing: Usual Oral:

Infants and Children:

Mycobacterium avium complex (MAC) (CDC, 2009):

Treatment, add-on therapy for severe infection: 10-20 mg/kg once daily (maximum: 300 mg)

Prophylaxis for first episode (HIV-positive/exposed patients ≥6 years): 300 mg once daily

Prophylaxis for recurrence (HIV positive-/exposed patients): 5 mg/kg (maximum dose: 300 mg) once daily as an optional add-on to primary therapy of clarithromycin and ethambutol

Tuberculosis, treatment (alternative to rifampin): 10-20 mg/kg (maximum dose: 300 mg) once daily or intermittently 2-3 times weekly

Adolescents and Adults (CDC, 2009a):

Disseminated MAC in advanced HIV infection:

Prophylaxis: 300 mg once daily or 150 mg twice daily to reduce gastrointestinal upset

Treatment: 300 mg once daily as an optional add-on to primary therapy of clarithromycin and ethambutol

Tuberculosis (alternative to rifampin):

Prophylaxis of LTBI: 300 mg once daily for 4 months

Treatment of active TB: 300 mg once daily or intermittently 2-3 times weekly as part of multidrug regimen

Dosage adjustment for concurrent efavirenz (no concomitant protease inhibitor): Adolescents and Adults: Increase rifabutin dose to 450-600 mg daily or 600 mg 3 times/week

Dosage adjustment for concurrent nelfinavir, amprenavir, indinavir: Adolescents and Adults: Reduce rifabutin dose to 150 mg/day; no change in dose if administered twice weekly

Dosage adjustment in renal impairment: CrCl <30 mL/minute: Reduce dose by 50%

Administration Oral: May administer with or without food or mix with applesauce if patient unable to swallow capsule; administer with food to decrease GI upset

Monitoring Parameters Periodic liver function tests, CBC with differential, platelet count, hemoglobin, hematocrit, ophthalmologic exam, number and type of stools/day for diarrhea

Dosage Forms Excipient information presented when available (limited, particularly for generics); consult specific product labeling.

Capsule, Oral:

Mycobutin: 150 mg

Generic: 150 mg

Extemporaneous Preparations A 20 mg/mL rifabutin oral suspension may be made with capsules and a 1:1 mixture of Ora-Sweet® and Ora-Plus®. Empty the the powder from eight 150 mg rifabutin capsules into a glass mortar; add 20 mL of vehicle and mix to a uniform paste. Mix while adding vehicle in incremental proportions to **almost** 60 mL; transfer to a calibrated bottle, rinse mortar with vehicle, and add quantity of vehicle sufficient to make 60 mL. Label "shake well". Stable for 12 weeks at 4°C, 25°C, 30°C, and 40°C.

Haslam JL, Egodage KL, Chen Y, et al, "Stability of Rifabutin in Two Extemporaneously Compounded Oral Liquids," *Am J Health Syst Pharm*, 1999, 56(4):333-6.

◆ **Rifadin** *see* Rifampin *on page 1858*

◆ **Rifampicin** *see* Rifampin *on page 1858*

Rifampin (rif AM pin)

Medication Safety Issues

Sound-alike/look-alike issues:

Rifadin may be confused with Rifater, Ritalin

Rifampin may be confused with ribavirin, rifabutin, Rifamate, rifapentine, rifaximin

Brand Names: US Rifadin

Brand Names: Canada Rifadin; Rofact

Therapeutic Category Antibiotic, Miscellaneous; Antitubercular Agent

Generic Availability (US) Yes

Use Management of active tuberculosis in combination with other agents [FDA approved in pediatric patients (age not specified) and adults]; elimination of meningococci from asymptomatic carriers [FDA approved in pediatric patients (age not specified) and adults]; has also been used for prophylaxis in contacts of patients with *Haemophilus influenzae* type B infection; used in combination with other anti-infectives in the treatment of staphylococcal infections

Pregnancy Risk Factor C

Pregnancy Considerations Teratogenic effects have been reported in animal studies. Rifampin crosses the human placenta. Due to the risk of tuberculosis to the fetus, treatment is recommended when the probability of maternal disease is moderate to high. Postnatal hemorrhages have been reported in the infant and mother with isoniazid administration during the last few weeks of pregnancy.

Breast-Feeding Considerations The manufacturer does not recommend breast-feeding due to tumorigenicity observed in animal studies; however, the CDC does not consider rifampin a contraindication to breast-feeding.

Contraindications Hypersensitivity to rifampin, any rifamycins, or any component of the formulation; concurrent use of atazanavir, darunavir, fosamprenavir, ritonavir/saquinavir, ritonavir, or tipranavir

Warnings/Precautions Use with caution and modify dosage in patients with liver impairment; observe for hyperbilirubinemia; discontinue therapy if this in conjunction with clinical symptoms or any signs of significant hepatocellular damage develop. Use with caution in patients receiving concurrent medications associated with hepatotoxicity. Use with caution in patients with a history of alcoholism (even if ethanol consumption is discontinued during therapy). Since rifampin since rifampin has enzyme-inducing properties, porphyria exacerbation is possible; use with caution in patients with porphyria; do not use for meningococcal disease, only for short-term treatment of asymptomatic carrier states

Regimens of >600 mg once or twice weekly in adults have been associated with a high incidence of adverse reactions including a flu-like syndrome, hypersensitivity, thrombocytopenia, leukopenia, and anemia. Urine, feces, saliva, sweat, tears, and CSF may be discolored to red/orange; remove soft contact lenses during therapy since permanent staining may occur. Do not administer IV form via IM or SubQ routes; restart infusion at another site if extravasation occurs. Prolonged use may result in fungal or bacterial superinfection, including *C. difficile*-associated diarrhea (CDAD) and pseudomembranous colitis; CDAD has been observed >2 months postantibiotic treatment. Monitor for compliance in patients on intermittent therapy.

Adverse Reactions

Cardiovascular: Edema, flushing

Central nervous system: Ataxia, behavioral changes, concentration impaired, confusion, dizziness, drowsiness, fatigue, fever, headache, numbness, psychosis

Dermatologic: Pemphigoid reaction, pruritus, rash, urticaria

Endocrine & metabolic: Adrenal insufficiency, menstrual disorders

Gastrointestinal: Anorexia, cramps, diarrhea, epigastric distress, flatulence, heartburn, nausea, pseudomembranous colitis, pancreatitis, vomiting

Hematologic: Agranulocytosis (rare), DIC, eosinophilia, hemoglobin decreased, hemolysis, hemolytic anemia, leukopenia, thrombocytopenia (especially with high-dose therapy)

Hepatic: Hepatitis (rare), jaundice, LFTs increased

Neuromuscular & skeletal: Myalgia, osteomalacia, weakness

Ocular: Exudative conjunctivitis, visual changes

Renal: Acute renal failure, BUN increased, hemoglobinuria, hematuria, interstitial nephritis, uric acid increased

Miscellaneous: Flu-like syndrome

Drug Interactions

Metabolism/Transport Effects **Substrate** of P-glycoprotein, SLCO1B1; **Inhibits** SLCO1B1; **Induces** CYP1A2 (strong), CYP2A6 (strong), CYP2B6 (strong), CYP2C19 (strong), CYP2C8 (strong), CYP2C9 (strong), CYP3A4 (strong), P-glycoprotein

Avoid Concomitant Use

Avoid concomitant use of Rifampin with any of the following: Abiraterone Acetate; Apixaban; Apremilast; Artemether; Atazanavir; Atovaquone; Axitinib; BCG; BCG (Intravesical); Bedaquiline; Boceprevir; Bortezomib; Bosutinib; Cabozantinib; Ceritinib; CloZAPine; Cobicistat; Crizotinib; Dabigatran Etexilate; Darunavir; Dasabuvir; Delavirdine; Dienogest; Diltiazem; Dronedarone; Edoxaban; Eliglustat; Elvitegravir; Enzalutamide; Esomeprazole; Etravirine; Everolimus; Fimasartan; Fosamprenavir; Ibrutinib; Idelalisib; Indinavir; Irinotecan; Isavuconazonium Sulfate; Itraconazole; Ivabradine; Ivacaftor; Lapatinib; Ledipasvir; Lopinavir; Lumefantrine; Lurasidone; Macitentan; Mifepristone; Mycophenolate; Naloxegol; Nelfinavir; Netupitant; NIFEdipine; Nilotinib; NiMODipine; Nintedanib; Nisoldipine; Olaparib; Ombitasvir; Omeprazole; Palbociclib; Panobinostat; Paritaprevir; PAZOPanib; Perampanel; Pirfenidone; PONATinib; Praziquantel; QuiNINE; Ranolazine; Regorafenib; Rilpivirine; Ritonavir; Rivaroxaban; Roflumilast; RomiDEPsin; Saquinavir; Simeprevir; Sofosbuvir; SORAfenib; Suvorexant; Tasimelteon; Telaprevir; Ticagrelor; Tipranavir; Tofacitinib; Tolvaptan; Toremifene; Trabectedin; Ulipristal; Vandetanib; Vemurafenib; VinCRIStine (Liposomal); Vorapaxar; Voriconazole

Increased Effect/Toxicity

Rifampin may increase the levels/effects of: Bosentan; Clarithromycin; Clopidogrel; Eluxadoline; Fexofenadine; Fimasartan; Isoniazid; Leflunomide; Lopinavir; Pitavastatin; Propofol; RomiDEPsin; Saquinavir

The levels/effects of Rifampin may be increased by: Antifungal Agents (Azole Derivatives, Systemic); Clarithromycin; Delavirdine; Eltrombopag; Macrolide Antibiotics; P-glycoprotein/ABCB1 Inhibitors; Pyrazinamide; Teriflunomide; Voriconazole

Decreased Effect

Rifampin may decrease the levels/effects of: Abiraterone Acetate; Afatinib; Alfentanil; Amiodarone; Antidiabetic Agents (Thiazolidinedione); Antiemetics (5HT3 Antagonists); Antifungal Agents (Azole Derivatives, Systemic); Apixaban; Apremilast; Aprepitant; ARIPiprazole; Artemether; Atazanavir; Atovaquone; Axitinib; Barbiturates; Bazedoxifene; BCG; BCG (Intravesical); BCG Vaccine (Immunization); Bedaquiline; Bendamustine; Beta-Blockers; Boceprevir; Bortezomib; Bosentan; Bosutinib; Brentuximab Vedotin; BusPIRone; Cabozantinib; Calcium Channel Blockers; Canagliflozin; Cannabidiol; Cannabis; Caspofungin; Ceritinib; Chloramphenicol; Citalopram; Clarithromycin; CloZAPine; Cobicistat; Contraceptives (Estrogens); Contraceptives (Progestins); Corticosteroids (Systemic); Crizotinib; CycloSPORINE (Systemic); CYP1A2 Substrates; CYP2A6 Substrates; CYP2B6 Substrates; CYP2C19 Substrates; CYP2C8 Substrates; CYP2C9 Substrates; CYP3A4 Substrates; Dabigatran Etexilate; Dapsone (Systemic); Darunavir; Dasabuvir; Dasatinib; Deferasirox; Delavirdine; Dexamethasone (Systemic); Diclofenac (Systemic); Dienogest; Diltiazem; Disopyramide; Dolutegravir; DOXOrubicin (Conventional); Doxycycline; Dronabinol; Dronedarone; Edoxaban; Efavirenz; Eliglustat; Elvitegravir; Enzalutamide; Erlotinib; Esomeprazole; Etravirine; Everolimus; Exemestane; FentaNYL; Fexofenadine; Fosamprenavir; Fosaprepitant; Fosphenytoin; Gefitinib; GuanFACINE; HMG-CoA Reductase Inhibitors; Hydrocodone; Hydrocortisone (Systemic); Ibrutinib; Idelalisib; Imatinib; Indinavir; Irinotecan; Isavuconazonium Sulfate; Itraconazole; Ivabradine; Ivacaftor; Ixabepilone; LamoTRIgine; Lapatinib; Ledipasvir; Linagliptin; Lopinavir; Losartan; Lumefantrine; Lurasidone; Macitentan; Maraviroc; Methadone; MethylPREDNISolone; Mifepristone; Mirabegron; Morphine (Systemic); Mycophenolate; Naloxegol; Nelfinavir; Netupitant; Nevirapine; NIFEdipine; Nilotinib; NiMODipine; Nintedanib; Nisoldipine; Nitrazepam; Olaparib; Ombitasvir; Omeprazole; OxyCODONE; Palbociclib; Paliperidone; Panobinostat; Paritaprevir; PAZOPanib; Perampanel; P-glycoprotein/ABCB1 Substrates; Phenytoin; Pirfenidone; PONATinib; Prasugrel; Praziquantel; PredniSOLONE (Systemic); PredniSONE; Propafenone; QUEtiapine; QuiNIDine; QuiNINE; Raltegravir; Ramelteon; Ranolazine; Regorafenib; Repaglinide; Rilpivirine; Ritonavir; Rivaroxaban; Roflumilast; Saquinavir; Saxagliptin;

Simeprevir; Sirolimus; Sodium Picosulfate; Sofosbuvir; SORAfenib; Sulfonylureas; SUNItinib; Suvorexant; Tacrolimus (Systemic); Tadalafil; Tamoxifen; Tasimelteon; Telaprevir; Temsirolimus; Terbinafine (Systemic); Tetrahydrocannabinol; Thyroid Products; Ticagrelor; Tipranavir; Tofacitinib; Tolvaptan; Toremifene; Trabectedin; Treprostinil; Typhoid Vaccine; Ulipristal; Valproic Acid and Derivatives; Vandetanib; Vemurafenib; Vilazodone; VinCRIStine (Liposomal); Vorapaxar; Voriconazole; Vortioxetine; Zaleplon; Zidovudine; Zolpidem; Zuclopenthixol

The levels/effects of Rifampin may be decreased by: P-glycoprotein/ABCB1 Inducers

Food Interactions Food decreases the extent of absorption; rifampin concentrations may be decreased if taken with food. Management: Administer on an empty stomach with a glass of water (ie, 1 hour prior to, or 2 hours after meals or antacids).

Storage/Stability Store capsules and intact vials at 25°C (77°F); excursions permitted to 15°C to 30°C (59°F to 86°F); avoid excessive heat (>40°C [104°F]). Protect the intact vials from light. Reconstituted vials are stable for 24 hours at room temperature.

Stability of parenteral admixture at room temperature (25°C [77°F]) is 4 hours for D_5W and 24 hours for NS.

Mechanism of Action Inhibits bacterial RNA synthesis by binding to the beta subunit of DNA-dependent RNA polymerase, blocking RNA transcription

Pharmacokinetics (Adult data unless noted)

Absorption: Oral: Well absorbed

Distribution: Highly lipophilic; crosses the blood-brain barrier and is widely distributed into body tissues and fluids such as the liver, lungs, gallbladder, bile, tears, and breast milk; distributes into CSF when meninges are inflamed

Protein binding: 80%

Metabolism: Undergoes enterohepatic recycling; metabolized in the liver to a deacetylated metabolite (active)

Half-life: 3-4 hours, prolonged with hepatic impairment

Time to peak serum concentration: Oral: Within 2-4 hours

Elimination: Principally in feces (60% to 65%) and urine (~30%)

Dialysis: Plasma rifampin concentrations are not significantly affected by hemodialysis or peritoneal dialysis

Dosing: Neonatal IV, Oral:

***H. influenzae* prophylaxis:** 10 mg/kg/day once daily for 4 days

Meningococcal prophylaxis: 10 mg/kg/day in divided doses every 12 hours for 2 days

***Staphylococcus aureus*, synergy for infections:** 5-20 mg/kg/day in divided doses every 12 hours with other antibiotics

Dosing: Usual Oral, IV:

Tuberculosis:

Active infection, treatment: **Note:** A four-drug regimen (isoniazid, rifampin, pyrazinamide, and ethambutol) is preferred for the initial, empiric treatment of TB. The regimen should be altered based on drug susceptibility results as appropriate. In HIV-exposed/positive patients, rifabutin may be used an alternative to rifampin. American Thoracic Society and CDC currently recommend twice weekly therapy as part of a short-course regimen, which follows 1-2 months of daily treatment of uncomplicated pulmonary tuberculosis in the compliant patient.

Daily therapy:

Infants and Children: 10-20 mg/kg/day (maximum dose: 600 mg)

Adults: 10 mg/kg/day administered once daily (maximum dose: 600 mg)

Directly observed therapy (DOT):

Infants and Children: 10-20 mg/kg (maximum dose: 600 mg) administered 2 times/week if HIV negative **or** administered 3 times weekly if HIV-exposed/positive.

Adults: 10 mg/kg (maximum dose: 600 mg) administered 2 or 3 times/week

Latent tuberculosis infection (LTBI) treatment (as an alternative to isoniazid): **Note:** Combination with pyrazinamide should not generally be offered (*MMWR*, Aug 8, 2003). In HIV-exposed/positive patients, isoniazid is preferred due to potential for drug interactions of rifampin with antiretroviral therapy.

Infants and Children: 10-20 mg/kg/day once daily for 4 months (maximum dose: 600 mg/day)

Adults: 10 mg/kg/dose once daily for 4 months (maximum dose: 600 mg/day)

Primary prophylaxis of isoniazid-resistant tuberculosis in HIV-exposed/positive patients: Infants and Children: 10-20 mg/kg/dose once daily for 4-6 months (maximum dose: 600 mg/day)

Endocarditis, prosthetic valve due to MRSA (Baddour, 2005; Lui, 2011):

Infants and Children: 15-20 mg/kg/day divided every 8 hours

Adults: 300 mg every 8 hours for at least 6 weeks (combine with vancomycin for the entire duration of therapy and gentamicin for the first 2 weeks)

***H. influenzae* prophylaxis:**

Infants and Children: 20 mg/kg/day once daily for 4 days, not to exceed 600 mg/dose

Adults: 600 mg once daily for 4 days

Meningococcal prophylaxis:

Infants and Children: 20 mg/kg/day in divided doses every 12 hours for 2 days, not to exceed 600 mg/dose

Adults: 600 mg every 12 hours for 2 days

***Staphylococcus aureus*, nasal carriers:**

Children: 15 mg/kg/day divided every 12 hours for 5-10 days; **Note: Must use in combination with at least one other systemic antistaphylococcal antibiotic.** Not recommended as first-line drug for decolonization; evidence is weak for use in patients with recurrent infections (Liu, 2011).

Adults: 600 mg/day for 5-10 days; **Note: Must use in combination with at least one other systemic antistaphylococcal antibiotic.** Not recommended as first-line drug for decolonization; evidence is weak for use in patients with recurrent infections (Liu, 2011).

***Staphylococcus aureus*, synergy for infections:** Adults: 600 mg once daily or 300-450 mg every 12 hours with other antibiotics. **Note:** Must be used in combination with another antistaphylococcal antibiotic to avoid rapid development of resistance (Liu, 2011).

Preparation for Administration Parenteral: Reconstitute vial with 10 mL SWFI. Prior to injection, further dilute in appropriate volume of a compatible solution (ie, D_5W, NS) at a final concentration not to exceed 6 mg/mL.

Administration

Oral: Administer on an empty stomach with a glass of water (ie, 1 hour prior to or 2 hours after meals or antacids) to increase total absorption (food may delay and reduce the amount of rifampin absorbed). The compounded oral suspension must be shaken well before using. May mix contents of capsule with applesauce or jelly

Parenteral: Administer by slow IV infusion over 30 minutes to 3 hours. Do not administer IM or SubQ. Avoid extravasation.

Monitoring Parameters Periodic monitoring of liver function (AST, ALT); bilirubin, CBC, platelet count

Test Interactions May interfere with urine detection of opioids (false-positive); positive Coombs' reaction [direct], rifampin inhibits standard assay's ability to measure serum folate and B_{12}; transient increase in LFTs and decreased biliary excretion of contrast media

Dosage Forms Excipient information presented when available (limited, particularly for generics); consult specific product labeling.

Capsule, Oral:
  Rifadin: 150 mg, 300 mg
  Generic: 150 mg, 300 mg

Solution Reconstituted, Intravenous:
  Rifadin: 600 mg (1 ea)
  Generic: 600 mg (1 ea)

Extemporaneous Preparations A rifampin 1% w/v suspension (10 mg/mL) may be made with capsules and one of four syrups (Syrup NF, simple syrup, Syrpalta® syrup, or raspberry syrup). Empty the contents of four 300 mg capsules or eight 150 mg capsules onto a piece of weighing paper. If necessary, crush contents to produce a fine powder. Transfer powder to a 4-ounce amber glass or plastic prescription bottle. Rinse paper and spatula with 20 mL of chosen syrup and add the rinse to bottle; shake vigorously. Add 100 mL syrup to the bottle and shake vigorously. Label "shake well". Stable for 4 weeks at room temperature or refrigerated.

A 25 mg/mL oral suspension may be made with capsules and cherry syrup concentrate diluted 1:4 with simple syrup, NF. Empty the contents of ten 300 mg capsules into a mortar and reduce to a fine powder. Add 20 mL of the vehicle and mix to a uniform paste; mix while adding the vehicle in incremental proportions to **almost** 120 mL; transfer to a calibrated bottle, rinse mortar with vehicle, and add quantity of vehicle sufficient to make 120 mL. Label "shake well" and "refrigerate". Stable for 28 days refrigerated (preferred) or at room temperature.

Nahata MC, Pai VB, and Hipple TF, *Pediatric Drug Formulations*, 5th ed, Cincinnati, OH: Harvey Whitney Books Co, 2004.

Rifaximin (rif AX i min)

Medication Safety Issues

Sound-alike/look-alike issues:
Rifaximin may be confused with rifampin

Brand Names: US Xifaxan

Therapeutic Category Antibiotic, Miscellaneous

Generic Availability (US) No

Use Treatment of travelers' diarrhea caused by noninvasive strains of *E. coli* (FDA approved in ages ≥12 years and adults); reduction in the risk of overt hepatic encephalopathy (HE) recurrence (FDA approved in ages ≥18 years and adults); has also been used in inflammatory bowel disease and irritable bowel syndrome

Pregnancy Considerations Adverse events have been observed in some animal reproduction studies. Due to the limited oral absorption of rifaximin in patients with normal hepatic function, exposure to the fetus is expected to be low.

Breast-Feeding Considerations It is not known if rifaximin is excreted in human milk. Due to the potential for serious adverse reactions in the nursing infant, the manufacturer recommends a decision be made whether to discontinue nursing or to discontinue the drug, taking into account the importance of treatment to the mother. Because of the limited oral absorption of rifaximin in patients with normal hepatic function, exposure to the nursing infant is expected to be low.

Contraindications Hypersensitivity to rifaximin, other rifamycin antibiotics, or any component of the formulation

Warnings/Precautions Hypersensitivity reactions (eg, exfoliative dermatitis, rash, urticaria, flushing, angioneurotic edema, pruritus, anaphylaxis) have occurred; these events have occurred as early as within 15 minutes of drug administration. Efficacy has not been established for the treatment of diarrhea due to pathogens other than *E. coli*, including *C. jejuni*, *Shigella* and *Salmonella*. Consider alternative therapy if symptoms persist or worsen after 24 to 48 hours of treatment. Not for treatment of systemic infections; <1% is absorbed orally. Prolonged use may result in fungal or bacterial superinfection, including *C. difficile*-associated diarrhea (CDAD) and pseudomembranous colitis; CDAD has been observed >2 months post-antibiotic treatment. Use caution in severe hepatic impairment (Child-Pugh class C); efficacy for prevention of encephalopathy has not been established in patients with a Model for End-Stage Liver Disease (MELD) score >25. Potentially significant drug-drug interactions may exist, requiring dose or frequency adjustment, additional monitoring, and/or selection of alternative therapy. Some dosage forms may contain propylene glycol; large amounts are potentially toxic and have been associated hyperosmolality, lactic acidosis, seizures, and respiratory depression; use caution (AAP 1997; Zar 2007).

Adverse Reactions

Cardiovascular: Chest pain, edema, hypotension, peripheral edema

Central nervous system: Attention disturbance, amnesia, confusion, depression, dizziness, fatigue, fever, headache, hypoesthesia, pain, tremor, vertigo

Dermatological: Cellulitis, pruritus, rash

Endocrine and metabolism: Hyper-/hypoglycemia, hyperkalemia, hyponatremia

Hepatic: Ascites

Gastrointestinal: Abdominal pain, abdominal tenderness, anorexia, dehydration, esophageal varices, nausea, weight gain, xerostomia

Hematologic: Anemia

Neuromuscular & skeletal: Arthralgia, muscle spasms, myalgia

Respiratory: Dyspnea, epistaxis, nasopharyngitis, pneumonia, rhinitis, upper respiratory tract infection

Miscellaneous: Influenza-like illness

All indications: Rare but important or life-threatening: Abnormal dreams, allergic dermatitis, anaphylaxis, angioneurotic edema, AST increased, choluria, CDAD, dry lips, dysuria, ear pain, exfoliative dermatitis, flushing, gingival disorder, hematuria, hot flashes, hypersensitivity reactions, lymphocytosis, migraine, monocytosis, motion sickness, nasal irritation, nasopharyngitis, neck pain, neutropenia, pharyngitis, pharyngolaryngeal pain, polyuria, proteinuria, sunburn, syncope, taste loss, tinnitus, urticaria, weakness, weight loss

Drug Interactions

Metabolism/Transport Effects Substrate of CYP3A4 (minor), P-glycoprotein, SLCO1B1; **Note:** Assignment of Major/Minor substrate status based on clinically relevant drug interaction potential; **Inhibits** P-glycoprotein, SLCO1B1

Avoid Concomitant Use

Avoid concomitant use of Rifaximin with any of the following: BCG; BCG (Intravesical)

Increased Effect/Toxicity

The levels/effects of Rifaximin may be increased by: CycloSPORINE (Systemic); P-glycoprotein/ABCB1 Inhibitors

Decreased Effect

Rifaximin may decrease the levels/effects of: BCG; BCG (Intravesical); BCG Vaccine (Immunization); Sodium Picosulfate

Storage/Stability Store at 20°C to 25°C (68°F to 77°F); excursions permitted to 15°C to 30°C (59°F to 86°F).

Mechanism of Action Rifaximin inhibits bacterial RNA synthesis by binding to bacterial DNA-dependent RNA polymerase.

Pharmacokinetics (Adult data unless noted)

Absorption: Low and variable; increased with worsening hepatic impairment (patients with Child-Pugh class C have greater exposure than Child-Pugh class A patients)

Ptrotein binding: Healthy subjects: ~68%; Hepatic impairment: 62%

Half-life elimination: Mean range: 2-5 hours

Time to peak serum concentration: 1 hour

Elimination: Feces (~97% as unchanged drug); urine (<1%)

Dosing: Usual

Pediatric:

Diarrhea, travelers': Oral: **Note:** Efficacy has not been established for the treatment of diarrhea due to pathogens other than *E. coli*, including *C. jejuni*, *Shigella*, and *Salmonella*; avoid use in diarrhea with fever or blood in the stool; consider alternative therapy if symptoms persist or worsen after 24 to 48 hours of treatment

Children 3 to 11 years: Limited data available: 100 mg 4 times daily for up to 5 days has been used in 38 children (age range: 3 to 8 years) to treat infectious diarrhea (Beseghi 1998; Frisari 1997)

Children ≥12 years and Adolescents: 200 mg 3 times daily for 3 days

Hepatic encephalopathy: Oral: Adolescents ≥18 years: Reduction of overt hepatic encephalopathy recurrence: 550 mg 2 times daily

Inflammatory bowel disease (IBD) (Crohn disease, ulcerative colitis): Limited data available: Oral: Children ≥8 years and Adolescents: 10 to 30 mg/kg/day in divided doses; maximum daily dose: 1200 mg/**day**. Dosing based on a retrospective experience of 23 pediatric patients (age range: 8 to 21 years) with IBD flare (Crohn disease, n=12; ulcerative colitis: n=11); patients received rifaximin 400 to 1200 mg/day (10 to 30 mg/kg/day); improvements in diarrhea and abdominal pain were reported within the first 4 weeks of therapy for the majority of patients (~74%), and within a week in some cases; higher total daily doses (1200 mg/day vs 400 mg/day) were associated with better symptom control (Muniyappa 2009).

Small intestinal bacterial overgrowth (SIBO) [eg, irritable bowel syndrome (IBS), chronic abdominal pain]: Limited data available; efficacy results variable: Oral: Children ≥3 years and Adolescents: 200 mg 3 times daily, dosing based on prospective study of 50 pediatric patients with IBS (age range: 3 to 15 years); results showed 7 days of therapy resulted in improved symptoms and a reduction in bacterial overgrowth based on lactulose breath test (LBT) results (Scarpellini 2013); however, a double-blind placebo-controlled trial in pediatric patients (n=75 including 49 who received rifaximin, age range: 8 to 18 years) with chronic abdominal pain showed very low efficacy in normalizing LBT (20% response rate) and treating SIBO compared to placebo at a higher dose of 550 mg 3 times daily for 7 days (Collins 2011).

Adults:

Hepatic encephalopathy: Oral: Reduction of overt hepatic encephalopathy recurrence: 550 mg 2 times daily

Travelers' diarrhea: Oral: 200 mg 3 times daily for 3 days

Dosing adjustment for renal impairment: There are no dosage adjustments provided in the manufacturer's labeling (has not been studied).

Dosing adjustment for hepatic impairment: No dosage adjustment necessary. Use with caution in patients with severe impairment (Child-Pugh class C) as systemic absorption does occur and pharmacokinetic parameters are highly variable.

Administration Oral: May be administered with or without food.

Monitoring Parameters Temperature, blood in stool, change in symptoms; monitor changes in mental status in hepatic encephalopathy

Dosage Forms Excipient information presented when available (limited, particularly for generics); consult specific product labeling.

Tablet, Oral:

Xifaxan: 200 mg, 550 mg [contains edetate disodium]

Extemporaneous Preparations A 20 mg/mL oral suspension may be made using tablets. Crush six 200 mg tablets and reduce to a fine powder. Add 30 mL of a 1:1 mixture of Ora-Sweet® and Ora-Plus® or a 1:1 mixture of Ora-Sweet® SF and Ora-Plus®; mix well while adding the vehicle in geometric proportions to **almost** 60 mL; transfer to a calibrated bottle, rinse mortar with vehicle, and add quantity of vehicle sufficient to make 60 mL. Label "shake well". Stable 60 days at room temperature.

Cober MP, Johnson CE, Lee J, et al, "Stability of Extemporaneously Prepared Rifaximin Oral Suspensions," *Am J Health Syst Pharm*, 2010, 67(4):287-89.

◆ **RIG** *see* Rabies Immune Globulin (Human) *on page 1830*

Rilonacept (ri LON a sept)

Brand Names: US Arcalyst

Therapeutic Category Interleukin-1 Receptor Antagonist

Generic Availability (US) No

Use Treatment of cryopyrin-associated periodic syndromes (CAPS), including familial cold autoinflammatory syndrome (FCAS) and Muckle-Wells syndrome (MWS) (FDA approved in ages ≥12 years and adults)

Pregnancy Risk Factor C

Pregnancy Considerations Adverse events have been observed in animal reproduction studies.

Breast-Feeding Considerations It is not known if rilonacept is excreted in breast milk. The manufacturer recommends that caution be exercised when administering rilonacept to nursing women.

Contraindications There are no contraindications listed in the manufacturer's labeling.

Warnings/Precautions May cause rare hypersensitivity reactions; discontinue use and initiate appropriate therapy if reaction occurs. Caution should be exercised when considering use in patients with a history of new/recurrent infections, with conditions that predispose them to infections, or with latent or localized infections. Therapy should not be initiated in patients with active or chronic infections. May increase risk of reactivation of latent tuberculosis; follow current guidelines for evaluation and treatment of latent tuberculosis prior to initiating rilonacept therapy. Use may impair defenses against malignancies; impact on the development and course of malignancies is not fully defined. Use may increase total cholesterol, HDL, LDL, and triglycerides; periodic assessment of lipid profile should occur. Tumor necrosis factor (TNF)-blocking agents should not be used in combination with rilonacept; risk of serious infection is increased. Immunizations should be up to date including pneumococcal and influenza vaccines before initiating therapy. Live vaccines should not be given concurrently. Administration of inactivated (killed) vaccines while on therapy may not be effective.

Adverse Reactions

Central nervous system: Hypoesthesia

Immunologic: Antibody development

Infection: Increased susceptibility to infection

Local: Injection site reaction (majority mild-moderate; typically lasting 1-2 days; characterized by bleeding, bruising, erythema, induration, inflammation, itching, pain, swelling, urticaria; other local reactions include dermatitis, vesicles)

Respiratory: Cough, sinusitis, upper respiratory tract infection

Rare but important or life-threatening: Bacterial meningitis (*Streptococcus pneumoniae*), bronchitis, colitis, gastrointestinal hemorrhage, hypercholesterolemia, hypersensitivity reaction, increased HDL cholesterol, increased LDL cholesterol, increased serum triglycerides, mycobacterium infection (*Mycobacterium intracellulare*), neutropenia (transient)

Drug Interactions

Metabolism/Transport Effects None known.

Avoid Concomitant Use

Avoid concomitant use of Rilonacept with any of the following: Anti-TNF Agents; BCG; BCG (Intravesical); Canakinumab; Natalizumab; Pimecrolimus; Tacrolimus (Topical); Tofacitinib; Vaccines (Live)

Increased Effect/Toxicity

Rilonacept may increase the levels/effects of: Canakinumab; Leflunomide; Natalizumab; Tofacitinib; Vaccines (Live)

The levels/effects of Rilonacept may be increased by: Anti-TNF Agents; Denosumab; Pimecrolimus; Roflumilast; Tacrolimus (Topical); Trastuzumab

Decreased Effect

Rilonacept may decrease the levels/effects of: BCG; BCG (Intravesical); Coccidioides immitis Skin Test; Sipuleucel-T; Vaccines (Inactivated); Vaccines (Live)

The levels/effects of Rilonacept may be decreased by: Echinacea

Storage/Stability Store intact vials in refrigerator at 2°C to 8°C (36°F to 46°F). Store in original carton; protect from light; do not freeze. Do not shake. After reconstitution, may be stored at controlled room temperature. Protect from light. Use within 3 hours of reconstitution.

Mechanism of Action Cryopyrin-associated periodic syndromes (CAPS) refers to rare genetic syndromes caused by mutations in the nucleotide-binding domain, leucine rich family (NLR), pyrin domain containing 3 (NLRP-3) gene or the cold-induced autoinflammatory syndrome-1 (*CIAS1*) gene. Cryopyrin, a protein encoded by this gene, regulates interleukin-1 beta (IL-1β) activation. Deficiency of cryopyrin results in excessive inflammation. Rilonacept reduces inflammation by binding to IL-1β (some binding of IL-1α and IL-1 receptor antagonist) and preventing interaction with cell surface receptors.

Pharmacodynamics Onset of action: Steady-state concentrations reached in ~6 weeks

Dosing: Usual SubQ: **Cryopyrin-associated periodic syndromes (CAPS):**

Children and Adolescents 12-17 years:

Initial: Loading dose 4.4 mg/kg; maximum dose: 320 mg/dose; **Note:** Loading dose may be divided into 1 or 2 separate injections (maximum injection volume: 2 mL/injection) and given on the same day at different sites

Maintenance dose: Begin 1 week after loading dose: 2.2 mg/kg/dose once weekly; maximum dose: 160 mg/dose; **Note:** Do not administer more frequently than once weekly.

Adolescents ≥18 years and Adults:

Initial: Loading dose: 320 mg administered as 2 separate injections (160 mg each) on the same day at different sites

Maintenance: Begin 1 week after loading dose: 160 mg once weekly; **Note:** Do not administer more frequently than once weekly.

Preparation for Administration SubQ: Reconstitute vial with 2.3 mL preservative free SWFI; quickly shake the vial back and forth for 1 minute, then allow solution to sit for 1 minute. If the powder is not completely dissolved, shake the vial for an additional 30 seconds, then allow solution to sit for 1 minute; repeat if necessary until powder is completely dissolved; resulting solution is 80 mg/mL. Each reconstituted vial allows for withdrawal of 2 mL (160 mg) for SubQ administration.

Administration SubQ: Administer subcutaneously; rotate injection sites (thigh, abdomen, upper arm); avoid sites that are bruised, red, tender, or hard. If total dose exceeds 2 mL, dose should be divided into 2 injections administered at different sites on the same day. Discard any unused portion.

Monitoring Parameters CBC with differential, C-reactive protein (CRP), serum amyloid A; signs or symptoms of infection; latent TB screening (prior to initiating therapy), lipid profile (2-3 months after initiating therapy and periodically thereafter)

Dosage Forms Excipient information presented when available (limited, particularly for generics); consult specific product labeling.

Solution Reconstituted, Subcutaneous [preservative free]:

Arcalyst: 220 mg (1 ea) [contains polyethylene glycol]

RimabotulinumtoxinB

(rime uh BOT yoo lin num TOKS in bee)

Medication Safety Issues

Other safety concerns:

Botulinum products are not interchangeable; potency differences may exist between the products.

Brand Names: US Myobloc

Therapeutic Category Muscle Contracture, Treatment

Generic Availability (US) No

Use Treatment of cervical dystonia (FDA approved in adults)

Medication Guide Available Yes

Pregnancy Risk Factor C (manufacturer)

Pregnancy Considerations Reproduction studies have not been conducted. Based on limited case reports using onabotulinumtoxinA, adverse fetal effects have not been observed with inadvertent administration during pregnancy. It is currently recommended to ensure adequate contraception in women of childbearing years.

Breast-Feeding Considerations It is not known if rimabotulinumtoxinB is excreted in breast milk. The manufacturer recommends that caution be exercised when administering rimabotulinumtoxinB to nursing women.

Contraindications Hypersensitivity to botulinum toxin or any component of the formulation; infection at the injection site(s)

Warnings/Precautions [U.S. Boxed Warning]: Distant spread of botulinum toxin beyond the site of injection has been reported; dysphagia and breathing difficulties have occurred and may be life threatening; other symptoms reported include blurred vision, diplopia, dysarthria, dysphonia, generalized muscle weakness, ptosis, and urinary incontinence which may develop within hours or weeks following injection. Risk likely greatest in children treated for the unapproved use of spasticity. Systemic effects have occurred following use in approved and unapproved uses, including low doses. Immediate medical attention required if respiratory, speech, or swallowing difficulties appear. Dysphagia may persist anywhere from 2 weeks up to 5 months after administration. In severe cases, patients may require alternative feeding methods. Risk factors include smaller neck muscle mass, bilateral injections into the sternocleidomastoid muscle, or injections into the levator scapulae. Use extreme caution in patients with pre-existing respiratory disease; use may weaken accessory muscles that are necessary for these patients to maintain adequate ventilation. Risk of aspiration resulting from severe dysphagia is increased in patients with decreased respiratory function.

Have appropriate support in case of anaphylactic reaction. Higher doses or more frequent administration may result in neutralizing antibody formation and loss of efficacy. Use caution if there is inflammation, excessive weakness, or atrophy at the proposed injection site(s). Concurrent use of onabotulinumtoxinA (or abobotulinumtoxinA) or use within <4 months of rimabotulinumtoxinB is not recommended. Use with caution in patients taking aminoglycosides or other drugs that interfere with neuromuscular transmission. Use with caution in patients with neuromuscular diseases (eg, myasthenia gravis, Eaton-Lambert syndrome) and neuropathic disorders (eg, amyotrophic lateral sclerosis. Rarely, arrhythmia and myocardial infarction have been reported with use of onabotulinumtoxinA (another botulinum toxin formulation), sometimes in patients with preexisting cardiovascular disease. Long-term effects of chronic therapy unknown. Product contains albumin and may carry a remote risk of virus transmission. Botulinum products (abobotulinumtoxinA, onabotulinumtoxinA, rimabotulinumtoxinB) are not interchangeable; potency units are specific to each preparation and cannot be compared or converted to any other botulinum product.

Warnings: Additional Pediatric Considerations The U.S. Food and Drug Administration (FDA) and Health Canada have issued respective communications to health care professionals alerting them of serious adverse events (including fatalities) in association with the use of onabotulinumtoxinA (Botox, Botox Cosmetic) and rimabotulinumtoxinB (Myobloc). Events reported are suggestive of botulism, indicating systemic spread of the botulinum toxin beyond the site of injection. Reactions were observed in both adult and pediatric patients treated for a variety of conditions with varying doses; however, the most serious outcomes, including respiratory failure and death, were associated with the use in children for cerebral palsy limb spasticity. The FDA has evaluated postmarketing cases and now reports that systemic and potentially fatal toxicity may result from local injection of the botulinum toxins in the treatment of other underlying conditions, such as cerebral palsy associated with limb spasticity. Monitor patients closely for signs/symptoms of systemic toxic effects (possibly occurring 1 day to several weeks after treatment) and instruct patients to seek immediate medical attention with worsening symptoms or dysphagia, dyspnea, muscle weakness, or difficulty speaking.

Adverse Reactions

Cardiovascular: Chest pain, edema, peripheral edema, vasodilation

Central nervous system: Anxiety, chills, confusion, dizziness, fever, headache, hyperesthesia, malaise, migraine, pain, somnolence, tremor, vertigo

Dermatologic: Bruising, pruritus

Endocrine & metabolic: Hypercholesterolemia

Gastrointestinal: Dyspepsia, dysphagia, glossitis, nausea, stomatitis, taste perversion, vomiting, xerostomia

Genitourinary: Cystitis, urinary tract infection, vaginal moniliasis

Hematologic: Serum neutralizing activity

Local: Injection site pain

Neuromuscular & skeletal: Arthralgia, arthritis, back pain, hernia, myasthenia, neck pain, torticollis, weakness

Ocular: Amblyopia, vision abnormal

Otic: Otitis media, tinnitus

Respiratory: Cough, dyspnea, pneumonia, rhinitis

Miscellaneous: Abscess, allergic reaction, antibody formation, cyst, flu-like syndrome, infection, neoplasm, viral infection

Rare but important or life-threatening: Constipation

Drug Interactions

Metabolism/Transport Effects None known.

Avoid Concomitant Use There are no known interactions where it is recommended to avoid concomitant use.

Increased Effect/Toxicity

The levels/effects of RimabotulinumtoxinB may be increased by: AbobotulinumtoxinA; Aminoglycosides; Anticholinergic Agents; Neuromuscular-Blocking Agents; OnabotulinumtoxinA

Decreased Effect There are no known significant interactions involving a decrease in effect.

Storage/Stability Store vials under refrigeration at 2°C to 8°C (36°F to 46°F) for up to 21 months. Protect from light. Once diluted, use within 4 hours. Does not contain preservative. Single use vial. Do not freeze.

Mechanism of Action RimabotulinumtoxinB (previously known as botulinum toxin type B) is a neurotoxin produced by *Clostridium botulinum*, spore-forming anaerobic bacillus. It cleaves synaptic Vesicle Association Membrane Protein (VAMP; synaptobrevin) which is a component of the protein complex responsible for docking and fusion of the synaptic vesicle to the presynaptic membrane. By blocking neurotransmitter release, rimabotulinumtoxinB paralyzes the muscle.

Pharmacodynamics Duration of paralysis: 12-16 weeks

Dosing: Usual IM: Adults: 2500-5000 units divided among affected muscles; patients without a prior history of tolerating botulinum toxin injections should receive a lower initial dose; subsequent doses should be individualized related to the patient's response; doses up to 10,000 units have been used

Preparation for Administration Parenteral: May be diluted with NS. Do not shake.

Administration Parenteral: For IM administration only by individuals understanding the relevant neuromuscular anatomy and any alterations to the anatomy due to prior surgical procedures and standard electromyographic techniques; solution may be diluted prior to administration

Monitoring Parameters Monitor patients closely for signs/symptoms of systemic toxic effects (possibly occurring 1 day to several weeks after treatment)

Toronto Western Spasmodic Torticollis Rating Scale (TWSTRS) which evaluates severity, disability, and pain

Dosage Forms Excipient information presented when available (limited, particularly for generics); consult specific product labeling.

Solution, Intramuscular [preservative free]:

Myobloc: 2500 units/0.5 mL (0.5 mL); 5000 units/mL (1 mL); 10,000 units/2 mL (2 mL) [contains albumin human]

Rimantadine (ri MAN ta deen)

Medication Safety Issues

Sound-alike/look-alike issues:

Rimantadine may be confused with amantadine, ranitidine, Rimactane

Flumadine® may be confused with fludarabine, flunisolide, flutamide

Brand Names: US Flumadine

Brand Names: Canada Flumadine®

Therapeutic Category Antiviral Agent, Oral

Generic Availability (US) Yes

Use Treatment of influenza A viral infection (FDA approved in ages ≥17 years and adults); prophylaxis of influenza A virus (FDA approved in ages ≥1 year and adults); please refer to current ACIP guidelines for recommendations during current flu season)

Pregnancy Risk Factor C

Pregnancy Considerations Animal data suggest embryotoxicity, maternal toxicity, and offspring mortality at doses 7-11 times the recommended human dose. There are no adequate and well-controlled studies in pregnant women.

Influenza infection may be more severe in pregnant women. Untreated influenza infection is associated with an increased risk of adverse events to the fetus and an increased risk of complications or death to the mother. Oseltamivir and zanamivir are currently recommended for the treatment or prophylaxis influenza in pregnant women and women up to 2 weeks postpartum. Appropriate antiviral agents are currently recommended as an adjunct to vaccination and should not be used as a substitute for vaccination in pregnant women (consult current CDC guidelines).

Healthcare providers are encouraged to refer women exposed to influenza vaccine, or who have taken an antiviral medication during pregnancy to the Vaccines and Medications in Pregnancy Surveillance System (VAMPSS) by contacting The Organization of Teratology Information Specialists (OTIS) at (877) 311-8972.

Breast-Feeding Considerations Do not use in nursing mothers due to potential adverse effect in infants. The CDC recommends that women infected with the influenza virus follow general precautions (eg, frequent hand washing) to decrease viral transmission to the child. Mothers with influenza-like illnesses at delivery should consider avoiding close contact with the infant until they have received 48 hours of antiviral medication, fever has resolved, and cough and secretions can be controlled. These measures may help decrease (but not eliminate) the risk of transmitting influenza to the newborn during breast-feeding. During this time, breast milk can be expressed and bottle-fed to the infant by another person who is not infected. Protective measures, such as wearing a face mask, changing into a clean gown or clothing, and strict hand hygiene should be continued by the mother for ≥7 days after the onset of symptoms or until symptom-free for 24 hours. Infant care should be performed by a non-infected person when possible (consult current CDC guidelines).

Contraindications Hypersensitivity to drugs of the adamantine class, including rimantadine and amantadine, or any component of the formulation

Warnings/Precautions Use with caution in patients with renal and hepatic dysfunction; avoid use, if possible, in patients with uncontrolled psychosis or severe psychoneurosis. An increase in seizure incidence may occur in patients with seizure disorders; discontinue drug if seizures occur; resistance may develop during treatment; viruses exhibit cross-resistance between amantadine and rimantadine. Due to increased resistance, the ACIP has recommended that rimantadine and amantadine no longer be used for the treatment or prophylaxis of influenza A in the United States until susceptibility has been re-established; consult current guidelines. Rimantadine is not effective in the prevention or treatment of influenza B virus infections. The elderly are at higher risk for CNS (eg, dizziness, headache, weakness) and gastrointestinal (eg, nausea/vomiting, abdominal pain) adverse events; dosage adjustment is recommended in elderly patients >65 years of age.

Adverse Reactions

Central nervous system: Concentration impaired, dizziness, headache, insomnia

Gastrointestinal: Abdominal pain, anorexia, nausea, vomiting, xerostomia

Neuromuscular & skeletal: Weakness

Rare but important or life-threatening: Agitation, ataxia, bronchospasm, cardiac failure, confusion, convulsions, depression, diarrhea, dyspnea, euphoria, gait abnormality, hallucinations, heart block, hyperkinesias, hypertension, lactation, palpitation, parosmia, pedal edema, rash, syncope, tachycardia, taste alteration, tremor

Drug Interactions

Metabolism/Transport Effects None known.

Avoid Concomitant Use There are no known interactions where it is recommended to avoid concomitant use.

Increased Effect/Toxicity

The levels/effects of Rimantadine may be increased by: MAO Inhibitors

Decreased Effect

Rimantadine may decrease the levels/effects of: Influenza Virus Vaccine (Live/Attenuated)

Food Interactions Food does not affect rate or extent of absorption.

Storage/Stability Store at 25°C (77°F); excursions permitted to 15°C to 30°C (59°F to 86°F).

Mechanism of Action Exerts its inhibitory effect on three antigenic subtypes of influenza A virus (H1N1, H2N2, H3N2) early in the viral replicative cycle, possibly inhibiting the uncoating process; it has no activity against influenza B virus and is two- to eightfold more active than amantadine

Pharmacokinetics (Adult data unless noted)

Absorption: Oral: Well absorbed

Distribution: 17-25 L/kg

Protein binding: ~40%

Metabolism: Extensively in the liver via hydroxylation and glucuronidation

Half-life:

- Children 4-8 years: 13-38 hours
- Adults: 25.4 hours

Time to peak serum concentration: 6 hours

Elimination: <25% excreted unchanged in the urine

Dialysis: Hemodialysis: Negligible effect

Dosing: Usual Oral:

Prophylaxis: Note: Monotherapy is not recommended. In order to control outbreaks in institutions, if influenza A virus subtyping is unavailable and oseltamivir-resistant viruses are circulating, rimantadine may be used in combination with oseltamivir if zanamivir cannot be used. Therapy should continue for ≥2 weeks and until ~10 days after illness onset in the last patient (CDC, 2011; Harper, 2009)

- Children 1-9 years: 5 mg/kg/day in 1-2 divided doses; maximum dose: 150 mg/day
- Children ≥10 years who weigh <40 kg: 5 mg/kg/day in 2 divided doses
- Children ≥10 years who weigh ≥40 kg and Adults: 100 mg twice daily

Treatment: Note: Dosages for treatment and prophylaxis are the same; duration of treatment: 5-7 days; optimal duration not established; discontinue as soon as clinically warranted to reduce the emergence of antiviral drug resistant viruses.

Dosage adjustment in renal impairment: Adults:

- CrCl ≥30 mL/minute: Dose adjustment not required
- CrCl <30 mL/minute: 100 mg/day

Dosage adjustment in hepatic impairment: Adults:

- Severe dysfunction: 100 mg/day

Administration Oral: May administer with food

Additional Information Not active against influenza B; treatment or prophylaxis in immunosuppressed patients has not been fully evaluated; duration of fever and other symptoms can be reduced if rimantadine therapy is started within the first 48 hours of influenza A illness

During an outbreak of influenza, administer rimantadine prophylaxis for 2-3 weeks after influenza vaccination until vaccine antibody titers are sufficient to provide protection

Dosage Forms Excipient information presented when available (limited, particularly for generics); consult specific product labeling.

Tablet, Oral, as hydrochloride:

- Flumadine: 100 mg [contains fd&c yellow #6 (sunset yellow), fd&c yellow #6 aluminum lake]
- Generic: 100 mg

Extemporaneous Preparations Rimantadine 10 mg/mL Suspension:

To prepare suspension, 10 mL of Ora-Sweet® will be required for every 100 mg tablet of rimantadine. (Do not prepare more than a 14-day supply).

- Calculate the total dose needed (daily dose x number of days = mg of rimantadine needed) and round the final mg of rimantadine needed up to the next 100 mg (eg, 750 mg would be 800 mg, or eight 100 mg tablets).
- Calculate the total volume of Ora-Sweet® by taking the rounded mg of rimantadine and dividing by 10 mg/mL (eg, 800 mg divided by 10 mg/mL = 80 mL).
- Grind required number of tablets in mortar and triturate to a fine powder. Slowly add 1/3 of the total volume of Ora-Sweet® to the mortar and triturate until a uniform suspension is achieved.
- Transfer to an amber glass or PET plastic bottle. Slowly add another 1/3 of the total volume of Ora-Sweet® to the mortar, rinsing the mortar, then transferring the contents into the bottle. Repeat using the final 1/3 of Ora-Sweet®. Add additional vehicle to bottle, if needed, to achieve the total calculated volume.
- Shake well to ensure homogeneous suspension. Some inert ingredients in the tablet may be insoluble.
- Label: Shake gently prior to each use.
- Suspension is stable for 14 days when stored at room temperature (25°C/77°F).

◆ **Rimantadine Hydrochloride** *see* Rimantadine *on page 1864*

◆ **Rimso-50** *see* Dimethyl Sulfoxide *on page 667*

◆ **Riomet** *see* MetFORMIN *on page 1375*

◆ **RisaQuad™ [OTC]** *see Lactobacillus on page 1203*

◆ **RisaQuad®-2 [OTC]** *see Lactobacillus on page 1203*

◆ **RisperDAL** *see* RisperiDONE *on page 1866*

◆ **Risperdal (Can)** *see* RisperiDONE *on page 1866*

◆ **Risperdal M-Tab** *see* RisperiDONE *on page 1866*

◆ **RisperDAL M-TAB** *see* RisperiDONE *on page 1866*

◆ **RisperDAL Consta** *see* RisperiDONE *on page 1866*

◆ **Risperdal Consta (Can)** *see* RisperiDONE *on page 1866*

RisperiDONE (ris PER i done)

Medication Safety Issues

Sound-alike/look-alike issues:

RisperiDONE may be confused with reserpine, rOPINIRole

RisperDAL may be confused with lisinopril, reserpine, Restoril

BEERS Criteria medication:

This drug may be potentially inappropriate for use in geriatric patients (Quality of evidence - moderate; Strength of recommendation - strong).

Related Information

Oral Medications That Should Not Be Crushed or Altered *on page 2476*

Safe Handling of Hazardous Drugs *on page 2455*

Brand Names: US RisperDAL; RisperDAL Consta; RisperDAL M-TAB; RisperiDONE M-TAB

Brand Names: Canada ACT Risperidone; Apo-Risperidone; Ava-Risperidone; Dom-Risperidone; JAMP-Risperidone; Mar-Risperidone; Mint-Risperidone; Mylan-Risperidone; Mylan-Risperidone ODT; PHL-Risperidone; PMS-Risperidone; PMS-Risperidone ODT; PRO-Risperidone; RAN-Risperidone; ratio-Risperidone; Risperdal; Risperdal Consta; Risperdal M-Tab; Riva-Risperidone; Sandoz-Risperidone; Teva-Risperidone

Therapeutic Category Antipsychotic Agent, Benzisoxazole; Second Generation (Atypical) Antipsychotic

Generic Availability (US) May be product dependent

Use

Oral: Management of schizophrenia (FDA approved in ages ≥13 years and adults); treatment of acute mania or mixed episodes associated with bipolar I disorder (FDA approved as monotherapy in ages ≥10 years and adults; FDA approved in combination with lithium or valproate in adults); treatment of irritability (including aggression, temper tantrums, self-injurious behavior, and quickly changing moods) associated with autistic disorder in children and adolescents (FDA approved in ages 5-16 years); has also been used for treatment of Tourette syndrome (tics), disruptive behavior disorders, and delirium and irritability in the management of pervasive development disorders.

IM: Management of schizophrenia (FDA approved in adults); maintenance treatment of bipolar I disorder as monotherapy or in combination with lithium or valproate (FDA approved in adults)

Pregnancy Risk Factor C

Pregnancy Considerations Adverse events were observed in animal reproduction studies. In human studies, risperidone and its metabolite cross the placenta (Newport, 2007). An increased risk of teratogenic effects has not been observed following maternal use of risperidone (limited data) (Coppola, 2007). Agenesis of the corpus callosum has been noted in one case report of an infant exposed *in utero*; relationship to risperidone exposure is not known. Antipsychotic use during the third trimester of pregnancy has a risk for extrapyramidal symptoms (EPS) and/or withdrawal symptoms in newborns following delivery. Symptoms in the newborn may include agitation, feeding disorder, hypertonia, hypotonia, respiratory distress, somnolence, and tremor. These effects may be self-limiting and allow recovery within hours or days with no specific treatment, or they may be severe requiring prolonged hospitalization. When using Risperdal® Consta®, patients should notify healthcare provider if they become or intend to become pregnant during therapy or within 12 weeks of last injection. Risperidone may cause hyperprolactinemia, which may decrease reproductive function in both males and females.

The ACOG recommends that therapy during pregnancy be individualized; treatment with psychiatric medications during pregnancy should incorporate the clinical expertise of the mental health clinician, obstetrician, primary healthcare provider, and pediatrician. Safety data related to atypical antipsychotics during pregnancy is limited and routine use is not recommended. However, if a woman is inadvertently exposed to an atypical antipsychotic while pregnant, continuing therapy may be preferable to switching to a typical antipsychotic that the fetus has not yet been exposed to; consider risk:benefit (ACOG, 2008).

Healthcare providers are encouraged to enroll women 18 to 45 years of age exposed to risperidone during pregnancy in the Atypical Antipsychotics Pregnancy Registry (1-866-961-2388 or http://www.womensmentalhealth.org/pregnancyregistry).

Breast-Feeding Considerations Risperidone and its metabolite are excreted in breast milk. Due to the potential for serious adverse reactions in the nursing infant, the manufacturer recommends a decision be made whether to discontinue nursing or to discontinue the drug, taking into account the importance of treatment to the mother. It is also recommended that women using Risperdal Consta not breast-feed during therapy or for 12 weeks after the last injection.

Contraindications Hypersensitivity to risperidone or any component of the formulation

Warnings/Precautions Hazardous agent - use appropriate precautions for handling and disposal (NIOSH 2014 [group 2]).

[US Boxed Warning]: Elderly patients with dementia-related psychosis treated with antipsychotics are at an increased risk of death compared to placebo. Most deaths appeared to be either cardiovascular (eg, heart failure, sudden death) or infectious (eg, pneumonia) in nature. In addition, an increased incidence of cerebrovascular effects (eg, transient ischemic attack, cerebrovascular accidents) has been reported in studies of placebo-controlled trials of risperidone in elderly patients with dementia-related psychosis. Use with caution in dementia with Lewy bodies; antipsychotics may worsen dementia symptoms and patients with dementia with Lewy bodies are more sensitive to the extrapyramidal side effects (APA [Rabins, 2007]). Risperidone is not approved for the treatment of dementia-related psychosis. The Canadian labeling indicates risperidone (oral) for short-term use in severe Alzheimer dementia to manage aggression and psychotic symptoms. Careful assessment of risk factors for stroke or existing cardiovascular morbidities is required prior to initiation.

Leukopenia, neutropenia, and agranulocytosis (sometimes fatal) have been reported in clinical trials and postmarketing reports with antipsychotic use; presence of risk factors (eg, pre-existing low WBC or history of drug-induced leuko-/neutropenia) should prompt periodic blood count assessment. Discontinue therapy at first signs of blood dyscrasias or if absolute neutrophil count <1,000/mm^3.

Low to moderately sedating, use with caution in disorders where CNS depression is a feature. Use with caution in Parkinson disease; antipsychotics may aggravate the motor disturbances of Parkinson disease (APA [Rabins, 2007]). Caution in patients with predisposition to seizures. Use with caution in renal or hepatic dysfunction; dose reduction recommended. Esophageal dysmotility and aspiration have been associated with antipsychotic use; use with caution in patients at risk of aspiration pneumonia (ie, Alzheimer's disease). Risperidone is associated with greater increases in prolactin levels as compared to other antipsychotic agents; clinical significance of hyperprolactinemia in patients with breast cancer or other prolactin-dependent tumors is unknown. May alter temperature regulation. May mask toxicity of other drugs or conditions (eg, intestinal obstruction, Reyes syndrome, brain tumor) due to antiemetic effects. Neutropenia has been reported with antipsychotic use, including fatal cases of agranulocytosis. Pre-existing myelosuppression (disease or drug-induced) increases risk and these patients should have frequent CBC monitoring; decreased blood counts in absence of other causative factors should prompt discontinuation of therapy.

Use with caution in patients with cardiovascular diseases (eg, heart failure, history of myocardial infarction or ischemia, cerebrovascular disease, conduction abnormalities). May cause orthostatic hypotension; use with caution in patients at risk of this effect (eg, concurrent medication use which may predispose to hypotension/bradycardia or presence of hypovolemia) or in those who would not tolerate transient hypotensive episodes. May alter cardiac conduction (low risk relative to other neuroleptics); life-threatening arrhythmias have occurred with therapeutic doses of neuroleptics.

May cause anticholinergic effects (confusion, agitation, constipation, xerostomia, blurred vision, urinary retention); therefore, they should be used with caution in patients with decreased gastrointestinal motility, urinary retention, BPH, xerostomia, or visual problems (including narrow-angle glaucoma). Relative to other neuroleptics, risperidone has a low potency of cholinergic blockade. Few case reports describe intraoperative floppy iris syndrome (IFIS) in patients receiving risperidone and undergoing cataract surgery (Ford, 2011). Prior to cataract surgery, evaluate for prior or current risperidone use. The benefits or risks of interrupting risperidone prior to surgery have not been established; clinicians are advised to proceed with surgery cautiously.

May cause extrapyramidal symptoms, including pseudoparkinsonism, acute dystonic reactions, akathisia, and tardive dyskinesia. Risk of dystonia (and possibly other EPS) may be greater with increased doses, use of conventional antipsychotics, males, and younger patients. Risk of tardive dyskinesia and potential for irreversibility may be increased in elderly patients (particularly women), prolonged therapy, and higher total cumulative dose. Risk of neuroleptic malignant syndrome (NMS) may be increased in patients with Parkinson's disease or Lewy body dementia; monitor for symptoms of confusion, obtundation, postural instability and extrapyramidal symptoms. May cause hyperglycemia; in some cases may be extreme and associated with ketoacidosis, hyperosmolar coma, or death. Use with caution in patients with diabetes or other disorders of glucose regulation; monitor for worsening of glucose control. Dyslipidemia has been reported with atypical antipsychotics; risk profile may differ between agents. Discrepant results have been reported in clinical trials, regarding lipid changes associated with risperidone (American Diabetes Association, 2004). Significant weight gain has been observed with antipsychotic therapy; incidence varies with product. Monitor waist circumference and BMI. Rare cases of priapism have been reported.

Use in elderly patients with dementia is associated with an increased risk of mortality and cerebrovascular accidents; avoid antipsychotic use for behavioral problems associated with dementia unless alternative nonpharmacologic therapies have failed and patient may harm self or others. In addition, use may cause or exacerbate syndrome of inappropriate antidiuretic hormone secretion or hyponatremia; monitor sodium closely with initiation or dosage adjustments in older adults (Beers Criteria).

The possibility of a suicide attempt is inherent in psychotic illness or bipolar disorder; use caution in high-risk patients during initiation of therapy. Prescriptions should be written for the smallest quantity consistent with good patient care. Long-term effects on growth or sexual maturation have not been evaluated. Vehicle used in injectable (polylactide-co-glycolide microspheres) has rarely been associated with retinal artery occlusion in patients with abnormal arterio-venous anastomosis.

Potentially significant drug-drug interactions may exist, requiring dose or frequency adjustment, additional monitoring, and/or selection of alternative therapy. Benzyl alcohol and derivatives: Some dosage forms may contain sodium benzoate/benzoic acid; benzoic acid (benzoate) is a metabolite of benzyl alcohol; large amounts of benzyl alcohol (≥99 mg/kg/day) have been associated with a potentially fatal toxicity ("gasping syndrome") in neonates; the "gasping syndrome" consists of metabolic acidosis, respiratory distress, gasping respirations, CNS dysfunction (including convulsions, intracranial hemorrhage), hypotension, and cardiovascular collapse (AAP, 1997; CDC, 1982); some data suggests that benzoate displaces bilirubin from protein binding sites (Ahlfors, 2001); avoid or use dosage forms containing benzyl alcohol derivative with caution in neonates. See manufacturer's labeling.

Warnings: Additional Pediatric Considerations Use with caution in children and adolescents; adverse effects due to elevated prolactin levels have been observed; long-term effects on growth or sexual maturation have not been evaluated.

Risperidone may cause a higher than normal weight gain in children and adolescents; monitor growth (including weight, height, BMI, and waist circumference) in pediatric patients receiving risperidone; compare weight gain to standard growth curves. Risperidone may cause increases in metabolic indices (eg, serum cholesterol, triglycerides). **Note:** A prospective, nonrandomized cohort study followed 338 antipsychotic naive pediatric patients (age 4 to 19 years) for a median 10.8 weeks (range 10.5 to 11.2 weeks) and reported the following significant mean increases in weight in kg (and % change from baseline): Olanzapine: 8.5 kg (15.2%), quetiapine: 6.1 kg (10.4%), risperidone: 5.3 kg (10.4%), and aripiprazole: 4.4 kg (8.1%) compared to the control cohort: 0.2 kg (0.65%). Increases in metabolic indices (eg, serum cholesterol, triglycerides, glucose) were also reported; a significant increase in serum triglycerides of 9.7 mg/mL was observed for patients receiving risperidone. Biannual monitoring of cardiometabolic indices after the first 3 months of therapy is suggested (Correll, 2009).

Children may experience a higher frequency of certain adverse effects than adults, particularly fatigue (18% to 42% vs ≤3%), somnolence (12% to 67% vs ≤14%), fever (20% vs 2%), constipation (21% vs 9%), increased salivation (22% vs 3%), abdominal pain (18% vs 4%), and dry mouth (13% vs 4%).

Adverse Reactions

Cardiovascular: Bradycardia, bundle branch block, buttock pain, chest pain, ECG changes, facial edema, first degree atrioventricular block, hypertension, hypotension, orthostatic hypotension, palpitations, paresthesia, peripheral edema, prolonged Q-T interval on ECG, syncope, tachycardia (more common in adults)

Central nervous system: Abnormal gait, agitation, akathisia, anxiety, ataxia, decreased attention span, depression, disturbed sleep, dizziness, drooling (more common in children), drowsiness (more common in adults), dystonia, falling, fatigue (more common in children), headache, hypoesthesia, insomnia, lethargy, malaise, nervousness, orthostatic dizziness, pain, parkinsonian-like syndrome (more common in children), sedation (more common in children), seizure, tardive dyskinesia, vertigo

Dermatologic: Acne vulgaris, eczema, pruritus, skin sclerosis, skin rash, xeroderma

Endocrine & metabolic: Amenorrhea, decreased libido, galactorrhea, gynecomastia, hyperglycemia, hyperprolactinemia, increased gamma-glutamyl transferase, increased thirst (more common in children), oligomenorrhea, weight gain (more common in children), weight loss

Gastrointestinal: Abdominal pain (more common in children), anorexia, constipation, decreased appetite, diarrhea, dyspepsia, gastritis, gastroenteritis, increased appetite (more common in children), nausea, sialorrhea, toothache, vomiting (more common in children), xerostomia

Genitourinary: Cystitis, ejaculatory disorder, erectile dysfunction, glycosuria, irregular menses, mastalgia, menstruation, sexual disorder, urinary incontinence (more common in children), urinary tract infection

Hematologic & oncologic: Anemia, neutropenia

Hepatic: Increased serum ALT, increased serum AST

Hypersensitivity: Hypersensitivity

Infection: Infection, influenza, localized infection, subcutaneous abscess, viral infection

Local: Induration at injection site, injection site reaction, pain at injection site, swelling at injection site

Neuromuscular & skeletal: Abnormal posture, akinesia, arthralgia, back pain, dyskinesia (more common in adults), hypokinesia, increased creatine phosphokinase, limb pain, musculoskeletal chest pain, myalgia, neck pain, tremor (more common in adults), weakness

Ophthalmic: Blurred vision, conjunctivitis, reduced visual acuity

Otic: Otalgia, otic infection

Respiratory: bronchitis, cough (more common in children), dyspnea, epistaxis, flu-like symptoms, nasal congestion, nasopharyngitis (more common in children), pharyngitis, pharyngolaryngeal pain, pneumonia, respiratory tract infection, rhinitis, rhinorrhea (more common in children), sinus congestion, sinusitis

Miscellaneous: Fever (more common in children)

Rare but important or life-threatening: Abnormal erythrocytes, abscess at injection site, acariasis, agranulocytosis, alopecia, anaphylaxis, angioedema, apnea, aspiration, atrial fibrillation, atrial premature contractions, cardiorespiratory arrest, cerebral ischemia, cerebrovascular accident, cholestatic hepatitis, cholinergic syndrome, coma, cyst, delirium, depression of ST segment on ECG, dermal ulcer, diabetes mellitus, diabetic coma, diabetic ketoacidosis, disruption of body temperature regulation, diverticulitis, esophageal motility disorder, eye infection, fecal incontinence, fecaloma, glaucoma, granulocytopenia, hematoma, hemorrhage, hepatic failure, hepatic injury, hyperkeratosis, hyperthermia, hypertonia, hypertriglyceridemia, hyperuricemia, hypoglycemia, hypokalemia, hyponatremia, hypothermia, impaired consciousness, increased serum cholesterol, intestinal obstruction, intraoperative floppy iris syndrome, leukocytosis, leukopenia, leukorrhea, lower respiratory tract infection, lymphadenopathy, mania, migraine, myocardial infarction, myocarditis, neuroleptic malignant syndrome, nystagmus, ocular hyperemia, pancreatitis, Pelger-Huët anomaly, phlebitis, pituitary neoplasm, precocious puberty, priapism, pulmonary embolism, renal insufficiency, retinal artery occlusion, retrograde ejaculation, rhabdomyolysis, SIADH, sleep apnea, swelling of eye, synostosis, thrombocytopenia, thrombophlebitis, thrombotic thrombocytopenic purpura, tissue necrosis, tongue paralysis, torticollis, transient ischemic attacks, unresponsive to stimuli, urinary retention, ventricular premature contractions, ventricular tachycardia, water intoxication, withdrawal syndrome

Drug Interactions

Metabolism/Transport Effects Substrate of CYP2D6 (major), CYP3A4 (minor), P-glycoprotein; **Note:** Assignment of Major/Minor substrate status based on clinically relevant drug interaction potential; **Inhibits** CYP2D6 (weak)

Avoid Concomitant Use

Avoid concomitant use of RisperiDONE with any of the following: Aclidinium; Amisulpride; Azelastine (Nasal); Eluxadoline; Glucagon; Ipratropium (Oral Inhalation); Metoclopramide; Orphenadrine; Paraldehyde; Potassium Chloride; Sulpiride; Thalidomide; Tiotropium; Umeclidinium

Increased Effect/Toxicity

RisperiDONE may increase the levels/effects of: AbobotulinumtoxinA; Alcohol (Ethyl); Amisulpride; Analgesics (Opioid); Anticholinergic Agents; ARIPiprazole; Azelastine (Nasal); Buprenorphine; CNS Depressants; Eluxadoline; Glucagon; Highest Risk QTc-Prolonging Agents; Hydrocodone; Mequitazine; Methotrimeprazine; Methylphenidate; Metyrosine; Mirabegron; Mirtazapine; Moderate Risk QTc-Prolonging Agents; OnabotulinumtoxinA; Orphenadrine; Paliperidone; Paraldehyde; Potassium Chloride; RimabotulinumtoxinB; Selective Serotonin Reuptake Inhibitors; Serotonin Modulators; Sulpiride; Suvorexant; Thalidomide; Tiotropium; Topiramate; Zolpidem

The levels/effects of RisperiDONE may be increased by: Abiraterone Acetate; Acetylcholinesterase Inhibitors (Central); Aclidinium; Brimonidine (Topical); Cannabis; Cobicistat; CYP2D6 Inhibitors (Moderate); CYP2D6 Inhibitors (Strong); Darunavir; Doxylamine; Dronabinol; Droperidol; HydrOXYzine; Hypotensive Agents; Ipratropium (Oral Inhalation); Kava Kava; Lithium; Loop Diuretics; Magnesium Sulfate; Methotrimeprazine; Methylphenidate; Metoclopramide; Metyrosine;

Mianserin; Mifepristone; Nabilone; Panobinostat; Peginterferon Alfa-2b; Perampanel; P-glycoprotein/ABCB1 Inhibitors; Pramlintide; Rufinamide; Selective Serotonin Reuptake Inhibitors; Serotonin Modulators; Sodium Oxybate; Tapentadol; Tetrahydrocannabinol; Umeclidinium; Valproic Acid and Derivatives; Verapamil

Decreased Effect

RisperiDONE may decrease the levels/effects of: Acetylcholinesterase Inhibitors; Amphetamines; Antidiabetic Agents; Anti-Parkinson's Agents (Dopamine Agonist); Itopride; Quinagolide; Secretin

The levels/effects of RisperiDONE may be decreased by: Acetylcholinesterase Inhibitors; CarBAMazepine; Lithium; Peginterferon Alfa-2b; P-glycoprotein/ABCB1 Inducers

Food Interactions Oral solution is not compatible with beverages containing tannin or pectinate (cola or tea). Management: Administer oral solution with water, coffee, orange juice, or low-fat milk.

Storage/Stability

Injection: Risperdal® Consta®: Store in refrigerator at 2°C to 8°C (36°F to 46°F) and protect from light. May be stored at room temperature of 25°C (77°F) for up to 7 days prior to administration. Following reconstitution, store at room temperature and use within 6 hours. Suspension settles in ~2 minutes; shake vigorously to resuspend prior to administration.

Oral solution, tablet: Store at 15°C to 25°C (59°F to 77°F). Protect from light and moisture. Keep orally-disintegrating tablets sealed in foil pouch until ready to use. Do not freeze solution.

Mechanism of Action Risperidone is a benzisoxazole atypical antipsychotic with mixed serotonin-dopamine antagonist activity that binds to 5-HT_2-receptors in the CNS and in the periphery with a very high affinity; binds to dopamine-D_2 receptors with less affinity. The binding affinity to the dopamine-D_2 receptor is 20 times lower than the 5-HT_2 affinity. The addition of serotonin antagonism to dopamine antagonism (classic neuroleptic mechanism) is thought to improve negative symptoms of psychoses and reduce the incidence of extrapyramidal side effects. $Alpha_1$, $alpha_2$ adrenergic, and histaminergic receptors are also antagonized with high affinity. Risperidone has low to moderate affinity for 5-HT_{1C}, 5-HT_{1D}, and 5-HT_{1A} receptors, weak affinity for D_1 and no affinity for muscarinics or $beta_1$ and $beta_2$ receptors

Pharmacokinetics (Adult data unless noted) Note: Following oral administration, the pharmacokinetics of risperidone and 9-hydroxyrisperidone in children were found to be similar to values in adults (after adjusting for differences in body weight).

Absorption:

Oral: Well absorbed

IM: Initial: <1% of dose released from microspheres; main release starts at ≥3 weeks; release is maintained from 4-6 weeks; release ends by 7 weeks

Distribution: Distributes into breast milk; breast milk to plasma ratio (n=1): Risperidone: 0.42; 9-hydroxyrisperidone: 0.24 (Hill, 2000)

V_d: Risperidone: 1-2 L/kg

Protein binding: Risperidone: 90%, plasma protein binding increases with increasing concentrations of $alpha_1$-acid glycoprotein; 9-hydroxyrisperidone: 77%; **Note:** Risperidone free fraction may be increased by ~35% in patients with hepatic impairment due to decreased concentrations of albumin and $alpha_1$-acid glycoprotein

Metabolism: Extensive in the liver via cytochrome P450 CYP2D6 to 9-hydroxyrisperidone (major active metabolite); also undergoes N-dealkylation (minor pathway); **Note:** 9-hydroxyrisperidone is the predominant circulating form and is approximately equal to risperidone in receptor binding activity; clinical effects are from combined concentrations of risperidone and 9-hydroxyrisperidone; clinically important differences between CYP2D6 poor and extensive metabolizers are not expected (pharmacokinetics of the sum of risperidone and 9-hydroxyrisperidone were similar in poor and extensive metabolizers)

Bioavailability:

Oral: 70%; tablet (relative to solution): 94%; **Note:** Orally-disintegrating tablets and oral solution are bioequivalent to tablets.

IM: Deltoid IM injection is bioequivalent to gluteal IM injection

Half-life (apparent):

Oral:

Risperidone: Extensive metabolizers: 3 hours; poor metabolizers: 20 hours

9-hydroxyrisperidone: Extensive metabolizers: 21 hours; poor metabolizers: 30 hours

Sum of risperidone and 9-hydroxyrisperidone: Overall mean: 20 hours

IM: 3-6 days (due to extended release of drug from microspheres and subsequent absorption)

Time to peak serum concentration: Oral: Solution or tablet:

Risperidone: 1 hour

9-hydroxyrisperidone: Extensive metabolizers: 3 hours; poor metabolizers: 17 hours

Elimination: Excreted as risperidone and metabolites in urine (70%) and feces (14%)

Clearance: Moderate to severe renal impairment (sum of risperidone and 9-hydroxyrisperidone): Decreased by 60%

Dosing: Usual

Pediatric:

Autism, associated irritability, including aggression, temper, tantrums, self-injurious behavior, and quickly changing moods:

Children ≥5 years and Adolescents: **Note:** Individualize dose according to patient response and tolerability:

15 to 20 kg: Oral: Initial: 0.25 mg/day; after ≥4 days, may increase dose to 0.5 mg/day; maintain this dose for ≥14 days. In patients not achieving sufficient clinical response, may increase dose in increments of 0.25 mg/day at ≥2-week intervals. Doses ranging from 0.5 to 3 mg/day have been evaluated; however, therapeutic effect reached plateau at 1 mg/day in clinical trials. Following clinical response, consider gradually decreasing dose to lowest effective dose. May be administered once daily or in divided doses twice daily.

≥20 kg: Oral: Initial: 0.5 mg/day; after ≥4 days, may increase dose to 1 mg/day; maintain this dose for ≥14 days. In patients not achieving sufficient clinical response, may increase dose in increments of 0.5 mg/day at ≥2-week intervals. Doses ranging from 0.5-3 mg/day have been evaluated; however, therapeutic effect reached plateau at 2.5 mg/day (3 mg/day in pediatric patients >45 kg) in clinical trials. Following clinical response, consider gradually decreasing to lowest effective dose. May be administered once daily or in divided doses twice daily.

Bipolar mania: Children and Adolescents 10 to 17 years: Oral: Initial: 0.5 mg once daily; dose may be adjusted if needed, in increments of 0.5 to 1 mg/day at intervals ≥24 hours, as tolerated, to a dose of 2.5 mg/day. Doses ranging from 0.5 to 6 mg/day have been evaluated; however, doses >2.5 mg/day do not confer additional benefit and are associated with increased adverse events; doses >6 mg/day have not been studied. **Note:** May administer 1/2 the daily dose twice daily in patients who experience persistent somnolence.

Delirium: Limited data available:

Children <5 years: Oral: Initial: 0.1 to 0.2 mg once daily at bedtime; dosing based on retrospective review of 10 pediatric patients (ages: 4 months to 16 years) which included three patients <5 years of age (Schieveld 2007)

Children ≥5 years and Adolescents: Oral: Initial: 0.2 to 0.5 mg once daily at bedtime; may titrate to lowest effective dose every 1 to 2 days; usual range: 0.2 to 2.5 mg/day in divided doses 2 to 4 times daily; maximum daily dose dependent upon patient weight: <20 kg: 1 mg/day; 20 to 45 kg: 2.5 mg/day, >45 kg: 3 mg/day (Karnik 2007; Schieveld 2007; Silver 2010)

Disruptive behavior disorders (eg, conduct disorder, oppositional defiant disorder): Limited data available: Children ≥4 years and Adolescents: Oral: Initial: 0.01 mg/kg/dose once daily for 2 days, then 0.02 mg/kg/dose once daily, may further increase on weekly basis as tolerated to 0.06 mg/kg/dose once daily; usual maximum daily dose: 2 mg/**day**; improvement in target symptoms typically within 1 to 4 weeks (Aman 2002; Findling 2004; Kutcher 2004; Pandina 2006). **Note:** May administer 1/2 the daily dose twice daily if breakthrough symptoms occur in the afternoon or evening.

Pervasive developmental disorders (PDD) (eg, disruptive behavior, aggression, irritability): Limited data available: Children ≥5 years and Adolescents: Oral: Initial: 0.01 mg/kg/dose once daily for 2 days, then 0.02 mg/kg/dose once daily; may further increase on weekly basis by ≤0.02 mg/kg/day increments as tolerated to 0.06 mg/kg/dose once daily; reported mean dose: 0.05 mg/kg/day (1.48 mg/day); other trials have reported similar optimal doses: 0.75 to 1.8 mg/day; improvement in target symptoms typically within 2 to 4 weeks (Fisman 1996; McDougle 1997; Shea 2004). **Note:** May administer 1/2 the daily dose twice daily if breakthrough symptoms occur in the afternoon or evening.

Schizophrenia: Adolescents 13 to 17 years: Oral: Initial: 0.5 mg once daily; dose may be adjusted if needed, in increments of 0.5 to 1 mg/day at intervals ≥24 hours, as tolerated, to a dose of 3 mg/day. Doses ranging from 1 to 6 mg/day have been evaluated; however, doses >3 mg/day do not confer additional benefit and are associated with increased adverse events. **Note:** May administer 1/2 the daily dose twice daily in patients who experience persistent somnolence.

Tourette syndrome, tics: Limited data available: Children ≥7 years and Adolescents: Oral: Initial: 0.25 to 0.5 mg once daily at night; may gradually titrate every 4 to 5 days in 0.25 to 0.5 mg increments to usual reported therapeutic range: 0.25 to 6 mg/day divided in twice daily doses (Dion 2002; Roessner 2011; Scahill 2003; Singer 2010)

Adult: **Note:** When reinitiating treatment after discontinuation, the initial titration schedule should be followed.

Bipolar mania: Oral: Initial: 2 to 3 mg/dose once daily; adjust dose as needed, by 1 mg/day increments at intervals ≥24 hours; dosing range: 1 to 6 mg/day; no dosing recommendation available for treatment >3 weeks duration

Bipolar I, maintenance: IM (RisperDAL Consta): 25 mg every 2 weeks; if unresponsive, some may benefit from larger doses (37.5 to 50 mg); maximum dose: 50 mg every 2 weeks. Dosage adjustments should not be made more frequently than every 4 weeks. A lower initial dose of 12.5 mg may be appropriate in some patients (eg, demonstrated poor tolerability to other psychotropic medications).

Note: Oral risperidone (or other antipsychotic) should be administered with the initial injection of RisperDAL Consta and continued for 3 weeks (then discontinued) to maintain adequate therapeutic plasma concentrations prior to main release phase of risperidone from injection site. When switching from depot administration to a short-acting formulation, administer short-acting agent in place of the next regularly scheduled depot injection.

Schizophrenia:

Oral: Initial: 2 mg/day in 1 to 2 divided doses; may be increased by 1 to 2 mg/day at intervals ≥24 hours to a recommended dosage range of 4 to 8 mg/day; may be given as a single daily dose once maintenance dose is achieved; daily dosages >6 mg do not appear to confer any additional benefit and the incidence of extrapyramidal symptoms is higher than with lower doses. Further dose adjustments should be made in increments/decrements of 1 to 2 mg/day on a weekly basis. Dose range studied in clinical trials: 4 to 16 mg/day. Maintenance: Recommended dosage range: 2 to 8 mg/day

IM: (RisperDAL Consta): Initial: 25 mg every 2 weeks; if unresponsive, some may benefit from larger doses (37.5 to 50 mg); maximum dose: 50 mg every 2 weeks. Dosage adjustments should not be made more frequently than every 4 weeks. A lower initial dose of 12.5 mg may be appropriate in some patients (eg, demonstrated poor tolerability to psychotropic medications).

Note: Oral risperidone (or other antipsychotic) should be administered with the initial injection of RisperDAL Consta and continued for 3 weeks (then discontinued) to maintain adequate therapeutic plasma concentrations prior to main release phase of risperidone from injection site. When switching from depot administration to a short-acting formulation, administer short-acting agent in place of the next regularly scheduled depot injection.

Dosing adjustment in renal impairment:

Children and Adolescents: There are no dosage adjustments provided in manufacturer's labeling.

Adults:

Oral: CrCl <30 mL/minute: Initial: 0.5 mg twice daily; increase (as tolerated) in increments of ≤0.5 mg twice daily; increases to dosages >1.5 mg twice daily should be made at intervals of ≥1 week; slower titration may be required in some patients. Clearance of the active moiety (sum of parent drug and active metabolite) is decreased by 60% in patients with moderate to severe renal disease (CrCl <60 mL/minute) compared to healthy subjects.

IM: Initiate with **oral** dosing (0.5 mg twice daily for 1 week, then 2 mg/day for 1 week); if tolerated, begin 25 mg **IM** every 2 weeks; continue oral dosing for 3 weeks after the first IM injection. An initial IM dose of 12.5 mg may also be considered.

Dosing adjustment in hepatic impairment:

Children and Adolescents: There are no dosage adjustments provided in manufacturer's labeling.

Adults:

Oral: Child-Pugh Class C: Initial: 0.5 mg twice daily; increase (as tolerated) in increments of ≤0.5 mg twice daily; increases to dosages >1.5 mg twice daily should be made at intervals of ≥1 week; slower titration may be required in some patients. The mean free fraction of risperidone in plasma was increased by 35% in patients with hepatic impairment compared to healthy subjects.

IM: Initiate with **oral** dosing (0.5 mg twice daily for 1 week, then 2 mg/day for 1 week); if tolerated, begin 25 mg **IM** every 2 weeks; continue oral dosing for 3 weeks after the first IM injection. An initial IM dose of 12.5 mg may also be considered.

Preparation for Administration Hazardous agent; use appropriate precautions for handling and disposal (NIOSH 2014 [group 2]).

IM: Risperdal Consta: Bring to room temperature prior to reconstitution. Reconstitute with provided diluent only. Shake vigorously to mix; will form thick, milky suspension. Following reconstitution, store at room temperature and use within 6 hours. Suspension settles in ~2 minutes; shake vigorously to resuspend prior to administration.

Administration Hazardous agent; use appropriate precautions for handling and disposal (NIOSH 2014 [group 2]).

Oral: May be administered without regard to meals.

Oral solution: May administer directly from the manufacturer provided calibrated pipette or may mix with water, coffee, orange juice, or low-fat milk; do not mix with cola or tea; **Note:** Manufacturer provided calibrated pipette is calibrated in milligrams and milliliters; minimum calibrated volume: 0.25 mL; maximum calibrated volume: 3 mL

Orally-disintegrating tablets: Do not remove tablet from blister pack until ready to administer; do not push tablet through foil (tablet may become damaged); peel back foil to expose tablet; use dry hands to remove tablet and place immediately on tongue; tablet will dissolve within seconds and may be swallowed with or without liquid; do not split or chew tablet

IM: After reconstitution, shake vial vigorously for a minimum of 10 seconds to properly mix; suspension should appear thick, milky, and uniform; use immediately (or within 6 hours of reconstitution); if suspension settles prior to use, shake vigorously to resuspend. Administer deep IM into either the deltoid muscle or the upper-outer quadrant of the gluteal area; avoid inadvertent injection into blood vessel; **do not administer IV;** alternate injection site between the two arms or buttocks; do not combine two different dosage strengths into one single administration; administer with needle provided (1-inch needle for deltoid administration or 2-inch needle for gluteal administration); do not substitute any components of the dose pack.

Monitoring Parameters Blood pressure (including orthostatic) and heart rate, particularly during dosage titration; mental status, abnormal involuntary movement scale (AIMS), and extrapyramidal symptoms; growth, BMI, waist circumference, and weight (in adults, weight should be assessed prior to treatment and at 4 weeks, 8 weeks, 12 weeks, and then at quarterly intervals; consider titrating to a different antipsychotic agent for a weight gain ≥5% of the initial weight); CBC with differential; liver enzymes in children (especially obese children or those who are rapidly gaining weight while receiving therapy); lipid profile; fasting blood glucose/Hgb A_{1c} (prior to treatment, at 3 months, then annually); prolactin serum concentrations

Additional Information Long-term usefulness of risperidone should be periodically re-evaluated in patients receiving the drug for extended periods of time. Risperdal® Consta® is a long-acting injection comprised of an extended release microsphere formulation; prior to injection, the microspheres are suspended in the provided diluent; the small polymeric microspheres degrade slowly, releasing the medication at a controlled rate.

Dosage Forms Excipient information presented when available (limited, particularly for generics); consult specific product labeling.

Solution, Oral:
- RisperDAL: 1 mg/mL (30 mL) [contains benzoic acid]
- Generic: 1 mg/mL (30 mL)

Suspension Reconstituted, Intramuscular:
- RisperDAL Consta: 12.5 mg (1 ea); 25 mg (1 ea); 37.5 mg (1 ea); 50 mg (1 ea)

Tablet, Oral:
- RisperDAL: 0.25 mg, 0.5 mg, 1 mg
- RisperDAL: 2 mg [contains fd&c yellow #6 aluminum lake]
- RisperDAL: 3 mg [contains fd&c yellow #10 (quinoline yellow)]
- RisperDAL: 4 mg [contains fd&c blue #2 aluminum lake, fd&c yellow #10 (quinoline yellow)]
- Generic: 0.25 mg, 0.5 mg, 1 mg, 2 mg, 3 mg, 4 mg

Tablet Dispersible, Oral:
- RisperDAL M-TAB: 0.5 mg, 1 mg, 2 mg, 3 mg, 4 mg [contains aspartame, peppermint oil (mentha piperita oil)]
- RisperiDONE M-TAB: 0.5 mg, 1 mg, 2 mg, 3 mg, 4 mg [contains aspartame]
- Generic: 0.25 mg, 0.5 mg, 1 mg, 2 mg, 3 mg, 4 mg

◆ **RisperiDONE M-TAB** *see* RisperiDONE *on page 1866*

◆ **Ritalin** *see* Methylphenidate *on page 1402*

◆ **Ritalin LA** *see* Methylphenidate *on page 1402*

◆ **Ritalin SR [DSC]** *see* Methylphenidate *on page 1402*

◆ **Ritalin SR (Can)** *see* Methylphenidate *on page 1402*

Ritonavir (ri TOE na veer)

Medication Safety Issues

Sound-alike/look-alike issues:

Ritonavir may be confused with Retrovir

Norvir may be confused with Norvasc

High alert medication:

This medication is in a class the Institute for Safe Medication Practices (ISMP) includes among its list of drug classes that have a heightened risk of causing significant patient harm when used in error.

Related Information

Adult and Adolescent HIV *on page 2392*

Oral Medications That Should Not Be Crushed or Altered *on page 2476*

Pediatric HIV *on page 2380*

Perinatal HIV *on page 2400*

Brand Names: US Norvir

Brand Names: Canada Norvir

Therapeutic Category Antiretroviral Agent; HIV Agents (Anti-HIV Agents); Protease Inhibitor

Generic Availability (US) No

Use Treatment of HIV infection in combination with other antiretroviral agents (FDA approved in ages >1 month and adults); has also been used as a pharmacokinetic "booster" for other protease inhibitors. **Note:** HIV regimens consisting of **three** antiretroviral agents are strongly recommended.

Pregnancy Risk Factor B

Pregnancy Considerations Adverse events were observed in animal reproduction studies only with doses which were also maternally toxic. Ritonavir has a low level of transfer across the human placenta; no increased risk of overall birth defects has been observed following first trimester exposure according to data collected by the antiretroviral pregnancy registry. Early studies have shown lower plasma levels during pregnancy compared to postpartum, however dosage adjustment is not needed when used as a low-dose booster in pregnant women. The DHHS Perinatal HIV Guidelines consider ritonavir to be a preferred protease inhibitor (PI) for use during pregnancy when used as a booster for other Pis (not recommended as a single protease inhibitor in ART naïve pregnant women). The oral solution contains alcohol and therefore may not be the best formulation for use in pregnancy. A small increased risk of preterm birth has been associated with maternal use of protease inhibitor-based combination antiretroviral (ARV) therapy during pregnancy; however, the benefits of use generally outweigh this risk and PIs should not be withheld if otherwise recommended.

Hyperglycemia, new onset of diabetes mellitus, or diabetic ketoacidosis have been reported with protease inhibitors; it is not clear if pregnancy increases this risk.

Regardless of CD4 count or HIV RNA copy number, all HIV-infected pregnant women should receive a combination antiretroviral ARV drug regimen. A combination of antepartum, intrapartum, and infant ARV prophylaxis is recommended. ARV therapy should be started as soon as possible in women with symptomatic infection. Although earlier initiation may be more effective in reducing the perinatal transmission of HIV, initiation may be delayed until after 12 weeks gestation in women who do not require immediate treatment after careful consideration of maternal conditions (eg, nausea and vomiting) and the potential risks of first trimester fetal exposure for specific agents. A scheduled cesarean delivery at 38 weeks gestation is recommended for all women with HIV RNA >1000 copies/mL or unknown concentrations near delivery in order to decrease transmission. If ARV therapy must be interrupted for <24 hours during the peripartum period, stop then restart all medications simultaneously in order to decrease the chance of developing resistance. Long-term follow-up is recommended for all infants exposed to ARV medications. In couples who want to conceive, the HIV-infected partner should attain maximum viral suppression prior to conception.

Health care providers are encouraged to enroll pregnant women exposed to antiretroviral medications in the Antiretroviral Pregnancy Registry (1-800-258-4263 or www.APRegistry.com). Health care providers caring for HIV-infected women and their infants may contact the National Perinatal HIV Hotline (888-448-8765) for clinical consultation (HHS [perinatal], 2014).

Breast-Feeding Considerations It is not known if ritonavir is excreted into breast milk; serum concentrations in nursing infants were undetectable at 12 weeks of age. Maternal or infant antiretroviral therapy does not completely eliminate the risk of postnatal HIV transmission. In addition, multiclass-resistant virus has been detected in breast-feeding infants despite maternal therapy. Therefore, in the United States, where formula is accessible, affordable, safe, and sustainable, and the risk of infant mortality due to diarrhea and respiratory infections is low, complete avoidance of breast-feeding by HIV-infected women is recommended to decrease potential transmission of HIV (HHS [perinatal], 2014).

Contraindications Hypersensitivity to ritonavir or any component of the formulation; concurrent alfuzosin, amiodarone, cisapride, dihydroergotamine, ergonovine, ergotamine, flecainide, lovastatin, methylergonovine, midazolam (oral), pimozide, propafenone, quinidine, sildenafil (when used for the treatment of pulmonary arterial hypertension [eg, Revatio®]), simvastatin, St John's wort, triazolam, and voriconazole (when ritonavir ≥800 mg/day)

Canadian labeling: Additional contraindications (not in U.S. labeling): Concurrent use with rivaroxaban, voriconazole (regardless of ritonavir dose), salmeterol, vardenafil, bepridil, astemizole, or terfenadine

Warnings/Precautions [U.S. Boxed Warning]: Ritonavir may interact with many medications, including antiarrhythmics, ergot alkaloids, and sedatives/hypnotics, resulting in potentially serious and/or life-threatening adverse events. Some interactions may require dose or frequency adjustment, additional monitoring, and/or selection of alternative therapy. Pancreatitis has been observed (including fatalities); use with caution in patients with increased triglycerides; monitor serum lipase and amylase and for gastrointestinal symptoms. Increases in total cholesterol and triglycerides have been reported; screening should be done prior to therapy and periodically throughout treatment. Temporary or permanent discontinuation may be clinically indicated.

Protease inhibitors have been associated with a variety of hypersensitivity events (some severe), including rash, anaphylaxis (rare), angioedema, bronchospasm, erythema multiforme, toxic epidermal necrolysis, and/or Stevens-Johnson syndrome (rare). It is generally recommended to discontinue treatment if severe rash or moderate symptoms accompanied by other systemic symptoms occur. Use with caution in patients with cardiomyopathy, ischemic heart disease, preexisting conduction abnormalities, or structural heart disease; may be at increased risk of conduction abnormalities (eg, second- or third-degree AV block). Ritonavir has been associated with AV block due to prolongation of PR interval; use caution with drugs that prolong the PR interval. Use with caution in patients with hemophilia A or B; increased bleeding during protease inhibitor therapy has been reported and additional Factor VIII may be needed. Changes in glucose tolerance, hyperglycemia, exacerbation of diabetes, DKA, and new-onset diabetes mellitus have been reported in patients receiving protease inhibitors. May be associated with fat redistribution (buffalo hump, increased abdominal girth, breast engorgement, facial atrophy, and dyslipidemia). Immune reconstitution syndrome may develop resulting in the occurrence of an inflammatory response to an indolent or residual opportunistic infection during initial HIV treatment or activation of autoimmune disorders (eg, Graves' disease, polymyositis, Guillain-Barré syndrome) later in therapy; further evaluation and treatment may be required. May cause hepatitis or exacerbate pre-existing hepatic dysfunction (including fatalities); use with caution in patients with hepatitis B or C, cirrhosis, or those with high baseline transaminases; consider increased monitoring of transaminases in these patients. Norvir® tablets are **not** bioequivalent to Norvir® capsules. Gastrointestinal side effects (eg, nausea, vomiting, abdominal pain, diarrhea) or paresthesias may be more common when patients are switching from the capsule to the tablet formulation due to a higher C_{max} (26% increase) observed with the tablet formulation compared to the capsule. These side effects should decrease as therapy is continued.

Oral solution contains ethanol and propylene glycol; healthcare providers should pay special attention to accurate calculation, measurement, and administration of dose; ethanol competitively inhibits propylene glycol metabolism; preterm infants may be at increased risk of toxicity due to decreased ability to metabolize propylene glycol. Postmarketing adverse reactions (cardiac toxicity, lactic acidosis, renal failure, CNS depression, respiratory complications, acute renal failure including fatalities) have been reported in preterm neonates receiving ritonavir-containing solutions. Do not use in neonates with a postmenstrual age (first day of mother's last menstrual period to birth plus elapsed time after birth) <44 weeks, unless benefit outweighs risk and neonate is closely monitored (serum creatinine and osmolality, CNS depression, renal toxicity, lactic acidosis, cardiac conduction abnormalities, hemolysis).

Warnings: Additional Pediatric Considerations Ritonavir oral solution contains 43% ethanol (v/v) and 26.6% propylene glycol (w/v); accidental ingestion could result in alcohol-related toxicity. Ethanol competitively inhibits propylene glycol metabolism, which may lead to propylene glycol toxicity in neonates due to impaired elimination. Preterm neonates may be at increased risk of adverse events from propylene glycol toxicity, including cardiotoxicity (complete AV block, bradycardia, cardiomyopathy), lactic acidosis, CNS depression, respiratory complications, acute renal failure, and death. Do not use oral solution in neonates with a PMA <44 weeks, unless benefit outweighs risk and neonate is closely monitored for increases in serum osmolality, serum creatinine, and other signs of propylene glycol toxicity (eg, CNS depression, seizures, cardiac arrhythmias, hemolysis); in neonates particularly, symptoms should be distinguished from sepsis. Toxicities have been reported with the use of products containing propylene glycol in all ages, including hyperosmolality, lactic acidosis, seizures, and respiratory depression. Due to concentration of ethanol in oral solution, an overdose in a child may cause potentially lethal alcohol toxicity. Treatment for overdose should be supportive and include general poisoning management; activated charcoal may help remove unabsorbed medication; dialysis unlikely to be of benefit; however, dialysis can remove alcohol and propylene glycol. In pediatric patients <6 months of age, the total amounts of ethanol and propylene glycol delivered from all medications should be considered to avoid toxicity.

Adverse Reactions

Cardiovascular: Edema (including peripheral edema), flushing, hypertension, syncope, vasodilatation

Central nervous system: Anxiety, confusion, depression, disturbance in attention, dizziness, drowsiness, fatigue, headache, insomnia, malaise, paresthesia, peripheral neuropathy

Dermatologic: Acne vulgaris, diaphoresis, pruritus, skin rash

Endocrine & metabolic: Hypercholesterolemia, increased serum triglycerides, increased uric acid, lipodystrophy (acquired)

Gastrointestinal: Abdominal pain, anorexia, diarrhea, dysgeusia, dyspepsia, flatulence, gastrointestinal hemorrhage, increased serum amylase (pediatric), nausea, throat irritation (local), vomiting

Hematologic & oncologic: Anemia (pediatric), neutropenia (pediatric), thrombocytopenia (pediatric)

Hepatic: Hepatitis, increased gamma-glutamyl transferase, increased serum ALT, increased serum AST

Hypersensitivity: Hypersensitivity reaction

Neuromuscular & skeletal: Increased creatine phosphokinase, musculoskeletal pain (arthralgia and back pain), myalgia, weakness

Ophthalmic: Blurred vision

Renal: Polyuria

Respiratory: Cough, oropharyngeal pain, pharyngitis

Miscellaneous: Fever

Rare but important or life-threatening: Adrenal suppression, adrenocortical cortex insufficiency, anaphylaxis, amnesia, angioedema, aphasia, asthma, atrioventricular block (first, second, or third degree), cachexia, cerebral ischemia, chest pain, cholestatic jaundice, coma, Cushing's syndrome, dementia, depersonalization, diabetes mellitus, diabetic ketoacidosis, esophageal ulcer, gastroenteritis, gastroesophageal reflux disease, gout, hallucination, hematologic disease (myeloproliferative), hemorrhage (in patients with hemophilia A or B), hepatic coma, hepatitis, hepatomegaly, hepatosplenomegaly, hyperglycemia, hypotension, hypothermia, hypoventilation, immune reconstitution syndrome, intestinal obstruction, leukemia (acute myeloblastic), leukopenia, lymphadenopathy, lymphocytosis, malignant melanoma, manic behavior, myocardial infarction, neuropathy, orthostatic hypotension, palpitations, pancreatitis, paralysis, pneumonia, prolongation P-R interval on ECG, prolonged Q-T interval on ECG, pseudomembranous colitis, rectal hemorrhage, redistribution of body fat, renal failure, renal insufficiency, right bundle branch block, seizure, Stevens-Johnson syndrome, subdural hematoma, syncope, tachycardia, torsades de pointes, toxic epidermal necrolysis, ulcerative colitis, vasospasm, venous thrombosis (cerebral)

Drug Interactions

Metabolism/Transport Effects **Substrate** of CYP1A2 (minor), CYP2B6 (minor), CYP2D6 (minor), CYP3A4 (major), P-glycoprotein; **Note:** Assignment of Major/Minor substrate status based on clinically relevant drug interaction potential; **Inhibits** CYP2C19 (weak), CYP2C8 (strong), CYP2C9 (weak), CYP2D6 (strong), CYP2E1 (weak), CYP3A4 (strong), P-glycoprotein, SLCO1B1; **Induces** CYP1A2 (weak/moderate), CYP2C9 (weak/moderate), CYP3A4 (weak)

Avoid Concomitant Use

Avoid concomitant use of Ritonavir with any of the following: Ado-Trastuzumab Emtansine; Alfuzosin; Amiodarone; Amodiaquine; Apixaban; Astemizole; Atovaquone; Avanafil; Axitinib; Barnidipine; Bosutinib; Cabozantinib; Ceritinib; Cisapride; Conivaptan; Crizotinib; Dapoxetine; Dasabuvir; Disulfiram; Domperidone; Dronedarone; Enzalutamide; Eplerenone; Ergot Derivatives; Etravirine; Everolimus; Flecainide; Fluticasone (Nasal); Fusidic Acid (Systemic); Halofantrine; Ibrutinib; Irinotecan; Isavuconazonium Sulfate; Ivabradine; Lapatinib; Lercanidipine; Lomitapide; Lovastatin; Lurasidone; Macitentan; Mequitazine; MetroNIDAZOLE (Systemic); Midazolam; Naloxegol; Nilotinib; NiMODipine; Nisoldipine; Olaparib; Palbociclib; PAZOPanib; Pimozide; Propafenone; QuiNIDine; QuiNINE; Ranolazine; Red Yeast Rice; Regorafenib; Rifampin; Rivaroxaban; Salmeterol; Silodosin; Simeprevir; Simvastatin; St Johns Wort; Suvorexant; Tamoxifen; Tamsulosin; Terfenadine; Thioridazine; Ticagrelor; Tolvaptan; Topotecan; Toremifene; Trabectedin; Triazolam; Ulipristal; Vemurafenib; VinCRIStine (Liposomal); Vorapaxar; Voriconazole

Increased Effect/Toxicity

Ritonavir may increase the levels/effects of: Ado-Trastuzumab Emtansine; Afatinib; Alfuzosin; Almotriptan; Alosetron; ALPRAZolam; Amiodarone; Amodiaquine; Apixaban; ARIPiprazole; Astemizole; AtoMOXetine; AtorvaSTATin; Avanafil; Axitinib; Barnidipine; Bedaquiline; Bortezomib; Bosentan; Bosutinib; Brentuximab Vedotin; Brinzolamide; Budesonide (Nasal); Budesonide (Systemic, Oral Inhalation); Budesonide (Topical); Cabazitaxel; Cabozantinib; Calcium Channel Blockers (Dihydropyridine); Calcium Channel Blockers (Nondihydropyridine); Cannabis; CarBAMazepine; Ceritinib; Cilostazol; Cisapride; Clarithromycin; Clorazepate; Colchicine; Conivaptan; Corticosteroids (Orally Inhaled); Corticosteroids (Systemic); Crizotinib; Cyclophosphamide; CycloSPORINE (Systemic); CYP2C8 Substrates; CYP2D6 Substrates; CYP3A4 Substrates; Dabigatran Etexilate; Dapoxetine; Dasabuvir; Dasatinib; Diazepam; Dienogest; Digoxin; Disulfiram; Domperidone; DOXOrubicin (Conventional); Dronabinol; Dronedarone; Drospirenone; Dutasteride; Edoxaban; Efavirenz; Eliglustat; Eluxadoline; Enfuvirtide; Enzalutamide; Eplerenone; Ergot Derivatives; Erlotinib; Estazolam; Etizolam; Everolimus; FentaNYL; Fesoterodine; Flecainide; Flurazepam; Fluticasone (Nasal); Fluticasone (Oral Inhalation); Fusidic Acid (Systemic); GuanFACINE; Halofantrine; Highest Risk QTc-Prolonging Agents; Hydrocodone; Ibrutinib; Idelalisib; Iloperidone; Imatinib; Imidafenacin; Irinotecan; Isavuconazonium Sulfate; Itraconazole; Ivabradine; Ivacaftor; Ixabepilone; Ketoconazole (Systemic); Lacosamide; Lapatinib; Ledipasvir; Lercanidipine; Levobupivacaine; Levomilnacipran; Linagliptin; Lomitapide; Lovastatin; Lurasidone; Macitentan; Maraviroc; MedroxyPROGESTERone; Meperidine; Mequitazine; MethylPREDNISolone; Metoprolol; MetroNIDAZOLE (Systemic); Midazolam; Mifepristone; Moderate Risk QTc-Prolonging Agents; Naloxegol; Nebivolol; Nefazodone; Nilotinib; NiMODipine; Nintedanib; Nisoldipine; Olaparib; Ospemifene; Oxybutynin; OxyCODONE; Palbociclib; Panobinostat; Parecoxib; Paricalcitol; PAZOPanib; P-glycoprotein/ABCB1 Substrates; Pimecrolimus; Pimozide; Pioglitazone; PONATinib; Pranlukast; PrednisoLONE (Systemic); PredniSONE; Propafenone; Protease Inhibitors; Prucalopride; QUEtiapine; QuiNIDine; QuiNINE; Ramelteon; Ranolazine; Red Yeast Rice;

Regorafenib; Retapamulin; Rifabutin; Rifaximin; Rilpivirine; Riociguat; Rivaroxaban; RomiDEPsin; Rosuvastatin; Ruxolitinib; Salmeterol; Saxagliptin; Sildenafil; Silodosin; Simeprevir; Simvastatin; SORAfenib; Suvorexant; Tacrolimus (Systemic); Tacrolimus (Topical); Tadalafil; Tamsulosin; Tasimelteon; Telaprevir; Temsirolimus; Terfenadine; Tetrabenazine; Tetrahydrocannabinol; Thioridazine; Ticagrelor; Tofacitinib; Tolterodine; Tolvaptan; Topotecan; Toremifene; Trabectedin; TraMADol; TraZODone; Treprostinil; Triamcinolone (Systemic); Triazolam; Ulipristal; Vardenafil; Vemurafenib; Vilazodone; VinBLAStine; VinCRIStine; VinCRIStine (Liposomal); Vorapaxar; Vortioxetine; Zopiclone; Zuclopenthixol

The levels/effects of Ritonavir may be increased by: ARIPiprazole; Clarithromycin; Delavirdine; Efavirenz; Enfuvirtide; Fusidic Acid (Systemic); Mifepristone; P-glycoprotein/ABCB1 Inhibitors; Posaconazole; QuiNINE; Simeprevir

Decreased Effect

Ritonavir may decrease the levels/effects of: Abacavir; Antidiabetic Agents; Atovaquone; Boceprevir; BuPROPion; Canagliflozin; Clarithromycin; Codeine; Contraceptives (Estrogens); Deferasirox; Delavirdine; Etravirine; Fosphenytoin; Hydrocodone; Ifosfamide; Iloperidone; LamoTRIgine; Meperidine; Methadone; OLANZapine; Phenytoin; Prasugrel; Proguanil; QuiNINE; Tamoxifen; Telaprevir; Ticagrelor; TraMADol; Valproic Acid and Derivatives; Voriconazole; Warfarin; Zidovudine

The levels/effects of Ritonavir may be decreased by: Boceprevir; CarBAMazepine; CYP3A4 Inducers (Moderate); CYP3A4 Inducers (Strong); Dabrafenib; Fosphenytoin; Garlic; Mitotane; Phenytoin; Rifampin; Siltuximab; St Johns Wort; Tocilizumab

Food Interactions Food enhances absorption. Management: Manufacturer recommends taking with food. Maintain adequate hydration, unless instructed to restrict fluid intake.

Storage/Stability

Capsule: Store under refrigeration at 2°C to 8°C (36°F to 46°F); may be left out at room temperature of <25°C (<77°F) if used within 30 days. Protect from light. Avoid exposure to excessive heat.

Solution: Store at room temperature at 20°C to 25°C (68°F to 77°F); do not refrigerate. Avoid exposure to excessive heat. Keep cap tightly closed.

Tablet: Store at ≤30°C (86°F); exposure to temperatures ≤50°C (122°F) permitted for ≤7 days. Exposure to high humidity outside of the original container (or a USP equivalent container) for >2 weeks is not recommended.

Mechanism of Action Binds to the site of HIV-1 protease activity and inhibits cleavage of viral Gag-Pol polyprotein precursors into individual functional proteins required for infectious HIV. This results in the formation of immature, noninfectious viral particles.

Pharmacokinetics (Adult data unless noted)

Absorption: Well absorbed

Distribution: High concentrations in serum and lymph nodes; V_d (apparent): 0.41 ± 0.25 L/kg

Protein binding: 98% to 99%

Metabolism: In the liver by cytochrome P450 isoenzyme CYP3A and (to a lesser extent) CYP2D6; five metabolites have been identified; the major metabolite (M-2), an isopropylthiazole oxidation metabolite, is active at a level similar to ritonavir, but is found in low concentrations in the plasma

Bioavailability: Absolute bioavailability unknown; tablets are **not** bioequivalent to capsules; mean peak concentration of tablet was found to be 26% higher than capsule in a single dose study, in patients fed a moderate-fat meal

Half-life:

Children: 2 to 4 hours

Adults: 3 to 5 hours

Time to peak serum concentration: Oral solution: Fasting: 2 hours; nonfasting: 4 hours

Elimination: Renal clearance is negligible; 3.5% of dose is excreted as unchanged drug in the urine; 34% excreted as unchanged drug in the feces

Clearance: Pediatric patients: 1.5 to 1.7 times faster than adults

Dosing: Neonatal PMA <44 weeks: Do not use due to potential toxicity from excipients; no data about appropriate dose or safety exists (DHHS [pediatric], 2014)

Dosing: Usual

Pediatric: **HIV infection, treatment: Note:** Use in combination with other antiretroviral agents: Oral:

Ritonavir as sole protease inhibitor: **Note:** Not recommended as the sole protease inhibitor in any regimen (DHHS [pediatric], 2014)

Infants >1 month (PMA ≥44 weeks) and Children:

Initial: 250 mg/m²/dose every 12 hours; titrate upward at 2- to 3-day intervals by 50 mg/m²/dose twice daily increments to 350 to 400 mg/m²/dose twice daily; maximum dose: 600 mg/dose twice daily; **Note:** Patients who do not tolerate 400 mg/m² twice daily (due to adverse effects) may be treated with the highest tolerated dose; however, an alternative antiretroviral agent should be considered.

Serum concentrations comparable to those seen in adults receiving standard doses were obtained in children >2 years of age who received 350 to 400 mg/m² twice daily. In younger patients (1 month to 2 years of age) who received 350 or 450 mg/m²/dose twice daily, ritonavir AUCs were 16% lower and trough concentrations were 60% lower than those observed in adults receiving standard doses; higher ritonavir AUCs were not observed with the 450 mg/m²/dose twice daily compared to the 350 mg/m²/dose twice daily dosing.

Adolescents: **Note:** Ritonavir as sole protease inhibitor is no longer commonly used in clinical practice and is not recommended in any initial antiretroviral regimen (DHHS [adults], 2014): 600 mg twice daily; may use a dose titration schedule to reduce adverse events (nausea/vomiting) by initiating therapy at 300 mg twice daily; increase dose at 2- to 3-day intervals by 100 mg twice daily increments up to a maximum dose of 600 mg twice daily

Ritonavir as pharmacokinetic enhancer ("booster doses" of ritonavir): **Note:** Ritonavir is used at lower doses to increase the serum concentrations of other protease inhibitors; the recommended dose of ritonavir varies when used with different protease inhibitors; see monographs for individual protease inhibitors for recommended doses; appropriate pediatric "booster doses" of ritonavir have not been established for use with every protease inhibitor or for all pediatric age groups.

Adult: **HIV infection, treatment: Note:** Use in combination with other antiretroviral agents: Oral:

Ritonavir as sole protease inhibitor: **Note:** Ritonavir as sole protease inhibitor is no longer commonly used in clinical practice and is not recommended in any initial antiretroviral regimen (DHHS [adults], 2014): 600 mg twice daily; may use a dose titration schedule to reduce adverse events (nausea/vomiting) by initiating therapy at 300 mg twice daily; increase dose at 2- to 3-day intervals by 100 mg twice daily increments up to a maximum dose of 600 mg twice daily

Ritonavir as pharmacokinetic enhancer ("booster doses" of ritonavir): **Note:** Ritonavir is used at lower doses to increase the serum concentrations of other protease inhibitors; the recommended dose of ritonavir varies when used with different protease inhibitors; see monographs for individual protease inhibitors for recommended doses

Usual dose: 100 to 400 mg/day, as 100 to 200 mg once or twice daily; range: 100 to 800 mg/day; dose depends on the protease inhibitor. In patients without evidence of PI resistance, once daily booster-dosing of 100 mg ritonavir may be preferred to 200 mg/day due to less gastrointestinal and metabolic adverse events.

Dosing adjustment in renal impairment: No adjustment recommended; renal clearance is negligible (DHHS [adult], 2014)

Dosing adjustment in hepatic impairment:

Mild to moderate hepatic impairment: No adjustment recommended; lower ritonavir serum concentrations have been reported in patients with moderate hepatic impairment (use with caution; monitor closely for adequate response)

Severe hepatic impairment: Use not recommended; pharmacokinetics of ritonavir has not been studied in these patients

Administration Administer with meals to improve tolerability. Swallow tablets whole; do not chew, break, or crush. Consider reserving liquid formulation for use in patients receiving tube feeding due to its bad taste. Shake liquid well before use. May mix liquid formulation with milk, chocolate milk, vanilla or chocolate pudding or ice cream, or a liquid nutritional supplement. Other techniques used to increase tolerance in children include dulling the taste buds by chewing ice, giving popsicles or spoonfuls of partially frozen orange or grape juice concentrates before administration of ritonavir; coating the mouth with peanut butter to eat before the dose; administration of strong-tasting foods such as maple syrup, cheese, or strong-flavored chewing gum immediately after a dose. Oral solution is highly concentrated; use a calibrated oral dosing syringe to measure and administer. Separate administration of ritonavir and didanosine by 2 hours (DHHS [pediatric], 2014).

Monitoring Parameters Note: Monitor CD4 percentage (if <5 years of age) or CD4 count (if ≥5 years of age) at least every 3 to 4 months (DHHS [pediatric], 2014).

Prior to initiation of therapy: Genotypic resistance testing, CD4 and viral load (every 3 to 4 months), CBC with differential, LFTs, BUN, creatinine, electrolytes, glucose, and urinalysis (every 6 to 12 months), and assessment of readiness for adherence with medication regimen. At initiation and with any change in treatment regimen: CBC with differential, electrolytes, calcium, phosphate, glucose, LFTs, bilirubin, urinalysis (at initiation), BUN, creatinine, albumin, total protein, lipid panel (at initiation), CD4, and viral load. After 1 to 2 weeks of therapy: Signs of medication toxicity and adherence. After 2 to 4 weeks of therapy: CBC with differential, viral load, signs of medication toxicity, and adherence; then every 3 to 4 months: CBC with differential, electrolytes, glucose, LFTs, bilirubin, BUN, creatinine, CD4, viral load, signs of medication toxicity, and adherence. Every 6 to 12 months: Lipid panel and urinalysis. CD4 monitoring frequency may be decreased to every 6 to 12 months in children who are adherent to therapy if the value is well above the threshold for opportunistic infections, viral suppression is sustained, and the clinical status is stable for more than 2 to 3 years (DHHS [pediatric], 2014). Monitor for growth and development, signs of HIV-specific physical conditions, HIV disease progression, opportunistic infections, hepatitis, or pancreatitis.

Dosage Forms Excipient information presented when available (limited, particularly for generics); consult specific product labeling.

Capsule, Oral:

Norvir: 100 mg [contains alcohol, usp]

Solution, Oral:

Norvir: 80 mg/mL (240 mL) [contains alcohol, usp, fd&c yellow #6 (sunset yellow), propylene glycol, saccharin sodium; peppermint-caramel flavor]

Tablet, Oral:

Norvir: 100 mg

- **Ritonavir and Lopinavir** *see* Lopinavir and Ritonavir *on page 1291*
- **Rituxan** *see* RiTUXimab *on page 1875*

RiTUXimab (ri TUK si mab)

Medication Safety Issues

Sound-alike/look-alike issues:

Rituxan may be confused with Remicade

RiTUXimab may be confused with brentuximab, bevacizumab, inFLIXimab, ramucirumab, ruxolitinib

High alert medication:

This medication is in a class the Institute for Safe Medication Practices (ISMP) includes among its list of drug classes that have a heightened risk of causing significant patient harm when used in error.

Administration issues:

The rituximab dose for rheumatoid arthritis is a flat dose (1000 mg) and is not based on body surface area (BSA).

Related Information

Prevention of Chemotherapy-Induced Nausea and Vomiting in Children *on page 2368*

Brand Names: US Rituxan

Brand Names: Canada Rituxan

Therapeutic Category Antineoplastic Agent, Anti-CD20; Antineoplastic Agent, Monoclonal Antibody; Antirheumatic Miscellaneous; Immunosuppressant Agent; Monoclonal Antibody

Generic Availability (US) No

Use Treatment of CD20-positive, B-cell non-Hodgkin's lymphoma (NHL) [including relapsed or refractory, low-grade or follicular B-cell NHL (as a single agent); follicular B-cell NHL, previously untreated (in combination with first-line chemotherapy, and as single-agent maintenance therapy if response to first-line rituximab with chemotherapy); non-progressing, low-grade B-cell NHL (as a single agent after first-line CVP treatment), diffuse large B-cell NHL, previously untreated (in combination with CHOP chemotherapy or other anthracycline-based regimen)]; treatment of CD20-positive chronic lymphocytic leukemia (CLL) (in combination with cyclophosphamide and fludarabine); treatment of moderately- to severely-active rheumatoid arthritis (in combination with methotrexate) in patients with inadequate response to one or more TNF antagonists; treatment of granulomatosis with polyangiitis (GPA; Wegener's Granulomatosis) and microscopic polyangiitis (MPA) in combination with glucorticoids (FDA approved in adults); has also been used for the treatment of systemic autoimmune disorders (other than rheumatoid arthritis; ie, autoimmune hemolytic anemia in children); refractory systemic lupus erythematosus; steroid-refractory chronic graft-versus-host disease (GVHD); refractory nephrotic syndrome, chronic immune thrombocytopenia (ITP); post-transplant lymphoproliferative disorder (PTLD)

Medication Guide Available Yes

Pregnancy Risk Factor C

Pregnancy Considerations Animal reproduction studies have demonstrated adverse effects including decreased (reversible) B-cells and immunosuppression. Rituximab crosses the placenta and can be detected in the newborn. In one infant born at 41 weeks gestation, *in utero* exposure occurred from week 16-37; rituximab concentrations were higher in the neonate at birth (32,095 ng/mL) than the mother (9750 ng/mL) and still measurable at 18 weeks of age (700 ng/mL infant; 500 ng/mL mother) (Friedrichs, 2006).

B-cell lymphocytopenia lasting <6 months may occur in exposed infants. Limited information is available following maternal use of rituximab for the treatment of lymphomas and hematologic disorders (Ton, 2011). Retrospective case reports of inadvertent pregnancy during rituximab treatment collected by the manufacturer (often combined with concomitant teratogenic therapies) describe premature births and infant hematologic abnormalities and infections; no specific pattern of birth defects has been observed (limited data) (Chakravarty, 2010). Use is not recommended to treat non-life-threatening maternal conditions (eg, rheumatoid arthritis) during pregnancy (Makol, 2011; Østensen, 2008) and other agents are preferred for treating lupus nephritis in pregnant women (Hahn, 2012).

Effective contraception should be used during and for 12 months following treatment. Healthcare providers are encouraged to enroll women with rheumatoid arthritis exposed to rituximab during pregnancy in the MotherToBabyAutoImmune Diseases Study by contacting the Organization of Teratology Information Specialists (OTIS) (877-311-8972).

Breast-Feeding Considerations It is not known if rituximab is excreted in human milk. However, human IgG is excreted in breast milk, and therefore, rituximab may also be excreted in milk. Although rituximab would not be expected to enter the circulation of a nursing infant in significant amounts, the decision to discontinue rituximab or discontinue breast-feeding should take into account the benefits of treatment to the mother.

Contraindications There are no contraindications listed in the FDA-approved manufacturer's labeling.

Canadian labeling (not in U.S. labeling): Type 1 hypersensitivity or anaphylactic reaction to murine proteins, Chinese Hamster Ovary (CHO) cell proteins, or any component of the formulation; patients who have or have had progressive multifocal leukoencephalopathy (PML)

Warnings/Precautions [U.S. Boxed Warning]: Severe (occasionally fatal) infusion-related reactions have been reported, usually with the first infusion; fatalities have been reported within 24 hours of infusion; monitor closely during infusion; discontinue for severe reactions and provide medical intervention for grades 3 or 4 infusion reactions. Reactions usually occur within 30-120 minutes and may include hypotension, angioedema, bronchospasm, hypoxia, urticaria, and in more severe cases pulmonary infiltrates, acute respiratory distress syndrome, myocardial infarction, ventricular fibrillation, cardiogenic shock and/or anaphylaxis. Risk factors associated with fatal outcomes include chronic lymphocytic leukemia, female gender, mantle cell lymphoma, or pulmonary infiltrates. Closely monitor patients with a history of prior cardiopulmonary reactions or with pre-existing cardiac or pulmonary conditions and patients with high numbers of circulating malignant cells (>25,000/mm^3). Prior to infusion, premedicate patients with acetaminophen and an antihistamine (and methylprednisolone for patients with RA). Discontinue infusion for severe reactions; treatment is symptomatic. Medications for the treatment of hypersensitivity reactions (eg, bronchodilators, epinephrine, antihistamines, corticosteroids) should be available for immediate use. Discontinue infusion for serious or life-threatening cardiac arrhythmias. Perform cardiac monitoring during and after the infusion in patients who develop clinically significant arrhythmias or who have a history of arrhythmia or angina. Mild-to-moderate infusion-related reactions (eg, chills, fever, rigors) occur frequently and are typically managed through slowing or interrupting the infusion. Infusion may be resumed at a 50% infusion rate reduction upon resolution of symptoms. Due to the potential for hypotension, consider withholding antihypertensives 12 hours prior to treatment.

[U.S. Boxed Warning]: Hepatitis B virus (HBV) reactivation may occur with use and may result in fulminant hepatitis, hepatic failure, and death. Screen all patients for HBV infection by measuring hepatitis B surface antigen (HBsAG) and hepatitis B core antibody (anti-HBc) prior to therapy initiation; monitor patients for clinical and laboratory signs of hepatitis or HBV during and for several months after treatment. Discontinue rituximab (and concomitant medications) if viral hepatitis develops and initiate appropriate antiviral therapy. Reactivation has occurred in patients who are HBsAg positive as well as in those who are HBsAg negative but are anti-HBc positive; HBV reactivation has also been observed in patients who had previously resolved HBV infection. HBV reactivation has been reported up to 24 months after therapy discontinuation. Use cautiously in patients who show evidence of prior HBV infection (eg, HBsAg positive [regardless of antibody status] or HBsAG negative but anti-HBc positive); consult with appropriate clinicians regarding monitoring and consideration of antiviral therapy before and/or during rituximab treatment. The safety of resuming rituximab treatment following HBV reactivation is not known; discuss reinitiation of therapy in patients with resolved HBV reactivation with physicians experienced in HBV management.

[U.S. Boxed Warning]: Progressive multifocal leukoencephalopathy (PML) due to JC virus infection has been reported with rituximab use; may be fatal. Cases were reported in patients with hematologic malignancies receiving rituximab either with combination chemotherapy, or with hematopoietic stem cell transplant. Cases were also reported in patients receiving rituximab for autoimmune diseases who had received prior or concurrent immunosuppressant therapy. Onset may be delayed, although most cases were diagnosed within 12 months of the last rituximab dose. A retrospective analysis of patients (n=57) diagnosed with PML following rituximab therapy, found a median of 16 months (following rituximab initiation), 5.5 months (following last rituximab dose), and 6 rituximab doses preceded PML diagnosis. Clinical findings included confusion/disorientation, motor weakness/hemiparesis, altered vision/speech, and poor motor coordination with symptoms progressing over weeks to months (Carson, 2009). Promptly evaluate any patient presenting with neurological changes; consider neurology consultation, brain MRI and lumbar puncture for suspected PML. Discontinue rituximab in patients who develop PML; consider reduction/discontinuation of concurrent chemotherapy or immunosuppressants. Avoid use if severe active infection is present. Serious and potentially fatal bacterial, fungal, and either new or reactivated viral infections may occur during treatment and after completing rituximab. Infections have been observed in patients with prolonged hypogammaglobulinemia, defined as hypogammaglobulinemia >11 months after rituximab exposure; monitor immunoglobulin levels as necessary. Associated new or reactivated viral infections have included cytomegalovirus, herpes simplex virus, parvovirus B19, varicella zoster virus, West Nile virus, and hepatitis B and C. Discontinue rituximab in patients who develop other serious infections and initiate appropriate anti-infective treatment.

Tumor lysis syndrome leading to acute renal failure requiring dialysis (some fatal) may occur 12-24 hours following the first dose when used as a single agent in the treatment of NHL. Hyperkalemia, hypocalcemia, hyperuricemia, and/or hyperphosphatemia may occur. Administer prophylaxis (antihyperuricemic therapy, hydration) in patients at high risk (high numbers of circulating malignant cells ≥25,000/mm^3 or high tumor burden). May cause fatal renal toxicity in patients with hematologic malignancies. Patients who received combination therapy with cisplatin and rituximab for NHL experienced renal toxicity during clinical trials; this combination is not an approved treatment regimen. Monitor for signs of renal failure; discontinue rituximab with increasing serum creatinine or oliguria. Correct electrolyte abnormalities; monitor hydration status.

[U.S. Boxed Warning]: Severe and sometimes fatal mucocutaneous reactions (lichenoid dermatitis, paraneoplastic pemphigus, Stevens-Johnson syndrome, toxic epidermal necrolysis and vesiculobullous dermatitis) have been reported; onset has been variable but has occurred as early as the first day of exposure. Discontinue in patients experiencing severe mucocutaneous skin reactions; the safety of re-exposure following mucocutaneous reactions has not been evaluated. Use caution with pre-existing cardiac or pulmonary disease, or prior cardiopulmonary events. Rheumatoid arthritis patients are at increased risk for cardiovascular events; monitor closely during and after each infusion. Elderly patients are at higher risk for cardiac (supraventricular arrhythmia) and pulmonary adverse events (pneumonia, pneumonitis). Abdominal pain, bowel obstruction, and perforation (rarely fatal) have been reported with an average onset of symptoms of ~6 days (range: 1-77 days); complaints of abdominal pain or repeated vomiting should be evaluated, especially if early in the treatment course. Live vaccines should not be given concurrently with rituximab; there is no data available concerning secondary transmission of live vaccines with or following rituximab treatment. RA patients should be brought up to date with nonlive immunizations (following current guidelines) at least 4 weeks before initiating therapy; evaluate risks of therapy delay versus benefit (of nonlive vaccines) for NHL patients. Safety and efficacy of rituximab in combination with biologic agents or disease-modifying antirheumatic drugs (DMARDs) other than methotrexate have not been established. Rituximab is not recommended for use in RA patients who have not had prior inadequate response to TNF antagonists. Safety and efficacy of re-treatment for RA have not been established. The safety of concomitant immunosuppressants other than corticosteroids has not been evaluated in patients with granulomatosis with polyangiitis (GPA; Wegener's granulomatosis) or microscopic polyangiitis (MPA) after rituximab-induced B-cell depletion. There are only limited data on subsequent courses of rituximab for GPA or MPA; safety and efficacy of re-treatment have not been established.

Some dosage forms may contain polysorbate 80 (also known as Tweens). Hypersensitivity reactions, usually a delayed reaction, have been reported following exposure to pharmaceutical products containing polysorbate 80 in certain individuals (Isaksson, 2002; Lucente 2000; Shelley, 1995). Thrombocytopenia, ascites, pulmonary deterioration, and renal and hepatic failure have been reported in premature neonates after receiving parenteral products containing polysorbate 80 (Alade, 1986; CDC, 1984). See manufacturer's labeling.

Adverse Reactions Note: Patients treated with rituximab for rheumatoid arthritis (RA) may experience fewer adverse reactions.

Cardiovascular: Flushing, hyper-/hypotension, peripheral edema

Central nervous system: Anxiety, chills, dizziness, fatigue, fever, headache, insomnia, migraine, pain

Dermatologic: Angioedema, pruritus, rash, urticaria

Endocrine & metabolic: Hyperglycemia

Gastrointestinal: Abdominal pain, diarrhea, dyspepsia, nausea, vomiting, weight gain

Hematologic: Anemia, cytopenia, lymphopenia, leukopenia, neutropenia, neutropenic fever, thrombocytopenia

Hepatic: ALT increased

Neuromuscular & skeletal: Arthralgia, back pain, muscle spasm, myalgia, neuropathy, paresthesia, weakness

Respiratory: Bronchospasm, cough, dyspnea, epistaxis, rhinitis, sinusitis, throat irritation, upper respiratory tract infection

Miscellaneous: Infusion-related reactions (may include angioedema, bronchospasm, chills, dizziness, fever, headache, hyper-/hypotension, myalgia, nausea, pruritus, rash, rigors, urticaria, and vomiting); infection (including bacterial, viral, fungal); night sweats; human antichimeric antibody (HACA) positive

Rare but important or life-threatening: Acute renal failure, anaphylactoid reaction/anaphylaxis, angina, aplastic anemia, ARDS, arrhythmia, bowel obstruction/perforation, bronchiolitis obliterans, cardiac failure, cardiogenic shock, encephalomyelitis, fatal infusion-related reactions, fulminant hepatitis, gastrointestinal perforation, hemolytic anemia, hepatic failure, hepatitis, hepatitis B reactivation, hyperviscosity syndrome (in Waldenström's macroglobulinemia), hypogammaglobulinemia (prolonged), hypoxia, interstitial pneumonitis, laryngeal edema, lichenoid dermatitis, lupus-like syndrome, marrow hypoplasia, MI, mucositis, mucocutaneous reaction, neutropenia (late-onset occurring >40 days after last dose), optic neuritis, pancytopenia (prolonged), paraneoplastic pemphigus (uncommon), pleuritis, pneumonia, pneumonitis, polyarticular arthritis, polymyositis, posterior reversible encephalopathy syndrome (PRES), progressive multifocal leukoencephalopathy (PML), pure red cell aplasia, renal toxicity, reversible posterior leukoencephalopathy syndrome (RPLS), serum sickness, Stevens-Johnson syndrome, supraventricular arrhythmia, systemic vasculitis, toxic epidermal necrolysis, tuberculosis reactivation, tumor lysis syndrome, uveitis, vasculitis with rash, ventricular fibrillation, ventricular tachycardia, vesiculobullous dermatitis, viral reactivation (includes JC virus, cytomegalovirus, herpes simplex virus, parvovirus B19, varicella zoster virus, West Nile virus, and hepatitis C), wheezing

Drug Interactions

Metabolism/Transport Effects None known.

Avoid Concomitant Use

Avoid concomitant use of RiTUXimab with any of the following: Abatacept; BCG; BCG (Intravesical); Belimumab; Certolizumab Pegol; CloZAPine; Dipyrone; Natalizumab; Pimecrolimus; Tacrolimus (Topical); Tofacitinib; Vaccines (Live)

Increased Effect/Toxicity

RiTUXimab may increase the levels/effects of: Abatacept; Belimumab; Certolizumab Pegol; CloZAPine; Leflunomide; Natalizumab; Tofacitinib; Vaccines (Live)

The levels/effects of RiTUXimab may be increased by: Antihypertensives; Denosumab; Dipyrone; Pimecrolimus; Roflumilast; Tacrolimus (Topical); Trastuzumab

Decreased Effect

RiTUXimab may decrease the levels/effects of: BCG; BCG (Intravesical); Coccidioides immitis Skin Test; Sipuleucel-T; Vaccines (Inactivated); Vaccines (Live)

The levels/effects of RiTUXimab may be decreased by: Echinacea

Storage/Stability Store intact vials refrigerated at 2°C to 8°C (36°F to 46°F); do not freeze. Do not shake. Protect vials from direct sunlight. Solutions for infusion are stable at 2°C to 8°C (36°F to 46°F) for 24 hours and at room temperature for an additional 24 hours.

Mechanism of Action Rituximab is a monoclonal antibody directed against the CD20 antigen on B-lymphocytes. CD20 regulates cell cycle initiation; and, possibly, functions as a calcium channel. Rituximab binds to the antigen on the cell surface, activating complement-dependent B-cell cytotoxicity; and to human Fc receptors, mediating cell killing through an antibody-dependent cellular toxicity. B-cells are believed to play a role in the development and progression of rheumatoid arthritis. Signs and symptoms of RA are reduced by targeting B-cells and the progression of structural damage is delayed.

Pharmacodynamics Duration: B-cell recovery begins ~6 months following completion of treatment; medium B-cell levels return to normal by 12 months

Pharmacokinetics (Adult data unless noted)

Distribution: Binds to lymphoid cells in the thymus, spleen, and B lymphocytes in peripheral blood and lymph nodes

Half-life: Adults:

NHL: Median terminal half-life: 22 days (range: 6-52 days)

CLL: Median terminal half-life: 32 days (range: 14-62 days)

Rheumatoid arthritis: 18 days (range: 5-78 days)

Dosing: Usual Refer to individual protocols. Pretreatment with acetaminophen and an antihistamine is recommended for all indications. For oncology uses, a uricostatic agent (eg, allopurinol) and aggressive hydration is recommended for patients at risk for tumor lysis syndrome (high tumor burden or lymphocytes >25,000/mm^3). In patients with CLL, *pneumocystis jiroveci* pneumonia (PCP) and antiherpetic viral prophylaxis is recommended during treatment (and for up to 12 months following treatment). In patients with WG and MPA, PCP prophylaxis is recommended during and for 6 months after rituximab treatment.

Infants, Children, and Adolescents:

Autoimmune hemolytic anemia: Infants ≥4 months, Children, and Adolescents: IV infusion: 375 mg/m^2 once weekly for 2-4 doses (Zecca, 2003)

Chronic ITP: Children and Adolescents: IV infusion: 375 mg/m^2 once weekly for 4 doses (Parodi, 2009; Wang, 2005)

Post-transplant lymphoproliferative disorder: Infants ≥11 months, Children, and Adolescents: IV infusion: 375 mg/m^2 once weekly for 3-4 doses (Milpied, 2000; Serinet, 2002)

Refractory SLE: Children ≥8 years and Adolescents: IV infusion: 375 mg/m^2 once weekly for 2-4 doses; or 750 mg/m^2 on days 1 and 15 (maximum dose: 1000 mg) (Marks, 2005)

Refractory severe nephrotic syndrome: Infants ≥11 months, Children, and Adolescents: IV infusion: 375 mg/m^2 once weekly for 1-4 doses has been used in small case series, case reports, and retrospective analyses, including reports of successful remission induction of severe or refractory nephrotic syndromes that are poorly responsive to standard therapies (Della Strologo, 2009; Fujinaga, 2010; Gugonis, 2008; Kaito, 2010; Prytula, 2010)

Adults:

CLL: IV infusion: 375 mg/m^2 on the day prior to fludarabine/cyclophosphamide in cycle 1, then 500 mg/m^2 on day 1 (every 28 days) of cycles 2-6

Granulomatosis with polyangiitis (GPA; Wegener's granulomatosis) and Microscopic polyangiitis (MPA): IV infusion: 375 mg/m^2 once weekly for 4 doses (in combination with methylprednisolone IV for 1-3 days followed by daily prednisone)

NHL (relapsed/refractory, low-grade or follicular CD20-positive, B-cell): IV infusion: 375 mg/m^2 once weekly for 4 or 8 doses

Retreatment following disease progression: IV infusion: 375 mg/m^2 once weekly for 4 doses

NHL (diffuse large B-cell): IV infusion: 375 mg/m^2 given on day 1 of each chemotherapy cycle for up to 8 doses

NHL (follicular, CD20-positive, B-cell, previously untreated): IV infusion: 375 mg/m^2 given on day 1 of each chemotherapy cycle for up to 8 doses

Maintenance therapy (as a single agent, in patients with partial or complete response to rituximab plus chemotherapy; begin 8 weeks after completion of combination chemotherapy): IV infusion: 375 mg/m^2 every 8 weeks for 12 doses

NHL (nonprogressing, low-grade, CD20-positive, B-cell, after first-line CVP): IV infusion: 375 mg/m^2 once weekly for 4 doses every 6 months for up to 4 cycles (initiate after 6-8 cycles of chemotherapy are completed)

NHL: Combination therapy with ibritumomab: IV infusion: 250 mg/m^2 IV day 1; repeat in 7-9 days with ibritumomab

Rheumatoid arthritis: IV infusion: 1000 mg on days 1 and 15 in combination with methotrexate; subsequent courses may be administered every 24 weeks (based on clinical evaluation), if necessary may be repeated no sooner than every 16 weeks. **Note:** Premedication with methylprednisolone 100 mg IV (or equivalent) is recommended 30 minutes prior to each dose.

Preparation for Administration IV infusion: Withdraw necessary amount of rituximab and dilute to a final concentration of 1 to 4 mg/mL with NS or D_5W. Gently invert the bag to mix the solution. Do not shake.

Administration IV infusion: **DO NOT ADMINISTER UNDILUTED OR as an IV push or rapid injection:**

Note: Some pediatric protocols utilize an alternate rituximab administration rate. Refer to specific protocol for administration rate guidelines.

Initial infusion: Start at a rate of 50 mg/hour. If no hypersensitivity or infusion-related reactions occur, increase infusion rate in 50 mg/hour increments every 30 minutes to a maximum infusion rate of 400 mg/hour as tolerated.

Subsequent infusions:

Standard infusion rate: If patient tolerated initial infusion, start at 100 mg/hour and increased by 100 mg/hour increments at 30 minute intervals to a maximum infusion rate of 400 mg/hour. If hypersensitivity or infusion-related reactions occur, slow or interrupt the infusion. If symptoms completely resolve, resume infusion at 50% of the previous rate.

Accelerated infusion rate (90 minutes): For adult patients with previously untreated follicular NHL and diffuse large B-cell NHL who are receiving a corticosteroid as part of their combination chemotherapy regimen, have a circulating lymphocyte count <5,000/mm^3, or have no significant cardiovascular disease. After tolerance has been established (no grade 3 or 4 infusion-related event) at the recommended infusion rate in cycle 1, a rapid infusion rate may be used beginning with cycle 2. The daily corticosteroid, acetaminophen, and diphenhydramine are administered prior to treatment, then the rituximab dose is administered over 90 minutes, with 20% of the dose administered over the first 30 minutes and the remaining 80% is given over 60 minutes (Sehn 2007). If the 90-minute infusion in cycle 2 is tolerated, the same rate may be used for the remainder of the treatment regimen (through cycles 6 or 8).

Monitoring Parameters Vital signs, CBC with differential and platelet counts (obtain at weekly to monthly intervals and more frequently in patients with cytopenias, or at 2-4 month intervals in rheumatoid arthritis patients, WG and MPA), serum electrolytes, uric acid, renal function tests, liver function tests, fluid balance; monitor for infusion reactions, cardiac monitoring for patients with pre-existing cardiac condition; peripheral CD20$^+$ cells; human antimurine antibody and human antichimeric antibody titers (high levels may increase the risk of allergic reactions); screening for hepatitis B, signs or symptoms of PML, signs or symptoms of bowel obstruction/perforation

Dosage Forms Excipient information presented when available (limited, particularly for generics); consult specific product labeling.

Concentrate, Intravenous [preservative free]:
Rituxan: 10 mg/mL (10 mL, 50 mL) [contains polysorbate 80]

- ◆ **RIV** *see* Influenza Virus Vaccine (Recombinant) *on page 1116*
- ◆ **RIV$_3$** *see* Influenza Virus Vaccine (Recombinant) *on page 1116*
- ◆ **Riva-Amiodarone (Can)** *see* Amiodarone *on page 125*
- ◆ **Riva-Amlodipine (Can)** *see* AmLODIPine *on page 133*
- ◆ **Riva-Atenolol (Can)** *see* Atenolol *on page 215*
- ◆ **RIVA-Atomoxetine (Can)** *see* AtoMOXetine *on page 217*
- ◆ **Riva-Atorvastatin (Can)** *see* AtorvaSTATin *on page 220*
- ◆ **Riva-Azithromycin (Can)** *see* Azithromycin (Systemic) *on page 242*
- ◆ **Riva-Baclofen (Can)** *see* Baclofen *on page 254*
- ◆ **Riva-Buspirone (Can)** *see* BusPIRone *on page 328*
- ◆ **Riva-Celecoxib (Can)** *see* Celecoxib *on page 418*
- ◆ **Riva-Ciprofloxacin (Can)** *see* Ciprofloxacin (Systemic) *on page 463*
- ◆ **Riva-Citalopram (Can)** *see* Citalopram *on page 476*
- ◆ **Riva-Clarithromycin (Can)** *see* Clarithromycin *on page 482*
- ◆ **Riva-Clindamycin (Can)** *see* Clindamycin (Systemic) *on page 487*
- ◆ **Riva-Clonazepam (Can)** *see* ClonazePAM *on page 506*
- ◆ **Rivacocet (Can)** *see* Oxycodone and Acetaminophen *on page 1594*
- ◆ **Riva-Cycloprine (Can)** *see* Cyclobenzaprine *on page 548*
- ◆ **Riva-Dicyclomine (Can)** *see* Dicyclomine *on page 645*
- ◆ **Riva-Enalapril (Can)** *see* Enalapril *on page 744*
- ◆ **Riva-Escitalopram (Can)** *see* Escitalopram *on page 786*
- ◆ **Riva-Ezetimibe (Can)** *see* Ezetimibe *on page 832*
- ◆ **Riva-Fluconazole (Can)** *see* Fluconazole *on page 881*
- ◆ **Riva-Fluoxetine (Can)** *see* FLUoxetine *on page 906*
- ◆ **Riva-Fluvox (Can)** *see* FluvoxaMINE *on page 928*
- ◆ **Riva-Fosinopril (Can)** *see* Fosinopril *on page 943*
- ◆ **Riva-Gabapentin (Can)** *see* Gabapentin *on page 954*
- ◆ **Riva-Glyburide (Can)** *see* GlyBURIDE *on page 975*
- ◆ **Riva-Hydroxyzine (Can)** *see* HydrOXYzine *on page 1058*
- ◆ **Riva-Lansoprazole (Can)** *see* Lansoprazole *on page 1219*
- ◆ **Riva-Letrozole (Can)** *see* Letrozole *on page 1224*
- ◆ **Riva-Lisinopril (Can)** *see* Lisinopril *on page 1280*
- ◆ **Riva-Loperamide (Can)** *see* Loperamide *on page 1288*
- ◆ **Riva-Lovastatin (Can)** *see* Lovastatin *on page 1305*
- ◆ **Riva-Metformin (Can)** *see* MetFORMIN *on page 1375*
- ◆ **Riva-Metoprolol-L (Can)** *see* Metoprolol *on page 1418*
- ◆ **Riva-Montelukast FC (Can)** *see* Montelukast *on page 1459*
- ◆ **Rivanase AQ (Can)** *see* Beclomethasone (Nasal) *on page 260*
- ◆ **Riva-Olanzapine (Can)** *see* OLANZapine *on page 1546*
- ◆ **Riva-Olanzapine ODT (Can)** *see* OLANZapine *on page 1546*
- ◆ **Riva-Omeprazole DR (Can)** *see* Omeprazole *on page 1555*
- ◆ **Riva-Ondansetron (Can)** *see* Ondansetron *on page 1564*
- ◆ **Riva-Oxybutynin (Can)** *see* Oxybutynin *on page 1588*
- ◆ **Riva-Pantoprazole (Can)** *see* Pantoprazole *on page 1618*
- ◆ **Riva-Paroxetine (Can)** *see* PARoxetine *on page 1634*
- ◆ **Riva-Pravastatin (Can)** *see* Pravastatin *on page 1749*
- ◆ **Riva-Quetiapine (Can)** *see* QUEtiapine *on page 1815*
- ◆ **Riva-Rabeprazole EC (Can)** *see* RABEprazole *on page 1828*
- ◆ **Riva-Ranitidine (Can)** *see* Ranitidine *on page 1836*
- ◆ **Riva-Risperidone (Can)** *see* RisperiDONE *on page 1866*
- ◆ **Riva-Rizatriptan ODT (Can)** *see* Rizatriptan *on page 1879*
- ◆ **Riva-Rosuvastatin (Can)** *see* Rosuvastatin *on page 1886*
- ◆ **Riva-Sertraline (Can)** *see* Sertraline *on page 1916*
- ◆ **Riva-Simvastatin (Can)** *see* Simvastatin *on page 1928*
- ◆ **Rivasol (Can)** *see* Zinc Sulfate *on page 2214*
- ◆ **Rivasone (Can)** *see* Betamethasone (Topical) *on page 280*
- ◆ **Riva-Sotalol (Can)** *see* Sotalol *on page 1963*
- ◆ **Riva-Terbinafine (Can)** *see* Terbinafine (Systemic) *on page 2021*
- ◆ **Riva-Valacyclovir (Can)** *see* ValACYclovir *on page 2138*
- ◆ **Riva-Venlafaxine XR (Can)** *see* Venlafaxine *on page 2166*
- ◆ **Riva-Verapamil SR (Can)** *see* Verapamil *on page 2170*
- ◆ **Rivotril (Can)** *see* ClonazePAM *on page 506*
- ◆ **Rixubis** *see* Factor IX (Recombinant) *on page 842*

Rizatriptan (rye za TRIP tan)

Brand Names: US Maxalt; Maxalt-MLT

Brand Names: Canada ACT Rizatriptan; ACT Rizatriptan ODT; Apo-Rizatriptan; Apo-Rizatriptan RPD; Dom-Rizatriptan RDT; JAMP-Rizatriptan; JAMP-Rizatriptan IR; Mar-Rizatriptan; Maxalt; Maxalt RPD; Mylan-Rizatriptan ODT; PMS-Rizatriptan RDT; Riva-Rizatriptan ODT; Rizatriptan RDT; Sandoz-Rizatriptan ODT

Therapeutic Category Antimigraine Agent; Serotonin 5-HT_{1D} Receptor Agonist

Generic Availability (US) Yes

Use Acute treatment of migraine with or without aura (FDA approved in ages ≥6 years and adults)

Pregnancy Risk Factor C

Pregnancy Considerations Adverse events were observed in animal reproduction studies. Information related to rizatriptan use in pregnancy is limited (Källén, 2011; Nezvalová-Henriksen, 2010; Nezvalová-Henriksen, 2012).

A pregnancy registry has been established to monitor outcomes of women exposed to rizatriptan during pregnancy (800-986-8999). Preliminary data from the pregnancy registry (prospectively collected from 65 live births 1998-2004) does not show an increased risk of congenital malformations (Fiore, 2005). Until additional information is available, other agents are preferred for the initial treatment of migraine in pregnancy (Da Silva, 2012; MacGregor, 2012; Williams, 2012).

Breast-Feeding Considerations It is not known if rizatriptan is excreted in breast milk. The manufacturer recommends that caution be exercised when administering rizatriptan to nursing women.

Contraindications Hypersensitivity to rizatriptan or any component of the formulation; documented ischemic heart disease or other significant cardiovascular disease; coronary artery vasospasm (including Prinzmetal's angina);

history of stroke or transient ischemic attack; peripheral vascular disease; ischemic bowel disease; uncontrolled hypertension; basilar or hemiplegic migraine; during or within 2 weeks of MAO inhibitors; during or within 24 hours of treatment with another 5-HT_1 agonist, or an ergot-containing or ergot-type medication (eg, methysergide, dihydroergotamine)

Warnings/Precautions Only indicated for treatment of acute migraine; not for the prevention of migraines or the treatment of cluster headache. If a patient does not respond to the first dose, the diagnosis of migraine should be reconsidered. Coronary artery vasospasm, transient ischemia, myocardial infarction, ventricular tachycardia/ fibrillation, cardiac arrest, and death have been reported with 5-HT_1 agonist administration. Patients who experience sensations of chest pain/pressure/tightness or symptoms suggestive of angina following dosing should be evaluated for coronary artery disease or Prinzmetal's angina before receiving additional doses; if dosing is resumed and similar symptoms recur, monitor with ECG. Should not be given to patients who have risk factors for CAD (eg, hypertension, hypercholesterolemia, smoker, obesity, diabetes, strong family history of CAD, menopause, male >40 years of age) without adequate cardiac evaluation. Patients with suspected CAD should have cardiovascular evaluation to rule out CAD before considering use; if cardiovascular evaluation is "satisfactory," first dose should be given in the healthcare provider's office (consider ECG monitoring). Periodic evaluation of cardiovascular status should be done in all patients. Significant elevation in blood pressure, including hypertensive crisis, has also been reported on rare occasions in patients with and without a history of hypertension. Cerebral/subarachnoid hemorrhage, stroke, peripheral vascular ischemia, gastrointestinal ischemia/infarction, splenic infarction and Raynaud's syndrome have been reported with 5-HT_1 agonist administration. Use is contraindicated in patients with a history of stroke or transient ischemic attack. Rarely, partial vision loss and blindness (transient and permanent) have been reported with 5-HT_1 agonists.

Use with caution in elderly or patients with hepatic or renal impairment (including dialysis patients). Symptoms of agitation, confusion, hallucinations, hyper-reflexia, myoclonus, shivering, and tachycardia may occur with concomitant proserotonergic drugs (eg, SSRIs/SNRIs or triptans) or agents which reduce rizatriptan's metabolism. Concurrent use of serotonin precursors (eg, tryptophan) is not recommended. If concomitant administration with SSRIs is warranted, monitor closely, especially at initiation and with dose increases. Acute migraine agents (eg, triptans, opioids, ergotamine, or a combination of the agents) used for 10 or more days per month may lead to worsening of headaches (medication overuse headache); withdrawal treatment may be necessary in the setting of overuse. Maxalt-MLT tablets contain phenylalanine.

Adverse Reactions

Cardiovascular: Chest pain, flushing, palpitation

Central nervous system: Dizziness, euphoria, fatigue (dose related; more common in adults), headache, hypoesthesia, pain, somnolence

Dermatologic: Skin flushing

Gastrointestinal: Abdominal discomfort, diarrhea, nausea, vomiting, xerostomia

Neuromuscular & skeletal: Neck, throat, and jaw pain/ tightness/pressure; paresthesia; tremor; weakness

Respiratory: Dyspnea

Miscellaneous: Feeling of heaviness

Rare but important or life-threatening: Anaphylaxis/anaphylactoid reactions, angina, angioedema, blurred vision, bradycardia, confusion, edema, hallucination (children), hearing impairment, hypertensive crisis, memory impairment, MI, myocardial ischemia, pruritus, seizure, syncope, tachycardia, tinnitus, tongue edema, toxic epidermal necrolysis, vasospasm, vertigo, wheezing

Drug Interactions

Metabolism/Transport Effects None known.

Avoid Concomitant Use

Avoid concomitant use of Rizatriptan with any of the following: Dapoxetine; Ergot Derivatives; MAO Inhibitors

Increased Effect/Toxicity

Rizatriptan may increase the levels/effects of: Antipsychotic Agents; Droxidopa; Ergot Derivatives; Metoclopramide; Serotonin Modulators

The levels/effects of Rizatriptan may be increased by: Antiemetics (5HT3 Antagonists); Antipsychotic Agents; Dapoxetine; Ergot Derivatives; MAO Inhibitors; Propranolol

Decreased Effect There are no known significant interactions involving a decrease in effect.

Food Interactions Food delays absorption. Management: Administer without regard to meals.

Storage/Stability Store at room temperature of 15°C to 30°C (59°F to 86°F); orally disintegrating tablets should be stored in blister pack until administration.

Mechanism of Action Selective agonist for serotonin (5-HT_{1B} and 5-HT_{1D} receptors) in cranial arteries; causes vasoconstriction and reduces sterile inflammation associated with antidromic neuronal transmission correlating with relief of migraine

Pharmacokinetics (Adult data unless noted)

Absorption: Complete

Distribution: V_d: 110-140 L

Protein binding: 14%

Metabolism: Via monoamine oxidase-A to a major inactive and a minor (14%) active metabolite; first-pass effect

Bioavailability: ~45%; AUC in females reported to be 30% higher than males

Half-life: 2-3 hours

Time to peak serum concentration: Maxalt®: 1-1.5 hours; Maxalt-MLT®: 1.6-2.5 hours

Elimination: Urine (82%, ~14% as unchanged drug); feces (12%)

Dialysis: Reported AUC 44% higher in dialysis patients compared to normal renal function; effects of hemodialysis or peritoneal dialysis are unknown

Dosing: Usual Oral: **Migraine, acute treatment:**

Children and Adolescents ≥6 years: **Note:** Safety and efficacy of multiple rizatriptan doses in a 24-hour period has not been established for pediatric patients.

<40 kg: 5 mg as a single dose

≥40 kg: 10 mg as a single dose

Adults: 5-10 mg, repeat after 2 hours if significant relief is not attained; maximum: 30 mg in a 24-hour period; **Note:** In patients with risk factors for coronary artery disease, following adequate evaluation to establish the absence of coronary artery disease, the initial dose should be administered in a setting where response may be evaluated (physician's office or similarly staffed setting). ECG monitoring may be considered.

Dosage adjustment with concomitant propranolol:

Children and Adolescents 6-17 years:

<40 kg: Do not use rizatriptan

≥40 kg: 5 mg as a single dose; maximum: 5 mg in a 24-hour period

Adults: 5 mg; may repeat after 2 hours; maximum daily dose: 15 mg in a 24-hour period

Administration Oral: Orally disintegrating tablets (Maxalt-MLT®): Do not remove the blister from the pouch until ready to use; blister pouch should be opened by peeling back (not pushing through foil) and with dry hands; place tablet on the tongue to dissolve; do not crush, break, or chew; additional liquids are not necessary.

Monitoring Parameters Headache severity

Additional Information Safety of treating >4 migraines per month is not established; rizatriptan is not indicated for migraine prophylaxis; safety and efficacy for cluster headaches has not been established.

Dosage Forms Excipient information presented when available (limited, particularly for generics); consult specific product labeling.

Tablet, Oral:
- Maxalt: 5 mg, 10 mg
- Generic: 5 mg, 10 mg

Tablet Dispersible, Oral:
- Maxalt-MLT: 5 mg, 10 mg [contains aspartame; peppermint flavor]
- Generic: 5 mg, 10 mg

- ◆ **Rizatriptan RDT (Can)** *see* Rizatriptan *on page* 1879
- ◆ **rLFN-α2** *see* Interferon Alfa-2b *on page* 1148
- ◆ **rLP2086** *see* Meningococcal Group B Vaccine *on page* 1351
- ◆ **Ro 5488** *see* Tretinoin (Systemic) *on page* 2108
- ◆ **RoActemra** *see* Tocilizumab *on page* 2079
- ◆ **Robafen [OTC]** *see* GuaiFENesin *on page* 988
- ◆ **Robafen AC** *see* Guaifenesin and Codeine *on page* 990
- ◆ **Robafen Cough [OTC]** *see* Dextromethorphan *on page* 631
- ◆ **Robafen DM [OTC]** *see* Guaifenesin and Dextromethorphan *on page* 992
- ◆ **Robaxin** *see* Methocarbamol *on page* 1387
- ◆ **Robaxin® (Can)** *see* Methocarbamol *on page* 1387
- ◆ **Robaxin-750** *see* Methocarbamol *on page* 1387
- ◆ **Robidrine® (Can)** *see* Pseudoephedrine *on page* 1801
- ◆ **Robinul** *see* Glycopyrrolate *on page* 979
- ◆ **Robinul-Forte** *see* Glycopyrrolate *on page* 979
- ◆ **Robitussin® (Can)** *see* GuaiFENesin *on page* 988
- ◆ **Robitussin AC** *see* Guaifenesin and Codeine *on page* 990
- ◆ **Robitussin Chest Congestion [OTC]** *see* GuaiFENesin *on page* 988
- ◆ **Robitussin Childrens Cough LA [OTC]** *see* Dextromethorphan *on page* 631
- ◆ **Robitussin CoughGels [OTC]** *see* Dextromethorphan *on page* 631
- ◆ **Robitussin Lingering CoughGels [OTC]** *see* Dextromethorphan *on page* 631
- ◆ **Robitussin Lingering LA Cough [OTC]** *see* Dextromethorphan *on page* 631
- ◆ **Robitussin Maximum Strength [OTC]** *see* Dextromethorphan *on page* 631
- ◆ **Robitussin Maximum Strength Cough + Congestion DM [OTC]** *see* Guaifenesin and Dextromethorphan *on page* 992
- ◆ **Robitussin Mucus+Chest Congest [OTC]** *see* GuaiFENesin *on page* 988
- ◆ **Robitussin Peak Cold Cough + Chest Congestion DM [OTC]** *see* Guaifenesin and Dextromethorphan *on page* 992
- ◆ **Robitussin Peak Cold Maximum Strength Cough + Chest Congestion DM [OTC]** *see* Guaifenesin and Dextromethorphan *on page* 992
- ◆ **Robitussin Peak Cold Sugar-Free Cough + Chest Congestion DM [OTC]** *see* Guaifenesin and Dextromethorphan *on page* 992
- ◆ **Rocaltrol** *see* Calcitriol *on page* 338
- ◆ **Rocephin** *see* CefTRIAXone *on page* 410

Rocuronium (roe kyoor OH nee um)

Medication Safety Issues

Sound-alike/look-alike issues:

Zemuron may be confused with Remeron

High alert medication:

The Institute for Safe Medication Practices (ISMP) includes this medication among its list of drugs which have a heightened risk of causing significant patient harm when used in error.

Other safety concerns:

United States Pharmacopeia (USP) 2006: The Interdisciplinary Safe Medication Use Expert Committee of the USP has recommended the following:

- Hospitals, clinics, and other practice sites should institute special safeguards in the storage, labeling, and use of these agents and should include these safeguards in staff orientation and competency training.
- Healthcare professionals should be on high alert (especially vigilant) whenever a neuromuscular-blocking agent (NMBA) is stocked, ordered, prepared, or administered.

Brand Names: US Zemuron

Brand Names: Canada Rocuronium Bromide Injection; Zemuron

Therapeutic Category Neuromuscular Blocker Agent, Nondepolarizing; Skeletal Muscle Relaxant, Paralytic

Generic Availability (US) Yes

Use Adjunct to general anesthesia, to facilitate endotracheal intubation, and provide skeletal muscle relaxation during surgery or mechanical ventilation (FDA approved in all ages); to facilitate rapid sequence intubation (FDA approved in adults)

Pregnancy Risk Factor C

Pregnancy Considerations Teratogenic effects were not observed in animal reproduction studies. Rocuronium crosses the placenta; umbilical venous plasma levels are ~18% of the maternal concentration following a maternal dose of 0.6 mg/kg (Abouleish, 1994). The manufacturer does not recommend use for rapid sequence induction during cesarean section.

Breast-Feeding Considerations Information related to rocuronium use and breast-feeding has not been located. If present in breast milk, oral absorption by a nursing infant would be expected to be minimal (Lee, 1993).

Contraindications Hypersensitivity (eg, anaphylaxis) to rocuronium, other neuromuscular-blocking agents, or any component of the formulation

Warnings/Precautions Use with caution in patients with cardiovascular disease and pulmonary disease; ventilation must be supported during neuromuscular blockade; certain clinical conditions may result in potentiation or antagonism of neuromuscular blockade:

Potentiation: Electrolyte abnormalities (eg, severe hypocalcemia, severe hypokalemia, hypermagnesemia), cachexia, neuromuscular diseases, metabolic acidosis, metabolic alkalosis, respiratory acidosis, Eaton-Lambert syndrome, and myasthenia gravis

Antagonism: Respiratory alkalosis, hypercalcemia, demyelinating lesions, peripheral neuropathies, denervation, and muscle trauma

Use with caution in patients with hepatic impairment; clinical duration may be prolonged. Resistance may occur in burn patients (≥20% of total body surface area), usually several days after the injury, and may persist for several months after wound healing. Cross-sensitivity with other neuromuscular-blocking agents may occur; use is contraindicated in patients with previous anaphylactic reactions to other neuromuscular blockers. Use with caution in patients with pulmonary hypertension or valvular heart disease. Use caution in the elderly. Should be administered by adequately trained individuals familiar with its use. Use appropriate anesthesia, pain control, and sedation. In patients requiring long-term administration in the ICU, tolerance to rocuronium may develop; use of a peripheral nerve stimulator to monitor drug effects is strongly recommended. Additional doses of rocuronium or any other neuromuscular-blocking agent should be avoided unless definite excessive response to nerve stimulation is present.

Some patients may experience prolonged recovery of neuromuscular function after administration (especially after prolonged use). Patients should be adequately recovered prior to extubation. Other factors associated with prolonged recovery should be considered (eg, corticosteroid use, patient condition). In addition to prolonging recovery from neuromuscular blockade, concomitant use with corticosteroids has been associated with development of acute quadriplegic myopathy syndrome (AQMS). Current guidelines recommend neuromuscular blockers be discontinued as soon as possible in patients receiving corticosteroids or interrupted daily until necessary to restart them based on clinical condition (Murray, 2002). Numerous drugs either *antagonize* (eg, acetylcholinesterase inhibitors) or *potentiate* (eg, calcium channel blockers, certain antimicrobials, inhalation anesthetics, lithium, magnesium salts, procainamide, and quinidine) the effects of neuromuscular blockade; use with caution in patients receiving these agents. Immediate treatment (including epinephrine 1:1000) for anaphylactoid and/or hypersensitivity reactions should be available during use. Not recommended by the manufacturer for rapid sequence intubation in pediatric patients; however, it has been used successfully in clinical trials for this indication. If extravasation occurs, local irritation may ensue; discontinue administration immediately and restart in another vein.

Adverse Reactions

Cardiovascular: Increased peripheral vascular resistance (abdominal aortic surgery: 24%, frequency not defined during other procedures), tachycardia (≤5%; incidence greater in children), hypertension, transient hypotension

Hypersensitivity: Anaphylaxis

Rare but important or life-threatening: Anaphylactoid reaction, asthma, cardiac arrhythmia, ECG abnormality, hiccups, injection site edema, nausea, vomiting

Drug Interactions

Metabolism/Transport Effects None known.

Avoid Concomitant Use

Avoid concomitant use of Rocuronium with any of the following: QuiNINE

Increased Effect/Toxicity

Rocuronium may increase the levels/effects of: Cardiac Glycosides; Corticosteroids (Systemic); OnabotulinumtoxinA; RimabotulinumtoxinB

The levels/effects of Rocuronium may be increased by: AbobotulinumtoxinA; Aminoglycosides; Calcium Channel Blockers; Capreomycin; Clindamycin (Topical); Colistimethate; CycloSPORINE (Systemic); Fosphenytoin-Phenytoin; Inhalational Anesthetics; Ketorolac (Nasal); Ketorolac (Systemic); Lincosamide Antibiotics; Lithium; Loop Diuretics; Magnesium Salts; Polymyxin B; Procainamide; QuiNIDine; QuiNINE; Spironolactone; Tetracycline Derivatives; Vancomycin

Decreased Effect

The levels/effects of Rocuronium may be decreased by: Acetylcholinesterase Inhibitors; Fosphenytoin-Phenytoin; Loop Diuretics

Storage/Stability Store unopened/undiluted vials under refrigeration at 2°C to 8°C (36°F to 46°F); do not freeze. When stored at room temperature (25°C [77°F]), it is stable for 60 days; once opened, use within 30 days. Dilutions up to 5 mg/mL in 0.9% sodium chloride, dextrose 5% in water, 5% dextrose in sodium chloride 0.9%, or lactated Ringer's are stable for up to 24 hours at room temperature.

Mechanism of Action Blocks acetylcholine from binding to receptors on motor endplate inhibiting depolarization

Pharmacodynamics

Maximum effect:
- Infants ≥3 months and Children: 30 seconds to 1 minute
- Adults: 1-3.7 minutes

Duration:
- Infants: 3-12 months: 40 minutes
- Children: 1-12 years: 26-30 minutes
- Adults: 20-94 minutes (dose-related) (most prolonged in elderly ≥65 years of age)

Pharmacokinetics (Adult data unless noted)

Distribution: V_d:
- Children: 0.21-0.3 L/kg
- Adults: 0.22-0.26 L/kg
  - Hepatic dysfunction: 0.53 L/kg
  - Renal dysfunction: 0.34 L/kg

Protein binding: ~30%

Half-life:
- Alpha elimination: 1-2 minutes
- Beta elimination:
  - Infants 3-12 months: 1.3 ± 0.5 hours
  - Children 1 to <3 years: 1.1 ± 0.7 hours
  - Children 3 to <8 years: 0.8 ± 0.3 hours
  - Adults: 1.4-2.4 hours
  - Hepatic dysfunction: 4.3 hours
  - Renal dysfunction: 2.4 hours

Elimination: Primarily biliary excretion (70%); up to 30% of dose excreted unchanged in urine

Clearance: Pediatric patients:
- Infants 3 to <12 months: 0.35 L/kg/hour
- Children 1 to <3 years: 0.32 L/kg/hour
- Children 3 to <8 years: 0.44 L/kg/hour

Dosing: Neonatal Note: Dose to effect; doses will vary due to interpatient variability. Dosing also dependent on anesthetic technique and age of patient. In general, the onset of effect is shortened and duration is prolonged as the dose increases. The time to maximum nerve block is longest in neonates.

Tracheal intubation, surgical:

Initial: IV: 0.45-0.6 mg/kg

Maintenance for continued surgical relaxation:
- IV: 0.075-0.15 mg/kg; dosing interval as determined by monitoring
- Continuous IV infusion: 7-10 **mcg**/kg/minute

Dosing: Usual Note: Dose to effect; doses will vary due to interpatient variability. Dosing also dependent on anesthetic technique and age of patient. The manufacturer recommends dosing based on actual body weight in all obese patients; however, may use ideal body weight (IBW) for morbidly obese (BMI >40 kg/m^2) adult patients (Leykin, 2004); onset time may be slightly delayed using IBW. In general, the onset of effect is shortened and duration is prolonged as the dose increases. The time to maximum nerve block is shortest in infants 1-3 months; the duration of relaxation is shortest in children 2-11 years and longest in infants.

Rapid sequence intubation: Children, Adolescents, and Adults: IV: 0.6-1.2 mg/kg; (Cheng, 2002; Fuchs-Buder, 1996; Mazurek, 1998; Naguib, 1997)

Tracheal intubation, surgical: Infants, Children, Adolescents, and Adults: **Note:** Inhaled anesthetic agents prolong the duration of action of rocuronium; use lower end of the dosing range; dosing interval guided by monitoring with a peripheral nerve stimulator.

Initial:
- IV: 0.45-0.6 mg/kg
- IM (Kaplan, 1999):
  - Infants ≥3 months: 1 mg/kg administered as a single dose

Children 1-6 years: 1.8 mg/kg administered as a single dose

Maintenance for continued surgical relaxation:

IV:

Infants, Children, and Adolescents: 0.075-0.15 mg/kg; repeat as needed

Adults: 0.1-0.2 mg/kg; repeat as needed

Continuous IV infusion:

Infants, Children, and Adolescents: 7-12 **mcg**/kg/minute; use the lower end of dosing range for infants and upper end for children >2 to ≤11 years of age

Adults: 4-16 mcg/kg/minute

Preparation for Administration Continuous IV infusion: Dilute with NS, D_5W, D_5NS or LR to a final concentration of 0.5 to 5 mg/mL; use within 24 hours of preparation

Administration Parenteral: IV: May be administered undiluted by rapid IV injection; or further diluted and infused as a continuous IV infusion

Monitoring Parameters Peripheral nerve stimulator measuring twitch response, heart rate, blood pressure, assisted ventilation status

Dosage Forms Excipient information presented when available (limited, particularly for generics); consult specific product labeling.

Solution, Intravenous, as bromide:

Zemuron: 50 mg/5 mL (5 mL); 100 mg/10 mL (10 mL)

Generic: 50 mg/5 mL (5 mL); 100 mg/10 mL (10 mL)

Solution, Intravenous, as bromide [preservative free]:

Generic: 50 mg/5 mL (5 mL); 100 mg/10 mL (10 mL)

- **Rocuronium Bromide** *see* Rocuronium *on page 1881*
- **Rocuronium Bromide Injection (Can)** *see* Rocuronium *on page 1881*
- **Rofact (Can)** *see* Rifampin *on page 1858*
- **Rogitine (Can)** *see* Phentolamine *on page 1684*
- **Rolene (Can)** *see* Betamethasone (Topical) *on page 280*
- **Romazicon (Can)** *see* Flumazenil *on page 892*
- **Romycin [DSC]** *see* Erythromycin (Ophthalmic) *on page 782*

Ropivacaine (roe PIV a kane)

Medication Safety Issues

Sound-alike/look-alike issues:

Ropivacaine may be confused with bupivacaine, rOPINIRole

Infusion bottles of Naropin (ropivacaine) and Ofirmev (acetaminophen) look similar. Potentially fatal mix-ups have been reported in which a glass bottle of Naropin was mistaken for Ofirmev in perioperative areas.

High alert medication:

The Institute for Safe Medication Practices (ISMP) includes this medication (epidural administration) among its list of drug classes which have a heightened risk of causing significant patient harm when used in error.

Brand Names: US Naropin

Brand Names: Canada Naropin; Ropivacaine Hydrochloride Injection, USP

Therapeutic Category Local Anesthetic, Injectable

Generic Availability (US) Yes

Use Production of local or regional anesthesia for surgery, obstetrical procedures, and for acute pain management: peripheral nerve block, local infiltration, sympathetic block, caudal or epidural block

Pregnancy Risk Factor B

Pregnancy Considerations Teratogenic events were not observed in animal studies. When used for epidural block during labor and delivery, systemically absorbed ropivacaine may cross the placenta, resulting in varying degrees of fetal or neonatal effects (eg, CNS or cardiovascular depression). Fetal or neonatal adverse events include fetal bradycardia (12%), neonatal jaundice (8%), low Apgar scores (3%), fetal distress (2%), neonatal respiratory disorder (3%). Maternal hypotension may also result from systemic absorption. In cases of hypotension, position pregnant woman in left lateral decubitus position to prevent aortocaval compression by the gravid uterus. Epidural anesthesia may prolong the second stage of labor.

Breast-Feeding Considerations It is not known if ropivacaine is excreted into breast milk; however, exposure to a nursing infant is expected to be low. The manufacturer recommends that caution be exercised when administering ropivacaine to nursing women.

Contraindications

Hypersensitivity to ropivacaine, amide-type local anesthetics (eg, bupivacaine, mepivacaine, lidocaine), or any component of the formulation

Canadian labeling: Additional contraindications (not in US labeling): Intravenous regional anesthesia (Bier block); obstetric paracervical block anesthesia

Warnings/Precautions Careful and constant monitoring of the patient's state of consciousness should be done following each local anesthetic injection; at such times, restlessness, anxiety, tinnitus, dizziness, blurred vision, tremors, depression, or drowsiness may be early warning signs of CNS toxicity. Treatment is primarily symptomatic and supportive. Intravascular injections should be avoided. Continuous intra-articular infusion of local anesthetics after arthroscopic or other surgical procedures is **not** an approved use; chondrolysis (primarily in the shoulder joint) has occurred following infusion, with some cases requiring arthroplasty or shoulder replacement. Local anesthetics have been associated with rare occurrences of sudden respiratory arrest, seizures, and cardiac arrest. When administering this agent, have ready access to drugs and equipment for resuscitation. Use with caution in patients with liver disease, severe renal impairment, cardiovascular disease, neurological or psychiatric disorders, acute porphyria, and in the elderly or debilitated; these patients may be at greater risk for toxicity. Cardiovascular adverse events (bradycardia, hypotension) may be age-related (more common in patients >61 years of age). Use caution in patients on type III antiarrhythmics (eg, amiodarone); consider ECG monitoring since cardiac effects may be additive. Use cautiously in hypotension, hypovolemia, or heart block. Ropivacaine is not recommended for use in emergency situations where rapid administration is necessary. Potentially significant drug-drug interactions may exist, requiring dose or frequency adjustment, additional monitoring, and/or selection of alternative therapy.

Adverse Reactions

Cardiovascular: Bradycardia, chest pain, hypo- or hypertension, tachycardia

Central nervous system: Anxiety, chills, dizziness, headache, lightheadedness

Dermatologic: Pruritus

Endocrine & metabolic: Hypokalemia

Gastrointestinal: Nausea, vomiting

Hematologic: Anemia

Neuromuscular & skeletal: Back pain, circumoral paresthesia, hypoesthesia, rigors, paresthesia

Renal: Oliguria

Respiratory: Dyspnea

Miscellaneous: Shivering

Rare but important or life-threatening: Angioedema, apnea (usually associated with epidural block in head/neck region), bronchospasm, cardiac arrest, cardiovascular collapse, chondrolysis (continuous intra-articular administration), dyskinesia, hallucinations, hyperthermia, myocardial depression, MI, rash, seizure, syncope, tinnitus, ventricular arrhythmia

Drug Interactions

Metabolism/Transport Effects Substrate of CYP1A2 (major), CYP2B6 (minor), CYP2D6 (minor), CYP3A4 (minor); **Note:** Assignment of Major/Minor substrate status based on clinically relevant drug interaction potential

Avoid Concomitant Use There are no known interactions where it is recommended to avoid concomitant use.

Increased Effect/Toxicity

The levels/effects of Ropivacaine may be increased by: Abiraterone Acetate; Ciprofloxacin (Systemic); CYP1A2 Inhibitors (Moderate); CYP1A2 Inhibitors (Strong); Deferasirox; FluvoxaMINE; Hyaluronidase; Peginterferon Alfa-2b; Propofol; Vemurafenib

Decreased Effect

Ropivacaine may decrease the levels/effects of: Technetium Tc 99m Tilmanocept

Storage/Stability Store at 20°C to 25°C (68°F to 77°F). Infusions should be discarded after 24 hours.

Mechanism of Action Blocks both the initiation and conduction of nerve impulses by decreasing the neuronal membrane's permeability to sodium ions, which results in inhibition of depolarization with resultant blockade of conduction

Pharmacodynamics

Onset of anesthetic action (dependent on dose and route of administration):
- Epidural block (100-200 mg): T10 sensory block: 10 minutes (range: 5-13 minutes)
- Epidural block, Cesarean section (up to 150 mg): T6 sensory block: 11-26 minutes

Duration (dependent upon dose and route of administration):
- Epidural block (100-200 mg): 4 hours (range: 3-5 hours)
- Epidural block, Cesarean section (up to 150 mg):
  - Sensory block: 1.7-3.2 hours
  - Motor block: 1.4-2.9 hours

Pharmacokinetics (Adult data unless noted)

Absorption: Well absorbed systemically in a biphasic manner following epidural administration; addition of epinephrine has no affect on the absorption of ropivacaine

Distribution: Distributes into breast milk
- V_d (after intravascular infusion):
  - Children: 2.1-4.2 L/kg
  - Adults: 41 ± 7 L

Protein binding: 94%

Metabolism: In the liver via cytochrome P450 isoenzyme, predominantly CYP1A2 and CYP3A4 (10 metabolites with 2 active)

Bioavailability: 87% to 98% (epidural)

Half-life:
- Epidural: Terminal phase:
  - Children: 4.9 hours (range: 3-6.7 hours)
  - Adults: 4.2 ± 1 hour
- IV: Adults: 1.9 ± 0.5 hours

Time to peak serum concentration (dose and route dependent):
- Caudal (children): 0.33-2.05 hours
- Cesarean section: 14-65 minutes
- Epidural (adults): 17-97 minutes

Elimination: 1% to 2% excreted unchanged in urine

Dosing: Usual Dose varies with procedure, depth of anesthesia, vascularity of tissues, duration of anesthesia, and condition of patient

Caudal block: Children (limited data): 2 mg/kg

Epidural block (other than caudal block): Children: 1.7 mg/kg

Lumbar epidural surgery: Adults: 75-150 mg (15-30 mL 0.5%); maximum: 200 mg (40 mL 0.5%)

Lumbar epidural Cesarean section: Adults: 100-150 mg (20-30 mL 0.5% **or** 15-20 mL 0.75%)

Thoracic epidural surgery: Adults: 25-75 mg (5-15 mL 0.5%)

Epidural continuous infusion:
- Children 4 months to 7 years (limited data) (Hansen 2000): 1 mg/kg loading dose followed by 0.4 mg/kg/hour continuous **epidural** infusion
- Adults: 10-14 mg loading dose (5-7 mL 0.2%) followed by 12-28 mg/hour (6-14 mL/hour 0.2%) continuous **epidural** infusion

Major nerve block (eg, brachial plexus block): Adults: 75-300 mg (10-40 mL 0.75%)

Minor nerve block and infiltration: Adults: 5-200 mg (1-40 mL 0.5%)

Administration Parenteral: Administer in small incremental doses; when using continuous intermittent catheter techniques, use frequent aspirations before and during the injection to avoid intravascular injection

Monitoring Parameters After epidural or subarachnoid administration: Blood pressure, heart rate, respiration, signs of CNS toxicity (lightheadedness, dizziness, tinnitus, restlessness, tremors, twitching, drowsiness, circumoral paresthesia)

Dosage Forms Excipient information presented when available (limited, particularly for generics); consult specific product labeling.

Solution, Injection, as hydrochloride [preservative free]:
- Naropin: 2 mg/mL (10 mL, 20 mL, 100 mL, 200 mL); 5 mg/mL (20 mL, 30 mL, 100 mL, 200 mL); 7.5 mg/mL (20 mL); 10 mg/mL (10 mL, 20 mL)
- Generic: 2 mg/mL (10 mL, 20 mL); 5 mg/mL (30 mL); 7.5 mg/mL (20 mL); 10 mg/mL (10 mL, 20 mL)

◆ **Ropivacaine Hydrochloride** *see* Ropivacaine *on page 1883*

◆ **Ropivacaine Hydrochloride Injection, USP (Can)** *see* Ropivacaine *on page 1883*

◆ **Rosadan** *see* MetroNIDAZOLE (Topical) *on page 1425*

◆ **Rosasol (Can)** *see* MetroNIDAZOLE (Topical) *on page 1425*

Rosiglitazone (roh si GLI ta zone)

Medication Safety Issues

Sound-alike/look-alike issues:

Avandia may be confused with Avalide, Coumadin, Prandin

High alert medication:

The Institute for Safe Medication Practices (ISMP) includes this medication among its list of drug classes which have a heightened risk of causing significant patient harm when used in error.

International issues:

Avandia [US, Canada, and multiple international markets] may be confused with Avanza brand name for mirtazapine [Australia]

Brand Names: US Avandia

Brand Names: Canada Avandia

Therapeutic Category Antidiabetic Agent, Oral; Antidiabetic Agent, Thiazolidinedione

Generic Availability (US) No

Use Adjunct treatment of type 2 diabetes mellitus (non-insulin-dependent, NIDDM) to improve glycemic control in patients who do not achieve control with diet and exercise alone or diet and exercise in combination with diabetic medication and for whom pioglitazone therapy is not an option (FDA approved in adults)

Prescribing and Access Restrictions Health Canada requires written informed consent for new and current patients receiving rosiglitazone.

Medication Guide Available Yes

Pregnancy Risk Factor C

Pregnancy Considerations Adverse effects were observed in initial animal reproduction studies.

Rosiglitazone has been found to cross the placenta during the first trimester of pregnancy. Inadvertent use early in pregnancy has not been shown to increase the risk of adverse fetal effects, although in the majority of cases, the medication was stopped as soon as pregnancy was detected (Chan 2005; Kalyoncu 2005; Yaris 2004).

Thiazolidinediones may cause ovulation in anovulatory premenopausal women, increasing the risk of pregnancy. Adequate contraception in premenopausal women is recommended. Due to long-term safety concerns associated with their use, thiazolidinediones should be avoided in women of reproductive age (Fauser 2012).

In women with diabetes, maternal hyperglycemia can be associated with congenital malformations as well as adverse effects in the fetus, neonate, and the mother (ACOG 2005; ADA 2015; Kitzmiller 2008; Metzger 2007). To prevent adverse outcomes, prior to conception and throughout pregnancy maternal blood glucose and HbA_{1c} should be kept as close to target goals as possible but without causing significant hypoglycemia (ACOG 2013; ADA 2015; Blumer 2013; Kitzmiller 2008). Prior to pregnancy, effective contraception should be used until glycemic control is achieved (Kitzmiller 2008)

Other agents are currently recommended to treat diabetes in pregnant women (ACOG 2013; Blumer 2013); rosiglitazone should not be used for the treatment of PCOS (Legro 2013).

Breast-Feeding Considerations It is not known if rosiglitazone is excreted in breast milk. Although breast-feeding is encouraged for all women, including those with diabetes, the safety of rosiglitazone during breast-feeding has not yet been established (Metzger 2007). The manufacturer recommends a decision be made whether to discontinue nursing or to discontinue the drug, taking into account the importance of treatment to the mother.

Contraindications

US labeling: Hypersensitivity to rosiglitazone or any component of the formulation; NYHA Class III/IV heart failure (initiation of therapy)

Canadian labeling: Hypersensitivity to rosiglitazone or any component of the formulation; any stage of heart failure (eg, NYHA Class I, II, III, IV); serious hepatic impairment; pregnancy

Warnings/Precautions [US Boxed Warning]: Thiazolidinediones, including rosiglitazone, may cause or exacerbate congestive heart failure; closely monitor for signs/symptoms of congestive heart failure (eg, rapid weight gain, dyspnea, edema), particularly after initiation or dose increases. If heart failure develops, treat accordingly and consider dose reduction or discontinuation. Not recommended for use in any patient with symptomatic heart failure. In the US, initiation of therapy is contraindicated in patients with NYHA class III or IV heart failure; in Canada use is contraindicated in patients with any stage of heart failure (NYHA class I, II, III, IV). Use with caution in patients with edema; may increase plasma volume and/or cause fluid retention, leading to heart failure. Monitor for signs/symptoms of heart failure. Dose-related weight gain observed with use; mechanism unknown but likely associated with fluid retention and fat accumulation. Use may also be associated with an increased risk of angina and MI. Use caution in patients at risk for cardiovascular events and monitor closely. Discontinue if any deterioration in cardiac status occurs.

The risk of hypoglycemia is increased when rosiglitazone is combined with other hypoglycemic agents; dosage adjustment of concomitant hypoglycemic agents may be necessary. Monitor blood glucose and HbA1c as clinically necessary. Should not be used in diabetic ketoacidosis. Mechanism requires the presence of endogenous insulin; therefore, use in type 1 diabetes (insulin dependent, IDDM) is not recommended. Use with insulin is not recommended; may increase the risk of heart failure. It may be necessary to discontinue therapy and administer insulin if the patient is exposed to stress (fever, trauma, infection, surgery). Do not initiate in patients with stable ischemic heart disease due to an increased risk of cardiovascular complications (Fihn 2012).

Potentially significant drug-drug interactions may exist, requiring dose or frequency adjustment, additional monitoring, and/or selection of alternative therapy.

Use with caution in patients with elevated transaminases (AST or ALT); do not initiate in patients with active liver disease or ALT >2.5 times ULN at baseline; evaluate patients with ALT ≤2.5 times ULN at baseline or during therapy for cause of enzyme elevation; during therapy, if ALT >3 times ULN, reevaluate levels promptly and discontinue if elevation persists or if jaundice occurs at any time during use. Idiosyncratic hepatotoxicity has been reported with another thiazolidinedione agent (troglitazone); avoid use in patients who previously experienced jaundice during troglitazone therapy. Increased incidence of bone fractures in females treated with rosiglitazone was observed during analysis of long-term trial; majority of fractures occurred in the upper arm, hand, and foot (differing from the hip or spine fractures usually associated with postmenopausal osteoporosis). According to the American Diabetes Association guidelines, thiazolidinediones should be avoided in patients with fracture risk factors (ADA 2015). May decrease hemoglobin/hematocrit and/or WBC count (slight); effects may be related to increased plasma volume and/or dose related. Changes in hemoglobin and hematocrit generally occurred during the first 3 months after initiation of therapy and after dose increases. Use with caution in patients with anemia.

Macular edema has been reported with thiazolidinedione use, including rosiglitazone; some patients with macular edema presented with blurred vision or decreased visual acuity, and most had peripheral edema at time of diagnosis. In addition, ophthalmological consultation should be initiated in these patients. Improvement in macular edema may occur with discontinuation of therapy. Use with caution in premenopausal, anovulatory women; may result in resumption of ovulation, increasing the risk of pregnancy. Use of adequate contraception in premenopausal women is recommended.

Additional Canadian warnings (not included in US labeling): If glycemic control is inadequate, rosiglitazone may be added to metformin or a sulfonylurea (if metformin use is contraindicated or not tolerated); use of triple therapy (rosiglitazone in combination with both metformin and a sulfonylurea) is not indicated due to increased risks of heart failure and fluid retention.

Adverse Reactions Note: As reported in monotherapy studies. Rare cases of hepatocellular injury have been reported in men in their 60s within 2 to 3 weeks after initiation of rosiglitazone therapy. LFTs in these patients revealed severe hepatocellular injury which responded with rapid improvement of liver function and resolution of symptoms upon discontinuation of rosiglitazone. Patients were also receiving other potentially hepatotoxic medications (Al-Salman, 2000; Freid, 2000).

Cardiovascular: Cardiac failure (incidence likely higher in patients with pre-existing cardiac failure), edema, hypertension, ischemic heart disease (incidence likely higher in patients with pre-existing CAD)

Central nervous system: Headache

Endocrine & metabolic: hypoglycemia, increased HDL cholesterol, increased LDL cholesterol, increased serum cholesterol (total), weight gain

Gastrointestinal: Diarrhea

Hematologic & oncologic: Anemia

Neuromuscular & skeletal: Arthralgia, back pain, bone fracture (incidence greater in females; usually upper arm, hand, or foot)

Respiratory: Nasopharyngitis, upper respiratory tract infection

Miscellaneous: Trauma

Rare but important or life-threatening: Anaphylaxis, angina pectoris, angioedema, cardiac arrest, coronary artery disease, coronary thrombosis, decreased HDL cholesterol, decreased hematocrit, decreased hemoglobin, decreased visual acuity, decreased white blood cell count, dyspnea, hepatic failure, hepatitis, increased serum bilirubin, increased serum transaminases, jaundice (reversible), macular edema, myocardial infarction, pleural effusion, pulmonary edema, Stevens-Johnson syndrome, thrombocytopenia, weight gain (rapid, excessive; usually due to fluid accumulation)

Drug Interactions

Metabolism/Transport Effects Substrate of CYP2C8 (major), CYP2C9 (minor); **Note:** Assignment of Major/Minor substrate status based on clinically relevant drug interaction potential; **Inhibits** CYP2C19 (weak), CYP2C8 (moderate), CYP2C9 (weak)

Avoid Concomitant Use

Avoid concomitant use of Rosiglitazone with any of the following: Amodiaquine; Insulin

Increased Effect/Toxicity

Rosiglitazone may increase the levels/effects of: Amodiaquine; CYP2C8 Substrates; Hypoglycemia-Associated Agents; Sulfonylureas

The levels/effects of Rosiglitazone may be increased by: Abiraterone Acetate; Alpha-Lipoic Acid; Androgens; Atazanavir; CYP2C8 Inhibitors (Moderate); CYP2C8 Inhibitors (Strong); Deferasirox; Gemfibrozil; Insulin; MAO Inhibitors; Mifepristone; Pegvisomant; Pregabalin; Quinolone Antibiotics; Salicylates; Selective Serotonin Reuptake Inhibitors; Trimethoprim; Vasodilators (Organic Nitrates)

Decreased Effect

The levels/effects of Rosiglitazone may be decreased by: Cholestyramine Resin; CYP2C8 Inducers (Strong); Dabrafenib; Hyperglycemia-Associated Agents; Quinolone Antibiotics; Rifampin; Thiazide Diuretics

Storage/Stability Store at 25°C (77°F); excursions are permitted between 15°C and 30°C (59°F and 86°F). Protect from light.

Mechanism of Action Thiazolidinedione antidiabetic agent that lowers blood glucose by improving target cell response to insulin, without increasing pancreatic insulin secretion. It has a mechanism of action that is dependent on the presence of insulin for activity. Rosiglitazone is an agonist for peroxisome proliferator-activated receptor-gamma (PPARgamma). Activation of nuclear PPAR-gamma receptors influences the production of a number of gene products involved in glucose and lipid metabolism. PPARgamma is abundant in the cells within the renal collecting tubules; fluid retention results from stimulation by thiazolidinediones which increases sodium reabsorption.

Pharmacodynamics Maximum effect: Up to 12 weeks

Pharmacokinetics (Adult data unless noted)

Distribution: V_{dss} (apparent): 17.6 L

Protein binding: 99.8%; primarily albumin

Metabolism: Hepatic (99%), metabolism by cytochrome P450 isoenzyme CYP2C8, minor metabolism via CYP2C9

Bioavailability: 99%

Half-life: 3-4 hours

Time to peak serum concentration: 1 hour, delayed with food

Elimination: Urine (64%) and feces (23%) as metabolites

Dosing: Usual Type 2 diabetes:

Children ≥10 years and Adolescents: Limited data available: Oral: Initial: 2 mg twice daily; then increase to 4 mg twice daily after 8 weeks; in combination with metformin; dosing presented was used 233 pediatric patients as part of a larger multicenter comparative trial of treatments (n=699) and results showed rosiglitazone and metformin more effective than other treatment arms (ie, metformin alone or metformin and lifestyle changes) at maintaining glycemic control (Copeland, 2011; The TODAY Study Group, 2007; The TODAY Study Group, 2012).

Adults: **Note:** All patients should be initiated at the lowest recommended dose:

Monotherapy: Oral: Initial: 4 mg as a single daily dose or in divided doses twice daily; if response is inadequate after 8-12 weeks of treatment the dosage may be increased to 8 mg daily as a single daily dose or in divided doses twice daily

Combination therapy (with sulfonylureas, metformin, or sulfonylurea plus metformin): Oral: Initial: 4 mg daily as a single daily dose or in divided doses twice daily. If response is inadequate after 8-12 weeks of treatment, the dosage may be increased to 8 mg daily as a single daily dose or in divided doses twice daily. Reduce dose of sulfonylurea if hypoglycemia occurs. It is unlikely that the dose of metformin will need to be reduced due to hypoglycemia.

Dosage adjustment in renal impairment: No dosage adjustment is required

Dosage adjustment in hepatic impairment: Clearance is significantly lower in hepatic impairment. Therapy should not be initiated if the patient exhibits active liver disease or increased transaminases (>2.5 times the upper limit of normal) at baseline

Administration Oral: May be taken without regard to meals

Monitoring Parameters Signs and symptoms of hypoglycemia, fluid retention, or heart failure, fasting blood glucose, hemoglobin A_{1c}; liver enzymes: Baseline, every 2 months for the first 12 months of therapy, and periodically thereafter; patients with an elevation in ALT >3 times the upper limit of normal should be rechecked as soon as possible; if the ALT levels remain >3 times the upper limit of normal, therapy with rosiglitazone should be discontinued; ophthalmic exams

Reference Range Indicators of optimal glycemic control in children and adolescents (IDF/ISPAD, 2011; Rewers, 2009): **Note:** Targets must be adjusted based on individual needs/circumstances (eg, patients who experience severe hypoglycemia, patients with hypoglycemic unawareness):

Blood glucose:

Fasting/Preprandial: 90-145 mg/dL

Postprandial: 90-180 mg/dL

Bedtime: 120-180 mg/dL

Hb A_{1C}: <7.5%

Dosage Forms Excipient information presented when available (limited, particularly for generics); consult specific product labeling.

Tablet, Oral:

Avandia: 2 mg, 4 mg, 8 mg

◆ **Rosone (Can)** *see* Betamethasone (Topical) *on page 280*

Rosuvastatin (roe soo va STAT in)

Medication Safety Issues

Sound-alike/look-alike issues:

Rosuvastatin may be confused with atorvaSTATin, nystatin, pitavastatin

Brand Names: US Crestor

Brand Names: Canada Apo-Rosuvastatin; CO Rosuvastatin; Crestor; Dom-Rosuvastatin; Jamp-Rosuvastatin;

Med-Rosuvastatin; Mint-Rosuvastatin; Mylan-Rosuvastatin; PMS-Rosuvastatin; RAN-Rosuvastatin; Riva-Rosuvastatin; Sandoz-Rosuvastatin; Teva-Rosuvastatin

Therapeutic Category Antilipemic Agent, HMG-CoA Reductase Inhibitor

Generic Availability (US) No

Use Adjunct to dietary therapy to reduce elevated total-C, LDL-C, and apo-B levels in patients with heterozygous familial hypercholesterolemia (HeFH) [FDA approved in ages 10-17 years (girls ≥1 year postmenarche)]. Adjunct to dietary therapy for hyperlipidemias to reduce elevations in total cholesterol (TC), LDL-C, apo-B, nonHDL-C, and triglycerides (TG) in patients with primary hypercholesterolemia (elevations of 1 or more components are present in Fredrickson type IIa, IIb, and IV hyperlipidemias) (FDA approved in adults); treatment of hypertriglyceridemia (FDA approved in adults); treatment of primary dysbetalipoproteinemia (Fredrickson type III hyperlipidemia) (FDA approved in adults); treatment of homozygous familial hypercholesterolemia (FH) (FDA approved in adults); to slow progression of atherosclerosis as an adjunct to diet to lower TC and LDL-C (FDA approved in adults)

Pregnancy Risk Factor X

Pregnancy Considerations Adverse events have been observed in some animal reproduction studies. There are reports of congenital anomalies following maternal use of HMG-CoA reductase inhibitors in pregnancy; however, maternal disease, differences in specific agents used, and the low rates of exposure limit the interpretation of the available data (Godfrey 2012; Lecarpentier 2012). Cholesterol biosynthesis may be important in fetal development; serum cholesterol and triglycerides increase normally during pregnancy. The discontinuation of lipid lowering medications temporarily during pregnancy is not expected to have significant impact on the long term outcomes of primary hypercholesterolemia treatment.

Use of rosuvastatin is contraindicated in pregnancy. HMG-CoA reductase inhibitors should be discontinued prior to pregnancy (ADA 2013). If treatment of dyslipidemias is needed in pregnant women or in women of reproductive age, other agents are preferred (Berglund 2012; Stone 2013). The manufacturer recommends administration to women of childbearing potential only when conception is highly unlikely and patients have been informed of potential hazards.

Breast-Feeding Considerations It is not known if rosuvastatin is excreted in breast milk. Due to the potential for serious adverse reactions in a nursing infant, use while breast-feeding is contraindicated by the manufacturer.

Contraindications

Known hypersensitivity to any component of the formulation; active liver disease or unexplained persistent elevations of serum transaminases; pregnancy; breast-feeding.

Canadian labeling: Additional contraindications (not in US labeling): Concomitant administration of cyclosporine; use of 40 mg dose in Asian patients, patients with predisposing risk factors for myopathy/rhabdomyolysis (eg, hereditary muscle disorders, history of myotoxicity with other HMG-CoA reductase inhibitors, concomitant use with fibrates or niacin, severe hepatic impairment, severe renal impairment [CrCl <30 mL/minute/1.73 m^2], hypothyroidism, alcohol abuse)

Warnings/Precautions Secondary causes of hyperlipidemia should be ruled out prior to therapy. Rosuvastatin has not been studied when the primary lipid abnormality is chylomicron elevation (Fredrickson types I and V). Postmarketing reports of fatal and nonfatal hepatic failure are rare. If serious hepatotoxicity with clinical symptoms and/or hyperbilirubinemia or jaundice occurs during treatment, interrupt therapy. If an alternate etiology is not identified, do not restart rosuvastatin. Liver enzyme tests should be obtained at baseline and as clinically indicated; routine periodic monitoring of liver enzymes is not necessary. Use with caution in patients who consume large amounts of ethanol or have a history of liver disease; use is contraindicated with active liver disease or unexplained transaminase elevations. Hematuria (microscopic) and proteinuria have been observed; more commonly reported in adults receiving rosuvastatin 40 mg daily, but typically transient and not associated with a decrease in renal function. Consider dosage reduction if unexplained hematuria and proteinuria persists. HMG-CoA reductase inhibitors may cause rhabdomyolysis with acute renal failure and/or myopathy. Discontinue in any patient in which CPK levels are markedly elevated (>10 times ULN) or if myopathy is suspected/diagnosed. This risk is dose-related and is increased with concurrent use of other lipid-lowering medications (fibric acid derivatives or niacin doses ≥1 g/day), other interacting drugs, drugs associated with myopathy (eg, colchicine), age ≥65 years, female gender, certain subgroups of Asian ancestry, uncontrolled hypothyroidism, and renal dysfunction. Dose reductions may be necessary. Immune-mediated necrotizing myopathy (IMNM), an autoimmune-mediated myopathy, has been reported (rarely) with HMG-CoA reductase inhibitor therapy. IMNM presents as proximal muscle weakness with elevated CPK levels, which persists despite discontinuation of HMG-CoA reductase inhibitor therapy; additionally, muscle biopsy may show necrotizing myopathy with limited inflammation; immunosuppressive therapy (eg, corticosteroids, azathioprine) may be useful for treatment.

The manufacturer recommends temporary discontinuation for elective major surgery, acute medical or surgical conditions, or in any patient experiencing an acute or serious condition predisposing to renal failure (eg, sepsis, dehydration, electrolyte disorders, hypotension, trauma, uncontrolled seizures). Based on current research and clinical guidelines (Fleisher 2009), HMG-CoA reductase inhibitors should be continued in the perioperative period. Patients should be instructed to report unexplained muscle pain, tenderness, weakness, or dark urine; in Canada, concomitant use with cyclosporine or niacin is contraindicated, and rosuvastatin at a dose of 40 mg/day in Asian patients is contraindicated. Small increases in HbA_{1c} (mean: ~0.1%) and fasting blood glucose have been reported with rosuvastatin; however, the benefits of statin therapy far outweigh the risk of dysglycemia.

Potentially significant interactions may exist, requiring dose or frequency adjustment, additional monitoring, and/or selection of alternative therapy. Consult drug interactions database for more detailed information. Dosage adjustment required in patients with a CrCl <30 mL/minute/1.73 m^2 and not receiving hemodialysis (contraindicated in the Canadian labeling. Use with caution in elderly patients as they are more predisposed to myopathy.

Adverse Reactions

Central nervous system: Dizziness, headache

Endocrine & metabolic: Diabetes mellitus (new onset)

Gastrointestinal: Abdominal pain, constipation, nausea

Hepatic: Increased serum ALT (>3 times ULN)

Neuromuscular & skeletal: Arthralgia, increased creatine phosphokinase, myalgia, weakness

Rare but important or life-threatening: Abnormal thyroid function test, cognitive dysfunction (reversible; includes amnesia, confusion, memory impairment), depression, elevated glycosylated hemoglobin (HbA_{1c}), gynecomastia, hematuria (microscopic), hepatic failure, hepatitis, hypersensitivity reaction (including angioedema, pruritus, skin rash, urticaria), immune-mediated necrotizing myopathy, increased gamma-glutamyl transferase, increased serum alkaline phosphatase, increased serum bilirubin, increased serum glucose, increased serum transaminases, jaundice, myoglobinuria, myopathy, myositis, pancreatitis, peripheral neuropathy, proteinuria (dose related), renal failure, rhabdomyolysis, sleep disorder (including insomnia and nightmares), thrombocytopenia

Drug Interactions

Metabolism/Transport Effects Substrate of CYP2C9 (minor), CYP3A4 (minor), SLCO1B1; **Note:** Assignment of Major/Minor substrate status based on clinically relevant drug interaction potential

Avoid Concomitant Use

Avoid concomitant use of Rosuvastatin with any of the following: Fusidic Acid (Systemic); Gemfibrozil; Ledipasvir; Red Yeast Rice

Increased Effect/Toxicity

Rosuvastatin may increase the levels/effects of: DAPTOmycin; PAZOPanib; Trabectedin; Vitamin K Antagonists

The levels/effects of Rosuvastatin may be increased by: Acipimox; Amiodarone; Bezafibrate; Boceprevir; Ciprofibrate; Clopidogrel; Colchicine; CycloSPORINE (Systemic); Dronedarone; Eltrombopag; Eluxadoline; Fenofibrate and Derivatives; Fusidic Acid (Systemic); Gemfibrozil; Itraconazole; Ledipasvir; Niacin; Niacinamide; Paritaprevir; Protease Inhibitors; Raltegravir; Red Yeast Rice; Simeprevir; Telaprevir; Teriflunomide

Decreased Effect

Rosuvastatin may decrease the levels/effects of: Lanthanum

The levels/effects of Rosuvastatin may be decreased by: Antacids; Eslicarbazepine

Storage/Stability Store between 20°C and 25°C (68°F to 77°F). Protect from moisture.

Mechanism of Action Inhibitor of 3-hydroxy-3-methylglutaryl coenzyme A (HMG-CoA) reductase, the rate-limiting enzyme in cholesterol synthesis (reduces the production of mevalonic acid from HMG-CoA); this then results in a compensatory increase in the expression of LDL receptors on hepatocyte membranes and a stimulation of LDL catabolism. In addition to the ability of HMG-CoA reductase inhibitors to decrease levels of high-sensitivity C-reactive protein (hsCRP), they also possess pleiotropic properties including improved endothelial function, reduced inflammation at the site of the coronary plaque, inhibition of platelet aggregation, and anticoagulant effects (de Denus 2002; Ray 2005).

Pharmacodynamics

Onset of action: Within 1 week

Maximum effect: 4 weeks

Pharmacokinetics (Adult data unless noted) Note: In pediatric patients (10-17 years of age), maximum serum concentration and AUC have been shown to be similar to adult values.

Distribution: V_d: 134 L

Protein binding: 88%, mostly to albumin

Metabolism: Hepatic (10%), via CYP2C9; N-desmethyl rosuvastatin, one-sixth to one-half the HMG-CoA reductase activity of the parent compound

Bioavailability: ~20% (high first-pass extraction by liver); increased in Asian patients (twofold increase in median exposure)

Half-life elimination: ~19 hours

Time to peak serum concentration: 3-5 hours

Elimination: Feces (90%), primarily as unchanged drug

Dosing: Usual Doses should be individualized according to the baseline LDL-cholesterol levels, the recommended goal of therapy, and patient response; adjustments should be made at intervals of 4 weeks or more.

Children and Adolescents: **Note:** A lower, conservative dosing regimen may be necessary in patient populations predisposed to myopathy, including patients of Asian descent or concurrently receiving other lipid-lowering agents (eg, gemfibrozil, niacin, fibric acid derivatives), amiodarone, atazanavir/ritonavir, cyclosporine, lopinavir/ritonavir, or indinavir (see conservative, maximum adult doses below).

Heterozygous familial hypercholesterolemia: Children and Adolescents 10-17 years: Oral: 5-20 mg once daily; may titrate dose at 4-week intervals; maximum daily dose: 20 mg/**day**

Homozygous familial hypercholesterolemia: Limited data available: Children and Adolescents (≥8 years and ≥32 kg): Oral: Initial dose: 20 mg once daily; titrate at 6-week intervals to 40 mg once daily. Although higher doses have been used (ie, 80 mg/day), additional benefit has not been reported. Dosing based on an open-label, forced-titration study of 44 patients (n=8 pediatric patients ≥8 years) which reported 72% of patients responded to rosuvastatin treatment (Marias, 2008).

Adults:

Hyperlipidemia, mixed dyslipidemia, hypertriglyceridemia, primary dysbetalipoproteinemia, slowing progression of atherosclerosis: Oral:

Initial dose:

General dosing: 10 mg once daily; 20 mg once daily may be used in patients with severe hyperlipidemia (LDL >190 mg/dL) and aggressive lipid targets

Conservative dosing: Patients requiring less aggressive treatment or predisposed to myopathy (including patients of Asian descent): 5 mg once daily

Titration: After 2 weeks, may be increased by 5-10 mg once daily; dosing range: 5-40 mg/day; maximum daily dose: 40 mg/**day**

Note: The 40 mg dose should be reserved for patients who have not achieved goal cholesterol levels on a dose of 20 mg/day, including patients switched from another HMG-CoA reductase inhibitor.

Homozygous familial hypercholesterolemia (FH): Initial: 20 mg once daily; maximum dose: 40 mg/day

Dosing adjustment with concomitant medications:

Adults:

Atazanavir/ritonavir or lopinavir/ritonavir: Initiate rosuvastatin at 5 mg once daily; rosuvastatin dose should not exceed 10 mg/day

Cyclosporine: Rosuvastatin dose should not exceed 5 mg/day

Gemfibrozil: Avoid concurrent use; if unable to avoid concurrent use, initiate rosuvastatin at 5 mg once daily; rosuvastatin dose should not exceed 10 mg/day

Dosing adjustment in renal impairment: Adults:

Mild to moderate impairment: No dosage adjustment required.

CrCl <30 mL/minute/1.73 m^2 and not receiving hemodialysis: Initial: 5 mg once daily; do not exceed 10 mg once daily

Dosing adjustments in hepatic impairment: There are no dosage adjustments provided in the manufacturer labeling; systemic exposure may be increased in patients with liver disease; use is contraindicated in patients with active liver disease or unexplained transaminase elevations.

Administration May be taken with or without food; may be taken at any time of the day.

Monitoring Parameters

Pediatric patients: Baseline: ALT, AST, and creatine phosphokinase levels (CPK); fasting lipid panel (FLP) and repeat ALT and AST should be checked after 4 weeks of therapy; if no myopathy symptoms or laboratory abnormalities, then monitor FLP, ALT, and AST every 3-4 months during the first year and then every 6 months thereafter (NHLBI, 2011).

Adults:

2013 ACC/AHA Blood Cholesterol Guideline recommendations (Stone, 2013):

Lipid panel (total cholesterol, HDL, LDL, triglycerides): Baseline lipid panel; fasting lipid profile within 4 to 12 weeks after initiation or dose adjustment and every 3 to 12 months (as clinically indicated) thereafter. If 2 consecutive LDL levels are <40 mg/dL, consider decreasing the dose.

Hepatic transaminase levels: Baseline measurement of hepatic transaminase levels (ie, ALT); measure hepatic function if symptoms suggest hepatotoxicity (eg, unusual fatigue or weakness, loss of appetite, abdominal pain, dark-colored urine or yellowing of skin or sclera) during therapy.

CPK: CPK should not be routinely measured. Baseline CPK measurement is reasonable for some individuals (eg, family history of statin intolerance or muscle disease, clinical presentation, concomitant drug therapy that may increase risk of myopathy). May measure CPK in any patient with symptoms suggestive of myopathy (pain, tenderness, stiffness, cramping, weakness, or generalized fatigue).

Evaluate for new-onset diabetes mellitus during therapy; if diabetes develops, continue statin therapy and encourage adherence to a heart-healthy diet, physical activity, a healthy body weight, and tobacco cessation.

If patient develops a confusional state or memory impairment, may evaluate patient for nonstatin causes (eg, exposure to other drugs), systemic and neuropsychiatric causes, and the possibility of adverse effects associated with statin therapy.

Manufacturer recommendations: Liver enzyme tests at baseline and repeated when clinically indicated. Upon initiation or titration, lipid panel should be analyzed within 2 to 4 weeks.

Dosage Forms Excipient information presented when available (limited, particularly for generics); consult specific product labeling.

Tablet, Oral:

Crestor: 5 mg, 10 mg, 20 mg, 40 mg

◆ **Rosuvastatin Calcium** *see* Rosuvastatin *on page 1886*

◆ **Rotarix** *see* Rotavirus Vaccine *on page 1889*

◆ **RotaTeq** *see* Rotavirus Vaccine *on page 1889*

Rotavirus Vaccine (ROE ta vye rus vak SEEN)

Medication Safety Issues

Administration issues:

Rotavirus vaccines (Rotarix and RotaTeq) are only available for **ORAL** administration. The live oral rotavirus vaccines have been inadvertently administered as an injection, thereby making the vaccine ineffective (ISMP, 2014). Avoid the administration of oral rotavirus vaccines as an injection. An oral dose should still be given if the dose was inadvertently administered as an injection (JAMA, 2014).

Related Information

Centers for Disease Control and Prevention (CDC) and Other Links *on page 2424*

Immunization Administration Recommendations *on page 2411*

Immunization Schedules *on page 2416*

Brand Names: US Rotarix; RotaTeq

Brand Names: Canada Rotarix; RotaTeq

Therapeutic Category Vaccine; Vaccine, Live Virus

Generic Availability (US) No

Use Routine immunization to prevent rotavirus gastroenteritis caused by serotypes G1, G2, G3, and G4 (RotaTeq) or serotypes G1, G3, G4, and G9 (Rotarix) (Rotarix: FDA approved in ages 6 to24 weeks; RotaTeq: FDA approved in ages 6 to 32 weeks)

The Advisory Committee on Immunization Practices (ACIP) recommends routine vaccination of all infants (CDC/ACIP [Cortese, 2009]).

Medication Guide Available Yes

Pregnancy Risk Factor C

Pregnancy Considerations Reproduction studies have not been conducted. Not indicated for use in women of reproductive age. Infants living in households with pregnant women may be vaccinated (CDC/ACIP [Cortese, 2009]).

Breast-Feeding Considerations Infants receiving vaccine may be breast fed (CDC/ACIP [Cortese, 2009]).

Contraindications Hypersensitivity to rotavirus vaccine or any component of the formulation; history of uncorrected congenital malformation of the GI tract (such as Meckel diverticulum) that would predispose the infant for intussusception (Rotarix only); history of intussusception; severe combined immunodeficiency disease

Warnings/Precautions Information is not available for use in postexposure prophylaxis. The decision to administer or delay vaccination because of current or recent febrile illness depends on the severity of symptoms and the etiology of the disease. Consider deferring administration in patients with moderate or severe acute illness (with or without fever); vaccination should not be delayed for patients with mild acute illness (with or without fever) (NCIRD/ACIP, 2011). Vaccination may not result in effective immunity in all patients. Response depends upon multiple factors (eg, type of vaccine, age of patient) and may be improved by administering the vaccine at the recommended dose, route, and interval. Vaccines may not be effective if administered during periods of altered immune competence (NCIRD/ACIP, 2011). Use caution with history of GI disorders, acute mild GI illness, chronic diarrhea, failure to thrive, congenital abdominal disorders, and abdominal surgery. Vaccine may be used with controlled gastroesophageal reflux disease. ACIP recommends that the vaccine should generally not be administered to infants with acute moderate or severe gastroenteritis. (CDC/ACIP [Cortese, 2009]). Rotarix is contraindicated with a history of an uncorrected congenital malformation of the GI tract; RotaTeq and Rotarix are contraindicated with a history of intussusception. An increased risk of intussusception was observed with a previously licensed rotavirus vaccine. Cases have been noted in postmarketing reports and a temporal association has been observed in postmarketing observational studies with current vaccines. Cases were noted within 21 to 31 days of the first dose, with a clustering of cases within the first 7 days following administration. An increased risk was also observed within the first 7 days of the second dose. Use of RotaTeq and Rotarix is contraindicated with a history of intussusception. In postmarketing experience, intussusception resulting in death following a second dose has been reported following a history of intussusception after the first dose.

Virus from live virus vaccines may be transmitted to nonvaccinated contacts; use caution in presence immunocompromised family members. Viral shedding occurs within the first weeks of administration; peak viral shedding generally occurs ~7 days after the first dose. The ACIP recommends vaccination of infants living in households with persons who are immunocompromised (CDC/ACIP [Cortese, 2009]). Safety and efficacy have not been established for use in immunocompromised infants (including blood dyscrasias, leukemia, lymphoma, malignant neoplasms affecting bone marrow or lymphatic system), infants on immunosuppressants (including high-dose corticosteroids; may be administered with topical corticosteroids or inhaled steroids), or infants with primary and acquired ▶

immunodeficiencies (including HIV/AIDS, cellular immune deficiencies, hypogammaglobulinemic and dysgammaglobulinemic states). The ACIP recommendations support vaccination of HIV-exposed or infected infants, since the diagnosis of infection may not be made prior to the first dose of the vaccine and also because strains of rotavirus vaccine are considerably attenuated (CDC/ACIP [Cortese, 2009]). In general, live vaccines should be administered ≥4 weeks prior to planned immunosuppression and avoided within 2 weeks of immunosuppression when feasible. Specific recommendations for use of this vaccine in immunocompromised patients with asplenia, cancer, HIV infection, cerebrospinal fluid leaks, cochlear implants, hematopoietic stem cell transplant (prior to or after), sickle cell disease, solid organ transplant (prior to or after), or those receiving immunosuppressive therapy for chronic conditions as well as contacts of immunocompromised patients are available from the IDSA (Rubin, 2014).

Immediate treatment (including epinephrine 1:1,000) for anaphylactoid and/or hypersensitivity reactions should be available during vaccine use (NCIRD/ACIP, 2011). Some packaging may contain natural latex/natural rubber. Not intended for use in adults. In order to maximize vaccination rates, the ACIP recommends simultaneous administration (ie, >1 vaccine on the same day at different anatomic sites) of all age-appropriate vaccines (live or inactivated) for which a person is eligible at a single clinic visit, unless contraindications exist. The ACIP prefers each dose of a specific vaccine in a series come from the same manufacturer when possible (NCIRD/ACIP, 2011). Administration errors have been reported. This vaccine is for oral administration only; doses inadvertently administered by injection are not considered valid and an oral replacement dose should be given according to the appropriate age and schedule (CDC [Hibbs, 2014]). Antipyretics have not been shown to prevent febrile seizures; antipyretics may be used to treat fever or discomfort following vaccination (NCIRD/ACIP, 2011). One study reported that routine prophylactic administration of acetaminophen to prevent fever prior to vaccination decreased the immune response of some vaccines; the clinical significance of this reduction in immune response has not been established (Prymula, 2009).

Warnings: Additional Pediatric Considerations Safety data with Rotarix in preterm neonates (≤36 weeks GA) showed a similar incidence of serious adverse effects compared to placebo (5.2% vs 5%); no deaths or cases of intussusception were reported in this population. Eye splashes to the provider, parent, or infant have been reported; to minimize risk of coughing, sneezing, and spitting, administer gently inside the cheek (CDC [Hibbs 2014]).

Adverse Reactions All serious adverse reactions must be reported to the U.S. Department of Health and Human Services (DHHS) Vaccine Adverse Event Reporting System (VAERS) 1-800-822-7967 or online at https://vaers.hhs.gov/esub/index.

Central nervous system: Fever >38.1°C, fussiness, irritability

Gastrointestinal: Diarrhea, flatulence, vomiting

Otic: Otitis media

Respiratory: Bronchospasm, nasopharyngitis

Rare but important or life-threatening: Anaphylaxis, angioedema, gastroenteritis with severe diarrhea and prolonged vaccine viral shedding in infants with SCID, hematochezia, immune thrombocytopenia (ITP), intussusception, Kawasaki disease, seizure, transmission of vaccine virus from recipient to nonvaccinated contacts, urticaria

Drug Interactions

Metabolism/Transport Effects None known.

Avoid Concomitant Use

Avoid concomitant use of Rotavirus Vaccine with any of the following: Belimumab; Fingolimod; Immunosuppressants

Increased Effect/Toxicity

The levels/effects of Rotavirus Vaccine may be increased by: AzaTHIOprine; Belimumab; Corticosteroids (Systemic); Dimethyl Fumarate; Fingolimod; Immunosuppressants; Leflunomide; Mercaptopurine; Methotrexate

Decreased Effect

Rotavirus Vaccine may decrease the levels/effects of: Tuberculin Tests

The levels/effects of Rotavirus Vaccine may be decreased by: AzaTHIOprine; Corticosteroids (Systemic); Dimethyl Fumarate; Fingolimod; Immunosuppressants; Leflunomide; Mercaptopurine; Methotrexate

Storage/Stability

Rotarix: Store intact vials under refrigeration at 2°C to 8°C (36°F to 46°F); diluent may be stored under refrigeration at 2°C to 8°C (36°F to 46°F) or at room temperature up to 25°C (77°F). Protect vaccine from light; discard diluent if frozen. Following reconstitution, may be refrigerated at 2°C to 8°C (36°F to 46°F) or stored at room temperature up to 25°C (77°F) for up to 24 hours. Discard if frozen. **Note:** In Canada, Rotarix is available as an oral suspension ready for use and does not need to be reconstituted. The oral suspension may be stored at 2°C to 8°C (36°F to 46°F); do not freeze. Protect from light.

RotaTeq: Store and transport under refrigeration at 2°C to 8°C (36°F to 46°F). Use as soon as possible once removed from refrigerator. Protect from light. Canadian labeling suggests that once the vaccine is removed from refrigeration, it may be stored at temperatures up to 25°C (77°F) for up to 4 hours; do not freeze. Protect from light.

Mechanism of Action A live vaccine; replicates in the small intestine and promotes active immunity to rotavirus gastroenteritis. Rotarix is specifically indicated for prevention of rotavirus gastroenteritis caused by serotypes G1, G3, G4, and G9 and RotaTeq is specifically indicated for prevention of rotavirus gastroenteritis caused by serotypes G1, G2, G3, and G4. However, these vaccines may provide immunity to other rotavirus serotypes.

Pharmacodynamics Note: There is no established relationship between antibody response and protection against gastroenteritis.

Seroconversion:

Rotarix: Antirotavirus IgA antibodies were noted 1 to 2 months following completion of the 2-dose series in 77% to 87% of infants.

RotaTeq: A threefold increase in antirotavirus IgA was noted following completion of the 3-dose regimen in 93% to 100% of infants.

Duration: Following administration of rotavirus vaccine, efficacy of protecting against any grade of rotavirus gastroenteritis through two seasons was 71% to 79%.

Dosing: Usual

Pediatric: **Note:** The ACIP recommends completing the vaccine se ries with the same product whenever possible. If continuing with same product will cause vaccination to be deferred, or if product used previously is unknown, vaccination should be completed with the product available. If RotaTeq was used in any previous doses, or if the specific product used was unknown, a total of 3 doses should be given (CDC/ACIP [Cortese 2009]).

Primary immunization:

Manufacturer's labeling:

Rotarix: Infants 6 to 24 weeks of age: Oral: 1 mL per dose for 2 doses, the first dose given at 6 weeks of age, followed by the second dose given ≥4 weeks later. The 2-dose series should be completed by 24 weeks of age.

RotaTeq: Infants 6 to 32 weeks of age: Oral: 2 mL per dose for 3 doses, the first dose given at 6 to 12 weeks of age, followed by subsequent doses at 4- to 10-week intervals. Administer all doses by 32 weeks of age.

ACIP recommendations (CDC/ACIP [Cortese 2009]): The first dose can be given at 6 weeks through 14 weeks 6 days of age. The series should not be started in infants ≥15 weeks. The final dose in the series should be administered by 8 months 0 days of age. The minimum interval between doses is 4 weeks. Rotarix should be given in 2 doses administered at 2- and 4 months of age. RotaTeq should be given in 3 doses administered at 2-, 4-, and 6 months of age. For infants inadvertently administered rotavirus vaccine at ≥15 weeks of age, the vaccine series may be completed according to schedule. Infants who have had rotavirus gastroenteritis before getting the full course of vaccine should still initiate or complete the recommended schedule; initial infection provides only partial immunity.

Catch-up immunization: CDC (ACIP) Recommendations (Strikas 2015): **Note:** Do not restart the series. If doses have been given, begin the below schedule at the applicable dose number. The series should not be started in infants ≥15 weeks. The final dose in the series should be administered by 8 months 0 days of age. For infants inadvertently administered rotavirus vaccine at ≥15 weeks of age, the vaccine series may be completed according to schedule and prior to 8 months and 0 days of age. If RotaTeq was used in any previous doses, or if the specific product used was unknown, a total of 3 doses should be given. Oral:

First dose given at <15 weeks of age

Second dose given at least 4 weeks after the first dose

Third dose given at least 4 weeks after the second dose (not needed if first 2 doses were Rotarix)

Dosing adjustment in renal impairment: There are no dosage adjustments provided in the manufacturer's labeling.

Dosing adjustment in hepatic impairment: There are no dosage adjustments provided in the manufacturer's labeling.

Preparation for Administration Oral:

Rotarix: Reconstitute only with provided diluent and transfer adapter. Connect transfer adapter onto vial and push downwards until transfer adapter is in place. Shake oral applicator containing liquid diluent (suspension will be a turbid liquid). Connect oral applicator to transfer adapter and transfer entire contents of oral applicator into the lyophilized vaccine. With transfer adapter in place, shake vigorously. Withdraw entire mixture back into oral applicator.

RotaTeq: Clear the fluid from the dispensing tip by holding the tube vertically and tapping the cap. Puncture the dispensing tip by screwing the cap clockwise until it becomes tight and then remove the cap by turning it counterclockwise.

Administration Oral use only; **not for injection**. May be administered before or after food, milk, or breast milk. To avoid potential eye splashes caused by coughing, sneezing, and spitting, administer gently inside the cheek (CDC [Hibbs 2014]). US law requires that the date of administration, the vaccine manufacturer, lot number of vaccine, and the administering person's name, title, and address be entered into the patient's permanent medical record.

Note: Although the Rotarix prescribing information states that a regurgitated or spit out dose may be repeated, the ACIP, AAP, and the RotaTeq prescribing information do not recommend readministering doses. Any remaining dose(s) should be administered on schedule (AAP 2009; CDC/ACIP [Cortese 2009]).

Rotarix: Reconstitute vaccine prior to administration. Infant should be in reclining position. Using oral applicator, administer contents into infant's inner cheek. If most of dose is spit out or regurgitated, may administer a replacement dose at the same visit. Dispose of applicator and vaccine vial in biologic waste container.

RotaTeq: Gently squeeze dose from ready-to-use dosing tube into infant's mouth toward the inner cheek until dosing tube is empty. After use, dispose of the empty tube and cap in a biologic waste container. If an incomplete dose is given (eg, infant spits or regurgitates dose), do not administer replacement dose. The infant can continue to receive any remaining doses of the series at the designated time interval. Do not mix or dilute vaccine with any other vaccine or solution.

Test Interactions Tuberculin tests: Rotavirus vaccine may diminish the diagnostic effect of tuberculin tests.

Additional Information Diphtheria and tetanus antigens in DTaP, HIB, IPV, hepatitis B vaccine, and pneumococcal conjugate vaccine may be given concurrently with rotavirus vaccine.

In the United States, rotavirus outbreaks occur from late fall to early spring. In the Southwest, the peak rotavirus season is November through December; the peak epidemic travels across the United States from west to east terminating in April through May in the Northeast.

Dosage Forms Excipient information presented when available (limited, particularly for generics); consult specific product labeling.

Powder, for suspension, oral [preservative free; human derived]:

Rotarix: G1P[8] ≥10^6 $CCID_{50}$ per 1 mL [contains sorbitol, sucrose; supplied with diluent which may contain natural rubber/natural latex in packaging]

Solution, oral [preservative free; bovine and human derived]:

RotaTeq: G1 ≥2.2 x 10^6 infectious units, G2 ≥2.8 x 10^6 infectious units, G3 ≥2.2 x 10^6 infectious units, G4 ≥2 x 10^6 infectious units, and P1A [8] ≥2.3 x 10^6 infectious units per 2 mL (2 mL) [contains sucrose]

- ◆ **Rotavirus Vaccine, Pentavalent** *see* Rotavirus Vaccine *on page 1889*
- ◆ **Rowasa** *see* Mesalamine *on page 1368*
- ◆ **Roxanol** *see* Morphine (Systemic) *on page 1461*
- ◆ **Roxicet** *see* Oxycodone and Acetaminophen *on page 1594*
- ◆ **Roxicodone** *see* OxyCODONE *on page 1590*
- ◆ **Roychlor (Can)** *see* Potassium Chloride *on page 1736*
- ◆ **RP-6976** *see* DOCEtaxel *on page 692*
- ◆ **RP-59500** *see* Quinupristin and Dalfopristin *on page 1827*
- ◆ **RS-25259** *see* Palonosetron *on page 1609*
- ◆ **RS-25259-197** *see* Palonosetron *on page 1609*
- ◆ **RTCA** *see* Ribavirin *on page 1851*
- ◆ **Rubella, Measles and Mumps Vaccines** *see* Measles, Mumps, and Rubella Virus Vaccine *on page 1327*
- ◆ **Rubella, Varicella, Measles, and Mumps Vaccine** *see* Measles, Mumps, Rubella, and Varicella Virus Vaccine *on page 1330*
- ◆ **Rubidomycin Hydrochloride** *see* DAUNOrubicin (Conventional) *on page 592*
- ◆ **RUF 331** *see* Rufinamide *on page 1891*

Rufinamide (roo FIN a mide)

Brand Names: US Banzel
Brand Names: Canada Banzel

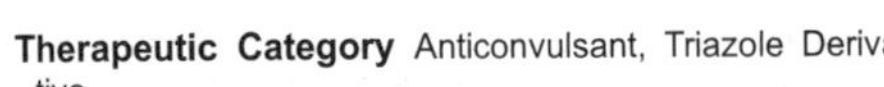

Therapeutic Category Anticonvulsant, Triazole Derivative

Generic Availability (US) No

Use Adjunctive therapy of seizures associated with Lennox-Gastaut syndrome (FDA approved in ages ≥4 years and adults)

Medication Guide Available Yes

Pregnancy Risk Factor C

Pregnancy Considerations Adverse effects were seen in animal reproduction studies. Hormonal contraceptives may be less effective with concurrent rufinamide use; additional forms of nonhormonal contraceptives should be used.

Patients exposed to rufinamide during pregnancy are encouraged to enroll themselves into the AED Pregnancy Registry by calling 1-888-233-2334. Additional information is available at www.aedpregnancyregistry.org.

Breast-Feeding Considerations Excretion into breast milk is unknown, but may be expected. Due to the potential for serious adverse reactions in the nursing infant, the manufacturer recommends a decision be made whether to discontinue nursing or to discontinue the drug, taking into account the importance of treatment to the mother.

Contraindications Patients with familial short QT syndrome

Canadian labeling: Additional contraindications (not in U.S. labeling): Family history of short QT syndrome; presence or history of short QT interval; hypersensitivity to rufinamide, triazole derivatives, or any component of the formulation

Warnings/Precautions Has been associated with shortening of the QT interval. Use caution in patients receiving concurrent medications that shorten the QT interval. Contraindicated in patients with familial short-QT syndrome (Canadian labeling also contraindicates use in patients with a family history of short QT syndrome or presence or history of short QT interval). Use has been associated with CNS-related adverse events, most significant of these were cognitive symptoms (including somnolence or fatigue) and coordination abnormalities (including ataxia, dizziness, and gait disturbances). Caution patients about performing tasks which require mental alertness (eg, operating machinery or driving).

Potentially serious, sometimes fatal, multiorgan hypersensitivity reactions (also known as drug reaction with eosinophilia and systemic symptoms [DRESS]) have been reported. Monitor for signs and symptoms (eg, fever, rash, lymphadenopathy, eosinophilia) in association with other organ system involvement (eg, hepatitis, nephritis, hematological abnormalities, myocarditis, myositis). Evaluate immediately if signs or symptoms are present. Discontinuation and conversion to alternate therapy may be required. Potentially serious, sometimes fatal, dermatologic reactions including Stevens-Johnson syndrome (SJS) have been reported; monitor for signs and symptoms of skin reactions; discontinuation and conversion to alternate therapy may be required. Potentially significant drug-drug interactions may exist, requiring dose or frequency adjustment, additional monitoring, and/or selection of alternative therapy.

Antiepileptics are associated with an increased risk of suicidal behavior/thoughts with use (regardless of indication); patients should be monitored for signs/symptoms of depression, suicidal tendencies, and other unusual behavior changes during therapy and instructed to inform their healthcare provider immediately if symptoms occur. Use with caution in patients with mild-to-moderate hepatic impairment; use in not recommended in patients with severe hepatic impairment. Anticonvulsants should not be discontinued abruptly because of the possibility of increasing seizure frequency; therapy should be withdrawn gradually to minimize the potential of increased seizure frequency, unless safety concerns require a more rapid withdrawal. Reducing dose by ~25% every two days was effective in trials. Decreased white blood cell count has been reported during treatment. Some dosage forms may contain propylene glycol; large amounts are potentially toxic and have been associated hyperosmolality, lactic acidosis, seizures, and respiratory depression; use caution (AAP, 1997; Zar, 2007).

Warnings: Additional Pediatric Considerations Case reports of possibly fatal multiorgan hypersensitivity reactions (including severe hepatitis) with rufinamide occurred in children <12 years and presented within the first 4 weeks of therapy. Children may experience some adverse effects not reported in adults, including aggression, attention disturbance, hyperactivity, pruritus, rash, nasopharyngitis, and seizures.

Some dosage forms may contain propylene glycol; in neonates large amounts of propylene glycol delivered orally, intravenously (eg, >3,000 mg/day), or topically have been associated with potentially fatal toxicities which can include metabolic acidosis, seizures, renal failure, and CNS depression; toxicities have also been reported in children and adults including hyperosmolality, lactic acidosis, seizures, and respiratory depression; use caution (AAP, 1997; Shehab, 2009).

Adverse Reactions

Cardiovascular: Shortened QT interval (dose related)

Central nervous system: Abnormal gait, aggressive behavior (children), anxiety (adults), ataxia, convulsions (children), disturbance in attention (children), dizziness, drowsiness, fatigue, headache (more common in adults), hyperactivity (children), status epilepticus, vertigo (adults)

Dermatologic: Pruritus (children), skin rash (children)

Gastrointestinal: Constipation (adults), decreased appetite (children), dyspepsia (adults), increased appetite, nausea, upper abdominal pain, vomiting (more common in children)

Hematologic & oncologic: Anemia, leukopenia

Infection: Influenza (children)

Neuromuscular & skeletal: Back pain (adults), tremor (adults)

Ophthalmic: Blurred vision (adults), diplopia, nystagmus (adults)

Otic: Otic infection (children), pollakiuria

Respiratory: Bronchitis (children), nasopharyngitis (children), sinusitis (children)

Rare but important or life-threatening: Atrioventricular block (first degree), bundle branch block (right), dysuria, hematuria, hypersensitivity (multiorgan), iron-deficiency anemia, lymphadenopathy, nephrolithiasis, neutropenia, nocturia, polyuria, Stevens-Johnson syndrome, suicidal ideation, thrombocytopenia, urinary incontinence

Drug Interactions

Metabolism/Transport Effects Inhibits CYP2E1 (weak); **Induces** CYP3A4 (weak)

Avoid Concomitant Use There are no known interactions where it is recommended to avoid concomitant use.

Increased Effect/Toxicity

Rufinamide may increase the levels/effects of: CNS Depressants; Fosphenytoin; PHENobarbital; Phenytoin

The levels/effects of Rufinamide may be increased by: Alcohol (Ethyl); Valproic Acid and Derivatives

Decreased Effect

Rufinamide may decrease the levels/effects of: ARIPiprazole; CarBAMazepine; Ethinyl Estradiol; Hydrocodone; NiMODipine; Norethindrone; Saxagliptin

The levels/effects of Rufinamide may be decreased by: CarBAMazepine; Fosphenytoin; PHENobarbital; Phenytoin; Primidone

Food Interactions Food increases the absorption of rufinamide. Management: Take with food.

Storage/Stability Store at 25°C (77°F); excursions permitted to 15°C to 30°C (59°F to 86°F). Protect tablets from moisture. Discard oral suspension within 90 days after opening; cap of bottle fits over the adapter.

Mechanism of Action A triazole-derivative antiepileptic whose exact mechanism is unknown. *In vitro*, it prolongs the inactive state of the sodium channels, thereby limiting repetitive firing of sodium-dependent action potentials mediating anticonvulsant effects.

Pharmacokinetics (Adult data unless noted) Note: Pharmacokinetic data in pediatric patients (4-17 years) has been shown to be similar to adult data.

Absorption: Slow; extensive ≥85%

Distribution: Apparent V_d: ~50 L (dose-dependent, dose: 3200 mg/day)

Protein binding: 34%, primarily to albumin

Metabolism: Extensively via carboxylesterase-mediated hydrolysis of the carboxylamide group to CGP 47292 (inactive metabolite); weak inhibitor of CYP2E1 and weak inducer of CYP3A4

Bioavailability: Extent decreased with increased dose; oral tablets and oral suspension are bioequivalent

Half-life: ~6-10 hours

Time to peak serum concentration: 4-6 hours

Elimination: Urine [85%, ~66% as CGP 47292 (inactive metabolite), <2% as unchanged drug]

Dialysis: Decreased AUC by 30% and maximum serum concentration by 16%; consider dosage adjustment

Dosing: Usual Oral: Lennox-Gastaut syndrome:

Children ≥4 years: Initial: 10 mg/kg/day in 2 equally divided doses; increase dose by ~10 mg/kg increments every other day to a target dose of 45 mg/kg/day in 2 equally divided doses (maximum dose: 3200 mg/day); effectiveness of doses lower than the target dose is unknown.

Adults: Initial: 400-800 mg/day in 2 equally divided doses; increase dose by 400-800 mg/day every other day to a maximum dose of 3200 mg/day in 2 equally divided doses; effectiveness of doses lower than 3200 mg/day is unknown.

Dosage adjustment for concomitant medications: Valproate: Initial rufinamide dose should be <10 mg/kg/day (children) or 400 mg/day (adults)

Dosage adjustment in renal impairment:

CrCl <30 mL/minute: No dosage adjustment needed

Hemodialysis: No specific guidelines available; consider dosage adjustment for loss of drug

Dosage adjustment in hepatic impairment:

Mild to moderate impairment: Use with caution

Severe impairment: Use in severe impairment has not been studied and is not recommended

Administration Administer with food.

Tablets: May be swallowed whole, split in half, or crushed.

Oral suspension: Shake well; use provided adapter and calibrated oral syringe to measure dose.

Monitoring Parameters Seizure frequency, duration, and severity; CBC; signs and symptoms of suicidality (eg, anxiety, depression, behavior changes); consider ECG (with concurrent medications that can shorten QT interval)

Dosage Forms Excipient information presented when available (limited, particularly for generics); consult specific product labeling.

Suspension, Oral:

Banzel: 40 mg/mL (460 mL) [contains methylparaben, propylene glycol, propylparaben; orange flavor]

Tablet, Oral:

Banzel: 200 mg, 400 mg [scored]

Extemporaneous Preparations A 40 mg/mL oral suspension may be made using tablets. Crush twelve 400 mg tablets (or twenty-four 200 mg tablets) and reduce to a fine powder. Add 60 mL of Ora-Plus® in incremental proportions until a smooth suspension is obtained; then mix well while adding 60 mL of Ora-Sweet® or Ora-Sweet® SF; transfer to a calibrated bottle. Label "shake well". Stable 90 days at room temperature.

Hutchinson DJ, Liou Y, Best R, et al, "Stability of Extemporaneously Prepared Rufinamide Oral Suspensions," *Ann Pharmacother*, 2010, 44(3):462-5.

- ◆ **RV1 (Rotarix)** *see* Rotavirus Vaccine *on page 1889*
- ◆ **RV5 (RotaTeq)** *see* Rotavirus Vaccine *on page 1889*
- ◆ **RWJ-270201** *see* Peramivir *on page 1672*
- ◆ **Ryanodex** *see* Dantrolene *on page 576*
- ◆ **Rylosol (Can)** *see* Sotalol *on page 1963*
- ◆ **Rynex PSE [OTC]** *see* Brompheniramine and Pseudoephedrine *on page 305*
- ◆ **Rythmodan (Can)** *see* Disopyramide *on page 689*
- ◆ **Rythmodan-LA (Can)** *see* Disopyramide *on page 689*
- ◆ **S2 [OTC]** *see* EPINEPHrine (Systemic, Oral Inhalation) *on page 760*
- ◆ **S2 (Can)** *see* EPINEPHrine (Systemic, Oral Inhalation) *on page 760*
- ◆ **Sabril** *see* Vigabatrin *on page 2174*

Sacrosidase (sak ROE si dase)

Brand Names: US Sucraid

Brand Names: Canada Sucraid®

Therapeutic Category Sucrase Deficiency, Treatment Agent

Generic Availability (US) No

Use Replacement therapy in congenital sucrase-isomaltase deficiency (CSID) [FDA approved in pediatric patients (age not specified) and adults]

Prescribing and Access Restrictions Sucraid® is not available in retail pharmacies or via mail-order pharmacies. To obtain the product, please refer to http://www.sucraid.net/how-to-order-sucraid or call 1-866-740-2743.

Pregnancy Risk Factor C

Pregnancy Considerations Animal reproduction studies have not been conducted. Use is not expected to cause fetal harm when used during pregnancy; administer to a pregnant woman only when indicated.

Breast-Feeding Considerations Sacrosidase is broken down in the stomach and intestines and the component amino acids and peptides are then absorbed as nutrients.

Contraindications Hypersensitivity to yeast, yeast products, glycerin (glycerol), or papain

Warnings/Precautions Hypersensitivity reactions to sacrosidase, including bronchospasm, have been reported. Administer initial doses in a setting where acute hypersensitivity reactions may be treated within a few minutes. Skin testing for hypersensitivity may be performed prior to administration to identify patients at risk. Product may contain papain. Severe hypersensitivity reactions, including anaphylaxis, have been observed with papain exposure. Tachycardia and hypotension, in association with some papain-induced hypersensitivity reactions, has also been observed. In addition, inconclusive data suggests a possible cross-sensitivity may exist between patients with natural rubber latex hypersensitivity and papaya, the source of papain. Use with caution in patients with diabetes; sacrosidase enables absorption of fructose and glucose.

Warnings: Additional Pediatric Considerations Oral solution contains 50% glycerol.

Adverse Reactions

Central nervous system: Headache, insomnia, nervousness

Endocrine & metabolic: Dehydration

Gastrointestinal: Abdominal pain, constipation, diarrhea, nausea, vomiting

Rare but important or life-threatening: Hypersensitivity reactions, wheezing

Drug Interactions

Metabolism/Transport Effects None known.

Avoid Concomitant Use There are no known interactions where it is recommended to avoid concomitant use.

Increased Effect/Toxicity There are no known significant interactions involving an increase in effect.

Decreased Effect There are no known significant interactions involving a decrease in effect.

Food Interactions May be inactivated or denatured if administered with fruit juice or warm or hot food/liquids. Isomaltase deficiency is not addressed by supplementation of sacrosidase. Management: Administer with 2-4 oz of water, milk, or formula. Because isomaltase deficiency is not addressed by supplementation of sacrosidase, adherence to a low-starch diet may be required.

Storage/Stability Store under refrigeration at 2°C to 8°C (36°F to 46°F); protect from heat. Protect from light. After initial opening, discard any unused product after 4 weeks.

Mechanism of Action Sacrosidase is a naturally-occurring gastrointestinal enzyme derived from baker's yeast (*Saccharomyces cerevisiae*) which breaks down the disaccharide sucrose to its monosaccharide components. Hydrolysis is necessary to allow absorption of these nutrients.

Pharmacokinetics (Adult data unless noted) Metabolism: Sacrosidase is metabolized in the GI tract to individual amino acids which are systemically absorbed

Dosing: Usual Congenital sucrose-isomaltase deficiency (CSID) or sucrase deficiency; oral replacement (CSID): Oral:

Infants and Children ≤15 kg: 8500 units (1 mL) per meal or snack

Children >15 kg, Adolescents, and Adults: 17,000 units (2 mL) per meal or snack

Preparation for Administration Oral: Dilute dose in 2 to 4 ounces of cold or room temperature water, milk, or formula

Administration Oral: Dilute dose prior to administration; approximately 1/2 of the dose may be taken before each meal or snack, and the remainder of the dose at the completion; do not administer with fruit juices, warm or hot food or liquids (may lower potency)

Monitoring Parameters Breath hydrogen test, oral sucrose tolerance test, urinary disaccharides, intestinal disaccharidases (measured from small bowel biopsy)

CSID symptomatology: Diarrhea, abdominal pain, gas, and bloating

Additional Information 1 mL = 22 drops from sacrosidase container tip

Dosage Forms Excipient information presented when available (limited, particularly for generics); consult specific product labeling.

Solution, Oral:

Sucraid: 8500 units/mL (118 mL) [contains papain]

- ◆ **Safe Tussin DM [OTC]** *see* Guaifenesin and Dextromethorphan *on page 992*
- ◆ **Safe Wash [OTC]** *see* Sodium Chloride *on page 1938*
- ◆ **Saizen** *see* Somatropin *on page 1957*
- ◆ **Saizen Click.Easy** *see* Somatropin *on page 1957*
- ◆ **SalAc [OTC]** *see* Salicylic Acid *on page 1894*
- ◆ **Salactic Film [OTC]** *see* Salicylic Acid *on page 1894*
- ◆ **Salacyn** *see* Salicylic Acid *on page 1894*
- ◆ **Salagen** *see* Pilocarpine (Systemic) *on page 1701*
- ◆ **Salagen® (Can)** *see* Pilocarpine (Systemic) *on page 1701*
- ◆ **Salazopyrin (Can)** *see* SulfaSALAzine *on page 1990*
- ◆ **Salazopyrin En-Tabs (Can)** *see* SulfaSALAzine *on page 1990*
- ◆ **Salbutamol** *see* Albuterol *on page 81*
- ◆ **Salbutamol HFA (Can)** *see* Albuterol *on page 81*
- ◆ **Salbutamol Sulphate** *see* Albuterol *on page 81*
- ◆ **Salcatonin** *see* Calcitonin *on page 337*
- ◆ **Salex** *see* Salicylic Acid *on page 1894*
- ◆ **Salicylazosulfapyridine** *see* SulfaSALAzine *on page 1990*

Salicylic Acid (sal i SIL ik AS id)

Medication Safety Issues

Sound-alike/look-alike issues:

Occlusal-HP may be confused with Ocuflox

Other safety concerns:

Transdermal patch may contain conducting metal (eg, aluminum); remove patch prior to MRI.

Brand Names: US Bensal HP; Betasal [OTC]; Calicylic [OTC]; Clear Away 1-Step Wart Remover [OTC]; Corn Remover One Step [OTC]; Corn Remover Ultra Thin [OTC]; DHS Sal [OTC]; Exuviance Blemish Treatment [OTC]; Gordofilm; Hydrisalic [OTC] [DSC]; Ionil [OTC]; Keralyt; Keralyt Scalp; Keralyt [OTC]; Mediplast [OTC]; Neutrogena Oil-Free Acne Wash [OTC]; One Step Callus Remover [OTC]; P & S [OTC]; Psoriasin [OTC]; Sal-Plant [OTC]; SalAc [OTC]; Salactic Film [OTC]; Salacyn; Salex; Salicylic Acid Wart Remover; Salkera; Salvax; Scalpicin 2 in 1 [OTC]; Scholls Callus Removers [OTC] [DSC]; Scholls Corn Removers Extra [OTC] [DSC]; Scholls Corn Removers Small [OTC] [DSC]; Scholls Corn Removers [OTC] [DSC]; Sebasorb [OTC]; Stri-Dex Maximum Strength [OTC]; Stri-Dex Sensitive Skin [OTC]; Stridex Essential [OTC]; Tinamed Corn/Callus Remover [OTC]; Tinamed Wart Remover [OTC]; Trans-Ver-Sal AdultPatch [OTC]; Trans-Ver-Sal PediaPatch [OTC]; Trans-Ver-Sal PlantarPatch [OTC]; UltraSal-ER; Virasal

Brand Names: Canada Duofilm; Duoforte 27; Occlusal-HP; Sebcur; Soluver; Soluver Plus; Trans-Plantar; Trans-Ver-Sal

Therapeutic Category Keratolytic Agent

Generic Availability (US) May be product dependent

Use Topically for its keratolytic effect in controlling seborrheic dermatitis or psoriasis of body and scalp, dandruff, and other scaling dermatoses; removing excessive keratin in hyperkeratotic skin disorders (eg, verrucae, ichthyoses, keratosis palmaris and plantaris, keratosis pilaris, and pityriasis rubra pilaris); removing warts, corns, calluses; used in the treatment of acne

Pregnancy Risk Factor C

Pregnancy Considerations Adverse events have been observed in animal reproduction studies when administered orally. Salicylates cross the placenta (Østensen 1998). Systemic absorption of topical salicylic acid occurs and varies depending on duration and vehicle (~9% to 25%) and is increased with occlusion (Akhavan 2003). Current guidelines do not recommend salicylic acid for the treatment of psoriasis in pregnant women due to limited safety data and the potential for systemic absorption (Bae 2012). For the topical treatment of acne or warts, salicylic acid can be used in pregnant women if the area of exposure and duration of therapy is limited, although other agents may be preferred (Murase, 2014). Consider maternal/fetal adverse events associated with aspirin if significant systemic exposure occurs (Akhavan 2003).

Breast-Feeding Considerations Salicylates are excreted in breast milk after oral administration (Bar-Oz 2003). Systemic absorption of topical salicylic acid occurs and varies depending on duration and vehicle (~9% to 25%) and is increased with occlusion. Consider adverse events associated with aspirin in nursing infants if significant systemic exposure occurs (Akhavan 2003). For the topical treatment of warts, salicylic acid can be used in breast-feeding women (systemic absorption is usually minimal) (Butler 2014). Breast-feeding women should avoid use around the chest area to prevent exposure to the nursing child. Due to the potential for serious adverse reactions in the nursing infant, the manufacturer recommends a decision be made whether to discontinue nursing or the drug, taking into account the importance of treatment to the mother.

Contraindications

Hypersensitivity to salicylic acid or any component of the formulation

Additional contraindications:

Bensal HP: Hypersensitivity to topical polyethylene glycols

Keralyt, Salex: Children <2 years

UltraSal-ER, Virasal: Impaired circulation or diabetes; moles, birthmarks; warts with hair growth or on face

OTC labeling: Corns/Warts: When used for self-medication, do not use if you have diabetes or have poor blood circulation; do not use on irritated skin, on any area that is infected or reddened, on moles, birthmarks, warts with hair growing from them, genital warts, or warts on the face or mucous membranes

Documentation of allergenic cross-reactivity for salicylates is limited. However, because of similarities in chemical structure and/or pharmacologic actions, the possibility of cross-sensitivity cannot be ruled out with certainty.

Warnings/Precautions Rare but serious and potentially life-threatening allergic reactions or severe irritation have been reported with use of topical OTC benzoyl peroxide or salicylic acid containing products; it has not been determined if the reactions are due to the active ingredients (benzoyl peroxide or salicylic acid), the inactive ingredients, or a combination of both. Hypersensitivity reactions may occur within minutes to a day or longer after product use and differ from local skin irritation (redness, burning, dryness, itching, peeling or slight swelling) that may occur at the site of product application. Treatment should be discontinued if hives or itching develop; patients should seek emergency medical attention if reactions such as throat tightness, difficulty breathing, feeling faint, or swelling of the eyes, face, lips, or tongue develop. Before using a topical OTC acne product for the first time, consumers should apply a small amount to 1 or 2 small affected areas for 3 days to make sure hypersensitivity symptoms do not develop (FDA Drug Safety Communication, 2014).

Do not combine use of topical salicylic acid with use of other salicylates or drugs that can increase salicylate serum concentrations; systemic absorption following topical use may occur and lead to toxicity. May decrease the efficacy of UVB phototherapy; do not use before therapy (Menter 2009).

Products are for external use only. Avoid prolonged use over large areas in children or patients with significant hepatic or renal impairment; may result in salicylism. Limit application area in children <12 years of age. Use may be associated with Reye syndrome; use caution in children or adolescents with varicella or influenza. Some products are contraindicated in children <2 years.

Self-medication (OTC use): Acne: Apply to affected areas only. Do not apply to broken skin or large areas of body. Dryness or irritation may be increased if other topical acne products are used at the same time. If irritation occurs, use only one topical acne product at a time. New users may test for sensitivity by applying the product sparingly to 1 to 2 affected areas for the first 3 days; if no discomfort occurs, may continue with directions on product labeling. May increase skin sensitivity to sunburn; use sunscreen and limit sun exposure during use and for 1 week afterward.

Self-medication (OTC use): Hyperkeratotic skin disorders: Prior to self-medication, patients should contact a health care provider if the condition covers a large area of the body and if the condition worsens or does not improve after regular use.

Self-medication (OTC use): Warts: Prior to OTC use, consult with a health care provider if you have diabetes or poor circulation. For external use only; not for application to areas that are irritated, infected, reddened, birthmarks, genital or facial warts, eyes, or mucous membranes.

Warnings: Additional Pediatric Considerations Some dosage forms may contain propylene glycol; in neonates large amounts of propylene glycol delivered orally, intravenously (eg, >3,000 mg/day), or topically have been associated with potentially fatal toxicities which can include metabolic acidosis, seizures, renal failure, and CNS depression; toxicities have also been reported in children and adults including hyperosmolality, lactic acidosis, seizures, and respiratory depression; use caution (AAP, 1997; Shehab, 2009).

Adverse Reactions

Central nervous system: Dizziness, headache, mental confusion

Local: Burning and irritation at site of exposure on normal tissue, peeling, scaling

Otic: Tinnitus

Respiratory: Hyperventilation

Drug Interactions

Metabolism/Transport Effects None known.

Avoid Concomitant Use There are no known interactions where it is recommended to avoid concomitant use.

Increased Effect/Toxicity There are no known significant interactions involving an increase in effect.

Decreased Effect There are no known significant interactions involving a decrease in effect.

Storage/Stability

Bensal HP: Store at 20°C to 25°C (68°F to 77°F); excursions are permitted between 15°C and 30°C (59°F and 86°F). Brief exposure up to 40°C (104°F) may be tolerated if the mean temperature does not exceed 25°C (77°F).

Keralyt gel, UltraSal-ER, Virasal: Store at 15°C to 30°C (59°F to 86°F). Flammable; keep away from heat and flame.

Keralyt shampoo: Store at 15°C to 30°C (59°F to 86°F).

Salex shampoo: Store at 20°C to 25°C (68°F to 77°F); do not freeze.

Salvax foam: Store at 15°C to 25°C (15°F to 30°F). Flammable; do not expose to temperatures >48°C (120°F) even when empty; do not puncture.

OTC products: Store at room temperature; may vary by product.

Mechanism of Action Produces desquamation of hyperkeratotic epithelium via dissolution of the intercellular cement which causes the cornified tissue to swell, soften, macerate, and desquamate. Salicylic acid is used for keratolytic skin disorders at concentrations of 3% to 6%; concentrations of 5% to 40% are used to remove corns and warts; concentrations up to 2% are used for acne (Akhavan 2003).

Pharmacokinetics (Adult data unless noted)

Absorption: Topical: Readily absorbed

Time to peak serum concentration: Within 5 hours when applied with an occlusive dressing

Elimination: Salicyluric acid (52%), salicylate glucuronides (42%), and salicylic acid (6%) are the major metabolites identified in urine after percutaneous absorption

Dosing: Usual Children ≥2 years and Adults: Topical:

Foam: Apply to the affected area twice daily. Rub into skin until completely absorbed.

Lotion, cream, gel: Apply a thin layer to the affected area once or twice daily

Shampoo: Initial: Use daily or every other day; apply to wet hair and massage vigorously into the scalp; rinse hair thoroughly after shampooing; 1-2 treatments/week will usually maintain control

Solution: Apply a thin layer directly to wart using brush applicator once daily as directed for 1 week or until the wart is removed

Administration Topical: For external use only. Not for ophthalmic, oral, anal, or intravaginal use. When applying in concentrations >10%, protect surrounding normal tissue with petrolatum

Monitoring Parameters Signs and symptoms of salicylate toxicity: Nausea, vomiting, dizziness, tinnitus, loss of hearing, lethargy, diarrhea, psychic disturbances

Dosage Forms Excipient information presented when available (limited, particularly for generics); consult specific product labeling. [DSC] = Discontinued product

Cream, External:
- Calicylic: 10% (60 g)
- Salacyn: 6% (400 g) [contains cetyl alcohol, disodium edta, methylparaben, propylparaben, trolamine (triethanolamine)]
- Generic: 6% (400 g, 454 g)

Foam, External:
- SalAc: 2% (100 g) [contains alcohol, usp]
- Salkera: 6% (60 g) [contains cetostearyl alcohol, edetate disodium dihydrate, methylparaben, propylene glycol, propylparaben]
- Salvax: 6% (70 g, 200 g) [contains ethylparaben, methylparaben, polysorbate 80, propylene glycol, propylparaben, trolamine (triethanolamine)]
- Generic: 6% (70 g, 200 g)

Gel, External:
- Exuviance Blemish Treatment: 2% (15 g) [contains denatured alcohol, peanut oil, propylene glycol]
- Hydrisalic: 17% (14 g [DSC]) [contains fd&c red #40, isopropyl alcohol]
- Keralyt: 3% (28.4 g) [contains alcohol, usp]
- Keralyt: 6% (40 g, 100 g) [contains hydroxypropyl cellulose, propylene glycol, sd alcohol 40]
- Sal-Plant: 17% (14 g)
- Generic: 6% (40 g)

Kit, External:
- Keralyt Scalp: 6% [contains edetate sodium (tetrasodium), propylene glycol, sd alcohol 40]
- Salex: 6% [contains cetyl alcohol, disodium edta, methylparaben, propylparaben, trolamine (triethanolamine)]
- Generic: 6%

Liquid, External:
- Neutrogena Oil-Free Acne Wash: 2% (124 mL) [contains benzalkonium chloride, disodium edta, fd&c red #40, propylene glycol]
- Psoriasin: 3% (177 mL) [dye free, fragrance free]
- Salicylic Acid Wart Remover: 27.5% (10 mL) [contains isopropyl alcohol]
- Scalpicin 2 in 1: 3% (44 mL) [fragrance free; contains menthol, propylene glycol]
- Tinamed Corn/Callus Remover: 17% (14.8 mL)
- Tinamed Wart Remover: 17% (14.8 mL) [contains alcohol, usp]
- Virasal: 27.5% (10 mL) [contains isopropyl alcohol, isopropyl-metacresol (isopropyl-m-cresol]
- Generic: 26% (10 mL); 27.5% (10 mL)

Lotion, External:
- Salacyn: 6% (414 mL) [contains cetyl alcohol, disodium edta, methylparaben, propylparaben, trolamine (triethanolamine)]
- Sebasorb: Attapulgite 10% and salicylic acid 2% (42 g)
- Generic: 6% (400 g, 414 mL, 473 mL)

Ointment, External:
- Bensal HP: 3% (4 g [DSC], 15 g [DSC], 30 g)

Pad, External:
- Clear Away 1-Step Wart Remover: 40% (14 ea)
- Corn Remover One Step: 40% (6 ea)
- Corn Remover Ultra Thin: 40% (9 ea)
- Mediplast: 40% (1 ea, 25 ea)
- One Step Callus Remover: 40% (4 ea)
- Scholls Callus Removers: 40% (4 ea [DSC], 6 ea [DSC])
- Scholls Corn Removers: 40% (9 ea [DSC])
- Scholls Corn Removers Extra: 40% (9 ea [DSC])
- Scholls Corn Removers Small: 40% (9 ea [DSC])
- Stri-Dex Maximum Strength: 2% (55 ea, 90 ea) [alcohol free]
- Stri-Dex Sensitive Skin: 0.5% (55 ea, 90 ea) [alcohol free]
- Stridex Essential: 1% (55 ea) [alcohol free; contains menthol, tetrasodium etidronate]

Patch, External:
- Trans-Ver-Sal AdultPatch: 15% (12 ea, 40 ea)
- Trans-Ver-Sal PediaPatch: 15% (15 ea, 40 ea)
- Trans-Ver-Sal PlantarPatch: 15% (10 ea)

Shampoo, External:
- Betasal: 3% (480 mL)
- DHS Sal: 3% (120 mL)
- DHS Sal: 3% (120 mL) [contains disodium edta]
- Ionil: 2% (120 mL)
- P & S: 2% (236 mL) [contains edetate sodium (tetrasodium), methylparaben, propylparaben, trolamine (triethanolamine)]
- Salex: 6% (177 mL) [contains methylparaben, propylparaben, trolamine (triethanolamine)]
- Generic: 6% (177 mL)

Solution, External:
- Gordofilm: 16.7% (15 mL)
- Salactic Film: 17% (15 mL)
- UltraSal-ER: 28.5% (10 mL) [contains isopropyl alcohol, phenol, polysorbate 80]
- Generic: 28.5% (10 mL)

- ◆ **Salicylic Acid and Sulfur** *see* Sulfur and Salicylic Acid *on page 1993*
- ◆ **Salicylic Acid Wart Remover** *see* Salicylic Acid *on page 1894*
- ◆ **Saline** *see* Sodium Chloride *on page 1938*
- ◆ **Saline Flush ZR** *see* Sodium Chloride *on page 1938*
- ◆ **Saline Mist Spray [OTC]** *see* Sodium Chloride *on page 1938*
- ◆ **Saljet [OTC]** *see* Sodium Chloride *on page 1938*
- ◆ **Saljet Rinse [OTC]** *see* Sodium Chloride *on page 1938*
- ◆ **Salkera** *see* Salicylic Acid *on page 1894*
- ◆ **Salk Vaccine** *see* Poliovirus Vaccine (Inactivated) *on page 1721*

Salmeterol (sal ME te role)

Medication Safety Issues

Sound-alike/look-alike issues:

Salmeterol may be confused with Salbutamol, Solu-Medrol

Serevent may be confused with Atrovent, Combivent, sertraline, Sinemet, Spiriva, Zoloft

Brand Names: US Serevent Diskus

Brand Names: Canada Serevent Diskhaler Disk; Serevent Diskus

Therapeutic Category Adrenergic Agonist Agent; Antiasthmatic; $Beta_2$-Adrenergic Agonist; Bronchodilator

Generic Availability (US) No

Use Concomitant therapy with inhaled corticosteroids for maintenance treatment of asthma and prevention of bronchospasm in patients with reversible obstructive airway disease, including patients with nocturnal symptoms (FDA approved in ages ≥4 years and adults); prevention of exercise-induced bronchospasm as concomitant therapy in patients with persistent asthma and as monotherapy in those without persistent asthma (FDA approved in ages ≥4 years and adults); maintenance treatment of bronchospasm associated with COPD (FDA approved in adults); **NOT** indicated for the relief of acute bronchospasm

Medication Guide Available Yes

Pregnancy Risk Factor C

Pregnancy Considerations Adverse events were observed in some animal reproduction studies. Beta-agonists have the potential to affect uterine contractility if administered during labor.

Uncontrolled asthma is associated with adverse events on pregnancy (increased risk of perinatal mortality, pre-eclampsia, preterm birth, low birth weight infants). Although data related to its use in pregnancy is limited, salmeterol may be used when a long-acting beta agonist is needed to treat moderate persistent or severe persistent asthma in pregnant women (NAEPP, 2005).

Breast-Feeding Considerations It is not known if salmeterol is excreted into breast milk. The manufacturer recommends that caution be exercised when administering salmeterol to nursing women. The use of beta$_2$-receptor agonists are not considered a contraindication to breast-feeding (NAEPP, 2005).

Contraindications

Hypersensitivity to salmeterol or any component of the formulation (milk proteins); monotherapy in the treatment of asthma (ie, use without a concomitant long-term asthma control medication, such as an inhaled corticosteroid); treatment of status asthmaticus or other acute episodes of asthma or COPD

Canadian labeling: Additional contraindications (not in U.S. labeling): Presence of tachyarrhythmias

Documentation of allergenic cross-reactivity for sympathomimetics is limited. However, because of similarities in chemical structure and/or pharmacologic actions, the possibility of cross-sensitivity cannot be ruled out with certainty.

Warnings/Precautions Asthma treatment: [U.S. Boxed Warning]: Long-acting beta$_2$-agonists (LABAs) increase the risk of asthma-related deaths. Salmeterol should only be used in asthma patients as adjuvant therapy in patients who are currently receiving but are not adequately controlled on a long-term asthma control medication (ie, an inhaled corticosteroid). Monotherapy with an LABA is contraindicated in the treatment of asthma. In a large, randomized, placebo-controlled U.S. clinical trial (SMART, 2006), salmeterol was associated with an increase in asthma-related deaths (when added to usual asthma therapy); risk is considered a class effect among all LABAs. Data are not available to determine if the addition of an inhaled corticosteroid lessens this increased risk of death associated with LABA use. Assess patients at regular intervals once asthma control is maintained on combination therapy to determine if step-down therapy is appropriate and the LABA can be discontinued (without loss of asthma control), and the patient can be maintained on an inhaled corticosteroid. LABAs are not appropriate in patients whose asthma is adequately controlled on low- or medium-dose inhaled corticosteroids. Do **not** use for acute bronchospasm. Short-acting beta$_2$-agonist (eg, albuterol) should be used for acute symptoms and symptoms occurring between treatments. Do **not** initiate in patients with significantly worsening or acutely deteriorating asthma; reports of severe (sometimes fatal) respiratory events have been reported when salmeterol has been initiated in this situation. Corticosteroids should not be stopped or reduced when salmeterol is initiated. During initiation, watch for signs of worsening asthma. Patients must be instructed to use short-acting beta$_2$-agonists (eg, albuterol) for acute asthmatic or COPD symptoms and to seek medical attention in cases where acute symptoms are not relieved or a previous level of response is diminished. The need to increase frequency of use of short-acting beta$_2$-agonist may indicate deterioration of asthma, and treatment must not be delayed. Because LABAs may disguise poorly controlled persistent asthma, frequent or chronic use of LABAs for exercise-induced bronchospasm is discouraged by the NIH Asthma Guidelines (NIH, 2007). Salmeterol should not be used more than twice daily; do not use with other long-acting beta$_2$-agonists. **[U.S. Boxed Warning]: LABAs may increase the risk of asthma-related hospitalization in pediatric and adolescent patients.** In general, a combination product containing a LABA and an inhaled corticosteroid is preferred in patients <18 years of age to ensure compliance.

COPD treatment: Appropriate use: Do **not** use for acute episodes of COPD. Do **not** initiate in patients with significantly worsening or acutely deteriorating COPD. Data are not available to determine if LABA use increases the risk of death in patients with COPD. Canadian labeling suggest concurrent use of oral or inhaled corticosteroids may not be necessary in COPD because the role of inhaled corticosteroids is less well established; concurrent use should be determined by the treating physician.

Use caution in patients with cardiovascular disease (eg, arrhythmia, coronary insufficiency, or hypertension), seizure disorders, diabetes, hyperthyroidism, hepatic impairment, or hypokalemia. Beta-agonists may cause elevation in blood pressure, heart rate, CNS stimulation/excitation, increase serum glucose, decrease serum potassium, increase risk of arrhythmia, and electrocardiogram (ECG) changes, such as flattening of the T wave, prolongation of the QTc interval, and ST segment depression.

Immediate hypersensitivity reactions (urticaria, angioedema, rash, bronchospasm) bronchospasm, hypotension) including anaphylaxis have been reported. There have been reports of laryngeal spasm, irritation, swelling (stridor, choking) with use. Salmeterol should not be used more than twice daily; do not exceed recommended dose; do not use with other long-acting beta$_2$-agonists; serious adverse events have been associated with excessive use of inhaled sympathomimetics. Rarely, paradoxical bronchospasm, which may be life threatening, may occur with use of inhaled bronchodilating agents; this should be distinguished from inadequate response. Potentially significant drug-drug interactions may exist, requiring dose or frequency adjustment, additional monitoring, and/or selection of alternative therapy (consult drug interactions database for more detailed information). Powder for oral inhalation contains lactose; very rare anaphylactic reactions have been reported in patients with severe milk protein allergy.

Adverse Reactions

Cardiovascular: Edema, hypertension, pallor

Central nervous system: Anxiety, dizziness, fever, headache, migraine, sleep disturbance

Dermatologic: Contact dermatitis, eczema, photodermatitis, rash, urticaria

Endocrine & metabolic: Hyperglycemia

Gastrointestinal: Dental pain, dyspepsia, gastrointestinal infection, nausea, oropharyngeal candidiasis, throat irritation, xerostomia

Hepatic: Liver enzymes increased

Neuromuscular & skeletal: Arthralgia, articular rheumatism, joint pain, muscular cramps/spasm/stiffness, pain, paresthesia, rigidity

Ocular: Keratitis/conjunctivitis

Respiratory: Asthma, cough, influenza, nasal congestion, pharyngitis, rhinitis, sinusitis, tracheitis/bronchitis, viral respiratory tract infection

Rare but important or life-threatening: Abdominal pain, agitation, aggression, anaphylactic reaction (some in patients with severe milk allergy [Diskus®]), angioedema, aphonia, arrhythmia, atrial fibrillation, cataracts, chest congestion, chest tightness, choking, contusions, Cushing syndrome, Cushingoid features, depression, dysmenorrhea, dyspnea, earache, ecchymoses, edema (facial, oropharyngeal), eosinophilic conditions, glaucoma, growth velocity reduction in children/adolescents, hypercorticism, hypersensitivity reaction (immediate and delayed), hypokalemia, hypothyroidism, intraocular pressure increased, laryngeal spasm/irritation, irregular menstruation, myositis, oropharyngeal irritation, osteoporosis, pallor, paradoxical bronchospasm, paradoxical tracheitis, paranasal sinus pain, PID, QTc prolongation, restlessness, stridor, supraventricular tachycardia, syncope, tremor, vaginal candidiasis, vaginitis, vulvovaginitis, rare cases of vasculitis (Churg-Strauss syndrome), ventricular tachycardia, weight gain

Drug Interactions

Metabolism/Transport Effects Substrate of CYP3A4 (major); **Note:** Assignment of Major/Minor substrate status based on clinically relevant drug interaction potential

Avoid Concomitant Use

Avoid concomitant use of Salmeterol with any of the following: Beta-Blockers (Nonselective); Conivaptan; CYP3A4 Inhibitors (Strong); Fusidic Acid (Systemic); Idelalisib; Iobenguane I 123; Long-Acting Beta2-Agonists; Loxapine; Telaprevir; Tipranavir

Increased Effect/Toxicity

Salmeterol may increase the levels/effects of: Atosiban; Highest Risk QTc-Prolonging Agents; Long-Acting Beta2-Agonists; Loop Diuretics; Loxapine; Moderate Risk QTc-Prolonging Agents; Sympathomimetics; Thiazide Diuretics

The levels/effects of Salmeterol may be increased by: Aprepitant; AtoMOXetine; Cannabinoid-Containing Products; Conivaptan; CYP3A4 Inhibitors (Moderate); CYP3A4 Inhibitors (Strong); Dasatinib; Fosaprepitant; Fusidic Acid (Systemic); Idelalisib; Ivacaftor; Linezolid; Luliconazole; MAO Inhibitors; Mifepristone; Netupitant; Palbociclib; Simeprevir; Stiripentol; Tedizolid; Telaprevir; Tipranavir; Tricyclic Antidepressants

Decreased Effect

Salmeterol may decrease the levels/effects of: Iobenguane I 123

The levels/effects of Salmeterol may be decreased by: Beta-Blockers (Beta1 Selective); Beta-Blockers (Nonselective); Betahistine

Storage/Stability Store at 68°F and 77°F (20°C and 25°C); excursions are permitted between 59°F and 86°F (15°C and 30°C). Protect from direct heat or sunlight. Store Diskus in the unopened foil pouch and only open when ready for use; stable for 6 weeks after removal from foil pouch.

Mechanism of Action Relaxes bronchial smooth muscle by selective action on beta$_2$-receptors with little effect on heart rate; salmeterol acts locally in the lung.

Pharmacodynamics

Onset of action: Asthma: 30-48 minutes; COPD: 2 hours

Peak effect: Asthma: 3 hours; COPD: 2-5 hours

Duration: Up to 12 hours

Pharmacokinetics (Adult data unless noted)

Protein binding: 96%

Metabolism: Extensive hydroxylation via CYP3A4

Half-life: 5.5 hours

Elimination: 60% in feces and 25% in urine over a 7-day period

Dosing: Usual Children ≥4 years and Adults:

Asthma, maintenance treatment; prevention: Inhalation, oral: 50 mcg (1 actuation/puff) twice daily, 12 hours apart; **Note:** For long-term asthma control, long-acting beta$_2$-agonists should be used in combination with inhaled corticosteroids and **not** as monotherapy.

Exercise-induced bronchospasm, prevention: Inhalation: 50 mcg (1 inhalation/puff) 30 minutes prior to exercise; additional doses should not be used for 12 hours; patients who are using salmeterol twice daily should **not** use an additional salmeterol dose prior to exercise; if twice daily use is not effective during exercise, consider other appropriate therapy; **Note:** Because long-acting beta$_2$-agonists (LABAs) may disguise poorly-controlled persistent asthma, frequent or chronic use of LABAs for exercise-induced bronchospasm is discouraged by the NAEPP Asthma Guidelines (NAEPP, 2007).

COPD, maintenance treatment: Adults: 50 mcg (1 inhalation/puff) twice daily (~12 hours apart); maximum: 1 inhalation twice daily

Administration Inhalation: Not for use with a spacer

Monitoring Parameters Pulmonary function tests, vital signs, CNS stimulation, serum glucose, serum potassium

Additional Information When salmeterol is initiated in patients previously receiving a short-acting beta agonist, instruct the patient to discontinue the regular use of the short-acting beta agonist and to utilize the shorter-acting agent for symptomatic or acute episodes only.

Dosage Forms Excipient information presented when available (limited, particularly for generics); consult specific product labeling.

Aerosol Powder Breath Activated, Inhalation:

Serevent Diskus: 50 mcg/dose (28 ea, 60 ea) [contains lactose]

◆ **Salmeterol and Fluticasone** *see* Fluticasone and Salmeterol *on page* 923
◆ **Salmeterol Xinafoate** *see* Salmeterol *on page* 1896
◆ **Salofalk (Can)** *see* Mesalamine *on page* 1368
◆ **Salonpas Gel-Patch Hot [OTC]** *see* Capsaicin *on page* 362
◆ **Salonpas Hot [OTC] [DSC]** *see* Capsaicin *on page* 362
◆ **Sal-Plant [OTC]** *see* Salicylic Acid *on page* 1894
◆ **Salt** *see* Sodium Chloride *on page* 1938
◆ **Salt Poor Albumin** *see* Albumin *on page* 79
◆ **Salvax** *see* Salicylic Acid *on page* 1894
◆ **Sancuso** *see* Granisetron *on page* 981
◆ **SandIMMUNE** *see* CycloSPORINE (Systemic) *on page* 556
◆ **Sandimmune I.V. (Can)** *see* CycloSPORINE (Systemic) *on page* 556
◆ **SandoSTATIN** *see* Octreotide *on page* 1539
◆ **Sandostatin (Can)** *see* Octreotide *on page* 1539
◆ **Sandostatin LAR (Can)** *see* Octreotide *on page* 1539
◆ **SandoSTATIN LAR Depot** *see* Octreotide *on page* 1539
◆ **Sandoz-Almotriptan (Can)** *see* Almotriptan *on page* 98
◆ **Sandoz-Amiodarone (Can)** *see* Amiodarone *on page* 125
◆ **Sandoz Amlodipine (Can)** *see* AmLODIPine *on page* 133
◆ **Sandoz-Anagrelide (Can)** *see* Anagrelide *on page* 163
◆ **Sandoz-Atenolol (Can)** *see* Atenolol *on page* 215
◆ **Sandoz-Atomoxetine (Can)** *see* AtoMOXetine *on page* 217
◆ **Sandoz-Atorvastatin (Can)** *see* AtorvaSTATin *on page* 220
◆ **Sandoz-Azithromycin (Can)** *see* Azithromycin (Systemic) *on page* 242
◆ **Sandoz-Betaxolol (Can)** *see* Betaxolol (Ophthalmic) *on page* 283

◆ **Sandoz-Bosentan (Can)** *see* Bosentan *on page 294*

◆ **Sandoz-Brimonidine (Can)** *see* Brimonidine (Ophthalmic) *on page 301*

◆ **Sandoz-Bupropion SR (Can)** *see* BuPROPion *on page 324*

◆ **Sandoz-Candesartan (Can)** *see* Candesartan *on page 358*

◆ **Sandoz-Carbamazepine (Can)** *see* CarBAMazepine *on page 367*

◆ **Sandoz-Cefprozil (Can)** *see* Cefprozil *on page 405*

◆ **Sandoz-Celecoxib (Can)** *see* Celecoxib *on page 418*

◆ **Sandoz-Ciprofloxacin (Can)** *see* Ciprofloxacin (Systemic) *on page 463*

◆ **Sandoz-Citalopram (Can)** *see* Citalopram *on page 476*

◆ **Sandoz-Clarithromycin (Can)** *see* Clarithromycin *on page 482*

◆ **Sandoz-Clonazepam (Can)** *see* ClonazePAM *on page 506*

◆ **Sandoz-Clopidogrel (Can)** *see* Clopidogrel *on page 513*

◆ **Sandoz-Cyclosporine (Can)** *see* CycloSPORINE (Systemic) *on page 556*

◆ **Sandoz-Diclofenac (Can)** *see* Diclofenac (Systemic) *on page 641*

◆ **Sandoz-Diclofenac Rapide (Can)** *see* Diclofenac (Systemic) *on page 641*

◆ **Sandoz-Diclofenac SR (Can)** *see* Diclofenac (Systemic) *on page 641*

◆ **Sandoz-Diltiazem CD (Can)** *see* Diltiazem *on page 661*

◆ **Sandoz-Diltiazem T (Can)** *see* Diltiazem *on page 661*

◆ **Sandoz-Dimenhydrinate [OTC] (Can)** *see* DimenhyDRINATE *on page 664*

◆ **Sandoz-Dorzolamide (Can)** *see* Dorzolamide *on page 706*

◆ **Sandoz-Enalapril (Can)** *see* Enalapril *on page 744*

◆ **Sandoz Escitalopram (Can)** *see* Escitalopram *on page 786*

◆ **Sandoz-Estradiol Derm 50 (Can)** *see* Estradiol (Systemic) *on page 795*

◆ **Sandoz-Estradiol Derm 75 (Can)** *see* Estradiol (Systemic) *on page 795*

◆ **Sandoz-Estradiol Derm 100 (Can)** *see* Estradiol (Systemic) *on page 795*

◆ **Sandoz Ezetimibe (Can)** *see* Ezetimibe *on page 832*

◆ **Sandoz-Famciclovir (Can)** *see* Famciclovir *on page 846*

◆ **Sandoz-Felodipine (Can)** *see* Felodipine *on page 855*

◆ **Sandoz Fentanyl Patch (Can)** *see* FentaNYL *on page 857*

◆ **Sandoz-Fluoxetine (Can)** *see* FLUoxetine *on page 906*

◆ **Sandoz-Fluvoxamine (Can)** *see* FluvoxaMINE *on page 928*

◆ **Sandoz-Glyburide (Can)** *see* GlyBURIDE *on page 975*

◆ **Sandoz-Indomethacin (Can)** *see* Indomethacin *on page 1101*

◆ **Sandoz-Irbesartan (Can)** *see* Irbesartan *on page 1158*

◆ **Sandoz-Lansoprazole (Can)** *see* Lansoprazole *on page 1219*

◆ **Sandoz-Letrozole (Can)** *see* Letrozole *on page 1224*

◆ **Sandoz-Levobunolol (Can)** *see* Levobunolol *on page 1238*

◆ **Sandoz-Levofloxacin (Can)** *see* Levofloxacin (Systemic) *on page 1243*

◆ **Sandoz-Linezolid (Can)** *see* Linezolid *on page 1268*

◆ **Sandoz-Lisinopril (Can)** *see* Lisinopril *on page 1280*

◆ **Sandoz-Loperamide (Can)** *see* Loperamide *on page 1288*

◆ **Sandoz Losartan (Can)** *see* Losartan *on page 1302*

◆ **Sandoz-Lovastatin (Can)** *see* Lovastatin *on page 1305*

◆ **Sandoz-Metformin FC (Can)** *see* MetFORMIN *on page 1375*

◆ **Sandoz-Methylphenidate SR (Can)** *see* Methylphenidate *on page 1402*

◆ **Sandoz-Metoprolol SR (Can)** *see* Metoprolol *on page 1418*

◆ **Sandoz-Metoprolol (Type L) (Can)** *see* Metoprolol *on page 1418*

◆ **Sandoz-Minocycline (Can)** *see* Minocycline *on page 1440*

◆ **Sandoz-Montelukast (Can)** *see* Montelukast *on page 1459*

◆ **Sandoz-Montelukast Granules (Can)** *see* Montelukast *on page 1459*

◆ **Sandoz-Morphine SR (Can)** *see* Morphine (Systemic) *on page 1461*

◆ **Sandoz-Mycophenolate Mofetil (Can)** *see* Mycophenolate *on page 1473*

◆ **Sandoz-Olanzapine (Can)** *see* OLANZapine *on page 1546*

◆ **Sandoz-Olanzapine ODT (Can)** *see* OLANZapine *on page 1546*

◆ **Sandoz-Omeprazole (Can)** *see* Omeprazole *on page 1555*

◆ **Sandoz-Ondansetron (Can)** *see* Ondansetron *on page 1564*

◆ **Sandoz-Oxycodone/Acetaminophen (Can)** *see* Oxycodone and Acetaminophen *on page 1594*

◆ **Sandoz-Pantoprazole (Can)** *see* Pantoprazole *on page 1618*

◆ **Sandoz-Paroxetine (Can)** *see* PARoxetine *on page 1634*

◆ **Sandoz-Pravastatin (Can)** *see* Pravastatin *on page 1749*

◆ **Sandoz Prednisolone (Can)** *see* PrednisoLONE (Ophthalmic) *on page 1758*

◆ **Sandoz-Prochlorperazine (Can)** *see* Prochlorperazine *on page 1774*

◆ **Sandoz-Quetiapine (Can)** *see* QUEtiapine *on page 1815*

◆ **Sandoz-Quetiapine XRT (Can)** *see* QUEtiapine *on page 1815*

◆ **Sandoz-Rabeprazole (Can)** *see* RABEprazole *on page 1828*

◆ **Sandoz-Ranitidine (Can)** *see* Ranitidine *on page 1836*

◆ **Sandoz-Risperidone (Can)** *see* RisperiDONE *on page 1866*

◆ **Sandoz-Rizatriptan ODT (Can)** *see* Rizatriptan *on page 1879*

◆ **Sandoz-Rosuvastatin (Can)** *see* Rosuvastatin *on page 1886*

◆ **Sandoz-Salbutamol (Can)** *see* Albuterol *on page 81*

◆ **Sandoz-Sertraline (Can)** *see* Sertraline *on page 1916*

◆ **Sandoz-Sildenafil (Can)** *see* Sildenafil *on page 1921*

◆ **Sandoz-Simvastatin (Can)** *see* Simvastatin *on page 1928*

◆ **Sandoz-Sotalol (Can)** *see* Sotalol *on page 1963*

Sapropterin (sap roe TER in)

Medication Safety Issues

Sound-alike/look-alike issues:

Sapropterin may be confused with cyproterone

Brand Names: US Kuvan

Brand Names: Canada Kuvan

Generic Availability (US) No

Use Reduction of blood phenylalanine (PHE) levels in patients with hyperphenylalaninemia caused by tetrahydrobiopterin (BH4)-responsive phenylketonuria (PKU) in conjunction with a PHE-restricted diet (FDA approved in ages ≥1 month and adults)

Pregnancy Risk Factor C

Pregnancy Considerations Adverse events have been observed in some animal reproduction studies. High levels of maternal phenylalanine are associated with congenital heart disease, developmental delay, facial dysmorphism, learning difficulties, and microcephaly. Phenylalanine (PHE) concentrations should be normalized prior to conception. Fetal development is optimal when PHE concentrations <360 micromol/L are achieved prior to conception (Vockley, 2014). Dietary control with proper supplementation is recommended during pregnancy. Maternal PHE requirements may change throughout pregnancy; frequent testing and dietary modifications may be necessary (Vockley, 2014). Some clinicians recommend that dietary control be achieved for at least 4 weeks prior to conception; however, studies suggest that as long as control is achieved by 10 weeks of pregnancy, teratogenic effects of untreated maternal phenylketonuria can be decreased (Koch, 2003; Maillot, 2007). In addition to standard fetal monitoring, fetal echocardiography is recommended at 18-22 weeks gestation (Vockley, 2014). Pregnant women exposed to sapropterin are encouraged to enroll in the Kuvan pregnancy registry (866-906-6100).

Breast-Feeding Considerations It is not known if sapropterin is excreted in breast milk. The US labeling recommends that caution be exercised when administering sapropterin to nursing women. The Canadian labeling does not recommend use in nursing women. Infants unaffected by phenylalanine hydroxylase (PHA) deficiency are able to metabolize the slightly higher PHE concentrations from breast milk of mothers with PHA deficiency (Vockley, 2014).

Contraindications

There are no contraindications listed in the manufacturer's labeling.

Canadian labeling: Hypersensitivity to sapropterin or any component of the formulation

Warnings/Precautions Phenylalanine (PHE) levels should be monitored and maintained within the target range during sapropterin treatment. Upon diagnosis, blood PHE levels should be lowered into the desired treatment range (120 to 360 micromol/L) as quickly as possible; infants with levels >600 micromol/L require treatment, although treatment may be initiated at ≥360 micromol/L; if testing is done in early infancy, it is recommended to initially lower blood PHE to 480 to 600 micromol/L (Vockley, 2014). Prolonged high levels of phenylalanine can result in severe neurologic damage, including behavioral abnormalities, delayed speech, microcephaly, seizures, and severe mental retardation. Low levels of phenylalanine are associated with catabolism and protein breakdown. Dietary management of phenylalanine intake is required to ensure nutritional balance and adequate phenylalanine control. Monitor blood PHE levels during treatment (frequently in children). Some patients my experience low blood phenylalanine levels. Children younger than 7 years treated with doses of 20 mg/kg/day are at increased risk for low levels of blood phenylalanine (hypophenylalaninemia). PHE blood level testing at doses <20 mg/kg may underestimate response rate (Vockley, 2014). Response to sapropterin treatment is established through treatment (cannot be predetermined by lab testing). Patients whose phenylalanine levels do not decrease after treatment at 20 mg/kg/day for 1 month are considered nonresponders.

Hypersensitivity reactions, including anaphylaxis and rash, have occurred; not recommended for use in patients with a history of anaphylaxis to sapropterin. Discontinue use and initiate appropriate medical treatment in patients who experience anaphylaxis. Dietary PHE restrictions should be continued in patients who experience anaphylaxis. Gastritis and hyperactivity have been reported; monitor patients for these adverse effects.

Has not been studied in patients with renal or hepatic impairment; monitor carefully; hepatic damage has been associated with impaired phenylalanine metabolism. Potentially significant drug-drug interactions may exist, requiring dose or frequency adjustment, additional monitoring, and/or selection of alternative therapy.

Adverse Reactions

Central nervous system: Headache

Gastrointestinal: Diarrhea, vomiting

Respiratory: Cough, nasal congestion, pharyngolaryngeal pain, rhinorrhea

Rare but important or life-threatening: Anaphylaxis, gastritis, gastrointestinal hemorrhage, hemorrhage (postprocedural), hyperactivity, increased gamma-glutamyl transferase, myocardial infarction, peripheral edema, seizure (including seizure exacerbation), upper respiratory tract infection

Drug Interactions

Metabolism/Transport Effects None known.

Avoid Concomitant Use There are no known interactions where it is recommended to avoid concomitant use.

Increased Effect/Toxicity

Sapropterin may increase the levels/effects of: Levodopa; Phosphodiesterase 5 Inhibitors

Decreased Effect

The levels/effects of Sapropterin may be decreased by: Methotrexate; PRALAtrexate

Storage/Stability Store at 20°C to 25°C (68°F to 77°F); excursions to 15°C to 30°C (59°F to 86°F) permitted. Protect from moisture.

Mechanism of Action Sapropterin is a synthetic form of the cofactor BH4 (tetrahydrobiopterin) for the enzyme phenylalanine hydroxylase (PAH). PAH hydroxylates phenylalanine to form tyrosine. BH4 activates residual PAH enzyme, improving normal phenylalanine metabolism and decreasing phenylalanine levels in sapropterin responders. Approximately 25% to 50% of patients with PAH deficiency are responsive to sapropterin (Vockley, 2014).

Pharmacodynamics

Onset of action: Within 24 hours of initial dose, decreases in serum Phe concentrations

Maximum effect: 1 month

Duration: 24 hours

Pharmacokinetics (Adult data unless noted)

Absorption: Enhanced with food (high-fat/high-calorie); absorption via intact tablet administration is greater than dissolved tablet administration

Metabolism: The enzymes dihydrofolate reductase and dihydropteridine reductase are responsible for the metabolism and recycling of BH4.

Half-life: 6.7 hours (range: ~4 to 17 hours)

Dosing: Usual

Pediatric: **Phenylalanine hydroxylase (PAH) deficiency disorders (eg, hyperphenylalaninemia, phenylketonuria [PKU]), adjunct treatment:** Oral:

Infants and Children ≤6 years:

Initial: 10 mg/kg/dose once daily; adjust dose after 1 month based on phenylalanine levels; if phenylalanine levels have not decreased from baseline after 1 month of therapy, increase dose to 20 mg/kg/dose once daily; if still no response after 1 month of therapy at the higher dose (20 mg/kg/day) then discontinue sapropterin (nonresponder)

Usual maintenance range: 5 to 20 mg/kg/dose once daily, dosage should be individualized based on patient response. **Note:** In clinical trials of patients ≥7 months, doses were rounded to the nearest 100 mg increment so dosages up to 24 mg/kg/day were used (Burton 2011)

Children ≥7 years and Adolescents:

Initial: 10 to 20 mg/kg/dose once daily; adjust dose after 1 month based on phenylalanine levels:

Initial dose 10 mg/kg/dose: If phenylalanine levels have not decreased from baseline after 1 month of therapy, increase dose to 20 mg/kg/dose once daily; if still no response after 1 month of therapy at the higher dose (20 mg/kg/day) then discontinue sapropterin (nonresponder)

Initial dose 20 mg/kg/dose: If no response after 1 month of therapy, discontinue sapropterin (nonresponder)

Usual maintenance range: 5 to 20 mg/kg/dose once daily; dosage should be individualized based on patient response. **Note:** In clinical trials of patients ≥7 months, doses were rounded to the nearest 100 mg increment so dosages up to 24 mg/kg/day were used (Burton 2011)

Adult: Phenylalanine hydroxylase (PAH) deficiency disorders (eg, hyperphenylalaninemia, phenylketonuria [PKU]), adjunct treatment: Oral: Initial: 10 to 20 mg/kg once daily; adjust after 1 month based on blood phenylalanine levels (if phenylalanine levels do not decrease from baseline after initiating 10 mg/kg, increase dose to 20 mg/kg once daily); discontinue if phenylalanine levels do not decrease after 1 month of treatment at 20 mg/kg/day (nonresponder). Maintenance range: 5 to 20 mg/kg once daily

Preparation for Administration

Oral:

Powder for oral solution:

Patients weighing ≤10 kg: Dissolve one packet in 5 or 10 mL of water or apple juice (refer to prescribing information for dilution and administration volumes); then withdraw dose volume into oral syringe. **Note:** For use in infants and young children, sapropterin has shown similar stability when mixed with phenylalanine-free formula (Burton 2011a).

Patients weighing >10 kg: Dissolve appropriate number of packets in 120 to 240 mL (4 to 8 oz) water or apple juice or in a small amount of soft foods, such as apple sauce or pudding, and mix thoroughly.

Tablets: Dissolve tablets in 120 to 240 mL (4 to 8 oz) water or apple juice; may crush or stir to aid in dissolution; dissolution may take several minutes and may not be complete (eg, small piece floating on surface of liquid); this is expected.

Administration Oral: Administer with food, preferably at the same time each day; a missed dose should be taken as soon as possible, but 2 doses should not be taken on the same day.

Powder for oral solution: Dissolve powder for oral solution in water or apple juice or mix in a small amount of soft foods, such as apple sauce or pudding, prior administration. Take within 30 minutes of dissolution. **Note:** For use in infants and young children, sapropterin has shown similar stability when mixed with phenylalanine-free formula, applesauce, and pudding (Burton 2011a).

Tablets: Swallow tablets whole or dissolve tablets in water or apple juice. Dose should be consumed within 15 minutes of dissolution; may rinse remaining tablet residue (with more water or apple juice) and drink. Tablets may also be crushed and then mixed in a small amount of soft food, such as apple sauce or pudding.

Monitoring Parameters Blood phenylalanine levels (baseline, after 1 week of treatment, periodically for first month, regularly thereafter); children may require more frequent monitoring; blood pressure in patients taking concomitant PDE-5 inhibitors (eg, sildenafil, vardenafil, tadalafil); patients with renal or hepatic impairment; change in neurologic status in patients taking concurrent levodopa; signs and symptoms of gastritis; hyperactivity

Guideline recommended monitoring for patients with phenylalanine hydroxylase deficiency (Vockley 2014):

Newly diagnosed infants: Monitor phenylalanine (PHE) and tyrosine (TYR) frequently until the PHE concentrations stabilize, then monitor PHE weekly until age 1 (increase frequency during rapid growth or dietary transitions)

Adolescents and Adults who are stable: Monitor PHE monthly

If formal nutritional assessment suggests suboptimal dietary intake or for over reliance on nutritionally incomplete medical foods: Consider monitoring plasma amino acids (full panel), transthyretin, albumin, CBC, ferritin, 25-OH vitamin D, vitamin B_{12}, red blood cell essential fatty acids, trace minerals (copper, selenium, zinc), vitamin A, comprehensive metabolic panel, and folic acid.

Reference Range Phenylalanine hydroxylase deficiency, blood phenylalanine goal range: 120 to 360 micromol/L (Vockley 2014)

Dosage Forms Excipient information presented when available (limited, particularly for generics); consult specific product labeling.

Packet, Oral, as dihydrochloride:

Kuvan: 100 mg (1 ea, 30 ea); 500 mg (1 ea, 30 ea)

Tablet Soluble, Oral, as dihydrochloride:

Kuvan: 100 mg

◆ **Sapropterin Dihydrochloride** *see* Sapropterin *on page 1900*

Saquinavir (sa KWIN a veer)

Medication Safety Issues

Sound-alike/look-alike issues:

Saquinavir may be confused with SINEquan

High alert medication:

This medication is in a class the Institute for Safe Medication Practices (ISMP) includes among its list of drug classes that have a heightened risk of causing significant patient harm when used in error.

Related Information

Adult and Adolescent HIV *on page 2392*
Pediatric HIV *on page 2380*
Perinatal HIV *on page 2400*

Brand Names: US Invirase

Brand Names: Canada Invirase

Therapeutic Category Antiretroviral Agent; HIV Agents (Anti-HIV Agents); Protease Inhibitor

Generic Availability (US) No

Use Treatment of HIV infection in combination with other antiretroviral agents (FDA approved in ages ≥16 years and adults); **Note:** HIV regimens consisting of three antiretroviral agents are strongly recommended; due to its low bioavailability, Invirase must only be used in combination regimens that include ritonavir "booster doses" so that adequate plasma saquinavir concentrations are attained

Medication Guide Available Yes

Pregnancy Risk Factor B

Pregnancy Considerations Adverse events were not observed in animal reproduction studies. Saquinavir has a low level of transfer across the human placenta. Based on available data, saquinavir administered twice daily with ritonavir 100 mg twice daily provide adequate levels in pregnant women. The DHHS Perinatal HIV Guidelines consider saquinavir and ritonavir to be an alternative combination for use in antiretroviral-naive pregnant women; use without ritonavir is **not** recommended. A small increased risk of preterm birth has been associated with maternal use of protease inhibitor-based combination antiretroviral (ARV) therapy during pregnancy; however, the benefits of use generally outweigh this risk and protease inhibitors (PIs) should not be withheld if otherwise recommended. Hyperglycemia, new onset of diabetes mellitus, or diabetic ketoacidosis have been reported with PIs; it is not clear if pregnancy increases this risk.

Regardless of CD4 count or HIV RNA copy number, all HIV-infected pregnant women should receive a combination antiretroviral ARV drug regimen. A combination of antepartum, intrapartum, and infant ARV prophylaxis is recommended. ARV therapy should be started as soon as possible in women with symptomatic infection. Although earlier initiation may be more effective in reducing the perinatal transmission of HIV, initiation may be delayed until after 12 weeks gestation in women who do not require immediate treatment after careful consideration of maternal conditions (eg, nausea and vomiting) and the potential risks of first trimester fetal exposure for specific agents. A scheduled cesarean delivery at 38 weeks gestation is recommended for all women with HIV RNA >1000 copies/mL or unknown concentrations near delivery in order to decrease transmission. If ARV therapy must be interrupted for <24 hours during the peripartum period, stop then restart all medications simultaneously in order to decrease the chance of developing resistance. Long-term follow-up is recommended for all infants exposed to ARV medications. In couples who want to conceive, the HIV-infected partner should attain maximum viral suppression prior to conception.

Health care providers are encouraged to enroll pregnant women exposed to antiretroviral medications in the Antiretroviral Pregnancy Registry (1-800-258-4263 or www.APRegistry.com). Health care providers caring for HIV-infected women and their infants may contact the National Perinatal HIV Hotline (888-448-8765) for clinical consultation (HHS [perinatal], 2014).

Breast-Feeding Considerations It is not known if saquinavir is excreted into breast milk. Maternal or infant antiretroviral therapy does not completely eliminate the risk of postnatal HIV transmission. In addition, multiclass-resistant virus has been detected in breast-feeding infants despite maternal therapy. Therefore, in the United States, where formula is accessible, affordable, safe, and sustainable, and the risk of infant mortality due to diarrhea and respiratory infections is low, complete avoidance of breast-feeding by HIV-infected women is recommended to decrease potential transmission of HIV (HHS [perinatal], 2014).

Contraindications

Hypersensitivity to saquinavir or any component of the formulation; congenital or acquired QT prolongation, refractory hypokalemia or hypomagnesemia, concomitant use of other medications that both increase saquinavir plasma concentrations and prolong the QT interval; complete AV block (without implanted ventricular pacemaker) or patients at high risk of complete AV block; severe hepatic impairment; coadministration of saquinavir/ritonavir with alfuzosin, amiodarone, bepridil, cisapride, dofetilide, ergot derivatives, flecainide, lidocaine (systemic), lovastatin, midazolam (oral), pimozide, propafenone, quinidine, rifampin, sildenafil (when used for pulmonary artery hypertension [eg, Revatio]), simvastatin, trazodone, or triazolam

Canadian labeling: Additional contraindications (not in U.S. labeling): Concurrent use with quetiapine, procainamide, sotalol, astemizole, or terfenadine; concurrent use with medications that both increase saquinavir plasma concentrations and prolong the PR interval

Warnings/Precautions Use caution in patients with hepatic insufficiency. May exacerbate pre-existing hepatic dysfunction; use with caution in patients with hepatitis B or C and in cirrhosis. May be associated with fat redistribution (buffalo hump, increased abdominal girth, breast engorgement, facial atrophy). Use caution in hemophilia. May increase cholesterol and/or triglycerides. Changes in glucose tolerance, hyperglycemia, exacerbation of diabetes, DKA, and new-onset diabetes mellitus have been reported in patients receiving protease inhibitors.

Photosensitivity reactions: May cause photosensitivity reactions (eg, exposure to sunlight may cause severe sunburn, skin rash, redness, or itching); advise patient to avoid exposure to sunlight and artificial light sources (eg, sunlamps, tanning bed/booth) and to wear protective clothing, wide-brimmed hats, sunglasses, and lip sunscreen (SPF ≥15). Sunscreen should be used (broad-spectrum sunscreen or physical sunscreen [preferred] or sunblock with SPF ≥15) (DHHS [pediatric], 2014).

Altered cardiac conduction: Saquinavir/ritonavir prolongs the QT interval, potentially leading to torsade de pointes, and prolongs the PR interval, potentially leading to heart block. Second- or third-degree AV block has been reported (rare). An ECG should be performed for all patients prior to starting saquinavir/ritonavir therapy; do not initiate therapy in patients with a baseline QT interval >450 msec or diagnosed with long QT syndrome. If baseline QT interval <450 msec, may initiate therapy but a subsequent ECG is recommended (U.S. labeling recommends an ECG after ~3 to 4 days of therapy; Canadian labeling recommends an ECG after ~10 days of therapy). If subsequent QT interval is >480 msec or is prolonged over baseline by >20 msec, therapy should be discontinued. Patients who may be at increased risk for QT- or PR-interval prolongation include those with heart failure, bradyarrhythmias, hepatic impairment, electrolyte abnormalities, ischemic heart disease, cardiomyopathy, structural heart disease, or those with pre-existing cardiac conduction abnormalities; ECG monitoring is recommended for these patients.

Must be used in combination with ritonavir. Continued administration after loss of viral suppression efficacy may increase the likelihood of cross-resistance to other protease inhibitors. Promptly discontinue therapy if viral suppression response is lost. High potential for drug interactions; concomitant use of saquinavir with some drugs may require cautious use, may not be recommended, may require dosage adjustments, or may be contraindicated. Consult drug interactions database for more detailed information. Patients may develop immune reconstitution syndrome resulting in the occurrence of an inflammatory response to an indolent or residual opportunistic infection during initial HIV treatment or activation of autoimmune disorders (eg, Graves' disease, polymyositis, Guillain-Barré syndrome) later in therapy; further evaluation and treatment may be required. Formulation contains lactose; Canadian product labeling recommends against use in patients with galactose intolerance, Lapp lactase deficiency or glucose-galactose malabsorption.

Adverse Reactions

Incidence data shown for saquinavir soft gel capsule formulation (no longer available) in combination with ritonavir.

Cardiovascular: Chest pain

Central nervous system: Anxiety, depression, fatigue, fever, headache, insomnia, pain

Dermatologic: Dry lips/skin, eczema, pruritus, rash, verruca

Endocrine & metabolic: Hyper-/hypoglycemia, hyperkalemia, libido disorder, lipodystrophy, serum amylase increased

Gastrointestinal: Abdominal discomfort, abdominal pain, appetite decreased, buccal mucosa ulceration, constipation, diarrhea, dyspepsia, flatulence, nausea, taste alteration, vomiting

Hepatic: AST increased, ALT increased, bilirubin increased

Neuromuscular & skeletal: Back pain, CPK increased, paresthesia, weakness

Renal: Creatinine kinase increased

Respiratory: Bronchitis, pneumonia, sinusitis

Miscellaneous: Influenza

Incidence not currently defined (limited to significant reactions; reported for hard or soft gel capsule with/without ritonavir)

Cardiovascular: Cyanosis, heart valve disorder (including murmur), hyper-/hypotension, peripheral vasoconstriction, prolonged QT interval, prolonged PR interval, syncope, thrombophlebitis

Central nervous system: Agitation, amnesia, ataxia, confusion, hallucination, hyper-/hyporeflexia, myelopolyradiculoneuritis, neuropathies, poliomyelitis, progressive multifocal encephalopathy, psychosis, seizures, somnolence, speech disorder, suicide attempt

Dermatologic: Alopecia, bullous eruption, dermatitis, erythema, maculopapular rash, photosensitivity, Stevens-Johnson syndrome, skin ulceration, urticaria

Endocrine & metabolic: Dehydration, diabetes, electrolyte changes, TSH increased

Gastrointestinal: Ascites, colic, dysphagia, esophagitis, bloody stools, gastritis, intestinal obstruction, hemorrhage (rectal), pancreatitis, stomatitis

Genitourinary: impotence, prostate enlarged, hematuria, UTI

Hematologic; Acute myeloblastic leukemia, anemia (including hemolytic), leukopenia, neutropenia, pancytopenia, splenomegaly, thrombocytopenia

Hepatic: Alkaline phosphatase increased, GGT increased, hepatitis, hepatomegaly, hepatosplenomegaly, jaundice, liver disease exacerbation

Neuromuscular & skeletal: Arthritis, LDH increased

Ocular: Blepharitis, visual disturbance

Otic: Otitis, hearing decreased, tinnitus

Renal: Nephrolithiasis, renal calculus

Respiratory: Dyspnea, hemoptysis, pharyngitis, upper respiratory tract infection

Miscellaneous: Immune reconstitution syndrome, infections (bacterial, fungal, viral)

Postmarketing and/or case reports: AV block (second or third degree), torsade de pointes

Drug Interactions

Metabolism/Transport Effects Substrate of CYP2D6 (minor), CYP3A4 (major), P-glycoprotein; **Note:** Assignment of Major/Minor substrate status based on clinically relevant drug interaction potential; **Inhibits** CYP2C19 (weak), CYP2C9 (weak), CYP2D6 (weak), CYP3A4 (strong), P-glycoprotein, SLCO1B1

Avoid Concomitant Use

Avoid concomitant use of Saquinavir with any of the following: Ado-Trastuzumab Emtansine; Alfuzosin; Amiodarone; Apixaban; Astemizole; Avanafil; Axitinib; Barnidipine; Bepridil; Bosutinib; Cabozantinib; Ceritinib; Cisapride; Conivaptan; Crizotinib; Dapoxetine; Darunavir; Dofetilide; Domperidone; Dronedarone; Eplerenone; Ergot Derivatives; Everolimus; Flecainide; Fusidic Acid (Systemic); Halofantrine; Highest Risk QTc-Prolonging Agents; Ibrutinib; Irinotecan; Isavuconazonium Sulfate; Ivabradine; Lapatinib; Lercanidipine; Lidocaine (Systemic); Lomitapide; Lopinavir; Lovastatin; Lurasidone; Macitentan; Midazolam; Mifepristone; Naloxegol; Nilotinib; NiMODipine; Nisoldipine; Olaparib; Palbociclib; PAZOPanib; Pimozide; Propafenone; QuiNIDine; Ranolazine; Red Yeast Rice; Regorafenib; Rifampin; Rivaroxaban; Salmeterol; Silodosin; Simeprevir; Simvastatin; St Johns Wort; Suvorexant; Tamsulosin; Terfenadine; Ticagrelor; Tipranavir; Tolvaptan; Topotecan; Toremifene; Trabectedin; TraZODone; Triazolam; Ulipristal; Vemurafenib; VinCRIStine (Liposomal); Vorapaxar

Increased Effect/Toxicity

Saquinavir may increase the levels/effects of: Ado-Trastuzumab Emtansine; Afatinib; Alfuzosin; Almotriptan; Alosetron; ALPRAZolam; Amiodarone; Apixaban; ARIPiprazole; Astemizole; AtorvaSTATin; Avanafil; Axitinib; Barnidipine; Bedaquiline; Bepridil; Bortezomib; Bosentan; Bosutinib; Brentuximab Vedotin; Brinzolamide; Budesonide (Nasal); Budesonide (Systemic, Oral Inhalation); Budesonide (Topical); Cabazitaxel; Cabozantinib; Calcium Channel Blockers (Dihydropyridine); Calcium Channel Blockers (Nondihydropyridine); Cannabis; CarBAMazepine; Ceritinib; Cilostazol; Cisapride; Clarithromycin; Clorazepate; Colchicine; Conivaptan; Corticosteroids (Orally Inhaled); Corticosteroids (Systemic); Crizotinib; Cyclophosphamide; CycloSPORINE (Systemic); CYP3A4 Substrates; Dabigatran Etexilate; Dapoxetine; Dasatinib; Diazepam; Digoxin; Dofetilide; Domperidone; DOXOrubicin (Conventional); Dronabinol; Dronedarone; Dutasteride; Edoxaban; Efavirenz; Eluxadoline; Enfuvirtide; Eplerenone; Ergot Derivatives; Erlotinib; Etizolam; Everolimus; FentaNYL; Fesoterodine; Flecainide; Flurazepam; Fluticasone (Nasal); Fluticasone (Oral Inhalation); Fusidic Acid (Systemic); GuanFACINE; Halofantrine; Highest Risk QTc-Prolonging Agents; Hydrocodone; Ibrutinib; Idelalisib; Imatinib; Imidafenacin; Irinotecan; Isavuconazonium Sulfate; Itraconazole; Ivabradine; Ivacaftor; Ixabepilone; Ketoconazole (Systemic); Lacosamide; Lapatinib; Ledipasvir; Lercanidipine; Levobupivacaine; Levomilnacipran; Lidocaine (Systemic); Lomitapide; Lopinavir; Lovastatin; Lurasidone; Macitentan; Maraviroc; Meperidine; MethylPREDNISolone;

Midazolam; Moderate Risk QTc-Prolonging Agents; Naloxegol; Nefazodone; Nilotinib; NiMODipine; Nintedanib; Nisoldipine; Olaparib; Ospemifene; Oxybutynin; OxyCODONE; Palbociclib; Panobinostat; Parecoxib; Paricalcitol; PAZOPanib; P-glycoprotein/ABCB1 Substrates; Pimecrolimus; Pimozide; PONATinib; Pranlukast; PrednisoLONE (Systemic); PredniSONE; Propafenone; Protease Inhibitors; Prucalopride; QuiNIDine; Ramelteon; Ranolazine; Red Yeast Rice; Regorafenib; Repaglinide; Retapamulin; Rifabutin; Rifaximin; Rilpivirine; Riociguat; Rivaroxaban; RomiDEPsin; Rosuvastatin; Ruxolitinib; Salmeterol; Saxagliptin; Sildenafil; Silodosin; Simeprevir; Simvastatin; SORAfenib; Suvorexant; Tacrolimus (Systemic); Tacrolimus (Topical); Tadalafil; Tamsulosin; Tasimelteon; Temsirolimus; Terfenadine; Tetrahydrocannabinol; Ticagrelor; Tofacitinib; Tolterodine; Tolvaptan; Topotecan; Toremifene; Trabectedin; TraMADol; TraZODone; Triazolam; Tricyclic Antidepressants; Ulipristal; Vardenafil; Vemurafenib; Vilazodone; VinCRIStine (Liposomal); Vorapaxar; Warfarin; Zopiclone

The levels/effects of Saquinavir may be increased by: Bepridil; Bitter Orange; Clarithromycin; CycloSPORINE (Systemic); Delavirdine; Enfuvirtide; Etravirine; Fusidic Acid (Systemic); H2-Antagonists; Itraconazole; Ivabradine; Ketoconazole (Systemic); Methadone; Mifepristone; P-glycoprotein/ABCB1 Inhibitors; Proton Pump Inhibitors; QTc-Prolonging Agents (Indeterminate Risk and Risk Modifying); Rifampin; Simeprevir

Decreased Effect

Saquinavir may decrease the levels/effects of: Abacavir; Antidiabetic Agents; Boceprevir; Clarithromycin; Contraceptives (Estrogens); Contraceptives (Progestins); Darunavir; Delavirdine; Etravirine; Ifosfamide; Meperidine; Methadone; Prasugrel; Pravastatin; Ticagrelor; Valproic Acid and Derivatives; Zidovudine

The levels/effects of Saquinavir may be decreased by: Boceprevir; Bosentan; CarBAMazepine; CYP3A4 Inducers (Moderate); CYP3A4 Inducers (Strong); Dabrafenib; Deferasirox; Efavirenz; Garlic; Mitotane; Nevirapine; Rifabutin; Rifampin; Siltuximab; St Johns Wort; Tipranavir; Tocilizumab

Food Interactions A high-fat meal maximizes bioavailability. Saquinavir levels may increase if taken with grapefruit juice. Management: Administer within 2 hours of a full meal. Monitor closely with concurrent grapefruit juice use.

Storage/Stability Store at 25°C (77°F); excursions permitted to 15°C to 30°C (59°F to 86°F).

Mechanism of Action Binds to the site of HIV-1 protease activity and inhibits cleavage of viral Gag-Pol polyprotein precursors into individual functional proteins required for infectious HIV. This results in the formation of immature, noninfectious viral particles.

Pharmacokinetics (Adult data unless noted)

Distribution: CSF concentration is negligible when compared to concentrations from matched plasma samples; partitions into tissues

V_d: 700 L

Protein binding: 98%

Metabolism: Extensive first-pass effect; hepatic metabolism by cytochrome P450 3A system to inactive mono- and dihydroxylated metabolites

Bioavailability:

Invirase capsules: 4% (increased in the presence of food); bioavailability of Invirase® capsules and tablets are similar when administered with low dose ritonavir (ie, booster doses of ritonavir)

Half-life, serum: 1 to 2 hours

Elimination: 81% to 88% of dose eliminated in feces; 1% to 3% excreted in urine within 5 days

Clearance: Children: Significantly higher than adults

Dosing: Neonatal Not approved for use; appropriate dose is unknown.

Dosing: Usual

Pediatric: **HIV Infection, treatment:** Oral: Use in combination with other antiretroviral agents. **Note:** ECG should be done prior to starting therapy; do not initiate therapy if pretreatment QT interval >450 msec or if there is a diagnosis of long QT syndrome. Saquinavir must only be used in regimens that include ritonavir "booster doses" so that adequate saquinavir serum concentrations are attained; do not use without ritonavir booster doses.

Infants and Children <2 years: Not approved for use; appropriate dose is unknown.

Children ≥2 years and Adolescents <16 years: Limited data available (DHHS [pediatric], 2014): Oral:

Treatment-experienced, ritonavir-boosted regimen: Children ≥2 years and Adolescents <16 years:

5 kg to <15 kg: Saquinavir 50 mg/kg/dose (maximum dose: 1000 mg) twice daily **plus** ritonavir 3 mg/kg/dose twice daily

15 kg to <40 kg: Saquinavir 50 mg/kg/dose (maximum dose: 1000 mg) twice daily **plus** ritonavir 2.5 mg/kg/dose twice daily

≥40 kg: Saquinavir 1000 mg **plus** ritonavir 100 mg twice daily

Salvage therapy, lopinavir/ritonavir-boosted regimen: Children ≥7 years and Adolescents <16 years: Saquinavir 750 mg/m^2/dose or 50 mg/kg/dose **plus** lopinavir/ritonavir twice daily; maximum single saquinavir dose: 1600 mg

Adolescents ≥16 years: Oral:

Ritonavir-boosted regimen: Saquinavir 1000 mg (five 200 mg capsules or two 500 mg tablets) **plus** ritonavir 100 mg twice daily

Lopinavir/ritonavir-boosted regimen: Saquinavir 1000 mg **plus** lopinavir 400 mg/ritonavir 100 mg twice daily; no additional ritonavir is necessary

Adult: **HIV Infection, treatment:** Oral: Use in combination with other antiretroviral agents. **Note:** ECG should be done prior to starting therapy; do not initiate therapy if pretreatment QT interval >450 msec or if there is a diagnosis of long QT syndrome. Saquinavir must only be used in regimens that include ritonavir "booster doses" so that adequate saquinavir serum concentrations are attained; do not use without ritonavir booster doses.

Ritonavir-boosted regimen: Saquinavir 1000 mg (five 200 mg capsules or two 500 mg tablets) **plus** ritonavir 100 mg twice daily

Lopinavir/ritonavir-boosted regimen: Saquinavir 1000 mg **plus** lopinavir 400 mg/ritonavir 100 mg twice daily; no additional ritonavir is necessary

Dosing adjustment in renal impairment:

Mild to moderate renal impairment: No initial dosage adjustment needed

Severe renal impairment or end-stage renal disease: Studies have not been conducted; use with caution; serum concentrations may be elevated

Dosing adjustment in hepatic impairment: Mild or moderate hepatic impairment: No dosage adjustment needed; use with caution; **Note:** Worsening of liver disease may occur in patients with underlying hepatitis B or C, cirrhosis, chronic alcoholism, or other underlying liver abnormalities. Use is contraindicated in severe hepatic impairment.

Administration Oral: Administer saquinavir (along with ritonavir) within 2 hours after a full meal to increase absorption; administer at same time as ritonavir-containing products. For patients unable to swallow a capsule, open the capsule and place the contents into an empty container. Add 15 mL of either sugar syrup or sorbitol syrup **or** 3 teaspoons of jam, stir for 30 to 60 seconds, and immediately administer full amount; mixture should be at room temperature before administration.

Monitoring Parameters Note: Monitor CD4 percentage (if <5 years of age) or CD4 count (if ≥5 years of age) at least every 3 to 4 months (DHHS [pediatric], 2014).

ECG (baseline and after 3 to 4 days of therapy); Prior to initiation of therapy: Genotypic resistance testing, CD4 and viral load (every 3 to 4 months), CBC with differential, LFTs, BUN, creatinine, lipid panel, electrolytes, glucose, and urinalysis (every 6 to 12 months), and assessment of readiness for adherence with medication regimen. At initiation and with any change in treatment regimen: CBC with differential, electrolytes, calcium, phosphate, glucose, LFTs, bilirubin, urinalysis (at initiation), BUN, creatinine, albumin, total protein, lipid panel (at initiation), CD4, and viral load. After 1 to 2 weeks of therapy: Signs of medication toxicity and adherence. After 2 to 4 weeks of therapy: CBC with differential, viral load, signs of medication toxicity, and adherence; then every 3 to 4 months: CBC with differential, electrolytes, glucose, LFTs, bilirubin, BUN, creatinine, CD4, viral load, signs of medication toxicity, and adherence. Every 6 to 12 months: Lipid panel and urinalysis. CD4 monitoring frequency may be decreased to every 6 to 12 months in children who are adherent to therapy if the value is well above the threshold for opportunistic infections, viral suppression is sustained, and the clinical status is stable for more than 2 to 3 years (DHHS [pediatric], 2014). Monitor for growth and development, signs of HIV-specific physical conditions, HIV disease progression, opportunistic infections or arrhythmias.

Reference Range Plasma trough concentration: 100 to 250 ng/mL (DHHS [adult/pediatric], 2014)

Additional Information Fortovase (saquinavir soft gel capsules) has been discontinued in the U.S. because ritonavir-boosted Invirase tablet-containing regimens result in fewer GI side effects and a lower pill burden compared to ritonavir-boosted Fortovase regimens.

Dosage Forms Excipient information presented when available (limited, particularly for generics); consult specific product labeling.

Capsule, Oral:
  Invirase: 200 mg

Tablet, Oral:
  Invirase: 500 mg

◆ **Saquinavir Mesylate** *see* Saquinavir *on page* 1902

◆ **Sarafem** *see* FLUoxetine *on page* 906

Sargramostim (sar GRAM oh stim)

Medication Safety Issues

Sound-alike/look-alike issues:

Leukine may be confused with Leukeran, leucovorin

Brand Names: US Leukine

Brand Names: Canada Leukine

Therapeutic Category Colony-Stimulating Factor; Hematopoietic Agent

Generic Availability (US) No

Use Accelerates myeloid recovery in patients undergoing autologous or allogeneic BMT, mobilizes hematopoietic progenitor cells into peripheral blood for collection by leukapheresis, and accelerates myeloid recovery following autologous peripheral stem cell transplantation and prolong survival in patients with graft failure or engraftment delay after BMT (FDA approved in adults); shortens time to neutrophil recovery and reduces the incidence of severe and life-threatening infections and infections resulting in death following induction chemotherapy in older adults with acute myelogenous leukemia (AML) (FDA approved in adults ≥55 years of age). Has also been used to increase neutrophil counts in patients with malignancies receiving myelosuppressive chemotherapy (beginning >24 hour after chemotherapy) and for management of neonatal neutropenia.

Pregnancy Risk Factor C

Pregnancy Considerations Animal reproduction studies have not been conducted.

Breast-Feeding Considerations It is not known if sargramostim is excreted in breast milk. Breast-feeding is not recommended by the manufacturer.

Contraindications Hypersensitivity to sargramostim, yeast-derived products, or any component of the formulation; concurrent (24 hours preceding/following) use with myelosuppressive chemotherapy or radiation therapy; patients with excessive (≥10%) leukemic myeloid blasts in bone marrow or peripheral blood

Warnings/Precautions Simultaneous administration or administration 24 hours preceding/following cytotoxic chemotherapy or radiotherapy is contraindicated due to the sensitivity of rapidly dividing hematopoietic progenitor cells. If there is a rapid increase in blood counts (ANC >20,000/mm^3, WBC >50,000/mm^3, or platelets >500,000/mm^3), decrease the dose by 50% or discontinue therapy. Excessive blood counts should fall to normal within 3 to 7 days after the discontinuation of therapy. Monitor CBC with differential twice weekly during treatment. Limited response to sargramostim may be seen in patients who have received bone marrow purged by chemical agents which do not preserve an adequate number of responsive hematopoietic progenitors (eg, <1.2 x 10^4/kg progenitors). In patients receiving autologous bone marrow transplant, response to sargramostim may be limited if extensive radiotherapy to the abdomen or chest or multiple myelotoxic agents were administered prior to transplantation. May potentially act as a growth factor for any tumor type, particularly myeloid malignancies; caution should be exercised when using in any malignancy with myeloid characteristics. Discontinue use if disease progression occurs during treatment.

Anaphylaxis or other serious allergic reactions have been reported; discontinue immediately and initiate appropriate therapy if a serious allergic or anaphylactic reaction occurs. A "first-dose effect", characterized by respiratory distress, hypoxia, flushing, hypotension, syncope, and/or tachycardia, may occur (rarely) with the first dose of a cycle and resolve with appropriate symptomatic treatment; symptoms do not usually occur with subsequent doses within that cycle. Sequestration of granulocytes in pulmonary circulation and dyspnea have been reported; monitor respiratory symptoms during and following IV infusion. Decrease infusion rate by 50% if dyspnea occurs; discontinue the infusion if dyspnea persists despite reduction in the rate of administration. Subsequent doses may be administered at the standard rate with careful monitoring. Use with caution in patients with hypoxia or pre-existing pulmonary disease. Edema, capillary leak syndrome, pleural and/or pericardial effusion have been reported; fluid retention has been shown to be reversible with dosage reduction or discontinuation of sargramostim with or without concomitant use of diuretics. Use with caution in patients with pre-existing fluid retention, pulmonary infiltrates, or congestive heart failure; may exacerbate fluid retention.

Use with caution in patients with preexisting cardiac disease. Reversible transient supraventricular arrhythmias have been reported, especially in patients with a history of arrhythmias. Use with caution in patients with hepatic impairment (hyperbilirubinemia and elevated transaminases have been observed) or renal impairment (serum creatinine elevations have been observed). Monitor hepatic and renal function at least every other week in patients with history of impairment.

Benzyl alcohol and derivatives: Some dosage forms may contain benzyl alcohol; large amounts of benzyl alcohol (≥99 mg/kg/day) have been associated with a potentially fatal toxicity ("gasping syndrome") in neonates; the "gasping syndrome" consists of metabolic acidosis, respiratory distress, gasping respirations, CNS dysfunction (including convulsions, intracranial hemorrhage), hypotension, and cardiovascular collapse (AAP, 1997; CDC, 1982); some data suggests that benzoate displaces bilirubin from protein binding sites (Ahlfors, 2001); avoid or use dosage forms containing benzyl alcohol with caution in neonates. See manufacturer's labeling.

Adverse Reactions

Cardiovascular: Chest pain, edema, hypertension, pericardial effusion, peripheral edema, tachycardia, thrombosis

Central nervous system: Anxiety, chills, headache, insomnia, malaise

Dermatologic: Pruritus, skin rash

Endocrine & metabolic: Hypercholesterolemia, hyperglycemia, hypomagnesemia, weight loss

Gastrointestinal: Abdominal pain, anorexia, diarrhea, dysphagia, gastric ulcer, gastrointestinal hemorrhage, hematemesis, nausea, vomiting

Hepatic: Hyperbilirubinemia

Immunologic: Antibody development

Neuromuscular & skeletal: Arthralgia, myalgia, ostealgia, weakness

Ophthalmic: Retinal hemorrhage

Renal: Increased blood urea nitrogen, increased serum creatinine

Respiratory: Dyspnea, epistaxis, pharyngitis, pleural effusion

Miscellaneous: Fever

Rare but important or life-threatening: Anaphylaxis, capillary leak syndrome, cardiac arrhythmia, eosinophilia, hypoxia, leukocytosis, liver function impairment (transient), pericarditis, prolonged prothrombin time, respiratory distress, rigors, sore throat, supraventricular cardiac arrhythmia, syncope, thrombocythemia, thrombophlebitis

Drug Interactions

Metabolism/Transport Effects None known.

Avoid Concomitant Use There are no known interactions where it is recommended to avoid concomitant use.

Increased Effect/Toxicity

Sargramostim may increase the levels/effects of: Bleomycin

The levels/effects of Sargramostim may be increased by: Cyclophosphamide

Decreased Effect There are no known significant interactions involving a decrease in effect.

Storage/Stability Store intact vials at 2°C to 8°C (36°F to 46°F); do not freeze. Do not shake.

Solution for injection: May be stored for up to 20 days at 2°C to 8°C (36°F to 46°F) once the vial has been entered. Discard remaining solution after 20 days.

Powder for injection: Preparations made with SWFI should be administered as soon as possible, and discarded within 6 hours of reconstitution. Solutions reconstituted with bacteriostatic water may be stored for up to 20 days at 2°C to 8°C (36°F to 46°F); do not freeze. When combining previously reconstituted solutions with freshly reconstituted solutions, administer within 6 hours following preparation; the contents of vials reconstituted with different diluents should not be mixed together.

Mechanism of Action Stimulates proliferation, differentiation and functional activity of neutrophils, eosinophils, monocytes, and macrophages.

Pharmacodynamics

Onset of action: Increase in WBC in 7-14 days

Duration: WBC will return to baseline within 1 week after discontinuing drug

Pharmacokinetics (Adult data unless noted)

Half-life:

Pediatric patients 6 months to 15 years: IV: Median: 1.6 hours; range: 0.9-2.5 hours; SubQ: Median: 2.3 hours (0.3-3.8 hours) (Stute, 1995)

Adults: IV: 60 minutes: SubQ: 2.7 hours

Time to peak serum concentration: SubQ: 1-3 hours

Dosing: Neonatal Neutropenia: Limited data available; efficacy result variable: SubQ: 10 mcg/kg/dose once daily for 5 days. The PROGRAMS trial (single-blind, multicenter) evaluated use in 280 premature neonates (GA: ≤31 weeks; weight: ≤10th percentile body weight) and showed a correction of neutropenia but no reduction in sepsis or improved survival (Carr, 2009); an extension study also reported no difference in developmental, neurological, or general health outcomes in former premature neonates who received sargramostim compared to placebo (Marlow, 2013)

Dosing: Usual

Infants, Children, and Adolescents: **Neutrophil recovery following bone marrow transplant:** Limited data available: IV: 250 mcg/m^2/day (infused over 2-4 hours or SubQ) once daily for 21 days to begin 2-4 hours after the marrow infusion on day 0 of BMT or not less than 24 hours after chemotherapy (Trigg, 2000; Nemunaitis, 1991)

Adults: **Note:** May round the dose to the nearest vial size (Ozer, 2000).

Acute myeloid leukemia (AML), neutrophil recovery following chemotherapy: Adults ≥55 years: IV: 250 mcg/m^2/day (infused over 4 hours) starting approximately on day 11 or 4 days following the completion of induction chemotherapy (if day 10 bone marrow is hypoplastic with <5% blasts), continue until ANC >1500/mm^3 for 3 consecutive days or a maximum of 42 days.

If a second cycle of chemotherapy is necessary, administer ~4 days after the completion of chemotherapy if the bone marrow is hypoplastic with <5% blasts.

Discontinue sargramostim immediately if leukemic regrowth occurs.

Bone marrow transplant (BMT), failure or engraftment delay: IV: 250 mcg/m^2/day (infused over 2 hours) for 14 days; if engraftment has not occurred after 7 days off sargramostim, may repeat. If engraftment still has not occurred after 7 days off sargramostim, a third course of 500 mcg/m^2/day for 14 days may be attempted. If there is still no improvement, it is unlikely that further dose escalation will be of benefit. If blast cells appear or disease progression occurs, discontinue treatment.

Myeloid reconstitution after allogeneic or autologous bone marrow transplant: IV: 250 mcg/m^2/day (infused over 2 hours), begin 2-4 hours after the marrow infusion and ≥24 hours after chemotherapy or radiotherapy, when the post marrow infusion ANC is <500/mm^3, and continue until ANC >1500/mm^3 for 3 consecutive days. If blast cells appear or progression of the underlying disease occurs, discontinue treatment.

Peripheral stem cell transplant, mobilization of peripheral blood progenitor cells (PBPC): IV, SubQ: 250 mcg/m^2/day IV (infused over 24 hours) or SubQ once daily; continue the same dose throughout PBPC collection.

Postperipheral blood progenitor cell transplantation: IV, SubQ: 250 mcg/m^2/day IV (infused over 24 hours) or

SubQ once daily beginning immediately following infusion of progenitor cells; continue until ANC is >1500/mm^3 for 3 consecutive days.

Dosing adjustment for adverse effects (hematologic) or "first dose" effect: Infants, Children, Adolescents, and Adults: If WBC > 50,000/mm^3, ANC is >20,000/mm^3, or platelets >500,000/mm^3, or severe adverse reaction occurs: Decrease dose by 50% or discontinue drug (based on protocol or patient's clinical condition).

Preparation for Administration

Parenteral: Powder for injection: Reconstitute with 1 mL of preservative free SWFI or bacteriostatic water for injection. Direct the diluent toward the side of the vial and gently swirl to reconstitute; do not shake. Do not mix the contents of vials which have been reconstituted with different diluents.

IV: Further dilution with NS is required. If the final sargramostim concentration is <10 mcg/mL, 1 mg of human albumin per 1 mL of NS should be added (eg, add 1 mL of 5% human albumin per 50 mL of NS). Albumin acts as a carrier molecule to prevent drug adsorption to the IV tubing. Albumin should be added to NS prior to addition of GM-CSF.

SubQ: May be administered without further dilution.

Administration Parenteral:

IV: Administer as 2-hour, 4-hour, or 24-hour infusion (indication specific). An in-line membrane filter should **not** be used for intravenous administration. Do not shake solution to avoid foaming.

SubQ: Administer reconstituted solution without further dilution; rotate injection sites; avoiding navel/waistline

Monitoring Parameters CBC with differential (at least twice weekly during therapy), platelets; renal/liver function tests (at least every 2 weeks); vital signs, weight; hydration status; pulmonary function

Test Interactions May interfere with bone imaging studies; increased hematopoietic activity of the bone marrow may appear as transient positive bone imaging changes

Additional Information Produced by recombinant DNA technology using a yeast-derived expression system

Dosage Forms Excipient information presented when available (limited, particularly for generics); consult specific product labeling. [DSC] = Discontinued product

Solution, Injection:

Leukine: 500 mcg/mL (1 mL [DSC]) [contains benzyl alcohol]

Solution Reconstituted, Intravenous [preservative free]:

Leukine: 250 mcg (1 ea)

- **Sarna® HC (Can)** *see* Hydrocortisone (Topical) *on page 1041*
- **Sarnol-HC [OTC]** *see* Hydrocortisone (Topical) *on page 1041*
- **Saturated Potassium Iodide Solution** *see* Potassium Iodide *on page 1740*
- **Saturated Solution of Potassium Iodide** *see* Potassium Iodide *on page 1740*
- **SC 33428** *see* IDArubicin *on page 1071*
- **Scalacort** *see* Hydrocortisone (Topical) *on page 1041*
- **Scalacort DK** *see* Hydrocortisone (Topical) *on page 1041*
- **Scalpicin 2 in 1 [OTC]** *see* Salicylic Acid *on page 1894*
- **Scalpicin Maximum Strength [OTC]** *see* Hydrocortisone (Topical) *on page 1041*
- **SCH 52365** *see* Temozolomide *on page 2012*
- **SCH 56592** *see* Posaconazole *on page 1730*
- **ScheinPharm Ranitidine (Can)** *see* Ranitidine *on page 1836*
- **Scholls Callus Removers [OTC] [DSC]** *see* Salicylic Acid *on page 1894*
- **Scholls Corn Removers [OTC] [DSC]** *see* Salicylic Acid *on page 1894*
- **Scholls Corn Removers Extra [OTC] [DSC]** *see* Salicylic Acid *on page 1894*
- **Scholls Corn Removers Small [OTC] [DSC]** *see* Salicylic Acid *on page 1894*
- **SCIG** *see* Immune Globulin *on page 1089*
- **S-Citalopram** *see* Escitalopram *on page 786*

Scopolamine (Systemic) (skoe POL a meen)

Medication Safety Issues

BEERS Criteria medication:

This drug may be potentially inappropriate for use in geriatric patients (Quality of evidence - moderate; Strength of recommendation - strong).

Other safety concerns:

Transdermal patch may contain conducting metal (eg, aluminum); remove patch prior to MRI.

Brand Names: US Transderm-Scop

Brand Names: Canada Buscopan; Scopolamine Hydrobromide Injection; Transderm-V

Therapeutic Category Anticholinergic Agent; Anticholinergic Agent, Transdermal

Generic Availability (US) May be product dependent

Use Transdermal: Prevention of nausea/vomiting associated with motion sickness and recovery from anesthesia and surgery (FDA approved in adults)

Pregnancy Risk Factor C

Pregnancy Considerations Adverse events were observed in some animal reproduction studies. Scopolamine crosses the placenta; may cause respiratory depression and/or neonatal hemorrhage when used during pregnancy. Transdermal scopolamine has been used as an adjunct to epidural anesthesia for cesarean delivery without adverse CNS effects on the newborn. Parenteral administration does not increase the duration of labor or affect uterine contractions. Except when used prior to cesarean section, use during pregnancy only if the benefit to the mother outweighs the potential risk to the fetus.

Breast-Feeding Considerations Scopolamine is excreted into breast milk. The manufacturer recommends caution be used if scopolamine is administered to a nursing woman.

Contraindications

Transdermal, oral: Hypersensitivity to scopolamine, other belladonna alkaloids, or any component of the formulation; narrow-angle glaucoma

Injection: Hypersensitivity to scopolamine, other belladonna alkaloids, or any component of the formulation; narrow-angle glaucoma; chronic lung disease (repeated administration)

Canadian labeling: Additional contraindications (not in U.S. labeling):

Oral: Glaucoma, megacolon, myasthenia gravis, obstructive prostatic hypertrophy

Injection:

Hyoscine butylbromide: Untreated narrow-angle glaucoma; megacolon, prostatic hypertrophy with urinary retention; stenotic lesions of the GI tract; myasthenia gravis; tachycardia, angina, or heart failure; IM administration in patients receiving anticoagulant therapy

Scopolamine hydrobromide: Glaucoma or predisposition to narrow-angle glaucoma; paralytic ileus; prostatic hypertrophy; pyloric obstruction; tachycardia secondary to cardiac insufficiency or thyrotoxicosis

Warnings/Precautions Use with caution in patients with coronary artery disease, tachyarrhythmias, heart failure, hypertension, or hyperthyroidism; evaluate tachycardia prior to administration. Use caution in hepatic or renal impairment; adverse CNS effects occur more often in these patients. Use injectable and transdermal products with caution in patients with prostatic hyperplasia or urinary retention. Discontinue if patient reports unusual visual disturbances or pain within the eye. Use caution in GI obstruction, hiatal hernia, reflux esophagitis, and ulcerative colitis. Use with caution in patients with a history of seizure or psychosis; may exacerbate these conditions. Lower doses (0.1mg) may have vagal mimetic effects (eg, increase vagal tone causing paradoxical bradycardia).

Anaphylaxis including episodes of shock has been reported following parenteral administration; observe for signs/symptoms of hypersensitivity following parenteral administration. Patients with a history of allergies or asthma may be at increased risk of hypersensitivity reactions. Adverse events (including dizziness, headache, nausea, vomiting) may occur following abrupt discontinuation of large doses or in patients with Parkinson's disease; adverse events may also occur following removal of the transdermal patch although symptoms may not appear until ≥24 hours after removal.

Idiosyncratic reactions may rarely occur; patients may experience acute toxic psychosis, agitation, confusion, delusions, hallucinations, paranoid behavior, and rambling speech. May cause CNS depression, which may impair physical or mental abilities; patients must be cautioned about performing tasks which require mental alertness (eg, operating machinery or driving). Effects with other sedative drugs or ethanol may be potentiated.

Transdermal patch may contain conducting metal (eg, aluminum); remove patch prior to MRI. Use of the transdermal product in patients with open-angle glaucoma may necessitate adjustments in glaucoma therapy.

Scopolamine (hyoscine) hydrobromide should not be interchanged with scopolamine butylbromide formulations; dosages are not equivalent.

Avoid use in the elderly due to potent anticholinergic adverse effects and uncertain effectiveness (Beers Criteria). Use with caution in infants and children since they may be more susceptible to adverse effects of scopolamine. Tablets may contain sucrose; avoid use of tablets in patients who are fructose intolerant.

Adverse Reactions

Cardiovascular: Bradycardia, flushing, orthostatic hypotension, tachycardia

Central nervous system: Acute toxic psychosis (rare), agitation (rare), ataxia, confusion, delusion (rare), disorientation, dizziness, drowsiness, fatigue, hallucination (rare), headache, irritability, loss of memory, paranoid behavior (rare), restlessness, sedation

Dermatologic: Drug eruptions, dry skin, dyshidrosis, erythema, pruritus, rash, urticaria

Endocrine & metabolic: Thirst

Gastrointestinal: Constipation, diarrhea, dry throat, dysphagia, nausea, vomiting, xerostomia

Genitourinary: Dysuria, urinary retention

Neuromuscular & skeletal: Tremor, weakness

Ocular: Accommodation impaired, blurred vision, conjunctival infection, cycloplegia, dryness, glaucoma (narrow-angle), increased intraocular pain, itching, photophobia, pupil dilation, retinal pigmentation

Respiratory: Dry nose, dyspnea

Miscellaneous: Anaphylaxis (rare), anaphylactic shock (rare), angioedema, diaphoresis decreased, heat intolerance, hypersensitivity reactions

Drug Interactions

Metabolism/Transport Effects None known.

Avoid Concomitant Use

Avoid concomitant use of Scopolamine (Systemic) with any of the following: Aclidinium; Azelastine (Nasal); Eluxadoline; Glucagon; Ipratropium (Oral Inhalation); Orphenadrine; Paraldehyde; Potassium Chloride; Thalidomide; Tiotropium; Umeclidinium

Increased Effect/Toxicity

Scopolamine (Systemic) may increase the levels/effects of: AbobotulinumtoxinA; Alcohol (Ethyl); Analgesics (Opioid); Anticholinergic Agents; Azelastine (Nasal); Buprenorphine; CNS Depressants; Eluxadoline; Glucagon; Hydrocodone; Methotrimeprazine; Metyrosine; Mirabegron; Mirtazapine; OnabotulinumtoxinA; Orphenadrine; Paraldehyde; Potassium Chloride; Pramipexole; RimabotulinumtoxinB; ROPINIRole; Rotigotine; Selective Serotonin Reuptake Inhibitors; Suvorexant; Thalidomide; Thiazide Diuretics; Tiotropium; Topiramate; Zolpidem

The levels/effects of Scopolamine (Systemic) may be increased by: Aclidinium; Brimonidine (Topical); Cannabis; Doxylamine; Dronabinol; Droperidol; HydrOXYzine; Ipratropium (Oral Inhalation); Kava Kava; Magnesium Sulfate; Methotrimeprazine; Mianserin; Nabilone; Perampanel; Pramlintide; Rufinamide; Sodium Oxybate; Tapentadol; Tetrahydrocannabinol; Umeclidinium

Decreased Effect

Scopolamine (Systemic) may decrease the levels/effects of: Acetylcholinesterase Inhibitors; Itopride; Metoclopramide; Secretin

The levels/effects of Scopolamine (Systemic) may be decreased by: Acetylcholinesterase Inhibitors

Storage/Stability

Solution for injection:

Butylbromide [Canadian product]: Store at room temperature. Do not freeze. Protect from light and heat. Stable in D_5W, $D_{10}W$, NS, Ringer's solution, and LR for up to 8 hours.

Hydrobromide: Store at room temperature of 20°C to 25°C (68°F to 77°F). Protect from light. Avoid acid solutions; hydrolysis occurs at pH <3.

Tablet [Canadian product]: Store at room temperature. Protect from light and heat.

Transdermal system: Store at 20°C to 25°C (68°F to 77°F).

Mechanism of Action Blocks the action of acetylcholine at parasympathetic sites in smooth muscle, secretory glands and the CNS; increases cardiac output, dries secretions, antagonizes histamine and serotonin; at usual recommended doses, causes blockade of muscarinic receptors at the cardiac SA-node and is parasympatholytic (ie, blocks vagal activity increasing heart rate)

Pharmacodynamics

Onset of action:

IM: 30 minutes to 1 hour

IV: 10 minutes

Transdermal: 4 hours

Duration:

IM: 4 to 6 hours

IV: 2 hours

Transdermal: 72 hours

Pharmacokinetics (Adult data unless noted)

Absorption: Well absorbed by all routes of administration

Metabolism: In the liver

Half-life: 9.5 hours

Elimination: <5% excreted unchanged in the urine

Dosing: Usual Note: Scopolamine injection is no longer available in the US.

Pediatric:

Preoperatively and antiemetic: Children: Scopolamine hydrobromide: IM, IV, SubQ: 6 mcg/kg/dose (maximum dose: 0.3 mg/dose); may be repeated every 6 to 8 hours

Motion sickness: Limited data available: Adolescents: Scopolamine base: Transdermal: Apply 1 disc behind the ear at least 4 hours prior to exposure every 3 days as needed (Kliegman 2007)

Adult:

Scopolamine base:

Preoperative: Transdermal patch: Apply 1 patch to hairless area behind ear the night before surgery or 1 hour prior to cesarean section (apply no sooner than 1 hour before surgery to minimize newborn exposure); remove 24 hours after surgery

Motion sickness: Transdermal patch: Apply 1 patch to hairless area behind the ear at least 4 hours prior to exposure and every 3 days as needed; effective if applied as soon as 2 to 3 hours before anticipated need, best if 12 hours before

Scopolamine hydrobromide:

Antiemetic: SubQ: 0.6 to 1 mg

Preoperative: IM, IV, SubQ: 0.3 to 0.65 mg

Sedation, tranquilization: IM, IV, SubQ: 0.6 mg 3 to 4 times daily

Preparation for Administration Parenteral: IV: Hydrobromide: Dilute with an equal volume of SWFI

Administration

Parenteral: IV: Administer by direct IV injection over 2 to 3 minutes

Transdermal: Apply patch to hairless area behind one ear. Wash hands before and after application of disc to avoid drug contact with eyes. Do not use any patch that has been damaged, cut, or manipulated in any way. Transdermal patch is programmed to deliver 1 mg over 3 days. Once applied, do not remove the patch for 3 full days (motion sickness). When used postoperatively for nausea/vomiting, the patch should be removed 24 hours after surgery. If patch becomes dislodged, discard and apply new patch.

Test Interactions Interferes with gastric secretion test

Product Availability Scopolamine injection is no longer available in the US.

Dosage Forms Excipient information presented when available (limited, particularly for generics); consult specific product labeling.

Patch 72 Hour, Transdermal:

Transderm-Scop: 1.5 mg (1 ea, 4 ea, 10 ea, 24 ea)

Solution, Injection, as hydrobromide:

Generic: 0.4 mg/mL (1 mL)

Scopolamine (Ophthalmic) (skoe POL a meen)

Brand Names: US Isopto Hyoscine

Therapeutic Category Anticholinergic Agent, Ophthalmic; Ophthalmic Agent, Mydriatic

Generic Availability (US) No

Use To produce cycloplegia and mydriasis; treatment of iridocyclitis

Pregnancy Considerations When administered intravenously or transdermally, scopolamine crosses the placenta; refer to Scopolamine (Systemic) monograph for details. Scopolamine is rapidly absorbed systemically after ocular application (Lahdes, 1990).

Contraindications Hypersensitivity to scopolamine or any component of the formulation; narrow-angle glaucoma

Warnings/Precautions For ophthalmic use only. To avoid precipitating angle closure glaucoma, an estimation of the depth of the anterior chamber angle should be made prior to use. Discontinue if patient reports unusual visual disturbances or pain within the eye. May cause drowsiness and/or blurred vision, which may impair physical or mental abilities; patients must be cautioned about performing tasks which require mental alertness (eg, operating machinery, driving). Some products contain benzalkonium chloride which may be absorbed by soft contact lenses; contact lenses should not be worn during treatment of ophthalmologic infections. Inadvertent contamination of multiple-dose ophthalmic solutions has caused bacterial keratitis.

Adverse Reactions Note: Systemic adverse effects have been reported following ophthalmic administration.

Central nervous system: Drowsiness, somnolence, visual hallucination

Dermatologic: Eczematoid dermatitis

Gastrointestinal: Xerostomia

Ocular: Blurred vision, edema, exudate, follicular conjunctivitis, increased intraocular pressure, local irritation, photophobia, vascular congestion

Drug Interactions

Metabolism/Transport Effects None known.

Avoid Concomitant Use

Avoid concomitant use of Scopolamine (Ophthalmic) with any of the following: Aclidinium; Azelastine (Nasal); Eluxadoline; Glucagon; Ipratropium (Oral Inhalation); Orphenadrine; Paraldehyde; Potassium Chloride; Thalidomide; Tiotropium; Umeclidinium

Increased Effect/Toxicity

Scopolamine (Ophthalmic) may increase the levels/effects of: AbobotulinumtoxinA; Alcohol (Ethyl); Analgesics (Opioid); Anticholinergic Agents; Azelastine (Nasal); Buprenorphine; CNS Depressants; Eluxadoline; Glucagon; Hydrocodone; Methotrimeprazine; Metyrosine; Mirabegron; Mirtazapine; OnabotulinumtoxinA; Orphenadrine; Paraldehyde; Potassium Chloride; Pramipexole; RimabotulinumtoxinB; ROPINIRole; Rotigotine; Selective Serotonin Reuptake Inhibitors; Suvorexant; Thalidomide; Thiazide Diuretics; Tiotropium; Topiramate; Zolpidem

The levels/effects of Scopolamine (Ophthalmic) may be increased by: Aclidinium; Brimonidine (Topical); Cannabis; Doxylamine; Dronabinol; Droperidol; HydrOXYzine; Ipratropium (Oral Inhalation); Kava Kava; Magnesium Sulfate; Methotrimeprazine; Mianserin; Nabilone; Perampanel; Pramlintide; Rufinamide; Sodium Oxybate; Tapentadol; Tetrahydrocannabinol; Umeclidinium

Decreased Effect

Scopolamine (Ophthalmic) may decrease the levels/effects of: Acetylcholinesterase Inhibitors; Itopride; Metoclopramide; Secretin

The levels/effects of Scopolamine (Ophthalmic) may be decreased by: Acetylcholinesterase Inhibitors

Storage/Stability Store at 8°C to 27°C (46°F to 80°F). Protect from light.

Mechanism of Action Blocks the action of acetylcholine at parasympathetic sites in sphincter muscle of the iris and the accommodative muscle of the ciliary body; prevents accommodation; dilates pupils

Dosing: Usual

Refraction:

Children: Instill 1 drop of 0.25% to eye(s) twice daily for 2 days before procedure

Adults: Instill 1-2 drops of 0.25% to eye(s) 1 hour before procedure

Iridocyclitis:

Children: Instill 1 drop of 0.25% to eye(s) up to 3 times/day

Adults: Instill 1-2 drops of 0.25% to eye(s) up to 3 times/day

Administration Instill drops to conjunctival sac of affected eye(s); avoid contact of bottle tip with skin or eye; finger pressure should be applied to lacrimal sac during and for 1-2 minutes after instillation to decrease risk of absorption and systemic reactions. Remove contact lenses prior to administration; wait 15 minutes before reinserting if using products containing benzalkonium chloride. Wash hands following administration.

Dosage Forms Excipient information presented when available (limited, particularly for generics); consult specific product labeling.

Solution, Ophthalmic, as hydrobromide:
Isopto Hyoscine: 0.25% (5 mL)

- ◆ **Scopolamine Base** *see* Scopolamine (Systemic) *on page 1907*
- ◆ **Scopolamine Butylbromide** *see* Scopolamine (Systemic) *on page 1907*
- ◆ **Scopolamine Hydrobromide** *see* Scopolamine (Ophthalmic) *on page 1909*
- ◆ **Scopolamine Hydrobromide** *see* Scopolamine (Systemic) *on page 1907*
- ◆ **Scopolamine Hydrobromide Injection (Can)** *see* Scopolamine (Systemic) *on page 1907*
- ◆ **Scopolamine, Hyoscyamine, Atropine, and Phenobarbital** *see* Hyoscyamine, Atropine, Scopolamine, and Phenobarbital *on page 1062*
- ◆ **Scorpion Antivenin** *see Centruroides* Immune $F(ab')_2$ (Equine) *on page 421*
- ◆ **Scorpion Antivenom** *see Centruroides* Immune $F(ab')_2$ (Equine) *on page 421*
- ◆ **Scot-Tussin Allergy Relief [OTC]** *see* DiphenhydrAMINE (Systemic) *on page 668*
- ◆ **Scot-Tussin Diabetes CF [OTC]** *see* Dextromethorphan *on page 631*
- ◆ **Scot-Tussin Expectorant [OTC]** *see* GuaiFENesin *on page 988*
- ◆ **Scot-Tussin Senior [OTC]** *see* Guaifenesin and Dextromethorphan *on page 992*
- ◆ **Scytera [OTC]** *see* Coal Tar *on page 523*
- ◆ **SD/01** *see* Pegfilgrastim *on page 1641*
- ◆ **Se-100 [OTC]** *see* Selenium *on page 1912*
- ◆ **Sea-Clens Wound Cleanser [OTC]** *see* Sodium Chloride *on page 1938*
- ◆ **Sea Soft Nasal Mist [OTC]** *see* Sodium Chloride *on page 1938*
- ◆ **Se Aspartate [OTC]** *see* Selenium *on page 1912*
- ◆ **Sebasorb [OTC]** *see* Salicylic Acid *on page 1894*
- ◆ **Sebcur (Can)** *see* Salicylic Acid *on page 1894*
- ◆ **Sebex [OTC]** *see* Sulfur and Salicylic Acid *on page 1993*
- ◆ **SE BPO Wash [DSC]** *see* Benzoyl Peroxide *on page 270*
- ◆ **Seb-Prev [DSC]** *see* Sulfacetamide (Topical) *on page 1982*
- ◆ **Seb-Prev Wash** *see* Sulfacetamide (Topical) *on page 1982*
- ◆ **Sebulex [OTC]** *see* Sulfur and Salicylic Acid *on page 1993*

Secobarbital (see koe BAR bi tal)

Medication Safety Issues

Sound-alike/look-alike issues:

Seconal® may be confused with Sectral®

BEERS Criteria medication:

This drug may be potentially inappropriate for use in geriatric patients (Quality of evidence - high; Strength of recommendation - strong).

Brand Names: US Seconal

Therapeutic Category Barbiturate; Hypnotic; Sedative

Generic Availability (US) No

Use Short-term treatment of insomnia; preanesthetic agent

Pregnancy Risk Factor D

Pregnancy Considerations Barbiturates can be detected in the placenta, fetal liver, and fetal brain. Fetal and maternal blood concentrations may be similar following parenteral administration. An increased incidence of fetal abnormalities may occur following maternal use. When used during the third trimester of pregnancy, withdrawal symptoms may occur in the neonate including seizures and hyperirritability; symptoms may be delayed up to 14 days. Use during labor does not impair uterine activity; however, respiratory depression may occur in the newborn; resuscitation equipment should be available, especially for premature infants.

Breast-Feeding Considerations Small amounts of barbiturates are found in breast milk.

Contraindications Hypersensitivity to barbiturates or any component of the formulation; marked hepatic impairment; dyspnea or airway obstruction; porphyria

Warnings/Precautions Should be used only after evaluation of potential causes of sleep disturbance. Failure of sleep disturbance to resolve after 7-10 days may indicate psychiatric or medical illness. Potential for drug dependency exists, abrupt cessation may precipitate withdrawal, including status epilepticus in epileptic patients. Do not administer to patients in acute pain. Use caution in elderly, debilitated, renally impaired, or pediatric patients. Avoid use in the elderly due to risk of overdose with low dosages, tolerance to sleep effects, and increased risk of physical dependence (Beers Criteria).

May cause paradoxical responses, including agitation and hyperactivity, particularly in acute pain and pediatric patients. Use with caution in patients with depression or suicidal tendencies, or in patients with a history of drug abuse. Tolerance, psychological and physical dependence may occur with prolonged use. Use with caution in patients with hepatic function impairment. May cause CNS depression, which may impair physical or mental abilities. Patients must cautioned about performing tasks which require mental alertness (eg, operating machinery or driving). Postmarketing studies have indicated that the use of hypnotic/sedative agents for sleep has been associated with hypersensitivity reactions including anaphylaxis as well as angioedema. An increased risk for hazardous sleep-related activities such as sleep-driving; cooking and eating food, and making phone calls while asleep have also been noted. Effects with other sedative drugs or ethanol may be potentiated. May cause respiratory depression or hypotension, Use with caution in patients with cardiovascular or respiratory disease.

Adverse Reactions

Central nervous system: Somnolence

Rare but important or life-threatening: Abnormal thinking, agitation, angioedema, anxiety, apnea, ataxia, bradycardia, CNS depression, complex sleep-related behavior (sleep-driving, cooking or eating food, making phone calls), confusion, constipation, dizziness, exfoliative dermatitis, fever, hallucinations, headache, hyperkinesis, hypotension, hypoventilation, insomnia, liver injury, megaloblastic anemia, nausea, nervousness, nightmares, pain at injection site, rash, syncope, unusual excitement, vomiting

Drug Interactions

Metabolism/Transport Effects **Induces** CYP2A6 (strong), CYP2C8 (strong), CYP2C9 (strong)

Avoid Concomitant Use

Avoid concomitant use of Secobarbital with any of the following: Azelastine (Nasal); Enzalutamide; Mianserin; Orphenadrine; Paraldehyde; Somatostatin Acetate; Thalidomide; Ulipristal

Increased Effect/Toxicity

Secobarbital may increase the levels/effects of: Alcohol (Ethyl); Azelastine (Nasal); Buprenorphine; CNS Depressants; Hydrocodone; Hypotensive Agents; Meperidine; Methotrimeprazine; Metyrosine; Mirtazapine; Orphenadrine; Paraldehyde; Pramipexole; ROPINIRole; Rotigotine; Selective Serotonin Reuptake Inhibitors; Suvorexant; Thalidomide; Thiazide Diuretics; Zolpidem

The levels/effects of Secobarbital may be increased by: Brimonidine (Topical); Cannabis; Chloramphenicol; Doxylamine; Dronabinol; Droperidol; Felbamate; HydrOXYzine; Kava Kava; Magnesium Sulfate; Methotrimeprazine; Mianserin; Nabilone; Perampanel; Primidone; Rufinamide; Sodium Oxybate; Somatostatin Acetate; Tapentadol; Tetrahydrocannabinol; Valproic Acid and Derivatives

Decreased Effect

Secobarbital may decrease the levels/effects of: Acetaminophen; Beta-Blockers; Calcium Channel Blockers; Chloramphenicol; Contraceptives (Estrogens); Contraceptives (Progestins); CycloSPORINE (Systemic); CYP2A6 Substrates; CYP2C8 Substrates; CYP2C9 Substrates; Diclofenac (Systemic); Doxycycline; Enzalutamide; Etoposide; Etoposide Phosphate; Felbamate; Griseofulvin; LamoTRIgine; Mianserin; Teniposide; Theophylline Derivatives; Treprostinil; Tricyclic Antidepressants; Ulipristal; Valproic Acid and Derivatives; Vitamin K Antagonists

The levels/effects of Secobarbital may be decreased by: Mianserin; Multivitamins/Minerals (with ADEK, Folate, Iron); Pyridoxine; Rifamycin Derivatives

Storage/Stability Store at controlled room temperature of 20°C to 25°C (68°F to 77°F).

Mechanism of Action Depresses CNS activity by binding to barbiturate site at GABA-receptor complex enhancing GABA activity, depressing reticular activity system; higher doses may be gabamimetic

Pharmacodynamics

Onset of action: Hypnosis: Oral: 15-30 minutes

Duration: Hypnosis: Oral: 3-4 hours with 100 mg dose

Pharmacokinetics (Adult data unless noted)

Absorption: Oral: Well absorbed (90%)

Distribution: V_d: Adults: 1.5 L/kg; crosses the placenta; appears in breast milk

Protein binding: 45% to 60%

Metabolism: In the liver by the microsomal enzyme system

Half-life:

- Children: 2-13 years: 2.7-13.5 hours
- Adults: 15-40 hours; mean 28 hours

Time to peak serum concentration: Oral: Within 2-4 hours

Elimination: Renally as inactive metabolites and small amounts as unchanged drug

Dialysis: Hemodialysis: Slightly dialyzable (5% to 20%)

Dosing: Usual Oral:

Children:

- Preoperative sedation: 2-6 mg/kg (maximum dose: 100 mg/dose) 1-2 hours before procedure
- Sedation: 6 mg/kg/day divided every 8 hours

Adults:

- Hypnotic: Usual: 100 mg/dose at bedtime; range 100-200 mg/dose
- Preoperative sedation: 100-300 mg 1-2 hours before procedure

Monitoring Parameters Blood pressure, heart rate, respiratory rate, pulse oximetry, CNS status

Additional Information Effectiveness for insomnia decreases greatly after 2 weeks of use; alkalinization of urine does not significantly increase excretion; withdraw slowly over 5-6 days after prolonged use to avoid sleep disturbances and rapid eye movement (REM) rebound

In March 2007, the FDA requested that all manufacturers of sedative-hypnotic drug products, including Seconal® (secobarbital), revise the labeling to include a greater emphasis on the risks of adverse events. The events include severe hypersensitivity reactions including anaphylaxis and/or angioedema, as well as hazardous sleep-related activities (eg, sleep-driving - driving while not fully awake after consumption of sedative-hypnotic drug, with no recollection of the event). Other activities may include preparing and ingesting food, and the use of the telephone, while asleep. These events may occur at any time during therapy including with the first dose administered.

Manufacturers must provide written notification to healthcare providers regarding the new warnings. In addition, manufacturers are to develop "Patient Medication Guides" designed to educate consumers about the potential risks and to advise them of precautionary measures that can be taken. This advice will contain recommendations on correct utilization of the medication as well as the avoidance of the consumption of ethanol and/or other CNS-depressant agents. The FDA is also recommending manufacturers conduct studies evaluating the frequencies of sleep-driving (and other sleep-related behaviors) with the individual products.

Patients should be instructed not to discontinue these medications without first speaking with their healthcare provider. Patients should also be informed of the potential for an allergic reaction, the signs and symptoms of anaphylaxis, and the appropriate emergency self-treatment of an anaphylactic reaction.

Additional information on the sedative-hypnotic products and sleep disorders is available at http://www.fda.gov/NewsEvents/Newsroom/PressAnnouncements/2007/ucm108868.htm

Controlled Substance C-II

Dosage Forms Excipient information presented when available (limited, particularly for generics); consult specific product labeling.

Capsule, Oral, as sodium:

Seconal: 100 mg [contains fd&c yellow #10 (quinoline yellow)]

◆ **Secobarbital Sodium** *see* Secobarbital *on page 1910*

◆ **Seconal** *see* Secobarbital *on page 1910*

◆ **SecreFlo** *see* Secretin *on page 1911*

Secretin (SEE kr tin)

Brand Names: US ChiRhoStim; SecreFlo

Therapeutic Category Diagnostic Agent, Gastrinoma (Zollinger-Ellison Syndrome); Diagnostic Agent, Pancreatic Exocrine Insufficiency

Generic Availability (US) No

Use Diagnosis of gastrinoma (Zollinger-Ellison syndrome) and diagnosis of pancreatic exocrine dysfunction (chronic pancreatitis); facilitation of endoscopic retrograde cholangiopancreatography (ERCP) visualization

Pregnancy Risk Factor C

Pregnancy Considerations Reproduction studies have not been conducted.

Breast-Feeding Considerations It is not known if secretin is excreted in breast milk. The manufacturer recommends that caution be exercised when administering secretin to nursing women.

Contraindications Hypersensitivity to secretin or any component of the formulation; acute pancreatitis

Warnings/Precautions Administer test dose to evaluate possible allergy to secretin, particularly in patients with a history of asthma or atopy; medications for the treatment of hypersensitivity should be available for immediate use. Use caution in patients with hepatic disease (including ethanol-induced disease); volume response to secretin may be exaggerated. Response may be blunted in the presence of anticholinergic agents, inflammatory bowel disease, or following vagotomy; blunted response is not indicative of pancreatic disease.

Adverse Reactions

Cardiovascular: Flushing

Gastrointestinal: Abdominal discomfort/pain, nausea, vomiting

Miscellaneous: Bleeding (sphincterectomy)

Rare but important or life-threatening: Abdominal cramps, anxiety, bloating, bradycardia (mild), diaphoresis, diarrhea, dyspepsia, faintness, fatigue, fever, headache, heart rate increased, hypotension, leukocytoplastic vasculitis, lightheadedness, numbness/tingling in the extremities, oral secretions increased, oxygen saturation decreased, pallor, pancreatitis (mild), rash (abdominal), respiratory distress (transient), sedation, seizure, warm sensation (abdomen/face)

Drug Interactions

Metabolism/Transport Effects None known.

Avoid Concomitant Use There are no known interactions where it is recommended to avoid concomitant use.

Increased Effect/Toxicity There are no known significant interactions involving an increase in effect.

Decreased Effect

The levels/effects of Secretin may be decreased by: Anticholinergic Agents

Storage/Stability Prior to reconstitution, store frozen at -20°C. Protect from light. Human product may also be stored under refrigeration for up to 1 year or at room temperature for up to 6 months.

Mechanism of Action Human and porcine secretin are both synthetically derived products and are equally potent on an osmolar basis. Secretin is a hormone which is normally secreted by duodenal mucosa and upper jejunal mucosa. It increases the volume and bicarbonate content of pancreatic juice; stimulates the flow of hepatic bile with a high bicarbonate concentration; stimulates gastrin release in patients with Zollinger-Ellison syndrome.

Pharmacodynamics

Maximum output of pancreatic secretions: Within 30 minutes

Duration: At least 2 hours

Pharmacokinetics (Adult data unless noted)

Distribution: V_d: Porcine formulation: 2 L (approximately); human formulation: 2.7 L

Protein binding: 40%

Inactivated by proteolytic enzymes if administered orally

Metabolism: Metabolic fate is thought to be hydrolysis to smaller peptides

Half-life: Porcine formulation: 27 minutes; human formulation: 45 minutes

Elimination: Clearance: Porcine formulation: 487 ± 136 mL/minute; human formulation: 580.9 ± 51.3 mL/minute

Dosing: Usual Children and Adults: IV:

Diagnostic agent for pancreatic function: 0.2 mcg/kg as single dose

Diagnostic agent for gastrinoma (Zollinger-Ellison): 0.4 mcg/kg as single dose

Facilitation of ERCP visualization: 0.2 mcg/kg as a single dose

Preparation for Administration Parenteral: Reconstitute 16 mcg vial with 8 mL NS to yield concentration of 2 mcg/mL; add 10 mL NS to the 40 mcg vial to yield a concentration of 4 mcg/mL; shake vigorously to ensure dissolution. Use immediately.

Administration Parenteral: Administer by direct IV injection slowly over 1 minute

Monitoring Parameters Peak bicarbonate concentration of duodenal fluid aspirate (chronic pancreatitis); serum gastrin (gastrinoma)

Reference Range

Peak gastric bicarbonate concentration:

Normal: 94-134 mEq/L

Chronic pancreatitis: <80 mEq/L

Severe pancreatitis: <50 mEq/L

Serum gastrin:

Normal: ≤110 pg/mL

Gastrinoma: >110 pg/mL

Additional Information SecreFlo™ is available currently as an orphan drug by contacting the manufacturer Repligen; a double-blind crossover study of secretin 0.2 clinical units/kg versus placebo in 56 autistic children revealed no significant differences between the 2 groups (1 clinical unit is equivalent to 0.2 mcg) (Owley, 2001)

Dosage Forms Excipient information presented when available (limited, particularly for generics); consult specific product labeling.

Solution Reconstituted, Intravenous:

ChiRhoStim: 16 mcg (1 ea)

SecreFlo: 16 mcg (1 ea)

◆ **Secretin, Human** *see* Secretin *on page 1911*

◆ **Secretin, Porcine** *see* Secretin *on page 1911*

◆ **Secura Antifungal [OTC]** *see* Miconazole (Topical) *on page 1431*

◆ **Secura Antifungal Extra Thick [OTC]** *see* Miconazole (Topical) *on page 1431*

◆ **Seebri Breezhaler (Can)** *see* Glycopyrrolate *on page 979*

◆ **Selax [OTC] (Can)** *see* Docusate *on page 697*

◆ **Selenicaps-200 [OTC]** *see* Selenium *on page 1912*

◆ **Selenimin [OTC]** *see* Selenium *on page 1912*

◆ **Selenimin-200 [OTC]** *see* Selenium *on page 1912*

Selenium (se LEE nee um)

Related Information

Safe Handling of Hazardous Drugs *on page 2455*

Brand Names: US Aqueous Selenium [OTC]; Oceanic Selenium [OTC]; Se Aspartate [OTC]; Se-100 [OTC]; Se-Plus Protein [OTC]; Selenicaps-200 [OTC]; Selenimin [OTC]; Selenimin-200 [OTC]

Therapeutic Category Trace Element, Parenteral

Generic Availability (US) May be product dependent

Use Prevention of selenium deficiency as an additive to parenteral nutrition (FDA approved in pediatric patients [age not specified] and adults)

Pregnancy Risk Factor C

Pregnancy Considerations Adverse events were seen with high doses in animal studies. Selenium is found in the placenta and cord blood. Teratogenic effects have not been observed with nontoxic doses in humans (IOM, 2000).

Breast-Feeding Considerations Selenium is found in breast milk. Concentrations vary based on maternal intake and time postpartum. Adverse events have not been observed with nontoxic maternal intake in humans (IOM, 2000).

Contraindications Undiluted administration into peripheral vein

Warnings/Precautions Use with caution in patients with GI or renal impairment. The parenteral product may contain aluminum; toxic aluminum concentrations may be seen with high doses, prolonged use, or renal dysfunction. Premature neonates are at higher risk due to immature renal function and aluminum intake from other parenteral sources. Parenteral aluminum exposure of >4 to 5 mcg/kg/day is associated with CNS and bone toxicity; tissue loading may occur at lower doses (Federal Register, 2002). See manufacturer's labeling.

Adverse Reactions Local: Irritation

Drug Interactions

Metabolism/Transport Effects None known.

Avoid Concomitant Use There are no known interactions where it is recommended to avoid concomitant use.

Increased Effect/Toxicity There are no known significant interactions involving an increase in effect.

Decreased Effect

Selenium may decrease the levels/effects of: Dolutegravir; Eltrombopag

Storage/Stability Prior to use, store at 20°C to 25°C (68°F to 77°F); excursions permitted to 15°C to 30°C (59°F to 86°F).

Mechanism of Action Part of glutathione peroxidase which protects cell components from oxidative damage due to peroxidases produced in cellular metabolism

Pharmacokinetics (Adult data unless noted) Elimination: Urine (primarily), feces, lungs, skin

Dosing: Neonatal

Adequate intake (AI): Oral: 15 mcg/day (IOM, 2000)

Parenteral nutrition, maintenance requirement: IV:

Manufacturer's labeling: 3 mcg/kg/day

ASPEN recommendations (ASPEN Pediatric Nutrition Support Core Curriculum [Corkins, 2010]; Mirtallo, 2004; Vanek, 2012):

<3 kg: 1.5 to 3 mcg/kg/day

≥3 kg: 2 to 3 mcg/kg/day

Dosing: Usual

Pediatric:

Adequate intake (AI) (IOM, 2000): Oral:

1 to 6 months: 15 mcg/day

7 to 12 months: 20 mcg/day

Recommended daily allowance (RDA) (IOM, 2000): Oral:

1 to 3 years: 20 mcg/day

4 to 8 years: 30 mcg/day

9 to 13 years 40 mcg/day

14 to 18 years: 55 mcg/day

Parenteral nutrition, maintenance requirement: IV: Infants, Children, and Adolescents:

Manufacturer's labeling: 3 mcg/kg/day; maximum daily dose: 40 mcg/**day**

ASPEN recommendations:

Age-directed dosing (Vanek, 2012): Infants, Children, and Adolescents: 1 to 3 mcg/kg/day; maximum daily dose: 100 mcg/**day**

Weight-directed dosing (ASPEN Pediatric Nutrition Support Core Curriculum [Corkins, 2010]; Mirtallo, 2004):

Infants <10 kg: 2 mcg/kg/day

Children 10 to 40 kg: 1 to 2 mcg/kg/day; maximum daily dose: 60 mcg/**day**

Adolescents >40 kg: 40 to 60 mcg/day

Adult:

Recommended daily allowance (RDA) (IOM, 2000): Oral:

Males and nonpregnant females: 55 mcg/day

Pregnancy: 60 mcg/day

Lactation: 70 mcg/day

Parenteral nutrition, maintenance requirement: IV:

Metabolically stable: 20 to 40 mcg/day

Deficiency from prolonged TPN support: 100 mcg/day

Dosing adjustment in renal impairment: Infants, Children, Adolescents and Adults: Use with caution; dose reduction or discontinuation may be necessary.

Dosing adjustment in hepatic impairment: Infants, Children, Adolescents, and Adults: There are no dosage adjustments in the manufacturer's labeling.

Administration Not for direct IV or IM injection; must be diluted; direct administration of solution causes tissue irritation

Monitoring Parameters Plasma selenium concentration for patients receiving long term TPN (every 3 to 6 months; some patients (ie, HSCT) may require more frequent monitoring) (ASPEN Pediatric Nutrition Support Core Curriculum [Corkins, 2010])

Reference Range Normal whole blood range: ~10 to 37 mcg/dL

Dosage Forms Excipient information presented when available (limited, particularly for generics); consult specific product labeling.

Capsule, Oral:

Selenicaps-200: 200 mcg [corn free, no artificial color(s), rye free, sugar free, wheat free, yeast free]

Capsule, Oral [preservative free]:

Se-100: 100 mcg [dye free, yeast free]

Liquid, Oral:

Aqueous Selenium: 95 mcg/drop (15 mL) [contains sodium benzoate]

Solution, Intravenous:

Generic: 40 mcg/mL (10 mL)

Tablet, Oral:

Oceanic Selenium: 50 mcg, 200 mcg [animal products free, gelatin free, gluten free, kosher certified, lactose free, no artificial color(s), no artificial flavor(s), starch free, sugar free, yeast free]

Se Aspartate: 50 mcg

Se-Plus Protein: 200 mcg

Selenimin: 125 mcg [corn free, rye free, starch free, sugar free, wheat free]

Selenimin-200: 200 mcg [corn free, rye free, starch free, sugar free, wheat free, yeast free]

Generic: 50 mcg, 200 mcg

Tablet, Oral [preservative free]:

Generic: 50 mcg, 200 mcg

Tablet Extended Release, Oral [preservative free]:

Generic: 200 mcg

◆ **Selenium** *see* Trace Elements *on page* 2097

Selenium Sulfide (se LEE nee um SUL fide)

Brand Names: US Anti-Dandruff [OTC]; Dandrex [OTC]; Selsun [DSC]; Tersi

Brand Names: Canada Versel®

Therapeutic Category Antiseborrheic Agent, Topical; Shampoos

Generic Availability (US) May be product dependent

Use To treat itching and flaking of the scalp associated with dandruff; to control scalp seborrheic dermatitis; treatment of tinea versicolor

Pregnancy Risk Factor C

Pregnancy Considerations Animal reproduction studies have not been conducted.

Breast-Feeding Considerations It is not known if selenium sulfide is found in breast milk following topical application. The manufacturer recommends that caution be used if administered to nursing women.

Contraindications Hypersensitivity to selenium or any component of the formulation

Warnings/Precautions Hazardous agent - use appropriate precautions for handling and disposal (EPA, U-listed). For external use only; avoid contact with eyes and genital areas. Due to the risk of systemic toxicity, do not use on damaged skin or mucous membranes. Discontinue use if irritation occurs. Avoid topical use in very young children; safety of topical in infants has not been established.

Adverse Reactions

Central nervous system: Lethargy

Dermatologic: Alopecia, hair discoloration, unusual dryness or oiliness of scalp

Gastrointestinal: Abdominal pain, garlic breath, vomiting following long-term use on damaged skin

Local: Burning, itching, irritation, stinging (transient)

Neuromuscular & skeletal: Tremor

Miscellaneous: Diaphoresis

Drug Interactions

Metabolism/Transport Effects None known.

Avoid Concomitant Use There are no known interactions where it is recommended to avoid concomitant use.

Increased Effect/Toxicity There are no known significant interactions involving an increase in effect.

Decreased Effect There are no known significant interactions involving a decrease in effect.

Storage/Stability

Foam, shampoo: Store at controlled room temperature of 15°C to 25°C (59°F to 77°F).

Lotion: Store below 30°C (86°F)

Mechanism of Action May block the enzymes involved in growth of epithelial tissue

Pharmacokinetics (Adult data unless noted) Absorption: Not absorbed topically through intact skin, but can be absorbed topically through damaged skin

Dosing: Usual Children ≥2 years and Adults: Topical:

Dandruff, seborrhea: Massage 5-10 mL into wet scalp, leave on scalp 2-3 minutes, rinse thoroughly and repeat application; alternatively, 5-10 mL of shampoo is applied and allowed to remain on scalp for 5-10 minutes before being rinsed off thoroughly without a repeat application; shampoo twice weekly for 2 weeks initially, then use once every 1-4 weeks as indicated depending upon control

Tinea versicolor: Apply the 2.5% lotion in a thin layer covering the body surface from the face to the knees; leave on skin for 10 minutes, then rinse thoroughly; apply every day for 7 days; then follow with monthly applications for 3 months to prevent recurrences

Administration Topical: For external use only; avoid contact with eyes or acutely inflamed skin

Dosage Forms Excipient information presented when available (limited, particularly for generics); consult specific product labeling. [DSC] = Discontinued product

Foam, External:

Tersi: 2.25% (70 g) [contains trolamine (triethanolamine)]

Lotion, External:

Selsun: 2.5% (120 mL [DSC])

Generic: 2.5% (118 mL, 120 mL)

Shampoo, External:

Anti-Dandruff: 1% (207 mL) [contains brilliant blue fcf (fd&c blue #1), menthol]

Dandrex: 1% (240 mL)

◆ **Selsun [DSC]** *see* Selenium Sulfide *on page 1913*

◆ **Selzentry** *see* Maraviroc *on page 1324*

◆ **Senexon [OTC]** *see* Senna *on page 1914*

◆ **Senexon-S [OTC]** *see* Docusate and Senna *on page 698*

Senna (SEN na)

Medication Safety Issues

Sound-alike/look-alike issues:

Perdiem may be confused with Pyridium

Senexon may be confused with Cenestin

Senokot may be confused with Depakote

Brand Names: US Ex-Lax Maximum Strength [OTC]; Ex-Lax [OTC]; Geri-kot [OTC]; GoodSense Senna Laxative [OTC]; Perdiem Overnight Relief [OTC]; Senexon [OTC]; Senna Lax [OTC]; Senna Laxative [OTC]; Senna Maximum Strength [OTC]; Senna Smooth [OTC]; Senna-Gen [OTC] [DSC]; Senna-GRX [OTC]; Senna-Lax [OTC]; Senna-Tabs [OTC]; Senna-Time [OTC]; SennaCon [OTC]; Senno [OTC]; Senokot To Go [OTC] [DSC]; Senokot XTRA [OTC]; Senokot [OTC]

Therapeutic Category Laxative, Stimulant

Generic Availability (US) May be product dependent

Use Short-term treatment of constipation (OTC products; FDA approved in ages ≥2 years and adults; consult specific product formulations for appropriate age groups)

Pregnancy Considerations An increased risk of congenital abnormalities was not observed following maternal use of senna during pregnancy (Acs, 2009). Short-term use of senna is generally considered safe during pregnancy (Mahadevan, 2006).

Breast-Feeding Considerations Maternal use of senna is considered compatible with breast-feeding (Mahadevan, 2006).

Contraindications Per Commission E: Intestinal obstruction, acute intestinal inflammation (eg, Crohn disease), colitis ulcerosa, appendicitis, abdominal pain of unknown origin

Warnings/Precautions Not recommended for over-the-counter (OTC) use in patients experiencing stomach pain, nausea, vomiting, or a sudden change in bowel movements which lasts >2 weeks. Not recommended for OTC use in children <2 years of age.

Benzyl alcohol and derivatives: Some dosage forms may contain sodium benzoate/benzoic acid; benzoic acid (benzoate) is a metabolite of benzyl alcohol; large amounts of benzyl alcohol (≥99 mg/kg/day) have been associated with a potentially fatal toxicity ("gasping syndrome") in neonates; the "gasping syndrome" consists of metabolic acidosis, respiratory distress, gasping respirations, CNS dysfunction (including convulsions, intracranial hemorrhage), hypotension, and cardiovascular collapse (AAP, 1997; CDC, 1982); some data suggests that benzoate displaces bilirubin from protein binding sites (Ahlfors, 2001); avoid or use dosage forms containing benzyl alcohol derivative with caution in neonates. See manufacturer's labeling.

Adverse Reactions Gastrointestinal: Abdominal cramps, diarrhea, nausea, vomiting

Drug Interactions

Metabolism/Transport Effects None known.

Avoid Concomitant Use There are no known interactions where it is recommended to avoid concomitant use.

Increased Effect/Toxicity There are no known significant interactions involving an increase in effect.

Decreased Effect There are no known significant interactions involving a decrease in effect.

Pharmacodynamics Onset of action:

Oral: Within 6 to 24 hours

Rectal: Evacuation occurs in 30 minutes to 2 hours

Pharmacokinetics (Adult data unless noted)

Metabolism: In the liver

Elimination: In the feces (via bile) and in urine

Dosing: Usual

Pediatric:

Constipation: Oral:

Concentrated liquid (Fletcher's Laxative for Kids; 167 mg/5mL senna concentrate):

Children 2 to <6 years: 5 to 10 mL (167 to 333 mg senna concentrate) once or twice daily

Children and Adolescents 6 to 15 years: 10 to 15 mL (333 to 500 mg senna concentrate) once or twice daily

Syrup (8.8 mg sennosides/5mL):

Children 2 to <6 years: 2.5 to 3.75 mL (4.4 to 6.6 mg sennosides) at bedtime, not to exceed 3.75 mL (6.6 mg sennosides) twice daily

Children 6 to <12 years: 5 to 7.5 mL (8.8 to 13.2 mg sennosides) at bedtime, not to exceed 7.5 mL (13.2 mg sennosides) twice daily

Children ≥12 years and Adolescents: 10 to 15 mL (17.6 mg to 26.4 mg sennosides) at bedtime, not to exceed 15 mL (26.4 mg sennosides) twice daily.

Tablets:

8.6 mg sennosides/tablet:

Children 2 to <6 years: 1/2 tablet (4.3 mg sennosides) at bedtime, not to exceed 1 tablet (8.6 mg sennosides) twice daily

Children 6 to <12 years: 1 tablet (8.6 mg sennosides) at bedtime, not to exceed 2 tablets (17.2 mg sennosides) twice daily
Children ≥12 years and Adolescents: 2 tablets (17.2 mg sennosides) at bedtime, not to exceed 4 tablets (34.4 mg sennosides) twice daily
15 mg sennosides/tablet:
Children 6 to <12 years: 1 tablet (15 mg sennosides) once or twice daily
Children ≥12 years and Adolescents: 2 tablets (30 mg sennosides) once or twice daily
25 mg sennosides/tablet
Children 6 to <12 years: 1 tablet (25 mg sennosides) once or twice daily
Children ≥12 years and Adolescents: 2 tablets (50 mg sennosides) once or twice daily
Bowel evacuation: Children ≥12 years and Adolescents: Oral: 130 mg sennosides between 2:00 PM to 4:00 PM on the day prior to procedure
Adult:
Constipation: Oral: OTC ranges: Sennosides 15 mg once daily (maximum: 70 to 100 mg/day, divided twice daily)
Bowel evacuation: Oral: Usual dose: Sennosides 130 mg between 2:00 PM to 4:00 PM on the day prior to procedure

Administration Oral: Administer with water; syrup can be taken with juice or milk or mixed with ice cream to mask taste.

Monitoring Parameters Fluid status, frequency of bowel movements, serum electrolytes if severe diarrhea occurs

Dosage Forms Excipient information presented when available (limited, particularly for generics); consult specific product labeling. [DSC] = Discontinued product
Leaves, Oral:
Generic: (454 g)
Liquid, Oral:
Senexon: 8.8 mg/5 mL (237 mL) [contains methylparaben, propylene glycol, propylparaben]
Syrup, Oral:
Senna-GRX: 8.8 mg/5 mL (15 mL, 236 mL) [contains parabens]
Generic: 8.8 mg/5 mL (236 mL, 237 mL); 176 mg/5 mL (15 mL, 237 mL)
Tablet, Oral:
Ex-Lax: 15 mg [sodium free]
Ex-Lax Maximum Strength: 25 mg [sodium free]
Geri-kot: 8.6 mg
GoodSense Senna Laxative: 8.6 mg
Perdiem Overnight Relief: 15 mg
Senexon: 8.6 mg
Senna Lax: 8.6 mg
Senna Laxative: 8.6 mg
Senna Maximum Strength: 25 mg
Senna Smooth: 15 mg [contains sodium benzoate]
Senna-Gen: 8.6 mg [DSC]
Senna-Lax: 8.6 mg
Senna-Tabs: 8.6 mg
Senna-Time: 8.6 mg
SennaCon: 8.6 mg
Senno: 8.6 mg
Senokot: 8.6 mg
Senokot To Go: 8.6 mg [DSC]
Senokot XTRA: 17.2 mg
Generic: 8.6 mg, 15 mg
Tablet Chewable, Oral:
Ex-Lax: 15 mg
Ex-Lax: 15 mg [chocolate flavor]

- **Senna and Docusate** *see* Docusate and Senna *on page 698*
- **SennaCon [OTC]** *see* Senna *on page 1914*
- **Senna-Gen [OTC] [DSC]** *see* Senna *on page 1914*
- **Senna-GRX [OTC]** *see* Senna *on page 1914*
- **Senna Lax [OTC]** *see* Senna *on page 1914*
- **Senna Laxative [OTC]** *see* Senna *on page 1914*
- **SennaLax-S [OTC]** *see* Docusate and Senna *on page 698*
- **Senna Maximum Strength [OTC]** *see* Senna *on page 1914*
- **Senna Plus [OTC]** *see* Docusate and Senna *on page 698*
- **Senna-S** *see* Docusate and Senna *on page 698*
- **Senna Smooth [OTC]** *see* Senna *on page 1914*
- **Senna-Tabs [OTC]** *see* Senna *on page 1914*
- **Senna-Time [OTC]** *see* Senna *on page 1914*
- **Senno [OTC]** *see* Senna *on page 1914*
- **Sennosides** *see* Senna *on page 1914*
- **Sennosides and Docusate** *see* Docusate and Senna *on page 698*
- **Senokot [OTC]** *see* Senna *on page 1914*
- **Senokot-S [OTC]** *see* Docusate and Senna *on page 698*
- **Senokot To Go [OTC] [DSC]** *see* Senna *on page 1914*
- **Senokot XTRA [OTC]** *see* Senna *on page 1914*
- **SenoSol-SS [OTC]** *see* Docusate and Senna *on page 698*
- **Sensodyne Repair & Protect [OTC]** *see* Fluoride *on page 899*
- **Sensorcaine** *see* Bupivacaine *on page 316*
- **Sensorcaine® (Can)** *see* Bupivacaine *on page 316*
- **Sensorcaine-MPF** *see* Bupivacaine *on page 316*
- **Sensorcaine-MPF Spinal** *see* Bupivacaine *on page 316*
- **Se-Plus Protein [OTC]** *see* Selenium *on page 1912*
- **Septa-Amlodipine (Can)** *see* AmLODIPine *on page 133*
- **Septa-Atenolol (Can)** *see* Atenolol *on page 215*
- **Septa-Ciprofloxacin (Can)** *see* Ciprofloxacin (Systemic) *on page 463*
- **Septa-Citalopram (Can)** *see* Citalopram *on page 476*
- **Septa Losartan (Can)** *see* Losartan *on page 1302*
- **Septa-Metformin (Can)** *see* MetFORMIN *on page 1375*
- **Septa-Ondansetron (Can)** *see* Ondansetron *on page 1564*
- **Septra** *see* Sulfamethoxazole and Trimethoprim *on page 1986*
- **Septra DS** *see* Sulfamethoxazole and Trimethoprim *on page 1986*
- **Septra Injection (Can)** *see* Sulfamethoxazole and Trimethoprim *on page 1986*
- **Serevent Diskhaler Disk (Can)** *see* Salmeterol *on page 1896*
- **Serevent Diskus** *see* Salmeterol *on page 1896*
- **Seromycin [DSC]** *see* CycloSERINE *on page 555*
- **SEROquel** *see* QUEtiapine *on page 1815*
- **Seroquel (Can)** *see* QUEtiapine *on page 1815*
- **SEROquel XR** *see* QUEtiapine *on page 1815*
- **Seroquel XR (Can)** *see* QUEtiapine *on page 1815*
- **Serostim** *see* Somatropin *on page 1957*

Sertaconazole (ser ta KOE na zole)

Brand Names: US Ertaczo
Therapeutic Category Antifungal Agent, Topical
Generic Availability (US) No

Use Topical treatment of interdigital tinea pedis in immunocompetent patients (FDA approved in ages ≥12 years and adults); has also been used for diaper dermatitis and tinia corporis

Pregnancy Risk Factor C

Pregnancy Considerations Adverse events were not observed in animal reproduction studies following oral administration.

Breast-Feeding Considerations It is not known if sertaconazole is excreted in breast milk. The manufacturer recommends that caution be exercised when administering sertaconazole to nursing women.

Contraindications There are no contraindications listed in the manufacturer's labeling.

Warnings/Precautions Discontinue drug if sensitivity or irritation occurs. For topical use only; avoid ophthalmologic, oral, or intravaginal use. Re-evaluate use if no response within 2 weeks.

Adverse Reactions

Dermatologic: Burning, contact dermatitis, dry skin, tenderness

Postmarketing and/or case reports: Desquamation, erythema, hyperpigmentation, pruritus, vesiculation

Drug Interactions

Metabolism/Transport Effects None known.

Avoid Concomitant Use There are no known interactions where it is recommended to avoid concomitant use.

Increased Effect/Toxicity There are no known significant interactions involving an increase in effect.

Decreased Effect There are no known significant interactions involving a decrease in effect.

Storage/Stability Store at 20°C to 25°C (68°F to 77°F); excursions are permitted between 15°C and 30°C (59°F and 86°F).

Mechanism of Action Alters fungal cell wall membrane permeability; inhibits the CYP450-dependent synthesis of ergosterol

Pharmacokinetics (Adult data unless noted)

Absorption: Topical: Minimal; serum concentrations below the limit of quantitation (< 2.5 ng/mL)

Dosing: Usual

Pediatric:

Diaper dermatitis, candida: Limited data available: Infants and Children 2 to 24 months: Topical: Apply twice daily for 2 weeks; dosing based on an open-label, noncomparative study (n=27, mean age: 5.7 months, range: 2 to 22 months), 88.8% had complete cure; one patient had increased erythema but continued treatment (Bonifaz, 2013.)

Tinia corporis: Limited data available: Children ≥2 years and Adolescents: Topical: Apply once daily for 2 weeks; dosing based on an open-label study (n=16 patients age: 2 to 16 years, including 14 patients with tinia corporis); clinical cure was achieved in 75% of patients at 2 weeks and 100% of patients at 4 weeks (2 weeks post therapy follow-up assessment); no adverse effects were reported (Van Esso, 1995)

Tinea pedis: Children ≥12 years and Adolescents: Topical: Apply between toes and to surrounding healthy skin twice daily for 4 weeks

Adult: **Tinea pedis:** Topical: Apply between toes and to surrounding healthy skin twice daily for 4 weeks

Dosing adjustment in renal impairment: There are no dosage adjustments provided in the manufacturer's labeling; however, dosage adjustment unlikely necessary due to low systemic absorption.

Dosing adjustment in hepatic impairment: There are no dosage adjustments provided in the manufacturer's labeling; however dosage adjustment unlikely necessary due to low systemic absorption.

Administration For external use only. Apply to affected area between toes and to surrounding healthy skin. Make sure skin is dry before applying; wash hands after application. Avoid use of occlusive dressing. Avoid contact with eyes, nose, mouth, and other mucous membranes.

Monitoring Parameters Reassess diagnosis if no clinical improvement after 2 weeks.

Dosage Forms Excipient information presented when available (limited, particularly for generics); consult specific product labeling.

Cream, External, as nitrate:

Ertaczo: 2% (60 g) [contains methylparaben]

◆ **Sertaconazole Nitrate** *see* Sertaconazole *on page 1915*

Sertraline (SER tra leen)

Medication Safety Issues

Sound-alike/look-alike issues:

Sertraline may be confused with cetirizine, selegiline, Serevent, Soriatane

Zoloft may be confused with Zocor

BEERS Criteria medication:

This drug may be potentially inappropriate for use in geriatric patients with a history of falls or fractures (Quality of evidence - high [moderate for SIADH]; Strength of recommendation - strong).

Related Information

Antidepressant Agents *on page 2257*

Brand Names: US Zoloft

Brand Names: Canada ACT Sertraline; Apo-Sertraline; Auro-Sertraline; Dom-Sertraline; GD-Sertraline; JAMP-Sertraline; Mar-Sertraline; MINT-Sertraline; Mylan-Sertraline; PHL-Sertraline; PMS-Sertraline; Q-Sertraline; Ran-Sertraline; ratio-Sertraline; Riva-Sertraline; Sandoz-Sertraline; Teva-Sertraline; Zoloft

Therapeutic Category Antidepressant, Selective Serotonin Reuptake Inhibitor (SSRI)

Generic Availability (US) Yes

Use Treatment of obsessive-compulsive disorder (FDA approved in ages ≥6 years and adults); treatment of major depressive disorder, panic disorder (with or without agoraphobia), post-traumatic stress disorder, premenstrual dysphoric disorder, and social anxiety disorder (social phobia) (FDA approved in adults)

Medication Guide Available Yes

Pregnancy Risk Factor C

Pregnancy Considerations Adverse events have been observed in animal reproduction studies. Sertraline crosses the human placenta. An increased risk of teratogenic effects, including cardiovascular defects, may be associated with maternal use of sertraline or other SSRIs; however, available information is conflicting. Nonteratogenic effects in the newborn following SSRI/SNRI exposure late in the third trimester include respiratory distress, cyanosis, apnea, seizures, temperature instability, feeding difficulty, vomiting, hypoglycemia, hypo- or hypertonia, hyper-reflexia, jitteriness, irritability, constant crying, and tremor. Symptoms may be due to the toxicity of the SSRIs/SNRIs or a discontinuation syndrome and may be consistent with serotonin syndrome associated with SSRI treatment. Persistent pulmonary hypertension of the newborn (PPHN) has also been reported with SSRI exposure. The long-term effects of *in utero* SSRI exposure on infant development and behavior are not known.

Due to pregnancy-induced physiologic changes, women who are pregnant may require adjusted doses of sertraline to achieve euthymia. The ACOG recommends that therapy with SSRIs or SNRIs during pregnancy be individualized; treatment of depression during pregnancy should incorporate the clinical expertise of the mental health clinician, obstetrician, primary healthcare provider, and pediatrician. According to the American Psychiatric Association (APA), the risks of medication treatment should be weighed against other treatment options and untreated depression. For women who discontinue antidepressant medications during pregnancy and who may be at high risk for postpartum depression, the medications can be restarted following delivery. Treatment algorithms have been developed by the ACOG and the APA for the management of depression in women prior to conception and during pregnancy.

Breast-Feeding Considerations Sertraline and desmethylsertraline are excreted in breast milk. Adverse events have been reported in nursing infants exposed to some SSRIs. The American Academy of Breastfeeding Medicine suggests that sertraline may be considered for the treatment of postpartum depression in appropriately selected women who are nursing. Infants exposed to sertraline while breast-feeding generally receive a low relative dose and serum concentrations are not detectable in most infants. Sertraline concentrations in the hindmilk are higher than in foremilk. If the benefits of the mother receiving the sertraline and breast-feeding outweigh the risks, the mother may consider pumping and discarding breast milk with the feeding 7-9 hours after the daily dose to decrease sertraline exposure to the infant. The long-term effects on development and behavior have not been studied. The manufacturer recommends that caution be exercised when administering sertraline to nursing women. Maternal use of an SSRI during pregnancy may cause delayed milk secretion.

Contraindications

Use of MAOIs intended to treat psychiatric disorders (concurrently or within 14 days of stopping an MAOI or sertraline); concurrent use with pimozide; initiation in patients treated with linezolid or methylene blue IV; hypersensitivity to sertraline or any component of the formulation; concurrent use with disulfiram (oral concentrate only).

Documentation of allergenic cross-reactivity for SSRIs is limited. However, because of similarities in chemical structure and/or pharmacologic actions, the possibility of cross-sensitivity cannot be ruled out with certainty.

Warnings/Precautions [U.S. Boxed Warning]: Antidepressants increase the risk of suicidal thinking and behavior in children, adolescents, and young adults (18 to 24 years of age) with major depressive disorder (MDD) and other psychiatric disorders; consider risk prior to prescribing. Short-term studies did not show an increased risk in patients >24 years of age and showed a decreased risk in patients ≥65 years. Closely monitor patients for clinical worsening, suicidality, or unusual changes in behavior, particularly during the initial 1 to 2 months of therapy or during periods of dosage adjustments (increases or decreases); the patient's family or caregiver should be instructed to closely observe the patient and communicate condition with healthcare provider. A medication guide concerning the use of antidepressants should be dispensed with each prescription. **Sertraline is not FDA approved for use in children with major depressive disorder (MDD). However, it is approved for the treatment of obsessive-compulsive disorder (OCD) in children ≥6 years of age.**

The possibility of a suicide attempt is inherent in major depression and may persist until remission occurs. Use caution in high-risk patients. Worsening depression and severe abrupt suicidality that are not part of the presenting symptoms may require discontinuation or modification of drug therapy. The patient's family or caregiver should be alerted to monitor patients for the emergence of suicidality and associated behaviors (such as agitation, irritability, hostility, impulsivity, and hypomania) and call healthcare provider.

May precipitate a mixed/manic episode in patients at risk for bipolar disorder. Use with caution in patients with a family history of bipolar disorder, mania, or hypomania. Patients presenting with depressive symptoms should be screened for bipolar disorder. **Sertraline is not FDA approved for the treatment of bipolar depression.**

Potentially life-threatening serotonin syndrome (SS) has occurred with serotonergic agents (eg, SSRIs, SNRIs), particularly when used in combination with other serotonergic agents (eg, triptans, TCAs, fentanyl, lithium, tramadol, buspirone, St John's wort, tryptophan) or agents that impair metabolism of serotonin (eg, MAO inhibitors intended to treat psychiatric disorders, other MAO inhibitors [ie, linezolid and intravenous methylene blue]). Discontinue treatment (and any concomitant serotonergic agent) immediately if signs/symptoms arise. Has a very low potential to impair cognitive or motor performance. However, caution patients regarding activities requiring alertness until response to sertraline is known. Does not appear to potentiate the effects of alcohol, however, ethanol use is not advised.

Use caution in patients with a previous seizure disorder or condition predisposing to seizures such as brain damage, alcoholism, or concurrent therapy with other drugs which lower the seizure threshold. May increase the risks associated with electroconvulsive therapy. May cause mild pupillary dilation which in susceptible individuals can lead to an episode of narrow-angle glaucoma. Consider evaluating patients who have not had an iridectomy for narrow-angle glaucoma risk factors. Use with caution in patients with hepatic dysfunction and in elderly patients. May cause hyponatremia/SIADH (elderly at increased risk); volume depletion (diuretics may increase risk). Use caution in elderly patients; may be potentially inappropriate in patients with a history of falls or fractures, and may cause or exacerbate syndrome of inappropriate antidiuretic hormone secretion or hyponatremia; monitor sodium closely with initiation or dosage adjustments in older adults (Beers Criteria). Sertraline acts as a mild uricosuric; use with caution in patients at risk of uric acid nephropathy. Use with caution in patients where weight loss is undesirable. May cause or exacerbate sexual dysfunction. Potentially significant drug-drug interactions may exist, requiring dose or frequency adjustment, additional monitoring, and/or selection of alternative therapy.

Use oral concentrate formulation with caution in patients with latex sensitivity; dropper dispenser contains dry natural rubber. Some dosage forms may contain polysorbate 80 (also known as Tweens). Hypersensitivity reactions, usually a delayed reaction, have been reported following exposure to pharmaceutical products containing polysorbate 80 in certain individuals (Isaksson, 2002; Lucente 2000; Shelley, 1995). Thrombocytopenia, ascites, pulmonary deterioration, and renal and hepatic failure have been reported in premature neonates after receiving parenteral products containing polysorbate 80 (Alade, 1986; CDC, 1984). See manufacturer's labeling.

Monitor growth in pediatric patients. Given their lower body weight, lower doses are advisable in pediatric patients in order to avoid excessive plasma levels, despite slightly greater metabolism efficiency than adults.

Abrupt discontinuation or interruption of antidepressant therapy has been associated with a discontinuation syndrome. Symptoms arising may vary with antidepressant however commonly include nausea, vomiting, diarrhea, headaches, lightheadedness, dizziness, diminished appetite, sweating, chills, tremors, paresthesias, fatigue, somnolence, and sleep disturbances (eg, vivid dreams, insomnia). Greater risks for developing a discontinuation syndrome have been associated with antidepressants with shorter half-lives, longer durations of treatment, and abrupt discontinuation. For antidepressants of short or intermediate half-lives, symptoms may emerge within 2 to 5 days after treatment discontinuation and last 7 to 14 days (APA, 2010; Fava, 2006; Haddad, 2001; Shelton, 2001; Warner, 2006).

Warnings: Additional Pediatric Considerations SSRI-associated behavioral activation (ie, restlessness, hyperkinesis, hyperactivity, agitation) is two- to threefold more prevalent in children compared to adolescents; it is more prevalent in adolescents compared to adults. Somnolence (including sedation and drowsiness) is more common in adults compared to children and adolescents and SSRI-associated vomiting is two- to threefold more prevalent in children compared to adolescents; it is more prevalent in adolescents compared to adults (Safer, 2006).

Adverse Reactions

Cardiovascular: Chest pain, palpitations

Central nervous system: Agitation, aggressive behavior (children ≥2%), anxiety, dizziness, drowsiness, fatigue, headache, hypertonia, hypoesthesia, insomnia, malaise, nervousness, pain, paresthesia, yawning

Dermatologic: Diaphoresis, skin rash

Endocrine & metabolic: Decreased libido, weight gain

Gastrointestinal: Abdominal pain, anorexia, constipation, diarrhea, dyspepsia, increased appetite, nausea, vomiting, xerostomia

Genitourinary: Ejaculatory disorder, impotence, urinary incontinence (children ≥2%)

Hematologic & oncologic: Purpura (children)

Neuromuscular & skeletal: Back pain (≥1%), hyperkinesia (children ≥2%), myalgia(≥1%), tremor, weakness

Ophthalmic: Visual disturbance

Otic: Tinnitus

Respiratory: Epistaxis (children ≥2%), rhinitis, sinusitis (children ≥2%)

Miscellaneous: Fever (children ≥2%)

Rare but important or life-threatening: Acute renal failure, agranulocytosis, altered platelet function, anaphylactoid reaction, angle-closure glaucoma, aplastic anemia, apnea, ataxia, atrial arrhythmia, atrioventricular block, bradycardia, cerebrovascular spasm, choreoathetosis, colitis, coma, cystitis, depression, diverticulitis, dystonia, edema, esophagitis, extrapyramidal reaction, hematuria, hemoptysis, hepatic failure, hepatitis, hepatomegaly, hypertension, hypoglycemia, hyponatremia, increased INR, increased serum bilirubin, increased serum transaminases, leukopenia, myocardial infarction, neuroleptic malignant syndrome (Stevens, 2008), oculogyric crisis, orthostatic hypotension, pancreatitis, peptic ulcer bleed, peripheral ischemia, proctitis, prolonged Q-T interval on ECG, pulmonary hypertension, pyelonephritis, rectal hemorrhage, serotonin syndrome, SIADH, Stevens-Johnson syndrome, suicidal ideation, thrombocytopenia, torsades de pointes, urinary frequency, ventricular tachycardia, withdrawal syndrome

Drug Interactions

Metabolism/Transport Effects **Substrate** of CYP2B6 (minor), CYP2C19 (minor), CYP2C9 (minor), CYP2D6 (minor), CYP3A4 (minor); **Note:** Assignment of Major/Minor substrate status based on clinically relevant drug interaction potential; **Inhibits** CYP1A2 (weak), CYP2B6 (moderate), CYP2C19 (moderate), CYP2C8 (weak), CYP2C9 (weak), CYP2D6 (moderate)

Avoid Concomitant Use

Avoid concomitant use of Sertraline with any of the following: Amodiaquine; Dapoxetine; Disulfiram; Dosulepin; Iobenguane I 123; Linezolid; MAO Inhibitors; Methylene Blue; Pimozide; Thioridazine; Tryptophan; Urokinase

Increased Effect/Toxicity

Sertraline may increase the levels/effects of: Agents with Antiplatelet Properties; Amodiaquine; Anticoagulants; Antidepressants (Serotonin Reuptake Inhibitor/Antagonist); Antipsychotic Agents; Apixaban; ARIPiprazole; Aspirin; Beta-Blockers; Blood Glucose Lowering Agents; BusPIRone; CarBAMazepine; Cilostazol; Citalopram; CloZAPine; Collagenase (Systemic); CYP2B6 Substrates; CYP2C19 Substrates; CYP2D6 Substrates; Dabigatran Etexilate; Deoxycholic Acid; Desmopressin; Dextromethorphan; Dosulepin; DOXOrubicin (Conventional); Eliglustat; Fesoterodine; Fosphenytoin; Galantamine; Highest Risk QTc-Prolonging Agents; Ibritumomab; Methadone; Methylene Blue; Metoprolol; Moderate Risk QTc-Prolonging Agents; Nebivolol; NSAID (COX-2 Inhibitor); NSAID (Nonselective); Obinutuzumab; Phenytoin; Pimozide; Propafenone; RisperiDONE; Rivaroxaban; Salicylates; Serotonin Modulators; Thiazide Diuretics; Thioridazine; Thrombolytic Agents; TiZANidine; Tositumomab and Iodine I 131 Tositumomab; TraMADol; Tricyclic Antidepressants; Urokinase; Vitamin K Antagonists

The levels/effects of Sertraline may be increased by: Alcohol (Ethyl); Analgesics (Opioid); Antiemetics (5HT3 Antagonists); Antipsychotic Agents; BusPIRone; Cimetidine; CNS Depressants; Dapoxetine; Dasatinib; Disulfiram; Glucosamine; Grapefruit Juice; Herbs (Anticoagulant/Antiplatelet Properties); Ibrutinib; Limaprost; Linezolid; Lithium; Macrolide Antibiotics; MAO Inhibitors; Metoclopramide; Metyrosine; Mifepristone; Multivitamins/Fluoride (with ADE); Multivitamins/Minerals (with ADEK, Folate, Iron); Multivitamins/Minerals (with AE, No Iron); Omega-3 Fatty Acids; Pentosan Polysulfate Sodium; Pentoxifylline; Prostacyclin Analogues; Tedizolid; Tipranavir; TraMADol; Tryptophan; Vitamin E

Decreased Effect

Sertraline may decrease the levels/effects of: Clopidogrel; Codeine; Iobenguane I 123; Ioflupane I 123; Tamoxifen; Thyroid Products

The levels/effects of Sertraline may be decreased by: CarBAMazepine; Cyproheptadine; Darunavir; Efavirenz; Fosphenytoin; NSAID (COX-2 Inhibitor); NSAID (Nonselective); Phenytoin

Food Interactions Sertraline average peak serum levels may be increased if taken with food. Management: Administer consistently with or without food.

Storage/Stability Store at 25°C (77°F); excursions are permitted between 15°C and 30°C (59°F and 86°F).

Mechanism of Action Antidepressant with selective inhibitory effects on presynaptic serotonin (5-HT) reuptake and only very weak effects on norepinephrine and dopamine neuronal uptake. *In vitro* studies demonstrate no significant affinity for adrenergic, cholinergic, GABA, dopaminergic, histaminergic, serotonergic, or benzodiazepine receptors.

Pharmacodynamics Maximum effect may take several weeks

Pharmacokinetics (Adult data unless noted)

Protein binding: 98%

Metabolism: Significant first pass effect; undergoes N-demethylation to N-desmethylsertraline (significantly less active than sertraline); both parent and metabolite undergo oxidative deamination, followed by reduction, hydroxylation and conjugation with glucuronide (**Note:** Children 6-17 years may metabolize sertraline slightly better than adults, as pediatric AUCs and peak concentrations were 22% lower than adults when adjusted for weight; however, lower doses are recommended for younger pediatric patients to avoid excessive drug levels)

Bioavailability: Tablets approximately equal to oral solution

Half-life: Parent: Mean: 26 hours; metabolite (N-desmethylsertraline): 62-104 hours

Children: 6-12 years: Mean: 26.2 hours

Children: 13-17 years: Mean: 27.8 hours

Adults: 18-45 years: Mean: 27.2 hours

Elimination: 40% to 45% of dose eliminated in urine (none as unchanged drug); 40% to 45% eliminated in feces (12% to 14% as unchanged drug)

Clearance: May be decreased in patients with hepatic impairment

Dialysis: Not likely to remove significant amount of drug due to large V_d

Dosing: Usual Oral:

Children 6-12 years:

Depression: **Note:** Not FDA approved: Initial: 12.5-25 mg once daily; titrate dose upwards if clinically needed; may increase by 25-50 mg/day increments at intervals of at least 1 week; mean final dose in 21 children (8-18 years of age) was 100 ± 53 mg or 1.6 mg/kg/day (n=11); range: 25-200 mg/day; maximum dose: 200 mg/day (Dopheide, 2006; Tierney, 1995); avoid excessive dosing

Obsessive-compulsive disorder: Initial: 25 mg once daily; titrate dose upwards if clinically needed; increase by 25-50 mg/day increments at intervals of at least 1 week; range: 25-200 mg/day; maximum dose: 200 mg/day; avoid excessive dosing

Adolescents 13-17 years:

Depression: Initial 25-50 mg once daily; titrate dose upwards if clinically needed; may increase by 50 mg/day increments at intervals of at least 1 week; mean final dose in 13 adolescents was 110 ± 50 mg or about 2 mg/kg/day (McConville, 1996); in another study using a slower titration, the mean dose at week 6 was 93 mg (n=41) and at week 10 was 127 mg (n=34) (Ambrosini, 1999); range: 25-200 mg/day; maximum dose: 200 mg/day (Dopheide, 2006).

Obsessive-compulsive disorder: Initial: 50 mg once daily; titrate dose upwards if clinically needed; increase by 50 mg/day increments at intervals of at least 1 week; range: 25-200 mg/day; maximum dose: 200 mg/day

Adults:

Depression and obsessive-compulsive disorder: Initial: 50 mg once daily; titrate dose upwards if clinically needed; increase by 50 mg/day increments at intervals of at least 1 week; range: 50-200 mg/day; maximum dose: 200 mg/day

Panic disorder, post-traumatic stress disorder, and social anxiety disorder: Initial: 25 mg once daily; increase dose after 1 week to 50 mg once daily; titrate dose further if clinically needed; increase by 50 mg/day increments at intervals of at least 1 week; range: 50-200 mg/day; maximum dose: 200 mg/day

Premenstrual dysphoric disorder: Initial: 50 mg/day given daily throughout the menstrual cycle **or** only during the luteal phase of the menstrual cycle (depending on assessment of physician); may increase if needed by 50 mg increments per menstrual cycle; maximum dose when using daily dosing throughout the menstrual cycle: 150 mg/day; maximum dose when dosing only during the luteal phase of the menstrual cycle: 100 mg/day. **Note:** If using a 100 mg/day dose with luteal phase dosing, use a 50 mg/day titration step for 3 days at the beginning of each luteal phase dosing period.

Dosing adjustment in renal impairment: None needed

Dosing adjustment in hepatic impairment: Use with caution and in reduced doses

Preparation for Administration Oral concentrate: Must be diluted before use. **Immediately before administration**, use the dropper provided to measure the required amount of concentrate; mix with 4 ounces (1/2 cup) of water, ginger ale, lemon/lime soda, lemonade, or orange juice only. Do not mix with any other liquids than these. The dose should be taken immediately after mixing; do not mix in advance. A slight haze may appear after mixing; this is normal.

Administration

Oral: May be administered without regard to food; do not administer with grapefruit juice; administer once daily dosage either in morning or evening.

Oral concentrate: Must dilute oral concentrate before use; measure dose with dropper provided and mix with 4 ounces of water, orange juice, lemonade, ginger ale, or lemon/lime soda; do not mix with other liquids; take dose immediately after mixing, do not mix ahead of time; sometimes a slight haze may be seen after mixing (this is normal). **Note:** Use with caution in patients with latex sensitivity; dropper dispenser contains dry natural rubber.

Monitoring Parameters Weight and growth in children if long-term therapy; uric acid, CBC, liver function, serum sodium, urine output. Monitor patient periodically for symptom resolution; monitor for worsening depression, suicidality, and associated behaviors (especially at the beginning of therapy or when doses are increased or decreased)

Test Interactions May interfere with urine detection of benzodiazepines (false-positive)

Additional Information Two larger studies of children and adolescents with depression and obsessive-compulsive disorder utilized a forced upward dosage titration of sertraline to 200 mg/day; these studies conclude that the adult dosage titration regimen can be used in children ≥6 years and adolescents (Alderman, 1998; March, 1998); however, other studies in adults (Fabre, 1995) demonstrate that lower sertraline doses (50 mg/day) are as effective as higher doses with fewer adverse effects and discontinuations of therapy.

A recent report (Lake, 2000) describes 5 children (age 8-15 years) who developed epistaxis (n=4) or bruising (n=1) while receiving sertraline therapy. Another recent report describes the SSRI discontinuation syndrome in 6 children; the syndrome was similar to that reported in adults (Diler, 2002). Due to limited long-term studies, the clinical usefulness of sertraline should be periodically reevaluated in patients receiving the drug for extended intervals; effects of long term use of sertraline on pediatric growth, development, and maturation have not been directly assessed.

Neonates born to women receiving SSRIs late during the third trimester may experience respiratory distress, apnea, cyanosis, temperature instability, vomiting, feeding difficulty, hypoglycemia, constant crying, irritability, hypotonia, hypertonia, hyper-reflexia, tremor, jitteriness, and seizures; these symptoms may be due to a direct toxic effect, withdrawal syndrome, or (in some cases) serotonin syndrome. Withdrawal symptoms occur in 30% of neonates exposed to SSRIs *in utero*; monitor newborns for at least 48 hours after birth; long-term effects of *in utero* exposure to SSRIs are unknown (Levinson-Castiel, 2006).

Dosage Forms Excipient information presented when available (limited, particularly for generics); consult specific product labeling.

Concentrate, Oral:

Zoloft: 20 mg/mL (60 mL) [contains alcohol, usp, menthol]

Generic: 20 mg/mL (60 mL)

Tablet, Oral:

Zoloft: 25 mg [scored; contains fd&c blue #1 aluminum lake, fd&c red #40 aluminum lake, fd&c yellow #10 aluminum lake, polysorbate 80]

Zoloft: 50 mg [scored; contains fd&c blue #2 aluminum lake]

Zoloft: 100 mg [scored; contains polysorbate 80]

Generic: 25 mg, 50 mg, 100 mg

◆ **Sertraline Hydrochloride** *see* Sertraline *on page 1916*

◆ **Serzone** *see* Nefazodone *on page 1493*

Sevelamer (se VEL a mer)

Medication Safety Issues

Sound-alike/look-alike issues:

Renagel may be confused with Reglan, Regonol, Renvela

Renvela may be confused with Reglan, Regonol, Renagel

Sevelamer may be confused with Savella®

International issues:

Renagel [U.S., Canada, and multiple international markets] may be confused with Remegel brand name for aluminium hydroxide and magnesium carbonate [Netherlands] and for calcium carbonate [Hungary, Great Britain and Ireland] and with Remegel Wind Relief brand name for calcium carbonate and simethicone [Great Britain]

Related Information

Oral Medications That Should Not Be Crushed or Altered *on page 2476*

Brand Names: US Renagel; Renvela

Brand Names: Canada Renagel; Renvela

Therapeutic Category Phosphate Binder

Generic Availability (US) May be product dependent

Use Reduction of serum phosphorus in patients with chronic kidney disease on hemodialysis (FDA approved in adults)

Pregnancy Risk Factor C

Pregnancy Considerations Adverse events were observed in animal reproduction studies. Sevelamer is not absorbed systemically; however, it may cause a reduction in the absorption of some vitamins.

Breast-Feeding Considerations Sevelamer is not absorbed systemically; however, it may cause a reduction in the absorption of some vitamins.

Contraindications Bowel obstruction

Warnings/Precautions Use with caution in patients with gastrointestinal disorders including dysphagia, swallowing disorders, severe gastrointestinal motility disorders (including constipation), or major gastrointestinal surgery. May cause reductions in vitamin D, E, K, or folic acid absorption. May bind to some drugs in the gastrointestinal tract and decrease their absorption; when changes in absorption of oral medications may have significant clinical consequences (such as antiarrhythmic and antiseizure medications), these medications should be taken at least 1 hour before or 3 hours after a dose of sevelamer. Tablets should not be taken apart or chewed; broken or crushed tablets will rapidly expand in water/saliva and may be a choking hazard.

Warnings: Additional Pediatric Considerations In a trial conducted in pediatric patients (n=18; age range: 10 months to 18 years), an increase in metabolic acidosis was noted in the sevelamer treatment group (incidence: 34.4%) (Pieper, 2006); in another pediatric trial (n=17, age range: 2 to 18 years), no untoward effects were reported (Mahdavi, 2003). Patients should be closely monitored.

Adverse Reactions

Endocrine & metabolic: Hypercalcemia, metabolic acidosis (more common in children)

Gastrointestinal: Abdominal pain, constipation, diarrhea, dyspepsia, flatulence, nausea, peritonitis (peritoneal dialysis), vomiting

Rare but important or life-threatening: Fecal impaction, intestinal obstruction (rare), intestinal perforation (rare)

Drug Interactions

Metabolism/Transport Effects None known.

Avoid Concomitant Use There are no known interactions where it is recommended to avoid concomitant use.

Increased Effect/Toxicity There are no known significant interactions involving an increase in effect.

Decreased Effect

Sevelamer may decrease the levels/effects of: Calcitriol (Systemic); Cholic Acid; CycloSPORINE (Systemic); Levothyroxine; Mycophenolate; Quinolone Antibiotics; Tacrolimus (Systemic)

Food Interactions May cause reductions in vitamin D, E, K, or folic acid absorption. Management: Must be administered with meals. Consider vitamin supplementation.

Storage/Stability Store at controlled room temperature of 25°C (77°F); excursions permitted to 15°C to 30°C (59°F to 86°F). Protect from moisture.

Mechanism of Action Sevelamer (a polymeric compound) binds phosphate within the intestinal lumen, limiting absorption and decreasing serum phosphate concentrations without altering calcium, aluminum, or bicarbonate concentrations.

Pharmacodynamics Onset of Action: Reduction in serum phosphorus: 1-2 weeks (Burke, 1997; Chertow, 1997)

Pharmacokinetics (Adult data unless noted)

Absorption: Not systemically absorbed

Elimination: Feces 100%

Dosing: Usual Note: Phosphate binding capacity: Sevelamer HCl 400 mg binds 32 mg of phosphate; 800 mg binds 64 mg of phosphate.

Infants, Children, and Adolescents:

Hyperphosphatemia: Limited data available: Oral:

Infants ≥10 months and Children < 2 years: Sevelamer HCl (Renagel): Mean final dose: 140 ± 86 mg/kg/day (5.38 ± 3.24 **g**/day) was reported in a small trial (n=18, age range: 10 months to 18 years) to achieve the targeted serum phosphorus level. Initial dosing was based upon prior phosphate binder dose and serum phosphorus concentrations (Pieper, 2006). In a case report of a 19-month old, an initial dose of 100 mg/kg/day divided every 8 hours with titration up to 130 mg/kg/day was reported to effectively lower serum phosphorus levels (Storms, 2006).

Children ≥2 years and Adolescents: Sevelamer HCl (Renagel): Initial dose: 400 or 800 mg three times daily administered with meals; titrate at monthly intervals in 1200 mg/day increments (ie, 400 mg at each meal) to target phosphorus level; final mean range: 140-163 mg/kg/day (5.38-6.7 **g**/day); dosing based on experience in 46 patients; prior or final comparative calcium salt phosphate-binder dose: 4 ± 3 **g**/day (Gulati, 2010; Mahdavi, 2003; Pieper, 2006). Sevelamer carbonate (Renvela) has also been used in pediatric patients with similar efficacy as sevelamer hydrochloride (Renagel) (Gonzalez, 2010).

Hyperphosphatemia, pretreatment of oral and enteral nutrition: Limited data available: Oral: 800 mg (tablets or powder) added to up to 400 mL of breast milk or 100 mL of infant formula, tube feeding, and cow's milk; after sitting for 10 minutes, decant liquid from the precipitate at the bottom; reported experience has shown a decrease in phosphate of >85% in breast milk, 42% in cow's milk, 48% in tube feeding, and 68% in infant formula (KDOQI, 2009; Raaijmakers, 2013)

Adults: **Control of serum phosphorus:** Oral:

Patients not taking a phosphate binder: 800-1600 mg 3 times daily with meals; the initial dose may be based on the serum phosphorus:

Serum phosphorus >5.5 mg/dL and <7.5 mg/dL: 800 mg 3 times daily

Serum phosphorus ≥7.5 mg/dL and <9 mg/dL: 1200-1600 mg 3 times daily

Serum phosphorus ≥9 mg/dL: 1600 mg 3 times daily

Maintenance dose adjustment based on serum phosphorous concentration [goal range: 3.5-5.5 mg/dL; maximum dose studied was equivalent to 13 **g**/day (sevelamer hydrochloride) or 14 **g**/day (sevelamer carbonate)]:
  Serum phosphorus >5.5 mg/dL: Increase by 400-800 mg per meal at 2-week intervals
  Serum phosphorus 3.5-5.5 mg/dL: Maintain current dose
  Serum phosphorus <3.5 mg/dL: Decrease by 400-800 mg per meal
Dosage adjustment when switching between phosphate-binder products: 667 mg of calcium acetate is equivalent to ~800 mg sevelamer (carbonate or hydrochloride); conversion based on dose per meal:
  Calcium acetate 667 mg: Convert to 800 mg Renagel/Renvela
  Calcium acetate 1334 mg: Convert to 1600 mg as Renagel/Renvela (800 mg tablets x 2) **or** 1200 mg as Renagel (400 mg tablets x 3)
  Calcium acetate 2001 mg: Convert to 2400 mg as Renagel/Renvela (800 mg tablets x 3) **or** 2000 mg as Renagel (400 mg tablets x 5)

Preparation for Administration Powder for oral suspension: Mix powder with water prior to administration. The 800 mg packet should be mixed with 30 mL of water and the 2,400 mg packet should be mixed with 60 mL of water (multiple packets may be mixed together using the appropriate amount of water).

Administration
Oral: Administer with meals, at least 1 hour before or 3 hours after other medications.
Tablets: Swallow tablets whole; do not break, chew, or crush; contents will expand with water.
Packets for oral suspension: Mix powder with water prior to administration. The 800 mg packet should be mixed with 30 mL of water and the 2,400 mg packet should be mixed with 60 mL of water (multiple packets may be mixed together using the appropriate amount of water). Stir vigorously to suspend mixture just prior to drinking; powder does not dissolve. Drink within 30 minutes of preparing or resuspend just prior to drinking.

Monitoring Parameters
Serum chemistries, including bicarbonate and chloride
Serum calcium and phosphorus: Frequency of measurement may be dependent upon the presence and magnitude of abnormalities, the rate of progression of CKD, and the use of treatments for CKD-mineral and bone disorders. In children initial assessment should occur at CKD stage 2 (KDIGO, 2009):
  CKD stage 3: Every 6-12 months
  CKD stage 4: Every 3-6 months
  CKD stage 5 and 5D: Every 1-3 months
Periodic 24-hour urinary calcium and phosphorus; magnesium; alkaline phosphatase every 12 months or more frequently in the presence of elevated PTH; creatinine, BUN, albumin; intact parathyroid hormone (iPTH) every 3-12 months depending on CKD severity

Reference Range
Corrected total serum calcium: Children, Adolescents, and Adults: CKD stages 2-5D: Maintain normal ranges; preferably on the lower end for stage 5 (KDIGO, 2009; KDOQI, 2005)
Phosphorus (KDIGO, 2009):
  CKD stages 3-5: Maintain normal ranges
  CKD stage 5D: Lower elevated phosphorus levels toward the normal range

Additional Information Chronic kidney disease (CKD) (KDIGO, 2013; KDOQI, 2002): Children ≥2 years, Adolescents, and Adults: GFR <60 mL/minute/1.73 m^2 or kidney damage for >3 months; stages of CKD are described below:
  CKD Stage 1: Kidney damage with normal or increased GFR; GFR >90 mL/minute/1.73 m^2
  CKD Stage 2: Kidney damage with mild decrease in GFR; GFR 60-89 mL/minute/1.73 m^2
  CKD Stage 3: Moderate decrease in GFR; GFR 30-59 mL/minute/1.73 m^2
  CKD Stage 4: Severe decrease in GFR; GFR 15-29 mL/minute/1.73 m^2
  CKD Stage 5: Kidney failure; GFR <15 mL/minute/1.73 m^2 or dialysis

Dosage Forms Excipient information presented when available (limited, particularly for generics); consult specific product labeling. [DSC] = Discontinued product
Packet, Oral, as carbonate:
  Renvela: 0.8 g (1 ea, 90 ea); 2.4 g (1 ea, 90 ea) [citrus flavor]
Tablet, Oral, as carbonate:
  Renvela: 800 mg
  Generic: 800 mg [DSC]
Tablet, Oral, as hydrochloride:
  Renagel: 400 mg, 800 mg

◆ **Sevelamer Carbonate** *see* Sevelamer *on page 1920*
◆ **Sevelamer Hydrochloride** *see* Sevelamer *on page 1920*
◆ **SfRowasa** *see* Mesalamine *on page 1368*
◆ **S/GSK1349572** *see* Dolutegravir *on page 701*
◆ **Sharobel** *see* Norethindrone *on page 1530*
◆ **Shohl's Solution (Modified)** *see* Sodium Citrate and Citric Acid *on page 1942*
◆ **Shopko Athletes Foot [OTC]** *see* Clotrimazole (Topical) *on page 518*
◆ **Shopko Nasal Decongestant [OTC]** *see* Pseudoephedrine *on page 1801*
◆ **Shopko Nasal Decongestant Max [OTC]** *see* Pseudoephedrine *on page 1801*
◆ **Sig-Enalapril (Can)** *see* Enalapril *on page 744*
◆ **Silace [OTC]** *see* Docusate *on page 697*
◆ **Siladryl Allergy [OTC]** *see* DiphenhydrAMINE (Systemic) *on page 668*
◆ **Silapap Children's [OTC]** *see* Acetaminophen *on page 44*
◆ **Silapap Infant's [OTC]** *see* Acetaminophen *on page 44*

Sildenafil (sil DEN a fil)

Medication Safety Issues
Sound-alike/look-alike issues:
  Revatio may be confused with ReVia, Revonto
  Sildenafil may be confused with silodosin, tadalafil, vardenafil
  Viagra may be confused with Allegra, Vaniqa

Brand Names: US Revatio; Viagra

Brand Names: Canada ACT-Sildenafil; Apo-Sildenafil; GD-Sildenafil; Jamp-Sildenafil; M-Sildenafil; Mint-Sildenafil; MYL-Sildenafil; PMS-Sildenafil; RAN-Sildenafil; ratio-Sildenafil R; Revatio; Sandoz-Sildenafil; Teva-Sildenafil; Viagra

Therapeutic Category Phosphodiesterase Type-5 (PDE5) Inhibitor

Generic Availability (US) May be product dependent

Use Treatment of WHO Group I pulmonary arterial hypertension (PAH) (Revatio: FDA approved in adults); treatment of erectile dysfunction (Viagra: FDA approved in male adults). Has also been used for treatment of persistent pulmonary hypertension of the newborn (PPHN)

refractory to treatment with inhaled nitric oxide; facilitation of weaning from nitric oxide (ie, to attenuate rebound effects after discontinuing inhaled nitric oxide); secondary pulmonary hypertension following cardiac surgery; **Note:** Use of Revatio, especially chronic use, is not recommended in pediatric patients due to a dose-dependent increased mortality risk observed in trials; however, situations may exist in which the benefit-risk profile of Revatio may make its use, with close monitoring, acceptable in individual pediatric patients, for example, when other treatment options are limited.

Pregnancy Risk Factor B

Pregnancy Considerations Adverse events were not observed in animal reproduction studies. Information related to the use of sildenafil for the treatment of pulmonary arterial hypertension (PAH) in pregnant women is limited (Hsu, 2011). Current guidelines recommend that women with PAH use effective contraception and avoid pregnancy (Badesch, 2007; McLaughlin, 2009). Less than 0.001% appears in the semen.

Breast-Feeding Considerations It is not known if sildenafil is excreted in breast milk. The manufacturer recommends that caution be exercised when administering sildenafil to nursing women.

Contraindications

Hypersensitivity to sildenafil or any component of the formulation; concurrent use (regularly/intermittently) of organic nitrates in any form (eg, nitroglycerin, isosorbide dinitrate); concomitant use of riociguat (a guanylate cyclase stimulator).

According to the manufacturers of protease inhibitors (atazanavir, darunavir, fosamprenavir, indinavir, lopinavir/ritonavir, nelfinavir, ritonavir, saquinavir, tipranavir): Concurrent use with a protease inhibitor regimen when sildenafil is used for pulmonary artery hypertension (eg, Revatio).

Warnings/Precautions Decreases in blood pressure may occur due to vasodilator effects; use with caution in patients with left ventricular outflow obstruction (aortic stenosis, hypertrophic obstructive cardiomyopathy), those on antihypertensive therapy, with resting hypotension (BP <90/50 mm Hg), fluid depletion, or autonomic dysfunction; may be more sensitive to hypotensive actions. Patients should be hemodynamically stable prior to initiating therapy at the lowest possible dose. Use with caution in patients with uncontrolled hypertension (>170/110 mm Hg); life-threatening arrhythmias, stroke or MI within the last 6 months; cardiac failure or coronary artery disease causing unstable angina; safety and efficacy have not been studied in these patients. There is a degree of cardiac risk associated with sexual activity; therefore, physicians should consider the cardiovascular status of their patients prior to initiating any treatment for erectile dysfunction. If pulmonary edema occurs when treating pulmonary arterial hypertension (PAH), consider the possibility of pulmonary veno-occlusive disease (PVOD); continued use is not recommended in patient with PVOD. Substantial consumption of ethanol may increase the risk of hypotension and orthostasis. Lower ethanol consumption has not been associated with significant changes in blood pressure or increase in orthostatic symptoms. Have patients avoid or limit ethanol consumption.

Sildenafil should be used with caution in patients with anatomical deformation of the penis (angulation, cavernosal fibrosis, or Peyronie's disease) and in patients who have conditions which may predispose them to priapism (sickle cell anemia, multiple myeloma, leukemia). All patients should be instructed to seek medical attention if erection persists >4 hours. Painful erection >6 hours in duration has been reported rarely.

Vision loss, including permanent loss of vision, may occur and be a sign of nonarteritic anterior ischemic optic neuropathy (NAION). Risk may be increased with history of vision loss. Other risk factors for NAION include low cup-to-disc ratio ("crowded disc"), coronary artery disease, diabetes, hypertension, hyperlipidemia, smoking, and age >50 years. May cause dose-related impairment of color discrimination. Use caution in patients with retinitis pigmentosa; a minority have genetic disorders of retinal phosphodiesterases (no safety information available). Sudden decrease or loss of hearing has been reported; hearing changes may be accompanied by tinnitus and dizziness. A direct relationship between therapy and vision or hearing loss has not been determined.

The potential underlying causes of erectile dysfunction should be evaluated prior to treatment. Potentially significant drug-drug interactions may exist, requiring dose or frequency adjustment, additional monitoring, and/or selection of alternative therapy. Use of sildenafil is contraindicated in patients currently taking nitrate preparations. However, when nitrate administration becomes medically necessary, the ACCF/AHA 2013 guidelines on treatment of ST-segment elevation MI and the ACCF/AHA 2012 guidelines on treatment of unstable angina/non ST-segment elevation MI support administration of nitrates only if 24 hours have elapsed after use of sildenafil (ACCF/AHA [Anderson, 2013]; ACCF/AHA [O'Gara, 2013]). Hypersensitivity reactions, including anaphylactic reaction and anaphylactic shock, have been reported.

Avoid abrupt discontinuation, especially if used as monotherapy in PAH as exacerbation may occur. Use caution in patients with bleeding disorders or with active peptic ulcer disease; safety has not been established. Efficacy has not be established for treatment of pulmonary hypertension associated with sickle cell disease. Use with caution in the elderly, or patients with renal or hepatic dysfunction; dose adjustment may be needed. Use of Revatio, especially chronic use, is not recommended in children. After 2 years of treatment, increased mortality was seen in a long-term (median treatment exposure: 4.6 years) study at higher doses (20-80 mg [depending upon weight] 3 times/day) (Barst, 2012a; Barst, 2012b).

Benzyl alcohol and derivatives: Some dosage forms may contain sodium benzoate/benzoic acid; benzoic acid (benzoate) is a metabolite of benzyl alcohol; large amounts of benzyl alcohol (≥99 mg/kg/day) have been associated with a potentially fatal toxicity ("gasping syndrome") in neonates; the "gasping syndrome" consists of metabolic acidosis, respiratory distress, gasping respirations, CNS dysfunction (including convulsions, intracranial hemorrhage), hypotension, and cardiovascular collapse (AAP, 1997; CDC, 1982); some data suggests that benzoate displaces bilirubin from protein binding sites (Ahlfors, 2001); avoid or use dosage forms containing benzyl alcohol derivative with caution in neonates. See manufacturer's labeling. Oral suspensions may be available in multiple concentrations (commercially available: 10 mg/mL; extemporaneous preparation: 2.5 mg/mL); dosing should be presented in mg of sildenafil; use extra precaution when verifying product formulation and calculation of dose volumes. The 2 mL oral syringe provided by the manufacturer only provides measurements for fixed doses of 5 mg and 20 mg; for patients not receiving either of these fixed doses, an appropriate-size calibrated oral syringe will need to be dispensed.

Adverse Reactions Based upon normal doses for either indication or route. (Adverse effects such as flushing, diarrhea, myalgia, and visual disturbances may be increased with adult doses >100 mg/24 hours.)

Cardiovascular: Flushing

Central nervous system: Dizziness, headache, insomnia, paresthesia

Dermatologic: Erythema, skin rash

Gastrointestinal: Diarrhea, dyspepsia, gastritis, nausea
Genitourinary: Urinary tract infection
Hepatic: Increased liver enzymes
Neuromuscular & skeletal: Back pain, myalgia
Ophthalmic: Visual disturbance (including vision color changes, blurred vision, and photophobia)
Respiratory: Epistaxis, exacerbation of dyspnea, nasal congestion, rhinitis, sinusitis
Miscellaneous: Fever
Rare but important or life-threatening: Abnormal hepatic function tests, absent reflexes, amnesia (transient global), anemia, anorgasmia, anterior chamber eye hemorrhage, anterior ischemic optic neuropathy, arthritis, auditory impairment, breast hypertrophy, burning sensation of eyes, cardiac failure, cataract, cerebrovascular hemorrhage, colitis, cystitis, depression, diaphoresis, diplopia, dry eye syndrome, dysphagia, ECG abnormality, ejaculatory disorder, exfoliative dermatitis, falling, gastroenteritis, genital edema, gingivitis, glossitis, gout, herpes simplex infection, hyperglycemia, hypernatremia, hypersensitivity reaction, hypertension, hypertonia, hypoglycemia, increased bronchial secretions, increased intraocular pressure, ischemic heart disease, laryngitis, leukopenia, malignant melanoma (Li, 2014), migraine, myasthenia, mydriasis, myocardial infarction, neuralgia, neuropathy, orthostatic hypotension, otalgia, peripheral edema, pharyngitis, photophobia, priapism, prolonged erection, pulmonary hemorrhage, rectal hemorrhage, retinal edema, retinal hemorrhage, retinal vascular disease, rupture of tendon, seizure, severe sickle cell crisis (vasoocclusive crisis in patients with pulmonary hypertension associated with sickle cell disease), skin photosensitivity, stomatitis, syncope, synovitis, tachycardia, transient ischemic attacks, unstable diabetes, urinary incontinence, ventricular arrhythmia, vitreous detachment, vitreous traction

Drug Interactions

Metabolism/Transport Effects **Substrate** of CYP1A2 (minor), CYP2C19 (minor), CYP2C9 (minor), CYP2D6 (minor), CYP2E1 (minor), CYP3A4 (major); **Note:** Assignment of Major/Minor substrate status based on clinically relevant drug interaction potential; **Inhibits** CYP2C9 (weak)

Avoid Concomitant Use

Avoid concomitant use of Sildenafil with any of the following: Alprostadil; Amyl Nitrite; Boceprevir; Conivaptan; Dapoxetine; Fusidic Acid (Systemic); Idelalisib; Phosphodiesterase 5 Inhibitors; Riociguat; Telaprevir; Vasodilators (Organic Nitrates)

Increased Effect/Toxicity

Sildenafil may increase the levels/effects of: Alpha1-Blockers; Alprostadil; Amyl Nitrite; Antihypertensives; Bosentan; HMG-CoA Reductase Inhibitors; Phosphodiesterase 5 Inhibitors; Riociguat; Vasodilators (Organic Nitrates)

The levels/effects of Sildenafil may be increased by: Alcohol (Ethyl); Aprepitant; Boceprevir; Conivaptan; CYP3A4 Inhibitors (Moderate); CYP3A4 Inhibitors (Strong); Dapoxetine; Dasatinib; Erythromycin (Systemic); Fluconazole; Fosaprepitant; Fusidic Acid (Systemic); Idelalisib; Itraconazole; Ivacaftor; Ketoconazole (Systemic); Lorcaserin; Luliconazole; Mifepristone; Netupitant; Palbociclib; Posaconazole; Protease Inhibitors; Sapropterin; Simeprevir; Stiripentol; Telaprevir; Voriconazole

Decreased Effect

The levels/effects of Sildenafil may be decreased by: Bosentan; CYP3A4 Inducers (Moderate); CYP3A4 Inducers (Strong); Dabrafenib; Deferasirox; Etravirine; Mitotane; Siltuximab; St Johns Wort; Tocilizumab

Food Interactions Grapefruit juice may increase serum levels/toxicity of sildenafil. Management: Avoid grapefruit juice.

Storage/Stability

Tablets/injection: Store at 20°C to 25°C (68°F to 77°F); excursions are permitted to 15°C to 30°C (59°F to 86°F).
Oral suspension: Store unreconstituted powder below 30°C (86°F); protect from moisture. Store reconstituted oral suspension below 30°C (86°F) or at 2°C to 8°C (36°F to 46°F). Do not freeze. Discard unused Revatio oral suspension after 60 days.

Mechanism of Action

Erectile dysfunction: Does not directly cause penile erections, but affects the response to sexual stimulation. The physiologic mechanism of erection of the penis involves release of nitric oxide (NO) in the corpus cavernosum during sexual stimulation. NO then activates the enzyme guanylate cyclase, which results in increased levels of cyclic guanosine monophosphate (cGMP), producing smooth muscle relaxation and inflow of blood to the corpus cavernosum. Sildenafil enhances the effect of NO by inhibiting phosphodiesterase type 5 (PDE-5), which is responsible for degradation of cGMP in the corpus cavernosum; when sexual stimulation causes local release of NO, inhibition of PDE-5 by sildenafil causes increased levels of cGMP in the corpus cavernosum, resulting in smooth muscle relaxation and inflow of blood to the corpus cavernosum; at recommended doses, it has no effect in the absence of sexual stimulation.
Pulmonary arterial hypertension (PAH): Inhibits phosphodiesterase type 5 (PDE-5) in smooth muscle of pulmonary vasculature where PDE-5 is responsible for the degradation of cyclic guanosine monophosphate (cGMP). Increased cGMP concentration results in pulmonary vasculature relaxation; vasodilation in the pulmonary bed and the systemic circulation (to a lesser degree) may occur.

Pharmacodynamics

Maximum effect: Decrease blood pressure: Oral: 1 to 2 hours
Duration of Action: Decrease blood pressure: <8 hours

Pharmacokinetics (Adult data unless noted)

Absorption: Oral: Rapid; slower with a high-fat meal; tablet and suspension are bioequivalent
Distribution: Distributes into tissues
V_d total: Neonates: 22.4 L (or 456 L/70 kg) (Mukherjee, 2009)
V_{dss}: Adults: 105 L
Protein binding:
Neonates: Sildenafil: 93.9% ± 2.5%; N-desmethyl metabolite: 92% ± 3% (Mukherjee, 2009)
Adults: Sildenafil and N-desmethyl metabolite: ~96%
Metabolism: Via the liver via cytochrome P450 isoenzyme CYP3A4 (major route) and CYP2C9 (minor route). Major metabolite (UK-103320 or desmethylsildenafil) is formed via N-desmethylation pathway and has 50% of the activity as sildenafil.
Bioavailability: Oral: Mean: 41%; range: 25% to 63%; may be higher in patients with PAH compared to healthy volunteers; **Note:** A 10 mg dose of the injection is predicted to have an effect equal to a 20 mg oral dose taking into consideration the parent drug and active metabolite
Half-life (terminal):
Sildenafil:
Neonates: PNA 1 day: 55.9 hours (Mukherjee, 2009)
Neonates: PNA 7 days: 47.7 hours (Mukherjee, 2009)
Adults: 4 hours
Active N-desmethyl metabolite:
Neonates: 11.9 hours (Mukherjee, 2009)
Adults: 4 hours

Time to peak serum concentration: Oral: Fasting: 30 to 120 minutes (median 60 minutes); delayed by 60 minutes with a high-fat meal

Elimination: Excreted as metabolites; 80% of dose excreted in feces, 13% in urine

Clearance: Decreased in patients with hepatic cirrhosis or severe renal impairment; clearance may be lower in patients with PAH compared to normal volunteers. Sildenafil clearance in newborns is significantly decreased compared to adults, but approaches adult (allometrically scaled) values by the first week of life (Mukherjee, 2009). Clearance of N-desmethyl active metabolite is decreased in patients with severe renal impairment.

Dosing: Neonatal

Note: In pediatric patients (1 to 17 years of age) with PAH, an increased mortality risk was associated with long-term use (>2 years) at dosage levels of 0.88 to 2.5 mg/kg/dose administered three times daily (Barst, 2012; Barst, 2012a); use of Revatio, especially chronic use, is not recommended in pediatric patients due to a dose-dependent increased mortality risk observed in trials; however, situations may exist in which the benefit-risk profile of Revatio may make its use, with close monitoring, acceptable in individual pediatric patients, for example, when other treatment options are limited. Oral suspensions may be available in multiple concentrations (commercially available: 10 mg/mL; extemporaneous preparation: 2.5 mg/mL); dosing should be presented in mg of sildenafil; use extra precaution when verifying product formulation and calculation of dose volumes.

Pulmonary hypertension: Note: Limited data available; dose not established; a wide range of doses and interpatient variability has been reported; careful dose titration is necessary; most literature consists of case reports or small studies.

Oral: Full-term neonates: Usual range: 0.5 to 3 mg/kg/dose every 6 to 12 hours; the largest study was a double-blind, randomized, placebo-controlled trial and used an initial dose of 3 mg/kg/dose every 6 hours in 31 patients (Vargas-Origel, 2010); earlier studies used 0.3 to 2 mg/kg/dose every 6 to 24 hours; optimal duration not established (Ahsman, 2009; Baquero, 2006; Noori, 2007)

IV: GA >34 weeks and PNA <72 hours: PPHN: 0.4 mg/kg loading dose administered over 3 hours followed by continuous infusion of 1.6 mg/kg/**day** for up to 7 days was used in four patients in an open-label, dose-escalation trial of 36 neonates with an oxygenation index (OI) ≥15 on two occasions at least 30 minutes apart; 29 patients were also receiving iNO (Steinhorn, 2009); **Note:** The dose listed here is the dose recommended by the authors for use in future clinical trials.

Pulmonary hypertension, facilitation of inhaled nitric oxide (iNO) wean (in patients who previously failed iNO wean): Note: Limited information exists; a wide range of doses and interpatient variability has been reported; careful dose titration is necessary; most literature consists of case reports or small studies.

Oral: Full-term neonates:

Single dose: ~0.3 mg/kg/dose given once 70 to 90 minutes prior to iNO discontinuation was used in three patients (3 days, 6 weeks, and 4 months of age) (Atz, 1999)

Multiple dose: Initial: 0.3 mg/kg/dose (range: 0.22 to 0.47 mg/kg/dose) every 6 hours (average duration: 28 days) was used in seven patients (median age: 12 months; range: 3 days to 21 months); optimal duration of treatment not established (Lee, 2008).

Dosing: Usual

Pediatric: **Note:** In pediatric patients (1 to 17 years of age) with PAH, an increased mortality risk was associated with long-term use (>2 years) at dosage levels of 0.88 to 2.5 mg/kg/dose administered three times daily (Barst, 2012; Barst, 2012a); use of Revatio, especially chronic use, is not recommended in pediatric patients due to a dose-dependent increased mortality risk observed in trials; however, situations may exist in which the benefit-risk profile of Revatio may make its use, with close monitoring, acceptable in individual pediatric patients, for example, when other treatment options are limited. Oral suspensions may be available in multiple concentrations (commercially available: 10 mg/mL; extemporaneous preparation: 2.5 mg/mL); dosing should be presented in mg of sildenafil; use extra precaution when verifying product formulation and calculation of dose volumes.

Pulmonary hypertension: Limited data available; dose and duration of therapy not established; interpatient variability has been reported; Oral:

Infants: Initial: 0.25 mg/kg/dose every 6 hours **or** 0.5 mg/kg/dose every 8 hours; titrate as needed; maximum reported dose range: 1 to 2 mg/kg/dose every 6 to 8 hours (Humpl, 2011; Mourani, 2009).

An open-label, prospective trial of 25 pediatric patients <5 years of age (median age: 6 months; age range: 10 days to 4.9 years) reported statistically significant improvement in echocardiography outcome measures; in 15 patients, sildenafil abolished rebound pulmonary hypertension following NO withdrawal; the initial dose of 0.25 mg/kg/dose four times daily was titrated as tolerated to a target of 1 mg/kg/dose four times daily; the reported median dose was 0.7 mg/kg/dose four times daily (range: 0.5 to 2.25 mg/kg/dose); reported duration of therapy was 9 days to 4.3 years (n=25); 11 patients were discontinued on sildenafil therapy due to clinical resolution; nine deaths were reported [severe lung hypoplasia (n=3); veno-occlusive disease post-chemotherapy (n=1); severe BPD (n=1); cause of death unrelated to pulmonary vascular disease (n=4)] (Humpl, 2011).

A retrospective trial of 25 pediatric patients <2 years of age (which included at least 16 infants) evaluated long-term safety and efficacy in patients with chronic lung disease (72% with BPD); at therapy initiation, the subject ages ranged from 14 days to 96 weeks (median: ~6 months); the initial dose of 0.5 mg/kg/dose every 8 hours was titrated as tolerated; the majority of patients were treated with 8 mg/kg/**day** (2 mg/kg/dose four times daily); echocardiogram showed clinical improvement in 88% of patients; reported duration of therapy was 28 to 950 days (median: 241 days); five deaths were reported during therapy (day 25 to 241 of therapy; median: 135 days); causes of death included sepsis, meningitis, and refractory respiratory disease (Mourani, 2009).

Children and Adolescents <18 years of age: **Note:** Dosage should not be increased; higher doses and long-term use are associated with an increased mortality risk (Barst, 2012; Barst, 2012a).

8 to 20 kg: 10 mg three times daily

>20 kg to 45 kg: 20 mg three times daily

>45 kg: 40 mg three times daily

Dosing based on the STARTS-1 and 2 trial, a randomized, double-blind, placebo-controlled study in 235 pediatric patients (1 to 17 years of age) which evaluated short-term and long-term safety and efficacy of 3 dose levels (low, medium, and high-dose); results suggested that the medium dose level (shown above) is efficacious at improving exercise capacity, functional class and hemodynamic status in the short-term (16 weeks duration); the low dosage level was not shown to be efficacious. The long-term safety and efficacy data showed a dose-dependent increased risk of mortality which was highest among the high-dose group. It was estimated that the dosing presented will produce serum concentration of 140 ng/mL and would be expected to inhibit 77% of phosphodiesterase type 5 activity *in vitro* (Barst, 2012; Barst, 2012a).

Pulmonary hypertension, congenital heart surgery (postoperative): Limited data available; dosing regimens variable:

Oral (or nasogastric tube): Infants, Children, and Adolescents: Initial: 0.5 mg/kg/dose upon admission to ICU; increase in 0.5 mg/kg/dose increments every 4 to 6 hours up to a maximum dose of 2 mg/kg/dose as tolerated; upon discontinuation of mechanical ventilation, sildenafil therapy can be tapered over 5 to 7 days; dosing based on a retrospective report of 100 pediatric patients (including neonates through >10 years of age) which showed reduction in pulmonary arterial pressures and/or prevention of severe pulmonary hypertension (Nemoto, 2010). A lower dose of 0.35 mg/kg/dose every 4 hours for 1 week postoperatively was used in a retrospective, case-controlled trial of 38 pediatric patients (age range: 5 to 33 months) (Palma, 2011). In another retrospective report (n=45, median age: 32.6 months; range: 6 days to 17 years), a mean dose of 0.9 ± 0.3 mg/kg/dose four times daily was reported (Uhm, 2010). **Note:** Use of preoperative sildenafil therapy for the prevention of pulmonary hypertension following congenital heart surgery has produced variable efficacy results (Palma, 2011); a double-blind, placebo-controlled trial showed a negative impact on oxygenation and ventricular function (Vassalos, 2011).

IV: Infants >60 days and Children: Loading dose: Range: 0.04 to 0.35 mg/kg administered over 5 minutes, followed by a maintenance infusion: Reported range: 0.015 to 0.4 mg/kg/**hour** continued for 24 to 72 hours was used for pulmonary hypertension occurring within 48 hours of the end of cardiac surgery in a multicenter, randomized, double-blind, placebo-controlled dose-finding trial (n=17; median age: 5 months; age range: 3 months to 14 years; neonates and infants <60 days were excluded from the trial); dosages were either low, medium, or high dose (n=4 each treatment group; n=5 placebo) designed to attain serum concentrations of 40, 120, and 360 ng/mL, respectively; patients receiving sildenafil at all dosages were found to have lower pulmonary artery pressure and when compared to placebo, shorter duration of mechanical ventilation (median: 3 days vs 8 days), shorter ICU stay (median: 6 days vs 15 days), and shorter hospitalization (median: 12 days vs 21 days); study closed early due to slow patient accrual leading to underpowered results; no conclusions about dosage were able to be determined (Fraisse, 2011).

Pulmonary hypertension, facilitation of inhaled nitric oxide (iNO) wean (in patients who have not previously failed iNO wean): Limited data available: Infants and Children ≤15 months: Oral: Single dose: 0.4 mg/kg/dose (range: 0.3 to 0.5 mg/kg/dose) given once 60 minutes prior to iNO discontinuation; dosing based on a randomized, double-blind, placebo-controlled trial in 29 infants and young children (median age: 5.6 months; age range: 1 to 15 months; n=15 treatment arm) (Namachivayam, 2006).

Adult:

Erectile dysfunction (Viagra): Oral: Usual: 50 mg taken as needed, ~1 hour before sexual activity (dose may be taken 30 minutes to 4 hours before sexual activity); dosing range: 25 to 100 mg once daily; maximum recommended dose: 100 mg once daily

Pulmonary arterial hypertension (Revatio):

Oral: 5 mg or 20 mg 3 times daily taken at least 4-6 hours apart; maximum recommended dose: 20 mg 3 times daily

IV: 2.5 mg or 10 mg 3 times daily

Dosage considerations for patients taking alpha blockers: Adults: Viagra: Initial: 25 mg

Dosage adjustment for concomitant use of potent CYP34A inhibitors: Adults:

Revatio:

Strong CYP3A inhibitors (eg, itraconazole, ketoconazole): Not recommended

Protease inhibitors: Concurrent use is contraindicated

Viagra: Strong CYP3A inhibitors (eg, itraconazole, ketoconazole) or erythromycin: Starting dose of 25 mg should be considered

Dosing adjustment in renal impairment: Adults:

CrCl ≥30 mL/minute:

Revatio: No dosage adjustment necessary.

Viagra: No dosage adjustment recommended.

CrCl <30 mL/minute:

Revatio: No dosage adjustment necessary.

Viagra: Starting dose of 25 mg should be considered.

Dosing adjustment in hepatic impairment: Adults:

Mild to moderate impairment (Child-Pugh classes A and B):

Revatio: No dosage adjustment necessary.

Viagra: Starting dose of 25 mg should be considered.

Severe impairment (Child-Pugh class C):

Revatio: There are no dosage adjustments provided in manufacturer's labeling (has not been studied).

Viagra: Starting dose of 25 mg should be considered.

Administration

Oral:

Revatio: Administer doses at least 4 to 6 hours apart; may be administered without regard to meals; shake oral suspension well prior to use; **Note:** Oral suspensions may be available in multiple concentrations (commercially available: 10 mg/mL; extemporaneous preparation: 2.5 mg/mL); use extra precaution when verifying product formulation and calculation of dose volumes. The 2 mL oral syringe provided by the manufacturer only provides measurements for fixed doses of 5 mg and 20 mg; for patients not receiving either of these fixed doses, an appropriate-size calibrated oral syringe will need to be dispensed.

Viagra: Administer with or without food 30 minutes to 4 hours before sexual activity

IV: Revatio:

Neonates: In clinical trials, loading dose was administered over 3 hours, followed by a continuous IV infusion (Steinhorn, 2009)

Infant, Children, and Adolescents: In clinical trials, loading dose was administered as a bolus over 5 minutes, followed by a continuous IV infusion (Fraisse, 2011)

Adults: Administer as an IV bolus

Monitoring Parameters Heart rate, blood pressure, oxygen saturation, PaO_2

Additional Information Sildenafil is ~10 times more selective for PDE-5 as compared to PDE-6. PDE-6 is found in the retina and is involved in phototransduction. At higher plasma levels, inhibition of PDE-6 may occur and may account for the abnormalities in color vision noted in some patients.

Dosage Forms Excipient information presented when available (limited, particularly for generics); consult specific product labeling.

Solution, Intravenous:

Revatio: 10 mg/12.5 mL (12.5 mL)

Generic: 10 mg/12.5 mL (12.5 mL)

Suspension Reconstituted, Oral:

Revatio: 10 mg/mL (112 mL) [contains sodium benzoate]

Tablet, Oral:

Revatio: 20 mg

Viagra: 25 mg, 50 mg, 100 mg [contains fd&c blue #2 aluminum lake]

Generic: 20 mg

Extemporaneous Preparations A 2.5 mg/mL sildenafil citrate oral suspension may be made with tablets and either a 1:1 mixture of methylcellulose 1% and simple syrup NF or a 1:1 mixture of Ora-Sweet and Ora-Plus. Crush thirty sildenafil 25 mg tablets (Viagra) in a mortar and reduce to a fine powder. Add small portions of chosen vehicle and mix to a uniform paste; mix while adding vehicle in incremental proportions to **almost** 300 mL; transfer to a graduated cylinder, rinse mortar with vehicle, and add quantity of vehicle sufficient to make 300 mL. Store in amber plastic bottles and label "shake well". Stable for 90 days at room temperature or refrigerated.

Nahata MC, Morosco RS, and Brady MT, "Extemporaneous Sildenafil Citrate Oral Suspensions for the Treatment of Pulmonary Hypertension in Children," *Am J Health-Syst Pharm*, 2006, 63(3):254-7.

◆ **Sildenafil Citrate** *see* Sildenafil *on page 1921*

◆ **Silenor** *see* Doxepin (Systemic) *on page 711*

◆ **Silexin [OTC]** *see* Guaifenesin and Dextromethorphan *on page 992*

◆ **Silkis (Can)** *see* Calcitriol *on page 338*

◆ **Silphen Cough [OTC]** *see* DiphenhydrAMINE (Systemic) *on page 668*

◆ **Silphen DM Cough [OTC]** *see* Dextromethorphan *on page 631*

◆ **Siltussin DAS [OTC]** *see* GuaiFENesin *on page 988*

◆ **Siltussin DM [OTC]** *see* Guaifenesin and Dextromethorphan *on page 992*

◆ **Siltussin DM DAS [OTC]** *see* Guaifenesin and Dextromethorphan *on page 992*

◆ **Siltussin SA [OTC]** *see* GuaiFENesin *on page 988*

◆ **Silvadene** *see* Silver Sulfadiazine *on page 1926*

◆ **Silver Bullet Suppository [OTC] (Can)** *see* Bisacodyl *on page 289*

Silver Nitrate (SIL ver NYE trate)

Therapeutic Category Ophthalmic Agent, Miscellaneous; Topical Skin Product

Generic Availability (US) Yes

Use Astringent; cauterization of wounds; germicidal; removal of granulation tissue, corns, and warts

Contraindications Hypersensitivity to silver nitrate or any component of the formulation; not for use on broken skin, cuts, or wounds

Warnings/Precautions Do not use applicator sticks on the eyes. Prolonged use may result in skin discoloration. Silver nitrate is a caustic agent and inappropriate use may cause chemical burns. Skin contact time with applicator sticks should be extremely short when used in neonates or on thin delicate skin contact.

Adverse Reactions

Dermatologic: Burning and skin irritation, staining of the skin

Hematologic: Methemoglobinemia

Drug Interactions

Metabolism/Transport Effects None known.

Avoid Concomitant Use

Avoid concomitant use of Silver Nitrate with any of the following: BCG; BCG (Intravesical)

Increased Effect/Toxicity There are no known significant interactions involving an increase in effect.

Decreased Effect

Silver Nitrate may decrease the levels/effects of: BCG; BCG (Intravesical); BCG Vaccine (Immunization); Sodium Picosulfate

Storage/Stability Must be stored in a dry place. Store in a tight, light-resistant container. Exposure to light causes silver to oxidize and turn brown. Dipping in water causes oxidized film to readily dissolve.

Mechanism of Action Free silver ions precipitate bacterial proteins by combining with chloride in tissue forming silver chloride; coagulates cellular protein to form an eschar; silver ions or salts or colloidal silver preparations can inhibit the growth of both gram-positive and gram-negative bacteria. This germicidal action is attributed to the precipitation of bacterial proteins by liberated silver ions. Silver nitrate coagulates cellular protein to form an eschar, and this mode of action is the postulated mechanism for control of benign hematuria, rhinitis, and recurrent pneumothorax.

Pharmacokinetics (Adult data unless noted) Absorption: Not readily absorbed from mucous membranes

Dosing: Usual Children and Adults:

Sticks: Apply to mucous membranes and other moist skin surfaces only on area to be treated

Topical solution: Apply a cotton applicator dipped in solution on the affected area 2-3 times/week for 2-3 weeks

Dosage Forms Excipient information presented when available (limited, particularly for generics); consult specific product labeling.

Applicator sticks, topical: Silver nitrate 75% and potassium nitrate 25%

Solution, topical: 0.5% (960 mL); 10% (30 mL); 25% (30 mL); 50% (30 mL)

Silver Sulfadiazine (SIL ver sul fa DYE a zeen)

Brand Names: US Silvadene; SSD; Thermazene [DSC]

Brand Names: Canada Flamazine®

Therapeutic Category Antibiotic, Topical

Generic Availability (US) Yes

Use Adjunct in the prevention and treatment of infection in second and third degree burns

Pregnancy Risk Factor B

Pregnancy Considerations Adverse events were not observed in animal reproduction studies. Because of the theoretical increased risk for hyperbilirubinemia and kernicterus, sulfadiazine is contraindicated for use near term, on premature infants, or on newborn infants during the first 2 months of life (refer to Sulfadiazine monograph).

Breast-Feeding Considerations It is not known if sulfadiazine is found in breast milk following topical application; however, sulfonamide serum concentrations may reach therapeutic levels following application to extensive areas. Oral sulfadiazine is contraindicated in nursing mothers since sulfonamides cross into the milk and may cause kernicterus in the newborn (refer to Sulfadiazine monograph).

Contraindications Hypersensitivity to silver sulfadiazine or any component of the formulation; premature infants or neonates <2 months of age (sulfonamides may displace bilirubin and cause kernicterus); pregnancy (approaching or at term)

Warnings/Precautions Use with caution in patients with G6PD deficiency, renal impairment, or history of allergy to other sulfonamides; sulfadiazine may accumulate in patients with impaired hepatic or renal function. Prolonged use may result in fungal or bacterial superinfection, including *C. difficile*-associated diarrhea (CDAD) and pseudomembranous colitis; CDAD has been observed >2 months postantibiotic treatment. Use of analgesic might be needed before application; systemic absorption may be significant and adverse reactions may occur

Warnings: Additional Pediatric Considerations Some dosage forms may contain propylene glycol; in neonates large amounts of propylene glycol delivered orally, intravenously (eg, >3,000 mg/day), or topically have been associated with potentially fatal toxicities which can include metabolic acidosis, seizures, renal failure, and CNS depression; toxicities have also been reported in children and adults including hyperosmolality, lactic acidosis, seizures, and respiratory depression; use caution (AAP, 1997; Shehab, 2009).

Adverse Reactions

Dermatologic: Discoloration of skin, erythema multiforme, itching, photosensitivity, rash

Hematologic: Agranulocytosis, aplastic anemia, hemolytic anemia, leukopenia

Hepatic: Hepatitis

Renal: Interstitial nephritis

Miscellaneous: Allergic reactions may be related to sulfa component

Drug Interactions

Metabolism/Transport Effects None known.

Avoid Concomitant Use

Avoid concomitant use of Silver Sulfadiazine with any of the following: BCG; BCG (Intravesical)

Increased Effect/Toxicity There are no known significant interactions involving an increase in effect.

Decreased Effect

Silver Sulfadiazine may decrease the levels/effects of: BCG; BCG (Intravesical); BCG Vaccine (Immunization); Sodium Picosulfate

Storage/Stability Discard if cream is darkened (reacts with heavy metals resulting in release of silver).

Mechanism of Action Acts upon the bacterial cell wall and cell membrane. Bactericidal for many gram-negative and gram-positive bacteria and is effective against yeast. Active against *Pseudomonas aeruginosa*, *Pseudomonas maltophilia*, *Enterobacter* species, *Klebsiella* species, *Serratia* species, *Escherichia coli*, *Proteus mirabilis*, *Morganella morganii*, *Providencia rettgeri*, *Proteus vulgaris*, *Providencia* species, *Citrobacter* species, *Acinetobacter calcoaceticus*, *Staphylococcus aureus*, *Staphylococcus epidermidis*, *Enterococcus* species, *Candida albicans*, *Corynebacterium diphtheriae*, and *Clostridium perfringens*

Pharmacokinetics (Adult data unless noted)

Absorption: Significant percutaneous absorption of sulfadiazine can occur especially when applied to extensive burns

Half-life: 10 hours and is prolonged in patients with renal insufficiency

Time to peak serum concentration: Within 3-11 days of continuous topical therapy

Elimination: ~50% excreted unchanged in urine

Dosing: Usual Children and Adults: Topical: Apply once or twice daily with a sterile gloved hand; apply to a thickness of 1/16"; burned area should be covered with cream at all times

Administration Topical: Apply to cleansed, debrided burned areas

Monitoring Parameters Serum electrolytes, UA, renal function test, CBC in patients with extensive burns on long-term treatment

Additional Information Contains methylparaben

Dosage Forms Excipient information presented when available (limited, particularly for generics); consult specific product labeling. [DSC] = Discontinued product

Cream, External:

Silvadene: 1% (20 g, 25 g, 50 g, 85 g, 400 g, 1000 g) [contains methylparaben, propylene glycol]

SSD: 1% (25 g, 50 g, 85 g, 400 g) [contains cetyl alcohol, methylparaben, propylene glycol]

Thermazene: 1% (20 g [DSC], 50 g [DSC], 85 g [DSC], 400 g [DSC], 1000 g [DSC]) [contains methylparaben, propylene glycol]

Generic: 1% (20 g, 25 g, 50 g, 85 g, 400 g)

◆ **Simbrinza** *see* Brinzolamide and Brimonidine *on page 302*

Simethicone (sye METH i kone)

Medication Safety Issues

Sound-alike/look-alike issues:

Simethicone may be confused with cimetidine

Mylanta may be confused with Mynatal

Mylicon may be confused with Modicon, Myleran

Brand Names: US Equalizer Gas Relief [OTC]; Gas Free Extra Strength [OTC]; Gas Relief Extra Strength [OTC]; Gas Relief Maximum Strength [OTC]; Gas Relief Ultra Strength [OTC]; Gas Relief [OTC]; Gas-X Childrens [OTC]; Gas-X Extra Strength [OTC]; Gas-X Infant Drops [OTC]; Gas-X Ultra Strength [OTC]; Gas-X [OTC]; GasAid [OTC]; Infants Gas Relief [OTC]; Infants Simethicone [OTC]; Mi-Acid Gas Relief [OTC]; Mytab Gas Maximum Strength [OTC]; Mytab Gas [OTC]; Phazyme Maximum Strength [OTC]; Phazyme Ultra Strength [OTC]; Phazyme [OTC]

Brand Names: Canada Ovol; Phazyme

Therapeutic Category Antiflatulent

Generic Availability (US) May be product dependent

Use Relieve flatulence, functional gastric bloating, and postoperative gas pains

Pregnancy Considerations Simethicone is not absorbed systemically following oral administration. Systemic absorption would be required in order for simethicone to cross the placenta and reach the fetus (Mahadevan 2006).

Breast-Feeding Considerations Due to lack of systemic absorption, simethicone is not expected to be excreted in breast milk (Hagemann 1998).

Contraindications Hypersensitivity to simethicone or any component of the formulation

Warnings/Precautions Benzyl alcohol and derivatives: Some dosage forms may contain sodium benzoate/benzoic acid; benzoic acid (benzoate) is a metabolite of benzyl alcohol; large amounts of benzyl alcohol (≥99 mg/kg/day) have been associated with a potentially fatal toxicity ("gasping syndrome") in neonates; the "gasping syndrome" consists of metabolic acidosis, respiratory distress, gasping respirations, CNS dysfunction (including convulsions, intracranial hemorrhage), hypotension, and cardiovascular collapse (AAP, 1997; CDC, 1982); some data suggests that benzoate displaces bilirubin from protein binding sites (Ahlfors, 2001); avoid or use dosage forms containing benzyl alcohol derivative with caution in neonates. See manufacturer's labeling.

Adverse Reactions Gastrointestinal: Loose stools

Drug Interactions

Metabolism/Transport Effects None known.

Avoid Concomitant Use There are no known interactions where it is recommended to avoid concomitant use.

Increased Effect/Toxicity There are no known significant interactions involving an increase in effect.

Decreased Effect There are no known significant interactions involving a decrease in effect.

Food Interactions Avoid carbonated beverages and gas-forming foods.

Storage/Stability Store at 20°C to 25°C (68°F to 77°F). Protect from moisture. Avoid high humidity and excessive heat.

Oral suspension: Do not freeze.

Mechanism of Action Decreases the surface tension of gas bubbles thereby disperses and prevents gas pockets in the GI system

Pharmacokinetics (Adult data unless noted) Elimination: In feces

Dosing: Usual Oral:

Infants and Children <2 years: 20 mg 4 times/day

Children 2-12 years: 40 mg 4 times/day

Children >12 years and Adults: 40-250 mg after meals and at bedtime as needed, not to exceed 500 mg/day

Administration Oral: Administer after meals or at bedtime; chew tablets thoroughly before swallowing; mix with water, infant formula or other liquid; place strips (Gas-X® Children's Tongue Twisters™ or Gas-X® Thin Strips™) directly on the tongue

Dosage Forms Excipient information presented when available (limited, particularly for generics); consult specific product labeling.

Capsule, Oral:

Gas Free Extra Strength: 125 mg [contains brilliant blue fcf (fd&c blue #1), fd&c red #40, fd&c yellow #10 (quinoline yellow)]

Gas Relief Extra Strength: 125 mg [contains brilliant blue fcf (fd&c blue #1), fd&c red #40, fd&c yellow #10 (quinoline yellow)]

Gas Relief Ultra Strength: 180 mg [contains fd&c red #40, fd&c yellow #6 (sunset yellow)]

Gas Relief Ultra Strength: 180 mg [contains fd&c yellow #6 (sunset yellow)]

Gas-X Extra Strength: 125 mg [contains brilliant blue fcf (fd&c blue #1), fd&c red #40, fd&c yellow #10 (quinoline yellow)]

Gas-X Ultra Strength: 180 mg [contains fd&c yellow #6 (sunset yellow)]

GasAid: 125 mg

Phazyme: 180 mg

Phazyme Maximum Strength: 250 mg [contains brilliant blue fcf (fd&c blue #1)]

Phazyme Ultra Strength: 180 mg [contains fd&c yellow #6 (sunset yellow)]

Generic: 125 mg, 180 mg

Liquid, Oral:

Gas-X Infant Drops: 20 mg/0.3 mL (30 mL) [alcohol free, no artificial color(s), no artificial flavor(s), saccharin free; contains polyethylene glycol, sodium benzoate]

Strip, Oral:

Gas-X Childrens: 40 mg (16 ea) [contains alcohol, usp, fd&c red #40; sweet cinnamon flavor]

Gas-X Extra Strength: 62.5 mg (18 ea, 30 ea) [contains alcohol, usp, brilliant blue fcf (fd&c blue #1); peppermint flavor]

Gas-X Extra Strength: 62.5 mg (18 ea) [contains alcohol, usp, fd&c red #40]

Suspension, Oral:

Equalizer Gas Relief: 40 mg/0.6 mL (30 mL) [vanilla flavor]

Gas Relief: 20 mg/0.3 mL (30 mL) [dye free; contains sodium benzoate; fruit flavor]

Infants Gas Relief: 20 mg/0.3 mL (30 mL) [contains sodium benzoate]

Infants Simethicone: 20 mg/0.3 mL (30 mL) [alcohol free, no artificial color(s), no artificial flavor(s), saccharin free; contains polyethylene glycol, sodium benzoate]

Generic: 40 mg/0.6 mL (30 mL)

Tablet Chewable, Oral:

Gas Relief: 80 mg [lactose free]

Gas Relief Maximum Strength: 125 mg [lactose free]

Gas-X: 80 mg [scored; cherry creme flavor]

Gas-X: 80 mg [scored; peppermint creme flavor]

Gas-X Extra Strength: 125 mg

Gas-X Extra Strength: 125 mg [scored; peppermint creme flavor]

Gas-X Extra Strength: 125 mg [contains fd&c yellow #10 aluminum lake; peppermint creme flavor]

Gas-X Extra Strength: 125 mg [contains soy protein; cherry cream flavor]

Mi-Acid Gas Relief: 80 mg

Mytab Gas: 80 mg [peppermint flavor]

Mytab Gas Maximum Strength: 125 mg [scored; peppermint flavor]

Phazyme: 125 mg [cool mint flavor]

Phazyme: 125 mg [contains aspartame; cool mint flavor]

Generic: 80 mg, 125 mg

◆ **Simply Allergy [OTC]** *see* DiphenhydrAMINE (Systemic) *on page 668*

◆ **Simply Cough [OTC]** *see* Dextromethorphan *on page 631*

◆ **Simply Sleep [OTC]** *see* DiphenhydrAMINE (Systemic) *on page 668*

◆ **Simply Sleep (Can)** *see* DiphenhydrAMINE (Systemic) *on page 668*

◆ **Simply Stuffy [OTC]** *see* Pseudoephedrine *on page 1801*

◆ **Simulect** *see* Basiliximab *on page 258*

Simvastatin (sim va STAT in)

Medication Safety Issues

Sound-alike/look-alike issues:

Simvastatin may be confused with atorvaSTATin, nystatin, pitavastatin

Zocor may be confused with Cozaar, Lipitor, Zoloft, ZyrTEC

International issues:

Cardin [Poland] may be confused with Cardem brand name for celiprolol [Spain]; Cardene brand name for nicardipine [U.S., Great Britain, Netherlands]

Brand Names: US Zocor

Brand Names: Canada ACT-Simvastatin; Apo-Simvastatin; Auro-Simvastatin; Dom-Simvastatin; JAMP-Simvastatin; Mar-Simvastatin; Mint-Simvastatin; Mylan-Simvastatin; PHL-Simvastatin; PMS-Simvastatin; Q-Simvastatin; RAN-Simvastatin; Riva-Simvastatin; Sandoz-Simvastatin; Simvastatin-Odan; Teva-Simvastatin; Zocor

Therapeutic Category Antilipemic Agent; HMG-CoA Reductase Inhibitor

Generic Availability (US) Yes

Use Adjunct to dietary therapy to decrease elevated serum total (total-C) and low density lipoprotein cholesterol (LDL-C), and apolipoprotein B (apo-B) in patients with heterozygous familial hypercholesterolemia if LDL-C remains ≥190 mg/dL, if ≥160 mg/dL with family history of premature cardiovascular disease (CVD) or presence of ≥2 cardiovascular risk factors (FDA approved in boys and postmenarcheal girls 10-17 years); adjunct to dietary therapy to decrease elevated serum total-C, LDL-C, apo-B, and triglyceride (TG) levels and to increase high-density lipoprotein cholesterol (HDL-C) in patients with primary hypercholesterolemia (heterozygous, familial, and nonfamilial) and mixed dyslipidemia (Fredrickson types IIa and IIb) (FDA approved in adults); reduce elevated TG in patients with hypertriglyceridemia (Fredrickson type IV) (FDA approved in adults); reduce elevated TG and VLDL-C in patients with primary dysbetalipoproteinemia (Fredrickson Type III) (FDA approved in adults); reduce elevated total-C and LDL-C in patients with homozygous familial hypercholesterolemia (FDA approved in adults)

Secondary prevention of cardiovascular events in hypercholesterolemic patients with established coronary heart disease (CHD) or at high risk for CHD: To reduce cardiovascular morbidity (myocardial infarction, coronary/noncoronary revascularization procedures) and mortality; to reduce the risk of stroke (FDA approved in adults)

Pregnancy Risk Factor X

Pregnancy Considerations Adverse events were not observed in animal reproduction studies. There are reports of congenital anomalies following maternal use of HMG-CoA reductase inhibitors in pregnancy; however, maternal disease, differences in specific agents used, and the low rates of exposure limit the interpretation of the available data (Godfrey, 2012; Lecarpentier, 2012). Cholesterol biosynthesis may be important in fetal development; serum cholesterol and triglycerides increase normally during pregnancy. The discontinuation of lipid lowering medications temporarily during pregnancy is not expected to have significant impact on the long term outcomes of primary hypercholesterolemia treatment.

Use of simvastatin is contraindicated in pregnancy. HMG-CoA reductase inhibitors should be discontinued prior to pregnancy (ADA, 2013). If treatment of dyslipidemias is needed in pregnant women or in women of reproductive age, other agents are preferred (Berglund, 2012; Stone, 2013). The manufacturer recommends administration to women of childbearing potential only when conception is highly unlikely and patients have been informed of potential hazards.

Breast-Feeding Considerations It is not known if simvastatin is excreted into breast milk. Due to the potential for serious adverse reactions in a nursing infant, breast-feeding is contraindicated by the manufacturer.

Contraindications Hypersensitivity to simvastatin or any component of the formulation; active liver disease; unexplained persistent elevations of serum transaminases; concomitant use of strong CYP3A4 inhibitors (eg, clarithromycin, erythromycin, itraconazole, ketoconazole, nefazodone, posaconazole, voriconazole, protease inhibitors [including boceprevir and telaprevir], telithromycin, cobicistat-containing products), cyclosporine, danazol, and gemfibrozil; pregnancy; breast-feeding

Warnings/Precautions Secondary causes of hyperlipidemia should be ruled out prior to therapy. Liver enzyme tests should be obtained at baseline and as clinically indicated; routine periodic monitoring of liver enzymes is not necessary. Use with caution in patients who consume large amounts of ethanol or have a history of liver disease; use is contraindicated with active liver disease and with unexplained transaminase elevations. Rhabdomyolysis with acute renal failure has occurred. Risk of rhabdomyolysis is dose-related and increased with high doses (80 mg), concurrent use of lipid-lowering agents which may also cause rhabdomyolysis (other fibrates or niacin doses ≥1 g/day), or moderate-to-strong CYP3A4 inhibitors (eg, amiodarone, grapefruit juice in large quantities, or verapamil), age ≥65 years, female gender, uncontrolled hypothyroidism, and renal dysfunction. In Chinese patients, do not use high-dose simvastatin (80 mg) if concurrently taking niacin ≥1 g/day; may increase risk of myopathy. Immune-mediated necrotizing myopathy (IMNM), an autoimmune-mediated myopathy, has been reported (rarely) with HMG-CoA reductase inhibitor therapy. IMNM presents as proximal muscle weakness with elevated CPK levels, which persists despite discontinuation of HMG-CoA reductase inhibitor therapy; additionally, muscle biopsy may show necrotizing myopathy with limited inflammation; immunosuppressive therapy (eg, corticosteroids, azathioprine) may be used for treatment. Concomitant use of simvastatin with some drugs may require cautious use, may not be recommended, may require dosage adjustments, or may be contraindicated. If concurrent use of a contraindicated interacting medication is unavoidable, treatment with simvastatin should be suspended during use or consider the use of an alternative HMG-CoA reductase inhibitor void of CYP3A4 metabolism. Monitor closely if used with other drugs associated with myopathy (eg, colchicine). Increases in HbA_{1c} and fasting blood glucose have been reported with HMG-CoA reductase inhibitors; however, the benefits of statin therapy far outweigh the risk of dysglycemia. The manufacturer recommends temporary discontinuation for elective major surgery, acute medical or surgical conditions, or in any patient experiencing an acute or serious condition predisposing to renal failure (eg, sepsis, hypotension, trauma, uncontrolled seizures). Based on current research and clinical guidelines (Fleisher, 2009), HMG-CoA reductase inhibitors should be continued in the perioperative period. Use with caution in patients with severe renal impairment; initial dosage adjustment is necessary; monitor closely.

Adverse Reactions

Cardiovascular: Atrial fibrillation, edema

Central nervous system: Headache, vertigo

Dermatologic: Eczema

Gastrointestinal: Abdominal pain, constipation, gastritis, nausea

Hepatic: Transaminases increased (>3 x ULN)

Neuromuscular & skeletal: CPK increased (>3 x normal), myalgia

Respiratory: Bronchitis, upper respiratory infections

Rare but important or life-threatening: Alkaline phosphatase increased, alopecia, amnesia (reversible), anaphylaxis, anemia, angioedema, arthralgia, arthritis, blood glucose increased, chills, cognitive impairment (reversible), confusion (reversible), depression, dermatomyositis, diabetes mellitus (new onset), diarrhea, dizziness, dryness of skin/mucous membranes, dyspepsia, dyspnea, eosinophilia, erythema multiforme, ESR increased, fever, flatulence, flushing, glycosylated hemoglobin (Hb A_{1c}) increased, GGT increased, hemolytic anemia, hepatic failure, hepatitis, hypersensitivity reaction, jaundice, leukopenia, malaise, memory disturbance (reversible), memory impairment (reversible), muscle cramps, nail changes, nodules, pancreatitis, paresthesia, peripheral neuropathy, photosensitivity, polymyalgia rheumatica, positive ANA, pruritus, purpura, rash, rhabdomyolysis, skin discoloration, Stevens-Johnson syndrome, systemic lupus erythematosus-like syndrome, thrombocytopenia, toxic epidermal necrolysis, urticaria, vasculitis, vomiting, weakness

Additional class-related events or case reports (not necessarily reported with simvastatin therapy): Alteration in taste, anorexia, anxiety, bilirubin increased, cataracts, cholestatic jaundice, cirrhosis, decreased libido, depression, erectile dysfunction/impotence, facial paresis, fatty liver, fulminant hepatic necrosis, gynecomastia, hepatoma, hyperbilirubinemia, immune-mediated necrotizing myopathy (IMNM), impaired extraocular muscle movement, increased CPK (>10 x normal), interstitial lung disease, ophthalmoplegia, peripheral nerve palsy, psychic disturbance, renal failure (secondary to rhabdomyolysis), thyroid dysfunction, tremor, vertigo

Drug Interactions

Metabolism/Transport Effects Substrate of CYP3A4 (major), SLCO1B1; **Note:** Assignment of Major/Minor substrate status based on clinically relevant drug interaction potential; **Inhibits** CYP2C8 (weak), CYP2C9 (weak), CYP2D6 (weak)

Avoid Concomitant Use

Avoid concomitant use of Simvastatin with any of the following: Amodiaquine; Boceprevir; Clarithromycin; Conivaptan; CycloSPORINE (Systemic); CYP3A4 Inhibitors (Strong); Danazol; Erythromycin (Systemic); Fusidic Acid (Systemic); Gemfibrozil; Grapefruit Juice; Idelalisib; Mifepristone; Protease Inhibitors; Red Yeast Rice; Telaprevir; Telithromycin

Increased Effect/Toxicity

Simvastatin may increase the levels/effects of: Amodiaquine; ARIPiprazole; DAPTOmycin; Diltiazem; PAZOPanib; Trabectedin; Vitamin K Antagonists

The levels/effects of Simvastatin may be increased by: Acipimox; Amiodarone; AmLODIPine; Aprepitant; Azithromycin (Systemic); Bezafibrate; Boceprevir;

Ciprofibrate; Clarithromycin; Colchicine; Conivaptan; CycloSPORINE (Systemic); CYP3A4 Inhibitors (Moderate); CYP3A4 Inhibitors (Strong); Cyproterone; Danazol; Dasatinib; Diltiazem; Dronedarone; Eltrombopag; Erythromycin (Systemic); Fenofibrate and Derivatives; Fluconazole; Fosaprepitant; Fusidic Acid (Systemic); Gemfibrozil; Grapefruit Juice; Green Tea; Idelalisib; Imatinib; Ivacaftor; Lercanidipine; Lomitapide; Luliconazole; Mifepristone; Netupitant; Niacin; Niacinamide; Palbociclib; Protease Inhibitors; QuiNINE; Raltegravir; Ranolazine; Red Yeast Rice; Sildenafil; Simeprevir; Stiripentol; Telaprevir; Telithromycin; Teriflunomide; Ticagrelor; Verapamil

Decreased Effect

Simvastatin may decrease the levels/effects of: Lanthanum

The levels/effects of Simvastatin may be decreased by: Antacids; Bosentan; CYP3A4 Inducers (Moderate); CYP3A4 Inducers (Strong); Dabrafenib; Deferasirox; Efavirenz; Eslicarbazepine; Etravirine; Fosphenytoin; Mitotane; Phenytoin; Rifamycin Derivatives; Siltuximab; St Johns Wort; Tocilizumab

Food Interactions Simvastatin serum concentration may be increased when taken with grapefruit juice. Management: Avoid concurrent intake of large quantities of grapefruit juice (>1 quart/day).

Storage/Stability Tablets should be stored in tightly-closed containers at temperatures between 5°C to 30°C (41°F to 86°F).

Mechanism of Action Simvastatin is a methylated derivative of lovastatin that acts by competitively inhibiting 3-hydroxy-3-methylglutaryl-coenzyme A (HMG-CoA) reductase, the enzyme that catalyzes the rate-limiting step in cholesterol biosynthesis. In addition to the ability of HMG-CoA reductase inhibitors to decrease levels of high-sensitivity C-reactive protein (hsCRP), they also possess pleiotropic properties including improved endothelial function, reduced inflammation at the site of the coronary plaque, inhibition of platelet aggregation, and anticoagulant effects (de Denus, 2002; Ray, 2005).

Pharmacodynamics

Onset of action: >3 days

Maximum effect: After 2 weeks

LDL-C reduction: 20-40 mg/day: 35% to 41% (for each doubling of this dose, LDL-C is lowered ~6%)

Average HDL-C increase: 5% to 15%

Average triglyceride reduction: 7% to 30%

Pharmacokinetics (Adult data unless noted)

Absorption: Oral: Although 85% is absorbed following administration, <5% reaches the general circulation due to an extensive first-pass effect

Protein binding: ~95%

Metabolism: Hepatic via CYP3A4; extensive first-pass effect

Time to peak serum concentration: 1.3-2.4 hours

Elimination: 13% excreted in urine and 60% in feces

Dosing: Usual

Children and Adolescents: **Note:** A lower, conservative dosing regimen may be necessary in patient populations predisposed to myopathy including patients of Chinese descent or those concurrently receiving other lipid-lowering agents (eg, niacin, fibric acid derivatives), amiodarone, amlodipine, diltiazem, dronedarone, ranolazine, verapamil (see the following conservative, maximum adult doses)

Heterozygous familial hypercholesterolemia: Children and Adolescents 10-17 years: Oral: Initial: 10 mg once daily in the evening; may increase dose in intervals of 4 weeks or more to a maximum daily dose: 40 mg/**day**

Hyperlipidemia: Limited data available: Children and Adolescents: Oral:

Children <10 years: Initial: 5 mg once daily in the evening increasing to 10 mg once daily after 4 weeks and to 20 mg once daily after another 4 weeks as tolerated; dosing based on initial compassionate use study (Ducobu, 1992)

Children ≥10 years and Adolescents: Initial: 10 mg once daily in the evening increasing to 20 mg once daily after 6 weeks and to 40 mg once daily after another 6 weeks as tolerated

Adults: **Note:** Doses should be individualized according to the baseline LDL-cholesterol levels, the recommended goal of therapy, and the patient's response; adjustments should be made at intervals of 4 weeks or more; doses may need adjusted based on concomitant medications

Note: Dosing limitation: **Simvastatin 80 mg is limited to patients that have been taking this dose for >12 consecutive months without evidence of myopathy and are not currently taking or beginning to take a simvastatin dose-limiting or contraindicated interacting medication.** If patient is unable to achieve LDL-C goal using the 40 mg dose of simvastatin, increasing to 80 mg dose is not recommended. Instead, switch patient to an alternative LDL-C-lowering treatment providing greater LDL-C reduction.

Homozygous familial hypercholesterolemia: Oral: 40 mg once daily in the evening

Prevention of cardiovascular events, hyperlipidemias: Oral: 10-20 mg once daily in the evening (range: 5-40 mg/day)

Patients requiring only moderate reduction of LDL-cholesterol: May be started at 5-10 mg once daily in the evening; adjust to achieve recommended LDL-C goal

Patients requiring reduction of >40% in low-density lipoprotein (LDL) cholesterol: May be started at 40 mg once daily in the evening; adjust to achieve recommended LDL-C goal

Patients with CHD or at high risk for cardiovascular events (patients with diabetes, PVD, history of stroke, or other cerebrovascular disease): Dosing should be started at 40 mg once daily in the evening; simvastatin should be started simultaneously with diet therapy

Dosing adjustment in patients receiving concomitant diltiazem, dronedarone, or verapamil: Adults: Dose should not exceed 10 mg/day

Dosing adjustment in patients receiving concomitant amiodarone, amlodipine, or ranolazine: Adults: Dose should not exceed 20 mg/day

Dosing adjustment in patients receiving concomitant lomitapide: Adults: Simvastatin dose should not exceed 20 mg/day (or 40 mg daily for those who previously tolerated simvastatin 80 mg daily for ≥1 year without evidence of muscle toxicity)

Dosing adjustment in Chinese patients on niacin doses ≥1 g/day: Adults: Use caution with simvastatin doses exceeding 20 mg/day; because of an increased risk of myopathy, do not increase simvastatin dose to 80 mg.

Dosing adjustment in renal impairment: Adults:

Manufacturer's recommendations:

Mild to moderate renal impairment: No dosage adjustment necessary; simvastatin does not undergo significant renal excretion

Severe renal impairment: CrCl <30 mL/minute; Initial: 5 mg/day with close monitoring

Alternative recommendation: No dosage adjustment necessary for any degree of renal impairment (Aronoff, 2007)

Dosing adjustments in hepatic impairment: Contraindicated in patients with active liver disease, including unexplained persistent elevations in hepatic transaminases.

Administration Oral: May be taken without regard to meals. Administration with the evening meal or at bedtime has been associated with somewhat greater LDL-C reduction

Monitoring Parameters

Pediatric patients: Baseline: ALT, AST, and creatine phosphokinase levels (CPK); fasting lipid panel (FLP) and repeat ALT and AST should be checked after 4 weeks of therapy; if no myopathy symptoms or laboratory abnormalities, then monitor FLP, ALT, and AST every 3 to 4 months during the first year and then every 6 months thereafter (NHLBI, 2011)

Adults:

2013 ACC/AHA Blood Cholesterol Guideline recommendations (Stone, 2013):

Lipid panel (total cholesterol, HDL, LDL, triglycerides): Baseline lipid panel; fasting lipid profile within 4 to 12 weeks after initiation or dose adjustment and every 3 to 12 months (as clinically indicated) thereafter. If 2 consecutive LDL levels are <40 mg/dL, consider decreasing the dose.

Hepatic transaminase levels: Baseline measurement of hepatic transaminase levels (ie, ALT); measure hepatic function if symptoms suggest hepatotoxicity (eg, unusual fatigue or weakness, loss of appetite, abdominal pain, dark-colored urine or yellowing of skin or sclera) during therapy.

CPK: CPK should not be routinely measured. Baseline CPK measurement is reasonable for some individuals (eg, family history of statin intolerance or muscle disease, clinical presentation, concomitant drug therapy that may increase risk of myopathy). May measure CPK in any patient with symptoms suggestive of myopathy (pain, tenderness, stiffness, cramping, weakness, or generalized fatigue).

Evaluate for new-onset diabetes mellitus during therapy; if diabetes develops, continue statin therapy and encourage adherence to a heart-healthy diet, physical activity, a healthy body weight, and tobacco cessation.

If patient develops a confusional state or memory impairment, may evaluate patient for nonstatin causes (eg, exposure to other drugs), systemic and neuropsychiatric causes, and the possibility of adverse effects associated with statin therapy.

Manufacturer recommendations: Liver enzyme tests at baseline and repeated when clinically indicated. Measure CPK when myopathy is being considered or may measure CPK periodically in high risk patients (eg, drug-drug interaction). Lipid panel should be analyzed after 4 weeks of therapy and periodically thereafter.

Dosage Forms Excipient information presented when available (limited, particularly for generics); consult specific product labeling.

Tablet, Oral:

Zocor: 5 mg, 10 mg, 20 mg, 40 mg, 80 mg

Generic: 5 mg, 10 mg, 20 mg, 40 mg, 80 mg

◆ **Simvastatin and Ezetimibe** *see* Ezetimibe and Simvastatin *on page 833*

◆ **Simvastatin-Odan (Can)** *see* Simvastatin *on page 1928*

◆ **Sinelee** *see* Capsaicin *on page 362*

◆ **Sinequan (Can)** *see* Doxepin (Systemic) *on page 711*

◆ **Singulair** *see* Montelukast *on page 1459*

◆ **Sinus Nasal Spray [OTC]** *see* Oxymetazoline (Nasal) *on page 1599*

Sirolimus (sir OH li mus)

Medication Safety Issues

Sound-alike/look-alike issues:

Rapamune may be confused with Rapaflo

Sirolimus may be confused with everolimus, pimecrolimus, silodosin, tacrolimus, temsirolimus

High alert medication:

This medication is in a class the Institute for Safe Medication Practices (ISMP) includes among its list of drug classes that have a heightened risk of causing significant patient harm when used in error.

Related Information

Oral Medications That Should Not Be Crushed or Altered *on page 2476*

Safe Handling of Hazardous Drugs *on page 2455*

Brand Names: US Rapamune

Brand Names: Canada Rapamune

Therapeutic Category Immunosuppressant Agent; mTOR Kinase Inhibitor

Generic Availability (US) May be product dependent

Use Prophylaxis of organ rejection in renal transplant patients at low-moderate immunologic risk in combination with corticosteroids and cyclosporine (cyclosporine may be withdrawn after 2-4 months in conjunction with an increase in sirolimus dosage) (FDA approved in ages ≥13 years and adults); prophylaxis of organ rejection in renal transplant patients at high immunologic risk in combination with cyclosporine and corticosteroids for the first year (FDA approved in ages ≥18 years and adults); has also been used for primary immunosuppression in heart and intestinal transplantation (given in conjunction with a calcineurin inhibitor, as a substitute for a calcineurin inhibitor to reduce side effects, or to eliminate steroid use); rescue agent for acute and chronic organ rejection (rescue due to calcineurin toxicity or to treat resistant acute or chronic rejection despite calcineurin inhibitor therapy); prevention of acute graft-versus-host disease (GVHD) in allogeneic stem cell transplantation; treatment of refractory acute or chronic GVHD; treatment of vascular anomalies

Medication Guide Available Yes

Pregnancy Risk Factor C

Pregnancy Considerations Adverse events have been observed in animal reproduction studies. Effective contraception must be initiated before therapy with sirolimus and continued for 12 weeks after discontinuation.

The National Transplantation Pregnancy Registry (NTPR, Temple University) is a registry for pregnant women taking immunosuppressants following any solid organ transplant. The NTPR encourages reporting of all immunosuppressant exposures during pregnancy in transplant recipients at 877-955-6877.

Breast-Feeding Considerations It is not known if sirolimus is excreted in breast milk. Due to the potential for adverse reactions in the breast-fed infant, including possible immunosuppression, breast-feeding is not recommended.

Contraindications Hypersensitivity to sirolimus or any component of the formulation

Warnings/Precautions Hazardous agent - use appropriate precautions for handling and disposal (NIOSH 2014 [group 2]).

[US Boxed Warning]: Immunosuppressive agents, including sirolimus, increase the risk of infection and may be associated with the development of lymphoma. Immune suppression may also increase the risk of opportunistic infections including activation of latent viral infections (including BK virus-associated nephropathy), fatal infections, and sepsis. Prophylactic treatment for *Pneumocystis jirovecii* pneumonia (PCP) should be administered for 1 year post-transplant; prophylaxis for cytomegalovirus (CMV) should be taken for 3 months post-transplant in patients at risk for CMV. Progressive multifocal leukoencephalopathy (PML), an opportunistic CNS infection caused by reactivation of the JC virus, has been reported in patients receiving immunosuppressive therapy, including sirolimus. Clinical findings of PML include apathy, ataxia, cognitive deficiency, confusion, and hemiparesis; promptly evaluate any patient presenting with neurological changes; consider decreasing the degree of immunosuppression with consideration to the risk of organ rejection in transplant patients.

[US Boxed Warning]: Sirolimus is not recommended for use in liver or lung transplantation. Bronchial anastomotic dehiscence cases have been reported in lung transplant patients when sirolimus was used as part of an immunosuppressive regimen; most of these reactions were fatal. Studies indicate an association with an increased risk of hepatic artery thrombosis (HAT), graft failure, and increased mortality (with evidence of infection) in liver transplant patients when sirolimus is used in combination with cyclosporine and/or tacrolimus. Most cases of HAT occurred within 30 days of transplant.

In renal transplant patients, *de novo* use without cyclosporine has been associated with higher rates of acute rejection. Sirolimus should be used in combination with cyclosporine (and corticosteroids) initially when used in renal transplant patients. Cyclosporine may be withdrawn in low-to-moderate immunologic risk patients after 2 to 4 months, in conjunction with an increase in sirolimus dosage. In high immunologic risk patients, use in combination with cyclosporine and corticosteroids is recommended for the first year. Safety and efficacy of combination therapy with cyclosporine in high immunologic risk patients has not been studied beyond 12 months of treatment; adjustment of immunosuppressive therapy beyond 12 months should be considered based on clinical judgment. Monitor renal function closely when combined with cyclosporine; consider dosage adjustment or discontinue in patients with increasing serum creatinine.

May increase serum creatinine and decrease GFR. Use caution when used concurrently with medications which may alter renal function. May delay recovery of renal function in patients with delayed allograft function. Increased urinary protein excretion has been observed when converting renal transplant patients from calcineurin inhibitors to sirolimus during maintenance therapy. A higher level of proteinuria prior to sirolimus conversion correlates with a higher degree of proteinuria after conversion. In some patients, proteinuria may reach nephrotic levels; nephrotic syndrome (new onset) has been reported. Increased risk of BK viral-associated nephropathy which may impair renal function and cause graft loss; consider decreasing immunosuppressive burden if evidence of deteriorating renal function.

Use caution with hepatic impairment; a reduction in the maintenance dose is recommended. Has been associated with an increased risk of fluid accumulation and lymphocele; peripheral edema, lymphedema, ascites, and pleural and pericardial effusions (including significant effusions and tamponade) were reported; use with caution in patients in whom fluid accumulation may be poorly tolerated, such as in cardiovascular disease (heart failure or hypertension) and pulmonary disease. Cases of interstitial lung disease (eg, pneumonitis, bronchiolitis obliterans organizing pneumonia [BOOP], pulmonary fibrosis) have been observed; risk may be increased with higher trough levels. Potentially significant drug-drug interactions may exist, requiring dose or frequency adjustment, additional monitoring, and/or selection of alternative therapy. Concurrent use with a calcineurin inhibitor (cyclosporine, tacrolimus) may increase the risk of calcineurin inhibitor-induced hemolytic uremic syndrome/thrombotic thrombocytopenic purpura/thrombotic microangiopathy (HUS/TTP/TMA). Immunosuppressants may affect response to vaccination. Therefore, during treatment with sirolimus, vaccination may be less effective. The use of live vaccines should be avoided.

Hypersensitivity reactions, including anaphylactic/anaphylactoid reactions, angioedema, exfoliative dermatitis, and hypersensitivity vasculitis have been reported. Concurrent use with other drugs known to cause angioedema (eg, ACE inhibitors) may increase risk. Immunosuppressant therapy is associated with an increased risk of skin cancer; limit sun and ultraviolet light exposure; use appropriate sun protection. May increase serum lipids (cholesterol and triglycerides); use with caution in patients with hyperlipidemia; monitor cholesterol/lipids; if hyperlipidemia occurs, follow current guidelines for management (diet, exercise, lipid lowering agents); antihyperlipidemic therapy may not be effective in normalizing levels. May be associated with wound dehiscence and impaired healing; use caution in the perioperative period. Patients with a body mass index (BMI) >30 kg/m^2 are at increased risk for abnormal wound healing.

Sirolimus tablets and oral solution are not bioequivalent, due to differences in absorption. Clinical equivalence was seen using 2 mg tablet and 2 mg solution. It is not known if higher doses are also clinically equivalent. Monitor sirolimus levels if changes in dosage forms are made. Some dosage forms may contain propylene glycol; large amounts are potentially toxic and have been associated hyperosmolality, lactic acidosis, seizures, and respiratory depression; use caution (AAP, 1997; Zar 2007). **[US Boxed Warning]: Should only be used by physicians experienced in immunosuppressive therapy and management of transplant patients. Adequate laboratory and supportive medical resources must be readily available.** Sirolimus concentrations are dependent on the assay method (eg, chromatographic and immunoassay) used; assay methods are not interchangeable. Variations in methods to determine sirolimus whole blood concentrations, as well as interlaboratory variations, may result in improper dosage adjustments, which may lead to subtherapeutic or toxic levels. Determine the assay method used to assure consistency (or accommodations if changes occur), and for monitoring purposes, be aware of alterations to assay method or reference range and that values from different assays may not be interchangeable.

Warnings: Additional Pediatric Considerations Animal studies have indicated that sirolimus may inhibit skeletal and muscle growth. There has been at least one human case report of growth failure in a child (Hymes, 2011).

Adverse Reactions Incidence of many adverse effects is dose related. Reported events exclusive to renal transplant patients unless otherwise noted. Frequency not always defined.

Cardiovascular: Chest pain (LAM), deep vein thrombosis, edema, hypertension, peripheral edema (LAM and renal transplants), pulmonary embolism, tachycardia

Central nervous system: Dizziness (LAM), headache (LAM and renal transplants), pain

Dermatologic: Acne vulgaris (LAM and renal transplants), skin rash

Endocrine & metabolic: Amenorrhea, diabetes mellitus, hypercholesterolemia (LAM and renal transplants), hypermenorrhea, hypertriglyceridemia, hypervolemia, hypokalemia, increased lactate dehydrogenase, menstrual disease, ovarian cyst

Gastrointestinal: Abdominal pain (LAM and renal transplants), constipation, diarrhea (LAM and renal transplants), nausea (LAM and renal transplants), stomatitis

Genitourinary: Urinary tract infection

Hematologic & oncologic: Anemia, hemolytic-uremic syndrome, leukopenia, lymphocele, lymphoproliferative disorder (including lymphoma), skin carcinoma (includes basal cell carcinoma, squamous cell carcinoma, melanoma), thrombocytopenia, thrombotic thrombocytopenic purpura

Infection: Herpes simplex infection, herpes zoster, sepsis

Neuromuscular & skeletal: Arthralgia, myalgia (LAM), osteonecrosis

Renal: Increased serum creatinine, pyelonephritis

Respiratory: Epistaxis, nasopharyngitis (LAM), pneumonia, upper respiratory tract infection (LAM)

Miscellaneous: Wound healing impairment

Rare but important or life-threatening: Ascites, azoospermia, cardiac tamponade, cytomegalovirus, dehiscence (fascial), Epstein-Barr infection, exfoliative dermatitis, focal segmental glomerulosclerosis, hepatic necrosis, hepatotoxicity, hyperglycemia, hypersensitivity angiitis, hypersensitivity reaction, hypophosphatemia, incisional hernia, interstitial pulmonary disease (dose related; includes pneumonitis, pulmonary fibrosis, and bronchiolitis obliterans organizing pneumonia with no identified infectious etiology), lymphedema, mycobacterium infection, nephrotic syndrome, neutropenia, pancreatitis, pancytopenia, pericardial effusion, pleural effusion, pneumonia due to *Pneumocystis carinii*, progressive multifocal leukoencephalopathy, proteinuria, pseudomembranous colitis, pulmonary alveolitis, pulmonary hemorrhage, renal disease (BK virus-associated), reversible posterior leukoencephalopathy syndrome, tuberculosis, weight loss, wound dehiscence

Drug Interactions

Metabolism/Transport Effects Substrate of CYP3A4 (major), P-glycoprotein; **Note:** Assignment of Major/Minor substrate status based on clinically relevant drug interaction potential

Avoid Concomitant Use

Avoid concomitant use of Sirolimus with any of the following: BCG; BCG (Intravesical); CloZAPine; Conivaptan; Crizotinib; Dipyrone; Enzalutamide; Fusidic Acid (Systemic); Idelalisib; Mifepristone; Natalizumab; Pimecrolimus; Posaconazole; Tacrolimus (Systemic); Tacrolimus (Topical); Tofacitinib; Vaccines (Live); Voriconazole

Increased Effect/Toxicity

Sirolimus may increase the levels/effects of: ACE Inhibitors; CloZAPine; CycloSPORINE (Systemic); Leflunomide; Natalizumab; Tacrolimus (Systemic); Tacrolimus (Topical); Tofacitinib; Vaccines (Live)

The levels/effects of Sirolimus may be increased by: Aprepitant; Boceprevir; Clotrimazole (Topical); Conivaptan; Crizotinib; CycloSPORINE (Systemic); CYP3A4 Inhibitors (Moderate); CYP3A4 Inhibitors (Strong); Dasatinib; Denosumab; Dipyrone; Fluconazole; Fosaprepitant; Fusidic Acid (Systemic); Idelalisib; Itraconazole; Ivacaftor; Ketoconazole (Systemic); Luliconazole; Macrolide Antibiotics; Mifepristone; Nelfinavir; Netupitant; Palbociclib; P-glycoprotein/ABCB1 Inhibitors; Pimecrolimus; Posaconazole; Roflumilast; Stiripentol; Tacrolimus (Systemic); Tacrolimus (Topical); Telaprevir; Trastuzumab; Voriconazole

Decreased Effect

Sirolimus may decrease the levels/effects of: Antidiabetic Agents; BCG; BCG (Intravesical); Coccidioides immitis Skin Test; Sipuleucel-T; Tacrolimus (Systemic); Vaccines (Inactivated); Vaccines (Live)

The levels/effects of Sirolimus may be decreased by: Bosentan; CYP3A4 Inducers (Moderate); CYP3A4 Inducers (Strong); Dabrafenib; Deferasirox; Echinacea; Efavirenz; Enzalutamide; Fosphenytoin; Mitotane; P-glycoprotein/ABCB1 Inducers; Phenytoin; Rifampin; Siltuximab; St Johns Wort; Tocilizumab

Food Interactions Grapefruit juice may decrease clearance of sirolimus. Ingestion with high-fat meals decreases peak concentrations but increases AUC by 23% to 35%. Management: Avoid grapefruit juice. Take consistently (either with or without food) to minimize variability.

Storage/Stability

Oral solution: Store at 2°C to 8°C (36°F to 46°F). Protect from light. A slight haze may develop in refrigerated solutions, but the quality of the product is not affected. After opening, solution should be used within 1 month. If necessary, may be stored at temperatures up to 25°C (77°F) for ≤15 days after opening. Product may be stored in amber syringe for a maximum of 24 hours (at room temperature or refrigerated). Discard syringe after single use. Solution should be used immediately following dilution.

Tablet: Store at 20°C to 25°C (68°F to 77°F). Protect from light.

Mechanism of Action Sirolimus inhibits T-lymphocyte activation and proliferation in response to antigenic and cytokine stimulation and inhibits antibody production. Its mechanism differs from other immunosuppressants. Sirolimus binds to FKBP-12, an intracellular protein, to form an immunosuppressive complex which inhibits the regulatory kinase, mTOR (mechanistic target of rapamycin). This inhibition suppresses cytokine mediated T-cell proliferation, halting progression from the G1 to the S phase of the cell cycle. It inhibits acute rejection of allografts and prolongs graft survival.

In lymphangioleiomyomatosis, the mTOR signaling pathway is activated through the loss of the tuberous sclerosis complex (TSC) gene function (resulting in cellular proliferation and release of lymphangiogenic growth factors). By inhibiting the mTOR pathway, sirolimus prevents the proliferation of lymphangioleiomyomatosis cells.

Pharmacokinetics (Adult data unless noted)

Absorption: Rapid

Distribution: V_{dss}: 12 ± 8 L/kg

Protein binding: ~92%; primarily to albumin

Metabolism: Extensive; in intestinal wall via P-glycoprotein and hepatic via CYP3A4; to 7 major metabolites

Bioavailability: Oral solution: 14%; tablet: 27% (relative to the oral solution); oral solution and tablets are not bioequivalent however, clinical equivalence shown at 2 mg dose

Half-life:

Children: 13.7 ± 6.2 hours

Adults: 62 ± 16 hours; extended in hepatic impairment (Child-Pugh class A or B) to 113 hours

Time to peak serum concentration: Oral solution: 1-3 hours; tablet: 1-6 hours

Elimination: Primarily eliminated via feces (91%) and urine (2.2%)

Dosing: Usual Note: Sirolimus tablets and oral solution are not bioequivalent due to differences in absorption; however, clinical equivalence has been demonstrated at the 2 mg dose

Pediatric: **Note:** Dosage should be individualized and based on monitoring of serum trough concentrations; target range is variable and may depend upon transplantation type, length of time since transplant, renal function, infection, rejection history, drug combinations used, and side effects of individual agents.

Heart transplantation: Limited data available: Children and Adolescents: Oral: **Note:** Not used first-line; most data describes as alternative immunosuppression in combination with either cyclosporine or tacrolimus in patients for renal-sparing effects, following retransplantation (treatment of rejection) or to prevent or promote regression of transplant coronary artery disease (Denfield, 2010)

BSA/weight-directed dosing:

Loading dose: 3 mg/m^2 on day 1 (Balfour, 2006; Denfield, 2010)

Maintenance dose: Evaluate serum trough concentrations and adjust dose to overall target range: 4-12 ng/mL (ISHLT, Costanzo 2010). Some trials report using lower target ranges of 4-10 ng/mL (Chinnock, 2011; Lobach, 2005; Matthews, 2010). In children, a specific maintenance dose has not been reported in the majority of trials. In 16 pediatric patients (age range: 2-18 years), the mean reported dose to reach target serum concentration of 5-10 ng/mL was 7 mg/m^2 (or 0.25 mg/kg) (Lobach, 2005). One trial used an initial median dose of 1 mg once daily (range: 0.3-2 mg once daily) and adjusted to achieve target concentration of 4-8 ng/mL (final dosage range 0.3-4 mg once daily) (Matthews, 2010). In adolescents <40 kg, an initial maintenance dose of 1 mg/m^2/day in 1-2 divided doses has been suggested (Denfield, 2010).

Alternative fixed dosing: Adolescents with weight ≥40 kg: Loading dose: 6 mg on day 1; then maintenance: 2 mg once daily; evaluate serum trough concentrations and adjust dose to overall target range: 4-12 ng/mL (Denfield, 2010; ISHLT Costanzo, 2010); some suggest higher initial targets when sirolimus therapy initiated and then decrease to 4-8 ng/mL (Balfour, 2005; Chinnock, 2011; Lobach, 2005).

Renal transplantation, prophylaxis of organ rejection (low to moderate immunologic risk): Oral:

Conversion from tacrolimus in patients with stable graft function: Children and Adolescents: Limited data available: Initial maintenance dose: 3 mg/m^2/day divided every 12 hours; adjust dose to achieve target sirolimus serum trough concentration (Hymes, 2008; Hymes, 2011). In one trial, a loading dose of 5 mg/m^2 on day 1 was used, followed by maintenance doses of 3 mg/m^2/day divided every 12 hours (Hymes, 2008).

Manufacturer's recommendations: Adolescents:

Weight <40 kg: Loading dose: 3 mg/m^2 on day 1; initial maintenance dose: 1 mg/m^2/day divided every 12 hours or once daily; adjust dose to achieve target sirolimus trough blood concentration

Weight ≥40 kg: Loading dose: 6 mg on day 1; maintenance: 2 mg once daily; adjust dose to achieve target sirolimus trough blood concentration.

Dosage adjustment: Sirolimus dosages should be adjusted to maintain trough concentrations within desired range based on risk and concomitant therapy; maximum daily dose: 40 mg/**day**. Dosage should be adjusted at intervals of 7-14 days to account for the long half-life of sirolimus; in children receiving twice-daily dosing, serum concentrations should be checked earlier due to pharmacokinetic differences. In general, dose proportionality may be assumed. New sirolimus dose **equals** current dose **multiplied by** (target concentration/current concentration). **Note:** If large dose increase is required, consider loading dose calculated as:

Loading dose **equals** (new maintenance dose **minus** current maintenance dose) **multiplied by** 3

Maximum daily dose: 40 mg/day; if required dose is >40 mg (due to loading dose), divide over 2 days. Serum concentrations should not be used as the sole basis for dosage adjustment (monitor clinical signs/symptoms, tissue biopsy, and laboratory parameters).

Maintenance therapy after withdrawal of cyclosporine: Following 2-4 months of combined therapy, withdrawal of cyclosporine may be considered in low to moderate risk patients. Cyclosporine should be discontinued over 4-8 weeks, and a necessary increase in the dosage of sirolimus (up to fourfold) should be anticipated due to removal of metabolic inhibition by cyclosporine and to maintain adequate immunosuppressive effects.

Vascular anomalies/tumors (eg, Kaposiform hemangioendothelioma); refractory: Very limited data available: Infants ≥7 months, Children, and Adolescents ≤14 years: Oral: Oral solution: Initial: 0.8 mg/m^2 twice daily (approximately every 12 hours); titrate to a serum trough concentration of 10-15 ng/mL; dosing based on a pilot case series (n=6), the mean response time was 25 days (range: 8-65 days) (Hammill, 2011).

Adults: **Renal transplantation, prophylaxis of organ rejection:** Oral:

Low- to moderate-immunologic risk patients: Dosing by body weight:

<40 kg: Loading dose: 3 mg/m^2 on day 1, followed by maintenance dosing of 1 mg/m^2 once daily

≥40 kg: Loading dose: 6 mg on day 1; maintenance: 2 mg once daily

High-immunologic risk patients: Oral: Loading dose: Up to 15 mg on day 1; maintenance: 5 mg/day; obtain trough concentration between days 5-7 and adjust accordingly. Continue concurrent cyclosporine/sirolimus therapy for 1 year following transplantation. Further adjustment of the regimen must be based on clinical status.

Dosage adjustment: Sirolimus dosages should be adjusted to maintain trough concentrations within desired range based on risk and concomitant therapy. Maximum daily dose: 40 mg. Dosage should be adjusted at intervals of 7-14 days to account for the long half-life of sirolimus. In general, dose proportionality may be assumed. New sirolimus dose **equals** current dose **multiplied by** (target concentration/current concentration). **Note:** If large dose increase is required, consider loading dose calculated as:

Loading dose **equals** (new maintenance dose **minus** current maintenance dose) **multiplied by** 3

Maximum daily dose: 40 mg/**day**; if required dose is >40 mg (due to loading dose), divide over 2 days. Serum concentrations should not be used as the sole basis for dosage adjustment (monitor clinical signs/symptoms, tissue biopsy, and laboratory parameters).

Maintenance therapy after withdrawal of cyclosporine: Cyclosporine withdrawal is not recommended in high-immunological risk patients. Following 2-4 months of combined therapy, withdrawal of cyclosporine may be considered in low-to-moderate risk patients. Cyclosporine should be discontinued over 4-8 weeks, and a necessary increase in the dosage of sirolimus (up to fourfold) should be anticipated due to removal of metabolic inhibition by cyclosporine and to maintain adequate immunosuppressive effects. Dose-adjusted trough target concentrations are typically 16-24 ng/mL for the first year post-transplant and 12-20 ng/mL thereafter (measured by chromatographic methodology).

Dosing adjustment in renal impairment: No dosage adjustment necessary (in loading or maintenance dose); however, adjustment of regimen (including discontinuation of therapy) should be considered when used concurrently with cyclosporine and elevated or increasing serum creatinine is noted.

Dosing adjustment in hepatic impairment:

Loading dose: No dosage adjustment required

Maintenance dose:

Mild to moderate hepatic impairment (Child-Pugh classes A and B): Reduce maintenance dose by ~33%

Severe hepatic impairment (Child-Pugh class C): Reduce maintenance dose by ~50%

Administration Hazardous agent; use appropriate precautions for handling and disposal (NIOSH 2014 [group 2]). May be taken with or without food, but take medication consistently with respect to meals to minimize absorption variability. Initial dose should be administered as soon as possible after transplant. Sirolimus should be taken 4 hours after oral cyclosporine (Neoral or Gengraf).

Oral solution: Use amber oral syringe to withdraw solution from the bottle. Empty dose from syringe into a glass or plastic cup and mix with at least 2 ounces of water or orange juice. No other liquids should be used for dilution. Patient should stir vigorously and drink the diluted sirolimus solution immediately. Then refill cup with an additional 4 ounces of water or orange juice; stir contents vigorously and have patient drink solution at once.

Oral tablets: Do not crush, split, or chew.

Monitoring Parameters Monitor LFTs and CBC during treatment. Monitor sirolimus levels in all patients (especially in pediatric patients, patients ≥13 years of age weighing <40 kg, patients with hepatic impairment, or on concurrent potent inhibitors or inducers of CYP3A4 or P-gp, and/or if cyclosporine dosing is markedly reduced or discontinued), and when changing dosage forms of sirolimus. Also monitor serum cholesterol and triglycerides, blood pressure, serum creatinine, and urinary protein. Serum drug concentrations should be determined 3-4 days after loading doses and 7-14 days after dosage adjustments; however, these concentrations should not be used as the sole basis for dosage adjustment, especially during withdrawal of cyclosporine (monitor clinical signs/symptoms, tissue biopsy, and laboratory parameters). **Note:** Concentrations and ranges are dependent on and will vary with assay methodology (chromatographic or immunoassay); assay methods are not interchangeable.

Reference Range Note: Sirolimus concentrations are dependent on the assay method (eg, chromatographic and immunoassay) used; assay methods are not interchangeable. Determine the assay method used to assure consistency (or accommodations if changes occur) and for monitoring purposes, be aware of alterations to assay method or reference range.

Children and Adolescents: **Note:** See institution specific guidelines:

- Target serum trough concentration for heart transplantation: 4-12 (ISHLT, Costanzo 2010)
- Target serum trough concentration for renal transplantation (based on HPLC methods):
  - Low to moderate immunologic risk (after cyclosporine withdrawal):
    - First year after transplant:16-24 ng/mL
    - After 1 year: 12-20 ng/mL
  - High immunologic risk (with cyclosporine): 10-15 ng/mL
- Target serum trough concentration for vascular anomalies: 10-15 ng/mL (Hammill, 2011)

Adults: **Note:** Trough concentrations vary based on clinical context and use of additional immunosuppressants. The following represents typical adult ranges.

- When combined with tacrolimus and mycophenolate mofetil (MMF) without steroids: 6-8 ng/mL
- As a substitute for tacrolimus (starting 4-8 weeks post-transplant), in combination with MMF and steroids: 8-12 ng/mL
- Following conversion from tacrolimus to sirolimus >6 months post-transplant due to chronic allograft nephropathy: 4-6 ng/mL

Dosage Forms Excipient information presented when available (limited, particularly for generics); consult specific product labeling.

Solution, Oral:
  Rapamune: 1 mg/mL (60 mL) [contains alcohol, usp]

Tablet, Oral:
  Rapamune: 0.5 mg, 1 mg, 2 mg
  Generic: 0.5 mg, 1 mg, 2 mg

- ◆ **Sirop Docusate De Sodium [OTC] (Can)** *see* Docusate *on page 697*
- ◆ **Sitavig** *see* Acyclovir (Topical) *on page 65*
- ◆ **SKF 104864** *see* Topotecan *on page 2092*
- ◆ **SKF 104864-A** *see* Topotecan *on page 2092*
- ◆ **Sklice** *see* Ivermectin (Topical) *on page 1183*
- ◆ **Sleep Aid [OTC]** *see* Doxylamine *on page 721*
- ◆ **Sleep Tabs [OTC]** *see* DiphenhydrAMINE (Systemic) *on page 668*
- ◆ **S-leucovorin** *see* LEVOleucovorin *on page 1248*
- ◆ **6S-leucovorin** *see* LEVOleucovorin *on page 1248*
- ◆ **Slo-Niacin [OTC]** *see* Niacin *on page 1511*
- ◆ **Slo-Pot (Can)** *see* Potassium Chloride *on page 1736*
- ◆ **Slow Fe [OTC]** *see* Ferrous Sulfate *on page 871*
- ◆ **Slow Iron [OTC]** *see* Ferrous Sulfate *on page 871*
- ◆ **Slow-K (Can)** *see* Potassium Chloride *on page 1736*
- ◆ **Slow-Mag [OTC]** *see* Magnesium Chloride *on page 1310*
- ◆ **Slow Magnesium/Calcium [OTC]** *see* Magnesium Chloride *on page 1310*
- ◆ **Slow Release Iron [OTC] [DSC]** *see* Ferrous Sulfate *on page 871*
- ◆ **SMX-TMP** *see* Sulfamethoxazole and Trimethoprim *on page 1986*
- ◆ **SMZ-TMP** *see* Sulfamethoxazole and Trimethoprim *on page 1986*
- ◆ **Snake Antivenin, FAB (Ovine)** *see Crotalidae* Polyvalent Immune Fab (Ovine) *on page 543*
- ◆ **Snake Antivenom, FAB (Ovine)** *see Crotalidae* Polyvalent Immune Fab (Ovine) *on page 543*
- ◆ **Sochlor [OTC]** *see* Sodium Chloride *on page 1938*
- ◆ **Sodium 2-Mercaptoethane Sulfonate** *see* Mesna *on page 1371*
- ◆ **Sodium *L*-Triiodothyronine** *see* Liothyronine *on page 1272*

Sodium Acetate (SOW dee um AS e tate)

Medication Safety Issues

Sound-alike/look-alike issues:

Sodium acetate may be confused with potassium acetate

Therapeutic Category Alkalinizing Agent, Parenteral; Electrolyte Supplement, Parenteral; Sodium Salt

Generic Availability (US) Yes

Use Sodium salt replacement; correction of acidosis through conversion of acetate to bicarbonate

Pregnancy Risk Factor C

Pregnancy Considerations Animal reproduction studies have not been conducted. Sodium requirements do not change during pregnancy (IOM, 2004).

Breast-Feeding Considerations Sodium is found in breast milk. Sodium requirements do not change during lactation (IOM, 2004).

Contraindications Hypernatremia and fluid retention

Warnings/Precautions Avoid extravasation, use with caution in patients with edema, heart failure, severe hepatic failure, or renal impairment. Use with caution in patients with acid/base alterations; contains acetate, monitor closely during acid/base correction. Close monitoring of serum sodium concentrations is needed to avoid hypernatremia. The parenteral product may contain aluminum; toxic aluminum concentrations may be seen with high doses, prolonged use, or renal dysfunction. Premature neonates are at higher risk due to immature renal function and aluminum intake from other parenteral sources. Parenteral aluminum exposure of >4 to 5 mcg/kg/day is associated with CNS and bone toxicity; tissue loading may occur at lower doses (Federal Register, 2002). See manufacturer's labeling.

Adverse Reactions

Cardiovascular: Hypervolemia, thrombosis

Dermatologic: Chemical cellulitis at injection site (extravasation)

Endocrine & metabolic: dilution of serum electrolytes, hypernatremia, hypocalcemia, hypokalemia, metabolic alkalosis, overhydration

Gastrointestinal: Flatulence, gastric distension

Local: Phlebitis

Respiratory: Pulmonary edema

Miscellaneous: Congestive conditions

Drug Interactions

Metabolism/Transport Effects None known.

Avoid Concomitant Use There are no known interactions where it is recommended to avoid concomitant use.

Increased Effect/Toxicity There are no known significant interactions involving an increase in effect.

Decreased Effect There are no known significant interactions involving a decrease in effect.

Storage/Stability Store at room temperature of 20°C to 25°C (68°F to 77°F).

Dosing: Neonatal Sodium acetate is metabolized to bicarbonate on an equimolar basis outside the liver; administer in large volume IV fluids as a sodium source. Dosage is dependent upon the clinical condition, fluid, electrolytes and acid-base balance of the patient.

Maintenance sodium requirements: IV: 3-4 mEq/kg/day; maximum dose: 100-150 mEq/day

Dosing: Usual Sodium acetate is metabolized to bicarbonate on an equimolar basis outside the liver; administer in large volume IV fluids as a sodium source. Dosage is dependent upon the clinical condition, fluid, electrolytes, and acid-base balance of the patient.

Maintenance sodium requirements: IV:

Infants and Children: 3-4 mEq/kg/day; maximum dose: 100-150 mEq/day

Adults: 154 mEq/day

Metabolic acidosis: If sodium acetate is desired over sodium bicarbonate, the amount of acetate may be dosed utilizing the equation found in the sodium bicarbonate monograph as each mEq acetate is converted to a mEq of HCO_3; see Sodium Bicarbonate monograph

Administration Parenteral: Must be diluted prior to IV administration; dose and rate of administration are dependent on patient condition. Consult individual institutional policies and procedures; in general, central-line administration is preferred for hypertonic solutions (>0.9%) if available and/or if infusion is to be continued; peripheral administration may be necessary for initiation of treatment in critical patients; use of peripheral administration should be limited (Luu, 2011). Some suggest central line administration is not needed until infusing solutions >2.8% sodium acetate in sterile water (2.8% sodium acetate in sterile water has osmolarity approximately equivalent to 2% sodium chloride) (Mortimer, 2006; Suarez, 2004). If diluted in D_5W or other solution, the osmolarity may be higher requiring central line administration at a lower sodium acetate concentration.

Monitoring Parameters Serum electrolytes including calcium, arterial blood gases (if indicated)

Additional Information Sodium and acetate content of 1 g: 7.3 mEq

Dosage Forms Excipient information presented when available (limited, particularly for generics); consult specific product labeling.

Solution, Intravenous, as anhydrous:

Generic: 2 mEq/mL (20 mL, 50 mL, 100 mL); 4 mEq/mL (50 mL, 100 mL)

◆ **Sodium Acid Carbonate** *see* Sodium Bicarbonate *on page 1936*

Sodium Benzoate (SOW dee um BENZ oh ate)

Therapeutic Category Ammonium Detoxicant; Hyperammonemia Agent; Urea Cycle Disorder (UCD) Treatment Agent

Use Adjunctive therapy for the prevention and treatment of hyperammonemia due to suspected or proven urea cycle disorders

Drug Interactions

Metabolism/Transport Effects None known.

Avoid Concomitant Use There are no known interactions where it is recommended to avoid concomitant use.

Increased Effect/Toxicity

The levels/effects of Sodium Benzoate may be increased by: Probenecid

Decreased Effect There are no known significant interactions involving a decrease in effect.

Mechanism of Action Assists in lowering serum ammonia levels by activation of a nonurea cycle pathway (the benzoate-hippurate pathway); ammonia in the presence of benzoate will conjugate with glycine to form hippurate which is excreted by the kidney

Pharmacokinetics (Adult data unless noted)

Half-life: 0.75-7.4 hours

Elimination: Clearance is largely attributable to metabolism with urinary excretion of hippurate, the major metabolite

Dosing: Neonatal Oral: Investigational use (not an FDA-approved drug): Initial loading dose: 0.25 g/kg/dose followed by 0.25 g/kg/day divided every 6-8 hours (Enns, 2007). **Note:** If IV administration is necessary, see the Sodium Phenylacetate and Sodium Benzoate monograph for information about a commercially available parenteral product.

Dosing: Usual Oral: Investigational use (not an FDA-approved drug): **Note:** If IV administration is necessary, see the Sodium Phenylacetate and Sodium Benzoate monograph for information about a commercially available parenteral product.

Infants and Children: Initial loading dose: 0.25 g/kg/dose followed by 0.25 g/kg/day divided every 6-8 hours (Enns, 2007).

Adolescents and Adults: Initial 5.5 g/m^2 followed by 5.5 g/m^2/day divided every 6-8 hours

Administration Not available commercially; Oral: Must be compounded using chemical powder

Monitoring Parameters Plasma ammonia and amino acids

Additional Information Used to treat urea cycle enzyme deficiency in combination with arginine; a maximum of 1 mole nitrogen is removed for every 1 mole of benzoate administered

Dosage Forms Powder: 454 g

◆ **Sodium Benzoate and Caffeine** *see* Caffeine *on page 335*

◆ **Sodium Benzoate and Sodium Phenylacetate** *see* Sodium Phenylacetate and Sodium Benzoate *on page 1947*

Sodium Bicarbonate (SOW dee um bye KAR bun ate)

Related Information

Management of Drug Extravasations *on page 2298*

Brand Names: US Neut

Therapeutic Category Alkalinizing Agent, Oral; Alkalinizing Agent, Parenteral; Antacid; Electrolyte Supplement, Oral; Electrolyte Supplement, Parenteral; Sodium Salt

Generic Availability (US) Yes

Use Management of metabolic acidosis; antacid; alkalinization of urine; stabilization of acid base status in cardiac arrest and treatment of life-threatening hyperkalemia

Pregnancy Risk Factor C

Pregnancy Considerations Animal reproduction studies have not been conducted. The use of sodium bicarbonate in pregnant women for the management of cardiac arrest and metabolic acidosis is the same as in nonpregnant women (Campbell, 2009; Vanden Hoek, 2010). Antacids containing sodium bicarbonate should not be used during pregnancy due to their potential to cause metabolic alkalosis and fluid overload (Mahadevan, 2007).

Breast-Feeding Considerations Sodium is found in breast milk (IOM, 2004).

Contraindications

Alkalosis, hypernatremia, severe pulmonary edema, hypocalcemia, unknown abdominal pain

Neutralizing additive (dental use): Not for use as a systemic alkalizer

Warnings/Precautions Rapid administration in neonates, infants, and children <2 years of age has led to hypernatremia, decreased CSF pressure, and intracranial hemorrhage. **Use of IV $NaHCO_3$ should be reserved for documented metabolic acidosis and for hyperkalemia-induced cardiac arrest.** Routine use in cardiac arrest is not recommended. Vesicant (at concentrations ≥8.4%); ensure proper catheter or needle position prior to and during infusion; avoid extravasation (tissue necrosis may occur due to hypertonicity). May cause sodium retention especially if renal function is impaired; not to be used in treatment of peptic ulcer; use with caution in patients with HF, edema, cirrhosis, or renal failure. Not the antacid of choice for the elderly because of sodium content and potential for systemic alkalosis.

Adverse Reactions

Cardiovascular: Cerebral hemorrhage, CHF (aggravated), edema

Central nervous system: Tetany

Gastrointestinal: Belching, flatulence (with oral), gastric distension

Endocrine & metabolic: Hypernatremia, hyperosmolality, hypocalcemia, hypokalemia, increased affinity of hemoglobin for oxygen-reduced pH in myocardial tissue necrosis when extravasated, intracranial acidosis, metabolic alkalosis, milk-alkali syndrome (especially with renal dysfunction)

Respiratory: Pulmonary edema

Drug Interactions

Metabolism/Transport Effects None known.

Avoid Concomitant Use There are no known interactions where it is recommended to avoid concomitant use.

Increased Effect/Toxicity

Sodium Bicarbonate may increase the levels/effects of: Alpha-/Beta-Agonists (Indirect-Acting); Amphetamines; Calcium Polystyrene Sulfonate; Dexmethylphenidate; Flecainide; Mecamylamine; Memantine; Methylphenidate; QuiNIDine; QuiNINE

The levels/effects of Sodium Bicarbonate may be increased by: AcetaZOLAMIDE

Decreased Effect

Sodium Bicarbonate may decrease the levels/effects of: Antipsychotic Agents (Phenothiazines); Atazanavir; Bisacodyl; Bismuth Subcitrate; Bosutinib; Captopril; Cefditoren; Cefpodoxime; Cefuroxime; Chloroquine; Corticosteroids (Oral); Dabigatran Etexilate; Dabrafenib; Dasatinib; Delavirdine; Elvitegravir; Erlotinib; Flecainide; Fosinopril; Gabapentin; HMG-CoA Reductase Inhibitors; Hyoscyamine; Iron Salts; Isoniazid; Itraconazole; Ketoconazole (Systemic); Ledipasvir; Lithium; Mesalamine; Methenamine; Multivitamins/Minerals (with ADEK, Folate, Iron); Nilotinib; PAZOPanib; PenicillAMINE; Phosphate Supplements; Potassium Acid Phosphate; Rilpivirine; Riociguat; Sotalol; Sulpiride; Tetracycline Derivatives; Trientine

Storage/Stability

Store injection at room temperature. Protect from heat and from freezing. Use only clear solutions.

Neutralizing additive (dental use): Store at 20°C to 25°C (68°F to 77°F).

Mechanism of Action

Dissociates to provide bicarbonate ion which neutralizes hydrogen ion concentration and raises blood and urinary pH

Neutralizing additive (dental use): Increases pH of lidocaine and epinephrine solution to improve tolerability and increase tissue uptake

Pharmacodynamics

Onset of action:

Oral, as antacid: 15 minutes

IV: Rapid

Duration:

Oral: 1-3 hours

IV: 8-10 minutes

Pharmacokinetics (Adult data unless noted)

Absorption: Oral: Well absorbed

Elimination: Reabsorbed by kidney and <1% is excreted in urine

Dosing: Neonatal Note: Rapid administration at a high concentration may be associated with fluctuation in cerebral blood flow and possibly ICH; carefully consider clinical need before administering (Aschner, 2008).

Metabolic acidosis: Dosage should be based on the following formula if blood gases and pH measurements are available: HCO_3^-(mEq) = 0.3 x weight (kg) x base deficit (mEq/L) **or** HCO_3^-(mEq) = 0.5 x weight (kg) x [24 - serum HCO_3^-(mEq/L)]; usual dosage: 1-2 mEq/kg/dose (Berg, 2010)

Note: In 55 asphyxiated neonates, a fixed dose of 1.8 mEq/kg/dose over 3-5 minutes administered within first 5 minutes of life did not show clinical benefit (eg, survival, acid-base status, neurodevelopmental outcomes) compared to control group (Lokesh, 2004; Murki, 2004).

Dosing: Usual

Cardiac arrest: Patient should be adequately ventilated before administering $NaHCO_3$

Infants: 1 mEq/kg slow IVP initially; may repeat with 0.5 mEq/kg in 10 minutes one time, or as indicated by the patient's acid-base status

Children and Adults: 1 mEq/kg IVP initially; may repeat with 0.5 mEq/kg in 10 minutes one time, or as indicated by the patient's acid-base status

Metabolic acidosis: Dosage should be based on the following formula if blood gases and pH measurements are available:

Infants and Children: HCO_3^-(mEq) = 0.3 x weight (kg) x base deficit (mEq/L) **or** HCO_3^-(mEq) = 0.5 x weight (kg) x [24 - serum HCO_3^-(mEq/L)]

Adults: HCO_3^-(mEq) = 0.2 x weight (kg) x base deficit (mEq/L) **or** HCO_3^-(mEq) = 0.5 x weight (kg) x [24 - serum HCO_3^-(mEq/L)]

If acid-base status is not available: Dose for older Children and Adults: 2-5 mEq/kg IV infusion over 4-8 hours; subsequent doses should be based on patient's acid-base status

Prevention of hyperuricemia secondary to tumor lysis syndrome (urinary alkalinization) (refer to individual protocols):

Infants and Children:

IV: 120-200 mEq/m^2/day diluted in maintenance IV fluids of 3000 mL/m^2/day; titrate to maintain urine pH between 6-7

Oral: 12 g/m^2/day divided into 4 doses; titrate to maintain urine pH between 6-7

Chronic renal failure: Oral: Initiate when plasma HCO_3^- <15 mEq/L:
Children: 1-3 mEq/kg/day in divided doses
Adults: 20-36 mEq/day in divided doses
Renal tubular acidosis: Oral:
Distal:
Children: 2-3 mEq/kg/day in divided doses
Adults: 0.5-2 mEq/kg/day given in 4-5 divided doses
Proximal: Children and Adults: Initial: 5-10 mEq/kg/day in divided doses; maintenance: Increase as required to maintain serum bicarbonate in the normal range
Urine alkalinization: Oral:
Children: 1-10 mEq (84-840 mg)/kg/day in divided doses; dose should be titrated to desired urinary pH
Adults: 48 mEq (4 g) initially, then 12-24 mEq (1-2 g) every 4 hours; dose should be titrated to desired urinary pH; doses up to 16 g/day have been used
Antacid: Oral: Adults: 325 mg to 2 grams 1-4 times/day

Preparation for Administration
Parenteral:
Direct IV injection: For neonates and infants, may dilute the 1 mEq/mL solution 1:1 with SWFI
IV infusion: Dilute in a dextrose solution (eg, D5W) to a maximum concentration of 0.5 mEq/mL
Prevention of hyperuricemia secondary to tumor lysis syndrome: Dilute in maintenance IV fluids of 3000 mL/m^2/day; refer to individual protocols

Administration
Oral: Administer 1 to 3 hours after meals
Parenteral:
Direct IV injection:
Neonates and Infants: Administer 0.5 mEq/mL solution (either using the 0.5 mEq/mL solution undiluted or dilute the 1 mEq/mL solution 1:1 with SWFI); administer slowly, maximum rate: 10 mEq/minute
Children, Adolescents, and Adults: Administer 1 mEq/mL solution; administer slowly
IV infusion: Must be diluted prior to administration; infusion time variable based upon use; for metabolic acidosis, infusions over 2 to 8 hours have been suggested; maximum rate of administration: 1 mEq/kg/hour
Vesicant (at concentrations ≥8.4%); ensure proper needle or catheter placement prior to and during IV infusion. Avoid extravasation. If extravasation occurs, stop infusion immediately and disconnect (leave needle/cannula in place); gently aspirate extravasated solution (do **NOT** flush the line); initiate hyaluronidase antidote (see Management of Drug Extravasations for more details); remove needle/cannula; apply dry cold compresses (Hurst, 2004); elevate extremity.

Vesicant/Extravasation Risk Vesicant (at concentrations ≥8.4%)

Monitoring Parameters Serum electrolytes including calcium, urinary pH, arterial blood gases (if indicated)

Additional Information 1 mEq $NaHCO_3$ is equivalent to 84 mg; each g of $NaHCO_3$ provides 12 mEq each of sodium and bicarbonate ions; the osmolarity of 0.5 mEq/mL is 1000 mOsm/L and 1 mEq/mL is 2000 mOsm/L

Dosage Forms Considerations
Sodium bicarbonate solution 4.2% [42 mg/mL] provides 0.5 mEq/mL each of sodium and bicarbonate
Sodium bicarbonate solution 7.5% [75 mg/mL] provides 0.9 mEq/mL each of sodium and bicarbonate
Sodium bicarbonate solution 8.4% [84 mg/mL] provides 1 mEq/mL each of sodium and bicarbonate

Dosage Forms Excipient information presented when available (limited, particularly for generics); consult specific product labeling.
Powder, Oral:
Generic: (1 g, 120 g, 454 g, 500 g, 1000 g, 2500 g, 12000 g, 25000 g, 45000 g)
Solution, Intravenous:
Neut: 4% (5 mL)
Generic: 4.2% (5 mL, 10 mL); 7.5% (50 mL); 8.4% (10 mL, 50 mL)
Tablet, Oral:
Generic: 325 mg, 650 mg

◆ **Sodium Bicarbonate and Omeprazole** *see* Omeprazole and Sodium Bicarbonate *on page 1558*

Sodium Chloride (SOW dee um KLOR ide)

Medication Safety Issues
Sound-alike/look-alike issues:
Afrin (saline) may be confused with Afrin (oxymetazoline)
High alert medication:
The Institute for Safe Medication Practices (ISMP) includes this medication (IV formulation >0.9% concentration) among its list of drugs which have a heightened risk of causing significant patient harm when used in error.
Other safety concerns:
Per The Joint Commission (TJC) recommendations, concentrated electrolyte solutions (eg, NaCl >0.9%) should not be available in patient care areas.

Inappropriate use of low sodium or sodium-free intravenous fluids (eg, D_5W, hypotonic saline) in pediatric patients can lead to significant morbidity and mortality due to hyponatremia (ISMP, 2009).

Related Information
Management of Drug Extravasations *on page 2298*
Pediatric Parenteral Nutrition *on page 2359*

Brand Names: US 4-Way Saline [OTC]; Afrin Saline Nasal Mist [OTC]; Altachlore [OTC]; Altamist Spray [OTC]; Ayr Nasal Mist Allergy/Sinus [OTC]; Ayr Saline Nasal Drops [OTC]; Ayr Saline Nasal Gel [OTC]; Ayr Saline Nasal No-Drip [OTC]; AYR Saline Nasal Rinse [OTC]; Ayr Saline Nasal [OTC]; Ayr [OTC]; Baby Ayr Saline [OTC]; Broncho Saline [OTC]; Deep Sea Nasal Spray [OTC]; Entsol Nasal Wash [OTC]; Entsol Nasal [OTC]; Entsol [OTC]; Humist [OTC]; HyperSal; Muro 128 [OTC]; Na-Zone [OTC]; Nasal Moist [OTC]; Nebusal; Ocean Complete Sinus Rinse [OTC]; Ocean for Kids [OTC]; Ocean Nasal Spray [OTC]; Ocean Ultra Saline Mist [OTC]; Pretz Irrigation [OTC]; Pretz [OTC]; PulmoSal; Rhinaris [OTC]; Safe Wash [OTC]; Saline Flush ZR; Saline Mist Spray [OTC]; Saljet Rinse [OTC]; Saljet [OTC]; Sea Soft Nasal Mist [OTC]; Sea-Clens Wound Cleanser [OTC]; Sochlor [OTC]; Sodium Chloride Thermoject Sys; Swab-Flush Saline Flush; Wound Wash Saline [OTC]

Therapeutic Category Electrolyte Supplement, Oral; Electrolyte Supplement, Parenteral; Lubricant, Ocular; Sodium Salt

Generic Availability (US) May be product dependent

Use Restoration of sodium ion in hyponatremia [FDA approved in pediatric patients (age not specified) and adults], restores moisture to nasal membranes [FDA approved in pediatric patients (age not specified) and adults], source of electrolytes and water for expansion of the extracellular fluid compartment [FDA approved in pediatric patients (age not specified) and adults], diluent and delivery system of compatible drug additives [FDA approved in pediatric patients (age not specified) and adults]; has also been used for reduction of intracranial pressure (ICP), improvement of mucociliary clearance and airway hydration in CF and acute viral bronchiolitis, reduction of corneal edema, and prevention of muscle cramps and heat prostration

Pregnancy Risk Factor C

Pregnancy Considerations Animal reproduction studies have not been conducted. Sodium requirements do not change during pregnancy (IOM, 2004). Nasal saline rinses may be used for the treatment of pregnancy rhinitis (Wallace, 2008)

Breast-Feeding Considerations Sodium is found in breast milk. Sodium requirements do not change during lactation (IOM, 2004).

Contraindications Hypersensitivity to sodium chloride or any component of the formulation; hypertonic uterus, hypernatremia, fluid retention

Warnings/Precautions The use of hypotonic saline solutions (eg, 0.225% sodium chloride) may result in hemolysis if administered rapidly and for prolonged periods. If hypotonic saline solutions become necessary, administration as D_5W/0.2% NaCl or 0.45% NaCl is recommended for most patients (eg, those without hyperglycemia). Use with caution in patients with HF, renal insufficiency, liver cirrhosis, hypertension, edema.

Administration of low sodium or sodium-free IV solutions may result in significant hyponatremia or water intoxication; monitor serum sodium concentration closely. In the treatment of acute hypernatremia (ie, development over a couple of hours), serum sodium concentration should be corrected no faster than 1-2 mEq/L per hour. If patient has been chronically hypernatremic, correct serum sodium no faster than 0.5 mEq/L per hour and by no more than 10-12 mEq/L in a given 24-hour period; use extreme caution since rapid correction may result in cerebral edema, herniation, coma, and death (Adrogue, 2000; Kraft, 2005).

When treating hyponatremia, rate of correction is dependent upon whether or not it is acute or chronic. Sodium toxicity (eg, osmotic demyelination syndrome) is almost exclusively related to how fast a sodium deficit is corrected; both rate and magnitude are extremely important. For patients with acute (<24 hours) or chronic (>48 hours), severe (<120 mEq/L) hyponatremia, a serum sodium concentration increase of 4-6 mEq/L within a 24-hour period is sufficient for most patients. In chronic severe hyponatremia, overcorrection risks iatrogenic osmotic demyelination syndrome. For patients with severe symptoms or other need for urgent correction, may increase by 4-6 mEq/L within the first 6 hours and postpone any further correction until the next day at a correction rate of 4-6 mEq/L per day. Choice of infusate sodium concentration is dependent upon the severity of the hyponatremia with more concentrated solutions (eg, 3% NaCl) for more severe cases; monitor serum sodium closely during administration (Sterns, 2013).

Benzyl alcohol and derivatives: Bacteriostatic sodium chloride contains benzyl alcohol; large amounts of benzyl alcohol (≥99 mg/kg/day) have been associated with a potentially fatal toxicity ("gasping syndrome") in neonates; the "gasping syndrome" consists of metabolic acidosis, respiratory distress, gasping respirations, CNS dysfunction (including convulsions, intracranial hemorrhage), hypotension, and cardiovascular collapse (AAP, 1997; CDC, 1982); some data suggests that benzoate displaces bilirubin from protein binding sites (Ahlfors, 2001); avoid or use dosage forms containing benzyl alcohol with caution in neonates. See manufacturer's labeling.

Wound Wash Saline is for single-patient use only.

Irrigants: For external use only; not for parenteral use. Do not use during electrosurgical procedures. Irrigating fluids may be absorbed into systemic circulation; monitor for fluid or solute overload.

Concentrated solutions of sodium chloride (>1%) are vesicants; ensure proper needle or catheter placement prior to and during infusion; avoid extravasation.

Warnings: Additional Pediatric Considerations In neonates, maximum serum concentration correction rate should generally not exceed 10 mEq/L/day; in infants, children, adolescents, and adults, do not exceed a maximum serum concentration correction rate of 12 mEq/L/day. Administration of low sodium or sodium free IV solutions may result in significant hyponatremia or water intoxication in pediatric patients; monitor serum sodium concentration.

Some dosage forms may contain propylene glycol; in neonates large amounts of propylene glycol delivered orally, intravenously (eg, >3,000 mg/day), or topically have been associated with potentially fatal toxicities which can include metabolic acidosis, seizures, renal failure, and CNS depression; toxicities have also been reported in children and adults including hyperosmolality, lactic acidosis, seizures, and respiratory depression; use caution (AAP, 1997; Shehab, 2009).

Adverse Reactions

Cardiovascular: Congestive heart failure, transient hypotension (especially with adult administration of 23.4% NaCl)

Central nervous system: Central pontine myelinolysis (due to rapid correction of hyponatremia)

Endocrine & metabolic: Dilution of serum electrolytes, extravasation, hypernatremia, hypervolemia, hypokalemia, overhydration

Gastrointestinal: Nausea, vomiting (oral use)

Local: Thrombosis, phlebitis, extravasation

Respiratory: Bronchospasm (inhalation with hypertonic solutions), pulmonary edema

Drug Interactions

Metabolism/Transport Effects None known.

Avoid Concomitant Use

Avoid concomitant use of Sodium Chloride with any of the following: Tolvaptan

Increased Effect/Toxicity

Sodium Chloride may increase the levels/effects of: Tolvaptan

Decreased Effect

Sodium Chloride may decrease the levels/effects of: Lithium

Storage/Stability Store injection at room temperature; do not freeze. Protect from heat. Use only clear solutions.

Mechanism of Action Principal extracellular cation; functions in fluid and electrolyte balance, osmotic pressure control, and water distribution

Pharmacokinetics (Adult data unless noted)

Absorption: Oral, IV: Rapid

Distribution: Widely distributed

Elimination: Mainly in urine but also in sweat, tears, and saliva

Dosing: Neonatal Dosage depends upon clinical condition, fluid, electrolyte, and acid-base balance of patient.

Normal daily requirement:

Premature neonates: Oral, IV: 2-5 mEq/kg/day (Mirtallo, 2004); infants born at ≤32 weeks gestation may require higher dosage (up to 8 mEq/kg/day) for the first 2 weeks of life (Al-Dahhan, 2002)

Term neonates: Oral, IV: 2-5 mEq/kg/day (Mirtallo, 2004)

Hyponatremia: IV: **0.9% isotonic solution:**

Dose (mEq sodium) = [desired serum sodium (mEq/L) – actual serum sodium (mEq/L)] x 0.6 x wt (kg)

Note: For acute correction, use 125 mEq/L as the "desired serum sodium"; acutely correct serum sodium by 5 mEq/L/dose increments (eg, from a serum concentration of 120 mEq/L to 125 mEq/L) using a serum correction rate of <0.4-0.5 mEq/L/hour; goal serum correction rate: ≤8-10 mEq/L/day. Hypertonic saline should be used with caution and only for severe cases of hyponatremia with a serum sodium <120 mEq/L and patient experiencing symptoms (Marcialis, 2011).

Nasal dryness/congestion: Intranasal: 0.9% intranasal solution: 2-6 drops per nostril as needed

Ocular dryness:

Ophthalmic, ointment: Apply once daily or more often as needed

Ophthalmic solution: Instill 1-2 drops into affected eye(s) every 3-4 hours

Volume expansion, resuscitation: AHA, AAP: Neonatal resuscitation recommendation: IV: **0.9% isotonic solution:** 10 mL/kg; may repeat (Kattwinkel, 2010); in a retrospective analysis of neonates requiring CPR at birth, 21 ± 14 mL/kg was the effective dose (n=13, GA: ≥34 weeks) (Wyckoff, 2005)

Dosing: Usual Dosage depends upon clinical condition, fluid, electrolyte, and acid-base balance of patient; systemic hypertonic solutions (>0.9%) should only be used for the initial treatment of acute serious symptomatic hyponatremia or increased intracranial pressure.

Pediatric:

Normal daily requirements:

Infants and Children ≤50 kg: Oral, IV: 2-5 mEq/kg/day (Mirtallo, 2004)

Children >50 kg and Adolescents: Oral, IV: 1-2 mEq/kg/day (Mirtallo, 2004)

Bronchiolitis, viral (inpatient): Infants and Children 1-24 months: Inhalation: **3% solution**: 4 mL inhaled every 2 hours for 3 doses followed by every 4 hours for 5 doses and continued every 6 hours until discharge (Kuzik, 2007); pretreatment with a bronchodilator may be necessary to prevent potential bronchospasm

Bronchodilator diluent: Infants, Children, and Adolescents: Inhalation: 1-3 sprays (1-3 mL) to dilute bronchodilator solution in nebulizer before administration

Cystic fibrosis: Children ≥6 years and Adolescents: Inhalation: **7% solution**: 4 mL inhaled twice daily. **Note:** Clinically, some CF centers use 3% or 3.5% inhaled solutions if patients cannot tolerate 7%; pretreatment with a bronchodilator is recommended to prevent potential bronchospasm

Dehydration: Infants, Children, and Adolescents: IV: **0.9% isotonic solution:** Initial: 20 mL/kg/dose; maximum dose: 1000 mL followed by remaining replacement using sodium chloride concentration appropriate for age over 24 hours for dehydration (Meyers, 2009)

Hyponatremia: Infants, Children, and Adolescents: IV: **Note:** Use **0.9% isotonic solution or 3% hypertonic solution** depending on clinical severity and etiology.

Dose (mEq sodium) = [desired serum sodium (mEq/L) - actual serum sodium (mEq/L)] x 0.6 x wt (kg)

Note: For acute correction, use 125 mEq/L as the "desired serum sodium"; acutely correct serum sodium by 5 mEq/L/dose increments (eg, from a serum concentration of 120 mEq/L to 125 mEq/L) using a serum correction rate of ≤2 mEq/L/hour for the first few hours followed by a serum correction rate of ≤0.5 mEq/L/hour; goal serum correction rate: ≤12 mEq/L/day; more gradual correction in increments of 10 mEq/L/day is indicated in the asymptomatic patient

Hypovolemic shock: Infants, Children, and Adolescents: IV: **0.9% isotonic solution:** 20 mL/kg/dose; may repeat up to ≥60 mL/kg until capillary perfusion improves or signs of fluid overload occur (Ceneviva, 1998; Parker, 2004)

Increased intracranial pressure (ICP): Infants, Children, and Adolescents: IV: **3% hypertonic solution:**

Bolus: Limited data available; dosing regimens variable:

Traumatic brain injury guidelines: 6.5-10 mL/kg/dose (Fisher, 1992; Kochanek, 2012)

Alternate dosing: 5 mL/kg/dose administered early in presentation (during critical care transport) was reported in a retrospective trial of 101 pediatric patients (age range: 2 months to 17 years) with suspected increased ICP (Luu, 2011); some centers use 2-5 mL/kg/dose; boluses are typically infused over 30 minutes but are occasionally administered more rapidly depending on the clinical scenario (Abd-Allah, 2012)

Continuous IV infusion: 0.1-1 mL/kg/hour titrated to maintain ICP <20 mm Hg (Kochanek, 2012); monitor serum sodium concentration closely; some centers utilize titration protocols with rate adjustments varying with serum sodium concentration; maintain serum osmolarity <360 mOsmol/L

Nasal dryness/congestion:

Infants: Intranasal: **0.9% intranasal solution:** 2-6 drops per nostril as needed

Children and Adolescents: Intranasal: Use as often as needed

Ocular dryness: Infants, Children, and Adolescents:

Ophthalmic, ointment: Apply once daily or more often as needed

Ophthalmic, solution: Instill 1-2 drops into affected eye(s) every 3-4 hours

Adult:

Bronchodilator diluent: Inhalation: 1-3 sprays (1-3 mL) to dilute bronchodilator solution in nebulizer before administration

Chloride maintenance electrolyte requirement in parenteral nutrition: IV: As needed to maintain acid-base balance with parenteral nutrition; use equal amounts of chloride and acetate to maintain balance and adjust ratio based on individual patient needs (Mirtallo, 2004).

GU irrigant: Irrigation: 1-3 L/day by intermittent irrigation

Hyponatremia: IV: To correct acute (<24 hours) or chronic (>48 hours), severe (<120 mEq/L) hyponatremia: In general, a serum sodium concentration increase of 4-6 mEq/L within a 24-hour period is sufficient to improve most symptoms of hyponatremia. In chronic severe hyponatremia, overcorrection risks iatrogenic osmotic demyelination syndrome. For patients with severe symptoms or other need for urgent correction, one approach is to increase serum sodium concentration by 4-6 mEq/L within the first 6 hours and postpone any further correction until the next day at a correction rate of 4-6 mEq/L per day. Choice of sodium correction fluid concentration is dependent upon the severity of the hyponatremia with more concentrated solutions (eg, 3% NaCl) for more severe cases; monitor serum sodium closely during administration (Sterns, 2013).

Irrigation: Spray affected area

Nasal congestion: Intranasal: 2-3 sprays in each nostril as needed

Ophthalmic:

Ointment: Apply once daily or more often

Solution: Instill 1-2 drops into affected eye(s) every 3-4 hours

Replacement: IV: Determined by laboratory determinations mEq

Sodium maintenance electrolyte requirement in parenteral nutrition: IV: 1-2 mEq/kg/24 hours; customize amounts based on individual patient needs (Mirtallo, 2004).

Administration

Inhalation: Nebulization; studies administering hypertonic saline utilized varying types of nebulizers, including jet and ultrasonic

Nasal: Spray into 1 nostril while gently occluding other

Ophthalmic: Apply to affected eye(s); avoid contact of bottle tip with eye or skin

Oral: Administer with full glass of water

Parenteral: Central-line administration is preferred for hypertonic saline (>0.9%) if available and/or if infusion is to be continued; peripheral administration may be necessary for initiation of treatment in critical patients; use of peripheral administration should be limited;

intraosseous administration may be used if unable to obtain intravenous access (Luu, 2011)
Rate of administration:
Bolus:
0.9% isotonic solution:
Hypotension, shock:
Neonates: Published data not available; consider slower administration to avoid IVH (Kattwinkel, 2010)
Infants, Children, and Adolescents: Administer boluses over 5 minutes (Brierley, 2009)
Dehydration: Bolus: Administer over 20-60 minutes
3% hypertonic solution: In pediatric patients, typically infused over 30 minutes (Abd-Allah, 2012); some trials have described administering at a rate of 10 mEq/kg/hour when treating acute, life-threatening ICP elevation (Kamat, 2003)
Continuous IV infusion: Maximum rate: 1 mEq/kg/hour
Vesicant at higher concentrations (>1%); ensure proper needle or catheter placement prior to and during infusion; avoid extravasation. If extravasation occurs, stop infusion immediately and disconnect (leave cannula/needle in place); gently aspirate extravasated solution (do **NOT** flush the line); remove needle/cannula; elevate extremity. Apply dry warm compresses (Hastings-Tolsma, 1993).

Vesicant/Extravasation Risk Vesicant (at concentrations >1%)

Monitoring Parameters Serum sodium, chloride, I & O, weight; ICP, serum osmolarity (when used to treat increased ICP), capillary perfusion, MAP, CVP (fluid resuscitation)

Reference Range Serum/plasma sodium concentration:
Premature neonates: 132-140 mEq/L
Full-term neonates: 133-142 mEq/L
Infants ≥2 months to Adults: 135-145 mEq/L

Additional Information
IV solutions: NS (0.9%) = 154 mEq/L; 3% NaCl = 513 mEq/L; 5% NaCl = 856 mEq/L
Tablet 1 g = 17.1 mEq
3% NaCl: Osmolarity: 1027 mOsm/L

Dosage Forms Considerations 1 g sodium chloride = elemental sodium 393.3 mg = 17.1 mEq sodium = sodium 17.1 mmol

Dosage Forms Excipient information presented when available (limited, particularly for generics); consult specific product labeling.
Aerosol Solution, Inhalation:
Broncho Saline: 0.9% (90 mL, 240 mL)
Aerosol Solution, Nasal [preservative free]:
Ocean Complete Sinus Rinse: (177 mL) [drug free]
Gel, Nasal:
Ayr Saline Nasal: (14.1 g) [contains aloe barbadensis, brilliant blue fcf (fd&c blue #1), methylparaben, propylparaben, soybean oil]
Ayr Saline Nasal No-Drip: (22 mL) [contains aloe barbadensis, benzalkonium chloride, benzyl alcohol, soybean oil]
Entsol Nasal: (20 g)
Rhinaris: 0.2% (28.4 g) [contains benzalkonium chloride, propylene glycol]
Liquid, External:
Sea-Clens Wound Cleanser: (355 mL)
Nebulization Solution, Inhalation:
Generic: 0.9% (3 mL)
Nebulization Solution, Inhalation [preservative free]:
HyperSal: 3.5% (4 mL) [latex free]
HyperSal: 7% (4 mL)
Nebusal: 3% (4 mL); 6% (4 mL)
PulmoSal: 7% (4 mL)
Generic: 0.9% (3 mL, 5 mL, 15 mL); 3% (4 mL, 15 mL); 7% (4 mL); 10% (4 mL, 15 mL)
Ointment, Ophthalmic:
Altachlore: 5% (3.5 g)
Muro 128: 5% (3.5 g)
Generic: 5% (3.5 g)
Packet, Nasal [preservative free]:
AYR Saline Nasal Rinse: 1.57 g (50 ea, 100 ea) [iodine free]
Solution, External:
Saljet: 0.9% (30 mL)
Wound Wash Saline: 0.9% (210 mL)
Solution, External [preservative free]:
Safe Wash: 0.9% (210 mL) [drug free, latex free]
Saljet Rinse: 0.9% (30 mL)
Solution, Injection:
Sodium Chloride Thermoject Sys: 0.9% (10 mL)
Generic: 0.9% (2 mL, 2.5 mL, 3 mL, 5 mL, 10 mL, 20 mL, 100 mL); 14.6% (20 mL, 40 mL)
Solution, Injection [preservative free]:
Generic: 0.9% (1 mL, 2 mL, 2.5 mL, 3 mL, 5 mL, 10 mL, 20 mL, 50 mL)
Solution, Intravenous:
SwabFlush Saline Flush: 0.9% (10 mL)
Generic: 0.45% (25 mL, 50 mL, 100 mL, 250 mL, 500 mL, 1000 mL); 0.9% (2.5 mL, 3 mL, 10 mL, 25 mL, 50 mL, 100 mL, 150 mL, 250 mL, 500 mL, 1000 mL); 3% (500 mL); 5% (500 mL); 23.4% (30 mL, 100 mL, 200 mL, 250 mL)
Solution, Intravenous [preservative free]:
Saline Flush ZR: 0.9% (2.5 mL, 5 mL, 10 mL) [latex free]
Generic: 0.9% (1 mL, 2 mL, 2.5 mL, 3 mL, 5 mL, 10 mL, 50 mL, 100 mL, 125 mL, 500 mL, 1000 mL)
Solution, Irrigation:
Generic: 0.9% (250 mL, 500 mL, 1000 mL, 1500 mL, 2000 mL, 3000 mL, 4000 mL, 5000 mL)
Solution, Nasal:
4-Way Saline: (29.6 mL)
Afrin Saline Nasal Mist: 0.65% (30 mL, 45 mL)
Altamist Spray: 0.65% (45 mL, 60 mL)
Ayr: 0.65% (50 mL)
Ayr Nasal Mist Allergy/Sinus: 2.65% (50 mL) [contains benzalkonium chloride]
Ayr Saline Nasal Drops: 0.65% (50 mL)
Baby Ayr Saline: 0.65% (30 mL)
Deep Sea Nasal Spray: 0.65% (44 mL) [contains benzalkonium chloride]
Entsol: (30 mL)
Humist: 0.65% (45 mL)
Na-Zone: 0.65% (59 mL)
Nasal Moist: 0.65% (15 mL, 45 mL)
Ocean for Kids: 0.65% (37.5 mL) [alcohol free, drug free; contains benzalkonium chloride]
Ocean Nasal Spray: 0.65% (45 mL, 66 mL, 104 mL, 480 mL) [contains benzalkonium chloride]
Pretz: (50 mL, 946 mL)
Pretz Irrigation: (237 mL)
Rhinaris: 0.2% (30 mL) [contains benzalkonium chloride, propylene glycol]
Saline Mist Spray: 0.65% (45 mL) [contains benzalkonium chloride]
Sea Soft Nasal Mist: 0.65% (45 mL)
Generic: 0.65% (44 mL, 45 mL)
Solution, Nasal [preservative free]:
Entsol Nasal: 3% (100 mL) [drug free]
Entsol Nasal Wash: (237 mL)
Ocean Ultra Saline Mist: (90 mL) [drug free]
Solution, Ophthalmic:
Altachlore: 5% (15 mL, 30 mL)
Muro 128: 2% (15 mL); 5% (15 mL, 30 mL)
Sochlor: 5% (15 mL)
Generic: 5% (15 mL)

Swab, Nasal:
Ayr Saline Nasal Gel: (20 ea) [contains methylparaben, propylparaben, soybean oil, trolamine (triethanolamine)]
Tablet, Oral:
Generic: 1 g

◆ **Sodium Chloride Thermoject Sys** *see* Sodium Chloride *on page 1938*

Sodium Citrate and Citric Acid

(SOW dee um SIT rate & SI trik AS id)

Medication Safety Issues

Sound-alike/look-alike issues:

Bicitra may be confused with Polycitra

Brand Names: US Cytra-2; Oracit®; Shohl's Solution (Modified); Virtrate-2

Brand Names: Canada PMS-Dicitrate

Therapeutic Category Alkalinizing Agent, Oral

Generic Availability (US) Yes

Use As long-term therapy to alkalinize the urine for control and/or dissolution of uric acid and cystine calculi of the urinary tract (FDA approved in children and adults); treatment of chronic metabolic acidosis secondary to chronic renal insufficiency or syndrome of renal tubular acidosis when use of potassium salt is contraindicated or undesirable (FDA approved in children and adults); buffer and neutralize gastric hydrochloric acid (FDA approved in adults).

Pregnancy Risk Factor Not established

Pregnancy Considerations Use caution with toxemia of pregnancy.

Contraindications Hypersensitivity to sodium citrate, citric acid, or any component of the formulation; severe renal insufficiency; sodium-restricted diet

Warnings/Precautions Conversion to bicarbonate may be impaired in patients with hepatic failure, in shock, or who are severely ill. Use caution with cardiac failure, hypertension, impaired renal function, and peripheral or pulmonary edema; contains sodium.

Benzyl alcohol and derivatives: Some dosage forms may contain sodium benzoate/benzoic acid; benzoic acid (benzoate) is a metabolite of benzyl alcohol; large amounts of benzyl alcohol (≥99 mg/kg/day) have been associated with a potentially fatal toxicity ("gasping syndrome") in neonates; the "gasping syndrome" consists of metabolic acidosis, respiratory distress, gasping respirations, CNS dysfunction (including convulsions, intracranial hemorrhage), hypotension, and cardiovascular collapse (AAP, 1997; CDC, 1982); some data suggests that benzoate displaces bilirubin from protein binding sites (Ahlfors, 2001); avoid or use dosage forms containing benzyl alcohol derivative with caution in neonates. See manufacturer's labeling.

Propylene glycol: Some dosage forms may contain propylene glycol; large amounts are potentially toxic and have been associated hyperosmolality, lactic acidosis, seizures, and respiratory depression; use caution (AAP, 1997; Zar, 2007).

Warnings: Additional Pediatric Considerations Some dosage forms may contain propylene glycol; in neonates large amounts of propylene glycol delivered orally, intravenously (eg, >3,000 mg/day), or topically have been associated with potentially fatal toxicities which can include metabolic acidosis, seizures, renal failure, and CNS depression; toxicities have also been reported in children and adults including hyperosmolality, lactic acidosis, seizures, and respiratory depression; use caution (AAP, 1997; Shehab, 2009).

Adverse Reactions Generally well tolerated with normal renal function.

Central nervous system: Tetany
Endocrine & metabolic: Metabolic alkalosis
Gastrointestinal: Diarrhea, nausea, vomiting

Drug Interactions

Metabolism/Transport Effects None known.

Avoid Concomitant Use There are no known interactions where it is recommended to avoid concomitant use.

Increased Effect/Toxicity

Sodium Citrate and Citric Acid may increase the levels/effects of: Aluminum Hydroxide

Decreased Effect There are no known significant interactions involving a decrease in effect.

Storage/Stability Store at controlled room temperature of 15°C to 30°C (59°F to 86°F); do not freeze. Protect from excessive heat.

Pharmacokinetics (Adult data unless noted)

Metabolism: ≥95% via hepatic oxidation to bicarbonate; may be impaired in patients with hepatic failure, shock, or severe illness
Elimination: Urine (<5% as sodium citrate)

Dosing: Neonatal Oral: **Note:** 1 mL of oral solution contains 1 mEq of bicarbonate:

Systemic alkalinization: 2-3 mEq bicarbonate/kg/day (2-3 mL/kg/day) in 3-4 divided doses

Dosing: Usual Oral: **Note:** 1 mL of oral solution contains 1 mEq of bicarbonate:

Systemic alkalinization:

Manufacturer's recommendation: Children ≥2 years: 5-15 mL (5-15 mEq bicarbonate) per dose after meals and at bedtime

Alternative recommendation: Dosing per mEq of bicarbonate: Infants and Children: 2–3 mEq bicarbonate/kg/**day** (2-3 mL/kg/**day**) in 3-4 divided doses

Adults: 10-30 mL (10-30 mEq bicarbonate) per dose after meals and at bedtime

Preparation for Administration Oral: Dilute each dose with 30 to 90 mL of water

Administration Oral: Shake well before use. Dose must be diluted prior to administration; administer after meals and at bedtime to avoid saline laxative effect; chilling solution prior to dosing helps to enhance palatability.

Monitoring Parameters Periodic serum (sodium, potassium, calcium, bicarbonate)

Dosage Forms Considerations Each mL provides 1 mEq sodium, and is equivalent to 1 mEq bicarbonate

Dosage Forms Excipient information presented when available (limited, particularly for generics); consult specific product labeling.

Solution, oral:

Cytra-2: Sodium citrate 500 mg and citric acid 334 mg per 5 mL (480 mL) [alcohol free, dye free, sugar free; contains propylene glycol and sodium benzoate; grape flavor]

Oracit®: Sodium citrate 490 mg and citric acid 640 mg per 5 mL (15 mL, 30 mL, 500 mL, 3840 mL)

Shohl's Solution (Modified): Sodium citrate 500 mg and citric acid 300 mg per 5 mL (480 mL) [contains alcohol]

Virtrate-2: Sodium citrate 500 mg and citric acid 334 mg per 5 mL (480 mL) [contains propylene glycol and sodium benzoate; grape flavor]

Generic: Sodium citrate 500 mg and citric acid 334 mg per 5 mL (480 mL)

◆ **Sodium Citrate, Citric Acid, and Potassium Citrate** *see* Citric Acid, Sodium Citrate, and Potassium Citrate *on page 479*

◆ **Sodium Cromoglicate** *see* Cromolyn (Nasal) *on page 542*

◆ **Sodium Cromoglicate** *see* Cromolyn (Ophthalmic) *on page 543*

◆ **Sodium Cromoglicate** *see* Cromolyn (Systemic, Oral Inhalation) *on page 541*

◆ **Sodium Diuril** *see* Chlorothiazide *on page 439*

◆ **Sodium Edecrin** *see* Ethacrynic Acid *on page 809*

◆ **Sodium Etidronate** *see* Etidronate *on page 815*

◆ **Sodium Ferric Gluconate** *see* Ferric Gluconate *on page 867*

◆ **Sodium Ferric Gluconate Complex** *see* Ferric Gluconate *on page 867*

◆ **Sodium Fluoride** *see* Fluoride *on page 899*

Sodium Glycerophosphate Pentahydrate

(SOE dee um glis er oh FOS fate pen ta HYE drate)

Related Information

Potassium Phosphate *on page 1743*

Sodium Phosphates *on page 1949*

Brand Names: US Glycophos

Therapeutic Category Electrolyte Supplement, Parenteral

Generic Availability (US) No

Use Supplement in parenteral nutrition to meet the requirements of phosphate; has also been used for general phosphate repletion during sodium phosphate and potassium phosphate shortages

Pregnancy Considerations Animal reproduction studies have not been conducted. Phosphorus requirements are similar in pregnant and nonpregnant women (IOM, 1997).

Breast-Feeding Considerations Phosphorus is a normal constituent of human milk (IOM, 1997).

Contraindications Patients in a state of dehydration or with hypernatremia, hyperphosphatemia, severe renal insufficiency, or shock

Warnings/Precautions Use with caution in patients with pre-existing electrolyte disturbances or risk of electrolyte disturbances and in patients with renal impairment due to risk of hypernatremia and hyperphosphatemia. Unlike phosphate products available in the U.S., sodium glycerophosphate pentahydrate is an organic phosphate product and varies from other phosphate products in terms of concentration, dosing, and preservative content; use caution when switching between products.

Adverse Reactions None reported by manufacturer.

Adverse drug reactions listed have been reported in one small clinical trial (n=27) (Topp, 2011a).

Central nervous system: Headache

Endocrine & metabolic: Hypocalcemia

Gastrointestinal: Nausea, xerostomia

Drug Interactions

Metabolism/Transport Effects None known.

Avoid Concomitant Use There are no known interactions where it is recommended to avoid concomitant use.

Increased Effect/Toxicity There are no known significant interactions involving an increase in effect.

Decreased Effect There are no known significant interactions involving a decrease in effect.

Storage/Stability Store intact vials at ≤25°C (77°F); do not freeze.

Mechanism of Action Phosphorous participates in bone deposition, calcium metabolism, utilization of B complex vitamins, and as a buffer in acid-base equilibrium.

Pharmacokinetics (Adult data unless noted)

Metabolism: Hydrolyzed to inorganic phosphate

Half-life elimination: Inorganic phosphate: 2.06 hours (Topp, 2011a)

Time to peak serum concentration: 4 hours (Topp, 2011a)

Elimination: Inorganic phosphate: Urine

Note: One study involving 27 healthy adult volunteers compared pharmacokinetic data from infusions of 80 mmol sodium phosphate and 80 mmol sodium glycerophosphate pentahydrate delivered over a 4-hour period in a randomized, double-blind, crossover study. Bioequivalence was demonstrated between the two drugs in terms of serum AUC (0-24 hours) and C_{max} levels of inorganic phosphate; however, the corrected excretion of inorganic phosphate in a 24-hour urine collection failed to demonstrate bioequivalence between sodium phosphate and sodium glycerophosphate pentahydrate. It is suggested that a small amount of unhydrolyzed sodium glycerophosphate in the urine, undetectable by the assay, is responsible for this discrepancy (Topp, 2011a).

Inorganic phosphate is released from the glycerophosphate molecule by hydrolysis. The maximum amount of glycerophosphate that can be hydrolyzed per day is dependent on serum alkaline phosphatase activity; use caution in patients with reduced alkaline phosphatase activity.

Dosing: Neonatal Note: When converting from inorganic phosphate products (ie, sodium phosphate and potassium phosphate), maintain the same mmol amount of phosphate. Doses are listed as mmol of phosphate. Sodium glycerophosphate pentahydrate 306.1 mg = sodium glycerophosphate 216 mg = phosphate 1 **mmol**. Sodium glycerophosphate pentahydrate will provide 2 mEq of sodium for every 1 mmol of phosphate delivered.

Caution: With orders for IV phosphate, there is considerable confusion associated with the use of millimoles (mmol) versus milliequivalents (mEq) to express the phosphate requirement. The most reliable method of ordering IV phosphate is by millimoles.

Parenteral nutrition, maintenance requirement: IV:

Manufacturer's labeling: 1-1.5 mmol/kg/day admixed within parenteral nutrition solution. Dosage should be individualized.

ASPEN recommendations (Mirtallo, 2004): 1-2 mmol/kg/day

Dosing: Usual Note: When converting from inorganic phosphate products (ie, sodium phosphate and potassium phosphate), maintain the same mmol amount of phosphate. Doses are listed as mmol of phosphate. Sodium glycerophosphate pentahydrate 306.1 mg = sodium glycerophosphate 216 mg = phosphate 1 **mmol**. Sodium glycerophosphate pentahydrate will provide 2 mEq of sodium for every 1 mmol of phosphate delivered.

Caution: With orders for IV phosphate, there is considerable confusion associated with the use of millimoles (mmol) versus milliequivalents (mEq) to express the phosphate requirement. The most reliable method of ordering IV phosphate is by millimoles.

Infants, Children, and Adolescents:

Parenteral nutrition, maintenance requirement: IV:

Manufacturer's labeling: Infants: 1-1.5 mmol/kg/day admixed within parenteral nutrition solution. Dosage should be individualized.

ASPEN recommendations (Mirtallo, 2004):

Infants and Children ≤50 kg: 0.5-2 mmol/kg/day

Children >50 kg and Adolescents: 10-40 mmol/day

Hypophosphatemia, acute: Hypophosphatemia does not necessarily equate with phosphate depletion. Hypophosphatemia may occur in the presence of low, normal, or high total body phosphate and conversely, phosphate depletion may exist with normal, low, or elevated levels of serum phosphate (Gaasbeek, 2005). It is difficult to provide concrete guidelines for the treatment of severe hypophosphatemia because the extent of total body deficits and response to therapy are difficult to predict. Aggressive doses of phosphate may result in a transient serum elevation followed by redistribution into intracellular compartments or bone tissue. Intermittent IV infusion should be reserved for severe depletion situations; requires continuous cardiac monitoring. Guidelines differ based on degree of illness, need/use of TPN, and severity of hypophosphatemia. If hyperkalemia exists, consider phosphate replacement strategy without potassium (eg, sodium phosphates). Various regimens for replacement of phosphate in adults have been studied. The regimens below have only been studied in adult patients, however, many institutions have used them in children safely and successfully. Obese patients and/or severe renal impairment were excluded from phosphate supplement trials. **Note:** 1 mmol phosphate = 31 mg phosphorus; 1 mg phosphorus = 0.032 mmol phosphate.

IV doses may be incorporated into the patient's maintenance IV fluids; intermittent IV infusion should be reserved for severe depletion situations. **Note:** Doses listed as mmol of phosphate.

Infants, Children, and Adolescents: **Note:** There are no prospective studies of parenteral phosphate replacement in children. The following weight-based guidelines for adult dosing may be cautiously employed in pediatric patients. Guidelines differ based on degree of illness, use of TPN, and severity of hypophosphatemia.

General replacement guidelines (Lentz, 1978): **Note:** The initial dose may be increased by 25% to 50% if the patient is symptomatic secondary to hypophosphatemia and lowered by 25% to 50% if the patient is hypercalcemic.

Low dose: 0.08 mmol/kg over 6 hours; use if losses are recent and uncomplicated

Intermediate dose: 0.16-0.24 mmol/kg over 4-6 hours; use if serum phosphorus level 0.5-1 mg/dL (0.16-0.32 mmol/L)

High dose: 0.36 mmol/kg over 6 hours; use if serum phosphorus <0.5 mg/dL (<0.16 mmol/L)

Patients receiving TPN (Clark, 1995):

Low dose: 0.16 mmol/kg over 4-6 hours; use if serum phosphorus level 2.3-3 mg/dL (0.73-0.96 mmol/L)

Intermediate dose: 0.32 mmol/kg over 4-6 hours; use if serum phosphorus level 1.6-2.2 mg/dL (0.51-0.72 mmol/L)

High dose: 0.64 mmol/kg over 8-12 hours; use if serum phosphorus <1.5 mg/dL (<0.5 mmol/L)

Critically ill adult trauma patients receiving TPN (Brown, 2006):

Low dose: 0.32 mmol/kg over 4-6 hours; use if serum phosphorus level 2.3-3 mg/dL (0.73-0.96 mmol/L)

Intermediate dose: 0.64 mmol/kg over 4-6 hours; use if serum phosphorus level 1.6-2.2 mg/dL (0.51-0.72 mmol/L)

High dose: 1 mmol/kg over 8-12 hours; use if serum phosphorus <1.5 mg/dL (<0.5 mmol/L)

Alternative method in critically ill patients (Kingston, 1985):

Low dose: 0.25 mmol/kg over 4 hours; use if serum phosphorus level 0.5-1 mg/dL (0.16-0.32 mmol/L)

Moderate dose: 0.5 mmol/kg over 4 hours; use if serum phosphorus level <0.5 mg/dL (<0.16 mmol/L)

Adults:

Phosphate replacement, parenteral nutrition: Manufacturer's labeling: IV: 10-20 mmol/day admixed within parenteral nutrition solution. Dosage should be individualized.

Phosphate repletion, general (off-label use):

Hypophosphatemia, acute treatment: IV: It is difficult to provide concrete guidelines for the treatment of severe hypophosphatemia because the extent of total body deficits and response to therapy are difficult to predict. Aggressive doses of phosphate may result in a transient serum elevation followed by redistribution into intracellular compartments or bone tissue. It is recommended that repletion of severe hypophosphatemia be done IV because large doses of oral phosphate may cause diarrhea and intestinal absorption may be unreliable. Intermittent IV infusion should be reserved for severe depletion situations; requires continuous cardiac monitoring. Guidelines differ based on degree of illness, need/use of TPN, and severity of hypophosphatemia. Obese patients and/or severe renal impairment were excluded from phosphate supplement trials. **Note:** 1 mmol phosphate = 31 mg phosphorus; 1 mg phosphorus = 0.032 mmol phosphate.

Critically ill adult patients receiving concurrent enteral/parenteral nutrition (Brown, 2006; Clark, 1995): **Note:** Round doses to the nearest 7.5 mmol for ease of preparation. If administering with phosphate-containing parenteral nutrition, do not exceed 15 mmol/L within parenteral nutrition. May use adjusted body weight for patients weighing >130% of ideal body weight (and BMI <40 kg/m^2) by using [IBW + 0.25 (ABW-IBW)]:

Low dose, serum phosphorus level 2.3-3 mg/dL (0.74-0.96 mmol/L): 0.16-0.32 mmol/kg over 4-6 hours

Intermediate dose, serum phosphorus level 1.6-2.2 mg/dL (0.51-0.71 mmol/L): 0.32-0.64 mmol/kg over 4-6 hours

High dose, serum phosphorus <1.5 mg/dL (<0.5 mmol/L): 0.64-1 mmol/kg over 8-12 hours

Parenteral nutrition: IV: 10-15 mmol/1000 kcal (Hicks, 2001) **or** 20-40 mmol/24 hours (Mirtallo, 2004)

Dosing adjustment in renal impairment: There are no dosing adjustments provided in the manufacturer's labeling (has not been studied); use with caution since phosphate excretion is primarily renal.

Dosing adjustments in hepatic impairment: There are no dosing adjustments provided in the manufacturer's labeling (has not been studied); however, phosphate excretion is primarily renal.

Preparation for Administration Must be diluted before administration; appropriate volume of diluent and maximum concentration have not been determined for intermittent phosphate repletion. Administer within 24 hours of preparation due to risk of microbial contamination.

Administration Must be diluted prior to parenteral administration. In general, the dose, concentration of infusion, and rate of administration may be dependent on patient condition and specific institution policy. Per the manufacturer, infusion time should not be <8 hours and not >24 hours.

Monitoring Parameters Serum sodium, calcium, and phosphorus concentrations; renal function; in pediatric patients after IV phosphate repletion, repeat serum phosphorus concentration should be checked 2 hours later (ASPEN Pediatric Nutrition Support Core Curriculum, 2010)

Reference Range Note: There is a diurnal variation with the nadir at 1100, plateau at 1600, and peak in the early evening (Gaasbeek, 2005); 1 mmol/L phosphate = 3.1 mg/dL phosphorus

Newborn 0-5 days: 4.8-8.2 mg/dL

1-3 years: 3.8-6.5 mg/dL

4-11 years: 3.7-5.6 mg/dL

12-15 years: 2.9-5.4 mg/dL

16-19 years: 2.7-4.7 mg/dL

Additional Information Cow's milk is a good source of phosphate with 1 mg elemental (0.032 mmol) elemental phosphate per mL.

Dosage Forms Excipient information presented when available (limited, particularly for generics); consult specific product labeling.

Solution, Intravenous:

Glycophos: 1 mmol/mL (20 mL)

◆ **Sodium Hydrogen Carbonate** *see* Sodium Bicarbonate *on page 1936*

◆ **Sodium Hyposulfate** *see* Sodium Thiosulfate *on page 1955*

◆ **Sodium Nafcillin** *see* Nafcillin *on page 1481*

Sodium Nitrite and Sodium Thiosulfate

(SOW dee um NYE trite & SOW dee um thye oh SUL fate)

Brand Names: US Nithiodote

Therapeutic Category Antidote

Use Treatment of acute, life-threatening cyanide poisoning (FDA approved in all ages)

Pregnancy Risk Factor C

Pregnancy Considerations Teratogenic effects have been observed following maternal exposure to high concentrations of sodium nitrite in drinking water. Teratogenic effects were not observed in animal reproduction studies of sodium nitrite or sodium thiosulfate. Embryotoxic and non-teratogenic effects were observed in animal reproduction studies of sodium nitrite. Methemoglobin reductase is lower in the fetus compared to adults and may result in adverse effects due to nitrite-induced prenatal hypoxia. There are no adequate and well-controlled studies of Nithiodote in pregnant women. In general, medications used as antidotes should take into consideration the health and prognosis of the mother; antidotes should be administered to pregnant women if there is a clear indication for use and should not be withheld because of fears of teratogenicity (Bailey, 2003).

Breast-Feeding Considerations It is not known if sodium nitrite or sodium thiosulfate is excreted in breast milk. The manufacturer recommends that caution be exercised when administering sodium nitrite and sodium thiosulfate to nursing women.

Contraindications There are no contraindications listed within the manufacturer's labeling.

Warnings/Precautions [U.S. Boxed Warning]: Sodium nitrite may cause methemoglobin formation and severe hypotension resulting in diminished oxygen-carrying capacity; serious adverse effects may occur at doses less than twice the recommended therapeutic dose. Monitor for adequate perfusion and oxygenation; ensure patient is euvolemic. Use with caution in patients where the diagnosis of cyanide poisoning is uncertain, patients with pre-existing diminished oxygen or cardiovascular reserve (eg, smoke inhalation victims, anemia, substantial blood loss, and cardiac or respiratory compromise), in patients at greater risk for developing methemoglobinemia (eg, congenital methemoglobin reductase deficiency), and in patients who may be susceptible to injury from vasodilation; the use of hydroxocobalamin is recommended in these patients. Sodium nitrite is generally discontinued for methemoglobin levels >30%. Intravenous methylene blue and exchange transfusion have been used to treat life-threatening methemoglobinemia. Use with caution with concomitant medications known to cause methemoglobinemia (eg, nitroglycerin, phenazopyridine). Collection of pretreatment blood cyanide concentrations does not preclude administration and should not delay administration in the emergency management of highly suspected or confirmed cyanide toxicity. Pretreatment levels may be useful as postinfusion levels may be inaccurate. Signs of cyanide poisoning may include altered mental status, cardiovascular collapse, chest tightness, mydriasis, nausea/vomiting, dyspnea, hyper-/hypotension, plasma lactate ≥8 mmol/L. Treatment of cyanide poisoning should include external decontamination and supportive therapy. Monitor patients for return of symptoms for 24-48 hours; repeat treatment (one-half the original dose) should be administered if symptoms return. Fire victims and patients with cyanide poisoning related to smoke inhalation may present with both cyanide and carbon monoxide poisoning. In these patients, the induction of methemoglobinemia (due to sodium nitrite) is contraindicated until carbon monoxide levels return to normal due to the risk of tissue hypoxia. Methemoglobinemia decreases the oxygen-carrying capacity of hemoglobin and the presence of carbon monoxide prevents hemoglobin from releasing oxygen to the tissues. In this scenario, sodium thiosulfate may be used alone to promote the clearance of cyanide. Hydroxocobalamin, however, should be considered to avoid the nitrite-related problems and because sodium thiosulfate has a slow onset of action. Consider consultation with a poison control center at 1-800-222-1222.

Patients with anemia will form more methemoglobin; dosage reduction in proportion to oxygen-carrying capacity is recommended. Patients with G6PD deficiency are at an increased risk for hemolytic crisis following sodium nitrite administration; monitor for an acute drop in hematocrit or if possible, consider alternative treatment options. The presence of sulfite hypersensitivity should not preclude the use of this medication.

Methemoglobin reductase, which is responsible for converting methemoglobin back to hemoglobin, has reduced activity in pediatric patients. In addition, infants and young children have some proportion of fetal hemoglobin which forms methemoglobin more readily than adult hemoglobin. Therefore, pediatric patients (eg, neonates and infants <6 months of age) are more susceptible to excessive nitrite-induced methemoglobinemia. Hydroxocobalamin may be a more effective and rapid alternative. Nitrites should be avoided in pregnant patients due to fetal hemoglobin's susceptibility to oxidative stress. Hydroxocobalamin will circumvent this problem and may be a more effective and rapid alternative. Use with caution in renal impairment and the elderly. Potentially significant drug-drug interactions may exist, requiring dose or frequency adjustment, additional monitoring, and/or selection of alternative therapy.

Adverse Reactions

Sodium nitrite:

Cardiovascular: Arrhythmias, cyanosis, flushing, hypotension, palpitations, syncope, tachycardia

Central nervous system: Anxiety, coma, confusion, dizziness, fatigue, headache, lightheadedness, seizure

Dermatologic: Urticaria

Endocrine & metabolic: Acidosis

Gastrointestinal: Abdominal pain, nausea, vomiting

Hematologic: Methemoglobinemia

Local: Injection site tingling

Neuromuscular & skeletal: Numbness, paresthesia, weakness

Ocular: Blurred vision

Respiratory: Dyspnea, tachypnea

Miscellaneous: Diaphoresis

Sodium thiosulfate:

Cardiovascular: Hypotension

Central nervous system: Disorientation, headache

Gastrointestinal: Nausea, salty taste, vomiting

Hematologic: Bleeding time prolonged

Miscellaneous: Warmth

Drug Interactions

Metabolism/Transport Effects None known.

Avoid Concomitant Use There are no known interactions where it is recommended to avoid concomitant use.

Increased Effect/Toxicity

Sodium Nitrite and Sodium Thiosulfate may increase the levels/effects of: Prilocaine

The levels/effects of Sodium Nitrite and Sodium Thiosulfate may be increased by: Methemoglobinemia Associated Agents; Nitric Oxide

Decreased Effect There are no known significant interactions involving a decrease in effect.

Storage/Stability Store at 20°C to 25°C (68°F to 77°F); excursions permitted to 15°C to 30°C (59°F to 86°F); do not freeze. Protect from direct light.

Mechanism of Action

Sodium nitrite: Promotes the formation of methemoglobin which competes with cytochrome oxidase for the cyanide ion. Cyanide combines with methemoglobin to form cyanomethemoglobin, thereby freeing the cytochrome oxidase and allowing aerobic metabolism to continue.

Sodium thiosulfate: Serves as a sulfur donor in rhodanese-catalyzed formation of thiocyanate (much less toxic than cyanide).

Pharmacodynamics

Sodium nitrite:

Onset: Peak effect: Methemoglobinemia: 30-60 minutes

Duration: Methemoglobinemia: ~55 minutes

Pharmacokinetics (Adult data unless noted)

Sodium nitrite:

Metabolism: To ammonia and other metabolites

Excretion: Urine (~40% as unchanged drug)

Sodium thiosulfate:

Half-life elimination:

Thiosulfate: ~3 hours (Howland, 2011)

Thiocyanate: ~3 hours; renal impairment: ≤9 days

Elimination: Urine (~20% to 50% as unchanged drug)

Dosing: Neonatal Cyanide poisoning: Refer to Infant, Children, and Adolescent dosing.

Dosing: Usual

Pediatric: **Note:** Dosing in pediatric patients expressed in multiple units (mg/kg, mL/kg, mL/m²), use extra precaution.

Cyanide poisoning: Infants, Children, and Adolescents: **Note:** Administer sodium nitrite first, followed immediately by the administration of sodium thiosulfate. Monitor the patient for 24 to 48 hours following doses. Sodium nitrite is generally discontinued for methemoglobin levels >30%.

Sodium nitrite:

Manufacturer's labeling: IV: 6 mg/kg (0.2 mL/kg or 6 to 8 mL/m² of a 3% solution); maximum dose: 300 mg (10 mL of a 3% solution); may repeat at one-half the original dose if symptoms of cyanide toxicity return

Alternate dosing: Hemoglobin-dependent dosing: IV: For patients who are unable to tolerate significant methemoglobinemia (eg, patients with comorbidities that compromise oxygen delivery, such as heart disease, lung disease, etc), dosing may be based on hemoglobin levels (when rapid bedside testing is available) to prevent fatal methemoglobinemia; see table (Berlin, 1970).

Dosing Based on Hgb Level	
Hemoglobin Level (g/dL)	**Dose of 3% Sodium Nitrite Solution (Maximum dose: 10 mL)**
7	0.19 mL/kg
8	0.22 mL/kg
9	0.25 mL/kg
10	0.27 mL/kg
11	0.3 mL/kg
12	0.33 mL/kg
13	0.36 mL/kg
14	0.39 mL/kg

Sodium thiosulfate:

Manufacturer's labeling: IV 250 mg/kg (1 mL/kg of a 25% solution); maximum dose 12.5 g (50mL of a 25% solution). Monitor the patient for 24 to 48 hours; if symptoms return, repeat both sodium nitrite and sodium thiosulfate at one-half the original doses.

Alternate dosing: IV: 500 mg/kg (2 mL/kg of a 25% solution); maximum dose: 12.5 g (50 mL of a 25% solution). Monitor the patient for 24 to 48 hours; if symptoms return, repeat both sodium nitrite and sodium thiosulfate at one-half the original doses (Howland, 2011).

Adult:

Cyanide poisoning: IV: **Note:** Administer sodium nitrite first, followed immediately by the administration of sodium thiosulfate. Monitor the patient for 24 to 48 hours following doses. Sodium nitrite is generally discontinued for methemoglobin levels >30%.

Sodium nitrite:

Manufacturer's labeling: 300 mg (10 mL of a 3% solution); may repeat at one-half the original dose if symptoms of cyanide toxicity return

Alternate dosing: For patients who are unable to tolerate significant methemoglobinemia (eg, patients with comorbidities that compromise oxygen delivery such as heart disease, lung disease), dosing may be based on hemoglobin levels (when rapid bedside testing is available) to prevent fatal methemoglobinemia; see table (Berlin, 1970).

Dosing Based on Hgb Level	
Hemoglobin Level (g/dL)	**Dose of 3% Sodium Nitrite Solution (Maximum dose: 10 mL)**
7	0.19 mL/kg
8	0.22 mL/kg
9	0.25 mL/kg
10	0.27 mL/kg
11	0.3 mL/kg
12	0.33 mL/kg
13	0.36 mL/kg
14	0.39 mL/kg

Sodium thiosulfate: 12.5 g (50 mL of a 25% solution); may repeat at one-half the original dose if symptoms of cyanide toxicity return

Note: Monitor the patient for 24 to 48 hours; if symptoms return, repeat both sodium nitrite and sodium thiosulfate at one-half the original doses

Dosing adjustment in renal impairment: There are no dosage adjustments provided in the manufacturer's labeling; however, renal elimination of sodium nitrite and sodium thiosulfate is significant and risk of adverse effects may be increased in patients with renal impairment.

Dosing adjustment in hepatic impairment: There are no dosage adjustments provided in the manufacturer's labeling (has not been studied).

Administration Administer both components undiluted via slow IV injection as soon as possible after diagnosis of acute, life-threatening cyanide poisoning. Administer sodium nitrite at a rate of 2.5 to 5 mL/minute, followed immediately by the administration of sodium thiosulfate over 10 to 30 minutes (Howland, 2011). Decrease rate of infusion in the event of significant hypotension, nausea, or vomiting.

Monitoring Parameters Monitor for at least 24 to 48 hours after administration; blood pressure and heart rate during and after infusion; hemoglobin/hematocrit; co-oximetry; serum lactate levels; venous-arterial PO_2 gradient; serum methemoglobin and oxyhemoglobin. Pretreatment cyanide levels may be useful diagnostically.

Dosage Forms Excipient information presented when available (limited, particularly for generics); consult specific product labeling.

Injection, solution [combination package]:

Nithiodote: Sodium nitrite 300 mg/10 mL (10 mL) and sodium thiosulfate 12.5 g/50 mL (50 mL)

◆ **Sodium Nitroferricyanide** *see* Nitroprusside *on page 1526*

◆ **Sodium Nitroprusside** *see* Nitroprusside *on page 1526*

Sodium Phenylacetate and Sodium Benzoate

(SOW dee um fen il AS e tate & SOW dee um BENZ oh ate)

Brand Names: US Ammonul®

Therapeutic Category Ammonium Detoxicant; Hyperammonemia Agent; Urea Cycle Disorder (UCD) Treatment Agent

Generic Availability (US) No

Use Adjunct to treatment of acute hyperammonemia and encephalopathy in patients with urea cycle disorders involving partial or complete deficiencies of carbamylphosphate synthetase (CPS), ornithine transcarbamoylase (OTC), argininosuccinate lysase (ASL), or argininosuccinate synthetase (ASS); for use with hemodialysis in acute neonatal hyperammonemic coma, moderate-to-severe hyperammonemic encephalopathy and hyperammonemia which fails to respond to initial therapy

Pregnancy Risk Factor C

Pregnancy Considerations In animal studies, phenylacetate was shown to cause neurological toxicity. Reproduction studies have not been conducted with this combination.

Contraindications Hypersensitivity to sodium phenylacetate, sodium benzoate, or any component of the formulation

Warnings/Precautions Nausea and vomiting may occur; premedication with antiemetics may be required. Severity of hyperammonemia may require hemodialysis, as well as nutritional management and medical support. Use caution with congestive heart failure, renal or hepatic dysfunction, or sodium retention associated with edema. Administer through a central line; peripheral administration may result in burning. Must be diluted prior to administration; avoid extravasation (may cause necrosis).

Warnings: Additional Pediatric Considerations Enhanced potassium excretion may occur with treatment of hyperammonemia, monitor serum potassium concentration closely. Repeat loading doses of drug are not indicated due to prolonged plasma levels noted in pharmacokinetic studies. Maintain caloric intake at 80 cal/kg/day.

Adverse Reactions Nonspecific adverse reactions include: Nervous system disorders; metabolism and nutrition disorders; respiratory, thoracic, and mediastinal disorders; general disorders and injection site reactions; gastrointestinal disorders; blood and lymphatic system disorders; cardiac disorders; skin and subcutaneous tissue disorders; vascular disorders; psychiatric disorders; injury, poisoning, and procedural complications; renal and urinary disorders

More blood and lymphatic system, and vascular disorders were reported for patients ≤30 days of age; more gastrointestinal disorders were reported for patients >30 days.

Cardiovascular: Hypotension

Central nervous system: Agitation, brain edema, coma, mental impairment, pyrexia, seizures

Endocrine & metabolic: Acidosis, hyperammonemia, hyperglycemia, hypocalcemia, hypokalemia, metabolic acidosis

Gastrointestinal: Diarrhea, nausea, vomiting

Genitourinary: Urinary tract infection

Hematologic: Anemia, disseminated intravascular coagulation (DIC)

Local: Injection site reaction

Respiratory: Respiratory distress

Miscellaneous: Infection

Rare but important or life-threatening: Abdominal distention, acute psychosis, acute respiratory distress syndrome, aggression, alkalosis, alopecia, anuria, areflexia, ataxia, atrial rupture, blindness, blood carbon dioxide changes, blood glucose changes, blood pH increased, bradycardia, brain death, brain hemorrhage, brain herniation, brain infarction, cardiac arrest/failure, cardiac output decreased, cardiogenic shock, cardiomyopathy, cardiopulmonary arrest/failure, cerebral atrophy, chest pain, cholestasis, clonus, coagulopathy, confusion, consciousness depressed, dehydration, dyspnea, edema, encephalopathy, fluid overload/retention, flushing, gastrointestinal hemorrhage, hallucinations, hemangioma, hemorrhage, hepatic artery stenosis, hepatic failure, hepatotoxicity, hypercapnia, hyperkalemia, hypernatremia, hypertension, hyperventilation, injection site reaction (blistering, extravasation, hemorrhage), intracranial pressure increased, jaundice, Kussmaul respiration, maculopapular rash, multiorgan failure, nerve paralysis, pancytopenia, pCO2 changes, pericardial effusion, phlebothrombosis, pneumonia aspiration, pneumothorax, pruritus, pulmonary edema, pulmonary hemorrhage, rash, renal failure, respiratory alkalosis/acidosis, respiratory arrest/failure, respiratory rate increased, sepsis, septic shock, subdural hematoma, tetany, thrombocytopenia, thrombosis, tremor, urinary retention, urticaria, weakness

Drug Interactions

Metabolism/Transport Effects None known.

Avoid Concomitant Use There are no known interactions where it is recommended to avoid concomitant use.

Increased Effect/Toxicity

The levels/effects of Sodium Phenylacetate and Sodium Benzoate may be increased by: Probenecid

Decreased Effect There are no known significant interactions involving a decrease in effect.

Storage/Stability Prior to dilution, store at room temperature of 25°C (77°F); excursions permitted to 15°C to 30°C (59°F to 86°F). Following dilution, solution for infusion may be stored at room temperature for up to 24 hours.

Mechanism of Action Sodium phenylacetate and sodium benzoate provide alternate pathways for the removal of ammonia through the formation of their metabolites. One mole of sodium phenylacetate removes two moles of nitrogen; one mole of sodium benzoate removes one mole of nitrogen.

Pharmacokinetics (Adult data unless noted)

Metabolism: Hepatic and renal; sodium phenylacetate conjugates with glutamine, forming the active metabolite, phenylacetylglutamine (PAG); sodium benzoate combines with glycine to form the active metabolite hippuric acid (HIP)

Excretion: Urine

Dosing: Neonatal IV: Administer as a loading dose over 90-120 minutes, followed by an equivalent dose as a maintenance infusion over 24 hours. Arginine HCl is administered concomitantly. Dosage based on weight and specific enzyme deficiency; therapy should continue until ammonia levels are in normal range. Do not repeat loading dose.

CPS and OTC deficiency: Ammonul® 2.5 mL/kg and arginine 10% 2 mL/kg (provides sodium phenylacetate 250 mg/kg, sodium benzoate 250 mg/kg **and** arginine hydrochloride 200 mg/kg)

ASS and ASL deficiency: Ammonul® 2.5 mL/kg and arginine 10% 6 mL/kg (provides sodium phenylacetate 250 mg/kg, sodium benzoate 250 mg/kg **and** arginine hydrochloride 600 mg/kg)

Note: Pending a specific diagnosis, the bolus and maintenance dose of arginine should be 6 mL/kg. If ASS or ASL are excluded as diagnostic possibilities, reduce dose of arginine to 2 mL/kg/day.

Dosing: Usual IV: Administer as a loading dose over 90-120 minutes, followed by an equivalent dose as a maintenance infusion over 24 hours. Arginine HCl is administered concomitantly. Dosage based on weight and specific enzyme deficiency; therapy should continue until ammonia levels are in normal range. Do not repeat loading dose.

Infants and Children ≤20 kg:

CPS and OTC deficiency: Ammonul® 2.5 mL/kg and arginine 10% 2 mL/kg (provides sodium phenylacetate 250 mg/kg, sodium benzoate 250 mg/kg **and** arginine hydrochloride 200 mg/kg)

ASS and ASL deficiency: Ammonul® 2.5 mL/kg and arginine 10% 6 mL/kg (provides sodium phenylacetate 250 mg/kg, sodium benzoate 250 mg/kg **and** arginine hydrochloride 600 mg/kg)

Note: Pending a specific diagnosis in infants, the bolus and maintenance dose of arginine should be 6 mL/kg. If ASS or ASL are excluded as diagnostic possibilities, reduce dose of arginine to 2 mL/kg/day.

Children >20 kg:

CPS and OTC deficiency: Ammonul® 55 mL/m^2 and arginine 10% 2 mL/kg (provides sodium phenylacetate 5.5 g/m^2, sodium benzoate 5.5 g/m^2 **and** arginine hydrochloride 200 mg/kg)

ASS and ASL deficiency: Ammonul® 55 mL/m^2 and arginine 10% 6 mL/kg (provides sodium phenylacetate 5.5 g/m^2, sodium benzoate 5.5 g/m^2, **and** arginine hydrochloride 600 mg/kg)

Dosage adjustment in renal impairment: Use with caution; monitor closely

Dialysis: Ammonia clearance is ~10 times greater with hemodialysis than by peritoneal dialysis or hemofiltration. Exchange transfusion is ineffective.

Dosage adjustment in hepatic impairment: Use with caution

Preparation for Administration IV: Dilute in $D_{10}W$ at ≥25 mL/kg; may mix with arginine HCl.

Administration IV: Must be administered via central line; administration via peripheral line may cause burns. Dilute in $D_{10}W$ prior to administration. May mix with arginine HCl. Infuse loading dose over 90 to 120 minutes; maintenance dose is a continuous infusion infused over 24 hours. In case of extravasation, discontinue infusion and resume at new injection site. Antiemetics may be needed to decrease nausea during infusion.

Monitoring Parameters Neurologic status, plasma ammonia, plasma glutamine, clinical response, serum electrolytes (potassium or bicarbonate supplementation may be required), acid-base balance, infusion site

Reference Range Long-term target levels (may not be appropriate for every patient):

Plasma ammonia: <40 µmol/L

Plasma glutamine: <1000 µmol/L

Normal plasma levels of alanine, glycine, lysine, arginine (except in arginase deficiency); normal urinary orotate excretion; normal plasma protein concentration

Additional Information Ucephan® (sodium phenylacetate and sodium benzoate), was previously available as an oral liquid for chronic treatment of urea cycle disorders. Although no longer commercially available, this combination may be compounded for patients not responsive to or tolerant of other treatments.

Dosage Forms Excipient information presented when available (limited, particularly for generics); consult specific product labeling.

Injection, solution [concentrate]:

Ammonul®: Sodium phenylacetate 100 mg and sodium benzoate 100 mg per 1 mL (50 mL)

Sodium Phenylbutyrate

(SOW dee um fen il BYOO ti rate)

Brand Names: US Buphenyl

Brand Names: Canada Pheburane

Therapeutic Category Ammonium Detoxicant; Hyperammonemia Agent; Urea Cycle Disorder (UCD) Treatment Agent

Generic Availability (US) May be product dependent

Use Adjunctive therapy in the chronic management of patients with urea cycle disorder involving deficiencies of carbamoylphosphate synthetase, ornithine transcarbamylase, or argininosuccinic acid synthetase; provides an alternative pathway for waste nitrogen excretion

Pregnancy Risk Factor C

Pregnancy Considerations Animal reproduction studies have not been conducted.

Breast-Feeding Considerations It is not known if sodium phenylbutyrate is excreted in breast milk. The manufacturer recommends that caution be exercised when administering sodium phenylbutyrate to nursing women.

Contraindications Should not be used in the treatment of acute hyperammonemia

Warnings/Precautions May cause sodium and fluid retention; use with caution in patients where fluid accumulation may be poorly tolerated. Contains sodium 125 mg per gram; use with caution, if at all, in patients who must maintain a low sodium intake. Hyperammonemia and hyperammonemic encephalopathy may still occur while on therapy; hyperammonemia should be managed as a medical emergency. Use with caution in patients with hepatic and renal impairment. The use of sodium phenylbutyrate tablets in children weighing <20 kg is not recommended.

Adverse Reactions

Cardiovascular: Syncope

Central nervous system: Depression, headache

Dermatologic: Rash

Endocrine & metabolic: Acidosis, alkalosis, amenorrhea/menstrual dysfunction, hyperbilirubinemia, hyperchloremia, hyper-/hypophosphatemia, hypernatremia, hyperuricemia, hypokalemia, total protein decreased

Gastrointestinal: Abdominal pain, abnormal taste, anorexia, gastritis, nausea, vomiting

Hematologic: Anemia, leukocytosis, leukopenia, thrombocytopenia, thrombocytosis

Hepatic: Alkaline phosphatase increased, transaminases increased

Renal: Renal tubular acidosis

Miscellaneous: Offensive body odor

Rare but important or life-threatening: Aplastic anemia, arrhythmia, bruising, constipation, edema, fatigue, lightheadedness, memory impairment, neuropathy (exacerbation), pancreatitis, peptic ulcer disease, rectal bleeding, somnolence

Drug Interactions

Metabolism/Transport Effects **Inhibits** CYP1A2 (weak), CYP2C19 (weak), CYP2C8 (weak), CYP2C9 (weak), CYP2D6 (weak)

Avoid Concomitant Use

Avoid concomitant use of Sodium Phenylbutyrate with any of the following: Amodiaquine

Increased Effect/Toxicity

Sodium Phenylbutyrate may increase the levels/effects of: Amodiaquine; ARIPiprazole; TiZANidine

The levels/effects of Sodium Phenylbutyrate may be increased by: Probenecid

Decreased Effect

The levels/effects of Sodium Phenylbutyrate may be decreased by: Corticosteroids (Systemic); Haloperidol; Valproic Acid and Derivatives

Storage/Stability Store at room temperature of 15°C to 30°C (59°F to 86°F). After opening, containers should be kept tightly closed.

Powder for oral solution: Use immediately after mixing powder with food, but stable up to 1 week if dissolved in water (5 g/10 mL) and stored at room temperature or in refrigerator.

Mechanism of Action Sodium phenylbutyrate is a prodrug which is rapidly converted to phenylacetate, followed by conjugation with glutamine to form phenylacetylglutamine; phenylacetylglutamine serves as a substitute for urea as it is clears nitrogenous waste from the body when excreted in the urine.

Pharmacokinetics (Adult data unless noted)

Distribution: V_d: 0.2 L/kg

Metabolism: conjugation to phenylacetylglutamine (active form); undergoes nonlinear Michaelis-Menten elimination kinetics

Half-life: 0.8 hours (parent compound); 1.2 hours (phenylacetate)

Time to peak serum concentration:

Powder: 1 hour

Tablet: 1.35 hours

Elimination: 80% of metabolite excreted in urine in 24 hours

Dosing: Neonatal Oral: 300-600 mg/kg/day divided 4-6 times daily dependent upon deficiency type (Berry, 2001)

Arginase deficiency: 300-600 mg/kg/day divided 4 times daily

Argininosuccinic acid lyase (ASL), argininosuccinic synthetase (ASS), carbamyl phosphate synthetase I (CPS), or ornithine transcarbamylase (OTC) deficiency: 450-600 mg/kg/day divided 4 times daily

Dosing: Usual Oral:

Infants and Children <20 kg: 300-600 mg/kg/day divided 4-6 times daily dependent upon on deficiency type; maximum daily dose: 20 g/day (Berry, 2001)

Arginase deficiency: 300-600 mg/kg/day divided 4 times daily

Argininosuccinic acid lyase (ASL), argininosuccinic synthetase (ASS), carbamyl phosphate synthetase I (CPS), or ornithine transcarbamylase (OTC) deficiency: 450-600 mg/kg/day divided 4 times daily

Children >20 kg and Adults: 9.9-13 g/m^2/day, divided 4-6 times daily; maximum daily dose: 20 g/day (Berry, 2001)

Administration Oral: Administer with meals or feedings; mix powder with food or drink; avoid mixing with acidic beverages (eg, most fruit juices or colas)

Monitoring Parameters Plasma ammonia and glutamine concentrations, serum electrolytes, proteins, hepatic and renal function tests, physical signs/symptoms of hyperammonemia (ie, lethargy, ataxia, confusion, vomiting, seizures, and memory impairment)

Additional Information Teaspoon and tablespoon measuring devices are provided with the powder; each 1 g powder contains 0.94 g sodium phenylbutyrate = 125 mg sodium; each tablet contains 0.5 g sodium phenylbutyrate = 62 mg sodium

Dosage Forms Considerations Powder products: 1 level teaspoon provides 3 g sodium phenylbutyrate, 1 level tablespoon provides 8.6 g sodium phenylbutyrate. Measurers provided with the product.

Dosage Forms Excipient information presented when available (limited, particularly for generics); consult specific product labeling.

Powder, Oral:

Buphenyl: (250 g) [contains sodium 125 mg/g]

Generic: (250 g)

Tablet, Oral:

Buphenyl: 500 mg [contains sodium 62 mg/tablet]

Extemporaneous Preparations A 200 mg/mL oral suspension may be prepared with sodium phenylbutyrate powder, USP; Ora-Plus®; and either Ora-Sweet® or Ora-Sweet® SF. Place 12 g of sodium phenylbutyrate in a glass mortar and reduce to a fine powder. Separately, mix 30 mL Ora-Plus® and 30 mL of either Ora-Sweet® or Ora-Sweet® SF for a total volume of 60 mL. Add 30 mL of the vehicle mixture to the powder and mix to a uniform smooth suspension. Transfer the mixture into a 2 oz amber prescription bottle; rinse mortar with vehicle, and add quantity of vehicle sufficient to make 60 mL. Label "shake well". Stable for 90 days at room temperature. **Note:** Authors recommend administering a masking agent such as chocolate syrup or peanut butter, before and after medication administration, to mask the bitter taste.

Caruthers RL and Johnson CE, "Stability of Extemporaneously Prepared Sodium Phenylbutyrate Oral Suspensions," *Am J Health Syst Pharm*, 2007, 64(14):1513-5.

◆ **Sodium Phosphate and Potassium Phosphate** *see* Potassium Phosphate and Sodium Phosphate *on page 1746*

Sodium Phosphates (SOW dee um FOS fates)

Medication Safety Issues

Administration issues:

Enemas and oral solution are available in pediatric and adult sizes; prescribe by "volume" not by "bottle."

Because inorganic phosphate exists as monobasic and dibasic anions, with the mixture of valences dependent on pH, ordering by mEq amounts is unreliable and may lead to large dosing errors. In addition, IV phosphate is available in the sodium and potassium salt; therefore, the content of these cations must be considered when ordering phosphate. The most reliable method of ordering IV phosphate is by millimoles, then specifying the potassium or sodium salt.

Brand Names: US Fleet Enema Extra [OTC]; Fleet Enema [OTC]; Fleet Pedia-Lax Enema [OTC]; LaCrosse Complete [OTC]; OsmoPrep

Brand Names: Canada Fleet Enema

Therapeutic Category Electrolyte Supplement, Oral; Electrolyte Supplement, Parenteral; Laxative, Saline; Sodium Salt

Generic Availability (US) Yes: Enema, injection, oral solution

Use

Injection: Treatment and prevention of hypophosphatemia; source of phosphate in large-volume IV fluids (FDA approved in all ages)

Oral:

Solution: Treatment of occasional constipation (OTC product: FDA approved in ages ≥5 years and adults)

Tablets (OsmoPrep): Bowel cleansing for colonoscopy (FDA approved in adults)

Rectal: Treatment of occasional constipation (OTC product: Fleet Pedia-Lax Enema: FDA approved in ages 2-11 years; Fleet Enema, Fleet Enema Extra: FDA approved in ages ≥12 years and adults. Refer to product-specific information to determine FDA approved ages for additional products).

Medication Guide Available Yes

Pregnancy Risk Factor C

Pregnancy Considerations Reproduction studies have not been conducted with these products. Use with caution in pregnant women.

Breast-Feeding Considerations Phosphorus, sodium, and potassium are normal constituents of human milk.

Contraindications Hypersensitivity to sodium phosphate salts or any component of the formulation; additional contraindications vary by product:

Enema: Ascites, clinically significant renal impairment, heart failure, imperforate anus, known or suspected GI obstruction, megacolon (congenital or acquired)

Intravenous preparation: Diseases with hyperphosphatemia, hypocalcemia, or hypernatremia

Tablets: Acute phosphate nephropathy (biopsy proven), bowel obstruction, bowel perforation, gastric bypass or stapling surgery, toxic colitis, toxic megacolon

OTC labeling (Oral Solution): When used for self-medication: Dehydration, heart failure, renal impairment, electrolyte abnormalities; use for bowel cleansing, use in children <5 years

Warnings/Precautions [U.S. Boxed Warning]: Acute phosphate nephropathy has been reported (rarely) with use of oral products as a colon cleanser prior to colonoscopy. Some cases have resulted in permanent renal impairment (some requiring dialysis). Risk factors for acute phosphate nephropathy may include increased age (>55 years of age), pre-existing renal dysfunction, bowel obstruction, active colitis, or dehydration, and the use of medicines that affect renal perfusion or function (eg, ACE inhibitors, angiotensin receptor blockers, diuretics, and possibly NSAIDs), although some cases have been reported in patients without apparent risk factors. Other preventive measures may include avoid exceeding maximum recommended doses and concurrent use of other laxatives containing sodium phosphate; encourage patients to adequately hydrate before, during, and after use; obtain baseline and postprocedure labs in patients at risk; consider hospitalization and intravenous hydration during bowel cleansing for patients unable to hydrate themselves (eg, frail patients). Use is contraindicated in patients with acute phosphate nephropathy (biopsy proven).

Use with caution in patients with impaired renal dysfunction, pre-existing electrolyte imbalances, risk of electrolyte disturbance (hypocalcemia, hyperphosphatemia, hypernatremia), or dehydration. If using as a bowel evacuant, correct electrolyte abnormalities before administration. Use caution in patients with unstable angina, history of myocardial infarction arrhythmia, cardiomyopathy; use caution in patients with or at risk for arrhythmias (eg, cardiomyopathy, prolonged QT interval, history of uncontrolled arrhythmias, recent MI) or with concurrent use of other QT-prolonging medications; pre-/postdose ECGs should be considered in high-risk patients.

Use caution in inflammatory bowel disease or severe active ulcerative colitis; may induce colonic aphthous ulceration and ischemic colitis (some requiring hospitalization). Use caution in patients with any of the following: Gastric retention or hypomotility, ileus, severe, chronic constipation, colitis. Use is contraindicated in patients with bowel obstruction (including pseudo) or perforation, congenital megacolon, gastric bypass or bariatric surgery, toxic colitis, or toxic megacolon. Use with caution in patients with impaired gag reflex and those prone to regurgitation or aspiration.

Use with caution in patients with a history of seizures and those at higher risk of seizures. Ensure adequate clear liquid intake prior to and during bowel evacuation regimens; inadequate fluid intake may lead to dehydration. Other oral medications may not be well absorbed when given during bowel evacuation because of rapid intestinal peristalsis. Use with caution in debilitated patients; consider each patient's ability to hydrate properly. Use with caution in geriatric patients. Laxatives and purgatives have the potential for abuse by bulimia nervosa patients.

Enemas and oral solution are available in pediatric and adult sizes; prescribe by "volume" not by "bottle."

Rare but potentially serious adverse effects (including death) may occur when exceeding recommended doses of over-the-counter (OTC) sodium phosphate preparations to treat constipation. Severe dehydration and alterations in serum electrolytes (eg, calcium, sodium, phosphate) leading to renal/cardiac adverse effects have been reported, mostly when single maximum doses were exceeded or when more than 1 dose was taken per day. Patients should be advised to adhere to the product labeling and not exceed maximum recommended doses. Health care providers should use caution when recommending doses for oral sodium phosphate preparations for children younger than 5 years of age. Rectal preparations should never be administered to children younger than 2 years of age (FDA Drug Safety Communication, 2014).

Aluminum: The parenteral product may contain aluminum; toxic aluminum concentrations may be seen with high doses, prolonged use, or renal dysfunction. Premature neonates are at higher risk due to immature renal function and aluminum intake from other parenteral sources. Parenteral aluminum exposure of >4 to 5 mcg/kg/day is associated with CNS and bone toxicity; tissue loading may occur at lower doses (Federal Register, 2002). See manufacturer's labeling.

Benzyl alcohol and derivatives: Some dosage forms may contain sodium benzoate/benzoic acid; benzoic acid (benzoate) is a metabolite of benzyl alcohol; large amounts of benzyl alcohol (≥99 mg/kg/day) have been associated with a potentially fatal toxicity ("gasping syndrome") in neonates; the "gasping syndrome" consists of metabolic acidosis, respiratory distress, gasping respirations, CNS dysfunction (including convulsions, intracranial hemorrhage), hypotension, and cardiovascular collapse (AAP, 1997; CDC, 1982); some data suggests that benzoate displaces bilirubin from protein binding sites (Ahlfors, 2001); avoid or use dosage forms containing benzyl alcohol derivative with caution in neonates. See manufacturer's labeling.

Adverse Reactions

Central nervous system: Dizziness, headache

Gastrointestinal: Abdominal pain, bloating, mucosal bleeding, nausea, superficial mucosal ulcerations, vomiting

Endocrine & metabolic: Hypernatremia, hyperphosphatemia, hypocalcemia (on colonoscopy day), hypokalemia (on colonoscopy day), hypophosphatemia (2-3 days postcolonoscopy)

Postmarketing and/or case reports: Acute phosphate nephropathy, anaphylaxis, bronchospasm, calcium nephrolithiasis, cardiac arrhythmia, dehydration, dysphagia, dyspnea, facial edema, increased blood urea nitrogen, increased serum creatinine, ischemic colitis, lip edema, paresthesia, pharyngeal edema, pruritus, rectal bleeding, renal failure, renal insufficiency, renal tubular necrosis, seizure, skin rash, tightness in throat, tongue edema, urticaria

Drug Interactions

Metabolism/Transport Effects None known.

Avoid Concomitant Use There are no known interactions where it is recommended to avoid concomitant use.

Increased Effect/Toxicity

Sodium Phosphates may increase the levels/effects of: Nonsteroidal Anti-Inflammatory Agents

The levels/effects of Sodium Phosphates may be increased by: ACE Inhibitors; Angiotensin II Receptor Blockers; Diuretics; Tricyclic Antidepressants

Decreased Effect

The levels/effects of Sodium Phosphates may be decreased by: Antacids; Calcium Salts; Iron Salts; Magnesium Salts; Multivitamins/Minerals (with ADEK, Folate, Iron); Sucralfate

Storage/Stability

Enema: Store at room temperature.

Oral solution: Store at room temperature.

Solution for injection: Store intact vials at 20°C to 25°C (68°F to 77°F); excursions permitted between 15°C and 30°C (59°F and 86°F).

Tablet: Store at 25°C (77°F); excursions permitted between 15°C and 30°C (59°F and 86°F).

Mechanism of Action As a laxative, exerts osmotic effect in the small intestine by drawing water into the lumen of the gut, producing distention and promoting peristalsis and evacuation of the bowel; phosphorous participates in bone deposition, calcium metabolism, utilization of B complex vitamins, and as a buffer in acid-base equilibrium

Pharmacodynamics Onset of action (catharsis):

Oral: 3-6 hours

Rectal: 2-5 minutes

Pharmacokinetics (Adult data unless noted)

Absorption: Oral: 1% to 20%

Elimination: Oral forms excreted in feces; IV forms are excreted in the urine with over 80% to 90% of dose reabsorbed by the kidney

Dosing: Neonatal Note: If phosphate repletion is required and a phosphate product is not available at your institution, consider the use of sodium glycerophosphate pentahydrate (Glycophos) as a suitable substitute. Concentration and dosing are different from FDA approved products; use caution when switching between products. Refer to Sodium Glycerophosphate Pentahydrate monograph.

Caution: With orders for IV phosphate, there is considerable confusion associated with the use of millimoles (mmol) versus milliequivalents (mEq) to express the phosphate requirement. The most reliable method of ordering IV phosphate is by millimoles, then specifying the potassium or sodium salt. Intravenous doses listed as mmol of phosphate. **Note:** Consider the contribution of sodium when determining the appropriate phosphate replacement.

Phosphorus Estimated Average Requirement (EAR): Dietary Intake Reference (DIR) (1997 National Academy of Science Recommendations) (**Note:** DIR is under review as of March 2009): Oral: 3.2 mmol/day (adequate intake)

Parenteral nutrition, maintenance requirement (Mirtallo, 2004): IV: 1-2 mmol/kg/day

Dosing: Usual Note: If phosphate repletion is required and a phosphate product is not available at your institution, consider the use of sodium glycerophosphate pentahydrate (Glycophos) as a suitable substitute. Concentration and dosing are different from FDA approved products; use caution when switching between products. Refer to Sodium Glycerophosphate Pentahydrate monograph.

Caution: With orders for IV phosphate, there is considerable confusion associated with the use of millimoles (mmol) versus milliequivalents (mEq) to express the phosphate requirement. The most reliable method of ordering IV phosphate is by millimoles, then specifying the potassium or sodium salt. Intravenous doses listed as mmol of phosphate. **Note:** Consider the contribution of sodium when determining the appropriate phosphate replacement.

Infants, Children, and Adolescents: Phosphorus: Oral: See table.

Phosphorus – Recommended Daily Allowance (RDA) and Estimated Average Requirement (EAR)

Age	RDA (mmol/day)	EAR (mmol/day)
1-6 mo	–	3.2[A]
7-12 mo	–	8.9[A]
1-3 y	14.8	12.3
4-8 y	16.1	13.1
9-18 y	40.3	34
19-30 y	22.6	18.7

[A]Adequate intake (AI)

Hypophosphatemia, acute: Hypophosphatemia does not necessarily equate with phosphate depletion. Hypophosphatemia may occur in the presence of low, normal, or high total body phosphate and conversely, phosphate depletion may exist with normal, low, or elevated levels of serum phosphate (Gaasbeek, 2005). It is difficult to provide concrete guidelines for the treatment of severe hypophosphatemia because the extent of total body deficits and response to therapy are difficult to predict. Aggressive doses of phosphate may result in a transient serum elevation followed by redistribution into intracellular compartments or bone tissue. Intermittent IV infusion should be reserved for severe depletion situations; requires continuous cardiac monitoring. Guidelines differ based on degree of illness, need/use of TPN, and severity of hypophosphatemia. If hypokalemia exists, consider phosphate replacement strategy with potassium (eg, potassium phosphates). Various regimens for replacement of phosphate in adults have been studied. The regimens below have only been studied in adult patients; however, many institutions have used them in children safely and successfully. Obese patients and/or severe renal impairment were excluded from phosphate supplement trials. **Note:** 1 mmol phosphate = 31 mg phosphorus; 1 mg phosphorus = 0.032 mmol phosphate.

IV doses may be incorporated into the patient's maintenance IV fluids; intermittent IV infusion should be reserved for severe depletion situations. **Note:** Doses listed as mmol of **phosphate**.

Children and Adolescents: **Note:** There are no prospective studies of parenteral phosphate replacement in children. The following weight-based guidelines for adult dosing may be cautiously employed in pediatric patients. Guidelines differ based on degree of illness, use of TPN, and severity of hypophosphatemia.

General replacement guidelines (Lentz, 1978): **Note:** The initial dose may be increased by 25% to 50% if the patient is symptomatic secondary to hypophosphatemia and lowered by 25% to 50% if the patient is hypercalcemic.

Low dose: 0.08 mmol/kg over 6 hours; use if losses are recent and uncomplicated

Intermediate dose: 0.16-0.24 mmol/kg over 4-6 hours; use if serum phosphorus level 0.5-1 mg/dL (0.16-0.32 mmol/L)

High dose: 0.36 mmol/kg over 6 hours; use if serum phosphorus <0.5 mg/dL (<0.16 mmol/L)

Patients receiving TPN (Clark, 1995):

Low dose: 0.16 mmol/kg over 4-6 hours; use if serum phosphorus level 2.3-3 mg/dL (0.73- 0.96 mmol/L)

Intermediate dose: 0.32 mmol/kg over 4-6 hours; use if serum phosphorus level 1.6-2.2 mg/dL (0.51-0.72 mmol/L)

High dose: 0.64 mmol/kg over 8-12 hours; use if serum phosphorus <1.5 mg/dL (<0.5 mmol/L)

Critically ill adult trauma patients receiving TPN (Brown, 2006):

Low dose: 0.32 mmol/kg over 4-6 hours; use if serum phosphorus level 2.3-3 mg/dL (0.73-0.96 mmol/L)

Intermediate dose: 0.64 mmol/kg over 4-6 hours; use if serum phosphorus level 1.6-2.2 mg/dL (0.51-0.72 mmol/L)

High dose: 1 mmol/kg over 8-12 hours; use if serum phosphorus <1.5 mg/dL (<0.5 mmol/L)

Alternative method in critically ill patients (Kingston, 1985):

Low dose: 0.25 mmol/kg over 4 hours; use if serum phosphorus level 0.5-1 mg/dL (0.16-0.32 mmol/L)

Moderate dose: 0.5 mmol/kg over 4 hours; use if serum phosphorus level <0.5 mg/dL (<0.16 mmol/L)

Maintenance: Oral: 2-3 mmol/kg/day in divided doses (including dietary intake)

Parenteral nutrition, maintenance requirement (Mirtallo, 2004): IV:

Infants and Children ≤50 kg: 0.5-2 mmol/kg/day

Children >50 kg and Adolescents: 10-40 mmol/day

Constipation:

Oral, solution (Monobasic sodium phosphate monohydrate 2.4 g and dibasic sodium phosphate heptahydrate 0.9 g per 5 mL): **Note:** Must be diluted in a full glass of water:

Children 5-9 years: 7.5 mL as a single dose

Children 10-11 years: 15 mL as a single dose

Children ≥12 years and Adolescents: 15 mL as a single dose; maximum single daily dose: 45 mL/**day**

Rectal: Fleet Enema:

Children 2-4 years: Administer **one half** contents of one 2.25 ounce pediatric enema

Children 5-11 years: Administer the contents of one 2.25 ounce pediatric enema

Children ≥12 years and Adolescents: Administer the contents of one 4.5 ounce enema as a single dose

Adults:

Hypophosphatemia, acute treatment: IV: It is difficult to provide concrete guidelines for the treatment of severe hypophosphatemia because the extent of total body deficits and response to therapy are difficult to predict. Aggressive doses of phosphate may result in a transient serum elevation followed by redistribution into intracellular compartments or bone tissue. It is recommended that repletion of severe hypophosphatemia be done IV because large doses of oral phosphate may cause diarrhea and intestinal absorption may be unreliable. Intermittent IV infusion should be reserved for severe depletion situations; requires continuous cardiac monitoring. Guidelines differ based on degree of illness, need/use of TPN, and severity of hypophosphatemia. If hypokalemia exists (some clinicians recommend threshold of <4 mmol/L), consider phosphate replacement strategy with potassium (eg, potassium phosphates). Obese patients and/or severe renal impairment patients were excluded from phosphate supplement trials. **Note:** 1 mmol phosphate = 31 mg phosphorus; 1 mg phosphorus = 0.032 mmol phosphate.

General replacement guidelines (Lentz, 1978):

Low dose, serum phosphorus losses are recent and uncomplicated: 0.08 mmol/kg over 6 hours

Intermediate dose, serum phosphorus level 0.5-1 mg/dL (0.16-0.32 mmol/L): 0.16-0.24 mmol/kg over 6 hours

Note: The initial dose may be increased by 25% to 50% if the patient is symptomatic secondary to hypophosphatemia and lowered by 25% to 50% if the patient is hypercalcemic.

Critically ill adult patients receiving concurrent enteral/parenteral nutrition (Brown, 2006; Clark, 1995): **Note:** Round doses to the nearest 7.5 mmol for ease of preparation. If administering with phosphate-containing parenteral nutrition, do not exceed 15 mmol/L within parenteral nutrition. May use adjusted body weight for patients weighing >130% of ideal body weight (and BMI <40 kg/m^2) by using [IBW + 0.25 (ABW-IBW)]:

Low dose, serum phosphorus level 2.3-3 mg/dL (0.74-0.96 mmol/L): 0.16-0.32 mmol/kg over 4-6 hours

Intermediate dose, serum phosphorus level 1.6-2.2 mg/dL (0.51-0.71 mmol/L): 0.32-0.64 mmol/kg over 4-6 hours

High dose, serum phosphorus <1.5 mg/dL (<0.5 mmol/L): 0.64-1 mmol/kg over 8-12 hours

Parenteral nutrition: IV: 10-15 mmol/1000 kcal (Hicks, 2001) **or** 20-40 mmol/24 hours (Mirtallo, 2004)

Laxative (Fleet): Rectal: Contents of one 4.5 oz enema as a single dose

Laxative: Oral solution: 15 mL as a single dose; maximum single daily dose: 45 mL

Bowel cleansing prior to colonoscopy: Oral tablets: **Note:** Do not use additional agents, especially other sodium phosphate products.

OsmoPrep: A total of 32 tablets and 2 quarts of clear liquids (8 ounces of clear liquids with each dose) divided as follows:

Evening before colonoscopy: 4 tablets every 15 minutes for 5 doses (total of 20 tablets)

3-5 hours prior to colonoscopy: 4 tablets every 15 minutes for 3 doses (total of 12 tablets)

Preparation for Administration Parenteral: Observe the vial for the presence of crystals. Do not use vial if crystals are present. Injection must be diluted in appropriate IV solution and volume prior to administration. **Note:** Due to the potential for solution crystallization, American Regent, Inc recommends the use of a 5 micron filter when preparing IV sodium phosphate containing solutions (Important Drug Safety Information, American Regent 2011); a similar recommendation has not been noted by other manufacturers.

Intermittent IV infusion: In general, the dose, concentration of infusion, and rate of administration may be dependent on patient condition and specific institution policy. Intermittent infusion doses of sodium phosphate for adults are typically prepared in 100 to 250 mL of NS or D_5W (usual phosphate concentration range: 0.15 to 0.6 mmol/mL) (Charron 2003; Rosen 1995).

Pediatric suggested maximum concentrations used by some centers:

Central line administration: 12 mmoL sodium phosphate/100 mL

Peripheral line administration: 5 mmoL sodium phosphate/100 mL

Adult suggested maximum concentrations:

Central line administration: 26.8 mmoL sodium phosphate/100 mL

Peripheral line administration: 6.7 mmoL sodium phosphate/100 mL

Administration

Oral: Maintain adequate fluid intake

Constipation (oral solution): Take on an empty stomach; dilute dose in 8 ounces of cool water, follow with an additional 8 ounces of water; **do not repeat dose within 24 hours**.

Bowel cleansing (OsmoPrep): Administer each dose with at least 8 ounces of clear liquids; have patient rehydrate before and after colonoscopy. Clear liquids may include water, flavored water, pulp-free lemonade, ginger ale, or apple juice; purple or red colored liquids should be avoided.

Parenteral: **Note:** In general, the dose, concentration of infusion, and rate of administration may be dependent on patient condition and specific institution policy. Due to the potential for solution crystallization, American Regent, Inc recommends the use of a 0.22-micron in-line filter for IV administration (1.2-micron filter if admixture contains lipids) (Important Drug Safety Information, American Regent 2011); a similar recommendation has not been noted by other manufacturers.

Intermittent IV infusion: Must be diluted in appropriate IV solution and volume prior to administration and infused slowly to avoid toxicity; in pediatric patients, suggested maximum concentrations used by some centers: Peripheral line: 0.05 mmol/mL; Central line: 0.12 mmol/mL (maximum concentrations were determined with consideration for maximum sodium concentration). Infusion of doses over 4 to 6 hours for mild/moderate hypophosphatemia or 8 to 12 hours for severe hypophosphatemia has been recommended (Brown 2006; Clark 1995; Lentz 1978); for adult patients with severe symptomatic hypophosphatemia (ie, <1.5 mg/dL), may administer at rates up to 15 mmol phosphate/hour (Charron 2003; Rosen 1995). Maximum rate of infusion: 0.06 mmol/kg/hour; do not infuse with calcium-containing IV fluids.

Parenteral nutrition solution: Calcium-phosphate stability in parenteral nutrition solutions is dependent upon the pH of the solution, temperature, and relative concentration of each ion. The pH of the solution is primarily dependent upon the amino acid concentration. The higher the percentage amino acids the lower the pH, the more soluble the calcium and phosphate. Individual commercially available amino acid solutions vary significantly with respect to pH lowering potential and subsequent calcium phosphate compatibility; consult product specific labeling for additional information.

Rectal: Gently insert enema tip into rectum with a slight side-to-side movement and tip pointing toward the navel; have patient bear down. Administer with patient lying on left side and knees bent or with patient kneeling and head and chest leaning forward until left side of face is resting comfortably. **Note:** Preparation for **one half** bottle administration: Unscrew cap and remove 30 mL of liquid; replace cap and administer as usual.

Monitoring Parameters

IV: Serum sodium, calcium, and phosphorus concentrations; renal function; in pediatric patients after IV phosphate repletion, repeat serum phosphorus concentration should be checked 2 hours later (ASPEN Pediatric Nutrition Support Core Curriculum, 2010)

Oral: Bowel cleansing: Baseline and postprocedure labs (electrolytes, calcium, phosphorus, BUN, creatinine) in patients at risk for acute renal nephropathy, seizure, or who have a history of electrolyte abnormality; ECG in patients with risks for prolonged QT or arrhythmias. Ensure euvolemia before initiating bowel preparation.

Rectal: Stool output

Reference Range Note: There is a diurnal variation with the nadir at 1100, plateau at 1600, and peak in the early evening (Gaasbeek, 2005); 1 mmol/L phosphate = 3.1 mg/dL phosphorus

Newborn 0-5 days: 4.8-8.2 mg/dL

1-3 years: 3.8-6.5 mg/dL

4-11 years: 3.7-5.6 mg/dL

12-15 years: 2.9-5.4 mg/dL

16-19 years: 2.7-4.7 mg/dL

Additional Information Cow's milk is a good source of phosphate with 1 mg elemental (0.032 mmol) elemental phosphate per mL

Fleet Pedia-Lax Enema: 2.25 oz bottle administers 59 mL

Fleet Enema: 4.5 oz bottle administers 118 mL

Dosage Forms Considerations

Sodium 4 mEq is equivalent to sodium 92 mg

Phosphorous 3 mmol is equivalent to phosphorus 93 mg

Dosage Forms Excipient information presented when available (limited, particularly for generics); consult specific product labeling.

Injection, solution [concentrate; preservative free]: Phosphorus 3 mmol and sodium 4 mEq per 1 mL (5 mL, 15 mL, 50 mL) [equivalent to phosphorus 93 mg and sodium 92 mg per 1 mL; source of electrolytes: monobasic and dibasic sodium phosphate]

Solution, oral: Monobasic sodium phosphate monohydrate 2.4 g and dibasic sodium phosphate heptahydrate 0.9 g per 5 mL (45 mL) [sugar free; contains sodium 556 mg/5 mL, sodium benzoate; ginger-lemon flavor]

Solution, rectal [enema]: Monobasic sodium phosphate monohydrate 19 g and dibasic sodium phosphate heptahydrate 7 g per 118 mL delivered dose (133 mL)

Fleet Enema: Monobasic sodium phosphate monohydrate 19 g and dibasic sodium phosphate heptahydrate 7 g per 118 mL delivered dose (133 mL) [contains sodium 4.4 g/118 mL]

Fleet Enema Extra: Monobasic sodium phosphate monohydrate 19 g and dibasic sodium phosphate heptahydrate 7 g per 197 mL delivered dose (230 mL) [contains sodium 4.4 g/197 mL]

Fleet Pedia-Lax™ Enema: Monobasic sodium phosphate monohydrate 9.5 g and dibasic sodium phosphate heptahydrate 3.5 g per 59 mL delivered dose (66 mL) [contains sodium 2.2 g/59 mL]

LaCrosse Complete: Monobasic sodium phosphate monohydrate 19 g and dibasic sodium phosphate heptahydrate 7 g per 118 mL delivered dose (133 mL) [contains sodium 4.4 g/118 mL]

Tablet, oral [scored]:

OsmoPrep: Monobasic sodium phosphate monohydrate 1.102 g and dibasic sodium phosphate anhydrous 0.398 g [sodium phosphate 1.5 g per tablet; gluten free]

Sodium Polystyrene Sulfonate

(SOW dee um pol ee STYE reen SUL fon ate)

Medication Safety Issues

Sound-alike/look-alike issues:

Kayexalate® may be confused with Kaopectate®

Sodium polystyrene sulfonate may be confused with calcium polystyrene sulfonate

Administration issues:

Always prescribe either one-time doses or as a specific number of doses (eg, 15 g q6h x 2 doses). Scheduled doses with no dosage limit could be given for days leading to dangerous hypokalemia.

International issues:

Kionex [U.S.] may be confused with Kinex brand name for biperiden [Mexico]

Brand Names: US Kalexate; Kayexalate; Kionex; SPS

Brand Names: Canada Kayexalate®; PMS-Sodium Polystyrene Sulfonate

Therapeutic Category Antidote, Hyperkalemia

Generic Availability (US) Yes

Use Treatment of hyperkalemia (FDA approved in adults)

Pregnancy Risk Factor C

Pregnancy Considerations Animal reproduction studies have not been conducted. There are no adequate and well-controlled studies in pregnant women. Use during pregnancy only if benefits outweigh the risks.

Breast-Feeding Considerations It is not known if sodium polystyrene sulfonate is excreted in breast milk. The manufacturer recommends that caution be exercised when administering sodium polystyrene sulfonate to nursing women.

Contraindications Hypersensitivity to sodium polystyrene sulfonate or any component of the formulation; hypokalemia; obstructive bowel disease; neonates with reduced gut motility (postoperatively or drug-induced); oral administration in neonates

Additional contraindications: Sodium polystyrene sulfonate suspension (**with** sorbitol): Rectal administration in neonates (particularly in premature infants); any postoperative patient until normal bowel function resumes

Warnings/Precautions Intestinal necrosis (including fatalities) and other serious gastrointestinal events (eg, bleeding, ischemic colitis, perforation) have been reported, especially when administered with sorbitol. Increased risk may be associated with a history of intestinal disease or surgery, hypovolemia, prematurity, and renal insufficiency or failure; use with sorbitol is not recommended. Avoid use in any postoperative patient until normal bowel function resumes or in patients at risk for constipation or impaction; discontinue use if constipation occurs. Oral or rectal administration of sorbitol-containing sodium polystyrene sulfonate suspensions is contraindicated in neonates (particularly with prematurity). Use with caution in patients with severe HF, hypertension, or edema; sodium load may exacerbate condition. Effective lowering of serum potassium from sodium polystyrene sulfonate may take hours to days after administration; consider alternative measures (eg, dialysis) or concomitant therapy (eg, IV sodium bicarbonate) in situations where rapid correction of severe hyperkalemia is required. Severe hypokalemia may occur; frequent monitoring of serum potassium is recommended within each 24-hour period; ECG monitoring may be appropriate in select patients. In addition to serum potassium-lowering effects, cation-exchange resins may also affect other cation concentrations possibly resulting in decreased serum magnesium and calcium. Large oral doses may cause fecal impaction (especially in elderly).

Concomitant administration of oral sodium polystyrene sulfonate with nonabsorbable cation-donating antacids or laxatives (eg, magnesium hydroxide) may result in systemic alkalosis and may diminish ability to reduce serum potassium concentrations; use with such agents is not recommended. In addition, intestinal obstruction has been reported with concomitant administration of aluminum hydroxide due to concretion formation. Enema will reduce the serum potassium faster than oral administration, but the oral route will result in a greater reduction over several hours. Oral administration in neonates and use in neonates with reduced gut motility (postoperatively or drug-induced) is contraindicated. Oral or rectal administration of sorbitol-containing sodium polystyrene sulfonate suspensions in neonates (particularly with prematurity) is also contraindicated due to propylene glycol content and risk of intestinal necrosis and digestive hemorrhage. Use sodium polystyrene sulfonate (**without** sorbitol) with caution in premature or low-birth-weight infants. Use with caution in children when administering rectally; excessive dosage or inadequate dilution may result in fecal impaction. Propylene glycol: Some dosage forms may contain propylene glycol; large amounts are potentially toxic and have been associated hyperosmolality, lactic acidosis, seizures, and respiratory depression; use caution (AAP, 1997; Zar, 2007).

Warnings: Additional Pediatric Considerations Some dosage forms may contain propylene glycol; in neonates large amounts of propylene glycol delivered orally, intravenously (eg, >3,000 mg/day), or topically have been associated with potentially fatal toxicities which can include metabolic acidosis, seizures, renal failure, and CNS depression; toxicities have also been reported in children and adults including hyperosmolality, lactic acidosis, seizures, and respiratory depression; use caution (AAP, 1997; Shehab, 2009).

Adverse Reactions

Endocrine & metabolic: Hypernatremia, hypocalcemia, hypokalemia, hypomagnesemia, sodium retention

Gastrointestinal: Anorexia, constipation, diarrhea, fecal impaction, intestinal necrosis (rare), intestinal obstruction (due to concretions in association with aluminum hydroxide), nausea, vomiting

Rare but important or life-threatening: Acute bronchitis (rare; associated with inhalation of particles), concretions, gastrointestinal bleeding, gastrointestinal ulceration, intestinal perforation, ischemic colitis

Drug Interactions

Metabolism/Transport Effects None known.

Avoid Concomitant Use

Avoid concomitant use of Sodium Polystyrene Sulfonate with any of the following: Laxatives (Magnesium Containing); Meloxicam; Sorbitol

Increased Effect/Toxicity

Sodium Polystyrene Sulfonate may increase the levels/effects of: Aluminum Hydroxide; Digoxin

The levels/effects of Sodium Polystyrene Sulfonate may be increased by: Antacids; Laxatives (Magnesium Containing); Meloxicam; Sorbitol

Decreased Effect

Sodium Polystyrene Sulfonate may decrease the levels/effects of: Lithium; Thyroid Products

Food Interactions Some liquids may contain potassium: Management: Do not mix in orange juice or in any fruit juice known to contain potassium.

Storage/Stability Store at 25°C (77°F); excursions permitted to 15°C to 30°C (59°F to 86°F). Store repackaged product in refrigerator and use within 14 days. Freshly prepared suspensions should be used within 24 hours. Do not heat resin suspension.

Mechanism of Action Removes potassium by exchanging sodium ions for potassium ions in the intestine (especially the large intestine) before the resin is passed from the body; exchange capacity is 1 mEq/g *in vivo*, and *in vitro* capacity is 3.1 mEq/g, therefore, a wide range of exchange capacity exists such that close monitoring of serum electrolytes is necessary

Pharmacodynamics Onset of action: Within 2-24 hours

Pharmacokinetics (Adult data unless noted) Elimination: Remains in the GI tract to be completely excreted in the feces (primarily as potassium polystyrene sulfonate)

Dosing: Neonatal Hyperkalemia (not preferred): Rectal: 1 g/kg/dose every 2-6 hours (Malone, 1991; Yaseen 2008); may employ lower doses by using the practical exchange ratio of 1 mEq K^+/g of resin as the basis for calculation. **Note:** Due to complications of hypernatremia and NEC, use in neonates should be reserved for refractory cases.

Dosing: Usual Hyperkalemia:

Infants and Children:

Oral: 1 g/kg/dose every 6 hours

Rectal: 1 g/kg/dose every 2-6 hours; in small children and infants, employ lower doses by using the practical exchange ratio of 1 mEq K^+/g of resin as the basis for calculation.

Adults:

Oral: 15 g 1-4 times/day

Rectal: 30-50 g every 6 hours

Preparation for Administration

Oral or NG: Powder for suspension: For each 1 g of the powdered resin, add 3 to 4 mL of water or syrup (amount of fluid usually ranges from 20 to 100 mL); use within 24 hours after preparation.

Enema: Powder for suspension: Suspend dose in 100 mL of an aqueous vehicle

Administration

Oral or NG:

Oral suspension: Shake commercially available suspension well before use. **Do not mix in orange juice.** Chilling the oral mixture will increase palatability.

Powder for suspension: Powdered resin must be mixed with water or syrup prior to administration.

Rectal: Route is less effective than oral administration. Administer cleansing enema first. Each dose of the powder for suspension should be suspended in an aqueous vehicle and administered as a warm emulsion (body temperature). The commercially available suspension should also be warmed to body temperature. During administration, the solution should be agitated gently. Retain enema in colon for at least 30-60 minutes and for several hours, if possible. Once retention time is complete, irrigate colon with a nonsodium-containing solution to remove resin

Monitoring Parameters Serum sodium, potassium, calcium, magnesium, ECG (if applicable)

Additional Information 1 g of resin binds ~1 mEq of potassium; 4.1 mEq sodium per g of powder; 1 level teaspoon contains 3.5 g polystyrene sulfonate

Dosage Forms Excipient information presented when available (limited, particularly for generics); consult specific product labeling.

Powder, Oral:

Kalexate: (454 g) [sorbitol free; contains sodium 100 mg (4.1 mEq)/g]

Kayexalate: (453.6 g) [contains sodium 100 mg (4.1 mEq)/g]

Kionex: (454 g) [contains sodium 100 mg (4.1 mEq)/g]

Generic: (15 g, 453.6 g, 454 g)

Suspension, Oral:

Kionex: 15 g/60 mL (60 mL, 473 mL) [contains alcohol, usp, methylparaben, propylene glycol, propylparaben, saccharin sodium, sodium 1500 mg (65 mEq)/60 mL, sorbitol; raspberry flavor]

SPS: 15 g/60 mL (60 mL, 120 mL, 473 mL) [contains alcohol, usp, methylparaben, propylene glycol, propylparaben, saccharin sodium, sodium 1500 mg (65 mEq)/60 mL, sorbitol; cherry flavor]

Generic: 15 g/60 mL (60 mL, 480 mL, 500 mL)

Suspension, Rectal:

Generic: 30 g/120 mL (120 mL); 50 g/200 mL (200 mL)

◆ **Sodium Sulamyd (Can)** *see* Sulfacetamide (Ophthalmic) *on page 1981*

◆ **Sodium Sulfacetamide** *see* Sulfacetamide (Ophthalmic) *on page 1981*

◆ **Sodium Sulfacetamide** *see* Sulfacetamide (Topical) *on page 1982*

Sodium Thiosulfate (SOW dee um thye oh SUL fate)

Related Information

Management of Drug Extravasations *on page 2298*

Therapeutic Category Antidote, Cyanide; Antidote, Extravasation

Generic Availability (US) Yes

Use Treatment of cyanide poisoning [FDA approved in pediatric patients (age not specified) and adults]; has also been used for used in the management of mechlorethamine extravasation, management of concentrated cisplatin (≥0.4 mg/mL) extravasation; management of bendamustine extravasation

Pregnancy Risk Factor C

Pregnancy Considerations Teratogenic effects were not observed in animal reproduction studies of sodium thiosulfate. In general, medications used as antidotes should take into consideration the health and prognosis of the mother; antidotes should be administered to pregnant women if there is a clear indication for use and should not be withheld because of fears of teratogenicity (Bailey 2003).

Breast-Feeding Considerations It is not known if sodium thiosulfate is excreted in breast milk. Because sodium thiosulfate may be used as an antidote in life-threatening situations, breast-feeding is not a contraindication to use. It is not known when breast-feeding may safely be restarted following administration; the manufacturer recommends caution be used following administration to nursing women.

Contraindications There are no contraindications listed within the manufacturer's labeling.

Warnings/Precautions Due to the risk for serious adverse effects, use with caution in patients where the diagnosis of cyanide poisoning is uncertain. However, if clinical suspicion of cyanide poisoning is high, treatment should not be delayed. Treatment of cyanide poisoning should include external decontamination and supportive therapy. Collection of pretreatment blood cyanide concentrations does not preclude administration and should not delay administration in the emergency management of highly suspected or confirmed cyanide toxicity. Pretreatment levels may be useful as postinfusion levels may be inaccurate. Monitor patients for return of symptoms for 24-48 hours; repeat treatment (one-half the original dose) should be administered if symptoms return. Fire victims may present with both cyanide and carbon monoxide poisoning. In these patients, the induction of methemoglobinemia with amyl nitrite or sodium nitrite is contraindicated until carbon monoxide levels return to normal due to the risk of tissue hypoxia. Methemoglobinemia decreases the oxygen-carrying capacity of hemoglobin and the presence of carbon monoxide prevents hemoglobin from releasing oxygen to the tissues. In this scenario, sodium thiosulfate may be used alone to promote the clearance of cyanide. Hydroxocobalamin, however, should be considered to avoid the nitrite-related problems and because sodium thiosulfate has a slow onset of action. Hydroxocobalamin, however, should be considered to avoid the nitrite-related problems and because sodium thiosulfate has a slow onset of action. Consider consultation with a poison control center at 1-800-222-1222.

The presence of sulfite hypersensitivity should not preclude the use of this medication.

Adverse Reactions

Cardiovascular: Hypotension

Central nervous system: Disorientation, headache

Gastrointestinal: Nausea, salty taste, vomiting

Hematologic: Bleeding time prolonged

Miscellaneous: Warmth

Drug Interactions

Metabolism/Transport Effects None known.

Avoid Concomitant Use There are no known interactions where it is recommended to avoid concomitant use.

Increased Effect/Toxicity There are no known significant interactions involving an increase in effect.

Decreased Effect There are no known significant interactions involving a decrease in effect.

Storage/Stability Store at 20°C to 25°C (68°F to 77°F); excursions permitted to 15°C to 30°C (59°F to 86°F). Protect from light. Do not freeze.

Extravasation management (off-label use/route): Store the 1/6 M solution for SubQ administration at 15°C to 30°C (59°F to 86°F) (Polovich 2009).

Mechanism of Action

Cyanide toxicity: Serves as a sulfur donor in rhodanese-catalyzed formation of thiocyanate (much less toxic than cyanide)

Extravasation management: Neutralizes the reactive species of mechlorethamine; reduces the formation of hydroxyl radicals which cause tissue injury

Pharmacokinetics (Adult data unless noted)

Half-life, elimination:

Thiosulfate: ~3 hours (Howland, 2011)

Thiocyanate: ~3 hours; renal impairment: ≤9 days

Elimination: Urine (~20% to 50% as unchanged drug)

Dosing: Usual

Pediatric:

Cyanide poisoning: Infant, Children, and Adolescents: **Note:** Administer in conjunction with sodium nitrite. Administer sodium nitrite first, followed immediately by the administration of sodium thiosulfate.

Manufacturer's labeling: IV 250 mg/kg (1 mL/kg of a 25% solution); maximum dose 12.5 **g** (50 mL of a 25% solution). Monitor patients for 24 to 48 hours; if symptoms return, repeat both sodium nitrite and sodium thiosulfate at one-half the original doses.

Alternate dosing: IV: 500 mg/kg (2 mL/kg of a 25% solution); maximum dose: 12.5 **g** (50 mL of a 25% solution). Monitor the patient for 24 to 48 hours; if symptoms return, repeat both sodium nitrite and sodium thiosulfate at one-half the original doses (Howland, 2011).

Extravasation management: Limited data available:

Mechlorethamine extravasation: Children and Adolescents, SubQ: 1/6 M (~4%) solution: Inject 2 mL for each mg of mechlorethamine suspected to have extravasated (Pérez Fidalgo, 2012; Polovich, 2009)

Cisplatin extravasation, concentrated: Infants, Children, and Adolescents: Inject 2 mL of a 1/6 M (~4%) sodium thiosulfate solution into existing IV line for each 100 mg of cisplatin extravasated; consider also injecting 1 mL of a 1/6 M (~4%) sodium thiosulfate solution as 0.1 mL subcutaneous injections (clockwise) into the area around the extravasation, may repeat subcutaneous injections several times over the next 3 to 4 hours (Ener, 2004)

Adult:

Cyanide poisoning: IV: **Note:** Administer in conjunction with sodium nitrite. Administer sodium nitrite first, followed immediately by the administration of sodium thiosulfate: 12.5 g (50 mL of a 25% solution); may repeat at one-half the original dose if symptoms of cyanide toxicity return.

Extravasation management: Limited data available:

Mechlorethamine extravasation: SubQ: Inject 2 mL of a 1/6 M (~4%) sodium thiosulfate solution (into the extravasation site) for each mg of mechlorethamine suspected to have extravasated (Pérez Fidalgo, 2012; Polovich, 2009)

Cisplatin extravasation, concentrated: Inject 2 mL of a 1/6 M (~4%) sodium thiosulfate solution into existing IV line for each 100 mg of cisplatin extravasated; consider also injecting 1 mL of a 1/6 M (~4%) sodium thiosulfate solution as 0.1 mL subcutaneous injections (clockwise) into the area around the extravasation, may repeat subcutaneous injections several times over the next 3 to 4 hours (Ener, 2004)

Bendamustine extravasation: SubQ: Bendamustine extravasation may be managed with 1/6 M (~4%) sodium thiosulfate solution in the same manner as mechlorethamine extravasation (Schulmeister, 2011)

Dosing adjustment in renal impairment: There are no dosage adjustments provided in the manufacturer's labeling; however, renal elimination of sodium thiosulfate is significant and risk of adverse effects may be increased in patients with renal impairment.

Dosing adjustment in hepatic impairment: There are no dosage adjustments provided in the manufacturer's labeling (has not been studied).

Preparation for Administration SubQ: Solution for extravasation management: Final concentration: 1/6 M (~4%) solution: Add 1.6 mL of 25% solution to 8.4 mL (Polovich 2009)

Administration Route of administration dependent upon use.

IV: **Cyanide poisoning:** Administer undiluted (25% solution) by IV infusion over 10 to 30 minutes immediately after the administration of sodium nitrite (Howland, 2011). Decrease rate of infusion in the event of significant hypotension.

SubQ: **Extravasation management:** Stop vesicant infusion immediately and disconnect IV line (leave needle/cannula in place); gently aspirate extravasated solution from the IV line (do **NOT** flush the line); remove needle/cannula (temporarily keep in place for cisplatin extravasation to allow for sodium thiosulfate administration through the needle/cannula); elevate extremity.

Mechlorethamine: Inject subcutaneously 1/6 M (~4%) sodium thiosulfate solution into the extravasation site using ≤25-gauge needle; change needle with each injection (Pérez Fidalgo 2012; Polovich 2009)

Cisplatin, concentrated: Inject 1/6 M (~4%) sodium thiosulfate solution into the existing IV line; also consider administering subcutaneous injections (clockwise) into the area around the extravasation using a new 25- or 27-gauge needle for each injection (Ener 2004)

Monitoring Parameters

Cyanide poisoning: Monitor for at least 24-48 hours after administration; blood pressure and heart rate during and after infusion; hemoglobin/hematocrit; co-oximetry; serum lactate levels; venous-arterial PO_2 gradient; serum methemoglobin and oxyhemoglobin. Pretreatment cyanide levels may be useful diagnostically.

Extravasation management: Monitor and document extravasation site for pain, blister formation, skin sloughing, arm/hand swelling/stiffness; monitor for fever, chills, or worsening pain

Dosage Forms Excipient information presented when available (limited, particularly for generics); consult specific product labeling. [DSC] = Discontinued product

Solution, Intravenous:

Generic: 10% [100 mg/mL] (10 mL [DSC]); 25% [250 mg/mL] (50 mL)

◆ **Sodium Thiosulfate and Sodium Nitrite** *see* Sodium Nitrite and Sodium Thiosulfate *on page* 1945

◆ **Sodium Thiosulphate** *see* Sodium Thiosulfate *on page* 1955

◆ **Sof-Lax [OTC]** *see* Docusate *on page* 697

◆ **Soflax [OTC] (Can)** *see* Docusate *on page* 697

◆ **Soflax C [OTC] (Can)** *see* Docusate *on page* 697

◆ **Soflax EX [OTC] (Can)** *see* Bisacodyl *on page* 289

◆ **Soflax Pediatric Drops [OTC] (Can)** *see* Docusate *on page 697*
◆ **Solaice** *see* Capsaicin *on page 362*
◆ **Solodyn** *see* Minocycline *on page 1440*
◆ **Soltamox** *see* Tamoxifen *on page 2005*
◆ **Solu-CORTEF** *see* Hydrocortisone (Systemic) *on page 1038*
◆ **Solu-Cortef (Can)** *see* Hydrocortisone (Systemic) *on page 1038*
◆ **Solugel® (Can)** *see* Benzoyl Peroxide *on page 270*
◆ **Solumedrol** *see* MethylPREDNISolone *on page 1409*
◆ **Solu-MEDROL** *see* MethylPREDNISolone *on page 1409*
◆ **Solu-Medrol (Can)** *see* MethylPREDNISolone *on page 1409*
◆ **Soluver (Can)** *see* Salicylic Acid *on page 1894*
◆ **Soluver Plus (Can)** *see* Salicylic Acid *on page 1894*

Somatropin (soe ma TROE pin)

Medication Safety Issues

Sound-alike/look-alike issues:

Humatrope may be confused with homatropine
Somatrem may be confused with somatropin
Somatropin may be confused with homatropine, sumatriptan

BEERS Criteria medication:

This drug may be potentially inappropriate for use in geriatric patients (Quality of evidence - high; Strength of recommendation - strong).

Brand Names: US Genotropin; Genotropin MiniQuick; Humatrope; Norditropin FlexPro; Norditropin NordiFlex Pen; Nutropin AQ NuSpin 10; Nutropin AQ NuSpin 20; Nutropin AQ NuSpin 5; Nutropin AQ Pen; Nutropin [DSC]; Omnitrope; Saizen; Saizen Click.Easy; Serostim; Tev-Tropin [DSC]; Zomacton; Zorbtive

Brand Names: Canada Genotropin GoQuick; Genotropin MiniQuick; Humatrope; Norditropin Nordiflex; Norditropin Simplexx; Nutropin AQ NuSpin; Nutropin AQ Pen; Omnitrope; Saizen; Serostim

Therapeutic Category Growth Hormone

Generic Availability (US) No

Use

Children:

Treatment of growth failure due to inadequate endogenous growth hormone secretion (Genotropin®, Humatrope®, Norditropin®, Nutropin®, Nutropin AQ®, Omnitrope®, Saizen®, Tev-Tropin®: FDA approved in children)

Treatment of short stature associated with Turner syndrome (Genotropin®, Humatrope®, Norditropin®, Nutropin®, Nutropin AQ®, Omnitrope®: FDA approved in children)

Treatment of Prader-Willi syndrome (Genotropin®, Omnitrope®: FDA approved in ages > 2 years)

Treatment of growth failure associated with chronic renal insufficiency (CRI) up until the time of renal transplantation (Nutropin®, Nutropin AQ®: FDA approved in children)

Treatment of growth failure in children born small for gestational age (SGA) who fail to manifest catch-up growth by 2-4 years of age (Genotropin®, Humatrope®, Norditropin® Omnitrope®: FDA approved in children)

Treatment of idiopathic short stature (nongrowth hormone-deficient short stature) defined by height standard deviation score (SDS) ≤2.25 and growth rate not likely to attain normal adult height (Genotropin®, Humatrope®, Nutropin®, Nutropin AQ®, Omnitrope®: FDA approved in children)

Treatment of short stature or growth failure associated with short stature homeobox gene (SHOX) deficiency (Humatrope®: FDA approved in children)

Treatment of short stature associated with Noonan syndrome (Norditropin®: FDA approved in children)

Adults: All indications: FDA approved in adults

HIV patients with wasting or cachexia with concomitant antiviral therapy (Serostim®)

Replacement of endogenous growth hormone in patients with adult growth hormone deficiency who meet both of the following criteria (Genotropin®, Humatrope®, Norditropin®, Nutropin®, Nutropin AQ®, Omnitrope®, Saizen®):

Biochemical diagnosis of adult growth hormone deficiency by means of a subnormal response to a standard growth hormone stimulation test (peak growth hormone ≤5 mcg/L). Confirmatory testing may not be required in patients with congenital/genetic growth hormone deficiency or multiple pituitary hormone deficiencies due to organic diseases.

and

Adult-onset: Patients who have adult growth hormone deficiency whether alone or with multiple hormone deficiencies (hypopituitarism) as a result of pituitary disease, hypothalamic disease, surgery, radiation therapy, or trauma

or

Childhood-onset: Patients who were growth hormone-deficient during childhood, confirmed as an adult before replacement therapy is initiated

Treatment of short-bowel syndrome (Zorbtive®)

Pregnancy Risk Factor B/C (depending upon manufacturer)

Pregnancy Considerations Teratogenic effects were not observed in animal studies. Reproduction studies have not been conducted with all agents. During normal pregnancy, maternal production of endogenous growth hormone decreases as placental growth hormone production increases. Data with somatropin use during pregnancy is limited.

Breast-Feeding Considerations It is not known if somatropin is excreted in breast milk. The manufacturer recommends that caution be exercised when administering somatropin to nursing women.

Contraindications Hypersensitivity to growth hormone or any component of the formulation; growth promotion in pediatric patients with closed epiphyses; progression or recurrence of any underlying intracranial lesion or actively growing intracranial tumor; acute critical illness due to complications following open heart or abdominal surgery; multiple accidental trauma or acute respiratory failure; evidence of active malignancy; active proliferative or severe nonproliferative diabetic retinopathy; use in patients with Prader-Willi syndrome **without** growth hormone deficiency (except Genotropin) or in patients with Prader-Willi syndrome **with** growth hormone deficiency who are severely obese, have a history of upper airway obstruction or sleep apnea, or have severe respiratory impairment

Warnings/Precautions Initiation of somatropin is contraindicated with acute critical illness due to complications following open heart or abdominal surgery, multiple accidental trauma, or acute respiratory failure; mortality may be increased. The safety of continuing somatropin in patients who develop these illnesses during therapy has not been established; use with caution. Use in contraindicated with active malignancy; monitor patients with pre-existing tumors or growth failure secondary to an intracranial lesion for recurrence or progression of underlying disease; discontinue therapy with evidence of recurrence. An increased risk of second neoplasm has been reported in childhood cancer survivors treated with somatropin; the most common second neoplasms were meningiomas in patients treated with radiation to the head for their first neoplasm. Patients with HIV and pediatric patients with short stature (genetic cause) have increased baseline risk of developing malignancies; consider risk/benefits prior to initiation of therapy and monitor these patients carefully. Monitor all patients for any malignant transformation of skin lesions.

Somatropin may decrease insulin sensitivity; use with caution in patients with diabetes or with risk factors for impaired glucose tolerance. Adjustment of antidiabetic medications may be necessary. Pancreatitis has been rarely reported; incidence in children (especially girls) with Turner syndrome may be greater than adults. Monitor for hypersensitivity reactions. Patients with hypoadrenalism may require increased dosages of glucocorticoids (especially cortisone acetate and prednisone) due to somatropin-mediated inhibition of 11 beta-hydroxysteroid dehydrogenase type 1; undiagnosed central hypoadrenalism may be unmasked. Excessive glucocorticoid therapy may inhibit the growth promoting effects of somatropin in children; monitor and adjust glucocorticoids carefully. Untreated/undiagnosed hypothyroidism may decrease response to therapy; monitor thyroid function test periodically and initiate/adjust thyroid replacement therapy as needed. Closely monitor other hormonal replacement treatments in patients with hypopituitarism. Obese patients may experience an increased incidence of adverse events when using a weight-based dosing regimen. Intracranial hypertension (IH) with headache, nausea, papilledema, visual changes, and/or vomiting has been reported with somatropin; funduscopic examination prior to initiation of therapy and periodically thereafter is recommended. Treatment should be discontinued in patients who develop papilledema; resuming treatment at a lower dose may be considered once IH-associated signs and symptoms have resolved. Patients with Turner syndrome, chronic renal failure and Prader-Willi syndrome may be at increased risk for IH. Progression of scoliosis may occur in children experiencing rapid growth. Patients with growth hormone deficiency may develop slipped capital epiphyses more frequently, evaluate any child with new onset of a limp or with complaints of hip or knee pain. Patients with Turner syndrome are at increased risk for otitis media and other ear/hearing disorders, cardiovascular disorders (including stroke, aortic aneurysm, hypertension), and thyroid disease, monitor carefully. Fluid retention may occur frequently in adults during use; manifestations of fluid retention (eg, edema, arthralgia, myalgia, nerve compression syndromes/paresthesias) are generally transient and dose dependent. Potentially significant drug-drug interactions may exist, requiring dose or frequency adjustment, additional monitoring, and/or selection of alternative therapy. Products may contain m-cresol. Not for IV injection. According to the Centers for Disease Control and Prevention (CDC), pen-shaped injection devices should never be used for more than one person (even when the needle is changed) because of the risk of infection. The injection device should be clearly labeled with individual patient information to ensure that the correct pen is used (CDC, 2012).

Benzyl alcohol and derivatives: Diluent may contain benzyl alcohol; large amounts of benzyl alcohol (≥99 mg/kg/day) have been associated with a potentially fatal toxicity ("gasping syndrome") in neonates; the "gasping syndrome" consists of metabolic acidosis, respiratory distress, gasping respirations, CNS dysfunction (including convulsions, intracranial hemorrhage), hypotension, and cardiovascular collapse (AAP, 1997; CDC, 1982); some data suggests that benzoate displaces bilirubin from protein binding sites (Ahlfors, 2001); avoid or use dosage forms containing benzyl alcohol with caution in neonates. See manufacturer's labeling.

Fatalities have been reported in pediatric patients with Prader-Willi syndrome following the use of growth hormone. The reported fatalities occurred in patients with one or more risk factors, including severe obesity, sleep apnea, respiratory impairment, or unidentified respiratory infection; male patients with one or more of these factors may be at greater risk. Treatment interruption is recommended in patients who show signs of upper airway obstruction, including the onset of, or increased, snoring. In addition, evaluation of and/or monitoring for sleep apnea and respiratory infections are recommended.

Patients with HIV infection should be maintained on antiretroviral therapy to prevent the potential increase in viral replication.

Avoid use in the elderly, except as hormone replacement following pituitary gland removal; use results in minimal effect on body composition and is associated with edema, arthralgia, carpal tunnel syndrome, gynecomastia, and impaired fasting glucose (Beers Criteria). Elderly may be more sensitive to the actions of somatropin; consider lower starting doses.

Safety and efficacy have not been established for the treatment of Noonan syndrome in children with significant cardiac disease. Children with epiphyseal closure who are treated for adult GHD need reassessment of therapy and dose. Administration site rotation is necessary to prevent tissue atrophy.

Adverse Reactions

Growth hormone deficiency: Adverse reactions reported with growth hormone deficiency vary greatly by age. Generally, percentages are less in pediatric patients than adults, and many of the reactions reported in adults are dose related. Percentages reported also vary by product. Below is a listing by age group; events reported more commonly overall are noted with an asterisk (*).

Children: Antibodies development, arthralgia, benign intracranial hypertension, edema, eosinophilia, glycosuria, Hb A_{1c} increased, headache, hematoma, hematuria, hyperglycemia (mild), hypertriglyceridemia, hypoglycemia, hypothyroidism, injection site reaction, intracranial tumor, leg pain, lipoatrophy, leukemia, meningioma, muscle pain, papilledema, pseudotumor cerebri, psoriasis exacerbation, rash, scoliosis progression, seizure, slipped capital femoral epiphysis, weakness

Adults: Acne, ALT increased, AST increased, arthralgia*, back pain, bronchitis, carpal tunnel syndrome, chest pain, cough, depression, diabetes mellitus (type 2), diaphoresis, dizziness, edema*, fatigue, flu-like syndrome*, gastritis, glucose intolerance, glucosuria, headache*, hyperglycemia (mild), hypertension, hypoesthesia, hypothyroidism, infection, insomnia, insulin resistance, joint disorder, leg edema, muscle pain, myalgia*, nausea, pain in extremities, paresthesia*, peripheral edema*, pharyngitis, retinopathy, rhinitis, skeletal pain*, stiffness in extremities, surgical procedure, upper respiratory tract infection, weakness

Additional/postmarketing reactions observed with growth hormone deficiency: Gynecomastia, increased growth of pre-existing nevi, pancreatitis

HARS: Serostim®: Arthrlagia, blood glucose increased, edema (peripheral), headache, hypoesthesia, myalgia, pain (extremity), paresthesia

Idiopathic short stature: Humatrope®: Arthralgia, arthrosis, gynecomastia, hip pain, hyperlipidemia, hypertension, myalgia, otitis media, scoliosis. Additional adverse reactions listed as reported using other products from ISS NCGS Cohort: Aggressiveness, benign intracranial hypertension, diabetes, edema, hair loss, headache, injection site reaction

Prader-Willi syndrome: Genotropin®: Aggressiveness, arthralgia, edema, hair loss, headache, benign intracranial hypertension, myalgia; fatalities associated with use in this population have been reported

Turner syndrome: Humatrope®: Ear disorders, otitis media, joint pain, respiratory illness, surgical procedures, urinary tract infection

HIV patients with wasting or cachexia: Serostim®: Edema, gynecomastia, headache, hypoesthesial; musculoskeletal disorders (arthralgia, arthrosis, myalgia); nausea, paresthesia, peripheral edema,

Short-bowel syndrome: Zorbtive®: Abdominal pain, arthralgia, chest pain, dehydration, diaphoresis, dizziness, facial edema,flatulence, generalized edema, hearing symptoms, infection, injection site pain, injection site reaction, malaise, moniliasis, myalgia, nausea, pain, peripheral edema,rash, rhinitis, vomiting

SHOX deficiency: Humatrope®: Arthralgia, excessive cutaneous nevi, gynecomastia, scoliosis

Small for gestational age: Genotropin®, Humatrope®: Mild, transient hyperglycemia; benign intracranial hypertension (rare); central precocious puberty; jaw prominence (rare); aggravation of pre-existing scoliosis (rare); injection site reactions; progression of pigmented nevi; carpal tunnel syndrome (rare) diabetes mellitus (rare); otitis media; headache; slipped capital femoral epiphysis

Drug Interactions

Metabolism/Transport Effects None known.

Avoid Concomitant Use There are no known interactions where it is recommended to avoid concomitant use.

Increased Effect/Toxicity There are no known significant interactions involving an increase in effect.

Decreased Effect

Somatropin may decrease the levels/effects of: Antidiabetic Agents; Cortisone; PredniSONE

The levels/effects of Somatropin may be decreased by: Estrogen Derivatives

Storage/Stability

Genotropin: Store at 2°C to 8°C (36°F to 46°F); do not freeze. Protect from light. Following reconstitution of 5.8 mg and 13.8 mg cartridge, store under refrigeration and use within 28 days.

Genotropin Miniquick: Store in refrigerator prior to dispensing, but may be stored ≤25°C (77°F) for up to 3 months after dispensing. Once reconstituted, solution must be refrigerated and used within 24 hours. Discard unused portion.

Humatrope:

Vial: Before and after reconstitution, store at 2°C to 8°C (36°F to 46°F); do not freeze. When reconstituted with provided diluent or bacteriostatic water for injection, use within 14 days. When reconstituted with sterile water for injection, use within 24 hours and discard unused portion.

Cartridge: Before and after reconstitution, store at 2°C to 8°C (36°F to 46°F); do not freeze. Following reconstitution with provided diluent, stable for 28 days under refrigeration.

Norditropin: Store at 2°C to 8°C (36°F to 46°F); do not freeze. Avoid direct light. When refrigerated, prefilled pen must be used within 4 weeks after initial injection. Orange and blue prefilled pens may also be stored up to 3 weeks at ≤25°C (77°F).

Nutropin: Before and after reconstitution, store at 2°C to 8°C (36°F to 46°F); do not freeze.

Nutropin vial: Use reconstituted vials within 14 days. When reconstituted with sterile water for injection, use immediately and discard unused portion.

Nutropin AQ formulations: Use within 28 days following initial use.

Omnitrope:

Powder for injection: Prior to reconstitution, store under refrigeration at 2°C to 8°C (36°F to 46°F); do not freeze. Protect from light. Reconstitute with provided diluent. Swirl gently; do not shake. Following reconstitution with the provided diluents, the 5.8 mg vial may be stored under refrigeration for up to 3 weeks. Store vial in carton to protect from light.

Solution: Prior to use, store under refrigeration at 2°C to 8°C (36°F to 46°F). Once the cartridge is loaded into the pen delivery system, store under refrigeration for up to 28 days after first use.

Saizen: Prior to reconstitution, store at room temperature 15°C to 30°C (59°F to 86°F). Following reconstitution with bacteriostatic water for injection, reconstituted solution should be refrigerated and used within 14 days. When reconstituted with sterile water for injection, use immediately and discard unused portion. The Saizen easy click cartridge, when reconstituted with the provided bacteriostatic water, should be stored under refrigeration and used within 21 days.

Serostim: Prior to reconstitution, store at room temperature 15°C to 30°C (59°F to 86°F). When reconstituted with sterile water for injection, use immediately and discard unused portion.

Tev-Tropin, Zomacton: Prior to reconstitution, store at 2°C to 8°C (36°F to 46°F). Following reconstitution with the provided diluents, should be refrigerated and used within 14 days (5 mg vial) or 28 days (10 mg vial); do not freeze. Some cloudiness may occur; do not use if cloudiness persists after warming to room temperature.

Zorbtive: Store unopened vials and diluent at room temperature of 15°C to 30°C (59°F to 86°F). Store reconstituted vial under refrigeration at 2°C to 8°C (36°F to 46°F) for up to 14 days; do not freeze.

Mechanism of Action Somatropin is a purified polypeptide hormones of recombinant DNA origin; somatropin contains the identical sequence of amino acids found in human growth hormone; human growth hormone assists growth of linear bone, skeletal muscle, and organs by stimulating chondrocyte proliferation and differentiation, lipolysis, protein synthesis, and hepatic glucose output; stimulates erythropoietin which increases red blood cell mass; exerts both insulin-like and diabetogenic effects; enhances the transmucosal transport of water, electrolytes, and nutrients across the gut

Pharmacokinetics (Adult data unless noted)

Absorption: IM, SubQ: Well absorbed

Distribution: V_d:

- Somatrem: 50 mL/kg
- Somatropin: 70 mL/kg

Metabolism: ~90% of dose metabolized in the liver and kidney cells

Bioavailability:

- SubQ:
  - Somatrem: 81% ± 20%
  - Somatropin: 75%
- IM: Somatropin: 63%

Half-life:

- SubQ:
  - Somatrem: 2.3 ± 0.42 hours
  - Somatropin: 3.8 hours
- IM: Somatropin: 4.9 hours

Elimination: 0.1% of dose excreted in urine unchanged

Dosing: Usual Note: Nutropin (lyophilized powder) has been discontinued in the US for more than 1 year.

Children:

AIDS-related wasting or cachexia: Serostim®: Children ≥6 years and Adolescents: Limited data available: SubQ: 0.04-0.07 mg/kg/day for 4 weeks; dosing based on two small trials of pediatric patients (n=11; age: 6-17 years)

Chronic renal insufficiency: Nutropin®, Nutropin® AQ: SubQ: 0.35 mg/kg **weekly** divided into daily injections; continue until the time of renal transplantation

Dosage recommendations in patients treated for CRI who require dialysis:

Hemodialysis: Administer dose at night prior to bedtime or at least 3-4 hours after hemodialysis to prevent hematoma formation from heparin

CCPD: Administer dose in the morning following dialysis

CAPD: Administer dose in the evening at the time of overnight exchange

Growth hormone inadequacy: Note: Therapy should be discontinued when patient has reached satisfactory adult height, when epiphyses have fused, or when the patient ceases to respond. Growth of 5 cm/year or more is expected; if growth rate does not exceed 2.5 cm in a 6-month period, double the dose for the next 6 months; if there is still no satisfactory response, discontinue therapy.

Genotropin®, Omnitrope®: SubQ: 0.16-0.24 mg/kg **weekly** divided into daily doses (6-7 doses)

Humatrope®: SubQ: 0.18-0.3 mg/kg **weekly** divided into equal doses 6-7 days/week

Norditropin®: SubQ: 0.024-0.034 mg/kg/dose 6-7 times per week

Nutropin®, Nutropin® AQ: SubQ: 0.3 mg/kg **weekly** divided into daily doses; in pubertal patients, dosage may be increased to 0.7 mg/kg **weekly** divided into daily doses

Saizen®: IM, SubQ: 0.18 mg/kg **weekly** divided into equal daily doses **or** as 0.06 mg/kg/dose administered 3 days per week **or** as 0.03 mg/kg/dose administered 6 days per week

Tev-Tropin™: SubQ: 0.3 mg/kg divided 3 times per week

Idiopathic short stature:

Genotropin®, Omnitrope®: SubQ: 0.47 mg/kg **weekly** divided into equal doses 6-7 days/week

Humatrope®: SubQ: 0.37 mg/kg **weekly** divided into daily doses (6-7 doses)

Nutropin®, Nutropin® AQ: SubQ: Up to 0.3 mg/kg **weekly** divided into daily doses

Noonan syndrome: Norditropin®: SubQ: Up to 0.066 mg/kg/day

Prader-Willi syndrome: Genotropin®, Omnitrope®: SubQ: 0.24 mg/kg **weekly** divided daily into 6-7 doses per week

SGA at birth who fail to catch-up by 2-4 years of age:

Genotropin®, Omnitrope: 0.48 mg/kg **weekly** divided daily into 6-7 doses per week

Humatrope®: SubQ: 0.47 mg/kg **weekly**divided into equal doses 6-7 days/week

Norditropin®: SubQ: Up to 0.469 mg/kg **weekly** divided into equal doses 7 days/week

Alternate dosing (small for gestational age): In older/early pubertal children or children with very short stature, consider initiating therapy at higher doses (0.469 mg/kg weekly divided into equal doses 7 days/week); then consider reducing the dose (0.231 mg/kg weekly) if substantial catch-up growth observed. In younger children (<4 years) with less severe short stature, consider initiating therapy with lower doses (0.231 mg/kg weekly) and then titrating the dose upwards as needed.

SHOX deficiency: Humatrope®: SubQ: 0.35 mg/kg **weekly** divided into equal doses 6-7 days per week

Turner syndrome:

Genotropin®; Omnitrope®: SubQ: 0.33 mg/kg **weekly** divided into 6-7 doses/week

Humatrope®: SubQ: 0.375 mg/kg **weekly** divided into equal doses 6-7 days/week

Nutropin®, Nutropin® AQ: SubQ: Up to 0.375 mg/kg **weekly** divided into equal doses 3-7 times/week

Adults:

AIDS-related wasting or cachexia: Serostim®: SubQ: Administered once daily at bedtime:

<35 kg: 0.1 mg/kg

35-44 kg: 4 mg

45-55 kg: 5 mg

>55 kg: 6 mg

Growth hormone deficiency: Note: To minimize adverse events in older or overweight patients, reduced dosages may be necessary. During therapy, dosage should be decreased if required by the occurrence of side effects or excessive IGF-1 levels.

Weight-based dosing:

Norditropin®: SubQ: Initial dose ≤0.028 mg/kg **weekly** divided into equal doses 7 days/week; after 6 weeks of therapy, may increase dose to 0.112 mg/kg weekly divided into equal doses 7 days/week

Nutropin®, Nutropin® AQ: SubQ: ≤0.006 mg/kg/day; dose may be increased according to individual requirements, up to a maximum of 0.025 mg/kg/day in patients <35 years of age, or up to a maximum of 0.0125 mg/kg/day in patients ≥35 years of age

Humatrope®: SubQ: ≤0.006 mg/kg/day; dose may be increased according to individual requirements, up to a maximum of 0.0125 mg/kg/day

Genotropin®, Omnitrope®: SubQ: ≤0.04 mg/kg **weekly** divided into 6-7 doses; dose may be increased at 4- to 8-week intervals according to individual requirements, to a maximum of 0.08 mg/kg/week

Saizen®: SubQ: ≤0.005 mg/kg/day; dose may be increased to not more than 0.01 mg/kg/day after 4 weeks, based on individual requirements

Nonweight-based dosing: SubQ: Initial: 0.2 mg/day (range: 0.15-0.3 mg/day); may increase every 1-2 months by 0.1-0.2 mg/day based on response and/or serum IGF-I levels

Dosage adjustment with estrogen supplementation (growth hormone deficiency): Larger doses of somatropin may be needed for women taking oral estrogen replacement products; dosing not affected by topical products

Short-bowel syndrome: Zorbtive®: SubQ: 0.1 mg/kg daily not to exceed 8 mg/day; treatment >4 weeks has not been studied adequately. Excessive fluid retention or arthralgias may be treated symptomatically or by a 50% dosage reduction; stop therapy for up to 5 days prior to lowering dosage if symptoms are severe; if symptoms do not resolve after 5 days or recur with the lowered dosage, discontinue treatment.

Dosage adjustment in renal impairment: Reports indicate patients with chronic renal failure tend to have decreased clearance; specific dosing suggestions not available

Dosage adjustment in hepatic impairment: Clearance may be reduced in patients with severe hepatic dysfunction; specific dosing suggestions not available

Preparation for Administration

Genotropin: Reconstitute with diluent provided.

Genotropin MiniQuick: Reconstitute with diluent provided. Consult the instructions provided with the reconstitution device.

Humatrope:

Cartridge: Consult HumatroPen User Guide for complete instructions for reconstitution. **Reconstitute with diluent syringe provided with cartridges ONLY; do not use diluent provided with vials or any other solutions.**

Vial: 5 mg: Reconstitute with 1.5 to 5 mL diluent provided. Inject diluent gently against the side of the vial and swirl gently until completely dissolved; do not shake. Solution should be clear; if solution is cloudy, do not use. If sensitivity to diluent should occur, may reconstitute using bacteriostatic water for injection (contains benzyl alcohol) or SWFI.

Nutropin: Vial:

5 mg: Reconstitute with 1 to 5 mL bacteriostatic water for injection. Swirl gently; do not shake.

10 mg: Reconstitute with 1-10 mL bacteriostatic water for injection. Swirl gently; do not shake.

Omnitrope powder: Reconstitute with provided diluent (contains benzyl alcohol). Swirl gently; do not shake. Solution should be clear; if cloudy or contains particulate matter do not use.

Saizen:

Click.easy cartridge: 8.8 mg: Reconstitute with the provided diluent (contains metacresol) using the click.easy reconstitution device. Consult click.easy reconstitution device instructions for use for details.

Vial:

5 mg: Reconstitute with 1 to 3 mL bacteriostatic water for injection (provided, contains benzyl alcohol); if sensitivity occurs to diluent may reconstitute with SWFI. Inject diluent gently against the side of the vial and gently swirl until dissolved; do not shake. Solution should be clear; if cloudy or contains particulate matter do not use. If reconstituted with SWFI, use immediately and discard any unused portion.

8.8 mg: Reconstitute with 2 to 3 mL bacteriostatic water for injection (provided, contains benzyl alcohol); if sensitivity occurs to diluent may reconstitute with SWFI. Inject diluent gently against the side of the vial and gently swirl until dissolved; do not shake. Solution should be clear; if cloudy or contains particulate matter do not use. If reconstituted with SWFI, use immediately and discard any unused portion.

Serostim: Vial:

4 mg: Reconstitute with 0.5 to 1 mL bacteriostatic water for injection (contains benzyl alcohol); inject diluent down side of vial and gently swirl until dissolved; do not shake. Solution should be clear; if cloudy or contains particulate matter do not use. For patients with benzyl alcohol sensitivity may reconstitute with SWFI, use immediately and discard any unused portion

5 mg or 6 mg: Reconstitute with 0.5 to 1 mL SWFI; inject diluent down side of vial and gently swirl until dissolved; do not shake. Solution should be clear; if cloudy or contains particulate matter do not use. Use immediately and discard any unused portion

Tev-Tropin: **Note:** Only use the provided diluent for the 5 mg and 10 mg vial; diluents differ between products and should not be interchanged. Once reconstituted, solution should be clear; if solution is cloudy or contains particulate matter do not use. Cloudiness may occur when stored in the refrigerator after reconstitution. Allow solution to warm to room temperature. If cloudiness persists, do not use.

5 mg vial: Reconstitute with 1 to 5 mL of provided diluent (bacteriostatic NS, contains benzyl alcohol). Aim diluent down side vial when injecting to prevent foaming; swirl gently until dissolved; do not shake. Use preservative-free NS for injection for use in newborns; when reconstituting with preservative-free NS for injection, use only one dose per vial; discard unused portion.

10 mg vial: Reconstitute with 1 mL of provided diluent (bacteriostatic water for injection, contains metacresol). Use the 25-gauge mixing needle provided. Aim diluent down side vial when injecting to prevent foaming; swirl gently until dissolved; do not shake.

Zorbtive: 8.8 mg vial: Reconstitute with 1 to 2 mL bacteriostatic water for injection (provided, contains benzyl alcohol). Inject diluent down the side of the vial and swirl gently until dissolved. May administer immediately or refrigerate for up to 14 days. For patients who are sensitive to benzyl alcohol, may reconstitute with SWFI per the manufacturer; must be administered immediately; discard any unused portion.

Administration

Parenteral: Administer SubQ notfor IV injection; do not shake vial. Administer into the thigh, buttock, or abdomen; rotate administration sites to avoid tissue atrophy. **Note:** Some products previously approved for IM administration; however, this route has been replaced with SubQ.

Product-specific information:

Norditropin cartridge must be administered using the corresponding color-coded NordiPen injection pen; do not interchange.

Omnitrope: Solution in the Omnitrope cartridges must be administered using the Omnitrope pen; when installing a new cartridge, prime pen prior to first use.

Tev-Tropin: When administering Tev-Tropin, use a standard sterile disposable needle or Tjet Needle-Free injection device for SubQ injection.

Timing of administration for chronic renal insufficiency:

Hemodialysis (HD): Administer at night just prior to sleeping and at least 3 to 4 hours after dialysis

Peritoneal dialysis (PD):

Chronic cycling: Administer in the morning after dialysis

Continuous ambulatory peritoneal dialysis (CAPD): Administer in the evening at the time of the overnight exchange

Monitoring Parameters Growth curve, periodic thyroid function tests, bone age (annually), periodical urine testing for glucose, somatomedin C levels; fundoscopic exams; progression of scoliosis and clinical evidence of slipped capital femoral epiphysis such as a limp or hip or knee pain

Product Availability

Nutropin (lyophilized powder) has been discontinued in the US for more than 1 year.

Zomacton: Ferring Pharmaceuticals acquired Tev-Tropin from Teva Pharmaceuticals in December 2014 and received FDA approval for a name change from Tev-Tropin to Zomacton. Zomacton became commercially available in June 2015. A needle-free administration device for Zomacton, ZOMA-Jet Needle-Free, is expected to be available for the 5 mg dose and in a new 10 mg dose later in 2015.

Dosage Forms Excipient information presented when available (limited, particularly for generics); consult specific product labeling. [DSC] = Discontinued product

Solution, Subcutaneous:

Norditropin FlexPro: 5 mg/1.5 mL (1.5 mL); 10 mg/1.5 mL (1.5 mL); 15 mg/1.5 mL (1.5 mL); 30 mg/3 mL (3 mL) [contains phenol]

Norditropin NordiFlex Pen: 30 mg/3 mL (3 mL) [contains phenol]

Nutropin AQ NuSpin 5: 5 mg/2 mL (2 mL) [contains phenol]

Nutropin AQ NuSpin 10: 10 mg/2 mL (2 mL) [contains phenol]

Nutropin AQ NuSpin 20: 20 mg/2 mL (2 mL) [contains phenol]

Nutropin AQ Pen: 10 mg/2 mL (2 mL)

Nutropin AQ Pen: 20 mg/2 mL (2 mL) [contains phenol]

Omnitrope: 5 mg/1.5 mL (1.5 mL) [contains benzyl alcohol]

Omnitrope: 10 mg/1.5 mL (1.5 mL) [contains phenol]

Solution Reconstituted, Injection:

Humatrope: 5 mg (1 ea)

Humatrope: 6 mg (1 ea); 12 mg (1 ea); 24 mg (1 ea) [contains glycerin, metacresol]

Saizen: 5 mg (1 ea); 8.8 mg (1 ea)

Saizen Click.Easy: 8.8 mg (1 ea)

Solution Reconstituted, Subcutaneous:

Genotropin: 5 mg (1 ea); 12 mg (1 ea) [contains metacresol]

Nutropin: 10 mg (1 ea [DSC]) [contains benzyl alcohol]

Omnitrope: 5.8 mg (1 ea)

Serostim: 4 mg (1 ea); 5 mg (1 ea); 6 mg (1 ea)
Tev-Tropin: 5 mg (1 ea [DSC])
Zomacton: 5 mg (1 ea) [contains benzyl alcohol]
Zomacton: 10 mg (1 ea) [contains metacresol]
Zorbtive: 8.8 mg (1 ea) [contains benzyl alcohol]
Solution Reconstituted, Subcutaneous [preservative free]:
Genotropin MiniQuick: 0.2 mg (1 ea); 0.4 mg (1 ea); 0.6 mg (1 ea); 0.8 mg (1 ea); 1 mg (1 ea); 1.2 mg (1 ea); 1.4 mg (1 ea); 1.6 mg (1 ea); 1.8 mg (1 ea); 2 mg (1 ea)

- ◆ **Sominex [OTC]** *see* DiphenhydrAMINE (Systemic) *on page 668*
- ◆ **Sominex (Can)** *see* DiphenhydrAMINE (Systemic) *on page 668*
- ◆ **Sominex Maximum Strength [OTC]** *see* DiphenhydrAMINE (Systemic) *on page 668*
- ◆ **Som Pam (Can)** *see* Flurazepam *on page 913*
- ◆ **Soolantra** *see* Ivermectin (Topical) *on page 1183*
- ◆ **Soothe® [OTC]** *see* Artificial Tears *on page 201*
- ◆ **Soothe & Cool INZO Antifungal [OTC]** *see* Miconazole (Topical) *on page 1431*
- ◆ **Soothe® Hydration [OTC]** *see* Artificial Tears *on page 201*

Sorbitol (SOR bi tole)

Therapeutic Category Laxative, Hyperosmolar; Laxative, Osmotic

Generic Availability (US) Yes

Use

Solution:

Oral: Hyperosmotic laxative; sweetening agent (OTC product: FDA approved in ages ≥12 years and adults); has also been used to facilitate the passage of charcoal-toxin complex through the intestinal tract

Rectal: Hyperosmotic laxative (OTC product: FDA approved in ages ≥2 years and adults); refer to product specific information for detail on ages for pediatric patients

Irrigation solution: Genitourinary irrigant in transurethral prostatic resection or other transurethral resection or other transurethral surgical procedures; irrigant for indwelling catheter to maintain patency (FDA approved in adults)

Pregnancy Risk Factor C

Pregnancy Considerations Animal reproduction studies have not been conducted.

Breast-Feeding Considerations The manufacturer recommends that caution be exercised when administering sorbitol to nursing women.

Contraindications Anuria

Warnings/Precautions Use with caution in patients with severe cardiopulmonary or renal impairment and in patients unable to metabolize sorbitol; large volumes may result in fluid overload and/or electrolyte changes.

Warnings: Additional Pediatric Considerations Excessive amounts of sorbitol may cause hypernatremic dehydration in pediatric patients; use with caution in infants; other causes of constipation should be evaluated prior to initiating therapy.

Adverse Reactions

Cardiovascular: Edema

Endocrine & metabolic: Fluid and electrolyte losses, hyperglycemia, lactic acidosis

Gastrointestinal: Abdominal discomfort, diarrhea, dry mouth, nausea, vomiting, xerostomia

Drug Interactions

Metabolism/Transport Effects None known.

Avoid Concomitant Use

Avoid concomitant use of Sorbitol with any of the following: Calcium Polystyrene Sulfonate; Sodium Polystyrene Sulfonate

Increased Effect/Toxicity

Sorbitol may increase the levels/effects of: Calcium Polystyrene Sulfonate; Sodium Polystyrene Sulfonate

Decreased Effect There are no known significant interactions involving a decrease in effect.

Storage/Stability

Irrigation solution: Avoid storage in temperatures >150°F; do not freeze.

Oral solution: Store at 15°C to 30°C (59°F to 86°F); do not freeze; below 15°C (59°F) cloudiness and thickening may occur; warming will restore clarity and fluidity without affecting product quality.

Mechanism of Action A polyalcoholic sugar with osmotic cathartic actions

Pharmacodynamics Onset of action: Rectal: 0.25 to 1 hour

Pharmacokinetics (Adult data unless noted)

Absorption: Oral, rectal: Poor

Metabolism: Mainly hepatic to fructose

Dosing: Usual

Pediatrics:

Constipation:

Oral: 70% solution:

Manufacturer's labeling: Children ≥12 years and Adolescents: Usual dose: 30 to 45 mL once daily as needed; maximum dose: 60 mL/dose; higher daily doses (60 to 90 mL in divided doses) may be necessary in some patients. **Note:** Consult product-specific labeling for detailed information.

Alternate dosing: Limited data available: Infants, Children and Adolescents: 1 to 3 mL/kg/day in divided doses, once or twice daily (Wyllie 2011). Usual range in adolescents: 30 to 90 mL/day

Rectal enema: 25% to 30% solution:

Children 2 to <12 years: 30 to 60 mL once daily as needed

Children ≥12 years and Adolescents: 120 mL once daily as needed

Fecal disimpaction, slow disimpaction: Oral: 70% solution: Limited data available: Infants, Children, and Adolescents: 2 mL/kg twice daily for 7 days (Pashankar 2005; Wyllie 2011)

Toxic ingestion, adjunct with charcoal: Children and Adolescents: Oral: 35% solution: 4.3 mL/kg; **Note:** Current guidelines recommend limiting use to a single dose administered with the initial charcoal dose of 1 g/kg (AACT/EAPCCT 2004).

Adult:

Hyperosmotic laxative (as single dose, at infrequent intervals):

Oral: 70% solution: 30 to 150 mL

Rectal enema: 25% to 30% solution: 120 mL

Transurethral surgical procedures: Irrigation: Topical: 3% to 3.3% as transurethral surgical procedure irrigation

Preparation for Administration Rectal enema: To prepare a 25% to 30% weight to volume solution, dilute 1 part 70% commercially available solution with 2.3 parts water.

Monitoring Parameters Stool output, fluid status, serum electrolytes (changes may be delayed due to slow absorption)

Dosage Forms Excipient information presented when available (limited, particularly for generics); consult specific product labeling.

Solution, Irrigation:

Generic: 3% (3000 mL); 3.3% (2000 mL, 4000 mL)

Solution, Oral:
Generic: 70% (30 mL, 473 mL, 474 mL, 480 mL, 3840 mL)
Solution, Rectal:
Generic: 70% (473 mL)

◆ **Sorbulax [OTC]** *see* Psyllium *on page 1804*
◆ **Sore Throat Relief [OTC]** *see* Benzocaine *on page 268*
◆ **Sorine** *see* Sotalol *on page 1963*

Sotalol (SOE ta lole)

Medication Safety Issues

Sound-alike/look-alike issues:

Sotalol may be confused with Stadol, Sudafed
Betapace may be confused with Betapace AF

BEERS Criteria medication:

This drug may be potentially inappropriate for use in geriatric patients (Quality of evidence - high; Strength of recommendation - strong).

Brand Names: US Betapace; Betapace AF; Sorine; Sotylize

Brand Names: Canada Apo-Sotalol; CO Sotalol; Dom-Sotalol; Med-Sotalol; Mylan-Sotalol; Novo-Sotalol; Nu-Sotalol; PHL-Sotalol; PMS-Sotalol; PRO-Sotalol; ratio-Sotalol; Rhoxal-sotalol; Riva-Sotalol; Rylosol; Sandoz-Sotalol; ZYM-Sotalol

Therapeutic Category Antiarrhythmic Agent, Class II; Antiarrhythmic Agent, Class III; Beta-Adrenergic Blocker

Generic Availability (US) Yes

Use

Betapace, Sorine, Sotylize: Treatment of life-threatening ventricular arrhythmias (eg, sustained ventricular tachycardia) (FDA approved in ages ≥3 days and adults)

Betapace AF, Sotylize: Maintenance of normal sinus rhythm in patients who have highly symptomatic atrial fibrillation and atrial flutter, but who are currently in normal sinus rhythm [not usually for use in patients with paroxysmal atrial fibrillation/flutter that is easily reversed (eg, by Valsalva maneuver)] (FDA approved in ages ≥3 days and adults)

Note: According to the American Heart Association/American College of Cardiology/Heart Rhythm Society (AHA/ACC/HRS), sotalol is not effective for conversion of atrial fibrillation to sinus rhythm but may be used to prevent atrial fibrillation (AHA/ACC/HRS [January, 2014]).

Pregnancy Risk Factor B

Pregnancy Considerations Adverse events were not observed in the initial animal reproduction studies; therefore, the manufacturer classifies sotalol as pregnancy category B. Sotalol crosses the placenta and is found in amniotic fluid. In a cohort study, an increased risk of cardiovascular defects was observed following maternal use of beta-blockers during pregnancy (Lennestål 2009). Intrauterine growth restriction (IUGR), small placentas, as well as fetal/neonatal bradycardia, hypoglycemia, and/or respiratory depression have been observed following *in utero* exposure to beta-blockers as a class. Adequate facilities for monitoring infants at birth should be available. Untreated chronic maternal hypertension and pre-eclampsia are also associated with adverse events in the fetus, infant, and mother; however, sotalol is currently not recommended for the initial treatment of hypertension in pregnancy (ACOG 2013). Because sotalol crosses the placenta in concentrations similar to the maternal serum, it has been used for the treatment of fetal atrial flutter or fetal supraventricular tachycardia without hydrops (Sonesson 1998). The clearance of sotalol is increased during the third trimester of pregnancy, but other pharmacokinetic parameters do not significantly differ from nonpregnant values (O'Hare 1983).

Breast-Feeding Considerations Sotalol is excreted in breast milk in concentrations higher than those found in the maternal serum (O'Hare 1980). Although adverse events in nursing infants have not been observed in case reports, close monitoring for bradycardia, hypotension, respiratory distress, and hypoglycemia is advised. Due to the potential for serious adverse reactions in the nursing infant, the manufacturer recommends a decision be made whether to discontinue nursing or to discontinue the drug, taking into account the importance of treatment to the mother.

Contraindications

Hypersensitivity to sotalol or any component of the formulation; bronchial asthma; sinus bradycardia (<50 bpm during waking hours [Betapace AF, Sotylize]); second- or third-degree AV block (unless a functioning pacemaker is present); congenital or acquired long QT syndromes; cardiogenic shock; uncontrolled heart failure

Additional contraindications (Betapace AF, Sotylize): Baseline QTc interval >450 msec; bronchospastic conditions; CrCl <40 mL/minute; serum potassium <4 mEq/L; sick sinus syndrome

Warnings/Precautions [U.S. Boxed Warning]: Sotalol can cause life-threatening ventricular tachycardia associated with QT interval prolongation (ie, torsades de pointes). Do not initiate if baseline QTc interval is >450 msec (Betapace AF, Sotylize). If QTc interval prolongs to 500 msec or exceeds 500 msec during therapy, reduce the dose, prolong the interval between doses, or discontinue use (Betapace AF, Sotylize). QTc prolongation is directly related to the concentration of sotalol; reduced creatinine clearance (CrCl), female gender, and large doses increase the risk of QTc prolongation and subsequent torsades de pointes. Manufacturer recommends initiation (or reinitiation) and dose increases be done in a hospital setting with continuous monitoring and staff familiar with the recognition and treatment of life-threatening arrhythmias. Some experts will initiate therapy on an outpatient basis in patients if in sinus rhythm provided the QT interval and serum potassium are normal and the patient is not receiving any other QT-interval prolonging medications but require inpatient hospitalization if patient is in atrial fibrillation (AHA/ACC/HRS [January, 2014]). Calculation of CrCl must occur prior to administration of the first dose. Dosage should be adjusted gradually with 3 days between dosing increments to achieve steady-state concentrations, and to allow time to monitor QT intervals. Monitor and adjust dose to prevent QTc prolongation. Potentially significant drug-drug interactions may exist, requiring dose or frequency adjustment, additional monitoring, and/or selection of alternative therapy.

Correct electrolyte imbalances before initiating (especially hypokalemia and hypomagnesemia) since these conditions increase the risk of torsades de pointes. Consider preexisting conditions such as sick sinus syndrome before initiating. May cause bradycardia (including heart block) and hypotension. Dose adjustments of agents that slow AV nodal conduction may be necessary when sotalol is initiated. Use cautiously within the first 2 weeks post-MI especially in patients with markedly impaired ventricular function (experience limited). Administer cautiously in compensated heart failure and monitor for a worsening of the condition. Use is contraindicated in patients with uncontrolled (or decompensated) heart failure. May precipitate or aggravate symptoms of arterial insufficiency in patients with PVD and Raynaud's disease; use with caution and monitor for progression of arterial obstruction. Bradycardia may be observed more frequently in elderly patients (>65 years of age); dosage reductions may be necessary. In the treatment of atrial fibrillation in the elderly, avoid antiarrhythmics as first-line treatment. In older adults, data suggests rate control may provide more benefits than risks compared to rhythm control for most patients (Beers Criteria). Beta-blocker therapy should not be withdrawn abruptly (particularly in patients with CAD), but gradually tapered to avoid acute tachycardia, hypertension, and/or ischemia. Severe exacerbation of angina, ventricular arrhythmias, and myocardial infarction (MI) have been reported following abrupt withdrawal of beta-blocker therapy. Temporary but prompt resumption of beta-blocker therapy may be indicated with worsening of angina or acute coronary insufficiency. When QTc prolongation occurs, consider weighing the risk of abrupt withdrawal of sotalol with the risk of QTc prolongation. Chronic beta-blocker therapy should not be routinely withdrawn prior to major surgery. Use cautiously in diabetics because it can mask prominent hypoglycemic symptoms. Use with caution in patients with bronchospastic disease, myasthenia gravis, or psychiatric disease. Adequate alpha-blockade is required prior to use of any beta-blocker for patients with untreated pheochromocytoma. May mask signs of hyperthyroidism (eg, tachycardia); if hyperthyroidism is suspected, carefully manage and monitor; abrupt withdrawal may exacerbate symptoms of hyperthyroidism or precipitate thyroid storm. Use caution with history of severe anaphylaxis to allergens; patients taking beta-blockers may become more sensitive to repeated challenges. Treatment of anaphylaxis (eg, epinephrine) in patients taking beta-blockers may be ineffective or promote undesirable effects.

[U.S. Boxed Warning]: Sotalol is indicated for both the treatment of documented life-threatening ventricular arrhythmias (marketed as Betapace, Sorine, and Sotylize) and for the maintenance of normal sinus rhythm in patients with symptomatic atrial fibrillation/flutter who are currently in sinus rhythm (marketed as Betapace AF and Sotylize). Betapace should not be substituted for Betapace AF; Betapace AF is distributed with an educational insert specifically for patients with atrial fibrillation/flutter.

Adverse Reactions

Cardiovascular: Angina pectoris, bradycardia (dose related), cardiac failure, cardiovascular signs and symptoms, cerebrovascular accident, chest pain, ECG abnormality, edema, hypertension, hypotension, palpitations, peripheral vascular disease, presyncope, proarrhythmia, prolonged Q-T interval on ECG (dose related), syncope, torsades de pointes (dose related), vasodilation, worsened ventricular tachycardia

Central nervous system: Anxiety, confusion, depression, dizziness, fatigue (dose related), headache, impaired consciousness, insomnia, mood changes, sensation of cold, sleep disorder

Dermatologic: Diaphoresis, hyperhidrosis, skin rash

Endocrine & metabolic: Sexual disorder, weight changes

Gastrointestinal: Abdominal distention, abdominal pain, change in appetite, colonic disease, decreased appetite, diarrhea, dyspepsia, flatulence, nausea and vomiting, stomach pain

Genitourinary: Genitourinary complaint, impotence

Hematologic & oncologic: Hemorrhage

Infection: Infection, influenza

Local: Local pain

Neuromuscular & skeletal: Back pain, limb pain, musculoskeletal chest pain, musculoskeletal pain, weakness

Ophthalmic: Visual disturbance

Respiratory: Asthma, dyspnea (dose related), pulmonary disease, tracheobronchitis, upper respiratory complaint

Miscellaneous: AICD discharge, fever, laboratory test abnormality

Rare but important or life-threatening: Alopecia, bronchiolitis obliterans organizing pneumonia, crusted skin (red), eosinophilia, hypersensitivity angiitis, increased liver enzymes, increased serum transaminases, leukopenia, paralysis, phlebitis, pruritus, pulmonary edema, Raynaud's phenomenon, retroperitoneal fibrosis, serum transaminases increased, skin necrosis (after extravasation), skin photosensitivity, thrombocytopenia

Drug Interactions

Metabolism/Transport Effects

None known.

Avoid Concomitant Use

Avoid concomitant use of Sotalol with any of the following: Beta2-Agonists; Ceritinib; Fingolimod; Floctafenine; Highest Risk QTc-Prolonging Agents; Ivabradine; Methacholine; Mifepristone; Moderate Risk QTc-Prolonging Agents; Propafenone; Rivastigmine

Increased Effect/Toxicity

Sotalol may increase the levels/effects of: Alpha-/Beta-Agonists (Direct-Acting); Alpha1-Blockers; Alpha2-Agonists; Amifostine; Antihypertensives; Antipsychotic Agents (Phenothiazines); Bradycardia-Causing Agents; Bupivacaine; Cardiac Glycosides; Ceritinib; Cholinergic Agonists; DULoxetine; Ergot Derivatives; Grass Pollen Allergen Extract (5 Grass Extract); Highest Risk QTc-Prolonging Agents; Hypotensive Agents; Insulin; Lacosamide; Levodopa; Lidocaine (Systemic); Lidocaine (Topical); Mepivacaine; Methacholine; Midodrine; Obinutuzumab; RiTUXimab; Sulfonylureas

The levels/effects of Sotalol may be increased by: Acetylcholinesterase Inhibitors; Alpha2-Agonists; Anilidopiperidine Opioids; Antipsychotic Agents (Phenothiazines); Barbiturates; Bretylium; Brimonidine (Topical); Calcium Channel Blockers (Nondihydropyridine); Diazoxide; Dipyridamole; Fingolimod; Floctafenine; Herbs (Hypotensive Properties); Ivabradine; Lidocaine (Topical); MAO Inhibitors; Mifepristone; Moderate Risk QTc-Prolonging Agents; Nicorandil; NIFEdipine; Pentoxifylline; Phosphodiesterase 5 Inhibitors; Propafenone; Prostacyclin Analogues; QTc-Prolonging Agents (Indeterminate Risk and Risk Modifying); Regorafenib; Reserpine; Rivastigmine; Ruxolitinib; Tofacitinib

Decreased Effect

Sotalol may decrease the levels/effects of: Beta2-Agonists; Theophylline Derivatives

The levels/effects of Sotalol may be decreased by: Antacids; Barbiturates; Herbs (Hypertensive Properties); Methylphenidate; Nonsteroidal Anti-Inflammatory Agents; Rifamycin Derivatives; Yohimbine

Food Interactions

Sotalol peak serum concentrations may be decreased if taken with food. Management: Administer without regard to meals.

Storage/Stability

Store at ~25°C (77°F); excursions are permitted between 15°C and 30°C (59°F and 86°F).

Mechanism of Action

Beta-blocker which contains both beta-adrenoreceptor-blocking (Vaughan Williams Class II) and cardiac action potential duration prolongation (Vaughan Williams Class III) properties

Class II effects: Increased sinus cycle length, slowed heart rate, decreased AV nodal conduction, and increased AV nodal refractoriness Sotalol has both $beta_1$- and $beta_2$-receptor blocking activity. The beta-blocking effect of sotalol is a noncardioselective (half maximal at about 80 mg/day and maximal at doses of 320-640 mg/day). Significant beta-blockade occurs at oral doses as low as 25 mg/day.

Class III effects: Prolongation of the atrial and ventricular monophasic action potentials, and effective refractory prolongation of atrial muscle, ventricular muscle, and atrioventricular accessory pathways in both the antegrade and retrograde directions. Sotalol is a racemic mixture of *d*- and *l*-sotalol; both isomers have similar Class III antiarrhythmic effects while the *l*-isomer is responsible for virtually all of the beta-blocking activity.

The Class III effects are seen only at oral doses ≥160 mg/day

Pharmacodynamics Onset of action: Oral: Rapid: 1 to 2 hours (Winters 1993)

Pharmacokinetics (Adult data unless noted)

Absorption: Decreased 20% by meals compared to fasting

Distribution: V_d: 1.2 to 2.4 L/kg (Hanyok 1993)

Protein binding: None

Metabolism: None

Bioavailability: 90% to 100%

Half-life elimination:

Neonates ≤1 month: 8.4 hours (Saul 2001b)

Infants and children >1 month to 24 months: 7.4 hours (Saul 2001b)

Children >2 years to <7 years: 9.1 hours (Saul 2001b)

Children 7 to 12 years: 9.2 hours (Saul 2001b)

Adults: 12 hours

Adults with renal failure (anuric): Up to 69 hours

Time to peak serum concentration:

Infants and children 3 days to 12 years: Mean range: 2 to 3 hours

Adults: 2.5 to 4 hours

Elimination: Urine (as unchanged drug)

Clearance (apparent) (Saul 2001b):

Neonates ≤1 month: 11 mL/minute

Infants and children >1 month to 24 months: 32 mL/minute

Children >2 years to <7 years: 63 mL/minute

Children 7 to 12 years: 95 mL/minute

Dosing: Neonatal Arrhythmias: Sotalol is indicated for both the treatment of documented life-threatening ventricular arrhythmias (marketed as Betapace/Sorine/Sotylize) and for the maintenance of normal sinus rhythm in patients with symptomatic atrial fibrillation/flutter who are currently in sinus rhythm (marketed as Betapace/Sotylize).

PNA ≥ 3 days: Oral: **Note:** Baseline QTc interval and CrCl must be determined prior to initiation. Dosage must be adjusted to individual response and tolerance; doses should be initiated or increased in a hospital facility that can provide continuous ECG monitoring, recognition and treatment of life-threatening arrhythmias, and CPR.

Note: Manufacturer's dosing recommendations are based on doses per m^2 (that are equivalent to the doses recommended in adults) and on pediatric pharmacokinetic and pharmacodynamic studies (Saul, 2001a; Saul, 2001b). BSA, rather than body weight, better predicted apparent clearance of sotalol; however, for a given dose per m^2, a larger drug exposure (larger AUC) and greater pharmacologic effects were observed in smaller subjects (ie, those with BSA <0.33 m^2 versus those with BSA ≥0.33 m^2). For infants and children ≤2 years of age, the manufacturer recommends a dosage reduction based on an age factor determined from a graph (see below).

Manufacturer's labeling: The manufacturer recommended pediatric dosage of 30 mg/**m**^{2}/dose given every 8 hours must be **REDUCED** by an age-related factor that is obtained from the graph (see graph). First, obtain the patient's age in months; use the graph to determine where the patient's age (on the logarithmic scale) intersects the age factor curve; read the age factor from the Y-axis; then multiply the age factor by the pediatric dose listed below (ie, the dose for children >2 years); this will result in the proper reduction in dose for age. For example, the age factor for a neonate (PNA: 14 days) is 0.5, so the initial dosage would be (0.5 x 30 mg/m^2/dose) = 15 mg/m^2/dose given every 8 hours. Similar calculations should be made for dosage titrations; increase dosage gradually, if needed; allow adequate time between dosage increments to achieve new steady-state and to monitor clinical response, heart rate and QTc intervals; half-life is prolonged with decreasing age (<2 years), so time to reach new steady-state will increase; for example, the time to reach steady-state in a neonate may be ≥1 week.

Sotalol Age Factor Nomogram for Patients ≤2 Years of Age

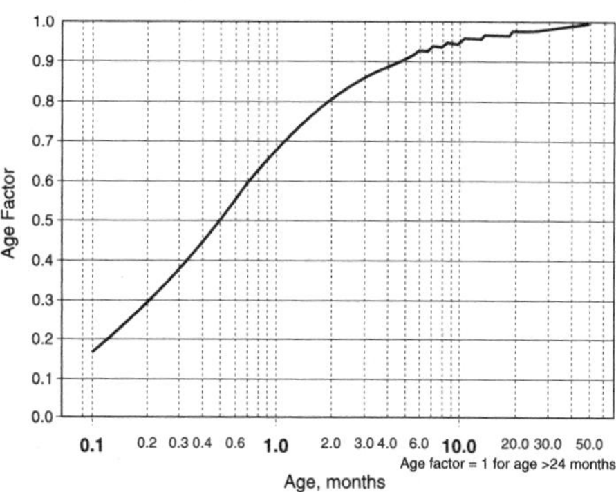

Adapted from U.S. Food and Drug Administration. http://www.fda.gov/cder/foi/label/2001/2115s3lbl.PDF

Alternate dosing: Limited data available:

Initial: 2 mg/kg/day divided every 8 hours; if needed, increase dosage gradually by 1-2 mg/kg/day increments; allow at least 3 days between dosage increments to achieve new steady-state and to monitor clinical response, heart rate, and QTc intervals (Läer, 2005)

Proposed target dose: 4 mg/kg/day divided every 8 hours; **Note:** It is not necessary to increase to target dosage if desired clinical effect has been achieved at a lower dosage

Dosing adjustment for toxicity: QTc ≥500 msec during initiation period (Betapace AF): Reduce dose or discontinue sotalol.

Dosing adjustment in renal impairment: There are no dosage adjustments provided in manufacturer's labeling; dosing in neonates with renal impairment has not been investigated; use lower doses or increased dosing intervals; closely monitor clinical response, heart rate and QTc interval; allow adequate time between dosage increments to achieve new steady-state, since half-life will be prolonged with renal impairment

Dosing: Usual Note: Baseline QTc interval and CrCl must be determined prior to initiation. Dosage must be adjusted to individual response and tolerance; doses should be initiated or increased in a hospital facility that can provide continuous ECG monitoring, recognition and treatment of life-threatening arrhythmias, and CPR:

Pediatric: **Note:** In pediatric patients, dosing may be based on either BSA (mg/m^2) or weight (mg/kg); use extra precaution to verify dosing parameters during calculations. Sotalol is indicated for both the treatment of documented life-threatening ventricular arrhythmias (marketed as Betapace/Sorine/Sotylize) and for the maintenance of normal sinus rhythm in patients with symptomatic atrial fibrillation/flutter who are currently in sinus rhythm (marketed as Betapace AF/Sotylize).

Arrhythmias: Oral: Manufacturer's dosing recommendations are based on doses per m^2 (that are equivalent to the doses recommended in adults) and on pediatric pharmacokinetic and pharmacodynamic studies (Saul 2001a; Saul 2001b). BSA, rather than body weight, better predicted apparent clearance of sotalol; however, for a given dose per m^2, a larger drug exposure (larger AUC) and greater pharmacologic effects were observed in smaller subjects (ie, those with BSA <0.33 m^2 versus those with BSA ≥0.33 m^2). For infants and children ≤2 years of age, the manufacturer recommends a dosage reduction based on an age factor determined from a graph (see below).

Manufacturer's labeling: **Note:** Use with extreme caution if QTc is >500 msec while receiving sotalol; reduce the dose or discontinue drug if QTc >550 msec.

Infants and Children ≤2 years: The manufacturer recommended pediatric dosage of 30 mg/**m^2**/dose every 8 hours must be **REDUCED** using an age-related factor that is obtained from the graph (see graph). First, obtain the patient's age in months; use the graph to determine where the patient's age (on the logarithmic scale) intersects the age factor curve; read the age factor from the Y-axis; then multiply the age factor by the pediatric dose listed below (ie, the dose for children >2 years); this will result in the proper reduction in dose for age. For example, the age factor for an infant 1 month of age is 0.68, so the initial dosage would be (0.68 x 30 mg/m^2/dose) = 20 mg/m^2/dose given every 8 hours. Similar calculations should be made for dosage titrations; increase dosage gradually, if needed; allow adequate time between dosage increments to achieve new steady-state and to monitor clinical response, heart rate and QTc intervals; half-life is prolonged with decreasing age (<2 years), so time to reach new steady-state will increase.

Sotalol Age Factor Nomogram for Patients ≤2 Years of Age

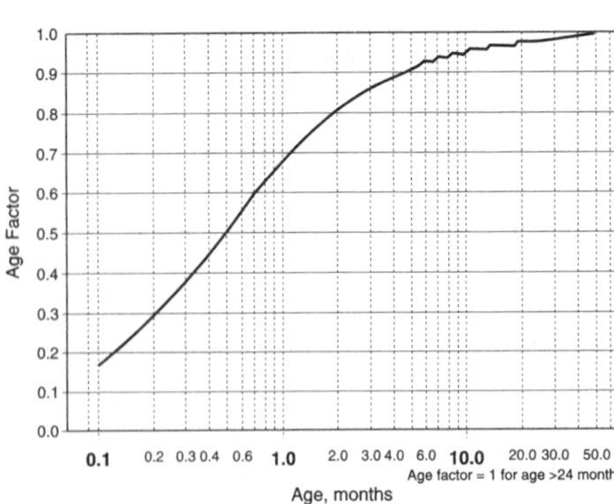

Adapted from U.S. Food and Drug Administration. http://www.fda.gov/cder/foi/label/2001/2115s3lbl.PDF

Children >2 years and Adolescents: Initial: 30 mg/**m^2**/dose given every 8 hours; increase dosage gradually if needed; allow at least 36 hours between dosage increments to achieve new steady-state and to monitor clinical response, heart rate, and QTc intervals; may increase gradually to a maximum of 60 mg/**m^2**/dose given every 8 hours; not to exceed adult doses (usual maximum adult daily dose: 320 mg/**day**)

Alternate dosing: Limited data available:

Initial: Infants, Children, and Adolescents: 2 mg/kg/day divided every 8 hours; if needed, increase dosage gradually by 1 to 2 mg/kg/day increments; allow 3 days between dosage increments to achieve new steady-state and to monitor clinical response, heart rate, and QTc intervals; maximum: 10 mg/kg/day (if no limiting side effects occur) (Beaufort-Krol 1997; Colloridi 1992; Läer 2005; Maragnes 1992; Pfammatter 1995; Pfammatter 1997; Tipple 1991); do not exceed adult doses (usual maximum adult daily dose: 320 mg/**day**)

Proposed target doses: **Note:** It is not necessary to increase to target dosage if desired clinical effect has been achieved at a lower dosage.

Infants and Children 1 month to 6 years: 6 mg/kg/day divided every 8 hours

Children >6 years and Adolescents: 4 mg/kg/day divided every 8 hours not to exceed adult doses (usual maximum adult daily dose: 320 mg/**day**)

Adult:

Ventricular arrhythmias (Betapace, Sorine, Sotylize):

Oral:

Initial: 80 mg twice daily; dose may be increased gradually (in increments of 80 mg/day [Sotalize]) to 160 to 320 mg daily; allow 3 days between dosing increments in order to attain steady-state plasma concentrations and to allow for monitoring of QT intervals

Usual range: Most patients respond to a total daily dose of 160 to 320 mg daily in 2 to 3 divided doses

Maximum: Some patients with life-threatening refractory ventricular arrhythmias may require total daily doses as high as 480 to 640 mg; however, these doses should only be prescribed when the potential benefit outweighs the increased risk of adverse events.

Atrial fibrillation or atrial flutter (Betapace AF, Sotylize): Oral: Initial: 80 mg twice daily. If the frequency of relapse does not reduce and excessive QTc prolongation does not occur after 3 days, the dose may be increased to 120 mg twice daily; may further increase to a maximum dose of 160 mg twice daily if response is inadequate and QTc prolongation is not excessive.

Dosing adjustment for toxicity: All patients:

QTc ≥500 msec during initiation period (Betapace AF, Sotylize): Reduce dose, prolong the dosing interval (Sotylize), or discontinue sotalol.

QTc ≥520 msec (or JT interval ≥430 msec if the QRS >100 msec) during maintenance therapy (Betapace AF): Reduce dose and carefully monitor QTc until <520 msec. If QTc interval ≥520 msec on the lowest maintenance dose, discontinue sotalol.

QTc ≥550 msec (Betapace, Sorine): Reduce dose or discontinue sotalol.

Dosing adjustment in renal impairment:

Infants, Children, and Adolescents: There are no dosage adjustments provided in manufacturer's labeling; dosing in children with renal impairment has not been investigated; use lower doses or increased dosing intervals; closely monitor clinical response, heart rate and QTc interval; allow adequate time between dosage increments to achieve new steady-state, since half-life will be prolonged with renal impairment

Adults: **Note:** Impaired renal function can increase the terminal half-life, resulting in increased drug accumulation. Dose escalations in renal impairment should be done after administration of at least 5 to 6 doses at appropriate intervals.

Betapace, Sorine, generic:

CrCl >60 mL/minute: Administer every 12 hours

CrCl 30 to 60 mL/minute: Administer every 24 hours

CrCl 10 to 29 mL/minute: Administer every 36 to 48 hours

CrCl <10 mL/minute: Individualize dose

Betapace AF, Sotylize:

CrCl >60 mL/minute: Administer every 12 hours

CrCl 40 to 60 mL/minute: Administer every 24 hours

CrCl <40 mL/minute: Use is contraindicated

Hemodialysis: Hemodialysis would be expected to reduce sotalol plasma concentrations because sotalol is not bound to plasma proteins and does not undergo extensive metabolism. According to the manufacturers of Betapace and Sorine, extreme caution should be employed if sotalol is used in patients with renal failure undergoing hemodialysis. According to the manufacturer of Betapace AF and Sotylize, use is contraindicated. Multiple cases of torsades de pointes have been reported when sotalol was used even at low dosages (eg, 80 mg daily) in patients with end-stage renal disease treated with hemodialysis (Huynh-Do 1996).

Peritoneal dialysis: Peritoneal dialysis does not remove sotalol; supplemental dose is not necessary (Aronoff 2007). Cases of torsades de pointes have been reported when sotalol was used even at low dosages (eg, 80 mg daily) in patients with end-stage renal disease treated with peritoneal dialysis (Dancey 1997; Tang 1997).

Dosing adjustment in hepatic impairment: All patients: There are no dosage adjustments provided in the manufacturer's labeling; however, dosage adjustment unlikely needed because sotalol is not metabolized by the liver.

Administration Oral: May be administered without regard to meals, but should be administered at the same time each day

Monitoring Parameters Serum creatinine, magnesium, potassium; heart rate, blood pressure; ECG (eg, QTc interval, PR interval); **Note:** Continuous ECG for a minimum of 3 days with initiation of therapy or dosage increase is suggested; however, patients with an increased sotalol half-life (eg, pediatric patients, especially those <2 years of age, or patients with renal impairment) may require longer monitoring to allow time to achieve steady-state concentrations and observe ECG effect. If baseline QTc >450 msec (or JT interval >330 msec if QRS over 100 msec), sotalol (Betapace AF, Sotylize) is contraindicated.

Betapace AF, Sotylize: In addition, during initiation and dosage titration, monitor the QT interval 2 to 4 hours after each dose. If QTc interval is ≥500 msec, reduce dose, prolong the dosing interval (Sotylize), or discontinue sotalol. If the QTc interval is <500 msec after 3 days (after fifth or sixth dose in patient receiving once-daily dosing), patient may be discharged on current regimen. Monitor QTc interval periodically thereafter.

Consult individual institutional policies and procedures.

Test Interactions May falsely increase urinary metanephrine values when fluorimetric or photometric methods are used; does not interact with HPLC assay with solid phase extraction for determination of urinary catecholamines

Additional Information Betapace AF: Do not discharge patients from the hospital within 12 hours of electrical or pharmacological conversion from atrial fibrillation/flutter to normal sinus rhythm.

Dosage Forms Excipient information presented when available (limited, particularly for generics); consult specific product labeling.

Solution, Intravenous, as hydrochloride:
 Generic: 150 mg/10 mL (10 mL)

Solution, Oral, as hydrochloride:
 Sotylize: 5 mg/mL (250 mL, 480 mL) [contains sodium benzoate; grape flavor]

Tablet, Oral, as hydrochloride:
 Betapace: 80 mg, 120 mg, 160 mg [scored; contains fd&c blue #2 aluminum lake]
 Betapace AF: 80 mg, 120 mg, 160 mg [scored]
 Sorine: 80 mg, 120 mg, 160 mg, 240 mg [scored]
 Generic: 80 mg, 120 mg, 160 mg, 240 mg

Extemporaneous Preparations Note: Commercial oral solution is available (5 mg/mL)

A 5 mg/mL sotalol syrup may be made with Betapace, Sorine, or Betapace AF tablets and Simple Syrup containing sodium benzoate 0.1% (Syrup, NF). Place 120 mL Syrup, NF in a 6-ounce amber plastic (polyethylene terephthalate) prescription bottle; add five Betapace, Sorine, or Betapace AF 120 mg tablets and shake the bottle to wet the tablets. Allow tablets to hydrate for at least 2 hours, then shake intermittently over ≥2 hours until the tablets are completely disintegrated; a dispersion of fine particles (water-insoluble inactive ingredients) in syrup should be obtained. **Note:** To simplify the disintegration process, tablets can hydrate overnight; tablets may also be crushed, carefully transferred into the bottle and shaken well until a dispersion of fine particles in syrup is obtained. Label "shake well". Stable for 3 months at 15°C to 30°C (59°F to 86°F) and ambient humidity.

Betapace prescribing information, Bayer HealthCare Pharmaceuticals Inc, Wayne, NJ, 2011.
Betapace AF prescribing information, Bayer HealthCare Pharmaceuticals Inc, Wayne, NJ, 2011.
Sorine prescribing information, Upsher-Smith, Minneapolis, MN, 2012.

◆ **Sotalol Hydrochloride** *see* Sotalol *on page 1963*
◆ **Sotylize** *see* Sotalol *on page 1963*
◆ **SPA** *see* Albumin *on page 79*
◆ **SPD417** *see* CarBAMazepine *on page 367*
◆ **Spectracef** *see* Cefditoren *on page 391*

Spinosad (SPIN oh sad)

Brand Names: US Natroba

Therapeutic Category Antiparasitic Agent, Topical; Pediculocide

Generic Availability (US) Yes

Use Topical treatment of head lice (*Pediculosis capitis*) infestation (FDA approved in ages ≥4 years and adults)

Pregnancy Risk Factor B

Pregnancy Considerations Adverse events were not observed in animal reproduction studies. The amount of spinosad absorbed systemically following topical administration is expected to be <3 ng/mL. Human studies did not assess the absorption of benzyl alcohol, an ingredient in the product.

Breast-Feeding Considerations Spinosad used topically is not systemically absorbed and will not be present in human milk. The formulation does include benzyl alcohol, which may be systemically absorbed and may be excreted in human milk. The manufacturer recommends that caution be exercised when administering spinosad to nursing women. Lactating women may choose to pump and discard breast milk for five benzyl alcohol half-lives (8 hours) after use to avoid ingestion of benzyl alcohol by an infant.

Contraindications There are no contraindications listed in the manufacturer's labeling

Warnings/Precautions For topical use on scalp and scalp hair only; not for oral, ophthalmic, or intravaginal use. Avoid contact with eyes. Wash hands after application. Should be used as a part of an overall lice management program.

Benzyl alcohol and derivatives: Some dosage forms may contain benzyl alcohol; large amounts of benzyl alcohol (≥99 mg/kg/day) have been associated with a potentially fatal toxicity ("gasping syndrome") in neonates; the "gasping syndrome" consists of metabolic acidosis, respiratory distress, gasping respirations, CNS dysfunction (including convulsions, intracranial hemorrhage), hypotension, and cardiovascular collapse (AAP, 1997; CDC, 1982); some data suggests that benzoate displaces bilirubin from protein binding sites (Ahlfors, 2001); avoid or use dosage forms containing benzyl alcohol with caution in neonates. See manufacturer's labeling.

Warnings: Additional Pediatric Considerations Some dosage forms may contain propylene glycol; in neonates large amounts of propylene glycol delivered orally, intravenously (eg, >3,000 mg/day), or topically have been associated with potentially fatal toxicities which can include metabolic acidosis, seizures, renal failure, and CNS depression; toxicities have also been reported in children and adults including hyperosmolality, lactic acidosis, seizures, and respiratory depression; use caution (AAP, 1997; Shehab, 2009).

Adverse Reactions

Dermatologic: Application site erythema, application site irritation, erythema of eyelid

Rare: Alopecia, application site reactions (dryness, exfoliation), dry skin

Drug Interactions

Metabolism/Transport Effects None known.

Avoid Concomitant Use There are no known interactions where it is recommended to avoid concomitant use.

Increased Effect/Toxicity There are no known significant interactions involving an increase in effect.

Decreased Effect There are no known significant interactions involving a decrease in effect.

Storage/Stability Store at 25°C (77°F); excursions permitted between 15°C to 30°C (59°F to 86°F).

Mechanism of Action Insect paralysis and death is caused by central nervous system excitation and involuntary muscle contractions. Spinosad is thought to be both pediculicidal and ovicidal (Stough, 2009).

Pharmacokinetics (Adult data unless noted) Absorption: Not absorbed topically [not detectable in a plasma sampling study of pediatric patients (4-15 years of age); absorption of the benzyl alcohol was not analyzed in the study].

Dosing: Usual Head lice: Infants ≥6 months, Children, Adolescents and Adults: Topical: Apply sufficient amount to cover dry scalp and completely cover dry hair (maximum dose: 120 mL); if live lice are seen after 7 days after first treatment, repeat with second application (Stough, 2009)

Administration For external use only. Shake bottle well. Apply to dry scalp and rub gently until the scalp is thoroughly moistened, then apply to dry hair, completely covering scalp and hair. Leave on for 10 minutes (start timing treatment after the scalp and hair have been completely covered). The hair should then be rinsed thoroughly with warm water. Shampoo may be used immediately after the product is completely rinsed off. If live lice are seen 7 days after the first treatment, repeat with second application. Avoid contact with the eyes; wash hands after use. Nit combing is not required, although a fine-tooth comb may be used to remove treated lice and nits from hair and scalp.

Dosage Forms Excipient information presented when available (limited, particularly for generics); consult specific product labeling.

Suspension, External:

Natroba: 0.9% (120 mL) [contains benzyl alcohol, cetearyl alcohol, fd&c yellow #6 (sunset yellow), isopropyl alcohol, propylene glycol]

Generic: 0.9% (120 mL)

Spironolactone (speer on oh LAK tone)

Medication Safety Issues

Sound-alike/look-alike issues:

Aldactone may be confused with Aldactazide

BEERS Criteria medication:

This drug may be potentially inappropriate for use in geriatric patients (Quality of evidence - moderate; Strength of recommendation - strong).

International issues:

Aldactone: Brand name for spironolactone [U.S., Canada, multiple international markets], but also the brand name for potassium canrenoate [Austria, Czech Republic, Germany, Hungary, Poland]

Aldactone [U.S., Canada, multiple international markets] may be confused with Aldomet brand name for methyldopa [multiple international markets]

Related Information

Safe Handling of Hazardous Drugs *on page 2455*

Brand Names: US Aldactone

Brand Names: Canada Aldactone; Teva-Spironolactone

Therapeutic Category Antihypertensive Agent; Diuretic, Potassium Sparing

Generic Availability (US) Yes

Use Management of edema associated with CHF, cirrhosis of the liver accompanied by edema or ascites, and nephrotic syndrome; treatment of primary hypertension, primary hyperaldosteronism, hypokalemia, and hirsutism; treatment of severe heart failure (NYHA class III-IV) to increase survival and reduce hospitalizations when used in addition to standard therapy

Pregnancy Risk Factor C

Pregnancy Considerations Adverse events were observed in some animal reproduction studies. The antiandrogen effects of spironolactone have been shown to cause feminization of the male fetus in animal studies. Spironolactone crosses the placenta (Regitz-Zagrosek, 2011).

The treatment of heart failure is generally the same in pregnant and nonpregnant women; however, spironolactone should be avoided in the first trimester due to its antiandrogenic effects (Regitz-Zagrosek, 2011). The use of mineralocorticoid receptor antagonists is not recommended to treat chronic uncomplicated hypertension in pregnant women and should generally be avoided in women of reproductive potential. When treatment for hypertension in pregnancy is needed, other agents are preferred (ACOG, 2013). Use of diuretics to treat edema during normal pregnancies is not appropriate; use may be considered when edema is due to pathologic causes (as in the nonpregnant patient); monitor.

Breast-Feeding Considerations The active metabolite of spironolactone (canrenone) has been found in breast milk. Information is available from a case report following maternal use of spironolactone 25 mg twice daily throughout pregnancy, then 4 times daily after delivery. Milk and maternal serum samples were obtained 17 days after birth. Two hours after the maternal dose, canrenone concentrations were ~144 ng/mL (serum) and ~104 ng/mL (milk). When measured 14.5 hours after the dose, canrenone concentrations were ~92 ng/mL (serum) and ~47 ng/mL (milk). The authors calculated the estimated maximum amount of canrenone to the nursing infant to be ~0.2% of the maternal dose (Phelps, 1977). Effects to humans are not known; however, this metabolite was found to be carcinogenic in rats. Diuretics have the potential to decrease milk volume and suppress lactation. According to the manufacturer, the decision to continue or discontinue breast-feeding during therapy should take into account the risk of exposure to the infant and the benefits of treatment to the mother; if use of spironolactone is essential, an alternative method of feeding should be used.

Contraindications

Anuria; acute renal insufficiency; significant impairment of renal excretory function; hyperkalemia; Addison's disease; concomitant use with eplerenone

Canadian labeling: Additional contraindications (not in U.S. labeling): Hypersensitivity to spironolactone or any component of the formulation; concomitant use with heparin or low molecular weight heparin

Warnings/Precautions Hazardous agent - use appropriate precautions for handling and disposal (NIOSH 2014 [group 2]).

[U.S. Boxed Warning]: Shown to be a tumorigen in chronic toxicity animal studies. Avoid unnecessary use.

Monitor closely for hyperkalemia; increases in serum potassium are dose related and rates of hyperkalemia also increase with declining renal function. The concurrent use of larger doses of ACE inhibitors (eg, ≥ lisinopril 10 mg daily in adults) also increases the risk of hyperkalemia (ACCF/AHA [Yancy, 2013]). Dose reduction or interruption of therapy may be necessary with development of hyperkalemia. Use is contraindicated in patients with hyperkalemia; use caution in conditions known to cause hyperkalemia. Risk of hyperkalemia is increased with declining renal function. Use with caution in patients with mild renal impairment; contraindicated with anuria, acute renal insufficiency, or significant impairment of renal excretory function. Potentially significant drug-drug interactions may exist, requiring dose or frequency adjustment, additional monitoring, and/or selection of alternative therapy. Somnolence and dizziness have been reported with use; advise patients to use caution when driving or operating machinery until response to initial treatment has been determined. Concurrent use with ethanol may Increase risk of orthostasis. Excess amounts can lead to profound diuresis with fluid and electrolyte loss; close medical supervision and dose evaluation are required. Watch for and correct electrolyte disturbances; adjust dose to avoid dehydration. In cirrhosis, avoid electrolyte and acid/base imbalances that might lead to hepatic encephalopathy. Gynecomastia is related to dose and duration of therapy; typically is reversible following discontinuation of therapy but may persist (rare). Discontinue use prior to adrenal vein catheterization. When evaluating a heart failure patient for spironolactone treatment, eGFR should be >30 mL/minute/1.73 m^2 or creatinine should be ≤2.5 mg/dL (men) or ≤2 mg/dL (women) with no recent worsening and potassium <5 mEq/L with no history of severe hyperkalemia (ACCF/AHA [Yancy, 2013]). Serum potassium levels require close monitoring and management if elevated. The manufacturer recommends to discontinue or interrupt therapy if serum potassium >5 mEq/L or serum creatinine >4 mg/dL. The ACCF/AHA recommends considering discontinuation upon the development of serum potassium >5.5 mEq/L or worsening renal function with careful evaluation of the entire medical regimen. Avoid routine triple therapy with the combined use of an ACE inhibitor, ARB, and spironolactone. Instruct patients with heart failure to discontinue use during an episode of diarrhea or dehydration or when loop diuretic therapy is interrupted (ACCF/AHA [Yancy, 2013]).

In the elderly, avoid use of doses >25 mg/day in patients with heart failure or with reduced renal function (eg, CrCl <30 mL/minute or eGFR ≤30 mL/minute/1.73 m^2 [Yancy, 2013]); risk of hyperkalemia is increased for heart failure patients receiving >25 mg/day, particularly if taking concomitant medications such as NSAIDS, ACE inhibitor, angiotensin receptor blocker, or potassium supplements (Beers Criteria).

Adverse Reactions

Cardiovascular: Vasculitis

Central nervous system: Ataxia, confusion, drowsiness, headache, lethargy

Dermatologic: Erythematous maculopapular rash, Stevens-Johnson syndrome, toxic epidermal necrolysis, urticaria

Endocrine & metabolic: Amenorrhea, gynecomastia, hyperkalemia

Gastrointestinal: Abdominal cramps, diarrhea, gastritis, gastrointestinal hemorrhage, gastrointestinal ulcer, nausea, vomiting

Genitourinary: Impotence, irregular menses, postmenopausal bleeding

Hematologic & oncologic: Agranulocytosis, malignant neoplasm of breast

Hepatic: Hepatotoxicity

Hypersensitivity: Anaphylaxis

Immunologic: DRESS syndrome

Renal: Increased blood urea nitrogen, renal failure, renal insufficiency

Miscellaneous: Fever

Drug Interactions

Metabolism/Transport Effects None known.

Avoid Concomitant Use

Avoid concomitant use of Spironolactone with any of the following: AMILoride; CycloSPORINE (Systemic); Tacrolimus (Systemic); Triamterene

Increased Effect/Toxicity

Spironolactone may increase the levels/effects of: ACE Inhibitors; Amifostine; Ammonium Chloride; Antihypertensives; Cardiac Glycosides; Ciprofloxacin (Systemic); CycloSPORINE (Systemic); Digoxin; DULoxetine; Hypotensive Agents; Levodopa; Neuromuscular-Blocking Agents (Nondepolarizing); Obinutuzumab; RisperiDONE; RiTUXimab; Sodium Phosphates; Tacrolimus (Systemic)

The levels/effects of Spironolactone may be increased by: Alfuzosin; AMILoride; Analgesics (Opioid); Angiotensin II Receptor Blockers; AtorvaSTATin; Barbiturates; Brimonidine (Topical); Canagliflozin; Cholestyramine Resin; Diazoxide; Drospirenone; Eplerenone; Heparin; Heparin (Low Molecular Weight); Herbs (Hypotensive Properties); MAO Inhibitors; Nicorandil; Nitrofurantoin; Nonsteroidal Anti-Inflammatory Agents; Pentoxifylline; Phosphodiesterase 5 Inhibitors; Potassium Salts; Prostacyclin Analogues; Tolvaptan; Triamterene; Trimethoprim

Decreased Effect

Spironolactone may decrease the levels/effects of: Abiraterone Acetate; Alpha-/Beta-Agonists; Cardiac Glycosides; Mitotane; QuiNIDine

The levels/effects of Spironolactone may be decreased by: Herbs (Hypertensive Properties); Methylphenidate; Nonsteroidal Anti-Inflammatory Agents; Yohimbine

Food Interactions Food increases absorption. Management: Administer with food to increase absorption and decrease GI upset.

Storage/Stability Store below 25°C (77°F).

Mechanism of Action Competes with aldosterone for receptor sites in the distal renal tubules, increasing sodium chloride and water excretion while conserving potassium and hydrogen ions; may block the effect of aldosterone on arteriolar smooth muscle as well

Pharmacokinetics (Adult data unless noted)

Distribution: V_d: Breast milk to plasma ratio: 0.51-0.72

Protein binding: 91% to 98%

Metabolism: In the liver to multiple metabolites, including canrenone (active)

Half-life:

- Spironolactone: 78-84 minutes
- Canrenone: 13-24 hours

Time to peak serum concentration: Within 1-3 hours (primarily as the active metabolite)

Elimination: Urinary and biliary

Dosing: Neonatal Oral: Diuretic: 1-3 mg/kg/day divided every 12-24 hours

Dosing: Usual Oral:

Children:

- Diuretic, hypertension: 1-3.3 mg/kg/day or 60 mg/m^2/day in divided doses every 6-12 hours; not to exceed 100 mg/day
- Diagnosis of primary aldosteronism: 100-400 mg/m^2/day in 1-2 divided doses

Adults:

- Edema, hypokalemia: 25-200 mg/day in 1-2 divided doses
- Hypertension (JNC 7): 25-50 mg/day divided once or twice daily
- Heart failure, severe (NYHA class III-IV; with ACE inhibitor and a loop diuretic ± digoxin): 12.5-25 mg/day;

maximum daily dose: 50 mg. If 25 mg once daily not tolerated, reduction to 25 mg every other day was the lowest maintenance dose possible.

Diagnosis of primary aldosteronism: 100-400 mg/day in 1-2 divided doses

Acne in women: 25-200 mg once daily

Hirsutism in women: 50-200 mg/day in 1-2 divided doses

CHF: Patients with severe heart failure already using an ACE inhibitor and a loop diuretic ± digoxin: 12.5-25 mg/day, increase or reduce depending on individual response and evidence of hyperkalemia; maximum daily dose: 50 mg

Dosing interval in renal impairment:

CrCl 10-50 mL/minute: Administer every 12-24 hours

CrCl <10 mL/minute: Avoid use

Administration Hazardous agent; use appropriate precautions for handling and disposal (NIOSH 2014 [group 2]).

Oral: Administer with food

Monitoring Parameters Serum potassium, sodium, and renal function

Test Interactions May interfere with the radioimmunoassay for digoxin.

Dosage Forms Excipient information presented when available (limited, particularly for generics); consult specific product labeling.

Tablet, Oral:

Aldactone: 25 mg

Aldactone: 50 mg, 100 mg [scored]

Generic: 25 mg, 50 mg, 100 mg

Extemporaneous Preparations Hazardous agent; use appropriate precautions for handling and disposal (NIOSH 2014 [group 2]).

A 1 mg/mL oral suspension may be made with tablets. Crush ten 25 mg tablets in a mortar and reduce to a fine powder. Add a small amount of purified water and soak for 5 minutes; add 50 mL 1.5% carboxymethylcellulose, 100 mL syrup NF, and mix to a uniform paste; mix while adding purified water in incremental proportions to **almost** 250 mL; transfer to a calibrated bottle, rinse mortar with purified water, and add quantity of purified water sufficient to make 250 mL. Label "shake well". Stable for 3 months at room temperature or refrigerated (Nahata, 1993).

A 2.5 mg/mL oral suspension may be made with tablets. Crush twelve 25 mg tablets in a mortar and reduce to a fine powder. Add small portions of distilled water or glycerin and mix to a uniform paste; mix while adding cherry syrup to **almost** 120 mL; transfer to a calibrated bottle, rinse mortar with cherry syrup, and add quantity of cherry syrup sufficient to make 120 mL. Label "shake well" and "refrigerate". This method may also be used with twenty-four 25 mg tablets for a 5 mg/mL oral suspension. Both concentrations are stable for 28 days refrigerated (Mathur, 1989).

A 25 mg/mL oral suspension may be made with tablets and either a 1:1 mixture of Ora-Sweet and Ora-Plus or a 1:1 mixture of Ora-Sweet SF and Ora-Plus. Crush one-hundred-twenty 25 mg tablets in a mortar and reduce to a fine powder. Add small portions of chosen vehicle and mix to a uniform paste; mix while adding vehicle in incremental proportions to **almost** 120 mL; transfer to a calibrated bottle, rinse mortar with vehicle, and add quantity of vehicle sufficient to make 120 mL. Store in amber bottles; label "shake well" and "refrigerate". Stable for 60 days refrigerated (Allen, 1996).

Allen LV Jr and Erickson MA 3rd, "Stability of Ketoconazole, Metolazone, Metronidazole, Procainamide Hydrochloride, and Spironolactone in Extemporaneously Compounded Oral Liquids," *Am J Health Syst Pharm*, 1996, 53(17):2073-8.

Mathur LK and Wickman A, "Stability of Extemporaneously Compounded Spironolactone Suspensions," *Am J Hosp Pharm*, 1989, 46(10):2040-2.

Nahata MC, Morosco RS, and Hipple TF, "Stability of Spironolactone in an Extemporaneously Prepared Suspension at Two Temperatures," *Ann Pharmacother*, 1993, 27(10):1198-9.

◆ **Spironolactone and Hydrochlorothiazide** *see* Hydrochlorothiazide and Spironolactone *on page 1030*

◆ **SPM 927** *see* Lacosamide *on page 1200*

◆ **Sporanox** *see* Itraconazole *on page 1176*

◆ **Sporanox Pulsepak** *see* Itraconazole *on page 1176*

◆ **SPS** *see* Sodium Polystyrene Sulfonate *on page 1953*

◆ **SQV** *see* Saquinavir *on page 1902*

◆ **SS734** *see* Besifloxacin *on page 276*

◆ **SSD** *see* Silver Sulfadiazine *on page 1926*

◆ **SSKI** *see* Potassium Iodide *on page 1740*

◆ **Stagesic [DSC]** *see* Hydrocodone and Acetaminophen *on page 1032*

◆ **StanGard Perio** *see* Fluoride *on page 899*

◆ **Stannous Fluoride** *see* Fluoride *on page 899*

◆ **Statex (Can)** *see* Morphine (Systemic) *on page 1461*

Stavudine (STAV yoo deen)

Medication Safety Issues

Sound-alike/look-alike issues:

Stavudine may be confused with cetirizine

Zerit may be confused with Zestril, Ziac, ZyrTEC

High alert medication:

This medication is in a class the Institute for Safe Medication Practices (ISMP) includes among its list of drug classes that have a heightened risk of causing significant patient harm when used in error.

Related Information

Adult and Adolescent HIV *on page 2392*

Pediatric HIV *on page 2380*

Perinatal HIV *on page 2400*

Brand Names: US Zerit

Brand Names: Canada Zerit

Therapeutic Category Antiretroviral Agent; HIV Agents (Anti-HIV Agents); Nucleoside Reverse Transcriptase Inhibitor (NRTI)

Generic Availability (US) Yes

Use Treatment of HIV infection in combination with other antiretroviral agents (FDA approved in all ages). **Note:** HIV regimens consisting of **three** antiretroviral agents are strongly recommended.

Medication Guide Available Yes

Pregnancy Risk Factor C

Pregnancy Considerations Adverse events were observed in some animal reproduction studies. Stavudine has a high level of transfer across the human placenta. No increased risk of overall birth defects has been observed following first trimester exposure according to data collected by the antiretroviral pregnancy registry. Pharmacokinetics of stavudine are not significantly altered during pregnancy; dose adjustments are not needed. Cases of lactic acidosis/hepatic steatosis syndrome related to mitochondrial toxicity have been reported in pregnant women with prolonged use of nucleoside analogues. It is not known if pregnancy itself potentiates this known side effect; however, women may be at increased risk of lactic acidosis and liver damage. In addition, these adverse events are similar to other rare but life-threatening syndromes that occur during pregnancy (eg, HELLP syndrome). Combination treatment with didanosine may also contribute to the risk of lactic acidosis and is not recommended. Hepatic enzymes and electrolytes should be monitored in women receiving nucleoside analogues and clinicians should watch for early signs of the syndrome. In addition, mitochondrial dysfunction may develop in infants following *in utero* exposure. The DHHS Perinatal HIV Guidelines recommend stavudine to be used only in special circumstances during pregnancy; do not use with didanosine or zidovudine; not recommended for initial therapy in antiretroviral-naïve pregnant women due to toxicity (HHS [perinatal], 2014).

Regardless of CD4 count or HIV RNA copy number, all HIV-infected pregnant women should receive a combination antiretroviral (ARV) drug regimen. A combination of antepartum, intrapartum, and infant ARV prophylaxis is recommended. ARV therapy should be started as soon as possible in women with symptomatic infection. Although earlier initiation may be more effective in reducing the perinatal transmission of HIV, initiation may be delayed until after 12 weeks' gestation in women who do not require immediate treatment after careful consideration of maternal conditions (eg, nausea and vomiting) and the potential risks of first trimester fetal exposure for specific agents. A scheduled cesarean delivery at 38 weeks' gestation is recommended for all women with HIV RNA >1000 copies/mL or unknown concentrations near delivery in order to decrease transmission. If ARV therapy must be interrupted for <24 hours during the peripartum period, stop then restart all medications simultaneously in order to decrease the chance of developing resistance. Long-term follow-up is recommended for all infants exposed to ARV medications. In couples who want to conceive, the HIV-infected partner should attain maximum viral suppression prior to conception.

Health care providers are encouraged to enroll pregnant women exposed to antiretroviral medications in the Antiretroviral Pregnancy Registry (1-800-258-4263 or www.APRegistry.com). Health care providers caring for HIV-infected women and their infants may contact the National Perinatal HIV Hotline (888-448-8765) for clinical consultation (HHS [perinatal], 2014).

Breast-Feeding Considerations Stavudine is excreted into breast milk; concentrations in nursing infants are negligible. Maternal or infant antiretroviral therapy does not completely eliminate the risk of postnatal HIV transmission. In addition, multiclass-resistant virus has been detected in breast-feeding infants despite maternal therapy. Therefore, in the United States, where formula is accessible, affordable, safe, and sustainable, and the risk of infant mortality due to diarrhea and respiratory infections is low, complete avoidance of breast-feeding by HIV-infected women is recommended to decrease potential transmission of HIV (HHS [perinatal], 2014).

Contraindications Hypersensitivity to stavudine or any component of the formulation

Warnings/Precautions Use with caution in patients who demonstrate previous hypersensitivity to zidovudine, didanosine, zalcitabine, pre-existing bone marrow suppression, renal insufficiency (dosage adjustment recommended), hepatic impairment, or peripheral neuropathy. Peripheral neuropathy may be a treatment-limiting side effect; consider permanent discontinuation. Zidovudine should not be used in combination with stavudine. **[U.S. Boxed Warning]: Lactic acidosis and severe hepatomegaly with steatosis have been reported with stavudine use, including fatal cases;** combination therapy with didanosine may increase risk; use with caution in patients with risk factors for liver disease (although acidosis has occurred in patients without known risk factors, risk may be increased with female gender, obesity, pregnancy, or prolonged exposure). Suspend treatment in any patient who develops clinical or laboratory findings suggestive of lactic acidosis or hepatotoxicity. Mortality of 50% associated in some case series, notably with serum lactate >10 mmol/L (DHHS [adult], 2014). Severe motor weakness (resembling Guillain-Barré syndrome) has been reported (including fatal cases, usually in association with lactic acidosis); manufacturer recommends discontinuation if motor weakness develops (with or without lactic acidosis). May cause redistribution of fat (eg, buffalo hump, peripheral wasting with increased abdominal girth, cushingoid appearance). Patients may develop immune reconstitution syndrome resulting in the occurrence of an inflammatory response to an indolent or residual opportunistic infection during initial HIV treatment or activation of autoimmune disorders (eg, Graves' disease, polymyositis, Guillain-Barré syndrome) later in therapy; further evaluation and treatment may be required. **[U.S. Boxed Warning]: Pancreatitis (including some fatal cases) has occurred during combination therapy with didanosine.** Suspend stavudine and didanosine combination therapy, and any other agents toxic to the pancreas, in patients with suspected pancreatitis. If pancreatitis diagnosis confirmed, use extreme caution if reinitiating stavudine; monitor closely and do not use didanosine in regimen. Use with caution in combination with interferon alfa with or without ribavirin in HIV/HBV coinfected patients; monitor closely for hepatic decompensation, anemia, or neutropenia; dose reduction or discontinuation of interferon and/or ribavirin may be required if toxicity evident. Combination therapy with didanosine or hydroxyurea may increase risk of hepatotoxicity, pancreatitis, or severe peripheral neuropathy; avoid stavudine or hydroxyurea combination.

Adverse Reactions Adverse reactions reported below represent experience with combination therapy with other nucleoside analogues and protease inhibitors.

Central nervous system: Headache

Dermatologic: Rash

Gastrointestinal: Diarrhea, nausea, vomiting

Hepatic: ALT increased, AST increased, GGT increased, hyperbilirubinemia

Neuromuscular & skeletal: Peripheral neuropathy

Miscellaneous: Amylase increased, lipase increased

Rare but important or life-threatening: Abdominal pain, allergic reaction, anemia, anorexia, chills, diabetes mellitus, fever, hepatic failure, hepatitis, hepatomegaly (with steatosis; some fatal), hyperglycemia, hyperlactatemia (symptomatic), hyperlipidemia, immune reconstitution syndrome, insomnia, insulin resistance, lactic acidosis (some fatal), leukopenia, macrocytosis, myalgia, neuromuscular weakness (severe-resembling Guillain-Barré), neutropenia, pancreatitis (some fatal), redistribution/accumulation/atrophy of body fat, thrombocytopenia

Drug Interactions

Metabolism/Transport Effects None known.

Avoid Concomitant Use

Avoid concomitant use of Stavudine with any of the following: Hydroxyurea; Zidovudine

Increased Effect/Toxicity

Stavudine may increase the levels/effects of: Didanosine; Hydroxyurea

The levels/effects of Stavudine may be increased by: Hydroxyurea; Ribavirin

Decreased Effect

The levels/effects of Stavudine may be decreased by: DOXOrubicin (Conventional); DOXOrubicin (Liposomal); Zidovudine

Storage/Stability Capsules and powder for reconstitution may be stored at controlled room temperature of 25°C (77°F). Reconstituted oral solution should be stored in refrigerator at 2°C to 8°C (36°F to 46°F) and is stable for 30 days.

Mechanism of Action Stavudine is a thymidine analog which interferes with HIV viral DNA dependent DNA polymerase resulting in inhibition of viral replication; nucleoside reverse transcriptase inhibitor

Pharmacokinetics (Adult data unless noted)

Absorption: Rapid

Distribution: Penetrates into the CSF achieving 16% to 97% (mean: 59%) of concomitant plasma concentrations; distributes into extravascular spaces and equally between RBCs and plasma

V_d:

Children: 0.73 ± 0.32 L/kg

Adults: 46 ± 21 L

Protein binding: Negligible

Metabolism: Converted intracellularly to active triphosphate form; metabolism of stavudine plays minimal role in its clearance; minor metabolites include oxidized stavudine and its glucuronide conjugate, glucuronide conjugate of stavudine, N-acetylcysteine conjugate of the ribose after glycosidic cleavage

Bioavailability: Capsule and solution are bioequivalent

Children: 77%

Adults: 86%

Half-life, elimination:

Newborns (at birth): 5.3 ± 2 hours

Neonates 14 to 28 days old: 1.6 ± 0.3 hours

Pediatric patients 5 weeks to 15 years: 0.9 ± 0.3 hours

Adults: 1.6 ± 0.2 hours

Note: Half-life is prolonged with renal dysfunction

Half-life, intracellular: Adults: 3.5 to 7 hours

Time to peak serum concentration: Within 1 hour

Elimination: Urine: 95% of dose (74% as unchanged drug); feces: 3% (62% as unchanged drug); undergoes glomerular filtration and active tubular secretion

Dialysis: 31 ± 5% of the dose is removed by hemodialysis; hemodialysis clearance (n=12) (mean ± SD): 120 ± 18 mL/minute

Dosing: Neonatal HIV infection, treatment: Use in combination with other antiretroviral agents.

PNA 0 to 13 days: Oral: 0.5 mg/kg/dose every 12 hours

PNA ≥14 days: Oral: 1 mg/kg/dose every 12 hours

Dosing: Usual

Pediatric: **HIV infection, treatment:** Use in combination with other antiretroviral agents.

Infants and Children <30 kg: Oral: 1 mg/kg/dose every 12 hours; maximum dose: 30 mg/dose

Children and Adolescents weighing 30 to 59 kg: Oral: 30 mg every 12 hours

Adolescents weighing ≥60 kg: Oral:

AIDS*Info* and WHO recommendations: 30 mg every 12 hours (DHHS [pediatric], 2014)

Manufacturer's labeling: 40 mg every 12 hours

Adult: **HIV infection, treatment:** Use in combination with other antiretroviral agents.

30 to 59 kg: Oral: 30 mg every 12 hours

≥60 kg: Oral: 40 mg every 12 hours

Note: The World Health Organization recommends 30 mg every 12 hours in all adult patients regardless of body weight (DHHS, [adult], 2014).

Dosing adjustment in renal impairment:

Infants, Children, and Adolescents: Insufficient data exists to recommend a specific dosage adjustment; however, a decrease in the dose should be considered in pediatric patients with renal impairment. The following guidelines have been used by some clinicians (Aronoff, 2007):

Weight <30 kg:

GFR >50 mL/minute/1.73 m^2: No adjustment required

GFR 30-50 mL/minute/1.73 m^2: 0.5 mg/kg/dose every 12 hours

GFR <30 mL/minute/1.73 m^2: 0.25 mg/kg/dose every 24 hours

Hemodialysis or peritoneal dialysis: 0.25 mg/kg/dose every 24 hours

Continuous renal replacement therapy (CRRT): 0.5 mg/kg/dose every 12 hours

Weight 30-59 kg:

GFR >50 mL/minute/1.73 m^2: No adjustment required

GFR 30-50 mL/minute/1.73 m^2: 15 mg every 12 hours

GFR <30 mL/minute/1.73 m^2: 7.5 mg every 24 hours

Hemodialysis or peritoneal dialysis: 7.5 mg every 24 hours

Continuous renal replacement therapy (CRRT): 15 mg every 12 hours

Adults:

Weight <60 kg:

CrCl ≥50 mL/minute: No dosage adjustment required

CrCl 26-50 mL/minute: 15 mg every 12 hours

CrCl 10-25 mL/minute: 15 mg every 24 hours

Hemodialysis: 15 mg every 24 hours

Weight ≥60 kg:

CrCl ≥50 mL/minute: No dosage adjustment required

CrCl 26-50 mL/minute: 20 mg every 12 hours

CrCl 10-25 mL/minute: 20 mg every 24 hours

Hemodialysis: 20 mg every 24 hours

Dosing adjustment in hepatic impairment: There are no dosage adjustments provided in the manufacturer labeling.

Preparation for Administration Oral solution: Reconstitute powder for oral solution with 202 mL of purified water as specified on the bottle. Shake vigorously until powder completely dissolves. Final suspension will be 1 mg/mL (200 mL).

Administration

Oral: Administer with or without food

Oral capsule: May be opened and dispersed in a small amount of water; administer immediately (DHHS [pediatric] 2014).

Oral solution: Shake well before using

Monitoring Parameters Note: Monitor CD4 percentage (if <5 years of age) or CD4 count (if ≥5 years of age) at least every 3-4 months (DHHS [pediatric], 2014).

Prior to initiation of therapy: Genotypic resistance testing, CD4 and viral load (every 3 to 4 months), CBC with differential, LFTs, BUN, creatinine, electrolytes, glucose, urinalysis (every 6 to 12 months), and assessment of readiness for adherence with medication regimen. At initiation and with any change in treatment regimen: CBC with differential, electrolytes, calcium, phosphate, glucose, LFTs, bilirubin, urinalysis (at initiation), BUN, creatinine, albumin, total protein, lipid panel (at initiation), CD4, and viral load. After 1 to 2 weeks of therapy: Signs of medication toxicity and adherence. After 2 to 4 weeks of therapy: CBC with differential, viral load, signs of medication toxicity, and adherence; then every 3 to 4 months: CBC with differential, electrolytes, glucose, LFTs, bilirubin, BUN, creatinine, CD4, viral load, signs of medication toxicity, and adherence. Lipid panel and urinalysis every 6 to 12 months. CD4 monitoring frequency may be decreased to every 6 to 12 months in children who are adherent to therapy if the value is well above the threshold for opportunistic infections, viral suppression is sustained, and the clinical status is stable for more than 2 to 3 years (DHHS [pediatric], 2014). Monitor for growth and development, signs of HIV-specific physical conditions, HIV disease progression, opportunistic infections peripheral neuropathy, pancreatitis, hepatotoxicity, or lactic acidosis.

Dosage Forms Excipient information presented when available (limited, particularly for generics); consult specific product labeling.

Capsule, Oral:

Zerit: 15 mg, 20 mg, 30 mg, 40 mg

Generic: 15 mg, 20 mg, 30 mg, 40 mg

Solution Reconstituted, Oral:

Zerit: 1 mg/mL (200 mL) [dye free; fruit flavor]

Generic: 1 mg/mL (200 mL)

◆ **Stavzor** *see* Valproic Acid and Derivatives *on page 2143*

◆ **Stay Awake [OTC]** *see* Caffeine *on page 335*

◆ **Stay Awake Maximum Strength [OTC]** *see* Caffeine *on page 335*

◆ **Stelazine** *see* Trifluoperazine *on page 2122*

◆ **Sterile Vancomycin Hydrochloride, USP (Can)** *see* Vancomycin *on page 2151*

◆ **STI-571** *see* Imatinib *on page 1078*

◆ **Stieprox (Can)** *see* Ciclopirox *on page 458*

◆ **Stieva-A (Can)** *see* Tretinoin (Topical) *on page 2111*

◆ **Stimate** *see* Desmopressin *on page 607*

◆ **Stimulant Laxative [OTC]** *see* Bisacodyl *on page 289*

◆ **St Joseph Adult Aspirin [OTC]** *see* Aspirin *on page 206*

◆ **Stomach Relief [OTC]** *see* Bismuth Subsalicylate *on page 290*

◆ **Stomach Relief Max St [OTC]** *see* Bismuth Subsalicylate *on page 290*

◆ **Stomach Relief Plus [OTC]** *see* Bismuth Subsalicylate *on page 290*

◆ **Stool Softener [OTC]** *see* Docusate *on page 697*

◆ **Stool Softener Laxative DC [OTC]** *see* Docusate *on page 697*

◆ **Stop** *see* Fluoride *on page 899*

◆ **Strattera** *see* AtoMOXetine *on page 217*

Streptomycin (strep toe MYE sin)

Medication Safety Issues

Sound-alike/look-alike issues:

Streptomycin may be confused with streptozocin

Brand Names: Canada Streptomycin for Injection

Therapeutic Category Antibiotic, Aminoglycoside; Antitubercular Agent

Generic Availability (US) Yes

Use Combination therapy for active tuberculosis (FDA approved in pediatric patients [age not specified] and adults); combination therapy with other agents for treatment of bacteremia caused by susceptible gram-negative bacilli, brucellosis, chancroid granuloma inguinale, *H. influenzae* (respiratory, endocardial, meningeal infections), *K. pneumoniae*, plague, streptococcal or enterococcal endocarditis, tularemia, urinary tract infections (caused by *A. aerogenes*, *E. coli*, *E. faecalis*, *K. pneumoniae*, *Proteus spp*) (FDA approved in pediatric patients [age not specified] and adults)

Pregnancy Risk Factor D

Pregnancy Considerations Streptomycin crosses the placenta. Many case reports of hearing impairment in children exposed *in utero* have been published. Impairment has ranged from mild hearing loss to bilateral deafness. Because of several reports of total irreversible bilateral congenital deafness in children whose mothers received streptomycin during pregnancy, the manufacturer classifies streptomycin as pregnancy risk factor D.

Breast-Feeding Considerations Streptomycin is excreted into breast milk; however, it is not well absorbed when taken orally. This limited oral absorption may minimize exposure to the nursing infant. Nondose-related effects could include modification of bowel flora. Breast-feeding is not recommended by the manufacturer.

Contraindications Hypersensitivity to streptomycin, other aminoglycosides, or any component of the formulation

Warnings/Precautions [U.S. Boxed Warnings]: May cause neurotoxicity, nephrotoxicity, and/or neuromuscular blockade and respiratory paralysis; usual risk factors include pre-existing renal impairment, concomitant neuro-/nephrotoxic medications, advanced age and dehydration. The drug's neurotoxicity can result in respiratory paralysis from neuromuscular blockade, especially when the drug is given soon after anesthesia or muscle relaxants. Use with caution in patients with pre-existing vertigo, tinnitus, hearing loss, neuromuscular disorders, or renal impairment; modify dosage in patients with renal impairment; ototoxicity is directly proportional to the amount of drug given and the duration of treatment; tinnitus or vertigo are indications of vestibular injury and impending bilateral irreversible damage; renal damage is usually reversible. Monitor renal function closely; peak serum concentrations should not surpass 20-25 mcg/mL in patients with renal impairment. Formulation contains metabisulfite; may cause allergic reactions in patients with sulfite sensitivity. **[U.S. Boxed Warning]: Parenteral form should be used only where appropriate audiometric and laboratory testing facilities are available.** Prolonged use may result in fungal or bacterial superinfection, including *C. difficile*-associated diarrhea (CDAD) and pseudomembranous colitis; CDAD has been observed >2 months postantibiotic treatment. IM injections should be administered in a large muscle well within the body to avoid peripheral nerve damage and local skin reactions.

Adverse Reactions

Cardiovascular: Hypotension

Central nervous system: Drug fever, headache, neurotoxicity, paresthesia of face

Dermatologic: Angioedema, exfoliative dermatitis, skin rash, urticaria

Gastrointestinal: Nausea, vomiting

Hematologic: Eosinophilia, hemolytic anemia, leukopenia, pancytopenia, thrombocytopenia

Neuromuscular & skeletal: Arthralgia, tremor, weakness

Ocular: Amblyopia

Otic: Ototoxicity (auditory), ototoxicity (vestibular)

Renal: Azotemia, nephrotoxicity

Respiratory: Difficulty in breathing

Miscellaneous: Anaphylaxis

Rare but important or life-threatening: Drug reaction with eosinophilia and systemic symptoms (DRESS), toxic epidermal necrolysis

Drug Interactions

Metabolism/Transport Effects None known.

Avoid Concomitant Use

Avoid concomitant use of Streptomycin with any of the following: Bacitracin (Systemic); BCG; BCG (Intravesical); Foscarnet; Mannitol; Mecamylamine

Increased Effect/Toxicity

Streptomycin may increase the levels/effects of: AbobotulinumtoxinA; Bacitracin (Systemic); Bisphosphonate Derivatives; CARBOplatin; Colistimethate; CycloSPORINE (Systemic); Mecamylamine; Neuromuscular-Blocking Agents; OnabotulinumtoxinA; RimabotulinumtoxinB; Tenofovir

The levels/effects of Streptomycin may be increased by: Amphotericin B; Capreomycin; Cephalosporins (2nd Generation); Cephalosporins (3rd Generation); Cephalosporins (4th Generation); CISplatin; Foscarnet; Loop Diuretics; Mannitol; Nonsteroidal Anti-Inflammatory Agents; Tenofovir; Vancomycin

Decreased Effect

Streptomycin may decrease the levels/effects of: BCG; BCG (Intravesical); BCG Vaccine (Immunization); Sodium Picosulfate; Typhoid Vaccine

The levels/effects of Streptomycin may be decreased by: Penicillins

Storage/Stability

Lyophilized powder: Store dry powder at controlled room temperature 20°C to 25°C (68°F to 77°F). Protect from light.

Solution: Store in refrigerator at 2°C to 8°C (36°F to 46°F).

Depending upon manufacturer, reconstituted solution remains stable for 24 hours at room temperature. Exposure to light causes darkening of solution without apparent loss of potency.

Mechanism of Action Inhibits bacterial protein synthesis by binding directly to the 30S ribosomal subunits causing faulty peptide sequence to form in the protein chain

Pharmacokinetics (Adult data unless noted)

Distribution: Distributes into most body tissues and fluids except the brain; small amounts enter the CSF only with inflamed meninges; crosses the placenta; small amounts appear in breast milk

Protein binding: 34%

Half-life (prolonged with renal impairment):

Newborns: 4 to 10 hours

Adults: 2 to 4.7 hours

Time to peak serum concentration: IM: Within 1 to 2 hours

Elimination: 30% to 90% of dose excreted as unchanged drug in urine, with small amount (1%) excreted in bile, saliva, sweat, and tears

Dosing: Neonatal Tuberculosis; multidrug-resistant (MDR): Limited data available: **Note:** Streptomycin is not recommended for initial treatment of tuberculosis and should be reserved for use as part of multidrug-resistant (MDR) TB regimens; usefulness limited by high rates of resistance (Blumberg 2003; WHO 2010); monitor plasma concentrations: IM, IV: **Note:** IM route preferred; consider use of IV route if IM therapy not tolerated (Bradley 2015; Morris 1994; Perez Tanoira 2014)

Daily therapy: 20 to 40 mg/kg/day (Abughali 1994; Cantwell 1994; Okascharoen 2003; Skevaki 2005)

Twice weekly: 20 to 40 mg/kg/dose twice weekly (Skevaki 2005)

Dosing: Usual

Pediatric: **Note:** Monitor serum drug concentrations.

General dosing, combination therapy for susceptible infection: Infants, Children, and Adolescents:

Manufacturer's labeling: IM: 20 to 40 mg/kg/day in divided doses every 6 to 12 hours; maximum dose: 1,000 mg/dose; maximum daily dose: 2,000 mg/**day**

Alternate dosing: IM, IV: 20 to 30 mg/kg/day divided every 12 hours; maximum daily dose: 1,000 mg/**day** (Bradley 2015)

Endocarditis, *Enterococcal*, resistant to gentamicin: Infants, Children, and Adolescents: IM, IV: 20 to 30 mg/kg/day divided every 12 hours; maximum daily dose: 2,000 mg/**day**; used in combination with other antibiotics, adjust dose to target concentrations (AHA [Baddour] 2005)

***Mycobacterium avium* complex, treatment:** Limited data available: Adolescents: IM, IV: 1,000 mg once daily as part of combination therapy (DHHS [Adult] 2015)

***Mycobacterium ulcerans* (Buruli ulcers):** Limited data available: Infants, Children, and Adolescents: IM: 15 mg/kg once daily; maximum daily dose: 1,000 mg/day; used in combination with rifampin for 8 weeks, or may use this combination for 4 weeks, followed by 4 weeks of rifampin-claithromycin combination therapy (WHO 2012)

Plague: Infants, Children, and Adolescents: IM, IV: 30 mg/kg/day divided every 12 hours for 10 days; maximum daily dose: 2,000 mg/**day** (*Red Book* [AAP] 2015; WHO 2009)

Tuberculosis: Note: Streptomycin is not recommended for initial treatment of tuberculosis and should be reserved for use as part of multidrug-resistant (MDR) TB regimens; usefulness limited by high rates of resistance (Blumberg 2003; WHO 2010); monitor plasma concentrations

Primary pulmonary disease:

Daily therapy:

Infants, Children weighing ≤40 kg, and Adolescents <15 years or weighing ≤40 kg: IM, IV: 20 to 40 mg/kg/day divided every 12 hours; maximum daily dose: 1,000 mg/**day** (Blumberg 2003; Bradley 2015; WHO, 2009a)

Children weighing >40 kg or Adolescents >40 kg or ≥15 years: IM, IV: 15 mg/kg/day once daily; maximum daily dose: 1,000 mg/**day** (Blumberg 2003; Pérez Tanoira 2014)

Directly observed therapy (DOT), twice weekly:

Infants, Children weighing ≤40 kg, and Adolescents <15 years or weighing ≤40 kg: IM, IV: 20 mg/kg/dose; maximum dose: 1,000 mg/dose (Blumberg 2003)

Children weighing >40 kg or Adolescents >40 kg or ≥15 years: IM, IV: 15 mg/kg/dose; maximum dose: 1,000 mg/dose (Blumberg 2003)

Meningitis (independent of HIV-status): Infants, Children, and Adolescents: IM, IV: 20 to 40 mg/kg/day once daily; maximum daily dose: 1,000 mg/**day** (DHHS [pediatric] 2013; *Red Book* [AAP] 2015)

Tularemia: Infants, Children, and Adolescents: IM: 15 mg/kg/dose twice daily for 10 days; maximum daily dose: 2,000 mg/**day** (WHO 2007)

Adult:

Usual dosage range: IM: 15 to 30 mg/kg/day or 1,000 to 2,000 mg daily

Indication-specific dosing:

Tuberculosis: IM:

Daily therapy: 15 mg/kg/day once daily (maximum dose: 1,000 mg)

Directly observed therapy (DOT), twice weekly: 25 to 30 mg/kg/dose twice weekly (maximum dose: 1,500 mg)

Directly observed therapy (DOT), 3 times weekly: 25 to 30 mg/kg 3 times weekly (maximum dose: 1,500 mg)

Endocarditis:

Enterococcal: IM: 1,000 mg every 12 hours for 2 weeks, then 500 mg every 12 hours for 4 weeks in combination with penicillin

Streptococcal: IM: 1,000 mg every 12 hours for 1 week, then 500 mg every 12 hours for 1 week in combination with penicillin

Tularemia: IM: 1,000 to 2,000 mg daily in divided doses every 12 hours (maximum daily dose: 2,000 mg/day) for 7 to 14 days until patient is afebrile for 5 to 7 days

Plague: IM: 30 mg/kg/day (or 2,000 mg) divided every 12 hours until the patient is afebrile for at least 3 days. **Note:** Full course is considered 10 days (WHO 2009).

Dosing adjustment in renal impairment: There are no adjustments provided in the manufacturer's labeling; however, the following adjustments have been recommended (Aronoff 2007):

Infants, Children, and Adolescents: **Note:** Renally adjusted dose recommendations are based on doses of 20 to 40 mg/kg/day every 24 hours.

GFR 30 to 50 mL/minute/1.73 m^2: Administer 7.5 mg/kg/dose every 24 hours

GFR 10 to 29 mL/minute/1.73 m^2: Administer 7.5 mg/kg/dose every 48 hours

GFR <10 mL/minute/1.73 m^2: Administer 7.5 mg/kg/dose every 72 to 96 hours

Intermittent hemodialysis (IHD): Administer 7.5 mg/kg/dose every 72 to 96 hours

Peritoneal dialysis (PD): Administer 7.5 mg/kg/dose every 72 to 96 hours

Continuous renal replacement therapy (CRRT): Administer every 24 hours; monitor levels. **Note:** Drug clearance is highly dependent on the method of renal replacement, filter type, and flow rate. Appropriate dosing requires close monitoring of pharmacologic response, signs of adverse reactions due to drug accumulation, as well as drug concentrations in relation to target trough (if appropriate).

Adults: **Note:** Renally adjusted dose recommendations are based on doses of 1,000 to 2,000 mg every 6 to 12 hours; tuberculosis dosing of 1,000 mg once daily.

CrCl 10 to 50 mL/minute: Administer every 24 to 72 hours

CrCl <10 mL/minute: Administer every 72 to 96 hours

Intermittent hemodialysis (IHD): One-half the dose administered after hemodialysis on dialysis days. **Note:** Dosing dependent on the assumption of 3 times weekly complete IHD sessions.

Peritoneal dialysis (PD): Administration via PD fluid: 20 to 40 mg/L (20 to 40 mcg/mL) of PD fluid

Continuous renal replacement therapy (CRRT): Administer every 24 to 72 hours; monitor levels. **Note:** Drug clearance is highly dependent on the method of renal replacement, filter type, and flow rate. Appropriate dosing requires close monitoring of pharmacologic response, signs of adverse reactions due to drug accumulation, as well as drug concentrations in relation to target trough (if appropriate).

Dosing adjustment in hepatic impairment: There are no adjustments provided in the manufacturer's labeling.

Preparation for Administration

Parenteral:

IM: Reconstitute 1,000 mg vial of lyophilized powder with appropriate volume of SWFI for desired final concentration: 1.8 mL to make 400 mg/mL, 3.2 mL for 250 mg/mL, or 4.2 mL for 200 mg/mL

IV: Further dilution of dose to concentration of 5 to 10 mg/mL in D_5W or NS (eg, adult doses of 12 to 15 mg/kg [maximum dose is 1,000 mg] added to NS (Morris 1994; Peloquin 1992; Pérez Tanoira 2014)

Administration

Parenteral:

IM: Inject deep IM into a large muscle mass; rotate injection sites

IV: After further dilution, infuse over 30 to 60 minutes (Morris 1994; Peloquin 1992; Pérez Tanoira 2014)

Monitoring Parameters Audiometric measurements and vestibular function (baseline, monthly while on therapy, and at 6 months following discontinuation of therapy); renal function (baseline, weekly during therapy or monthly for first 6 months of therapy, then every 3 months and at 6 months following discontinuation of therapy); baseline and frequent assessment of serum electrolytes (including calcium, magnesium, and potassium), liver function tests, growth parameters (CDC 2003; Seddon 2012).

Reference Range Therapeutic: Peak: 20 to 30 mcg/mL; Trough: <5 mcg/mL; Toxic: Peak: >50 mcg/mL; Trough: >10 mcg/mL

Additional Information For use by patients with active tuberculosis that is resistant to isoniazid and rifampin or patients with active tuberculosis in areas where resistance is common and whose drug susceptibility is not yet known. Pfizer will distribute streptomycin directly to physicians and health clinics at no charge. Call Pfizer at 1-800-254-4445.

Dosage Forms Excipient information presented when available (limited, particularly for generics); consult specific product labeling.

Solution Reconstituted, Intramuscular:

Generic: 1 g (1 ea)

- ◆ **Streptomycin for Injection (Can)** *see* Streptomycin *on page 1973*
- ◆ **Streptomycin Sulfate** *see* Streptomycin *on page 1973*
- ◆ **Striant** *see* Testosterone *on page 2025*
- ◆ **Stridex Essential [OTC]** *see* Salicylic Acid *on page 1894*
- ◆ **Stri-Dex Maximum Strength [OTC]** *see* Salicylic Acid *on page 1894*
- ◆ **Stri-Dex Sensitive Skin [OTC]** *see* Salicylic Acid *on page 1894*
- ◆ **Stromectol** *see* Ivermectin (Systemic) *on page 1181*
- ◆ **Strong Iodine Solution** *see* Potassium Iodide and Iodine *on page 1742*
- ◆ **Sublinox (Can)** *see* Zolpidem *on page 2220*
- ◆ **Suboxone** *see* Buprenorphine and Naloxone *on page 322*
- ◆ **Subsys** *see* FentaNYL *on page 857*

Succimer (SUKS si mer)

Brand Names: US Chemet

Brand Names: Canada Chemet

Therapeutic Category Antidote, Lead Toxicity; Chelating Agent, Oral

Generic Availability (US) No

Use Treatment of lead poisoning in children with blood levels >45 mcg/dL; not indicated for prophylaxis of lead poisoning in a lead-containing environment

Pregnancy Risk Factor C

Pregnancy Considerations Adverse events were observed in animal reproduction studies.

Lead poisoning: Lead is known to cross the placenta in amounts related to maternal plasma levels. Prenatal lead exposure may be associated with adverse events such as spontaneous abortion, preterm delivery, decreased birth weight, and impaired neurodevelopment. Some adverse outcomes may occur with maternal blood lead levels <10 mcg/dL. In addition, pregnant women exposed to lead may have an increased risk of gestational hypertension. Consider chelation therapy in pregnant women with confirmed blood lead levels ≥45 mcg/dL (pregnant women with blood lead levels ≥70 mcg/dL should be considered for chelation regardless of trimester); consultation with experts in lead poisoning and high-risk pregnancy is recommended. Encephalopathic pregnant women should be chelated regardless of trimester (CDC, 2010).

Breast-Feeding Considerations It is not known if succimer is excreted in breast milk. When used for the treatment of lead poisoning, the amount of lead in breast milk may range from 0.6% to 3% of the maternal serum concentration. Women with confirmed blood lead levels ≥40 mcg/dL should not initiate breast-feeding; pumping and discarding breast milk is recommended until blood lead levels are <40 mcg/dL, at which point breast-feeding may resume (CDC, 2010). Calcium supplementation may reduce the amount of lead in breast milk.

Contraindications Hypersensitivity to succimer or any component of the formulation

Warnings/Precautions Investigate, identify, and remove sources of lead exposure prior to treatment; do not permit patients to re-enter the contaminated environment until lead abatement has been completed. Primary care providers should consult experts in chemotherapy of heavy metal toxicity before using chelation drug therapy. Succimer is not used to prevent lead poisoning. A rebound rise in serum lead levels may occur after treatment as lead is released from storage sites into blood. The severity of rebound may guide the frequency of future monitoring and the need for additional chelation therapy. Succimer does not cross blood-brain barrier and should not be used to treat encephalopathy associated with lead toxicity. Adequate hydration should be maintained during therapy.

Transient elevations in serum transaminases have been reported. Evaluate serum transaminases at baseline and weekly during treatment; more frequent monitoring may be required in patients with a history of liver disease. Use with caution in patients with renal impairment. Succimer is dialyzable; however, the lead chelates are not. Mild-to-moderate neutropenia has been reported; evaluate CBC with differential at baseline, weekly during treatment, and immediately upon the development of any sign of infection. The manufacturer recommends withholding treatment for ANC <1200/mm^3; treatment may be cautiously resumed when ANC returns to baseline or >1500/mm^3. Consultation with a medical toxicologist to determine the risk versus benefit of withholding treatment is recommended. Monitor for the development of allergic or other mucocutaneous reactions. A reversible mucocutaneous vesicular eruption of the oral mucosa, external urethral meatus, or perianal area has been reported (rarely).

Adverse Reactions

Cardiovascular: Arrhythmia (adults)

Central nervous system: Chills, dizziness, drowsiness, fatigue, fever, headache, sleepiness

Dermatologic: Rash (including papular rash, herpetic rash and mucocutaneous eruptions); pruritus

Endocrine & metabolic: Cholesterol increased

Gastrointestinal: Abdominal cramps, appetite decreased, diarrhea, hemorrhoid symptoms, metallic taste, loose stools, mucosal irritation, nausea, sore throat, vomiting

Genitourinary: Proteinuria (adults), urine output decreased (adults), voiding difficulty (adults)

Hematologic & oncologic: Eosinophilia, increased platelet count

Hepatic: Alkaline phosphatase increased, ALT increased, AST increased

Infection: Common cold

Neuromuscular & skeletal: Back pain, flank pain, knee pain (adults), leg pain (adults), neuropathy, paresthesia, rib pain

Ocular: Cloudy film in eye, watery eyes

Otic: Otitis media, plugged ears

Respiratory: Cough, nasal congestion, rhinorrhea

Miscellaneous: Flu-like syndrome, moniliasis

Rare but important or life-threatening: Allergic reactions (especially with retreatment), neutropenia (causal relationship not established)

Drug Interactions

Metabolism/Transport Effects None known.

Avoid Concomitant Use There are no known interactions where it is recommended to avoid concomitant use.

Increased Effect/Toxicity There are no known significant interactions involving an increase in effect.

Decreased Effect There are no known significant interactions involving a decrease in effect.

Storage/Stability Store between 15°C to 25°C (59°F to 77°F); avoid excessive heat.

Mechanism of Action Succimer is an analog of dimercaprol. It forms water soluble chelates with heavy metals which are subsequently excreted renally. Succimer binds heavy metals; however, the chemical form of these chelates is not known.

Pharmacokinetics (Adult data unless noted)

Absorption: Oral: Rapid, variable

Metabolism: Extensive to mixed succimer-cysteine disulfides

Half-life, elimination: 2 days

Time to peak serum concentration: ~1-2 hours

Elimination: ~25% in urine with peak urinary excretion occurring between 2-4 hours after dosing; of the total amount of succimer eliminated in urine, 90% is eliminated as mixed succimer-cysteine disulfide conjugates; 10% is excreted unchanged; fecal excretion of succimer probably represents unabsorbed drug

Dialysis: Succimer is dialyzable but lead chelates are not

Dosing: Usual Children and Adults: Oral: 10 mg/kg/dose (or 350 mg/m^2/dose) every 8 hours for 5 days followed by 10 mg/kg/dose (or 350 mg/m^2/dose) every 12 hours for 14 days

Succimer Dosing

Weight		Dosage[1] (mg)
18-35 lbs	8-15 kg	100
36-55 lbs	16-23 kg	200
56-75 lbs	24-34 kg	300
76-100 lbs	35-44 kg	400
>100 lbs	>45 kg	500

[1]To be administered every 8 hours.

Note: Concomitant iron therapy has been reported in a small number of children without the formation of a toxic complex with iron (as seen with dimercaprol); courses of therapy may be repeated if indicated by weekly monitoring of blood lead levels; lead levels should be stabilized to <15 mcg/dL; 2 weeks between courses is recommended unless more timely treatment is indicated by lead levels; patients who have received calcium disodium EDTA with or without BAL may be treated with succimer after at least 4 weeks have passed since treatment

Dosing adjustment in renal/hepatic impairment: Administer with caution and monitor closely

Administration Oral: Ensure adequate patient hydration; for patients who cannot swallow the capsule, sprinkle the medicated beads on a small amount of soft food or administer with a fruit juice to mask the odor

Monitoring Parameters Blood lead levels; liver enzymes and CBC with differential (prior to therapy and weekly during therapy)

Test Interactions False-positive ketones (U) using nitroprusside methods, falsely decreased serum CPK; falsely decreased uric acid measurement

Dosage Forms Excipient information presented when available (limited, particularly for generics); consult specific product labeling.

Capsule, Oral:

Chemet: 100 mg

Succinylcholine (suks in il KOE leen)

Medication Safety Issues

High alert medication:

The Institute for Safe Medication Practices (ISMP) includes this medication among its list of drugs which have a heightened risk of causing significant patient harm when used in error.

Other safety concerns:

United States Pharmacopeia (USP) 2006: The Interdisciplinary Safe Medication Use Expert Committee of the USP has recommended the following:

- Hospitals, clinics, and other practice sites should institute special safeguards in the storage, labeling, and use of these agents and should include these safeguards in staff orientation and competency training.
- Healthcare professionals should be on high alert (especially vigilant) whenever a neuromuscular-blocking agent (NMBA) is stocked, ordered, prepared, or administered.

International issues:

Quelicin [U.S., Brazil, Canada, Indonesia] may be confused with Keflin brand name for cefalotin [Argentina, Brazil, Mexico, Netherlands, Norway]

Related Information

Serotonin Syndrome *on page 2447*

Brand Names: US Anectine; Quelicin; Quelicin-1000

Brand Names: Canada Quelicin®

Therapeutic Category Neuromuscular Blocker Agent, Depolarizing; Skeletal Muscle Relaxant, Paralytic

Generic Availability (US) No

Use Adjunct to anesthesia, to facilitate endotracheal intubation, and to provide skeletal muscle relaxation during surgery or mechanical ventilation (FDA approved in all ages)

Pregnancy Risk Factor C

Pregnancy Considerations Reproduction studies have not been conducted. Small amounts cross the placenta. Sensitivity to succinylcholine may be increased due to a ~24% decrease in plasma cholinesterase activity during pregnancy and several days postpartum.

Breast-Feeding Considerations It is not known if succinylcholine is excreted in breast milk. The manufacturer recommends that caution be exercised when administering succinylcholine to nursing women.

Contraindications Hypersensitivity to succinylcholine or any component of the formulation; personal or familial history of malignant hyperthermia; myopathies associated with elevated serum creatine phosphokinase (CPK) values; acute phase of injury following major burns, multiple trauma, extensive denervation of skeletal muscle or upper motor neuron injury

Warnings/Precautions [U.S. Boxed Warning]: Use caution in children and adolescents. Acute rhabdomyolysis with hyperkalemia, ventricular arrhythmias and cardiac arrest have been reported (rarely) in children with undiagnosed skeletal muscle myopathy. Use in children should be reserved for emergency intubation or where immediate airway control is necessary. Use with caution in patients with pre-existing hyperkalemia, extensive or severe burns; severe hyperkalemia may develop in patients with chronic abdominal infections, burn injuries, children with skeletal muscle myopathy, subarachnoid hemorrhage, or conditions which cause degeneration of the nervous system. Alkalosis, hypercalcemia, demyelinating lesions, peripheral neuropathies, denervation, infection, muscle trauma, and diabetes mellitus may result in antagonism of neuromuscular blockade. Electrolyte abnormalities, severe hyponatremia, severe hypocalcemia, severe hypokalemia, hypermagnesemia, neuromuscular diseases, acidosis, acute intermittent porphyria, Eaton-Lambert syndrome, myasthenia gravis, renal failure, and hepatic failure may result in potentiation of neuromuscular blockade. May increase vagal tone.

Succinylcholine is metabolized by plasma cholinesterase; use with caution (if at all) in patients suspected of being homozygous for the atypical plasma cholinesterase gene.

Use with caution in patients with extensive or severe burns; risk of hyperkalemia is increased following injury. May increase intraocular pressure; use caution with narrow angle glaucoma or penetrating eye injuries. Risk of bradycardia may be increased with second dose and may occur more in children. Use may be associated with acute onset of malignant hyperthermia; risk may be increased with concomitant administration of volatile anesthetics. Use with caution in the elderly; effects and duration are more variable.

Maintenance of an adequate airway and respiratory support is critical. Should be administered by adequately trained individuals familiar with its use.

Warnings: Additional Pediatric Considerations
In children and adolescents, rare reports of acute rhabdomyolysis with hyperkalemia followed by ventricular dysrhythmias, cardiac arrest, and death have been reported in children with undiagnosed skeletal muscle myopathy, most frequently Duchenne muscular dystrophy. This syndrome presents as peaked T-waves and sudden cardiac arrest within minutes after the administration of succinylcholine. Bradycardia and rarely asystole have been reported; higher incidence in children, particularly those receiving doses >1.5 mg/kg, and following repeat dosing in both children and adults. Also, if sudden cardiac arrest occurs immediately after administration of succinylcholine, consider hyperkalemia as potential etiology and manage accordingly.

Adverse Reactions

Cardiovascular: Arrhythmias, bradycardia (higher with second dose, more frequent in children), cardiac arrest, hyper-/hypotension, tachycardia

Dermatologic: Rash

Endocrine & metabolic: Hyperkalemia

Gastrointestinal: Salivation (excessive)

Neuromuscular & skeletal: Jaw rigidity, muscle fasciculation, postoperative muscle pain, rhabdomyolysis (with possible myoglobinuric acute renal failure)

Ocular: Intraocular pressure increased

Renal: Acute renal failure (secondary to rhabdomyolysis)

Respiratory: Apnea, respiratory depression (prolonged)

Miscellaneous: Anaphylaxis, malignant hyperthermia

Rare but important or life-threatening: Acute quadriplegic myopathy syndrome (prolonged use), myositis ossificans (prolonged use)

Drug Interactions

Metabolism/Transport Effects None known.

Avoid Concomitant Use

Avoid concomitant use of Succinylcholine with any of the following: QuiNINE

Increased Effect/Toxicity

Succinylcholine may increase the levels/effects of: Analgesics (Opioid); Cardiac Glycosides; OnabotulinumtoxinA; RimabotulinumtoxinB

The levels/effects of Succinylcholine may be increased by: AbobotulinumtoxinA; Acetylcholinesterase Inhibitors; Aminoglycosides; Bambuterol; Capreomycin; Clindamycin (Topical); Colistimethate; Cyclophosphamide; CycloSPORINE (Systemic); Echothiophate Iodide; Lincosamide Antibiotics; Lithium; Loop Diuretics; Magnesium Salts; Phenelzine; Polymyxin B; Procainamide; QuiNIDine; QuiNINE; Tetracycline Derivatives; Vancomycin

Decreased Effect

The levels/effects of Succinylcholine may be decreased by: Loop Diuretics

Storage/Stability Manufacturer recommends refrigeration at 2°C to 8°C (36°F to 46°F) and may be stored at room temperature for 14 days; however, additional testing has demonstrated stability for ≤6 months unrefrigerated (25°C) (Ross, 1988; Roy, 2008). Stability in polypropylene syringes (20 mg/mL) at room temperature (25°C) is 45 days (Storms, 2003). Stability of parenteral admixture (1-2 mg/mL) at refrigeration temperature (4°C) is 24 hours in D_5W or NS.

Mechanism of Action Acts similar to acetylcholine, produces depolarization of the motor endplate at the myoneural junction which causes sustained flaccid skeletal muscle paralysis produced by state of accommodation that develops in adjacent excitable muscle membranes

Pharmacodynamics

IM:
- Onset of action: 2-3 minutes
- Duration: 10-30 minutes

IV:
- Onset of action: Within 30-60 seconds
- Duration: ~4-6 minutes

Pharmacokinetics (Adult data unless noted)

Metabolism: Succinylcholine is rapidly hydrolyzed by plasma pseudocholinesterase to inactive metabolites

Elimination: 10% excreted unchanged in urine

Dosing: Neonatal Note: Because of the risk of malignant hyperthermia, use of continuous IV infusion is **not** recommended.

Endotracheal intubation, nonemergent (Kumar, 2010):
IM: 2 mg/kg/dose if no IV access
IV: 1-2 mg/kg/dose

Dosing: Usual

Paralysis/skeletal muscle relaxation: Infants, Children, and Adolescents: **Note:** Because of the risk of malignant hyperthermia, use of continuous IV infusion is **not** recommended in infants and children.
IM: 3-4 mg/kg; maximum dose: 150 mg
IV:
Infants: Initial: 2 mg/kg; maintenance: 0.3-0.6 mg/kg every 5-10 minutes as needed
Children and Adolescents: Initial: 1 mg/kg; maintenance: 0.3-0.6 mg/kg every 5-10 minutes as needed

Adults:
IM: Up to 3-4 mg/kg; total dose should not exceed 150 mg
IV: Intubation: 0.6 mg/kg (range: 0.3-1.1 mg/kg; rapid sequence intubation: 1-1.5 mg/kg
Note: Pretreatment with atropine may reduce occurrence of bradycardia. Initial dose of succinylcholine must be increased when nondepolarizing agent pretreatment used because of the antagonism between succinylcholine and nondepolarizing neuromuscular-blocking agents.

Dosing adjustment in renal impairment: Use carefully and/or consider dose reduction; prolonged neuromuscular blockade may occur if reduced plasma cholinesterase activity coexists.

Dosing adjustment in hepatic impairment: Use carefully and/or consider dose reduction; prolonged neuromuscular blockade may occur if reduced plasma cholinesterase activity coexists.

Administration Parenteral:
IM: Injection should be made deeply. Use only when IV access is not available.
IV: May be administered undiluted by rapid IV injection.

Monitoring Parameters Heart rate, blood pressure, serum potassium, assisted ventilator status, peripheral nerve stimulator measuring twitch response

Dosage Forms Excipient information presented when available (limited, particularly for generics); consult specific product labeling.
Solution, Injection, as chloride:
Anectine: 20 mg/mL (10 mL) [contains methylparaben]
Quelicin: 20 mg/mL (10 mL) [contains methylparaben, propylparaben]
Quelicin-1000: 100 mg/mL (10 mL)

◆ **Succinylcholine Chloride** *see* Succinylcholine *on page 1976*

◆ **Sucraid** *see* Sacrosidase *on page 1893*

◆ **Sucraid® (Can)** *see* Sacrosidase *on page 1893*

Sucralfate (soo KRAL fate)

Medication Safety Issues

Sound-alike/look-alike issues:
Sucralfate may be confused with salsalate
Carafate may be confused with Cafergot

Administration issues:
For oral administration only. Fatal pulmonary or cerebral embolism has been reported following inadvertent IV administration of sucralfate.

Brand Names: US Carafate

Brand Names: Canada Apo-Sucralfate; Dom-Sucralfate; Novo-Sucralate; Nu-Sucralate; PMS-Sucralate; Sucralfate-1; Sulcrate®; Sulcrate® Suspension Plus; Teva-Sucralfate

Therapeutic Category Gastrointestinal Agent, Gastric or Duodenal Ulcer Treatment

Generic Availability (US) May be product dependent

Use Short-term management of duodenal ulcers; gastric ulcers; suspension may be used topically for treatment of stomatitis due to cancer chemotherapy or other causes of esophageal, gastric, and rectal erosions; treatment of NSAID mucosal damage; prevention of stress ulcers

Pregnancy Risk Factor B

Pregnancy Considerations Adverse events were not observed in animal reproduction studies. Sucralfate is only minimally absorbed following oral administration. Based on available data, use of sucralfate does not appear to increase the risk of adverse fetal events when used during the first trimester (Mahadevan, 2006).

Breast-Feeding Considerations It is not known if sucralfate is excreted in breast milk. Sucralfate is only minimally absorbed following oral administration. The manufacturer recommends that caution be exercised when administering sucralfate to nursing women.

Contraindications Hypersensitivity to sucralfate or any component of the formulation

Warnings/Precautions Because sucralfate acts locally at the ulcer site, successful therapy with sucralfate should not be expected to alter the posthealing frequency of recurrence or the severity of duodenal ulceration. Use with caution in patients with chronic renal failure; sucralfate is an aluminum complex, small amounts of aluminum are absorbed following oral administration. Excretion of aluminum may be decreased in patients with chronic renal failure. Use tablets with caution in patients with conditions that may impair swallowing; aspiration has been reported. Potentially significant interactions may exist, requiring dose or frequency adjustment, additional monitoring, and/or selection of alternative therapy.

Adverse Reactions
Gastrointestinal: Constipation
Rare but important or life-threatening: Anaphylaxis, bezoar formation; hypersensitivity (urticaria, angioedema, facial swelling, laryngospasm, respiratory difficulty, rhinitis)

Drug Interactions

Metabolism/Transport Effects None known.

Avoid Concomitant Use
Avoid concomitant use of Sucralfate with any of the following: Multivitamins/Minerals (with ADEK, Folate, Iron); Vitamin D Analogs

Increased Effect/Toxicity
The levels/effects of Sucralfate may be increased by: Multivitamins/Fluoride (with ADE); Multivitamins/Minerals (with ADEK, Folate, Iron); Vitamin D Analogs

Decreased Effect
Sucralfate may decrease the levels/effects of: Antifungal Agents (Azole Derivatives, Systemic); Cholic Acid; Digoxin; Dolutegravir; Eltrombopag; Furosemide; Levothyroxine; Multivitamins/Fluoride (with ADE); Phosphate Supplements; QuiNIDine; Quinolone Antibiotics; Sulpiride; Tetracycline Derivatives; Vitamin K Antagonists

Storage/Stability Suspension: Shake well. Store at 20°C to 25°C (68°F to 77°F); do **not** freeze.

Mechanism of Action Forms a complex by binding with positively charged proteins in exudates, forming a viscous paste-like, adhesive substance. This selectively forms a protective coating that acts locally to protect the gastric lining against peptic acid, pepsin, and bile salts.

Pharmacodynamics GI protection effect:
Acid neutralizing capacity: 14-17 mEq/1 g dose of sucralfate
Onset of action: 1-2 hours
Duration: Up to 6 hours

Pharmacokinetics (Adult data unless noted)
Absorption: Oral: <5%
Metabolism: Not metabolized
Elimination: 90% excreted in stool; small amounts that are absorbed are excreted in the urine as unchanged compounds

Dosing: Usual Oral:
Children: Dose not established; doses of 40-80 mg/kg/day divided every 6 hours have been used
Stomatitis: 5-10 mL (1 g/10 mL); swish and spit or swish and swallow 4 times/day
Adults:
Stress ulcer prophylaxis: 1 g 4 times/day
Stress ulcer treatment: 1 g every 4 hours
Duodenal ulcer:
Treatment: 1 g 4 times/day for 4-8 weeks, or alternatively 2 g twice daily; treatment is recommended for 4-8 weeks in adults
Maintenance: Prophylaxis: 1 g twice daily
Stomatitis: 1 g/10 mL suspension, swish and spit or swish and swallow 4 times/day
Proctitis: Rectal enema: 2 g/20 mL once or twice daily
Dosage comment in renal impairment: Aluminum salt is minimally absorbed (<5%), however, may accumulate in renal failure

Administration
Oral: Administer on an empty stomach 1 hour before meals and at bedtime; tablet may be broken or dissolved in water before ingestion; do not administer antacids within 30 minutes of administration; shake suspension well before use
Rectal: May administer oral suspension as rectal enema; shake suspension well before use

Additional Information There is approximately 14-16 mEq acid neutralizing capacity per 1 g sucralfate

Dosage Forms Excipient information presented when available (limited, particularly for generics); consult specific product labeling.
Suspension, Oral:
Carafate: 1 g/10 mL (420 mL) [contains fd&c red #40, methylparaben; cherry flavor]
Tablet, Oral:
Carafate: 1 g [scored; contains fd&c blue #1 aluminum lake]
Generic: 1 g

Extemporaneous Preparations Note: Commercial oral suspension is available (100 mg/mL).

A 66.67 mg/mL oral suspension may be made with tablets. Add eight 1 g tablets to a 120 mL glass bottle. Add 40 mL of SWFI and allow tablets to dissolve (~2 minutes). Add 40 mL of sorbitol 70% solution and shake well. In a separate container, dissolve 2 flavor packets (Vari-Flavors; Ross Laboratories) with 10 mL of water, and swirl until dissolved then add to drug mixture. Add SWFI to make 120 mL. Label "shake well" and "refrigerate". Use within 2 weeks.

Ferraro JM. Sucralfate suspension for mouth ulcers. *Drug Intell Clin Pharm*. 1985;19(6):480.

- **Sucralfate-1 (Can)** *see* Sucralfate *on page 1978*
- **Sucrets® Children's [OTC]** *see* Dyclonine *on page 725*
- **Sucrets® Maximum Strength [OTC]** *see* Dyclonine *on page 725*
- **Sucrets® Regular Strength [OTC]** *see* Dyclonine *on page 725*

Sucrose (SOO krose)

Brand Names: US Sweet-Ease® [OTC]; TootSweet™ [OTC]

Therapeutic Category Analgesic, Nonopioid

Generic Availability (US) No

Use Provide short-term analgesia in neonates during minor procedures (eg, heel stick, eye exam for retinopathy of prematurity, circumcision, immunization, venipuncture, ET intubation and suctioning, NG tube insertion, IM or subcutaneous injection); provide short-term analgesia in infants during immunization administration

Contraindications Hypersensitivity to sucrose, corn, corn products, or any component of the formulation

Warnings/Precautions Patients should have a functioning gastrointestinal tract; avoid use in patients with gastrointestinal tract abnormalities (eg, esophageal atresia or tracheal esophageal fistula); while necrotizing enterocolitis (NEC) has not been reported with sucrose administration, risk:benefit assessment should be considered in patients at high risk for NEC. Avoid use in patients at risk for aspiration; sucrose should not be used for patients requiring ongoing analgesia. Concentration of some products has been shown to increase (up to 40%) when stored over a 6-month period. Efficacy in unstable or extremely low birthweight, premature neonates has not been established.

Adverse Reactions
Cardiovascular: Bradycardia (self-limiting)
Respiratory: Oxygen desaturation or brief apnea in premature neonates (spontaneous resolution)

Storage/Stability Store at 4°C to 32°C (40°F to 90°F). For some products, concentration may increase (up to 40%) when stored over a 6-month period. Unused portion should be discarded.

Mechanism of Action Exact mechanism is not known; it has been proposed that sucrose induces endogenous opioid release.

Pharmacodynamics
Maximum effect: 2 minutes
Duration: 3-5 minutes

Dosing: Neonatal Oral: 0.1-0.2 mL of 24% solution placed on the tongue or buccal surface 2 minutes prior to procedure; various regimens reported, effective range: 0.05-0.5 mL (maximum dose: 2 mL). For doses >0.1 mL, some studies have administered in aliquots with first dose 2 minutes prior to procedure and remainder of dose given intermittently (typically 3 times) during or after procedure (Johnston, 1999; Stevens, 2010).

Dosing: Usual Oral: Infants prior to immunization: 2 mL of 24% solution administered 1-2 minutes prior to vaccine administration has been used; others have shown 10 mL of 25% effective in infants receiving their 2-month vaccinations (Reis, 2003). For older infants, higher concentration of solution for analgesic effect: 2 mL of 50% or 75% solution has been shown effective (Harrison, 2010; Shah, 2009)

Administration For single oral use only. May be administered directly into baby's mouth or via a pacifier dipped into solution. Do not reuse or sterilize; dispose product after use.

Monitoring Parameters Heart rate, respiratory rate, pain relief

Dosage Forms Excipient information presented when available (limited, particularly for generics); consult specific product labeling.
Solution, oral:
Sweet-Ease® Preserved: 24% (15 mL)
TootSweet™: 24% (0.5 mL, 1 mL, 2 mL, 12 mL)
Solution, oral [preservative free]:
Sweet-Ease Natural®: 24% (15 mL)

- **Sudafed** *see* Pseudoephedrine *on page 1801*
- **Sudafed [OTC]** *see* Pseudoephedrine *on page 1801*
- **Sudafed 12 Hour [OTC]** *see* Pseudoephedrine *on page 1801*
- **Sudafed 24 Hour [OTC]** *see* Pseudoephedrine *on page 1801*
- **Sudafed Childrens [OTC]** *see* Pseudoephedrine *on page 1801*
- **Sudafed® Decongestant (Can)** *see* Pseudoephedrine *on page 1801*
- **Sudafed PE Childrens [OTC]** *see* Phenylephrine (Systemic) *on page 1685*

- ◆ **Sudafed PE Maximum Strength [OTC]** *see* Phenylephrine (Systemic) *on page 1685*
- ◆ **Sudafed® Sinus Advance (Can)** *see* Pseudoephedrine and Ibuprofen *on page 1803*
- ◆ **Sudanyl [OTC]** *see* Pseudoephedrine *on page 1801*
- ◆ **SudoGest [OTC]** *see* Pseudoephedrine *on page 1801*
- ◆ **SudoGest 12 Hour [OTC]** *see* Pseudoephedrine *on page 1801*
- ◆ **Sudogest PE [OTC]** *see* Phenylephrine (Systemic) *on page 1685*
- ◆ **Sufenta** *see* SUFentanil *on page 1980*

SUFentanil (soo FEN ta nil)

Medication Safety Issues

Sound-alike/look-alike issues:

SUFentanil may be confused with alfentanil, fentaNYL

Sufenta® may be confused with Alfenta, Sudafed, Survanta

High alert medication:

The Institute for Safe Medication Practices (ISMP) includes this medication among its list of drugs which have a heightened risk of causing significant patient harm when used in error.

Brand Names: US Sufenta

Brand Names: Canada Sufenta; Sufentanil Citrate Injection, USP

Therapeutic Category Analgesic, Narcotic; General Anesthetic

Generic Availability (US) Yes

Use Analgesia; analgesia adjunct; anesthetic agent

Pregnancy Risk Factor C

Pregnancy Considerations Adverse event were observed in some animal reproduction studies. Administration of epidural sufentanil with bupivacaine with or without epinephrine is indicated in labor and delivery. Intravenous use or larger epidural doses are not recommended in pregnant women. When used for pain relief during labor, opioids may temporarily affect the heart rate of the fetus (ACOG, 2002).

Breast-Feeding Considerations It is not known if sufentanil is excreted in breast milk. The manufacturer recommends that caution be exercised when administering sufentanil to nursing women. Parenteral opioids used during labor have the potential to interfere with a newborns natural reflex to nurse within the first few hours after birth. When needed, a short-acting opioid such as sufentanil is preferred for women who will be nursing. Nursing infants exposed to large doses of opioids should be monitored for apnea and sedation (Montgomery, 2012).

Contraindications

Hypersensitivity to sufentanil or any component of the formulation, or known intolerance to other opioid agonists

Documentation of allergenic cross-reactivity for opioids is limited. However, because of similarities in chemical structure and/or pharmacologic actions, the possibility of cross-sensitivity cannot be ruled out with certainty.

Warnings/Precautions Sufentanil shares the toxic potentials of opioid agonists, and precautions of opioid agonist therapy should be observed. Use with caution in patients with bradyarrhythmias, hepatic impairment, or renal impairment. Use with extreme caution in patients with head injury, intracranial lesions, or elevated ICP; exaggerated elevation of ICP may occur. Use with caution in patients with pre-existing respiratory compromise (hypoxia and/or hypercapnia), COPD or other obstructive pulmonary disease, and kyphoscoliosis or other skeletal disorder which may alter respiratory function; critical respiratory depression may occur, even at therapeutic dosages. Use caution in patients who are morbidly obese, debilitated, or elderly. Use caution in neonates as sufentanil clearance is slow much slower than adults; neonates with cardiovascular disease have an even slower clearance. The clearance of sufentanil in children 2 to 8 years of age was shown to be twice as rapid as that seen in adults and adolescents (Lundberg, 2011). Inject slowly over at least 2 minutes (Sebel, 1982); rapid IV infusion may result in skeletal muscle and chest wall rigidity, impaired ventilation, or respiratory distress/arrest; nondepolarizing skeletal muscle relaxant may be required. Due to the high incidence of apnea, hypotension, tachycardia, and muscle rigidity, it should be administered by individuals specifically trained in the use of anesthetic agents and should not be used in diagnostic or therapeutic procedures outside the monitored anesthesia setting; resuscitative and intubation equipment should be readily available.

Adverse Reactions

Cardiovascular: Bradycardia, cardiac arrhythmia, hyper-/hypotension

Central nervous system: CNS depression, confusion, somnolence

Dermatologic: Pruritus

Gastrointestinal: Nausea, vomiting

Ocular: Blurred vision

Neuromuscular & Skeletal: Chest wall rigidity

Rare but important or life-threatening: Anaphylaxis, apnea, arrhythmia, biliary spasm, bronchospasm, cardiac arrest, chills, circulatory depression; cold, clammy skin; dizziness, dysesthesia, erythema, itching, laryngospasm, mental depression, paradoxical CNS excitation or delirium, physical and psychological dependence with prolonged use, respiratory depression (dose related), seizure, skeletal muscle rigidity, skin rash, tachycardia, urinary retention, urinary tract spasm, urticaria

Drug Interactions

Metabolism/Transport Effects **Substrate** of CYP3A4 (major); **Note:** Assignment of Major/Minor substrate status based on clinically relevant drug interaction potential

Avoid Concomitant Use

Avoid concomitant use of SUFentanil with any of the following: Azelastine (Nasal); Ceritinib; Conivaptan; Eluxadoline; Fusidic Acid (Systemic); Idelalisib; MAO Inhibitors; Mixed Agonist / Antagonist Opioids; Orphenadrine; Paraldehyde; Thalidomide

Increased Effect/Toxicity

SUFentanil may increase the levels/effects of: Alcohol (Ethyl); Alvimopan; Azelastine (Nasal); Beta-Blockers; Bradycardia-Causing Agents; Calcium Channel Blockers (Nondihydropyridine); Ceritinib; CNS Depressants; Desmopressin; Diuretics; Eluxadoline; Hydrocodone; Ivabradine; Lacosamide; MAO Inhibitors; Methotrimeprazine; Metyrosine; Mirtazapine; Orphenadrine; Paraldehyde; Pramipexole; ROPINIRole; Rotigotine; Selective Serotonin Reuptake Inhibitors; Suvorexant; Thalidomide; Zolpidem

The levels/effects of SUFentanil may be increased by: Amphetamines; Anticholinergic Agents; Antipsychotic Agents (Phenothiazines); Aprepitant; Bretylium; Brimonidine (Topical); Cannabis; Conivaptan; CYP3A4 Inhibitors (Moderate); CYP3A4 Inhibitors (Strong); Dasatinib; Doxylamine; Dronabinol; Droperidol; Fosaprepitant; Fusidic Acid (Systemic); HydrOXYzine; Idelalisib; Ivacaftor; Kava Kava; Luliconazole; Magnesium Sulfate; Methotrimeprazine; Mifepristone; Nabilone; Netupitant; Palbociclib; Perampanel; Rufinamide; Ruxolitinib; Simeprevir; Sodium Oxybate; Stiripentol; Succinylcholine; Tapentadol; Tetrahydrocannabinol; Tofacitinib

Decreased Effect

SUFentanil may decrease the levels/effects of: Pegvisomant

The levels/effects of SUFentanil may be decreased by: Ammonium Chloride; Mixed Agonist / Antagonist Opioids; Naltrexone

Storage/Stability Store at 20°C to 25°C (68°F to 77°F). Protect from light.

Mechanism of Action Binds to opioid receptors throughout the CNS. Once receptor binding occurs, effects are exerted by opening K+ channels and inhibiting Ca++ channels. These mechanisms increase pain threshold, alter pain perception, inhibit ascending pain pathways; short-acting opioid; dose-related inhibition of catecholamine release (up to 30 mcg/kg) controls sympathetic response to surgical stress.

Pharmacodynamics

Onset of action: 1-3 minutes

Duration: Dose dependent; anesthesia adjunct doses: 5 minutes

Pharmacokinetics (Adult data unless noted)

Distribution: V_{dss}:

Children 2-8 years: 2.9 ± 0.6 L/kg

Adults: 1.7 ± 0.2 L/kg

Protein binding (alpha$_1$-acid glycoprotein):

Neonates: 79%

Adults:

Male: 93%

Postpartum women: 91%

Metabolism: Primarily by the liver via demethylation and dealkylation

Half-life, elimination:

Neonates: 382-1162 minutes

Children 2-8 years: 97 ± 42 minutes

Adolescents 10-15 years: 76 ± 33 minutes

Adults: 164 ± 22 minutes

Elimination: ~2% excreted unchanged in the urine; 80% of dose excreted in urine (mostly as metabolites) within 24 hours

Clearance:

Children 2-8 years: 30.5 ± 8.8 mL/minute/kg

Adolescents: 12.8 ± 12 mL/minute/kg

Adults: 12.7 ± 0.8 mL/minute/kg

Dosing: Neonatal Doses should be titrated to appropriate effects; wide range of doses, dependent upon desired degree of analgesia or anesthesia.

General anesthesia, adjunct (deep intraoperative anesthesia for neonatal cardiac surgery): Full-term neonates: IV: 5-10 mcg/kg/dose as needed; followed by a continuous IV infusion (for postoperative anesthesia): 2 mcg/kg/**hour** for 24 hours (Anand, 1992)

Analgesia/sedation in mechanically ventilated patients: Preterm neonates: IV: Loading dose: 0.5 mcg/kg/dose administered over 10 minutes, followed by 0.2 mcg/kg/**hour** continuous infusion was used in 15 mechanically ventilated premature neonates (mean GA: 29.1 weeks (26-34 weeks) and produced "burst-suppression-like" EEG patterns (Tich, 2010)

Dosing: Usual Doses should be titrated to appropriate effects; wide range of doses, dependent upon desired degree of analgesia or anesthesia; use lean body weight to dose patients who are >20% above ideal body weight.

Children <12 years: Anesthesia: IV: Initial: 10-25 mcg/kg; maintenance: Up to 25-50 mcg as needed

Adults: IV:

Adjunct to general anesthesia:

Low dose: Initial: 0.5-1 mcg/kg; maintenance: 10-25 mcg as needed

Moderate dose: Initial: 2-8 mcg/kg; maintenance: 10-50 mcg as needed

Anesthesia: Initial: 8-30 mcg/kg; maintenance: 10-50 mcg as needed

Preparation for Administration IV: May further dilute in an appropriate fluid to a concentration <50 mcg/mL

Administration

Parenteral: IV: Administer at a concentration ≤ 50 mcg/mL (undiluted)

Intermittent IV: May be administered by either slow injection or as an infusion.

Slow IV injection: Administer over at least 2 minutes (Moore 1985; Sebel 1982); in adults, a range of 2 to 10 minutes has been used [Miller 2010].

Continuous IV infusion: Administer as a continuous infusion via an infusion pump

Monitoring Parameters Respiratory rate, blood pressure, heart rate, oxygen saturation, neurological status (for degree of analgesia/anesthesia)

Controlled Substance C-II

Dosage Forms Excipient information presented when available (limited, particularly for generics); consult specific product labeling.

Solution, Intravenous [preservative free]:

Sufenta: 50 mcg/mL (1 mL); 100 mcg/2 mL (2 mL); 250 mcg/5 mL (5 mL)

Generic: 50 mcg/mL (1 mL); 100 mcg/2 mL (2 mL); 250 mcg/5 mL (5 mL)

- ◆ **Sufentanil Citrate** *see* SUFentanil *on page 1980*
- ◆ **Sufentanil Citrate Injection, USP (Can)** *see* SUFentanil *on page 1980*
- ◆ **Sulamyd** *see* Sulfacetamide (Ophthalmic) *on page 1981*
- ◆ **Sulamyd** *see* Sulfacetamide (Topical) *on page 1982*
- ◆ **Sulbactam and Ampicillin** *see* Ampicillin and Sulbactam *on page 159*
- ◆ **Sulcrate® (Can)** *see* Sucralfate *on page 1978*
- ◆ **Sulcrate® Suspension Plus (Can)** *see* Sucralfate *on page 1978*

Sulfacetamide (Ophthalmic) (sul fa SEE ta mide)

Medication Safety Issues

Sound-alike/look-alike issues:

Bleph-10 may be confused with Blephamide

Brand Names: US Bleph-10

Brand Names: Canada AK Sulf Liq; Bleph 10 DPS; Diosulf; PMS-Sulfacetamide; Sodium Sulamyd

Therapeutic Category Antibiotic, Ophthalmic; Antibiotic, Sulfonamide Derivative

Generic Availability (US) Yes

Use Ophthalmic: Treatment of conjunctivitis and other superficial ocular infections due to susceptible organisms (Ointment; solution: FDA approved in ages ≥2 months and adults); adjunctive treatment with systemic sulfonamides for therapy of trachoma (Solution: FDA approved in ages ≥ 2 months and adults)

Pregnancy Risk Factor C

Pregnancy Considerations Animal reproduction studies have not been conducted. Use of systemic sulfonamides during pregnancy may cause kernicterus in the newborn.

Breast-Feeding Considerations The amount of systemic absorption following ophthalmic administration is not known. Use of systemic sulfonamides while breastfeeding may cause kernicterus in the newborn; the amount of systemic absorption following ophthalmic administration is not known. According to the manufacturer, the decision to continue or discontinue breast-feeding during therapy should take into account the risk of exposure to the infant and the benefits of treatment to the mother.

Contraindications

Hypersensitivity to sulfonamides or any component of the formulation.

Documentation of allergenic cross-reactivity for sulfonamides is limited. However, because of similarities in chemical structure and/or pharmacologic actions, the possibility of cross-sensitivity cannot be ruled out with certainty.

Warnings/Precautions Severe reactions (rare fatalities) to sulfonamides have been reported, regardless of route of administration; reactions may include Stevens-Johnson syndrome, toxic epidermal necrolysis, fulminant hepatic necrosis, or blood dyscrasias. Discontinue at first sign of serious reaction. Chemical similarities are present among sulfonamides, sulfonylureas, carbonic anhydrase inhibitors, thiazides, and loop diuretics (except ethacrynic acid). Use in patients with sulfonamide allergy is specifically contraindicated in product labeling; however, a risk of cross-reaction exists in patients with allergy to any of these compounds; avoid use when previous reaction has been severe. Prolonged use may lead to overgrowth of nonsusceptible organisms, including fungi. If superinfection is suspected, institute appropriate alternative therapy.

May be inactivated by purulent exudates containing PABA. For topical application to the eye only; not for injection. To avoid contamination, do not touch tip of container to any surface. Do not use concurrently with silver preparations.

Adverse Reactions

Cardiovascular: Edema

Ocular (following ophthalmic application): Burning, conjunctivitis, conjunctival hyperemia, corneal ulcers, irritation, stinging

Miscellaneous: Allergic reactions, systemic lupus erythematosus

Drug Interactions

Metabolism/Transport Effects None known.

Avoid Concomitant Use There are no known interactions where it is recommended to avoid concomitant use.

Increased Effect/Toxicity There are no known significant interactions involving an increase in effect.

Decreased Effect There are no known significant interactions involving a decrease in effect.

Storage/Stability

Solution: Store at 8°C to 25°C (46°F to 77°F); protect from light. Darkened solutions should not be used.

Ointment: Store at 20°C to 25°C (68°F to 77°F).

Mechanism of Action Interferes with bacterial growth by inhibiting bacterial folic acid synthesis through competitive antagonism of PABA

Pharmacodynamics Onset of action: Improvement of conjunctivitis is usually seen within 3-6 days

Dosing: Usual Infants ≥2 months, Children, Adolescents, and Adults:

Conjunctivitis: Ophthalmic:

Ointment: Instill 1/2" ribbon into the lower conjunctival sac of affected eye(s) every 3-4 hours and at bedtime; increase dosing interval as condition responds. Ointment may be used as an adjunct to the solution; usual duration of treatment: 7-10 days

Solution: Instill 1-2 drops into the lower conjunctival sac of affected eye(s) every 2-3 hours initially; increase dosing interval as condition responds; usual duration of treatment: 7-10 days

Trachoma: Ophthalmic: Solution: Instill 2 drops into the conjunctival sac of affected eye(s) every 2 hours; must be used in conjunction with systemic therapy

Administration For topical application to the eye only; not for injection. Avoid contact of tube or bottle tip with skin or eye. Apply finger pressure to lacrimal sac during and for 1-2 minutes after instillation to decrease risk of absorption and systemic effects.

Monitoring Parameters Response to therapy

Dosage Forms Excipient information presented when available (limited, particularly for generics); consult specific product labeling.

Ointment, Ophthalmic, as sodium:

Generic: 10% (3.5 g)

Solution, Ophthalmic, as sodium:

Bleph-10: 10% (5 mL)

Generic: 10% (5 mL, 15 mL)

Sulfacetamide (Topical) (sul fa SEE ta mide)

Medication Safety Issues

Sound-alike/look-alike issues:

Klaron may be confused with Klor-Con

Brand Names: US APOP [DSC]; Klaron; Ovace Plus; Ovace Plus Wash; Ovace Wash; Seb-Prev Wash; Seb-Prev [DSC]

Brand Names: Canada Sulfacet-R

Therapeutic Category Acne Products; Antibiotic, Sulfonamide Derivative; Topical Skin Product

Generic Availability (US) May be product dependent

Use Treatment of seborrheic dermatitis, seborrhea sicca, acne vulgaris, and secondary cutaneous bacterial infections due to organisms susceptible to sulfonamides (FDA approved in ages ≥12 years and adults; refer to product specific information for FDA approved indications)

Pregnancy Risk Factor C

Pregnancy Considerations Animal reproduction studies have not been conducted. The amount of sulfacetamide available systemically following topical administration is unknown. Use of systemic sulfonamides during pregnancy may cause kernicterus in the newborn.

Breast-Feeding Considerations Small amounts of sulfonamides administered orally are excreted in breast milk; it is not known if sulfacetamide administered topically is excreted in breast milk. Use of systemic sulfonamides while breast-feeding may cause kernicterus in the newborn.

Contraindications

Known or suspected hypersensitivity to sulfonamides or any component of the formulation; kidney disease (Ovace Plus Wash and Ovace Plus lotion)

Note: Although the FDA approved product labeling states this medication is contraindicated with other sulfonamide-containing drug classes, the scientific basis of this statement has been challenged. See "Warnings/Precautions" for more detail.

Warnings/Precautions Severe reactions to sulfonamides have been reported, regardless of route of administration. Reactions may include Stevens-Johnson syndrome, toxic epidermal necrolysis, fulminant hepatic necrosis, or blood dyscrasias; fatalities have occurred. Fatalities associated with severe reactions, including drug-induced systemic lupus erythematosus, have occurred with sulfonamides (regardless of route). Skin rash or other reactions have occurred in patients with no prior history of sulfonamide hypersensitivity. Discontinue use at the first sign of hypersensitivity or rash. Monitor closely for local irritation and/or sensitization during long-term therapy. Systemic absorption is increased with application to large, infected, abraded, denuded, or burned skin. Application to infected area containing nonsusceptible organisms may cause proliferation of the organism.

For external use only; avoid contact with eyes and mucous membranes. Discontinue use if irritation, rash, or signs of hypersensitivity occur. Some products contain sodium metabisulfite which may cause allergic reactions in certain individuals (eg, asthmatic patients). Products are not compatible with silver-containing products.

Benzyl alcohol and derivatives: Some dosage forms may contain benzyl alcohol; large amounts of benzyl alcohol (≥99 mg/kg/day) have been associated with a potentially fatal toxicity ("gasping syndrome") in neonates; the "gasping syndrome" consists of metabolic acidosis, respiratory distress, gasping respirations, CNS dysfunction (including convulsions, intracranial hemorrhage), hypotension, and cardiovascular collapse (AAP, 1997; CDC, 1982); some data suggests that benzoate displaces bilirubin from protein binding sites (Ahlfors, 2001); avoid or use dosage forms containing benzyl alcohol with caution in neonates. See manufacturer's labeling.

Sulfonamide ("sulfa") allergy: Traditionally, concerns for cross-reactivity have extended to all compounds containing the sulfonamide structure (SO_2NH_2). An expanded understanding of allergic mechanisms indicates cross-reactivity between antibiotic sulfonamides and nonantibiotic sulfonamides may not occur, or at the very least this potential is extremely low (Brackett 2004; Johnson 2005; Slatore 2004; Tornero 2004). In particular, mechanisms of cross-reaction due to antibody production (anaphylaxis) are unlikely to occur with nonantibiotic sulfonamides and antibiotic sulfonamides. A nonantibiotic sulfonamide compound which contains the arylamine structure and therefore may cross-react with antibiotic sulfonamides is sulfasalazine (Zawodniak 2010). T-cell-mediated (type IV) reactions (eg, maculopapular rash) are less understood and it is not possible to completely exclude this potential based on current insights. In cases where prior reactions were severe (Stevens-Johnson syndrome/TEN), some clinicians choose to avoid exposure to these classes.

Warnings: Additional Pediatric Considerations Some dosage forms may contain propylene glycol; in neonates large amounts of propylene glycol delivered orally, intravenously (eg, >3,000 mg/day), or topically have been associated with potentially fatal toxicities which can include metabolic acidosis, seizures, renal failure, and CNS depression; toxicities have also been reported in children and adults including hyperosmolality, lactic acidosis, seizures, and respiratory depression; use caution (AAP, 1997; Shehab, 2009).

Adverse Reactions

Dermatologic: Burning sensation of skin, erythema, pruritus, Stevens-Johnson syndrome, stinging of the skin, toxic epidermal necrolysis

Hematologic & oncologic: Agranulocytosis, aplastic anemia, hematologic abnormality

Hepatic: Fulminant hepatic necrosis

Hypersensitivity: Hypersensitivity reaction

Local: Local irritation, localized edema

Neuromuscular & skeletal: Systemic lupus erythematosus

Drug Interactions

Metabolism/Transport Effects None known.

Avoid Concomitant Use

Avoid concomitant use of Sulfacetamide (Topical) with any of the following: BCG; BCG (Intravesical)

Increased Effect/Toxicity There are no known significant interactions involving an increase in effect.

Decreased Effect

Sulfacetamide (Topical) may decrease the levels/effects of: BCG; BCG (Intravesical); BCG Vaccine (Immunization); Sodium Picosulfate

Storage/Stability

Cream, shampoo, Ovace Plus lotion: Store at 25°C (77°F); excursions permitted to 15°C to 30°C (59°F to 86°F). Protect from freezing and excess heat. May darken slightly on storage; efficacy or safety is not affected. Keep tightly closed.

Klaron lotion, topical suspension: Store at 20°C to 25°C (68°F to 77°F). Keep tightly closed.

Wash: May darken slightly on storage; efficacy or safety is not affected. Keep tightly closed.

Ovace Plus Wash cleansing gel: Store at 25°C (77°F); excursions permitted to 15°C to 30°C (59°F to 86°F). Protect from freezing and excess heat.

Ovace Wash, Ovace Plus Wash liquid: Store at 20°C to 25°C (68°F to 77°F); excursions permitted to 15°C to 30°C (59°F to 86°F). Brief exposures to temperatures up to 40°C (104°F) may be tolerated provided the mean temperature does not exceed 25°C (77°F); however, such exposure should be minimized.

SEB-Prev: Store at 20°C to 25°C (68°F to 77°F). Protect from freezing and excess heat.

Mechanism of Action Interferes with bacterial growth by inhibiting bacterial folic acid synthesis through competitive antagonism of PABA

Pharmacokinetics (Adult data unless noted) Absorption: Poor through intact skin

Dosing: Usual Children ≥12 years and Adults:

Acne: Topical: Klaron® Lotion: Apply thin film to affected area twice daily

Seborrheic dermatitis, including seborrhea sicca: Topical:

Ovace® Plus Wash; Ovace® Wash: Wash affected area twice daily; repeat application for 8-10 days. Dosing interval may be increased as eruption subsides. Applications once or twice weekly, or every other week may be used for prevention. If treatment needs to be reinitiated, start therapy as a twice daily regimen.

Ovace® Plus Shampoo: Wash hair at least twice weekly

Secondary cutaneous bacterial infections: Topical: Ovace® Plus Wash; Ovace® Wash: Wash affected area once daily for 8-10 days

Administration For external use only; avoid contact with eyes and mucous membranes.

Lotion: Shake lotion well before using; apply a thin film to affected area.

Shampoo: Apply to wet hair and massage vigorously into scalp; thoroughly rinse hair.

Wash: Apply to wet hair or skin and massage into a full lather; rinse thoroughly and pat dry; repeat after 10-20 seconds (for seborrheic dermatitis). If skin dryness occurs, rinse off early or use less frequently. Regular shampooing after use on hair is not necessary; however, hair should be shampooed at least once weekly.

Monitoring Parameters Response to therapy

Dosage Forms Considerations APOP gel is formulated in a vehicle containing 0.5% bakuchiol, a natural compound extracted from *Psoralea corylifolia* purported to exert antimicrobial and anti-inflammatory activity, as well as reduce scarring from acne lesions.

Dosage Forms Excipient information presented when available (limited, particularly for generics); consult specific product labeling. [DSC] = Discontinued product

Cream, External, as sodium:

Ovace Plus: 10% (57 g) [contains benzyl alcohol, butylparaben, cetyl alcohol, disodium edta, ethylparaben, methylparaben, propylparaben]

Foam, External:

Ovace Plus: 9.8% (100 g) [contains benzyl alcohol, cetyl alcohol, propylene glycol]

Gel, External, as sodium:

APOP: 10% (57 g [DSC]) [contains benzyl alcohol, cetyl alcohol, disodium edta]

Ovace Plus Wash: 10% (355 mL) [contains cetearyl alcohol, edetate disodium dihydrate, methylparaben]

Generic: 10% (355 mL); 10% (355 mL)

Liquid, External, as sodium:

Ovace Plus Wash: 10% (180 mL, 473 mL) [contains cetearyl alcohol, edetate disodium, methylparaben]

Ovace Wash: 10% (180 mL, 355 mL, 480 mL) [contains edetate disodium, methylparaben]

Seb-Prev Wash: 10% (340 mL) [contains edetate disodium, methylparaben]

Generic: 10% (177 mL, 180 mL, 354.8 mL, 355 mL, 480 mL)

Lotion, External, as sodium:

Klaron: 10% (118 mL)

Klaron: 10% (118 mL) [contains disodium edta, methylparaben, propylene glycol, sodium metabisulfite]

Ovace Plus: 9.8% (57 g, 113 g) [contains benzyl alcohol, cetyl alcohol, disodium edta]

Seb-Prev: 10% (118 mL [DSC]) [contains methylparaben, sodium metabisulfite]
Generic: 10% (118 mL)
Shampoo, External, as sodium:
Ovace Plus: 10% (237 mL) [contains cetearyl alcohol, methylparaben, propylparaben]
Generic: 10% (237 mL)
Suspension, External, as sodium:
Generic: 10% (118 mL)

◆ **Sulfacetamide Sodium** *see* Sulfacetamide (Ophthalmic) *on page 1981*

◆ **Sulfacetamide Sodium** *see* Sulfacetamide (Topical) *on page 1982*

◆ **Sulfacet-R (Can)** *see* Sulfacetamide (Topical) *on page 1982*

SulfADIAZINE (sul fa DYE a zeen)

Medication Safety Issues

Sound-alike/look-alike issues:

SulfADIAZINE may be confused with sulfaSALAzine

Therapeutic Category Antibiotic, Sulfonamide Derivative

Generic Availability (US) Yes

Use Adjunctive treatment in toxoplasmosis with pyrimethamine [FDA approved in ages ≥2 months and adults (may be used in ages <2 months for treatment of congenital toxoplasmosis)]

Treatment of chancroid, trachoma, inclusion conjunctivitis, urinary tract infections, and nocardiosis (not first line), treatment and prophylaxis of meningococcal meningitis, treatment of *H. influenza* meningitis, prophylaxis of rheumatic fever prophylaxis in penicillin-allergic patient, treatment of uncomplicated attack of malaria due to chloroquine-resistant *Plasmodium falciparum* (FDA approved in ages ≥2 months and adults)

Pregnancy Risk Factor C

Pregnancy Considerations Adverse events have been observed in animal reproduction studies. Sulfadiazine crosses the placenta (Speert, 1943). Available studies and case reports have failed to show an increased risk for congenital malformations after sulfadiazine use (Heinonen, 1977); however, studies with sulfonamides as a class have shown mixed results (ACOG, 2011).

Sulfadiazine is recommended for use in pregnant women to prevent *T. gondii* infection of the fetus, for the maternal treatment of *Toxoplasmic gondii* encephalitis, and as an alternative agent for the secondary prevention of rheumatic fever (CDC, 2009; DHHS, 2013; Gerber, 2009). Sulfonamides may be used to treat other infections in pregnant women when clinically appropriate for confirmed infections caused by susceptible organisms; use during the first trimester should be limited to situations where no alternative therapies are available (ACOG, 2011). Because safer options are available for the treatment of urinary tract infections in pregnant women, use of sulfonamide-containing products >32 weeks gestation should be avoided (Lee, 2008). Due to the theoretical increased risk for hyperbilirubinemia and kernicterus, sulfadiazine is contraindicated by the manufacturer for use near term. Neonatal healthcare providers should be informed if maternal sulfonamide therapy is used near the time of delivery (DHHS, 2013).

Breast-Feeding Considerations Sulfadiazine distributes into human milk. Sulfonamides should not be used while nursing an infant with G6PD deficiency or hyperbilirubinemia (Della-Giustina, 2003). Per the manufacturer, sulfadiazine is contraindicated in nursing mothers since sulfonamides cross into the milk and may cause kernicterus in the newborn. Nondose-related effects could include modification of bowel flora.

Contraindications Hypersensitivity to any sulfa drug or any component of the formulation; infants <2 months of age unless indicated for the treatment of congenital toxoplasmosis; pregnancy (at term); breast-feeding

Warnings/Precautions Fatalities associated with severe reactions including agranulocytosis, aplastic anemia and other blood dyscrasias, hepatic necrosis, Stevens-Johnson syndrome, and toxic epidermal necrolysis have occurred; discontinue use at first sign of rash or signs of serious adverse reactions. Use with caution in patients with allergies or asthma.

Not for the treatment of group A beta-hemolytic streptococcal infections. Prolonged use may result in fungal or bacterial superinfection, including *C. difficile*-associated diarrhea (CDAD) and pseudomembranous colitis; CDAD has been observed >2 months postantibiotic treatment. Use with caution in patients with G6PD deficiency; hemolysis may occur. Use with caution in patients with hepatic impairment. Use with caution in patients with renal impairment; dosage modification required. Maintain adequate hydration to prevent crystalluria. Sulfa antibiotics have been shown to displace bilirubin from protein binding sites which may potentially lead to hyperbilirubinemia and kernicterus in neonates and young infants; do not use in neonates; avoid use in infants <2 months unless other options are not available.

Benzyl alcohol and derivatives: Some dosage forms may contain sodium benzoate/benzoic acid; benzoic acid (benzoate) is a metabolite of benzyl alcohol; large amounts of benzyl alcohol (≥99 mg/kg/day) have been associated with a potentially fatal toxicity ("gasping syndrome") in neonates; the "gasping syndrome" consists of metabolic acidosis, respiratory distress, gasping respirations, CNS dysfunction (including convulsions, intracranial hemorrhage), hypotension, and cardiovascular collapse (AAP, 1997; CDC, 1982); some data suggests that benzoate displaces bilirubin from protein binding sites (Ahlfors, 2001); avoid or use dosage forms containing benzyl alcohol derivative with caution in neonates. See manufacturer's labeling.

Sulfonamide ("sulfa") allergy: Traditionally, concerns for cross-reactivity have extended to all compounds containing the sulfonamide structure (SO_2NH_2). An expanded understanding of allergic mechanisms indicates cross-reactivity between antibiotic sulfonamides and nonantibiotic sulfonamides may not occur, or at the very least this potential is extremely low (Brackett 2004; Johnson 2005; Slatore 2004; Tornero 2004). In particular, mechanisms of cross-reaction due to antibody production (anaphylaxis) are unlikely to occur with nonantibiotic sulfonamides and antibiotic sulfonamides. A nonantibiotic sulfonamide compound which contains the arylamine structure and therefore may cross-react with antibiotic sulfonamides is sulfasalazine (Zawodniak 2010). T-cell-mediated (type IV) reactions (eg, maculopapular rash) are less understood and it is not possible to completely exclude this potential based on current insights. In cases where prior reactions were severe (Stevens-Johnson syndrome/TEN), some clinicians choose to avoid exposure to these classes.

Adverse Reactions

Cardiovascular: Allergic myocarditis, periarteritis nodosa

Central nervous system: Ataxia, chills, convulsions, depression, fever, hallucinations, headache, insomnia, vertigo

Dermatologic: Epidermal necrolysis, erythema multiforme, exfoliative dermatitis, photosensitivity, pruritus, purpura, rash, skin eruptions, Stevens-Johnson syndrome, urticaria

Endocrine & metabolic: Hypoglycemia, thyroid function disturbance

Gastrointestinal: Abdominal pain, anorexia, diarrhea, nausea, pancreatitis, stomatitis, vomiting
Genitourinary: Crystalluria, stone formation, toxic nephrosis with oliguria and anuria
Hematologic: Agranulocytopenia, aplastic anemia, hemolytic anemia, hypoprothrombinemia, leukopenia, methemoglobinemia, thrombocytopenia
Hepatic: Hepatitis
Neuromuscular & skeletal: Arthralgia, peripheral neuritis
Ocular: Conjunctival/scleral injection, periorbital edema
Otic: Tinnitus
Renal: Diuresis
Miscellaneous: Anaphylactoid reactions, lupus erythematosus, serum sickness-like reactions

Drug Interactions

Metabolism/Transport Effects **Substrate** of CYP2C9 (major), CYP2E1 (minor), CYP3A4 (minor); **Note:** Assignment of Major/Minor substrate status based on clinically relevant drug interaction potential; **Inhibits** CYP2C9 (strong)

Avoid Concomitant Use

Avoid concomitant use of SulfADIAZINE with any of the following: BCG; BCG (Intravesical); Mecamylamine; Methenamine; Potassium P-Aminobenzoate; Procaine

Increased Effect/Toxicity

SulfADIAZINE may increase the levels/effects of: Bosentan; Carvedilol; CycloSPORINE (Systemic); CYP2C9 Substrates; Diclofenac (Systemic); Dronabinol; Hypoglycemia-Associated Agents; Lacosamide; Mecamylamine; Methotrexate; Ospemifene; Parecoxib; Porfimer; Prilocaine; Ramelteon; Sodium Nitrite; Sulfonylureas; Tetrahydrocannabinol; Verteporfin; Vitamin K Antagonists

The levels/effects of SulfADIAZINE may be increased by: Androgens; Antidiabetic Agents; Cannabis; Ceritinib; CYP2C9 Inhibitors (Moderate); CYP2C9 Inhibitors (Strong); Dexketoprofen; Herbs (Hypoglycemic Properties); MAO Inhibitors; Methenamine; Mifepristone; Nitric Oxide; Pegvisomant; Quinolone Antibiotics; Salicylates; Selective Serotonin Reuptake Inhibitors

Decreased Effect

SulfADIAZINE may decrease the levels/effects of: BCG; BCG (Intravesical); BCG Vaccine (Immunization); CycloSPORINE (Systemic); Sodium Picosulfate; Typhoid Vaccine

The levels/effects of SulfADIAZINE may be decreased by: CYP2C9 Inducers (Strong); Dabrafenib; Potassium P-Aminobenzoate; Procaine; Quinolone Antibiotics

Food Interactions Vitamin C or acidifying agents (cranberry juice) may cause crystalluria. Management: Avoid large quantities of vitamin C or acidifying agents (cranberry juice).

Storage/Stability Store at controlled room temperature of 20°C to 25°C (68°F to 77°F). Protect from light.

Mechanism of Action Interferes with bacterial growth by inhibiting bacterial folic acid synthesis through competitive antagonism of PABA

Pharmacokinetics (Adult data unless noted)

Absorption: Oral: Well absorbed
Distribution: Excreted in breast milk; diffuses into CSF with higher concentrations reached when meninges are inflamed; distributed into most body tissues
Protein binding: 38% to 48%
Metabolism: Metabolized by N-acetylation
Half-life: 10 hours
Time to peak serum concentration: Within 4 hours
Elimination: In urine as metabolites (15% to 40%) and as unchanged drug (43% to 60%)

Dosing: Neonatal **Congenital toxoplasmosis:** Oral: 100 mg/kg/day divided every 12 hours for 12 months in conjunction with pyrimethamine and supplemental leucovorin (CDC, 2009)

Dosing: Usual

Infants <2 months: **Congenital toxoplasmosis:** Oral: 100 mg/kg/day divided every 12 hours for 12 months in conjunction with pyrimethamine and supplemental leucovorin (CDC, 2009)

Infants ≥2 months, Children, and Adolescents:

General dosing, susceptible infection: Oral:
Manufacturer's labeling: Initial: 75 mg/kg/dose or 2000 mg/m^2/dose once followed by maintenance: 150 mg/kg/day or 4000 mg/m^2/day divided every 4-6 hours; maximum daily dose: 6 **g/day**
Alternate dosing: 120-150 mg/kg/day in divided doses 4-6 times daily; maximum daily dose: 6 g/**day** (*Red Book*, 2012)

Toxoplasmosis (CDC, 2009; *Red Book*, 2012): Oral:
Congenital: Infants: 100 mg/kg/day divided every 12 hours for 12 months in conjunction with pyrimethamine
Acquired: Acute induction therapy: Infants ≥2 months, Children, and Adolescents: 100-200 mg/kg/day divided every 4-6 hours in conjunction with pyrimethamine and supplemental leucovorin; maximum daily dose: 6 g/**day**. Continue acute induction therapy for at least 6 weeks, then follow with chronic suppressive therapy.
Secondary prophylaxis (HIV-exposed/-positive): Infants ≥2 months and Children: 85-120 mg/kg/day divided every 6-12 hours; in combination with pyrimethamine and leucovorin; maximum daily dose: 4000 mg/**day**
Encephaltitis; Toxoplasma gondii; treatment (HIV-exposed/-positive) (CDC, 2013): Adolescents: Oral:
Acute therapy: At least 6 weeks of therapy recommended; use in conjunction with pyrimethamine and supplemental leucovorin combination therapy or with atovaquone
Patient weight <60 kg: 1000 mg every 6 hours
Patient weight ≥60 kg: 1500 mg every 6 hours
Chronic maintenance therapy: 2000-4000 mg/day in divided doses 2-4 times daily in conjunction with pyrimethamine and leucovorin or with atovaquone; begin after completion of acute therapy

Rheumatic fever; secondary prophylaxis: Oral:
Manufacturer's labeling:
≤30 kg: 500 mg once daily
≥30 kg: 1000 mg/day
Alternate dosing (Gerber, 2009; *Red Book*, 2012):
Patient weight ≤27 kg: 500 mg once daily
Patient weight >27 kg: 1000 mg once daily

Adults:

General dosing: Oral: Initial 2000-4000 mg once, followed by 2000-4000 mg/day in divided doses 3-6 times daily

***Toxoplasma gondii* encephalitis (HIV-exposed/-positive patients)** (CDC, 2013a): Oral:
Acute therapy: At least 6 weeks of therapy necessary; use in conjunction with pyrimethamine and leucovorin combination therapy or with atovaquone
Patient weight <60 kg: 1000 mg every 6 hours
Patient weight ≥60 kg: 1500 mg every 6 hours
Chronic maintenance therapy: 2000-4000 mg/day in divided doses 2-4 times daily in conjunction with pyrimethamine and leucovorin or with atovaquone; begin after completion of acute therapy

Rheumatic fever prophylaxis: Oral:
<30 kg: 500 mg/day
≥30 kg: 1000 mg/day

Dosing adjustment in renal impairment: There are no dosage adjustments in the manufacturer's labeling.

Dosing adjustment in hepatic impairment: There are no dosage adjustments in the manufacturer's labeling.

Administration Oral: Administer with at least 8 ounces of water and around-the-clock to promote less variation in peak and trough serum levels. In adults, oral sodium bicarbonate may be used to alkalinize the urine of patients unable to maintain adequate fluid intake (in order to prevent crystalluria, azotemia, oliguria) (Lerner, 1996)

Monitoring Parameters CBC, renal function tests, urinalysis; signs of serious blood disorders (sore throat, fever, pallor, purpura, jaundice); CD4+ count in HIV-exposed/-positive patients treated for toxoplasmosis; sulfonamide blood concentrations may be monitored for severe infections (target: 12-15 mg/100 mL); observe for change in bowel frequency

Additional Information Sulfadiazine plus pyrimethamine confers protection against *Pneumocystis jirovecii* so additional PCP prophylaxis not required (CDC, 2009).

Dosage Forms Excipient information presented when available (limited, particularly for generics); consult specific product labeling.

Tablet, Oral:

Generic: 500 mg

Extemporaneous Preparations A 200 mg/mL oral suspension may be made with sulfadiazine powder and sterile water. Place 50 g sulfadiazine powder in a glass mortar. Add small portions of sterile water and mix to a uniform paste; mix while incrementally adding sterile water to **almost** 250 mL; transfer to a calibrated bottle, rinse mortar with sterile water, and add sufficient quantity of sterile water to make 250 mL. Label "shake well" and "refrigerate". Stable for 3 days refrigerated. **Note:** Suspension may also be prepared by crushing one-hundred 500 mg tablets; however, it is stable for only 2 days.

Pathmanathan U, Halgrain D, Chiadmi F, et al, "Stability of Sulfadiazine Oral Liquids Prepared From Tablets and Powder," *J Pharm Pharm Sci*, 2004, 7(1):84-7.

Sulfamethoxazole and Trimethoprim

(sul fa meth OKS a zole & trye METH oh prim)

Medication Safety Issues

Sound-alike/look-alike issues:

Bactrim may be confused with bacitracin, Bactine, Bactroban

Co-trimoxazole may be confused with clotrimazole

Septra may be confused with Ceptaz, Sectral

Septra DS may be confused with Semprex-D

Brand Names: US Bactrim; Bactrim DS; Septra DS; Sulfatrim

Brand Names: Canada Apo-Sulfatrim; Apo-Sulfatrim DS; Apo-Sulfatrim Pediatric; Protrin DF; Septra Injection; Teva-Trimel; Teva-Trimel DS; Trisulfa; Trisulfa DS; Trisulfa S

Therapeutic Category Antibiotic, Sulfonamide Derivative

Generic Availability (US) Yes

Use

Oral: Treatment of urinary tract infections caused by susceptible *E. coli*, *Klebsiella* and *Enterobacter* sp., *M. morganii*, *P. mirabilis* and *P. vulgaris* (FDA approved in ages ≥2 months and adults); single course treatment of acute otitis media due to *H. influenzae*, *S. pneumoniae*, and *M. catarrhalis* (FDA approved in ages ≥2 months and adults); prophylaxis and treatment of *Pneumocystis jirovecii* pneumonitis (PCP) [FDA approved in pediatric patients (age not specified) and adults]; treatment of enteritis caused by *Shigella flexneri* or *Shigella sonnei* (FDA approved in ages ≥2 months and adults); acute exacerbations of chronic bronchitis due to susceptible strains of *H. influenzae* or *S. pneumoniae* (FDA approved in adults); traveler's diarrhea due to enterotoxigenic *E. coli* (FDA approved in adults). Has also been used for treatment of typhoid fever, *Nocardia asteroids*, MRSA, and *Stenotrophomonas maltophilia* infections

Parenteral: Treatment of *Pneumocystis jirovecii* pneumonitis (PCP), *Shigella*, and severe urinary tract infections due to *E. coli*, *Klebsiella*, and *Enterobacter* spp, *M. morganii*, *P. mirabilis*, and *P. vulgaris* (FDA approved in children and adults); has also been used in treatment of severe or complicated infections caused by susceptible bacteria when oral therapy is not feasible, including typhoid fever and *Nocardia asteroides* infection

Pregnancy Risk Factor D

Pregnancy Considerations Adverse events have been observed in animal reproduction studies. Trimethoprim-sulfamethoxazole (TMP-SMX) crosses the placenta and distributes to amniotic fluid (Ylikorkala, 1973). An increased risk of congenital malformations (neural tube defects, cardiovascular malformations, urinary tract defects, oral clefts, club foot) following maternal use of TMP-SMX during pregnancy has been observed in some studies. Folic acid supplementation may decrease this risk (Crider 2009; Czeizel 2001; Hernandez-Diaz 2000; Hernandez-Diaz 2001; Matok 2009). Due to theoretical concerns that sulfonamides pass the placenta and may cause kernicterus in the newborn, neonatal healthcare providers should be informed if maternal sulfonamide therapy is used near the time of delivery (DHHS 2013).

The pharmacokinetics of TMP-SMX are similar to nonpregnant values in early pregnancy (Ylikorkala, 1973). TMP-SMX is recommended for the prophylaxis or treatment of *Pneumocystis jirovecii* pneumonia (PCP), prophylaxis of *Toxoplasmic gondii* encephalitis (TE), and for the acute and chronic treatment of Q fever in pregnancy (CDC 2013; DHHS 2013). Sulfonamides may also be used to treat other infections in pregnant women when clinically appropriate; use during the first trimester should be limited to situations where no alternative therapies are available (ACOG 2011). Because safer options are available for the treatment of urinary tract infections in pregnant women, use of TMP-containing products in the first trimester and sulfonamide-containing products >32 weeks gestation should be avoided (Lee 2008).

Breast-Feeding Considerations Small amounts of TMP and SMX are transferred into breast milk. The manufacturer recommends that caution be used if administered to nursing women, especially if breast-feeding ill, jaundiced, premature, or stressed infants due to the potential risk of bilirubin displacement and kernicterus. Sulfonamides should not be used while nursing an infant with G6PD deficiency or hyperbilirubinemia (Della-Giustina, 2003). Maternal indications for TMP-SMX must also be considered prior to nursing. Nondose-related effects could include modification of bowel flora.

Contraindications

Hypersensitivity to any sulfa drug, trimethoprim, or any component of the formulation; history of drug induced-immune thrombocytopenia with use of sulfonamides or trimethoprim; megaloblastic anemia due to folate deficiency; infants <2 months of age (manufacturer's labeling), infants <4 weeks of age (CDC 2009); marked hepatic damage or severe renal disease (if patient not monitored)

Note: Although the FDA approved product labeling states this medication is contraindicated with other sulfonamide-containing drug classes, the scientific basis of this statement has been challenged. See "Warnings/Precautions" for more detail.

Warnings/Precautions Use with caution in patients with G6PD deficiency, impaired renal or hepatic function or potential folate deficiency (malnourished, chronic anticonvulsant therapy, or elderly); maintain adequate hydration to prevent crystalluria; adjust dosage in patients with renal impairment.

Fatalities associated with severe reactions including Stevens-Johnson syndrome, toxic epidermal necrolysis, hepatic necrosis, agranulocytosis, aplastic anemia, thrombocytopenia and other blood dyscrasias have been reported; discontinue use at first sign of rash or serious adverse reactions. Elderly patients appear at greater risk for more severe adverse reactions. May cause hypoglycemia, particularly in malnourished, or patients with renal or hepatic impairment. Use with caution in patients with porphyria or thyroid dysfunction. Potentially significant interactions may exist, requiring dose or frequency adjustment, additional monitoring, and/or selection of alternative therapy. Slow acetylators may be more prone to adverse reactions. Caution in patients with allergies or asthma. Incidence of adverse effects appears to be increased in patients with AIDS. Prolonged use may result in fungal or bacterial superinfection, including *C. difficile*-associated diarrhea (CDAD) and pseudomembranous colitis; CDAD has been observed >2 months postantibiotic treatment. Avoid concomitant use with leucovorin when treating *Pneumocystis jirovecii* pneumonia (PCP) in HIV patients; may increase risk of treatment failure and death.

When used for uncomplicated urinary tract infections, this combination should not be used if a single agent is effective. Additionally, sulfonamides should not be used to treat group A beta-hemolytic streptococcal infections.

May cause hyponatremia or hyperkalemia. Potential risk factors for trimethoprim-induced hypokalemia include high dosage (20 mg/kg/day of trimethoprim), renal impairment, older age, hypoaldosteronism, and concomitant use of medications causing or exacerbating hyperkalemia (Perazella, 2000). Elderly patients are at an increased risk for severe and potentially life-threatening hyperkalemia when trimethoprim is used concomitantly with spironolactone, ACE inhibitors, or ARBs (Antoniou 2010; Antoniou 2011; Antoniou 2015).

Injection vehicle may contain and sodium metabisulfite.

Benzyl alcohol and derivatives: Some dosage forms may contain benzyl alcohol; large amounts of benzyl alcohol (≥99 mg/kg/day) have been associated with a potentially fatal toxicity ("gasping syndrome") in neonates; the "gasping syndrome" consists of metabolic acidosis, respiratory distress, gasping respirations, CNS dysfunction (including convulsions, intracranial hemorrhage), hypotension, and cardiovascular collapse (AAP 1997; CDC 1982); some data suggests that benzoate displaces bilirubin from protein binding sites (Ahlfors 2001); avoid or use dosage forms containing benzyl alcohol with caution in neonates. See manufacturer's labeling.

Propylene glycol: Some dosage forms may contain propylene glycol; large amounts are potentially toxic and have been associated hyperosmolality, lactic acidosis, seizures, and respiratory depression; use caution (AAP 1997; Zar 2007).

Sulfonamide ("sulfa") allergy: Traditionally, concerns for cross-reactivity have extended to all compounds containing the sulfonamide structure (SO_2NH_2). An expanded understanding of allergic mechanisms indicates cross-reactivity between antibiotic sulfonamides and nonantibiotic sulfonamides may not occur, or at the very least this potential is extremely low (Brackett 2004; Johnson 2005; Slatore 2004; Tornero 2004). In particular, mechanisms of cross-reaction due to antibody production (anaphylaxis) are unlikely to occur with nonantibiotic sulfonamides and antibiotic sulfonamides. A nonantibiotic sulfonamide compound which contains the arylamine structure and therefore may cross-react with antibiotic sulfonamides is sulfasalazine (Zawodniak 2010). T-cell-mediated (type IV) reactions (eg, maculopapular rash) are less understood and it is not possible to completely exclude this potential based on current insights. In cases where prior reactions were severe (Stevens-Johnson syndrome/TEN), some clinicians choose to avoid exposure to these classes.

Warnings: Additional Pediatric Considerations Sulfa antibiotics have been shown to displace bilirubin from protein binding sites which may potentially lead to hyperbilirubinemia and kernicterus in neonates and young infants; do not use in neonates; avoid use in infants <2 months unless other options are not available (eg, *Pneumocystis*).

Some dosage forms may contain propylene glycol; in neonates large amounts of propylene glycol delivered orally, intravenously (eg, >3,000 mg/day), or topically have been associated with potentially fatal toxicities which can include metabolic acidosis, seizures, renal failure, and CNS depression; toxicities have also been reported in children and adults including hyperosmolality, lactic acidosis, seizures and respiratory depression; use caution (AAP, 1997; Shehab, 2009).

Adverse Reactions

Cardiovascular: Allergic myocarditis, periarteritis nodosa (rare)

Central nervous system: Apathy, aseptic meningitis, ataxia, chills, depression, fatigue, hallucination, headache, insomnia, nervousness, peripheral neuritis, seizure, vertigo

Dermatologic: Erythema multiforme (rare), exfoliative dermatitis (rare), pruritus, skin photosensitivity, skin rash, Stevens-Johnson syndrome (rare), toxic epidermal necrolysis (rare), urticaria

Endocrine & metabolic: Hyperkalemia (generally at high dosages), hypoglycemia (rare), hyponatremia

Gastrointestinal: Abdominal pain, anorexia, diarrhea, glottis edema, kernicterus (in neonates), nausea, pancreatitis, pseudomembranous colitis, stomatitis, vomiting

Genitourinary: Crystalluria, diuresis (rare), nephrotoxicity (in association with cyclosporine), toxic nephrosis (with anuria and oliguria)

Hematologic & oncologic: Agranulocytosis, anaphylactoid purpura (IgA vasculitis; rare), aplastic anemia, eosinophilia, hemolysis (with G6PD deficiency), hemolytic anemia, hypoprothrombinemia, leukopenia, megaloblastic anemia, methemoglobinemia, neutropenia, thrombocytopenia

Hepatic: Cholestatic jaundice, hepatotoxicity (including hepatitis, cholestasis, and hepatic necrosis), hyperbilirubinemia, increased transaminases

Hypersensitivity: Anaphylaxis, angioedema, hypersensitivity reaction, serum sickness

Neuromuscular & skeletal: Arthralgia, myalgia, rhabdomyolysis (mainly in AIDS patients), systemic lupus erythematosus (rare), weakness

Ophthalmic: Conjunctival injection, injected sclera

Otic: Tinnitus

Renal: Increased blood urea nitrogen, increased serum creatinine, interstitial nephritis, renal failure

Respiratory: Cough, dyspnea, pulmonary infiltrates

Miscellaneous: Fever

Rare but important or life-threatening: Idiopathic thrombocytopenic purpura, prolonged Q-T interval on ECG, thrombotic thrombocytopenic purpura

Drug Interactions

Metabolism/Transport Effects Refer to individual components.

Avoid Concomitant Use

Avoid concomitant use of Sulfamethoxazole and Trimethoprim with any of the following: Amodiaquine; BCG; BCG (Intravesical); Dofetilide; Leucovorin Calcium-Levoleucovorin; Mecamylamine; Methenamine; Potassium P-Aminobenzoate; Procaine

Increased Effect/Toxicity

Sulfamethoxazole and Trimethoprim may increase the levels/effects of: ACE Inhibitors; Amantadine; Amodiaquine; Angiotensin II Receptor Blockers; Antidiabetic Agents (Thiazolidinedione); AzaTHIOprine; Bosentan; Cannabis; Carvedilol; CycloSPORINE (Systemic); CYP2C8 Substrates; CYP2C9 Substrates; Dapsone (Systemic); Dapsone (Topical); Digoxin; Dofetilide; Dronabinol; Eplerenone; Fosphenytoin; Highest Risk QTc-Prolonging Agents; Hypoglycemia-Associated Agents;

LamiVUDine; Mecamylamine; Memantine; Mercaptopurine; MetFORMIN; Methotrexate; Moderate Risk QTc-Prolonging Agents; Phenytoin; Porfimer; PRALAtrexate; Prilocaine; Procainamide; Repaglinide; Sodium Nitrite; Spironolactone; Sulfonylureas; Tetrahydrocannabinol; Varenicline; Verteporfin; Vitamin K Antagonists

The levels/effects of Sulfamethoxazole and Trimethoprim may be increased by: Amantadine; Androgens; Antidiabetic Agents; Ceritinib; CYP2C9 Inhibitors (Moderate); CYP2C9 Inhibitors (Strong); Dapsone (Systemic); Dexketoprofen; Herbs (Hypoglycemic Properties); MAO Inhibitors; Memantine; Methenamine; Mifepristone; Nitric Oxide; Pegvisomant; Quinolone Antibiotics; Salicylates; Selective Serotonin Reuptake Inhibitors

Decreased Effect

Sulfamethoxazole and Trimethoprim may decrease the levels/effects of: BCG; BCG (Intravesical); BCG Vaccine (Immunization); CycloSPORINE (Systemic); Sodium Picosulfate; Typhoid Vaccine

The levels/effects of Sulfamethoxazole and Trimethoprim may be decreased by: Bosentan; CYP2C9 Inducers (Strong); CYP3A4 Inducers (Moderate); CYP3A4 Inducers (Strong); Dabrafenib; Deferasirox; Fosphenytoin; Leucovorin Calcium-Levoleucovorin; Mitotane; Phenytoin; Potassium P-Aminobenzoate; Procaine; Quinolone Antibiotics; Siltuximab; St Johns Wort; Tocilizumab

Storage/Stability

Injection: Store at room temperature; do not refrigerate. Less soluble in more alkaline pH. Protect from light. Solution must be diluted prior to administration. Following dilution, store at room temperature; do not refrigerate. Manufacturer recommended dilutions and stability of parenteral admixture at room temperature (25°C):
- 5 mL/125 mL D_5W; stable for 6 hours.
- 5 mL/100 mL D_5W; stable for 4 hours.
- 5 mL/75 mL D_5W; stable for 2 hours.
- Studies have also confirmed limited stability in NS; detailed references should be consulted.

Suspension, tablet: Store at controlled room temperature of 15°C to 25°C (59°F to 77°F). Protect from light.

Mechanism of Action Sulfamethoxazole interferes with bacterial folic acid synthesis and growth via inhibition of dihydrofolic acid formation from para-aminobenzoic acid; trimethoprim inhibits dihydrofolic acid reduction to tetrahydrofolate resulting in sequential inhibition of enzymes of the folic acid pathway

Pharmacokinetics (Adult data unless noted)

Absorption: Oral: Almost completely (90% to 100%)

Distribution: Joint fluid, sputum, middle ear fluid, bile, and CSF

V_d: TMP:
- Newborns: ~2.7 L/kg (range: 1.3-4.1 hours) (Springer, 1982)
- Infants: 1.5 L/kg (Hoppu, 1989)
- Children 1-10 years: 0.86-1 L/kg (Hoppu, 1987)
- Adults: ~1.3 L/kg (Hoppu, 1987)

Protein binding:
- TMP: ~44%
- SMX: 68%

Metabolism: Hepatic, both to multiple metabolites; SMX to hydroxy (via CYP2C9) and acetyl derivatives, and also conjugated with glucuronide; TMP to oxide and hydroxy derivatives; the free forms of both SMX and TMP are therapeutically active

Half-life:
- TMP: Prolonged in renal failure
  - Newborns: ~19 hours; range: 11-27 hours (Springer, 1982)
  - Infants 2 months to 1 year: ~4.6 hours; range: 3-6 hours (Hoppu, 1989)
  - Children 1-10 years: 3.7-5.5 hours (Hoppu, 1987)
  - Children and Adolescents >10 years: 8.19 hours
  - Adults: 6-11 hours
- SMX: 9-12 hours, prolonged in renal failure

Time to peak serum concentration: Oral: Within 1-4 hours

Elimination: Both excreted in urine as metabolites and unchanged drug

Dosing: Usual Note: Dosage recommendations are based on the trimethoprim (TMP) component:

Infants 4 weeks to <2 months (HIV-exposed/-positive):
- ***Pneumocystis* prophylaxis:** Oral: 150 mg TMP/**m²**/day or 5 mg TMP/kg/day for 3-7 days of every week; total daily dose may be given in divided doses every 12 hours for 3 consecutive or alternating days, in divided doses every 12 hours every day or as a single daily dose for 3 consecutive days (CDC, 2009; *Red Book*, 2012)

Infants ≥2 months, Children, and Adolescents:
- **General dosing, susceptible infection:** Oral, IV: 8-12 mg TMP/kg/day in divided doses every 12 hours; maximum single dose: 160 mg TMP (*Red Book*, 2012)
- **Blastomycosis; South African (Paracoccidioiodomycosis):** IV: 8-10 mg TMP/kg/day in divided doses 3 times daily for 3-6 weeks; after clinical improvement, may transition to oral therapy: 10 mg TMP/kg/day in divided doses 2 times daily for 2 years or longer (*Red Book*, 2012)
- ***Cyclosporiasis*:** Limited data available: Oral: 10 mg TMP/kg/day in divided doses twice daily for 7-10 days; maximum single dose: 160 mg TMP (*Red Book*, 2012)
- **Meningitis:** IV: 10-20 mg TMP/kg/day divided every 6-12 hours for 7-21 days; duration dependent on the pathogen and clinical course (Tunkel, 2004)
- **MRSA, community-acquired mild to moderate skin/soft tissue infection:** Oral: 8-12 mg TMP/kg/day in divided doses every 12 hours (Liu, 2011); alternatively, use of 20 mg TMP/kg/day in divided doses every 6 hours has been reported (Norrby-Teglund, 2008). If using empirically, consider addition of group A streptococcal coverage.
- **Otitis media, acute:** Oral: 6-10 mg TMP/kg/day in divided doses every 12 hours for 10 days. **Note:** Due to resistance of *S. pneumoniae*, should not be used in patients that fail first-line amoxicillin therapy (AAP, [Lieberthal, 2013]).
- ***Pneumocystis jirovecii* pneumonia (PCP) (HIV-exposed/-positive):**
  - Infants ≥2 months and Children (CDC, 2009):
    - Treatment: Oral, IV: 15-20 mg TMP/kg/day in divided doses every 6-8 hours for 21 days (CDC, 2009)
    - Prophylaxis: Oral: 150 mg TMP/**m²**/day or 5 mg TMP/kg/day for 3-7 days of every week; total daily dose may be given in divided doses every 12 hours for 3 consecutive or alternating days, in divided doses every 12 hours every day or as a single daily dose for 3 consecutive days; maximum daily dose: TMP 320 mg/**day** (CDC, 2009)
  - Adolescents (DHHS, 2013):
    - Treatment:
      - Mild to moderate: Oral: 15-20 mg TMP/kg/day in 3 divided doses for 21 days **or** alternatively, 320 mg TMP 3 times daily for 21 days
      - Moderate to severe: Initial: IV: 15-20 mg TMP/kg/day in 3-4 divided doses for 21 days; may switch to oral after clinical improvement
    - Prophylaxis: Oral: 80-160 mg TMP daily **or** alternatively, 160 mg TMP 3 times weekly
- **Q-Fever (*Coxiella burnetii*); mild infection (doxycycline therapeutic failure):** Children <8 years: Oral: 8 mg TMP/kg/day in divided doses twice daily for 14 days; maximum daily dose 320 mg TMP/**day** (CDC, 2013)
- **Shigellosis: Note:** Due to reported widespread resistance empiric therapy with sulfamethoxazole and

trimethoprim is not recommended (CDC-NARMS, 2010; WHO, 2005)

Oral:

Manufacturer's labeling: 8 mg TMP/kg/day in divided doses every 12 hours for 5 days; maximum single dose: 160 mg TMP

Alternate dosing: IDSA recommendations for infectious diarrhea: 10 mg TMP/kg/day in divided doses every 12 hours for 3 days (for immunocompetent patients) or 7-10 days (for immunocompromised patients); maximum single dose: 160 mg TMP (Guerrant, 2001)

IV: 8-10 mg TMP/kg/day in divided doses every 6, 8, or 12 hours for up to 5 days

Toxoplasmosis (HIV-exposed/infected):

Prophylaxis, primary:

Infants ≥2 months and Children: Oral: 150 mg TMP/**m^2**/day for 3-7 days of every week; total daily dose may be given in divided doses every 12 hours for 3 consecutive or alternating days, in divided doses every 12 hours every day or as a single daily dose for 3 consecutive days (CDC, 2009)

Adolescents: Oral: 160 mg TMP daily (preferred) **or** 160 mg TMP 3 times weekly **or** 80 mg TMP daily (DHHS, 2013)

Treatment, encephalitis: Adolescents: Oral, IV: 10 mg/kg/day TMP in two divided doses for at least 6 weeks; longer duration may be required in some patients followed by chronic maintenance therapy (DHHS, 2013)

Chronic maintenance therapy; postencephalitis treatment: Adolescents: Oral: 160 mg TMP twice daily (DHHS, 2013)

Urinary tract infection:

Treatment:

Oral:

Infants and Children 2-24 months: 6-12 mg TMP/kg/day in divided doses every 12 hours for 7-14 days (AAP, 2011)

Children >24 months and Adolescents: 8 mg TMP/kg/day in divided doses every 12 hours for 3 days; longer duration may be required in some patients; maximum single dose: 160 mg TMP

IV: 8-10 mg TMP/kg/day in divided doses every 6, 8, or 12 hours for up to 14 days with serious infections

Prophylaxis: Oral: 2 mg TMP/kg/dose once daily (Mattoo, 2007; *Red Book*, 2012)

Adults:

General dosing, susceptible infection:

Oral: 1-2 double strength tablets (sulfamethoxazole 800 mg; trimethoprim 160 mg) every 12-24 hours

IV: 8-20 mg TMP/kg/day divided every 6-12 hours

Chronic bronchitis, acute exacerbation: Oral: One double strength tablet every 12 hours for 10-14 days

Dialysis-related infections:

Exit-site and tunnel infections: Oral: One single-strength tablet daily (Li, 2010)

Peritonitis:

Oral: One double-strength tablet twice daily (Li, 2010)

Intraperitoneal: Loading dose: TMP 320 mg/L; Maintenance: TMP 80 mg/L (Aronoff, 2007; Warady, 2000)

Meningitis, bacterial: IV: 10-20 mg TMP/kg/day in divided doses every 6-12 hours

***Nocardia*:** Oral, IV:

Cutaneous infections: 5-10 mg TMP/kg/day in 2-4 divided doses

Severe infections (pulmonary/cerebral): 15 mg TMP/kg/day in 2-4 divided doses for 3-4 weeks, then 10 mg TMP/kg/day in 2-4 divided doses. Treatment duration is controversial; an average of 7 months has been reported.

Note: Therapy for severe infection may be initiated IV and converted to oral therapy (frequently converted to approximate dosages of oral solid dosage forms: 2 DS tablets every 8-12 hours). Although not widely available, sulfonamide levels should be considered in patients with questionable absorption, at risk for dose-related toxicity or those with poor therapeutic response.

***Pneumocystis jirovecii* pneumonia (PCP) prophylaxis and treatment in HIV-positive patients** (DHHS, 2013):

Prophylaxis: Oral: 80-160 mg TMP daily or alternatively, 160 mg TMP 3 times weekly

Treatment:

Mild to moderate: Oral: 15-20 mg TMP/kg/day in 3 divided doses for 21 days **or** alternatively, 320 mg TMP 3 times daily for 21 days

Moderate to severe: Oral, IV: 15-20 mg TMP/kg/day in 3-4 divided doses for 21 days

Sepsis: IV: 20 mg TMP/kg/day divided every 6 hours

Shigellosis: Note: Due to reported widespread resistance, empiric therapy with sulfamethoxazole and trimethoprim is not recommended (CDC-NARMS, 2010; WHO, 2005).

Oral: One double strength tablet every 12 hours for 5 days

IV: 8-10 mg TMP/kg/day in divided doses every 6, 8, or 12 hours for up to 5 days

Skin/soft tissue infection due to community-acquired MRSA: Oral: 1-2 double strength tablets every 12 hours (Liu, 2011; Stevens, 2005); **Note:** If beta-hemolytic *Streptococcus* spp are also suspected, a beta-lactam antibiotic should be added to the regimen (Liu, 2011)

***Toxoplasma gondii* encephalitis** (DHHS, 2013):

Primary prophylaxis: Oral: 160 mg TMP daily (preferred) **or** 160 mg TMP 3 times weekly **or** 80 mg TMP daily

Treatment (alternative to sulfadiazine, pyrimethamine, and leucovorin calcium): Oral, IV: 5 mg/kg TMP twice daily

Travelers' diarrhea: Oral: One double strength tablet every 12 hours for 5 days

Urinary tract infection:

Oral: One double strength tablet every 12 hours

Duration of therapy: Uncomplicated: 3-5 days; Complicated: 7-10 days

Pyelonephritis: 14 days

Prostatitis: Acute: 2 weeks; Chronic: 2-3 months

IV: 8-10 mg TMP/kg/day in divided doses every 6, 8, or 12 hours for up to 14 days with severe infections

Dosing adjustment in renal impairment:

Manufacturer's labeling: Infants ≥2 months, Children, Adolescents, and Adults: Oral, IV:

CrCl >30 mL/minute: No adjustment required

CrCl 15-30 mL/minute: Administer 50% of recommended dose

CrCl <15 mL/minute: Use is not recommended

Alternate recommendations:

CrCl 15-30 mL/minute:

Treatment: Children, Adolescents, and Adults: Oral, IV: Administer full daily dose (divided every 12 hours) for 24-48 hours, then decrease daily dose by 50% and administer every 24 hours; **Note:** For serious infections, including *Pneumocystis jirovecii* pneumonia (PCP), full daily dose is given in divided doses every 6-8 hours for 2 days, followed by reduction to 50% daily dose divided every 12 hours (Nahata, 1995).

PCP prophylaxis: Adolescents and Adults: Oral: One-half single-strength tablet (40 mg trimethoprim) daily **or** one single-strength tablet (80 mg trimethoprim) daily **or** 3 times weekly (Masur, 2002).

CrCl <15 mL/minute:

Treatment: Children, Adolescents, and Adults: Oral, IV: Administer 50% of the daily dose every 48 hours (Nahata, 1995); **Note:** In pediatric patients with GFR <10 mL/minute/1.73 m^2, use is not recommended by some clinicians; if use is required, administer 5-10 mg trimethoprim/kg every 24 hours (Aronoff, 2007).

PCP prophylaxis: Adolescents and Adults: Oral: One-half single-strength tablet (40 mg trimethoprim) daily **or** one single-strength tablet (80 mg trimethoprim) 3 times weekly (Masur, 2002). While the guidelines do acknowledge the alternative of giving one single-strength tablet daily, this may be inadvisable in the uremic/ESRD patient.

Hemodialysis:

Treatment:

Infants, Children, and Adolescents: Not recommended, but if required, administer 5-10 mg TMP/kg every 24 hours (Aronoff, 2007)

Adults: 2.5-10 mg/kg trimethoprim every 24 hours **or** 5-20 mg/kg trimethoprim 3 times weekly after IHD. **Note:** Dosing is highly dependent upon indication for use (eg, treatment of cystitis versus treatment of PCP pneumonia (Heinz, 2009).

PCP prophylaxis: Adolescents and Adults: Oral: One single-strength tablet (80 mg trimethoprim) after each dialysis session (Masur, 2002)

Note: Dosing dependent on the assumption of 3 times/week, complete IHD sessions.

Peritoneal dialysis (PD): Not significantly removed by CAPD; supplemental dosing is not required (Aronoff, 2007):

Treatment: Children, Adolescents, and Adults: Oral, IV: Administer 50% of daily dose every 48 hours (Nahata, 1995); **Note:** In pediatric PD patients, use is not recommended by some clinicians, if use is required, administer 5-10 mg trimethoprim/kg every 24 hours (Aronoff, 2007).

PCP prophylaxis: Adolescents and Adults: Oral: One-half single-strength tablet (40 mg trimethoprim) daily **or** 1 single-strength tablet (80 mg trimethoprim) 3 times weekly (Masur, 2002). While the guidelines do acknowledge the alternative of giving 1 single-strength tablet daily, this may be inadvisable in the uremic/ESRD patient.

CRRT:

Infants, Children, and Adolescents: 5 mg TMP/kg/dose every 8 hours (Aronoff, 2007)

Adults (Heintz, 2009; Trotman, 2005): Drug clearance is highly dependent on the method of renal replacement, filter type, and flow rate. Appropriate dosing requires close monitoring of pharmacologic response, signs of adverse reactions due to drug accumulation, as well as drug concentrations in relation to target trough (if appropriate). The following are general recommendations only (based on dialysate flow/ultrafiltration rates of 1-2 L/hour and minimal residual renal function) and should not supersede clinical judgment:

CVVH/CVVHD/CVVHDF: 2.5-7.5 mg/kg of TMP every 12 hours. **Note:** Dosing regimen dependent on clinical indication. Critically-ill patients with *P. jirovecii* pneumonia receiving CVVHDF may require up to 10 mg/kg every 12 hours (Heintz, 2009).

Dosing adjustment in hepatic impairment: There are no dosage adjustments provided in the manufacturer's labeling.

Preparation for Administration IV: Must dilute in D_5W prior to administration.

Usual preparation: Dilute to 1:25 dilution (5 mL drug to 125 mL diluent, ie, D_5W)

Fluid restriction: Dilute to 1:15 dilution (5 mL drug to 75 mL diluent, ie, D_5W) or a 1:10 dilution (5 mL drug to 50 mL diluent, ie, D_5W)

Administration

Oral: Administer without regard to meals. Shake suspension well before use.

Parenteral: **Do not administer IM**. IV infusion: Inspect solution for evidence of cloudiness or precipitation prior to administration; infuse diluted solution over 60 to 90 minutes.

Monitoring Parameters CBC, renal function test, liver function test, urinalysis; observe for change in bowel frequency

Test Interactions Increased creatinine (Jaffé alkaline picrate reaction); increased serum methotrexate by dihydrofolate reductase method

Additional Information Leucovorin calcium should be given if bone marrow suppression occurs. Guidelines for prophylaxis of *Pneumocystis jirovecii* pneumonia: Initiate PCP prophylaxis in the following patients (CDC, 2009):

- All infants born to HIV-infected mothers should be given prophylaxis with TMP-SMZ beginning at 4-6 weeks of age and continue until HIV infection has been reasonably excluded
- All HIV-infected infants <12 months, regardless of CD4+ count or percentage, should continue prophylaxis through the first year of life and reassess based on defined thresholds
- Children 1-5 years of age with CD4+ count <500/mm^3 or CD4+ percentage <15%
- Children ≥6 years of age with CD4+ count <200 or CD4+ percentage <15%
- Adolescents and Adults with CD4+ count <200 or oropharyngeal candidiasis

Dosage Forms Excipient information presented when available (limited, particularly for generics); consult specific product labeling. **Note:** The 5:1 ratio (SMX:TMP) remains constant in all dosage forms.

Injection, solution: Sulfamethoxazole 80 mg and trimethoprim 16 mg per mL (5 mL, 10 mL, 30 mL)

Suspension, oral: Sulfamethoxazole 200 mg and trimethoprim 40 mg per 5 mL (20 mL, 480 mL)

Sulfatrim: Sulfamethoxazole 200 mg and trimethoprim 40 mg per 5 mL (480 mL) [contains alcohol <0.5%, propylene glycol; cherry flavor]

Tablet, oral: Sulfamethoxazole 400 mg and trimethoprim 80 mg

Bactrim: Sulfamethoxazole 400 mg and trimethoprim 80 mg

Tablet, double-strength, oral: Sulfamethoxazole 800 mg and trimethoprim 160 mg

Bactrim DS: Sulfamethoxazole 800 mg and trimethoprim 160 mg

Septra DS: Sulfamethoxazole 800 mg and trimethoprim 160 mg

◆ **Sulfamylon** *see* Mafenide *on page 1308*

SulfaSALAzine (sul fa SAL a zeen)

Medication Safety Issues

Sound-alike/look-alike issues:

SulfaSALAzine may be confused with salsalate, sulfADIAZINE

Azulfidine may be confused with Augmentin, azaTHIOprine

Related Information

Oral Medications That Should Not Be Crushed or Altered *on page 2476*

Brand Names: US Azulfidine; Azulfidine EN-tabs; Sulfazine; Sulfazine EC

Brand Names: Canada Apo-Sulfasalazine; PMS-Sulfasalazine; Salazopyrin; Salazopyrin En-Tabs

Therapeutic Category 5-Aminosalicylic Acid Derivative; Anti-inflammatory Agent

Generic Availability (US) Yes

Use Oral:

Tablet: Treatment of mild to moderate ulcerative colitis, adjunct therapy for severe ulcerative colitis and prolongation of remission of ulcerative colitis episodes (FDA approved in ages ≥6 years and adults)

Enteric coated tablet: Management of ulcerative colitis (FDA approved in ages ≥6 years and adults); treatment of juvenile idiopathic arthritis (JIA) in patients with an inadequate response to NSAIDs or salicylates (FDA approved in ages 6-16 years), and treatment of rheumatoid arthritis in an inadequate response to, or intolerance of, an adequate trial of full doses of one or more NSAIDs (FDA approved in adults); has also been used for induction therapy for Crohn's disease. **Note:** Although it is an FDA-labeled indication, the use of sulfasalazine for treatment of JIA is not recommended (per manufacturer; Ringold, 2013).

Pregnancy Risk Factor B

Pregnancy Considerations Adverse events have not been observed in animal reproduction studies. Sulfasalazine and sulfapyridine cross the placenta; a potential for kernicterus in the newborn exists. Agranulocytosis was noted in an infant following maternal use of sulfasalazine during pregnancy. Additionally, cases of neural tube defects have been reported (causation undetermined); sulfasalazine is known to inhibit the absorption and metabolism of folic acid and may diminish the effects of folic acid supplementation. Based on available data, an increase in fetal malformations has not been observed following maternal use of sulfasalazine for the treatment of inflammatory bowel disease or ulcerative colitis. When treatment for inflammatory bowel disease is needed during pregnancy, sulfasalazine may be used, although supplementation with folic acid is recommended (Habal, 2012; Mahadevan, 2009; Mottet, 2007).

Breast-Feeding Considerations Sulfasalazine is excreted in breast milk; sulfapyridine concentrations are ~30% to 60% of the maternal serum. Bloody stools or diarrhea have been reported in nursing infants. Although sulfapyridine has poor bilirubin-displacing ability, exposure may cause kernicterus in the newborn. The manufacturer recommends that caution be used in women who are breast-feeding. Other sources consider use of sulfasalazine to be safe while breast-feeding; monitoring of the infant is recommended (Habal, 2012; Mahadevan, 2009; Mottet, 2007).

Contraindications

Hypersensitivity to sulfasalazine, sulfa drugs, salicylates, or any component of the formulation; intestinal or urinary obstruction; porphyria

Note: Although the FDA approved product labeling states this medication is contraindicated with other sulfonamide-containing drug classes, the scientific basis of this statement has been challenged. See "Warnings/Precautions" for more detail.

Canadian labeling: Additional contraindications (not in U.S. labeling): Severe renal impairment (GFR <30 mL/minute/1.73 m^2); severe hepatic impairment; use in pediatric patients <2 years of age; patients in whom acute asthmatic attacks, urticaria, rhinitis or other allergic manifestations are precipitated by acetyl salicylic acid (ASA) or other NSAIDs

Warnings/Precautions Use with extreme caution in patients with renal impairment (Canadian labeling contraindicates use in severe impairment [GFR <30 mL/minute/1.73 m^2]), impaired hepatic function (Canadian labeling contraindicates use in severe impairment), or blood dyscrasias. Fatalities associated with severe reactions including agranulocytosis, aplastic anemia, and other blood dyscrasias have occurred; discontinue use at first sign of rash or signs of serious adverse reactions. The presence of clinical signs such as sore throat, fever, pallor, or purpura may be indicative of a serious blood disorder; monitor complete blood counts frequently. Serious infections (some fatal), including sepsis and pneumonia, have been reported. Infections may be associated with agranulocytosis, neutropenia, or myelosuppression. Monitor for signs/symptoms of infection during and after sulfasalazine therapy and promptly evaluate if infection occurs; discontinue therapy for serious infections. Use cautiously in patients with a history of recurring or chronic infections or with underlying conditions or concomitant therapy which may predispose them to infectious complications.

Use caution in patients with severe allergies or bronchial asthma. Hemolytic anemia may occur when used in patients with G6PD deficiency; use cautiously. May decrease folic acid absorption. Deaths from irreversible neuromuscular or central nervous system changes, fibrosing alveolitis, agranulocytosis, aplastic anemia, and other blood dyscrasias have been reported. In males, oligospermia (rare) and infertility has been reported. Slow acetylators may be more prone to adverse reactions. Discontinue enteric coated tablets if noted to pass without disintegrating.

Severe skin reactions (some fatal), including Stevens-Johnson syndrome (SJS), exfoliative dermatitis, and toxic epidermal necrolysis (TEN) have occurred with sulfonamides (including sulfasalazine), most commonly during the first month of treatment; discontinue use at first sign of skin rash, mucosal lesions, or any other sign of dermatologic toxicity. Severe and life-threatening hypersensitivity reactions, including drug rash with eosinophilia and systemic symptoms (DRESS) syndrome have been reported. Fever or lymphadenopathy may be present prior to rash development. Other severe hypersensitivity reactions may include internal organ involvement, such as hepatitis, nephritis, myocarditis, mononucleosis-like syndrome, hematologic abnormalities (including hematophagic histiocytosis), and/or pneumonitis including eosinophilic infiltration. Discontinue treatment for severe reactions and evaluate promptly.

Sulfonamide ("sulfa") allergy: Traditionally, concerns for cross-reactivity have extended to all compounds containing the sulfonamide structure (SO_2NH_2). An expanded understanding of allergic mechanisms indicates cross-reactivity between antibiotic sulfonamides and nonantibiotic sulfonamides may not occur, or at the very least this potential is extremely low (Brackett 2004; Johnson 2005; Slatore 2004; Tornero 2004). In particular, mechanisms of cross-reaction due to antibody production (anaphylaxis) are unlikely to occur with nonantibiotic sulfonamides and antibiotic sulfonamides. A nonantibiotic sulfonamide compound which contains the arylamine structure and therefore may cross-react with antibiotic sulfonamides is sulfasalazine (Zawodniak 2010). T-cell-mediated (type IV) reactions (eg, maculopapular rash) are less understood and it is not possible to completely exclude this potential based on current insights. In cases where prior reactions were severe (Stevens-Johnson syndrome/TEN), some clinicians choose to avoid exposure to these classes.

Warnings: Additional Pediatric Considerations Pediatric patients treated with sulfasalazine for JIA have a high incidence of adverse events, including a serum-sickness-like reaction which presents with fever, nausea, vomiting, headache, rash, and altered LFTs; discontinue treatment if these occur; use of sulfasalazine for treatment of JIA is not recommended (per manufacturer; Ringold, 2013).

Adverse Reactions

Central nervous system: Dizziness, headache

Dermatologic: Pruritus, skin rash, urticaria

Gastrointestinal: Abdominal pain, anorexia, dyspepsia, gastric distress, nausea, stomatitis, vomiting
Genitourinary: Oligospermia (reversible)
Hematologic & oncologic: Heinz body anemia, hemolytic anemia, leukopenia, thrombocytopenia
Hepatic: Abnormal hepatic function tests
Respiratory: Cyanosis
Miscellaneous: Fever
Rare but important or life-threatening (includes reactions reported with mesalamine or other sulfonamides): Agranulocytosis, alopecia, anaphylaxis, angioedema, aplastic anemia, arthralgia, cauda equina syndrome, cholestatic hepatitis, cholestatic jaundice, conjunctival injection, crystalluria, depression, diarrhea, DRESS syndrome, drowsiness, eosinophilia, exfoliative dermatitis, folate deficiency, fulminant hepatitis, Guillain-Barré syndrome, hallucination, hearing loss, hematologic abnormality, hematologic disease (pseudomononucleosis), hematuria, hemolytic-uremic syndrome, hepatic cirrhosis, hepatic failure, hepatic necrosis, hepatitis, hepatotoxicity (idiosyncratic) (Chalasani, 2014), hypoglycemia, hypoprothrombinemia, injected sclera, insomnia, interstitial nephritis, interstitial pulmonary disease, jaundice, Kawasaki syndrome (single case report), lupus-like syndrome, megaloblastic anemia, meningitis, methemoglobinemia, myelitis, myelodysplastic syndrome, myocarditis (allergic), nephritis, nephrolithiasis, nephrotic syndrome, neutropenia (congenital), neutropenic enterocolitis, oropharyngeal pain, pancreatitis, parapsoriasis varioliformis acuta, periarteritis nodosa, pericarditis, periorbital edema, peripheral neuropathy, pleurisy, pneumonia, pneumonitis, proteinuria, pulmonary alveolitis, purpura, renal disease (acute), rhabdomyolysis, seizure, sepsis, serum sickness-like reaction (children with JRA have frequent and severe reaction), skin discoloration, skin photosensitivity, Stevens-Johnson syndrome, thyroid function impairment, toxic epidermal necrolysis, toxic nephrosis, urine discoloration, vasculitis

Drug Interactions

Metabolism/Transport Effects None known.

Avoid Concomitant Use There are no known interactions where it is recommended to avoid concomitant use.

Increased Effect/Toxicity

SulfaSALAzine may increase the levels/effects of: Heparin; Heparin (Low Molecular Weight); Methotrexate; Prilocaine; Sodium Nitrite; Thiopurine Analogs; Varicella Virus-Containing Vaccines

The levels/effects of SulfaSALAzine may be increased by: Nitric Oxide; Nonsteroidal Anti-Inflammatory Agents

Decreased Effect

SulfaSALAzine may decrease the levels/effects of: Cardiac Glycosides; Folic Acid; Methylfolate

Storage/Stability Store at 25°C (77°F); excursions permitted to 15°C to 30°C (59°F to 86°F).

Mechanism of Action 5-aminosalicylic acid (5-ASA) is the active component of sulfasalazine; the specific mechanism of action of 5-ASA is unknown; however, it is thought that it modulates local chemical mediators of the inflammatory response, especially leukotrienes, and is also postulated to be a free radical scavenger or an inhibitor of tumor necrosis factor (TNF); action appears topical rather than systemic

Pharmacodynamics Onset of action:
JIA: Minimum trial of 3 months is necessary
Ulcerative colitis: >3-4 weeks

Pharmacokinetics (Adult data unless noted)

Absorption: Oral: 10% to 15% as unchanged drug from the small intestine; upon administration, the drug is split into sulfapyridine and 5-aminosalicylic acid (5-ASA) in the colon
Bioavailability: Sulfasalazine: <15%; sulfapyridine: ~60%; 5-aminosalicylic acid: ~10% to 30%
Distribution: Breast milk to plasma ratio: 0.09-0.17
Metabolism: Both components are metabolized in the liver; slow acetylators have higher plasma sulfapyridine concentrations
Half-life:
- Sulfasalazine:
  - Single dose: 5.7 hours
  - Multiple doses: 7.6 hours
- Sulfapyridine:
  - Single dose: 8.4 hours
  - Multiple doses: 10.4 hours

Time to peak serum concentration:
- Serum sulfasalazine: Within 1.5-6 hours
- Serum sulfapyridine (active metabolite): Within 6-24 hours

Elimination: Primarily in urine (as unchanged drug, components, and acetylated metabolites); small amounts appear in feces

Dosing: Usual

Children and Adolescents:

Inflammatory bowel disease (eg, ulcerative colitis; Crohn's disease): Oral:
Weight-based dosing:
Manufacturer's labeling: Ulcerative colitis: Children ≥6 years and Adolescents:
Induction: 40-60 mg/kg/day in 3-6 divided doses; maximum daily dose: 4000 mg/**day**
Maintenance: 30 mg/kg/day in 4 divided doses; maximum daily dose: 2000 mg/**day**
Alternate dosing:
Induction: Crohn disease, ulcerative colitis: 40-70 mg/kg/day in 4-6 divided doses; in some cases, higher induction doses up to 100 mg/kg/day may be required; maximum daily dose: 4000 mg/**day** (Rufo, 2012; Sandu, 2010; Turner, 2012)
Maintenance: Ulcerative colitis: 30-70 mg/kg/day in 2-6 divided doses; maximum daily dose: 4000 mg/**day** (Sandu, 2010; Turner, 2012)
Fixed dosing [Salazopyrin prescribing information (Canada), 2013]: Children ≥25 kg and Adolescents: **Note:** Consider dose reduction or use of enteric coated tablet in patients experiencing adverse gastrointestinal effects with uncoated tablet.
Acute attacks:
- 25 to <35 kg: 500 mg 3 times daily
- 35-50 kg: 1000 mg 2-3 times daily

Maintenance of remission:
- 25 to <35 kg: 500 mg 2 times daily
- 35-50 kg: 500 mg 2-3 times daily

Desensitization regimen: Children ≥6 years and Adolescents: For patients who may be sensitive to treatment, it is suggested to start with a total dose of 50-250 mg daily and double it every 4-7 days until the desired dose is achieved. Discontinue if symptoms of sensitivity occur. Do not attempt in patients with a history of agranulocytosis or those who have had a previous anaphylactoid reaction on sulfasalazine therapy.

Juvenile idiopathic arthritis: Children and Adolescents 6-16 years: Oral: Enteric coated tablet: 30-50 mg/kg/day in 2 divided doses; maximum daily dose: 2000 mg/**day** (Beukelman, 2011); **Note:** Although it is an FDA-labeled indication, the use of sulfasalazine for treatment of JIA is not recommended (per manufacturer; Ringold, 2013).

Adults:

Rheumatoid arthritis: Oral: Enteric coated tablet: Initial: 0.5-1 g daily; increase weekly to maintenance dose of 2 g daily in 2 divided doses; maximum: 3 g daily (if response to 2 g daily is inadequate after 12 weeks of treatment)

Ulcerative colitis: Oral:

Initial: 3-4 g daily in evenly divided doses at ≤8-hour intervals; may initiate therapy with 1-2 g daily to reduce GI intolerance. **Note:** American College of Gastroenterology guideline recommendations: Titrate to 4-6 g daily in 4 divided doses (Kornbluth, 2010)

Maintenance dose: 2 g daily in evenly divided doses at ≤8-hour intervals; if GI intolerance occurs reduce dosage by 50% and gradually increase to target dose after several days. If GI intolerance persists, stop drug for 5-7 days and reintroduce at a lower daily dose.

Desensitization regimen: For patients who may be sensitive to treatment, it is suggested to start with a total dose of 50-250 mg daily and double it every 4-7 days until the desired dose is achieved. Discontinue if symptoms of sensitivity occur. Do not attempt in patients with a history of agranulocytosis or those who have had a previous anaphylactoid reaction on sulfasalazine therapy.

Dosing adjustment in renal impairment: There are no dosage adjustments provided in manufacturer's labeling; use with extreme caution.

Dosing adjustment in hepatic impairment: There are no dosage adjustments provided in manufacturer's labeling; use with extreme caution.

Administration Tablets should be administered in evenly divided doses, preferably after meals. Do not crush enteric coated tablets.

Monitoring Parameters CBC, liver function tests (prior to therapy, then every other week for first 3 months of therapy, followed by every month for the second 3 months, then once every 3 months thereafter), urinalysis, renal function tests, liver function tests, stool frequency, hematocrit, reticulocyte count

Test Interactions Reports of possible interference with measurements, by liquid chromatography, of urinary normetanephrine causing a false-positive test result have been observed in patients exposed to sulfasalazine or its metabolite, mesalamine/mesalazine.

Dosage Forms Excipient information presented when available (limited, particularly for generics); consult specific product labeling.

Tablet, Oral:

Azulfidine: 500 mg [scored]

Sulfazine: 500 mg [scored]

Generic: 500 mg

Tablet Delayed Release, Oral:

Azulfidine EN-tabs: 500 mg

Sulfazine EC: 500 mg

Generic: 500 mg

Extemporaneous Preparations A 100 mg/mL oral suspension may be made with tablets. Place twenty 500 mg tablets in a mortar and add a small amount of a 1:1 mixture of Ora-Sweet® and Ora-Plus® to cover the tablets. Let soak for 20-30 minutes. Crush the tablets and mix to a uniform paste; mix while adding the vehicle in equal proportions to **almost** 100 mL; transfer to a calibrated bottle, rinse mortar with vehicle, and add sufficient quantity of vehicle to make 100 mL. Label "shake well". Stable 91 days under refrigeration or at room temperature.

Lingertat-Walsh K, Walker SE, Law S, et al, "Stability of Sulfasalazine Oral Suspension," *Can J Hosp Pharm*, 2006, 59(4):194-200.

◆ **Sulfatrim** *see* Sulfamethoxazole and Trimethoprim *on page 1986*

◆ **Sulfazine** *see* SulfaSALAzine *on page 1990*

◆ **Sulfazine EC** *see* SulfaSALAzine *on page 1990*

◆ **Sulfisoxazole and Erythromycin** *see* Erythromycin and Sulfisoxazole *on page 784*

Sulfur and Salicylic Acid

(SUL fyoor & sal i SIL ik AS id)

Brand Names: US ala seb [OTC]; Pernox Lemon [OTC]; Pernox Regular [OTC]; Sebex [OTC]; Sebulex [OTC]

Therapeutic Category Antiseborrheic Agent, Topical

Generic Availability (US) Yes

Use Therapeutic shampoo for dandruff and seborrheal dermatitis; acne skin cleanser

Pregnancy Considerations Refer to Salicylic Acid monograph.

Breast-Feeding Considerations Refer to Salicylic Acid monograph.

Contraindications Contraindicated in patients allergic to sulfur

Warnings/Precautions For external use only; avoid contact with eyes; discontinue use if skin irritation develops; infants are more sensitive to sulfur than adults; do not use in children <2 years.

Rare but serious and potentially life-threatening allergic reactions or severe irritation have been reported with use of topical OTC benzoyl peroxide or salicylic acid containing products; it has not been determined if the reactions are due to the active ingredients (benzoyl peroxide or salicylic acid), the inactive ingredients, or a combination of both. Hypersensitivity reactions may occur within minutes to a day or longer after product use and differ from local skin irritation (redness, burning, dryness, itching, peeling or slight swelling) that may occur at the site of product application. Treatment should be discontinued if hives or itching develop; patients should seek emergency medical attention if reactions such as throat tightness, difficulty breathing, feeling faint, or swelling of the eyes, face, lips, or tongue develop. Before using a topical OTC acne product for the first time, consumers should apply a small amount to 1 or 2 small affected areas for 3 days to make sure hypersensitivity symptoms do not develop (FDA Drug Safety Communication, 2014).

Adverse Reactions Local: Topical preparations containing 2% to 5% sulfur generally are well tolerated, local irritation may occur, concentration >15% is very irritating to the skin, higher concentration (eg, 10% or higher) may cause systemic toxicity (eg, headache, vomiting, muscle cramps, dizziness, collapse)

Storage/Stability Preparations containing sulfur may react with metals including silver and copper, resulting in discoloration of the metal

Mechanism of Action Salicylic acid works synergistically with sulfur in its keratolytic action to break down keratin and promote skin peeling

Pharmacokinetics (Adult data unless noted) Absorption: 1% of topically applied sulfur is absorbed; sulfur is reduced to hydrogen sulfide

Dosing: Usual General guidelines; consult specific product labeling. Children ≥2 years and Adults: Topical:

Shampoo: Initial: Massage onto wet scalp; leave lather on scalp for 5 minutes, rinse, repeat application, then rinse thoroughly; use daily or every other day; 1-2 treatments/week will usually maintain control

Soap: Use daily or every other day

Administration Topical: Avoid contact with the eyes; for external use only

Dosage Forms Excipient information presented when available (limited, particularly for generics); consult specific product labeling.

Cleanser, topical [scrub]:

Pernox® Lemon: Sulfur 2% and salicylic acid 1.5% (56 g, 113 g)

Pernox® Regular: Sulfur 2% and salicylic acid 1.5% (113 g)

Shampoo, topical:
ala seb: Sulfur 2% and salicylic acid 2% (118 mL, 355 mL) [contains soya lecithin]
Sebex: Sulfur 2% and salicylic acid 2% (118 mL)
Sebulex®: Sulfur 2% and salicylic acid 2% (200 g)

Sulindac (SUL in dak)

Medication Safety Issues

Sound-alike/look-alike issues:

Clinoril may be confused with Cleocin, Clozaril

BEERS Criteria medication:

This drug may be potentially inappropriate for use in geriatric patients (Quality of evidence - moderate; Strength of recommendation - strong).

Brand Names: Canada Apo-Sulin; Teva-Sulindac

Therapeutic Category Analgesic, Non-narcotic; Anti-inflammatory Agent; Nonsteroidal Anti-inflammatory Drug (NSAID), Oral

Generic Availability (US) Yes

Use Management of inflammatory diseases including osteoarthritis, rheumatoid arthritis, acute gouty arthritis, ankylosing spondylitis, and acute painful shoulder (acute subacromial bursitis/supraspinatus tendonitis) (FDA approved in adults)

Medication Guide Available Yes

Pregnancy Risk Factor C

Pregnancy Considerations Adverse events were not observed in the initial animal reproduction studies; therefore, the manufacturer classifies sulindac as pregnancy category C. Sulindac and the sulfide metabolite have been found to cross the placenta. NSAID exposure during the first trimester is not strongly associated with congenital malformations; however, cardiovascular anomalies and cleft palate have been observed following NSAID exposure in some studies. The use of an NSAID in the first trimester may be associated with an increased risk of miscarriage. Nonteratogenic effects have been observed following NSAID administration during the third trimester including myocardial degenerative changes, prenatal constriction of the ductus arteriosus, failure of the ductus arteriosus to close postnatally, and fetal tricuspid regurgitation; renal dysfunction or failure, oligohydramnios; gastrointestinal bleeding or perforation, increased risk of necrotizing enterocolitis; intracranial bleeding, platelet dysfunction with resultant bleeding; or pulmonary hypertension. Because they may cause premature closure of the ductus arteriosus, use of NSAIDs late in pregnancy should be avoided (use after 31-32 weeks gestation is not recommended by some clinicians). Sulindac has been used in the management of preterm labor. The chronic use of NSAIDs in women of reproductive age may be associated with infertility that is reversible upon discontinuation of the medication. A registry is available for pregnant women exposed to autoimmune medications including sulindac. For additional information contact the Organization of Teratology Information Specialists, OTIS Autoimmune Diseases Study, at (877) 311-8972.

Breast-Feeding Considerations It is not known if sulindac is excreted into breast milk. Breast-feeding is not recommended by the manufacturer.

Contraindications Hypersensitivity or allergic-type reactions to sulindac, aspirin, other NSAIDs, or any component of the formulation; perioperative pain in the setting of coronary artery bypass graft (CABG) surgery

Warnings/Precautions [U.S. Boxed Warning]: NSAIDs are associated with an increased risk of adverse cardiovascular thrombotic events, including MI and stroke. Use caution with fluid retention. Avoid use in heart failure (ACCF/AHA [Yancy, 2013]). Concurrent administration of ibuprofen, and potentially other nonselective NSAIDs, may interfere with aspirin's cardioprotective effect. May cause new-onset hypertension or worsening of existing hypertension. NSAID use may compromise existing renal function; dose-dependent decreases in prostaglandin synthesis may result from NSAID use, reducing renal blood flow which may cause renal decompensation. NSAID use may increase the risk for hyperkalemia. Patients with impaired renal function, dehydration, heart failure, liver dysfunction, those taking diuretics, and ACE inhibitors, and the elderly are at greater risk of renal toxicity and hyperkalemia. Rehydrate patient before starting therapy; monitor renal function closely. Not recommended for use in patients with advanced renal disease. Long-term NSAID use may result in renal papillary necrosis. Use caution in patients with renal lithiasis; sulindac metabolites have been reported as components of renal stones. Maintain adequate hydration in patients with a history of renal stones. Use with caution in patients with decreased hepatic function. May require dosage adjustment in hepatic dysfunction; sulfide and sulfone metabolites may accumulate. The elderly are at increased risk for adverse effects. **[U.S. Boxed Warning]: Use is contraindicated for treatment of perioperative pain in the setting of coronary artery bypass graft (CABG) surgery.** Risk of MI and stroke may be increased with use following CABG surgery.

[U.S. Boxed Warning]: NSAIDs may increase risk of gastrointestinal irritation, inflammation, ulceration, bleeding, and perforation. Use the lowest effective dose for the shortest duration of time, consistent with individual patient goals, to reduce risk of cardiovascular or GI adverse events. When used concomitantly with aspirin, a substantial increase in the risk of gastrointestinal complications (eg, ulcer) occurs; concomitant gastroprotective therapy (eg, proton pump inhibitors) is recommended (Bhatt, 2008). Pancreatitis has been reported; discontinue with suspected pancreatitis.

Avoid chronic use in the elderly (unless alternative agents ineffective and patient can receive concomitant gastroprotective agent); nonselective oral NSAID use is associated with an increased risk of GI bleeding and peptic ulcer disease in older adults in high risk category (eg, >75 years or age or receiving concomitant oral/parenteral corticosteroids, anticoagulants, or antiplatelet agents) (Beers Criteria).

NSAIDS may cause drowsiness, dizziness, blurred vision and other neurologic effects which may impair physical or mental abilities; patients must be cautioned about performing tasks which require mental alertness (eg, operating machinery or driving). Discontinue use with blurred or diminished vision and perform ophthalmologic exam. Monitor vision with long-term therapy.

Platelet adhesion and aggregation may be decreased, may prolong bleeding time; patients with coagulation disorders or who are receiving anticoagulants should be monitored closely. Anemia may occur; patients on long-term NSAID therapy should be monitored for anemia. Rarely, NSAID use may cause severe blood dyscrasias (eg, agranulocytosis, aplastic anemia, thrombocytopenia). NSAIDs may cause serious skin adverse events including exfoliative dermatitis, Stevens-Johnson syndrome (SJS) and toxic epidermal necrolysis (TEN); discontinue use at first sign of skin rash or hypersensitivity. Anaphylactoid reactions may occur. Do not use in patients who experience bronchospasm, asthma, rhinitis, or urticaria with NSAID or aspirin therapy. Use caution in other forms of asthma. May increase the risk of aseptic meningitis, especially in patients with systemic lupus erythematosus (SLE) and mixed connective tissue disorders.

Withhold for at least 4-6 half-lives prior to surgical or dental procedures.

Adverse Reactions

Cardiovascular: Edema

Central nervous system: Dizziness, headache, nervousness

Dermatologic: Pruritus, rash

Gastrointestinal: Abdominal cramps, anorexia, constipation, diarrhea, flatulence, GI pain, heartburn, nausea, vomiting

Otic: Tinnitus

Rare but important or life-threatening: Agranulocytosis, ageusia, alopecia, anaphylaxis, angioneurotic edema, aplastic anemia, arrhythmia, aseptic meningitis, bitter taste, blurred vision, bone marrow depression, bronchial spasm, bruising, CHF, cholestasis, colitis, conjunctivitis, crystalluria, depression, dry mucous membranes, dyspnea, dysuria, epistaxis, erythema multiforme, exfoliative dermatitis, fever, gastritis, GI bleeding, GI perforation, glossitis, gynecomastia, hearing decreased, hematuria, hemolytic anemia, hepatic failure, hepatitis, hepatotoxicity (idiosyncratic) (Chalasani, 2014), hyperglycemia, hyperkalemia, hypersensitivity reaction, hypersensitivity syndrome (includes chills, diaphoresis, fever, flushing), hypersensitivity vasculitis, hypertension, insomnia, intestinal stricture, interstitial nephritis, jaundice, leukopenia, liver function abnormal, metallic taste, necrotizing fasciitis, nephrotic syndrome, neuritis, neutropenia, palpitation, pancreatitis, paresthesia, peptic ulcer, photosensitivity, proteinuria, psychosis, purpura, renal calculi, renal failure, renal impairment, retinal disturbances, seizure, somnolence, Stevens-Johnson syndrome, stomatitis, syncope, thrombocytopenia, toxic epidermal necrolysis, urine discoloration, urticaria, vaginal bleeding, vertigo, visual disturbance, weakness

Drug Interactions

Metabolism/Transport Effects None known.

Avoid Concomitant Use

Avoid concomitant use of Sulindac with any of the following: Dexketoprofen; Floctafenine; Ketorolac (Nasal); Ketorolac (Systemic); Morniflumate; NSAID (COX-2 Inhibitor); Omacetaxine; Urokinase

Increased Effect/Toxicity

Sulindac may increase the levels/effects of: 5-ASA Derivatives; Agents with Antiplatelet Properties; Aliskiren; Aminoglycosides; Anticoagulants; Apixaban; Bisphosphonate Derivatives; Collagenase (Systemic); CycloSPORINE (Systemic); Dabigatran Etexilate; Deferasirox; Deoxycholic Acid; Desmopressin; Digoxin; Drospirenone; Eplerenone; Haloperidol; Ibritumomab; Methotrexate; Nonsteroidal Anti-Inflammatory Agents; NSAID (COX-2 Inhibitor); Obinutuzumab; Omacetaxine; PEMEtrexed; Porfimer; Potassium-Sparing Diuretics; PRALAtrexate; Quinolone Antibiotics; Rivaroxaban; Salicylates; Tacrolimus (Systemic); Tenofovir; Thrombolytic Agents; Tositumomab and Iodine I 131 Tositumomab; Urokinase; Vancomycin; Verteporfin; Vitamin K Antagonists

The levels/effects of Sulindac may be increased by: ACE Inhibitors; Angiotensin II Receptor Blockers; Antidepressants (Tricyclic, Tertiary Amine); Corticosteroids (Systemic); CycloSPORINE (Systemic); Dasatinib; Dexketoprofen; Diclofenac (Systemic); Dimethyl Sulfoxide; Floctafenine; Glucosamine; Herbs (Anticoagulant/Antiplatelet Properties); Ibrutinib; Ketorolac (Nasal); Ketorolac (Systemic); Limaprost; Morniflumate; Multivitamins/Fluoride (with ADE); Multivitamins/Minerals (with ADEK, Folate, Iron); Multivitamins/Minerals (with AE, No Iron); Omega-3 Fatty Acids; Pentosan Polysulfate Sodium; Pentoxifylline; Probenecid; Prostacyclin Analogues; Selective Serotonin Reuptake Inhibitors; Serotonin/Norepinephrine Reuptake Inhibitors; Sodium Phosphates; Tipranavir; Treprostinil; Vitamin E

Decreased Effect

Sulindac may decrease the levels/effects of: ACE Inhibitors; Aliskiren; Angiotensin II Receptor Blockers; Beta-Blockers; Eplerenone; HydrALAZINE; Loop Diuretics; Potassium-Sparing Diuretics; Prostaglandins (Ophthalmic); Salicylates; Selective Serotonin Reuptake Inhibitors; Thiazide Diuretics

The levels/effects of Sulindac may be decreased by: Bile Acid Sequestrants; Salicylates

Storage/Stability Store at room temperature of 15°C to 30°C (59°F to 86°F).

Mechanism of Action Reversibly inhibits cyclooxygenase-1 and 2 (COX-1 and 2) enzymes, which results in decreased formation of prostaglandin precursors; has antipyretic, analgesic, and anti-inflammatory properties

Other proposed mechanisms not fully elucidated (and possibly contributing to the anti-inflammatory effect to varying degrees), include inhibiting chemotaxis, altering lymphocyte activity, inhibiting neutrophil aggregation/activation, and decreasing proinflammatory cytokine levels.

Pharmacokinetics (Adult data unless noted)

Absorption: 90%

Distribution: Crosses blood-brain barrier (brain concentrations <4% of plasma concentrations)

Protein binding: Sulindac: 93%, sulfone metabolite: 95%, sulfide metabolite: 98%; primarily to albumin

Metabolism: Hepatic; prodrug metabolized to sulfide metabolite (active) for therapeutic effects and to sulfone metabolites (inactive); parent and inactive sulfone metabolite undergo extensive enterohepatic recirculation; metabolites undergo glucuronide conjugation

Half-life elimination: Sulindac: ~8 hours; sulfide metabolite: ~16 hours

Time to peak serum concentration: Sulindac: 3-4 hours; sulfide and sulfone metabolites: 5-6 hours

Elimination: Urine (~50%, primarily as inactive metabolites, <1% as active metabolite); feces (~25%, primarily as metabolites); **Note:** Metabolites appear principally as glucuronide conjugates in urine and bile.

Dosing: Usual Oral:

Children: Limited information exists; some centers use the following: 2-4 mg/kg/day in 2 divided doses; maximum: 6 mg/kg/day; do not exceed 400 mg/day (Giannini, 1995; Skeith, 1991)

Adults: 150-200 mg twice daily; not to exceed 400 mg/day

Dosing adjustment in renal impairment: Not recommended with advanced renal impairment; if required, decrease dose and monitor closely.

Dosing adjustment in hepatic impairment: Dose reduction is necessary; discontinue if abnormal liver function tests occur.

Administration Oral: Administer with food or milk to decrease GI upset

Monitoring Parameters Liver enzymes, BUN, serum creatinine, CBC with differential, platelet count; periodic ophthalmologic exams with chronic use

Test Interactions Increased chloride (S), increased sodium (S), increased bleeding time

Dosage Forms Excipient information presented when available (limited, particularly for generics); consult specific product labeling.

Tablet, Oral:

Generic: 150 mg, 200 mg

SUMAtriptan (soo ma TRIP tan)

Medication Safety Issues

Sound-alike/look-alike issues:

SUMAtriptan may be confused with saxagliptin, sitaGLIPtin, somatropin, ZOLMitriptan

Brand Names: US Alsuma; Imitrex; Imitrex STATdose Refill; Imitrex STATdose System; Sumavel DosePro

Brand Names: Canada ACT-Sumatriptan; Apo-Sumatriptan; Ava-Sumatriptan; Dom-Sumatriptan; Imitrex DF; Imitrex Injection; Imitrex Nasal Spray; Mylan-Sumatriptan; PHL-Sumatriptan; PMS-Sumatriptan; Sandoz-Sumatriptan; Sumatriptan DF; Taro-Sumatriptan; Teva-Sumatriptan; Teva-Sumatriptan DF

Therapeutic Category Antimigraine Agent

Generic Availability (US) May be product dependent

Use

Injection, intranasal, and tablets: Acute treatment of migraine with or without aura (FDA approved in adults)

Injection: Acute treatment of cluster headaches (FDA approved in adults)

Pregnancy Risk Factor C

Pregnancy Considerations Adverse events were observed in animal reproduction studies. In a study using full term healthy human placentas, limited amounts of sumatriptan were found to cross the placenta (Schenker, 1995).

An overall increased risk of major congenital malformations has not been observed following first trimester exposure to sumatriptan in several studies. Pregnancy outcome information for sumatriptan is available from a pregnancy registry sponsored by GlaxoSmithKline. As of October 2008, data was available for 558 infants/fetuses exposed to sumatriptan, and seven exposed to both sumatriptan and naratriptan. The risk of major birth defects following sumatriptan exposure was 4.6% (95% CI: 2.9-7.2) (Cunnington, 2009). The pregnancy registry was closed in January, 2012 and additional information may be obtained from the manufacturer (800-336-2176). An analysis of data collected between 1995-2008 using the Swedish Medical Birth Register reported pregnancy outcomes following 5-$HT_{1B/1D}$ agonist exposure. An increased risk of major congenital malformations was not observed following sumatriptan exposure (2229 exposed during the first trimester) (Källén, 2011). An increased risk of major congenital malformations was not observed in the prospective Norwegian Mother and Child Cohort Study. The study included women with 5-$HT_{1B/1D}$ agonist exposure between 1999-2006 (n=455); of these, 217 were exposed to sumatriptan (Nezvalová-Henriksen, 2010; Nezvalová-Henriksen, 2012).

If treatment for cluster headaches is needed during pregnancy, sumatriptan may be used (Jürgens, 2009). Other agents are preferred for the initial treatment of migraine in pregnancy (Da Silva, 2012; MacGregor, 2012; Williams, 2012); however, sumatriptan may be considered if first-line agents fail (MacGregor, 2012).

Breast-Feeding Considerations The excretion of sumatriptan into breast milk was studied in five lactating women, 10-28 weeks postpartum (mean: 22.2 weeks). Sumatriptan 6 mg SubQ was administered and maternal milk and blood samples were collected over 8 hours after the dose. Sumatriptan was detected in breast milk. Maximum concentrations in the maternal blood (mean: 80.2 mcg/L; 0.25 hours after the dose) and milk (mean: 87.2 mcg/L; 2.5 hours after the dose) were similar. However, the amount of sumatriptan an infant would be exposed to following breast-feeding is considered to be small (although the mean milk-to-plasma ratio is ~4.9, weight-adjusted doses estimates suggest breast-fed infants receive 3.5% of a maternal dose). Expressing and discarding the milk for 8-12 hours after a single dose is suggested to reduce the amount present even further (Wojnar-Horton, 1996). Breast-feeding is not recommended by some manufacturers; however, according to other sources if treatment is needed, breast-feeding does not need to be discontinued (Jürgens, 2009; MacGregor, 2012).

Contraindications Hypersensitivity to sumatriptan or any component of the formulation, including allergic contact dermatitis to the transdermal patch; ischemic heart disease or signs or symptoms of ischemic heart disease (including Prinzmetal's angina, angina pectoris, myocardial infarction, silent myocardial ischemia); cerebrovascular syndromes (including strokes, transient ischemic attacks); peripheral vascular disease (including ischemic bowel disease); uncontrolled hypertension; use within 24 hours of ergotamine derivatives; use within 24 hours of another 5-HT_1 agonist; concurrent administration or within 2 weeks of discontinuing an MAO type A inhibitors; management of hemiplegic or basilar migraine; Wolff-Parkinson-White syndrome or arrhythmias associated with other cardiac accessory conduction pathway disorders; severe hepatic impairment (not Sumavel)

Warnings/Precautions Anaphylactic, anaphylactoid, and hypersensitivity reactions (including angioedema) have been reported; may be life threatening or fatal. Sumatriptan is only indicated for the acute treatment of migraine or cluster headache (product dependent); not indicated for migraine prophylaxis, or for the treatment of hemiplegic or basilar migraine. Acute migraine agents (eg, 5-HT_1 agonists, opioids, ergotamine, or a combination of the agents) used for 10 or more days per month may lead to worsening of headaches (medication overuse headache); withdrawal treatment may be necessary in the setting of overuse. May cause CNS depression, such as dizziness, weakness, or drowsiness, which may impair physical or mental abilities; patients must be cautioned about performing tasks which require mental alertness (eg, operating machinery or driving). If a patient does not respond to the first dose, the diagnosis of migraine or cluster headache should be reconsidered; rule out underlying neurologic disease in patients with atypical headache and in patients with no prior history of migraine or cluster headache. Cardiac events (coronary artery vasospasm, transient ischemia, myocardial infarction, ventricular tachycardia/fibrillation, cardiac arrest and death), cerebral/subarachnoid hemorrhage, and stroke have been reported with 5-HT_1 agonist administration (some occurring within a few hours of administration). Discontinue sumatriptan if these events occur. Patients who experience sensations of chest pain/pressure/tightness or symptoms suggestive of angina following dosing should be evaluated for coronary artery disease or Prinzmetal's angina before receiving additional doses; if dosing is resumed and similar symptoms recur, monitor with ECG. Perform a cardiovascular evaluation in 5-HT_1 agonists-naive patients who have risk factors for CAD prior to initiation of therapy. Patients with suspected CAD should have cardiovascular evaluation to rule out CAD before considering use; if cardiovascular evaluation is "satisfactory," first dose should be given in the health care provider's office (consider ECG monitoring). Periodic evaluation of cardiovascular status should be done in these patients during intermittent long-term use.

Significant elevation in blood pressure, including hypertensive crisis, has been reported on rare occasions in patients with and without a history of hypertension; use is contraindicated in patients with uncontrolled hypertension. Peripheral vascular ischemia, GI vascular ischemia and infarction, splenic infarction, and Raynaud syndrome been reported with 5-HT_1 agonists. Transient and permanent blindness and significant partial vision loss have been very rarely reported. Use with caution in patients with a history of seizure disorder or in patients with a lowered seizure threshold; seizures have been reported after sumatriptan administration in patients with or without a history of seizures. Use the oral formulation with caution (and with dosage limitations) in patients with mild to moderate hepatic impairment where treatment is necessary and advisable. Presystemic clearance of orally administered sumatriptan is reduced in hepatic impairment, leading to increased plasma concentrations; dosage reduction of the oral product is recommended. Non-oral routes of administration (intranasal, subcutaneous) do not undergo similar hepatic first-pass metabolism and are not expected to result in significantly altered pharmacokinetics in patients with hepatic impairment. Use of the oral, intranasal, transdermal, or Imitrex injectable is contraindicated in severe hepatic impairment; Sumavel is not recommended in severe hepatic impairment. Allergic contact dermatitis may occur with use of transdermal patch; erythematous plaque and/or erythemato-vesicular or erythemato-bullous eruptions may develop. Erythema alone is common and not by itself an indication of sensitization. Discontinue use if allergic contact dermatitis is suspected. Patients sensitized from use of transdermal system may develop systemic sensitization or other systemic reactions if sumatriptan-containing products are taken by other routes (oral, subcutaneous); if treatment with sumatriptan by other routes is required, first dose should be taken under close medical supervision. Do not apply transdermal patch in areas near or over electrically-active implantable or body-worn medical devices (eg, implantable cardiac pacemaker, body-worn insulin pump, implantable deep brain stimulator); patch contains metal parts and must be removed before magnetic resonance imaging (MRI) procedures.

Potentially significant drug-drug interactions may exist, requiring dose or frequency adjustment, additional monitoring, and/or selection of alternative therapy. Serotonin syndrome may occur with 5-HT_1 agonists, particularly when used concomitantly with other serotonergic drugs; symptoms (eg, mental status changes, tachycardia, hyperthermia, nausea, vomiting, diarrhea, hyperreflexia, incoordination) typically occur minutes to hours after initiation/ dose increase of a serotonergic drug. Discontinue use if serotonin syndrome is suspected. Use with caution in the elderly; perform a cardiovascular evaluation prior to initiation of therapy in elderly patients with cardiovascular risk factors (eg, diabetes, hypertension, smoking, obesity, strong family history of coronary artery disease) and periodically during intermittent long-term use.

Warnings: Additional Pediatric Considerations Serious adverse effects, such as MI, stroke, visual loss, and death, have been reported in pediatric patients after sumatriptan use by the oral, intranasal, and/or SubQ routes; frequency of such adverse effects cannot currently be determined, monitor patients closely.

Adverse Reactions

Injection:

Cardiovascular: Chest discomfort, flushing

Central nervous system: Anxiety, burning sensation, cold sensation, dizziness, drowsiness, feeling of heaviness, feeling of tightness, feeling strange, headache, localized warm feeling, malaise, nasal cavity pain, paresthesia, pressure sensation, tight feeling in head

Dermatologic: Diaphoresis

Gastrointestinal: Abdominal distress, dysphagia, nausea and vomiting, sore throat

Local: Injection site reaction (includes bleeding, bruising, swelling, and erythema)

Neuromuscular & skeletal: Jaw pain, muscle cramps, myalgia, neck pain, numbness, weakness

Ophthalmic: Visual disturbance

Respiratory: Bronchospasm, nasal signs and symptoms, sinus discomfort

Nasal spray:

Central nervous system: Dizziness

Gastrointestinal: Nausea, sore throat, unpleasant taste, vomiting

Respiratory: Nasal signs and symptoms

Tablet:

Cardiovascular: Chest pain, hot and cold flashes, palpitations, syncope

Central nervous system: Burning sensation, dizziness, drowsiness, headache, hyperacusis, malaise, migraine, numbness, pain (nonspecified), paresthesia, sensation of pressure (neck/throat/jaw or nonspecified), sleepiness, vertigo

Gastrointestinal: Diarrhea, nausea, reduced salivation, vomiting

Genitourinary: Hematuria

Hematologic & oncologic: Hemolytic anemia, hemorrhage (ear or nose/throat)

Hypersensitivity: Hypersensitivity reaction

Neuromuscular & skeletal: Myalgia

Otic: Hearing loss, tinnitus

Respiratory: Allergic rhinitis, dyspnea, rhinitis, sinusitis, upper respiratory tract inflammation

Transdermal system:

Central nervous system: Feeling abnormal (paresthesia, warm/cold sensation), localized warm feeling, sensation of pressure (chest/neck/throat/jaw)

Dermatologic: Allergic contact dermatitis, skin discoloration (application site), skin vesicle (application site)

Hematologic & oncologic: Bruise (application site)

Local: Localized irritation, localized pain, localized pruritus

Rare but important or life-threatening: Skin erosion (application site)

Route unspecified: Rare but important or life-threatening: Abdominal aortic aneurysm, abnormal hepatic function tests, accommodation disturbance, acute renal failure, anemia, cardiac arrhythmia, cardiomyopathy, cerebrovascular accident, colonic ischemia, coronary artery vasospasm, cyanosis, deafness, dystonic reaction, giant-cell arteritis, hallucination, hematuria, hemorrhage (nose/ throat), hypersensitivity reaction, increased intracranial pressure, increased thyroid stimulating hormone level, intestinal obstruction, myocardial infarction, optic neuropathy (ischemic), pancytopenia, Prinzmetal angina, psychomotor disturbance, pulmonary embolism, Raynaud's phenomenon, retinal blood vessel occlusion (artery), seizure, serotonin syndrome, skin photosensitivity, subarachnoid hemorrhage, thrombosis, vasculitis

Drug Interactions

Metabolism/Transport Effects None known.

Avoid Concomitant Use

Avoid concomitant use of SUMAtriptan with any of the following: Dapoxetine; Ergot Derivatives; MAO Inhibitors

Increased Effect/Toxicity

SUMAtriptan may increase the levels/effects of: Antipsychotic Agents; Droxidopa; Ergot Derivatives; Metoclopramide; Serotonin Modulators

The levels/effects of SUMAtriptan may be increased by: Antiemetics (5HT3 Antagonists); Antipsychotic Agents; Dapoxetine; Ergot Derivatives; MAO Inhibitors

Decreased Effect There are no known significant interactions involving a decrease in effect.

Storage/Stability

Alsuma: Store at 25°C (77°F); excursions are permitted between 15°C and 30°C (59°F and 86°F); do not refrigerate. Protect from light.

Imitrex injectable, tablet, intranasal: Store at 2°C to 30°C (36°F to 86°F). Protect from light.

Sumavel DosePro: Store at 20°C to 25°C (68°F to 77°F); excursions are permitted between 15°C and 30°C (59°F and 86°F); do not freeze. Protect from light.

Zecuity: Store at 20°C to 25°C (68°F to 77°F); excursions are permitted between 15°C and 30°C (59°F and 86°F); do not refrigerate or freeze.

Mechanism of Action Selective agonist for serotonin (5-HT_{1B} and 5-HT_{1D} receptors) on intracranial blood vessels and sensory nerves of the trigeminal system; causes vasoconstriction and reduces neurogenic inflammation associated with antidromic neuronal transmission correlating with relief of migraine

Pharmacodynamics Migraine pain relief:

Onset of action:

Oral: 1-1.5 hours

Nasal: ~15-30 minutes

SubQ: 10 minutes to 2 hours

Maximum effect: Oral: 2-4 hours

Pharmacokinetics (Adult data unless noted)

Distribution: Distributes to breast milk following SubQ administration

V_d (central): 50 L

V_d (apparent): 2.4 L/kg

Protein binding: 14% to 21%

Metabolism: In the liver to an indole acetic acid metabolite (inactive) which then undergoes ester glucuronide conjugation; may be metabolized by monoamine oxidase (MAO); extensive first-pass metabolism following oral administration

Bioavailability:

Oral: ~15%; may be significantly increased with liver disease

Intranasal: 17% (compared to SubQ)

SubQ: 97%; **Note:** Sumavel® DosePro® is bioequivalent to sumatriptan SubQ injection via needle when administered into the thigh or abdomen

Half-life:

Distribution: 15 minutes

Terminal: 2 hours; range: 1-4 hours

Time to peak serum concentration:

Oral: Healthy adults: 2 hours; during migraine attacks: 2.5 hours

SubQ: Range: 5-20 minutes; mean: 12 minutes

Elimination: 60% of an oral dose is renally excreted (primarily as metabolites), 40% is eliminated via the feces, and only 3% as unchanged drug; 42% of an intranasal dose is excreted as the indole acetic acid metabolite with 3% excreted in the urine unchanged; 22% of a SubQ dose is excreted in urine unchanged and 38% as the indole acetic acid metabolite

Dosing: Usual Note: Use in children and adolescents <18 years of age not recommended by manufacturer. Results of clinical studies are mixed with regards to efficacy, particularly with oral and injectable sumatriptan; a 2004 practice parameter concluded that sumatriptan nasal spray was effective for the acute treatment of migraines in adolescent patients (Lewis, 2004); additional studies are needed.

Intranasal:

Children 5-12 years: 5 mg, 10 mg, or 20 mg administered in one nostril **as a single dose**, given as soon as possible after the onset of migraine; dose should be selected on an individual basis; optimal dose not established. A double-blind, placebo controlled study of 129 patients (8-17 years; mean 12.4 years) used a weight-based dosing regimen: Body weight: 20-39 kg: 10 mg/dose; body weight ≥40 kg: 20 mg/dose; however, relatively few children <12 years old were included in the study (Ahonen, 2004). A small, randomized, double-blind, placebo-controlled study of 14 children (6-9 years; median: 8.2 years) used intranasal doses of 20 mg/dose (Ueberall, 1999). A small, retrospective review of 10 children (5-12 years; mean: 9.9 years), used intranasal doses of 5 mg (n=2) or 20 mg (n=8) (Hershey, 2001).

Adolescents ≥12 years: 5 mg, 10 mg, or 20 mg administered in one nostril **as a single dose** given as soon as possible after the onset of migraine; dose should be selected on an individual basis (Lewis, 2004; Rothner, 2000; Winner, 2000; Winner, 2006)

Adults: Initial single dose: 5 mg, 10 mg, or 20 mg administered in one nostril, given as soon as possible after the onset of migraine; dose should be selected on an individual basis; 10 mg dose may be administered as 5 mg in each nostril; may repeat after 2 hours; maximum: 40 mg/day

SubQ:

Children and Adolescents 6-18 years: 3-6 mg single dose. An open-labeled prospective trial of 17 children 6-16 years with juvenile migraine used SubQ doses of 6 mg in 15 children (30-70 kg), and 3 mg/dose in two children (22 kg and 30 kg) (MacDonald, 1994). Another open-label prospective trial in 50 consecutive children (ages 6-18 years) with severe migraine used SubQ doses of 0.06 mg/kg/dose. Relief was reported as good/excellent in 84% of the patients; 16% reported fair to poor relief; additional studies are needed (Linder, 1996).

Adults: Initial: 4-6 mg; may repeat if needed ≥1 hour after initial dose; maximum: 12 mg/day

Oral:

Adolescents: Efficacy of oral sumatriptan was **not** established in five controlled trials in adolescent patients; frequency of adverse events was dose-related and age-dependent (ie, younger patients reported more adverse events)

Adults: Initial single dose: 25 mg given as soon as possible after the onset of a migraine; range 25-100 mg/dose; dose should be selected on an individual basis; maximum single dose: 100 mg; may repeat after 2 hours; maximum: 200 mg/day

Dosing adjustment in hepatic impairment: Adults:

Mild to moderate hepatic impairment:

Oral: Bioavailability of oral sumatriptan is increased with liver disease. If treatment is needed, do not exceed single doses of 50 mg.

Intranasal: Has not been studied in patients with hepatic impairment; however, because the intranasally administered drug does not undergo first-pass metabolism, serum concentrations would not be expected to be altered.

SubQ: Has been studied and pharmacokinetics were not altered in patients with hepatic impairment compared to healthy patients.

Severe hepatic impairment: Oral, nasal, and SubQ (limited to Imitrex® injection, per prescribing information) formulations are contraindicated with severe hepatic impairment.

Dosing adjustment in renal impairment: No dosage adjustments are recommended.

Administration

Intranasal: Each nasal spray unit is preloaded with 1 dose; **do not** test the spray unit before use; remove unit from plastic pack when ready to use; while sitting down, gently blow nose to clear nasal passages; keep head upright and close one nostril gently with index finger; hold container with other hand, with thumb supporting bottom and index and middle fingers on either side of nozzle; insert nozzle into nostril about 1/2 inch; close mouth; take a breath through nose while releasing spray into nostril by pressing firmly on blue plunger; remove nozzle from nostril; keep head level for 10-20 seconds and gently breathe in through nose and out through mouth; **do not breathe deeply**

Oral: Administer with water or other fluids; swallow tablet whole; do not split tablet

Parenteral: SubQ use only; do **not** administer IM; do **not** administer IV (may cause coronary vasospasm). Needle penetrates 1/4 inch of skin; use in areas of the body with adequate skin and subcutaneous thickness.

Alsuma™ is a prefilled single use autoinjector device; product information suggests SubQ administration into lateral thigh or upper arm (adults). Discard after use.

Needleless administration (Sumavel® DosePro®): Do **not** administer IM; do **not** administer IV (may cause coronary vasospasm). Administer SubQ to the abdomen (>2 inches from the navel) or thigh; do not administer to other areas of the body (eg, arm). Sumavel® DosePro® device is for single use only; discard after use; do not use if the tip of the device is tilted or broken; **Note:** A loud burst of air will be heard and a sensation in the skin will be felt at the time a dose is delivered with this device.

Additional Information The safety of treating an average of >4 headaches in a 30-day period has not been established. Sumatriptan is **not** indicated for migraine prophylaxis.

Sumavel® DosePro® is a single-use, prefilled, disposable, needle-free SubQ delivery system; it uses pressure from a compressed nitrogen gas source to deliver medication via a small, precise hole in the glass medication chamber; medication is propelled through the skin and delivered SubQ without a needle.

Product Availability Zecuity (transdermal system): FDA approved January 2013; anticipated availability is currently unknown. Refer to prescribing information for additional information.

Dosage Forms Excipient information presented when available (limited, particularly for generics); consult specific product labeling.

Solution, Nasal:
- Imitrex: 5 mg/actuation (1 ea); 20 mg/actuation (1 ea)
- Generic: 5 mg/actuation (1 ea); 20 mg/actuation (1 ea)

Solution, Subcutaneous, as succinate [strength expressed as base]:
- Alsuma: 6 mg/0.5 mL (0.5 mL)
- Imitrex: 6 mg/0.5 mL (0.5 mL)
- Imitrex STATdose Refill: 4 mg/0.5 mL (0.5 mL)
- Imitrex STATdose System: 4 mg/0.5 mL (0.5 mL)
- Generic: 4 mg/0.5 mL (0.5 mL); 6 mg/0.5 mL (0.5 mL)

Solution, Subcutaneous, as succinate [strength expressed as base, preservative free]:
- Generic: 6 mg/0.5 mL (0.5 mL)

Solution Auto-injector, Subcutaneous, as succinate [strength expressed as base]:
- Imitrex STATdose System: 6 mg/0.5 mL (0.5 mL)
- Generic: 6 mg/0.5 mL (0.5 mL)

Solution Cartridge, Subcutaneous, as succinate [strength expressed as base]:
- Imitrex STATdose Refill: 6 mg/0.5 mL (0.5 mL)

Solution Jet-injector, Subcutaneous, as succinate [strength expressed as base]:
- Sumavel DosePro: 4 mg/0.5 mL (0.5 mL); 6 mg/0.5 mL (0.5 mL)

Solution Prefilled Syringe, Subcutaneous, as succinate [strength expressed as base, preservative free]:
- Generic: 6 mg/0.5 mL (0.5 mL)

Tablet, Oral, as succinate [strength expressed as base]:
- Imitrex: 25 mg, 50 mg, 100 mg
- Generic: 25 mg, 50 mg, 100 mg

Extemporaneous Preparations A 5 mg/mL oral liquid preparation made from tablets and one of three different vehicles (Ora-Sweet®, Ora-Sweet® SF, or Syrpalta® syrups). **Note:** Ora-Plus® Suspending Vehicle is used with Ora-Sweet® or Ora-Sweet® SF to facilitate dispersion of the tablets (Ora-Plus® is not necessary if Syrpalta® is the vehicle). Crush nine 100 mg tablets in a mortar and reduce to a fine powder. Add 40 mL of Ora-Plus® in 5 mL increments and mix thoroughly between each addition; rinse mortar and pestle 5 times with 10 mL of Ora-Plus®, pouring into bottle each time, and add quantity of appropriate syrup (Ora-Sweet® or Ora-Sweet® SF) sufficient to make 180 mL. Store in amber glass bottles in the dark; label "shake well", "refrigerate", and "protect from light". Stable for 21 days refrigerated.

Fish DN, Beall HD, Goodwin SD, et al, "Stability of Sumatriptan Succinate in Extemporaneously Prepared Oral Liquids," *Am J Health Syst Pharm*, 1997, 54(14):1619-22.

Tacrolimus (Systemic) (ta KROE li mus)

Medication Safety Issues

Sound-alike/look-alike issues:

Prograf may be confused with Gengraf, PROzac

Tacrolimus may be confused with everolimus, pimecrolimus, sirolimus, temsirolimus

High alert medication:

This medication is in a class the Institute for Safe Medication Practices (ISMP) includes among its list of drug classes that have a heightened risk of causing significant patient harm when used in error.

Other safety concerns:

The immediate release (Hecoria, Prograf) and extended release (Astagraf XL, Advagraf [Canadian product]) oral formulations are not interchangeable and are not substitutable.

Related Information

Safe Handling of Hazardous Drugs *on page 2455*

Brand Names: US Astagraf XL; Hecoria [DSC]; Prograf

Brand Names: Canada Advagraf; Prograf; Sandoz-Tacrolimus

Therapeutic Category Immunosuppressant Agent

Generic Availability (US) May be product dependent

Use Prevention of organ rejection in solid organ transplantation patients (FDA approved in children and adults) or prevention and treatment of graft-versus-host disease (GVHD) in allogeneic stem cell transplantation patients

Medication Guide Available Yes

Pregnancy Risk Factor C

Pregnancy Considerations Adverse events were observed in animal reproduction studies. Tacrolimus crosses the human placenta and is measurable in the cord blood, amniotic fluid, and newborn serum. Tacrolimus concentrations in the placenta may be higher than the maternal serum (Jain, 1997). Infants with lower birth weights have been found to have higher tacrolimus concentrations (Bramham, 2013). Transient neonatal hyperkalemia and renal dysfunction have been reported.

Tacrolimus pharmacokinetics are altered during pregnancy. Whole blood concentrations decrease as pregnancy progresses; however, unbound concentrations increase. Measuring unbound concentrations may be preferred, especially in women with anemia or hypoalbuminemia. If unbound concentration measurement is not available, interpretation of whole blood concentrations should account for RBC count and serum albumin concentration (Hebert, 2013; Zheng, 2012).

In general, women who have had a kidney transplant should be instructed that fertility will be restored following the transplant but that pregnancy should be avoided for ~2 years. Tacrolimus may be used as an immunosuppressant during pregnancy. The risk of infection, hypertension, and pre-eclampsia may be increased in pregnant women who have had a kidney transplant (EPBG, 2002).

The National Transplantation Pregnancy Registry (NTPR) is a registry which follows pregnancies which occur in maternal transplant recipients or those fathered by male transplant recipients. The NTPR encourages reporting of pregnancies following solid organ transplant by contacting them at 877-955-6877.

Breast-Feeding Considerations Tacrolimus is excreted into breast milk; concentrations are variable and lower than that of the maternal serum. The low bioavailability of tacrolimus following oral absorption may also decrease the amount of exposure to a nursing infant (Bramham, 2013; French, 2003; Gardiner, 2006). In one study, tacrolimus serum concentrations in the infants did not differ between those who were bottle fed or breast-fed (all infants were exposed to tacrolimus throughout pregnancy) (Bramham, 2013). Available information suggests that tacrolimus exposure to the nursing infant is ≤0.5% of the weight-adjusted maternal dose (Bramham, 2013; French, 2003; Gardiner, 2006). The manufacturer recommends that nursing be discontinued, taking into consideration the importance of the drug to the mother.

Contraindications Hypersensitivity to tacrolimus, polyoxyl 60 hydrogenated castor oil (HCO-60), or any other component of the formulation.

Warnings/Precautions Hazardous agent - use appropriate precautions for handling and disposal (NIOSH 2014 [group 2]).

[U.S. Boxed Warning]: Risk of developing infections (including bacterial, viral [including CMV], fungal, and protozoal infections [including opportunistic infections]) is increased. Latent viral infections may be activated, including BK virus (associated with polyoma virus-associated nephropathy [PVAN]) and JC virus (associated with progressive multifocal leukoencephalopathy [PML]); may result in serious adverse effects. Immunosuppression increases the risk for CMV viremia and/or CMV disease; the risk of CMV disease is increased for patients who are CMV-seronegative prior to transplant and receive a graft from a CMV-seropositive donor. Consider reduction in immunosuppression if PVAN, PML, CMV viremia and/or CMV disease occurs. **[U.S. Boxed Warning]: Immunosuppressive therapy may result in the development of lymphoma and other malignancies (predominantly skin malignancies).** The risk for new-onset diabetes and insulin-dependent post-transplant diabetes mellitus (PTDM) is increased with tacrolimus use after transplantation, including in patients without pretransplant history of diabetes mellitus; insulin dependence may be reversible; monitor blood glucose frequently; risk is increased in African-American and Hispanic kidney transplant patients. Nephrotoxicity (acute or chronic) has been reported, especially with higher doses; to avoid excess nephrotoxicity do not administer simultaneously with other nephrotoxic drugs (eg, sirolimus, cyclosporine). Neurotoxicity may occur especially when used in high doses; tremor headache, coma and delirium have been reported and are associated with serum concentrations. Seizures may also occur. Posterior reversible encephalopathy syndrome (PRES) has been reported; symptoms (altered mental status, headache, hypertension, seizures, and visual disturbances) are reversible with dose reduction or discontinuation of therapy; stabilize blood pressure and reduce dose with suspected or confirmed PRES diagnosis.

Pure red cell aplasia (PRCA) has been reported in patients receiving tacrolimus. Use with caution in patients with risk factors for PRCA including parvovirus B19 infection, underlying disease, or use of concomitant medications associated with PRCA (eg, mycophenolate). Discontinuation of therapy should be considered with diagnosis of PRCA. Monitoring of serum concentrations (trough for oral therapy) is essential to prevent organ rejection and reduce drug-related toxicity. Use caution in renal or hepatic dysfunction, dosing adjustments may be required. Delay initiation of therapy in kidney transplant patients if postoperative oliguria occurs; begin therapy no sooner than 6 hours and within 24 hours post-transplant, but may be delayed until renal function has recovered. Mild-to-severe hyperkalemia may occur; monitor serum potassium levels. Hypertension may commonly occur; antihypertensive treatment may be necessary; avoid use of potassium-sparing diuretics due to risk of hyperkalemia; concurrent use of calcium channel blockers may require tacrolimus dosage adjustment. Gastrointestinal perforation may occur; all reported cases were considered to be a complication of transplant surgery or accompanied by infection, diverticulum, or malignant neoplasm. Myocardial hypertrophy has been reported (rare). Prolongation of the QT/QTc and torsade de pointes may occur; avoid use in patients with congenital long QT syndrome. Consider obtaining electrocardiograms and monitoring electrolytes (magnesium, potassium, calcium) periodically during treatment in patients with congestive heart failure, bradyarrhythmias, those taking certain antiarrhythmic medications or other medicinal products that lead to QT prolongation, and those with electrolyte disturbances such as hypokalemia, hypocalcemia, or hypomagnesemia. Potentially significant drug-drug/drug-food interactions may exist, requiring dose or frequency adjustment, additional monitoring, and/or selection of alternative therapy. In liver transplantation, the tacrolimus dose and target range should be reduced to minimize the risk of nephrotoxicity when used in combination with everolimus. Extended release tacrolimus in combination with sirolimus is not recommended in renal transplant patients; the safety and efficacy of immediate release tacrolimus in combination with sirolimus has not been established in this patient population. Concomitant use was associated with increased mortality, graft loss, and hepatic artery thrombosis in liver transplant patients, as well as increased risk of renal impairment, wound healing complications, and PTDM in heart transplant recipients.

Immediate release and extended release capsules are NOT interchangeable or substitutable. The extended release formulation is a once daily preparation; and immediate release is intended for twice daily administration. Serious adverse events, including organ rejection may occur if inadvertently substituted. **[U.S. Boxed Warning]: Extended release tacrolimus was associated with increased mortality in female liver transplant recipients; the use of extended release tacrolimus is not recommended in liver transplantation.** Mortality at 12 months was 18% in females who received extended release tacrolimus compared to 8% for females who received regular release tacrolimus. Each mL of injection contains polyoxyl 60 hydrogenated castor oil (HCO-60) (200 mg) and dehydrated alcohol USP 80% v/v.

Hypersensitivity reactions, including anaphylaxis, have been reported with tacrolimus injection. Tacrolimus injection contains polyoxyl 60 hydrogenated castor oil (HCO-60), a castor oil derivative. HCO-60 is a solubilizer similar to polyoxyethylated castor oil (also known as polyoxyl 35 castor oil or Cremophor EL); polyoxyethylated castor oil is associated with hypersensitivity reactions (Nicolai, 2012). Tacrolimus intravenous (IV) use should be limited to patients unable to take oral capsules. Monitor patient for a minimum of 30 minutes after initiation of infusion and then at frequent intervals; discontinue infusion if anaphylaxis occurs. Patients should be transitioned from IV to oral tacrolimus as soon as the patient can tolerate oral administration. Patients should not be immunized with live vaccines during or shortly after treatment and should avoid close contact with recently vaccinated (live vaccine) individuals. Oral formulations contain lactose; the Canadian labeling does not recommend use of these products in patients who may be lactose intolerant (eg, Lapp lactase deficiency, glucose-galactose malabsorption, galactose intolerance). **[U.S. Boxed Warning]: Should be administered under the supervision of a physician experienced in immunosuppressive therapy and organ transplantation in a facility appropriate for monitoring and managing therapy.**

Adverse Reactions As reported for kidney, liver, and heart transplantation:

Cardiovascular: Angina pectoris, atrial fibrillation, atrial flutter, bradycardia, cardiac arrest, cardiac arrhythmia, cardiac failure, cardiorespiratory arrest, cerebral infarction, cerebral ischemia, chest pain, decreased heart rate, deep vein thrombophlebitis, deep vein thrombosis, ECG abnormality (QRS or ST segment or T wave), edema, flushing, hemorrhagic stroke, hypertension, hypertrophic cardiomyopathy, hypotension, ischemic heart disease, myocardial infarction, orthostatic hypotension, pericardial effusion (heart transplant), peripheral edema, peripheral vascular disease, phlebitis, syncope, tachycardia, thrombosis, vasodilatation, ventricular premature contractions

Central nervous system: Abnormal dreams, abnormality in thinking, agitation, amnesia, anxiety, aphasia, ataxia, brain disease, carpal tunnel syndrome, chills, confusion, convulsions, depression, dizziness, drowsiness, emotional lability, excessive crying, falling, fatigue, flaccid paralysis, hallucinations, headache, hypertonia, hypoesthesia, insomnia, mental status changes, mood elevation, myasthenia, myoclonus, nervousness, neurotoxicity, nightmares, pain, paresis, paresthesia, peripheral neuropathy, psychosis, seizure, vertigo, voice disorder, writing difficulty

Dermatologic: Acne vulgaris, alopecia, bruise, cellulitis, condyloma acuminatum, dermal ulcer, dermatological reaction, dermatitis (including fungal), diaphoresis, exfoliative dermatitis, hypotrichosis, pruritus, skin discoloration, skin photosensitivity, skin rash

Endocrine & metabolic: Acidosis, albuminuria, alkalosis, anasarca, Cushing's syndrome, decreased serum bicarbonate, decreased serum iron, dehydration, diabetes mellitus (post-transplant), gout, hirsutism, hypercalcemia, hypercholesterolemia, hyperglycemia, hyperkalemia, hyperlipidemia, hypertriglyceridemia, hyperuricemia, hypervolemia, hypocalcemia, hypoglycemia, hypokalemia, hypomagnesemia, hyponatremia, hypophosphatemia, increased gamma-glutamyl transferase, increased lactate dehydrogenase, weight changes

Gastrointestinal: Abdominal pain, anorexia, aphthous stomatitis, cholangitis, colitis, constipation, delayed gastric emptying, diarrhea, duodenitis, dyspepsia, dysphagia, enlargement of abdomen, esophagitis (including ulcerative), flatulence, gastric ulcer, gastritis, gastroenteritis, gastroesophageal reflux disease, gastrointestinal hemorrhage, gastrointestinal perforation, hernia, hiccups, increased appetite, intestinal obstruction, nausea, oral candidiasis, pancreatic disease (pseudocyst), pancreatitis (including hemorrhagic and necrotizing), peritonitis, rectal disease, stomach cramps, stomatitis, vomiting

Genitourinary: Anuria, bladder spasm, cystitis, dysuria, hematuria, nocturia, oliguria, proteinuria, toxic nephrosis, urinary frequency, urinary incontinence, urinary retention, urinary tract infection, urinary urgency, vaginitis

Hematologic & oncologic: Anemia, blood coagulation disorder, decreased prothrombin time, hemolytic anemia, hemorrhage, hypochromic anemia, hypoproteinemia, increased hematocrit, increased INR, Kaposi's sarcoma, leukocytosis, leukopenia, malignant neoplasm of bladder, malignant neoplasm of thyroid (papillary), neutropenia, pancytopenia, polycythemia, skin neoplasm, thrombocytopenia

Hepatic: Abnormal hepatic function tests, ascites, cholestatic jaundice, hepatic injury, hepatitis (including acute, chronic, and granulomatous), hyperbilirubinemia, increased liver enzymes, increased serum alkaline phosphatase, jaundice

Hypersensitivity: Hypersensitivity reaction

Infection: Abscess, bacterial infection, cytomegalovirus disease, Epstein Barr virus infection, herpes simplex infection, infection, polyoma virus infection, sepsis, serious infection, tinea versicolor

Local: Localized phlebitis, postoperative wound complication

Neuromuscular & skeletal: Arthralgia, arthropathy, back pain, leg cramps, muscle spasm, muscle weakness of the extremities, myalgia, neuropathy (including compression), osteopenia, osteoporosis, tremor, weakness

Ophthalmic: Amblyopia, blurred vision, conjunctivitis, visual disturbance

Otic: Hearing loss, otalgia, otitis externa, otitis media, tinnitus

Renal: Acute renal failure, hydronephrosis, increased blood urea nitrogen, increased serum creatinine, renal disease (BK nephropathy), renal function abnormality, renal tubular necrosis

Respiratory: Allergic rhinitis, asthma, atelectasis, bronchitis, cough, dyspnea, emphysema, flu-like symptoms, pharyngitis, pleural effusion, pneumonia, pneumothorax, pulmonary disease, pulmonary edema, pulmonary infiltrates, respiratory depression, respiratory failure, respiratory tract infection, rhinitis, sinusitis

Miscellaneous: Fever, graft complications, postoperative pain, wound healing impairment

Rare but important or life-threatening: Adult respiratory distress syndrome, agranulocytosis, anaphylactoid reaction, anaphylaxis, angioedema, basal cell carcinoma, biliary tract disease (stenosis), blindness, cerebrovascular accident, coma, deafness, decreased serum fibrinogen, delirium, disseminated intravascular coagulation, dysarthria, graft versus host disease (acute and chronic), hemiparesis, hemolytic-uremic syndrome, hemorrhagic cystitis, hepatic cirrhosis, hepatic failure, hepatic necrosis, hepatic veno-occlusive disease, hepatosplenic T-cell lymphomas, hepatotoxicity, hyperpigmentation, interstitial pulmonary disease, leukemia, leukoencephalopathy, liver steatosis, lymphoproliferative disorder (post-transplant or related to EBV), malignant melanoma, multi-organ failure, mutism, optic atrophy, osteomyelitis, photophobia, polyarthritis, progressive multifocal leukoencephalopathy (PML), prolonged partial thromboplastin time, prolonged Q-T interval on ECG, pulmonary hypertension, pure red cell aplasia, quadriplegia, reversible posterior leukoencephalopathy syndrome, rhabdomyolysis, septicemia, squamous cell carcinoma, status epilepticus, Stevens-Johnson syndrome, supraventricular extrasystole, supraventricular tachycardia, thrombocytopenic purpura, thrombotic thrombocytopenic purpura, torsades de pointes, toxic epidermal necrolysis, venous thrombosis, ventricular fibrillation

Note: Calcineurin inhibitor-induced hemolytic uremic syndrome/thrombotic thrombocytopenic purpura/thrombotic microangiopathy (HUS/TTP/TMA) have been reported (with concurrent sirolimus).

Drug Interactions

Metabolism/Transport Effects Substrate of CYP3A4 (major), P-glycoprotein; **Note:** Assignment of Major/Minor substrate status based on clinically relevant drug interaction potential; **Inhibits** P-glycoprotein

Avoid Concomitant Use

Avoid concomitant use of Tacrolimus (Systemic) with any of the following: BCG; BCG (Intravesical); Bosutinib; CloZAPine; Conivaptan; Crizotinib; CycloSPORINE (Systemic); Dipyrone; Enzalutamide; Eplerenone; Foscarnet; Fusidic Acid (Systemic); Grapefruit Juice; Idelalisib; Mifepristone; Natalizumab; PAZOPanib; Pimecrolimus; Potassium-Sparing Diuretics; Silodosin; Sirolimus; Tacrolimus (Topical); Temsirolimus; Tofacitinib; Topotecan; Vaccines (Live); VinCRIStine (Liposomal)

Increased Effect/Toxicity

Tacrolimus (Systemic) may increase the levels/effects of: Afatinib; Bosutinib; Brentuximab Vedotin; CloZAPine; Colchicine; CycloSPORINE (Systemic); Dabigatran Etexilate; DOXOrubicin (Conventional); Dronedarone; Edoxaban; Everolimus; Fenofibrate and Derivatives; Fosphenytoin; Highest Risk QTc-Prolonging Agents; Ledipasvir; Leflunomide; Moderate Risk QTc-Prolonging Agents; Naloxegol; Natalizumab; PAZOPanib; P-glycoprotein/ABCB1 Substrates; Phenytoin; Prucalopride; Rifaximin; Rivaroxaban; Silodosin; Sirolimus; Temsirolimus; Tofacitinib; Topotecan; Vaccines (Live); VinCRIStine (Liposomal)

The levels/effects of Tacrolimus (Systemic) may be increased by: Alcohol (Ethyl); Antidepressants (Serotonin Reuptake Inhibitor/Antagonist); Aprepitant; Boceprevir; Calcium Channel Blockers (Dihydropyridine); Calcium Channel Blockers (Nondihydropyridine); Chloramphenicol; Clotrimazole (Oral); Clotrimazole (Topical); Conivaptan; Crizotinib; CycloSPORINE (Systemic); CYP3A4 Inhibitors (Moderate); CYP3A4 Inhibitors (Strong); Danazol; Dasatinib; Denosumab; Dipyrone; Dronedarone; Efonidipine; Eplerenone; Ertapenem; Fluconazole; Fosaprepitant; Foscarnet; Fusidic Acid (Systemic); Grapefruit Juice; Idelalisib; Itraconazole; Ivacaftor; Ketoconazole (Systemic); Levofloxacin (Systemic); Luliconazole; Macrolide Antibiotics; Mifepristone; Netupitant; Nonsteroidal Anti-Inflammatory Agents; Palbociclib; P-glycoprotein/ABCB1 Inhibitors; Pimecrolimus; Posaconazole; Potassium-Sparing Diuretics; Protease Inhibitors; Proton Pump Inhibitors; Ranolazine; Ritonavir; Roflumilast; Schisandra; Sirolimus; Stiripentol; Tacrolimus (Topical); Telaprevir; Temsirolimus; Trastuzumab; Voriconazole

Decreased Effect

Tacrolimus (Systemic) may decrease the levels/effects of: Antidiabetic Agents; BCG; BCG (Intravesical); Coccidioides immitis Skin Test; Sipuleucel-T; Vaccines (Inactivated); Vaccines (Live)

The levels/effects of Tacrolimus (Systemic) may be decreased by: Bosentan; Caspofungin; Cinacalcet; CYP3A4 Inducers (Moderate); CYP3A4 Inducers (Strong); Dabrafenib; Deferasirox; Echinacea; Efavirenz; Enzalutamide; Fosphenytoin; Mitotane; P-glycoprotein/ABCB1 Inducers; Phenytoin; Rifamycin Derivatives; Sevelamer; Siltuximab; Sirolimus; St Johns Wort; Temsirolimus; Tocilizumab

Food Interactions

Ethanol: Alcohol may increase the rate of release of extended-release tacrolimus and adversely affect tacrolimus safety and/or efficacy. Management: Avoid alcohol.

Food: Food decreases rate and extent of absorption. High-fat meals have most pronounced effect (37% and 25% decrease in AUC, respectively, and 77% and 25% decrease in C_{max}, respectively, for immediately release and extended release formulations). Grapefruit juice, a CYP3A4 inhibitor, may increase serum level and/or toxicity of tacrolimus. Management: Administer with or without food (immediate release), but be consistent. Administer extended release on an empty stomach. Avoid concurrent use of grapefruit juice.

Storage/Stability

Injection: Prior to dilution, store at 5°C to 25°C (41°F to 77°F). Following dilution, stable for 24 hours in D_5W or NS in glass or polyethylene containers. Do not store in polyvinyl chloride containers since the polyoxyl 60 hydrogenated castor oil injectable vehicle may leach phthalates from polyvinyl chloride containers.

Capsules:

Astagraf XL, Prograf: Store at 25°C (77°F); excursions permitted between 15°C and 30°C (59°F and 86°F).

Hecoria: Store at 20°C to 25°C (68°F to 77°F).

Mechanism of Action Suppresses cellular immunity (inhibits T-lymphocyte activation), by binding to an intracellular protein, FKBP-12 and complexes with calcineurin dependent proteins to inhibit calcineurin phosphatase activity

Pharmacokinetics (Adult data unless noted)

Absorption: Erratic and incomplete oral absorption (5% to 67%); food within 15 minutes of administration decreases absorption (27%)

Distribution: Distributes to erythrocytes, breast milk, lung, kidneys, pancreas, liver, placenta, heart, and spleen:

Children: 2.6 L/kg (mean)

Adults: 0.85-1.41 L/kg (mean) in liver and renal transplant patients

Protein binding: 99% to alpha-acid glycoprotein (some binding to albumin)

Metabolism: Hepatic metabolism through the cytochrome P450 system (CYP3A) to eight possible metabolites

(major metabolite: 31-demethyl tacrolimus has same activity as tacrolimus *in vitro*)

Bioavailability: Oral:

Children: 7% to 55%

Adults: 7% to 32%

Half-life:

Children: 7.7-15.3 hours

Adults: 23-46 hours (in healthy volunteers)

Time to peak serum concentration: Oral: 0.5-6 hours

Elimination: Primarily in bile; <1% excreted unchanged in urine

Clearance: 7-103 mL/minute/kg (average: 30 mL/minute/kg); clearance higher in children

Dosing: Usual

Children: **Note:** Younger children generally require higher maintenance doses on a mg/kg basis than older children, adolescents, or adults (Kim, 2005; Montini, 2006)

Oral:

Liver transplant: Initial: 0.15-0.2 mg/kg/day divided every 12 hours

Heart transplant: Initial: 0.1-0.3 mg/kg/day divided every 12 hours (Pollock-Barziv, 2005; Swenson, 1995)

Kidney transplant: Initial: 0.2-0.3 mg/kg/day divided every 12 hours (Filler, 2005; Kim, 2005; Montini, 2006)

Prevention of graft-vs-host disease (off-label use): Convert from IV to oral dose (1:4 ratio): Multiply total daily IV dose times 4 and administer in 2 divided oral doses per day, every 12 hours (Yanik, 2000)

IV:

Liver transplant: 0.03-0.05 mg/kg/day as a continuous infusion

Heart transplant: 0.01-0.03 mg/kg/day as a continuous infusion (Groetzner, 2005)

Kidney transplant: 0.06 mg/kg/day as a continuous infusion (Trompeter, 2002)

Prevention of graft-vs-host disease (off-label use): Initial: 0.03 mg/kg/day (based on lean body weight) as continuous infusion. Treatment should begin at least 24 hours prior to stem cell infusion and continued only until oral medication can be tolerated (Yanik, 2000).

Adults:

Oral: 0.075-0.2 mg/kg/day divided every 12 hours

Liver transplant: Initial: 0.1-0.15 mg/kg/day divided every 12 hours

Heart transplant: Initial: 0.075 mg/kg/day divided every 12 hours

Kidney transplant: Initial: 0.2 mg/kg/day in combination with azathioprine or 0.1 mg/kg/day in combination with mycophenolate mofetil. Administer in 2 divided doses every 12 hours.

Prevention of graft-vs-host disease (off-label use): Convert from IV to oral dose (1:4 ratio): Multiply total daily IV dose times 4 and administer in 2 divided oral doses per day, every 12 hours (Uberti, 1999)

IV continuous infusion: 0.01-0.05 mg/kg/day

Liver or kidney transplant: Initial: 0.03-0.05 mg/kg/day

Heart transplant: Initial: 0.01 mg/kg/day

Graft-vs-host disease (off-label use):

Prevention: 0.03 mg/kg/day (based on lean body weight) as continuous infusion. Treatment should begin at least 24 hours prior to stem cell infusion and continued only until oral medication can be tolerated (Przepiorka, 1999).

Treatment: Initial: 0.03 mg/kg/day (based on lean body weight) as continuous infusion (Furlong, 2000; Przepiorka, 1999)

Dosing adjustment in renal or hepatic impairment: Patients with renal or hepatic impairment should receive the lowest dose in the recommended dosage range; further reductions in dose below these ranges may be required

Hemodialysis: Not removed by hemodialysis

Preparation for Administration Hazardous agent; use appropriate precautions for handling and disposal (NIOSH 2014 [group 2]).

Parenteral: IV infusion: Dilute with D_5W or NS to a final concentration between 0.004 mg/mL and 0.02 mg/mL. Tacrolimus adsorbs to PVC so diluted solutions should be prepared in glass or polyethylene containers.

Administration Hazardous agent; use appropriate precautions for handling and disposal (NIOSH 2014 [group 2]).

Note: Administration should begin no sooner than 6 hours post-transplant in liver and heart transplant patients; in kidney transplant patients the initial dose may be administered within 24 hours of transplant, but should be delayed until renal function has recovered.

Oral: Immediate release: Administer with or without food; be consistent with timing and composition of meals if GI intolerance occurs and administration with food becomes necessary (per manufacturer); do not administer with grapefruit juice; do not administer within 2 hours before or after antacids

Parenteral: Administer by continuous IV infusion; Must be diluted prior to administration. Do not use PVC tubing when administering diluted solutions; polyvinyl chloride-free administration tubing should be used to minimize the potential for significant drug absorption onto the tubing; adsorption of the drug to PVC tubing may become clinically significant with low concentrations. Do not mix with solutions with a pH ≥9 (eg, acyclovir or ganciclovir) due to chemical degradation of tacrolimus (use different ports in multilumen lines). Do not alter dose with concurrent T-tube clamping. Continue only until oral medication can be tolerated.

Monitoring Parameters Liver enzymes, BUN, serum creatinine, glucose, potassium, magnesium, phosphorus, blood tacrolimus concentrations, CBC with differential; blood pressure, neurologic status, ECG

Reference Range Limited data correlating serum concentration to therapeutic efficacy/toxicity:

Trough (whole blood ELISA): 5-20 ng/mL

Trough (HPLC): 0.5-1.5 ng/mL

Heart transplant: Typical whole blood trough concentrations:

Months 1-3: 10-20 ng/mL

Months ≥4: 6-18 ng/mL

Kidney transplant: Whole blood trough concentrations:

In combination with azathioprine:

Months 1-3: 7-20 ng/mL

Months 4-12: 5-15 ng/mL

In combination with mycophenolate mofetil/IL-2 receptor antagonist (eg, daclizumab): Months 1-12: 4-11 ng/mL

Liver transplant: Whole blood trough concentrations: Months 1-12: 5-20 ng/mL

Prevention of graft-vs-host disease: 10-20 ng/mL (Uberti, 1999); although some institutions use a lower limit of 5 ng/mL and an upper limit of 15 ng/mL (Przepiorka, 1999; Yanik, 2000)

Additional Information Tacrolimus should be initiated no sooner than 6 hours after transplant; convert IV tacrolimus to oral form as soon as possible or within 2-3 days (the oral formulation should be started 8-12 hours after stopping the IV infusion); when switching a patient from cyclosporine to tacrolimus, allow at least 24 hours after discontinuing cyclosporine before initiating tacrolimus therapy to minimize the risk of nephrotoxicity

Additional dosing considerations:

Switch from IV to oral therapy: Approximately threefold increase in dose compared to IV

Pediatric patients: Approximately two times higher dose compared to adults

Product Availability Envarsus XR: FDA approved July 2015; availability anticipated in the fourth quarter of 2015. Envarsus XR is administered once daily and indicated for the prophylaxis of organ rejection in kidney transplant patients converted from tacrolimus immediate-release formulations. Refer to the prescribing information for additional information.

Dosage Forms Excipient information presented when available (limited, particularly for generics); consult specific product labeling. [DSC] = Discontinued product

Capsule, Oral:
- Hecoria: 0.5 mg [DSC], 1 mg [DSC], 5 mg [DSC]
- Prograf: 0.5 mg, 1 mg, 5 mg
- Generic: 0.5 mg, 1 mg, 5 mg

Capsule Extended Release 24 Hour, Oral:
- Astagraf XL: 0.5 mg, 1 mg, 5 mg

Solution, Intravenous:
- Prograf: 5 mg/mL (1 mL) [contains alcohol, usp]

Extemporaneous Preparations Hazardous agent; use appropriate precautions for handling and disposal (NIOSH 2014 [group 2]). When manipulating capsules, NIOSH recommends double gloving, a protective gown, and preparation in a controlled device; if not prepared in a controlled device, respiratory and eye protection as well as ventilated engineering controls are recommended (NIOSH, 2014).

A 0.5 mg/mL tacrolimus oral suspension may be made with immediate release capsules and a 1:1 mixture of Ora-Plus and Simple Syrup, N.F. Mix the contents of six 5 mg tacrolimus capsules with quantity of vehicle sufficient to make 60 mL. Store in glass or plastic amber prescription bottles; label "shake well". Stable for 56 days at room temperature (Esquivel, 1996; Foster, 1996).

A 1 mg/mL tacrolimus oral suspension may be made with immediate release capsules, sterile water, Ora-Plus, and Ora-Sweet. Pour the contents of six 5 mg capsules into a plastic amber prescription bottle. Add ~5 mL of sterile water and agitate bottle until drug disperses into a slurry. Add equal parts Ora-Plus and Ora-Sweet in sufficient quantity to make 30 mL. Store in plastic amber prescription bottles; label "shake well". Stable for 4 months at room temperature (Elefante, 2006).

Elefante A, Muindi J, West K, et al, "Long-Term Stability of a Patient-Convenient 1 mg/mL Suspension of Tacrolimus for Accurate Maintenance of Stable Therapeutic Levels," *Bone Marrow Transplant*, 2006, 37(8):781-4.

Esquivel C, So S, McDiarmid S, Andrews W, and Colombani PM, "Suggested Guidelines for the Use of Tacrolimus in Pediatric Liver Transplant Patients," *Transplantation*, 1996, 61(5):847-8.

Foster JA, Jacobson PA, Johnson CE, et al, "Stability of Tacrolimus in an Extemporaneously Compounded Oral Liquid (Abstract of Meeting Presentation)," *American Society of Health-System Pharmacists Annual Meeting*, 1996, 53:P-52(E).

Tacrolimus (Topical) (ta KROE li mus)

Medication Safety Issues

Sound-alike/look-alike issues:

Tacrolimus may be confused with everolimus, pimecrolimus, sirolimus, temsirolimus

High alert medication:

This medication is in a class the Institute for Safe Medication Practices (ISMP) includes among its list of drug classes that have a heightened risk of causing significant patient harm when used in error.

Related Information

Safe Handling of Hazardous Drugs *on page 2455*

Brand Names: US Protopic

Brand Names: Canada Protopic®

Generic Availability (US) Yes

Use Second-line agent for short-term and intermittent treatment of moderate to severe atopic dermatitis in nonimmunocompromised patients not responsive to conventional therapy or when conventional therapy is not appropriate (0.03% ointment: FDA approved in ages ≥2 years and adults; 0.1% ointment: FDA approved in ages ≥16 years and adults)

Medication Guide Available Yes

Pregnancy Risk Factor C

Pregnancy Considerations Adverse events were observed in animal reproduction studies. Tacrolimus crosses the human placenta and is measurable in the cord blood, amniotic fluid, and newborn serum following systemic use. Refer to the Tacrolimus (Systemic) monograph for additional information.

Breast-Feeding Considerations Tacrolimus is excreted into breast milk following systemic administration. Refer to the Tacrolimus (Systemic) monograph for additional information.

Contraindications Hypersensitivity to tacrolimus or any component of the formulation

Warnings/Precautions Hazardous agent - use appropriate precautions for handling and disposal (NIOSH 2014 [group 2]).

[U.S. Boxed Warning]: Topical calcineurin inhibitors have been associated with rare cases of malignancy (including skin and lymphoma); therefore, it should be limited to short-term and intermittent treatment using the minimum amount necessary for the control of symptoms and only on involved areas. Use in children <2 years of age is not recommended, children ages 2-15 should only use the 0.03% ointment. Avoid use on malignant or premalignant skin conditions (eg cutaneous T-cell lymphoma). Should not be used in immunocompromised patients. Do not apply to areas of active bacterial or viral infection; infections at the treatment site should be cleared prior to therapy. Topical calcineurin agents are considered second-line therapies in the treatment of atopic dermatitis/eczema, and should be limited to use in patients who have failed treatment with other therapies. Patients with atopic dermatitis are predisposed to skin infections, and tacrolimus therapy has been associated with risk of developing eczema herpeticum, varicella zoster, and herpes simplex. If atopic dermatitis is not improved in <6 weeks, re-evaluate to confirm diagnosis. May be associated with development of lymphadenopathy; possible infectious causes should be investigated. Discontinue use in patients with unknown cause of lymphadenopathy or acute infectious mononucleosis. Acute renal failure has been observed (rarely) with topical use. Not recommended for use in patients with skin disease which may increase systemic absorption (eg, Netherton's syndrome). Minimize sunlight exposure during treatment. Safety not established in patients with generalized erythroderma. Safety of intermittent use for >1 year has not been established, particularly since the effect on immune system development is unknown. Should not be used in immunocompromised patients; safety and efficacy have not been evaluated.

Adverse Reactions As reported in children and adults, unless otherwise noted.

Cardiovascular: Peripheral edema (adults), hypertension (adults)

Central nervous system: Depression (adults), headache (adults), hyperesthesia (adults), insomnia (adults), pain, paresthesia (adults), tingling of skin

Dermatologic: Acne vulgaris (adults), alopecia (adults), burning sensation of skin, contact eczema herpeticum (children), contact dermatitis, dermatological disease (children), erythema, folliculitis, fungal dermatitis (adults), pruritus, pustular rash (adults), skin infection (adults), skin rash (adults), sunburn (adults), urticaria (adults), vesiculobullous dermatitis (children), xeroderma (children)

Gastrointestinal: Abdominal pain (children), diarrhea, dyspepsia (adults), gastroenteritis (adults), nausea (children), vomiting (adults)

Genitourinary: Dysmenorrhea (adults), urinary tract infection (adults)

Hematologic & oncologic: Lymphadenopathy (children), malignant lymphoma, malignant neoplasm of skin
Hypersensitivity: Hypersensitivity reaction (adults)
Infection: Herpes zoster, infection, varicella zoster infection
Neuromuscular & skeletal: Arthralgia (adults), back pain (adults), myalgia (adults), weakness (adults)
Ocular: Conjunctivitis (adults)
Otic: Otalgia (children), otitis media (children)
Respiratory: Asthma (adults), bronchitis (adults), flu-like symptoms, increased cough (children), pharyngitis (adults), pneumonia (adults), rhinitis (children), sinusitis (adults)
Miscellaneous: Accidental injury, alcohol intolerance (adults), allergic reaction, cyst (adults), fever (children)
Rare but important or life-threatening: Abnormality in thinking, abscess, acne rosacea, acute renal failure, aggravated tooth caries, anaphylactoid reaction, anemia, anorexia, anxiety, application site edema, arthropathy, basal cell carcinoma, benign neoplasm (breast), blepharitis, bursitis, cataract, chest pain, chills, colitis, conjunctival edema, cutaneous candidiasis, cystitis, dehydration, dermal ulcer, diaphoresis, dry nose, dysgeusia, dyspnea, ecchymoses, edema, epistaxis, furunculosis, gastritis, heart valve disease, hernia, hyperbilirubinemia, hypercholesterolemia, hypertonia, hypothyroidism, impetigo (bullous), laryngitis, leukoderma, malaise, malignant lymphoma, malignant melanoma, migraine, muscle cramps, nail disease, neck pain, neoplasm (benign), oral candidiasis, osteoarthritis, osteomyelitis, otitis externa, pulmonary disease, rectal disease, renal insufficiency, seborrhea, seizure, septicemia, skin discoloration, skin photosensitivity, squamous cell carcinoma, stomatitis, syncope, tachycardia, tendon disease, unintended pregnancy, vaginitis, vasodilatation, vertigo, visual disturbance, vulvovaginal candidiasis, xerophthalmia, xerostomia

Drug Interactions

Metabolism/Transport Effects **Substrate** of CYP3A4 (minor), P-glycoprotein; **Note:** Assignment of Major/Minor substrate status based on clinically relevant drug interaction potential

Avoid Concomitant Use

Avoid concomitant use of Tacrolimus (Topical) with any of the following: CycloSPORINE (Systemic); Immunosuppressants; Sirolimus; Temsirolimus

Increased Effect/Toxicity

Tacrolimus (Topical) may increase the levels/effects of: Alcohol (Ethyl); CycloSPORINE (Systemic); Immunosuppressants; Sirolimus; Temsirolimus

The levels/effects of Tacrolimus (Topical) may be increased by: Antidepressants (Serotonin Reuptake Inhibitor/Antagonist); Antifungal Agents (Azole Derivatives, Systemic); Calcium Channel Blockers (Nondihydropyridine); CycloSPORINE (Systemic); Danazol; Grapefruit Juice; Macrolide Antibiotics; Protease Inhibitors; Sirolimus; Temsirolimus

Decreased Effect There are no known significant interactions involving a decrease in effect.

Storage/Stability Store at room temperature of 25°C (77°F); excursions permitted to 15°C to 30°C (59°F to 86°F).

Mechanism of Action Suppresses cellular immunity (inhibits T-lymphocyte activation), by binding to an intracellular protein, FKBP-12 and complexes with calcineurin dependent proteins to inhibit calcineurin phosphatase activity

Pharmacokinetics (Adult data unless noted)

Absorption: Minimally absorbed
Bioavailability: <0.5%

Dosing: Usual Moderate to severe atopic dermatitis: **Note:** Discontinue use when symptoms have cleared. If no improvement occurs within 6 weeks, patients should be re-examined to confirm diagnosis.

Children and Adolescents ≥2-15 years: Apply a thin layer of 0.03% ointment to affected area twice daily; rub in gently and completely

Adolescents ≥16 years and Adults: Apply a thin layer of 0.03% or 0.1% ointment to affected area twice daily; rub in gently and completely

Administration Hazardous agent; use appropriate precautions for handling and disposal (NIOSH 2014 [group 2]). For external use only; do not cover with occlusive dressings; apply thin layer and rub ointment in gently and completely onto clean, dry skin. Do not bathe, shower, or swim right after ointment application. Moisturizers can be applied after ointment application.

Dosage Forms Excipient information presented when available (limited, particularly for generics); consult specific product labeling.

Ointment, External:
Protopic: 0.03% (30 g, 60 g, 100 g); 0.1% (30 g, 60 g, 100 g)
Generic: 0.03% (30 g, 60 g, 100 g); 0.1% (30 g, 60 g, 100 g)

- **Tactuo™ (Can)** *see* Adapalene and Benzoyl Peroxide *on page 71*
- **Tagamet HB [OTC]** *see* Cimetidine *on page 461*
- **Talwin** *see* Pentazocine *on page 1664*
- **Tambocor [DSC]** *see* Flecainide *on page 879*
- **Tambocor™ (Can)** *see* Flecainide *on page 879*
- **Tamiflu** *see* Oseltamivir *on page 1572*

Tamoxifen (ta MOKS i fen)

Medication Safety Issues

Sound-alike/look-alike issues:

Tamoxifen may be confused with pentoxifylline, Tambocor, tamsulosin, temazepam

Related Information

Oral Medications That Should Not Be Crushed or Altered *on page 2476*
Safe Handling of Hazardous Drugs *on page 2455*

Brand Names: US Soltamox

Brand Names: Canada Apo-Tamox; Mylan-Tamoxifen; Nolvadex-D; PMS-Tamoxifen; Teva-Tamoxifen

Therapeutic Category Antineoplastic Agent, Estrogen Receptor Antagonist

Generic Availability (US) May be product dependent

Use Treatment of metastatic (female and male) breast cancer; adjuvant treatment of breast cancer after primary treatment with surgery and radiation; reduce risk of invasive breast cancer in women with ductal carcinoma *in situ* (DCIS) after surgery and radiation; reduce the incidence of breast cancer in women at high risk (all indications: FDA approved in adults); has also been used in treatment of McCune-Albright Syndrome (MAS) in girls associated with precocious puberty

Medication Guide Available Yes

Pregnancy Risk Factor D

Pregnancy Considerations Animal reproduction studies have demonstrated fetal adverse effects and fetal loss. There have been reports of vaginal bleeding, birth defects and fetal loss in pregnant women. Tamoxifen use during pregnancy may have a potential long term risk to the fetus of a DES-like syndrome. For sexually-active women of childbearing age, initiate during menstruation (negative β-hCG immediately prior to initiation in women with irregular cycles). Tamoxifen may induce ovulation. Barrier or nonhormonal contraceptives are recommended. Pregnancy should be avoided during treatment and for 2 months after treatment has been discontinued.

Breast-Feeding Considerations It is not known if tamoxifen is excreted in breast milk, however, it has been shown to inhibit lactation. Due to the potential for adverse reactions, women taking tamoxifen should not breast-feed.

Contraindications Hypersensitivity to tamoxifen or any component of the formulation; concurrent warfarin therapy or history of deep vein thrombosis or pulmonary embolism (when tamoxifen is used for breast cancer risk reduction in women at high risk for breast cancer or with ductal carcinoma *in situ* [DCIS])

Warnings/Precautions Hazardous agent - use appropriate precautions for handling and disposal (NIOSH 2014 [group 1]). **[U.S. Boxed Warning]: Serious and life-threatening events (some fatal), including stroke, pulmonary emboli, and uterine or endometrial malignancies, have occurred at an incidence greater than placebo during use for breast cancer risk reduction in women at high-risk for breast cancer and in women with ductal carcinoma *in situ* (DCIS). In women already diagnosed with breast cancer, the benefits of tamoxifen treatment outweigh risks; evaluate risks versus benefits (and discuss with patients) when used for breast cancer risk reduction.** An increased incidence of thromboembolic events, including DVT and pulmonary embolism, has been associated with use for breast cancer; risk is increased with concomitant chemotherapy; use with caution in individuals with a history of thromboembolic events. Thrombocytopenia and/or leukopenia may occur; neutropenia and pancytopenia have been reported rarely. Although the relationship to tamoxifen therapy is uncertain, rare hemorrhagic episodes have occurred in patients with significant thrombocytopenia. Use with caution in patients with hyperlipidemias; infrequent postmarketing cases of hyperlipidemias have been reported. Decreased visual acuity, retinal vein thrombosis, retinopathy, corneal changes, color perception changes, and increased incidence of cataracts (and the need for cataract surgery), have been reported. Hypercalcemia has occurred in some patients with bone metastasis, usually within a few weeks of therapy initiation; institute appropriate hypercalcemia management; discontinue if severe. Local disease flare and increased bone and tumor pain may occur in patients with metastatic breast cancer; may be associated with (good) tumor response.

Potentially significant drug-drug interactions may exist, requiring dose or frequency adjustment, additional monitoring, and/or selection of alternative therapy. Decreased efficacy and an increased risk of breast cancer recurrence has been reported with concurrent moderate or strong CYP2D6 inhibitors (Aubert, 2009; Dezentje, 2009). Concomitant use with select SSRIs may result in decreased tamoxifen efficacy. Strong CYP2D6 inhibitors (eg, fluoxetine, paroxetine) and moderate CYP2D6 inhibitors (eg, sertraline) are reported to interfere with transformation to the active metabolite endoxifen; when possible, select alternative medications with minimal or no impact on endoxifen levels (NCCN Breast Cancer Risk Reduction Guidelines v.1.2013; Sideras, 2010). Weak CYP2D6 inhibitors (eg, venlafaxine, citalopram) have minimal effect on the conversion to endoxifen (Jin, 2005; NCCN Breast Cancer Risk Reduction Guidelines v.1.2013); escitalopram is also a weak CYP2D6 inhibitor. In a retrospective analysis of breast cancer patients taking tamoxifen and SSRIs, concomitant use of paroxetine and tamoxifen was associated with an increased risk of death due to breast cancer (Kelly, 2010). Lower plasma concentrations of endoxifen have been observed in patients associated with reduced CYP2D6 activity (Jin, 2005; Schroth, 2009) and may be associated with reduced efficacy, although data is conflicting. Routine CYP2D6 testing is not recommended at this time in order to determine optimal endocrine therapy (NCCN Breast Cancer Guidelines v.2.2013; Visvana than, 2009).

Tamoxifen use may be associated with changes in bon mineral density (BMD) and the effects may be depender upon menstrual status. In postmenopausal women, tamox ifen use is associated with a protective effect on bon mineral density (BMD), preventing loss of BMD which last over the 5-year treatment period. In premenopausa women, a decline (from baseline) in BMD mineral densit has been observed in women who continued to menstru ate; may be associated with an increased risk of fractures Liver abnormalities such as cholestasis, fatty liver, hepat tis, and hepatic necrosis have occurred. Hepatocellula carcinomas have been reported in some studies; relation ship to treatment is unclear. Tamoxifen is associated wit an increased incidence of uterine or endometrial cancers Endometrial hyperplasia, polyps, endometriosis, uterin fibroids, and ovarian cysts have occurred. Monitor an promptly evaluate any report of abnormal vaginal bleeding Amenorrhea and menstrual irregularities have bee reported with tamoxifen use.

Warnings: Additional Pediatric Considerations Som dosage forms may contain propylene glycol; in neonate large amounts of propylene glycol delivered orally, intra venously (eg, >3,000 mg/day), or topically have bee associated with potentially fatal toxicities which can includ metabolic acidosis, seizures, renal failure, and CN depression; toxicities have also been reported in childre and adults including hyperosmolality, lactic acidosis, seiz ures and respiratory depression; use caution (AAP, 1997 Shehab, 2009).

Adverse Reactions

Cardiovascular: Angina, cardiovascular ischemia, ches pain, deep venous thrombus, edema, flushing, hype tension, MI, peripheral edema, vasodilation, venou thrombotic events

Central nervous system: Anxiety, depression, dizziness fatigue, headache, insomnia, mood changes, pain

Dermatologic: Alopecia, rash, skin changes

Endocrine & metabolic: Altered menses, amenorrhea breast neoplasm, breast pain, fluid retention, hot flashes hypercholesterolemia, menstrual disorder, oligome norrhea

Gastrointestinal: Abdominal cramps, abdominal pain, anc rexia, constipation, diarrhea, dyspepsia, nausea, throa irritation (oral solution), vomiting, weight gain/loss

Genitourinary: Leukorrhea, ovarian cyst, urinary tract infec tion, vaginal bleeding, vaginal discharge, vaginal hemo rhage, vaginitis, vulvovaginitis

Hematologic: Anemia, thrombocytopenia

Hepatic: AST increased, serum bilirubin increased

Neuromuscular & skeletal: Arthralgia, arthritis, arthrosis back pain, bone pain, fracture, joint disorder, musculos keletal pain, myalgia, osteoporosis, paresthesia weakness

Ocular: Cataract

Renal: Serum creatinine increased

Respiratory: Bronchitis, cough, dyspnea, pharyngitis sinusitis

Miscellaneous: Allergic reaction, cyst, diaphoresis, flu-lik syndrome, infection/sepsis, lymphedema, neoplasm

Rare but important or life-threatening: Angioedema, bu lous pemphigoid, cholestasis, corneal changes, endome trial cancer, endometrial hyperplasia, endometrial polyps endometriosis, erythema multiforme, fatty liver, hepati necrosis, hepatitis, hypercalcemia, hyperlipidemia hypersensitivity reactions, hypertriglyceridemia, impc tence (males), interstitial pneumonitis, loss of libid (males), pancreatitis, phlebitis, pruritus vulvae, pulmc nary embolism, retinal vein thrombosis, retinopathy, sec ond primary tumors, Stevens-Johnson syndrome, stroke tumor pain and local disease flare (including increase i lesion size and erythema) during treatment of metastatic breast cancer (generally resolves with continuation); uterine fibroids, vaginal dryness, visual color perception changes

Drug Interactions

Metabolism/Transport Effects Substrate of CYP2A6 (minor), CYP2B6 (minor), CYP2C9 (major), CYP2D6 (major), CYP2E1 (minor), CYP3A4 (major); **Note:** Assignment of Major/Minor substrate status based on clinically relevant drug interaction potential; **Inhibits** CYP2B6 (weak), CYP2C8 (moderate), CYP2C9 (weak), P-glycoprotein

Avoid Concomitant Use

Avoid concomitant use of Tamoxifen with any of the following: Amodiaquine; Bosutinib; Conivaptan; CYP2D6 Inhibitors (Strong); Fusidic Acid (Systemic); Idelalisib; Ospemifene; PAZOPanib; Silodosin; Topotecan; VinCRIStine (Liposomal); Vitamin K Antagonists

Increased Effect/Toxicity

Tamoxifen may increase the levels/effects of: Afatinib; Amodiaquine; Bosutinib; Brentuximab Vedotin; Colchicine; CYP2C8 Substrates; Dabigatran Etexilate; DOXOrubicin (Conventional); Edoxaban; Everolimus; Highest Risk QTc-Prolonging Agents; Ledipasvir; Mipomersen; Moderate Risk QTc-Prolonging Agents; Naloxegol; Ospemifene; PAZOPanib; P-glycoprotein/ABCB1 Substrates; Prucalopride; Rifaximin; Rivaroxaban; Silodosin; Topotecan; VinCRIStine (Liposomal); Vitamin K Antagonists

The levels/effects of Tamoxifen may be increased by: Abiraterone Acetate; Conivaptan; CYP2C9 Inhibitors (Moderate); CYP2C9 Inhibitors (Strong); CYP3A4 Inhibitors (Moderate); CYP3A4 Inhibitors (Strong); Dasatinib; Fosaprepitant; Fusidic Acid (Systemic); Idelalisib; Ivacaftor; Luliconazole; Mifepristone; Netupitant; Palbociclib; Panobinostat; Peginterferon Alfa-2b; Simeprevir

Decreased Effect

Tamoxifen may decrease the levels/effects of: Anastrozole; Letrozole; Ospemifene

The levels/effects of Tamoxifen may be decreased by: Bexarotene (Systemic); Bosentan; CYP2C9 Inducers (Strong); CYP2D6 Inhibitors (Moderate); CYP2D6 Inhibitors (Strong); CYP3A4 Inducers (Moderate); CYP3A4 Inducers (Strong); Dabrafenib; Deferasirox; Mitotane; Peginterferon Alfa-2b; Rifamycin Derivatives; Siltuximab; St Johns Wort; Tocilizumab

Food Interactions Grapefruit juice may decrease the metabolism of tamoxifen. Management: Avoid grapefruit juice.

Storage/Stability

Oral solution: Store at ≤25°C (77°F); do not freeze or refrigerate. Protect from light. Discard opened bottle after 3 months.

Tablets: Store at 20°C to 25°C (68°F to 77°F). Protect from light.

Mechanism of Action Competitively binds to estrogen receptors on tumors and other tissue targets, producing a nuclear complex that decreases DNA synthesis and inhibits estrogen effects; nonsteroidal agent with potent antiestrogenic properties which compete with estrogen for binding sites in breast and other tissues; cells accumulate in the G_0 and G_1 phases; therefore, tamoxifen is cytostatic rather than cytocidal.

Pharmacokinetics (Adult data unless noted)

Absorption: Well absorbed

Distribution: High concentrations found in uterus, endometrial, and breast tissue

Protein binding: 99%

Metabolism: Hepatic; via CYP2D6 to 4-hydroxytamoxifen and via CYP3A4/5 to N-desmethyl-tamoxifen. Each is then further metabolized into endoxifen (4-hydroxy-tamoxifen via CYP3A4/5 and N-desmethyl-tamoxifen via CYP2D6); both 4-hydroxy-tamoxifen and endoxifen are 30- to 100-fold more potent than tamoxifen.

Half-life elimination: Tamoxifen: ~5-7 days; N-desmethyl tamoxifen: ~14 days

Time to peak, serum concentrations:

Children 2-10 years (female): ~8 hours

Adults: ~5 hours

Elimination: Feces (26% to 51%); urine (9% to 13%)

Clearance: Higher (~2.3 fold) in female pediatric patients (2-10 years) compared to adult breast cancer patients; within pediatric population, clearance faster in children 2-6 years compared to older children

Dosing: Usual

Pediatric: **McCune-Albright syndrome; precocious puberty:** Limited data available: Children 2 to 10 years: Oral: 20 mg once daily; dosing based on a trial of 25 girls ≤10 years of age (range: 2.9 to 10.9 years) who received treatment for 1 year; frequency of vaginal bleeding episodes were decreased; growth velocity was significantly decreased prior to pretreatment rates as was skeletal maturation; ovarian and uterine volumes were increased; further studies are needed (Eugester 2003)

Adult: **Note:** For the treatment of breast cancer, patients receiving both tamoxifen and chemotherapy should receive treatment sequentially, with tamoxifen following completion of chemotherapy.

Breast cancer treatment:

Adjuvant therapy (females): 20 mg once daily for 5 years

Metastatic (males and females): 20 to 40 mg/day (doses >20 mg should be given in 2 divided doses). **Note:** Although the FDA-approved labeling recommends dosing up to 40 mg/day, clinical benefit has not been demonstrated with doses above 20 mg/day (Bratherton 1984).

Premenopausal women: Duration of treatment is 5 years (NCCN Breast Cancer guidelines v.1.2011)

Postmenopausal women: Duration of tamoxifen treatment is 2 to 3 years followed by an aromatase inhibitor (AI) to complete 5 years; if contraindications or intolerant to AI, may take tamoxifen for the full 5 years **or** extended therapy: 4.5-6 years of tamoxifen followed by 5 years of an AI (NCCN Breast Cancer guidelines v.1.2011)

DCIS (females), to reduce the risk for invasive breast cancer: 20 mg once daily for 5 years

Breast cancer risk reduction (pre- and postmenopausal high-risk females): 20 mg once daily for 5 years

Dosing adjustment in renal impairment: There are no dosage adjustments provided in the manufacturer's labeling (not studied).

Dosing adjustment in hepatic impairment: There are no dosage adjustments provided in the manufacturer's labeling; the effect of hepatic dysfunction on tamoxifen pharmacokinetics has not been determined.

Administration Hazardous agent; use appropriate precautions for handling and disposal (NIOSH 2014 [group 1]). Administer tablets or oral solution with or without food; use supplied dosing cup for oral solution.

Monitoring Parameters CBC with platelets, serum calcium, LFTs; triglycerides and cholesterol (in patients with pre-existing hyperlipidemias); INR and PT (in patients on vitamin K antagonists); abnormal vaginal bleeding; breast and gynecologic exams (baseline and routine), mammogram (baseline and routine); signs/symptoms of DVT (leg swelling, tenderness) or PE (shortness of breath); ophthalmic exam (if vision problem or cataracts); bone mineral density (premenopausal women)

McCune-Albright syndrome: In the pediatric clinical trial (study duration: 12 months), the following were monitored: Serum estradiol, estrone, DHEAS, LH, FSH, and IGF-1 (baseline, and at 6 and 12 months of therapy); liver function test (baseline and at 3, 6, and 12 months of therapy); CBC and INR at baseline; assessments of puberty status and growth at baseline and periodically during therapy (6 and 12 months): Height, weight, Tanner stage, bone age (radiographs), vaginal bleeding data, and pelvic ultrasounds (Eugester, 2003)

Test Interactions T_4 elevations (which may be explained by increases in thyroid-binding globulin) have been reported; not accompanied by clinical hyperthyroidism

Dosage Forms Excipient information presented when available (limited, particularly for generics); consult specific product labeling.

Solution, Oral:

Soltamox: 10 mg/5 mL (150 mL) [sugar free; contains alcohol, usp, propylene glycol; licorice-aniseed flavor]

Tablet, Oral:

Generic: 10 mg, 20 mg

Extemporaneous Preparations Hazardous agent: Use appropriate precautions for handling and disposal (NIOSH 2014 [group 1]).

A 0.5 mg/mL oral suspension may be prepared with tablets. Place two 10 mg tablets into 40 mL purified water and let stand ~2-5 minutes. Stir until tablets are completely disintegrated (dispersion time for each 10 mg tablet is ~2-5 minutes). Administer immediately after preparation. To ensure the full dose is administered, rinse glass several times with water and administer residue.

Lam MS, "Extemporaneous Compounding of Oral Liquid Dosage Formulations and Alternative Drug Delivery Methods for Anticancer Drugs," *Pharmacotherapy*, 2011, 31(2):164-92.

- **Tamoxifen Citras** *see* Tamoxifen *on page 2005*
- **Tamoxifen Citrate** *see* Tamoxifen *on page 2005*

Tamsulosin (tam SOO loe sin)

Medication Safety Issues

Sound-alike/look-alike issues:

Flomax may be confused with Flonase, Flovent, Foltx, Fosamax

Tamsulosin may be confused with tacrolimus, tamoxifen, terazosin

International issues:

Flomax [U.S., Canada, and multiple international markets] may be confused with Flomox brand name for cefcapene [Japan]; Volmax brand name for salbutamol [multiple international markets]

Flomax: Brand name for tamsulosin [U.S., Canada, and multiple international markets], but also the brand name for morniflumate [Italy]

Related Information

Oral Medications That Should Not Be Crushed or Altered *on page 2476*

Brand Names: US Flomax

Brand Names: Canada Apo-Tamsulosin CR; Flomax CR; Mylan-Tamsulosin; ratio-Tamsulosin; Sandoz-Tamsulosin; Tamsulosin CR; Teva-Tamsulosin; Teva-Tamsulosin CR

Therapeutic Category Alpha$_1$ Blocker

Generic Availability (US) Yes

Use Treatment of signs and symptoms of benign prostatic hyperplasia (BPH) (FDA approved in adult males); has also been used for nephrolithiasis and for management of primary bladder neck dysfunction.

Pregnancy Risk Factor B

Pregnancy Considerations Adverse events were not observed in animal reproduction studies. For pregnant women with kidney stones, other treatments such as stents or ureteroscopy, are recommended if stone removal is needed (Preminger, 2007; Tan, 2013).

Contraindications Hypersensitivity to tamsulosin or any component of the formulation

Warnings/Precautions Not intended for use as an antihypertensive drug. May cause significant orthostatic hypotension and syncope, especially with first dose; anticipate a similar effect if therapy is interrupted for a few days, if dosage is rapidly increased, or if another antihypertensive drug (particularly vasodilators) or a PDE-5 inhibitor (eg, sildenafil, tadalafil, vardenafil) is introduced. "First-dose" orthostatic hypotension may occur 4 to 8 hours after dosing; may be dose related. Patients should be cautioned about performing hazardous tasks, driving, or operating heavy machinery when starting new therapy or adjusting dosage upward. Discontinue if symptoms of angina occur or worsen. Rule out prostatic carcinoma with screening before beginning therapy with tamsulosin and then screen at regular intervals.

Intraoperative floppy iris syndrome (IFIS) is characterized by a combination of flaccid iris that billows with intraoperative currents, progressive intraoperative miosis despite dilation, and potential iris prolapse. IFIS has been observed in cataract and glaucoma surgery patients who were on or were previously treated with alpha$_1$-blockers, particularly with tamsulosin use (Abdel-Aziz, 2009); in some cases, patients had discontinued the alpha$_1$-blocker 5 weeks to 9 months prior to the surgery. The benefit of discontinuing alpha-blocker therapy prior to cataract or glaucoma surgery has not been established. IFIS may increase the risk of ocular complications during and after surgery. May require modifications to surgical technique; instruct patients to inform ophthalmologist of current or previous alpha$_1$-blocker use when considering eye surgery. Initiation of tamsulosin therapy in patients with planned cataract or glaucoma surgery is not recommended. Priapism has been associated with use (rarely). Rarely, patients with a sulfa allergy have also developed an allergic reaction to tamsulosin; avoid use when previous reaction has been severe or life-threatening. Potentially significant drug-drug interactions may exist, requiring dose or frequency adjustment, additional monitoring, and/or selection of alternative therapy.

Warnings: Additional Pediatric Considerations Tamsulosin has been well tolerated in pediatric patients during trials when used for management of nephrolithiasis and primary bladder neck dysfunction (Donohoe 2005; Mokhless 2012; Tasian 2014; Van Batavia 2010). Studies using tamsulosin for the management of elevated detrusor leak point pressure in pediatric patients (ages 2 to 16 years) with a known neurological disorder (eg, spina bifida) failed to show efficacy. In two pooled trials, adverse events occurring in ≥5% of patients included urinary tract infection, vomiting, pyrexia, headache, nasopharyngitis, cough, pharyngitis, influenza, diarrhea, abdominal pain, and constipation.

Adverse Reactions

Cardiovascular: Orthostatic hypotension

Central nervous system: Dizziness, drowsiness, headache, insomnia, vertigo

Endocrine & metabolic: Loss of libido

Gastrointestinal: Diarrhea, nausea

Genitourinary: Ejaculation failure

Infection: Infection

Neuromuscular & skeletal: Back pain, weakness

Ophthalmic: Blurred vision

Respiratory: Cough, pharyngitis, rhinitis, sinusitis

Rare but important or life-threatening): Epistaxis, exfoliative dermatitis, hypersensitivity reaction, hypotension, intraoperative floppy iris syndrome, palpitation, priapism, syncope

Drug Interactions

Metabolism/Transport Effects **Substrate** of CYP2D6 (minor), CYP3A4 (major); **Note:** Assignment of Major/Minor substrate status based on clinically relevant drug interaction potential

Avoid Concomitant Use

Avoid concomitant use of Tamsulosin with any of the following: Alpha1-Blockers; Conivaptan; CYP3A4 Inhibitors (Strong); Fusidic Acid (Systemic); Idelalisib

Increased Effect/Toxicity

Tamsulosin may increase the levels/effects of: Alpha1-Blockers; Calcium Channel Blockers

The levels/effects of Tamsulosin may be increased by: Aprepitant; Beta-Blockers; Cimetidine; Conivaptan; CYP2D6 Inhibitors (Strong); CYP3A4 Inhibitors (Moderate); CYP3A4 Inhibitors (Strong); Dapoxetine; Dasatinib; Fosaprepitant; Fusidic Acid (Systemic); Idelalisib; Ivacaftor; Luliconazole; MAO Inhibitors; Mifepristone; Netupitant; Palbociclib; Phosphodiesterase 5 Inhibitors; Simeprevir; Stiripentol

Decreased Effect

Tamsulosin may decrease the levels/effects of: Alpha-/Beta-Agonists; Alpha1-Agonists

The levels/effects of Tamsulosin may be decreased by: Bosentan; CYP3A4 Inducers (Moderate); CYP3A4 Inducers (Strong); Dabrafenib; Deferasirox; Mitotane; Siltuximab; St Johns Wort; Tocilizumab

Food Interactions Fasting increases bioavailability by 30% and peak concentration 40% to 70%. Management: Administer 30 minutes after the same meal each day.

Storage/Stability Store at 25°C (77°F); excursions are permitted between 15°C and 30°C (59°F and 86°F).

Mechanism of Action Tamsulosin is an antagonist of $alpha_{1A}$-adrenoreceptors in the prostate. Smooth muscle tone in the prostate is mediated by $alpha_{1A}$-adrenoreceptors; blocking them leads to relaxation of smooth muscle in the bladder neck and prostate causing an improvement of urine flow and decreased symptoms of BPH. Approximately 75% of the $alpha_1$-receptors in the prostate are of the $alpha_{1A}$ subtype.

Pharmacokinetics (Adult data unless noted) Note: Pharmacokinetics in pediatric patients (ages 2 to 16 years) were found to be similar to adult values (Tsuda 2010).

Absorption: >90%

Distribution: V_{dss}: 16 L

Protein binding: 94% to 99%, primarily to alpha-1 acid glycoprotein (AAG)

Metabolism: Hepatic via CYP3A4 and CYP2D6; metabolites undergo extensive conjugation to glucuronide or sulfate

Half-life elimination: Healthy volunteers: 9 to 13 hours; Target population: 14 to 15 hours

Time to peak serum concentration: Fasting: 4 to 5 hours; with food: 6 to 7 hours

Elimination: Urine (76%, <10% as unchanged drug); feces (21%)

Dosing: Usual

Pediatric:

Nephrolithiasis, distal stones: Limited data available; optimal dose not established (Mokhless 2012; Tasian 2014):

Children 2 to 4 years: Oral: 0.2 or 0.4 mg once daily at bedtime

Children >4 years and Adolescents: Oral: 0.4 mg once daily at bedtime

Dosing based on two studies. The larger was a multi-institutional retrospective cohort study of pediatric patients with stones up to 10 mm; patients received either tamsulosin 0.4 mg once daily (n=99, median age: 14.8 years) or analgesics alone (n=175). Spontaneous stone passage was higher in the treatment group (55% vs 44%, p=0.03); treatment group was older and had smaller, more distal stones. When adjusted for stone size and location as part of analysis of 99 case matched pairs, success was also higher in the treatment group (OR 3.31, 95% CI: 1.49 to 7.34) (Tasian 2014). The smaller study was a prospective, randomized controlled trial of pediatric patients with stones up to 12 mm; patients received either tamsulosin 0.4 mg once daily (0.2 mg if ≤4 years old) (n=33, age: 2 to 15 years) or placebo (n=28). In this study, 45% of the treatment group had previously received either extracorporeal shock wave lithotripsy (ESWL) or percutaneous nephrolithotomy, but none in the control group had received these therapies; however, stone size at the start of treatment was similar between groups. Treatment resulted in higher expulsion rate (87.8% vs 64.2%, p<0.01), less days to expulsion (mean: 8.2 vs 14.5 days, p<0.001), less pain episodes (mean: 1.4 vs 2.2, p<0.02) and less need for analgesia (mean: 0.7 vs 1.4, p<0.02) (Mokhless 2012). In both studies, tamsulosin was well tolerated and there were no reported adverse effects.

Primary bladder neck dysfunction: Limited data available: Children ≥3 years and Adolescents: Oral: Initial dose: 0.2 mg once daily, increase by 0.2 mg increments based on response (symptoms and urodynamic studies) and tolerability. Mean effective dose: 0.4 mg daily; maximum reported daily dose: 0.8 mg/**day**. Dosing based on two trials evaluating treatment with alpha blockers, including over 50 pediatric patients who received tamsulosin. Treatment resulted in improved urine flow rates and decreased post-void residual urine volume; values returned to pretreatment levels when therapy was discontinued. Tamsulosin was well tolerated with no major adverse effects and benefits continued for at least 3 years (Donohoe 2005; Van Batavia 2010).

Adult: **Benign prostatic hyperplasia (BPH):** Males: Oral: 0.4 mg once daily ~30 minutes after the same meal each day; dose may be increased after 2 to 4 weeks to 0.8 mg once daily in patients who fail to respond. If therapy is discontinued or interrupted for several days, restart with 0.4 mg once daily.

Dosing adjustment in renal impairment: Adult males:

CrCl ≥10 mL/minute: No adjustment needed

CrCl <10 mL/minute: There are no dosage adjustments provided in the manufacturer's labeling (has not been studied)

Dosing adjustment in hepatic impairment: Adult males:

Mild to moderate impairment: No dosage adjustment is necessary.

Severe impairment: There are no dosage adjustments provided in the manufacturer's labeling (has not been studied).

Administration Per the manufacturer, capsules should be swallowed whole; do not crush, chew, or open. In pediatric trials, capsules were opened and the contents mixed with food (eg, yogurt or pudding) or juice (Donohoe 2005; Tasian 2014).

Monitoring Parameters Blood pressure, urinary symptoms

Dosage Forms Excipient information presented when available (limited, particularly for generics); consult specific product labeling.

Capsule, Oral, as hydrochloride:

Flomax: 0.4 mg [contains fd&c blue #2 (indigotine)]

Generic: 0.4 mg

- **Tamsulosin CR (Can)** *see* Tamsulosin *on page 2008*
- **Tamsulosin Hydrochloride** *see* Tamsulosin *on page 2008*
- **Tanta-Orciprenaline® (Can)** *see* Metaproterenol *on page 1374*

- ◆ **TAP-144** *see* Leuprolide *on page 1229*
- ◆ **Tapazole** *see* Methimazole *on page 1386*
- ◆ **TargaDOX** *see* Doxycycline *on page 717*
- ◆ **Targel® [OTC] (Can)** *see* Coal Tar *on page 523*
- ◆ **Taro-Carbamazepine Chewable (Can)** *see* CarBAMazepine *on page 367*
- ◆ **Taro-Ciclopirox (Can)** *see* Ciclopirox *on page 458*
- ◆ **Taro-Ciprofloxacin (Can)** *see* Ciprofloxacin (Systemic) *on page 463*
- ◆ **Taro-Clindamycin (Can)** *see* Clindamycin (Topical) *on page 491*
- ◆ **Taro-Clobetasol (Can)** *see* Clobetasol *on page 498*
- ◆ **Taro-Docusate [OTC] (Can)** *see* Docusate *on page 697*
- ◆ **Taro-Enalapril (Can)** *see* Enalapril *on page 744*
- ◆ **Taro-Fluconazole (Can)** *see* Fluconazole *on page 881*
- ◆ **Taro-Mometasone (Can)** *see* Mometasone (Topical) *on page 1456*
- ◆ **Taro-Phenytoin (Can)** *see* Phenytoin *on page 1690*
- ◆ **Taro-Sone (Can)** *see* Betamethasone (Topical) *on page 280*
- ◆ **Taro-Sumatriptan (Can)** *see* SUMAtriptan *on page 1995*
- ◆ **Taro-Warfarin (Can)** *see* Warfarin *on page 2195*
- ◆ **Tavist Allergy [OTC]** *see* Clemastine *on page 486*
- ◆ **Tavist ND** *see* Loratadine *on page 1296*
- ◆ **Taxol** *see* PACLitaxel (Conventional) *on page 1602*
- ◆ **Taxotere** *see* DOCEtaxel *on page 692*

Tazarotene (taz AR oh teen)

Brand Names: US Avage; Fabior; Tazorac

Brand Names: Canada Tazorac

Therapeutic Category Acne Products; Keratolytic Agent

Generic Availability (US) No

Use

Cream: Treatment of acne vulgaris [Tazorac (0.1%): FDA approved in ages ≥12 years and adults]; treatment of plaque psoriasis [Tazorac (0.05% and 0.1%): FDA approved in ages ≥18 years and adults]; mitigation (palliation) of facial skin wrinkling, facial mottled hyper-/hypopigmentation, and benign facial lentigines as adjunct to comprehensive skin care and sunlight avoidance [Avage (0.1%): FDA approved in ages ≥17 years and adults]

Gel: Treatment of mild to moderate facial acne vulgaris [Tazorac (0.1%): FDA approved in ages ≥12 years and adults]; treatment of stable plaque psoriasis of up to 20% body surface area involvement [Tazorac (0.05% and 0.1%): FDA approved in ages ≥12 years and adults]

Pregnancy Risk Factor X

Pregnancy Considerations Adverse events were observed in animal reproduction studies. Use in pregnancy is contraindicated. A negative pregnancy test should be obtained within 2 weeks prior to treatment; treatment should begin during a normal menstrual period.

Breast-Feeding Considerations It is not known if tazarotene is excreted in breast milk; recommendations for use differ by manufacturers' labeling. Systemic absorption depends on formulation and size of surface area.

Contraindications

Hypersensitivity to tazarotene or any component of the formulation; women who are or may become pregnant

Documentation of allergenic cross-reactivity for retinoids is limited. However, because of similarities in chemical structure and/or pharmacologic actions, the possibility of cross-sensitivity cannot be ruled out with certainty.

Warnings/Precautions Women of childbearing potential must consider the possibility of pregnancy prior to initiation of therapy; a negative pregnancy test should be obtained within 2 weeks prior to treatment and treatment should begin during a normal menstrual period. Adequate contraceptive measures must be used to avoid pregnancy during treatment. Use with caution in patients with a history of local tolerability reactions or local hypersensitivity; burning, excessive pruritus, peeling, and skin redness may occur. Treatment can increase skin sensitivity to weather extremes of wind or cold. Concomitant topical medications (eg, medicated or abrasive soaps, cleansers, or cosmetics with a strong drying effect) should be avoided due to increased skin irritation. Reduce frequency or discontinue use until irritation disappears. May cause photosensitivity; exposure to sunlight/sunlamps should be avoided unless deemed medically necessary, and in such cases, exposure should be minimized (including use of sunscreens, protective clothing) during use of tazarotene. Risk may be increased by concurrent therapy with known photosensitizers (thiazides, tetracyclines, fluoroquinolones, phenothiazines, sulfonamides). Use with caution in patients with a personal or family history of skin cancer. Daily sunscreen use and other protective measures recommended. Patients with sunburn should discontinue use until sunburn has healed. For external use only; avoid contact with eyes, eyelids, and mouth. Not for use on eczematous, abraded, broken, or sunburned skin; not for treatment of lentigo maligna. The efficacy of tazarotene gel in the treatment of acne previously treated with other retinoids or resistant to oral antibiotics has not been established. Avoid application over extensive areas; specifically, safety and efficacy of gel applied over >20% of BSA have not been established. Propellant in foam formulation is flammable; avoid fire and smoking during and immediately after use.

Benzyl alcohol and derivatives: Some dosage forms may contain benzyl alcohol; large amounts of benzyl alcohol (≥99 mg/kg/day) have been associated with a potentially fatal toxicity ("gasping syndrome") in neonates; the "gasping syndrome" consists of metabolic acidosis, respiratory distress, gasping respirations, CNS dysfunction (including convulsions, intracranial hemorrhage), hypotension, and cardiovascular collapse (AAP, 1997; CDC, 1982); some data suggests that benzoate displaces bilirubin from protein binding sites (Ahlfors, 2001); avoid or use dosage forms containing benzyl alcohol with caution in neonates. See manufacturer's labeling.

Adverse Reactions

Cardiovascular: Peripheral edema

Dermatologic: Burning sensation of skin, cheilitis, contact dermatitis, dermatitis, desquamation, eczema, erythema, exacerbation of psoriasis, pruritus, skin discoloration, skin fissure, skin irritation, skin pain, skin photosensitivity, skin rash, stinging of the skin, xeroderma

Endocrine & metabolic: Hypertriglyceridemia

Local: Application site pain, local hemorrhage

Ophthalmic: Ocular irritation (including edema, irritation and inflammation of the eye or eyelid)

Rare but important or life-threatening: Impetigo, skin blister

Drug Interactions

Metabolism/Transport Effects None known.

Avoid Concomitant Use There are no known interactions where it is recommended to avoid concomitant use.

Increased Effect/Toxicity There are no known significant interactions involving an increase in effect.

Decreased Effect There are no known significant interactions involving a decrease in effect.

Storage/Stability

Cream: Store at 25°C (77°F); excursions are permitted between -5°C to 30°C (23°F to 86°F).

Foam: Store at 20°C to 25°C (68°F to 77°F); excursions are permitted between 15°C to 30°C (59°F to 86°F).

Protect from freezing. Foam is flammable; avoid high temperatures.

Gel: Store at 25°C (77°F); excursions are permitted between 15°C to 30°C (59°F to 86°F).

Mechanism of Action Synthetic, acetylenic retinoid which modulates differentiation and proliferation of epithelial tissue and exerts some degree of anti-inflammatory and immunological activity

Pharmacodynamics

Onset of action: Psoriasis: 1 week

Duration: Psoriasis: Up to 12 weeks after discontinuation when initially treated for 2-3 months (duration may be less if initial treatment was shorter)

Pharmacokinetics (Adult data unless noted)

Absorption: Minimal following cutaneous application (≤6% of dose)

Protein binding: Metabolite: >99%

Metabolism: Prodrug, rapidly metabolized via esterases to an active metabolite (tazarotenic acid) following topical application and systemic absorption; tazarotenic acid undergoes further hepatic metabolism

Half-life: Metabolite: 18 hours

Elimination: Urine and feces as metabolites

Dosing: Usual

Children and Adolescents:

Acne vulgaris: Children ≥12 years and Adolescents: Topical: Tazorac (0.1% cream or gel): Apply as a thin film (2 mg/cm^2) to affected areas once daily in the evening for up to 12 weeks

Psoriasis: Topical:

Cream: Adolescents ≥18 years: Tazorac (0.05%): Initial: Apply a thin film (2 mg/cm^2) to affected area once daily in the evening; may increase strength to 0.1% if tolerated and necessary

Gel: Children ≥12 years and Adolescents: Tazorac (0.05%): Initial: Apply a thin film (2 mg/cm^2) to affected area once daily in the evening for up to 12 months; may increase strength to 0.1% if tolerated and necessary; apply to no more than 20% of the body surface area

Palliation of fine facial wrinkles, facial mottled hyper-/hypopigmentation, benign facial lentigines: Adolescents ≥17 years: Topical: Avage: Apply a pea-sized amount once daily at bedtime; lightly cover entire face including eyelids if desired

Adults:

Acne vulgaris: Topical: Tazorac (0.1% cream or gel): Apply as a thin film (2 mg/cm^2) to affected areas once daily in the evening for up to 12 weeks

Psoriasis: Topical:

Cream: Tazorac (0.05%): Initial: Apply a thin film (2 mg/cm^2) to affected area once daily in the evening; may increase strength to 0.1% if tolerated and necessary

Gel: Tazorac (0.05%): Initial: Apply a thin film (2 mg/cm^2) to affected area once daily in the evening for up to 12 months; may increase strength to 0.1% if tolerated and necessary; apply to no more than 20% of the body surface area

Palliation of fine facial wrinkles, facial mottled hyper-/hypopigmentation, benign facial lentigines: Topical: Avage: Apply a pea-sized amount once daily at bedtime; lightly cover entire face including eyelids if desired

Dosing adjustment in renal impairment: There are no dosage adjustments provided in the manufacturer's labeling; however, dosage adjustment unlikely necessary due to low systemic absorption.

Dosing adjustment in hepatic impairment: There are no dosage adjustments provided in the manufacturer's labeling; however, dosage adjustment unlikely necessary due to low systemic absorption.

Administration For external use only; avoid contact with eyes and mouth; also avoid contact with the eyelids when used for acne or psoriasis. Do not apply to eczematous or sunburned skin.

Acne: Apply in evening after gently cleansing and drying face; apply enough to cover entire affected area.

Palliation of fine facial wrinkles, facial mottled hyper-/hypopigmentation, benign facial lentigines: Apply to clean, dry face at bedtime; lightly cover entire face including eyelids if desired. Emollients or moisturizers may be applied before or after; if applied before tazarotene, ensure cream or lotion has absorbed into the skin and has dried completely.

Psoriasis: Apply in evening. If a bath or shower is taken prior to application, dry the skin before applying. If emollients are used, apply them at least 1 hour prior to application. Unaffected skin may be more susceptible to irritation; avoid application to these areas.

Monitoring Parameters Disease severity in plaque psoriasis (reduction in erythema, scaling, induration); pregnancy test prior to treatment of females of childbearing age

Dosage Forms Excipient information presented when available (limited, particularly for generics); consult specific product labeling.

Cream, External:

Avage: 0.1% (30 g) [contains benzyl alcohol]

Tazorac: 0.05% (30 g, 60 g); 0.1% (30 g, 60 g) [contains benzyl alcohol]

Foam, External:

Fabior: 0.1% (50 g, 100 g)

Gel, External:

Tazorac: 0.05% (30 g, 100 g); 0.1% (30 g, 100 g) [contains benzyl alcohol]

- **Tazicef** *see* CefTAZidime *on page 407*
- **Tazobactam and Piperacillin** *see* Piperacillin and Tazobactam *on page 1706*
- **Tazocin (Can)** *see* Piperacillin and Tazobactam *on page 1706*
- **Tazorac** *see* Tazarotene *on page 2010*
- **Taztia XT** *see* Diltiazem *on page 661*
- **Tbo-Filgrastim** *see* Filgrastim *on page 876*
- **3TC** *see* LamiVUDine *on page 1205*
- **3TC, Abacavir, and Zidovudine** *see* Abacavir, Lamivudine, and Zidovudine *on page 38*
- **T-Cell Growth Factor** *see* Aldesleukin *on page 89*
- **TCGF** *see* Aldesleukin *on page 89*
- **TCN** *see* Tetracycline *on page 2035*
- **Td** *see* Diphtheria and Tetanus Toxoids *on page 674*
- **Td Adsorbed (Can)** *see* Diphtheria and Tetanus Toxoids *on page 674*
- **Tdap** *see* Diphtheria and Tetanus Toxoids, and Acellular Pertussis Vaccine *on page 681*
- **TDF** *see* Tenofovir *on page 2017*
- **Teardrops® (Can)** *see* Artificial Tears *on page 201*
- **Tears Again® [OTC]** *see* Artificial Tears *on page 201*
- **Tears Naturale® II [OTC]** *see* Artificial Tears *on page 201*
- **Tears Naturale® Forte [OTC]** *see* Artificial Tears *on page 201*
- **Tears Naturale® Free [OTC]** *see* Artificial Tears *on page 201*
- **Tears Naturale PM [OTC]** *see* Artificial Tears *on page 201*
- **Tears Renewed® [OTC]** *see* Ocular Lubricant *on page 1542*
- **Tebrazid™ (Can)** *see* Pyrazinamide *on page 1807*
- **Tecnu First Aid [OTC]** *see* Lidocaine (Topical) *on page 1258*

- ◆ **Tecta (Can)** *see* Pantoprazole *on page 1618*
- ◆ **Tegaderm CHG Dressing [OTC]** *see* Chlorhexidine Gluconate *on page 434*
- ◆ **TEGretol** *see* CarBAMazepine *on page 367*
- ◆ **Tegretol (Can)** *see* CarBAMazepine *on page 367*
- ◆ **TEGretol-XR** *see* CarBAMazepine *on page 367*
- ◆ **Telzir (Can)** *see* Fosamprenavir *on page 936*
- ◆ **Temodal (Can)** *see* Temozolomide *on page 2012*
- ◆ **Temodar** *see* Temozolomide *on page 2012*
- ◆ **Temovate** *see* Clobetasol *on page 498*
- ◆ **Temovate E** *see* Clobetasol *on page 498*

Temozolomide (te moe ZOE loe mide)

Medication Safety Issues

Sound-alike/look-alike issues:

Temodar may be confused with Tambocor

Temozolomide may be confused with temsirolimus

High alert medication:

This medication is in a class the Institute for Safe Medication Practices (ISMP) includes among its list of drug classes which have a heightened risk of causing significant patient harm when used in error.

Related Information

Oral Medications That Should Not Be Crushed or Altered *on page 2476*

Prevention of Chemotherapy-Induced Nausea and Vomiting in Children *on page 2368*

Safe Handling of Hazardous Drugs *on page 2455*

Brand Names: US Temodar

Brand Names: Canada ACH-Temozolomide; ACT Temozolomide; Temodal

Therapeutic Category Antineoplastic Agent, Alkylating Agent

Generic Availability (US) May be product dependent

Use Treatment of refractory anaplastic astrocytoma with progression after initial therapy with a nitrosourea and procarbazine (FDA approved in adults); treatment of newly-diagnosed glioblastoma multiforme (initially in combination with radiotherapy, then as maintenance treatment) (FDA approved in adults)

Active against recurrent glioblastoma multiforme, low-grade astrocytoma, low-grade oligodendroglioma, metastatic CNS lesions, refractory primary CNS lymphoma, anaplastic oligodendroglioma, primitive neuroectodermal tumors (PNET), including medulloblastoma, pediatric neuroblastoma, advanced or metastatic melanoma, cutaneous T-cell lymphomas [mycosis fungoides (MF) and Sezary Syndrome (SS)], carcinoid tumors, advanced neuroendocrine tumors (carcinoid or islet cell), Ewing's sarcoma (recurrent or progressive), soft tissue sarcomas (extremity/retroperitoneal/intra-abdominal or hemangiopericytoma/solitary fibrous tumor)

Pregnancy Risk Factor D

Pregnancy Considerations Adverse events were observed in animal reproduction studies. May cause fetal harm when administered to pregnant women. Male and female patients should avoid pregnancy while receiving temozolomide.

Breast-Feeding Considerations It is not known if temozolomide is excreted in breast milk. Due to the potential for serious adverse reactions in the nursing infant, a decision should be made to discontinue nursing or to discontinue temozolomide, taking into account the importance of treatment to the mother.

Contraindications Hypersensitivity (eg, allergic reaction, anaphylaxis, urticaria, Stevens-Johnson syndrome, toxic epidermal necrolysis) to temozolomide or any component of the formulation; hypersensitivity to dacarbazine (both drugs are metabolized to MTIC)

Canadian labeling: Additional contraindications (not in U.S. labeling): Not recommended in patients with severe myelosuppression

Warnings/Precautions Hazardous agent - use appropriate precautions for handling and disposal (NIOSH 2014 [group 1]). *Pneumocystis jirovecii* pneumonia (PCP) may occur; risk is increased in those receiving steroids or longer dosing regimens; monitor all patients for development of PCP (particularly if also receiving corticosteroids); PCP prophylaxis is required in patients receiving radiotherapy in combination with the 42-day temozolomide regimen. Myelosuppression may occur; may require treatment interruption, dose reduction, and/or discontinuation; monitor blood counts; an increased incidence has been reported in geriatric and female patients. Prolonged pancytopenia resulting in aplastic anemia has been reported (may be fatal); concurrent use of temozolomide with medications associated with aplastic anemia (eg, carbamazepine, co-trimoxazole, phenytoin) may obscure assessment for development of aplastic anemia. ANC should be $\geq$1,500/mm^3 and platelets $\geq$100,000/mm^3 prior to treatment. Rare cases of myelodysplastic syndrome and secondary malignancies, including acute myeloid leukemia, have been reported. Use caution in patients with severe hepatic or renal impairment; has not been studied in dialysis patients. Hepatotoxicity has been reported; may be severe or fatal. Monitor liver function tests at baseline, halfway through the first cycle, prior to each subsequent cycle, and at ~2 to 4 weeks after the last dose. Postmarketing reports of hepatotoxicity have included liver function abnormalities, hepatitis, hepatic failure, cholestasis, hepatitis cholestasis, jaundice, cholelithiasis, hepatic steatosis, hepatic necrosis, hepatic lesion, and hepatic encephalopathy (Sarganas, 2012).

Temozolomide is associated with a moderate emetic potential (Dupuis, 2011; Roila, 2010); antiemetics are recommended to prevent nausea and vomiting. Increased MGMT (O-6-methylguanine-DNA methyltransferase) activity/levels within tumor tissue is associated with temozolomide resistance. Glioblastoma patients with decreased levels (due to methylated MGMT promoter) may be more likely to benefit from the combination of radiation therapy and temozolomide (Hegi, 2008; Stupp, 2009). Determination of MGMT status may be predictive for response to alkylating agents. Potentially significant drug-drug interactions may exist, requiring dose or frequency adjustment, additional monitoring, and/or selection of alternative therapy. Bioequivalence has only been established when IV temozolomide is administered over 90 minutes; shorter or longer infusion times may result in suboptimal dosing.

Polysorbate 80: Some dosage forms may contain polysorbate 80 (also known as Tweens). Hypersensitivity reactions, usually a delayed reaction, have been reported following exposure to pharmaceutical products containing polysorbate 80 in certain individuals (Isaksson, 2002; Lucente 2000; Shelley, 1995). Thrombocytopenia, ascites, pulmonary deterioration, and renal and hepatic failure have been reported in premature neonates after receiving parenteral products containing polysorbate 80 (Alade, 1986; CDC, 1984). See manufacturer's labeling.

Adverse Reactions

Cardiovascular: Peripheral edema

Central nervous system: Abnormal gait, amnesia, anxiety, ataxia, confusion, convulsions, depression, dizziness, drowsiness, fatigue, headache, hemiparesis, insomnia, memory impairment, paresis, paresthesia

Dermatologic: Alopecia, erythema, pruritus, skin rash, xeroderma

Endocrine & metabolic: Hypercorticoidism, weight gain

Gastrointestinal: Abdominal pain, anorexia, constipation, diarrhea, dysgeusia, dysphagia, nausea (less common in grades 3/4), stomatitis, vomiting (less common in grades 3/4)
Genitourinary: Mastalgia (less common in females), urinary frequency, urinary incontinence, urinary tract infection
Hematologic & oncologic: Anemia (less common in grades 3/4), leukopenia (more common in grades 3/4), lymphocytopenia (more common in grades 3/4), neutropenia (more common in grades 3/4), thrombocytopenia (more common in grades 3/4)
Hypersensitivity: Hypersensitivity reaction
Infection: Viral infection
Neuromuscular & skeletal: Arthralgia, back pain, myalgia, weakness
Ophthalmic: Blurred vision, diplopia, visual disturbance (visual deficit/vision changes)
Respiratory: Cough, dyspnea, pharyngitis, upper respiratory tract infection, sinusitis
Miscellaneous: Fever, radiation injury (less common in maintenance phase after radiotherapy)
Rare by important or life-threatening: Alveolitis, anaphylaxis, aplastic anemia, cytomegalovirus disease (reactivation), diabetes insipidus, emotional lability, erythema multiforme, febrile neutropenia, flu-like symptoms, hallucination, hematoma, hemorrhage, hepatitis, hepatitis B (reactivation), hepatotoxicity, herpes simplex infection, herpes zoster, hyperbilirubinemia, hyperglycemia, hypersensitivity pneumonitis, hypokalemia, metastases (including myeloid leukemia) myelodysplastic syndrome, opportunistic infection (including pneumocystosis), oral candidiasis, pancytopenia (may be prolonged), peripheral neuropathy, petechia, pneumonitis, pulmonary fibrosis, Stevens-Johnson syndrome

Drug Interactions

Metabolism/Transport Effects None known.

Avoid Concomitant Use

Avoid concomitant use of Temozolomide with any of the following: BCG; BCG (Intravesical); CloZAPine; Dipyrone; Natalizumab; Pimecrolimus; Tacrolimus (Topical); Tofacitinib; Vaccines (Live)

Increased Effect/Toxicity

Temozolomide may increase the levels/effects of: CloZAPine; Leflunomide; Natalizumab; Tofacitinib; Vaccines (Live)

The levels/effects of Temozolomide may be increased by: Denosumab; Dipyrone; Pimecrolimus; Roflumilast; Tacrolimus (Topical); Trastuzumab; Valproic Acid and Derivatives

Decreased Effect

Temozolomide may decrease the levels/effects of: BCG; BCG (Intravesical); Coccidioides immitis Skin Test; Sipuleucel-T; Vaccines (Inactivated); Vaccines (Live)

The levels/effects of Temozolomide may be decreased by: Echinacea

Food Interactions Food reduces rate and extent of absorption. Management: Administer consistently either with food or without food (was administered in studies under fasting and nonfasting conditions).

Storage/Stability

Capsule: Store at room temperature of 25°C (77°F); excursions permitted to 15°C to 30°C (59°F to 86°F).
Injection: Store intact vials refrigerated at 2°C to 8°C (36°F to 46°F). Reconstituted vials may be stored for up to 14 hours at room temperature of 25°C (77°F); infusion must be completed within 14 hours of reconstitution.

Mechanism of Action Temozolomide is a prodrug which is rapidly and nonenzymatically converted to the active alkylating metabolite MTIC [(methyl-triazene-1-yl)-imidazole-4-carboxamide]; this conversion is spontaneous, nonenzymatic, and occurs under physiologic conditions in all tissues to which it distributes. The cytotoxic effects of MTIC are manifested through alkylation (methylation) of DNA at the O^6, N^7 guanine positions which lead to DNA double strand breaks and apoptosis. Non-cell cycle specific.

Pharmacokinetics (Adult data unless noted)

Absorption: Oral: Rapidly and completely absorbed
Distribution: Extensive tissue distribution; crosses the blood brain barrier; V_d: 0.4 L/kg
Protein binding: 14%
Bioavailability: Oral: 100% (on a mg-per-mg basis, IV temozolomide, infused over 90 minutes, is bioequivalent to an oral dose)
Metabolism: At a neutral or alkaline pH, hydrolyzes to active MTIC (3-methyl-(triazen-1-yl) imidazole-4-carboxamide) and temozolomide acid metabolite; MTIC is further metabolized to 5-amino-imidazole-4-carboxamide (AIC) and methylhydrazine (active alkylating agent); CYP isoenzymes play only a minor role in metabolism (of temozolomide and MTIC)
Half-life:
Children: 1.7 hours
Adults: 1.6-1.8 hours
Time to peak serum concentration: Oral: 1 hour; 2.3 hours after high fat meal
Elimination: <1% excreted in feces; 5% to 7% of unchanged temozolomide excreted renally
Clearance: 5.5 L/hour/m²; women have a ~5% lower clearance than men (adjusted for body surface area); children 3-17 years have similar temozolomide clearance as adults

Dosing: Usual Note: Temozolomide is associated with a moderate emetic potential (Roila 2010); antiemetics are recommended to prevent nausea and vomiting. Prior to dosing, ANC should be ≥1,500/mm³ and platelets ≥100,000/mm³.

Pediatric: **Note:** Dose, frequency, number of doses, and start date may vary by protocol and treatment phase. Refer to individual protocols.

Neuroblastoma, relapsed or refractory: Infants, Children, and Adolescents: Oral: 100 mg/m²/dose once daily for 5 days, repeat cycle every 21 days for up to 6 cycles; use in combination with irinotecan; administer 1 hour prior to irinotecan (Bagatell 2011). **Note:** Temozolomide doses were rounded to the nearest capsule size.

Ewing's sarcoma, recurrent or progressive: Children ≥2 years and Adolescents: Oral: 100 mg/m²/dose once daily for 5 days, repeat cycle every 21 days (in combination with irinotecan; administer 1 hour prior to irinotecan) (Casey 2009); dosing based on a retrospective review

Solid tumors, relapsed or refractory [including but not limited to brain tumor (astrocytomas, gliomas, medulloblastoma), neuroblastoma, and sarcomas]: Infants, Children, and Adolescents: Oral:
Manufacturer's labeling: Children ≥3 years and Adolescents: 160 to 200 mg/m²/dose once daily for 5 days every 28 days
Alternative dosing: 200 to 215 mg/m²/dose days 1 to 5 every 21 to 28 days; dose was decreased to 180 mg/m²/dose for patients who received prior craniospinal irradiation or relapsed after bone marrow transplant (De Sio 2006; Nicholson 2007)

Adult:

Anaplastic astrocytoma (refractory): Oral, IV: Initial dose: 150 mg/m² once daily for 5 consecutive days of a 28-day treatment cycle. If ANC ≥1,500/mm³ and platelets ≥100,000/mm³, on day 1 of subsequent cycles, may increase to 200 mg/m² once daily for 5 consecutive days of a 28-day treatment cycle. May continue until disease progression.

Dosage modification for toxicity:

ANC <1,000/mm^3 or platelets <50,000/mm^3 on day 22 or day 29 (day 1 of next cycle): Postpone therapy until ANC >1,500/mm^3 and platelets >100,000/mm^3; reduce dose by 50 mg/m^2/day (but not below 100 mg/m^2) for subsequent cycle

ANC 1000 to 1500/mm^3 or platelets 50,000-100,000/mm^3 on day 22 or day 29 (day 1 of next cycle): Postpone therapy until ANC >1500/mm^3 and platelets >100,000/mm^3; maintain initial dose

Glioblastoma multiforme (newly diagnosed, high-grade glioma): Oral, IV:

Concomitant phase: 75 mg/m^2/day for 42 days with focal radiotherapy (60 Gy administered in 30 fractions). **Note:** PCP prophylaxis is required during concomitant phase and should continue in patients who develop lymphocytopenia until lymphocyte recovery to ≤ grade 1. Obtain weekly CBC.

Continue at 75 mg/m^2/day throughout the 42-day concomitant phase (up to 49 days) as long as ANC ≥1,500/mm^3, platelet count ≥100,000/mm^3, and nonhematologic toxicity ≤ grade 1 (excludes alopecia, nausea/vomiting)

Dosage modification for toxicity:

ANC ≥500/mm^3 but <1,500/mm^3 **or** platelet count ≥10,000/mm^3 but <100,000/mm^3 **or** grade 2 nonhematologic toxicity (excludes alopecia, nausea/vomiting): Interrupt therapy

ANC <500/mm^3 **or** platelet count <10,000/mm^3 **or** grade 3/4 nonhematologic toxicity (excludes alopecia, nausea/vomiting): Discontinue therapy

Maintenance phase (consists of 6 treatment cycles): Begin 4 weeks after concomitant phase completion. **Note:** Each subsequent cycle is 28 days (consisting of 5 days of drug treatment followed by 23 days without treatment). Draw CBC within 48 hours of day 22; hold next cycle and do weekly CBC until ANC >1500/mm^3 and platelet count >100,000/mm3; dosing modification should be based on lowest blood counts and worst nonhematologic toxicity during the previous cycle.

Cycle 1: 150 mg/m^2 once daily for 5 days of a 28-day treatment cycle

Cycles 2 to 6: May increase to 200 mg/m^2 once daily for 5 days; repeat every 28 days (if ANC ≥1,500/mm^3, platelets ≥100,000/mm^3 and nonhematologic toxicities for cycle 1 are ≤ grade 2 [excludes alopecia, nausea/vomiting]); **Note:** If dose was not escalated at the onset of cycle 2, do not increase for cycles 3 to 6).

Dosage modification (during maintenance phase) for toxicity:

ANC <1,000/mm^3, platelet count <50,000/mm^3, or grade 3 nonhematologic toxicity (excludes alopecia, nausea/vomiting) during previous cycle: Decrease dose by 1 dose level (by 50 mg/m^2/day for 5 days), unless dose has already been lowered to 100 mg/m^2/day, then discontinue therapy.

If dose reduction <100 mg/m^2/day is required or grade 4 nonhematologic toxicity (excludes alopecia, nausea/vomiting), or if the same grade 3 nonhematologic toxicity occurs after dose reduction: Discontinue therapy.

Dosage adjustment in renal impairment: Adults: Oral:

CrCl ≥36 mL/minute/m^2: No effect on temozolomide clearance was demonstrated

Severe renal impairment (CrCl <36 mL/minute/m^2): Use with caution; no dosage adjustments provided in manufacturers labeling

Dialysis patients: Use has not been studied

Dosage adjustment in hepatic impairment: Adults: Severe hepatic impairment: Use with caution; no dosage adjustments provided in manufacturer's labeling

Preparation for Administration Hazardous agent; use appropriate precautions for handling and disposal (NIOSH 2014 [group 1]).

Parenteral: IV: Bring to room temperature prior to reconstitution. Reconstitute each 100 mg vial with 41 mL SWFI to a final concentration of 2.5 mg/mL. Swirl gently; do not shake. Place dose without further dilution into an empty sterile infusion bag. Infusion must be completed within 14 hours of reconstitution.

Administration Hazardous agent; use appropriate precautions for handling and disposal (NIOSH 2014 [group 1]). Temozolomide is associated with a moderate emetic potential (Dupuis 2011; Roila 2010); antiemetics are recommended to prevent nausea and vomiting.

Oral: Swallow capsule intact with a glass of water; do not chew; if patient is unable to swallow capsule, open capsule and dissolve in apple juice or applesauce taking precautions to avoid exposure to the cytotoxic agent; administer on an empty stomach or at bedtime to reduce the incidence of nausea and vomiting; absorption is affected by food; may administer with food as long as food intake and administration are performed at the same time each day to ensure consistent bioavailability. Do not repeat if vomiting occurs after dose is administered; wait until the next scheduled dose.

Parenteral: IV: Infuse over 90 minutes. Infusion must be completed within 14 hours of reconstitution. Flush line before and after administration; may be administered through the same IV line as NS. Do not administer other medications through the same IV line.

Monitoring Parameters CBC with ANC (absolute neutrophil count) and platelet count; monitor for CNS effects, gastrointestinal disturbance, myelosuppression, opportunistic infection, vision disturbance, and cough on a regular basis; dosage adjustments may be necessary for toxicity.

Additional Information To minimize the risk of a wrong dose error, each strength of temozolomide must be packaged and dispensed in a separate vial or in its original glass bottle. Label each container with the appropriate number of capsules to be taken each day.

Increased MGMT (O-6-methylguanine-DNA methyltransferase) activity/levels within tumor tissue is associated with temozolomide resistance. Glioblastoma patients with decreased levels (due to methylated MGMT promoter) may be more likely to benefit from the combination of radiation therapy and temozolomide (Hegi, 2008; Stupp, 2009). Determination of MGMT status may be predictive for response to alkylating agents.

Dosage Forms Excipient information presented when available (limited, particularly for generics); consult specific product labeling.

Capsule, Oral:

Temodar: 5 mg [contains fd&c blue #2 (indigotine)]

Temodar: 20 mg, 100 mg

Temodar: 140 mg [contains fd&c blue #2 (indigotine)]

Temodar: 180 mg, 250 mg

Generic: 5 mg, 20 mg, 100 mg, 140 mg, 180 mg, 250 mg

Solution Reconstituted, Intravenous:

Temodar: 100 mg (1 ea) [pyrogen free; contains polysorbate 80]

Extemporaneous Preparations Hazardous agent: Use appropriate precautions for handling and disposal (NIOSH 2014 [group 1]).

A 10 mg/mL temozolomide oral suspension may be compounded in a vertical flow hood. Mix the contents of ten 100 mg capsules and 500 mg of povidone K-30 powder in a glass mortar; add 25 mg anhydrous citric acid dissolved in 1.5 mL purified water and mix to a uniform paste; mix while adding 50 mL Ora-Plus® in incremental proportions. Transfer to an amber plastic bottle, rinse mortar 4 times with small portions of either Ora-Sweet® or Ora-Sweet®

SF, and add quantity of Ora-Sweet® or Ora-Sweet® SF sufficient to make 100 mL. Store in plastic amber prescription bottles; label "shake well" and "refrigerate"; include the beyond-use date. Stable for 7 days at room temperature or 60 days refrigerated (preferred).

Trissel LA, Yanping Z, and Koontz SE, "Temozolomide Stability in Extemporaneously Compounded Oral Suspension," *Int J Pharm Compound*, 2006, 10(5):396-9.

◆ **Tempra (Can)** *see* Acetaminophen *on page 44*

◆ **Tenex** *see* GuanFACINE *on page 993*

Teniposide (ten i POE side)

Medication Safety Issues

Sound-alike/look-alike issues:

Teniposide may be confused with etoposide

High alert medication:

This medication is in a class the Institute for Safe Medication Practices (ISMP) includes among its list of drug classes which have a heightened risk of causing significant patient harm when used in error.

Other safety concerns:

A solvent in teniposide, N,N-dimethylacetamide, is incompatible with many closed system transfer devices (CSTDs) used for preparing injectable antineoplastics. The plastic components of CSTDs may dissolve and result in subsequent leakage and potential infusion of dissolved plastic into the patient (ISMP [Smetzer 2015]).

Related Information

Management of Drug Extravasations *on page 2298*

Prevention of Chemotherapy-Induced Nausea and Vomiting in Children *on page 2368*

Safe Handling of Hazardous Drugs *on page 2455*

Brand Names: Canada Vumon

Therapeutic Category Antineoplastic Agent, Podophyllotoxin Derivative; Antineoplastic Agent, Topoisomerase II Inhibitor

Generic Availability (US) Yes

Use Treatment of childhood acute lymphoblastic leukemia (ALL) refractory to induction with other therapy (FDA approved in pediatric patients ages ≥6 months)

Pregnancy Risk Factor D

Pregnancy Considerations Adverse effects were observed in animal reproduction studies. May cause fetal harm if administered during pregnancy. Women of childbearing potential should avoid becoming pregnant during teniposide treatment.

Breast-Feeding Considerations It is not known if teniposide is excreted in breast milk. Due to the potential for serious adverse reactions in the nursing infant, a decision should be made to discontinue teniposide or to discontinue breast-feeding, taking into account the importance of treatment to the mother.

Contraindications Hypersensitivity to teniposide, polyoxyl 35/polyoxyethylated castor oil (Cremophor EL), or any component of the formulation

Warnings/Precautions Hazardous agent - use appropriate precautions for handling and disposal (NIOSH 2014 [group 1]).

[US Boxed Warning]: Severe myelosuppression resulting in infection or bleeding may occur; may be dose-limiting; monitor blood counts. Patients with Down syndrome and leukemia may be more sensitive to the myelosuppressive effects; reduced initial doses are recommended. Contains polyoxyl 35/polyoxyethylated castor oil (Cremophor EL), which is associated with hypersensitivity reactions. **[US Boxed Warning]: Hypersensitivity reactions, including anaphylaxis-like reactions, have been reported; may occur with initial dosing or with repeated exposure to teniposide. Epinephrine, with or without corticosteroids and antihistamines, has been employed to alleviate hypersensitivity reaction symptoms.** Hypersensitivity reactions may include bronchospasm, dyspnea, hypertension, hypotension, tachycardia, flushing, chills, fever, or urticaria. Monitor closely during infusion (observe continuously for first 60 minutes, frequently thereafter). Stop infusion for signs of anaphylaxis; immediate treatment for anaphylactic reaction should be available during administration (may require treatment with epinephrine, corticosteroids, antihistamines, pressors, or volume expanders). Patients experiencing prior hypersensitivity are at risk for recurrence; re-treat only if the potential benefit outweighs the risk of hypersensitivity; premedication (with corticosteroids and antihistamines) is recommended for re-treatment. Hypotension may occur with rapid infusion; infuse slowly over at least 30 to 60 minutes; discontinue for clinically significant hypotension; if infusion is restarted after being withheld for hypotension, reinitiate at a slower infusion rate.

Use with caution in patients with renal or hepatic impairment; may require dosage reduction in patients with significant impairment. Teniposide is considered an irritant (Perez Fidalgo, 2012). For IV use only; ensure proper catheter/needle position prior to infusion; monitor infusion site; may cause local tissue necrosis and/or thrombophlebitis if extravasation occurs. Since teniposide is highly bound to plasma proteins, carefully monitor patients with hypoalbuminemia. Product contains about 43% alcohol. Acute CNS depression, hypotension and metabolic acidosis have been reported; these events occurred in patients who received high-dose teniposide (investigation protocol) and were premedicated with antiemetics, which along with the alcohol content of teniposide, may have contributed to the CNS depression. **[US Boxed Warning]: Should be administered under the supervision of an experienced cancer chemotherapy physician. Appropriate management of therapy and complications is possible only when adequate treatment facilities are readily available.** Potentially significant drug-drug interactions may exist, requiring dose or frequency adjustment, additional monitoring, and/or selection of alternative therapy.

Benzyl alcohol and derivatives: Some dosage forms may contain benzyl alcohol; large amounts of benzyl alcohol (≥99 mg/kg/day) have been associated with a potentially fatal toxicity ("gasping syndrome") in neonates; the "gasping syndrome" consists of metabolic acidosis, respiratory distress, gasping respirations, CNS dysfunction (including convulsions, intracranial hemorrhage), hypotension, and cardiovascular collapse (AAP, 1997; CDC, 1982); some data suggests that benzoate displaces bilirubin from protein binding sites (Ahlfors, 2001); avoid or use dosage forms containing benzyl alcohol with caution in neonates. See manufacturer's labeling.

N,N-dimethylacetamide: Teniposide contains N,N-dimethylacetamide, which is incompatible with many closed system transfer devices (CSTDs); the plastic components of CSTDs may dissolve and result in subsequent leakage and potential infusion of dissolved plastic into the patient (ISMP [Smetzer 2015]).

Adverse Reactions

Cardiovascular: Hypotension (associated with rapid [<30 minutes] infusions)

Central nervous system: Fever

Dermatologic: Alopecia (usually reversible), rash

Gastrointestinal: Diarrhea, mucositis, nausea/vomiting (mild to moderate)

Hematologic: Anemia, leukopenia, myelosuppression, neutropenia, thrombocytopenia

Hematologic: Bleeding

Miscellaneous: Hypersensitivity reactions (includes bronchospasm, chills, dyspnea, fever, flushing, hyper-/hypotension, tachycardia, or urticaria); infection

Rare but important or life-threatening: Arrhythmia, CNS depression, confusion, headache, hepatic dysfunction, intractable hypotension, metabolic abnormality, metabolic acidosis, neuropathy (severe), neurotoxicity, renal dysfunction, thrombophlebitis, tissue necrosis (upon extravasation), weakness

Drug Interactions

Metabolism/Transport Effects **Substrate** of CYP3A4 (major), P-glycoprotein; **Note:** Assignment of Major/Minor substrate status based on clinically relevant drug interaction potential; **Inhibits** CYP2C9 (weak)

Avoid Concomitant Use

Avoid concomitant use of Teniposide with any of the following: BCG; BCG (Intravesical); CloZAPine; Conivaptan; Dipyrone; Fusidic Acid (Systemic); Idelalisib; Natalizumab; Pimecrolimus; Tacrolimus (Topical); Tofacitinib; Vaccines (Live)

Increased Effect/Toxicity

Teniposide may increase the levels/effects of: CloZAPine; Leflunomide; Natalizumab; Tofacitinib; Vaccines (Live); VinCRIStine; VinCRIStine (Liposomal)

The levels/effects of Teniposide may be increased by: Aprepitant; Conivaptan; CYP3A4 Inhibitors (Moderate); CYP3A4 Inhibitors (Strong); Dasatinib; Denosumab; Dipyrone; Fosaprepitant; Fusidic Acid (Systemic); Idelalisib; Ivacaftor; Luliconazole; Mifepristone; Netupitant; Palbociclib; P-glycoprotein/ABCB1 Inhibitors; Pimecrolimus; Roflumilast; Simeprevir; Stiripentol; Tacrolimus (Topical); Trastuzumab

Decreased Effect

Teniposide may decrease the levels/effects of: BCG; BCG (Intravesical); Coccidioides immitis Skin Test; Sipuleucel-T; Vaccines (Inactivated); Vaccines (Live)

The levels/effects of Teniposide may be decreased by: Barbiturates; Bosentan; CYP3A4 Inducers (Moderate); CYP3A4 Inducers (Strong); Dabrafenib; Deferasirox; Echinacea; Fosphenytoin; Mitotane; P-glycoprotein/ABCB1 Inducers; Phenytoin; Siltuximab; St Johns Wort; Tocilizumab

Storage/Stability Store ampuls in refrigerator at 2°C to 8°C (36°F to 46°F). Protect from light. Solutions diluted for infusion to a concentration of 0.1, 0.2, or 0.4 mg/mL are stable at room temperature for up to 24 hours after preparation; solutions diluted to 1 mg/mL should be used within 4 hours of preparation. Because precipitation may occur at any concentration, the manufacturer recommends administrating as soon as possible after preparation. Use appropriate precautions for handling and disposal. Do not refrigerate solutions prepared for infusion.

Mechanism of Action Teniposide does not inhibit microtubular assembly; it has been shown to delay transit of cells through the S phase and arrest cells in late S or early G_2 phase, preventing cells from entering mitosis. Teniposide is a topoisomerase II inhibitor, and appears to cause DNA strand breaks by inhibition of strand-passing and DNA ligase action.

Pharmacokinetics (Adult data unless noted)

Distribution: Mainly into liver, kidneys, small intestine, and adrenals; limited distribution into CSF <1%

Children: V_d: 3-11 L/m^2

Adults: V_d: 8-44 L/m^2

Protein binding: >99%; primarily albumin

Metabolism: Hepatic, extensive

Half-life: Children: 5 hours

Elimination: Urine (44%, 4% to 12% as unchanged drug); feces (≤10%)

Clearance: Renal: 10% of total body clearance

Dosing: Usual Note: Patients with Down syndrome may be more sensitive to the myelosuppressive effects; administer the first course at half the usual dose and adjust dose in subsequent cycles upward based on degree of toxicities (myelosuppression and mucositis) in the previous course(s).

Infants ≥6 months, Children, and Adolescents: **Acute lymphoblastic leukemia (ALL; combination therapy):**

Manufacturer's labeling: Regimens may vary: IV: 165 mg/m^2 twice weekly for 8-9 doses or 250 mg/m^2 weekly for 4-8 weeks

Alternate dosing: IV: 165 mg/m^2/dose days 1 and 2 of weeks 3, 13, and 23 (Lauer, 2001)

Dosing adjustment in renal or hepatic impairment: No specific recommendation (insufficient data). Dose adjustments may be necessary in patient with significant renal or hepatic impairment.

Preparation for Administration Hazardous agent; use appropriate precautions for handling and disposal (NIOSH 2014 [group 1]).

Parenteral: IV infusion: Teniposide must be diluted with either D_5W or NS to a final concentration of 0.1, 0.2, 0.4, or 1 mg/mL. Precipitation may occur at any concentration; inspect closely for particulates and administer as soon as possible after preparation. **Solutions should be prepared in non-DEHP-containing containers, such as glass or polyolefin containers.** The use of polyvinyl chloride (PVC) containers is not recommended. Teniposide contains N,N-dimethylacetamide, which is incompatible with many closed system transfer devices (CSTDs); the plastic components of CSTDs may dissolve and result in subsequent leakage and potential infusion of dissolved plastic into the patient (ISMP [Smetzer 2015]).

Administration Hazardous agent; use appropriate precautions for handling and disposal (NIOSH 2014 [group 1]).

Parenteral: IV infusion: Administer slowly by IV infusion over at least 30 to 60 minutes to minimize the risk of hypotensive reactions; do not administer by rapid IV injection. Administer through non-DEHP-containing administration sets; flush infusion line with D_5W or NS before and after infusion; incompatible with heparin. Precipitation may occur at any concentration; administer as soon as possible after preparation; inspect solution prior to administration. Observe patient continuously for at least the first 60 minutes of infusion, observe frequently thereafter. Stop infusion and treat accordingly for signs of anaphylaxis or clinically significant hypotension; if infusion is restarted after being withheld for hypotension, reinitiate at a slower infusion rate.

Teniposide contains N, N-dimethylacetamide, which is incompatible with many closed system transfer devices (CSTDs); the plastic components of CSTDs may dissolve and result in subsequent leakage and potential infusion of dissolved plastic into the patient (ISMP [Smetzer 2015]).

Vesicant/Extravasation Risk Irritant

Monitoring Parameters CBC, platelet count, renal and hepatic function tests; blood pressure; monitor for hypersensitivity reaction (observe continuously for first 60 minutes of infusion, frequently thereafter)

Dosage Forms Excipient information presented when available (limited, particularly for generics); consult specific product labeling.

Solution, Intravenous:

Generic: 10 mg/mL (5 mL)

◆ **Tenivac** *see* Diphtheria and Tetanus Toxoids *on page 674*

Tenofovir (ten OF oh vir)

Medication Safety Issues

High alert medication:

This medication is in a class the Institute for Safe Medication Practices (ISMP) includes among its list of drug classes that have a heightened risk of causing significant patient harm when used in error.

Related Information

Adult and Adolescent HIV *on page 2392*
Pediatric HIV *on page 2380*
Perinatal HIV *on page 2400*

Brand Names: US Viread

Brand Names: Canada Viread

Therapeutic Category Antiretroviral Agent; HIV Agents (Anti-HIV Agents); Nucleotide Reverse Transcriptase Inhibitor (NRTI)

Generic Availability (US) No

Use Treatment of HIV-1 infection in combination with other antiretroviral agents (FDA approved in ages ≥2 years and adults); **Note:** HIV regimens consisting of three antiretroviral agents are strongly recommended; treatment of chronic hepatitis B virus (HBV) (FDA approved in ages ≥12 years and adults)

Pregnancy Risk Factor B

Pregnancy Considerations Adverse events were observed in some animal reproduction studies. Tenofovir has a high level of transfer across the human placenta. Intrauterine growth has not been affected in human studies, but one study found lower length and head circumference. Clinical studies in children have shown bone demineralization with chronic use. No increased risk of overall birth defects has been observed following first trimester exposure according to data collected by the antiretroviral pregnancy registry. Limited data indicate decreased maternal bioavailability during the third trimester; dose adjustments are not needed. Cases of lactic acidosis/hepatic steatosis syndrome related to mitochondrial toxicity have been reported in pregnant women with prolonged use of nucleoside analogues. It is not known if pregnancy itself potentiates this known side effect; however, women may be at increased risk of lactic acidosis and liver damage. In addition, these adverse events are similar to other rare but life-threatening syndromes which occur during pregnancy (eg, HELLP syndrome). Hepatic enzymes and electrolytes should be monitored in women receiving nucleoside analogues and clinicians should watch for early signs of the syndrome. In addition, mitochondrial dysfunction may develop in infants following *in utero* exposure. Renal function should also be monitored. The DHHS Perinatal HIV Guidelines consider tenofovir in combination with either emtricitabine or lamivudine to be a preferred NRTI backbone for use in antiretroviral-naïve pregnant women. The DHHS Perinatal HIV Guidelines consider emtricitabine plus tenofovir, or lamivudine plus tenofovir as recommended dual NRTI/NtRTI backbones for HIV/HBV coinfected pregnant women. Hepatitis B flare may occur if tenofovir is discontinued postpartum.

Regardless of CD4 count or HIV RNA copy number, all HIV-infected pregnant women should receive a combination antiretroviral (ARV) drug regimen. A combination of antepartum, intrapartum, and infant ARV prophylaxis is recommended. ARV therapy should be started as soon as possible in women with symptomatic infection. Although earlier initiation may be more effective in reducing the perinatal transmission of HIV, also consider maternal conditions (eg, nausea and vomiting) and the potential risks of first trimester fetal exposure for specific agents. A scheduled cesarean delivery at 38 weeks' gestation is recommended for all women with HIV RNA >1000 copies/mL or unknown concentrations near delivery in order to decrease transmission. If ARV therapy must be interrupted for <24 hours during the peripartum period, stop then restart all medications simultaneously in order to decrease the chance of developing resistance. Long-term follow-up is recommended for all infants exposed to ARV medications. In couples who want to conceive, the HIV-infected partner should attain maximum viral suppression prior to conception.

Health care providers are encouraged to enroll pregnant women exposed to antiretroviral medications in the Antiretroviral Pregnancy Registry (1-800-258-4263 or www.APRegistry.com). Health care providers caring for HIV-infected women and their infants may contact the National Perinatal HIV Hotline (888-448-8765) for clinical consultation (HHS [perinatal], 2014).

Breast-Feeding Considerations Tenofovir is excreted in breast milk. Maternal or infant antiretroviral therapy does not completely eliminate the risk of postnatal HIV transmission. In addition, multiclass-resistant virus has been detected in breast-feeding infants despite maternal therapy. Therefore, in the United States, where formula is accessible, affordable, safe, and sustainable, and the risk of infant mortality due to diarrhea and respiratory infections is low, complete avoidance of breast-feeding by HIV-infected women is recommended to decrease potential transmission of HIV (HHS [perinatal], 2014).

Contraindications

U.S. labeling: There are no contraindications listed in the manufacturer's labeling.

Canadian labeling: Hypersensitivity to tenofovir or any component of the formulation; concurrent use with fixed-dose combination products that contain tenofovir (Truvada, Atripla, Complera, or Stribild); concurrent use with adefovir (Hepsera)

Warnings/Precautions **[U.S Boxed Warning]: Lactic acidosis and severe hepatomegaly with steatosis have been reported with tenofovir and other nucleoside analogues, including fatal cases;** use with caution in patients with risk factors for liver disease (risk may be increased in obese patients or prolonged exposure) and suspend treatment in any patient who develops clinical or laboratory findings suggestive of lactic acidosis (transaminase elevation may/may not accompany hepatomegaly and steatosis). May cause redistribution of fat (eg, buffalo hump, peripheral wasting with increased abdominal girth, cushingoid appearance). Immune reconstitution syndrome may develop resulting in the occurrence of an inflammatory response to an indolent or residual opportunistic infection during initial HIV treatment or activation of autoimmune disorders (eg, Graves' disease, polymyositis, Guillain-Barré syndrome) later in therapy; further evaluation and treatment may be required. Use caution in hepatic impairment; limited data supporting treatment of chronic hepatitis B in patients with decompensated liver disease; observe for increased adverse reactions, including renal dysfunction.

In clinical trials, use has been associated with decreases in bone mineral density in HIV-1 infected adults and increases in bone metabolism markers. Serum parathyroid hormone and 1,25 vitamin D levels were also higher. Decreases in bone mineral density have also been observed in clinical trials of HIV-1 infected pediatric patients. Observations in chronic hepatitis B infected pediatric patients (aged 12-18 years) were similar. Consider monitoring of bone density in adult and pediatric patients with a history of pathologic fractures or with other risk factors for bone loss or osteoporosis. Consider calcium and vitamin D supplementation for all patients; effect of supplementation has not been studied but may be beneficial. Long-term bone health and fracture risk unknown. Skeletal growth (height) appears to be unaffected in tenofovir-treated children and adolescents.

May cause osteomalacia with proximal renal tubulopathy. Bone pain, extremity pain, fractures, arthralgias, weakness and muscle pain have been reported. In patients at risk for renal dysfunction, persistent or worsening bone or muscle symptoms should be evaluated for hypophosphatemia and osteomalacia.

Do not use as monotherapy in treatment of HIV. Clinical trials in HIV-infected patients whose regimens contained only three nucleoside reverse transcriptase inhibitors (NRTI) show less efficacy, early virologic failure and high rates of resistance substitutions. Use three NRTI regimens with caution and monitor response carefully. Triple drug regimens with two NRTIs in combination with a non-nucleoside reverse transcriptase inhibitor or a HIV-1 protease inhibitor are usually more effective. Treatment of HIV in patients with unrecognized/untreated hepatitis B virus (HBV) may lead to rapid HBV resistance. Patients should be tested for presence of chronic hepatitis B infection prior to initiation of therapy. In patients coinfected with HIV and HBV, an appropriate antiretroviral combination should be selected due to HIV resistance potential; these patients should receive tenofovir dosed for HIV therapy.

Tenofovir is predominately eliminated renally; use caution in renal impairment. May cause acute renal failure or Fanconi syndrome; use caution with other nephrotoxic agents (including high dose or multiple NSAID use or those which compete for active tubular secretion). Acute renal failure has occurred in HIV-infected patients with risk factors for renal impairment who were on a stable tenofovir regimen to which a high dose or multiple NSAID therapy was added. Consider alternatives to NSAIDS in patients taking tenofovir and at risk for renal impairment. Calculate creatinine clearance prior to initiation of therapy and monitor renal function (including recalculation of creatinine clearance and serum phosphorus) during therapy. Dosage adjustment required in patients with CrCl <50 mL/minute. IDSA guidelines recommend avoiding tenofovir in HIV patients with preexisting kidney disease (CrCl <50 mL/minute and not on hemodialysis or GFR <60 mL/minute/1.73 m^2) when other effective HIV treatment options exist because data suggest risk of chronic kidney disease (CKD) is increased (IDSA [Lucas 2014]). IDSA guidelines also recommend discontinuing tenofovir (and substituting with alternative antiretroviral therapy) in HIV-infected patients who develop a decline in GFR (a >25% decrease in GFR from baseline and to a level of <60 mL/minute/1.73 m^2) during use, particularly in presence of proximal tubular dysfunction (eg, euglycemic glycosuria, increased urinary phosphorus excretion and hypophosphatemia, proteinuria [new onset or worsening]) (IDSA [Lucas 2014]). Use caution in patients with low body weight, or concurrent medications which increase tenofovir levels. Use caution in the elderly; dosage adjustment based on renal function may be required. Pancreatitis has been reported; use with caution in patients with a prior history or risk factors for pancreatitis. Discontinue if pancreatitis is suspected.

[U.S. Boxed Warning]: If treating HBV, acute exacerbation of hepatitis B may occur upon discontinuation. Monitor liver function closely for several months after discontinuing treatment; reinitiation of antihepatitis B therapy may be required. Treatment of HBV in patients with unrecognized/untreated HIV may lead to HIV resistance; patients should be tested for presence of HIV infection prior to initiating therapy. Do not use as monotherapy in treatment of HIV. Treatment of HIV in patients with unrecognized/untreated HBV may lead to rapid HBV resistance. Patients should be tested for presence of chronic hepatitis B prior to initiation of therapy. Potentially significant drug-drug interactions may exist, requiring dose or frequency adjustment, additional monitoring, and/or selection of alternative therapy. Do not use concurrently with adefovir or tenofovir combination products.

Warnings: Additional Pediatric Considerations Osteomalacia and reduced bone mineral density (BMD) may occur; long-term effects in humans are not known. Postmarketing cases of osteomalacia which may increase risk of bone fractures have also been reported in association with proximal renal tubulopathy. Recent studies suggest that tenofovir-related bone loss may be greater in children who are less mature (eg, Tanner stage 1 to 2) than in those who are more physically mature (Tanner ≥3). A significant decrease in lumbar spine BMD (>6%) was reported in five of 15 pediatric patients who received a tenofovir-containing regimen for 48 weeks. No orthopedic fractures occurred, but two patients required discontinuation of tenofovir. All five patients with a decrease in BMD were virologic responders and prepubertal (Tanner Stage 1). This study found a moderately strong correlation between decreases in bone mineral density z scores at week 48 and age at baseline. No correlation between decreases in bone mineral density z scores and tenofovir dose or pharmacokinetics was observed; BMD loss may limit the usefulness of tenofovir in prepubertal children [DHHS (pediatric), 2014; Giacomet, 2005; Hazra, 2005; Purdy, 2008].

Adverse Reactions Includes data from both treatment-naive and treatment-experienced HIV patients and in chronic hepatitis B.

Cardiovascular: Chest pain

Central nervous system: Anxiety, depression, dizziness, fatigue, headache, insomnia, pain, peripheral neuropathy

Dermatologic: Diaphoresis, pruritus, skin rash (includes maculopapular, pustular, or vesiculobullous rash; pruritus; or urticaria)

Endocrine & metabolic: Glycosuria, hypercholesterolemia, hyperglycemia, increased serum triglycerides, lipodystrophy, weight loss

Gastrointestinal: Abdominal pain, anorexia, diarrhea, dyspepsia, flatulence, increased serum amylase, nausea, vomiting

Genitourinary: Hematuria

Hematologic & oncologic: Neutropenia

Hepatic: Increased serum alkaline phosphatase, increased serum ALT, increased serum AST, increased serum transaminases

Neuromuscular & skeletal: Arthralgia, back pain, decreased bone mineral density, increased creatine phosphokinase, myalgia, weakness

Renal: Increased serum creatinine, renal failure

Respiratory: Nasopharyngitis, pneumonia, sinusitis, upper respiratory tract infection

Miscellaneous: Fever

Rare but important or life-threatening: Angioedema, exacerbation of hepatitis B (following discontinuation), Fanconi's syndrome, hepatitis, hypersensitivity reaction, hypokalemia, hypophosphatemia, immune reconstitution syndrome, increased gamma-glutamyl transferase, interstitial nephritis, lactic acidosis, myopathy, nephrogenic diabetes insipidus, nephrotoxicity, osteomalacia, pancreatitis, polyuria, proteinuria, proximal tubular nephropathy, renal insufficiency, renal tubular necrosis, rhabdomyolysis, severe hepatomegaly with steatosis

Drug Interactions

Metabolism/Transport Effects **Substrate** of BCRP, P-glycoprotein; **Inhibits** CYP1A2 (weak)

Avoid Concomitant Use

Avoid concomitant use of Tenofovir with any of the following: Adefovir; Didanosine

Increased Effect/Toxicity

Tenofovir may increase the levels/effects of: Adefovir; Aminoglycosides; Darunavir; Didanosine; Ganciclovir-Valganciclovir; TiZANidine

The levels/effects of Tenofovir may be increased by: Acyclovir-Valacyclovir; Adefovir; Aminoglycosides; Atazanavir; Cidofovir; Cobicistat; Darunavir; Diclofenac (Systemic); Ganciclovir-Valganciclovir; Ledipasvir; Lopinavir; Nonsteroidal Anti-Inflammatory Agents; Simeprevir; Telaprevir

Decreased Effect

Tenofovir may decrease the levels/effects of: Atazanavir; Didanosine; Simeprevir; Tipranavir

The levels/effects of Tenofovir may be decreased by: Adefovir; Tipranavir

Food Interactions Fatty meals may increase the bioavailability of tenofovir. Management: May administer with or without food.

Storage/Stability Store at 25°C (77°F); excursions are permitted between 15°C and 30°C (59°F and 86°F). Dispense only in original container.

Mechanism of Action Tenofovir disoproxil fumarate (TDF), a nucleotide reverse transcriptase inhibitor, is an analog of adenosine 5'-monophosphate; it interferes with the HIV viral RNA dependent DNA polymerase resulting in inhibition of viral replication. TDF is first converted intracellularly by hydrolysis to tenofovir and subsequently phosphorylated to the active tenofovir diphosphate. Tenofovir inhibits replication of HBV by inhibiting HBV polymerase.

Pharmacokinetics (Adult data unless noted)

Distribution: V_d: 1.2 to 1.3 L/kg

Protein binding: Minimal (7.2% to serum proteins)

Metabolism: Not metabolized by CYP isoenzymes; tenofovir disoproxil fumarate (a prodrug) undergoes diester hydrolysis to tenofovir; tenofovir undergoes phosphorylation to the active tenofovir diphosphate

Bioavailability: Oral:

Tablets: 25% (fasting); high-fat meals will increase AUC by 40%

Powder: Peak serum concentrations are 26% lower compared to tablet, but the mean AUCs are similar

Half-life: Serum: 17 hours; intracellular: 10 to 50 hours

Time to peak serum concentration: Fasting: 1 hour

Elimination: Excreted via glomerular filtration and active tubular secretion; after IV administration: 70% to 80% is excreted in the urine as unchanged drug within 72 hours; after multiple oral doses (administered with food): 32% ± 10% is excreted in the urine within 24 hours

Clearance: Total body clearance is decreased in patients with renal impairment

Dosing: Usual

Pediatric:

HIV infection, treatment: Use in combination with other antiretroviral agents: **Note:** Some experts recommend avoiding tenofovir (especially for initial therapy) in prepubertal patients and those in early puberty (Tanner stages 1 and 2), due to concerns about the potential increased risk of bone mineral density loss. Other experts recommend measuring bone mineral density prior to initiation of therapy and 6 months later in these patients [DHHS (pediatric), 2014]:

Infants and Children <2 years: Not approved for use; dose is unknown

Children 2 to <12 years; weighing <35 kg: Oral: 8 mg/kg/dose once daily; maximum daily dose: 300 mg/**day**

Dosage form specific:

Oral powder: **Note:** One level scoop = 40 mg tenofovir disoproxil fumarate

10 to <12 kg: 80 mg (2 scoops) once daily
12 to <14 kg: 100 mg (2.5 scoops) once daily
14 to <17 kg: 120 mg (3 scoops) once daily
17 to <19 kg: 140 mg (3.5 scoops) once daily
19 to <22 kg: 160 mg (4 scoops) once daily
22 to <24 kg: 180 mg (4.5 scoops) once daily
24 to <27 kg: 200 mg (5 scoops) once daily
27 to <29 kg: 220 mg (5.5 scoops) once daily
29 to <32 kg: 240 mg (6 scoops) once daily
32 to <34 kg: 260 mg (6.5 scoops) once daily
34 to <35 kg: 280 mg (7 scoops) once daily
≥35 kg: 300 mg (7.5 scoops) once daily

Oral tablets:

17 to <22 kg: 150 mg once daily
22 to <28 kg: 200 mg once daily
28 to <35 kg: 250 mg once daily
≥35 kg: 300 mg once daily

Children ≥12 years and Adolescents; weight ≥35 kg: Oral: 300 mg once daily

Hepatitis B infection, chronic: Children and Adolescents ≥12 years weighing ≥35 kg: Oral: 300 mg once daily; **Note:** Optimal duration of therapy is unknown.

Adult:

HIV infection, treatment: Oral: 300 mg once daily; **Note:** Use in combination with other antiretroviral agents

Hepatitis B infection, chronic: Oral: 300 mg once daily; **Note:** Tenofovir is recommended for first-line treatment of HBV (Lok, 2009). Concurrent use with adefovir and/or tenofovir combination products should be avoided.

Treatment duration (AASLD practice guidelines; Lok, 2009): **Note:** Patients not achieving <2 log decrease in serum HBV DNA after at least 6 months of therapy should either receive additional treatment or be switched to an alternative therapy.

Hepatitis Be antigen (HBeAg) positive chronic hepatitis: Treat ≥1 year until HBeAg seroconversion and undetectable serum HBV DNA; continue therapy for ≥6 months after HBeAg seroconversion

HBeAg negative chronic hepatitis: Treat >1 year until hepatitis B surface antigen (HB_sAg) clearance

Decompensated liver disease: Lifelong treatment is recommended

Dosing adjustment in renal impairment:

Children and Adolescents: There are no dosage adjustments provided in manufacturer's labeling; has not been studied. Dosage should be decreased in patients with CrCl <50 mL/minute (DHHS [pediatric], 2014)

Adult: Oral: **Note:** Use of powder formulation has not been evaluated in renal impairment. Closely monitor clinical response and renal function in these patients; clinical effectiveness and safety of these guidelines have not been evaluated.

CrCl ≥50 mL/minute: No adjustment necessary
CrCl 30 to 49 mL/minute: 300 mg every 48 hours
CrCl 10 to 29 mL/minute: 300 mg every 72 to 96 hours
CrCl <10 mL/minute without dialysis: There are no dosage adjustments provided in manufacturer's labeling; has not been studied.

Hemodialysis: 4 hours of hemodialysis removed ~10% of a single 300 mg dose; 300 mg every 7 days or after a total of ~12 hours of dialysis (eg, once weekly with 3 hemodialysis sessions of ~4 hours in length); administer dose after completion of dialysis

Dosing adjustment in hepatic impairment: No dosage adjustment required; in adults, limited number of patients have been studied (especially HBV patients with decompensated liver disease); observe for increased adverse reactions, including renal dysfunction.

Administration Oral:

Powder: Must administer with food. Measure dose only using the supplied dosing scoop. Mix powder well with 2-4 ounces of soft food (applesauce, baby food, yogurt) and swallow immediately (avoids bitter taste); ensure that entire mixture is ingested. Do **not** mix in liquid (powder may float on top of the liquid even after stirring).

Tablets: May be administered without regard to meals

Monitoring Parameters

Hepatitis B, treatment: Test patients for HIV prior to starting therapy; CBC with differential, hemoglobin, MCV, reticulocyte count, liver enzymes, bilirubin, renal and hepatic function tests, and HBV RNA plasma levels. Monitor for potential bone and renal abnormalities. Calculate creatinine clearance in all patients prior to starting tenofovir therapy and as clinically needed; monitor for alterations in calculated creatinine clearance and serum phosphorus in patients at risk or with a history of renal dysfunction and patients receiving concurrent nephrotoxic agents. Monitor weight and growth in children. Consider bone mineral density assessment for all patients with a history of pathologic bone fractures or other risk factors for osteoporosis or bone loss. Monitor hepatic function closely (clinically and with laboratory tests) for at least several months after discontinuing tenofovir therapy.

HIV treatment: Note: Monitor CD4 percentage (if <5 years of age) or CD4 count (if ≥5 years of age) at least every 3 to 4 months (DHHS [pediatric], 2014). Screen for hepatitis B before starting tenofovir. Also prior to initiation of therapy: Genotypic resistance testing, CD4 and viral load (every 3 to 4 months), CBC with differential, LFTs, BUN, creatinine, urine dipstick for protein and glucose, electrolytes, and glucose, urinalysis (every 6 to 12 months), and assessment of readiness for adherence with medication regimen. At initiation and with any change in treatment regimen: CBC with differential, electrolytes, calcium, phosphate, glucose, LFTs, bilirubin, urinalysis (at initiation), BUN, creatinine, albumin, total protein, lipid panel (at initiation), CD4, and viral load. After 1 to 2 weeks of therapy: Signs of medication toxicity and adherence. After 2 to 4 weeks of therapy: CBC with differential, viral load, and signs of medication toxicity, and adherence; then every 3 to 4 months: CBC with differential, electrolytes, glucose, LFTs, bilirubin, BUN, creatinine, CD4, viral load, signs of medication toxicity, and adherence. Every 6 to 12 months: Lipid panel and urinalysis. CD4 monitoring frequency may be decreased to every 6 to 12 months in children who are adherent to therapy if the value is well above the threshold for opportunistic infections, viral suppression is sustained, and the clinical status is stable for more than 2 to 3 years (DHHS [pediatric], 2014). Monitor for growth and development, signs of HIV-specific physical conditions, HIV disease progression, opportunistic infections, bone loss, or lactic acidosis. Consider bone mineral density assessment for all patients with a history of pathologic bone fractures or other risk factors for osteoporosis or bone loss. Some experts recommend obtaining a DXA scan prior to therapy and 6 months into therapy, especially for patients in pre- and early puberty (Tanner stages 1 and 2) (DHHS [pediatric], 2014).

Additional Information Long term studies demonstrating a decrease of clinical progression of HIV in patients receiving tenofovir are needed. Consider tenofovir in patients with HIV strains that would be susceptible as assessed by treatment history or laboratory tests. Mutation of reverse transcriptase at the 65 codon (K65R mutation) confers *in vitro* resistance to tenofovir; the K65R mutation is selected in some patients after treatment with didanosine, zalcitabine, or abacavir; thus, cross-resistance may occur. Multiple nucleoside mutations with a T69S double insertion showed decreased *in vitro* susceptibility to tenofovir; patients with HIV strains that had ≥3 zidovudine-associated mutations that included M41L or L210W showed decreased responses to tenofovir (but these responses were still better than placebo); patients with mutations at K65R, or L74V without zidovudine-associated mutations seemed to have a decreased response to tenofovir

A high rate of early virologic failure in therapy-naïve adult HIV patients has been observed with the once-daily three-drug combination therapy of didanosine enteric-coated beadlets (Videx EC), lamivudine, and tenofovir and the once-daily three-drug combination therapy of abacavir, lamivudine, and tenofovir. These combinations should not be used as a new treatment regimen for naïve or pretreated patients. Any patient currently receiving either of these regimens should be closely monitored for virologic failure and considered for treatment modification. Early virologic failure was also observed in therapy-naïve adult HIV patients treated with tenofovir, didanosine enteric-coated beadlets (Videx EC) and either efavirenz or nevirapine; rapid emergence of resistant mutations has also been reported with this combination; the combination of tenofovir, didanosine, and any non-nucleoside reverse transcriptase inhibitor is **not** recommended as initial antiretroviral therapy. Current guidelines warn **not** to use tenofovir concurrently with didanosine for the treatment of HIV infection; risk of didanosine toxicity (including pancreatitis and lactic acidosis) is increased and virologic failures have been reported (DHHS [adult], 2014).

Dosage Forms Excipient information presented when available (limited, particularly for generics); consult specific product labeling.

Powder, Oral, as disoproxil fumarate:
- Viread: 40 mg/g (60 g)

Tablet, Oral, as disoproxil fumarate:
- Viread: 150 mg, 200 mg, 250 mg
- Viread: 300 mg [contains fd&c blue #2 aluminum lake]

- ◆ **Tenofovir and Emtricitabine** *see* Emtricitabine and Tenofovir *on page* *742*
- ◆ **Tenofovir Disoproxil Fumarate** *see* Tenofovir *on page* *2017*
- ◆ **Tenofovir Disoproxil Fumarate, Efavirenz, and Emtricitabine** *see* Efavirenz, Emtricitabine, and Tenofovir *on page* *734*
- ◆ **Tenormin** *see* Atenolol *on page* *215*
- ◆ **Tensilon® (Can)** *see* Edrophonium *on page* *729*
- ◆ **Tera-Gel Tar [OTC]** *see* Coal Tar *on page* *523*

Terazosin (ter AY zoe sin)

Medication Safety Issues

BEERS Criteria medication:

This drug may be potentially inappropriate for use in geriatric patients (Quality of evidence - moderate; Strength of recommendation - strong).

Brand Names: Canada Apo-Terazosin; Dom-Terazosin; Hytrin; Nu-Terazosin; PHL-Terazosin; PMS-Terazosin; ratio-Terazosin; Teva-Terazosin

Therapeutic Category Alpha-Adrenergic Blocking Agent, Oral; Antihypertensive Agent; Vasodilator

Generic Availability (US) Yes

Use Treatment of benign prostate hyperplasia (BPH) (FDA approved in adults); treatment of hypertension alone or in combination with other agents, such as diuretics or beta-blockers (FDA approved in adults)

Pregnancy Risk Factor C

Pregnancy Considerations Teratogenic effects have not been observed in animal studies. Decreased fetal weight and increased risk of fetal mortality were noted in some animal reproduction studies. There are no adequate and well-controlled studies in pregnant women. Use only if benefit outweighs risk.

Untreated chronic maternal hypertension is associated with adverse events in the fetus, infant, and mother. If treatment for hypertension during pregnancy is needed, other agents are generally preferred (ACOG, 2013).

Breast-Feeding Considerations It is not known if terazosin is excreted in breast milk. The manufacturer recommends that caution be exercised when administering terazosin to nursing women.

Contraindications Hypersensitivity to terazosin or any component of the formulation

Warnings/Precautions Can cause significant orthostatic hypotension and syncope, especially with first dose; anticipate a similar effect if therapy is interrupted for a few days, if dosage is rapidly increased, or if another antihypertensive drug (particularly vasodilators) or a PDE-5 inhibitor is introduced. Discontinue if symptoms of angina occur or worsen. Patients should be cautioned about performing hazardous tasks when starting new therapy or adjusting dosage upward. Prostate cancer should be ruled out before starting for BPH. Intraoperative floppy iris syndrome has been observed in cataract surgery patients who were on or were previously treated with $alpha_1$-blockers. Causality has not been established and there appears to be no benefit in discontinuing alpha-blocker therapy prior to surgery. Priapism has been associated with use (rarely). In the elderly, avoid use as an antihypertensive due to high risk of orthostatic hypotension; alternative agents preferred due to a more favorable risk/benefit profile (Beers Criteria).

Adverse Reactions

Cardiovascular: Orthostatic hypotension, palpitation, peripheral edema, syncope, tachycardia

Central nervous system: Dizziness, somnolence, vertigo

Gastrointestinal: Nausea, weight gain

Genitourinary: Impotence, libido decreased

Neuromuscular & skeletal: Back pain, extremity pain, muscle weakness, paresthesia

Ocular: Blurred vision

Respiratory: Dyspnea, nasal congestion, sinusitis

Rare but important or life-threatening: Abdominal pain, abnormal vision, allergic reactions, anaphylaxis, anxiety, arrhythmia, arthralgia, arthritis, atrial fibrillation, bronchitis, chest pain, conjunctivitis, constipation, cough, diaphoresis, diarrhea, dyspepsia, epistaxis, facial edema, fever, flatulence, flu-like syndrome, gout, insomnia, intraoperative floppy iris syndrome (IFIS), joint disorder, myalgia, neck pain, pharyngitis, polyuria, priapism, pruritus, rash, rhinitis, shoulder pain, thrombocytopenia, tinnitus, urinary incontinence, urinary tract infection, vasodilation, vomiting, xerostomia

Drug Interactions

Metabolism/Transport Effects None known.

Avoid Concomitant Use

Avoid concomitant use of Terazosin with any of the following: Alpha1-Blockers

Increased Effect/Toxicity

Terazosin may increase the levels/effects of: Alpha1-Blockers; Amifostine; Antihypertensives; Calcium Channel Blockers; DULoxetine; Hypotensive Agents; Levodopa; Obinutuzumab; RisperiDONE; RiTUXimab

The levels/effects of Terazosin may be increased by: Barbiturates; Beta-Blockers; Brimonidine (Topical); Dapoxetine; Diazoxide; Herbs (Hypotensive Properties); MAO Inhibitors; Nicorandil; Pentoxifylline; Phosphodiesterase 5 Inhibitors; Prostacyclin Analogues

Decreased Effect

Terazosin may decrease the levels/effects of: Alpha-/Beta-Agonists; Alpha1-Agonists

The levels/effects of Terazosin may be decreased by: Herbs (Hypertensive Properties); Methylphenidate; Yohimbine

Storage/Stability Store at 20°C to 25°C (68°F to 77°F); protect from light and moisture.

Mechanism of Action $Alpha_1$-specific blocking agent with minimal $alpha_2$ effects; this allows peripheral postsynaptic blockade, with the resultant decrease in arterial tone, while preserving the negative feedback loop which is mediated by the peripheral presynaptic $alpha_2$-receptors; terazosin relaxes the smooth muscle of the bladder neck, thus reducing bladder outlet obstruction

Pharmacodynamics

Onset of action: Antihypertensive effect: 15 minutes

Maximum effect: Antihypertensive effect: 2-3 hours

Duration: Antihypertensive effect: 24 hours

Pharmacokinetics (Adult data unless noted)

Absorption: Rapid, complete

Protein binding: 90% to 94%

Metabolism: Hepatic; minimal first pass

Half-life: ~12 hours

Time to peak serum concentration: ~1 hour

Elimination: Feces (~60%, ~20% as unchanged drug); urine (~40%, ~10% as unchanged drug)

Dialysis: ~10% removed during hemodialysis

Dosing: Usual Note: If drug is discontinued for greater than several days, consider beginning with initial dose and retitrate as needed.

Children and Adolescents: **Hypertension:** Oral: Initial: 1 mg once daily typically administered at bedtime; slowly increase dose to achieve desired blood pressure as tolerated; maximum daily dose: 20 mg/**day** (NHBPEP, 2004; NHLBI, 2011)

Adults:

Benign prostatic hyperplasia: Oral: Initial: 1 mg at bedtime; thereafter, titrate upwards, if needed, over several weeks, balancing therapeutic benefit with terazosin-induced postural hypotension; most patients require 10 mg day; if no response after 4-6 weeks of 10 mg/day, may increase to 20 mg/day

Hypertension: Oral: Initial: 1 mg at bedtime; slowly increase dose to achieve desired blood pressure, up to 20 mg/day; usual dose range (JNC 7): 1-20 mg once daily. **Note:** Dosage may be given on a twice-daily regimen if response is diminished at 24 hours.

Administration Oral: Administer without regard to meals at the same time each day.

Monitoring Parameters Standing and sitting/supine blood pressure, especially 2-3 hours after the initial dose, then prior to doses (to ensure adequate control throughout the dosing interval); urinary symptoms if used for BPH treatment

Dosage Forms Excipient information presented when available (limited, particularly for generics); consult specific product labeling.

Capsule, Oral:

Generic: 1 mg, 2 mg, 5 mg, 10 mg

Terbinafine (Systemic) (TER bin a feen)

Medication Safety Issues

Sound-alike/look-alike issues:

Terbinafine may be confused with terbutaline

LamISIL may be confused with LaMICtal, Lomotil

Brand Names: US LamISIL; Terbinex

Brand Names: Canada Apo-Terbinafine; Auro-Terbinafine; CO Terbinafine; Dom-Terbinafine; GD-Terbinafine; JAMP-Terbinafine; Lamisil; Mylan-Terbinafine; PHL-Terbinafine; PMS-Terbinafine; Q-Terbinafine; Riva-Terbinafine; Sandoz-Terbinafine; Teva-Terbinafine

Generic Availability (US) May be product dependent

Use Oral:

Granules: Treatment of tinea capitis (FDA approved in ages ≥4 years and adults)

Tablet: Treatment of onychomycosis of the toenail or fingernail due to susceptible dermatophytes (FDA approved in adults)

Pregnancy Risk Factor B

Pregnancy Considerations Adverse events were not observed in animal reproduction studies. Avoid use in pregnancy since treatment of onychomycosis is postponable.

Breast-Feeding Considerations Terbinafine is excreted in breast milk; the milk/plasma ratio is 7:1. Breast-feeding is not recommended by the manufacturer.

Contraindications Hypersensitivity to terbinafine or any component of the formulation

Warnings/Precautions Due to potential toxicity, confirmation of diagnostic testing of nail or skin specimens prior to treatment of onychomycosis or dermatomycosis is recommended. Use caution in patients sensitive to allylamine antifungals (eg, naftifine, butenafine); cross sensitivity to terbinafine may exist. Transient decreases in absolute lymphocyte counts were observed in clinical trials; severe neutropenia (reversible upon discontinuation) has also been reported. Monitor CBC in patients with pre-existing immunosuppression if therapy is to continue >6 weeks and discontinue therapy if ANC ≤1000/mm^3.

Serious skin and hypersensitivity reactions (eg, Stevens-Johnson syndrome, toxic epidermal necrolysis, erythema multiforme, exfoliative dermatitis, bullous dermatitis, drug reaction with eosinophilia and systemic symptoms [DRESS] syndrome) have occurred. If progressive skin rash or signs and symptoms of a hypersensitivity reaction occur, discontinue treatment. Cases of hepatic failure, some leading to liver transplant or death, have been reported; not recommended for use in patients with active or chronic liver disease. If clinical evidence of liver injury develops (eg, nausea, anorexia, fatigue, vomiting, right upper abdominal pain, jaundice, dark urine, pale stools), assess hepatic function immediately; discontinue therapy in cases of elevated liver function tests. Use with caution in patients with renal dysfunction (CrCl ≤50 mL/minute) (per Canadian labeling, not recommended for use); clearance is reduced by ~50%.

Disturbances of taste and/or smell may occur; resolution may be delayed (eg, >1 year) following discontinuation of therapy or in some cases, disturbance may be permanent. Discontinue therapy in patients with symptoms of taste or smell disturbance.

Adverse Reactions Adverse events listed for tablets unless otherwise specified. Granules were studied in patients 4-12 years of age.

Central nervous system: Headache

Dermatologic: Pruritus, skin rash, urticaria

Gastrointestinal: Abdominal pain, diarrhea, dysgeusia, dyspepsia, flatulence, nausea, sore throat (granules), toothache (granules), vomiting

Hepatic: Liver enzyme disorder

Infection: Influenza (granules)

Ophthalmic: Visual disturbance

Respiratory: Cough (granules), nasal congestion (granules), nasopharyngitis (granules), rhinorrhea (granules), upper respiratory tract infection (children, granules)

Miscellaneous: Fever (granules)

Rare but important or life-threatening: Acute generalized exanthematous pustulosis, acute pancreatitis, agranulocytosis, alopecia, altered sense of smell, anaphylaxis, angioedema, depression, DRESS syndrome, exacerbation of psoriasis, exacerbation of systemic lupus erythematosus, hepatic disease, hepatic failure, hypersensitivity reaction, pancytopenia, rhabdomyolysis, severe neutropenia, Stevens-Johnson syndrome, thrombocytopenia, toxic epidermal necrolysis, vasculitis, visual field loss

Drug Interactions

Metabolism/Transport Effects Substrate of CYP1A2 (minor), CYP2C19 (minor), CYP2C9 (minor), CYP3A4 (minor); **Note:** Assignment of Major/Minor substrate status based on clinically relevant drug interaction potential; **Inhibits** CYP2D6 (strong); **Induces** CYP3A4 (weak)

Avoid Concomitant Use

Avoid concomitant use of Terbinafine (Systemic) with any of the following: Mequitazine; Pimozide; Saccharomyces boulardii; Tamoxifen; Thioridazine

Increased Effect/Toxicity

Terbinafine (Systemic) may increase the levels/effects of: ARIPiprazole; AtoMOXetine; CYP2D6 Substrates; DOXOrubicin (Conventional); Eliglustat; Fesoterodine; Iloperidone; Mequitazine; Metoprolol; Nebivolol; Pimozide; Propafenone; Tamsulosin; Tetrabenazine; Thioridazine; TraMADol; Tricyclic Antidepressants; Vortioxetine

Decreased Effect

Terbinafine (Systemic) may decrease the levels/effects of: ARIPiprazole; Codeine; Hydrocodone; Iloperidone; NiMODipine; Saccharomyces boulardii; Saxagliptin; Tamoxifen; TraMADol

The levels/effects of Terbinafine (Systemic) may be decreased by: Rifampin

Storage/Stability

Granules: Store at 25°C (77°F); excursions permitted between 15°C to 30°C (59°F to 86°F).

Tablet: Store below 25°C (77°F). Protect from light.

Mechanism of Action Synthetic allylamine derivative which inhibits squalene epoxidase, a key enzyme in sterol biosynthesis in fungi. This results in a deficiency in ergosterol within the fungal cell wall and results in fungal cell death.

Pharmacokinetics (Adult data unless noted)

Absorption: Children and Adults: >70%

Distribution: Distributed to sebum and skin predominantly

Protein binding: Plasma: >99%

Metabolism: Hepatic predominantly via CYP1A2, 3A4, 2C8, 2C9, and 2C19 to inactive metabolites

Bioavailability:

Children: 36% to 64%

Adults: 40%

Half-life, terminal: 200-400 hours; very slow release of drug from skin and adipose tissues occurs; effective half-life: Children: 27-31 hours; Adults: ~36 hours

Time to peak serum concentration: Children and Adults: 1-2 hours

Elimination: Children and Adults: 70% in urine

Clearance: Children (14-68 kg): 15.6-26.7 L/hour

Dosing: Usual

Children and Adolescents:

Tinea capitis: Children ≥4 years and Adolescents: Oral: Granules:

<25 kg: 125 mg once daily for 6 weeks

25-35 kg: 187.5 mg once daily for 6 weeks

>35 kg: 250 mg once daily for 6 weeks

Onychomycosis (Gupta, 1997): Limited data available: Children and Adolescents: Oral: Tablets:

10-20 kg: 62.5 mg once daily for 6 weeks (fingernails) or 12 weeks (toenails)

20-40 kg: 125 mg once daily for 6 weeks (fingernails) or 12 weeks (toenails)

>40 kg: 250 mg once daily for 6 weeks (fingernails) or 12 weeks (toenails)

Adults: **Onychomycosis:** Oral: Tablet: Fingernail: 250 mg once daily for 6 weeks; Toenail: 250 mg once daily for 12 weeks

Dosing adjustment in renal impairment: No dosage adjustment provided in manufacturer's U.S. labeling; however, clearance is decreased 50% in patients with CrCl ≤50 mL/minute.

Dosing adjustment in hepatic impairment: Hepatic cirrhosis: Use is not recommended in chronic or active hepatic disease.

Administration Tablets may be administered without regard to meals. Granules should be taken with food; sprinkle on a spoonful of nonacidic food (eg, pudding, mashed potatoes); do not use applesauce or fruit-based foods; swallow granules whole without chewing

Monitoring Parameters AST/ALT prior to initiation, repeat if used >6 weeks; CBC

Additional Information Patients should not be considered therapeutic failures until they have been symptom-free for 2-4 weeks following a course of treatment; GI complaints usually subside with continued administration.

Dosage Forms Considerations Terbinex Kit contains terbinafine 250 mg tablets and hydroxypropyl-chitosan 1% nail lacquer

Dosage Forms Excipient information presented when available (limited, particularly for generics); consult specific product labeling.

Kit, Combination:
- Terbinex: 250 mg & 1%

Packet, Oral:
- LamISIL: 125 mg (1 ea, 14 ea); 187.5 mg (1 ea, 14 ea) [contains polyethylene glycol]

Tablet, Oral:
- LamISIL: 250 mg
- Generic: 250 mg

Extemporaneous Preparations A 25 mg/mL oral suspension may be made using tablets. Crush twenty 250 mg tablets and reduce to a fine powder. Add small amount of a 1:1 mixture of Ora-Sweet® and Ora-Plus® and mix to a uniform paste; mix while adding the vehicle in geometric proportions to **almost** 200 mL; transfer to a calibrated bottle, rinse mortar with vehicle, and add quantity of vehicle sufficient to make 200 mL. Label "shake well" and "refrigerate". Stable 42 days.

Nahata MC, Pai VB, and Hipple TF, *Pediatric Drug Formulations*, 5th ed, Cincinnati, OH: Harvey Whitney Books Co, 2004.

Terbinafine (Topical) (TER bin a feen)

Medication Safety Issues

Sound-alike/look-alike issues:

Terbinafine may be confused with terbutaline

Brand Names: US LamISIL Advanced [OTC]; LamISIL AT Jock Itch [OTC]; LamISIL AT Spray [OTC]; LamISIL AT [OTC]; LamISIL Spray

Brand Names: Canada Lamisil

Therapeutic Category Antifungal Agent, Topical

Generic Availability (US) May be product dependent

Use Antifungal for the treatment of tinea pedis (athlete's foot), tinea cruris (jock itch), and tinea corporis (ringworm) (OTC/prescription formulations); tinea versicolor (prescription formulations)

Pregnancy Considerations Adverse events were not observed in animal reproduction studies with systemic terbinafine. Systemic absorption is limited following topical application.

Breast-Feeding Considerations Following oral administration, terbinafine is excreted into breast milk. (Refer to the Terbinafine (Systemic) monograph for additional information). Systemic absorption is limited following topical application. Nursing mothers should not apply topical formulations to the breast.

Contraindications Hypersensitivity to terbinafine or any component of the formulation

Warnings/Precautions For topical use only. Not intended for ophthalmologic, oral, or vaginal administration. Do not use on nails or scalp. If irritation/sensitivity develops, discontinue therapy and institute appropriate alternative therapy.

Benzyl alcohol and derivatives: Some dosage forms may contain benzyl alcohol; large amounts of benzyl alcohol (≥99 mg/kg/day) have been associated with a potentially fatal toxicity ("gasping syndrome") in neonates; the "gasping syndrome" consists of metabolic acidosis, respiratory distress, gasping respirations, CNS dysfunction (including convulsions, intracranial hemorrhage), hypotension, and cardiovascular collapse (AAP, 1997; CDC, 1982); some data suggests that benzoate displaces bilirubin from protein binding sites (Ahlfors, 2001); avoid or use dosage forms containing benzyl alcohol with caution in neonates. See manufacturer's labeling.

Warnings: Additional Pediatric Considerations Some dosage forms may contain propylene glycol; in neonates large amounts of propylene glycol delivered orally, intravenously (eg, >3,000 mg/day), or topically have been associated with potentially fatal toxicities which can include metabolic acidosis, seizures, renal failure, and CNS depression; toxicities have also been reported in children and adults including hyperosmolality, lactic acidosis, seizures and respiratory depression; use caution (AAP, 1997; Shehab, 2009).

Adverse Reactions

Dermatologic: Burning, contact dermatitis, dryness, exfoliation, irritation, pruritus, rash

Local: Irritation, stinging

Drug Interactions

Metabolism/Transport Effects None known.

Avoid Concomitant Use There are no known interactions where it is recommended to avoid concomitant use.

Increased Effect/Toxicity There are no known significant interactions involving an increase in effect.

Decreased Effect There are no known significant interactions involving a decrease in effect.

Storage/Stability

Cream: Store at 20°C to 25°C (68°F to 77°F).

Gel: Store at ≤30°C (≤86°F).

Solution: Store at 8°C to 25°C (46°F to 77°F).

Mechanism of Action Synthetic allylamine derivative which inhibits squalene epoxidase, a key enzyme in sterol biosynthesis in fungi. This results in a deficiency in ergosterol within the fungal cell wall and results in fungal cell death.

Pharmacokinetics (Adult data unless noted)

Absorption: Children and Adults: Limited (<5%)

Distribution: Distributed to sebum and skin predominantly

Half-life: 14-35 hours

Dosing: Usual

Cream, gel, solution: Children ≥12 years and Adults:

- Athlete's foot (tinea pedis): OTC/prescription formulations: Apply to affected area twice daily for at least 1 week, not to exceed 4 weeks
- Ringworm (tinea corporis) and jock itch (tinea cruris): OTC formulations: Apply cream to affected area once or twice daily for at least 1 week, not to exceed 4 weeks; apply gel or solution once daily for 7 days

Cream, solution: Adults: Tinea versicolor: Prescription formulation: Apply to affected area twice daily for 1 week

Administration Apply to clean, dry affected area in sufficient quantity to cover; avoid contact with eyes, nose, mouth, or other mucous membranes. Do not use occlusive dressings.

Dosage Forms Excipient information presented when available (limited, particularly for generics); consult specific product labeling.

Cream, External, as hydrochloride:
- LamISIL AT: 1% (12 g, 24 g, 30 g, 36 g, 42 g) [contains benzyl alcohol, cetyl alcohol]
- LamISIL AT Jock Itch: 1% (12 g) [contains benzyl alcohol, cetyl alcohol]
- Generic: 1% (12 g, 15 g, 24 g, 30 g)

Gel, External:
- LamISIL Advanced: 1% (12 g) [contains alcohol, usp]

Solution, External, as hydrochloride:
- LamISIL AT Spray: 1% (30 mL, 125 mL) [contains alcohol, usp, propylene glycol]
- LamISIL Spray: 1% (30 mL) [contains alcohol, usp]

◆ **Terbinafine Hydrochloride** *see* Terbinafine (Systemic) *on page 2021*

◆ **Terbinafine Hydrochloride** *see* Terbinafine (Topical) *on page 2023*

◆ **Terbinex** *see* Terbinafine (Systemic) *on page 2021*

Terbutaline (ter BYOO ta leen)

Medication Safety Issues

Sound-alike/look-alike issues:

Brethine may be confused with Methergine

Terbutaline may be confused with terbinafine, TOLBUTamide

Terbutaline and methylergonovine parenteral dosage forms look similar. Due to their contrasting indications, use care when administering these agents.

Related Information

Management of Drug Extravasations *on page 2298*

Brand Names: Canada Bricanyl® Turbuhaler®

Therapeutic Category Adrenergic Agonist Agent; Antiasthmatic; Beta$_2$-Adrenergic Agonist; Bronchodilator; Sympathomimetic; Tocolytic Agent

Generic Availability (US) Yes

Use Bronchodilator for relief of reversible bronchospasm in patients with asthma, bronchitis, and emphysema

Pregnancy Risk Factor C

Pregnancy Considerations Adverse events have been observed in animal reproduction studies. Terbutaline crosses the placenta; umbilical cord concentrations are ~11% to 48% of maternal blood levels.

Uncontrolled asthma is associated with adverse events on pregnancy (increased risk of perinatal mortality, preeclampsia, preterm birth, low birth weight infants). Terbutaline is not recommended for the treatment of asthma during pregnancy; inhaled beta$_2$-receptor agonists are preferred (NAEPP, 2005).

[U.S. Boxed Warning]: Terbutaline is not FDA approved for and should not be used for prolonged tocolysis (>48-72 hours). Use for maintenance tocolysis should not be done in the outpatient setting. Adverse events observed in pregnant women include arrhythmias, increased heart rate, hyperglycemia (transient), hypokalemia, myocardial ischemia, and pulmonary edema. Heart rate may be increased in the fetus and hypoglycemia may occur in the neonate. Terbutaline has been used in the management of preterm labor. Tocolytics may be used for the short-term (48 hour) prolongation of pregnancy to allow for the administration of antenatal steroids and should not be used prior to fetal viability or when the risks of use to the fetus or mother are greater than the risk of preterm birth (ACOG, 2012).

Breast-Feeding Considerations Terbutaline is excreted in breast milk; concentrations are similar to or higher than those in the maternal plasma. Based on information from four cases, exposure to the breast-fed infant would be <1% of the weight-adjusted maternal dose. Adverse events were not observed in nursing infants (Boréus, 1982; Lönnerholm, 1982). The manufacturer recommends that terbutaline be used in breast-feeding women only if the potential benefit to the mother outweighs the possible risk to the infant. The use of beta$_2$-receptor agonists are not considered a contraindication to breast-feeding (NAEPP, 2005).

Contraindications

Hypersensitivity to terbutaline, sympathomimetic amines, or any component of the formulation

Injection: Additional contraindications: Prolonged (>72 hours) prevention or management of preterm labor

Oral: Additional contraindications: Prevention or treatment of preterm labor

Warnings/Precautions [U.S. Boxed Warning]: Terbutaline is not FDA approved for and should not be used for prolonged tocolysis (>48-72 hours). Use for maintenance tocolysis should not be done in the outpatient setting. Adverse events observed in pregnant women include arrhythmias, increased heart rate, hyperglycemia (transient), hypokalemia, myocardial ischemia, and pulmonary edema. Heart rate may be increased in the fetus and hypoglycemia may occur in the neonate. Oral terbutaline is contraindicated for acute or chronic use in the management of preterm labor.

Use caution in patients with cardiovascular disease (arrhythmia or hypertension or HF), convulsive disorders, diabetes, glaucoma, hyperthyroidism, or hypokalemia. Beta-agonists may cause elevation in blood pressure, heart rate, and result in CNS stimulation/excitation. Beta$_2$-agonists may increase risk of arrhythmia, increase serum glucose, or decrease serum potassium.

When used as a bronchodilator, optimize anti-inflammatory treatment before initiating maintenance treatment with terbutaline. Do not use as a component of chronic therapy without an anti-inflammatory agent. Only the mildest form of asthma (Step 1 and/or exercise-induced) would not require concurrent use based upon asthma guidelines. Patient must be instructed to seek medical attention in cases where acute symptoms are not relieved or a previous level of response is diminished. The need to increase frequency of use may indicate deterioration of asthma, and treatment must not be delayed.

Immediate hypersensitivity reactions (urticaria, angioedema, rash, bronchospasm) have been reported. Do not exceed recommended dose; serious adverse events including fatalities, have been associated with excessive use of inhaled sympathomimetics. Rarely, paradoxical bronchospasm may occur with use of inhaled bronchodilating agents; this should be distinguished from inadequate response.

Warnings: Additional Pediatric Considerations Children may experience a higher frequency of some adverse effects than adults, including congestion, cough, fever, nasopharyngitis, pharyngeal pain, rhinorrhea, toothache, and vomiting.

Adverse Reactions

Cardiovascular: Hypertension, pounding heartbeat, tachycardia

Central nervous system: Nervousness, restlessness

Endocrine & metabolic: Decreased serum potassium, increased serum glucose

Gastrointestinal: Bad taste in mouth, dry mouth, nausea, vomiting

Neuromuscular & skeletal: Dizziness, drowsiness, headache, insomnia, lightheadedness, muscle cramps, trembling, weakness

Miscellaneous: Diaphoresis

Rare but important or life-threatening: Arrhythmia, cardiac arrest (preterm labor), chest pain, hyperglycemia (preterm labor), hypokalemia (preterm labor), hypotension (preterm labor), paradoxical bronchospasm, myocardial infarction (preterm labor), myocardial ischemia (preterm labor), pulmonary edema (preterm labor)

Drug Interactions

Metabolism/Transport Effects None known.

Avoid Concomitant Use

Avoid concomitant use of Terbutaline with any of the following: Beta-Blockers (Nonselective); Iobenguane I 123; Loxapine

Increased Effect/Toxicity

Terbutaline may increase the levels/effects of: Atosiban; Highest Risk QTc-Prolonging Agents; Loop Diuretics; Loxapine; Moderate Risk QTc-Prolonging Agents; Sympathomimetics; Thiazide Diuretics

The levels/effects of Terbutaline may be increased by: AtoMOXetine; Cannabinoid-Containing Products; Linezolid; MAO Inhibitors; Mifepristone; Tedizolid; Tricyclic Antidepressants

Decreased Effect

Terbutaline may decrease the levels/effects of: Iobenguane I 123

The levels/effects of Terbutaline may be decreased by: Beta-Blockers (Beta1 Selective); Beta-Blockers (Nonselective); Betahistine

Storage/Stability Store injection at room temperature; do not freeze. Protect from heat and light. Use only clear solutions. Store powder for inhalation (Bricanyl® Turbuhaler [Canadian availability]) at room temperature between 15°C and 30°C (58°F and 86°F).

Mechanism of Action Relaxes bronchial and uterine smooth muscle by action on beta$_2$-receptors with less effect on heart rate

Pharmacodynamics

Onset of action:
- Oral: 30 minutes
- Oral inhalation: 5-30 minutes
- SubQ: 6-15 minutes

Duration:
- Oral: 4-8 hours
- Oral inhalation: 3-6 hours
- SubQ: 1.5-4 hours

Pharmacokinetics (Adult data unless noted)

Absorption: 33% to 50%

Distribution: Breast milk to plasma ratio: <2.9

Metabolism: Possible first-pass metabolism after oral use

Half-life: 5.7 hours (range: 2.9-14 hours)

Time to peak serum concentration: SubQ: 0.5 hours

Elimination: Primarily (60%) unchanged in urine after parenteral use

Dosing: Usual

Children <12 years:

Oral: Initial: 0.05 mg/kg/dose every 8 hours, increase gradually, up to 0.15 mg/kg/dose; maximum daily dose: 5 mg

SubQ: 0.005-0.01 mg/kg/dose to a maximum of 0.4 mg/dose every 15-20 minutes for 3 doses; may repeat every 2-6 hours as needed

Note: Continuous IV infusion has been used successfully in children with asthma; a 2-10 mcg/kg loading dose followed by an 0.08-0.4 mcg/kg/minute continuous infusion; depending upon the clinical response, the dosage may require titration in increments of 0.1-0.2 mcg/kg/minute every 30 minutes; doses as high as 10 mcg/kg/minute have been used.

Children ≥12 years and Adults:

Oral: 2.5-5 mg/dose every 6-8 hours; maximum daily dose:
- 12-15 years: 7.5 mg
- >15 years: 15 mg

SubQ: 0.25 mg/dose repeated in 20 minutes for 3 doses; a total dose of 0.75 mg should not be exceeded

Preparation for Administration Parenteral: Continuous IV infusion: Pediatric patients (asthma): May dilute in D$_5$W or NS to a concentration <1 mg/mL (Murray 2014)

Administration

Oral: May administer without regard to food; administer around-the-clock to promote less variation in peak and trough serum levels.

Parenteral:

Direct IV injection: Administer undiluted over 5 to 10 minutes

Continuous IV infusion: Administer via an infusion pump at a concentration ≤1 mg/mL (Bogie 2007; Murray 2014; Sinclair-Pingel 2006)

Monitoring Parameters Heart rate, blood pressure, respiratory rate, serum potassium, arterial or capillary blood gases (if applicable)

Dosage Forms Excipient information presented when available (limited, particularly for generics); consult specific product labeling.

Solution, Injection, as sulfate:
- Generic: 1 mg/mL (1 mL)

Tablet, Oral, as sulfate:
- Generic: 2.5 mg, 5 mg

Extemporaneous Preparations A 1 mg/mL oral suspension may be made with tablets. Crush twenty-four 5 mg tablets in a mortar and reduce to a fine powder. Add 5 mL purified water USP and mix to a uniform paste; mix while adding simple syrup, NF in incremental proportions to **almost** 120 mL; transfer to a calibrated bottle, rinse mortar with vehicle, and add quantity of simple syrup, NF sufficient to make 120 mL. Label "shake well" and "refrigerate". Stable for 30 days.

Nahata MC, Pai VB, and Hipple TF, *Pediatric Drug Formulations*, 5th ed, Cincinnati, OH: Harvey Whitney Books Co, 2004.

◆ **Terbutaline Sulfate** *see* Terbutaline *on page* 2024

◆ **Tersa Tar Shp [OTC] (Can)** *see* Coal Tar *on page* 523

◆ **Tersi** *see* Selenium Sulfide *on page* 1913

◆ **TESPA** *see* Thiotepa *on page* 2053

◆ **Testim** *see* Testosterone *on page* 2025

◆ **Testopel** *see* Testosterone *on page* 2025

Testosterone (tes TOS ter one)

Medication Safety Issues

Sound-alike/look-alike issues:

Testosterone may be confused with testolactone

Testoderm may be confused with Estraderm

AndroGel 1% may be confused with AndroGel 1.62%

Bio-T-Gel may be confused with T-Gel

BEERS Criteria medication:

This drug may be potentially inappropriate for use in geriatric patients (Quality of evidence - moderate; Strength of recommendation - weak).

Other safety concerns:

Transdermal patch may contain conducting metal (eg, aluminum); remove patch prior to MRI.

Related Information

Safe Handling of Hazardous Drugs *on page* 2455

Brand Names: US Androderm; AndroGel; AndroGel Pump; Aveed; Axiron; Depo-Testosterone; First-Testosterone; First-Testosterone MC; Fortesta; Natesto; Striant; Testim; Testopel; Vogelxo; Vogelxo Pump

Brand Names: Canada Andriol; Androderm; AndroGel; Andropository; Axiron; Delatestryl; Depotest 100; Everone 200; PMS-Testosterone; Testim

Therapeutic Category Androgen

Generic Availability (US) May be product dependent

Use

Parenteral:

Cypionate injection: Testosterone hormone replacement therapy in males for conditions associated with a deficiency or absence of endogenous testosterone; primary hypogonadism (congenital or acquired) and hypogonadotropic hypogonadism (congenital or acquired) (All indications: FDA approved in ages ≥12 years and adults)

Enanthate injection:

Male patients: Testosterone hormone replacement therapy in males for conditions associated with a deficiency or absence of endogenous testosterone; primary hypogonadism (congenital or acquired) and hypogonadotropic hypogonadism (congenital or acquired); delayed puberty (All indications: FDA approved in adolescents and adults)

Female patients: Inoperable metastatic breast cancer (FDA approved in adults)

Pellet (subcutaneous implant): Testosterone hormone replacement therapy in males for conditions associated with a deficiency or absence of endogenous testosterone; primary hypogonadism (congenital or acquired) and hypogonadotropic hypogonadism (congenital or acquired) (All indications: FDA approved in adolescents and adults)

Buccal system, topical gel, topical solution, transdermal system: Testosterone hormone replacement therapy in males for conditions associated with a deficiency or absence of endogenous testosterone; primary hypogonadism (congenital or acquired) and hypogonadotropic hypogonadism(congenital or acquired) (All indications: FDA approved in ages ≥18 years and adults)

Medication Guide Available Yes

Pregnancy Risk Factor X

Pregnancy Considerations Testosterone may cause adverse effects, including masculinization of the female fetus, if used during pregnancy. Females who are or may become pregnant should also avoid skin-to-skin contact to areas where testosterone has been applied topically on another person.

Breast-Feeding Considerations High levels of endogenous maternal testosterone, such as those caused by certain ovarian cysts, suppress milk production. Maternal serum testosterone levels generally fall following pregnancy and return to normal once breast-feeding is stopped. The amount of testosterone present in breast milk or the effect to the nursing infant following maternal supplementation is not known. Some products are contraindicated while breast-feeding. Females who are nursing should avoid skin-to-skin contact to areas where testosterone has been applied topically on another person.

Contraindications

Hypersensitivity to testosterone or any component of the formulation; males with carcinoma of the breast or known or suspected carcinoma of the prostate; women who are breast-feeding, pregnant, or who may become pregnant.

Depo-Testosterone: Also contraindicated in serious hepatic, renal, or cardiac disease

Documentation of allergenic cross-reactivity for androgens is limited. However, because of similarities in chemical structure and/or pharmacologic actions, the possibility of cross-sensitivity cannot be ruled out with certainty.

Warnings/Precautions Hazardous agent; use appropriate precautions for handling and disposal (NIOSH 2014 [group 3]).

When used to treat delayed male puberty, perform radiographic examination of the hand and wrist every 6 months to determine the rate of bone maturation. May cause hypercalcemia in patients with prolonged immobilization or cancer. May accelerate bone maturation without producing compensating gain in linear growth. May decrease glucose levels. May alter serum lipid profile; use caution with history of MI or coronary artery disease. Androgens may worsen BPH; patients may also be at an increased risk of prostate cancer. Use caution in elderly patients or patients with other demographic factors which may increase the risk of prostatic carcinoma; careful monitoring is required. Discontinue therapy if urethral obstruction develops in patients with BPH (use lower dose if restarted). Withhold therapy pending urological evaluation in patients with palpable prostate nodule or induration, PSA >4 ng/mL, or PSA >3 ng/mL in men at high risk of prostate cancer (Bhasin, 2010). Venous thromboembolic events including deep vein thrombosis (DVT) and pulmonary embolism (PE) have been reported with testosterone products. Evaluate patients with symptoms of pain, edema, warmth and erythema in the lower extremity for DVT and those with acute shortness of breath for PE. Discontinue therapy if a venous thromboembolism is suspected. Use with caution in patients with diseases that may be exacerbated by fluid retention including cardiac, hepatic, or renal dysfunction; testosterone may cause fluid retention. May cause gynecomastia. Large doses may suppress spermatogenesis. During treatment for metastatic breast cancer, women should be monitored for signs of virilization; discontinue if mild virilization is present to prevent irreversible symptoms.

May be inappropriate in the elderly due to potential risk of cardiac problems and contraindication for use in men with prostate cancer; in general, avoid use in older adults except in the setting of moderate-to-severe hypogonadism (Beers Criteria). In addition, elderly patients may be at greater risk for prostatic hyperplasia, prostate cancer, fluid retention, and transaminase elevations.

Prolonged use of high doses of oral androgens has been associated with serious hepatic effects (peliosis hepatis, hepatic neoplasms, cholestatic hepatitis, jaundice). Prolonged use of intramuscular testosterone enanthate has been associated with multiple hepatic adenomas. Discontinue therapy if signs or symptoms of hepatic dysfunction (such as jaundice) develop.

May potentiate sleep apnea in some male patients (obesity or chronic lung disease). May increase hematocrit requiring dose adjustment or discontinuation; discontinue therapy if hematocrit exceeds 54%; may reinitiate at lower dose (Bhasin, 2010). Oligospermia may occur after prolonged administration or excessive dosage; discontinue therapy if this occurs, if restarted, a lower dose should be used. Priapism or excessive sexual stimulation may occur; discontinue therapy if this occurs, if restarted, a lower dose should be used.

Testosterone undecanoate injection: **[US Boxed Warning]: Serious pulmonary oil microembolism (POME) reactions and anaphylaxis have been reported with testosterone undecanoate injection. Reactions include anaphylaxis, chest pain, urge to cough, dizziness, dyspnea, throat tightening, and syncope; may be life threatening. Reactions may occur after any injection during the course of therapy, including the first dose. Patients must be monitored for 30 minutes after injection. Due to the risk of serious POME reactions, Aveed is only available through the Aveed REMS program.** To minimize risk of adverse reactions, inject deeply into gluteal muscle.

[US Boxed Warning]: Virilization in children has been reported following contact with unwashed or unclothed application sites of men using topical testosterone. Patients should strictly adhere to instructions for use in order to prevent secondary exposure. Virilization of female sexual partners has also been reported with male use of topical testosterone. Symptoms of virilization generally regress following removal of exposure; however, in some children, enlarged genitalia and bone age did not fully return to age appropriate normal. Signs of inappropriate virilization in women or children following secondary exposure to topical testosterone should be brought to the attention of a healthcare provider. Topical testosterone products (gels and solution) may have different doses, strengths, or application instructions that may result in different systemic exposure; these products are not interchangeable. Use of the intranasal gel is not recommended in patients with sinus disease, mucosal inflammatory disorders (eg, Sjogren syndrome), or with a history of nasal disorders, nasal or sinus surgery, nasal fracture within the previous 6 months, or nasal fracture that caused a deviated anterior nasal septum. Safety and efficacy have not been established in males with a BM

>35 kg/m^2. Transdermal patch may contain conducting metal (eg, aluminum); remove patch prior to MRI. Gels, solution, transdermal, and buccal system have not been evaluated in males <18 years of age; safety and efficacy of injection have not been established in males <12 years of age. Some testosterone products may be chemically synthesized from soy. Some products may contain castor oil. Use of Axiron in males with BMI >35 kg/m2 has not been established. Anabolic steroids may be abused; abuse may be associated with adverse physical and psychological effects. Dependance may occur when used outside of approved dosage/indications.

Studies have suggested an increased risk of cardiovascular events among groups of men prescribed testosterone therapy (Basaria, 2010; Finkle, 2014; Vigen, 2013). The Endocrine Society suggests it may be prudent to avoid testosterone therapy in men who have experienced a cardiovascular event (eg, MI, stroke, acute coronary syndrome) in the past six months (The Endocrine Society, 2014). These risks are currently under review by the FDA (Drug Safety Communication, 2014).

Benzyl alcohol and derivatives: Some dosage forms may contain benzyl alcohol; large amounts of benzyl alcohol (≥99 mg/kg/day) have been associated with a potentially fatal toxicity ("gasping syndrome") in neonates; the "gasping syndrome" consists of metabolic acidosis, respiratory distress, gasping respirations, CNS dysfunction (including convulsions, intracranial hemorrhage), hypotension, and cardiovascular collapse (AAP, 1997; CDC, 1982); some data suggests that benzoate displaces bilirubin from protein binding sites (Ahlfors, 2001); avoid or use dosage forms containing benzyl alcohol with caution in neonates. See manufacturer's labeling. Testosterone cypionate should not be used interchangeably with testosterone propionate because of differences in duration of action. Potentially significant interactions may exist, requiring dose or frequency adjustment, additional monitoring, and/or selection of alternative therapy.

Warnings: Additional Pediatric Considerations Some dosage forms may contain propylene glycol; in neonates large amounts of propylene glycol delivered orally, intravenously (eg, >3,000 mg/day), or topically have been associated with potentially fatal toxicities which can include metabolic acidosis, seizures, renal failure, and CNS depression; toxicities have also been reported in children and adults including hyperosmolality, lactic acidosis, seizures and respiratory depression; use caution (AAP, 1997; Shehab, 2009).

Adverse Reactions

Cardiovascular: Decreased blood pressure, deep vein thrombosis, edema, hypertension, increased blood pressure, vasodilatation

Central nervous system: Abnormal dreams, aggressive behavior, altered sense of smell, amnesia, anxiety, chills, depression, dizziness, emotional lability, excitement, fatigue, headache, hostility, insomnia, irritability, malaise, mood swings, nervousness, outbursts of anger, paresthesia, seizure, sleep apnea, suicidal ideation, taste disorder

Dermatologic: Acne vulgaris, alopecia, contact dermatitis, diaphoresis, erythema, folliculitis, hair discoloration, hyperhidrosis, pruritus, seborrhea, skin rash, xeroderma

Endocrine & metabolic: Change in libido, decreased gonadotropin, fluid retention, gynecomastia, hirsutism (increase in pubic hair growth), hot flash, hypercalcemia, hyperchloremia, hypercholesterolemia, hyperglycemia, hyperkalemia, hyperlipidemia, hypernatremia, hypoglycemia, hypokalemia, increased plasma estradiol concentration, inorganic phosphate retention, menstrual disease (including amenorrhea), weight gain

Gastrointestinal: Diarrhea, gastroesophageal reflux disease, gastrointestinal hemorrhage, gastrointestinal irritation, increased appetite, nausea, vomiting

Following buccal administration (most common): Dysgeusia, gingival pain, gingival swelling, mouth irritation (including gums), unpleasant taste

Genitourinary: Benign prostatic hypertrophy, difficulty in micturition, ejaculatory disorder, hematuria, impotence, irritable bladder, mastalgia, oligospermia, priapism, prostate induration, prostate specific antigen increase, prostatitis, spontaneous erections, testicular atrophy, urinary tract infection, virilization

Hepatic: Abnormal hepatic function tests, cholestatic hepatitis, cholestatic jaundice, hepatic insufficiency, hepatic necrosis, hepatocellular neoplasms, increased serum bilirubin, peliosis hepatis

Hematologic & oncologic: Anemia, clotting factors suppression, hemorrhage, increased hematocrit, increased hemoglobin, leukopenia, malignant neoplasm of prostate, polycythemia, prostate carcinoma

Hypersensitivity: Anaphylactoid reaction, hypersensitivity reaction (including pulmomary oil microembolism)

Local: Application site reaction (gel, solution), erythema at injection site, inflammation at injection site, pain at injection site

Transdermal system: Application site burning, application site erythema, application site induration, application site pruritus, application site vesicles (including burn-like blisters under system), local allergic contact dermatitis, local skin exfoliation

Neuromuscular & skeletal: Abnormal bone growth (accelerated), arthralgia, back pain, hemarthrosis, hyperkinesia, weakness

Ophthalmic: Increased lacrimation

Renal: Increased serum creatinine, polyuria

Respiratory: Bronchitis (≥3%), nasopharyngitis (≥3%), sinusitis (≥3%), upper respiratory tract infection (≥3%), dyspnea

Rare but important or life-threatening: Injection, gel: Abnormal erythropoiesis, abscess at injection site, anaphylaxis, androgenetic alopecia, asthma, cardiac arrest, cardiac failure, cerebrovascular accident, chronic obstructive pulmonary disease, cognitive dysfunction, diabetes mellitus, epididymitis, hearing loss (sudden), hematoma at injection site, hepatotoxicity (idiosyncratic) (Chalasani, 2014), hyperparathyroidism, hypersensitivity angiitis, increased intraocular pressure, Korsakoff's psychosis (nonalcoholic), migraine, myocardial infarction, personality disorder, prolonged prothrombin time, prostatic intraepithelial neoplasia, reversible ischemic neurological deficit, spermatocele, systemic lupus erythematosus, tachycardia, thrombocytopenia, thrombosis, urinary incontinence, venous insufficiency, vesicobullous rash, virilization (of children, following secondary exposure to topical gel [advanced bone age, aggressive behavior, enlargement of clitoris requiring surgery, enlargement of penis, increased erections, increased libido, pubic hair development]), vitreous detachment

Drug Interactions

Metabolism/Transport Effects Substrate of CYP2B6 (minor), CYP2C19 (minor), CYP2C9 (minor), CYP3A4 (minor); **Note:** Assignment of Major/Minor substrate status based on clinically relevant drug interaction potential

Avoid Concomitant Use

Avoid concomitant use of Testosterone with any of the following: Dehydroepiandrosterone

Increased Effect/Toxicity

Testosterone may increase the levels/effects of: Blood Glucose Lowering Agents; C1 inhibitors; CycloSPORINE (Systemic); Vitamin K Antagonists

The levels/effects of Testosterone may be increased by: Corticosteroids (Systemic); Dehydroepiandrosterone

Decreased Effect There are no known significant interactions involving a decrease in effect.

Storage/Stability

Androderm: Store at 20°C to 25°C (68°F to 77°F). Do not store outside of pouch. Excessive heat may cause system to burst.

AndroGel 1%, AndroGel 1.62%, Axiron: Store at 25°C (77°F); excursions are permitted between 15°C and 30°C (59°F and 86°F).

Fortesta, Testim: Store at 20°C to 25°C (68°F to 77°F); excursions are permitted between 15°C and 30°C (59°F and 86°F). Do not freeze.

Aveed: Store at 25°C (77°F); excursions are permitted between 15°C and 30°C (59°F and 86°F) Store in original container.

Depo-Testosterone: Store at 20°C to 25°C (68°F to 77°F). Protect from light.

Natesto, Vogelxo: Store at 20°C and 25°C (68°F to 77°F); excursions are permitted between 15°C and 30°C (59°F and 86°F).

Striant: Store at 20°C to 25°C (68°F to 77°F). Protect from heat and moisture.

Testopel: Store in a cool location.

Mechanism of Action Principal endogenous androgen responsible for promoting the growth and development of the male sex organs and maintaining secondary sex characteristics in androgen-deficient males

Pharmacodynamics Duration (route and ester dependent): Cypionate and enanthate esters (IM administration) have the longest duration: ≤2-4 weeks; pellets: 3-4 months; gel: 24-48 hours

Pharmacokinetics (Adult data unless noted)

Absorption: Transdermal gel: ~10%

Protein binding: 98%, bound to sex hormone-binding globulin (40%) and albumin

Metabolism: Hepatic; forms metabolites including estradiol and dihydrotestosterone (DHT); both are active

Half-life: Variable: 10-100 minutes; Cypionate: IM: 8 days

Elimination: Urine (90%), feces (6%)

Dosing: Usual

Infants, Children ≥12 years, and Adolescents <18 years:

Note: Dosage and duration of therapy depend upon age, sex, diagnosis, patient's response to therapy, and appearance of adverse effects; in general total doses >400 mg/month are not required due to the prolonged action of the drug.

Delayed puberty: Children ≥12 years and Adolescents: Typically not recommended for use before 14 years of age (Palmert, 2012)

IM:

Manufacturer labeling: Enanthate: 50-200 mg every 2-4 weeks; usual duration 4-6 months; various regimens evaluated, some begin with high initial doses and taper down as puberty progresses, and others begin low and titrate upward to effect and then taper

Alternate dosing: Initial: Enanthate or cypionate: 50 mg/dose every 4 weeks for 3-6 months; may increase dose in 25-50 mg increments for another 3-6 months to effect; maximum dose: 100 mg; typical duration of therapy: 12 months; if no response or inadequate response after 1 year of treatment, diagnosis should be reconsidered and additional testing performed (Palmert, 2012)

Subcutaneous implant: Pellet: Usual range: 150-450 mg every 3-6 months; usual duration: 4-6 months; dosing typically on the lower end of range; various regimens have been used

Male hypogonadism: Children ≥12 years and Adolescents:

IM: Enanthate or cypionate:

Initiation of pubertal growth: 25-75 mg every 3-4 weeks, gradually titrate dose every 6-9 months to 100-150 mg; typical duration of initiation therapy 3-4 years (Han, 2010; Wales, 2011)

Maintenance therapy: 200-250 mg every 3-4 weeks; once expected adult height and adequate virilization achieved, may convert to other testosterone replacement dosage form (eg, patch, gel, etc) (Han, 2010; Wales, 2011)

Subcutaneous implant: Pellet:

Manufacturer's labeling: Usual range: 150-450 mg every 3-6 months; various regimens have been used

Alternate dosing: 8-10 mg/kg/dose every 6 months (Zacharin, 1997)

Multiple pituitary hormone deficiency (with microphallus): Limited data available: Infants: IM: Enanthate or cypionate: 25 mg every 4 weeks for 1-3 months

Adolescents ≥18 years and Adults:

Inoperable metastatic breast cancer (females): IM: Enanthate: 200-400 mg every 2-4 weeks

Hypogonadism or hypogonadotropic hypogonadism (males):

IM: Enanthate or cypionate: 50-400 mg every 2-4 weeks (FDA-approved dosing range); 75-100 mg/week or 150-200 mg every 2 weeks (Bhasin, 2010)

Subcutaneous implant: Pellet: 150-450 mg every 3-6 months

Topical:

Buccal: 30 mg twice daily (every 12 hours) applied to the gum region above the incisor tooth

Gel: Apply to clean, dry, intact skin. **Do not apply testosterone gel to the genitals.**

AndroGel® 1%: 50 mg applied once daily in the morning to the shoulder and upper arms or abdomen. Dosage may be increased to a maximum of 100 mg.

Dose adjustment based on testosterone levels:

Less than normal range: Increase dose from 50 mg to 75 mg or from 75 mg to 100 mg once daily

Greater than normal range: Decrease dose. Discontinue if consistently above normal at 50 mg daily

AndroGel® 1.62%: 40.5 mg applied once daily in the morning to the shoulder and upper arms. Dosage may be increased to a maximum of 81 mg

Dose adjustment based on testosterone levels:

>750 ng/dL: Decrease dose by 20.25 mg/day

350-750 ng/dL: Maintain current dose

<350 ng/dL: Increase dose by 20.25 mg/day

Fortesta™: 40 mg once daily in the morning. Apply to the thighs. Dosing range: 10-70 mg/day

Dose adjustment based on serum testosterone levels:

≥2500 ng/dL: Decrease dose by 20 mg/day

1250 to <2500 ng/dL: Decrease dose by 10 mg/day

500 and <1250 ng/dL: Maintain current dose

<500 ng/dL: Increase dose by 10 mg/day

Testim®: 5 g (containing 50 mg of testosterone) applied once daily (preferably in the morning) to the shoulder and upper arms. Dosage may be increased to a maximum of 10 g (containing 100 mg of testosterone) daily.

Dose adjustment based on testosterone levels:

Less than normal range: Increase dose from 5 g (50 mg testosterone) to 10 g (100 mg testosterone) once daily

Greater than normal range: Decrease dose. Discontinue if consistently above normal at 5 g (50 mg testosterone) daily

Solution (Axiron®): 60 mg once daily; dosage range 30-120 mg/day. Apply to the axilla at the same time each morning; do not apply to other parts of the body

Apply to clean, dry, intact skin. **Do not apply testosterone solution to the genitals.**

Dose adjustment based on serum testosterone levels:

>1050 ng/dL: Decrease 60 mg/day dose to 30 mg/day; if levels >1050 ng/dL persist after dose reduction discontinue therapy

<300 ng/dL: Increase 60 mg/day dose to 90 mg/day, or increase 90 mg/day dose to 120 mg/day

Transdermal system (Androderm®): **Note:** Initial dose is either 4 mg/day or 5 mg/day and dose adjustment varies as follows:

Initial: 4 mg/day (as one 4 mg/day patch; do **not** use two 2 mg/day patches)

Dose adjustment based on testosterone levels:

>930 ng/dL: Decrease dose to 2 mg/day

400-930 ng/dL: Continue 4 mg/day

<400 ng/dL: Increase dose to 6 mg/day (as one 4 mg/day and one 2 mg/day patch)

Initial: 5 mg/day (as one 5 mg/day or two 2.5 mg/day patches)

Dose adjustment based on testosterone levels:

>1030 ng/dL: Decrease dose to 2.5 mg/day

300-1030 ng/dL: Continue 5 mg/day

<300 ng/dL: Increase dose to 7.5 mg/day (as one 5 mg/day and one 2.5 mg/day patch)

Dosing conversion: If needed, patients may be switched from the 2.5 mg/day, 5 mg/day, and 7.5 mg/day patches as follows. Patch change should occur at their next scheduled dosing. Measure early morning testosterone concentrations ~2 weeks after switching therapy:

From 2.5 mg/day patch to 2 mg/day patch

From 5 mg/day patch to 4 mg/day patch

From 7.5 mg/day patch to 6 mg/day patch (one 2 mg/day and one 4 mg/day patch)

Delayed puberty (males):

IM: Enanthate: 50-200 mg every 2-4 weeks for a limited duration

Pellet (for subcutaneous implantation): 150-450 mg every 3-6 months

Dosing adjustment in renal impairment: No dosage adjustment provided in manufacturer's labeling (has not been studied). Use with caution; may enhance edema formation.

Dosing adjustment in hepatic impairment: No dosage adjustment provided in manufacturer's labeling (has not been studied). Use with caution; may enhance edema formation.

Administration Hazardous agent; use appropriate precautions for handling and disposal (NIOSH 2014 [group 3]).

Oral, buccal: Striant™: One mucoadhesive for buccal application (buccal system) should be applied to a comfortable area above the incisor tooth. Apply flat side of system on fingertip. Gently push the curved side against upper gum. Rotate to alternate sides of mouth with each application. Hold buccal system firmly in place for 30 seconds to ensure adhesion. The buccal system should adhere to gum for 12 hours. If the buccal system falls out, replace with a new system. If the system falls out within 4 hours of next dose, the new buccal system should remain in place until the time of the following scheduled dose. System will soften and mold to shape of gum as it absorbs moisture from mouth. Do not chew or swallow the buccal system; check to ensure buccal system is in place following toothbrushing, use of mouthwash, and consumption of food or beverages. The buccal system will not dissolve; gently remove by sliding downwards from gum; avoid scratching gum.

Parenteral: IM (cypionate, enanthate): Warming injection to room temperature and shaking vial will help redissolve crystals that have formed after storage. Administer by deep IM injection into the gluteal muscle.

Topical:

Transdermal patch: Androderm®: Apply patch to clean, dry area of skin on the back, abdomen, upper arms, or thigh. Do not apply to bony areas or parts of the body that are subject to prolonged pressure while sleeping or sitting. **Do not apply to the scrotum.** Avoid showering, washing the site, or swimming for 3 hours after application. Following patch removal, mild skin irritation may be treated with OTC hydrocortisone cream. A small amount of triamcinolone acetonide 0.1% cream may be applied under the system to decrease irritation; do not use ointment. Patch should be applied nightly. Rotate administration sites, allowing 7 days between applying to the same site.

Topical gel and solution: Apply to clean, dry, intact skin. Application sites should be allowed to dry for a few minutes prior to dressing. Hands should be washed with soap and water after application. **Do not apply testosterone gel or solution to the genitals.** Alcohol-based gels and solutions are flammable; avoid fire or smoking until dry. Testosterone may be transferred to another person following skin-to-skin contact with the application site. Strict adherence to application instructions is needed in order to decrease secondary exposure. Thoroughly wash hands after application and cover application site with clothing (ie, shirt) once gel or solution has dried, or clean application site thoroughly with soap and water prior to contact in order to minimize transfer. In addition to skin-to-skin contact, secondary exposure has also been reported following exposure to secondary items (eg, towel, shirt, sheets). If secondary exposure occurs, the other person should thoroughly wash the skin with soap and water as soon as possible.

AndroGel® 1%, AndroGel® 1.62%, Testim®: Apply (preferably in the morning) to clean, dry, intact skin of the shoulder and upper arms. AndroGel® 1% may also be applied to the abdomen; do not apply AndroGel® 1.62% or Testim® to the abdomen. Area of application should be limited to what will be covered by a short-sleeve t-shirt. Apply at the same time each day. Upon opening the packet(s), the entire contents should be squeezed into the palm of the hand and immediately applied to the application site(s). Alternatively, a portion may be squeezed onto palm of hand and applied, repeating the process until entire packet has been applied. Application site should not be washed for ≥2 hours following application of AndroGel® 1.62% or Testim®, or >5 hours for AndroGel® 1%.

AndroGel® 1% multidose pump: Prime pump 3 times (and discard this portion of product) prior to initial use. Each actuation delivers 12.5 mg of testosterone (4 actuations = 50 mg; 6 actuations = 75 mg; 8 actuations = 100 mg); each actuation may be applied individually or all at the same time. Application site should not be washed for >5 hours following application.

AndroGel® 1.62% multidose pump: Prime pump 3 times (and discard this portion of product) prior to initial use. Each actuation delivers 20.25 mg of gel (2 actuations = 40.5 mg; 3 actuations = 60.75 mg; 4 actuations = 81 mg); each actuation may be applied individually or all at the same time.

Axiron®: Apply using the applicator to the axilla at the same time each morning. Do not apply to other parts of the body (eg, abdomen, genitals, shoulders, upper arms). Avoid washing the site or swimming for 2 hours after application. Prior to first use, prime the applicator pump by depressing it 3 times (discard this portion of the product). After priming, position the nozzle over the applicator cup and depress pump fully one time; ensure liquid enters cup. Each pump actuation delivers testosterone 30 mg. No more than 30 mg (one pump) should be added to the cup at one time. The total dose should be divided between axilla (eg, 30 mg/day: Apply to one axilla only; 60 mg/day: Apply 30 mg to each axilla; 90 mg/day: Apply 30 mg to each axilla, allow to dry, then apply an additional 30 mg to one axilla; etc). To apply dose, keep applicator upright and wipe into the axilla; if solution runs or drips, use cup to wipe. Do not rub into skin with fingers or hand. If more than one 30 mg dose is needed, repeat process. Apply roll-on or stick antiperspirants or deodorants prior to testosterone. Once application site is dry, cover with clothing. After use, rinse applicator under running water and pat dry with a tissue. The application site and dose of this product are not interchangeable with other topical testosterone products.

Fortesta™: Apply to skin of front and inner thighs. Do not apply to other parts of the body. Use one finger to rub gel evenly onto skin of each thigh. Avoid showering, washing the site, or swimming for 2 hours after application. Prior to first dose, prime the pump by holding canister upright and fully depressing the pump 8 times (discard this portion of the product). Each pump actuation delivers testosterone 10 mg. The total dose should be divided between thighs (eg, 10 mg/day: Apply 10 mg to one thigh only; 20 mg/day: Apply 10 mg to each thigh; 30 mg/day: Apply 20 mg to one thigh and 10 mg to the other thigh; etc). Once application site is dry, cover with clothing. The application site and dose of this product are not interchangeable with other topical testosterone products.

Monitoring Parameters Periodic liver function tests, cholesterol, hemoglobin and hematocrit (prior to therapy, at 3-6 months, then annually); radiologic examination of wrist and hand every 6 months (when using in prepubertal children). Withhold initial treatment with hematocrit >50%, hyperviscosity, untreated obstructive sleep apnea, or uncontrolled severe heart failure. Monitor urine and serum calcium and signs of virilization in women treated for breast cancer. Serum glucose (may be decreased by testosterone, monitor patients with diabetes). Evaluate males for response to treatment and adverse events 3-6 months after initiation and then annually.

Bone mineral density: Monitor after 1-2 years of therapy in hypogonadal men with osteoporosis or low trauma fracture (Bhasin, 2010)

Adults:

PSA: In men >40 years of age with baseline PSA >0.6 ng/mL, PSA and prostate exam (prior to therapy, at 3-6 months, then as based on current guidelines). Withhold treatment pending urological evaluation in patients with palpable prostate nodule or induration or PSA >4 ng/mL or if PSA >3 ng/mL in men at high risk of prostate cancer (Bhasin, 2010).

Do not treat with severe untreated BPH with IPSS symptom score >19.

Serum testosterone: After initial dose titration (if applicable), monitor 3-6 months after initiating treatment, then annually

Injection: Measure midway between injections. Adjust dose or frequency if testosterone concentration is <400 ng/dL or >700 ng/dL (Bhasin, 2010)

AndroGel® 1%, Testim®: Morning serum testosterone levels ~14 days after start of therapy or dose adjustments

AndroGel® 1.62%: Morning serum testosterone levels after 14 and 28 days of starting therapy or dose adjustments and periodically thereafter

Androderm®: Morning serum testosterone levels (following application the previous evening) ~14 days after start of therapy or dose adjustments

Axiron®: Serum testosterone levels can be measured 2-8 hours after application and after 14 days of starting therapy or dose adjustments

Fortesta™: Serum testosterone levels can be measured 2 hours after application and after 14 and 35 days of starting therapy or dose adjustments

Striant®: Application area of gums; total serum testosterone 4-12 weeks after initiating treatment, prior to morning dose

Testopel®: Measure at the end of the dosing interval (Bhasin, 2010)

Reference Range Total testosterone, males:

12-13 years: <800 ng/dL
14 years: <1200 ng/dL
15-16 years: 100-1200 ng/dL
17-18 years: 300-1200 ng/dL
19-40 years: 300-950 ng/dL
>40 years: 240-950 ng/dL
Free testosterone, males: 9-30 ng/dL

Test Interactions Testosterone may decrease thyroxine-binding globulin, resulting in decreased total T_4; free thyroid hormone levels are not changed.

Controlled Substance C-III

Dosage Forms Excipient information presented when available (limited, particularly for generics); consult specific product labeling.

Cream, Transdermal:
First-Testosterone MC: 2% (60 g) [contains benzyl alcohol, sesame oil]

Gel, Nasal:
Natesto: 5.5 mg/actuation (7.32 g)

Gel, Transdermal:
AndroGel: 25 mg/2.5 g (1%) (2.5 g); 50 mg/5 g (1%) (5 g); 20.25 mg/1.25 g (1.62%) (1.25 g); 40.5 mg/2.5 g (1.62%) (2.5 g) [contains alcohol, usp]
AndroGel Pump: 12.5 mg/actuation (1%) (75 g); 20.25 mg/actuation (1.62%) (75 g) [contains alcohol, usp]
Fortesta: 10 mg/actuation (2%) (60 g) [odorless; contains propylene glycol, trolamine (triethanolamine)]
Testim: 50 mg/5 g (1%) (5 g) [contains alcohol, usp, propylene glycol, tromethamine]
Vogelxo: 50 MG/5GM (1%) (5 g) [contains alcohol, usp, tromethamine]
Vogelxo Pump: 12.5 mg/actuation (1%) (75 g) [contains alcohol, usp, tromethamine]
Generic: 25 mg/2.5 g (1%) (2.5 g); 50 mg/5 g (1%) (5 g); 10 mg/actuation (2%) (60 g); 12.5 mg/actuation (1%) (75 g); 50 MG/5GM (1%) (5 g)

Miscellaneous, Buccal:
Striant: 30 mg (60 ea)

Ointment, Transdermal:
First-Testosterone: 2% (60 g) [contains benzyl alcohol, butylated hydroxytoluene (bht), petrolatum, sesame oil]

Patch 24 Hour, Transdermal:
Androderm: 2 mg/24 hr (1 ea, 60 ea); 4 mg/24 hr (1 ea, 30 ea)

Pellet, Implant:
Testopel: 75 mg (10 ea, 100 ea)

Solution, Transdermal:
Axiron: 30 mg/actuation (90 mL)

Solution, Intramuscular, as cypionate:
Depo-Testosterone: 100 mg/mL (10 mL); 200 mg/mL (1 mL, 10 mL) [contains benzyl alcohol, benzyl benzoate]
Generic: 100 mg/mL (10 mL); 200 mg/mL (1 mL, 10 mL)

Solution, Intramuscular, as enanthate:
Generic: 200 mg/mL (5 mL)

Solution, Intramuscular, as undecanoate:
Aveed: 750 mg/3 mL (3 mL) [contains benzyl benzoate, castor oil (ricine oil)]

◆ **Testosterone Cypionate** *see* Testosterone *on page 2025*

◆ **Testosterone Enanthate** *see* Testosterone *on page 2025*

◆ **Testosterone Undecanoate** *see* Testosterone *on page 2025*

◆ **Tetanus and Diphtheria Toxoid** *see* Diphtheria and Tetanus Toxoids *on page 674*

Tetanus Immune Globulin (Human)

(TET a nus i MYUN GLOB yoo lin HYU man)

Related Information

Centers for Disease Control and Prevention (CDC) and Other Links *on page 2424*

Immunization Administration Recommendations *on page 2411*

Immunization Schedules *on page 2416*

Brand Names: US HyperTET S/D

Brand Names: Canada HyperTET S/D

Therapeutic Category Immune Globulin

Generic Availability (US) No

Use Prophylaxis for tetanus following injury in patients whose immunization for tetanus is incomplete or uncertain [FDA approved in pediatric patients (age not specified) and adults]

The Advisory Committee on Immunization Practices (ACIP) recommends passive immunization with tetanus immune globulin (TIG) for the following:

- Persons with a wound that is not clean or minor and who have received ≤2 or an unknown number of adsorbed tetanus toxoid doses (CDC/ACIP [Broder 2006]; CDC/ACIP [Kretsinger 2006]).
- Persons who are wounded in bombings or similar mass casualty events if no reliable history of completed primary vaccination with tetanus exists. In case of shortage, use should be reserved for persons ≥60 years of age and immigrants from regions other than Europe or North America (CDC/ACIP [Chapman 2008]).

Pregnancy Risk Factor C

Pregnancy Considerations Animal reproduction studies have not been conducted. Tetanus immune globulin and a tetanus toxoid containing vaccine are recommended by the ACIP as part of the standard wound management to prevent tetanus in pregnant women (CDC 57[RR6], 2008; CDC 62[7], 2013).

Contraindications There are no contraindications listed in the manufacturer's labeling.

Warnings/Precautions Hypersensitivity and anaphylactic reactions can occur; immediate treatment (including epinephrine 1:1000) should be available. Use caution in patients with isolated immunoglobulin A deficiency or a history of systemic hypersensitivity to human immunoglobulins. Use with caution in patients with thrombocytopenia or coagulation disorders; IM injections may be contraindicated. Product of human plasma; may potentially contain infectious agents which could transmit disease. Screening of donors, as well as testing and/or inactivation or removal of certain viruses, reduces the risk. Infections thought to be transmitted by this product should be reported to the manufacturer. Skin testing should not be performed as local irritation can occur and be misinterpreted as a positive allergic reaction. When used for the treatment of tetanus infection, TIG removes circulating toxin, but does not remove toxin bound to nerve endings (CDC 2012). Not for intravenous administration.

Adverse Reactions

Central nervous system: Temperature increased

Dermatologic: Angioneurotic edema (rare)

Local: Injection site: Pain, soreness, tenderness

Renal: Nephritic syndrome (rare)

Miscellaneous: Anaphylactic shock (rare)

Drug Interactions

Metabolism/Transport Effects None known.

Avoid Concomitant Use There are no known interactions where it is recommended to avoid concomitant use.

Increased Effect/Toxicity There are no known significant interactions involving an increase in effect.

Decreased Effect

Tetanus Immune Globulin (Human) may decrease the levels/effects of: Vaccines (Live)

Storage/Stability Store at 2°C to 8°C (26°F to 46°F). Do not use if frozen.

Mechanism of Action Provides passive immunity towards tetanus by supplying antibodies to neutralize the free form of toxins produced by *Clostridium tetani*.

Pharmacokinetics (Adult data unless noted)

Half-life elimination: Individuals with normal IgG concentration: ~23 days

Time to peak serum concentration: 2 days

Dosing: Neonatal

Prophylaxis of tetanus: IM: 250 units regardless of weight or age (Bradley 2015; CDC/ACIP [Chapman 2008]; *Red Book* [AAP 2012]); may also calculate 4 units/kg; however, most experts recommend using full vial dose.

Treatment of tetanus: IM: 3,000 to 6,000 units. Infiltration of part of the dose around the wound is recommended. Some experts recommend a lower 500 unit dose which appears to be as effective as higher doses and may cause less discomfort (Bradley 2015; *Red Book* [AAP 2012]; WHO 2010).

Dosing: Usual

Prophylaxis of tetanus:

Infants and Children <7 years: I.M.: 250 units regardless of weight or age (*Red Book* [AAP 2012]); may also calculate 4 units/kg; however, most experts recommend using full vial dose.

Children ≥7 years, Adolescents, and Adults: IM: 250 units as a single dose; may be increased to 500 units if there has been a delay in initiating prophylaxis or when the wound is considered very tetanus prone

Tetanus prophylaxis in wound management (CDC/ACIP [Broder 2006]): Infants, Children, Adolescents, and Adults: IM: Tetanus prophylaxis in patients with wounds should be based on if the wound is clean or contaminated and the immunization status of the patient. Wound management includes proper use of tetanus toxoid and/or tetanus immune globulin (TIG), wound cleaning, and (if required) surgical debridement and the proper use of antibiotics. Patients with an uncertain or incomplete tetanus immunization status should have additional follow-up to ensure a series is completed. Patients with a history of Arthus reaction following a previous dose of a tetanus toxoid-containing vaccine should not receive a tetanus toxoid-containing vaccine until >10 years after the most recent dose even if they have a wound that is neither clean nor minor. See table on next page.

Tetanus Prophylaxis Wound Management

History of Tetanus Immunization (Doses)	Clean, Minor Wounds		All Other Wounds[1]	
	Tetanus toxoid[2]	TIG	Tetanus toxoid[2]	TIG
Uncertain or <3 doses	Yes	No	Yes	Yes
3 or more doses	No[3]	No	No[4]	No

[1]Such as, but not limited to, wounds contaminated with dirt, feces, soil, and saliva; puncture wounds; wounds from crushing, tears, burns, and frostbite.

[2]Tetanus toxoid in this chart refers to a tetanus toxoid containing vaccine. For children <7 years old DTaP (DT, if pertussis vaccine contraindicated) is preferred to tetanus toxoid alone. For children ≥7 years of age, Adolescents, and Adults, Td preferred to tetanus toxoid alone; Tdap may be preferred if the patient has not previously been vaccinated with Tdap.

[3]Yes, if ≥10 years since last dose.

[4]Yes, if ≥5 years since last dose.

Abbreviations: **DT** = Diphtheria and Tetanus Toxoids (formulation for age ≤6 years); **DTaP** = Diphtheria and Tetanus Toxoids, and Acellular Pertussis (formulation for age ≤6 years; Daptacel®, Infanrix®); **Td** = Diphtheria and Tetanus Toxoids (formulation for age ≥7 years; Decavac®, Tenivac™); **TT** = Tetanus toxoid (adsorbed [formulation for age ≥7 years]); **Tdap** = Diphtheria and Tetanus Toxoids, and Acellular Pertussis (Adacel® or Boostrix® [formulations for age ≥7 years]); **TIG** = Tetanus Immune Globulin

Treatment of tetanus: Infants, Children, Adolescents, and Adults: IM: 3,000 to 6,000 units. Infiltration of part of the dose around the wound is recommended. Some experts recommend a lower 500 unit dose which appears to be as effective as higher doses and may cause less discomfort (Bradley 2015; *Red Book* [AAP 2012]; WHO 2010).

Dosing adjustment in renal impairment: There are no dosage adjustments provided in the manufacturer's labeling.

Dosing adjustment in hepatic impairment: There are no dosage adjustments provided in the manufacturer's labeling.

Administration IM: Administer into lateral aspect of mid-thigh or deltoid muscle of upper arm; not for IV administration. Avoid gluteal region due to risk of injury to sciatic nerve; if gluteal region is used, administer only in the upper outer quadrant. When administered for treatment of tetanus, may be infiltrated locally around the wound site. Do not administer tetanus toxoid and TIG in same syringe (toxoid will be neutralized); tetanus toxoid may be administered at the same time at a separate site. To prevent syncope-related injuries, adolescents and adults should be vaccinated while seated or lying down (NCIRD/ACIP 2011).

Dosage Forms Excipient information presented when available (limited, particularly for generics); consult specific product labeling.

Injectable, Intramuscular:

HyperTET S/D: 250 units/mL (1 ea)

◆ **Tetanus Toxoid** *see* Diphtheria and Tetanus Toxoids, Acellular Pertussis, Poliovirus and *Haemophilus* b Conjugate Vaccine *on page 679*

Tetanus Toxoid (Adsorbed)

(TET a nus TOKS oyd, ad SORBED)

Medication Safety Issues

Sound-alike/look-alike issues:

Tetanus toxoid products may be confused with influenza virus vaccine and tuberculin products. Medication errors have occurred when tetanus toxoid products have been inadvertently administered instead of tuberculin skin tests (PPD) and influenza virus vaccine. These products are refrigerated and often stored in close proximity to each other.

Related Information

Centers for Disease Control and Prevention (CDC) and Other Links *on page 2424*

Immunization Administration Recommendations *on page 2411*

Immunization Schedules *on page 2416*

Therapeutic Category Vaccine; Vaccine, Inactivated Bacteria

Generic Availability (US) Yes

Use Indicated as booster dose in the active immunization against tetanus when combined antigen preparations are not indicated (FDA approved in ages ≥7 years and adults). **Note:** Tetanus and diphtheria toxoids for adult use (Td) is the preferred immunizing agent for most adults and for children after their seventh birthday. Young children should receive trivalent DTaP (diphtheria and tetanus toxoids, and acellular pertussis vaccine) as part of their childhood immunization program, unless pertussis is contraindicated, then DT is warranted.

Pregnancy Risk Factor C

Pregnancy Considerations Animal studies have not been conducted. Inactivated bacterial vaccines have not been shown to cause increased risks to the fetus (CDC, 2011). The ACIP recommends vaccination in previously unvaccinated women or in women with an incomplete vaccination series, whose child may be born in unhygienic conditions. Tetanus immune globulin and a tetanus toxoid-containing vaccine are recommended by the ACIP as part of the standard wound management to prevent tetanus in pregnant women. Vaccination using Td is preferred.

Breast-Feeding Considerations Inactivated vaccines do not affect the safety of breast-feeding for the mother or the infant. Breast-feeding infants should be vaccinated according to the recommended schedules (CDC, 2011).

Contraindications Hypersensitivity to tetanus toxoid or any component of the formulation

Warnings/Precautions Avoid injection into a blood vessel; allergic reactions may occur; epinephrine 1:1000 must be available. Patients who are immunocompromised may have reduced response; may be used in patients with HIV infection. In general, household and close contacts of persons with altered immunocompetence may receive all age appropriate vaccines (CDC, 2011); inactivated vaccines should be administered ≥2 weeks prior to planned immunosuppression when feasible (Rubin, 2014). May defer elective immunization during febrile illness or acute infection. In patients with a history of severe local reaction (Arthus-type) following previous dose, do not give further routine or emergency doses of tetanus and diphtheria toxoids for 10 years. Use caution in patients on anticoagulants, with thrombocytopenia, or bleeding disorders (bleeding may occur following intramuscular injection). Use with caution if Guillain-Barré syndrome occurred within 6 weeks of prior tetanus toxoid. Syncope has been reported with use of injectable vaccines and may be accompanied by transient visual disturbances, weakness, or tonic-clonic movements. Procedures should be in place to avoid injuries from falling and to restore cerebral perfusion if syncope occurs. Contains thimerosal. In order to maximize vaccination rates, the ACIP recommends simultaneous administration of all age-appropriate vaccines (live or inactivated) for which a person is eligible at a single clinic visit, unless contraindications exist. The use of combination vaccines is generally preferred over separate injections, taking into consideration provider assessment, patient preference, and adverse events. When using combination vaccines, the minimum age for administration is the oldest minimum age for any individual component; the minimum interval between dosing is the greatest minimum interval between any individual component.

Vaccination may not result in effective immunity in all patients. Response depends upon multiple factors (eg, type of vaccine, age of patient) and may be improved by administering the vaccine at the recommended dose, route, and interval. Vaccines may not be effective if administered during periods of altered immune competence (CDC, 2011).

Warnings: Additional Pediatric Considerations Antipyretics have not been shown to prevent febrile seizures; antipyretics may be used to treat fever or discomfort following vaccination (CDC/ACIP [Kroger, 2011]). One study reported that routine prophylactic administration of acetaminophen to prevent fever prior to vaccination decreased the immune response of some vaccines; the clinical significance of this reduction in immune response has not been established (Prymula, 2009).

Adverse Reactions All serious adverse reactions must be reported to the U.S. Department of Health and Human Services (DHHS) Vaccine Adverse Event Reporting System (VAERS) 1-800-822-7967 or online at https://vaers.hhs.gov/esub/index.

Cardiovascular: Hypotension

Central nervous system: Brachial neuritis, fever, malaise, pain

Gastrointestinal: Nausea

Local: Edema, induration (with or without tenderness), rash, redness, urticaria, warmth

Neuromuscular: Arthralgia, Guillain-Barré syndrome

Miscellaneous: Anaphylactic reaction, Arthus-type hypersensitivity reaction

Drug Interactions

Metabolism/Transport Effects None known.

Avoid Concomitant Use There are no known interactions where it is recommended to avoid concomitant use.

Increased Effect/Toxicity There are no known significant interactions involving an increase in effect.

Decreased Effect

The levels/effects of Tetanus Toxoid (Adsorbed) may be decreased by: Belimumab; Fingolimod; Immunosuppressants; Meningococcal Polysaccharide (Groups A / C / Y and W-135) Tetanus Toxoid Conjugate Vaccine

Storage/Stability Store at 2°C to 8°C (26°F to 46°F); do not freeze.

Mechanism of Action Tetanus toxoid preparations contain the toxin produced by virulent tetanus bacilli (detoxified growth products of *Clostridium tetani*). The toxin has been modified by treatment with formaldehyde so that it has lost toxicity but still retains ability to act as antigen and produce active immunity; the aluminum salt, a mineral adjuvant, delays the rate of absorption and prolongs and enhances its properties; duration ~10 years.

Pharmacodynamics Duration: Primary immunization: ~10 years

Dosing: Usual

Children ≥7 years, Adolescents, and Adults:

Primary immunization: Not indicated for this use; combined antigen vaccines are recommended. **Note:** In most patients, Td is the recommended product for primary immunization, booster doses, and tetanus immunization in wound management (refer to Diphtheria and Tetanus Toxoid monograph):

Booster doses: I.M: 0.5 mL every 10 years

Tetanus prophylaxis in wound management: Tetanus prophylaxis in patients with wounds should consider if the wound is clean or contaminated, the immunization status of the patient, proper use of tetanus toxoid and/or tetanus immune globulin (TIG), wound cleaning, and (if required) surgical debridement and the proper use of antibiotics. Patients with an uncertain or incomplete tetanus immunization status should have additional follow-up to ensure a series is completed. Patients with a history of Arthus reaction following a previous dose of a tetanus toxoid-containing vaccine should not receive a tetanus toxoid-containing vaccine until >10 years after the most recent dose even if they have a wound that is neither clean nor minor. See table.

Tetanus Prophylaxis Wound Management

History of Tetanus Immunization (Doses)	Clean, Minor Wounds		All Other Wounds[1]	
	Tetanus toxoid[2]	TIG	Tetanus toxoid[2]	TIG
Uncertain or <3 doses	Yes	No	Yes	Yes
3 or more doses	No[3]	No	No[4]	No

[1]Such as, but not limited to, wounds contaminated with dirt, feces, soil, and saliva; puncture wounds; wounds from crushing, tears, burns, and frostbite.

[2]Tetanus toxoid in this chart refers to a tetanus toxoid containing vaccine. For children <7 years old DTaP (DT, if pertussis vaccine contraindicated) is preferred to tetanus toxoid alone. For children ≥7 years of age and Adults, Td preferred to tetanus toxoid alone; Tdap may be preferred if the patient has not previously been vaccinated with Tdap.

[3]Yes, if ≥10 years since last dose.

[4]Yes, if ≥ 5 years since last dose.

Abbreviations: **DT** = Diphtheria and Tetanus Toxoids (formulation for age ≤6 years); **DTaP** = Diphtheria and Tetanus Toxoids, and Acellular Pertussis (formulation for age ≤6 years; Daptacel®, Infanrix®); **Td** = Diphtheria and Tetanus Toxoids (formulation for age ≥7 years; Decavac®, Tenivac™); **TT** = Tetanus toxoid (adsorbed [formulation for age ≥7 years]); **Tdap** = Diphtheria and Tetanus Toxoids, and Acellular Pertussis (Adacel® or Boostrix® [formulations for age ≥7 years]); **TIG** = Tetanus Immune Globulin

Adapted from the Yellow Book 2010, Chapter 2, *Routine Vaccine-Preventable Diseases, Tetanus*; Available at www.cdc.gov/yellowbook; and *MMWR*, 2006, 55:RR-17.

Administration IM: Shake well prior to use. Administer into lateral aspect of midthigh or deltoid muscle of upper arm; may be administered SubQ if intramuscular route cannot be used; **not for IV administration**. Adolescents and adults should be vaccinated while seated or lying down. U.S. law requires that the date of administration, the vaccine manufacturer, lot number of vaccine, and the administering person's name, title, and address be entered into the patient's permanent medical record.

Monitoring Parameters Observe for syncope for 15 minutes following administration. If seizure-like activity associated with syncope occurs, maintain patient in supine or Trendelenburg position to reestablish adequate cerebral perfusion.

Additional Information In order to maximize vaccination rates, the ACIP recommends simultaneous administration (ie, >1 vaccine on the same day at different anatomic sites) of all age-appropriate vaccines (live or inactivated) for which a person is eligible at a single visit, unless contraindications exist. If available, the use of combination vaccines is generally preferred over separate injections, taking into consideration provider assessment, patient preference, and potential adverse events. If separate vaccines being used, evaluate product information regarding same syringe compatibility of vaccines. Separate needles and syringes should be used for each injection. The ACIP prefers each dose of specific vaccine in a series come from the same manufacturer if possible (CDC, 2011).

For additional information, please refer to the following website: http://www.cdc.gov/vaccines/vpd-vac/.

Dosage Forms Excipient information presented when available (limited, particularly for generics); consult specific product labeling. [DSC] = Discontinued product

Solution, Intramuscular:

Generic: 5 units (0.5 mL [DSC])

- ◆ **Tetanus Toxoid, Reduced Diphtheria Toxoid, and Acellular Pertussis, Adsorbed** *see* Diphtheria and Tetanus Toxoids, and Acellular Pertussis Vaccine *on page* 681
- ◆ **Tetcaine** *see* Tetracaine (Ophthalmic) *on page* 2034

Tetracaine (Systemic) (TET ra kane)

Brand Names: Canada Pontocaine
Therapeutic Category Local Anesthetic, Injectable
Generic Availability (US) Yes
Use Spinal anesthesia
Pregnancy Risk Factor C
Pregnancy Considerations Animal reproduction studies have not been conducted.
Breast-Feeding Considerations It is not known if tetracaine (systemic) is excreted in breast milk. The manufacturer recommends that caution be exercised when administering tetracaine (systemic) to nursing women.
Contraindications Hypersensitivity to tetracaine, ester-type anesthetics, aminobenzoic acid, or any component of the formulation; injection should not be used when spinal anesthesia is contraindicated
Warnings/Precautions Use with caution in patients with cardiac disease (especially rhythm disturbances, heart block, or shock), hyperthyroidism, and abnormal or decreased levels of plasma esterases. Use of the lowest effective dose is recommended. Acutely ill, elderly, debilitated, obstetric patients, or patients with increased intra-abdominal pressure may require decreased doses. Dental practitioners and/or clinicians using local anesthetic agents should be well-trained in diagnosis and management of emergencies that may arise from the use of these agents. Resuscitative equipment, oxygen, and other resuscitative drugs should be available for immediate use.
Adverse Reactions Note: Adverse effects listed are those characteristics of local anesthetics. Systemic adverse effects are generally associated with excessive doses or rapid absorption.
Cardiovascular: Cardiac arrest, hypotension
Central nervous system: Chills, convulsions, dizziness, drowsiness, nervousness, unconsciousness
Dermatologic: Urticaria
Gastrointestinal: Nausea, vomiting
Hematologic: Methemoglobinemia
Neuromuscular & skeletal: Tremors
Ocular: Blurred vision, pupil constriction
Otic: Tinnitus
Respiratory: Respiratory arrest
Miscellaneous: Allergic reaction, anaphylaxis
Drug Interactions
Metabolism/Transport Effects None known.
Avoid Concomitant Use There are no known interactions where it is recommended to avoid concomitant use.
Increased Effect/Toxicity
The levels/effects of Tetracaine (Systemic) may be increased by: Hyaluronidase
Decreased Effect
Tetracaine (Systemic) may decrease the levels/effects of: Technetium Tc 99m Tilmanocept
Storage/Stability Store solution under refrigeration. Protect from light.
Mechanism of Action Ester local anesthetic blocks both the initiation and conduction of nerve impulses by decreasing the neuronal membrane's permeability to sodium ions, which results in inhibition of depolarization with resultant blockade of conduction
Pharmacodynamics Duration: 1.5-3 hours
Pharmacokinetics (Adult data unless noted)
Metabolism: By the liver
Elimination: Metabolites are renally excreted
Dosing: Usual
Children: Safety and efficacy have not been established
Adults:
Injection: Dosage varies with the anesthetic procedure, the degree of anesthesia required, and the individual patient response; it is administered by subarachnoid injection for spinal anesthesia. High, medium, low, or saddle blocks use 0.2% or 0.3% solution. Prolonged effect (2-3 hours): Use 1% solution (a 1% solution should be diluted with an equal volume of CSF before administration)
Perineal anesthesia: 5 mg
Perineal and lower extremities: 10 mg
Anesthesia extending up to the costal margin: 15-20 mg
Low spinal anesthesia (saddle block): 2-5 mg
Preparation for Administration Solution: Hyperbaric solution: May be made by mixing equal volumes of the 1% solution and $D_{10}W$.
Administration Subarachnoid administration by experienced individuals only
Dosage Forms Excipient information presented when available (limited, particularly for generics); consult specific product labeling.
Solution, Injection, as hydrochloride [preservative free]:
Generic: 1% (2 mL)

Tetracaine (Ophthalmic) (TET ra kane)

Brand Names: US Altacaine; Tetcaine; TetraVisc; TetraVisc Forte
Therapeutic Category Local Anesthetic, Ophthalmic
Generic Availability (US) Yes
Use Local anesthesia for various ophthalmic procedures of short duration (eg, tonometry, gonioscopy), minor ophthalmic surgical procedures (eg, removal of corneal foreign bodies, suture removal), and for various diagnostic purposes (eg, conjunctival scrapings) (FDA approved in adults)
Pregnancy Risk Factor C
Pregnancy Considerations Animal reproduction studies have not been conducted.
Breast-Feeding Considerations It is not known if tetracaine (ophthalmic) is excreted in breast milk. The manufacturer recommends that caution be exercised when administering tetracaine (ophthalmic) to nursing women.
Contraindications Hypersensitivity to tetracaine or any component of the formulation
Warnings/Precautions For ophthalmic use only. May delay wound healing. Prolonged use is not recommended. The anesthetized eye should be protected from irritation, foreign bodies, and rubbing to prevent inadvertent damage. Immediate type allergic corneal reactions, characterized by epithelial keratitis/filament formation, necrotic epithelium sloughing, stromal edema, descemetitis, and iritis, have been reported rarely.

Some formulations may contain benzalkonium chloride which may be adsorbed by soft contact lenses; remove contacts prior to administration and wait 15 minutes before reinserting.
Adverse Reactions Ocular: Allergic corneal reaction (rare), burning (transient), chemosis, conjunctival redness (transient), lacrimation, photophobia, stinging (transient)
Drug Interactions
Metabolism/Transport Effects None known.
Avoid Concomitant Use There are no known interactions where it is recommended to avoid concomitant use
Increased Effect/Toxicity There are no known significant interactions involving an increase in effect.
Decreased Effect There are no known significant interactions involving a decrease in effect.
Storage/Stability Store at room temperature of 15°C to 30°C (59°F to 86°F). Protect from light; keep container closed tightly.
Mechanism of Action Ester local anesthetic blocks both the initiation and conduction of nerve impulses by decreasing the neuronal membrane's permeability to sodium

potassium, and other ions, which results in inhibition of depolarization with resultant blockade of conduction

Pharmacodynamics

Onset of action: Anesthetic effects: Within 30 seconds

Duration: 1.5-3 hours

Pharmacokinetics (Adult data unless noted)

Metabolism: Hepatic; detoxified by plasma esterases to aminobenzoic acid

Elimination: Urine

Dosing: Usual Adults:

Short-term (nonsurgical procedures) anesthesia: Instill 1-2 drops just prior to evaluation

Minor surgical procedures: Instill 1-2 drops every 5-10 minutes for up to 3 doses

Prolonged surgical procedures (such as cataract extraction): Instill 1-2 drops every 5-10 minutes for up to 5 doses

Administration Apply drops to conjunctiva of affected eye(s); avoid contact of bottle tip with skin or eye; finger pressure should be applied to lacrimal sac during and for 1-2 minutes after instillation to decrease risk of absorption and systemic reactions

Dosage Forms Excipient information presented when available (limited, particularly for generics); consult specific product labeling.

Solution, Ophthalmic, as hydrochloride:

Altacaine: 0.5% (1 ea, 15 mL, 30 mL)

Tetcaine: 0.5% (15 mL) [contains chlorobutanol (chlorobutol), edetate disodium]

TetraVisc: 0.5% (1 ea, 5 mL) [contains benzalkonium chloride]

TetraVisc Forte: 0.5% (1 ea, 5 mL) [contains benzalkonium chloride, edetate disodium]

Generic: 0.5% (1 mL, 2 mL, 15 mL)

Tetracaine (Topical) (TET ra kane)

Brand Names: Canada Ametop; Pontocaine

Therapeutic Category Analgesic, Topical; Local Anesthetic, Topical

Generic Availability (US) Yes

Use Local anesthesia for mucous membranes

Pregnancy Risk Factor C

Pregnancy Considerations Animal reproduction studies have not been conducted.

Contraindications Hypersensitivity to tetracaine, ester-type anesthetics, aminobenzoic acid, or any component of the formulation

Warnings/Precautions For topical use only. Use with caution in patients with cardiac disease, hyperthyroidism, and abnormal or decreased levels of plasma esterases. Use of the lowest effective dose is recommended. Use caution in acutely ill, elderly, debilitated, or obstetric patients. Dental practitioners and/or clinicians using local anesthetic agents should be well trained in diagnosis and management of emergencies that may arise from the use of these agents. Resuscitative equipment, oxygen, and other resuscitative drugs should be available for immediate use.

Adverse Reactions Note: Adverse effects listed are those characteristics of local anesthetics. Systemic adverse effects are generally associated with excessive doses or rapid absorption.

Cardiovascular: Cardiac arrest, hypotension

Central nervous system: Chills, convulsions, dizziness, drowsiness, nervousness, unconsciousness

Dermatologic: Urticaria

Gastrointestinal: Nausea, vomiting

Hematologic: Methemoglobinemia

Neuromuscular & skeletal: Tremors

Ocular: Blurred vision, pupil constriction

Otic: Tinnitus

Respiratory: Respiratory arrest

Miscellaneous: Allergic reaction, anaphylaxis

Drug Interactions

Metabolism/Transport Effects None known.

Avoid Concomitant Use There are no known interactions where it is recommended to avoid concomitant use.

Increased Effect/Toxicity There are no known significant interactions involving an increase in effect.

Decreased Effect There are no known significant interactions involving a decrease in effect.

Storage/Stability Store under refrigeration at 2°C to 8°C (36°F to 46°F).

Mechanism of Action Ester local anesthetic blocks both the initiation and conduction of nerve impulses by decreasing the neuronal membrane's permeability to sodium ions, which results in inhibition of depolarization with resultant blockade of conduction

Pharmacodynamics

Onset of action: Within 3 minutes when applied to mucous membranes

Duration: 1.5-3 hours

Pharmacokinetics (Adult data unless noted)

Metabolism: By the liver

Elimination: Metabolites are renally excreted

Dosing: Usual

Children: Safety and efficacy have not been established

Adults: Apply 2% solution as needed; do not exceed 20 mg (1 mL) per application

- ◆ **Tetracaine and Lidocaine** *see* Lidocaine and Tetracaine *on page 1266*
- ◆ **Tetracaine Hydrochloride** *see* Tetracaine (Ophthalmic) *on page 2034*
- ◆ **Tetracaine Hydrochloride** *see* Tetracaine (Systemic) *on page 2034*
- ◆ **Tetracaine Hydrochloride** *see* Tetracaine (Topical) *on page 2035*
- ◆ **Tetracosactide** *see* Cosyntropin *on page 539*

Tetracycline (tet ra SYE kleen)

Medication Safety Issues

Sound-alike/look-alike issues:

Tetracycline may be confused with tetradecyl sulfate

Achromycin may be confused with actinomycin, Adriamycin

Related Information

H. pylori Treatment in Pediatric Patients *on page 2358*

Oral Medications That Should Not Be Crushed or Altered *on page 2476*

Brand Names: Canada Apo-Tetra; Nu-Tetra

Therapeutic Category Acne Products; Antibiotic, Ophthalmic; Antibiotic, Tetracycline Derivative; Antibiotic, Topical

Generic Availability (US) Yes

Use

Children, Adolescents, and Adults: Treatment of Rocky Mountain spotted fever caused by susceptible *Rickettsia* or brucellosis

Adolescents and Adults: Presumptive treatment of chlamydial infection in patients with gonorrhea

Children >8 years, Adolescents, and Adults: Treatment of moderate to severe inflammatory acne vulgaris, Lyme disease, mycoplasmal disease or *Legionella*

Pregnancy Risk Factor D

Pregnancy Considerations Tetracyclines cross the placenta and accumulate in developing teeth and long tubular bones. Tetracyclines may discolor fetal teeth following maternal use during pregnancy; the specific teeth involved and the portion of the tooth affected depends on the timing and duration of exposure relative to tooth calcification. The pharmacokinetics of tetracycline are not altered in pregnant patients with normal renal function. Hepatic toxicity during pregnancy, potentially associated with tetracycline use, has been widely reported in the literature. As a class, tetracyclines are generally considered second-line antibiotics in pregnant women and their use should be avoided (Mylonas, 2011; Whalley, 1966; Whalley, 1970).

Breast-Feeding Considerations Tetracycline is excreted into breast milk (Matsuda, 1984). According to the manufacturer, the decision to continue or discontinue breast-feeding during therapy should take into account the risk of exposure to the infant and the benefits of treatment to the mother. Tetracycline binds to calcium. The calcium in the maternal milk will decrease the amount of tetracycline absorbed by the breast-feeding infant (Mitrano, 2009). Nondose-related effects could include modification of bowel flora.

Contraindications Hypersensitivity to tetracycline or any component of the formulation

Warnings/Precautions Use with caution in patients with renal or hepatic impairment (eg, elderly); dosage modification required in patients with renal impairment since it may increase BUN as an antianabolic agent. Hepatotoxicity has been reported rarely; risk may be increased in patients with preexisting hepatic or renal impairment. Pseudotumor cerebri has been reported with tetracycline use (usually resolves with discontinuation); outdated drug can cause nephropathy; use protective measure to avoid photosensitivity. Prolonged use may result in fungal or bacterial superinfection, including *C. difficile*-associated diarrhea (CDAD) and pseudomembranous colitis; CDAD has been observed >2 months postantibiotic treatment. May cause tissue hyperpigmentation, enamel hypoplasia, or permanent tooth discoloration; use of tetracyclines should be avoided during tooth development (children <8 years of age) unless other drugs are not likely to be effective or are contraindicated. Do not use during pregnancy. In addition to affecting tooth development, tetracycline use has been associated with retardation of skeletal development and reduced bone growth.

Warnings: Additional Pediatric Considerations Do not administer to children <8 years of age due to permanent discoloration of teeth and retardation of skeletal development and bone growth (risk being greatest for children <4 years and in those receiving high doses). Tetracyclines have been associated with increases in BUN secondary to antianabolic effects. Pseudotumor cerebri has been reported rarely in infants and adolescents; use with isotretinoin has been associated with cases of pseudotumor cerebri; avoid concomitant treatment with isotretinoin.

Adverse Reactions

Cardiovascular: Pericarditis

Central nervous system: Bulging fontanels in infants, increased intracranial pressure, paresthesia, pseudotumor cerebri

Dermatologic: Exfoliative dermatitis, photosensitivity, pigmentation of nails, pruritus

Gastrointestinal: Abdominal cramps, anorexia, antibiotic-associated pseudomembranous colitis, diarrhea, discoloration of teeth and enamel hypoplasia (young children), esophagitis, nausea, pancreatitis, staphylococcal enterocolitis, vomiting

Hematologic: Thrombophlebitis

Hepatic: Hepatotoxicity

Renal: Acute renal failure, azotemia, renal damage

Miscellaneous: Anaphylaxis, candidal superinfection, hypersensitivity reactions, superinfection

Drug Interactions

Metabolism/Transport Effects **Substrate** of CYP3A4 (major); **Note:** Assignment of Major/Minor substrate status based on clinically relevant drug interaction potential

Avoid Concomitant Use

Avoid concomitant use of Tetracycline with any of the following: BCG; BCG (Intravesical); Mecamylamine; Retinoic Acid Derivatives; Strontium Ranelate

Increased Effect/Toxicity

Tetracycline may increase the levels/effects of: Mecamylamine; Mipomersen; Neuromuscular-Blocking Agents; Porfimer; QuiNINE; Retinoic Acid Derivatives; Verteporfin; Vitamin K Antagonists

Decreased Effect

Tetracycline may decrease the levels/effects of: Atovaquone; BCG; BCG (Intravesical); BCG Vaccine (Immunization); Iron Salts; Penicillins; Sodium Picosulfate; Typhoid Vaccine

The levels/effects of Tetracycline may be decreased by: Antacids; Bile Acid Sequestrants; Bismuth Subcitrate; Bismuth Subsalicylate; Bosentan; Calcium Salts; CYP3A4 Inducers (Moderate); CYP3A4 Inducers (Strong); Dabrafenib; Deferasirox; Iron Salts; Lanthanum; Magnesium Salts; Mitotane; Multivitamins/Minerals (with ADEK, Folate, Iron); Multivitamins/Minerals (with AE, No Iron); Quinapril; Siltuximab; St Johns Wort; Strontium Ranelate; Sucralfate; Sucroferric Oxyhydroxide; Tocilizumab; Zinc Salts

Food Interactions Serum concentrations may be decreased if taken with dairy products. Management: Take on an empty stomach 1 hour before or 2 hours after meals to increase total absorption. Administer around-the-clock to promote less variation in peak and trough serum levels.

Storage/Stability Store at 20°C to 25°C (68°F to 77°F); protect oral forms from light. Use of outdated tetracyclines has caused a Fanconi-like syndrome (nausea, vomiting, acidosis, proteinuria, glycosuria, aminoaciduria, polydipsia, polyuria, hypokalemia).

Mechanism of Action Inhibits bacterial protein synthesis by binding with the 30S and possibly the 50S ribosomal subunit(s) of susceptible bacteria; may also cause alterations in the cytoplasmic membrane

Pharmacokinetics (Adult data unless noted)

Distribution: Widely distributed to most body fluids and tissues including ascitic, synovial and pleural fluids bronchial secretions; appears in breast milk; poor penetration into CSF

Absorption:

Oral: 75%

IM: Poor, with less than 60% of dose absorbed

Protein binding: 30% to 60%

Half-life: 6-12 hours with normal renal function and is prolonged with renal impairment

Time to peak serum concentration: Within 2-4 hours

Elimination: Primary route is the kidney, with 60% of a dose excreted as unchanged drug in urine, small amounts appear in bile

Dialysis: Slightly dialyzable (5% to 20%)

Dosing: Usual Oral:

Children >8 years: 25-50 mg/kg/day in divided doses every 6 hours; not to exceed 3 g/day

Adolescents and Adults: 250-500 mg/dose every 6-12 hours

Dosing adjustment in renal impairment:

CrCl 50-80 mL/minute: Administer every 8-12 hours

CrCl 10-50 mL/minute: Administer every 12-24 hours

CrCl <10 mL/minute: Administer every 24 hours

Administration

Oral: Administer 1 hour before or 2 hours after meals with adequate amounts of fluid; avoid taking antacids, calcium, iron, dairy products, or milk formulas within 3 hours of tetracyclines

Topical: Small amount of ointment should be applied to cleansed affected area.

Monitoring Parameters Renal, hepatic, and hematologic function tests; observe for changes in bowel frequency

Dosage Forms Excipient information presented when available (limited, particularly for generics); consult specific product labeling.

Capsule, Oral, as hydrochloride:

Generic: 250 mg, 500 mg

Extemporaneous Preparations A 25 mg/mL oral suspension may be made using capsules. Empty the contents of six 500 mg capsules into mortar. Add a small amount (~20 mL) of a 1:1 mixture of Ora-Sweet® and Ora-Plus® and mix to a uniform paste; mix while adding the vehicle in geometric proportions to **almost** 120 mL; transfer to a calibrated bottle, rinse mortar with vehicle, and add quantity of vehicle sufficient to make 120 mL. Label "shake well" and "refrigerate". Stable 28 days refrigerated.

Nahata MC, Pai VB, and Hipple TF, *Pediatric Drug Formulations*, 5th ed, Cincinnati, OH: Harvey Whitney Books Co, 2004.

- ◆ **Tetracycline Hydrochloride** *see* Tetracycline *on page 2035*
- ◆ **Tetra-Formula Nighttime Sleep [OTC]** *see* DiphenhydrAMINE (Systemic) *on page 668*
- ◆ **Tetrahydrobiopterin** *see* Sapropterin *on page 1900*
- ◆ **Tetrahydrocannabinol** *see* Dronabinol *on page 722*
- ◆ **Tetraiodothyronine and Triiodothyronine** *see* Thyroid, Desiccated *on page 2058*

Tetrastarch (TET ra starch)

Brand Names: US Voluven

Brand Names: Canada Volulyte; Voluven

Therapeutic Category Plasma Volume Expander, Colloid

Generic Availability (US) No

Use Treatment and prophylaxis of hypovolemia (FDA approved in all ages); **Note:** This is not a substitute for blood or plasma; does not have oxygen-carrying capacity.

Pregnancy Risk Factor C

Pregnancy Considerations Adverse events have been observed in animal reproduction studies.

Breast-Feeding Considerations It is not known if tetrastarch is excreted in breast milk. The manufacturer recommends that caution be exercised when administering tetrastarch to nursing women.

Contraindications Hypersensitivity to hydroxyethyl starch or any component of the formulation; renal failure with oliguria or anuria (not related to hypovolemia); dialysis; any fluid overload condition (eg, pulmonary edema, congestive heart failure); severe hypernatremia; severe hyperchloremia; patients with intracranial bleeding; critically ill adult patients, including patients with sepsis, due to increased risk of mortality and renal replacement therapy; severe liver disease; preexisting coagulation or bleeding disorders.

Warnings/Precautions [U.S. Boxed Warning]: HES solutions have been associated with mortality and renal injury requiring renal replacement therapy in critically-ill patients, including patients with sepsis; avoid use in critically-ill adult patients, including those with sepsis. Use should also be avoided in patients admitted to the ICU (Brunkhorst, 2008; Perel, 2011; Perner, 2012; Zarychanski, 2009). The Society of Critical Care Medicine (SCCM) also recommends against the use of HES solutions for fluid resuscitation of severe sepsis and septic shock; crystalloids (eg, sodium chloride) are recommended instead (Dellinger, 2013). If used in patients who are not critically ill, avoid use in patients with preexisting renal dysfunction and discontinue use at the first sign of renal injury. Since the need for renal replacement therapy has been reported up to 90 days after HES administration, continue to monitor renal function in all patients for at least 90 days.

Monitor the coagulation status in patients undergoing open heart surgery in association with cardiopulmonary bypass. HES solutions have been associated with excess bleeding in these patients. If used in other patient populations, discontinue use of HES at the first sign of coagulopathy. Use is contraindicated in patients with preexisting coagulation or bleeding disorders. Large volumes of pentastarch may cause reduction in hemoglobin concentration, coagulation factors, and other plasma proteins due to hemodilution; coagulation may be impaired (eg, prolonged PT, PTT, and clotting times) and a transient prolongation of bleeding time may be observed. Use caution in severe bleeding disorders (eg, von Willebrand's disease); may increase the risk of more bleeding. Use with caution in patients with active hemorrhage.

Anaphylactoid reactions have occurred; discontinue use immediately with signs of hypersensitivity and administer appropriate therapy. Use with caution in patients at risk from overexpansion of blood volume, including the very young or elderly patients; use is contraindicated in heart failure or any preexisting condition where volume overload is a potential concern. Adjust the dosage in patients with preexisting cardiac dysfunction. Use is contraindicated with oliguria or anuria unrelated to hypovolemia or patients receiving hemodialysis. Monitor liver function at baseline and periodically during treatment. Use is contraindicated in patients with severe liver disease; may result in further reduction of coagulation factors, increasing the risk of bleeding. Large volumes of tetrastarch may cause a reduction in hemoglobin concentration, coagulation factors, and other plasma proteins due to hemodilution; coagulation may be impaired (eg, prolonged PT, PTT, and clotting times) and a transient prolongation of bleeding time may be observed. May cause temporarily elevated serum amylase levels and interfere with pancreatitis diagnosis. Not a substitute for red blood cells or coagulation factors. Severely dehydrated patients should be infused with a sufficient volume of crystalloid solution prior to administering tetrastarch.

Warnings: Additional Pediatric Considerations HES use has also been associated with acute kidney injury in pediatric patients (Reinhart, 2012).

Adverse Reactions

Dermatologic: Pruritus (dose dependent; may be delayed), skin rash

Gastrointestinal: Increased serum amylase

Hematologic & oncologic: Anemia, coagulation time increased, decreased clotting factors, decreased hematocrit, prolonged prothrombin time, wound hemorrhage

Rare but important or life-threatening: Acute renal failure, anaphylactoid reaction, anaphylaxis, bradycardia, bronchospasm, circulatory shock, flu-like symptoms, hypersensitivity reaction, hypotension, non-cardiogenic pulmonary edema, shock, tachycardia

Drug Interactions

Metabolism/Transport Effects None known.

Avoid Concomitant Use There are no known interactions where it is recommended to avoid concomitant use.

Increased Effect/Toxicity There are no known significant interactions involving an increase in effect.

Decreased Effect There are no known significant interactions involving a decrease in effect.

Storage/Stability Store at 15°C to 25°C (59°F to 77°F); do not freeze.

Mechanism of Action Produces plasma volume expansion by virtue of its highly colloidal starch structure

Pharmacodynamics Duration of action: ≥6 hours

Pharmacokinetics (Adult data unless noted)

Distribution: 5.9 L

Metabolism: Molecules >50,000 daltons are metabolized by plasma α-amylase

Half-life: 12 hours

Elimination: Urine [smaller hydroxyethyl starch (<50,000 daltons) unchanged, metabolites]

Clearance: 31.4 mL/minute

Dosing: Neonatal Note: With severe dehydration, administer crystalloid first. Dose and rate of infusion dependent on amount of blood lost, on maintenance or restoration of hemodynamics, and on amount of hemodilution. Titrate to individual colloid needs, hemodynamics, and hydration status. Do not use in critically ill patients, those undergoing open heart surgery with cardiopulmonary bypass, or those with preexisting renal dysfunction.

Volume expansion: IV infusion: Usual range: 7-25 mL/kg/dose; maximum daily dose: 50 mL/kg/**day**; in clinical trials of intraoperative use, a dose of 10 mL/kg/dose has been reported (Osthaus, 2008; Witt, 2008)

Dosing: Usual Note: With severe dehydration, administer crystalloid first. Dose and rate of infusion dependent on amount of blood lost, on maintenance or restoration of hemodynamics, and on amount of hemodilution. Titrate to individual colloid needs, hemodynamics, and hydration status. Do not use in critically ill patients, those undergoing open heart surgery with cardiopulmonary bypass, or those with preexisting renal dysfunction.

Infants, Children, and Adolescents: **Volume expansion:**

Infants and Children <2 years: IV infusion: Usual range: 7-25 mL/kg/dose; mean reported dose: 16 ± 9 mL/kg/dose; maximum daily dose: 50 mL/kg/**day**; in clinical trials of intraoperative use, a dose of 10 mL/kg/dose has been reported (Chong Sung, 2006; Osthaus, 2008; Witt, 2008).

Children 2-12 years: IV infusion: Usual range: 25-47 mL/kg/dose; mean reported dose: 36 ± 11 mL/kg/dose; maximum daily dose: 50 mL/kg/**day**; in clinical trials of intraoperative use, a dose of 10 mL/kg/dose has been reported (Chong Sung, 2006; Osthaus, 2008; Witt, 2008).

Adolescents >12 years: IV Infusion: Administer up to 50 mL/kg/**day** (or up to 3500 mL daily in a 70 kg patient); may administer repetitively over several days.

Adults: **Volume expansion:** IV infusion: Administer up to 50 mL/kg/**day** (or up to 3500 mL daily in a 70 kg patient); may administer repetitively over several days.

Dosing adjustment in renal impairment: Avoid use in patients with pre-existing renal dysfunction; discontinue use at the first sign of renal injury.

Dosing adjustment in hepatic impairment: No dosage adjustments provided in manufacturer's labeling; use with caution in severe impairment.

Administration Administer IV only; may be administered via infusion pump or pressure infusion; if administered by pressure infusion, air should be withdrawn or expelled from bag prior to infusion to prevent air embolus. Infuse the first 10-20 mL slowly to observe for anaphylaxis; have epinephrine and resuscitative equipment available. Change IV tubing at least once every 24 hours.

Monitoring Parameters Blood pressure, heart rate, capillary refill time, CVP, RAP, MAP; if pulmonary artery catheter in place, monitor cardiac index, PCWP, SVR, and PVR; hemoglobin, coagulation parameters, renal function (continue to monitor for at least 90 days after administration), urine output, acid-base balance

Test Interactions

Serum amylase levels may be temporarily elevated following administration; could interfere with the diagnosis of pancreatitis.

Administration of large volumes may result in decreased coagulation factors, plasma proteins, and /or hematocrit due to dilutional effect.

Additional Information Voluven®: 6% hetastarch (130/0.4) in 0.9% sodium chloride

Molecular weight: ~130,000

Sodium: 154 mEq/L

Chloride: 154 mEq/L

Osmolarity: 308 mOsm/L

Dosage Forms Excipient information presented when available (limited, particularly for generics); consult specific product labeling.

Solution, Intravenous:

Voluven: 6% (500 mL) [dehp free, latex free, pvc free]

◆ **TetraVisc** *see* Tetracaine (Ophthalmic) *on page 2034*

◆ **TetraVisc Forte** *see* Tetracaine (Ophthalmic) *on page 2034*

◆ **Teva-5 ASA (Can)** *see* Mesalamine *on page 1368*

◆ **Teva-Acyclovir (Can)** *see* Acyclovir (Systemic) *on page 61*

◆ **Teva-Alprazolam (Can)** *see* ALPRAZolam *on page 100*

◆ **Teva-Amiodarone (Can)** *see* Amiodarone *on page 125*

◆ **Teva-Amlodipine (Can)** *see* AmLODIPine *on page 133*

◆ **Teva-Atenolol (Can)** *see* Atenolol *on page 215*

◆ **Teva-Atomoxetine (Can)** *see* AtoMOXetine *on page 217*

◆ **Teva-Azathioprine (Can)** *see* AzaTHIOprine *on page 236*

◆ **Teva-Bosentan (Can)** *see* Bosentan *on page 294*

◆ **Teva-Buprenorphine/Naloxone (Can)** *see* Buprenorphine and Naloxone *on page 322*

◆ **Teva-Buspirone (Can)** *see* BusPIRone *on page 328*

◆ **Teva-Candesartan (Can)** *see* Candesartan *on page 358*

◆ **Teva-Carbamazepine (Can)** *see* CarBAMazepine *on page 367*

◆ **Teva-Cefadroxil (Can)** *see* Cefadroxil *on page 387*

◆ **Teva-Celecoxib (Can)** *see* Celecoxib *on page 418*

◆ **Teva-Cephalexin (Can)** *see* Cephalexin *on page 422*

◆ **Teva-Chlorpromazine (Can)** *see* ChlorproMAZINE *on page 443*

◆ **Teva-Ciprofloxacin (Can)** *see* Ciprofloxacin (Systemic) *on page 463*

◆ **Teva-Citalopram (Can)** *see* Citalopram *on page 476*

◆ **Teva-Clarithromycin (Can)** *see* Clarithromycin *on page 482*

◆ **Teva-Clindamycin (Can)** *see* Clindamycin (Systemic) *on page 487*

◆ **Teva-Clonazepam (Can)** *see* ClonazePAM *on page 506*

◆ **Teva-Clopidogrel (Can)** *see* Clopidogrel *on page 513*

◆ **Teva-Diclofenac (Can)** *see* Diclofenac (Systemic) *on page 641*

◆ **Teva-Diclofenac EC (Can)** *see* Diclofenac (Systemic) *on page 641*

◆ **Teva-Diclofenac K (Can)** *see* Diclofenac (Systemic) *on page 641*

◆ **Teva-Diclofenac SR (Can)** *see* Diclofenac (Systemic) *on page 641*

◆ **Teva-Diltiazem (Can)** *see* Diltiazem *on page 661*

◆ **Teva-Diltiazem CD (Can)** *see* Diltiazem *on page 661*

◆ **Teva-Diltiazem HCL ER Capsules (Can)** *see* Diltiazem *on page 661*

◆ **Teva-Docusate Sodium [OTC] (Can)** *see* Docusate *on page 697*

◆ **Teva-Doxazosin (Can)** *see* Doxazosin *on page 709*

◆ **Teva-Doxycycline (Can)** *see* Doxycycline *on page 717*

◆ **Teva-Efavirenz (Can)** *see* Efavirenz *on page 731*

◆ **Teva-Enalapril (Can)** *see* Enalapril *on page 744*

◆ **Teva-Escitalopram (Can)** *see* Escitalopram *on page 786*

◆ **Teva-Ezetimibe (Can)** *see* Ezetimibe *on page 832*

◆ **Teva-Famotidine (Can)** *see* Famotidine *on page 847*

◆ **Teva-Fentanyl (Can)** *see* FentaNYL *on page 857*

Thalidomide (tha LI doe mide)

Medication Safety Issues

Sound-alike/look-alike issues:

Thalidomide may be confused with flutamide, lenalidomide, pomalidomide

Thalomid may be confused with Revlimid, thiamine

High alert medication:

This medication is in a class the Institute for Safe Medication Practices (ISMP) includes among its list of drug classes that have a heightened risk of causing significant patient harm when used in error.

International issues:

Thalomid [US, Canada] may be confused with Thilomide brand name for lodoxamide [Greece, Turkey]

Related Information

Oral Medications That Should Not Be Crushed or Altered *on page 2476*

Prevention of Chemotherapy-Induced Nausea and Vomiting in Children *on page 2368*

Safe Handling of Hazardous Drugs *on page 2455*

Brand Names: US Thalomid

Brand Names: Canada Thalomid

Therapeutic Category Angiogenesis Inhibitor; Immunosuppressant Agent; Tumor Necrosis Factor (TNF) Blocking Agent

Generic Availability (US) No

Use Treatment of and suppressive maintenance therapy for cutaneous manifestations of moderate to severe erythema nodosum leprosum (ENL) (FDA approved in ages ≥12 years and adults); treatment of newly diagnosed multiple myeloma in combination with dexamethasone (FDA approved in adults). Has also been used for treatment of Crohn's disease/ulcerative colitis when other therapies have failed, refractory chronic graft-versus-host disease (cGVHD), AIDS-related aphthous stomatitis, systemic juvenile idiopathic arthritis (SJIA), and various malignancies.

Prescribing and Access Restrictions US: As a requirement of the REMS program, access to this medication is restricted. Thalidomide is approved for marketing only under a special distribution program, the Thalomid REMS (https://www.celgeneriskmanagement.com or 1-888-423-5436), which has been approved by the FDA. Prescribers, patients, and pharmacies must be certified with the program to prescribe or dispense thalidomide. No more than a 4-week supply should be dispensed. Blister packs should be dispensed intact (do not repackage capsules). Prescriptions must be filled within 7 days (for females of reproductive potential) or within 30 days (for all other patients) after authorization number obtained. Subsequent prescriptions may be filled only if fewer than 7 days of therapy remain on the previous prescription. A new prescription is required for further dispensing (a telephone prescription may not be accepted.) Pregnancy testing is required for females of childbearing potential.

Canada: Access to thalidomide is restricted through a controlled distribution program called RevAid. Only physicians and pharmacists enrolled in this program are authorized to prescribe or dispense thalidomide. Patients must be enrolled in the program by their physicians. Further information is available at www.RevAid.ca or by calling 1-888-738-2431.

Medication Guide Available Yes

Pregnancy Risk Factor X

Pregnancy Considerations [US Boxed Warning]: Thalidomide may cause severe birth defects or embryo-fetal death if taken during pregnancy. Thalidomide cannot be used in women who are pregnant or may become pregnant during therapy as even a single dose may cause severe birth defects. In order to decrease the risk of fetal exposure, thalidomide is available only through a special restricted distribution program (Thalomid REMS). Reproduction studies in animals and data from pregnant women have shown evidence of fetal abnormalities; use is contraindicated in women who are or may become pregnant. Anomalies observed in humans include amelia, phocomelia, bone defects, ear and eye abnormalities, facial palsy, congenital heart defects, urinary and genital tract malformations; mortality in ~40% of infants at or shortly after birth has also been reported.

Women of reproductive potential must avoid pregnancy 4 weeks prior to therapy, during therapy, during therapy interruptions, and for ≥4 weeks after therapy is discontinued. Two forms of effective contraception or total abstinence from heterosexual intercourse must be used by females who are not infertile or who have not had a hysterectomy. A negative pregnancy test (sensitivity of at least 50 mIU/mL) 10 to 14 days prior to therapy, within 24 hours prior to beginning therapy, weekly during the first 4 weeks, and every 4 weeks (every 2 weeks for women with irregular menstrual cycles) thereafter is required for women of childbearing potential. Thalidomide must be immediately discontinued for a missed period, abnormal pregnancy test or abnormal menstrual bleeding; refer patient to a reproductive toxicity specialist if pregnancy occurs during treatment.

Females of reproductive potential (including health care workers and caregivers) must also avoid contact with thalidomide capsules.

Thalidomide is also present in the semen of males. Males (even those vasectomized) must use a latex or synthetic condom during any sexual contact with women of childbearing potential and for up to 28 days following discontinuation of therapy. Males taking thalidomide must not donate sperm.

The parent or legal guardian for patients between 12 to 18 years of age must agree to ensure compliance with the required guidelines.

If pregnancy occurs during treatment, thalidomide must be immediately discontinued and the patient referred to a reproductive toxicity specialist. Any suspected fetal exposure to thalidomide must be reported to the FDA via the MedWatch program (1-800-FDA-1088) and to Celgene Corporation (1-888-423-5436). In Canada, thalidomide is available only through a restricted-distribution program called RevAid (1-888-738-2431).

Breast-Feeding Considerations It is not known if thalidomide is excreted in breast milk. Due to the potential for serious adverse reactions in the infant, a decision should be made to discontinue nursing or discontinue treatment with thalidomide, taking into account the importance of treatment to the mother. Use in breast-feeding women is contraindicated in the Canadian labeling.

Contraindications

Hypersensitivity to thalidomide or any component of the formulation; pregnancy

Canadian labeling: Additional contraindications (not in US labeling): Hypersensitivity to lenalidomide or pomalidomide; both females at risk of becoming pregnant and male patients who are unable to follow or comply with conditions for use (refer to manufacturer labeling); breast-feeding

Warnings/Precautions Hazardous agent - use appropriate precautions for handling and disposal (NIOSH 2014 [group 2]).

Avoid exposure to non-intact capsules and body fluids of patients receiving thalidomide. If exposure occurs, wash area with soap and water. Wear gloves to prevent cutaneous exposure.

[US Boxed Warning]: Thalidomide use for the treatment of multiple myeloma is associated with an increased risk for venous thromboembolism (VTE), including deep vein thrombosis (DVT) and pulmonary embolism (PE); the risk is increased when used in combination with standard chemotherapy agents, including dexamethasone. In one controlled study, the incidence of VTE was 22.5% in patients receiving thalidomide in combination with dexamethasone, compared to 4.9% for dexamethasone alone. Monitor for signs and symptoms of thromboembolism (shortness of breath, chest pain, or arm or leg swelling) and instruct patients to seek prompt medical attention with development of these symptoms. Consider thromboprophylaxis based on risk factors. Ischemic heart disease, including MI and stroke, also occurred at a higher rate (compared to placebo) in myeloma patients receiving thalidomide plus dexamethasone who had not received prior treatment. Assess individual risk factors for thromboembolism and consider thromboprophylaxis. The American Society of Clinical Oncology guidelines for VTE prophylaxis and treatment recommend thromboprophylaxis for patients receiving thalidomide in combination with chemotherapy and/or dexamethasone; either aspirin or low molecular weight heparin (LMWH) are recommended for lower risk patient and LMWH is recommended for higher risk patients (Lyman 2013). Anticoagulant prophylaxis should be individualized and selected based on the venous thromboembolism risk of the combination treatment regimen, using the safest and easiest to administer (Palumbo 2008). The Canadian labeling recommends anticoagulant prophylaxis for at least the first 5 months of thalidomide-based therapy. Monitor for signs/symptoms of thromboembolism and advise patients to seek immediate care if symptoms (shortness of breath, chest pain, arm/leg swelling) develop. Other medications that are also associated with thromboembolism should be used with caution.

May cause leukopenia and neutropenia; avoid initiating therapy if ANC $<750/mm^3$; monitor blood counts. Persistent neutropenia may require treatment interruption. Anemia and thrombocytopenia have also been observed. May cause bradycardia; use with caution when administering concomitantly with medications that may also decrease heart rate. May require thalidomide dose reduction or discontinuation. Stevens-Johnson syndrome (SJS) and toxic epidermal necrolysis (TEN) have been reported (may be fatal); withhold therapy and evaluate if skin rash occurs; permanently discontinue if rash is exfoliative, purpuric, bullous or if SJS or TEN is suspected. Hypersensitivity, including erythematous macular rash, possibly associated with fever, tachycardia and hypotension has been reported. May require treatment interruption for severe reactions; discontinue if recurs with rechallenge. Hepatotoxicity (primarily abnormal hepatic function tests although some serious and fatal cases of hepatic injury) has been observed usually within the first 2 months of treatment (Thalomid Canadian labeling 2015); most events resolved without intervention after discontinuing thalidomide.

Increased incidence of second primary malignancies (SPMs), including acute myeloid leukemia (AML) and myelodysplastic syndrome (MDS), has been observed in previously untreated multiple myeloma patients receiving thalidomide in combination with melphalan, and prednisone. In addition to AML and MDS, solid tumors have been reported with thalidomide maintenance treatment for multiple myeloma (Usmani 2012). Carefully evaluate patients for SPMs prior to and during treatment and manage as clinically indicated.

Thalidomide is commonly associated with peripheral neuropathy; may be irreversible. Neuropathy generally occurs following chronic use (over months), but may occur with short-term use; onset may be delayed. Use caution with other medications that may also cause peripheral neuropathy. Monitor for signs/symptoms of neuropathy monthly for the first 3 months of therapy and regularly thereafter. Electrophysiological testing may be considered at baseline and every 6 months to detect asymptomatic neuropathy. To limit further damage, immediately discontinue (if clinically appropriate) in patients who develop neuropathy. Reinitiate therapy only if neuropathy returns to baseline; may require dosage reduction or permanent discontinuation. Seizures (including grand mal convulsions) have been reported in postmarketing data; monitor closely for clinical changes indicating potential seizure activity in patients with a history of seizures, concurrent therapy with drugs that alter seizure threshold, or conditions that predispose to seizures. May cause dizziness, drowsiness, and/or somnolence; caution patients about performing tasks that require mental alertness (eg, operating machinery or driving). Avoid ethanol and concomitant medications that may exacerbate these symptoms; dose reductions may be necessary for excessive drowsiness or somnolence. May cause orthostatic hypotension; use with caution in patients who would not tolerate transient hypotensive episodes. When arising from a recumbent position, advise patients to sit upright for a few minutes prior to standing. Constipation may commonly occur. May require treatment interruption or dosage reduction. Certain adverse reactions (constipation, fatigue, weakness, nausea, hypokalemia, hyperglycemia, DVT, pulmonary embolism, atrial fibrillation) are more likely in elderly patients. In studies conducted prior to the use of highly active antiretroviral therapy, thalidomide use was associated with increased viral loads in HIV infected patients. Monitor viral load after the 1st and 3rd months of therapy and every 3 months thereafter. Patients with a high tumor burden may be at risk for tumor lysis syndrome; monitor closely; institute appropriate management for hyperuricemia.

Potentially significant drug-drug interactions may exist, requiring dose or frequency adjustment, additional monitoring, and/or selection of alternative therapy. Patients should not donate blood during thalidomide treatment and for 1 month after therapy discontinuation

[US Boxed Warning]: Thalidomide may cause severe birth defects or embryo-fetal death if taken during pregnancy. Thalidomide cannot be used in women who are pregnant or may become pregnant during therapy as even a single dose may cause severe birth defects. In order to decrease the risk of fetal exposure, thalidomide is available only through a special restricted distribution program (Thalomid REMS). Use is contraindicated in women who are or may become pregnant. Pregnancy must be excluded prior to therapy initiation with 2 negative pregnancy tests. Women of reproductive potential must avoid pregnancy 4 weeks prior to therapy, during therapy, during therapy interruptions, and for ≥4 weeks after therapy is discontinued; two reliable methods of birth control, or abstinence from heterosexual intercourse, must be used. Males taking thalidomide (even those vasectomized) must use a latex or synthetic condom during any sexual contact with women of childbearing potential and for up to 28 days following discontinuation of therapy. Males taking thalidomide must not donate sperm. Some forms of contraception may not be appropriate in certain patients. An intrauterine device (IUD) or implantable contraceptive may increase the risk of infection or bleeding; estrogen containing products may increase the risk of thromboembolism.

Due to the embryo-fetal risk, thalidomide is only available through a restricted program under the Thalomid REMS program. Prescribers and pharmacies must be certified with the program to prescribe or dispense thalidomide. Patients must sign an agreement and comply with the REMS program requirements.

Adverse Reactions

Cardiovascular: Edema, facial edema, hypotension, peripheral edema, thrombosis/embolism

Central nervous system: Agitation/anxiety, confusion, dizziness, fatigue, fever, headache, insomnia, malaise, motor neuropathy, nervousness, pain, sensory neuropathy, somnolence, vertigo

Dermatologic: Acne, dermatitis (fungal), desquamation, dry skin, maculopapular rash, nail disorder, pruritus, rash

Endocrine & metabolic: Hyperlipemia, hypocalcemia

Gastrointestinal: Anorexia, constipation, diarrhea, flatulence, nausea, oral moniliasis, tooth pain, weight gain/loss, xerostomia

Genitourinary: Impotence

Hematologic: Anemia, leukopenia, lymphadenopathy, neutropenia

Hepatic: AST increased, bilirubin increased, LFTs abnormal

Neuromuscular & skeletal: Arthralgia, back pain, muscle weakness, myalgia, neck pain/rigidity, neuropathy, paresthesia, tremor, weakness

Renal: Albuminuria, hematuria

Respiratory: Dyspnea, pharyngitis, rhinitis, sinusitis

Miscellaneous: Diaphoresis, infection

Rare but important or life-threatening: Acute renal failure, alkaline phosphatase increased, ALT increased, amenorrhea, angioedema, aphthous stomatitis, arrhythmia, atrial fibrillation, bile duct obstruction, bradycardia, BUN increased, carpal tunnel, cerebral vascular accident, CML, creatinine clearance decreased, creatinine increased, deafness, depression, diplopia, dysesthesia, ECG abnormalities, enuresis, eosinophilia, epistaxis, erythema multiforme, erythema nodosum, erythroleukemia, exfoliative dermatitis, febrile neutropenia, foot drop, galactorrhea, granulocytopenia, gynecomastia, hearing loss, hepatomegaly, Hodgkin's disease, hypercalcemia, hyper-/hypokalemia, hypersensitivity, hypertension, hyper-/hypothyroidism, hypersensitivity, hyperuricemia, hypomagnesemia, hyponatremia, hypoproteinemia, intestinal obstruction, intestinal perforation, interstitial pneumonitis, LDH increased, lethargy, leukocytosis, loss of consciousness, lymphedema, lymphopenia, mental status changes, metrorrhagia, MI, myxedema, nystagmus, oliguria, orthostatic hypotension, pancytopenia, paresthesia, petechiae, peripheral neuritis, photosensitivity, pleural effusion, prothrombin time changes, psychosis, pulmonary embolus, pulmonary hypertension, purpura, Raynaud's syndrome, renal failure, secondary malignancy (AML, MDS, solid tumors), seizure, sepsis, septic shock, sexual dysfunction, sick sinus syndrome, status epilepticus, Stevens-Johnson syndrome, stomach ulcer, stupor, suicide attempt, syncope, tachycardia, thrombocytopenia, toxic epidermal necrolysis, transient ischemic attack, tumor lysis syndrome, urticaria

Drug Interactions

Metabolism/Transport Effects None known.

Avoid Concomitant Use

Avoid concomitant use of Thalidomide with any of the following: Abatacept; Anakinra; Azelastine (Nasal); BCG; BCG (Intravesical); Canakinumab; Certolizumab Pegol; CloZAPine; CNS Depressants; Dipyrone; Natalizumab; Orphenadrine; Paraldehyde; Pimecrolimus; Rilonacept; Tacrolimus (Topical); Tocilizumab; Tofacitinib; Vaccines (Live); Vedolizumab

Increased Effect/Toxicity

Thalidomide may increase the levels/effects of: Abatacept; Alcohol (Ethyl); Anakinra; Azelastine (Nasal); Bisphosphonate Derivatives; Canakinumab; Certolizumab Pegol; CloZAPine; Leflunomide; Metyrosine; Natalizumab; Orphenadrine; Pamidronate; Paraldehyde; Pramipexole; Rilonacept; ROPINIRole; Rotigotine; Selective Serotonin Reuptake Inhibitors; Tofacitinib; Vaccines (Live); Vedolizumab; Zoledronic Acid

The levels/effects of Thalidomide may be increased by: Brimonidine (Topical); Cannabis; CNS Depressants; Contraceptives (Estrogens); Contraceptives (Progestins); Denosumab; Dexamethasone (Systemic); Dipyrone; Dronabinol; Erythropoiesis-Stimulating Agents; Estrogen Derivatives; Kava Kava; Magnesium Sulfate; Nabilone; Pimecrolimus; Roflumilast; Rufinamide; Tacrolimus (Topical); Tetrahydrocannabinol; Tocilizumab; Trastuzumab

Decreased Effect

Thalidomide may decrease the levels/effects of: BCG; BCG (Intravesical); Coccidioides immitis Skin Test; Sipuleucel-T; Vaccines (Inactivated); Vaccines (Live)

The levels/effects of Thalidomide may be decreased by: Echinacea

Storage/Stability Store at 20°C to 25°C (68°F to 77°F); excursions are permitted between 15°C and 30°C (59°F and 86°F). Protect from light. Keep in original package.

Mechanism of Action Immunomodulatory and antiangiogenic characteristics; immunologic effects may vary based on conditions; may suppress excessive tumor necrosis factor-alpha production in patients with ENL, yet may increase plasma tumor necrosis factor-alpha levels in HIV-positive patients. In multiple myeloma, thalidomide is associated with an increase in natural killer cells and increased levels of interleukin-2 and interferon gamma. Other proposed mechanisms of action include suppression of angiogenesis, prevention of free-radical-mediated DNA damage, increased cell mediated cytotoxic effects, and altered expression of cellular adhesion molecules.

Pharmacokinetics (Adult data unless noted)

Absorption: Slow, good

Distribution: V_d: 1.1 L/kg

Protein binding: 55% to 66%

Metabolism: Minimal (unchanged drug is the predominant circulating component)

Half-life elimination: 5.5 to 7.3 hours

Time to peak, plasma concentration: 2 to 5 hours

Elimination: Urine (92%; <4% of the dose as unchanged drug); feces (<2%)

Dosing: Usual

Pediatric:

AIDS-related aphthous stomatitis: Limited data available: Adolescents ≥13 years: Oral: 200 mg once daily at bedtime for 4 weeks or sooner if resolution. May be increased to 200 mg twice daily if no improvement after 4 weeks. Dosing based on double-blind, placebo-controlled trial by AIDS Clinical Trials Group (n=57, age: ≥13 years) which showed 55% healing in treatment group vs 7% in placebo (Jacobson, 1997).

Chronic graft-versus-host disease (refractory), treatment: Limited data available: Children ≥2 years and Adolescents: Oral: Initial: 3 to 6 mg/kg/**day** (maximum initial daily dose: 100 mg/**day**) at bedtime or in 2 to 4 divided doses before meals; may be adjusted at ≥2 week intervals based on patient response up to 12 mg/kg/**day** in 3 to 4 divided doses (maximum daily dose: 800 mg/**day**) (Browne, 2000; Rovelli, 1998; Wolff, 2011); one trial using initial doses of 3 mg/kg/dose every 6 hours (dose adjusted to attain goal thalidomide concentration of ≥5 mcg/mL 2 hours postdose) (Vogelsang, 1992)

Crohn's disease/ulcerative colitis (refractory), treatment: Limited data available: Children ≥1 year and Adolescents: Oral: 0.5 to 3 mg/kg/**day** (maximum daily dose: 300 mg/**day**), usually dosed once daily in the evening; titrate to lowest effective dose after remission is achieved (Facchini, 2001; Lazzerini, 2007; Martelossi, 2004; Zheng, 2011)

Erythema nodosum leprosum (ENL), cutaneous: Children ≥12 years and Adolescents: Oral:

Acute: Initial: 100 to 300 mg once daily at bedtime; continue until signs/symptoms subside (usually ~2 weeks), then taper off in 50 mg decrements every 2 to 4 weeks. For severe cases with moderate to severe neuritis, corticosteroids may be initiated with thalidomide (taper off and discontinue corticosteroids when neuritis improves).

Patients weighing <50 kg: Initiate at lower end of dosage range

Severe cutaneous reaction or patients previously requiring high doses: May be initiated or increased to 400 mg/day at bedtime or in divided doses

Maintenance (prevention/suppression, or with flares during tapering attempts): Maintain on the minimum dosage necessary to control the reaction; efforts to taper should be repeated every 3 to 6 months, in decrements of 50 mg every 2 to 4 weeks

Systemic juvenile idiopathic arthritis (SJIA): Limited data available: Children ≥3 years and Adolescents: Oral: Initial 2 mg/kg/**day**, if necessary may increase at 2-week intervals to 3-5 mg/kg/**day**. Data based on a multicenter, open-labeled prospective study (n=13, age: 3-23 years); within 4 weeks, 11 of 13 patients showed improvement in JRA scores, significant decreases in ESR, and significant increase in hemoglobin (Lehman, 2004).

Adult:

Erythema nodosum leprosum, acute cutaneous: Oral: Initial: 100 to 300 mg once daily at bedtime, continue until signs/symptoms subside (usually ~2 weeks), then taper off in 50 mg decrements every 2 to 4 weeks. For severe cases with moderate to severe neuritis, corticosteroids may be initiated with thalidomide (taper off and discontinue corticosteroids when neuritis improves).

Patients weighing <50 kg: Initiate at lower end of the dosing range

Severe cutaneous reaction or patients previously requiring high doses: May be initiated at up to 400 mg once daily at bedtime or in divided doses

Erythema nodosum leprosum, maintenance (prevention/suppression, or with flares during tapering attempts): Oral: Maintain on the minimum dosage necessary to control the reaction; efforts to taper should be repeated every 3 to 6 months, in decrements of 50 mg every 2 to 4 weeks

Multiple myeloma: Oral: 200 mg once daily at bedtime (in combination with dexamethasone)

Dosing adjustment for toxicity: Children, Adolescents, and Adults: ANC ≤750/mm^3: Withhold treatment if clinically appropriate

Multiple myeloma: Adults: Constipation, oversedation, peripheral neuropathy: Temporarily withhold or continue with a reduced dose

Peripheral neuropathy (Richardson, 2012):

Grade 1: Reduce dose by 50%

Grade 2: Temporarily interrupt therapy; once resolved to ≤ grade 1, resume therapy with a 50% dosage reduction (if clinically appropriate)

Grade 3 or higher: Discontinue therapy

Dosing adjustment for renal impairment: Children, Adolescents, and Adults: No adjustment is required for patients with renal impairment and on dialysis (per manufacturer). In a study of six adult patients with end-stage renal disease on dialysis, although clearance was increased by dialysis, a supplemental dose was not needed (Eriksson, 2003).

Multiple myeloma: Adult: An evaluation of 29 newly diagnosed adult myeloma patients with renal failure (serum creatinine ≥2 mg/dL) treated with thalidomide and dexamethasone (some also received cyclophosphamide) found that toxicities and efficacy were similar to patients with normal renal function (Seol, 2010). A study evaluating induction therapy with thalidomide and dexamethasone in 31 newly diagnosed adult myeloma patients with renal failure (CrCl <50 mL/minute), including 16 patients with severe renal impairment (CrCl <30 mL/minute) and seven patients on chronic hemodialysis found that toxicities were similar to patients without renal impairment and that thalidomide and dexamethasone could be administered safely (Tosi, 2009).

Dosing adjustment for hepatic impairment: There are no dosage adjustments provided in manufacturer's labeling (has not been studied); however, thalidomide does not appear to undergo significant hepatic metabolism.

Administration Hazardous agent; use appropriate precautions for handling and disposal (NIOSH 2014 [group 2]). Wear gloves to prevent cutaneous exposure. Do not open or crush capsules. Avoid extensive handling of capsules; capsules should remain in blister pack until ingestion. If exposed to the powder content from broken capsules or body fluids from patients receiving thalidomide, the exposed area should be washed with soap and water. Administer with water, preferably at bedtime, once daily on an empty stomach, at least 1 hour after the evening meal. Doses >400 mg/day may be given in 2 to 3 divided doses. For missed doses, if <12 hours have passed, patient may receive dose; if >12 hours have passed, wait until next dose is due.

Monitoring Parameters CBC with differential, platelets; thyroid function tests (TSH at baseline then every 2 to 3 months during thalidomide treatment [Hamnvik, 2011]). In HIV-seropositive patients: Viral load after 1 and 3 months, then every 3 months. Pregnancy testing (sensitivity of at least 50 mIU/mL) is required within 24 hours prior to initiation of therapy, weekly during the first 4 weeks, then every 4 weeks in women with regular menstrual cycles or every 2 weeks in women with irregular menstrual cycles. Signs of neuropathy monthly for the first 3 months, then periodically during treatment; consider monitoring of sensory nerve application potential amplitudes (at baseline and every 6 months) to detect asymptomatic neuropathy. Monitor for signs and symptoms of thromboembolism (shortness of breath, chest pain, arm/leg swelling), tumor lysis syndrome, bradycardia, and syncope; monitor for clinical changes indicating potential seizure activity (in patients with a history of seizure).

Reference Range Graft vs host disease: Therapeutic plasma thalidomide levels are 5 to 8 mcg/mL(Vogelsang, 1992), although it has been suggested that lower plasma levels (0.5 to 1.5 mcg/mL) may be therapeutic; peak serum thalidomide level after a 200 mg dose: 1.8 mcg/mL

Dosage Forms Excipient information presented when available (limited, particularly for generics); consult specific product labeling.

Capsule, Oral:

Thalomid: 50 mg, 100 mg

Thalomid: 150 mg, 200 mg [contains fd&c blue #2 (indigotine)]

Extemporaneous Preparations Hazardous agent; use appropriate precautions for handling and disposal (NIOSH 2014 [group 2]). When manipulating capsules, NIOSH recommends double gloving, a protective gown, and preparation in a controlled device; if not prepared in a controlled device, respiratory and eye protection, as well as ventilated engineering controls, are recommended (NIOSH, 2014).

A 20 mg/mL oral suspension may be prepared with capsules and a 1:1 mixture of Ora-Sweet and Ora-Plus. Empty the contents of twelve 100 mg capsules into a glass mortar. Add small portions of the vehicle and mix to a uniform paste; mix while adding the vehicle in incremental proportions to almost 60 mL; transfer to an amber calibrated bottle, rinse mortar with vehicle, and add quantity of vehicle sufficient to make 60 mL. Label "shake well," "protect from light," and "refrigerate". Stable for 35 days refrigerated.

Kraft S, Johnson CE, and Tyler RP, "Stability of an Extemporaneously Prepared Thalidomide Suspension," *Am J Health Syst Pharm*, 2011, 69(1):56-8.

- **Thalomid** *see* Thalidomide *on page 2040*
- **Tham** *see* Tromethamine *on page 2131*
- **THC** *see* Dronabinol *on page 722*
- **The Magic Bullet [OTC]** *see* Bisacodyl *on page 289*
- **The Magic Bullett [OTC] (Can)** *see* Bisacodyl *on page 289*
- **Theo-24** *see* Theophylline *on page 2044*
- **Theochron** *see* Theophylline *on page 2044*
- **Theo ER (Can)** *see* Theophylline *on page 2044*
- **Theolair (Can)** *see* Theophylline *on page 2044*

Theophylline (thee OFF i lin)

Related Information

Oral Medications That Should Not Be Crushed or Altered *on page 2476*

Brand Names: US Elixophyllin; Theo-24; Theochron

Brand Names: Canada Apo-Theo LA®; Novo-Theophyl SR; PMS-Theophylline; Pulmophylline; ratio-Theo-Bronc; Teva-Theophylline SR; Theo ER; Theolair; Uniphyl

Therapeutic Category Antiasthmatic; Bronchodilator; Respiratory Stimulant; Theophylline Derivative

Generic Availability (US) May be product dependent

Use

Oral: Treatment of symptoms and reversible airway obstruction due to chronic asthma, chronic bronchitis, COPD, or other chronic lung diseases [Immediate release oral solution: FDA approved in all ages; Extended release 12 hour tablets: FDA approved in ages ≥ 6 years and adults; Extended release 24 hour capsules (Theo-24®) and tablets: FDA approved in ages ≥12 years and adults); has also been used for treatment of idiopathic apnea of prematurity and to increase diaphragmatic contractility

Note: The Global Initiative for Asthma Guidelines (2009) and the National Asthma Education and Prevention Program Guidelines (2007) do not recommend oral theophylline as a long-term control medication for asthma in children ≤5 years of age; use has been shown to be effective as an add-on (but not preferred) agent in older children, adolescents, and adults with severe asthma treated with inhaled or oral glucocorticoids. The guidelines do not recommend theophylline for the treatment of exacerbations of asthma.

Parenteral: Adjunctive treatment of acute exacerbations of asthma and other chronic lung diseases (eg, chronic bronchitis, emphysema) (FDA approved in all ages)

Pregnancy Risk Factor C

Pregnancy Considerations Teratogenic effects were observed in animal reproduction studies. Theophylline crosses the placenta; adverse effects may be seen in the newborn. Use is generally safe when used at the recommended doses (serum concentrations 5-12 mcg/mL) however maternal adverse events may be increased and efficacy may be decreased in pregnant women. Theophylline metabolism may change during pregnancy; the half-life is similar to that observed in otherwise healthy, nonsmoking adults with asthma during the first and second trimesters (~8.7 hours), but may increase to 13 hours (range: 8-18 hours) during the third trimester. The volume of distribution is also increased during the third trimester. Monitor serum levels. The recommendations for the use of theophylline in pregnant women with asthma are similar to those used in nonpregnant adults (National Heart, Lung, and Blood Institute Guidelines 2004).

Breast-Feeding Considerations The concentration of theophylline in breast milk is similar to the maternal serum concentration. Irritability may be observed in the nursing infant. Serious adverse events in the infant are unlikely unless toxic serum levels are present in the mother.

Contraindications Hypersensitivity to theophylline or any component of the formulation; premixed injection may contain corn-derived dextrose and its use is contraindicated in patients with allergy to corn-related products

Warnings/Precautions If a patient develops signs and symptoms of theophylline toxicity (eg, persistent, repetitive vomiting), a serum theophylline level should be measured and subsequent doses held. Serum theophylline monitoring may be lessened as lower therapeutic ranges are established. More intense monitoring may be required during acute illness or when interacting drugs are introduced into the regimen. Use with caution in patients with peptic ulcer, hyperthyroidism, seizure disorders, and patients with tachyarrhythmias (eg, sinus tachycardia, atrial fibrillation); use may exacerbate these conditions. Theophylline-induced nonconvulsive status epilepticus has been reported (rarely) and should be considered in patients who develop CNS abnormalities. Theophylline clearance may be decreased in patients with acute pulmonary edema, congestive heart failure, cor-pulmonale, fever, hepatic disease, acute hepatitis, cirrhosis, hypothyroidism, sepsis with multiorgan failure, and shock; clearance may also be decreased in neonates, infants <3 months of age with decreased renal function, infants <1 year of age, the elderly >60 years, and patients following cessation of smoking. Some dosage forms may contain propylene glycol; large amounts are potentially toxic and have been associated hyperosmolality, lactic acidosis, seizures, and respiratory depression; use caution (AAP, 1997; Zar 2007).

Adverse Reactions Adverse events observed at therapeutic serum levels:

Cardiovascular: Flutter, tachycardia

Central nervous system: Headache, hyperactivity (children), insomnia, restlessness, seizures, status epilepticus (nonconvulsive)

Endocrine & metabolic: Hypercalcemia (with concomitant hyperthyroid disease)

Gastrointestinal: Nausea, reflux or ulcer aggravation, vomiting

Genitourinary: Difficulty urinating (elderly males with prostatism)

Neuromuscular & skeletal: Tremor

Renal: Diuresis (transient)

Drug Interactions

Metabolism/Transport Effects Substrate of CYP1A2 (major), CYP2C9 (minor), CYP2D6 (minor), CYP2E1 (major), CYP3A4 (major); **Note:** Assignment of Major/Minor substrate status based on clinically relevant drug interaction potential; **Inhibits** CYP1A2 (weak)

Avoid Concomitant Use

Avoid concomitant use of Theophylline with any of the following: Conivaptan; Deferasirox; Fusidic Acid (Systemic); Idelalisib; Iobenguane I 123; Riociguat; Stiripentol

Increased Effect/Toxicity

Theophylline may increase the levels/effects of: Formoterol; Indacaterol; Olodaterol; Pancuronium; Riociguat; Sympathomimetics; TiZANidine

The levels/effects of Theophylline may be increased by: Abiraterone Acetate; Alcohol (Ethyl); Allopurinol; Antithyroid Agents; Aprepitant; AtoMOXetine; Cannabinoid-Containing Products; Cimetidine; Conivaptan; CYP1A2 Inhibitors (Moderate); CYP1A2 Inhibitors (Strong); CYP3A4 Inhibitors (Moderate); CYP3A4 Inhibitors (Strong); Dasatinib; Deferasirox; Disulfiram; Estrogen Derivatives; Febuxostat; FluvoxaMINE; Fosaprepitant; Fusidic Acid (Systemic); Idelalisib; Interferons; Isoniazid; Ivacaftor; Linezolid; Luliconazole; Macrolide Antibiotics; Methotrexate; Metreleptin; Mexiletine; Mifepristone; Netupitant; Palbociclib; Peginterferon Alfa-2b; Pentoxifylline; Propafenone; QuiNINE; Quinolone Antibiotics; Simeprevir; Stiripentol; Tedizolid; Thiabendazole; Ticlopidine; Vemurafenib; Zafirlukast; Zileuton

Decreased Effect

Theophylline may decrease the levels/effects of: Adenosine; Benzodiazepines; CarBAMazepine; Fosphenytoin; Iobenguane I 123; Lithium; Pancuronium; Phenytoin; Regadenoson; Zafirlukast

The levels/effects of Theophylline may be decreased by: Adalimumab; Barbiturates; Beta-Blockers (Beta1 Selective); Beta-Blockers (Nonselective); Bosentan; Cannabis; CarBAMazepine; CYP1A2 Inducers (Strong); CYP3A4 Inducers (Moderate); CYP3A4 Inducers (Strong); Cyproterone; Dabrafenib; Fosphenytoin; Isoproterenol; Metreleptin; Mitotane; Phenytoin; Protease Inhibitors; Siltuximab; St Johns Wort; Teriflunomide; Thyroid Products; Tocilizumab

Food Interactions

Ethanol: Ethanol may decrease theophylline clearance. Management: Avoid or limit ethanol.

Food: Food does not appreciably affect the absorption of liquid, fast-release products, and most sustained release products; however, food may induce a sudden release (dose-dumping) of once-daily sustained release products resulting in an increase in serum drug levels and potential toxicity. Changes in diet may affect the elimination of theophylline; charbroiled foods may increase elimination, reducing half-life by 50%. Management: Should be taken with water 1 hour before or 2 hours after meals. Avoid extremes of dietary protein and carbohydrate intake.

Storage/Stability Tablet, premixed infusion, solution: Store at controlled room temperature of 25°C (77°F).

Mechanism of Action Causes bronchodilatation, diuresis, CNS and cardiac stimulation, and gastric acid secretion by blocking phosphodiesterase which increases tissue concentrations of cyclic adenine monophosphate (cAMP) which in turn promotes catecholamine stimulation of lipolysis, glycogenolysis, and gluconeogenesis and induces release of epinephrine from adrenal medulla cells

Pharmacokinetics (Adult data unless noted)

Absorption: Oral: Rapid and complete with up to 100% absorption depending upon the formulation used

Distribution: V_d: 0.45 L/kg (range: 0.3-0.7 L/kg) based on ideal body weight; crosses into the CSF; poorly distributes into body fat

Protein binding: 40%; primarily to albumin; decreased protein binding in neonates (due to a greater percentage of fetal albumin), hepatic cirrhosis, uncorrected acidemia, third trimester of pregnancy, and geriatric patients

Metabolism: Hepatic via demethylation (CYP 1A2) and hydroxylation (CYP 2E1 and 3A4); theophylline is metabolized to active metabolites, caffeine and 3-methylxanthine; in neonates this theophylline-derived caffeine accumulates due to decreased hepatic metabolism and significant concentrations of caffeine may occur; a substantial decrease in serum caffeine concentrations occurs after 40 weeks postmenstrual age

Half-life: See table.

Theophylline Mean Clearance and Half-Life With Respect to Age and Altered Physiological States[A]

Patient Group	Clearance (mL/kg/minute)	Half-life (hours)
Premature infants		
postnatal age 3-15 days	0.29	30
postnatal age 25-57 days	0.64	20
Term infants		
postnatal age 1-2 days	Not reported[B]	25
postnatal age 3-30 weeks[C]	Not reported[B]	11
Children and Adolescents		
1-4 years	1.7	3.4
4-12 years	1.6	Not reported[B]
13-15 years	0.9	Not reported[B]
16-17 years	1.4	3.7 (range: 1.5-5.9)
≥18 years (nonsmoking asthmatic)	0.65	8.2
Adults		
≤60 years (nonsmoking asthmatic)	0.65	8.2
>60 years (nonsmoking, healthy)	0.41	9.8
Acute pulmonary edema	0.33	19
Cystic fibrosis (14-28 years)	1.25	6
Liver disease		
acute hepatitis	0.35	19.2
cholestasis	0.65	14.4
cirrhosis	0.31	32
Sepsis with multiorgan failure	0.46	18.8
Hypothyroid	0.38	11.6
Hyperthyroid	0.8	4.5

[A]From Hendeles L, 1995.

[B]Either not reported or not reported in a comparable format.

[C]Maturation of clearance in premature infants and term infants is most closely related to postmenstrual age (PMA); adult clearance values are reached at approximately 55 weeks PMA and higher pediatric values at approximately 60 weeks PMA (Kraus, 1993).

Elimination: Urine; neonates excrete approximately 50% of the dose unchanged in urine; Infants >3 months, children, adolescents, and adults excrete 10% in urine as unchanged drug

Dosing: Neonatal Note: Dose should be calculated using ideal body weight and individualized by serum concentrations. Due to the longer half-life compared to older patients, the time to achieve steady-state serum concentrations is prolonged in neonates (see theophylline half-life table); serum theophylline concentrations should be drawn after 48-72 hours of therapy (usually 72 hours in neonates); repeat values should be obtained 3 days after each change in dosage or weekly if on a stabilized dosage. If renal function decreased, consider dose reduction and additional monitoring.

Apnea of prematurity: Oral: Immediate release oral solution:

Loading dose: 5-6 mg/kg/dose (Bhatta-Metta, 2003)

Maintenance: 2-6 mg/kg/**day** divided every 8-12 hours (Bhatta-Mehta, 2003; Henderson-Smart, 2011; Skouroliakou, 2009)

Bronchospasm, neonatal lung disease: Oral:

Loading dose: 4.6 mg/kg/dose

Maintenance:

Premature neonates PNA <24 days: 1 mg/kg/dose every 12 hours

Premature neonates PNA ≥24 days: 1.5 mg/kg/dose every 12 hours

Full-term neonates: Total daily dose may be calculated using equation below; divide into 3 equal doses and administer at 8-hour intervals

Total daily dose (mg/**day**) = [(0.2 x age in weeks) +5] x (weight in kg)

Conversion from aminophylline (IV) to theophylline therapy: In premature neonates, the same dose may be used; evaluate serum concentrations at 48 hours or sooner if symptoms indicate.

Dosing adjustment in renal impairment: Dose reduction and frequent monitoring of serum theophylline concentrations are required in neonates with decreased renal function; 50% of dose is excreted unchanged in the urine of neonates.

Dosing: Usual Doses should be individualized based on steady-state serum concentrations; theophylline pharmacokinetics have age-dependent factors which may alter required doses particularly in pediatric patients. For obese patients, ideal body weight should be used for dosage calculation.

Infants, Children, and Adolescents:

Acute symptoms: Manufacturer's labeling: **Note:** Not recommended for the treatment of asthma exacerbations (NAEPP, 2007).

Loading dose: **Note:** Doses presented intended to achieve a serum level of approximately 10 mcg/mL; loading doses should be given intravenously (preferred) or with a rapidly absorbed oral product (not an extended release product). On the average, for every 1 mg/kg theophylline given, blood concentrations will rise 2 mcg/mL.

Patients **not** currently receiving methylxanthines:

IV: 4.6 mg/kg/dose

Oral: Immediate release product: 5 mg/kg

Patients currently receiving methylxanthines: A loading dose is not recommended without first obtaining a serum theophylline concentration in patients who have received aminophylline or theophylline within the past 24 hours. The loading dose should be calculated as follows:

Dose = (C desired – C measured) (V_d)

C desired = desired serum theophylline concentration

C measured = measured serum theophylline concentration

Maintenance dose: Continuous IV infusion: **Note:** Dosing presented is to achieve a target concentration of 10 mcg/mL. Lower initial doses may be required in patients with reduced theophylline clearance. Dosage should be adjusted according to serum concentration measurements during the first 12- to 24-hour period.

Infants 4-6 weeks: 1.5 mg/kg/dose every 12 hours

Infants 6-52 weeks: Dose (mg/kg/**hour**) = (0.008 X age in weeks) + 0.21

Children 1 to <9 years: 0.8 mg/kg/**hour**

Children 9 to <12 years: 0.7 mg/kg/**hour**

Adolescents 12 to <16 years (otherwise healthy, nonsmokers): 0.5 mg/kg/**hour**; maximum daily dose: 900 mg/**day** unless serum concentrations indicate need for larger dose

Adolescents 12 to <16 years (cigarette or marijuana smokers): 0.7 mg/kg/**hour**

Adolescents 16-18 years (otherwise healthy, nonsmokers): 0.4 mg/kg/**hour**; maximum dose: 900 mg/**day** unless serum concentrations indicate need for larger dose

Cardiac decompensation, cor pulmonale, hepatic dysfunction, sepsis with multiorgan failure, shock: Initial: 0.2 mg/kg/**hour**; maximum dose: 400 mg/**day** unless serum concentrations indicate need for larger dose

Chronic conditions: Note: Increase dose only if tolerated. Consider lowering dose or using a slower titration if caffeine-like adverse events occur. Smaller doses given more frequently may be used in patients with a more rapid metabolism to prevent breakthrough symptoms which could occur due to low trough concentration prior to the next dose.

Immediate release formulation: Oral: **Note:** If at risk for impaired clearance or not feasible to monitor serum theophylline concentrations: Do not exceed 16 mg/kg/**day**; maximum daily dose: 400 mg/**day**

Manufacturer's labeling: Frequency based upon age.

Infants: Total daily dose (mg/day) = [(0.2 x age in weeks) + 5] x (weight in kg); frequency is based on age

Dosing interval:

≤26 weeks: Divide in 3 equal doses and administer every 8 hours

>26 weeks: Divide in 4 equal doses and administer every 6 hours

Children and Adolescents 1-15 years and ≤45 kg:

Initial:

Days 1-3: 12-14 mg/kg/**day** in divided doses every 4-6 hours; maximum daily dose: 300 mg/**day**

Days 4-6: 16 mg/kg/**day** in divided doses every 4-6 hours; maximum daily dose: 400 mg/**day**

Maintenance: 20 mg/kg/**day** in divided doses every 4-6 hours; maximum daily dose: 600 mg/**day**

Children and Adolescents >45 kg or Adolescents ≥16 years:

Initial:

Days 1-3: 300 mg/**day** in divided doses every 6-8 hours

Days 4-6: 400 mg/**day** in divided doses every 6-8 hours

Maintenance: 600 mg/**day** in divided doses every 6-8 hour

Alternate dosing; age-directed: Some centers have used the following based on age-dependent pharmacokinetics of theophylline:

Children 1 to < 9 years: 20-24 mg/kg/**day**; maximum daily dose: 600 mg/**day**

Children 9-12 years: 16 mg/kg/**day**; maximum daily dose: 600 mg/**day**

Children and Adolescents >12-16 years (nonsmokers): 13 mg/kg/**day**; maximum daily dose: 600 mg/**day**

Children >12 years and Adolescents (smokers): 16 mg/kg/**day**; maximum daily dose: 600 mg/**day**

Adolescents >16 years (nonsmokers): 10 mg/kg/**day**; maximum daily dose: 600 mg/**day**

Extended release formulations: Oral: **Note:** If at risk for impaired clearance or not feasible to monitor serum theophylline concentrations: Do not exceed 16 mg/kg/**day**; maximum daily dose: 400 mg/day

Children ≥6 years and Adolescents <16 years, weighing ≤45 kg:

Initial:

Days 1-3: 12-14 mg/kg/**day**; maximum daily dose: 300 mg/**day**

Days 4-6: 16 mg/kg/**day**; maximum daily dose: 400 mg/**day**

Maintenance: 20 mg/kg/**day**; maximum daily dose: 600 mg/**day**

Dosing interval (product specific):

12-hour extended release tablets: Children ≥6 years and Adolescents: Divide in 2 equal doses and administer every 12 hours

24-hour extended release tablets: Children ≥12 years and Adolescents: Administer every 24 hours

Children ≥6 years and Adolescents, weighing >45 kg or Adolescents ≥16 years:

12-hour extended release tablets: Children ≥6 years and Adolescents, weighing >45 kg or Adolescents ≥16 years:

Initial:

Days 1-3: 300 mg/**day** in divided doses every 12 hours

Days 4-6: 400 mg/**day** in divided doses every 12 hours

Maintenance: 600 mg/**day** in divided doses every 12 hours

24-hour extended release tablets: Children ≥12 years and Adolescents, weighing >45 kg or Adolescents ≥16 years:

Initial:

Days 1-3: 300-400 mg once daily

Days 4-6: 400-600 mg once daily

Maintenance: Titrate according to serum concentrations

Alternate dosing: Age-directed: Some centers have used the following based on age-dependent pharmacokinetics of theophylline:

Children 6 to <9 years: 20-24 mg/kg/**day**; maximum daily dose: 600 mg/**day**

Children 9-12 years: 16 mg/kg/**day**; maximum daily dose: 600 mg/**day**

Children and Adolescents >12-16 years (nonsmokers): 13 mg/kg/**day**; maximum daily dose: 600 mg/**day**

Children >12 years and Adolescents (smokers): 16 mg/kg/**day**; maximum daily dose: 600 mg/**day**

Adolescents >16 years (nonsmokers): 10 mg/kg/**day**; maximum daily dose: 600 mg/**day**

Adults:

Acute symptoms: Manufacturer's labeling: **Note:** Not recommended for the treatment of asthma exacerbations (NAEPP, 2007).

Loading dose: **Note:** Doses presented intended to achieve a serum concentration of approximately 10 mcg/mL; loading doses should be given intravenously (preferred) or with a rapidly absorbed oral product (not an extended release product). On the average, for every 1 mg/kg theophylline given, blood concentrations will rise 2 mcg/mL.

Patients **not** currently receiving aminophylline or theophylline:

IV: 4.6 mg/kg/dose

Oral: Immediate release product: 5 mg/kg/dose

Patients currently receiving aminophylline or theophylline: A loading dose is not recommended without first obtaining a serum theophylline concentration in patients who have received aminophylline or theophylline within the past 24 hours. The loading dose should be calculated as follows:

Dose = (C desired – C measured) (V_d)

C desired = desired serum theophylline concentration

C measured = measured serum theophylline concentration

Maintenance dose: Continuous IV infusion: **Note:** Dosing presented is to achieve a target concentration of 10 mcg/mL. Lower initial doses may be required in patients with reduced theophylline clearance. Dosage should be adjusted according to serum concentration measurements during the first 12- to 24-hour period.

Adults ≤60 years (otherwise healthy, nonsmokers): 0.4 mg/kg/**hour**; maximum daily dose: 900 mg/**day** unless serum concentrations indicate need for larger dose

Adults >60 years: 0.3 mg/kg/**hour**; maximum daily dose: 400 mg/**day** unless serum levels indicate need for larger dose

Chronic conditions: Oral: **Note:** Increase dose only if tolerated. Consider lowering dose or using a slower titration if caffeine-like adverse events occur. Smaller doses given more frequently may be used in patients with a more rapid metabolism to prevent breakthrough symptoms which could occur due to low trough concentration prior to the next dose.

Immediate release oral solution: Initial dose: 300 mg/**day** administered in divided doses every 6-8 hours; maintenance: 400-600 mg/day (maximum daily dose: 600 mg/**day**)

Extended release formulations: Initial dose: 300-400 mg once daily; maintenance: 400-600 mg once daily (maximum daily dose: 600 mg/**day**)

Dosage adjustment based on serum theophylline concentrations: Infants, Children, Adolescents, and Adults: **Note:** Recheck serum theophylline concentrations after 3 days when using oral dosing, or after 12 hours (children) or 24 hours (adults) when dosing intravenously. Patients maintained with oral therapy should be reassessed at 6- to 12-month intervals, when clinically indicated or if concomitant medication is added which may affect theophylline serum concentration.

<9.9 mcg/mL: If tolerated, but symptoms remain, increase dose by ~25%. Recheck serum theophylline concentrations.

10-14.9 mcg/mL: Maintain dosage if tolerated. Recheck serum concentrations at 24-hour intervals (for acute IV dosing) or at 6- to 12-month intervals (for oral dosing).

15-19.9 mcg/mL: Consider 10% dose reduction to improve safety margin even if dose is tolerated.

20-24.9 mcg/mL: Decrease dose by ~25%. Recheck serum concentrations.

25-30 mcg/mL: Skip next dose (oral) or stop infusion for 12 hours (children) or 24 hours (adults) and decrease subsequent doses by at least 25%. Recheck serum concentrations.

>30 mcg/mL: Stop dosing and treat overdose; if resumed, decrease subsequent doses by at least 50%. Recheck serum concentrations.

Dosing adjustment in renal impairment: Oral, IV:

Infants 1-3 months: Consider dose reduction and frequent monitoring of serum theophylline concentrations

Infants >3 months, Children, Adolescents, and Adults: No adjustment necessary

Dosing adjustment in hepatic impairment:

Oral: Infants, Children, Adolescents, and Adults: Dose reduction and frequent monitoring of serum theophylline concentration are required in patients with decreased hepatic function (eg, cirrhosis, acute hepatitis, cholestasis)

IV: Manufacturer's labeling: Infants, Children, Adolescents, and Adults: Initial: 0.2 mg/kg/**hour**; maximum daily dose: 400 mg/**day** unless serum concentrations indicate need for larger dose

Administration

Oral: Administer on an empty stomach, 1 hour before or 2 hours after a meal. Sustained release preparations should be administered with a full glass of water, whole or cut by half only; do not crush; sustained release capsule forms may be opened and sprinkled on soft foods; do not chew or crush beads

Parenteral: Premix IV infusion bags available, administer loading dose over 30 minutes; rate for continuous IV infusion dependent upon dosage

Monitoring Parameters Respiratory rate, heart rate, serum theophylline concentration, pulmonary function tests, arterial or capillary blood gases (if applicable); number and severity of apnea spells (apnea of prematurity)

Reference Range

Therapeutic concentrations:

Asthma: 5-15 mcg/mL

Apnea of prematurity: 6-12 mcg/mL; goal concentration is reduced due to decreased protein binding and higher free fraction

Toxic concentration: >20 mcg/mL

Guidelines for Drawing Theophylline Serum Samples

Dosage Form	When to Obtain Sample[A]
IV bolus	30 minutes after end of 30-minute infusion
IV continuous infusion	12-24 hours after initiation of infusion
Oral immediate release formulations	Peak: 1 hour postdose after at least 1 day of therapy Trough: Just before a dose after at least 1 day of therapy

[A]The time to achieve steady-state serum concentrations is prolonged in patients with longer half-lives (eg, infants and adults with cardiac or liver failure (see theophylline half-life table). In these patients, serum theophylline concentrations should be drawn after 48-72 hours of therapy; serum concentrations may need to be done prior to steady-state to assess the patient's current progress or evaluate potential toxicity.

Test Interactions Plasma glucose, uric acid, free fatty acids, total cholesterol, HDL, HDL/LDL ratio, and urinary free cortisol excretion may be increased by theophylline. Theophylline may decrease triiodothyronine.

Additional Information Due to improved theophylline clearance during the first year of life, serum concentration determinations and dosage adjustments may be needed to optimize therapy

Dosage Forms Excipient information presented when available (limited, particularly for generics); consult specific product labeling.

Capsule Extended Release 24 Hour, Oral:
- Theo-24: 100 mg
- Theo-24: 200 mg [contains fd&c yellow #10 (quinoline yellow)]
- Theo-24: 300 mg [contains brilliant blue fcf (fd&c blue #1), fd&c red #40]
- Theo-24: 400 mg [contains fd&c red #40]

Elixir, Oral:
- Elixophyllin: 80 mg/15 mL (473 mL) [contains fd&c red #40, saccharin sodium; mixed fruit flavor]

Solution, Intravenous:
- Generic: 400 mg (250 mL, 500 mL); 800 mg (500 mL)

Solution, Oral:
- Generic: 80 mg/15 mL (473 mL)

Tablet Extended Release 12 Hour, Oral:
- Theochron: 100 mg, 200 mg, 300 mg [scored]
- Generic: 100 mg, 200 mg, 300 mg, 450 mg

Tablet Extended Release 24 Hour, Oral:
- Generic: 400 mg, 600 mg

Extemporaneous Preparations Note: An alcohol-containing commercial oral solution is available (80 mg/15mL).

A 5 mg/mL oral suspension may be made with tablets. Crush one 300 mg extended release tablet in a mortar and reduce to a fine powder. Add small portions of a 1:1 mixture of Ora-Sweet® and Ora-Plus® and mix to a uniform paste; mix while adding the vehicle in equal proportions to **almost** 60 mL; transfer to a calibrated bottle, rinse mortar with vehicle, and add sufficient quantity of vehicle to make 60 mL. Label "shake well". Stable for 90 days at room temperature.

Johnson CE, VanDeKoppel S, and Myers E, "Stability of Anhydrous Theophylline in Extemporaneously Prepared Alcohol-Free Oral Suspensions," *Am J Health-Syst Pharm*, 2005, 62(23):2518-20.

◆ **Theophylline Anhydrous** *see* Theophylline *on page 2044*

◆ **Theophylline Ethylenediamine** *see* Aminophylline *on page 122*

◆ **TheraCort [OTC]** *see* Hydrocortisone (Topical) *on page 1041*

◆ **Thera-Ear [OTC]** *see* Carbamide Peroxide *on page 371*

◆ **Therapeutic [OTC]** *see* Coal Tar *on page 523*

◆ **Theraplex T [OTC]** *see* Coal Tar *on page 523*

◆ **Thermazene [DSC]** *see* Silver Sulfadiazine *on page 1926*

◆ **Thiamazole** *see* Methimazole *on page 1386*

◆ **Thiamin** *see* Thiamine *on page 2048*

Thiamine (THYE a min)

Medication Safety Issues

Sound-alike/look-alike issues:

Thiamine may be confused with Tenormin, Thalomid, Thorazine

International issues:

Doxal [Brazil] may be confused with Doxil brand name for doxorubicin [U.S.]

Doxal: Brand name for pyridoxine/thiamine [Brazil], but also the brand name for doxepin [Finland]

Brand Names: Canada Betaxin

Therapeutic Category Nutritional Supplement; Vitamin, Water Soluble

Generic Availability (US) Yes

Use Treatment of thiamine deficiency including beriberi, Wernicke's encephalopathy syndrome, and peripheral neuritis associated with pellagra; alcoholic patients with altered sensorium; various genetic metabolic disorders

Pregnancy Risk Factor A

Pregnancy Considerations Water soluble vitamins cross the placenta. Thiamine requirements may be increased during pregnancy (IOM, 1998). Severe nausea and vomiting (hyperemesis gravidarum) may lead to thiamine deficiency manifested as Wernicke's encephalopathy (Chiossi, 2006).

Breast-Feeding Considerations Thiamine is found in breast milk and concentrations are similar in well-nourished mothers who use supplements and those that do not. Thiamine requirements may be increased in nursing women compared to non-nursing women (IOM, 1998).

Contraindications Hypersensitivity to thiamine or any component of the formulation

Warnings/Precautions Use with caution with parenteral route (especially IV) of administration. Hypersensitivity reactions have been reported following repeated parenteral doses; consider skin test in individuals with history of allergic reactions. Single vitamin deficiency is rare; evaluate for other deficiencies. Dextrose administration may precipitate acute symptoms of thiamine deficiency; use caution when thiamine status is marginal or suspect. The parenteral product may contain aluminum; toxic aluminum concentrations may be seen with high doses, prolonged use, or renal dysfunction. Premature neonates are at higher risk due to immature renal function and aluminum intake from other parenteral sources. Parenteral aluminum exposure of >4 to 5 mcg/kg/day is associated with CNS and bone toxicity; tissue loading may occur at lower doses (Federal Register, 2002). See manufacturer's labeling.

Adverse Reactions Adverse reactions reported with injection.

Cardiovascular: Cyanosis

Central nervous system: Restlessness

Dermatologic: Angioneurotic edema, pruritus, urticaria

Gastrointestinal: Hemorrhage into GI tract, nausea, tightness of the throat

Local: Induration and/or tenderness at the injection site (following IM administration)

Neuromuscular & skeletal: Weakness

Respiratory: Pulmonary edema

Miscellaneous: Anaphylactic/hypersensitivity reactions (following IV administration), diaphoresis, warmth

Drug Interactions

Metabolism/Transport Effects None known.

Avoid Concomitant Use There are no known interactions where it is recommended to avoid concomitant use.

Increased Effect/Toxicity There are no known significant interactions involving an increase in effect.

Decreased Effect There are no known significant interactions involving a decrease in effect.

Food Interactions

Ethanol: May decrease thiamine absorption. Management: Higher doses may be needed in patients with history of ethanol abuse.

Food: High carbohydrate diets may increase thiamine requirement.

Storage/Stability Injection: Store at 15°C to 30°C (59°F to 86°F). Protect from light.

Mechanism of Action An essential coenzyme in carbohydrate metabolism by combining with adenosine triphosphate to form thiamine pyrophosphate

Pharmacokinetics (Adult data unless noted)

Absorption:
- Oral: Poor
- IM: Rapid and complete

Metabolism: In the liver

Elimination: Renally as unchanged drug only after body storage sites become saturated

Dosing: Neonatal Adequate intake: Oral: 0.2 mg (0.03 mg/kg)

Dosing: Usual

Adequate intake: Oral: Infants:
- 1 to <6 months: 0.2 mg (0.03 mg/kg)
- 6-12 months: 0.3 mg (0.03 mg/kg)

Recommended daily allowance (RDA): Oral:
- 1-3 years: 0.5 mg
- 4-8 years: 0.6 mg
- 9-13 years: 0.9 mg
- 14-18 years:
  - Male: 1.2 mg
  - Female: 1 mg
- ≥19 years:
  - Male: 1.2 mg
  - Female: 1.1 mg

Dietary supplement (depends on caloric or carbohydrate content of the diet):
- Oral:
  - Infants: 0.3-0.5 mg/day
  - Children: 0.5-1 mg/day
  - Adults: 1-2 mg/day
- **Note:** The above doses can be found in multivitamin preparations

Thiamine deficiency (beriberi):
- Children: 10-25 mg/dose IM or IV daily (if critically ill), or 10-50 mg/dose orally every day for 2 weeks, then 5-10 mg/dose orally daily for 1 month
- Adults: 5-30 mg/dose IM or IV 3 times/day (if critically ill); then orally 5-30 mg/day in single or divided doses 3 times/day for 1 month

Wernicke's encephalopathy: Adults: Initial: 100 mg IV, then 50-100 mg/day IM or IV until consuming a regular, balanced diet

Metabolic disorders: Oral: Adults: 10-20 mg/day (dosages up to 4 g/day in divided doses have been used)

Administration

Oral: May administer with or without food

Parenteral: Administer by slow IV injection or IM

Reference Range Normal values: 1.6-4 mg/dL

Test Interactions False-positive for uric acid using the phosphotungstate method and for urobilinogen using the Ehrlich's reagent; large doses may interfere with the spectrophotometric determination of serum theophylline concentration

Additional Information Dietary sources include legumes, pork, beef, whole grains, yeast, fresh vegetables; a deficiency state can occur in as little as 3 weeks following total dietary absence

Dosage Forms Excipient information presented when available (limited, particularly for generics); consult specific product labeling.

Capsule, Oral, as hydrochloride:
- Generic: 50 mg

Solution, Injection, as hydrochloride:
- Generic: 100 mg/mL (2 mL)

Tablet, Oral, as hydrochloride:
- Generic: 50 mg, 100 mg, 250 mg

Tablet, Oral, as hydrochloride [preservative free]:
- Generic: 100 mg

Extemporaneous Preparations A 100 mg/mL oral suspension may be made with commercially available thiamine powder. Add 10 g of powder to a mortar. Add small portions of a 1:1 mixture of Ora-Sweet® and Ora-Plus® and mix to a uniform paste; mix while adding the vehicle in equal proportions to **almost** 100 mL; transfer to a calibrated bottle, rinse mortar with vehicle, and add sufficient quantity of vehicle to make 100 mL. Label "shake well". Stable 91 days under refrigeration or at room temperature.

Ensom MH and Decarie D, "Stability of Thiamine in Extemporaneously Compounded Suspensions," *Can J Hosp Pharm*, 2005, 58(1):26-30.

◆ **Thiamine Hydrochloride** *see* Thiamine *on page 2048*

◆ **Thiaminium Chloride Hydrochloride** *see* Thiamine *on page 2048*

Thioguanine (thye oh GWAH neen)

Medication Safety Issues

Sound-alike/look-alike issues:

Thioguanine may be confused with thiotepa

High alert medication:

This medication is in a class the Institute for Safe Medication Practices (ISMP) includes among its list of drug classes which have a heightened risk of causing significant patient harm when used in error.

Other safety concerns:

6-thioguanine and 6-TG are error-prone abbreviations (associated with sixfold overdoses of thioguanine)

International issues:

Lanvis [Canada and multiple international markets] may be confused with Lantus brand name for insulin glargine [U.S., Canada, and multiple international markets]

Related Information

Oral Medications That Should Not Be Crushed or Altered *on page 2476*

Prevention of Chemotherapy-Induced Nausea and Vomiting in Children *on page 2368*

Safe Handling of Hazardous Drugs *on page 2455*

Brand Names: US Tabloid

Brand Names: Canada Lanvis®

Therapeutic Category Antineoplastic Agent, Antimetabolite; Antineoplastic Agent, Antimetabolite (Purine Analog)

Generic Availability (US) No

Use Remission induction and remission consolidation treatment of acute nonlymphocytic leukemia (ANLL, AML) [FDA approved in pediatrics (age not specified) and adults]; has also been used for treatment of acute lymphoblastic leukemia (ALL)

Pregnancy Risk Factor D

Pregnancy Considerations Animal studies have demonstrated adverse effects. There are no adequate and well-controlled studies in pregnant women. May cause fetal harm if administered during pregnancy. Women of childbearing potential should avoid becoming pregnant during treatment.

Breast-Feeding Considerations Due to the potential for serious adverse reactions in the nursing infant, the manufacturer recommends to discontinue breast-feeding during therapy.

Contraindications Prior resistance to thioguanine (or mercaptopurine)

Canadian labeling: Additional contraindications (not in US labeling): Hypersensitivity to thioguanine or any component of the formulation

Warnings/Precautions Hazardous agent - use appropriate precautions for handling and disposal (NIOSH 2014 [group 1]).

Not recommended for maintenance therapy or long-term continuous treatment; long-term continuous therapy or maintenance treatment is associated with a high risk for hepatotoxicity, hepatic sinusoidal obstruction syndrome (SOS; formerly called veno-occlusive disease), or portal hypertension; monitor liver function carefully for liver toxicity and discontinue in patients with evidence of hepatic SOS (eg, hyperbilirubinemia, hepatomegaly [tender], and weight gain due to ascites and fluid retention) or portal hypertension (eg, splenomegaly, thrombocytopenia, esophageal varices); hepatotoxicity with or without transaminase elevations may occur; pathologic findings of hepatotoxicity include hepatoportal sclerosis, nodular regenerative hyperplasia, peliosis hepatitis, and periportal fibrosis. Advise patients to avoid alcohol; may increase the risk for hepatotoxicity.

Myelosuppression (anemia, leukopenia, and/or thrombocytopenia) is a common dose-related toxicity (may be delayed); monitor for infection (due to leukopenia) or bleeding(due to thrombocytopenia); withhold treatment with abnormally significant drop in blood counts. Patients with genetic enzyme deficiency of thiopurine methyltransferase (TPMT) or who are receiving drugs which inhibit this enzyme (mesalazine, olsalazine, sulfasalazine) may be highly sensitive to myelosuppressive effects and may require substantial dose reductions.

Hyperuricemia occurs commonly with treatment; institute adequate hydration and prophylactic allopurinol. Thioguanine is potentially carcinogenic. Cross resistance with mercaptopurine generally occurs. Avoid vaccination with live vaccines during treatment.

Warnings: Additional Pediatric Considerations Liver toxicity is particularly prevalent in children (up to 25%) receiving maintenance therapy for acute lymphoblastic leukemia and in males.

Adverse Reactions

Endocrine & metabolic: Fluid retention, hyperuricemia (common)

Gastrointestinal: Anorexia, intestinal necrosis, intestinal perforation, nausea, splenomegaly, stomatitis, vomiting, weight gain

Hematologic: Anemia (may be delayed), bleeding, granulocytopenia, leukopenia (common; may be delayed), marrow hypoplasia, pancytopenia, thrombocytopenia (common; may be delayed)

Hepatic: Ascites, esophageal varices, hepatic necrosis (centrilobular), hepatic sinusoidal obstruction syndrome (SOS; veno-occlusive disease), hepatitis, hepatomegaly [tender], hepatoportal sclerosis, hepatotoxicity, hyperbilirubinemia, jaundice, LFTs increased, nodular regenerative hyperplasia, peliosis hepatitis, periportal fibrosis, portal hypertension

Miscellaneous: Infection

Drug Interactions

Metabolism/Transport Effects None known.

Avoid Concomitant Use

Avoid concomitant use of Thioguanine with any of the following: BCG; BCG (Intravesical); CloZAPine; Dipyrone; Natalizumab; Pimecrolimus; Tacrolimus (Topical); Tofacitinib; Vaccines (Live)

Increased Effect/Toxicity

Thioguanine may increase the levels/effects of: CloZAPine; Leflunomide; Natalizumab; Tofacitinib; Vaccines (Live)

The levels/effects of Thioguanine may be increased by: 5-ASA Derivatives; Denosumab; Dipyrone; Pimecrolimus; Roflumilast; Tacrolimus (Topical); Trastuzumab

Decreased Effect

Thioguanine may decrease the levels/effects of: BCG; BCG (Intravesical); Coccidioides immitis Skin Test; Sipuleucel-T; Vaccines (Inactivated); Vaccines (Live)

The levels/effects of Thioguanine may be decreased by: Echinacea

Storage/Stability Store tablet at room temperature at 15°C to 25°C (59°F to 77°F). Protect from moisture.

Mechanism of Action Purine analog that is incorporated into DNA and RNA resulting in the blockage of synthesis and metabolism of purine nucleotides

Pharmacokinetics (Adult data unless noted)

Absorption: Oral: 30% (range: 14% to 46%), variable and incomplete

Distribution: Does not reach therapeutic concentrations in the CSF

Metabolism: Rapid and extensive hepatic metabolism by thiopurine methyltransferase (TPMT) to 2-amino-6-methylthioguanine (MTG; active) and inactive compounds

Half-life, terminal: 5-9 hours

Time to peak serum concentration: 8 hours

Elimination: Metabolites excreted in urine

Dosing: Usual Oral (refer to individual protocols): **Acute lymphoblastic leukemia (ALL); delayed intensification treatment phase (combination therapy):** Children ≥1 year: 60 mg/m^2/dose once daily for 14 days (Lange, 2002; Nachman, 1998)

Dosage adjustment in renal impairment: Children: No adjustment required (Aronoff, 2007).

Dosage adjustment in hepatic impairment: Deterioration in transaminases, alkaline phosphatase or bilirubin, toxic hepatitis, biliary stasis, clinical jaundice, evidence of hepatic sinusoidal obstruction syndrome (veno-occlusive disease), or evidence of portal hypertension: Discontinue treatment.

Administration Hazardous agent; use appropriate precautions for handling and disposal (NIOSH 2014 [group 1]).

Oral: Total daily dose can be given at one time.

Monitoring Parameters CBC with differential and platelet count, liver function tests (serum transaminases, alkaline phosphatase, bilirubin), hemoglobin, hematocrit, serum uric acid; testing for thiopurine methyltransferase (TPMT) deficiency is available; clinical signs of portal hypertension or hepatic sinusoidal obstruction syndrome (SOS; veno-occlusive disease)

Additional Information Myelosuppressive effects:

WBC: Moderate

Platelets: Moderate

Onset (days): 7-10

Nadir (days): 14

Recovery (days): 21

Note: Myelosuppressive effects may be delayed; continuation of treatment should be evaluated at first sign of decreased hematologic parameter.

Dosage Forms Excipient information presented when available (limited, particularly for generics); consult specific product labeling.

Tablet, Oral:

Tabloid: 40 mg

Extemporaneous Preparations Hazardous agent: Use appropriate precautions for handling and disposal (NIOSH 2014 [group 1]).

A 20 mg/mL oral suspension may be made with tablets, methylcellulose 1%, and simple syrup NF. Crush fifteen 40 mg tablets in a mortar and reduce to a fine powder. Add 10 mL methylcellulose 1% in incremental proportions and mix to a uniform paste. Transfer to a graduated cylinder, rinse mortar with simple syrup, and add quantity of simple syrup sufficient to make 30 mL. Label "shake well" and "refrigerate". Stable for 84 days refrigerated (preferred) or at room temperature.

Dressman JB and Poust RI, "Stability of Allopurinol and Five Antineoplastics in Suspension," *Am J Hosp Pharm*, 1983, 40(4):616-8.

Nahata MC, Pai VB, and Hipple TF, *Pediatric Drug Formulations*, 5th ed, Cincinnati, OH: Harvey Whitney Books Co, 2004.

◆ **6-Thioguanine (error-prone abbreviation)** *see* Thioguanine *on page 2049*

◆ **Thiophosphoramide** *see* Thiotepa *on page 2053*

◆ **Thioplex** *see* Thiotepa *on page 2053*

Thioridazine (thye oh RID a zeen)

Medication Safety Issues

Sound-alike/look-alike issues:

Thioridazine may be confused with thiothixene, Thorazine

Mellaril may be confused with Elavil, Mebaral®

BEERS Criteria medication:

This drug may be potentially inappropriate for use in geriatric patients (Quality of evidence - moderate; Strength of recommendation - strong).

Therapeutic Category Antipsychotic Agent, Typical, Phenothiazine; First Generation (Typical) Antipsychotic; Phenothiazine Derivative

Generic Availability (US) Yes

Use Due to prolongation of the QTc interval, thioridazine is currently indicated only for the treatment of refractory schizophrenic patients [FDA approved in pediatric patients (age not specified) and adults]; in the past, the drug had been used for management of psychotic disorders; depressive neurosis; dementia in elderly; severe behavioral problems in children

Pregnancy Considerations Jaundice or hyper- or hyporeflexia have been reported in newborn infants following maternal use of phenothiazines. Antipsychotic use during the third trimester of pregnancy has a risk for abnormal muscle movements (extrapyramidal symptoms [EPS]) and withdrawal symptoms in newborns following delivery. Symptoms in the newborn may include agitation, feeding disorder, hypertonia, hypotonia, respiratory distress, somnolence, and tremor; these effects may be self-limiting or require hospitalization.

Breast-Feeding Considerations Other phenothiazines are excreted in human milk; excretion of thioridazine is not known.

Contraindications Severe CNS depression; severe hyper-/hypotensive heart disease; coma; in combination with other drugs that are known to prolong the QTc interval, CYP2D6 inhibitors (fluoxetine, paroxetine), and/or fluvoxamine, propranolol, or pindolol; in patients with congenital long QT syndrome or a history of cardiac arrhythmias; patients known to have genetic defect leading to reduced levels of activity of CYP2D6

Warnings/Precautions **[US Boxed Warning]: Thioridazine has been shown to prolong the QTc interval in a dose-related manner; this may potentially cause Torsades de pointes and sudden death.** Therefore, thioridazine should be reserved for patients with schizophrenia who have failed to respond to adequate levels of other antipsychotic drugs. Risk of torsades de pointes and/or sudden death may be higher with in patients with bradycardia, hypokalemia, the presence of congenital prolongation of the QTc interval, reduced activity of cytochrome P450 (CYP-450) 2D6, or concomitant use of other drugs that prolong the QTc interval, inhibit CYP2D6, or interfere with the clearance of thioridazine. Consider a cardiac evaluation (including Holter monitoring) in patients who experience symptoms that may be associated with Torsades de Pointes (dizziness, palpitations, syncope). Discontinue therapy in patients with a QTc >500 msec. May cause orthostatic hypotension; use with caution in patients at risk of this effect or those who would tolerate transient hypotensive episodes (cerebrovascular disease, cardiovascular disease, or other medications which may predispose). **[US Boxed Warning]: Elderly patients with dementia-related psychosis treated with antipsychotics are at an increased risk of death compared to placebo.** Most deaths appeared to be either cardiovascular (eg, heart failure, sudden death) or infectious (eg, pneumonia) in nature. Thioridazine is not approved for the treatment of dementia-related psychosis.

Leukopenia, neutropenia, and agranulocytosis (sometimes fatal) have been reported in clinical trials and postmarketing reports with antipsychotic use; presence of risk factors (eg, preexisting low WBC or history of drug-induced leuko-/neutropenia) should prompt periodic blood count assessment. Discontinue therapy at first signs of blood dyscrasias or if absolute neutrophil count <1,000/mm^3.

May cause CNS depression, which may impair physical or mental abilities; patients must be cautioned about performing tasks that require mental alertness (eg, operating machinery, driving). Use with caution in Parkinson disease (APA [Lehman, 2004]). Use caution in patients with hemodynamic instability; predisposition to seizures; subcortical brain damage; severe cardiac, hepatic, or renal disease. Do not initiate therapy in patients with a QTc interval >450 msec. Esophageal dysmotility and aspiration have been associated with antipsychotic use; use with caution in patients at risk of pneumonia (ie, Alzheimer disease) (Maddalena, 2004). Use associated with increased prolactin levels; clinical significance of hyperprolactinemia in patients with breast cancer or other prolactin-dependent tumors is unknown. Impaired core body temperature regulation may occur; caution with strenuous exercise, heat exposure, dehydration, and concomitant medication possessing anticholinergic effects (Kowk, 2005; Martinez, 2002).

May cause anticholinergic effects (constipation, xerostomia, blurred vision, urinary retention); use with caution in patients with decreased gastrointestinal motility, paralytic ileus, urinary retention, BPH, xerostomia, or visual problems. Relative to other neuroleptics, thioridazine has a high potency of cholinergic blockade (APA [Lehman, 2004]).

May cause extrapyramidal symptoms, including pseudoparkinsonism, acute dystonic reactions, akathisia, and tardive dyskinesia. Risk of dystonia (and possibly other EPS) may be greater with increased doses, use of conventional antipsychotics, males, and younger patients (APA [Lehman, 2004]). Risk of tardive dyskinesia and potential for irreversibility may be increased in elderly patients (particularly women), prolonged therapy, and higher total cumulative dose; antipsychotics may also mask signs/symptoms of tardive dyskinesia. Consider therapy discontinuation with signs/symptoms of tardive dyskinesia. In elderly patients, avoid use; potent anticholinergic agent with potential to cause QT-interval prolongation. Use in elderly patients with dementia is associated with an increased risk of mortality and cerebrovascular accidents; avoid antipsychotic use for behavioral problems associated with dementia unless alternative nonpharmacologic therapies have failed and patient may harm self or others. In addition, use may cause or exacerbate syndrome of inappropriate antidiuretic hormone secretion or hyponatremia; monitor sodium closely with initiation or dosage adjustments in older adults (Beers Criteria). Use with caution in patients with narrow-angle glaucoma; condition may be exacerbated by cholinergic blockade (APA [Lehman, 2004]). May be associated with neuroleptic malignant syndrome (NMS); monitor for mental status changes, fever, muscle rigidity, and/or autonomic instability. Following recovery from NMS, reintroduction of drug therapy should be carefully considered; if an antipsychotic agent is resumed, monitor closely for NMS. May cause pigmentary retinopathy, characterized by diminution of visual acuity, brownish coloring of vision, and impairment of night vision, in patients exceeding recommended doses. Periodic eye examinations are recommended in patients receiving 600 mg/day or more (Oshika 1995). Potentially significant drug-drug interactions may exist, requiring dose or frequency adjustment, additional monitoring, and/or selection of alternative therapy.

Adverse Reactions

Cardiovascular: ECG changes, hypotension, orthostatic hypotension, peripheral edema, prolonged QT Interval on ECG, torsades de pointes

Central nervous system: Disruption of temperature regulation (Martinez 2002), drowsiness, drug-induced Parkinson disease, extrapyramidal reaction, headache, hyperactivity, lethargy, psychotic reaction, seizure, tardive dyskinesia (Lehman 2004)

Dermatologic: Dermatitis, hyperpigmentation (Lehman 2004), pallor, skin photosensitivity, skin rash, urticaria

Endocrine & metabolic: Amenorrhea, galactorrhea, weight gain (Lehman 2004)

Gastrointestinal: Constipation, diarrhea, nausea, parotid gland enlargement, vomiting, xerostomia

Genitourinary: Breast engorgement, ejaculatory disorder, priapism

Hematologic & oncologic: Agranulocytosis, leukopenia

Ophthalmic: Blurred vision, corneal opacity (Lehman 2004), retinitis pigmentosa

Respiratory: Nasal congestion

Drug Interactions

Metabolism/Transport Effects Substrate of CYP2C19 (minor), CYP2D6 (major); **Note:** Assignment of Major/Minor substrate status based on clinically relevant drug interaction potential; **Inhibits** CYP1A2 (weak), CYP2C9 (weak), CYP2D6 (strong), CYP2E1 (weak)

Avoid Concomitant Use

Avoid concomitant use of Thioridazine with any of the following: Aclidinium; Amisulpride; Azelastine (Nasal); CYP2D6 Inhibitors; Dapoxetine; Eluxadoline; FLUoxetine; FluvoxaMINE; Glucagon; Highest Risk QTc-Prolonging Agents; Ipratropium (Oral Inhalation); Ivabradine; Mequitazine; Metoclopramide; Mifepristone; Moclobemide; Moderate Risk QTc-Prolonging Agents; Orphenadrine; Paraldehyde; Pimozide; Potassium Chloride; Sulpiride; Tamoxifen; Thalidomide; Tiotropium; Umeclidinium

Increased Effect/Toxicity

Thioridazine may increase the levels/effects of: AbobotulinumtoxinA; Alcohol (Ethyl); Amisulpride; Analgesics (Opioid); Anticholinergic Agents; ARIPiprazole; AtoMOXetine; Azelastine (Nasal); Beta-Blockers; Buprenorphine; Chlorpheniramine; CNS Depressants; CYP2D6 Substrates; DOXOrubicin (Conventional); Eluxadoline; Fesoterodine; Glucagon; Highest Risk QTc-Prolonging Agents; Hydrocodone; Mequitazine; Methylphenidate; Metoprolol; Metyrosine; Nebivolol; OnabotulinumtoxinA; Orphenadrine; Paraldehyde; Pimozide; Porfimer; Potassium Chloride; RimabotulinumtoxinB; Selective Serotonin Reuptake Inhibitors; Serotonin Modulators; Sulpiride; Suvorexant; Tamsulosin; Thalidomide; Thiazide Diuretics; Thiopental; Tiotropium; TiZANidine; Topiramate; TraMADol; Verteporfin; Vortioxetine; Zolpidem

The levels/effects of Thioridazine may be increased by: Acetylcholinesterase Inhibitors (Central); Aclidinium; Antimalarial Agents; Beta-Blockers; Brimonidine (Topical); Cannabis; Chlorpheniramine; Cobicistat; CYP2D6 Inhibitors; Dapoxetine; Darunavir; Doxylamine; Dronabinol; FLUoxetine; FluvoxaMINE; Ipratropium (Oral Inhalation); Ivabradine; Kava Kava; Magnesium Sulfate; Methylphenidate; Metoclopramide; Metyrosine; Mifepristone; Moclobemide; Moderate Risk QTc-Prolonging Agents; Nabilone; Peginterferon Alfa-2b; Perampanel; Pramlintide; QTc-Prolonging Agents (Indeterminate Risk and Risk Modifying); Rufinamide; Serotonin Modulators; Sodium Oxybate; Tapentadol; Tetrahydrocannabinol; Umeclidinium

Decreased Effect

Thioridazine may decrease the levels/effects of: Acetylcholinesterase Inhibitors; Amphetamines; Anti-Parkinson's Agents (Dopamine Agonist); Codeine; Itopride; Quinagolide; Secretin; Tamoxifen; TraMADol

The levels/effects of Thioridazine may be decreased by: Acetylcholinesterase Inhibitors; Antacids; Anti-Parkinson's Agents (Dopamine Agonist); Peginterferon Alfa-2b

Storage/Stability Store at 20°C to 25°C (68°F to 77°F). Protect from light.

Mechanism of Action Thioridazine is a piperidine phenothiazine which blocks postsynaptic mesolimbic dopaminergic receptors in the brain; also has activity at serotonin, noradrenaline, and histamine receptors (Fenton, 2007).

Pharmacokinetics (Adult data unless noted)

Protein binding: 99%

Metabolism: In the liver to active and inactive metabolites

Bioavailability: 25% to 33%

Half-life: Adults: 9-30 hours

Dialysis: Not dialyzable: (0% to 5%)

Dosing: Usual Oral:

Children >2 years: Initial: 0.5 mg/kg/day in 2-3 divided doses; range: 0.5-3 mg/kg/day; usual: 1 mg/kg/day in 2-3 divided doses; maximum dose: 3 mg/kg/day

Behavior problems: Initial: 10 mg 2-3 times/day, increase gradually

Severe psychoses: Initial: 25 mg 2-3 times/day, increase gradually

Children >12 years and Adults:

Schizophrenia/psychoses: Initial: 25-100 mg 3 times/day with gradual increments as needed and tolerated; maximum daily dose: 800 mg/day in 2-4 divided doses; maintenance: 10-200 mg/dose 2-4 times/day

Depressive disorders, dementia: Initial: 25 mg 3 times/day; maintenance dose: 20-200 mg/day

Administration Oral: Administer with water, food, or milk to decrease GI upset; dilute the oral concentrate with water or juice before administration; do not administer liquid thioridazine simultaneously with carbamazepine suspension; do not mix liquid thioridazine with enteric formulas

Monitoring Parameters Baseline and periodic ECG and serum potassium; periodic eye exam, CBC with differential, blood pressure, liver enzyme tests

Test Interactions May interfere with urine detection of methadone and phencyclidine (false-positives) (Lancelin, 2005; Long, 1996).

Additional Information In cases of overdoses, cardiovascular monitoring and continuous ECG monitoring should be performed; avoid drugs (such as quinidine, disopyramide, and procainamide) that may further prolong the QT interval

Note: All Mellaril® (brand name) products have been discontinued; Mellaril® suspension was discontinued October, 2000; oral concentrate 100 mg/mL was discontinued March 2001; tablets and 30 mg/mL oral concentrate were discontinued in January 2002.

Dosage Forms Excipient information presented when available (limited, particularly for generics); consult specific product labeling.

Tablet, Oral, as hydrochloride:

Generic: 10 mg, 25 mg, 50 mg, 100 mg

◆ **Thioridazine Hydrochloride** *see* Thioridazine *on page 2051*

◆ **Thiosulfuric Acid Disodium Salt** *see* Sodium Thiosulfate *on page 1955*

Thiotepa (thye oh TEP a)

Medication Safety Issues

Sound-alike/look-alike issues:

Thiotepa may be confused with thioguanine

High alert medication:

This medication is in a class the Institute for Safe Medication Practices (ISMP) includes among its list of drug classes which have a heightened risk of causing significant patient harm when used in error.

Administration issues:

Product availability: Thiotepa is not currently available in the U.S. market. The FDA is allowing temporary importation of a European product (brand name Tepadina) through manufacturer Adienne SA (Italy) to fulfill clinical need. Indications and dosing vary greatly between the U.S. and European products; verify product, dosing, and preparation instructions prior to dispensation and administration.

Intrathecal medication safety: The American Society of Clinical Oncology (ASCO)/Oncology Nursing Society (ONS) chemotherapy administration safety standards (Jacobson, 2009) encourage the following safety measures for intrathecal chemotherapy:

- Intrathecal medication should not be prepared during the preparation of any other agents
- After preparation, keep in an isolated location or container clearly marked with a label identifying as "intrathecal" use only
- Delivery to the patient should only be with other medications intended for administration into the central nervous system

Related Information

Management of Drug Extravasations *on page 2298*

Prevention of Chemotherapy-Induced Nausea and Vomiting in Children *on page 2368*

Safe Handling of Hazardous Drugs *on page 2455*

Therapeutic Category Antineoplastic Agent, Alkylating Agent

Generic Availability (US) May be product dependent

Use Treatment of superficial tumors of the bladder; palliative treatment of adenocarcinoma of breast or ovary; control of pleural, pericardial, or peritoneal effusions caused by metastatic tumors (FDA approved in adults); has also been used for intrathecal treatment of leptomeningeal metastases (in adults) and as part of a conditioning regimen prior to autologous or allogeneic hematopoietic stem cell transplantation

Pregnancy Risk Factor D

Pregnancy Considerations Adverse events were observed in animal reproduction studies. May cause harm if administered during pregnancy. Effective contraception is recommended for men and women of childbearing potential.

Breast-Feeding Considerations It is not known if thiotepa is excreted in breast milk. Due to the potential for serious adverse reactions in the nursing infant, the manufacturer recommends a decision be made whether to discontinue nursing or to discontinue the drug, taking into account the importance of treatment to the mother.

Contraindications Hypersensitivity to thiotepa or any component of the formulation

Note: May be contraindicated in certain circumstances of hepatic, renal, and/or bone marrow failure; evaluate on an individual basis as lower dose treatment (with close monitoring) may still be appropriate if the potential benefit outweighs the risks

Warnings/Precautions Hazardous agent - use appropriate precautions for handling and disposal (NIOSH 2014 [group 1]). Myelosuppression is common; use with caution in patients with bone marrow damage, dosage reduction recommended. Use may be contraindicated with existing marrow damage and should be limited to cases where benefit outweighs risk. Monitor for infection or bleeding; death due to septicemia and hemorrhage has occurred. Myelosuppression (including fatal cases) has also been reported with intravesicular administration (due to systemic absorption). Monitor blood counts closely. Potentially teratogenic, mutagenic, and carcinogenic; myelodysplastic syndrome and acute myeloid leukemia (AML) have been reported. Reduce dosage and use extreme caution in patients with hepatic, renal, or bone marrow damage. Use may be contraindicated with impairment/damage and should be limited to cases where benefit outweighs risk. In children, thiotepa is associated with a high emetic potential at doses ≥300 mg/m^2; antiemetics are recommended to prevent nausea and vomiting (Dupuis, 2011).

When used for intrathecal administration (off-label route), should not be prepared during the preparation of any other agents; after preparation, keep intrathecal medications in an isolated location or container clearly marked with a label identifying as "intrathecal" use only; delivery of intrathecal medications to the patient should only be with other medications intended for administration into the central nervous system (Jacobson, 2009). Potentially significant drug-drug interactions may exist, requiring dose or frequency adjustment, additional monitoring, and/or selection of alternative therapy.

Due to the shortage of the U.S. generic product, the FDA is allowing temporary importation of a European product (brand name Tepadina) to fulfill clinical need. Indications and dosing vary greatly between the U.S. and European products; verify product, dosing, and preparation instructions prior to dispensation and administration.

Adverse Reactions

Central nervous system: Chills, dizziness, fatigue, fever, headache

Dermatologic: Alopecia, contact dermatitis, depigmentation (with topical treatment), dermatitis, rash, urticaria

Endocrine & metabolic: Amenorrhea, spermatogenesis inhibition

Gastrointestinal: Abdominal pain, anorexia, nausea, vomiting

Genitourinary: Dysuria, urinary retention

Hematologic: Anemia, bleeding, leukopenia, thrombocytopenia

Local: Injection site pain

Neuromuscular & skeletal: Weakness

Ocular: Blurred vision, conjunctivitis

Renal: Hematuria

Respiratory: Asthma, epistaxis, laryngeal edema, wheezing

Miscellaneous: Allergic reaction, anaphylactic shock, infection

Rare but important or life-threatening: Acute myeloid leukemia (AML), chemical cystitis (bladder instillation), hemorrhagic cystitis (bladder instillation), myelodysplastic syndrome

Drug Interactions

Metabolism/Transport Effects Inhibits CYP2B6 (moderate)

Avoid Concomitant Use

Avoid concomitant use of Thiotepa with any of the following: BCG; BCG (Intravesical); CloZAPine; Dipyrone; Natalizumab; Pimecrolimus; Tacrolimus (Topical); Tofacitinib; Vaccines (Live)

Increased Effect/Toxicity

Thiotepa may increase the levels/effects of: BuPROPion; CloZAPine; CYP2B6 Substrates; Leflunomide; Natalizumab; Tofacitinib; Vaccines (Live)

The levels/effects of Thiotepa may be increased by: Denosumab; Dipyrone; Pimecrolimus; Roflumilast; Tacrolimus (Topical); Trastuzumab

Decreased Effect

Thiotepa may decrease the levels/effects of: BCG; BCG (Intravesical); Coccidioides immitis Skin Test; Sipuleucel-T; Vaccines (Inactivated); Vaccines (Live)

The levels/effects of Thiotepa may be decreased by: Echinacea

Storage/Stability

Note: Due to drug shortage in the United States, the FDA is allowing temporary importation of a European product (Tepadina). Verify product, storage, and preparation instructions prior to dispensation and administration. Refer to specific product labeling for details.

Tepadina: Store intact vials under refrigeration at 2°C to 8°C (36°F to 46°F). Protect from light; do not freeze. Reconstituted solution (10 mg/mL) is stable for 8 hours when stored at 2°C to 8°C (36°F to 46°F). Solution further diluted for infusion is stable for 24 hours when stored at 2°C to 8°C (36°F to 46°F), or for 4 hours when stored at 25°C (77°F).

Generic product labeling (U.S.): Store intact vials under refrigeration at 2°C to 8°C (36°F to 46°F). Protect from light. Reconstituted solutions (10 mg/mL) are stable for up to 8 hours when stored under refrigeration. Solutions further diluted for infusion should be used immediately.

After preparation, keep intrathecal medications in an isolated location or container clearly marked with a label identifying as "intrathecal" use only.

Mechanism of Action Alkylating agent that reacts with DNA phosphate groups to produce cross-linking of DNA strands leading to inhibition of DNA, RNA, and protein synthesis; mechanism of action has not been explored as thoroughly as the other alkylating agents, it is presumed that the aziridine rings open and react as nitrogen mustard; reactivity is enhanced at a lower pH

Pharmacokinetics (Adult data unless noted)

Absorption: Variable absorption through serous membranes and from IM injection sites; bladder mucosa: 10% to 100% and is increased with mucosal inflammation or tumor infiltration

Distribution: V_{dss}: 0.7-1.6 L/kg; distributes into CSF

Protein binding: 8% to 13%

Metabolism: In the liver via oxidative desulfuration (cytochrome P450 microsomal enzyme system) primarily to TEPA (active metabolite)

Half-life, terminal:

- Thiotepa: 109 minutes (51.6-212 minutes) with dose-dependent clearance
- TEPA: 10-21 hours

Elimination: Very little thiotepa or active metabolite are excreted unchanged in urine (1.5% of thiotepa dose)

Dosing: Usual Refer to individual protocols

Infants, Children, and Adolescents: IV:

- HSCT for CNS malignancy (combination chemotherapy): 300 mg/m²/dose daily for 3 days (Dunkel, 2010; Finlay, 2008; Gilheeney, 2010; Grodman, 2009)
- HSCT for neuroblastoma/solid tumors (combination chemotherapy): Children and Adolescents: 300 mg/m²/dose daily for 3 days (Kletzel, 1998; Kushner, 2001; Kushner, 2006)

Adults:

- IV: Ovarian, breast cancer: 0.3-0.4 mg/kg/dose every 1-4 weeks
- Intracavitary: Effusions: 0.6-0.8 mg/kg/dose
- Intrathecal: Leptomeningeal metastases: 10 mg twice a week for 4 weeks, then weekly for 4 weeks, then monthly for 4 doses (NCCN CNS cancer guidelines v.1.2010)
- Intravesical: Bladder cancer: 60 mg in 30-60 mL NS retained for 2 hours once weekly for 4 weeks

Dosing adjustment in renal impairment: Use with extreme caution; reduced dose may be warranted. Use may be contraindicated with existing renal impairment and should be limited to cases where benefit outweighs risk.

Dosing adjustment in hepatic impairment: Use with extreme caution; reduced dose may be warranted. Use may be contraindicated with existing hepatic impairment and should be limited to cases where benefit outweighs risk.

Dosage adjustment for hematologic toxicity: IV:

- WBC ≤3000/mm³: Discontinue treatment
- Platelets ≤150,000/mm³: Discontinue treatment
- **Note:** Use may be contraindicated with pre-existing marrow damage and should be limited to cases where benefit outweighs risk.

Preparation for Administration Hazardous agent; use appropriate precautions for handling and disposal (NIOSH 2014 [group 1]). **Note:** Due to drug shortage in the US, the FDA is allowing temporary importation of a European product (Tepadina). Verify product, storage, and preparation instructions prior to dispensation and administration. Refer to specific product labeling for details.

Reconstitution:

- Tepadina: Reconstitute each 15 mg vial with 1.5 mL SWFI, or each 100 mg vial with 10 mL SWFI, to a concentration of 10 mg/mL. Gently mix by repeated inversions. Solution may be clear or opalescent; do not use if particulate matter is present.
- Generic product labeling (US): Reconstitute each 15 mg vial with 1.5 mL SWFI to a concentration of 10 mg/mL. Filter through a 0.22 micron filter (polysulfone membrane [eg, Sterile Aerodisc] or triton-free cellulose mixed ester [eg, Millex-GS]) prior to administration; do not use solutions which precipitate or remain opaque after filtering.

Route-specific preparations:

- Bladder instillation: Adults: After reconstitution, prepare with 60 mg diluted in 30 to 60 mL NS
- Intrapleural or pericardial: Adults: Further dilute dose to a volume of 10 to 20 mL in NS or D_5W
- Intrathecal: Adults: Further dilute to a final concentration of 1 mg/mL in preservative-free buffered solution (Grossman 1993) Intrathecal medications should not be prepared during the preparation of any other agents.
- IV: Further dilute dose in NS (product specific dilutions)
  - Tepadina: Further dilute reconstituted solution for IV infusion in 500 mL NS (1,000 mL NS if dose >500 mg). If dose is <250 mg, dilute in an appropriate volume of NS to achieve a final concentration of 0.5 to 1 mg/mL.
  - Generic product labeling (US): Solutions for IV use should be further diluted in NS

Administration Hazardous agent; use appropriate precautions for handling and disposal (NIOSH 2014 [group 1]). In children, thiotepa is associated with a high emetic potential at doses ≥300 mg/m²; antiemetics are recommended to prevent nausea and vomiting (Dupuis 2011).

Bladder instillation: Adults: Instill by catheter directly into the bladder and retain for 2 hours; patients should reposition every 15 to 30 minutes for maximal exposure.

Intrathecal: Adults: Intrathecal dilutions are preservative-free and should be used as soon as possible after preparation. After preparation, store intrathecal medications (until use) in an isolated location or container clearly marked with a label identifying as "intrathecal" use only.

IV: Further dilute reconstituted solution prior to administeration. Administer low doses (adult) as a rapid injection over 5 minutes; high doses (pediatric) have longer infusion times (eg, over 2- to 4-hour infusion); refer to specific protocols.

Vesicant/Extravasation Risk May be an irritant

Monitoring Parameters CBC with differential and platelet count, uric acid, urinalysis, renal and hepatic function tests

Additional Information Myelosuppressive effects:

WBC: Moderate
Platelets: Severe
Onset (days): 7-10
Nadir (days): 14-20
Recovery (days): 28

Thiothixene (thye oh THIKS een)

Medication Safety Issues

Sound-alike/look-alike issues:

Thiothixene may be confused with FLUoxetine, thioridazine

Navane may be confused with Norvasc, Nubain

BEERS Criteria medication:

This drug may be potentially inappropriate for use in geriatric patients (Quality of evidence - moderate; Strength of recommendation - strong).

Brand Names: Canada Navane

Therapeutic Category Antipsychotic Agent, Typical, Phenothiazine; First Generation (Typical) Antipsychotic; Phenothiazine Derivative

Generic Availability (US) Yes

Use Management of schizophrenia (FDA approved in ages ≥12 years and adults); also used for management of psychotic disorders

Pregnancy Considerations Adverse events were observed in some animal reproduction studies. Antipsychotic use during the third trimester of pregnancy has a risk for abnormal muscle movements (extrapyramidal symptoms [EPS]) and withdrawal symptoms in newborns following delivery. Symptoms in the newborn may include agitation, feeding disorder, hypertonia, hypotonia, respiratory distress, somnolence, and tremor; these effects may be self-limiting or require hospitalization. The ACOG recommends that therapy during pregnancy be individualized; treatment with psychiatric medications during pregnancy should incorporate the clinical expertise of the mental health clinician, obstetrician, primary healthcare provider, and pediatrician. When treating schizophrenia during pregnancy, atypical antipsychotics may be better tolerated by the mother however more information related to fetal effects may be available for agents considered typical (or first generation) antipsychotics (ACOG, 2008). Information related to the use of thiothixene in pregnancy is limited and other agents may be preferred.

Breast-Feeding Considerations It is not known if thiothixene is excreted into breast milk; other agents are preferred for use in nursing women (Klinger, 2013).

Contraindications Hypersensitivity to thiothixene or any component of the formulation; severe CNS depression; circulatory collapse; blood dyscrasias; coma

Warnings/Precautions [U.S. Boxed Warning]: Elderly patients with dementia-related psychosis treated with antipsychotics are at an increased risk of death compared to placebo. Most deaths appeared to be either cardiovascular (eg, heart failure, sudden death) or infectious (eg, pneumonia) in nature. Thiothixene is not approved for the treatment of dementia-related psychosis.

May alter cardiac conduction; life-threatening arrhythmias have occurred with therapeutic doses of antipsychotics. Avoid use in patients with underlying QT prolongation, in those taking medicines that prolong the QT interval, or cause polymorphic ventricular tachycardia; monitor ECG closely for dose-related QT effects (Haddad, 2002; Stollberger, 2005).

Leukopenia, neutropenia, and agranulocytosis (sometimes fatal) have been reported in clinical trials and postmarketing reports with antipsychotic use; presence of risk factors (eg, preexisting low WBC or history of drug-induced leuko-/neutropenia) should prompt periodic blood count assessment. Discontinue therapy at first signs of blood dyscrasias or if absolute neutrophil count <1000/mm^3.

Antipsychotic use has been associated with esophageal dysmotility and aspiration; use with caution in patients at risk of aspiration pneumonia (ie, Alzheimer disease) (Maddalena, 2004). May cause extrapyramidal symptoms, including pseudoparkinsonism, acute dystonic reactions, akathisia, and tardive dyskinesia. Risk of dystonia (and possibly other EPS) may be greater with increased doses, use of conventional antipsychotics, males, and younger patients. Risk of tardive dyskinesia and potential for irreversibility may be increased in elderly patients (particularly women), prolonged therapy, and higher total cumulative dose. Use may be associated with NMS; monitor for mental status changes, fever, muscle rigidity, and/or autonomic instability. May cause orthostatic hypotension; use with caution in patients at risk of this effect or in those who would not tolerate transient hypotensive episodes (cerebrovascular disease, cardiovascular disease, hypovolemia, or concurrent medication use which may predispose to hypotension/bradycardia). May rarely cause pigmentary retinopathy and lenticular pigmentation. Impaired core body temperature regulation may occur; caution with strenuous exercise, heat exposure, dehydration, and concomitant medication possessing anticholinergic effects.

Photosensitivity has been reported with thiothixene; avoid undue exposure to sunlight. May be sedating, use with caution in disorders where CNS depression is a feature; patients must be cautioned about performing tasks which require mental alertness (eg, operating machinery or driving). Effects may be potentiated when used with other sedative drugs or ethanol. May cause anticholinergic effects (constipation, xerostomia, blurred vision, urinary retention); use with caution in patients with decreased gastrointestinal motility, paralytic ileus, urinary retention, BPH, xerostomia, or visual problems. Relative to other neuroleptics, thiothixene has a low potency of cholinergic blockade. May mask toxicity of other drugs or conditions (eg, intestinal obstruction, Reye's syndrome, brain tumor) due to antiemetic effects. Use is associated with increased prolactin levels; clinical significance of hyperprolactinemia in patients with breast cancer or other prolactin-dependent tumors is unknown.

Use with caution in patients with severe cardiovascular disease, narrow-angle glaucoma, hepatic impairment, Parkinson disease, renal impairment, or seizure disorder. Potentially significant drug-drug interactions may exist, requiring dose or frequency adjustment, additional monitoring, and/or selection of alternative therapy.

Use in elderly patients with dementia is associated with an increased risk of mortality and cerebrovascular accidents; avoid antipsychotic use for behavioral problems associated with dementia unless alternative nonpharmacologic therapies have failed and patient may harm self or others. In addition, use may cause or exacerbate syndrome of inappropriate antidiuretic hormone secretion or hyponatremia; monitor sodium closely with initiation or dosage adjustments in older adults May also be inappropriate in older adults depending on comorbidities (eg, dementia, delirium) due to its potent anticholinergic effects (Beers Criteria). Increased risk for developing tardive dyskinesia, particularly elderly women.

Adverse Reactions

Cardiovascular: Cardiac arrest, ECG changes, hypotension, peripheral edema, syncope, tachycardia

Central nervous system: Abnormal cerebrospinal fluid, agitation, cerebral edema, dizziness, drowsiness, extrapyramidal reaction (akathisia, dystonias, pseudoparkinsonism, tardive dyskinesia), fatigue, hyperreflexia (infants), hypertonia (neonates), hypotonia (neonates), insomnia, Neuroleptic Malignant Syndrome, restlessness, seizure

Dermatologic: Contact dermatitis, diaphoresis, exfoliative dermatitis, pruritus, skin discoloration (blue-gray), skin photosensitivity, skin rash, urticaria

Endocrine & metabolic: Amenorrhea, change in libido, galactorrhea, glycosuria, gynecomastia, hyperglycemia, hyperprolactinemia, hypoglycemia, menstrual disease, polydipsia, weight gain

Gastrointestinal: Anorexia, constipation, diarrhea, increased appetite, nausea, paralytic ileus, sialorrhea, stomach pain, vomiting, xerostomia

Genitourinary: Breast hypertrophy, difficulty in micturition, ejaculatory disorder, impotence, lactation, mastalgia

Hematologic & oncologic: Leukocytosis, leukopenia

Hepatic: Increased serum alkaline phosphatase, increased serum transaminase

Hypersensitivity: Anaphylaxis (rare)

Neuromuscular & skeletal: Lupus-like syndrome, tremor, weakness

Ophthalmic: Blurred vision, miosis, mydriasis, retinitis pigmentosa

Respiratory: Asphyxia, nasal congestion, respiratory distress (neonates)

Miscellaneous: Fever, paradoxical reaction (excerbation of psychotic symptoms)

Drug Interactions

Metabolism/Transport Effects **Substrate** of CYP1A2 (major); **Note:** Assignment of Major/Minor substrate status based on clinically relevant drug interaction potential; **Inhibits** CYP2D6 (weak)

Avoid Concomitant Use

Avoid concomitant use of Thiothixene with any of the following: Aclidinium; Amisulpride; Azelastine (Nasal); Eluxadoline; Glucagon; Ipratropium (Oral Inhalation); Metoclopramide; Orphenadrine; Paraldehyde; Potassium Chloride; Sulpiride; Thalidomide; Tiotropium; Umeclidinium

Increased Effect/Toxicity

Thiothixene may increase the levels/effects of: AbobotulinumtoxinA; Alcohol (Ethyl); Amisulpride; Analgesics (Opioid); Anticholinergic Agents; ARIPiprazole; Azelastine (Nasal); Buprenorphine; CNS Depressants; Eluxadoline; Glucagon; Highest Risk QTc-Prolonging Agents; Hydrocodone; Mequitazine; Methotrimeprazine; Methylphenidate; Metyrosine; Mirabegron; Mirtazapine; Moderate Risk QTc-Prolonging Agents; OnabotulinumtoxinA; Orphenadrine; Paraldehyde; Potassium Chloride; RimabotulinumtoxinB; Selective Serotonin Reuptake Inhibitors; Serotonin Modulators; Sulpiride; Suvorexant; Thalidomide; Thiazide Diuretics; Tiotropium; Topiramate; Zolpidem

The levels/effects of Thiothixene may be increased by: Abiraterone Acetate; Acetylcholinesterase Inhibitors (Central); Aclidinium; Brimonidine (Topical); Cannabis; CYP1A2 Inhibitors (Moderate); CYP1A2 Inhibitors (Strong); Deferasirox; Doxylamine; Dronabinol; Droperidol; HydrOXYzine; Ipratropium (Oral Inhalation); Kava Kava; Lithium; Magnesium Sulfate; Methotrimeprazine; Methylphenidate; Metoclopramide; Metyrosine; Mianserin; Mifepristone; Nabilone; Peginterferon Alfa-2b; Perampanel; Pramlintide; Rufinamide; Serotonin Modulators; Sodium Oxybate; Tapentadol; Tetrahydrocannabinol; Umeclidinium; Vemurafenib

Decreased Effect

Thiothixene may decrease the levels/effects of: Acetylcholinesterase Inhibitors; Amphetamines; Anti-Parkinson's Agents (Dopamine Agonist); Itopride; Quinagolide; Secretin

The levels/effects of Thiothixene may be decreased by: Acetylcholinesterase Inhibitors; Anti-Parkinson's Agents (Dopamine Agonist); Cannabis; CYP1A2 Inducers (Strong); Cyproterone; Lithium; Teriflunomide

Storage/Stability Store at 20°C to 25°C (68°F to 77°F). Protect from moisture. Dispense in a tight, light-resistant container.

Mechanism of Action Thiothixene is a thioxanthene antipsychotic which elicits antipsychotic activity by postsynaptic blockade of CNS dopamine receptors resulting in inhibition of dopamine-mediated effects; also has alpha-adrenergic blocking activity

Dosing: Usual Oral:

Children <12 years: Dose not well established (use not recommended); 0.25 mg/kg/day in divided doses

Children ≥12 years and Adults: Initial: 2 mg 3 times/day, up to 20-30 mg/day; maximum dose: 60 mg/day

Administration Oral: Administer with food or water

Monitoring Parameters Periodic eye exam, CBC with differential, blood pressure, liver enzyme tests

Test Interactions May cause false-positive pregnancy test

Dosage Forms Excipient information presented when available (limited, particularly for generics); consult specific product labeling.

Capsule, Oral:

Generic: 1 mg, 2 mg, 5 mg, 10 mg

- ◆ **Thorazine** *see* ChlorproMAZINE *on page* *443*
- ◆ **Three-Factor PCC** *see* Factor IX Complex (Human) [(Factors II, IX, X)] *on page* *836*
- ◆ **Thrombi-Gel®** *see* Thrombin (Topical) *on page* *2056*
- ◆ **Thrombin-JMI®** *see* Thrombin (Topical) *on page* *2056*
- ◆ **Thrombin-JMI® Epistaxis Kit** *see* Thrombin (Topical) *on page* *2056*
- ◆ **Thrombin-JMI® Pump Spray Kit** *see* Thrombin (Topical) *on page* *2056*
- ◆ **Thrombin-JMI® Syringe Spray Kit** *see* Thrombin (Topical) *on page* *2056*

Thrombin (Topical) (THROM bin, TOP i kal)

Medication Safety Issues

Administration issues:

For topical use only. Do not administer intravenously or intra-arterially.

To reduce the risk of intravascular administration, the Institute for Safe Medication Practices (ISMP) has the following recommendations:

- Prepare, label, and dispense topical thrombin from the pharmacy department (including doses used in the operating room).
- Do not leave vial or syringe at bedside.
- Add auxiliary label to all labels and syringes stating "For topical use only - do not inject".
- When appropriate, use solutions which can be applied with an absorbable gelatin sponge or use a dry form on oozing surfaces.

- When appropriate, use spray kits to help differentiate between parenteral products.

Brand Names: US Evithrom®; Recothrom Spray Kit; Recothrom®; Thrombi-Gel®; Thrombi-Pad®; Thrombin-JMI®; Thrombin-JMI® Epistaxis Kit; Thrombin-JMI® Pump Spray Kit; Thrombin-JMI® Syringe Spray Kit

Therapeutic Category Hemostatic Agent

Generic Availability (US) No

Use Hemostasis aid whenever minor bleeding from capillaries and small venules is accessible and control by standard surgical techniques is ineffective or impractical (Evithrom: FDA approved in pediatric patients [age not specified] and adults; Recothrom: FDA approved in ages ≥1 month and adults; Thrombin-JMI: FDA approved in adults)

Trauma dressing for temporary control of moderate-to-severe bleeding wounds; control of surface bleeding from vascular access sites and percutaneous catheter/ tubes (Thrombi-Gel; Thrombi-Pad: FDA approved in adults)

Pregnancy Risk Factor C

Pregnancy Considerations Animal reproduction studies have not been conducted. Reproduction studies conducted with the solvent/detergent used in processing the human-derived product (Evithrom®) showed adverse events in animals. Only residual levels of the solvent/ detergent would be expected to remain in the finished product.

Breast-Feeding Considerations Breast feeding is not recommended by the manufacturer.

Contraindications Hypersensitivity to thrombin or any component of the formulation; not for direct injection into the circulatory system (for topical use only); additionally,

Evithrom® is also contraindicated in patients with known anaphylactic or severe systemic reactions to blood products; also contraindicated for the treatment of severe or brisk arterial bleeding

Recothrom® is also contraindicated in patients with hypersensitivity to hamster proteins; also contraindicated for the treatment of massive or brisk arterial bleeding

Thrombi-Gel®: Should not be used in closure of skin incisions, due to possible interference with healing of skin edges.

Thrombin-JMI® and Thrombi-Pad® are also contraindicated in patients with hypersensitivity to material of bovine origin.

Warnings/Precautions For topical use only. Do not inject intravenously or intra-arterially. Intravascular clotting, possibly leading to death, may occur following injection. Powder and solution formulations may be used in combination with absorbable gelatin sponges

[U.S. Boxed Warning]: Bovine-source topical thrombin may be associated with abnormal hemostasis, ranging from asymptomatic laboratory alterations to severe bleeding and/or thrombosis. Abnormalities appear to be immunologically mediated; repeated applications increase risk. Consult expert in coagulation disorders if laboratory evidence and/or signs and symptoms of bleeding are noted. Re-exposure of patients who develop antibodies to bovine thrombin preparations should be avoided. Evithrom® is a product of human plasma; may potentially contain infectious agents which could transmit disease. Screening of donors, as well as testing and/or inactivation or removal of certain viruses, reduces the risk. Infections thought to be transmitted by this product should be reported to the manufacturer. Recothrom® should be used with caution in patients with known hypersensitivity to snake proteins (manufacturing process uses an enzyme isolated from a snake protein); the potential for allergic reaction theoretically exists. Do not use Thrombi-Gel® or Thrombi-Pad® in the presence of infection; use caution in areas of contamination. Thrombi-Pad® is nonabsorbable; do not leave in the body.

Adverse Reactions

Cardiovascular: Thromboembolism

Dermatologic: Pruritus

Gastrointestinal: Nausea, vomiting

Hematologic and oncologic: Increased INR, increased neutrophils, lymphocytopenia, prolonged partial thromboplastin time, prolonged prothrombin time

Hypersensitivity: Hypersensitivity reaction

Immunologic: Antibody development

Local: Postoperative wound complication

Drug Interactions

Metabolism/Transport Effects None known.

Avoid Concomitant Use There are no known interactions where it is recommended to avoid concomitant use.

Increased Effect/Toxicity There are no known significant interactions involving an increase in effect.

Decreased Effect There are no known significant interactions involving a decrease in effect.

Storage/Stability

Evithrom®: Store frozen at -18°C or colder; must be thawed prior to use. Unopened vials may also be stored under refrigeration at 2°C to 8°C (36°F to 46°F) for up to 30 days. Stable for up to 24 hours at room temperature. Do not refreeze if thawed; do not refrigerate once at room temperature. Discard unused portion after 24 hours at room temperature.

Recothrom®: Store at 2°C to 25°C (36°F to 77°F). Following reconstitution, may store at this temperature for up to 24 hours. Vials are for single use only; discard any unused portion.

Thrombi-Gel®: Store at 2°C to 25°C (36°F to 77°F). After wetting with SWFI or 0.9% sodium chloride, use within 3 hours.

Thrombi-Pad®: Store at 2°C to 25°C (36°F to 77°F). If pad is wetted with 0.9% sodium chloride, use within 1 hour.

Thrombin-JMI®: Store at 2°C to 25°C (36°F to 77°F). Solutions may be stored at 2°C to 8°C (36°F to 46°F) for up to 24 hours or at room temperature for up to 8 hours

Mechanism of Action Activates platelets and catalyzes the conversion of fibrinogen to fibrin to promote hemostasis.

Dosing: Usual

Pediatric:

Hemostasis: Topical: **Note:** For topical use only; do not administer intravenously or intra-arterially:

Evithrom: Infants, Children, and Adolescents: Dose depends on area to be treated; may apply directly or in conjunction with an absorbable gelatin sponge; up to 10 mL was used with absorbable gelatin sponge in clinical studies

Recothrom: Infants ≥1 month, Children, and Adolescents: Dose depends on area to be treated including size of and number of bleeding sites; may apply directly or in conjunction with an absorbable gelatin sponge

Adult:

Hemostasis: Topical: **Note:** For topical use only; do not administer intravenously or intra-arterially:

Evithrom: Dose depends on area to be treated; up to 10 mL was used with absorbable gelatin sponge in clinical studies

Recothrom: Dose depends on area to be treated

Thrombi-Gel 10, 40, 100: Wet product with up to 3 mL, 10 mL, or 20 mL, respectively, NS or SWFI; apply directly over source of the bleeding with manual pressure

Thrombi-Pad: Apply pad directly over source of bleeding; may apply dry or wetted with up to 10 mL of NS. If desired, product may be left in place for up to 24 hours; do not leave in the body.

Thrombin-JMI:

Solution: Use 1,000 to 2,000 units/mL of solution where bleeding is profuse; use 100 units/mL for bleeding from skin or mucosal surfaces

Powder: May apply powder directly to the site of bleeding or on oozing surfaces

Preparation for Administration Topical solution:

Evithrom: May thaw in refrigerator (1 day) or at room temperature (1 hour). The 2 mL and 5 mL vials may also be thawed at 37°C (98.6°F) for up to 10 minutes.

Recothrom: Reconstitute using diluent provided in prefilled syringe. Gently swirl to dissolve powder; avoid excessive agitation; powder should dissolve within 1 minute; resulting in a concentration of 1,000 units/mL. Do not use diluent syringe to withdraw solution from vial.

Thrombin-JMI: Reconstitute using NS

Administration Topical: For topical use only; do not administer intravenously or intra-arterially.

Evithrom: Must be thawed prior to use. May apply thawed solution directly or in combination with absorbable gelatin sponge; when using with absorbable gelatin sponge, knead thoroughly to saturate the pad and remove trapped air bubbles.

Recothrom: May apply reconstituted solution directly or in combination with absorbable gelatin sponge.

Thrombi-Gel: May cut or roll to desired shape prior to wetting; once wetted and prior to applying, knead thoroughly to saturate the pad and remove trapped air bubbles.

Thrombi-Pad: May apply dry or wet.

Thrombin-JMI: May be applied directly as a powder or as reconstituted solution; sponge surface free of blood prior to application, if possible.

Additional Information One unit is amount required to clot 1 mL of standardized fibrinogen solution in 15 seconds

Dosage Forms Excipient information presented when available (limited, particularly for generics); consult specific product labeling.

Pad, topical [preservative free; bovine derived]:

Thrombi-Pad® 3x3: ≥200 units (10s)

Powder for reconstitution, topical [bovine derived]:

Thrombin-JMI®: 5000 units, 20,000 units [supplied with diluent]

Thrombin-JMI® Epistaxis kit: 5000 units [supplied with diluent]

Thrombin-JMI® Pump Spray Kit: 20,000 units [supplied with diluents]

Thrombin-JMI® Syringe Spray Kit: 5000 units; 20,000 units [supplied with diluent]

Powder for reconstitution, topical [preservative free; recombinant]:

Recothrom®: 5000 units; 20,000 units [production involves products derived from hamster and snake sources; supplied with diluent]

Recothrom Spray Kit: 20,000 units [production involves products derived from hamster and snake sources; supplied with diluent]

Solution, topical [human derived]:

Evithrom®: 800-1200 units/mL (2 mL, 5 mL, 20 mL)

Sponge, topical [preservative free; bovine derived]:

Thrombi-Gel® 10: ≥1000 units (10s)

Thrombi-Gel® 40: ≥1000 units (5s)

Thrombi-Gel® 100: ≥2000 units (5s)

◆ **Thrombi-Pad®** *see* Thrombin (Topical) *on page 2056*

◆ **Thymocyte Stimulating Factor** *see* Aldesleukin *on page 89*

◆ **Thymoglobulin** *see* Antithymocyte Globulin (Rabbit) *on page 180*

Thyroid, Desiccated (THYE roid DES i kay tid)

Medication Safety Issues

BEERS Criteria medication:

This drug may be potentially inappropriate for use in geriatric patients (Quality of evidence - low; Strength of recommendation - strong).

Brand Names: US Armour Thyroid; Nature-Throid; NP Thyroid; Westhroid; Westhroid-P [DSC]; WP Thyroid

Therapeutic Category Thyroid Product

Generic Availability (US) Yes

Use Replacement or supplemental therapy in hypothyroidism of any etiology (FDA approved in all ages); pituitary TSH suppressant for the treatment or prevention of various types of euthyroid goiter, thyroid nodules, thyroiditis, multinodular goiter, and thyroid cancer (FDA approved in adults); **Note:** Not indicated for treatment of transient hypothyroidism associated with subacute thyroiditis.

Pregnancy Risk Factor A

Pregnancy Considerations Endogenous thyroid hormones minimally cross the placenta; the fetal thyroid becomes active around the end of the first trimester. Liothyronine has not been found to increase the risk of teratogenic or adverse effects following maternal use during pregnancy.

Uncontrolled maternal hypothyroidism may result in adverse neonatal and maternal outcomes. To prevent adverse events, normal maternal thyroid function should be maintained prior to conception and throughout pregnancy. Levothyroxine is considered the treatment of choice for the control of hypothyroidism during pregnancy.

Breast-Feeding Considerations Endogenous thyroid hormones are minimally found in breast milk and are not associated with adverse events.

Contraindications Hypersensitivity to beef or pork or any component of the formulation; untreated thyrotoxicosis; uncorrected adrenal insufficiency

Warnings/Precautions [US Boxed Warning]: In euthyroid patients, thyroid supplements are ineffective and potentially toxic for weight reduction. High doses may produce serious or even life-threatening toxic effects particularly when used with some anorectic drugs. Thyroid supplements are not recommended for the treatment of female or male infertility, unless associated with hypothyroidism. Use with caution and reduce dosage in patients with angina pectoris or other cardiovascular disease and elderly since they may be more likely to have compromised cardiovascular function (Beers Criteria); chronic hypothyroidism predisposes patients to coronary artery disease. Use with caution in patients with adrenal insufficiency (contraindicated with uncorrected adrenal insufficiency), diabetes mellitus or insipidus, and myxedema; symptoms may be exaggerated or aggravated; initial dosage reduction is recommended in patients with long-standing myxedema. Treatment with glucocorticoids should precede thyroid replacement therapy in patients with adrenal insufficiency (ATA/AACE [Garber 2012]). Desiccated thyroid contains variable amounts of T_3, T_4, and other triiodothyronine compounds which are more likely to cause cardiac signs or symptoms due to fluctuating levels. Avoid use in the elderly due to risk of cardiac effects and the availability of safer alternatives (Beers Criteria). Many clinicians consider levothyroxine to be the drug of choice for thyroid replacement.

Warnings: Additional Pediatric Considerations Overtreatment may result in craniosynostosis in infants and premature closure of epiphyses in children; monitor use closely. May cause transient alopecia in children during the first few months of therapy. In neonates and infants, cardiac overload, arrhythmias, and aspiration from avid suckling may occur during initiation of therapy (eg, first 2 weeks); monitor closely.

Adverse Reactions Note: Adverse reactions often indicative of excess thyroid replacement and/or hyperthyroidism.

Rare but important or life-threatening: Alopecia, cardiac arrhythmia, chest pain, dyspnea, excessive bone loss with overtreatment (excess thyroid replacement), hand tremor, myalgia, palpitation, tachycardia, tremor

Drug Interactions

Metabolism/Transport Effects None known.

Avoid Concomitant Use

Avoid concomitant use of Thyroid, Desiccated with any of the following: Sodium Iodide I131

Increased Effect/Toxicity

Thyroid, Desiccated may increase the levels/effects of: Tricyclic Antidepressants; Vitamin K Antagonists

The levels/effects of Thyroid, Desiccated may be increased by: Piracetam

Decreased Effect

Thyroid, Desiccated may decrease the levels/effects of: Sodium Iodide I131; Theophylline Derivatives

The levels/effects of Thyroid, Desiccated may be decreased by: Bile Acid Sequestrants; Calcium Polystyrene Sulfonate; Calcium Salts; CarBAMazepine; Ciprofloxacin (Systemic); Estrogen Derivatives; Fosphenytoin; Lanthanum; Phenytoin; Rifampin; Selective Serotonin Reuptake Inhibitors; Sodium Polystyrene Sulfonate

Storage/Stability Store at 15°C to 30°C (59°F to 86°F).

Mechanism of Action The primary active compound is T_3 (triiodothyronine), which may be converted from T_4 (thyroxine) and then circulates throughout the body to influence growth and maturation of various tissues; exact mechanism of action is unknown; however, it is believed the thyroid hormone exerts its many metabolic effects through control of DNA transcription and protein synthesis; involved in normal metabolism, growth, and development; promotes gluconeogenesis, increases utilization and mobilization of glycogen stores and stimulates protein synthesis, increases basal metabolic rate

Pharmacodynamics Onset of action: Liothyronine (T_3): ~3 hours

Pharmacokinetics (Adult data unless noted)

Absorption: T_4: 40% to 80%; T_3: 95%; desiccated thyroid contains T_4, T_3, and iodine (primarily bound)

Protein binding: T_4: >99% bound to plasma proteins including thyroxine-binding globulin, thyroxine-binding prealbumin, and albumin

Metabolism: Hepatic to triiodothyronine (active); ~80% T_4 deiodinated in kidney and periphery; glucuronidation/conjugation also occurs; undergoes enterohepatic recirculation

Half-life elimination, serum:

- T_4: Euthyroid: 6-7 days; Hyperthyroid: 3-4 days; Hypothyroid: 9-10 days
- T_3: 0.75 days (Brent, 2011)

Time to peak serum concentration: T_4: 2-4 hours; T_3: 2-3 days

Elimination: Urine (major route of elimination); partially feces

Dosing: Neonatal Note: Doses presented as mg/kg/dose or mg/dose; closely review dosing units; adjust dose based upon clinical response and laboratory parameters

Congenital hypothyroidism: Oral: 4.8-6 mg/kg/dose or 15-30 mg/dose once daily. **Note:** AAP recommends levothyroxine as the preferred treatment for hypothyroidism in neonates (AAP, 2006). Neonates should have therapy initiated at full doses.

Dosing: Usual

Infants, Children, and Adolescents: **Note:** Doses presented as mg/kg/dose or mg/dose; closely review dosing units; adjust dose based upon clinical response and laboratory parameters.

Congenital Hypothyroidism: Note: Infants should have therapy initiated at full doses; Oral:

- Infants 1–6 months: 4.8-6 mg/kg/dose or 15-30 mg/dose once daily
- Infants >6-12 months: 3.6-4.8 mg/kg/dose or 30-45 mg/dose once daily
- Children 1-5 years: 3-3.6 mg/kg/dose or 45-60 mg/dose once daily
- Children 6-12 years: 2.4-3 mg/kg/dose or 60-90 mg/dose once daily
- Adolescents: Typical doses >1.2-1.8 mg/kg/dose or 90 mg/dose once daily

Adults: **Note:** The American Association of Clinical Endocrinologists does not recommend the use of desiccated thyroid for thyroid replacement therapy for hypothyroidism (Baskin, 2002).

Hypothyroidism: Oral: Initial: 15-30 mg; increase with 15 mg increments every 2-3 weeks; use 15 mg in patients with cardiovascular disease or long-standing myxedema. Maintenance dose: Usually 60-120 mg/day; monitor TSH and clinical symptoms.

Administration Oral: Administer on an empty stomach in the morning before breakfast.

Monitoring Parameters T_4, TSH, heart rate, blood pressure, clinical signs of hypo- and hyperthyroidism; growth, bone development (children); TSH is the most reliable guide for evaluating adequacy of thyroid replacement dosage. TSH may be elevated during the first few months of thyroid replacement despite patients being clinically euthyroid. In cases where T_4 remains low and TSH is within normal limits, an evaluation of "free" (unbound) T_4 is needed to evaluate further increase in dosage.

In congenital hypothyroidism, adequacy of replacement should be determined using both TSH and total- or free-T_4. During the first 3 years of life, total- or free-T_4 should be maintained in the upper 1/2 of the normal range; this should result in normalization of the TSH. In some patients, TSH may not normalize due to a resetting of the pituitary-thyroid feedback as a result of *in utero* hypothyroidism. Monitor closely for cardiac overload, arrhythmias and aspiration from avid suckling.

Pediatric patients: Monitor closely for under/overtreatment. Undertreatment may decrease intellectual development and linear growth, and lead to poor school performance due to impaired concentration and slowed mentation. Overtreatment may adversely affect brain maturation, accelerate bone age (leading to premature closure of the epiphyses and reduced adult height); craniosynostosis has been reported in infants. Perform routine clinical examinations at regular intervals (to assess mental and physical growth and development). Suggested frequency for monitoring thyroid function tests: Every 1-2 months during the first year of life, every 2-3 months between ages 1-3 years, and every 3-12 months thereafter until growth is completed; repeat tests 2 weeks after any change in dosage.

Reference Range

Thyroid Function Tests

Lab Parameters	Age	Normal Range
T_4 (thyroxine) serum concentration	1-7 days	10.1-20.9 mcg/dL
	8-14 days	9.8-16.6 mcg/dL
	1 month to 1 year	5.5-16.0 mcg/dL
	>1 year	4.0-12.0 mcg/dL
Free thyroxine index (FTI)	1-3 days	9.3-26.6
	1-4 weeks	7.6-20.8
	1-4 months	7.4-17.9
	4-12 months	5.1-14.5
	1-6 years	5.7-13.3
	>6 years	4.8-14.0
T_3 serum concentration	Newborns	100-470 ng/dL
	1-5 years	100-260 ng/dL
	5-10 years	90-240 ng/dL
	10 years to Adult	70-210 ng/dL
T_3 uptake		35%-45%
TSH serum concentration	Cord	3-22 micro international units/mL
	1-3 days	<40 micro international units/mL
	3-7 days	<25 micro international units/mL
	>7 days	0-10 micro international units/mL

Test Interactions

T_4-binding globulin (TBG): Factors that alter binding in serum (ATA/AACE [Garber 2012]):

Note: T_4 is ~99.97% protein bound. Factors that alter protein binding will affect serum total T_4 levels; however, measurement of serum free T_4 (the metabolically active moiety) has largely replaced serum total T_4 for thyroid status assessment.

Conditions/states that increase TBG binding: Pregnancy, hepatitis, porphyria, neonatal state

Medications that increase TBG binding: Estrogens, 5-fluorouracil, heroin, methadone, mitotane, perphenazine, selective estrogen receptor modulators (eg, tamoxifen, raloxifene)

Conditions/states that decrease TBG binding: Hepatic failure, nephrosis, severe illness

Medications that decrease TBG binding: Androgens, anabolic steroids, glucocorticoids, L-asparaginase, nicotinic acid

Thyroxine (T_4) and Triiodothyronine (T_3): Serum binding inhibitors (ATA/AACE [Garber 2012]):

Medications that inhibit T_4 and T_3 binding: Carbamazepine, furosemide, free fatty acids, heparin, NSAIDS (variable, transient), phenytoin, salicylates

Thyroid gland hormone: Interference with production and secretion (ATA/AACE [Garber 2012]):

Medications affecting iodine uptake: Amiodarone, iodinated contrast agents, iodine, ethionamide

Medications affecting hormone production: Amiodarone, ethionamide, iodinated contrast agents, iodine, sulfonylureas, sulfonamides, thionamides (carbimazole, methimazole, propylthiouracil)

Medications affecting secretion: Amiodarone, iodinated contrast agents, iodine, lithium

Medications inducing thyroiditis: Alemtuzumab, amiodarone, antiangiogenic agents (lenalidomide, thalidomide), denileukin diftitoxin, interferon alpha, interleukins, lithium, tyrosine kinase inhibitors (sunitinib, sorafenib)

Medications potentially causing the development of Graves': Alemtuzumab, interferon alpha, highly active antiretroviral therapy

Medications potentially ameliorating thyroiditis (if autoimmune) or Graves': Glucocorticoids

Hypothalamic-pituitary axis and TSH: Interference with secretion (ATA/AACE [Garber 2012]):

Medications decreasing TSH secretion: Bexarotene, dopamine, dopaminergic agonists (bromocriptine, cabergoline), glucocorticoids, interleukin-6, metformin, opiates, somatostatin analogues (octreotide, lanreotide), thyroid hormone analogues

Mediations increasing TSH secretion: Amphetamine, interleukin 2, metoclopramide, ritonavir, St John's wort

Medications potentially causing hypophysitis: Ipilimumab

Additional Information Tablet strengths may vary by manufacturer in terms of grains or mg; dosing recommendations are based on general clinical equivalencies that 1 grain = 60 mg or 65 mg; 1/2 grain = 30 mg or 32.5 mg; and 1/4 grain = 15 mg or 16.25 mg.

Dosage Forms Excipient information presented when available (limited, particularly for generics); consult specific product labeling. [DSC] = Discontinued product

Tablet, Oral:

Armour Thyroid: 15 mg, 30 mg, 60 mg, 90 mg, 120 mg
Armour Thyroid: 180 mg [scored]
Armour Thyroid: 240 mg
Armour Thyroid: 300 mg [scored]
Nature-Throid: 16.25 mg, 32.5 mg
Nature-Throid: 48.75 mg, 65 mg, 81.25 mg, 97.5 mg, 113.75 mg, 130 mg, 146.25 mg, 162.5 mg, 195 mg, 260 mg, 325 mg [scored]
NP Thyroid: 30 mg, 60 mg, 90 mg
Westhroid: 16.25 mg [DSC], 32.5 mg
Westhroid: 48.75 mg [DSC], 65 mg [scored]
Westhroid: 81.25 mg [DSC]
Westhroid: 97.5 mg, 113.75 mg [DSC], 130 mg, 146.25 mg [DSC], 162.5 mg [DSC], 195 mg, 260 mg [DSC], 325 mg [DSC] [scored]
Westhroid-P: 16.25 mg [DSC], 32.5 mg [DSC]
Westhroid-P: 48.75 mg [DSC], 65 mg [DSC], 97.5 mg [DSC], 130 mg [DSC] [scored]
WP Thyroid: 16.25 mg, 32.5 mg
WP Thyroid: 48.75 mg, 65 mg [scored]
WP Thyroid: 81.25 mg
WP Thyroid: 97.5 mg, 113.75 mg, 130 mg [scored]

- **Thyroid Extract** *see* Thyroid, Desiccated *on page* 2058
- **Thyroid USP** *see* Thyroid, Desiccated *on page* 2058
- **Thyrolar** *see* Liotrix *on page* 1276
- **ThyroShield [OTC]** *see* Potassium Iodide *on page* 1740

TiaGABine (tye AG a been)

Medication Safety Issues

Sound-alike/look-alike issues:

TiaGABine may be confused with tiZANidine

Brand Names: US Gabitril

Therapeutic Category Anticonvulsant, Miscellaneous

Generic Availability (US) Yes

Use Adjunctive therapy in the treatment of partial seizures (FDA approved in ages ≥12 years and adults)

Medication Guide Available Yes

Pregnancy Risk Factor C

Pregnancy Considerations Adverse events were observed in animal reproduction studies. Information specific to the use of tiagabine in pregnancy is limited (Leppik 1999; Neppe 2000). Patients exposed to tiagabine during pregnancy are encouraged to enroll themselves into the North American Antiepileptic Drug (NAAED) Pregnancy

Registry by calling 1-888-233-2334. Additional information is available at www.aedpregnancyregistry.org.

Breast-Feeding Considerations It is not known if tiagabine is excreted into breast milk. Information specific to the use of tiagabine while breast-feeding is limited (Neppe, 2000). According to the manufacturer, tiagabine should be used in breast-feeding women only when the benefits outweigh the potential risks.

Contraindications Hypersensitivity to tiagabine or any component of the formulation

Warnings/Precautions Antiepileptics are associated with an increased risk of suicidal behavior/thoughts with use (regardless of indication). Monitor all patients for notable changes in behavior that might indicate suicidal thoughts or depression; notify health care provider immediately if symptoms occur. New-onset seizures and status epilepticus have been associated with tiagabine use when taken for off-label indications. Seizures have occurred with doses as low as 4 mg/day and shortly after a dosage increase, even after stable therapy. In most cases, patients were using concomitant medications (eg, antidepressants, antipsychotics, stimulants, opioids). In these instances, the discontinuation of tiagabine, followed by an evaluation for an underlying seizure disorder, is suggested. Use for unapproved indications, however, has not been proven to be safe or effective and is not recommended. Anticonvulsants should not be discontinued abruptly because of the possibility of increasing seizure frequency; therapy should be withdrawn gradually to minimize the potential of increased seizure frequency, unless safety concerns require a more rapid withdrawal.

Use with caution in patients with hepatic impairment. Evidence of residual binding of tiagabine in the retina and uvea after 3 weeks has been observed in animal studies; although not directly measured, melanin binding is suggested. Long-term (up to 1 year) toxicological studies of tiagabine in animals showed no treatment-related ophthalmoscopic changes and macro- and microscopic examinations of the eye were unremarkable. The ability of available tests to detect potentially adverse consequences, if any, of the binding of tiagabine to melanin-containing tissue is unknown, and there was no systematic monitoring for relevant ophthalmological changes during the clinical development of tiagabine. Prescribers should be aware of the possibility of long-term ophthalmologic effects. Moderately severe to incapacitating generalized weakness has been reported after administration of tiagabine. The weakness resolved in all cases after a reduction in dose or discontinuation of tiagabine. Severe reactions, including Stevens-Johnson syndrome, although rarely reported, have resulted in fatalities. Experience in patients not receiving enzyme-inducing drugs has been limited; caution should be used in treating any patient who is not receiving one of these medications (decreased dose and slower titration may be required). May cause CNS depression, which may impair physical or mental abilities; patients must be cautioned about performing tasks that require mental alertness (eg, operating machinery or driving). Potentially significant interactions may exist, requiring dose or frequency adjustment, additional monitoring, and/or selection of alternative therapy.

Adverse Reactions

Cardiovascular: Chest pain, edema, hypertension, palpitations, peripheral edema, syncope, tachycardia, vasodilation

Central nervous system: Abnormal gait, agitation, ataxia, chills, confusion, depersonalization, depression, dizziness, drowsiness, dysarthria, emotional lability, euphoria, hallucination, hostility, hypertonia, hypoesthesia, hyporeflexia, hypotonia, insomnia, lack of concentration, malaise, memory impairment, migraine, myasthenia, myoclonus, nervousness, pain, paranoia, paresthesia, personality disorder, speech disturbance, status epilepticus, stupor, twitching, vertigo

Dermatologic: Alopecia, bruise, pruritus, skin rash, xeroderma

Endocrine & metabolic: Weight gain, weight loss

Gastrointestinal: Abdominal pain, diarrhea, gingivitis, increased appetite, nausea, oral mucosa ulcer, stomatitis, vomiting

Genitourinary: Abnormal uterine bleeding, dysmenorrhea, dysuria, urinary incontinence, urinary tract infection, vaginitis

Hematologic & oncologic: Lymphadenopathy

Hypersensitivity: Hypersensitivity reaction

Infection: Infection

Neuromuscular & skeletal: Arthralgia, hyperkinesia, hypokinesia, myalgia, neck pain, tremor, weakness

Ophthalmic: Amblyopia, nystagmus, visual disturbance

Otic: Otalgia, otitis media, tinnitus

Respiratory: Bronchitis, dyspnea, epistaxis, flu-like symptoms, pharyngitis, pneumonia

Miscellaneous: Accidental injury, cyst, diaphoresis, language problems

Rare but important or life-threatening: Abnormal electroencephalogram, abnormal erythrocytes, abnormal hepatic function tests, abnormal pap smear, abnormal stools, abscess, altered sense of smell, amenorrhea, anemia, angina pectoris, apathy, aphthous stomatitis, apnea, arthritis, asthma, benign skin neoplasm, blepharitis, blindness, brain disease, breast hypertrophy, bursitis, cellulitis, cerebral ischemia, cholecystitis, cholelithiasis, CNS neoplasm, coma, contact dermatitis, cutaneous nodule, cystitis, deafness, dehydration, delusions, dental caries, dermal ulcer, dysgeusia, dysphagia, ECG abnormality, eczema, eructation, exfoliative dermatitis, eye pain, facial edema, fecal incontinence, fibrocystic breast disease, furunculosis, gastritis, gastrointestinal hemorrhage, gingival hyperplasia, glossitis, goiter, hematuria, hemiplegia, hemoptysis, hemorrhage, hepatomegaly, hernia, herpes simplex infection, herpes zoster, hirsutism, hyperacusis, hypercholesteremia, hyperglycemia, hypermenorrhea, hyperreflexia, hyperventilation, hypoglycemia, hypokalemia, hyponatremia, hypotension, hypothyroidism, impotence, increased libido, keratoconjunctivitis, laryngitis, leg cramps, leukopenia, maculopapular rash, mastalgia, melena, movement disorder, muscle spasm, myocardial infarction, neuritis, oral paresthesia, orthostatic hypotension, osteoarthrosis, otitis externa, pallor, paralysis, pelvic pain, periodontal abscess, peripheral neuritis, peripheral vascular disease, petechia, phlebitis, photophobia, psoriasis, psychoneurosis, psychosis, pyelonephritis, rectal hemorrhage, renal failure, salpingitis, seizure (in patients with or without underlying seizure disorder), sepsis, sialorrhea, skin carcinoma, skin discoloration, skin photosensitivity, status epilepticus, Stevens-Johnson syndrome, subcutaneous nodule, suicidal ideation, suicidal tendencies, tendinous contracture, thrombocytopenia, thrombophlebitis, urethritis, urinary retention, urinary urgency, vaginal hemorrhage, vesiculobullous dermatitis, visual field defect, voice disorder, withdrawal seizures

Drug Interactions

Metabolism/Transport Effects Substrate of CYP3A4 (major); **Note:** Assignment of Major/Minor substrate status based on clinically relevant drug interaction potential

Avoid Concomitant Use

Avoid concomitant use of TiaGABine with any of the following: Azelastine (Nasal); Conivaptan; Fusidic Acid (Systemic); Idelalisib; Orphenadrine; Paraldehyde; Thalidomide

Increased Effect/Toxicity

TiaGABine may increase the levels/effects of: Alcohol (Ethyl); Azelastine (Nasal); Buprenorphine; CNS Depressants; Hydrocodone; Methotrimeprazine; Metyrosine;

Mirtazapine; Orphenadrine; Paraldehyde; Pramipexole; ROPINIRole; Rotigotine; Selective Serotonin Reuptake Inhibitors; Suvorexant; Thalidomide; Zolpidem

The levels/effects of TiaGABine may be increased by: Aprepitant; Brimonidine (Topical); Cannabis; Conivaptan; CYP3A4 Inhibitors (Moderate); CYP3A4 Inhibitors (Strong); Dasatinib; Doxylamine; Dronabinol; Droperidol; Fosaprepitant; Fusidic Acid (Systemic); HydrOXYzine; Idelalisib; Ivacaftor; Kava Kava; Luliconazole; Magnesium Sulfate; Methotrimeprazine; Mifepristone; Nabilone; Netupitant; Palbociclib; Perampanel; Rufinamide; Simeprevir; Sodium Oxybate; Stiripentol; Tapentadol; Tetrahydrocannabinol

Decreased Effect

The levels/effects of TiaGABine may be decreased by: Bosentan; CYP3A4 Inducers (Moderate); CYP3A4 Inducers (Strong); Dabrafenib; Deferasirox; Mefloquine; Mianserin; Mitotane; Orlistat; Siltuximab; St Johns Wort; Tocilizumab

Food Interactions Food reduces the rate but not the extent of absorption. Management: Administer with food.

Storage/Stability Store at controlled room temperature of 20°C to 25°C (68°F to 77°F). Protect from moisture and light.

Mechanism of Action The exact mechanism by which tiagabine exerts antiseizure activity is not definitively known; however, *in vitro* experiments demonstrate that it enhances the activity of gamma aminobutyric acid (GABA). It is thought that the binding of tiagabine to the GABA uptake carrier inhibits the uptake of GABA into presynaptic neurons, allowing an increased amount of GABA to be available to postsynaptic neurons; based on *in vitro* studies, tiagabine does not inhibit the uptake of dopamine, norepinephrine, serotonin, glutamate, or choline

Pharmacokinetics (Adult data unless noted)

Absorption: Rapid and nearly complete (>95%)

Distribution: Mean V_d:

Children 3-10 years: 2.4 L/kg

Adults: 1.3-1.6 L/kg

Note: V_d values are more similar between children and adults when expressed as L/m^2 (Gustavson, 1997)

Protein binding: 96%, mainly to albumin and alpha$_1$-acid glycoprotein

Metabolism: Extensive in the liver via oxidation and glucuronidation; undergoes enterohepatic recirculation

Bioavailability: Oral: 90%

Diurnal effect: Trough concentrations and AUC are lower in the evening versus morning

Half-life:

Children 3-10 years: Mean: 5.7 hours (range: 2-10 hours)

Children 3-10 years receiving enzyme-inducing AEDs: Mean: 3.2 hours (range: 2-7.8 hours)

Adults (normal volunteers): 7-9 hours

Adult patients receiving enzyme-inducing AEDs: 2-5 hours

Time to peak serum concentration: Fasting state: ~45 minutes

Elimination: ~2% excreted unchanged in urine; 25% excreted in urine and 63% excreted in feces as metabolites

Clearance:

Children 3-10 years: 4.2 ± 1.6 mL/minute/kg

Children 3-10 years receiving enzyme-inducing AEDs: 8.6 ± 3.3 mL/minute/kg

Adults (normal volunteers): 109 mL/minute

Adult patients: 1.9 ± 0.5 mL/minute/kg

Adult patients receiving enzyme-inducing AEDs: 6.3 ± 3.5 mL/minute/kg

Note: Clearance values are more similar between children and adults when expressed as mL/minute/m^2 (Gustavson, 1997)

Hepatic impairment: Clearance of unbound drug is decreased by 60%

Dosing: Usual Oral: **Note:** Doses were determined in patients receiving enzyme-inducing AEDs; use of these doses in patients **not** receiving enzyme-inducing AEDs may result in serum concentrations more than twice those of patients receiving enzyme-inducing AEDS; **lower doses are required in patients not receiving enzyme-inducing agents;** a slower titration may also be necessary in these patients. Consider tiagabine dosage adjustment if enzyme-inducing agent is added, discontinued, or dose is changed. Do **not** use loading doses of tiagabine in any patient; do **not** use a rapid dosage escalation or increase the dose in large increments.

Children <12 years: Only limited preliminary information is available; dosing guidelines are not established (Adkins, 1998; Pellock, 1999)

Children 12-18 years: Initial: 4 mg once daily for 1 week, then 8 mg/day given in 2 divided doses for 1 week, then increase weekly by 4-8 mg/day; administer in 2-4 divided doses per day; titrate dose to response; maximum dose: 32 mg/day (doses >32 mg/day have been used in select adolescent patients for short periods of time)

Adults: Initial: 4 mg once daily for 1 week, then increase weekly by 4-8 mg/day; administer in 2-4 divided doses per day; titrate dose to response; usual maintenance: 32-56 mg/day in 2-4 divided doses; maximum dose: 56 mg/day. **Note:** Twice daily dosing may not be well tolerated and dosing 3 times/day is the currently favored dosing frequency (Kalviainen, 1998).

Dosing adjustment in renal impairment: None needed

Dosing adjustment in hepatic impairment: Reduced doses and longer dosing intervals may be required

Administration Oral: Administer with food (to avoid rapid increase in plasma concentrations and adverse CNS effects)

Monitoring Parameters Seizure frequency, duration, and severity; signs and symptoms of suicidality (eg, anxiety, depression, behavior changes)

Reference Range Not established

Additional Information Population pharmacokinetic analysis suggests that tiagabine may be administered at similar doses without adjustment for age, gender, or body weight in epilepsy patients ≥11 years of age (Samara, 1998)

Dosage Forms Excipient information presented when available (limited, particularly for generics); consult specific product labeling.

Tablet, Oral, as hydrochloride:

Gabitril: 2 mg [contains fd&c yellow #6 (sunset yellow)]

Gabitril: 4 mg [contains fd&c yellow #10 (quinoline yellow)]

Gabitril: 12 mg [contains brilliant blue fcf (fd&c blue #1), fd&c yellow #10 (quinoline yellow)]

Gabitril: 16 mg [contains fd&c blue #2 (indigotine)]

Generic: 2 mg, 4 mg

Extemporaneous Preparations A 1 mg/mL tiagabine hydrochloride oral suspension may be made with tablets and a 1:1 mixture of Ora-Sweet® and Ora-Plus®. Crush ten 12 mg tablets in a mortar and reduce to a fine powder. Add small portions of the vehicle and mix to a uniform paste; mix while adding the vehicle in incremental proportions to **almost** 120 mL; transfer to a graduated cylinder; rinse mortar with vehicle, and add quantity of vehicle sufficient to make 120 mL. Label "shake well" and "refrigerate". Store in amber plastic prescription bottles; stable for 70 days at room temperature or 91 days refrigerated (preferred) (Nahata 2004).

A 1 mg/mL oral suspension may be made with tablets and a 6:1 mixture of simple syrup, NF and methylcellulose 1%. Crush ten 12 mg tablets in a mortar and reduce to a fine powder. Add 17 mL of methylcellulose 1% gel and mix to a uniform paste; mix while adding simple syrup, NF in incremental proportions to **almost** 120 mL; transfer to a graduated cylinder, rinse mortar with syrup, and add quantity of syrup sufficient to make 120 mL. Label "shake well" and "refrigerate". Store in amber plastic prescription bottles; stable for 42 days at room temperature or 91 days refrigerated (preferred) (Nahata 2004).

- **Tiagabine Hydrochloride** *see* TiaGABine *on page 2060*
- **Tiamol® (Can)** *see* Fluocinonide *on page 898*
- **Tiazac** *see* Diltiazem *on page 661*
- **Tiazac XC (Can)** *see* Diltiazem *on page 661*

Ticarcillin and Clavulanate Potassium

(tye kar SIL in & klav yoo LAN ate poe TASS ee um)

Brand Names: US Timentin [DSC]

Brand Names: Canada Timentin

Therapeutic Category Antibiotic, Beta-lactam and Beta-lactamase Combination; Antibiotic, Penicillin (Antipseudomonal)

Generic Availability (US) No

Use Treatment of infections caused by susceptible organisms involving the lower respiratory tract, urinary tract, skin and skin structures, bone and joint, gynecologic, intra-abdominal infections, and septicemia (FDA approved in ages ≥3 months and adults). Clavulanate expands activity of ticarcillin to include beta-lactamase producing strains of *S. aureus*, *H. influenzae*, *Moraxella catarrhalis*, *B. fragilis*, *Klebsiella*, *Prevotella*, *P. aeruginosa*, *Stenotrophomonas maltophilia*, *E. coli*, and *Proteus* species

Pregnancy Risk Factor B

Pregnancy Considerations Adverse events were not observed in animal reproduction studies. Ticarcillin and clavulanate cross the placenta (Maberry, 1992). Maternal use of penicillins has generally not resulted in an increased risk of adverse fetal effects (Crider, 2009; Santos, 2011). Ticarcillin/clavulanate is approved for the treatment of postpartum gynecologic infections, including endometritis, caused by susceptible organisms.

Breast-Feeding Considerations Small amounts of ticarcillin are found in breast milk (Matsuda, 1984; von Kobyletzki, 1983); however, it is not orally absorbed (Brogden, 1980). The manufacturer recommends that caution be exercised when administering ticarcillin/clavulanate to nursing women.

Contraindications Hypersensitivity (history of a serious reaction [eg, anaphylaxis, Stevens-Johnson syndrome]) to ticarcillin, clavulanate, or to other beta-lactams (eg, penicillins, cephalosporins)

Warnings/Precautions Serious and occasionally severe or fatal hypersensitivity (anaphylactic) reactions have been reported in patients on penicillin therapy (especially with a history of beta-lactam hypersensitivity and/or a history of sensitivity to multiple allergens); use with caution in patients with seizures and in patients with HF due to high sodium load. Hypokalemia has been reported; monitor serum potassium in patients with fluid and electrolyte imbalance and in patients receiving prolonged therapy. Use with caution and modify dosage in patients with renal impairment; Bleeding disorders have been observed (particularly in renal impairment); discontinue if thrombocytopenia or bleeding occurs. Prolonged use may result in fungal or bacterial superinfection, including *C. difficile*-associated diarrhea (CDAD) and pseudomembranous colitis; CDAD has been observed >2 months postantibiotic treatment.

Adverse Reactions

Cardiovascular: Local thrombophlebitis (with IV injection)

Central nervous system: Confusion, drowsiness, headache, seizure

Dermatologic: Skin rash

Endocrine & metabolic: Electrolyte disturbance, hypernatremia, hypokalemia

Gastrointestinal: *Clostridium difficile* diarrhea, diarrhea, nausea

Genitourinary: Proteinuria (false positive)

Hematologic & oncologic: Bleeding complication, eosinophilia, hemolytic anemia, positive direct Coombs' test (false positive)

Hepatic: Hepatotoxicity, increased serum ALT, increased serum AST, jaundice

Immunologic: Jarisch Herxheimer reaction

Infection: Superinfection (fungal or bacterial)

Renal: Interstitial nephritis (acute)

Miscellaneous: Anaphylaxis

Rare but important or life-threatening: Altered sense of smell, chest discomfort, chills, decreased hematocrit, decreased hemoglobin, decreased serum potassium, dizziness, dysgeusia, erythema multiforme, flatulence, headache, hemorrhagic cystitis, hypersensitivity reaction, hypouricemia, increased blood urea nitrogen, increased lactate dehydrogenase, increased serum alkaline phosphatase, increased serum creatinine, injection site reaction (burning, induration, pain, swelling), leukopenia, myalgia, myoclonus, neutropenia, prolonged prothrombin time, pruritus, pseudomembranous colitis (during or after antibacterial treatment), Stevens-Johnson syndrome, stomatitis, thrombocytopenia, toxic epidermal necrolysis, urticaria

Drug Interactions

Metabolism/Transport Effects None known.

Avoid Concomitant Use

Avoid concomitant use of Ticarcillin and Clavulanate Potassium with any of the following: BCG; BCG (Intravesical); Probenecid

Increased Effect/Toxicity

Ticarcillin and Clavulanate Potassium may increase the levels/effects of: Methotrexate; Vitamin K Antagonists

The levels/effects of Ticarcillin and Clavulanate Potassium may be increased by: Probenecid

Decreased Effect

Ticarcillin and Clavulanate Potassium may decrease the levels/effects of: Aminoglycosides; BCG; BCG (Intravesical); BCG Vaccine (Immunization); Mycophenolate; Sodium Picosulfate; Typhoid Vaccine

The levels/effects of Ticarcillin and Clavulanate Potassium may be decreased by: Tetracycline Derivatives

Storage/Stability

Vials: Store intact vials at ≤24°C (≤75°F). Reconstituted solution is stable for 6 hours at room temperature and 72 hours when refrigerated. IV infusion in NS or LR is stable for 24 hours at room temperature (21°C to 24°C [70°F to 75°F]), 7 days when refrigerated (4°C [39°F]), or 30 days when frozen (-18°C [0°F]). IV infusion in D_5W solution is stable for 24 hours at room temperature (21°C to 24°C [70°F to 75°F]), 3 days when refrigerated (4°C [39°F]), or 7 days when frozen (-18°C [0°F]. After freezing, thawed solution is stable for 8 hours at room temperature. Do not refreeze. Darkening of drug indicates loss of potency of clavulanate potassium.

Premixed solution: Store frozen at ≤-20°C (-4°F). Thawed solution is stable for 24 hours at room temperature (22°C [72°F]) or 7 days under refrigeration at (4°C [39°F]); do not refreeze.

Mechanism of Action Inhibits bacterial cell wall synthesis by binding to one or more of the penicillin-binding proteins (PBPs), which in turn inhibits the final transpeptidation step of peptidoglycan synthesis in bacterial cell walls, thus inhibiting cell wall biosynthesis. Bacteria eventually lyse due to ongoing activity of cell wall autolytic enzymes (autolysins and murein hydrolases) while cell wall assembly is arrested.

Pharmacokinetics (Adult data unless noted)

Distribution: Ticarcillin is distributed into tissue, interstitial fluid, pleural fluid, and bile; low concentrations of ticarcillin distribute into the CSF but increase when meninges are inflamed

V_{dss} ticarcillin: 0.22 L/kg

V_{dss} clavulanic acid: 0.4 L/kg

Protein binding:

Ticarcillin: 45%

Clavulanic acid: 25%

Metabolism: Clavulanic acid is metabolized hepatically

Half-life: In patients with normal renal function

Neonates:

Clavulanic acid: 1.9 hours

Ticarcillin: 4.4 hours

Children (1 month to 9.3 years):

Clavulanic acid: 54 minutes

Ticarcillin: 66 minutes

Adults:

Clavulanic acid: 66-90 minutes

Ticarcillin: 66-72 minutes; 13 hours (in patients with renal failure)

Clavulanic acid does not affect the clearance of ticarcillin

Elimination:

Children: 71% of the ticarcillin and 50% of the clavulanic acid dose are excreted unchanged in the urine over 4 hours

Adults: Ticarcillin: Urine (60% to 70% as unchanged drug); Clavulanic acid: Urine (35% to 45% as unchanged drug)

Dialysis: Removed by hemodialysis

Dosing: Neonatal IV: **Note:** Timentin® (ticarcillin/clavulanate) is a combination product; each 3.1 g contains 3 g ticarcillin disodium and 0.1 g clavulanic acid. Dosage recommendations are based on **ticarcillin** component:

General dosing, susceptible infection (*Red Book*, 2012): IV:

Body weight <1 kg:

PNA ≤14 days: 75 mg ticarcillin/kg/dose every 12 hours

PNA 15-28 days: 75 mg ticarcillin/kg/dose every 8 hours

Body weight ≥1 kg:

PNA ≤7 days: 75 mg ticarcillin/kg/dose every 12 hours

PNA 8-28 days: 75 mg ticarcillin/kg/dose every 8 hours

Dosing: Usual

Infants, Children, and Adolescents: **Note:** Timentin® (ticarcillin/clavulanate) is a combination product; each 3.1 g contains 3 g ticarcillin disodium and 0.1 g clavulanic acid. Dosage recommendations are based on **ticarcillin** component:

General dosing, susceptible infection: IV:

Mild to moderate infections: 200 mg ticarcillin/kg/day in divided doses every 6 hours; maximum daily dose: 12 **g** ticarcillin/**day**

Severe infections:

Manufacturer's labeling: 300 mg ticarcillin/kg/day in divided doses every 4 hours

AAP recommendations: 200-300 mg ticarcillin/kg/day in divided doses every 4-6 hours

Maximum daily dose: 18 **g** ticarcillin/**day**

Cystic fibrosis: IV: 400 mg ticarcillin/kg/day in divided doses every 6 hours; higher doses have been used: 400-750 mg ticarcillin/kg/day in divided doses every 6 hours (Zobell, 2013)

Adults:

Systemic infections: IV: 3.1 **g** (ticarcillin 3000 mg plus clavulanic acid 100 mg) every 4-6 hours (maximum: 24 g of ticarcillin/day)

Amnionitis, cholangitis, diverticulitis, endometritis, epididymo-orchitis, mastoiditis, orbital cellulitis, peritonitis, pneumonia (aspiration): IV: 3.1 **g** (ticarcillin 3000 mg plus clavulanic acid 100 mg) every 6 hours

Intra-abdominal infection, complicated, community-acquired, mild to moderate: IV: 3.1 **g** (ticarcillin 3000 mg plus clavulanic acid 100 mg) every 6 hours for 4-7 days (provided source controlled)

Liver abscess, parafascial space infections, septic thrombophlebitis: IV: 3.1 **g** (ticarcillin 3000 mg plus clavulanic acid 100 mg) every 4 hours

***Pseudomonas* infections:** IV: 3.1 **g** (ticarcillin 3000 mg plus clavulanic acid 100 mg) every 4 hours

Urinary tract infections: IV: 3.1 **g** (ticarcillin 3000 mg plus clavulanic acid 100 mg) every 6-8 hours

Dosing adjustment in renal impairment: Note: Dosage recommendations are based on **ticarcillin** component:

Infants, Children, and Adolescents: There are no dosage adjustments provided in the manufacturer's labeling; however, the following have been used by some clinicians (Aronoff, 2007): Dosing based on a usual dose of 200-300 ticarcillin mg/kg/day in divided doses every 6 hours.

GFR >30 mL/minute/1.73 m^2: No adjustment required.

GFR 10-29 mL/minute/1.73 m^2: 50-75 mg ticarcillin/kg every 8 hours

GFR <10 mL/minute/1.73 m^2 (without concomitant hepatic failure): 50-75 mg ticarcillin/kg every 12 hours

GFR <10 mL/minute/1.73 m^2 (with concomitant hepatic failure): 50-75 mg ticarcillin/kg every 24 hours

Intermittent hemodialysis (without concomitant hepatic failure): 50-75 mg ticarcillin/kg every 12 hours

Intermittent hemodialysis (with concomitant hepatic failure): 50-75 mg ticarcillin/kg every 24 hours

Peritoneal dialysis (without concomitant hepatic failure): 50-75 mg ticarcillin/kg every 12 hours

Peritoneal dialysis (with concomitant hepatic failure): 50-75 mg ticarcillin/kg every 24 hours

Continuous renal replacement therapy (CRRT): 50-75 mg ticarcillin/kg every 8 hours

Adults:

CrCl >60 mL/minute: No dosage adjustment required.

CrCl 30-60 mL/minute: 2000 mg ticarcillin component every 4 hours or 3.1 **g** (3000 mg ticarcillin component) every 8 hours

CrCl 10-30 mL/minute: 2000 mg ticarcillin component every 8 hours or 3.1 **g** (3000 mg ticarcillin component) every 12 hours

CrCl <10 mL/minute without concomitant hepatic dysfunction: 2000 mg ticarcillin component every 12 hours

CrCl <10 mL/minute with concomitant hepatic dysfunction: 2000 mg ticarcillin component every 24 hours

Intermittent hemodialysis (IHD) (administer after hemodialysis on dialysis days): Dialyzable (20% to 50%): 2000 mg of ticarcillin component every 12 hours; supplemented with 3.1 **g** (3000 mg ticarcillin component) after each dialysis session. Alternatively, administer 2000 mg of ticarcillin component every 8 hours without a supplemental dose for deep-seated infections (Heintz, 2009). **Note:** Dosing dependent on the assumption of 3 times/week, complete IHD sessions.

Peritoneal dialysis (PD): 3.1 **g** (3000 mg ticarcillin component) every 12 hours

Continuous renal replacement therapy (CRRT) (Heintz, 2009; Trotman, 2005): Drug clearance is highly dependent on the method of renal replacement, filter type, and flow rate. Appropriate dosing requires close monitoring of pharmacologic response, signs of adverse reactions due to drug accumulation, as well as drug concentrations in relation to target trough (if appropriate). The following are general recommendations only (based on dialysate flow/ultrafiltration rates of 1-2 L/hour and minimal residual renal function) and should not supersede clinical judgment:

CVVH: Loading dose of 3.1 **g** (3000 mg ticarcillin component) followed by 2000 mg ticarcillin component every 6-8 hours

CVVHD: Loading dose of 3.1 **g** (3000 mg ticarcillin component) followed by 3.1 **g** (3000 mg ticarcillin component) every 6-8 hours

CVVHDF: Loading dose of 3.1 **g** (3000 mg ticarcillin component) followed by 3.1 **g** (3000 mg ticarcillin component) every 6 hours

Note: Do not administer in intervals exceeding every 8 hours. Clavulanate component is hepatically eliminated; extending the dosing interval beyond 8 hours may result in loss of beta-lactamase inhibition.

CVVH: Dose as for CrCl 10-50 mL/minute

Hemodialysis: 2 g every 12 hours; supplement with 3 g after each dialysis

Peritoneal Dialysis: 3 g every 12 hours

Dosing in hepatic impairment: Adults: With concomitant renal dysfunction (CrCl <10 mL/minute) 2000 mg ticarcillin component every 24 hours

Preparation for Administration Parenteral: Reconstitute 3.1 g vials with 13 mL SWFI or NS; shake well; resulting concentration is ticarcillin 200 mg/mL and clavulanic acid 6.7 mg/mL. Reconstitute 31 g bulk vials with 76 mL SWFI or NS; shake well; resulting concentration is ticarcillin 300 mg/mL and clavulanic acid 10 mg/mL. Further dilute to a final concentration of 10 to 100 mg/mL in D_5W, LR, or NS.

Administration Parenteral: Administer by IV intermittent infusion over 30 minutes

Some penicillins (eg, carbenicillin, ticarcillin, and piperacillin) have been shown to inactivate aminoglycosides *in vitro*. This has been observed to a greater extent with tobramycin and gentamicin, while amikacin has shown greater stability against inactivation. Concurrent use of these agents may pose a risk of reduced antibacterial efficacy *in vivo*, particularly in the setting of profound renal impairment. However, definitive clinical evidence is lacking. If combination penicillin/aminoglycoside therapy is desired in a patient with renal dysfunction, separation of doses (if feasible), and routine monitoring of aminoglycoside levels, CBC, and clinical response should be considered.

Monitoring Parameters Serum electrolytes, periodic renal, hepatic and hematologic function tests; observe IV injection site for signs of extravasation; observe for signs and symptoms of anaphylaxis during first dose

Test Interactions Positive Coombs' test, false-positive urinary proteins

Some penicillin derivatives may accelerate the degradation of aminoglycosides *in vitro*, leading to a potential underestimation of aminoglycoside serum concentration.

Product Availability Not available in the US

Dosage Forms Excipient information presented when available (limited, particularly for generics); consult specific product labeling. [DSC] = discontinued product

Infusion [premixed, frozen]:

Timentin: Ticarcillin 3 g and clavulanic acid 0.1 g (100 mL [DSC]) [contains sodium 4.51 mEq and potassium 0.15 mEq per g]

Injection, powder for reconstitution:

Timentin: Ticarcillin 3 g and clavulanic acid 0.1 g (3.1 g [DSC], 31 g [DSC]) [contains sodium 4.51 mEq and potassium 0.15 mEq per g]

◆ **Ticarcillin and Clavulanic Acid** *see* Ticarcillin and Clavulanate Potassium *on page 2063*

◆ **TIG** *see* Tetanus Immune Globulin (Human) *on page 2031*

◆ **Tigan** *see* Trimethobenzamide *on page 2125*

Tigecycline (tye ge SYE kleen)

Brand Names: US Tygacil

Brand Names: Canada Tygacil

Therapeutic Category Antibiotic, Glycylcycline

Generic Availability (US) No

Use Treatment of complicated skin and skin structure infections, complicated intra-abdominal infections (eg, appendicitis, cholecystitis, peritonitis, liver abscess), and community-acquired bacterial pneumonia caused by susceptible organisms (FDA approved in ages ≥18 years and adults). **Note:** Not indicated for the treatment of diabetic foot infections nor hospital-acquired pneumonia (HAP), including ventilator-associated pneumonia (VAP). Subgroup of patients with ventilator-associated pneumonia who received tigecycline demonstrated inferior efficacy, including lower cure rates and increased mortality than the comparator group.

Pregnancy Risk Factor D

Pregnancy Considerations Because adverse effects were observed in animals and because of the potential for permanent tooth discoloration, tigecycline is classified pregnancy category D. Tigecycline frequently causes nausea and vomiting and, therefore, may not be ideal for use in a patient with pregnancy-related nausea.

Breast-Feeding Considerations It is not known if tigecycline is found in breast milk. The manufacturer recommends caution if giving tigecycline to a nursing woman. Nondose-related effects could include modification of bowel flora.

Contraindications

Hypersensitivity to tigecycline or any component of the formulation

Documentation of allergenic cross-reactivity for tetracyclines is limited. However, because of similarities in chemical structure and/or pharmacologic actions, the possibility of cross-sensitivity cannot be ruled out with certainty.

Canadian labeling: Additional contraindications (not in U.S. labeling): Hypersensitivity to tetracycline class of antibiotics

Warnings/Precautions [U.S. Boxed Warning]: In Phase 3 and 4 clinical trials, an increase in all-cause mortality was observed in patients treated with tigecycline compared to those treated with comparator antibiotics; cause has not been established. Use should be reserved for situations in which alternative treatments are not appropriate. In general, deaths were the result of worsening infection, complications of infection, or underlying comorbidity. May cause life-threatening anaphylaxis/anaphylactoid reactions. Due to structural similarity with tetracyclines, use caution in patients with prior hypersensitivity and/or severe adverse reactions associated with tetracycline use (Canadian labeling contraindicates use in patients with hypersensitivity to tetracyclines). Due to structural similarities with tetracyclines, may be associated with photosensitivity, pseudotumor cerebri, pancreatitis, and antianabolic effects (including increased BUN, azotemia, acidosis, and hyperphosphatemia) observed with this class. Acute pancreatitis (including fatalities) has been reported, including patients without known risk factors;

discontinue use when suspected. May cause fetal harm if used during pregnancy; patients should be advised of potential risks associated with use. Permanent discoloration of the teeth may occur if used during tooth development (fetal stage through children up to 8 years of age).

Safety and efficacy in children <18 years of age have not been established due to increased mortality observed in trials of adult patients. Use only if no alternative antibiotics are available. Because of effects on tooth development (yellow-gray-brown discoloration), use in patients <8 years is not recommended.

Use caution in hepatic impairment; dosage adjustment recommended in severe hepatic impairment. Abnormal liver function tests (increased total bilirubin, prothrombin time, transaminases) have been reported. Isolated cases of significant hepatic dysfunction and hepatic failure have occurred. Closely monitor for worsening hepatic function in patients that develop abnormal liver function tests during therapy. Adverse hepatic effects may occur after drug discontinuation.

Prolonged use may result in fungal or bacterial superinfection, including *C. difficile*-associated diarrhea (CDAD) and pseudomembranous colitis; CDAD has been observed >2 months postantibiotic treatment. Use with caution if using as monotherapy for patients with intestinal perforation (in the small sample of available cases, septic shock occurred more frequently than patients treated with imipenem/cilastatin comparator). Do not use for diabetic foot infections; non-inferiority was not demonstrated in studies. Do not use for healthcare-acquired pneumonia (HAP) or ventilator-associated pneumonia (VAP); increased mortality and decreased efficacy have been reported in HAP and VAP trials.

Adverse Reactions

Cardiovascular: Localized phlebitis
Central nervous system: Dizziness, headache
Dermatologic: Skin rash
Endocrine & metabolic: Hyponatremia, increased amylase
Gastrointestinal: Abdominal pain, diarrhea, dyspepsia, nausea, vomiting
Hematologic & oncologic: Anemia, hypoproteinemia
Hepatic: Hyperbilirubinemia, increased serum ALT, increased serum AST, increased serum alkaline phosphatase
Infection: Abscess, infection
Neuromuscular & skeletal: Weakness
Renal: Increased blood urea nitrogen
Respiratory: Pneumonia
Miscellaneous: Abnormal healing
Rare but important or life-threatening: Acute pancreatitis, allergic skin reaction, anaphylactoid reaction, anaphylaxis, anorexia, *Clostridium difficile* associated diarrhea, dysgeusia, eosinophilia, hepatic insufficiency, hepatic failure, hypocalcemia, hypoglycemia, increased INR, increased serum creatinine, increased serum transaminases, increased INR, increased serum creatinine, increased serum transaminases, prolonged partial thromboplastin time, prolonged prothrombin time, pruritus, septic shock, Stevens-Johnson syndrome, swelling at injection site, thrombocytopenia, thrombophlebitis, vaginal moniliasis, vaginitis

Drug Interactions

Metabolism/Transport Effects None known.

Avoid Concomitant Use There are no known interactions where it is recommended to avoid concomitant use.

Increased Effect/Toxicity

Tigecycline may increase the levels/effects of: Warfarin

Decreased Effect There are no known significant interactions involving a decrease in effect.

Storage/Stability Prior to reconstitution, store at 20°C to 25°C (68°F to 77°F); excursions are permitted between 15°C and 30°C (59°F and 86°F). Reconstituted solution may be stored at room temperature (not to exceed 25°C [77°F]) for up to 6 hours in the vial or up to 24 hours if further diluted in a compatible IV solution. Alternatively, may be stored refrigerated at 2°C to 8°C (36°F to 46°F) for up to 48 hours following immediate transfer of the reconstituted solution into NS or D_5W.

Mechanism of Action A glycylcycline antibiotic that binds to the 30S ribosomal subunit of susceptible bacteria, thereby, inhibiting protein synthesis. Generally considered bacteriostatic; however, bactericidal activity has been demonstrated against isolates of *S. pneumoniae* and *L. pneumophila*. Tigecycline is a derivative of minocycline (9-t-butylglycylamido minocycline), and while not classified as a tetracycline, it may share some class-associated adverse effects. Tigecycline has demonstrated activity against a variety of gram-positive and -negative bacterial pathogens including methicillin-resistant staphylococci.

Pharmacokinetics (Adult data unless noted)

Distribution: Extensive tissue distribution; distributes into gallbladder, lung, and colon
V_d:
- Children (8-11 years): 2.84 L/kg (range: 0.397-11.2 L/kg) (Purdy, 2012)
- Adults: 7-9 L/kg

Protein binding: 71% to 89%
Metabolism: Hepatic (not extensively), via glucuronidation, N-acetylation, and epimerization to several metabolites, each <10% of the dose. Clearance is reduced by 55% and half-life increased by 43% in moderate hepatic impairment.
Half-life elimination: Single dose: 27 hours; Multiple doses: 42 hours
Elimination: 22% excreted in urine as unchanged drug; 59% in feces, primarily as unchanged drug

Dosing: Usual Note: Duration of therapy dependent on severity/site of infection and clinical status and response to therapy.

Children ≥8 years and Adolescents: Limited data available: **Note:** Use should be reserved for situations when no effective alternative therapy is available; should not be used in pediatric patients <8 years due to adverse effects on tooth development.

General dosing, susceptible infection: IV: Dosing based on data from pharmacokinetic trials.
- Children 8-11 years: 1.2 mg/kg/dose every 12 hours; maximum single dose: 50 mg
- Children ≥12 years and Adolescents: 50 mg every 12 hours

Adults:

Intra-abdominal infection, complicated: IV: 100 mg as a single dose, then 50 mg every 12 hours for 5-14 days. **Note:** 2010 IDSA guidelines recommend a treatment duration of 4-7 days (provided source controlled) for community-acquired, mild to moderate infection (Solomkin, 2010).

Skin and skin structure infection, complicated: IV: 100 mg as a single dose, then 50 mg every 12 hours for 5-14 days

Pneumonia, community-acquired: IV: 100 mg as a single dose, then 50 mg every 12 hours for 7-14 days

Dosing adjustment in renal impairment: Not dialyzable; no dosage adjustment necessary.

Dosing adjustment in hepatic impairment:
- Mild to moderate impairment (Child-Pugh class A or B): No dosage adjustment needed.
- Severe impairment (Child-Pugh class C): Adults: 100 mg as a single dose, then 25 mg every 12 hours

Preparation for Administration IV: Reconstitute each vial with 5.3 mL NS, D_5W, or LR; swirl gently to dissolve; resulting solution is 10 mg/mL. Reconstituted solution must be further diluted to a final concentration not to exceed 1 mg/mL. Reconstituted solution should be yellow-orange; discard if not this color.

Administration IV: Infuse over 30 to 60 minutes through dedicated line or via Y-site.

Monitoring Parameters Periodic hepatic function tests; resolution of infection; observe patient for diarrhea

Dosage Forms Excipient information presented when available (limited, particularly for generics); consult specific product labeling.

Solution Reconstituted, Intravenous:

Tygacil: 50 mg (1 ea)

- **Tim-AK (Can)** *see* Timolol (Ophthalmic) *on page 2067*
- **Timentin [DSC]** *see* Ticarcillin and Clavulanate Potassium *on page 2063*
- **Timentin (Can)** *see* Ticarcillin and Clavulanate Potassium *on page 2063*

Timolol (Ophthalmic) (TIM oh lol)

Medication Safety Issues

Sound-alike/look-alike issues:

Timolol may be confused with atenolol, Tylenol®

Timoptic® may be confused with Betoptic S®, Talacen, Viroptic®

Other safety concerns:

Bottle cap color change: Timoptic®: Both the 0.25% and 0.5% strengths are now packaged in bottles with yellow caps; previously, the color of the cap on the product corresponded to different strengths.

International issues:

Betimol [U.S.] may be confused with Betanol brand name for metipranolol [Monaco]

Brand Names: US Betimol; Istalol; Timoptic; Timoptic Ocudose; Timoptic-XE

Brand Names: Canada Apo-Timop®; Dom-Timolol; Mylan-Timolol; Novo-Timol; PMS-Timolol; Sandoz-Timolol; Tim-AK; Timolol Maleate-EX; Timoptic-XE®; Timoptic®

Therapeutic Category Beta-Adrenergic Blocker; Beta-Adrenergic Blocker, Ophthalmic

Generic Availability (US) Yes

Use Treatment of elevated intraocular pressure in patients with open-angle glaucoma or ocular hypertension (Timolol GFS: FDA approved in pediatric patients [age not specified] and adults; other timolol products: FDA approved in adults); has also been used topically for treatment of infantile hemangioma

Pregnancy Risk Factor C

Pregnancy Considerations Adverse events were not observed in animal reproduction studies; therefore, the manufacturer classifies timolol ophthalmic as pregnancy category C. Timolol crosses the placenta. Decreased fetal heart rate has been observed following maternal use of oral and ophthalmic timolol during pregnancy. In a cohort study, an increased risk of cardiovascular defects was observed following maternal use of beta-blockers during pregnancy. Intrauterine growth restriction (IUGR), small placentas, as well as fetal/neonatal bradycardia, hypoglycemia, and/or respiratory depression have been observed following *in utero* exposure to beta-blockers as a class. Adequate facilities for monitoring infants at birth should be available. Untreated chronic maternal hypertension and pre-eclampsia are also associated with adverse events in the fetus, infant, and mother. If timolol is required for the treatment of glaucoma during pregnancy, the minimum effective dose should be used in combination with punctual occlusion to decrease exposure to the fetus.

Breast-Feeding Considerations Timolol is excreted into breast milk following ophthalmic administration. According to the manufacturer, the decision to continue or discontinue breast-feeding during therapy should take into account the risk of exposure to the infant and the benefits of treatment to the mother. Due to the potential for adverse events, nursing infants (especially those with cardiorespiratory problems) should be monitored.

Contraindications Hypersensitivity to timolol or any component of the formulation; sinus bradycardia; sinus node dysfunction; heart block greater than first degree (except in patients with a functioning artificial pacemaker); cardiogenic shock; uncompensated cardiac failure; bronchospastic disease

Warnings/Precautions Consider pre-existing conditions such as sick sinus syndrome before initiating. Use with caution in patients with compensated heart failure and monitor for a worsening of the condition. Use with caution in patients on concurrent digoxin, verapamil, or diltiazem; bradycardia or heart block can occur. Concomitant use with other topical beta-blockers should be avoided; monitor for increased effects (systemic or intraocular) with concomitant use of a systemic beta-blocker. Use with caution in patients receiving inhaled anesthetic agents known to depress myocardial contractility. In general, patients with bronchospastic disease should not receive beta-blockers; if used at all, should be used cautiously with close monitoring. Use with caution in patients with diabetes mellitus; may potentiate hypoglycemia and/or mask signs and symptoms. Can precipitate or aggravate symptoms of arterial insufficiency in patients with PVD and Raynaud's disease. Use with caution and monitor for progression of arterial obstruction. May mask signs of hyperthyroidism (eg, tachycardia); if hyperthyroidism is suspected, carefully manage and monitor; abrupt withdrawal may exacerbate symptoms of hyperthyroidism or precipitate thyroid storm. Use caution with history of severe anaphylaxis to allergens; patients taking beta-blockers may become more sensitive to repeated challenges. Treatment of anaphylaxis (eg, epinephrine) in patients taking beta-blockers may be ineffective or promote undesirable effects.

Should not be used alone in angle-closure glaucoma (has no effect on pupillary constriction). Multidose vials have been associated with development of bacterial keratitis; avoid contamination. Beta-blockade and/or other suppressive therapy have been associated with choroidal detachment following filtration procedures. Some products contain benzalkonium chloride which may be absorbed by soft contact lenses; remove lens prior to administration and wait 15 minutes before reinserting.

Warnings: Additional Pediatric Considerations Pediatric patients, particularly infants, may attain higher plasma concentrations compared to adults (Coppens 2004; Passo 1984); systemic adverse effects may occur (eg, hypotension, bradycardia, bronchospasm, and apnea); use the lowest effective dose; some experts advocate avoiding the use of ophthalmic beta-blockers in premature and small infants (Moore 2007).

Adverse Reactions

Cardiovascular: Angina pectoris, arrhythmia, bradycardia, cardiac arrest, cardiac failure, cerebral ischemia, cerebral vascular accident, edema, heart block, hypertension, hypotension, palpitation, Raynaud's phenomenon

Central nervous system: Anxiety, confusion, depression, disorientation, dizziness, hallucinations, headache, insomnia, memory loss, nervousness, nightmares, somnolence

Dermatologic: Alopecia, angioedema, pseudopemphigoid, psoriasiform rash, psoriasis exacerbation, rash, urticaria

Endocrine & metabolic: Hypoglycemia masked, libido decreased

Gastrointestinal: Anorexia, diarrhea, dyspepsia, nausea, xerostomia

Genitourinary: Impotence, retoperitoneal fibrosis

Hematologic: Claudication

Neuromuscular & skeletal: Myasthenia gravis exacerbation, paresthesia

Ocular: Blepharitis, blurred vision, burning, cataract, choroidal detachment (following filtration surgery), conjunctival injection, conjunctivitis, corneal sensitivity decreased, cystoid macular edema, diplopia, dry eyes, foreign body sensation, hyperemia, itching, keratitis, ocular discharge, ocular pain, ptosis, stinging, tearing, visual acuity decreased refractive changes, visual disturbances

Otic: Tinnitus

Respiratory: Bronchospasm, cough, dyspnea, nasal congestion, pulmonary edema, respiratory failure

Miscellaneous: Allergic reactions, cold hands/feet, Peyronie's disease, systemic lupus erythematosus

Drug Interactions

Metabolism/Transport Effects Substrate of CYP2D6 (major); **Note:** Assignment of Major/Minor substrate status based on clinically relevant drug interaction potential; **Inhibits** CYP2D6 (weak)

Avoid Concomitant Use

Avoid concomitant use of Timolol (Ophthalmic) with any of the following: Beta2-Agonists; Ceritinib; Floctafenine; Methacholine; Rivastigmine

Increased Effect/Toxicity

Timolol (Ophthalmic) may increase the levels/effects of: Alpha-/Beta-Agonists (Direct-Acting); Alpha1-Blockers; Alpha2-Agonists; Antipsychotic Agents (Phenothiazines); ARIPiprazole; Bradycardia-Causing Agents; Bupivacaine; Cardiac Glycosides; Ceritinib; Cholinergic Agonists; Disopyramide; DULoxetine; Ergot Derivatives; Fingolimod; Grass Pollen Allergen Extract (5 Grass Extract); Hypotensive Agents; Insulin; Ivabradine; Lacosamide; Levodopa; Lidocaine (Systemic); Lidocaine (Topical); Mepivacaine; Methacholine; Midodrine; RisperiDONE; Sulfonylureas

The levels/effects of Timolol (Ophthalmic) may be increased by: Abiraterone Acetate; Acetylcholinesterase Inhibitors; Alpha2-Agonists; Aminoquinolines (Antimalarial); Amiodarone; Anilidopiperidine Opioids; Antipsychotic Agents (Phenothiazines); Barbiturates; Bretylium; Calcium Channel Blockers (Nondihydropyridine); Cobicistat; CYP2D6 Inhibitors (Moderate); CYP2D6 Inhibitors (Strong); Darunavir; Dipyridamole; Disopyramide; Dronedarone; Floctafenine; MAO Inhibitors; Nicorandil; NIFEdipine; Panobinostat; Peginterferon Alfa-2b; Propafenone; Regorafenib; Reserpine; Rivastigmine; Ruxolitinib; Selective Serotonin Reuptake Inhibitors; Tofacitinib

Decreased Effect

Timolol (Ophthalmic) may decrease the levels/effects of: Beta2-Agonists; Theophylline Derivatives

The levels/effects of Timolol (Ophthalmic) may be decreased by: Barbiturates; Nonsteroidal Anti-Inflammatory Agents; Peginterferon Alfa-2b; Rifamycin Derivatives

Storage/Stability Drops: Store at room temperature of 15°C to 25°C (59°F to 77°F); do not freeze. Protect from light.

Timolol GFS: Store at 2°C to 25°C (36°F to 77°F). Protect from light.

Timoptic® in OcuDose®: Store in the protective foil wrap and use within 1 month after opening foil package.

Mechanism of Action Blocks both $beta_1$- and $beta_2$-adrenergic receptors, reduces intraocular pressure by reducing aqueous humor production or possibly outflow; reduces blood pressure by blocking adrenergic receptors and decreasing sympathetic outflow, produces a negative chronotropic and inotropic activity through an unknown mechanism

Pharmacodynamics Intraocular pressure reduction:

Onset of action: Within 30 minutes

Maximum effect: 1 to 2 hours

Duration: 24 hours

Pharmacokinetics (Adult data unless noted)

Absorption: Timolol is measurable in the serum following ophthalmic use.

Half life: 4 hours

Dosing: Usual

Pediatric:

Glaucoma: Infants, Children, and Adolescents: Use lowest effective dose; the gel formulation may be preferable due to decreased systemic absorption (Coppens 2009): Ophthalmic:

Gel-forming solution (Timolol GFS, Timoptic-XE): Instill 1 drop (either 0.25% or 0.5%) once daily into affected eye(s) (Coppens 2009; Moore 2007)

Solution: Limited data available: Initial: 0.25% solution instill 1 drop twice daily into affected eye(s); increase to 0.5% solution if response not adequate; decrease to 1 drop once daily into affected eye(s) if controlled maximum dose: 1 drop (0.5% solution)/dose (Hoskins 1985; Moore 2007)

Infantile hemangioma, superficial: Limited data available: Infants and Children: Topical: Gel-forming solution: Apply 1 drop of the 0.5% gel-forming solution twice daily to the site (Chakkittakandiyil 2012; Chan 2013 Chen 2013; Lee 2013; Pope 2010). The largest experience is a multicenter retrospective report describing use in over 60 patients which showed improvement in all but one patient with a mean duration of treatment of 3.4 ± 2.7 months (Chakkittakandiyil 2012). A smaller randomized trial compared timolol 0.5% gel (n=15) to placebo (n=17) on superficial infantile lesions covering various areas of the body; initial lesion improvements were observed after 12 to 16 weeks, and significant color changes reported at week 24 (Chan 2013). A smaller (n=13) retrospective, open-label trial also showed success with two drops of 0.25% timolol gel-forming solution twice daily on periocular infantile hemangiomas (Chambers 2012). Timolol was reported as being well tolerated in the trials.

Adult: **Glaucoma:** Ophthalmic:

Solution: Initial: 0.25% solution, instill 1 drop twice daily into affected eye(s); increase to 0.5% solution if response not adequate; decrease to 1 drop/day if controlled; do not exceed 1 drop twice daily of 0.5% solution.

Istalol: Instill 1 drop (0.5% solution) once daily into affected eye(s) in the morning

Gel-forming solution (Timolol GFS, Timoptic-XE): Instill 1 drop (either 0.25% or 0.5%) once daily into affected eye(s)

Dosing adjustment in renal impairment: There are no dosage adjustments provided in the manufacturer's labeling.

Dosing adjustment in hepatic impairment: There are no dosage adjustments provided in the manufacturer's labeling.

Administration Ophthalmic: Administer other topically applied ophthalmic mediations at least 10 minutes prior timolol

Wash hands before use; invert closed bottle and shake gel once before use; remove cap carefully so that tip does not touch anything; hold bottle between thumb and index finger; use index finger of other hand to pull down the lower eyelid to form a pocket for the eye drop and tilt head back; place the dispenser tip close to the eye and gently squeeze the bottle to administer 1 drop remove pressure on bottle after a single drop has been released; **do not allow the dispenser tip to touch the eye**; replace cap and store bottle in an upright position in a clean area; do **not** enlarge hole of dispenser; do **not** wash tip with water, soap, or any other cleaner Some solutions contain benzalkonium chloride; wait at least 15 minutes after instilling solution before inserting soft contact lenses. With solution, apply gentle pressure to lacrimal sac during and immediately following instillation (1 minute) or instruct patient to gently close eyelid after administration, to decrease systemic absorption of ophthalmic drops (Urtti 1993; Zimmerman 1982)

Topical: Wash hands. Apply drop to hemangioma site area and rub in gently to cover entire hemangioma (Chambers 2012; Chan 2013)

Monitoring Parameters Monitor IOP; systemic beta-blocker effects including vital signs (especially in younger patients)

Dosage Forms Excipient information presented when available (limited, particularly for generics); consult specific product labeling.

Gel Forming Solution, Ophthalmic, as maleate [strength expressed as base]:
Timoptic-XE: 0.25% (5 mL); 0.5% (5 mL)
Generic: 0.25% (5 mL); 0.5% (5 mL)

Solution, Ophthalmic, as hemihydrate [strength expressed as base]:
Betimol: 0.25% (5 mL); 0.5% (5 mL, 10 mL, 15 mL) [contains benzalkonium chloride]

Solution, Ophthalmic, as maleate [strength expressed as base]:
Istalol: 0.5% (2.5 mL, 5 mL) [contains benzalkonium chloride]
Timoptic: 0.25% (5 mL); 0.5% (5 mL, 10 mL) [contains benzalkonium chloride]
Generic: 0.25% (5 mL, 10 mL, 15 mL); 0.5% (5 mL, 10 mL, 15 mL)

Solution, Ophthalmic, as maleate [strength expressed as base, preservative free]:
Timoptic Ocudose: 0.25% (60 ea); 0.5% (60 ea)

- ◆ **Timolol Hemihydrate** *see* Timolol (Ophthalmic) *on page 2067*
- ◆ **Timolol Maleate** *see* Timolol (Ophthalmic) *on page 2067*
- ◆ **Timolol Maleate-EX (Can)** *see* Timolol (Ophthalmic) *on page 2067*
- ◆ **Timoptic** *see* Timolol (Ophthalmic) *on page 2067*
- ◆ **Timoptic® (Can)** *see* Timolol (Ophthalmic) *on page 2067*
- ◆ **Timoptic Ocudose** *see* Timolol (Ophthalmic) *on page 2067*
- ◆ **Timoptic-XE** *see* Timolol (Ophthalmic) *on page 2067*
- ◆ **Timoptic-XE® (Can)** *see* Timolol (Ophthalmic) *on page 2067*
- ◆ **Tinactin [OTC]** *see* Tolnaftate *on page 2083*
- ◆ **Tinactin Deodorant [OTC]** *see* Tolnaftate *on page 2083*
- ◆ **Tinactin Jock Itch [OTC]** *see* Tolnaftate *on page 2083*
- ◆ **Tinamed Corn/Callus Remover [OTC]** *see* Salicylic Acid *on page 1894*
- ◆ **Tinamed Wart Remover [OTC]** *see* Salicylic Acid *on page 1894*
- ◆ **Tinaspore [OTC]** *see* Tolnaftate *on page 2083*
- ◆ **Tincture of Opium** *see* Opium Tincture *on page 1569*
- ◆ **Tindamax** *see* Tinidazole *on page 2069*

Tinidazole (tye NI da zole)

Brand Names: US Tindamax

Therapeutic Category Amebicide; Antibiotic, Miscellaneous; Antiprotozoal, Nitroimidazole

Generic Availability (US) Yes

Use Treatment of giardiasis caused by *G. duodenalis* (*G. lamblia*) (FDA approved in ages > 3 years and adults); treatment of intestinal amebiasis and amebic liver abscess caused by *E. histolytica* (FDA approved in ages >3 years and adults); treatment of trichomoniasis caused by *T. vaginalis* (FDA approved in adults); treatment of bacterial vaginosis caused by *Bacteroides* spp, *Gardnerella vaginalis*, and *Prevotella* spp (FDA approved in nonpregnant adult females)

Pregnancy Risk Factor C

Pregnancy Considerations Adverse events have been observed in some animal reproduction studies. Tinidazole crosses the human placenta and enters the fetal circulation. The safety of tinidazole for the treatment of trichomoniasis caused by *T. vaginalis* in pregnant women has not been well evaluated. Other agents are preferred for the treatment of bacterial vaginosis during pregnancy (CDC, 2010). The manufacturer contraindicates use of tinidazole during the first trimester of pregnancy.

Breast-Feeding Considerations Tinidazole is excreted into breast milk in concentrations similar to those in the maternal serum and can be detected for up to 72 hours after administration. Tinidazole is contraindicated in nursing mothers unless breast-feeding is interrupted during therapy and for 3 days after the last dose.

Contraindications Hypersensitivity to tinidazole, nitroimidazole derivatives (including metronidazole), or any component of the formulation; pregnancy (1st trimester); breast-feeding

Warnings/Precautions Use caution with CNS diseases; seizures and peripheral neuropathy have been reported with tinidazole and other nitroimidazole derivatives. **[U.S. Boxed Warning]: Carcinogenicity has been observed with another nitroimidazole derivative (metronidazole) in animal studies;** use should be reserved for approved indications only. Use caution with current or history of blood dyscrasias or hepatic impairment. When used for amebiasis, not indicated for the treatment of asymptomatic cyst passage. Prolonged use may result in fungal or bacterial superinfection, including *C. difficile*-associated diarrhea (CDAD), pseudomembranous colitis, and/or vaginal candidiasis. CDAD has been observed >2 months postantibiotic treatment.

Adverse Reactions

Cardiovascular: Flushing, palpitation

Central nervous system: Ataxia, coma (rare), confusion (rare), depression (rare), dizziness, drowsiness, fatigue/malaise, fever, giddiness, headache, insomnia, seizure, vertigo

Dermatologic: Angioedema, pruritus, rash, urticaria

Endocrine & metabolic: Menorrhagia

Gastrointestinal: Abdominal pain, anorexia, appetite decreased, constipation, diarrhea, dyspepsia/cramps/epigastric discomfort, flatulence, furry tongue (rare), metallic/bitter taste, nausea, oral candidiasis, salivation, stomatitis, thirst, tongue discoloration, vomiting, xerostomia

Genitourinary: *Candida* vaginitis, painful urination, pelvic pain, urine abnormality/darkened, vaginal discharge increased, vaginal odor, vulvovaginal discomfort

Hematologic: Leukopenia (transient), neutropenia (transient), thrombocytopenia (reversible; rare)

Hepatic: Transaminases increased

Neuromuscular & skeletal: Arthralgia, arthritis, myalgia, peripheral neuropathy (transient, includes numbness and paresthesia), weakness

Renal: Urinary tract infection

Respiratory: Bronchospasm (rare), dyspnea (rare), pharyngitis (rare), upper respiratory tract infection

Miscellaneous: Burning sensation, *Candida* overgrowth, diaphoresis

Rare but important or life-threatening: Acute hypersensitivity reaction (severe), erythema multiforme, Stevens-Johnson syndrome

Drug Interactions

Metabolism/Transport Effects Substrate of CYP3A4 (minor); **Note:** Assignment of Major/Minor substrate status based on clinically relevant drug interaction potential

Avoid Concomitant Use

Avoid concomitant use of Tinidazole with any of the following: Alcohol (Ethyl); Disulfiram

Increased Effect/Toxicity

Tinidazole may increase the levels/effects of: Alcohol (Ethyl); Disulfiram

Decreased Effect There are no known significant interactions involving a decrease in effect.

Food Interactions

Ethanol: Concurrent ethanol use may cause a disulfiram-like reaction characterized by flushing, headache, nausea, vomiting, sweating or tachycardia. Management: The manufacturer recommends to avoid all ethanol or any ethanol-containing drugs during and for at least 3 days after completion of treatment.

Food: Peak antibiotic serum concentration lowered and delayed, but total drug absorbed not affected. Management: Administer with food.

Storage/Stability Store at controlled room temperature of 15°C to 30°C (59°F to 86°F). Protect from light.

Mechanism of Action After diffusing into the organism, it is proposed that tinidazole causes cytotoxicity by damaging DNA and preventing further DNA synthesis.

Pharmacokinetics (Adult data unless noted)

Absorption: Rapid and complete

Distribution: V_d: 50 L; distributes to most body tissues and fluids; crosses the blood-brain barrier

Protein binding: 12%

Metabolism: Hepatic via CYP3A4 (primarily); undergoes oxidation, hydroxylation and conjugation

Half-life elimination: 12-14 hours

Time to peak serum concentration: ~1.6 hours (fasting, delayed ~2 hours when given with food)

Excretion: Urine (20% to 25%); feces (12%)

Dosing: Usual

Pediatric:

Amebiasis, intestinal: Children >3 years and Adolescents: Oral: 50 mg/kg/day for 3 days; maximum daily dose: 2000 mg/**day**; for patients with severe and extra-intestinal disease, administer for 5 days (*Red Book* [AAP], 2012)

Amebiasis, liver abscess: Children >3 years and Adolescents: Oral: 50 mg/kg/day for 3 to 5 days; maximum daily dose: 2000 mg/**day**

Bacterial vaginosis: Adolescents: Oral: 2000 mg once daily for 2 days **or** 1000 mg once daily for 5 days (CDC, 2010)

Giardiasis: Children >3 years and Adolescents: Oral: 50 mg/kg as a single dose; maximum dose: 2000 mg

***Helicobacter pylori* infection:** Limited data available: Children >3 years and Adolescents: Oral: 20 mg/kg/day in 1 to 2 divided doses for 5 to 7 days in combination with other agents; some studies have used a longer duration of 2 to 6 weeks; maximum daily dose: 1000 mg/**day** (Francavilla, 2005; Moshkowitz, 1998; Nijevitch, 2000; Oderda, 1992)

Nongonococcal urethritis, recurrent/persistent: Adolescents: Oral: 2000 mg as a single dose in combination with azithromycin (CDC, 2010)

Trichomoniasis:

Children >3 years: Oral: 50 mg/kg as a single dose; maximum dose: 2000 mg (*Red Book* [AAP], 2012)

Adolescents: Oral: 2000 mg as a single dose; sexual partners should be treated at the same time; if treatment failure, can consider extended regimen of 2000 mg once daily for 5 days (CDC, 2010; *Red Book* [AAP], 2012)

Adult:

Amebiasis, intestinal: Oral: 2000 mg/day for 3 days

Amebiasis, liver abscess: Oral: 2000 mg/day for 3 to 5 days

Bacterial vaginosis: Oral: 2000 mg/day for 2 days **or** 1000 mg/day for 5 days

Giardiasis: Oral: 2000 mg as a single dose

Trichomoniasis: Oral: 2000 mg as a single dose; sexual partners should be treated at the same time

Dosing adjustment in renal impairment: Children >3 years, Adolescents, and Adults: No dosage adjustment necessary

Hemodialysis: Approximately 43% removed during a 6-hour session; an additional dose equal to 1/2 the usual dose should be administered at the end of hemodialysis if tinidazole is administered prior to hemodialysis on dialysis days

Dosing adjustment in hepatic impairment: There are no dosage adjustments provided in the manufacturer's labeling (has not been studied); use with caution.

Administration Oral: Administer with food to minimize gastrointestinal adverse effects.

Test Interactions May interfere with AST, ALT, triglycerides, glucose, and LDH testing

Dosage Forms Excipient information presented when available (limited, particularly for generics); consult specific product labeling.

Tablet, Oral:

Tindamax: 250 mg, 500 mg [scored; contains fd&c red #40 aluminum lake, fd&c yellow #6 aluminum lake]

Generic: 250 mg, 500 mg

Extemporaneous Preparations A 67 mg/mL suspension may be made with tablets and cherry syrup. Crush four 500 mg tablets in a mortar and reduce to a fine powder. Add 10 mL cherry syrup and mix to a uniform paste; mix while adding cherry syrup in incremental proportions to **almost** 30 mL; transfer to a calibrated bottle, rinse mortar with vehicle, and add quantity of vehicle sufficient to make 30 mL. Label "shake well". Stable for 7 days.

Tindamax® prescribing information, Mission Pharmacal Company, San Antonio, TX, 2007. Available at http://www.accessdata.fda.gov/drugsatfda_docs/label/2007/021618s003lbl.pdf

◆ **Tioguanine** *see* Thioguanine *on page* 2049

◆ **Tiotixene** *see* Thiothixene *on page* 2055

Tipranavir (tip RA na veer)

Medication Safety Issues

High alert medication:

This medication is in a class the Institute for Safe Medication Practices (ISMP) includes among its list of drug classes that have a heightened risk of causing significant patient harm when used in error.

Related Information

Adult and Adolescent HIV *on page* 2392

Oral Medications That Should Not Be Crushed or Altered *on page* 2476

Pediatric HIV *on page* 2380

Perinatal HIV *on page* 2400

Brand Names: US Aptivus

Brand Names: Canada Aptivus

Therapeutic Category Antiviral Agent; HIV Agents (Anti-HIV Agents); Protease Inhibitor

Generic Availability (US) No

Use Treatment of HIV-1 infections in combination with ritonavir and other antiretroviral agents in patients who are highly treatment-experienced or multiprotease inhibitor-resistant (FDA approved in ages ≥2 years and adults). **Note:** HIV regimens consisting of **three** antiretroviral agents are strongly recommended.

Pregnancy Risk Factor C

Pregnancy Considerations Adverse events were observed in some animal reproduction studies. Tipranavir crosses the human placenta. The DHHS Perinatal HIV Guidelines note there are insufficient data to recommend use during pregnancy; however, if used, tipranavir must be given with low-dose ritonavir boosting. A small increased risk of preterm birth has been associated with maternal use of protease inhibitor-based combination antiretroviral

(ARV) therapy during pregnancy; however, the benefits of use generally outweigh this risk and protease inhibitors (PIs) should not be withheld if otherwise recommended. Hyperglycemia, new onset of diabetes mellitus, or diabetic ketoacidosis have been reported with PIs; it is not clear if pregnancy increases this risk.

Regardless of CD4 count or HIV RNA copy number, all HIV-infected pregnant women should receive a combination ARV drug regimen. A combination of antepartum, intrapartum, and infant ARV prophylaxis is recommended. ARV therapy should be started as soon as possible in women with symptomatic infection. Although earlier initiation may be more effective in reducing the perinatal transmission of HIV, initiation may be delayed until after 12 weeks' gestation in women who do not require immediate treatment after careful consideration of maternal conditions (eg, nausea and vomiting) and the potential risks of first trimester fetal exposure for specific agents. A scheduled cesarean delivery at 38 weeks' gestation is recommended for all women with HIV RNA >1000 copies/mL or unknown concentrations near delivery in order to decrease transmission. If ARV therapy must be interrupted for <24 hours during the peripartum period, stop then restart all medications simultaneously in order to decrease the chance of developing resistance. Long-term follow-up is recommended for all infants exposed to ARV medications. In couples who want to conceive, the HIV-infected partner should attain maximum viral suppression prior to conception.

Health care providers are encouraged to enroll pregnant women exposed to antiretroviral medications in the Antiretroviral Pregnancy Registry (1-800-258-4263 or www.APRegistry.com). Health care providers caring for HIV-infected women and their infants may contact the National Perinatal HIV Hotline (888-448-8765) for clinical consultation (HHS [perinatal], 2014).

Women receiving estrogen (as hormonal contraception or replacement therapy) may have an increased incidence of rash.

Breast-Feeding Considerations It is not known if tipranavir is excreted into breast milk. Maternal or infant antiretroviral therapy does not completely eliminate the risk of postnatal HIV transmission. In addition, multiclass-resistant virus has been detected in breast-feeding infants despite maternal therapy. Therefore, in the United States, where formula is accessible, affordable, safe, and sustainable, and the risk of infant mortality due to diarrhea and respiratory infections is low, complete avoidance of breast-feeding by HIV-infected women is recommended to decrease potential transmission of HIV (HHS [perinatal], 2014).

Contraindications Concurrent therapy of tipranavir/ritonavir with alfuzosin, amiodarone, bepridil, cisapride, ergot derivatives (eg, dihydroergotamine, ergonovine, ergotamine, methylergonovine), flecainide, lovastatin, midazolam (oral), pimozide, propafenone, quinidine, rifampin, sildenafil (for pulmonary arterial hypertension [eg, Revatio®]), simvastatin, St John's wort, and triazolam; moderate-to-severe hepatic impairment (Child-Pugh class B or C)

Warnings/Precautions **[U.S. Boxed Warning]: In combination with ritonavir, may cause hepatitis (including fatalities) and/or exacerbate preexisting hepatic dysfunction (causal relationship not established); patients with chronic hepatitis B or C are at increased risk.** Monitor patients closely; discontinue use if signs or symptoms of toxicity occur or if asymptomatic AST/ALT elevations >10 times upper limit of normal or AST/ALT elevations >5-10 times upper limit of normal concurrently with total bilirubin >2.5 times the upper limit of normal occur. Use with caution in patients with mild hepatic impairment; contraindicated in moderate-to-severe impairment. May be associated with fat redistribution (buffalo hump, increased abdominal girth, breast engorgement, facial atrophy). Use caution in hemophilia. May increase cholesterol and/or triglycerides; hypertriglyceridemia may increase risk of pancreatitis. May cause hyperglycemia. Use with caution in patients with sulfonamide allergy. Protease inhibitors have been associated with a variety of hypersensitivity events (some severe), including rash, anaphylaxis (rare), angioedema, bronchospasm, erythema multiforme, and/or Stevens-Johnson syndrome (rare). It is generally recommended to discontinue treatment if severe rash or moderate symptoms accompanied by other systemic symptoms occur. Patients may develop immune reconstitution syndrome resulting in the occurrence of an inflammatory response to an indolent or residual opportunistic infection during initial HIV treatment or activation of autoimmune disorders (eg, Graves' disease, polymyositis, Guillain-Barré syndrome) later in therapy; further evaluation and treatment may be required.

[U.S. Boxed Warning]: Tipranavir in combination with ritonavir has been associated with rare reports of fatal and nonfatal intracranial hemorrhage; causal relationship not established. Events often occurred in patients with medical conditions (eg, CNS lesions, head trauma, recent neurosurgery, coagulopathy, alcohol abuse) or concurrent therapy which may have influenced these events. Tipranavir may inhibit platelet aggregation. Use with caution in patients who may be at risk for increased bleeding (trauma, surgery or other medical conditions) or in patients receiving concurrent medications which may increase the risk of bleeding, including antiplatelet agents and anticoagulants.

High potential for drug interactions; concomitant use of tipranavir with some drugs may require cautious use, may not be recommended, may require dosage adjustments, or may be contraindicated. Capsules contain dehydrated alcohol 7% w/w (0.1 g per capsule).

Warnings: Additional Pediatric Considerations Skin rash may occur with tipranavir plus ritonavir use, including urticarial rash, maculopapular rash, or photosensitivity; may be accompanied by joint pain or stiffness, throat tightness, or generalized pruritus; reported incidence (all grades): Pediatric patients: 21%, adults: 8% to 10%; median onset: 53 days; treatment may be continued if rash is mild to moderate (rash may resolve; median duration: 22 days); discontinue therapy in cases of severe rash.

Tipranavir oral solution contains vitamin E (116 units/mL), which is significantly higher than the RDA; avoid taking additional vitamin E (other than a daily multivitamin). The recommended pediatric dose of tipranavir (14 mg/kg body weight) results in a vitamin E dose of 16 units/kg body weight per day, significantly higher than the reference daily intake for vitamin E (10 units) and close to the upper limit of tolerability for children.

Some dosage forms may contain propylene glycol; in neonates large amounts of propylene glycol delivered orally, intravenously (eg, >3,000 mg/day), or topically have been associated with potentially fatal toxicities which can include metabolic acidosis, seizures, renal failure, and CNS depression; toxicities have also been reported in children and adults including hyperosmolality, lactic acidosis, seizures and respiratory depression; use caution (AAP, 1997; Shehab, 2009).

Adverse Reactions

Central nervous system: Fatigue, fever, headache

Dermatologic: Rash

Endocrine & metabolic: Dehydration, hypercholesterolemia, hypertriglyceridemia

Gastrointestinal: Abdominal pain, amylase increased, diarrhea, nausea, vomiting, weight loss
Hepatic: ALT increased, AST increased, GGT increased, transaminases increased
Hematologic: Anemia, bleeding, neutropenia, WBC decreased
Neuromuscular & skeletal: CPK increased, myalgia
Respiratory: Cough, dyspnea, epistaxis
Rare but important or life-threatening: Abdominal distension, anorexia, appetite decreased, diabetes mellitus, dizziness, dyspepsia, exanthem, facial wasting, flatulence, flu-like syndrome, gastroesophageal reflux, hepatic failure, hepatic steatosis, hepatitis, hyperbilirubinemia, hyperglycemia, hypersensitivity, immune reconstitution syndrome, insomnia, intracranial hemorrhage, lipase increased, lipoatrophy, lipodystrophy (acquired), lipohypertrophy, malaise, mitochondrial toxicity, muscle cramp, neuropathy (peripheral), pancreatitis, pruritus, renal insufficiency, sleep disorder, somnolence, thrombocytopenia

Drug Interactions

Metabolism/Transport Effects **Substrate** of CYP3A4 (major); **Note:** Assignment of Major/Minor substrate status based on clinically relevant drug interaction potential; **Inhibits** BSEP, CYP2D6 (strong); **Induces** P-glycoprotein

Avoid Concomitant Use

Avoid concomitant use of Tipranavir with any of the following: Alfuzosin; Amiodarone; AtorvaSTATin; Bepridil; Boceprevir; Cholic Acid; Cisapride; Dabigatran Etexilate; Ergot Derivatives; Etravirine; Flecainide; Fluticasone (Nasal); Fluticasone (Oral Inhalation); Ledipasvir; Lomitapide; Lovastatin; Mequitazine; Midazolam; Pimozide; Propafenone; Protease Inhibitors; QuiNIDine; Rifampin; Salmeterol; Simeprevir; Simvastatin; Sofosbuvir; St Johns Wort; Tadalafil; Tamoxifen; Telaprevir; Thioridazine; Triazolam; VinCRIStine (Liposomal)

Increased Effect/Toxicity

Tipranavir may increase the levels/effects of: Agents with Antiplatelet Properties; Alfuzosin; ALPRAZolam; Amiodarone; Anticoagulants; ARIPiprazole; AtoMOXetine; AtorvaSTATin; Bepridil; Bosentan; Calcium Channel Blockers (Dihydropyridine); Calcium Channel Blockers (Nondihydropyridine); CarBAMazepine; Cholic Acid; Cisapride; Clarithromycin; Colchicine; Contraceptives (Progestins); Cyclophosphamide; CycloSPORINE (Systemic); CYP2D6 Substrates; Digoxin; DOXOrubicin (Conventional); Eliglustat; Eluxadoline; Enfuvirtide; Ergot Derivatives; Fesoterodine; Flecainide; Fluticasone (Nasal); Fluticasone (Oral Inhalation); Iloperidone; Itraconazole; Ketoconazole (Systemic); Lomitapide; Lovastatin; Meperidine; Mequitazine; Metoprolol; Midazolam; Nebivolol; Nefazodone; Pimozide; Propafenone; Protease Inhibitors; QuiNIDine; Rifabutin; Riociguat; Rosuvastatin; Salmeterol; Sildenafil; Simeprevir; Simvastatin; Tacrolimus (Systemic); Tacrolimus (Topical); Tadalafil; Tamsulosin; Temsirolimus; Tetrabenazine; Thioridazine; TraMADol; TraZODone; Triazolam; Tricyclic Antidepressants; Vitamin E; Vortioxetine

The levels/effects of Tipranavir may be increased by: Clarithromycin; CycloSPORINE (Systemic); Delavirdine; Disulfiram; Enfuvirtide; Estrogen Derivatives; Fluconazole; MetroNIDAZOLE (Systemic); MetroNIDAZOLE (Topical); Simeprevir

Decreased Effect

Tipranavir may decrease the levels/effects of: Abacavir; Afatinib; Antidiabetic Agents; Boceprevir; Brentuximab Vedotin; Clarithromycin; Codeine; Dabigatran Etexilate; Delavirdine; Didanosine; Dolutegravir; DOXOrubicin (Conventional); Estrogen Derivatives; Etravirine; Fosphenytoin; Hydrocodone; Iloperidone; Ledipasvir; Linagliptin; Meperidine; Methadone; P-glycoprotein/ABCB1 Substrates; PHENobarbital; Phenytoin; Protease Inhibitors; Proton Pump Inhibitors; Raltegravir; Sofosbuvir; Tamoxifen; Telaprevir; Tenofovir; Theophylline Derivatives; TraMADol; Valproic Acid and Derivatives; VinCRIStine (Liposomal); Zidovudine

The levels/effects of Tipranavir may be decreased by: Boceprevir; Bosentan; CarBAMazepine; CYP3A4 Inducers (Moderate); CYP3A4 Inducers (Strong); Dabrafenib; Deferasirox; Fosphenytoin; Garlic; Mitotane; PHENobarbital; Phenytoin; Rifampin; Siltuximab; St Johns Wort; Tenofovir; Tocilizumab

Storage/Stability

Capsule: Prior to opening bottle, store under refrigeration at 2°C to 8°C (36°F to 46°F). After bottle is opened, may be stored at controlled room temperature of 25°C (77°F) for up to 60 days.
Oral solution: Store at 15°C to 30°C (59°F to 86°F). After bottle is open, use within 60 days. Do not refrigerate or freeze oral solution.

Mechanism of Action Binds to the site of HIV-1 protease activity and inhibits cleavage of viral Gag-Pol polyprotein precursors into individual functional proteins required for infectious HIV. This results in the formation of immature, noninfectious viral particles.

Pharmacokinetics (Adult data unless noted)

Absorption: Incomplete (percentage not established)
Distribution: V_d:
- Children:
  - 2 to <6 years: 4 L
  - 6 to <12 years: 4.7 L
- Children and Adolescents 12 to 18 years: 5.3 L
- Adults: 7.7 to 10.2 L

Protein binding: >99% (albumin, alpha$_1$-acid glycoprotein)
Metabolism: Hepatic, via CYP3A4 (minimal when coadministered with ritonavir)
Bioavailability: Not established
Half-life:
- Children:
  - 2 to <6 years of age: ~8 hours
  - 6 to <12 years of age: ~7 hours
- Children and Adolescents 12 to 18 years: ~5 hours
- Adults: Males: 6 hours; Females: 5.5 hours

Time to peak serum concentration:
- Children and Adolescents 2 to 18 years: 2.5 to 2.7 hours
- Adults: ~3 hours

Elimination: Feces (82%); urine (4%); primarily as unchanged drug (when coadministered with ritonavir)

Dosing: Usual

Pediatric: **HIV infection, treatment:** Oral: **Note:** Use in combination with other antiretroviral agents. Not recommended for treatment-naïve patients. Coadministration with ritonavir is required.
- Infants and Children <2 years: Not recommended for use
- Children ≥2 years and Adolescents:
  - Weight-directed dosing: Tipranavir 14 mg/kg (maximum: 500 mg) twice daily **plus** ritonavir 6 mg/kg (maximum: 200 mg) twice daily
    - If intolerance or toxicity develops and virus is not resistant to multiple protease inhibitors: May decrease dose to: Tipranavir 12 mg/kg **plus** ritonavir 5 mg/kg twice daily; do not exceed adult doses
  - BSA-directed dosing: Tipranavir 375 mg/m^2 (maximum: 500 mg) twice daily **plus** ritonavir 150 mg/m^2 (maximum: 200 mg) twice daily
    - If intolerance or toxicity develops and virus is not resistant to multiple protease inhibitors: May decrease dose to: Tipranavir 290 mg/m^2 **plus** ritonavir 115 mg/m^2 twice daily; do not exceed adult doses

Adult: **HIV infection, treatment:** Oral: Use in combination with other antiretroviral agents. Not recommended for treatment naïve patients. **Note:** Coadministration with ritonavir is required. Tipranavir 500 mg **plus** ritonavir 200 mg twice daily

Dosing adjustment in renal impairment: No adjustment required (DHHS [adult, pediatric], 2014)

Dosing adjustment in hepatic impairment:
Mild impairment (Child-Pugh class A): No adjustment required; use with caution
Moderate to severe impairment (Child-Pugh class B or C): Use is contraindicated

Administration Coadministration with ritonavir is required. In pediatric patients, may administer tipranavir **plus** ritonavir **capsules** or **solution** together with food (DHHS [pediatric], 2014) and in adults without regard to meals (DHHS [adult], 2014). Administer tipranavir **plus** ritonavir **tablets** at the same time with food.

Monitoring Parameters Note: Monitor CD4 percentage (if <5 years of age) or CD4 count (if ≥5 years of age) at least every 3 to 4 months (DHHS [pediatric], 2014).

Prior to initiation of therapy: Genotypic resistance testing, CD4 and viral load (every 3 to 4 months), CBC with differential, LFTs, BUN, creatinine, lipid panel, electrolytes, glucose, urinalysis (every 6 to 12 months), and assessment of readiness for adherence with medication regimen. At initiation and with any change in treatment regimen: CBC with differential, electrolytes, calcium, phosphate, glucose, LFTs, bilirubin, urinalysis (at initiation), BUN, creatinine, albumin, total protein, lipid panel (at initiation), CD4, and viral load. After 1 to 2 weeks of therapy: Signs of medication toxicity and adherence. After 2 to 4 weeks of therapy: CBC with differential, viral load, and signs of medication toxicity, and adherence; then every 3 to 4 months: CBC with differential, electrolytes, glucose, LFTs, bilirubin, BUN, creatinine, CD4, viral load, signs of medication toxicity, and adherence. Every 6 to 12 months: Lipid panel and urinalysis. CD4 monitoring frequency may be decreased to every 6 to 12 months in children who are adherent to therapy if the value is well above the threshold for opportunistic infections, viral suppression is sustained, and the clinical status is stable for more than 2 to 3 years (DHHS [pediatric], 2014). Monitor for growth and development, signs of HIV-specific physical conditions, HIV disease progression, opportunistic infections, hepatitis, or pancreatitis.

Reference Range Plasma trough concentration ≥20,500 ng/mL (based on data from treatment-experienced patient with resistant HIV-1 strains) (DHHS [adult, pediatric], 2014)

Dosage Forms Excipient information presented when available (limited, particularly for generics); consult specific product labeling.
Capsule, Oral:
Aptivus: 250 mg
Solution, Oral:
Aptivus: 100 mg/mL (95 mL) [contains polyethylene glycol, propylene glycol, tocophersolan; buttermint-butter toffee flavor]

- ◆ **Tirosint** *see* Levothyroxine *on page* 1250
- ◆ **Titralac [OTC]** *see* Calcium Carbonate *on page* 343
- ◆ **Tivicay** *see* Dolutegravir *on page* 701
- ◆ **Tivorbex** *see* Indomethacin *on page* 1101
- ◆ **TIV (Trivalent Inactivated Influenza Vaccine)** *see* Influenza Virus Vaccine (Inactivated) *on page* 1108
- ◆ **TMC-114** *see* Darunavir *on page* 588
- ◆ **TMC125** *see* Etravirine *on page* 823
- ◆ **TMP** *see* Trimethoprim *on page* 2126
- ◆ **TMP-SMX** *see* Sulfamethoxazole and Trimethoprim *on page* 1986
- ◆ **TMP-SMZ** *see* Sulfamethoxazole and Trimethoprim *on page* 1986
- ◆ **TMZ** *see* Temozolomide *on page* 2012
- ◆ **TNG** *see* Nitroglycerin *on page* 1523
- ◆ **Tobi** *see* Tobramycin (Systemic, Oral Inhalation) *on page* 2073
- ◆ **TOBI (Can)** *see* Tobramycin (Systemic, Oral Inhalation) *on page* 2073
- ◆ **Tobi Podhaler** *see* Tobramycin (Systemic, Oral Inhalation) *on page* 2073
- ◆ **TOBI Podhaler (Can)** *see* Tobramycin (Systemic, Oral Inhalation) *on page* 2073

Tobramycin (Systemic, Oral Inhalation)

(toe bra MYE sin)

Medication Safety Issues

Sound-alike/look-alike issues:
Tobramycin may be confused with Trobicin, vancomycin

International issues:
Nebcin [Multiple international markets] may be confused with Naprosyn brand name for naproxen [U.S., Canada, and multiple international markets]; Nubain brand name for nalbuphine [Multiple international markets]

High alert medication:
The Institute for Safe Medication Practices (ISMP) includes this medication (intrathecal administration) among its list of drug classes which have a heightened risk of causing significant patient harm when used in error.

Brand Names: US Bethkis; Kitabis Pak; Tobi; Tobi Podhaler

Brand Names: Canada JAMP-Tobramycin; TOBI; TOBI Podhaler; Tobramycin For Injection; Tobramycin For Injection, USP; Tobramycin Injection; Tobramycin Injection, USP

Therapeutic Category Antibiotic, Aminoglycoside

Generic Availability (US) May be product dependent

Use

Parenteral: Treatment of documented or suspected infections caused by susceptible gram-negative bacilli, including *Pseudomonas aeruginosa*; nonpseudomonal enteric bacillus infection which is more susceptible to tobramycin than gentamicin based on microbiology testing; susceptible organisms in lower respiratory tract infections (FDA approved in adults), serious central nervous system infection caused by susceptible organisms (FDA approved in adults), septicemia (FDA approved in all ages); intra-abdominal, skin, bone, soft tissue, and urinary tract infections (FDA approved in adults); has also been used for empiric therapy in cystic fibrosis and immunocompromised patients

Inhalation: Management of cystic fibrosis patients with *P. aeruginosa* (FDA approved in ages ≥6 years and adults)

Pregnancy Risk Factor D

Pregnancy Considerations [U.S. Boxed Warning]: Aminoglycosides may cause fetal harm if administered to a pregnant woman. There are several reports of total irreversible bilateral congenital deafness in children whose mothers received another aminoglycoside (streptomycin) during pregnancy; therefore, tobramycin is classified as pregnancy category D. Tobramycin crosses the placenta and produces detectable serum levels in the fetus. Although serious side effects to the fetus have not been reported following maternal use of tobramycin, a potential for harm exists.

Due to pregnancy-induced physiologic changes, some pharmacokinetic parameters of tobramycin may be altered. Pregnant women have an average-to-larger volume of distribution which may result in lower serum peak levels than for the same dose in nonpregnant women. Serum half-life is also shorter.

Breast-Feeding Considerations Tobramycin is excreted into breast milk and breast-feeding is not recommended by the manufacturer; however, tobramycin is not well absorbed when taken orally. This limited oral absorption may minimize exposure to the nursing infant. Nondose-related effects could include modification of bowel flora.

Contraindications Hypersensitivity to tobramycin, other aminoglycosides, or any component of the formulation

Warnings/Precautions **[U.S. Boxed Warning]: Aminoglycosides may cause neurotoxicity and/or nephrotoxicity;** usual risk factors include preexisting renal impairment, concomitant neuro-/nephrotoxic medications, advanced age, and dehydration. Ototoxicity may be directly proportional to the amount of drug given and the duration of treatment; tinnitus or vertigo are indications of vestibular injury and impending hearing loss; renal damage is usually reversible. Tinnitus and/or hearing loss have also been reported. May cause neuromuscular blockade, respiratory failure, and prolonged respiratory paralysis, especially when given soon after anesthesia or muscle relaxants. **[U.S. Boxed Warnings]: Aminoglycosides may cause fetal harm if administered to a pregnant woman.**

Not intended for long-term therapy due to toxic hazards associated with extended administration; use caution in pre-existing renal insufficiency, vestibular or cochlear impairment, myasthenia gravis, Parkinson's disease, hypocalcemia, and conditions which depress neuromuscular transmission. Dosage modification required in patients with impaired renal function during systemic therapy. Prolonged use may result in fungal or bacterial superinfection, including *C. difficile*-associated diarrhea (CDAD) and pseudomembranous colitis; CDAD has been observed >2 months postantibiotic treatment. Solution may contain sodium metabisulfate; use caution in patients with sulfite allergy. Solution for injection may contain sodium metabisulfate; use caution in patients with sulfite allergy. Bronchospasm may occur with tobramycin solution for inhalation; bronchospasm or wheezing should be treated appropriately if either arise. Safety and efficacy of the solution for inhalation have not been demonstrated in patients with FEV_1 <40% or >80% predicted (Bethkis, TOBI), or FEV_1 <25% or >80% predicted (TOBI Podhaler) or FEV_1 <25% or >75% predicted (Kitabis Pak), in patients colonized with *Burkholderia cepacia*, or in patients <6 years of age. With powder for inhalation, consider baseline audiogram in patients at increased risk of auditory dysfunction. If any patient experiences tinnitus or hearing loss during treatment, audiological assessment should be performed. Serum tobramycin concentrations do not need to be monitored; one hour after powder inhalation, serum concentrations of 1-2 mcg/mL have been observed. If ototoxicity or nephrotoxicity occur, discontinue therapy until serum concentrations fall below 2 mcg/mL.

Potentially significant drug-drug interactions may exist, requiring dose or frequency adjustment, additional monitoring, and/or selection of alternative therapy.

Warnings: Additional Pediatric Considerations Use with caution in premature infants and neonates; immature renal function may increase risk of accumulation and related toxicity. Use with caution in pediatric patients on extracorporeal membrane oxygenation (ECMO); pharmacokinetics of aminoglycosides may be altered; dosage adjustment and close monitoring necessary. With use of Tobi podhaler (oral capsule powder for inhalation), taste disturbance (dysgeusia) was reported more frequently in pediatric patients ≥6 years (7.4%) than adults (2.7%).

Adverse Reactions

Injection: Frequency not defined:

Central nervous system: Confusion, disorientation, dizziness, headache, lethargy, vertigo

Dermatologic: Exfoliative dermatitis, pruritus, skin rash, urticaria

Endocrine & metabolic: Decreased serum calcium, decreased serum magnesium, decreased serum potassium and/or decreased serum sodium, increased lactate dehydrogenase

Gastrointestinal: Diarrhea, nausea, vomiting

Genitourinary: Casts in urine, oliguria, proteinuria

Hematologic & oncologic: Anemia, eosinophilia, granulocytopenia, leukocytosis, leukopenia, thrombocytopenia

Hepatic: Increased serum ALT, increased serum AST, increased serum bilirubin

Local: Pain at injection site

Miscellaneous: Fever

Otic: Auditory ototoxicity, hearing loss, tinnitus, vestibular ototoxicity

Renal: Increased blood urea nitrogen, increased serum creatinine

Inhalation

Cardiovascular: Chest discomfort

Central nervous system: Headache, malaise, voice disorder

Dermatologic: Skin rash

Endocrine: Increased serum glucose

Gastrointestinal: Diarrhea, dysgeusia, nausea, vomiting, xerostomia

Hematologic & oncologic: Eosinophilia, increased erythrocyte sedimentation rate, increased serum immunoglobulins

Miscellaneous: Fever

Neuromuscular & skeletal: Musculoskeletal chest pain, myalgia

Otic: Deafness (including unilateral deafness, reported as mild to moderate hearing loss or increased hearing loss), hypoacusis, tinnitus

Respiratory: Bronchitis, bronchospasm, cough, discoloration of sputum, dyspnea, epistaxis, hemoptysis, laryngitis, nasal congestion, oropharyngeal pain, pharyngolaryngeal pain, productive cough, pulmonary disease (includes pulmonary or cystic fibrosis exacerbations), rales, reduced forced expiratory volume, respiratory depression, rhinitis, throat irritation, tonsillitis, upper respiratory tract infection, wheezing

Rare but important or life-threatening: Abnormal breath sounds, decreased exercise tolerance, decrease in forced vital capacity, hypersensitivity reaction, increased bronchial secretions, lower respiratory tract infection, obstructive pulmonary disease, oral candidiasis, pneumonitis, pruritus, pulmonary congestion, urticaria

Drug Interactions

Metabolism/Transport Effects None known.

Avoid Concomitant Use

Avoid concomitant use of Tobramycin (Systemic, Oral Inhalation) with any of the following: BCG; BCG (Intravesical); Foscarnet; Mannitol; Mecamylamine

Increased Effect/Toxicity

Tobramycin (Systemic, Oral Inhalation) may increase the levels/effects of: AbobotulinumtoxinA; Bisphosphonate Derivatives; CARBOplatin; Colistimethate; CycloSPORINE (Systemic); Mecamylamine; Neuromuscular-Blocking Agents; OnabotulinumtoxinA; RimabotulinumtoxinB; Tenofovir

The levels/effects of Tobramycin (Systemic, Oral Inhalation) may be increased by: Amphotericin B; Capreomycin; Cephalosporins (2nd Generation); Cephalosporins (3rd Generation); Cephalosporins (4th Generation); CISplatin; Foscarnet; Loop Diuretics; Mannitol; Nonsteroidal Anti-Inflammatory Agents; Tenofovir; Vancomycin

Decreased Effect

Tobramycin (Systemic, Oral Inhalation) may decrease the levels/effects of: BCG; BCG (Intravesical); BCG

Vaccine (Immunization); Sodium Picosulfate; Typhoid Vaccine

The levels/effects of Tobramycin (Systemic, Oral Inhalation) may be decreased by: Penicillins

Storage/Stability

Injection: Stable at room temperature both as the clear, colorless solution and as the dry powder. Reconstituted solutions remain stable for 24 hours at room temperature and 96 hours when refrigerated.

Powder, for inhalation (TOBI Podhaler): Store in original package at 25°C (77°F); excursions permitted to 15°C to 30°C (59°F to 86°F). Protect from moisture.

Solution, for inhalation (Bethkis, Kitabis Pak, TOBI): Store under refrigeration at 2°C to 8°C (36°F to 46°F). May be stored in foil pouch (opened or unopened) at room temperature of 25°C (77°F) for up to 28 days. Protect from light. The colorless to pale yellow solution may darken over time if not stored under refrigeration; however, the color change does not affect product quality. Do not use if solution has been stored at room temperature for >28 days.

Mechanism of Action Interferes with bacterial protein synthesis by binding to 30S and 50S ribosomal subunits, resulting in a defective bacterial cell membrane

Pharmacodynamics Displays concentration-dependent killing; bacteriocidal

Pharmacokinetics (Adult data unless noted)

Absorption:
- Oral: Poor
- IM: Rapid and complete
- Inhalation: Low systemic bioavailability; accumulation can occur in patients with a low glomerular filtration rate
  - Peak serum concentration following inhalation:
    - Solution for inhalation: ~1 mcg/mL following a 300 mg dose
    - Powder for inhalation: ~1 mcg/mL (range: 0.49 to 1.55 mcg/mL) following a 112 mg dose

Distribution: Distributes primarily in the extracellular fluid volume; poor penetration into the CSF; drug accumulates in the renal cortex; small amounts distribute into bile, sputum, saliva, and tears
- V_d: Higher in neonates than older pediatric and adult patients; also increased in patients with edema, ascites, fluid overload; decreased in patients with dehydration
  - Systemic:
    - Neonates: 0.45 ± 0.1 L/kg
    - Infants: 0.4 ± 0.1 L/kg
    - Children: 0.35 ± 0.15 L/kg
    - Adolescents: 0.3 ± 0.1 L/kg
    - Adults: 0.2 to 0.3 L/kg
  - Inhalation: Tobramycin remains concentrated primarily in the airways

Protein binding: <30%

Half-life:
- IV:
  - Neonates:
    - ≤1,200 g: 11 hours
    - >1,200 g: 2 to 9 hours
  - Infants: 4 ± 1 hour
  - Children: 2 ± 1 hour
  - Adolescents: 1.5 ± 1 hour
  - Adults with normal renal function: 2 to 3 hours, directly dependent upon glomerular filtration rate; impaired renal function: 5 to 70 hours
- Inhalation:
  - Bethkis: 4.4 hours
  - TOBI/TOBI podhaler: CF patients: 3 hours

Time to peak serum concentration:
- IM: Within 30 to 90 minutes
- IV: 30 minutes after a 30-minute infusion; **Note:** Distribution may be prolonged after larger doses. One study reported a 1.7-hour distribution period after a 60-minute, high-dose aminoglycoside infusion (Demczar 1997).
- Inhalation (TOBI podhaler): 60 minutes

Elimination: With normal renal function, 93% of dose excreted in urine within 24 hours

Dosing: Neonatal Note: Dosage should be based on actual weight unless the patient has hydrops fetalis. Dosage should be individualized based upon serum concentration monitoring.

General dosing; susceptible infection: Limited data available: IV: Dosing strategies may vary by institution as a wide variety of dosing regimens have been studied. Consider single-dose administration with serum concentration monitoring in patients with urine output <1 mL/kg/hour or serum creatinine >1.3 mg/dL rather than scheduled dosing. Consider prolongation of dosing interval when coadministered with ibuprofen or indomethacin or in neonates with history of the following: Birth depression, birth hypoxia/asphyxia, or cyanotic congenital heart disease. Some dosing based on gentamicin studies.

Age-directed dosing (de Hoog 2002; DiCenzo 2003; Hagen 2009; Hansen 2003; Ohler 2000; Serane 2009):
- GA <32 weeks: 4 to 5 mg/kg/dose every 48 hours
- GA 32 to 36 weeks: 4 to 5 mg/kg/dose every 36 hours
- GA ≥37 weeks: 4 to 5 mg/kg/dose every 24 hours
- **Note:** In some trials, a fixed interval of every 24 hours was used with dosages ranging from 2.5 to 4 mg/kg/dose based on GA (ie, lower doses were used for younger GA).

Weight-directed dosing (*Red Book*, 2012): IM, IV:
- Body weight <1 kg:
  - PNA ≤14 days: 5 mg/kg/dose every 48 hours
  - PNA 15 to 28 days: 4-5 mg/kg/dose every 24 to 48 hours
- Body weight 1 to 2 kg:
  - PNA ≤7 days: 5 mg/kg/dose every 48 hours
  - PNA 8 to 28 days: 4 to 5 mg/kg/dose every 24 to 48 hours
- Body weight >2 kg:
  - PNA ≤7 days: 4 mg/kg/dose every 24 hours
  - PNA 8 to 28 days: 4 mg/kg/dose every 12 to 24 hours

Dosing: Usual Note: Dosage should be based on an estimate of ideal body weight. Some dosing is based on gentamicin studies. In morbidly obese children, adolescents, and adults, dosage requirement may best be estimated using a dosing weight of IBW + 0.4 (TBW - IBW). Dosage should be individualized based upon serum concentration monitoring.

Pediatric:

General dosing, susceptible infection: Infants, Children, and Adolescents:
- Conventional dosing: IM, IV: 2.5 mg/kg/dose every 8 hours; some pediatric patients may require larger doses (ie, patients undergoing continuous hemofiltration, patients with major burns, febrile granulocytopenic patients); modify dose based on individual patient requirements as determined by renal function, serum drug concentrations, and patient-specific clinical parameters
- Manufacturer's labeling: IM, IV: 2 to 2.5 mg/kg/dose every 8 hours
- Extended-interval dosing: IV:
  - Weight-directed: 4.5 to 7.5 mg/kg/dose every 24 hours (Contopoulos-Ioannidis 2004; *Red Book* 2012)
  - Age-directed: Based on data from 114 patients, the following has been suggested (McDade 2010):
    - 3 months to <2 years: 9.5 mg/kg/dose every 24 hours
    - 2 to <8 years: 8.5 mg/kg/dose every 24 hours
    - ≥8 years: 7 mg/kg/dose every 24 hours

Cystic fibrosis, pulmonary infection: Infants, Children, and Adolescents:
- Conventional dosing: IM, IV: 3.3 mg/kg/dose every 8 hours
- Extended-interval dosing: IV: Initial: 10 to 12 mg/kg/dose every 24 hours (Flume 2009; Smyth 2005; Van Meter 2009); **Note:** The CF Foundation recommends extended-interval dosing as preferred over conventional dosing.

Intra-abdominal infection, complicated: Infants, Children, and Adolescents: IV: 3 to 7.5 mg/kg/**day** divided every 8 to 24 hours (Solomkin 2010)

CNS infection:
- Meningitis (Tunkel 2004):
  - Infants and Children: IV: 7.5 mg/kg/**day** divided every 8 hours
  - Adolescents: IV: 5 mg/kg/**day** divided every 8 hours
- VP-shunt infection, ventriculitis: Limited data available: Infants, Children, and Adolescents: Intraventricular/intrathecal **(use a preservative-free preparation)**: 5 to 20 mg/**day**

Peritonitis (CAPD) (Warady 2012):Infants, Children, and Adolescents: Intraperitoneal: Continuous: Loading dose: 8 mg per liter of dialysate; maintenance dose: 4 mg per liter

Pulmonary infection: Inhalation:
- Cystic fibrosis patients: Children ≥6 years and Adolescents:
  - Bethkis, Kitabis Pak, TOBI: 300 mg every 12 hours; administer in repeated cycles of 28 days on drug, followed by 28 days off drug
  - TOBI Podhaler: 112 mg (4 x 28 mg capsules) every 12 hours; administer in repeated cycles of 28 days on drug followed by 28 days off drug
- Noncystic fibrosis patients: Limited data available: **Note:** Used by some centers; no published data are available: Children and Adolescents: 40 to 80 mg/dose 2 to 3 times daily

Urinary tract infection:
- Traditional dosing: Infants and Children 2 to 24 months: IV: 5 mg/kg/**day** divided every 8 hours (AAP 2011)
- Extended-interval dosing: Limited data available: IV: Based on data from 179 patients, the following age-directed dosing has been suggested (Carapetis 2001):
  - 1 month to <5 years: 7.5 mg/kg/dose every 24 hours
  - 5 to 10 years: 6 mg/kg/dose every 24 hours
  - >10 years: 4.5 mg/kg/dose every 24 hours

Adult: In underweight and nonobese patients, use of total body weight (TBW) instead of ideal body weight for determining the initial mg/kg/dose is widely accepted (Nicolau, 1995). Ideal body weight (IBW) also may be used to determine doses for patients who are neither underweight nor obese (Gilbert 2009).

General dosing, susceptible infection:
- Conventional: IM, IV: 1 to 2.5 mg/kg/dose every 8 to 12 hours; to ensure adequate peak concentrations early in therapy, higher initial dosage may be considered in selected patients when extracellular water is increased (edema, septic shock, postsurgical, or trauma)
- Once daily: IV: 4 to 7 mg/kg/dose once daily; some clinicians recommend this approach for all patients with normal renal function; this dose is at least as efficacious with similar, if not less, toxicity than conventional dosing

Cystic fibrosis: Inhalation:
- Bethkis, Kitabis Pak, TOBI: 300 mg every 12 hours (do not administer doses <6 hours apart); administer in repeated cycles of 28 days on drug followed by 28 days off drug
- TOBI podhaler: 112 mg (4 x 28 mg capsules) every 12 hours (do not administer doses <6 hours apart); administer in repeated cycles of 28 days on drug followed by 28 days off drug

Dosage adjustment in renal impairment:

Inhalation: Children ≥6 years, Adolescents, and Adults: There are no dosage adjustments provided in manufacturer's labeling (has not been studied).

Parenteral:
- Infants, Children, and Adolescents: IM, IV:
  - The following adjustments have been recommended (Aronoff, 2007): **Note:** Renally adjusted dose recommendations are based on doses of 2.5 mg/kg/dose every 8 hours.
    - GFR >50 mL/minute/1.73 m^2: No adjustment required
    - GFR 30 to 50 mL/minute/1.73 m^2: Administer every 12 to 18 hours
    - GFR 10 to 29 mL/minute/1.73 m^2: Administer every 18 to 24 hours
    - GFR <10 mL/minute/1.73 m^2: Administer every 48 to 72 hours
  - Intermittent hemodialysis: Dialyzable (25% to 70%): 2 mg/kg/dose; redose as indicated by serum concentrations
  - Peritoneal dialysis (PD): 2 mg/kg/dose; redose as indicated by serum concentrations
  - Continuous renal replacement therapy (CRRT): 2 to 2.5 mg/kg/dose every 12 to 24 hours, monitor serum concentrations
- Adults:
  - Conventional dosing: IM, IV:
    - CrCl ≥60 mL/minute: Administer every 8 hours
    - CrCl 40 to 60 mL/minute: Administer every 12 hours
    - CrCl 20 to 40 mL/minute: Administer every 24 hours
    - CrCl 10 to 20 mL/minute: Administer every 48 hours
    - CrCl <10 mL/minute: Administer every 72 hours
  - High-dose therapy: IV: Interval may be extended (eg, every 48 hours) in patients with moderate renal impairment (CrCl 30 to 59 mL/minute) and/or adjusted based on serum concentration determinations.
  - Intermittent hemodialysis (IHD) (administer after hemodialysis on dialysis days) (Heintz 2009): Dialyzable (25% to 75%; variable; dependent on filter, duration, and type of IHD); **Note:** Dosing dependent on the assumption of 3 times/week, complete IHD sessions.
    - IV:
      - Loading dose of 2 to 3 mg/kg loading dose followed by:
        - Mild UTI or synergy: 1 mg/kg every 48 to 72 hours; consider redosing for pre-HD or post-HD serum concentrations <1 mcg/mL
        - Moderate to severe UTI: 1 to 1.5 mg/kg every 48 to 72 hours; consider redosing for pre-HD serum concentrations <1.5 to 2 mcg/mL or post-HD serum concentrations <1 mcg/mL
        - Systemic gram negative rod infection: 1.5 to 2 mg/kg every 48 to 72 hours; consider redosing for pre-HD concentrations <3 to 5 mcg/mL or post-HD serum concentrations <2 mcg/mL
  - Peritoneal dialysis (PD):
    - Administration via PD fluid:
      - Gram-positive infection (eg, synergy): 3 to 4 mg/L (3 to 4 mcg/mL) of PD fluid
      - Gram-negative infection: 4 to 8 mg/L (4 to 8 mcg/mL) of PD fluid
    - Administration via IV, IM route during PD: Dose as for CrCl <10 mL/minute and follow serum concentrations

Continuous renal replacement therapy (CRRT) (Heintz 2009; Trotman 2005): Drug clearance is highly dependent on the method of renal replacement, filter type, and flow rate. Appropriate dosing requires close monitoring of pharmacologic response, signs of adverse reactions due to drug accumulation, as well as drug concentrations in relation to target trough (if appropriate). The following are general recommendations only (based on dialysate flow/ultrafiltration rates of 1 to 2 L/hour and minimal residual renal function) and should not supersede clinical judgment:

CVVH/CVVHD/CVVHDF: IV: Loading dose of 2 to 3 mg/kg followed by:

Mild UTI or synergy: IV: 1 mg/kg every 24 to 36 hours (redose when serum concentration <1 mcg/mL)

Moderate to severe UTI: IV: 1 to 1.5 mg/kg every 24 to 36 hours (redose when serum concentration <1.5 to 2 mcg/mL)

Systemic gram-negative infection: IV: 1.5 to 2.5 mg/kg every 24 to 48 hours (redose when serum concentration <3 to 5 mcg/mL)

Dosage adjustment in hepatic impairment:

Inhalation: Children ≥6 years, Adolescents, and Adults: No dosage adjustment necessary

Parenteral: Adults: IM, IV: No dosage adjustment necessary

Preparation for Administration Parenteral: IV: May dilute in NS or D_5W for IV infusion. In adults, dilution in 50 to 100 mL is recommended; premix admixtures commercially available for some dosages. In infants and children, the volume should be less, but allow for accurate measurement and administration; final IV concentration for administration should not exceed 10 mg/mL.

Administration

Inhalation: Doses should be administered as close to a 12-hour schedule as possible; do not administer less than 6 hours apart

Bethkis, Kitabis Pak, TOBI: Use a PARI LC Plus reusable nebulizer and a PARI Vios air compressor (Bethkis) or a DeVilbiss Pulmo-Aide air compressor (Kitabis Pak, TOBI) for administration; patient should be sitting or standing upright and breathing normally through the mouthpiece of the nebulizer. Nebulizer treatment period is usually over 15 minutes. If patient receiving multiple inhalation products, administer bronchodilator first, followed by chest physiotherapy, any other nebulized medications, and then tobramycin last. Do not mix with other nebulizer medications.

TOBI Podhaler: Capsules should be administered by oral inhalation via Podhaler device following manufacturer recommendations for use and handling. Capsules should be removed from the blister packaging immediately prior to use and should not be swallowed. Patients requiring bronchodilator therapy should administer the bronchodilator 15-90 minutes prior to TOBI Podhaler. The sequence of chest physiotherapy and additional inhaled therapies is at the discretion of the healthcare provider; however, TOBI Podhaler should always be administered last. Use the new podhaler device provided with each weekly pack.

Parenteral:

IM: Administer undiluted by deep IM route if possible. Slower absorption and lower peak concentrations, probably due to poor circulation in the atrophic muscle, may occur following IM injection in paralyzed patients, suggest IV route.

IV: Administer by slow intermittent infusion over 30-60 minutes (administer higher doses over 60 minutes) or by direct injection over 15 minutes; administer beta-lactam antibiotics, such as penicillins and cephalosporins, at least 1 hour before or after tobramycin; simultaneous administration may result in reduced antibacterial efficacy

Monitoring Parameters Urinalysis, urine output, BUN, serum creatinine, peak and trough serum tobramycin concentrations; **Note:** Do not use fingerstick for obtaining blood sample in patients concurrently receiving inhaled tobramycin as it may result in falsely elevated drug concentrations); be alert to ototoxicity, audiograms

With conventional dosing, typically obtain serum concentration after the third dose; exceptions for earlier monitoring may include neonates, patients with rapidly changing renal function, or patients receiving extended-interval dosing. Not all pediatric patients who receive aminoglycosides require monitoring of serum aminoglycoside concentrations. Indications for use of aminoglycoside serum concentration monitoring include:

Treatment course >5 days

Patients with decreased or changing renal function

Patients with a poor therapeutic response

Neonates and Infants <3 months of age

Atypical body constituency (obesity, expanded extracellular fluid volume)

Clinical need for higher doses or shorter intervals (cystic fibrosis, burns, endocarditis, meningitis, relatively resistant organism)

Patients on hemodialysis or chronic ambulatory peritoneal dialysis

Signs of nephrotoxicity or ototoxicity

Concomitant use of other nephrotoxic agents

Patients on high-dose aerosolized tobramycin: The utility of monitoring serum concentrations in patients with renal impairment should be per clinician's discretion; serum concentrations achieved following inhalation are significantly less than those achieved following parenteral therapy in patients with normal renal function. Obtaining peak tobramycin concentration 1 hour following inhalation to identify patients who are significant absorbers, in patients with decreased glomerular filtration rate, in patients on concomitant parenteral therapy, and in infants have been recommended by some clinicians (Abdulhamid, 2008).

Reference Range

Traditional dosing: Timing of serum samples: Draw peak 30 minutes after 30-minute infusion has been completed or 1 hour following IM injection or beginning of infusion; draw trough immediately before next dose

Therapeutic concentrations:

Peak:

Serious infections: 6-8 mcg/mL (12-17 micromole/L)

Life-threatening infections: 8-10 mcg/mL (17-21 micromole/L)

Urinary tract infections: 4-6 mcg/mL

Synergy against gram-positive organisms: 3-5 mcg/mL

Trough:

Serious infections: 0.5-1 mcg/mL

Life-threatening infections: 1-2 mcg/mL

The American Thoracic Society (ATS) recommends trough levels of <1 mcg/mL for adult patients with hospital-acquired pneumonia.

Timing of serum samples: Draw peak 30 minutes after completion of 30-minute infusion or at 1 hour following initiation of infusion or IM injection; draw trough within 30 minutes prior to next dose; aminoglycoside levels measured from blood taken from Silastic® central catheters can sometimes give falsely elevated readings

Extended-interval: **Note:** Pediatric therapeutic monitoring protocols have not been standardized; peak values are 2-3 times greater with extended-interval dosing regimens compared to traditional dosing

Noncystic fibrosis patients: Consider monitoring tobramycin serum concentration 18-20 hours after the start of the infusion to ensure the drug-free interval does not exceed typical postantibiotic effect (PAE) duration.

Cystic fibrosis patients: Clinically two methods are utilized. Peak: 25-35 mcg/mL (some centers use 20-30 mcg/mL); 18- to 20-hour value: Detectable but <1 mcg/mL; trough: Nondetectable

Method A: Obtain two serum concentrations at least 1 half-life apart after distribution is complete (eg, obtain a serum concentration 2 hours and 10 hours after the start of the infusion), calculate elimination rate and extrapolate a C_{max} and C_{min}

Method B: Obtain a peak serum concentration 60 minutes after a 60-minute infusion and a serum concentration 18-20 hours after the start of the infusion to ensure the drug-free interval does not exceed typical postantibiotic effect (PAE) duration (4-6 hours)

Test Interactions Some penicillin derivatives may accelerate the degradation of aminoglycosides *in vitro*, leading to a potential underestimation of aminoglycoside serum concentration.

Additional Information Some penicillins (eg, carbenicillin, ticarcillin, and piperacillin) have been shown to inactivate aminoglycosides *in vitro*. This has been observed to a greater extent with tobramycin and gentamicin, while amikacin has shown greater stability against inactivation. Concurrent use of these agents may pose a risk of reduced antibacterial efficacy *in vivo*, particularly in the setting of profound renal impairment; however, definitive clinical evidence is lacking. If combination penicillin/aminoglycoside therapy is desired in a patient with renal dysfunction, separation of doses (if feasible), and routine monitoring of aminoglycoside levels, CBC, and clinical response should be considered.

Product Availability Kitabis Pak: FDA approved December 2014. Kitabis Pak is a co-packaged kit containing a reusable nebulizer and tobramycin inhalation solution.

Dosage Forms Excipient information presented when available (limited, particularly for generics); consult specific product labeling.

Capsule, Inhalation:
- Tobi Podhaler: 28 mg

Nebulization Solution, Inhalation [preservative free]:
- Bethkis: 300 mg/4 mL (4 mL)
- Kitabis Pak: 300 mg/5 mL (5 mL) [contains sodium chloride, sodium hydroxide, sulfuric acid]
- Tobi: 300 mg/5 mL (5 mL) [contains sodium chloride, sodium hydroxide, sulfuric acid]
- Generic: 300 mg/5 mL (5 mL)

Solution, Injection:
- Generic: 10 mg/mL (2 mL); 80 mg/2 mL (2 mL); 1.2 g/30 mL (30 mL); 2 g/50 mL (50 mL)

Solution, Intravenous:
- Generic: 80 mg (100 mL)

Solution Reconstituted, Injection:
- Generic: 1.2 g (1 ea)

Solution Reconstituted, Injection [preservative free]:
- Generic: 1.2 g (1 ea)

Tobramycin (Ophthalmic) (toe bra MYE sin)

Medication Safety Issues

Sound-alike/look-alike issues:

Tobramycin may be confused with Trobicin, vancomycin

Tobrex may be confused with TobraDex

Brand Names: US Tobrex

Brand Names: Canada PMS-Tobramycin; Sandoz-Tobramycin; Tobrex®

Therapeutic Category Antibiotic, Aminoglycoside; Antibiotic, Ophthalmic

Generic Availability (US) May be product dependent

Use Used topically to treat superficial ophthalmic infections caused by susceptible bacteria

Pregnancy Risk Factor B

Pregnancy Considerations Adverse events were not observed following systemic administration of tobramycin in animal reproduction studies; therefore, tobramycin ophthalmic is classified as pregnancy category B. When administered IM or IV, tobramycin crosses the placenta. Refer to the Tobramycin (Systemic, Oral Inhalation) monograph for details. The amount of tobramycin available systemically following topical application of the ophthalmic drops is undetectable (<0.2 mcg/mL). Systemic absorption would be required in order for tobramycin ophthalmic to cross the placenta and reach the fetus.

Breast-Feeding Considerations Due to undetectable (<0.2 mcg/mL) systemic absorption of tobramycin ophthalmic drops, excretion of tobramycin into breast milk would not be expected; however, because of the potential for adverse events in a nursing infant, breast-feeding is not recommended by the manufacturer. When administered IM or IV, tobramycin is detected in breast milk. Refer to the Tobramycin (Systemic, Oral Inhalation) monograph for details.

Contraindications Hypersensitivity to tobramycin, other aminoglycosides, or any component of the formulation

Warnings/Precautions For ophthalmic use only. Severe hypersensitivity reactions have occurred with ophthalmic administration of tobramycin. Prompt discontinuation of drug should occur if local reaction suggests hypersensitivity. Prolonged use may result in fungal or bacterial superinfection. If condition worsens and/or superinfection is suspected, appropriate therapy should be instituted. Some products contain benzalkonium chloride which may be absorbed by soft contact lenses; contact lens should not be worn during treatment of ophthalmologic infections.

Adverse Reactions Rare but important or life-threatening: Conjunctival erythema, lid itching, lid swelling

Drug Interactions

Metabolism/Transport Effects None known.

Avoid Concomitant Use There are no known interactions where it is recommended to avoid concomitant use.

Increased Effect/Toxicity There are no known significant interactions involving an increase in effect.

Decreased Effect There are no known significant interactions involving a decrease in effect.

Storage/Stability

Solution (Tobrex®): Store at 8°C to 27°C (46°F to 80°F).

Some product-specific storage recommendations are: Store at 25°C (77°F); excursions permitted to 15°C to 30°C (59°F to 86°F). Consult specific product labeling.

Mechanism of Action Interferes with bacterial protein synthesis by binding to 30S and 50S ribosomal subunits resulting in a defective bacterial cell membrane

Dosing: Usual

Children ≥2 months and Adults:

Ointment: Apply 0.5" ribbon into the affected eye 2-3 times/day; for severe infections, apply ointment every 3-4 hours

Solution:

Mild to moderate infections: Instill 1-2 drops every 4 hours

Severe infections: Instill 2 drops every 30-60 minutes initially, then reduce to less frequent intervals

Administration Avoid contact of tube or bottle tip with skin or eye; apply finger pressure to lacrimal sac during and for 1-2 minutes after instillation of drops to decrease risk of absorption and systemic effects.

Dosage Forms Excipient information presented when available (limited, particularly for generics); consult specific product labeling.

Ointment, Ophthalmic:
- Tobrex: 0.3% (3.5 g)

Solution, Ophthalmic:
Tobrex: 0.3% (5 mL)
Generic: 0.3% (5 mL)

- ◆ **Tobramycin For Injection (Can)** *see* Tobramycin (Systemic, Oral Inhalation) *on page 2073*
- ◆ **Tobramycin For Injection, USP (Can)** *see* Tobramycin (Systemic, Oral Inhalation) *on page 2073*
- ◆ **Tobramycin Injection (Can)** *see* Tobramycin (Systemic, Oral Inhalation) *on page 2073*
- ◆ **Tobramycin Injection, USP (Can)** *see* Tobramycin (Systemic, Oral Inhalation) *on page 2073*
- ◆ **Tobramycin Sulfate** *see* Tobramycin (Ophthalmic) *on page 2078*
- ◆ **Tobramycin Sulfate** *see* Tobramycin (Systemic, Oral Inhalation) *on page 2073*
- ◆ **Tobrex** *see* Tobramycin (Ophthalmic) *on page 2078*
- ◆ **Tobrex® (Can)** *see* Tobramycin (Ophthalmic) *on page 2078*

Tocilizumab (toe si LIZ oo mab)

Brand Names: US Actemra

Brand Names: Canada Actemra

Therapeutic Category Antirheumatic, Disease Modifying; Interleukin-6 Receptor Antagonist; Monoclonal Antibody

Generic Availability (US) No

Use Treatment of active systemic juvenile idiopathic arthritis (SJIA) (FDA approved in ages ≥2 years); treatment of active polyarticular juvenile idiopathic arthritis (PJIA) (FDA approved in ages ≥2 years); treatment of moderately- to severely-active rheumatoid arthritis in patients who have had an inadequate response to one or more disease-modifying antirheumatic drugs (DMARDs) (FDA approved in adults)

Medication Guide Available Yes

Pregnancy Risk Factor C

Pregnancy Considerations Adverse events have been observed in some animal reproduction studies. Monoclonal antibodies cross the placenta, with the largest amount transferred during the third trimester. A pregnancy registry has been established to monitor outcomes of women exposed to tocilizumab during pregnancy (877-311-8972).

Breast-Feeding Considerations It is not known if tocilizumab is excreted in human milk. Because many immunoglobulins are excreted in human milk and the potential for serious adverse reactions exists, a decision should be made whether to discontinue nursing or to discontinue the drug, taking into account the importance of the drug to the mother.

Contraindications

Hypersensitivity to tocilizumab or any component of the formulation

Canadian labeling: Additional contraindications (not in U.S. labeling): Active infections

Warnings/Precautions **[U.S. Boxed Warning]: Serious and potentially fatal infections (including active tuberculosis, invasive fungal, bacterial, viral, protozoal, and other opportunistic infections) have been reported in patients receiving tocilizumab; infection may lead to hospitalization or death. Most of the serious infections have occurred in patients on concomitant immunosuppressive therapy. Patients should be closely monitored for signs and symptoms of infection during and after treatment. If serious infection occurs during treatment, withhold tocilizumab until infection is controlled. Prior to treatment initiation, carefully consider risk versus benefit in patients with chronic or recurrent infections,** tuberculosis exposure, history of or current opportunistic infection, underlying conditions predisposing to infection, or patients residing in or with travel to areas of endemic tuberculosis or endemic mycosis, The most common serious infections occurring have included pneumonia, UTI, cellulitis, herpes zoster, gastroenteritis, diverticulitis, sepsis, and bacterial arthritis. Do not administer tocilizumab to a patient with an active infection, including localized infection. Interrupt treatment for opportunistic infection or sepsis. **[U.S. Boxed Warning]: Tuberculosis (pulmonary or extrapulmonary) has been reported in patients receiving tocilizumab; both reactivation of latent infection and new infections have been reported. Patients should be tested for latent tuberculosis infection before and during therapy; consider treatment of latent tuberculosis prior to tocilizumab treatment. Some patients who test negative prior to therapy may develop active infection; monitor for signs and symptoms of tuberculosis during and after treatment in all patients.** Patients should be evaluated for tuberculosis risk factors with a tuberculin skin test prior to starting therapy. Consider antituberculosis treatment in patients with a history of latent or active tuberculosis if adequate treatment course cannot be confirmed, and for patients with risk factors for tuberculosis despite a negative test. Rare reactivation of herpes zoster has been reported. Patients should be brought up to date with all immunizations before initiating therapy. Live vaccines should not be given concurrently; there is no data available concerning secondary transmission of infection from live vaccines in patients receiving therapy.

Use of tocilizumab may affect defenses against malignancies; impact on the development and course of malignancies is not fully defined, however, malignancies were observed in clinical trials. Use with caution in patients with pre-existing or recent onset CNS demyelinating disorders; rare cases of CNS demyelinating disorders (eg, multiple sclerosis) have occurred. All patients should be monitored for signs and symptoms of demyelinating disorders. May cause hypersensitivity or anaphylaxis; anaphylactic events including fatalities have been reported with IV administration; hypersensitivity reactions have occurred in patients who were premedicated, in patients with and without a prior history of hypersensitivity, and as early as the first infusion. Medications for the treatment of hypersensitivity reactions should be available for immediate use. Patients should seek medical attention if symptoms of hypersensitivity reaction occur with subcutaneous use. Stop infusion and permanently discontinue treatment in patients who develop a hypersensitivity reaction to tocilizumab. In clinical studies, reactions requiring treatment discontinuation included generalized erythema, rash, and urticaria. Use is not recommended in patients with active hepatic disease or hepatic impairment. Monitor ALT and AST. Do not initiate treatment if ALT or AST is >1.5 times ULN. Use with caution in patients at increased risk for gastrointestinal perforation; perforation has been reported, typically secondary to diverticulitis. Monitor for new-onset abdominal symptoms; promptly evaluate if new symptoms occur.

Use may cause increases in total cholesterol, triglycerides, LDL and HDL cholesterol; monitor ~4-8 weeks after initiation, then approximately every 6 months; hyperlipidemia should be managed according to current guidelines. Neutropenia and thrombocytopenia may occur; may require treatment interruption, dose or interval modification, or discontinuation. Monitor neutrophils and platelets. Do not initiate treatment in patients with an ANC <2000/mm^3 or platelet count <100,000/mm^3; discontinue treatment for ANC <500/mm^3 or platelet count <50,000/mm^3. Monitor transaminases; treatment should be discontinued in patients who develop elevated ALT or AST >5 x ULN. Patients receiving concomitant hepatotoxic drugs (eg, methotrexate) are at an increased risk of developing elevated transaminases; elevations are typically reversible and do not result in clinically evident hepatic injury.

Potentially significant drug/drug interactions may exist, requiring dose or frequency adjustment, additional monitoring, and/or selection of alternative therapy. Concomitant use with other biological DMARDs (eg, TNF blockers, IL-1 receptor blockers, anti-CD20 monoclonal antibodies, selective costimulation modulators) has not been studied and should should be avoided. Cautious use is recommended in elderly patients due to an increased incidence of serious infections. Subcutaneous administration is only indicated for adult patients with rheumatoid arthritis. Do not use subcutaneous injection for IV infusion.

Some dosage forms may contain polysorbate 80 (also known as Tweens). Hypersensitivity reactions, usually a delayed reaction, have been reported following exposure to pharmaceutical products containing polysorbate 80 in certain individuals (Isaksson, 2002; Lucente 2000; Shelley, 1995). Thrombocytopenia, ascites, pulmonary deterioration, and renal and hepatic failure have been reported in premature neonates after receiving parenteral products containing polysorbate 80 (Alade, 1986; CDC, 1984). See manufacturer's labeling.

Adverse Reactions As reported for monotherapy, except where noted. Combination therapy refers to use in rheumatoid arthritis with nonbiological DMARDs or use in SJIA or PJIA in trials where most patients (~70% to 80%) were taking methotrexate at baseline.

Cardiovascular: Hypertension, peripheral edema

Central nervous system: Dizziness, headache

Dermatologic: Dermatological reaction (combination therapy; includes pruritus, urticaria), skin rash

Endocrine & metabolic: Hypothyroidism, increased LDL cholesterol (>1.5-2 x ULN; combination therapy; children and adolescents), increased serum cholesterol (>240 mg/dL; >1.5-2 x ULN; combination therapy; children and adolescents)

Gastrointestinal: Abdominal pain, diarrhea (children and adolescents), gastric ulcer, gastritis, oral mucosa ulcer, stomatitis, weight gain

Hematologic & oncologic: Leukopenia, neutropenia (combination therapy), thrombocytopenia (combination therapy)

Hepatic: Increased serum ALT, increased serum AST, increased serum bilirubin

Immunologic: Antibody development

Infection: Herpes simplex infection

Local: Injection site reaction (SubQ: Including erythema, pruritus, pain, and hematoma)

Ophthalmic: Conjunctivitis

Renal: Nephrolithiasis

Respiratory: Bronchitis, cough, dyspnea, nasopharyngitis, upper respiratory tract infection

Miscellaneous: Infusion-related reaction (combination therapy)

Rare but important or life-threatening: Anaphylaxis, anaphylactoid reaction, angioedema, aspergillosis, candidiasis, cellulitis, chronic inflammatory demyelinating polyneuropathy, cryptococcosis, diverticulitis, gastroenteritis, gastrointestinal perforation, herpes zoster, hypersensitivity, hypersensitivity pneumonitis, hypertriglyceridemia, hypotension, increased HDL cholesterol, malignant neoplasm (including breast and colon cancer), multiple sclerosis, otitis media, pneumonia, pneumocystosis, reactivation of latent Epstein-Barr virus, septic arthritis, sepsis, Stevens-Johnson syndrome, tuberculosis, urinary tract infection, varicella

Drug Interactions

Metabolism/Transport Effects None known.

Avoid Concomitant Use

Avoid concomitant use of Tocilizumab with any of the following: Abatacept; Anti-TNF Agents; BCG; BCG (Intravesical); Belimumab; Natalizumab; Pimecrolimus; Tacrolimus (Topical); Tofacitinib; Vaccines (Live)

Increased Effect/Toxicity

Tocilizumab may increase the levels/effects of: Abatacept; Anti-TNF Agents; Belimumab; Leflunomide; Natalizumab; Tofacitinib; Vaccines (Live)

The levels/effects of Tocilizumab may be increased by: Denosumab; Pimecrolimus; Roflumilast; Tacrolimus (Topical); Trastuzumab

Decreased Effect

Tocilizumab may decrease the levels/effects of: BCG; BCG (Intravesical); Coccidioides immitis Skin Test; CYP3A4 Substrates; Sipuleucel-T; Vaccines (Inactivated); Vaccines (Live)

The levels/effects of Tocilizumab may be decreased by: Echinacea

Storage/Stability Store intact vials/syringes at 2°C to 8°C (36°F to 46°F). Do not freeze. Protect vials and syringes from light (store in the original package until time of use); keep syringes dry. Solutions diluted for IV infusion may be stored at 2°C to 8°C (36°F to 46°F) or room temperature for up to 24 hours and should be protected from light. Discard unused product remaining in the vials.

Mechanism of Action Antagonist of the interleukin-6 (IL-6) receptor. Endogenous IL-6 is induced by inflammatory stimuli and mediates a variety of immunological responses. Inhibition of IL-6 receptors by tocilizumab leads to a reduction in cytokine and acute phase reactant production.

Pharmacokinetics (Adult data unless noted)

Distribution: V_{dss}: Children: 2.54 L (SJIA), 4.08 L (PJIA); Adults: 6.4 L

Bioavailability: SubQ: 80%

Half-life elimination:

IV: Terminal, single dose: 6.3 days (concentration-dependent); may be increased at steady state up to: Children: 16 days (PJIA), 23 days (SJIA); Adults: 13 days

SubQ: Concentration dependent: Adults: Up to 5 days (every other week dosing) or 13 days (every week dosing)

Dosing: Usual Note: Do not initiate if ANC is <2000/mm^3, platelets are <100,000/mm^3 or if ALT or AST are >1.5 times ULN.

Pediatric: **Note:** Dose adjustment should not be made based solely on a single-visit body weight measurement due to fluctuations in body weight. May be used as monotherapy or in combination with methotrexate.

Polyarticular juvenile idiopathic arthritis (PJIA): Children ≥2 years and Adolescents:

<30 kg: IV: 10 mg/kg every 4 weeks

≥30 kg: IV: 8 mg/kg every 4 weeks; maximum single dose: 800 mg

Systemic juvenile idiopathic arthritis (SJIA): Children ≥2 years and Adolescents:

<30 kg: IV: 12 mg/kg/dose every 2 weeks

≥30 kg: IV: 8 mg/kg/dose every 2 weeks; maximum dose: 800 mg

Adult: **Rheumatoid arthritis: Note:** Methotrexate or other *nonbiologic* disease-modifying antirheumatic drugs (DMARDs) may be continued for the treatment of rheumatoid arthritis. Tocilizumab should not be used in combination with *biologic* DMARDs.

IV: Initial: 4 mg/kg/dose every 4 weeks; may be increased to 8 mg/kg/dose based on clinical response maximum single dose: 800 mg

SubQ:

<100 kg: 162 mg every other week; increase to every week based on clinical response

≥100 kg: 162 mg every week

Transitioning from IV therapy to SubQ therapy: Administer the first SubQ dose instead of the next scheduled IV dose.

Dosing adjustment in renal impairment: Children ≥2 years, Adolescents, and Adults:

Mild renal impairment: No dosage adjustment required.

Moderate to severe renal impairment: There are no dosage adjustments provided in the manufacturer labeling (not studied).

Dosing adjustment in hepatic impairment: Children ≥2 years, Adolescents, and Adults: There are no dosage adjustments provided in the manufacturer's labeling (not studied); not recommended for use in patients with active hepatic disease or hepatic impairment.

Dosing adjustment for toxicity:

Children ≥2 years and Adolescents: Polyarticular and systemic juvenile idiopathic arthritis (SJIA): Dose reductions have not been studied; however, dose interruptions are recommended for liver enzyme abnormalities, low neutrophil counts, and low platelets similar to recommendations provided for adult rheumatoid arthritis patients (see below). In addition, consider interrupting or discontinuing concomitant methotrexate and/or other medications and hold tocilizumab dosing until the clinical situation has been assessed.

Adults: Rheumatoid arthritis (RA):

Liver enzyme abnormalities:

>1 to 3 x ULN: For persistent increases in this range, reduce IV tocilizumab dose to 4 mg/kg or SubQ therapy to every other week or interrupt therapy until ALT/AST have normalized; adjust concomitant DMARDs as appropriate

>3 to 5 x ULN (confirm with repeat testing): Interrupt tocilizumab therapy until ALT/AST <3 x ULN, then resume tocilizumab IV dose at 4 mg/kg or resume SubQ therapy at every other week. For persistent increases in this range, discontinue therapy

>5 x ULN: Discontinue therapy

Low absolute neutrophil counts (ANC):

ANC >1000 cells/mm^3: Maintain dose

ANC 500-1000 cells/mm^3: Interrupt therapy; when ANC >1000 cells/mm^3, resume tocilizumab IV dose at 4 mg/kg or resume SubQ therapy at every other week dosing; may increase IV dose to 8 mg/kg or SubQ therapy to every week as clinically appropriate

ANC <500 cells/mm^3: Discontinue therapy

Low platelet counts:

Platelets 50,000-100,000 cells/mm^3: Interrupt therapy; when platelet count is >100,000 cells/mm^3, resume tocilizumab IV dose at 4 mg/kg or resume SubQ therapy at every other week dosing; may increase IV dose to 8 mg/kg or SubQ therapy to every week as clinically appropriate

Platelets <50,000 cells/mm^3: Discontinue therapy

Preparation for Administration IV: Use vials to prepare IV infusion solutions; do not use prefilled SubQ syringes to prepare IV solutions. Prior to administration, further dilute dose to 50 mL (children <30 kg) or 100 mL (children ≥30 kg and adults) by slowly adding to NS. Withdraw volume of NS equal to the volume of tocilizumab required for dose; slowly add tocilizumab dose into infusion bag or bottle. Gently invert to mix to avoid foaming. Diluted solutions may be stored under refrigeration or at room temperature for up to 24 hours (protected from light) and are compatible with polypropylene, polyethylene (PE), polyvinyl chloride (PVC), and glass infusion containers. Allow diluted solution to reach room temperature prior to infusion.

Administration

Intravenous: Allow diluted solution to reach room temperature prior to administration; infuse over 60 minutes using a dedicated IV line. Do not administer IV push or IV bolus. Do not use if opaque particles or discoloration are visible.

SubQ: Adults: Administer the full amount in the prefilled syringe. Allow to reach room temperature prior to use. Do not use if particulate matter or discoloration is visible; solution should be clear and colorless to pale yellow. Rotate injection sites; avoid injecting into moles, scars, or tender, bruised, red, or hard skin. Prefilled syringe is available for use by patients (self-administration).

Monitoring Parameters Latent TB screening prior to therapy initiation; neutrophils, platelets, ALT/AST (prior to therapy, 4-8 weeks after start of therapy, and every 3 months thereafter [RA]); neutrophils, platelets, ALT/AST (prior to therapy, at second infusion, and every 2-4 weeks [SJIA] or 4-8 weeks [PJIA] thereafter); additional liver function tests (eg, bilirubin) as clinically indicated; lipid panel (prior to, at 4-8 weeks following initiation, and every ~6 months during therapy); signs and symptoms of infection (prior to, during, and after therapy); signs and symptoms of CNS demyelinating disorder.

The following lab schedule has been used in patients with SJIA: 1-2 weeks, and 1, 2, 6, and 9 months: CBC with differential, C-reactive protein, erythrocyte sedimentation rate, ferritin, and LDH (Dewitt, 2012).

Dosage Forms Excipient information presented when available (limited, particularly for generics); consult specific product labeling.

Solution, Intravenous [preservative free]:

Actemra: 80 mg/4 mL (4 mL); 200 mg/10 mL (10 mL); 400 mg/20 mL (20 mL) [contains polysorbate 80]

Solution Prefilled Syringe, Subcutaneous [preservative free]:

Actemra: 162 mg/0.9 mL (0.9 mL) [contains polysorbate 80]

◆ **Tofranil** *see* Imipramine *on page 1086*

◆ **Tofranil-PM** *see* Imipramine *on page 1086*

◆ **Tolectin** *see* Tolmetin *on page 2081*

Tolmetin (TOLE met in)

Medication Safety Issues

Sound-alike/look-alike issues:

Tolmetin may be confused wit tolcapone

BEERS Criteria medication:

This drug may be potentially inappropriate for use in geriatric patients (Quality of evidence - moderate; Strength of recommendation - strong).

Therapeutic Category Analgesic, Non-narcotic; Nonsteroidal Anti-inflammatory Drug (NSAID), Oral

Generic Availability (US) Yes

Use Treatment of inflammatory and rheumatoid disorders, including juvenile idiopathic arthritis

Medication Guide Available Yes

Pregnancy Risk Factor C

Pregnancy Considerations Adverse events were not observed in the initial animal reproduction studies; therefore, the manufacturer classifies tolmetin as pregnancy category C. NSAID exposure during the first trimester is not strongly associated with congenital malformations; however, cardiovascular anomalies and cleft palate have been observed following NSAID exposure in some studies. The use of an NSAID close to conception may be associated with an increased risk of miscarriage. Nonteratogenic effects have been observed following NSAID administration during the third trimester including myocardial degenerative changes, prenatal constriction of the ductus arteriosus, fetal tricuspid regurgitation, failure of the ductus arteriosus to close postnatally; renal dysfunction or failure, oligohydramnios; gastrointestinal bleeding or perforation, increased risk of necrotizing enterocolitis; intracranial bleeding (including intraventricular hemorrhage), platelet dysfunction with resultant bleeding;

pulmonary hypertension. Because they may cause premature closure of the ductus arteriosus, use of NSAIDs late in pregnancy should be avoided (use after 31 or 32 weeks gestation is not recommended by some clinicians). The chronic use of NSAIDs in women of reproductive age may be associated with infertility that is reversible upon discontinuation of the medication.

Breast-Feeding Considerations Tolmetin is found in breast milk and breast-feeding is not recommended by the manufacturer.

Contraindications Hypersensitivity to tolmetin, aspirin, other NSAIDs, or any component of the formulation; perioperative pain in the setting of coronary artery bypass graft (CABG) surgery

Warnings/Precautions [U.S. Boxed Warning]: NSAIDs are associated with an increased risk of adverse cardiovascular thrombotic events, including MI and stroke. Risk may be increased with duration of use or pre-existing cardiovascular risk factors or disease. Carefully evaluate individual cardiovascular risk profiles prior to prescribing. May cause new-onset hypertension or worsening of existing hypertension. Use caution with fluid retention. Avoid use in heart failure (ACCF/AHA [Yancy, 2013]). Concurrent administration of ibuprofen, and potentially other nonselective NSAIDs, may interfere with aspirin's cardioprotective effect. **[U.S. Boxed Warning]: Use is contraindicated for treatment of perioperative pain in the setting of coronary artery bypass graft (CABG) surgery.** Risk of MI and stroke may be increased with use following CABG surgery.

Platelet adhesion and aggregation may be decreased; may prolong bleeding time; patients with coagulation disorders or who are receiving anticoagulants should be monitored closely. Anemia may occur; patients on long-term NSAID therapy should be monitored for anemia. Rarely, NSAID use may cause severe blood dyscrasias (eg, agranulocytosis, aplastic anemia, thrombocytopenia).

NSAID use may compromise existing renal function; dose-dependent decreases in prostaglandin synthesis may result from NSAID use, reducing renal blood flow which may cause renal decompensation. NSAID use may increase the risk for hyperkalemia. Patients with impaired renal function, dehydration, heart failure, liver dysfunction, those taking diuretics, and ACE inhibitors, and the elderly are at greater risk of renal toxicity and hyperkalemia. Rehydrate patient before starting therapy; monitor renal function closely. Not recommended for use in patients with advanced renal disease. Long-term NSAID use may result in renal papillary necrosis. Acute interstitial nephritis and nephritic syndrome have been reported with tolmetin.

In the elderly, avoid chronic use (unless alternative agents ineffective and patient can receive concomitant gastroprotective agent); nonselective oral NSAID use is associated with an increased risk of GI bleeding and peptic ulcer disease in older adults in high risk category (eg, >75 years or age or receiving concomitant oral/parenteral corticosteroids, anticoagulants, or antiplatelet agents) (Beers Criteria).

[U.S. Boxed Warning]: NSAIDs may increase risk of gastrointestinal irritation, inflammation, ulceration, bleeding, and perforation. These events may occur at any time during therapy and without warning. Use caution with a history of GI disease (bleeding or ulcers), concurrent therapy with aspirin, anticoagulants and/or corticosteroids, smoking, use of alcohol, the elderly or debilitated patients. When used concomitantly with aspirin, a substantial increase in the risk of gastrointestinal complications (eg, ulcer) occurs; concomitant gastroprotective therapy (eg, proton pump inhibitors) is recommended (Bhatt, 2008).

Use the lowest effective dose for the shortest duration of time, consistent with individual patient goals, to reduce risk of cardiovascular or GI adverse events. Alternate therapies should be considered for patients at high risk.

NSAIDs may cause serious skin adverse events including exfoliative dermatitis, Stevens-Johnson syndrome (SJS) and toxic epidermal necrolysis (TEN); discontinue use at first sign of skin rash or hypersensitivity. Anaphylactoid reactions may occur, even without prior exposure; patients with "aspirin triad" (bronchial asthma, aspirin intolerance, rhinitis) may be at increased risk. Do not use in patients who experience bronchospasm, asthma, rhinitis, or urticaria with NSAID or aspirin therapy.

Use with caution in patients with decreased hepatic function. Closely monitor patients with any abnormal LFT. Severe hepatic reactions (eg, fulminant hepatitis, liver failure) have occurred with NSAID use, rarely; discontinue if signs or symptoms of liver disease develop, or if systemic manifestations occur.

NSAIDS may cause drowsiness, dizziness, blurred vision, and other neurologic effects which may impair physical or mental abilities; patients must be cautioned about performing tasks which require mental alertness (eg, operating machinery or driving). Discontinue use with blurred or diminished vision and perform ophthalmologic exam. Monitor vision with long-term therapy.

The elderly are at increased risk for adverse effects (especially peptic ulceration, CNS effects, renal toxicity) from NSAIDs even at low doses.

Withhold for at least 4-6 half-lives prior to surgical or dental procedures.

Adverse Reactions

Cardiovascular: Chest pain, hypertension, edema

Central nervous system: Depression, dizziness, drowsiness, headache

Dermatologic: Skin irritation

Endocrine & metabolic: Weight gain/loss

Gastrointestinal: Abdominal pain, constipation, diarrhea, flatulence, gastritis, heartburn, nausea, peptic ulcer, vomiting

Genitourinary: Urinary tract infection

Hematologic: Hemoglobin/hematocrit decreases (transient)

Neuromuscular & skeletal: Weakness

Ocular: Visual disturbances

Otic: Tinnitus

Renal: BUN increased

Rare but important or life-threatening: Agranulocytosis anaphylactoid reactions, CHF, dysuria, epistaxis, erythema multiforme, exfoliative dermatitis, fever, fluid retention, GI bleeding, GI perforation, glossitis granulocytopenia, hematuria, hemolytic anemia, hepatic failure, hepatic necrosis, hepatitis, hepatitis (fulminant) hepatotoxicity (idiosyncratic) (Chalasani, 2014), interstitial nephritis, jaundice, liver function tests (abnormal) lymphadenopathy, macular changes, nephrotic syndrome, optic neuropathy, proteinuria, purpura, renal failure, retinal changes, serum sickness, stomatitis Stevens-Johnson syndrome, thrombocytopenia, toxic epidermal necrolysis, urticaria

Drug Interactions

Metabolism/Transport Effects None known.

Avoid Concomitant Use

Avoid concomitant use of Tolmetin with any of the following: Dexketoprofen; Floctafenine; Ketorolac (Nasal); Ketorolac (Systemic); Morniflumate; NSAID (COX-2 Inhibitor); Omacetaxine; Urokinase

Increased Effect/Toxicity

Tolmetin may increase the levels/effects of: 5-ASA Derivatives; Agents with Antiplatelet Properties; Aliskiren

Aminoglycosides; Anticoagulants; Apixaban; Bisphosphonate Derivatives; Collagenase (Systemic); CycloSPORINE (Systemic); Dabigatran Etexilate; Deferasirox; Deoxycholic Acid; Desmopressin; Digoxin; Drospirenone; Eplerenone; Haloperidol; Ibritumomab; Lithium; Methotrexate; Nonsteroidal Anti-Inflammatory Agents; NSAID (COX-2 Inhibitor); Obinutuzumab; Omacetaxine; PEMEtrexed; Porfimer; Potassium-Sparing Diuretics; PRALAtrexate; Quinolone Antibiotics; Rivaroxaban; Salicylates; Tacrolimus (Systemic); Tenofovir; Thrombolytic Agents; Tositumomab and Iodine I 131 Tositumomab; Urokinase; Vancomycin; Verteporfin; Vitamin K Antagonists

The levels/effects of Tolmetin may be increased by: ACE Inhibitors; Angiotensin II Receptor Blockers; Antidepressants (Tricyclic, Tertiary Amine); Corticosteroids (Systemic); CycloSPORINE (Systemic); Dasatinib; Dexketoprofen; Diclofenac (Systemic); Floctafenine; Glucosamine; Herbs (Anticoagulant/Antiplatelet Properties); Ibrutinib; Ketorolac (Nasal); Ketorolac (Systemic); Limaprost; Morniflumate; Multivitamins/Fluoride (with ADE); Multivitamins/Minerals (with ADEK, Folate, Iron); Multivitamins/Minerals (with AE, No Iron); Omega-3 Fatty Acids; Pentosan Polysulfate Sodium; Pentoxifylline; Probenecid; Prostacyclin Analogues; Selective Serotonin Reuptake Inhibitors; Serotonin/Norepinephrine Reuptake Inhibitors; Sodium Phosphates; Tipranavir; Treprostinil; Vitamin E

Decreased Effect

Tolmetin may decrease the levels/effects of: ACE Inhibitors; Aliskiren; Angiotensin II Receptor Blockers; Beta-Blockers; Eplerenone; HydrALAZINE; Loop Diuretics; Potassium-Sparing Diuretics; Prostaglandins (Ophthalmic); Salicylates; Selective Serotonin Reuptake Inhibitors; Thiazide Diuretics

The levels/effects of Tolmetin may be decreased by: Bile Acid Sequestrants; Salicylates

Food Interactions Tolmetin peak serum concentrations may be decreased if taken with food or milk. Management: May be administered with antacids to decrease GI upset.

Storage/Stability Store at 15°C to 30°C (59°F to 86°F). Protect from light.

Mechanism of Action Reversibly inhibits cyclooxygenase-1 and 2 (COX-1 and 2) enzymes, which results in decreased formation of prostaglandin precursors; has antipyretic, analgesic, and anti-inflammatory properties.

Other proposed mechanisms not fully elucidated (and possibly contributing to the anti-inflammatory effect to varying degrees) include inhibiting chemotaxis, altering lymphocyte activity, inhibiting neutrophil aggregation/activation, and decreasing proinflammatory cytokine levels.

Pharmacokinetics (Adult data unless noted)

Absorption: Oral: Well absorbed
Protein binding: 99%
Metabolism: In the liver via oxidation and conjugation
Half-life, elimination: 5 hours
Time to peak serum concentration: Within 30-60 minutes
Elimination: Excreted in the urine as metabolites or conjugates

Dosing: Usual Oral:

Children ≥2 years:
Anti-inflammatory: Initial: 20 mg/kg/day in 3-4 divided doses, then 15-30 mg/kg/day in 3-4 divided doses; maximum dose: 30 mg/kg/day in 4 divided doses; do not exceed 1800 mg/day
Analgesic: 5-7 mg/kg/dose every 6-8 hours
Adults: 400 mg 3 times/day; usual dose: 600 mg to 1.8 g/day; maximum dose: 2 g/day

Administration Oral: May administer with food, milk, or antacids to decrease GI adverse effects

Monitoring Parameters CBC with differential, liver enzymes, occult blood loss, BUN, serum creatinine; periodic ophthalmologic exams

Test Interactions Increased protein, bleeding time; may interfere with urine detection of cannabinoids (false-positive)

Dosage Forms Excipient information presented when available (limited, particularly for generics); consult specific product labeling.

Capsule, Oral:
Generic: 400 mg
Tablet, Oral:
Generic: 200 mg, 600 mg

◆ **Tolmetin Sodium** *see* Tolmetin *on page* 2081

Tolnaftate (tole NAF tate)

Medication Safety Issues

Sound-alike/look-alike issues:

Tinactin® may be confused with Talacen

Brand Names: US Anti-Fungal [OTC]; Antifungal [OTC]; Athletes Foot Spray [OTC]; Dr Gs Clear Nail [OTC]; Fungi-Guard [OTC]; Fungoid-D [OTC]; Jock Itch Spray [OTC]; LamISIL AF Defense [OTC]; Medi-First Anti-Fungal [OTC]; Mycocide Clinical NS [OTC]; Podactin [OTC]; Tinactin Deodorant [OTC]; Tinactin Jock Itch [OTC]; Tinactin [OTC]; Tinaspore [OTC]; Tolnaftate Antifungal [OTC]

Brand Names: Canada Pitrex

Therapeutic Category Antifungal Agent, Topical

Generic Availability (US) Yes

Use Treatment of tinea pedis, tinea cruris, tinea corporis, tinea manuum caused by *Trichophyton rubrum*, *T. mentagrophytes*, *T. tonsurans*, *M. canis*, *M. audouinii*, and *E. floccosum*; also effective in the treatment of tinea versicolor infections due to *Malassezia furfur*

Contraindications Hypersensitivity to tolnaftate or any component of the formulation; nail and scalp infections

Warnings/Precautions For topical use only; avoid contact with eyes. Apply to clean, dry skin. When used for self-medication (OTC use), contact healthcare provider if condition does not improve within 4 weeks. Discontinue if sensitivity or irritation occurs. Not for self-medication (OTC use) in children <2 years of age.

Warnings: Additional Pediatric Considerations Some dosage forms may contain propylene glycol; in neonates large amounts of propylene glycol delivered orally, intravenously (eg, >3,000 mg/day), or topically have been associated with potentially fatal toxicities which can include metabolic acidosis, seizures, renal failure, and CNS depression; toxicities have also been reported in children and adults including hyperosmolality, lactic acidosis, seizures and respiratory depression; use caution (AAP, 1997; Shehab, 2009).

Adverse Reactions

Dermatologic: Contact dermatitis, pruritus
Local: Irritation, stinging

Drug Interactions

Metabolism/Transport Effects None known.

Avoid Concomitant Use There are no known interactions where it is recommended to avoid concomitant use.

Increased Effect/Toxicity There are no known significant interactions involving an increase in effect.

Decreased Effect There are no known significant interactions involving a decrease in effect.

Mechanism of Action Distorts the hyphae and stunts mycelial growth in susceptible fungi

Pharmacodynamics Onset of action: Response may be seen 24-72 hours after initiation of therapy

Dosing: Usual Children and Adults: Topical: Spray aerosol or apply 1-3 drops of solution or a small amount of cream or powder and rub into the affected areas 2-3 times/day for 2-4 weeks

Administration Topical: Wash and dry affected area before drug application; avoid contact with eyes

Monitoring Parameters Resolution of skin infection

Additional Information Usually not effective alone for the treatment of infections involving hair follicles or nails

Dosage Forms Excipient information presented when available (limited, particularly for generics); consult specific product labeling.

Aerosol, External:
- Athletes Foot Spray: 1% (150 g) [contains sd alcohol 40]
- Tinactin: 1% (150 g)

Aerosol Powder, External:
- Jock Itch Spray: 1% (130 g) [contains sd alcohol 40b]
- LamISIL AF Defense: 1% (133 g)
- Tinactin: 1% (133 g)
- Tinactin Deodorant: 1% (133 g)

Cream, External:
- Antifungal: 1% (15 g) [odorless]
- Fungi-Guard: 1% (15 g)
- Fungoid-D: 1% (113 g) [contains cetyl alcohol, methylparaben, propylene glycol, propylparaben, trolamine (triethanolamine)]
- Medi-First Anti-Fungal: 1% (1 ea)
- Tinactin: 1% (15 g, 30 g)
- Tinactin Jock Itch: 1% (15 g)
- Tolnaftate Antifungal: 1% (114 g) [contains cetyl alcohol, methylparaben, polysorbate 80, propylene glycol, propylparaben]
- Generic: 1% (15 g, 20 g, 28.3 g, 30 g)

Powder, External:
- Anti-Fungal: 1% (45 g)
- LamISIL AF Defense: 1% (113 g)
- Podactin: 1% (45 g)
- Tinactin: 1% (108 g)
- Generic: 1% (45 g)

Solution, External:
- Dr Gs Clear Nail: 1% (18 mL) [contains propylene glycol]
- Mycocide Clinical NS: 1% (30 mL) [contains propylene glycol]
- Tinaspore: 1% (10 mL)
- Generic: 1% (10 mL)

◆ **Tolnaftate Antifungal [OTC]** *see* Tolnaftate *on page* 2083

◆ **Toloxin (Can)** *see* Digoxin *on page* 652

Tolterodine (tole TER oh deen)

Medication Safety Issues

Sound-alike/look-alike issues:

Tolterodine may be confused with fesoterodine, tolcapone

Detrol® may be confused with Ditropan

BEERS Criteria medication:

This drug may be potentially inappropriate for use in geriatric patients (Quality of evidence - varies based on comorbidity; Strength of recommendation - varies based on comorbidity)

Related Information

Oral Medications That Should Not Be Crushed or Altered *on page* 2476

Brand Names: US Detrol; Detrol LA

Brand Names: Canada Detrol®; Detrol® LA; Unidet®

Therapeutic Category Anticholinergic Agent

Generic Availability (US) Yes

Use Treatment of patients with an overactive bladder with symptoms of urinary frequency, urgency, or urge incontinence

Pregnancy Risk Factor C

Pregnancy Considerations Teratogenic effects were observed in some animal reproduction studies.

Breast-Feeding Considerations It is not known if tolterodine is excreted in breast milk. Due to the potential for serious adverse reactions in the nursing infant, a decision should be made whether to discontinue nursing or to discontinue the drug, taking into account the importance of treatment to the mother.

Contraindications Hypersensitivity to tolterodine or fesoterodine (both are metabolized to 5-hydroxymethyl tolterodine) or any component of the formulation; urinary retention; gastric retention; uncontrolled narrow-angle glaucoma

Warnings/Precautions Cases of angioedema have been reported; some cases have occurred after a single dose. Discontinue immediately if angioedema and associated difficulty breathing, airway obstruction, or hypotension develop. May cause drowsiness, dizziness, and/or blurred vision, which may impair physical or mental abilities; patients must be cautioned about performing tasks which require mental alertness (eg, operating machinery or driving). Consider dose reduction or discontinuation if CNS effects occur. Use with caution in patients with bladder flow obstruction, may increase the risk of urinary retention. Use with caution in patients with gastrointestinal obstructive disorders (ie, pyloric stenosis), may increase the risk of gastric retention. Use with caution in patients with myasthenia gravis and controlled (treated) narrow-angle glaucoma; metabolized in the liver and excreted in the urine and feces, dosage adjustment is required for patients with renal or hepatic impairment. Tolterodine has been associated with QTc prolongation at high (supratherapeutic) doses. The manufacturer recommends caution in patients with congenital prolonged QT or in patients receiving concurrent therapy with QTc-prolonging drugs (class Ia or III antiarrhythmics). However, the mean change in QTc even at supratherapeutic dosages was less than 15 msec. Individuals who are CYP2D6 poor metabolizers or in the presence of inhibitors of CYP2D6 and CYP3A4 may be more likely to exhibit prolongation. Dosage adjustment is recommended in patients receiving CYP3A4 inhibitors (a lower dose of tolterodine is recommended). This medication is associated with potent anticholinergic properties which may be inappropriate in older adults depending on comorbidities (eg, dementia, delirium) (Beers Criteria).

Adverse Reactions

Cardiovascular: Chest pain

Central nervous system: Anxiety, dizziness, fatigue, headache, somnolence

Dermatologic: Dry skin

Gastrointestinal: Dry mouth

Gastrointestinal: Abdominal pain, constipation, diarrhea, dyspepsia, weight gain

Genitourinary: Dysuria

Neuromuscular & skeletal: Arthralgia

Ocular: Abnormal vision, dry eyes

Respiratory: Bronchitis, sinusitis

Miscellaneous: Flu-like syndrome, infection

Rare but important or life-threatening: Anaphylaxis, angioedema, confusion, dementia aggravated, disorientation, hallucinations, memory impairment, palpitation, peripheral edema, QTc prolongation, tachycardia

Drug Interactions

Metabolism/Transport Effects Substrate of CYP2C19 (minor), CYP2C9 (minor), CYP2D6 (major), CYP3A4 (major); **Note:** Assignment of Major/Minor substrate status based on clinically relevant drug interaction potential

Avoid Concomitant Use

Avoid concomitant use of Tolterodine with any of the following: Aclidinium; Conivaptan; Eluxadoline; Fusidic Acid (Systemic); Glucagon; Idelalisib; Ipratropium (Oral Inhalation); Potassium Chloride; Tiotropium; Umeclidinium

Increased Effect/Toxicity

Tolterodine may increase the levels/effects of: AbobotulinumtoxinA; Analgesics (Opioid); Anticholinergic Agents; Cannabinoid-Containing Products; Eluxadoline; Glucagon; Highest Risk QTc-Prolonging Agents; Mirabegron; Moderate Risk QTc-Prolonging Agents; OnabotulinumtoxinA; Potassium Chloride; RimabotulinumtoxinB; Thiazide Diuretics; Tiotropium; Topiramate; Warfarin

The levels/effects of Tolterodine may be increased by: Abiraterone Acetate; Aclidinium; Aprepitant; Conivaptan; CYP2D6 Inhibitors (Moderate); CYP2D6 Inhibitors (Strong); CYP3A4 Inhibitors (Moderate); CYP3A4 Inhibitors (Strong); Dasatinib; Fosaprepitant; Fusidic Acid (Systemic); Idelalisib; Ipratropium (Oral Inhalation); Ivacaftor; Luliconazole; Mianserin; Mifepristone; Netupitant; Palbociclib; Panobinostat; Peginterferon Alfa-2b; Pramlintide; Simeprevir; Stiripentol; Umeclidinium; VinBLAStine

Decreased Effect

Tolterodine may decrease the levels/effects of: Acetylcholinesterase Inhibitors; Itopride; Metoclopramide; Secretin

The levels/effects of Tolterodine may be decreased by: Acetylcholinesterase Inhibitors; Bosentan; CYP3A4 Inducers (Moderate); CYP3A4 Inducers (Strong); Dabrafenib; Deferasirox; Mitotane; Peginterferon Alfa-2b; Siltuximab; St Johns Wort; Tocilizumab

Food Interactions Food increases bioavailability (~53% increase) of tolterodine tablets (dose adjustment not necessary); does not affect the pharmacokinetics of tolterodine extended release capsules. As a CYP3A4 inhibitor, grapefruit juice may increase the serum level and/or toxicity of tolterodine, but unlikely secondary to high oral bioavailability. Management: Monitor patients closely with concurrent grapefruit juice use.

Storage/Stability Store at 25°C (77°F); excursions permitted to 15°C to 30°C (59°F to 86°F). Protect from light.

Mechanism of Action Tolterodine is a competitive antagonist of muscarinic receptors. In animal models, tolterodine demonstrates selectivity for urinary bladder receptors over salivary receptors. Urinary bladder contraction is mediated by muscarinic receptors. Tolterodine increases residual urine volume and decreases detrusor muscle pressure.

Pharmacokinetics (Adult data unless noted)

Absorption: Immediate release tablet: Rapid; ≥77%

Distribution: IV: V_d: Adults: 113 ± 27 L

Protein binding: >96% (primarily bound to $alpha_1$-acid glycoprotein)

Metabolism: Extensively hepatic, primarily via CYP2D6 (some metabolites share activity) and CYP3A4 usually (minor pathway). In patients with a genetic deficiency of CYP2D6, metabolism via CYP3A4 predominates. Forms three active metabolites.

Half-life elimination:

Immediate release tablet: Extensive metabolizers: ~2 hours; poor metabolizers: ~10 hours

Extended release capsule: Extensive metabolizers: ~7 hours; poor metabolizers: ~18 hours

Time to peak serum concentration:

Immediate release tablet: 1-2 hours

Extended release capsule: 2-6 hours

Excretion: Urine (77%); feces (17%); excreted primarily as metabolites (<1% unchanged drug) of which the active 5-hydroxymethyl metabolite accounts for 5% to 14% (<1% in poor metabolizers)

Dosing: Usual Oral: Adults: Treatment of overactive bladder:

Immediate release tablet: 2 mg twice daily; the dose may be lowered to 1 mg twice daily based on individual response and tolerability

Dosing adjustment in patients concurrently taking strong CYP3A4 inhibitors (eg, ketoconazole, clarithromycin, ritonavir): 1 mg twice daily

Extended release capsule: 4 mg once daily; dose may be lowered to 2 mg once daily based on individual response and tolerability

Dosing adjustment in patients concurrently taking strong CYP3A4 inhibitors (eg, ketoconazole, clarithromycin, ritonavir): 2 mg once daily

Dosing adjustment in renal impairment:

Immediate release tablet: Significantly reduced renal function (studies conducted in patients with CrCl 10-30 mL/minute): 1 mg twice daily; use with caution

Extended release capsule:

CrCl 10-30 mL/minute: 2 mg once daily

CrCl <10 mL/minute: Use is not recommended; has not been studied

Dosing adjustment in hepatic impairment:

Immediate release tablet: Significantly reduced hepatic function: 1 mg twice daily; use with caution

Extended release capsule:

Mild to moderate impairment (Child-Pugh class A or B): 2 mg once daily

Severe impairment (Child-Pugh class C): Use is not recommended; has not been studied

Administration Oral: Administer without regard to food; do not break, crush, or chew extended release capsules.

Dosage Forms Excipient information presented when available (limited, particularly for generics); consult specific product labeling.

Capsule Extended Release 24 Hour, Oral, as tartrate:

Detrol LA: 2 mg, 4 mg

Generic: 2 mg, 4 mg

Tablet, Oral, as tartrate:

Detrol: 1 mg, 2 mg

Generic: 1 mg, 2 mg

- **Tolterodine Tartrate** *see* Tolterodine *on page 2084*
- **Tomoxetine** *see* AtoMOXetine *on page 217*
- **TootSweet™ [OTC]** *see* Sucrose *on page 1979*
- **Topactin (Can)** *see* Fluocinonide *on page 898*
- **Topamax** *see* Topiramate *on page 2085*
- **Topamax Sprinkle** *see* Topiramate *on page 2085*
- **Topex Topical Anesthetic** *see* Benzocaine *on page 268*
- **Topicaine [OTC]** *see* Lidocaine (Topical) *on page 1258*
- **Topicaine 5 [OTC]** *see* Lidocaine (Topical) *on page 1258*
- **Topiragen [DSC]** *see* Topiramate *on page 2085*

Topiramate (toe PYRE a mate)

Medication Safety Issues

Sound-alike/look-alike issues:

Topamax may be confused with Sporanox, TEGretol, TEGretol-XR, Toprol-XL

Administration issues

Bioequivalence has not been demonstrated between Trokendi XR and Qudexy XR.

Qudexy XR capsules may be opened to sprinkle the entire contents on a small amount (~1 teaspoon) of soft food. Do not open and sprinkle Trokendi XR capsules on food, chew, or crush; doing so may disrupt the triphasic release properties.

Avoid alcohol use with Trokendi XR within 6 hours prior to and 6 hours after administration; concurrent use may result in dose dumping.

Related Information

Oral Medications That Should Not Be Crushed or Altered *on page 2476*

Safe Handling of Hazardous Drugs *on page 2455*

Brand Names: US Qudexy XR; Topamax; Topamax Sprinkle; Topiragen [DSC]; Trokendi XR

Brand Names: Canada Abbott-Topiramate; ACT Topiramate; Apo-Topiramate; AURO-Topiramate; Dom-Topiramate; GD-Topiramate; Mint-Topiramate; Mylan-Topiramate; PHL-Topiramate; PMS-Topiramate; PRO-Topiramate; Q-Topiramate; RAN-Topiramate; Sandoz-Topiramate; TEVA-Topiramate; Topamax

Therapeutic Category Anticonvulsant, Miscellaneous

Generic Availability (US) May be product dependent

Use Oral:

Immediate release: Topamax: Initial monotherapy of primary generalized tonic-clonic seizures or partial onset seizures (FDA approved in ages ≥2 years and adults); adjunctive treatment of primary generalized tonic-clonic seizures or partial onset seizures (FDA approved in ages ≥2 years and adults); adjunctive treatment of seizures associated with Lennox-Gastaut syndrome (FDA approved in ages ≥2 years); prophylaxis of migraine headache (FDA approved in ages ≥12 years and adults); has also been used for infantile spasms

Extended release: Qudexy XR, Trokendi XR: Initial monotherapy of primary generalized tonic-clonic seizures or partial onset seizures (FDA approved in ages ≥10 years and adults); adjunctive treatment of primary generalized tonic-clonic seizures or partial onset seizures (Qudexy XR: FDA approved in ages ≥2 years and adults; Trokendi XR: FDA approved in ages ≥6 years and adults); adjunctive treatment of seizures associated with Lennox-Gastaut syndrome (Qudexy XR: FDA approved in ages ≥2 years and adults; Trokendi XR: FDA approved in ages ≥6 years)

Medication Guide Available Yes

Pregnancy Risk Factor D

Pregnancy Considerations Adverse events have been observed in animal reproduction studies. Based on limited data (n=5), topiramate was found to cross the placenta and could be detected in neonatal serum (Ohman, 2002). Topiramate may cause fetal harm if administered to a pregnant woman. An increased risk of oral clefts (cleft lip and/or palate) has been observed following first trimester exposure. Data from the North American Antiepileptic Drug (NAAED) Pregnancy Registry reported that the prevalence of oral clefts was 1.2% for infants exposed to topiramate during the first trimester of pregnancy, versus 0.39% to 0.46% for infants exposed to other antiepileptic drugs and 0.12% with no exposure. Although not evaluated during pregnancy, metabolic acidosis may be induced by topiramate. In general, metabolic acidosis during pregnancy may result in adverse effects and fetal death. Pregnant women and their newborns should be monitored for metabolic acidosis. Maternal serum concentrations may decrease during the second and third trimesters of pregnancy therefore therapeutic drug monitoring should be considered in pregnant women who require therapy (Ohman, 2009; Westin, 2009).

Use for migraine prophylaxis is contraindicated per the Canadian labeling in pregnant women or women of childbearing potential who are not using effective contraception.

Patients exposed to topiramate during pregnancy are encouraged to enroll themselves into the AED Pregnancy Registry by calling 1-888-233-2334. Additional information is available at www.aedpregnancyregistry.org.

Breast-Feeding Considerations Topiramate is excreted into breast milk. Based on information from five nursing infants, infant plasma concentrations of topiramate have been reported as 10% to 20% of the maternal plasma concentration. The manufacturer recommends that caution be used if administered to a nursing woman.

Contraindications

Extended release: Recent alcohol use (ie, within 6 hours prior to and 6 hours after administration) (Trokendi XR only); patients with metabolic acidosis who are taking concomitant metformin

Immediate release: There are no contraindications listed in the manufacturer's labeling.

Canadian labeling (not in U.S. labeling): Hypersensitivity to topiramate or any component of the formulation or container; pregnancy and women in childbearing years not using effective contraception (migraine prophylaxis only)

Warnings/Precautions Hazardous agent – use appropriate precautions for handling and disposal (NIOSH 2014 [group 3]).

Antiepileptics are associated with an increased risk of suicidal behavior/thoughts with use (regardless of indication); patients should be monitored for signs/symptoms of depression, suicidal tendencies, and other unusual behavior changes during therapy and instructed to inform their healthcare provider immediately if symptoms occur. Use with caution in patients with hepatic, respiratory, or renal impairment. Topiramate may decrease serum bicarbonate concentrations (up to 67% of epilepsy patients and 77% of migraine patients). Risk may be increased in patients with a predisposing condition (organ dysfunction, diarrhea, ketogenic diet, status epilepticus, or concurrent treatment with other drugs which may cause acidosis). Metabolic acidosis may occur at dosages as low as 50 mg/day. Monitor serum bicarbonate as well as potential complications of chronic acidosis (nephrolithiasis, nephrocalcinosis, osteomalacia/osteoporosis, and reduced growth rates and/or weight in children). Kidney stones have been reported in both children and adults; the risk of kidney stones is about 2-4 times that of the untreated population; consider avoiding use in patients on a ketogenic diet; the risk of kidney stones may be reduced by increasing fluid intake.

Cognitive dysfunction (confusion, psychomotor slowing, difficultly with concentration/attention, difficultly with memory, speech or language problems), psychiatric disturbances (depression or mood disorders), and sedation (somnolence or fatigue) may occur with topiramate use; incidence may be related to rapid titration and higher doses. Patients must be cautioned about performing tasks which require mental alertness (eg, operating machinery or driving). Effects with other sedative drugs or ethanol may be potentiated. Topiramate may also cause paresthesia, dizziness, and ataxia. Topiramate has been associated with acute myopia and secondary angle-closure glaucoma in adults and children, typically within 1 month of initiation; discontinue in patients with acute onset of decreased visual acuity and/or ocular pain. Visual field defects have also been reported independent of increased intraocular pressure; generally reversible upon discontinuation. Consider discontinuation if visual problems occur at any time during treatment. Hyperammonemia with or without encephalopathy may occur with or without concomitant valproate administration; valproic acid dose-dependency was observed in limited pediatric studies; use with caution in patients with inborn errors of metabolism or decreased hepatic mitochondrial activity. Hypothermia (core body temperature <35°C [95°F]) has been reported with concomitant use of topiramate and valproic acid; may occur with or without associated hyperammonemia and may develop after topiramate initiation or dosage increase; discontinuation of topiramate or valproic acid may be necessary. Topiramate may be associated with oligohydrosis and hyperthermia, most frequently in children; use caution and monitor closely during strenuous exercise, during exposure to high environmental temperature, or in patients receiving receiving other carbonic anhydrase inhibitors and drugs with anticholinergic activity. Use with caution in the elderly; dosage adjustment may be required.

The exacerbation and development of eating disorders, including anorexia nervosa and bulimia, has been reported in case reports of adolescents receiving topiramate for migraines or chronic headaches and an adult receiving topiramate for epilepsy. Prior to initiation of topiramate screen for a history of eating disorder symptoms, eating disorder risk factors (eg, history of dieting behavior), cognitive symptoms of eating disorders (eg, weigh or shape concerns, fear of gaining weight, drive for thinness), and any recent changes in social functioning including increased withdrawal or isolation. Inquire whether the patient has unrealistic or unhealthy weight goals. Evaluate exercise habits (eg, look for over-exercising or compulsive exercising above that of similarly athletic peers) and dietary intake; assess rigid patterns or avoidance of specific categories of foods and preoccupation with maintaining a "healthy diet" or experimentation with fad diets. In adolescents assess developmental weight history with growth curves. Monitor eating behaviors and weight closely in patients receiving topiramate who have eating disorder symptoms or risk factors (Lebow 2015; Rosenow 2002).

Potentially significant drug-drug interactions may exist, requiring dose or frequency adjustment, additional monitoring, and/or selection of alternative therapy. Avoid abrupt withdrawal of topiramate therapy; it should be withdrawn/tapered slowly to minimize the potential of increased seizure frequency. Doses were also gradually withdrawn in migraine prophylaxis studies.

Warnings: Additional Pediatric Considerations In pediatric clinical trials for adjunctive treatment of seizures, persistent decreases in serum bicarbonate occurred in 67% of patients receiving topiramate (versus 10% of those receiving placebo). Markedly low serum bicarbonate values were reported in 11% of pediatric patients receiving topiramate (versus 0% of those receiving placebo). In pediatric monotherapy trials, persistent decreases in serum bicarbonate occurred in 9% of patients receiving 50 mg/day and 25% of patients receiving 400 mg/day. Markedly low serum bicarbonate values were reported in 1% to 6% of pediatric patients receiving topiramate monotherapy. The risk of topiramate-induced metabolic acidosis may be increased in patients with predisposing conditions (eg, diarrhea, status epilepticus, hepatic impairment, renal dysfunction, severe respiratory disorders, ketogenic diet, surgery) or concurrent treatment with other drugs that may cause acidosis. Metabolic acidosis may be more common and more severe in infants and children <2 years of age with up to 45% of patients receiving 25 mg/kg/day developing metabolic acidosis in clinical trials. Monitor for potential complications of chronic acidosis including nephrolithiasis, nephrocalcinosis, osteomalacia/osteoporosis, and reduction in growth rates (including weight). Reductions in Z scores (from baseline) for length, weight, and head circumference were observed in infants and toddlers who received long-term topiramate (for up to 1 year) for intractable partial epilepsy; reductions in Z scores for length and weight correlated to the severity of metabolic acidosis. Serum bicarbonate should be monitored at baseline and periodically during topiramate therapy. The most common adverse effects of topiramate observed in children include the following: Anorexia, cognitive problems, dizziness, fatigue, fever, flushing, headache, mood problems, parethesia, somnolence, and weight loss; neuropsychiatric and cognitive adverse effects were reported with a lower incidence in children than adults. Pediatric patients <24 months of age may be at increased risk for topiramate-associated hyperammonemia, especially when used concurrently with valproic acid; monitor closely for lethargy, vomiting, or unexplained changes in mental status.

Risk of nephrolithiasis (kidney stones) is higher in children; reported incidence in adults: 1.5%; in pediatric patients <24 months with long-term use (up to 1 year): 7% (kidney or bladder stones); one retrospective study evaluating long-term use (1 year) in children with epilepsy (n=96; mean age: 6.9 ± 3.8 years) reported an incidence of 5.2% (Mahmoud, 2011); risk may be increased with ketogenic diet or concomitant drugs that produce metabolic acidosis; avoid use while on topiramate therapy; maintain adequate hydration during therapy; monitor for signs or symptoms of kidney or bladder or kidney stone development.

Extended release dosage forms (Qudexy XR and Trokendi XR) are not bioequivalent and should not be interchanged. Qudexy XR capsules may be opened and contents sprinkled on a small amount (~1 teaspoon) of soft food. Do not open and sprinkle Trokendi XR capsules on food, nor chew or crush; doing so may disrupt the triphasic release properties.

Adverse Reactions Adverse events are reported for adult and pediatric patients for various indications and regimens. **Note:** A wide range of dosages were studied. Incidence of adverse events was frequently lower in the pediatric population studied.

Cardiovascular: Angina pectoris, atrioventricular block, bradycardia (adjunctive therapy for epilepsy in children 2 to 16 years, chest pain, deep vein thrombosis, edema, facial edema, flushing, hypertension, hypotension, orthostatic hypotension, phlebitis, pulmonary embolism, syncope, vasodilatation

Central nervous system: Abnormal electroencephalogram, abnormal gait, aggressive behavior, agitation, altered sense of smell, anxiety, apathy, aphasia, apraxia, ataxia, behavioral problems (adjunctive therapy for epilepsy in children 2 to 16 years), brain disease, cognitive dysfunction, confusion, delirium, delusions, depersonalization, depression, dizziness, drowsiness, dysarthria, dystonia, emotional lability, euphoria, exacerbation of depression, exacerbation of migraine headache, fatigue, hallucination, headache, hyperesthesia, hypertonia, hypoesthesia, hyporeflexia (adjunctive therapy for epilepsy in children 2 to 16 years), insomnia, irritability, lack of concentration, language problems, memory impairment, mood disorder, nervousness, neuropathy, pain, paranoia, paresthesia, psychomotor retardation, psychosis, psychoneurosis (adjunctive therapy for epilepsy in children 2 to 16 years), rigors, sensory disturbance, speech disturbance, stupor, tonic-clonic seizures (adjunctive therapy for epilepsy in children 2 to 16 years), vertigo, voice disorder, weight loss

Dermatologic: Abnormal hair texture, acne vulgaris, alopecia, body odor, dermatitis (adjunctive therapy for epilepsy in children 2 to 16 years), dermatological disease, diaphoresis, eczema (adjunctive therapy for epilepsy in children 2 to 16 years), erythematous rash, hypertrichosis (adjunctive therapy for epilepsy in children 2 to 16 years), pallor (adjunctive therapy for epilepsy in children 2 to 16 years), pruritus, seborrhea (adjunctive therapy for epilepsy in children 2 to 16 years), skin discoloration (adjunctive therapy for epilepsy in children 2 to 16 years), skin photosensitivity, skin rash, urticaria

Endocrine & metabolic: Albuminuria, amenorrhea, decreased libido, decreased serum bicarbonate, decreased serum phosphate, dehydration, diabetes mellitus, hot flash, hyperammonemia with/without encephalopathy with/without valproate (migraine therapy in adolescents 12 to 17 years), hyperglycemia, hyperlipidemia, hypermenorrhea, hyperthyroidism (migraine therapy in adolescents 12 to 17 years), hypocalcemia, hypoglycemia (adjunctive therapy for epilepsy in children 2 to 16 years), increased gamma-glutamyl transferase, increased thirst, intermenstrual bleeding, menstrual disease, weight gain (adjunctive therapy for epilepsy in children 2 to 16 years)

Gastrointestinal: Abdominal pain, ageusia, anorexia, constipation, decreased appetite, diarrhea, dysgeusia, dyspepsia, dysphagia (adjunctive therapy for epilepsy in children 2 to 16 years), enlargement of abdomen, esophagitis, fecal incontinence (adjunctive therapy for epilepsy in children 2 to 16 years), flatulence (adjunctive therapy for epilepsy in children 2 to 16 years), gastritis, gastroenteritis, gastroesophageal reflux disease, gastrointestinal disease, gingival hemorrhage, gingival hyperplasia (adjunctive therapy for epilepsy in children 2 to 16 years), gingivitis, glossitis (adjunctive therapy for epilepsy in children 2 to 16 years), hemorrhoids, increased appetite (adjunctive therapy for epilepsy in children 2 to 16 years), melena, nausea, sialorrhea (adjunctive therapy for epilepsy in children 2 to 16 years), stomatitis, vomiting, xerostomia

Genitourinary: Cystitis, dysuria, ejaculatory disorder, genital candidiasis, hematuria, impotence, leukorrhea (adjunctive therapy for epilepsy in children 2 to 16 years), mastalgia, nipple discharge, nocturia (adjunctive therapy for epilepsy in children 2 to 16 years), oliguria, premature ejaculation, prostatic disease, urinary frequency, urinary incontinence, urinary retention, urinary tract infection, urine abnormality, vaginal hemorrhage

Hematologic & oncologic: Anemia, eosinophilia, granulocytopenia, hematoma (adjunctive therapy for epilepsy in children 2 to 16 years), hemorrhage, leukopenia, lymphadenopathy, lymphocytopenia, neoplasm, prolonged prothrombin time (adjunctive therapy for epilepsy in children 2 to 16 years), purpura (adjunctive therapy for epilepsy in children 2 to 16 years), thrombocythemia, thrombocytopenia (adjunctive therapy for epilepsy in children 2 to 16 years)

Hepatic: Increased serum alkaline phosphatase, increased serum ALT, increased serum AST

Hypersensitivity: Hypersensitivity reaction

Infection: Candidiasis, infection, viral infection

Neuromuscular & skeletal: Arthralgia, arthropathy, back pain, dyskinesia, hyperkinesia (adjunctive therapy for epilepsy in children 2 to 16 years), leg cramps, leg pain, muscle spasm, myalgia, skeletal pain, tremor, weakness

Ophthalmic: Abnormal lacrimation (adjunctive therapy for epilepsy in children 2 to 16 years), accommodation disturbance, blepharoptosis, blurred vision, conjunctivitis, diplopia, eye disease, eye pain, myopia (adjunctive therapy for epilepsy in children 2 to 16 years), nystagmus, photophobia, scotoma, strabismus, visual disturbance, visual field defect, xerophthalmia

Otic: Hearing loss, otitis media, tinnitus

Renal: Increased serum creatinine, nephrolithiasis, polyuria, renal pain

Respiratory: Asthma, bronchitis, cough, dyspnea, epistaxis, flu-like symptoms, laryngitis (migraine therapy in adolescents 12 to 17 years), pharyngeal edema (migraine therapy in adolescents 12 to 17 years), pharyngitis, pneumonia, respiratory tract disease (adjunctive therapy for epilepsy in children 2 to 16 years), rhinitis, sinusitis, upper respiratory tract infection

Miscellaneous: Fever, trauma

Rare but important or life-threatening: Acute myopia with secondary angle-closure glaucoma, bone marrow depression (epilepsy), cerebellar syndrome (epilepsy), decreased serum phosphate (migraine therapy in adolescents 12 to 17 years), erythema multiforme, hepatic failure (including fatalities), hyperthermia, hypohidrosis, hypothermia (with valproate, with or without hyperammonemia), hypokalemia (adjunctive therapy in adults with partial-onset seizures), lymphocytosis (epilepsy), maculopathy, metabolic acidosis (hyperchloremia, nonanion gap), pancreatitis, pancytopenia (epilepsy), pemphigus, renal tubular acidosis, Stevens-Johnson syndrome, suicidal ideation, tongue edema (epilepsy), upper motor neuron lesion (epilepsy), vasospasm (epilepsy)

Drug Interactions

Metabolism/Transport Effects **Inhibits** CYP2C19 (weak); **Induces** CYP3A4 (weak)

Avoid Concomitant Use

Avoid concomitant use of Topiramate with any of the following: Alcohol (Ethyl); Azelastine (Nasal); Carbonic Anhydrase Inhibitors; Orphenadrine; Paraldehyde; Thalidomide; Ulipristal

Increased Effect/Toxicity

Topiramate may increase the levels/effects of: Alpha-/Beta-Agonists (Indirect-Acting); Amitriptyline; Amphetamines; Azelastine (Nasal); Buprenorphine; Carbonic Anhydrase Inhibitors; CNS Depressants; Flecainide; Fosphenytoin; Hydrocodone; Lithium; Memantine; MetFORMIN; Methotrimeprazine; Metyrosine; Mirtazapine; Orphenadrine; Paraldehyde; Phenytoin; Pramipexole; Primidone; QuiNIDine; ROPINIRole; Rotigotine; Selective Serotonin Reuptake Inhibitors; Suvorexant; Thalidomide; Valproic Acid and Derivatives; Zolpidem

The levels/effects of Topiramate may be increased by: Alcohol (Ethyl); Anticholinergic Agents; Brimonidine (Topical); Cannabis; Doxylamine; Dronabinol; Droperidol; HydrOXYzine; Kava Kava; Loop Diuretics; Magnesium Sulfate; Methotrimeprazine; Nabilone; Perampanel; Rufinamide; Salicylates; Sodium Oxybate; Tapentadol; Tetrahydrocannabinol; Thiazide Diuretics

Decreased Effect

Topiramate may decrease the levels/effects of: ARIPiprazole; Contraceptives (Estrogens); Contraceptives (Progestins); Methenamine; NiMODipine; Primidone; Saxagliptin; Ulipristal

The levels/effects of Topiramate may be decreased by: CarBAMazepine; Fosphenytoin; Mefloquine; Mianserin; Orlistat; Phenytoin

Food Interactions Ketogenic diet may increase the possibility of acidosis and/or kidney stones. Management: Monitor for symptoms of acidosis or kidney stones.

Storage/Stability

Extended release capsules: Store at 15°C to 30°C (59°F to 86°F). Protect from moisture. Protect from light.

Sprinkle capsules: Store at or below 25°C (77°F). Protect from moisture.

Tablets: Store at 15°C to 30°C (59°F to 86°F). Protect from moisture.

Mechanism of Action Anticonvulsant activity may be due to a combination of potential mechanisms: Blocks neuronal voltage-dependent sodium channels, enhances GABA(A) activity, antagonizes AMPA/kainate glutamate receptors, and weakly inhibits carbonic anhydrase.

Pharmacokinetics (Adult data unless noted) Note: Immediate release preparations are bioequivalent (sprinkle capsule and tablet); extended release capsules (Trokendi XR) administered once daily is bioequivalent to twice daily administration of immediate release formulations.

Absorption: Rapid; Immediate release formulation: Unaffected by food; Extended release capsule: Qudexy XR: The T_{max} was delayed 4 hours by high-fat meal; however, the C_{max} and AUC were not; Trokendi XR: A single dose with a high-fat meal increased the C_{max} by 37%, shortened the T_{max} to approximately 8 hours; this effect is significantly reduced following repeat administrations.

Distribution:

V_d: 0.6 to 0.8 L/kg

Protein binding: 15% to 41%; percent protein bound decreases as blood concentrations increase

Metabolism: Minor amounts metabolized hepatically via hydroxylation, hydrolysis, and glucuronidation; percentage of dose metabolized in liver and clearance are increased in patients receiving enzyme inducers (eg, carbamazepine, phenytoin)

Bioavailability: Immediate release: Tablet: 80% (relative to a prepared solution)

Half-life:

Immediate release:

Not receiving concomitant enzyme inducers or valproic acid:

Neonates (full-term) with hypothermia: ~43 hours (Fillipi, 2009)

Infants and Children 9 months to <4 years: 10.4 hours (range: 8.5 to 15.3 hours) (Mikaeloff, 2004)

Children 4 to 7 years: Mean range: 7.7 to 8 hours (Rosenfeld, 1999)

Children 8 to 11 years: Mean range: 11.3 to 11.7 hours (Rosenfeld, 1999)

Children and Adolescents 12 to 17 years: Mean range: 12.3 to 12.8 hours (Rosenfeld, 1999)

Receiving concomitant enzyme inducers (eg, carbamazepine, phenytoin, phenobarbital):

Neonates (full-term) with hypothermia: 26.5 hours (Fillipi, 2009)

Infants and Children 9 months to <4 years: 6.5 hours (range: 3.75 to 10.2 hours) (Mikaeloff, 2004)

Children and Adolescents 4 to 17 years: 7.5 hours (Rosenfeld, 1999)

Receiving valproic acid: Infants and Children 9 months to 4 years: 9.2 hours (range: 7.23 to 12 hours) (Mikaeloff, 2004)

Adults: 19 to 23 hours (mean: 21 hours)

Adults with renal impairment: 59 ± 11 hours

Extended release: Qudexy XR: ~56 hours; Trokendi XR: ~31 hours

Time to peak serum concentration:

Immediate release:

Neonates (full-term) with hypothermia: 3.8 hours (Fillipi, 2009)

Infants and Children 9 months to <4 years: 3.7 hours (range: 1.5 to 10.2 hours) (Michealoff, 2004)

Children 4 to 17 years: Mean range: 1 to 2.8 hours (Rosenfeld, 1999)

Adults: 2 hours; range: 1.4 to 4.3 hours

Extended release: Qudexy XR: ~20 hours; Trokendi XR: ~24 hours

Elimination: Urine (~70% as unchanged drug); may undergo renal tubular reabsorption

Clearance:

Not receiving concomitant enzyme inducers or valproic acid:

Neonates (full-term) with hypothermia: 13.4 mL/kg/hour (Fillipi, 2009)

Infants and Children 9 months to <4 years: 46.5 mL/kg/hour (range: 30.5 to 70.9 mL/kg/hour) (Mikaeloff, 2004)

Children 4 to 17 years: 27.6 mL/kg/hour (Rosenfeld, 1999)

Receiving concomitant enzyme inducers:

Neonates (full-term) with hypothermia: 17.9 mL/kg/hour (Fillipi, 2009)

Infants and Children 9 months to <4 years: 85.4 mL/kg/hour (range: 46.2 to 135 mL/kg/hour) (Mikaeloff, 2004)

Children and Adolescents 4 to 17 years: 60.6 mL/kg/hour (Rosenfeld, 1999)

Receiving valproic acid: Infants and Children 9 months to <4 years: 49.6 mL/kg/hour (range: 26.6 to 60.2 mL/kg/h) (Mikaeloff, 2004)

Adults: 20 to 30 mL/minute

Dosing: Neonatal

Neonatal seizures; refractory: Limited data available; efficacy results variable: Term neonate: Oral: Immediate release: 10 mg/kg/day was used in five neonates and 3 mg/kg/day was used in one neonate who were refractory to phenobarbital. In four of the five patients who received the higher dose, an absence or reduction in seizure frequency was observed; the neonate who received low dose (3 mg/kg) had no apparent change in seizures; no adverse effects noted required discontinuation of therapy (Glass 2011).

Neuroprotectant following anoxic injury (with cooling): Limited data available; efficacy results variable: Term neonate: Oral: Immediate release: 5 mg/kg/dose on day 1 followed by 3 mg/kg/dose once daily on day 2 and 3 was used in 11 neonates in study of safety; no adverse effects were noted (Filippi 2010). In an earlier pharmacokinetic pilot study of 13 neonates, the same investigators used 5 mg/kg/dose once daily for 3 days; results showed targeted serum concentrations (5 to 20 ng/mL) were achieved in 11 of 13 patients with some accumulation in patients treated with deep hypothermia (Filippi 2009).

Dosing: Usual

Pediatric: **Note:** Do not abruptly discontinue therapy; taper dosage gradually to prevent rebound effects.

Infantile spasms: Oral: Limited data available; dosing regimens variable. Consider twice-daily therapy once dose titration begins:

Newly diagnosed infantile spasm: Weight-directed dosing: Infants and Children 3 to 24 months: Immediate release: Initial: 1 to 3 mg/kg/day administered as 1 or 2 daily doses; titrate every 3 to 7 days in 1 to 3 mg/kg/day increments as tolerated until seizures controlled; reported mean dose range: 9.1 to 14 mg/kg/day; reported range: 4 to 27 mg/kg/day. Dosing based on two small studies; first was an open-label trial of 15 pediatric patients (mean age: 8 months; age range: 4 to 14 months) with newly diagnosed infantile spasms which used an initial dose of 3 mg/kg/day in 2 divided doses; doses were increased by 3 mg/kg/day every 3 days until seizures were controlled or toxicity developed; mean dose required: 14 mg/kg/day (9 to 27 mg/kg/day); median rate of spasm reduction was 41% within the first 2 months of therapy with 20% of patients becoming spasm free (three of 15 patients) and 33% achieving a 50% reduction in spasm frequency (five of 15 patients) (Hosain, 2006). In another trial of 20 pediatric patients (median age: 6.5 months; range: 3 to 24 months) with newly diagnosed infantile spasms, an initial dose of 1 mg/kg/day was used; dose was increased by 1 mg/kg/day at weekly intervals until seizures were controlled up to a maximum daily dose: 12 mg/kg/day; reported mean stabilizing dose: 9.1 mg/kg/day (4 to 12 mg/kg/day); results showed 30% of patients became spasm free (six of 20 patients) and 70% achieved at least a 50% reduction in spasm frequency (Kwon, 2006)

Refractory: Fixed dosing: Infants ≥3 months to Children ≤4 years; weight ≥7 kg: Immediate release: Initial: 25 mg/day once daily; titrate in 25 mg/day increments every 2 to 3 days as tolerated until seizures controlled up to a maximum daily dose: 24 mg/kg/day; dosing is from an open-label trial of 11 pediatric patients (mean age: 24 months) which reported a mean stabilizing dose of 15 mg/kg/day (8.3 to 23.7 mg/kg/day); results showed statistically significant decrease in spasm frequency with 45% of patients becoming spasm free (Glauser, 1998). In an extension phase of this study in eight of the initial subjects, the mean dose was 29 mg/kg/day (maximum daily dose: 50 mg/kg/day); 50% of the remaining patients (four of eight) were seizure free and all patients except one maintained a ≥50% reduction in spasm frequency (Glauser, 2000)

Anticonvulsant, adjunctive therapy: Oral:

Children and Adolescents 2 to 16 years:

Partial onset seizures or Lennox-Gastaut syndrome:

Immediate release: Children and Adolescents 2 to 16 years: Initial: 1 to 3 mg/kg/day (maximum dose: 25 mg/dose) administered nightly for 1 week; increase at 1- to 2-week intervals in increments of 1 to 3 mg/kg/day in 2 divided doses; titrate dose to response; usual maintenance: 5 to 9 mg/kg/day in 2 divided doses

Extended release:

Qudexy XR: Children and Adolescents 2 to 16 years: Initial: 25 mg once daily (approximately 1 to 3 mg/kg/day) administered nightly for 1 week; increase at 1- to 2-week intervals in increments of 1 to 3 mg/kg/day rounded to the nearest appropriate capsule size administered once daily; titrate dose to response; usual maintenance: 5 to 9 mg/kg/dose once daily; range: 5 to 9 mg/kg/dose once daily

Trokendi XR: Children and Adolescents 6 to 16 years, able to swallow capsule whole: Initial: 25 mg once daily (approximately 1 to 3 mg/kg/day) administered nightly for 1 week; increase at 1- to 2-week intervals in increments of 1 to 3 mg/kg/day rounded to the nearest appropriate capsule size administered once daily; titrate dose to response; usual maintenance: 5 to 9 mg/kg/dose once daily

Primary generalized tonic-clonic seizures:

Immediate release: Children and Adolescents 2 to 16 years: Initial: 1 to 3 mg/kg/day (maximum dose: 25 mg/dose) administered nightly for 1 week; increase over 8 weeks in increments of 1 to 3 mg/kg/day in 2 divided doses to a target dose of 6 mg/kg/day in 2 divided doses

Extended release:

Qudexy XR: Children and Adolescents 2 to 16 years: Initial: 25 mg once daily (approximately 1 to 3 mg/kg/day) administered nightly for 1 week; increase over 8 weeks in increments of 1 to 3 mg/kg/day rounded to the nearest appropriate capsule size to a target dose of 6 mg/kg/day once daily; range: 5 to 9 mg/kg/dose once daily

Trokendi XR: Children and Adolescents 6 to 16 years, able to swallow capsule whole: Initial: 25 mg once daily (approximately 1 to 3 mg/kg/day) administered nightly for 1 week; increase over 8 weeks in increments of 1 to 3 mg/kg/day rounded to the nearest appropriate capsule size to a target dose of 6 mg/kg/day once daily

Adolescents ≥17 years:

Partial onset seizures or Lennox-Gastaut syndrome:

Immediate release: Initial: 25 to 50 mg/day administered daily for 1 week; increase at weekly intervals by 25 to 50 mg/day; administer in 2 divided doses; titrate dose to response; usual maintenance dose: 100 to 200 mg twice daily; maximum daily dose: 1600 mg/**day**; **Note:** Doses above 400 mg/day have not been shown to increase efficacy in dose-response studies in adults.

Extended release: Quedexy XR, Trokendi XR: Initial: 25 to 50 mg once daily for 1 week; increase at weekly intervals by 25 to 50 mg/day once daily; titrate dose to response; longer intervals between dosage adjustment may be used; usual maintenance dose: 200 to 400 mg once daily; maximum daily dose: 1600 mg/**day**; higher doses have not been studied

Primary generalized tonic-clonic seizures:

Immediate release: Initial: 25 to 50 mg/day once daily for 1 week; increase over 8 weeks in increments of 25 to 50 mg/day in 2 divided doses; titrate dose to response; usual maintenance dose: 200 mg twice daily; use slower initial titration rate (>2 week intervals); maximum daily dose: 1600 mg/**day**; **Note:** Doses above 400 mg/day have not been shown to increase efficacy in dose-response studies in adults.

Extended release: Qudexy XR, Trokendi XR: Initial: 25 mg to 50 mg once daily for 1 week; increase at weekly intervals by 25 to 50 mg/day increments once daily; titrate dose to response; usual maintenance dose: 400 mg once daily; maximum daily dose: 1600 mg/**day**; higher doses have not been studied

Anticonvulsant, monotherapy: Partial onset seizures or primary generalized tonic-clonic seizures: Oral:

Immediate release:

Children 2 to <10 years: Initial: 25 mg once daily (in evening); may increase if tolerated to 25 mg twice daily in week 2; thereafter, may increase by 25 to 50 mg/day at weekly intervals over 5 to 7 weeks up to the lower end of the target daily maintenance dosing range (ie, to the minimum recommended maintenance dose); if additional seizure control is needed and therapy is tolerated, may further increase by 25 to 50 mg/day at weekly intervals up to the upper end of the target daily maintenance dosing range (ie, to the maximum recommended maintenance dose):

Target daily maintenance dosing range:

≤11 kg: 150 to 250 mg/day in 2 divided doses

12 to 22 kg: 200 to 300 mg/day in 2 divided doses

23 to 31 kg: 200 to 350 mg/day in 2 divided doses

32 to 38 kg: 250 to 350 mg/day in 2 divided doses

>38 kg: 250 to 400 mg/day in 2 divided doses

Children ≥10 years and Adolescents: Initial: 25 mg twice daily; increase at weekly intervals by 50 mg/day increments up to a dose of 100 mg twice daily (week 4 dose); thereafter, may further increase at weekly intervals by 100 mg/day increments up to the recommended maximum dose of 200 mg twice daily

Extended release: Qudexy XR, Trokendi XR: Children ≥10 years and Adolescents: Initial: 50 mg once daily for 1 week; increase at weekly intervals by 50 mg/day increments up to a dose of 200 mg once daily (week 4 dose); thereafter, may increase at weekly intervals by 100 mg/day increments up to the recommended dose of 400 mg once daily

Migraine prophylaxis: Oral:

Children 6 to <12 years; weight: ≥20 kg: Limited data available: Immediate release: Initial: 15 mg once daily for 1 week; then increase to 15 mg twice daily for 1 week; then increase to 25 mg twice daily for 7 days; continue to gradually titrate to effect up to target dose of 2 to 3 mg/kg/day divided twice daily; maximum daily dose: 200 mg/**day**; dosing based on a double-randomized, placebo-controlled trial of 90 pediatric patients <12 years (treatment arm: n= 59; mean age: 11.3 years as part of a larger trial with a total of 108 pediatric patients receiving topiramate compared to 49 receiving placebo) which showed a mean reduction in migraine days/month with topiramate and significantly more topiramate patients experienced ≥75% reduction in mean monthly migraine days compared to placebo (32% vs 14%) for overall study population; mean maintenance dose: 2 mg/kg/day; treatment duration of maintenance dose: 12 weeks (Winner, 2005)

Children ≥12 years and Adolescents: Initial: 25 mg/day once daily at night for 1 week; increase at weekly intervals in 25 mg/day increments as tolerated and indicated to recommended dose of 50 mg twice daily; in a double-blind, placebo-controlled, dose-finding trial of 103 pediatric patients ≥12 years (mean age: 14.2 years), the daily dose of 100 mg/day was shown to significantly decrease frequency of migraine attacks compared to a lower dose of 50 mg/day (Lewis, 2009)

Adult: **Note:** Do not abruptly discontinue therapy; taper dosage gradually to prevent rebound effects. In clinical trials, adult doses were withdrawn by decreasing in weekly intervals of 50-100 mg/day gradually over 2 to 8 weeks for seizure treatment, and by decreasing in weekly intervals by 25-50 mg/day for migraine prophylaxis.

Epilepsy, monotherapy: Partial onset seizure and primary generalized tonic-clonic seizure: Oral:

Immediate release: Initial: 25 mg twice daily; may increase weekly by 50 mg daily up to 100 mg twice daily (week 4 dose); thereafter, may further increase weekly by 100 mg daily up to the recommended dose of 200 mg twice daily

Extended release: Initial: 50 mg daily for 1 week; may increase weekly by 50 mg daily up to 200 mg once daily (week 4 dose); thereafter, may further increase weekly by 100 mg daily up to the recommended dose of 400 mg once daily.

Epilepsy, adjunctive therapy: Partial onset seizure, primary generalized tonic-clonic seizure, Lennox-Gastaut syndrome: Oral: **Note**: Doses >1600 mg have not been studied.

Immediate release: Initial: 25 mg once or twice daily for 1 week; may increase weekly by 25 to 50 mg daily until response; usual maintenance dose: 100 to 200 mg twice daily (partial-onset seizures) or 200 mg twice daily (primary generalized tonic-clonic seizures). Doses >400 mg have not shown additional benefit for treatment of partial-onset seizures.

Extended release: Initial: 25 to 50 mg once daily for 1 week; may increase weekly by 25 to 50 mg daily until response; usual maintenance dose: 200 to 400 mg once daily (partial-onset seizures, Lennox-Gastaut syndrome) or 400 mg once daily (primary generalized tonic-clonic seizures). Doses >400 mg daily have not shown additional benefit for treatment of partial-onset seizure

Migraine prophylaxis: Oral: Immediate release: Initial: 25 mg once daily (in evening); may increase weekly by 25 mg daily up to the recommended dose of 100 mg daily in 2 divided doses. Increased intervals between dose adjustments may be considered. Doses >100 mg daily have shown no additional benefit.

Dosing adjustment in renal impairment: Oral:

Infants, Children, and Adolescents: There are no dosage adjustments provided in the manufacturer's labeling; however, the following guidelines have been used by some clinicians (Aronoff, 2007):

GFR >50 mL/minute/1.73 m^2: No dosage adjustment necessary

GFR 10 to 50 mL/minute/1.73 m^2: Administer 50% of dose

GFR <10 mL/minute/1.73 m^2: Administer 25% of dose

Hemodialysis/peritoneal dialysis (PD): Administer 25% of dose; supplemental dose after hemodialysis needed

Continuous renal replacement therapy (CRRT): Administer 50% of dose

Adults: Manufacturer's labeling: CrCl <70 mL/minute/1.73 m^2: Administer 50% of the usual dose; titrate more slowly due to prolonged half-life; significantly hemodialyzed; cleared by hemodialysis at a rate that is 4 to 6 times greater than a normal individual; supplemental doses may be required

Dosing adjustment in hepatic impairment: Children, Adolescents, and Adults: There are no dosage adjustments provided in the manufacturer's labeling; however, clearance may be reduced. Carefully adjust dose as plasma concentrations may be increased if normal dosing is used.

Administration Hazardous agent; use appropriate precautions for handling and disposal (NIOSH 2014 [group 3]). May be administered without regard to food.

Immediate release:

Tablets: Broken tablets have a bitter taste; tablets may be crushed, mixed with water, and administered immediately.

Sprinkle capsules: Swallow sprinkle capsules whole or open and sprinkle contents on small amount of soft food (eg, 1 teaspoonful of applesauce, oatmeal, ice cream, pudding, custard, or yogurt); swallow sprinkle/food mixture immediately; do not chew; do not store for later use; drink fluids after dose to make sure mixture is completely swallowed.

Extended release:

Qudexy XR: May be swallowed whole or may be opened and sprinkled on a small amount (~1 teaspoon) of soft food; swallow immediately and do not chew.

Trokendi XR: Swallow capsules whole; do not sprinkle capsules on food, chew, or crush. Avoid alcohol use with within 6 hours prior to and 6 hours after administration.

Monitoring Parameters Frequency, duration, and severity of seizure episodes or migraine headaches; renal function; monitor serum electrolytes including baseline and periodic serum bicarbonate, symptoms of metabolic acidosis, complications of chronic acidosis (eg, nephrolithiasis, rickets, and reduced growth rates); monitor body temperature and for decreased sweating, especially in warm or hot weather; monitor serum ammonia concentration in patients with unexplained lethargy, vomiting, or mental status changes; intraocular pressure, symptoms of secondary angle closure glaucoma; signs and symptoms of suicidality (eg, anxiety, depression, behavior changes)

Reference Range Not applicable; plasma topiramate concentrations have not been shown to correlate with clinical efficacy

Dosage Forms Excipient information presented when available (limited, particularly for generics); consult specific product labeling. [DSC] = Discontinued product

Capsule ER 24 Hour Sprinkle, Oral:

Qudexy XR: 25 mg (30 ea, 500 ea); 50 mg (30 ea, 500 ea); 100 mg (30 ea, 500 ea); 150 mg (30 ea, 500 ea); 200 mg (30 ea, 500 ea)

Generic: 25 mg (30 ea, 500 ea); 50 mg (30 ea, 500 ea); 100 mg (30 ea, 500 ea); 150 mg (30 ea, 500 ea); 200 mg (30 ea, 500 ea)

Capsule Extended Release 24 Hour, Oral:

Trokendi XR: 25 mg [contains brilliant blue fcf (fd&c blue #1), sodium benzoate]

Trokendi XR: 50 mg, 100 mg, 200 mg [contains brilliant blue fcf (fd&c blue #1), fd&c yellow #6 (sunset yellow), sodium benzoate]

Capsule Sprinkle, Oral:

Topamax Sprinkle: 15 mg, 25 mg

Generic: 15 mg, 25 mg

Tablet, Oral:

Topamax: 25 mg, 50 mg, 100 mg, 200 mg

Topiragen: 25 mg [DSC], 50 mg [DSC], 100 mg [DSC], 200 mg [DSC]

Generic: 25 mg, 50 mg, 100 mg, 200 mg

Extemporaneous Preparations Hazardous agent; use appropriate precautions for handling and disposal (NIOSH 2014 [group 3]).

A 6 mg/mL topiramate oral suspension may be made with tablets and one of two different vehicles (a 1:1 mixture of Ora-Sweet and Ora-Plus, or a mixture of Simple Syrup, NF and methylcellulose 1% with parabens). Crush six 100 mg tablets in a mortar and reduce to a fine powder. Add a small amount of methylcellulose gel and mix to a uniform paste (**Note:** Use a small amount of methylcellulose gel when using the 1:1 Ora-Sweet and Ora-Plus mixture as the vehicle; use 10 mL methylcellulose 1% with parabens when using Simple Syrup, NF as the vehicle); mix while adding the chosen vehicle in incremental proportions to **almost** 100 mL; transfer to a graduated cylinder; rinse mortar with vehicle, and add quantity of vehicle sufficient to make 100 mL. Store in plastic prescription bottles; label "shake well" and "refrigerate". Stable for 90 days refrigerated (preferred) or at room temperature.

Nahata MC, Pai VB, and Hipple TF, *Pediatric Drug Formulations*, 5th ed, Cincinnati, OH: Harvey Whitney Books Co, 2004.

◆ **Toposar** *see* Etoposide *on page 819*

Topotecan (toe poe TEE kan)

Medication Safety Issues

Sound-alike/look-alike issues:

Hycamtin may be confused with Mycamine

Topotecan may be confused with irinotecan

High alert medication:

This medication is in a class the Institute for Safe Medication Practices (ISMP) includes among its list of drug classes which have a heightened risk of causing significant patient harm when used in error.

Other safety concerns:

Topotecan overdoses have been reported; potential causes include omission of the leading zero and missing the decimal point when prescribing, preparing, and administering. Recommended intravenous doses should generally not exceed 4 mg; verify dose prior to administration.

Related Information

Management of Drug Extravasations *on page 2298*

Oral Medications That Should Not Be Crushed or Altered *on page 2476*

Prevention of Chemotherapy-Induced Nausea and Vomiting in Children *on page 2368*

Safe Handling of Hazardous Drugs *on page 2455*

Brand Names: US Hycamtin

Brand Names: Canada Hycamtin; Topotecan For Injection; Topotecan Hydrochloride For Injection

Therapeutic Category Antineoplastic Agent, Camptothecin; Antineoplastic Agent, Topoisomerase Inhibitor

Generic Availability (US) May be product dependent

Use Treatment of metastatic ovarian cancer; relapsed or refractory small cell lung cancer; recurrent or resistant (stage IVB) cervical cancer (in combination with cisplatin) (All indications: FDA approved in adults); has also been used in pediatric solid tumors including Ewing's sarcoma, osteosarcoma, rhabdomyosarcoma, and neuroblastoma and acute leukemias (ALL, AML)

Pregnancy Risk Factor D

Pregnancy Considerations Adverse effects were observed in animal reproduction studies. May cause fetal harm in pregnant women. Women of childbearing potential should use highly effective contraception to prevent pregnancy during treatment and for at least 1 month after therapy discontinuation.

Breast-Feeding Considerations It is not known if topotecan is excreted in breast milk. Due to the potential for serious adverse reactions in the nursing infant, the manufacturer recommends to discontinue breast-feeding in women who are receiving topotecan.

Contraindications

Hypersensitivity to topotecan or any component of the formulation; severe bone marrow depression (IV formulation)

Canadian labeling: Additional contraindications (not in U.S. labeling): Severe renal impairment (CrCl <20 mL/minute); pregnancy; breast-feeding

Warnings/Precautions Hazardous agent - use appropriate precautions for handling and disposal (NIOSH 2014 [group 1]). **[U.S. Boxed Warning]: May cause neutropenia, which may be severe or lead to infection or fatalities. Monitor blood counts frequently. Do NOT administer to patients with baseline neutrophils <1500/mm³ and platelets <100,000/mm³.** The dose-limiting toxicity is bone marrow suppression (primarily neutropenia); may also cause thrombocytopenia and anemia. Neutropenia is not cumulative overtime. Nadir neutrophil, platelet, and red blood cell counts occurred at a median of 12 days, 15 days, and 15 days, respectively. In a clinical study comparing IV to oral topotecan, G-CSF support was administered in a higher percentage of patients receiving oral topotecan (Eckardt, 2007). Bone marrow suppression may require dosage reduction and/or growth factor support. Topotecan-induced neutropenia may lead to neutropenic colitis (including fatalities); should be considered in patients presenting with neutropenia, fever and abdominal pain.

Diarrhea has been reported with oral topotecan; may be severe (requiring hospitalization); incidence may be higher in the elderly; educate patients on early recognition and proper management, including diet changes, increase in fluid intake, antidiarrheals, and antibiotics. The median time to onset of diarrhea (grade 2 or worse) was 9 days. The incidence of diarrhea may be higher in the elderly. Do not administer in patients with grade 3 or 4 diarrhea; reduce dose upon recovery to ≤ grade 1 toxicity. Interstitial lung disease (ILD) (with fatalities) has been reported; discontinue use in patients with confirmed ILD diagnosis; risk factors for ILD include a history of ILD, pulmonary fibrosis, lung cancer, thoracic radiation, and the use of colony-stimulating factors or medication with pulmonary toxicity; monitor pulmonary symptoms (cough, fever, dyspnea, and/or hypoxia). Use caution in renal impairment; may require dose adjustment (use in severe renal impairment is contraindicated in the Canadian labeling). Potentially significant drug-drug interactions may exist, requiring dose or frequency adjustment, additional monitoring, and/or selection of alternative therapy. Topotecan exposure is increased when oral topotecan is used concurrently with P-glycoprotein inhibitors; avoid concurrent use. Topotecan overdoses have been reported; potential causes include omission of the leading zero and missing the decimal point when prescribing, preparing, and administering. Recommended intravenous doses should generally not exceed 4 mg in adults; verify dose prior to administration.

Adverse Reactions

Central nervous system: Fatigue, fever, headache, pain

Dermatologic: Alopecia (reversible), rash

Gastrointestinal: Abdominal pain, anorexia, constipation, diarrhea, nausea, obstruction, stomatitis, vomiting

Hematologic: Anemia, leukopenia, neutropenia (nadir 8-11 days; recovery <21 days), neutropenic fever/sepsis, thrombocytopenia

Hepatic: BUN increased, liver enzymes increased (transient)

Neuromuscular & skeletal: Paresthesia, weakness

Respiratory: Cough, dyspnea, pneumonia

Miscellaneous: Infection, sepsis

Rare but important or life-threatening: Allergic reactions, anaphylactoid reactions, angioedema, bleeding (severe, associated with thrombocytopenia), dermatitis (severe), extravasation (inadvertent), interstitial lung disease (ILD), neutropenic colitis, pancytopenia, pruritus (severe)

Drug Interactions

Metabolism/Transport Effects Substrate of BCRP

Avoid Concomitant Use

Avoid concomitant use of Topotecan with any of the following: BCG; BCG (Intravesical); CloZAPine; Dipyrone; Natalizumab; P-glycoprotein/ABCB1 Inhibitors; Pimecrolimus; Tacrolimus (Topical); Tofacitinib; Vaccines (Live)

Increased Effect/Toxicity

Topotecan may increase the levels/effects of: CloZAPine; Leflunomide; Natalizumab; Tofacitinib; Vaccines (Live)

The levels/effects of Topotecan may be increased by: BCRP/ABCG2 Inhibitors; Denosumab; Dipyrone; Filgrastim; P-glycoprotein/ABCB1 Inhibitors; Pimecrolimus; Platinum Derivatives; Roflumilast; Tacrolimus (Topical); Trastuzumab

Decreased Effect

Topotecan may decrease the levels/effects of: BCG; BCG (Intravesical); Coccidioides immitis Skin Test; Sipuleucel-T; Vaccines (Inactivated); Vaccines (Live)

The levels/effects of Topotecan may be decreased by: Echinacea; Fosphenytoin-Phenytoin

Storage/Stability

IV:

Solution for injection: Store intact vials at 2°C to 8°C (36°F to 45°F). Protect from light. Single-use vials should be discarded after initial vial entry. Stability of solutions diluted for infusion is variable; refer to specific product information for details.

Lyophilized powder: Store intact vials at 20°C to 25°C (68°F to 77°F). Protect from light. Reconstituted solution is stable for up to 28 days at 20°C to 25°C (68°F to 77°F), although the manufacturer recommends use immediately after reconstitution. Solutions diluted in D_5W or NS are stable for 24 hours at room temperature (manufacturer's labeling) or up to 7 days under refrigeration (Craig, 1997). Reconstituted solution for injection (reconstituted with bacteriostatic SWFI to 1 mg/mL) for oral administration is stable for 14 days at 4°C in plastic syringes (Daw, 2004).

Oral: Store at 2°C to 8°C (36°F to 46°F). Protect from light.

Mechanism of Action Binds to topoisomerase I and stabilizes the cleavable complex so that religation of the cleaved DNA strand cannot occur. This results in the accumulation of cleavable complexes and single-strand DNA breaks. Topotecan acts in S phase of the cell cycle.

Pharmacokinetics (Adult data unless noted)

Note: Pharmacokinetic data in pediatric patients and young adults (0.4-22 years) demonstrated a high level of interpatient variability (43% to 57% dependent upon parameter evaluated) as well as intrapatient variability (20% to 22% dependent upon parameter evaluated) (Schaiquevich, 2007)

Absorption: Oral: Rapid

Distribution:

Pediatric patients and young adults (0.4-22 years): Mean range: 32.2-32.7 L/m^2 (Schaiquevich, 2007)

Adults: 25-75 L/m^2 (Hartmann, 2006)

Protein binding: 35%

Metabolism: Undergoes pH dependent hydrolysis of its active lactone moiety to yield a relatively inactive open-ring hydroxy acid form in plasma; metabolized in the liver to N-demethylated topotecan

Bioavailability: Oral: Capsule: Adults: ~40%; data from pediatric patients (1-18 years) showed that, while highly variable, the reported median oral bioavailability with oral administration of the reconstituted parenteral solution is similar to adults (Daw, 2004; Zamboni, 1999)

Half-life:

Pediatric patients (0-18 years): Lactone moiety: 2.58 hours ± 0.15 (range: 0.2-7.1 hours) (Santana, 2005)

Adults:

IV: 2-3 hours; renal impairment: ~5 hours

Oral: 3-6 hours

Time to peak serum concentration: Oral:

Pediatric patients (1-18 years): Parenteral formulation (reconstituted lyophilized formulation): 0.75-2 hours (Zamboni, 1999)

Adults: Capsules: 1-2 hours; delayed with high-fat meal (3-4 hours)

Elimination:

IV: Urine (51%; 3% as N-desmethyl topotecan); feces (18%; 2% as N-desmethyl topotecan)

Oral: Urine (20%; 2% as N-desmethyl topotecan); feces (33%; <2% as N-desmethyl topotecan)

Clearance:

Pediatric patients (0.4-18 years): GFR most significant determinant of clearance; a linear model with GFR has been observed; BSA is also a significant determinant of clearance and AUC more so than patient weight; infants <6 months have decreased clearance (Schaiquevich, 2007). However, pharmacokinetic data from six pediatric patients with severe renal impairment (n=5: Unilateral nephrectomy; n=1: Anephric on hemodialysis) suggests that other mechanisms than GFR may assist with renal clearance; in these patients, overall systemic clearance was shown to be similar to matched controls (age, BSA, and Scr) despite decreased GFR (Iacono, 2003; Iacono, 2004)

Adults: Topotecan plasma clearance is 24% higher in males than in female patients

Dosing: Usual Note: In adults, baseline neutrophil count should be ≥1500/mm^3 and platelets should be ≥100,000/mm^3 prior to treatment; for retreatment, neutrophil count should be >1000/mm^3; platelets >100,000/mm^3 and hemoglobin ≥9 g/dL; consult individual pediatric protocols for details regarding baseline neutrophil and platelet counts and hemoglobin.

Pediatric: **Note:** Dosing and frequency may vary by protocol and/or treatment phase; refer to specific protocol. In pediatric patients, dosing may be based on either BSA (mg/m^2) or weight (mg/kg); use extra precaution to verify dosing parameters during calculations.

Acute lymphoblastic leukemia; recurrent (first relapse): Children and Adolescents: Induction therapy: IV: 2.4 mg/m^2/dose once daily for 7 to 9 days (Furman 2002; Hijiya 2008)

Acute myeloid leukemia; recurrent, refractory: Children and Adolescents: IV: Initial: 4 mg/m^2/dose once on day 1; subsequent daily doses (days 2 to 5) determined by pharmacokinetic analysis (target AUC: 140 ± 20 ng/mL/hour) and administered once daily (in combination with cladribine); the median reported topotecan dose was 4 mg/m^2/day (range: 1.7 to 6 mg/m^2/day) (Inaba 2010)

CNS malignancies, including gliomas:

Fixed dosing: Infants, Children, and Adolescents: Oral (using reconstituted lyophilized parenteral formulation): 0.8 mg/m^2/dose once daily for 21 days of a 28-day cycle was used in 25 pediatric patients (median age: 9.2 years; range 0.8 to 23 years) with recurrent brain tumors, including gliomas, medulloblastoma, and ependymoma; the reported median number of cycles: 1.9 [range: 0.5 to 15 cycles (months)] (Minturn 2011)

Dose escalation: Children ≥3 years and Adolescents: Oral (using reconstituted lyophilized parenteral formulation): Initial: 0.4 mg/m^2/dose once daily was used in a trial of 32 pediatric patients (median age: 9.5 years, range: 3 to 18 years) with recurrent or progression of high-grade glioma; dosage was increased based upon patient tolerance and individual dose-limiting toxicity; doses were increased in 0.2 mg/m^2 increments at weekly intervals for the first 2 weeks of therapy and then increased in 0.1 mg/m^2 increments at weekly intervals up to the maximum dose of 2 mg/m^2/day; once the patient's maximum tolerated dose was reached, the daily dose was decreased until toxicity became acceptable; reported final median maximum tolerated dose: 0.9 mg/m²/day (range: 0.6 to 2 mg/m²/day); median duration of therapy: 3 months (range: 21 days to 1 year) (Wagner 2004)

Neuroblastoma:

Induction: Infants, Children, and Adolescents: IV:

Patient weight ≤12 kg: 0.04 mg/**kg**/dose once daily for 5 days (in combination with cyclophosphamide); repeat cycle every 21 days for 6 cycles (Park 2011)

Patient weight >12 kg: Initial: 1.2 mg/m²/dose once daily for 5 days (in combination with cyclophosphamide); repeat cycle every 21 days for 6 cycles (Park 2011)

Note: Pharmacokinetic analysis was used to guide topotecan therapy during the first 2 cycles using a target AUC: 50 to 70 ng/mL/hour; median dose for cycle 1 was 1.2 mg/m²/day (range: 0.75 to 2.1 mg/m²/day) and for cycle 2, the median dose was 1.3 mg/m²/day (range: 1.2 to 2.9 mg/m²/day) (Park 2011)

Recurrent, refractory, or untreated metastatic disease:

IV: Children and Adolescents:

Combination therapy: 0.75 mg/m²/dose once daily for 5 days (in combination with cyclophosphamide); repeat cycle every 21 days (Ashraf 2013; Kretschmar 2004; London 2010; Saylors 2001; Zage 2008)

Monotherapy: 2 mg/m²/day for 5 days (London 2010)

Oral (using reconstituted lyophilized parenteral formulation): Children ≥2 years and Adolescents: 0.8 mg/m²/dose once daily for 14 days (in combination with oral cyclophosphamide); repeat cycle every 21 to 28 days (Bowers 2004). In a Phase I dose escalation trial of 20 pediatric patients (median age: 10.6 years) with refractory solid tumors including neuroblastoma, a daily dose of 1.8 mg/m² once daily for 5 days, followed by 2 days rest, then another 5 days of therapy (one cycle: 10 doses over 12 days); repeat cycle every 28 days was shown to stabilize disease in some patients (Daw, 2004).

Hematopoietic stem-cell transplant; conditioning: Children and Adolescents: IV: 2 mg/m²/dose on days -8 through -4 prior to stem cell transfusion (total dose: 10 mg/m²), in combination with carboplatin and thiotepa, was used in 21 patients (median age: 4.1 years; range: 1-29 years) with refractory solid tumors (neuroblastoma: n=11) (Kushner, 2001). In a Phase I/II trial of 51 patients (median age: 5.1 years; range: 1.5 to 21 years), an initial dose of: 3 mg/m²/dose on day -11 was used with subsequent doses (days -10 through -2; 10 days total of topotecan therapy) determined by pharmacokinetic analysis (target AUC: 100 ± 20 ng/mL/hour) and administered once daily (in combination with cyclophosphamide on days -6 through -2); the median reported topotecan dose was 3.1 mg/m²/day (range: 1.1 to 4.6 mg/m²/day) (Kaskow 2012)

Pediatric solid tumors; recurrent or refractory or untreated metastatic including rhabdosarcoma, Ewing sarcoma:

IV: Infants, Children, and Adolescents:

Combination therapy: 0.75 mg/m²/dose once daily for 5 days every 21 days in combination with cyclophosphamide (Bernstien 2006; Hunhold 2006; Saylors 2001; Waterhouse 2004) or with cyclophosphamide and vincristine (VTC regimen) (Pappo 2001); this dosing has also been administered in combination with temozolomide in 28-day cycles (TOTEM regimen) (Rubie 2010)

Single-agent therapy (window therapy): 2-2.4 mg/m²/dose once daily for 5 days every 21 days (Pappo 2001)

Oral [using reconstituted lyophilized parenteral formulation or oral capsules (for patients able to swallow)]: Children ≥3 years and Adolescents: 1.8 mg/m² once daily for 5 days, followed by 2 days rest, then another 5 days of therapy (one cycle: 10 doses over 12 days); repeat cycle every 28 days; when using oral capsules, doses were rounded to the nearest 0.25 mg; dosing based on a Phase I trial dose escalation trial of 20 pediatric patients (median age: 10.6 years) with refractory solid tumors (Daw 2004)

Adults:

Cervical cancer, recurrent or resistant: IV: 0.75 mg/m²/day for 3 days [followed by cisplatin on day 1 only (with hydration)] every 21 days

Ovarian cancer, metastatic: IV: 1.5 mg/m²/day for 5 consecutive days every 21 days, minimum of 4 cycles recommended in the absence of tumor progression **or** (weekly administration) 4 mg/m² on days 1, 8, and 15 every 28 days until disease progression or unacceptable toxicity or a maximum of 12 months (Sehouli 2011)

Small cell lung cancer, relapsed or refractory:

IV: 1.5 mg/m²/day for 5 consecutive days every 21 days, minimum of 4 cycles recommended in the absence of tumor progression

Oral: 2.3 mg/m²/day for 5 consecutive days every 21 days (round dose to the nearest 0.25 mg); if patient vomits after dose is administered, do not give a replacement dose

Dosing adjustment in renal impairment:

Infants, Children, and Adolescents: Consult protocol for specific recommendations. Some centers have considered the following adjustments: IV:

Baseline: Initial dosing:

CrCl >40 mL/minute/1.73 m²: No adjustment necessary

CrCl 20 to 40 mL/minute/1.73 m²: Administer 50% of dose

CrCl <20 mL/minute/1.73 m²: Hold doses until renal function recovers (CrCl >20 mL/minute/1.73 m²)

During therapy:

CrCl >60 mL/minute/1.73 m²: No adjustment necessary

CrCl 40 to 60 mL/minute/1.73 m²: Administer 50% of dose

CrCl 20 to <40 mL/minute/1.73 m²: Administer 25% to 50% of dose

CrCl <20 mL/minute/1.73 m²: Hold doses until renal function recovers (CrCl >20 mL/minute/1.73 m²)

Hemodialysis: Very limited data available; some data suggest that clearance of the lactone metabolite is similar to pediatric patients with normal renal function; a case report describes topotecan use in an anephric 6-year old diagnosed with Wilms tumor; the patient received 0.75 mg/m²/dose once daily for 5 days every 21 days with hemodialysis on day 2 and 4; on dialysis days, topotecan was administered ~2 hours before the start of the dialysis session; dosage reductions required for toxicity (myelosuppression) after cycle 4 (Aronoff 2007; Iacono 2004)

Continuous renal replacement therapy (CRRT): Administer 50% of dose or reduce dose by 0.75 mg/m²/dose, if appropriate (Aronoff, 2007)

Adult:

Manufacturer's recommendations:

IV:

CrCl ≥40 mL/minute: No dosage adjustment necessary.

CrCl 20 to 39 mL/minute: Reduce dose to 0.75 mg/m²/dose

CrCl <20 mL/minute: There are no dosage adjustments provided in manufacturer's U.S. labeling (insufficient data available for dosing recommendation).

Note: For topotecan in combination with cisplatin for cervical cancer, do not initiate treatment in patients with serum creatinine >1.5 mg/dL; consider discontinuing treatment in patients with serum creatinine >1.5 mg/dL in subsequent cycles.

Oral:

CrCl ≥50 mL/minute: No dosage adjustment necessary

CrCl 30 to 49 mL/minute: Reduce dose to 1.8 mg/m²/day

CrCl <30 mL/minute: There are no dosage adjustments provided in manufacturer's U.S. labeling (insufficient data available for dosing recommendation).

Alternate recommendations:

Aronoff, 2007: IV:

CrCl >50 mL/minute: Administer 75% of dose

CrCl 10 to 50 mL/minute: Administer 50% of dose

CrCl <10 mL/minute: Administer 25% of dose

Hemodialysis: Avoid use

Continuous ambulatory peritoneal dialysis (CAPD): Avoid use

Continuous renal replacement therapy (CRRT): 0.75 mg/m²

Kintzel, 1995: IV:

CrCl 46 to 60 mL/minute: Administer 80% of dose

CrCl 31 to 45 mL/minute: Administer 75% of dose

CrCl ≤30 mL/minute: Administer 70% of dose

Dosing adjustment in hepatic impairment: Adults:

IV: Bilirubin 1.7 to 15 mg/dL: No adjustment necessary; the half-life is increased slightly; usual doses are generally tolerated

Oral: Bilirubin >1.5 mg/dL: No adjustment necessary

Dosing adjustment for toxicity: Adults:

Cervical cancer: IV: Severe febrile neutropenia (<1000/mm³ with temperature of 38°C) or platelet count <25,000/mm³: Reduce topotecan to 0.6 mg/m²/day for subsequent cycles [may consider GCSF support (beginning on day 4) prior to instituting dose reduction for neutropenic fever]. **Note:** Cisplatin may also require dose adjustment.

For neutropenic fever despite G-SCF use, reduce dose to 0.45 mg/m²/day for subsequent cycles.

Ovarian cancer: IV: Dosage adjustment for hematological effects: Severe neutropenia (<500/mm³) or platelet count <25,000/mm³: Reduce dose to 1.25 mg/m²/day for subsequent cycles [may consider G-CSF support (beginning on day 6) prior to instituting dose reduction for neutropenia]

Small cell lung cancer:

IV: Dosage adjustment for hematological effects: Severe neutropenia (<500/mm³) or platelet count <25,000/mm³: Reduce dose to 1.25 mg/m²/day for subsequent cycles [may consider G-CSF support (beginning on day 6) prior to instituting dose reduction for severe neutropenia]

Oral: Severe neutropenia (neutrophils <500/mm³ associated with fever or infection or lasting ≥7 days) or prolonged neutropenia (neutrophils ≥500/mm³ to ≤1000/mm³ lasting beyond day 21) or platelets <25,000/mm³ or grades 3 or 4 diarrhea: Reduce dose by 0.4 mg/m²/day for subsequent cycles (may consider same dosage reduction for grade 2 diarrhea if clinically indicated)

Preparation for Administration Hazardous agent; use appropriate precautions for handling and disposal (NIOSH 2014 [group 1]).

Parenteral: Reconstitute lyophilized powder with 4 mL SWFI. Further dilute reconstituted lyophilized powder and solution for injection in D_5W or NS.

Oral: Parenteral formulation (lyophilized powder) for oral use: Reconstitute with 4 mL SWFI to a final concentration of 1 mg/mL; mix dose in 30 mL of an acidic medium (eg, apple, grape, or orange juice). **Note:** The reconstituted injectable solution is tasteless; the acidic medium serves as the vehicle only, not to mask the taste (Bowers 2004; Daw 2004; Minturn 2001; Wagner 2004)

Administration Hazardous agent; use appropriate precautions for handling and disposal (NIOSH 2014 [group 1]).

Parenteral: IV: Administer by intermittent infusion over 30 minutes.

Oral:

Capsules: May administer with or without food. Swallow capsule whole; do not crush, chew, or divide capsule.

Parenteral formulation; lyophilized powder for oral use. After reconstitution, mix dose in 30 mL of an acidic medium (eg, apple, grape, or orange juice); **Note:** The reconstituted injectable solution is tasteless; the acidic medium serves as the vehicle only, not to mask the taste (Bowers 2004; Daw 2004; Minturn 2001; Wagner 2004)

Vesicant/Extravasation Risk Irritant

Monitoring Parameters CBC with differential and platelet count; renal function tests; bilirubin; monitor for signs and symptoms of interstitial lung disease; diarrhea symptoms/hydration status

Dosage Forms Excipient information presented when available (limited, particularly for generics); consult specific product labeling.

Capsule, Oral:

Hycamtin: 0.25 mg, 1 mg

Solution, Intravenous:

Generic: 4 mg/4 mL (4 mL)

Solution, Intravenous [preservative free]:

Generic: 4 mg/4 mL (4 mL)

Solution Reconstituted, Intravenous:

Hycamtin: 4 mg (1 ea)

Generic: 4 mg (1 ea)

Solution Reconstituted, Intravenous [preservative free]:

Generic: 4 mg (1 ea)

Extemporaneous Preparations

Hazardous agent; use appropriate precautions for handling and disposal (NIOSH 2014 [group 1]).

For patients unable to swallow capsules whole, reconstituted topotecan solution for injection (1 mg/mL concentration) may be mixed with up to 30 mL of acidic fruit juice (eg, apple, orange, grape) immediately prior to oral administration.

Daw NC, Santana VM, Iacono LC, et al. Phase I and pharmacokinetic study of topotecan administered orally once daily for 5 days for 2 consecutive weeks to pediatric patients with refractory solid tumors. *J Clin Oncol*. 2004;22(5):829-837.

- **Topotecan For Injection (Can)** *see* Topotecan *on page 2092*
- **Topotecan Hydrochloride** *see* Topotecan *on page 2092*
- **Topotecan Hydrochloride For Injection (Can)** *see* Topotecan *on page 2092*
- **Toprol XL** *see* Metoprolol *on page 1418*
- **Topsyn® (Can)** *see* Fluocinonide *on page 898*
- **Toradol** *see* Ketorolac (Systemic) *on page 1192*
- **Toradol® (Can)** *see* Ketorolac (Systemic) *on page 1192*
- **Toradol® IM (Can)** *see* Ketorolac (Systemic) *on page 1192*
- **Torasemide** *see* Torsemide *on page 2095*

Torsemide (TORE se mide)

Medication Safety Issues

Sound-alike/look-alike issues:

Torsemide may be confused with furosemide

Demadex may be confused with Denorex

Brand Names: US Demadex

Therapeutic Category Antihypertensive Agent; Diuretic, Loop

Generic Availability (US) Yes

Use Management of edema associated with CHF and hepatic or renal disease (including chronic renal failure); used alone or in combination with antihypertensives in treatment of hypertension (FDA approved in adults)

Pregnancy Risk Factor B

Pregnancy Considerations A decrease in fetal weight, an increase in fetal resorption, and delayed fetal ossification has occurred in animal studies.

Breast-Feeding Considerations It is not known if torsemide is excreted in breast milk. The manufacturer recommends that caution be exercised when administering torsemide to nursing women.

Contraindications Hypersensitivity to torsemide, any component of the formulation, or any sulfonylurea; anuria

Warnings/Precautions Loop diuretics are potent diuretics; excess amounts can lead to profound diuresis with fluid and electrolyte loss; close medical supervision and dose evaluation are required. Potassium supplementation and/or use of potassium-sparing diuretics may be necessary to prevent hypokalemia. In contrast to thiazide diuretics, a loop diuretic can also lower serum calcium concentrations. Electrolyte disturbances can predispose a patient to serious cardiac arrhythmias. Use with caution in patients with cirrhosis; avoid sudden changes in fluid and electrolyte balance and acid/base status which may lead to hepatic encephalopathy. Administration with an aldosterone antagonist or potassium-sparing diuretic may provide additional diuretic efficacy and maintain normokalemia. Coadministration of antihypertensives may increase the risk of hypotension.

Monitor fluid status and renal function in an attempt to prevent oliguria, azotemia, and reversible increases in BUN and creatinine; close medical supervision of aggressive diuresis required. Diuretic resistance may occur in some patients, despite higher doses of loop diuretic treatment, and can usually be overcome by intravenous administration, the use of two diuretics together (eg, furosemide and chlorothiazide), or the use of a diuretic with a positive inotropic agent. When such combinations are used, serum electrolytes need to be monitored even more closely (Cody, 1994; ACC/AHA [Yancy, 2013]; HFSA, 2010). Ototoxicity has been demonstrated following oral administration of torsemide and following rapid IV administration of other loop diuretics. Other possible risk factors may include use in renal impairment, excessive doses, and concurrent use of other ototoxins (eg, aminoglycosides). If given the morning of surgery, torsemide may render the patient volume depleted and blood pressure may be labile during general anesthesia.

Sulfonamide ("sulfa") allergy: The FDA-approved product labeling for many medications containing a sulfonamide chemical group includes a broad contraindication in patients with a prior allergic reaction to sulfonamides. There is a potential for cross-reactivity between members of a specific class (eg, two antibiotic sulfonamides). However, concerns for cross-reactivity have previously extended to all compounds containing the sulfonamide structure (SO_2NH_2). An expanded understanding of allergic mechanisms indicates cross-reactivity between antibiotic sulfonamides and nonantibiotic sulfonamides may not occur or at the very least this potential is extremely low (Brackett 2004; Johnson 2005; Slatore 2004; Tornero 2004). In particular, mechanisms of cross-reaction due to antibody production (anaphylaxis) are unlikely to occur with nonantibiotic sulfonamides. T-cell-mediated (type IV) reactions (eg, maculopapular rash) are less well understood and it is not possible to completely exclude this potential based on current insights. In cases where prior reactions were severe (Stevens-Johnson syndrome/TEN), some clinicians choose to avoid exposure to these classes.

Adverse Reactions

Cardiovascular: Chest pain, ECG abnormality

Central nervous system: Nervousness

Gastrointestinal: Constipation, diarrhea, dyspepsia, nausea, sore throat

Genitourinary: Excessive urination

Neuromuscular & skeletal: Arthralgia, myalgia, weakness

Respiratory: Cough, rhinitis

Rare but important or life-threatening: Angioedema, arthritis, atrial fibrillation, esophageal hemorrhage, GI hemorrhage, hyperglycemia, hyperuricemia, hypokalemia, hyponatremia, hypotension, hypovolemia, impotence, leukopenia, pancreatitis, rash, rectal bleeding, shunt thrombosis, Stevens-Johnson syndrome, syncope, thirst, thrombocytopenia, toxic epidermal necrolysis, ventricular tachycardia, vomiting

Drug Interactions

Metabolism/Transport Effects Substrate of CYP2C8 (minor), CYP2C9 (major), SLCO1B1; **Note:** Assignment of Major/Minor substrate status based on clinically relevant drug interaction potential

Avoid Concomitant Use

Avoid concomitant use of Torsemide with any of the following: Mecamylamine

Increased Effect/Toxicity

Torsemide may increase the levels/effects of: ACE Inhibitors; Allopurinol; Amifostine; Aminoglycosides; Antihypertensives; Cardiac Glycosides; CISplatin; Dofetilide; DULoxetine; Foscarnet; Hypotensive Agents; Ivabradine; Levodopa; Lithium; Mecamylamine; Methotrexate; Neuromuscular-Blocking Agents; Obinutuzumab; RisperiDONE; RiTUXimab; Salicylates; Sodium Phosphates; Topiramate; Warfarin

The levels/effects of Torsemide may be increased by: Alfuzosin; Analgesics (Opioid); Barbiturates; Beta2-Agonists; Brimonidine (Topical); Canagliflozin; Ceritinib; Corticosteroids (Orally Inhaled); Corticosteroids (Systemic); CycloSPORINE (Systemic); CYP2C9 Inhibitors (Moderate); CYP2C9 Inhibitors (Strong); Diazoxide; Eltrombopag; Herbs (Hypotensive Properties); Licorice; MAO Inhibitors; Methotrexate; Mifepristone; Nicorandil; Pentoxifylline; Phosphodiesterase 5 Inhibitors; Probenecid; Prostacyclin Analogues; Teriflunomide

Decreased Effect

Torsemide may decrease the levels/effects of: Antidiabetic Agents; Lithium; Neuromuscular-Blocking Agents

The levels/effects of Torsemide may be decreased by: Bile Acid Sequestrants; CYP2C9 Inducers (Strong); Dabrafenib; Herbs (Hypertensive Properties); Methotrexate; Methylphenidate; Nonsteroidal Anti-Inflammatory Agents; Probenecid; Salicylates; Yohimbine

Storage/Stability

IV: Store at 15°C to 30°C (59°F to 86°F). If torsemide is to be administered via continuous infusion, stability has been demonstrated through 24 hours at room temperature in plastic containers for the following fluids and concentrations:

200 mg torsemide (10 mg/mL) added to 250 mL D_5W, 250 mL NS or 500 mL 0.45% sodium chloride

50 mg torsemide (10 mg/mL) added to 500 mL D_5W, 500 mL NS, or 500 mL 0.45% sodium chloride

Tablets: Store at 15°C to 30°C (59°F to 86°F).

Mechanism of Action Inhibits reabsorption of sodium and chloride in the ascending loop of Henle and distal renal tubule, interfering with the chloride-binding cotransport system, thus causing increased excretion of water, sodium, chloride, magnesium, and calcium; does not alter GFR, renal plasma flow, or acid-base balance

Pharmacodynamics

Onset of action:

Oral: 60 minutes

IV: 10 minutes

Maximum effect:

Oral: 60-120 minutes

IV: Within 60 minutes

Duration: Oral, IV: 6-8 hours

Pharmacokinetics (Adult data unless noted)

Absorption: Oral: Rapid

Distribution: V_d: 12-15 L; cirrhosis: approximately doubled

Protein binding: Plasma: ≥99%

Metabolism: Hepatic by cytochrome P450, 80%

Bioavailability: ~80%

Half-life: 3.5 hours; 7-8 hours in cirrhosis (dose modification appears unnecessary)

Time to peak serum concentration: Oral: 1 hour; delayed ~30 minutes when administered with food

Elimination: 20% eliminated unchanged in urine

Dosing: Usual Note: Dose equivalency for adult patients with normal renal function (approximate): Torsemide 20 mg = Bumetanide 1 mg = furosemide 40 mg = ethacrynic acid 50 mg

Adults (**Note:** IV and oral dosing are equivalent):

Edema:

Chronic renal failure: Oral, IV: Initial: 20 mg once daily; may increase gradually by doubling dose until the desired diuretic response is obtained (maximum recommended daily dose: 200 mg)

Heart failure:

Oral: Initial: 10-20 mg once daily; may increase gradually by doubling dose until the desired diuretic response is obtained. **Note:** ACC/AHA 2009 guidelines for heart failure maximum daily dose: 200 mg (Hunt, 2009)

IV: Initial: 10-20 mg; may repeat every 2 hours with double the dose as needed. **Note:** ACC/AHA 2009 guidelines for heart failure recommend maximum single dose:100-200 mg (Hunt, 2009)

Hepatic cirrhosis: Oral: Initial: 5-10 mg once daily; may increase gradually by doubling dose until the desired diuretic response is obtained (maximum recommended single dose: 40 mg). **Note:** Administer with an aldosterone antagonist or a potassium-sparing diuretic.

Hypertension: Oral: Initial: 5 mg once daily; may increase to 10 mg once daily after 4-6 weeks if adequate antihypertensive response is not apparent; if still not effective, an additional antihypertensive agent may be added. Usual dosage range (JNC 7): 2.5-10 mg once daily. **Note:** Thiazide-type diuretics are preferred in the treatment of hypertension (Chobanian, 2003)

Administration

IV: Administer over ≥2 minutes; reserve IV administration for situations which require rapid onset of action

Oral: Administer without regard to meals; patients may be switched from the IV form to the oral (and vice-versa) with no change in dose

Monitoring Parameters Renal function, serum electrolytes, fluid balance, blood pressure, body weight

Dosage Forms Excipient information presented when available (limited, particularly for generics); consult specific product labeling. [DSC] = Discontinued product

Solution, Intravenous:

Generic: 20 mg/2 mL (2 mL [DSC]); 50 mg/5 mL (5 mL [DSC])

Tablet, Oral:

Demadex: 5 mg, 10 mg, 20 mg, 100 mg [scored]

Generic: 5 mg, 10 mg, 20 mg, 100 mg

◆ **Total Allergy [OTC]** *see* DiphenhydrAMINE (Systemic) *on page 668*

◆ **Total Allergy Medicine [OTC]** *see* DiphenhydrAMINE (Systemic) *on page 668*

◆ **Totect** *see* Dexrazoxane *on page 622*

◆ **Toujeo SoloStar** *see* Insulin Glargine *on page 1126*

◆ **tPA** *see* Alteplase *on page 105*

◆ **TPV** *see* Tipranavir *on page 2070*

◆ **tRA** *see* Tretinoin (Systemic) *on page 2108*

Trace Elements (trase EL e ments)

Related Information

Pediatric Parenteral Nutrition *on page 2359*

Brand Names: US Multitrace-4; Multitrace-4 Concentrate; Multitrace-4 Neonatal; Multitrace-4 Pediatric; Multitrace-5; Multitrace-5 Concentrate; Trace Elements 4 Pediatric

Therapeutic Category Mineral, Parenteral; Trace Element, Multiple, Neonatal; Trace Element, Parenteral

Generic Availability (US) Yes

Use Prevent and correct trace metal deficiencies (FDA approved in all ages)

Pregnancy Risk Factor C

Pregnancy Considerations Refer to individual elements for requirements in pregnancy.

Breast-Feeding Considerations Refer to individual elements for requirements while breast-feeding.

Warnings/Precautions Benzyl alcohol and derivatives: Some dosage forms may contain benzyl alcohol; large amounts of benzyl alcohol (≥99 mg/kg/day) have been associated with a potentially fatal toxicity ("gasping syndrome") in neonates; the "gasping syndrome" consists of metabolic acidosis, respiratory distress, gasping respirations, CNS dysfunction (including convulsions, intracranial hemorrhage), hypotension, and cardiovascular collapse (AAP, 1997; CDC, 1982); some data suggests that benzoate displaces bilirubin from protein binding sites (Ahlfors, 2001); avoid or use dosage forms containing benzyl alcohol with caution in neonates. See manufacturer's labeling.

Food Interactions Decreased absorption of oral zinc when administered with bran products, protein, and phytates.

Pharmacokinetics (Adult data unless noted)

Chromium: 10% to 20% oral absorption; excretion primarily via kidneys and bile

Copper: 30% oral absorption; 80% elimination via bile; intestinal wall 16% and urine 4%

Manganese: 10% oral absorption; excretion primarily via bile; ancillary routes via pancreatic secretions or reabsorption into the intestinal lumen occur during periods of biliary obstruction

Selenium: Very poor oral absorption; 75% excretion via kidneys, remainder via feces, lung, and skin

Zinc: 20% to 30% oral absorption; 90% excretion in stools, remainder via urine and perspiration

Dosing: Neonatal

ASPEN Guidelines: Trace Mineral Daily Requirements[1] (Mirtallo, 2004)

	Preterm Neonates (<3 kg)	Term Neonates (3-10 kg)
Chromium[2]	0.05-0.2 mcg/kg	0.2 mcg/kg
Copper[3]	20 mcg/kg	20 mcg/kg
Manganese[4]	1 mcg/kg	1 mcg/kg
Selenium[2,5]	1.5-2 mcg/kg	2 mcg/kg
Zinc	400 mcg/kg	50-250 mcg/kg

[1]Recommended intakes of trace elements **cannot** be achieved through the use of a commercially available combination trace element product. Only through the use of individualized trace element products can recommended intakes be achieved.

[2]Reduce dose in patients with renal dysfunction.

[3]Reduce dose by 50% in patients with impaired biliary excretion or cholestatic liver disease.

[4]Omit in patients with impaired biliary excretion or cholestatic liver disease.

[5]Indicated for use in long-term parenteral nutrition patients.

Dosing: Usual

Infants, Children, and Adolescents:

ASPEN Guidelines: Trace Mineral Daily Requirements[1] (Mirtallo, 2004)

	Infants 3-10 kg	Infants, Children, and Adolescents 10-40 kg	Adolescents >40 kg
Chromium[2]	0.2 mcg/kg	0.14-0.2 mcg/kg	5-15 mcg
Copper[3]	20 mcg/kg	5-20 mcg/kg	200-500 mcg
Manganese[4]	1 mcg/kg	1 mcg/kg	40-100 mcg
Selenium[2,5]	2 mcg/kg	1-2 mcg/kg	40-60 mcg
Zinc	50-250 mcg/kg	50-125 mcg/kg	2-5 **mg**

[1]Recommended intakes of trace elements **cannot** be achieved through the use of a commercially available combination trace element product. Only through the use of individualized trace element products can recommended intakes be achieved.

[2]Reduce dose in patients with renal dysfunction.

[3]Reduce dose by 50% in patients with impaired biliary excretion or cholestatic liver disease.

[4]Omit in patients with impaired biliary excretion or cholestatic liver disease.

[5]Indicated for use in long-term parenteral nutrition patients.

Adults: **Recommended daily parenteral dosage: Manufacturer labeling:**

Chromium: 10-15 mcg; use caution in renal dysfunction

Copper: 0.5-1.5 **mg**; decrease dose or omit in patients with severe liver dysfunction and/or biliary tract obstruction

Manganese: 150-800 mcg; decrease dose or omit in patients with severe liver dysfunction and/or biliary tract obstruction

Selenium: 20-40 mcg; decrease dose or omit in patients with renal dysfunction and/or gastrointestinal malfunction

Zinc: 2.5-4 **mg**

Administration Parenteral: Must be diluted prior to use and infused as component of parenteral nutrition or parenteral solutions

Reference Range

Chromium: 0.18-0.47 ng/mL (SI: 35-90 nmol/L); some laboratories report much higher

Copper: ~0.7-1.5 mcg/mL (SI: 11-24 micromoles/L); levels are higher in pregnant women and children; **Note:** May not be a meaningful measurement of body stores.

Manganese: 18-30 mcg/dL (SI: 2.3-3.8 micromoles/L)

Selenium: 95-165 ng/mL (SI: 120-209 nmol/L)

Zinc: 70-120 mcg/dL (SI: 10-18.4 micromoles/L)

Additional Information The following describe the symptomatology associated with excess trace elements:

Chromium: Nausea, vomiting, GI ulcers, renal and hepatic dysfunction, convulsions, coma

Copper: Prostration, behavioral changes, diarrhea, progressive marasmus, hypotonia, photophobia, hepatic dysfunction, peripheral edema

Manganese: Irritability, speech disturbances, abnormal gait, headache, anorexia, apathy, impotence, cholestatic jaundice, movement disorders

Selenium: Alopecia, weak nails, dermatitis, dental defects, GI disorders, nervousness, mental depression, metallic taste, garlic odor of breath and sweat

Zinc: Profuse diaphoresis, consciousness decreased, blurred vision, tachycardia, hypothermia

Dosage Forms Excipient information presented when available (limited, particularly for generics); consult specific product labeling.

Injection, solution:

Addamel N: Chromium 1 mcg, copper 0.13 mg, fluoride 0.095 mg, iodide 0.013 mg, iron 0.11 mg, manganese 0.027 mg, molybdenum 1.9 mcg, selenium, 3.2 mcg, and zinc 0.65 mg per 1 mL (20 mL)

Multitrace-4: Chromium 4 mcg, copper 0.4 mg, manganese 0.1 mg, and zinc 1 mg per 1 mL (10 mL) [contains aluminum, benzyl alcohol]

Multitrace-4 Concentrate: Chromium 10 mcg, copper 1 mg, manganese 0.5 mg, and zinc 5 mg per 1 mL (1 mL) [contains aluminum]; chromium 10 mcg, copper 1 mg, manganese 0.5 mg, and zinc 5 mg per 1 mL (10 mL) [contains benzyl alcohol]

Multitrace-4 Neonatal: Chromium 0.85 mcg, copper 0.1 mg, manganese 0.025 mg, and zinc 1.5 mg per 1 mL (2 mL) [contains aluminum]

Multitrace-5: Chromium 4 mcg, copper 0.4 mg, manganese 0.1 mg, selenium 20 mcg, and zinc 1 mg per 1 mL (10 mL) [contains aluminum, benzyl alcohol]

Multitrace-5 Concentrate: Chromium 10 mcg, copper 1 mg, manganese 0.5 mg, selenium 60 mcg, and zinc 5 mg per 1 mL (1 mL) [contains aluminum]; chromium 10 mcg, copper 1 mg, manganese 0.5 mg, selenium 60 mcg, and zinc 5 mg per 1 mL (10 mL) [contains benzyl alcohol]

Peditrace: Copper 20 mcg, iodide 1 mcg, fluoride 57 mcg, manganese 1 mcg, selenium 2 mcg, and zinc 250 mcg per 1 mL (10 mL)

Trace Elements 4 Pediatric: Chromium 1 mcg, copper 0.1 mg, manganese 0.03 mg, and zinc 0.5 mg per 1 mL (10 mL) [contains aluminum, benzyl alcohol]

Injection, solution [preservative free]:

Multitrace-4 Pediatric: Chromium 1 mcg, copper 0.1 mg, manganese 0.025 mg, and zinc 1 mg per 1 mL (3 mL) [contains aluminum]

◆ **Trace Elements 4 Pediatric** *see* Trace Elements *on page* 2097

◆ **Trace Metals** *see* Trace Elements *on page* 2097

◆ **Trace Minerals** *see* Trace Elements *on page* 2097

◆ **Tracleer** *see* Bosentan *on page* 294

TraMADol (TRA ma dole)

Medication Safety Issues

Sound-alike/look-alike issues:

TraMADol may be confused with tapentadol, Toradol, Trandate, traZODone, Voltaren

Ultram may be confused with lithium, Ultane, Ultracet, Voltaren

International issues:

Theradol [Netherlands] may be confused with Foradil brand name for formoterol [U.S., Canada, and multiple international markets], Terazol brand name for terconazole [U.S. and Canada], and Toradol brand name for ketorolac [Canada and multiple international markets]

Trexol [Mexico] may be confused with Trexall brand name for methotrexate [U.S.]; Truxal brand name for chlorprothixene [multiple international markets]

Related Information

Oral Medications That Should Not Be Crushed or Altered *on page 2476*

Brand Names: US Active-Tramadol; ConZip; EnovaRX-Tramadol; Synapryn FusePaq; Ultram; Ultram ER

Brand Names: Canada Apo-Tramadol; Durela; Ralivia; Tridural; Ultram; Zytram XL

Therapeutic Category Analgesic, Opioid

Generic Availability (US) May be product dependent

Use

Immediate release formulations: Relief of moderate to moderately-severe pain (Ultram: FDA approved in ages ≥17 years and adults; Rybix™ ODT: FDA approved in ages ≥16 years and adults), including postoperative, cancer, neuropathic, low back pain, and pain associated with orthopedic disorders)

Extended release formulations: For patients requiring around-the-clock management of moderate to moderately-severe pain for an extended period of time (Ultram ER: FDA approved in ages ≥18 years and adults)

Pregnancy Risk Factor C

Pregnancy Considerations Adverse events were observed in animal reproduction studies. Tramadol has been shown to cross the human placenta when administered during labor. Postmarketing reports following tramadol use during pregnancy include neonatal seizures, withdrawal syndrome, fetal death, and stillbirth. Tramadol is not recommended for use during labor and delivery. Some Canadian products are contraindicated for use in pregnant women.

If chronic opioid exposure occurs in pregnancy, adverse events in the newborn (including withdrawal) may occur; monitoring of the neonate is recommended (Chou, 2009). Neonatal abstinence syndrome following opioid exposure may present with autonomic (eg, fever, temperature instability), gastrointestinal (eg, diarrhea, vomiting, poor feeding/weight gain), or neurologic (eg, high-pitched crying, increased muscle tone, irritability, seizure, tremor) symptoms (Dow, 2012; Hudak, 2012).

Breast-Feeding Considerations Tramadol is excreted into breast milk. Sixteen hours following a single 100 mg IV dose, the amount of tramadol found in breast milk was 0.1% of the maternal dose. Use is not recommended by the manufacturer for postdelivery analgesia in nursing mothers. Some Canadian products are contraindicated for use in nursing women. Nursing infants exposed to large doses of opioids should be monitored for apnea and sedation (Montgomery, 2012).

Contraindications Hypersensitivity to tramadol, opioids, or any component of the formulation

Additional contraindications for Ultram®, Rybix™ ODT, and Ultram® ER: Any situation where opioids are contraindicated, including acute intoxication with alcohol, hypnotics, centrally-acting analgesics, opioids, or psychotropic drugs

Additional contraindications for ConZip: Severe/acute bronchial asthma, hypercapnia, or significant respiratory depression in the absence of appropriately monitored setting and/or resuscitative equipment

Canadian product labeling:

Tramadol is contraindicated during or within 14 days following MAO inhibitor therapy

Extended release formulations: Additional contraindications:

Ralivia™, Tridural™: Severe (CrCl <30 mL/minute) renal dysfunction, severe (Child-Pugh class C) hepatic dysfunction

Durela™ and Zytram® XL: Severe (CrCl <30 mL/minute) renal dysfunction, severe (Child-Pugh class C) hepatic dysfunction; known or suspected mechanical GI obstruction or any disease/condition that affects bowel transit; mild, intermittent or short-duration pain that can be managed with other pain medication; management of peri-operative pain; obstructive airway, acute respiratory depression, cor pulmonale, delirium tremens, seizure disorder, severe CNS depression, increased cerebrospinal or intracranial pressure, head injury, breast-feeding, pregnancy; use during labor and delivery

Warnings/Precautions Rare but serious anaphylactoid reactions (including fatalities) often following initial dosing have been reported. Pruritus, hives, bronchospasm, angioedema, toxic epidermal necrolysis (TEN) and Stevens-Johnson syndrome also have been reported with use. Previous anaphylactoid reactions to opioids may increase risks for similar reactions to tramadol. Caution patients to swallow extended release tablets whole. Rapid release and absorption of tramadol from extended release tablets that are broken, crushed, or chewed may lead to a potentially lethal overdose. May cause CNS depression, which may impair physical or mental abilities; patients must be cautioned about performing tasks which require mental alertness (eg, operating machinery or driving). Effects with other sedative drugs or ethanol may be potentiated. May cause CNS depression and/or respiratory depression, particularly when combined with other CNS depressants. Use with caution and reduce dosage when administered to patients receiving other CNS depressants. An increased risk of seizures may occur in patients receiving serotonin reuptake inhibitors (SSRIs or anorectics), tricyclic antidepressants or other cyclic compounds (including cyclobenzaprine, promethazine), neuroleptics, drugs which may lower seizure threshold, or drugs which impair metabolism of tramadol (ie, CYP2D6 and 3A4 inhibitors). Patients with a history of seizures, or with a risk of seizures (head trauma, metabolic disorders, CNS infection, or malignancy, or during ethanol/drug withdrawal) are also at increased risk. Potentially significant drug interactions may exist, requiring dose or frequency adjustment, additional monitoring, and/or selection of alternative therapy.

Elderly (particularly >75 years of age), debilitated patients and patients with chronic respiratory disorders may be at greater risk of adverse events. Use with caution in patients with increased intracranial pressure or head injury. Avoid use in patients who are suicidal or addiction prone; use with caution in patients taking tranquilizers and/or antidepressants, or those with an emotional disturbance including depression. Healthcare provider should be alert to problems of abuse, misuse, and diversion. Use caution in heavy alcohol users. Use caution in treatment of acute abdominal conditions; may mask pain. Use tramadol with caution and reduce dosage in patients with liver disease or renal dysfunction. Avoid using extended release tablets in severe hepatic impairment. Tolerance or drug dependence may result from extended use (withdrawal symptoms have been reported); abrupt discontinuation should be avoided. Tapering of dose at the time of discontinuation limits the risk of withdrawal symptoms. Some products may contain phenylalanine.

After chronic maternal exposure to opioids, neonatal withdrawal syndrome may occur in the newborn; monitor neonate closely. Signs and symptoms include irritability, hyperactivity and abnormal sleep pattern, high pitched cry, tremor, vomiting, diarrhea and failure to gain weight. Onset, duration and severity depend on the drug used, duration of use, maternal dose, and rate of drug elimination by the newborn. Opioid withdrawal syndrome in the neonate, unlike in adults, may be life-threatening and should be treated according to protocols developed by neonatology experts.

Adverse Reactions

Cardiovascular: Chest pain, flushing, hypertension, orthostatic hypotension, peripheral edema, vasodilation

Central nervous system: Agitation, anxiety, apathy, ataxia, central nervous system stimulation, chills, confusion, depersonalization, depression, dizziness, drowsiness, euphoria, fatigue, headache, hypertonia, hypoesthesia, insomnia, lethargy, malaise, nervousness, pain, paresthesia, restlessness, rigors, sleep disorder, vertigo, withdrawal syndrome

Dermatologic: Dermatitis, diaphoresis, pruritus, skin rash

Endocrine & metabolic: Hot flash, hyperglycemia, weight loss

Gastrointestinal: Abdominal pain, anorexia, constipation, decreased appetite, diarrhea, dyspepsia, flatulence, nausea, sore throat, vomiting, xerostomia

Genitourinary: Menopausal symptoms, pelvic pain, prostatic disease, urine abnormality, urinary frequency, urinary retention, urinary tract infection

Neuromuscular & skeletal: Arthralgia, back pain, increased creatine phosphokinase, myalgia, neck pain, tremor, weakness

Ophthalmic: Blurred vision, miosis, visual disturbance

Respiratory: Bronchitis, cough, dyspnea, nasopharyngitis, pharyngitis, respiratory congestion, rhinitis, rhinorrhea, sinusitis, sneezing, upper respiratory tract infection

Miscellaneous: Accidental injury, fever, flu-like syndrome

Rare but important or life-threatening: Abnormal gait, anemia, appendicitis, bradycardia, cataract, cellulitis, cholecystitis, cholelithiasis, cognitive dysfunction, deafness, dysphagia, dysuria, ECG abnormality, edema, fecal impaction, gastroenteritis, gastrointestinal hemorrhage, gout, hematuria, hepatic failure, hypersensitivity reaction, hypoglycemia, increased blood urea nitrogen, increased gamma-glutamyl transferase, increased liver enzymes, increased serum creatinine, ischemic heart disease, menstrual disease, migraine, muscle spasm, mydriasis, night sweats, otitis, palpitations, pancreatitis, peripheral ischemia, pneumonia, proteinuria, pulmonary edema, pulmonary embolism, sedation, seizure, serotonin syndrome, skin vesicle, speech disturbance, Stevens-Johnson syndrome, stomatitis, suicidal tendencies, syncope, tachycardia, thrombocytopenia

Drug Interactions

Metabolism/Transport Effects **Substrate** of CYP2B6 (minor), CYP2D6 (major), CYP3A4 (major); **Note:** Assignment of Major/Minor substrate status based on clinically relevant drug interaction potential

Avoid Concomitant Use

Avoid concomitant use of TraMADol with any of the following: Azelastine (Nasal); CarBAMazepine; Dapoxetine; Eluxadoline; Mixed Agonist / Antagonist Opioids; Orphenadrine; Paraldehyde; Thalidomide

Increased Effect/Toxicity

TraMADol may increase the levels/effects of: Alcohol (Ethyl); Alvimopan; Antipsychotic Agents; Azelastine (Nasal); CarBAMazepine; CNS Depressants; Desmopressin; Diuretics; Eluxadoline; Hydrocodone; MAO Inhibitors; Methotrimeprazine; Metoclopramide; Metyrosine; Orphenadrine; Paraldehyde; Pramipexole; ROPINIRole; Rotigotine; Selective Serotonin Reuptake Inhibitors; Serotonin Modulators; Suvorexant; Thalidomide; Tricyclic Antidepressants; Vitamin K Antagonists; Zolpidem

The levels/effects of TraMADol may be increased by: Amphetamines; Anticholinergic Agents; Antipsychotic Agents; Antipsychotic Agents (Phenothiazines); Brimonidine (Topical); Cannabis; Cyclobenzaprine; CYP2D6 Inhibitors (Strong); CYP3A4 Inhibitors (Strong); Dapoxetine; Doxylamine; Dronabinol; Droperidol; HydrOXYzine; Kava Kava; Magnesium Sulfate; Methotrimeprazine; Nabilone; Perampanel; Rufinamide; Selective Serotonin Reuptake Inhibitors; Sodium Oxybate; Succinylcholine; Tapentadol; Tetrahydrocannabinol; Tricyclic Antidepressants

Decreased Effect

TraMADol may decrease the levels/effects of: CarBAMazepine; Pegvisomant

The levels/effects of TraMADol may be decreased by: Ammonium Chloride; Antiemetics (5HT3 Antagonists); Bosentan; CarBAMazepine; CYP2D6 Inhibitors (Moderate); CYP2D6 Inhibitors (Strong); CYP3A4 Inducers (Moderate); CYP3A4 Inducers (Strong); Dabrafenib; Deferasirox; Mitotane; Mixed Agonist / Antagonist Opioids; Naltrexone; Siltuximab; St Johns Wort; Tocilizumab

Food Interactions

Immediate release tablet: Rate and extent of absorption were not significantly affected by food. Management: Administer without regard to meals.

Extended release:

ConZip™: Rate and extent of absorption were unaffected by food. Management: Administer without regard to meals.

Ultram® ER: High-fat meal reduced C_{max} and AUC, and increased T_{max} by 3 hours. Management: Administer with or without food, but keep consistent.

Orally disintegrating tablet: Food delays the time to peak serum concentration by 30 minutes; extent of absorption was not significantly affected. Management: Administer without regard to meals.

Storage/Stability Store at 25°C (77°F); excursions permitted to 15°C to 30°C (59°F to 86°F).

Mechanism of Action Tramadol and its active metabolite (M1) binds to μ-opiate receptors in the CNS causing inhibition of ascending pain pathways, altering the perception of and response to pain; also inhibits the reuptake of norepinephrine and serotonin, which are neurotransmitters involved in the descending inhibitory pain pathway responsible for pain relief (Grond, 2004)

Pharmacodynamics Immediate release formulations:

Onset of action: ~1 hour

Maximum effect: 2-4 hours

Duration: 3-6 hours

Pharmacokinetics (Adult data unless noted)

Absorption: Immediate release formulation: Rapid and complete; extended release formulation: Delayed

Distribution: V_d: 2.5-3 L/kg

Protein binding: 20%

Metabolism: Primarily hepatic via demethylation, glucuronidation, and sulfation; N-demethylation via CYP3A4; active O-desmethyltramadol metabolite formed by CYP2D6

Bioavailability: Immediate release: 75%; extended release: Ultram ER: 85% to 90% as compared to the immediate-release dosage form

Half-life:

Tramadol: ~6-8 hours

Active metabolite: 7-9 hours (prolonged in hepatic or renal impairment)

Time to peak serum concentration: Immediate release formulations: 2 hours; extended release (formulation specific): Ultram ER: ~12 hours; orally disintegrating tablet: Food delays the time to peak serum concentration by 30 minutes

Elimination: Excreted in urine as unchanged drug (30%) and metabolites (60%)

Dialysis: <7% removed in a 4-hour hemodialysis period

Dosing: Usual Moderate to severe pain: Oral:

Children and Adolescents 4 to <16 years: Immediate release tablet or liquid: 1-2 mg/kg/dose every 4-6 hours; maximum single dose: 100 mg; maximum total daily dose is the lesser of: 8 mg/kg/day **or** 400 mg/day (Finkel, 2002; Payne, 2002; Rose, 2003)

Adolescents ≥16 years and Adults:

Immediate release formulations:

Tablet: 50-100 mg every 4-6 hours; maximum total daily dose: 400 mg/day. For patients not requiring rapid onset of effect, tolerability to adverse effects may be improved by initiating therapy at 25 mg/day and titrating dose by 25 mg every 3 days until 25 mg 4 times/day is reached. Dose may then be increased by 50 mg every 3 days as tolerated to reach 50 mg 4 times/day.

Orally-disintegrating tablet (Rybix ODT): 50-100 mg every 4-6 hours; maximum total daily dose: 400 mg/day. For patients not requiring rapid onset of effect, tolerability to adverse effects may be improved by initiating therapy at 50 mg/day and titrating dose by 50 mg every 3 days until 50 mg 4 times/day is reached; maximum total daily dose: 400 mg/day

Extended release formulations: Ultram ER: Adults ≥18 years: 100 mg once daily; titrate by 100 mg increments every 5 days if needed for pain relief; maximum: 300 mg/day

Dosing adjustment in hepatic impairment:

Immediate release formulations: Adults: Cirrhosis: Recommended dose: 50 mg every 12 hours

Extended release formulations: Ultram ER: Do not use in patients with severe (Child-Pugh Class C) hepatic impairment

Dosing adjustment in renal impairment:

Immediate release formulations: Adults: CrCl <30 mL/minute: Administer 50-100 mg dose every 12 hours (maximum: 200 mg/day)

Extended release formulations: Do not use in patients with CrCl <30 mL/minute

Administration Oral:

Immediate release tablet: May administer with or without food, but it is recommended that it be administered in a consistent manner.

Extended release tablet: Swallow whole with a sufficient amount of liquid. Do not crush, cut, dissolve, or chew extended release tablet; tablet should be taken once daily at approximately the same time each day.

Orally disintegrating tablet: Remove from foil blister by peeling back (do not push tablet through the foil). Place tablet on tongue and allow to dissolve (may take ~1 minute); water is not needed but may be administered with water. Do not chew, break, or split tablet.

Monitoring Parameters Pain relief, respiratory rate, blood pressure, and pulse; signs of tolerance, oversedation, withdrawal, abuse or suicidal ideation; renal and hepatic function

Test Interactions May interfere with urine detection of phencyclidine (false-positive).

Controlled Substance C-IV

Dosage Forms Considerations

ConZip extended release capsules are formulated as a biphasic product, providing immediate and extended release components:

100 mg: 25 mg (immediate release) and 75 mg (extended release)

200 mg: 50 mg (immediate release) and 150 mg (extended release)

300 mg: 50 mg (immediate release) and 250 mg (extended release)

EnovaRX-Tramadol and Active-Tramadol creams are compounded from kits. Refer to manufacturer's labeling for compounding instructions.

Synapryn FusePaq is a compounding kit for the preparation of an oral suspension. Refer to manufacturer's labeling for compounding instructions.

Dosage Forms Excipient information presented when available (limited, particularly for generics); consult specific product labeling.

Capsule Extended Release 24 Hour, Oral, as hydrochloride:

ConZip: 100 mg, 200 mg, 300 mg [contains fd&c blue #2 aluminum lake, fd&c yellow #10 aluminum lake]

Generic: 100 mg, 150 mg, 200 mg, 300 mg

Cream, External, as hydrochloride:

Active-Tramadol: 8% (120 g) [contains chlorocresol (chloro-m-cresol)]

EnovaRX-Tramadol: 5% (60 g, 120 g) [contains cetyl alcohol]

Suspension Reconstituted, Oral, as hydrochloride:

Synapryn FusePaq: 10 mg/mL (500 mL) [contains saccharin sodium, sodium benzoate]

Tablet, Oral, as hydrochloride:

Ultram: 50 mg [scored]

Generic: 50 mg

Tablet Extended Release 24 Hour, Oral, as hydrochloride:

Ultram ER: 100 mg, 200 mg, 300 mg

Generic: 100 mg, 200 mg, 300 mg

Extemporaneous Preparations A 5 mg/mL oral suspension may be made with tablets and either Ora-Sweet® SF or a mixture of 30 mL Ora-Plus® and 30 mL strawberry syrup. Crush six 50 mg tramadol tablets in a mortar and reduce to a fine powder. Add small portions of the chosen vehicle and mix to a uniform paste; mix while adding vehicle in incremental proportions to **almost** 60 mL; transfer to a calibrated bottle, rinse mortar with vehicle, and add quantity of vehicle sufficient to make 60 mL. Label "shake well before use". Stable for 90 days refrigerated or at room temperature.

Wagner DS, Johnson CE, Cichon-Hensley BK, et al, "Stability of Oral Liquid Preparations of Tramadol in Strawberry Syrup and a Sugar-Free Vehicle," *Am J Health Syst Pharm*, 2003, 60(12):1268-70.

◆ **Tramadol Hydrochloride** *see* TraMADol *on page 2098*

◆ **Trandate** *see* Labetalol *on page 1197*

Tranexamic Acid (tran eks AM ik AS id)

Medication Safety Issues

Sound-alike/look-alike issues:

Cyklokapron may be confused with cycloSPORINE

Brand Names: US Cyklokapron; Lysteda

Brand Names: Canada Cyklokapron; Tranexamic Acid Injection BP

Therapeutic Category Antifibrinolytic Agent; Antihemophilic Agent; Hemostatic Agent

Generic Availability (US) Yes

Use

Oral: Tablet (Lysteda): Treatment of cyclic heavy menstrual bleeding (menorrhagia) (FDA approved in females ≥12 years)

Parenteral: Short-term use (2 to 8 days) in hemophilia patients to reduce or prevent hemorrhage and reduce need for blood factor replacement therapy during and following tooth extraction (FDA approved in pediatric patients [age not specified] and adults); has also been used to decrease perioperative blood loss and the need for transfusion in patients undergoing congenital heart disease corrective surgery, scoliosis-related surgery, craniosynostosis surgery and congenital diaphragmatic hernia repair with ECMO; orally administered for the prevention of hereditary angioedema attacks (HAE) (long and short-term) and for management of traumatic hyphema

Pregnancy Risk Factor B

Pregnancy Considerations Adverse events were not observed in animal reproduction studies. Tranexamic acid crosses the placenta and concentrations within cord blood are similar to maternal concentrations. Tranexamic acid has been evaluated for the treatment of postpartum hemorrhage (Ducloy-Bouthors 2011; Gungorduk 2011). Lysteda is not indicated for use in pregnant women.

Breast-Feeding Considerations Small amounts of tranexamic acid are excreted in breast milk. The manufacturer recommends that caution be used if administered to a nursing woman.

Contraindications

Injection: Hypersensitivity to tranexamic acid or any component of the formulation; acquired defective color vision; active intravascular clotting; subarachnoid hemorrhage

Oral: Hypersensitivity to tranexamic acid or any component of the formulation; active thromboembolic disease (eg, cerebral thrombosis, DVT, or PE); history of thrombosis or thromboembolism, including retinal vein or retinal artery occlusion; intrinsic risk of thrombosis or thromboembolism (eg, hypercoagulopathy, thrombogenic cardiac rhythm disease, thrombogenic valvular disease); concurrent use of combination hormonal contraception

Warnings/Precautions Venous and arterial thrombosis or thromboembolism, including central retinal artery/vein obstruction, has been reported. Use the injection with caution in patients with thromboembolic disease; oral formulation is contraindicated. Concomitant use with certain procoagulant agents (eg, anti-inhibitor coagulant complex/factor IX complex concentrates, oral tretinoin, hormonal contraceptives) may further increase the risk of thrombosis; concurrent use with either the oral or injectable formulation may be contraindicated, not recommended, or to be used with caution. Use the injection with caution in patients with upper urinary tract bleeding, ureteral obstruction due to clot formation has been reported. Use with extreme caution in patients with DIC requiring antifibrinolytic therapy; patients should be under strict supervision of a physician experienced in treating this disorder. Use with caution in patients with uncorrected cardiovascular or cerebrovascular disease due to complications of thrombosis.

Visual defects (eg, color vision change, visual loss) and retinal venous and arterial occlusions have been reported; discontinue treatment if changes in vision occur; prompt ophthalmic examination should be performed by an ophthalmologist. Use of the injection is contraindicated in patients with acquired defective color vision since this would prohibit monitoring one endpoint as a measure of ophthalmic toxicity. Seizures have been reported with use; most often with intraoperative use (eg, open chamber cardiac surgery) and in older patients. Ligneous conjunctivitis has been reported with the oral formulation, but resolved upon discontinuation of therapy. Severe hypersensitivity reactions have rarely been reported. A case of anaphylactic shock has also been reported in a patient who received an IV bolus of tranexamic acid. Use with caution in patients with renal impairment; dosage modification may be necessary. May cause CNS depression, which may impair physical or mental abilities; patients must be cautioned about performing tasks which require mental alertness (eg, operating machinery or driving).

Potentially significant drug-drug interactions may exist, requiring dose or frequency adjustment, additional monitoring, and/or selection of alternative therapy.

Adverse Reactions

Injection:

Cardiovascular: Hypotension (with rapid IV injection)

Central nervous system: Giddiness

Dermatologic: Allergic dermatitis

Endocrine & metabolic: Unusual menstrual discomfort

Gastrointestinal: Diarrhea, nausea, vomiting

Ocular: Blurred vision

Oral:

Central nervous system: Fatigue, headache

Gastrointestinal: Abdominal pain

Hematologic: Anemia

Neuromuscular & skeletal: Arthralgia, back pain, muscle cramps/spasms, muscle pain

Respiratory: Nasal/sinus symptoms

All formulations: Rare but important or life-threatening: Allergic skin reaction, anaphylactic shock, anaphylactoid reactions, cerebral thrombosis, deep vein thrombosis (DVT), diarrhea, dizziness, nausea, pulmonary embolism, renal cortical necrosis, retinal artery/vein obstruction, seizure, ureteral obstruction, visual disturbances (including impaired color vision and loss), vomiting

Drug Interactions

Metabolism/Transport Effects None known.

Avoid Concomitant Use

Avoid concomitant use of Tranexamic Acid with any of the following: Anti-inhibitor Coagulant Complex (Human); Contraceptives (Estrogens); Contraceptives (Progestins)

Increased Effect/Toxicity

Tranexamic Acid may increase the levels/effects of: Anti-inhibitor Coagulant Complex (Human); Fibrinogen Concentrate (Human)

The levels/effects of Tranexamic Acid may be increased by: Contraceptives (Estrogens); Contraceptives (Progestins); Fibrinogen Concentrate (Human); Tretinoin (Systemic)

Decreased Effect There are no known significant interactions involving a decrease in effect.

Storage/Stability Store at 25°C (77°F); excursions permitted to 15°C to 30°C (59°F to 86°F).

Injection: According to the manufacturer, the diluted mixture may be stored for up to 4 hours at room temperature. However, solutions prepared in NS are chemically stable for up to 180 days at room temperature (McCluskey 2014). Solutions prepared in D_5W should be used within the same day of preparation (Trissels 2015). In another study, tranexamic acid (undiluted) was shown to be chemically stable for up to 12 weeks when stored at -20°C, 4°C, 22°C, and 50°C; freezing tranexamic acid in original ampuls is unacceptable due to cracking of the ampuls (de Guzman 2013). Freezing tranexamic acid in original vials has not been evaluated.

Mechanism of Action Forms a reversible complex that displaces plasminogen from fibrin resulting in inhibition of fibrinolysis; it also inhibits the proteolytic activity of plasmin

With reduction in plasmin activity, tranexamic acid also reduces activation of complement and consumption of C1 esterase inhibitor (C1-INH), thereby decreasing inflammation associated with hereditary angioedema.

Pharmacokinetics (Adult data unless noted)

Distribution: V_d: 9 to 12 L; CSF levels are 10% of plasma

Protein binding: 3%

Bioavailability: Oral: ~45%

Half-life: IV: 2 hours; Oral: 11 hours

Time to peak serum concentration:

IV: 5 minutes

Oral: 2.5 hours (range: 1 to 5 hours)

Elimination: Urine (>95% as unchanged drug)

Dosing: Neonatal

Prevention of bleeding associated with ECMO during surgery for congenital diaphragmatic hernia repair: Limited data available: Term neonates: IV: Loading dose: 4 mg/kg as a single dose 30 to 60 minutes before repair, followed by a continuous infusion of 1 mg/kg/**hour** for 24 hours, was reported to reduce blood loss and hemorrhagic complications (Keijzer, 2012; van der Staak, 1997)

Prevention of perioperative bleeding associated with cardiac surgery: Limited data available; reported dosing regimens variable and ideal dose-response not established: Term neonates (GA >36 weeks at time of procedure): IV: Loading dose: 100 mg/kg over 15 minutes, priming dose: 100 mg/kg into the by-pass circuit followed by and infusion at 10 mg/kg/hour (Graham, 2012; Schindler, 2011)

Dosing: Usual

Pediatric:

Menorrhagia: Female Children ≥12 years and Adolescents: Oral: Tablet: 1,300 mg 3 times daily; maximum daily dose: 3900 mg/**day** for up to 5 days during monthly menstruation

Prevention of bleeding associated with tooth extraction in hemophilic patients (in combination with replacement therapy): Infants, Children, and Adolescents: IV: 10 mg/kg immediately before surgery, then 10 mg/kg/dose 3 to 4 times daily; may be used for 2 to 8 days

Prevention of bleeding associated with cardiac surgery: Limited data available; reported regimens variable and ideal dose-response not established: Infants, Children, and Adolescents ≤15 years: IV: 10 mg/kg into the by-pass circuit after induction, during cardiopulmonary bypass, and after protamine reversal of heparin for a total of 3 doses; regimen used in two separate trials (n=80, age range: 2 months to 15 years) (Chauhan, 2004; Chauhan, 2004a). Also reported in the younger patients undergoing cardiac surgery (typically <2 years or 20 kg): Loading dose: 100 mg/kg, followed by 10 mg/kg/hour IV infusion (continued until ICU transport) and 100 mg/kg priming dose into the circuit when by-pass initiated (Reid, 1997; Schindler, 2011). In children 1 to 12 years and weighing 5 to 40 kg, a pharmacokinetic analysis proposed the following regimen to achieve a target serum concentration range of 20 to 30 mcg/mL: IV: Loading dose: 6.4 mg/kg over 5 minutes followed by a weight-adjusted continuous infusion in the range of 2 to 3.1 mg/kg/hour; the pharmacokinetic data showed that patients weighing less should receive an initial infusion rate at the higher end of the range (ie, if patient weight =5 kg then initial infusion rate: 3.1 mg/kg/hour; or if patient weight =40 kg then initial infusion rate: 2 mg/kg/hour) (Grassin-Deyle, 2013)

Prevention of perioperative bleeding associated with spinal surgery (eg, idiopathic scoliosis): Limited data available; reported dosing regimens variable; ideal dose response not established: Children ≥8 years and Adolescents: IV: Loading dose: 100 mg/kg, followed by infusion at 10 mg/kg/hour until skin closure (Sethna, 2005; Shapiro 2007). Other reported regimens with positive results: Loading dose: 20 mg/kg, followed by 10 mg/kg/hour infusion (Grant, 2009) or loading dose: 10 mg/kg and 1 mg/kg/hour infusion (Grant, 2009; Neilipovitz, 2001)

Prevention of perioperative bleeding associated with craniosyntosis surgery: Limited data available; reported dosing regimens variable; ideal dose-response not established: Infants ≥2 months and Children ≤6 years: IV: Loading dose of 50 mg/kg over 15 minutes prior to incision, followed by infusion at 5 mg/kg/hour until skin closure (Goobie, 2011) **or** 15 mg/kg over 15 minutes prior to incision, followed by infusion at 10 mg/kg/hour until skin closure (Dadure, 2011)

Hereditary angioedema (HAE), prophylaxis: Limited data available: Children and Adolescents:

Long-term prophylaxis: Oral: 20 to 75 mg/kg/day in 2 to 3 divided doses; maximum daily dose range: 3,000 to 6,000 mg/**day** (Bowen, 2010; Farkas, 2007; Gompels, 2005; Zuraw, 2013) **or** 1,000 to 2,000 mg daily (~50 mg/kg/day; depending on age and size of patient); may consider alternate-day regimen or twice-weekly regimen when frequency of attacks reduces; diarrhea may be a dose-limiting side effect (Gompels, 2005)

Short-term prophylaxis (eg, prior to surgical or diagnostic interventions in head/neck region): Oral:

Weight-directed: 20 to 40 mg/kg/day in 2 to 3 divided doses; maximum daily dose: 6,000 mg/**day** (Bowen, 2010; Farkas, 2007); other guidelines suggest 50 to 75 mg/kg/day in 2 to 3 divided doses (Craig [WAO], 2012)

Fixed dosing: Patients with an adequate weight (eg, ≥50 kg): 500 mg 4 times daily (Gompels, 2005); therapy usually initiated 2 to 5 days before dental work and continue for 2 days after the procedure (Bowen, 2004; Gompels, 2005)

Traumatic hyphema: Limited data available: Children and Adolescents: Oral: 25 mg/kg/dose every 8 hours for 5 to 7 days (Rahmani, 1999; Vangsted, 1983). **Note:** This same regimen may also be used for secondary hemorrhage after an initial traumatic hyphema event.

Adult:

Tooth extraction in patients with hemophilia (in combination with replacement therapy): IV: 10 mg/kg immediately before surgery, then 10 mg/kg/dose 3 to 4 times daily; may be used for 2 to 8 days

Menorrhagia: Oral: 1300 mg 3 times daily (3,900 mg/day) for up to 5 days during monthly menstruation

Dosing adjustment in renal impairment: Note: Recommendations are dependent on use and route.

Oral: **Menorrhagia:** Female Children ≥12 years, Adolescents, and Adults:

S_{cr} >1.4 to 2.8 mg/dL: 1,300 mg twice daily (2,600 mg/day) for up to 5 days

S_{cr} 2.9 to 5.7 mg/dL: 1,300 mg once daily for up to 5 days

S_{cr} >5.7 mg/dL: 650 mg once daily for up to 5 days

IV: **Tooth extraction in patients with hemophilia:** Infants, Children, Adolescents, and Adults:

S_{cr} 1.36 to 2.83 mg/dL: Maintenance dose of 10 mg/kg/dose twice daily

S_{cr} >2.83 to 5.66 mg/dL: Maintenance dose of 10 mg/kg/dose once daily

S_{cr} >5.66 mg/dL: Maintenance dose of 10 mg/kg/dose every 48 hours **or** 5 mg/kg/dose once daily

Dosing adjustment in hepatic impairment: All patients: No adjustment is necessary.

Preparation for Administration

Parenteral: Continuous IV infusion:

Pediatric: In perioperative pediatric trials, loading doses may be further diluted in 1 mL/kg or 20 mL of NS (Goobie 2011; Grassin-Deyle 2013; Reid 1997; Schindler 2011). For intravenous infusion, tranexamic acid may be further diluted with D_5W, NS, or other compatible solutions to a concentration <100 mg/mL.

Adult: Tranexamic acid doses may be diluted in 50 to 250 mL of NS or D_5W (Trissels 2015). According to the manufacturer, tranexamic acid may be mixed with most solutions for infusion such as electrolyte solutions, carbohydrate solutions, amino acid solutions, and dextran solutions.

Administration

Oral: Administer without regard to meals; tablets should be swallowed whole; do not break, split, chew, or crush.

Parenteral:

Intermittent IV doses: May be administered undiluted (100 mg/mL) by direct IV injection; use plastic syringe only for IV push; or may further dilute dose and infuse over 5 to 30 minutes; maximum administration rate: 100 mg/minute

Continuous IV infusion:
Pediatric:
Loading doses: In perioperative pediatric trials, loading doses were administered either undiluted or diluted and infused over 15 minutes (Dadure 2011; Goobie 2011; Neilipovitz 2001; Reid 1997; Sethna 2005).
IV infusion: After dilution, administer by continuous IV infusion at a rate not to exceed 100 mg/minute.
Adult: Loading doses: Usually diluted and administered over 5 to 30 minutes. Maximum administration rate: 100 mg/minute

Monitoring Parameters Ophthalmic examination (visual acuity, color vision, eye-ground, and visual fields) at baseline and regular intervals during the course of therapy in patients being treated for longer than several days; signs/symptoms of hypersensitivity reactions, seizures, thrombotic events, and ureteral obstruction

Additional Information *In vitro* data suggests that neonates require a lower serum tranexamic acid concentration than adults (6.54 mcg/mL vs 17.5 mcg/mL) to completely prevent fibrinolysis (Yee, 2013). In pediatric patients weighing 5 to 40 kg undergoing cardiac surgery with bypass, a target serum concentration range of 20 to 30 mcg/mL has been used in pharmacokinetic analysis (Dowd, 2002; Grassin-Deyle, 2013).

Dosage Forms Excipient information presented when available (limited, particularly for generics); consult specific product labeling.
Solution, Intravenous:
Cyklokapron: 100 mg/mL (10 mL)
Generic: 100 mg/mL (10 mL)
Solution, Intravenous [preservative free]:
Generic: 100 mg/mL (10 mL)
Tablet, Oral:
Lysteda: 650 mg
Generic: 650 mg

Extemporaneous Preparations A 5% (50 mg/mL) oral solution may be prepared by diluting 5 mL of 10% (100 mg/mL) tranexamic acid injection with 5 mL sterile water. Label "refrigerate". Stable for 5 days refrigerated.

A 25 mg/mL oral suspension may be prepared with tablets. Place one 500 mg tablet (strength not available in U.S.) into 20 mL water and let stand ~2-5 minutes. Begin stirring and continue until the tablet is completely disintegrated, forming a fine particulate suspension (dispersion time for each 500 mg tablet is ~2-5 minutes). Administer immediately after preparation.

Lam MS, "Extemporaneous Compounding of Oral Liquid Dosage Formulations and Alternative Drug Delivery Methods for Anticancer Drugs," *Pharmacotherapy* 2011, 31(2):164-92.

◆ **Tranexamic Acid Injection BP (Can)** *see* Tranexamic Acid *on page 2101*
◆ **Transderm-V (Can)** *see* Scopolamine (Systemic) *on page 1907*
◆ **Transderm-Nitro (Can)** *see* Nitroglycerin *on page 1523*
◆ **Transderm-Scop** *see* Scopolamine (Systemic) *on page 1907*
◆ **Trans-Plantar (Can)** *see* Salicylic Acid *on page 1894*
◆ ***trans*-Retinoic Acid** *see* Tretinoin (Systemic) *on page 2108*
◆ ***trans*-Retinoic Acid** *see* Tretinoin (Topical) *on page 2111*
◆ **Trans-Ver-Sal (Can)** *see* Salicylic Acid *on page 1894*
◆ **Trans-Ver-Sal AdultPatch [OTC]** *see* Salicylic Acid *on page 1894*
◆ **Trans-Ver-Sal PediaPatch [OTC]** *see* Salicylic Acid *on page 1894*
◆ **Trans-Ver-Sal PlantarPatch [OTC]** *see* Salicylic Acid *on page 1894*
◆ ***trans* Vitamin A Acid** *see* Tretinoin (Systemic) *on page 2108*
◆ **Tranxene-T** *see* Clorazepate *on page 516*
◆ **Tranxene T-Tab** *see* Clorazepate *on page 516*
◆ **Travatan Z** *see* Travoprost *on page 2104*
◆ **Travel Sickness [OTC]** *see* Meclizine *on page 1337*
◆ **Travel Tabs [OTC] (Can)** *see* DimenhyDRINATE *on page 664*

Travoprost (TRA voe prost)

Medication Safety Issues
Sound-alike/look-alike issues:
Travatan may be confused with Xalatan

Brand Names: US Travatan Z

Brand Names: Canada Apo-Travoprost Z; Sandoz-Travoprost; Teva-Travoprost Z Ophthalmic Solution; Travatan Z

Therapeutic Category Ophthalmic Agent, Antiglaucoma; Prostaglandin, Ophthalmic

Generic Availability (US) Yes

Use Reduction of elevated intraocular pressure in patients with open-angle glaucoma or ocular hypertension (FDA approved in ages ≥16 years and adults)

Pregnancy Risk Factor C

Pregnancy Considerations Teratogenic effects were observed in animal studies following systemic administration. If ophthalmic agents are needed during pregnancy, the minimum effective dose should be used in combination with punctual occlusion to decrease potential exposure to the fetus (Samples, 1988).

Breast-Feeding Considerations It is not known if travoprost is excreted in breast milk. The manufacturer recommends that caution be exercised when administering travoprost to nursing women.

Contraindications There are no contraindications listed in the manufacturer's U.S. product labeling.

Canadian labeling: Hypersensitivity to travoprost or any component of the formulation; pregnancy or women attempting to become pregnant

Warnings/Precautions May permanently change/increase brown pigmentation of the iris, the eyelid skin, and eyelashes. In addition, may increase the length, thickness, and/or number of eyelashes (may vary between eyes); changes occur slowly and may not be noticeable for months or years. Bacterial keratitis, caused by inadvertent contamination of multiple-dose ophthalmic solutions, has been reported. Remove contact lens prior to instillation; may reinsert 15 minutes following administration. Use caution in patients with intraocular inflammation (eg, uveitis), aphakic patients, pseudophakic patients with a torn posterior lens capsule, or patients with risk factors for macular edema. Safety and efficacy have not been determined for use in patients with renal or hepatic impairment, angle-closure-, inflammatory-, or neovascular glaucoma. Use in pediatric patients (<16 years of age) is not recommended due to possible safety issues of increased pigmentation following long-term chronic use.

Adverse Reactions
Cardiovascular: Angina pectoris, bradycardia, chest pain, hypertension, hypotension
Central nervous system: Anxiety, depression, foreign body sensation of eye, headache, pain
Dermatologic: Hyperpigmentation of eyelashes, increased growth in number of eyelashes
Endocrine & metabolic: Hypercholesterolemia
Gastrointestinal: Dyspepsia, gastrointestinal distress
Genitourinary: Prostatic disease, urinary incontinence, urinary tract infection

Hypersensitivity: Hypersensitivity reaction
Infection: Infection
Neuromuscular & skeletal: Arthritis, back pain
Ophthalmic: Blepharitis, blurred vision, cataract, conjunctivitis, corneal staining, crusting of eyelid, decreased visual acuity, dry eye syndrome, eye discomfort, eye pain, eye pruritus, hyperpigmentation of eyelids, increased eyelash length, increased eyelash thickness, iris discoloration, keratitis, lacrimation, ocular hyperemia, ophthalmic inflammation, photophobia, subconjunctival hemorrhage, visual disturbance
Respiratory: Bronchitis, flu-like symptoms, sinusitis
Rare but important or life-threatening: Asthma, bacterial keratitis (due to solution contamination), corneal edema, cystoid macular edema, iritis, macular edema, tachycardia, uveitis

Drug Interactions

Metabolism/Transport Effects None known.

Avoid Concomitant Use There are no known interactions where it is recommended to avoid concomitant use.

Increased Effect/Toxicity There are no known significant interactions involving an increase in effect.

Decreased Effect

The levels/effects of Travoprost may be decreased by: Nonsteroidal Anti-Inflammatory Agents

Storage/Stability Store between 2°C and 25°C (36°F and 77°F).

Mechanism of Action A selective FP prostanoid receptor agonist which lowers intraocular pressure by increasing trabecular meshwork and outflow

Pharmacodynamics

Onset of action: ~2 hours
Maximum effect: 12 hours

Pharmacokinetics (Adult data unless noted)

Absorption: Absorbed via cornea
Metabolism: Hydrolyzed by esterases in the cornea to active free acid; systemically; the free acid is metabolized to inactive metabolites
Half-life elimination: 45 minutes (range: 17 to 86 minutes)

Dosing: Usual Note: Do not exceed once-daily dosing (may decrease IOP-lowering effect).

Pediatric: **Elevated intraocular pressure:** Ophthalmic: Children and Adolescents: Limited data available: 1 drop into affected eye(s) once daily in the evening (Yanovich, 2008)

Adult: **Elevated intraocular pressure:** Ophthalmic: Instill 1 drop into affected eye(s) once daily in the evening

Dosing adjustment in renal impairment: Adolescents ≥16 years and Adults: There are no dosage adjustments provided in the manufacturer's labeling; however, dosage adjustments are unlikely due to low systemic absorption.

Dosing adjustment in hepatic impairment: Adolescents ≥16 years and Adults: There are no dosage adjustments provided in the manufacturer's labeling; however, dosage adjustments are unlikely due to low systemic absorption.

Administration Travoprost may be used with other eye drops to lower intraocular pressure. If using more than one ophthalmic product, wait at least 5 minutes in between application of each medication. Apply gentle pressure to lacrimal sac immediately following instillation (1 minute) or instruct patient to gently close eyelid after administration to decrease systemic absorption of ophthalmic drops (Urtti, 1993; Zimmerman, 1982). Remove contact lenses prior to administration and wait 15 minutes (after administration) before reinserting. Avoid contact of bottle tip with skin or eye; ocular solutions can become contaminated by common bacteria known to cause ocular infections. Serious damage to the eye and subsequent loss of vision may occur from using contaminated solutions

Dosage Forms Excipient information presented when available (limited, particularly for generics); consult specific product labeling.

Solution, Ophthalmic:
Travatan Z: 0.004% (2.5 mL, 5 mL) [benzalkonium free]
Generic: 0.004% (2.5 mL, 5 mL)

TraZODone (TRAZ oh done)

Medication Safety Issues

Sound-alike/look-alike issues:

Desyrel may be confused with deferoxamine, Demerol, Delsym, SEROquel, Zestril
TraZODone may be confused with traMADol, ziprasidone

International issues:

Desyrel [Canada, Turkey] may be confused with Deseril brand name for methysergide [Australia, Belgium, Great Britain, Netherlands]

Related Information

Antidepressant Agents *on page 2257*
Oral Medications That Should Not Be Crushed or Altered *on page 2476*

Brand Names: US Oleptro

Brand Names: Canada Apo-Trazodone; Apo-Trazodone D; Dom-Trazodone; Mylan-Trazodone; Novo-Trazodone; Nu-Trazodone; Nu-Trazodone D; Oleptro; PHL-Trazodone; PMS-Trazodone; ratio-Trazodone; Teva-Trazodone; Trazorel; ZYM-Trazodone

Therapeutic Category Antidepressant, Serotonin Reuptake Inhibitor/Antagonist

Generic Availability (US) May be product dependent

Use Treatment of depression, including major depressive disorder (FDA approved in adults); has also been used for treatment of insomnia and prevention of migraines

Medication Guide Available Yes

Pregnancy Risk Factor C

Pregnancy Considerations Adverse effects were observed in some animal reproduction studies. When trazodone is taken during pregnancy, an increased risk of major malformations has not been observed in the limited number of pregnancies studied (Einarson, 2003; Einarson, 2009). The long-term effects of *in utero* trazodone exposure on infant development and behavior are not known.

The ACOG recommends that therapy with antidepressants during pregnancy be individualized; treatment of depression during pregnancy should incorporate the clinical expertise of the mental health clinician, obstetrician, primary healthcare provider, and pediatrician. According to the American Psychiatric Association (APA), the risks of medication treatment should be weighed against other treatment options and untreated depression. Consideration should be given to using agents with safety data in pregnancy. For women who discontinue antidepressant medications during pregnancy and who may be at high risk for postpartum depression, the medications can be restarted following delivery. Treatment algorithms have been developed by the ACOG and the APA for the management of depression in women prior to conception and during pregnancy (ACOG, 2008; APA, 2010; Yonkers, 2009).

Breast-Feeding Considerations Trazodone is excreted into breast milk; breast milk concentrations peak ~2 hours following administration. It is not known if the trazodone metabolite is found in breast milk (Verbeeck, 1986). The long-term effects on neurobehavior have not been studied. The manufacturer recommends that caution be exercised when administering trazodone to nursing women.

Contraindications Hypersensitivity to trazodone or any component of the formulation; use of MAO inhibitors intended to treat psychiatric disorders (concurrently or within 14 days of discontinuing either trazodone or the MAO inhibitor); initiation of trazodone in a patient receiving linezolid or intravenous methylene blue

Warnings/Precautions [U.S. Boxed Warning]: Antidepressants increase the risk of suicidal thinking and behavior in children, adolescents, and young adults (18 to 24 years of age) with major depressive disorder (MDD) and other psychiatric disorders; consider risk prior to prescribing. Short-term studies did not show an increased risk in patients >24 years of age and showed a decreased risk in patients ≥65 years of age. Closely monitor for clinical worsening, suicidality, or unusual changes in behavior, particularly during the initial 1 to 2 months of therapy or during periods of dosage adjustments (increases or decreases); the patient's family or caregiver should be instructed to closely observe the patient and communicate condition with healthcare provider. A medication guide should be dispensed with each prescription. **Trazodone is not FDA approved for use in children.**

The possibility of a suicide attempt is inherent in major depression and may persist until remission occurs. Worsening depression and severe abrupt suicidality that are not part of the presenting symptoms may require discontinuation or modification of drug therapy. The patient's family or caregiver should be alerted to monitor patients for the emergence of suicidality and associated behaviors (such as agitation, irritability, hostility, impulsivity, and hypomania) and call healthcare provider.

May worsen psychosis in some patients or precipitate a shift to mania or hypomania in patients with bipolar disorder. Patients presenting with depressive symptoms should be screened for bipolar disorder. Monotherapy in patients with bipolar disorder should be avoided. **Trazodone is not FDA approved for the treatment of bipolar depression.**

Priapism, including cases resulting in permanent dysfunction, has occurred with the use of trazodone. Instruct patient to seek medical assistance for erection lasting >4 hours; use with caution in patients who have conditions which may predispose them to priapism (eg, sickle cell anemia, multiple myeloma, leukemia). Not recommended for use in a patient during the acute recovery phase of MI. The risks of sedation, postural hypotension, and/or syncope are high relative to other antidepressants. Trazodone frequently causes sedation, which may result in impaired performance of tasks requiring alertness (eg, operating machinery or driving).

Use with caution in patients with a history of cardiovascular disease (including previous MI, stroke, tachycardia, or conduction abnormalities). Although the risk of conduction abnormalities with this agent is low relative to other antidepressants, QT prolongation (with or without torsade de pointes), ventricular tachycardia, and other arrhythmias have been observed with the use of trazodone (reports limited to immediate-release formulation); use with caution in patients with pre-existing cardiac disease. May impair platelet aggregation resulting in increased risk of bleeding events (eg, epistaxis, life threatening bleeding).

Potentially life-threatening serotonin syndrome (SS) has occurred with serotonergic agents (eg, SSRIs, SNRIs), particularly when used in combination with other serotonergic agents (eg, triptans, TCAs, fentanyl, lithium, tramadol, buspirone, St John's wort, tryptophan) or agents that impair metabolism of serotonin (eg, MAO inhibitors intended to treat psychiatric disorders, other MAO inhibitors [ie, linezolid and intravenous methylene blue]). Discontinue treatment (and any concomitant serotonergic agent) immediately if signs/symptoms arise.

Serotonin syndrome (SS)/neuroleptic malignant syndrome (NMS)-like reactions may occur with trazodone when used alone, particularly if used with other serotonergic agents (eg, serotonin/norepinephrine reuptake inhibitors [SNRIs], selective serotonin reuptake inhibitors [SSRIs], or triptans), drugs that impair serotonin metabolism (eg, MAO inhibitors), or antidopaminergic agents (eg, antipsychotics). If concurrent use is clinically warranted, carefully observe patient during treatment initiation and dose increases. Do not use concurrently with serotonin precursors (eg, tryptophan).

Use caution in patients with a previous seizure disorder or condition predisposing to seizures such as brain damage, or alcoholism. Bone fractures have been associated with antidepressant treatment. Consider the possibility of a fragility fracture if an antidepressant-treated patient presents with unexplained bone pain, point tenderness, swelling, or bruising (Rabenda, 2013; Rizzoli, 2012). Use with caution in patients with hepatic or renal dysfunction and in elderly patients. May cause SIADH and hyponatremia, predominantly in the elderly; volume depletion and/or concurrent use of diuretics likely increases risk. May cause mild pupillary dilation which in susceptible individuals can lead to an episode of narrow-angle glaucoma. Consider evaluating patients who have not had an iridectomy for narrow-angle glaucoma risk factors. Potentially significant drug-drug interactions may exist, requiring dose or frequency adjustment, additional monitoring, and/or selection of alternative therapy.

Abrupt discontinuation or interruption of antidepressant therapy has been associated with a discontinuation syndrome. Symptoms arising may vary with antidepressant however commonly include nausea, vomiting, diarrhea, headaches, lightheadedness, dizziness, diminished appetite, sweating, chills, tremors, paresthesias, fatigue, somnolence, and sleep disturbances (eg, vivid dreams, insomnia). Greater risks for developing a discontinuation syndrome have been associated with antidepressants with shorter half-lives, longer durations of treatment, and abrupt discontinuation. For antidepressants of short or intermediate half-lives, symptoms may emerge within 2 to 5 days after treatment discontinuation and last 7 to 14 days (APA, 2010; Fava, 2006; Haddad, 2001; Shelton, 2001; Warner, 2006).

Adverse Reactions

Cardiovascular: Edema

Central nervous system: Agitation, ataxia, confusion, disorientation, dizziness, fatigue, headache, memory impairment, migraine, sedation

Dermatologic: Night sweats

Endocrine & metabolic: Decreased libido

Gastrointestinal: Abdominal pain, constipation, dysgeusia, nausea, vomiting, xerostomia

Genitourinary: Ejaculatory disorder, urinary urgency

Neuromuscular & skeletal: Back pain, myalgia, tremor

Ophthalmic: Blurred vision, visual disturbance

Respiratory: Dyspnea

Rare but important and life-threatening: Abnormal dreams, abnormal orgasm, acne, akathisia, allergic reactions, alopecia, amylase increased, anemia, angle-closure glaucoma, anxiety, aphasia, apnea, appetite increased, arrhythmia, ataxia, atrial fibrillation, bladder pain, bradycardia, breast enlargement/engorgement, cardiac arrest, cardiospasm, cerebrovascular accident, chest pain, CHF, chills, cholestasis, clitorism, conduction block, diplopia, dry eyes, early menses, erectile dysfunction, extrapyramidal symptoms, eye pain, flushing, gait disturbance, hallucination, hearing loss (partial), hematuria, hemolytic anemia, hepatitis, hirsutism, hyperbilirubinemia, hyperhidrosis, hypersalivation, hypersensitivity, hypoesthesia, hypomania, impaired speech, impotence, insomnia, jaundice, lactation, leukocytosis, leukonychia, libido increased, liver enzyme alteration, methemoglobinemia, MI, muscle twitching, orthostatic hypotension, palpitation, paranoia, photophobia, photosensitivity reaction, priapism, pruritus, psoriasis, psychosis, QT prolongation, rash, reflux esophagitis, retrograde ejaculation, salivation increased, seizure, SIADH, speech impairment, stupor, tachycardia, tardive dyskinesia, tinnitus, torsade de pointes, urinary frequency increased, urinary incontinence, urinary retention, urticaria, vasodilation, ventricular ectopy, ventricular tachycardia, vertigo, weakness

Drug Interactions

Metabolism/Transport Effects **Substrate** of CYP2D6 (minor), CYP3A4 (major); **Note:** Assignment of Major/Minor substrate status based on clinically relevant drug interaction potential; **Induces** P-glycoprotein

Avoid Concomitant Use

Avoid concomitant use of TraZODone with any of the following: Conivaptan; Dapoxetine; Fusidic Acid (Systemic); Idelalisib; Linezolid; Lopinavir; MAO Inhibitors; Methylene Blue; Saquinavir

Increased Effect/Toxicity

TraZODone may increase the levels/effects of: Antipsychotic Agents; Antipsychotic Agents (Phenothiazines); Fosphenytoin; Highest Risk QTc-Prolonging Agents; Methylene Blue; Metoclopramide; Moderate Risk QTc-Prolonging Agents; Phenytoin; Serotonin Modulators

The levels/effects of TraZODone may be increased by: Alcohol (Ethyl); Antiemetics (5HT3 Antagonists); Antipsychotic Agents; Antipsychotic Agents (Phenothiazines); Aprepitant; Atazanavir; Boceprevir; BusPIRone; Conivaptan; CYP3A4 Inhibitors (Moderate); CYP3A4 Inhibitors (Strong); Dapoxetine; Darunavir; Dasatinib; Fosamprenavir; Fosaprepitant; Fusidic Acid (Systemic); Idelalisib; Indinavir; Ivacaftor; Linezolid; Lopinavir; Luliconazole; MAO Inhibitors; Mifepristone; Nelfinavir; Netupitant; Palbociclib; Ritonavir; Saquinavir; Selective Serotonin Reuptake Inhibitors; Simeprevir; Stiripentol; Tedizolid; Telaprevir; Tipranavir; Venlafaxine

Decreased Effect

TraZODone may decrease the levels/effects of: Warfarin

The levels/effects of TraZODone may be decreased by: Bosentan; CYP3A4 Inducers (Moderate); CYP3A4 Inducers (Strong); Dabrafenib; Deferasirox; Fosphenytoin; Mitotane; Phenytoin; Siltuximab; St Johns Wort; Tocilizumab

Food Interactions Time to peak serum levels may be increased if immediate release trazodone is taken with food. Management: Administer immediate release after meals to decrease lightheadedness and postural hypotension. Administer extended release on an empty stomach.

Storage/Stability

Immediate release tablet: Store at room temperature; avoid temperatures >40°C (>104°F). Protect from light.

Extended release tablet: Store at room temperature of 15°C to 30°C (59°F to 86°F). Protect from light.

Mechanism of Action Inhibits reuptake of serotonin, causes adrenoreceptor subsensitivity, and induces significant changes in 5-HT presynaptic receptor adrenoreceptors. Trazodone also significantly blocks histamine (H_1) and alpha$_1$-adrenergic receptors.

Pharmacodynamics Onset of action: Antidepressant effect:

Immediate release: 1-4 weeks

Extended release: ~6 weeks

Pharmacokinetics (Adult data unless noted)

Absorption: Well absorbed

Protein binding: 85% to 95%

Metabolism: Hepatic via hydroxylation and oxidation; metabolized extensively by CYP3A4 to active metabolite, m-chlorophenylpiperazine (mCPP)

Half-life, elimination: 5-9 hours, prolonged in obese patients

Time to peak serum concentration:

Immediate release: Fasting: 1 hour; food: 2 hours

Extended release: 9 hours; not significantly affected by food

Elimination: Primarily in urine (74%, <1% excreted unchanged) with ~21% excreted in feces

Dosing: Usual

Pediatric:

Depression: Limited data available; efficacy results variable (Dopheide 2006); **Note:** Not recommended for first- or second-line treatment of depression (AACAP 2007): Oral: Immediate release formulation:

Weight-based dosing: Children and Adolescents 6 to 18 years: Initial: 1.5 to 2 mg/kg/**day** in divided doses; increase gradually every 3 to 4 days as needed; maximum dose: 6 mg/kg/**day** in 3 divided doses

Fixed-dose: Adolescents: Initial: 25 to 50 mg/**day**; increase to 100 to 150 mg/**day** in divided doses

Insomnia; sleep disturbances (in children with comorbid psychiatric disorders): Limited data available; frequently used clinically in children with comorbid psychiatric disorders (eg, mood disorder, anxiety disorder, developmental delay with ADHD) (Owens 2010): Oral: Immediate release formulation:

Children 18 months to 5 years: Dosing based on a subset of a pediatric trial which included young children (n=16; range: 20 months to 5 years) with opsoclonus-myoclonus syndrome and used fixed doses (see below); however, the median overall dose (n=19) reported was 2.6 mg/kg/**day** (range: 1.2 to 6.9 mg/kg/**day**) (Pranzatelli 2005)

Children 18 months to <3 years: Initial: 25 mg/dose at bedtime; may increase dose at 2-week intervals in 25 mg increments; maximum dose: 100 mg/dose

Children 3 to 5 years: Initial 50 mg/dose at bedtime; may increase dose at 2-week intervals in 25 mg increments; maximum dose: 150 mg/dose

Children >5 years and Adolescents: Initial: 0.75 to 1 mg/kg/dose or 25 to 50 mg at bedtime; reported range: 0.5 to 2 mg/kg/**day** (do not to exceed adult dosing: 200 mg/day); reported trials conducted in pediatric patients with comorbid psychiatric disorders (eg, ADHD, autism, developmental delay), or sleep bruxism (Hollway 2011; Kratochvil 2005); when used for palliative care, multiple daily dosing may be necessary; 25 to 50 mg/dose increase gradually to twice or three times daily as needed (do not exceed adult dosing)

Migraine, prophylaxis: Children and Adolescents ≥7 years: Limited data available: Efficacy results variable: Oral: Immediate release formulation: 1 mg/kg/**day** in 3 divided doses; maximum dose: 150 mg/dose (Battistella 1993; Damen 2005; Lewis 2004)

Adult: **Depression: Note:** Therapeutic effects may take up to 6 weeks. Therapy is normally maintained for 6 to 12 months after optimum response is reached to prevent recurrence of depression.

Immediate release: Initial: 150 mg/day in 3 divided doses (may increase by 50 mg/day every 3 to 7 days); maximum dose: 600 mg/day

Extended release: Initial: 150 mg once daily at bedtime (may increase by 75 mg/day every 3 days); maximum dose: 375 mg/day; once adequate response obtained, gradually reduce with adjustment based on therapeutic response

Dosing adjustment in renal impairment: Has not been studied; use with caution.

Dosing adjustment in hepatic impairment: Has not been studied; use with caution.

Administration Oral:

Immediate release: Administer after meals or a snack to decrease lightheadedness, sedation, and postural hypotension

Extended release: Take on an empty stomach; swallow whole or as a half tablet without food. Tablet may be broken along the score line, but do not crush or chew.

Monitoring Parameters Blood pressure, mental status, liver enzymes. Monitor patient periodically for symptom resolution; monitor for worsening depression, suicidality, and associated behaviors (especially at the beginning of therapy or when doses are increased or decreased).

Reference Range Note: Plasma levels do not always correlate with clinical effectiveness.

Therapeutic: 0.5-2.5 mcg/mL (SI: 1-6 micromoles/L)

Potentially toxic: >2.5 mcg/mL (SI: >6 micromoles/L)

Toxic: >4 mcg/mL (SI: >10 micromoles/L)

Test Interactions May interfere with urine detection of amphetamine/methamphetamine (false-positive).

Dosage Forms Excipient information presented when available (limited, particularly for generics); consult specific product labeling.

Tablet, Oral, as hydrochloride:

Generic: 50 mg, 100 mg, 150 mg, 300 mg

Tablet Extended Release 24 Hour, Oral, as hydrochloride:

Oleptro: 150 mg, 300 mg [scored]

- ◆ **Trazodone Hydrochloride** *see* TraZODone *on page 2105*
- ◆ **Trazorel (Can)** *see* TraZODone *on page 2105*
- ◆ **Trecator** *see* Ethionamide *on page 813*
- ◆ **Trecator® (Can)** *see* Ethionamide *on page 813*
- ◆ **Tremytoine Inj (Can)** *see* Phenytoin *on page 1690*
- ◆ **TRENtal [DSC]** *see* Pentoxifylline *on page 1670*
- ◆ **Tretin-X** *see* Tretinoin (Topical) *on page 2111*

Tretinoin (Systemic) (TRET i noyn)

Medication Safety Issues

Sound-alike/look-alike issues:

Tretinoin may be confused with ISOtretinoin

Vesanoid may be confused with VESIcare

Other safety concerns:

Tretinoin (which is also called all-*trans* retinoic acid, or ATRA) may be confused with isotretinoin; while both products may have uses in cancer treatment, they are **not** interchangeable.

Related Information

Oral Medications That Should Not Be Crushed or Altered *on page 2476*

Prevention of Chemotherapy-Induced Nausea and Vomiting in Children *on page 2368*

Safe Handling of Hazardous Drugs *on page 2455*

Brand Names: Canada Vesanoid

Therapeutic Category Antineoplastic Agent, Miscellaneous; Antineoplastic Agent, Retinoic Acid Derivatives; Retinoic Acid Derivative

Generic Availability (US) Yes

Use Induction of remission in patients with acute promyelocytic leukemia (APL), French American British (FAB) classification M3 (including the M3 variant) characterized by t(15;17) translocation and/or PML/RARα gene presence (FDA approved in adults); has also been used in post consolidation and maintenance therapy in APL and combination therapy (with arsenic trioxide) for remission induction in APL

Pregnancy Risk Factor D

Pregnancy Considerations Adverse events were observed in animal reproduction studies. **[U.S. Boxed Warning]: High risk of teratogenicity; if treatment with tretinoin is required in women of childbearing potential, two reliable forms of contraception should be used simultaneously during and for 1 month after treatment, unless abstinence is the chosen method. Within 1 week prior to starting therapy, serum or urine pregnancy test (sensitivity at least 50 mIU/mL) should be collected. If possible, delay therapy until results are available. Repeat pregnancy testing and contraception counseling monthly throughout the period of treatment.** Contraception must be used even when there is a history of infertility or menopause, unless a hysterectomy has been preformed. Tretinoin was detected in the serum of a neonate at birth following maternal use of standard doses during pregnancy (Takitani, 2005). Use in humans for the treatment of acute promyelocytic leukemia (APL) is limited and exposure occurred after the first trimester in most cases (Valappil, 2007). However, major fetal abnormalities and spontaneous abortions have been reported with other retinoids; some of these abnormalities were fatal. If the clinical condition of a patient presenting with APL during pregnancy warrants immediate treatment, tretinoin use should be avoided in the first trimester; treatment with tretinoin may be considered in the second and third trimester with careful fetal monitoring, including cardiac monitoring (Sanz, 2009).

Breast-Feeding Considerations It is not known if tretinoin is excreted in breast milk. Due to the potential for serious adverse reactions in the nursing infant, breast-feeding should be discontinued prior to treatment initiation.

Contraindications Hypersensitivity to tretinoin, other retinoids, parabens, or any component of the formulation

Warnings/Precautions Hazardous agent: Use appropriate precautions for handling and disposal (NIOSH 2014 [group 3]).

[U.S. Boxed Warning]: About 25% of patients with APL treated with tretinoin have experienced APL differentiation syndrome (DS) (formerly called retinoic-acid-APL [RA-APL] syndrome), which is characterized by fever, dyspnea, acute respiratory distress, weight gain, radiographic pulmonary infiltrates and pleural or pericardial effusions, edema, and hepatic, renal, and/or multiorgan failure. DS usually occurs during the first month of treatment, with some cases reported following the first dose. DS has been observed with or without concomitant leukocytosis and has occasionally been accompanied by impaired myocardial contractility and episodic hypotension; endotracheal intubation and mechanical ventilation have been required in some cases due to progressive hypoxemia, and several patients have expired with multiorgan failure. About one-half of DS cases are severe, which is associated with increased mortality. Management has not been defined, although high-dose steroids given at the first suspicion appear to reduce morbidity and mortality. Regardless of the leukocyte count, at the first signs suggestive of DS, immediately initiate steroid therapy with dexamethasone 10 mg IV every 12 hours for 3-5 days; taper off over 2 weeks. Most patients do not require termination of tretinoin therapy during treatment of DS.

[U.S. Boxed Warning]: During treatment, ~40% of patients will develop rapidly evolving leukocytosis. A high WBC at diagnosis increases the risk for further leukocytosis and may be associated with a higher risk of life-threatening complications. If signs and symptoms of the APL-DS syndrome are present together with leukocytosis, initiate treatment with high-dose steroids immediately. Consider adding full-dose chemotherapy (including an anthracycline, if not contraindicated) to the tretinoin therapy on day 1 or 2 for patients presenting with a WBC count of >5 x 10^9/L. Consider adding chemotherapy immediately in patients who presented with a WBC count of <5 x 10^9/L, yet the WBC count reaches ≥6 x 10^9/L by day 5, or ≥10 x 10^9/L by day 10, or ≥15 x 10^9/L by day 28.

[U.S. Boxed Warning]: High risk of teratogenicity; if treatment with tretinoin is required in women of childbearing potential, two reliable forms of contraception should be used during and for 1 month after treatment. Microdosed progesterone products ("minipill") may provide inadequate pregnancy protection. Repeat pregnancy testing and contraception counseling monthly throughout the period of treatment. If possible, initiation of treatment with tretinoin should be delayed until negative pregnancy test result is confirmed.

Retinoids have been associated with pseudotumor cerebri (benign intracranial hypertension), especially in children. Concurrent use of other drugs associated with this effect (eg, tetracyclines) may increase risk. Early signs and symptoms include papilledema, headache, nausea, vomiting, visual disturbances, intracranial noises, or pulsate tinnitus.

Up to 60% of patients experienced hypercholesterolemia or hypertriglyceridemia, which were reversible upon completion of treatment. Venous thrombosis and MI have been reported in patient without risk factors for thrombosis or MI; the risk for thrombosis (arterial and venous) is increased during the first month of treatment. Use with caution with antifibrinolytic agents; thrombotic complications have been reported (rarely) with concomitant use. Elevated liver function test results occur in 50% to 60% of patients during treatment. Carefully monitor liver function test results during treatment and give consideration to a temporary withdrawal of tretinoin if test results reach >5 times the upper limit of normal. Most liver function test abnormalities will resolve without interruption of treatment or after therapy completion. May cause headache, malaise, and/or dizziness; caution patients about performing tasks which require mental alertness (eg, operating machinery or driving). Effects may be potentiated when used with other sedative drugs or ethanol. Patients with APL are at high risk and can have severe adverse reactions to tretinoin. **[U.S. Boxed Warning]: Should be administered under the supervision of an experienced cancer chemotherapy physician.** Tretinoin treatment for APL should be initiated early, discontinue if pending cytogenetic analysis does not confirm APL by t(15;17) translocation or the presence of the PML/RARα fusion protein (caused by translocation of the promyelocytic [PML] gene on chromosome 15 and retinoic acid receptor [RAR] alpha gene on chromosome 17).

Tretinoin (which is also known as all-*trans* retinoic acid, or ATRA) and isotretinoin may be confused, while both products may be used in cancer treatment, they are **not** interchangeable; verify product prior to dispensing and administration to prevent medication errors.

Adverse Reactions Most patients will experience drug-related toxicity, especially headache, fever, weakness and fatigue. These are seldom permanent or irreversible and do not typically require therapy interruption.

Cardiovascular: Arrhythmias, cardiac arrest, cardiac failure, cardiomyopathy, chest discomfort, cerebral hemorrhage, edema, facial edema, flushing, heart enlarged, heart murmur, hyper-/hypotension, ischemia, MI, myocarditis, pallor, pericarditis, peripheral edema, secondary cardiomyopathy, stroke

Central nervous system: Agitation, anxiety, aphasia, cerebellar edema, CNS depression, coma, confusion, dementia, depression, dizziness, encephalopathy, facial paralysis, fever, forgetfulness, hallucination, headache, hypotaxia, hypothermia, insomnia, Intracranial hypertension, light reflex absent, malaise, pain, seizure, slow speech, somnolence, spinal cord disorder, unconsciousness

Dermatologic: Alopecia, cellulitis, pruritus, rash, skin changes, skin/mucous membrane dryness

Endocrine & metabolic: Acidosis, fluid imbalance, hypercholesterolemia and/or hypertriglyceridemia

Gastrointestinal: Abdominal distention, abdominal pain, anorexia, constipation, diarrhea, dyspepsia, GI hemorrhage, hepatitis, hepatosplenomegaly, liver function tests increased, mucositis, nausea/vomiting, ulcer, weight gain/loss

Genitourinary: Dysuria, micturition frequency, prostate enlarged

Hematologic: Disseminated intravascular coagulation, hemorrhage, leukocytosis

Hepatic: Ascites, hepatitis, liver function tests increased

Local: Phlebitis

Neuromuscular & skeletal: Abnormal gait, asterixis, bone inflammation, bone pain, dysarthria, flank pain, hemiplegia hyporeflexia leg weakness, myalgia, paresthesia, tremor

Ocular: Agnosia, ocular disorder, visual acuity change, visual disturbance, visual field deficit

Otic: Earache/ear fullness, hearing loss

Renal: Acute renal failure, renal insufficiency, renal tubular necrosis

Respiratory: Bronchial asthma, dyspnea, expiratory wheezing, larynx edema, lower respiratory tract disorders, pleural effusion, pneumonia, pulmonary hypertension, pulmonary infiltration, rales, respiratory insufficiency, upper respiratory tract disorders

Miscellaneous: Diaphoresis, infection, lymph disorder, shivering, retinoic acid-acute promyelocytic leukemia syndrome/differentiation syndrome

Rare but important or life-threatening: Arterial thrombosis, basophilia, erythema nodosum, genital ulceration, hypercalcemia, hyperhistaminemia, irreversible hearing loss, myositis, organomegaly, pancreatitis, pseudotumor cerebri, renal infarct, Sweet's syndrome, thrombocytosis, vasculitis (skin), venous thrombosis

Drug Interactions

Metabolism/Transport Effects Substrate of CYP2A6 (minor), CYP2B6 (minor), CYP2C8 (major), CYP2C9 (minor); **Note:** Assignment of Major/Minor substrate status based on clinically relevant drug interaction potential; **Inhibits** CYP2C9 (weak); **Induces** CYP2E1 (weak/moderate)

Avoid Concomitant Use

Avoid concomitant use of Tretinoin (Systemic) with any of the following: BCG; BCG (Intravesical); Multivitamins/Fluoride (with ADE); Multivitamins/Minerals (with ADEK, Folate, Iron); Multivitamins/Minerals (with AE, No Iron); Natalizumab; Pimecrolimus; Tacrolimus (Topical); Tetracycline Derivatives; Tofacitinib; Vaccines (Live); Vitamin A

Increased Effect/Toxicity

Tretinoin (Systemic) may increase the levels/effects of: Antifibrinolytic Agents; Leflunomide; Natalizumab; Porfimer; Tofacitinib; Vaccines (Live); Verteporfin

The levels/effects of Tretinoin (Systemic) may be increased by: Abiraterone Acetate; CYP2C8 Inhibitors (Moderate); CYP2C8 Inhibitors (Strong); Deferasirox; Denosumab; Mifepristone; Multivitamins/Fluoride (with ADE); Multivitamins/Minerals (with ADEK, Folate, Iron); Multivitamins/Minerals (with AE, No Iron); Pimecrolimus; Roflumilast; Tacrolimus (Topical); Tetracycline Derivatives; Trastuzumab; Vitamin A

Decreased Effect

Tretinoin (Systemic) may decrease the levels/effects of: BCG; BCG (Intravesical); Coccidioides immitis Skin Test; Contraceptives (Estrogens); Contraceptives (Progestins); Sipuleucel-T; Vaccines (Inactivated); Vaccines (Live)

The levels/effects of Tretinoin (Systemic) may be decreased by: CYP2C8 Inducers (Strong); Dabrafenib; Echinacea

Food Interactions Absorption of retinoids has been shown to be enhanced when taken with food. Management: Administer with a meal.

Storage/Stability Store capsule at 20°C to 25°C (68°F to 77°F). Protect from light.

Mechanism of Action Tretinoin appears to bind one or more nuclear receptors and decreases proliferation and induces differentiation of APL cells; initially produces maturation of primitive promyelocytes and repopulates the marrow and peripheral blood with normal hematopoietic cells to achieve complete remission

Pharmacokinetics (Adult data unless noted) Note: Reported pediatric values similar to adult (Smith, 1992; Takitani, 2004)

Absorption: Well-absorbed

Protein binding: >95%, predominantly to albumin

Metabolism: Hepatic via CYP; primary metabolite: 4-oxo-all-*trans*-retinoic acid; displays autometabolism

Half-life: 0.5-2 hours

Time to peak serum concentration: 1-2 hours

Elimination: Urine (63%); feces (30%)

Dosing: Usual Refer to individual protocols: **Note:** Induction treatment of APL with tretinoin should be initiated early; discontinue if pending cytogenetic analysis does not confirm t(15;17) translocation or the presence of the PML/RARα fusion protein.

Acute promyelocytic leukemia (APL): Oral:

Children and Adolescents: Limited data available (de Botton, 2004; Gregory, 2009; Mann, 2001; Ortega, 2005; Sanz, 2009; Testi, 2005):

Remission induction: 45 mg/m^2/day in two equally divided doses until documentation of complete remission (CR); discontinue after CR or after 90 days of treatment, whichever occurs first

Remission induction (in combination with an anthracycline): 25 mg/m^2/day in two equally divided doses until complete remission or 90 days

Consolidation therapy, intermediate- and high-risk patients: 25 mg/m^2/day in two equally divided doses for 15 days each month for 3 months

Maintenance therapy, intermediate- and high-risk patients: 25 mg/m^2/day in two equally divided doses for 15 days every 3 months for 2 years

Adults:

Remission induction: 45 mg/m^2/day in two equally divided doses until documentation of complete remission (CR); discontinue 30 days after CR or after 90 days of treatment, whichever occurs first

Remission induction (in combination with an anthracycline +/- cytarabine): 45 mg/m^2/day in two equally divided doses until complete remission or 90 days (Powell, 2010) or until complete hematologic remission (Adès, 2008; Sanz, 2008; Sanz, 2010)

Remission induction (in combination with arsenic trioxide): 45 mg/m^2/day in two equally divided doses until <5% blasts in marrow and no abnormal promyelocytes or up to 85 days (Estey, 2006; Ravandi, 2009)

Consolidation therapy: 45 mg/m^2/day in two equally divided doses for 15 days each month for 3 months (in combination with chemotherapy) (Lo-Coco, 2010; Sanz, 2010) **or** 45 mg/m^2/day for 14 days every 4 weeks for 7 cycles (in combination with arsenic trioxide) (Ravandi, 2009)

Maintenance therapy, intermediate- and high-risk patients: 45 mg/m^2/day in two equally divided doses for 15 days every 3 months for 2 years (Sanz, 2004)

Dosing adjustment in renal impairment: There are no dosage adjustments provided in the manufacturer's labeling.

Dosing adjustment in hepatic impairment: Adults:

Hepatic impairment prior to treatment: There are no dosage adjustments provided in the manufacturer's labeling.

Hepatotoxicity during treatment: Liver enzymes may normalize with dosage reduction or with continued treatment; discontinue if normalization does not readily occur or if hepatitis is suspected.

Administration Hazardous agent; use appropriate precautions for handling and disposal (NIOSH 2014 [group 3]).

Oral: Administer with a meal; do not crush capsules. Although the manufacturer does not recommend the use of the capsule contents to extemporaneously prepare tretinoin suspension, there are limited case reports of use in patients who are unable to swallow the capsules whole. For pediatric patients unable to swallow capsules, some centers have suggested softening the capsule in warm milk (in a medicine cup) for 2 minutes then having the child either chew the capsule alone or placing in a spoonful of soft food (Alba 2013; Testi 2014).

NG tube: In a patient with a nasogastric (NG) tube, tretinoin capsules were cut open, with partial aspiration of the contents into a glass syringe, the residual capsule contents were mixed with soy bean oil and aspirated into the same syringe and administered (Shaw 1995). Tretinoin capsules have also been mixed with sterile water (~20 mL) and heated in a water bath (37°C) to melt the capsules and create an oily suspension for NG tube administration (Bargetzi 1996). Tretinoin has also been administered sublingually by squeezing the capsule contents beneath the tongue (Kueh 1999). For pediatric patients, some centers have suggested contents of capsule may be mixed with milk and administered NG (Alba 2013; Testi 2014). Low plasma levels have been reported when contents of tretinoin capsules were administered directly through a feeding tube, although patient-specific impaired absorption may have been a contributing factor (Takitani 2004).

Monitoring Parameters Bone marrow cytology to confirm t(15;17) translocation or the presence of the PML/RARα fusion protein (do not withhold treatment initiation for results); monitor CBC with differential, coagulation profile, liver function test results, and triglyceride and cholesterol levels frequently; monitor closely for signs of APL differentiation syndrome (eg, monitor volume status, pulmonary status, temperature, respiration)

Additional Information For management of APL differentiation syndrome, initiate at first signs of DS: Dexamethasone 10 mg IV every 12 hours for 3-5 days; consider interrupting tretinoin until resolution of hypoxia

Dosage Forms Excipient information presented when available (limited, particularly for generics); consult specific product labeling.

Capsule, Oral:

Generic: 10 mg

Extemporaneous Preparations Hazardous agent: Use appropriate precautions for handling and disposal (NIOSH 2014 [group 3]).

Although the manufacturer does not recommend the use of the capsule contents to extemporaneously prepare a suspension of tretinoin (due to reports of low plasma levels) (Vesanoid® data on file), there are limited case reports of use in patients who are unable to swallow the capsules whole. In a patient with a nasogastric (NG) tube, tretinoin capsules were cut open, with partial aspiration of the contents aspirated into a glass syringe. The residual capsule contents were mixed with soybean oil, aspirated into the syringe, and administered (Shaw, 1995). Tretinoin capsules have also been mixed with sterile water (~20 mL) and heated in a water bath to melt the capsules and create an oily suspension for NG tube administration (Bargetzi, 1996). Tretinoin has also been administered sublingually by squeezing the capsule contents beneath the tongue (Kueh, 1999).

Bargetzi MJ, Tichelli A, Gratwohl A, et al, "Oral All-Transretinoic Acid Administration in Intubated Patients With Acute Promyelocytic Leukemia," *Schweiz Med Wochenschr*, 1996, 126(45):1944-5.

Kueh YK, Liew PP, Ho PC, et al, "Sublingual Administration of All-*Trans*-Retinoic Acid to a Comatose Patient With Acute Promyelocytic Leukemia," *Ann Pharmacother*, 1999, 33(4):503-5.

Shaw PJ, Atkins MC, Nath CE, et al, "ATRA Administration in the Critically Ill Patient," *Leukemia*, 1995, 9(7):1288.
Vesanoid® data on file, Roche Pharmaceuticals

Tretinoin (Topical) (TRET i noyn)

Medication Safety Issues

Sound-alike/look-alike issues:

Tretinoin may be confused with ISOtretinoin, Tenormin, triamcinolone, trientine

International issues:

Renova [U.S., Canada] may be confused with Remov brand name for nimesulide [Italy]

Related Information

Safe Handling of Hazardous Drugs *on page 2455*

Brand Names: US Atralin; Avita; Refissa; Renova; Renova Pump; Retin-A; Retin-A Micro; Retin-A Micro Pump; Tretin-X

Brand Names: Canada Rejuva-A; Renova; Retin-A; Retin-A Micro; Retinova; Stieva-A; Vitamin A Acid

Therapeutic Category Acne Products; Retinoic Acid Derivative; Vitamin, Topical

Generic Availability (US) May be product dependent

Use Treatment of acne vulgaris, photodamaged skin, and some skin cancers

Pregnancy Risk Factor C

Pregnancy Considerations Adverse events were observed in animal reproduction studies following topical application of tretinoin. Teratogenic effects were also observed in pregnant women following topical use; however, a causal association has not been established. When treatment for acne is needed during pregnancy, other agents are preferred (Kong, 2013). These products should not be used for palliation of fine wrinkles, mottled hyperpigmentation, and tactile roughness of facial skin in women who are pregnant, attempting to conceive, or at high risk for pregnancy.

Breast-Feeding Considerations It is not known if tretinoin (topical) is excreted into breast milk. The manufacturer recommends that caution be exercised when administering tretinoin (topical) to nursing women.

Contraindications

Hypersensitivity to tretinoin or any component of the formulation

Documentation of allergenic cross-reactivity for retinoids is limited. However, because of similarities in chemical structure and/or pharmacologic actions, the possibility of cross-sensitivity cannot be ruled out with certainty.

Warnings/Precautions Hazardous agent - use appropriate precautions for handling and disposal of tretinoin (NIOSH 2014 [group 3]). Use with caution in patients with eczema; may cause severe irritation. Avoid or minimize excessive exposure to sunlight and sunlamps; avoid contact with abraded skin, sunburned skin, mucous membranes, eyes, mouth, angles of the nose. Use is associated with increased susceptibility/sensitivity to UV light; avoid or minimize excessive exposure to sunlamps or sunlight. Daily sunscreen (SPF 15 or higher) use and other protective measures (eg, clothing over treated areas) are recommended. Treatment can increase skin sensitivity to weather extremes of wind or cold. Excessive dryness, redness, and swollen or blistered skin may occur. Also, concomitant topical medications (eg, medicated or abrasive soaps, cleansers, or cosmetics with a strong drying effect) should be used with caution due to increased skin irritation. Reduce the amount, frequency, or discontinue use until irritation disappears. Discontinue tretinoin if drug sensitivity, chemical irritation, or a systemic adverse reaction occurs.

When used for palliation of fine wrinkles, mottled hyperpigmentation, or facial skin roughness, should be used as part of a comprehensive skincare and sun avoidance program. Atralin gel contains soluble fish proteins; use caution in patients with sensitivities or allergies to fish. Gel is flammable; do not expose to high temperatures or flame. Cream 0.02%: Do not use the 0.02% cream for longer than 52 weeks when using for palliation of fine wrinkles. Cream 0.05%: Do not use the 0.05% cream for longer than 48 weeks when using for palliation of fine wrinkles, mottled hyperpigmentation, and tactile roughness of facial skin.

Potentially significant interactions may exist, requiring dose or frequency adjustment, additional monitoring, and/or selection of alternative therapy.

Warnings: Additional Pediatric Considerations Some dosage forms may contain propylene glycol; in neonates large amounts of propylene glycol delivered orally, intravenously (eg, >3,000 mg/day), or topically have been associated with potentially fatal toxicities which can include metabolic acidosis, seizures, renal failure, and CNS depression; toxicities have also been reported in children and adults including hyperosmolality, lactic acidosis, seizures and respiratory depression; use caution (AAP, 1997; Shehab, 2009).

Adverse Reactions

Dermatologic: Burning sensation of the skin, dermatitis, erythema, skin irritation

Local: Skin edema

Drug Interactions

Metabolism/Transport Effects None known.

Avoid Concomitant Use

Avoid concomitant use of Tretinoin (Topical) with any of the following: Multivitamins/Fluoride (with ADE); Multivitamins/Minerals (with ADEK, Folate, Iron); Multivitamins/Minerals (with AE, No Iron)

Increased Effect/Toxicity

Tretinoin (Topical) may increase the levels/effects of: Porfimer; Verteporfin

The levels/effects of Tretinoin (Topical) may be increased by: Multivitamins/Fluoride (with ADE); Multivitamins/Minerals (with ADEK, Folate, Iron); Multivitamins/Minerals (with AE, No Iron)

Decreased Effect There are no known significant interactions involving a decrease in effect.

Food Interactions Vitamin A toxicity may rarely occur. Management: Avoid excessive intake of vitamin A (cod liver oil, halibut fish oil).

Storage/Stability

Atralin gel, Avita gel: Store at 20°C to 25°C (68°F to 77°F); excursions are permitted between 15°C and 30°C (59°F and 86°F). Protect from freezing.

Avita cream: Store below 30°C (86°F). Avoid freezing.

Refissa: Store at 20°C to 25°C (68°F to 77°F). Do not freeze.

Renova: Store at 25°C (77°F); excursions are permitted between 15°C and 30°C (59°F and 86°F).

Retin-A cream, Tretin-X cream: Store below 27°C (80°F).

Retin-A gel: Store below 30°C (86°F).

Retin-A Micro gel: Store at 20°C to 25°C (68°F to 77°F); excursions are permitted between 15°C and 30°C (59°F and 86°F). Store pump upright.

Mechanism of Action Tretinoin is a derivative of vitamin A. When used topically, it modifies epithelial growth and differentiation. In patients with acne, it decreases the cohesiveness of follicular epithelial cells and decreases micromedo formation. Additionally, tretinoin stimulates mitotic activity and increased turnover of follicular epithelial cells causing extrusion of the comedones.

Pharmacodynamics

Onset of action: 2-3 weeks

Maximum effect: May require 6 weeks or longer

Pharmacokinetics (Adult data unless noted)

Absorption: Topical: Minimum absorption

Metabolism: In the liver
Elimination: In bile and urine

Dosing: Usual Children >12 years and Adults: Topical: Begin therapy with a weaker formulation of tretinoin (0.025% cream or 0.01% gel) and increase the concentration as tolerated; apply once daily before retiring or on alternate days; if stinging or irritation develop, decrease frequency of application

Administration Hazardous agent; use appropriate precautions for handling and disposal (NIOSH 2014 [group 3]).

Topical: Apply to dry skin (wait at least 15-30 minutes to apply after cleansing); avoid contact with eyes, mucous membranes, mouth, or open wounds

Additional Information Liquid preparation generally is more irritating

Dosage Forms Excipient information presented when available (limited, particularly for generics); consult specific product labeling.

Cream, External:
- Avita: 0.025% (20 g, 45 g)
- Refissa: 0.05% (20 g, 40 g) [contains edetate disodium, methylparaben, propylparaben]
- Renova: 0.02% (40 g, 60 g) [contains benzyl alcohol, cetyl alcohol, edetate disodium, methylparaben, propylparaben]
- Renova Pump: 0.02% (44 g) [contains benzyl alcohol, cetyl alcohol, edetate disodium, methylparaben, propylparaben]
- Retin-A: 0.025% (20 g, 45 g); 0.05% (20 g, 45 g); 0.1% (20 g, 45 g)
- Tretin-X: 0.0375% (35 g); 0.075% (35 g)
- Generic: 0.025% (20 g, 45 g); 0.05% (20 g, 40 g, 45 g, 60 g); 0.1% (20 g, 45 g)

Gel, External:
- Atralin: 0.05% (45 g) [contains benzyl alcohol, butylparaben, ethylparaben, fish collagen hydrolyzates, isobutylparaben, methylparaben, propylparaben, trolamine (triethanolamine)]
- Avita: 0.025% (20 g, 45 g)
- Retin-A: 0.01% (15 g, 45 g); 0.025% (15 g, 45 g)
- Retin-A Micro: 0.04% (20 g, 45 g); 0.1% (20 g, 45 g) [contains benzyl alcohol, disodium edta, propylene glycol, trolamine (triethanolamine)]
- Retin-A Micro Pump: 0.04% (50 g); 0.08% (50 g); 0.1% (50 g) [contains benzyl alcohol, disodium edta, propylene glycol, trolamine (triethanolamine)]
- Generic: 0.01% (15 g, 45 g); 0.025% (15 g, 45 g); 0.04% (20 g, 45 g, 50 g); 0.1% (20 g, 45 g, 50 g)

Kit, External:
- Tretin-X: 0.025%, 0.05%, 0.1% [contains benzyl alcohol, cetearyl alcohol, disodium edta, fd&c red #40, methylparaben, propylparaben, tartrazine (fd&c yellow #5), trolamine (triethanolamine)]

◆ **Tretinoin and Clindamycin** *see* Clindamycin and Tretinoin *on page 494*

◆ **Tretinoinum** *see* Tretinoin (Systemic) *on page 2108*

◆ **Trexall** *see* Methotrexate *on page 1390*

◆ **Triaderm (Can)** *see* Triamcinolone (Topical) *on page 2117*

Triamcinolone (Systemic) (trye am SIN oh lone)

Medication Safety Issues

Sound-alike/look-alike issues:

Kenalog may be confused with Ketalar

Other safety concerns:

TAC (occasional abbreviation for triamcinolone) is an error-prone abbreviation (mistaken as tetracaine-adrenaline-cocaine)

Related Information

Corticosteroids Systemic Equivalencies *on page 2260*

Brand Names: US Aristospan Intra-Articular; Aristospan Intralesional; Kenalog

Brand Names: Canada Aristospan

Therapeutic Category Adrenal Corticosteroid; Anti-inflammatory Agent; Antiasthmatic; Corticosteroid, Systemic; Glucocorticoid

Generic Availability (US) No

Use

Intra-articular (Aristospan 20 mg/mL, Kenalog-10 and -40): Adjunct therapy for acute gouty arthritis, acute/subacute bursitis, acute tenosynovitis, epicondylitis, rheumatoid arthritis, synovitis, or osteoarthritis [FDA approved in pediatric patients (age not specified) and adults]; has also been used intrabursally and into tendon sheaths

Intralesional (Aristospan 5 mg/mL, Kenalog-10): Alopecia areata; discoid lupus erythematosus; infiltrated, inflammatory lesions associated with granuloma annulare, lichen planus, neurodermatitis, and psoriatic plaques; keloids; necrobiosis lipoidica diabeticorum; possibly helpful in cystic tumors of an aponeurosis or tendon (ganglia) [FDA approved in pediatric patients (age not specified) and adults]; has also been used for infantile hemangioma

Intramuscular: Kenalog-40: Anti-inflammatory or immunosuppressant agent in the treatment of a variety of diseases, including those of allergic, hematologic, dermatologic, neoplastic, nervous system, rheumatic, endocrine, gastrointestinal, ophthalmic, renal, or respiratory origin [FDA approved in pediatric patients (age not specified) and adults]

Pregnancy Risk Factor C

Pregnancy Considerations Adverse events have been observed with corticosteroids in animal reproduction studies. Some studies have shown an association between first trimester systemic corticosteroid use and oral clefts (Park-Wyllie, 2000; Pradat, 2003). Systemic corticosteroids may also influence fetal growth (decreased birth weight); however, information is conflicting (Lunghi, 2010). Hypoadrenalism may occur in newborns following maternal use of corticosteroids in pregnancy; monitor.

Breast-Feeding Considerations Corticosteroids are excreted in human milk; information specific to triamcinolone has not been located. The manufacturer notes that when used systemically, maternal use of corticosteroids have the potential to cause adverse events in a nursing infant (eg, growth suppression, interfere with endogenous corticosteroid production); therefore, caution should be used if administered to a nursing woman. A case report notes a decrease in milk production following a high-dose triamcinolone injection in a nursing mother with a previously abundant milk supply (McGuire, 2012).

Contraindications Hypersensitivity to triamcinolone or any component of the formulation; systemic fungal infections; cerebral malaria; immune thrombocytopenia (ITP) (IM injection)

Warnings/Precautions May cause hypercorticism or suppression of hypothalamic-pituitary-adrenal (HPA) axis, particularly in younger children or in patients receiving high doses for prolonged periods. HPA axis suppression may lead to adrenal crisis. Withdrawal and discontinuation of a corticosteroid should be done slowly and carefully. Particular care is required when patients are transferred from systemic corticosteroids to inhaled products due to possible adrenal insufficiency or withdrawal from steroids, including an increase in allergic symptoms. Patients receiving >20 mg per day of prednisone (or equivalent) may be most susceptible. Fatalities have occurred due to adrenal insufficiency in asthmatic patients during and after transfer from systemic corticosteroids to aerosol steroids; aerosol steroids do not provide the systemic steroid needed to treat patients having trauma, surgery, or infections.

Acute myopathy has been reported with high-dose corticosteroids, usually in patients with neuromuscular transmission disorders; may involve ocular and/or respiratory muscles; monitor creatine kinase; recovery may be delayed. Corticosteroid use may cause psychiatric disturbances, including depression, euphoria, insomnia, mood swings, and personality changes. Preexisting psychiatric conditions may be exacerbated by corticosteroid use. Prolonged use of corticosteroids may also increase the incidence of secondary infection, mask acute infection (including fungal infections), prolong or exacerbate viral infections, or limit response to vaccines. Exposure to chickenpox or measles should be avoided; corticosteroids should not be used to treat ocular herpes simplex. Corticosteroids should not be used for cerebral malaria, fungal infections, or viral hepatitis. Close observation is required in patients with latent tuberculosis and/or TB reactivity; restrict use in active TB (only fulminating or disseminated TB in conjunction with antituberculosis treatment). Amebiasis should be ruled out in any patient with recent travel to tropic climates or unexplained diarrhea prior to initiation of corticosteroids. Use with caution in patients with threadworm infection; may cause serious hyperinfection. Prolonged treatment with corticosteroids has been associated with the development of Kaposi sarcoma (case reports); if noted, discontinuation of therapy should be considered. Increased mortality was observed in patients receiving high-dose IV methylprednisolone; high-dose corticosteroids should not be used for the management of head injury.

Use with caution in patients with thyroid disease, hepatic impairment, renal impairment, cardiovascular disease, diabetes, myasthenia gravis, osteoporosis, patients at risk for seizures, or GI diseases (diverticulitis, intestinal anastomoses, peptic ulcer, ulcerative colitis). Use caution following acute MI (corticosteroids have been associated with myocardial rupture). Because of the risk of adverse effects, systemic corticosteroids should be used cautiously in the elderly in the smallest possible effective dose for the shortest duration. Use with caution in cataracts and/or glaucoma; increased intraocular pressure, open-angle glaucoma, and cataracts have occurred with prolonged use. Oral steroid treatment is not recommended for the treatment of acute optic neuritis; consider routine eye exams in chronic users.

Withdraw therapy with gradual tapering of dose. Administer products only via recommended route (depending on product used). Do **not** administer any triamcinolone product via the intrathecal route; serious adverse events, including fatalities, have been reported. Corticosteroids are not approved for epidural injection. Serious neurologic events (eg, spinal cord infarction, paraplegia, quadriplegia, cortical blindness, stroke), some resulting in death, have been reported with epidural injection of corticosteroids, with and without use of fluoroscopy.

Rare cases of anaphylactoid reactions have been observed in patients receiving corticosteroids. Use may affect growth velocity; growth should be routinely monitored in pediatric patients. Patients may require higher doses when subject to stress (ie, trauma, surgery, severe infection). Potentially significant drug-drug interactions may exist, requiring dose or frequency adjustment, additional monitoring, and/or selection of alternative therapy.

Benzyl alcohol and derivatives: Some dosage forms may contain benzyl alcohol; large amounts of benzyl alcohol (≥99 mg/kg/day) have been associated with a potentially fatal toxicity ("gasping syndrome") in neonates; the "gasping syndrome" consists of metabolic acidosis, respiratory distress, gasping respirations, CNS dysfunction (including convulsions, intracranial hemorrhage), hypotension, and cardiovascular collapse (AAP, 1997; CDC, 1982); some data suggests that benzoate displaces bilirubin from protein binding sites (Ahlfors, 2001); avoid or use dosage forms containing benzyl alcohol with caution in neonates. See manufacturer's labeling.

Polysorbate 80: Some dosage forms may contain polysorbate 80 (also known as Tweens). Hypersensitivity reactions, usually a delayed reaction, have been reported following exposure to pharmaceutical products containing polysorbate 80 in certain individuals (Isaksson, 2002; Lucente 2000; Shelley, 1995). Thrombocytopenia, ascites, pulmonary deterioration, and renal and hepatic failure have been reported in premature neonates after receiving parenteral products containing polysorbate 80 (Alade, 1986; CDC, 1984). See manufacturer's labeling.

Warnings: Additional Pediatric Considerations Adrenal suppression with failure to thrive has been reported in infants and young children receiving intralesional corticosteroid injections for the treatment of infantile hemangioma; failure to gain weight may persist until HPA axis recovers; time to recovery of adrenal function may be prolonged (mean: 19.5 weeks; range 4 to 65 weeks) (DeBoer, 2008; Morkane, 2011). May cause osteoporosis (at any age) or inhibition of bone growth in pediatric patients. Use with caution in patients with osteoporosis. In a population-based study of children, risk of fracture was shown to be increased with >4 courses of corticosteroids; underlying clinical condition may also impact bone health and osteoporotic effect of corticosteroids (Leonard, 2007). Tissue atrophy at the site of IM injection has been reported; avoid intramuscular injections into the deltoid area. Cutaneous atrophy was reported in 2.5% of pediatric patients when given intra-articularly (Bloom, 2011). Prevention of periarticular subcutaneous atrophy via injecting small amounts of saline into the joint and applying pressure following the injection has been recommended (Hashkas, 2005).

Adverse Reactions

Cardiovascular: Arrhythmia, bradycardia, cardiac arrest, cardiac enlargement, CHF, circulatory collapse, edema, hypertension, hypertrophic cardiomyopathy (premature infants), myocardial rupture (following recent MI), syncope, tachycardia, thromboembolism, vasculitis

Central nervous system: Arachnoiditis (intrathecal), depression, emotional instability, euphoria, headache, insomnia, intracranial pressure increased, malaise, meningitis (intrathecal), mood changes, neuritis, neuropathy, personality change, pseudotumor cerebri (with discontinuation), seizure, spinal cord infarction, stroke, vertigo

Dermatologic: Abscess (sterile), acne, allergic dermatitis, angioedema, atrophy (cutaneous/subcutaneous), bruising, dry skin, erythema, hair thinning, hirsutism, hyper-/hypopigmentation, hypertrichosis, impaired wound healing, lupus erythematosus-like lesions, petechiae, purpura, rash, skin test suppression, striae, thin skin

Endocrine & metabolic: Carbohydrate intolerance, Cushingoid state, diabetes mellitus, fluid retention, glucose intolerance, growth suppression (children), hypokalemia, hypokalemic alkalosis, menstrual irregularities, negative nitrogen balance, sodium retention, sperm motility altered

Gastrointestinal: Abdominal distention, appetite increased, GI hemorrhage, GI perforation, nausea, pancreatitis, peptic ulcer, ulcerative esophagitis, weight gain

Hepatic: Hepatomegaly, liver function tests increased

Local: Thrombophlebitis

Neuromuscular & skeletal: Aseptic necrosis of femoral and humeral heads, calcinosis, Charcot-like arthropathy, fractures, joint tissue damage, muscle mass loss, myopathy, osteoporosis, parasthesia, paraplegia, quadriplegia, tendon rupture, vertebral compression fractures, weakness

Ocular: Cataracts, cortical blindness, exophthalmos, glaucoma, ocular pressure increased, papilledema

Renal: Glycosuria

Respiratory: Pulmonary edema

Miscellaneous: Abnormal fat deposits, anaphylactoid reaction, anaphylaxis, diaphoresis, hiccups, infection, moon face

Drug Interactions

Metabolism/Transport Effects Substrate of CYP3A4 (minor); **Note:** Assignment of Major/Minor substrate status based on clinically relevant drug interaction potential

Avoid Concomitant Use

Avoid concomitant use of Triamcinolone (Systemic) with any of the following: Aldesleukin; BCG; BCG (Intravesical); Indium 111 Capromab Pendetide; Loxapine; Mifepristone; Natalizumab; Pimecrolimus; Tacrolimus (Topical); Tofacitinib

Increased Effect/Toxicity

Triamcinolone (Systemic) may increase the levels/effects of: Acetylcholinesterase Inhibitors; Amphotericin B; Androgens; Ceritinib; Deferasirox; Leflunomide; Loop Diuretics; Loxapine; Natalizumab; Nicorandil; NSAID (COX-2 Inhibitor); NSAID (Nonselective); Quinolone Antibiotics; Thiazide Diuretics; Tofacitinib; Vaccines (Live); Warfarin

The levels/effects of Triamcinolone (Systemic) may be increased by: Aprepitant; CYP3A4 Inhibitors (Strong); Denosumab; Estrogen Derivatives; Fosaprepitant; Indacaterol; Mifepristone; Neuromuscular-Blocking Agents (Nondepolarizing); Pimecrolimus; Ritonavir; Roflumilast; Salicylates; Tacrolimus (Topical); Telaprevir; Trastuzumab

Decreased Effect

Triamcinolone (Systemic) may decrease the levels/effects of: Aldesleukin; Antidiabetic Agents; BCG; BCG (Intravesical); Calcitriol (Systemic); Coccidioides immitis Skin Test; Corticorelin; Hyaluronidase; Indium 111 Capromab Pendetide; Isoniazid; Salicylates; Sipuleucel-T; Telaprevir; Urea Cycle Disorder Agents; Vaccines (Inactivated); Vaccines (Live)

The levels/effects of Triamcinolone (Systemic) may be decreased by: CYP3A4 Inducers (Strong); Echinacea; Mifepristone; Mitotane

Storage/Stability Injection, suspension:

Acetonide injectable suspension: Kenalog®: Store at 20°C to 25°C (68°F to 77°F); avoid freezing. Protect from light.

Hexacetonide injectable suspension: Store at 20°C to 25°C (68°F to 77°F); avoid freezing. Protect from light. Diluted suspension stable up to 1 week.

Mechanism of Action A long acting corticosteroid with minimal sodium-retaining potential. Decreases inflammation by suppression of migration of polymorphonuclear leukocytes and reversal of increased capillary permeability; suppresses the immune system by reducing activity and volume of the lymphatic system; suppresses adrenal function at high doses

Pharmacokinetics (Adult data unless noted)

Distribution: V_d: 99.5 ± 27.5 L

Protein binding: ~68%

Metabolism: Hepatic to 3 identified metabolites (significantly less active than parent drug)

Half-life: Elimination: 88 minutes; Biologic: 18-36 hours

Time to peak serum concentration: IM: Within 8-10 hours

Elimination: 40% of dose is excreted in urine; 60% in feces

Dosing: Usual Adjust dose depending upon condition being treated and response of patient. The lowest possible dose should be used to control the condition; when dose reduction is possible, the dose should be reduced gradually.

Pediatric:

General dosing, treatment of inflammatory and allergic conditions: Children and Adolescents:

Manufacturer's labeling: Acetonide (Kenolog-40): IM: Initial: 0.11 to 1.6 mg/kg/day (or 3.2 to 48 mg/m²/day) in 3 to 4 divided doses

Alternate dosing: Limited data available: Acetonide: Children 6 to 12 years: IM: 0.03 to 0.2 mg/kg/dose every 1 to 7 days (Kliegman, 2011)

Juvenile idiopathic arthritis (JIA), other rheumatic conditions:

Manufacturer's labeling: Children and Adolescents:

Acetonide (Kenalog-10 or -40): Intra-articular: Initial: Smaller joints: 2.5 to 5 mg, larger joints: 5 to 15 mg; maximum dose/treatment (several joints at one time): 20 to 80 mg

Hexacetonide (Aristospan 20 mg/mL): Intra-articular: Average dose: 2 to 20 mg; smaller joints: 2 to 6 mg; larger joints: 10 to 20 mg. Frequency of injection into a single joint is every 3 to 4 weeks as necessary; to avoid possible joint destruction use as infrequently as possible

Alternate dosing: Limited data available: Children and Adolescents: Hexacetonide: Intra-articular: Large joints (typically knees, ankles): 1 to 1.5 mg/kg/dose; maximum dose: 40 mg; doses greater than 1.5 mg/kg have not been associated with additional clinical benefit; similar dosing for the acetonide salt can be used; however, data shows that the response is greater and lasts longer with hexacetonide (Bloom, 2011; Hashkes, 2005; Zulian, 2003; Zulian 2004)

Infantile hemangioma, severe: Limited data available: Infants and Children ≤49 months: Intralesional: Dosage dependent upon size of lesion: Commonly reported: 1 to 2 mg/kg/dose of the acetonide suspension (either 10 mg/mL or 40 mg/mL) administered in divided doses along the lesion perimeter ~monthly (4 to 5 weeks most frequently reported interval); a maximum dose up to 30 mg/dose has been used; others have reported: 1 to 30 mg of the 10 mg/mL acetonide injection divided into multiple injections along the lesion; has also been used in combination with betamethasone intralesional injections (Chen, 2000; Maguiness, 2012; Pandey, 2009; Praseyono, 2011). From the largest reported experience (n=1514, age range: 1 to 49 months), triamcinolone (1 to 2 mg/kg once every month) alone or in combination with oral corticosteroid (if no response after 6 injections of monotherapy) showed lesion size decrease of 50% or more in 90.3% of infants (age <1 year) and 80% in those >1 year (Pandey, 2009). Another trial (n=155, age range at first injection: 2 to 12 months) which used 1 to 30 mg of a 10 mg/mL concentration administered approximately once monthly (mean interval: 5 weeks) for 3 to 6 months showed lesion size decreased by at least 50% in 85% of the patients (Chen, 2000)

Dermatoses (steroid-responsive, including contact/atopic dermatitis):

Acetonide (Kenalog-10): Intradermal: Adolescents: Up to 1 mg per injection site and may be repeated 1 or more times weekly; multiple sites may be injected if they are 1 cm or more apart, not to exceed 30 mg

Hexacetonide (Aristospan 5 mg/mL): Intralesional, sublesional: Adolescents: Up to 0.5 mg/square inch of affected skin; initial range: 2 to 48 mg; frequency of dose is determined by clinical response

Adult:

Dermatoses (steroid-responsive, including contact/atopic dermatitis):

Acetonide (Kenalog-10): Intradermal: Initial: 1 mg

Hexacetonide (Aristospan 5 mg/mL): Intralesional, sublesional: Up to 0.5 mg/square inch of affected skin; range: 2 to 48 mg/day

Hay fever/pollen asthma: Kenalog-40: IM: 40 to 100 mg as a single injection/season

Multiple sclerosis (acute exacerbation): Kenalog-40: IM: 160 mg daily for 1 week, followed by 64 mg every other day for 1 month

Rheumatic or arthritic disorders:

Intra-articular (or similar injection as designated):

Acetonide (Kenalog-10 or -40): Intra-articular, intrabursal, tendon sheaths: Initial: Smaller joints: 2.5 to 5 mg, larger joints: 5 to 15 mg; may require up to 10 mg for small joints and up to 40 mg for large joints; maximum dose/treatment (several joints at one time): 20 to 80 mg

Hexacetonide (Aristospan 20 mg/mL): Intra-articular: Average dose: 2 to 20 mg; smaller joints: 2 to 6 mg; larger joints: 10 to 20 mg. Frequency of injection into a single joint is every 3 to 4 weeks as necessary; to avoid possible joint destruction use as infrequently as possible

IM: Acetonide (Kenalog-40): Initial: 60 mg; range: 2.5 to 100 mg/day

Dosing adjustment in renal impairment: There are no dosage adjustments provided in the manufacturer's labeling.

Dosing adjustment in hepatic impairment: There are no dosage adjustments provided in the manufacturer's labeling.

Preparation for Administration Hexacetonide injectable suspension: Shake well before use to ensure suspension is uniform. Inspect visually to ensure no clumping; avoid diluents containing parabens, phenol, or other preservatives (may cause flocculation). Suspension for intralesional (5 mg/mL) administration may be diluted with D_5NS, D_{10}NS, NS, or SWFI to a 1:1, 1:2, or 1:4 concentration. Solutions for intra-articular (20 mg/mL) administration may be diluted with lidocaine 1% or 2%.

Administration Shake well before use to ensure suspension is uniform. Inspect visually to ensure no clumping; administer immediately after withdrawal so settling does not occur in the syringe. Do **not** administer any product IV or via the epidural or intrathecal route. Dilute hexacetonide injection with a compatible solution prior to administration.

Acetonide:

Kenalog-10 injection: For intra-articular or intralesional administration only. When administered intralesionally, inject directly into the lesion (ie, intradermally or subcutaneously). Tuberculin syringes with a 23- to 25-gauge needle are preferable for intralesional injections. For infantile hemangioma, 27- and 30-gauge needles have been used (Chen 2000; Prasetyono 2011).

Kenalog-40 injection: For intra-articular, soft tissue or IM administration. When administered IM, inject deep into the gluteal muscle using a minimum needle length of 1 1/2 inches for adults. Obese patients may require a longer needle. Alternate sites for subsequent injections. Avoid IM injections into deltoid area.

Hexacetonide:

Aristospan (5 mg/mL): For intralesional or sublesional administration only; use a ≥23-gauge needle

Aristospan (20 mg/mL): For intra-articular and soft tissue administration only; use a ≥23-gauge needle

Monitoring Parameters Intraocular pressure (if therapy >6 weeks); weight, height, and linear growth of pediatric patients (with chronic use); assess HPA suppression. Monitor blood pressure, serum glucose, potassium, calcium, hemoglobin, occult blood loss, and clinical presence of adverse effects.

Dosage Forms Excipient information presented when available (limited, particularly for generics); consult specific product labeling.

Suspension, Injection, as acetonide:

Kenalog: 10 mg/mL (5 mL); 40 mg/mL (1 mL, 5 mL, 10 mL) [contains benzyl alcohol, polysorbate 80]

Suspension, Injection, as hexacetonide:

Aristospan Intra-Articular: 20 mg/mL (1 mL, 5 mL) [contains benzyl alcohol]

Aristospan Intralesional: 5 mg/mL (5 mL) [contains benzyl alcohol]

Triamcinolone (Nasal) (trye am SIN oh lone)

Medication Safety Issues

Sound-alike/look-alike issues:

Nasacort may be confused with NasalCrom

Other safety concerns:

TAC (occasional abbreviation for triamcinolone) is an error-prone abbreviation (mistaken as tetracaine-adrenaline-cocaine)

Brand Names: US Nasacort Allergy 24HR [OTC]; Nasacort AQ

Brand Names: Canada Nasacort Allergy 24HR; Nasacort AQ

Therapeutic Category Anti-inflammatory Agent; Corticosteroid, Intranasal; Glucocorticoid

Generic Availability (US) Yes

Use Management of nasal symptoms associated with seasonal and perennial allergic rhinitis (FDA approved in ages ≥2 years and adults)

Intranasal corticosteroids have also been used as an adjunct to antibiotics in empiric treatment of acute bacterial rhinosinusitis primarily in patients with history of allergic rhinitis (Chow, 2012) and in pediatric patients with mild obstructive sleep apnea syndrome who cannot undergo adenotonsillectomy or who still have symptoms after surgery (Marcus, 2012).

Pregnancy Risk Factor C

Pregnancy Considerations Adverse events were observed in some animal reproduction studies. Intranasal corticosteroids are recommended for the treatment of rhinitis during pregnancy; the lowest effective dose should be used (NAEPP, 2005; Wallace, 2008).

Breast-Feeding Considerations Corticosteroids are excreted in human milk; information specific to triamcinolone has not been located. The use of inhaled corticosteroids is not considered a contraindication to breastfeeding (NAEPP, 2005). The manufacturer recommends that caution be used if administered to a nursing woman.

Contraindications

Hypersensitivity to triamcinolone or any component of the formulation

Documentation of allergenic cross-reactivity for corticosteroids is limited. However, because of similarities in chemical structure and/or pharmacologic actions, the possibility of cross-sensitivity cannot be ruled out with certainty.

Canadian labeling: Additional contraindications (not in US labeling): Active or quiescent tuberculosis, or untreated fungal, bacterial and viral infection.

Warnings/Precautions Avoid use in patients with recent nasal septal ulcers, nasal surgery, or nasal trauma until healing has occurred. Avoid using higher than recommended dosages; suppression of linear growth (ie, reduction of growth velocity), reduced bone mineral density, or hypercorticism (Cushing syndrome) may occur; titrate to lowest effective dose. Reduction in growth velocity may occur when corticosteroids are administered to pediatric patients, even at recommended doses via intranasal route (monitor growth). Nasal septal perforation, nasal ulceration, epistaxis, and localized *Candida albicans* infections of the nose and/or pharynx may occur; monitor patients periodically for adverse nasal effects. Use with caution in patients with cataracts and/or glaucoma; increased intraocular pressure, open-angle glaucoma, and cataracts have occurred with prolonged use. Consider routine eye exams in chronic users.

Prolonged use of corticosteroids may increase the incidence of secondary infection, mask acute infection (including fungal infections), prolong or exacerbate viral infections, or limit response to vaccines. Exposure to chickenpox and/or measles should be avoided; corticosteroids should be used with caution, if at all, in patients with ocular herpes simplex, latent tuberculosis, and/or TB reactivity, or in patients with untreated fungal, viral, or bacterial infections. Canadian labeling contraindicates in active or quiescent tuberculosis, or untreated fungal, bacterial, and viral infection. When used at excessive doses, may cause hypercorticism or suppression of hypothalamic-pituitary-adrenal (HPA) axis, particularly in younger children or in patients receiving high doses for prolonged periods. HPA axis suppression may lead to adrenal crisis. Withdrawal and discontinuation of a corticosteroid should be done slowly and carefully. Particular care is required when patients are transferred from systemic corticosteroids to inhaled products due to possible adrenal insufficiency or withdrawal from steroids, including an increase in allergic symptoms.

Adverse Reactions

Cardiovascular: Facial edema

Central nervous system: Headache, pain

Dermatologic: Photosensitivity, rash

Endocrine & metabolic: Dysmenorrhea

Gastrointestinal: Abdominal pain, diarrhea, dyspepsia, nausea, oral moniliasis, taste perversion, toothache, vomiting, weight gain, xerostomia

Genitourinary: Cystitis, urinary tract infection, vaginal moniliasis

Local: Nasal burning (transient), nasal stinging (transient)

Neuromuscular & skeletal: Back pain, bursitis, myalgia, tenosynovitis

Ocular: Conjunctivitis

Otic: Otitis media

Respiratory: Asthma, bronchitis, chest congestion, cough, epistaxis, pharyngitis, sinusitis

Miscellaneous: Allergic reaction, flu-like syndrome, infection, voice alteration

Rare but important or life-threatening: Anaphylaxis, blood cortisol decreased, bone mineral density loss (rare; prolonged use), cataracts, dizziness, dry throat, dyspnea, fatigue, glaucoma, growth suppression, hoarseness, hypersensitivity, insomnia, intraocular pressure increased, nasal septum perforation, oral candidiasis, osteoporosis (rare; prolonged use), pruritus, sneezing, throat irritation, urticaria (rare), wheezing, wound healing impaired

Drug Interactions

Metabolism/Transport Effects **Substrate** of CYP3A4 (minor); **Note:** Assignment of Major/Minor substrate status based on clinically relevant drug interaction potential

Avoid Concomitant Use There are no known interactions where it is recommended to avoid concomitant use.

Increased Effect/Toxicity

Triamcinolone (Nasal) may increase the levels/effects of: Ceritinib

Decreased Effect There are no known significant interactions involving a decrease in effect.

Storage/Stability Store at 20°C to 25°C (68°F to 77°F); do not freeze.

Mechanism of Action Suppresses the immune system by reducing activity and volume of the lymphatic system

Pharmacokinetics (Adult data unless noted)

Absorption: Systemic absorption may occur following intranasal administration.

Half-life:

Terminal (intranasal): 3.1 hours

Elimination: 40% of dose is excreted in urine; 60% in feces

Dosing: Usual

Children and Adolescents: **Seasonal or perennial rhinitis:** Intranasal: Nasacort® AQ: Discontinue treatment if adequate control of symptoms has not occurred after 3 weeks of use.

Children 2-5 years: 110 mcg once daily delivered as 55 mcg (1 spray) **per nostril** once daily

Children 6-11 years: Initial: 110 mcg once daily delivered as 55 mcg (1 spray) **per nostril** once daily; may increase to 220 mcg once daily delivered as 110 mcg (2 sprays) **per nostril** once daily if response not adequate; once symptoms are controlled, reduce to 110 mcg once daily delivered as 55 mcg (1 spray) **per nostril** once daily

Children ≥12 years and Adolescents: Initial: 220 mcg once daily delivered as 110 mcg (2 sprays) **per nostril** once daily; once symptoms are controlled, reduce dose to 110 mcg once daily delivered as 55 mcg (1 spray) **per nostril** once daily.

Adults: **Seasonal or perennial rhinitis:** Intranasal: Nasacort® AQ: Initial: 220 mcg once daily delivered as 110 mcg (2 sprays) **per nostril** once daily; once symptoms are controlled, reduce dose to 110 mcg once daily delivered as 55 mcg (1 spray) **per nostril** once daily

Administration Shake container well before each use. Before first use, prime by pressing pump 5 times or until a fine spray appears. Repeat priming with 1 spray if ≥14 days between use. Blow nose to clear nostrils. Insert applicator into nostril, keeping bottle upright, and close off the other nostril. Breathe in through nose. While inhaling, press pump to release spray. Avoid blowing nose for 15 minutes after use. Do not spray into eyes or mouth. Discard after labeled number of doses has been used, even if bottle is not completely empty.

Monitoring Parameters Mucous membranes for signs of fungal infection, growth (pediatric patients), signs/symptoms of HPA axis suppression/adrenal insufficiency; ocular changes

Additional Information When used short term as adjunctive therapy in acute bacterial rhinosinusitis (ABRS), intranasal steroids show modest symptomatic improvement and few adverse effects; improvement is primarily due to increased sinus drainage. Use should be considered optional in ABRS; however, intranasal corticosteroids should be routinely prescribed to ABRS patients who have a history of or concurrent allergic rhinitis (Chow, 2012).

Dosage Forms Considerations Nasacort AQ 16.5 g bottles contain 120 sprays.

Dosage Forms Excipient information presented when available (limited, particularly for generics); consult specific product labeling.

Aerosol, Nasal, as acetonide:

Nasacort Allergy 24HR: 55 mcg/actuation (10.8 mL, 16.9 mL) [contains benzalkonium chloride, edetate disodium, polysorbate 80]

Nasacort AQ: 55 mcg/actuation (16.5 g)

Generic: 55 mcg/actuation (16.5 g)

Triamcinolone (Ophthalmic)

(trye am SIN oh lone)

Medication Safety Issues

Other safety concerns:

TAC (occasional abbreviation for triamcinolone) is an error-prone abbreviation (mistaken as tetracaine-adrenaline-cocaine)

Brand Names: US Triesence

Therapeutic Category Anti-inflammatory Agent, Ophthalmic; Corticosteroid, Ophthalmic

Generic Availability (US) No

Use Intravitreal: Treatment of sympathetic ophthalmia, temporal arteritis, uveitis, ocular inflammatory conditions unresponsive to topical corticosteroids; visualization during vitrectomy

Pregnancy Risk Factor D

Pregnancy Considerations Triamcinolone was shown to be teratogenic in animal reproduction studies. Some studies have shown an association between first trimester corticosteroid use and oral clefts; adverse events in the fetus/neonate have been noted in case reports following large doses of systemic corticosteroids during pregnancy. The amount of triamcinolone absorbed systemically following ophthalmic administration is not known.

Breast-Feeding Considerations Corticosteroids are excreted in human milk; information specific to triamcinolone has not been located. The amount of triamcinolone absorbed systemically following ophthalmic administration is not known.

Contraindications Hypersensitivity to triamcinolone or any component of the formulation; cerebral malaria; idiopathic thrombocytopenia purpura; systemic fungal infections

Warnings/Precautions Use with caution in patients with cataracts and/or glaucoma; increased intraocular pressure, open-angle glaucoma, and cataracts have occurred with prolonged use. Monitor closely for increased intraocular pressure. Consider routine eye exams in chronic users. Do not use in patients with active ocular herpes simplex. Intravitreal injection has been associated with endophthalmitis and visual disturbances. Blindness has been reported following injection into nasal turbinates and intralesional injections into the head. Safety of intraturbinal, subconjunctival, subtenons, or retrobulbar injections has not been demonstrated.

May be absorbed systemically. Absorption may cause manifestations of Cushing's syndrome, hyperglycemia, or glycosuria. Other systemic effects include CNS/behavioral changes, hypertension, gastrointestinal perforation, acute myopathy, and osteoporosis. Prolonged use may cause hypercorticism or suppression of hypothalamic-pituitary-adrenal (HPA) axis, particularly in younger children or in patients receiving high doses for prolonged periods. HPA axis suppression may lead to adrenal crisis. Prolonged use may result in fungal or bacterial ocular superinfection; discontinue if infection persists despite appropriate antimicrobial therapy.

Some dosage forms may contain polysorbate 80 (also known as Tweens). Hypersensitivity reactions, usually a delayed reaction, have been reported following exposure to pharmaceutical products containing polysorbate 80 in certain individuals (Isaksson, 2002; Lucente 2000; Shelley, 1995). Thrombocytopenia, ascites, pulmonary deterioration, and renal and hepatic failure have been reported in premature neonates after receiving parenteral products containing polysorbate 80 (Alade, 1986; CDC, 1984). See manufacturer's labeling.

Adverse Reactions

Blurred vision, cataract progression, conjunctival hemorrhage, discomfort (transient), endophthalmitis, glaucoma, hypopyon, inflammation, intraocular pressure increase, optic disc vascular disorder, retinal detachment, vitreous floaters, visual acuity decreased

Rare but important or life-threatening: Exophthalmos

Drug Interactions

Metabolism/Transport Effects None known.

Avoid Concomitant Use There are no known interactions where it is recommended to avoid concomitant use.

Increased Effect/Toxicity

Triamcinolone (Ophthalmic) may increase the levels/effects of: Ceritinib

The levels/effects of Triamcinolone (Ophthalmic) may be increased by: NSAID (Ophthalmic)

Decreased Effect There are no known significant interactions involving a decrease in effect.

Storage/Stability Triesence™: Store at 4°C to 25°C (39°F to 77°F); do not freeze. Protect from light.

Mechanism of Action Suppresses the immune system by reducing activity and volume of the lymphatic system

Pharmacokinetics (Adult data unless noted) Half-life elimination: Biologic: 18-36 hours

Dosing: Usual Ophthalmic injection: Intravitreal: Children and Adults:

Ocular disease: Initial: 4 mg as a single dose; additional doses may be given as needed over the course of treatment

Visualization during vitrectomy: 1-4 mg

Administration Not for IV use. Shake vial well prior to use. Administer under controlled aseptic conditions (eg, sterile gloves, sterile drape, sterile eyelid speculum). Adequate anesthesia and a broad-spectrum bactericidal agent should be administered prior to injection. Inject immediately after withdrawing from vial. If administration is required in the second eye, a new vial should be used. Do not use if agglomerated (clumpy or granular appearance).

Monitoring Parameters Following injection, monitor for increased intraocular pressure and endophthalmitis; check for perfusion of optic nerve head immediately after injection, tonometry within 30 minutes, biomicroscopy between 2-7 days after injection.

Dosage Forms Excipient information presented when available (limited, particularly for generics); consult specific product labeling.

Suspension, Intraocular, as acetonide:

Triesence: 40 mg/mL (1 mL) [contains polysorbate 80]

Triamcinolone (Topical) (trye am SIN oh lone)

Medication Safety Issues

Sound-alike/look-alike issues:

Kenalog® may be confused with Ketalar®

Other safety concerns:

TAC (occasional abbreviation for triamcinolone) is an error-prone abbreviation (mistaken as tetracaine-adrenaline-cocaine)

Related Information

Topical Corticosteroids *on page 2262*

Brand Names: US Dermasorb TA; Kenalog; Oralone; Pediaderm TA; Trianex; Triderm

Brand Names: Canada Kenalog®; Oracort; Triaderm

Therapeutic Category Anti-inflammatory Agent, Topical; Corticosteroid, Topical; Glucocorticoid

Generic Availability (US) May be product dependent

Use

Cream, lotion, ointment, and spray: Relief of inflammation and pruritus associated with corticosteroid-responsive dermatoses [FDA approved in pediatric patients (age not specified) and adults]

Dental paste: Adjunctive treatment and temporary relief of symptoms related to oral inflammatory lesions and ulcerative lesions due to trauma (FDA approved in adults)

Pregnancy Risk Factor C

Pregnancy Considerations Corticosteroids were found to be teratogenic following topical application in animal reproduction studies. In general, the use of topical corticosteroids during pregnancy is not considered to have significant risk, however, intrauterine growth retardation in the infant has been reported (rare). The use of large amounts or for prolonged periods of time should be avoided.

Breast-Feeding Considerations Corticosteroids are excreted in human milk; information specific to triamcinolone has not been located. The amount of triamcinolone absorbed systemically following topical administration is variable. Hypertension in the nursing infant has been reported following corticosteroid ointment applied to the nipples. Use with caution.

Contraindications Hypersensitivity to triamcinolone or any component of the formulation; fungal, viral, or bacterial infections of the mouth or throat (oral topical formulation)

Warnings/Precautions Topical corticosteroids may be absorbed percutaneously. Absorption may cause manifestations of Cushing's syndrome, hyperglycemia, or glycosuria. Absorption is increased by the use of occlusive dressings, application to denuded skin, or application to large surface areas. Do not use occlusive dressings on weeping or exudative lesions and general caution with occlusive dressings should be observed; discontinue if skin irritation or contact dermatitis should occur; do not use in patients with decreased skin circulation. May cause hypercorticism or suppression of hypothalamic-pituitary-adrenal (HPA) axis, particularly in younger children or in patients receiving high doses for prolonged periods. HPA axis suppression may lead to adrenal crisis.

Prolonged use may result in fungal or bacterial superinfection; discontinue if dermatological infection persists despite appropriate antimicrobial therapy. Topical use has been associated with local sensitization (redness, irritation); discontinue if sensitization is noted. When used as a topical agent in the oral cavity, if significant regeneration or repair of oral tissues has not occurred in seven days, re-evaluation of the etiology of the oral lesion is advised.

Because of the risk of adverse effects associated with systemic absorption, topical corticosteroids should be used cautiously in the elderly in the smallest possible effective dose for the shortest duration. Children may absorb proportionally larger amounts after topical application and may be more prone to systemic effects. HPA axis suppression, intracranial hypertension, and Cushing's syndrome have been reported in children receiving topical corticosteroids. Prolonged use may affect growth velocity; growth should be routinely monitored in pediatric patients. Some dosage forms may contain polysorbate 80 (also known as Tweens). Hypersensitivity reactions, usually a delayed reaction, have been reported following exposure to pharmaceutical products containing polysorbate 80 in certain individuals (Isaksson, 2002; Lucente 2000; Shelley, 1995). Thrombocytopenia, ascites, pulmonary deterioration, and renal and hepatic failure have been reported in premature neonates after receiving parenteral products containing polysorbate 80 (Alade, 1986; CDC, 1984). See manufacturer's labeling.

Warnings: Additional Pediatric Considerations Topical corticosteroids may be absorbed percutaneously. The extent of absorption is dependent on several factors, including epidermal integrity (intact vs abraded skin), formulation, age of the patient, prolonged duration of use, and the use of occlusive dressings. Percutaneous absorption of topical steroids is increased in neonates (especially preterm neonates), infants, and young children. Hypothalamic-pituitary-adrenal (HPA) suppression may occur, particularly in younger children or in patients receiving high doses for prolonged periods; acute adrenal insufficiency (adrenal crisis) may occur with abrupt withdrawal after long-term therapy or with stress. Infants and small children may be more susceptible to HPA axis suppression or other systemic toxicities due to larger skin surface area to body mass ratio; use with caution in pediatric patients.

Some dosage forms may contain propylene glycol; in neonates large amounts of propylene glycol delivered orally, intravenously (eg, >3,000 mg/day), or topically have been associated with potentially fatal toxicities which can include metabolic acidosis, seizures, renal failure, and CNS depression; toxicities have also been reported in children and adults including hyperosmolality, lactic acidosis, seizures and respiratory depression; use caution (AAP, 1997; Shehab, 2009).

Adverse Reactions

Dermatologic: Acneiform eruptions, allergic contact dermatitis, dryness, folliculitis, hypertrichosis, hypopigmentation, miliaria, perioral dermatitis, pruritus, skin atrophy, skin infection (secondary), skin maceration, striae

Endocrine: HPA axis suppression; metabolic effects (hyperglycemia, hypokalemia)

Local: Burning, irritation

Drug Interactions

Metabolism/Transport Effects None known.

Avoid Concomitant Use

Avoid concomitant use of Triamcinolone (Topical) with any of the following: Aldesleukin

Increased Effect/Toxicity

Triamcinolone (Topical) may increase the levels/effects of: Ceritinib; Deferasirox

The levels/effects of Triamcinolone (Topical) may be increased by: Telaprevir

Decreased Effect

Triamcinolone (Topical) may decrease the levels/effects of: Aldesleukin; Corticorelin; Hyaluronidase; Telaprevir

Storage/Stability

Lotion/ointment: Store at room temperature.

Spray: Store at room temperature; avoid excessive heat.

Paste: Store at 20°C to 25°C (68°F to 77°F).

Mechanism of Action Topical corticosteroids have anti-inflammatory, antipruritic, and vasoconstrictive properties. May depress the formation, release, and activity of endogenous chemical mediators of inflammation (kinins, histamine, liposomal enzymes, prostaglandins) through the induction of phospholipase A_2 inhibitory proteins (lipocortins) and sequential inhibition of the release of arachidonic acid. Triamcinolone has intermediate to high range potency (dosage-form dependent).

Pharmacokinetics (Adult data unless noted)

Absorption: Topical corticosteroids are absorbed percutaneously. The extent is dependent on several factors, including epidermal integrity (intact vs abraded skin), formulation, and the use of occlusive dressings.

Metabolism: Hepatic

Half-life: Biologic: 18-36 hours

Elimination: 40% of dose is excreted in urine; 60% in feces

Dosing: Usual

Infants, Children, and Adolescents: **Dermatoses (steroid-responsive, including contact/atopic dermatitis):** Topical: **Note:** Frequency based upon severity of condition:

- Cream, Ointment:
  - 0.025% or 0.05%: Apply thin film to affected areas 2-4 times daily
  - 0.1% or 0.5%: Apply thin film to affected areas 2-3 times daily
- Lotion:
  - 0.025%: Apply 2-4 times daily
  - 0.1%: Apply 2-3 times daily
- Spray: Apply to affected area up to 3-4 times daily

Adult:

Dermatoses (steroid-responsive, including contact/atopic dermatitis): Topical:

- Cream, Ointment:
  - 0.025% or 0.05%: Apply thin film to affected areas 2-4 times/daily
  - 0.1% or 0.5%: Apply thin film to affected areas 2-3 times daily
- Spray: Apply to affected area 3-4 times daily

Oral inflammatory lesions/ulcers: Oral topical (dental paste): Press a small dab (about 1/4 inch) to the lesion 1-3 times daily until a thin film develops; a larger quantity may be required for coverage of some lesions. For optimal results, use only enough to coat the lesion with a thin film; do not rub in.

Administration

Topical: Apply sparingly to affected area and gently rub in until disappears; do not occlude area, unless directed; do not use on open skin; avoid contact with eyes

Dental: Apply small dab until thin, smooth film develops; do not rub in; spreading the paste may result in a granular, gritty sensation and crumbling; apply at bedtime to allow contact of the medication with the lesion overnight; if more frequent application is necessary, apply after meals.

Monitoring Parameters Growth in pediatric patients; assess HPA axis suppression (eg, ACTH stimulation test, morning plasma cortisol test, urinary free cortisol test)

Dosage Forms Excipient information presented when available (limited, particularly for generics); consult specific product labeling. [DSC] = Discontinued product

Aerosol Solution, External, as acetonide:
- Kenalog: (63 g, 100 g)
- Generic: (63 g, 100 g)

Cream, External, as acetonide:
- Triderm: 0.1% (28.4 g, 85.2 g) [contains propylene glycol]
- Generic: 0.025% (15 g, 80 g, 454 g); 0.1% (15 g, 30 g, 80 g, 453.6 g, 454 g); 0.5% (15 g)

Kit, External, as acetonide:
- Dermasorb TA: 0.1% [contains cetyl alcohol, milk protein, propylene glycol]
- Pediaderm TA: 0.1% [contains cetyl alcohol, methylparaben, polysorbate 80, propylene glycol, propylparaben]

Lotion, External, as acetonide:
- Generic: 0.025% (60 mL); 0.1% (60 mL)

Ointment, External, as acetonide:
- Trianex: 0.05% (17 g [DSC], 85 g [DSC], 430 g)
- Generic: 0.025% (15 g, 80 g, 454 g); 0.1% (15 g, 80 g, 453.6 g, 454 g); 0.5% (15 g)

Paste, Mouth/Throat, as acetonide:
- Oralone: 0.1% (5 g)
- Generic: 0.1% (5 g)

◆ **Triamcinolone Acetonide** *see* Triamcinolone (Nasal) *on page 2115*

◆ **Triamcinolone acetonide** *see* Triamcinolone (Ophthalmic) *on page 2116*

◆ **Triamcinolone Acetonide, Parenteral** *see* Triamcinolone (Systemic) *on page 2112*

◆ **Triamcinolone Hexacetonide** *see* Triamcinolone (Systemic) *on page 2112*

◆ **Triaminic Allerchews [OTC]** *see* Loratadine *on page 1296*

◆ **Triaminic Children's Fever Reducer Pain Reliever [OTC]** *see* Acetaminophen *on page 44*

◆ **Triaminic Cough & Congestion [OTC]** *see* Guaifenesin and Dextromethorphan *on page 992*

◆ **Triaminic Cough/Runny Nose [OTC]** *see* DiphenhydrAMINE (Systemic) *on page 668*

◆ **Triaminic Long Acting Cough [OTC]** *see* Dextromethorphan *on page 631*

Triamterene (trye AM ter een)

Medication Safety Issues

Sound-alike/look-alike issues:

Triamterene may be confused with trimipramine

Dyrenium may be confused with Pyridium

Brand Names: US Dyrenium

Therapeutic Category Antihypertensive Agent; Diuretic, Potassium Sparing

Generic Availability (US) No

Use Used alone or in combination with other diuretics to treat edema and hypertension; decreases potassium excretion caused by kaliuretic diuretics

Pregnancy Risk Factor C

Pregnancy Considerations Adverse events have not been observed in animal reproduction studies. Triamterene crosses the placenta and is found in cord blood. Use of triamterene to treat edema during normal pregnancies is not appropriate; use may be considered when edema is due to pathologic causes (as in the nonpregnant patient); monitor.

Breast-Feeding Considerations It is not known if triamterene is excreted in breast milk. Breast-feeding is not recommended by the manufacturer.

Contraindications Anuria; severe or progressive kidney disease or dysfunction with the possible exception of nephrosis; severe hepatic disease; hypersensitivity to the drug or any of its components; preexisting elevated serum potassium, as is sometimes seen in patients with impaired renal function or azotemia, or in patients who develop hyperkalemia while on the drug; coadministration with other potassium-sparing agents, such as spironolactone, amiloride, or other formulations containing triamterene

Warnings/Precautions [U.S. Boxed Warning]: Hyperkalemia can occur; patients at risk include those with renal impairment, diabetes, the elderly, and the severely ill. Serum potassium levels must be monitored at frequent intervals especially when dosages are changed or with any illness that may cause renal dysfunction. In patients who develop hyperkalemia or if hyperkalemia is suspected, obtain an electrocardiogram to rule out hyperkalemia-induced QRS prolongation or other cardiac arrhythmias. Discontinue triamterene and any potassium supplementation in patients who develop hyperkalemia; treat cardiac arrhythmias as clinically indicated. Triamterene can lead to profound diuresis with fluid and electrolyte loss; close medical supervision and dose evaluation are required. Patients with heart failure, renal disease, or cirrhosis may be particularly susceptible to fluid and electrolyte abnormalities. Watch for and correct electrolyte disturbances; adjust dose to avoid dehydration. Avoid potassium supplements, potassium-containing salt substitutes, a diet rich in potassium, or other drugs that can cause hyperkalemia. Use with caution in patients with severe hepatic dysfunction; in cirrhosis, avoid electrolyte and acid/base imbalances that might lead to hepatic encephalopathy Use with caution in patients with prediabetes or diabetes mellitus; may increase blood glucose concentrations and necessitate dosage adjustment of hypoglycemic agents. Use cautiously in patients with history of kidney stones and gout; may cause elevation in uric acid. Potentially significant drug-drug interactions may exist, requiring dose or frequency adjustment, additional monitoring, and/or selection of alternative therapy. Isolated occurrences of hypersensitively reactions have been reported. Observe for blood dyscrasias, liver damage or idiosyncratic reactions. Can cause photosensitivity. Withdraw triamterene gradually in patients who have received triamterene for prolonged periods of time.

Adverse Reactions

Central nervous system: Dizziness, fatigue, headache

Dermatologic: Skin photosensitivity, skin rash

Endocrine & metabolic: Hyperkalemia, hypokalemia, increased uric acid, metabolic acidosis

Gastrointestinal: Diarrhea, nausea, vomiting, xerostomia

Genitourinary: Azotemia

Hematologic & oncologic: Hematologic abnormality, megaloblastic anemia, thrombocytopenia

Hepatic: Jaundice, liver enzyme disorder

Hypersensitivity: Anaphylaxis

Neuromuscular & skeletal: Weakness

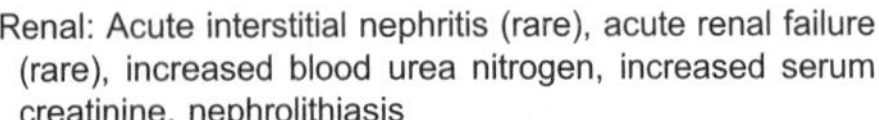

Renal: Acute interstitial nephritis (rare), acute renal failure (rare), increased blood urea nitrogen, increased serum creatinine, nephrolithiasis

Drug Interactions

Metabolism/Transport Effects None known.

Avoid Concomitant Use

Avoid concomitant use of Triamterene with any of the following: CycloSPORINE (Systemic); Spironolactone; Tacrolimus (Systemic)

Increased Effect/Toxicity

Triamterene may increase the levels/effects of: ACE Inhibitors; Amifostine; Ammonium Chloride; Antihypertensives; Cardiac Glycosides; CycloSPORINE (Systemic); Dofetilide; DULoxetine; Hypotensive Agents; Levodopa; Obinutuzumab; RisperiDONE; RiTUXimab; Sodium Phosphates; Spironolactone; Tacrolimus (Systemic)

The levels/effects of Triamterene may be increased by: Alfuzosin; Analgesics (Opioid); Angiotensin II Receptor Blockers; Barbiturates; Brimonidine (Topical); Canagliflozin; Diazoxide; Drospirenone; Eplerenone; Heparin; Heparin (Low Molecular Weight); Herbs (Hypotensive Properties); Indomethacin; MAO Inhibitors; Nicorandil; Nonsteroidal Anti-Inflammatory Agents; Pentoxifylline; Phosphodiesterase 5 Inhibitors; Potassium Salts; Prostacyclin Analogues; Tolvaptan

Decreased Effect

Triamterene may decrease the levels/effects of: Cardiac Glycosides; QuiNIDine

The levels/effects of Triamterene may be decreased by: Herbs (Hypertensive Properties); Methylphenidate; Nonsteroidal Anti-Inflammatory Agents; Yohimbine

Mechanism of Action Blocks epithelial sodium channels in the late distal convoluted tubule (DCT) and collecting duct which inhibits sodium reabsorption from the lumen. This effectively reduces intracellular sodium, decreasing the function of Na+/K+ ATPase, leading to potassium retention and decreased calcium, magnesium, and hydrogen excretion. As sodium uptake capacity in the DCT/collecting duct is limited, the natriuretic, diuretic, and antihypertensive effects are generally considered weak.

Pharmacodynamics

Onset of action: Diuresis occurs within 2-4 hours

Duration: 7-9 hours

Note: Maximum therapeutic effect may not occur until after several days of therapy

Pharmacokinetics (Adult data unless noted)

Absorption: Oral: Unreliably absorbed

Metabolism: Hepatic conjugation

Half-life: 100-150 minutes

Elimination: 21% excreted unchanged in urine

Dosing: Usual Oral:

Children: 1-2 mg/kg/day in 1-2 divided doses; maximum dose: 3-4 mg/kg/day and not to exceed 300 mg/day

Adults: 100-300 mg/day in 1-2 divided doses; usual dosage range (JNC 7): 50-100 mg/day

Dosage adjustment in renal impairment: CrCl <10 mL/minute: Avoid use

Dosage adjustment in hepatic impairment: Dose reduction is recommended in patients with cirrhosis

Administration Oral: Administer with food to avoid GI upset

Monitoring Parameters Electrolytes (sodium, potassium, magnesium, HCO_3, chloride), CBC, BUN, creatinine, platelets

Test Interactions Interferes with fluorometric assay of quinidine

Additional Information Abrupt discontinuation of therapy may result in rebound kaliuresis; taper off gradually

Dosage Forms Excipient information presented when available (limited, particularly for generics); consult specific product labeling.

Capsule, Oral:

Dyrenium: 50 mg [contains fd&c yellow #6 (sunset yellow)]

Dyrenium: 100 mg

- ◆ **Trianex** *see* Triamcinolone (Topical) *on page 2117*
- ◆ **Triatec-8 (Can)** *see* Acetaminophen and Codeine *on page 50*
- ◆ **Triatec-8 Forte (Can)** *see* Acetaminophen and Codeine *on page 50*
- ◆ **Triatec-30 (Can)** *see* Acetaminophen and Codeine *on page 50*

Triazolam (trye AY zoe lam)

Medication Safety Issues

Sound-alike/look-alike issues:

Triazolam may be confused with alPRAZolam

Halcion may be confused with halcinonide, Haldol

BEERS Criteria medication:

This drug may be potentially inappropriate for use in geriatric patients (Quality of evidence - high; Strength of recommendation - strong).

Brand Names: US Halcion

Therapeutic Category Benzodiazepine; Hypnotic; Sedative

Generic Availability (US) Yes

Use Short-term (generally 7-10 days) treatment of insomnia (FDA approved in ages ≥18 years and adults)

Medication Guide Available Yes

Pregnancy Risk Factor X

Pregnancy Considerations A case report describes placental transfer of triazolam following a maternal overdose. Teratogenic effects have been observed with some benzodiazepines; however, additional studies are needed. The incidence of premature birth and low birth weights may be increased following maternal use of benzodiazepines; hypoglycemia and respiratory problems in the neonate may occur following exposure late in pregnancy. Neonatal withdrawal symptoms may occur within days to weeks after birth and "floppy infant syndrome" (which also includes withdrawal symptoms) have been reported with some benzodiazepines (Bergman, 1992; Iqbal, 2002; Sakai, 1996; Wikner, 2007). Use of triazolam is contraindicated in pregnant women.

Breast-Feeding Considerations Although information specific to triazolam has not been located, all benzodiazepines are expected to be excreted into breast milk. Drowsiness, lethargy, or weight loss in nursing infants have been observed in case reports following maternal use of some benzodiazepines (Iqbal, 2002). Breast-feeding is not recommended by the manufacturer.

Contraindications Hypersensitivity to triazolam, other benzodiazepines, or any component of the formulation; concurrent therapy with cytochrome P450 3A (CYP 3A) inhibitors including itraconazole, ketoconazole, nefazodone, and several HIV protease inhibitors; pregnancy

Warnings/Precautions As a hypnotic, should be used only after evaluation of potential causes of sleep disturbance. Failure of sleep disturbance to resolve after 7 to 10 days may indicate psychiatric or medical illness. A worsening of insomnia or the emergence of new abnormalities of thought or behavior may represent unrecognized psychiatric or medical illness and requires immediate and careful evaluation. Prescription should be written for a maximum of 7 to 10 days and should not be prescribed in quantities exceeding a 1-month supply. Rebound insomnia or withdrawal symptoms may occur following abrupt discontinuation or large decreases in dose. Use caution when reducing dose or withdrawing therapy; decrease slowly and monitor for withdrawal symptoms. Flumazenil may cause withdrawal in patients receiving long-term benzodiazepine therapy. An increase in daytime anxiety may occur after as few as 10 days of continuous use, which may be related to withdrawal reaction in some patients.

Use with caution in elderly or debilitated patients, patients with hepatic disease (including alcoholics), or renal impairment. Use with caution in patients with respiratory compromise, COPD, or sleep apnea. In older adults, benzodiazepines increase the risk of impaired cognition, delirium, falls, fractures, and motor vehicle accidents. Due to increased sensitivity in this age group, avoid use for treatment of insomnia, agitation, or delirium. (Beers Criteria). Elderly also experience greater sedation and increased psychomotor impairment (Greenblatt, 1991). In debilitated patients, benzodiazepines increase the risk for oversedation, impaired coordination, and dizziness with use. Reports of hypersensitivity reactions, including anaphylaxis and angioedema, have been reported with triazolam.

Causes CNS depression (dose-related) resulting in sedation, dizziness, confusion, or ataxia which may impair physical and mental capabilities. Patients must be cautioned about performing tasks which require mental alertness (eg, operating machinery or driving). Abnormal thinking and behavior changes including symptoms of decreased inhibition (eg, excessive aggressiveness and extroversion), bizarre behavior, agitation, hallucinations, and depersonalization have been reported with the use of benzodiazepine hypnotics. Some evidence suggests symptoms may be dose-related. Anterograde amnesia may occur at a higher rate with triazolam than with other benzodiazepines. An increased risk for hazardous sleep-related activities such as sleep-driving; cooking and eating food, having sex, and making phone calls while asleep have also been noted. Concurrent use of alcohol and other CNS depressants as well as exceeding the maximum recommended dose may increase the risk of these behaviors. Patients will often not remember doing these activities. Consider discontinuation of therapy for patients who report sleep-driving episodes. Benzodiazepines have been associated with falls and traumatic injury and should be used with extreme caution in patients who are at risk of these events (especially the elderly).

Use caution in patients with suicidal risk. Minimize risks of overdose by prescribing the least amount of drug that is feasible in suicidal patients. Worsening of depressive symptoms has also been reported with use of benzodiazepines. Use with caution in patients with a history of drug dependence. Paradoxical reactions, including hyperactive or aggressive behavior have been reported with benzodiazepines, particularly in adolescent/pediatric or psychiatric patients. Evaluate any new changes in behavior. Triazolam is a short half-life benzodiazepine. Tolerance develops to the hypnotic effects (Vinkers, 2012). Chronic use of this agent may increase the perioperative benzodiazepine dose needed to achieve desired effect. Does not have analgesic, antidepressant, or antipsychotic properties. Potentially significant drug-drug interactions may exist, requiring dose or frequency adjustment, additional monitoring, and/or selection of alternative therapy.

Adverse Reactions

Central nervous system: Ataxia, dizziness, drowsiness, headache, lightheadedness, nervousness

Gastrointestinal: Nausea, vomiting

Rare but important or life-threatening: Anaphylaxis, angioedema, anterograde amnesia; complex sleep-related behavior (sleep-driving, cooking or eating food, making phone calls); confusion, cramps, depression, dermatitis, dreaming/nightmares, dysesthesia, euphoria, fatigue, hepatic failure (fulminant), memory impairment, pain, paresthesia, tachycardia, violent acts, visual disturbance, weakness, xerostomia

In addition, the following have been reported in association with triazolam and other benzodiazepines: Burning tongue/glossitis/stomatitis, chest pain, dysarthria, jaundice, libido changes, menstrual irregularities; paradoxical reactions (eg, aggressiveness, agitational state, delusions, falling, hallucination, mania, sleep disturbances, syncope); pruritus, sedation, slurred speech, urinary incontinence, urinary retention

Drug Interactions

Metabolism/Transport Effects Substrate of CYP3A4 (major); **Note:** Assignment of Major/Minor substrate status based on clinically relevant drug interaction potential; **Inhibits** CYP2C8 (weak), CYP2C9 (weak)

Avoid Concomitant Use

Avoid concomitant use of Triazolam with any of the following: Amodiaquine; Azelastine (Nasal); Boceprevir; Cobicistat; Conivaptan; Fusidic Acid (Systemic); Idelalisib; Itraconazole; Ketoconazole (Systemic); Methadone; OLANZapine; Orphenadrine; Paraldehyde; Protease Inhibitors; Sodium Oxybate; Telaprevir; Thalidomide

Increased Effect/Toxicity

Triazolam may increase the levels/effects of: Alcohol (Ethyl); Amodiaquine; Azelastine (Nasal); Buprenorphine; CloZAPine; CNS Depressants; Hydrocodone; Methadone; Methotrimeprazine; Metyrosine; Mirtazapine; Orphenadrine; Paraldehyde; Pramipexole; ROPINIRole; Rotigotine; Selective Serotonin Reuptake Inhibitors; Sodium Oxybate; Suvorexant; Thalidomide; Zolpidem

The levels/effects of Triazolam may be increased by: Aprepitant; Boceprevir; Brimonidine (Topical); Cannabis; Cobicistat; Conivaptan; CYP3A4 Inhibitors (Moderate); CYP3A4 Inhibitors (Strong); Dasatinib; Doxylamine; Dronabinol; Droperidol; Fosaprepitant; Fusidic Acid (Systemic); HydrOXYzine; Idelalisib; Itraconazole; Ivacaftor; Kava Kava; Ketoconazole (Systemic); Luliconazole; Macrolide Antibiotics; Magnesium Sulfate; Methotrimeprazine; Mifepristone; Nabilone; Netupitant; OLANZapine; Palbociclib; Perampanel; Protease Inhibitors; Rufinamide; Simeprevir; Stiripentol; Tapentadol; Teduglutide; Telaprevir; Tetrahydrocannabinol

Decreased Effect

The levels/effects of Triazolam may be decreased by: Bosentan; CYP3A4 Inducers (Moderate); CYP3A4 Inducers (Strong); Dabrafenib; Deferasirox; Dexamethasone (Systemic); Mitotane; Siltuximab; St Johns Wort; Theophylline Derivatives; Tocilizumab; Yohimbine

Food Interactions Benzodiazepine serum concentrations may be increased by grapefruit juice. Management: Limit or avoid grapefruit juice (Sugimoto, 2006).

Storage/Stability Store at 20°C to 25°C (68°F to 77°F).

Mechanism of Action Binds to stereospecific benzodiazepine receptors on the postsynaptic GABA neuron at several sites within the central nervous system, including the limbic system and reticular formation. Enhancement of the inhibitory effect of GABA on neuronal excitability results by increased neuronal membrane permeability to chloride ions. This shift in chloride ions results in hyperpolarization (a less excitable state) and stabilization. Benzodiazepine receptors and effects appear to be linked to the GABA-A receptors. Benzodiazepines do not bind to GABA-B receptors (Vinkers, 2012).

Pharmacodynamics Hypnotic effects:

Onset of action: Within 15-30 minutes

Duration: 6-7 hours

Pharmacokinetics (Adult data unless noted)

Distribution: V_d: 0.8-1.8 L/kg

Protein binding: 89%

Metabolism: Extensive in the liver; primary metabolites are conjugated glucuronides

Half-life: 1.5-5.5 hours
Time to peak serum concentration: Within 2 hours
Elimination: In urine as unchanged drug (minor amounts) and metabolites

Dosing: Usual
Pediatric:
Dental preprocedural sedation: Limited data available: Children and Adolescents <18 years: Oral: 0.02 mg/kg administered as an elixir has been used in children (n=20) for sedation prior to dental procedures (Meyer 1990); do not exceed adult doses
Insomnia: Adolescents ≥18 years: Oral: 0.125 to 0.25 mg at bedtime; the lower dose of 0.125 mg at bedtime may be sufficient in some patients, such as those with low body weight; maximum daily dose: 0.5 mg/day
Adult: **Insomnia (short-term use):** Usual dose: 0.25 mg at bedtime; 0.125 mg at bedtime may be sufficient in some patients, such as those with low body weight; maximum dose: 0.5 mg daily

Administration Oral: Administer dose in bed, since onset of hypnotic effect is rapid; tablet may be crushed or swallowed whole

Monitoring Parameters Daytime alertness; respiratory rate; behavior profile

Controlled Substance C-IV

Dosage Forms Excipient information presented when available (limited, particularly for generics); consult specific product labeling.
Tablet, Oral:
Halcion: 0.25 mg [scored]
Generic: 0.125 mg, 0.25 mg

- ◆ **Tribavirin** *see* Ribavirin *on page* 1851
- ◆ **Tri-Buffered Aspirin [OTC]** *see* Aspirin *on page* 206
- ◆ **Trichloroacetaldehyde Monohydrate** *see* Chloral Hydrate *on page* 429
- ◆ **Tricosal** *see* Choline Magnesium Trisalicylate *on page* 452
- ◆ **Triderm** *see* Triamcinolone (Topical) *on page* 2117
- ◆ **Tridil** *see* Nitroglycerin *on page* 1523
- ◆ **Tridural (Can)** *see* TraMADol *on page* 2098
- ◆ **Triesence** *see* Triamcinolone (Ophthalmic) *on page* 2116
- ◆ **Triethylenethiophosphoramide** *see* Thiotepa *on page* 2053

Trifluoperazine (trye floo oh PER a zeen)

Medication Safety Issues
Sound-alike/look-alike issues:
Trifluoperazine may be confused with trihexyphenidyl
Stelazine may be confused with selegiline
BEERS Criteria medication:
This drug may be potentially inappropriate for use in geriatric patients (Quality of evidence - moderate; Strength of recommendation - strong).

Therapeutic Category Antipsychotic Agent, Typical, Phenothiazine; First Generation (Typical) Antipsychotic; Phenothiazine Derivative

Generic Availability (US) Yes

Use Treatment of schizophrenia (FDA approved in ages ≥6 years and adults); short-term treatment of generalized nonpsychotic anxiety (not a drug of choice) (FDA approved in adults); also used for management of psychotic disorders

Pregnancy Considerations Adverse events have not been observed in animal reproduction studies, except when using doses that were also maternally toxic. Prolonged jaundice, extrapyramidal signs, or hyporeflexia have been reported in newborn infants following maternal use of phenothiazines. Antipsychotic use during the third trimester of pregnancy has a risk for extrapyramidal and/or withdrawal symptoms in newborns following delivery. Symptoms in the newborn may include agitation, feeding disorder, hypertonia, hypotonia, respiratory distress, somnolence, and tremor; these effects may be self-limiting or require hospitalization.

Breast-Feeding Considerations Trifluoperazine is excreted in breast milk and was measurable in the serum of three nursing infants (adverse events were not reported). Milk concentrations may be higher than those found in the maternal serum (Yoshida 1999). Infants should be monitored for signs of adverse events. Due to the potential for serious adverse reactions in the nursing infant, the manufacturer recommends a decision be made whether to discontinue nursing or to discontinue the drug, taking into account the importance of treatment to the mother.

Contraindications Hypersensitivity to trifluoperazine, phenothiazines, or any component of the formulation; comatose or greatly depressed states due to CNS depressants; bone marrow suppression; blood dyscrasias; hepatic disease

Warnings/Precautions [US Boxed Warning]: Elderly patients with dementia-related psychosis treated with antipsychotics are at an increased risk of death compared to placebo. Most deaths appeared to be either cardiovascular (eg, heart failure, sudden death) or infectious (eg, pneumonia) in nature. Trifluoperazine is not approved for the treatment of dementia-related psychosis.

Leukopenia, neutropenia, thrombocytopenia, anemia, agranulocytosis (sometimes fatal), and pancytopenia have been reported in clinical trials and postmarketing reports with antipsychotic use; presence of risk factors (eg, preexisting low WBC or history of drug-induced leuko-/neutropenia) should prompt periodic blood count assessment. Discontinue therapy at first signs of blood dyscrasias or if absolute neutrophil count <1,000/mm^3. Due to anticholinergic effects, should be used with caution in patients with decreased gastrointestinal motility, urinary retention, BPH, xerostomia, visual problems, or glaucoma. Relative to other antipsychotics, trifluoperazine has a low potency of cholinergic blockade (APA [Lehman 2004]). May cause extrapyramidal symptoms (EPS), including pseudoparkinsonism, acute dystonic reactions, akathisia, and tardive dyskinesia. Risk of dystonia (and possibly other EPS) may be greater with increased doses, use of conventional antipsychotics, males, and younger patients (APA [Lehman 2004]). Risk of tardive dyskinesia and potential for irreversibility may be increased in elderly patients (particularly women), prolonged therapy, and higher total cumulative dose. May be associated with neuroleptic malignant syndrome (NMS) or pigmentary retinopathy (Oshika 1995).

May cause CNS depression, which may impair physical or mental abilities; patients must be cautioned about performing tasks that require mental alertness (eg, operating machinery, driving). Use with caution in Parkinson's disease (APA [Lehman 2004]). Caution in patients with hemodynamic instability; predisposition to seizures; or cardiac disease; use is contraindicated in patients with hepatic disease. Esophageal dysmotility and aspiration have been associated with antipsychotic use - use with caution in patients at risk of aspiration pneumonia (ie, Alzheimer disease) (Maddalena 2004). Use associated with increased prolactin levels; clinical significance of hyperprolactinemia in patients with breast cancer or other prolactin-dependent tumors is unknown. May alter temperature regulation (Kowk 2005; Martinez 2002) or mask toxicity of other drugs due to antiemetic effects. May alter cardiac conduction; life-threatening arrhythmias have occurred with therapeutic doses of antipsychotics. Avoid use in patients with underlying QT prolongation, in those taking medicines that prolong the QT interval, or cause polymorphic ventricular tachycardia; monitor ECG closely for dose-related QT effects (Haddad 2002; Stollberger 2005). May cause orthostatic hypotension - use with caution in patients at risk of this effect or those who would tolerate transient hypotensive episodes (cerebrovascular disease, cardiovascular disease or other medications which may predispose) (APA [Lehman 2004]).

Use in elderly patients with dementia is associated with an increased risk of mortality and cerebrovascular accidents; avoid antipsychotic use for behavioral problems associated with dementia unless alternative nonpharmacologic therapies have failed and patient may harm self or others. In addition, use may cause or exacerbate syndrome of inappropriate antidiuretic hormone secretion or hyponatremia; monitor sodium closely with initiation or dosage adjustments in older adults. May also be inappropriate in older adults depending on comorbidities (eg, dementia, delirium) due to its potent anticholinergic effects (Beers Criteria). Increased risk for developing tardive dyskinesia, particularly elderly women.

Potentially significant drug-drug interactions may exist, requiring dose or frequency adjustment, additional monitoring, and/or selection of alternative therapy

Trifluoperazine is not the first drug of choice for most patients with nonpsychotic anxiety. Do not exceed recommended dose and duration; use of trifluoperazine at higher doses or for longer intervals may cause persistent tardive dyskinesia (may be irreversible).

Adverse Reactions

Cardiovascular: Cardiac arrest, hypotension, orthostatic hypotension

Central nervous system: Dizziness; extrapyramidal symptoms (akathisia, dystonias, pseudoparkinsonism, tardive dyskinesia); headache, impairment of temperature regulation, lowering of seizure threshold, neuroleptic malignant syndrome (NMS)

Dermatologic: Discoloration of skin (blue-gray), increased sensitivity to sun, photosensitivity, rash

Endocrine & metabolic: Breast pain, galactorrhea, gynecomastia, hyperglycemia, hypoglycemia, lactation, libido (changes in), menstrual cycle (changes in)

Gastrointestinal: Constipation, nausea, stomach pain, vomiting, weight gain, xerostomia

Genitourinary: Difficulty in urination, ejaculatory disturbances, priapism, urinary retention

Hematologic: Agranulocytosis, aplastic anemia, eosinophilia, hemolytic anemia, leukopenia, pancytopenia, thrombocytopenic purpura

Hepatic: Cholestatic jaundice, hepatotoxicity

Neuromuscular & skeletal: Tremor

Ocular: Cornea and lens changes, pigmentary retinopathy

Respiratory: Nasal congestion

Drug Interactions

Metabolism/Transport Effects Substrate of CYP1A2 (major); **Note:** Assignment of Major/Minor substrate status based on clinically relevant drug interaction potential

Avoid Concomitant Use

Avoid concomitant use of Trifluoperazine with any of the following: Aclidinium; Amisulpride; Azelastine (Nasal); Eluxadoline; Glucagon; Ipratropium (Oral Inhalation); Metoclopramide; Orphenadrine; Paraldehyde; Potassium Chloride; Sulpiride; Thalidomide; Tiotropium; Umeclidinium

Increased Effect/Toxicity

Trifluoperazine may increase the levels/effects of: AbobotulinumtoxinA; Alcohol (Ethyl); Amisulpride; Analgesics (Opioid); Anticholinergic Agents; Antidepressants (Serotonin Reuptake Inhibitor/Antagonist); Azelastine (Nasal); Beta-Blockers; Buprenorphine; CNS Depressants; Eluxadoline; Glucagon; Hydrocodone; Mequitazine; Methotrimeprazine; Methylphenidate; Metyrosine; Mirabegron; Mirtazapine; OnabotulinumtoxinA; Orphenadrine; Paraldehyde; Porfimer; Potassium Chloride; RimabotulinumtoxinB; Selective Serotonin Reuptake Inhibitors; Serotonin Modulators; Sulpiride; Suvorexant; Thalidomide; Thiazide Diuretics; Thiopental; Tiotropium; Topiramate; Verteporfin; Zolpidem

The levels/effects of Trifluoperazine may be increased by: Abiraterone Acetate; Acetylcholinesterase Inhibitors (Central); Aclidinium; Antidepressants (Serotonin Reuptake Inhibitor/Antagonist); Antimalarial Agents; Beta-Blockers; Brimonidine (Topical); Cannabis; CYP1A2 Inhibitors (Moderate); CYP1A2 Inhibitors (Strong); Deferasirox; Doxylamine; Dronabinol; Droperidol; HydrOXYzine; Ipratropium (Oral Inhalation); Kava Kava; Lithium; Magnesium Sulfate; Methotrimeprazine; Methylphenidate; Metoclopramide; Metyrosine; Mianserin; Nabilone; Peginterferon Alfa-2b; Perampanel; Pramlintide; Rufinamide; Serotonin Modulators; Sodium Oxybate; Tapentadol; Tetrabenazine; Tetrahydrocannabinol; Umeclidinium; Vemurafenib

Decreased Effect

Trifluoperazine may decrease the levels/effects of: Acetylcholinesterase Inhibitors; Amphetamines; Anti-Parkinson's Agents (Dopamine Agonist); Itopride; Quinagolide; Secretin

The levels/effects of Trifluoperazine may be decreased by: Acetylcholinesterase Inhibitors; Antacids; Anti-Parkinson's Agents (Dopamine Agonist); Cannabis; CYP1A2 Inducers (Strong); Cyproterone; Lithium; Teriflunomide

Storage/Stability Store at 20°C to 25°C (68°F to 77°F). Protect from moisture and light

Mechanism of Action Trifluoperazine is a piperazine phenothiazine antipsychotic which blocks dopamine, subtype 2 (D_2), receptors in mesolimbocortical and nigrostriatal areas of the brain (APA [Lehman, 2004]).

Pharmacodynamics

Onset of action: For control of agitation, aggression, hostility: 2-4 weeks; for control of psychotic symptoms (hallucinations, disorganized thinking or behavior, delusions): Within 1 week

Adequate trial: 6 weeks at moderate to high dose based on tolerability

Duration: Variable

Pharmacokinetics (Adult data unless noted)

Metabolism: Extensively hepatic

Half-life: >24 hours with chronic use

Dialysis: Not dialyzable (0% to 5%)

Dosing: Usual Oral:

Schizophrenia/psychoses (**Note:** Dosage should be individualized; use lowest effective dose and shortest effective duration; periodically reassess the need for continued treatment):

- Children <6 years: Dosage not established
- Children 6-12 years: Hospitalized or well-supervised patients: Initial: 1 mg 1-2 times/day; gradually increase dose until symptoms are controlled or adverse effects have become troublesome; maintenance: 1-15 mg/day in 1-2 divided doses (maximum: 15 mg/day)
- Children >12 years:
  - Inpatient: Initial: 2-5 mg twice daily; gradually increase dose; usual maintenance: 15-20 mg/day in 2 divided doses (maximum: 40 mg/day)
  - Outpatient: Initial: 1-3 mg twice daily (maximum: 6 mg/day)
- Adults:
  - Inpatient: Initial: 2-5 mg twice daily; gradually increase dose; usual maintenance: 15-20 mg/day in 2 divided doses (maximum dose: 40 mg/day)
  - Outpatient: Initial: 1-3 mg twice daily (maximum: 40 mg/day; exceptions occur-indication specific)

Nonpsychotic anxiety: Adults: 1-2 mg twice daily; maximum: 6 mg/day; therapy for anxiety should not exceed 12 weeks; do not exceed 6 mg/day for longer than 12 weeks when treating anxiety; agitation, jitteriness, or insomnia may be confused with original neurotic or psychotic symptoms

Administration May be taken with food to decrease GI upset; do not take within 2 hours of any antacids

Monitoring Parameters Vital signs; periodic eye exam, CBC with differential, liver enzyme tests; fasting blood glucose/Hgb A_{1c}; BMI; therapeutic response (mental status, mood, affect, gait), and adverse reactions at beginning of therapy and periodically with long-term use [eg, excess sedation, extrapyramidal symptoms, tardive dyskinesia, CNS changes, abnormal involuntary movement scale (AIMS)]

Test Interactions Phenothiazines may produce a false-positive for phenylketonuria

Additional Information Long-term usefulness of trifluoperazine should be periodically re-evaluated in patients receiving the drug for extended periods; consideration should be given whether to decrease the maintenance dose or discontinue drug therapy

Dosage Forms Excipient information presented when available (limited, particularly for generics); consult specific product labeling.

Tablet, Oral:

Generic: 1 mg, 2 mg, 5 mg, 10 mg

◆ **Trifluoperazine Hydrochloride** *see* Trifluoperazine *on page 2122*

◆ **Trifluorothymidine** *see* Trifluridine *on page 2124*

Trifluridine (trye FLURE i deen)

Medication Safety Issues

Sound-alike/look-alike issues:

Viroptic® may be confused with Timoptic®

Brand Names: US Viroptic

Brand Names: Canada Sandoz-Trifluridine; Viroptic®

Therapeutic Category Antiviral Agent, Ophthalmic

Generic Availability (US) Yes

Use Treatment of primary keratoconjunctivitis and recurrent epithelial keratitis caused by herpes simplex virus types I and II

Pregnancy Risk Factor C

Pregnancy Considerations Adverse effects were not observed during animal reproduction studies of the ophthalmic solution.

Breast-Feeding Considerations The amount of trifluridine available systemically following topical application of the ophthalmic drops is negligible.

Contraindications Hypersensitivity to trifluridine or any component of the formulation

Warnings/Precautions Mild local irritation of conjunctival and cornea may occur when instilled but usually transient effects.

Adverse Reactions Ocular: Burning or stinging (5%), palpebral edema (3%), epithelial keratopathy, hyperemia, hypersensitivity reactions, irritation, keratitis sicca, ocular pressure increased, stromal edema, superficial punctate keratopathy

Drug Interactions

Metabolism/Transport Effects None known.

Avoid Concomitant Use There are no known interactions where it is recommended to avoid concomitant use.

Increased Effect/Toxicity There are no known significant interactions involving an increase in effect.

Decreased Effect There are no known significant interactions involving a decrease in effect.

Storage/Stability Store refrigerated at 2°C to 8°C (36°F to 46°F).

Mechanism of Action Interferes with viral replication by inhibiting thymidylate synthetase and incorporating into viral DNA in place of thymidine.

Pharmacodynamics Onset of action: Response to treatment occurs within 2-7 days; epithelial healing is complete in 1-2 weeks

Pharmacokinetics (Adult data unless noted) Absorption: Ophthalmic: Systemic absorption is negligible, while corneal penetration is adequate

Dosing: Usual Children and Adults: Ophthalmic: Instill 1 drop into affected eye every 2 hours while awake, to a maximum of 9 drops/day, until re-epithelialization of corneal ulcer occurs; then use 1 drop every 4 hours for another 7 days; do **not** exceed 21 days of treatment

Administration Ophthalmic: Avoid contact of bottle tip with skin or eye; instill drops onto the cornea of the affected eye(s); apply finger pressure to lacrimal sac during and for 1-2 minutes after instillation to decrease risk of absorption and systemic effects

Monitoring Parameters Ophthalmologic exam (test for corneal staining with fluorescein or rose Bengal)

Additional Information Found to be effective in 138 of 150 patients unresponsive or intolerant to idoxuridine or vidarabine

Dosage Forms Excipient information presented when available (limited, particularly for generics); consult specific product labeling.

Solution, Ophthalmic:

Viroptic: 1% (7.5 mL) [contains thimerosal]

Generic: 1% (7.5 mL)

◆ **Triglycerides, Medium Chain** *see* Medium Chain Triglycerides *on page 1338*

Trihexyphenidyl (trye heks ee FEN i dil)

Medication Safety Issues

Sound-alike/look-alike issues:

Trihexyphenidyl may be confused with trifluoperazine

BEERS Criteria medication:

This drug may be potentially inappropriate for use in geriatric patients (Quality of evidence - moderate; Strength of recommendation - strong).

Brand Names: Canada PMS-Trihexyphenidyl; Trihexyphenidyl

Therapeutic Category Anti-Parkinson's Agent; Anticholinergic Agent; Antidote, Drug-induced Dystonic Reactions

Generic Availability (US) Yes

Use Adjunctive treatment of Parkinson's disease and treatment of drug-induced extrapyramidal symptoms (EPS) (FDA approved in adults); has also been used for treatment of dystonia in cerebral palsy

Pregnancy Risk Factor C

Pregnancy Considerations Animal reproduction studies have not been conducted. One case report did not show evidence of adverse events after trihexyphenidyl administration during pregnancy (Robottom, 2011).

Breast-Feeding Considerations It is not known if trihexyphenidyl is excreted in breast milk. The manufacturer recommends that caution be exercised when administering trihexyphenidyl to nursing women. Anticholinergic agents may suppress lactation.

Contraindications Hypersensitivity to trihexyphenidyl or any component of the formulation; narrow angle glaucoma.

Warnings/Precautions May cause anticholinergic effects (constipation, xerostomia, blurred vision, urinary retention); monitor patients on long-term use. May precipitate angle closure with an increase in intraocular pressure. If blurring of vision occurs, consider the possibility of narrow angle glaucoma; blindness because of aggravation of narrow angle glaucoma has been reported. Patients should have a gonioscope evaluation prior to initiation of therapy and close monitoring of IOP. Use with caution in hot weather or during exercise, especially when administered concomitantly with other atropine-like drugs to chronically ill patients, alcoholics, patients with CNS disease, or persons doing manual labor in a hot environment. Use with caution in patients with cardiovascular disease (including hypertension), glaucoma, prostatic hyperplasia or any tendency toward urinary retention, liver or kidney disorders, and obstructive disease of the GI tract. May impair memory and further exacerbate cognitive deficits in elderly patients; in high doses may cause confusion, delirium, and hallucinations (Holloman 1997; Tonda 1994). Dose reduction or discontinuation of trihexyphenidyl has been associated with neuroleptic malignant syndrome (NMS) and withdrawal symptoms including tension, irritability, perspiration, palpitations, headache, insomnia, abdominal distress, anorexia, faint or choking feelings, nausea, and photophobia (McInnis 1985). Withdraw trihexyphenidyl gradually; abrupt or rapid discontinuation may result in acute exacerbation of symptoms (Manos 1981a; Manos 1981b). May impair physical or mental abilities; patients must be cautioned about performing tasks that require mental alertness (eg, operating machinery, driving). Potentially significant interactions may exist, requiring dose or frequency adjustment, additional monitoring, and/or selection of alternative therapy. Not recommended for use in patients with tardive dyskinesia (unless concomitant Parkinson disease exists); trihexyphenidyl does not relieve symptoms of tardive dyskinesia and may potentially exacerbate symptoms. Avoid use in older adults; not recommended for prevention of extrapyramidal symptoms with antipsychotics; alternative agents preferred in the treatment of Parkinson disease. May be inappropriate in older adults depending on comorbidities (eg, dementia, delirium) because of its potent anticholinergic effects (Beers Criteria).

Adverse Reactions

Cardiovascular: Tachycardia

Central nervous system: Agitation, confusion, delusions, dizziness, drowsiness, euphoria, hallucination, headache, nervousness, paranoia, psychiatric disturbance

Dermatologic: Skin rash

Gastrointestinal: Constipation, intestinal obstruction, nausea, parotitis, toxic megacolon, vomiting, xerostomia

Genitourinary: Urinary retention

Neuromuscular & skeletal: Weakness

Ophthalmic: Blurred vision, glaucoma, increased intraocular pressure, mydriasis

Drug Interactions

Metabolism/Transport Effects None known.

Avoid Concomitant Use

Avoid concomitant use of Trihexyphenidyl with any of the following: Aclidinium; Eluxadoline; Glucagon; Ipratropium (Oral Inhalation); Potassium Chloride; Tiotropium; Umeclidinium

Increased Effect/Toxicity

Trihexyphenidyl may increase the levels/effects of: AbobotulinumtoxinA; Analgesics (Opioid); Anticholinergic Agents; Cannabinoid-Containing Products; Eluxadoline; Glucagon; Mirabegron; OnabotulinumtoxinA; Potassium Chloride; RimabotulinumtoxinB; Thiazide Diuretics; Tiotropium; Topiramate

The levels/effects of Trihexyphenidyl may be increased by: Aclidinium; Ipratropium (Oral Inhalation); Mianserin; Pramlintide; Umeclidinium

Decreased Effect

Trihexyphenidyl may decrease the levels/effects of: Acetylcholinesterase Inhibitors; Itopride; Metoclopramide; Secretin

The levels/effects of Trihexyphenidyl may be decreased by: Acetylcholinesterase Inhibitors

Storage/Stability Store at 20°C to 25°C (68°F to 77°F).

Mechanism of Action Exerts a direct inhibitory effect on the parasympathetic nervous system. It also has a relaxing effect on smooth musculature; exerted both directly on the muscle itself and indirectly through parasympathetic nervous system (inhibitory effect)

Pharmacokinetics (Adult data unless noted)

Metabolism: Hydroxylation of the alicyclic groups

Time to peak serum concentration: 1.3 hours

Half-life: 33 hours

Elimination: Urine and bile

Dosing: Usual Oral:

Children 2-17 years: Dystonia in cerebral palsy: Initial: 0.1-0.2 mg/kg/day in three divided doses for 1 week; increase by 0.05-0.3 mg/kg/day in three divided doses for the second week; thereafter, titrate up weekly by 0.05-0.5 mg/kg/day in three divided doses as clinically tolerated; dosage is based on a prospective trial of 23 patients (Sanger, 2007); maximum dose: 0.75 mg/kg/day; however, a double-blind, prospective crossover study of 16 patients evaluating the effects of higher dosage resulted in improved clinical outcomes with doses ranging between 0.05-2.6 mg/kg/day in three divided doses although adverse reactions were common per author report (n=8 doses ≥2 mg/kg/day; Rice, 2009)

Adults:

Parkinson's disease: Initial: 1 mg/day; increase by 2 mg increments at intervals of 3-5 days; usual dose: 6-10 mg/day in 3-4 divided doses; doses of 12-15 mg/day may be required

Drug-induced extrapyramidal symptoms: Initial: 1 mg/day; increase as necessary to usual range: 5-15 mg/day in 3-4 divided doses

Use in combination with levodopa: Usual range: 3-6 mg/day in divided doses

Administration Oral: May be taken before or after meals; tolerated best if given in 3 daily doses and with food. High doses (>10 mg/day) may be divided into 4 doses, at meal times and at bedtime.

Monitoring Parameters Intraocular pressure monitoring and gonioscopic evaluations (baseline and at regular intervals)

Dosage Forms Excipient information presented when available (limited, particularly for generics); consult specific product labeling.

Elixir, Oral, as hydrochloride:

Generic: 0.4 mg/mL (473 mL)

Tablet, Oral, as hydrochloride:

Generic: 2 mg, 5 mg

- **Trihexyphenidyl Hydrochloride** *see* Trihexyphenidyl *on page 2124*
- **Trilafon** *see* Perphenazine *on page 1676*
- **Trileptal** *see* OXcarbazepine *on page 1584*
- **Trilisate** *see* Choline Magnesium Trisalicylate *on page 452*
- **TriLyte** *see* Polyethylene Glycol-Electrolyte Solution *on page 1724*

Trimethobenzamide (trye meth oh BEN za mide)

Medication Safety Issues

Sound-alike/look-alike issues:

Tigan may be confused with Tiazac, Ticlid

Trimethobenzamide may be confused with metoclopramide, trimethoprim

BEERS Criteria medication:

This drug may be potentially inappropriate for use in geriatric patients (Quality of evidence - moderate; Strength of recommendation - strong).

Brand Names: US Tigan

Brand Names: Canada Tigan

Therapeutic Category Antiemetic

Generic Availability (US) Yes

Use Treatment of postoperative nausea and vomiting; treatment of nausea and vomiting associated with gastroenteritis

Pregnancy Considerations Teratogenic effects were not observed in animal reproduction studies. Trimethobenzamide has been used to treat nausea and vomiting of pregnancy (ACOG, 2004).

Breast-Feeding Considerations It is not known if trimethobenzamide is excreted in breast milk.

Contraindications Hypersensitivity to trimethobenzamide or any component of the formulation; injection contraindicated in children

Warnings/Precautions May mask toxicity of other drugs or conditions (eg, appendicitis, Reye syndrome, or other encephalopathy) due to antiemetic effects. May cause drowsiness; patient should avoid tasks requiring alertness (eg, driving, operating machinery). Effects may be potentiated when used with other sedative drugs or ethanol. May cause extrapyramidal symptoms (EPS) which may be confused with CNS symptoms of primary disease responsible for emesis. Avoid use in the elderly due to the risk of EPS adverse effects combined with lower efficacy, as compared to other antiemetics (Beers Criteria). Risk of CNS adverse effects (eg, coma, EPS, seizure) may be increased in patients with acute febrile illness, dehydration, electrolyte imbalance, encephalitis, or gastroenteritis; use caution. Allergic-type skin reactions have been reported with use; discontinue with signs of sensitization. Trimethobenzamide clearance is predominantly renal; dosage reductions may be recommended in patient with renal impairment. Use capsule formulation with caution in children; antiemetics are not recommended for uncomplicated vomiting in children, limit antiemetic use to prolonged vomiting of known etiology. Use of injection is contraindicated in children. Potentially significant drug-drug interactions may exist, requiring dose or frequency adjustment, additional monitoring, and/or selection of alternative therapy.

Adverse Reactions

Cardiovascular: Hypotension (IV administration)

Central nervous system: Coma, depression, disorientation, dizziness, drowsiness, EPS, headache, Parkinson-like symptoms, seizure

Dermatologic: Allergic-type skin reactions

Gastrointestinal: Diarrhea

Hematologic: Blood dyscrasias

Hepatic: Jaundice

Local: Injection site burning, pain, redness, stinging, or swelling

Neuromuscular & skeletal: Muscle cramps, opisthotonos

Ocular: Blurred vision

Miscellaneous: Hypersensitivity reactions

Drug Interactions

Metabolism/Transport Effects None known.

Avoid Concomitant Use

Avoid concomitant use of Trimethobenzamide with any of the following: Aclidinium; Eluxadoline; Glucagon; Ipratropium (Oral Inhalation); Potassium Chloride; Tiotropium; Umeclidinium

Increased Effect/Toxicity

Trimethobenzamide may increase the levels/effects of: AbobotulinumtoxinA; Analgesics (Opioid); Anticholinergic Agents; Cannabinoid-Containing Products; Eluxadoline; Glucagon; Mirabegron; OnabotulinumtoxinA; Potassium Chloride; RimabotulinumtoxinB; Thiazide Diuretics; Tiotropium; Topiramate

The levels/effects of Trimethobenzamide may be increased by: Aclidinium; Alcohol (Ethyl); Ipratropium (Oral Inhalation); Mianserin; Pramlintide; Umeclidinium

Decreased Effect

Trimethobenzamide may decrease the levels/effects of: Acetylcholinesterase Inhibitors; Itopride; Metoclopramide; Secretin

The levels/effects of Trimethobenzamide may be decreased by: Acetylcholinesterase Inhibitors

Storage/Stability Capsules and injection: Store at room temperature of 25°C (77°F); excursions are permitted between 15°C and 30°C (59°F and 86°F).

Mechanism of Action Acts centrally to inhibit the medullary chemoreceptor trigger zone by blocking emetic impulses to the vomiting center

Pharmacodynamics

Onset of action:
- Oral: 10-40 minutes
- IM: 15-35 minutes

Duration:
- Oral: 3-4 hours
- IM: 2-3 hours

Pharmacokinetics (Adult data unless noted)

Metabolism: Via oxidation, forms metabolite trimethobenzamide N-oxide

Bioavailability: Oral dose is 100% of IM dose

Half-life: Adults: 7-9 hours

Time to peak serum concentration:
- Oral: 45 minutes
- IM: 30 minutes

Elimination: 30% to 50% excreted unchanged in urine in 24 hours

Dosing: Usual

Children:
- Oral: 15-20 mg/kg/day (400-500 mg/m^2/day) divided into 3-4 doses; **or as an alternative**
  - <13.6 kg: 100 mg 3-4 times/day
  - 13.6-40 kg: 100-200 mg 3-4 times/day
  - >40 kg: 300 mg 3-4 times/day
- IM: Not recommended

Adults:
- Oral: 300 mg 3-4 times/day
- IM: 200 mg 3-4 times/day
- Postoperative nausea and vomiting (PONV): IM: 200 mg, followed 1 hour later by a second 200 mg dose

Dosage adjustment in renal impairment: CrCl ≤70 mL/minute: Consider dosage reduction or increasing dosing interval (specific adjustment guidelines are not provided in the manufacturer's labeling)

Administration

Oral: May administer without regard to food

Parenteral: IM use only by deep injection into upper outer quadrant of gluteal region; **not** for IV use

Additional Information Note: Less effective than phenothiazines but may be associated with fewer side effects

Dosage Forms Excipient information presented when available (limited, particularly for generics); consult specific product labeling. [DSC] = Discontinued product

Capsule, Oral, as hydrochloride:
- Tigan: 300 mg
- Generic: 300 mg

Solution, Intramuscular, as hydrochloride:
- Tigan: 100 mg/mL (2 mL)
- Tigan: 100 mg/mL (20 mL) [contains phenol]
- Generic: 100 mg/mL (2 mL [DSC], 20 mL [DSC])

◆ **Trimethobenzamide HCl** *see* Trimethobenzamide *on page* 2125

◆ **Trimethobenzamide Hydrochloride** *see* Trimethobenzamide *on page* 2125

Trimethoprim (trye METH oh prim)

Brand Names: US Primsol

Brand Names: Canada Apo-Trimethoprim®

Therapeutic Category Antibiotic, Miscellaneous

Generic Availability (US) May be product dependent

Use Treatment of otitis media caused by susceptible *Streptococcus pneumoniae* and *Haemophilus influenzae* (oral solution: FDA approved in pediatric patients ≥6 months); treatment of urinary tract infections caused by susceptible *Escherichia coli, Proteus mirabilis, Klebsiella pneumoniae, Enterobacter* spp, and coagulase-negative *Staphylococcus* (including *S. saprophyticus*) (FDA approved in adults). Has also been used in combination with other agents for treatment of *Pneumocystis jirovecii* pneumonia (PCP)

Pregnancy Risk Factor C

Pregnancy Considerations Adverse effects have been observed in animal reproduction studies. Trimethoprim crosses the placenta and can be detected in the fetal serum and amniotic fluid (Reid, 1975). Adverse events may be associated with trimethoprim use during pregnancy (Andersen, 2012; Andersen, 2013; Mølgaard-Nielsen, 2012). Untreated urinary tract infections may cause adverse pregnancy outcomes (Nicolle, 2005); because safer options are available for the treatment of UTIs in pregnant women, use of TMP containing products in the first trimester should be avoided (Lee, 2008). Studies evaluating the effects of trimethoprim administration in pregnancy have also been conducted with sulfamethoxazole/trimethoprim (see the Sulfamethoxazole and Trimethoprim monograph for details).

Breast-Feeding Considerations Trimethoprim is excreted in breast milk. The manufacturer recommends caution while using trimethoprim in a breast-feeding woman because trimethoprim may interfere with folic acid metabolism. Nondose-related effects could include modification of bowel flora. Also see the sulfamethoxazole/trimethoprim monograph for additional information.

Contraindications Hypersensitivity to trimethoprim or any component of the formulation; megaloblastic anemia due to folate deficiency

Warnings/Precautions Use with caution in patients with impaired renal or hepatic function or with possible folate deficiency. Prolonged use may result in fungal or bacterial superinfection, including *C. difficile*-associated diarrhea (CDAD) and pseudomembranous colitis; CDAD has been observed >2 months postantibiotic treatment.

Benzyl alcohol and derivatives: Some dosage forms may contain sodium benzoate/benzoic acid; benzoic acid (benzoate) is a metabolite of benzyl alcohol; large amounts of benzyl alcohol (≥99 mg/kg/day) have been associated with a potentially fatal toxicity ("gasping syndrome") in neonates; the "gasping syndrome" consists of metabolic acidosis, respiratory distress, gasping respirations, CNS dysfunction (including convulsions, intracranial hemorrhage), hypotension, and cardiovascular collapse (AAP 1997; CDC 1982); some data suggests that benzoate displaces bilirubin from protein binding sites (Ahlfors, 2001); avoid or use dosage forms containing benzyl alcohol derivative with caution in neonates. See manufacturer's labeling.

Propylene glycol: Some dosage forms may contain propylene glycol; large amounts are potentially toxic and have been associated hyperosmolality, lactic acidosis, seizures, and respiratory depression; use caution (AAP 1997; Zar 2007).

Trimethoprim may cause hyperkalemia; potential risk factors include high dosage (20 mg/kg/day), renal impairment, older age, hypoaldosteronism, and concomitant use of medications causing or exacerbating hyperkalemia (Perazella 2000). Elderly patients are at an increased risk for severe and potentially life-threatening hyperkalemia when trimethoprim is used concomitantly with spironolactone, ACE inhibitors, or ARBs (Antoniou 2010; Antoniou 2011; Antoniou 2015).

Warnings: Additional Pediatric Considerations Due to resistance, should not be used for treatment of acute otitis media caused by *Moraxella catarrhalis*. Trimethoprim is not indicated for prolonged administration or prophylaxis of otitis media in any age.

Adverse Reactions

Central nervous system: Aseptic meningitis (rare), fever

Dermatologic: Erythema multiforme (rare), exfoliative dermatitis (rare), maculopapular rash, phototoxic skin eruptions, pruritus (common), Stevens-Johnson syndrome (rare), toxic epidermal necrolysis (rare)

Endocrine & metabolic: Hyperkalemia, hyponatremia

Gastrointestinal: Epigastric distress, glossitis, nausea, vomiting

Hematologic: Leukopenia, megaloblastic anemia, methemoglobinemia, neutropenia, thrombocytopenia

Hepatic: Cholestatic jaundice (rare), liver enzymes increased

Renal: Increased BUN and creatinine

Miscellaneous: Anaphylaxis, hypersensitivity reactions

Drug Interactions

Metabolism/Transport Effects Substrate of CYP2C9 (major), CYP3A4 (major); **Note:** Assignment of Major/Minor substrate status based on clinically relevant drug interaction potential; **Inhibits** CYP2C8 (moderate), CYP2C9 (moderate)

Avoid Concomitant Use

Avoid concomitant use of Trimethoprim with any of the following: Amodiaquine; BCG; BCG (Intravesical); Dofetilide; Leucovorin Calcium-Levoleucovorin

Increased Effect/Toxicity

Trimethoprim may increase the levels/effects of: ACE Inhibitors; Amantadine; Amodiaquine; Angiotensin II Receptor Blockers; Antidiabetic Agents (Thiazolidinedione); AzaTHIOprine; Bosentan; Cannabis; Carvedilol; CYP2C8 Substrates; CYP2C9 Substrates; Dapsone (Systemic); Dapsone (Topical); Digoxin; Dofetilide; Dronabinol; Eplerenone; Fosphenytoin; Highest Risk QTc-Prolonging Agents; LamiVUDine; Memantine; Mercaptopurine; MetFORMIN; Methotrexate; Moderate Risk QTc-Prolonging Agents; Phenytoin; PRALAtrexate; Procainamide; Repaglinide; Spironolactone; Tetrahydrocannabinol; Varenicline

The levels/effects of Trimethoprim may be increased by: Amantadine; Ceritinib; CYP2C9 Inhibitors (Moderate); CYP2C9 Inhibitors (Strong); Dapsone (Systemic); Memantine; Mifepristone

Decreased Effect

Trimethoprim may decrease the levels/effects of: BCG; BCG (Intravesical); BCG Vaccine (Immunization); Sodium Picosulfate; Typhoid Vaccine

The levels/effects of Trimethoprim may be decreased by: Bosentan; CYP2C9 Inducers (Strong); CYP3A4 Inducers (Moderate); CYP3A4 Inducers (Strong); Dabrafenib; Deferasirox; Fosphenytoin; Leucovorin Calcium-Levoleucovorin; Mitotane; Phenytoin; Siltuximab; St Johns Wort; Tocilizumab

Storage/Stability

Solution: Store between 15°C to 25°C (59°F to 77°F). Protect from light.

Tablets: Store at 20°C to 25°C (68°F to 77°F). Protect from light.

Mechanism of Action Inhibits folic acid reduction to tetrahydrofolate, and thereby inhibits microbial growth

Pharmacokinetics (Adult data unless noted)

Absorption: Oral: Readily and extensively absorbed

Distribution: Penetrates into middle ear fluid with a mean peak middle ear fluid concentration in children 1-12 years of 2 mcg/mL after a single 4 mg/kg dose

V_d:
Newborns: 2.7 L/kg (range: 1.3-4.1 hours) (Springer, 1982)
Infants: 1.5 L/kg (Hoppu, 1989)
Children (Hoppu, 1987):
1-3 years: 0.86 L/kg
8-10 years: 1 L/kg
Adults: ~1.3 L/kg (Hoppu, 1987)
Protein binding: ~44%
Metabolism: Partially hepatic (10% to 20%) via demethylation, oxidation, and hydroxylation
Bioavailability: Similar for tablets and solution
Half-life: Prolonged with renal impairment
Newborns: 19 hours; range: 11-27 hours (Springer, 1982)
Infants 2 months to 1 year: 4.6 hours; range: 3-6 hours (Hoppu, 1989)
Children (Hoppu, 1987):
1-3 years: 3.7 hours
8-10 years: 5.4 hours
Adults, normal renal function: 8-10 hours
Time to peak serum concentration: 1-4 hours
Elimination: Significantly excreted in urine (50% to 60%); 80% as unchanged drug via glomerular filtration and tubular secretion
Dialysis: Moderately dialyzable (20% to 50%)

Dosing: Usual
Infants, Children, and Adolescents:
Otitis media, acute: Infants ≥6 months, Children, and Adolescents: Oral: 10 mg/kg/day in divided doses every 12 hours for 10 days; maximum daily dose: 400 mg/day
Urinary tract infection (uncomplicated), treatment: Infants ≥2 months, Children, and Adolescents: Oral: 4-6 mg/kg/day in divided doses every 12 hours; **Note:** Preferred therapy is sulfamethoxazole and trimethoprim combined product (AAP, 2011).
***Pneumocystis jirovecii* pneumonia (PCP), treatment:** Children and Adolescents: Oral: 15 mg/kg/day in 3 divided doses for 21 days; in combination with dapsone; data in children is limited; preferred therapy is sulfamethoxazole and trimethoprim combined product (DHHS [adult and pediatric], 2013)
Adults:
Urinary tract infection (uncomplicated), treatment: Oral: 100 mg every 12 hours or 200 mg every 24 hours for 10 days; alternative duration of 3 days has been recommended (Gupta, 2011)
***Pneumocystis jirovecii* pneumonia (PCP); treatment:** Oral: 15 mg/kg/day in 3 divided doses for 21 days in combination with dapsone (DHHS [adult], 2013)
Dosing adjustment in renal impairment: Manufacturer's recommendation: Children and Adults:
CrCl 15-30 mL/minute: Administer 50% of recommended dose.
CrCl <15 mL/minute: Use is not recommended.
Dosing adjustment in hepatic impairment: No dosage adjustments are provided in the manufacturer labeling.

Administration Oral: Administer on an empty stomach; may administer with milk or food if GI upset occurs

Monitoring Parameters CBC with differential, platelet count, liver enzyme tests, bilirubin, serum potassium, serum creatinine and BUN

Reference Range Therapeutic:
Peak: 5-15 mg/L
Trough: 2-8 mg/L

Test Interactions May falsely increase creatinine determination measured by the Jaffé alkaline picrate assay; may interfere with determination of serum methotrexate when measured by methods that use a bacterial dihydrofolate reductase as the binding protein (eg, the competitive binding protein technique); does **not** interfere with RIA for methotrexate

Dosage Forms Excipient information presented when available (limited, particularly for generics); consult specific product labeling.
Solution, Oral [strength expressed as base]:
Primsol: 50 mg/5 mL (473 mL) [alcohol free, dye free]
Tablet, Oral:
Generic: 100 mg

Extemporaneous Preparations Note: Commercial oral solution is available (10 mg/mL [dye free, ethanol free; contains propylene glycol, sodium benzoate; bubblegum flavor])

A 10 mg/mL oral suspension may be made with tablets. Crush ten 100 mg tablets in a mortar and reduce to a fine powder. Add 20 mL of a 1:1 mixture of Simple Syrup, NF, and Methylcellulose 1% and mix to a uniform paste; mix while adding the vehicle in incremental proportions to **almost** 100 mL; transfer to a calibrated bottle, rinse mortar with vehicle, and add quantity of vehicle sufficient to make 100 mL. Label "shake well" and "refrigerate". Stable for 91 days.

Nahata MC, Pai VB, and Hipple TF, *Pediatric Drug Formulations*, 5th ed, Cincinnati, OH: Harvey Whitney Books Co, 2004.

Trimethoprim and Polymyxin B

(trye METH oh prim & pol i MIKS in bee)

Brand Names: US Polytrim®
Brand Names: Canada PMS-Polytrimethoprim; Polytrim™
Therapeutic Category Antibiotic, Ophthalmic
Generic Availability (US) Yes
Use Treatment of surface ocular conjunctivitis and blepharoconjunctivitis caused by susceptible *S. aureus*, *S. epidermidis*, *S. pneumoniae*, *S. viridans*, *H. influenzae*, and *P. aeruginosa* (FDA approved in ages ≥2 months and adults)
Pregnancy Risk Factor C
Pregnancy Considerations Adverse events have been observed with trimethoprim in animal reproduction studies; animal reproduction studies have not been conducted with polymyxin B. See individual agents. If ophthalmic agents are needed during pregnancy, the minimum effective dose should be used in combination with punctual occlusion to decrease potential exposure to the fetus (Samples, 1988).
Breast-Feeding Considerations It is not known if trimethoprim or polymyxin B can be detected in breast milk following ophthalmic administration. The manufacturer recommends that caution be exercised when administering trimethoprim/polymyxin B to nursing women. See individual agents.
Contraindications Hypersensitivity to trimethoprim, polymyxin B, or any component of the formulation
Warnings/Precautions See individual agents.
Warnings: Additional Pediatric Considerations Not indicated for prophylaxis or treatment of ophthalmia neonatorum.
Adverse Reactions Ocular: Burning, itching, edema, rash, redness increased, stinging, tearing
Drug Interactions
Metabolism/Transport Effects Refer to individual components.
Avoid Concomitant Use
Avoid concomitant use of Trimethoprim and Polymyxin B with any of the following: Amodiaquine; Bacitracin (Systemic); BCG; BCG (Intravesical); Dofetilide; Leucovorin Calcium-Levoleucovorin; Mecamylamine
Increased Effect/Toxicity
Trimethoprim and Polymyxin B may increase the levels/effects of: ACE Inhibitors; Amantadine; Amodiaquine; Angiotensin II Receptor Blockers; Antidiabetic Agents (Thiazolidinedione); AzaTHIOprine; Bacitracin (Systemic); Bosentan; Cannabis; Carvedilol; Colistimethate; CYP2C8 Substrates; CYP2C9 Substrates; Dapsone

(Systemic); Dapsone (Topical); Digoxin; Dofetilide; Dronabinol; Eplerenone; Fosphenytoin; Highest Risk QTc-Prolonging Agents; LamiVUDine; Mecamylamine; Memantine; Mercaptopurine; MetFORMIN; Methotrexate; Moderate Risk QTc-Prolonging Agents; Neuromuscular-Blocking Agents; Phenytoin; PRALAtrexate; Procainamide; Repaglinide; Spironolactone; Tetrahydrocannabinol; Varenicline

The levels/effects of Trimethoprim and Polymyxin B may be increased by: Amantadine; Capreomycin; Ceritinib; CYP2C9 Inhibitors (Moderate); CYP2C9 Inhibitors (Strong); Dapsone (Systemic); Memantine; Mifepristone

Decreased Effect

Trimethoprim and Polymyxin B may decrease the levels/effects of: BCG; BCG (Intravesical); BCG Vaccine (Immunization); Sodium Picosulfate; Typhoid Vaccine

The levels/effects of Trimethoprim and Polymyxin B may be decreased by: Bosentan; CYP2C9 Inducers (Strong); CYP3A4 Inducers (Moderate); CYP3A4 Inducers (Strong); Dabrafenib; Deferasirox; Fosphenytoin; Leucovorin Calcium-Levoleucovorin; Mitotane; Phenytoin; Siltuximab; St Johns Wort; Tocilizumab

Storage/Stability Store at 15°C to 25°C (59°F to 77°F); protect from light.

Dosing: Usual Infants ≥2 months, Children, Adolescents, and Adults: Ophthalmic: Instill 1 drop in eye(s) every 3 hours (maximum: 6 doses/day) for 7-10 days (manufacturer's recommendation for mild to moderate infection)

Administration For topical use in eye only; avoid contamination of the applicator tip. Apply finger pressure to lacrimal sac during and for 1-2 minutes after instillation to decrease risk of absorption and systemic effects.

Additional Information Polytrim®: pH 4-6.2; osmolality: 270-310 mOsm/kg

Dosage Forms Excipient information presented when available (limited, particularly for generics); consult specific product labeling.

Solution, ophthalmic: Trimethoprim 1 mg and polymyxin B sulfate 10,000 units per 1 mL (10 mL)

Polytrim®: Trimethoprim 1 mg and polymyxin B sulfate 10,000 units per 1 mL (10 mL) [contains benzalkonium chloride]

- ◆ **Trimethoprim and Sulfamethoxazole** *see* Sulfamethoxazole and Trimethoprim *on page* *1986*
- ◆ **Trinipatch (Can)** *see* Nitroglycerin *on page* *1523*
- ◆ **Triostat** *see* Liothyronine *on page* *1272*
- ◆ **Tripedia** *see* Diphtheria and Tetanus Toxoids, and Acellular Pertussis Vaccine *on page* *681*
- ◆ **Triple Antibiotic** *see* Bacitracin, Neomycin, and Polymyxin B *on page* *253*
- ◆ **Triple Paste AF [OTC]** *see* Miconazole (Topical) *on page* *1431*
- ◆ **Trip-PSE** *see* Triprolidine and Pseudoephedrine *on page* *2129*

Triprolidine and Pseudoephedrine

(trye PROE li deen & soo doe e FED rin)

Medication Safety Issues

BEERS Criteria medication:

This drug may be potentially inappropriate for use in geriatric patients (Quality of evidence - moderate; Strength of recommendation - strong).

Brand Names: US Aprodine [OTC]; Ed A-Hist PSE [OTC]; Entre-Hist PSE; Genac; Hist-PSE; Histafed; Pediatex TD [DSC]; Trip-PSE

Brand Names: Canada Actifed

Therapeutic Category Antihistamine/Decongestant Combination; Sympathomimetic

Generic Availability (US) Yes

Use Temporary relief of nasal congestion, running nose, sneezing, itching of nose or throat and itchy, watery eyes due to common cold, hay fever or other upper respiratory allergies (OTC product: FDA approved in ages ≥6 years and adults). **Note:** Approved ages and uses for generic products may vary; consult labeling for specific information.

Pregnancy Considerations Maternal antihistamine use has generally not resulted in an increased risk of birth defects; however, information related to triprolidine is limited. Refer to the Pseudoephedrine monograph for information related to decongestants.

Breast-Feeding Considerations Triprolidine is excreted into breast milk. Based on data from three cases, the estimated exposure to the nursing infant is <1% of the weight-adjusted maternal dose. Antihistamines may decrease maternal serum prolactin concentrations when administered prior to the establishment of nursing. Pseudoephedrine is also excreted into breast milk. Refer to the Pseudoephedrine monograph for information related to decongestants.

Contraindications OTC labeling: When used for self-medication, do not use if you have hypersensitivity to pseudoephedrine, triprolidine or any component of the formulation; are taking MAO inhibitor therapy (concurrent or within 2 weeks); are taking sedatives or tranquilizers (without first consulting physician)

Warnings/Precautions May cause CNS depression, which may impair physical or mental abilities; patients must be cautioned about performing tasks which require mental alertness (eg, operating machinery or driving). Effects may be potentiated when used with other sedative drugs or ethanol. When used for self medication (OTC), do not exceed recommended doses; discontinue use and contact health care provider if symptoms do not improve within 7 days or are accompanied by fever, nervousness, dizziness or sleeplessness occur or if new symptoms occur. Consult health care provider prior to OTC use with heart disease, hypotension, thyroid disease, diabetes, asthma, emphysema, chronic bronchitis, glaucoma, or enlarged prostate. In the elderly, avoid use of triprolidine (potent anticholinergic agent) due to increased risk of confusion, dry mouth, constipation, and other anticholinergic effects; clearance decreases in patients of advanced age (Beers Criteria).

Warnings: Additional Pediatric Considerations Safety and efficacy for the use of cough and cold products in pediatric patients <4 years of age is limited; the AAP warns against the use of these products for respiratory illnesses in this age group. Serious adverse effects including death have been reported (in some cases, high blood concentrations of pseudoephedrine were found). Many of these products contain multiple active ingredients, increasing the risk of accidental overdose when used with other products. The FDA notes that there are no approved OTC uses for these products in pediatric patients <2 years of age. Health care providers are reminded to ask caregivers about the use of OTC cough and cold products in order to avoid exposure to multiple medications containing the same ingredient (AAP 2012; FDA 2008).

Adverse Reactions

Cardiovascular: Tachycardia

Central nervous system: Dizziness, drowsiness, fatigue, headache, insomnia, nervousness, transient stimulation

Gastrointestinal: Abdominal pain, appetite increase, diarrhea, nausea, weight gain, xerostomia

Genitourinary: Dysuria

Neuromuscular & skeletal: Arthralgia, weakness

Respiratory: Pharyngitis, thickening of bronchial secretions

Miscellaneous: Diaphoresis

Drug Interactions

Metabolism/Transport Effects Refer to individual components.

Avoid Concomitant Use

Avoid concomitant use of Triprolidine and Pseudoephedrine with any of the following: Aclidinium; Azelastine (Nasal); Eluxadoline; Ergot Derivatives; Glucagon; Iobenguane I 123; Ipratropium (Oral Inhalation); MAO Inhibitors; Orphenadrine; Paraldehyde; Potassium Chloride; Thalidomide; Tiotropium; Umeclidinium

Increased Effect/Toxicity

Triprolidine and Pseudoephedrine may increase the levels/effects of: AbobotulinumtoxinA; Alcohol (Ethyl); Analgesics (Opioid); Anticholinergic Agents; ARIPiprazole; Azelastine (Nasal); Buprenorphine; CNS Depressants; Eluxadoline; Glucagon; Hydrocodone; Methotrimeprazine; Metyrosine; Mirabegron; Mirtazapine; OnabotulinumtoxinA; Orphenadrine; Paraldehyde; Potassium Chloride; Pramipexole; RimabotulinumtoxinB; ROPINIRole; Rotigotine; Selective Serotonin Reuptake Inhibitors; Suvorexant; Sympathomimetics; Thalidomide; Thiazide Diuretics; Tiotropium; Topiramate; Zolpidem

The levels/effects of Triprolidine and Pseudoephedrine may be increased by: Aclidinium; Alkalinizing Agents; AtoMOXetine; Brimonidine (Topical); Cannabis; Carbonic Anhydrase Inhibitors; Doxylamine; Dronabinol; Droperidol; Ergot Derivatives; HydrOXYzine; Ipratropium (Oral Inhalation); Kava Kava; Linezolid; Magnesium Sulfate; MAO Inhibitors; Methotrimeprazine; Mianserin; Nabilone; Perampanel; Pramlintide; Rufinamide; Serotonin/Norepinephrine Reuptake Inhibitors; Sodium Oxybate; Tapentadol; Tedizolid; Tetrahydrocannabinol; Umeclidinium

Decreased Effect

Triprolidine and Pseudoephedrine may decrease the levels/effects of: Acetylcholinesterase Inhibitors; Benzylpenicilloyl Polylysine; Betahistine; FentaNYL; Hyaluronidase; Iobenguane I 123; Itopride; Metoclopramide; Secretin

The levels/effects of Triprolidine and Pseudoephedrine may be decreased by: Acetylcholinesterase Inhibitors; Alpha1-Blockers; Amphetamines; Spironolactone; Urinary Acidifying Agents

Storage/Stability Store at room temperature. Protect from light and freezing.

Mechanism of Action Refer to Pseudoephedrine monograph.

Triprolidine is a member of the propylamine (alkylamine) chemical class of H_1-antagonist antihistamines. As such, it is considered to be relatively less sedating than traditional antihistamines of the ethanolamine, phenothiazine, and ethylenediamine classes of antihistamines. Triprolidine has a shorter half-life and duration of action than most of the other alkylamine antihistamines. Like all H_1-antagonist antihistamines, the mechanism of action of triprolidine is believed to involve competitive blockade of H_1-receptor sites resulting in the inability of histamine to combine with its receptor sites and exert its usual effects on target cells. Antihistamines do not interrupt any effects of histamine which have already occurred. Therefore, these agents are used more successfully in the prevention rather than the treatment of histamine-induced reactions.

Pharmacokinetics (Adult data unless noted) Also see Pseudoephedrine monograph.

Metabolism: Triprolidine: Extensively hepatic (Simons 1986)

Half-life: Triprolidine: ~2 to 5 hours (Simons 1986)

Time to peak serum concentration: Triprolidine: ~2 hours (Simons 1986)

Elimination: Triprolidine: Urine (~1% as unchanged triprolidine) (Simons 1986)

Dosing: Usual

Pediatric: **Note:** Multiple concentrations of oral liquid formulations (liquid, syrup) exist; close attention must be paid to the concentration when ordering or administering.

Cold, allergy symptoms: Oral:

Liquid (Triprolodine 0.938 mg and pseudoephedrine 10 mg per **1 mL**):

Children 6 to <12 years: 1.33 mL every 6 hours, do not exceed 4 doses in 24 hours; maximum daily dose: 5.33 mL/24 hours

Children ≥12 years and Adolescents: 2.67 mL every 6 hours, do not exceed 4 doses in 24 hours; maximum daily dose: 10.68 mL/24 hours

Syrup (Triprolidine 1.25 mg and pseudoephedrine 30 mg per **5 mL**):

Children 6 to 12 years: 5 mL every 4 to 6 hours; do not exceed 4 doses in 24 hours; maximum daily dose: 20 mL/24 hours

Children ≥12 years and Adolescents: 10 mL every 6 hours; do not exceed 4 doses in 24 hours; maximum daily dose: 40 mL/24 hours

Tablet (Triprolidine 2.5 mg and pseudoephedrine 60 mg):

Children 6 to <12 years: 1/2 tablet every 4 to 6 hours; do not exceed 4 doses in 24 hours

Children ≥12 years and Adolescents: One tablet every 4 to 6 hours; do not exceed 4 doses in 24 hours

Adult:

Cold, allergy symptoms: Oral:

Liquid (triprolidine 0.938 mg and pseudoephedrine 10 mg per 1 mL): 2.67 mL every 6 hours; maximum daily dose: 4 doses [10.68 mL]/24 hours

Syrup (triprolidine 1.25 mg and pseudoephedrine 30 mg per 5 mL): 10 mL every 4 to 6 hours; maximum daily dose: 4 doses [40 mL]/24 hours

Tablet (triprolidine 2.5 mg and pseudoephedrine 60 mg): One tablet every 4 to 6 hours; maximum daily dose: 4 doses/24 hours)

Test Interactions

Pseudoephedrine: Interferes with urine detection of amphetamine (false-positive).

Triprolidine: May suppress the wheal and flare reactions to skin test antigens.

Dosage Forms Excipient information presented when available (limited, particularly for generics); consult specific product labeling. [DSC] = Discontinued product

Liquid, oral:

Entre-Hist PSE: Triprolidine hydrochloride 0.938 mg and pseudoephedrine hydrochloride 10 mg per 1 mL (30 mL) [cotton candy flavor]

Pediatex TD: Triprolidine hydrochloride 0.938 mg and pseudoephedrine hydrochloride 10 mg per 1 mL (30 mL [DSC]) [cotton candy flavor]

Syrup, oral: Triprolidine hydrochloride 1.25 mg and pseudoephedrine hydrochloride 30 mg per 5 mL (120 mL) [DSC]

Aprodine: Triprolidine hydrochloride 1.25 mg and pseudoephedrine hydrochloride 30 mg per 5 mL (120 mL)

Tablet, oral:

Aprodine: Triprolidine hydrochloride 2.5 mg and pseudoephedrine hydrochloride 60 mg

Ed A-Hist PSE: Triprolidine hydrochloride 2.5 mg and pseudoephedrine hydrochloride 60 mg

- ◆ **Tris Buffer** *see* Tromethamine *on page 2131*
- ◆ **Trisenox** *see* Arsenic Trioxide *on page 198*
- ◆ **Tris(hydroxymethyl)aminomethane** *see* Tromethamine *on page 2131*
- ◆ **Trisulfa (Can)** *see* Sulfamethoxazole and Trimethoprim *on page 1986*
- ◆ **Trisulfa DS (Can)** *see* Sulfamethoxazole and Trimethoprim *on page 1986*

- ◆ **Trisulfa S (Can)** *see* Sulfamethoxazole and Trimethoprim *on page 1986*
- ◆ **Trivagizole-3® (Can)** *see* Clotrimazole (Topical) *on page 518*
- ◆ **Trivalent Recombinant Hemagglutinin (rHA) Vaccine** *see* Influenza Virus Vaccine (Recombinant) *on page 1116*
- ◆ **Trixaicin [OTC]** *see* Capsaicin *on page 362*
- ◆ **Trixaicin HP [OTC]** *see* Capsaicin *on page 362*
- ◆ **Trizivir** *see* Abacavir, Lamivudine, and Zidovudine *on page 38*
- ◆ **Trocaine Throat [OTC]** *see* Benzocaine *on page 268*
- ◆ **Trocal Cough Suppressant [OTC]** *see* Dextromethorphan *on page 631*
- ◆ **Trokendi XR** *see* Topiramate *on page 2085*

Tromethamine (troe METH a meen)

Medication Safety Issues

Sound-alike/look-alike issues:

Tromethamine may be confused with TrophAmine

Related Information

Management of Drug Extravasations *on page 2298*

Brand Names: US Tham

Therapeutic Category Alkalinizing Agent, Parenteral

Generic Availability (US) No

Use Correction of severe metabolic acidosis in patients in whom sodium or carbon dioxide elimination is restricted (eg, infants needing alkalinization after receiving maximum sodium bicarbonate [8 to 10 mEq/kg/24 hours]) (FDA approved in pediatric patients [age not specified] and adults); correction of metabolic acidosis associated with cardiac bypass surgery or cardiac arrest (FDA approved in adults); to correct excess acidity of stored blood that is preserved with acid citrate dextrose (ACD) (FDA approved in adults)

Pregnancy Risk Factor C

Pregnancy Considerations Animal studies have not been conducted. There are no adequate and well-controlled studies in pregnant women. Use only if potential benefit outweighs possible risk to the fetus.

Breast-Feeding Considerations It is not known if tromethamine is excreted in breast milk. The manufacturer recommends that caution be exercised when administering tromethamine to nursing women.

Contraindications Hypersensitivity to tromethamine or any component of the formulation; uremia or anuria; chronic respiratory acidosis (neonates); salicylate intoxication (neonates)

Warnings/Precautions Reduce dose and monitor pH carefully in renal impairment; drug should not be given for a period of longer than 24 hours unless for a life-threatening situation. May cause respiratory depression; monitor closely especially if patient not intubated. May cause hypoglycemia with extremely large doses. Vesicant; ensure proper needle or catheter placement prior to and during administration; avoid extravasation; may cause inflammation and tissue necrosis.

Warnings: Additional Pediatric Considerations Avoid infusion via low-lying umbilical venous catheters (particularly with concentrations ≥1.2 M) due to associated risk of hepatocellular necrosis; severe local tissue necrosis and sloughing may occur if solution extravasates; administer via central line or large vein slowly. Due to the greater osmotic effects of tromethamine, use of sodium bicarbonate for the treatment of acidotic neonates and infants with RDS may be preferred; may cause prolonged hypoglycemia in neonates or with rapid IV infusion and overdosage. Monitor pH carefully as large doses may increase blood pH greater than normal which may result in depressed respiration.

Adverse Reactions

Cardiovascular: Hypervolemia, venospasm

Endocrine & metabolic: Hyperkalemia, hypoglycemia (usually doses >500 mg/kg administered over <1 hour)

Hepatic: Hepatic necrosis (resulted during delivery via umbilical venous catheter)

Local: Necrosis with extravasation, phlebitis, tissue irritation

Respiratory: Apnea, pulmonary edema, respiratory depression

Drug Interactions

Metabolism/Transport Effects None known.

Avoid Concomitant Use There are no known interactions where it is recommended to avoid concomitant use.

Increased Effect/Toxicity

Tromethamine may increase the levels/effects of: Alpha-/Beta-Agonists (Indirect-Acting); Amphetamines; Flecainide; Mecamylamine; Memantine; QuiNINE

Decreased Effect There are no known significant interactions involving a decrease in effect.

Storage/Stability Store at 20°C to 25°C (68°F to 77°F). Protect from freezing.

Mechanism of Action Acts as a proton acceptor, which combines with hydrogen ions, liberating bicarbonate buffer, to correct acidosis. It buffers both metabolic and respiratory acids, limiting carbon dioxide generation. Also an osmotic diuretic.

Pharmacokinetics (Adult data unless noted) 30% of dose is not ionized; rapidly eliminated by kidneys

Dosing: Neonatal Note: Dose dependent upon severity and progression of acidosis; doses should be administered slowly to prevent overtreatment. Tromethamine is available as a 0.3 M solution (THAM); doses are based on this concentration and expressed as volumes (mL/kg). Each mL of THAM = 0.3 mmol = 36 mg = 0.3 mEq

Metabolic acidosis with respiratory distress syndrome (RDS): IV:

Manufacturer's labeling: 1 mL/kg for each pH unit below 7.4; additional doses to be determined by changes in PaO_2, pH, and pCO_2

Alternate dosing (Nahas 1998): Limited data available:

Dose (mL) of THAM = body weight (kg) × base deficit (mEq/L)

Note: The maximum dose recommended for neonates with normal renal function is 5 to 7 mmol/kg/day; lower doses may be needed in patients with renal dysfunction. In general, dose should be delivered slowly, over 1 hour in premature neonates. Use of a small loading dose (25% of the calculated dose) over 5 to 10 minutes through an umbilical or peripheral vein followed by remainder of the dose over 1 hour has been reported (Gupta 1967; Nahas 1998; Strauss 1968).

Dosing: Usual Note: Dose dependent upon severity and progression of acidosis; doses should be administered slowly to prevent overtreatment. Tromethamine is available as a 0.3 M solution (THAM); doses are based on this concentration and expressed as volumes (mL/kg). Each mL of THAM = 0.3 mmol = 36 mg = 0.3 mEq

Pediatric:

Metabolic acidosis: Infants, Children, and Adolescents:

IV: Empiric dosage based upon base deficit: Dose (mL) of THAM = body weight (kg) x base deficit (mEq/L) x 1.1*

Usual range: 1 to 2 mEq/kg/dose; maximum dose in 24 hours: 15 mEq/kg/24 hours (15 mmol/kg/24 hours) (Kliegman 2007; Nahas 1998)

*Factor of 1.1 accounts for an approximate reduction of 10% in buffering capacity due to the presence of sufficient acetic acid to lower the pH of the 0.3 M solution to approximately 8.6

Metabolic acidosis with cardiac arrest: Limited data available: **Note:** Routine use of buffering agents during cardiac arrest not recommended (AHA [Klienman 2010]): Infants, Children, and Adolescents: THAM: IV: 1 mL/kg should raise bicarbonate concentration by 1 mEq/L (Fuhrman 2011)

Adult:

Metabolic acidosis with cardiac arrest:

IV: 3.6 to 10.8 g (111 to 333 mL); additional amounts may be required to control acidosis after arrest reversed

Open chest: Intraventricular: 2 to 6 g (62 to 185 mL). **Note:** Do not inject into cardiac muscle.

Acidosis associated with cardiac bypass surgery: IV: Average dose: 9 mL/kg (2.7 mEq/kg); 500 mL is adequate for most adults; maximum dose: 500 mg/kg over at least 1 hour

Excess acidity of acid citrate dextrose (ACD) blood in cardiac bypass surgery: 15 to 77 mL of 0.3 molar solution added to each 500 mL of ACD blood

Administration

Parenteral: IV infusion: Infuse undiluted solution (0.3 M) slowly

Pediatric: Metabolic acidosis: Administer over at least 1 hour

Adult:

Correction of metabolic acidosis in cardiac bypass surgery: Administer by slow IV infusion over at least 1 hour (maximum rate: 500 mg/kg over at least 1 hour); rapid administration may result in prolonged hypoglycemia.

Correction of metabolic acidosis in cardiac arrest: If chest is not open, inject into a large peripheral vein.

Vesicant (with IV administration); ensure proper needle or catheter placement prior to and during administration; avoid extravasation. If extravasation occurs, stop IV administration immediately and disconnect (leave cannula/needle in place); gently aspirate extravasated solution (do **NOT** flush the line); remove needle/cannula; elevate extremity.

Vesicant/Extravasation Risk Vesicant

Monitoring Parameters Serum electrolytes, arterial blood gases, serum pH, blood sugar, ECG monitoring, renal function tests

Dosage Forms Excipient information presented when available (limited, particularly for generics); consult specific product labeling.

Solution, Intravenous:

Tham: 30 mEq/100 mL (500 mL)

Tropicamide (troe PIK a mide)

Brand Names: US Mydral [DSC]; Mydriacyl

Brand Names: Canada Diotrope; Mydriacyl

Therapeutic Category Ophthalmic Agent, Mydriatic

Generic Availability (US) Yes

Use Short-acting mydriatic used in diagnostic procedures; as well as preoperatively and postoperatively; treatment of some cases of acute iritis, iridocyclitis, and keratitis

Pregnancy Risk Factor C

Pregnancy Considerations Animal reproduction studies have not been conducted. If ophthalmic agents are needed during pregnancy, the minimum effective dose should be used in combination with punctual occlusion to decrease potential exposure to the fetus (Samples, 1988).

Breast-Feeding Considerations It is not known if tropicamide is excreted in breast milk. The manufacturer recommends that caution be used if administered to nursing women.

Contraindications

Hypersensitivity to tropicamide or any component of the formulation

Documentation of allergenic cross-reactivity for belladonna alkaloids is limited. However, because of similarities in chemical structure and/or pharmacologic actions, the possibility of cross-sensitivity cannot be ruled out with certainty.

Warnings/Precautions May cause drowsiness and/or blurred vision, which may impair physical or mental abilities; patients must be cautioned about performing tasks that require mental alertness (eg, operating machinery, driving). May cause a transient increase in intraocular pressure. Use with caution in infants and children; may cause potentially dangerous CNS disturbances. Psychotic reactions, behavioral disturbances, and vasomotor or cardiorespiratory collapse in children have been reported with the use of anticholinergic drugs.

For topical ophthalmic use only. To avoid excessive systemic absorption, apply gentle finger pressure to lacrimal sac for 2 to 3 minutes following application. Do not touch dropper tip to eyelids or any surface. Contains benzalkonium chloride, which may be absorbed by soft contact lenses; remove lenses prior to administration.

Adverse Reactions

Cardiovascular: Central nervous system dysfunction, tachycardia

Central nervous system: Headache

Dermatologic: Pallor

Gastrointestinal: Nausea, vomiting, xerostomia

Hypersensitivity: Hypersensitivity reaction

Neuromuscular & skeletal: Muscle rigidity

Ophthalmic: Blurred vision, photophobia, stinging of eyes (transient), superficial punctate keratitis

Drug Interactions

Metabolism/Transport Effects None known.

Avoid Concomitant Use There are no known interactions where it is recommended to avoid concomitant use.

Increased Effect/Toxicity There are no known significant interactions involving an increase in effect.

Decreased Effect There are no known significant interactions involving a decrease in effect.

Storage/Stability Store at 8°C to 27°C (46°F to 80°F). Do not refrigerate or store at high temperatures.

Mechanism of Action Prevents the sphincter muscle of the iris and the muscle of the ciliary body from responding to cholinergic stimulation; produces dilation and prevents accommodation.

Pharmacodynamics

Maximum mydriatic effect: ~20-40 minutes

Duration: ~6-7 hours

Maximum cycloplegic effect:

Peak: 20-35 minutes

Duration: <6 hours

Dosing: Neonatal Ophthalmic: Mydriasis: Instill 1 drop (0.5%) 15-20 minutes prior to procedure (1% concentration may be required in patients with heavily pigmented irides); **Note:** In premature neonates, use of 1% solution, while effective, has been associated with significant increases in mean blood pressure when used simultaneously with phenylephrine eye drops (Chew, 2005).

Dosing: Usual Children and Adults: Ophthalmic:

Cycloplegia: Instill 1-2 drops (1%); may repeat in 5 minutes. The exam must be performed within 30 minutes after the repeat dose; if the patient is not examined within 20-30 minutes, instill an additional drop. Concentrations <1% are inadequate for producing satisfactory cycloplegia.

Mydriasis: Instill 1-2 drops (0.5%) 15-20 minutes before exam; may repeat every 30 minutes as needed

Administration Ophthalmic: To minimize systemic absorption, apply finger pressure on the lacrimal sac for 1-2 minutes following instillation of the ophthalmic solution; avoid contact of bottle tip with skin or eye

Dosage Forms Excipient information presented when available (limited, particularly for generics); consult specific product labeling. [DSC] = Discontinued product

Solution, Ophthalmic:

Mydral: 0.5% (15 mL [DSC]); 1% (15 mL [DSC])

Mydriacyl: 1% (3 mL, 15 mL)

Generic: 0.5% (15 mL); 1% (2 mL, 3 mL, 15 mL)

- ◆ **Trumenba** *see* Meningococcal Group B Vaccine *on page 1351*
- ◆ **Trusopt** *see* Dorzolamide *on page 706*
- ◆ **Truvada** *see* Emtricitabine and Tenofovir *on page 742*
- ◆ **TSPA** *see* Thiotepa *on page 2053*
- ◆ **TT** *see* Tetanus Toxoid (Adsorbed) *on page 2032*
- ◆ **Tums [OTC]** *see* Calcium Carbonate *on page 343*
- ◆ **Tums Chews Extra Strength (Can)** *see* Calcium Carbonate *on page 343*
- ◆ **Tums Chewy Delights [OTC]** *see* Calcium Carbonate *on page 343*
- ◆ **Tums E-X 750 [OTC]** *see* Calcium Carbonate *on page 343*
- ◆ **Tums Extra Strength (Can)** *see* Calcium Carbonate *on page 343*
- ◆ **Tums Freshers [OTC]** *see* Calcium Carbonate *on page 343*
- ◆ **Tums Kids [OTC]** *see* Calcium Carbonate *on page 343*
- ◆ **Tums Lasting Effects [OTC]** *see* Calcium Carbonate *on page 343*
- ◆ **Tums Regular Strength (Can)** *see* Calcium Carbonate *on page 343*
- ◆ **Tums Smoothies [OTC]** *see* Calcium Carbonate *on page 343*
- ◆ **Tums Smoothies (Can)** *see* Calcium Carbonate *on page 343*
- ◆ **Tums Ultra 1000 [OTC]** *see* Calcium Carbonate *on page 343*
- ◆ **Tums Ultra Strength (Can)** *see* Calcium Carbonate *on page 343*
- ◆ **TussiCaps** *see* Hydrocodone and Chlorpheniramine *on page 1034*
- ◆ **Tussigon** *see* Hydrocodone and Homatropine *on page 1036*
- ◆ **Tussin [OTC]** *see* GuaiFENesin *on page 988*
- ◆ **Tussionex** *see* Hydrocodone and Chlorpheniramine *on page 1034*
- ◆ **Tussionex Pennkinetic** *see* Hydrocodone and Chlorpheniramine *on page 1034*
- ◆ **Twinject (Can)** *see* EPINEPHrine (Systemic, Oral Inhalation) *on page 760*
- ◆ **Ty21a Vaccine** *see* Typhoid Vaccine *on page 2133*
- ◆ **Tygacil** *see* Tigecycline *on page 2065*
- ◆ **Tylenol [OTC]** *see* Acetaminophen *on page 44*
- ◆ **Tylenol (Can)** *see* Acetaminophen *on page 44*
- ◆ **Tylenol #2** *see* Acetaminophen and Codeine *on page 50*
- ◆ **Tylenol #3** *see* Acetaminophen and Codeine *on page 50*
- ◆ **Tylenol 8 Hour [OTC]** *see* Acetaminophen *on page 44*
- ◆ **Tylenol Arthritis Pain [OTC]** *see* Acetaminophen *on page 44*
- ◆ **Tylenol Children's [OTC]** *see* Acetaminophen *on page 44*
- ◆ **Tylenol Children's Meltaways [OTC] [DSC]** *see* Acetaminophen *on page 44*
- ◆ **Tylenol Codeine** *see* Acetaminophen and Codeine *on page 50*
- ◆ **Tylenol Extra Strength [OTC]** *see* Acetaminophen *on page 44*
- ◆ **Tylenol Jr. Meltaways [OTC]** *see* Acetaminophen *on page 44*
- ◆ **Tylenol No. 1 (Can)** *see* Acetaminophen and Codeine *on page 50*
- ◆ **Tylenol No. 1 Forte (Can)** *see* Acetaminophen and Codeine *on page 50*
- ◆ **Tylenol No. 2 with Codeine (Can)** *see* Acetaminophen and Codeine *on page 50*
- ◆ **Tylenol No. 3 with Codeine (Can)** *see* Acetaminophen and Codeine *on page 50*
- ◆ **Tylenol No. 4 with Codeine (Can)** *see* Acetaminophen and Codeine *on page 50*
- ◆ **Tylenol with Codeine #3** *see* Acetaminophen and Codeine *on page 50*
- ◆ **Tylenol with Codeine #4** *see* Acetaminophen and Codeine *on page 50*
- ◆ **Tylox** *see* Oxycodone and Acetaminophen *on page 1594*
- ◆ **Typherix (Can)** *see* Typhoid Vaccine *on page 2133*
- ◆ **Typhim Vi** *see* Typhoid Vaccine *on page 2133*

Typhoid Vaccine (TYE foid vak SEEN)

Related Information

Centers for Disease Control and Prevention (CDC) and Other Links *on page 2424*

Immunization Administration Recommendations *on page 2411*

Immunization Schedules *on page 2416*

Brand Names: US Typhim Vi; Vivotif

Brand Names: Canada Typherix; Typhim Vi; Vivotif

Therapeutic Category Vaccine; Vaccine, Inactivated Bacteria; Vaccine, Live Bacteria

Generic Availability (US) No

Use

Active immunization to prevent disease from exposure to *Salmonella typhi*

Parenteral (Typhim Vi): FDA approved in ages ≥2 years and adults

Oral: Live attenuated Ty21a vaccine (Vivotif): FDA approved in ages ≥6 years and adults

Not for routine vaccination. The Advisory Committee on Immunization Practices (ACIP) recommends vaccination for the following patients (CDC/ACIP [Jackson 2015]):

- Travelers to areas with a recognized risk of exposure to *S. typhi*
- Persons with intimate exposure (eg, household contact) to a person with *S. typhi* fever or a known carrier
- Laboratory technicians with frequent exposure to *S. typhi*

Medication Guide Available Yes

Pregnancy Risk Factor C

Pregnancy Considerations Animal reproduction studies have not been conducted. The manufacturer of the Typhim Vi injection suggests delaying vaccination until the second or third trimester if possible. Untreated typhoid fever may lead to miscarriage or vertical intrauterine transmission causing neonatal typhoid (rare).

Breast-Feeding Considerations It is not known if typhoid vaccine is excreted in breast milk.

Contraindications

Hypersensitivity to any component of the vaccine. In addition, the oral vaccine is contraindicated with congenital or acquired immunodeficient state, acute febrile illness

Canadian labeling: Additional contraindications (not in US labeling): Typherix: Acute severe febrile illness. **Note:** Canadian immunization guidelines also contraindicate oral typhoid vaccine in pregnancy, acute gastrointestinal condition or inflammatory bowel disease.

Warnings/Precautions Not all recipients of typhoid vaccine will be fully protected against typhoid fever. Travelers should take all necessary precautions to avoid contact or ingestion of potentially contaminated food or water sources. Should not be used to treat typhoid fever or a chronic typhoid carrier.

Injection: Administer at least 2 weeks prior to expected exposure. The decision to administer or delay vaccination because of current or recent febrile illness depends on the severity of symptoms and the etiology of the disease. Consider deferring administration in patients with moderate or severe acute illness (with or without fever); vaccination should not be delayed for patients with mild acute illness (with or without fever) (NCIRD/ACIP 2011). Use caution with coagulation disorders (including thrombocytopenia) and patients on anticoagulant therapy; bleeding/hematoma may occur from IM administration; if the patient receives antihemophilia or other similar therapy, IM injection can be scheduled shortly after such therapy is administered (NCIRD/ACIP 2011). Immediate treatment (including epinephrine 1:1000) for anaphylactoid and/or hypersensitivity reactions should be readily available (NCIRD/ACIP 2011). Syncope has been reported with use of injectable vaccines and may result in serious secondary injury (eg, skull fracture, cerebral hemorrhage); typically reported in adolescents and young adults and within 15 minutes after vaccination. Procedures should be in place to avoid injuries from falling and to restore cerebral perfusion if syncope occurs (NCIRD/ACIP 2011).

Oral: Full immunization schedule should be completed at least 1 week prior to expected exposure. The complete immunization schedule must be followed to achieve optimum immune response. Do not administer during acute GI illness; vaccination may be deferred with persistent diarrhea or vomiting.

In order to maximize vaccination rates, the ACIP recommends simultaneous administration of all age-appropriate vaccines (live or inactivated) for which a person is eligible at a single clinic visit, unless contraindications exist. Vaccination may not result in effective immunity in all patients. Response depends upon multiple factors (eg, type of vaccine, age of patient) and may be improved by administering the vaccine at the recommended dose, route, and interval. Use with caution in severely immunocompromised patients (eg, patients receiving chemo/radiation therapy or other immunosuppressive therapy [including high-dose corticosteroids]); may have a reduced response to vaccination. In general, household and close contacts of persons with altered immunocompetence may receive all age appropriate vaccines (IDSA [Rubin 2014]; NCIRD/ACIP 2011); inactivated vaccines should be administered ≥2 weeks prior to planned immunosuppression when feasible; live vaccines should be administered ≥4 weeks prior to planned immunosuppression and avoided within 2 weeks of immunosuppression when feasible (IDSA [Rubin 2014]).

Specific recommendations for vaccination in immunocompromised patients with asplenia, cancer, HIV infection, cerebrospinal fluid leaks, cochlear implants, hematopoietic stem cell transplant (prior to or after), sickle cell disease, solid organ transplant (prior to or after), or those receiving immunosuppressive therapy for chronic conditions as well as contacts of immunocompromised patients are available from the IDSA (Rubin 2014). Antipyretics have not been shown to prevent febrile seizures; antipyretics may be used to treat fever or discomfort following vaccination (NCIRD/ACIP 2011). One study reported that routine prophylactic administration of acetaminophen to prevent fever prior to vaccination decreased the immune response of some vaccines; the clinical significance of this reduction in immune response has not been established (Prymula 2009).

Adverse Reactions In the U.S., all serious adverse reactions must be reported to the Department of Health and Human Services (DHHS) Vaccine Adverse Event Reporting System (VAERS) 1-800-822-7967 or online at https://vaers.hhs.gov/esub/index. In Canada, adverse reactions may be reported to local provincial/territorial health agencies or to the Vaccine Safety Section at Public Health Agency of Canada (1-866-844-0018).

Injection:

Central nervous system: Generalized ache, headache, malaise

Dermatologic: Pruritus

Gastrointestinal: Nausea, vomiting

Local: Erythema at injection site, induration at injection site, pain at injection site, swelling at injection site, tenderness at injection site

Neuromuscular & skeletal: Muscle tenderness, myalgia

Miscellaneous: Fever greater than 100 to 101 degrees, fever (undefined)

Rare but important or life-threatening: Anaphylaxis, angioedema, asthma, diarrhea, flu-like symptoms, Guillain-Barré syndrome, hypersensitivity reaction, intestinal perforation (jejunum), loss of consciousness, lymphadenopathy, neck pain, serum sickness, skin rash, syncope (with and without convulsions)

Oral:

Central nervous system: Headache

Dermatologic: Skin rash

Gastrointestinal: Abdominal pain, diarrhea, nausea, vomiting

Miscellaneous: Fever

Rare but important or life-threatening: Anaphylaxis, demyelinating disease, myalgia, pain, rheumatoid arthritis, sepsis

Drug Interactions

Metabolism/Transport Effects None known.

Avoid Concomitant Use

Avoid concomitant use of Typhoid Vaccine with any of the following: Belimumab; Fingolimod; Immunosuppressants

Increased Effect/Toxicity

The levels/effects of Typhoid Vaccine may be increased by: AzaTHIOprine; Belimumab; Corticosteroids (Systemic); Dimethyl Fumarate; Fingolimod; Immunosuppressants; Leflunomide; Mercaptopurine; Methotrexate

Decreased Effect

Typhoid Vaccine may decrease the levels/effects of: Tuberculin Tests

The levels/effects of Typhoid Vaccine may be decreased by: Antibiotics; AzaTHIOprine; Corticosteroids (Systemic); Dimethyl Fumarate; Fingolimod; Immune Globulins; Immunosuppressants; Leflunomide; Mercaptopurine; Methotrexate; Proguanil

Storage/Stability

Typherix: Store between 2°C to 8°C (35°F to 46°F); do not freeze. Discard if vaccine has been frozen. Protect from light.

Typhim Vi: Store between 2°C to 8°C (35°F to 46°F); do not freeze.

Vivotif: Store between 2°C to 8°C (35°F to 46°F).

Mechanism of Action Virulent strains of *Salmonella typhi* cause disease by penetrating the intestinal mucosa and entering the systemic circulation via the lymphatic vasculature. One possible mechanism of conferring immunity may be the provocation of a local immune response in the intestinal tract induced by oral ingesting of a live strain with subsequent aborted infection. The ability of *S. typhi* to produce clinical disease (and to elicit an immune response) is dependent on the bacteria having a complete lipopolysaccharide. The live attenuate Ty21a strain lacks the enzyme UDP-4-galactose epimerase so that lipopolysaccharide is only synthesized under conditions that induce bacterial autolysis. Thus, the strain remains avirulent despite the production of sufficient lipopolysaccharide to evoke a protective immune response. Despite low levels of lipopolysaccharide synthesis, cells lyse before gaining a virulent phenotype due to the intracellular accumulation of metabolic intermediates.

Efficacy: Based on a systematic review and meta-analysis, the estimated 2.5 to 3 year cumulative efficacy was 55% (95% confidence interval [CI]: 30% to 70%) for the injectable vaccine and 48% (CI: 34% to 58%) for the oral vaccine (CDC/ACIP [Jackson 2015]).

Pharmacodynamics

Onset of action: Immunity to *Salmonella typhi*: Oral: ~1 week; IM: ~2 weeks

Duration: Immunity: Oral: ~5 years; IM: ~2 years

Dosing: Usual

Pediatric: **Immunization:**

Oral (Vivotif): Children ≥6 years and Adolescents:

Primary immunization: One capsule on alternate days (eg, day 1, 3, 5, and 7) for a total of 4 doses; all doses should be completed at least 1 week prior to potential exposure

Reimmunization: Optimal schedule has not been established; a full course of primary immunization every 5 years is currently recommended for repeated or continued exposure

IM (Typhim Vi): Children ≥2 years and Adolescents:

Primary immunization: 0.5 mL given at least 2 weeks prior to expected exposure

Reimmunization: 0.5 mL; optimal schedule has not been established; a single dose every 2 years is currently recommended for repeated or continued exposure

Adult: **Immunization:**

Oral (Vivotif):

Primary immunization: One capsule on alternate days (eg, day 1, 3, 5, and 7) for a total of 4 doses; all doses should be completed at least 1 week prior to potential exposure

Reimmunization: Optimal schedule has not been established; a full course of primary immunization every 5 years is currently recommended for repeated or continued exposure

IM (Typhim Vi):

Primary immunization: 0.5 mL given at least 2 weeks prior to expected exposure

Reimmunization: 0.5 mL; optimal schedule has not been established; a single dose every 2 years is currently recommended for repeated or continued exposure

Dosing adjustment in renal impairment: There are no dosage adjustments provided in manufacturer's labeling.

Dosing adjustment in hepatic impairment: There are no dosage adjustments provided in manufacturer's labeling.

Administration

Parenteral: Administer by IM injection into the anterolateral aspect of the thigh or into the deltoid muscle; not for IV or SubQ administration. To prevent syncope-related injuries, adolescents and adults should be vaccinated while seated or lying down (NCIRD/ACIP 2011). **Note:** For patients at risk of hemorrhage following intramuscular injection, the vaccine should be administered intramuscularly if, in the opinion of the physician familiar with the patient's bleeding risk, the vaccine can be administered by this route with reasonable safety. If the patient receives antihemophilia or other similar therapy, intramuscular vaccination can be scheduled shortly after such therapy is administered. A fine needle (23 gauge or smaller) can be used for the vaccination and firm pressure applied to the site (without rubbing) for at least 2 minutes. The patient should be instructed concerning the risk of hematoma from the injection. Patients on anticoagulant therapy should be considered to have the same bleeding risks and treated as those with clotting factor disorders (NCIRD/ACIP 2011).

Oral: Oral capsule should be taken 1 hour before a meal with cold or lukewarm drink on alternate days (days 1, 3, 5, and 7); swallow capsule whole, do not chew

U.S. law requires that the date of administration, the vaccine manufacturer, lot number of vaccine, and the administering person's name, title, and address be entered into the patient's permanent medical record.

Monitoring Parameters After injection, observe for syncope for 15 minutes following administration (NCIRD/ACIP 2011). If seizure-like activity associated with syncope occurs, maintain patient in supine or Trendelenburg position to reestablish adequate cerebral perfusion.

Dosage Forms Excipient information presented when available (limited, particularly for generics); consult specific product labeling.

Capsule, enteric coated [live]:

Vivotif: Viable *S. typhi* Ty21a 2-6.8 x 10^9 colony-forming units and nonviable *S. typhi* Ty21a 5-50 x 10^9 bacterial cells [contains lactose 100-180 mg/capsule and sucrose 26-130 mg/capsule]

Injection, solution [inactivated]:

Typhim Vi: Purified Vi capsular polysaccharide 25 mcg/0.5 mL (0.5 mL, 10 mL) [derived from *S. typhi* Ty2 strain]

◆ **Typhoid Vaccine Live Oral Ty21a** *see* Typhoid Vaccine *on page 2133*

◆ **506U78** *see* Nelarabine *on page 1496*

◆ **UCB-P071** *see* Cetirizine *on page 423*

◆ **Uceris** *see* Budesonide (Systemic, Oral Inhalation) *on page 307*

◆ **UK-427,857** *see* Maraviroc *on page 1324*

◆ **UK92480** *see* Sildenafil *on page 1921*

◆ **UK109496** *see* Voriconazole *on page 2190*

◆ **Ulcidine (Can)** *see* Famotidine *on page 847*

◆ **Ulesfia** *see* Benzyl Alcohol *on page 273*

◆ **Ultiva** *see* Remifentanil *on page 1843*

◆ **Ultiva® (Can)** *see* Remifentanil *on page 1843*

◆ **Ultram** *see* TraMADol *on page 2098*

◆ **Ultram ER** *see* TraMADol *on page 2098*

◆ **UltraSal-ER** *see* Salicylic Acid *on page 1894*

◆ **Ultrase (Can)** *see* Pancrelipase *on page 1614*

◆ **Ultrase MT (Can)** *see* Pancrelipase *on page 1614*

◆ **Ultravate** *see* Halobetasol *on page 1001*

◆ **Ultravate® (Can)** *see* Halobetasol *on page 1001*

◆ **Ultravate PAC [DSC]** *see* Halobetasol *on page 1001*

◆ **Ultresa** *see* Pancrelipase *on page 1614*

◆ **Unasyn** *see* Ampicillin and Sulbactam *on page 159*

Undecylenic Acid and Derivatives

(un de sil EN ik AS id & dah RIV ah tivs)

Brand Names: US Fungi-Nail® [OTC]

Therapeutic Category Antifungal Agent, Topical

Generic Availability (US) No

Use Treatment of athlete's foot (tinea pedis), ringworm (except nails and scalp), prickly heat, jock itch (tinea cruris), diaper rash, and other minor skin irritations due to superficial dermatophytes

Contraindications Hypersensitivity to undecylenic acid or any component of the formulation

Warnings/Precautions For topical use only; avoid contact with eyes. Apply to clean, dry skin. When used for self-medication (OTC use), contact health care provider if condition does not improve within 4 weeks. Discontinue if sensitivity or irritation occurs. Not for self-medication (OTC use) in children <2 years of age.

Drug Interactions

Metabolism/Transport Effects None known.

Avoid Concomitant Use There are no known interactions where it is recommended to avoid concomitant use.

Increased Effect/Toxicity There are no known significant interactions involving an increase in effect.

Decreased Effect There are no known significant interactions involving a decrease in effect.

Pharmacodynamics Onset of action: Improvement in erythema and pruritus may be seen within 1 week after initiation of therapy

Dosing: Usual Children and Adults: Topical: Apply as needed twice daily for 2-4 weeks

Administration Topical: Clean and dry the affected area before topical application; if the solution is sprayed or applied onto the affected area, allow area to air dry; ointment or cream should be applied at night, the powder may be applied during the day or used alone when a drying effect is needed

Monitoring Parameters Resolution of skin infection

Dosage Forms Excipient information presented when available (limited, particularly for generics); consult specific product labeling.

Solution, topical:

Fungi-Nail®: Undecylenic acid 25% (29.57 mL)

- **Unidet® (Can)** *see* Tolterodine *on page* 2084
- **Uniphyl (Can)** *see* Theophylline *on page* 2044
- **Unisom-2 (Can)** *see* Doxylamine *on page* 721
- **Unithroid** *see* Levothyroxine *on page* 1250
- **Unithroid Direct** *see* Levothyroxine *on page* 1250
- **UniVert** *see* Meclizine *on page* 1337
- **Urasal® (Can)** *see* Methenamine *on page* 1385
- **Urate Oxidase** *see* Rasburicase *on page* 1839
- **Urea Peroxide** *see* Carbamide Peroxide *on page* 371
- **Urecholine** *see* Bethanechol *on page* 284
- **Urex** *see* Methenamine *on page* 1385
- **Urex** *see* Methenamine *on page* 1385
- **Urinary Pain Relief [OTC]** *see* Phenazopyridine *on page* 1678
- **Uro-Mag [OTC]** *see* Magnesium Oxide *on page* 1316
- **Uromax (Can)** *see* Oxybutynin *on page* 1588
- **Uromitexan (Can)** *see* Mesna *on page* 1371
- **Urozide (Can)** *see* Hydrochlorothiazide *on page* 1028
- **Urso (Can)** *see* Ursodiol *on page* 2136
- **Urso 250** *see* Ursodiol *on page* 2136
- **Ursodeoxycholic Acid** *see* Ursodiol *on page* 2136
- **Ursodesoxycholic Acid** *see* Ursodiol *on page* 2136

Ursodiol (ur soe DYE ol)

Medication Safety Issues

Sound-alike/look-alike issues:

Ursodiol may be confused with ulipristal

Brand Names: US Actigall; Urso 250; Urso Forte

Brand Names: Canada Dom-Ursodiol C; PHL-Ursodiol C; PMS-Ursodiol C; Urso; Urso DS

Therapeutic Category Gallstone Dissolution Agent

Generic Availability (US) Yes

Use Gallbladder stone dissolution (FDA approved in adults); prevention of gallstone formation (obese patients experiencing rapid weight loss) (FDA approved in adults); primary biliary cirrhosis (Urso®) (FDA approved in adults). Other uses include facilitate bile excretion in infants with biliary atresia; treatment of cholestasis secondary to PN; improve the hepatic metabolism of essential fatty acids in patients with cystic fibrosis

Pregnancy Risk Factor B

Pregnancy Considerations Adverse events have not been observed in animal reproduction studies. Ursodiol (ursodeoxycholic acid) is the treatment of choice for intrahepatic cholestasis of pregnancy (Kremer, 2011).

Breast-Feeding Considerations It is not known if ursodiol is excreted in breast milk. The manufacturer recommends that caution be exercised when administering ursodiol to nursing women.

Contraindications Hypersensitivity to ursodiol or any component of the formulation; not to be used with cholesterol, radiopaque, bile pigment stones; patients with unremitting acute cholecystitis, cholangitis, biliary obstruction, gallstone pancreatitis, or biliary-gastrointestinal fistula; allergy to bile acids

Warnings/Precautions Gallbladder stone dissolution may take several months of therapy; complete dissolution may not occur and recurrence of stones within 5 years has been observed in 50% of patients. Patients should be cautiously selected for therapy, consider alternative treatments. Specific treatments should be initiated in patients with ascites, hepatic encephalopathy, variceal bleeding, or if an urgent liver transplant is necessary. Use with caution in patients with a nonvisualizing gallbladder; therapy should be discontinued if gallbladder nonvisualization occurs during treatment. Use with caution in patients with chronic liver disease; monitor liver function tests monthly for the first 3 months, and every six months thereafter or as clinically necessary. Discontinuation of therapy may be necessary with significant elevations in liver function tests. Maintain bile flow during therapy to prevent biliary obstruction.

Adverse Reactions

Central nervous system: Dizziness, headache

Dermatologic: Alopecia, rash

Endocrine & metabolic: Hyperglycemia

Gastrointestinal: Constipation, diarrhea, dyspepsia, nausea, peptic ulcer, vomiting

Genitourinary: Urinary tract infection

Hematologic & oncologic: Leukopenia, thrombocytopenia

Hepatic: Cholecystitis

Hypersensitivity: Hypersensitivity reaction

Infection: Viral infection

Neuromuscular & skeletal: Arthritis, back pain, musculoskeletal pain, myalgia

Renal: Increased serum creatinine

Respiratory: Bronchitis, cough, flu-like symptoms, pharyngitis, upper respiratory tract infection

Rare but important or life-threatening: Abdominal distress, abdominal pain, abnormal hepatic function tests, angioedema, anorexia, biliary colic, esophagitis, facial edema, fever, hepatobiliary disease, increased gamma-glutamyl transferase, increased liver enzymes, increased serum alkaline phosphatase, increased serum ALT, increased serum AST, increased serum bilirubin, jaundice, laryngeal edema, malaise, metallic taste, myalgia, peripheral edema, pruritus, transaminases increased, urticaria, weakness

Drug Interactions

Metabolism/Transport Effects None known.

Avoid Concomitant Use There are no known interactions where it is recommended to avoid concomitant use.

Increased Effect/Toxicity There are no known significant interactions involving an increase in effect.

Decreased Effect

Ursodiol may decrease the levels/effects of: Nitrendipine

The levels/effects of Ursodiol may be decreased by: Aluminum Hydroxide; Bile Acid Sequestrants; Estrogen Derivatives; Fibric Acid Derivatives

Storage/Stability

Actigall: Store at 25°C (77°F); excursions permitted to 15°C to 30°C (59°F to 86°F).

Urso: Store at 20°C to 25°C (68°F to 77°F).

Urso Forte: Store at 20°C to 25°C (68°F to 77°F). When broken in half, scored Urso Forte 500 mg tablets maintain quality for up to 28 days when kept in current packaging and stored at 20°C to 25°C (68°F to 77°F). Split tablets should be stored separately from whole tablets due to bitter taste.

Mechanism of Action Decreases the cholesterol content of bile and bile stones by reducing the secretion of cholesterol from the liver and the fractional reabsorption of cholesterol by the intestines. Mechanism of action in primary biliary cirrhosis is not clearly defined.

Pharmacokinetics (Adult data unless noted)

Absorption: 90%

Protein binding: 70%

Metabolism: Undergoes extensive enterohepatic recycling; following hepatic conjugation and biliary secretion, the drug is hydrolyzed to active ursodiol, where it is recycled or transformed to lithocholic acid by colonic microbial flora; during chronic administration, ursodiol becomes a major biliary and plasma bile acid constituting 30% to 50% of biliary and plasma bile acids

Elimination: In feces via bile

Dosing: Neonatal Oral:

Parenteral nutrition-induced cholestasis, treatment: 30 mg/kg/day in 3 divided doses (Chen, 2004); some centers divide in 2 daily doses

Parenteral nutrition-induced cholestasis, prevention: 5 mg/kg/day in 4 divided doses beginning on day of life 3 with initiation of parenteral nutrition; increase dose to 10 mg/kg/day in 4 divided doses with initiation of enteral feeding; increase dose to 20 mg/kg/day in 4 divided doses when full enteral feedings reached. Dosing based on a double-blind, placebo-controlled study of 30 premature neonates (birth weight ≤900 g; GA: <34 weeks) which showed earlier achievement of full feeds and slight decrease of fecal fat excretion in the treatment group (Arslanoglu, 2008)

Dosing: Usual Oral:

Biliary atresia: Infants: 10-15 mg/kg/day once daily

Improvement in the hepatic metabolism of essential fatty acids in cystic fibrosis: Children: 30 mg/kg/day in 2 divided doses

TPN-induced cholestasis, treatment: Infants and Children: 30 mg/kg/day in 3 divided doses (Spagnuolo, 1996)

Gallstone dissolution: Adults: 8-10 mg/kg/day in 2-3 divided doses; maintenance therapy: 250 mg/day at bedtime for 6 months to 1 year; use beyond 24 months is not established

Gallstone prevention: Adults: 300 mg twice daily

Primary biliary cirrhosis: Adults: 13-15 mg/kg/day in 4 divided doses

Administration Oral: Administer with food or, if a single dosage, at bedtime

Monitoring Parameters ALT, AST, sonogram, oral cholecystogram before therapy and every 6 months during therapy; obtain ultrasound images of gallbladder at 6-month intervals for the first year of therapy

Additional Information 30% to 50% of patients have stone recurrence after dissolution

Dosage Forms Excipient information presented when available (limited, particularly for generics); consult specific product labeling.

Capsule, Oral:

Actigall: 300 mg

Generic: 300 mg

Tablet, Oral:

Urso 250: 250 mg

Urso Forte: 500 mg [scored]

Generic: 250 mg, 500 mg

Extemporaneous Preparations A 20 mg/mL ursodiol oral suspension may be made with capsules and either a 1:1 mixture of Ora-Sweet and Ora-Plus or a 1:1 mixture of methylcellulose 1% and syrup NF. Empty the contents of seventeen 300 mg capsules into a mortar. Add small portions of the chosen vehicle and mix to a uniform paste; mix while adding the vehicle in incremental proportions to **almost** 255 mL; transfer to a calibrated bottle, rinse mortar with vehicle, and add quantity of vehicle sufficient to make 255 mL. Label "shake well" and "refrigerate". Stable for 91 days refrigerated (Nahata, 1999).

A 25 mg/mL ursodiol oral suspension may be made with capsules. Empty the contents of ten 300 mg capsules into a mortar; add 10 mL Glycerin, USP and mix until smooth. Mix while adding 60 mL Ora-Plus; transfer mixture to a light-resistant bottle, rinse mortar with a small amount of Orange Syrup, NF, and add quantity of syrup sufficient to make 120 mL. Label "shake well". Stable for 60 days at room temperature or refrigerated (Mallett, 1997).

A 50 mg/mL ursodiol oral suspension may be made with tablets and 60 mL of either a 1:1 mixture of Ora-Plus and strawberry syrup or a 1:1 mixture of Ora-Plus and Ora-Sweet SF. Crush twelve 250 mg tablets in a mortar and reduce to a fine powder. Add small portions of the chosen vehicle and mix to a uniform paste; mix while adding the vehicle in incremental proportions to **almost** 60 mL; transfer to a calibrated bottle, rinse mortar with vehicle, and add quantity of vehicle sufficient to make 60 mL. Label "shake well" and "refrigerate". Stable for 90 days refrigerated (Johnson, 2002).

A 60 mg/mL ursodiol oral suspension may be made with capsules. Empty the contents of twelve 300 mg capsules into a mortar. Add small portions of glycerin and mix to a uniform paste; mix while adding simple syrup in incremental proportions to **almost** 60 mL; transfer to a calibrated bottle, rinse mortar with vehicle, and add quantity of vehicle sufficient to make 60 mL. Label "shake well" and "refrigerate". Stable for 35 days refrigerated (Johnson, 1995).

Johnson CE and Nesbitt J, "Stability of Ursodiol in an Extemporaneously Compounded Oral Liquid," *Am J Health Syst Pharm*, 1995, 52 (16):1798-1800.

Johnson CE and Streetman DD, "Stability of Oral Suspensions of Ursodiol Made From Tablets," *Am J Health Syst Pharm*, 2002, 59 (4):361-3.

Mallett MS, Hagan RL, and Peters DA, "Stability of Ursodiol 25 mg/mL in an Extemporaneously Prepared Oral Liquid," *Am J Health Syst Pharm*, 1997, 54(12):1401-4.

Nahata MC, Morosco RS, and Hipple TF, "Stability of Ursodiol in Two Extemporaneously Prepared Oral Suspensions," *J Appl Ther Res*, 1999, 2:221-4.

◆ **Urso DS (Can)** *see* Ursodiol *on page 2136*

◆ **Urso Forte** *see* Ursodiol *on page 2136*

◆ **Utradol (Can)** *see* Etodolac *on page 816*

◆ **Vacuant Mini-Enema [OTC] [DSC]** *see* Docusate *on page 697*

◆ **Vagistat-3 [OTC]** *see* Miconazole (Topical) *on page 1431*

ValACYclovir (val ay SYE kloe veer)

Medication Safety Issues

Sound-alike/look-alike issues:

Valtrex may be confused with Keflex, Valcyte, Zovirax

ValACYclovir may be confused with acyclovir, valGANciclovir, vancomycin

Brand Names: US Valtrex

Brand Names: Canada Apo-Valacyclovir; CO Valacyclovir; DOM-Valacyclovir; Mylan-Valacyclovir; PHL-Valacyclovir; PMS-Valacyclovir; PRO-Valacyclovir; Riva-Valacyclovir; Valtrex

Therapeutic Category Antiviral Agent, Oral

Generic Availability (US) Yes

Use Treatment of herpes labialis (cold sores) (FDA approved in ages ≥12 years and adults); treatment of chickenpox in immunocompetent patients (FDA approved in ages 2 to <18 years); treatment of herpes zoster (shingles) in immunocompetent patients (FDA approved in adults); treatment of initial and recurrent episodes of genital herpes (FDA approved in adults); suppression of recurrent genital herpes and reduction of heterosexual transmission of genital herpes in immunocompetent patients (FDA approved in adults); has also been used for suppression of genital herpes in HIV-infected individuals; suppression and prevention of vertical transmission of recurrent genital herpes during labor and delivery; for prevention and treatment of herpes infections in both immunocompromised and immunocompetent patients

Pregnancy Risk Factor B

Pregnancy Considerations Adverse events were not observed in animal reproduction studies. Valacyclovir is metabolized to acyclovir. In a pharmacokinetic study, maternal acyclovir serum concentrations were higher in pregnant women receiving valacyclovir than those given acyclovir for the suppression of recurrent herpes simplex virus (HSV) infection late in pregnancy. Amniotic fluid concentrations were also higher; however, there was no evidence that fetal exposure differed between the groups (Kimberlin, 1998). Data from an acyclovir pregnancy registry has shown no increased rate of birth defects than that of the general population; however, the registry is small and the manufacturer notes that use during pregnancy is only warranted if the potential benefit to the mother justifies the risk of the fetus. Because more data is available for acyclovir, that agent is preferred for the treatment of genital herpes in pregnant women (ACOG, 2000; CDC, 2010); however, valacyclovir may be considered for use due to its simplified dosing schedule (DHHS, 2013). Pregnant women who have a history of genital herpes recurrence, suppressive therapy is recommended starting at 36 weeks gestation (ACOG, 2000; DHHS, 2013).

Breast-Feeding Considerations Valacyclovir is metabolized to acyclovir; acyclovir (but not unchanged valacyclovir) can be detected in breast milk. Peak concentrations in breast milk range from 0.5-2.3 times the corresponding maternal acyclovir serum concentration. This is expected to provide a nursing infant with a dose of acyclovir equivalent to ~0.6 mg/kg/day following ingestion of valacyclovir 500 mg twice daily by the mother. The manufacturer recommends that caution be used if administered to a nursing woman. Other sources note that women with HSV infection taking valacyclovir may breast-feed as long as there are not lesions on the breast, body lesions are covered, and strict hand hygiene is practiced (ACOG, 2000; Jaiyeoba, 2012). Women with HSV who also have HIV infection should not breast-feed; complete avoidance of breast-feeding by HIV-infected women is recommended to decrease potential transmission of HIV (DHHS [perinatal], 2012).

Contraindications Hypersensitivity to valacyclovir, acyclovir, or any component of the formulation

Warnings/Precautions Thrombotic thrombocytopenic purpura/hemolytic uremic syndrome has occurred in immunocompromised patients (at doses of 8 g/day). Safety and efficacy have not been established for treatment/suppression of recurrent genital herpes or disseminated herpes in patients with profound immunosuppression (eg, advanced HIV with CD4 <100 cells/mm^3). CNS adverse effects (including agitation, hallucinations, confusion, delirium, seizures, and encephalopathy) have been reported. Use caution in patients with renal impairment, the elderly, and/or those receiving nephrotoxic agents. Acute renal failure has been observed in patients with renal dysfunction; dose adjustment may be required. Precipitation in renal tubules may occur leading to urinary precipitation; adequately hydrate patient. For cold sores, treatment should begin at with earliest symptom (tingling, itching, burning). For genital herpes, treatment should begin as soon as possible after the first signs and symptoms (within 72 hours of onset of first diagnosis or within 24 hours of onset of recurrent episodes). For herpes zoster, treatment should begin within 72 hours of onset of rash. For chickenpox, treatment should begin with earliest sign or symptom. Use with caution in the elderly; CNS effects have been reported.

Warnings: Additional Pediatric Considerations CNS adverse events (eg, agitation, hallucinations, confusion, delirium, seizures, and encephalopathy) have been reported in children with and without renal dysfunction receiving doses exceeding those recommended for current renal function.

Adverse Reactions

Central nervous system: Depression, dizziness, fatigue, fever, headache

Dermatologic: Rash

Endocrine: Dehydration, dysmenorrhea

Gastrointestinal: Abdominal pain, diarrhea, nausea, vomiting

Hematologic: Mild leukopenia, thrombocytopenia

Hepatic: Alkaline phosphatase increased, ALT increased, AST increased

Neuromuscular & skeletal: Arthralgia

Respiratory: Nasopharyngitis, rhinorrhea

Miscellaneous: Herpes simplex

Rare but important or life-threatening: Acute hypersensitivity reactions (angioedema, anaphylaxis, dyspnea, pruritus, rash, urticaria); aggression, agitation, alopecia, anemia, aplastic anemia, ataxia, creatinine increased, coma, confusion, consciousness decreased, delirium, dysarthria, encephalopathy, erythema multiforme, facial edema, hallucinations (auditory and visual), hemolytic uremic syndrome (HUS), hepatitis, hypertension, leukocytoclastic vasculitis, mania, photosensitivity reaction, psychosis, renal failure, renal pain, seizure, tachycardia, thrombotic thrombocytopenic purpura (TTP), tremor, urinary precipitation, visual disturbances

Drug Interactions

Metabolism/Transport Effects None known.

Avoid Concomitant Use

Avoid concomitant use of ValACYclovir with any of the following: Foscarnet; Varicella Virus Vaccine; Zoster Vaccine

Increased Effect/Toxicity

ValACYclovir may increase the levels/effects of: Mycophenolate; Tenofovir; Zidovudine

The levels/effects of ValACYclovir may be increased by: Foscarnet; Mycophenolate

Decreased Effect

ValACYclovir may decrease the levels/effects of: Varicella Virus Vaccine; Zoster Vaccine

Storage/Stability Store at 15°C to 25°C (59°F to 77°F).

Mechanism of Action Valacyclovir is rapidly and nearly completely converted to acyclovir by intestinal and hepatic metabolism. Acyclovir is converted to acyclovir monophosphate by virus-specific thymidine kinase then further converted to acyclovir triphosphate by other cellular enzymes. Acyclovir triphosphate inhibits DNA synthesis and viral replication by competing with deoxyguanosine triphosphate for viral DNA polymerase and being incorporated into viral DNA.

Pharmacokinetics (Adult data unless noted)

Absorption: Rapid

Distribution: Acyclovir is widely distributed throughout the body including brain, kidney, lungs, liver, spleen, muscle, uterus, vagina, and CSF; CSF acyclovir concentration is 50% of serum concentration; crosses the placenta; excreted into breast milk

Protein binding: 13.5% to 17.9%

Metabolism: Valacyclovir is converted to acyclovir and L-valine by first-pass intestinal and/or hepatic metabolism; acyclovir is metabolized to a small extent by aldehyde oxidase, alcohol, and aldehyde dehydrogenase to inactive metabolites

Bioavailability: ~42% to 64%, decreased bioavailability with higher doses in children

Half-life:
- Normal renal function:
  - Acyclovir:
    - Children: 1.3-2.5 hours, slower clearance with increased age
    - Adults: 2-3.5 hours
  - Valacyclovir: Adults: ~30 minutes
- End-stage renal disease: Acyclovir: 14-20 hours

Time to peak serum concentration:
- Children: 1.4-2.6 hours
- Adults: 1.5 hours

Elimination: 88% as acyclovir in the urine. **Note:** Following oral radiolabeled valacyclovir administration, 46% of the label is eliminated in feces and 47% is eliminated in urine.

Dialysis: 33% removed during 4-hour hemodialysis session; administer dose postdialysis

Dosing: Usual Oral:

Infants, Children, and Adolescents:

Chickenpox, treatment (immunocompetent patients): 2 years to <18 years: 20 mg/kg/dose 3 times daily for 5 days (maximum: 1000 mg/dose), initiate within 24 hours of rash onset

Herpes labialis (cold sores), treatment: ≥12 years: 2000 mg every 12 hours for 1 day (2 doses), initiate at earliest symptom onset

HSV or VZV, prophylaxis (immunocompromised patients with normal renal function): Children and Adolescents: Limited data available: 15-30 mg/kg/dose given 3 times daily have been reported in pharmacokinetic studies (maximum: 2000 mg/dose)

HSV, treatment (immunocompetent patients): 3 months to 11 years: 20 mg/kg/dose twice daily (maximum: 1000 mg/dose) (Kimberlin, 2010)

Adults:

CMV prophylaxis in allogeneic HSCT recipients: 2000 mg 4 times daily

Herpes labialis (cold sores): 2000 mg every 12 hours for 1 day, initiate at earliest symptom onset

Herpes zoster (shingles): 1000 mg 3 times daily for 7 days

HSV, VZV in cancer patients:
- Prophylaxis: 500 mg 2-3 times daily
- Treatment: 1000 mg 3 times daily

Genital herpes:
- Initial episode: 1000 mg twice daily for 10 days
- Recurrent episode: 500 mg twice daily for 3 days
- Reduction of transmission: 500 mg once daily (source partner)
- Suppressive therapy:
  - Immunocompetent patients: 1000 mg once daily (500 mg once daily in patients with ≤9 recurrences/year)
  - HIV-infected patients (CD4 ≥100 cells/mm^3): 500 mg twice daily
  - Suppressive therapy during pregnancy: 500 mg twice daily from 36 weeks estimated gestational age until delivery

Dosing interval in renal impairment:
- Herpes labialis: Adolescents and Adults:
  - CrCl 30-49 mL/minute: 1000 mg every 12 hours for 2 doses
  - CrCl 10-29 mL/minute: 500 mg every 12 hours for 2 doses
  - CrCl <10 mL/minute: 500 mg as a single dose
- Herpes zoster: Adults:
  - CrCl 30-49 mL/minute: 1000 mg every 12 hours
  - CrCl 10-29 mL/minute: 1000 mg every 24 hours
  - CrCl <10 mL/minute: 500 mg every 24 hours
- Genital herpes: Adolescents and Adults:
  - Initial episode:
    - CrCl 10-29 mL/minute: 1000 mg every 24 hours
    - CrCl <10 mL/minute: 500 mg every 24 hours
  - Recurrent episode: CrCl ≤29 mL/minute: 500 mg every 24 hours
  - Suppressive therapy: CrCl ≤29 mL/minute:
    - For usual dose of 1000 mg every 24 hours, decrease dose to 500 mg every 24 hours
    - For usual dose of 500 mg every 24 hours, decrease dose to 500 mg every 48 hours
    - HIV-infected patients: 500 mg every 24 hours

Administration Oral: May administer with or without food

Monitoring Parameters Urinalysis, BUN, serum creatinine, liver enzymes, CBC

Additional Information

Nadal (2002) suggests the following dosage equivalency:
- 30 mg/kg/dose 3 times/day valacyclovir corresponds to IV acyclovir 250 mg/m^2 or 10 mg/kg/dose 3 times/day
- 20 mg/kg/dose 3 times/day valacyclovir corresponds to oral acyclovir 20 mg/kg 4-5 times/day

Eksborg, et al (2002) suggests the following dosage equivalency: 500 mg valacyclovir equivalent to 349 mg of IV acyclovir

Dosage Forms Excipient information presented when available (limited, particularly for generics); consult specific product labeling.

Tablet, Oral:
- Valtrex: 500 mg [contains fd&c blue #2 aluminum lake]
- Valtrex: 1 g [scored; contains fd&c blue #2 aluminum lake]
- Generic: 500 mg, 1 g

Extemporaneous Preparations A 50 mg/mL oral suspension may be made with caplets and either Ora-Sweet® or Ora-Sweet SF®. Crush eighteen 500 mg caplets in a mortar and reduce to a fine powder. Add 5 mL portions of chosen vehicle (40 mL total) and mix to a uniform paste; transfer to a 180 mL calibrated amber glass bottle, rinse mortar with 10 mL of vehicle 5 times, and add quantity of vehicle sufficient to make 180 mL. Label "shake well" and "refrigerate". Stable for 21 days refrigerated.

Fish DN, Vidaurri VA, and Deeter RG, "Stability of Valacyclovir Hydrochloride in Extemporaneously Prepared Oral Liquids," *Am J Health Syst Pharm*, 1999, 56(19):1957-60.

◆ **Valacyclovir Hydrochloride** *see* ValACYclovir *on page 2138*

◆ **Valcyte** *see* ValGANciclovir *on page 2139*

◆ **23-Valent Pneumococcal Polysaccharide Vaccine** *see* Pneumococcal Polysaccharide Vaccine (23-Valent) *on page 1718*

ValGANciclovir (val gan SYE kloh veer)

Medication Safety Issues

Sound-alike/look-alike issues:

Valcyte may be confused with Valium, Valtrex

ValGANciclovir may be confused with valACYclovir, ganciclovir

Related Information

Oral Medications That Should Not Be Crushed or Altered *on page 2476*

Safe Handling of Hazardous Drugs *on page 2455*

Brand Names: US Valcyte

Brand Names: Canada Apo-Valganciclovir; Valcyte

Therapeutic Category Antiviral Agent

Generic Availability (US) May be product dependent

Use Prevention of CMV disease in high-risk patients undergoing heart transplantation (FDA approved in ages 1 month to 16 years and adults); prevention of CMV disease in high-risk patients undergoing kidney transplantation (FDA approved in ages 4 months to 16 years and adults); treatment of cytomegalovirus (CMV) retinitis in patients with acquired immunodeficiency syndrome (AIDS) (FDA approved in adults); prevention of CMV disease in high-risk patients (donor CMV positive/recipient CMV negative) undergoing kidney/pancreas transplantation (FDA approved in adults); has also been used for prevention of CMV disease in high-risk pediatric patients undergoing BMT or hematopoietic stem cell transplant, solid organ transplants other than those indicated above, prevention of CMV disease in HIV-exposed/-positive patients, and treatment of congenital CMV disease

Pregnancy Considerations [U.S. Boxed Warning]: May cause temporary or permanent inhibition of spermatogenesis; has the potential to cause birth defects in humans. Valganciclovir is converted to ganciclovir and shares its reproductive toxicity. Ganciclovir crosses the placenta. Based on animal data, temporary or permanent impairment of fertility may occur in males and females. Ganciclovir is also teratogenic in animals. The manufacturer recommends females of reproductive potential undergo pregnancy testing prior to therapy. Females should use effective contraception during treatment and for 30 days after; males should use barrier contraception during treatment and for 90 days after.

Adverse events following congenital CMV infection may also occur. Hearing loss, mental retardation, microcephaly, seizures, and other medical problems have been observed. The indications for treating CMV retinitis during pregnancy are the same as in non-pregnant HIV infected woman; however systemic therapy should be avoided during the first trimester when possible. Use of valganciclovir is recommended to treat maternal infection, but not recommended for the treatment of asymptomatic maternal disease for the sole purpose of preventing infant infection. Monitoring of the fetus is recommended. Current recommendations for use of valganciclovir in HIV infected pregnant women are based on data from ganciclovir use in pregnant women following organ transplant or use late in pregnancy in non-HIV infected women [DHHS Adult OI, 2014].

Breast-Feeding Considerations It is not known if ganciclovir or valganciclovir are excreted into breast milk; breast feeding is not recommended. HIV-infected mothers are discouraged from breast-feeding to decrease the potential transmission of HIV. The manufacturer also notes the potential for hematologic toxicity or cancer to the nursing infant following exposure to ganciclovir.

Contraindications Hypersensitivity to valganciclovir, ganciclovir, or any component of the formulation

Warnings/Precautions Hazardous agent - use appropriate precautions for handling and disposal (NIOSH 2014 [group 2]).

[U.S. Boxed Warning]: Severe leukopenia, neutropenia, anemia, thrombocytopenia, pancytopenia, bone marrow aplasia and aplastic anemia have been reported; do not use in patients with an absolute neutrophil count <500/mm^3, platelet count <25,000/mm^3, or hemoglobin <8 g/dL. Use with caution in patients with impaired renal function (dose adjustment required). Acute renal failure (ARF) may occur; ensure adequate hydration and use with caution in patients receiving concomitant nephrotoxic agents. Elderly patients with or without pre-existing renal impairment may develop ARF; use with caution and adjust dose as needed. **[U.S. Boxed Warning]: May cause temporary or permanent inhibition of spermatogenesis; has the potential to cause birth defects and cancers in humans.** Due to its teratogenic potential, females should use effective contraception during treatment and for 30 days after; males should use barrier contraception during treatment and for 90 days after. Fertility may be temporarily or permanently impaired in males and females.

Due to differences in bioavailability, valganciclovir tablets cannot be substituted for ganciclovir capsules on a one-to-one basis. The preferred dosage form for pediatric patients is the oral solution; however, valganciclovir tablets may used so long as the calculated dose is within 10% of the available tablet strength (450 mg). Not indicated for use in liver transplant patients (higher incidence of tissue-invasive CMV relative to oral ganciclovir was observed in trials). Use of valganciclovir for the treatment of congenital CMV disease has not been evaluated.

Benzyl alcohol and derivatives: Some dosage forms may contain sodium benzoate/benzoic acid; benzoic acid (benzoate) is a metabolite of benzyl alcohol; large amounts of benzyl alcohol (≥99 mg/kg/day) have been associated with a potentially fatal toxicity ("gasping syndrome") in neonates; the "gasping syndrome" consists of metabolic acidosis, respiratory distress, gasping respirations, CNS dysfunction (including convulsions, intracranial hemorrhage), hypotension, and cardiovascular collapse (AAP, 1997; CDC, 1982); some data suggests that benzoate displaces bilirubin from protein binding sites (Ahlfors, 2001); avoid or use dosage forms containing benzyl alcohol derivative with caution in neonates. See manufacturer's labeling.

Warnings: Additional Pediatric Considerations The rates of certain adverse events and laboratory abnormalities, such as upper respiratory tract infection, pyrexia, nasopharyngitis, anemia, and neutropenia, were reported more frequently in pediatric patients than in adults in clinical trials. In a 6-month trial evaluating congenital CMV treatment in neonates and infants, the reported incidence of grade 3 or 4 neutropenia was similar between valganciclovir and placebo (21% vs 27%) (Kimberlin 2015).

Adverse Reactions

Cardiovascular: Edema, hypertension, hypotension, peripheral edema

Central nervous system: Agitation, confusion, depression, dizziness, fatigue, hallucination, headache, insomnia, pain, paresthesia, peripheral neuropathy, psychosis, seizure

Dermatologic: Acne vulgaris, dermatitis, increased wound secretion, pruritus

Endocrine & metabolic: Dehydration, hyperglycemia, hyperkalemia, hypocalcemia, hypokalemia, hypomagnesemia, hypophosphatemia

Gastrointestinal: Abdominal distention, abdominal pain, constipation, decreased appetite, diarrhea, dyspepsia, nausea, vomiting

Genitourinary: Dysuria, urinary tract infection

Hematologic: Anemia, aplastic anemia, bone marrow depression, neutropenia, pancytopenia, thrombocytopenia

Hepatic: Ascites, hepatic insufficiency

Hypersensitivity: Hypersensitivity reaction

Immunologic: Graft rejection, organ transplant rejection

Infection: Localized infection, sepsis, wound infection
Local: Catheter infection
Neuromuscular & skeletal: Arthralgia, back pain, limb pain, muscle cramps, tremor, weakness
Ophthalmic: Retinal detachment
Renal: Decreased creatinine clearance, increased serum creatinine, renal impairment
Respiratory: Cough, dyspnea, nasopharyngitis, pharyngitis, pleural effusion, rhinorrhea, upper respiratory tract infection
Miscellaneous: Fever, postoperative complication, postoperative pain, wound dehiscence
Rare but important or life-threatening: Acute renal failure, anaphylaxis, bone marrow aplasia, reduced fertility (males)

Drug Interactions

Metabolism/Transport Effects None known.

Avoid Concomitant Use

Avoid concomitant use of ValGANciclovir with any of the following: Imipenem

Increased Effect/Toxicity

ValGANciclovir may increase the levels/effects of: Imipenem; Mycophenolate; Reverse Transcriptase Inhibitors (Nucleoside); Tenofovir

The levels/effects of ValGANciclovir may be increased by: Mycophenolate; Probenecid; Tenofovir

Decreased Effect There are no known significant interactions involving a decrease in effect.

Food Interactions Coadministration with a high-fat meal increased AUC by 30%. Management: Valganciclovir should be taken with meals.

Storage/Stability

Oral solution: Store dry powder at 25°C (77°F); excursions permitted to 15°C to 30°C (59°F to 86°F). Store oral solution at 2°C to 8°C (36°F to 46°F); do not freeze. Discard any unused medication after 49 days.

Tablet: Store at 25°C (77°F); excursions permitted to 15°C to 30°C (59°F to 86°F).

Mechanism of Action Valganciclovir is rapidly converted to ganciclovir in the body. The bioavailability of ganciclovir from valganciclovir is increased 10-fold compared to oral ganciclovir. A dose of 900 mg achieved systemic exposure of ganciclovir comparable to that achieved with the recommended doses of intravenous ganciclovir of 5 mg/kg. Ganciclovir is phosphorylated to a substrate which competitively inhibits the binding of deoxyguanosine triphosphate to DNA polymerase resulting in inhibition of viral DNA synthesis.

Pharmacokinetics (Adult data unless noted)

Absorption: Well absorbed; high-fat meal increases AUC by 30%
Distribution: V_{dss}: Ganciclovir: 0.7 L/kg; distributes to most body fluids, tissues, and organs including CSF, ocular tissue, and brain
Protein binding: Ganciclovir: 1% to 2%
Metabolism: Prodrug converted to ganciclovir by intestinal mucosal cells and hepatocytes
Bioavailability: 60% (with food); similar in pediatric patients 4 months to 16 years; neonates: Initial data: 54% (Acosta, 2007)
Half-life: Ganciclovir:
- Pediatric patients (heart, kidney, or liver transplant): Mean range:
  - 4 months to 2 years: 2.8 to 4.5 hours
  - 2 to 12 years: 2.8 to 3.8 hours
  - 12 to 16 years: 4.9 to 6 hours
- Adults:
  - Healthy or HIV-positive/CMV-positive patients: 4.08 hours; prolonged with renal impairment
  - Heart, kidney, kidney-pancreas, or liver transplant patients: Mean range: 6.18 to 6.77 hours

Time to peak serum concentration: 1 to 3 hours as ganciclovir
Elimination: Majority (80% to 90%) excreted as ganciclovir in the urine

Dosing: Neonatal Congenital CMV infection; treatment: Limited data available: GA ≥32 weeks and ≥1.8 kg: Oral: 16 mg/kg/dose every 12 hours for 6 months (Acosta 2007; Bradley 2015; DHHS [pediatric] 2013; Kimberlin 2008, Kimberlin 2015, *Red Book* [AAP 2012]).

Initial neonatal dose determination based on pharmacokinetic studies of 24 neonates (GA: 34 to 41 weeks; PNA at time of therapy initiation: ≥6 days) which demonstrated that 16 mg/kg/dose twice daily produced similar serum concentrations to ganciclovir 6 mg/kg intravenously twice daily with a 6 week recommended duration of therapy based on ganciclovir experience (Acosta 2007; DHHS [pediatric] 2013, Kimberlin 2008, *Red Book* [AAP 2012). A longer duration of therapy (6 months) was evaluated in a randomized trial of 96 neonates (GA >32 weeks weighing ≥1,800 g; PNA at time of therapy initiation <30 days) which compared treatment with 6 weeks of therapy (n=47) to 6 months of therapy (n=49); results demonstrated a modest improvement in long-term hearing and developmental outcomes (evaluated at 12 and 24 months of age) with the longer duration of therapy (6 month course); however, short-term improvement (evaluated at 6 months of age) in hearing was not demonstrated (Kimberlin 2015).

Dosing: Usual

Pediatric: **Note:** Valganciclovir tablets and ganciclovir capsules cannot be substituted on a mg-per-mg basis since they are NOT BIOEQUIVALENT. In pediatric patients, valganciclovir oral solution is the preferred oral dosage form in pediatric patients for accuracy in dosing; valganciclovir tablets can be considered if the calculated dose is within 10% of the available tablet strength (450 mg). In pediatric patients, dosing may be based on either BSA (mg/m^2) or weight (mg/kg); use extra precaution to verify dosing parameters during calculations. Adolescents ≥17 years should use tablet formulation.

Congenital CMV infection; treatment (continuation from neonatal period): Limited data available: Infants 1 to 6 months of age: Oral: 16 mg/kg/dose every 12 hours for 6 months; dosing based on a pharmacokinetic study of 24 neonates demonstrated that 16 mg/kg/dose twice daily produced similar serum concentrations to ganciclovir 6 mg/kg intravenously twice daily with a 6 week recommended duration of therapy based on ganciclovir experience (Acosta 2007; DHHS [pediatric] 2013; Kimberlin 2008; *Red Book* [AAP 2012]). A longer duration of therapy (6 months) was evaluated in a randomized trial of 96 neonates (GA >32 weeks weighing ≥1.8 kg; PNA at time of therapy initiation <30 days) which compared treatment with 6 weeks of therapy (n=47) to 6 months of therapy (n=49); results demonstrated a modest improvement in long-term hearing and developmental outcomes (evaluated at 12 and 24 months of age) with the longer duration of therapy (6 month course); however, short-term improvement (evaluated at 6 months of age) in hearing was not demonstrated (Kimberlin 2015).

Prevention of CMV disease: Oral:

Following solid organ transplantation:

Heart transplantation: Begin therapy within 10 days of transplantation; continue therapy until 100 days post-transplantation. Doses should be rounded to the nearest 10 mg increment; maximum daily dose: 900 mg/**day**

Infants, Children, and Adolescents 1 month to 16 years:

Once daily dose (mg) = 7 x body surface area x creatinine clearance*

Adolescents ≥17 years: 900 mg once daily

Kidney transplantation: Begin therapy within 10 days of transplantation; continue therapy until 200 days post-transplantation or 100 days post-transplantation if kidney-pancreas transplant in adolescents ≥17 years. Doses should be rounded to the nearest 10 mg increment; maximum daily dose: 900 mg/**day**

Infants, Children, and Adolescents 4 months to 16 years:

Once daily dose (mg) = 7 x body surface area x creatinine clearance*

Adolescents ≥17 years: 900 mg once daily

Liver transplantation: Limited data available: Infants, Children, and Adolescents 4 months to 16 years (Kotton 2013; Lapidus-Krol 2010; Vaudry 2009): **Note:** In adults, studies in liver transplant patients reported a higher incidence of tissue-invasive CMV with valganciclovir relative to oral ganciclovir. In pediatric trials, therapy was initiated within 10 days of transplantation and continued therapy until 100 days post-transplantation (Vaundry 2009); maximum daily dose: 900 mg/**day**

Once daily dose (mg) = 7 x body surface area x creatinine clearance*

HIV-exposed/-positive: Infants, Children, and Adolescents 4 months to 16 years (DHHS [pediatric] 2013):

Once daily dose (mg) = 7 x body surface area x creatinine clearance*

Consider therapy initiation for children <6 years of age who are CMV-seropositive and have a CD4 percentage <5% of and for children ≥6 years of age who are CMV-seropositive and have CD4 cell counts <50 cells/mm^3. Consider cessation of therapy when CD4 cell count is >10% in children <6 years of age and >100 cells/mm^3 for children ≥6 years of age; maximum daily dose: 900 mg/**day**

* Creatinine clearance calculation (based on the modified Schwartz formula):

CrCl (mL/minute/1.73 m^2) = [k x height (cm)] ÷ serum creatinine (mg/dL)

Note: If the calculated CrCl is >150 mL/minute/1.73 m^2, then a maximum value of 150 mL/minute/1.73 m^2 should be used to calculate the dose.

Note: Calculated using a modified Schwartz formula where k =

- 0.33 in infants <1 year of age with low birthweight for gestational age
- 0.45 in infants <1 year of age with birthweight appropriate for gestational age
- 0.45 in children 1 year to <2 years
- 0.55 in boys age 2 to <13 years
- 0.55 in girls age 2 to <16 years
- 0.7 in boys age 13 to 16 years

CMV retinitis; treatment: Adolescents (DHHS [adult] 2013): Oral:

Induction (active retinitis): 900 mg twice daily for 14 to 21 days

Maintenance: Following induction treatment or for patients with inactive CMV retinitis who require maintenance therapy: 900 mg once daily for at least 3 to 6 months

Adult: **Note:** Manufacturer recommends that adult patients should use tablet formulation, **NOT** the oral solution.

CMV retinitis: Oral:

Induction: 900 mg twice daily for 21 days

Maintenance: Following induction treatment or for patients with inactive CMV retinitis who require maintenance therapy: 900 mg once daily

Prevention of CMV disease following transplantation: Oral: 900 mg once daily beginning within 10 days of transplantation; continue therapy until 100 days (heart or kidney-pancreas transplant) or 200 days (kidney transplant) post-transplantation

Dosing adjustment in renal impairment:

Infants, Children, and Adolescents 1 month to 16 years: No additional dosage adjustments required; use of equation adjusts for renal function.

Adolescents >16 years and Adults (tablet formulation):

Induction dose:

CrCl ≥60 mL/minute: No dosage adjustment necessary

CrCl 40 to 59 mL/minute: 450 mg twice daily

CrCl 25 to 39 mL/minute: 450 mg once daily

CrCl 10 to 24 mL/minute: 450 mg every 2 days

CrCl <10 mL/minute:

Manufacturer's labeling: Use not recommended; ganciclovir (with appropriately specified renal dosage adjustment) should be used instead of valganciclovir

Alternate recommendations: HIV-1 infected persons: Consider valganciclovir solution 200 mg 3 times weekly (Lucas 2014)

End stage renal disease (ESRD) on intermittent hemodialysis (IHD):

Manufacturer's labeling: Use not recommended; ganciclovir (with appropriately specified renal dosage adjustment) should be used instead of valganciclovir

Alternate recommendations: HIV-1 infected persons: Consider valganciclovir solution 200 mg 3 times weekly (Lucas 2014); valganciclovir is dialyzable and should be administered following dialysis

Maintenance/prevention dose:

CrCl ≥60 mL/minute: No dosage adjustment necessary

CrCl 40 to 59 mL/minute: 450 mg once daily

CrCl 25 to 39 mL/minute: 450 mg every 2 days

CrCl 10 to 24 mL/minute: 450 mg twice weekly

CrCl <10 mL/minute:

Manufacturer's labeling: Use not recommended; ganciclovir (with appropriately specified renal dosage adjustment) should be used instead of valganciclovir

Alternate recommendations: HIV-infected persons: Consider valganciclovir solution 100 mg 3 times weekly (Lucas 2014)

End stage renal disease (ESRD) on intermittent hemodialysis (IHD):

Manufacturer's labeling: Use not recommended; ganciclovir (with appropriately specified renal dosage adjustment) should be used instead of valganciclovir

Alternate recommendations: HIV-1 infected persons: Consider valganciclovir solution 100 mg 3 times weekly (Lucas 2014); valganciclovir is dialyzable and should be administered following dialysis

Dosing adjustment in hepatic impairment: There are no dosage adjustments provided in the manufacturer's labeling (has not been studied).

Preparation for Administration Hazardous agent; use appropriate precautions for handling and disposal (NIOSH 2014 [group 2]).

Oral solution: Prior to dispensing, prepare the oral solution by adding 91 mL of purified water to the bottle; shake well. Discard any unused medication after 49 days. A reconstituted 100 mL bottle will only provide 88 mL of solution for administration.

Administration Hazardous agent; use appropriate precautions for handling and disposal (NIOSH 2014 [group 2]). Due to the carcinogenic and mutagenic potential, avoid direct contact with broken or crushed tablets, powder for oral solution, and oral solution. Consideration should be given to handling and disposal according to guidelines issued for antineoplastic drugs; however, there is no consensus on the need for these precautions.

Oral: Administer with meals. The preferred dosage form for pediatric patients is the oral solution; however, valganciclovir tablets may be used as long as the calculated dose is within 10% of the available tablet strength (450 mg)

Oral solution: Prepare the oral solution by adding 91 mL of purified water to the bottle; shake well; a reconstituted 100 mL bottle will only provide 88 mL of solution for administration

Monitoring Parameters Retinal exam at least every 4 to 6 weeks when treating CMV retinitis; CBC with differential, platelet count, serum creatinine at baseline and periodically during therapy

Additional Information Note: A pharmacokinetic study of 10 solid organ and stem cell transplant patients (8 months to 13 years) found that 20 mg/kg/day of oral valganciclovir produced a similar ganciclovir exposure as 10 mg/kg/day of IV ganciclovir (Launay 2011).

Dosage Forms Excipient information presented when available (limited, particularly for generics); consult specific product labeling.

Solution Reconstituted, Oral:

Valcyte: 50 mg/mL (88 mL) [contains saccharin sodium, sodium benzoate; tutti-frutti flavor]

Tablet, Oral:

Valcyte: 450 mg

Generic: 450 mg

Extemporaneous Preparations Hazardous agent; use appropriate precautions for handling and disposal (NIOSH 2014 [group 2]).

Note: Commercial preparation is available (50 mg/mL)

A 60 mg/mL oral suspension may be with tablets and a 1:1 mixture of Ora-Sweet® and Ora-Plus®. Crush sixteen 450 mg tablets and reduce to a fine powder. Add 1 mL portions of chosen vehicle (10 mL total) and mix to a uniform paste; mix while adding the vehicle in incremental proportions to **almost** 120 mL; transfer to a calibrated amber glass bottle, rinse mortar with vehicle, and add quantity of vehicle sufficient to make 120 mL. Label "shake well" and "refrigerate". Stable for 35 days refrigerated.

Henkin CC, Griener JC, and Ten Eick AP, "Stability of Valganciclovir in Extemporaneously Compounded Liquid Formulations," *Am J Health Syst Pharm*, 2003, 60(7):687-90.

◆ **Valganciclovir Hydrochloride** *see* ValGANciclovir *on page 2139*

◆ **Valisone Scalp Lotion (Can)** *see* Betamethasone (Topical) *on page 280*

◆ **Valium** *see* Diazepam *on page 635*

◆ **Valorin [OTC]** *see* Acetaminophen *on page 44*

◆ **Valorin Extra [OTC]** *see* Acetaminophen *on page 44*

◆ **Valproate Semisodium** *see* Valproic Acid and Derivatives *on page 2143*

◆ **Valproate Sodium** *see* Valproic Acid and Derivatives *on page 2143*

◆ **Valproic Acid** *see* Valproic Acid and Derivatives *on page 2143*

◆ **Valproic Acid Derivative** *see* Valproic Acid and Derivatives *on page 2143*

Valproic Acid and Derivatives

(val PROE ik AS id & dah RIV ah tives)

Medication Safety Issues

Sound-alike/look-alike issues:

Depakene may be confused with Depakote

Depakote may be confused with Depakene, Depakote ER, Senokot

Depakote ER may be confused with divalproex enteric coated

Valproate sodium may be confused with vecuronium

Related Information

Oral Medications That Should Not Be Crushed or Altered *on page 2476*

Safe Handling of Hazardous Drugs *on page 2455*

Brand Names: US Depacon; Depakene; Depakote; Depakote ER; Depakote Sprinkles; Stavzor

Brand Names: Canada Apo-Divalproex; Apo-Valproic; Depakene; Dom-Divalproex; Dom-Valproic Acid; Dom-Valproic Acid E.C.; Epival; Epival ECT; Mylan-Divalproex; Mylan-Valproic; Novo-Divalproex; Novo-Valproic; PHL-Divalproex; PHL-Valproic Acid; PHL-Valproic Acid E.C.; PMS-Divalproex; PMS-Valproic Acid; PMS-Valproic Acid E.C.; ratio-Valproic; Sandoz-Valproic

Therapeutic Category Anticonvulsant, Miscellaneous; Infantile Spasms, Treatment

Generic Availability (US) May be product dependent

Use

Oral:

Immediate release capsules and syrup (Depakene®): Monotherapy and adjunctive therapy in the treatment of patients with complex partial seizures (FDA approved in ages ≥10 years and adults), monotherapy and adjunctive therapy of simple and complex absence seizures [FDA approved in pediatric patients (age not specified) and adults], and adjunctive therapy in patients with multiple seizure types that include absence seizures [FDA approved in pediatric patients (age not specified) and adults]; has also been used to treat mixed seizure types, myoclonic and generalized tonic-clonic (grand mal) seizures; may be effective in infantile spasms; oral syrup has also been used rectally for treatment of seizure disorders when oral route is not available

Delayed release capsules (Stavzor™): Monotherapy and adjunctive therapy in the treatment of patients with complex partial seizures (FDA approved in ages ≥10 years and adults); monotherapy and adjunctive therapy of simple and complex absence seizures and adjunctive therapy in patients with multiple seizure types that include absence seizures [FDA approved pediatric patients (age not specified) and adults]; prophylaxis of migraine headaches (FDA approved in ages ≥12 years and adults); treatment of manic episodes of bipolar disorders (FDA approved in adults)

Delayed release tablets (Depakote®): Monotherapy and adjunctive therapy in the treatment of patients with complex partial seizures, monotherapy and adjunctive therapy of simple and complex absence seizures and adjunctive therapy in patients with multiple seizure types that include absence seizures [FDA approved in pediatric patients (age not specified) and adults]; prophylaxis of migraine headaches (FDA approved in ages ≥16 years and adults); treatment of manic episodes of bipolar disorders (FDA approved in adults)

Extended release tablets (Depakote ER®): Monotherapy and adjunctive therapy in the treatment of patients with complex partial seizures; monotherapy and adjunctive therapy of simple and complex absence seizures and adjunctive therapy in patients with multiple seizure types that include absence seizures (all epilepsy types listed: FDA approved in ages ≥10 years and adults); prophylaxis of migraine headaches (FDA approved in ages ≥12 years and adults); treatment of manic episodes of bipolar disorders (FDA approved in adults)

Sprinkle capsules (Depakote®): Monotherapy and adjunctive therapy in the treatment of patients with complex partial seizures (FDA approved in ages ≥10 years and adults); monotherapy and adjunctive therapy of simple and complex absence seizures and adjunctive therapy in patients with multiple seizure types that include absence seizures [FDA approved in pediatric patients (age not specified) and adults]; has also been used to treat mixed seizure types, myoclonic and generalized tonic-clonic (grand mal) seizures; may be effective in infantile spasms

Parenteral: Injection (Depacon®): Monotherapy and adjunctive therapy in the treatment of patients with complex partial seizures (FDA approved in ages ≥10 years and adults); monotherapy and adjunctive therapy of simple and complex absence seizures, and adjunctive therapy in patients with multiple seizure types that include absence seizures [FDA approved in pediatric patients (age not specified) and adults]; has also been used to treat mixed seizure types, myoclonic and generalized tonic-clonic (grand mal) seizures; may be effective in infantile spasms. **Note:** Parenteral formulation is indicated for patients in whom oral administration of valproic acid or derivatives is temporarily not feasible; has also been used in patients with absence status epileptics.

Medication Guide Available Yes

Pregnancy Risk Factor X (migraine prophylaxis)/D (all other indications)

Pregnancy Considerations Adverse events have been observed in animal reproduction studies and in human pregnancies. **[U.S. Boxed Warning]: May cause major congenital malformations, such as neural tube defects (eg, spina bifida) and decreased IQ scores following in utero exposure. Use is contraindicated in pregnant women for the prevention of migraine. Use is not recommended in women of childbearing potential for any other condition unless valproate is essential to manage her condition and alternative therapies are not appropriate. Effective contraception should be used during therapy.**

Valproic acid crosses the placenta (Harden 2009b). Neural tube defects, craniofacial defects, cardiovascular malformations, hypospadias, and limb malformations have been reported. Information from the North American Antiepileptic Drug Pregnancy Registry notes the rate of major malformations to be 9% to 11% following an average exposure to valproate monotherapy 1,000 mg/day; this is an increase in congenital malformations when compared with monotherapy with other antiepileptic drugs (AED). Based on data from the CDC National Birth Defects Prevention Network, the risk of spinal bifida is approximately 1% to 2% following valproate exposure (general population risk estimated to be 0.06% to 0.07%).

Nonteratogenic adverse effects have also been reported. Decreased IQ scores have been noted in children exposed to valproate in utero when compared to children exposed to other antiepileptic medications or no antiepileptic medications; the risk of autism spectrum disorders may also be increased. Fatal hepatic failure and hypoglycemia in infants have been noted in case reports following in utero exposure to valproic acid.

Clotting factor abnormalities (hypofibrinogenemia, thrombocytopenia, or decrease in other coagulation factors) may develop in the mother following valproate use during pregnancy; close monitoring of coagulation factors is recommended.

Current guidelines recommend complete avoidance of valproic acid and derivatives for the treatment of epilepsy in pregnant women whenever possible (Harden 2009a), especially when used for conditions not associated with permanent injury or risk of death. Effective contraception should be used during treatment. When pregnancy is being planned, consider tapering off of therapy prior to conception if appropriate; abrupt discontinuation of therapy may cause status epilepticus and lead to maternal and fetal hypoxia. Folic acid decreases the risk of neural tube defects in the general population; supplementation with folic acid should be used prior to conception and during pregnancy in all women, including those taking valproate.

A pregnancy registry is available for women who have been exposed to valproic acid. Patients may enroll themselves in the North American Antiepileptic Drug (NAAED) Pregnancy Registry by calling (888) 233-2334. Additional information is available at www.aedpregnancyregistry.org.

Breast-Feeding Considerations Valproate is excreted into breast milk. Breast milk concentrations of valproic acid have been reported as 1% to 10% of maternal concentration. The weight-adjusted dose to the infant has been calculated to be ~4% (Hagg, 2000). The manufacturer recommends that caution be used if administered to nursing women.

Contraindications Hypersensitivity to valproic acid, divalproex, derivatives, or any component of the formulation; hepatic disease or significant impairment; urea cycle disorders; pregnant women for the prevention of migraine; known mitochondrial disorders caused by mutations in mitochondrial DNA polymerase gamma (POLG; eg, Alpers-Huttenlocher syndrome [AHS]) or children <2 years of age suspected of having a POLG-related disorder

Warnings/Precautions Hazardous agent - use appropriate precautions for handling and disposal (NIOSH 2014 [groups 2 and 3]).

[U.S. Boxed Warning]: Hepatic failure resulting in fatalities has occurred in patients, usually in the initial 6 months of therapy; children <2 years of age are at considerable risk. Risk is also increased in patients with hereditary neurometabolic syndromes caused by DNA mutations of the mitochondrial DNA polymerase gamma (POLG) gene (eg, Alpers-Huttenlocher syndrome [AHS]). Other risk factors include organic brain disease, mental retardation with severe seizure disorders, congenital metabolic disorders, and patients on multiple anticonvulsants. Monitor patients closely for appearance of malaise, weakness, facial edema, anorexia, jaundice, and vomiting; discontinue immediately with signs/symptom of significant or suspected impairment. Liver function tests should be performed at baseline and at regular intervals after initiation of therapy, especially within the first 6 months. Hepatic dysfunction may progress despite discontinuing treatment. Should only be used as monotherapy and with extreme caution in children <2 years of age and/or patients at high risk for hepatotoxicity. Contraindicated with significant hepatic impairment.

[U.S. Boxed Warning]: Risk of valproate-induced acute liver failure and death is increased in patients with hereditary neurometabolic syndromes caused by DNA mutations of the mitochondrial polymerase gamma (POLG) gene (eg, Alpers-Huttenlocher syndrome [AHS]). Use is contraindicated in patients with known mitochondrial disorders caused by POLG mutations and children <2 years of age suspected of having a POLG-related disorder. Use in children ≥2 years of age suspected of having a POLG-related disorder only after other anticonvulsants have failed and with close monitoring for the development of acute liver injury. POLG mutation testing should be performed in accordance with current clinical practice.

[U.S. Boxed Warning]: Cases of life-threatening pancreatitis, occurring at the start of therapy or following years of use, have been reported in adults and children. Some cases have been hemorrhagic with rapid progression of initial symptoms to death. Promptly evaluate symptoms of abdominal pain, nausea, vomiting, and/or anorexia; should generally be discontinued if pancreatitis is diagnosed.

[U.S. Boxed Warning]: May cause major congenital malformations such as neural tube defects (eg, spina bifida) and decreased IQ scores following in utero exposure. Use is contraindicated in pregnant women for the prevention of migraine. Use is not

recommended in women of childbearing potential for any other condition unless valproate is essential to manage her condition and alternative therapies are not appropriate. Effective contraception should be used during therapy.

Multiorgan hypersensitivity reactions (also known as drug reaction with eosinophilia and systemic symptoms [DRESS]): Potentially serious, sometimes fatal multiorgan hypersensitivity reactions have rarely been reported with some antiepileptic drugs including valproate therapy in adults and children; monitor for signs and symptoms of possible disparate manifestations associated with lymphatic, hepatic, renal, and/or hematologic organ systems; discontinuation and conversion to alternative therapy may be required.

May cause dose-related thrombocytopenia, inhibition of platelet aggregation, and bleeding. In some cases, platelet counts may be normalized with continued treatment; however, reduce dose or discontinue drug if patient develops evidence of hemorrhage, bruising, or a disorder of hemostasis/coagulation. Evaluate platelet counts prior to initiating therapy and periodically thereafter. In addition to platelets, valproate may be associated with a decrease in other cell lines and myelodysplasia.

Hyperammonemia and/or encephalopathy, sometimes fatal, have been reported following the initiation of valproate therapy and may be present with normal transaminase levels. Ammonia levels should be measured in patients who develop unexplained lethargy and vomiting, changes in mental status, or in patients who present with hypothermia (unintentional drop in core body temperature to <35°C/95°F). Discontinue therapy if ammonia levels are increased and evaluate for possible urea cycle disorder (UCD). Hyperammonemic encephalopathy has been reported in patients with UCD, particularly ornithine transcarbamylase deficiency. Use is contraindicated in patients with known UCD. Evaluation of UCD should be considered for the following patients prior to the start of therapy: History of unexplained encephalopathy or coma; encephalopathy associated with protein load; pregnancy or postpartum encephalopathy; unexplained mental retardation; history of elevated plasma ammonia or glutamine; history of cyclical vomiting and lethargy; episodic extreme irritability, ataxia; low BUN or protein avoidance; family history of UCD or unexplained infant deaths (particularly male); or signs or symptoms of UCD (hyperammonemia, encephalopathy, respiratory alkalosis). Hypothermia has been reported with valproate therapy; hypothermia may or may not be associated with hyperammonemia; may also occur with concomitant topiramate therapy following topiramate initiation or dosage increase. Hyperammonemia and/or encephalopathy may also occur with concomitant topiramate therapy in patients who previously tolerated monotherapy with either medication.

In vitro studies have suggested valproate stimulates the replication of HIV and CMV viruses under experimental conditions. The clinical consequence of this is unknown, but should be considered when monitoring affected patients.

Antiepileptics are associated with an increased risk of suicidal behavior/thoughts with use (regardless of indication); patients should be monitored for signs/symptoms of depression, suicidal tendencies, and other unusual behavior changes during therapy and instructed to inform their healthcare provider immediately if symptoms occur.

Intravenous valproate is not recommended for post-traumatic seizure prophylaxis in patients with acute head trauma; study results for this indication suggested increased mortality with IV valproate use compared to IV phenytoin. Anticonvulsants should not be discontinued abruptly because of the possibility of increasing seizure frequency; valproate should be withdrawn gradually to minimize the potential of increased seizure frequency, unless safety concerns require a more rapid withdrawal. Patients treated for bipolar disorder should be monitored closely for clinical worsening or suicidality; prescriptions should be written for the smallest quantity consistent with good patient care.

Reversible and irreversible cerebral and cerebellar atrophy have been reported; motor and cognitive function should be routinely monitored to assess for signs and symptoms of brain atrophy. CNS depression may occur with valproate use. Patients must be cautioned about performing tasks which require mental alertness (operating machinery or driving). Effects with other sedative drugs or ethanol may be potentiated. Use with caution in the elderly as the elderly may be more sensitive to sedating effects and dehydration; in some elderly patients with somnolence, concomitant decreases in nutritional intake and weight loss were observed. Reduce initial dosages in elderly and closely monitor fluid status, nutritional intake, somnolence, and other adverse events. Potentially significant drug-drug interactions may exist, requiring dose or frequency adjustment, additional monitoring, and/or selection of alternative therapy.

Medication residue in stool has been reported (rarely) with oral Depakote (divalproex sodium) formulations; some reports have occurred in patients with shortened GI transit times (eg, diarrhea) or anatomic GI disorders (eg, ileostomy, colostomy). In patients reporting medication residue in stool, it is recommended to monitor valproate level and clinical condition.

Warnings: Additional Pediatric Considerations Neonates, infants, and children <2 years of age are at considerably increased risk for hepatotoxicity/hepatic failure, especially those on anticonvulsant polytherapy, with congenital metabolic disorders, with severe seizure disorders and mental retardation, or with organic brain disease; monitor patients closely for appearance of malaise, loss of seizure control, weakness, facial edema, anorexia, jaundice, and vomiting; monitor liver enzymes prior to therapy and at frequent intervals, especially during the first 6 months. Although carnitine is clearly indicated for the management of valproic acid overdose and hepatotoxicity (and strongly recommended for select patients at high risk of valproic acid-associated hepatotoxicity), the role of routine prophylactic carnitine supplementation is unclear (Freeman, 1994; Raskind, 2000). A case of a fatal hepatotoxic reaction has been reported in a child receiving valproic acid despite carnitine supplementation (Murphy, 1993). A valproic acid-associated Reye's-like syndrome has also been reported (Hilmas, 2000).

Rare multiorgan hypersensitivity reactions have been reported pediatric patients in association with initiation of valproic acid and derivatives; at least one death has been reported; patient may present with fever and rash in association with symptoms of organ system dysfunction [eg, lymphadenopathy, hepatitis, abnormalities in liver function tests, hematologic abnormalities (eosinophilia, neutropenia, thrombocytopenia), pruritus, oliguria, nephritis, arthralgia, asthenia]; valproic acid and derivatives should be discontinued in patients suspected of having multiorgan hypersensitivity reactions. Medication residue in stool has been reported (rarely) with oral Depakote (divalproex sodium) formulations; some reports have occurred in patients with shortened GI transit times (eg, diarrhea) or anatomic GI disorders (eg, ileostomy, colostomy). In patients reporting medication residue in stool, it is recommended to monitor valproate level and clinical condition.

Adverse Reactions

Cardiovascular: Chest pain, edema, facial edema, hypertension, hypotension, orthostatic hypotension, palpitations, peripheral edema, tachycardia, vasodilatation

Central nervous system: Abnormal dreams, abnormal gait, abnormality in thinking, agitation, amnesia, anxiety, ataxia, catatonia, chills, confusion, depression, dizziness, drowsiness, dyskinesia, emotional lability, hallucination, headache, hyper-reflexia, hypertonia, insomnia, malaise, myasthenia, nervousness, pain, paresthesia, personality disorder, sleep disorder, speech disturbance, tardive dyskinesia, twitching, vertigo

Dermatologic: Alopecia, diaphoresis, erythema nodosum, furunculosis, maculopapular rash, pruritus, seborrhea, skin rash, vesiculobullous dermatitis, xeroderma

Endocrine & metabolic: Amenorrhea, menstrual disease, weight gain, weight loss

Gastrointestinal: Abdominal pain, anorexia, constipation, diarrhea, dysgeusia, dyspepsia, dysphagia, eructation, fecal incontinence, flatulence, gastroenteritis, gingival hemorrhage, glossitis, hematemesis, hiccups, increased appetite, nausea, oral mucosa ulcer, pancreatitis, periodontal abscess, stomatitis, vomiting, xerostomia

Genitourinary: Cystitis, dysmenorrhea, dysuria, urinary frequency, urinary incontinence, vaginal hemorrhage, vaginitis

Hematologic & oncologic: Ecchymoses, hypoproteinemia, petechia, prolonged bleeding time, thrombocytopenia (dose related)

Hepatic: Increased serum ALT, increased serum AST

Infection: Fungal infection, infection, viral infection

Local: Injection site reaction, pain at injection site

Neuromuscular & skeletal: Arthralgia, back pain, discoid lupus erythematosus, dysarthria, hypokinesia, leg cramps, myalgia, neck pain, neck stiffness, osteoarthritis, tremor, weakness

Ophthalmic: Conjunctivitis, diplopia, dry eye syndrome, eye pain, nystagmus, photophobia, visual disturbance (amblyopia, blurred vision)

Otic: Deafness, otitis media, tinnitus

Respiratory: Bronchitis, cough, dyspnea, epistaxis, flu-like symptoms, pharyngitis, pneumonia, rhinitis, sinusitis

Miscellaneous: Accidental injury, fever

Rare but important or life-threatening: Abnormal thyroid function tests, acute porphyria, aggressive behavior, agranulocytosis, anemia, aplastic anemia, bradycardia, brain disease (rare), breast hypertrophy, cerebral atrophy (reversible or irreversible), coma (rare), decreased bone mineral density, decreased plasma carnitine concentrations, decreased platelet aggregation, dementia, eosinophilia, Fanconi-like syndrome (rare, in children), galactorrhea, hemorrhage, hepatic failure, hepatotoxicity, hostility, hyperactivity, hyperammonemia, hyperammonemic encephalopathy (in patients with UCD), hyperandrogenism, hyperglycinemia, hypersensitivity angiitis, hypersensitivity reaction, hypofibrinogenemia, hyponatremia, hypothermia, leukopenia, lymphocytosis, macrocytosis, ostealgia, osteopenia, pancytopenia, parotid gland enlargement, polycystic ovary syndrome (rare), psychosis, severe hypersensitivity (with multiorgan dysfunction), SIADH, Stevens-Johnson syndrome, suicidal ideation, suicidal tendencies, toxic epidermal necrolysis (rare), urinary tract infection

Drug Interactions

Metabolism/Transport Effects **Substrate** of CYP2A6 (minor), CYP2B6 (minor), CYP2C19 (minor), CYP2C9 (minor), CYP2E1 (minor); **Note:** Assignment of Major/Minor substrate status based on clinically relevant drug interaction potential; **Inhibits** CYP2C9 (weak); **Induces** CYP2A6 (weak/moderate)

Avoid Concomitant Use

Avoid concomitant use of Valproic Acid and Derivatives with any of the following: Cosyntropin

Increased Effect/Toxicity

Valproic Acid and Derivatives may increase the levels/effects of: Barbiturates; CarBAMazepine; Ethosuximide; LamoTRIgine; LORazepam; Minoxidil (Systemic); Paliperidone; Primidone; RisperiDONE; Rufinamide; Sodium Oxybate; Temozolomide; Tricyclic Antidepressants; Vorinostat; Zidovudine

The levels/effects of Valproic Acid and Derivatives may be increased by: ChlorproMAZINE; Cosyntropin; Felbamate; GuanFACINE; Primidone; Salicylates; Topiramate

Decreased Effect

Valproic Acid and Derivatives may decrease the levels/effects of: Fosphenytoin-Phenytoin; OLANZapine; OXcarbazepine; Urea Cycle Disorder Agents

The levels/effects of Valproic Acid and Derivatives may be decreased by: Barbiturates; CarBAMazepine; Carbapenems; Ethosuximide; Fosphenytoin-Phenytoin; Mefloquine; Methylfolate; Mianserin; Orlistat; Protease Inhibitors; Rifampin

Food Interactions Food may delay but does not affect the extent of absorption. Management: May administer with food if GI upset occurs.

Storage/Stability

Oral capsules:

Depakene: Store at 15°C to 25°C (59°F to 77°F).

Stavzor: Store at 25°C (77° F); excursions are permitted between 15°C and 30°C (59°F and 86°F).

Oral sprinkle capsules (Depakote): Store below 25°C (77°F).

Oral solution (Depakene): Store below 30°C (86°F).

Oral tablets:

Depakote: Store below 30°C (86°F).

Depakote ER: Store tablets at 25°C (77°F); excursions are permitted between 15°C and 30°C (59°F and 86°F).

IV: Store at controlled room temperature 15°C to 30°C (59°F to 86°F). Stable in D_5W, NS, and LR for at least 24 hours when stored in glass or PVC.

Mechanism of Action Causes increased availability of gamma-aminobutyric acid (GABA), an inhibitory neurotransmitter, to brain neurons or may enhance the action of GABA or mimic its action at postsynaptic receptor sites. Divalproex sodium is a compound of sodium valproate and valproic acid; divalproex dissociates to valproate in the GI tract.

Pharmacokinetics (Adult data unless noted)

Protein binding: 80% to 90% (concentration dependent); free fraction: ~10% at serum concentration at 40 mcg/mL and ~18.5% at 130 mcg/mL; decreased protein binding in neonates and patients with renal impairment or chronic hepatic disease

Distribution: Distributes into CSF at concentrations similar to unbound concentration in plasma (ie, ~10% of total plasma concentration)

V_d:

Total valproate: 11 L/1.73 m^2

Free valproate: 92 L/1.73 m^2

Metabolism: Extensively hepatic via glucuronide conjugation (30% to 50% of administered dose) and 40% via mitochondrial beta-oxidation; other oxidative metabolic pathways occur to a lesser extent. The relationship between dose and total valproate concentration is nonlinear; concentration does not increase proportionally with the dose, but increases to a lesser extent due to saturable plasma protein binding. The kinetics of unbound drug are linear.

Bioavailability: Oral: All products, except Depakote®-ER, are equivalent to IV **Depakote®-ER tablets are not equivalent to Depakote® delayed release tablets and are not interchangeable**; mean bioavailability of Depakote®-ER tablets is 89%, relative to Depakote® delayed release tablets. In pediatric patients 10-17 years of age, once-daily administration of Depakote®-ER produced valproate plasma concentration-time profiles similar to adults.

Half-life: Increased with liver disease

Newborns (exposed to VPA *in utero*): 30-60 hours

Neonates 1st week of life: 40-45 hours

Neonates <10 days: 10-67 hours

Infants and Children >2 months: 7-13 hours

Children and Adolescents 2-14 years: 9 hours (Range: 3.5-20 hours) (Cloyd, 1993)

Adults: 9-16 hours

Time to peak serum concentration:

Oral: Depakote ® tablet and sprinkle capsules: ~4 hours; Depakote® ER: 4-17 hours; Stavzor™: 2 hours

Rectal: 1-3 hours (Graves, 1987)

IV: End of the infusion

Elimination: Urine (30% to 50% as glucuronide conjugate, <3% as unchanged drug); faster clearance in children who receive other antiepileptic drugs and those who are younger; age and polytherapy explain 80% of interpatient variability in total clearance; children >10 years of age have pharmacokinetic parameters similar to adults

Dialysis: Hemodialysis reduces valproate concentrations by ~20%

Dosing: Neonatal Note: Due to the increased risk of valproic acid and derivatives-associated hepatotoxicity, valproic acid and derivatives are not preferred agents for use in neonates.

Refractory seizures: Limited data available: Oral: Loading dose: 20 mg/kg, followed by a maintenance dose of 5 to 10 mg/kg/dose every 12 hours; adjust dose according to serum concentrations; dosing based on a report of six neonates (GA: 30 to 41 weeks) that showed oral valproic acid effectively controlled seizure activity in five of six patients; however, therapy was discontinued in 50% of the patients due to hyperammonemia; frequent monitoring is recommended (Evans 1998; Gal 1988).

Refractory status epilepticus: Limited data available: IV: Loading dose: 20 to 40 mg/kg followed by a continuous IV infusion of 5 mg/kg/**hour** was used in five neonates; once patients were seizure-free for 12 hours and no longer had seizure activity on EEG, the infusion rate was decreased every 2 hours by 1 mg/kg/**hour** (Uberall 2000).

Dosing: Usual

Pediatric: **Note:** Use of Depakote-ER in pediatric patients <10 years of age is not recommended; do not confuse Depakote-ER with Depakote. **Erroneous substitution of Depakote® (delayed release tablets) for Depakote-ER has resulted in toxicities; only Depakote-ER is intended for once daily administration.**

Migraine prophylaxis:

Depakote: Adolescents ≥16 years: Oral: 250 mg twice daily; adjust dose based on patient response; maximum daily dose: 1,000 mg/**day**

Stavzor: Children and Adolescents ≥12 years: Oral: 250 mg twice daily; adjust dose based on patient response; maximum daily dose: 1,000 mg/**day**

Depakote ER: Children and Adolescents ≥12 years: Oral: 500 mg once daily for 7 days, may increase to 1,000 mg once daily; adjust dose based on patient response; usual dosage range: 500 to 1000 mg/day; dose should be individualized; if smaller dosage adjustments are needed, use Depakote delayed release tablets

Seizures disorders: Infants, Children, and Adolescents: **Note:** Due to the increased risk of valproic acid and derivatives-associated hepatotoxicity in patients <2 years, valproic acid and derivatives are not preferred agents in this population.

Oral:

General dosing (including complex partial seizures): Initial: 10 to 15 mg/kg/day in 1 to 3 divided doses; increase by 5 to 10 mg/kg/day at weekly intervals until seizures are controlled or side effects preclude further increases; daily doses >250 mg should be given in divided doses; maintenance: 30 to 60 mg/kg/day in 2 to 3 divided doses; Depakote and Depakote Sprinkle can be given twice daily; **Note:** Children receiving more than 1 anticonvulsant (ie, polytherapy) may require doses up to 100 mg/kg/day in 3 to 4 divided doses.

Simple and complex absence seizures: Initial: 15 mg/kg/day in 1 to 3 divided doses; increase by 5 to 10 mg/kg/day at weekly intervals until seizures are controlled or side effects preclude further increases; daily doses >250 mg should be given in divided doses; maintenance: 30 to 60 mg/kg/day in 2 to 3 divided doses; Depakote and Depakote Sprinkle can be given twice daily

Conversion to Depakote ER from a stable dose of Depakote®: May require an increase in the total daily dose between 8% and 20% to maintain similar serum concentrations

Conversion to monotherapy from adjunctive therapy: The concomitant antiepileptic drug (AED) can be decreased by ~25% every 2 weeks; dosage reduction of the concomitant AED may begin when valproate or derivative therapy is initiated or 1 to 2 weeks following valproate or derivative initiation

Parenteral: IV: Total daily IV dose is equivalent to the total daily oral dose; however, IV dose should be divided with a frequency of every 6 hours; if IV form is administered 2 to 3 times/day, close monitoring of trough concentrations is recommended; switch patients to oral product as soon as clinically possible as IV use >14 days has not been studied.

Rectal: Dilute oral syrup 1:1 with water for use as a retention enema (Graves 1987):

Loading dose: 17 to 20 mg/kg once

Maintenance: 10 to 15 mg/kg/dose every 8 hours

Status epilepticus; refractory: Limited data available; Infants, Children, and Adolescents:

IV:

Loading dose: Initial: 20 to 40 mg/kg; some experts recommend an additional 20 mg/kg after 10 to 15 minutes if needed (Brophy 2012); there is limited experience with loading doses >40 mg/kg in infants.

In one retrospective study, an initial loading dose of 25 mg/kg was effective in stopping seizure activity within 20 minutes after the end of the infusion in all 18 patients treated for status epilepticus (Yu 2003). A separate retrospective trial found a higher efficacy rate in pediatric patients who received an initial loading dose of 30 to 40 mg/kg (73.3%, n=15) compared to 20 to 30 mg/kg (46.2%, n=26) or >40 mg/kg (40%, n=10) (Uberall 2000). In an open-label, randomized comparative trial, an initial loading dose of 30 mg/kg was administered (n=20; age range: 7 months to 10 years of age; mean age: 3 years); a repeat bolus of 10 mg/kg could be administered if seizures were not controlled within 10 minutes; mean required dose: 37.5 ± 4.4 mg/kg; median required dose: 40 mg/kg (Mehta 2007).

Maintenance dose: IV infusion: 5 mg/kg/**hour** after the loading dose was used in pediatric continuous IV infusion studies (Mehta 2007; Uberall 2000); once patients were seizure-free for 6 hours, the infusion rate was decreased by 1 mg/kg/**hour** every 2 hours (Mehta 2007).

Rectal: Dilute oral syrup 1:1 with water for use as a retention enema (Snead 1985):

Loading dose: 15 to 20 mg/kg once

Maintenance: 10 to 15 mg/kg/dose every 8 hours

Adult:

Seizures: Note: Administer doses >250 mg/day in divided doses.

Oral:

Simple and complex absence seizure: Initial: 15 mg/kg/day; increase by 5 to 10 mg/kg/day at weekly intervals until therapeutic concentrations are achieved; maximum daily dose: 60 mg/kg/**day**

Complex partial seizure: Initial: 10 to 15 mg/kg/day; increase by 5 to 10 mg/kg/day at weekly intervals until therapeutic concentrations are achieved; maximum daily dose: 60 mg/kg/**day**

Note: Regular release and delayed release formulations are usually given in 2 to 4 divided doses per day; extended release formulation (Depakote ER) is usually given once daily. In patients previously maintained on regular release valproic acid therapy (Depakene) who convert to delayed release divalproex sodium tablets (Depakote) or valproic acid capsules (Stavzor), the same daily dose and frequency as the regular release should be used; once therapy is stabilized, the frequency of Depakote or Stavzor may be adjusted to 2 to 3 times daily.

Conversion to Depakote ER from a stable dose of Depakote: May require an increase in the total daily dose between 8% and 20% to maintain similar serum concentrations

Conversion to monotherapy from adjunctive therapy: The concomitant antiepileptic drug (AED) can be decreased by ~25% every 2 weeks; dosage reduction of the concomitant AED may begin when the valproic acid or derivative is initiated or 1 to 2 weeks following valproic acid or derivative initiation

IV: Total daily IV dose should be equivalent to the total daily dose of the oral valproic acid or derivative; administer dose with the same frequency as oral products; switch patient to oral products as soon as possible.

Status epilepticus:

Loading dose: IV: 20 to 40 mg/kg administered at 3 to ≤6 mg/kg/minute; after 10 minutes an additional 20 mg/kg dose may be given if clinically indicated (Brophy 2012)

Maintenance dose: IV infusion: 1 to 4 mg/kg/hour; titrate dose as needed based upon patient response and evaluation of drug-drug interactions

Mania: Oral:

Depakote tablet, Stavzor: Initial: 750 mg/day in divided doses; adjust dose as rapidly as possible to desired clinical effect; maximum daily dose: 60 mg/kg/**day**

Depakote ER: Initial: 25 mg/kg/day given once daily; adjust dose as rapidly as possible to desired clinical effect; maximum daily dose: 60 mg/kg/**day**

Migraine prophylaxis: Oral:

Depakote tablet, Stavzor: Initial: 250 mg twice daily; adjust dose based on patient response, maximum daily dose: 1,000 mg/day

Depakote ER: Initial: 500 mg once daily for 7 days, may increase to 1000 mg once daily; adjust dose based on patient response; usual dosage range 500 to 1,000 mg/day; dose should be individualized; if smaller dosage adjustments are needed, use Depakote delayed release tablets

Dosing adjustment in renal impairment: No dosage adjustment required; however, protein binding is reduced in patients with renal impairment; monitoring **only** total valproate serum concentrations may be misleading.

Dosing adjustment in hepatic impairment: Valproic acid and derivatives are contraindicated in patients with hepatic disease or significant hepatic dysfunction. Potentially fatal hepatotoxicity may occur with valproic acid or derivative use. Clearance is decreased in patients with liver impairment. Hepatic disease is also associated with decreased albumin concentrations and 2- to 2.6-fold increase in the unbound fraction of valproate. Free concentrations of valproate may be elevated while total concentrations appear normal; therefore, monitoring **only** total valproate concentrations may be misleading.

Preparation for Administration Hazardous agent; use appropriate precautions for handling and disposal (NIOSH 2014 [group 2]).

Parenteral: IV: Manufacturer's labeling recommends diluting dose in 50 mL of D_5W, NS, or LR for patients ≥10 years of age. In pediatric clinical trials doses were usually diluted 1:1 with NS or D_5W (Mehta 2007; Uberall 2000).

Rectal: Dilute oral solution or syrup 1:1 with an equal volume of water prior to administration (Graves 1987)

Administration Hazardous agent; use appropriate precautions for handling and disposal (NIOSH 2014 [group 2]).

Oral: May administer with food to decrease adverse GI effects; do not administer with carbonated drinks.

Depakote ER: Swallow whole; do not crush or chew.

Depakote sprinkle capsules: May be swallowed whole or capsule may be opened and sprinkled on small amount (1 teaspoonful) of soft food (eg, pudding, applesauce) to be used immediately; do not crush or chew sprinkle beads; do not store drug food mixture for later use.

Depakene capsule, Stavzor: Swallow whole; do not break, crush, or chew.

Parenteral: IV:

Manufacturer recommendations: Dilute dose prior to administration; infuse over 60 minutes; maximum infusion rate: 20 mg/minute; **Note:** Rapid infusions may be associated with an increase in adverse effects; infusions of ≤15 mg/kg administered over 5 to 10 minutes (1.5 to 3 mg/kg/minute) were generally well tolerated (Ramsay, 2003). In pediatric patients, an infusion rate of 1.5 to 3 mg/kg/minute has been recommended (Brophy 2012).

Rapid IV loading doses:

Infants and Children: Dilute dose prior to administration; administer at 1.5 to 3 mg/kg/minute (Brophy 2012; Yu 2003). Faster infusion rates have been used in some studies; doses of 20 to 40 mg/kg have been administered over 1 to 5 minutes (Meht, 2007; Uberall 2000).

Adults: The European Federation of Neurological Societies (EFNS) recommends maximum administration rates of 6 mg/kg/minute (Meierkord 2006). **Note:** In two adult studies, the drug was administered undiluted at rates as high as 10 mg/kg/minute (Limdi 2007) and 500 mg/minute (Limdi 2005).

Rectal: Dilute oral solution or syrup prior to rectal administration (Graves 1987)

Monitoring Parameters Liver enzymes (prior to therapy and at frequent intervals, especially during the first 6 months), bilirubin, serum ammonia (with symptoms of lethargy, mental status change), CBC with platelets (prior to initiation and periodically during therapy), serum concentrations, PT/PTT (especially prior to surgery); signs and symptoms of suicidality (eg, anxiety, depression, behavior changes), motor and cognitive function

Reference Range Note: In general, trough concentrations should be used to assess adequacy of therapy; peak concentrations may also be drawn if clinically necessary (eg, concentration-related toxicity). Additional patient-specific factors must be taken into consideration when interpreting drug concentrations, including indication, age, clinical response, pregnancy status, adherence, comorbidities, adverse effects, and concomitant medications (Patsalos, 2008; Reed, 2006).

Seizure disorder:

Therapeutic: 50-100 mcg/mL (SI: 350-690 micromoles/L); the relationship between plasma concentration and therapeutic response is not well documented; some patients may require lower concentrations to achieve therapeutic effect, and others may require higher concentration, but have a higher risk of toxicity

Toxic: >100-150 mcg/mL (SI: >690-1040 micromoles/L); probability of thrombocytopenia increases with total valproate concentrations ≥110 mcg/mL (SI: ≥760 micromoles/L) in females or ≥135 mcg/mL (SI: ≥930 micromoles/L) in males

Seizure control may improve at concentrations >100 mcg/mL (SI: >690 micromoles/L), but toxicity may occur.

Mania: Therapeutic trough: 50-125 mcg/mL (SI: 350-860 micromoles/L); risk of toxicity increases at concentrations >125 mcg/mL (SI: 875 micromole/L)

Test Interactions May cause a false-positive result for urine ketones (valproate partially eliminated as a keto-metabolite in the urine); may alter thyroid function tests

Additional Information Acute intoxications: Naloxone may reverse the CNS depressant effects but may also block the action of other anticonvulsants; carnitine may reduce the ammonia concentration

Dosage Forms Considerations Strengths of divalproex sodium and valproate sodium products are expressed in terms of valproic acid

Dosage Forms Excipient information presented when available (limited, particularly for generics); consult specific product labeling.

Capsule, Oral, as valproic acid:
- Depakene: 250 mg
- Generic: 250 mg

Capsule Delayed Release, Oral, as valproic acid:
- Stavzor: 125 mg, 250 mg, 500 mg [contains fd&c yellow #6 (sunset yellow)]

Capsule Sprinkle, Oral, as divalproex sodium:
- Depakote Sprinkles: 125 mg [contains brilliant blue fcf (fd&c blue #1)]
- Generic: 125 mg

Solution, Intravenous, as valproate sodium:
- Depacon: 100 mg/mL (5 mL)

Solution, Intravenous, as valproate sodium [preservative free]:
- Generic: 100 mg/mL (5 mL); 500 mg/5 mL (5 mL)

Solution, Oral, as valproate sodium:
- Generic: 250 mg/5 mL (473 mL)

Syrup, Oral, as valproate sodium:
- Depakene: 250 mg/5 mL (480 mL)
- Generic: 250 mg/5 mL (5 mL, 10 mL, 473 mL)

Tablet Delayed Release, Oral, as divalproex sodium:
- Depakote: 125 mg [contains brilliant blue fcf (fd&c blue #1), fd&c red #40]
- Depakote: 250 mg [contains fd&c yellow #6 (sunset yellow)]
- Depakote: 500 mg [contains fd&c blue #2 (indigotine)]
- Generic: 125 mg, 250 mg, 500 mg

Tablet Extended Release 24 Hour, Oral, as divalproex sodium:
- Depakote ER: 250 mg, 500 mg
- Generic: 250 mg, 500 mg

Valsartan (val SAR tan)

Medication Safety Issues

Sound-alike/look-alike issues:

Valsartan may be confused with losartan, Valstar, Valturna

Diovan may be confused with Zyban

International issues:

Diovan [U.S., Canada, and multiple international markets] may be confused with Dianben, a brand name for metformin [Spain]

Brand Names: US Diovan

Brand Names: Canada ACT Valsartan; Apo-Valsartan; Auro-Valsartan; Ava-Valsartan; Diovan; Mylan-Valsartan; PMS-Valsartan; Ran-Valsartan; Sandoz-Valsartan; Teva-Valsartan

Therapeutic Category Angiotensin II Receptor Blocker; Antihypertensive Agent

Generic Availability (US) Yes

Use Treatment of primary hypertension alone or in combination with other antihypertensive agents (FDA approved in ages 6-16 years and adults); reduction of cardiovascular mortality in clinically stable patients with left ventricular failure or left ventricular dysfunction postmyocardial infarction (FDA approved in adults); treatment of heart failure (NYHA Class II-IV) (FDA approved in adults)

Pregnancy Risk Factor D

Pregnancy Considerations **[U.S. Boxed Warning]: Drugs that act on the renin-angiotensin system can cause injury and death to the developing fetus. Discontinue as soon as possible once pregnancy is detected.** The use of drugs which act on the renin-angiotensin system are associated with oligohydramnios. Oligohydramnios, due to decreased fetal renal function, may lead to fetal lung hypoplasia and skeletal malformations. Use is also associated with anuria, hypotension, renal failure, skull hypoplasia, and death in the fetus/neonate. in The exposed fetus should be monitored for fetal growth, amniotic fluid volume, and organ formation. Infants exposed *in utero* should be monitored for hyperkalemia, hypotension, and oliguria (exchange transfusions or dialysis may be needed). These adverse events are generally associated with maternal use in the second and third trimesters.

Untreated chronic maternal hypertension is also associated with adverse events in the fetus, infant, and mother. The use of angiotensin II receptor blockers is not recommended to treat chronic uncomplicated hypertension in pregnant women and should generally be avoided in women of reproductive potential (ACOG, 2013).

Breast-Feeding Considerations It is not known if valsartan is found in breast milk. Due to the potential for serious adverse reactions in the nursing infant, the manufacturer recommends a decision be made whether to discontinue nursing or to discontinue the drug, taking into account the importance of treatment to the mother. The Canadian labeling contraindicates use in nursing women.

Contraindications Hypersensitivity to valsartan or any component of the formulation; concomitant use with aliskiren in patients with diabetes mellitus

Canadian labeling: Additional contraindications (not in U.S. labeling): Concomitant use with aliskiren in patients with moderate-to-severe renal impairment (GFR <60 mL/minute/1.73 m^2); pregnancy; breastfeeding

Warnings/Precautions **[U.S. Boxed Warning]: Drugs that act on the renin-angiotensin system can cause injury and death to the developing fetus. Discontinue as soon as possible once pregnancy is detected.** May cause hyperkalemia; avoid potassium supplementation unless specifically required by healthcare provider. During the initiation of therapy, hypotension may occur, particularly in patients with heart failure or post-MI patients. Use extreme caution with concurrent administration of potassium-sparing diuretics or potassium supplements, in patients with mild-to-moderate hepatic dysfunction (adjust dose), in those who may be sodium/water depleted (eg, on high-dose diuretics), and in the elderly; correct depletion first.

Use caution with unstented unilateral/bilateral renal artery stenosis. When unstented bilateral renal artery stenosis is present, use is generally avoided due to the elevated risk of deterioration in renal function unless possible benefits outweigh risks. Use with caution with preexisting renal insufficiency; significant aortic/mitral stenosis. May be associated with deterioration of renal function and/or increases in serum creatinine, particularly in patients with low renal blood flow (eg, renal artery stenosis, heart failure) whose glomerular filtration rate (GFR) is dependent on efferent arteriolar vasoconstriction by angiotensin II. Use caution in patients with severe renal impairment or significant hepatic dysfunction. Monitor renal function closely in patients with severe heart failure; changes in renal function should be anticipated and dosage adjustments of valsartan or concomitant medications may be needed. Potentially significant drug-drug interactions may exist, requiring dose or frequency adjustment, additional monitoring, and/or selection of alternative therapy. In surgical patients on chronic angiotensin receptor blocker (ARB) therapy, intraoperative hypotension may occur with induction and maintenance of general anesthesia.

Angioedema has been reported rarely with some angiotensin II receptor antagonists (ARBs) and may occur at any time during treatment (especially following first dose). It may involve the head and neck (potentially compromising airway) or the intestine (presenting with abdominal pain). Patients with idiopathic or hereditary angioedema or previous angioedema associated with ACE-inhibitor therapy may be at an increased risk. Prolonged frequent monitoring may be required, especially if tongue, glottis, or larynx are involved, as they are associated with airway obstruction. Patients with a history of airway surgery may have a higher risk of airway obstruction. Discontinue therapy immediately if angioedema occurs. Aggressive early management is critical. Intramuscular (IM) administration of epinephrine may be necessary. Do not readminister to patients who have had angioedema with ARBs.

Warnings: Additional Pediatric Considerations In a hypertension clinical trial of 90 children <6 years if age, five severe adverse events occurred in the treatment group, including two deaths (causes were identified as viral gastroenteritis and pneumonia) and three cases of increased liver enzymes; all patients also had significant comorbidities (primarily renal or urinary abnormalities); a causal relationship to valsartan could not be established nor excluded; use not recommended in this age group per manufacturer labeling (Flynn, 2008). Small increases in serum creatinine may occur following initiation; consider discontinuation in patients with progressive and/or significant deterioration in renal function. Not recommended for use in children with GFR <30 mL/minute/1.73 m^2; has not been studied.

Adverse Reactions

Cardiovascular: Hypotension, orthostatic hypotension, syncope

Central nervous system: Dizziness, fatigue, headache, orthostatic dizziness, vertigo

Endocrine & metabolic: Serum potassium increased, hyperkalemia

Gastrointestinal: Abdominal pain (including upper), diarrhea, nausea

Hematologic & oncologic: Neutropenia

Infection: Viral infection

Neuromuscular & skeletal: Arthralgia, back pain

Ophthalmic: Blurred vision

Otic: Vertigo

Renal: Increased blood urea nitrogen, increased serum creatinine, renal insufficiency

Respiratory: Cough

All indications: Rare but important or life-threatening: Alopecia, anaphylaxis, anemia, angioedema, anorexia, bullous dermatitis, decreased hematocrit, decreased hemoglobin, dyspepsia, flatulence, hepatitis (rare), hypersensitivity reaction, impotence, insomnia, liver function tests increased, microcytic anemia, myalgia, palpitation, paresthesia, photosensitivity, pruritus, renal failure, rhabdomyolysis, skin rash, taste disorder, thrombocytopenia (very rare), vasculitis, xerostomia

Drug Interactions

Metabolism/Transport Effects Substrate of MRP2, SLCO1B1; **Inhibits** CYP2C9 (weak)

Avoid Concomitant Use There are no known interactions where it is recommended to avoid concomitant use.

Increased Effect/Toxicity

Valsartan may increase the levels/effects of: ACE Inhibitors; Amifostine; Antihypertensives; Ciprofloxacin (Systemic); CycloSPORINE (Systemic); Drospirenone; DULoxetine; Hydrochlorothiazide; Hypotensive Agents; Levodopa; Lithium; Nonsteroidal Anti-Inflammatory Agents; Obinutuzumab; Potassium-Sparing Diuretics; RisperiDONE; RiTUXimab; Sodium Phosphates

The levels/effects of Valsartan may be increased by: Alfuzosin; Aliskiren; Barbiturates; Brimonidine (Topical); Canagliflozin; Dapoxetine; Diazoxide; Eltrombopag; Eplerenone; Heparin; Heparin (Low Molecular Weight); Herbs (Hypotensive Properties); Hydrochlorothiazide; MAO Inhibitors; Nicorandil; Pentoxifylline; Phosphodiesterase 5 Inhibitors; Potassium Salts; Prostacyclin Analogues; Teriflunomide; Tolvaptan; Trimethoprim

Decreased Effect

The levels/effects of Valsartan may be decreased by: Herbs (Hypertensive Properties); Methylphenidate; Nonsteroidal Anti-Inflammatory Agents; Yohimbine

Food Interactions Food decreases the peak plasma concentration and extent of absorption by 50% and 40%, respectively. Management: Administer consistently with regard to food.

Storage/Stability Store at 25°C (77°F); excursions permitted to 15°C to 30°C (59°F to 86°F). Protect from moisture.

Mechanism of Action Valsartan produces direct antagonism of the angiotensin II (AT2) receptors, unlike the ACE inhibitors. It displaces angiotensin II from the AT1 receptor and produces its blood pressure-lowering effects by antagonizing AT1-induced vasoconstriction, aldosterone release, catecholamine release, arginine vasopressin release, water intake, and hypertrophic responses. This action results in more efficient blockade of the cardiovascular effects of angiotensin II and fewer side effects than the ACE inhibitors.

Pharmacodynamics

Antihypertensive effect:

- Onset of action: 2 hours postdose
- Maximum effect: Within 6 hours postdose; with chronic dosing, substantial hypotensive effects are seen within 2 weeks; maximum effect: After 4 weeks
- Duration: 24 hours

Pharmacokinetics (Adult data unless noted)

Distribution: V_d: 17 L

Protein binding: 95%, primarily albumin

Metabolism: To inactive metabolite (valeryl 4-hydroxy valsartan) via unidentified enzyme(s)

Bioavailability:

- Tablet: 25% (range: 10% to 35%)
- Suspension: ~40% (~1.6 times more than tablet)

Half-life, elimination:

- Pediatric patients:
  - 1-5 years: ~4 hours (Blumer, 2009)
  - 6-16 years: ~5 hours (Blumer, 2009)
- Adults: ~6 hours

Time to peak serum concentration:

- Pediatric patients 1-16 years: Oral suspension: 2 hours (Blumer, 2009)
- Adults: Tablets: 2-4 hours

Elimination: Feces (83%) and urine (13%) primarily as unchanged drug; 20% of dose is recovered as metabolites

- Clearance: Found to be similar per kg bodyweight in children vs adults receiving a single dose of the suspension (Blumer, 2009)

Dialysis: Not removed by hemodialysis

Dosing: Usual

Children and Adolescents: **Hypertension:** Oral: **Note:** Due to increased bioavailability of extemporaneously prepared oral suspension (not commercially available), patients may require a higher dose when converting from oral suspension to tablet dosage form.

Children 1-5 years, weighing ≥8 kg: Limited data available: Reported dosage range: 0.4-3.4 mg/kg/dose once daily; maximum daily dose dependent upon patient weight: <18 kg: 40 mg/**day**; ≥18 kg: 80 mg/**day**. Dosing based on a single multicenter, international, placebo-controlled, dose-finding, crossover trial of 90 children 1-5 years (mean age: 3.2 years; minimum patient weight: 8 kg) which randomized patients to receive low, medium, or high doses according to patient body weight. Patients <18 kg received low dose: 5 mg once daily; medium dose: 20 mg once daily; or high dose: 40 mg once daily. Patients ≥18 kg received low dose: 10 mg once daily; medium dose: 40 mg once daily; or high dose: 80 mg once daily. Results showed significant antihypertensive effects in all dose level groups; five severe adverse events were reported during treatment (Flynn, 2008).

Children and Adolescents 6-16 years: Initial: 1.3 mg/kg once daily; maximum initial daily dose: 40 mg/**day**; may titrate to effect up to a maximum dose of 2.7 mg/kg/dose once daily or maximum daily dose: 160 mg/**day**, whichever is lower; doses greater than this have not been studied

Adolescents ≥17 years: Initial: 80 mg or 160 mg once daily (in patients who are not volume depleted); dose may be increased to achieve desired effect; maximum daily dose: 320 mg/**day**; in adults, usual dosage range (JNC 7): 80-320 mg once daily

Adults:

Hypertension: Oral: Initial: 80 mg or 160 mg once daily (in patients who are not volume depleted); dose may be increased to achieve desired effect; maximum recommended dose: 320 mg once daily; usual dosage range (JNC 7): 80-320 mg once daily

Heart failure: Oral: Initial: 40 mg twice daily; titrate dose to 80-160 mg twice daily, as tolerated; maximum dose: 320 mg/day in divided doses

Left ventricular dysfunction after MI: Initial: 20 mg twice daily; titrate dose to target of 160 mg twice daily as tolerated; may initiate ≥12 hours following MI

Dosing adjustment in renal impairment:

Children ≥ 6 years and Adolescents:

CrCl ≥30 mL/minute: No dosage adjustment necessary.

CrCl <30 mL/minute or Dialysis: There are no dosage adjustments provided in manufacturer's labeling; has not been studied; use not recommended.

Adults:

CrCl ≥30 mL/minute: No dosage adjustment necessary.

CrCl <30 mL/minute: There are no dosage adjustments provided in manufacturer's labeling; safety and efficacy have not been established.

Dialysis: Not significantly removed.

Dosing adjustment in hepatic impairment: Children ≥6 years, Adolescents, and Adults:

Mild to moderate impairment: No dosage adjustment necessary; use caution in patients with liver disease. Patients with mild to moderate chronic disease have twice the exposure as healthy volunteers.

Severe impairment: There are no dosage adjustments provided in manufacturer's labeling; has not been studied.

Administration May be administered without regard to food

Monitoring Parameters Blood pressure, BUN, serum creatinine, renal function, baseline and periodic serum electrolytes

Dosage Forms Excipient information presented when available (limited, particularly for generics); consult specific product labeling.

Tablet, Oral:

Diovan: 40 mg [scored]

Diovan: 80 mg, 160 mg, 320 mg

Generic: 40 mg, 80 mg, 160 mg, 320 mg

Extemporaneous Preparations A 4 mg/mL oral suspension may be made from tablets, Ora-Plus®, and Ora-Sweet® SF. Add 80 mL of Ora-Plus® to an 8-ounce amber glass bottle containing eight valsartan 80 mg tablets. Shake well for ≥2 minutes. Allow the suspension to stand for a minimum of 1 hour, then shake for ≥1 minute. Add 80 mL of Ora-Sweet SF® to the bottle and shake for ≥10 seconds. Store in amber glass prescription bottles; label "shake well". Stable for 30 days at room temperature or 75 days refrigerated.

Diovan® prescribing information, Novartis Pharmaceuticals Corp, East Hanover, NJ, 2012.

- ◆ **Valtrex** *see* ValACYclovir *on page 2138*
- ◆ **Val-Vancomycin (Can)** *see* Vancomycin *on page 2151*
- ◆ **Vanceril** *see* Beclomethasone (Oral Inhalation) *on page 262*
- ◆ **Vancocin (Can)** *see* Vancomycin *on page 2151*
- ◆ **Vancocin HCl** *see* Vancomycin *on page 2151*

Vancomycin (van koe MYE sin)

Medication Safety Issues

Sound-alike/look-alike issues:

IV vancomycin may be confused with INVanz

Vancomycin may be confused with clindamycin, gentamicin, tobramycin, valACYclovir, vecuronium, Vibramycin

High alert medication:

The Institute for Safe Medication Practices (ISMP) includes this medication (intrathecal administration) among its list of drug classes which have a heightened risk of causing significant patient harm when used in error.

Related Information

Prevention of Infective Endocarditis *on page 2378*

Brand Names: US First-Vancomycin 25; First-Vancomycin 50; Vancocin HCl

Brand Names: Canada JAMP-Vancomycin; PMS-Vancomycin; Sterile Vancomycin Hydrochloride, USP; Val-Vancomycin; Vancocin; Vancomycin Hydrochloride for Injection; Vancomycin Hydrochloride for Injection, USP

Therapeutic Category Antibiotic, Miscellaneous

Generic Availability (US) Yes

Use

Parenteral: Treatment of patients with the following infections or conditions: Infections due to documented or suspected methicillin-resistant *S. aureus* or beta-lactam resistant coagulase negative *Staphylococcus*; serious or life-threatening infections (eg, endocarditis, meningitis, osteomyelitis) due to documented or suspected staphylococcal or streptococcal infections in patients who are allergic to penicillins and/or cephalosporins; empiric therapy of infections associated with central lines, VP shunts, hemodialysis shunts, vascular grafts, prosthetic heart valves (FDA approved in all ages)

Oral: Treatment of *C. difficile*-associated diarrhea and enterocolitis caused by *Staphylococcus aureus* (including methicillin-resistant strains) (FDA approved in pediatric patients [age not specified0 and adults)

Pregnancy Risk Factor B (oral); C (injection)

Pregnancy Considerations Adverse events have not been observed in animal reproduction studies. Vancomycin crosses the placenta and can be detected in fetal serum, amniotic fluid, and cord blood (Bourget 1991; Reyes 1989). Adverse fetal effects, including sensorineural hearing loss or nephrotoxicity, have not been reported following maternal use during the second or third trimesters of pregnancy.

The pharmacokinetics of vancomycin may be altered during pregnancy and pregnant patients may need a higher dose of vancomycin. Maternal half-life is unchanged, but the volume of distribution and the total plasma clearance may be increased (Bourget 1991). Individualization of therapy through serum concentration monitoring may be warranted. Vancomycin is recommended for the treatment of mild, moderate, or severe *Clostridium difficile* infections in pregnant women (ACG [Surawicz 2013]). Vancomycin is recommended as an alternative agent to prevent the transmission of group B streptococcal (GBS) disease from mothers to newborns (ACOG 2011; CDC 2010).

Breast-Feeding Considerations Vancomycin is excreted in human milk following IV administration. If given orally to the mother, the minimal systemic absorption of the dose would limit the amount available to pass into the milk. Vancomycin is recommended for the treatment of mild, moderate, or severe *Clostridium difficile* infections in breast-feeding women (ACG [Surawicz 2013]). Due to the potential for serious adverse reactions in the nursing infant, the manufacturer recommends a decision be made whether to discontinue nursing or to discontinue the drug, taking into account the importance of treatment to the mother. Nondose-related effects could include modification of bowel flora.

Contraindications Hypersensitivity to vancomycin or any component of the formulation

Warnings/Precautions May cause nephrotoxicity although limited data suggest direct causal relationship; usual risk factors include preexisting renal impairment, concomitant nephrotoxic medications, advanced age, and dehydration (nephrotoxicity has also been reported following treatment with oral vancomycin, typically in patients >65 years of age). If multiple sequential (≥2) serum creatinine concentrations demonstrate an increase of 0.5 mg/dL or ≥50% increase from baseline (whichever is greater) in the absence of an alternative explanation, the patient should be identified as having vancomycin-induced nephrotoxicity (Rybak, 2009). Discontinue treatment if signs of nephrotoxicity occur; renal damage is usually reversible.

May cause neurotoxicity; usual risk factors include preexisting renal impairment, concomitant neuro-/nephrotoxic medications, advanced age, and dehydration. Ototoxicity, although rarely associated with monotherapy, is proportional to the amount of drug given and the duration of treatment. Tinnitus or vertigo may be indications of vestibular injury and impending bilateral irreversible damage. Discontinue treatment if signs of ototoxicity occur. Prolonged therapy (>1 week) or total doses exceeding 25 g may increase the risk of neutropenia; prompt reversal of neutropenia is expected after discontinuation of therapy. Prolonged use may result in fungal or bacterial superinfection, including *C. difficile*-associated diarrhea (CDAD) and pseudomembranous colitis; CDAD has been observed >2 months postantibiotic treatment. Use with caution in patients with renal impairment or those receiving other nephrotoxic or ototoxic drugs; dosage modification required in patients with impaired renal function (especially elderly). Accumulation may occur after multiple oral doses of vancomycin in patients with renal impairment; consider monitoring trough concentrations in this circumstance.

Rapid IV administration may result in hypotension, flushing, erythema, urticaria, and/or pruritus. Oral vancomycin is only indicated for the treatment of pseudomembranous colitis due to *C. difficile* and enterocolitis due to *S. aureus* and is not effective for systemic infections; parenteral vancomycin is not effective for the treatment of colitis due to *C. difficile* and enterocolitis due to *S. aureus*. Clinically significant serum concentrations have been reported in patients with inflammatory disorders of the intestinal mucosa who have taken oral vancomycin (multiple doses) for the treatment of *C. difficile*-associated diarrhea. Although use may be warranted, the risk for adverse reactions may be higher in this situation; consider monitoring serum trough concentrations, especially with renal insufficiency, severe colitis, concurrent rectal vancomycin administration, and/or concomitant IV aminoglycosides. The Society for Healthcare Epidemiology of America (SHEA) and the Infectious Diseases Society of America (IDSA) suggest that it is appropriate to obtain trough concentrations when a patient is receiving long courses of ≥2 g/day in adults (SHEA/IDSA [Cohen, 2010]). **Note:** The SHEA, the IDSA, and the American College of Gastroenterology (ACG) recommend the use of oral metronidazole for initial treatment of mild to moderate *C. difficile* infection and the use of oral vancomycin for initial treatment of severe *C. difficile* infection (SHEA/IDSA [Cohen, 2010]; ACG [Surawicz, 2013]).

Adverse Reactions

Injection:

Cardiovascular: Hypotension accompanied by flushing

Central nervous system: Chills, drug fever

Dermatologic: Erythematous rash on face and upper body (red neck or red man syndrome)

Hematologic: Eosinophilia, reversible neutropenia

Local: Phlebitis

Rare but important or life-threatening: Drug rash with eosinophilia and systemic symptoms (DRESS), ototoxicity (rare; use of other ototoxic agents may increase risk), renal failure (limited data suggesting direct relationship), Stevens-Johnson syndrome, thrombocytopenia, vasculitis

Oral:

Cardiovascular: Peripheral edema

Central nervous system: Fatigue, fever, headache

Gastrointestinal: Abdominal pain, bad taste (with oral solution), diarrhea, flatulence, nausea, vomiting

Genitourinary: Urinary tract infection

Neuromuscular & skeletal: Back pain

Rare but important or life-threatening: Creatinine increased, interstitial nephritis, ototoxicity, renal failure, renal impairment, thrombocytopenia, vasculitis

Drug Interactions

Metabolism/Transport Effects None known.

Avoid Concomitant Use

Avoid concomitant use of Vancomycin with any of the following: BCG; BCG (Intravesical)

Increased Effect/Toxicity

Vancomycin may increase the levels/effects of: Aminoglycosides; Colistimethate; Neuromuscular-Blocking Agents

The levels/effects of Vancomycin may be increased by: Nonsteroidal Anti-Inflammatory Agents; Piperacillin

Decreased Effect

Vancomycin may decrease the levels/effects of: BCG; BCG (Intravesical); BCG Vaccine (Immunization); Sodium Picosulfate; Typhoid Vaccine

The levels/effects of Vancomycin may be decreased by: Bile Acid Sequestrants

Storage/Stability

Capsules: Store at controlled room temperature of 15°C to 30°C (59°F to 86°F).

Injection: Reconstituted 500 mg and 1 g vials are stable for at either room temperature or under refrigeration for 14 days. **Note:** Vials contain no bacteriostatic agent. Solutions diluted for administration in either D_5W or NS are stable under refrigeration for 14 days or at room temperature for 7 days.

Premixed solution (manufacturer premixed): Store at -20°C (-4°F); once thawed, solutions are stable for 72 hours at room temperature or for 30 days refrigerated. Do not refreeze.

Mechanism of Action Inhibits bacterial cell wall synthesis by blocking glycopeptide polymerization through binding tightly to D-alanyl-D-alanine portion of cell wall precursor

Pharmacodynamics Displays time-dependent antimicrobial killing; slowly bacteriocidal

Pharmacokinetics (Adult data unless noted)

Absorption:
- Oral: Poor; may be enhanced with bowel inflammation
- IM: Erratic
- Intraperitoneal: Can result in 38% systemic absorption

Distribution: Wide and variable distribution in body tissues and fluids including pericardial, pleural, ascites, and synovial fluids; low concentration in CSF

V_d:
- Neonate, term: 0.57 to 0.69 L/kg (de Hoog 2004)
- Neonates, receiving ECMO (mean age: ~39 weeks): Variable; 1.1 L/kg (range: 0.6 to 2.1 L/kg) (Amaker 1996); others have reported lower values: 0.45 ± 0.18 L/kg (Buck 1998)
- Pediatric patients: Median: 0.57 L/kg (range: 0.26 to 1.05 L/kg) (Marsot 2012)
- Adult: 0.4 to 1 L/kg (Rybak 2009)

Relative diffusion from blood into CSF: Distribution improved with inflamed meninges and typically exceeds usual MICs

Children:
- CSF concentrations: 0.2 to 17.3 mcg/mL (de Hoog 2004)
- CSF:blood level ratio: Normal meninges: Nil; Inflamed meninges: 7.1% to 68% (de Hoog 2004)

Adults:
- Uninflamed meninges: 0 to 4 mcg/mL; serum concentration dependent (Rybak 2009)
- Inflamed meninges: 6 to 11 mcg/mL; serum concentration dependent (Rybak 2009)
- CSF:blood level ratio: Normal meninges: Nil; Inflamed meninges: 20% to 30%

Protein binding: 55%

Metabolism: <3%

Half-life, biphasic: Prolonged significantly with reduced renal function

Terminal:
- Newborns: 6 to 10 hours
- 3 months to 4 years: 4 hours
- >3 years: 2.2 to 3 hours
- Adults: 5 to 8 hours

Elimination: Primarily via glomerular filtration; excreted as unchanged drug in the urine (80% to 90%); oral doses are excreted primarily in the feces; presence of malignancy in children is associated with an increase in vancomycin clearance

Clearance:
- Neonates: 0.63 to 1.5 mL/minute/kg; dependent on GA and/or PMA (de Hoog 2004)
- Neonates, receiving ECMO: 0.78 mL/minute/kg (range: 0.49 to 1.07 mL/minute/kg) (Amaker 1996)
- Pediatric patients: Median: 1.1 mL/minute/kg (range: 0.33 to 1.87 mL/minute/kg) (Marsot 2012)
- Adults: 0.71 to 1.31 mL/minute/kg (de Hoog 2004)

Dialysis: Poorly dialyzable by intermittent hemodialysis (0% to 5%); however, use of high-flux membranes and continuous renal replacement therapy (CRRT) increases vancomycin clearance, and generally requires replacement dosing

Dosing: Neonatal

General dosing, susceptible infection: Note: Consider single-dose administration with serum concentration monitoring rather than scheduled dosing in patients with urine output <1 mL/kg/hour or if serum creatinine significantly increases from baseline (eg, doubles). Consider prolongation of dosing interval when coadministered with ibuprofen or indomethacin or in neonates with history of the following: Birth depression, birth hypoxia/asphyxia, or cyanotic congenital heart disease.

Initial dosage recommendation:

Renal function-based dosing (Capparelli 2001; *Nelson's Pocket Book of Pediatric Antimicrobial Therapy* 2012): IV:

PNA ≤60 days:

≤28 weeks GA:
- S_{cr} <0.5 mg/dL: 15 mg/kg/dose every 12 hours
- S_{cr} 0.5 to 0.7 mg/dL: 20 mg/kg/dose every 24 hours
- S_{cr} 0.8 to 1 mg/dL: 15 mg/kg/dose every 24 hours
- S_{cr} 1.1 to 1.4 mg/dL: 10 mg/kg/dose every 24 hours
- S_{cr} >1.4 mg/dL: 15 mg/kg/dose every 48 hours

>28 weeks GA:
- S_{cr} <0.7 mg/dL: 15 mg/kg/dose every 12 hours
- S_{cr} 0.7 to 0.9 mg/dL: 20 mg/kg/dose every 24 hours
- S_{cr} 1 to 1.2 mg/dL: 15 mg/kg/dose every 24 hours
- S_{cr} 1.3 to 1.6 mg/dL: 10 mg/kg/dose every 24 hours
- S_{cr} >1.6 mg/dL: 15 mg/kg/dose every 48 hours

PNA >60 days: 30 to 40 mg/kg/**day** divided every 6 to 8 hours

Weight-based dosing (*Red Book* 2009): IV:

PNA <7 days:
- <1,200 g: 15 mg/kg/dose every 24 hours
- 1,200 to 2,000 g: 10 to 15 mg/kg/dose every 12 to 18 hours
- >2,000 g: 10 to 15 mg/kg/dose every 8 to 12 hours

PNA ≥7 days:
- <1,200 g: 15 mg/kg/dose every 24 hours
- 1,200 to 2,000 g: 10 to 15 mg/kg/dose every 8 to 12 hours
- >2,000 g: 10 to 15 mg/kg/dose every 6 to 8 hours

ECMO, initial dosing in full-term neonates: IV: 15 to 20 mg/kg/dose every 18 to 24 hours (Buck 2003); closely monitor serum concentrations; more frequent dosing may be needed for some patients

CNS Infection:

Meningitis (Tunkel 2004): **Note:** Maintain trough serum concentrations of 15 to 20 mcg/mL; for neonates <2 kg, consider use of smaller doses and longer intervals. IV:
- PNA ≤7 days and ≥2 kg: 20 to 30 mg/kg/**day** divided every 8 to 12 hours
- PNA >7days and ≥2 kg: 30 to 45 mg/kg/**day** divided every 6 to 8 hours

VP-shunt infection, ventriculitis: Limited data available: Intrathecal/intraventricular (**use a preservative-free preparation**): 5 to 10 mg/day (Tunkel 2004)

Dosing adjustment in renal impairment: Monitor vancomycin serum concentrations and adjust accordingly.

Dosing: Usual Initial dosage recommendation: **Note:** Doses require adjustment in renal impairment. Consider single-dose administration with serum concentration monitoring rather than scheduled dosing in patients with urine output <1 mL/kg/hour or if serum creatinine significantly increases from baseline (eg, doubles):

Pediatric:

General dosing, susceptible infection:

Infants ≤2 months:

Weight-based dosing (*Red Book* 2012): **Note:** Every 6 hour dosing recommended as initial dosage regimen if targeting trough serum concentrations >10 mcg/mL (Benner 2009; Frymoyer 2009) in patients with normal renal function. Close monitoring of serum concentrations and assurance of adequate hydration status is recommended.

Mild to moderate infection: IV: 40 to 45 mg/kg/**day** divided every 6 to 8 hours; dose and frequency should be individualized based on serum concentrations; usual maximum daily dose: 2,000 mg/**day**

Severe infection: IV: 45 to 60 mg/kg/**day** divided every 6 to 8 hours; dose and frequency should be individualized based on serum concentrations; usual maximum daily dose: 4,000 mg/**day**

Renal function-based dosing (Capparelli 2001; *Nelson's Pocket Book of Pediatric Antimicrobial Therapy* 2012):

>28 weeks GA:

S_{cr} <0.7 mg/dL: 15 mg/kg/dose every 12 hours

S_{cr} 0.7 to 0.9 mg/dL: 20 mg/kg/dose every 24 hours

S_{cr} 1 to 1.2 mg/dL: 15 mg/kg/dose every 24 hours

S_{cr} 1.3 to 1.6 mg/dL: 10 mg/kg/dose every 24 hours

S_{cr} >1.6 mg/dL: 15 mg/kg/dose every 48 hours

Infants >2 months, Children, and Adolescents (*Red Book* 2012): **Note:** Every 6 hour dosing recommended as initial dosage regimen if targeting trough serum concentrations >10 mcg/mL (Benner 2009; Frymoyer 2009) in patients with normal renal function. Close monitoring of serum concentrations and assurance of adequate hydration status is recommended.

Mild to moderate infection: IV: 40 to 45 mg/kg/**day** divided every 6 to 8 hours; dose and frequency should be individualized based on serum concentrations; usual maximum daily dose: 2,000 mg/**day**

Severe infection: IV: 45 to 60 mg/kg/**day** divided every 6 to 8 hours; dose and frequency should be individualized based on serum concentrations; usual maximum daily dose: 4,000 mg/**day**

Bacteremia [*S. aureus* (methicillin-resistant)]: Infants, Children, and Adolescents: IV: 15 mg/kg/dose every 6 hours for 2 to 6 weeks depending on severity (Liu 2011)

Bone and joint infection:

Osteomyelitis [*S. aureus* (methicillin-resistant)]: Infants, Children, and Adolescents: IV: 15 mg/kg/dose every 6 hours for a minimum of 4 to 6 weeks (Liu 2011)

Septic arthritis [*S. aureus* (methicillin-resistant)]: Infants, Children, and Adolescents: IV: 15 mg/kg/dose every 6 hours for minimum of 3 to 4 weeks (Liu 2011)

***C. difficile*-associated diarrhea (CDAD):**

Manufacturer's labeling: Infants, Children, and Adolescents: Oral: 40 mg/kg/day divided every 6 to 8 hours for 7 to 10 days; maximum daily dose: 2,000 mg/day

Alternate dosing: Severe or recurrent infection: Infants, Children, and Adolescents: Oral, rectal enema: 40 mg/kg/day in 4 divided doses for ≥10 days; maximum daily dose: 2,000 mg/**day**; if complete ileus, rectal enema dosage form may be preferable (*Red Book* [AAP] 2012; Schutze 2013)

CNS infection:

Brain abscess, subdural empyema, spinal epidural abscess [*S. aureus* (methicillin-resistant)]: Infants, Children, and Adolescents: IV: 15 mg/kg/dose every 6 hours for 4 to 6 weeks (some experts combine with rifampin) (Lui 2011)

Meningitis: Infants, Children, and Adolescents: IV: 15 mg/kg/dose every 6 hours; **Note:** Maintain trough serum concentrations of 15 to 20 mcg/mL (Tunkel 2004)

S. aureus (methicillin-resistant): Infants, Children, and Adolescents: 15 mg/kg/dose every 6 hours for 2 weeks (some experts combine with rifampin) (Liu 2011)

VP-shunt infection, ventriculitis: Limited data available: Infants, Children, and Adolescents: Intrathecal/intraventricular **(use a preservative-free preparation)**: 5 to 20 mg/**day**; usual dose: 10 or 20 mg/**day** (Tunkel 2004)

Endocarditis:

Treatment: Infants, Children, and Adolescents: IV: 40 mg/kg/**day** divided every 6 to 12 hours for 4 to 6 weeks; dosage should be adjusted to target peak serum concentrations of 30 to 45 mcg/mL and trough serum concentrations of 10 to 15 mcg/mL; may combine with gentamicin for 2 to 6 weeks based on organism, resistance pattern, and type of valve (Baddour 2005; Ferrieri 2002). **Note:** Recommended by the AHA as an alternative agent in β-lactam allergic patients.

S. aureus (methicillin-resistant):

AHA Guidelines: Infants, Children, and Adolescents: IV: 40 mg/kg/**day** divided every 6 to 12 hours for at least 6 weeks; dosage should be adjusted to target peak serum concentrations of 30 to 45 mcg/mL and trough serum concentrations of 10 to 15 mcg/mL; **Note:** For prosthetic valves, combination with rifampin for the entire duration of therapy and gentamicin for the first 2 weeks has been recommended (Baddour 2005; Ferrieri 2002).

IDSA Guidelines: Infants, Children, and Adolescents: IV: 60 mg/kg/**day** divided every 6 hours for at least 6 weeks (Liu 2011)

Prophylaxis, GI, or genitourinary procedures: Infants, Children, and Adolescents: IV: 20 mg/kg over 1 hour; complete infusion 30 minutes prior to the procedure (Wilson 2007). **Note:** Recommended by the AHA as an alternative agent in β-lactam allergic patients. As of April 2007, routine prophylaxis for GI/GU procedures is no longer recommended by the AHA.

Enterocolitis (*S. aureus*): Infants, Children, and Adolescents: Oral: 40 mg/kg/**day** divided every 6 to 8 hours for 7 to 10 days; maximum daily dose: 2,000 mg/**day**

Intra-abdominal infection, complicated (MRSA): Infants, Children, and Adolescents: IV: 40 mg/kg/**day** divided every 6 to 8 hours (Solomkin 2010)

Peritonitis (CAPD) (Warady 2012):

Prophylaxis: Infants, Children, and Adolescents:

Touch contamination of PD line (if known MRSA colonization): Intraperitoneal: 25 mg per liter

High-risk gastrointestinal procedures: **Note:** Use should be reserved for patients at high risk for MRSA: IV: 10 mg/kg administered 60 to 90 minutes before procedure; maximum dose: 1,000 mg

Treatment: Infants, Children, and Adolescents: Intraperitoneal:

Intermittent: Initial dose: 30 mg/kg in the long dwell; subsequent doses: 15 mg/kg/dose every 3 to 5 days during the long dwell; **Note:** Increased clearance may occur in patients with residual renal function; subsequent doses should be based on serum concentration obtained 2 to 4 days after the previous dose; redosing should occur when serum concentration <15 mcg/mL.

Continuous: Loading dose: 1,000 mg per liter of dialysate; maintenance dose: 25 mg per liter

Pneumonia:

Community-acquired pneumonia (CAP): Infants ≥3 months, Children, and Adolescents: IV: 40 to 60 mg/kg/**day** every 6 to 8 hours; dosing to achieve AUC/MIC >400 has been recommended for treating moderate to severe MRSA infections (Bradley 2011)

Alternate regimen: *S. aureus* (methicillin-resistant): Infants, Children, and Adolescents: IV: 60 mg/kg/**day** divided every 6 hours for 7 to 21 days depending on severity (Liu 2011)

Healthcare-associated pneumonia (HAP), *S. aureus* (methicillin-resistant): Infants, Children, and Adolescents: IV: 60 mg/kg/**day** divided every 6 hours for 7 to 21 days depending on severity (Liu 2011)

Septic thrombosis of cavernous or dural venous sinus [*S. aureus* (methicillin-resistant)]: Infants

Children, and Adolescents: IV: 15 mg/kg/dose every 6 hours for 4 to 6 weeks (some experts combine with rifampin) (Lui 2011)

Skin and skin structure infections, complicated: [MRSA or *S. aureus* (methicillin sensitive) in penicillin allergic patients]: Infants, Children, and Adolescents: IV: 40 mg/kg/**day** divided every 6 hours (Stevens 2005)

Alternate regimen: *S. aureus* (methicillin-resistant): Infants, Children, and Adolescents: IV: 60 mg/kg/**day** divided every 6 hours for 7 to 14 days (Liu 2011)

Adult:

Usual dosage range: Initial intravenous dosing should be based on actual body weight; subsequent dosing adjusted based on serum trough vancomycin concentrations.

IV: 2,000 to 3,000 mg/**day** (or 30 to 60 mg/kg/**day**) in divided doses every 8 to 12 hours (Rybak 2009); **Note:** Dose requires adjustment in renal impairment.

Oral: 500 to 2,000 mg/**day** in divided doses every 6 hours

Indication-specific dosing:

Catheter-related infections: Antibiotic lock technique (Mermel 2009): 2 mg/mL ± 10 units heparin/mL **or** 2.5 mg/mL ± 2,500 **or** 5,000 units heparin/mL **or** 5 mg/mL ± 5,000 units heparin/mL (preferred regimen); instill into catheter port with a volume sufficient to fill the catheter (2 to 5 mL). **Note:** May use SWI/NS or D_5W as diluents. Do not mix with any other solutions. Dwell times generally should not exceed 48 hours before renewal of lock solution. Remove lock solution prior to catheter use, then replace.

***C. difficile*-associated diarrhea (CDAD):** Oral:

Manufacturer recommendations: 125 mg 4 times daily for 10 days

IDSA guideline recommendations: Severe infection: 125 mg every 6 hours for 10 to 14 days; Severe, complicated infection: 500 mg every 6 hours with or without concurrent IV metronidazole. May consider vancomycin retention enema (in patients with complete ileus) (Cohen 2010)

Complicated infections in seriously ill patients: IV: Loading dose: 25 to 30 mg/kg (based on actual body weight) may be used to rapidly achieve target concentration; then 15 to 20 mg/kg/dose every 8 to 12 hours (Rybak 2009)

Endocarditis:

Treatment: IV: 1,000 mg every 12 hours for 4 to 6 weeks; may combine with gentamicin for 2 to 6 weeks based on organism, resistance pattern, and type of valve (Gould 2012)

Prophylaxis (Wilson 2007):

Dental, oral, or upper respiratory tract surgery: IV: 1,000 mg 1 hour before surgery. **Note:** AHA guidelines now recommend prophylaxis only in patients undergoing invasive procedures and in whom underlying cardiac conditions may predispose to a higher risk of adverse outcomes should infection occur.

GI/GU procedure: IV: 1,000 mg 1 hour prior to surgery; must be used in combination with gentamicin. **Note:** As of April 2007, routine prophylaxis for GI/GU procedures no longer recommended by the AHA.

Enterocolitis (*S. aureus*): Oral: 500 to 2,000 mg/**day** in 3 to 4 divided doses for 7 to 10 days (usual dose: 125 to 500 mg every 6 hours)

Group B streptococcus (neonatal prophylaxis): IV: 1,000 mg every 12 hours until delivery. **Note:** Reserved for penicillin allergic patients at high risk for anaphylaxis if organism is resistant to clindamycin or where no susceptibility data are available (CDC 2010).

Meningitis:

IV: 30 to 60 mg/kg/**day** in divided doses every 8 to 12 hours (Rybak 2009) **or** 500 to 750 mg every 6 hours (with third generation cephalosporin for PCN-resistant *Streptococcus pneumoniae*)

Intrathecal, intraventricular: 5 to 20 mg/day

MRSA infections (Liu 2011): IV: 15 to 20 mg/kg/dose every 8 to 12 hours; duration of therapy dependent upon site of infection and clinical response

Susceptible (MIC ≤1 mcg/mL) gram-positive infections: IV: 15 to 20 mg/kg/dose (usual: 750 to 1,500 mg) every 8 to 12 hours. **Note:** If MIC ≥2 mcg/mL, alternative therapies are recommended (Rybak 2009)

Dosing adjustment in renal impairment:

Oral: No dosage adjustment provided in manufacturer's labeling; however, dosage adjustment unlikely due to low systemic absorption.

IV: **Vancomycin levels should be monitored in patients with any renal impairment:**

Infants, Children, and Adolescents: The following adjustments have been recommended (Aronoff 2007): **Note:** Renally adjusted dose recommendations are based on doses of 10 mg/kg/dose every 6 hours or 15 mg/kg/dose every 8 hours:

GFR 30 to 50 mL/minute/1.73 m^2: 10 mg/kg/dose every 12 hours

GFR 10 to 29 mL/minute/1.73 m^2: 10 mg/kg/dose every 18 to 24 hours

GFR <10 mL/minute/1.73 m^2: 10 mg/kg/dose; redose based on serum concentrations

Intermittent hemodialysis: 10 mg/kg/dose; redose based on serum concentrations

Peritoneal dialysis (PD): 10 mg/kg/dose; redose based on serum concentrations

Continuous renal replacement therapy (CRRT): 10 mg/kg/dose every 12 to 24 hours; monitor serum concentrations

Adults: Some experts suggest:

CrCl >50 mL/minute: Start with 15 to 20 mg/kg/dose (usual: 750 to 1,500 mg) every 8 to 12 hours

CrCl 20 to 49 mL/minute: Start with 15 to 20 mg/kg/dose (usual: 750 to 1,500 mg) every 24 hours

CrCl <20 mL/minute: Will need longer intervals; determine by serum concentration monitoring

Note: In the critically ill patient with renal insufficiency, the initial loading dose (25 to 30 mg/kg) should not be reduced; however, subsequent dosage adjustments should be made based on renal function and trough serum concentrations.

Poorly dialyzable by intermittent hemodialysis (0% to 5%); however, use of high-flux membranes and continuous renal replacement therapy (CRRT) increases vancomycin clearance and generally requires replacement dosing.

Intermittent hemodialysis (IHD) (administer after hemodialysis on dialysis days): Following loading dose of 15 to 25 mg/kg, give either 500 to 1,000 mg or 5 to 10 mg/kg after each dialysis session (Heintz 2009). **Note:** Dosing dependent on the assumption of 3 times/week, complete IHD sessions.

Redosing based on pre-HD serum concentrations:

<10 mg/L: Administer 1,000 mg after HD

10 to 25 mg/L: Administer 500 to 750 mg after HD

>25 mg/L: Hold vancomycin

Redosing based on post-HD serum concentrations:

<10 to 15 mg/L: Administer 500 to 1,000 mg

Peritoneal dialysis (PD):

Administration via PD fluid: 15 to 30 mg/L (15 to 30 mcg/mL) of PD fluid

Systemic: Loading dose of 1,000 mg, followed by 500 to 1,000 mg every 48 to 72 hours with close monitoring of levels

Continuous renal replacement therapy (CRRT) (Heintz 2009; Trotma, 2005): Drug clearance is highly dependent on the method of renal replacement, filter type, and flow rate. Appropriate dosing requires close monitoring of pharmacologic response, signs of adverse reactions due to drug accumulation, as well as drug concentrations in relation to target trough (if appropriate). The following are general recommendations only (based on dialysate flow/ultrafiltration rates of 1 to 2 L/hour and minimal residual renal function) and should not supersede clinical judgment:

CVVH: Loading dose of 15 to 25 mg/kg, followed by either 1,000 mg every 48 hours or 10 to 15 mg/kg every 24 to 48 hours

CVVHD: Loading dose of 15 to 25 mg/kg, followed by either 1,000 mg every 24 hours or 10 to 15 mg/kg every 24 hours

CVVHDF: Loading dose of 15 to 25 mg/kg, followed by either 1,000 mg every 24 hours or 7.5 to 10 mg/kg every 12 hours

Note: Consider redosing patients receiving CRRT for vancomycin serum concentrations <10 to 15 mg/L.

Dosing adjustment in hepatic impairment: Degrees of hepatic dysfunction do not affect the pharmacokinetics of vancomycin (Marti 1996)

Preparation for Administration

Oral: Reconstitute powder for injection; flavoring syrups maybe added to improve taste. See Extemporaneous Preparations section for details. **Note:** Multiple concentrations described (25 mg/mL, 50 mg/mL); use caution when determining dose volume.

Parenteral: Reconstitute vials with SWFI to a final concentration of 50 mg/mL (see manufacturer's labeling for specific details). Further dilute the reconstituted solution to a final concentration ≤5 mg/mL). In fluid restricted patients, a concentration of 10 mg/mL may be used, but the risk of infusion reactions increases.

Intrathecal/intraventricular: Dilute to 1 to 5 mg/mL concentration in preservative free NS for administration into the CSF (Al-Jeraisy 2004; Pfausler 1997).

Rectal enema: Reconstitute powder for injection; further dilution of dose in NS to prepare either a 1 mg/mL or 5 mg/mL enema solution have been used in adults (eg, 500 mg in 100 mL or 500 mL NS) (SHEA/IDSA [Cohen 2010]); the more dilute solutions (1 mg/mL) have been suggested to ensure delivery to the ascending and transverse colon (Surawicz 2013). If sodium chloride causes hyperchloremia, a solution with lower chloride concentration (eg, LR) could be considered (Surawicz 2013).

Administration

Oral: Oral solution may be compounded or vancomycin powder for injection may be reconstituted and used for oral administration (SHEA/IDSA [Cohen 2010]). The unflavored, diluted solution may also be administered via nasogastric tube.

Parenteral: Administer intermittent IV infusion over 60 minutes. Red man syndrome may occur if the infusion is too rapid. It is not an allergic reaction, but may be characterized by hypotension and/or a maculopapular rash appearing on the face, neck, trunk, and/or upper extremities; if this should occur, slow the infusion rate to administer dose over 90 to 120 minutes and increase the dilution volume; the reaction usually dissipates in 30 to 60 minutes; administration of antihistamines just before the infusion may also prevent or minimize this reaction.

Extravasation treatment: Monitor IV site closely; extravasation will cause serious injury with possible necrosis and tissue sloughing. Rotate infusion site frequently.

Intrathecal/Intraventricular: Administer as diluted solution (1 to 5 mg/mL)

Rectal: Instill vancomycin enema solution via rectal foley; retain for 1 hour

Monitoring Parameters Periodic renal function tests (especially when targeting higher serum concentrations), urinalysis, serum vancomycin concentrations, WBC; audiogram (in patients who concurrently receive ototoxic chemotherapy); fluid status

Reference Range Measure trough serum concentrations to assess efficacy. Peak concentrations may be helpful in the setting of atypical pharmacokinetic profile. Trough serum concentration typically obtained at steady state (ie, prior to the fourth dose). Target trough serum concentration may vary depending on organism, MIC, source of infection, and/or other patient factors (Rybak 2009).

15 to 20 mcg/mL: For organisms with an MIC = 1 mcg/mL or complicated infections (bacteremia, endocarditis, osteomyelitis, meningitis, and hospital-acquired pneumonia caused by *Staphylococcus* spp.) (Rybak 2009)

10 to 15 mcg/mL: Current recommendation for all other infections with an organism with an MIC <1 mcg/mL

5 to 10 mcg/mL: Traditional recommendation; may be adequate to treat some infections based on site and MIC; however, this range is not recommended in the adult guidelines for vancomycin use due to resistance development potential

Note: Although AUC/MIC is the preferred method to determine clinical effectiveness, trough serum concentrations may be used as a surrogate marker and is recommended as the most accurate and practical method of vancomycin monitoring.

Additional Information "Red man syndrome," characterized by skin rash and hypotension, is not an allergic reaction but rather is associated with too rapid infusion of the drug. To alleviate or prevent the reaction, infuse vancomycin at a rate of ≥30 minutes for each 500 mg of drug being administered (eg, 1 g over ≥60 minutes); 1.5 g over ≥90 minutes. When treating pathogens with a vancomycin MIC ≥2 mcg/mL, alternative antibiotics should be considered.

Dosage Forms Excipient information presented when available (limited, particularly for generics); consult specific product labeling.

Capsule, Oral:

Vancocin HCl: 125 mg, 250 mg [contains fd&c blue #2 (indigotine)]

Generic: 125 mg, 250 mg

Solution, Intravenous:

Generic: 500 mg/100 mL (100 mL); 750 mg/150 mL (150 mL); 1 g/200 mL (200 mL)

Solution, Oral:

First-Vancomycin 25: 25 mg/mL (150 mL, 300 mL) [contains fd&c red #40, fd&c yellow #10 (quinoline yellow), sodium benzoate; white grape flavor]

First-Vancomycin 50: 50 mg/mL (150 mL, 210 mL, 300 mL) [contains fd&c red #40, fd&c yellow #10 (quinoline yellow), sodium benzoate; white grape flavor]

Solution Reconstituted, Intravenous:

Generic: 500 mg (1 ea); 750 mg (1 ea); 1000 mg (1 ea); 5000 mg (1 ea); 10 g (1 ea)

Solution Reconstituted, Intravenous [preservative free]:

Generic: 1000 mg (1 ea); 5000 mg (1 ea); 10 g (1 ea)

Extemporaneous Preparations Note: A vancomycin (25 mg/mL or 50 mg/mL) suspension is commercially available as a compounding kit (First-Vancomycin).

Using a vial of vancomycin powder for injection (reconstituted to 50 mg/mL), add the appropriate volume for the dose to 30 mL of water and administer orally or via NG tube. For oral administration, common flavoring syrups may be added to improve taste.

Vancomycin Hydrochloride for Injection, USP (prescribing information), Schaumburg, Il, APP Pharmaceuticals, LLC, 2011.

A vancomycin 25 mg/mL solution in Ora-Sweet® and water (1:1) may be prepared by reconstituting vancomycin for injection with sterile water, then dilute with a 1:1 mixture of Ora-Sweet® and distilled water to a final concentration of 25 mg/mL; transfer to amber prescription bottle. Stable for 75 days refrigerated or for 26 days at room temperature.

Ensom MH, Decarie D, and Lakhani A, "Stability of Vancomycin 25 mg/mL in Ora-Sweet and Water in Unit-Dose Cups and Plastic Bottles at 4°C and 25°C," *Can J Hosp Pharm*, 2010, 63(5):366-72.

- ◆ **Vancomycin Hydrochloride** *see* Vancomycin *on page 2151*
- ◆ **Vancomycin Hydrochloride for Injection (Can)** *see* Vancomycin *on page 2151*
- ◆ **Vancomycin Hydrochloride for Injection, USP (Can)** *see* Vancomycin *on page 2151*
- ◆ **Vandazole** *see* MetroNIDAZOLE (Topical) *on page 1425*
- ◆ **Vaniqa** *see* Eflornithine *on page 737*
- ◆ **Vaniqa® (Can)** *see* Eflornithine *on page 737*
- ◆ **Van-Letrozole (Can)** *see* Letrozole *on page 1224*
- ◆ **Vanos** *see* Fluocinonide *on page 898*
- ◆ **Vantas** *see* Histrelin *on page 1022*
- ◆ **Vantin** *see* Cefpodoxime *on page 404*
- ◆ **VAQTA** *see* Hepatitis A Vaccine *on page 1011*
- ◆ **VAR** *see* Varicella Virus Vaccine *on page 2157*
- ◆ **Varicella, Measles, Mumps, and Rubella Vaccine** *see* Measles, Mumps, Rubella, and Varicella Virus Vaccine *on page 1330*

Varicella Virus Vaccine

(var i SEL a VYE rus vak SEEN)

Medication Safety Issues

Sound-alike/look-alike issues:

Varicella virus vaccine has been given in error (instead of the indicated varicella immune globulin) to pregnant women exposed to varicella.

Other safety concerns:

Both varicella vaccine and zoster vaccine are live, attenuated strains of varicella-zoster virus. Their indications, dosing, and composition are distinct. Varicella is indicated in children to prevent chickenpox, while zoster vaccine is indicated in older individuals to prevent reactivation of the virus which causes shingles. Zoster vaccine is **not** a substitute for varicella vaccine and should not be used in children.

Related Information

Centers for Disease Control and Prevention (CDC) and Other Links *on page 2424*

Immunization Administration Recommendations *on page 2411*

Immunization Schedules *on page 2416*

Brand Names: US Varivax

Brand Names: Canada Varilrix; Varivax III

Therapeutic Category Vaccine; Vaccine, Live Virus

Generic Availability (US) No

Use Immunization against varicella in individuals who do not have evidence of immunity (FDA approved in ages ≥12 months and adults).

The ACIP (CDC/ACIP [Marin 2007]) recommends vaccination for all children, adolescents, and adults who do not have evidence of immunity. Vaccination is especially important for:

- Health care personnel
- Persons with close contact to those at high risk for severe disease
- Persons living or working in environments where transmission is likely (teachers, childcare workers, residents, and staff of institutional settings)
- Persons in environments where transmission has been reported
- Nonpregnant women of childbearing age
- Adolescents and adults in households with children
- International travelers

Postexposure prophylaxis: Vaccination within 3 days (possibly 5 days) after exposure to rash is effective in preventing illness or modifying severity of disease (CDC/ACIP [Marin 2007]).

Medication Guide Available Yes

Pregnancy Considerations Varicella virus vaccine is contraindicated for use in pregnant females and pregnancy should be avoided for 3 months (per manufacturer labeling; 1 month per ACIP) following vaccination. Varicella disease during the 1st or 2nd trimesters may result in congenital varicella syndrome. The onset of maternal varicella infection from 5 days prior to 2 days after delivery may cause varicella infection in the newborn. All women should be assessed for immunity during a prenatal visit; those without evidence of immunity should be vaccinated upon completion or termination of pregnancy (CDC/ACIP [Marin, 2007]). Based on information collected from 1995-2013 using the manufacturer's pregnancy registry, of 820 women who received a varicella containing vaccine, there were no infants born with abnormalities consistent with congenital varicella syndrome. Any exposures to the vaccine during pregnancy or within 3 months prior to pregnancy should be reported to the manufacturer (Merck & Co, 877-888-4231) or to VAERS (800-822-7967) as suspected adverse reactions.

Breast-Feeding Considerations Following immunization, varicella virus was not detected in the milk samples of 12 breast-feeding women and none of the breast-fed infants seroconverted. Immunization should not be delayed due to breast-feeding (CDC/ACIP [Marin, 2007]). The manufacturer recommends that caution be exercised when administering varicella virus vaccine to nursing women. Breast-feeding infants should be vaccinated according to the recommended schedules (NCIRD/ACIP, 2011).

Contraindications

U.S. labeling: Severe allergic or anaphylactic reaction to the vaccine, neomycin, gelatin, or any component of the formulation; immunosuppressed or immunodeficient individuals including individuals with leukemia, lymphomas, or other malignant neoplasms affecting the bone marrow or lymphatic systems; persons with AIDs or other clinical manifestations of HIV; those receiving immunosuppressive therapy (including immunosuppressive doses of corticosteroids); history of primary and acquired immunodeficiency states; active, untreated tuberculosis; current febrile illness (per manufacturer labeling); pregnancy

Canadian labeling: Additional contraindications (not in U.S. labeling): Varivax III: Family history of congenital or hereditary immunodeficiency (unless immune competence of vaccine recipient is demonstrated); Varilrix: Primary or acquired immunodeficiency with a total lymphocyte count <1200/mm^3

Warnings/Precautions Immediate treatment (including epinephrine 1:1,000) for anaphylactoid reaction should be available during vaccine use (NCIRD/ACIP, 2011). Varicella vaccine and antibody-containing products (eg, immune globulin, blood products) should **not** be administered simultaneously. Guidelines with suggested administration intervals are available (NCIRD/ACIP, 2011). Vaccination may not result in effective immunity in all patients. Response depends upon multiple factors (eg, type of vaccine, age of patient) and may be improved by administering the vaccine at the recommended dose, route, and interval. Vaccines may not be effective if administered during periods of altered immune competence (NCIRD/ACIP, 2011). The manufacturer notes that vaccinated individuals should not have close association with susceptible high-risk individuals for 6 weeks following vaccination. High-risk individuals include immunocompromised persons, pregnant women without evidence of immunity, newborns of mothers without evidence of immunity, and all infants born <28 weeks' gestation (regardless of maternal immunity). However, the CDC notes that transmission of the virus is rare and recommends that vaccine recipients who develop a vaccine-related rash avoid contact with susceptible individuals at high risk for complications until the lesions are resolved (crusted over or fade away) or until no new lesions appear for 24 hours. According to the CDC guidelines, having a pregnant household member is not a contraindication to vaccination (CDC/ACIP [Marin, 2007]). Although fever is a contraindication per the manufacturer, current guidelines allow for administration to patients with mild acute illness with or without low grade fever (CDC/ACIP [Marin, 2007]). Syncope has been reported with use of injectable vaccines and may result in serious secondary injury (eg, skull fracture, cerebral hemorrhage); typically reported in adolescents and young adults and within 15 minutes after vaccination. Procedures should be in place to avoid injuries from falling and to restore cerebral perfusion if syncope occurs (NCIRD/ACIP, 2011). Although the manufacturer contraindicates administration to persons with HIV, guidelines for use are available. Children with HIV infection with age-specific CD4+ T-lymphocyte percentages ≥15% may receive live attenuated varicella vaccine. Vaccination may be considered for children >8 years, adolescents, and adults with CD4+ T-lymphocyte counts ≥200 cells/microliter (CDC/ACIP [Marin, 2007]). Defer use in patients with a family history of congenital or hereditary immunodeficiency until immune competence in the vaccine recipient is demonstrated (CDC/ACIP [Marin, 2007]).

Products may contain gelatin, neomycin, or albumin; patients with history of anaphylaxis should not receive vaccine (CDC/ACIP [Marin, 2007]). Contact dermatitis to neomycin is not a contraindication to the vaccine. Avoid salicylates in children and adolescents 12 months through 17 years for 6 weeks after vaccination; varicella may increase the risk of Reye's syndrome. In order to maximize vaccination rates, the ACIP recommends simultaneous (ie, >1 vaccine on the same day at different anatomic sites) administration of all age-appropriate vaccines (live or inactivated) for which a person is eligible at a single clinic visit, unless contraindications exist. The use of combination vaccines is generally preferred over separate injections, taking into consideration provider assessment, patient preference, and adverse events. When using combination vaccines, the minimum age for administration is the oldest minimum age for any individual component; the minimum interval between dosing is the greatest minimum interval between any individual components (NCIRD/ACIP, 2011). Use of this vaccine is contraindicated in persons who are immunosuppressed or immunodeficient. In general, live vaccines should be administered ≥4 weeks prior to planned immunosuppression and avoided within 2 weeks of immunosuppression when feasible (Rubin, 2014). Use of this vaccine for specific medical and/or other indications (eg, immunocompromising conditions, hepatic or kidney disease, diabetes) is also addressed in the ACIP Recommended Adult Immunization Schedule (CDC/ACIP [Kim, 2015]). Specific recommendations for use of this vaccine in immunocompromised patients with asplenia, cancer, HIV infection, cerebrospinal fluid leaks, cochlear implants, hematopoietic stem cell transplant (prior to or after), sickle cell disease, solid organ transplant (prior to or after), or those receiving immunosuppressive therapy for chronic conditions as well as contacts of immunocompromised patients are available from the IDSA (Rubin, 2014).

Medications active against the herpesvirus family (eg, acyclovir, famciclovir, valacyclovir) may interfere with the varicella vaccine; avoid varicella vaccination to a patient who has received these antivirals 24 hours before vaccination; avoid use of these antiviral agents for 14 days after varicella vaccination (CDC/ACIP [Kim, 2015]).

Antipyretics have not been shown to prevent febrile seizures; antipyretics may be used to treat fever or discomfort following vaccination (NCIRD/ACIP, 2011). One study reported that routine prophylactic administration of acetaminophen to prevent fever prior to vaccination decreased the immune response of some vaccines; the clinical significance of this reduction in immune response has not been established (Prymula, 2009).

Varilrix (Canadian availability; not available in U.S.): Approved for use in high-risk patients (eg, acute leukemia, chronic disease, organ transplantation) if complete remission ≥12 months (acute leukemia), lymphocyte count ≥1200/mm^3 and evidence of immune competence can be demonstrated prior to vaccination. Canadian National Advisory Committee on Immunization (NACI) suggests that Varivax® III may also be used for select groups (NACI, 2012). Consult product labeling and/or NACI for specific recommendations regarding appropriate use in high risk patients.

Adverse Reactions All serious adverse reactions must be reported to the U.S. Department of Health and Human Services (DHHS) Vaccine Adverse Event Reporting System (VAERS) 1-800-822-7967 or online at https://vaers.hhs.gov/esub/index. In Canada, adverse reactions may be reported to local provincial/territorial health agencies or to the Vaccine Safety Section at Public Health Agency of Canada (1-866-844-0018).

Central nervous system: Chills, disturbed sleep, fatigue, headache, irritability, malaise, nervousness

Dermatologic: Contact dermatitis, dermatitis, diaper rash, eczema, miliaria, pruritus, rash at injection site (varicella-like), urticaria, varicella-like rash, xeroderma

Gastrointestinal: Abdominal pain, constipation, decreased appetite, diarrhea, nausea, period of tooth development, vomiting

Genitourinary: Herpes labialis

Hematologic & oncologic: Lymphadenopathy

Hypersensitivity: Hypersensitivity reaction

Local: Injection site reaction

Neuromuscular & skeletal: Arthralgia, myalgia, neck stiffness

Otic: Otitis

Respiratory: Cough, respiratory tract disease (lower/upper)

Miscellaneous: Fever

Rare but important or life-threatening: Anaphylactic shock, anaphylaxis, aplastic anemia, aseptic meningitis, ataxia, Bell's palsy, cerebrovascular accident, encephalitis, erythema multiforme, febrile seizures, Guillain-Barre syndrome, hemiparesis (acute), hepatitis, herpes zoster, IgA vasculitis, necrotizing retinitis (immunocompromised patients), pneumonitis, seizure (nonfebrile), Stevens-Johnson syndrome, thrombocytopenia (including immune thrombocytopenia), transverse myelitis, varicella (disseminated or vaccine strain)

Drug Interactions

Metabolism/Transport Effects None known.

Avoid Concomitant Use

Avoid concomitant use of Varicella Virus Vaccine with any of the following: Acyclovir-Valacyclovir; Belimumab; Famciclovir; Fingolimod; Immunosuppressants

Increased Effect/Toxicity

The levels/effects of Varicella Virus Vaccine may be increased by: 5-ASA Derivatives; AzaTHIOprine; Belimumab; Corticosteroids (Systemic); Dimethyl Fumarate;

Fingolimod; Immunosuppressants; Leflunomide; Mercaptopurine; Methotrexate; Salicylates; Smallpox Vaccine

Decreased Effect

Varicella Virus Vaccine may decrease the levels/effects of: Tuberculin Tests

The levels/effects of Varicella Virus Vaccine may be decreased by: Acyclovir-Valacyclovir; AzaTHIOprine; Corticosteroids (Systemic); Dimethyl Fumarate; Famciclovir; Fingolimod; Immune Globulins; Immunosuppressants; Leflunomide; Mercaptopurine; Methotrexate

Storage/Stability Prior to reconstitution and during shipping, store vaccine in freezer at -50°C to -15°C (-58°F to 5°F). Use of dry ice may subject vaccine to temperatures colder than -58°F (-50°C). Vaccine may be stored under refrigeration at 2°C to 8°C (36°F to 46°F) for up to 72 hours. Protect from light. Store diluent at room temperature of 20°C to 25°C (68°F to 77°F) or in refrigerator. Gently agitate to mix thoroughly. (Total volume of reconstituted vaccine will be ~0.5 mL.) Administer immediately following reconstitution, discard reconstituted vaccine if not used within 30 minutes.

Canadian formulations:

Varilrix: Prior to reconstitution, store vaccine under refrigeration at 2°C to 8°C (36°F to 46°F). Vaccine not affected by freezing. Store diluent at 25°C (77°F) or under refrigeration. Following reconstitution, vaccine may be stored for 90 minutes at 25°C (77°F) or up to 8 hours under refrigeration. Discard if not used within recommended times.

Varivax III: Maintain vaccine at -50°C to 8°C (-58°F to 46°F) during transport. Prior to reconstitution, vaccine may be stored in a freezer at temperatures above -50°C (-58°F) or under refrigeration at 2°C to 8°C (36°F to 46°F). Vials transferred from freezer to a refrigerator may be placed back in freezer as long as they have not been reconstituted. Store diluent at room temperature 20°C to 25°C (68°F to 77°F) or under refrigeration. Administer immediately following reconstitution; discard reconstituted vaccine if not administered within 90 minutes.

Mechanism of Action As a live, attenuated vaccine, varicella virus vaccine offers active immunity to disease caused by the varicella-zoster virus by inducing cell mediated and humoral immune responses

Pharmacodynamics

Onset of action: Seroconversion occurred in 97% of healthy children ~4 to 6 weeks following a one-dose regimen; using a two-dose regimen, the seroconversion rate was 99.9% 6 weeks after the second dose. In adolescents ≥13 years of age and adults, the seroconversion rate was ~75% 4 weeks after the first dose and 99% 4 weeks after the second dose

Duration: Antibody titers detectable at 10 years postvaccination. Actual antibody titers vary by year and age group but are ~99% to 100% for children at 10 years and 100% for adolescents and adults at 6 years postvaccination. Exposure to wild-type varicella may boost antibody levels.

Dosing: Usual

Pediatric:

Primary immunization: Children ≥12 months:

CDC/ACIP recommendations: SubQ: 0.5 mL per dose for a total of 2 doses administered as follows: 12 to 15 months of age and 4 to 6 years of age. The second dose may be administered earlier provided ≥3 months have elapsed after the first dose (CDC/ACIP [Marin 2007]). If the second dose was administered ≥4 weeks after the first dose, it may be considered as valid (CDC/ACIP [Strikas 2015]).

Manufacturer's labeling: SubQ: 0.5 mL per dose; a second dose may be administered ≥3 months later

Catch-up immunization: Children and Adolescents: CDC (ACIP) recommendations (Strikas 2015): **Note:** Do not restart the series. If doses have been given, begin the below schedule at the applicable dose number. SubQ: 0.5 mL per dose for a total of 2 doses administered as follows:

First dose given on the elected date

Second dose given at least 3 months after the first dose (if age <13 years) or at least 4 weeks after the first dose (if age ≥13 years)

Postexposure prophylaxis (healthy, previously unvaccinated individuals): Children (≥12 months) and Adolescents: SubQ: 0.5 mL administered ideally within 72 hours postexposure but may be used up to 120 hours (5 days) postexposure (CDC/ACIP [Marin, 2007])

Adult:

Primary immunization: All patients without evidence of immunity (CDC/ACIP [Kim 2015):

Varicella vaccine-naïve: SubQ: 0.5 mL per dose, followed by a second dose at least 4 to 8 weeks later

Previously received 1 dose of varicella vaccine: SubQ: 0.5 mL as a single dose

Postexposure prophylaxis (healthy, previously unvaccinated individuals): SubQ: 0.5 mL administered ideally within 72 hours postexposure but may be used up to 120 hours (5 days) postexposure (CDC/ACIP [Marin 2007])

Dosing adjustment in renal impairment: There are no dosage adjustments provided in manufacturer's labeling.

Dosing adjustment in hepatic impairment: There are no dosage adjustments provided in manufacturer's labeling.

Preparation for Administration SubQ: Reconstitute vaccine with total volume of the provided diluent. Gently agitate to mix thoroughly. Total volume of reconstituted vaccine will be ~0.5 mL. Administer vaccine within 30 minutes of preparation.

Administration SubQ: Inject subcutaneously into the outer aspect of the upper arm or anterolateral aspect of the thigh; not for IV or IM administration. To prevent syncope related injuries, adolescents and adults should be vaccinated while seated or lying down (NCIRD/ACIP 2011). US law requires that the date of administration, the vaccine manufacturer, lot number of vaccine, and the administering person's name, title, and address be entered into the patient's permanent medical record.

Monitoring Parameters Rash, fever; observe for syncope for 15 minutes following administration (NCIRD/ACIP 2011). If seizure-like activity associated with syncope occurs, maintain patient in supine or Trendelenburg position to re-establish adequate cerebral perfusion.

Additional Information Evidence of immunity to varicella includes any of the following (CDC/ACIP [Marin, 2007]):

Documentation of age-appropriate vaccination with varicella vaccine.

Laboratory evidence of immunity or laboratory confirmation of disease.

Birth in the United States prior to 1980 (except for health care personnel, pregnant women, and the immunocompromised).

Diagnosis or verification of varicella disease by health care provider.

Diagnosis or verification of herpes zoster by health care provider.

Dosage Forms Excipient information presented when available (limited, particularly for generics); consult specific product labeling.

Injectable, Subcutaneous [preservative free]:

Varivax: 1350 PFU/0.5 mL (1 ea)

◆ **Varicella Zoster** *see* Varicella-Zoster Immune Globulin (Human) *on page 2160*

Varicella-Zoster Immune Globulin (Human)

(var i SEL a- ZOS ter i MYUN GLOB yoo lin HYU man)

Medication Safety Issues

Sound-alike/look-alike issues:

Varicella virus vaccine has been given in error (instead of the indicated varicella immune globulin) to pregnant women exposed to varicella.

Other safety concerns:

ALERT: Canadian Boxed Warning: Health Canada-approved labeling includes a boxed warning. See Warnings/Precautions section for a concise summary of this information. For verbatim wording of the boxed warning, consult the product labeling.

Related Information

Centers for Disease Control and Prevention (CDC) and Other Links *on page 2424*

Immunization Administration Recommendations *on page 2411*

Immunization Schedules *on page 2416*

Brand Names: US VariZIG

Brand Names: Canada VariZIG

Therapeutic Category Immune Globulin

Generic Availability (US) No

Use Postexposure prophylaxis of varicella in high-risk individuals including: Immunocompromised children and adults; newborns of mothers with varicella shortly before or after delivery; premature infants, neonates, and infants <1 year of age; adults without evidence of immunity; pregnant women (FDA approved in all ages)

The Advisory Committee on Immunization Practices (ACIP) recommends varicella-zoster immune globulin (VZIG) for patients who are at high risk for severe varicella infection and complications, patients who were exposed to varicella or herpes zoster, and patients for whom varicella vaccine is contraindicated. The decision to use VZIG should take into consideration if the patient lacks evidence of immunity, if exposure is likely to result in an infection, and if the patient is at greater risk for varicella complications than the general population. The following are patient groups for whom VZIG is recommended (CDC, 2013):

- Immunocompromised patients without evidence of immunity, including those with neoplastic disease (eg, leukemia or lymphoma), primary or acquired immunodeficiency, and immunosuppressive therapy (including steroid therapy equivalent to prednisone ≥2 mg/kg or 20 mg/day)
- Newborn of mother who had onset of chickenpox within 5 days before delivery or within 48 hours after delivery
- Hospitalized premature infants (≥28 weeks gestation) who were exposed during the neonatal period and whose mother has no history of chickenpox
- Hospitalized premature infants (<28 weeks gestation or ≤1000 g) regardless of maternal history and who were exposed during the neonatal period
- Pregnant women without evidence of immunity who have been exposed

Pregnancy Risk Factor C

Pregnancy Considerations Animal reproduction studies have not been conducted. Endogenous immune globulins cross the placenta. Clinical use of other immunoglobulins suggest that there are no adverse effects on the fetus. Women who do not have evidence of immunity to varicella may be at increased risk of complications if infected during pregnancy. Varicella infection in the mother can also lead to intrauterine infection in the fetus. VZIG is primarily used to prevent maternal complications, not fetal infection (CDC, 2007).

Breast-Feeding Considerations It is not known if this preparation is excreted into breast milk; endogenous immune globulins can be found in breast milk (Agarwal, 2011). The manufacturer recommends that caution be used if administered to breast-feeding women.

Contraindications *U.S. labeling:* History of anaphylaxis or other severe reaction associated with past human immune globulin administration; IgA deficiency

Canadian labeling: Additional contraindications (not in US labeling): Hypersensitivity to any component of the formulation; patients with evidence of immunity to varicella zoster virus (ie, with previous varicella infection or vaccination)

Warnings/Precautions [Canadian Boxed Warning]: Hypersensitivity and anaphylactic reactions can occur; immediate treatment (including epinephrine 1:1000) should be available. Reactions can occur in patients with IgA deficiency or hypersensitivity reactions to human globulin.

Noncardiogenic pulmonary edema has been reported with intravenous administration of immune globulin. Monitor for symptoms of transfusion-related acute lung injury (TRALI) including severe respiratory distress, hypoxemia, fever, and pulmonary edema which typically occur within 1-6 hours after administration. Use caution with preexisting respiratory conditions. Per Canadian labeling, IM administration may be preferred in this patient population. Acute renal dysfunction (increased serum creatinine, oliguria, acute renal failure) can rarely occur; usually within 7 days of use (more likely with products stabilized with sucrose). Use with caution in patients with renal disease, diabetes mellitus, volume depletion, sepsis, paraproteinemia, nephrotoxic medications, and in the elderly due to risk of renal dysfunction. Thrombotic events have been reported with administration of intravenous immune globulin; use with caution in patients with cardiovascular risk factors, history of atherosclerosis, advanced age, impaired cardiac output, coagulation disorders, prolonged periods of immobilization, and/or known hyperviscosity disorders. Per Canadian labeling, IM administration may be preferred in this patient population. Use with caution in patients with a history of bleeding disorders (including thrombocytopenia) and/or patients on anticoagulant therapy; bleeding/hematoma may occur from IM administration.

[Canadian Boxed Warnings]: Product of human plasma; may potentially contain infectious agents which could transmit disease. Screening of donors, as well as testing and/or inactivation or removal of certain viruses, reduces the risk. Infections thought to be transmitted by this product should be reported to the manufacturer (Cangene Corporation 800-768-2304).

Some dosage forms may contain polysorbate 80 (also known as Tweens). Hypersensitivity reactions, usually a delayed reaction, have been reported following exposure to pharmaceutical products containing polysorbate 80 in certain individuals (Isaksson, 2002; Lucente 2000; Shelley, 1995). Thrombocytopenia, ascites, pulmonary deterioration, and renal and hepatic failure have been reported in premature neonates after receiving parenteral products containing polysorbate 80 (Alade, 1986; CDC, 1984). See manufacturer's labeling.

Varicella zoster immune globulin should be administered as soon as possible following exposure (within 96 hours, preferred) to reduce the severity of varicella. There is no evidence which shows therapy will reduce the incidence of chickenpox infection after exposure to varicella zoster virus, or that it will effect established varicella zoster virus infections. According to the U.S. CDC guidelines, healthy and immunocompromised patients (except bone marrow transplant recipients [BMT]) with positive history of varicella infection are considered immune. BMT patients who had varicella infection *prior* to transplant are **not** considered immune. BMT patients who develop varicella infection *after* transplant **are** considered immune. Patients who are fully vaccinated, but later became immunocompromised should be monitored closely; treatment with VZIG is not indicated, but other therapy may be needed if disease occurs (CDC, 2007). The American Society for Blood and Marrow Transplantation (ASBMT) also has guidelines for use of varicella zoster immune globulin in highly immunosuppressed hematopoietic cell transplant (HCT) recipients who are exposed to varicella or zoster or to a varicella zoster vaccinee who has a varicella-like rash. Highly-immunosuppressed patients include those <24 months after HCT or ≥24 months post HCT and on immune suppressive therapy or have chronic graft-versus-host disease (Tomblyn, 2009).

Adverse Reactions

U.S. labeling:

Central nervous system: Chills, fatigue. headache
Dermatologic: Skin rash
Gastrointestinal: Nausea
Local: Pain at injection site
Rare but important or life-threatening: Deep vein thrombosis, hypersensitivity reaction, serum sickness, thrombosis

Canadian labeling:

Cardiovascular: Flushing
Central nervous system: Chills, dizziness, fatigue, headache, insomnia, pain
Dermatologic: Dermatitis, skin rash (including erythematous)
Gastrointestinal: Dysgeusia, nausea
Local: Injection site reaction (bruising, itching, pain, or tenderness), pain at injection site
Neuromuscular & skeletal: Myalgia, neck pain
Miscellaneous: Fever

Drug Interactions

Metabolism/Transport Effects None known.

Avoid Concomitant Use There are no known interactions where it is recommended to avoid concomitant use.

Increased Effect/Toxicity There are no known significant interactions involving an increase in effect.

Decreased Effect

Varicella-Zoster Immune Globulin (Human) may decrease the levels/effects of: Vaccines (Live)

Storage/Stability Prior to reconstitution, store at 2°C to 8°C (36°F to 46°F); do not freeze. Following reconstitution, may store at 2°C to 8°C (36°F to 46°F) for up to 12 hours.

Mechanism of Action Antibodies obtained from pooled human plasma of individuals with high titers of varicella-zoster provide passive immunity.

Pharmacodynamics Duration: 3 weeks

Pharmacokinetics (Adult data unless noted)

Half-life: 26.2 ± 4.6 days
Time to peak serum concentration: Within 5 days

Dosing: Neonatal Postexposure prophylaxis, varicella: IM: **Note:** Administration should begin as soon as possible and within 10 days after exposure (CDC, 2013). High-risk, susceptible patients who are re-exposed >3 weeks after a prior dose of VZIG should receive another full dose; there is no evidence VZIG modifies established varicella-zoster infections. The minimum dose is 62.5 units.
≤2 kg: 62.5 units
2.1 to 10 kg: 125 units

Dosing: Usual Note: Administration should begin as soon as possible and within 10 days after exposure (CDC, 2013). In hematopoietic cell transplant (HCT) recipients who are exposed to varicella or zoster or a varicella zoster vaccine vaccinee who develops a varicella-like rash, administration should occur within 96 hours, ideally within 48 hours (Tomblyn, 2009). High-risk, susceptible patients who are re-exposed >3 weeks after a prior dose of VZIG should receive another full dose; there is no evidence VZIG modifies established varicella-zoster infections. The minimum dose is 62.5 units and the maximum dose is 625 units.

Pediatric: **Postexposure prophylaxis, varicella:** Infants, Children, and Adolescents: IM:
2.1 to 10 kg: 125 units
10.1 to 20 kg: 250 units
20.1 to 30 kg: 375 units
30.1 to 40 kg: 500 units
>40 kg: 625 units

Adult: **Postexposure prophylaxis, varicella:** Patient weight >40 kg: IM: 625 units; **Note:** Refer to pediatric dosing for weight based dosing in adults ≤40 kg.

Preparation for Administration IM: Reconstitute with 1.25 mL of diluent to a final concentration of 100 units/mL; use only the provided diluent. Inject diluent slowly and at an angle onto the inside glass wall of the vial. Gently invert vial and swirl to dissolve; do not shake.

Administration For IM administration only. Administer into deltoid muscle or anterolateral aspect of upper thigh; avoid gluteal region; may require ≥2 injections depending on patient size. Do not exceed 3 mL per injection site.

Monitoring Parameters Observe for adverse effects following administration; baseline assessment of blood viscosity in patients at risk for hyperviscosity; signs and symptoms of varicella infection for 28 days after VZIG administration (CDC, 2013).

Test Interactions May cause false-positive test for immunity to VZV for 3 months following administration. May cause a false-positive Coomb's test.

Additional Information In susceptible children and adults for whom the varicella vaccine is not contraindicated, live varicella virus vaccine can be given within 3-5 days after exposure to prevent or modify infection severity. There is no evidence VZIG modifies established varicella-zoster infections.

VZIG contains <40 mcg/mL of IgA

Dosage Forms Excipient information presented when available (limited, particularly for generics); consult specific product labeling.

Solution, Intramuscular [preservative free]:
VariZIG: 125 units/1.2 mL (1.2 mL) [contains polysorbate 80]

Solution Reconstituted, Intramuscular [preservative free]:
VariZIG: 125 units (1 ea) [contains polysorbate 80]

◆ **Varicella-Zoster Virus (VZV) Vaccine (Varicella)** *see* Varicella Virus Vaccine *on page 2157*

◆ **Varilrix (Can)** *see* Varicella Virus Vaccine *on page 2157*

◆ **Varivax** *see* Varicella Virus Vaccine *on page 2157*

◆ **Varivax III (Can)** *see* Varicella Virus Vaccine *on page 2157*

◆ **VariZIG** *see* Varicella-Zoster Immune Globulin (Human) *on page 2160*

◆ **VasoClear [OTC]** *see* Naphazoline (Ophthalmic) *on page 1488*

◆ **VasoClear-A [OTC]** *see* Naphazoline (Ophthalmic) *on page 1488*

◆ **Vasocon® (Can)** *see* Naphazoline (Ophthalmic) *on page 1488*

Vasopressin (vay soe PRES in)

Medication Safety Issues

Sound-alike/look-alike issues:

Vasopressin may be confused with desmopressin

High alert medication:

The Institute for Safe Medication Practices (ISMP) includes this medication (IV or intraosseous administration) among its list of drugs which have a heightened risk of causing significant patient harm when used in error.

Administration issues:

Use care when prescribing and/or administering vasopressin solutions. Close attention should be given to concentration of solution, route of administration, dose, and rate of administration (units/minute, units/kg/minute, units/kg/hour).

Related Information

Adult ACLS Algorithms *on page 2236*

Management of Drug Extravasations *on page 2298*

Brand Names: US Pitressin Synthetic [DSC]; Vasostrict

Brand Names: Canada Pressyn; Pressyn AR

Therapeutic Category Antidiuretic Hormone Analog; Hormone, Posterior Pituitary

Generic Availability (US) Yes

Use Treatment of diabetes insipidus; prevention and treatment of postoperative abdominal distention; differential diagnosis of diabetes insipidus [FDA approved in pediatric patients (age not specified) and adults]. Has also been used as an adjunct in the treatment of acute massive hemorrhage of GI tract or esophageal varices; treatment of pulseless arrest, ventricular fibrillation or tachycardia, and asystole/pulseless electrical activity; vasodilatory/septic shock with hypotension unresponsive to fluid resuscitation or exogenous catecholamines; cardiac arrest secondary to anaphylaxis (unresponsive to epinephrine); and donor management of brain-dead patients (hormone replacement therapy).

Pregnancy Risk Factor C

Pregnancy Considerations Animal reproduction studies have not been conducted. Vasopressin may produce tonic uterine contractions; however, doses sufficient for diabetes insipidus are not likely to produce this effect.

Breast-Feeding Considerations It is not known if vasopressin is excreted in breast milk. Oral absorption by a nursing infant is unlikely because vasopressin is rapidly destroyed in the GI tract; however, consider pumping and discarding breast milk for 1.5 hours after receiving vasopressin (Vasostrict only) to minimize potential exposure to the breast-fed infant. The manufacturer recommends that caution be exercised when administering vasopressin to nursing women.

Contraindications Hypersensitivity to vasopressin or any component of the formulation; hypersensitivity to chlorobutanol (Vasostrict only); uncorrected chronic nephritis with nitrogen retention (Pitressin Synthetic only)

Warnings/Precautions Use with caution in patients with seizure disorders, migraine, asthma, vascular disease, renal disease, cardiovascular disease, including arteriosclerosis; goiter with cardiac complications. IV administration (off-label route): Vesicant; ensure proper needle or catheter placement prior to and during infusion; extravasation may lead to severe vasoconstriction and localized tissue necrosis, gangrene of extremities, tongue, and ischemic colitis; avoid extravasation. May cause water intoxication; early signs include drowsiness, listlessness, and headache, these should be recognized to prevent coma and seizures. Elderly patients should be cautioned not to increase their fluid intake beyond that sufficient to satisfy their thirst in order to avoid water intoxication and hyponatremia; under experimental conditions, the elderly have shown to have a decreased responsiveness to vasopressin with respect to its effects on water homeostasis.

Adverse Reactions

Cardiovascular: Angina pectoris, atrial fibrillation, bradycardia, cardiac arrest, cardiac arrhythmia, ischemic heart disease, limb ischemia (distal), localized blanching, low cardiac output, myocardial infarction, right heart failure, shock, vasoconstriction (peripheral)

Central nervous system: Headache (pounding), vertigo

Dermatologic: Circumoral pallor, diaphoresis, gangrene of skin or other tissues, skin lesion (ischemic), urticaria

Endocrine & metabolic: Hyponatremia, hypovolemic shock, water intoxication

Gastrointestinal: Abdominal cramps, flatulence, mesenteric ischemia, nausea, vomiting

Hematologic & oncologic: Decreased platelet count, hemorrhage (intractable)

Hepatic: Increased serum bilirubin

Hypersensitivity: Anaphylaxis

Neuromuscular & skeletal: Tremor

Renal: Renal insufficiency

Respiratory: Bronchoconstriction

Drug Interactions

Metabolism/Transport Effects None known.

Avoid Concomitant Use There are no known interactions where it is recommended to avoid concomitant use.

Increased Effect/Toxicity There are no known significant interactions involving an increase in effect.

Decreased Effect There are no known significant interactions involving a decrease in effect.

Food Interactions Ethanol may decrease the antidiuretic effect. Management: Avoid ethanol.

Storage/Stability

Store intact vials between 2°C and 8°C (36°F and 46°F). Do not freeze.

Vasostrict: May also remove intact vials from refrigeration and store at 20°C to 25°C (68°F to 77°F) for up to 12 months or manufacturer expiration date, whichever is earlier (indicate date of removal on the vial). Discard unused diluted solution after 18 hours at room temperature or 24 hours under refrigeration. Discard vial after 48 hours after first entry.

Mechanism of Action Increases cyclic adenosine monophosphate (cAMP) which increases water permeability at the renal tubule resulting in decreased urine volume and increased osmolality; causes peristalsis by directly stimulating the smooth muscle in the GI tract; direct vasoconstrictor without inotropic or chronotropic effects. In vasodilatory shock, vasopressin increases systemic vascular resistance and mean arterial blood pressure and decreases heart rate and cardiac output.

Pharmacodynamics IM, SubQ:

Onset of action: 1 hour

Duration: 2-8 hours

Pharmacokinetics (Adult data unless noted)

Destroyed by trypsin in GI tract, must be administered parenterally

Metabolism: Most of dose is rapidly metabolized in liver and kidney

Half-life: 10-35 minutes

Dosing: Neonatal IV: **Note:** Units of measure vary by indication and age (ie, milliunits/kg/**hour**, units/kg/**hour**, milliunits/kg/minute, units/kg/minute); extra precautions should be taken.

Vasodilatory shock with hypotension unresponsive to fluid resuscitation and exogenous catecholamines: Note: Limited information available; efficacy results variable; optimal dose and timing have not been clearly established: Continuous IV infusion: 0.17 to 10 milliunits/kg/minute (0.01 to 0.6 units/kg/**hour**) have been used; doses were initiated at the lower end of the range and titrated to effect in most studies. Dosing based on retrospective reviews and case reports that have shown increases in arterial blood pressure and urine output and also allowed for dosage reductions of additional vasopressors (Bidegain 2010; Brierley 2009; Choong 2008; Ikegami 2010; Meyer 2008).

Dosing: Usual Note: Units of measure vary by indication and age (ie, milliunits/kg/**hour**, units/kg/**hour**, milliunits/kg/minute, units/kg/minute); extra precautions should be taken.

Diabetes insipidus:

IM, SubQ: (Highly variable dosage; titrate dosage based upon serum and urine sodium and osmolality in addition to fluid balance and urine output)

Children: 2.5 to 10 units 2 to 4 times/day

Adults: 5 to 10 units 2 to 4 times/day as needed

Continuous IV infusion: Children and Adults: Initial: 0.5 milliunits/kg/**hour** (0.0005 units/kg/**hour**); double dosage as needed every 30 minutes to a maximum of 10 milliunits/kg/**hour** (0.01 units/kg/**hour**)

Donor management in brain-dead patients (hormone replacement therapy): Continuous IV infusion:

Infants, Children, and Adolescents: (Nakagawa/NATCO Guidelines 2008): 0.5 to 1 milliunits/kg/**hour** (0.0005 to 0.001 units/kg/**hour**); titrate dose to maintain urine output at 3 to 4 mL/kg/**hour**. In one retrospective case-controlled study (n=34, age: 8.2 ± 6.2 years), the average dose was 41 milliunits/kg/**hour** (0.041 units/kg/**hour**) (Katz 2000).

Adults: Initial: 1 unit bolus, followed by 0.5 to 4 units/**hour** (Rosendale 2003; UNOS Critical Pathway 2002)

GI hemorrhage: Continuous IV infusion (may also be infused directly into the superior mesenteric artery):

Children: Initial: 2 to 5 milliunits/kg/minute (0.002 to 0.005 units/kg/minute); titrate dose as needed; maximum dose: 10 milliunits/kg/minute (0.01 units/kg/minute) (Tuggle 1988)

Alternative: Initial: 0.1 units/minute; increase by 0.05 units/minute to a maximum of:

<5 year: 0.2 units/minute

5 to 12 years: 0.3 units/minute

>12 years: 0.4 units/minute

If bleeding stops for 12 hours, then taper off over 24 to 48 hours.

Adults: Initial: 0.2 to 0.4 units/minute, then titrate dose as needed (maximum dose: 0.8 units/minute); if bleeding stops, continue at same dose for 12 hours, then taper off over 24 to 48 hours

Pulseless arrest, ventricular fibrillation, ventricular tachycardia:

Infants, Children, and Adolescents: IV: Limited data available: 0.4 units/kg after traditional resuscitation methods and at least two doses of epinephrine have been administered; **Note:** Due to insufficient evidence, no formal recommendations for or against the routine use of vasopressin during pediatric cardiac arrest are provided (Duncan 2009; Mann 2002; PALS 2010).

Adults: IV, I.O.: 40 units; may give one dose to replace first or second dose of epinephrine. IV/I.O. drug administration is preferred, but if no access, may give endotracheally. ACLS guidelines do not recommend a specific endotracheal dose; however, may be given endotracheally using the same IV dose (ACLS 2010; Wenzel 1997).

Vasodilatory shock with hypotension unresponsive to fluid resuscitation and exogenous catecholamines: Continuous IV infusion:

Infants and Children: 0.17 to 8 milliunits/kg/minute (0.01 to 0.48 units/kg/**hour** has been used; efficacy results have varied; optimal dose and timing has not been established. Dosing based on retrospective reviews and case reports that have shown increases in arterial blood pressure and urine output and also allowed for dosage reductions of additional vasopressors (Brierley 2009; Choong 2008; Meyer 2008). The only double-blind, placebo-controlled trial (n=65, age: 3 to 14 years) evaluated a dose of 0.5 to 2 milliunits/kg/minute (0.03 to 0.12 units/kg/**hour**) at multiple centers and found no significant difference in the time to reach hemodynamic stability and a trend toward increased mortality in the vasopressin group was noted. Based on these findings, the authors did not recommend routine use of vasopressin; further evaluations of dosing regimens needed (Choong 2009)

Adults: Initial: 0.01 to 0.04 units/minute; titrate to effect (doses >0.04 units/minute have been associated with increased risk of cardiovascular side effects); most case reports have used 0.04 units/minute continuous infusion as a fixed dose

Note: Abrupt discontinuation of infusion may result in hypotension; to discontinue gradually taper infusion

Dosing adjustment in hepatic impairment: Some patients with cirrhosis respond to much lower doses

Preparation for Administration Parenteral: Continuous IV infusion: Dilute in NS or D_5W to a final concentration of 0.1 to 1 unit/mL. Use of a diluted solution (0.04 units/mL) was described in a pediatric clinical trial that utilized lower dosing (eg, 0.0005 units/kg/**hour**) (Wise-Faberowski 2004).

Administration Parenteral:

Continuous IV infusion: Dilute prior to administration. Infusion through central line is strongly recommended.

Vesicant; ensure proper needle or catheter placement prior to and during infusion; avoid extravasation. If extravasation occurs, stop infusion immediately and disconnect (leave cannula/needle in place); gently aspirate extravasated solution (do **NOT** flush the line); remove needle/cannula; elevate extremity. Initiate phentolamine (or alternative antidote) (see Management of Drug Extravasations for more details).

IM: Administer without further dilution.

Endotracheal: Administer, then flush with 5 to 10 mL NS, followed by several manual ventilations.

Vesicant/Extravasation Risk Vesicant

Monitoring Parameters Fluid intake and output, urine specific gravity, urine and serum osmolality, serum and urine sodium; hemoglobin and hematocrit (GI bleeding)

Reference Range Vasopressin concentration:

Basal: <4 pg/mL

Water deprivation: 10 pg/mL

Shock: 100-1000 pg/mL (biphasic response)

Dosage Forms Excipient information presented when available (limited, particularly for generics); consult specific product labeling. [DSC] = Discontinued product

Solution, Injection:

Pitressin Synthetic: 20 units/mL (1 mL [DSC]) [contains chlorobutanol (chlorobutol)]

Generic: 20 units/mL (0.5 mL [DSC], 1 mL, 10 mL [DSC])

Solution, Intravenous:

Vasostrict: 20 units/mL (1 mL) [contains chlorobutanol (chlorobutol)]

- ◆ **Vasostrict** *see* Vasopressin *on page* *2161*
- ◆ **Vasotec** *see* Enalapril *on page* *744*
- ◆ **Vasotec IV (Can)** *see* Enalaprilat *on page* *748*
- ◆ **Vaxigrip (Can)** *see* Influenza Virus Vaccine (Inactivated) *on page* *1108*
- ◆ **Vazculep** *see* Phenylephrine (Systemic) *on page* *1685*
- ◆ **Vectical** *see* Calcitriol *on page* *338*

Vecuronium (vek ue ROE nee um)

Medication Safety Issues

Sound-alike/look-alike issues:

Vecuronium may be confused with valproate sodium, vancomycin

Norcuron may be confused with Narcan

High alert medication:

The Institute for Safe Medication Practices (ISMP) includes this medication among its list of drugs which have a heightened risk of causing significant patient harm when used in error.

Other safety concerns:

United States Pharmacopeia (USP) 2006: The Interdisciplinary Safe Medication Use Expert Committee of the USP has recommended the following:

- Hospitals, clinics, and other practice sites should institute special safeguards in the storage, labeling, and use of these agents and should include these safeguards in staff orientation and competency training.
- Healthcare professionals should be on high alert (especially vigilant) whenever a neuromuscular-blocking agent (NMBA) is stocked, ordered, prepared, or administered.

Brand Names: Canada Norcuron®

Therapeutic Category Neuromuscular Blocker Agent, Nondepolarizing; Skeletal Muscle Relaxant, Paralytic

Generic Availability (US) Yes

Use Adjunct to anesthesia, to facilitate endotracheal intubation, and provide skeletal muscle relaxation during surgery or mechanical ventilation (FDA approved in ages >7 weeks to 16 years and adults)

Pregnancy Risk Factor C

Pregnancy Considerations Animal reproduction studies have not been conducted. The pharmacokinetics of vecuronium are altered during pregnancy. Use in cesarean section has been reported; umbilical venous concentrations were 11% of maternal values at delivery.

Breast-Feeding Considerations It is not known if vecuronium is excreted in breast milk. The manufacturer recommends that caution be exercised when administering vecuronium to nursing women.

Contraindications Hypersensitivity to vecuronium or any component of the formulation

Warnings/Precautions Ventilation must be supported during neuromuscular blockade. Vecuronium does not relieve pain or produce sedation; use should include appropriate anesthesia, pain control, and sedation. In patients requiring long-term administration, use of a peripheral nerve stimulator to monitor drug effects is strongly recommended. Additional doses of vecuronium or any other neuromuscular-blocking agent should be avoided unless nerve stimulation response suggests inadequate neuromuscular blockade. Certain clinical conditions may result in potentiation (dosage reduction may be necessary) or antagonism (dosage increase may be necessary) of neuromuscular blockade:

Antagonism: Respiratory alkalosis, hypercalcemia, demyelinating lesions, peripheral neuropathies, denervation, and muscle trauma

Potentiation: Electrolyte abnormalities (eg, severe hypocalcemia, severe hypokalemia, hypermagnesemia), neuromuscular diseases, metabolic acidosis, metabolic alkalosis, respiratory acidosis, Eaton-Lambert syndrome, and myasthenia gravis

Resistance may occur in burn patients (≥20% of total body surface area), usually several days after the injury, and may persist for several months after wound healing. Resistance may occur in patients who are immobilized. Hypothermia may prolong the duration of action. Use with caution in patients with hepatic impairment; clinical duration may be prolonged. Use with caution in patients who are anephric; clinical duration may be prolonged. Use with caution in patients who have underlying respiratory disease. Some patients may experience delayed recovery of neuromuscular function after administration (especially after prolonged use). Other factors associated with delayed recovery should be considered (eg, corticosteroid use, disease-related conditions). Cross-sensitivity with other neuromuscular-blocking agents may occur; use extreme caution in patients with previous anaphylactic reactions. Use caution in the elderly; dosage reduction may be considered. Children 1-10 years of age may require slightly higher initial doses and slightly more frequent supplementation. **[U.S. Boxed Warning]: Should be administered by adequately trained individuals familiar with its use.**

Benzyl alcohol and derivatives: Diluent may contain benzyl alcohol; large amounts of benzyl alcohol (≥99 mg/kg/day) have been associated with a potentially fatal toxicity ("gasping syndrome") in neonates; the "gasping syndrome" consists of metabolic acidosis, respiratory distress, gasping respirations, CNS dysfunction (including convulsions, intracranial hemorrhage), hypotension, and cardiovascular collapse (AAP, 1997; CDC, 1982); some data suggests that benzoate displaces bilirubin from protein binding sites (Ahlfors, 2001); avoid or use dosage forms containing benzyl alcohol with caution in neonates. See manufacturer's labeling.

Adverse Reactions Rare but important or life-threatening: Acute quadriplegic myopathy syndrome (prolonged use), Bradycardia, circulatory collapse, edema, flushing; hypersensitivity reaction (hypotension, tachycardia, erythema, rash, urticaria); itching, myositis ossificans (prolonged use), rash

Drug Interactions

Metabolism/Transport Effects None known.

Avoid Concomitant Use

Avoid concomitant use of Vecuronium with any of the following: QuiNINE

Increased Effect/Toxicity

Vecuronium may increase the levels/effects of: Cardiac Glycosides; Corticosteroids (Systemic); OnabotulinumtoxinA; RimabotulinumtoxinB

The levels/effects of Vecuronium may be increased by: AbobotulinumtoxinA; Aminoglycosides; Calcium Channel Blockers; Capreomycin; Clindamycin (Topical); Colistimethate; CycloSPORINE (Systemic); Dantrolene; Fosphenytoin-Phenytoin; Inhalational Anesthetics; Ketorolac (Nasal); Ketorolac (Systemic); Lincosamide Antibiotics; Lithium; Loop Diuretics; Magnesium Salts; Piperacillin; Polymyxin B; Procainamide; QuiNIDine; QuiNINE; Spironolactone; Tetracycline Derivatives; Vancomycin

Decreased Effect

The levels/effects of Vecuronium may be decreased by: Acetylcholinesterase Inhibitors; CarBAMazepine; Fosphenytoin-Phenytoin; Loop Diuretics

Storage/Stability Store intact vials of powder for injection at room temperature 20°C to 25°C (68°F to 77°F). Vials reconstituted with bacteriostatic water for injection (BWFI) may be stored for 5 days under refrigeration or at room temperature. Vials reconstituted with other compatible diluents (nonbacteriostatic) should be stored under refrigeration and used within 24 hours.

Mechanism of Action Blocks acetylcholine from binding to receptors on motor endplate inhibiting depolarization

Pharmacodynamics

Onset of action: Within 1-3 minutes

Duration (dose dependent): 30-40 minutes

Pharmacokinetics (Adult data unless noted)

Distribution: V_d:

- Infants: 0.36 L/kg
- Children: 0.2 L/kg
- Adults: 0.27 L/kg

Protein binding: 60% to 80%

Half-life, distribution: Adults: 4 minutes

Half-life, elimination:

- Infants: 65 minutes
- Children: 41 minutes
- Adults: 65-75 minutes

Elimination: Vecuronium bromide and its metabolite(s) appear to be excreted principally in feces via biliary elimination (50%); the drug and its metabolite(s) are also excreted in urine (25%); the rate of elimination is appreciably reduced with hepatic dysfunction but not with renal dysfunction

Dosing: Neonatal Paralysis/skeletal muscle relaxation: IV: 0.1 mg/kg/dose; maintenance: 0.03-0.15 mg/kg/dose every 1-2 hours as needed

Dosing: Usual Paralysis/skeletal muscle relaxation:

Infants >7 weeks to 1 year:

IV: 0.1 mg/kg/dose; repeat every hour as needed

Continuous IV infusion: 1-1.5 **mcg**/kg/minute (0.06-0.09 mg/kg/**hour**)

Children and Adolescents >1-16 years:

IV: 0.1 mg/kg/dose; repeat every hour as needed

Continuous IV infusion: 1.5-2.5 **mcg**/kg/minute (0.09-0.15 mg/kg/**hour**)

Adults:

IV: 0.1 mg/kg/dose; repeat every hour as needed

Continuous IV infusion: 0.8-1.7 **mcg**/kg/minute (0.05-0.1 mg/kg/**hour**)

Dosing adjustment in hepatic impairment: Dose reductions are necessary in patients with cirrhosis or cholestasis

Usual Infusion Concentrations: Neonatal IV infusion: 1 mg/mL

Usual Infusion Concentrations: Pediatric IV infusion: 0.1 mg/mL, 0.2 mg/mL, 1 mg/mL

Preparation for Administration

Parenteral:

IV bolus: Reconstitute with provided diluent or compatible solution for injection to final concentration of 1 mg/mL; for neonatal use, reconstitute with SWFI instead of provided diluent (contains benzyl alcohol).

Continuous IV infusion: Further dilute reconstituted vial in a compatible solution for IV infusion; the manufacturer suggests a final concentration range of 0.1 to 0.2 mg/mL; however, concentrations as high as 1 mg/mL have been reported (Murray 2014; Phillips 2011; Sinclair-Pingel 2006).

Administration

Parenteral:

IV bolus: Administer undiluted (reconstituted solution at 1 mg/mL) by rapid direct injection

Continuous IV infusion: Administer via an infusion pump at a concentration not to exceed 1 mg/mL

Monitoring Parameters Assisted ventilation status, heart rate, blood pressure, peripheral nerve stimulator measuring twitch response

Additional Information Produces minimal, if any, histamine release

Dosage Forms Excipient information presented when available (limited, particularly for generics); consult specific product labeling.

Solution Reconstituted, Intravenous, as bromide:

Generic: 10 mg (1 ea); 20 mg (1 ea)

Solution Reconstituted, Intravenous, as bromide [preservative free]:

Generic: 10 mg (1 ea); 20 mg (1 ea)

Velaglucerase Alfa (vel a GLOO ser ase AL fa)

Brand Names: US Vpriv

Brand Names: Canada VPRIV

Therapeutic Category Enzyme, Glucocerebrosidase; Gaucher's Disease, Treatment Agent

Generic Availability (US) No

Use Long-term enzyme replacement therapy (ERT) for patients with Type 1 Gaucher's disease (FDA approved in ages ≥4 years and adults)

Pregnancy Risk Factor B

Pregnancy Considerations Teratogenic effects were not observed in animal reproduction studies. Pregnancy may exacerbate existing type I Gaucher disease or result in new symptoms. Women with type I Gaucher disease have an increased risk of spontaneous abortion if disease is not well controlled. Adverse pregnancy outcomes, including hepatosplenomegaly and thrombocytopenia, may occur.

Breast-Feeding Considerations It is not known if velaglucerase alfa is excreted in breast milk. The manufacturer recommends that caution be used if administered to nursing women.

Contraindications There are no contraindications listed in the manufacturer's labeling.

Warnings/Precautions Use with caution in patients who have exhibited hypersensitivity reactions to velaglucerase alfa or other enzyme replacement therapies. Anaphylaxis has occurred; appropriate medical support should be readily available in the event of a serious reaction. The most common hypersensitivity reactions reported in clinical trials include asthenia, dizziness, fatigue, fever, headache, hyper-/hypotension, nausea, and pyrexia. Most reactions were mild and occurred during the first 6 months of treatment. Management strategies of more severe reactions include symptomatic treatment, pretreatment with antihistamines, antipyretics, and/or corticosteroids, and slowing of the infusion rate. Treatment should be discontinued if anaphylaxis or other acute reactions occur. The development of IgG antibodies has been reported; monitor antibodies in those patients who developed antibodies to other enzyme replacement therapies.

Warnings: Additional Pediatric Considerations Pediatric patients (4 to 17 years) may experience a higher frequency of some adverse effects than adults (>10% difference in incidence), including fever, rash, prolonged aPTT, and upper respiratory tract infection.

Adverse Reactions

Cardiovascular: Flushing, hypertension, hypotension, tachycardia

Central nervous system: Dizziness, fatigue, headache, weakness

Dermatologic: Skin rash (more common in children), urticaria

Gastrointestinal: Abdominal pain, nausea

Hematologic & oncologic: Prolonged partial thromboplastin time (more common in children)

Hypersensitivity: Hypersensitivity reaction

Immunologic: Immunogenicity

Neuromuscular & skeletal: Arthralgia (knee), back pain, ostealgia

Miscellaneous: Fever (more common in children)

Rare but important or life-threatening: Anaphylaxis, chest discomfort, dyspnea

Drug Interactions

Metabolism/Transport Effects None known.

Avoid Concomitant Use There are no known interactions where it is recommended to avoid concomitant use.

Increased Effect/Toxicity There are no known significant interactions involving an increase in effect.

Decreased Effect There are no known significant interactions involving a decrease in effect.

Storage/Stability Store intact vials at 2°C to 8°C (36°F to 46°F). Once reconstituted, the product should be used immediately. If immediate use is not possible, the reconstituted or diluted product may be stored for up to 24 hours at 2°C to 8°C (36°F to 46°F). The infusion should be completed within 24 hours of reconstitution. Do not freeze. Protect from light. Discard any unused solution.

Mechanism of Action Velaglucerase alfa, which contains the same amino acid sequence as endogenous glucocerebrosidase, catalyzes the hydrolysis of glucocerebroside to glucose and ceramide in the lysosome. In patients with type 1 Gaucher's disease, glucocerebrosidase deficiency results in accumulation of glucocerebroside in macrophages, thereby causing the associated signs and symptoms. Velaglucerase alfa is used to diminish hepatosplenomegaly and improve anemia, thrombocytopenia, and bone disease.

Pharmacokinetics (Adult data unless noted) Note: Values reported below based on combined pediatric patient (4-17 years) and adult data.

Distribution: V_{dss}: 0.08-0.11 L/kg

Half-life: 11-12 minutes

Dosing: Usual Note: Pretreatment with antihistamines and/or corticosteroids can be considered for prevention of subsequent infusion reactions in patients with hypersensitivity reactions requiring symptomatic treatment; during clinical studies, patients were not routinely premedicated prior to infusion.

Pediatric: **Gaucher's disease (type 1):** Children and Adolescents 4 to 17 years: IV: 60 units/kg every other week; adjust based upon disease activity; dosing range: 15 to 60 units/kg every other week. **Note:** When switching from imiglucerase to velaglucerase alfa, initiate velaglucerase alfa treatment 2 weeks after the last imiglucerase dose and at the same dose as stable imiglucerase therapy.

Adult: **Gaucher's disease (type 1):** IV: 60 units/kg administered every 2 weeks; adjust dose based upon disease activity (range: 15 to 60 units/kg evaluated in clinical trials). **Note:** When switching from imiglucerase to velaglucerase alfa in stable patients, initiate treatment 2 weeks after the last imiglucerase dose and at the same dose.

Dosing adjustment in renal impairment: There are no dosage adjustments provided in manufacturer's labeling.

Dosing adjustment in hepatic impairment: There are no dosage adjustments provided in manufacturer's labeling.

Preparation for Administration Parenteral: Reconstitute vial with 4.3 mL of SWFI to a final concentration of 100 units/mL. Gently mix vials; do not shake. The solution for infusion should be further diluted in 100 mL of NS. Slight flocculation (white irregular-shaped particles) may occur; this is acceptable for administration.

Administration Parenteral: For IV administration. Infuse over 60 minutes through an in-line low protein-binding 0.2 micron filter. Do not infuse other products in the same infusion tubing.

Monitoring Parameters CBC, liver enzymes, IgG antibodies; MRI, CT, or US of liver and spleen; bone density studies; monitor antibodies in those patients who developed antibodies to other enzyme replacement therapies

Additional Information Gaucher Disease Registry: https://www.registrynxt.com/Gaucher/Pages/Home.aspx

Dosage Forms Excipient information presented when available (limited, particularly for generics); consult specific product labeling.

Solution Reconstituted, Intravenous [preservative free]:
Vpriv: 400 units (1 ea)

◆ **Velban** *see* VinBLAStine *on page 2177*

◆ **Veletri** *see* Epoprostenol *on page 769*

◆ **Veltin** *see* Clindamycin and Tretinoin *on page 494*

◆ **Veltin** *see* Clindamycin and Tretinoin *on page 494*

Venlafaxine (ven la FAX een)

Medication Safety Issues

Sound-alike/look-alike issues:

Effexor may be confused with Effexor XR

Effexor XR may be confused with Enablex

BEERS Criteria medication:

This drug may be potentially inappropriate for use in geriatric patients (Quality of evidence - moderate; Strength of recommendation - strong).

Related Information

Antidepressant Agents *on page 2257*

Oral Medications That Should Not Be Crushed or Altered *on page 2476*

Brand Names: US Effexor XR

Brand Names: Canada ACT Venlafaxine XR; Apo-Venlafaxine XR; Dom-Venlafaxine XR; Effexor XR; GD-Venlafaxine XR; Mylan-Venlafaxine XR; PMS-Venlafaxine XR; Ran-Venlafaxine XR; Riva-Venlafaxine XR; Sandoz-Venlafaxine XR; Teva-Venlafaxine XR; Venlafaxine XR

Therapeutic Category Antidepressant, Serotonin/Norepinephrine Reuptake Inhibitor

Generic Availability (US) Yes

Use Treatment of major depressive disorder, generalized anxiety disorder, social anxiety disorder (social phobia), and panic disorder (all indications: FDA approved in adults); has also been used to treat ADHD and autism in children and obsessive-compulsive disorder and chronic fatigue syndrome in adults

Medication Guide Available Yes

Pregnancy Risk Factor C

Pregnancy Considerations Adverse events have been observed in some animal reproduction studies. Venlafaxine and its active metabolite ODV cross the human placenta. An increased risk of teratogenic effects following venlafaxine exposure during pregnancy has not been observed, based on available data. The risk of spontaneous abortion may be increased. Neonatal seizures and neonatal abstinence syndrome have been noted in case reports following maternal use of venlafaxine during pregnancy. Nonteratogenic effects in the newborn following SSRI/SNRI exposure late in the third trimester include respiratory distress, cyanosis, apnea, seizures, temperature instability, feeding difficulty, vomiting, hypoglycemia, hyper- or hypotonia, hyper-reflexia, jitteriness, irritability, constant crying, and tremor. Symptoms may be due to the toxicity of the SNRI or a discontinuation syndrome and may be consistent with serotonin syndrome associated with treatment. The long-term effects of *in utero* SNRI/SSRI exposure on infant development and behavior are not known.

Due to pregnancy-induced physiologic changes, some pharmacokinetic parameters of venlafaxine may be altered. Women should be monitored for decreased efficacy. The ACOG recommends that therapy with SSRIs or SNRIs during pregnancy be individualized; treatment of depression during pregnancy should incorporate the clinical expertise of the mental health clinician, obstetrician, primary healthcare provider, and pediatrician. According to the American Psychiatric Association (APA), the risks of medication treatment should be weighed against other treatment options and untreated depression. For women who discontinue antidepressant medications during pregnancy and who may be at high risk for postpartum depression, the medications can be restarted following delivery. Treatment algorithms have been developed by the ACOG and the APA for the management of depression in women prior to conception and during pregnancy.

Breast-Feeding Considerations Venlafaxine and ODV are found in breast milk and the serum of nursing infants. Adverse events have not been observed; however, it is recommended to monitor the infant for adverse events if the decision to breast-feed has been made. The long-term effects on neurobehavior have not been studied, thus one should prescribe venlafaxine to a mother who is breast-feeding only when the benefits outweigh the potential risks. The manufacturer does not recommend breast-feeding during therapy.

Contraindications Hypersensitivity to venlafaxine or any component of the formulation; use of MAOIs intended to treat psychiatric disorders (concurrently or within 14 days of discontinuing the MAOI); initiation of MAOI intended to treat psychiatric disorders within 7 days of discontinuing venlafaxine; initiation in patients receiving linezolid or IV methylene blue

Warnings/Precautions [U.S. Boxed Warning]: Antidepressants increase the risk of suicidal thinking and behavior in children, adolescents, and young adults (18-24 years of age) with major depressive disorder (MDD) and other psychiatric disorders; consider risk prior to prescribing. Short-term studies did not show an increased risk in patients >24 years of age and showed a decreased risk in patients ≥65 years. Closely monitor for clinical worsening, suicidality, or unusual changes in behavior, particularly during the first few months of therapy or during periods of dosage adjustments (increases or decreases); the patient's family or caregiver should be instructed to closely observe the patient and communicate condition with healthcare provider. Reduced growth rate has been observed with venlafaxine therapy in children. A medication guide should be dispensed with each prescription.

The possibility of a suicide attempt is inherent in major depression and may persist until remission occurs. Use caution in high-risk patients. Worsening depression and severe abrupt suicidality that are not part of the presenting symptoms may require discontinuation or modification of drug therapy. The patient's family or caregiver should be alerted to monitor patients for the emergence of suicidality and associated behaviors (such as agitation, irritability, hostility, impulsivity, and hypomania) and call healthcare provider.

May precipitate a shift to mania or hypomania in patients with bipolar disorder. Patients presenting with depressive symptoms should be screened for bipolar disorder, including details regarding family history of suicide, bipolar disorder, and depression. Monotherapy in patients with bipolar disorder should be avoided. **Venlafaxine is not FDA approved for the treatment of bipolar depression.**

Potentially life-threatening serotonin syndrome (SS) has occurred with serotonergic agents (eg, SSRIs, SNRIs), particularly when used in combination with other serotonergic agents (eg, triptans, TCAs, fentanyl, lithium, tramadol, buspirone, St John's wort, tryptophan) or agents that impair metabolism of serotonin (eg, MAO inhibitors intended to treat psychiatric disorders, other MAO inhibitors [ie, linezolid and intravenous methylene blue]). Discontinue treatment (and any concomitant serotonergic agent) immediately if signs/symptoms arise.

May cause sustained increase in blood pressure or tachycardia; dose related and increases are generally modest (12-15 mm Hg diastolic). Control preexisting hypertension prior to initiation of venlafaxine. Use caution in patients with recent history of MI, unstable heart disease, cerebrovascular conditions, or hyperthyroidism; may cause increase in anxiety, nervousness, insomnia; may cause weight loss (use with caution in patients where weight loss is undesirable); may cause increases in serum cholesterol and triglycerides; monitor during long-term treatment. Use caution with hepatic or renal impairment; dosage adjustments recommended. May cause hyponatremia/SIADH, age (the elderly), volume depletion and/or concurrent use of diuretics likely increases risk. Discontinue treatment in patients with symptomatic hyponatremia.

May impair platelet aggregation resulting in increased risk of bleeding events, particularly if used concomitantly with aspirin, or NSAIDs, warfarin, or other anticoagulants. Bleeding related to SSRI or SNRI use has been reported to range from relatively minor bruising and epistaxis to life-threatening hemorrhage. Interstitial lung disease and eosinophilic pneumonia have been rarely reported; may present as progressive dyspnea, cough, and/or chest pain. Prompt evaluation and possible discontinuation of therapy may be necessary. Venlafaxine may increase the risks associated with electroconvulsive therapy. Use cautiously in patients with previous seizure disorder. The risks of cognitive or motor impairment, as well as the potential for anticholinergic effects are very low. May cause or exacerbate sexual dysfunction. Bone fractures have been associated with antidepressant treatment. Consider the possibility of a fragility fracture if an antidepressant-treated patient presents with unexplained bone pain, point tenderness, swelling, or bruising (Rabenda, 2013; Rizzoli, 2012).

Use caution in elderly patients; may cause or exacerbate syndrome of inappropriate antidiuretic hormone secretion or hyponatremia; monitor sodium closely with initiation or dosage adjustments in older adults (Beers Criteria). Use caution in patients with increased intraocular pressure or at risk of acute narrow-angle glaucoma (angle-closure glaucoma). Potentially significant drug-drug interactions may exist, requiring dose or frequency adjustment, additional monitoring, and/or selection of alternative therapy.

Abrupt discontinuation or interruption of antidepressant therapy has been associated with a discontinuation syndrome. Symptoms arising may vary with antidepressant however commonly include nausea, vomiting, diarrhea, headaches, lightheadedness, dizziness, diminished appetite, sweating, chills, tremors, paresthesias, fatigue, somnolence, and sleep disturbances (eg, vivid dreams, insomnia). Greater risks for developing a discontinuation syndrome have been associated with antidepressants with shorter half-lives, longer durations of treatment, and abrupt discontinuation. For antidepressants of short or intermediate half-lives, symptoms may emerge within 2-5 days after treatment discontinuation and last 7-14 days (APA, 2010; Fava, 2006; Haddad, 2001; Shelton, 2001; Warner, 2006).

Warnings: Additional Pediatric Considerations May cause anxiety, nervousness, and insomnia; in children treated for ADHD, an increase in hyperactivity (behavioral activation) was reported (Olvera, 1996). May cause anorexia and significant, dose related weight loss; use with caution in patients where weight loss is undesirable; may adversely affect weight and height in children; monitor closely in pediatric patients; weight loss in pediatric patients was not limited to those with venlafaxine-associated anorexia; reduction in growth rate, as assessed by height, was greater in children <12 years of age than in adolescents. A case of priapism has been reported in an adolescent patient (Samuel, 2000).

Adverse Reactions

Cardiovascular: Chest pain, edema, hypertension (dose related), palpitations, tachycardia, vasodilation

Central nervous system: Abnormal dreams, abnormality in thinking, agitation, amnesia, anorgasmia (female), anxiety, chills, confusion, depersonalization, depression, dizziness, drowsiness, headache, hypertonia, hypoesthesia, insomnia, migraine, nervousness, paresthesia, trismus, twitching, vertigo, yawning

Dermatologic: Diaphoresis, ecchymoses, pruritus

Endocrine & metabolic: Albuminuria, decreased libido, hypercholesterolemia, increased serum triglycerides, orgasm abnormal, weight gain, weight loss (more common in children & adolescents)

Gastrointestinal: Abdominal pain, anorexia, constipation, diarrhea, dysgeusia, dyspepsia, flatulence, increased appetite, nausea, vomiting, xerostomia

Genitourinary: Abnormal ejaculation, impotence, urinary disorder

Neuromuscular & skeletal: Neck pain, tremor, weakness

Ophthalmic: Accommodation disturbance, mydriasis, visual disturbance

Respiratory: Dyspnea, increased cough, pharyngitis

Miscellaneous: Accidental injury, fever

Rare but important or life-threatening: Abnormal behavior, abnormal gait, abnormal healing, abortion, acne vulgaris, adjustment disorder, ageusia, agranulocytosis, alcohol abuse, alcohol intolerance, alcohol intoxication, alopecia, altered sense of smell, amenorrhea, anaphylaxis, anemia, aneurysm, angina pectoris, angle-closure glaucoma, apathy, aphasia, appendicitis, arthritis, arthropathy, asthma, atelectasis, atrophic striae, attempted suicide, bacteremia, balanitis, basophilia, bigeminy, biliary colic, bladder pain, blepharitis, bone spur, bradycardia, bruxism, buccoglossal syndrome, bundle branch block, bursitis, candidiasis, carcinoma, cardiac arrhythmia (including atrial fibrillation, supraventricular tachycardia, ventricular extrasystoles, ventricular fibrillation, ventricular tachycardia, and torsades de pointes), cardiovascular disease (mitral valve and circulatory disturbance), cataract, cellulitis, central nervous system stimulation, cerebrovascular accident, cervicitis, changes in LDH, cheilitis, chest congestion, cholecystitis, cholelithiasis, chromatopsia, colitis, congenital anomalies, congestive heart failure, conjunctival edema, conjunctivitis, corneal lesion, coronary artery disease, crystalluria, cystitis, deafness, decreased pupillary reflex, deep vein thrombosis, dehydration, delirium, delusions, dementia, diabetes mellitus, diplopia, duodenitis, dysphagia, dysuria, eczema, electric shock-like sensation, emotional lability, endometriosis, eosinophilia, erythema multiforme, esophagitis, extrapyramidal reaction, eye pain, facial paralysis, first degree atrioventricular block, furunculosis, gastroenteritis, gastroesophageal reflux disease, gastrointestinal ulcer, gingivitis, glossitis, glycosuria, goiter, gout, granuloma, Guillain-Barré syndrome, hair discoloration, hematoma, hemochromatosis, hemorrhage (eye, GI, gum, mucocutaneous, rectal, retinal, subconjunctival, uterine, vaginal), hemorrhoids, hepatic effects (including GGT elevation; abnormalities of unspecified liver function tests; liver damage, necrosis, or failure; and fatty liver), hepatitis, homicidal ideation, hostility, hyperacidity, hyperacusis, hypercalciuria, hyperesthesia, hyperreflexia, hyperthyroidism, hyperuricemia, hyperventilation, hypoglycemia, hypohidrosis, hypokalemia, hypokinesia, hypomenorrhea, hyponatremia, hypophosphatemia, hyporeflexia, hypotension, hypothyroidism, hypotonia, hypoventilation, hysteria, ileitis, impulse control disorder, increased energy, increased libido, increased serum prolactin, interstitial pulmonary disease (including eosinophilic pneumonia), intestinal obstruction, keratitis, labyrinthitis, laryngismus, laryngitis, leukocytosis, leukoderma, leukopenia, leukorrhea, lichenoid dermatitis, loss of consciousness, lymphadenopathy, lymphocytosis, melena, menopause, miliaria, miosis, multiple myeloma, muscle spasm, myasthenia, nephrolithiasis, neuralgia, neuritis, neuropathy, neutropenia, night sweats, nystagmus, oliguria, onychia sicca, oral candidiasis, oral mucosa ulcer, oral paresthesia, orchitis, ostealgia, osteoporosis, osteosclerosis, otitis externa, otitis media, ovarian cyst, pancreatitis, pancytopenia, panic, papilledema, paranoia, paresis, parotitis, pathological fracture, pelvic pain, periodontitis, peripheral vascular disease, petechial rash, plantar fasciitis, pleurisy, pneumonia, polyuria, proctitis, prolonged bleeding time, prolonged erection, prostatic disease, pruritic rash, psoriasis, psychosis, psychotic depression, pulmonary embolism, purpura, pustular rash, pyelonephritis, pyuria, rectal disease, renal failure, renal function abnormality, renal pain, rhabdomyolysis, rheumatoid arthritis, rupture of tendon, salpingitis, scleritis, seborrhea, seizure, serotonin syndrome, SIADH, sialorrhea, sinus arrhythmia, skin atrophy, skin discoloration, skin hypertrophy, skin photosensitivity, sleep apnea, speech disturbance, Stevens-Johnson syndrome, stomatitis, stupor, suicidal ideation (reported at a frequency up to 2% in children/ adolescents with major depressive disorder), tenosynovitis, thrombocythemia, thrombocytopenia, thyroiditis, thyroid nodule, tongue discoloration, uremia, urinary incontinence, urinary urgency, urolithiasis, urticaria, uterine spasm, uveitis, vaginal dryness, vaginitis, vesicobullous dermatitis, visual field defect, voice disorder, withdrawal syndrome, xeroderma, xerophthalmia

Drug Interactions

Metabolism/Transport Effects Substrate of CYP2C19 (minor), CYP2C9 (minor), CYP2D6 (major), CYP3A4 (major); **Note:** Assignment of Major/Minor substrate status based on clinically relevant drug interaction potential; **Inhibits** CYP2B6 (weak), CYP2D6 (weak)

Avoid Concomitant Use

Avoid concomitant use of Venlafaxine with any of the following: Conivaptan; Dapoxetine; Fusidic Acid (Systemic); Idelalisib; Iobenguane I 123; Linezolid; MAO Inhibitors; Methylene Blue; Urokinase

Increased Effect/Toxicity

Venlafaxine may increase the levels/effects of: Agents with Antiplatelet Properties; Alpha-/Beta-Agonists; Anticoagulants; Antipsychotic Agents; Apixaban; ARIPiprazole; Aspirin; Collagenase (Systemic); Dabigatran Etexilate; Deoxycholic Acid; Highest Risk QTc-Prolonging Agents; Ibritumomab; Methylene Blue; Moderate Risk QTc-Prolonging Agents; NSAID (Nonselective); Obinutuzumab; Rivaroxaban; Salicylates; Serotonin Modulators; Thrombolytic Agents; Tositumomab and Iodine I 131 Tositumomab; TraZODone; Urokinase; Vitamin K Antagonists

The levels/effects of Venlafaxine may be increased by: Abiraterone Acetate; Alcohol (Ethyl); Antiemetics (5HT3 Antagonists); Antipsychotic Agents; Aprepitant; Conivaptan; CYP2D6 Inhibitors (Moderate); CYP2D6 Inhibitors (Strong); CYP3A4 Inhibitors (Moderate); CYP3A4 Inhibitors (Strong); Dapoxetine; Dasatinib; Fosaprepitant; Fusidic Acid (Systemic); Glucosamine; Herbs (Anticoagulant/Antiplatelet Properties); Ibrutinib; Idelalisib; Ivacaftor; Limaprost; Linezolid; Luliconazole; MAO Inhibitors; Metoclopramide; Mifepristone; Multivitamins/Fluoride (with ADE); Multivitamins/Minerals (with ADEK, Folate, Iron); Multivitamins/Minerals (with AE, No Iron); Netupitant; Omega-3 Fatty Acids; Palbociclib; Panobinostat; Peginterferon Alfa-2b; Pentosan Polysulfate Sodium; Pentoxifylline; Propafenone; Prostacyclin Analogues; Simeprevir; Stiripentol; Tedizolid; Vitamin E; Voriconazole

Decreased Effect

Venlafaxine may decrease the levels/effects of: Alpha2-Agonists; Indinavir; Iobenguane I 123; Ioflupane I 123

The levels/effects of Venlafaxine may be decreased by: Bosentan; CYP3A4 Inducers (Moderate); CYP3A4 Inducers (Strong); Dabrafenib; Deferasirox; Mitotane; Peginterferon Alfa-2b; Siltuximab; St Johns Wort; Tocilizumab

Storage/Stability Store immediate-release tablets and extended-release capsules at 20°C to 25°C (68°F to 77°F). Store extended-release tablets at 25°C (77°F); excursions are permitted between 15°C and 30°C (59°F and 86°F).

Mechanism of Action Venlafaxine and its active metabolite, O-desmethylvenlafaxine (ODV), are potent inhibitors of neuronal serotonin and norepinephrine reuptake and weak inhibitors of dopamine reuptake. Venlafaxine and ODV have no significant activity for muscarinic cholinergic, H_1-histaminergic, or alpha$_2$-adrenergic receptors. Venlafaxine and ODV do not possess MAO-inhibitory activity. Venlafaxine functions like an SSRI in low doses (37.5 mg/day) and as a dual mechanism agent affecting serotonin and norepinephrine at doses above 225 mg/day (Harvey, 2000; Kelsey, 1996).

Pharmacokinetics (Adult data unless noted)

Absorption: Oral: ≥92%

Distribution: Distributes into breast milk; breast milk to plasma ratio: Venlafaxine: 2.8-4.8 (mean: 4.1); ODV: 2.8-3.8 (mean: 3.1) (Ilett, 1998)
Mean V_d (apparent): Adults:
Venlafaxine: 7.5 ± 3.7 L/kg
ODV: 5.7 ± 1.8 L/kg
Protein binding: Venlafaxine: 27%; ODV: 30%
Metabolism: Extensive in the liver, primarily via cytochrome P450 CYP2D6 to o-desmethylvenlafaxine (ODV; active metabolite); also metabolized to N-desmethylvenlafaxine, N,O-desmethylvenlafaxine, and other minor metabolites. **Note:** Clinically important differences between CYP2D6 poor and extensive metabolizers is not expected (sum of venlafaxine and ODV serum concentrations is similar in poor and extensive metabolizers; ODV is approximately equal in activity and potency to venlafaxine)
Bioavailability: Oral: 45%
Half-life:
Adults: Venlafaxine: 5 ± 2 hours; ODV: 11 ± 2 hours
Adults with cirrhosis: Venlafaxine: Half-life prolonged by ~30%; ODV: Half-life prolonged by ~60%
Adults with renal impairment (GFR: 10-70 mL/minute): Venlafaxine: Half-life prolonged by ~50%; ODV: Half-life prolonged by ~40%
Adults on dialysis: Venlafaxine: Half-life prolonged by ~180%; ODV: Half-life prolonged by 142%
Time to peak serum concentration:
Immediate release: Venlafaxine: 2 hours; ODV: 3 hours
Extended release: Venlafaxine: 5.5 hours; ODV: 9 hours
Elimination: ~87% of dose is excreted in urine within 48 hours; 5% as unchanged drug, 29% as unconjugated ODV, 26% as conjugated ODV, and 27% as other minor metabolites
Clearance:
Adults with cirrhosis: Venlafaxine: Clearance is decreased by ~50%; ODV: Clearance is decreased by ~30%
Adults with more severe cirrhosis: Venlafaxine: Clearance is decreased by ~90%
Adults with renal impairment (GFR: 10-70 mL/minute): Venlafaxine: Clearance is decreased by ~24%; ODV: Clearance unchanged versus normal subjects
Adults on dialysis: Venlafaxine: Clearance decreased by ~57%; ODV: Clearance decreased by ~56%
Dialysis: Not likely to significantly remove drug due to large volume of distribution

Dosing: Usual

Pediatric:

Attention-deficit/hyperactivity disorder (ADHD): Limited data available: Children and Adolescents 8 to <17 years: Oral: Immediate release: Initial: 12.5 mg then titrate: Children <40 kg: Increase by 12.5 mg/week to maximum daily dose: 50 mg/day in 2 divided doses or Children ≥40 kg: Increase by 25 mg/week to maximum daily dose: 75 mg/day in 3 divided doses. Dosing based on an open-label clinical 5-week trial of 16 children and adolescents (mean age: 11.6 ± 2.3 years); mean dose: 60 mg/day (1.4 mg/kg/day) in 2 to 3 divided doses; ten patients completed the study [2 were lost to follow-up; 5 discontinued therapy due to adverse effects (4 had an increase in hyperactivity; 1 had severe nausea)]; venlafaxine decreased behavioral symptoms (but not cognitive symptoms) in 7 of 16 subjects (44%) (Olvera 1996). An initial dose of 37.5 mg given 3 times/day was used in an 11-year-old female with ADHD; the dose was slowly titrated to 100 mg given 3 times/day; after 6 weeks the patient showed moderate to marked improvement in symptoms, but developed hypertension; the dose was then decreased to 75 mg given 3 times/day with normalization of blood pressure (Pleak 1995).

Autism spectrum disorders: Limited data available: Children ≥ 3 years and Adolescents: Oral: Immediate release: One retrospective report is available; 10 patients (3 to 21 years of age; mean 10.5 ± 5.6 years) with autism spectrum disorders (autism, Asperger's syndrome, and pervasive developmental disorders not otherwise specified) received initial doses of 12.5 mg/day administered once daily at breakfast; doses were gradually titrated based on clinical response and side effects; mean final dose: 24.4 mg/day; range: 6.25 to 50 mg/day; 6 of the 10 patients were sustained-treatment responders (Hollander 2000).

Depression: Limited data available: Children ≥7 years and Adolescents ≤17 years: **Note:** Due to the lack of demonstrated efficacy and concerns about an increased risk for suicidal behavior, venlafaxine should be reserved for pediatric patients with major depression who do not respond to fluoxetine or sertraline (Dopheide 2006). Oral:

Immediate release: One double-blind, placebo-controlled, 6-week study is available; 33 children and adolescents (8 to 17 years of age) with major depression completed the trial (16 received venlafaxine; for children 8 to 12 years, doses were initiated at 12.5 mg once daily for 3 days, then increased to 12.5 mg twice daily for 3 days, then increased to 12.5 mg given 3 times/day for the rest of the study; for adolescents 13 to 17 years, doses were initiated at 25 mg once daily for 3 days, then increased to 25 mg twice daily for 3 days, then increased to 25 mg given 3 times/day for the rest of the study; both venlafaxine and placebo patients improved over time; however, no significant difference in symptoms was noted between groups (ie, venlafaxine did not have a significant effect on symptoms or specific behaviors); the authors suggest this lack of efficacy may be due to the low doses used and short duration of treatment (Mandoki 1997).

Extended release: A large multicenter double-blind, placebo-controlled study of venlafaxine-ER in children and adolescents 7 to 17 years of age with major depression is ongoing; this study is using higher doses; initial: 37.5 mg/day for 1 week; with increases to 75 mg/day for weeks 2 to 8; results are not yet available (Weller 2000). One report of two 16-year-old patients used higher doses of venlafaxine (final doses: 112.5 mg/day and 150 mg/day) in combination with lithium to successfully treat major depression (Walter 1998).

Adult:

Immediate release: Depression: Initial: 75 mg/day in 2 t 3 divided doses; dose may be increased (if needed) by increments of up to 75 mg/day at intervals of ≥4 days as tolerated, up to 225 mg/day. **Note:** Doses >225 mg/day for outpatients (moderately depressed patients) were not more effective; more severely depressed patients may require 350 mg/day; maximum: 375 mg/day in 3 divided doses

Extended release:

Depression: Initial: Usual: 75 mg/day; may start with 37.5 mg/day for 4 to 7 days to allow patient to adjust to medication, then increase to 75 mg/day; dose may be increased (if needed) by increments of up to 75 mg/day at intervals of ≥4 days as tolerated, up to a maximum of 225 mg/day. **Note:** Although higher doses of the immediate release tablets have been used in more severely depressed inpatients (see above), experience with extended release capsule in doses >225 mg/day is very limited.

Generalized anxiety disorder and social anxiety disorder: 75 mg/day; may start with 37.5 mg/day for 4 to 7 days to allow patient to adjust to medication, then increase to 75 mg/day. **Note:** Although a dose-response relationship has not been clearly established, certain patients may benefit from doses >75 mg/day; dose may be increased (if needed) by increments of up to 75 mg/day at intervals of ≥4 days as tolerated, up to a maximum of 225 mg/day.

Panic disorder: Initial: 37.5 mg once daily for 7 days; may increase to 75 mg daily; dose may be increased further (if needed) by increments of up to 75 mg/day at intervals of ≥7 days; maximum dose: 225 mg/day

Dosing adjustment in renal impairment: Adults: GFR 10 to 70 mL/minute: Decrease total daily dose by 25% to 50%

Dosing adjustment in patients on dialysis: Decrease total daily dose by 50%; withhold dose until completion of dialysis treatment; further individualization of dose may be needed

Dosing adjustment in hepatic impairment: Moderate hepatic impairment: Decrease total daily dose by 50%; further individualization of dose may be needed

Administration

Immediate release tablet: Administer with food

Extended release capsule: Administer with food once daily at about the same time each day; swallow whole with fluid; do not crush, chew, divide, or place in water; capsule may be opened and entire contents sprinkled on spoonful of applesauce; swallow drug/food mixture immediately. Do not store for future use; do not chew contents (ie, pellets) of capsule; follow drug/food mixture with water to ensure complete swallowing of pellets.

Monitoring Parameters Monitor blood pressure regularly, especially in patients with high baseline blood pressure; monitor renal and hepatic function (for possible dose reductions), heart rate, weight, height, serum cholesterol and sodium. Monitor patient periodically for symptom resolution; monitor for worsening depression, suicidality, and associated behaviors (especially at the beginning of therapy or when doses are increased or decreased)

Test Interactions May interfere with urine detection of phencyclidine and amphetamine (false-positives).

Additional Information Drug release from extended release capsules is not pH dependent (it is controlled by diffusion through the coating membrane on the spheroids); patients with depression who are receiving immediate release tablets may be switched to Effexor XR® using the nearest mg/day equivalent dose (dosing may need further individualization)

Long-term usefulness of venlafaxine should be periodically re-evaluated in patients receiving the drug for extended periods of time. Neonates born to women receiving venlafaxine, other SNRIs (serotonin and norepinephrine reuptake inhibitors), and SSRIs late during the third trimester may experience respiratory distress, apnea, cyanosis, temperature instability, vomiting, feeding difficulty, hypoglycemia, constant crying, irritability, hypotonia, hypertonia, hyper-reflexia, tremor, jitteriness, and seizures; these symptoms may be due to a direct toxic effect, withdrawal syndrome, or (in some cases) serotonin syndrome. Withdrawal symptoms occur in 30% of neonates exposed to SSRIs and SNRIs *in utero*; monitor newborns for at least 48 hours after birth; long-term effects of *in utero* exposure to SSRIs and SNRIs are unknown (Levinson-Castiel, 2006).

Dosage Forms Excipient information presented when available (limited, particularly for generics); consult specific product labeling.

Capsule Extended Release 24 Hour, Oral:

Effexor XR: 37.5 mg, 75 mg, 150 mg

Generic: 37.5 mg, 75 mg, 150 mg

Tablet, Oral:

Generic: 25 mg, 37.5 mg, 50 mg, 75 mg, 100 mg

Tablet Extended Release 24 Hour, Oral:

Generic: 37.5 mg, 75 mg, 150 mg, 225 mg

- ◆ **Venlafaxine XR (Can)** *see* Venlafaxine *on page 2166*
- ◆ **Venofer** *see* Iron Sucrose *on page 1166*
- ◆ **Ventolin Diskus (Can)** *see* Albuterol *on page 81*
- ◆ **Ventolin HFA** *see* Albuterol *on page 81*
- ◆ **Ventolin I.V. Infusion (Can)** *see* Albuterol *on page 81*
- ◆ **Ventolin Nebules P.F. (Can)** *see* Albuterol *on page 81*
- ◆ **Ventolin Respirator (Can)** *see* Albuterol *on page 81*
- ◆ **VePesid** *see* Etoposide *on page 819*
- ◆ **Vepesid (Can)** *see* Etoposide *on page 819*
- ◆ **Veramyst** *see* Fluticasone (Nasal) *on page 917*

Verapamil (ver AP a mil)

Medication Safety Issues

Sound-alike/look-alike issues:

Calan may be confused with Colace, diltiazem

Covera-HS may be confused with Covaryx HS, Provera

Isoptin may be confused with Isopto Tears

Verelan may be confused with Voltaren

High alert medication:

The Institute for Safe Medication Practices (ISMP) includes this medication (IV formulation) among its list of drug classes which have a heightened risk of causing significant patient harm when used in error.

Administration issues:

Significant differences exist between oral and IV dosing. Use caution when converting from one route of administration to another.

International issues:

Dilacor [Brazil] may be confused with Dilacor XR brand name for diltiazem [U.S.]

Related Information

Oral Medications That Should Not Be Crushed or Altered *on page 2476*

Brand Names: US Calan; Calan SR; Isoptin SR; Verelan; Verelan PM

Brand Names: Canada Apo-Verap; Apo-Verap SR; Dom-Verapamil SR; Isoptin SR; Mylan-Verapamil; Mylan-Verapamil SR; Novo-Veramil; Novo-Veramil SR; PHL-Verapamil SR; PMS-Verapamil SR; PRO-Verapamil SR; Riva-Verapamil SR; Verapamil Hydrochloride Injection, USP; Verapamil SR; Verelan

Therapeutic Category Antianginal Agent; Antiarrhythmic Agent, Class IV; Antihypertensive Agent; Calcium Channel Blocker; Calcium Channel Blocker, Nondihydropyridine

Generic Availability (US) Yes

Use

Oral: Treatment of hypertension (all oral products) (FDA approved in adults); angina pectoris (vasospastic, chronic stable, unstable) (Calan®, Covera-HS®) (FDA approved in adults); supraventricular tachyarrhythmia [PSVT (prophylaxis), atrial fibrillation/flutter (rate control)] (Calan®) (FDA approved in adults)

IV: Supraventricular tachyarrhythmia [PSVT; atrial fibrillation/flutter (rate control)] (FDA approved in all ages)

Pregnancy Risk Factor C

Pregnancy Considerations Adverse events were observed in some animal reproduction studies in doses which also caused maternal toxicity. Verapamil crosses the placenta. Use during pregnancy may cause adverse fetal effects (bradycardia, heart block, hypotension) (Tan, 2001). Women with hypertrophic cardiomyopathy who are controlled with verapamil prior to pregnancy may continue therapy, but increased fetal monitoring is recommended (Gersh, 2011). Verapamil is not the preferred treatment for paroxysmal supraventricular tachycardia (PSVT) in pregnant women (Blomström-Lundqvist, 2003). Untreated chronic maternal hypertension is associated with adverse events in the fetus, infant, and mother. If treatment for hypertension during pregnancy is needed, other agents are preferred (ACOG, 2013).

Breast-Feeding Considerations Verapamil is excreted into breast milk; the estimated exposure to the nursing infant is <1% of the maternal dose. Breast-feeding is not recommended by some manufacturers.

Contraindications Hypersensitivity to verapamil or any component of the formulation; severe left ventricular dysfunction; hypotension (systolic pressure <90 mm Hg) or cardiogenic shock; sick sinus syndrome (except in patients with a functioning artificial ventricular pacemaker); second- or third-degree AV block (except in patients with a functioning artificial ventricular pacemaker); atrial flutter or fibrillation and an accessory bypass tract (Wolff-Parkinson-White [WPW] syndrome, Lown-Ganong-Levine syndrome)

IV: Additional contraindications include concurrent use of IV beta-blocking agents; ventricular tachycardia

Warnings/Precautions Avoid use in heart failure; can exacerbate condition; use is contraindicated in severe left ventricular dysfunction. Symptomatic hypotension with or without syncope can rarely occur; blood pressure must be lowered at a rate appropriate for the patient's clinical condition. Rare increases in hepatic enzymes can be observed. Can cause first-degree AV block or sinus bradycardia; use is contraindicated in patients with sick sinus syndrome, second- or third-degree AV block (except in patients with a functioning artificial pacemaker), or an accessory bypass tract (eg, WPW syndrome). Other conduction abnormalities are rare. Considered contraindicated in patients with wide complex tachycardias unless known to be supraventricular in origin; severe hypotension likely to occur upon administration (ACLS, 2010). Use caution when using verapamil together with a beta-blocker. Administration of IV verapamil and an IV beta-blocker within a few hours of each other may result in asystole and should be avoided; simultaneous administration is contraindicated. Use with other agents known to reduce SA node function and/or AV nodal conduction (eg, digoxin) or reduce sympathetic outflow (eg, clonidine) may increase the risk of serious bradycardia. Verapamil significantly increases digoxin serum concentrations; adjust digoxin dose. Use with caution in patients with HCM with outflow tract obstruction (especially those with high gradients, advanced heart failure, or sinus bradycardia); may be used in patients who cannot tolerate beta-blockade. Verapamil should not be used in those with systemic hypotension or severe dyspnea at rest (Gersh, 2011; Nishimura, 2004).

Decreased neuromuscular transmission has been reported with verapamil; use with caution in patients with attenuated neuromuscular transmission (Duchenne's muscular dystrophy, myasthenia gravis); dosage reduction may be required. Use with caution in renal impairment; monitor hemodynamics and possibly ECG if severe impairment, particularly if concomitant hepatic impairment. Use with caution in patients with hepatic impairment; dosage reduction may be required; monitor hemodynamics and possibly ECG if severe impairment. May prolong recovery from nondepolarizing neuromuscular-blocking agents. Use Covera-HS (extended-release delivery system) with caution in patients with severe GI narrowing. In patients with extremely short GI transit times (eg, <7 hours), dosage adjustment may be required; inadequate pharmacokinetic data. In neonates and young infants, avoid IV use for SVT due to severe apnea, bradycardia, hypotensive reactions, and cardiac arrest; in children, use IV with caution as myocardial depression and hypotension may occur.

Warnings: Additional Pediatric Considerations Although effective in terminating SVT in older children, verapamil is not the drug of choice (due to adverse effects) and is not included in the current PALS tachyarrhythmia algorithm.

Adverse Reactions

Cardiovascular: AV block, bradycardia, CHF/pulmonary edema, flushing, hypotension, peripheral edema

Central nervous system: Dizziness, fatigue, headache, lethargy, pain, sleep disturbance

Dermatologic: Rash

Gastrointestinal: Constipation, diarrhea, dyspnea, gingival hyperplasia, nausea

Hepatic: Liver enzymes increased

Neuromuscular & skeletal: Myalgia, paresthesia

Respiratory: Dyspnea

Miscellaneous: Flu-like syndrome

Rare but important or life-threatening:

Oral: Abdominal discomfort, alopecia, angina, arthralgia, atrioventricular dissociation, blurred vision, bruising, cerebrovascular accident, chest pain, claudication, confusion, diaphoresis, ECG abnormal, equilibrium disorders, erythema multiforme, exanthema, extrapyramidal symptoms, galactorrhea/hyperprolactinemia, gastrointestinal distress, gynecomastia, hyperkeratosis, impotence, insomnia, macules, MI, muscle cramps, palpitation, psychosis, purpura (vasculitis), shakiness, somnolence, spotty menstruation, Stevens-Johnson syndrome, syncope, tinnitus, urination increased, urticaria, weakness, xerostomia

IV: Bronchi/laryngeal spasm, depression, diaphoresis, itching, muscle fatigue, respiratory failure, rotary nystagmus, seizure, sleepiness, urticaria, vertigo

Postmarketing and/or case reports: Asystole, eosinophilia, EPS, exfoliative dermatitis, GI obstruction, hair color change, paralytic ileus, Parkinsonian syndrome, pulseless electrical activity, shock, ventricular fibrillation

Drug Interactions

Metabolism/Transport Effects **Substrate** of CYP1A2 (minor), CYP2B6 (minor), CYP2C9 (minor), CYP2E1 (minor), CYP3A4 (major), P-glycoprotein; **Note:** Assignment of Major/Minor substrate status based on clinically relevant drug interaction potential; **Inhibits** CYP1A2 (weak), CYP2C9 (weak), CYP2D6 (weak), CYP3A4 (moderate), P-glycoprotein

Avoid Concomitant Use

Avoid concomitant use of Verapamil with any of the following: Bosutinib; Ceritinib; Conivaptan; Dantrolene; Disopyramide; Dofetilide; Domperidone; Fusidic Acid (Systemic); Ibrutinib; Idelalisib; Ivabradine; Lomitapide; Naloxegol; Olaparib; PAZOPanib; Pimozide; Silodosin; Simeprevir; Tolvaptan; Topotecan; Trabectedin; Ulipristal; VinCRIStine (Liposomal)

Increased Effect/Toxicity

Verapamil may increase the levels/effects of: Afatinib; Alcohol (Ethyl); Aliskiren; Amifostine; Amiodarone; Antihypertensives; ARIPiprazole; AtorvaSTATin; Atosiban; Avanafil; Beta-Blockers; Bosentan; Bosutinib; Bradycardia-Causing Agents; Brentuximab Vedotin; Budesonide (Systemic, Oral Inhalation); Budesonide (Topical); BusPIRone; Calcium Channel Blockers (Dihydropyridine); Cannabis; CarBAMazepine; Cardiac Glycosides; Ceritinib; Cilostazol; Colchicine; CycloSPORINE (Systemic); CYP3A4 Substrates; Dabigatran Etexilate; Dapoxetine; Disopyramide; Dofetilide; Domperidone; DOXOrubicin (Conventional); Dronabinol; Dronedarone; DULoxetine; Edoxaban; Eletriptan; Eliglustat; Eplerenone; Everolimus; FentaNYL; Fexofenadine; Fingolimod; Flecainide; Fosphenytoin; Halofantrine; Hydrocodone; Hypotensive Agents; Ibrutinib; Imatinib; Ivabradine; Ivacaftor; Lacosamide; Ledipasvir; Levodopa; Lithium; Lomitapide; Lovastatin; Lurasidone; Magnesium Salts; Midodrine; Naloxegol; Neuromuscular-Blocking Agents

(Nondepolarizing); NiMODipine; Nintedanib; Nitroprusside; Obinutuzumab; Olaparib; OxyCODONE; PAZOPanib; P-glycoprotein/ABCB1 Substrates; Phenytoin; Pimecrolimus; Pimozide; Propafenone; Prucalopride; QuiNIDine; Ranolazine; Red Yeast Rice; Rifaximin; RisperiDONE; RiTUXimab; Rivaroxaban; Salicylates; Salmeterol; Saxagliptin; Silodosin; Simeprevir; Simvastatin; Suvorexant; Tacrolimus (Systemic); Tacrolimus (Topical); Tetrahydrocannabinol; TiZANidine; Tolvaptan; Topotecan; Trabectedin; Ulipristal; Vilazodone; VinCRIStine (Liposomal); Zopiclone; Zuclopenthixol

The levels/effects of Verapamil may be increased by: Alfuzosin; Alpha1-Blockers; Anilidopiperidine Opioids; Antifungal Agents (Azole Derivatives, Systemic); Aprepitant; AtorvaSTATin; Barbiturates; Bretylium; Brimonidine (Topical); Calcium Channel Blockers (Dihydropyridine); Cimetidine; CloNIDine; Conivaptan; CycloSPORINE (Systemic); CYP3A4 Inhibitors (Moderate); CYP3A4 Inhibitors (Strong); Dantrolene; Dasatinib; Diazoxide; Dronedarone; Fluconazole; Fosaprepitant; Fusidic Acid (Systemic); Grapefruit Juice; Herbs (Hypotensive Properties); Idelalisib; Ivabradine; Luliconazole; Macrolide Antibiotics; Magnesium Salts; MAO Inhibitors; Mifepristone; Netupitant; Nicorandil; Palbociclib; Pentoxifylline; P-glycoprotein/ABCB1 Inhibitors; Phosphodiesterase 5 Inhibitors; Prostacyclin Analogues; Protease Inhibitors; QuiNIDine; Regorafenib; Ruxolitinib; Stiripentol; Telithromycin; Tofacitinib

Decreased Effect

Verapamil may decrease the levels/effects of: Clopidogrel; Ifosfamide; MetFORMIN

The levels/effects of Verapamil may be decreased by: Barbiturates; Bosentan; Calcium Salts; CarBAMazepine; CYP3A4 Inducers (Moderate); CYP3A4 Inducers (Strong); Dabrafenib; Deferasirox; Efavirenz; Herbs (Hypertensive Properties); Methylphenidate; Mitotane; Nafcillin; P-glycoprotein/ABCB1 Inducers; Rifamycin Derivatives; Siltuximab; St Johns Wort; Tocilizumab; Yohimbine

Food Interactions

Ethanol: Verapamil may increase ethanol levels. Management: Monitor patients and caution about increased effects.

Food: Grapefruit juice may increase the serum concentration of verapamil. Management: Avoid grapefruit juice or use with caution and monitor for effects.

Storage/Stability Store at controlled room temperature of 15°C to 30°C (59°F to 86°F). Protect from light.

Mechanism of Action Inhibits calcium ion from entering the "slow channels" or select voltage-sensitive areas of vascular smooth muscle and myocardium during depolarization; produces relaxation of coronary vascular smooth muscle and coronary vasodilation; increases myocardial oxygen delivery in patients with vasospastic angina; slows automaticity and conduction of AV node.

Pharmacodynamics

Maximum effect:
- Oral (nonsustained tablets): 2 hours
- IV: 1-5 minutes

Duration:
- Oral: 6-8 hours
- IV: 10-20 minutes

Pharmacokinetics (Adult data unless noted)

Absorption: Well-absorbed

Distribution: V_d: 3.89 L/kg (Storstein, 1984)

Protein binding:
- Neonates: ~60%
- Adults: ~90%

Metabolism: Extensive first-pass effect, metabolized in the liver to several inactive dealkylated metabolites; major metabolite is norverapamil which possesses weak hemodynamic effects (20% that of verapamil)

Bioavailability: Oral: 20% to 30%

Half-life:
- Infants: 4.4-6.9 hours
- Adults (single dose): 2-8 hours, increased up to 12 hours with multiple dosing
- Adults: Severe hepatic impairment: 14-16 hours

Elimination: 70% of dose excreted in urine as metabolites (3% to 4% as unchanged drug), and 16% in feces

Dialysis: Not removed by hemodialysis

Dosing: Usual

IV: **Note:** Although verapamil is effective in the treatment of SVT, it is not included in the PALS tachyarrhythmia algorithm due to its adverse effects (PALS, 2010).

Infants: **Should not be used in infants without expert consultation and is generally not recommended**; administer with continuous ECG monitoring, have IV calcium available at bedside: 0.1-0.2 mg/kg/dose (usual: 0.75-2 mg/dose) may repeat dose in 30 minutes if adequate response not achieved; **Note:** Optimal interval for subsequent doses is unknown and must be individualized for each specific patient.

Children 1-15 years: 0.1-0.3 mg/kg/dose; maximum dose: 5 mg/dose; may repeat dose in 30 minutes if adequate response not achieved; maximum for second dose: 10 mg/dose; **Note:** Optimal interval for subsequent doses is unknown and must be individualized for each specific patient.

Oral: Dose not well established:

Children: 4-8 mg/kg/day in 3 divided doses

or

1-5 years: 40-80 mg every 8 hours

>5 years: 80 mg every 6-8 hours

Note: A mean daily dose of ~5 mg/kg/day (range: 2.3-8.1 mg/kg/day) was used in 22 children 15 days to 17 years of age receiving chronic oral therapy for SVT (n=20) or hypertrophic cardiomyopathy (n=2) (Piovan, 1995).

Adults:

IV (ACLS 2010 guidelines): PSVT (narrow complex, unresponsive to vagal maneuvers and adenosine, in patients with preserved cardiac function): Initial: 2.5-5 mg; if no response in 15-30 minutes and no adverse effects seen, give 5-10 mg every 15-30 minutes to a maximum total dose of 20-30 mg

IV: Manufacturer's recommendations: 5-10 mg (0.075-0.15 mg/kg); may repeat 10 mg (0.15 mg/kg) 30 minutes after the initial dose if needed and if patient tolerated initial dose; **Note:** Optimal interval for subsequent doses is unknown and must be individualized for each specific patient.

Angina: Oral: **Note:** When switching from immediate release to extended/sustained release formulations, the total daily dose remains the same unless formulation strength does not allow for equal conversion.

Immediate release: Initial: 80-120 mg 3 times/day (small stature: 40 mg 3 times/day); usual dose range (Gibbons, 2003): 80-160 mg 3 times/day

Extended release: Covera-HS®: Initial: 180 mg once daily at bedtime; if inadequate response, may increase dose at weekly intervals to 240 mg once daily, then 360 mg once daily, then 480 mg once daily; maximum dose: 480 mg/day

Chronic atrial fibrillation (rate control), PSVT prophylaxis: Oral: Immediate release: 240-480 mg/day in 3-4 divided doses; usual dose range (European Heart Rhythm Association, 2006): 120-360 mg/day

Hypertension: Oral: **Note:** When switching from immediate release to extended/sustained release formulations, the total daily dose remains the same unless formulation strength does not allow for equal conversion.

Immediate release: 80 mg 3 times/day; usual dose range (JNC 7): 80-320 mg/day in 2 divided doses

Sustained release: Usual dose range (JNC 7): 120-480 mg/day in 1-2 divided doses; **Note:** There is no evidence of additional benefit with doses >360 mg/day.

Calan® SR, Isoptin® SR: Initial: 180 mg once daily in the morning (small stature: 120 mg/day); if inadequate response, may increase dose at weekly intervals to 240 mg once daily, then 180 mg twice daily (or 240 mg in the morning followed by 120 mg in the evening); maximum dose: 240 mg twice daily

Verelan®: Initial: 180 mg once daily in the morning (small stature: 120 mg/day); if inadequate response, may increase dose at weekly intervals to 240 mg once daily, then 360 mg once daily, then 480 mg once daily; maximum dose: 480 mg/day

Extended release: Usual dose range (JNC 7): 120-360 mg once daily (once daily dosing is recommended at bedtime)

Covera-HS®: Initial: 180 mg once daily at bedtime; if inadequate response, may increase dose at weekly intervals to 240 mg once daily, then 360 mg once daily, then 480 mg once daily; maximum dose: 480 mg/day

Verelan® PM: Initial: 200 mg once daily at bedtime (small stature: 100 mg once daily); if inadequate response, may increase dose at weekly intervals to 300 mg once daily, then 400 mg once daily; maximum dose: 400 mg/day

Dosing adjustment in renal impairment: Children and Adults: Use with caution and closely monitor ECG for PR prolongation, blood pressure, and other signs of overdose; dosage reduction may be needed. The manufacturer of Verelan® PM recommends an initial adult dose of 100 mg/day at bedtime. **Note:** A number of studies show no difference in verapamil (or norverapamil metabolite) disposition between chronic renal failure and control patients, suggesting that dosage adjustment is not required in renal impairment (Beyerlein, 1990; Hanyok, 1988; Mooy, 1985; Zachariah, 1991). However, a study in adults suggests reduced renal clearance of verapamil and its metabolite (norverapamil) with advanced renal failure (Storstein, 1984). Additionally, several clinical papers report adverse effects of verapamil in patients with chronic renal failure receiving recommended doses of verapamil (Pritza, 1991; Váquez, 1996). Thus, prudence dictates cautious use, close monitoring, and dosage adjustment if needed.

Dosing adjustment in hepatic impairment: Children and Adults: In patients with cirrhosis, reduce dose to 20% and 50% of normal dose for oral and intravenous administration, respectively; monitor blood pressure for hypotension and ECG for prolongation of PR interval (Somogyi, 1981). The manufacturer of Verelan PM® recommends an initial adult dose of 100 mg/day at bedtime. The manufacturers of Calan®, Calan® SR, Covera-HS®, Isoptin® SR, and Verelan® recommend giving 30% of the normal dose to patients with severe hepatic impairment.

Administration

Oral:

Immediate release: Can be administered with or without food.

Extended and sustained release preparations: Swallow whole; do not break, chew, or crush.

Calan SR, Isoptin SR: Administer with food; other formulations may be administered without regard to meals

Verelan, Verelan PM: Capsule may be opened and contents sprinkled on one tablespoonful of applesauce; swallow immediately, do not chew; do not store for future use; follow with water to ensure complete swallowing of capsule pellets; do not subdivide contents of capsule

Parenteral: IV: Administer undiluted dose over 2 to 3 minutes; infuse over 3 to 4 minutes if blood pressure is in the lower range of normal

Monitoring Parameters ECG, blood pressure, heart rate; hepatic enzymes with long-term use

Test Interactions May interfere with urine detection of methadone (false-positive).

Dosage Forms Excipient information presented when available (limited, particularly for generics); consult specific product labeling. [DSC] = Discontinued product

Capsule Extended Release 24 Hour, Oral, as hydrochloride:

Verelan: 120 mg [DSC]

Verelan: 120 mg [contains fd&c red #40, methylparaben, propylparaben]

Verelan: 180 mg [DSC]

Verelan: 180 mg [contains fd&c red #40, methylparaben, propylparaben]

Verelan: 240 mg [DSC]

Verelan: 240 mg [contains brilliant blue fcf (fd&c blue #1), fd&c red #40, methylparaben, propylparaben]

Verelan: 360 mg [DSC]

Verelan: 360 mg [contains brilliant blue fcf (fd&c blue #1), fd&c red #40, methylparaben, propylparaben]

Verelan PM: 100 mg [DSC]

Verelan PM: 100 mg [contains brilliant blue fcf (fd&c blue #1), fd&c red #40]

Verelan PM: 200 mg [DSC]

Verelan PM: 200 mg [contains brilliant blue fcf (fd&c blue #1), fd&c red #40]

Verelan PM: 300 mg [DSC]

Verelan PM: 300 mg [contains brilliant blue fcf (fd&c blue #1), fd&c red #40]

Generic: 100 mg, 120 mg, 180 mg, 200 mg, 240 mg, 300 mg, 360 mg

Solution, Intravenous, as hydrochloride:

Generic: 2.5 mg/mL (2 mL, 4 mL)

Tablet, Oral, as hydrochloride:

Calan: 80 mg, 120 mg [scored]

Generic: 40 mg, 80 mg, 120 mg

Tablet Extended Release, Oral, as hydrochloride:

Calan SR: 120 mg

Calan SR: 180 mg [scored]

Calan SR: 240 mg [scored; contains fd&c blue #2 aluminum lake, fd&c yellow #10 aluminum lake]

Isoptin SR: 120 mg

Isoptin SR: 180 mg [scored]

Isoptin SR: 240 mg [scored; contains fd&c blue #2 aluminum lake, fd&c yellow #10 aluminum lake]

Generic: 120 mg, 180 mg, 240 mg

Extemporaneous Preparations A 50 mg/mL oral suspension may be made with immediate release tablets and either a 1:1 mixture of Ora-Sweet and Ora-Plus or a 1:1 mixture of Ora-Sweet SF and Ora-Plus or cherry syrup. When using cherry syrup, dilute cherry syrup concentrate 1:4 with simple syrup, NF. Crush seventy-five verapamil hydrochloride 80 mg tablets in a mortar and reduce to a fine powder. Add small portions of chosen vehicle (40 mL total) and mix to a uniform paste; mix while adding the vehicle in incremental proportions to **almost** 120 mL; transfer to a calibrated bottle, rinse mortar with vehicle, and add quantity of vehicle sufficient to make 120 mL. Label "shake well", "refrigerate", and "protect from light". Stable for 60 days refrigerated (preferred) or at room temperature (Allen, 1996).

A 50 mg/mL oral suspension may be made with immediate release tablets, a 1:1 preparation of methylcellulose 1% and simple syrup, and purified water. Crush twenty 80 mg verapamil tablets in a mortar and reduce to a fine powder. Add 3 mL purified water USP and mix to a uniform paste; mix while adding the vehicle incremental proportions to **almost** 32 mL; transfer to a calibrated bottle, rinse mortar with vehicle, and add quantity of vehicle sufficient to make 32 mL. Label "shake well" and "refrigerate". Stable for 91 days refrigerated (preferred) or at room temperature (Nahata, 1997).

Allen LV Jr and Erickson MA 3rd, "Stability of Labetalol Hydrochloride, Metoprolol Tartrate, Verapamil Hydrochloride, and Spironolactone With Hydrochlorothiazide in Extemporaneously Compounded Oral Liquids," *Am J Health Syst Pharm*, 1996, 53(19):304-9.

Nahata MC, "Stability of Verapamil in an Extemporaneous Liquid Dosage Form," *J Appl Ther Res*, 1997,1(3):271-3.

◆ **Verapamil Hydrochloride** *see* Verapamil *on page 2170*

◆ **Verapamil Hydrochloride Injection, USP (Can)** *see* Verapamil *on page 2170*

◆ **Verapamil SR (Can)** *see* Verapamil *on page 2170*

◆ **Verdrocet** *see* Hydrocodone and Acetaminophen *on page 1032*

◆ **Verelan** *see* Verapamil *on page 2170*

◆ **Verelan PM** *see* Verapamil *on page 2170*

◆ **Veripred 20** *see* PrednisoLONE (Systemic) *on page 1755*

◆ **Vermox** *see* Mebendazole *on page 1333*

◆ **Versacloz** *see* CloZAPine *on page 519*

◆ **Versed** *see* Midazolam *on page 1433*

◆ **Versel® (Can)** *see* Selenium Sulfide *on page 1913*

◆ **Vertin-32 [OTC] [DSC]** *see* Meclizine *on page 1337*

◆ **Vesanoid** *see* Tretinoin (Systemic) *on page 2108*

◆ **Vfend** *see* Voriconazole *on page 2190*

◆ **VFEND (Can)** *see* Voriconazole *on page 2190*

◆ **Vfend IV** *see* Voriconazole *on page 2190*

◆ **VFEND For Injection (Can)** *see* Voriconazole *on page 2190*

◆ **Viagra** *see* Sildenafil *on page 1921*

◆ **Vibramycin** *see* Doxycycline *on page 717*

◆ **Vibra-Tabs (Can)** *see* Doxycycline *on page 717*

◆ **Vicks 44E [OTC]** *see* Guaifenesin and Dextromethorphan *on page 992*

◆ **Vicks DayQuil Mucus Control DM [OTC]** *see* Guaifenesin and Dextromethorphan *on page 992*

◆ **Vicks Nature Fusion Cough [OTC]** *see* Dextromethorphan *on page 631*

◆ **Vicks Nature Fusion Cough & Chest Congestion [OTC]** *see* Guaifenesin and Dextromethorphan *on page 992*

◆ **Vicks Pediatric Formula 44E [OTC]** *see* Guaifenesin and Dextromethorphan *on page 992*

◆ **Vicodin®** *see* Hydrocodone and Acetaminophen *on page 1032*

◆ **Vicodin ES** *see* Hydrocodone and Acetaminophen *on page 1032*

◆ **Vicodin HP** *see* Hydrocodone and Acetaminophen *on page 1032*

◆ **ViCPS** *see* Typhoid Vaccine *on page 2133*

◆ **Vidaza** *see* AzaCITIDine *on page 233*

◆ **Videx** *see* Didanosine *on page 646*

◆ **Videx EC** *see* Didanosine *on page 646*

Vigabatrin (vye GA ba trin)

Medication Safety Issues

Sound-alike/look-alike issues:

Vigabatrin may be confused with Vibativ

Related Information

Safe Handling of Hazardous Drugs *on page 2455*

Brand Names: US Sabril

Brand Names: Canada Sabril

Therapeutic Category Anticonvulsant, Miscellaneous; Infantile Spasms, Treatment

Generic Availability (US) No

Use

Monotherapy for treatment of infantile spasms in patients for whom the potential benefits outweigh the potential risk of vision loss (FDA approved in ages 1 month to 2 years)

Adjunct therapy for refractory complex partial seizures in patients with inadequate response to several alternative treatments and for whom the potential benefits outweigh the potential risk of vision loss (FDA approved in ages ≥10 years and adults)

Prescribing and Access Restrictions As a requirement of the REMS program, access to this medication is restricted. Vigabatrin is only available in the U.S. under a special restricted distribution program (SHARE). Under the SHARE program, only prescribers and pharmacies registered with the program are able to prescribe and distribute vigabatrin. Vigabatrin may only be dispensed to patients who are enrolled in and meet all conditions of SHARE. Contact the SHARE program at 1-888-45-SHARE.

Medication Guide Available Yes

Pregnancy Risk Factor C

Pregnancy Considerations Adverse events were observed in animal reproduction studies. Vigabatrin crosses the placenta in humans (Tran, 1998). Birth defects have been reported following use in pregnancy and include: cardiac defects, limb defects, male genital malformations, fetal anticonvulsant syndrome, renal and ear abnormalities. Time of exposure or maternal dosage was not reported and information is not available relating to the incidence or types of these outcomes in comparison to the general epilepsy population. Visual field examinations have been conducted following in utero exposure in a limited number of children tested at ≥6 years of age; no visual field loss was observed in 4 children and results were inconclusive in 2 others (Lawthorn, 2009; Sorri 2005). Use during pregnancy is contraindicated in Canadian product labeling.

Patients exposed to vigabatrin during pregnancy are encouraged to enroll in the North American Antiepileptic Drug (NAAED) Pregnancy Registry by calling 1-888-233-2334. Additional information is available at www.aedpregnancyregistry.org.

Breast-Feeding Considerations Small amounts of vigabatrin are found in human milk (≤4% of the weight-adjusted maternal dose based on 2 cases) (Tran, 1998). Due to the potential for serious adverse reactions in the nursing infants, the manufacturer recommends a decision be made whether to discontinue nursing or to discontinue the drug, taking into account the importance of the drug to the mother.

Use while breast-feeding is contraindicated in Canadian product labeling.

Contraindications

There are no contraindications listed in the manufacturer's labeling.

Canadian labeling: Hypersensitivity to vigabatrin or any component of the formulation; pregnancy; breast-feeding

Warnings/Precautions Hazardous agent - use appropriate precautions for handling and disposal (NIOSH 2014 [group 3]).

Use has been associated with decreased hemoglobin and hematocrit; cases of significantly reduced hemoglobin (<8 g/dL) and/or hematocrit (<24%) have been reported. Somnolence and fatigue can occur with use; patients must be cautioned about performing tasks which require mental alertness (eg, operating machinery or driving). Peripheral edema and edema independent of hypertension, heart failure, weight gain, renal or hepatic dysfunction has been reported. Patients must be closely monitored for potential neurotoxicity (observed in animal models but not established in adults). Peripheral neuropathy and manifesting as numbness or tingling in the toes or feet, reduced distal lower limb vibration or position sensation, or progressive loss of reflexes, starting at the ankles has been reported in adult patients. Pooled analysis of trials involving various antiepileptics (regardless of indication) showed an increased risk of suicidal thoughts/behavior (incidence rate: 0.43% treated patients compared to 0.24% of patients receiving placebo); risk observed as early as 1 week after initiation and continued through duration of trials (most trials ≤24 weeks). Monitor all patients for notable changes in behavior that might indicate suicidal thoughts or depression; notify healthcare provider immediately if symptoms occur. Use has been associated with an average weight gain of 3.5 kg in adults and ≥7% of baseline body weight in pediatric patients.

[U.S. Boxed Warning]: Vigabatrin causes permanent vision loss in infants, children and adults. Due to the risk of vision loss and because vigabatrin, provides an observable symptomatic benefit when it is effective, the patient who fails to show substantial clinical benefit within a short period of time after initiation of treatment (2-4 weeks for infantile spasms; <3 months for refractory complex partial seizures), should be withdrawn from therapy. If in the clinical judgment of the prescriber evidence of treatment failure becomes obvious earlier in treatment, vigabatrin should be discontinued at that time. Patient response to and continued need for treatment should be periodically assessed. The onset of vision loss is unpredictable, and can occur within weeks of starting treatment or sooner, or at any time during treatment, even after months or years. The risk of vision loss increases with increasing dose and cumulative exposure, but there is no dose or exposure known to be free of risk of vision loss. It is possible that vision loss can worsen despite discontinuation. Assessment of vision loss is difficult in children and the frequency and extent of vision loss in infants and children is poorly characterized. Most data are available in adult patients. Vigabatrin causes permanent bilateral concentric visual field constriction in >30% of patients ranging in severity from mild to severe, including tunnel vision to within 10 degrees of visual fixation, and can result in disability. In some cases, vigabatrin can damage the central retina and may decrease visual acuity. In infants and children, symptoms of vision loss are unlikely to be recognized by the parent or caregiver before loss is severe. Vision loss of milder severity, although potentially unrecognized by the parent or caregiver, may still adversely affect function. Vision should be assessed to the extent possible at baseline (no later than 4 weeks after initiation), at least every 3 months during therapy and at 3-6 months after discontinuation. Once detected, vision loss is not reversible; even with frequent monitoring, it is expected that some patients will develop severe vision loss. Vigabatrin should not be used in patients with, or at high risk of, other types of irreversible vision loss unless the benefits of treatment clearly outweigh the risks. The interaction of other types of irreversible vision damage with vision damage from vigabatrin has not been well-characterized, but is likely adverse. Vigabatrin should not be used with other drugs associated with serious adverse ophthalmic effects such as retinopathy or glaucoma unless the benefits clearly outweigh the risks. The lowest dose and shortest exposure should be used that is consistent with clinical objectives. The possibility that vision loss from vigabatrin may be more common, more severe or have more severe functional consequences in infants and children than in adults cannot be excluded.

Use with caution in patients with a history of psychosis (psychotic/agitated reactions may occur more frequently), depression, or behavioral problems. Use with caution in patients with renal impairment; modify dose children (≥10 years) and adults with in renal impairment (CrCl <80 mL/minute). May cause an increase in seizure frequency in some patients; use with particular caution in patients with myoclonic seizures, which may be more prone to this effect. Potentially significant drug-drug interactions may exist, requiring dose or frequency adjustment, additional monitoring, and/or selection of alternative therapy. Effects with other sedative drugs or ethanol may be potentiated. Use with caution in the elderly as severe sedation and confusion have been reported; consider dose and/or frequency adjustments as renal clearance may be decreased.

Abnormal MRI changes have been reported in some infants. Resolution of MRI changes usually occurs with discontinuation of therapy. MRI changes were not seen in older children and adult patients. **[U.S. Boxed Warning]: Because of the risk of permanent vision loss, vigabatrin is only available through a restricted distribution program (SHARE) under a Risk Evaluation and Mitigation Strategy (REMS) program. Under the SHARE program, only prescribers and pharmacies registered with the program are able to prescribe and distribute vigabatrin. Vigabatrin may only be dispensed to patients who are enrolled in and meet all conditions of SHARE. Call 888-45-SHARE or visit http://sabril.net/ for further information.** Anticonvulsants should not be discontinued abruptly because of the possibility of increasing seizure frequency; therapy should be withdrawn gradually to minimize the potential of increased seizure frequency, unless safety concerns require a more rapid withdrawal. Vigabatrin is not indicated as a first-line agent for complex partial seizures.

Warnings: Additional Pediatric Considerations Dose dependent, asymptomatic MRI abnormalities have been reported in infants treated with vigabatrin for infantile spasms; resolution of abnormalities generally occurs upon vigabatrin discontinuation; abnormalities resolved in a few infants, despite continued use; some infants displayed coincident motor abnormalities, but no causal relationship has been established; risk for long-term clinical sequelae has not been studied. Animal models have shown intramyelinic edema in the brain; current evidence suggests that this does not occur in humans; however, patients should be monitored for neurotoxicity. A relationship between MRI abnormalities in infants and animal model findings has not been established. Somnolence and fatigue occurs at a higher incidence in infants compared to adults (infants: ≤45%; adults: ≤24%). May cause fever; higher incidence reported in infants than adults (≤30% vs 6%). May cause vomiting; higher incidence in infants (up to 20%). Infants may experience a higher frequency of other adverse effects than adults, including vomiting and upper respiratory tract infections.

Adverse Reactions

Cardiovascular: Edema, peripheral edema

Central nervous system: Abnormal behavior, abnormal thinking, aggression, anxiety, confusion, coordination impaired, depression, disturbance in attention, dizziness, fatigue, fever, headache, hypoesthesia, hypotonia, insomnia, irritability, lethargy, memory impairment, postictal state, sedation, seizure, sensory disturbance, somnolence, status epilepticus, vertigo

Dermatologic: Contusion, rash

Endocrine & metabolic: Dysmenorrhea, fluid retention

Gastrointestinal: Abdominal distention, abdominal pain, appetite decreased/increased, constipation, diarrhea, dyspepsia, hemorrhoidal symptoms, nausea, viral gastroenteritis, vomiting, weight gain

Genitourinary: Urinary tract infection

Neuromuscular & skeletal: Arthralgia, back pain, dysarthria, extremity pain, hyper-reflexia, hyporeflexia, joint swelling, muscle spasms, myalgia, paresthesia, shoulder pain, tremor, weakness

Ocular: Blurred vision, conjunctivitis, diplopia, eye strain, nystagmus, strabismus, visual field constriction

Otic: Otitis media, tinnitus

Respiratory: Bronchitis, cough, dyspnea, nasal congestion, pharyngitis, pharyngolaryngeal pain, pneumonia, sinus headache, sinusitis, upper respiratory tract infection

Miscellaneous: Candidiasis, croup, influenza, thirst, viral infection

Rare but important or life-threatening: Acute psychosis, angioedema, cholestasis, deafness, delayed puberty, delirium, encephalopathy, facial edema, gastrointestinal hemorrhage, hypomania, laryngoedema, malignant hyperthermia, multiorgan failure, optic neuritis, pruritus, psychotic disorder, pulmonary embolism, respiratory failure, Stevens-Johnson syndrome, toxic epidermal necrolysis

Drug Interactions

Metabolism/Transport Effects **Induces** CYP2C9 (weak/moderate)

Avoid Concomitant Use

Avoid concomitant use of Vigabatrin with any of the following: Azelastine (Nasal); Orphenadrine; Paraldehyde; Thalidomide

Increased Effect/Toxicity

Vigabatrin may increase the levels/effects of: Alcohol (Ethyl); Azelastine (Nasal); Buprenorphine; ClonazePAM; CNS Depressants; Hydrocodone; Methotrimeprazine; Metyrosine; Mirtazapine; Orphenadrine; Paraldehyde; Pramipexole; ROPINIRole; Rotigotine; Selective Serotonin Reuptake Inhibitors; Suvorexant; Thalidomide; Zolpidem

The levels/effects of Vigabatrin may be increased by: Brimonidine (Topical); Cannabis; Doxylamine; Dronabinol; Droperidol; HydrOXYzine; Kava Kava; Magnesium Sulfate; Methotrimeprazine; Nabilone; Perampanel; Rufinamide; Sodium Oxybate; Tapentadol; Tetrahydrocannabinol

Decreased Effect

Vigabatrin may decrease the levels/effects of: Fosphenytoin; Phenytoin

The levels/effects of Vigabatrin may be decreased by: Mefloquine; Mianserin; Orlistat

Storage/Stability Store at 20°C to 25°C (68°F to 77°F).

Mechanism of Action Irreversibly inhibits gamma-aminobutyric acid transaminase (GABA-T), increasing the levels of the inhibitory compound gamma amino butyric acid (GABA) within the brain. Duration of effect is dependent upon rate of GABA-T resynthesis.

Pharmacodynamics Note: A correlation between serum concentrations and efficacy has not been established.

Duration of action: Variable; dependent on rate of GABA-T resynthesis

Pharmacokinetics (Adult data unless noted)

Absorption: Rapid, complete

Distribution: V_{dss}: 1.1 L/kg

Protein binding: Does not bind to plasma proteins

Metabolism: Minimal

Bioavailability: Oral: Tablet and oral solution are bioequivalent

Half-life: Prolonged in renal impairment

Infants and Children 5 months to 2 years: 5.7 hours

Children 10 to 16 years: 9.5 hours

Adults: 10.5 hours

Time to peak serum concentration:

Infants and Children 5 months to 2 years: 2.5 hours

Children 10 to 16 years and Adults: 1 hour

Note: Under fed conditions, T_{max} delayed by 2 hours and the maximum serum concentration decreased by 33%; the AUC remained unchanged.

Elimination: Urine (80% as unchanged drug)

Clearance:

Infants: 2.4 ± 0.8 L/hour

Children: 5.7 ± 2.5 L/hour

Adults: 7 L/hour

Dosing: Usual

Pediatric:

Infantile spasms: Infants and Children 1 month to 2 years of age: Oral: Powder for oral solution: Initial: 50 mg/kg/day divided twice daily; may titrate upwards by 25 to 50 mg/kg/day increments every 3 days based on response and tolerability; maximum daily dose: 150 mg/kg/**day** divided twice daily; **Note:** To taper, decrease dose by 25 to 50 mg/kg/day every 3 to 4 days.

Refractory complex partial seizures; adjunctive treatment: Oral:

Manufacturer's labeling: Children ≥10 years and Adolescents: Dose dependent upon weight and/or age.

Patient weight 25 to 60 kg and age 10 to 16 years: Initial: 250 mg twice daily; increase daily dose at weekly intervals based on response and tolerability. Recommended maintenance dose: 1000 mg twice daily; **Note**: To taper, decrease daily dose by one-third every week for 3 weeks.

Patient weight >60 kg (regardless of age), or age >16 years (regardless of weight): Initial: 500 mg twice daily; increase daily dose in 500 mg increments at weekly intervals based on response and tolerability. Recommended dose: 1500 mg twice daily. **Note:** To taper, decrease dose by 1000 mg daily on a weekly basis.

Alternate dosing: Limited data available: Children weighing ≥10 **kg** and Adolescents ≤16 years: Initial: 40 mg/kg/day divided twice daily; maintenance dosages based on patient weight (Camposano, 2008; Coppola, 2004; Sabril prescribing information (Canada), 2012; Willmore, 2009):

10 to 15 kg: 500 to 1000 mg/day divided twice daily

16 to 30 kg: 1000 to 1500 mg/day divided twice daily

31 to 50 kg: 1500 to 3000 mg/day divided twice daily

>50 kg: 2000 to 3000 mg/day divided twice daily

Adult: **Refractory complex partial seizures; adjunctive treatment:** Oral: Initial: 500 mg twice daily; increase daily dose by 500 mg increments at weekly intervals based on response and tolerability; recommended maintenance dose: 1500 mg twice daily; **Note:**To taper, decrease dose by 1000 mg/day on a weekly basis.

Dosing adjustment in renal impairment:

Infants and Children ≤2 years: There are no dosage adjustment provided in U.S. manufacturer's labeling; data is not available; vigabatrin is primarily eliminated through the kidney; use with caution; consider dosage reduction in patients with any degree of renal impairment (Sabril prescribing information [Canada], 2012)

Children >2 to <10 years: Limited data available: patients with any degree of renal impairment should have dosage reduction (Sabril prescribing information [Canada], 2012)

Children ≥10 years, Adolescents, and Adults: **Note:** Manufacturer recommends estimating renal function using the Schwartz equation (children 10 to <12 years) and the Cockcroft-Gault formula (children ≥12 years, adolescents, and adults)

CrCl >80 mL/minute: No dosage adjustment necessary

CrCl >50 to 80 mL/minute: Decrease dose by 25%

CrCl >30 to 50 mL/minute: Decrease dose by 50%

CrCl >10 to 30 mL/minute: Decrease dose by 75%

Hemodialysis: Reduces vigabatrin plasma concentration by 40 to 60%.

Dosing adjustment in hepatic impairment: There are no dosage adjustment provided in manufacturer's labeling; has not been studied; however, does not undergo appreciable hepatic metabolism.

Preparation for Administration Hazardous agent; use appropriate precautions for handling and disposal (NIOSH 2014 [group 3]).

Powder for oral solution: Dissolve each 500 mg powder packet in 10 mL (may use provided syringe to measure) of cold or room temperature water to make a 50 mg/mL solution; discard solution if it is not clear (or free of particles) and colorless

Administration Hazardous agent; use appropriate precautions for handling and disposal (NIOSH 2014 [group 3]).

Oral: May be administered without regard to food.

Powder for oral solution: Reconstitute powder packet prior to administration. The appropriate dose aliquot should be administered immediately after reconstitution; may use provided oral syringe. Any remaining liquid should be discarded.

Monitoring Parameters Ophthalmologic examination by an ophthalmic professional with expertise in visual field interpretation and the ability to perform dilated indirect ophthalmoscopy of the retina at baseline (no later than 4 weeks after therapy initiation), periodically during therapy (every 3 months), and 3-6 months after discontinuation of therapy; assessment should include visual acuity and visual field whenever possible including mydriatic peripheral fundus examination and visual field perimetry. Observe patient for excessive sedation, especially when instituting or increasing therapy; frequency, duration, and severity of seizure episodes; hemoglobin and hematocrit; renal function; weight; signs and symptoms of suicidality (eg, anxiety, depression, behavior changes), neurotoxicity, peripheral neuropathy, and edema.

Reference Range A correlation between serum concentrations and efficacy has not been established.

Test Interactions Vigabatrin has been reported to decrease AST and ALT activity in the plasma in up to 90% of patients, causing the enzymes to become undetectable in some patients; this may preclude use of AST and ALT as markers for hepatic injury. Vigabatrin may increase amino acids in the urine leading to false-positive tests for rare genetic metabolic disorders

Dosage Forms Excipient information presented when available (limited, particularly for generics); consult specific product labeling.

Packet, Oral:

Sabril: 500 mg (50 ea)

Tablet, Oral:

Sabril: 500 mg [scored]

◆ **Vigamox** *see* Moxifloxacin (Ophthalmic) *on page 1470*

◆ **Vimizim** *see* Elosulfase Alfa *on page 738*

◆ **Vimpat** *see* Lacosamide *on page 1200*

VinBLAStine (vin BLAS teen)

Medication Safety Issues

Sound-alike/look-alike issues:

VinBLAStine may be confused with vinCRIStine, vinorelbine

High alert medication:

This medication is in a class the Institute for Safe Medication Practices (ISMP) includes among its list of drug classes which have a heightened risk of causing significant patient harm when used in error.

Administration issues:

For IV use only. Fatal if administered by other routes. To prevent fatal inadvertent intrathecal injection, it is strongly recommended that vinblastine doses be dispensed in a small minibag (25 to 50 mL of a compatible solution), and **NOT** a syringe (ISMP, 2014). Vinblastine should **NOT** be prepared during the preparation of any intrathecal medications. After preparation, keep vinblastine in a location **away** from the separate storage location recommended for intrathecal medications. Vinblastine should **NOT** be delivered to the patient at the same time with any medications intended for central nervous system administration.

Related Information

Management of Drug Extravasations *on page 2298*

Prevention of Chemotherapy-Induced Nausea and Vomiting in Children *on page 2368*

Safe Handling of Hazardous Drugs *on page 2455*

Brand Names: Canada Vinblastine Sulphate Injection

Therapeutic Category Antineoplastic Agent, Antimicrotubular; Antineoplastic Agent, Mitotic Inhibitor; Antineoplastic Agent, Vinca Alkaloid

Generic Availability (US) Yes

Use Treatment of Hodgkin lymphoma, lymphocytic lymphoma, histiocytic lymphoma, testicular germinal-cell cancers, Langerhans cell histiocytosis (histiocytosis X; Letterer-Siwe disease), choriocarcinoma, breast cancer (refractory/resistant), mycosis fungoides, and Kaposi's sarcoma (All indications: FDA approved in pediatrics [age not specified] and adults)

Pregnancy Risk Factor D

Pregnancy Considerations Adverse effects were observed in animal reproduction studies. May cause fetal harm if administered during pregnancy. Women of childbearing potential should avoid becoming pregnant during vinblastine treatment. Aspermia has been reported in males who have received treatment with vinblastine.

Breast-Feeding Considerations It is not known if vinblastine is excreted in breast milk. Due to the potential for serious adverse reactions in the nursing infant, a decision should be made whether to discontinue vinblastine or to discontinue breast-feeding, taking into account the importance of treatment to the mother.

Contraindications Significant granulocytopenia (unless as a result of condition being treated); presence of bacterial infection

Warnings/Precautions Hazardous agent - use appropriate precautions for handling and disposal (NIOSH 2014 [group 1]). Avoid eye contamination (exposure may cause severe irritation). **[U.S. Boxed Warning]: For IV use only. Intrathecal administration may result in death.** To prevent administration errors, the Institute for Safe Medication Practices (ISMP) Targeted Medication Safety Best Practices for Hospitals initiative strongly recommends dispensing vinblastine diluted in a minibag (ISMP, 2014). **If not dispensed in a minibag, affix an auxiliary label stating "For intravenous use only - fatal if given by other routes" and also place in an overwrap labeled "Do not remove covering until moment of injection."** Vinblastine should **NOT** be prepared during the preparation of any intrathecal medications. After preparation, keep vinblastine in a location **away** from the separate storage location recommended for intrathecal medications. Vinblastine should **NOT** be delivered to the patient at the same time with any medications intended for central nervous system administration.

[U.S. Boxed Warning]: Vinblastine is a vesicant; ensure proper needle or catheter placement prior to and during infusion. Avoid extravasation. Extravasation may cause significant irritation. Individuals

administering should be experienced in vinblastine administration. If extravasation occurs, discontinue immediately and initiate appropriate extravasation management, including local injection of hyaluronidase and moderate heat application to the affected area. Use a separate vein to complete administration.

Leukopenia commonly occurs; granulocytopenia may be severe with higher doses. The leukocyte nadir generally occurs 5 to 10 days after administration; recovery typically occurs 7 to 14 days later. Monitor for infections if WBC <2,000/mm^3. Leukopenia may be more pronounced in cachectic patients and patients with skin ulceration and may be less pronounced with lower doses used for maintenance therapy. Leukocytes and platelets may fall considerably with moderate doses when marrow is infiltrated with malignant cells (further use in this situation is not recommended). Thrombocytopenia and anemia may occur rarely.

May rarely cause disabling neurotoxicity; usually reversible. Seizures and severe and permanent CNS damage has occurred with higher then recommended doses and/or when administered more frequently than recommended. Acute shortness of breath and severe bronchospasm have been reported, most often in association with concurrent administration of mitomycin; may occur within minutes to several hours following vinblastine administration or up to 14 days following mitomycin administration; use caution in patients with preexisting pulmonary disease. Use with caution in patients with hepatic impairment; toxicity may be increased; may require dosage modification. Use with caution in patients with ischemic heart disease. Stomatitis may occur (rare); may be disabling, but is usually reversible.

Potentially significant drug-drug interactions may exist, requiring dose or frequency adjustment, additional monitoring, and/or selection of alternative therapy. **[U.S. Boxed Warning]: Should be administered under the supervision of an experienced cancer chemotherapy physician.**

Benzyl alcohol and derivatives: Some dosage forms may contain benzyl alcohol; large amounts of benzyl alcohol (≥99 mg/kg/day) have been associated with a potentially fatal toxicity ("gasping syndrome") in neonates; the "gasping syndrome" consists of metabolic acidosis, respiratory distress, gasping respirations, CNS dysfunction (including convulsions, intracranial hemorrhage), hypotension, and cardiovascular collapse (AAP, 1997; CDC, 1982); some data suggests that benzoate displaces bilirubin from protein binding sites (Ahlfors, 2001); avoid or use dosage forms containing benzyl alcohol with caution in neonates. See manufacturer's labeling.

Adverse Reactions

Common:

Cardiovascular: Hypertension
Central nervous system: Malaise
Dermatologic: Alopecia
Gastrointestinal: Constipation
Hematologic: Myelosuppression, leukopenia/granulocytopenia (nadir: 5-10 days; recovery: 7-14 days; dose-limiting toxicity)
Neuromuscular & skeletal: Bone pain, jaw pain, tumor pain

Less common:

Cardiovascular: Angina, cerebrovascular accident, coronary ischemia, ECG abnormalities, limb ischemia, MI, myocardial ischemia, Raynaud's phenomenon
Central nervous system: Depression, dizziness, headache, neurotoxicity (duration: >24 hours), seizure, vertigo
Dermatologic: Dermatitis, photosensitivity (rare), rash, skin blistering
Endocrine & metabolic: Aspermia, hyperuricemia, SIADH
Gastrointestinal: Abdominal pain, anorexia, diarrhea, gastrointestinal bleeding, hemorrhagic enterocolitis, ileus, metallic taste, nausea (mild), paralytic ileus, rectal bleeding, stomatitis, toxic megacolon, vomiting (mild)
Genitourinary: Urinary retention
Hematologic: Anemia, thrombocytopenia (recovery within a few days), thrombotic thrombocytopenic purpura
Local: Cellulitis (with extravasation), irritation, phlebitis (with extravasation), radiation recall
Neuromuscular & skeletal: Deep tendon reflex loss, myalgia, paresthesia, peripheral neuritis, weakness
Ocular: Nystagmus
Otic: Auditory damage, deafness, vestibular damage
Renal: Hemolytic uremic syndrome
Respiratory: Bronchospasm, dyspnea, pharyngitis

Drug Interactions

Metabolism/Transport Effects **Substrate** of CYP2D6 (minor), CYP3A4 (major), P-glycoprotein; **Note:** Assignment of Major/Minor substrate status based on clinically relevant drug interaction potential; **Inhibits** CYP2D6 (weak); **Induces** P-glycoprotein

Avoid Concomitant Use

Avoid concomitant use of VinBLAStine with any of the following: BCG; BCG (Intravesical); CloZAPine; Conivaptan; Dabigatran Etexilate; Dipyrone; Fusidic Acid (Systemic); Idelalisib; Ledipasvir; Natalizumab; Pimecrolimus; Sofosbuvir; Tacrolimus (Topical); Tofacitinib; Vaccines (Live); VinCRIStine (Liposomal)

Increased Effect/Toxicity

VinBLAStine may increase the levels/effects of: ARIPiprazole; CloZAPine; Leflunomide; MitoMYcin (Systemic); Natalizumab; Tofacitinib; Tolterodine; Vaccines (Live)

The levels/effects of VinBLAStine may be increased by: Aprepitant; Conivaptan; CYP3A4 Inhibitors (Moderate); CYP3A4 Inhibitors (Strong); Dasatinib; Denosumab; Dipyrone; Fosaprepitant; Fusidic Acid (Systemic); Idelalisib; Itraconazole; Ivacaftor; Lopinavir; Luliconazole; Macrolide Antibiotics; MAO Inhibitors; Mifepristone; Netupitant; Palbociclib; P-glycoprotein/ABCB1 Inhibitors; Pimecrolimus; Posaconazole; Ritonavir; Roflumilast; Simeprevir; Stiripentol; Tacrolimus (Topical); Trastuzumab; Voriconazole

Decreased Effect

VinBLAStine may decrease the levels/effects of: Afatinib; BCG; BCG (Intravesical); Brentuximab Vedotin; Coccidioides immitis Skin Test; Dabigatran Etexilate; DOXOrubicin (Conventional); Ledipasvir; Linagliptin; P-glycoprotein/ABCB1 Substrates; Sipuleucel-T; Sofosbuvir; Vaccines (Inactivated); Vaccines (Live); VinCRIStine (Liposomal)

The levels/effects of VinBLAStine may be decreased by: Bosentan; CYP3A4 Inducers (Moderate); CYP3A4 Inducers (Strong); Dabrafenib; Deferasirox; Echinacea; Mitotane; P-glycoprotein/ABCB1 Inducers; Siltuximab; St Johns Wort; Tocilizumab

Storage/Stability Note: Dispense in an overwrap which bears the statement "Do not remove covering until the moment of injection. Fatal if given intrathecally. For IV use only." If dispensing in a syringe (minibag is preferred) should be labeled: "Fatal if given intrathecally. For IV use only."

Store intact vials under refrigeration at 2°C to 8°C (36°F to 46°F). Protect from light.

Mechanism of Action Vinblastine binds to tubulin and inhibits microtubule formation, therefore, arresting the cell at metaphase by disrupting the formation of the mitotic spindle; it is specific for the M and S phases. Vinblastine may also interfere with nucleic acid and protein synthesis by blocking glutamic acid utilization.

Pharmacokinetics (Adult data unless noted)
Metabolism: Hepatic (via CYP3A4) to an active metabolite
Half-life, terminal: 24.8 hours
Elimination: Feces (10%); urine (14%)

Dosing: Usual Note: Dosing and frequency may vary by indication, protocol, and/or treatment phase and hematologic response; refer to specific protocol. **For IV use only.** In order to prevent inadvertent intrathecal administration, the Institute for Safe Medication Practices (ISMP) strongly recommends dispensing vinblastine in a minibag (**NOT** a syringe).

Pediatric:

Hodgkin lymphoma: Infants, Children, and Adolescents: IV:

Manufacturer's labeling: Initial dose: 6 mg/m²/dose; do not administer more frequently than every 7 days

ABVD regimen: 6 mg/m²/dose administered on days 1 and 15 of a 28 day cycle in combination with doxorubicin, bleomycin, and darcarbazine (Hutchinson, 1989)

ChlVPP regimen: 6 mg/m²/dose administered on days 1 and 8 of a 28 day cycle in combination with chlorambucil, procarbazine, and prednisolone; minimum reported age: 7 months (Atra, 2002; Capra, 2007; Hall, 2007; Stoneham, 2007)

Langerhans cell histiocytosis; multisystem (Letterer-Siwe disease; Histiocytosis X): Infants, Children, and Adolescents: IV:

Manufacturer's labeling: Initial dose: 6.5 mg/m²/dose; do not administer more frequently than every 7 days

Alternate dosing: Limited data available: Induction: 6 mg/m²/dose every 7 days in combination with prednisone for 6 to 12 weeks depending upon clinical response; then begin maintenance therapy of 6 mg/m²/dose every 3 weeks in combination with prednisone, continue for a total duration of vinblastine therapy of 12 months (Gadner, 2013; Haupt, 2013)

Germ cell tumors; extracranial (eg, testicular, ovarian, mediastinal): Infants, Children, and Adolescents: IV: Initial dose: 3 mg/m²/dose; per the manufacturer, do not administer more frequently than every 7 days; however, in some trials, a single dose was used (Lopes, 2009) and others used a daily dose of vinblastine administered over 1 hour for 2 days (Göbel, 2001; Schneider, 2000)

Adult: **Hodgkin lymphoma, lymphocytic lymphoma, histiocytic lymphoma, mycosis fungoides, testicular cancer, Kaposi sarcoma, histiocytosis X (Letterer-Siwe disease):** IV: Initial: 3.7 mg/m²; adjust dose every 7 days (based on white blood cell response) up to 5.5 mg/m² (second dose); 7.4 mg/m² (third dose); 9.25 mg/m² (fourth dose); and 11.1 mg/m² (fifth dose); do not administer more frequently than every 7 days. Usual dosage range: 5.5 to 7.4 mg/m² every 7 days; maximum dose: 18.5 mg/m²; dosage adjustment goal is to reduce white blood cell count to ~3,000/mm³

Dosing adjustment in renal impairment: No dosage adjustment necessary.

Dosing adjustment in hepatic impairment: All patients: The manufacturer's labeling recommends the following adjustment: Serum bilirubin >3 mg/dL: Administer 50% of dose

The following adjustments have also been recommended (Floyd, 2006; Superfin, 2007):

Serum bilirubin 1.5 to 3 mg/dL or transaminases 2 to 3 times ULN: Administer 50% of dose

Serum bilirubin >3 times ULN: Avoid use.

Preparation for Administration Hazardous agent; use appropriate precautions for handling and disposal (NIOSH 2014 [group 1]).

IV infusion: May dilute dose in 25 to 50 mL NS or D_5W; dilution in larger volumes (≥100 mL) of IV fluids is not recommended as this may increase the risk of vein irritation and extravasation. **In order to prevent inadvertent intrathecal administration, the Institute for Safe Medication Practices (ISMP) strongly recommends dispensing vinblastine in a minibag (NOT in a syringe)** (ISMP 2014). Vinblastine should **NOT** be prepared during the preparation of any intrathecal medications. If dispensing vinblastine in a syringe, affix an auxiliary label stating "For intravenous use only - fatal if given by other routes" to the syringe, and the syringe must also be packaged in the manufacturer-provided overwrap which bears the statement "Do not remove covering until the moment of injection. For intravenous use only. Fatal if given intrathecally." After preparation, keep vinblastine in a location away from the separate storage location recommended for intrathecal medications. Vinblastine should **NOT** be delivered to the patient at the same time with any medications intended for central nervous system administration.

Administration Hazardous agent; use appropriate precautions for handling and disposal (NIOSH 2014 [group 1]). **In order to prevent inadvertent intrathecal administration, the Institute for Safe Medication Practices (ISMP) strongly recommends dispensing vinblastine in a minibag (NOT in a syringe).**

IV infusion: For IV administration only. **Fatal if given intrathecally.** The preferred administration is as a short infusion in a minibag. If administration via a minibag is not possible, vinblastine may also be administered undiluted (1 mg/mL) over 1 minute into a free flowing IV line to prevent venous irritation/extravasation. Prolonged administration times (≥30 to 60 minutes) and/or increased administration volumes may increase the risk of vein irritation and extravasation.

Vesicant; ensure proper needle or catheter placement prior to and during infusion. Avoid extravasation. If extravasation occurs, stop infusion immediately and disconnect (leave cannula/needle in place); gently aspirate extravasated solution (do **NOT** flush the line); initiate hyaluronidase antidote (see Management of Drug Extravasations for more details); remove needle/cannula; apply dry warm compresses for 20 minutes 4 times a day for 1 to 2 days; elevate extremity (Pérez Fidalgo 2012). Remaining portion of the vinblastine dose should be infused through a separate vein.

Vesicant/Extravasation Risk Vesicant

Monitoring Parameters CBC with differential and platelet count, serum uric acid, hepatic function tests

Dosage Forms Excipient information presented when available (limited, particularly for generics); consult specific product labeling.

Solution, Intravenous, as sulfate:
Generic: 1 mg/mL (10 mL)

Solution Reconstituted, Intravenous, as sulfate:
Generic: 10 mg (1 ea)

◆ **Vinblastine Sulfate** *see* VinBLAStine *on page 2177*

◆ **Vinblastine Sulphate Injection (Can)** *see* VinBLAStine *on page 2177*

◆ **Vincaleukoblastine** *see* VinBLAStine *on page 2177*

◆ **Vincasar PFS** *see* VinCRIStine *on page 2179*

VinCRIStine (vin KRIS teen)

Medication Safety Issues

Sound-alike/look-alike issues:

VinCRIStine may be confused with vinBLAStine, vinorelbine

VinCRIStine conventional may be confused with vinCRIStine liposomal

Oncovin may be confused with Ancobon

High alert medication:

This medication is in a class the Institute for Safe Medication Practices (ISMP) includes among its list of drug classes which have a heightened risk of causing significant patient harm when used in error.

BEERS Criteria medication:

This drug may be potentially inappropriate for use in geriatric patients (Quality of evidence - moderate; Strength of recommendation - strong).

Administration issues:

For IV use only. Fatal if administered by other routes. To prevent fatal inadvertent intrathecal injection, it is strongly recommended that vincristine doses be dispensed in a small minibag (25 to 50 mL of a compatible solution), and **NOT** a syringe (ISMP, 2014). Vincristine should **NOT** be prepared during the preparation of any intrathecal medications. After preparation, keep vincristine in a location **away** from the separate storage location recommended for intrathecal medications. Vincristine should **NOT** be delivered to the patient at the same time with any medications intended for central nervous system administration.

Related Information

Management of Drug Extravasations *on page 2298*

Prevention of Chemotherapy-Induced Nausea and Vomiting in Children *on page 2368*

Safe Handling of Hazardous Drugs *on page 2455*

Brand Names: US Vincasar PFS

Brand Names: Canada Vincristine Sulfate Injection; Vincristine Sulfate Injection USP

Therapeutic Category Antineoplastic Agent, Antimicrotubular; Antineoplastic Agent, Mitotic Inhibitor; Antineoplastic Agent, Vinca Alkaloid

Generic Availability (US) Yes

Use Treatment of acute lymphocytic leukemia (ALL), Hodgkin lymphoma, neuroblastoma, non-Hodgkin lymphomas, Wilms' tumor, and rhabdomyosarcoma [FDA approved in pediatrics (age not specified) and adults]; has also been used in the treatment of central nervous system tumors, chronic lymphocytic leukemia (CLL), Ewing's sarcoma, gestational trophoblastic tumors (high-risk), multiple myeloma, retinoblastoma, and small cell lung cancer

Pregnancy Risk Factor D

Pregnancy Considerations Animal reproduction studies have demonstrated teratogenicity and fetal loss. May cause fetal harm if administered during pregnancy. Women of childbearing potential should avoid becoming pregnant during treatment.

Breast-Feeding Considerations It is not known if vincristine is excreted in breast milk. Due to the potential for serious adverse reactions in the nursing infant, the decision to discontinue vincristine or to discontinue breastfeeding should take into account the benefits of treatment to the mother.

Contraindications Patients with the demyelinating form of Charcot-Marie-Tooth syndrome

Warnings/Precautions Hazardous agent - use appropriate precautions for handling and disposal (NIOSH 2014 [group 1]); avoid eye contamination.

[U.S. Boxed Warning]: For IV administration only; inadvertent intrathecal administration usually results in death. To prevent administration errors, the Institute for Safe Medication Practices (ISMP) Targeted Medication Safety Best Practices for Hospitals initiative and the World Health Organization strongly recommend dispensing vincristine diluted in a minibag (ISMP, 2014; WHO, 2007), **if not dispensed in a minibag, affix an auxiliary label stating "For intravenous use only - fatal if given by other routes" and also place in an overwrap labeled "Do not remove covering until moment of injection."** Vincristine should **NOT** be prepared during the preparation of any intrathecal medications. After preparation, keep vincristine in a location **away** from the separate storage location recommended for intrathecal medications. Vincristine should **NOT** be delivered to the patient at the same time with any medications intended for central nervous system administration.

[U.S. Boxed Warning]: Vincristine is a vesicant; ensure proper needle or catheter placement prior to and during infusion. Avoid extravasation. Individuals administering should be experienced in vincristine administration. Extravasation may cause significant irritation. If extravasation occurs, discontinue immediately and initiate appropriate extravasation management, including local injection of hyaluronidase and moderate heat application to the affected area. Use a separate vein to complete administration.

Neurotoxicity, including alterations in mental status such as depression, confusion, or insomnia may occur; neurologic effects are dose-limiting (may require dosage reduction) and may be additive with those of other neurotoxic agents and spinal cord irradiation. Use with caution in patients with preexisting neuromuscular disease and/or with concomitant neurotoxic agents. Constipation, paralytic ileus, intestinal necrosis and/or perforation may occur; constipation may present as upper colon impaction with an empty rectum (may require flat film of abdomen for diagnosis); generally responds to high enemas and laxatives. All patients should be on a prophylactic bowel management regimen.

Potentially significant drug-drug interactions may exist, requiring dose or frequency adjustment, additional monitoring, and/or selection of alternative therapy. Acute shortness of breath and severe bronchospasm have been reported with vinca alkaloids, usually when used in combination with mitomycin. Onset may be several minutes to hours after vincristine administration and up to 2 weeks after mitomycin. Progressive dyspnea may occur. Permanently discontinue vincristine if pulmonary dysfunction occurs.

Use with caution in patients with hepatic impairment; dosage modification required. May be associated with hepatic sinusoidal obstruction syndrome (SOS; formerly called veno-occlusive disease), increased risk in children <3 years of age; use with caution in hepatobiliary dysfunction. Monitor for signs or symptoms of hepatic SOS, including bilirubin >1.4 mg/dL, unexplained weight gain, ascites, hepatomegaly, or unexplained right upper quadrant pain (Arndt, 2004). Acute uric acid nephropathy has been reported with vincristine. Use with caution in the elderly; may cause or exacerbate syndrome of inappropriate antidiuretic hormone secretion or hyponatremia; monitor sodium closely with initiation or dosage adjustments in older adults (Beers Criteria).

Adverse Reactions

Cardiovascular: Edema, hyper-/hypotension, MI, myocardial ischemia

Central nervous system: Ataxia, coma, cranial nerve dysfunction (auditory damage, extraocular muscle impairment, laryngeal muscle impairment, paralysis, paresis, vestibular damage, vocal cord paralysis), dizziness, fever, headache, neurotoxicity (dose-related), neuropathic pain (common), seizure, vertigo

Dermatologic toxicity: Alopecia (common), rash

Endocrine & metabolic: Hyperuricemia, parotid pain, SIADH (rare)

Gastrointestinal: Abdominal cramps, abdominal pain, anorexia, constipation (common), diarrhea, intestinal necrosis, intestinal perforation, nausea, oral ulcers, paralytic ileus, vomiting, weight loss

Genitourinary: Bladder atony, dysuria, polyuria, urinary retention

Hematologic: Anemia (mild), leukopenia (mild), thrombocytopenia (mild), thrombotic thrombocytopenic purpura
Hepatic: Hepatic sinusoidal obstruction syndrome (SOS; veno-occlusive liver disease)
Local: Phlebitis, tissue irritation/necrosis (if infiltrated)
Neuromuscular & skeletal: Back pain, bone pain, deep tendon reflex loss, difficulty walking, foot drop, gait changes, jaw pain, limb pain, motor difficulties, muscle wasting, myalgia, paralysis, paresthesia, peripheral neuropathy (common), sensorimotor dysfunction, sensory loss
Ocular: Cortical blindness (transient), nystagmus, optic atrophy with blindness
Otic: Deafness
Renal: Acute uric acid nephropathy, hemolytic uremic syndrome
Respiratory: Bronchospasm, dyspnea, pharyngeal pain
Miscellaneous: Allergic reactions (rare), anaphylaxis (rare), hypersensitivity (rare)

Drug Interactions

Metabolism/Transport Effects **Substrate** of CYP3A4 (major), P-glycoprotein; **Note:** Assignment of Major/Minor substrate status based on clinically relevant drug interaction potential

Avoid Concomitant Use

Avoid concomitant use of VinCRIStine with any of the following: BCG; BCG (Intravesical); Conivaptan; Fusidic Acid (Systemic); Idelalisib; Natalizumab; Pimecrolimus; Tacrolimus (Topical); Tofacitinib; Vaccines (Live)

Increased Effect/Toxicity

VinCRIStine may increase the levels/effects of: Leflunomide; MitoMYcin (Systemic); Natalizumab; Tofacitinib; Vaccines (Live)

The levels/effects of VinCRIStine may be increased by: Aprepitant; Conivaptan; CYP3A4 Inhibitors (Moderate); CYP3A4 Inhibitors (Strong); Dasatinib; Denosumab; Fosaprepitant; Fusidic Acid (Systemic); Idelalisib; Itraconazole; Ivacaftor; Lopinavir; Luliconazole; Macrolide Antibiotics; MAO Inhibitors; Mifepristone; Netupitant; NIFEdipine; Palbociclib; P-glycoprotein/ABCB1 Inhibitors; Pimecrolimus; Posaconazole; Ritonavir; Roflumilast; Simeprevir; Stiripentol; Tacrolimus (Topical); Teniposide; Trastuzumab; Voriconazole

Decreased Effect

VinCRIStine may decrease the levels/effects of: BCG; BCG (Intravesical); Coccidioides immitis Skin Test; Fosphenytoin; Phenytoin; Sipuleucel-T; Vaccines (Inactivated); Vaccines (Live)

The levels/effects of VinCRIStine may be decreased by: Bosentan; CYP3A4 Inducers (Moderate); CYP3A4 Inducers (Strong); Dabrafenib; Deferasirox; Echinacea; Fosphenytoin; Mitotane; P-glycoprotein/ABCB1 Inducers; Phenytoin; Siltuximab; St Johns Wort; Tocilizumab

Storage/Stability Store intact vials refrigerated at 2°C to 8°C (36°F to 46°F). Protect from light.

IV solution: Diluted in 25 to 50 mL NS or D_5W, stable for 7 days under refrigeration, or 2 days at room temperature. In ambulatory pumps, solution is stable for 7 days at room temperature. After preparation, keep vincristine in a location away from the separate storage location recommended for intrathecal medications.

Mechanism of Action Binds to tubulin and inhibits microtubule formation, therefore, arresting the cell at metaphase by disrupting the formation of the mitotic spindle; it is specific for the M and S phases. Vincristine may also interfere with nucleic acid and protein synthesis by blocking glutamic acid utilization.

Pharmacokinetics (Adult data unless noted) **Note:** In pediatric patients, significant intrapatient and interpatient variability has been reported (Gidding, 1999).

Distribution: Rapidly removed from bloodstream and tightly bound to tissues; poor penetration into the CSF
Metabolism: Extensive in the liver via CYP3A
Half-life, terminal: 85 hours (range: 19 to 155 hours)
Elimination: Primarily in feces (~80%); urine (10% to 20%; <1% as unchanged drug)

Clearance: In pediatric patients, correlation with diagnosis has been reported; clearance in patients with ALL and non-Hodgkin lymphoma higher than Wilms' tumor (Gidding, 1999):

Infants: Vincristine clearance is lower compared to children; more closely related to body weight than to body surface area (Crom, 1994)

Children and Adolescents 2 to 18 years: Reported means: 357 to 482 mL/minute/m²; some suggest faster clearance in children <10 years of age than in adolescents (Crom, 1994); however, more recent data does not support this finding nor a dosage reduction in adolescent patients (Frost, 2003; Gidding, 1999)

Dosing: Neonatal **Note:** Dosing and frequency may vary by protocol and/or treatment phase; refer to specific protocol. In pediatric patients, dosing may be based on either BSA (mg/m²) or weight (mg/kg); use extra precaution to verify dosing parameters during calculations.

Neuroblastoma (CE-CAdO regimen): IV:

Newborns: 0.035 mg/**kg** on day 1 every 21 days for 2 cycles (Rubie, 1998) or on days 1 and 5 for 2 cycles (Rubie, 2001)

Older neonates: 0.75 mg/m² to 1.05 mg/m² on days 1 and 5 every 21 days for 2 cycles (Rubie, 1998) or 0.05 mg/**kg** on days 1 and 5 for 2 cycles (Rubie, 2001)

Dosing: Usual **Note:** Doses may be capped at a maximum of 2 mg/dose. Dosing and frequency may vary by protocol and/or treatment phase; refer to specific protocol.

Pediatric: **Note:** In pediatric patients, dosing may be based on either BSA (mg/m²) or weight (mg/kg); use extra precaution to verify dosing parameters during calculations.

Malignancy, general dosing: Manufacturer's labeling: IV:

≤10 kg: 0.05 mg/**kg**/dose once weekly

>10 kg: 1.5 to 2 mg/m²/dose; frequency may vary based on protocol; maximum dose: 2 mg

Acute lymphocytic leukemia (ALL): IV: Children: 1.5 mg/m²/dose; maximum dose: 2 mg; reported frequency variable; both regimens studied in children ≤10 years:

Bostrom, 2003: Administer dose on the following days: Induction phase: Days 0, 7, 14, and 21; Consolidation phase: Days 0, 28, and 56; Delayed intensification phase: Days 0, 7, and 14; Maintenance phase: Days 0, 28, and 56

Avramis, 2003: Administer dose on the following days: Induction phase: Days 0, 7, 14, and 21; Consolidation phase: Days 0, 28, and 56; Interim maintenance phases: Days 0 and 28; Delayed intensification phase: Days 0, 7, and 14; Maintenance phase: Every 4 weeks

Burkitt lymphoma and B-cell ALL: IV: Children and Adolescents: 1.5 mg/m²/dose; maximum dose: 2 mg; reported frequency variable

Bowman, 1996: Administer dose on days 4 and 11 of initial phase cycle; initial phase is in combination with cyclophosphamide, doxorubicin, and CNS prophylaxis (alternates with secondary phase) for a total of 4 cycles of each phase

Reiter, 1999: Administer dose on day 1 of cycle AA in combination with dexamethasone, ifosfamide, methotrexate, cytarabine, etoposide, and CNS prophylaxis and of cycle BB in combination with dexamethasone, cyclophosphamide, methotrexate, doxorubicin, and CNS prophylaxis

Ewing sarcoma: Limited data available: IV: Children and Adolescents: Dose and frequency regimens variable:
Grier, 2003: 2 mg/m²/dose on day 1 of a 21 day cycle, administer either every cycle or during odd-numbered cycles; maximum dose: 2 mg
Kolb, 2003: 0.67 mg/m²/**day** as a continuous IV infusion on days 1, 2, and 3; total dose for cycle: 2 mg/m²/**cycle** (maximum dose/cycle: 2 mg) during cycles 1, 2, 3, and 6
Hodgkin lymphoma: IV: Children and Adolescents: BEACOPP regimen: 2 mg/m² on day 7 of a 21-day treatment cycle; maximum dose: 2 mg (Kelly, 2002)
Neuroblastoma: IV:
Infants: CE-CAdO regimen:
Body surface area-directed (Rubie, 1998):
<10 kg: 0.75 mg/m² to 1.05 mg/m² on days 1 and 5 every 21 days for 2 cycles; some infants may only receive on day 1. **Note:** This dosing equates to a 30% to 50% reduction in the dose used for patients ≥10 kg.
≥10 kg: 1.5 mg/m² on days 1 and 5 every 21 days for 2 cycles; maximum dose: 2 mg
Weight-based: 0.05 mg/**kg** on days 1 and 5 for 2 cycles (Rubie, 2001)
Children and Adolescents:
CE-CAdO regimen (Rubie, 1998):
<10 kg: 0.75 mg/m² to 1.05 mg/m² on days 1 and 5 every 21 days for 2 cycles
≥10 kg: 1.5 mg/m² on days 1 and 5 every 21 days for 2 cycles; maximum dose: 2 mg
CAV-P/VP regimen: 0.033 mg/**kg/day** as a continuous infusion days 1, 2, and 3 (total dose: 0.1 mg/**kg**), then 1.5 mg/m² bolus day 9 of courses 1, 2, 4, and 6; maximum dose: 2 mg/dose (Kushner, 1994)
Retinoblastoma: Limited data available: IV:
Infants and Children ≤36 months: 0.05 mg/**kg**/dose; maximum dose: 2 mg; reported frequency variable
Rodriguez-Galindo, 2003: Administer dose on day 1 every 21 days in combination with carboplatin for 8 cycles
Freidman, 2000: Administer dose day 0 every 28 days in combination with carboplatin and etoposide for 6 cycles
Children >36 months: 1.5 mg/m² on day 0 every 28 days in combination with carboplatin and etoposide for 6 cycles; maximum dose: 2 mg (Friedman, 2000)
Rhabdomyosarcoma: Infants, Children, and Adolescents (Crist, 2001):
VA regimen:
Infants: Initial: 0.75 mg/m²/dose as a single dose during week 1; if tolerated, may increase to dose to 1.13 mg/m²/dose as a single dose for week 2 and further increase to 1.5 mg/m²/dose weekly for weeks 3 to 8, weeks 13 to 20, and weeks 25 to 32
Children and Adolescents: 1.5 mg/m²/dose weekly (maximum dose: 2 mg/dose) for weeks 1 to 8, weeks 13 to 20, and weeks 25 to 32
VAC regimen:
Infants: 0.75 mg/m²/dose weekly for weeks 0 to 12, week 16, and weeks 20 to 25; continuation therapy: Weeks 29 to 34 and weeks 38 to 43
Children and Adolescents: 1.5 mg/m²/dose weekly (maximum dose: 2 mg/dose) for weeks 0 to 12, week 16, and weeks 20 to 25; continuation therapy: weeks 29 to 34 and weeks 38 to 43
Wilm's tumor: Dose and frequency regimens variable; regimens studies in infants, children, and adolescents
Pritchard, 1995:
Infants: 0.75 mg/m²/dose weekly for 10 to 11 weeks then every 3 weeks for 15 additional weeks
Children and Adolescents: 1.5 mg/m²/dose weekly for 10 to 11 weeks then every 3 weeks for 15 additional weeks
Green, 2007:
Infants and Children ≤30 kg: 0.05 mg/**kg**/dose (maximum dose: 2 mg) weeks 1, 2, 4, 5, 6, 7, 8, 10, and 11, followed by 0.067 mg/**kg**/dose (maximum dose: 2 mg) weeks 12, 13, 18, and 24
Children and Adolescents >30 kg: 1.5 mg/m²/dose (maximum dose: 2 mg) weeks 1, 2, 4, 5, 6, 7, 8, 10, and 11, followed by 2 mg/m²/dose (maximum dose: 2 mg) weeks 12, 13, 18, and 24

Adult:
General dosing: Manufacturer's labeling: 1.4 mg/m²/dose; frequency may vary based on protocol; maximum dose: 2 mg/dose
ALL:
Hyper-CVAD regimen: 2 mg/dose days 4 and 11 during odd-numbered cycles (cycles 1, 3, 5, 7) of an 8-cycle phase, followed by maintenance treatment (if needed) of 2 mg monthly for 2 years (Kantarjian, 2004)
Larson (CALBG 8811) regimen: Induction phase: 2 mg/dose days 1, 8, 15, and 22 (4-week treatment cycle); Early intensification phase: 2 mg/dose days 15 and 22 (4-week treatment cycle, repeat once); Late intensification phase: 2 mg/dose days 1, 8, 15 (8-week treatment cycle); Maintenance phase: 2 mg/dose day 1 every 4 weeks until 24 months from diagnosis (Larson, 1995)
Central nervous system tumors: IV: PCV regimen: 1.4 mg/m²/dose (maximum dose: 2 mg) on days 8 and 29 of a 6-week treatment cycle for a total of 6 cycles (van de Bent, 2006) **or** 1.4 mg/m²/dose (no maximum dose) on days 8 and 29 of a 6-week treatment cycle for up to 4 cycles (Cairncross, 2006)
Hodgkin lymphoma:
BEACOPP regimen: 1.4 mg/m²/dose (maximum dose: 2 mg) on day 8 of a 21-day treatment cycle (Diehl, 2003)
Stanford V regimen: 1.4 mg/m²/dose (maximum dose: 2 mg) in weeks 2, 4, 6, 8, 10, and 12 (Horning, 2000; Horning, 2002)
Non-Hodgkin lymphoma:
Burkitt lymphoma:
CODOX-M/IVAC: Cycles 1 and 3 (CODOX-M): 1.5 mg/m² (no maximum dose) days 1 and 8 of cycle 1 and days 1, 8, and 15 of cycle 3 (Magrath, 1996) **or** 1.5 mg/m² (maximum dose: 2 mg) days 1 and 8 of cycles 1 and 3 (Mead, 2002; Mead, 2008); CODOX-M is in combination with cyclophosphamide, doxorubicin, methotrexate, and CNS prophylaxis and alternates with IVAC (etoposide, ifosfamide, and cytarabine) for a total of 4 cycles
Hyper-CVAD: 2 mg (flat dose) days 4 and 11 of courses 1, 3, 5, and 7 (in combination with cyclophosphamide, doxorubicin, and dexamethasone) and alternates with even courses 2, 4, 6, and 8 (methotrexate and cytarabine) (Thomas, 2006)
Follicular lymphoma: CVP regimen: 1.4 mg/m²/dose (maximum dose: 2 mg) on day 1 of a 21-day treatment cycle for 8 cycles (Marcus, 2005)
Large B-cell lymphoma:
CHOP regimen: 1.4 mg/m²/dose (maximum dose: 2 mg) on day 1 of a 21-day treatment cycle for 8 cycles (Coiffier, 2002)
EPOCH regimen: 0.4 mg/m²/day continuous infusion for 4 days (over 96 hours) (total 1.6 mg/m²/cycle; dose not usually capped) of a 21-day treatment cycle (Wilson, 2002)

Dosing adjustment for renal impairment: Adults: No dosage adjustment necessary (Kintzel, 1995)
Dosing adjustment for hepatic impairment: All patients: The manufacturer's labeling recommends the following adjustment: Serum bilirubin >3 mg/dL: Administer 50% of normal dose.

The following adjustments have also been recommended:

Floyd, 2006: Serum bilirubin 1.5 to 3 mg/dL or transaminases 2 to 3 times ULN or alkaline phosphatase increased: Administer 50% of dose.

Superfin, 2007:

Serum bilirubin 1.5-3 mg/dL: Administer 50% of dose.

Serum bilirubin >3 mg/dL: Avoid use.

Preparation for Administration Hazardous agent; use appropriate precautions for handling and disposal (NIOSH 2014 [group 1]).

IV infusion: May be diluted in 25 to 50 mL NS or D_5W. **In order to prevent inadvertent intrathecal administration the World Health Organization (WHO) and the Institute for Safe Medication Practices (ISMP) strongly recommend dispensing vincristine in a minibag (NOT in a syringe).** Vincristine should **NOT** be prepared during the preparation of any intrathecal medications. If dispensing vincristine in a syringe, affix an auxiliary label stating **"For intravenous use only - fatal if given by other routes"** to the syringe, and the syringe must also be packaged in the manufacturer-provided overwrap which bears the statement **"Do not remove covering until the moment of injection. For intravenous use only. Fatal if given intrathecally."** After preparation, keep vincristine in a location away from the separate storage location recommended for intrathecal medications. Vincristine should **NOT** be delivered to the patient at the same time with any medications intended for central nervous system administration.

Administration Hazardous agent; use appropriate precautions for handling and disposal (NIOSH 2014 [group 1]). **Note: For IV administration only; fatal if given intrathecally;** vincristine should **NOT** be delivered to the patient with any medications intended for central nervous system administration. **Note: In order to prevent inadvertent intrathecal administration, the World Health Organization (WHO) and the Institute for Safe Medical Practices (ISMP) recommend dispensing vincristine in a minibag (rather than a syringe).** Vincristine should **NOT** be prepared during the preparation of any intrathecal medication. After preparation, keep vincristine in a location away from the separate storage location recommended for intrathecal medications. If dispensing vincristine in a syringe, affix an auxiliary label stating **"For intravenous use only - fatal if given by other routes"** to the syringe and the syringe must be packaged in the manufacturer-provided overwrap which bears the statement **"Do not remove covering until the moment of injection. For intravenous use only. Fatal if given intrathecally."**

IV infusion: Fatal if given intrathecally. The preferred administration is as a short infusion over 5 to 10 minutes in a minibag. If administration via a minibag is not possible, vincristine may also be administered undiluted (1 mg/mL) over 1 minute into a free flowing IV line to prevent venous irritation/extravasation. Some protocols utilize a 24-hour continuous IV infusion

Vincristine is a vesicant; ensure proper needle or catheter placement prior to and during infusion; avoid extravasation. If extravasation occurs, stop infusion immediately and disconnect (leave cannula/needle in place); gently aspirate extravasated solution (do **NOT** flush the line); initiate hyaluronidase antidote (see Management of Drug Extravasations for more details); apply dry warm compresses for 20 minutes 4 times a day for 1 to 2 days; elevate extremity (Pérez Fidalgo 2012). Remaining portion of the vincristine dose should be infused through a separate vein.

Note: Do not administer to patients while they are receiving radiation therapy through ports that include the liver. If used in combination with L-asparaginase, administer vincristine 12 to 24 hours before L-asparaginase to minimize toxicity.

Vesicant/Extravasation Risk Vesicant

Monitoring Parameters Serum electrolytes (sodium), hepatic function tests, neurologic examination, CBC with differential, serum uric acid, monitor infusion site, monitor for constipation/ileus and for signs/symptoms of peripheral neuropathy

Additional Information Ten times the usual recommended dose of vincristine in children <13 years of age has been lethal; doses of 3 to 4 mg/m^2 can be expected to produce severe toxic manifestations. Treatment is supportive and symptomatic, including anticonvulsants, fluid restriction, and diuretics to prevent adverse effects from SIADH and enemas or cathartics to prevent ileus. Use of leucovorin calcium may be helpful in treating vincristine overdose. Leucovorin calcium 100 mg IV every 3 hours for 24 hours, then every 6 hours for at least 48 hours has been administered in case reports.

Dosage Forms Excipient information presented when available (limited, particularly for generics); consult specific product labeling.

Solution, Intravenous, as sulfate:

Vincasar PFS: 1 mg/mL (1 mL, 2 mL)

Solution, Intravenous, as sulfate [preservative free]:

Generic: 1 mg/mL (1 mL, 2 mL)

◆ **Vincristine (Conventional)** *see* VinCRIStine *on page 2179*

◆ **Vincristine Sulfate** *see* VinCRIStine *on page 2179*

◆ **Vincristine Sulfate Injection (Can)** *see* VinCRIStine *on page 2179*

◆ **Vincristine Sulfate Injection USP (Can)** *see* VinCRIStine *on page 2179*

Vinorelbine (vi NOR el been)

Medication Safety Issues

Sound-alike/look-alike issues:

Vinorelbine may be confused with vinBLAStine, vinCRIStine

High alert medication:

This medication is in a class the Institute for Safe Medication Practices (ISMP) includes among its list of drug classes which have a heightened risk of causing significant patient harm when used in error.

Administration issues:

Vinorelbine is intended **for IV use only**: Inadvertent intrathecal administration of other vinca alkaloids has resulted in death. Syringes containing vinorelbine should be labeled **"For IV use only. Fatal if given intrathecally."** Vinorelbine should **NOT** be prepared during the preparation of any intrathecal medications. After preparation, keep vinorelbine in a location **away** from the separate storage location recommended for intrathecal medications.

Related Information

Management of Drug Extravasations *on page 2298*

Prevention of Chemotherapy-Induced Nausea and Vomiting in Children *on page 2368*

Safe Handling of Hazardous Drugs *on page 2455*

Brand Names: US Navelbine

Brand Names: Canada Navelbine; Vinorelbine Injection, USP; Vinorelbine Tartrate for Injection

Therapeutic Category Antineoplastic Agent, Antimicrotubular; Antineoplastic Agent, Vinca Alkaloid

Generic Availability (US) Yes

Use Treatment of non-small cell lung cancer (FDA approved in adults); has also been used for refractory/recurrent solid tumors, Hodgkin's lymphoma, and leukemias

Pregnancy Risk Factor D

Pregnancy Considerations Animal reproduction studies have demonstrated embryotoxicity, fetotoxicity, decreased fetal weight, and delayed ossification. May cause fetal harm if administered during pregnancy. Women of childbearing potential should avoid becoming pregnant during vinorelbine treatment.

Breast-Feeding Considerations It is not known if vinorelbine is excreted in breast milk. Due to the potential for serious adverse reactions in the nursing infant, breastfeeding should be discontinued during treatment.

Contraindications Pretreatment granulocyte counts <1000/mm^3

Warnings/Precautions Hazardous agent - use appropriate precautions for handling and disposal (NIOSH 2014 [group 1]). **[U.S. Boxed Warning]: For IV use only; intrathecal administration of other vinca alkaloids has resulted in death. If dispensed in a syringe, should be labeled "for intravenous use only - fatal if given intrathecally". [U.S. Boxed Warning]: Vesicant; ensure proper needle or catheter placement prior to and during infusion. Avoid extravasation. Extravasation may cause local tissue necrosis and/or thrombophlebitis. [U.S. Boxed Warning]: Severe granulocytopenia may occur with treatment (may lead to infection); granulocyte counts should be ≥1000 cells/mm^3 prior to treatment initiation; dosage adjustment may be required based on blood counts (monitor blood counts prior to each dose).** Granulocytopenia is a dose-limiting toxicity; nadir is generally 7-10 days after administration and recovery occurs within the following 7-14 days. Monitor closely for infections and/or fever in patients with severe granulocytopenia. Use with extreme caution in patients with compromised marrow reserve due to prior chemotherapy or radiation therapy.

Fatal cases of interstitial pulmonary changes and ARDS have been reported (with single-agent therapy (mean onset of symptoms: 1 week); promptly evaluate changes in baseline pulmonary symptoms or any new onset pulmonary symptoms (eg, dyspnea, cough, hypoxia). Acute shortness of breath and severe bronchospasm have been reported with vinca alkaloids; usually associated with the concurrent administration of mitomycin.

Vinorelbine should **NOT** be prepared during the preparation of any intrathecal medications. After preparation, keep vinorelbine in a location **away** from the separate storage location recommended for intrathecal medications. Elimination is predominantly hepatic; while there is no evidence that toxicity is enhanced in patients with elevated transaminases, use with caution in patients with severe hepatic injury or impairment; dosage modification required for elevated total bilirubin. May cause new onset or worsening of pre-existing neuropathy; use with caution in patients with neuropathy; monitor for new or worsening sign/symptoms of neuropathy; dosage adjustment required. May cause severe constipation (grade 3-4), paralytic ileus, intestinal obstruction, necrosis, and/or perforation; some events were fatal. Oral vinorelbine (not available in the U.S.) is associated with a moderate antiemetic potential; antiemetics are recommended to prevent nausea/vomiting (Dupuis, 2011; Roila, 2010); IV vinorelbine has a minimal emetic potential (Dupuis, 2011; Roila, 2010). Potentially significant drug-drug interactions may exist, requiring dose or frequency adjustment, additional monitoring, and/or selection of alternative therapy. May have radiosensitizing effects with prior or concurrent radiation therapy; radiation recall reactions may occur in patients who have received prior radiation therapy. Avoid eye contamination (exposure may cause severe irritation). **[U.S. Boxed Warning]: Should be administered under the supervision of an experienced cancer chemotherapy physician.**

Adverse Reactions

Cardiovascular: Chest pain

Central nervous system: Fatigue

Dermatologic: Alopecia, rash

Gastrointestinal: Constipation, diarrhea, nausea, paralytic ileus, vomiting

Hematologic: Anemia, granulocytopenia (nadir: 7-10 days; recovery 14-21 days), leukopenia, neutropenia, neutropenic fever/sepsis, thrombocytopenia

Hepatic: AST increased, total bilirubin increased

Local: Injection site pain, injection site reaction (includes erythema and vein discoloration), phlebitis

Neuromuscular & skeletal: Arthralgia, jaw pain, myalgia, peripheral neuropathy, loss of deep tendon reflexes, weakness

Otic: Ototoxicity

Respiratory: Dyspnea

Rare but important or life-threatening: Abdominal pain, allergic reactions, anaphylaxis, angioedema, back pain, DVT, dysphagia, esophagitis, flushing, gait instability, headache, hemolytic uremic syndrome, hemorrhagic cystitis, hyper-/hypotension, hyponatremia, intestinal necrosis, intestinal obstruction, intestinal perforation, interstitial pulmonary changes, local rash, local urticaria, MI (rare), mucositis, muscle weakness, myocardial ischemia, pancreatitis, paralytic ileus, pneumonia, pruritus, pulmonary edema, pulmonary embolus, radiation recall (dermatitis, esophagitis), skin blistering, syndrome of inappropriate ADH secretion, tachycardia, thromboembolic events, thrombotic thrombocytopenic purpura, tumor pain, urticaria, vasodilation

Drug Interactions

Metabolism/Transport Effects Substrate of CYP2D6 (minor), CYP3A4 (major); **Note:** Assignment of Major/Minor substrate status based on clinically relevant drug interaction potential; **Inhibits** CYP2D6 (weak)

Avoid Concomitant Use

Avoid concomitant use of Vinorelbine with any of the following: BCG; BCG (Intravesical); CloZAPine; Conivaptan; Dipyrone; Fusidic Acid (Systemic); Idelalisib; Natalizumab; Pimecrolimus; Tacrolimus (Topical); Tofacitinib; Vaccines (Live)

Increased Effect/Toxicity

Vinorelbine may increase the levels/effects of: ARIPiprazole; CloZAPine; Leflunomide; MitoMYcin (Systemic); Natalizumab; Tofacitinib; Vaccines (Live)

The levels/effects of Vinorelbine may be increased by: Aprepitant; CISplatin; Conivaptan; CYP3A4 Inhibitors (Moderate); CYP3A4 Inhibitors (Strong); Dasatinib; Denosumab; Dipyrone; Fosaprepitant; Fusidic Acid (Systemic); Gefitinib; Idelalisib; Itraconazole; Ivacaftor; Luliconazole; Macrolide Antibiotics; Mifepristone; Netupitant; PACLitaxel (Conventional); PACLitaxel (Protein Bound); Palbociclib; Pimecrolimus; Posaconazole; Roflumilast; Simeprevir; Stiripentol; Tacrolimus (Topical); Trastuzumab; Voriconazole

Decreased Effect

Vinorelbine may decrease the levels/effects of: BCG; BCG (Intravesical); Coccidioides immitis Skin Test; Sipuleucel-T; Vaccines (Inactivated); Vaccines (Live)

The levels/effects of Vinorelbine may be decreased by: Bosentan; CYP3A4 Inducers (Moderate); CYP3A4 Inducers (Strong); Dabrafenib; Deferasirox; Echinacea; Mitotane; Siltuximab; St Johns Wort; Tocilizumab

Storage/Stability Store intact vials refrigerated at 2°C to 8°C (36°F to 46°F); do not freeze. Protect from light. Intact vials are stable at room temperature of 25°C (77°F) for up to 72 hours. Solutions diluted for infusion in polypropylene syringes or polyvinyl chloride bags are stable for 24 hours at 5°C to 30°C (41°F to 86°F). After preparation, keep vinorelbine in a location **away** from the separate storage location recommended for intrathecal medications.

Mechanism of Action Semisynthetic vinca alkaloid which binds to tubulin and inhibits microtubule formation, therefore, arresting the cell at metaphase by disrupting the formation of the mitotic spindle; it is specific for the M and S phases. Vinorelbine may also interfere with nucleic acid and protein synthesis by blocking glutamic acid utilization.

Pharmacokinetics (Adult data unless noted)

Distribution: Binds extensively to human platelets and lymphocytes (80% to 91%); V_d:

Children and Adolescents 2-17 years: 21.1 ± 12.2 L/kg (Johansen, 2006)

Adults: 25-40 L/kg

Protein binding: 80% to 91%

Metabolism: Extensively hepatic, via CYP3A4, to two metabolites, deacetylvinorelbine (active) and vinorelbine N-oxide

Half-life elimination: Triphasic:

Children and Adolescents 2-17 years: Terminal: 16.5 ± 9.7 hours (Johansen, 2006)

Adults: Terminal: 28-44 hours

Elimination: Feces (46%); urine (18%, 10% to 12% as unchanged drug)

Dosing: Usual

Infants, Children, and Adolescents:

Hodgkin's lymphoma; refractory or recurrent: Limited data available: IV: Children ≥10 years and Adolescents: 25 mg/m^2 once weekly on days 1 and 8 of a 21-day cycle in combination with gemcitabine (Cole, 2009)

Leukemias; acute (ALL, AML), refractory, or recurrent: Limited data available: IV:

Infants: 0.67 mg/**kg** once weekly on days 0, 7, 14 of a 14-day cycle in combination with topotecan, clofarabine, and thiotepa (TVTC regimen) (Steinherz, 2010)

Children and Adolescents: 20 mg/m^2 once weekly on days 0, 7, and 14 of a 14-day cycle in combination with topotecan, clofarabine, and thiotepa (TVTC regimen) (Shuka, 2014; Steinherz, 2010)

Solid tumors; refractory or recurrent: Limited data available: Children and Adolescents: IV:

Monotherapy: 30 mg/m^2 once weekly for weeks 1-6 of an 8-week cycle for 10 courses; may reduce dosage to 27 mg/m^2 for Grade 3 or 4 hematologic toxicity in patients who demonstrate objective response or who have had treatment delay beyond 63 days (week 9) from the previous course (Kuttesch, 2009)

Combination therapy: 25 mg/m^2 once weekly for 3 weeks on days 1, 8, and 15 of each 28-day cycle in combination with cyclophosphamide (Casanova, 2004; Minard-Colin, 2012)

Adults: **Non-small cell lung cancer (NSCLC):** IV: **Note:** Utilize patient's actual body weight (full weight) for calculation of body surface area- or weight-based dosing, particularly when the intent of therapy is curative; manage regimen-related toxicities in the same manner as for nonobese patients; if a dose reduction is utilized due to toxicity, consider resumption of full weight-based dosing with subsequent cycles, especially if cause of toxicity (eg, hepatic or renal impairment) is resolved (Griggs, 2012).

Monotherapy: 30 mg/m^2 every 7 days until disease progression or unacceptable toxicity

Combination therapy: 25-30 mg/m^2 every 7 days in combination with cisplatin

Dosing adjustment in hematological toxicity: Adults: **Note:** In patients with concurrent hematologic toxicity and hepatic impairment, administer the lower of the doses determined from the adjustment recommendations.

Granulocyte counts should be ≥1000 cells/mm^3 prior to the administration of vinorelbine. Adjustments in the dosage of vinorelbine should be based on granulocyte counts obtained on the day of treatment as follows:

Granulocytes ≥1500 cells/mm^3 on day of treatment: Administer 100% of starting dose

Granulocytes 1000-1499 cells/mm^3 on day of treatment: Administer 50% of starting dose

Granulocytes <1000 cells/mm^3 on day of treatment: Do not administer. Repeat granulocyte count in 1 week; if 3 consecutive doses are held because granulocyte count is <1000 cells/mm^3, discontinue vinorelbine.

For patients who, during treatment, have experienced fever and/or sepsis while granulocytopenic or had 2 consecutive weekly doses held due to granulocytopenia, subsequent doses of vinorelbine should be:

75% of starting dose for granulocytes ≥1500 cells/mm^3

37.5% of starting dose for granulocytes 1000-1499 cells/mm^3

Dosage adjustment for neurotoxicity: Adults: Neurotoxicity ≥ grade 2: Discontinue treatment

Dosage adjustment for other adverse events: Adults: Severe adverse events: Reduce dose or discontinue treatment

Dosing adjustment in renal impairment: Adults:

Renal insufficiency: No dosage adjustment necessary

Hemodialysis: Initial: IV: Reduce dose to 20 mg/m^2/week; administer either after dialysis (on dialysis days) or on nondialysis days (Janus, 2010)

Dosing adjustment in hepatic impairment: All patients: **Note:** In patients with concurrent hematologic toxicity and hepatic impairment, administer the lower of the doses determined from the adjustment recommendations. Administer with caution in patients with hepatic insufficiency. In patients who develop hyperbilirubinemia during treatment with vinorelbine, the dose should be adjusted for total bilirubin as follows:

Serum bilirubin ≤2 mg/dL: Administer 100% of dose

Serum bilirubin 2.1-3 mg/dL: Administer 50% of dose (Ecklund, 2005; Floyd, 2006; Superfin, 2006)

Serum bilirubin >3 mg/dL: Administer 25% of dose (Ecklund, 2005; Floyd, 2006; Superfin, 2006)

Preparation for Administration Hazardous agent; use appropriate precautions for handling and disposal (NIOSH 2014 [group 1]).

IV: **Note: Vinorelbine should NOT be prepared during the preparation of any intrathecal medications.** After preparation, keep vinorelbine in a location away from the separate storage location recommended for intrathecal medications. Vinorelbine should **NOT** be delivered to the patient at the same time with any medications intended for central nervous system administration.

Syringe: Dilute in D_5W or NS to a final concentration of 1.5 to 3 mg/mL; syringes containing vinorelbine should be labeled **"For IV use only. Fatal if given intrathecally"**

IV bag: Dilute in D_5W, NS, ½NS, D_5½NS, LR, or Ringer's to a final concentration of 0.5 to 2 mg/mL

Administration Hazardous agent; use appropriate precautions for handling and disposal (NIOSH 2014 [group 1]).

IV: **For IV use only; FATAL IF GIVEN INTRATHECALLY.** Administer as a direct intravenous push or rapid bolus, over 6 to 10 minutes (up to 30 minutes); in pediatric trials, vinorelbine typically administered over 6 to 10 minutes. Longer infusions may increase the risk of pain and phlebitis. Intravenous doses should be followed by at least 75 to 125 mL of NS or D_5W to reduce the incidence of phlebitis and inflammation.

Vesicant; avoid extravasation. Assure proper needle or catheter position prior to administration. If extravasation occurs, stop infusion immediately and disconnect (leave cannula/needle in place); gently aspirate extravasated solution (do **NOT** flush the line); initiate hyaluronidase antidote (See Management of Drug Extravasations for more details); apply dry warm compresses for 20 minutes 4 times a day for 1 to 2 days; elevate extremity (Pérez Fidalgo 2012). Remaining portion of the vinorelbine dose should be infused through a separate vein.

Vesicant/Extravasation Risk Vesicant.

Monitoring Parameters CBC with differential and platelet count (prior to each dose, and after treatment), hepatic function tests; monitor for new-onset pulmonary symptoms (or worsening from baseline); monitor for neuropathy (new or worsening symptoms; monitor infusion site; monitor for signs symptoms of constipation/ileus

Dosage Forms Excipient information presented when available (limited, particularly for generics); consult specific product labeling.

Solution, Intravenous:

Navelbine: 10 mg/mL (1 mL); 50 mg/5 mL (5 mL)

Generic: 10 mg/mL (1 mL); 50 mg/5 mL (5 mL)

Solution, Intravenous [preservative free]:

Generic: 10 mg/mL (1 mL); 50 mg/5 mL (5 mL)

◆ **Vinorelbine Injection, USP (Can)** *see* Vinorelbine *on page 2183*
◆ **Vinorelbine Tartrate** *see* Vinorelbine *on page 2183*
◆ **Vinorelbine Tartrate for Injection (Can)** *see* Vinorelbine *on page 2183*
◆ **Viokace** *see* Pancrelipase *on page 1614*
◆ **Viokase (Can)** *see* Pancrelipase *on page 1614*
◆ **Viosterol** *see* Ergocalciferol *on page 772*
◆ **Viracept** *see* Nelfinavir *on page 1497*
◆ **Viramune** *see* Nevirapine *on page 1507*
◆ **Viramune XR** *see* Nevirapine *on page 1507*
◆ **Virasal** *see* Salicylic Acid *on page 1894*
◆ **Virazole** *see* Ribavirin *on page 1851*
◆ **Viread** *see* Tenofovir *on page 2017*
◆ **Viroptic** *see* Trifluridine *on page 2124*
◆ **Viroptic® (Can)** *see* Trifluridine *on page 2124*
◆ **Virt-Phos 250 Neutral** *see* Potassium Phosphate and Sodium Phosphate *on page 1746*
◆ **Virtrate-2** *see* Sodium Citrate and Citric Acid *on page 1942*
◆ **Virtrate-3** *see* Citric Acid, Sodium Citrate, and Potassium Citrate *on page 479*
◆ **Virtrate-K** *see* Potassium Citrate and Citric Acid *on page 1738*
◆ **Virtussin A/C** *see* Guaifenesin and Codeine *on page 990*
◆ **Viscous Lidocaine** *see* Lidocaine (Topical) *on page 1258*
◆ **Visine-LR [OTC]** *see* Oxymetazoline (Ophthalmic) *on page 1600*
◆ **Visipaque** *see* Iodixanol *on page 1154*
◆ **Vistaril** *see* HydrOXYzine *on page 1058*
◆ **Vistide** *see* Cidofovir *on page 459*
◆ **Vita-C [OTC]** *see* Ascorbic Acid *on page 202*
◆ **Vitamin C** *see* Ascorbic Acid *on page 202*

Vitamin A (VYE ta min aye)

Medication Safety Issues

Sound-alike/look-alike issues:

Aquasol may be confused with Anusol

Related Information

Multivitamin Product Table *on page 2266*

Brand Names: US A-25 [OTC]; AFirm 1X [OTC]; AFirm 2X [OTC]; AFirm 3X [OTC]; Aquasol A; Gordons-Vite A [OTC]; Vitamin A Fish [OTC]

Therapeutic Category Nutritional Supplement; Vitamin, Fat Soluble

Generic Availability (US) May be product dependent

Use Treatment of vitamin A deficiency (injection: FDA approved in all ages; oral: FDA approved in adults); has also been used for prevention of vitamin A deficiency, supplementation in infants and children ≤5 years with measles, and prevention of chronic lung disease in premature neonates

Pregnancy Risk Factor X

Pregnancy Considerations Adverse events have been observed in animal reproduction studies. In humans, the critical period of exposure is the first trimester of pregnancy. Excess vitamin A during pregnancy may cause craniofacial malformations, as well as CNS, heart, and thymus abnormalities. Maternal vitamin A deficiency also causes adverse effects in the fetus, and vitamin A requirements are increased in pregnant women (IOM, 2000). The manufacturer notes that the safety of doses >6000 units/day in pregnant women has not been established and doses greater than the RDA are contraindicated in pregnant women or those who may become pregnant. High doses are used in some areas of the world for supplementation where deficiency is a public health problem (eg, to prevent night blindness); however, single doses >25,000 units should be avoided within 60 days of conception. High-dose supplementation is otherwise not recommended as part of routine antenatal care (WHO, 2011c).

Breast-Feeding Considerations Vitamin A requirements are increased in breast-feeding women (IOM, 2000). High-dose supplementation (eg, doses higher than the RDA) is not recommended in otherwise healthy women who receive adequate nutrition (WHO, 2011b)

Contraindications Hypersensitivity to vitamin A or any component of the formulation; hypervitaminosis A; pregnancy (dose exceeding RDA); intravenous administration of Aquasol A®

Warnings/Precautions Evaluate other sources of vitamin A while receiving this product. Patients receiving >25,000 units/day should be closely monitored for toxicity. Parenteral vitamin A: In low birth weight infants, polysorbates have been associated with thrombocytopenia, renal dysfunction, hepatomegaly, cholestasis, ascites, hypotension, and metabolic acidosis (E-Ferol syndrome).

Some dosage forms may contain polysorbate 80 (also known as Tweens). Hypersensitivity reactions, usually a delayed reaction, have been reported following exposure to pharmaceutical products containing polysorbate 80 in certain individuals (Isaksson, 2002; Lucente 2000; Shelley, 1995). Thrombocytopenia, ascites, pulmonary deterioration, and renal and hepatic failure have been reported in premature neonates after receiving parenteral products containing polysorbate 80 (Alade, 1986; CDC, 1984). See manufacturer's labeling.

Benzyl alcohol and derivatives: Some dosage forms may contain benzyl alcohol; large amounts of benzyl alcohol (≥99 mg/kg/day) have been associated with a potentially fatal toxicity ("gasping syndrome") in neonates; the "gasping syndrome" consists of metabolic acidosis, respiratory distress, gasping respirations, CNS dysfunction (including convulsions, intracranial hemorrhage), hypotension, and cardiovascular collapse (AAP, 1997; CDC, 1982); some data suggests that benzoate displaces bilirubin from protein binding sites (Ahlfors, 2001); avoid or use dosage forms containing benzyl alcohol with caution in neonates. See manufacturer's labeling.

Adverse Reactions Miscellaneous: Allergic reactions (rare), anaphylactic shock (following IV administration)

Drug Interactions

Metabolism/Transport Effects None known.

Avoid Concomitant Use

Avoid concomitant use of Vitamin A with any of the following: Retinoic Acid Derivatives

Increased Effect/Toxicity

Vitamin A may increase the levels/effects of: Bexarotene (Topical); Retinoic Acid Derivatives

Decreased Effect

The levels/effects of Vitamin A may be decreased by: Orlistat

Food Interactions Excessive ethanol intake depletes the liver of vitamin A and may enhance vitamin A toxicity (IOM, 2000)

Storage/Stability Injection: Store at 2°C to 8°C (36°F to 46°F); do not freeze. Protect from light. The following stability information has also been reported for Aquasol A® injection: May be stored at room temperature for up to 4 weeks (Cohen, 2007).

Mechanism of Action Vitamin A is a fat soluble vitamin needed for visual adaptation to darkness, maintenance of epithelial cells, immune function and embryonic development.

Pharmacokinetics (Adult data unless noted)

Absorption: Vitamin A in dosages **not** exceeding physiologic replacement is well absorbed in the small intestine after oral administration; water miscible preparations are absorbed more rapidly than oil preparations; large oral doses, conditions of fat malabsorption, low protein intake, or hepatic or pancreatic disease reduce oral absorption

Distribution: Large amounts concentrate for storage in the liver

Metabolism: Converted in the small intestine to retinol and further metabolized in the liver; conjugated with glucuronide, undergoes enterohepatic circulation

Elimination: In feces via biliary elimination

Dosing: Neonatal 1 unit vitamin A = 0.3 mcg retinol

Adequate Intake (AI): 400 mcg (1330 units)

Chronic lung disease, prevention in ELBW: IM: 5000 units/dose 3 times weekly (ie, MWF) initiated within the first 96 hours of life and continued for 4 weeks was used in 405 neonates (mean GA: 26.8 weeks; mean birth weight: 770 g; range: 400-1000 g) (Tyson, 1999).

Dosing: Usual 1 unit vitamin A = 0.3 mcg retinol

Dietary Reference Intake for vitamin A (presented as retinol activity equivalent [RAE]) (IOM, 2000): Oral:

Adequate Intake (AI) (IOM, 2000):

1-6 months: 400 mcg/day (1330 units/day)

6-12 months: 500 mcg/day (1670 units/day)

Recommended Daily Allowance (RDA) (IOM, 2000): Oral:

1-3 years: 300 mcg/day (1000 units/day)

4-8 years: 400 mcg/day (1330 units/day)

9-13 years: 600 mcg/day (2000 units/day)

>13 years and Adults: Female: 700 mcg/day (2330 units/day); Male: 900 mcg/day (3000 units/day)

Pregnant females:

14-18 years: 750 mcg/day (2500 units/day)

≥19 years: 770 mcg/day (2560 units/day)

Lactating females:

14-18 years: 1200 mcg/day (4000 units/day)

≥19 years: 1300 mcg/day (4330 units/day)

Measles infection, supplementation (WHO, 2004; WHO, 2010): Infants and Children: Oral:

Infants <6 months: 50,000 units daily for 2 days

Infants 6-11 months: 100,000 units daily for 2 days

Children ≥12 months to 5 years: 200,000 units daily for 2 days

Note: If severe malnutrition or ophthalmologic evidence of vitamin A deficiency is present, repeat a single dose 2-4 weeks after the second dose.

Vitamin A deficiency (varying recommendations available):

Prophylaxis for at-risk populations (eg, potential HIV infection, local prevalence of nightblindness >1% in ages 24-59 months or prevalence of serum retinol ≤0.7 mmol/L is ≥20% in ages 6-59 months) (WHO, 2008; WHO, 2010; WHO, 2011a; WHO, 2011b; WHO, 2011c; WHO, 2011d): Oral:

Infants <6 months: Not recommended

Infants 6-12 months: 100,000 units; administer as a single dose; repeat every 4-6 months, but do not readminister within 30 days of previous dose

Children and Adolescents: 200,000 units; administer as a single dose; repeat every 4-6 months, but do not readminister within 30 days of previous dose

Adults: 200,000 units/dose every 6 months

Pregnant women: Maximum 10,000 units once daily or 25,000 units once weekly. Administer for a minimum of 12 weeks during pregnancy or until delivery.

Postpartum women: 200,000 units at delivery or within 8 weeks of delivery

Treatment:

Infants:

IM: 7500-15,000 units once daily for 10 days followed by oral supplementation

Oral: 5000-10,000 units daily for 2 months following IM dosing

Children 1-8 years:

IM: 17,500-35,000 units once daily for 10 days followed by oral supplementation

Oral: 5000-10,000 units once daily for 2 months following IM dosing

Children >8 years and Adults:

IM: 100,000 units once daily for 3 days; then 50,000 units once daily for 14 days followed by oral supplementation

Oral: 10,000-20,000 units once daily for 2 months following IM dosing

Xerophthalmia (WHO, 1997; WHO, 2010): Oral:

Infants <6 months: 50,000 units administered as a single dose; repeat the next day and again after at least 2 weeks for a total of 3 doses

Infants 6-12 months: 100,000 units administered as a single dose; repeat the next day and again after at least 2 weeks for a total of 3 doses

Children and Adolescents: 200,000 units administered as a single dose; repeat the next day and again after at least 2 weeks for a total of 3 doses

Adults: 200,000 units once daily for 2 days; repeat with single dose in 2 weeks. **Note:** Females of reproductive age with night blindness or Bitot's spots should receive 5000-10,000 units daily or ≤25,000 units once weekly; if severe xerophthalmia, females of reproductive age may receive high dose (ie, 200,000 unit regimen) regardless of pregnancy status.

Malabsorption syndrome (prophylaxis): Children >8 years and Adults: Oral: 10,000-50,000 units/day of water miscible product

Administration

Oral: Administer with food or milk; for infants and children <24 months of age, capsules may be cut open and contents squeezed into the mouth

Parenteral: **For IM use only**; for neonatal patients, a 0.3 mL syringe and 29-gauge needle should be used for IM dose administration

Additional Information 1 USP vitamin A unit = 0.3 mcg of all-*trans* isomer of retinol; 1 RAE (retinol activity equivalent) = 1 mcg of all-*trans*-retinol = 12 mcg of dietary beta-carotene (IOM, 2000)

Dosage Forms Excipient information presented when available (limited, particularly for generics); consult specific product labeling.

Capsule, Oral:
A-25: 25,000 units
Vitamin A Fish: 7500 units
Generic: 10,000 units
Capsule, Oral [preservative free]:
A-25: 25,000 units [dye free]
Generic: 8000 units
Cream, External:
AFirm 1X: 0.15% (30 g) [fragrance free; contains benzyl alcohol, cetyl alcohol, disodium edta, methylparaben, peg-10 soya sterol, trolamine (triethanolamine)]
AFirm 2X: 0.3% (30 g) [fragrance free; contains benzyl alcohol, cetyl alcohol, disodium edta, methylparaben, peg-10 soya sterol, trolamine (triethanolamine)]
AFirm 3X: 0.6% (30 g) [fragrance free; contains benzyl alcohol, cetyl alcohol, disodium edta, methylparaben, peg-10 soya sterol, trolamine (triethanolamine)]
Gordons-Vite A: 100,000 units/g (75 g, 120 g, 480 g, 2400 g)
Lotion, External:
Gordons-Vite A: 100,000 units (120 mL, 4000 mL)
Solution, Intramuscular:
Aquasol A: 50,000 units/mL (2 mL) [contains chlorobutanol (chlorobutol)]
Tablet, Oral:
Generic: 10,000 units, 15,000 units, Vitamin A 10000 units and beta carotene 1000 units

- **Vitamin A Acid** *see* Tretinoin (Topical) *on page 2111*
- **Vitamin A Fish [OTC]** *see* Vitamin A *on page 2186*
- **Vitamin B_1** *see* Thiamine *on page 2048*
- **Vitamin B_2** *see* Riboflavin *on page 1856*
- **Vitamin B_3** *see* Niacin *on page 1511*
- **Vitamin B_6** *see* Pyridoxine *on page 1810*
- **Vitamin B_{12}** *see* Cyanocobalamin *on page 545*
- **Vitamin B_{12a}** *see* Hydroxocobalamin *on page 1050*
- **Vitamin Bw** *see* Biotin *on page 289*
- **Vitamin D2** *see* Ergocalciferol *on page 772*
- **Vitamin D3 Super Strength [OTC]** *see* Cholecalciferol *on page 448*

Vitamin E (VYE ta min ee)

Medication Safety Issues
Sound-alike/look-alike issues:
Aquasol E may be confused with Anusol

Related Information
Multivitamin Product Table *on page 2266*

Brand Names: US Alph-E [OTC]; Alph-E-Mixed 1000 [OTC]; Alph-E-Mixed [OTC]; Aquasol E [OTC]; Aquavit-E [OTC]; Aqueous Vitamin E [OTC]; E-400 [OTC]; E-400-Clear [OTC]; E-400-Mixed [OTC]; E-Max-1000 [OTC]; E-Pherol [OTC]; Formula E 400 [OTC]; Gordons-Vite E [OTC]; Natural Vitamin E [OTC]; Nutr-E-Sol [OTC]; Vita-Plus E [OTC]; Vitamin E Beauty [OTC]; Vitec [OTC]; Xtra-Care [OTC]

Therapeutic Category Nutritional Supplement; Vitamin, Fat Soluble; Vitamin, Topical

Generic Availability (US) May be product dependent

Use Prevention and treatment of vitamin E deficiency

Pregnancy Considerations Vitamin E crosses the placenta. Maternal serum concentrations of α tocopherol increase with lipid concentrations as pregnancy progresses; however, placental transfer remains constant. Additional supplementation is not needed in pregnant women without deficiency (IOM, 2000).

Breast-Feeding Considerations Vitamin E is found in breast milk; concentrations decrease over time and are highest immediately postpartum. Breast milk concentrations may be affected by maternal intake; however, additional supplementation is not needed in nursing women (IOM, 2000).

Contraindications Hypersensitivity to vitamin E or any component of the formulation

Warnings/Precautions May induce vitamin K deficiency (Corkins, 2010). Necrotizing enterocolitis has been associated with oral administration of large dosages (eg, >200 units/day) of a hyperosmolar vitamin E preparation in low birth weight infants.

Some dosage forms may contain polysorbate 80 (also known as Tweens). Hypersensitivity reactions, usually a delayed reaction, have been reported following exposure to pharmaceutical products containing polysorbate 80 in certain individuals (Isaksson, 2002; Lucente 2000; Shelley, 1995). Thrombocytopenia, ascites, pulmonary deterioration, and renal and hepatic failure have been reported in premature neonates after receiving parenteral products containing polysorbate 80 (Alade, 1986; CDC, 1984). See manufacturer's labeling.

Warnings: Additional Pediatric Considerations Excessive intake of vitamin E may be associated with adverse effects, including hemorrhagic effects; use caution when total daily intake from all sources exceeds the recommended age-based daily upper limit: 1 to 3 years: 200 mg; 4 to 8 years: 300 mg; 9 to 13 years: 600 mg; 14 to 18 years: 800 mg; ≥19 years: 1,000 mg; monitor serum concentrations (IOM, 2000).

Some dosage forms may contain propylene glycol; in neonates large amounts of propylene glycol delivered orally, intravenously (eg, >3,000 mg/day), or topically have been associated with potentially fatal toxicities which can include metabolic acidosis, seizures, renal failure, and CNS depression; toxicities have also been reported in children and adults including hyperosmolality, lactic acidosis, seizures and respiratory depression; use caution (AAP, 1997; Shehab, 2009).

Adverse Reactions
Central nervous system: Fatigue, headache
Dermatologic: Contact dermatitis with topical preparation, rash
Endocrine & metabolic: Creatinuria, gonadal dysfunction, hypercholesterolemia, hypertriglyceridemia, serum thyroxine decreased, serum triiodothyronine decreased
Gastrointestinal: Diarrhea, intestinal cramps, nausea, necrotizing enterocolitis (infants)
Neuromuscular & skeletal: CPK increased, weakness
Ocular: Blurred vision
Renal: Serum creatinine increased

Drug Interactions
Metabolism/Transport Effects None known.
Avoid Concomitant Use There are no known interactions where it is recommended to avoid concomitant use.
Increased Effect/Toxicity
Vitamin E may increase the levels/effects of: Agents with Antiplatelet Properties; Anticoagulants; Ibrutinib

The levels/effects of Vitamin E may be increased by: Tipranavir

Decreased Effect
Vitamin E may decrease the levels/effects of: CycloSPORINE (Systemic)

The levels/effects of Vitamin E may be decreased by: Orlistat

Storage/Stability Protect from light.

Mechanism of Action Prevents oxidation of vitamin A and C; protects polyunsaturated fatty acids in membranes from attack by free radicals and protects red blood cells against hemolysis

Pharmacokinetics (Adult data unless noted)
Absorption: Oral: Depends upon the presence of bile; absorption is reduced in conditions of malabsorption, in

low birth weight premature infants, and as dosage increases; water miscible preparations are better absorbed than oil preparations

Metabolism: Hepatic to glucuronides

Elimination: Feces

Dosing: Neonatal

Adequate intake (AI): Oral: 4 mg/day; **Note:** Adequate intake represents α-tocopherol intake from dietary consumption.

Cholestasis, chronic; supplementation: Oral: 25 to 50 units/day; a water soluble formulation is preferred (Kleigman, 2011)

Deficiency, vitamin E: Oral:

Treatment: 25 to 50 units/day for 1 week, followed by adequate dietary intake (Kleigman, 2011)

Prevention: Aquasol E drops: 5 units/day

Cystic fibrosis supplementation: Oral: 40 to 50 units/day (Borowitz, 2002)

Dosing: Usual

Infants, Children, and Adolescents:

Adequate intake (AI): Oral: **Note:** Adequate intake represents α-tocopherol intake from dietary consumption

1 to 6 months: 4 mg/day

7 to 12 months: 5 mg/day

Recommended daily allowance (RDA): Oral: **Note:** Recommended daily allowance represents α-tocopherol intake from dietary consumption.

1 to 3 years: 6 mg/day

4 to 8 years: 7 mg/day

9 to 13 years: 11 mg/day

14 to 18 years: 15 mg/day

Cholestasis, chronic; supplementation: Oral:

Infants: 20 to 50 units/kg/day; in the trials, a water soluble formulation was used (Corkins, 2010; Sokol, 1993)

Biliary atresia, post-hepatoportoenterostomy (HPE): Initial: 100 units/day using AquaADEK (2 mL); titrate dose based upon serum concentrations in 25 units/kg/day increments up to 100 units/kg/day to target α-tocopherol serum concentration range: 3.8 to 20.3 mcg/mL, vitamin E:total serum lipids ratio of 0.6 mg/g; patients with a total bilirubin <2 mg/dL may require lower doses (Shneider, 2012)

Children: 1 unit/kg/day; a water soluble formulation is preferred (Kleigman, 2011)

Deficiency, vitamin E: Oral:

Treatment (associated with malabsorption): Children: 1 unit/kg/day; adjust dose based on serum concentrations; a water soluble formulation is preferred (Kleigman, 2011)

Prevention: Aquasol E:

Infants: 5 units/day

Children <4 years: 10 units/day

Children ≥4 years and Adolescents: 15 units/day

Cystic fibrosis supplementation (Borowitz, 2002): Oral:

1 to 12 months: 40 to 50 units/day

1 to 3 years: 80 to 150 units/day

4 to 8 years: 100 to 200 units/day

>8 years: 200 to 400 units/day

Superficial dermatologic irritation: Children and Adolescents: Topical: Apply a thin layer over affected area

Adults:

Recommended daily allowance (RDA): Oral: **Note:** Recommended daily allowance represents α-tocopherol intake from dietary consumption. 15 mg/day

Lactating female: 19 mg/day

Superficial dermatologic irritation: Topical: Apply a thin layer over affected area

Administration Oral: May administer with or without food. Swallow capsules whole; do not crush or chew.

Monitoring Parameters Plasma tocopherol concentrations

Reference Range Plasma tocopherol: 6-14 mcg/mL

Additional Information Vitamin E, also known as α-tocopherol, occurs as several different isomers: RRR-α-tocopherol (the only form of α-tocopherol that occurs naturally in foods) and the *2,S* and *2,R* sterioisomers that occur in fortified foods and supplements [also known as all racemic (*all rac*)-α-tocopherol]. Only the *2,R*-stereoisomeric forms of α-tocopherol are biologically active, thus a higher amount of all racemic (*all rac*)-α-tocopherol is needed than the vitamin E found naturally in foods (based on milligram amount) (IOM, 2000).

In the past, the recommended daily allowance (RDA) for vitamin E had been expressed in units. The term units has been replaced by milligrams (mg) of α-tocopherol or may also be expressed as alpha tocopherol equivalents (ATE), which refer to the biologically active (R) stereoisomer content. While international units are no longer recognized, many fortified foods and supplements continue to use this term. USP units are now used by the pharmaceutical industry when labeling vitamin E supplements. Both IUs and USP units are based on the same equivalency. One unit of vitamin E=1 mg of all racemic (*all-rac*)-α-tocopheryl acetate (synthetic Vitamin E; also known as dl-α-tocopherol acetate) or 0.67 mg RRR-α-tocopherol (naturally occurring vitamin E; also known as d-α-tocopherol) (IOM, 2000).

Dosage Forms Excipient information presented when available (limited, particularly for generics); consult specific product labeling.

Capsule, Oral:

Alph-E: 400 units

Alph-E-Mixed: 200 units

Alph-E-Mixed 1000: 1000 units

Alph-E-Mixed: 400 units [corn free, milk free, sugar free, wheat free, yeast free]

Formula E 400: 400 units

Vita-Plus E: 400 units

Generic: 100 units, 200 units, 400 units, 1000 units

Capsule, Oral [preservative free]:

E-400: 400 units [corn free, gluten free, milk derivatives/products, no artificial color(s), no artificial flavor(s), sodium free, soy free, starch free, sugar free, yeast free]

E-400-Clear: 400 units [dye free]

E-400-Mixed: 400 units [dye free]

E-Max-1000: 1000 units [dye free]

Generic: 100 units, 400 units

Cream, External:

Gordons-Vite E: 1500 units/30 g (15 g, 75 g, 480 g, 2400 g)

Generic: 1000 units (112 g)

Liquid, External:

Generic: 920 units/mL (28.5 mL, 57 mL, 114 mL)

Liquid, Oral:

Nutr-E-Sol: 400 units/15 mL (473 mL) [color free, starch free, sugar free]

Lotion, External:

Vitec: (113 g)

Xtra-Care: (2 mL, 59 mL, 118 mL, 237 mL, 621 mL, 1000 mL, 3840 mL)

Oil, External:

Vitamin E Beauty: 24,000 units/52 mL (52 mL); 49,000 units/52 mL (52 mL)

Solution, Oral:

Aquasol E: 15 units/0.3 mL (12 mL, 30 mL) [contains polysorbate 80, propylene glycol, saccharin]

Aquavit-E: 15 units/0.3 mL (30 mL) [butterscotch flavor]

Aqueous Vitamin E: 15 units/0.3 mL (30 mL) [anise-butterscotch flavor]

Generic: 15 units/0.3 mL (12 mL)

Tablet, Oral:
E-Pherol: 400 units
Natural Vitamin E: 200 units, 400 units [animal products free, gelatin free, gluten free, kosher certified, lactose free, no artificial color(s), no artificial flavor(s), starch free, sugar free, yeast free]
Generic: 100 units, 200 units, 400 units

- ◆ **Vitamin E Beauty [OTC]** *see* Vitamin E *on page 2188*
- ◆ **Vitamin G** *see* Riboflavin *on page 1856*
- ◆ **Vitamin H** *see* Biotin *on page 289*
- ◆ **Vitamin K** *see* Phytonadione *on page 1698*
- ◆ **Vitamin K_1** *see* Phytonadione *on page 1698*
- ◆ **Vita-Plus E [OTC]** *see* Vitamin E *on page 2188*
- ◆ **Vitec [OTC]** *see* Vitamin E *on page 2188*
- ◆ **Vitrase** *see* Hyaluronidase *on page 1025*
- ◆ **Vitrasert [DSC]** *see* Ganciclovir (Ophthalmic) *on page 959*
- ◆ **Vituz** *see* Hydrocodone and Chlorpheniramine *on page 1034*
- ◆ **Vi Vaccine** *see* Typhoid Vaccine *on page 2133*
- ◆ **Vivactil [DSC]** *see* Protriptyline *on page 1798*
- ◆ **Viva-Drops® [OTC]** *see* Artificial Tears *on page 201*
- ◆ **Vivarin [OTC]** *see* Caffeine *on page 335*
- ◆ **Vivelle-Dot** *see* Estradiol (Systemic) *on page 795*
- ◆ **Vivotif** *see* Typhoid Vaccine *on page 2133*
- ◆ **VLB** *see* VinBLAStine *on page 2177*
- ◆ **VM-26** *see* Teniposide *on page 2015*
- ◆ **Vogelxo** *see* Testosterone *on page 2025*
- ◆ **Vogelxo Pump** *see* Testosterone *on page 2025*
- ◆ **Voltaren** *see* Diclofenac (Systemic) *on page 641*
- ◆ **Voltaren Rapide (Can)** *see* Diclofenac (Systemic) *on page 641*
- ◆ **Voltaren SR (Can)** *see* Diclofenac (Systemic) *on page 641*
- ◆ **Voltaren-XR [DSC]** *see* Diclofenac (Systemic) *on page 641*
- ◆ **Volulyte (Can)** *see* Tetrastarch *on page 2037*
- ◆ **Voluven** *see* Tetrastarch *on page 2037*
- ◆ **von Willebrand Factor/Factor VIII Complex** *see* Antihemophilic Factor/von Willebrand Factor Complex (Human) *on page 173*
- ◆ **Voraxaze** *see* Glucarpidase *on page 974*

Voriconazole (vor i KOE na zole)

Medication Safety Issues

Sound-alike/look-alike issues:

Voriconazole may be confused with fluconazole, itraconazole, posaconazole

Related Information

Safe Handling of Hazardous Drugs *on page 2455*

Brand Names: US Vfend; Vfend IV

Brand Names: Canada Apo-Voriconazole; Sandoz-Voriconazole; Teva-Voriconazole; VFEND; VFEND For Injection; Voriconazole For Injection

Therapeutic Category Antifungal Agent, Systemic; Antifungal Agent, Triazole

Generic Availability (US) Yes

Use Treatment of invasive aspergillosis; treatment of candidemia in non-neutropenic patients, deep tissue *Candida* infections and esophageal candidiasis; treatment of serious fungal infections caused by *Scedosporium apiospermum* or *Fusarium* spp (including *Fusarium solanae*) (All indications: FDA approved in ages ≥12 years and adults)

Pregnancy Risk Factor D

Pregnancy Considerations Voriconazole can cause fetal harm when administered to a pregnant woman. Voriconazole was teratogenic and embryotoxic in animal studies, and lowered plasma estradiol in animal models. Women of childbearing potential should use effective contraception during treatment. Should be used in pregnant woman only if benefit to mother justifies potential risk to the fetus.

Breast-Feeding Considerations It is not known if voriconazole is excreted in breast milk. Due to the potential for serious adverse reactions in the nursing infant, the manufacturer recommends a decision be made whether to discontinue nursing or to discontinue the drug, taking into account the importance of treatment to the mother.

Contraindications Hypersensitivity to voriconazole or any component of the formulation; coadministration with astemizole, barbiturates (long acting), carbamazepine, cisapride, efavirenz (≥400 mg daily), ergot derivatives (ergotamine and dihydroergotamine), pimozide, quinidine, rifampin, rifabutin, ritonavir (≥800 mg daily; also avoid low dose [eg, 200 mg daily] dosing if possible), sirolimus, St John's wort, terfenadine

Documentation of allergenic cross-reactivity for imidazole antifungals is limited. However, because of similarities in chemical structure and/or pharmacologic actions, the possibility of cross-sensitivity cannot be ruled out with certainty.

Warnings/Precautions Hazardous agent - use appropriate precautions for handling and disposal (NIOSH 2014 [group 3]).

Visual changes, including blurred vision, changes in visual acuity, color perception, and photophobia, are commonly associated with treatment; postmarketing cases of optic neuritis and papilledema (lasting >1 month) have also been reported. Patients should be warned to avoid tasks which depend on vision, including operating machinery or driving. Changes are reversible on discontinuation following brief exposure/treatment regimens (≤28 days).

Serious (and rarely fatal) hepatic reactions (eg, hepatitis, cholestasis, fulminant failure) have been observed with voriconazole. In lung transplant recipients, median time to hepatic toxicity was 14 days with the majority occurring within 30 days of therapy initiation (Luong, 2012). Use with caution in patients with serious underlying medical conditions (eg, hematologic malignancy); hepatic reactions have occurred in patients with no identifiable underlying risk factors. Liver dysfunction is usually reversible upon therapy discontinuation. Monitor serum transaminase and bilirubin at baseline and at least weekly for the first month of treatment. Monitoring frequency can then be reduced to monthly during continued use if no abnormalities are noted. If marked elevations occur compared to baseline, discontinue unless benefit/risk of treatment justifies continued use.

Voriconazole tablets contain lactose; avoid administration in hereditary galactose intolerance, Lapp lactase deficiency, or glucose-galactose malabsorption. Suspension contains sucrose; use caution with fructose intolerance, sucrase-isomaltase deficiency, or glucose-galactose malabsorption. Avoid/limit use of intravenous formulation in patients with moderate to severe renal impairment (CrCl <50 mL/minute); injection contains excipient cyclodextrin (sulfobutyl ether beta-cyclodextrin [SBECD]), which may accumulate, although the clinical significance of this finding is uncertain (Luke, 2010); consider using oral voriconazole in these patients unless benefit of injection outweighs the risk. If injection is used in patients CrCl

<50 mL/minute, monitor serum creatinine closely; if increases occur, consider changing therapy to oral voriconazole.

Anaphylactoid-type reactions (eg, flushing, fever, sweating, tachycardia, chest tightness, dyspnea, nausea, pruritus, rash) may occur with IV infusion. Consider discontinuation of infusion should these reactions occur. Acute renal failure has been observed in severely ill patients; use with caution in patients receiving concomitant nephrotoxic medications. Evaluate renal function (particularly serum creatinine) at baseline and periodically during therapy.

Potentially significant drug-drug interactions may exist, requiring dose or frequency adjustment, additional monitoring, and/or selection of alternative therapy. QT interval prolongation has been associated with voriconazole use; rare cases of arrhythmia (including torsade de pointes), cardiac arrest, and sudden death have been reported, usually in seriously ill patients with comorbidities and/or risk factors (eg, prior cardiotoxic chemotherapy, cardiomyopathy [especially with concomitant heart failure], electrolyte imbalance, or concomitant QTc-prolonging drugs). Also use with caution in patients with potentially proarrhythmic conditions (eg, congenital or acquired QT syndrome, sinus bradycardia, or preexisting symptomatic arrhythmias); correct electrolyte abnormalities (eg, hypokalemia, hypomagnesemia, hypocalcemia) prior to initiating and during therapy. Do not infuse concomitantly with blood products or short-term concentrated electrolyte solutions, even if the two infusions are running in separate intravenous lines (or cannulas).

Rare cases of malignancy (melanoma, squamous cell carcinoma [SCC]) have been reported in patients with prior onset of severe photosensitivity reactions or exposure to standard dose long-term voriconazole therapy (in lung transplant recipients, SCC increased by ~6% per 60 days with a 28% absolute risk increase at 5 years [Singer, 2012]). Other serious exfoliative cutaneous reactions, including Stevens-Johnson syndrome, have also been reported. Patients, including children, should avoid exposure to direct sunlight and should use protective clothing and high SPF sunscreen; may cause photosensitivity, especially with long-term use. If phototoxic reactions occur, referral to a dermatologist and voriconazole discontinuation should be considered. If therapy is continued, dermatologic evaluation should be performed on a systematic and regular basis to allow early detection and management of premalignant lesions. Pediatric patients are at particular risk for phototoxicity; stringent photoprotective measures are necessary in children due to the risk of squamous cell carcinoma. In children experiencing photoaging injuries (eg lentigines or ephelides), avoidance of sun and dermatologic follow-up are warranted even after treatment is discontinued. Discontinue use in patients who develop an exfoliative cutaneous reaction or a skin lesion consistent with squamous cell carcinoma or melanoma. Periodic total body skin examinations should be performed, particularly with prolonged use. Fluorosis and/or periostitis may occur during long-term therapy. If patient develops skeletal pain and radiologic findings of fluorosis or periostitis, discontinue therapy.

Voriconazole demonstrates nonlinear pharmacokinetics. Dose modifications may result in unpredictable changes in serum concentrations and contribute to toxicity. It is important to note that cutoff trough threshold values ranged widely among studies; however, an upper limit of <5.0 mg/L would be reasonable for most disease states (see CDC recommendations for *Exserohilum rostratum* in Reference Range section) (CDC, 2012). In patients >14 years of age or 12-14 years and weighing >50 kg, data suggest that pharmacokinetics are similar to adults (Friberg, 2012). In patients <12 years of age, the full pharmacokinetic profile for voriconazole is not completely defined, and for patients <2 years, the data are sparse. In children 2 to <12 years, current data suggests voriconazole undergoes a high degree of variability in exposure with linear elimination at lower doses and nonlinear elimination at higher doses; therefore, to achieve similar AUC as adults, increased dosage is necessary in children (Friberg, 2012; Karlsson, 2009; Walsh, 2004).

Correct electrolyte abnormalities (eg, hypokalemia, hypomagnesemia, hypocalcemia) prior to initiating and during therapy. Monitor pancreatic function in patients (children and adults) at risk for acute pancreatitis (eg, recent chemotherapy or hematopoietic stem cell transplantation). Pancreatitis has occurred in pediatric patients.

Benzyl alcohol and derivatives: Some dosage forms may contain sodium benzoate/benzoic acid; benzoic acid (benzoate) is a metabolite of benzyl alcohol; large amounts of benzyl alcohol (≥99 mg/kg/day) have been associated with a potentially fatal toxicity ("gasping syndrome") in neonates; the "gasping syndrome" consists of metabolic acidosis, respiratory distress, gasping respirations, CNS dysfunction (including convulsions, intracranial hemorrhage), hypotension, and cardiovascular collapse (AAP, 1997; CDC, 1982); some data suggests that benzoate displaces bilirubin from protein binding sites (Ahlfors, 2001); avoid or use dosage forms containing benzyl alcohol derivative with caution in neonates. See manufacturer's labeling.

Warnings: Additional Pediatric Considerations

Unlike adults, a correlation between liver function test abnormalities and higher plasma drug concentrations and/or doses has not been clearly observed in pediatric patients (Driscoll, 2011; Neely, 2010; Soler-Palacín, 2012). Monitor liver function and bilirubin at baseline and periodically during therapy; if abnormal LFT's occur during therapy, additional close monitoring for more severe hepatic injury recommended; if more severe hepatic injury develops, discontinuation of therapy should be considered. With serious exfoliative cutaneous reactions (eg, Stevens Johnson syndrome), reports of a causal relationship to dose and/or serum concentration have been mixed in pediatric patients with a dose- and/or concentration-dependent relationship reported in some cases (Bernhard, 2012; Soler-Palacín, 2012) and others have reported phototoxicities without any relation to dose and/or concentration (Frick, 2010; Hansford, 2012). In pediatric patients, an increased risk and earlier onset of photosensitivity reactions have been observed with concurrent methotrexate therapy (van Hasselt, 2013).

In pediatric patients <12 years, bioequivalence between the oral tablet and suspension has not been determined; due to possible shortened gastric transit time in infants and children, absorption of tablets may be different than adults; it is recommended that infants and children <12 years only receive oral suspension formulation. Additionally, data suggests that children <12 years have approximately a 50% reduction in bioavailability than adults; in some pediatric patients, voriconazole therapy should be initiated with the parenteral formulation with conversion to oral therapy once significant clinical improvement has been observed (Karlsson, 2009; Vfend prescribing information [Europe Medicines Agency], 2013); consider monitoring serum concentrations (Chen, 2012).

Adverse Reactions

Cardiovascular: Tachycardia
Central nervous system: Chills, hallucinations, headache
Dermatologic: Skin rash
Endocrine & metabolic: Hypokalemia
Gastrointestinal: Nausea, vomiting

Hepatic: Cholestatic jaundice, increased serum alkaline phosphatase, increased serum ALT, increased serum AST

Ophthalmic: Photophobia, visual disturbance

Renal: Increased serum creatinine

Miscellaneous: Fever

Rare but important or life-threatening: Acute renal failure, adrenocortical insufficiency, agranulocytosis, alopecia, anaphylactoid reaction, anemia (aplastic, hemolytic, macrocytic, megaloblastic, or microcytic), angioedema, anorexia, anuria, arthritis, ascites, ataxia, atrial arrhythmia, atrial fibrillation, atrioventricular block, bacterial infection, bigeminy, blighted ovum, bone marrow depression, bradycardia, brain disease, bundle branch block, cardiac arrest, cardiac failure, cardiomegaly, cardiomyopathy, cellulitis, cerebral edema, cerebral hemorrhage, cerebral ischemia, cerebrovascular accident, chest pain, cholecystitis, cholelithiasis, cholestasis, chromatopsia, color blindness, coma, confusion, convulsions, corneal opacity, cyanosis, deafness, deep vein thrombophlebitis, deep vein thrombosis, delirium, dementia, dental fluorosis, depersonalization, depression, diabetes insipidus, diarrhea, discoid lupus erythematosus, disseminated intravascular coagulation, drowsiness, duodenal ulcer (active), duodenitis, dyspnea, eczema, edema, encephalitis, endocarditis, eosinophilia, erythema multiforme, esophageal ulcer, exfoliative dermatitis, extrapyramidal reaction, extrasystoles, fixed drug eruption, fungal infection, gastric ulcer, gastrointestinal hemorrhage, glucose tolerance decreased, graft versus host disease, Guillain-Barre syndrome, hematemesis, hemorrhagic cystitis, hepatic coma, hepatic failure, hepatitis, hepatomegaly, herpes simplex infection, hydronephrosis, hyperbilirubinemia, hypercholesterolemia, hyper-/hypocalcemia, hyper-/hypoglycemia, hyper-/hypomagnesemia, hyper-/hyponatremia, hyper-/hypotension, hyper-/hypothyroidism, hyperkalemia, hypersensitivity reaction, hyperuricemia, hypophosphatemia, hypoxia, impotence, increased blood urea nitrogen, increased gamma-glutamyl transferase, increased lactate dehydrogenase, increased susceptibility to infection, intestinal perforation, intracranial hypertension, jaundice, leukopenia, lymphadenopathy, lymphangitis, maculopapular rash, malignant melanoma, melanosis, multi-organ failure, myasthenia, myocardial infarction, myopathy, nephritis, nephrosis, neuropathy, nocturnal amblyopia, nodal arrhythmia, nodule, nystagmus, oculogyric crisis, optic atrophy, optic neuritis, orthostatic hypotension, osteomalacia, osteonecrosis, osteoporosis, otitis externa, palpitations, pancreatitis, pancytopenia, papilledema, paresthesia, perforated duodenal ulcer, periosteal disease, peripheral edema, peritonitis, petechia, pleural effusion, pneumonia, prolonged bleeding time, prolonged QT interval on ECG, pruritus, pseudomembranous colitis, pseudoporphyria, psoriasis, psychosis, pulmonary edema, pulmonary embolism, purpura, rectal hemorrhage, renal insufficiency, renal tubular necrosis, respiratory distress syndrome, respiratory tract infection, retinal hemorrhage, retinitis, seizure, sepsis, skin discoloration, skin photosensitivity, splenomegaly, squamous cell carcinoma, Stevens-Johnson syndrome, subconjunctival hemorrhage, substernal pain, suicidal ideation, supraventricular extrasystole, supraventricular tachycardia, syncope, thrombocytopenia, thrombophlebitis, thrombotic thrombocytopenic purpura, tongue edema, tonic-clonic seizures, torsades de pointes, toxic epidermal necrolysis, uremia, urinary incontinence, urinary retention, urinary tract infection, urticaria, uterine hemorrhage, uveitis, vaginal hemorrhage, vasodilation, ventricular arrhythmia, ventricular fibrillation, ventricular tachycardia, visual field defect

Drug Interactions

Metabolism/Transport Effects Substrate of CYP2C19 (major), CYP2C9 (major), CYP3A4 (minor); **Note:** Assignment of Major/Minor substrate status based on clinically relevant drug interaction potential; **Inhibits** CYP2C19 (moderate), CYP2C9 (moderate), CYP3A4 (strong)

Avoid Concomitant Use

Avoid concomitant use of Voriconazole with any of the following: Ado-Trastuzumab Emtansine; Alfuzosin; Apixaban; Astemizole; Atazanavir; Avanafil; Axitinib; Barbiturates; Barnidipine; Bosutinib; Cabozantinib; CarBAMazepine; Ceritinib; Cisapride; Conivaptan; Crizotinib; Dapoxetine; Darunavir; Dihydroergotamine; Dofetilide; Domperidone; Dronedarone; Eletriptan; Eplerenone; Ergoloid Mesylates; Ergonovine; Ergotamine; Everolimus; Fluconazole; Halofantrine; Ibrutinib; Irinotecan; Isavuconazonium Sulfate; Ivabradine; Lapatinib; Lercanidipine; Lomitapide; Lopinavir; Lovastatin; Lurasidone; Macitentan; Methylergonovine; Naloxegol; Nilotinib; NiMODipine; Nisoldipine; Olaparib; Palbociclib; Pimozide; QuiNIDine; Ranolazine; Red Yeast Rice; Regorafenib; Rifamycin Derivatives; Ritonavir; Rivaroxaban; Saccharomyces boulardii; Salmeterol; Silodosin; Simeprevir; Simvastatin; Sirolimus; St Johns Wort; Suvorexant; Tamsulosin; Terfenadine; Ticagrelor; Tolvaptan; Toremifene; Trabectedin; Ulipristal; Vemurafenib; VinCRIStine (Liposomal); Vorapaxar

Increased Effect/Toxicity

Voriconazole may increase the levels/effects of: Ado-Trastuzumab Emtansine; Alfuzosin; Almotriptan; Alosetron; Antineoplastic Agents (Vinca Alkaloids); Apixaban; ARIPiprazole; Astemizole; AtorvaSTATin; Avanafil; Axitinib; Barnidipine; Bedaquiline; Boceprevir; Bortezomib; Bosentan; Bosutinib; Brentuximab Vedotin; Brinzolamide; Budesonide (Nasal); Budesonide (Systemic, Oral Inhalation); Budesonide (Topical); BusPIRone; Busulfan; Cabazitaxel; Cabozantinib; Calcium Channel Blockers; Cannabis; Carvedilol; Ceritinib; Cilostazol; Cisapride; Citalopram; Cobicistat; Colchicine; Conivaptan; Contraceptives (Estrogens); Contraceptives (Progestins); Corticosteroids (Orally Inhaled); Corticosteroids (Systemic); Crizotinib; CycloSPORINE (Systemic); CYP2C19 Substrates; CYP2C9 Substrates; CYP3A4 Substrates; Dapoxetine; Dasatinib; Diclofenac (Systemic); Diclofenac (Topical); Dienogest; Dihydroergotamine; DOCEtaxel; Dofetilide; Domperidone; DOXOrubicin (Conventional); Dronabinol; Dronedarone; Drospirenone; Dutasteride; Efavirenz; Eletriptan; Eliglustat; Elvitegravir; Enzalutamide; Eplerenone; Ergoloid Mesylates; Ergonovine; Ergotamine; Erlotinib; Etizolam; Etravirine; Everolimus; FentaNYL; Fesoterodine; Fluticasone (Nasal); Fluticasone (Oral Inhalation); Fosamprenavir; Fosphenytoin; GuanFACINE; Halofantrine; Highest Risk QTc-Prolonging Agents; Hydrocodone; Ibrutinib; Ibuprofen; Idelalisib; Iloperidone; Imatinib; Imidafenacin; Irinotecan; Isavuconazonium Sulfate; Ivabradine; Ivacaftor; Ixabepilone; Lacosamide; Lapatinib; Lercanidipine; Levobupivacaine; Levomilnacipran; Lomitapide; Losartan; Lovastatin; Lurasidone; Macitentan; Maraviroc; MedroxyPROGESTERone; Meloxicam; Methadone; Methylergonovine; MethylPREDNISolone; Mifepristone; Moderate Risk QTc-Prolonging Agents; Naloxegol; Nelfinavir; Nilotinib; NiMODipine; Nisoldipine; Olaparib; Ospemifene; Oxybutynin; OxyCODONE; Palbociclib; Panobinostat; Parecoxib; Paricalcitol; PAZOPanib; Phenytoin; Pimecrolimus; Pimozide; PONATinib; Porfimer; Pranlukast; PrednisoLONE (Systemic); PredniSONE; Propafenone; Proton Pump Inhibitors; QUEtiapine; QuiNIDine; Ramelteon; Ranolazine; Red Yeast Rice; Regorafenib; Repaglinide; Retapamulin; Reverse Transcriptase Inhibitors (Non-Nucleoside); Rifamycin Derivatives; Rilpivirine; Rivaroxaban; RomiDEPsin; Ruxolitinib; Salmeterol;

Saxagliptin; Sildenafil; Silodosin; Simeprevir; Simvastatin; Sirolimus; Solifenacin; SORAfenib; Sulfonylureas; SUNItinib; Suvorexant; Tacrolimus (Systemic); Tacrolimus (Topical); Tadalafil; Tamsulosin; Tasimelteon; Telaprevir; Terfenadine; Tetrahydrocannabinol; Ticagrelor; Tofacitinib; Tolterodine; Tolvaptan; Toremifene; Trabectedin; TraMADol; Ulipristal; Vardenafil; Vemurafenib; Venlafaxine; Verteporfin; Vilazodone; VinCRIStine (Liposomal); Vitamin K Antagonists; Vorapaxar; Zolpidem; Zopiclone; Zuclopenthixol

The levels/effects of Voriconazole may be increased by: Atazanavir; Boceprevir; Chloramphenicol; Cobicistat; Contraceptives (Estrogens); Contraceptives (Progestins); CYP2C19 Inhibitors (Moderate); CYP2C19 Inhibitors (Strong); CYP2C9 Inhibitors (Moderate); CYP2C9 Inhibitors (Strong); Etravirine; Fluconazole; Fosamprenavir; Luliconazole; Mifepristone; Proton Pump Inhibitors; Telaprevir

Decreased Effect

Voriconazole may decrease the levels/effects of: Amphotericin B; Atazanavir; Clopidogrel; Ifosfamide; Prasugrel; Saccharomyces boulardii; Ticagrelor

The levels/effects of Voriconazole may be decreased by: Atazanavir; Barbiturates; CarBAMazepine; CYP2C9 Inducers (Strong); Dabrafenib; Darunavir; Didanosine; Efavirenz; Etravirine; Fosphenytoin; Lopinavir; Phenytoin; Reverse Transcriptase Inhibitors (Non-Nucleoside); Rifamycin Derivatives; Ritonavir; St Johns Wort; Sucralfate; Telaprevir

Food Interactions Food may decrease voriconazole absorption. Management: Oral voriconazole should be taken 1 hour before or 1 hour after a meal. Maintain adequate hydration unless instructed to restrict fluid intake.

Storage/Stability

Powder for injection: Store vials between 15°C to 30°C (59°F to 86°F). Reconstituted solutions are stable for up to 24 hours under refrigeration at 2°C to 8°C (36°F to 46°F).

Powder for oral suspension: Store at 2°C to 8°C (36°F to 46°F). Reconstituted oral suspension is stable for up to 14 days if stored at 15°C to 30°C (59°F to 86°F). Do not refrigerate or freeze.

Tablets: Store at 15°C to 30°C (59°F to 86°F).

Mechanism of Action Interferes with fungal cytochrome P450 activity (selectively inhibits 14-alpha-lanosterol demethylation), decreasing ergosterol synthesis (principal sterol in fungal cell membrane) and inhibiting fungal cell membrane formation.

Pharmacokinetics (Adult data unless noted) Note: Overall, in pediatric patients, voriconazole pharmacokinetics are complex. In adolescents >14 years and pediatric patients 12-14 years and weighing >50 kg, data suggests that pharmacokinetics are similar to adults (Friberg, 2012). In pediatric patients <12 years, the full pharmacokinetic profile for voriconazole is not completely defined and for patients <2 years, the data is sparse. In children 2 to <12 years, current data suggests voriconazole undergoes a high degree of variability in exposure with linear elimination at lower doses and nonlinear at higher doses; therefore, to achieve similar AUC as adults, higher mg/kg dosing is necessary in children (Friberg, 2012; Karlsson, 2009; Walsh, 2010).

Absorption: Oral: Rapid and complete

Distribution: Extensive tissue distribution; CSF concentration ~50% of plasma concentration (Walsh, 2008)

Children 2 to <12 years: Biphasic, V_d (central): 0.81 L/kg; V_d (peripheral): 2.2 L/kg (Karlsson, 2009)

Adults: V_d: 4.6 L/kg

Protein binding: 58%

Metabolism: Metabolized by cytochrome P450 enzymes CYP2C19, CYP2C9, and CYP3A4 to voriconazole N-oxide (minimal antifungal activity); CYP2C19 is significantly involved in metabolism of voriconazole; CYP2C19 exhibits genetic polymorphism (15% to 20% Asians may be poor metabolizers of voriconazole; 3% to 5% Caucasians and African Americans may be poor metabolizers). In children 2 to 12 years, metabolic clearance is faster than in adults (Walsh, 2010). In children 2 to 12 years, the majority of data has shown that the pharmacokinetic parameters of voriconazole are affected by a patient's CYP2C19 genotype (Hicks, 2014; Narita, 2013; Wang 2014) although, an initial report suggested CYP2C19 genotype had no apparent effect on exposure in children (Driscoll, 2011).

Bioavailability: Oral:

Children 2 to <12 years: Reported range highly variable: ~45% to 64% (Friberg, 2012; Karlsson, 2009) and values as high as 80% have been reported (Neely, 2010)

Adults: 96%

Half-life: Variable, dose dependent

Time to peak serum concentration: Oral:

Children 2 to <12 years: Median: 1.1 hours (range: 0.73-8.03 hours) (Driscoll, 2011)

Adults: 1-2 hours

Elimination: Urine (as inactive metabolites; <2% as unchanged drug)

Dosing: Neonatal Fungal infection, severe; treatment: Limited data available (case series and reports); dosing regimens variable: IV: Usual reported dose: 12-20 mg/kg/day divided every 8-12 hours; doses up to 24 mg/kg/day have been used; dosing based on experience in 23 neonates of which the majority were premature (minimum GA: 24 weeks) (Celik, 2013; Doby, 2012; Turan, 2011); earlier data describes lower daily doses of 4-8 mg/kg/day divided every 12 hours (Celik, 2013; Frankenbusch, 2006; Kohli, 2008; Santos, 2007). In the rare instance in which conversion to oral therapy described, oral therapy was initiated at same IV dose. **Note:** Pharmacokinetic neonatal data is sparse; consider monitoring serum concentrations (trough); the frequency dependent upon several factors and some suggest more frequent monitoring in neonates (Chen, 2012).

Dosing: Usual

Pediatric: **Note:** In pediatric patients <12 years, bioequivalence between the oral tablet and suspension has not been determined; due to possible shortened gastric transit time in infants and children, absorption of tablets may be different than adults; it is recommended that infants and children <12 years only receive oral suspension formulation [Vfend prescribing information (Europe Medicines Agency), 2013].

Infants and Children <2 years: **Fungal infection; treatment, including empiric therapy:** Limited data available (small case series, n=17 patients): IV, Oral suspension: Initial: 9 mg/kg/dose every 12 hours followed by monitoring of serum trough concentrations typically initiated after 3 doses; adjust dose to achieve target value (>1 mcg/mL); median final dosage: 31.5 mg/kg/**day** (12-71 mg/kg/**day**) divided every 12 hours; dosing based on experience which showed lower initial regimens (7 mg/kg/dose every 12 hours) achieved therapeutic troughs in only 14% of infants and children <2 years (Bartenlink, 2013; Gerin, 2011)

Children 2 to <12 years: Limited data available:

General dosing, susceptible infection (*Red Book*, 2012):

IV:

Loading dose: 9 mg/kg/dose every 12 hours for 2 doses on day 1

Maintenance: 9 mg/kg/dose every 12 hours; maximum single dose: 350 mg

Oral: 9 mg/kg/dose every 12 hours; maximum single dose: 350 mg; **Note:** In most patients, oral therapy has not been recommended as initial therapy for treatment; it has been recommended to convert parenteral to oral therapy only after significant clinical improvement has been observed [Vfend prescribing information (Europe Medicines Agency), 2013]. Earlier data had suggested a fixed dose (200 mg twice daily) in children 2-12 years (Karlsson, 2009); however, additional trials have shown interpatient variability and low drug exposure in older or heavier children within this age range; weight-based dosing is now recommended (Driscoll, 2011; Frieberg, 2012); **Note:** Clinical trials have only used the oral suspension product in this population; due to difference in GI transit time and lack of data with the tablet dosage form in these patients, only the oral suspension is recommended [Vfend prescribing information (Europe Medicines Agency), 2013].

Aspergillosis, invasive, including disseminated and extrapulmonary infection; treatment: Duration of therapy should be a minimum of 6-12 weeks or throughout period of immunosuppression (Walsh, 2008):

IV: **Note:** Recent data suggest higher doses (mg/kg) are required; consider using a loading dose: 9 mg/kg/dose every 12 hours for 2 doses on day 1, followed by a maintenance dose: 8-9 mg/kg/dose every 12 hours; maximum dose: 350 mg. Monitoring of concentrations may be warranted (Driscoll, 2011; *Red Book*, 2012)

Non-HIV-exposed/-positive: 5-7 mg/kg/dose every 12 hours (Walsh, 2008); see Note regarding higher dose recommendations (Walsh, 2008)

HIV-exposed/-positive (CDC, 2009): See Note regarding higher dose recommendations.

Loading dose: 6-8 mg/kg/dose (maximum: 400 mg/dose) every 12 hours for 2 doses on day 1

Maintenance dose: 7 mg/kg/dose (maximum: 200 mg/dose) every 12 hours; change to oral administration when able; duration of therapy (IV and oral combined): ≥12 weeks but should be individualized

Oral suspension: May consider oral therapy once patient stable

Non-HIV-exposed/-positive: 9 mg/kg/dose every 12 hours (*Red Book*, 2012)

HIV-exposed/-positive (CDC, 2009): **Note:** Recent data suggest higher doses (mg/kg) are required (9 mg/kg every 12 hours) (*Red Book*, 2012)

Loading dose: 8 mg/kg/dose (maximum: 400 mg/dose) every 12 hours for 2 doses on day 1

Maintenance dose: 7 mg/kg/dose (maximum: 200 mg/dose) every 12 hours

Candidiasis or other serious fungal infection, treatment: IV: Loading dose: 9 mg/kg/dose every 12 hours for 2 doses on day 1, followed by a maintenance dose: 8-9 mg/kg/dose every 12 hours; maximum dose: 350 mg (Driscoll, 2011; *Red Book*, 2012)

Children ≥12 years and Adolescents:

Aspergillosis, invasive, including disseminated and extrapulmonary infection; treatment: Duration of therapy should be a minimum of 6-12 weeks or throughout period of immunosuppression (Walsh, 2008):

IV: Initial: Loading dose: 6 mg/kg every 12 hours for 2 doses; followed by maintenance dose of 4 mg/kg every 12 hours

Oral: Maintenance dose:

Manufacturer's labeling: Patient weight:

<40 kg: 100 mg every 12 hours; maximum daily dose: 300 mg/**day**

≥40 kg: 200 mg every 12 hours; maximum daily dose: 600 mg/**day**

IDSA recommendations (Walsh, 2008): May consider oral therapy in place of IV with dosing of 4 mg/kg (rounded up to convenient tablet dosage form) every 12 hours; however, IV administration is preferred in serious infections since comparative efficacy with the oral formulation has not been established.

Candidemia and other deep tissue *Candida* infections; non-neutropenic patient: Treatment should continue for a minimum of 14 days following resolution of symptoms or following last positive culture, whichever is longer.

IV: Initial: Loading dose 6 mg/kg every 12 hours for 2 doses; followed by maintenance dose of 3-4 mg/kg every 12 hours

Oral:

Manufacturer's labeling: Maintenance dose: Patient weight:

<40 kg: 100 mg every 12 hours; maximum daily dose: 300 mg/**day**

≥40 kg: 200 mg every 12 hours; maximum daily dose: 600 mg/**day**

IDSA recommendations (Pappas, 2009): Initial: Loading dose: 400 mg every 12 hours for 2 doses; followed by 200 mg every 12 hours

Candidiasis, esophageal: Treatment should continue for a minimum of 14 days, and for at least 7 days following resolution of symptoms: Oral: Patient weight:

<40 kg: 100 mg every 12 hours; maximum daily dose: 300 mg/**day**

≥40 kg: 200 mg every 12 hours; maximum daily dose: 600 mg/**day**

Endophthalmitis, fungal: IV: 6 mg/kg every 12 hours for 2 doses, then 3-4 mg/kg every 12 hours (Pappas, 2009)

Scedosporiosis, fusariosis:

IV: Initial: Loading dose: 6 mg/kg every 12 hours for 2 doses; followed by maintenance dose of 4 mg/kg every 12 hours

Oral: Maintenance dose: Patient weight:

<40 kg: 100 mg every 12 hours; maximum daily dose 300 mg/**day**

≥40 kg: 200 mg every 12 hours; maximum daily dose: 600 mg/**day**

Adult:

Candidemia and other deep tissue *Candida* infections: Treatment should continue for a minimum of 14 days following resolution of symptoms or following last positive culture, whichever is longer.

IV: Initial: Loading dose 6 mg/kg every 12 hours for 2 doses; followed by maintenance dose of 3-4 mg/kg every 12 hours

Oral: Manufacturer's labeling: Maintenance dose: Patient weight:

<40 kg: 100 mg every 12 hours; maximum: 300 mg/day

≥40 kg: 200 mg every 12 hours; maximum: 600 mg/day

Esophageal candidiasis: Oral: Treatment should continue for a minimum of 14 days, and for at least 7 days following resolution of symptoms: Patient weight:

<40 kg: 100 mg every 12 hours; maximum: 300 mg/day

≥40 kg: 200 mg every 12 hours; maximum: 600 mg/day

Scedosporiosis, fusariosis:

IV: Initial: Loading dose: 6 mg/kg every 12 hours for 2 doses; followed by maintenance dose of 4 mg/kg every 12 hours

Oral: Maintenance dose: Patient weight:

<40 kg: 100 mg every 12 hours; maximum 300 mg/day

≥40 kg: 200 mg every 12 hours; maximum: 600 mg/day

Dosage adjustment in patients unable to tolerate treatment: Children ≥12 years, Adolescents, and Adults:

IV: Dose may be reduced to 3 mg/kg every 12 hours

Oral: Patient weight:

<40 kg: Dose may be reduced in 50 mg decrements to a minimum 100 mg every 12 hours

≥40 kg: Dose may be reduced in 50 mg decrements to a minimum dosage of 200 mg every 12 hours

Dosage adjustment in patients receiving concomitant CYP450 enzyme inducers or substrates: Children ≥12 years, Adolescents, and Adults:

Efavirenz: Oral: Increase maintenance dose of voriconazole to 400 mg every 12 hours and reduce efavirenz dose to 300 mg once daily; upon discontinuation of voriconazole, return to the initial dose of efavirenz

Phenytoin:

IV: Increase voriconazole maintenance dosage to 5 mg/kg every 12 hours

Oral: Patient weight:

<40 kg: Increase voriconazole dose to 200 mg every 12 hours

≥40 kg: Increase voriconazole dose to 400 mg every 12 hours

Dosing adjustment in renal impairment: Children ≥12 years, Adolescents, and Adults:

Oral: No adjustment necessary

Parenteral: IV:

Mild (CrCl ≥50 mL/minute): No adjustment necessary

Moderate to severe (CrCl <50 mL/minute): Accumulation of the intravenous vehicle occurs. After initial IV loading dose, oral voriconazole should be administered, unless an assessment of the risk:benefit justifies the use of IV voriconazole. Monitor serum creatinine and change to oral voriconazole therapy when possible.

Dialysis: Poorly dialyzed; no supplemental dose or dosage adjustment necessary, including patients on intermittent hemodialysis, peritoneal dialysis, or continuous renal replacement therapy (eg, CVVHD)

Dosing adjustment in hepatic impairment: Children ≥12 years, Adolescents, and Adults:

Mild to moderate hepatic dysfunction (Child-Pugh Class A and B): Use standard loading dose regimen, then decrease maintenance dose by 50%

Severe hepatic impairment (Child-Pugh Class C): Not recommended for use unless benefit outweighs the risk; monitor closely for toxicity; not studied

Preparation for Administration Hazardous agent; use appropriate precautions for handling and disposal (NIOSH 2014 [group 3])

Oral: Powder for oral suspension: Add 46 mL of water to the bottle to make 40 mg/mL suspension. Shake vigorously for ~1 minute. Do not refrigerate or freeze.

Parenteral: Reconstitute 200 mg vial with 19 mL of SWFI resulting in a concentration of 10 mg/mL; use of automated syringe during reconstitution is not recommended. IV infusion: Further dilute reconstituted solution with NS, LR, D_5WLR, $D_5W^{1/2}NS$, D_5W, D_5W with KCl 20 mEq/L, $^{1/2}NS$, or D_5WNS to a final concentration of ≤5 mg/mL. Do not dilute with 4.2% sodium bicarbonate infusion.

Administration Hazardous agent; use appropriate precautions for handling and disposal (NIOSH 2014 [group 3])

Oral: Administer at least one hour before or one hour after a meal; maintain adequate hydration unless instructed to restrict fluid intake

Oral suspension: Shake suspension for approximately 10 seconds before use; do not mix suspension with other medications, flavoring agents, or other fluids.

Parenteral: IV infusion: **Do not administer IV push**; voriconazole must be administered by IV infusion over 1 to 2 hours at a rate not to exceed 3 mg/kg/hour. Do not infuse concomitantly into same line or cannula with other drug infusions, including TPN.

Monitoring Parameters Serum electrolytes, periodic renal function tests (particularly serum creatinine), hepatic function tests, and bilirubin; monitor visual activity, visual field, and color perception if treatment course continues >28 days; ECG in select patients; pancreatic function in patients at risk for acute pancreatitis; voriconazole trough levels in patients exhibiting signs of toxicity or not responding to treatment; total body skin examination yearly or more frequently if lesions occur

Reference Range Trough: 1-6 mcg/mL; some have suggested a higher minimum trough (2 mcg/mL) for disseminated infections or those in isolated sites (Chen, 2012)

Dosage Forms Excipient information presented when available (limited, particularly for generics); consult specific product labeling.

Solution Reconstituted, Intravenous:

Generic: 200 mg (1 ea)

Solution Reconstituted, Intravenous [preservative free]:

Vfend IV: 200 mg (1 ea) [latex free]

Vfend IV: 200 mg (1 ea)

Suspension Reconstituted, Oral:

Vfend: 40 mg/mL (75 mL) [contains sodium benzoate; orange flavor]

Generic: 40 mg/mL (75 mL)

Tablet, Oral:

Vfend: 50 mg, 200 mg

Generic: 50 mg, 200 mg

- ◆ **Voriconazole For Injection (Can)** *see* Voriconazole *on page 2190*
- ◆ **VoSolHC [DSC]** *see* Acetic Acid, Propylene Glycol Diacetate, and Hydrocortisone *on page 56*
- ◆ **VoSpire ER** *see* Albuterol *on page 81*
- ◆ **VP-16** *see* Etoposide *on page 819*
- ◆ **VP-16-213** *see* Etoposide *on page 819*
- ◆ **VPI-Baclofen Intrathecal (Can)** *see* Baclofen *on page 254*
- ◆ **Vpriv** *see* Velaglucerase Alfa *on page 2165*
- ◆ **VPRIV (Can)** *see* Velaglucerase Alfa *on page 2165*
- ◆ **VSL #3® [OTC]** *see Lactobacillus on page 1203*
- ◆ **VSL #3®-DS** *see Lactobacillus on page 1203*
- ◆ **Vumon (Can)** *see* Teniposide *on page 2015*
- ◆ **VWF/FVIII Concentrate** *see* Antihemophilic Factor/von Willebrand Factor Complex (Human) *on page 173*
- ◆ **VWF:RCo** *see* Antihemophilic Factor/von Willebrand Factor Complex (Human) *on page 173*
- ◆ **vWF:RCof** *see* Antihemophilic Factor/von Willebrand Factor Complex (Human) *on page 173*
- ◆ **VX-770** *see* Ivacaftor *on page 1180*
- ◆ **Vytorin** *see* Ezetimibe and Simvastatin *on page 833*
- ◆ **Vyvanse** *see* Lisdexamfetamine *on page 1278*
- ◆ **VZIG** *see* Varicella-Zoster Immune Globulin (Human) *on page 2160*
- ◆ **VZV Vaccine (Varicella)** *see* Varicella Virus Vaccine *on page 2157*

Warfarin (WAR far in)

Medication Safety Issues

Sound-alike/look-alike issues:

Coumadin may be confused with Avandia, Cardura, Compazine, Kemadrin

Jantoven may be confused with Janumet, Januvia

High alert medication:

The Institute for Safe Medication Practices (ISMP) includes this medication among its list of drugs which have a heightened risk of causing significant patient harm when used in error.

National Patient Safety Goals:

The Joint Commission on Accreditation of Healthcare Organizations requires healthcare organizations that provide anticoagulant therapy to have a process in place to reduce the risk of anticoagulant-associated patient harm. Patients receiving anticoagulants should receive individualized care through a defined process that includes standardized ordering, dispensing, administration, monitoring and education. This does not apply to routine short-term use of anticoagulants for prevention of venous thromboembolism when the expectation is that the patient's laboratory values will remain within or close to normal values (NPSG.03.05.01).

Brand Names: US Coumadin; Jantoven

Brand Names: Canada Apo-Warfarin; Coumadin; Mylan-Warfarin; Novo-Warfarin; Taro-Warfarin

Therapeutic Category Anticoagulant

Generic Availability (US) May be product dependent

Use Prophylaxis and treatment of venous thrombosis, pulmonary embolism, and thromboembolic disorders; prevention and treatment of thromboembolic complications in patients with prosthetic heart valves or atrial fibrillation; reduction of the risk of death, recurrent MI, and thromboembolic events such as systemic embolization or stroke after MI; has also been used for the prevention of recurrent arterial ischemic stroke and TIAs.

Medication Guide Available Yes

Pregnancy Risk Factor D (women with mechanical heart valves)/X (other indications)

Pregnancy Considerations Warfarin crosses the placenta; concentrations in the fetal plasma are similar to maternal values. Teratogenic effects have been reported following first trimester exposure and may include coumarin embryopathy (nasal hypoplasia and/or stippled epiphyses; limb hypoplasia may also be present). Adverse CNS events to the fetus have also been observed following exposure during any trimester and may include CNS abnormalities (including ventral midline dysplasia, dorsal midline dysplasia). Spontaneous abortion, fetal hemorrhage, and fetal death may also occur. Use is contraindicated during pregnancy (or in women of reproductive potential) except in women with mechanical heart valves who are at high risk for thromboembolism; use is also contraindicated in women with threatened abortion, eclampsia, or preeclampsia. Frequent pregnancy tests are recommended for women who are planning to become pregnant and adjusted-dose heparin or low molecular weight heparin (LMWH) should be substituted as soon as pregnancy is confirmed or adjusted-dose heparin or LMWH should be used instead of warfarin prior to conception.

In pregnant women with high-risk mechanical heart valves, the benefits of warfarin therapy should be discussed with the risks of available treatments (ACCP [Bates, 2012]; AHA/ACC [Nishimura, 2014]); when possible avoid warfarin use during the first trimester (ACCP [Bates, 2012]) and close to delivery (ACCP [Bates, 2012]; AHA/ACC [Nishimura, 2014]). Use of warfarin during the first trimester may be considered if the therapeutic INR can be achieved with a dose ≤5 mg/day (AHA/ACC [Nishimura, 2014]). Adjusted-dose LMWH or adjusted-dose heparin may be used throughout pregnancy or until week 13 of gestation when therapy can be changed to warfarin. LMWH or heparin should be resumed close to delivery. In women who are at a very high risk for thromboembolism (older generation mechanical prosthesis in mitral position or history of thromboembolism), warfarin can be used throughout pregnancy and replaced with LMWH or heparin near term; the use of low-dose aspirin is also recommended (ACCP [Bates, 2012] AHA/ACC [Nishimura, 2014]). Women who require long-term anticoagulation with warfarin and who are considering pregnancy, LMWH substitution should be done prior to conception when possible. If anti-Xa monitoring cannot be done, do not use LMWH therapy in pregnant patients with a mechanical prosthetic valve (AHA/ACC [Nishimura, 2014]). When choosing therapy, fetal outcomes (ie, pregnancy loss, malformations), maternal outcomes (ie, VTE, hemorrhage), burden of therapy, and maternal preference should be considered (ACCP [Bates, 2012]).

Breast-Feeding Considerations Breast-feeding women may be treated with warfarin. Based on available data, warfarin does not pass into breast milk. Women who are breast-feeding should be carefully monitored to avoid excessive anticoagulation. According to the American College of Chest Physicians (ACCP), warfarin may be used in lactating women who wish to breast-feed their infants (Bates, 2012). Monitor nursing infants for bruising or bleeding (per manufacturer).

Contraindications Hypersensitivity to warfarin or any component of the formulation; hemorrhagic tendencies (eg, patients bleeding from the GI, respiratory, or GU tract; cerebral aneurysm; cerebrovascular hemorrhage; dissecting aortic aneurysm; spinal puncture and other diagnostic or therapeutic procedures with potential for significant bleeding; history of bleeding diathesis); recent or potential surgery of the eye or CNS; major regional lumbar block anesthesia or traumatic surgery resulting in large, open surfaces; blood dyscrasias; severe uncontrolled or malignant hypertension; pericarditis or pericardial effusion; bacterial endocarditis; unsupervised patients with conditions associated with a high potential for noncompliance; eclampsia/pre-eclampsia, threatened abortion, pregnancy (except in women with mechanical heart valves at high risk for thromboembolism)

Warnings/Precautions Hazardous agent; use appropriate precautions for handling and disposal (NIOSH 2014 [group 3]).

Use care in the selection of patients appropriate for this treatment. Ensure patient cooperation especially from the alcoholic, illicit drug user, demented, or psychotic patient; ability to comply with routine laboratory monitoring is essential. Use with caution in trauma, acute infection, moderate-severe renal insufficiency, prolonged dietary insufficiencies, moderate-severe hypertension, polycythemia vera, vasculitis, open wound, active TB, any disruption in normal GI flora, history of PUD, anaphylactic disorders, indwelling catheters, severe diabetes, and menstruating and postpartum women. Use with caution in patients with thyroid disease; warfarin responsiveness may increase (Ageno, 2012). Use with caution in protein C deficiency. Use with caution in patients with heparin-induced thrombocytopenia and DVT. Warfarin monotherapy is contraindicated in the initial treatment of active HIT. Reduced liver function, regardless of etiology, may impair synthesis of coagulation factors leading to increased warfarin sensitivity.

[U.S. Boxed Warning]: May cause major or fatal bleeding. Risk factors for bleeding include high intensity anticoagulation (INR >4), age (>65 years), variable INRs, history of GI bleeding, hypertension, cerebrovascular disease, serious heart disease, anemia, malignancy, trauma, renal insufficiency, drug-drug interactions, long duration of therapy, or known genetic deficiency in CYP2C9 activity. Patient must be instructed to report bleeding, accidents, or falls. Unrecognized bleeding sites (eg, colon cancer) may be uncovered by anticoagulation. Patient must also report any new or discontinued medications, herbal or alternative products used, or significant changes in smoking or dietary habits. Necrosis or gangrene of the skin and other tissue can occur, usually in conjunction with protein C or S deficiency. Consider alternative therapies if anticoagulation is necessary. Warfarin therapy may release atheromatous plaque emboli; symptoms depend on site of embolization, most commonly kidneys, pancreas, liver, and spleen. In some cases may lead to necrosis or death. "Purple toes syndrome," due to cholesterol microembolization, may rarely occur. The elderly may be more sensitive to anticoagulant therapy.

Presence of the CYP2C9*2 or *3 allele and/or polymorphism of the vitamin K oxidoreductase (VKORC1) gene may increase the risk of bleeding. Lower doses may be required in these patients; genetic testing may help determine appropriate dosing.

When temporary interruption is necessary before surgery, discontinue for approximately 5 days before surgery; when there is adequate hemostasis, may reinstitute warfarin therapy ~12-24 hours after surgery (evening of or next morning). Decision to safely continue warfarin therapy through the procedure and whether or not bridging of anticoagulation is necessary is dependent upon risk of perioperative bleeding and risk of thromboembolism, respectively. If risk of thromboembolism is elevated, consider bridging warfarin therapy with an alternative anticoagulant (eg, unfractionated heparin, LMWH) (Guyatt, 2012).

Warnings: Additional Pediatric Considerations Oral anticoagulant therapy is usually avoided in neonates due to a greater potential risk of bleeding (Monagle, 2001) and other problems (Monagle, 2008). If used in pediatric patients, monitor closely; rare hair loss and tracheal calcification have been reported in children.

Adverse Reactions Bleeding is the major adverse effect of warfarin. Hemorrhage may occur at virtually any site. Risk is dependent on multiple variables, including the intensity of anticoagulation and patient susceptibility.

Cardiovascular: Vasculitis

Central nervous system: Signs/symptoms of bleeding (eg, dizziness, fatigue, fever, headache, lethargy, malaise, pain)

Dermatologic: Alopecia, bullous eruptions, dermatitis, rash, pruritus, urticaria

Gastrointestinal: Abdominal pain, diarrhea, flatulence, gastrointestinal bleeding, nausea, taste disturbance, vomiting

Genitourinary: Hematuria

Hematologic: Anemia, retroperitoneal hematoma, unrecognized bleeding sites (eg, colon cancer) may be uncovered by anticoagulation

Hepatic: Hepatitis (including cholestatic hepatitis), transaminases increased

Neuromuscular & skeletal: Osteoporosis (potential association with long-term use), paralysis, paresthesia, weakness

Respiratory: Respiratory tract bleeding, tracheobronchial calcification

Miscellaneous: Anaphylactic reaction, hypersensitivity/allergic reactions, skin necrosis, gangrene, "purple toes" syndrome

Drug Interactions

Metabolism/Transport Effects **Substrate** of CYP1A2 (minor), CYP2C19 (minor), CYP2C9 (major), CYP3A4 (minor); **Note:** Assignment of Major/Minor substrate status based on clinically relevant drug interaction potential; **Inhibits** CYP2C19 (weak), CYP2C9 (weak)

Avoid Concomitant Use

Avoid concomitant use of Warfarin with any of the following: Apixaban; Dabigatran Etexilate; Edoxaban; Enzalutamide; Omacetaxine; Rivaroxaban; Streptokinase; Tamoxifen; Urokinase; Vorapaxar

Increased Effect/Toxicity

Warfarin may increase the levels/effects of: Anticoagulants; Collagenase (Systemic); Deferasirox; Deoxycholic Acid; Ethotoin; Fosphenytoin; Ibritumomab; Nintedanib; Obinutuzumab; Omacetaxine; Phenytoin; Regorafenib; Rivaroxaban; Sulfonylureas; Tositumomab and Iodine I 131 Tositumomab

The levels/effects of Warfarin may be increased by: Acetaminophen; Agents with Antiplatelet Properties; Allopurinol; Amiodarone; Androgens; Apixaban; Atazanavir; Bicalutamide; Boceprevir; Capecitabine; Cephalosporins; Ceritinib; Chloral Hydrate; Chloramphenicol; Chondroitin Sulfate; Cimetidine; Clopidogrel; Cloxacillin; Cobicistat; Corticosteroids (Systemic); Cranberry; CYP2C9 Inhibitors (Moderate); CYP2C9 Inhibitors (Strong); Dabigatran Etexilate; Dasatinib; Desvenlafaxine; Dexmethylphenidate; Disulfiram; Dronedarone; Econazole; Edoxaban; Efavirenz; Erlotinib; Erythromycin (Ophthalmic); Esomeprazole; Ethacrynic Acid; Ethotoin; Etoposide; Exenatide; Fenofibrate and Derivatives; Fenugreek; Fibric Acid Derivatives; Fluconazole; Fluorouracil (Systemic); Fluorouracil (Topical); Fosamprenavir; Fosphenytoin; Fusidic Acid (Systemic); Gefitinib; Gemcitabine; Ginkgo Biloba; Glucagon; Glucosamine; Green Tea; Herbs (Anticoagulant/Antiplatelet Properties); HMG-CoA Reductase Inhibitors; Ibrutinib; Ifosfamide; Imatinib; Itraconazole; Ivermectin (Systemic); Ketoconazole (Systemic); Lansoprazole; Leflunomide; LevOCARNitine; Levomilnacipran; Limaprost; Lomitapide; Macrolide Antibiotics; Methylphenidate; Metreleptin; MetroNIDAZOLE (Systemic); Miconazole (Oral); Miconazole (Topical); Mifepristone; Milnacipran; Mirtazapine; Multivitamins/Fluoride (with ADE); Multivitamins/Minerals (with ADEK, Folate, Iron); Multivitamins/Minerals (with AE, No Iron); Nelfinavir; Neomycin; Nonsteroidal Anti-Inflammatory Agents; NSAID (COX-2 Inhibitor); NSAID (Nonselective); Omega-3 Fatty Acids; Omeprazole; Oritavancin; Orlistat; Penicillins; Pentosan Polysulfate Sodium; Pentoxifylline; Phenytoin; Posaconazole; Proguanil; Propafenone; Prostacyclin Analogues; QuiNIDine; QuiNINE; Quinolone Antibiotics; Ranitidine; RomiDEPsin; Salicylates; Saquinavir; Selective Serotonin Reuptake Inhibitors; Sitaxentan; SORAfenib; Streptokinase; Sugammadex; Sulfinpyrazone; Sulfonamide Derivatives; Sulfonylureas; Tamoxifen; Tegafur; Telaprevir; Tetracycline Derivatives; Thrombolytic Agents; Thyroid Products; Tibolone; Tigecycline; Tipranavir; Tolterodine; Toremifene; Torsemide; TraMADol; Tricyclic Antidepressants; Urokinase; Vemurafenib; Venlafaxine; Vitamin E; Vorapaxar; Voriconazole; Vorinostat; Zafirlukast; Zileuton

Decreased Effect

The levels/effects of Warfarin may be decreased by: Adalimumab; Alcohol (Ethyl); Antithyroid Agents; Aprepitant; AzaTHIOprine; Barbiturates; Bile Acid Sequestrants; Boceprevir; Bosentan; CarBAMazepine; Cloxacillin; Coenzyme Q-10; Contraceptives (Estrogens); Contraceptives (Progestins); CYP2C9 Inducers (Strong); Dabrafenib; Darunavir; Dicloxacillin; Efavirenz; Elvitegravir; Enzalutamide; Eslicarbazepine; Estrogen Derivatives; Flucloxacillin [Floxacillin]; Fosaprepitant; Ginseng (American); Glutethimide; Green Tea; Griseofulvin; Lixisenatide; Lopinavir; Mercaptopurine; Metreleptin; Multivitamins/Minerals (with ADEK, Folate, Iron); Nafcillin; Nelfinavir; Phytonadione; Progestins; Rifamycin Derivatives; Ritonavir; St Johns Wort; Sucralfate; Telaprevir; Teriflunomide; TraZODone

Food Interactions

Ethanol: Acute ethanol ingestion (binge drinking) decreases the metabolism of oral anticoagulants and increases PT/INR. Chronic daily ethanol use increases the metabolism of oral anticoagulants and decreases PT/INR. Management: Avoid ethanol.

Food: The anticoagulant effects of warfarin may be decreased if taken with foods rich in vitamin K. Vitamin E may increase warfarin effect. Cranberry juice may increase warfarin effect. Management: Maintain a consistent diet; consult prescriber before making changes in diet. Take warfarin at the same time each day.

Storage/Stability

Injection: Prior to reconstitution, store at 15°C to 30°C (59°F to 86°F). Following reconstitution with 2.7 mL of sterile water (yields 2 mg/mL solution), stable for 4 hours at 15°C to 30°C (59°F to 86°F). Protect from light.

Tablet: Store at 15°C to 30°C (59°F to 86°F). Protect from light.

Mechanism of Action Hepatic synthesis of coagulation factors II (half-life 42 to 72 hours), VII (half-life 4 to 6 hours), IX, and X (half-life 27 to 48 hours), as well as proteins C and S, requires the presence of vitamin K. These clotting factors are biologically activated by the addition of carboxyl groups to key glutamic acid residues within the proteins' structure. In the process, "active" vitamin K is oxidatively converted to an "inactive" form, which is then subsequently reactivated by vitamin K epoxide reductase complex 1 (VKORC1). Warfarin competitively inhibits the subunit 1 of the multi-unit VKOR complex, thus depleting functional vitamin K reserves and hence reduces synthesis of active clotting factors.

Pharmacodynamics Anticoagulation effects:

Onset of action: 24-72 hours

Maximum effect: Within 5-7 days

Duration of action (single dose): 2-5 days

Pharmacokinetics (Adult data unless noted)

Absorption: Oral: Rapid

Distribution: Adults: V_d: 0.14 L/kg

Protein binding: 99%

Metabolism: Hepatic, primarily via CYP2C9; minor pathways include CYP2C19, 1A2, and 3A4

Genomic variants: Clearance of S-warfarin is reduced by ~37% in patients heterozygous for 2C9 (*1/*2 or *1/*3), and reduced by ~70% in patients homozygous for reduced function alleles (*2/*2, *2/*3, or *3/*3)

Half-life, elimination: Adults: 20-60 hours; mean: 40 hours; highly variable among individuals

Elimination: Urine (92%, primarily as metabolites; very little warfarin is excreted unchanged in the urine)

Dosing: Usual Note: Dosing must be individualized. **Note:** New product labeling identifies genetic factors which may increase patient sensitivity to warfarin. Specifically, genetic variations in the proteins CYP2C9 and VKORC1, responsible for warfarin's primary metabolism and pharmacodynamic activity, respectively, have been identified as predisposing factors associated with decreased dose requirement and increased bleeding risk. A genotyping test is available and may provide important guidance on initiation of anticoagulant therapy.

Oral:

Infants and Children: **To maintain an International Normalized Ratio (INR) between 2-3**:

Initial loading dose on day 1 (if baseline INR is 1-1.3): 0.2 mg/kg (maximum dose: 10 mg); use initial loading dose of 0.1 mg/kg if patient has liver dysfunction or has undergone a Fontan procedure (Streif, 1999)

Loading dose for days 2-4: doses are dependent upon patient's INR

- if INR is 1.1-1.3, repeat the initial loading dose
- if INR is 1.4-1.9, give 50% of the initial loading dose
- if INR is 2-3, give 50% of the initial loading dose
- if INR is 3.1-3.5, give 25% of the initial loading dose
- if INR is >3.5, hold the drug until INR <3.5, then restart at 50% of previous dose

Maintenance dose guidelines for day 5 of therapy and beyond: Doses are dependent upon patient's INR

- if INR is 1.1-1.4, increase dose by 20% of previous dose
- if INR is 1.5-1.9, increase dose by 10% of previous dose
- if INR is 2-3, do not change the dose
- if INR is 3.1-3.5, decrease dose by 10% of previous dose
- if INR is >3.5, hold the drug and check INR daily until INR <3.5, then restart at 20% less than the previous dose

Usual maintenance dose: ~0.1 mg/kg/day; range: 0.05-0.34 mg/kg/day; the dose in mg/kg/day is inversely related to age. In the largest pediatric study (n=319; Streif, 1999), infants <12 months of age required a mean dose of 0.33 mg/kg/day, but children 13-18 years required a mean dose of 0.09 mg/kg/day; a target INR of 2-3 was used for a majority of these patients (75% of warfarin courses). Overall, children required a mean dose of 0.16 mg/kg/day to achieve a target INR of 2-3. In another study (Andrew, 1994), to attain an INR of 1.3-1.8, infants <12 months (n=2) required 0.24 and 0.27 mg/kg/day, but children >1 year required a mean of 0.08 mg/kg/day (range: 0.03-0.17 mg/kg/day). Consistent anticoagulation may be difficult to maintain in children <5 years of age. Children receiving phenobarbital, carbamazepine, or enteral nutrition may require higher maintenance doses (Streif, 1999).

Adults: **Note:** Initial dosing must be individualized. Consider patient factors (hepatic function, cardiac function, age, nutritional status, concurrent therapy, risk of bleeding) in addition to prior dose response (if available) and the clinical situation. Initial dose: 2-5 mg daily for 2 days **or** 5-10 mg daily for 1-2 days (Ansell, 2008); then adjust dose according to results of INR; usual maintenance dose ranges from 2-10 mg daily; individual patients may require loading and maintenance doses outside these general guidelines.

Note: Lower starting doses may be required for patients with hepatic impairment, poor nutrition, CHF, elderly, high risk of bleeding, patients who are debilitated, or those with reduced function genomic variants of the catabolic enzymes CYP2C9 (*2 or *3 alleles) or VKORC1 (-1639 polymorphism); see table. Higher initial doses may be reasonable in selected patients (ie, receiving enzyme-inducing agents and with low risk of bleeding). Overlapping a parenteral anticoagulant and warfarin therapy by at least 5 days is necessary in treatment of DVT/PE even if the INR is therapeutic earlier. Although an elevation in INR (due to factor VII depletion) may be seen early (within the first 24 to 48 hours) in warfarin therapy, it does not represent adequate anticoagulation. Factors II and X must also be depleted which takes considerably longer (ACCP [Guyatt 2012]).

Range[1] of Expected Therapeutic Maintenance Dose Based on CYP2C9[2] and VKORC1[3] Genotypes

VKORC1	CYP2C9					
	*1/*1	*1/*2	*1/*3	*2/*2	*2/*3	*3/*3
GG	5-7 mg	5-7 mg	3-4 mg	3-4 mg	3-4 mg	0.5-2 mg
AG	5-7 mg	3-4 mg	3-4 mg	3-4 mg	0.5-2 mg	0.5-2 mg
AA	3-4 mg	3-4 mg	0.5-2 mg	0.5-2 mg	0.5-2 mg	0.5-2 mg

Note: Must also take into account other patient-related factors when determining initial dose (eg, age, body weight, concomitant medications, comorbidities)

[1]Ranges derived from multiple published clinical studies.

[2]Patients with CYP2C9 *1/*3, *2/*2, *2/*3, and *3/*3 alleles may take up to 4 weeks to achieve maximum INR with a given dose regimen.

[3]VKORC1 -1639G>A (rs 9923231) variant is used in this table; other VKORC1 variants may also be important determinants of dose.

IV: (For patients who cannot take oral form): IV dose is equal to oral dose

Dosing adjustment in renal disease: No adjustment required; however, patients with renal failure have an increased risk of bleeding complications. Monitor closely.

Dosing adjustment in hepatic disease: Monitor effect at usual doses; the response to oral anticoagulants may be markedly enhanced in obstructive jaundice (due to reduced vitamin K absorption) and also in hepatitis and cirrhosis (due to decreased production of vitamin K-dependent clotting factors); INR should be closely monitored

Preparation for Administration Hazardous agent; use appropriate precautions for handling and disposal (NIOSH 2014 [group 3]).

Parenteral: Reconstitute with 2.7 mL of SWFI (yields 2 mg/mL solution).

Administration Hazardous agent; use appropriate precautions for handling and disposal (NIOSH 2014 [group 3]).

Oral: Administer with or without food. Take at the same time each day.

Parenteral: For IV use only; do not administer IM. Administer by slow IV injection over 1 to 2 minutes into peripheral vein

Monitoring Parameters INR (preferred) or prothrombin time; hemoglobin, hematocrit, signs and symptoms of bleeding; consider genotyping of CYP2C9 and VKORC1 prior to initiation of therapy, if available.

Reference Range The INR is now the standard test used to monitor warfarin anticoagulation; the desired INR is based upon indication; due to the lack of pediatric clinical trials assessing optimal INR ranges and clinical outcomes, the desired INR ranges for children are extrapolated from adult studies; the optimal therapeutic INR ranges may possibly be lower in children versus adults. Further pediatric studies are needed (Monagle, 2008). **Note:** If INR is not available, prothrombin time should be 1½ to 2 times the control.

Targeted INR and Ranges for Children, Based on Indication[a,b,c]

Indication	Targeted INR	Targeted INR Range
Systemic venous thromboembolism[d]	2.5	2-3
Central venous line-related thrombosis, initial 3 months of therapy	2.5	2-3
Central venous line-related thrombosis after first 3 months of warfarin therapy (**Note:** This is a prophylactic dose)	1.7	1.5-1.9
Central venous line, long-term home TPN (prophylactic dose) (Not recommended routinely)		2-3
Primary prophylaxis following Fontan procedure	2.5	2-3
Primary prophylaxis for dilated cardiomyopathy	2.5	2-3
Primary prophylaxis for biological prosthetic heart valves in children	Follow adult guidelines in table below	
Primary prophylaxis for mechanical prosthetic heart valves in children	Follow adult guidelines in table below	
Kawasaki disease with giant coronary aneurysms	2.5	2-3
Cerebral sinovenous thrombosis **Note:** INR recommendations from 2004 Chest guidelines	2.5	2-3

[a]Information from Monagle, 2004 and Monagle, 2008.

[b]Children are defined in the Chest guidelines as patients aged 28 days to 16 years of age.

[c]See Monagle, 2008 for timing of initiation and adjunct antithrombotic and antiplatelet therapy.

[d]Anticoagulant therapy with UFH or LMWH is recommended for children with first episode of venous thromboembolism (central venous line and noncentral venous line related).

Adult Target INR Ranges Based Upon Indication

Indication	Targeted INR	Targeted INR Range
Cardiac		
Acute myocardial infarction (high risk)[a]	2.5	2-3[b,c]
Atrial fibrillation or atrial flutter	2.5	2-3
Valvular		
Bileaflet or Medtronic Hall tilting disk mechanical aortic valve in normal sinus rhythm and normal LA size	2.5	2-3
Bileaflet or tilting disk mechanical mitral valve	3	2.5-3.5
Caged ball or caged disk mechanical valve	3	2.5-3.5
Mechanical prosthetic valve with systemic embolism despite adequate anticoagulation	3 **or** 3.5[d]	2.5-3.5[d] **or** 3-4[d]
Mechanical valve and risk factors for thromboembolism (eg, AF, MI[e], LA enlargement, hypercoagulable state, low EF) or history of atherosclerotic vascular disease	3	2.5-3.5[f]
Bioprosthetic mitral valve	2.5	2-3[g]
Bioprosthetic mitral or aortic valve with prior history of systemic embolism	2.5	2-3[g]
Bioprosthetic mitral or aortic valve with evidence of LA thrombus at surgery	2.5	2-3[h]
Bioprosthetic mitral or aortic valve with risk factors for thromboembolism (eg, AF, hypercoagulable state or low EF)	2.5	2-3[i]
Prosthetic mitral valve thrombosis (resolved)	4	3.5-4.5[c]
Prosthetic aortic valve thrombosis (resolved)	3.5	3-4[c]
Rheumatic mitral valve disease and normal sinus rhythm (LA diameter >5.5 cm), AF, previous systemic embolism, or LA thrombus	2.5	2-3
Thromboembolism Treatment		
Venous thromboembolism	2.5	2-3[j,k]
Thromboprophylaxis		
Chronic thromboembolic pulmonary hypertension (CTPH)	2.5	2-3
Lupus inhibitor (no other risk factors)	2.5	2-3
Lupus inhibitor and recurrent thromboembolism	3	2.5-3.5
Major trauma patients with impaired mobility undergoing rehabilitation	2.5	2-3
Spinal cord injury (acute) undergoing rehabilitation	2.5	2-3
Total hip or knee replacement (elective) or hip fracture surgery	2.5	2-3[l]
Other Indications		
Cerebral venous sinus thrombosis	2.5	2-3[m]
Ischemic stroke due to AF	2.5	2-3

[a]High-risk includes large anterior MI, significant heart failure, intracardiac thrombus, atrial fibrillation, history of thromboembolism.

[b]Maintain anticoagulation for 3 months.

[c]Combine with aspirin 81 mg/day.

(footnotes continued on next page)

Adult Target INR Ranges Based Upon Indication *(continued)*

[d]Combine with aspirin 81 mg/day, if not previously receiving, **and/or** if previous target INR was 2.5, then new target INR should be 3 (2.5-3.5). If previous target INR was 3, then new target INR should be 3.5 (3-4).

[e]MI refers to anterior-apical ST-segment elevation myocardial infarction.

[f]Combine with aspirin 81 mg/day unless patient is at high risk of bleeding (eg, history of GI bleed, age >80 years).

[g]Maintain anticoagulation for 3 months after valve insertion, then switch to aspirin 81 mg/day if no other indications for warfarin exist or clinically reassess need for warfarin in patients with prior history of systemic embolism.

[h]Maintain anticoagulation with warfarin until thrombus resolution.

[i]If patient has history of atherosclerotic vascular disease, combine with aspirin 81 mg/day unless patient is at high risk of bleeding (eg, history of GI bleed, age >80 years).

[j]Treat for 3 months in patients with VTE due to transient reversible risk factor. Treat for a minimum of 3 months in patients with unprovoked VTE and evaluate for long-term therapy. Other risk groups (eg, cancer) may require >3 months of therapy.

[k]In patients with unprovoked VTE who prefer less frequent INR monitoring, low-intensity therapy (INR range: 1.5-1.9) with less frequent monitoring is recommended over stopping treatment.

[l]Continue for at least 10 days and up to 35 days after surgery.

[m]Continue for up to 12 months.

Warfarin levels are not used for monitoring degree of anticoagulation. They may be useful if a patient with unexplained coagulopathy is using the drug surreptitiously or if it is unclear whether clinical resistance is due to true drug resistance or lack of drug intake.

Normal prothrombin time (PT): 10.9-12.9 seconds. Healthy premature newborns have prolonged coagulation test screening results (eg, PT, aPTT, TT) which return to normal adult values at approximately 6 months of age. However, healthy premature newborns (ie, those not receiving antithrombotic agents), do not develop spontaneous hemorrhage or thrombotic complications because of a balance between procoagulants and inhibitors.

Additional Information Usual duration of therapy in children (Monagle, 2008):

DVT:
- Idiopathic TE: ≥6 months
- Recurrent idiopathic TE: Indefinite
- Secondary thrombosis (with resolved risk factors): ≥3 months
- Recurrent secondary TE: Anticoagulate until removal of precipitating factor (≥3 months)

Primary prophylaxis for Glenn or Bilateral Cavopulmonary Shunts (BCPS): Continue until ready for Fontan surgery

Post-Fontan surgery: Optimal duration not defined

Cardiomyopathy in children eligible for transplant: Until transplant

Primary pulmonary hypertension: Duration not listed

Biological prosthetic heart valves: Follow adult recommendations

Mechanical prosthetic heart valves: Follow adult recommendations

Ventricular assist device (VAD) placement: Until transplant or weaned from VAD

Kawasaki disease: Treatment depends on severity of coronary involvement

Cerebral sinovenous thrombosis (CSVT) in neonates: 6 weeks-3 months

CSVT in children: ≥3 months

Neonates with homozygous protein C deficiency: Long-term

Note: Overdoses of warfarin may be treated with vitamin K, to reverse warfarin's anticoagulation effect. Prospective genotyping is available and may provide important guidance on initiation of anticoagulant therapy. Commercial testing with PGxPredict™:WARFARIN is now available from PGxHealth™ (Division of Clinical Data, Inc, New Haven, CT). The test genotypes patients for presence of the CYP2C9*2 or *3 alleles and the VKORC1 -1639G>A polymorphism. The results of the test allow patients to be phenotyped as extensive, intermediate, or poor metabolizers (CYP2C9) and as low, intermediate, or high warfarin sensitivity (VKORC1). Ordering information is available at 888-592-7327 or warfarininfo@pgxhealth.com.

Dosage Forms Excipient information presented when available (limited, particularly for generics); consult specific product labeling. [DSC] = Discontinued product

Solution Reconstituted, Intravenous, as sodium:
- Coumadin: 5 mg (1 ea [DSC])

Tablet, Oral, as sodium:
- Coumadin: 1 mg [scored]
- Coumadin: 2 mg [scored; contains fd&c blue #2 aluminum lake, fd&c red #40 aluminum lake]
- Coumadin: 2.5 mg [scored; contains fd&c blue #1 aluminum lake, fd&c yellow #10 aluminum lake]
- Coumadin: 3 mg [scored; contains fd&c blue #2 aluminum lake, fd&c red #40 aluminum lake, fd&c yellow #6 aluminum lake]
- Coumadin: 4 mg [scored; contains fd&c blue #1 aluminum lake]
- Coumadin: 5 mg [scored; contains fd&c yellow #6 aluminum lake]
- Coumadin: 6 mg [scored; contains fd&c blue #1 aluminum lake, fd&c yellow #6 aluminum lake]
- Coumadin: 7.5 mg [scored; contains fd&c yellow #10 aluminum lake, fd&c yellow #6 aluminum lake]
- Coumadin: 10 mg [scored; dye free]
- Jantoven: 1 mg [scored; contains fd&c red #40 aluminum lake]
- Jantoven: 2 mg [scored; contains fd&c blue #2 aluminum lake, fd&c red #40 aluminum lake]
- Jantoven: 2.5 mg [scored; contains fd&c blue #1 aluminum lake, fd&c yellow #10 aluminum lake]
- Jantoven: 3 mg [scored]
- Jantoven: 4 mg [scored; contains fd&c blue #1 aluminum lake]
- Jantoven: 5 mg [scored; contains fd&c yellow #6 aluminum lake]
- Jantoven: 6 mg [scored; contains fd&c blue #1 aluminum lake]
- Jantoven: 7.5 mg [scored; contains fd&c yellow #10 aluminum lake, fd&c yellow #6 aluminum lake]
- Jantoven: 10 mg [scored]
- Generic: 1 mg, 2 mg, 2.5 mg, 3 mg, 4 mg, 5 mg, 6 mg, 7.5 mg, 10 mg

- ◆ **Warfarin Sodium** *see* Warfarin *on page 2195*
- ◆ **4-Way Fast Acting [OTC]** *see* Phenylephrine (Nasal) *on page 1688*
- ◆ **4-Way Menthol [OTC]** *see* Phenylephrine (Nasal) *on page 1688*
- ◆ **4-Way Saline [OTC]** *see* Sodium Chloride *on page 1938*
- ◆ **Welchol** *see* Colesevelam *on page 530*
- ◆ **Wellbutrin** *see* BuPROPion *on page 324*
- ◆ **Wellbutrin XL** *see* BuPROPion *on page 324*
- ◆ **Wellbutrin SR** *see* BuPROPion *on page 324*
- ◆ **Westcort** *see* Hydrocortisone (Topical) *on page 1041*
- ◆ **Westcort® (Can)** *see* Hydrocortisone (Topical) *on page 1041*

- ◆ **Westhroid** *see* Thyroid, Desiccated *on page 2058*
- ◆ **Westhroid-P [DSC]** *see* Thyroid, Desiccated *on page 2058*
- ◆ **White Mineral Oil** *see* Mineral Oil *on page 1439*
- ◆ **Wilate** *see* Antihemophilic Factor/von Willebrand Factor Complex (Human) *on page 173*
- ◆ **Winpred (Can)** *see* PredniSONE *on page 1760*
- ◆ **WinRho SDF** *see* Rh_o(D) Immune Globulin *on page 1847*
- ◆ **Woman's Laxative [OTC] (Can)** *see* Bisacodyl *on page 289*
- ◆ **Womens Laxative [OTC]** *see* Bisacodyl *on page 289*
- ◆ **Wound Wash Saline [OTC]** *see* Sodium Chloride *on page 1938*
- ◆ **WP Thyroid** *see* Thyroid, Desiccated *on page 2058*
- ◆ **WR-2721** *see* Amifostine *on page 115*
- ◆ **WR-139007** *see* Dacarbazine *on page 572*
- ◆ **WR-139013** *see* Chlorambucil *on page 430*
- ◆ **WR-139021** *see* Carmustine *on page 377*
- ◆ **Wycillin** *see* Penicillin G Procaine *on page 1659*
- ◆ **Wycillin® (Can)** *see* Penicillin G Procaine *on page 1659*
- ◆ **Wydase** *see* Hyaluronidase *on page 1025*
- ◆ **Xanax** *see* ALPRAZolam *on page 100*
- ◆ **Xanax® (Can)** *see* ALPRAZolam *on page 100*
- ◆ **Xanax TS™ (Can)** *see* ALPRAZolam *on page 100*
- ◆ **Xanax XR** *see* ALPRAZolam *on page 100*
- ◆ **Xartemis XR** *see* Oxycodone and Acetaminophen *on page 1594*
- ◆ **Xerclear** *see* Acyclovir and Hydrocortisone *on page 66*
- ◆ **Xerese™** *see* Acyclovir and Hydrocortisone *on page 66*
- ◆ **Xifaxan** *see* Rifaximin *on page 1861*
- ◆ **Xilep** *see* Rufinamide *on page 1891*
- ◆ **Ximino** *see* Minocycline *on page 1440*
- ◆ **Xodol 5/300** *see* Hydrocodone and Acetaminophen *on page 1032*
- ◆ **Xodol 7.5/300** *see* Hydrocodone and Acetaminophen *on page 1032*
- ◆ **Xodol 10/300** *see* Hydrocodone and Acetaminophen *on page 1032*
- ◆ **Xolair** *see* Omalizumab *on page 1553*
- ◆ **Xolegel** *see* Ketoconazole (Topical) *on page 1191*
- ◆ **Xolido XP [OTC]** *see* Lidocaine (Topical) *on page 1258*
- ◆ **Xolox [DSC]** *see* Oxycodone and Acetaminophen *on page 1594*
- ◆ **Xopenex** *see* Levalbuterol *on page 1233*
- ◆ **Xopenex Concentrate** *see* Levalbuterol *on page 1233*
- ◆ **Xopenex HFA** *see* Levalbuterol *on page 1233*
- ◆ **Xpect [OTC]** *see* GuaiFENesin *on page 988*
- ◆ **X-Pur Chlorhexidine (Can)** *see* Chlorhexidine Gluconate *on page 434*
- ◆ **X-Seb T Pearl [OTC]** *see* Coal Tar *on page 523*
- ◆ **X-Seb T Plus [OTC]** *see* Coal Tar *on page 523*
- ◆ **Xtra-Care [OTC]** *see* Vitamin E *on page 2188*
- ◆ **Xylocaine** *see* Lidocaine (Systemic) *on page 1255*
- ◆ **Xylocaine** *see* Lidocaine (Topical) *on page 1258*
- ◆ **Xylocaine (Cardiac)** *see* Lidocaine (Systemic) *on page 1255*
- ◆ **Xylocaine-MPF** *see* Lidocaine (Systemic) *on page 1255*
- ◆ **Xylocaine® MPF With Epinephrine** *see* Lidocaine and Epinephrine *on page 1262*
- ◆ **Xylocaine Viscous** *see* Lidocaine (Topical) *on page 1258*
- ◆ **Xylocaine® With Epinephrine** *see* Lidocaine and Epinephrine *on page 1262*
- ◆ **Xylocard (Can)** *see* Lidocaine (Systemic) *on page 1255*
- ◆ **Xyntha** *see* Antihemophilic Factor (Recombinant) *on page 168*
- ◆ **Xyntha Solofuse** *see* Antihemophilic Factor (Recombinant) *on page 168*
- ◆ **Xyzal** *see* Levocetirizine *on page 1241*

Yellow Fever Vaccine (YEL oh FEE ver vak SEEN)

Related Information

Centers for Disease Control and Prevention (CDC) and Other Links *on page 2424*

Immunization Administration Recommendations *on page 2411*

Immunization Schedules *on page 2416*

Brand Names: US YF-VAX

Brand Names: Canada YF-VAX

Therapeutic Category Vaccine; Vaccine, Live (Viral)

Generic Availability (US) No

Use To provide active immunity to yellow fever virus to individuals who are either traveling to or living in endemic yellow fever areas (FDA approved in ages ≥9 months and adults)

The Advisory Committee on Immunization Practices (ACIP) recommends vaccination for: Persons traveling to or living in areas at risk for yellow fever transmission; persons traveling to countries which require vaccination for international travel; laboratory personnel who may be exposed to the yellow fever virus or concentrated preparations of the vaccine.

Although the vaccine is approved for use in children ≥9 months of age, the CDC recommends use in children as young as 6 months under unusual circumstances (eg, travel to an area where exposure is unavoidable). Children <6 months of age should **never** receive the vaccine.

Medication Guide Available Yes

Pregnancy Risk Factor C

Pregnancy Considerations Animal reproduction studies have not been conducted. Adverse events were not observed in the mother or fetus following vaccination during the third trimester of pregnancy in Nigerian women; however, maternal seroconversion was reduced. Inadvertent exposure early in the first trimester of pregnancy in Brazilian women did not show decreased maternal seroconversion; no major congenital abnormalities were noted. Cord blood from an infant whose mother was vaccinated during the first trimester tested positive for IgM antibodies; no adverse events were noted in the infant. Vaccine should be administered if travel to an endemic area is unavoidable and the infant should be monitored after birth. Tests to verify maternal immune response may be considered. If a pregnant woman is to be vaccinated only to satisfy an international requirement (as opposed to decreasing risk of infection), efforts should be made to obtain a waiver letter. Women should wait 4 weeks after receiving vaccine before conceiving (CDC, 2010).

Breast-Feeding Considerations Laboratory confirmed transmission of 17DD yellow fever vaccine virus via breast-feeding has been documented. Yellow fever vaccine was administered to a nursing mother 15 days postpartum. She was exclusively breast-feeding her newborn. Eight days after maternal vaccination, the infant developed a fever, was irritable, refused to nurse, then was hospitalized for seizures the next day. Yellow fever virus specific to the vaccine and IgM antibodies were detected in the newborn CSF. The child was discharged after 24 days in the hospital; growth and neurodevelopment were normal through 6 months of age. Breast-feeding is contraindicated by the manufacturer, particularly in infants <9 months of age. If travel to an endemic area cannot be avoided or postponed, women who are nursing should be vaccinated. Breast-feeding does not adversely affect immunization (CDC, 2010; WHO, 2013).

Contraindications Hypersensitivity to egg or chick embryo protein, or any component of the formulation; children <9 months of age (per manufacturer); children <6 months of age (CDC guidelines); acute or febrile disease; immunosuppressed patients (eg HIV infection, leukemia, lymphoma, thymic disease, generalized malignancy, or immunosuppression due to drugs or radiation); breast-feeding women

Warnings/Precautions Vaccination may not result in effective immunity in all patients. Response depends upon multiple factors (eg, type of vaccine, age of patient) and may be improved by administering the vaccine at the recommended dose, route, and interval. Vaccines may not be effective if administered during periods of altered immune competence (CDC, 2011). Malnourished persons may have a decreased response to vaccination (CDC, 2010). Patients who are immunosuppressed have a theoretical risk of encephalitis with yellow fever vaccine administration; consider delaying travel or obtaining a waiver letter. Patients on low-dose or short-term corticosteroids are not considered immunosuppressed and may be offered the vaccine. If vaccination is only to satisfy an international requirement (as opposed to decreasing risk of infection), efforts should be made to obtain a waiver letter. Per the ACIP guidelines, use is contraindicated in patients with symptomatic HIV infection or patients with CD4+ counts <200/mm^3 (or <15% of total lymphocytes in children <6 years of age); use caution when administering the vaccine to patients with asymptomatic infection with CD4+ counts 200-499/mm^3 (or 15% to 24% of total lymphocytes in children <6 years of age) (CDC, 2010). In general, household and close contacts of persons with altered immunocompetence may receive all age appropriate vaccines (CDC, 2011); live vaccines should be administered ≥4 weeks prior to planned immunosuppression and avoided within 2 weeks of immunosuppression when feasible. Specific recommendations for use of this vaccine in immunocompromised patients considering international travel as well as contacts of immunocompromised patients are available from the IDSA (Rubin, 2014).

Immediate treatment (including epinephrine 1:1000) for anaphylactoid and/or hypersensitivity reactions should be available during vaccine use. Use is contraindicated in patients with immediate-type hypersensitivity reactions to eggs. Less severe or localized manifestations of allergy are not contraindications; in general, persons who are able to eat eggs or egg products may receive the vaccine. A hypersensitivity screening test and desensitization procedure is available for persons with suspected or known severe egg sensitivity. Consult manufacturer's labeling for details. Syncope has been reported with use of injectable vaccines and may be accompanied by transient visual disturbances, weakness, or tonic-clonic movements. Procedures should be in place to avoid injuries from falling and to restore cerebral perfusion if syncope occurs.

The vial stopper contains latex; product may contain gelatin. Immunization should be delayed during the course of an acute or febrile illness. The presence of a low-grade fever is generally not a reason to postpone vaccination (CDC, 2011). Due to an increased incidence of serious adverse events observed in older adults compared to younger adults, use with caution in the elderly ≥65 years (per manufacturer) or ≥60 years (per ACIP guidelines), particularly in patients who have not previously received the vaccine. The risk for vaccine-associated neurologic disease (YEL-AND) and vaccine-associated viscerotropic disease (YEL-AVD) is also increased. The ACIP guidelines note that if travel is unavoidable, the decision to vaccinate travelers ≥60 years should be made after weighing the risks vs benefits (CDC, 2011). Avoid use in pregnant women unless travel to high-risk areas is unavoidable. The manufacturer contraindicates use in infants <9 months of age due to risk of encephalitis. The CDC allows for use in infants 6-8 months of age when possible exposure with the yellow fever virus is unavoidable and the risk of infection exists. Infants <6 months of age should never be vaccinated (CDC, 2010). Transfusion-related transmission of yellow fever vaccine virus has been reported; wait 2 weeks after immunization with yellow fever vaccine to donate blood (CDC, 2010). In order to maximize vaccination rates, the ACIP recommends simultaneous administration of all age-appropriate vaccines (live or inactivated) for which a person is eligible at a single clinic visit, unless contraindications exist (CDC, 2011).

Warnings: Additional Pediatric Considerations Antipyretics have not been shown to prevent febrile seizures; antipyretics may be used to treat fever or discomfort following vaccination (CDC, 2011). One study reported that routine prophylactic administration of acetaminophen to prevent fever prior to vaccination decreased the immune response of some vaccines; the clinical significance of this reduction in immune response has not been established (Prymula, 2009).

Adverse Reactions All serious adverse reactions must be reported to the U.S. Department of Health and Human Services (DHHS) Vaccine Adverse Event Reporting System (VAERS) 1-800-822-7967 or online at https://vaers.hhs.gov/esub/index. In Canada, adverse reactions may be reported to local provincial/territorial health agencies or to the Vaccine Safety Section at Public Health Agency of Canada (1-866-844-0018).

Adverse reactions may be increased in patients <9 months or ≥60 years of age):

Central nervous system: Chills, fever, focal neurological defects, headache, malaise, seizure

Dermatologic: Rash, urticaria

Local: Injection site reactions (edema, erythema, hypersensitivity, mass, pain, pruritus, rash, warmth)

Neuromuscular & skeletal: Myalgia, weakness

Miscellaneous: Guillain-Barré syndrome (GBS), hypersensitivity (immediate), vaccine-associated neurotropic disease (rare), viscerotropic disease (rare; may be associated with multiorgan failure)

Vaccine-associated neurologic disease (YEL-AND) may manifest as meningoencephalitis (neurotropic disease), GBS, acute disseminated encephalomyelitis, and bulbar palsy. Vaccine-associated viscerotropic disease (YEL-AVD) mimics naturally-acquired yellow fever disease; risk may be increased in older patients and those with a history of thymus disease or thymectomy.

Drug Interactions

Metabolism/Transport Effects None known.

Avoid Concomitant Use

Avoid concomitant use of Yellow Fever Vaccine with any of the following: Belimumab; Fingolimod; Immunosuppressants

Increased Effect/Toxicity

The levels/effects of Yellow Fever Vaccine may be increased by: AzaTHIOprine; Belimumab; Corticosteroids (Systemic); Dimethyl Fumarate; Fingolimod; Immunosuppressants; Leflunomide; Mercaptopurine; Methotrexate

Decreased Effect

Yellow Fever Vaccine may decrease the levels/effects of: Tuberculin Tests

The levels/effects of Yellow Fever Vaccine may be decreased by: AzaTHIOprine; Corticosteroids (Systemic); Dimethyl Fumarate; Fingolimod; Immunosuppressants; Leflunomide; Mercaptopurine; Methotrexate

Storage/Stability Store at 2°C to 8°C (35°F to 46°F); do not freeze. Vaccine must be used within 60 minutes of reconstitution. Keep suspension refrigerated until used.

Pharmacodynamics Onset of action: Seroconversion: 10-14 days

Dosing: Usual Children ≥6 months and Adults: SubQ: One dose (0.5 mL) ≥10 days before travel; Booster: Repeat same dosage every 10 years if at continued risk of exposure (CDC, 2010).

Preparation for Administration Parenteral: SubQ: Reconstitute only with diluent provided; use entire contents of provided diluent. Inject diluent slowly into vial and allow to stand for 1 to 2 minutes. Gently swirl until a uniform suspension forms; swirl well before withdrawing dose. Avoid vigorous shaking to prevent foaming of suspension. Use within 60 minutes following reconstitution; keep suspension refrigerated until used.

Administration Parenteral: SubQ: Use within 60 minutes following reconstitution; keep suspension refrigerated until used. Swirl well before withdrawing dose; avoid vigorous shaking to prevent foaming of suspension. Administer by SubQ injection into the anterolateral aspect of the thigh or arm; **not for IV or IM administration**. If inadvertently administered IM, the dose does not need to be repeated. Use of expired vaccine is not considered a valid dose and should be repeated after 28 days. For booster doses, if the date of previous vaccination cannot be determined and the patient requires vaccination, the booster dose can be given (CDC 2010). Adolescents and adults should be vaccinated while seated or lying down.

Monitoring Parameters Observe for syncope for 15 minutes following administration. If seizure-like activity associated with syncope occurs, maintain patient in supine or Trendelenburg position to reestablish adequate cerebral perfusion.

Additional Information A desensitization procedure is available for persons with severe egg sensitivity. Consult manufacturer's labeling for details. Some countries require a valid International Certification of Vaccination or Prophylaxis (ICVP) showing receipt of vaccine. Certificate is valid beginning 10 days after and for 10 years following vaccination (booster doses received within 10 years are valid from the date of vaccination). The WHO requires revaccination every 10 years to maintain traveler's vaccination certificate. Current requirements and recommendations for immunization related to travel destination can be obtained from the CDC Travelers' Health Web site (www.cdc.gov/travel). All travelers to endemic areas should be advised of the risks of yellow fever disease and all available methods to prevent it. All travelers should take protective measures to avoid mosquito bites.

In order to maximize vaccination rates, the ACIP recommends simultaneous administration (ie, >1 vaccine on the same day at different anatomic sites) of all age-appropriate vaccines (live or inactivated) for which a person is eligible at a single visit, unless contraindications exist. If available, the use of combination vaccines is generally preferred over separate injections, taking into consideration provider assessment, patient preference, and potential adverse events. If separate vaccines being used, evaluate product information regarding same syringe compatibility of vaccines. Separate needles and syringes should be used for each injection. The ACIP prefers each dose of specific vaccine in a series come from the same manufacturer if possible (CDC, 2011).

The following CDC agencies may be contacted if serologic testing is needed or for advice when administering yellow fever vaccine to pregnant women, children < 9 months, or patients with altered immune status:

Division of Vector-Borne Infectious Diseases: 970-221-6400

Division of Global Migration and Quarantine: 404-498-1600

Dosage Forms Excipient information presented when available (limited, particularly for generics); consult specific product labeling.

Injection, powder for reconstitution [17D-204 strain]:

YF-VAX®: ≥4.74 Log_{10} plaque-forming units (PFU) per 0.5 mL dose [single-dose or 5-dose vial; produced in chicken embryos; contains gelatin; packaged with diluent; vial stopper contains latex]

- ◆ **YF-VAX** *see* Yellow Fever Vaccine *on page 2201*
- ◆ **YM-08310** *see* Amifostine *on page 115*
- ◆ **Yodoxin** *see* Iodoquinol *on page 1155*
- ◆ **Z4942** *see* Ifosfamide *on page 1075*
- ◆ **Zaclir Cleansing** *see* Benzoyl Peroxide *on page 270*
- ◆ **Zaditor [OTC]** *see* Ketotifen (Ophthalmic) *on page 1196*
- ◆ **Zaditor® (Can)** *see* Ketotifen (Ophthalmic) *on page 1196*

Zafirlukast (za FIR loo kast)

Medication Safety Issues

Sound-alike/look-alike issues:

Accolate may be confused with Accupril, Accutane, Aclovate

Brand Names: US Accolate

Brand Names: Canada Accolate

Therapeutic Category Antiasthmatic; Leukotriene Receptor Antagonist

Generic Availability (US) Yes

Use Prophylaxis and chronic treatment of asthma (FDA approved in ages ≥5 years and adults)

Pregnancy Risk Factor B

Pregnancy Considerations Adverse events were not observed in animal reproduction studies except with doses that were also maternally toxic. Based on limited data, an increased risk of teratogenic effects has not been observed with zafirlukast use in pregnancy (Bakhireva, 2007). Uncontrolled asthma is associated with adverse events on pregnancy (increased risk of perinatal mortality, pre-eclampsia, preterm birth, low birth weight infants). Zafirlukast may be considered for use in women who had a favorable response prior to becoming pregnant; however, initiating a leukotriene receptor antagonist during pregnancy is an alternative (but not preferred) treatment option for mild persistent asthma (NAEPP, 2005).

Breast-Feeding Considerations Zafirlukast is excreted into breast milk. In women receiving zafirlukast 40 mg twice daily, maternal serum concentrations were 225 ng/mL and breast milk concentrations were 50 ng/mL. Due to the potential for adverse reactions in the nursing infant, breast-feeding is not recommended by the manufacturer.

Contraindications Hypersensitivity to zafirlukast or any component of the formulation; hepatic impairment (including hepatic cirrhosis)

Canadian labeling: Additional contraindications (not in U.S. labeling): Patients in whom zafirlukast was discontinued due to treatment related hepatotoxicity

Warnings/Precautions Zafirlukast is not approved for use in the reversal of bronchospasm in acute asthma attacks, including status asthmaticus. Therapy with zafirlukast can be continued during acute exacerbations of asthma.

Hepatic adverse events (including hepatitis, hyperbilirubinemia, and hepatic failure) have been reported; female patients may be at greater risk. Periodic testing of liver function may be considered (early detection coupled with therapy discontinuation is generally believed to improve the likelihood of recovery). Advise patients to be alert for and to immediately report symptoms (eg, anorexia, right upper quadrant abdominal pain, nausea). If hepatic dysfunction is suspected (due to clinical signs/symptoms), discontinue use immediately and measure liver function tests (particularly ALT); resolution observed in most but not all cases upon discontinuation of therapy. Do not resume or restart if hepatic function studies indicate dysfunction. Use in patients with hepatic impairment (including hepatic cirrhosis) is contraindicated. Postmarketing reports of behavioral changes (ie, depression, insomnia) have been noted. Instruct patients to report neuropsychiatric symptoms/events during therapy.

Monitor INR closely with concomitant warfarin use. Rare cases of eosinophilic vasculitis (Churg-Strauss) have been reported in patients receiving zafirlukast (usually, but not always, associated with reduction in concurrent steroid dosage). No causal relationship established. Monitor for eosinophilic vasculitis, rash, pulmonary symptoms, cardiac symptoms, or neuropathy.

Clearance is decreased in elderly patients; C_{max} and AUC are increased approximately two- to threefold in adults ≥65 years compared to younger adults; however, no dosage adjustments are recommended in this age group. An increased proportion of zafirlukast patients >55 years of age reported infections as compared to placebo-treated patients. These infections were mostly mild or moderate in intensity and predominantly affected the respiratory tract. Infections occurred equally in both sexes, were dose-proportional to total milligrams of zafirlukast exposure, and were associated with coadministration of inhaled corticosteroids.

Adverse Reactions

Central nervous system: Dizziness, fever, headache, pain
Gastrointestinal: Abdominal pain, diarrhea, dyspepsia, nausea, vomiting
Hepatic: ALT increased
Neuromuscular & skeletal: Back pain, myalgia, weakness
Miscellaneous: Infection
Rare but important or life-threatening: Agranulocytosis, angioedema, arthralgia, bleeding, bruising, depression, edema, eosinophilia (systemic), eosinophilic pneumonia, hepatic failure, hepatitis, hyperbilirubinemia, hypersensitivity reactions, insomnia, malaise, pruritus, rash, urticaria, vasculitis with clinical features of Churg-Strauss syndrome (rare)

Drug Interactions

Metabolism/Transport Effects Substrate of CYP2C9 (major); **Note:** Assignment of Major/Minor substrate status based on clinically relevant drug interaction potential; **Inhibits** CYP1A2 (weak), CYP2C19 (weak), CYP2C8 (weak), CYP2C9 (moderate), CYP2D6 (weak)

Avoid Concomitant Use

Avoid concomitant use of Zafirlukast with any of the following: Amodiaquine; Loxapine

Increased Effect/Toxicity

Zafirlukast may increase the levels/effects of: Amodiaquine; ARIPiprazole; Bosentan; Cannabis; Carvedilol; CYP2C9 Substrates; Dronabinol; Loxapine; Tetrahydrocannabinol; Theophylline Derivatives; TiZANidine; Vitamin K Antagonists

The levels/effects of Zafirlukast may be increased by: Ceritinib; CYP2C9 Inhibitors (Moderate); CYP2C9 Inhibitors (Strong); Mifepristone

Decreased Effect

The levels/effects of Zafirlukast may be decreased by: CYP2C9 Inducers (Strong); Dabrafenib; Erythromycin (Systemic); Theophylline Derivatives

Food Interactions Food decreases bioavailability of zafirlukast by 40%. Management: Take on an empty stomach 1 hour before or 2 hours after meals.

Storage/Stability Store tablets at controlled room temperature of 20°C to 25°C (68°F to 77°F). Protect from light and moisture; dispense in original airtight container.

Mechanism of Action Zafirlukast is a selectively and competitive leukotriene-receptor antagonist (LTRA) of leukotriene D4 and E4 (LTD4 and LTE4), components of slow-reacting substance of anaphylaxis (SRSA). Cysteinyl leukotriene production and receptor occupation have been correlated with the pathophysiology of asthma, including airway edema, smooth muscle constriction, and altered cellular activity associated with the inflammatory process, which contribute to the signs and symptoms of asthma.

Pharmacodynamics Asthma symptom improvement:
Maximum effect: 2-6 weeks
Duration: 12 hours

Pharmacokinetics (Adult data unless noted)

Absorption: Rapid
Bioavailability: Food decreases bioavailability by ~40%
Distribution: Extensively excreted into breast milk; breast milk to plasma ratio: 0.15
V_{dss}: ~70 L
Protein binding: ≥99%, predominantly albumin
Metabolism: Extensively metabolized by liver via cytochrome P450 isoenzyme CYP2C9 pathway
Half-life, elimination: ~10 hours (range: 8-16 hours)
Time to peak serum concentration:
Children: 2-2.5 hours
Adults: 3 hours
Elimination: Fecal (~90%) and urine (~10%)
Clearance:
Children 5-6 years: 9.2 L/hour
Children 7-11 years: 11.4 L/hour
Adults: 20 L/hour

Dosing: Usual Oral:
Children 5-11 years: 10 mg twice daily
Children ≥12 years and Adults: 20 mg twice daily
Dosing adjustment in renal impairment: Dosage adjustment is not necessary.
Dosing adjustment in hepatic impairment: Use is contraindicated.

Administration Oral: Administer at least 1 hour before or 2 hours after a meal

Monitoring Parameters Pulmonary function tests (FEV-1, PEF), improvement in asthma symptoms, periodic liver function tests

Reference Range Obtaining plasma concentrations not clinically indicated; plasma zafirlukast serum concentrations exceeding 5 ng/mL at 12-14 hours following oral doses have correlated with activity; mean trough serum levels at doses of 20 mg twice daily were 20 ng/mL

Dosage Forms Excipient information presented when available (limited, particularly for generics); consult specific product labeling.
Tablet, Oral:
Accolate: 10 mg, 20 mg
Generic: 10 mg, 20 mg

◆ **Zamicet [DSC]** *see* Hydrocodone and Acetaminophen *on page 1032*

Zanamivir (za NA mi veer)

Medication Safety Issues

Sound-alike/look-alike issues:
Relenza® may be confused with Albenza®, Aplenzin™

Brand Names: US Relenza Diskhaler

Brand Names: Canada Relenza®

Therapeutic Category Antiviral Agent; Neuraminidase Inhibitor

Generic Availability (US) No

Use Treatment of influenza A or B infection in patients who have been symptomatic for no more than 2 days (FDA approved in children ≥7 years and adults); prophylaxis of influenza A or B infection (FDA approved in children ≥5 years and adults); has also been used for treatment of patients symptomatic for >2 days with severe illness (CDC, 2010)

The Advisory Committee on Immunization Practices (ACIP) recommends that antiviral **treatment** be considered for the following (see specific antiviral product monograph for appropriate patient selection):

- Persons with severe, complicated or progressive illness
- Hospitalized persons
- Persons at higher risk for influenza complications:
  - Children <2 years of age (highest risk in children <6 months of age)
  - Adults ≥65 years of age
  - Persons with chronic disorders of the pulmonary (including asthma) or cardiovascular systems (except hypertension)
  - Persons with chronic metabolic diseases (including diabetes mellitus), hepatic disease, renal dysfunction, hematologic disorders (including sickle cell disease), or immunosuppression (including immunosuppression caused by medications or HIV)
  - Persons with neurologic/neuromuscular conditions (including conditions such as spinal cord injuries, seizure disorders, cerebral palsy, stroke, mental retardation, moderate-to-severe developmental delay, or muscular dystrophy) which may compromise respiratory function, the handling of respiratory secretions, or that can increase the risk of aspiration
  - Pregnant or postpartum women (≤2 weeks after delivery)
  - Persons <19 years of age on long-term aspirin therapy
  - American Indians and Alaskan Natives
  - Persons who are morbidly obese (BMI ≥40)
  - Residents of nursing homes or other chronic care facilities
- Use may also be considered for previously healthy, nonhigh risk outpatients with confirmed or suspected influenza based on clinical judgment when treatment can be started within 48 hours of illness onset.

The ACIP recommends that **prophylaxis** be considered for the following (see specific antiviral product monograph for appropriate patient selection):

- Postexposure prophylaxis may be considered for family or close contacts of suspected or confirmed cases, who are at higher risk of influenza complications, and who have not been vaccinated against the circulating strain at the time of the exposure or if exposure occurred within 2 weeks of vaccination.
- Postexposure prophylaxis may be considered for unvaccinated healthcare workers who had occupational exposure without protective equipment.
- Pre-exposure prophylaxis should only be used for persons at very high risk of influenza complications and who cannot be otherwise protected at times of high risk for exposure. Prophylaxis should also be administered to all eligible residents of institutions that house patients at high risk when needed to control outbreaks.

Prescribing and Access Restrictions Zanamivir *aqueous solution* intended for nebulization or intravenous (IV) administration is **not** currently approved for use. Data on safety and efficacy via these routes of administration are limited. However, limited supplies of zanamivir aqueous solution may be made available through the Zanamivir Compassionate Use Program for qualifying patients for the treatment of serious influenza illness. For information, contact the GlaxoSmithKline Clinical Support Help Desk at 1-866-341-9160 or gskclinicalsupportHD@gsk.com.

Pregnancy Risk Factor C

Pregnancy Considerations Adverse events were not observed in animal reproduction studies. An increased risk of adverse neonatal or maternal outcomes has not been observed following use of zanamivir during pregnancy. Untreated influenza infection is associated with an increased risk of adverse events to the fetus and an increased risk of complications or death to the mother. Neuraminidase inhibitors are currently recommended for the treatment or prophylaxis of influenza in pregnant women and women up to 2 weeks postpartum (CDC 60 [1], 2011; CDC March 13, 2014; January 2015).

Breast-Feeding Considerations It is not known if zanamivir is found in human milk and the manufacturer recommends that caution be exercised when administering zanamivir to nursing women. Influenza may cause serious illness in postpartum women and prompt evaluation for febrile respiratory illnesses is recommended (Louie, 2011).

Contraindications Hypersensitivity to zanamivir or any component of the formulation (contains milk proteins)

Warnings/Precautions Allergic-like reactions, including anaphylaxis, oropharyngeal edema, and serious skin rashes have been reported. Rare occurrences of neuropsychiatric events (including confusion, delirium, hallucinations, and/or self-injury) have been reported from postmarketing surveillance; direct causation is difficult to establish (influenza infection may also be associated with behavioral and neurologic changes). Patients must be instructed in the use of the delivery system. Antiviral treatment should begin within 48 hours of symptom onset. However, the CDC recommends that treatment may still be beneficial and should be started in hospitalized patients with severe, complicated or progressive illness if >48 hours. Treatment should not be delayed while awaiting results of laboratory tests for influenza. Nonhospitalized persons who are not at high risk for developing severe or complicated illness and who have a mild disease are not likely to benefit if treatment is started >48 hours after symptom onset. Nonhospitalized persons who are already beginning to recover do not need treatment. Effectiveness has not been established in patients with significant underlying medical conditions or for prophylaxis of influenza in nursing home patients (per manufacturer). The CDC recommends zanamivir to be used to control institutional outbreaks of influenza when circulating strains are suspected of being resistant to oseltamivir (refer to current guidelines). Not recommended for use in patients with underlying respiratory disease, such as asthma or COPD, due to lack of efficacy and risk of serious adverse effects. Bronchospasm, decreased lung function, and other serious adverse reactions, including those with fatal outcomes, have been reported in patients with and without airway disease; discontinue with bronchospasm or signs of decreased lung function. For a patient with an underlying airway disease where a medical decision has been made to use zanamivir, a fast-acting bronchodilator should be made available, and used prior to each dose. Not a substitute for annual flu vaccination; has not been shown to reduce risk of transmission of influenza to others. Consider primary or concomitant bacterial infections. Powder for oral inhalation contains lactose; use contraindicated in patients allergic to milk proteins. The inhalation powder should only be administered via inhalation using the provided Diskhaler® delivery device. The commercially available formulation is **not** intended to be solubilized or administered via any nebulizer/mechanical ventilator; inappropriate administration has resulted in death. Safety and efficacy of repeated courses or use with hepatic impairment or severe renal impairment have not been established. Indicated for children ≥5 years of age (for influenza prophylaxis) and children ≥7 years of age (for influenza treatment); children ages 5-6 years may have inadequate inhalation (via Diskhaler®) for the treatment of influenza.

Warnings: Additional Pediatric Considerations Pediatric patients with influenza may be at increased risk for neuropsychiatric events (confusion, abnormal behavior) and seizures early in their illness; monitor closely.

Adverse Reactions

Central nervous system: Dizziness, fatigue, fever/chills, headache, malaise

Dermatologic: Urticaria

Gastrointestinal: Abdominal pain, anorexia, appetite decreased, diarrhea, nausea, throat/tonsil discomfort/pain, vomiting

Neuromuscular & skeletal: Arthralgia, articular rheumatism, muscle pain, musculoskeletal pain

Respiratory: Bronchitis, cough, infection, nasal inflammation, nasal signs and symptoms, sinusitis

Miscellaneous: Viral infection

Rare but important or life-threatening: Allergic or allergic-like reaction (including oropharyngeal edema), arrhythmia, bronchospasm, consciousness altered, delusions, dyspnea, hallucinations, neuropsychiatric events (self-injury, confusion, delirium), nightmares, rash (including serious cutaneous reactions [eg, erythema multiforme, Stevens-Johnson syndrome, toxic epidermal necrolysis]), seizure, syncope

Drug Interactions

Metabolism/Transport Effects None known.

Avoid Concomitant Use There are no known interactions where it is recommended to avoid concomitant use.

Increased Effect/Toxicity There are no known significant interactions involving an increase in effect.

Decreased Effect

Zanamivir may decrease the levels/effects of: Influenza Virus Vaccine (Live/Attenuated)

Storage/Stability Store at 25°C (77°F); excursions permitted to 15°C to 30°C (59°F to 86°F). Do not puncture blister until taking a dose using the Diskhaler®.

Mechanism of Action Zanamivir inhibits influenza virus neuraminidase enzymes, potentially altering virus particle aggregation and release.

Pharmacokinetics (Adult data unless noted)

Absorption: Systemic: 4% to 17%

Protein binding: <10%

Metabolism: None

Half-life: 2.5-5.1 hours; mild-to-moderate renal impairment: 4.7 hours; severe renal impairment: 18.5 hours

Time to peak serum concentration: 1-2 hours

Elimination: Urine (as unchanged drug); feces (unabsorbed drug)

Dosing: Usual Note: 10 mg dose is provided by 2 inhalations (one 5 mg blister per inhalation):

Pediatric:

Influenza virus A and B; treatment: Oral inhalation: Children ≥7 years and Adolescents: Two inhalations (10 mg) twice daily for 5 days; doses on first day should be separated by at least 2 hours; on subsequent days, doses should be spaced by ~12 hours. Begin within 2 days of signs or symptoms. Longer treatment may be considered for patients who remain severely ill after 5 days.

Influenza virus A and B; prophylaxis: Oral inhalation:

Manufacturer's labeling:

Household setting: Children ≥5 years and Adolescents: Two inhalations (10 mg) once daily for 10 days; begin within 36 hours following onset of signs or symptoms of index case

Community outbreak: Adolescents: Two inhalations (10 mg) once daily for 28 days; begin within 5 days of outbreak

Alternate dosing: Children ≥5 years and Adolescents:

Household setting: CDC Recommendation: Two inhalations (10 mg) once daily for 7 days after last known exposure (CDC, 2012)

Community outbreak: IDSA/PIDS recommendations: Two inhalations (10 mg) once daily; continue until influenza activity in community subsides or immunity obtained from immunization; up to 28 days has been well tolerated (Bradley, 2011; CDC, 2011)

Institutional outbreak: CDC recommendations: Two inhalations (10 mg) once daily; continue for ≥2 weeks and until ~7 days after identification of illness onset in the last patient. Zanamivir is to be used to control institutional outbreaks of influenza when circulating strains are suspected of being resistant to oseltamivir (CDC, 2012).

HIV-exposed/-positive: Two inhalations (10 mg) once daily for 10 days after last known exposure (DHHS [pediatric], 2013)

Adult: **Influenza virus A and B:**

Manufacturer's labeling: Oral inhalation:

Prophylaxis, household setting: Two inhalations (10 mg) once daily for 10 days. Begin within 36 hours following onset of signs or symptoms of index case.

Prophylaxis, community outbreak: Two inhalations (10 mg) once daily for 28 days. Begin within 5 days of outbreak.

Treatment: Two inhalations (10 mg total) twice daily for 5 days. Doses on first day should be separated by at least 2 hours; on subsequent days, doses should be spaced by ~12 hours. Begin within 2 days of signs or symptoms. Longer treatment may be considered for patients who remain severely ill after 5 days.

Alternate dosing: Oral inhalation:

Prophylaxis, household exposure: Two inhalations (10 mg) once daily for 7 days after last known exposure (CDC, 2012)

Prophylaxis, institutional outbreak: Two inhalations (10 mg) once daily; continue for ≥2 weeks and until ~7 days after identification of illness onset in the last patient. Zanamivir is to be used to control institutional outbreaks of influenza when circulating strains are suspected of being resistant to oseltamivir (CDC, 2012).

Prophylaxis, community outbreak (IDSA/PIDS, 2011): Two inhalations (10 mg) once daily; continue until influenza activity in community subsides or immunity obtained from immunization; up to 28 days has been well tolerated (CDC, 2011)

Dosing adjustment in renal impairment: Children, Adolescents, and Adults: Adjustment not necessary following a 5-day course of treatment due to low systemic absorption; however, the potential for drug accumulation should be considered.

Administration Oral Inhalation: **Inhalation powder not for use via nebulizer:** Use a Diskhaler® delivery device (a special breath-activated plastic inhaler). The foil blister disk containing zanamivir inhalation powder should not be manipulated or solubilized. Load Relenza® Rotadisk® into the diskhaler; a blister that contains medication is pierced and the drug is dispersed into the air stream created when the patient inhales through the mouthpiece. Patients scheduled to take inhaled bronchodilators at the same time as zanamivir should be advised to use their bronchodilator before taking zanamivir.

Monitoring Parameters Monitor respiratory function changes in behavior; if used for prophylaxis, signs/symptoms of influenza infection

Dosage Forms Excipient information presented when available (limited, particularly for generics); consult specific product labeling.

Aerosol Powder Breath Activated, Inhalation:

Relenza Diskhaler: 5 mg/blister (20 ea) [contains lactose]

◆ **Zantac** *see* Ranitidine *on page* 1836

◆ **Zantac 75 [OTC]** *see* Ranitidine *on page* 1836

◆ **Zantac 75 (Can)** *see* Ranitidine *on page* 1836

- ◆ **Zantac 150 Maximum Strength [OTC]** *see* Ranitidine *on page 1836*
- ◆ **Zantac Maximum Strength Non-Prescription (Can)** *see* Ranitidine *on page 1836*
- ◆ **Zarontin** *see* Ethosuximide *on page 814*
- ◆ **Zarontin® (Can)** *see* Ethosuximide *on page 814*
- ◆ **Zaroxolyn [DSC]** *see* Metolazone *on page 1416*
- ◆ **Zaroxolyn (Can)** *see* Metolazone *on page 1416*
- ◆ **Zarxio** *see* Filgrastim *on page 876*
- ◆ **ZD9238** *see* Fulvestrant *on page 950*
- ◆ **ZDV** *see* Zidovudine *on page 2207*
- ◆ **ZDV, Abacavir, and Lamivudine** *see* Abacavir, Lamivudine, and Zidovudine *on page 38*
- ◆ **Zeasorb-AF [OTC]** *see* Miconazole (Topical) *on page 1431*
- ◆ **Zecuity** *see* SUMAtriptan *on page 1995*
- ◆ **Zegerid** *see* Omeprazole and Sodium Bicarbonate *on page 1558*
- ◆ **Zegerid OTC [OTC]** *see* Omeprazole and Sodium Bicarbonate *on page 1558*
- ◆ **Zeldox** *see* Ziprasidone *on page 2216*
- ◆ **Zemplar** *see* Paricalcitol *on page 1632*
- ◆ **Zemuron** *see* Rocuronium *on page 1881*
- ◆ **Zenatane** *see* ISOtretinoin *on page 1171*
- ◆ **Zenhale (Can)** *see* Mometasone and Formoterol *on page 1457*
- ◆ **Zenpep** *see* Pancrelipase *on page 1614*
- ◆ **Zenzedi** *see* Dextroamphetamine *on page 625*
- ◆ **Zephrex-D [OTC]** *see* Pseudoephedrine *on page 1801*
- ◆ **Zerit** *see* Stavudine *on page 1970*
- ◆ **Zestril** *see* Lisinopril *on page 1280*
- ◆ **Zetia** *see* Ezetimibe *on page 832*
- ◆ **Zetonna** *see* Ciclesonide (Nasal) *on page 454*
- ◆ **Ziagen** *see* Abacavir *on page 34*
- ◆ **Ziana** *see* Clindamycin and Tretinoin *on page 494*

Zidovudine (zye DOE vyoo deen)

Medication Safety Issues

Sound-alike/look-alike issues:

Azidothymidine may be confused with azaTHIOprine, aztreonam

Retrovir may be confused with acyclovir, ritonavir

High alert medication:

This medication is in a class the Institute for Safe Medication Practices (ISMP) includes among its list of drug classes that have a heightened risk of causing significant patient harm when used in error.

Other safety concerns:

AZT is an error-prone abbreviation (mistaken as azathioprine, aztreonam)

Related Information

Adult and Adolescent HIV *on page 2392*

Pediatric HIV *on page 2380*

Perinatal HIV *on page 2400*

Safe Handling of Hazardous Drugs *on page 2455*

Brand Names: US Retrovir

Brand Names: Canada Apo-Zidovudine; AZT; Novo-AZT; Retrovir; Retrovir (AZT)

Therapeutic Category Antiretroviral Agent; HIV Agents (Anti-HIV Agents); Nucleoside Reverse Transcriptase Inhibitor (NRTI)

Generic Availability (US) May be product dependent

Use Treatment of HIV-1 infection in combination with other antiretroviral agents [Oral: FDA approved in ages ≥4 weeks and adults; Injection (short-term use): FDA approved in adults] (**Note:** HIV regimens consisting of three antiretroviral agents are strongly recommended); chemoprophylaxis to reduce perinatal HIV-1 transmission [Oral, injection: FDA approved in ages 0 days to 6 weeks (postpartum therapy of HIV-1 exposed neonate) and adults (antepartum and intrapartum therapy of HIV-1 infected mother)]; has also been used as HIV postexposure prophylaxis (eg, chemoprophylaxis after occupational exposure to HIV)

Pregnancy Risk Factor C

Pregnancy Considerations Adverse events have been observed in some animal reproduction studies. Zidovudine has a high level of transfer across the human placenta and the placenta also metabolizes zidovudine to the active metabolite. No increased risk of overall birth defects has been observed following first trimester exposure according to data collected by the antiretroviral pregnancy registry. The pharmacokinetics of zidovudine are not significantly altered in pregnancy and dosing adjustment is not needed. The HHS Perinatal HIV Guidelines consider zidovudine in combination with lamivudine to be a preferred NRTI backbone for use in antiretroviral-naive pregnant women. Zidovudine should be administered IV near delivery regardless of antepartum regimen or mode of delivery in women with HIV RNA >1000 copies/mL or unknown HIV RNA status.

Cases of lactic acidosis/hepatic steatosis syndrome related to mitochondrial toxicity have been reported in pregnant women with prolonged use of nucleoside analogues. It is not known if pregnancy itself potentiates this known side effect; however, women may be at increased risk of lactic acidosis and liver damage. In addition, these adverse events are similar to other rare but life-threatening syndromes which occur during pregnancy (eg, HELLP syndrome). Hepatic enzymes and electrolytes should be monitored in women receiving nucleoside analogues and clinicians should watch for early signs of the syndrome. In addition, mitochondrial dysfunction may develop in infants following *in utero* exposure.

Regardless of CD4 count or HIV RNA copy number, all HIV-infected pregnant women should receive a combination antiretroviral (ARV) drug regimen. A combination of antepartum, intrapartum, and infant ARV prophylaxis is recommended. ARV therapy should be started as soon as possible in women with symptomatic infection. Although earlier initiation may be more effective in reducing the perinatal transmission of HIV, initiation may be delayed until after 12 weeks' gestation in women who do not require immediate treatment after careful consideration of maternal conditions (eg, nausea and vomiting) and the potential risks of first trimester fetal exposure for specific agents. A scheduled cesarean delivery at 38 weeks' gestation is recommended for all women with HIV RNA >1000 copies/mL or unknown concentrations near delivery in order to decrease transmission. If ARV therapy must be interrupted for <24 hours during the peripartum period, stop then restart all medications simultaneously in order to decrease the chance of developing resistance. Long-term follow-up is recommended for all infants exposed to ARV medications. In couples who want to conceive, the HIV-infected partner should attain maximum viral suppression prior to conception.

Health care providers are encouraged to enroll pregnant women exposed to antiretroviral medications in the Antiretroviral Pregnancy Registry (1-800-258-4263 or www.APRegistry.com). Health care providers caring for HIV-infected women and their infants may contact the National Perinatal HIV Hotline (888-448-8765) for clinical consultation (HHS [perinatal], 2014).

Breast-Feeding Considerations Zidovudine is excreted into breast milk. Concentrations of zidovudine in breast milk are similar to those in the maternal serum. Maternal or infant antiretroviral therapy does not completely eliminate the risk of postnatal HIV transmission. In addition, multi-class-resistant virus has been detected in breast-feeding infants despite maternal therapy. Therefore, in the United States, where formula is accessible, affordable, safe, and sustainable, and the risk of infant mortality due to diarrhea and respiratory infections is low, complete avoidance of breast-feeding by HIV-infected women is recommended to decrease potential transmission of HIV (HHS [perinatal], 2014).

Contraindications

Potentially life-threatening hypersensitivity to zidovudine or any component of the formulation

Canadian labeling: Additional contraindications (not in U.S. labeling): Neutrophil count <750/mm^3 or hemoglobin <7.5 g/dL (4.65 mmol/L)

Warnings/Precautions Hazardous agent - use appropriate precautions for handling and disposal (NIOSH 2014 [group 2]).

[U.S. Boxed Warning]: Hematologic toxicity, including neutropenia and severe anemia have been reported with use, especially with advanced HIV-1 disease. Toxicity may be related to duration of use and prior bone marrow reserve. Hemoglobin reduction may occur in as early as 2 to 4 weeks; neutropenia usually occurs after 6 to 8 weeks. Pancytopenia has been reported (usually reversible). Use with caution in patients with bone marrow compromise (granulocytes <1,000 cells/mm^3 or hemoglobin <9.5 mg/dL); dose interruption may be required in patients who develop anemia or neutropenia. **[U.S. Boxed Warning]: Lactic acidosis and severe hepatomegaly with steatosis have been reported, including fatal cases.** Risks may be increased with liver disease, obesity, pregnancy, prolonged exposure, or in females. Suspend treatment with zidovudine in any patient who develops clinical or laboratory findings suggestive of lactic acidosis (transaminase elevation may/may not accompany hepatomegaly and steatosis). Use caution in combination with interferon alfa with or without ribavirin in HIV/HCV coinfected patients; monitor closely for hepatic decompensation, anemia, or neutropenia; dose reduction or discontinuation of interferon and/or ribavirin may be required if toxicity evident.

Zidovudine newborn prophylaxis may affect diagnostic virologic assays in HIV-exposed infants. If a virologic assay result is negative while the infant is receiving combination antiretroviral prophylaxis, repeat virologic testing should be considered 2 to 4 weeks after cessation of antiretroviral prophylaxis (HHS [pediatric], 2014).

[U.S. Boxed Warning]: Prolonged use has been associated with symptomatic myopathy and myositis. Pathological changes observed are similar to that produced by HIV-1 disease. May cause redistribution of fat (eg, buffalo hump, peripheral wasting with increased abdominal girth, cushingoid appearance). Immune reconstitution syndrome may develop resulting in the occurrence of an inflammatory response to an indolent or residual opportunistic infection during initial HIV treatment or activation of autoimmune disorders (eg, Graves disease, polymyositis, Guillain-Barré syndrome) later in therapy; further evaluation and treatment may be required. Hematologic toxicity may be increased due to increased serum concentrations in patients with severe hepatic impairment. Use with caution in patients with severe renal impairment; dosage adjustment recommended. Reduce dose in patients with severe renal impairment. Potentially significant interactions may exist, requiring dose or frequency adjustment, additional monitoring, and/or selection of alternative therapy. Latex is used in injection vial stopper and may cause allergic reactions in latex-sensitive individuals.

Benzyl alcohol and derivatives: Some dosage forms may contain sodium benzoate/benzoic acid; benzoic acid (benzoate) is a metabolite of benzyl alcohol; large amounts of benzyl alcohol (≥99 mg/kg/day) have been associated with a potentially fatal toxicity ("gasping syndrome") in neonates; the "gasping syndrome" consists of metabolic acidosis, respiratory distress, gasping respirations, CNS dysfunction (including convulsions, intracranial hemorrhage), hypotension, and cardiovascular collapse (AAP, 1997; CDC, 1982); some data suggests that benzoate displaces bilirubin from protein binding sites (Ahlfors, 2001); avoid or use dosage forms containing benzyl alcohol derivative with caution in neonates. See manufacturer's labeling.

Warnings: Additional Pediatric Considerations Use with caution in patients with ANC <1000 cells/mm^3 or hemoglobin <9.5 g/dL; consider interruption of therapy for significant anemia (Hgb <7.5 g/dL or reduction >25% of baseline; neonates: Hgb <7 g/dL) or neutropenia (ANC <750 cells/mm^3 or reduction >50% from baseline; neonates ANC <500 cells/mm^3); use of erythropoietin or filgrastim may be necessary in some patients. In perinatally HIV-exposed infants, the sensitivity of diagnostic virologic assays, particularly HIV RNA assays, may be affected by combination antiretroviral prophylactic therapy in the infant. Thus, a negative result of a diagnostic virologic assay should be repeated 2 to 4 weeks after cessation of neonatal combination antiretroviral prophylactic therapy (HHS [pediatric], 2015).

Adverse Reactions

Cardiovascular: ECG abnormality (children), edema (children), heart failure (children), left ventricular dilation (children)

Central nervous system: Chills, fatigue, fever (children), headache, insomnia, irritability (children), malaise, nervousness (children)

Dermatologic: Rash (more common in children)

Gastrointestinal: Abdominal cramps, abdominal pain, anorexia, constipation (adults), diarrhea (children), dyspepsia, nausea (more common in adults), vomiting (more common in adults), weight loss (children)

Genitourinary: Hematuria (children)

Hematologic: Anemia (more common in neonates), granulocytopenia, macrocytosis (children), neutropenia (children), thrombocytopenia (children)

Hepatic: Hepatomegaly (children), transaminases increased

Neuromuscular & skeletal: Arthralgia, musculoskeletal pain, myalgia, neuropathy, weakness

Otic: Hearing loss

Respiratory: Cough (children)

Rare but important or life-threatening: Allergic reactions, amblyopia, anaphylaxis, angioedema, anxiety, aplastic anemia, back pain, body fat redistribution, cardiomyopathy, confusion, CPK increased, depression, diabetes, dizziness, dyslipidemias, dyspnea, gynecomastia, hearing loss, hemolytic anemia, hepatitis, hepatomegaly with steatosis, immune reconstitution syndrome, insulin resistance, jaundice, lactic acidosis, LDH increased, leukopenia, loss of mental acuity, lymphadenopathy, macular edema, mania, myopathy, myositis, oral mucosa pigmentation, pancreatitis, pancytopenia with marrow hypoplasia, paresthesia, photophobia, pruritus, pure red cell aplasia, rhabdomyolysis, seizure, skin/nail pigmentation changes (blue), Stevens-Johnson syndrome, syncope, taste perversion, toxic epidermal necrolysis, tremor, urticaria, vertigo

Drug Interactions

Metabolism/Transport Effects **Substrate** of CYP2A6 (minor), CYP2C19 (minor), CYP2C9 (minor), CYP3A4 (minor), OAT3; **Note:** Assignment of Major/Minor substrate status based on clinically relevant drug interaction potential

Avoid Concomitant Use

Avoid concomitant use of Zidovudine with any of the following: Amodiaquine; BCG (Intravesical); CloZAPine; Dipyrone; Stavudine

Increased Effect/Toxicity

Zidovudine may increase the levels/effects of: Amodiaquine; CloZAPine; Ribavirin

The levels/effects of Zidovudine may be increased by: Acyclovir-Valacyclovir; Clarithromycin; Dexketoprofen; Dipyrone; DOXOrubicin (Conventional); DOXOrubicin (Liposomal); Fluconazole; Ganciclovir-Valganciclovir; Interferons; Methadone; Probenecid; Raltegravir; Teriflunomide; Valproic Acid and Derivatives

Decreased Effect

Zidovudine may decrease the levels/effects of: BCG (Intravesical); Stavudine

The levels/effects of Zidovudine may be decreased by: Clarithromycin; DOXOrubicin (Conventional); DOXOrubicin (Liposomal); Protease Inhibitors; Rifamycin Derivatives

Storage/Stability

IV: Store undiluted vials at 15°C to 25°C (59°F to 77°F). Protect from light. When diluted, solution is physically and chemically stable for 24 hours at room temperature and 48 hours if refrigerated. Attempt to administer diluted solution within 8 hours if stored at room temperature or 24 hours if refrigerated to minimize potential for microbial-contaminated solutions (vials are single-use and do not contain preservative).

Tablets, capsules, syrup: Store at 15°C to 25°C (59°F to 77°F). Protect capsules from moisture.

Mechanism of Action Zidovudine is a thymidine analog which interferes with the HIV viral RNA-dependent DNA polymerase resulting in inhibition of viral replication; nucleoside reverse transcriptase inhibitor

Pharmacokinetics (Adult data unless noted) **Note:** In general, pharmacokinetic data for pediatric patients >3 months to 12 years of age are similar to data in adult patients.

Absorption: Oral: Well absorbed

Distribution: Significant penetration into the CSF

CSF/plasma ratio:

Infants 3 months to Children 12 years (n=38): Median: 0.68; range: 0.03 to 3.25

Adults (n=39): Median: 0.6; range: 0.04 to 2.62

V_d: 1.6 L/kg

Protein binding: 25% to 38%

Metabolism: Extensive first-pass effect; hepatic via glucuronidation to inactive metabolites

Bioavailability: Oral: Similar for tablets, capsules, and syrup

Neonates <14 days: 89%

Infants 14 days to 3 months: 61%

Infants 3 months to Children 12 years: 65%

Adults: 64% ± 10%

Half-life, terminal:

Premature neonate: 6.3 hours

Full-term neonates: 3.1 hours

Infants 14 days to 3 months: 1.9 hours

Infants 3 months to Children 12 years: 1.5 hours

Adults: 0.5 to 3 hours (mean: 1.1 hours)

Time to peak serum concentration: Within 30 to 90 minutes

Elimination: Urinary excretion (63% to 95%)

Oral: 72% to 74% of drug excreted in urine as metabolites and 14% to 18% as unchanged drug

IV: 45% to 60% excreted in urine as metabolites and 18% to 29% as unchanged drug

Dosing: Neonatal

HIV-1 infection, treatment (HHS [pediatric] 2015): Use in combination with other antiretroviral agents; standard neonatal doses may be excessive in premature neonates; evaluation of hepatic and renal function should be performed prior to final dose increases: **Note:** Use IV route only until oral therapy can be administered:

Oral:

GA <30 weeks: 2 mg/kg/dose every 12 hours; at 4 weeks of age, increase dose to 3 mg/kg/dose every 12 hours; at >8 to 10 weeks of age, increase to 12 mg/kg/dose every 12 hours

GA ≥30 weeks and <35 weeks: 2 mg/kg/dose every 12 hours; at PNA 15 days, increase dose to 3 mg/kg/dose every 12 hours; at >6 to 8 weeks of age, increase to 12 mg/kg/dose every 12 hours

GA ≥35 weeks: 4 mg/kg/dose every 12 hours; at >4 weeks of age, increase to 12 mg/kg/dose every 12 hours

IV: **Note:** The IV dose is 75% of the oral dose administered at the same interval

GA <30 weeks: 1.5 mg/kg/dose every 12 hours; at 4 weeks of age, increase dose to 2.3 mg/kg/dose every 12 hours; at >8 to 10 weeks of age, increase to 9 mg/kg/dose every 12 hours

GA ≥30 weeks and <35 weeks: 1.5 mg/kg/dose every 12 hours; at PNA 15 days, increase dose to 2.3 mg/kg/dose every 12 hours; at >6 to 8 weeks of age, increase to 9 mg/kg/dose every 12 hours

GA ≥35 weeks: 3 mg/kg/dose every 12 hours; at >4 weeks of age, increase to 9 mg/kg/dose every 12 hours

Perinatal HIV-1 transmission, prevention: Note: A 6-week course of zidovudine in the neonate is generally recommended for all HIV-exposed neonates to prevent perinatal transmission of HIV; a shorter 4-week course may be considered for neonates ≥35 weeks' gestation at birth if the mother received standard combination antiretroviral therapy during pregnancy, viral suppression was consistent, and maternal adherence is not a concern. In addition, the recommended regimen in the US to prevent perinatal transmission of HIV also includes maternal antepartum oral zidovudine and maternal intrapartum IV zidovudine. Use of zidovudine in combination with nevirapine is recommended in the neonate in select situations (eg, infants born to HIV-infected mothers with no antepartum antiretroviral therapy prior to labor or during labor; or infants born to mothers with only intrapartum antiretroviral therapy) and may be considered in other situations (eg, infants born to mothers with suboptimal viral suppression at delivery; or infants born to mothers with known antiretroviral drug-resistant virus). **Note:** Zidovudine dosing should begin as soon as possible after birth (within 6 to 12 hours after delivery) and continue for the first 6 weeks of life. If neonate is diagnosed as HIV positive, discontinue prevention (prophylaxis) dosing and begin treatment regimen (see above) (HHS [perinatal] 2014).

Premature neonates (HHS [perinatal], 2014): **Note:** Standard neonatal doses may be excessive in premature neonates.

Oral:

GA <30 weeks: 2 mg/kg/dose every 12 hours; at 4 weeks of age, increase dose to 3 mg/kg/dose every 12 hours

GA ≥30 weeks and <35 weeks: 2 mg/kg/dose every 12 hours; at PNA 15 days, increase dose to 3 mg/kg/dose every 12 hours

GA ≥35 weeks: 4 mg/kg/dose every 12 hours

IV: **Note:** Use IV route only until oral therapy can be administered:

GA <30 weeks: 1.5 mg/kg/dose every 12 hours; at 4 weeks of age, increase dose to 2.3 mg/kg/dose every 12 hours

GA ≥30 weeks and <35 weeks: 1.5 mg/kg/dose every 12 hours; at PNA 15 days, increase dose to 2.3 mg/kg/dose every 12 hours

GA ≥35 weeks: 3 mg/kg/dose every 12 hours

Full-term neonates:

Oral:

Manufacturer's labeling: 2 mg/kg/dose every 6 hours

AIDS*info* recommendation: 4 mg/kg/dose every 12 hours (HHS [perinatal], 2014)

World Health Organization simplified dosing regimen: For use in low resource settings: **Note:** With the WHO regimen, neonates who weigh >3.75 kg at birth will receive a smaller zidovudine dose (compared with the mg/kg/dose method) and infants <3.75 kg will receive a larger zidovudine dose (WHO, 2010)

Birth weight <2 kg: Use weight based dosing

Birth weight 2 to <2.5 kg: 10 mg twice daily

Birth weight ≥2.5 kg: 15 mg twice daily

IV: **Note**: Use IV route only until oral therapy can be administered:

Manufacturer's labeling: 1.5 mg/kg/dose every 6 hours

AIDS*info* recommendation: 3 mg/kg/dose every 12 hours (HHS [perinatal], 2014)

Dosage adjustment for hematologic toxicity: Consider interruption of therapy for significant anemia (Hgb <7.5 g/dL or >25% decrease from baseline; neonates: HgB < 7 g/dL) and/or significant neutropenia (ANC <750 cells/mm^3 or >50% decrease from baseline; neonates ANC < 500 cells/mm^3) until evidence of bone marrow recovery occurs; once bone marrow recovers, dose may be resumed using appropriate adjunctive therapy (eg, epoetin alfa) (HHS [pediatric], 2015).

Dosing: Usual

Pediatric:

HIV-1 infection, treatment: Use in combination with other antiretroviral agents.

Oral:

Infants born prematurely (PCA <35 weeks): Refer to Dosing-Neonatal

Infants (born at or near term with PCA ≥35 weeks and at least 4 weeks of age), Children, and Adolescents: **Note:** The 3-times-daily dosing is approved but rarely used in practice (HHS [pediatric], 2015).

Weight-directed dosing:

4 to <9 kg: 12 mg/kg/dose twice daily **or** 8 mg/kg/dose 3 times daily

9 to <30 kg: 9 mg/kg/dose twice daily **or** 6 mg/kg/dose 3 times daily

≥30 kg: 300 mg twice daily **or** 200 mg 3 times daily

BSA-directed dosing: 240 mg/**m^2**/dose every 12 hours (maximum dose: 300 mg/dose) or 160 mg/**m^2**/dose every 8 hours (maximum dose: 200 mg/dose)

IV: **Note:** Use IV route only until oral therapy can be administered:

Infants ≥3 months, Children, and Adolescents weighing <30 kg: 120 mg/m^2/dose every 6 hours; maximum dose: 160 mg/dose (Retrovir prescribing information [Canada] 2014)

Adolescents ≥30 kg: 1 to 2 mg/kg every 4 hours around the clock (Retrovir prescribing information [Canada] 2014)

HIV postexposure prophylaxis: Children ≥12 years and Adolescents: Oral: 300 mg twice daily **or** 200 mg 3 times daily (with food) in combination with lamivudine or emtricitabine, with or without a protease inhibitor depending on risk; begin therapy within 2 hours of exposure if possible; continue for four weeks (CDC 2005).

Perinatal transmission, prevention: Note: A 6-week course of zidovudine in the neonate is generally recommended for all HIV-exposed neonates to prevent perinatal transmission of HIV; a shorter 4-week course may be considered for infants ≥35 weeks' gestation at birth if the mother received standard combination antiretroviral therapy during pregnancy, viral suppression was consistent, and maternal adherence is not a concern. In addition, the recommended regimen in the US to prevent perinatal transmission of HIV also includes maternal antepartum oral zidovudine and maternal intrapartum IV zidovudine. Use of zidovudine in combination with nevirapine is recommended in the neonate in select situations (eg, infants born to HIV-infected mothers with no antepartum antiretroviral therapy) prior to labor or during labor; or infants born to mothers with only intrapartum antiretroviral therapy) and may be considered in other situations (eg, infants born to mothers with suboptimal viral suppression at delivery; or infants born to mothers with known antiretroviral drug-resistant virus). **Note:** Zidovudine dosing should begin as soon as possible after birth (within 6 to 12 hours after delivery) and continue for the first 6 weeks of life. If neonate is diagnosed as HIV positive, discontinue prevention (prophylaxis) dosing and begin treatment regimen (see above) (HHS [perinatal] 2014).

Infants <6 weeks and full-term at birth:

Oral:

Manufacturer's labeling: 2 mg/kg/dose every 6 hours

AIDS*info* recommendation: 4 mg/kg/dose every 12 hours (DHHS [perinatal], 2014)

IV: **Note:** Use IV route only until oral therapy can be administered:

Manufacturer's labeling: 1.5 mg/kg/dose every 6 hours

AIDS*info* recommendation: 3 mg/kg/dose every 12 hours (DHHS [pediatric, perinatal], 2014)

Adult:

HIV infection, treatment:

Oral: 300 mg twice daily

IV: 1 mg/kg/dose administered every 4 hours around-the-clock (5 to 6 doses daily)

HIV postexposure prophylaxis: Oral: 300 mg twice daily **or** 200 mg 3 times daily (with food) in combination with lamivudine or emtricitabine. A third agent may be added for high risk exposures. Therapy should be started within 2 hours of exposure and continued for 4 weeks (CDC, 2005).

Perinatal transmission, prevention: Maternal dose **Note:** Dose adjustment not required in pregnant women. Begin oral therapy with usual recommended doses based on current guidelines. Zidovudine should be administered by continuous IV infusion during labor and delivery regardless of antepartum regimen or mode of delivery in women with HIV RNA >1,000 copies/mL or unknown HIV RNA status. If oral zidovudine was part of the antepartum regimen, discontinue during intrapartum IV infusion. Other antiretroviral agents should be continued orally. Zidovudine IV is not required in women receiving combination antiretroviral therapy who have HIV RNA ≤1000 copies/mL consistently in late pregnancy and/or near delivery and have no adherence or tolerance concerns (HHS [perinatal], 2014).

During labor and delivery, administer zidovudine IV 2 mg/kg as loading dose, followed by a continuous IV infusion of 1 mg/kg/hour until delivery. For scheduled cesarean delivery, begin IV zidovudine 3 hours before surgery.

Dosing adjustment in renal impairment:

Infants >6 weeks, Children, and Adolescents:

The following adjustments have been recommended (Aronoff 2007): **Note:** Renally adjusted dose recommendations are based on oral doses of 160 mg/$\mathbf{m^2}$/dose every 8 hours and IV dose of 120 mg/$\mathbf{m^2}$/dose every 6 hours.

GFR ≥10 mL/minute/1.73 m^2: No dosage adjustment required

GFR <10 mL/minute/1.73 m^2: Administer 50% of dose every 8 hours

Intermittent hemodialysis (IHD): Administer 50% of dose every 8 hours

Peritoneal dialysis (PD): Administer 50% of dose every 8 hours

Continuous renal replacement therapy (CRRT): No adjustment required

Adults:

CrCl ≥15 mL/minute: No dosage adjustment necessary

End-stage renal disease patients (CrCl <15 mL/minute) and patients receiving hemodialysis:

Oral:

Manufacturer's labeling: 100 mg every 6 to 8 hours

AIDS*info* guidelines: 100 mg every 8 hours or 300 mg once daily (HHS [adult] 2014)

IV: 1 mg/kg/dose every 6 to 8 hours

Peritoneal dialysis:

Oral: 100 mg every 6 to 8 hours

IV: 1 mg/kg/dose every 6 to 8 hours

Continuous renal replacement therapy (CRRT): No adjustment needed (Aronoff, 2007)

Dosing adjustment in hepatic impairment: All patients: There are no specific dosage adjustments provided in the manufacturer's labeling (has not been studied); however, adjustment may be necessary due to extensive hepatic metabolism; dosage reduction may be required; use with caution; monitor for hematologic toxicities frequently.

Dosing adjustment for hematologic toxicity: Consider interruption of therapy for significant anemia (Hgb <7.5 g/dL or >25% decrease from baseline) and/or significant neutropenia (ANC <750 cells/mm^3 or >50% decrease from baseline) until evidence of bone marrow recovery occurs; once bone marrow recovers, dose may be resumed using appropriate adjunctive therapy (eg, epoetin alfa).

Preparation for Administration Hazardous agent; use appropriate precautions for handling and disposal (NIOSH 2014 [group 2]).

Parenteral: Dilute with D_5W to a final concentration ≤4 mg/mL.

Administration Hazardous agent; use appropriate precautions for handling and disposal (NIOSH 2014 [group 2]).

Oral: May be administered without regard to meals

Parenteral: IV infusion: Administer over 1 hour; in neonates dose may be infused over 30 minutes. Do not administer IM; do not administer IV push or by rapid infusion.

Monitoring Parameters Note: The absolute CD4 cell count is currently recommended to monitor immune status in children of all ages; CD4 percentage can be used as an alternative. This recommendation is based on the use of absolute CD4 cell counts in the current pediatric HIV infection stage classification and as thresholds for initiation of antiretroviral treatment (HHS [pediatric] 2015).

Prior to initiation of therapy: Genotypic resistance testing, CD4 and viral load (every 3 to 4 months), CBC with differential, LFTs, BUN, creatinine, electrolytes, glucose, urinalysis (every 6 to 12 months), and assessment of readiness for adherence with medication regimen. At initiation and with any change in treatment regimen: CBC with differential, electrolytes, calcium, phosphate, glucose, LFTs, bilirubin, urinalysis (at initiation), BUN, creatinine, albumin, total protein, lipid panel (at initiation), CD4, and viral load. After 1 to 2 weeks of therapy: Signs of medication toxicity and adherence. After 2 to 4 weeks of therapy: CBC with differential, viral load, signs of medication toxicity and adherence; then every 3 to 4 months: CBC with differential, electrolytes, glucose, LFTs, bilirubin, BUN, creatinine, CD4, viral load, signs of medication toxicity, and adherence. Lipid panel and urinalysis every 6 to 12 months. CD4 monitoring frequency may be decreased to every 6 to 12 months in children who are adherent to therapy if the value is well above the threshold for opportunistic infections, viral suppression is sustained, and the clinical status is stable for more than 2 to 3 years (HHS [pediatric] 2015). Monitor for growth and development, signs of HIV-specific physical conditions, HIV disease progression, opportunistic infections, hepatotoxicity, anemia, or lactic acidosis.

Dosage Forms Excipient information presented when available (limited, particularly for generics); consult specific product labeling.

Capsule, Oral:

Retrovir: 100 mg [contains soybean lecithin]

Generic: 100 mg

Solution, Intravenous [preservative free]:

Retrovir: 10 mg/mL (20 mL)

Syrup, Oral:

Retrovir: 50 mg/5 mL (240 mL) [contains sodium benzoate; strawberry flavor]

Generic: 50 mg/5 mL (240 mL)

Tablet, Oral:

Generic: 300 mg

◆ **Zidovudine, Abacavir, and Lamivudine** *see* Abacavir, Lamivudine, and Zidovudine *on page* *38*

◆ **Zidovudine and Lamivudine** *see* Lamivudine and Zidovudine *on page* *1209*

◆ **Zilactin [OTC]** *see* Benzyl Alcohol *on page* *273*

◆ **Zilactin-B® (Can)** *see* Benzocaine *on page* *268*

◆ **Zilactin Baby [OTC]** *see* Benzocaine *on page* *268*

◆ **Zilactin Baby® (Can)** *see* Benzocaine *on page* *268*

Zileuton (zye LOO ton)

Related Information

Oral Medications That Should Not Be Crushed or Altered *on page* *2476*

Brand Names: US Zyflo; Zyflo CR

Therapeutic Category 5-Lipoxygenase Inhibitor

Generic Availability (US) No

Use For prophylaxis and chronic treatment of asthma (FDA approved in ages ≥12 years and adults); **NOT** indicated for the relief of acute bronchospasm; therapy may continue during asthma exacerbations

Pregnancy Risk Factor C

Pregnancy Considerations Adverse events were observed in animal reproduction studies. If a leukotriene modifier is needed during pregnancy, other agents are preferred (ACOG, 2008).

Breast-Feeding Considerations It is not known if zileuton is excreted into breast milk. Due to the potential tumorigenicity of zileuton in animal studies, the manufacturer does not recommend breast-feeding.

Contraindications Hypersensitivity to zileuton or any component of the formulation; active liver disease or transaminase elevations ≥3 times ULN

Warnings/Precautions Not indicated for the reversal of bronchospasm in acute asthma attacks, including status asthmaticus; therapy may be continued during acute asthma exacerbations. Hepatic adverse effects have been reported (elevated transaminase levels); females >65 years and patients with pre-existing elevated transaminases may be at greater risk. Serum ALT should be monitored. Discontinue zileuton and follow transaminases until normal if patients develop clinical signs/symptoms of liver dysfunction or with transaminase levels >5 times ULN (use caution with history of liver disease and/or in those patients who consume substantial quantities of ethanol). Due to the risk of hepatotoxicity, the manufacturer does not recommend use of zileuton in children <12 years of age. Postmarketing reports of behavioral changes and sleep disorders have been noted. CNS effects may be potentiated when used with other sedative drugs or ethanol.

Adverse Reactions

Cardiovascular: Chest pain

Central nervous system: Dizziness, fever, headache, insomnia, malaise, nervousness, pain, somnolence

Dermatologic: Pruritus, rash

Gastrointestinal: Abdominal pain, constipation, diarrhea, dyspepsia, flatulence, nausea, vomiting

Genitourinary: Urinary tract infection, vaginitis

Hematologic: Leukopenia

Hepatic: ALT increased, hepatotoxicity

Neuromuscular & skeletal: Arthralgia, hypertonia, myalgia, neck pain/rigidity

Ocular: Conjunctivitis

Respiratory: Pharyngolaryngeal pain, sinusitis, upper respiratory tract infection

Miscellaneous: Hypersensitivity reactions, lymphadenopathy

Rare but important or life-threatening: Behavior/mood changes, hepatitis, hyperbilirubinemia, jaundice, liver failure, suicidality, suicide

Drug Interactions

Metabolism/Transport Effects **Substrate** of CYP1A2 (minor), CYP2C9 (minor), CYP3A4 (minor); **Note:** Assignment of Major/Minor substrate status based on clinically relevant drug interaction potential; **Inhibits** CYP1A2 (weak)

Avoid Concomitant Use

Avoid concomitant use of Zileuton with any of the following: Loxapine; Pimozide

Increased Effect/Toxicity

Zileuton may increase the levels/effects of: Loxapine; Pimozide; Propranolol; Theophylline; TiZANidine; Warfarin

Decreased Effect There are no known significant interactions involving a decrease in effect.

Food Interactions Zyflo CR®: Improved absorption when administered with food. Management: Administer with food.

Storage/Stability Store tablets at 20°C to 25°C (68°F to 77°F). Protect from light.

Mechanism of Action Specific 5-lipoxygenase inhibitor which inhibits leukotriene formation. Leukotrienes augment neutrophil and eosinophil migration, neutrophil and monocyte aggregation, leukocyte adhesion, increased capillary permeability, and smooth muscle contraction (which contribute to inflammation, edema, mucous secretion, and bronchoconstriction in the airway of the asthmatic.)

Pharmacokinetics (Adult data unless noted)

Absorption: Well-absorbed

Distribution: 1.2 L/kg

Protein binding: 93%, primarily albumin

Metabolism: Hepatic and gastrointestinal; zileuton and N-dehydroxylated metabolite can be metabolized by CYP1A2, 2C9, and 3A4

Half-life, elimination: ~3 hours

Time to peak serum concentration: Immediate release: 1.7 hours

Elimination: Urine (~95% primarily as metabolites); feces (~2%)

Dialysis: <0.5% removed by hemodialysis

Dosing: Usual Oral: Children, Adolescents ≥12 years, and Adults:

Immediate release: 600 mg 4 times/day

Extended release: 1200 mg twice daily

Dosing adjustment in renal impairment: No dosage adjustment necessary in renal impairment or with hemodialysis.

Dosing adjustment in hepatic impairment: Contraindicated with hepatic impairment.

Administration Extended release: Do not crush, cut, or chew tablet; administer within 1 hour after morning and evening meals.

Monitoring Parameters Hepatic transaminases (prior to initiation and during therapy), specifically monitor serum ALT (prior to initiation, once a month for the first 3 months, every 2-3 months for the remainder of the first year, and periodically thereafter for patients receiving long-term therapy). Monitor vital signs and lung sounds prior to and periodically during therapy.

Dosage Forms Excipient information presented when available (limited, particularly for generics); consult specific product labeling.

Tablet, Oral:

Zyflo: 600 mg [scored]

Tablet Extended Release 12 Hour, Oral:

Zyflo CR: 600 mg

- ◆ **Zinacef** *see* Cefuroxime *on page 414*
- ◆ **Zinacef in Sterile Water** *see* Cefuroxime *on page 414*
- ◆ **Zinc** *see* Trace Elements *on page 2097*
- ◆ **Zinc 15 [OTC]** *see* Zinc Sulfate *on page 2214*
- ◆ **Zinc-220 [OTC]** *see* Zinc Sulfate *on page 2214*

Zinc Acetate (zink AS e tate)

Related Information

Oral Medications That Should Not Be Crushed or Altered *on page 2476*

Brand Names: US Galzin

Therapeutic Category Trace Element

Generic Availability (US) No

Use Maintenance treatment of Wilson's disease following initial chelation therapy (FDA approved in ages ≥10 years and adults)

Pregnancy Risk Factor A

Pregnancy Considerations The risk of fetal harm appears remote with use of zinc acetate during pregnancy. An increased risk of fetal abnormalities has not been observed in pregnant women receiving zinc acetate (regardless of trimester).

Breast-Feeding Considerations Women receiving zinc therapy should avoid nursing due to risks for zinc-induced copper deficiency in nursing infants.

Contraindications Hypersensitivity to zinc salts or any component of the formulation.

Warnings/Precautions Not recommended for initial treatment of Wilson's disease in symptomatic patients. May be used as maintenance therapy after patient has been stabilized on initial chelation therapy. Neurological deterioration may occur with initial therapy as copper stores are mobilized. Hepatic copper levels should not be used to manage therapy as they do not differentiate between potentially toxic free copper and safely bound copper. Gastric irritation/upset may occur particularly with morning dose. Use in hepatic and/or renal impairment has not been studied.

Adverse Reactions

Central nervous system: Neurologic deterioration (uncommon)

Endocrine & metabolic: Amylase increased, lipase increased

Gastrointestinal: Gastric irritation
Hepatic: Alkaline phosphatase increased, hepatic function decreased (rare)

Drug Interactions

Metabolism/Transport Effects None known.

Avoid Concomitant Use There are no known interactions where it is recommended to avoid concomitant use.

Increased Effect/Toxicity There are no known significant interactions involving an increase in effect.

Decreased Effect

Zinc Acetate may decrease the levels/effects of: Ceftibuten; Cephalexin; Deferiprone; Dolutegravir; Eltrombopag; Quinolone Antibiotics; Tetracycline Derivatives; Trientine

The levels/effects of Zinc Acetate may be decreased by: Trientine

Food Interactions Food and beverages other than water may interfere with zinc absorption. Management: Administer on empty stomach at least 1 hour before or 2-3 hours after meals and 1 hour away from beverages other than water. Can give 1 hour after breakfast if GI irritation occurs.

Storage/Stability Store at 25°C (77°F); excursions permitted to 15°C to 30°C (59°F to 86°F). Protect from light.

Mechanism of Action Zinc induces production of the copper binding protein metallothionein in enterocytes. Copper binding within enterocytes results in an impairment of the intestinal absorption of dietary copper and reabsorption of endogenously secreted copper in saliva, bile, gastric acid. Following enterocyte desquamation, bound copper is eliminated in the feces.

Pharmacodynamics

Onset of action: Slow
Duration of action: Inhibition of copper uptake: ~11 days following cessation of therapy (Anderson, 1998)

Pharmacokinetics (Adult data unless noted)

Absorption: pH dependent (enhanced at pH ≤3); impaired by food (Anderson, 1998)
Elimination: Primarily in feces

Dosing: Usual Note: Dose expressed in mg **elemental** zinc

Children and Adolescents: **Wilson's disease:** Oral:

Manufacturer labeling: Children ≥10 years and Adolescents: 25 mg 3 times daily; may increase to 50 mg 3 times daily if inadequate response to lower dose

AASLD recommendations (Roberts, 2008): **Note:** Three times daily dosing recommended; doses must be administered at least twice daily to be effective:

Children >5 years and <50 kg: Limited data available: 25 mg 3 times daily

Children >50 kg and Adolescents: 50 mg 3 times daily

Adults: **Wilson's disease:** Oral:

Males and nonpregnant females: 50 mg 3 times daily

Pregnant females: 25 mg 3 times daily; may increase to 50 mg 3 times daily if inadequate response to lower dose

Administration Administer on empty stomach at least 1 hour before or 2-3 hours after meals, and 1 hour away from beverages other than water. Gastric irritation most commonly associated with morning dose; may administer 1 hour after breakfast if gastric irritation occurs. Swallow capsule whole; do not chew or open.

Monitoring Parameters Serum non-ceruloplasmin bound copper, 24-hour urinary copper excretion, 24-hour urinary zinc levels, LFTs, iron and/or other trace minerals, neurologic evaluation including speech, periodic ophthalmic exam

Reference Range Target ranges for patients with Wilson's disease on zinc acetate therapy:

24-hour urinary copper excretion: ≤75 mcg/24 hours (patients on chelation therapy will have increased urinary copper due to chelated copper)

Non-ceruloplasmin plasma copper (free copper): <20 mcg/dL

Dosage Forms Considerations

Strength of Galzin capsule is expressed as elemental zinc

Dosage Forms Excipient information presented when available (limited, particularly for generics); consult specific product labeling.

Capsule, Oral:

Galzin: 25 mg, 50 mg

◆ **Zincate [DSC]** *see* Zinc Sulfate *on page* 2214

Zinc Chloride (zink KLOR ide)

Therapeutic Category Trace Element

Generic Availability (US) Yes

Use Prevention of zinc deficiency as an additive to parenteral nutrition (FDA approved in all ages)

Pregnancy Risk Factor C

Pregnancy Considerations Zinc crosses the placenta and can be measured in the cord blood and placenta. Fetal concentrations are regulated by the placenta (de Moraes, 2011).

Breast-Feeding Considerations Zinc is found in breast milk; concentrations decrease over the first 6 months of lactation. Concentrations are generally not affected by dietary supplementation (IOM, 2000)

Warnings/Precautions Use with caution in patients with renal impairment. IV administration of zinc without copper may cause a decrease in copper serum concentrations. The parenteral product may contain aluminum; toxic aluminum concentrations may be seen with high doses, prolonged use, or renal dysfunction. Premature neonates are at higher risk due to immature renal function and aluminum intake from other parenteral sources. Parenteral aluminum exposure of >4 to 5 mcg/kg/day is associated with CNS and bone toxicity; tissue loading may occur at lower doses (Federal Register, 2002). See manufacturer's labeling.

Adverse Reactions Rare but important or life-threatening: Hypotension, indigestion, jaundice, leukopenia, nausea, neutropenia, pulmonary edema, vomiting

Drug Interactions

Metabolism/Transport Effects None known.

Avoid Concomitant Use There are no known interactions where it is recommended to avoid concomitant use.

Increased Effect/Toxicity There are no known significant interactions involving an increase in effect.

Decreased Effect

Zinc Chloride may decrease the levels/effects of: Dolutegravir; Eltrombopag; Trientine

The levels/effects of Zinc Chloride may be decreased by: Trientine

Storage/Stability Store intact vial at 20°C to 25°C (68°F to 77°F).

Pharmacokinetics (Adult data unless noted)

Distribution: Storage sites are liver and skeletal muscle; serum levels do not adequately reflect whole-body zinc status

Protein binding: 55% bound to albumin; 40% bound to alpha 1-macroglobulin

Elimination: Primarily in feces (Anderson, 1998)

Dosing: Neonatal Parenteral nutrition, maintenance requirement: IV: **Note:** Dosage expressed in terms of **elemental** zinc:

ASPEN recommendations:

Premature neonates <3 kg: 400 mcg/kg/day (Mirtallo, 2004); higher doses have been suggested in premature neonates: 450-500 mcg/kg/day (Vanek, 2012)

Term neonates ≥3 kg: 50-250 mcg/kg/day (Mirtallo, 2004; Vanek, 2012)

Manufacturer's labeling:
Premature neonates <3 kg: 300 mcg/kg/day
Term neonates ≥3 kg: 100 mcg/kg/day

Dosing: Usual Note: Dosages may be presented in units of mcg or mg, use caution to ensure correct units. Clinical response may not occur for up to 6-8 weeks:

Infants, Children, and Adolescents: **Parenteral nutrition, maintenance requirement:** IV: **Note:** Dosage expressed in terms of **elemental** zinc; higher doses may be needed if impaired intestinal absorption or an excessive loss of zinc (eg, excessive, prolonged diarrhea, high-output intestinal fistula, burns)

ASPEN recommendations:
Age-directed dosing (Vanek, 2012):
Infants <3 months: 250 mcg/kg/day
Infants ≥3 months: 50 mcg/kg/day
Children: 50 mcg/kg/day; maximum daily dose: 5000 mcg/**day**
Weight-directed dosing (Mirtallo, 2004):
Infants <10 kg: 50-250 mcg/kg/day
Children 10-40 kg: 50-125 mcg/kg/day; maximum daily dose: 5000 mcg/**day**
Adolescents >40 kg: 2-5 mg/day
Manufacturer labeling: Infants >3 kg and Children ≤5 years: 100 mcg/kg/day

Adults: **Parenteral nutrition, maintenance requirement:** IV: **Note:** Dosage expressed in terms of **elemental** zinc:
Acute metabolic states: 4.5-6 mg/day
Metabolically stable: 2.5-4 mg/day
Replacement for small bowel fluid loss (metabolically stable): An additional 12.2 mg zinc/L of fluid lost or an additional 17.1 mg zinc per kg of stool or ileostomy output

Preparation for Administration IV: Must dilute in at least 100 mL prior to administration; usually diluted in parenteral nutrition or maintenance fluids

Administration IV: Dilute as component of daily parenteral nutrition or maintenance fluids; do not give undiluted by direct injection into a peripheral vein due to potential for phlebitis and tissue irritation and potential to increase renal losses of minerals from a bolus injection

Monitoring Parameters Patients on parenteral nutrition should have periodic serum copper and serum zinc levels; alkaline phosphatase, taste acuity, mental depression

Dosage Forms Considerations Strength of zinc chloride injection is expressed as elemental zinc

Dosage Forms Excipient information presented when available (limited, particularly for generics); consult specific product labeling.
Solution, Intravenous:
Generic: 1 mg/mL (10 mL)

◆ **Zincofax® (Can)** *see* Zinc Oxide *on page* 2214

Zinc Oxide (zink OKS ide)

Brand Names: US Ammens® Original Medicated [OTC]; Ammens® Shower Fresh [OTC]; Balmex® [OTC]; Boudreaux's® Butt Paste [OTC]; Critic-Aid Skin Care® [OTC]; Desitin® Creamy [OTC]; Desitin® [OTC]; Dr. Smith's Diaper Rash [OTC]; Elta Seal Moisture Barrier [OTC]; Pharmabase Barrier [OTC]

Brand Names: Canada Zincofax®

Therapeutic Category Topical Skin Product

Generic Availability (US) Yes: Ointment

Use Protective coating for mild skin irritations and abrasions; soothing and protective ointment to promote healing of chapped skin, diaper rash

Pregnancy Considerations Zinc oxide is not expected to be absorbed systemically following topical administration to healthy skin (Newman, 2009). Systemic absorption would be required in order for zinc oxide to cross the placenta and reach the fetus.

Contraindications Hypersensitivity to zinc oxide or any component of the formulation

Adverse Reactions Local: Irritation, skin sensitivity

Drug Interactions

Metabolism/Transport Effects None known.

Avoid Concomitant Use There are no known interactions where it is recommended to avoid concomitant use.

Increased Effect/Toxicity There are no known significant interactions involving an increase in effect.

Decreased Effect There are no known significant interactions involving a decrease in effect.

Storage/Stability Avoid prolonged storage at temperatures >30°C.

Mechanism of Action Mild astringent with weak antiseptic properties

Dosing: Neonatal Topical: Apply several times daily to affected area

Dosing: Usual Infants, Children, and Adults: Topical: Apply several times daily to affected area

Administration Topical: For external use only; do not use in the eyes

Dosage Forms Excipient information presented when available (limited, particularly for generics); consult specific product labeling.
Cream, topical:
Balmex®: 11.3% (60 g, 120 g, 480 g) [contains aloe, benzoic acid, soybean oil, and vitamin E]
Elta Seal Moisture Barrier: 6% (114 g)
Cream, topical [stick]:
Balmex®: 11.3% (56 g) [contains aloe, benzoic acid, soybean oil, and vitamin E]
Ointment, topical: 20% (30 g, 60 g, 454 g); 40% (120 g)
Desitin®: 40% (30 g, 60 g, 90 g, 120 g, 270 g, 480 g) [contains cod liver oil and lanolin]
Desitin® Creamy: 10% (60 g, 120 g)
Dr. Smith's Diaper Rash: 10% (57 g, 85 g, 27 g)
Pharmabase Barrier: 9.38% (500 g)
Paste, topical:
Boudreaux's® Butt Paste: 16% (30 g, 60 g, 120 g, 480 g) [contains castor oil, boric acid, mineral oil, and Peruvian balsam]
Critic-Aid Skin Care®: 20% (71 g, 170 g)
Powder, topical:
Ammens® Original Medicated: 9.1% (312 g)
Ammens® Shower Fresh: 9.1% (312 g)

Zinc Sulfate (zink SUL fate)

Medication Safety Issues

Sound-alike/look-alike issues:
$ZnSO_4$ is an error-prone abbreviation (mistaken as morphine sulfate)

Brand Names: US Eye-Sed [OTC]; Orazinc [OTC]; Zinc 15 [OTC]; Zinc-220 [OTC]; Zincate [DSC]

Brand Names: Canada Anuzinc; Rivasol

Therapeutic Category Mineral, Oral; Mineral, Parenteral; Trace Element

Generic Availability (US) Yes

Use
Oral: Dietary supplementation of zinc (OTC: FDA approved in adults); has also been used to help reduce the duration and severity of diarrhea in malnourished patients
Parenteral: Prevention of zinc deficiency as an additive to parenteral nutrition (FDA approved in all ages)

Pregnancy Risk Factor C

Pregnancy Considerations Zinc crosses the placenta and can be measured in the cord blood and placenta. Fetal concentrations are regulated by the placenta (de Moraes, 2011).

Breast-Feeding Considerations Zinc is found in breast milk; concentrations decrease over the first 6 months of lactation. Concentrations are generally not affected by dietary supplementation (IOM, 2000).

Contraindications Injection: Do not administer undiluted into peripheral vein

Warnings/Precautions Use with caution in patients with renal impairment. IV administration of zinc without copper may cause a decrease in copper serum concentrations. The parenteral product may contain aluminum; toxic aluminum concentrations may be seen with high doses, prolonged use, or renal dysfunction. Premature neonates are at higher risk due to immature renal function and aluminum intake from other parenteral sources. Parenteral aluminum exposure of >4 to 5 mcg/kg/day is associated with CNS and bone toxicity; tissue loading may occur at lower doses (Federal Register, 2002). See manufacturer's labeling.

Adverse Reactions

Central nervous system: Dizziness, headache

Gastrointestinal: Abdominal cramps, diarrhea, nausea, vomiting

Drug Interactions

Metabolism/Transport Effects None known.

Avoid Concomitant Use There are no known interactions where it is recommended to avoid concomitant use.

Increased Effect/Toxicity There are no known significant interactions involving an increase in effect.

Decreased Effect

Zinc Sulfate may decrease the levels/effects of: Ceftibuten; Cephalexin; Deferiprone; Dolutegravir; Eltrombopag; Quinolone Antibiotics; Tetracycline Derivatives; Trientine

The levels/effects of Zinc Sulfate may be decreased by: Trientine

Food Interactions Avoid foods high in calcium or phosphorus.

Storage/Stability

Capsule: Store at 15°C to 30°C (59°F to 86°F).

Tablet (Orazinc®): Store at 13°C to 24°C (55°F to 76°F).

Injection: Prior to use, store at room temperature of 20°C to 25°C (68°F to 77°F); excursions permitted to 15°C to 30°C (59°F to 86°F).

Pharmacokinetics (Adult data unless noted)

Absorption: pH-dependent; enhanced at lower pH; (pH <3); impaired by food (Anderson, 1998)

Distribution: Storage sites are liver and skeletal muscle; serum levels do not adequately reflect whole-body zinc status

Protein binding: 55% bound to albumin; 40% bound to alpha 1-macroglobulin

Elimination: Primarily in feces (Anderson, 1998)

Dosing: Neonatal Note: Clinical response may not occur for up to 6-8 weeks.

Adequate intake (AI): Oral: 2 mg **elemental** zinc/day

Parenteral nutrition, maintenance requirement: IV: **Note:** Dosage expressed in terms of **elemental** zinc:

ASPEN recommendations:

Premature neonates <3 kg: 400 mcg/kg/day (Mirtallo, 2004); higher doses have been suggested in premature neonates: 450-500 mcg/kg/day (Vanek, 2012)

Term neonates ≥3 kg: 50-250 mcg/kg/day (Mirtallo, 2004; Vanek, 2012)

Manufacturer's labeling:

Premature neonates <3 kg: 300 mcg/kg/day

Term neonates ≥3 kg: 100 mcg/kg/day

Dosing: Usual Note: Dosages may be presented in units of mcg or mg; use caution to ensure correct units. Clinical response may not occur for up to 6-8 weeks:

Infants, Children, and Adolescents:

Adequate intake (AI): Oral: Infants 1-6 months: 2 mg **elemental** zinc/day

Recommended daily allowance (RDA): Oral:

Infants 7-12 months and Children 1-3 years: 3 mg **elemental** zinc/day

Children 4-8 years: 5 mg **elemental** zinc/day

Children and Adolescents 9-13 years: 8 mg **elemental** zinc/day

Adolescents 14-18 years:

Female: 9 mg **elemental** zinc/day

Male: 11 mg **elemental** zinc/day

Zinc deficiency, treatment: Oral:

Infants and Children: 0.5-1 mg **elemental** zinc/kg/day in divided doses 1-3 times daily; higher doses may be needed if impaired intestinal absorption or an excessive loss of zinc (eg, excessive, prolonged diarrhea, high-output intestinal fistula, burns)

Adolescents: 25-50 mg **elemental** zinc (110-220 mg zinc sulfate) 3 times daily; higher doses may be needed if impaired intestinal absorption or an excessive loss of zinc (eg, excessive, prolonged diarrhea, high-output intestinal fistula, burns)

Parenteral nutrition, maintenance requirement: IV: **Note:** Dosage expressed in terms of **elemental** zinc; higher doses may be needed if impaired intestinal absorption or an excessive loss of zinc (eg, excessive, prolonged diarrhea, high-output intestinal fistula, burns)

ASPEN recommendations:

Age-directed dosing (Vanek, 2012):

Infants <3 months: 250 mcg/kg/day

Infants ≥3 months: 50 mcg/kg/day

Children: 50 mcg/kg/day; maximum daily dose: 5000 mcg/**day**

Weight-directed dosing (Mirtallo, 2004):

Infants <10 kg: 50-250 mcg/kg/day

Children 10-40 kg: 50-125 mcg/kg/day; maximum daily dose: 5000 mcg/**day**

Adolescents >40 kg: 2-5 mg/day

Manufacturer labeling: Infants >3 kg and Children ≤5 years: 100 mcg/kg/day; maximum daily dose: 5000 mcg/**day**

Diarrhea, treatment; malnourished patient (WHO/UNICEF, 2004): Oral: **Note:** Dosage expressed in terms of **elemental** zinc; **Note:** Zinc should be started in conjunction with oral rehydration solutions at first sign of diarrhea:

Infants <6 months: 10 mg once daily for 10-14 days

Infants >6 months and Children: 20 mg once daily for 10-14 days

Adults:

Recommended daily allowance (RDA): Oral:

Female: 8 mg **elemental** zinc/day

Male: 11 mg **elemental** zinc/day

Zinc deficiency, treatment: Oral: 25-50 mg **elemental** zinc/dose (110-220 mg zinc sulfate) 3 times daily

Parenteral nutrition, maintenance requirement: IV: **Note:** Dosage expressed in terms of **elemental** zinc:

Acute metabolic states: 4.5-6 mg/day

Metabolically stable: 2.5-4 mg/day

Replacement for small bowel fluid loss (metabolically stable): An additional 12.2 mg zinc/L of fluid lost, or an additional 17.1 mg zinc per kg of stool or ileostomy output

Administration

Oral: Administer with food if GI upset occurs

Parenteral: Dilute as component of daily parenteral nutrition or maintenance fluids; do not give undiluted by direct injection into a peripheral vein due to potential for phlebitis and tissue irritation and potential to increase renal losses of minerals from a bolus injection

Monitoring Parameters Patients on parenteral nutrition or chronic therapy should have periodic serum copper and serum zinc levels; alkaline phosphatase, taste acuity, mental depression

Dosage Forms Considerations
Strength of zinc sulfate injection is expressed as elemental zinc
Oral zinc sulfate is approximately 23% elemental zinc

Dosage Forms Excipient information presented when available (limited, particularly for generics); consult specific product labeling. [DSC] = Discontinued product
Capsule, Oral:
Orazinc: 220 mg
Zinc-220: 220 mg
Zincate: 220 mg [DSC]
Generic: 220 mg
Solution, Intravenous:
Generic: 1 mg/mL (10 mL [DSC]); 5 mg/mL (5 mL)
Solution, Ophthalmic:
Eye-Sed: 0.217% (15 mL) [contains benzalkonium chloride, boric acid]
Tablet, Oral:
Orazinc: 110 mg
Zinc 15: 66 mg
Generic: 220 mg
Tablet, Oral [preservative free]:
Generic: 220 mg

◆ **Zinc Undecylenate** *see* Undecylenic Acid and Derivatives *on page 2135*
◆ **Zinda-Letrozole (Can)** *see* Letrozole *on page 1224*
◆ **Zinecard** *see* Dexrazoxane *on page 622*
◆ **Zingo** *see* Lidocaine (Topical) *on page 1258*

Ziprasidone (zi PRAS i done)

Medication Safety Issues
Sound-alike/look-alike issues:
Ziprasidone may be confused with TraZODone
BEERS Criteria medication:
This drug may be potentially inappropriate for use in geriatric patients (Quality of evidence - moderate; Strength of recommendation - strong).

Related Information
Oral Medications That Should Not Be Crushed or Altered *on page 2476*
Safe Handling of Hazardous Drugs *on page 2455*

Brand Names: US Geodon
Brand Names: Canada Zeldox
Therapeutic Category Second Generation (Atypical) Antipsychotic
Generic Availability (US) May be product dependent
Use Due to its greater capacity to prolong the QT interval, ziprasidone is generally not considered to be a first-line agent.
Oral: Treatment of schizophrenia (FDA approved in adults); treatment as monotherapy of acute manic or mixed episodes associated with bipolar disorder with or without psychosis (FDA approved in adults); maintenance adjunctive therapy (to lithium or valproate) for bipolar I disorder (FDA approved in adults). **Note:** In June 2009, an FDA advisory panel advised that ziprasidone is effective in patients 10-17 years of age for the treatment of mixed and manic episodes of bipolar disorder, but did not conclude that it was safe due to large number of subjects lost to follow-up and ambiguity within QTc prolongation data. Has also been used in children and adolescents for treatment of Tourette's syndrome, tic disorders, irritability associated with autism, and pervasive development disorders not otherwise specified (PDD-NOS).
Injection: Acute agitation in patients with schizophrenia (FDA approved in adults)

Pregnancy Risk Factor C

Pregnancy Considerations Adverse events were observed in animal reproduction studies. Antipsychotic use during the third trimester of pregnancy has a risk for abnormal muscle movements (extrapyramidal symptoms [EPS]) and/or withdrawal symptoms in newborns following delivery. Symptoms in the newborn may include agitation, feeding disorder, hypertonia, hypotonia, respiratory distress, somnolence, and tremor; these effects may be self-limiting or require hospitalization. Ziprasidone may cause hyperprolactinemia, which may decrease reproductive function in both males and females.

The ACOG recommends that therapy during pregnancy be individualized; treatment with psychiatric medications during pregnancy should incorporate the clinical expertise of the mental health clinician, obstetrician, primary healthcare provider, and pediatrician. Safety data related to atypical antipsychotics during pregnancy is limited and routine use is not recommended. However, if a woman is inadvertently exposed to an atypical antipsychotic while pregnant, continuing therapy may be preferable to switching to a typical antipsychotic that the fetus has not yet been exposed to; consider risk:benefit (ACOG, 2008).

Healthcare providers are encouraged to enroll women 18-45 years of age exposed to ziprasidone during pregnancy in the Atypical Antipsychotics Pregnancy Registry (1-866-961-2388 or http://www.womensmentalhealth.org/pregnancyregistry).

Breast-Feeding Considerations It is not known if ziprasidone is excreted into breast milk. Breast-feeding is not recommended by the manufacturer.

Contraindications Hypersensitivity to ziprasidone or any component of the formulation; history of (or current) prolonged QT; congenital long QT syndrome; recent myocardial infarction; uncompensated heart failure; concurrent use of other QTc-prolonging agents including arsenic trioxide, chlorpromazine, class Ia antiarrhythmics (eg, disopyramide, quinidine, procainamide), class III antiarrhythmics (eg, amiodarone, dofetilide, ibutilide, sotalol), dolasetron, droperidol, gatifloxacin, halofantrine, levomethadyl, mefloquine, mesoridazine, moxifloxacin, pentamidine, pimozide, probucol, sparfloxacin, tacrolimus, and thioridazine

Warnings/Precautions Hazardous agent - use appropriate precautions for handling and disposal (NIOSH 2014 [group 3]). **[US Boxed Warning]: Elderly patients with dementia-related behavioral disorders treated with antipsychotics are at an increased risk of death compared to placebo.** Most deaths appeared to be either cardiovascular (eg, heart failure, sudden death) or infectious (eg, pneumonia) in nature. Use with caution in dementia with Lewy bodies; antipsychotics may worsen dementia symptoms and patients with dementia with Lewy bodies are more sensitive to the extrapyramidal side effects (APA [Rabins, 2007]). Ziprasidone is not approved for the treatment of dementia-related psychosis.

May result in QTc prolongation (dose related), which has been associated with the development of malignant ventricular arrhythmias (torsade de pointes) and sudden death. Note contraindications related to this effect. Observed prolongation was greater than with other atypical antipsychotic agents (risperidone, olanzapine, quetiapine), but less than with thioridazine. Correct electrolyte disturbances, especially hypokalemia or hypomagnesemia, prior to use and throughout therapy. Use caution in patients with bradycardia. Discontinue in patients found to have persistent QTc intervals >500 msec. Patients with symptoms of dizziness, palpitations, or syncope should receive further cardiac evaluation. May cause orthostatic hypotension. Use is contraindicated in patients with recent acute myocardial infarction (MI), QT prolongation, or uncompensated heart failure. Avoid use in patients with a history of cardiac arrhythmias; use with caution in patients with history of MI or unstable heart disease. Dyslipidemia has been reported with atypical antipsychotics; risk profile may differ between agents.

Leukopenia, neutropenia, and agranulocytosis (sometimes fatal) have been reported in clinical trials and postmarketing reports with antipsychotic use; presence of risk factors (eg, preexisting low WBC or history of drug-induced leuko-/neutropenia) should prompt periodic blood count assessment. Discontinue therapy at first signs of blood dyscrasias or if absolute neutrophil count <1000/mm^3. Potentially serious, sometimes fatal drug reaction with eosinophilia and systemic symptoms (DRESS), also known as multiorgan hypersensitivity reactions, have also been reported with ziprasidone. Monitor for signs and symptoms of possible disparate manifestations associated with lymphatic, hepatic, renal, cardiovascular, and/or hematologic organ systems; discontinuation and conversion to alternate therapy may be required.

May cause extrapyramidal symptoms (EPS). Risk of dystonia (and probably other EPS) may be greater with increased doses, use of conventional antipsychotics, males, and younger patients. Impaired core body temperature regulation may occur; caution with strenuous exercise, heat exposure, dehydration, and concomitant medication possessing anticholinergic effects; not reported in premarketing trials of ziprasidone. Antipsychotic use may also be associated with neuroleptic malignant syndrome (NMS). Use with caution in patients at risk of seizures.

Atypical antipsychotics have been associated with development of hyperglycemia. There is limited documentation with ziprasidone and specific risk associated with this agent is not known. Use caution in patients with diabetes or other disorders of glucose regulation; monitor for worsening of glucose control. May increase prolactin levels; clinical significance of hyperprolactinemia in patients with breast cancer or other prolactin-dependent tumors is unknown.

Use in elderly patients with dementia is associated with an increased risk of mortality and cerebrovascular accidents; avoid antipsychotic use for behavioral problems associated with dementia unless alternative nonpharmacologic therapies have failed and patient may harm self or others. In addition, use may cause or exacerbate syndrome of inappropriate antidiuretic hormone secretion or hyponatremia; monitor sodium closely with initiation or dosage adjustments in older adults (Beers Criteria).

Cognitive and/or motor impairment (sedation) is common with ziprasidone. CNS effects may be potentiated when used with other sedative drugs or ethanol. Use with caution in disorders where CNS depression is a feature. Use with caution in Parkinson disease; antipsychotics may aggravate the motor disturbances of Parkinson disease (APA [Rabins, 2007]). Antipsychotic use has been associated with esophageal dysmotility and aspiration; use with caution in patients at risk of pneumonia (ie, Alzheimer's disease). Use caution in hepatic impairment. Ziprasidone has been associated with a fairly high incidence of rash (5%). Significant weight gain has been observed with antipsychotic therapy; incidence varies with product. Monitor waist circumference and BMI. Rare cases of priapism have been reported. Use the intramuscular formulation with caution in patients with renal impairment; formulation contains cyclodextrin, an excipient which may accumulate in renal insufficiency, although the clinical significance of this finding is uncertain (Luke, 2010).

The possibility of a suicide attempt is inherent in psychotic illness or bipolar disorder; use caution in high-risk patients during initiation of therapy. Prescriptions should be written for the smallest quantity consistent with good patient care.

Warnings: Additional Pediatric Considerations

Observed QTc prolongation with ziprasidone was greater than with other atypical antipsychotic agents (eg, risperidone, olanzapine, quetiapine), but less than with thioridazine. A prospective study followed 20 children (mean age: 13.2 years) for an average of 4.6 months and reported significant QTc prolongation at relatively low ziprasidone doses (mean daily dose: 30 mg ± 13 mg/day); the authors suggest the effect is not dose dependent in children unlike adults and recommend reserving ziprasidone use as second- or third-line for patients at risk for QTc prolongation or when using doses >40 mg/day (Blair, 2005). Use with caution during diarrheal illnesses; monitor electrolytes closely, particularly K and Mg (Blair, 2004). May cause hyperprolactinemia; use with caution in children and adolescents; adverse effects due to increased prolactin concentrations have been observed; long-term effects on growth or sexual maturation have not been evaluated.

Pediatric psychiatric disorders are frequently serious mental disorders which present with variable symptoms that do not always match adult diagnostic criteria. Conduct a thorough diagnostic evaluation and carefully consider risks of psychotropic medication before initiation in pediatric patients. Medication therapy for pediatric patients with bipolar disorder is indicated as part of a total treatment program that frequently includes educational, psychological, and social interventions.

Adverse Reactions

Cardiovascular: Bradycardia, chest pain, facial edema, hypertension, orthostatic hypotension, tachycardia, vasodilatation

Central nervous system: Agitation, akathisia, akinesia, amnesia, anxiety, ataxia, chills, confusion, delirium, dizziness, drowsiness, dystonia, extrapyramidal symptoms, fever, headache, hostility, hypothermia, insomnia, oculogyric crisis, personality disorder, psychosis, speech disturbance, vertigo

Dermatologic: Fungal dermatitis, photosensitivity reaction, skin rash

Endocrine & metabolic: Dysmenorrhea

Gastrointestinal: Abdominal pain, anorexia, buccoglossal syndrome, constipation, diarrhea, dyspepsia, dysphagia, nausea, rectal hemorrhage, sialorrhea, tongue edema, vomiting, weight gain, xerostomia

Genitourinary: Priapism

Local: Pain at injection site

Neuromuscular & skeletal: Abnormal gait, back pain, choreoathetosis, cogwheel rigidity, dysarthria, dyskinesia, hyperkinesia, hypertonia, hypoesthesia, hypokinesia, hypotonia, myalgia, neuropathy, paresthesia, tremor, twitching, weakness

Ophthalmic: Diplopia, visual disturbance

Respiratory: Cough, dyspnea, infection, pharyngitis, rhinitis

Miscellaneous: Diaphoresis, flank pain, flu-like syndrome, furunculosis, withdrawal syndrome

Rare but important or life-threatening: Abnormal ejaculation, albuminuria, alkaline phosphatase increased, alopecia, amenorrhea, anemia, angina pectoris, angioedema, atrial fibrillation, basophilia, blepharitis, bruising, bundle branch block, cardiomegaly, cataract, cerebrovascular accident, cholestatic jaundice, circumoral paresthesia, conjunctivitis, contact dermatitis, creatinine (serum) increased, depression, DRESS syndrome, dry eyes, eczema, eosinophilia, epistaxis, exfoliative dermatitis, facial droop, fecal impaction, first degree atrioventricular, galactorrhea, gingival bleeding, gynecomastia, hematemesis, hematuria, hemoptysis, hepatitis, hepatomegaly, hyperchloremia, hypercholesterolemia, hyperglycemia, hyperkalemia, hypermenorrea, hyperreflexia, hypersensitivity reaction, hyperthyroidism, hyperuricemia, hypocalcemia, hypochloremia, hypocholesterolemia, hypoglycemia, hypokalemia, hypomagnesemia, hypomania, hyponatremia, hypoproteinemia, hypothyroidism, impotence, increased blood urea nitrogen, increased creatine phosphokinase, increased gamma-glutamyl transferase, increased monocytes, jaundice, keratitis, keratoconjunctivitis, ketosis, lactation (female), laryngismus, LDH increased, leukocytosis, leukopenia, leukoplakia (mouth), liver steatosis, lymphadenopathy, lymphedema, lymphocytosis, maculopapular rash, mania, melena, myocarditis, myoclonus, myopathy, neuroleptic malignant syndrome, nocturia, nystagmus, ocular hemorrhage, oliguria, paralysis, peripheral edema, phlebitis, photophobia, pneumonia, polycythemia, polyuria, prolonged Q-T interval on ECG (>500 msec), pulmonary embolism, respiratory alkalosis, seizure, serotonin syndrome, sexual dysfunction (male and female), syncope, tardive dyskinesia, tenosynovitis, thirst, thrombocythemia, thrombocytopenia, thrombophlebitis, thyroiditis, tinnitus, torsade de pointes, torticollis, transaminases increased, trismus, urinary incontinence, urinary retention, urticaria, uterine hemorrhage, vaginal hemorrhage, vesiculobullous dermatitis, visual field defect

Drug Interactions

Metabolism/Transport Effects Substrate of CYP1A2 (minor), CYP3A4 (minor); **Note:** Assignment of Major/Minor substrate status based on clinically relevant drug interaction potential; **Inhibits** CYP2D6 (weak)

Avoid Concomitant Use

Avoid concomitant use of Ziprasidone with any of the following: Amisulpride; Azelastine (Nasal); FLUoxetine; Highest Risk QTc-Prolonging Agents; Ivabradine; Metoclopramide; Mifepristone; Moderate Risk QTc-Prolonging Agents; Orphenadrine; Paraldehyde; Sulpiride; Thalidomide

Increased Effect/Toxicity

Ziprasidone may increase the levels/effects of: Alcohol (Ethyl); Amisulpride; Azelastine (Nasal); Buprenorphine; CNS Depressants; FLUoxetine; Highest Risk QTc-Prolonging Agents; Hydrocodone; Methotrimeprazine; Methylphenidate; Metyrosine; Orphenadrine; Paraldehyde; Selective Serotonin Reuptake Inhibitors; Serotonin Modulators; Sulpiride; Suvorexant; Thalidomide; Zolpidem

The levels/effects of Ziprasidone may be increased by: Acetylcholinesterase Inhibitors (Central); Brimonidine (Topical); Cannabis; Doxylamine; Dronabinol; FLUoxetine; Ivabradine; Kava Kava; Magnesium Sulfate; Methotrimeprazine; Methylphenidate; Metoclopramide; Metyrosine; Mifepristone; Moderate Risk QTc-Prolonging Agents; Nabilone; Perampanel; QTc-Prolonging Agents (Indeterminate Risk and Risk Modifying); Rufinamide; Serotonin Modulators; Sodium Oxybate; Tapentadol; Tetrahydrocannabinol

Decreased Effect

Ziprasidone may decrease the levels/effects of: Amphetamines; Antidiabetic Agents; Anti-Parkinson's Agents (Dopamine Agonist); Quinagolide

The levels/effects of Ziprasidone may be decreased by: CarBAMazepine

Food Interactions Administration with a meal containing at least 500 calories increases serum levels ~80%. Management: Administer with a meal containing at least 500 calories (Lincoln, 2010).

Storage/Stability

Capsule: Store at 25°C (77°F); excursion permitted to 15°C to 30°C (59°F to 86°F).

Vials for injection: Store at 25°C (77°F); excursion permitted to 15°C to 30°C (59°F to 86°F). Protect from light. Following reconstitution, injection may be stored at room temperature up to 24 hours or under refrigeration for up to 7 days. Protect from light.

Mechanism of Action Ziprasidone is a benzylisothiazolylpiperazine antipsychotic. The exact mechanism of action is unknown. However, *in vitro* radioligand studies show that ziprasidone has high affinity for D_2, D_3, 5-HT_{2A}, 5-HT_{1A}, 5-HT_{2C}, 5-HT_{1D}, and alpha$_1$-adrenergic; moderate affinity for histamine H_1 receptors; and no appreciable affinity for alpha$_2$-adrenergic receptors, beta-adrenergic, 5-HT_3, 5-HT_4, cholinergic, mu, sigma, or benzodiazepine receptors. Ziprasidone functions as an antagonist at the D_2, 5-HT_{2A}, and 5-HT_{1D} receptors and as an agonist at the 5-HT_{1A} receptor. Ziprasidone moderately inhibits the reuptake of serotonin and norepinephrine.

Pharmacokinetics (Adult data unless noted)

Absorption: Well absorbed; presence of food increases by up to twofold

Distribution: Apparent V_d: 1.5 L/kg

Protein binding: 99%, primarily to albumin and alpha$_1$-acid glycoprotein

Metabolism: Extensively hepatic, primarily chemical and enzymatic reductions via glutathione and aldehyde oxidase, respectively; less than 1/3 of total metabolism via CYP3A4 and CYP1A2 (minor)

Bioavailability: IM: 100%, Oral: ~60% under fed conditions

Half-life:
- IM: 2-5 hours
- Oral:
  - Children: Mean: 3.3-4.1 hours (Sallee, 2006)
  - Adult: 7 hours

Time to peak serum concentration:
- IM: ≤60 minutes
- Oral:
  - Children: Mean: 5-5.5 hours (Sallee, 2006)
  - Adult: 6-8 hours

Elimination: Feces (66%) and urine (20%) as metabolites; little as unchanged drug (<1% urine, <4% feces)
- Clearance:
  - Children: Mean: 11.5-13.1 mL/minute/kg (Sallee, 2006)
  - Adult: Mean: 7.5 mL/minute/kg
- Dialysis: Not removed by hemodialysis

Dosing: Usual

Children and Adolescents:

Acute agitation (schizophrenia): Limited data available (Barzman, 2007; Khan, 2006; Staller, 2004): IM:
- Children 5-11 years: 10 mg
- Adolescents ≥12 years: 10-20 mg; **Note:** One study (n=59; age range: 5-19 years) reported that 69% of 20 mg doses surpassed the desired calming therapeutic effect and caused varying degrees of sedation (4% of patients were unable to be aroused) (Barzman, 2007)

Autism and PDD-NOS irritability: Limited data available: Oral: Children ≥8 years and Adolescents: Reported final dose range: 20-160 mg/day divided twice daily

A prospective, open-labeled study of 12 patients (12-18 years) used the following individually titrated doses (Malone, 2007)
- Patient weight ≤35 kg: Initial: 20 mg every other day given at bedtime for 2 doses; then increase dose in weekly increments based on clinical response and tolerability: Week 1: 10 mg twice daily (20 mg/day) Week 2: 20 mg twice daily (40 mg/day); Week 3 40 mg twice daily (80 mg/day); Week 4: 80 mg twice daily (160 mg/day)
- Patient weight >35 kg: Initial: 20 mg/day at bedtime for 3 doses; then increase dose in weekly increments based on clinical response and tolerability: Week 1: 20 mg twice daily (40 mg/day); Week 2: 40 mg twice daily (80 mg/day); Week 4: 80 mg twice daily (160 mg/day)

A case series of 12 patients (8-20 years) initiated therapy at 20 mg/day given at bedtime and then increased by 10-20 mg/week divided twice daily based on clinical response and tolerability; final ziprasidone dosage ranged between 20-120 mg/day (mean: ~60 mg/day) divided twice daily (McDougle, 2002)

Bipolar I disorder: Oral: Children and Adolescents 10-17 years: **Note:** In June 2009, an FDA advisory panel advised that ziprasidone is effective in patients 10-17 years of age for the treatment of mixed and manic episodes of bipolar disorder, but did not conclude that it was safe due to large number of subjects lost to follow-up and ambiguity within QTc prolongation data; limited data available (DelBello, 2008; DelBello, 2008a; Elbe, 2008; Findling, 2008; Mechcatie, 2009)

Initial dose: 20 mg/day; titrate dose upwards as tolerated, using twice daily dosing over a 2-week period to the weight-based target range: 60-80 mg/day (≤45 kg) divided into twice daily doses or 120-160 mg/day (>45 kg) divided into twice daily doses.

Alternate dosing: An open-label, 8-week study of 21 patients [6-17 years (mean: 10.3 years)] with bipolar disorder and comorbid conditions (eg, ADHD, depression, conduct disorder) used the following weight-based dosing regimen (Biederman, 2007):

Initial dose: 1 mg/kg/day divided twice daily; increase to 1.5 mg/kg/day divided twice daily by Week 2 and increase to 2 mg/kg/day divided twice daily by Week 3 if tolerated; maximum dose: 160 mg/day; **Note:** Only 14 of the 21 patients completed the study; five dropped out due to lack of efficacy; two dropped out due to adverse reactions; patients experienced a high incidence of sedation (46%) and headaches (38%).

Tourette's syndrome, tic disorder: Limited data available: Oral: Children and Adolescents 7-16 years: Initial dose: 5 mg/day for 3 days then using twice daily dosing, titrate dose as tolerated up to 40 mg/day divided twice daily. Dosing is based on a double-blind, placebo-controlled pilot study (n=28), mean daily dose at the end of trial: 28.2 + 9.6 mg/day (Sallee, 2000).

Adults:

Acute agitation (schizophrenia): IM: 10 mg every 2 hours **or** 20 mg every 4 hours; maximum: 40 mg/day; oral therapy should replace IM administration as soon as possible. Use >3 days has not been studied.

Bipolar mania: Oral: Initial: 40 mg twice daily; adjustment: May increase to 60 or 80 mg twice daily on second day of treatment; average dose 40-80 mg twice daily

Schizophrenia: Oral: Initial: 20 mg twice daily; adjustment: Increases (if indicated) should be made no more frequently than every 2 days; ordinarily patients should be observed for improvement over several weeks before adjusting the dose. Maintenance: Range: 20-100 mg twice daily; however, dosages >80 mg twice daily are generally not recommended

Dosing adjustment in renal impairment: Adults:

Oral: No dosage adjustment is recommended

IM: Cyclodextrin, an excipient in the IM formulation, is cleared by renal filtration; use with caution

Ziprasidone is not removed by hemodialysis.

Dosing adjustment in hepatic impairment: No dosage adjustment is recommended; however, drug undergoes extensive hepatic metabolism and systemic exposure may be increased. Use with caution.

Preparation for Administration Hazardous agent; use appropriate precautions for handling and disposal (NIOSH 2014 [group 3]).

Parenteral: IM: Reconstitute with 1.2 mL SWFI. Shake vigorously; forms a pale, pink solution containing 20 mg/mL ziprasidone.

Administration Hazardous agent; use appropriate precautions for handling and disposal (NIOSH 2014 [group 3]).

Oral: Administer with food.

Parenteral: For IM use only; do not administer IV

Monitoring Parameters Vital signs; serum potassium and magnesium; CBC with differential; fasting lipid profile and fasting blood glucose/Hb A_{1c} (prior to treatment, at 3 months, then annually); weight, BMI, waist circumference; personal/family history of diabetes; blood pressure; mental status, abnormal involuntary movement scale (AIMS), extrapyramidal symptoms. Weight should be assessed prior to treatment, at 4 weeks, 8 weeks, 12 weeks, and then at quarterly intervals. Consider titrating to a different antipsychotic agent for a weight gain ≥5% of the initial weight. Monitor patient periodically for symptom resolution. In children, baseline and periodic (eg, when initially reach steady state, with dose changes or addition of an interacting drug) ECG monitoring in children has been recommended by several pediatric clinicians (Blair, 2004; Blair, 2005; Elbe, 2008). Discontinue drug in patients found to have persistent QTc intervals >500 msec.

Additional Information Long-term usefulness of ziprasidone should be periodically re-evaluated in patients receiving the drug for extended periods of time. A Phase III trial designed to evaluate ziprasidone in adolescents with schizophrenia was terminated early due to lack of efficacy; no safety concerns were noted.

Agitation and/or aggression after traumatic brain injury (TBI): A case series of 20 patients [ages: 9 months to 17 years (median: 8 years)] reported using age-based ziprasidone dosing during the immediate TBI recovery phase with a total duration of therapy range of 3-8 days. To discontinue, ziprasidone dose was tapered over ~2 days. Doses were initiated at a low dose and titrated up based on agitation level and Riker SAS score; however, minimal dosage adjustments were required during the study. The drug appeared to be safe and effective (Scott, 2009). Initial dosing:

<2 years: 1.7 mg/kg/day divided 2-3 times/day (final dose: 1.8 mg/kg/day)

2-6 years: 0.9 mg/kg/day divided twice daily (final dose: 1.5 mg/kg/day)

7-12 years: 0.7 mg/kg/day divided twice daily (final dose: 1.5 mg/kg/day)

≥13 years: 0.6 mg/kg/day divided twice daily (final dose: 0.7 mg/kg/day)

Dosage Forms Excipient information presented when available (limited, particularly for generics); consult specific product labeling.

Capsule, Oral, as hydrochloride:

Geodon: 20 mg, 40 mg, 60 mg, 80 mg

Generic: 20 mg, 40 mg, 60 mg, 80 mg

Solution Reconstituted, Intramuscular, as mesylate [strength expressed as base]:

Geodon: 20 mg (1 ea)

Extemporaneous Preparations Hazardous agent: Use appropriate precautions for handling and disposal (NIOSH 2014 [group 3]).

A 2.5 mg/mL oral solution may be made with the injection. Use 8 vials of the 20 mg injectable powder. Add 1.2 mL of distilled water to each vial to make a 20 mg/mL solution. Once dissolved, transfer 7.5 mL to a calibrated bottle and add quantity of vehicle (Ora-Sweet®) sufficient to make 60 mL. Label "shake well" and "refrigerate". Stable for 14 days at room temperature or 42 days refrigerated (preferred).

Green K and Parish RC, "Stability of Ziprasidone Mesylate in an Extemporaneously Compounded Oral Solution," *J Pediatr Pharmacol Ther*, 2010, 15:138-41.

◆ **Ziprasidone Hydrochloride** *see* Ziprasidone *on page 2216*

◆ **Ziprasidone Mesylate** *see* Ziprasidone *on page 2216*

- **Zipsor** *see* Diclofenac (Systemic) *on page 641*
- **Zirgan** *see* Ganciclovir (Ophthalmic) *on page 959*
- **Zithromax** *see* Azithromycin (Systemic) *on page 242*
- **Zithromax For Intravenous Injection (Can)** *see* Azithromycin (Systemic) *on page 242*
- **Zithromax TRI-PAK** *see* Azithromycin (Systemic) *on page 242*
- **Zithromax Tri-Pak** *see* Azithromycin (Systemic) *on page 242*
- **Zithromax Z-PAK** *see* Azithromycin (Systemic) *on page 242*
- **Zmax** *see* Azithromycin (Systemic) *on page 242*
- **Zmax SR (Can)** *see* Azithromycin (Systemic) *on page 242*
- **$ZnSO_4$ (error-prone abbreviation)** *see* Zinc Sulfate *on page 2214*
- **Zocor** *see* Simvastatin *on page 1928*
- **Zofran** *see* Ondansetron *on page 1564*
- **Zofran ODT** *see* Ondansetron *on page 1564*
- **Zoloft** *see* Sertraline *on page 1916*

Zolpidem (zole PI dem)

Medication Safety Issues

Sound-alike/look-alike issues:

Ambien may be confused with Abilify, Ativan, Ambi 10

Sublinox may be confused with Suboxone

Zolpidem may be confused with lorazepam, zaleplon, Zyloprim

BEERS Criteria medication:

This drug may be potentially inappropriate for use in geriatric patients (Quality of evidence - moderate; Strength of recommendation - strong).

International issues:

Ambien [U.S., Argentina, Israel] may be confused with Amyben brand name for amiodarone [Great Britain]

Related Information

Oral Medications That Should Not Be Crushed or Altered *on page 2476*

Brand Names: US Ambien; Ambien CR; Edluar; Intermezzo; Zolpimist

Brand Names: Canada Sublinox

Therapeutic Category Hypnotic, Nonbenzodiazepine

Generic Availability (US) May be product dependent

Use Oral:

Tablets:

Ambien: Short-term treatment of insomnia (with difficulty of sleep onset) (FDA approved in age ≥18 years and adults)

Ambien CR: Treatment of insomnia (with difficulty of sleep onset and/or sleep maintenance) (FDA approved in age ≥18 years and adults)

Sublingual:

Edluar: Short-term treatment of insomnia (with difficulty of sleep onset) (FDA approved in age ≥18 years and adults)

Intermezzo: "As needed" treatment of middle-of-the-night insomnia with ≥4 hours of sleep time remaining (FDA approved in age age ≥18 years and adults)

Oral spray: Zolpimist: Short-term treatment of insomnia (with difficulty of sleep onset) (FDA approved in age ≥18 years and adults)

Medication Guide Available Yes

Pregnancy Risk Factor C

Pregnancy Considerations Adverse events were observed in some animal reproduction studies. Zolpidem crosses the placenta (Juric, 2009). Severe neonatal respiratory depression has been reported when zolpidem was used at the end of pregnancy, especially when used concurrently with other CNS depressants. Children born of mothers taking sedative/hypnotics may be at risk for withdrawal; neonatal flaccidity has been reported in infants following maternal use of sedative/hypnotics during pregnancy. Additional adverse effects to the fetus/newborn have been noted in some studies (Wang, 2010; Wikner, 2011).

Breast-Feeding Considerations Zolpidem is excreted in breast milk. The manufacturer recommends that caution be exercised when administering zolpidem to nursing women.

Contraindications

Hypersensitivity to zolpidem or any component of the formulation

Canadian labeling: Additional contraindications (not in U.S. labeling): Significant obstructive sleep apnea syndrome and acute and/or severe impairment of respiratory function; myasthenia gravis; severe hepatic impairment; personal or family history of sleepwalking

Warnings/Precautions Should be used only after evaluation of potential causes of sleep disturbance. Failure of sleep disturbance to resolve after 7-10 days may indicate the need for psychiatric and/or medical illness reevaluation. Hypnotics/sedatives have been associated with abnormal thinking and behavior changes including decreased inhibition, aggression, bizarre behavior, agitation, visual and auditory hallucinations, and depersonalization. These changes may occur unpredictably and may indicate previously unrecognized psychiatric disorders; evaluate appropriately. Sedative/hypnotics may produce withdrawal symptoms following abrupt discontinuation. Use with caution in patients with depression; worsening of depression, including suicide or suicidal ideation has been reported with the use of hypnotics. Intentional overdose may be an issue in this population. The minimum dose that will effectively treat the individual patient should be used. Prescriptions should be written for the smallest quantity consistent with good patient care. May cause CNS depression impairing physical and mental capabilities; patients must be cautioned about performing tasks which require mental alertness (operating machinery or driving). Drowsiness and a decreased level of consciousness may lead to falls and severe injuries; hip fractures and intracranial hemorrhage have been reported. Zolpidem should only be administered when the patient is able to stay in bed a full night (7 to 8 hours) before being active again. Intermezzo should be taken in bed if patient awakens in the middle of the night (ie, if ≥4 hours left before waking) and there is difficulty in returning to sleep.

Potentially significant drug-drug interactions may exist, requiring dose or frequency adjustment, additional monitoring, and/or selection of alternative therapy.

Use caution in patients with myasthenia gravis (contraindicated in the Canadian labeling). Avoid use in patients with sleep apnea or a history of sedative-hypnotic abuse. Postmarketing studies have indicated that the use of hypnotic/sedative agents (including zolpidem) for sleep has been associated with hypersensitivity reactions including anaphylaxis as well as angioedema. Do not rechallenge patient if such reactions occur. An increased risk for hazardous sleep-related activities such as sleep-driving, cooking and eating food, making phone calls or having sex while asleep have also been noted; amnesia, anxiety, and other neuropsychiatric symptoms may also occur. Discontinue treatment in patients who report any sleep-related episodes. Canadian labeling recommends avoiding use in patients with disorders (eg, restless legs syndrome, periodic limb movement disorder, sleep apnea) that may disrupt sleep and cause frequent awakenings, potentially increasing the risk of complex sleep-related behaviors. Use with caution in patients with a history of drug dependence. Risk of abuse is increased in patients with a history or family history of alcohol or drug abuse or mental illness.

Use caution with respiratory disease (Canadian labeling contraindicates use with acute and/or severe impairment of respiratory function). Use caution with hepatic impairment (Canadian labeling contraindicates use in severe impairment); dose adjustment required. Because of the rapid onset of action, administer immediately prior to bedtime, after the patient has gone to bed and is having difficulty falling asleep, or during the middle of the night when at least 4 hours are left before waking (Intermezzo).

Use caution in the elderly; dose adjustment recommended. Closely monitor elderly or debilitated patients for impaired cognitive and/or motor performance, confusion, and potential for falling. Avoid chronic use (>90 days) in older adults; adverse events, including delirium, falls, fractures, have been observed with nonbenzodiazepine hypnotic use in the elderly similar to events observed with benzodiazepines. Data suggests improvements in sleep duration and latency are minimal (Beers Criteria).

Dosage adjustment is recommended for females; pharmacokinetic studies involving zolpidem showed a significant increase in maximum concentration and exposure in females compared to males at the same dose. When studied for the unapproved use of insomnia associated with ADHD in children, a higher incidence (~7%) of hallucinations was reported. In addition, sleep latency did not decrease compared to placebo.

Some dosage forms may contain polysorbate 80 (also known as Tweens). Hypersensitivity reactions, usually a delayed reaction, have been reported following exposure to pharmaceutical products containing polysorbate 80 in certain individuals (Isaksson, 2002; Lucente 2000; Shelley, 1995). Thrombocytopenia, ascites, pulmonary deterioration, and renal and hepatic failure have been reported in premature neonates after receiving parenteral products containing polysorbate 80 (Alade, 1986; CDC, 1984). See manufacturer's labeling.

Warnings: Additional Pediatric Considerations The most common adverse effects observed in children include the following: Dizziness, headache, hallucinations, affect lability, enuresis, gastroenteritis, and anxiety (Blumer, 2009).

Some dosage forms may contain propylene glycol; in neonates large amounts of propylene glycol delivered orally, intravenously (eg, >3,000 mg/day), or topically have been associated with potentially fatal toxicities which can include metabolic acidosis, seizures, renal failure, and CNS depression; toxicities have also been reported in children and adults including hyperosmolality, lactic acidosis, seizures and respiratory depression; use caution (AAP, 1997; Shehab, 2009).

Adverse Reactions

Cardiovascular: Chest discomfort, increased blood pressure, palpitations

Central nervous system: Abnormal dreams, amnesia, anxiety, apathy, ataxia, burning sensation, confusion, depersonalization, depression, disinhibition, disorientation, dizziness, drowsiness, drugged feeling, eating disorder (binge eating), emotional lability, equilibrium disturbance, euphoria, fatigue, hallucination, headache, hypoesthesia, increased body temperature, insomnia, lack of concentration, lethargy, memory impairment, paresthesia, psychomotor retardation, sleep disorder, stress, vertigo

Dermatologic: Skin rash, urticaria, wrinkling of skin

Endocrine & metabolic: Hypermenorrhea

Gastrointestinal: Abdominal distress, abdominal tenderness, change in appetite, constipation, diarrhea, dyspepsia, flatulence, frequent bowel movements, gastroenteritis, gastroesophageal reflux disease, hiccups, nausea, vomiting, xerostomia

Genitourinary: Dysuria, urinary tract infection, vaginal dryness

Hypersensitivity: Hypersensitivity reaction

Neuromuscular & skeletal: Arthralgia, back pain, muscle cramps, muscle spasm, myalgia, neck pain, tremor, weakness

Ophthalmic: Accommodation disturbance, asthenopia, blurred vision, diplopia, eye redness, visual disturbance (including altered depth perception)

Otic: Labyrinthitis, tinnitus

Respiratory: Dry throat, flu-like symptoms, lower respiratory tract infection, pharyngitis, sinusitis, throat irritation, upper respiratory tract infection

Miscellaneous: Fever

Rare but important or life-threatening: Abnormal hepatic function tests, acute renal failure, aggressive behavior, anaphylaxis, anemia, angina pectoris, angioedema, anorexia, arteritis, arthritis, breast fibroadenosis, breast neoplasm, bronchitis, cardiac arrhythmia, cerebrovascular disease, circulatory shock, cognitive dysfunction, corneal ulcer, delusions, dementia, dermatitis, drug tolerance, dysarthria, dysphagia, edema, extrasystoles, glaucoma, hepatic insufficiency, hyperbilirubinemia, hyperglycemia, hyperlipidemia, hypertension, hypotension, hysteria, illusion, impotence, leukopenia, lymphadenopathy, migraine, myocardial infarction, neuralgia, neuritis, neuropathy, orthostatic hypotension, panic disorder, personality disorder, psychoneurosis, pulmonary edema, pulmonary embolism, pyelonephritis, respiratory depression, restless leg syndrome, rhinitis, scleritis, somnambulism, syncope, tachycardia, tenesmus, tetany, thrombosis, urinary incontinence, vaginitis, ventricular tachycardia

Drug Interactions

Metabolism/Transport Effects Substrate of CYP1A2 (minor), CYP2C19 (minor), CYP2C9 (minor), CYP2D6 (minor), CYP3A4 (major); **Note:** Assignment of Major/Minor substrate status based on clinically relevant drug interaction potential

Avoid Concomitant Use

Avoid concomitant use of Zolpidem with any of the following: Azelastine (Nasal); Conivaptan; Fusidic Acid (Systemic); Idelalisib; Orphenadrine; Paraldehyde; Sodium Oxybate; Thalidomide

Increased Effect/Toxicity

Zolpidem may increase the levels/effects of: Alcohol (Ethyl); Azelastine (Nasal); Buprenorphine; CarBAMazepine; Hydrocodone; Methotrimeprazine; Metyrosine; Orphenadrine; Paraldehyde; Pramipexole; ROPINIRole; Rotigotine; Selective Serotonin Reuptake Inhibitors; Sodium Oxybate; Suvorexant; Thalidomide

The levels/effects of Zolpidem may be increased by: Antifungal Agents (Azole Derivatives, Systemic); Aprepitant; Brimonidine (Topical); Cannabis; CNS Depressants; Conivaptan; CYP3A4 Inhibitors (Moderate); CYP3A4 Inhibitors (Strong); Dasatinib; Dronabinol; Droperidol; FluvoxaMINE; Fosaprepitant; Fusidic Acid (Systemic); Idelalisib; Ivacaftor; Kava Kava; Luliconazole; Magnesium Sulfate; Methotrimeprazine; Mifepristone; Nabilone; Netupitant; Palbociclib; Perampanel; Rufinamide; Simeprevir; Stiripentol; Tapentadol; Tetrahydrocannabinol

Decreased Effect

The levels/effects of Zolpidem may be decreased by: Bosentan; CarBAMazepine; CYP3A4 Inducers (Moderate); CYP3A4 Inducers (Strong); Dabrafenib; Deferasirox; Flumazenil; Mitotane; Rifamycin Derivatives; Siltuximab; St Johns Wort; Telaprevir; Tocilizumab

Food Interactions Maximum plasma concentration and bioavailability are decreased with food; time to peak plasma concentration is increased; half-life remains unchanged. Grapefruit juice may decrease the metabolism of zolpidem. Management: Do not administer with (or immediately after) a meal. Avoid grapefruit juice.

Storage/Stability

Ambien, Edluar, Intermezzo: Store at 20°C to 25°C (68°F to 77°F). Protect sublingual tablets from light and moisture.

Ambien CR: Store at 15°C to 25°C (59°F to 77°F); limited excursions permitted up to 30°C (86°F).

Zolpimist: Store upright at 25°C (77°F); excursions are permitted to 15°C to 30°C (59°F to 86°F). Do not freeze. Avoid prolonged exposure to temperatures >30°C (86°F).

Sublinox [Canadian product]: Store at 15°C to 30°C (59°F to 86°F); protect from light and moisture.

Mechanism of Action Zolpidem, an imidazopyridine hypnotic that is structurally dissimilar to benzodiazepines, enhances the activity of the inhibitory neurotransmitter, γ-aminobutyric acid (GABA), via selective agonism at the benzodiazepine-1 (BZ_1) receptor; the result is increased chloride conductance, neuronal hyperpolarization, inhibition of the action potential, and a decrease in neuronal excitability leading to sedative and hypnotic effects. Because of its selectivity for the BZ_1 receptor site over the BZ_2 receptor site, zolpidem exhibits minimal anxiolytic, myorelaxant, and anticonvulsant properties (effects largely attributed to agonism at the BZ_2 receptor site).

Pharmacodynamics

Onset of action: Immediate release: 30 minutes

Duration: Immediate release: 6-8 hours

Pharmacokinetics (Adult data unless noted) Note: C_{max} and AUC are increased by ~45% in female patients

Absorption: Oral:

Immediate release and sublingual: Rapid

Extended release: Biphasic absorption; rapid initial absorption (similar to immediate release product); then provides extended concentrations in the plasma beyond 3 hours postadministration

Distribution: V_d, apparent:

Children 2-6 years: 1.8 ± 0.8 L/kg (Blumer, 2008)

Children >6-12 years: 2.2 ± 1.7 L/kg (Blumer, 2008)

Adolescents: 1.2 ± 0.4 L/kg (Blumer, 2008)

Adults: 0.54 L/kg (Holm, 2004)

Protein binding: ~93%

Metabolism: Hepatic methylation and hydroxylation via CYP3A4 (~60%), CYP2C9 (~22%), CYP1A2 (~14%), CYP2D6 (~3%), and CYP2C19 (~3%) to three inactive metabolites

Bioavailability: 70% (Holm, 2004)

Half-life elimination:

Children 2-6 years: Tablet (immediate release): 1.8 hours (Blumer, 2008)

Children >6 years and Adolescents: Tablet (immediate release): 2.3 hours (Blumer, 2008)

Adults:

Spray (Zolpimist): ~3 hours (range: 1.7-8.4 hours)

Sublingual tablet (Edluar, Intermezzo): ~3 hours (range: 1.4-6.7 hours)

Tablet (immediate release, extended release): ~2.5 hours (range: 1.4-4.5 hours); Cirrhosis: 9.9 hours (range: 4.1-25.8 hours)

Time to peak serum concentration:

Children 2-6 years: Tablet (immediate release): 0.9 hours (Blumer, 2008)

Children >6-12 years: Tablet (immediate release): 1.1 hours (Blumer, 2008)

Adolescents: Tablet (immediate release): 1.3 hours (Blumer, 2008)

Adults:

Spray (Zolpimist): ~0.9 hours

Sublingual tablet:

Edluar: ~1.4 hours; with food: ~1.8 hours

Intermezzo: 0.6-1.3 hours; with food: ~3 hours

Tablet: Immediate release: 1.6 hours; with food: 2.2 hours; Extended release: 1.5 hours; with food: 4 hours

Elimination: Urine (48% to 67%, primarily as metabolites); feces (29% to 42%, primarily as metabolites)

Clearance, apparent:

Children and Adolescents (Blumer, 2008):

Children 2-6 years: 11.7 ± 7.9 mL/minute/kg

Children >6-12 years: 9.7 ± 10.3 mL/minute/kg

Adolescents: 4.8 ± 2 mL/minute/kg

Adults: Intermezzo: Males: 4 mL/minute/kg; Females: 2.7 mL/minute/kg

Dosing: Usual Note: The lowest effective dose should be used; higher doses may be more likely to impair next-morning activities.

Children and Adolescents ≤17 years: **Insomnia:** Oral: Limited data available; efficacy results variable and have **not** been demonstrated in randomized placebo-controlled trials. An open-label, dose escalation pharmacokinetic evaluation showed zolpidem was well-tolerated in pediatric patients 2-18 years of age and recommended a dose of 0.25 mg/kg at bedtime for evaluation in future efficacy trials (Blumer, 2008). A single case report describes an 18-month-old infant who was effectively treated with zolpidem for primary insomnia (Bhat, 2008). However, zolpidem has **not** been shown to be effective in a randomized placebo-controlled trial (n=201) of children aged 6-17 years with ADHD-associated insomnia; zolpidem 0.25 mg/kg/dose (maximum dose: 10 mg) administered nightly did **not** decrease sleep latency; in addition, hallucinations occurred in 7.4% of patients (Blumer, 2009). A comparative, randomized controlled trial of zolpidem and haloperidol in pediatric burn patients (n=40, mean age: 9.4 ± 0.7 years) showed zolpidem dosed at 0.5 mg/kg nightly for one week (maximum dose: 20 mg) minimally increased Stage 3/4 sleep and REM but not total sleep time; the authors no longer use zolpidem to try to improve sleep in their pediatric burn patients (Armour, 2008).

Adolescents ≥18 years and Adults: **Insomnia:** Oral:

Immediate release tablet, spray: 5 mg (females) or 5-10 mg (males) immediately before bedtime; maximum dose: 10 mg

Extended release tablet: 6.25 mg (females) or 6.25-12.5 mg (males) immediately before bedtime; maximum dose: 12.5 mg

Sublingual tablet:

Edluar: 5 mg (females) or 5-10 mg (males) immediately before bedtime; maximum dose: 10 mg daily

Intermezzo: **Note:** Should be taken if patient awakens in middle of night, has difficulty returning to sleep, and has at least 4 hours left before waking.

Females: 1.75 mg once per night as needed; maximum dose: 1.75 mg/night

Males: 3.5 mg once per night as needed; maximum dose: 3.5 mg/night

Dosage adjustment with concomitant CNS depressants: Females and males: 1.75 mg once per night as needed; dose adjustment of concomitant CNS depressant(s) may be necessary

Dosing adjustment for renal impairment: Adults: There are no dosage adjustments provided in manufacturer's labeling; however, some zolpidem labeling recommends monitoring patients with renal impairment closely.

Dosing adjustment for hepatic impairment: Adults:

Immediate release tablet, spray: 5 mg immediately before bedtime

Extended release tablet: 6.25 mg immediately before bedtime

Sublingual tablet:

Edluar: 5 mg immediately before bedtime

Intermezzo: Females and males: 1.75 mg once per night as needed. **Note:** Take only if ≥4 hours left before waking.

Administration

All formulations (excluding Intermezzo): Administer immediately before bedtime due to rapid onset of action. For faster sleep onset, do not administer with (or immediately after) a meal.

Sublingual tablets (Edluar, Intermezzo): Examine blister-pack before use; do not use if blisters are broken, torn, or missing. Separate individual blisters at perforation; peel off top layer of paper; push tablet through foil. Place under the tongue and allow to disintegrate; do not swallow or administer with water. Intermezzo should be taken in bed if patient awakens in the middle of the night and has at least 4 hours left before waking.

Oral spray (Zolpimist): Spray directly into the mouth over the tongue. Prior to initial use, pump should be primed by spraying 5 times. If pump is not used for at least 14 days, reprime pump with 1 spray.

Extended release tablets (Ambien CR): Swallow whole; do not divide, crush, or chew.

Monitoring Parameters Daytime alertness; respiratory rate; behavior profile

Test Interactions Increased aminotransferase [ALT/AST], bilirubin (S); decreased RAI uptake

Controlled Substance C-IV

Dosage Forms Excipient information presented when available (limited, particularly for generics); consult specific product labeling.

Solution, Oral, as tartrate:
- Zolpimist: 5 mg/actuation (7.7 mL) [contains benzoic acid, propylene glycol; cherry flavor]

Tablet, Oral, as tartrate:
- Ambien: 5 mg [contains fd&c red #40, polysorbate 80]
- Ambien: 10 mg
- Generic: 5 mg, 10 mg

Tablet Extended Release, Oral, as tartrate:
- Ambien CR: 6.25 mg
- Ambien CR: 12.5 mg [contains fd&c blue #2 (indigotine)]
- Generic: 6.25 mg, 12.5 mg

Tablet Sublingual, Sublingual, as tartrate:
- Edluar: 5 mg, 10 mg [contains saccharin sodium]
- Intermezzo: 1.75 mg, 3.5 mg

◆ **Zolpidem Tartrate** *see* Zolpidem *on page 2220*

◆ **Zolpimist** *see* Zolpidem *on page 2220*

◆ **Zolvit [DSC]** *see* Hydrocodone and Acetaminophen *on page 1032*

◆ **Zomacton** *see* Somatropin *on page 1957*

◆ **Zonalon (Can)** *see* Doxepin (Systemic) *on page 711*

◆ **Zonegran** *see* Zonisamide *on page 2223*

Zonisamide (zoe NIS a mide)

Medication Safety Issues

Sound-alike/look-alike issues:

Zonegran may be confused with SINEquan
Zonisamide may be confused with lacosamide

Related Information

Safe Handling of Hazardous Drugs *on page 2455*

Brand Names: US Zonegran

Therapeutic Category Anticonvulsant, Miscellaneous

Generic Availability (US) Yes

Use Adjunctive treatment of partial seizures (FDA approved in ages >16 years and adults); has been used investigationally for the treatment of generalized epilepsies including, generalized tonic-clonic seizures, absence seizures, infantile spasms, myoclonic epilepsies, and Lennox-Gastaut syndrome (Leppik, 1999; Oommen, 1999)

Medication Guide Available Yes

Pregnancy Risk Factor C

Pregnancy Considerations Teratogenic effects were observed in animal reproduction studies. Zonisamide crosses the placenta and can be detected in the newborn following delivery. Although adverse fetal events have been reported, the risk of teratogenic effects following maternal use of zonisamide in not clearly defined. Other agents may be preferred until additional data is available. Newborns should be monitored for transient metabolic acidosis after birth. Zonisamide clearance may increase in the second trimester of pregnancy, requiring dosage adjustment. Women of childbearing potential are advised to use effective contraception during therapy.

Patients exposed to zonisamide during pregnancy are encouraged to enroll themselves into the AED Pregnancy Registry by calling 1-888-233-2334. Additional information is available at http://www.aedpregnancyregistry.org.

Breast-Feeding Considerations Zonisamide is excreted in breast milk in concentrations similar to those in the maternal plasma and has been detected in the plasma of a nursing infant. Due to the potential for serious adverse reactions in the nursing infant, the manufacturer recommends a decision be made whether to discontinue nursing or to discontinue the drug, taking into account the importance of treatment to the mother.

Contraindications

Hypersensitivity to zonisamide, sulfonamides, or any component of the formulation

Note: Although the FDA approved product labeling states this medication is contraindicated with other sulfonamide-containing drug classes, the scientific basis of this statement has been challenged. See "Warnings/Precautions" for more detail.

Warnings/Precautions Hazardous agent - use appropriate precautions for handling and disposal (NIOSH 2014 [group 3]).

Use may be associated with the development of metabolic acidosis (generally dose-dependent) in certain patients; predisposing conditions/therapies include renal disease, severe respiratory disease, diarrhea, status epilepticus, ketogenic diet, and other medications. Metabolic acidosis can occur at doses as low as 25 mg daily. Pediatric patients may also be at an increased risk for and may have more severe metabolic acidosis. Serum bicarbonate should be monitored in all patients prior to and during use; if metabolic acidosis occurs, consider decreasing the dose or tapering the dose to discontinue. If use continued despite acidosis, alkali treatment should be considered. Untreated metabolic acidosis may increase the risk of developing nephrolithiasis, nephrocalcinosis, osteomalacia (or rickets in children), or osteoporosis; pediatric patients may also have decreased growth rates.

Pooled analysis of trials involving various antiepileptics (regardless of indication) showed an increased risk of suicidal thoughts/behavior (incidence rate: 0.43% treated patients compared to 0.24% of patients receiving placebo); risk observed as early as 1 week after initiation and continued through duration of trials (most trials ≤24 weeks). Monitor all patients for notable changes in behavior that might indicate suicidal thoughts or depression; notify healthcare provider immediately if symptoms occur.

Discontinue zonisamide in patients who develop acute renal failure or a significant sustained increase in creatinine/BUN concentration. Kidney stones have been reported. Do not use in patients with renal impairment (GFR <50 mL/minute); use with caution in patients with hepatic impairment. Use with caution in patients with hepatic impairment.

Significant CNS effects include psychiatric symptoms (eg, depression, psychosis), psychomotor slowing (eg, difficulty with concentration, speech or language problems), and fatigue or somnolence; may occur within the first month of treatment, most commonly at doses of ≥300 mg/day. ▶

May cause sedation, which may impair physical or mental abilities; patients must be cautioned about performing tasks which require mental alertness (eg, operating machinery or driving). Anticonvulsants should not be discontinued abruptly because of the possibility of increasing seizure frequency; therapy should be withdrawn gradually to minimize the potential of increased seizure frequency, unless safety concerns require a more rapid withdrawal.

Decreased sweating (oligohydrosis) and hyperthermia requiring hospitalization have been reported in children; use with caution when used in combination with other drugs that may predispose patients to heat-related disorders (eg, anticholinergics). Potentially significant interactions may exist, requiring dose or frequency adjustment, additional monitoring, and/or selection of alternative therapy. Consult drug interactions database for more detailed information.

Sulfonamide ("sulfa") allergy: The FDA-approved product labeling for many medications containing a sulfonamide chemical group includes a broad contraindication in patients with a prior allergic reaction to sulfonamides. There is a potential for cross-reactivity between members of a specific class (eg, two antibiotic sulfonamides). However, concerns for cross-reactivity have previously extended to all compounds containing the sulfonamide structure (SO_2NH_2). An expanded understanding of allergic mechanisms indicates cross-reactivity between antibiotic sulfonamides and nonantibiotic sulfonamides may not occur or at the very least this potential is extremely low (Brackett 2004; Johnson 2005; Slatore 2004; Tornero 2004). In particular, mechanisms of cross-reaction due to antibody production (anaphylaxis) are unlikely to occur with nonantibiotic sulfonamides. T-cell-mediated (type IV) reactions (eg, maculopapular rash) are less well understood and it is not possible to completely exclude this potential based on current insights. In cases where prior reactions were severe (Stevens-Johnson syndrome/TEN), some clinicians choose to avoid exposure to these classes.

Warnings: Additional Pediatric Considerations Pediatric patients may also be at an increased risk and may have more severe metabolic acidosis. Untreated metabolic acidosis may increase the risk of developing nephrolithiasis, nephrocalcinosis, osteomalacia (or rickets in children), or osteoporosis; pediatric patients may also have decreased growth rates. Oligohydrosis (decreased sweating) and hyperthermia have been reported in 40 pediatric patients; many cases occurred after exposure to elevated environmental temperatures; some cases resulted in heat stroke requiring hospitalization; pediatric patients may be at an increased risk; monitor patients, especially pediatric patients, for decreased sweating and hyperthermia, especially in warm or hot weather; use zonisamide with caution in patients receiving drugs that predispose to heat-related disorders (eg, anticholinergic agents, carbonic anhydrase inhibitors). In children, agitation, anxiety, ataxia, and behavior disorders have been reported (Kimura, 1994).

Adverse Reactions

Cardiovascular: Facial edema

Central nervous system: Agitation, anxiety, ataxia, confusion, convulsions, decreased mental acuity, depression, dizziness, drowsiness, fatigue, headache, hyperesthesia, hyperthermia, hypotonia, insomnia, irritability, lack of concentration, memory impairment, nervousness, schizophreniform disorder, seizure, speech decreased, speech disturbance, status epilepticus, tiredness

Dermatologic: Bruising, hypohidrosis (children), pruritus, skin rash, Stevens-Johnson syndrome, toxic epidermal necrolysis

Endrocrine & metabolic: Metabolic acidosis

Gastrointestinal: Abdominal pain, anorexia, constipation, diarrhea, dysgeusia, dyspepsia, nausea, vomiting, weight loss, xerostomia

Hematologic & oncologic: Agranulocytosis, aplastic anemia

Neuromuscular & skeletal: Abnormal gait, paresthesia, tremor, weakness

Ophthalmic: Amblyopia, diplopia, nystagmus

Otic: Tinnitus

Renal: Increased blood urea nitrogen, nephrolithiasis

Respiratory: Increased cough, pharyngitis, rhinitis

Miscellaneous: Accidental injury, flu-like syndrome

Rare (but important or life threatening symptoms): Alopecia, amenorrhea, apnea, arthritis, atrial fibrillation, bladder calculus, bradycardia, brain disease, cardiac failure, cerebrovascular accident, cholangitis, cholecystitis, cholestatic jaundice, colitis, deafness, duodenitis, fecal incontinence, gastrointestinal ulcer, gingivitis, glaucoma, hematemesis, hematuria, hemoptysis, hirsutism, hypermenorrhea, hypersensitivity reaction, hypertension, hypoglycemia, hyponatremia, hypotension, immunodeficiency, impotence, iritis, leukopenia, lupus erythematosus, lymphadenopathy, mastitis, neuropathy, oculogyric crisis, pancreatitis, photophobia, psychomotor disturbance, pulmonary embolism, rectal hemorrhage, stroke, suicidal behavior, suicidal ideation, syncope, thrombocytopenia, thrombophlebitis, urinary incontinence, ventricular premature contractions

Drug Interactions

Metabolism/Transport Effects Substrate of CYP2C19 (minor), CYP3A4 (major); **Note:** Assignment of Major/Minor substrate status based on clinically relevant drug interaction potential

Avoid Concomitant Use

Avoid concomitant use of Zonisamide with any of the following: Azelastine (Nasal); Carbonic Anhydrase Inhibitors; Conivaptan; Fusidic Acid (Systemic); Idelalisib; Orphenadrine; Paraldehyde; Thalidomide

Increased Effect/Toxicity

Zonisamide may increase the levels/effects of: Alcohol (Ethyl); Alpha-/Beta-Agonists (Indirect-Acting); Amphetamines; Azelastine (Nasal); Buprenorphine; Carbonic Anhydrase Inhibitors; CNS Depressants; Flecainide; Hydrocodone; Memantine; MetFORMIN; Methotrimeprazine; Metyrosine; Mirtazapine; Orphenadrine; Paraldehyde; Pramipexole; QuiNIDine; ROPINIRole; Rotigotine; Selective Serotonin Reuptake Inhibitors; Suvorexant; Thalidomide; Zolpidem

The levels/effects of Zonisamide may be increased by: Aprepitant; Brimonidine (Topical); Cannabis; Conivaptan; CYP3A4 Inhibitors (Moderate); CYP3A4 Inhibitors (Strong); Dasatinib; Doxylamine; Dronabinol; Droperidol; Fosaprepitant; Fusidic Acid (Systemic); HydrOXYzine; Idelalisib; Ivacaftor; Kava Kava; Luliconazole; Magnesium Sulfate; Methotrimeprazine; Mifepristone; Nabilone; Netupitant; Palbociclib; Perampanel; Rufinamide; Salicylates; Simeprevir; Sodium Oxybate; Stiripentol; Tapentadol; Tetrahydrocannabinol

Decreased Effect

Zonisamide may decrease the levels/effects of: Lithium; Methenamine

The levels/effects of Zonisamide may be decreased by: Bosentan; CYP3A4 Inducers (Moderate); CYP3A4 Inducers (Strong); Dabrafenib; Deferasirox; Fosphenytoin; Mefloquine; Mianserin; Mitotane; Orlistat; PHENobarbital; Phenytoin; Siltuximab; St Johns Wort; Tocilizumab

Food Interactions Food delays time to maximum concentration, but does not affect bioavailability. Management: Administer without regard to meals.

Storage/Stability Store at 25°C (77°F) excursions are permitted between 15°C and 30°C (59°F and 86°F). Protect from moisture and light.

Mechanism of Action Stabilizes neuronal membranes and suppresses neuronal hypersynchronization through action at sodium and calcium channels; does not affect GABA activity.

Pharmacokinetics (Adult data unless noted)

Absorption: Oral: Rapid and complete

Distribution: V_d (apparent): 1.45 L/kg; highly concentrated in erythrocytes

Protein binding: 40%

Metabolism: Hepatic; undergoes acetylation to form N-acetyl zonisamide and reduction via cytochrome P450 isoenzyme CYP3A4 to 2-sulfamoylacetylphenol (SMAP); SMAP then undergoes conjugation with glucuronide

Half-life: ~63 hours (range: 50-68 hours)

Time to peak serum concentration: 2-6 hours

Elimination: Urine: 62% (35% as unchanged drug, 15% as N-acetyl zonisamide, 50% as SMAP glucuronide); feces (3%); **Note:** Of the dose recovered in Japanese patients, 28% is as unchanged drug, 52% is as N-acetyl zonisamide, and 19% is as SMAP glucuronide (Glauser, 2002)

Dosing: Usual

Pediatric:

Partial seizures; adjunct therapy:

Infants, Children, and Adolescents ≤16 years: Limited data available; dosing regimens variable: Initial: 1 to 2 mg/kg/day given in two divided doses/day; increase dose in increments of 0.5 to 1 mg/kg/day every 2 weeks; usual dose: 5 to 8 mg/kg/day; dosing based on a review article of the literature (primarily Japanese experience) (Glauser 2002).Others have recommended higher initial and maximum doses: Initial: 2 to 4 mg/kg/day given in two divided doses/day; titrate dose upwards if needed every 2 weeks; usual dose: 4 to 8 mg/kg/day; maximum daily dose: 12 mg/kg/day (Leppik 1999; Oommen 1999)

Adolescents >16 years: Initial: 100 mg once daily; dose may be increased to 200 mg/day after 2 weeks; further increases in dose should be made in increments of 100 mg/day and only after a minimum of 2 weeks between adjustments; usual effective dose: 100 to 600 mg/day. **Note:** There is no evidence of increased benefit with doses >400 mg/day. Steady-state serum concentrations fluctuate 27% with once daily dosing, and 14% with twice daily dosing; patients may benefit from divided doses given twice daily (Leppik 1999)

Infantile spasms: Limited data available: Faster titration of zonisamide has been used to control infantile spasms. Suzuki treated 11 newly diagnosed infants (mean age: ~6 months) with zonisamide monotherapy starting at doses of 3 to 5 mg/kg/day given in 2 divided doses/day; doses were increased every 4th day until seizures were controlled or a maximum dose of 10 mg/kg/day was attained; four of 11 patients responded at doses of 4 to 5 mg/kg/day (Suzuki 1997). Yanai treated 27 newly diagnosed infantile spasm patients with zonisamide add-on or monotherapy starting at doses of 2 to 4 mg/kg/day given in 2 divided doses/day; doses were increased by 2 to 5 mg/kg every 2 to 4 days until seizures were controlled or a maximum of 10 to 20 mg/kg/day was attained; nine of 27 patients responded at a mean effective dose of 7.8 mg/kg/day (range: 5 to 12.5 mg/kg/day); non-responders received doses of 8 to 20 mg/kg/day (mean: 10.8 mg/kg/day) (Yania 1999). Suzuki treated 54 newly diagnosed infants (11 of which were previously reported) with zonisamide monotherapy starting at doses of 3 to 4 mg/kg/day given in 2 divided doses; doses were increased every 4th day until seizures were controlled or a maximum dose of 10 to 13 mg/kg/day was attained; 11 of 54 infants responded at a mean effective dose of 7.2 mg/kg/day (range: 4 to 12 mg/kg/day); the majority of infants who responded did so at a dose of 4 to 8 mg/kg/day and within 1 to 2 weeks of starting therapy (Suzuki 2001).

Adult: **Adjunctive treatment of partial seizures:** Oral: Initial: 100 mg/day. Dose may be increased to 200 mg/day after 2 weeks. Further dosage increases to 300 mg and 400 mg/day can then be made with a minimum of 2 weeks between adjustments, in order to reach steady state at each dosage level. Doses of up to 600 mg/day have been studied, however, there is no evidence of increased response with doses >400 mg/day.

Dosage adjustment in renal impairment: Slower dosage titration and more frequent monitoring are recommended. Do not use if GFR <50 mL/minute. Marked renal impairment (CrCl <20 mL/minute) was associated with a 35% increase in AUC.

Dosage adjustment in hepatic impairment: Slower titration and frequent monitoring are indicated.

Administration Hazardous agent; use appropriate precautions for handling and disposal (NIOSH 2014 [group 3]). May be administered without regard to meals; swallow capsule whole; do not crush, chew, or break capsule.

Monitoring Parameters Seizure frequency, duration, and severity; symptoms of CNS adverse effects; skin rash; periodic BUN and serum creatinine; serum bicarbonate prior to initiation and periodically during therapy; serum electrolytes, including chloride, phosphorus, and calcium; alkaline phosphatase; serum albumin; symptoms of metabolic acidosis; monitor patients, especially pediatric patients, for decreased sweating and hyperthermia, especially in warm or hot weather; signs and symptoms of suicidality (eg, anxiety, depression, behavior changes)

Reference Range Monitoring of plasma concentrations may be useful; proposed therapeutic range: 10-20 mcg/mL; patients may benefit from higher concentrations (ie, up to 30 mcg/mL), but concentrations >30 mcg/mL have been associated with adverse effects (Leppik, 1999; Oommen, 1999)

Dosage Forms Excipient information presented when available (limited, particularly for generics); consult specific product labeling.

Capsule, Oral:

Zonegran: 25 mg, 100 mg

Generic: 25 mg, 50 mg, 100 mg

Extemporaneous Preparations Hazardous agent; use appropriate precautions during preparation and disposal (NIOSH 2014 [group 3]).

A 10 mg/mL suspension may be made using capsules and either simple syrup or methylcellulose 0.5%. Empty contents of ten 100 mg capsules into glass mortar. Reduce to a fine powder and add a small amount of Simple Syrup, NF and mix to a uniform paste; mix while adding the chosen vehicle in incremental proportions to **almost** 100 mL; transfer to an amber calibrated plastic bottle, rinse mortar with vehicle, and add quantity of vehicle sufficient to make 100 mL. Label "shake well" and "refrigerate". When using simple syrup vehicle, stable 28 days at room temperature or refrigerated (preferred). When using methylcellulose vehicle, stable 7 days at room temperature or 28 days refrigerated. **Note:** Although no visual evidence of microbial growth was observed, storage under refrigeration would be recommended to minimize microbial contamination.

Abobo CV, Wei B, and Liang D, "Stability of Zonisamide in Extemporaneously Compounded Oral Suspensions," *Am J Health Syst Pharm*, 2009, 66(12):1105-9.

◆ **Zorbtive** *see* Somatropin *on page 1957*

◆ **Zortress** *see* Everolimus *on page 825*

◆ **Zorvolex** *see* Diclofenac (Systemic) *on page 641*

APPENDIX TABLE OF CONTENTS

EMERGENCY DRIP CALCULATIONS

The availability of a limited number of standard concentrations for emergency medications (eg, vasopressors) within an institution is required by The Joint Commission (JCAHO 2004). With standardized concentrations, the equation below can be used to calculate the rate of infusion (mL/hour) for a given dose (mcg/kg/minute):

$$\text{Rate (mL/hour)} = \frac{\text{dose (mcg/kg/minute)} \times \text{weight (kg)} \times 60 \text{ minute/hour}}{\text{concentration (mcg/mL)}}$$

If a standardized concentration delivers the dose in too low of a volume (eg, <1 mL/hour) then a lower standardized concentration (ie, more dilute) is used. If a standardized concentration delivers the dose in too high of a volume (depending on patient's size and fluid status), a higher standardized concentration (ie, more concentrated) is used.

In 2011, the Institute for Safe Medication Practices (ISMP) and the Vermont Oxford Network (VON), a group of health care professionals working to improve neonatal care, collaborated along with US neonatal intensive care units to identify and recommend standard concentrations for use in neonatal patients. The following table represents their recommendations for emergency medications. For a complete list of all their recommended standard concentrations, go to www.ismp.org/Tools/PediatricConcentrations.pdf

ISMP/VON Recommended Standardized Neonatal Concentrations for Emergency Medications

Drug	Concentration (mcg/mL)
Alprostadil	10
DOBUTamine	2,000
DOPamine	1,600
EPINEPHrine	10
Norepinephrine	16

Some centers use the following pediatric standardized concentrations according to patient weight (Campbell 1994):

Standardized Concentrations by Patient Weight

Drug	Patient Weight (kg)	Concentration (mcg/mL)
DOPamine	2 to 3 4 to 8 9 to 15 >15	200 400 800 1,600
EPINEPHrine, Isoproterenol, or Norepinephrine	2 to 3 4 to 8 ≥9	5 10 20

Other centers use the following standardized concentrations depending on both patient weight and dose (Hodding 2010):

Drug	Standardized Concentrations (mcg/mL)			
DOBUTamine	800	1,600	3,200	6,400
DOPamine	800	1,600	3,200	6,400
EPINEPHrine	20	40	60	120
Norepinephrine	20	40	60	120
Isoproterenol	20	40	60	120

Some centers also limit the number of standardized concentrations to only two per emergency medication (Larsen 2005)

Drug	Standardized Concentrations (mcg/mL)	
DOBUTamine	1,000	4,000
DOPamine	800	3,200
EPINEPHrine	8	64
Norepinephrine	8	64
Isoproterenol	8	64

An example of how different standardized concentrations are used for different patient weights and doses is given below for dopamine. Each table lists the dopamine infusion rate in mL/hour for a specific patient weight (in kg) and dose (in mcg/kg/minute) for a specific standardized concentration. The first table is for dopamine **1,600** mcg/mL and the second table for **800** mcg/mL.

DOPamine Infusion Rate (mL/hour) According to Patient Weight (kg) and Dose (mcg/kg/minute) Using Standardized Concentration of 1,600 mcg/mL

Weight (kg)	Dose (mcg/kg/minute)				
	5	7.5	10	15	20
2	0.4*	0.6*	0.8*	1.1	1.5
3	0.6*	0.8*	1.1	1.7	2.3
4	0.8*	1.1	1.5	2.3	3
5	0.9*	1.4	1.9	2.8	3.8
7	1.3	2.0	2.6	3.9	5.3
10	1.9	2.8	3.8	5.6	7.5
12	2.3	3.4	4.5	6.8	9.0
14	2.6	3.9	5.3	7.9	10.5
16	3	4.5	6	9	12
18	3.4	5.1	6.8	10.1	13.5
20	3.8	5.6	7.5	11.3	15
25	4.7	7	9.4	14.1	18.8
30	5.6	8.4	11.3	16.9	22.5
35	6.6	9.8	13.1	19.7	26.3
40	7.5	11.3	15	22.5	30
45	8.4	12.7	16.9	25.3	33.8
50	9.4	14.1	18.8	28.1	37.5

*For rates <1 mL/hour, use 800 mcg/mL concentration

DOPamine Infusion Rate (mL/hour) According to Patient Weight (kg) and Dose (mcg/kg/minute) Using Standardized Concentration of 800 mcg/mL

Weight (kg)	Dose (mcg/kg/minute)				
	5	7.5	10	15	20
2	0.8	1.1	1.5	2.3	3
3	1.1	1.7	2.3	3.4	4.5
4	1.5	2.3	3	4.5	6
5	1.9	2.8	3.8	5.6	7.5

BACKGROUND INFORMATION

The Joint Commission (formerly called JCAHO) and the "Rule of Six"

In its 2004 National Patient Safety Goals (NPSG), The Joint Commission (TJC) required organizations to "standardize and limit the number of drug concentrations available in the organization" to meet patient safety goal # 3 ("Improve the safety of using high-alert medications"). High-alert medications are drugs that possess a great risk of causing significant injury to patients when they are used in error. Emergency medications (eg, vasopressors) qualify as high-alert drugs.

Historically, the "Rule of Six" was used to calculate patient-specific IV concentrations of emergency medication infusions, so that 1 mL/hour would deliver a set mcg/kg/minute dose.

TJC has determined that using the "Rule of Six" or other methods to individualize a concentration of a high-alert drug for a specific patient (ie, use of a nonstandardized concentration) is **not** in compliance with the requirement of the above NPSG goal. In addition, the "Rule of Six" is not recommended by the Institute for Safe Medication Practices (ISMP). Limiting and standardizing the number of drug concentrations (as opposed to using the "Rule of Six") is thought to be safer and less error prone.

REFERENCES

Campbell MM, Taeubel MA, Kraus DM. Updated bedside charts for calculating pediatric doses of emergency medications. *Am J Hosp Pharm.* 1994;51(17):2147-2152.

Hodding JH, Executive Director, Pharmacy and Nutritional Services, Long Beach Memorial Medical Center and Miller Children's Hospital, Long Beach, CA, personal correspondence, April 2010.

Joint Commission on Accreditation of Healthcare Organizations (JCAHO). 2004 national patient safety goals, frequently asked questions: updated 8/30/04. August 30, 2004.

Joint Commission on Accreditation of Healthcare Organizations (JCAHO). Transition plan from 'rule of 6'. JCAHOnline, December 2004/January 2005.

Larsen GY, Parker HB, Cash J, O'Connell M, Grant MC. Standard drug concentrations and smart-pump technology reduce continuous-medication-infusion errors in pediatric patients. *Pediatrics.* 2005;116(1):e21-e25.

NEWBORN RESUSCITATION ALGORITHM

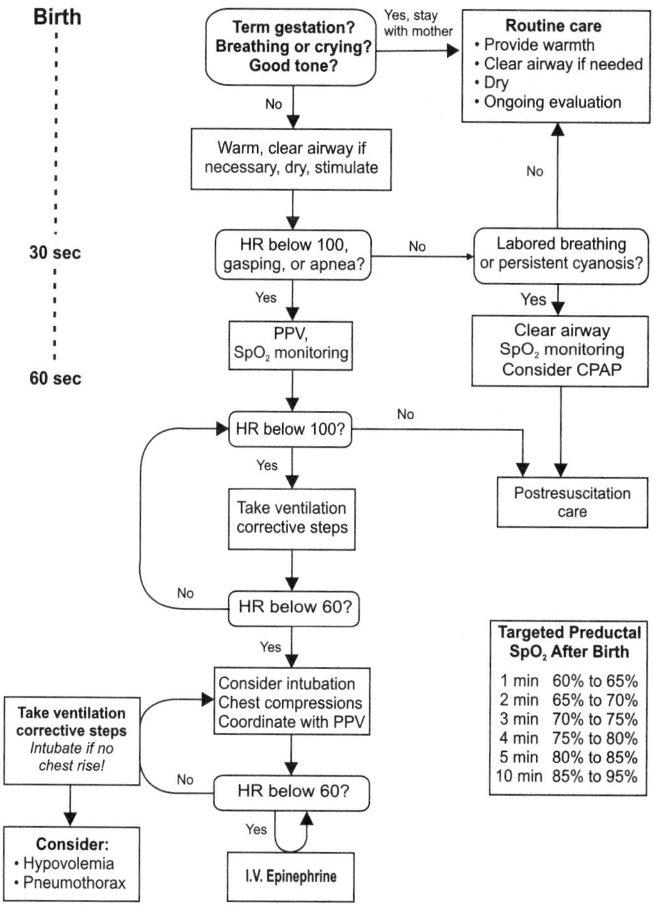

Targeted Preductal SpO_2 After Birth	
1 min	60% to 65%
2 min	65% to 70%
3 min	70% to 75%
4 min	75% to 80%
5 min	80% to 85%
10 min	85% to 95%

Epinephrine dose for neonatal resuscitation: I.V.: 0.01-0.03 mg/kg (0.1-0.3 mL/kg of **1:10,000** solution) every 3-5 minutes. **Note:** I.V. is the preferred neonatal route. While obtaining I.V. access, one may consider higher doses via E.T.: 0.05-0.1 mg/kg (0.5-1 mL/kg of **1:10,000** solution).

MATERNAL CARDIAC ARREST

First Responder

- Activate maternal cardiac arrest team
- Document time of onset of maternal cardiac arrest
- Place the patient supine
- Start chest compressions as per BLS algorithm; place hands slightly higher on sternum than usual

Subsequent Responders

Maternal Interventions

Treat per BLS and ACLS Algorithms

- Do not delay defibrillation
- Give typical ACLS drugs and doses
- Ventilate with 100% oxygen
- Monitor waveform capnography and CPR quality
- Provide post-cardiac arrest care as appropriate

Maternal Modifications

- Start I.V. above the diaphragm
- Assess for hypovolemia and give fluid bolus when required
- Anticipate difficult airway; experienced provider preferred for advanced airway placement
- If patient receiving I.V./I.O. magnesium prearrest, stop magnesium and give I.V./I.O. calcium chloride 10 mL in 10% solution, or calcium gluconate 30 mL in 10% solution
- Continue all maternal resuscitative interventions (CPR, positioning, defribrillation, drugs, and fluids) during and after cesarean section

Obstetric Interventions for Patient With an Obviously Gravid Uterus*

- Perform manual left uterine displacement (LUD) - displace uterus to the patient's left to relieve aortocaval compression
- Remove both internal and external fetal monitors if present

Obstetric and neonatal teams should immediately prepare for possible emergency cesarean section

- If no ROSC by 4 minutes of resuscitative efforts, consider performing immediate emergency cesarean section
- Aim for delivery within 5 minutes of onset of resuscitative efforts

*An obviously gravid uterus is a uterus that is deemed clinically to be sufficiently large to cause aortocaval compression

Search for and Treat Possible Contributing Factors (BEAU-CHOPS)

Bleeding/DIC
Embolism: Coronary/pulmonary/amniotic fluid embolism
Anesthetic complications
Uterine atony
Cardiac disease (MI/ischemia/aortic dissection/cardiomyopathy)
Hypertension/pre-eclampsia/eclampsia
Other: Differential diagnosis of standard ACLS guidelines
Placenta abruptio/previa
Sepsis

PEDIATRIC ALS (PALS) ALGORITHMS

Pediatric Bradycardia
With a Pulse and Poor Perfusion

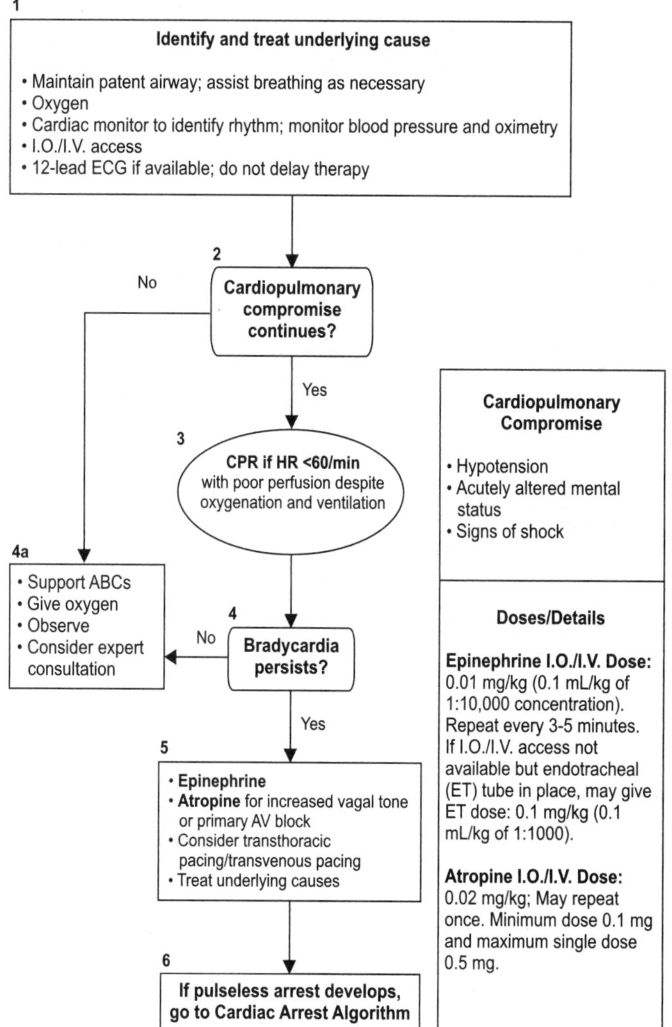

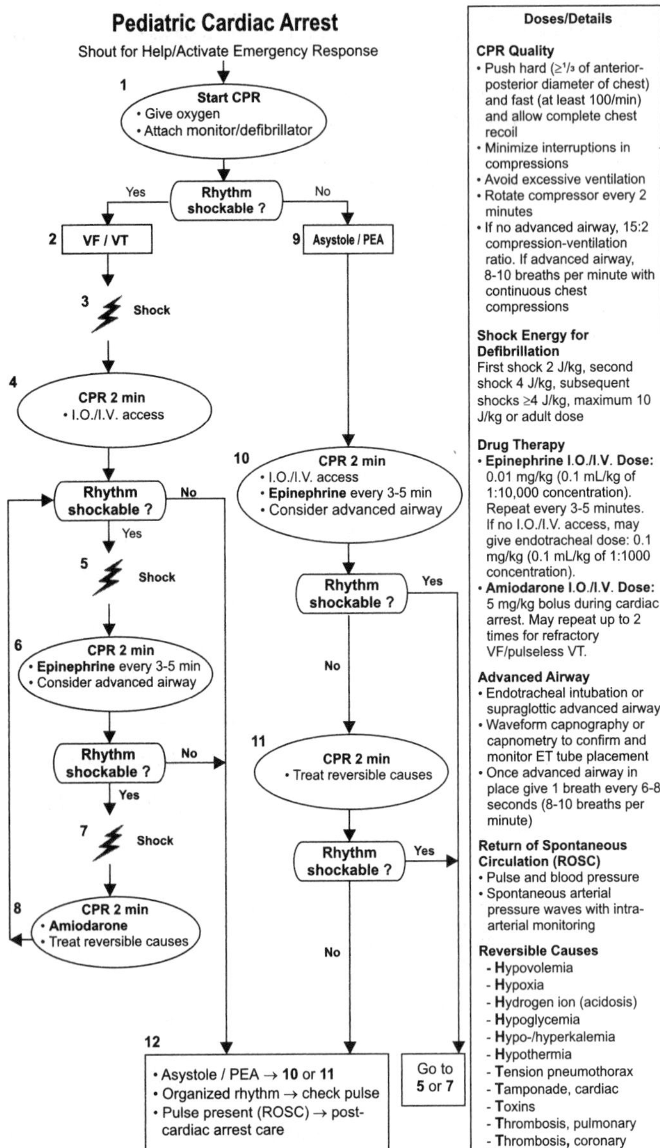
Pediatric Cardiac Arrest
Shout for Help/Activate Emergency Response
1 Start CPR
• Give oxygen
• Attach monitor/defibrillator
Rhythm shockable ?
Yes
No
2 VF / VT
3 Shock
4 CPR 2 min
• I.O./I.V. access
Rhythm shockable ?
No
Yes
5 Shock
6 CPR 2 min
• Epinephrine every 3-5 min
• Consider advanced airway
Rhythm shockable ?
No
Yes
7 Shock
8 CPR 2 min
• Amiodarone
• Treat reversible causes
9 Asystole / PEA
10 CPR 2 min
• I.O./I.V. access
• Epinephrine every 3-5 min
• Consider advanced airway
Rhythm shockable ?
Yes
No
11 CPR 2 min
• Treat reversible causes
Rhythm shockable ?
Yes
No
12
• Asystole / PEA → 10 or 11
• Organized rhythm → check pulse
• Pulse present (ROSC) → post-cardiac arrest care
Go to 5 or 7
Doses/Details
CPR Quality
• Push hard (≥1/3 of anterior-posterior diameter of chest) and fast (at least 100/min) and allow complete chest recoil
• Minimize interruptions in compressions
• Avoid excessive ventilation
• Rotate compressor every 2 minutes
• If no advanced airway, 15:2 compression-ventilation ratio. If advanced airway, 8-10 breaths per minute with continuous chest compressions
Shock Energy for Defibrillation
First shock 2 J/kg, second shock 4 J/kg, subsequent shocks ≥4 J/kg, maximum 10 J/kg or adult dose
Drug Therapy
• Epinephrine I.O./I.V. Dose: 0.01 mg/kg (0.1 mL/kg of 1:10,000 concentration). Repeat every 3-5 minutes. If no I.O./I.V. access, may give endotracheal dose: 0.1 mg/kg (0.1 mL/kg of 1:1000 concentration).
• Amiodarone I.O./I.V. Dose: 5 mg/kg bolus during cardiac arrest. May repeat up to 2 times for refractory VF/pulseless VT.
Advanced Airway
• Endotracheal intubation or supraglottic advanced airway
• Waveform capnography or capnometry to confirm and monitor ET tube placement
• Once advanced airway in place give 1 breath every 6-8 seconds (8-10 breaths per minute)
Return of Spontaneous Circulation (ROSC)
• Pulse and blood pressure
• Spontaneous arterial pressure waves with intra-arterial monitoring
Reversible Causes
- Hypovolemia
- Hypoxia
- Hydrogen ion (acidosis)
- Hypoglycemia
- Hypo-/hyperkalemia
- Hypothermia
- Tension pneumothorax
- Tamponade, cardiac
- Toxins
- Thrombosis, pulmonary
- Thrombosis, coronary

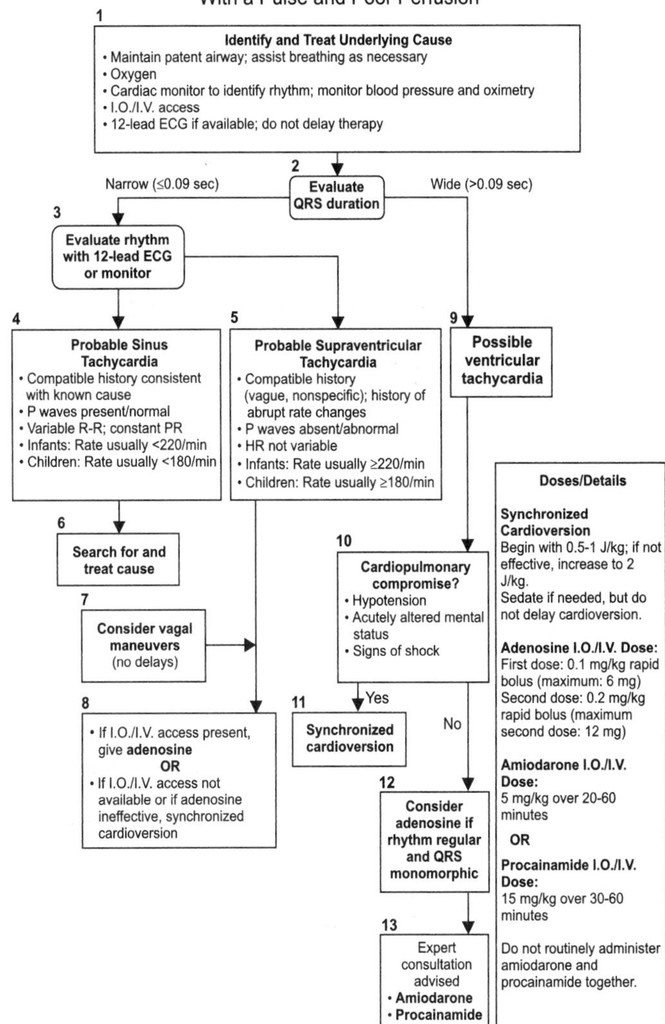
Pediatric Tachycardia
With a Pulse and Poor Perfusion
1
Identify and Treat Underlying Cause
• Maintain patent airway; assist breathing as necessary
• Oxygen
• Cardiac monitor to identify rhythm; monitor blood pressure and oximetry
• I.O./I.V. access
• 12-lead ECG if available; do not delay therapy
2
Evaluate QRS duration
Narrow (≤0.09 sec)
Wide (>0.09 sec)
3
Evaluate rhythm with 12-lead ECG or monitor
4
Probable Sinus Tachycardia
• Compatible history consistent with known cause
• P waves present/normal
• Variable R-R; constant PR
• Infants: Rate usually <220/min
• Children: Rate usually <180/min
5
Probable Supraventricular Tachycardia
• Compatible history (vague, nonspecific); history of abrupt rate changes
• P waves absent/abnormal
• HR not variable
• Infants: Rate usually ≥220/min
• Children: Rate usually ≥180/min
9
Possible ventricular tachycardia
6
Search for and treat cause
7
Consider vagal maneuvers (no delays)
8
• If I.O./I.V. access present, give adenosine
OR
• If I.O./I.V. access not available or if adenosine ineffective, synchronized cardioversion
10
Cardiopulmonary compromise?
• Hypotension
• Acutely altered mental status
• Signs of shock
Yes
No
11
Synchronized cardioversion
12
Consider adenosine if rhythm regular and QRS monomorphic
13
Expert consultation advised
• Amiodarone
• Procainamide
Doses/Details
Synchronized Cardioversion
Begin with 0.5-1 J/kg; if not effective, increase to 2 J/kg.
Sedate if needed, but do not delay cardioversion.
Adenosine I.O./I.V. Dose:
First dose: 0.1 mg/kg rapid bolus (maximum: 6 mg)
Second dose: 0.2 mg/kg rapid bolus (maximum second dose: 12 mg)
Amiodarone I.O./I.V. Dose:
5 mg/kg over 20-60 minutes
OR
Procainamide I.O./I.V. Dose:
15 mg/kg over 30-60 minutes
Do not routinely administer amiodarone and procainamide together.

ADULT ACLS ALGORITHMS

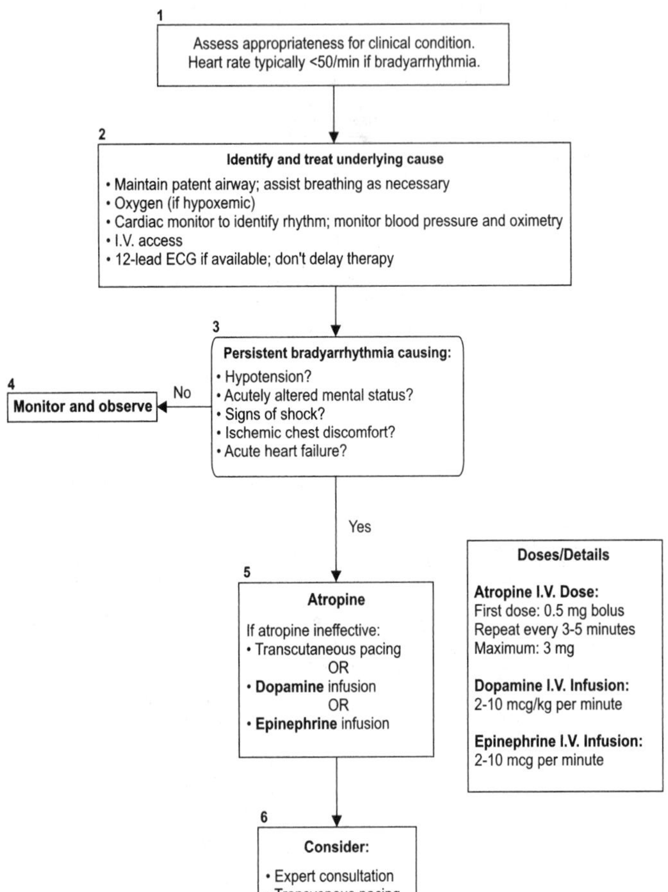
Adult Bradycardia
(With Pulse)
1
Assess appropriateness for clinical condition.
Heart rate typically <50/min if bradyarrhythmia.
2
Identify and treat underlying cause
• Maintain patent airway; assist breathing as necessary
• Oxygen (if hypoxemic)
• Cardiac monitor to identify rhythm; monitor blood pressure and oximetry
• I.V. access
• 12-lead ECG if available; don't delay therapy
3
Persistent bradyarrhythmia causing:
• Hypotension?
• Acutely altered mental status?
• Signs of shock?
• Ischemic chest discomfort?
• Acute heart failure?
No
4
Monitor and observe
Yes
5
Atropine
If atropine ineffective:
• Transcutaneous pacing
OR
• Dopamine infusion
OR
• Epinephrine infusion
6
Consider:
• Expert consultation
• Transvenous pacing
Doses/Details
Atropine I.V. Dose:
First dose: 0.5 mg bolus
Repeat every 3-5 minutes
Maximum: 3 mg
Dopamine I.V. Infusion:
2-10 mcg/kg per minute
Epinephrine I.V. Infusion:
2-10 mcg per minute

Adult Cardiac Arrest

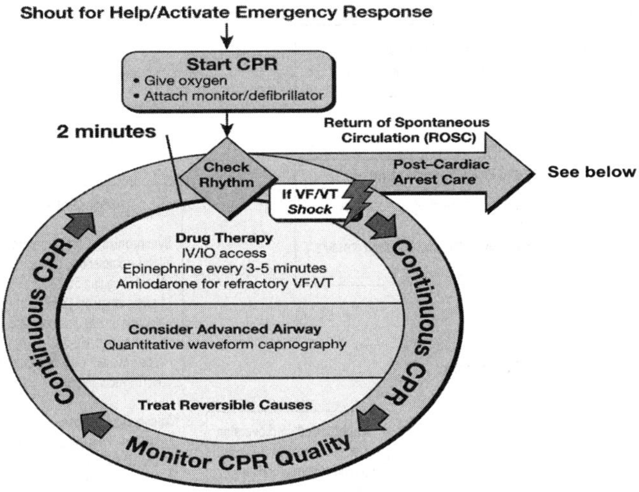

Shout for Help/Activate Emergency Response

Start CPR
- Give oxygen
- Attach monitor/defibrillator

2 minutes

Check Rhythm

Return of Spontaneous Circulation (ROSC)

Post–Cardiac Arrest Care

See below

If VF/VT *Shock*

Drug Therapy
IV/IO access
Epinephrine every 3-5 minutes
Amiodarone for refractory VF/VT

Consider Advanced Airway
Quantitative waveform capnography

Treat Reversible Causes

Continuous CPR

Continuous CPR

Monitor CPR Quality

CPR Quality

- Push hard (≥2 inches [5 cm]) and fast (≥100/min) and allow complete chest recoil
- Minimize interruptions in compressions
- Avoid excessive ventilation
- Rotate compressor every 2 minutes
- If no advanced airway, 30:2 compression-ventilation ratio
- Quantitative waveform capnography
  - If $PETCO_2$ <10 mm Hg, attempt to improve CPR quality
- Intra-arterial pressure
  - If relaxation phase (diastolic) pressure <20 mm Hg, attempt to improve CPR quality

Return of Spontaneous Circulation (ROSC)

- Pulse and blood pressure
- Abrupt sustained increase in $PETCO_2$ (typically ≥40 mm Hg)
- Spontaneous arterial pressure waves with intra-arterial monitoring

Shock Energy

- **Biphasic:** Manufacturer recommendation (120 to 200 J); if unknown, use maximum available. Second and subsequent doses should be equivalent, and higher doses may be considered.
- **Monophasic:** 360 J

Drug Therapy

- Epinephrine IV/I.O. Dose: 1 mg every 3 to 5 minutes
- Vasopressin IV/I.O. Dose: 40 units can replace first or second dose of epinephrine
- Amiodarone IV/I.O. Dose: First dose: 300 mg bolus; Second dose: 150 mg

Advanced Airway

- Supraglottic advanced airway or endotracheal intubation
- Waveform capnography to confirm and monitor ET tube placement
- 8 to 10 breaths per minute with continuous chest compressions

Reversible Causes

- **H**ypovolemia; **H**ypoxia; **H**ydrogen ion (acidosis); **H**ypo-/hyperkalemia; **H**ypothermia
- **T**ension pneumothorax; **T**amponade, cardiac; **T**oxins; **T**hrombosis, pulmonary; **T**hrombosis, coronary

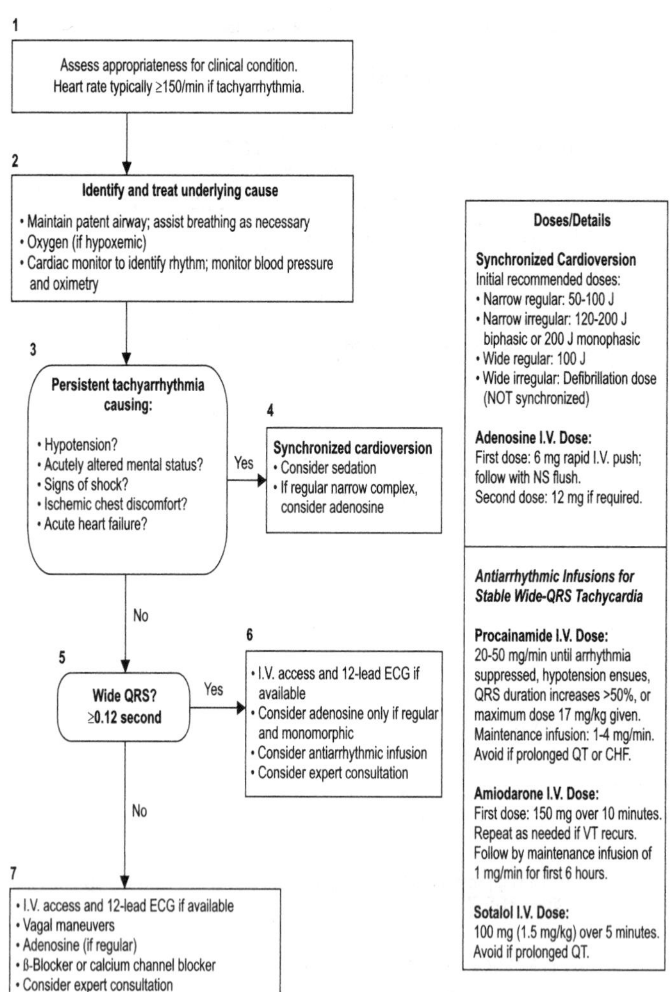

Adult Tachycardia
(With Pulse)
1
Assess appropriateness for clinical condition.
Heart rate typically ≥150/min if tachyarrhythmia.
2
Identify and treat underlying cause
• Maintain patent airway; assist breathing as necessary
• Oxygen (if hypoxemic)
• Cardiac monitor to identify rhythm; monitor blood pressure and oximetry
3
Persistent tachyarrhythmia causing:
• Hypotension?
• Acutely altered mental status?
• Signs of shock?
• Ischemic chest discomfort?
• Acute heart failure?
Yes
4
Synchronized cardioversion
• Consider sedation
• If regular narrow complex, consider adenosine
No
5
Wide QRS?
≥0.12 second
Yes
6
• I.V. access and 12-lead ECG if available
• Consider adenosine only if regular and monomorphic
• Consider antiarrhythmic infusion
• Consider expert consultation
No
7
• I.V. access and 12-lead ECG if available
• Vagal maneuvers
• Adenosine (if regular)
• ß-Blocker or calcium channel blocker
• Consider expert consultation
Doses/Details
Synchronized Cardioversion
Initial recommended doses:
• Narrow regular: 50-100 J
• Narrow irregular: 120-200 J biphasic or 200 J monophasic
• Wide regular: 100 J
• Wide irregular: Defibrillation dose (NOT synchronized)
Adenosine I.V. Dose:
First dose: 6 mg rapid I.V. push; follow with NS flush.
Second dose: 12 mg if required.
Antiarrhythmic Infusions for Stable Wide-QRS Tachycardia
Procainamide I.V. Dose:
20-50 mg/min until arrhythmia suppressed, hypotension ensues, QRS duration increases >50%, or maximum dose 17 mg/kg given.
Maintenance infusion: 1-4 mg/min.
Avoid if prolonged QT or CHF.
Amiodarone I.V. Dose:
First dose: 150 mg over 10 minutes.
Repeat as needed if VT recurs.
Follow by maintenance infusion of 1 mg/min for first 6 hours.
Sotalol I.V. Dose:
100 mg (1.5 mg/kg) over 5 minutes.
Avoid if prolonged QT.

Note: Sotalol injection is no longer available.

Reprinted with permission: 2010 American Heart Association guidelines for cardiopulmonary resuscitation and emergency cardiovascular care – Part 8: adult advanced cardiovascular life support. *Circulation*. 2010;122(Suppl 3):S729-S767. ©2010 American Heart Association, Inc.

See http://circ.ahajournals.org/cgi/content/full/122/18_suppl_3/S729.

All requests to use this information must go through the AHA.

NORMAL PEDIATRIC HEART RATES

Age	Mean Heart Rate (beats/minute)	Heart Rate Range (2nd to 98th percentile)
<1 d	123	93 to 154
1 to 2 d	123	91 to 159
3 to 6 d	129	91 to 166
1 to 3 wk	148	107 to 182
1 to 2 mo	149	121 to 179
3 to 5 mo	141	106 to 186
6 to 11 mo	134	109 to 169
1 to 2 y	119	89 to 151
3 to 4 y	108	73 to 137
5 to 7 y	100	65 to 133
8 to 11 y	91	62 to 130
12 to 15 y	85	60 to 119

Adapted from: *The Harriet Lane Handbook*. 12th ed. Greene MG, ed. St Louis, MO: Mosby Yearbook; 1991.

Normal QRS Axes (in degrees)

Age	Mean	Range
1 wk to 1 mo	+110	+30 to +180
1 to 3 mo	+70	+10 to +125
3 mo to 3 y	+60	+10 to +110
>3 y	+60	+20 to +120
Adults	+50	–30 to +105

INTERVALS AND SEGMENTS OF AN ECG CYCLE

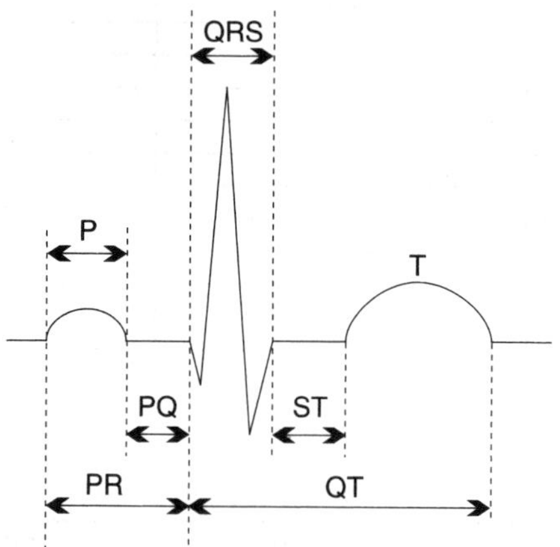

HEXAXIAL REFERENCE SYSTEM

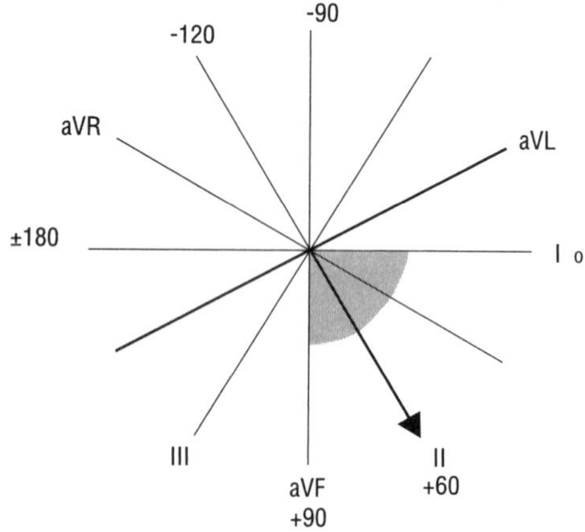

NORMAL RESPIRATORY RATES

Hour After Birth	Average Respiratory Rate	Range
1st hour	60 breaths/minute	20 to 100
2 to 6 hours	50 breaths/minute	20 to 80
>6 hours	30 to 40 breaths/minute	20 to 60

Age (years)	Mean RR (breaths/minute)
0 to 2	25 to 30
3 to 9	20 to 25
10 to 18	16 to 20

MEASURING PEDIATRIC BLOOD PRESSURE

Figure 1. Determination of Proper Cuff Size, Step 1

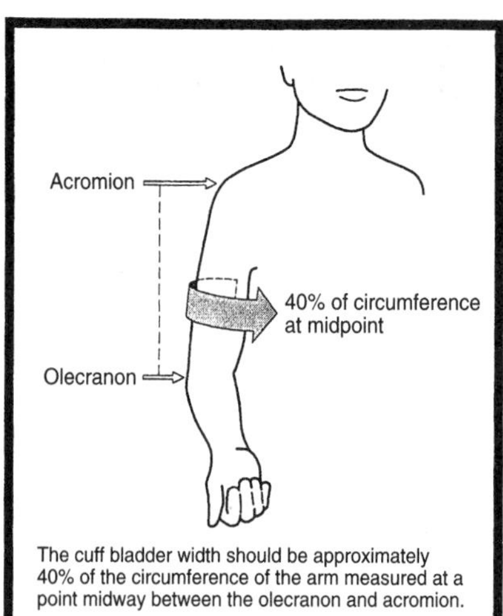
Acromion
40% of circumference
at midpoint
Olecranon
The cuff bladder width should be approximately
40% of the circumference of the arm measured at a
point midway between the olecranon and acromion.

Figure 2. Determination of Proper Cuff Size, Step 2

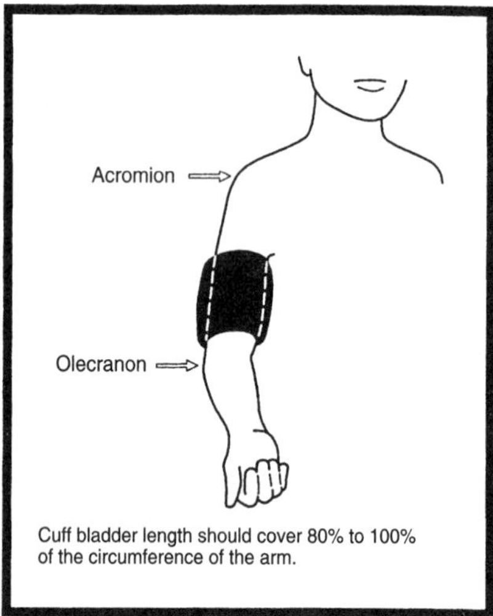
Acromion
Olecranon
Cuff bladder length should cover 80% to 100%
of the circumference of the arm.

Figure 3. Blood Pressure Measurement

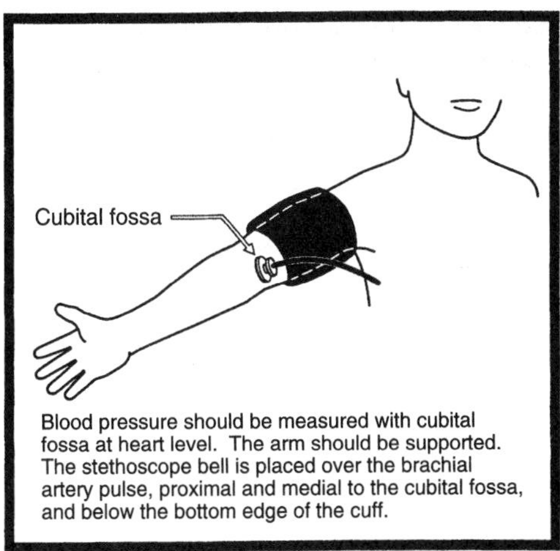

Blood pressure should be measured with cubital fossa at heart level. The arm should be supported. The stethoscope bell is placed over the brachial artery pulse, proximal and medial to the cubital fossa, and below the bottom edge of the cuff.

Used with permission: Perloff D, Grim C, Flack J, et al, "Human Blood Pressure Determination by Sphygmomanometry," *Circulation*, 1993, 88:2460-7.

HYPOTENSION, DEFINITIONS BY AGE GROUP

Hypotension is a *systolic* blood pressure <5th percentile of normal for age, namely:

- <60 mm Hg in term neonates (0 to 28 days)
- <70 mm Hg in infants (1 to 12 months)
- <70 mm Hg + (2 x age in years) in children 1 to 10 years
- <90 mm Hg in children ≥10 years of age

REFERENCE

American Heart Association Emergency Cardiovascular Care Committee. 2005 American Heart Association (AHA) guidelines for cardiopulmonary resuscitation (CPR) and emergency cardiovascular care (ECC). *Circulation*. 2005;112(24 Suppl):IV-167.

HYPERTENSION, CLASSIFICATION BY AGE GROUP[1]

Age Group	Significant Hypertension (mm Hg)	Severe Hypertension (mm Hg)
Newborn (7 d)		
systolic BP	≥96	≥106
Newborn (8 to 30 d)		
systolic BP	≥104	≥110
Infant (<2 y)		
systolic BP	≥112	≥118
diastolic BP	≥74	≥82
Children (3 to 5 y)		
systolic BP	≥116	≥124
diastolic BP	≥76	≥84
Children (6 to 9 y)		
systolic BP	≥122	≥130
diastolic BP	≥78	≥86
Children (10 to 12 y)		
systolic BP	≥126	≥134
diastolic BP	≥82	≥90
Adolescents (13 to 15 y)		
systolic BP	≥136	≥144
diastolic BP	≥86	≥92
Adolescents (16 to 18 y)		
systolic BP	≥142	≥150
diastolic BP	≥92	≥98

Adapted from Horan MJ. *Pediatrics*. 1987;79:1-25.

[1]See also Blood Pressure Measurement, Age Specific Percentiles, and 90th and 95th Percentiles of Blood Pressure by Percentiles of Height

BLOOD PRESSURE IN PREMATURE INFANTS, NORMAL

(Birth weight 600 to 1,750 g)[1]

Day	600 to 999 g		1,000 to 1,249 g	
	S (± 2SD)	D (± 2SD)	S (± 2SD)	D (± 2SD)
1	37.9 (17.4)	23.2 (10.3)	44 (22.8)	22.5 (13.5)
3	44.9 (15.7)	30.6 (12.3)	48 (15.4)	36.5 (9.6)
7	50 (14.8)	30.4 (12.4)	57 (14)	42.5 (16.5)
14	50.2 (14.8)	37.4 (12)	53 (30)	
28	61 (23.5)	45.8 (27.4)	57 (30)	
Day	**1,250 to 1,499 g**		**1,500 to 1,750 g**	
	S (± 2SD)	D (± 2SD)	S (± 2SD)	D (± 2SD)
1	48 (18)	27 (12.4)	47 (15.8)	26 (15.6)
3	59 (21.1)	40 (13.7)	51 (18.2)	35 (10)
7	68 (14.8)	40 (11.3)	66 (23)	41 (24)
14	64 (21.2)	36 (24.2)	76 (34.8)	42 (20.3)
28	69 (31.4)	44 (26.2)	73 (5.6)	50 (9.9)

[1]Blood pressure was obtained by the Dinamap method

S = systolic, D = diastolic, SD = standard deviation

Modified from Ingelfinger JR, Powers L, Epstein MF. Blood pressure norms in low-weight infants: birth through four weeks. *Pediatr Res.* 1983;17:319A.

BLOOD PRESSURE MEASUREMENTS, AGE-SPECIFIC PERCENTILES

Blood Pressure Measurements: Ages 0 to 12 Months, BOYS

Korotkoff phase IV (K4) used for diastolic BP. Reproduced with permission from Horan MJ. *Pediatrics*. 1987;79:11-25.

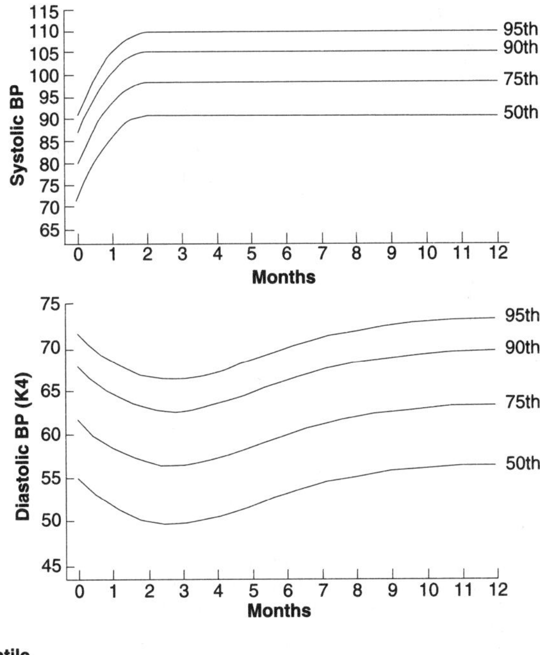

90th Percentile													
Systolic BP	87	101	106	106	106	105	105	105	105	105	105	105	105
Diastolic BP	68	65	63	63	63	65	66	67	68	68	69	69	69
Height cm	51	59	63	66	68	70	72	73	74	76	77	78	80
Weight kg	4	4	5	5	6	7	8	9	9	10	10	11	11

Blood Pressure Measurements: Ages 0 to 12 Months, GIRLS

Korotkoff phase IV (K4) used for diastolic BP. Reproduced with permission from Horan MJ. *Pediatrics*. 1987;79:11-25.

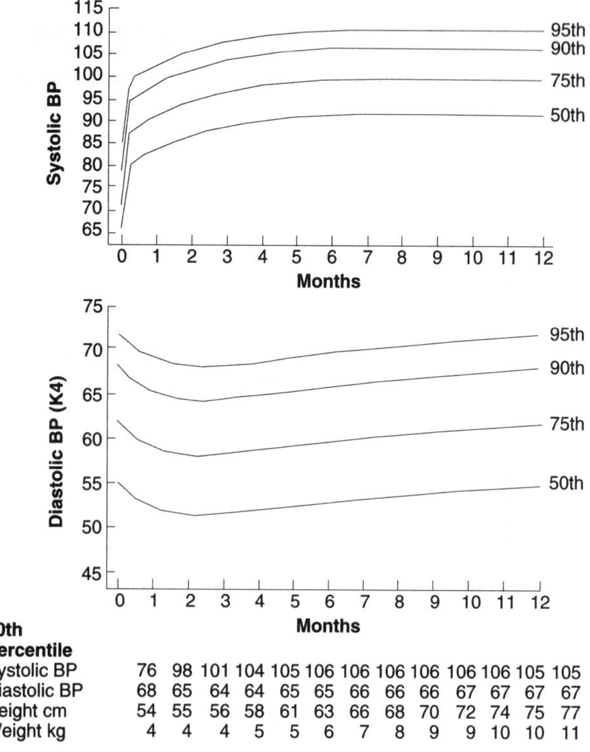

90th Percentile													
Systolic BP	76	98	101	104	105	106	106	106	106	106	106	105	105
Diastolic BP	68	65	64	64	65	65	66	66	66	67	67	67	67
Height cm	54	55	56	58	61	63	66	68	70	72	74	75	77
Weight kg	4	4	4	5	5	6	7	8	9	9	10	10	11

Blood Pressure Levels for BOYS by Age and Height Percentile

Age (y)	BP Percentile[1]	Systolic BP (mm Hg)							Diastolic BP (mm Hg)[2]						
		Height Percentile[3]													
		5%	10%	25%	50%	75%	90%	95%	5%	10%	25%	50%	75%	90%	95%
1	50th	80	81	83	85	87	88	89	34	35	36	37	38	39	39
	90th	94	95	97	99	100	102	103	49	50	51	52	53	53	54
	95th	98	99	101	103	104	106	106	54	54	55	56	57	58	58
	99th	105	106	108	110	112	113	114	61	62	63	64	65	66	66
2	50th	84	85	87	88	90	92	92	39	40	41	42	43	44	44
	90th	97	99	100	102	104	105	106	54	55	56	57	58	58	59
	95th	101	102	104	106	108	109	110	59	59	60	61	62	63	63
	99th	109	110	111	113	115	117	117	66	67	68	69	70	71	71
3	50th	86	87	89	91	93	94	95	44	44	45	46	47	48	48
	90th	100	101	103	105	107	108	109	59	59	60	61	62	63	63
	95th	104	105	107	109	110	112	113	63	63	64	65	66	67	67
	99th	111	112	114	116	118	119	120	71	71	72	73	74	75	75
4	50th	88	89	91	93	95	96	97	47	48	49	50	51	51	52
	90th	102	103	105	107	109	110	111	62	63	64	65	66	66	67
	95th	106	107	109	111	112	114	115	66	67	68	69	70	71	71
	99th	113	114	116	118	120	121	122	74	75	76	77	78	78	79
5	50th	90	91	93	95	96	98	98	50	51	52	53	54	55	55
	90th	104	105	106	108	110	111	112	65	66	67	68	69	69	70
	95th	108	109	110	112	114	115	116	69	70	71	72	73	74	74
	99th	115	116	118	120	121	123	123	77	78	79	80	81	81	82
6	50th	91	92	94	96	98	99	100	53	53	54	55	56	57	57
	90th	105	106	108	110	111	113	113	68	68	69	70	71	72	72
	95th	109	110	112	114	115	117	117	72	72	73	74	75	76	76
	99th	116	117	119	121	123	124	125	80	80	81	82	83	84	84
7	50th	92	94	95	97	99	100	101	55	55	56	57	58	59	59
	90th	106	107	109	111	113	114	115	70	70	71	72	73	74	74
	95th	110	111	113	115	117	118	119	74	74	75	76	77	78	78
	99th	117	118	120	122	124	125	126	82	82	83	84	85	86	86
8	50th	94	95	97	99	100	102	102	56	57	58	59	60	60	61
	90th	107	109	110	112	114	115	116	71	72	72	73	74	75	76
	95th	111	112	114	116	118	119	120	75	76	77	78	79	79	80
	99th	119	120	122	123	125	127	127	83	84	85	86	87	87	88

Blood Pressure Levels for BOYS by Age and Height Percentile *continued*

Age (y)	BP Percentile[1]	Systolic BP (mm Hg)							Diastolic BP (mm Hg)[2]						
		Height Percentile[3]													
		5%	10%	25%	50%	75%	90%	95%	5%	10%	25%	50%	75%	90%	95%
9	50th	95	96	98	100	102	103	104	57	58	59	60	61	61	62
	90th	109	110	112	114	115	117	118	72	73	74	75	76	76	77
	95th	113	114	116	118	119	121	121	76	77	78	79	80	81	81
	99th	120	121	123	125	127	128	129	84	85	86	87	88	88	89
10	50th	97	98	100	102	103	105	106	58	59	60	61	61	62	63
	90th	111	112	114	115	117	119	119	73	73	74	75	76	77	78
	95th	115	116	117	119	121	122	123	77	78	79	80	81	81	82
	99th	122	123	125	127	128	130	130	85	86	86	88	88	89	90
11	50th	99	100	102	104	105	107	107	59	59	60	61	62	63	63
	90th	113	114	115	117	119	120	121	74	74	75	76	77	78	78
	95th	117	118	119	121	123	124	125	78	78	79	80	81	82	82
	99th	124	125	127	129	130	132	132	86	86	87	88	89	90	90
12	50th	101	102	104	106	108	109	110	59	60	61	62	63	63	64
	90th	115	116	118	120	121	123	123	74	75	75	76	77	78	79
	95th	119	120	122	123	125	127	127	78	79	80	81	82	82	83
	99th	126	127	129	131	133	134	135	86	87	88	89	90	90	91
13	50th	104	105	106	108	110	111	112	60	60	61	62	63	64	64
	90th	117	118	120	122	124	125	126	75	75	76	77	78	79	79
	95th	121	122	124	126	128	129	130	79	79	80	81	82	83	83
	99th	128	130	131	133	135	136	137	87	87	88	89	90	91	91
14	50th	106	107	109	111	113	114	115	60	61	62	63	64	65	65
	90th	120	121	123	125	126	128	128	75	76	77	78	79	79	80
	95th	124	125	127	128	130	132	132	80	80	81	82	83	84	84
	99th	131	132	134	136	138	139	140	87	88	89	90	91	92	92
15	50th	109	110	112	113	115	117	117	61	62	63	64	65	66	66
	90th	122	124	125	127	129	130	131	76	77	78	79	80	80	81
	95th	126	127	129	131	133	134	135	81	81	82	83	84	85	85
	99th	134	135	136	138	140	142	142	88	89	90	91	92	93	93
16	50th	111	112	114	116	118	119	120	63	63	64	65	66	67	67
	90th	125	126	128	130	131	133	134	78	78	79	80	81	82	82
	95th	129	130	132	134	135	137	137	82	83	83	84	85	86	87
	99th	136	137	139	141	143	144	145	90	90	91	92	93	94	94

Blood Pressure Levels for BOYS by Age and Height Percentile *continued*

Age (y)	BP Percentile[1]	Systolic BP (mm Hg)							Diastolic BP (mm Hg)[2]						
		Height Percentile[3]													
		5%	10%	25%	50%	75%	90%	95%	5%	10%	25%	50%	75%	90%	95%
17	50th	114	115	116	118	120	121	122	65	66	66	67	68	69	70
	90th	127	128	130	132	134	135	136	80	80	81	82	83	84	84
	95th	131	132	134	136	138	139	140	84	85	86	87	87	88	89
	99th	139	140	141	143	145	146	147	92	93	93	94	95	96	97

[1]Blood pressure percentile determined by a single measurement

[2]Korotkoff phase V (K5) used for diastolic BP

[3]Height percentile determined by standard growth curves

Source: National High Blood Pressure Education Program Working Group on High Blood Pressure in Children and Adolescents. The fourth report on the diagnosis, evaluation, and treatment of high blood pressure in children and adolescents. *Pediatrics*. 2004;114(2 Suppl 4th report):555-576.

Blood Pressure Levels for GIRLS by Age and Height Percentile

Age (y)	BP Percentile[1]	Systolic BP (mm Hg)							Diastolic BP (mm Hg)[2]						
		Height Percentile[3]													
		5%	10%	25%	50%	75%	90%	95%	5%	10%	25%	50%	75%	90%	95%
1	50th	83	84	85	86	88	89	90	38	39	39	40	41	41	42
	90th	97	97	98	100	101	102	103	52	53	53	54	55	55	56
	95th	100	101	102	104	105	106	107	56	57	57	58	59	59	60
	99th	108	108	109	111	112	113	114	64	64	65	65	66	67	67
2	50th	85	85	87	88	89	91	91	43	44	44	45	46	46	47
	90th	98	99	100	101	103	104	105	57	58	58	59	60	61	61
	95th	102	103	104	105	107	108	109	61	62	62	63	64	65	65
	99th	109	110	111	112	114	115	116	69	69	70	70	71	72	72
3	50th	86	87	88	89	91	92	93	47	48	48	49	50	50	51
	90th	100	100	102	103	104	106	106	61	62	62	63	64	64	65
	95th	104	104	105	107	108	109	110	65	66	66	67	68	68	69
	99th	111	111	113	114	115	116	117	73	73	74	74	75	76	76
4	50th	88	88	90	91	92	94	94	50	50	51	52	52	53	54
	90th	101	102	103	104	106	107	108	64	64	65	66	67	67	68
	95th	105	106	107	108	110	111	112	68	68	69	70	71	71	72
	99th	112	113	114	115	117	118	119	76	76	76	77	78	79	79
5	50th	89	90	91	93	94	95	96	52	53	53	54	55	55	56
	90th	103	103	105	106	107	109	109	66	67	67	68	69	69	70
	95th	107	107	108	110	111	112	113	70	71	71	72	73	73	74
	99th	114	114	116	117	118	120	120	78	78	79	79	80	81	81
6	50th	91	92	93	94	96	97	98	54	54	55	56	56	57	58
	90th	104	105	106	108	109	110	111	68	68	69	70	70	71	72
	95th	108	109	110	111	113	114	115	72	72	73	74	74	75	76
	99th	115	116	117	119	120	121	122	80	80	80	81	82	83	83
7	50th	93	93	95	96	97	99	99	55	56	56	57	58	58	59
	90th	106	107	108	109	111	112	113	69	70	70	71	72	72	73
	95th	110	111	112	113	115	116	116	73	74	74	75	76	76	77
	99th	117	118	119	120	122	123	124	81	81	82	82	83	84	84
8	50th	95	95	96	98	99	100	101	57	57	57	58	59	60	60
	90th	108	109	110	111	113	114	114	71	71	71	72	73	74	74
	95th	112	112	114	115	116	118	118	75	75	75	76	77	78	78
	99th	119	120	121	122	123	125	125	82	82	83	83	84	85	86

Blood Pressure Levels for GIRLS by Age and Height Percentile *continued*

Age (y)	BP Percentile[1]	Systolic BP (mm Hg)							Diastolic BP (mm Hg)[2]						
		Height Percentile[3]													
		5%	10%	25%	50%	75%	90%	95%	5%	10%	25%	50%	75%	90%	95%
9	50th	96	97	98	100	101	102	103	58	58	58	59	60	61	61
	90th	110	110	112	113	114	116	116	72	72	72	73	74	75	75
	95th	114	114	115	117	118	119	120	76	76	76	77	78	79	79
	99th	121	121	123	124	125	127	127	83	83	84	84	85	86	87
10	50th	98	99	100	102	103	104	105	59	59	59	60	61	62	62
	90th	112	112	114	115	116	118	118	73	73	73	74	75	76	76
	95th	116	116	117	119	120	121	122	77	77	77	78	79	80	80
	99th	123	123	125	126	127	129	129	84	84	85	86	86	87	88
11	50th	100	101	102	103	105	106	107	60	60	60	61	62	63	63
	90th	114	114	116	117	118	119	120	74	74	74	75	76	77	77
	95th	118	118	119	121	122	123	124	78	78	78	79	80	81	81
	99th	125	125	126	128	129	130	131	85	85	86	87	87	88	89
12	50th	102	103	104	105	107	108	109	61	61	61	62	63	64	64
	90th	116	116	117	119	120	121	122	75	75	75	76	77	78	78
	95th	119	120	121	123	124	125	126	79	79	79	80	81	82	82
	99th	127	127	128	130	131	132	133	86	86	87	88	88	89	90
13	50th	104	105	106	107	109	110	110	62	62	62	63	64	65	65
	90th	117	118	119	121	122	123	124	76	76	76	77	78	79	79
	95th	121	122	123	124	126	127	128	80	80	80	81	82	83	83
	99th	128	129	130	132	133	134	135	87	87	88	89	89	90	91
14	50th	106	106	107	109	110	111	112	63	63	63	64	65	66	66
	90th	119	120	121	122	124	125	125	77	77	77	78	79	80	80
	95th	123	123	125	126	127	129	129	81	81	81	82	83	84	84
	99th	130	131	132	133	135	136	136	88	88	89	90	90	91	92
15	50th	107	108	109	110	111	113	113	64	64	64	65	66	67	67
	90th	120	121	122	123	125	126	127	78	78	78	79	80	81	81
	95th	124	125	126	127	129	130	131	82	82	82	83	84	85	85
	99th	131	132	133	134	136	137	138	89	89	90	91	91	92	93
16	50th	108	108	110	111	112	114	114	64	64	65	66	66	67	68
	90th	121	122	123	124	126	127	128	78	78	79	80	81	81	82
	95th	125	126	127	128	130	131	132	82	82	83	84	85	85	86
	99th	132	133	134	135	137	138	139	90	90	90	91	92	93	93

Blood Pressure Levels for GIRLS by Age and Height Percentile *continued*

Age (y)	BP Percentile[1]	Systolic BP (mm Hg)							Diastolic BP (mm Hg)[2]						
		Height Percentile[3]													
		5%	10%	25%	50%	75%	90%	95%	5%	10%	25%	50%	75%	90%	95%
17	50th	108	109	110	111	113	114	115	64	65	65	66	67	67	68
	90th	122	122	123	125	126	127	128	78	79	79	80	81	81	82
	95th	125	126	127	129	130	131	132	82	83	83	84	85	85	86
	99th	133	133	134	136	137	138	139	90	90	91	91	92	93	93

[1]Blood pressure percentile determined by a single measurement

[2]Korotkoff phase V (K5) used for diastolic BP

[3]Height percentile determined by standard growth curves

Source: National High Blood Pressure Education Program Working Group on High Blood Pressure in Children and Adolescents. The fourth report on the diagnosis, evaluation, and treatment of high blood pressure in children and adolescents. *Pediatrics*. 2004;114(2 Suppl 4th report):555-576.

NEW YORK HEART ASSOCIATION (NYHA) CLASSIFICATION OF FUNCTIONAL CAPACITY OF PATIENTS WITH DISEASES OF THE HEART, 1994 REVISIONS

Class I

Patients with cardiac disease but without resulting limitation of physical activity. Ordinary physical activity does not cause undue fatigue, palpitation, dyspnea, or anginal pain.

Class II

Patients with cardiac disease resulting in slight limitation of physical activity. They are comfortable at rest. Ordinary physical activity results in fatigue, palpitation, dyspnea, or anginal pain.

Class III

Patients with cardiac disease resulting in marked limitation of physical activity. They are comfortable at rest. Less than ordinary activity causes fatigue, palpitation, dyspnea, or anginal pain.

Class IV

Patients with cardiac disease resulting in inability to carry on any physical activity without discomfort. Symptoms of heart failure or the anginal syndrome may be present even at rest. If any physical activity is undertaken, discomfort increases.

REFERENCE

The Criteria Committee of the New York Heart Association. *Nomenclature and Criteria for Diagnosis of Diseases of the Heart and Great Vessels.* 9th ed. Boston, MA: Little, Brown & Co; 1994;253-256.

WORLD HEALTH ORGANIZATION (WHO) FUNCTIONAL CLASSIFICATION OF PULMONARY HYPERTENSION

Class I

Patients with pulmonary hypertension but without resulting limitation of physical activity. Ordinary physical activity does not cause undue dyspnea or fatigue, chest pain, or near syncope.

Class II

Patients with pulmonary hypertension resulting in slight limitation of physical activity. They are comfortable at rest. Ordinary physical activity causes undue dyspnea or fatigue, chest pain, or near syncope.

Class III

Patients with pulmonary hypertension resulting in marked limitation of physical activity. They are comfortable at rest. Less than ordinary activity causes undue dyspnea or fatigue, chest pain, or near syncope.

Class IV

Patients with pulmonary hypertension with inability to carry out any physical activity without symptoms. These patients manifest signs of right heart failure. Dyspnea and/or fatigue may be present even at rest. Discomfort is increased by any physical activity.

REFERENCE

Widlitz A, Barst RJ. Pulmonary arterial hypertension in children. *Eur Respir J.* 2003;21(1):155-176.

ANTIDEPRESSANT AGENTS

Comparison of Usual Adult Dosage, Mechanism of Action, and Adverse Effects

Drug	Initial Adult Dose	Usual Adult Dosage (mg/d)	Dosage Forms	Adverse Effects						Comments
				ACH	Drowsiness	Orthostatic Hypotension	Conduction Abnormalities	GI Distress	Weight Gain	
Tricyclic Antidepressants and Related Compounds[1]										
Amitriptyline	25 to 75 mg qhs	100 to 300	T	4+	4+	3+	3+	1+	4+	Also used in chronic pain, migraine, and as a hypnotic; contraindicated with cisapride
Amoxapine	50 mg 1 to 3 times daily	100 to 400	T	2+	2+	2+	2+	0	2+	May cause extrapyramidal symptom (EPS)
ClomiPRAMINE[2] (Anafranil)	25 to 75 mg qhs	100 to 250	C	4+	4+	2+	3+	1+	4+	Only approved for OCD
Desipramine (Norpramin)	25 to 50 mg/d	100 to 300	T	1+	2+	2+	2+	0	1+	Blood levels useful for therapeutic monitoring
Doxepin	25 to 75 mg qhs	100 to 300	C, L, T	3+	4+	2+	2+	0	4+	
Imipramine (Tofranil, Tofranil-PM)	25 to 75 mg qhs	100 to 300	T, C	3+	3+	4+	3+	1+	4+	Blood levels useful for therapeutic monitoring
Maprotiline	25 to 75 mg qhs	100 to 225	T	2+	3+	2+	2+	0	2+	
Nortriptyline (Pamelor)	25 to 50 mg qhs	50 to 150	C, L	2+	2+	1+	2+	0	1+	Blood levels useful for therapeutic monitoring
Protriptyline (Vivactil)	10 to 20 mg divided in 3 to 4 doses	15 to 60	T	2+	1+	2+	3+	1+	1+	
Trimipramine (Surmontil)	25 to 50 mg qhs	75 to 300	C	4+	4+	3+	3+	0	4+	
Selective Serotonin Reuptake Inhibitors[3]										
Citalopram (Celexa)	20 mg qAM	20 to 60	T, L	0	0	0	0	3+[4]	1+	
Escitalopram (Lexapro)	10 mg qAM	10 to 20	T, L	0	0	0	0	3+	1+	S-enantiomer of citalopram
FLUoxetine (PROzac, PROzac Weekly, Sarafem, Selfemra)	10 to 20 mg qAM	20 to 80	C, CDR, L, T	0	0	0	0	3+[4]	1+	CYP2B6 and 2D6 inhibitor
FluvoxaMINE[2] (Luvox CR)	50 to 100 mg qhs	100 to 300	T, CXR	0	0	0	0	3+[4]	1+	Contraindicated with pimozide, thioridazine, mesoridazine, CYP1A2, 2B6, 2C19, and 3A4 inhibitors
PARoxetine (Paxil, Paxil CR, Pexeva)	10 to 20 mg qAM	20 to 50	T, CXR, L	1+	1+	0	0	3+[4]	2+	CYP2B6 and 2D6 inhibitor
Sertraline (Zoloft)	25 to 50 mg qAM	50 to 200	T, L	0	0	0	0	3+[4]	1+	CYP2B6 and 2C19 inhibitor
Vilazodone (Viibryd)	10 mg qAM	10 to 40	T	0	0	0	0	3+	0	CYP2C8, 2C19, and 2D6 inhibitor; also is a 5-HT_{1A} partial agonist

Comparison of Usual Adult Dosage, Mechanism of Action, and Adverse Effects *continued*

Drug	Initial Adult Dose	Usual Adult Dosage (mg/d)	Dosage Forms	Adverse Effects: ACH	Drowsiness	Orthostatic Hypotension	Conduction Abnormalities	GI Distress	Weight Gain	Comments
Dopamine-Reuptake Blocking Compounds										
BuPROPion (Aplenzin, Buproban, Budeprion SR, Budeprion XL, Forfivo XL, Wellbutrin, Wellbutrin SR, Wellbutrin XL, Zyban)	100 mg bid-tid IR[5] 150 mg qAM-bid SR[6] 150 to 174 mg daily XR[7]	300 to 450	T, TSR, TXR	0	0	0	1+/0	1+	0	Contraindicated with seizures, bulimia, and anorexia; low incidence of sexual dysfunction IR: A 6-h interval between doses preferred SR: An 8-h interval between doses preferred XR: Administer once daily
Serotonin/Norepinephrine Reuptake Inhibitors[8]										
Desvenlafaxine (Pristiq)	50 mg/d	50 to 100	TXR	0	1+	1+	0	3+[4]	0	Active metabolite of venlafaxine
DULoxetine (Cymbalta)	40 to 60 mg/d	40 to 60	CDR	1+	1+	0	1+	3+	0	Also indicated for GAD, management of pain associated with diabetic neuropathy, and management of fibromyalgia
Levomilnacipran (Fetzima)	20 mg/d	20 to 120	CXR	1+	0	2+	1+	2+	0	1S,2R-enantiomer of milnacipram
Milnacipran[9] (Savella)	12.5 mg/d	100 to 200	T	2+	1+	0	1+	3+	0	Only indicated for fibromyalgia
Venlafaxine (Effexor, Effexor XR)	25 mg bid-tid IR 37.5 mg qd XR	75 to 375 IR 75 to 225 XR	T, TXR, CXR	1+	1+	0	1+	3+[4]	0	High-dose may be useful to treat refractory depression; frequency of hypertension increases with dosage >225 mg/d
5-HT_2 Receptor Antagonist Properties										
Nefazodone	25 to 100 mg bid	150 to 600	T	1+	1+	2+	1+	1+	0	Contraindicated with carbamazepine, pimozide, astemizole, cisapride, and terfenadine; caution with triazolam and alprazolam; low incidence of sexual dysfunction
TraZODone (Oleptro)	50 mg tid IR 150 mg qhs XR	150 to 600 IR 150 to 375 XR	T, TXR	0	4+	3+	1+	1+	2+	
5-HT_3 Receptor Antagonist Properties										
Vortioxetine (Brintellix)	10 mg/d	5 to 20	T	0	0	0	0	3+	0	Also is a 5-HT_{1A} agonist; moderate incidence of sexual dysfunction
Noradrenergic Antagonist										
Mirtazapine (Remeron, Remeron SolTab)	15 mg qhs	15 to 45	T, TOD	1+	3+	1+	1+	0	3+	Dose >15 mg/d less sedating, low incidence of sexual dysfunction

Comparison of Usual Adult Dosage, Mechanism of Action, and Adverse Effects *continued*

Drug	Initial Adult Dose	Usual Adult Dosage (mg/d)	Dosage Forms	Adverse Effects						Comments
				ACH	Drowsiness	Orthostatic Hypotension	Conduction Abnormalities	GI Distress	Weight Gain	
Monoamine Oxidase Inhibitors										
Isocarboxazid (Marplan)	10 mg tid	10 to 30	T	2+	2+	2+	1+	1+	2+	Diet must be low in tyramine; contraindicated with sympathomimetics and other antidepressants
Phenelzine (Nardil)	15 mg tid	15 to 90	T	2+	2+	2+	0	1+	3+	
Tranylcypromine (Parnate)	10 mg bid	10 to 60	T	2+	1+	2+	1+	1+	2+	
Selegiline (EmSam)	6 mg/d	6 to 12	Transdermal	2+	1+	2+	0	1+	0	Low tyramine diet not required for 6 mg/d dosage

ACH = anticholinergic effects (dry mouth, blurred vision, urinary retention, constipation); 0 - 4+ = absent or rare - relatively common; T = tablet; TSR = tablet, sustained release; TXR = tablet, extended release; TOD = tablet, orally disintegrating; L = liquid; C = capsule; CDR = capsule, delayed release; CXR = capsule, extended release; IR = immediate release; SR = sustained release; XR = extended release

[1]**Important note:** A 1-week supply taken all at once in a patient receiving the maximum dose can be fatal.

[2]Not approved by FDA for depression; approved for OCD

[3]Flat dose response curve, headache, nausea, and sexual dysfunction are common side effects for SSRIs.

[4]Nausea is usually mild and transient.

[5]IR: 100 mg bid; may be increased to 100 mg tid no sooner than 3 days after beginning therapy

[6]SR: 150 mg qAM; may be increased to 150 mg bid as early as day 4 of dosing. To minimize seizure risk, do not exceed SR 200 mg/dose.

[7]May be increased day 4 (treatment of depression) or after 1 week (treatment of SAD) of dosing.

[8]Do not use with sibutramine; relatively safe in overdose

[9]Milnacipran is only approved for fibromyalgia.

CORTICOSTEROIDS SYSTEMIC EQUIVALENCIES

Glucocorticoid	Approximate Equivalent Dose (mg)	Routes of Administration	Relative Anti-inflammatory Potency	Relative Mineralocorticoid Potency	Protein Binding (%)	Half-life Plasma (min)
Short-Acting						
Cortisone	25	PO, IM	0.8	0.8	90	30
Hydrocortisone	20	IM, IV	1	1	90	90
Intermediate-Acting						
MethylPREDNISolone[1]	4	PO, IM, IV	5	0	—	180
PrednisoLONE	5	PO, IM, IV, intra-articular, intradermal, soft tissue injection	4	0.8	90 to 95	200
PredniSONE	5	PO	4	0.8	70	60
Triamcinolone[1]	4	IM, intra-articular, intradermal, intrasynovial, soft tissue injection	5	0	—	300
Long-Acting						
Betamethasone	0.75	PO, IM, intra-articular, intradermal, intrasynovial, soft tissue injection	25	0	64	100 to 300
Dexamethasone	0.75	PO, IM, IV, intra-articular, intradermal, soft tissue injection	25 to 30	0	—	100 to 300
Mineralocorticoids						
Fludrocortisone	—	PO	10	125	42	200

[1]May contain propylene glycol as an excipient in injectable forms

Asare K. Diagnosis and treatment of adrenal insufficiency in the critically ill patient. *Pharmacotherapy.* 2007;27(11):1512-1528.

INHALED CORTICOSTEROIDS

Estimated Comparative Daily Dosage

Children ≥12 Years of Age and Adults

Drug	Low Daily Dose	Medium Daily Dose	High Daily Dose
Beclomethasone aerosol solution inhalation	80 to 240 mcg	>240 to 480 mcg	>480 mcg
Budesonide aerosol powder breath-activated inhalation	180 to 600 mcg	>600 to 1,200 mcg	>1,200 mcg
Ciclesonide HFA	160 to 320 mcg	>320 to 640 mcg	>640 mcg
Flunisolide aerosol solution inhalation	320 mcg	>320 to 640 mcg	>640 mcg
Fluticasone HFA	88 to 264 mcg	>264 to 440 mcg	>440 mcg
Fluticasone aerosol powder breath-activated inhalation	100 to 300 mcg	>300 to 500 mcg	>500 mcg
Mometasone aerosol powder breath-activated inhalation	200 mcg	400 mcg	>400 mcg

HFA = hydrofluoroalkane

Children <12 Years of Age

Drug	Low Daily Dose	Medium Daily Dose	High Daily Dose
Beclomethasone inhalation	0 to 4 years: NA 5 to 11 years: 80 to 160 mcg	0 to 4 years: NA 5 to 11 years: >160 to 320 mcg	0 to 4 years: NA 5 to 11 years: >320 mcg
Budesonide aerosol powder breath-activated inhalation	0 to 4 years: NA 5 to 11 years: 180 to 400 mcg	0 to 4 years: NA 5 to 11 years: >400 to 800 mcg	0 to 4 years: NA 5 to 11 years: >800 mcg
Budesonide nebulized	0 to 4 years: 0.25 to 0.5 mg 5 to 11 years: 0.5 mg	0 to 4 years: >0.5 to 1 mg 5 to 11 years: 1 mg	0 to 4 years: >1 mg 5 to 11 years: 2 mg
Ciclesonide HFA	0 to 4 years: NA 5 to 11 years: 80 to 160 mcg	0 to 4 years: NA 5 to 11 years: >160 to 320 mcg	0 to 4 years: NA 5 to 11 years: >320 mcg
Flunisolide aerosol solution inhalation	0 to 4 years: NA 5 to 11 years: 160 mcg	0 to 4 years: NA 5 to 11 years: 320 mcg	0 to 4 years: NA 5 to 11 years: ≥640 mcg
Fluticasone HFA	0 to 4 years: 176 mcg 5 to 11 years: 88 to 176 mcg	0 to 11 years: >176 to 352 mcg	0 to 11 years: >352 mcg
Fluticasone aerosol powder breath-activated inhalation	0 to 4 years: NA 5 to 11 years: 100 to 200 mcg	0 to 4 years: NA 5 to 11 years: >200 to 400 mcg	0 to 4 years: NA 5 to 11 years: >400 mcg
Mometasone aerosol powder breath-activated inhalation	NA	NA	NA

HFA = hydrofluoroalkane, NA = not approved for use in this age group or no data available

REFERENCE

Expert Panel Report 3. Guidelines for the diagnosis and management of asthma. *Clinical Practice Guidelines*, National Institutes of Health, National Heart, Lung, and Blood Institute, NIH Publication No. 08-4051. Available at http://www.nhlbi.nih.gov/guidelines/asthma/asthgdln.htm

TOPICAL CORTICOSTEROIDS

GUIDELINES FOR SELECTION AND USE OF TOPICAL CORTICOSTEROIDS

The quantity prescribed and the frequency of refills should be monitored to reduce the risk of adrenal suppression. In general, short courses of high-potency agents are preferable to prolonged use of low potency. After control is achieved, control should be maintained with a low potency preparation.

1. Low- to medium-potency agents are usually effective for treating thin, acute, inflammatory skin lesions; whereas, high or super-potent agents are often required for treating chronic, hyperkeratotic, or lichenified lesions.
2. Since the stratum corneum is thin on the face and intertriginous areas, low-potency agents are preferred but a higher potency agent may be used for 2 weeks.
3. Because the palms and soles have a thick stratum corneum, high or super-potent agents are frequently required.
4. Low potency agents are preferred for infants and the elderly. Infants have a high body surface area to weight ratio; elderly patients have thin, fragile skin.
5. The vehicle in which the topical corticosteroid is formulated influences the absorption and potency of the drug. Ointment bases are preferred for thick, lichenified lesions; they enhance penetration of the drug. Creams are preferred for acute and subacute dermatoses; they may be used on moist skin areas or intertriginous areas. Solutions, gels, and sprays are preferred for the scalp or for areas where a nonoil-based vehicle is needed.
6. In general, super-potent agents should not be used for longer than 2 to 3 weeks unless the lesion is limited to a small body area. Medium- to high-potency agents usually cause only rare adverse effects when treatment is limited to 3 months or less, and use on the face and intertriginous areas are avoided. If long-term treatment is needed, intermittent vs continued treatment is recommended.
7. Most preparations are applied once or twice daily. More frequent application may be necessary for the palms or soles because the preparation is easily removed by normal activity and penetration is poor due to a thick stratum corneum. Every-other-day or weekend-only application may be effective for treating some chronic conditions.

Relative Potency of Selected Topical Corticosteroids

Steroid		Dosage Form
	Very High Potency	
0.05%	Betamethasone dipropionate, augmented	Gel, lotion, ointment
0.05%	Clobetasol propionate	Cream, foam, gel, lotion, ointment, shampoo, spray
0.05%	Diflorasone diacetate	Ointment
0.05%	Halobetasol propionate	Cream, ointment
	High Potency	
0.1%	Amcinonide	Cream, ointment, lotion
0.05%	Betamethasone dipropionate, augmented	Cream
0.05%	Betamethasone dipropionate	Cream, ointment
0.1%	Betamethasone valerate	Ointment
0.05%	Desoximetasone	Gel
0.25%	Desoximetasone	Cream, ointment
0.05%	Diflorasone diacetate	Cream, ointment
0.05%	Fluocinonide	Cream, ointment, gel
0.1%	Halcinonide	Cream, ointment
0.5%	Triamcinolone acetonide	Cream, spray
	Intermediate Potency	
0.05%	Betamethasone dipropionate	Lotion
0.1%	Betamethasone valerate	Cream
0.1%	Clocortolone pivalate	Cream
0.05%	Desoximetasone	Cream
0.1%	Diflucortolone	Cream, oily cream, ointment
0.02%	Flumethasone pivalate	Cream
0.025%	Fluocinolone acetonide	Cream, ointment
0.05%	Flurandrenolide	Cream, ointment, lotion, tape
0.005%	Fluticasone propionate	Ointment
0.05%	Fluticasone propionate	Cream, lotion
0.1%	Hydrocortisone butyrate[1]	Ointment, solution
0.2%	Hydrocortisone valerate[1]	Cream, ointment
0.1%	Mometasone furoate[1]	Cream, ointment, lotion

Relative Potency of Selected Topical Corticosteroids *(continued)*

Steroid		Dosage Form
0.1%	Prednicarbate	Cream, ointment
0.025%	Triamcinolone acetonide	Cream, ointment, lotion
0.1%	Triamcinolone acetonide	Cream, ointment, lotion
	Low Potency	
0.05%	Alclometasone dipropionate[1]	Cream, ointment
0.05%	Desonide	Cream, ointment
0.01%	Fluocinolone acetonide	Cream, solution
0.5%	Hydrocortisone[1]	Cream, ointment, lotion
0.5%	Hydrocortisone acetate[1]	Cream, ointment
1%	Hydrocortisone acetate[1]	Cream, ointment
1%	Hydrocortisone[1]	Cream, ointment, lotion, solution
2.5%	Hydrocortisone[1]	Cream, ointment, lotion

[1]Not fluorinated

IMMUNE GLOBULIN PRODUCT COMPARISON

Brand Name	Concentration	pH	Initial Rate		Max Rate		IgA Content (mcg/mL)	Osmolarity/ Osmolality (mOsmol/kg)	Comments
			IV	SubQ[1]	IV[2]	SubQ[1]			
Bivigam	10%	4 to 4.6	0.3 mL/kg/h	–	3.6 mL/kg/h	–	≤200	Not available	Contains polysorbate 80
Carimune NF[3]	3%	6.4 to 6.8	1 mL/kg/h	–	6 mL/kg/h	–	Trace[4]	192 to 498[5]	Contains sucrose
	12%		0.24 mL/kg/h		1.5 mL/kg/h			768 to 1074[5]	
Flebogamma DIF	5%	5 to 6	0.6 mL/kg/h	–	6 mL/kg/h	–	<50	240 to 370	
	10%		0.6 mL/kg/h		4.8 mL/kg/h		<100		
GamaSTAN S/D	15% to 18%	6.4 to 7.2	–	–	–	–	Not available	Not available	For IM use
Gammagard S/D	5%	6.4 to 7.2	0.5 mL/kg/h	–	4 mL/kg/h	–	≤1[6]	636	Contains polysorbate 80
	10%		0.5 mL/kg/h		8 mL/kg/h		≤2[6]	1,250	
Gammagard Liquid	10%	4.6 to 5.1	0.5 mL/kg/h	<40 kg: 15 mL/h/site with a maximum of 8 sites ≥40 kg: 20 mL/h/site with a maximum of 8 sites	5 mL/kg/h 5.4 mL/kg/h (MMN only)	<40 kg: 20 mL/h/site with a maximum of 8 sites; maximum **total** rate: 160 mL/h ≥40 kg: 30 mL/h/site with a maximum of 8 sites; maximum **total** rate: 240 mL/h	37	240 to 300	
Gammaked	10%	4 to 4.5	0.6 mL/kg/h 1.2 mL/kg/h (CIDP only)	20 mL/h/site with a maximum of 8 sites	4.8 mL/kg/h	Not determined	46	258	
Gammaplex	5%	4.8 to 5	0.6 mL/kg/h	–	4.8 mL/kg/h	–	<10	420 to 500	Contains polysorbate 80
Gamunex-C	10%	4 to 4.5	0.6 mL/kg/h 1.2 mL/kg/h (CIDP only)	20 mL/h/site with a maximum of 8 sites	4.8 mL/kg/h	Not determined	46	258	
Hizentra	20%	4.6 to 5.2	–	15 mL/h/site with a maximum of 4 sites	–	Up to 25 mL/h/site with a maximum of 4 sites; maximum **total** rate: 50 mL/h	≤50	380	Contains L-proline and polysorbate 80

continued

Brand Name	Concentration	pH	Initial Rate		Max Rate		IgA Content (mcg/mL)	Osmolarity/ Osmolality (mOsmol/kg)	Comments
			IV	SubQ[1]	IV[2]	SubQ[1]			
HyQvia	10%	4.6 to 5.1	–	*First 2 infusions:* <40 kg: 5 mL/h for 5 to 15 min; 10 mL/h for 5 to 15 min; 20 mL/h for 5 to 15 min; 40 mL/h for 5 to 15 min; then 80 mL/h for remainder of infusion ≥40 kg: 10 mL/h for 5 to 15 min; 30 mL/h for 5 to 15 min; 60 mL/h for 5 to 15 min; 120 mL/h for 5 to 15 min; then 240 mL/h for remainder of infusion *Next 2 or 3 infusions:* <40 kg: 10 mL/h for 5 to 15 min; 20 mL/h for 5 to 15 min; 40 mL/h for 5 to 15 min; 80 mL/h for 5 to 15 min; then 160 mL/h for remainder of infusion ≥40 kg: 10 mL/h for 5 to 15 min; 30 mL/h for 5 to 15 min; 120 mL/h for 5 to 15 min; 240 mL/h for 5 to 15 min; then 300 mL/h for remainder of infusion	–	<40 kg: 160 mL/h ≥40 kg: 300 mL/h	37	240 to 300	Supplied with hyaluronidase (human recombinant)
Octagam	5%	5.1 to 6	0.6 mL/kg/h	–	4 mL/kg/h	–	≤200	310 to 380	Contains maltose
Octagam	10%	4.5 to 5	0.6 mL/kg/h	–	7.2 mL/kg/h	–	106	310 to 380	Sucrose-free
Privigen	10%	4.6 to 5	0.3 mL/kg/h	–	2.4 mL/kg/h (ITP) 4.8 mL/kg/h	–	≤25	240 to 440	Contains L-proline

CIDP = chronic inflammatory demyelinating polyneuropathy, ITP = immune (idiopathic) thrombocytopenic purpura, MMN = multifocal motor neuropathy

[1]Subcutaneous administration **only** for the treatment of primary humoral immunodeficiency (PI)

[2]Lower infusion rates should be used in patients at risk for renal dysfunction or thrombotic complications; see specific product information for details.

[3]Other concentrations may be prepared; see product information for additional details.

[4]Per product information; other sources list IgA content as 1,000 to 2,000 mcg/mL for 6% solution (Siegel J. Immune globulins: therapeutic, pharmaceutical, cost, and administration considerations. *Pharm Prac News.* 2013).

[5]Osmolarity depends on concentration and diluent used; see product information for details.

[6]Data presented is based on the maximum concentration that can be prepared. The 5% solution with IgA content <2.2 mcg/mL has been discontinued. The lower IgA product (ie, IgA <1 mcg/mL for the 5% prepared solution) is available by special request; contact manufacturer or see specific product information for details.

MULTIVITAMIN PRODUCT TABLE

Injectable Formulations

Product	A (units)	B_1 (mg)	B_2 (mg)	B_6 (mg)	B_{12} (mcg)	C (mg)	D (units)	E (units)	K (mcg)	Additional Information
Solution										
Infuvite Adult (***per 10 mL***)	3,300	6	3.6	6	5	200	200	10	150	Supplied as two 5 mL vials. Biotin 60 mcg, folic acid 600 mcg, niacinamide 40 mg, dexpanthenol 15 mg
Infuvite Pediatric (***per 5 mL***)	2,300	1.2	1.4	1	1	80	400	7	200	Supplied as one 4 mL vial and one 1 mL vial. Biotin 20 mcg, folic acid 140 mcg, niacinamide 17 mg, dexpanthenol 5 mg
M.V.I.-12 (***per 10 mL***)	3,300	6	3.6	6	5	200	200	10		Supplied as a single 2-chambered 10 mL vial. Biotin 60 mcg, folic acid 600 mcg, niacinamide 40 mg, dexpanthenol 15 mg
M.V.I. Adult (***per 10 mL***)	3,300	6	3.6	6	5	200	200	10	150	Supplied as two 5 mL vials or a single 2-chambered 10 mL vial. Also available in a pharmacy bulk package (two 50 mL vials). Biotin 60 mcg, folic acid 600 mcg, niacinamide 40 mg, dexpanthenol 15 mg
Powder for Reconstitution										
M.V.I. Pediatric	2,300	1.2	1.4	1	1	80	400	7	200	Biotin 20 mcg, folic acid 140 mcg, niacinamide 17 mg, dexpanthenol 5 mg, aluminum, polysorbate 80

Adult Formulations

Product	A (units)	B_1 (mg)	B_2 (mg)	B_6 (mg)	B_{12} (mcg)	C (mg)	D (units)	E (units)	Additional Information
Caplet									
Folinic-Plus				50	2,000 (methylcobalamin)				Folinic acid 4 mg
Glutofac-ZX	5,000	20	20	25	2,500	200	400	100	Biotin 200 mcg, Cr 200 mcg, Cu 2.5 mg, folic acid 2,800 mcg, lutein 500 mcg, lycopene 500 mcg, Mg 100 mg, Mn 2.5 mg, niacinamide 100 mg, pantothenic acid 10 mg, Se 100 mcg, Zn 15 mg
Strovite Forte	4,000	20	20	25	50	500	400	60	Biotin 0.15 mg, Cr 0.05 mg, Cu 3 mg, Fe (as ferrous fumarate) 10 mg, folic acid 1 mg, Mg 50 mg, Mo 20 mcg, niacinamide 100 mg, pantothenic acid 25 mg, Se 50 mcg, Zn 15 mg; contains soy products
Strovite Plus	5,000	20	20	25	50	500		30	Biotin 0.15 mg, Cr 0.1 mcg, Cu 3 mg, Fe (as ferrous fumarate) 27 mg, folic acid 0.8 mg, Mg 50 mg, Mn 5 mg, niacinamide 100 mg, pantothenic acid 25 mg, Zn 22.5 mg; contains soy products
Capsule									
BP Vit 3 Plus				12.5	500		1,000		Folic acid 1 mg, omega-3 fatty acids 500 mg (including DHA 350 mg and EPA 35 mg), phytosterol 200 mg; contains soy products
FeRiva					12	152			Biotin 300 mcg, docusate sodium 25 mg, Fe 75 mg (as ferrous bisglycinate chelate and carbonyl iron), folic acid 1 mg
FeRivaFA					12	175			Biotin 300 mcg, Cu 1.5 mg, docusate sodium 50 mg, Fe 110 mg (as ferrous asparto glycinate, ferrous bisglycinate chelate, and ferrous fumarate), folate 1 mg (as L-methylfolate calcium [molar equivalent to folic acid 600 mcg] and folic acid 400 mcg)
Ferrex 150 Forte Plus					25	60 mg ascorbic acid 0.8 mg threonic acid			Fe [elemental] 150 mg, folic acid 1 mg, succinic acid 50 mg
Foltrin					15	75			Fe [elemental] 110 mg, folic acid 0.5 mg, special liver-stomach concentrate 240 mg
Fusion						25			Iron 130 mg (as ferrous fumarate 65 mg and polysaccharide iron complex 65 mg), *lactobacillus casei* 30 mg
Fusion Plus		2	3	10	12	75			Biotin 300 mcg, iron 130 mg (as ferrous fumarate 65 mg and polysaccharide iron complex 65 mg), folic acid 1,250 mcg, *lactobacillus casei* 30 mg, niacin 10 mg, pantothenic acid 6 mg
Hemocyte Plus		10	6	5	15	200			Cu 0.8 mg, Fe [elemental] 106 mg, folic acid 1 mg, Mg 6.9 mg, Mn 1.3 mg, niacinamide 30 mg, pantothenic acid 10 mg, Zn 18.2 mg
Integra						40			Fe [elemental] 125 mg; niacin 3 mg
Integra F						40			Fe [elemental] 125 mg; folic acid 1 mg; niacin 3 mg
Integra Plus		5	5	25	10	210			Biotin 300 mcg; Fe [elemental] 125 mg; folic acid 1 mg; niacin 20 mg; pantothenic acid 7 mg
K-Tan Plus		10	6	5	15	200			Cu 0.8 mg, Fe (as ferrous fumarate and polysaccharide iron complex) 106 mg, folic acid 1 mg, Mn 1.3 mg, niacinamide 30 mg, pantothenic acid 10 mg, Zn 18.2 mg
Ocuvel						250		200	Cu 1 mg, folic acid 0.5 mg, lutein 5 mg, zeaxanthin 1 mg, Zn 40 mg
Ocuvite Lutein [OTC]						60		30	Cu 2 mg, lutein 6 mg, Zn 15 mg
Tandem Plus		10	6	5	15	200			Cu 0.8 mg, Fe (as ferrous fumarate) 162 mg, Fe (as polysaccharide) 115.2 mg, folic acid 1 mg, Mn 1.3 mg, niacinamide 30 mg, pantothenic acid 10 mg, Zn 18.2 mg

Adult Formulations *continued*

Product	A (units)	B_1 (mg)	B_2 (mg)	B_6 (mg)	B_{12} (mcg)	C (mg)	D (units)	E (units)	Additional Information
Capsule, Softgel									
Ocuvite Adult 50+ [OTC]						150		30	Cu 1 mg, lutein 6 mg, omega-3 fatty acids 250 mg (as DHA 90 mg and EPA 160 mg), Zn 9 mg; contains soy products
PreserVision Lutein [OTC]						226		200	Cu 0.8 mg, lutein 5 mg, Zn 34.8 mg; contains soy products
Gummy									
One A Day VitaCraves Gummies [OTC] (**2 per serving**)	4,000			2	10	60	400	40	Biotin 150 mcg, choline 60 mcg, folic acid 400 mcg, inositol 40 mcg, iodine 80 mcg, pantothenic acid 10 mg, Zn 5 mg
One A Day VitaCraves Sour Gummies [OTC] (**2 per serving**)	4,000			2	10	60	400	40	Biotin 150 mcg, choline 60 mcg, folic acid 400 mcg, inositol 40 mcg, iodine 80 mcg, pantothenic acid 10 mg, Zn 5 mg
One A Day VitaCraves Gummies Plus Immunity Support [OTC] (**2 per serving**)	4,000			2	10	125	400	40	Biotin 150 mcg, folic acid 400 mcg, iodine 80 mcg, pantothenic acid 20 mg, Se 35 mcg, Zn 5 mg
Liquid									
Centamin [OTC] (***per 15 mL***)	1,300	1.5	1.7	2	6	60	400	30	Biotin 300 mcg, Cr 25 mcg, Fe 9 mg, iodine 150 mcg, Mo 25 mcg, niacin 20 mg, pantothenic acid 10 mg, Zn 3 mg (237 mL)
Centrum [OTC] (***per 15 mL***)		1.5	1.7	2	6	60		30	Biotin 300 mcg, Cr 25 mcg, Fe 9 mg, iodine 150 mcg, Mn 2 mg, Mo 25 mcg, niacin 20 mg, pantothenic acid 10 mg, Zn 3 mg; contains alcohol 5.7%, sodium benzoate (236 mL)
Drinkables Fruits and Vegetables [OTC] (***per 1 oz***)	1,812	100 mcg	100 mcg	100 mcg	0.2	38	142	11	Biotin 30 mcg, Ca 10 mg, choline 1 mg, Cr 43 mcg, Fe 180 mcg, folic acid 142 mcg, inositol 1 mg, lutein 100 mcg, lycopene 100 mcg, Mg 3 mg, Mn 0.7 mg, niacin 1 mg, PABA 1 mg, pantothenic acid 4 mg, phosphorus 7 mg, potassium 35 mg, sodium 10 mg, Stevia extract 18 mg, vitamin K 28 mcg, proprietary blend 22 g (887 mL)
Drinkables Multi Vitamins [OTC] (***per 1 oz***)	5,000	1.5	1.7	2	6	80	400	30	Biotin 300 mcg, choline 3 mg, Cr 120 mcg, folic acid 400 mcg, inositol 3 mg, lutein 250 mcg, lycopene 300 mcg, Mn 2 mg, niacin 20 mg, PABA 3 mg, pantothenic acid 10 mg, vitamin K 80 mcg, proprietary trace mineral blend 252 mg (444 mL, 976 mL)
Geriation [OTC] (***per 30 mL***)		5	2.5	1	1				Choline 100 mg, Fe 15 mg, iodine 100 mcg, Mg 2 mg, Mn 2 mg, niacinamide 50 mg, pantothenic acid 10 mg, Zn 2 mg (473 mL); contains alcohol 18%
Geritol Tonic [OTC] (***per 15 mL***)		2.5	2.5	0.5					Choline 50 mg, Fe 18 mg, methionine 25 mg, niacin 50 mg, pantothenic acid 2 mg (120 mL, 360 mL)
Multi-Delyn [OTC] (***per 5 mL***)	2,250	0.8	1	0.9	4	54	360	13.5	Niacin 12 mg; alcohol-free, sugar-free (240 mL, 473 mL)
Soft Chews									
Viactiv [OTC]	2,500	1.5	1.7	2	6	60	400	33	Biotin 30 mcg, Ca 200 mg, folic acid 400 mcg, niacin 15 mg, pantothenic acid 10 mg; sodium 10 mg; contains soy products
Viactiv With Calcium [OTC]							500		Ca 500 mg, sodium 10 mg, vitamin K 40 mcg; contains soy products
Tablet									
Androvite [OTC] (***per 6 tablets***)	25,000	50	50	100	125	1000	400	400	Betaine 100 mg, biotin 125 mcg, boron 3 mg, Cr 200 mcg, Cu 2 mg, Fe (as amino acid chelate) 18 mg, folic acid 400 mcg, hesperidin 35 mg, inositol 36 mg, iodine 150 mcg, Mg 500 mg, Mn 10 mg, niacinamide 50 mg, PABA 25 mg, pancreatin 4X 75 mg, pantothenic acid 100 mg, rutin 25 mg, Se 200 mcg, Zn 50 mg

Adult Formulations *continued*

Product	A (units)	B_1 (mg)	B_2 (mg)	B_6 (mg)	B_{12} (mcg)	C (mg)	D (units)	E (units)	Additional Information
Centrum [OTC]	3,500	1.5	1.7	2	6	60	400	30	Biotin 30 mcg, boron 75 mcg, Ca 200 mg, chloride 72 mg, Cr 35 mcg, Cu 0.5 mg, Fe 18 mg, folic acid 400 mcg, iodine 150 mcg, Mg 50 mg, Mn 2.3 mg, Mo 45 mcg, niacin 20 mg, nickel 5 mcg, pantothenic acid 10 mg, phosphorus 20 mg, potassium 80 mg, Se 55 mcg, silicon 2 mg, tin 10 mcg, vanadium 10 mcg, vitamin K 25 mcg, Zn 11 mg; contains sodium benzoate
Centrum Cardio [OTC] (***per tablet; dose: 2 tablets daily***)	1,750	0.75	0.85	2.5	100	30	200	15	Biotin 15 mcg, boron 16 mcg, Ca 54 mg, chloride 29 mg, Cr 60 mcg, Cu 0.35 mg, Fe 3 mg, folic acid 200 mcg, iodine 75 mcg, Mg 20 mg, Mn 1 mg, Mo 37.5 mcg, niacin 10 mg, nickel 2.5 mcg, pantothenic acid 5 mg, phosphorus 40 mg, phytosterols 400 mg, potassium 32 mg, Se 10 mcg, silicon 1 mg, tin 5 mcg, vanadium 5 mcg, vitamin K 12.5 mcg, Zn 3.75 mg; contains sodium benzoate, soy products
Centrum Performance [OTC]	3,500	4.5	5.1	6	18	120	400	60	Biotin 50 mcg, boron 60 mcg, Ca 100 mg, chloride 72 mg, Cr 120 mcg, Cu 0.9 mg, Fe 18 mg, folic acid 400 mcg, ginseng root 50 mg, iodine 150 mcg, Mg 40 mg, Mn 4 mg, Mo 75 mcg, niacin 40 mg, nickel 5 mcg, pantothenic acid 12 mg, phosphorus 48 mg, potassium 80 mg, Se 70 mcg, silicon 4 mg, tin 10 mcg, vanadium 10 mcg, vitamin K 25 mcg, Zn 11 mg; contains sodium benzoate
Centrum Silver [OTC]	2,500	1.5	1.7	3	25	60	500	50	Biotin 30 mcg, boron 150 mcg, Ca 220 mg, chloride 72 mg, Cr 45 mcg, Cu 0.5 mg, folic acid 400 mcg, iodine 150 mcg, lutein 250 mcg, lycopene 300 mcg, Mg 50 mg, Mn 2.3 mg, Mo 45 mcg, niacin 20 mg, nickel 5 mcg, pantothenic acid 10 mg, phosphorus 20 mg, potassium 80 mg, Se 55 mcg, silicon 2 mg, vanadium 10 mcg, vitamin K 30 mcg, Zn 11 mg; contains sodium benzoate
Centrum Silver Ultra Men's [OTC]	3,500	1.5	1.7	6	100	120	600	60	Biotin 30 mcg, boron 150 mcg, Ca 250 mg, chloride 72 mg, Cr 60 mcg, Cu 0.7 mg, folic acid 300 mcg, iodine 150 mcg, lutein 300 mcg, lycopene 600 mcg, Mg 50 mg, Mn 4 mg, Mo 50 mcg, niacin 20 mg, nickel 5 mcg, pantothenic acid 10 mg, phosphorus 20 mg, potassium 80 mg, Se 100 mcg, silicon 2 mg, vanadium 10 mcg, vitamin K 60 mcg, Zn 15 mg; contains soy products
Centrum Silver Ultra Women's [OTC]	3,500	1.1	1.1	5	50	100	800	35	Biotin 30 mcg, boron 150 mcg, Ca 500 mg, chloride 72 mg, Cr 50 mcg, Cu 0.5 mg, Fe (as ferrous fumarate) 8 mg, folic acid 400 mcg, iodine 150 mcg, lutein 300 mcg, Mg 50 mg, Mn 2.3 mg, Mo 50 mcg, niacin 14 mg, nickel 5 mcg, pantothenic acid 5 mg, phosphorus 20 mg, potassium 80 mg, Se 55 mcg, silicon 2 mg, vanadium 10 mcg, vitamin K 50 mcg, Zn 15 mg; contains soy products
Centrum Ultra Men's [OTC]	3,500	1.2	1.3	2	6	90	600	45	Biotin 40 mcg, boron 150 mcg, Ca 210 mg, chloride 72 mg, Cr 35 mcg, Cu 0.9 mg, Fe (as ferrous fumarate) 8 mg, folic acid 200 mcg, iodine 150 mcg, lycopene 600 mcg, Mg 100 mg, Mn 2.3 mg, Mo 50 mcg, niacin 16 mg, nickel 5 mcg, pantothenic acid 15 mg, phosphorus 20 mg, potassium 80 mg, Se 100 mcg, silicon 2 mg, tin 10 mcg, vanadium 10 mcg, vitamin K 60 mcg, Zn 11 mg; contains soy products
Centrum Ultra Women's [OTC]	3,500	1.1	1.1	2	6	75	800	35	Biotin 40 mcg, boron 150 mcg, Ca 500 mg, chloride 72 mg, Cr 25 mcg, Cu 0.9 mg, Fe (as ferrous fumarate) 18 mg, folic acid 400 mcg, iodine 150 mcg, Mg 100 mg, Mn 1.8 mg, Mo 50 mcg, niacin 14 mg, nickel 5 mcg, pantothenic acid 15 mg, phosphorus 20 mg, potassium 80 mg, Se 55 mcg, silicon 2 mg, tin 10 mcg, vanadium 10 mcg, vitamin K 50 mcg, Zn 8 mg; contains soy products
DiatxZN		1.5	1.5	50	2 mg	60			Biotin 300 mcg, Cu 1.5 mg, folic acid 5 mg, niacinamide 20 mg, pantothenic acid 10 mg, Zn 25 mg; gluten-free, sugar-free
FeRiva 21/7					12	175			Docusate sodium 50 mg, Fe 75 mg (as ferrous asparto glycinate), folate 1 mg (as L-methylfolate calcium [molar equivalent to folic acid 600 mcg] and folic acid 400 mcg), succinic acid 150 mg, Zn 10 mg
Freedavite [OTC]	5,000	1.5	1.7	2	6	60	400	30	Biotin 30 mcg, Ca 20 mg, Cu 0.1 mg, Fe (as ferrous fumarate) 1.8 mg, folic acid 400 mcg, iodine 75 mcg, Mg 8 mg, Mn 0.625 mg, niacinamide 20 mg, pantothenic acid 10 mg, Se 35 mcg, Zn 1.5 mg

Adult Formulations *continued*

Product	A (units)	B_1 (mg)	B_2 (mg)	B_6 (mg)	B_{12} (mcg)	C (mg)	D (units)	E (units)	Additional Information
Geri-Freeda [OTC]	5,000	15	15	15	15	150	400	15	Betaine 10 mg, biotin 15 mcg, Ca 50 mg, choline 10 mg, Cr 60 mcg, Cu 0.5 mg, folic acid 400 mcg, hesperidin 10 mg, inositol 10 mg, iodine 150 mcg, L-lysine 25 mg, Mg 25 mg, Mn 1 mg, niacinamide 50 mg, PABA 10 mg, pantothenic acid 15 mg, Se 35 mcg, Zn 7.5 mg
Geritol Complete [OTC]	6,100	1.5	1.7	2	6.7	57	400	30	Biotin 44 mcg, Ca 148 mg, chloride 20 mg, Cr 12 mcg, Cu 1.8 mg, Fe 16 mg, folic acid 0.38 mg, iodine 120 mcg, Mg 86 mg, Mn 2.4 mg, Mo 1 mcg, niacin 20 mg, pantothenic acid 13 mg, phosphorus 118 mg, potassium 36 mg, selenium 1 mcg, vitamin K 24 mcg, Zn 13.5 mg
Gynovite Plus [OTC] (***per 6 tablets***)	5,000	10	10	20	125	180	400	400	Betaine 100 mg, biotin 125 mcg, boron 3 mg, Ca 500 mg, Cr 200 mcg, Cu 2 mg, Fe (as amino acid chelate) 18 mg, folic acid 400 mcg, hesperidin 35 mg, inositol 50 mg, iodine 150 mcg, Mg 600 mg, Mn 10 mg, niacinamide 20 mg, PABA 25 mg, pancreatin 4X 93 mg, pantothenic acid 10 mg, rutin 25 mg, Se 200 mcg, Zn 15 mg
Hi-Kovite [OTC] (***per contents of 1 vitamin tablet plus 1 mineral tablet***)	5,000	10	10	10	10	200	400	30	Bioflavonoids 10 mg, biotin 30 mcg, Ca 120 mg, Cu 0.5 mg, Fe (as ferrous fumarate) 9 mg, folic acid 400 mcg, inositol 10 mg, iodine 75 mcg, L-lysine 10 mg, Mg 60 mg, Mn 1 mg, niacinamide 100 mg, PABA 10 mg, pantothenic acid 10 mg, potassium 35 mg, Se 17.5 mcg, Zn 7.5 mg
Iberet-500		6	6	5	25	500			Iron 105 mg, niacin 30 mg, pantothenic acid 10 mg
ICaps AREDS Formula [OTC] (**per 2 tablets**)	28,640					452		400	Cu 1.6 mg, Zn 69.6 mg
ICaps Lutein and Zeaxanthin Formula [OTC] (**per 2 tablets**)	6,600		10			400		150	Cu 4 mg, lutein/zeaxanthin 4 mg, Mn 10 mg, Se 40 mcg, Zn 60 mg
ICaps Multivitamin [OTC] (**per 4 tablets**)		1.5	10	2	6	512	400	430	Biotin 30 mcg, Ca 333 mg, Cr 120 mcg, Cu 3.6 mg, folic acid 400 mcg, iodine 150 mcg, lutein 6.67 mg, lycopene 0.3 mg, Mg 100 mg, Mn 2 mg, Mo 75 mcg, niacin 10 mg, pantothenic acid 10 mg, phosphorus 140 mg, Se 40 mg, vitamin K 25 mcg, zeaxanthin 3.3 mg, Zn 84.6 mg
Maxaron Forte					250 (methylcobalamin)	200			Fe (as ferrous fumarate) 70 mg, Fe (as iron glycinate sulfate) 80 mg, L-methylfolate calcium 1.13 mg
Monocaps [OTC]	5,000	15	15	15	15	120	400	15	Biotin 15 mcg, Ca 50 mg, Cu 0.1 mg, Fe (as ferrous fumarate) 14 mg, folic acid 400 mcg, iodine 150 mcg, lecithin 10 mg, L-lysine 10 mg, Mg 30 mg, Mn 1 mg, niacinamide 40 mg, pantothenic acid 15 mg, Se 35 mcg, Zn 3.75 mg
Multilex [OTC]	10,000	10	5	1.7	3	100	400	5.5	Ca 10 mg, Cu 1 mg, Fe 15 mg, Mg 5 mg, Mn 1 mg, niacinamide 30 mg, potassium iodide 0.15 mg, Zn 1.5 mg
Multilex-T&M [OTC]	10,000	15	10	2	7.5	150	400	5.5	Ca 10 mg, Cu 1 mg, Fe 15 mg, Mg 5 mg, Mn 1 mg, niacinamide 100 mg, potassium iodide 0.15 mg, Zn 1.5 mg
Myadec [OTC]	5,000	1.7	2	3	6	60	400	30	Biotin 30 mcg, boron 150 mcg, Ca 162 mg, chloride 36 mg, Cr 25 mcg, Cu 2 mg, Fe 18 mg, folic acid 400 mcg, iodine 150 mcg, Mg 100 mg, Mn 2.5 mg, Mo 25 mcg, niacin 20 mg, nickel 5 mcg, pantothenic acid 10 mg, phosphorus 125 mg, potassium 40 mg, Se 25 mcg, silicon 10 mcg, tin 10 mcg, vanadium 10 mcg, vitamin K 25 mcg, Zn 15 mg; contains soy products
NicAzel Forte				8					Azerizin 700 mg (proprietary blend of nicotinamide, azelaic acid, quercetin, and curcumin), Cu 2 mg, folic acid 500 mcg, Zn 12 mg; contains tartrazine
Nicomide									Cr 100 mcg, Cu 2 mg, folate 500 mcg (as L-methylfolate calcium), niacinamide 750 mg, Se 50 mcg, Zn 27 mg
Ocuvite [OTC]	1,000					200		60	Cu 2 mg, lutein 2 mg, Se 55 mcg, Zn 40 mg

Adult Formulations *continued*

Product	A (units)	B_1 (mg)	B_2 (mg)	B_6 (mg)	B_{12} (mcg)	C (mg)	D (units)	E (units)	Additional Information
One A Day Cholesterol Plus [OTC]	2,500	1.5	1.7	2	6	60	400	30	Biotin 50 mcg, boron 150 mcg, Ca 100 mg, Cr 120 mcg, Cu 2 mg, folic acid 400 mcg, iodine 150 mcg, Mg 100 mg, Mn 2 mg, Mo 75 mcg, niacin 20 mg, pantothenic acid 10 mg, phytosterols 100 mg, potassium 99 mg, Se 70 mcg, Zn 15 mg; contains soy products
One A Day Energy [OTC]	3,500	3	3.4	4	12	60	400	22.5	Biotin 300 mcg, boron 150 mcg, caffeine 90 mg, Ca 250 mg, Cr 100 mcg, Cu 2 mg, Fe 9 mg, folic acid 400 mcg, guarana seed powder 110 mg, iodine 150 mcg, Mg 40 mg, Mn 2 mg, Mo 25 mcg, niacin 40 mg, nickel 5 mcg, pantothenic acid 10 mg, potassium 99 mg, Se 45 mcg, silicon 5 mg, tin 10 mcg, vitamin K 25 mcg, Zn 15 mg; contains tartrazine
One A Day Essential [OTC]	3,000	1.5	1.7	2	6	60	400	30	Ca 45 mg, folic acid 400 mcg, niacin 20 mg, pantothenic acid 10 mg; contains soy products
One A Day Maximum [OTC]	2,500	1.5	1.7	2	6	60	400	30	Biotin 30 mcg, boron 150 mcg, Ca 162 mg, chloride 72 mg, Cr 65 mcg, Cu 2 mg, Fe 18 mg, folic acid 400 mcg, iodine 150 mcg, Mg 100 mg, Mn 3.5 mg, Mo 160 mcg, niacin 20 mg, nickel 5 mcg, pantothenic acid 10 mg, phosphorus 109 mg, potassium 80 mg, Se 20 mcg, silicon 2 mg, tin 10 mcg, vanadium 10 mcg, vitamin K 25 mcg, Zn 15 mg; contains soy products
One A Day Menopause Formula [OTC]	2,500	3	3.4	8	12	60	800	33	Biotin 300 mcg, boron 1,500 mcg, Ca 300 mg, Cr 120 mcg, Cu 1 mg, folic acid 400 mcg, iodine 150 mcg, Mg 50 mg, Mn 2 mg, Mo 37.5 mg, niacin 20 mg, pantothenic acid 15 mg, Se 20 mcg, soybean extract 60 mg, Zn 15 mg; contains soy products
One A Day Men's 50+ Advantage [OTC]	2,500	4.5	3.4	6	25	60	700	22.5	Biotin 30 mcg, Ca 120 mg, Cr 180 mcg, Cu 2 mg, folic acid 400 mcg, ginko biloba extract 120 mg, iodine 150 mcg, lycopene 300 mcg, Mg 100 mg, Mn 4 mg, molybdenum 90 mcg, niacin 20 mg, pantothenic acid 15 mg, Se 110 mcg, vitamin K 20 mcg, Zn 22.5 mg
One A Day Men's Health Formula [OTC]	3,500	1.2	1.7	3	18	60	700	22.5	Biotin 30 mcg, Ca 210 mg, Cr 120 mcg, Cu 2 mg, folic acid 400 mcg, lycopene 300 mcg, Mg 120 mg, Mn 2 mg, niacin 16 mg, pantothenic acid 5 mg, Se 110 mcg, vitamin K 20 mcg, Zn 15 mg
One A Day Men's Pro Edge [OTC]	3,500	3	3.4	4	12	80	800	33	Biotin 300 mcg, Ca 200 mg, Cr 120 mcg, Cu 2 mg, folic acid 400 mcg, Mg 200 mg, Mn 2 mg, niacin 25 mg, pantothenic acid 15 mg, Se 70 mcg, vitamin K 20 mcg, Zn 15 mg; contains tartrazine
One A Day Teen Advantage for Her [OTC]	2,500	2.3	2.6	3	9	120	800	30	Biotin 300 mcg, Ca 300 mg, Cr 120 mcg, Cu 2 mg, Fe 18 mg, folic acid 400 mcg, Mg 50 mg, Mn 2 mg, niacin 30 mg, pantothenic acid 10 mg, Se 20 mcg, vitamin K 25 mcg, Zn 15 mg
One A Day Teen Advantage for Him [OTC]	2,500	3.75	4.25	5	15	120	400	30	Biotin 300 mcg, Ca 200 mg, Cr 120 mcg, Cu 2 mg, Fe 9 mg, folic acid 400 mcg, Mg 100 mg, Mn 2 mg, niacin 30 mg, pantothenic acid 10 mg, Se 20 mcg, vitamin K 25 mcg, Zn 15 mg
One A Day Women's [OTC]	2,500	1.5	1.7	2	6	60	1,000	22.5	Biotin 30 mcg, Ca 500 mg, Cr 120 mcg, Cu 2 mg, Fe 18 mg, folic acid 400 mcg, Mg 50 mg, Mn 2 mg, niacin 10 mg, pantothenic acid 5 mg, Se 20 mcg, vitamin K 25 mcg, Zn 15 mg; contains tartrazine
One A Day Women's 50+ Advantage [OTC]	2,500	4.5	3.4	6	25	60	1,000	22.5	Biotin 30 mcg, Ca 500 mg, Cr 180 mcg, Cu 2 mg, folic acid 400 mcg, ginkgo biloba extract 120 mg, iodine 150 mcg, Mg 50 mg, Mn 4 mg, Mo 90 mcg, niacin 20 mg, pantothenic acid 15 mg, Se 20 mcg, vitamin K 20 mcg, Zn 22.5 mg; contains tartrazine
One A Day Women's Active Metabolism [OTC]	2,500	2.4	2.7	3.2	9.5	60	800	22.5	Biotin 30 mcg, Ca 300 mg, caffeine 120 mg, Cr 120 mcg, Cu 2 mg, Fe 18 mg, folic acid 400 mcg, guarana seed 50 mg, Mg 50 mg, Mn 2 mg, niacin 10 mg, pantothenic acid 5 mg, Se 20 mcg, vitamin K 25 mcg, Zn 15 mg; contains soy products
One A Day Women's Active Mind & Body [OTC]	2,500	2.4	2.7	3.2	9.5	60	800	30	Biotin 30 mcg, Ca 300 mg, Cr 120 mcg, Cu 2 mg, Fe 18 mg, folic acid 400 mcg, guarana blend 180 mg, Mg 50 mg, Mn 2 mg, niacin 10 mg, pantothenic acid 5 mg, Se 20 mcg, vitamin K 25 mcg, Zn 15 mg; contains tartrazine

Adult Formulations *continued*

Product	A (units)	B_1 (mg)	B_2 (mg)	B_6 (mg)	B_{12} (mcg)	C (mg)	D (units)	E (units)	Additional Information
Optivite P.M.T. [OTC] ***(per 6 tablets)***	12,500	25	25	300	60	1,500	100	100	Betaine 100 mg, bioflavonoids 250 mg, biotin 60 mcg, Ca 125 mg, choline 313 mg, Cr 100 mcg, Fe (as amino acid chelate) 15 mg, folic acid 200 mcg, inositol 24 mg, iodine 75 mcg, Mg 250 mg, Mn 10 mg, niacinamide 25 mg, PABA 25 mg, pancreatin 4X 93 mg, pantothenic acid 25 mg, potassium 48 mg, rutin 25 mg, Se 100 mcg, Zn 25 mg
PreserVision AREDS [OTC] (***per 2 tablets***)	14,320					226		200	Cu 0.8 mg, Zn 34.8 mg
Quintabs [OTC]	5,000	30	30	30	30	300	400	50	Biotin 30 mcg, folic acid 400 mcg, niacinamide 100 mg, pantothenic acid 30 mg
Quintabs-M [OTC]	5,000	30	30	30	30	300	400	50	Biotin 30 mcg, Ca 30 mg, Cu 0.2 mg, Fe (as ferrous fumarate) 10 mg, folic acid 400 mcg, iodine 150 mcg, Mg 15 mg, Mn 2 mg, niacinamide 100 mg, pantothenic acid 30 mg, Se 35 mcg, Zn 7.5 mg
Quintabs-M Iron-Free [OTC]	5,000	30	30	30	30	300	400	50	Biotin 30 mcg, Ca 30 mg, Cu 0.2 mg, folic acid 400 mcg, iodine 150 mcg, Mg 15 mg, Mn 2 mg, niacinamide 100 mg, pantothenic acid 30 mg, Se 35 mcg, Zn 7.5 mg
Repliva 21/7					10	140 mg as ascorbic acid 60 mg as Ester-C supplement			Fe [elemental] 151 mg, folic acid 1 mg, succinic acid 150 mg
Theragran-M	5,000	3	3.4	6	12	90	400	60	Biotin 30 mcg, boron 150 mcg, Ca 40 mg, chloride 7.5 mg, Cr 50 mcg, Cu 2 mg, Fe 9 mg, folic acid 400 mcg, iodine 150 mcg, Mg 100 mg, Mn 2 mg, Mo 75 mcg, Ni 5 mcg, niacin 20 mg, pantothenic acid 10 mg, phosphorous 31 mg, potassium 7.5 mg, Se 70 mg, silicon 2 mg, tin 10 mcg, vanadium 10 mcg, vitamin K 28 mcg, Zn 15 mg; contains soy products
Thera-M [OTC]	5,000	3	3.4	6	12	90	400		Biotin 30 mcg, boron 150 mcg, Ca 40 mg, chloride 7.5 mg, Cr 50 mcg, Cu 2 mg, Fe (as ferrous fumarate) 9 mg, folic acid 400 mcg, iodine 150 mcg, Mg 100 mg, Mn 2 mg, Mo 75 mcg, Ni 5 mcg, niacinamide 20 mg, pantothenic acid 10 mg, phosphorous 31 mg, potassium 7.5 mg, Se 70 mcg, silicon 2 mg, tin 10 mcg, vanadium 10 mcg, vitamin K 28 mcg, Zn 15 mg; contains soy products
T-Vites [OTC]		25	25	25	30	100	400		Biotin 30 mcg, folic acid 400 mcg, Mg 100 mg, Mn 0.5 mg, niacinamide 150 mg, pantothenic acid 25 mg, potassium 35 mg, Zn 3.75 mg
Ultra Freeda A-Free [OTC] (***per 3 tablets***)		50	50	50	100	1,000	400	200	Base (choline, inositol, PABA) 100 mg, bioflavonoids 100 mg, biotin 300 mcg, Ca 250 mg, Cr 200 mcg, Fe (as ferrous fumarate) 18 mg, folic acid 800 mcg, iodine 150 mcg, Mg 100 mg, Mn 10 mg, Mo 12.5 mcg, niacinamide and niacin 100 mg, pantothenic acid 100 mg, potassium 35 mg, Se 100 mcg, Zn 22.5 mg
Ultra Freeda Iron-Free [OTC] (***per 3 tablets***)	5,000	50	50	50	100	1,000	400	200	Base (choline, inositol) 100 mg, bioflavonoids 100 mg, biotin 300 mcg, Ca 250 mg, Cr 200 mcg, folic acid 800 mcg, iodine 150 mcg, Mg 100 mg, Mn 10 mg, Mo 12.5 mcg, niacinamide and niacin 100 mg, pantothenic acid 100 mg, potassium 35 mg, Se 100 mcg, Zn 22.5 mg
Ultra Freeda With Iron [OTC] (***per 3 tablets***)	5,000	50	50	50	100	1,000	400	200	Base (choline, inositol) 100 mg, bioflavonoids 100 mg, biotin 300 mcg, Ca 250 mg, Cr 200 mcg, Fe (as ferrous fumarate) 18 mg, folic acid 800 mcg, iodine 150 mcg, Mg 100 mg, Mn 10 mg, Mo 12.5 mcg, niacinamide and niacin 100 mg, pantothenic acid 100 mg, potassium 35 mg, Se 100 mcg, Zn 22.5 mg
Xtramins [OTC]	1,000	5	2	5	10	50	100	10	Boron 1 mg, Ca 250 mg, Cr 40 mcg, Cu 500 mcg, Fe (as iron gluconate) 10 mg, folic acid 400 mcg, iodine 150 mcg, Mg 20 mg, Mn 2 mg, niacinamide 15 mg, PABA 5 mg, pantothenic acid 5 mg, potassium 45 mg, Se 30 mcg, Zn 10 mg; gluten-free, sugar-free

Adult Formulations *continued*

Product	A (units)	B_1 (mg)	B_2 (mg)	B_6 (mg)	B_{12} (mcg)	C (mg)	D (units)	E (units)	Additional Information
Yelets [OTC]	5,000	10	10	10	10	100	400	30	Biotin 30 mcg, Ca 60 mg, Fe (as ferrous fumarate) 18 mg, folic acid 400 mcg, iodine 150 mcg, L-lysine 10 mg, Mg 20 mg, Mn 1 mg, niacinamide 25 mg, pantothenic acid 10 mg, Se 17.5 mcg, Zn 7.5 mg
Tablet, Chewable									
Centrum [OTC]	3,500	1.5	1.7	2	6	60	400	30	Biotin 45 mcg, Ca 108 mg, Cr 20 mcg, Cu 2 mg, Fe 18 mg, folic acid 400 mcg, iodine 150 mcg, Mg 40 mg, Mn 1 mg, Mo 20 mcg, niacin 20 mg, pantothenic acid 10 mg, phosphorus 50 mg, vitamin K 10 mcg, Zn 15 mg; contains sodium benzoate, soy products
Centrum Flavor Burst [OTC] (***per 4 tablets***)	2,000			2	10	60	800	40	Biotin 150 mcg, choline 76 mg, folic acid 400 mcg, inositol 40 mcg, iodine 80 mcg, pantothenic acid 10 mg, Zn 5 mg; grape, mixed fruit, and tropical fruit flavors
Centrum Silver [OTC]	4,000	2.2	2.7	7	25	75	400	70	Biotin 45 mcg, Ca 200 mg, Cr 100 mcg, Cu 2 mg, folic acid 400 mcg, iodine 100 mcg, lutein 250 mcg, Mg 50 mg, Mn 4.5 mg, Mo 25 mcg, niacin 12 mg, nickel 5 mcg, pantothenic acid 10 mg, phosphorus 125 mg, Se 22.5 mcg, silicon 4 mg, tin 10 mcg, vanadium 10 mcg, Zn 15 mg; contains phenylalanine, sodium benzoate, soy products
Wafers									
CalciFol				10	25		200		Boron 1 mg, Ca 1342 mg, folic acid 1.6 mg, magnesium 50 mg
Calcifolic-D				10	125		300		Boron 250 mcg, Ca 1342 mg, folic acid 1 mg, magnesium 50 mg

ALA = α-linolenic acid, Ca = calcium, Cr = chromium, Cu = copper, DHA = docosahexaenoic acid, EPA = eicosapentaenoic acid, Fe = iron, Mg = magnesium, Mn = manganese, Mo = molybdenum, Se = selenium, Zn = zinc

Pediatric Formulations

Product	A (units)	B_1 (mg)	B_2 (mg)	B_6 (mg)	B_{12} (mcg)	C (mg)	D (units)	E (units)	Additional Information
Capsule, softgel									
AquADEKs [OTC]	18,167 (92% as beta carotene)	1.5	1.7	1.9	12	75	1,200	150 units as d-alpha tocopherol and 80 mg as mixed tocopherols	Biotin 100 mcg, coenzyme Q_{10} 10 mg, folic acid 100 mcg, niacinamide 10 mg, pantothenic acid 12 mg, selenium 75 mcg, sodium 10 mg, vitamin K 700 mcg, Zn 10 mg; contains sodium benzoate; casein-free, gluten-free
Drops									
AquADEKs [OTC] (**per mL**)	5,751 (87% as beta carotene)	0.6	0.6	0.6		45	600	50 units as d-alpha tocopherol and 15 mg as mixed tocopherols	Biotin 15 mcg, coenzyme Q_{10} 2 mg, niacinamide 6 mg, pantothenic acid 3 mg, selenium 10 mcg, sodium 10 mg, vitamin K 400 mcg, Zn 5 mg; contains sodium benzoate; dye-free, casein-free, gluten-free
MyKidz Iron [OTC] (***per 2 mL***)	1,500					35	400		Fe [elemental] 10 mg; alcohol-free, sugar-free, dye-free
MyKidz Iron FL (***per 2 mL***)	1,500					35	400		Fe [elemental] 10 mg, fluoride 0.25 mg; alcohol-free, sugar-free, dye-free 118 mL)
Poly-Vi-Sol [OTC] (***per mL***)	1,500	0.5	0.6	0.4	2	35	400	5	Niacin 8 mg; gluten-free (50 mL)
Poly-Vi-Sol With Iron [OTC] (***per mL***)	1,500	0.5	0.6	0.4		35	400	5	Fe [elemental] 10 mg, niacin 8 mg; gluten-free (50 mL)
Quflora 0.25 mg/mL fluoride drops (***per mL***)	1,000	0.5	0.6	0.4	2	35	400	5	Cu 1 mg, fluoride 0.25 mg, folic acid 35 mcg, Mg 10 mg, niacinamide 0.8 mg
Quflora 0.5 mg/mL fluoride drops (***per mL***)	1,100	1	1	1	3	45	400	12	Cu 1 mg, fluoride 0.5 mg, folic acid 81 mcg, Mg 12 mg, niacinamide 2 mg
Tri-Vi-Sol [OTC] (***per mL***)	1,500					35	400		Gluten-free (50 mL)
Gummy									
Flintstones Gummies [OTC] (***per 2 gummies***)	2,000			1	5	30	200	20	Biotin 75 mcg, choline 38 mcg, folic acid 200 mcg, inositol 20 mcg, iodine 40 mcg, pantothenic acid 5 mg, zinc 2.5 mg
Flintstones Gummies Plus Immunity Support [OTC] (***per 2 gummies***)	2,000			1	5	125	200	20	Biotin 75 mcg, folic acid 200 mcg, inositol 20 mcg, iodine 40 mcg, pantothenic acid 5 mg, Zn 2.5 mg
Flintstones Gummies Plus Bone Building Support [OTC] (***per 2 gummies***)	1,600			1	5	30	400	20	Biotin 75 mcg, Ca 100 mg, iodine 40 mcg, pantothenic acid 5 mg, Zn 2.5 mg
Flintstones Sour Gummies [OTC] (***per 2 gummies***)	2,000			1	5	30	200	20	Biotin 75 mcg, choline 38 mcg, folic acid 200 mcg, inositol 20 mcg, iodine 40 mcg, pantothenic acid 5 mg, zinc 2.5 mg; contains tartrazine
One A Day Kids Jolly Rancher Gummies [OTC] (***per 2 gummies***)	2,000			1	5	30	200	20	Biotin 75 mcg, choline 30 mcg, folic acid 200 mcg, inositol 20 mcg, iodine 40 mcg, pantothenic acid 5 mg, Zn 2.5 mg; contains tartrazine

Pediatric Formulations *continued*

Product	A (units)	B_1 (mg)	B_2 (mg)	B_6 (mg)	B_{12} (mcg)	C (mg)	D (units)	E (units)	Additional Information
One A Day Kids Jolly Rancher Sour Gummies [OTC] (***per 2 gummies***)	2,000			1	5	30	200	20	Biotin 75 mcg, choline 30 mcg, folic acid 200 mcg, inositol 20 mcg, iodine 40 mcg, pantothenic acid 5 mg, Zn 2.5 mg; contains tartrazine
One A Day Kids Scooby-Doo! Gummies [OTC] (***per 2 gummies***)	2,000			1	5	30	200	20	Biotin 75 mcg, choline 30 mcg, folic acid 200 mcg, inositol 20 mcg, iodine 40 mcg, pantothenic acid 5 mg, zinc 2.5 mg
Strip									
Poly-Vi-Flor FS		0.5	0.6	0.4			400	5	Flouride 1 mg, folate 200 mcg (as L-methylfolate calcium), niacinamide 8 mg; contains polysorbate 80, sodium benzoate, soy products; gluten-free; berry flavor
Tablet									
Floriva	2,000 (50% as beta carotene)	1.3	1.5	1.8	6	75	600	20	Biotin 40 mcg, Cu 1 mg, folate 262 mcg (as L-methylfolate glucosamine [molar equivalent to folic acid 162 mcg] and folic acid 100 mcg), niacinamide 15 mg, Zn 5 mg; dye-free, gluten-free, sugar-free. Available in two fluoride strengths: 0.5 mg, 1 mg
Tablet, Chewable									
AquADEKs [OTC] (***per 2 tablets***)	18,167 (92% as beta carotene)	1.5	1.7	1.9	12	70	1,200	100 units as d-alpha tocopherol and 30 mg as mixed tocopherols	Biotin 100 mcg, coenzyme Q_{10} 10 mg, folic acid 200 mcg, niacinamide 10 mg, pantothenic acid 12 mg, selenium 75 mcg, sodium 10 mg, vitamin K 700 mcg, Zn 10 mg; contains sodium benzoate; casein-free, gluten-free
Centrum Flavor Burst Kids [OTC] **(per 2 tablets)**	1,000			1	5	30	400	20	Biotin 75 mcg, choline 38 mg, folic acid 200 mcg, inositol 20 mcg, iodine 40 mcg, pantothenic acid 5 mg, Zn 2.5 mg; grape and blue raspberry and tropical burst flavors
Centrum Kids [OTC]	3,500	1.5	1.7	2	6	60	400	30	Biotin 45 mcg, Ca 108 mg, Cr 20 mcg, Cu 2 mg, Fe 18 mg, folic acid 400 mcg, iodine 150 mcg, Mg 40 mg, Mn 1 mg, Mo 20 mcg, niacin 20 mg, pantothenic acid 10 mg, phosphorus 50 mg, vitamin K 10 mcg, Zn 15 mg; contains phenylalanine, sodium benzoate, soy products
Flintstones Complete [OTC]	3,000	1.5	1.7	2	6	60	600	30	Biotin 40 mcg, Ca 100 mg, Cu 2 mg, Fe 18 mg, folic acid 400 mcg, iodine 150 mcg, niacin 15 mg, pantothenic acid 10 mg, sodium 10 mg, vitamin K 55 mcg, Zn 12 mg; contains sucralose, soy products
Flintstones Plus Bone Building Support [OTC]	2,500	1.05	1.2	1.05	4.5	60	400	15	Calcium 200 mg, folic acid 300 mcg, niacin 13.5 mg, sodium 10 mg; contains phenylalanine, soy products
Flintstones Plus Immunity Support [OTC]	2,500	1.05	1.2	1.05	4.5	250	400	15	Folic acid 300 mcg, niacin 13.5 mg, sodium 25 mg
Flintstones Plus Iron [OTC]	2,500	1.05	1.2	1.05	4.5	60	400	15	Fe 15 mg, folic acid 300 mcg, niacin 13.5 mg, sodium 10 mg; contains soy products
My First Flintstones [OTC]	1,998	1.05	1.2	1.05	4.5	60	400	15	Folic acid 300 mcg, niacin 10 mg, sodium 10 mg; contains soy products
One A Day Kids Scooby-Doo! Complete [OTC]	3,000	1.5	1.7	2	6	60	400	30	Biotin 40 mcg, Ca 100 mg, Cu 2 mg, Fe 18 mg, folic acid 400 mcg, iodine 150 mcg, Mg 20 mg, niacin 15 mg, pantothenic acid 10 mg, phosphorus 100 mg, sodium 10 mg, Zn 12 mg; contains phenylalanine; sugar-free
Quflora	1,200	1.2	1.3	1.5	4	60	400	15	Cu 1 mg, folate 208 mcg (as L-methylfolate glucosamine [molar equivalent to folic acid 108 mcg] and folic acid 100 mcg), Mg 15 mg, niacinamide 5 mg; grape flavor. Available in three fluoride strengths: 0.25 mg, 0.5 mg, 1 mg

Pediatric Formulations *continued*

Product	A (units)	B_1 (mg)	B_2 (mg)	B_6 (mg)	B_{12} (mcg)	C (mg)	D (units)	E (units)	Additional Information
SourceCF [OTC]	16,000	1.5	1.7	1.9	6	100	1,000	200	Biotin 100 mcg, folic acid 200 mcg, niacinamide 10 mg, pantothenic acid 12 mg, vitamin K 800 mcg, Zn 15 mg
Vitalets [OTC]	2,500	0.75	0.85	1	3	40	200	15	Biotin 150 mcg, Ca 80 mg, Fe (as ferrous fumarate) 10 mg, folic acid 200 mcg, Mg 20 mg, Mn 0.1 mg, niacinamide 10 mg, pantothenic acid 5 mg, phosphorus 60 mg, Zn 0.8 mg

Ca = calcium, Cr = chromium, Cu = copper, Fe = iron, Mg = magnesium, Mn = manganese, Mo = molybdenum, Zn = zinc

Prenatal Formulations

Product	A (units)	B_1 (mg)	B_2 (mg)	B_6 (mg)	B_{12} (mcg)	C (mg)	D (units)	E (units)	Additional Information
Caplet									
Néevo		3	3.4	2.6	0.5	80	400	30	Biotin 30 mcg, Ca 200 mg, Cu 2 mg, Fe (as polysaccharide iron complex) 29 mg, folic acid 0.4 mg, L-methylfolate calcium (molar equivalent to folic acid 1 mg), Mg 40 mg, niacinamide 20 mg, pantothenic acid 7 mg, Zn 15 mg; contains sodium benzoate
Prenate chewable				10	125		300		Biotin 280 mcg, blueberry extract 25 mg, boron 250 mcg, Ca 500 mg, folate 1 mg (as L-methylfolate glucosamine [molar equivalent to folic acid 600 mcg] and folic acid 400 mcg), Mg 50 mg
Select-OB [OTC]	1,700	1.6	1.8	2.5	5	60	400	30	Fe (as polysaccharide iron complex) 29 mg, folic acid 1 mg, Mg 25 mg, niacinamide 15 mg, Zn 15 mg; gluten-free
Vitafol-OB [OTC]	2,700	1.6	1.8	2.5	12	70	400	30	Ca 100 mg, Cu 2 mg, Fe [elemental] 65 mg, folic acid 1 mg, Mg 25 mg, niacinamide 18 mg, Zn 25 mg; gluten-free, sugar-free
Vitafol-PN	1,700	1.6	1.8	2.5	5	60	400	30	Ca 125 mg, Fe [elemental] 65 mg, folic acid 1 mg, Mg 25 mg, niacinamide 15 mg, Zn 15 mg
Capsule									
Concept OB		5	5	25	10	210			Biotin 300 mcg, Cu 0.8 mg, DHA 156 mg, EPA 39 mg, Fe (as ferrous fumarate) 130 mg, Fe (as polysaccharide iron complex) 92.4 mg, folic acid 1 mg, Mg 6.9 mg, Mn 1.3 mg, niacin 20 mg, pantothenic acid 7 mg, Zn 18.2 mg
Folet One				30	15	18	250	15	DHA 225 mg, docusate sodium 25 mg, Fe 38 mg, folate 1 mg, Mg 15 mg, Zn 20 mg; contains soy products
Nexa Plus				25		28	800	30	Biotin 250 mcg, Ca 160 mg, DHA 350 mg, docusate calcium 55 mg, Fe 29 mg, folic acid 1.25 mg; contains soy products
PreFol-DHA				25		28	400	30	Ca 160 mg, docusate sodium 55 mg, Fe (as ferrous fumarate) 26 mg, folic acid 1.2 mg, DHA 300 mg; contains soy products
Prenate Pixie				5	13	30	500	10	Biotin 75 mcg, blueberry extract (*vaccinium angustifolium*) 5 mg, DHA 200 mg, Fe 10 mg (as ferrous aspartoglycinate), folate 1 mg, potassium iodide 150 mcg; contains soy products
Provida DHA		2	3	25	10	30	400		Biotin 300 mcg, Cu 1 mg, DHA 110 mg, Fe (as ferrous fumarate and polysaccharide iron complex) 32 mg, folic acid 1.25 mg, *lactobacillus casei* 30 mg, Mg 7 mg, niacinamide 2 mg, pantothenic acid 5 mg, Zn 6 mg
R-Natal OB		2	4	20	30	100	400	30	Cu 2 mg, DHA 320 mg, Fe (as carbonyl iron) 20 mg, folic acid 1 mg, Zn 30 mg; contains soy products
Triveen-PRx RNF				25		28	400	30	Ca 160 mg, docusate sodium 55 mg, Fe (as ferrous fumarate) 26 mg, folic acid 1.2 mg, DHA 300 mg; contains soy products
Virt-Care One				25		25	170	30	Calcium 150 mg, Fe (as carbonyl iron 20 mg and ferrous aspartate glycinate 7 mg), folic acid 1 mg, linoleic acid 30 mg, omega-3 fatty acids 330 mg (including DHA 260 mg, EPA 40 mg, and ALA 30 mg); contains soy products

Prenatal Formulations *continued*

Product	A (units)	B_1 (mg)	B_2 (mg)	B_6 (mg)	B_{12} (mcg)	C (mg)	D (units)	E (units)	Additional Information
Virt-PN DHA				25	12	85	200	10	Ca 140 mg, DHA 300 mg, Fe 27 mg, folate 1 mg (as L-methylfolate calcium [molar equivalent to folic acid 600 mcg] and folic acid 400 mcg), Mg 45 mg; contains soy products
VirtPrex				25		28	400	30	Calcium phosphate tribasic 160 mg, DHA 300 mg, docusate sodium 55 mg, Fe 26 mg (as ferrous fumarate), folic acid 1.2 mg; contains soy products
Vitafol Ultra	1,100 (as beta carotene)	1.6	1.8	2.5	12	30	1,000	20	Algal oil 415 mg, Cu 2 mg, DHA 200 mg, Fe (as polysaccharide iron complex) 29 mg, folate 1 mg (as L-methylfolate calcium [molar equivalent to folic acid 0.6 mg] and folic acid 0.4 mg), Mg 20 mg, niacinamide 15 mg, potassium iodide 150 mcg, Zn 25 mg; contains soy products
Capsule, Softgel									
CitraNatal Harmony				25			400	30	Algal oil 650 mg, Ca 104 mg, DHA 265 mg, docusate sodium 50 mg, Fe (as carbonyl iron) 29 mg, folic acid 1 mg
Concept DHA		2	3	25	12.5	25			Biotin 300 mcg, Cu 2 mg, Fe (as ferrous fumarate) 53.5 mg, Fe (as polysaccharide iron complex) 38 mg, folic acid 1 mg, Mg 5 mg, niacin 1.8 mg, pantothenic acid 5 mg, Zn 10 mg
EnBrace HR		25 mcg (thiamine pyrophosphate)	25 mcg (flavin adenine dinucleotide)	25 mcg (pyridoxal 5' phosphate)	50 mcg (adenosylcobalamin)				Ascorbates (as magnesium ascorbate 24 mg and zinc ascorbate 1 mg), betaine 500 mcg, Fe 1.5 mg (as ferrous glycine cysteinate), flavin adenine dinucleotide 25 mcg, folate (as folic acid 1 mg, folinic acid 2.5 mg, and L-methylfolate magnesium 5.23 mg), L-threonate magnesium 1 mg, nicotinamide adenine dinucleotide hydride 25 mcg,omega-3 fatty acids (as phosphatidylserine-DHA 6.4 mg and phosphatidylserine-EPA 800 mcg), phosphatidylserine 12 mg; contains bovine gelatin; dye-free, gluten-free
Infanate Plus				25			400	30	Ca 104 mg, DHA 260 mg, docusate sodium 50 mg, Fe (as ferrous fumarate and carbonyl iron) 27 mg, folic acid 1 mg; contains soy products
Natelle One				25		30		30	Ca 102 mg, DHA 250 mg, EPA not more than 0.625 mg, Fe (as ferrous fumarate) 28 mg, folic acid 1 mg; contains soy products
NéevoDHA				25	1	40		30	Ca 75 mg, DHA 250 mg, Fe (as ferrous fumarate) 27 mg, folic acid 400 mcg, L-methylfolate calcium (molar equivalent to folic acid 1 mg); contains soy products
PreferaOB One				50	12	25	400	10	Biotin 30 mcg, DHA 200 mg, Fe 28 mg (22 mg as polysaccharide complex and 6 mg as heme iron polypeptide), folic acid 1 mg, iodine 175 mcg, niacinamide 17 mg, pantothenic acid 10 mg, Zn 15 mg; contains soy products
Prenate DHA				26	25	90	400	40	Ca 155 mg, DHA 300 mg, Fe (as ferrous asparto glycinate) 18 mg, folate 1 mg (as L-methylfolate calcium [molar equivalent to folic acid 600 mcg] and folic acid 400 mcg), Mg 50 mg; contains soy products; gluten-free
Prenate Essential				26	13	90	220	10	Biotin 280 mcg, Ca 145 mg, DHA 300 mg, EPA 40 mg, Fe (as ferrous fumarate) 29 mg, folate 1 mg (as L-methylfolate glucosamine [molar equivalent to folic acid 600 mcg] and folic acid 400 mcg), iodine 150 mcg, Mg 50 mg; contains soy products, tartrazine

Prenatal Formulations *continued*

Product	A (units)	B_1 (mg)	B_2 (mg)	B_6 (mg)	B_{12} (mcg)	C (mg)	D (units)	E (units)	Additional Information
Prenate Mini				26	13	60	1,000	10	Biotin 280 mcg, blueberry extract (*vaccinium* spp) 25 mg, Ca 80 mg, DHA 350 mg, Fe (as carbonyl iron and ferrous asparto glycinate) 18 mg, folate 1 mg (as L-methylfolate calcium [molar equivalent to folic acid 400 mcg] and folic acid 400 mcg), iodine 150 mcg, Mg 25 mg; contains soy products, tartrazine; gluten-free, lactose-free
PreNexa Premier				25		28	800	30	Ca 160 mg, DHA 310 mg, docusate sodium 55 mg, Fe 27 mg, folic acid 1.25 mg; contains soy products
TriCare Prenatal DHA One		3	3.4	25	100	60	800	30	Biotin 300 mcg, Cu 2 mg, DHA 215 mg, docusate sodium 25 mg, EPA 45 mg, Fe (as ferrous fumarate) 27 mg, folic acid 1 mg, niacin 20 mg, Zn 10 mg
Virt-C DHA		2	3	25	12.5	25			Biotin 300 mcg, Cu 2 mg, Fe [elemental] 35 mg (as ferrous fumarate 53.5 mg and polysaccharide iron complex 38 mg), folic acid 1 mg, Mg 5 mg, niacin 1.8 mg, omega-3 fatty acids 200 mg (including DHA 156 mg and EPA 39 mg), pantothenic acid 5 mg, Zn 10 mg; contains soy products
vitaMedMD One Rx		1.5	1.7	25	8	60	400	21	Biotin 300 mcg, DHA 200 mg, Fe 30 mg, folate 1 mg (as L-methylfolate glucosamine [molar equivalent to folic acid 600 mcg] and folic acid 400 mcg), niacinamide 20 mg, pantothenic acid 10 mg, Zn 7.5 mg
vitaPearl		1.7	2	25	8	30	400	30	Biotin 300 mcg, DHA 200 mg, Fe 30 mg, folic acid 1.4 mg, niacinamide 20 mg, pantothenic acid 10 mg, potassium iodide 150 mcg, zinc 7.5 mg; gluten-free, lactose-free, sugar-free
Tablet									
A-Free Prenatal [OTC] (***per 3 tablets***)		6	6	3	6	100	400	30	Biotin 30 mcg, calcium 1,000 mg, Cu 0.3 mg, Fe (as ferrous fumarate) 27 mg, folic acid 800 mcg, Mg 100 mg, Mn 0.3 mg, niacinamide 30 mg, pantothenic acid 15 mg, Zn 22.5 mg; natural base contains bioflavonoids and hesperidin 66 mg
B-Nexa				42					Calcium 124 mg, folic acid 1.22 mg, ginger root powder extract 100 mg
CitraNatal Rx		3	3.4	20		120	400	30	Ca 125 mg, Cu 2 mg, docusate sodium 50 mg, Fe (as carbonyl iron, ferrous gluconate) 27 mg, folic acid 1 mg, iodine 150 mcg, niacinamide 20 mg, Zn 25 mg
Femecal OB		1.5	1.6	50	12		400	10	Biotin 30 mcg, Cu 0.8 mg, Fe 28 mg (22 mg as polysaccharide iron complex and 6 mg as ferrous aspartate and iron glycinate), folic acid 1 mg, iodine 175 mcg, niacinamide 17 mg, pantothenic acid 10 mg, Se 65 mcg, Zn 15 mg
Focalgin-B				42					Ca 124.23 mg, folic acid 1.22 mg, ginger 100 mg
Foltabs Prenatal		3	3.4	20		120	400	30	Ca 125 mg, Cu 2 mg, docusate sodium 50 mg, Fe 27 mg, folic acid 1 mg, iodine 150 mcg, niacinamide 20 mg, Zn 25 mg
Gesticare		3	3	50	8	120	420	30	Ca 200 mg, choline 55 mg, Fe (as ferrous fumarate) 28 mg, folic acid 1 mg, iodine 150 mcg, niacinamide 20 mg, Zn 15 mg
KPN Prenatal [OTC] (***per 3 tablets***)	2,000	6	6	3	6	100	400	30	Biotin 30 mcg, Ca 1,000 mg, Cu 0.3 mg, Fe (as ferrous fumarate) 27 mg, folic acid 800 mcg, Mg 100 mg, Mn 0.3 mg, niacinamide 30 mg, pantothenic acid 15 mg, Zn 22.5 mg; natural base contains 66 mg bioflavonoids and hesperidin

Prenatal Formulations *continued*

Product	A (units)	B_1 (mg)	B_2 (mg)	B_6 (mg)	B_{12} (mcg)	C (mg)	D (units)	E (units)	Additional Information
Mini-Prenatal [OTC]	2,000	2	3	3	10	100	400	15	Biotin 100 mcg, Ca 200 mg, Cu 2 mg, Fe (as ferrous fumarate) 27 mg, folic acid 800 mcg, Mg 60 mg, Mn 2 mg, niacinamide 20 mg, pantothenic acid 10 mg, Zn 15 mg
Multi-Nate 30	3,000	1.8	4	25	12	120	400	30	Ca 200 mg, Cu 2 mg, Fe 29 mg, folic acid 1 mg, Mg 25 mg, niacin 20 mg, Zn 25 mg; contains soy products
Niva-Plus	4,000	1.84	3	10	12	120	400	22	Ca 200 mg, Cu 2 mg, Fe (as ferrous fumarate) 27 mg, folic acid 1 mg, niacinamide 20 mg, Zn 25 mg
PreferaOB		1.5	1.6	50	12		400	10	Biotin 30 mcg, Cu 0.8 mg, Fe 34 mg (28 mg as polysaccharide complex and 6 mg as heme iron polypeptide), folic acid 1 mg, iodine 250 mcg, niacin 17 mg, pantothenic acid 10 mg, Se 65 mg, Zn 4.5 mg
Prenaissance Next-B				42					Ca 124.23 mg, folic acid 1.22 mg, ginger 100 mg; contains tartrazine
Prenatabs FA	4,000	3	3	3	8	120	400	30	Ca 200 mg, Fe (as ferrous fumarate) 29 mg, folic acid 1 mg, iodine 150 mcg, niacin 20 mg, Zn 15 mg
Prenatabs Rx	4,000 (beta carotene)	3	3	3	8	120	400	30	Biotin 30 mcg, Ca 200 mg, Cu 3 mg, Fe (as iron carbonyl) 29 mg, folic acid 1 mg, Mg 100 mg, niacinamide 20 mg, pantothenic acid 7 mg, potassium iodide 150 mcg, Zn 15 mg; contains soy products
Prenatal 19	1,000	3	3	20	12	100	400	30	Ca 200 mg, docusate sodium 25 mg, Fe (as ferrous fumarate) 29 mg, folic acid 1 mg, niacinamide 15 mg, pantothenic acid 7 mg, Zn 20 mg; contains soy products
Prenatal One Daily [OTC]	2,000	2	3	3	10	100	400	15	Biotin 100 mcg, Ca 200 mg, Cu 2 mg, Fe (as ferrous fumarate) 27 mg, folic acid 800 mcg, Mg 60 mg, Mn 2 mg, niacinamide 20 mg, pantothenic acid 10 mg, Zn 15 mg
Prenatal Rx 1	4,000	1.5	1.6	4	2.5	80	400	15	Biotin 30 mg, Ca 200 mg, Cu 3 mg, Fe (as ferrous fumarate) 60 mg, folic acid 1 mg, Mg 100 mg, niacinamide 17 mg, pantothenic acid 7 mg, Zn 25 mg
Prenate Elite	2,600	3	3.5	21	13	75	450	10	Biotin 330 mcg, Ca 100 mg, Cu 1.5 mg, Fe (as ferrous fumarate) 26 mg, folate 1 mg (as L-methylfolate glucosamine [molar equivalent to folic acid 600 mcg] and folic acid 400 mcg), iodine 150 mcg, Mg 25 mg, niacinamide 21 mg, pantothenic acid 6 mg, Zn 15 mg
TriCare Prenatal		1.6	1.6	3.1	12	100	400	30	Ca 200 mg, Cu 2 mg, Fe (as ferrous fumarate) 27 mg, folic acid 1 mg, niacinamide 20 mg, Zn 10 mg
Virt-Advance	2,700 (as beta carotene)	3	3.4	20	12	120	400	30	Ca 200 mg, Cu 2 mg, docusate sodium 50 mg, Fe 90 mg (as iron carbonyl), folic acid 1 mg, Mg 30 mg, niacinamide 20 mg, Zn 25 mg; contains tartrazine
Virt Nate	3,000 (as beta carotene)	1.8	4	25	12	120	400	22	Ca 200 mg, Cu 2 mg, Fe 28 mg (as ferrous fumarae), folic acid 1 mg, Mg 25 mg, niacinamide 20 mg, Zn 25 mg
Virt-Vite GT	2,700 (as beta carotene)	3	3.4	20	12	120	400	10	Biotin 30 mcg, Ca 200 mg, Cu 2 mg, docusate sodium 50 mg, Fe 90 mg (as iron carbonyl), folic acid 1 mg, Mg 30 mg, niacinamide 20 mg, pantothenic acid 6 mg, Zn 15 mg
Vitafol-Nano				2.5	12		1,000		Fe (as ferrous fumarate) 18 mg, folate 1 mg (as L-methylfolate calcium [molar equivalent to folic acid 0.6 mg] and folic acid 0.4 mg), potassium iodide 150 mcg

Prenatal Formulations *continued*

Product	A (units)	B_1 (mg)	B_2 (mg)	B_6 (mg)	B_{12} (mcg)	C (mg)	D (units)	E (units)	Additional Information
Vol-Tab Rx	4,000 (beta carotene)	3	3	3	8	120	400	30	Biotin 30 mcg, Ca 200 mg, Cu 3 mg, Fe (as iron carbonyl) 29 mg, folic acid 1 mg, Mg 100 mg, niacinamide 20 mg, pantothenic acid 7 mg, potassium iodide 150 mcg, Zn 15 mg
VP-Heme OB		1.5	1.6	50	12		400	10	Biotin 30 mcg, Ca 10 mg, Cu 0.8 mg, Fe 34 mg (28 mg as polysaccharide iron complex and 6 mg as heme iron polypeptide), folic acid 1 mg, niacinamide 17 mg, potassium iodide 250 mcg, selenium 65 mcg, Zn 4.5 mg
Tablet, Chewable									
NataChew [OTC]	1,000	2	3	10	12	120	400	11	Fe (as ferrous fumarate) 29 mg, folic acid 1 mg, niacinamide 20 mg
PreCare				2		50	6 mcg	3.5	Ca 250 mg, Cu 2 mg, Fe (as ferrous fumarate) 40 mg, folic acid 1 mg, Mg 50 mg, Zn 15 mg
Prena1			1.7	2	8		400		Folic acid 1.4 mg
Prenatal 19 Chewable	1,000	3	3	20	12	100	400	30	Ca 200 mg, Fe (as ferrous fumarate) 29 mg, folic acid 1 mg, niacinamide 15 mg, pantothenic acid 7 mg, Zn 20 mg
Select-OB	1,700	1.6	1.8	2.5	5	60	400	30	Fe 29 mg, folic acid 1 mg, Mg 25 mg, niacin 15 mg, Zn 15 mg
Vinate Care				2		50	6 mcg	3.5	Ca 250 mg, Cu 2 mg, Fe (as ferrous fumarate) 40 mg, folic acid 1 mg, Mg 50 mg, Zn 15 mg
vitaMedMD RediChew Rx			1.7	2	8		400		Folic acid 1.4 mg
Combination Package									
CitraNatal 90 DHA (***tablet***)		3	3.4	20		120	400	30	Ca 159 mg, Cu 2 mg, docusate sodium 50 mg, Fe 90 mg (as carbonyl iron and ferrous gluconate), folic acid 1 mg, iodine 150 mcg, niacinamide 20 mg, Zn 25 mg Packaged with ***gelatin capsule*** containing DHA 300 mg and EPA 0.75 mg
CitraNatal Assure		3	3.4	25		120	400	30	Ca 125 mg, Cu 2 mg, docusate sodium 50 mg, Fe (as carbonyl iron and ferrous gluconate) 35 mg, folic acid 1 mg, iodine 150 mcg, niacin 20 mg, Zn 25 mg Packaged with ***softgel capsule*** containing DHA 300 mg
CitraNatal B-Calm				25		120	400		Ca 125 mg, Fe (as carbonyl iron) 20 mg, folic acid 1 mg Packaged with two B_6 25 mg tablets
CitraNatal DHA (***tablet***)		3	3.4	20		120	400	30	Ca 125 mg, Cu 2 mg, docusate sodium 50 mg, Fe 27 mg (as carbonyl iron and ferrous gluconate), folic acid 1 mg, iodine 150 mcg, niacinamide 20 mg, Zn 25 mg. Packaged with ***gelatin capsule*** containing DHA 250 mg.
CitraNatal 90 DHA (***tablet***)		3	3.4	20		120	400	30	Ca 200 mg, Cu 2 mg, docusate sodium 50 mg, Fe 90 mg (as carbonyl iron), folic acid 1 mg, iodine 150 mcg, niacinamide 20 mg, Zn 25 mg. Packaged with ***gelatin capsule*** containing DHA 250 mg.
Duet DHA Balanced (***tablet***)	2,840	1.5	4	50	12	120	840	2	Ca 215 mg, Cu 2 mg, Fe 26 mg, folic acid 1 mg, iodine 210 mcg, Mg 25 mg, niacinamide 20 mg, Zn 25 mg Packaged with ***softgel capsule*** containing omega-3 fatty acids 267 mg
Folet DHA (***tablet***)	2,700	3	3.4	40	12	120	400	18	Docusate sodium 50 mg, Fe 38 mg (as ferrous bisglycinate chelate and iron carbonyl), folate 1 mg, Mg 30 mg, niacinamide 20 mg, Se 65 mcg, Zn 10 mg Packaged with ***softgel capsule*** containing DHA 350 mg

Prenatal Formulations *continued*

Product	A (units)	B_1 (mg)	B_2 (mg)	B_6 (mg)	B_{12} (mcg)	C (mg)	D (units)	E (units)	Additional Information
Foltabs Prenatal Plus DHA		3	3.4	20		120	400	30	Ca 125 mg, Cu 2 mg, docusate sodium 50 mg, Fe 27 mg, folic acid 1 mg, iodine 150 mcg, niacinamide 20 mg, Zn 25 mg Packaged with ***gelatin capsule*** containing DHA 250 mg
Gesticare DHA		3	3	50	8	120	410	30	Ca 200 mg, choline 55 mg, Fe (as ferrous fumarate) 27 mg, folic acid 1 mg, iodine 150 mcg, niacinamide 20 mg, Zn 15 mg Packaged with ***gelatin capsule*** containing DHA 250 mg and EPA not more than 0.625 mg
One A Day Women's Prenatal [OTC] (***tablet***)	4,000	1.7	2	2.5	8	60	400	30	Biotin 300 mcg, Ca 300 mg, Cu 2 mg, Fe 28 mg, folic acid 800 mcg, iodine 150 mcg, Mg 50 mg, niacin 20 mg, pantothenic acid 10 mg, Zn 15 mg Packaged with ***softgel capsule*** containing omega-3 fatty acids 223 mg (as DHA 200 mg and EPA 23 mg); contains soy products.
Paire OB Plus DHA		1.5	1.6	50	12		400	10	Biotin 30 mcg, Cu 0.8 mg, Fe 28 mg, folic acid 1 mg, iodine 175 mcg, niacinamide 17 mg, pantothenic acid 10 mg, Se 65 mcg, Zn 15 mg Packaged with ***softgel capsule*** containing DHA 200 mg
PreferaOB + DHA		1.5	1.6	50	12		400	10	Biotin 30 mcg, Cu 0.8 mg, Fe 34 mg (28 mg as polysaccharide complex and 6 mg as heme iron polypeptide), folic acid 1 mg, iodine 250 mcg, niacin 17 mg, pantothenic acid 10 mg, Se 65 mg, Zn 4.5 mg Packaged with ***softgel*** containing DHA 200 mg
Vitafol-OB+DHA (***caplet***)	2,700	1.6	1.8	2.5	12	70	400	30	Ca 100 mg, Cu 2 mg, Fe [elemental] 65 mg, folic acid 1 mg, Mg 25 mg, niacinamide 18 mg, Zn 25 mg; gluten-free, sugar-free Packaged with ***gelatin capsule*** containing DHA 250 mg
vitaMedMD Plus Rx		3	3.4	25	12	60	600	30	Biotin 300 mcg, calcium 150 mg, Cu 2 mg, Fe 30 mg, folate 1 mg (as L-methylfolate glucosamine [molar equivalent to folic acid 600 mcg] and folic acid 400 mcg), iodine 150 mcg, niacinamide 20 mg, pantothenic acid 10 mg, Zn 15 mg Packaged with ***softgel capsule*** containing DHA 300 mg
VitaPhil + DHA	2,600	3	3.5	30	12	120	420	20	Biotin 30 mcg, Ca 8 mg, choline 60 mg, Cu 2 mg, Fe 26 mg, folic acid 1 mg, niacinamide 20 mg, Mg 50 mg, Se 50 mg, Zn 15 mg; contains soy products Packaged with ***softgel capsule*** containing DHA 200 mg
VP-Heme OB + DHA (**tablet**)		1.5	1.6	50	12		400	10	Biotin 30 mcg, Ca 10 mg, Cu 0.8 mg, Fe 34 mg (28 mg as polysaccharide iron complex and 6 mg as heme iron polypeptide), folic acid 1 mg, niacinamide 17 mg, potassium iodide 250 mcg, selenium 65 mcg, Zn 4.5 mg Packaged with **softgel capsule** containing omega-3 fatty acids 203 mg (as DHA 200 mg, ALA 0.5 mg, and DPA 2.5 mg)

Ca = calcium, Cr = chromium, Cu = copper, DHA = docosahexaenoic acid (from omega-3 fatty acids), Fe = iron, Mg = magnesium, Mn = manganese, Mo = molybdenum, Se = selenium, Zn = zinc

Vitamin B Complex Combinations

Product	B_1 (mg)	B_2 (mg)	B_6 (mg)	B_{12} (mcg)	C (mg)	E (units)	Additional Information
Caplet							
Allbee with C [OTC]	15	10.2	5		300		Biotin 300 mcg, folic acid 400 mcg, niacinamide 50 mg, pantothenic acid 10 mg
Allbee C-800 [OTC]	15	17	25	12	800	45	Biotin 300 mcg, folic acid 400 mcg, niacinamide 100 mg, pantothenic acid 25 mg
Allbee C-800 + Iron [OTC]	15	17	25	12	800	45	Biotin 300 mcg, Fe 27 mg, folic acid 0.4 mg, niacinamide 100 mg, pantothenic acid 25 mg
Nephronex	1.5	1.7	10	10	60		Biotin 300 mcg, folic acid 1 mg, nicotinic acid 20 mg, pantothenic acid 10 mg
Capsule							
Virt-Caps	1.5	1.7	10	6	100		Biotin 150 mcg, folic acid 1 mg, niacinamide 20 mg, pantothenic acid 5 mg
Elixir							
Eldertonic **(per 15 mL)**	0.5	0.6	0.7	2			Mg 0.7 mg, Mn 0.7 mg, niacin 7 mg, pantothenic acid 3 mg, Zn 5 mg [contains alcohol 13.5%]
Liquid							
Gevrabon [OTC] **(per 30 mL)**	5	2.5	1	1			Choline 10 mg, Fe 15 mg, iodine 100 mcg, Mn 2 mg, niacinamide 50 mg, pantothenic acid 10 mg, Zn 2 mg; alcohol, benzoic acid; sherry wine flavor (480 mL)
Nephronex **(per 5 mL)**	1.5	1.7	10	10	60		Biotin 300 mcg, folic acid 900 mcg, nicotinic acid 20 mg, pantothenic acid 10 mg
Softgel							
Nephrocaps	1.5	1.7	10	6	100		Biotin 150 mcg, folate 1 mg, niacinamide 20 mg, pantothenic acid 5 mg
Renal Caps	1.5	1.7	10	6	100		Biotin 150 mcg, folic acid 1 mg, niacinamide 20 mg, pantothenic acid 5 mg
Tablet							
Bee Zee [OTC]	15	10.2	10	6	600	45	Biotin 300 mcg, folic acid 400 mcg, niacinamide 100 mg, pantothenic acid 25 mg, Zn 22.5 mg
DexFol	1.5	1.5	50	1	60		Biotin 300 mcg, cobalamin 1 mg, folacin 5 mg, niacinamide 20 mg, pantothenic acid 10 mg; dye-free, sugar-free, lactose-free
Kobee [OTC]	10	10	10	10			Biotin 10 mcg, choline citrate 10 mg, folic acid 400 mcg, inositol 10 mg, niacinamide 50 mg, PABA 10 mg, pantothenic acid 10 mg
NephPlex Rx	1.5	1.7	10	6	60		Biotin 300 mcg, folic acid 1 mg, niacinamide 20 mg, pantothenic acid 10 mg, zinc 12.5 mg
Nephro-Vite [OTC]	1.5	1.7	10	6	60		Biotin 300 mcg, folic acid 0.8 mg, niacinamide 20 mg, pantothenic acid 10 mg
Nephro-Vite Rx	1.5	1.7	10	6	60		Biotin 300 mcg, folic acid 1 mg, niacinamide 20 mg, pantothenic acid 10 mg
Nephron FA	1.5	1.7	10	6	40		Biotin 300 mcg, docusate sodium 75 mg, ferrous fumarate 200 mg, folic acid 1 mg, niacinamide 20 mg, pantothenic acid 10 mg
Quin B Strong [OTC]	25	25	25	25			Biotin 25 mcg, folic acid 400 mcg, niacinamide 100 mg, pantothenic acid 25 mg (in a base containing 25 mg of choline citrate and inositol)
Quin B Strong with C and Zinc [OTC]	25	25	25	25	500		Biotin 25 mcg, folic acid 400 mcg, niacinamide 100 mg, pantothenic acid 25 mg, Zn 15 mg (in a base containing 25 mg of choline citrate and inositol)
Rena-Vite [OTC]	1.5	1.7	10	6	60		Biotin 300 mcg, folic acid 800 mcg, niacin 20 mg, pantothenic acid 10 mg
Rena-Vite RX	1.5	1.7	10	6	60		Biotin 300 mcg, folate 1 mg, niacin 20 mg, pantothenic acid 10 mg
Stresstabs High Potency Advanced [OTC]	10	10	5	12	250	30	Biotin 45 mcg, Ca 70 mg, Cu 3 mg, folic acid 400 mcg, niacinamide 100 mg, pantothenic acid 20 mg, phosphorus 30 mg, Zn 23.9 mg
Stresstabs High Potency Energy [OTC]	10	10	5	5	300	30	Biotin 45 mcg, Ca 20 mg, Fe 4 mg, folic acid 400 mcg, niacinamide 100 mg, pantothenic acid 20 mg, phosphorus 15 mg
Stresstabs High Potency Weight [OTC]	10	10	5	12	300	30	Biotin 45 mcg, Ca 44 mg, chronium 200 mcg, EGCG 32 mg, folic acid 400 mcg, niacinamide 100 mg, pantothenic acid 20 mg, phosphorus 32 mg

Vitamin B Complex Combinations *continued*

Product	B_1 (mg)	B_2 (mg)	B_6 (mg)	B_{12} (mcg)	C (mg)	E (units)	Additional Information
Super Dec B 100 [OTC]	100	100	100	100			Biotin 100 mcg, folic acid 400 mcg, niacinamide 100 mg, pantothenic acid 100 mg (in a base containing 100 mg of choline citrate and inositol)
Superplex-T [OTC]	15	10	5	10	500		Niacinamide 100 mg, pantothenic acid 18.3 mg, sodium 70 mg
Super Quints 50 [OTC]	50	50	50	50			Biotin 50 mcg, folic acid 400 mcg, niacinamide 50 mg, pantothenic acid 50 mg (in a base containing 50 mg of choline citrate, glutaminic acid, glutamine, glycine, inositol, and lysine)
Surbex-T [OTC]	12.4	9	3.7	9	450		Niacinamide 90.7 mg, pantothenic acid 16.6 mg, sodium 65 mg
Vita-Bee/C [OTC]	15	10.2	5		300		Biotin 300 mcg, folic acid 400 mcg, niacinamide 50 mg, pantothenic acid 10 mg
Z-Bec [OTC]	15	10.2	10	6	600	45	Biotin 300 mcg, folic acid 400 mcg, niacinamide 100 mg, pantothenic acid 25 mg, Zn 22.5 mg
Tablet, Dissolving							
Nephrocaps QT	1.5	1.7	10	6	100		Biotin 150 mcg; cholecalciferol 1,750 units; folic acid 1 mg; niacin 20 mg; pantothenic acid 5 mg; fruit-punch flavor

Ca = calcium, Cu = copper, Fe = iron, Mg = magnesium, Mn = manganese, Se = selenium, Zn = zinc

OPIOID CONVERSION TABLE

This table serves as a general guide to opioid conversion. Utilization of a direct conversion without a detailed patient and medication assessment is not recommended and may result in over- or underdosing. Values are based on single-dose adult studies. Duration of action may be shorter in children due to faster elimination (in general) compared to adults. The pharmacokinetics of opioids in children and infants >6 months of age are similar to adults, but infants <6 months of age, especially those who are premature or physically compromised, may demonstrate decreased clearance and are at risk of apnea.

Drug	Onset (min)	Duration (h)	Equianalgesic IM Dose (mg)	Equianalgesic PO Dose[1] (mg)	Parenteral Oral Ratio
Alfentanil	IV: Immediate	<0.25 to 0.33	No data	—	—
Codeine[2]	IM: 10 to 30 PO: 30 to 60	4 to 6	100 to 130	200	1/2 to 2/3
FentaNYL	IM: 7 to 15 IV: Immediate	IM: 1 to 2 IV: 0.5 to 1	0.1	—	—
HYDROcodone	PO: 10 to 20	3 to 6	—	30 to 45	—
HYDROmorphone	PO: 15 to 30	4 to 5	1.5	7.5	1/5
Meperidine[3]	PO, IM, SubQ: 10 to 15 IV: ≤5	PO, IM, SubQ: 2 to 4 IV: 2 to 3	75	300	1/3 to 1/2
Methadone[4]	PO: 30 to 60 IV: 10 to 20	Acute: 4 to 6 Chronic: >8	*Pediatrics:* Acute: 10 Chronic: Not established[5]	*Pediatrics:* Acute: 20 Chronic: Not established[5] *Adults*[6]: See Guidelines for Conversion to Oral Methadone in Adults	—
Morphine	PO (immediate release): 15 to 60 IV: ≤5	PO (immediate release), IV, IM, SubQ: 3 to 5 Extended release tablets: 8 to 12	10	30	1/6; ratio decreases to 1/1.5 to 2.5 upon chronic dosing
OxyCODONE	PO (immediate release): 15 to 30	PO: Immediate release: 4 to 5 Controlled release: 12	—	20	—
Pentazocine	PO, IM, SubQ: 15 to 30 IV: ≤2 to 3	PO: 4 to 5 IV, IM, SubQ: 2 to 3	30	50	1/3

Guidelines for Conversion to Oral Methadone in Adults[6]

Oral Morphine Dose or Equivalent (mg/day)	Oral Morphine:Oral Methadone (Conversion Ratio)
<90	4:1
90 to 300	8:1
>300	12:1

[1]Chronic administration may alter pharmacokinetics and change parenteral oral ratio.

[2]Codeine should not be used in infants <6 months of age due to slow metabolism, accumulation of morphine (major metabolite), and risk of apnea/death. In addition, 10% of the population cannot convert codeine to morphine and therefore will not experience analgesia. Conversely, ultra-rapid metabolizers may have an exaggerated opioid response.

[3]Not recommended for routine use due to potential accumulation of a neurotoxic metabolite

[4]Conversion to methadone requires close observation for delayed sedation which may occur 3 to 5 days postconversion. Dosing interval needs to be increased after the initial 1 to 2 days of treatment to avoid late sedation.

[5]A conversion factor for pediatric patients receiving chronic opioids has not been identified; doses lower than those listed for acute opioid administration would be recommended based on adult data. Some experts recommend against the use of an "equianalgesic" dosage of methadone (to prevent or treat opioid withdrawal) because calculated methadone doses may be unnecssarily high for this indication (Lugo 2001).

[6]Conversion of higher doses may be guided by the following (consult a pain or palliative care specialist if unfamiliar with methadone prescribing): As the total daily dose of morphine increases, the equianalgesic dose ratio (methadone:morphine) changes in adults (American Pain Society 2008). Total daily dose should be divided by 3 and administered every 8 hours. Methadone is significantly more potent with repetitive dosing. Begin methadone at lower doses and gradually titrate. Use these conversion guidelines only in adult patients; do not use in pediatric patients; applicability to pediatric patients is unknown and may be dangerous or potentially lethal.

REFERENCES

Friedrichsdorf SJ, Kang TI. The management of pain in children with life-limiting illnesses. *Pediatr Clin North Am.* 2007;54(5):645-672.

Lugo RA, MacLaren R, Cash J, Pribble CG, Vernon DD. Enteral methadone to expedite fentanyl discontinuation and prevent opioid abstinence syndrome in the PICU. *Pharmacotherapy.* 2001;21(12):1566-1573.

National Cancer Institute. Pain (PDQ). Available at http://www.cancer.gov/cancertopics/pdq/supportivecare/pain/HealthProfessional/page1. Accessed May 7, 2009.

National Comprehensive Cancer Network (NCCN). Clinical practice guidelines in oncology: adult cancer pain. Version 1, 2009. Available at http://www.nccn.org/professionals/physician_gls/PDF/pain.pdf

Patanwala AE, Duby J, Waters D, Erstad BL. Opioid conversions in acute care. *Ann Pharmacother.* 2007;41(2):255-266.

Principles of Analgesic Use in the Treatment of Acute Pain and Cancer Pain. 6th ed. Glenview, IL: American Pain Society; 2008.

APOTHECARY/METRIC EQUIVALENTS

Apothecary-Metric Exact Equivalents

1 gram (g)	=	15.43 grains (gr)	0.1 mg	=	1/600 gr
1 milliliter (mL)	=	16.23 minims	0.12 mg	=	1/500 gr
1 minim	=	0.06 mL	0.15 mg	=	1/400 gr
1 gr	=	64.8 milligrams (mg)	0.2 mg	=	1/300 gr
1 fluid ounce (fl oz)	=	29.57 mL	0.3 mg	=	1/200 gr
1 pint (pt)	=	473.2 mL	0.4 mg	=	1/150 gr
1 ounce (oz)	=	28.35 g	0.5 mg	=	1/120 gr
1 pound (lb)	=	453.6 g	0.6 mg	=	1/100 gr
1 kilogram (kg)	=	2.2 lb	0.8 mg	=	1/80 gr
1 quart (qt)	=	946.4 mL	1 mg	=	1/65 gr

Apothecary-Metric Approximate Equivalents[1]

Liquids

1 teaspoonful	=	5 mL
1 tablespoonful	=	15 mL

Solids

1/4 grain	=	15 mg
1/2 grain	=	30 mg
1 grain	=	60 mg
1 1/2 grain	=	100 mg
5 grains	=	300 mg
10 grains	=	600 mg

[1]Use exact equivalents for compounding and calculations requiring a high degree of accuracy.

POUNDS/KILOGRAMS CONVERSION

1 pound = 0.45359 kilograms
1 kilogram = 2.2 pounds

lb	=	kg	lb	=	kg	lb	=	kg
1 lb		0.45 kg	70 lbs		31.75 kg	140 lbs		63.5 kg
5 lbs		2.27 kg	75 lbs		34.02 kg	145 lbs		65.77 kg
10 lbs		4.54 kg	80 lbs		36.29 kg	150 lbs		68.04 kg
15 lbs		6.8 kg	85 lbs		38.56 kg	155 lbs		70.31 kg
20 lbs		9.07 kg	90 lbs		40.82 kg	160 lbs		72.58 kg
25 lbs		11.34 kg	95 lbs		43.09 kg	165 lbs		74.84 kg
30 lbs		13.61 kg	100 lbs		45.36 kg	170 lbs		77.11 kg
35 lbs		15.88 kg	105 lbs		47.63 kg	175 lbs		79.38 kg
40 lbs		18.14 kg	110 lbs		49.9 kg	180 lbs		81.65 kg
45 lbs		20.41 kg	115 lbs		52.16 kg	185 lbs		83.92 kg
50 lbs		22.68 kg	120 lbs		54.43 kg	190 lbs		86.18 kg
55 lbs		24.95 kg	125 lbs		56.7 kg	195 lbs		88.45 kg
60 lbs		27.22 kg	130 lbs		58.91 kg	200 lbs		90.72 kg
65 lbs		29.48 kg	135 lbs		61.24 kg			

TEMPERATURE CONVERSION

Celsius to Fahrenheit = (°C x 9/5) + 32 = °F
Fahrenheit to Celsius = (°F - 32) x 5/9 = °C

°C	=	°F
100		212
50		122
41		105.8
40.8		105.4
40.6		105.1
40.4		104.7
40.2		104.4
40		104
39.8		103.6
39.6		103.3
39.4		102.9
39.2		102.6

°C	=	°F
39		102.2
38.8		101.8
38.6		101.5
38.4		101.1
38.2		100.8
38		100.4
37.8		100.1
37.6		99.7
37.4		99.3
37.2		99
37		98.6

°C	=	°F
36.8		98.2
36.6		97.9
36.4		97.5
36.2		97.2
36		96.8
35.8		96.4
35.6		96.1
35.4		95.7
35.2		95.4
35		95
0		32

CYTOCHROME P450 ENZYMES: SUBSTRATES, INHIBITORS, AND INDUCERS

INTRODUCTION

Most drugs are eliminated from the body, at least in part, by being chemically altered to less lipid-soluble products (ie, metabolized), and thus are more likely to be excreted via the kidneys or the bile. Phase I metabolism includes drug hydrolysis, oxidation, and reduction, and results in drugs that are more polar in their chemical structure, while Phase II metabolism involves the attachment of an additional molecule onto the drug (or partially metabolized drug) in order to create an inactive and/or more water soluble compound. Phase II processes include (primarily) glucuronidation, sulfation, glutathione conjugation, acetylation, and methylation.

Virtually any of the Phase I and II enzymes can be inhibited by some xenobiotic or drug. Some of the Phase I and II enzymes can be induced. Inhibition of the activity of metabolic enzymes will result in increased concentrations of the substrate (drug), whereas induction of the activity of metabolic enzymes will result in decreased concentrations of the substrate. For example, the well-documented enzyme-inducing effects of phenobarbital may include a combination of Phase I and II enzymes. Phase II glucuronidation may be increased via induced UDP-glucuronosyltransferase (UGT) activity, whereas Phase I oxidation may be increased via induced cytochrome P450 (CYP) activity. However, for most drugs, the primary route of metabolism (and the primary focus of drug-drug interaction) is Phase I oxidation.

CYP enzymes may be responsible for the metabolism (at least partial metabolism) of ~75% of all drugs, with the CYP3A subfamily responsible for nearly half of this activity. Found throughout plant, animal, and bacterial species, CYP enzymes represent a superfamily of xenobiotic metabolizing proteins. There have been several hundred CYP enzymes identified in nature, each of which has been assigned to a family (1, 2, 3, etc), subfamily (A, B, C, etc), and given a specific enzyme number (1, 2, 3, etc) according to the similarity in amino acid sequence that it shares with other enzymes. Of these many enzymes, only a few are found in humans, and even fewer appear to be involved in the metabolism of xenobiotics (eg, drugs). The key human enzyme subfamilies include CYP1A, CYP2A, CYP2B, CYP2C, CYP2D, CYP2E, and CYP3A. However, the number of distinct isozymes (eg, CYP2C9) found to be functionally active in humans, as well as, the number of genetically variant forms of these isozymes (eg, CYP2C9*2) in individuals continues to expand.

CYP enzymes are found in the endoplasmic reticulum of cells in a variety of human tissues (eg, skin, kidneys, brain, lungs), but their predominant sites of concentration and activity are the liver and intestine. Though the abundance of CYP enzymes throughout the body is relatively equally distributed among the various subfamilies, the relative contribution to drug metabolism is (in decreasing order of magnitude) CYP3A4 (nearly 50%), CYP2D6 (nearly 25%), CYP2C8/9 (nearly 15%), then CYP1A2, CYP2C19, CYP2A6, and CYP2E1. Owing to their potential for numerous drug-drug interactions, those drugs that are identified in preclinical studies as substrates of CYP3A enzymes are often given a lower priority for continued research and development in favor of drugs that appear to be less affected by (or less likely to affect) this enzyme subfamily.

Each enzyme subfamily possesses unique selectivity toward potential substrates. For example, CYP1A2 preferentially binds medium-sized, planar, lipophilic molecules, while CYP2D6 preferentially binds molecules that possess a basic nitrogen atom. Some CYP subfamilies exhibit polymorphism (ie, genetic variation that results in a modified enzyme with small changes in amino acid sequences that may manifest differing catalytic properties). The best described polymorphisms involve CYP2C9, CYP2C19, and CYP2D6. Individuals possessing "wild type" genes exhibit normal functioning CYP capacity. Others, however, possess genetic variants that leave the person with a subnormal level of catalytic potential (so called "poor metabolizers"). Poor metabolizers would be more likely to experience toxicity from drugs metabolized by the affected enzymes (or less effects if the enzyme is responsible for converting a prodrug to it's active form as in the case of codeine). The percentage of people classified as poor metabolizers varies by enzyme and population group. As an example, ~7% of Caucasians and only about 1% of Asians appear to be CYP2D6 poor metabolizers.

CYP enzymes can be both inhibited and induced by other drugs, leading to increased or decreased serum concentrations (along with the associated effects), respectively. Induction occurs when a drug causes an increase in the amount of smooth endoplasmic reticulum, secondary to increasing the amount of the affected CYP enzymes in the tissues. This "revving up" of the CYP enzyme system may take several days to reach peak activity, and likewise, may take several days, even months, to return to normal following discontinuation of the inducing agent.

CYP inhibition occurs via several potential mechanisms. Most commonly, a CYP inhibitor competitively (and reversibly) binds to the active site on the enzyme, thus preventing the substrate from binding to the same site, and preventing the substrate from being metabolized. The affinity of an inhibitor for an enzyme may be expressed by an inhibition constant (Ki) or IC50 (defined as the concentration of the inhibitor required to cause 50% inhibition under a given set of conditions). In addition to reversible competition for an enzyme site, drugs may inhibit enzyme activity by binding to sites on the enzyme other than that to which the substrate would bind, and thereby cause a change in the functionality or physical structure of the enzyme. A drug may also bind to the enzyme in an irreversible (ie, "suicide") fashion. In such a case, it is not the concentration of drug at the enzyme site that is important (constantly binding and releasing), but the number of molecules available for binding (once bound, always bound).

Although an inhibitor or inducer may be known to affect a variety of CYP subfamilies, it may only inhibit one or two in a clinically important fashion. Likewise, although a substrate is known to be at least partially metabolized by a variety of CYP enzymes, only one or two enzymes may contribute significantly enough to its overall metabolism to warrant concern when used with potential inducers or inhibitors. Therefore, when attempting to predict the level of risk of using two drugs that may affect each other via altered CYP function, it is important to identify the relative effectiveness of the inhibiting/inducing drug on the CYP subfamilies that significantly contribute to the metabolism of the substrate. The contribution of a specific CYP pathway to substrate metabolism should be considered not only in light of other known CYP pathways, but also other nonoxidative pathways for substrate metabolism (eg, glucuronidation) and transporter proteins (eg, P-glycoprotein) that may affect the presentation of a substrate to a metabolic pathway.

HOW TO USE THIS TABLE

The following table provides a clinically relevant perspective on drugs that are affected by, or affect, cytochrome P450 (CYP) enzymes. Not all human, drug-metabolizing CYP enzymes are specifically (or separately) included in the table. Some enzymes have been excluded because they do not appear to significantly contribute to the metabolism of marketed drugs (eg, CYP2C18). In the case of CYP3A4, the industry routinely uses this single enzyme designation to represent all enzymes in the CYP3A subfamily. CYP3A7 is present in fetal livers. It is effectively absent from adult livers. CYP3A4 (adult) and CYP3A7 (fetal) appear to share similar properties in their respective hosts. The impact of CYP3A7 in fetal and neonatal drug interactions has not been investigated.

An enzyme that appears to play a clinically significant (major) role in a drug's metabolism is indicated by "S". A clinically significant designation is the result of a two-phase review. The first phase considered the contribution of each CYP enzyme to the overall metabolism of the drug. The enzyme pathway was considered potentially clinically relevant if it was responsible for at least 30% of the metabolism of the drug. If so, the drug was subjected to a second phase. The second phase considered the clinical relevance of a substrate's concentration being increased twofold, or decreased by one-half (such as might be observed if combined with an effective CYP inhibitor or inducer, respectively). If either of these changes was considered to present a clinically significant concern, the CYP pathway for the drug was designated "major." If neither change would appear to present a clinically significant concern, or if the CYP enzyme was responsible for a smaller portion of the overall metabolism (ie, <30%), then no association between the enzyme and the drug will appear in the table.

Enzymes that are strongly or moderately inhibited by a drug are indicated by "↓". Enzymes that are weakly inhibited are not identified in the table. The designations are the result of a review of published clinical reports, available Ki data, and assessments published by other experts in the field. As it pertains to Ki values set in a ratio with achievable serum drug concentrations ([I]) under normal dosing conditions, the following parameters were employed: $[I]/Ki \geq 1$ = strong; [I]/Ki 0.1 to 1 = moderate; $[I]/Ki < 0.1$ = weak.

Enzymes that appear to be effectively induced by a drug are indicated by "↑". This designation is the result of a review of published clinical reports and assessments published by experts in the field.

In general, clinically significant interactions are more likely to occur between substrates ("S") and either inhibitors or inducers of the same enzyme(s), which have been indicated by "↓" and "↑", respectively. However, these assessments possess a degree of subjectivity, at times based on limited indications regarding the significance of CYP effects of particular agents. An attempt has been made to balance a conservative, clinically-sensitive presentation of the data with a desire to avoid the numbing effect of a "beware of everything" approach. It is important to note that information related to CYP metabolism of drugs is expanding at a rapid pace, and thus, the contents of this table should only be considered to represent a "snapshot" of the information available at the time of publication.

SELECTED READINGS

Bjornsson TD, Callaghan JT, Einolf HJ, et al. The conduct of *in vitro* and *in vivo* drug-drug interaction studies: a PhRMA perspective. *J Clin Pharmacol.* 2003;43(5):443-469.

Drug-Drug Interactions. Rodrigues AD, ed. New York, NY: Marcel Dekker, Inc; 2002.

Metabolic Drug Interactions. Levy RH, Thummel KE, Trager WF, et al, eds. Philadelphia, PA: Lippincott Williams & Wilkins; 2000.

Michalets EL. Update: clinically significant cytochrome P-450 drug interactions. *Pharmacotherapy.* 1998;18(1):84-112.

Thummel KE, Wilkinson GR. *In vitro* and *in vivo* drug interactions involving human CYP3A. *Annu Rev Pharmacol Toxicol.* 1998;38:389-430.

Zhang Y, Benet LZ. The gut as a barrier to drug absorption: combined role of cytochrome P450 3A and P-Glycoprotein. *Clin Pharmacokinet.* 2001;40(3):159-168.

SELECTED WEBSITES

http://www.cypalleles.ki.se/
http://www.fda.gov/Drugs/DevelopmentApprovalProcess/DevelopmentResources/DrugInteractionsLabeling/ucm080499.htm

CYP: Substrates, Inhibitors, Inducers

S = substrate; ↓ = inhibitor; ↑ = inducer

Drug	1A2	2A6	2B6	2C8	2C9	2C19	2D6	2E1	3A4
Acenocoumarol	S				S				
Alfentanil									S
Alfuzosin									S
Alosetron	S								
ALPRAZolam									S
Ambrisentan						S			S
Aminophylline	S								
Amiodarone		↓		S	↓		↓		S, ↓
Amitriptyline							S		
AmLODIPine	↓								S
Amobarbital		↑							
Amoxapine							S		
Aprepitant									S, ↓
ARIPiprazole							S		S

CYP: Substrates, Inhibitors, Inducers *(continued)*

Drug	1A2	2A6	2B6	2C8	2C9	2C19	2D6	2E1	3A4
Armodafinil						↓			S, ↑
Atazanavir									S, ↓
Atomoxetine							S		
Atorvastatin									S
Benzphetamine									S
Betaxolol	S						S		
Bisoprolol									S
Bortezomib						S, ↓			S
Bosentan					S, ↑				S, ↑
Bromazepam									S
Bromocriptine									S
Budesonide									S
Buprenorphine									S
BuPROPion			S						
BusPIRone									S
Busulfan									S
Caffeine	S								↓
Captopril							S		
CarBAMazepine	↑		↑	↑	↑	↑			S, ↑
Carisoprodol						S			
Carvedilol					S		S		
Celecoxib				↓	S				
ChlordiazePOXIDE									S
Chloroquine							S, ↓		S
Chlorpheniramine									S
ChlorproMAZINE							S, ↓		
Chlorzoxazone								S	
Ciclesonide									S
Cilostazol									S
Cimetidine	↓					↓	↓		↓
Cinacalcet							↓		
Ciprofloxacin	↓								
Cisapride									S
Citalopram						S			S
Clarithromycin									S, ↓
Clobazam						S			S
ClomiPRAMINE	S					S	S, ↓		
ClonazePAM									S
Clorazepate									S
Clotrimazole									↓
CloZAPine	S						↓		
Cobicistat									S, ↓
Cocaine							↓		S
Codeine[1]							S		
Colchicine									S
Conivaptan									S, ↓
Cyclobenzaprine	S								
Cyclophosphamide[2]			S						S
CycloSPORINE									S, ↓
Dacarbazine	S							S	
Dantrolene									S
Dapsone					S				S

CYP: Substrates, Inhibitors, Inducers *(continued)*

Drug	1A2	2A6	2B6	2C8	2C9	2C19	2D6	2E1	3A4
Darifenacin							↓		S
Darunavir									S
Dasabuvir				S					
Dasatinib									S
Delavirdine					↓	↓	↓		S, ↓
Desipramine		↓	↓				S, ↓		↓
Desogestrel						S			
Dexamethasone									S, ↑
Dexlansoprazole						S, ↓			S
Dexmedetomidine		S					↓		
Dextromethorphan							S		
Diazepam						S			S
Diclofenac	↓								
Dihydroergotamine									S
Diltiazem									S, ↓
DiphenhydrAMINE							↓		
Disopyramide									S
Disulfiram								↓	
DOCEtaxel									S
Doxepin							S		
DOXOrubicin			↓				S		S
Doxycycline									↓
DULoxetine	S						S, ↓		
Efavirenz[3]			S		↓	↓			S, ↓, ↑
Eletriptan									S
Enflurane								S	
Eplerenone									S
Ergoloid mesylates									S
Ergonovine									S
Ergotamine									S
Erlotinib									S
Erythromycin									S, ↓
Escitalopram						S			S
Esomeprazole						S, ↓			S
Estradiol	S								S
Estrogens, conjugated A/synthetic	S								S
Estrogens, conjugated equine	S								S
Estrogens, esterified	S								S
Estropipate	S								S
Eszopiclone									S
Ethinyl estradiol									S
Ethosuximide									S
Etoposide									S
Exemestane									S
Felbamate									S
Felodipine				↓					S
FentaNYL									S
Flecainide							S		
Fluconazole					↓	↓			↓
Flunisolide									S
FLUoxetine	↓				S	↓	S, ↓		
FluPHENAZine							S		

CYP: Substrates, Inhibitors, Inducers *(continued)*

Drug	1A2	2A6	2B6	2C8	2C9	2C19	2D6	2E1	3A4
Flurazepam									S
Flurbiprofen					↓				
Flutamide	S								S
Fluticasone									S
Fluvastatin					S, ↓				
FluvoxaMINE	S, ↓					↓	S		
Fosamprenavir (as amprenavir)									S, ↓
Fosaprepitant									S, ↓
Fosphenytoin (as phenytoin)			↑	↑	S, ↑	S, ↑			↑
Fospropofol	↓		S		S	↓			↓
Gefitinib									S
Gemfibrozil	↓			↓	↓	↓			
Glimepiride					S				
GlipiZIDE					S				
Guanabenz	S								
Haloperidol							S, ↓		S, ↓
Halothane								S	
Ibuprofen					↓				
Ifosfamide[4]		S				S			S
Imatinib							↓		S, ↓
Imipramine						S	S, ↓		
Indinavir									S, ↓
Indomethacin					↓				
Irbesartan				↓	↓				
Irinotecan			S						S
Isoflurane								S	
Isoniazid		↓				↓	↓	S, ↓	
Isosorbide dinitrate									S
Isosorbide mononitrate									S
Isradipine									S
Itraconazole									S, ↓
Ixabepilone									S
Ketamine			S		S				S
Ketoconazole	↓	↓			↓	↓	↓		S, ↓
Lansoprazole						S, ↓			S
Lapatinib									S
Letrozole		↓							
Levonorgestrel									S
Lidocaine							S, ↓		S, ↓
Lomustine							S		
Lopinavir									S
Loratadine						↓			
Losartan				↓	S, ↓				S
Lovastatin									S
Maprotiline							S		
Maraviroc									S
MedroxyPROGESTERone									S
Mefenamic acid					↓				
Mefloquine									S
Mephobarbital						S			
Mestranol[5]					S				S
Methadone							↓		S

CYP: Substrates, Inhibitors, Inducers *(continued)*

Drug	1A2	2A6	2B6	2C8	2C9	2C19	2D6	2E1	3A4
Methamphetamine							S		
Methoxsalen	↓	↓							
Methsuximide						S			
Methylergonovine									S
MethylPREDNISolone									S
Metoprolol							S		
MetroNIDAZOLE									↓
Mexiletine	S, ↓						S		
Miconazole	↓	↓			↓	↓	↓	↓	S, ↓
Midazolam									S
Mirtazapine	S						S		S
Moclobemide						S	S		
Modafinil						↓			S
Montelukast					S				S
Nafcillin									↑
Nateglinide					S				S
Nebivolol							S		
Nefazodone							S		S, ↓
Nelfinavir						S			S, ↓
Nevirapine			↑						S, ↑
NiCARdipine					↓	↓	↓		S, ↓
NIFEdipine	↓								S
Nilotinib									S
Nilutamide						S			
NiMODipine									S
Nisoldipine									S
Norethindrone									S
Norfloxacin	↓								↓
Norgestrel									S
Nortriptyline							S		
Ofloxacin	↓								
OLANZapine	S								
Omeprazole					↓	S, ↓			S
Ondansetron									S
OXcarbazepine									↑
PACLitaxel				S	S				S
Pantoprazole						S, ↓			
Paricalcitol									S
Paritaprevir									S
PARoxetine			↓				S, ↓		
PAZOPanib									S
Pentamidine						S			
PENTobarbital		↑							↑
Perphenazine							S		
PHENobarbital	↑	↑	↑	↑	↑	S			↑
Phenytoin			↑	↑	S, ↑	S, ↑			↑
Pimozide	S								S
Pindolol							S		
Pioglitazone				S, ↓					
Piroxicam					↓				
Posaconazole									↓
Primaquine	↓								S

CYP: Substrates, Inhibitors, Inducers *(continued)*

Drug	1A2	2A6	2B6	2C8	2C9	2C19	2D6	2E1	3A4
Primidone	↑		↑	↑	↑				↑
Procainamide							S		
Progesterone						S			S
Promethazine			S				S		
Propafenone							S		
Propofol	↓		S		S	↓			↓
Propranolol	S						S		
Protriptyline							S		
Pyrimethamine					↓				
Quazepam						S			S
QUEtiapine									S
QuiNIDine							↓		S, ↓
QuiNINE				↓	↓		↓		S
RABEprazole				↓		S, ↓			S
Ramelteon	S								
Ranolazine							↓		S
Rasagiline	S								
Repaglinide				S					S
Rifabutin									S, ↑
Rifampin	↑	↑	↑	↑	↑	↑			↑
Rifapentine				↑	↑				↑
Riluzole	S								
RisperiDONE							S		
Ritonavir				↓			S, ↓		S, ↓
ROPINIRole	S								
Ropivacaine	S								
Rosiglitazone				S, ↓					
Salmeterol									S
Saquinavir									S, ↓
Secobarbital		↑		↑	↑				
Selegiline			S						
Sertraline			↓			S, ↓	S, ↓		↓
Sevoflurane								S	
Sibutramine									S
Sildenafil									S
Simvastatin									S
Sirolimus									S
Sitaxsentan					↓	↓			↓
Solifenacin									S
SORAfenib			↓	↓	↓				
Spiramycin									S
SUFentanil									S
SulfADIAZINE					S, ↓				
Sulfamethoxazole					S, ↓				
SUNItinib									S
Tacrine	S								
Tacrolimus									S
Tadalafil									S
Tamoxifen				↓	S		S		S
Tamsulosin							S		S
Telithromycin									S, ↓
Temsirolimus									S

CYP: Substrates, Inhibitors, Inducers *(continued)*

Drug	1A2	2A6	2B6	2C8	2C9	2C19	2D6	2E1	3A4
Teniposide									S
Terbinafine							↓		
Tetracycline									S, ↓
Theophylline	S							S	S
Thiabendazole	↓								
Thioridazine							S, ↓		
Thiotepa			↓						
Thiothixene	S								
TiaGABine									S
Ticlopidine						↓	↓		S
Timolol							S		
Tinidazole									S
Tipranavir									S
TiZANidine	S								
TOLBUTamide					S, ↓				
Tolterodine							S		S
Toremifene									S
Torsemide					S				
TraMADol[1]							S		S
Tranylcypromine	↓	↓				↓	↓		
TraZODone									S
Tretinoin				S					
Triazolam									S
Trifluoperazine	S								
Trimethoprim				↓	S, ↓				S
Trimipramine						S	S		S
Vardenafil									S
Venlafaxine							S		S
Verapamil									S, ↓
VinBLAStine									S
VinCRIStine									S
Vinorelbine									S
Voriconazole					S	S			↓
Warfarin					S, ↓				
Zafirlukast					S, ↓				
Zileuton	↓								
Zolpidem									S
Zonisamide									S
Zopiclone					S				S
Zuclopenthixol							S		

[1]This opioid analgesic is bioactivated *in vivo* via CYP2D6. Inhibiting this enzyme would decrease the effects of the analgesic. The active metabolite might also affect, or be affected by, CYP enzymes.

[2]Cyclophosphamide is bioactivated *in vivo* to acrolein via CYP2B6 and 3A4. Inhibiting these enzymes would decrease the effects of cyclophosphamide.

[3]Data have shown both induction (*in vivo*) and inhibition (*in vitro*) of CYP3A4.

[4]Ifosfamide is bioactivated *in vivo* to acrolein via CYP3A4. Inhibiting this enzyme would decrease the effects of ifosfamide.

[5]Mestranol is bioactivated *in vivo* to ethinyl estradiol via CYP2C8/9. See Ethinyl Estradiol for additional CYP information.

MANAGEMENT OF DRUG EXTRAVASATIONS

A potential complication of drug therapy is extravasation. A variety of symptoms, including erythema, ulceration, pain, tissue sloughing, and necrosis, are possible. A variety of drugs have been reported to cause tissue damage if extravasated.

DEFINITIONS

- **Extravasation:** Unintentional or inadvertent leakage (or instillation) of fluid out of a blood vessel into surrounding tissue
- **Irritant:** An agent that causes aching, tightness, and phlebitis with or without inflammation, but does not typically cause tissue necrosis. Irritants can cause necrosis if the extravasation is severe or left untreated.
- **Vesicant:** An agent that has the potential to cause blistering, severe tissue injury, or tissue necrosis when extravasated
- **Flare:** Local, nonpainful, possibly allergic reaction often accompanied by reddening along the vein

PREVENTING EXTRAVASATIONS

Although it is not possible to prevent all extravasations, a few precautions can minimize the risk to the patient. The vein used should be a large, intact vessel with good blood flow. Veins in the forearm (ie, basilic, cephalic, and median antebrachial) are usually good options for peripheral infusions. To minimize the risk of dislodging the catheter, avoid using veins in the hands, dorsum of the foot, and any joint space (eg, antecubital). It is important to remember to not administer chemotherapy distal to a recent venipuncture.

A frequently recommended precaution against drug extravasation is the use of a central venous catheter. Use of a central line has several advantages, including high patient satisfaction, reliable venous access, high flow rates, and rapid dilution of the drug. Many institutions encourage or require use of a vascular access device for administration of vesicant agents. Despite their benefit, central lines are not an absolute solution. Vascular access devices are subject to a number of complications. Misplacement/migration of the catheter or improper placement of the needle in accessing injection ports, and cuts, punctures, infections, or rupture of the catheter itself have all been reported.

Education of both the patient and practitioner is imperative. Educate the patient to immediately report any signs of pain, itching, tingling, burning, redness, swelling, or discomfort, all of which could be early signs of extravasation. Symptoms of extravasation which may appear later include blistering, ulceration, and necrosis. Ensure the health care team is informed of the risks and management strategies for both prevention and treatment of extravasations. Absence of blood return, resistance upon administration, or interruption of the IV flow should raise suspicion of potential extravasation.

INITIAL EXTRAVASATION MANAGEMENT

1. **Stop the infusion:** At the first suspicion of extravasation, the drug infusion and IV fluids should be stopped.
2. **Do NOT remove the catheter/needle:** The IV tubing should be disconnected, but the catheter/needle should be left in place to facilitate aspiration of fluid from the extravasation site and, if appropriate, administration of an antidote.
3. **Aspirate fluid:** To the extent possible, the extravasated drug solution should gently be removed from the subcutaneous tissues. It is important to avoid any friction or pressure to the area.
4. **Do NOT flush the line:** Flooding the infiltration site with saline or dextrose in an attempt to dilute the drug solution is not recommended.
5. **Remove the catheter/needle:** If an antidote is not going to be administered into the extravasation site, the catheter/needle should be removed. If an antidote is to be injected into the area, it should be injected through the catheter to ensure delivery of the antidote to the extravasation site. When this has been accomplished, the catheter should then be removed.
6. **Elevate:** The affected extremity should be elevated.
7. **Compresses:** If indicated, apply dry compress to area of extravasation (either cold or warm, depending on vesicant extravasated).
8. **Monitor and document:** Mark the extravasation site (using a surgical felt pen, gently draw an outline on the skin of the extravasation area) and photograph if possible. Monitor and document the event and follow-up activities according to institutional policy.

Table 1: Vesicant Agents and Extravasation Management

Extravasated Medication	Preferred Antidote	Antidote Administration	Supportive Management	Comments
Amino Acids (4.25%)/parenteral nutrition	Hyaluronidase	Hyaluronidase: Intradermal or SubQ: Inject a total of 1 mL (15 units/mL) as five separate 0.2 mL injections (using a 25-gauge needle) into area of extravasation at the leading edge in a clockwise manner (MacCara 1983; Zenk 1981)	Apply dry cold compresses (Hurst 2004)	
Aminophylline	Hyaluronidase	Hyaluronidase: Intradermal or SubQ: Inject a total of 1 mL (15 units/mL) as five separate 0.2 mL injections (using a 25-gauge needle) into area of extravasation at the leading edge in a clockwise manner (MacCara 1983; Zenk 1981)	Apply dry cold compresses (Hurst 2004)	
Amsacrine	No known antidote	No known antidote	Apply dry warm compresses (Schulmeister 2011)	Not commercially available in the US
Bendamustine	Sodium Thiosulfate	May be managed in the same manner as mechlorethamine extravasation (Schulmeister 2011): Sodium thiosulfate $^1/_6$ M solution: Inject subcutaneously into extravasation area using 2 mL for each mg of mechlorethamine suspected to have extravasated (Pérez Fidalgo 2012; Polovich 2009)	Apply dry cold compresses for 20 minutes 4 times/day for 1 to 2 days (Pérez Fidalgo 2012)	Irritant with vesicant-like properties (reports of both irritant and vesicant reactions)
Calcium Chloride (≥10%)	Hyaluronidase	Hyaluronidase: Intradermal or SubQ: Inject a total of 1 mL (15 units/mL) as five separate 0.2 mL injections (using a 25-gauge needle) into area of extravasation at the leading edge in a clockwise manner (MacCara 1983; Zenk 1981)	Apply dry cold compresses (Hurst 2004)	
Calcium Gluconate	Hyaluronidase	Hyaluronidase: Intradermal or SubQ: Inject a total of 1 mL (15 units/mL) as five separate 0.2 mL injections (using a 25-gauge needle) into area of extravasation at the leading edge in a clockwise manner (MacCara 1983; Zenk 1981)	Apply dry cold compresses (Hurst 2004)	
CISplatin (>0.4 mg/mL)	Sodium Thiosulfate	Sodium thiosulfate $^1/_6$ M solution: Inject 2 mL into existing IV line for each 100 mg of cisplatin extravasated; then consider also injecting 1 mL as 0.1 mL subcutaneous injections (clockwise) around the area of extravasation; may repeat subcutaneous injections several times over the next 3 to 4 hours (Ener 2004) Dimethyl sulfoxide (DMSO) may also be considered an option. Apply topically to a region covering twice the affected area every 8 hours for 7 days; begin within 10 minutes of extravasation; do not cover with a dressing (Pérez Fidalgo 2012).	Information conflicts regarding use of warm or cold compresses	
Contrast Media	Hyaluronidase	Hyaluronidase: Intradermal or SubQ: Inject a total of 1 mL (15 units/mL) as five separate 0.2 mL injections (using a 25-gauge needle) into area of extravasation at the leading edge in a clockwise manner (MacCara 1983; Zenk 1981) The injection of a total of 5 mL (150 units/mL) as five separate 1 mL injections around the extravasation site has been also used successfully (Rowlett 2012)	Apply dry cold compresses (Hurst 2004)	
DACTINomycin	No known antidote	No known antidote	Apply dry cold compress for 20 minutes 4 times/day for 1 to 2 days (Pérez Fidalgo 2012)	
Dantrolene	No known antidote	No known antidote	No recommendation	
DAUNOrubicin (Conventional)	Dexrazoxane or topical Dimethyl Sulfoxide (DMSO)	Adults: Dexrazoxane 1,000 mg/m^2 (maximum dose: 2,000 mg) IV (administer in a large vein remote from site of extravasation) over 1 to 2 hours days 1 and 2, then 500 mg/m^2 (maximum dose: 1,000 mg) IV over 1 to 2 hours day 3; begin within 6 hours after extravasation (Mouridsen 2007; Pérez Fidalgo 2012). **Note:** Reduce dexrazoxane dose by 50% in patients with moderate to severe renal impairment (CrCl <40 mL/min). Pediatrics and Adults: DMSO: Apply topically to a region covering twice the affected area every 8 hours for 7 days; begin within 10 minutes of extravasation; do not cover with a dressing (Pérez Fidalgo 2012)	Apply dry cold compress for 20 minutes 4 times/day for 1 to 2 days (Pérez Fidalgo 2012). Withhold cooling for 15 minutes before and after dexrazoxane.	If using dexrazoxane, do not use DMSO. Administer dexrazoxane through a large vein remote from area of the extravasation.

Table 1: Vesicant Agents and Extravasation Management *continued*

Extravasated Medication	Preferred Antidote	Antidote Administration	Supportive Management	Comments
Dextrose (≥10%)	Hyaluronidase	Hyaluronidase: **Dextrose 10%:** Intradermal or SubQ: Inject a total of 1 mL (15 units/mL) as five separate 0.2 mL injections (using a 25-gauge needle) into area of extravasation at the leading edge in a clockwise manner (MacCara 1983; Zenk 1981) **Dextrose 50%:** Injection of a total of 1 mL (150 units/mL) as five separate 0.2 mL injections administered along the leading edge of erythema has been used successfully (Wiegand 2010)	Apply dry cold compresses (Hurst 2004)	
Diazepam	No known antidote	No known antidote	Apply dry cold compresses (Hurst 2004)	
Digoxin	No known antidote	No known antidote	No recommendation	
DOCEtaxel	No known antidote	No known antidote	Information conflicts regarding use of warm or cold compresses	Irritant with vesicant-like properties (reports of both irritant and vesicant reactions)
DOPamine	Phentolamine	Phentolamine: Dilute 5 to 10 mg in 10 to 15 mL NS and administer into extravasation site as soon as possible after extravasation (Peberdy 2010) *Alternatives to phentolamine (due to shortage):* Nitroglycerin topical 2% ointment (based on limited case reports in neonates/ infants): Apply 4 mm/kg as a thin ribbon to the affected areas; may repeat after 8 hours if needed (Wong 1992) **or** apply a 1-inch strip on the affected site (Denkler 1989) Terbutaline (based on limited case reports): Infiltrate extravasation area using a solution of terbutaline 1 mg diluted to 10 mL in NS (large extravasation site; administration volume varied from 3 to 10 mL) **or** 1 mg diluted in 1 mL 0.9% NS (small/distal extravasation site; administration volume varied from 0.5 to 1 mL) (Stier 1999)	Apply dry warm compresses (Hurst 2004)	
DOXOrubicin (Conventional)	Dexrazoxane or topical DMSO	Adults: Dexrazoxane 1,000 mg/m^2 (maximum dose: 2,000 mg) IV (administer in a large vein remote from site of extravasation) over 1 to 2 hours days 1 and 2, then 500 mg/m^2 (maximum dose: 1,000 mg) IV over 1 to 2 hours day 3; begin within 6 hours after extravasation (Mouridsen 2007; Pérez Fidalgo 2012). **Note:** Reduce dexrazoxane dose by 50% in patients with moderate to severe renal impairment (CrCl <40 mL/min). Pediatrics and Adults: DMSO: Apply topically to a region covering twice the affected area every 8 hours for 7 days; begin within 10 minutes of extravasation; do not cover with a dressing (Pérez Fidalgo 2012)	Apply dry cold compress for 20 minutes 4 times/day for 1 to 2 days (Pérez Fidalgo 2012). Withhold cooling for 15 minutes before and after dexrazoxane.	If using dexrazoxane, do not use DMSO. Administer dexrazoxane through a large vein remote from area of the extravasation.
EPINEPHrine	Phentolamine	Phentolamine: Dilute 5 to 10 mg in 10 to 15 mL NS and administer into extravasation site as soon as possible after extravasation (Peberdy 2010) *Alternatives to phentolamine (due to shortage):* Nitroglycerin topical 2% ointment (based on limited case reports in neonates/ infants): Apply 4 mm/kg as a thin ribbon to the affected areas; may repeat after 8 hours if needed (Wong 1992) **or** apply a 1-inch strip on the affected site (Denkler 1989) Terbutaline (based on limited case reports): Infiltrate extravasation area using a solution of terbutaline 1 mg diluted to 10 mL in NS (large extravasation site; administration volume varied from 3 to 10 mL) **or** 1 mg diluted in 1 mL NS (small/ distal extravasation site; administration volume varied from 0.5 to 1 mL) (Stier 1999)	Apply dry warm compresses (Hurst 2004)	

Table 1: Vesicant Agents and Extravasation Management *continued*

Extravasated Medication	Preferred Antidote	Antidote Administration	Supportive Management	Comments
EPIrubicin	Dexrazoxane or topical DMSO	Adults: Dexrazoxane 1,000 mg/m^2 (maximum dose: 2,000 mg) IV (administer in a large vein remote from site of extravasation) over 1 to 2 hours days 1 and 2, then 500 mg/m^2 (maximum dose: 1,000 mg) IV over 1 to 2 hours day 3; begin within 6 hours after extravasation (Mouridsen 2007; Pérez Fidalgo 2012). **Note:** Reduce dexrazoxane dose by 50% in patients with moderate to severe renal impairment (CrCl <40 mL/min). Pediatrics and Adults: DMSO: Apply topically to a region covering twice the affected area every 8 hours for 7 days; begin within 10 minutes of extravasation; do not cover with a dressing (Pérez Fidalgo 2012)	Apply dry cold compress for 20 minutes 4 times/day for 1 to 2 days (Pérez Fidalgo 2012). Withhold cooling for 15 minutes before and after dexrazoxane.	If using dexrazoxane, do not use DMSO. Administer dexrazoxane through a large vein remote from area of the extravasation.
Esmolol	No known antidote	No known antidote	No recommendation	
HydrOXYzine	No known antidote	No known antidote	No recommendation	**Note:** Labeled route of administration for parenteral hydroxyzine is by IM injection only; IV administration is contraindicated.
IDArubicin	Dexrazoxane or topical DMSO	Adults: Dexrazoxane 1,000 mg/m^2 (maximum dose: 2,000 mg) IV (administer in a large vein remote from site of extravasation) over 1 to 2 hours days 1 and 2, then 500 mg/m^2 (maximum dose: 1,000 mg) IV over 1 to 2 hours day 3; begin within 6 hours after extravasation (Mouridsen 2007; Pérez Fidalgo 2012). **Note:** Reduce dexrazoxane dose by 50% in patients with moderate to severe renal impairment (CrCl <40 mL/min). Pediatrics and Adults: DMSO: Apply topically to a region covering twice the affected area every 8 hours for 7 days; begin within 10 minutes of extravasation; do not cover with a dressing (Pérez Fidalgo 2012)	Apply dry cold compress for 20 minutes 4 times/day for 1 to 2 days (Pérez Fidalgo 2012). Withhold cooling for 15 minutes before and after dexrazoxane.	If using dexrazoxane, do not use DMSO. Administer dexrazoxane through a large vein remote from area of the extravasation.
Mannitol (>5%)	Hyaluronidase	Hyaluronidase: SubQ: Administer multiple 0.5 to 1 mL injections of a 15 units/mL solution around the periphery of the extravasation (Kumar 2003)	No recommendation	
Mechlorethamine	Sodium Thiosulfate	Sodium thiosulfate $^1/_6$ M solution: Inject subcutaneously into extravasation area using 2 mL for each mg of mechlorethamine suspected to have extravasated (Pérez Fidalgo 2012; Polovich 2009)	Apply ice for 6 to 12 hours after sodium thiosulfate administration (Mustargen prescribing information 2012; Polovich 2009) **or** may apply dry cold compresses for 20 minutes 4 times/day for 1 to 2 days (Perez Fidalgo 2012)	
Methylene Blue	Nitroglycerin topical 2% ointment	Nitroglycerin topical 2% ointment (based on mechanism of extravasation injury **[has not been clinically evaluated]**): Apply a 1-inch strip on the site of ischemia; may redose every 8 hours as necessary (Reynolds 2014)	Apply dry, warm compresses (based on mechanism of extravasation injury **(has not been clinically evaluated)** proximal to the infection site (Reynolds 2014)	
MitoMYcin	Topical DMSO	DMSO: Apply topically to a region covering twice the affected area every 8 hours for 7 days; begin within 10 minutes of extravasation; do not cover with a dressing (Pérez Fidalgo 2012)	Apply dry cold compress for 20 minutes 4 times/day for 1 to 2 days (Pérez Fidalgo 2012)	

Table 1: Vesicant Agents and Extravasation Management *continued*

Extravasated Medication	Preferred Antidote	Antidote Administration	Supportive Management	Comments
MitoXANtrone	Dexrazoxane or topical DMSO	Adults: Dexrazoxane 1,000 mg/m² (maximum dose: 2,000 mg) IV (administer in a large vein remote from site of extravasation) over 1 to 2 hours days 1 and 2, then 500 mg/m² (maximum dose: 1,000 mg) IV over 1 to 2 hours day 3; begin within 6 hours after extravasation (Mouridsen 2007; Pérez Fidalgo 2012). **Note:** Reduce dexrazoxane dose by 50% in patients with moderate to severe renal impairment (CrCl <40 mL/min). Pediatrics and Adults: DMSO: Apply topically to a region covering twice the affected area every 8 hours for 7 days; begin within 10 minutes of extravasation; do not cover with a dressing (Pérez Fidalgo 2012)	Apply dry cold compress for 20 minutes 4 times/day for 1 to 2 days (Pérez Fidalgo 2012)	Irritant with vesicant-like properties (reports of both irritant and vesicant reactions). Administer dexrazoxane through a large vein remote from area of the extravasation.
Nafcillin	Hyaluronidase	Hyaluronidase: Intradermal or SubQ: Inject a total of 1 mL (15 units/mL) as five separate 0.2 mL injections (using a 25-gauge needle) into area of extravasation at the leading edge in a clockwise manner (MacCara 1983; Zenk 1981)	Apply dry cold compresses (Hurst 2004)	
Norepinephrine	Phentolamine	Phentolamine: Dilute 5 to 10 mg in 10 to 15 mL NS and administer into extravasation site as soon as possible after extravasation (Peberdy 2010) **or** dilute 5 to 10 mg in 10 mL NS and administer into extravasation area (within 12 hours of extravasation) (Phentolamine product information 1999) *Alternatives to phentolamine (due to shortage):* Nitroglycerin topical 2% ointment (based on limited case reports in neonates/ infants): Apply 4 mm/kg as a thin ribbon to the affected areas; may repeat after 8 hours if needed (Wong 1992) **or** apply a 1-inch strip on the affected site (Denkler 1989) Terbutaline (based on limited case reports): Infiltrate extravasation area using a solution of terbutaline 1 mg diluted to 10 mL in NS (large extravasation site; administration volume varied from 3 to 10 mL) **or** 1 mg diluted in 1 mL NS (small/ distal extravasation site; administration volume varied from 0.5 to 1 mL) (Stier 1999)	Apply dry warm compresses (Hurst 2004)	
Oxaliplatin	No known antidote	No known antidote	Information conflicts regarding use of warm or cold compresses Cold compresses could potentially precipitate or exacerbate peripheral neuropathy (de Lemos 2005)	Irritant with vesicant-like properties (reports of both irritant and vesicant reactions)
PACLitaxel	Hyaluronidase	Hyaluronidase: *If needle/cannula still in place:* Administer 1 to 6 mL (150 units/mL) into existing IV line; usual dose is 1 mL for each 1 mL of extravasated drug; if needle/ cannula has been removed, inject subcutaneously in a clockwise manner around area of extravasation; may repeat several times over the next 3 to 4 hours (Ener 2004)	Information conflicts regarding use of warm or cold compresses	Irritant with vesicant-like properties (reports of both irritant and vesicant reactions)
Pentamidine	No known antidote	No known antidote	Dry warm compresses (Reynolds 2014)	Irritant with vesicant-like properties (reports of both irritant and vesicant reactions)

Table 1: Vesicant Agents and Extravasation Management *continued*

Extravasated Medication	Preferred Antidote	Antidote Administration	Supportive Management	Comments
Phenylephrine	Phentolamine	Phentolamine: Dilute 5 to 10 mg in 10 to 15 mL NS and administer into extravasation site as soon as possible after extravasation (Peberdy 2010) *Alternatives to phentolamine (due to shortage):* Nitroglycerin topical 2% ointment (based on limited case reports in neonates/ infants): Apply 4 mm/kg as a thin ribbon to the affected areas; may repeat after 8 hours if needed (Wong 1992) **or** apply a 1-inch strip on the affected site (Denkler 1989) Terbutaline (based on limited case reports): Infiltrate extravasation area using a solution of terbutaline 1 mg diluted to 10 mL in NS (large extravasation site; administration volume varied from 3 to 10 mL) **or** 1 mg diluted in 1 mL NS (small/ distal extravasation site; administration volume varied from 0.5 to 1 mL) (Stier 1999)	Apply dry warm compresses (Hurst 2004)	
Phenytoin	No antidote **or** Hyaluronidase	Conflicting information: Do not use antidotes (pediatrics) (Montgomery 1999) Hyaluronidase: SubQ: Inject four separate 0.2 mL injections of 15 units/mL (using a 25-gauge needle) into area of extravasation (Sokol 1998)	No recommendation	
Potassium Acetate (>0.1 mEq/mL)	Hyaluronidase	Hyaluronidase: Intradermal or SubQ: Inject a total of 1 mL (15 units/mL) as five separate 0.2 mL injections (using a 25-gauge needle) into area of extravasation at the leading edge in a clockwise manner (MacCara 1983; Zenk 1981)	Apply dry cold compresses (Hurst 2004)	Reports of both irritant and vesicant reactions
Potassium Chloride (>0.1 mEq/mL)	Hyaluronidase	Hyaluronidase: Intradermal or SubQ: Inject a total of 1 mL (15 units/mL) as five separate 0.2 mL injections (using a 25-gauge needle) into area of extravasation at the leading edge in a clockwise manner (MacCara 1983; Zenk 1981)	Apply dry cold compresses (Hurst 2004)	Reports of both irritant and vesicant reactions
Potassium Phosphate (may depend on concentration)	Hyaluronidase	Hyaluronidase: Intradermal or SubQ: Inject a total of 1 mL (15 units/mL) as five separate 0.2 mL injections (using a 25-gauge needle) into area of extravasation at the leading edge in a clockwise manner (MacCara 1983; Zenk 1981)	Apply dry cold compresses (Hurst 2004)	May be an irritant
Promethazine	No known antidote	No known antidote	Apply dry cold compresses (Hurst 2004)	**Note:** Preferred route of administration for promethazine is by deep intramuscular (IM) injection. If IV route is used, discontinue infusion immediately with onset of burning/pain; evaluate for inadvertent arterial injection or extravasation.
Sodium Bicarbonate (≥8.4%)	Hyaluronidase	Hyaluronidase: SubQ: Inject four to five separate 0.2 mL injections of 15 units/mL around area of extravasation (Hurst 2004)	Apply dry cold compresses (Hurst 2004)	
Sodium Chloride (>1%)	No known antidote	No known antidote	Apply dry warm compresses (Hastings-Tolsma 1993)	
Streptozocin	No known antidote	No known antidote	No recommendation	Irritant with vesicant-like properties (reports of both irritant and vesicant reactions)
Trabectedin	No known antidote	No known antidote	No recommendation	Not commercially available in the US
Tromethamine	No known antidote	No known antidote	No recommendation	

Table 1: Vesicant Agents and Extravasation Management *continued*

Extravasated Medication	Preferred Antidote	Antidote Administration	Supportive Management	Comments
Vasopressin	Phentolamine	Phentolamine: Dilute 5 to 10 mg in 10 to 15 mL NS and administer into extravasation site as soon as possible after extravasation (Peberdy 2010) *Alternatives to phentolamine (due to shortage):* Nitroglycerin topical 2% ointment (based on limited case reports in neonates/infants): Apply 4 mm/kg as a thin ribbon to the affected areas; may repeat after 8 hours if needed (Wong 1992) **or** apply a 1-inch strip on the affected site (Denkler 1989) Terbutaline (based on limited case reports): Infiltrate extravasation area using a solution of terbutaline 1 mg diluted to 10 mL in NS (large extravasation site; administration volume varied from 3 to 10 mL) **or** 1 mg diluted in 1 mL NS (small/distal extravasation site; administration volume varied from 0.5 to 1 mL) (Stier 1999)	No recommendation	
VinBLAStine	Hyaluronidase	Hyaluronidase: *If needle/cannula still in place:* Administer 1 to 6 mL (150 units/mL) into existing IV line; usual dose is 1 mL for each 1 mL of extravasated drug (Pérez Fidalgo 2012; Schulmeister 2011) *If needle/cannula was removed:* Inject 1 to 6 mL (150 units/mL) subcutaneously in a clockwise manner using 1 mL for each 1 mL of drug extravasated (Schulmeister 2011) or administer 1 mL (150 units/mL) as five separate 0.2 mL injections (using a 25-gauge needle) into the extravasation site (Polovich 2009)	Apply dry warm compress for 20 minutes 4 times/day for 1 to 2 days (Pérez Fidalgo 2012)	
VinCRIStine	Hyaluronidase	Hyaluronidase: *If needle/cannula still in place:* Administer 1 to 6 mL (150 units/mL) into existing IV line; usual dose is 1 mL for each 1 mL of extravasated drug (Pérez Fidalgo 2012; Schulmeister 2011) *If needle/cannula was removed:* Inject 1 to 6 mL (150 units/mL) subcutaneously in a clockwise manner using 1 mL for each 1 mL of drug extravasated (Schulmeister 2011) **or** administer 1 mL (150 units/mL) as five separate 0.2 mL injections (using a 25-gauge needle) into the extravasation site (Polovich 2009)	Apply dry warm compress for 20 minutes 4 times/day for 1 to 2 days (Pérez Fidalgo 2012)	
Vindesine	Hyaluronidase	Hyaluronidase: *If needle/cannula still in place:* Administer 1 to 6 mL (150 units/mL) into existing IV line; usual dose is 1 mL for each 1 mL of extravasated drug (Pérez Fidalgo 2012; Schulmeister 2011) *If needle/cannula was removed:* Inject 1 to 6 mL (150 units/mL) subcutaneously in a clockwise manner using 1 mL for each 1 mL of drug extravasated (Schulmeister 2011) **or** administer 1 mL (150 units/mL) as five separate 0.2 mL injections (using a 25-gauge needle) into the extravasation site (Polovich 2009)	Apply dry warm compress for 20 minutes 4 times/day for 1 to 2 days (Pérez Fidalgo 2012)	Not commercially available in the US
Vinorelbine	Hyaluronidase	Hyaluronidase: *If needle/cannula still in place:* Administer 1 to 6 mL (150 units/mL) into existing IV line; usual dose is 1 mL for each 1 mL of extravasated drug (Pérez Fidalgo 2012; Schulmeister 2011) *If needle/cannula was removed:* Inject 1 to 6 mL (150 units/mL) subcutaneously in a clockwise manner using 1 mL for each 1 mL of drug extravasated (Schulmeister 2011) **or** administer 1 mL (150 units/mL) as five separate 0.2 mL injections (using a 25-gauge needle) into the extravasation site (Polovich 2009)	Apply dry warm compress for 20 minutes 4 times/day for 1 to 2 days (Pérez Fidalgo 2012)	

SUPPORTIVE MANAGEMENT

Compresses: Two issues for which there is less consensus are the application of warm or cold compresses and the use of various antidotes for extravasation management. A variety of recommendations exists for each of these concerns; however, there is no consensus concerning the proper approach.

Cold: Intermittent cooling of the area of extravasation results in vasoconstriction, potentially restricting the spread of the drug and decreasing the pain and inflammation in the area. Application of dry cold compresses for 20 minutes 4 times/day for 1 to 2 days is usually recommended as immediate treatment for most drug extravasations, including anthracycline, antibiotic (eg, mitomycin or dactinomycin), or alkylating agent extravasation (Pérez Fidalgo 2012). Cold dry compresses may also be utilized in the management of nonvesicant extravasations.

Warm: Application of dry warm compresses results in a localized vasodilation and increased blood flow. Increased circulation is believed to facilitate removal of the drug from the area of extravasation. Application of dry warm compresses for 20 minutes 4 times/day for 1 to 2 days is generally recommended for extravasation of vinca alkaloid, taxane, and platinum derivatives (Pérez Fidalgo 2012). Avoid moist heat. Most data are from animal studies with relatively few human case reports. Animal models indicate application of heat exacerbates the damage from anthracycline extravasations.

For some agents, such as oxaliplatin and taxanes, there are conflicting recommendations. Some reports recommend application of cold; others recommend warm.

For most vasopressors (dopamine, ephedrine, norepinephrine, and phenylephrine), dry, warm compresses may be applied (Hurst 2004). Cool compresses should be avoided with vasopressor extravasation as cooling may exacerbate vasoconstrictive effects (Reynolds 2014).

Table 2: Antineoplastic Agents Associated With Irritation or Occasional Extravasation Reactions

Arsenic Trioxide	Gemcitabine
Bendamustine[1]	Ibritumomab
Bleomycin	Ifosfamide
Bortezomib	Irinotecan
Busulfan	Ixabepilone
CARBOplatin	Melphalan
Carmustine	MitoXANtrone[1]
CISplatin (≤0.4 mg/mL)	Oxaliplatin[1]
Cladribine	PACLitaxel[1]
Cyclophosphamide	PACLitaxel (Protein Bound)
Dacarbazine	Pentamidine[1]
DAUNOrubicin Citrate (Liposomal)	Streptozocin[1]
DOCEtaxel[1]	Teniposide
DOXOrubicin (Liposomal)	Thiopental[1]
Etoposide	Thiotepa
Etoposide Phosphate	Topotecan
Fluorouracil	

[1]Irritant with vesicant-like properties (there have been reports of both irritant and vesicant reactions)

The nurse administering the vesicant agent should monitor the patient and IV site frequently. Prior to drug administration, verify the patency of the IV line. The line should be flushed with 5 to 10 mL of a saline or dextrose solution (depending on compatibility) and the drug(s) infused through the side of a free-flowing IV line over 2 to 5 minutes. If an extravasation occurs, it is important to monitor the site closely at 24 hours, 1 week, 2 weeks, and as necessary for any signs and symptoms of extravasation.

EXTRAVASATION-SPECIFIC ANTIDOTES

Dexrazoxane: Dexrazoxane, a derivative of EDTA, is an intracellular chelating agent initially approved as a cardioprotective agent in patients receiving anthracycline therapy. It is believed that the cardioprotective effect of dexrazoxane is a result of chelating iron following intracellular hydrolysis. Dexrazoxane is not an effective chelator itself but is hydrolyzed intracellularly to an open-ring chelator form, which complexes with iron, other heavy metals, and doxorubicin complexes to inhibit the generation of free radicals. In the management of anthracycline-induced extravasation, dexrazoxane may act by reversibly inhibiting topoisomerase II, protecting tissue from anthracycline cytotoxicity, thereby decreasing tissue damage.

Dexrazoxane is administered as 3 IV infusions over 1 to 2 hours through a different venous access location: 1,000 mg/m^2 within 6 hours, 1,000 mg/m^2 after 24 hours, and 500 mg/m^2 after 48 hours of the actual extravasation up to a maximum total dose of 2,000 mg on days 1 and 2 and 1,000 mg on day 3, respectively (Mouridsen 2007). Localized cooling was permitted (except within 15 minutes before and after dexrazoxane infusion). Prior to administering dexrazoxane, discontinue DMSO as studies suggest the single agent is more effective than when used in combination with DMSO. **Note:** Reduce dexrazoxane dose by 50% in patients with moderate to severe renal impairment (CrCl <40 mL/minute).

Dimethyl sulfoxide (DMSO): Case reports and small studies have suggested that DMSO is an effective treatment for certain chemotherapy extravasations (anthracyclines, mitomycin, and mitoxantrone). DMSO has free-radical scavenger properties, which increases removal of vesicant drugs from tissues to minimize tissue damage in extravasation management (Pérez Fidalgo 2012). Common dosing is to apply topically by gently painting DMSO 50% solution onto an area twice the size of the extravasation with a saturated gauze pad or cotton swab every 8 hours for 7 days (Pérez Fidalgo 2012). Allow the site to dry. Do not cover with a dressing, as severe blistering may result. During application, DMSO may cause local erythema. Clinical reports of DMSO use are difficult to interpret due to variations in DMSO concentration (50% to 99%); the product is only commercially available in the United States at a concentration of 50% (vol/vol) solution in water.

Hyaluronidase: Hyaluronidase is an enzyme that destroys hyaluronic acid, an essential component of connective tissue. This results in increased permeability of the tissue, facilitating diffusion and absorption of fluids. It is postulated that increasing the diffusion of extravasated fluids results in more rapid absorption, thereby limiting tissue damage. In individual case reports, hyaluronidase has been reported effective in preventing tissue damage from a wide variety of agents, including vinca alkaloids, epipodophyllotoxins, and taxanes. The ESMO/EONS guidelines suggest that 150 to 900 units may be administered subcutaneously around the area of chemotherapy extravasation (Pérez Fidalgo 2012). Administration as 5 separate 0.2 mL (15 units/mL) SubQ or intradermal injections into the extravasation site has been reported (MacCara 1983). A 24-gauge or smaller needle should be used. It is recommended to use a new syringe for each injection site. If needle/cannula still in place, administration of a 1 to 6 mL hyaluronidase (150 units/mL) has been reported in the management of plant alkaloid extravasation (Pérez Fidalgo 2012; Schulmeister 2011) and paclitaxel extravasation (Ener 2004). Refer to Table 1 for vesicant-specific management.

Phentolamine: Phentolamine minimizes tissue injury due to extravasation of norepinephrine and other sympathomimetic vasoconstrictors. Inject 5 to 10 mg diluted in 10 to 15 mL normal saline and inject/infiltrate into the extravasation area; begin as soon as possible after extravasation but within 12 hours. ***Note:*** *Phentolamine is currently not manufactured/distributed in the United States, although it is available in other countries.*

Topical nitroglycerin or terbutaline (alternatives to phentolamine): Terbutaline and topical nitroglycerin have been used (case reports) as alternatives to phentolamine in the event of phentolamine supply shortages. Topical nitroglycerin (2% ointment) is reported to reverse the vasoconstriction at the extravasation site caused by infiltration of sympathomimetic vasoconstrictors; case reports for use in neonates/infants suggest resolution of ischemia (Denkler 1989; Wong 1992).

Sodium thiosulfate: Sodium thiosulfate (1/6 molar) has been recommended for treatment of mechlorethamine, concentrated cisplatin, and bendamustine extravasations. Sodium thiosulfate provides a substrate for alkylation by mechlorethamine, preventing the alkylation and subsequent destruction in subcutaneous tissue.

Preparation of a 1/6 molar solution of sodium thiosulfate:

- Dilute 4 mL of a sodium thiosulfate 10% solution into a syringe with 6 mL of sterile water for injection, resulting in 10 mL of 1/6 molar solution

  or

- Dilute 1.6 mL of a sodium thiosulfate 25% solution with 8.4 mL of sterile water for injection, resulting in 10 mL of 1/6 molar solution

Inject the 1/6 molar sodium thiosulfate solution either into the existing needle/cannula or subcutaneously around the edge of the extravasation site using a tuberculin syringe, using a new syringe for each injection site. The dose of sodium thiosulfate and route of administration depend on the amount of drug extravasated. Refer to Table 1 for vesicant-specific dosing.

REFERENCES

Albanell J, Baselga J. Systemic therapy emergencies. *Semin Oncol.* 2000;27(3):347-361.

Bellin MF, Jakobsen JA, Tomassin I, et al. Contrast medium extravasation injury: guidelines for prevention and management. *Eur Radiol.* 2002;12 (11):2807-2812.

Bertelli G. Prevention and management of extravasation of cytotoxic drugs. *Drug Saf.* 1995;12(4):245-255.

Boyle DM, Engelking C. Vesicant extravasation: myths and realities. *Oncol Nurs Forum.* 1995;22(1):57-67.

de Lemos ML. Role of dimethylsulfoxide for mangement of chemotherapy extravasation. *J Oncol Pharm Practice.* 2004;10(4):197-200.

de Lemos ML, Walisser S. Management of extravasation of oxaliplatin. *J Oncol Pharm Pract.* 2005;11(4):159-162.

Denkler KA, Cohen BE. Reversal of dopamine extravasation injury with topical nitroglycerin ointment. *Plast Reconstr Surg.* 1989;84(5):811-813.

Doellman D, Hadaway L, Bowe-Geddes LA, et al. Infiltration and extravasation: update on prevention and management. *J Infus Nurs.* 2009;32 (4):203-211.

Dorr RT. Antidotes to vesicant chemotherapy extravasations. *Blood Rev.* 1990;4(1):41-60.

Dorr RT, Soble M, Alberts DS. Efficacy of sodium thiosulfate as a local antidote to mechlorethamine skin toxicity in the mouse. *Cancer Chemother Pharmacol.* 1988;22(4):299-302.

Dumbarton TC, Gorman SK, Minor S, Loubani O, White F, Green R. Local cutaneous necrosis secondary to a prolonged peripheral infusion of methylene blue in vasodilatory shock. *Ann Pharmacother.* 2012;46(3):e6.

Ener RA, Meglathery SB, Styler M. Extravasation of systemic hemato-oncological therapies. *Ann Oncol.* 2004;15(6):858-862.

Hadaway L. Infiltration and extravasation. *Am J Nurs.* 2007;107(8):64-72.

Hastings-Tolsma MT, Yucha CB, Tompkins J, Robson L, Szeverenyi N. Effect of warm and cold applications on the resolution of I.V. infiltrations. *Res Nurs Health.* 1993;16(3):171-178.

Hurst S, McMillan M. Innovative solutions in critical care units: extravasation guidelines. *Dimens Crit Care Nurs.* 2004;23(3):125-128.

Kumar MM, Sprung J. The use of hyaluronidase to treat mannitol extravasation. *Anesth Analg.* 2003;97(4):1199-1200.

Kurul S, Saip P, Aydin T. Totally implantable venous-access ports: local problems and extravasation injury. *Lancet Oncol.* 2002;3(11):684-692.

Larson DL. Alterations in wound healing secondary to infusion injury. *Clin Plast Surg.* 1990;17(3):509-517.

Larson DL. Treatment of tissue extravasation by antitumor agents. *Cancer.* 1982;49(9):1796-1799.

Larson DL. What is the appropriate management of tissue extravasation by antitumor agents? *Plast Reconstr Surg.* 1985;75(3):397-405.

MacCara ME. Extravasation: a hazard of intravenous therapy. *Drug Intell Clin Pharm.* 1983;17(10):713-717.

Montgomery LA, Hanrahan K, Kottman K, Otto A, Barrett T, Hermiston B. Guideline for I.V. infiltrations in pediatric patients. *Pediatr Nurs.* 1999;25 (2):167-169, 173-180.

Mouridsen HT, Langer SW, Buter J, et al. Treatment of anthracycline extravasation with savene (dexrazoxane): results from two prospective clinical multicentre studies. *Ann Oncol.* 2007;18(3):546-550.

Mustargen product information, Lundbeck, 2012

Peberdy MA, Callaway CW, Neumar RW, et al. Part 9: post-cardiac arrest care: 2010 American Heart Association guidelines for cardiopulmonary resuscitation and emergency cardiovascular care. *Circulation.* 2010;122(18 Suppl 3):S768-S786.

Pérez Fidalgo JA, García Fabregat L, Cervantes A, et al. Management of chemotherapy extravasation: ESMO-EONS clinical practice guidelines. *Ann Oncol.* 2012;23(Suppl 7):vii167-173.

Perry MC. Extravasation. *The Chemotherapy Source Book.* 4th ed. Philadelphia, PA; 2008.

Phentolamine product information, Bedford Laboratories, 1999

Polovich M, Whitford JN, Olsen M. *Chemotherapy and Biotherapy Guidelines and Recommendations for Practice.* 3rd ed. Pittsburgh, PA: Oncology Nursing Society; 2009.

Reynolds PM, Maclaren R, Mueller SW, Fish DN, Kiser TH. Management of extravasation injuries: a focused evaluation of noncytotoxic medications. *Pharmacotherapy*. 2014;34(6):617-632.
Rowlett J. Extravasation of contrast media managed with recombinant human hyaluronidase. *Am J Emerg Med*. 2012;30(9):2102.
Schrijvers DL. Extravasation: a dreaded complication of chemotherapy. *Ann Oncol*. 2003;14(Suppl 3):iii26-iii30.
Schulmeister L, Camp-Sorrell D. Chemotherapy extravasation from implanted ports. *Oncol Nurs Forum*. 2000;27(3):531-538.
Schulmeister L. Extravasation management: clinical update. *Semin Oncol Nurs*. 2011;27(1):82-90.
Schulmeister L. Preventing and managing vesicant chemotherapy extravasations. *J Support Oncol*. 2010;8(5):212-215.
Sokol DK, Dahlmann A, Dunn DW. Hyaluronidase treatment for intravenous phenytoin extravasation. *J Child Neurol*. 1998;13(5):246-247.
Stanford BL, Hardwicke F. A review of clinical experience with paclitaxel extravasations. *Support Care Cancer*. 2003;11(5):270-277.
Stier PA, Bogner MP, Webster K, Leikin JB, Burda A. Use of subcutaneous terbutaline to reverse peripheral ischemia. *Am J Emerg Med*. 1999;17(1):91-94.
Wang CL, Cohan RH, Ellis JH, Adusumilli S, Dunnick NR. Frequency, management, and outcome of extravasation of nonionic iodinated contrast medium in 69,657 intravenous injections. *Radiology*. 2007;243(1):80-87.
Wiegand R, Brown J. Hyaluronidase for the management of dextrose extravasation. *Am J Emerg Med*. 2010;28(2):257.
Wong AF, McCulloch LM, Sola A. Treatment of peripheral tissue ischemia with topical nitroglycerin ointment in neonates. *J Pediatr*. 1992;121(6):980-983.
Zenk KE. Management of intravenous extravasations. *Infusion*. 1981;5(4):77-79.

BURN MANAGEMENT

Modified Lund-Browder Burn Assessment Chart Estimation of Total Body Surface Area of Burn Involvement[1] (% by site and age)

Site[2]	0 to 1 years	1 to 4 years	5 to 9 years	10 to 14 years	15 years	Adult
Head	9.5	8.5	6.5	5.5	4.5	3.5
Neck	0.5	0.5	0.5	0.5	0.5	0.5
Trunk	13	13	13	13	13	13
Upper arm	2	2	2	2	2	2
Forearm	1.5	1.5	1.5	1.5	1.5	1.5
Hand	1.5	1.5	1.5	1.5	1.5	1.5
Perineum	1	1	1	1	1	1
Buttock (each)	2.5	2.5	2.5	2.5	2.5	2.5
Thigh	2.75	3.25	4	4.25	4.5	4.75
Leg	2.5	2.5	2.75	3	3.25	3.5
Foot	1.75	1.75	1.75	1.75	1.75	1.75

[1]Applies only to second- and third-degree burns.

[2]Percentage for each site is only for **a single extremity with** anterior **OR** posterior involvement. Percentage should be **doubled if both anterior and posterior** involvement of a single extremity.

The total body surface area of burn involvement is determined by the sum of the percentages of each site.

Adapted from: Coren CV. Burn injuries in children. *Pediatric Annals*. 1987;16(4):328-339.

Parkland Fluid Replacement Formula

A guideline for replacement of deficits and ongoing losses (**Note:** For infants, maintenance fluids may need to be added to this): Administer 4 mL/kg/% burn of Ringer's lactate (glucose may be added but beware of stress hyperglycemia) over the first 24 hours; half of this total is given over the first 8 hours **calculated from the time of injury**; the remaining half is given over the next 16 hours. The second 24-hour fluid requirements average 50% to 75% of first day's requirement. Concentrations and rates best determined by monitoring weight, serum electrolytes, urine output, NG losses, etc.

Colloid may be added after 18 to 24 hours (1 g/kg/day of albumin) to maintain serum albumin >2 g per 100 mL.

Potassium is generally withheld for the first 48 hours due to the large amount of potassium that is released from damaged tissues. To manage serum electrolytes, monitor urine electrolytes twice weekly and replace calculated urine losses.

CONTRACEPTIVE COMPARISON TABLE

Combination Oral Contraceptive Categories and Regimens

Monophasic contraceptives: Constant dose of estrogen and progestin provided in the active pills per cycle

Biphasic and triphasic contraceptive: Dose of estrogen and progestin vary in the active pills. Decreases the total doses of hormones per cycle; however, may not be associated with a significant increase in safety or efficacy

21/7 regimen: Considered to be the "conventional" regimen; consists of 21 days of active tablets, followed by 7 days of inactive tablets; provides monthly withdrawal bleeding. Symptoms of hormone withdrawal may occur during the hormone-free (inactive) interval and include bloating, breast tenderness, headaches, pelvic pain, and swelling

24/4 regimen: Consists of 24 days of active tablets, followed by 4 days of inactive tablets. Decreases the hormone-free interval from 7 to 4 days to decrease the symptoms associated with hormone withdrawal; provides monthly withdrawal bleeding with decreased duration and lighter blood flow as compared to 21/7 regimens

24/2/2 and 21/2/5 regimens: Multiphasic contraceptive. Decreases the hormone-free interval from 7 to 0 to 2 days by providing a lower, noncontraceptive dose of ethinyl estradiol (0.01 mg) in place of some or all of the placebo tablets to decrease the symptoms associated with hormone withdrawal. Provides monthly withdrawal bleeding with decreased duration and lighter blood flow as compared to 21/7 regimens

84/7 regimen: Extended-cycle contraceptive. Consists of 84 days of active tablets, followed by 7 days of inactive tablets. Decreases withdrawal bleeding to 4 times/year

365-day regimen: Extended-cycle contraceptive. Consists of 365 days of active tablets; eliminates withdrawal bleeding

Ferrous fumarate may be provided in place of placebo tablets in some formulations to facilitate ease of administration; not for therapeutic purposes.

Levomefolate may be provided in place of placebo tablets in some formulations to reduce the risk of neural tube defects if pregnancy occurs during or shortly after use.

Combination Oral Contraceptive Formulations – Monophasic

Brand Name	Regimen (# of pills/pack)	Formulation Content			Additional Information
		Estrogen	Progestin	Other	
Gianvi Loryna Vestura Yaz	24/4 regimen (28)	Day 1 to 24: Ethinyl estradiol 0.02 mg	Day 1 to 24: Drospirenone 3 mg	Day 25 to 28: Inactive tablets	
Beyaz	24/4 regimen (28)	Day 1 to 24: Ethinyl estradiol 0.02 mg	Day 1 to 24: Drospirenone 3 mg	Day 1 to 28: Levomefolate calcium 0.451 mg	
Loestrin 24 Fe Lomedia 24 Fe Minastrin 24 Fe	24/4 regimen (28)	Day 1 to 24: Ethinyl estradiol 0.02 mg	Day 1 to 24: Norethindrone acetate 1 mg	Day 25 to 28: Ferrous fumarate 75 mg	
Generess Fe Layolis Fe	24/4 regimen (28)	Day 1 to 24: Ethinyl estradiol 0.025 mg	Day 1 to 24: Norethindrone 0.8 mg	Day 25 to 28: Ferrous fumarate 75 mg	Chewable tablet; efficacy in women with a BMI >35 kg/m^2 has not been evaluated
Gildess 1/20 Junel 1/20 Larin 1/20 Loestrin 21 1/20 Microgestin 1/20	21/7 regimen (21)	Day 1 to 21: Ethinyl estradiol 0.02 mg	Day 1 to 21: Norethindrone acetate 1 mg		
Aviane 28 Falmina Lessina Lutera Orsythia Sronyx	21/7 regimen (28)	Day 1 to 21: Ethinyl estradiol 0.02 mg	Day 1 to 21: Levonorgestrel 0.1 mg	Day 22 to 28: Inactive tablets	
Gildess Fe 1/20 Junel Fe 1/20 Larin Fe 1/20 Loestrin Fe 1/20 Microgestin Fe 1/20 Tarina FE 1/20	21/7 regimen (28)	Day 1 to 21: Ethinyl estradiol 0.02 mg	Day 1 to 21: Norethindrone acetate 1 mg	Day 22 to 28: Ferrous fumarate 75 mg	
Apri Desogen Emoquette Ortho-Cept Reclipsen Solia	21/7 regimen (28)	Day 1 to 21: Ethinyl estradiol 0.03 mg	Day 1 to 21: Desogestrel 0.15 mg	Day 22 to 28: Inactive tablets	
Safyral	21/7 regimen (28)	Day 1 to 21: Ethinyl estradiol 0.03 mg	Day 1 to 21: Drospirenone 3 mg	Day 1 to 28: Levomefolate calcium 0.451 mg	
Ocella Syeda Yasmin Zarah	21/7 regimen (28)	Day 1 to 21: Ethinyl estradiol 0.03 mg	Day 1 to 21: Drospirenone 3 mg		
Altavera Kurvelo Levora Marlissa Nordette 28 Portia 28	21/7 regimen (28)	Day 1 to 21: Ethinyl estradiol 0.03 mg	Day 1 to 21: Levonorgestrel 0.15 mg	Day 22 to 28: Inactive tablets	

Combination Oral Contraceptive Formulations – Monophasic *continued*

Brand Name	Regimen (# of pills/pack)	Formulation Content			Additional Information
		Estrogen	Progestin	Other	
Gildess 1.5/30 Junel 1.5/30 Larin 1.5/30 Loestrin 21 1.5/30 Microgestin 1.5/30	21/7 regimen (21)	Day 1 to 21: Ethinyl estradiol 0.03 mg	Day 1 to 21: Norethindrone acetate 1.5 mg		
Gildess Fe 1.5/30 Junel Fe 1.5/30 Larin Fe 1.5/30 Loestrin Fe 1.5/30 Microgestin Fe 1.5/30	21/7 regimen (28)	Day 1 to 21: Ethinyl estradiol 0.03 mg	Day 1 to 21: Norethindrone acetate 1.5 mg	Day 22 to 28: Ferrous fumarate 75 mg	
Low-Ogestrel 21	21/7 regimen (28)	Day 1 to 21: Ethinyl estradiol 0.03 mg	Day 1 to 21: Norgestrel 0.3 mg		
Cryselle 28 Elinest Low-Ogestrel 28 Lo/Ovral 28	21/7 regimen (28)	Day 1 to 21: Ethinyl estradiol 0.03 mg	Day 1 to 21: Norgestrel 0.3 mg	Day 22 to 28: Inactive tablets	
Zovia 1/35	21/7 regimen (21)	Day 1 to 21: Ethinyl estradiol 0.035 mg	Day 1 to 21: Ethynodiol diacetate 1 mg		
Kelnor 1/35 Zovia 1/35	21/7 regimen (28)	Day 1 to 21: Ethinyl estradiol 0.035 mg	Day 1 to 21: Ethynodiol diacetate 1 mg	Day 22 to 28: Inactive tablets	
Balziva Briellyn Femcon Fe (chewable) Gildagia Ovcon 35 Philith Vyfemla Zenchent (28s) Zeosa (chewable)	21/7 regimen (28)	Day 1 to 21: Ethinyl estradiol 0.035 mg	Day 1 to 21: Norethindrone 0.4 mg	Day 22 to 28: Inactive tablets	
Femcon Fe Wymzya Fe Zenchent Fe	21/7 regimen (28)	Day 1 to 21: Ethinyl estradiol 0.035 mg	Day 1 to 21: Norethindrone 0.4 mg	Day 22 to 28: Ferrous fumarate 75 mg	Chewable tablets
Brevicon 28 Modicon 28 Necon 0.5/35 Nortrel 0.5/35 Wera	21/7 regimen (28)	Day 1 to 21: Ethinyl estradiol 0.035 mg	Day 1 to 21: Norethindrone 0.5 mg	Day 22 to 28: Inactive tablets	
Alyacen 1/35 Cyclafem 1/35 Dasetta 1/35 Necon 1/35 Norinyl 1+35 Nortrel 1/35 Ortho-Novum 1/35	21/7 regimen (28)	Day 1 to 21: Ethinyl estradiol 0.035 mg	Day 1 to 21: Norethindrone 1 mg	Day 22 to 28: Inactive tablets	
Nortrel 1/35	21/7 regimen (21)	Day 1 to 21: Ethinyl estradiol 0.035 mg	Day 1 to 21: Norethindrone 1 mg		

Combination Oral Contraceptive Formulations – Monophasic *continued*

Brand Name	Regimen (# of pills/pack)	Formulation Content			Additional Information
		Estrogen	Progestin	Other	
Estarylla Mono-Linyah MonoNessa Ortho-Cyclen 28 Previfem Sprintec	21/7 regimen (28)	Day 1 to 21: Ethinyl estradiol 0.035 mg	Day 1 to 21: Norgestimate 0.25 mg	Day 22 to 28: Inactive tablets	
Zovia 1/50	21/7 regimen (21)	Day 1 to 21: Ethinyl estradiol 0.05 mg	Day 1 to 21: Ethynodiol diacetate 1 mg		
Zovia 1/50	21/7 regimen (28)	Day 1 to 21: Ethinyl estradiol 0.05 mg	Day 1 to 21: Ethynodiol diacetate 1 mg	Day 22 to 28: Inactive tablets	
Ovcon 50	21/7 regimen (28)	Day 1 to 21: Ethinyl estradiol 0.05 mg	Day 1 to 21: Norethindrone 1 mg	Day 22 to 28: Inactive tablets	
Ogestrel	21/7 regimen (28)	Day 1 to 21: Ethinyl estradiol 0.05 mg	Day 1 to 21: Norgestrel 0.5 mg	Day 22 to 28: Inactive tablets	
Necon 1/50 Norinyl 1+50	21/7 regimen (28)	Day 1 to 21: Mestranol 0.05 mg	Day 1 to 21: Norethindrone 1 mg	Day 22 to 28: Inactive tablets	

Combination Oral Contraceptive Formulations – Multiphasic

Brand Name	Regimen (# of pills/pack)	Formulation Content			Additional Information
		Estrogen	Progestin	Other	
Lo Loestrin Fe Lo Minastrin Fe	24/2/2 regimen (28)	Day 1 to 24: Ethinyl estradiol 0.01 mg	Day 1 to 24: Norethindrone acetate 1 mg		Efficacy in women with a BMI >35 kg/m^2 has not been evaluated
		Day 25 to 26: Ethinyl estradiol 0.01 mg			
				Day 27 to 28: Ferrous fumarate 75 mg	
Azurette Kariva Mircette	21/2/5 regimen (28)	Day 1 to 21: Ethinyl estradiol 0.02 mg	Day 1 to 21: Desogestrel 0.15 mg		
				Day 22 to 23: Inactive tablets	
		Day 24 to 28: Ethinyl estradiol 0.01 mg			

Combination Oral Contraceptive Formulations – Biphasic

Brand Name	Regimen (# of pills/pack)	Formulation Content			Additional Information
		Estrogen	Progestin	Other	
Azurette Kariva Mircette Viorele	21/7 regimen (28)	Day 1 to 21: Ethinyl estradiol 0.02 mg	Day 1 to 21: Desogestrel 0.15 mg		
		Day 24 to 28: Ethinyl estradiol 0.01 mg			
				Day 22 to 23: Inactive tablets	
Necon 10/11	21/7 regimen (28)	Day 1 to 10: Ethinyl estradiol 0.035 mg	Day 1 to 10: Norethindrone 0.5 mg		
		Day 11 to 21: Ethinyl estradiol 0.035 mg	Day 11 to 21: Norethindrone 1 mg		
				Day 22 to 28: Inactive tablets	

Combination Oral Contraceptive Formulations – Triphasic

Brand Name	Regimen (# of pills/pack)	Formulation Content			Additional Information
		Estrogen	Progestin	Other	
Estrostep Fe Tilia Tilia Fe Tri-Legest Fe	21/7 regimen (28)	Day 1 to 5: Ethinyl estradiol 0.02 mg	Day 1 to 5: Norethindrone acetate 1 mg		Escalating dose of estrogen; constant dose of progestin
		Day 6 to 12: Ethinyl estradiol 0.03 mg	Day 6 to 12: Norethindrone acetate 1 mg		
		Day 13 to 21: Ethinyl estradiol 0.035 mg	Day 13 to 21: Norethindrone acetate 1 mg		
Caziant Cesia Cyclessa Velivet	21/7 regimen (28)	Day 1 to 7: Ethinyl estradiol 0.025 mg	Day 1 to 7: Desogestrel 0.1 mg		Constant dose of estrogen; escalating dose of progestin
		Day 8 to 14: Ethinyl estradiol 0.025 mg	Day 8 to 14: Desogestrel 0.125 mg		
		Day 15 to 21: Ethinyl estradiol 0.025 mg	Day 15 to 21: Desogestrel 0.15 mg		
				Day 22 to 28: Inactive tablets	
Ortho Tri-Cyclen Lo Tri Lo Sprintec	21/7 regimen (28)	Day 1 to 7: Ethinyl estradiol 0.025 mg	Day 1 to 7: Norgestimate 0.18 mg		Constant dose of estrogen; escalating dose of progestin
		Day 8 to 14: Ethinyl estradiol 0.025 mg	Day 8 to 14: Norgestimate 0.215 mg		
		Day 15 to 21: Ethinyl estradiol 0.025 mg	Day 15 to 21: Norgestimate 0.25 mg		
				Day 22 to 28: Inactive tablets	
Enpresse Levonest Myzilra Trivora	21/7 regimen (28)	Day 1 to 6: Ethinyl estradiol 0.03 mg	Day 1 to 6: Levonorgestrel 0.05 mg		Escalating doses of estrogen and progestin
		Day 7 to 11: Ethinyl estradiol 0.04 mg	Day 7 to 11: Levonorgestrel 0.075 mg		
		Day 12 to 21: Ethinyl estradiol 0.03 mg	Day 12 to 21: Levonorgestrel 0.125 mg		
				Day 22 to 28: Inactive tablets	
Alyacen 7/7/7 Cyclafem 7/7/7 Dasetta 7/7/7 Necon 7/7/7 Nortrel 7/7/7 Ortho-Novum 7/7/7	21/7 regimen (28)	Day 1 to 7: Ethinyl estradiol 0.035 mg	Day 1 to 7: Norethindrone 0.5 mg		Constant dose of estrogen; escalating dose of progestin
		Day 8 to 14: Ethinyl estradiol 0.035 mg	Day 8 to 14: Norethindrone 0.75 mg		
		Day 15 to 21: Ethinyl estradiol 0.035 mg	Day 15 to 21: Norethindrone 1 mg		
				Day 22 to 28: Inactive tablets	
Aranelle Leena Tri-Norinyl	21/7 regimen (28)	Day 1 to 7: Ethinyl estradiol 0.035 mg	Day 1 to 7: Norethindrone 0.5 mg		
		Day 8 to 16: Ethinyl estradiol 0.035 mg	Day 8 to 16: Norethindrone 1 mg		
		Day 17 to 21: Ethinyl estradiol 0.035 mg	Day 17 to 21: Norethindrone 0.5 mg		
				Day 22 to 28: inactive tablets	
Ortho Tri-Cyclen Tri-Estarylla Tri-Linyah TriNessa Tri-Previfem Tri-Sprintec	21/7 regimen (28)	Day 1 to 7: Ethinyl estradiol 0.035 mg	Day 1 to 7: Norgestimate 0.18 mg		Constant dose of estrogen; escalating dose of progestin
		Day 8 to 14: Ethinyl estradiol 0.035 mg	Day 8 to 14: Norgestimate 0.215 mg		
		Day 15 to 21: Ethinyl estradiol 0.035 mg	Day 15 to 21: Norgestimate 0.25 mg		
				Day 22 to 28: Inactive tablets	

Combination Oral Contraceptive Formulations – Four-phase

Brand Name	Regimen (# of pills/pack)	Formulation Content			Additional Information
		Estrogen	Progestin	Other	
Natazia	26/2 regimen (28)	Day 1 to 2: Estradiol valerate 3 mg			Efficacy in women with BMI >30 kg/m^2 has not been evaluated; not recommended for women who are taking strong CYP3A4 inducers
		Day 3 to 7: Estradiol valerate 2 mg	Day 3 to 7: Dienogest 2 mg		
		Day 8 to 24: Estradiol valerate 2 mg	Day 8 to 24: Dienogest 3 mg		
		Day 25 to 26: Estradiol valerate 1 mg			
				Days 27 to 28: Inactive tablets	

Combination Oral Contraceptive Formulations – Extended cycle

Brand Name	Regimen (# of pills/pack)	Formulation Content			Additional Information
		Estrogen	Progestin	Other	
Amethyst	365-day regimen (28)	Daily: Ethinyl estradiol 0.02 mg	Daily: Levonorgestrel 0.09 mg		No hormone-free interval; no withdrawal bleeding episodes; 365 days of active pills
Introvale Jolessa Quasense Seasonale	84/7 regimen (91)	Day 1 to 84: Ethinyl estradiol 0.03 mg	Day 1 to 84: Levonorgestrel 0.15 mg		Four withdrawal bleeding episodes/year
				Days 85 to 91: Inactive tablets	

Combination Oral Contraceptive Formulations – Extended cycle/multiphasic

Brand Name	Regimen (# of pills/pack)	Formulation Content			Additional Information
		Estrogen	Progestin	Other	
Amethia Lo LoSeasonique	(91)	Day 1 to 84: Ethinyl estradiol 0.02 mg	Day 1 to 84: Levonorgestrel 0.1 mg		No hormone-free interval; four withdrawal bleeding episodes/year
		Day 85 to 91: Ethinyl estradiol 0.01 mg			
Amethia Seasonique	(91)	Day 1 to 84: Ethinyl estradiol 0.03 mg	Day 1 to 84: Levonorgestrel 0.15 mg		No hormone-free interval; four withdrawal bleeding episodes/year
		Day 85 to 91: Ethinyl estradiol 0.01 mg			
Quartette	(91)	Day 1 to 42: Ethinyl estradiol 0.02 mg	Day 1 to 84: Levonorgestrel 0.15 mg		No hormone-free interval; four withdrawal bleeding episodes/year
		Day 43 to 63: Ethinyl estradiol 0.025 mg			
		Day 64 to 84: Ethinyl estradiol 0.03 mg			
		Day 85 to 91: Ethinyl estradiol 0.01 mg			

Progestin-Only Oral Contraceptives

Brand Name	Progestin	Additional Information
Camila Errin Heather Jolivette Micronor Nora-BE Nor-QD	Norethindrone 0.35 mg	No hormone-free interval
Plan B	Levonorgestrel 0.75 mg	For emergency contraception
EContra EZ Plan B One Step Take Action	Levonorgestrel 1.5 mg	For emergency contraception

Additional Hormonal Contraceptive Products[1]

Brand Name	Route	Formulation Content			Additional Information
		Estrogen	Progestin	Other	
Depo-Provera CI	IM		Medroxyprogesterone 150 mg		Dosed every 3 months
Depo-subQ Provera 104	SubQ		Medroxyprogesterone 104 mg		Dosed every 3 months
ella	Oral			Ulipristal acetate 30 mg	Selective progesterone receptor modulator for emergency contraception
Implanon, Nexplanon	Subdermal		Etonogestrel 68 mg; 60 to 70 µg/day initially (week 5 to 6) and decreases to ~25 to 30 µg/day at the end of the third year		Long-acting reversible contraception (up to 3 years)
Liletta	Intrauterine		Levonorgestrel ~15.6 mcg/day		Long-acting reversible contraception (up to 3 years)
Mirena	Intrauterine		Levonorgestrel 20 mcg/day		Long-acting reversible contraception (up to 5 years)
NuvaRing	Vaginal	Day 1 to 21: Ethinyl estradiol 0.015 mg	Day 1 to 21: Etonogestrel 0.12 mg		21/7 regimen
Ortho Evra Xulane	Transdermal	Day 1 to 21: Ethinyl estradiol 0.02 mcg	Day 1 to 21: Norelgestromin 0.15 mg		21/7 regimen
Skyla	Intrauterine		Levonorgestrel ~6 mcg/day		Long-acting reversible contraception (up to 3 years)

[1]Products presented in alphabetical order by brand name

Estrogens Used for Contraception

Ethinyl estradiol (EE)	Low-dose combination hormonal contraceptives contain ≤35 mcg EE Original combination oral contraceptive pills contained EE in doses ≤150 mcg; the highest dose currently available is EE 50 mcg and should not be used unless medically indicated Decreasing doses of EE decrease the risk of VTE, MI; also associated with bleeding irregularities (amenorrhea, infrequent bleeding, prolonged or frequent bleeding, unscheduled bleeding, spotting) Increased doses of EE are associated with bloating, breast tenderness, and nausea
Estradiol valerate (E2V)	Metabolized to EE ~3% of the dose is directly bioavailable as estradiol
Mestranol	Original estrogen used in oral contraceptives Metabolized to EE (large variability)

Progestins Used for Contraception

Desogestrel	Structurally related to testosterone Converted into etonogestrel
Dienogest	Structurally related to testosterone Antiandrogenic activity and is devoid of estrogenic, androgenic, glucocorticoid, and mineralocorticoid activities Potential uses include hormone replacement therapy or endometriosis
Drospirenone	Spironolactone analogue with antimineralocorticoid and antiandrogenic activity When combined with ethinyl estradiol, used to treat premenstrual dysphoric disorder and acne
Ethynodiol diacetate	Structurally related to testosterone
Etonogestrel	Biologically active metabolite of desogestrel Progestational activity with minimal intrinsic androgenicity
Levonorgestrel	Structurally related to testosterone
Medroxyprogesterone acetate	Structurally related to progesterone
Norelgestromin	Biologically active metabolite of norgestimate
Norethindrone	Structurally related to testosterone
Norethindrone acetate	Structurally related to testosterone Converted to norethindrone
Norgestimate	Structurally related to testosterone High progestational activity with minimal intrinsic androgenicity

CLINICAL PRACTICE GUIDELINES

Centers for Disease Control and Prevention (CDC). US medical eligibility criteria for contraceptive use, 2010. *MMWR*. May 2010.
Centers for Disease Control and Prevention (CDC). US medical eligibility criteria for contraceptive use, 2010, update. *MMWR*. July 2011.
Centers for Disease Control and Prevention (CDC). US selected practice recommendations for contraceptive use, 2013. *MMWR*. June 2013.

PATIENT INFORMATION

Food and Drug Administration (FDA) Office of Women's Health – Birth Control Poster
Food and Drug Administration (FDA) Office of Women's Health – Emergency Contraception (Emergency Birth Control) Fact Sheet
Food and Drug Administration (FDA) Office of Women's Health – Birth Control Methods Fact Sheet

REFERENCES

Burkman R, Bell C, Serfaty D. The evolution of combined oral contraception: improving the risk-to-benefit ratio. *Contraception*. 2011;84(1):19-34.
Centers for Disease Control and Prevention (CDC). Update to CDC's US medical eligibility criteria for contraceptive use, 2010: revised recommendations for the use of contraceptive methods during the postpartum period. *MMWR Morb Mortal Wkly Rep*. 2011;60(26):878-883.
Centers for Disease Control and Prevention (CDC). US medical eligibility criteria for contraceptive use, 2010. *MMWR Recomm Rep*. 2010;59(RR-4):1-86.
Choice of contraceptives. *Treat Guidel Med Lett*. 2010;8(100):89-96.
Cremer M, Phan-Weston S, Jacobs A. Recent innovations in oral contraception. *Semin Reprod Med*. 2010;28(2):140-146.
Goldzieher JW, Brody SA. Pharmacokinetics of ethinyl estradiol and mestranol. *Am J Obstet Gynecol*. 1990;163(6 Pt 2):2114-2119.
Grossman Barr N. Managing adverse effects of hormonal contraceptives. *Am Fam Physician*. 2010;82(12):1499-1506.
Practice Committee of American Society for Reproductive Medicine. Hormonal contraception: recent advances and controversies. *Fertil Steril*. 2008;90(5 Suppl):S103-S113.
Read CM. New regimens with combined oral contraceptive pills – moving away from traditional 21/7 cycles. *Eur J Contracept Reprod Health Care*. 2010;15(Suppl 2):S32-S41.
Sitruk-Ware R, Nath A. The use of newer progestins for contraception. *Contraception*. 2010;82(5):410-417.

INSULIN PRODUCTS

Types of Insulin	Onset (h)	Peak Glycemic Effect (h)	Duration (h)
Rapid-Acting			
Insulin lispro (HumaLOG)	0.25 to 0.5	0.5 to 2.5	≤5
Insulin aspart (NovoLOG)	0.2 to 0.3	1 to 3	3 to 5
Insulin glulisine (Apidra)	0.2 to 0.5	1.6 to 2.8	3 to 4
Insulin (oral inhalation) (Afrezza)	~0.25	~0.88	2.5 to 3 hours
Short-Acting			
Insulin regular (systemic) (HumuLIN R, NovoLIN R)	0.5	2.5 to 5	4 to 12 (up to 24 hours for U-500)
Intermediate-Acting			
Insulin NPH (isophane suspension) (HumuLIN N, NovoLIN N)	1 to 2	4 to 12	14 to 24
Long-Acting			
Insulin detemir (Levemir)	3 to 4	3 to 9	6 to 23 (duration is dose dependent)
Insulin glargine (Lantus)	3 to 4	*	~11 to >24
Combinations			
Insulin aspart protamine suspension and insulin aspart (NovoLOG Mix 70/30)	0.17 to 0.33	1 to 4	18 to 24
Insulin lispro protamine and insulin lispro (HumaLOG Mix 75/25)	0.25 to 0.5	1 to 6.5	14 to 24
Insulin NPH suspension and insulin regular solution (NovoLIN 70/30)	0.5	2 to 12	18 to 24

*Insulin glargine has no pronounced peak.

ENTERAL NUTRITION PRODUCT COMPARISON

PREMATURE NEONATAL PRODUCTS

Premature Formula[1,2] – Initial Hospitalization

Indication: Premature infant formulas designed for rapidly growing LBW infants

	Preterm Human Milk	Enfamil Premature 20 Cal[3]	Enfamil Premature 24 Cal[3,4]	Enfamil Premature 30 Cal[3,5]	Similac Special Care 20 With Iron[6]	Similac Special Care 24 With Iron[4,6]	Similac Special Care 30 With Iron[6]	Gerber Good Start Premature 20	Gerber Good Start Premature 24[4]
Calories per 100 mL	67	68	81	100	68	81	101	68	81
Protein g per 100 mL	1.62	2	2.48 (2.8)[4]	3	2.03	2.43 (2.68)[4]	3.04	2	2.4 (2.9)[4]
Protein source	Preterm human milk	Nonfat milk and whey protein concentrate	Nonfat milk and whey protein concentrate	Nonfat milk and whey protein concentrate	Nonfat milk and whey protein concentrate	Nonfat milk and whey protein concentrate	Nonfat milk and whey protein concentrate	100% enzymatically hydrolyzed whey protein isolate (milk)	100% enzymatically hydrolyzed whey protein isolate (milk)
Carbohydrate g per 100 mL	6.64	7.4	8.9 (8.5)[4]	11.2	6.97	8.4 (8.1)[4]	7.84	7.1	8.5 (7.9)[4]
Carbohydrate source	Lactose	Corn syrup solids and lactose	Corn syrup solids and lactose	Maltodextrin	Corn syrup solids and lactose (50:50)	Corn syrup solids and lactose	Corn syrup solids and lactose (50:50)	Lactose, maltodextrin (50:50)	Lactose, maltodextrin (50:50)
Fat g per 100 mL	3.89	3.4	4.1	5.2	3.67	4.41	6.71	3.5	4.2
Fat source (essential fatty acid amounts are per 100 kcal)	Preterm human milk	40% MCT, soy, and high oleic vegetable oils (sunflower/ safflower); DHA[7] (17 mg); ARA[7] (34 mg); linoleic acid (810 mg); linolenic acid (90 mg)	40% MCT, soy, and high oleic vegetable oils (sunflower/ safflower); DHA[7] (17 mg); ARA[7] (34 mg); linoleic acid (810 mg); linolenic acid (90 mg)	40% MCT, soy, and high oleic vegetable oils (sunflower/ safflower); DHA[7] (17 mg); ARA[7] (34 mg); linoleic acid (810 mg); linolenic acid (90 mg); soy lecithin	MCT, soy, and coconut oils (50:30:18) with DHA and ARA[7]	MCT, soy, and coconut oils (50:30:18) with DHA and ARA[7]; soy lecithin	MCT, soy, and coconut oils (50:30:18) with DHA and ARA[7]; soy lecithin	MCT, high oleic sunflower or safflower, soy oils, single cell DHA[7] (0.32%), ARA[7] (0.64%), linoleic acid (950 mg), linolenic acid (100 mg) (40:29:29:2)	MCT, high oleic sunflower or safflower, soy oils, single cell DHA[7] (0.32%), ARA[7] (0.64%), linoleic acid (950 mg), linolenic acid (100 mg) (40:29:29:2)
Osmolality mOsm/kg H_2O	290	240	300	320	235	280	325	229	275
Osmolarity mOsm/L		220	260	270	188	240	282	187	225
Sodium mEq/L (mg/L)	10.8 (248)	(390)	(470)	(590)	12.6 (291)	15.2 (349)	19 (436)	(370)	(450)
Potassium mEq/L (mg/L)	14.6 (570)	(660)	(800)	(1,030)	22.3 (872)	26.8 (1,047)	33.5 (1,308)	(810)	(970)
Chloride mEq/L (mg/L)	15.6 (550)	(610)	(730)	(860)	15.5 (548)	18.6 657	23.2 (821)	(570)	(690)
Calcium mEq/L (mg/L)	12.4 (248)	(1,120)	(1,340)	(1,670)	60.7 (1,217)	72.9 (1,461)	91.3 (1,826)	(1,110)	(1,330)
Phosphorus mEq/L (mg/L)	(128)	(560)	(670)	(840)	(676)	(812)	(1,014)	(570)	(690)
Iron mg/L	1	12.2 (3.4)[8]	14.6 (4.1)[8]	18.3	12.2 (2.5)[8]	14.6	18.3	12	15
% free water		90	88	85	90	89	85		

Premature Formula[1,2] – Initial Hospitalization *continued*

	Preterm Human Milk	Enfamil Premature 20 Cal[3]	Enfamil Premature 24 Cal[3,4]	Enfamil Premature 30 Cal[3,5]	Similac Special Care 20 With Iron[6]	Similac Special Care 24 With Iron[4,6]	Similac Special Care 30 With Iron[6]	Gerber Good Start Premature 20	Gerber Good Start Premature 24[4]
Manufacturer	Mothers	Mead Johnson	Mead Johnson	Mead Johnson	Abbott	Abbott	Abbott	Gerber	Gerber
Special information		Gluten-free	Gluten-free	Gluten-free	Kosher, Halal	Kosher, Halal	Kosher, Halal		

[1]Information based on manufacturer's literature as of 2013 and is subject to change

[2]To approximate values of 24-cal/oz formulation, multiply the values desired, found in the 20-cal/oz formula, by 1.2.

[3]Not recommended for use in patients >2.5 kg because may receive excessive fat soluble vitamin quantities with continued use

[4]Also available as high-protein formula; carbohydrate and protein amounts for the high-protein formulas are listed in parentheses

[5]Can use as a ready-to-feed formula, mix with Enfamil Premature 24 kcal/oz to make 25 to 29 kcal/oz, or mix with Enfamil Premature 24 kcal/oz high-protein to increase protein and kcal/oz

[6]Provides 2 mg of elemental iron per kg/day if providing 120 kcal/kg/day; not recommended for use in patients >3.6 kg

[7]DHA (docosahexaenoic acid) and ARA (arachidonic acid) are fatty acids found naturally in breast milk. DHA is provided via *Crypthecodinium cohnii* oil. ARA is provided via *Mortienella alphia* oil.

[8]Low-iron formulation in parentheses

Human Milk Fortifiers[1,2]

Indication: Add to human milk as a supplement for premature and low birth weight infants

	Enfamil Human Milk Fortifier	Enfamil Human Milk Fortifier Acidified Liquid[3]	Similac Human Milk Fortifier
Calories /packet	3.5	7.5 per 5 mL vial	3.5
Protein g/packet	0.28	0.55	0.25
Protein source	Milk protein isolate and whey protein hydrolysate	Wey protein isolate hydrolysate (milk)	Nonfat milk and whey protein concentrate
Carbohydrate g/packet	<0.1	<0.3	0.45
Carbohydrate source	Corn syrup solids	Pectin	Corn syrup solids
Fat g/packet	0.25	0.58	0.09
Fat source (essential fatty acid amounts are per 100 kcal)	MCT and soybean oils and soy lecithin (140 mg of linoleic acid and 17 mg of linolenic acid per 4 packets)	MCT, vegetable oils (soy, high oleic sunflower oils), DHA[3,5] (24 mg), ARA[3,5] (38 mg), linoleic acid (730 mg), linolenic acid (60 mg)	MCT oil and soy lecethin
Osmolality mOsm/kg H_2O	Additional 35 when added to breast milk	Additional 36 when added to human milk	
Sodium mEq/packet (mg/packet)	(4)	(6.75)	0.16 (3.75)
Potassium mEq/packet (mg/packet)	(7.25)	(11.3)	0.4 (15.8)
Chloride mEq/packet (mg/packet)	(3.25)	(7)	0.27 (9.5)
Calcium mEq/packet (mg/packet)	(22.5)	(29)	1.46 (29.3)
Phosphorus mEq/packet (mg/packet)	(12.5)	(16)	0.54 (16.8)
Iron mg/packet	0.36	0.44	0.088
Manufacturer	Mead Johnson	Mead Johnson	Abbott
Special information	Gluten-free	Gluten-free	Kosher, Halal

[1]Information based on manufacturer's literature as of 2013 and is subject to change

[2]May be mixed with human milk or fed alternatively with human milk to low birth weight infants.

[3]Meets ADA and CDC feeding preparation guidelines. Contains 4 g of protein per 100 kcal with human milk; pH of 4.3 by itself; pH of 4.7 with human milk. Four 5 mL vials contain 12 mg of DHA, 188 international units of vitamin D, and 1.76 mg of elemental iron. One 5 mL vial + 25 mL of human milk per 100 kcal would provide 24 mg of DHA and 38 mg of ARA. One 5 mL vial + 50 mL of human milk increases caloric content by 2 kcal/oz. Two 5 mL vials + 25 mL of human milk increases caloric content by 4 kcal/oz.

[4]Not recommended for use in patients >3.6 kg

[5]DHA (docosahexaenoic acid) and ARA (arachidonic acid) are fatty acids found naturally in breast milk. DHA is provided via *Crypthecodinium cohnii* oil. ARA is provided via *Mortienella alphia* oil.

Premature Formula – Enhanced Caloric Preparations

Indications: Premature Neonates Who Need High Calorie Low Volume Feedings

Similac Special Care Liqui-Mix System[1]

	22 calorie/oz formula	26 calorie/oz formula	27 calorie/oz formula	27 calorie/oz formula	28 calorie/oz formula
Base formula to begin with	Similac Special Care 20 With Iron (SSC 20)	Similac Special Care 24 With Iron[2] (SSC 24)	Similac Special Care 20 With Iron (SSC 20)	Similac Special Care 24 With Iron[2] (SSC 24)	Similac Special Care 24 With Iron[2] (SSC 24)
Formula used to increase caloric content	Similac Special Care 24 With Iron[2] (SSC 24)	Similac Special Care 30 With Iron (SSC 30)	Similac Special Care 30 With Iron (SSC 30)	Similac Special Care 30 With Iron (SSC 30)	Similac Special Care 30 With Iron (SSC 30)
Mixing instructions	15 mL SSC 20 + 15 mL SSC 24	20 mL SSC 24 + 10 mL SSC 30	10 mL SSC 20 + 20 mL SSC 30	15 mL SSC 24 + 15 mL SSC 30	10 mL SSC 24 + 20 mL SSC 30
Ratio	1:1	2:1	1:2	1:1	1:2
Calories per 100 mL	74	88	90	91	95
Protein g per 100 mL	2.23 (2.35)[2]	2.64 (2.8)[2]	2.71	2.74 (2.86)[2]	2.84 (2.92)[2]
Protein source	Nonfat milk and whey protein concentrate	Nonfat milk and whey protein concentrate	Nonfat milk and whey protein concentrate	Nonfat milk and whey protein concentrate	Nonfat milk and whey protein concentrate
Carbohydrate g per 100 mL	7.7 (7.5)[2]	8.2 (8)[2]	7.5	8.1 (8)[2]	8 (7.9)[2]
Carbohydrate source	Corn syrup solids and lactose (50:50)	Corn syrup solids and lactose (50:50)	Corn syrup solids and lactose (50:50)	Corn syrup solids and lactose (50:50)	Corn syrup solids and lactose (50:50)
Fat g per 100 mL	4.04	5.17	5.69	5.56	5.94
Fat source (essential fatty acid amounts are per 100 kcal)	MCT, soy, and coconut oils (50:30:18) with DHA and ARA[3]; soy lecithin	MCT, soy, and coconut oils (50:30:18) with DHA and ARA[3]; soy lecithin	MCT, soy, and coconut oils (50:30:18) with DHA and ARA[3]; soy lecithin	MCT, soy, and coconut oils (50:30:18) with DHA and ARA[3]; soy lecithin	MCT, soy, and coconut oils (50:30:18) with DHA and ARA[3]; soy lecithin
Osmolality mOm/kg H_2O	258	295	295	305	310
Sodium mEq/L (mg/L)	13.9 (320)	16 (380)	16.9 (390)	17 (390)	18 (410)
Potassium mEq/L (mg/L)	24.5 (960)	29 (1,130)	29.7 (1,160)	30 (1,180)	31 (1,220)
Chloride mEq/L (mg/L)	17 (600)	20 (710)	20.6 (730)	21 (740)	22 (770)
Calcium mEq/L (mg/L)	(1,340)	(1,580)	(1,620)	(1,640)	(1,700)
Phosphorus mEq/L (mg/L)	(740)	(880)	(900)	(910)	(950)
Iron mg/L	13	15.8	13.5	16.4	17
Manufacturer	Abbott	Abbott	Abbott	Abbott	Abbott

[1]Information based on manufacturer's literature as of 2011 and is subject to change

[2]Also available as high-protein formula; carbohydrate and protein amounts for the high-protein formula are listed in parentheses

[3]DHA (docosahexaenoic acid) and ARA (arachidonic acid) are fatty acids found naturally in breast milk. DHA is provided via *Crypthecodinium cohnii* oil. ARA is provided via *Mortienella alphia* oil.

Enfamil Mixing Instructions[1]

	26 calorie/oz formula	27 calorie/oz formula	28 calorie/oz formula
Base formula to begin with	Enfamil Premature High Protein 24 Cal (EPHP 24)	Enfamil Premature High Protein 24 Cal (EPHP 24)	Enfamil Premature High Protein 24 Cal (EPHP 24)
Formula used to increase caloric content	Enfamil Premium Infant Concentrate (EPIC)	Enfamil Premium Infant Concentrate (EPIC)	Enfamil Premium Infant Concentrate (EPIC)
Mixing instructions	60 mL EPHP 24 + 8 mL EPIC	60 mL EPHP 24 + 14 mL EPIC	60 mL EPHP 24 + 20 mL EPIC
Calories per 100 mL	88	92	95
Protein g per 100 mL	2.9	2.9	2.9
Protein source	Nonfat milk and whey protein concentrate	Nonfat milk and whey protein concentrate	Nonfat milk and whey protein concentrate
Carbohydrate g per 100 mL	9.3	9.7	10.1
Carbohydrate source	Corn syrup soids, lactose, galactooligosaccharides[2,3], polydextrose	Corn syrup soids, lactose, galactooligosaccharides[2,3], polydextrose	Corn syrup soids, lactose, galactooligosaccharides[2,3], polydextrose
Fat g per 100 mL	4.5	4.7	4.8
Fat source (essential fatty acid amounts are per 100 kcal)	MCT, soy, high oleic vegetable (sunflower/safflower), palm olein, and coconut oils; DHA[4] (14.9 mg); ARA[4] (30 mg); linoleic acid; linolenic acid; and soy lecithin	MCT, soy, high oleic vegetable (sunflower/safflower), palm olein, and coconut oils; DHA[4] (15.6 mg); ARA[4] (32 mg); linoleic acid; linolenic acid; and soy lecithin	MCT, soy, high oleic vegetable (sunflower/safflower), palm olein, and coconut oils; DHA[4] (16.2 mg); ARA[4] (33 mg); linoleic acid; linolenic acid; and soy lecithin
Sodium mEq/L (mg/L)	(460)	(450)	(440)
Potassium mEq/L (mg/L)	(880)	(920)	(960)
Chloride mEq/L (mg/L)	(750)	(750)	(760)
Calcium mEq/L (mg/L)	(1,300)	(1,290)	(1,270)
Phosphorus mEq/L (mg/L)	(670)	(660)	(660)
Iron mg/L	15.8	16.4	17.1
Manufacturer	Mead Johnson	Mead Johnson	Mead Johnson

[1]Information based on manufacturer's literature as of 2011 and is subject to change

[2]Contains Bifidus BL, beneficial cultures like those found in breast milk to help support a healthy immune system

[3]Prebiotic

[4]DHA (docosahexaenoic acid) and ARA (arachidonic acid) are fatty acids which are found naturally in breast milk. DHA is provided via *Crypthecodinium cohnii* oil. ARA is provided via *Mortienella alphia* oil.

Premature Formula[1,2] – At Discharge

Indication: Premature infant formulas designed for rapidly growing LBW infants

	Enfamil EnfaCare[3]	Similac Expert Care Neosure	Gerber Good Start Nourish
Calories per 100 mL	73	74	74
Protein g per 100 mL	2.1	2.08	2.1
Protein source	Nonfat milk and whey protein concentrate	Nonfat milk and whey protein concentrate	100% enzymatically hydrolyzed whey protein isolate (milk)
Carbohydrate g per 100 mL	7.7	7.51	7.8
Carbohydrate source	Powder: Corn syrup solids, lactose Liquid: Maltodextrin, lactose	Corn syrup solids, lactose	Lactose, maltodextrin (60:40)
Fat g per 100 mL	3.9	4.09	3.9
Fat source (essential fatty acid amounts are per 100 kcal)	High oleic vegetable (sunflower/ safflower), soy, 20% MCT, and coconut oils; DHA[4] (17 mg); ARA[4] (34 mg); linoleic acid (860 to 950 mg)[5]; linolenic acid (90 to 95 mg)[6]	Soy, high oleic safflower, MCT, and coconut oils with DHA and ARA[4]; soy lecithin	High oleic sunflower or safflower, MCT, and soy oils; single cell DHA[4] (0.32%); ARA[4] (0.64%); linoleic acid (900 mg); linolenic acid (60 mg); soy lecithin
Osmolality mOsm/kg H_2O	250 (liquid) 310 (powder)	250	275
Osmolarity mOsm/L	220 (liquid) 280 (powder)	187	180
Sodium mEq/L (mg/L)	(260 – liquid) (280 – powder)	10.7 (245)	(260)
Potassium mEq/L (mg/L)	(780)	27 (1,056)	(781)
Chloride mEq/L (mg/L)	(580)	15.7 (558)	(551)
Calcium mEq/L (mg/L)	(890)	39 (781)	(893)
Phosphorus mEq/L (mg/L)	(490)	(461)	(484)
Iron mg/L	13.3	13.4	13
% free water	89	89	
Manufacturer	Mead Johnson	Abbott	Gerber
Special information	Gluten-free	Kosher, Halal	

[1]Information based on manufacturer's literature as of 2013 and is subject to change

[2]To approximate values of 24-cal/oz formulation, multiply the values desired found in the 20-cal/oz formula by 1.2.

[3]Recommended minimum patient weight >1.8 kg

[4]DHA (docosahexaenoic acid) and ARA (arachidonic acid) are fatty acids found naturally in breast milk. DHA is provided via *Crypthecodinium cohnii* oil. ARA is provided via *Mortienella alphia* oil.

[5]Amount of linoleic acid varies depending on product and size: 860 mg in the powder, 900 mg in the 2 fl oz ready-to-feed, 950 mg in the 32 fl oz ready-to-feed

[6]Amount of linolenic acid varies depending on product and size: 90 mg in the 2 fl oz ready-to-feed, 95 mg in the 32 fl oz ready-to-feed and the powder

INFANT PRODUCTS

Infant Milk-Based Formulas[1,2]

Indications: Feeding normal term infants or sick infants without special nutritional requirements

	Human Milk	Enfamil Premium[3]	Similac Advance[4]	Similac Advance Organic[5]	Gerber Good Start Gentle	Gerber Good Start Protect[6]	Enfamil A.R.[7]	Similac Sensitive RS
Calories per 100 mL	68	67	68	68	68	68	68	68
Protein g per 100 mL	1	1.4	1.4	1.4	1.49	1.49	1.67	1.5
Protein source	Mature Term human milk	Nonfat milk, whey protein concentrate	Nonfat milk, whey protein concentrate	Organic nonfat milk	100% whey protein concentrate (milk)	100% whey protein concentrate (milk)	Nonfat milk	Milk protein isolate
Carbohydrate g per 100 mL	7.2	7.5	7.2	7.1	7.85	7.58	7.5	7.2
Carbohydrate source	Lactose	Lactose, galactooligosaccharides[8,9], polydextrose	Lactose and galactooligosaccharides[8]	Organic maltodextrin, organic sugar, fructooligosaccharides[8]	Corn (30%) maltodextrin, lactose (70%), galactooligosaccharides[8] (4 g/L)	Lactose and corn maltodextrin	Rice starch, lactose, maltodextrin, galactooligiosaccharides[8,9], polydextrose	Corn syrup, rice starch, sugar (50:30:20)
Fat g per 100 mL	3.91	3.5	3.78	3.8	3.45	3.42	3.4	3.7
Fat source (essential fatty acid amounts are per 100 kcal)	Human milk, fat	Vegetable oil (palm olein, coconut, soy, and high oleic sunflower oils), DHA[10] (17 mg), ARA[10] (34 mg), linoleic acid (860 mg), linoleic acid (80 mg), soy lecithin	High oleic safflower, soy, and coconut oils (40:30:29) DHA: 0.15%[10] ARA: 0.40%[10]	Organic high oleic sunflower, organic soy, and organic coconut oils (40:30:29), DHA & ARA[10]	Vegetable oil (palm, soy, coconut, and high oleic safflower or sunflower oils), DHA[10] (0.32%), ARA[10] (0.64%), linoleic acid (900 mg), linolenic acid (85 mg) (46:26:20:6:2), soy lecithin	Vegetable oil, (palm, soy, coconut, and high oleic safflower or sunflower oils), DHA[10] (0.32%), ARA[10] (0.64%), linoleic acid (900 mg), linolenic acid (85 mg) (46:26:20:6:2), soy lecithin	Vegetable oils (palm olein, soy, coconut, and high oleic safflower oils), DHA[10] (17 mg), ARA[10] (34 mg), linoleic acid (860 mg), linolenic acid (85 mg)	High oleic safflower, soy, and coconut oils; DHA and ARA[10] (40:30:29)
Osmolality mOsm/kg H_2O	286	300	310	225	250	250	240 (liquid) 230 (powder)	270
Osmolarity mOsm/L		270	127	127	133	133	220 (liquid) 210 (powder)	240
Sodium mEq/L (mg/L)	7.7 (177)	(180)	7.1 (162)	7.1 (163)	(183)	(183)	(267)	(240)
Potassium mEq/L (mg/L)	13.6 (531)	(720)	18.2 (710)	18.1 (710)	(730)	(730)	(720)	(867)
Chloride mEq/L (mg/L)	11.9 (422)	(420)	12.4 (440)	12.4 (442)	(440)	(440)	(500)	(534)
Calcium mEq/L (mg/L)	16 (280)	27 (520)	26.3 (528)	26.3 (530)	(453)	(453)	(520)	(1301)
Phosphorus mEq/L (mg/L)	9 (143)	(287)	18.8 (284)	(285)	(257)	(257)	(354)	(867)
Iron mg/L	0.27	12	12.2	12.2	10.1	10.1	12	12.2
% free water	80 to 90	89	90	90	90	90	89	90
Manufacturer	Mothers	Mead Johnson	Abbott	Abbott	Gerber	Gerber	Mead Johnson	Abbott

Infant Milk-Based Formulas[1,2] *continued*

	Human Milk	Enfamil Premium[3]	Similac Advance[4]	Similac Advance Organic[5]	Gerber Good Start Gentle	Gerber Good Start Protect[6]	Enfamil A.R.[7]	Similac Sensitive RS
Special information							Gluten-free	
Special uses							Thickened with added rice starch for babies who spit up frequently	With added rich starch to help reduce spit-up; milk-based, lactose-free formula

[1]Information based on manufacturer's literature as of 2013 and is subject to change

[2]To approximate values for the content of a 24-, 27-, or 30-cal/oz formula (made by dilution of a powder-based formulation), multiply the value desired, found in the above 20-cal/oz formula, by the following factors: 1.2 (24-cal/oz), 1.35 (27-cal/oz), or 1.5 (30-cal/oz).

[3]Available as newborn and infant products. Newborn product is for birth to 3 months of age and provides 400 international units of vitamin D in 27 fl oz and is similar to breast milk 3 to 5 days after initiation of lactation. Infant product is for 0 to 12 months of age.

[4]Contains nucleotides and prebiotics for enhanced immune function.

[5]Certified USDA organic

[6]Contains Bifidus BL, beneficial cultures like those found in breast milk to help support a healthy immune system

[7]Viscosity in the bottle is 10 times routine formula, yet it flows freely through a standard nipple

[8]Prebiotic

[9]Polydextrose + galactooligosaccharides = Natural Defense Dual Prebiotics from Mead Johnson. They support the growth of healthy gut bacteria which help support immune function.

[10]DHA (docosahexaenoic acid) and ARA (arachidonic acid) are fatty acids which are found naturally in breast milk. DHA is provided via *Crypthecodinium cohnii* oil. ARA is provided via *Mortienella alphia* oil.

Infant Milk-Based Formulas – Reduced Lactose and Lactose Free[1,2]

Indications: Feeding normal term infants or sick infants without special nutritional requirements

	Enfamil Gentlease[3]	Similac Sensitive	Gerber Good Start Soothe[4]
Calories per 100 mL	67	68	68
Protein g per 100 mL	1.5	1.45	1.5
Protein source	Partially hydrolyzed nonfat milk and whey protein concentrate (soy)	Milk protein isolate	100% whey partially hydrolyzed
Carbohydrate g per 100 mL	7.2	7.5	7.58
Carbohydrate source	Corn syrup solids	Corn maltodextrin, sugar, galactooligosaccaharides[5] (55:43:4)	Maltodextrin, lactose (70:30)
Fat g per 100 mL	3.5	3.65	3.45
Fat source (essential fatty acid amounts are per 100 kcal)	Vegetable oil (palm olein, soy, coconut, and high oleic sunflower oils), DHA[6] (17 mg), ARA[6] (34 mg), linoleic acid (860 mg), linolenic acid (80 mg)	High oleic safflower, soy, and coconut oils (40:30:29) DHA: 0.15% ARA: 0.40%[6]	Vegetable oil (palm olein, soy, coconut, and high oleic safflower or sunflower oils), DHA[6] (0.32%), ARA[6] (0.64%), linoleic acid (900 mg), linolenic acid (85 mg)
Osmolality mOsm/kg H_2O	230 (powder) 220 (liquid)	200	132
Osmolarity mOsm/L	210 (powder) 200 (liquid)	135	195
Sodium mEq/L (mg/L)	(240)	8.8 (203)	(183)
Potassium mEq/L (mg/L)	(720)	18.5 (724)	(730)
Chloride mEq/L (mg/L)	(420)	12.4 (440)	(440)
Calcium mEq/L (mg/L)	(547)	28.3 (568)	(487)
Phosphorus mEq/L (mg/L)	(307)	21.6 (379)	(271)
Iron mg/L	12	12.2	10
% free water	89	90	90
Manufacturer	Mead Johnson	Abbott	Gerber
Special information	Gluten-free	Kosher, Halal	

[1]Information based on manufacturer's literature as of 2013 and is subject to change

[2]To approximate values for the content of a 24-, 27-, or 30-cal/oz formula (made by dilution of a powder-based formulation), multiply the value desired, found in the above 20-cal/oz formula, by the following factors: 1.2 (24-cal/oz), 1.35 (27-cal/oz), or 1.5 (30-cal/oz).

[3]Previous product Enfamil LactoFree LIPIL discontinued. Recommend using Enfamil Gentlease instead. Enfamil Gentlease contains 1/5 the lactose of regular milk-based formulas and is for infants who have shown transient intolerance to lactose and is marketed for fussiness/gas.

[4]30% lactose of regular milk-based formulas

[5]Prebiotic

[6]DHA (docosahexaenoic acid) and ARA (arachidonic acid) are fatty acids found naturally in breast milk. DHA is provided via *Crypthecodinium cohnii* oil. ARA is provided via *Mortienella alphia* oil.

Casein Hydrolysate Formulas[1,2]

Indication: For infants requiring low molecular weight peptides or amino acids

	Nutramigen[3]	Pregestimil[4]	Pregestimil 24	Similac Expert Care Alimentum
Calories per 100 mL	67	68	81	68
Protein g per 100 mL	1.87	1.89	2.3	1.86
Protein source	Casein hydrolysate, L-cystine, L-tyrosine, L-tryptophan, taurine	Casein hydrolysate (milk), L-cystine, L-tyrosine, L-tryptophan, taurine	Casein hydrolysate (milk), L-cystine, L-tyrosine, L-tryptophan, taurine	Casein hydrolysate, L-cystine, L-tyrosine, L-tryptophan
Carbohydrate g per 100 mL	6.87	6.9	8.3	6.9
Carbohydrate source	Corn syrup solids and modified corn starch	Corn syrup solids and modified corn starch	Corn syrup solids and modified cornstarch	Corn maltodextrin and sugar (70:30)
Fat g per 100 mL	3.54	3.78	4.5	3.75
Fat source (essential fatty acid amounts are per 100 kcal)	Vegetable oils (palm olein, soy, coconut, and high oleic sunflower oils), DHA[4] (17 mg), ARA[4] (34 mg), linoleic acid (940 mg), linolenic acid (80 to 85 mg)[5]	55% MCT, soy, and high oleic vegetable (sunflower/safflower) oils; DHA[4] (17 mg); ARA[4] (34 mg); linoleic acid (940 mg); linolenic acid (95 to 120 mg)[6]	55% MCT, soy, corn, and high oleic vegetable (sunflower/safflower) oils; DHA[4] (17 mg); ARA[4] (34 mg); linoleic acid (940 mg); linolenic acid (120 mg)	High oleic safflower, 33% medium chain triglycerides, and soy oils; DHA[4] (0.15%); ARA[4] (0.4%) (35:33:28:4); DATEM[7]
Osmolality mOsm/kg H_2O	260 to 320[8] (liquid) 300 (powder)	290 (liquid) 320 (powder)	340	370
Osmolarity mOsm/L	230 to 290[9] (liquid) 270 (powder)	260 (liquid) 280 (powder)	300	171
Sodium mEq/L (mg/L)	(313)	(313)	(373)	12.9 (298)
Potassium mEq/L (mg/L)	(734)	(733)	(872)	20.3 (798)
Chloride mEq/L (mg/L)	(574)	(574)	(682)	15.5 (541)
Calcium mEq/L (mg/L)	(627)	(627)	(743)	35.4 (710)
Phosphorus mEq/L (mg/L)	(347)	(347)	(412)	(507)
Iron mg/L	12	12	14.3	12.2
% free water	89	89	86	90
Manufacturer	Mead Johnson	Mead Johnson	Mead Johnson	Abbott
Special information	Lactose-free, gluten-free, galactose-free, sucrose-free	Lactose-free, gluten-free, galactose-free, sucrose-free	Lactose-free, gluten-free, galactose-free, sucrose-free	Ready-to-feed is corn-free
Special uses	Sensitivity to intact proteins found in milk and soy formulas, patients with colic, and patients with galactosemia	Fat malabsorption or sensitivity to intact proteins; may be used in cystic fibrosis, short bowel syndrome, intractable diarrhea, severe protein calorie malnutrition, and patients with galactosemia	Fat malabsorption or sensitivity to intact proteins; may be used in cystic fibrosis, short bowel syndrome, intractable diarrhea, severe protein calorie malnutrition, and patients with galactosemia	Severe food allergies, sensitivity (including colic) to intact proteins, protein maldigestion or fat malabsorption

[1]Information based on manufacturer's literature as of 2013 and is subject to change

[2]To approximate values for the content of a 24-, 27-, or 30-cal/oz formula (made by dilution of a powder-based formulation), multiply the value desired, found in the above 20-cal/oz formula, by the following factors: 1.2 (24-cal/oz), 1.35 (27-cal/oz), or 1.5 (30-cal/oz)

[3]Also available with EnfloraLGG, which is a probiotic to support the strength of the intestinal barrier and to support digestive health

[4]DHA (docosahexaenoic acid) and ARA (arachidonic acid) are fatty acids found naturally in breast milk. DHA is provided via *Crypthecodinium cohnii* oil. ARA is provided via *Mortienella alphia* oil.

[5]Amount of linolenic acid varies depending on product and size: 80 mg in the 8 fl oz concentrate and 2, 8, and 32 fl oz ready-to-feed; 85 mg in the 6 fl oz ready-to-feed and the 13 fl oz concentrate

[6]Amount of linolenic acid varies depending on product and size: 95 mg in the powder; 120 mg in the ready-to-feed

[7]Diacetyl tartaric acid esters of mono-diglycerides is an emulsifier derived from soy, palm, or canola oil.

[8]Osmolality varies depending on product and size: 260 mOsm/kg H_2O for the 13 fl oz concentrates and the 6 fl oz ready-to-feed; 270 mOsm/kg H_2O for the 8 and 32 fl oz ready-to-feed; 320 mOsm/kg H_2O for the 2 fl oz ready-to-feed

[9]Osmolarity varies depending on product and size: 230 mOsm/L for the 6 oz ready-to-feed and the 13 fl oz concentrate; 240 mOsm/L for the 8 and 32 fl oz ready-to-feeds; 290 mOsm/L for the 2 fl oz ready-to-feed

Infant Soy Formulas[1,2]

Indications: Lactase deficiency, milk intolerance, or galactosemia; not recommended for premature infants with birthweight <1.8 kg

	Enfamil ProSobee	Similac Soy Isomil	Gerber Good Start Soy
Calories per 100 mL	68	67.6	67.6
Protein g per 100 mL	1.67	1.66	1.69
Protein source	Soy protein isolate, L-methionine, taurine	Soy protein isolate, L-methionine	Enzymatically hydrolyzed soy protein isolate, L-methionine, taurine
Carbohydrate g per 100 mL	7.1	7	7.51
Carbohydrate source	Corn syrup solids	Corn syrup solids, sugar, fructoolgiosaccharide[3] (78:19:3)	Corn maltodextrin sucrose (79:21)
Fat g per 100 mL	3.5	3.69	3.45
Fat source (essential fatty acid amounts are per 100 kcal)	Vegetable oils (palm olein, soy, coconut, and high oleic sunflower oils), DHA[4] (17 mg), ARA[4] (34 mg), linoleic acid (860 mg), linolenic acid (80 to 85 mg)[5]	High oleic safflower, soy, and coconut oils (41:30:28); DHA[4] (0.15%), ARA[4] (0.4%)	Vegetable oils (palm olein, soy, coconut, and high oleic safflower or sunflower oils), DHA[4] (0.32%), ARA[4] (0.64%), linoleic acid (920 mg), linolenic acid (85 mg), soy lecithin
Osmolality mOsm/kg H_2O	170 to 200[6]	200	180
Osmolarity mOsm/L	153 to 180[7]	155	156
Sodium mEq/L (mg/L)	(240)	12.9 (298)	(271)
Potassium mEq/L (mg/L)	(800)	18.7 (730)	(785)
Chloride mEq/L (mg/L)	(533)	11.8 (419)	(473)
Calcium mEq (mg/L)	(700)	35.4 (710)	(710)
Phosphorus mEq/L (mg/L)	(460)	32.9 (507)	(426)
Iron mg/L	12	12.2	12.1
% free water	89	90	90
Manufacturer	Mead Johnson	Abbott	Gerber
Special information	Gluten-free, lactose-free, galactose-free		Kosher, Halal

[1]Information based on manufacturer's literature as of 2013 and is subject to change

[2]To approximate values for the content of a 24-, 27-, or 30-cal/oz formula (made by dilution of a powder-based formulation), multiply the value desired, found in the above 20-cal/oz formula, by the following factors: 1.2 (24-cal/oz), 1.35 (27-cal/oz), or 1.5 (30-cal/oz).

[3]Prebiotic

[4]DHA (docosahexaenoic acid) and ARA (arachidonic acid) are fatty acids found naturally in breast milk. DHA is provided via *Crypthecodinium cohnii* oil. ARA is provided via *Mortienella alphia* oil.

[5]Amount of linolenic acid varies depending on product and size: 80 mg in the powder, 8 and 13 fl oz concentrates, and 2 and 8 fl oz ready-to-feed; 85 mg in the 6 and 32 fl oz ready-to-feed

[6]Osmolality varies depending on product and size: 170 mOsm/kg H_2O for the 8 and 13 fl oz concentrates and the 6, 8, and 32 fl oz ready-to-feed; 180 mOsm/kg H_2O for the powder; 190 mOsm/kg H_2O for the 2 fl oz ready-to-feed

[7]Osmolarity varies depending on product and size: 153 mOsm/L for the 6 and 32 fl oz ready-to-feed; 155 mOsm/L for the 8 and 13 fl oz concentrates and the 8 fl oz ready-to-feed; 162 mOsm/L for the powder; 180 mOsm/L for the 2 fl oz ready-to-feed

Infant Elemental Enteral Formulas[1]

	EleCare DHA/ARA[2,3] (20 kcal/oz)	Neocate Infant DHA & ARA[2,3] (20 kcal/oz)	Neocate Nutra[4]	PurAmino
Calories/mL	0.68	0.67	4.7/g	0.68
Carbohydrate g per 100 mL	7.2	7.8	67.4 per 100 g	6.9
Carbohydrate source	Corn syrup solids	Corn syrup solids		Corn syrup solids
Protein g per 100 mL	2.09	2.1	8.2 per 100 g	1.87
Protein source	Free amino acids	Free L-amino acids	Free L-amino acids	Free L-amino acids
Fat g per 100 mL	3.24	3	18.8 per 100 g	3.53
Fat source (essential fatty acid amounts are per 100 kcal)	High oleic safflower, MCT, and soy oils (39:33:28)	33% MCT (palm kernel/ coconut), high oleic sunflower, and soy oils; DHA and ARA[2]	4% MCT refined vegetable oils (fractionated coconut, high oleic sunflower, canola, and sunflower oils)	Vegetable oil (palm olein, coconut, soy, and high oleic sunflower oils), DHA and ARA[2], linoleic acid (860 mg)
Osmolality mOsm/kg	350 unflavored	375		350
Osmolarity mOsm/L	187			320
Sodium mEq/L (mg/L)	13.5 (304)	(250)	(38 per 100 g)	(313)
Potassium mEq/L (mg/L)	26.4 (1014)	(1,033)	(<20 per 100 g)	(734)
Chloride mEq/L (mg/L)	11.5 (405)	(517)	(44 per 100 g)	(574)
Calcium mEq/L (mg/L)	39.2 (784)	(831)	(667 per 100 g)	(627)
Phosphorus mg/L	548	624	(340 per 100 g)	347
Iron mg/L	9.9	12.4	5.9 per 100 g	12
% Free water	90			89
Manufacturer	Abbott	Nutricia	Nutricia	Mead Johnson

[1]Information based on manufacturer's literature as of 2013 and is subject to change

[2]DHA (docosahexaenoic acid) and ARA (arachidonic acid) are fatty acids which are found naturally in breast milk. DHA is provided via *Crypthecodinium cohnii* oil. ARA is provided via *Mortienella alphia* oil.

[3]Indicated for 0 to 12 month olds

[4]First and only amino acid-based semi-solid medical food

OLDER INFANT/TODDLER PRODUCTS

Older Infant/Toddler Milk-Based Formulas[1]

	Enfagrow Premium Next Step[2]	Enfagrow Gentlease Next Step[3]	Similac Go & Grow Milk-Based formula	Gerber Graduates Gentle	Gerber Graduates Protect[4]
Calories per 100 mL	67	67	65	68	68
Protein g per 100 mL	1.73	1.73	1.95	1.47	1.47
Protein source	Nonfat milk	Partially hydrolyzed nonfat milk and whey protein concentrate solids (soy)	Nonfat milk, lactose	100% whey protein concentrate (milk)	100% whey protein concentrate (milk)
Carbohydrate g per 100 mL	7	7	6.6	7.73	7.47
Carbohydrate source	Corn syrup solids, lactose, galactoolgiosaccharides[5], polydextrose[5]	Corn syrup solids, galactoolgiosaccharides[5], polydextrose[5]	Lactose, galactoolgiosaccharides[5]	Lactose, maltodextrin (70:30), and galactooligosaccharides[5] (4 g/L)	Lactose and maltodextrin (70:30)
Fat g per 100 mL	3.54	3.5	3.5	3.4	3.4
Fat source	Vegetable oils (palm olein, soy, coconut, and high oleic sunflower oils), DHA[6] (17 mg), ARA[6] (34 mg), linoleic acid (860 mg), linolenic acid (85 mg)	Vegetable oils (palm olein, soy, coconut, and high oleic sunflower oils), DHA[6] (17 mg), ARA[6] (34 mg), linoleic acid (860 mg), linolenic acid (85 mg)	High oleic safflower, soy, and coconut oil; DHA and ARA[6]	Palm olein, soy, coconut, and high oleic safflower or sunflower oils; DHA[6] (0.32%); ARA[6] (0.64%); linoleic acid (900 mg); linolenic acid (85 mg); soy lecithin	Palm olein, soy, coconut, and high oleic safflower or sunflower oils; DHA[6] (0.32%); ARA[6] (0.64%); linoleic acid (900 mg); linolenic acid (85 mg); soy lecithin
Osmolality mOsm/kg H_2O	270	230	300	180	250
Osmolarity mOsm/L	240	210	135	148	148
Sodium mEq/L (mg/L)	(240)	(267)	(195)	(180)	(180)
Potassium mEq/L (mg/L)	(867)	(867)	(975)	(720)	(720)
Chloride mEq/L (mg/L)	(534)	(534)	(520)	(434)	(434)
Calcium mEq/L (mg/L)	(1,301)	(1,301)	(1,268)	(1,267)	(1,267)
Phosphorus mEq/L (mg/L)	(867)	(867)	(845)	(707)	(707)
Iron mg/L	13.3	13.3	13.5	13.3	13.3
% free water	89	89	90	89	89
Manufacturer	Mead Johnson	Mead Johnson	Abbott	Gerber	Gerber

Older Infant/Toddler Milk-Based Formulas[1] *continued*

	Enfagrow Premium Next Step[2]	Enfagrow Gentlease Next Step[3]	Similac Go & Grow Milk-Based formula	Gerber Graduates Gentle	Gerber Graduates Protect[4]
Special information	Gluten-free	Gluten-free	Gluten-free, Kosher, Halal		
Special uses	Infants and toddlers 9 to 36 months	Infants 9 to 36 months	Infants and toddlers 9 to 24 months; specifically formulated to help bridge nutritional gaps that can be associated with transition to table foods.	Infants 9 to 24 months	Infants 9 to 24 months

[1]Information based on manufacturer's literature as of 2013 and is subject to change

[2]Also available as Enfagrow Premium Older Toddler for 12 to 36 months in either vanilla or natural milk flavor. Contains polydextrose + galactooligosaccharides – Natural Defense Dual Prebiotics from Mead Johnson. They support the growth of healthy gut bacteria which help support immune function.

[3]Contains $^{1}/_{2}$ the lactose of other milk-based infant/toddler formulas. Contains polydextrose + galactooligosaccharides – Natural Defense Dual Prebiotics from Mead Johnson. They support the growth of healthy gut bacteria which help support immune function.

[4]Contains Bifidus BL, beneficial cultures like those found in breast milk to help support a healthy immune system

[5]Prebiotic

[6]DHA (docosahexaenoic acid) and ARA (arachidonic acid) are fatty acids found naturally in breast milk. DHA is provided via *Crypthecodinium cohnii* oil. ARA is provided via *Mortienella alphia* oil.

Older Infant/Toddler Soy Formulas[1,2]

Indications: Lactase deficiency, milk intolerance, or galactosemia

	Enfagrow Soy Next Step[3]	Gerber Graduates Soy[4]	Similac Go & Grow Soy-Based formula[4]
Calories per 100 mL	67	68	68
Protein g per 100 mL	2.2	1.87	1.89
Protein source	Soy protein isolate, L-methionine, taurine	Enzymatically hydrolyzed soy protein isolate, L-methionine, taurine	Soy protein isolate, L-methionine, taurine
Carbohydrate g per 100 mL	7.87	7.3	6.96
Carbohydrate source	Corn syrup solids	Corn maltodextrin, sucrose (79:21)	Corn syrup solids, sugar, fructooligosaccharides[5]
Fat g per 100 mL	2.93	3.3	3.7
Fat source	Vegetable oils (palm olein, soy, coconut, and high oleic sunflower oils), DHA[6] (17 mg), ARA[6] (34 mg), linoleic acid (720 mg), linolenic acid (70 mg)	Vegetable oils (palm olein, soy, coconut, and high oleic sunflower oils), DHA[6], ARA[6] (46:26:20:6:2), linoleic acid (920 mg), soy lecithin	High oleic safflower, soy, and coconut oils; DHA[6]; ARA[6]
Osmolality mOsm/kg H_2O	230	180	200
Osmolarity mOsm/L	200	156	160
Sodium mEq/L (mg/L)	(240)	(269)	12.9 (298)
Potassium mEq/L (mg/L)	(800)	(774)	(811)
Chloride mEq/L (mg/L)	(534)	(474)	11.8 (419)
Calcium mEq/L (mg/L)	(1,301)	(1,267)	(1,318)
Phosphorus mEq/L (mg/L)	56 (867)	(707)	(879)
Iron mg/L	13.3	13.3	13.5
% free water	88	89	90
Manufacturer	Mead Johnson	Gerber	Abbott
Special information	Gluten-free, lactose-free, galactose-free	Lactose-free	

[1]Information based on manufacturer's literature as of 2013 and is subject to change

[2] To approximate values for the content of a 24-, 27-, or 30-cal/oz formula (made by dilution of a powder-based formulation), multiply the value desired, found in the above 20-cal/oz formula, by the following factors: 1.2 (24-cal/oz), 1.35 (27-cal/oz), or 1.5 (30-cal/oz)

[3]Indicated for infants and toddlers ≥9 months

[4]Indicated for infants and toddlers 9 to 24 months

[5]Prebiotic

[6]DHA (docosahexaenoic acid) and ARA (arachidonic acid) are fatty acids which are found naturally in breast milk. DHA is provided via *Crypthecodinium cohnii* oil. ARA is provided via *Mortienella alphia* oil.

Soy Formula[1] – Special Indications

Indications: Dietary management of diarrhea in infants >6 months and toddlers

	Similac Expert Care for Diarrhea
Calories per 100 mL	68
Protein g per 100 mL	1.8
Protein source	Soy protein isolate, L-methionine
Carbohydrate g per 100 mL	6.83
Carbohydrate source	Corn syrup solids and sugar (60:40)
Fat g per 100 mL	3.69
Fat source	Soy and coconut oils (60:40)
Osmolality mOsm/kg H_2O	240
Osmolarity mOsm/L	163
Sodium mEq/L (mg/L)	12.9 (298)
Potassium mEq/L (mg/L)	18.7 (730)
Chloride mEq/L (mg/L)	11.8 (419)
Calcium mEq/L (mg/L)	35.4 (710)
Phosphorus mEq/L (mg/L)	(507)
Iron mg/L	12.2
% free water	90
Manufacturer	Abbott
Special information	Lactose-free, gluten-free, Kosher, Halal

[1]Information based on manufacturer's literature as of 2013 and is subject to change

PEDIATRIC PRODUCTS

Pediatric Enteral Formulas[1]

A selection of the commonly used enteral feedings for children 1 to 13 years of age

	PediaSure Enteral Formula[2]	PediaSure Enteral Formula With Fiber[2]	Peptamen Junior[3-6]	Compleat Pediatric[4,6]	Compleat Pediatric Reduced Calorie[4,8]
Calories/oz	30	30	30	30	18
Calories/mL	1	1	1	1	0.6
Carbohydrate g per 100 mL	13.9	14.3	13.6	13.2	7.5
Carbohydrate source	Corn maltodextrin, sugar	Corn maltodextrin, sugar	Maltodextrin, sugar, corn starch, guar gum, sucralose	Corn syrup, green pea and green bean puree, peach and cranberry juice, maltodextrin	Corn syrup, green pea, green bean, and peach puree; tomato, carrot, and cranberry juice
Protein g per 100 mL	3	3	3	3.76	3
Protein source	Milk protein concentrate	Milk protein concentrate	Enzymatically hydrolyzed whey protein (milk)	Chicken, sodium caseinate, and pea puree	Chicken, sodium caeinate, and pea puree
Fat g per 100 mL	3.8	3.8	3.8	3.9	2
Fat source	High oleic safflower, soy, and MCT oils; soy lecithin	High oleic safflower, soy, and MCT oils; soy lecithin	MCT (coconut and/or palm kernel), soybean, and canola oils; lecithin	Canola and MCT (coconut and/or palm kernel) oils; hydroxylated soy lecithin	Canola and MCT (coconut and/or palm kernel) oils, hydroxylated soy lecithin
Osmolality mOsm/kg	335 vanilla	350 vanilla	260 unflavored 380 vanilla/chocolate 400 strawberry	380	300
Osmolarity mOsm/L	278	278	255		
Sodium mEq/L (mg/L)	17 (380)	17 (380)	20 (460)	33 (760)	33.5 (770)
Potassium mEq/L (mg/L)	33 (1,308)	34 (1,310)	33.8 (1,320)	42 (1,640)	45.1 (1,760)
Chloride mEq/L (mg/L)	32 (1,139)	32 (1,140)	30.4 (1,080)	15.7 (560)	15.7 (560)
Calcium mEq/L (mg/L)	53 (1,055)	53 (1,055)	(1,120)	(1,440)	(1,440)
Phosphorus mEq/L (mg/L)	(844)	(844)	(840)	(1,000)	(1,050)
Iron (mg/L)	11	11	14	14	13
% Free water	84	85	85	82	87
Fiber (g/unit dose)		Dietary: 0.8 scFOS: 2		Dietary: 1.7[9]	Dietary: 1.7[9]
Manufacturer	Abbott	Abbott	Nestle	Nestle	Nestle

Pediatric Enteral Formulas[1] *continued*

	PediaSure Enteral Formula[2]	PediaSure Enteral Formula With Fiber[2]	Peptamen Junior[3-6]	Compleat Pediatric[4,6]	Compleat Pediatric Reduced Calorie[4,8]
Indication			For patients with impaired GI function, short bowel syndrome, cerebral palsy, cystic fibrosis, Crohn disease, malabsorption, chronic diarrhea, delayed gastric emptying, growth failure, transitioning from parenteral nutrition		For patients with decreased caloric needs
Special information	Gluten-free, lactose-free, Kosher, Halal (not for galactosemia)		Gluten-free, lactose-free (not Kosher)	Blenderized tube feeding formula containing real food; equivalent to 2 servings of fruits/vegetables for patients 1 to 4 years of age; equivalent to 1.6 servings of fruits/vegetables for patients >4 years of age; lactose-free, gluten-free (not for galactosemia)	Equivalent to 3 servings of fruits/vegetables for patients 1 to 4 years of age; equivalent to 2 servings of fruits/vegetables for patients >4 years of age

[1]Information based on manufacturer's literature as of 2013 and is subject to change

[2]Prebiotic Nutraflora scFOS (short chain fructooligosaccaharides) provides fuel for beneficial bacteria in the digestive tract that help to support a healthy immune system.

[3]Also available with Prebio (3.6 g/L) prebiotic formulation

[4]Contains CalciLock blend of essential nutrients to help support healthy bone development

[5]Closed system with SpikeRight PLUS port, the first available proximal-end enteral connector system designed to be incompatible with IV equipment

[6]Meets or exceed 100% DRIs for protein and 25 key vitamins and minerals in 1,000 mL for patients 1 to 8 years of age and in 1,500 mL for patients 9 to 13 years of age

[7]1.7 oz dry packet mixed with 220 mL of water produces 250 mL of formula.

[8]Meets or exceed 100% DRIs for protein and 25 key vitamins and minerals in 1,000 mL for patients 1 to 8 years of age and in 1,200 mL for patients 9 to 13 years of age

[9]Nutrisource fiber is a soluble fiber (6.8 g/L), PHGG

Pediatric Enteral Formulas[1]

A selection of the commonly used enteral feedings for children 1 to 13 years of age

	Peptamen Junior with Fiber[2-4]	Nutren Junior[2,3,5]	Nutren Junior with Fiber[2-5]	Pediasure Peptide 1.0 Cal[3,6]
Calories/oz	30	30	30	30
Calories/mL	1	1	1	1
Carbohydrate g per 100 mL	13.6	11	11	13.4
Carbohydrate source	Maltodextrin, sugar, corn starch, pea fiber, fructooligosaccharide[6,8], inulin	Maltodextrin, sugar	Maltodextrin, sugar, pea fiber, fructooligosaccharide[6], inulin	Corn maltodextrin
Protein g per 100 mL	3	3	3	3
Protein source	Enzymatically hydrolyzed whey protein (milk)	Milk protein concentrate, 50% whey protein concentrate	Milk protein concentrate, 50% whey protein concentrate	Whey protein hydrolysate, hydrolyzed sodium caseinate
Fat g per 100 mL	3.8	5	5	4.05
Fat source	MCT (coconut and/or palm kernel), soybean, and canola oils; soy lecithin	Soybean, canola, and MCT (coconut and/or palm kernel) oils; soy lecithin	Soybean, canola, and MCT (coconut and/or palm kernel) oils; soy lecithin	Structured lipid (interesterified canola and MCTs), MCTs, canola oils, soy lecithin
Osmolality mOsm/kg	390 vanilla	350 vanilla	350 vanilla	390 vanilla, strawberry 250 unflavored
Osmolarity mOsm/L	255	256	256	
Sodium mEq/L (mg/L)	20 (460)	20 (460)	20 (460)	31.2 (717)
Potassium mEq/L (mg/L)	33.8 (1,320)	33.8 (1,320)	33.8 (1,320)	34.6 (1,350)
Chloride mEq/L (mg/L)	30.4 (1,080)	30.4 (1,080)	30.4 (1,080)	28.5 (1,010)
Calcium mEq/L (mg/L)	(1,120)	(1,200)	(1,200)	(1,060)
Phosphorus mEq/L (mg/L)	(840)	(840)	(840)	(844)
Iron (mg/L)	14	14	14	14
% Free water	84	85	85	84.5
Fiber (g/unit dose)	Dietary 1.85 Soluble: 0.9 Insoluble: 0.95		Dietary 1.5 Soluble: 0.55 Insoluble: 0.95	Dietary: 0.7 scFOS: 0.7
Manufacturer	Nestle	Nestle	Nestle	Abbott
Special information	(not Kosher)	Gluten-free, lactose-free, Kosher	Gluten-free, lactose-free, Kosher	

[1]Information based on manufacturer's literature as of 2013 and is subject to change

[2]Contains CalciLock blend of essential nutrients to help support healthy bone development

[3]Meets or exceed 100% DRIs for protein and 25 key vitamins and minerals in 1,000 mL for patients 1 to 8 years of age and in 1,500 mL for patients 9 to 13 years of age

[4]Contains Prebio, a soluble fiber (3.6 g/L) to help promote the growth of beneficial bacteria and 3.8 g/L insoluble fiber to help support normal bowel function

[5]Closed system with SpikeRight PLUS port, the first available proximal-end enteral connector system designed to be incompatible with IV equipment

[6]Prebiotic Nutraflora scFOS (short chain fructooligosaccaharides) provides fuel for beneficial bacteria in the digestive tract that help to support a healthy immune system.

[7]Meets or exceed 100% DRIs for protein and 25 key vitamins and minerals in 667 mL (1,000 kcal) for patients 1 to 8 years of age and in 1,000 mL (1,500 kcal) for patients 9 to 13 years of age

[8]Prebiotic

[9]Lipid blend provides 720 mg/L of EPA and DHA to help modulate pro-inflammatory mediators

Pediatric Elemental Enteral Formulas[1]

	EleCare Jr (30 kcal/oz)	Neocate Junior[2,3] (30 kcal/oz)	Vivonex Pediatric[4-7]
Calories/mL	1.01	1	0.8
Carbohydrate g per 100 mL	10.7	10.4	13
Carbohydrate source	Corn syrup solids	Corn syrup solids	Maltodextrin, modified cornstarch
Protein g per 100 mL	3.1	3.3	2.4
Protein source	Free amino acids	Free L-amino acids	100% free L-amino acids
Fat g per 100 mL	4.91	5	2.3
Fat source (essential fatty acid amounts are per 100 kcal)	High oleic safflower, MCT, and soy oils (39:33:28)	35% MCT, refined vegetable oils (palm kernel and/or coconut, canola, and high oleic safflower oils)	MCT (coconut and/or palm kernel) and soybean oils
Osmolality mOm/kg	590 unflavored/vanilla	550 unflavored 630 tropical 650 chocolate/vanilla[3]	360
Osmolarity mOsm/L	280		
Sodium mEq/L (mg/L)	20 (459)	(500)	17 (400)
Potassium mEq/L (mg/L)	39 (1,526)	(1,370)	31 (1,200)
Chloride mEq/L (mg/L)	17 (608)	(762)	28 (1,000)
Calcium mEq/L (mg/L)	58.7 (1,174)	(1,180)	(1,120)
Phosphorus mg/L	822	799	(840)
Iron mg/L	14.9	16	10
% free water	84		89
Manufacturer	Abbott	Nutricia	Nestle

[1]Information based on manufacturer's literature as of 2013 and is subject to change

[2]Indicated for 1- to 10-year-olds

[3]Also available in product containing prebiotics

[4]For patients with severe impaired GI function, transitioning from parenteral nutrition, severe short bowel syndrome, malabsorption syndrome, Crohn disease, intestinal failure, status post-GI trauma/surgery, or burns; not for children <1 year of age; gluten-free, lactose-free, Kosher

[5]Contains CalciLock blend of essential nutrients to help support healthy bone development

[6]Meets or exceeds 100% DRIs for protein and 25 key vitamins and minerals in 1,000 mL for patients 1 to 8 years of age and in 1,500 mL for patients 9 to 13 years of age

[7]1.7 oz dry packet mixed with 220 mL of water produces 250 mL of formula

Pediatric High Caloric Density Enteral Formulas[1]

	Pediasure 1.5 Cal[2]	Pediasure 1.5 Cal With Fiber[2]	Peptamen Junior 1.5[2,4]	Pediasure Peptide 1.5 Cal[3,7]
Calories/mL	1.5	1.5	1.5	1.5
Carbohydrate g per 100 mL	16	16.5	18	20.1
Carbohydrate source	Corn maltodextrin	Corn maltodextrin	Maltodextrin, cornstarch, fructooligosaccharide[3,5], inulin, guar gum	Corn maltodextrin
Protein g per 100 mL	5.9	5.9	4.5	4.51
Protein source	Milk protein concentrate	Milk protein concentrate	Enzymatically, hydrolyzed whey protein (milk)	Whey protein hydrolysate, hydrolyzed sodium caseinate
Fat g per 100 mL	6.8	6.8	6.8	6
Fat source	High oleic safflower, soy, and MCT oils; soy lecithin; DHA (from *cohnii* oil)	High oleic safflower, soy, and MCT oils; soy lecithin; DHA (from *cohnii* oil)	60% MCT (coconut and/or palm kernel), soybean, and canola oils; soy lecithin[6]	Structured lipid (interesterified canola and MCTs), MCTs, canola oils, soy lecithin
Osmolality mOsm/kg	370 vanilla	390 vanilla	450 unflavored	450 vanilla
Osmolarity mOsm/L	278	278	385	
Sodium mEq/L (mg/L)	16.5 (380)	16.5 (380)	30 (692)	46.7 (1,075)
Potassium mEq/L (mg/L)	42 (1,650)	42 (1,650)	50.8 (1,980)	51.9 (2,025)
Chloride mEq/L (mg/L)	32 (1,140)	32 (1,140)	45.6 (1,620)	42.8 (1,520)
Calcium mEq/L (mg/L)	74 (1,480)	74 (1,480)	(1,650)	(1,580)
Phosphorus mEq/L (mg/L)	(1,055)	(1,055)	(1,352)	(1,265)
Iron (mg/L)	11	11	21	21
% free water	78.1	78.1	77	76.8
Fiber (g/unit dose)		Dietary: 3 scFOS: 1.5[3]	Soluble: 1.34	Dietary: 1.1 scFOS: 1.1[3]
Manufacturer	Abbott	Abbott	Nestle	Abbott
Special uses/ information	For patients 1 to 13 years of age Gluten-free, lactose-free, Kosher, Halal	For patients 1 to 13 years of age Gluten-free, lactose-free, Kosher, Halal	For patients who need volume/fluid restriction with impaired GI function, short bowel syndrome, cerebral palsy, cystic fibrosis, Crohn disease, malabsorption, chronic diarrhea, growth failure, transitioning from parenteral nutrition, critical illness/trauma, transplant	

[1]Information based on manufacturer's literature as of 2013 and is subject to change

[2]Meets or exceeds 100% DRIs for protein and 25 key vitamins and minerals in 1,000 mL for patients 1 to 8 years of age and in 1,500 mL for patients 9 to 13 years of age

[3]Prebiotic Nutraflora scFOS (short chain fructooligosacchardies) provides fuel for beneficial bacteria in the digestive tract that helps to supprot a healthy immune system.

[4]Contains CalciLock blend of essential nutrients to help support healthy bone development

[5]Prebiotic

[6]Lipid blend provides 720 mg/L of EPA and DHA to help modulate pro-inflammatory mediators

[7][illegible] exceeds 100% DRIs for protein and 25 key vitamins and minerals in 667 mL (1,000 kcal) for patients 1 to 8 years of age and in 1,000 mL (1,500 kcal) for patients 9 to 13 years of age

Pediatric Nutritionally Complete Drinks[1]

A selection of the commonly used supplemental drinks

	Boost Kid Essentials[2,3]	Boost Kid Essentials 1.5[2,4]	Boost Kid Essentials 1.5 with Fiber[2,4]	Resource Breeze	Carnation Breakfast Essentials (ready-to-drink)	Carnation Breakfast Essentials[5] (powder)	PediaSure	PediaSure with Fiber	PediaSure SideKicks	PediaSure Sidekicks Clear	EO28 Splash
Calories/oz	30	45	45	30	24	24	30	30	18.9	17.6	30
Calories/mL	1	1.5	1.5	1.06	0.8	0.8	1	1	0.63	0.6	1
Carbohydrate g per 100 mL	13.4	16.4	16.4	22.8	10.3	3.9	13.9	13.9	8.9	12	14.6
Carbohydrate source	Maltodextrin, sugar	Maltodextrin, sugar	Maltodextrin, sugar	Sugar, corn syrup, maltodextrin	Sugar, maltodextrin, sucralose	Sugar, maltodextrin, lactose	Sucrose and corn maltodextrin	Sucrose and corn maltodextrin	Sugar	Corn maltodextrin, sugar	Maltodextrin and sugar
Protein g per 100 mL	2.8	4.2	4.2	3.8	3.5	13	3	3	3	3	2.5
Protein source	Sodium and calcium caseinates, whey protein concentrate	Sodium and calcium caseinates, whey protein concentrate	Sodium and calcium caseinates, whey protein concentrate	Whey protein isolate (milk)	Calcium caseinate	Nonfat milk	Milk protein concentrate, whey protein concentrate, soy protein isolate	Milk protein concentrate and soy protein isolate	Milk protein concentrate, soy protein isolate, whey protein concentrate	Whey protein isolate	Free L-amino acids
Fat g per 100 mL	3.8	7.6	7.6		1.5	0.5 g/serving	3.8	3.8	2.1		3.5
Fat source	High oleic sunflower, soybean, MCT (coconut and/or palm kernel), and soy oils; soy lecithin	MCT, soy, and sunflower oils, soy lecithin	Soybean, high oleic sunflower, MCT (coconut and/or palm kernel), soy, and sunflower oils; soy lecithin		Corn oil	Trace butterfat	High oleic safflower oil, canola oil	High oleic safflower oil, canola oil	Soy oil, soy lecithin		Fractionated coconut, canola, and high oleic sunflower oils
Osmolality mOsm/kg	550 vanilla 600 chocolate 570 strawberry	390 vanilla	405 vanilla	750 orange	480 classic French vanilla 490 chocolate splash		480 vanilla, strawberry, banana, berry 540 chocolate	480 vanilla	420 vanilla	325 tropical fruit, wild berry	820 grape, tropical fruit, and orange-pineapple
Osmolarity mOsm/L							278	278	278	278	
Sodium mEq/L (mg/L)	23.7 (546)	30.1 (693)	30.1 (693)	14.8 (338)	23.6 (545)	8.3/serving (190/serving)	17 (380)	17 (380)	17 (380)	(175)	(200)
Potassium mEq/L (mg/L)	29 (1,134)	33.3 (1,302)	33.3 (1,302)	0.4 (21.1)	25.8 (1,000)	18 (700)	33 (1,308)	33 (1,308)	41.5 (1,646)	(150)	(930)
Chloride mEq/L (mg/L)	15.4 (546)	21 (748)	21 (748)				32 (1,139)	32 (1,139)	32 (1,139)		(350)
Calcium mEq/L (mg/L)	(1,260)	(1,470)	(1,470)		(1,515)	(500)	53 (1,055)	53 (1,055)	53 (1,055)	(175)	(620)

Pediatric Nutritionally Complete Drinks[1] *continued*

	Boost Kid Essentials[2,3]	Boost Kid Essentials 1.5[2,4]	Boost Kid Essentials 1.5 with Fiber[2,4]	Resource Breeze	Carnation Breakfast Essentials (ready-to-drink)	Carnation Breakfast Essentials[5] (powder)	PediaSure	PediaSure with Fiber	PediaSure SideKicks	PediaSure Sidekicks Clear	EO28 Splash
Phosphorus mEq/L (mg/L)	(882)	(1,260)	(1,260)	(633)	(1,515)	(500)	(844)	(844)	(844)	(750)	(620)
Iron (mg/L)	13.9	13.9	13.9	11.4	13.6		11	11	11	9	7.7
% Free water	84	72	71	83	86		84	84	89.5	90	80
Fiber (g/unit dose)			Dietary: 2.1 Insoluble: 0.5			Dietary: <1/ serving	Dietary: 1 scFOS: 1[6]	Dietary: 3 scFOS: 1.8[6]	Dietary: 3 scFOS: 2.4[6]		
Indication	1 to 13 years old	1 to 13 years old	1 to 13 years old			Reduced calorie	1 to 13 years old	1 to 13 years old	All the nutrition of Pediasure with less calories and less fat than Pediasure	For supplemental use in 1- to 3-year-olds only; no more than 1 serving per day	>1 year old; nutritionally complete, ready-to-drink amino acid-based
Manufacturer	Nestle	Nestle	Nestle	Nestle	Nestle	Nestle	Abbott	Abbott	Abbott	Abbott	Nutricia
Special information	Gluten-free, lactose-free, Kosher	Gluten-free, lactose-free, Kosher		Fruit-flavored, clear liquid; gluten-free, lactose-free, Kosher, Halal (all flavors)	Available in sugar-free form; Kosher, cholesterol-restricted	Available in sugar-free form; Kosher, cholesterol-restricted	Gluten-free, lactose-free, Kosher, contains DHA (from tuna oil) of 32 mg per 8 fl oz			Suitable for clear liquid diet and fat-restricted diet	

[1]Information based on manufacturer's literature as of 2013 and is subject to change

[2]Contains CalciLock blend of essential nutrients to help support healthy bone development

[3]Meets or exceed 100% DRIs for protein and 25 key vitamins and minerals in 1,000 mL for patients 1 to 8 years of age and in 1,500 mL for patients 9 to 13 years of age

[4]Meets or exceed 100% DRIs for protein and 25 key vitamins and minerals in 750 mL for patients 1 to 8 years of age and in 1,000 mL for patients 9 to 13 years of age

[5]One envelope (6 level tablespoons) added to 8 oz of fat-free milk; mix with soy or lactose-reduced milk for decreased lactose content

[6]Prebiotic Nutraflora scFOS (short chain fructooligosaccaharides) provides fuel for beneficial bacteria in the digestive tract that help to support a healthy immune system.

ADOLESCENT/ADULT PRODUCTS

Adolescent and Adult Enteral Formulas[1]

	Osmolite 1 Cal	Jevity	Nutren 1[2]	Ensure	Boost[3]
Calories/mL	1.06	1.06	1	1.05	1
Carbohydrate g per 100 mL	14.4	15.5	12.8	16.9	17.1
Carbohydrate source	Corn maltodextrin, corn syrup solids	Corn maltodextrin, corn syrup solids, soy fiber	Maltodextrin, sugar	Sugar, corn maltodextrin	Corn syrup solids, sugar
Protein g per 100 mL	4.43	4.43	4	3.8	4.2
Protein source	Sodium and calcium caseinate, soy protein isolate	Sodium and calcium caseinates, soy protein isolate	Calcium-potassium caseinate (milk)	Milk protein concentrate and soy protein concentrate	Milk protein concentrate, soy protein isolate
Fat g per 100 mL	3.47	3.47	3.8	2.5	1.7
Fat source	Canola, corn, and MCT oils, and soy lecithin	Canola, corn, and MCT oils, and soy lecithin	Canola, MCT (coconut and/or palm kernel), and corn oils; soy lecithin	Soy, canola, and corn oils, soy lecithin	Vegetable oils (canola, high oleic sunflower, and corn); soy lecithin
Osmolality mOsm/kg H_2O	300 unflavored	300 unflavored	370 vanilla	620 strawberry, vanilla, butter pecan 640 creamy milk chocolate, rich dark chocolate	625 vanilla, chocolate, or strawberry
Osmolarity mOsm/L	374	370	370	329	
Sodium mEq/L (mg/L)	40.4 (930)	40.4 (930)	38 (880)	36.7 (844)	27.1 (625)
Potassium mEq/L (mg/L)	40.2 (1,570)	40.2 (1,570)	31.7 (1,240)	40 (1,561)	49.2 (1,917)
Chloride mEq/L (mg/L)	40.7 (1,440)	37 (1,310)	33.8 (1,200)	33.3 (1,181)	31.7 (1,133)
Calcium mEq/L (mg/L)	(760)	(910)	(668)	(1,266)	(1,250)
Phosphorus mEq/L (mg/L)	(760)	(760)	(668)	(1,055)	(1,250)
Iron (mg/L)	14	14	12	19	18.8
% free water	84	84	85	83	85
Fiber (g/unit dose)		Dietary: 1.4 per 100 mL	Also available with fiber[4]		
Manufacturer	Abbott	Abbott	Nestle	Abbott	Nestle
Special uses	Low residue, isotonic formula	Isotonic formula with fiber	Normal protein/normal calorie requirements	Supplement; for interim sole-source feeding	Nutritionally complete drink
Special information			Gluten-free, lactose-free, Kosher		Gluten-free, lactose-free, Kosher (not for galactosemia)

[1]Information based on manufacturer's literature as of 2013 and is subject to change

[2]Also available with fiber with Prebio (prebiotics)

[3]Contains CalciLock blend of essential nutrients to help support healthy bone development

[4]Prebio is a fiber blend to help promote healthy microbiota and contains 3.5 g of dietary fiber with 1.3 g of soluble fiber and 2.2 g of insoluble fiber.

Adolescent and Adult Elemental Enteral Formulas With Modified Protein[1]

	Peptamen	Peptamen 1.5[2]	Tolerex[3] (powder)	Vivonex Plus[4] (powder)	Vivonex RFT[2]	Vivonex T.E.N.[5] (powder)	Vital 1.0 Cal[6]	Vital 1.5 Cal[6]
Calories/mL	1	1.5	1	1	1	1	1	1.5
Carbohydrate g per 100 mL	12.8	18.4	22.6	18.8	17.6	20.4	13	18.7
Carbohydrate source	Maltodextrin, cornstarch, guar gum	Maltodextrin, cornstarch, guar gum	Maltodextrin, modified corn starch	Maltodextrin (corn), modified cornstarch	Maltodextrin, modified corn starch	Maltodextrin (corn), modified cornstarch	Maltodextrin, sugar, scFOS[5], sucralose	Maltodextrin, sugar, scFOS[5], sucralose
Protein g per 100 mL	4	6.8	2.1	4.5	5	3.8	4	6.75
Protein source	Enzymatically hydrolyzed whey (milk)	Enzymatically hydrolyzed whey (milk)	Free L-amino acids	Free L-amino acids (30% from branched chain amino acids)	Free L-amino acids (29% from branched chain amino acids)	Free L-amino acids	Whey protein hydrolysate, partially hydrolyzed sodium caseinate	Whey protein hydrolysate, partially hydrolyzed sodium caseinate
Fat g per 100 mL	3.9	5.6	0.2	0.66	1.2	0.26	3.8	5.71
Fat source	70% MCT (coconut and/or palm kernel) and soybean oils; soy lecithin	70% MCT (coconut and/or palm kernel) and soybean oils; soy lecithin	Safflower oil	Soybean oil	Soybean oil	Safflower oil	Structured lipid (interesterified canola oil and MCT), canola oil, and MCT	Structured lipid (interesterified canola oil and MCT), canola oil, and MCT
Osmolality mOsm/kg	270 unflavored 380 vanilla	550 unflavored, vanilla	550 unflavored	650	630 unflavored	630 unflavored	390 vanilla	610 vanilla
Osmolarity mOsm/L							340	544
Sodium mEq/L (mg/L)	24.3 (560)	44.3 (1,020)	22 (500)	26 (605)	30.4 (700)	26 (610)	(1,055)	(1,500)
Potassium mEq/L (mg/L)	38.5 (1,500)	48 (1,860)	30 (1,167)	25 (969)	31 (1,200)	23 (928)	(1,400)	(2,000)
Chloride mEq/L (mg/L)	28.2 (1,000)	49 (1,740)	26 (935)	26 (933)	23 (800)	24 (841)	(1,055)	(1,500)
Calcium mEq/L (mg/L)	(800)	(1,000)	(550)	(550)	(668)	(500)	(705)	(1,000)
Phosphorus mg/L	(700)	(1,000)	(551)	(550)	(668)	(500)	(705)	(1,000)
Fiber g/unit dose							Dietary: 1 scFOS: 1[6]	Dietary: 1 scFOS: 1[6]
Iron mg/L	18	27	10	10	12	9	13	18
% Free water	85	77	84	83	85	83	84.2	76.4
Manufacturer	Nestle	Nestle	Nestle	Nestle	Nestle	Nestle	Abbott	Abbott

Adolescent and Adult Elemental Enteral Formulas With Modified Protein[1] *continued*

	Peptamen	Peptamen 1.5[2]	Tolerex[3] (powder)	Vivonex Plus[4] (powder)	Vivonex RFT[2]	Vivonex T.E.N.[5] (powder)	Vital 1.0 Cal[6]	Vital 1.5 Cal[6]
Indication	For patients with impaired GI function related to: Malabsorption, pancreatitis, short bowel syndrome, chronic diarrhea, cystic fibrosis, delayed gastric emptying, cerebral palsy, Crohn disease/IBD, malabsorption related to cancer treatment, malnutrition, and Celiac disease with malabsorption; also for early enteral feeding and transition from or dual feeding with parenteral nutrition	For patients with impaired GI function related to: Malabsorption, pancreatitis, short bowel syndrome, chronic diarrhea, cystic fibrosis, delayed gastric emptying, cerebral palsy, Crohn disease/IBD, malabsorption related to cancer treatment; also for early enteral feeding, transition from parenteral nutrition, shortened feeding schedules, elevated protein requirements, and fluid/volume restrictions	For patients with severely impaired GI function related to: Severe protein and fat malabsorption and specialized nutrient needs	Provides nutrition to patients with severely impaired GI function, severe protein and fat malabsorption, extensive bowel resection, malabsorption syndrome, select trauma/surgery, intestinal failure, chylothorax, and pancreatitis; also for parenteral nutrition alternative, dual feeding with parenteral nutrition, transitional feeding, early postoperative feeding, and trophic feeding	Provides nutrition to patients with severely impaired GI function, severe protein and fat malabsorption, extensive bowel resection, malabsorption syndrome, select trauma/surgery, intestinal failure, chylothorax, and pancreatitis; also for parenteral nutrition alternative, dual feeding with parenteral nutrition, transitional feeding, early postoperative feeding, and trophic feeding	Provides nutrition to patients with severely impaired GI function, severe protein and fat malabsorption, extensive bowel resection, malabsorption syndrome, select trauma/surgery, intestinal failure, chylothorax, and pancreatitis; also for parenteral nutrition alternative, dual feeding with parenteral nutrition, transitional feeding, early postoperative feeding, and trophic feeding	Peptide-based elemental formula for malabsorption, maldigestion, or impaired GI function or for symptoms of GI intolerance	Peptide-based elemental formula for malabsorption, maldigestion, or impaired GI function or for symptoms of GI intolerance
Special information	Gluten-free, lactose-free, low residue (not for galactosemia)	Gluten-free, lactose-free, low residue (not for galactosemia)	100% free amino acids with only 2% of calories from fat Gluten-free, lactose-free, low residue, Kosher (not for galactosemia)	Gluten-free, lactose-free, low residue, Kosher	Gluten-free, lactose-free, low residue, Kosher (not for galactosemia)	Gluten-free, lactose-free, low-residue, Kosher	Gluten-free, lactose-free, low-residue	Gluten-free, lactose-free, low-residue

[1]Information based on manufacturer's literature as of 2013 and is subject to change

[2]Closed system with SpikeRight PLUS port, the first available proximal-end enteral connector system designed to be incompatible with IV equipment

[3]2.82 oz dry packet mixed with 255 mL of water produces 300 mL of formula

[4]2.8 oz dry packet mixed with 250 mL of water produces 300 mL of formula; not for children 0 to 3 years of age

[5]2.84 oz dry packet mixed with 250 mL of water produces 300 mL of formula

[6]Prebiotic Nutraflora scFOS (short chain fructooligosaccharides) provide fuel for beneficial bacteria in the digestive tract that help to support a healthy immune system

Adolescent and Adult High Caloric Density Enteral Formulas[1]

	Ensure Plus	Osmolite 1.2 Cal	Osmolite 1.5 Cal	Nutren 1.5[2]	Nutren 2[2]	Jevity 1.2 Cal	Jevity 1.5 Cal	Isosource 1.5 Cal[2]	Hi-Cal
Calories/mL	1.5	1.2	1.5	1.5	2	1.2	1.5	1.5	2
Carbohydrate g per 100 mL	21.5	15.8	20.4	16.8	19.6	16.9	21.6	16.8	21.6
Carbohydrate source	Corn, maltodextrin, sugar, scFOS[3]	Corn, maltodextrin	Corn, maltodextrin	Maltodextrin	Corn syrup solids, maltodextrin, sugar	Corn, maltodextrin, corn syrup solids, fructooligosaccharides, soy fiber, and oat fiber	Corn, maltodextrin, corn syrup solids, fructooligosaccharides, soy fiber, and oat fiber	Maltodextrin, sugar, soy fiber, and partially hydrolyzed guar gum	Corn syrup solids, sugar, corn maltodextrin
Protein g per 100 mL	5.5	5.55	6.27	6	8	5.6	6.4	6.8	8.4
Protein source	Milk protein, caseinate, soy protein concentrate, whey protein concentrate	Sodium and calcium caseinates	Sodium and calcium caseinates, soy protein isolate	Calcium-potassium caseinate (milk)	Calcium-potassium caseinate (milk)	Sodium and calcium caseinates, soy protein isolate	Sodium and calcium caseinates, soy protein isolate	Sodium and calcium caseinates (milk)	Sodium and calcium caseinates
Fat g per 100 mL	4.6	3.93	4.91	6.8	10.4	3.9	5	6.5	8.9
Fat source	Canola, and corn oils, soy lecithin	High oleic safflower, canola, and MCT oils, soy lecithin	High oleic safflower, canola, and MCT oils; soy lecithin	50% MCT (coconut and/or palm kernel), canola, and corn oils; soy lecithin	75% MCT (coconut and/or palm kernel), canola, and corn oils; soy lecithin	Canola, corn, and MCT oils; soy lecithin	Canola, corn, and MCT oils, soy lecithin	Canola, MCT (coconut and/or palm kernel), and soy oils; hydroxylated soy lecithin	Corn oil and soy lecithin
Osmolality mOsm/kg	680 vanilla, strawberry, butter pecan, milk chocolate	360 unflavored	525 unflavored	430 unflavored 510 vanilla	745 vanilla	450 unflavored	525 unflavored	650 unflavored 585 vanilla	705 vanilla
Osmolarity mOsm/L		465	512			465	518		
Sodium mEq/L (mg/L)	40.5 (928)	58.3 (1,340)	60.9 (1,400)	50.4 (1,160)	56.5 (1,300)	58.7 (1,350)	60.9 (1,400)	56.5 (1,300)	63 (1,456)
Potassium mEq/L (mg/L)	45 (1,772)	46.4 (1,810)	46 (1,800)	48.2 (1,880)	49.2 (1,920)	47.3 (1,850)	55.1 (2,150)	55 (2,140)	62 (2,447)
Chloride mEq/L (mg/L)	32 (1,139)	43.5 (1,540)	48 (1,700)	49 (1,740)	52.8 (1,876)	42.4 (1,500)	38.4 (1,360)	45 (1,610)	40.5 (1,435)
Calcium mEq/L (mg/L)	(1,266)	(1,200)	(1,000)	(1,000)	(1,340)	(1,200)	(1,200)	(1,072)	(844)
Phosphorus mEq/L (mg/L)	(1,266)	(1,200)	(1,000)	(1,000)	(1,340)	(1,200)	(1,200)	(1,020)	(844)
Iron (mg/L)	19	18	18	18	24	18	18	19	15.2
% free water	75.9	82	76.2	76	70	80.7	76	78	70

Adolescent and Adult High Caloric Density Enteral Formulas[1] *continued*

	Ensure Plus	Osmolite 1.2 Cal	Osmolite 1.5 Cal	Nutren 1.5[2]	Nutren 2[2]	Jevity 1.2 Cal	Jevity 1.5 Cal	Isosource 1.5 Cal[2]	Hi-Cal
Fiber (g/unit dose)	Dietary: 3 scFOS: 3[3]					Dietary: 1.8 scFOS: 8[3]	Dietary: 2.2 scFOS: 1[3]	Dietary: 2/can[4] Soluble: 1.1/can Insoluble: 0.9/can	
Manufacturer	Abbott	Abbott	Abbott	Nestle	Nestle	Abbott	Abbott	Nestle	Abbott
Special uses/ information	For those with fluid restrictions or require volume-limited feedings; supplement; for interim sole-source feeding	Increased calories, increased protein, decreased residue	Increased calories, increased protein, decreased residue	Increased calories Gluten-free, lactose-free, Kosher	Calorically dense Gluten-free, lactose-free, Kosher	Increased protein with fiber Gluten-free, lactose-free, Kosher, Halal	Increased protein with fiber Gluten-free, lactose-free, Kosher, Halal	High calorie, high nitrogen formula with fiber Gluten-free, lactose-free, Kosher	Increased calories fortified with vitamins and minerals

[1]Information based on manufacturer's literature as of 2013 and is subject to change

[2]Closed system with SpikeRight PLUS port, the first available proximal-end enteral connector system designed to be incompatible with IV equipment

[3]Prebiotic Nutraflora scFOS (short chain fructooligosaccaharides) provides fuel for beneficial bacteria in the digestive tract that helps to support a healthy immune system.

[4]NUTRISOURCE FIBER (soy)

SPECIALTY PRODUCTS

Casein Hydrolysate Formulas[1,2]

Indication: For infants predisposed to or being treated for hypocalcemia due to hyperphosphatemia whose renal or cardiovascular functions would benefit from lowered mineral concentrations

	Similac PM 60/40
Calories per 100 mL	68
Protein g per 100 mL	1.5
Protein source	Whey protein caseinate, sodium caseinate
Carbohydrate g per 100 mL	6.9
Carbohydrate source	Lactose
Fat g per 100 mL	3.79
Fat source	High oleic safflower, soy, coconut oils (41:30:29)
Osmolality mOsm/kg H_2O	280
Osmolarity mOsm/L	124
Sodium mEq/L (mg/L)	7.1 (162)
Potassium mEq/L (mg/L)	13.8 (541)
Chloride mEq/L (mg/L)	11.3 (399)
Calcium mEq/L (mg/L)	18.9 (379)
Phosphorus mEq/L (mg/L)	(189)
Iron mg/L	4.7
% free water	90
Manufacturer	Abbott
Special information	Gluten-free, Kosher, Halal
Special uses	Renal and cardiovascular disease

[1]Information based on manufacturer's literature as of 2013 and is subject to change

Nutrition for the Ketogenic Diet[1]

Indications: Dietary management of intractable epilepsy, pyruvate dehydrogenase deficiency, glucose transport type-1 deficiency

	KetoCal 3:1[2,3]	KetoCal 4:1[2,4]	KetoCal 4:1 LQ[2,5]
Calories /mL	1	1.44	1.5
Protein g per 100 mL	2.2	3	3.1
Protein source	Milk protein, L-cystine, L-tryptophan, taurine	Dry whole milk, L-isoleucine, L-tryptophan, taurine	Sodium caseinate (milk), L-cystine, L-tryptophan, whey protein concentrate (milk)
Carbohydrate g per 100 mL	1	0.6	1.73
Carbohydrate source	Lactose	Corn syrup solids	Soy fiber, cornstartch, inulin
Fat g per 100 mL	9.7	14.4	14.8
Fat source (essential fatty acid amounts are per 100 kcal)	Refined vegetable oil (palm and soy oils)	Hydrogenated soybean oil, refined soybean oil, soy lecithin	Refined vegetable oil (high oleic sunflower, soy, and palm oils), soy lecithin, DHA[6] (37 mg), ARA[6] (37 mg), linoleic acid (2152 mg), linolenic acid (209 mg)
Osmolality mOsm/kg H_2O	180	197	260 vanilla 280 unflavored
Sodium mEq/L (mg/L)	(411)	(600)	(1,030)
Potassium mEq/L (mg/L)	(1,290)	(2,160)	(1,650)
Chloride mEq/L (mg/L)	(629)	(1,000)	(1,550)
Calcium mEq/L (mg/L)	(1,090)	(1,600)	(884)
Phosphorus mEq/L (mg/L)	(730)	(1,300)	(884)
Iron mg/L	16	22	15
% free water			77.8
Manufacturer	Nutricia	Nutricia	Nutricia
Special information		Recommend reconstitution ratio of 4 mL of water for each 1 g of powder	

[1]Information based on manufacturer's literature as of 2013 and is subject to change

[2]Ratio represents fats to carbohydrates plus protein

[3]For patients up to 8 years of age; powder formulation to initiate the ketogenic diet

[4]For patients >1 year of age; powder formulation

[5]For patients ≤13 years of age; ready-to-use formulation

[6]DHA (docosahexaenoic acid) and ARA (arachidonic acid) are fatty acids which are found naturally in breast milk. DHA is provided via *Crypthecodinium cohnii* oil. ARA is provided via *Mortienella alphia* oil.

Low Long Chain Fatty Acids Formulas[1]

	Portagen	Enfaport
Calories per 100 mL	100	100
Protein g per 100 mL	3.5	3.6
Protein source	Sodium caseinate	Calcium and sodium caseinates (milk)
Carbohydrate g per 100 mL	11.5	10.3
Carbohydrate source	75% corn syrup solids and 25% sugar	Corn syrup solids
Fat g per 100 mL	4.8	5.5
Fat source (essential fatty acid amounts are per 100 kcal)	87% MCT, 13% corn oils, soy lecithin	84% MCT and 13% soy oils, 3% DHA[2] (17 mg), ARA[2] (34 mg), linoleic acid (350 mg), linolenic acid (50 mg), soy lecithin
Osmolality mOsm/kg	350	280
Osmolarity mOsm/L	300	240
Sodium mEq/L (mg/L)	(552)	(300)
Potassium mEq/L (mg/L)	(1,250)	(1,170)
Chloride mEq/L (mg/L)	(865)	(880)
Calcium mEq/L (mg/L)	(938)	(950)
Phosphorus mEq/L (mg/L)	(708)	(530)
Iron mg/L	18.8	18.3
% free water	87	84
Manufacturer	Mead Johnson	Mead Johnson
Indication	For children and adults with defects in the intraluminal hydrolysis of fats (decreased bile salts, decreased pancreatic lipase); defective mucosal fat absorption (decreased mucosal permeability, decreased absorptive surface); and/or defective lymphatic transport of fat (ie, intestinal lymphatic obstruction); if used long-term, not nutritionally complete and will require supplementation of essential fatty acids and ultra trace minerals	Iron-fortified, milk-based infant formula with 84% of fat as MCT for infants with chylothorax or LCHAD deficiency (long chain 3-hydroxyacyl CoA dehydrogenase – inherited disorder of fat oxidation)
Special information	Gluten-free, lactose-free	Gluten-free, lactose-free, sucrose-free

[1]Information based on manufacturer's literature as of 2013 and is subject to change

[2]DHA (docosahexaenoic acid) and ARA (arachidonic acid) are fatty acids which are found naturally in breast milk. DHA is provided via *Crypthecodinium cohnii* oil. ARA is provided via *Mortienella alphia* oil.

NUTRITIONAL MODULARS

Nutritional Modulars – Carbohydrate and Protein Supplements[1]

	Polycose Powder	ProMod Liquid Protein[2,3]	Benecalorie (liquid)	Beneprotein (powder)	Liquid Protein Fortifier	Resource Benefiber	Duocal
Indication	Carbohydrate additive for use as a caloric supplement which is readily mixable in most foods, enteral formulas or beverages without appreciably altering their taste	Protein supplement which mixes readily in enteral formulas, most foods, or beverages without appreciably altering their taste; indicated for wounds, protein-energy malnutrition, involuntary weight loss, pre- and postsurgery anorexia, stress, trauma, cancer, burns	Calorie and protein supplement which mixes well into most foods and beverages	Protein supplement; 100% high quality whey proteins; mixes instantly in a variety of foods/beverages without compromising taste or texture	Protein supplement for preterm infants; peptides and amino acids for easy digestion and absorption; for use with breast milk or infant formula	For dietary management of occasional constipation; mixes instantly in a variety of foods/beverages without compromising taste or texture	To increase calories by adding to food and beverages; contains no protein; neutral flavor
Calories	3.8/g[4]	3.3/mL	7.5/mL[5]	3.6/g[6]	0.67/mL	4/g[7]	4.9/g[8]
Protein (g)		0.33/mL	0.16/mL	0.86/g	0.17/mL		
Protein source		Hydrolyzed beef collagen	Calcium caseinate (milk)	Whey protein isolate (milk)	Casein hydrolysate (milk)		
Carbohydrate (g)	0.94/g	0.47/mL				1/g	0.73/g
Carbohydrate source	Glucose polymers derived from controlled hydrolysis of corstarch	Glycerin	Sucralose			Partially hydrolyzed guar gum	Hydrolyzed corn starch
Fat (g)			0.75/mL				0.22/g
Fat source			High oleic sunflower oil	Soy lecithin			Corn/coconut oil and MCT oils (fractionated coconut, palm kernel)
Osmolality mOsm/kg					1 mL contributes 12 for 100 mL feeding		1 scoop = 5 g; for 1:3 dilution, 310; 0.93 mOsm/g powder
Osmolarity mOsm/L	247[9]	59.9					
Sodium mEq/L (mg/L)	<0.057/g (<1.3/g)	(<0.0018/mL)		2.1/g (0.09/g)		3.76/g (0.175/g)	<0.2/g
Potassium mEq/L (mg/L)	<0.003/g (<0.1/g)	(<0.0007/mL)		4.3/g (0.11/g)		3.76/g (0.1/g)	<0.05/g
Chloride mEq/L (mg/L)	<0.063/g (<2.23/g)						<0.2/g
Calcium mEq/L (mg/L)	<0.015/g (<0.3/g)		(0.002)	(2.9/g)			<0.05/g
Phosphorus mEq/L (mg/L)	(<0.15/g)	(<0.003/mL)					<0.05/g

Nutritional Modulars – Carbohydrate and Protein Supplements[1] *continued*

	Polycose Powder	ProMod Liquid Protein[2,3]	Benecalorie (liquid)	Beneprotein (powder)	Liquid Protein Fortifier	Resource Benefiber	Duocal
Manufacturer	Abbott	Abbott	Nestle	Nestle	Abbott	Nestle	Nutricia
Special information		Powder displacement is 0.63 mL/g Gluten-free, Kosher	Gluten-free, lactose-free, cholesterol-free, Kosher	Gluten-free, lactose-free, Kosher	The first and only commercially sterile, extensively hydrolyzed liquid protein designed for preterm infant feedings Eliminates the need for powder mixing and meets ADA and CDC recommendations to reduce risk of contamination		Milk protein-free

[1]These products are not complete formulations and should not be used as a sole source of nutrition; information based on manufacturer's literature as of 2013 and is subject to change

[2]Comes in fruit punch flavor

[3]Promod Powder is no longer commercially available.

[4]1 teaspoon (2 g) = 8 calories, 1 tablespoon (6 g) = 23 calories, 1/4 cup (24 g) = 91 calories.

[5]Serving is a 1.5 fl oz package

[6]1 scoop = 7 g packet = 1.5 tablespoons

[7]1 tbsp = 4 g packet, usually mix with 2 to 4 fl oz. This provides 3 g of soluble dietary fiber.

[8]42 cal/tablespoon

[9]Approximate osmotic contribution to solution mixed into is 1.6 mOsm/g with a low renal solute load of 0.13 mOsm/g

Nutritional Modulars – Fat Supplement[1]

	Vegetable Oil[2]	Microlipid	MCT Oil[3]	Whole Milk
Indications	Inexpensive fat source for calories and essential fatty acids	50% fat emulsion for use as a source of calories or essential fatty acids; it mixes easily and stays in emulsion	Fat supplement for use in patients who cannot efficiently digest and absorb long-chain fats	For children >1 year of age
Calories	8.3/mL	4.5/mL	7.7/mL	157 per 8 oz
Protein (g)	—	—	—	8.2 per 8 oz
Protein source	—	—	—	82% casein, 18% whey
Carbohydrate (g)	—	—	—	11.5 per 8 oz
Carbohydrate source	—	—	—	Lactose
Fat (g)	0.93/mL	0.5/mL	0.93/mL	8.2 per 8 oz
Fat source	Corn, soybean, sunflower or safflower oils[5]	Safflower oil[4], polyglycerol esters, soy lecithin	Modified coconut/palm kernel oils	Butter fat
Osmolality mOsm/kg	—	62	—	285
Sodium mEq/L (mg/L)	—	—	—	5.3 per 8 oz (120 per 8 oz)
Potassium mEq/L (mg/L)	—	—	—	9.6 per 8 oz (377 per 8 oz)
Calcium mEq/L (mg/L)	—	—	—	14.9 per 8 oz (295 per 8 oz)
Phosphorus mEq/L (mg/L)	—	—	—	(230 per 8 oz)
Iron mg/L	—	—	—	Trace
% free water	—	45	—	91
Manufacturer		Nestle	Nestle	
Special information		Can administer 15 mL via syringe through the feeding tube and flush afterwards with 30 mL water Gluten-free, lactose-free, Kosher	Recommended initial volume is 15 mL administrated gradually. Recommended max volume over 24 hrs is 100 mL as indicated, given in divided doses not to exceed 15 to 20 mL. Can administer 15 mL via syringe through the feeding tube and flush afterwards with 30 mL water. For oral consumption, may mix with juice, milk, sauces, salad dressings, or other foods. Gluten-free, lactose-free, Kosher	

[1]These products are not complete formulations and should not be used as a sole source of nutrition; information based on manufacturer's literature as of 2013 and is subject to change

[2]1 tablespoon = 14 g

[3]Does not contain essential fatty acids

[4]Rich source of polyunsaturated fat

[5]% of linoleic from fat: Soybean oil 51%, corn oil 58%, sunflower oil 65%, safflower oil 77%

ELECTROLYTE REPLACEMENT

Oral Electrolyte Maintenance Solution[1]

	Pedialyte[2]	Pedialyte Freezer Pop[3]	Enfamil Enfalyte[4,5]
Indications	Replace fluids and electrolytes lost during diarrhea and vomiting to prevent dehydration in infants/ children	Replace fluids and electrolytes lost during diarrhea and vomiting to prevent dehydration in infants/ children	Oral electrolyte maintenance solution using rice syrup solids as carbohydrate source to help replace electrolytes and water one might lose from vomiting and diarrhea; for infants and children
Calories	0.1/mL	0.1/mL	0.126/mL
Protein (g)			
Protein source			
Carbohydrate (g)	25	25	30
Carbohydrate source	Dextrose	Dextrose	Rice syrup solids
Fat (g)			
Fat source			
Osmolality mOsm/kg	250 unflavored 270 flavored	270 flavored	160
Osmolarity mOsm/L			168
Sodium mEq/L (mg/L)	45	45	50 (1,150)
Potassium mEq/L (mg/L)	20	20	25 (980)
Chloride mEq/L (mg/L)	35	35	45 (160)
Calcium mEq/L (mg/L)			
Phosphorus mEq/L (mg/L)			
Iron mg/L			
Manufacturer	Abbott	Abbott	Mead Johnson
Special information	Kosher, Halal (only certain flavors)		

[1]These products are not complete formulations and should not be used as a sole source of nutrition; information based on manufacturer's literature as of 2013 and is subject to change

[2]Unflavored but available as grape, fruit, bubblegum, strawberry, and apple

[3]Each freezer pop is 2.1 fl oz. Grape, cherry, orange, and blue raspberry are not Kosher.

[4]Cherry

[5]Contains citrate 34 mEq/L

FLUID AND ELECTROLYTE REQUIREMENTS IN CHILDREN

Maintenance Fluids (Two methods)

Surface area method (most commonly used in children >10 kg): 1,500 to 2,000 mL/m²/day

Body weight method[A]

Weight	Daily Fluids (Holliday-Segar Method)	Hourly Rate (Holliday-Segar Estimate)
<10 kg	100 mL/kg/day	4 mL/kg/hour
11 to 20 kg	1,000 mL + 50 mL/kg (for each kg >10)	40 mL/hour + 2 mL/kg/hour (for each kg >10)
>20 kg	1,500 mL + 20 mL/kg (for each kg >20)	60 mL/hour + 1 mL/kg/hour (for each kg >20)

[A]Should not be used in patients <14 days; generally overestimates needs.

Maintenance Electrolytes (See specific monographs for more detailed information)

Sodium: 3 to 4 mEq/kg/day
Potassium: 2 to 3 mEq/kg/day

Alterations of Maintenance Fluid Requirements

Fever	Increase maintenance fluids by 5 mL/kg/day for each degree of temperature above 38°C
Hyperventilation	Increase maintenance fluids by 10 to 60 mL/100 kcal BEE (basal energy expenditure)
Sweating	Increase maintenance fluids by 10 to 25 mL/100 kcal BEE (basal energy expenditure)
Hyperthyroidism	Variable increase in maintenance fluids: 25% to 50%
Renal disease	Monitor and analyze output; adjust therapy accordingly
Renal failure	Maintenance fluids are equal to insensible losses (300 mL/m²) + urine replacement (mL for mL)
Diarrhea	Increase maintenance fluids on a mL/mL loss basis

Dehydration Fluid Therapy

Goals of therapy:

- Restore circulatory volume to prevent shock (10% to 15% dehydration)
- Restore combined intracellular and extracellular deficits of water and electrolytes within 24 hours for isotonic or hyponatremic dehydration. For hypertonic dehydration restore over 48 hours.
- Maintain adequate water and electrolytes
- Resolve homeostatic distortions (eg, acidosis)
- Replace ongoing losses

Analysis of the Severity of Dehydration by Physical Signs

Clinical Sign	Mild	Moderate	Severe
Degree of dehydration Infant Child/Adult	 <5% <3%	 5% to 10% 3% to 6%	 >10% >6%
Skin turgor	Normal	Decreased	Markedly decreased
Mucous membranes	Thirsty	Dry	Parched
Skin color	Normal	Pale	Mottled
Urine output	Decreased	Oliguria	Anuria
Blood pressure	Normal	Normal, ↓	↓↓
Heart rate	Normal, ↑	↑	↑↑
Capillary refill	Normal	Delayed (>1.5 seconds)	Very delayed (>3 seconds)
Fontanelle (<7 mo)	Flat	Sunken	Very sunken
CNS	Consolable	Irritable/lethargic	Limp, depressed consciousness

Adapted from *Nelson's Textbook of Pediatrics*. 19th ed. Saunders; 2011 and *Current Pediatric Diagnosis & Treatment*. 20th ed. McGraw Hill; 2011.

Classification of Dehydration (based upon the serum sodium concentration)

Isotonic	130 to 150 mEq/L
Hypotonic	<130 mEq/L
Hypertonic	>150 mEq/L

Water deficit may also be calculated (in isotonic dehydration):

$$\text{Water deficit (mL)} = \frac{\text{\% dehydration x wt (kg) x 1,000 g/kg}}{100}$$

Fluid Replacement

Rehydration begins with a fluid bolus if adequate perfusion is not present. Fluid boluses of 20 mL/kg (maximum single dose: 1,000 mL) using crystalloids (eg, normal saline or lactated Ringers) are administered over 20 to 60 minutes or as rapidly as possible if necessary; repeat doses until circulation is improved [eg, warm skin, decreased heart rate (towards normal), improved capillary refill time, urine output restored]. Once perfusion has been restored then fluid replacement (maintenance plus deficit) is continued over the next 24 hours (isotonic/hypotonic dehydration) or 48 hours (hypertonic dehydration).

For 24 hour replacement, half the deficit fluid is given in the first 8 hours and the second half is given over the last 16 hours. Although $D_5$1/4NS provides the estimated sodium requirement for most patients when used as a maintenance fluid, there is a risk of developing iatrogenic hyponatremia. To prevent hyponatremia, many clinicians use 1/2NS instead. Some clinicians have suggested NS should be used for maintenance fluids.

For hypernatremic dehydration the total deficit volume plus the maintenance volume for 48 hours should be combined and the total administered over 48 hours. This is done to prevent osmotic fluid shifts which could lead to cerebral edema and possibly seizures. The fluid used for replacement should be hypotonic (eg, $D_5$1/4 NS) to ensure sodium is not corrected by more than 10 mEq/L/day.

Example of Fluid Replacement (assume 10 kg infant with 10% isotonic dehydration)

	Water	Sodium (mEq)	Potassium (mEq)
Maintenance	1,000 mL	40	20
Deficit[A]	1,000 mL	80	80
Total	2,000 mL	120	100

[A]Reduce this total by any fluid boluses given initially.

First 8 hours:

Replace 1/3 maintenance water = 330 mL

Replace 1/2 deficit water = 500 mL

Total 830 mL/8 h = 103 mL/h

Replace 1/2 of Na^+ & K^+ = 60 mEq sodium/803 mL; 50 mEq potassium/803 mL (It is suggested that the maximum initial potassium concentration used is 40 mEq/L and is **not** started until urine output has been established.)

The actual order would appear as: $D_5$1/2NS at 103 mL/hour for 8 hours; add 40 mEq/L KCl after patient voids.

Second 16 hours:

Replace 2/3 maintenance water = 670 mL

Replace 1/2 deficit water = 500 mL

Total 1,260 mL/16 h = 79 mL/h

Replace remainder of sodium and potassium.

The actual order would appear as: $D_5$1/2NS with KCl 40 mEq/L at 79 mL/hour for 16 hours.

Analysis of Ongoing Losses

Electrolyte Composition of Biological Fluids (mEq/L)

Fluid Type	Sodium	Potassium	HCO_3^-
Gastric	20 to 80	5 to 20	0
Small intestine	100 to 140	5 to 15	40
Diarrheal stool	10 to 90	10 to 80	40
Ileostomy	45 to 135	3 to 15	40

CURRENT Diagnosis and Treatment Pediatrics, 20th ed, McGraw-Hill, 2011.

Because of the wide range of normal values, specific analyses are suggested in individual cases.

Oral Rehydration

Due to the high worldwide incidence of dehydration from infantile diarrhea, effective, inexpensive oral rehydration solutions have been developed. In the US, a typical effective solution for rehydration contains 45 to 75 mEq/L sodium, 20 to 25 mEq/L potassium, 30 to 34 mEq/L bicarbonate or its equivalent, and sufficient chloride to provide electroneutrality. Two percent to 3% glucose helps facilitate electrolyte and water absorption in the intestine and provides short-term calories. Oral replacement fluids should be administered frequently in small quantities (5 to 15 mL) to provide 50 mL/kg over 4 hours in mild dehydration and 100 mL/kg over 6 hours for moderate dehydration. Oral rehydration should **not** be used if any of the following exists: Altered level of consciousness, respiratory distress, acute surgical abdomen, >10% volume depletion in infants, hemodynamic instability, severe hyponatremia (Na <120 mEq/L) or severe hypernatremia (Na >160 mEq/L). Clear liquids such as broth, juice, tea, and soda are not appropriate for fluid replacement due to high osmolarity and limited electrolytes and should be avoided. The following table describes the electrolyte/sugar content of commonly used oral rehydration solutions.

Composition of Frequently Used Oral Electrolyte Replacement Solutions

Solutions	Carbohydrate (g/L)	Na^+ (mEq/L)	K^+ (mEq/L)	Cl^- (mEq/L)	Base[A] (mEq/L)
WHO solution, modified	13.5	75	20	65	30
Pedialyte	25	45	20	35	30
Enfalyte	30	50	25	45	34
Oralyte	25	45	20	35	30

[A]Actual or potential bicarbonate (eg, acetate, citrate, or lactate)

Adapted from Centers for Disease Control and Prevention (CDC). Managing acute gastroenteritis among children: oral rehydration, maintenance, and nutritional therapy. *MMWR*. 2003;52(RR-16):1-16 and manufacturer's labeling.

REFERENCES

Centers for Disease Control and Prevention (CDC). Managing acute gastroenteritis among children: oral rehydration, maintenance, and nutritional therapy. *MMWR Recomm R.* 2003;52(RR-16):1-16.

Ford DM. Fluid, electrolyte, & acid-base disorders & therapy. *CURRENT Diagnosis and Treatment Pediatrics.* 20th ed. Hay WW, Levin MJ, Sondheimer JM, et al, eds. New York: McGraw-Hill; 2011;1299-1307.

Greenbaum LA. Deficit therapy. *Nelson Textbook of Pediatrics.* 19th ed. Kliegman RM, Stanton BF, St. Geme JW, et al, eds. Philadelphia, PA: Saunders; 2011;245-249.

Meyers RS. Pediatric fluid and electrolyte therapy. *J Pediatr Pharmacol Ther.* 2009;14(4):204-211.

H. PYLORI TREATMENT IN PEDIATRIC PATIENTS

First-Line Therapies

Triple therapy: Duration of therapy is 7 to 14 days

1. Proton pump inhibitor (PPI) + Amoxicillin + MetroNIDAZOLE
2. PPI + Amoxicillin + Clarithromycin*
3. Bismuth salts + Amoxicillin + MetroNIDAZOLE

Sequential therapy: PPI + Amoxicillin for 5 days, followed by PPI + Clarithromycin* + MetroNIDAZOLE for 5 days

*Clarithromycin-based therapy should only be considered first-line if local clarithromycin resistance rates are known to be low or susceptibility testing reveals the patient has a clarithromycin-susceptible strain.

Second-Line (Salvage) Therapies

Quadruple therapy: PPI + Amoxicillin + MetroNIDAZOLE + Bismuth salts for up to 14 days

Triple therapy: PPI + Levofloxacin (or Moxifloxacin) + Amoxicillin for up to 14 days

Recommended Dosages

Omeprazole: 0.5 to 1 mg/kg/dose twice daily (maximum dose: 20 mg/dose)
Note: For other PPIs, comparable acid inhibitory doses suggested (Gold 2000)

Amoxicillin: 25 mg/kg/dose twice daily (maximum dose: 1,000 mg/dose)

Clarithromycin*: 10 mg/kg/dose twice daily (maximum dose: 500 mg/dose)

MetroNIDAZOLE: 10 mg/kg/dose twice daily (maximum dose: 500 mg/dose)

Bismuth subsalicylate: 2 mg/kg/dose 4 times daily

Levofloxacin or moxifloxacin: No dose provided in guidelines; data is limited

REFERENCE

Koletzko S, Jones NL, Goodman KJ, et al. Evidence-based guidelines from ESPGHAN and NASPGHAN for *Helicobacter pylori* infection in children. *J Pediatr Gastroenterol Nutr.* 2011;53(2):230-243.

Gold BD, Colletti RB, Abbott M, et al. *Helicobacter pylori* infection in children: recommendations for diagnosis and treatment. *J Pediatr Gastroenterol Nutr.* 2000;31(5):490-497.

PEDIATRIC PARENTERAL NUTRITION

The following information is intended as a brief overview of the use of PN in infants and children.

Goal: The therapeutic goal of PN in infants and children is both to maintain nutrition status and to achieve balanced somatic growth; in premature infants, the goal is to mimic intrauterine growth.

General Indications for Use: PN is the provision of required nutrients by the intravenous route to replenish, optimize, or maintain nutritional status.

Specific Indications

PN of **all** required nutrients (total parenteral nutrition) is indicated in patients for whom it is expected that it would be impossible or dangerous to enterally administer nutrition. PN in combination with enteral nutrition is indicated in patients who are expected to be unable to meet their nutritional needs by the enteral route alone within 5 days. Peripheral PN is indicated only for partial nutritional supplementation or as bridge therapy for patients awaiting central venous access.

1. Patients with an inability to absorb nutrients via the gastrointestinal tract, which may include the following: Severe diarrhea, short bowel syndrome, developmental anomalies of the GI tract, inflammatory bowel disease, cystic fibrosis, or anatomic or functional loss of GI integrity
2. Severe malnutrition
3. Severe catabolic states, such as burns, trauma, or sepsis
4. Patients undergoing high dose chemotherapy, radiation, and bone marrow transplantation
5. Patients whose clinical condition may necessitate complete bowel rest (eg, necrotizing enterocolitis, pancreatitis, GI fistulas, or recent GI surgery)
6. Intensive care low-birth-weight infants
7. Neonatal asphyxia
8. Meconium ileus
9. Respiratory distress syndrome (RDS)

Nutritional Assessment

Nutritional screening may be done on admission by staff nurses or dietitian to identify patients who are malnourished or at risk of malnutrition. Patients identified through the screening process as being at risk should receive a complete nutritional assessment which may include anthropometric measurements, diet history, laboratory values, and physical exam. As many as 44% of hospitalized pediatric patients are malnourished and require nutritional therapy. The type of nutritional support indicated depends on the underlying disease, the degree of gastrointestinal function, and the severity of malnutrition. Acutely malnourished patients have an increased risk for serious infection, postoperative complications, and death. Indicators of acute protein-calorie malnutrition include low weight for height, low serum albumin, lymphopenia, decreased body fat folds, and decreased arm muscle area.

Nutritional Requirements

Energy requirements vary based on age. The following table provides an estimate for caloric and protein requirements at various ages for normal subjects.

Daily Caloric and Protein Requirements for Pediatric Patients

Age	kcal/kg/day	Protein g/kg/day
Preterm neonate	90 to 120	3 to 4
Term infant <1 year	85 to 105	2 to 3
1 to 7 years	75 to 90	1.5 to 3
7 to 10 years	50 to 75	1.5 to 3
11 to 12 years	50 to 75	0.8 to 2.5
>12 to 18 years	30 to 50	0.8 to 2.5

Patients who are severely malnourished or markedly catabolic may require higher levels to achieve catch-up growth or meet increased requirements. Patients who are well-nourished and/or inactive may require less.

During parenteral nutrition, 10% to 16% of calories should be in the form of amino acids to achieve optimal benefit (~3 to 4 g/kg/day in preterm infants, 2 to 3 g/kg/day in infants, 1.5 to 3 g/kg/day in children (1 to 10 years), and 0.8 to 2.5 g/kg/day in adolescents). Exceptions include patients with renal or hepatic failure (where less protein is indicated), or in the treatment of severe trauma, head injury, or sepsis (where more protein may be indicated).

PN ORDERING

Fluid Intake

The patient should be given a total volume of fluid reasonable for his/her age and cardiovascular status. It is generally safe to start with the fluid maintenance level of 1,500 mL/m^2/day in children >10 kg or use the Holliday-Segar weight-based method in children >2 weeks (see Fluid and Electrolyte Requirements in Children). The fluid requirements in preterm infants are extremely variable due to much greater insensible water losses from radiant warmers and bili-lights. While the standard fluid maintenance of 100 mL/kg/day may be sufficient for term infants, intakes of up to 150 mL/kg/day may be necessary in the very low birth weight infants. Be sure to consider significant fluid intake from medications or other IV fluids and enteral diets in planning the fluids available for PN.

Amino Acids

Amino acids may be described as either a "standard" mixture of essential and nonessential amino acids or "specialized" mixtures. Specialized mixtures are intended for use in patients whose physiologic or metabolic needs may not be met with the "standard" amino acid compositions. Examples of specialized solutions include:

TrophAmine, Aminosyn PF, PremaSol	Indicated for use in premature infants and young children due to addition of taurine, L-glutamic acid, L-aspartic acid, increased amounts of histidine, and reduction in amounts of methionine, alanine, phenylalanine, and glycine. Supplementation with a cysteine[1] additive has been recommended.
HepatAmine	Indicated for treatment in patients with hepatic encephalopathy due to cirrhosis or hepatitis or in patients with liver disease who are intolerant of standard amino acid solutions. Contains higher percentage of branched-chain amino acids and a lower percentage of aromatic amino acids than standard mixtures.
NephrAmine, Aminosyn RF	Indicated for use in patients with compromised renal function who are intolerant of standard amino acid solutions. Contains a mixture of essential amino acids and histidine.

[1]Supplementation is usually provided as a fixed ratio to the amino acid solution: 40 mg of cysteine per gram of amino acid; duration of supplementation is usually for the first year of life, but practice varies widely.

Protein provides 4 kcal per gram.

Amino acid calculations:

% amino acid = amino acid (g) per 100 mL

Grams of protein = grams of nitrogen x 6.25

$$\text{\% amino acid desired} = \frac{\text{(g amino acid/kg)} \times \text{weight (kg)} \times 100}{\text{total PN fluid volume (mL)}}$$

Dextrose

For central PN, dextrose is usually begun with a 10% to 12.5% solution or a solution providing dextrose at no more than 5 mg/kg/minute (in neonates and premature infants). The concentration is advanced, if tolerated, by 2.5% to 5% per day (2 to 2.5 mg/kg/minute increments in neonates and premature infants) to the desired caloric density, usually 20% to 25% dextrose. Fluid restricted patients often need 30% to 35% dextrose to meet their energy needs. For peripheral PN, 5% to 12.5% dextrose is utilized.

Dextrose provides 3.4 kcal per gram.

Dextrose calculations:

% Dextrose = dextrose (g) per 100 mL

$$\text{Dextrose infusion rate (mg/kg/minute)} = \frac{\text{rate (mL/h)} \times \text{\% dextrose} \times 0.166}{\text{weight (kg)}}$$

$$\text{\% Dextrose desired}^{1} = \frac{\text{desired rate (mg/kg/min)} \times \text{weight (kg)}}{0.166 \times \text{rate (mL/h)}}$$

[1]Do not use dextrose concentrations <5% due to hypotonicity.

Fat Emulsion (FE)

There are three roles for intravenous fat in parenteral nutrition:

1. To provide nonprotein calories
2. To provide essential fatty acids and a "balanced" calorie source
3. To provide calories in catabolic patients with limited ability to excrete CO_2

The FE dosage is increased as tolerated daily (see General Guidelines for Initiation and Advancement for PN following). The maximum fat intake is 3.5 g/kg/day and no more than 60% of the total daily caloric intake. It is administered as a continuous infusion over 24 hours or at a rate no greater than 0.15 to 0.17 g/kg/hour via a Y-connector with the dextrose-amino acid IV line. In patients receiving cyclic PN, the FE should be administered over the duration of the PN infusion. The triglyceride concentration should be checked on initiation and then weekly. Triglyceride concentrations should be maintained at <200 mg/dL in neonates, <350 mg/dL in renal patients, and <250 mg/dL in other patients. FE should be used cautiously in neonates with hyperbilirubinemia due to displacement of bilirubin from albumin by the free fatty acids. An increase in free bilirubin may increase the risk of kernicterus. Significant displacement occurs when the free fatty acid to serum albumin molar ratio (FFA/SA) >6. For example, infants with a total bilirubin >8 to 10 mg/dL (assuming an albumin concentration of 2.5 to 3 g/dL) should not receive more parenteral FE than required to meet the essential fatty acid requirement of 0.5 to 1 g/kg/day.

Note: Avoid use of 10% FE in preterm infants because a greater accumulation of plasma lipids occurs due to the greater phospholipid load of the 10% concentration.

Fat emulsion 10% provides 1.1 kcal/mL or 11 kcal/g

Fat emulsion 20% provides 2 kcal/mL or 10 kcal/g

Fat emulsion calculations:

20% FE = 20 g fat per 100 mL = 2 kcal/mL

$$\text{Desired 20\% FE (mL)} = \frac{\text{(\% total kcal as fat) x (total kcal)}}{\text{2 kcal/mL}}$$

or as an alternative

Desired 20% FE (mL) = FE (g/kg) x weight (kg) x 5 mL/g

General Guidelines for Initiation and Advancement of PN[1]

Age	Initiation and Advancement[2]	Protein (g/kg/day)	Dextrose	Fat (g/kg/day)
Premature infant	Initial	1.5 to 3	5 to 7 mg/kg/min	1 to 2
	Daily increase	1	1 to 2.5 mg/kg/min or 1% to 2.5% increments	0.5 to 1
	Goal	3 to 4	8 to 12 mg/kg/min (max: 14 to 18 mg/kg/min)	3 to 3.5
Term infant <1 y	Initial	1 to 3	6 to 9 mg/kg/min	1 to 2
	Daily increase	1	1 to 2 mg/kg/min or 2.5% to 5% increments	0.5 to 1
	Goal	2 to 3	12 mg/kg/min (max: 14 to 18 mg/kg/min)	3
Children 1 to 10 y	Initial	1 to 2	10%	1 to 2
	Daily increase	1	1 to 2 mg/kg/min or 5% increments	0.5 to 1
	Goal	1.5 to 3	8 to 10 mg/kg/min	2 to 3
>10 y	Initial	0.8 to 1.5	3.5 mg/kg/min or 10%	1
	Daily increase	1	1 to 2 mg/kg/min or 5% increments	1
	Goal	0.8 to 2.5	5 to 6 mg/kg/min	1 to 2.5

[1]Rate of advancement may be limited by metabolic tolerance (eg, hyperglycemia, azotemia, hypertriglyceridemia)

[2]Timely intervention in premature infants is essential with initiation of dextrose as soon as possible after birth, amino acids within the first 12 hours, and fat emulsion within 24 to 48 hours of life.

ELECTROLYTES AND MINERALS

Guideline for Daily Electrolyte and Mineral Requirements

	Preterm Neonates (mEq/kg)	Infants/Children (mEq/kg)	Adolescents/Children >50 kg
Sodium	2 to 5[1]	2 to 5	1 to 2 mEq/kg
Potassium	2 to 4	2 to 4	1 to 2 mEq/kg
Calcium gluconate[2]	2 to 4[3]	0.5 to 4	10 to 20 mEq/day
Magnesium	0.3 to 0.5	0.3 to 0.5	10 to 30 mEq/day
Phosphate[2]	1 to 2 mmol/kg[3]	0.5 to 2 mmol/kg	10 to 40 mmol/day

[1]Premature infants lose sodium in urine due to the immature resorptive function of kidney and diuretic use. Hyponatremia may lead to poor tissue growth and adverse developmental outcomes. Sodium content in PN may be adjusted to a maximum of 154 mEq/L (NS) to achieve normal sodium serum levels.

[2]Calcium-phosphate stability in parenteral nutrition solutions is dependent upon the pH of the solution, temperature, and relative concentration of each ion. The pH of the solution is primarily dependent upon the amino acid concentration. The higher the percentage amino acids the lower the pH, the more soluble the calcium and phosphate. Individual commercially available amino acid solutions vary significantly with respect to pH lowering potential and consequent calcium phosphate compatibility. See the pharmacist for specific calcium phosphate stability information.

[3]A 1.7:1 calcium to phosphate ratio in PN allows for the highest absolute retention of both minerals and simulates the *in utero* accretion of calcium and phosphate.

VITAMINS AND TRACE ELEMENTS

Vitamins

A pediatric parenteral multivitamin product is indicated for children <11 years of age and <40 kg. Children >40 kg or >11 years of age may receive adult multivitamin formulations.

Dosage:

Pediatric MVI[1]:
Neonates: 2 mL/kg/day; maximum 5 mL/day
Infants and Children ≤11 years: 5 mL/day
Children >40 kg or >11 years and Adults: Use adult formulation[2] 10 mL/day

Trace Element Daily Requirements[1]

	Preterm Neonates <3 kg (mcg/kg/day)	Term Neonates 3 to 10 kg (mcg/kg/day)	Children 10 to 40 kg (mcg/kg/day)	Adolescents >40 kg (per day)
Chromium[2]	0.05 to 0.2	0.2	0.14 to 0.2	5 to 15 mcg
Copper[3]	20	20	5 to 20	200 to 500 mcg
Manganese[4]	1	1	1	40 to 100 mcg
Selenium[2,5]	1.5 to 2	2	1 to 2	40 to 60 mcg
Zinc	400	50 to 250	50 to 125	2 to 5 mg

[1]Recommended intakes of trace elements cannot be achieved through the use of a single pediatric trace element product. Only through the use of individualized trace element products can recommended intakes be achieved.

[2]Reduce dose in patients with renal dysfunction.

[3]Reduce dose by 50% in patients with impaired biliary excretion or cholestatic liver disease.

[4]Omit in patient with impaired biliary excretion or cholestatic liver disease.

[5]Indicated for use in long-term parenteral nutrition patients.

These are recommended daily trace element requirements. Additional supplementation may be indicated in clinical conditions resulting in excessive losses. For example, additional zinc may be needed in situations of excessive gastrointestinal losses.

DEVELOPING THE PN GOAL REGIMEN

The purpose of this example is to illustrate the thought process in determining what dextrose and amino acid solution and fat emulsion intake would provide the desired daily fluid calorie and protein goals. The following example utilizes the method of calculating calories from protein, dextrose, and fat. However, some clinicians do not include protein calories since protein is used as a building block for adequate growth and development, rather than a calorie source.

1. Calculate the fluid, protein, and caloric goals. Example:

   Weight = 10 kg

   Fluids = 100 mL/kg/day = 1,000 mL

   Calories = 100 kcal/kg/day = 1,000 kcal

   Protein = 2.5 g/kg/day = 25 g

2. If fat emulsion (FE) comprises 30% to 35% of the total daily calories, using the above example: 30% of 1,000 kcal = 300 kcal
   300 kcal ÷ 2 kcal/mL (20% FE) = 150 mL

3. Calculate percent amino acid solution to achieve goal protein intake. Example:
   [25 g (total protein) ÷ 850 mL (total fluid)] x 100 = 2.9%

4. Determine the calories from protein. Example:
   25 g x 4 kcal/g = 100 kcal

5. To determine the goal dextrose concentration calculate the total daily calories remaining. Example:

1,000 kcal	(total daily calories)
-100 kcal	(daily calories from protein)
-300 kcal	(daily calories from fats)
600 kcal	(total daily calories remaining)

6. Determine the concentration of dextrose to achieve the total daily calories remaining. Example:
   600 kcal ÷ 3.4 kcal/g x [100 ÷ 850 mL[1]] = 21%
   [1]Total daily fluids desired minus that from fats.

7. Calculate the goal dextrose infusion rate (DIR) in mg/kg/minute. Example:
   (850 mL ÷ 24 hours) x 21% x 0.166 ÷ 10 kg = 12.3 mg/kg/minute
   This patient's goal regimen would be: Dextrose 21%, amino acid 2.9%, 850 mL/day plus fat emulsion 20% 150 mL/day.

Suggested PN Monitoring Guidelines

Parameter	Suggested Frequency	
	Initial/Hospitalized	**Follow-up/Outpatient**
Growth		
Weight	Daily	Daily to every visit
Height/length	Weekly	Weekly to every visit
Body composition (triceps skinfold, bone age)	Initially	Monthly to annually
Metabolic (Serum[1])		
Electrolytes	Daily to twice weekly	Weekly to every visit
Magnesium	Daily to weekly	Weekly to every visit
Phosphorus	Daily to weekly	Weekly to every visit
BUN/creatinine	Weekly	Weekly to every visit
Acid-base status	Until stable	As indicated
Prealbumin	Weekly	Weekly to every visit
Glucose	Daily to weekly	Weekly to every visit
Triglyceride	Weekly	Weekly to every visit
Liver function tests	Weekly	Weekly to every visit
Complete blood count/differential	Weekly	Weekly to every visit
Platelets, PT/PTT	Weekly	As indicated
Iron indices	As indicated	Biannually to annually
Trace elements	As indicated	Annually
Carnitine	As indicated	As indicated
Folate/vitamin B_{12}	As indicated	As indicated
Ammonia	As indicated	As indicated
Bilirubin, direct	Weekly	As indicated
Clinical Calculations		
Fluid balance	Daily	As indicated
Projected vs actual intake	Daily	Weekly to every visit
Calorie/protein intake	Daily	As indicated

Frequency depends on clinical condition

[1]For metabolically unstable patients, need to check more frequently

Adapted from: Guidelines for the use of parenteral and enteral nutrition in adult and pediatric patients. ASPEN board of directors and the clinical guidelines task force. *JPEN J Parenter Enteral Nutr.* 2002;26(1 Suppl):1-138SA.

Pharmacologic considerations of mixing medications with PN solutions include:

- Adsorption — bag, bottle, tubing, filter
- Blood levels
- Site of injection/administration
- Flush
- Amino acid-dextrose concentrations
- pH factors
- Temperature
- Additives in solution
- Heparin dose

REFERENCES

ASPEN Board of Directors and The Clinical Guidelines Task Force. Guidelines for the use of parenteral and enteral nutrition in adult and pediatric patients. *JPEN J Parenter Enteral Nutr.* 2002;26(1 Suppl):1-138SA.

Carney LN, Nepa A, Cohen SS, et al. Parenteral and enteral nutrition support: determining the best way to feed. *The A.S.P.E.N Pediatric Nutrition Support Core Curriculum.* Corkins MR, Balint J, Bobo E, et al, eds. Silver Spring, MD: American Society of Parenteral and Enteral Nutrition. 2010;433-447.

Mirtallo J, Canada T, Johnson D, et al. Safe practices for parenteral nutrition. *JPEN J Parenter Enteral Nutr.* 2004;28(6):S39-S70.

IDEAL BODY WEIGHT CALCULATION

Adults (18 years and older)

IBW (male) = 50 + (2.3 x height in inches over 5 feet)

IBW (female) = 45.5 + (2.3 x height in inches over 5 feet)

IBW is in kg.

Children

a. 1 to 18 years (Traub 1980)

$$\text{IBW} = \frac{(\text{height}^2 \times 1.65)}{1{,}000}$$

IBW is in kg.

Height is in cm.

b. 5 feet and taller (Traub 1980)

IBW (male) = 39 + (2.27 x height in inches over 5 feet)

IBW (female) = 42.2 + (2.27 x height in inches over 5 feet)

IBW is in kg.

c. 1 to 17 years (Traub 1983)

$\text{IBW} = 2.396e^{0.01863\ (\text{height})}$

IBW is in kg.

Height is in cm.

REFERENCES

Traub SL, Johnson CE. Comparison of methods of estimating creatinine clearance in children. *Am J Hosp Pharm.* 1980;37(2):195-201.

Traub SL, Kichen L. Estimating ideal body mass in children. *Am J Hosp Pharm.* 1983;40(1):107-110.

BODY SURFACE AREA OF CHILDREN AND ADULTS

Calculating Body Surface Area in Children

In a child of average size, find weight and corresponding surface area on the boxed scale to the left or use the nomogram to the right. Lay a straightedge on the correct height and weight points for the child, then read the intersecting point on the surface area scale. (**Note:** 2.2 lb = 1 kg)

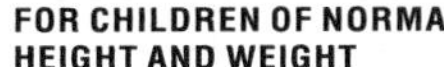

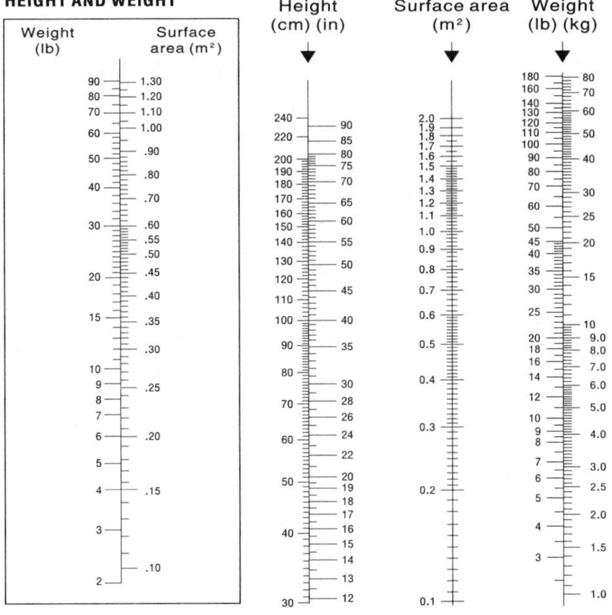

BODY SURFACE AREA FORMULA
(Adult and Pediatric)

$$BSA\ (m^2) = \sqrt{\frac{Ht\ (in) \times Wt\ (lb)}{3131}}$$ or, in metric: $$BSA\ (m^2) = \sqrt{\frac{Ht\ (cm) \times Wt\ (kg)}{3600}}$$

References

Lam TK and Leung DT, "More on Simplified Calculation of Body Surface Area," *N Engl J Med*, 1988, 318(17):1130 (Letter).

Mosteller RD, "Simplified Calculation of Body Surface Area", *N Engl J Med*, 1987, 317(17):1098 (Letter).

AVERAGE WEIGHTS AND SURFACE AREAS

Average Height, Weight, and Surface Area by Age and Gender

Age	Girls			Boys		
	Height (cm)	Weight (kg)	BSA (m^2)	Height (cm)	Weight (kg)	BSA (m^2)
Birth	49.5	3.4	0.22	50	3.6	0.22
3 mo	59	5.6	0.3	61	6	0.32
6 mo	65	7.2	0.36	67	7.9	0.38
9 mo	70	8.3	0.4	72	9.3	0.43
12 mo	74.5	9.5	0.44	75.5	10.3	0.46
15 mo	77	10.3	0.47	79	11.1	0.49
18 mo	80	11	0.49	82	11.7	0.52
21 mo	83	11.6	0.52	85	12.2	0.54
2 y	86	12	0.54	87.5	12.6	0.55
2.5 y	91	13	0.57	92	13.5	0.59
3 y	94.5	13.8	0.6	96	14.3	0.62
3.5 y	97	15	0.64	98	15	0.64
4 y	101	16	0.67	102	16	0.67
4.5 y	104	17	0.7	105	17	0.7
5 y	107.5	18	0.73	109	18.5	0.75
6 y	115	20	0.8	115	21	0.82
7 y	121.5	23	0.88	122	23	0.88
8 y	127.5	25.5	0.95	127.5	26	0.96
9 y	133	29	1.04	133.5	28.5	1.03
10 y	138	33	1.12	138.5	32	1.1
11 y	144	37	1.22	143.5	36	1.2
12 y	151	41.5	1.32	149	40.5	1.29
13 y	157	46	1.42	156	45.5	1.4
14 y	160.5	49.5	1.49	163.5	51	1.52
15 y	162	52	1.53	170	56	1.63
16 y	162.5	54	1.56	173.5	61	1.71
17 y	163	55	1.58	175	64.5	1.77
Adult[1]	163.5	58	1.62	177	83.5	2.03

Data extracted from the CDC growth charts based on the 50th percentile height and weight for a given age[2]

Body surface area calculation[3]: Square root of [(Ht x Wt) / 3,600]

[1]McDowell MA, Fryar CD, Hirsch R, Ogden CL. Anthropometric reference data for children and adults: US population, 1999-2002. *Adv Data*. 2005;(361):1-5.

[2]Centers for Disease Control and Prevention (CDC). 2000 CDC growth charts: United States. Available at http://www.cdc.gov/growthcharts. Accessed November 16, 2007.

[3]Mosteller RD. Simplified calculation of body-surface area *N Engl J Med*. 1987;317(17):1098.

PHYSICAL DEVELOPMENT

Weight gain first 6 weeks

20 g/day

Birth weight

regained by day 14
doubles by age 4 months
triples by age 12 months
quadruples by age 2 years

Teeth

1st tooth 6 to 18 months
teeth = age (months) – 6 (until 30 months)

Head circumference

35 cm at birth
44 cm by 6 months
47 cm by 1 year
1 cm/month for 1st year
0.25 cm/month 2nd year

Length

increases 50% by age 1 year
doubles by age 4 years
triples by age 13 years

Tanner Stages of Sexual Development

Stage	Characteristics	Age at Onset (mean ± SD)
Genital stages: Male		
1	Prepubertal	
2	Scrotum and testes enlarge; skin of scrotum reddens and rugations appear	11.4 ± 1.1 y
3	Penis lengthens; testes enlarge further	12.9 ± 1 y
4	Penis growth continues in length and width; glans develops adult form	13.8 ± 1 y
5	Development completed; adult appearance	14.9 ± 1.1 y
Breast development: Female		
1	Prepubertal	
2	Breast buds appear; areolae enlarge	11.2 ± 1.1 y
3	Elevation of breast contour; areolae enlarge	12.2 ± 1.1 y
4	Areolae and papilla form a secondary mound on breast	13.1 ± 1.2 y
5	Adult form	15.3 ± 1.7 y
Menarche		
Pubic hair: Both sexes		13.5 ± 1 y
1	Prepubertal, no coarse hair	
2	Longer, silky hair appears at base of penis or along labia	F: 11.7 ± 1.2 y M: 12 ± 1 y
3	Hair coarse, kinky, spreads over pubic bone	F: 12.4 ± 1.1 y M: 13.9 ± 1 y
4	Hair of adult quality but not spread to junction of medial thigh with perineum	F: 13 ± 1 y M: 14.4 ± 1.1 y
5	Spread to medial thigh	F: 14.4 ± 1.1 y M: 15.2 ± 1.1 y
6	"Male escutcheon"	Variable if occurs
Maximum growth rate		
Male at 14.1 ± 0.9 y		
Female at 12.1 ± 0.9 y		

PREVENTION OF CHEMOTHERAPY-INDUCED NAUSEA AND VOMITING IN CHILDREN

Note: Unless otherwise specified, emetogenic potential listed is for single agent treatment. For multi-agent regimens, if not otherwise specified, emetogenic potential should be based on the component with the higher emetic potential.

Highly Emetogenic Chemotherapy (Frequency of Emesis: >90%)

Altretamine
CARBOplatin
Carmustine >250 mg/m^2
CISplatin
Cyclophosphamide ≥1,000 mg/m^2
Cytarabine 3,000 mg/m^2
Dacarbazine
DACTINomycin
Mechlorethamine
Methotrexate ≥12 g/m^2
Procarbazine (oral)
Streptozocin
Thiotepa ≥300 mg/m^2
Multi-agent regimens:
- Cyclophosphamide + Anthracycline (doxorubicin or epirubicin)
- Cyclophosphamide + Etoposide
- Cytarabine 150 to 200 mg/m^2 + Daunorubicin
- Cytarabine 300 mg/m^2 + Etoposide
- Cytarabine 300 mg/m^2 + Teniposide
- Doxorubicin + Ifosfamide
- Doxorubicin + Methotrexate 5 g/m^2
- Etoposide + Ifosfamide

Moderately Emetogenic Chemotherapy (Frequency of Emesis: 30% to 90%)

Aldesleukin >12 to 15 million units/m^2
Amifostine >300 mg/m^2
Arsenic trioxide
AzaCITIDine
Bendamustine
Busulfan (IV)
Carmustine ≤250 mg/m^2
Clofarabine
Cyclophosphamide <1,000 mg/m^2 (IV)
Cyclophosphamide (oral)
Cytarabine >200 mg/m^2 to <3,000 mg/m^2
DAUNOrubicin
DOXOrubicin
EPIrubicin
Etoposide (oral)
IDArubicin
Ifosfamide
Imatinib
Intrathecal treatment (methotrexate and/or cytarabine ± hydrocortisone)
Irinotecan
Lomustine
Melphalan >50 mg/m^2
Methotrexate ≥250 **mg**/m^2 to <12 **g**/m^2
Mitotane
Oxaliplatin ≥75 mg/m^2
Temozolomide (IV)
Temozolomide (oral)

Low Emetogenic Chemotherapy (Frequency of Emesis: 10% to <30%)

Aldesleukin ≤12 million units/m^2
Amifostine ≤300 mg/m^2
Bexarotene (oral)
Busulfan (oral)
Capecitabine
Cytarabine ≤200 mg/m^2
DOCEtaxel
DOXOrubicin (liposomal)
Etoposide (IV)
Everolimus
Fludarabine (oral)
Fluorouracil
Gemcitabine
Ixabepilone
Methotrexate >50 to <250 mg/m^2
MitoMYcin
MitoXANtrone
Nilotinib
PACLitaxel
PACLitaxel (protein bound)
PEMEtrexed
Teniposide
Thiotepa <300 mg/m^2
Topotecan
Tretinoin
Vorinostat

Minimal Emetogenic Chemotherapy (Frequency of Emesis: <10%)

Alemtuzumab
Asparaginase
Bevacizumab
Bleomycin
Bortezomib
Cetuximab
Chlorambucil
Cladribine
Dasatinib
Decitabine
Denileukin diftitox
Dexrazoxane
Erlotinib
Fludarabine (IV)
Gefitinib
Gemtuzumab ozogamicin
Hydroxyurea
Interferon alfa
Lapatinib
Lenalidomide
Melphalan (oral, low dose)
Mercaptopurine (oral)
Methotrexate ≤50 mg/m^2
Methotrexate (oral)
Nelarabine
Panitumumab
Pegaspargase
Peginterferon alfa
Pentostatin
RiTUXimab
SORAfenib
SUNItinib
Temsirolimus
Thalidomide
Thioguanine (oral)
Trastuzumab
Valrubicin
VinBLAStine
VinCRIStine
Vinorelbine (IV)

Prevention of Acute Nausea and Vomiting

Acute nausea and vomiting includes vomiting, retching, or nausea which occurs within 24 hours of administration of chemotherapeutic agents. Guidelines for prevention of acute nausea and vomiting from the Pediatric Oncology Group of Ontario (POGO) recommend the following for pediatric patients ages 1 month to 18 years (Dupuis 2013):

For prevention of acute nausea and vomiting due to chemotherapy with **highly** emetogenic risk:
- Children ≥12 years and Adolescents receiving chemotherapy agents that do **not** potentially interact with aprepitant: Ondansetron or granisetron plus dexamethasone plus aprepitant
- Children ≥12 years and Adolescents receiving chemotherapy agents that **potentially** interact with aprepitant: Ondansetron or granisetron plus dexamethasone
- Infants and Children <12 years: Ondansetron or granisetron plus dexamethasone
- Pediatric patients receiving highly emetogenic chemotherapeutic agents who cannot receive corticosteroids (due to contraindications): Ondansetron or granisetron plus chlorpromazine or nabilone

For prevention of acute nausea and vomiting due to chemotherapy with **moderately** emetogenic risk:
- Infants, Children, and Adolescents: Ondansetron or granisetron plus dexamethasone
- Pediatric patients receiving moderately emetogenic chemotherapeutic agents who cannot receive corticosteroids (due to contraindications): Ondansetron or granisetron plus chlorpromazine or metoclopramide or nabilone

For prevention of acute nausea and vomiting due to chemotherapy with **low** emetogenic risk:
- Infants, Children, and Adolescents: Ondansetron or granisetron

For prevention of acute nausea and vomiting due to chemotherapy with **minimal** emetogenic risk: No routine prophylaxis

Pediatric Antiemetic Dosing Based on Emetogenic Potential

Name	Chemotherapy Emetogenic Potential	Route/Dose
Serotonin Antagonists		
Granisetron	High	IV: 40 mcg/kg/dose as a single daily dose
	Moderate or low	IV: 40 mcg/kg/dose as a single daily dose Oral: 40 mcg/kg/dose every 12 hours
Ondansetron	High	IV, Oral: 0.15 mg/kg/dose (5 mg/m^2/dose); prior to chemotherapy and then every 8 hours (maximum recommended IV dose: 16 mg)
	Moderate	IV, Oral: 0.15 mg/kg/dose (5 mg/m^2/dose); prior to chemotherapy and then every 12 hours (maximum: 8 mg/dose)
	Low	IV, Oral: 0.3 mg/kg/dose (10 mg/m^2/dose); prior to chemotherapy (maximum IV dose: 16 mg)
Substance P/Neurokinin 1 Receptor Antagonist		
Aprepitant	High	Children ≥12 years and Adolescents: Oral: 125 mg on day 1, followed by 80 mg once daily on days 2 and 3
Corticosteroid		
Dexamethasone	High	IV, Oral: 6 mg/m^2/dose every 6 hours **Note:** If administering with aprepitant, reduce dexamethasone dose by 50%
	Moderate	IV, Oral: ≤0.6 m^2: 2 mg every 12 hours >0.6 m^2 4 mg every 12 hours **Note:** If administering with aprepitant, reduce dexamethasone dose by 50%
Phenothiazine		
ChlorproMAZINE	High or moderate	IV: 0.5 mg/kg/dose every 6 hours
Dopamine Receptor Antagonist		
Metoclopramide	Moderate	IV, Oral: 1 mg/kg/dose IV prior to chemotherapy, then 0.0375 mg/kg/dose orally every 6 hours (administer concomitantly with diphenhydramine or benztropine)
Cannabinoid		
Nabilone	High or moderate	Oral: <18 kg: 0.5 mg twice daily 18 to 30 kg: 1 mg twice daily >30 kg: 1 mg 3 times daily Maximum daily dose: 0.06 mg/kg/**day**

Prevention and Treatment of Anticipatory Nausea and Vomiting

The risk for anticipatory nausea and vomiting will be minimized if acute and delayed nausea and vomiting associated with chemotherapy are optimally managed. If anticipatory nausea and vomiting develop, interventions including hypnosis and/or systematic desensitization (eg, deep muscle relaxation with imagery) may be offered to help manage symptoms (Dupuis 2014; Roila 2010). Guidelines for prevention and treatment of anticipatory nausea and vomiting from POGO recommend the following for pediatric patients ages 1 month to 18 years (Dupuis 2014): Lorazepam 0.04 to 0.08 mg/kg/dose (maximum dose: 2 mg) administered orally once at bedtime the evening prior to chemotherapy and once prior to chemotherapy the next day may be used to prevent or treat anticipatory nausea and vomiting.

REFERENCES

Basch E, Prestrud AA, Hesketh PJ, et al. Antiemetics: American Society of Clinical Oncology clinical practice guideline update. *J Clin Oncol.* 2011;29(31):4189-4198.

Dupuis LL, Boodhan S, Holdsworth M, et al. Guideline for the prevention of acute nausea and vomiting due to antineoplastic medication in pediatric cancer patients. *Pediatr Blood Cancer.* 2013;60(7):1073-1082.

Dupuis LL, Boodhan S, Sung L, et al. Guideline for the classification of the acute emetogenic potential of antineoplastic medication in pediatric cancer patients. *Pediatr Blood Cancer.* 2011;57(2):191-198.

Dupuis LL, Robinson PD, Boodhan S, et al. Guideline for the prevention and treatment of anticipatory nausea and vomiting due to chemotherapy in pediatric cancer patients. *Pediatr Blood Cancer.* 2014;61(8):1506-1512.

Multinational Association of Supportive Care in Cancer. MASCC/ESMO antiemetic guideline 2013. http://www.mascc.org/assets/documents/mascc_guidelines_english_2013.pdf. Accessed October 2013.

National Comprehensive Cancer Network (NCCN). Clinical practice guidelines in oncology: antiemesis. v.2.2014. http://www.nccn.org/professionals/physician_gls/PDF/antiemesis.pdf

Roila F, Herrstedt J, Aapro M, et al. Guideline update for MASCC and ESMO in the prevention of chemotherapy- and radiotherapy-induced nausea and vomiting: results of the Perugia consensus conference. *Ann Oncol.* 2010;21(Suppl 5):v232-v243.

TUMOR LYSIS SYNDROME

INTRODUCTION

Tumor lysis syndrome (TLS) is a potentially life-threatening disorder that is characterized as an acute metabolic disturbance resulting from the rapid destruction of tumor cells. Cellular destruction releases intracellular constituents (nucleic acids, anions, cations, peptides) that overwhelm the body's normal mechanisms for their utilization, excretion, and elimination. Signs and symptoms of TLS often develop within 72 hours of beginning cytotoxic chemotherapy in patients with newly diagnosed acute leukemias (acute lymphoblastic leukemia [ALL] and acute myeloid leukemia [AML]) or lymphoproliferative malignancies (Burkitt's and non-Burkitt's lymphomas). Moreover, TLS can occur spontaneously in malignant diseases with vigorous cell turnover. Although most commonly reported in patients with hematologic and lymphoid malignancies, TLS has also been reported with solid tumors such as breast cancer, colon cancer, melanoma, ovarian cancer, prostate cancer, small cell lung cancer, and testicular cancer. Acute TLS attributed to administration of a corticosteroid, imatinib, rituximab, sorafenib, and zoledronic acid in patients with treatment-sensitive tumors have been reported in the medical literature. Additional treatment and diagnostic procedures attributed with causing tumor lysis syndrome include total body irradiation, splenic irradiation, staging laparotomy, laparoscopic splenectomy preceded by splenic artery embolization, and radiofrequency interstitial thermal ablation of metastatic hepatic lesions. Metabolic abnormalities associated with acute TLS include hyperphosphatemia, hyperkalemia, hyperuricemia, azotemia, hypocalcemia, and metabolic acidosis. Cardiac arrhythmias, seizures, and major organ failure can occur in severe cases of TLS. Hyperkalemia, hyperuricemia, and hypocalcemia can produce cardiac arrhythmias, tetany, and sudden death. Acute renal failure can occur due to precipitation of uric acid and calcium phosphate in the renal tubules.

PREDISPOSING FACTORS

1. Leukemia with high white blood cell count (>25,000/mm^3) or rapidly increasing peripheral blast count
2. Solid tumors with bulky disease (>10 cm), high tumor cell proliferation rate, wide metastatic dispersal, and/or bone marrow involvement
3. Acute myeloid leukemia with history of chronic myelomonocytic leukemia
4. Marked sensitivity of the tumor to a particular treatment modality
5. Renal impairment, including pre-existing volume depletion
6. Elevated pretreatment lactic dehydrogenase (LDH) serum concentrations (>2 times ULN)
7. Elevated pretreatment uric acid (>7.5 mg/dL), potassium, and/or phosphate serum concentrations independent of renal impairment

CLINICAL FEATURES AND TREATMENT

Classification and Risk Stratification

TLS can be described as either laboratory (LTLS) or clinical (CTLS) type. LTLS is the presence of 2 or more abnormal lab values or a 25% change in lab values within 3 days before or 7 days after chemotherapy. Laboratory values to monitor include uric acid, potassium, phosphorus, and calcium. CTLS is defined as LTLS with at least one clinical manifestation such as renal insufficiency, seizures, cardiac arrhythmias, or sudden death.

Certain patients have greater risk for developing LTLS and/or CTLS and should be treated more aggressively to prevent its occurrence. Risk stratification guides what type of prophylaxis and management therapies should be used for which patients. Patients classified as high risk should have aggressive prophylactic treatment with hydration and rasburicase while being monitored closely in an ICU or similarly monitored setting. Intermediate risk patients should receive prophylactic treatment with hydration and allopurinol; if hyperuricemia does develop in these patients, consider rasburicase. Initial management of pediatric patients at intermediate risk may include rasburicase. Patients at low risk for developing TLS require no prophylactic therapy but should be monitored closely and treated as necessary.

Risk Stratification

Type of Cancer	High Risk	Intermediate Risk	Low Risk
Non-Hodgkin lymphoma (NHL)	Burkitt's, Burkitt's-ALL (B-ALL), lymphoblastic lymphoma	Diffuse large B-cell lymphoma (DLBCL)	Indolent NHL
Acute lymphoblastic leukemia (ALL)	WBC ≥100,000 cells/mm^3	WBC 50,000 to 100,000 cells/mm^3	WBC ≤50,000 cells/mm^3
Acute myeloid leukemia (AML)	WBC ≥50,000 cells/mm^3; monoblastic; rapidly increasing peripheral blast count	WBC 10,000 to 50,000 cells/mm^3	WBC ≤10,000 cells/mm^3
Chronic lymphocytic leukemia (CLL)		WBC 10,000 to 100,000 cells/mm^3; treatment with fludarabine	WBC ≤10,000 cells/mm^3
Other hematologic malignancies (chronic myeloid leukemia [CML], multiple myeloma) and solid tumors		Rapid proliferation with expected rapid response to therapy	Remainder of patients

LDH ≥2 x ULN, renal impairment, or elevated uric acid, potassium, or phosphate serum concentrations increases risk level (Sarno 2013)

Monitoring

High risk patients should have laboratory and clinical parameters (serum uric acid, phosphate, calcium, creatinine, LDH, and fluid input and output) monitored 4 to 6 hours after initiating chemotherapy. For all patients treated with rasburicase, monitor serum uric acid 4 hours after administration, then every 6 to 8 hours thereafter until resolution of TLS occurs. Frequent assessment of serum chemistries and fluid balance is necessary to avert pathophysiologic adverse events and guide the duration of rasburicase therapy. Electrolyte and fluid abnormalities must be addressed at the time that they are identified. However, rasburicase is administered no more frequently than once daily to achieve uric acid control for a duration of 5 to 7 doses (has also been administered as a single dose schedule with repeat doses, if needed, based on serum uric acid level).

Intermediate risk patients should be monitored throughout and for at least 24 hours after completion of chemotherapy. If rasburicase is not used, laboratory parameters should be monitored 8 hours after initiation of chemotherapy and regularly thereafter according to the patient's clinical condition and institutional practice.

Low risk patients should be monitored as determined by the institution and patient factors. If TLS has not occurred within 2 days, development is very unlikely.

General Principles

Prevention and early management of TLS are aimed at decreasing the risk of morbidity and mortality from cardiac arrhythmias, seizures, and organ failure. In patients with high or intermediate risk, vigorous hydration is the cornerstone of the initial management for acute or potential TLS. Patients should be hydrated with 2 to 3 L/m^2/day (200 mL/kg/day if ≤10 kg) intravenous fluid (Children: $D_5W^1/_4NS$; Adults: Not specified) to maintain urine output of 80 to 100 mL/m^2/hour (4 to 6 mL/kg/hour if ≤10 kg), with diuretic use if necessary (avoid or minimize diuretic use in patients with hypovolemia or obstructive uropathy). Due to the tendency for calcium phosphate nephrocalcinosis and the potential for metabolic alkalosis, urinary alkalinization with sodium bicarbonate is no longer universally recommended for the treatment and prevention of TLS (Coiffier 2008).

Allopurinol should be administered to intermediate risk patients to decrease endogenous uric acid production and reduce associated urinary obstruction; dose reductions may be required for renal dysfunction (Coiffier 2008). In adult or pediatric patients, give 150 to 300 mg/m^2/day (or 10 mg/kg/day in pediatric patients) divided every 8 hours (maximum: 800 mg/day) orally or 200 to 400 mg/m^2/day IV (in 1 to 3 divided doses; maximum: 600 mg/day). The time to maximum effect of allopurinol is 27 hours. While allopurinol decreases uric acid production, it is ineffective in reducing markedly elevated uric acid concentrations which may allow renotubular crystal formation and obstruction despite its administration. In addition, allopurinol impedes the clearance of purine analogues such as mercaptopurine and azathioprine.

Rasburicase is administered to rapidly reduce uric acid concentrations; significant reduction in plasma uric acid concentrations is measurable four hours following drug administration. Rasburicase, which is a recombinant form of urate oxidase produced in *Saccharomyces cerevisiae*, catalyzes the degradation of uric acid to allantoin, which is more soluble and readily excreted by the kidneys. Rasburicase is reserved for patients at high risk for TLS (or considered in intermediate risk pediatric patients), patients with elevated uric acid concentrations, or patients with signs of moderate to severe renal impairment or other major organ dysfunction. The major risks associated with administration of rasburicase include anaphylaxis, hypersensitivity reactions, methemoglobinemia, and hemolysis. Rasburicase is contraindicated in patients with glucose-6-phosphate dehydrogenase deficiency due to an increased risk of hemolysis. An additional concern with rasburicase administration is the development of neutralizing antibodies. This phenomenon was observed in 64% of 28 normal, healthy volunteers studied; the effect of neutralizing antibodies on the efficacy of this product with repeated usage is unknown. Rasburicase appears to be less immunogenic in patients with hematologic or lymphoid malignancies receiving chemotherapy. One study reported detection of neutralizing antibodies in 2% of 184 patients with hematologic or lymphoid malignancies treated with rasburicase before and throughout chemotherapy (Cortes 2010).

Rasburicase is approved for use in pediatric and adult patients, with the labeled dose of 0.2 mg/kg/dose daily for up to five days. Due to the costs and risks of therapy plus the immediate and measurable effects of rasburicase, some centers administer a single dose which is repeated daily as warranted by plasma uric acid concentrations. The following doses (based on risk for TLS) and duration of treatment based on plasma uric acid concentrations have been recommended for children: 0.2 mg/kg once daily (duration based on plasma uric acid concentrations) for high risk patients, 0.15 mg/kg once daily (duration based on plasma uric acid concentrations) for intermediate risk, and 0.05 to 0.1 mg/kg once daily (duration based on clinical judgment) if used for low-risk patients (Coiffier 2008). Weight- and risk-based dosing as detailed above has been reported in adults. Fixed-dose rasburicase, ranging from 3 to 7.5 mg as a single dose (Hutcherson 2006; McDonnell 2006; Reeves 2008; Trifilio 2006) with doses (1.5 to 6 mg) repeated if needed (based on serum uric acid concentrations) has also been reported in adults. The optimal timing of rasburicase administration (with respect to chemotherapy administration) is not specified in the manufacter's labeling. In some studies, chemotherapy was administered 4 to 24 hours after the first rasburicase dose (Cortes 2010; Kikuchi 2009; Vadhan-Raj 2012); however, rasburicase generally may be administered irrespective of chemotherapy timing.

Upon rasburicase administration, serum uric acid levels generally decrease within 4 hours. In order to allow for appropriate therapeutic effect and to accurately assess the need for a repeat dose, repeat uric acid levels should be drawn no earlier than 4 hours post-rasburicase dose. Rasburicase will degrade uric acid *in vitro* when the blood sample is stored at room temperature. Consequently, to prevent artifactually depressed uric acid concentrations, plasma samples must be collected in prechilled tubes, then immediately placed in an ice water bath until centrifuged at 4°C. Plasma must be analyzed within four hours of collection.

Clinical features and treatment for specific metabolic disorders are discussed in the following sections.

Hyperuricemia

Cytolysis during TLS releases purine and pyrimidine nucleotides into the bloodstream and extracellular tissues. Oxidation of the purines hypoxanthine and xanthine yields uric acid, which can precipitate in the renal tubules and cause oliguric renal failure. A high concentration of uric acid and an acidic urine pH promote uric acid crystallization and renotubular precipitation. Maintenance of urine flow is utilized to reduce purine precipitation and preserve renal function. Allopurinol blocks the endogenous production of uric acid by inhibiting the enzyme xanthine oxidase, which oxidizes hypoxanthine and xanthine to uric acid. Allopurinol is used prophylactically during the early management of TLS in intermediate risk patients. Rasburicase decreases existing uric acid concentrations by conversion of this molecule to the inactive and soluble metabolite allantoin, which is readily excreted by the kidneys. Rasburicase should be used prophylactically in high risk patients or in patients with preexisting hyperuricemia or acute renal impairment.

Hyperkalemia

Potassium is primarily an intracellular ion that is released during massive cellular breakdown. Increasing concentrations of serum potassium can be dangerous, leading to cardiac arrhythmias or sudden death, especially in the presence of hypocalcemia (see following discussion). Standard treatments to remove potassium from the blood stream and extracellular fluids should be initiated as warranted by the patient's serum potassium concentration and electrocardiographic abnormalities. Other sources of potassium intake (including nutritional sources, medications, and intravenous solutions) should be eliminated in patients at risk for or with TLS. Pharmaceutical measures routinely used to manage hyperkalemia in patients with TLS include volume expansion with forced diuresis, administration of insulin with glucose, and the cation exchange product sodium polystyrene sulfonate. Sodium bicarbonate can be administered IV push to induce influx of potassium into cells. Textbook algorithms for management of hyperkalemia include instructions for administration of calcium as a cardioprotective measure; however, this is **not** a standard intervention in the setting of TLS. Calcium gluconate administration must be done judiciously in the patient with TLS as it can precipitate as calcium phosphate in highly perfused tissues. Monitor patient ECG and cardiac rhythm closely for arrhythmias.

Hyperphosphatemia

The release of intracellular inorganic phosphate following massive cellular breakdown sets into motion several important clinical features. Serum phosphate concentrations will quickly exceed the threshold for normal renal excretion, with phosphate excretion becoming limited by the glomerular filtration rate. Any azotemia that develops during therapy will hinder phosphate excretion. Treatment includes the use of phosphate binders such as aluminum hydroxide, sevelamer, calcium carbonate (avoid use in patients with hypercalcemia and limit use to pediatric patients), or lanthanum carbonate (avoid use in pediatric patients). In severe cases of hyperphosphatemia, hemodialysis or hemofiltration may be necessary.

Hypocalcemia

High phosphate concentrations will also cause reciprocal hypocalcemia. Although generally asymptomatic, hypocalcemia may cause neuromuscular irritation, tetany, and cardiac dysrhythmias. Symptomatic patients may receive calcium gluconate intravenously (slowly, with ECG monitoring) to increase serum calcium concentrations. Unfortunately, despite hypocalcemia, the solubility product of calcium and phosphate may be exceeded in acute TLS due to high concentrations of phosphate, resulting in tissue calcification and organ failure. For this reason, calcium gluconate should be administered cautiously and only if necessary.

Hemodialysis/Hemofiltration

Due to the unpredictability of TLS, renal replacement therapy may be needed and can be lifesaving. Hemodialysis or hemofiltration may be used to control and maintain fluid volume and/or to remove uric acid, phosphate, and potassium from serum. Intermittent hemodialysis, continuous arteriovenous hemodialysis, or continuous veno-venous hemodiafiltration should be considered as warranted by the severity of serum chemistry abnormalities, major organ dysfunction, and the patient's response to pharmaceutical treatments.

Leukoreduction/Plasmapheresis

Leukoreduction, which utilizes plasmapheresis and hydroxyurea to rapidly decrease the peripheral white blood cell count, is performed in some cases of acute myeloid leukemia. The primary goal of leukoreduction is to reduce the risk of complications from serum hyperviscosity syndrome consequent to a very high white blood cell count. However, leukoreduction can indirectly reduce the risk of TLS as removal of circulating blasts diminishes the primary source of cells undergoing lysis in patients with acute myeloid leukemia. Plasmapheresis is used infrequently and very cautiously in patients with acute promyelocytic leukemia due to the inherent disease-related risks of coagulopathy, hemorrhage, and hypotension in this population. Plasmapheresis is rarely used for leukoreduction in patients with lymphocytic or lymphoblastic leukemias as these patients are at lower risk for hyperviscosity syndrome despite a high white blood cell count. This is because lymphocytes do not have the same 'sticky' quality as myeloid cells. Hydroxyurea can be used without plasmapheresis to achieve leukoreduction.

REFERENCES

Abu-Alfa AK, Younes A. Tumor lysis syndrome and acute kidney injury: evaluation, prevention, and management. *Am J Kidney Dis*. 2010;55(5 Suppl 3): S1-S13.

Al-Kali A, Farooq S, Tfayli A. Tumor lysis syndrome after starting treatment with gleevec in a patient with chronic myelogenous leukemia. *J Clin Pharm Ther*. 2009;34(5):607-610.

Arnold TM, Reuter JP, Delman BS, Shanholtz CB. Use of single-dose rasburicase in an obese female. *Ann Pharmacother*. 2004;38(9):1428-1431.

Barry BD, Kell MR, Redmond HP. Tumor lysis syndrome following endoscopic radiofrequency interstitial thermal ablation of colorectal liver metastases. *Surg Endosc*. 2002;16(7):1109.

Cairo MS, Bishop M. Tumour lysis syndrome: new therapeutic strategies and classification. *Br J Haematol*. 2004;127(1):3-11.

Cairo MS, Coiffier B, Reiter A, Younes A; TLS Expert Panel. Recommendations for the evaluation of risk and prophylaxis of tumour lysis syndrome (TLS) in adults and children with malignant diseases: an expert TLS panel consensus. *Br J Haematol*. 2010;149(4):578-586.

Chen SW, Hwang WS, Tsao CJ, Liu HS, Huang GC. Hydroxyurea and splenic irradiation-induced tumour lysis syndrome: a case report and review of the literature. *J Clin Pharm Ther*. 2005;30(6):623-625.

Coiffier B, Altman A, Pui CH, Younes A, Cairo MS. Guidelines for the management of pediatric and adult tumor lysis syndrome: an evidence-based review. *J Clin Oncol*. 2008;26(16):2767-2778.

Coiffier B, Mounier N, Bologna S, et al. Efficacy and safety of rasburicase (recombinant urate oxidase) for the prevention and treatment of hyperuricemia during induction chemotherapy of aggressive non-hodgkin's lymphoma: results of the GRAAL1 (Groupe d'Etude Des Lymphomes De l'Adulte trial on rasburicase activity in adult lymphoma) study. *J Clin Oncol*. 2003;21(23):4402-4406.

Cortes J, Moore JO, Maziarz RT, et al. Control of plasma uria acid in adults at risk for tumor lysis syndrome: efficacy and safety of rasburicase alone and rasburicase followed by allopurinol compared with allopurinol alone – results of a multicenter phase III study. *J Clin Oncol*. 2010;28(27):4207-4213.

Duzova A, Cetin M, Gümrük F, Yetgin S. Acute tumour lysis syndrome following a single-dose corticosteroid in children with acute lymphoblastic leukaemia. *Eur J Haematol*. 2001;66(6):404-407.

Gemici C. Tumour lysis syndrome in solid tumours. *Clin Oncol (R Coll Radiol)*. 2006;18(10):773-780.

Habib GS, Saliba WR. Tumor lysis syndrome after hydrocortisone treatment in metastatic melanoma: a case report and review of the literature. *Am J Med Sci.* 2002;323(3):155-157.
Huang WS, Yang CH. Sorafenib induced tumor lysis syndrome in an advanced hepatocellular carcinoma patient. *World J Gastroenterol.* 2009;15(35):4464-4466.
Hutcherson DA, Gammon DC, Bhatt MS, Faneuf M. Reduced-dose rasburicase in the treatment of adults with hyperuricemia associated with malignancy. *Pharmacotherapy.* 2006;26(2):242-247.
Jabr FI. Acute tumor lysis syndrome induced by rituximab in diffuse large B-cell lymphoma. *Int J Hematol.* 2005;82(4):312-314.
Kikuchi A, Kigasawa H, Tsurusawa M, et al. A study of rasburicase for the management of hyperuricemia in pediatric patients with newly diagnosed hematologic malignancies at high risk for tumor lysis syndrome. *Int J Hematol.* 2009;90(4):492-500.
Kurt M, Onal IK, Elkiran T, Altun B, Altundag K, Gullu I. Acute tumor lysis syndrome triggered by zoledronic acid in patient with metastatic lung adenocarcinoma. *Med Oncol.* 2005;22(2):203-206.
Lee MH, Cheng KI, Jang RC, Hsu JH, Dai ZK, Wu JR. Tumour lysis syndrome developing during an operation. *Anaesthesia.* 2007;62(1):85-87.
Lee AC, Li CH, So KT, Chan R. Treatment of impending tumor lysis with single-dose rasburicase. *Ann Pharmacother.* 2003;37(11):1614-1617.
Leibowitz AB, Adamsky C, Gabrilove J, Labow DM. Intraoperative acute tumor lysis syndrome during laparoscopic splenectomy preceded by splenic artery embolization. *Surg Laparosc Endosc Percutan Tech.* 2007;17(3):210-211.
Lerza R, Botta M, Barsotti B, et al. Dexamethazone-induced acute tumor lysis syndrome in a T-cell malignant lymphoma. *Leuk Lymphoma.* 2002;43(5):1129-1132.
Linck D, Basara N, Tran V, et al. Peracute onset of severe tumor lysis syndrome immediately after 4 Gy fractionated TBI as part of reduced intensity preparative regimen in a patient with T-ALL with high tumor burden. *Bone Marrow Transplant.* 2003;31(10):935-937.
Liu CY, Sims-McCallum RP, Schiffer CA. A single dose of rasburicase is sufficient for the treatment of hyperuricemia in patients receiving chemotherapy. *Leuk Res.* 2005;29(4):463-465.
Mato AR, Riccio BE, Qin L, et al. A predictive model for the detection of tumor lysis syndrome during AML induction therapy. *Leuk Lymphoma.* 2006;47(5):877-883.
McBride A, Westervelt P. Recognizing and managing the expanded risk of tumor lysis syndrome in hematologic and solid malignancies. *J Hematol Oncol.* 2012;5:75.
McDonnell AM, Lenz KL, Frei-Lahr DA, Hayslip J, Hall PD. Single-dose rasburicase 6 mg in the management of tumor lysis syndrome in adults. *Pharmacotherapy.* 2006;26(6):806-812.
National Comprehensive Cancer Network (NCCN). Practice guidelines in oncology: acute myeloid leukemia, version 1.2011. http://www.nccn.org/professionals/physician_gls/PDF/aml.pdf
Oztop I, Demirkan B, Yaren A, et al. Rapid tumor lysis syndrome in a patient with metastatic colon cancer as a complication of treatment with 5-fluorouracil/leucoverin and irinotecan. *Tumori.* 2004;90(5):514-516.
Reeves DJ, Bestul DJ. Evaluation of a single fixed dose of rasburicase 7.5 mg for the treatment of hyperuricemia in adults with cancer. *Pharmacother.* 2008;28(6):685–690.
Riccio B, Mato A, Olson EM, Berns JS, Luger S. Spontaneous tumor lysis syndrome in acute myeloid leukemia: two cases and a review of the literature. *Cancer Biol Ther.* 2006;5(12):1614-1617.
Rostom AY, El-Hussainy G, Kandil A, Allam A. Tumor lysis syndrome following hemi-body irradiation for metastatic breast cancer. *Ann Oncol.* 2000;11(10):1349-1351.
Sarno J. Prevention and management of tumor lysis syndrome in adults with malignancy. *J Adv Pract Oncol.* 2013;4(2):101-106.
Sorscher SM. Tumor lysis syndrome following docetaxel therapy for extensive metastatic prostate cancer. *Cancer Chemother Pharmacol.* 2004;54(2):191-192.
Theodorou D, Lagoudianakis E, Pattas M, et al. Pretreatment tumor lysis syndrome associated with bulky retroperitoneal tumors. Recognition is the mainstay of therapy. *Tumori.* 2006;92(6):540-541.
Trifilio S, Gordon L, Singhal S, et al. Reduced-dose rasburicase (recombinant xanthine oxidase) in adult cancer patients with hyperuricemia. *Bone Marrow Transplant.* 2006;37(11):997-1001.
Vadhan-Raj S, Fayad LE, Fanale MA, et al. A randomized trial of a single-dose rasburicase versus five-daily doses in patients at risk for tumor lysis syndrome. *Ann Oncol.* 2012;23(6):1640-1645.
Wagner J, Arora S. Oncologic metabolic emergencies. *Emerg Med Clin North Am.* 2014;32(3):509-525.
Yahata T, Nishikawa N, Aoki Y, Tanaka K. Tumor lysis syndrome associated with weekly paclitaxel treatment in a case with ovarian cancer. *Gynecol Oncol.* 2006;103(2):752-754.
Zigrossi P, Brustia M, Bobbio F, Campanini M. Flare and tumor lysis syndrome with atypical features after letrozole therapy in advanced breast cancer. A case report. *Ann Ital Med Int.* 2001;16(2):112-117.

TOTAL BLOOD VOLUME

Age	Example Weight (kg) [age]	Approximate Total Blood Volume (mL/kg)[1]	Estimated Total Blood Volume (mL)
Premature infant	1.5	89 to 105	134 to 158
Term newborn	3.4	78 to 86	265 to 292
1 to 12 months	7.6 (6 months)	73 to 78	555 to 593
1 to 3 years	12.4 (2 years)	74 to 82	918 to 1,017
4 to 6 years	18.2 (5 years)	80 to 86	1,456 to 1,565
7 to 18 years	45.5 (13 years)	83 to 90	3,777 to 4,095
Adults	70	68 to 88	4,760 to 6,160

[1]Approximate total blood volume information compiled from: *Nathan and Oski's Hematology of Infancy and Childhood*. 5th ed. Nathan DG, Orkin SH, eds. Philadelphia, PA: WB Saunders; 1998.

ASSESSMENT OF LIVER FUNCTION

Child-Pugh Score

Component	Score Given for Observed Findings		
	1	2	3
Encephalopathy grade[1]	None	1 to 2	3 to 4
Ascites	None	Mild or controlled by diuretics	Moderate or refractory despite diuretics
Albumin (g/dL)	>3.5	2.8 to 3.5	<2.8
Total bilirubin (mg/dL)	<2 (<34 micromoles/L)	2 to 3 (34 to 50 micromoles/L)	>3 (>50 micromoles/L)
or			
Modified total bilirubin[2]	<4	4 to 7	>7
Prothrombin time (seconds prolonged)	<4	4 to 6	>6
or			
INR	<1.7	1.7 to 2.3	>2.3

[1]**Encephalopathy Grades**

Grade 0: Normal consciousness, personality, neurological examination, electroencephalogram
Grade 1: Restless, sleep disturbed, irritable/agitated, tremor, impaired handwriting, 5 cps waves
Grade 2: Lethargic, time-disoriented, inappropriate, asterixis, ataxia, slow triphasic waves
Grade 3: Somnolent, stuporous, place-disoriented, hyperactive reflexes, rigidity, slower waves
Grade 4: Unrousable coma, no personality/behavior, decerebrate, slow 2 to 3 cps delta activity

Alternative Encephalopathy Grades

Grade 1: Mild confusion, anxiety, restlessness, fine tremor, slowed coordination
Grade 2: Drowsiness, disorientation, asterixis
Grade 3: Somnolent but rousable, marked confusion, incomprehensible speech, incontinent, hyperventilation
Grade 4: Coma, decerebrate posturing, flaccidity

[2]Modified total bilirubin used to score patients who have Gilbert syndrome or who are taking indinavir.

CHILD-PUGH CLASSIFICATION

Class A (mild hepatic impairment): Score 5 to 6
Class B (moderate hepatic impairment): Score 7 to 9
Class C (severe hepatic impairment): Score 10 to 15

REFERENCES

Centers for Disease Control and Prevention (CDC). Report of the NIH panel to define principles of therapy of HIV infection and guidelines for the use of antiretroviral agents in HIV-infected adults and adolescents. March 2004. Available at http://www.aidsinfo.nih.gov

US Department of Health and Human Services Food and Drug Administration. Guidance for industry, pharmacokinetics in patients with impaired hepatic function: study design, data analysis, and impact on dosing and labeling. May 2003. Available at http://www.fda.gov/OHRMS/DOCKETS/98fr/99D-5047-GDL00002.pdf

HOTLINE AND IMPORTANT PHONE NUMBERS

AIDS Hotline (National)	(800) 232-4636
American Association of Poison Control Centers (AAPCC)	(800) 222-1222
American College of Clinical Pharmacy (ACCP)	(913) 492-3311
American Dental Association (ADA)	(312) 440-2500
American Medical Association (AMA)	(800) 621-8335
American Pharmacists Association (APhA)	(202) 628-4410
American Society of Health-System Pharmacists	(866) 279-0681
Animal Poison Control Center (24-hours)	(888) 426-4435
Canadian Pharmacists Association	(613) 523-7877
Center for Disease Control	(800) CDC-INFO
FDA (Rare Diseases/Orphan Drugs)	(301) 796-8660
National Cancer Institute	(800) 4-CANCER
Asthma and Allergy Foundation of America	(800) 7-ASTHMA
Epilepsy Foundation	(800) 332-1000
National Council on Patient Information & Education	(301) 340-3940
National Institute of Health	(301) 496-4000
National Capital Poison Center	(800) 222-1222
Pediatric Pharmacy Advocacy Group (PPAG) Membership Information	(901) 380-3617
National Pesticide Information Center	(800) 858-7378
Rocky Mountain Poison Control Information	(800) 222-1222

PREVENTION OF INFECTIVE ENDOCARDITIS

Recommendations by the American Heart Association

(*Circulation*. 2007;116(15):1736-1754.)

The recommendations were formulated by a writing group under the auspices of the American Heart Association (AHA), and included representation from the Infectious Diseases Society of America (IDSA), the American Academy of Pediatrics (AAP), and the American Dental Association (ADA). Additionally, input was received from both national and international experts on infective endocarditis (IE). These guidelines are based on expert interpretation and review of scientific literature from 1950 through 2006. The consensus statement was subsequently reviewed by outside experts not affiliated with the writing group and by the Science Advisory and Coordinating Committee of the American Heart Association. These guidelines are meant to aid practitioners but are not intended as the standard of care or as a substitute for clinical judgment.

In a major departure from the former recommendations, the current guidelines have been greatly simplified to place a much greater emphasis on a very limited number of underlying cardiac conditions (see Table 1). These specific conditions have been associated with the highest risk of adverse outcomes due to IE. Patients should receive IE prophylaxis only if they are undergoing certain invasive procedures (see Table 2) and have at least one of the underlying cardiovascular conditions specified below.

Common situations for which routine prophylaxis was previously, but no longer recommended, include mitral valve prolapse, general dental cleanings and local anesthetic administration (noninfected tissue), and bronchoscopy (see Table 2).

Table 1. Cardiac Conditions Associated With the Highest Risk of Adverse Outcome From Endocarditis

Prophylaxis With Dental Procedures Is Recommended
Previous infective endocarditis
Prosthetic cardiac valves
Congenital heart disease (CHD)
Unrepaired cyanotic CHD, including palliative shunts and conduits
Completely repaired congenital heart defect with prosthetic material or device, whether placed by surgery or by catheter intervention, during the first 6 months after the procedure[1]
Repaired CHD with residual defects at the site or adjacent to the site of a prosthetic patch or prosthetic device (which inhibit endothelialization)
Cardiac transplantation recipients who develop cardiac valvulopathy

[1]Prophylaxis is recommended because endothelialization of prosthetic material occurs within 6 months after the procedure.

Table 2. Guidance for Use of Prophylactic Antibiotic Therapy Based on Procedure or Condition[1]

Location of Procedure	Prophylaxis Recommended	Prophylaxis NOT Recommended
Dental	All invasive manipulations of the gingival or periapical region or perforation of oral mucosa (includes biopsies, suture removal, placement of orthodontic bands)	Anesthetic injections through noninfected tissue, radiographs, placement/adjustment/removal prosthodontics/orthodontic appliances or brackets, shedding of deciduous teeth, trauma-induced bleeding from lips, gums, or oral mucosa
Respiratory tract	Biopsy/incision of respiratory mucosa (eg, tonsillectomy/adenoidectomy); drainage of abscess or empyema[2]	Bronchoscopy (unless incision of mucosa required)
Gastrointestinal (GI) or genitourinary (GU) tract	Established GI/GU infection or prevention of infectious sequelae[3]; elective cystoscopy or other urinary tract procedure with established enterococci infection/ colonization[3,4]	Routine diagnostic procedures, including esophagogastroduodenoscopy or colonoscopy in the absence of active infection; vaginal delivery and hysterectomy
Skin, skin structure, or musculoskeletal	Any surgical procedure involving infected tissue	Procedures conducted in noninfected tissue; tattoos and ear/body piercing

[1]Patients should receive prophylactic antibiotic therapy if they meet the criteria for a specified procedure/condition in this table and they have a high-risk cardiovascular condition listed in the preceding text.

[2]If infection is known or suspected to be caused by *Staphylococcus aureus*, consider antistaphylococcal penicillin or cephalosporin, or vancomycin in beta-lactam-sensitive patients.

[3]Consider alternate agents with activity against enterococci (ampicillin, penicillin, piperacillin); vancomycin (for beta-lactam-sensitive patients)

[4]Eradication of enterococci from the urinary tract should be considered.

Table 3. Prophylactic Regimens for Dental Procedures

Situation	Agent	Regimen to Be Given 30 to 60 Minutes Before Procedure	
		Adults	Children[1]
Standard general prophylaxis	Amoxicillin	2,000 mg PO	50 mg/kg PO
Unable to take oral medications	Ampicillin **or**	2,000 mg IM/IV	50 mg/kg IM/IV
	CeFAZolin or cefTRIAXone	1,000 mg IM/IV	50 mg/kg IM/IV
Allergic to penicillin	Clindamycin **or**	600 mg PO	20 mg/kg PO
	Cephalexin[2] or other dose-equivalent first/second generation cephalosporin[2] **or**	2,000 mg PO	50 mg/kg PO
	Azithromycin or clarithromycin	500 mg PO	15 mg/kg PO
Allergic to penicillin and unable to take oral medications	Clindamycin **or**	600 mg IM/IV	20 mg/kg IM/IV
	CeFAZolin[2] or cefTRIAXone[2]	1,000 mg IM/IV	50 mg/kg IM/IV

[1]Total children's dose should not exceed adult dose.

[2]Cephalosporins should not be used in individuals with immediate-type hypersensitivity reaction (urticaria, angioedema, or anaphylaxis) to penicillins.

Gastrointestinal/Genitourinary/Respiratory Procedures and Surgery Involving Skin, Skin Structure, or Musculoskeletal Tissue

In general, antibiotic prophylaxis solely to prevent IE is **not** recommended in patients undergoing GI/GU procedures or surgery involving skin, skin structure, or musculoskeletal tissue, unless infection is present at the site where the procedure is to occur. For patients with conditions listed in Table 1 undergoing an invasive respiratory tract procedure to treat an established infection (eg, drainage of an abscess or empyema) and the infection is known or suspected to be caused by *Staphlococcus aureus* (*S. aureus*), an antistaphlococcal penicillin or cephalosporin is recommended. In those patients with infections of the GI or GU tract undergoing GI/GU procedures, it may be reasonable to administer an agent with activity against enterococci (eg, ampicillin, penicillin, piperacillin); amoxicillin or ampicillin is preferred. In patients with a condition listed in Table 1 undergoing surgery involving infected skin, skin structure, or musculoskeletal tissue, it is reasonable that the regimen contain an agent with activity against staphylococci and beta-hemolytic streptococci (eg, antistaphlococcal penicillin or cephalosporin). In any case, vancomycin (or clindamycin in the setting of infected skin, skin structure, or musculoskeletal tissue) may be administered to patients unable to tolerate a beta-lactam (eg, ampicillin). Vancomycin should be administered with any infection known or suspected to be caused by a methicillin-resistant *S. aureus*.

Table 4. Vancomycin Dosing

	Dosage for Adults	Dosage for Children
Vancomyin	1,000 mg IV infused **slowly over 1 hour**; complete infusion within 30 minutes before procedure	20 mg/kg (maximum: 1,000 mg) IV infused **slowly over 1 hour**; complete infusion within 30 minutes before procedure

If infection is caused by a known or suspected strain of resistant enterococcus, consult with an infectious diseases expert.

REFERENCE

Wilson W, Taubert KA, Gewitz M, et al. Prevention of infective endocarditis. Guidelines from the American Heart Association. A guideline from the American Heart Association Rheumatic Fever, Endocarditis, and Kawasaki Disease Committee, Council on Cardiovascular Disease in the Young, and the Council on Clinical Cardiology, Council on Cardiovascular Surgery and Anesthesia, and the Quality of Care and Outcomes Research Interdisciplinary Working Group. *Circulation*. 2007;116(15):1736-1754.

PEDIATRIC HIV

Selected information from: The Panel on Antiretroviral Therapy and Medical Management of HIV-Infected Children. Guidelines for the use of antiretroviral agents in pediatric HIV infection. March 5, 2015. Available at http://aidsinfo.nih.gov/contentfiles/PediatricGuidelines.pdf

Human Immunodeficiency Virus (HIV) Infection Stage[1] Based on Age-Specific CD4 Cell Count or Percentage[2]

Stage	<1 year		1 to <6 years		≥6 years	
	Cells/mm³	%	Cells/mm³	%	Cells/mm³	%
1	≥1,500	≥34	≥1,000	≥30	≥500	≥26
2	750 to 1,499	26 to 33	500 to 999	22 to 29	200 to 499	14 to 25
3	<750	<26	<500	<22	<200	<14

[1]The stage is based primarily on the CD4 count; the CD4 count takes precedence over the CD4 percentage, and the percentage is considered only if the count is missing. If a Stage 3-defining opportunistic illness has been diagnosed (see next table), then the stage is 3, regardless of the CD4 test results.

[2]Modified from: Centers for Disease Control and Prevention (CDC). Revised Surveillance Definition for HIV Infection – United States, 2014. *MMWR*. 2014;63(RR-3):1-10.

HIV-Related Symptoms

Mild HIV-Related Symptoms

Children with **two** or more of the conditions listed but none of the conditions listed in Moderate Symptoms category:

- Lymphadenopathy (≥0.5 cm at more than two sites; bilateral at one site)
- Hepatomegaly
- Splenomegaly
- Dermatitis
- Parotitis
- Recurrent or persistent upper respiratory infection, sinusitis, or otitis media

Moderate HIV-Related Symptoms

- Anemia (Hgb <8 g/dL), neutropenia (WBC <1,000/mm^3), and/or thrombocytopenia (platelet count <100,000/mm^3) persisting ≥30 days
- Bacterial meningitis, pneumonia, or sepsis (single episode)
- Candidiasis, oropharyngeal (thrush), persisting (>2 months) in children >6 months of age
- Cardiomyopathy
- Cytomegalovirus infection with onset before 1 month of age
- Diarrhea, recurrent or chronic
- Hepatitis
- Herpes simplex virus (HSV) stomatitis, recurrent (>2 episodes within 1 year)
- HSV bronchitis, pneumonitis, or esophagitis with onset before 1 month of age
- Herpes zoster (shingles) involving at least two distinct episodes or more than one dermatome
- Leiomyosarcoma
- Lymphoid interstitial pneumonia (LIP) or pulmonary lymphoid hyperplasia complex
- Nephropathy
- Nocardiosis
- Persistent fever (lasting >1 month)
- Toxoplasmosis with onset before 1 month of age
- Varicella, disseminated (complicated chickenpox)

Stage 3-Defining Opportunistic Illnesses in HIV Infection

- Bacterial infections, multiple or recurrent (only among children <6 years of age)
- Candidiasis of bronchi, trachea, or lungs
- Candidiasis of esophagus
- Cervical cancer, invasive (only among adults, adolescents, and children ≥6 years of age)
- Coccidioidomycosis, disseminated or extrapulmonary

- Cryptococcosis, extrapulmonary
- Cryptococcosis, chronic intestinal (>1 month duration)
- Cytomegalovirus disease (other than liver, spleen, or lymph nodes), onset at >1 month of age
- Cytomegalovirus retinitis (with loss of vision)
- Encephalopathy attributed to HIV (ie, at least one of the following progressive findings present for at least 2 months in the absence of a concurrent illness other than HIV infection that could explain the findings):
  - Failure to attain or loss of developmental milestones or loss of intellectual ability, verified by standard developmental scale or neuropsychological tests;
  - Impaired brain growth or acquired microcephaly demonstrated by head circumference measurements or brain atrophy demonstrated by CT or MRI (serial imaging is required for children <2 years of age);
  - Acquired symmetric motor deficit manifested by two or more of the following: Paresis, pathologic reflexes, ataxia, or gait disturbance
- HSV: Chronic ulcers (>1 month duration) or bronchitis, pneumonitis, or esophagitis (onset at >1 month of age)
- Histoplasmosis, disseminated or extrapulmonary
- Isosporiasis, chronic intestinal (>1 month duration)
- Kaposi's sarcoma
- Lymphoma, Burkitt (or equivalent term)
- Lymphoma, immunoblastic (or equivalent term)
- Lymphoma, primary, of brain
- *Mycobacterium avium* complex or *Mycobacterium kansasii*, disseminated or extrapulmonary
- Mycobacterium tuberculosis of any site, pulmonary (only among adults, adolescents, or children ≥6 years of age), disseminated or extrapulmonary
- Mycobacterium, other species or unidentified species, disseminated or extrapulmonary
- *Pneumocystis jiroveci* (previously known as *Pneumocystis carini*) pneumonia
- Pneumonia, recurrent (only among adults, adolescents, and children ≥6 years of age)
- Progressive multifocal leukoencephalopathy
- Salmonella septicemia, recurrent
- Toxoplasmosis of the brain, onset at >1 month of age
- Wasting syndrome attributed to HIV, ie, in the absence of a concurrent illness other than HIV infection that could explain the following findings:
  - Persistent weight loss >10% of baseline; **OR**
  - Downward crossing of at least two of the following percentile lines on the weight-for-age chart (eg, 95th, 75th, 50th, 25th, 5th) in a child ≥1 year of age; **OR**
  - <5th percentile on weight-for-height chart on two consecutive measurements, ≥30 days apart **PLUS**
    - Chronic diarrhea (ie, ≥two loose stools per day for >30 days); **OR**
    - Documented fever (for ≥30 days, intermittent or constant)

REFERENCES

Centers for Disease Control and Prevention (CDC). 1994 revised classification system for human immunodeficiency virus infection in children less than 13 years of age. *MMWR*. 1994;43(RR-12):1-10.

Centers for Disease Control and Prevention (CDC). Revised surveillance case definition for HIV infection – United States, 2014. *MMWR Recomm Rep.* 2014;63(RR-03):1-10.

INDICATIONS FOR INITIATION OF ANTIRETROVIRAL THERAPY IN HIV-INFECTED CHILDREN

This table provides general guidance rather than absolute recommendations for an individual patient. Factors to be considered in decisions about initiation of therapy include the risk of disease progression as determined by CD4 percentage or count and plasma HIV RNA copy number, the potential benefits and risks of therapy, and the ability of the caregiver to adhere to administration of the therapeutic regimen. **Urgent treatment** should be initiated within 1 to 2 weeks, including an expedited discussion on adherence. In nonurgent settings, more time can be taken to fully assess and address issues associated with adherence with the caregivers and the child prior to initiating therapy.

Patients/caregivers may choose to postpone therapy, and on a case-by-case basis, providers may elect to defer therapy based on clinical and/or psychosocial factors. Children in whom antiretroviral therapy is deferred need close follow-up. Factors to consider in deciding when to initiate therapy in children in whom treatment was deferred include: Increasing HIV RNA levels (such as HIV RNA levels approaching 100,000 copies/mL); CD4 cell count or percentage values approaching the age-related threshold for treatment; development of clinical symptoms; and the ability of caregiver and child to adhere to the prescribed regimen.

Age/Criteria	Recommendation
<12 months	
Regardless of clinical symptoms, immune status, or viral load	Urgent treatment
1 to <6 years	
CDC stage 3-defining opportunistic illnesses[a]	Urgent treatment
CDC stage 3 immunodeficiency[b]: CD4 <500 cells/mm^3	Urgent treatment
Moderate HIV-related symptoms[a]	Treat
HIV RNA >100,000 copies/mL[c]	Treat
CD4 cell count[b] 500 to 999 cells/mm^3	Treat
Asymptomatic or mild symptoms[a] **and** CD4 cell count[b] ≥1,000 cells/mm^3	Consider treatment
≥6 years	
CDC stage 3-defining opportunistic illnesses[a]	Urgent treatment
CDC stage 3 immunodeficiency[b]: CD4 cell count <200 cells/mm^3	Urgent treatment
Moderate HIV-related symptoms[a]	Treat
HIV RNA >100,000 copies/mL[c]	Treat
CD4 cell count[b] 200 to 499 cells/mm^3	Treat
Asymptomatic or mild symptoms[a] **and** CD4 cell count ≥500 cells/mm^3	Consider treatment

[a]See above list of HIV-related symptoms

[b]Laboratory data should be confirmed with a second test to meet the treatment criteria before initiation of antiretroviral therapy.

[c]To avoid overinterpretation of temporary blips in viral load (eg, which can occur during intercurrent illnesses), plasma HIV RNA level >100,000 copies/mL should be confirmed by a second level before initiating antiretroviral therapy.

[d]The guidelines recommend treatment for patients in this group when CD4 cell count is ≤500 cells/mm^3; rating of evidence is strongest for treatment when CD4 cell count is <350 cells/mm^3.

ANTIRETROVIRAL REGIMENS RECOMMENDED FOR INITIAL THERAPY FOR HIV INFECTION IN CHILDREN

A combination antiretroviral regimen in treatment-naïve children generally contains 1 NNRTI plus a 2-NRTI backbone or 1 PI (generally with low-dose ritonavir boosting) plus a 2-NRTI backbone. Regimens should be individualized based on advantages and disadvantages of each combination.

Preferred Regimen	
Children ≥14 days to <3 years of age[1]	2 NRTIs **plus** lopinavir/ritonavir
Children ≥3 years to <6 years of age	2 NRTIs **plus** efavirenz[2]
	2 NRTIs **plus** lopinavir/ritonavir
Children ≥6 years of age	2 NRTIs **plus** atazanavir **plus** low-dose ritonavir
	2 NRTIs **plus** efavirenz[2]
	2 NRTIs **plus** lopinavir/ritonavir
Alternative Regimens	
Children >14 days of age	2 NRTIs **plus** nevirapine[3]
Children ≥3 months to <6 years and weighing ≥10 kg	2 NRTIs **plus** atazanavir **plus** low-dose ritonavir
Children ≥2 years	2 NRTIs **plus** raltegravir[4]
Children ≥3 years to <12 years of age	2 NRTIs **plus** twice-daily darunavir **plus** low-dose ritonavir
Children ≥12 years of age and weighing ≥40 kg	2 NRTIs **plus** once-daily darunavir **plus** low-dose ritonavir[5]
	2 NRTIs **plus** dolutegravir
Regimens for Use in Special Circumstances	
Children ≥4 weeks to <2 years of age and weighing ≥3 kg	2 NRTIs **plus** raltegravir[4]
Children ≥6 months of age[6]	2 NRTIs **plus** fosamprenavir **plus** low-dose ritonavir
Children ≥2 years of age	2 NRTIs **plus** nelfinavir
Children ≥12 years of age and ≥40 kg	2 NRTIs **plus** dolutegravir
Treatment-naïve adolescents ≥13 years of age and weighing >39 kg	2 NRTIs **plus** atazanavir unboosted
Preferred 2-NRTI Backbone Options for Use in Combination With Additional Drugs	
Children birth to 3 months of age	Zidovudine **plus** (lamiVUDine **or** emtricitabine)
Children ≥3 months and ≤12 years of age	Abacavir **plus** (lamiVUDine **or** emtricitabine)
	Zidovudine **plus** (lamiVUDine **or** emtricitabine)
Adolescents ≥13 years of age at Tanner stage 3	Abacavir **plus** (lamiVUDine **or** emtricitabine)
Adolescents at Tanner stage 4 or 5	Abacavir **plus** (lamiVUDine **or** emtricitabine)
	Tenofovir **plus** (lamiVUDine **or** emtricitabine)
Alternative 2-NRTI Backbone Options for Use in Combination With Additional Drugs	
Children ≥2 weeks of age	Didanosine **plus** (lamiVUDine **or** emtricitabine)
	Zidovudine **plus** didanosine
Children ≥3 months of age	Zidovudine **plus** abacavir
Children and adolescents at Tanner stage 3	Tenofovir **plus** (lamiVUDine **or** emtricitabine)
Adolescents ≥13 years of age	Zidovudine **plus** (lamiVUDine **or** emtricitabine)
2-NRTI Regimens for Use in Special Circumstances in Combination With Additional Drugs	
	Stavudine **plus** (lamiVUDine **or** emtricitabine)
	Tenofovir **plus** (lamiVUDine **or** emtricitabine) (prepubertal children ≥2 years of age and adolescents, Tanner stage 1 or 2)

NRTI = nucleoside analogue reverse transcriptase inhibitor, NNRTI = non-nucleoside analogue reverse transcriptase inhibitor, PI = protease inhibitor

[1]Lopinavir/ritonavir should not be administered to neonates before a postmenstrual age (first day of the mother's last menstrual period to birth plus the time elapsed after birth) of 42 weeks and a postnatal age of at least 14 days.

[2]Efavirenz is licensed for use in children ≥3 months of age with weight ≥3.5 kg but is not recommended by the panel as initial therapy in children ≥3 months to 3 years of age. Unless adequate contraception can be assured, efavirenz-based therapy is not recommended for adolescent females who are sexually active and may become pregnant.

[3]Nevirapine should not be used in postpubertal girls with CD4 count >250/mm^3, unless the benefit clearly outweighs the risk. Nevirapine is FDA approved for treatment of infants ≥15 days of age.

[4]Raltegravir pills or chewable tablets can be used in children ≥2 years of age as an alternate integrase strand transfer inhibitor. Use of granules or chewable tablets in infants and children 4 weeks to 2 years of age can be considered in special circumstances.

[5]Darunavir once daily should not be used if any one of the following resistance-associated substitutions is present (V11I, V32I, L33F, I47V, I50V, I54L, I54M, T74P, L76V, I84V, and L89V).

[6]Fosamprenavir with low-dose ritonavir should only be administered to infants born at ≥38 weeks GA who have attained a PNA of 28 days and to infants born before 38 weeks GA who have reached a PMA of 42 weeks.

Antiretroviral Regimens or Components Not Recommended for Initial Treatment of HIV Infection in Children

Regimen or Antiretroviral Component	Rationale for Being Not Recommended
Unboosted atazanavir-containing regimens in children <13 years of age and/or <39 kg	Reduced exposure
Darunavir-based regimens once-daily in children ≥3 years to <12 years of age	Insufficient data to recommend
Unboosted darunavir	Use without ritonavir has not been studied
Dual (full-dose) PI regimens	Insufficient data to recommend
Dual NRTI combination of abacavir **plus** didanosine	Insufficient data to recommend
Dual NRTI combination of abacavir **plus** tenofovir	Insufficient data to recommend
Dual NRTI combination of stavudine **plus** didanosine	Significant toxicities
Dual NRTI combination of tenofovir **plus** didanosine	Increase in concentrations; high rate of virologic failure
Dolutegravir-based regimens for children <12 years of age or body weight <40 kg	Insufficient data to recommend
Efavirenz-based regimens for children <3 years of age	Appropriate dose not determined
Enfuvirtide (T-20)-containing regimens	Insufficient data to recommend; injectable preparation
Etravirine-based regimens	Insufficient data to recommend
Elvitegravir-based regimens	Insufficient data to recommend
Fosamprenavir without ritonavir boosting	Reduced exposure; medication burden
Indinavir-based regimens	Renal toxicities
Once-daily lopinavir/ritonavir	Reduced drug exposure
Maraviroc-based regimens	Insufficient data to recommend
Nelfinavir-containing regimens for children <2 years of age	Appropriate dose not determined
Regimens containing only NRTIs	Inferior virologic efficacy
Regimens containing three drug classes	Insufficient data to recommend
Full-dose ritonavir or use of ritonavir as the sole PI	GI intolerance; metabolic toxicity
Regimens containing three NRTIs and an NNRTI	Insufficient data to recommend
Rilpivirine-based regimens	Insufficient data to recommend
Saquinavir-based regimens	Limited dosing and outcome data burden
Tenofovir-containing regimens in children <2 years of age	Potential bone toxicity; appropriate dose has yet to be determined
Tipranvir-based regimens	Increased dose of ritonavir for boosting; reported cases of intracranial hemorrhage

NNRTI = non-nucleoside analogue reverse transcriptase inhibitor, NRTI = nucleoside analogue reverse transcriptase inhibitor, PI = protease inhibitor

Antiretroviral Regimens or Components That Should Never Be Recommended or Treatment of HIV Infection in Children

	Rationale	Exception
Antiretroviral Regimens Never Recommended for Children		
One antiretroviral drug alone (monotherapy)	Rapid development of resistance Inferior antiretroviral activity compared to combination with ≥3 antiretroviral drugs Monotherapy "holding" regimens associated with more rapid CD4 decline compared to nonsuppressive combination antiretroviral therapy	HIV-exposed infants (with negative viral testing) during 6-week period of prophylaxis to prevent perinatal transmission
Two NRTIs alone	Rapid development of resistance Inferior antiretroviral activity compared to combination with ≥3 antiretroviral drugs	Not recommended for initial therapy; for patients currently on this treatment, some clinicians may opt to continue if virologic goals are achieved
Tenofovir **plus** abacavir **plus** lamiVUDine **or** emtricitabine as triple NRTI regimen	High rate of early virologic failure when this triple NRTI regimen used as initial therapy in treatment-naïve adults	No exception
Tenofovir **plus** didanosine **plus** lamiVUDine **or** emtricitabine as triple NRTI regimen	High rate of early virologic failure when this triple NRTI regimen used as initial therapy in treatment-naïve adults	No exception
Antiretroviral Components Never Recommended as Part of Antiretroviral Regimen for Children		
Atazanavir **plus** indinavir	Potential additive hyperbilirubinemia	No exception
Dual NNRTI combinations	Enhanced toxicity	No exception
Dual NRTI combinations:		
LamiVUDine **plus** emtricitabine	Similar resistance profile and no additive benefit	No exception
Stavudine **plus** zidovudine	Antagonistic effect on HIV	No exception
Efavirenz in 1st trimester of pregnancy or in sexually active adolescent girls of childbearing potential when reliable contraception cannot be ensured	Potential for teratogenicity	When no other antiretroviral option is available and potential benefits outweigh risks
Nevirapine as initial therapy in adolescent girls with CD4 count >250 cells/mm^3 or adolescent boys with CD4 count >400 cells/mm^3	Increased incidence of symptomatic (including serious and potentially fatal) hepatic events in these patient groups	Only if benefit clearly outweighs the risk
Unboosted saquinavir, darunavir, or tipranavir	Poor oral bioavailability Inferior virologic activity compared to other protease inhibitors	No exception

NNRTI = non-nucleoside analogue reverse transcriptase inhibitor, NRTI = nucleoside analogue reverse transcriptase inhibitor

DEFINITIONS OF TREATMENT FAILURE IN HIV-INFECTED CHILDREN

Treatment failure can be categorized as virologic failure, immunologic failure, clinical failure, or some combination of the three. Laboratory results must be confirmed with repeat testing before a final assessment of virologic or immunologic treatment failure is made. Almost all antiretroviral management decisions for treatment failure are based on addressing virologic failure.

Virologic failure occurs as an incomplete initial response to therapy or as a viral rebound after virologic suppression is achieved. **Virologic suppression** is defined as having plasma viral load below the lower level of quantification (LLQ) using the most sensitive assay (LLQ 20 to 75 copies/mL). Older assays with LLQ of 400 copies/mL are not recommended.

Virologic failure is defined for all children as a repeated plasma viral load >200 copies/mL after 6 months of therapy. Because infants with high plasma viral loads at initiation of therapy occasionally take longer than 6 months to achieve viral suppression, some experts continue the treatment regimen for such infants if viral load is declining but is still >200 copies/mL at 6 months and monitor closely for continued decline to virologic suppression soon thereafter. However, ongoing nonsuppression, especially with NNRTI-based regimens, increases the risk of drug resistance. There is controversy regarding the clinical implication of HIV RNA levels between the LLQ and <200 copies/mL in patients on combination antiretroviral therapy (cART). HIV-infected adults with detectable viral loads and a quantified result <200 copies/mL after 6 months of cART often ultimately achieve virologic suppression without regimen change.

Viral rebound is defined as repeated detection of plasma viral load above the level of quantification after a person had achieved virologic suppression in response to therapy. "Blips," defined as isolated episodes of plasma viral load detectable at low levels (<500 copies/mL), followed by return to viral suppression, are common and not generally reflective of virologic failure. However, repeated or persistent plasma viral load detection above 200 (especially if >500 copies/mL) after having achieved virologic suppression usually represents viral failure.

Immunologic failure is defined as a suboptimal immunologic response to therapy or an immunologic decline while on therapy. While there is no standardized definition, many experts would consider a suboptimal immunologic response to therapy as the failure to maintain or achieve a CD4 cell count or percentage that is at least above the age-specific range for severe immunodeficiency. Evaluation of immune response in children is complicated by the normal age-related changes in CD4 cell count. Thus, the normal decline in CD4 values with age needs to be considered when evaluating declines in CD4 parameters. CD4 percentage tends to vary less with age. At about 5 years of age, absolute CD4 cell count values in children approach those of adults; consequently, changes in absolute count can be used in children ≥5 years of age.

Clinical failure is defined as the occurrence of new opportunistic infections (OIs) and/or other clinical evidence of HIV disease progression during therapy. Clinical failure represents the most urgent and concerning type of treatment failure and should prompt an immediate evaluation. Clinical evidence of HIV disease progression during therapy includes:

- **Severe or recurrent infection or illness:** Recurrence or persistence of AIDS-defining conditions or other serious infections
- **Progressive neurodevelopmental deterioration:** Two or more of the following on repeated assessments:
  - Impairment in brain growth
  - Decline of cognitive function documented by psychometric testing
  - Clinical motor dysfunction
- **Growth failure:** Persistent decline in weight-growth velocity despite adequate nutritional support and without other explanation

Assessment of Causes of Virologic Antiretroviral Treatment Failure

Assessment	Assessment Method	Intervention
Nonadherence	1. Interview child and caretaker • Take 24-hour or 7-day recall • Obtain description of: – WHO gives medication – WHAT is given (names, doses) – WHERE medications are kept, administered – WHEN they are taken/given – HOW medications make child feel • Conduct open-ended discussion of experiences taking/giving medications and barriers/challenges	Identify or re-engage family members to support/supervise adherence. Establish fixed daily times and routines for medication administration. Avoid confusion with drug names by explaining that drug therapies have generic names, trade names, and many agents are coformulated under a third or fourth name. Explore opportunities for facility or home-based DOT.
	2. Review pharmacy records • Assess timeliness of refills	
	3. Observe medication administration • Observe dosing/administration in clinic • Conduct home-based observation by visiting health professional • Admit to hospital for trial of therapy – Observe administration/tolerance monitor treatment response	Simplify medication regimen if feasible. Substitute new agents if single ARV is poorly tolerated. Consider DOT Use tools to simplify administration (pill boxes, reminders including alarms, integrated medication packaging for AM or PM dosing). As a last resort, consider gastric tube placement to facilitate adherence.
	4. Conduct psychosocial assessment • Make a comprehensive family-focused assessment of factors likely to impact adherence with particular attention toward recent changes in: – Status of caregiver, financial stability, housing, child/caretaker relationships – School and achievement – Substance abuse (child, caretaker, family members) – Mental health and behavior – Child/youth and caretaker beliefs toward antiretroviral therapy – Disclosure status (to child and others) – Peer pressure	Address competing needs through appropriate social services. Address and treat concomitant mental illness and behavioral disorders. Initiate disclosure discussions with family/child. Initiate disclosure discussions with family/child. Consider need for child protection services and alternate care settings when necessary.
Pharmacokinetics and Dosing Issues	1. Recalculate doses for individual medications using weight or body surface area. 2. Identify concomitant medications including prescription, over-the-counter, and recreational substances; assess for drug-drug interactions. 3. Consider drug levels for specific antiretroviral drugs	Adjust drug doses. Discontinue or substitute competing medications. Reinforce applicable food restrictions.
Antiretroviral Resistance Testing	1. Perform genotypic and phenotypic resistance assays 2. Perform tropism assay, as appropriate.	If no resistance detected to current drugs, focus on improving adherence. If resistance to current regimen detected, optimize adherence and evaluate potential for new regimen.

Options for Regimens With at Least Two Fully Active Agents With Goal of Virologic Suppression in Patients With Failed Antiretroviral Therapy and Evidence of Viral Resistance[1]

Prior Regimen	Recommended Change (in order of relative preference)[1]
2 NRTIs + NNRTI	• 2 NRTIs + PI
	• 2 NRTIs + integrase inhibitor
2 NRTIs + PI	• 2 NRTIs + NNRTI
	• 2 NRTIs + integrase inhibitor
	• 2 NRTIs + different ritonavir-boosted PI
	• NRTI(s) + integrase inhibitor + (NNRTI **or** different ritonavir-boosted PI)
3 NRTIs	• 2 NRTIs + NNRTI
	• 2 NRTIs + PI
	• 2 NRTIs + integrase inhibitor
	• Integrase inhibitor + 2 other active agents [chosen from NNRTI, PI, NRTI(s)]
Failed regimen(s) that included NRTI(s), NNRTI(s), and PI(s)	• 2 NRTIs + integrase inhibitor (+ ritonavir-boosted PI if additional active drug needed)
	• NRTI(s) + ritonavir-boosted PI + integrase inhibitor [consider adding enfuvirtide and/or maraviroc[2] if additional active drug(s) are needed]
	• NRTI(s) + ritonavir-boosted darunavir, lopinavir, or saquinavir + etravirine [consider adding one or more of maraviroc[2], enfuvirtide, or integrase inhibitor if additional active drug(s) are needed]
	• >1 NRTI + 2 ritonavir-boosted PIs (lopinavir/ritonavir + saquinavir **or** lopinavir/ritonavir + atazanavir) [consider adding enfuvirtide or an integrase inhibitor if additional active drug(s) are needed]

[1]Antiretroviral therapy regimens should be chosen based on treatment history and drug-resistance testing to optimize antiretroviral drug effectiveness in the subsequent regimen. This is particularly important in selecting NRTI components of an NNRTI-based regimen where drug resistance may occur rapidly to the NNRTI if the virus is not sufficiently sensitive to the NRTIs. Regimens should contain at least two, but preferably three, fully active drugs for durable, potent virologic suppression. Please see individual drug monographs for information about drug interactions and dose adjustment when designing a regimen for children with multiclass drug resistance. Collaboration with a pediatric HIV specialist is especially important when choosing regimens for children with multiclass drug resistance. Regimens in this table are listed in relative order of preference and are provided as examples, but this list in not exhaustive.

[2]No current Food and Drug Administration (FDA)-approved pediatric indication for maraviroc

ROLE OF THERAPEUTIC DRUG MONITORING IN MANAGEMENT OF PEDIATRIC HIV INFECTION

Evaluation of antiretroviral drug plasma concentrations is not routinely required in the management of pediatric HIV but should be considered in children receiving combination antiretroviral therapy in the following scenarios:

- Use of antiretroviral drugs with limited pharmacokinetic data and therapeutic experience in children (eg, for use of efavirenz in children <3 years of age and darunavir with once-daily dosing in children <12 years of age)
- Significant drug-drug interactions and food-drug interactions
- Unexpected suboptimal treatment response (eg, lack of virologic suppression with history of medical adherence and lack of resistance mutations)
- Suspected suboptimal absorption of the drug
- Suspected dose-dependent toxicity

Evaluation of the genetic G516T polymorphism of drug metabolizing enzyme cytochrome P450 (CYP450) 2B6 in combination with the evaluation of plasma efavirenz concentrations is recommended for children <3 years of age receiving efavirenz because the dosing recommendation depends on the result, given the significant association between this polymorphism and efavirenz concentrations.

Target Trough Concentrations of Antiretroviral Drugs[a]

Drug	Concentration (ng/mL)
Established Efficacy Plasma Trough Concentrations	
Atazanavir	150
Fosamprenavir	400[b]
Indinavir	100
Lopinavir	1,000
Nelfinavir[2]	800
Saquinavir	100 to 250
Efavirenz	1,000
Nevirapine	3,000
Maraviroc	>50[c]
Tipranavir	20,500[c]
Median (Range) Plasma Trough Concentrations From Clinical Trials	
Darunavir (600 mg twice daily)	3,300 (1,255 to 7,368)
Etravirine	275 (81 to 2,980)
Raltegravir	72 (29 to 118)

[a]Measurable amprenavir concentration

[b]Measurable active M8 metabolite

[c]Suggested median plasma trough concentration in treatment-experienced patients with resistant HIV-1 strain only

ANTIRETROVIRAL DRUG RESISTANCE TESTING

- Antiretroviral drug resistance testing is recommended at the times of HIV diagnosis, before initiation of therapy, in all treatment-naïve patients. Genotypic resistance testing is preferred for this purpose.
- Antiretroviral drug resistance testing is recommended prior to changing therapy for treatment failure.
- Resistance testing in the setting of virological failure should be obtained while the patient is still on the failing regimen, or within 4 weeks of discontinuation of the regimen.
- Phenotypic resistance testing should be used (usually in addition to genotypic resistance testing) for patients with known or suspected complex drug resistance mutation patterns, which generally arise after virologic failure of successive antiretroviral therapy regimens.
- The absence of detectable resistance to a drug does not ensure that its use will be successful as mutations may not be detected once the drug has been discontinued. A history of all previously used antiretroviral agents and previous resistance test results must be reviewed when making decisions regarding the choice of new agents for patients with virologic failure.
- Viral Coreceptor (tropism) assays should be used whenever the use of a CCR5 antagonist is being considered. Tropism assays should also be considered for patients who demonstrate virologic failure while receiving therapy that contains a CCR5 antagonist.
- Consultation with a pediatric HIV specialist is recommended for interpretation of resistance assays when considering initiating or changing an antiretroviral regimen in a pediatric patient.

STRATEGIES TO IMPROVE ADHERENCE TO ANTIRETROVIRAL MEDICATIONS

Initial Intervention Strategies

- Establish trust and identify mutually acceptable goals for care with patient and caregiver.
- Obtain explicit agreement on need for treatment and adherence with patient and caregiver.
- Identify depression, low self-esteem, substance abuse, or other mental health issues for the child/adolescent and/or caregiver that may decrease adherence. Treat prior to starting therapy, if possible.
- Identify family, friends, health team members, or others who can help with adherence support.
- Educate patient and family about the critical role of adherence in therapy outcome.
- Specify the adherence target: ≥95% of prescribed doses.
- Educate patient and family about the relationship between partial adherence and resistance.
- Educate patient and family about resistance and constraint of later choices of antiretroviral drug; explain that while a failure of adherence may be temporary, the effects on treatment choice may be permanent.
- Develop a treatment plan that the patient and family understand and to which they feel committed.

- Establish readiness to take medication by practice sessions or other means.
- For patient education and to assess tolerability of medications chosen, consider a brief period of hospitalization at start c therapy in selected circumstances.

Medication Strategies

- Choose the simplest regimen possible, reducing dosing frequency and number of pills.
- Choose a regimen with dosing requirements that best conform to daily and weekly routines and variations in patient an family activities.
- Choose the most palatable medicine possible (pharmacists may be able to add syrups or flavoring agents to increas palatability).
- Choose drugs with the fewest side effects; provide anticipatory guidance for management of side effects.
- Simplify food requirements for medication administration.
- Prescribe drugs carefully to avoid adverse drug-drug interactions.
- Assess pill swallowing capacity and offer pill-swallowing training.

Follow-up Intervention Strategies

- Monitor adherence at each visit, as well as in between visits by telephone, email, text, and social media as needed.
- Provide ongoing support, encouragement, and understanding of the difficulties of the demands of attaining 95% adherence with medication doses.
- Use patient education aids including pictures, calendars, and stickers.
- Encourage use of pillboxes, reminders, alarms, pagers, and timers.
- Provide follow-up clinic visits, telephone calls, and SMS text messages to support and assess adherence.
- Provide access to support groups, peer groups, or one-on-one counseling for caregivers and patients especially for those with known depression or drug use issues, which are known to decrease adherence.
- Provide pharmacist-based adherence support, such as medication education counseling, blister packs, refill reminders automatic refills, and home delivery of medications.
- Consider directly observed therapy (DOT) at home, in the clinic, or in select circumstances, during a brief inpatien hospitalization.
- Consider gastrostomy tube use in selected circumstances.

Modifying Antiretroviral Regimens in Children With Sustained Virologic Suppression on Antiretroviral Therapy

For children who have sustained virologic suppression on their current regimen, changing to a new antiretroviral regimen with improved pill burden or tolerance can be considered in order to facilitate continued adherence, decrease drug-associated toxicities, or improve safety.

Examples of Changes in Antiretroviral Regimen Components That Are Made for Reasons of Simplification, Convenience, and Safety Profile in Children Who Have Sustained Virologic Suppression on Their Current Regimen[1]

Antiretroviral Drug(s)	Current Age	Body Size Attained	Potential Antiretroviral Regimen Change	Comment[2]
NRTIs				
Abacavir twice daily	≥1 year	Any	Abacavir once daily	
Zidovudine or didanosine (or stavudine)[3]	≥1 year	N/A	Abacavir	Once-daily dosing; less long-term mitochondrial toxicity
	Adolescence	Pubertal maturity (Tanner stage IV or V)	Tenofovir Abacavir	Once-daily dosing; less long-term mitochondrial toxicity; coformulation with other ARVs can further reduce pill burden
PIs				
Lopinavir/ritonavir twice daily	≥1 year	≥3 kg	Raltegravir or ritonavir-boosted atazanavir	Better palatability; less adverse lipid effect; lower pill burden; once-daily dosing with ritonavir-boosted atazanavir
	≥3 years	N/A	Ritonavir-boosted atazanavir Efavirenz Ritonavir-boosted darunavir Raltegravir	Once-daily dosing with ritonavir-boosted atazanavir and efavirenz; better palatability; less adverse lipid effect
	≥12 years	≥40 kg	Ritonavir-boosted darunavir Ritonavir-boosted atazanavir Dolutegravir	Once-daily dosing possible; lower pill burden
Other				
Any multi-pill and/or twice-daily regimen	Adolescence	Pubertal maturity (Tanner stage IV or V)	Co-formulated: • Efavirenz/emtricitabine/ tenofovir (Atripla) • Elvitegravir/cobicistat/ emtricitabine/tenofovir (Stribild) • Emtricitabine/rilpivirine/ tenofovir (Complera) • Abacavir/dolutegravir/ lamivudine (Triumeq)	Once-daily dosing; single pill; alignment with adult regimens

[1]This list is not exhaustive in that it does not necessarily list all potential options, but instead, shows examples of what kinds of changes can be made.

[2]Comments relevant to the potential ARV change listed. Does not include all relevant information. Please refer to individual drug monograph for full information.

[3]Because of concerns about long-term adverse effects, stavudine may be replaced with a safer drug even before sustained virologic suppression is achieved.

ADULT AND ADOLESCENT HIV

Selected information from the Panel on Antiretroviral Guidelines for Adults and Adolescents. Guidelines for the use of antiretroviral agents in HIV-1-infected adults and adolescents. Department of Health and Human Services. April 8, 2015. Available at http://www.aidsinfo.nih.gov/ContentFiles/AdultandAdolescentGL.pdf

Goals of HIV Therapy and Strategies to Achieve Them

Goals of Therapy

- Maximal and durable suppression of viral load
- Restoration and/or preservation of immunologic function
- Improvement of quality of life
- Reduction of HIV-related morbidity and mortality
- Prevention of HIV transmission

Strategies to Achieve Goals of Therapy

- Rational sequencing of drugs
- Preservation of future treatment options
- Selection of appropriate combination therapy
- Maximize adherence to the antiretroviral regimen
- Optimize initial regimen with use of pretreatment genotypic drug resistance testing
- Optimize antiretroviral regimen with use of therapeutic drug monitoring in selected clinical settings

Recommendations on the Indications and Frequency of Viral Load and CD4 Count Monitoring[1]

Clinical Scenario	Viral Load Monitoring	CD4 Count Monitoring
Before initiating ART	At entry into care If ART initiation is deferred, repeat viral load before initiating ART In patients not initiating ART, repeat testing is optional	At entry into care If ART is deferred, repeat CD4 count every 3 to 6 months[2]
After initiating ART	Preferably within 2 to 4 weeks (and no later than 8 weeks) after initiation of ART; thereafter, repeat every 4 to 8 weeks until viral load is suppressed	3 months after initiation of ART
After modifying ART because of drug toxicities or for regimen simplification in a patient with viral suppression	4 to 8 weeks after modification of ART to confirm effectiveness of new regimen	Monitor according to prior CD4 count and duration on ART, as outlined below
After modifying ART because of virologic failure	Preferably within 2 to 4 weeks (but no later than 8 weeks) after modification; thereafter, repeat every 4 to 8 weeks until viral load is suppressed. If viral suppression is not possible, repeat viral load every 3 months or more frequently if indicated	Every 3 to 6 months
During the first 2 years of ART	Every 3 to 4 months	Every 3 to 6 months[1]
After 2 years of ART (viral load consistently suppressed, CD4 consistently 300 to 500 cells/mm^3)	Can extend to every 6 months for patients with consistent viral suppression for ≥2 years	Every 12 months
After 2 years of ART (viral load consistently suppressed, CD4 consistently >500 cells/mm^3)	Can extend to every 6 months for patients with consistent viral suppression for ≥2 years	Optional
While on ART with detectable viremia (viral load repeatedly >200 copies/mL)	Every 3 months or more frequently if clinical indicated	Every 3 to 6 months
Change in clinical status (eg, new HIV clinical symptom or initiation of interferon, chronic systemic corticosteroids, or antineoplastic therapy	Every 3 months	Perform CD4 count and repeat ad clinically indicated[3]

ART = antiretroviral therapy

[1]Monitoring of lymphocyte subsets other than CD4 (eg, CD8, CD19) has not proven clinically useful, adds to costs, and is not routinely recommended

[2]Some experts may repeat CD4 count every 3 months in patients with low baseline CD4 count (<200 to 300 cells/mm^3) before ART but every 6 months in those who initiated ART at higher CD4 cell count (eg, >300 cells/mm^3)

[3]The following are examples of clinically indicated scenarios: Changes in a patient's clinical status that may decrease CD4 count and thus prompt initiation of prophylaxis for opportunistic infections, such as new HIV-associated symptoms, or initiation of treatment with medications which are known to reduce CD4 cell count

Initiating Antiretroviral Therapy in Treatment-Naïve HIV-1-Infected Patient[1,2]

Clinical Condition	Recommendations
HIV-infected patient	Antiretroviral therapy is recommended for all HIV-infected individuals[3]
Patients who are at risk of transmitting HIV to sexual partners	Antiretroviral therapy is recommended for HIV-infected individuals for prevention of transmission of HIV
AIDS-defining illness, including HIV-associated dementia Pregnant women[4] Acute opportunistic infections Lower CD4 counts (<200 cells/mm^3) Patients with HIV-associated nephropathy Acute/recent infection Patients coinfected with hepatitis B virus (HBV) Patients coinfected with hepatitis C virus (HCV) Rapidly declining CD4 counts (>100 cells/mm^3 decrease per year) Higher viral loads (>100,000 copies/mL)	Antiretroviral therapy is strongly recommended regardless of CD4 count; these conditions favor more rapid initiation of therapy

[1]Patients initiating antiretroviral therapy should be willing and able to commit to lifelong treatment, and should understand the benefits and risks of therapy and the importance of adherence.

[2]Patients may choose to postpone therapy, and providers, on a case-by-case basis, may elect to defer therapy based on clinical and/or psychosocial factors.

[3]The strength of this recommendation varies on the basis of pretreatment CD4 cell count:

CD4 count <350 cells/mm^3: Strong recommendation with evidence from randomized controlled trials

CD4 count 350 to 500 cells/mm^3: Strong recommendation with evidence from well-designed nonrandomized trials or observational cohort studies with long-term clinical outcomes

CD4 count >500 cells/mm^3: Moderate recommendation; expert opinion

[4]Combination antiretroviral therapy is recommended for all HIV-infected pregnant women to prevent maternal-to-child transmission, even if the mother does not require antiretroviral therapy for her own health. Following delivery, considerations regarding continuation of the maternal antiretroviral regimen for therapeutic indications are the same as for other nonpregnant individuals. For more detailed discussion, please refer to: Recommendations for use of antiretroviral drugs in pregnant HIV-1-infected women for maternal health and interventions to reduce perinatal HIV transmission in the United States. Available at http://www.aidsinfo.nih.gov/guidelines/

Conditions in Which Deferral of Therapy Might Be Considered

Some patients and their clinicians may decide to defer therapy for a period of time based on clinical or personal circumstances. The degree to which these factors might support deferral of therapy depends on the CD4 count and viral load. Although deferring therapy for the reasons listed below may be reasonable for patients with high CD4 counts (eg, >500 cells/mm^3), deferral for patients with much lower CD4 counts (eg, <200 cells/mm^3) should be considered only in rare situations and should be undertaken with close clinical follow-up. A brief delay in initiating therapy may be considered to allow a patient more time to prepare for lifelong treatment. Deferral may be considered in the following conditions:

- When there are significant barriers to adherence.
- Presence of comorbidities that complicate or prohibit antiretroviral therapy.
  Examples include:
  - Patients requiring surgery that might result in an extended interruption of antiretroviral therapy.
  - Patients taking medications that have clinically significant drug interactions with antiretroviral agents and for whom alternative therapy is not available.
  - Patients with a poor prognosis due to a concomitant medical condition who would not be expected to derive survival or quality-of-life benefits from antiretroviral therapy.
- Elite HIV controllers or long-term nonprogressors (**Note:** Antiretroviral therapy is recommended for nonprogressors who have consistently detectable viremia (HIV >200 to 1,000 copies/mL) and elite controllers who exhibit evidence of disease progression (as defined by declining CD4 counts or development of HIV-related complications).

Antiretroviral Regimens for Treatment-Naïve Patients

Patients who are naïve to antiretroviral therapy should be started on one of the following types of combination regimens:

- **INSTI + 2 NRTIs; or**
- **NNRTI + 2 NRTIs; or**
- **PI (boosted with ritonavir or cobicistat) + 2 NRTIs**

Selection of a regimen should be individualized based on virologic efficacy, toxicity, pill burden, dosing frequency, drug-drug interaction potential, resistance testing results, and comorbid conditions. Drug classes and regimens within each class are listed in alphabetical order.

For more detailed recommendations on antiretroviral choices and dosing in HIV-infected pregnant women, please refer to: Recommendations for use of antiretroviral drugs in pregnant HIV-1-infected women for maternal health and interventions to reduce perinatal HIV transmission in the United States. Available at http://www.aidsinfo.nih.gov/guidelines

Recommended, Alternative, and Other ART Regimen Options for Treatment-Naïve Patients

Recommended Regimen Options
INSTI-based Regimens • DTG/ABC/3TC[1] – **only** for patients who are HLA-B*5701 negative • DTG plus TDF/FTC[1] • EVG/COBI/TDF/FTC – **only** for patients with pretreatment estimated CrCl ≥70 mL/min • RAL + TDF/FTC[1]
PI-based Regimen • DRV/r + TDF/FTC[1]
Alternative Regimen Options
Regimens that are effective and tolerable but that have potential disadvantages when compared with the recommended regimens listed above, have limitations for use in certain patient populations, or have less supporting data from randomized clinical trials. **An alternative regimen may be the preferred regimen for some patients.**
NNRTI-based Regimens • EFV/TDF/FTC[1] • RPV/TDF/FTC[1] – **only** for patients with pretreatment HIV RNA <100,000 copies/mL and CD4 cell count >200 cells/mm^3
PI-based Regimens • ATV/COBI plus TDF/FTC[1] – **only** for patients with pretreatment estimated CrCl ≥70 mL/min • ATV/r plus TDF/FTC[1] • (DRV/COBI or DRV/r) + ABC/3TC[1] – **only** for patients who are HLA-B*5701 negative • DRV/COBI plus TDF/FTC[1] – **only** for patients with pretreatment estimated CrCl ≥70 mL/min
Other Regimen Options
Regimens that, in comparison with Recommended and Alternative regimens, may have reduced virologic activity, limited supporting data from large comparative clinical trials, or other factors, such as greater toxicities, higher pill burden, drug interaction potential, or limitations for use in certain patient populations.
INSTI-based Regimen • RAL + ABC/3TC[1] – **only** for patients who are HLA-B*5701 negative
NNRTI-based Regimen • EFV plus ABC/3TC[1] – **only** for patients who are HLA-B*5701 negative and with pretreatment HIV RNA <100,000 copies/mL
PI-based Regimens • (ATV/COBI or ATV/r) plus ABC/3TC[1] – **only** for patients who are HLA-B*5701 negative and with pretreatment HIV RNA <100,000 copies/mL • LPV/r (once[2] or twice daily) plus ABC/3TC[1] – **only** for patients who are HLA-B*5701 negative • LPV/r (once[2] or twice daily) plus TDF/FTC[1]
Other Regimens When TDF or ABC Cannot Be Used • DRV/r plus RAL – **only** for patients with pretreatment HIV RNA <100,000 copies/mL and CD4 cell count >200 cells/mm^3 • LPV/r (twice daily) plus 3TC (twice daily)

3TC = lamiVUDine, ABC = abacavir, ART = antiretroviral therapy, ATV/COBI = cobicistat-boosted atazanavir, ATV/r = ritonavir-boosted atazanavir, COBI = cobicistat, DRV/COBI = cobicistat-boosted darunavir, DRV/r = ritonavir-boosted darunavir, DTG = dolutegravir, EFV = efavirenz, EVG = elvitegravir, FTC = emtricitabine, INSTI = integrase strand transfer inhibitor, LPV/r = ritonavir-boosted lopinavir, NNRTI = nonnucleoside reverse transcriptase inhibitor, NRTI = nucleos(t)ide reverse transcriptase inhibitor, PI = protease inhibitor, RAL = raltegravir, RPV = rilpivirine, TDF = tenofovir

The following combinations in the lists above are available as fixed-dose combination formulations: ABC/3TC, ATV/COBI, DRV/COBI, DTG/ABC/3TC, EFV/TDF/FTC, EVG/COBI/TDF/FTC, LPV/r, RPV/TDF/FTC, and TDF/FTC

[1]3TC may substitute for FTC or vice versa.

[2]Once daily LPV/r is not recommended for pregnant patients.

Antiretroviral Components Not Recommended as Initial Therapy

Antiretroviral Drugs or Components (in alphabetical order)	Reasons for Not Recommending as Initial Therapy
Abacavir/lamivudine/zidovudine (coformulated) as triple-NRTI combination regimen	Inferior virologic efficacy
Abacavir + lamiVUDine + zidovudine + tenofovir as quadruple NRTI combination	Inferior virologic efficacy
Atazanavir (unboosted)	Less potent than boosted atazanavir
Darunavir (unboosted)	Usage without ritonavir has not been studied
Delavirdine	Inferior virologic efficacy Inconvenient dosing (3 times/day)
Didanosine + lamiVUDine (or emtricitabine)	Inferior virologic efficacy Limited clinical trial experience in treatment-naïve patients Didanosine toxicity, such as pancreatitis and peripheral neuropathy
Didanosine + tenofovir	High rate of early virologic failure Rapid selection of resistant mutations Potential for immunologic nonresponse/$CD4^+$ decline Increased didanosine drug exposure and toxicities
Enfuvirtide	No clinical trial experience in treatment-naïve patients Requires twice daily subcutaneous injections
Etravirine	Insufficient data in treatment-naïve patients
Fosamprenavir (unboosted or ritonavir-boosted)	Virologic failure with unboosted fosamprenavir-based regimen may select mutations that confer resistance to fosamprenavir and darunavir Less clinical trial data for ritonavir-boosted fosamprenavir than for other ritonavir-boosted protease inhibitors
Indinavir (unboosted)	Inconvenient dosing (3 times/day with meal restrictions) Fluid requirement Indinavir toxicities, such as nephrolithiasis and crystalluria
Indinavir (ritonavir-boosted)	Fluid requirement Indinavir toxicities, such as nephrolithiasis and crystalluria
Maraviroc	Requires testing for CCR5 tropism before initiation of therapy No virologic benefit when compared with other recommended regimens Requires twice-daily dosing
Nelfinavir	Inferior virologic efficacy Diarrhea
Nevirapine	Associated with serious and potentially fatal toxicity (hepatic events and severe rash, including Stevens-Johnson syndrome and toxic epidermal necrolysis) When compared to efavirenz, nevirapine did not meet noninferiority criteria
Ritonavir as sole PI	High pill burden Gastrointestinal intolerance Metabolic toxicity
Saquinavir (unboosted)	Inadequate bioavailability Inferior virologic efficacy
Saquinavir (ritonavir-boosted)	High pill burden Can cause QT and PR prolongation; requires pretreatment and follow-up ECG
Stavudine + lamiVUDine	Significant toxicities including lipoatrophy, peripheral neuropathy, and hyperlactatemia, including symptomatic and life-threatening lactic acidosis, hepatic steatosis, and pancreatitis
Tipranavir (ritonavir-boosted)	Inferior virologic efficacy Higher rate of adverse events than other ritonavir-boosted protease inhibitors Higher dose of ritonavir required for boosting than with other protease inhibitors
Zidovudine + lamiVUDine	Greater toxicities (including bone marrow suppression; GI toxicities; mitochondrial toxicities, such as lipoatrophy, lactic acidosis, and hepatic steatosis; skeletal muscle myopathy; and cardiomyopathy) compared to recommended NRTIs

Antiretroviral Regimens or Components That Should Not Be Offered at Any Time

	Rationale	Exception
Antiretroviral Regimens Not Recommended		
Monotherapy with NRTI	Rapid development of resistance Inferior antiretroviral activity when compared to combination with three or more antiretrovirals	No exception
Dual-NRTI regimens	Rapid development of resistance Inferior antiretroviral activity when compared to combination with three or more antiretrovirals	No exception
Triple-NRTI regimens except for abacavir/zidovudine/lamivudine or possibly tenofovir + zidovudine/lamivudine	High rate of early virologic nonresponse seen when triple NRTI combinations including ABC/TDF/3TC or TDF/ddl/3TC were used as initial regimen in treatment-naive patients Other triple-NRTI regimens have not been evaluated	Abacavir/zidovudine/lamivudine; and possibly tenofovir + zidovudine/lamivudine in selected patients where other combinations are not desirable
Antiretroviral Components Not Recommended as Part of Antiretroviral Regimen		
Atazanavir + indinavir	Potential additive hyperbilirubinemia	No exception
Didanosine + stavudine	High incidence of toxicities – peripheral neuropathy, pancreatitis, and hyperlactatemia Reports of serious, even fatal, cases of lactic acidosis with hepatic steatosis with or without pancreatitis in pregnant women	No exception
Didanosine + tenofovir	Increased didanosine concentrations and serious didanosine-associated toxicities Potential for immunologic nonresponse and/or CD4 cell count decline High rate of virologic failure Rapid selection of resistance mutations at failure	Clinicians caring for patients who are clinically stable on regimens containing tenofovir + didanosine should consider altering the NRTIs to avoid this combination
2-NNRTI combination	When EFV combined with NVP, higher incidence of clinical adverse events seen when compared to either EFV- or NVP-based regimen Both EFV and NVP may induce metabolism and may lead to reductions in etravirine (ETR) exposure; thus, should not be used in combination	No exception
Efavirenz in first trimester of pregnancy or in women with significant childbearing potential	Teratogenic in nonhuman primates	When no other antiretroviral options are available and potential benefits outweigh the risks
Emtricitabine + lamiVUDine	Similar resistance profile No potential benefit	No exception
Etravirine + unboosted PI	Etravirine may induce metabolism of these PIs, appropriate doses not yet established.	No exception
Etravirine + ritonavir-boosted atazanavir or fosamprenavir	Etravirine may alter the concentrations of these PIs, appropriate doses not yet established.	No exception
Etravirine + ritonavir-boosted tipranavir	Etravirine concentration may be significantly reduced by RTV-boosted tipranavir	No exception
Nevirapine in treatment-naïve women with CD4 >250 or men with CD4 >400	High incidence of symptomatic hepatotoxicity	If no other antiretroviral option available, if used, patients should be closely monitored
Stavudine + zidovudine	Antagonistic effect on HIV-1	No exception
Unboosted darunavir, saquinavir, or tipranavir	Inadequate bioavailability	No exception

Recommendations for Using Drug-Resistance Assays

Clinical Setting/Recommendation	Rationale
Drug-Resistance Assay Recommended	
In acute HIV infection: Drug resistance testing is recommended, regardless of whether treatment will be initiated immediately or deferred. A genotypic assay is generally preferred.	If treatment is to be initiated, drug resistance testing will determine whether drug-resistant virus was transmitted and will help in the design of initial or changed (if therapy was initiated prior to test results) regimens. Genotypic testing is preferable to phenotypic testing because of lower cost, faster turnaround time, and greater sensitivity for detecting mixtures of wild-type and resistant virus.
If treatment is deferred, repeat resistance testing should be considered at the time ART is initiated. A genotypic assay is generally preferred.	If treatment is deferred, testing still should be performed because of the greater likelihood that transmitted resistance-associated mutations will be detected earlier in the course of HIV infection; results of testing may be important when treatment is eventually initiated. Repeat testing at the time ART is initiated should be considered because of the possibility that the patient may have acquired drug-resistant virus.
In treatment-naïve patients with chronic HIV infection: Drug resistance testing is recommended at the time of entry into HIV care, regardless of whether therapy is initiated immediately or deferred. A genotypic assay is generally preferred. If therapy is deferred, repeat resistance testing should be considered at the time ART is initiated. A genotypic assay is generally preferred.	Transmitted HIV with baseline resistance to at least one drug may be seen in 6% to 16% of patients. Suboptimal virologic responses may be seen in patients with baseline resistant mutations. Some drug resistance mutations can remain detectable for years in untreated chronically infected patients. Repeat testing prior to initiation of ART should be considered because that the patient may have acquired a drug-resistant virus. Genotypic testing is preferred for the reasons noted previously.
If an INSTI is considered for an ART-naïve patient and transmitted INSTI resistance is a concern, providers may wish to supplement standard resistance testing with a specific INSTI genotypic resistance assay	Standard genotypic drug-resistance assays test only for mutations in the RT and PR genes.
If use of a CCR5 antagonist is being considered, a coreceptor tropism assay should be performed.	A phenotypic tropism assay is preferred to determine HIV-1 coreceptor usage. A genotypic tropism assay should be considered as an alternative test to predict HIV-1 coreceptor usage.
In patients with virologic failure: Drug resistance testing is recommended in persons on combination antiretroviral therapy with HIV RNA levels >1,000 copies/mL. In persons with HIV RNA levels >500 but <1,000 copies/mL, testing may be unsuccessful but should still be considered.	Testing can help determine the role of resistance in drug failure and maximize the clinician's ability to select active drugs for the new regimen. Drug resistance testing should be performed while the patient is taking prescribed antiretroviral drugs or, if not possible, within 4 weeks after discontinuing therapy.
A genotypic assay is generally preferred in those experiencing virologic failure on their first or second regimens.	Genotypic testing is generally preferred for the reasons noted previously.
In patients failing INSTI-based regimens, genotypic testing for INSTI resistance should be performed to determine whether to include drugs from this class in subsequent regimens.	Standard genotypic drug-resistance assays test only for mutations in the RT and PR genes.
If use of a CCR5 antagonist is being considered, a coreceptor tropism assay should be performed.	A phenotypic tropism assay is preferred to determine HIV-1 coreceptor usage. A genotypic tropism assay should be considered as an alternative test to predict HIV-1 coreceptor usage.
Addition of phenotypic assay to genotypic assay is generally preferred for those with known or suspected complex drug resistance patterns, particularly to protease inhibitors.	Phenotypic testing can provide useful additional information for those with complex drug resistance mutation patterns, particularly to protease inhibitors.
In patients with suboptimal suppression of viral load: Drug resistance testing is recommended in persons with suboptimal suppression of viral load after initiation of antiretroviral therapy.	Testing can help determine the role of resistance and thus assist in identifying the number of active drugs available for a new regimen.
In HIV-infected pregnant women: Genotypic resistance testing is recommended for all pregnant women prior to initiation of therapy and for those entering pregnancy with detectable HIV RNA levels while on therapy.	The goals of antiretroviral therapy in HIV-infected pregnant women are to achieve maximal viral suppression for treatment of maternal HIV infection as well as for prevention of perinatal HIV transmission. Genotypic resistance testing will assist the clinician in selecting the optimal regimen for the patient.
Drug-Resistance Assay Not Usually Recommended	
After therapy discontinued: Drug resistance testing is not usually recommended after discontinuation (>4 weeks) of antiretroviral drugs.	Drug-resistance mutations may become minor species in the absence of selective drug pressure, and available assays may not detect minor drug-resistant species. If testing is performed in this setting, the detection of drug resistance may be of value, but its absence does not rule out the presence of minor drug-resistant species.
In patients with low HIV RNA levels: Drug resistance testing is not usually recommended in persons with a plasma viral load <500 copies/mL.	Resistance assays cannot be consistently performed because of low HIV RNA levels

Identifying, Diagnosing, and Managing Acute and Recent HIV-1 Infection

- **Suspicion of acute HIV infection:** Signs or symptoms of acute HIV infection with recent (within 2 to 6 weeks) high HIV risk exposure[1]
  - Signs/symptoms/laboratory findings may include but are not limited to one or more of the following: Fever, lymphadenopathy, skin rash, myalgia/arthralgia, headache, diarrhea, oral ulcers, leucopenia, thrombocytopenia, transaminase elevation
  - High-risk exposures include sexual contact with a person infected with HIV or at risk for HIV, sharing of injection drug use paraphernalia, or contact of mucous membranes or breaks in skin with potentially infectious fluids[1]
- **Differential diagnosis:** Includes but is not limited to viral illnesses, such as EBV- and non-EBV (eg, CMV)-related infectious mononucleosis syndromes, influenza, viral hepatitis, streptococcal infection, syphilis
- **Evaluation/diagnosis of acute HIV infection:**
  - Acute infection is defined as detectable HIV RNA or p24 antigen [the antigen used in currently available HIV antigen/antibody (Ag/Ab) combination assays], in serum or plasma in the setting of a negative or indeterminate HIV antibody test result.
    - A reactive HIV antibody test or Ag/Ab combination test must be followed by supplemental confirmatory testing.
    - A negative or indeterminate HIV antibody test in a person with a positive Ag/Ab test or in whom acute HIV infection is suspected requires assessment of plasma HIV RNA to diagnose acute HIV infection.
    - A positive result on an FDA-approved quantitative or qualitative plasma HIV RNA test in the setting of a negative or indeterminate antibody result is consistent with acute HIV infection.
  - Patients presumptively diagnosed with acute HIV infection should have serologic testing repeated over the next 3 to 6 months to document seroconversion.
- **Considerations for antiretroviral therapy during early HIV infection:**
  - All pregnant women with early HIV infection should start on a combination ARV regimen as soon as possible to prevent perinatal transmission of HIV
  - Treatment for early HIV infection should be offered to all nonpregnant people
  - The risks of antiretroviral therapy during early infection are consistent with those for initiating antiretroviral therapy in chronically infected asymptomatic patients with high CD4 counts
  - If therapy is initiated, the goal should be for sustained plasma virologic suppression

[1]In some settings, behaviors conducive to acquisition of HIV infection might not be ascertained or might not be perceived as "high-risk" by the health care provider or the patient or both. Thus, symptoms and signs consistent with acute retroviral syndrome should motivate consideration of this diagnosis, even in the absence of reported high-risk behaviors.

Associated Signs and Symptoms of Acute Retroviral Syndrome and Percentage of Expected Frequency

- Fever (96%)
- Lymphadenopathy (74%)
- Pharyngitis (70%)
- Rash (70%)
  - Erythematous maculopapular with lesions on face and trunk and sometimes extremities, including palms and soles
  - Mucocutaneous ulceration involving mouth, esophagus, or genitals
- Myalgia or arthralgia (54%)
- Diarrhea (32%)
- Headache (32%)
- Nausea and vomiting (27%)
- Hepatosplenomegaly (14%)
- Weight loss (13%)
- Thrush (12%)
- Neurologic symptoms (12%)
  - Meningoencephalitis or aseptic meningitis
  - Peripheral neuropathy or radiculopathy
  - Facial palsy
  - Guillain-Barré syndrome
  - Brachial neuritis
  - Cognitive impairment or psychosis

REFERENCE

Niu MT, Stein DS, Schnittman SM. Primary human immunodeficiency virus type 1 infection: review of pathogenesis and early treatment intervention in humans and animal retrovirus infections. *J Infect Dis*. 1993;168(6):1490-1501.

PERINATAL HIV

Overview and Rationale of Perinatal Antiretroviral Therapy

Antiretroviral agents are used during pregnancy for two reasons: 1) To treat maternal human immunodeficiency virus (HIV) infection and 2) To reduce the risk of perinatal HIV transmission. The pivotal clinical trial that demonstrated the benefits of antiretroviral prophylaxis to decrease the risk of perinatal HIV transmission was the Pediatric AIDS Clinical Trials Group (PACTG) 076 (Connor 1994). In this randomized, double-blind, placebo-controlled trial, zidovudine monotherapy was administered in three phases: 1) Antepartum (to the pregnant woman), 2) Intrapartum (during labor to the pregnant woman) and 3) Postpartum (to the newborn infant for 6 weeks). A relative reduction of 67.5% in the risk of perinatal HIV transmission was observed in this study; the mother to infant HIV transmission rate decreased from 25.5% in the placebo group to 8.3% in the zidovudine group.

Many studies have been conducted and much has been learned since publication of that pivotal study. Currently, antiretroviral monotherapy is **not** considered to be appropriate for the treatment of HIV infection. Maternal use of combination highly active antiretroviral therapy (ie, HAART) is considered to be the standard of care, both for the treatment of maternal HIV infection and to reduce the risk of perinatal HIV transmission. Optimal reduction of the risk of perinatal HIV transmission still includes a three-phase approach with appropriate antiretroviral medications administered 1) Antepartum (to the pregnant woman), 2) Intrapartum (during labor to the pregnant woman) and 3) Postpartum (to the newborn infant). The antepartum HAART regimen should contain at least three antiretroviral agents (see below) and include one or more nucleoside reverse transcriptase inhibitor (NRTI) drugs with a high placental transfer rate (eg, zidovudine, lamivudine, emtricitabine, tenofovir, abacavir). Intrapartum zidovudine is recommended for HIV-infected pregnant women with HIV RNA >1,000 copies/mL (or unknown HIV RNA) near delivery, regardless of their antiretroviral regimen or mode of delivery. A 6-week course of zidovudine is generally recommended for all newborns born to women who are HIV positive; however, a 4-week course of zidovudine may be considered in the infant when the mother has received standard combination antiretroviral therapy during pregnancy with consistent viral suppression and there are no concerns related to maternal adherence (see Table 3). A two-drug postpartum regimen, consisting of a 6-week course of zidovudine plus a three-dose course of nevirapine, is recommended for newborns whose mothers have not received antepartum antiretroviral therapy (see Table 4). Use of combination antiretroviral prophylaxis may be considered on a case-by-case basis in newborns in special circumstances who are at higher risk of HIV perinatal transmission (eg, infants born to HIV-infected mothers with no antiretroviral therapy prior to labor or during labor; infants born to mothers with only intrapartum antiretroviral therapy; infants born to mothers with suboptimal viral suppression at delivery; or infants born to mothers with known antiretroviral drug-resistant virus). Today, with the use of antepartum HAART therapy, prenatal HIV counseling and testing, antiretroviral prophylaxis, scheduled cesarean delivery, and avoidance of breastfeeding, the perinatal transmission rate of HIV infection has decreased to <2% in the United States and Europe.

Specific recommendations for the use of antiretroviral drugs during pregnancy are updated regularly by the Department of Health and Human Services Panel on Treatment of HIV-Infected Pregnant Women and Prevention of Perinatal Transmission. The latest guidelines are available at http://AIDSinfo.nih.gov. Health care professionals are encouraged to contact the antiretroviral pregnancy registry to monitor outcomes of pregnant women exposed to antiretroviral medications – (800) 258-4263 or http://www.APRegistry.com).

The 2014 Panel recommendations include the following (information is summarized here for the reader):

General Principles

Note: Combined antepartum, intrapartum and infant antiretroviral prophylaxis is recommended for the prevention of perinatal HIV.

Preconception:

- Discussion of childbearing intentions with all women of childbearing age should be conducted on an ongoing basis throughout the course of their care.
- Effective and appropriate contraception should be selected to avoid unintended pregnancy.
- Preconception counseling concerning safer sexual practices (and elimination of alcohol, illicit drug use, and smoking) should be conducted.
- All HIV-infected women who wish to become pregnant should be receiving a maximally suppressive antiretroviral regimen.
- Evaluation or selection of antiretroviral therapy should consider efficacy for maternal treatment, hepatitis B virus disease status, the potential for teratogenicity if pregnancy should occur, and possible adverse outcomes for mother and fetus.
- Peri-contraception administration of antiretroviral pre-exposure prophylaxis (PrEP) for HIV-uninfected partners may offer an additional tool to reduce the risk of sexual transmission. The utility of PrEP of the uninfected partner when the infected partner is receiving ART and has a suppressed viral load has not been studied.
- For both concordant and discordant couples, the HIV-infected partner should attain maximum viral suppression before attempting conception. Refer to Perinatal Guidelines for additional information about reproductive options for HIV-concordant and serodiscordant couples.

Antepartum:

- Known risks and benefits of antiretroviral therapy during pregnancy should be discussed with all HIV-infected women.
- Combined antepartum, intrapartum, and infant antiretroviral prophylaxis is recommended because antiretroviral drugs reduce perinatal transmission by several mechanisms, including lowering maternal antepartum viral load and providing infant pre- and post-exposure prophylaxis.

- Assessment of HIV disease status and recommendations about initial antiretroviral therapy or changes to current regimen should be included in initial evaluation of pregnant women infected with HIV. The National Perinatal HIV Hotline provides free clinical consultation on all aspects of perinatal HIV care – (888) 448-8765.
- All HIV-infected pregnant women should receive a combination antepartum antiretroviral drug regimen containing at least three agents regardless of plasma HIV RNA copy number or CD4 count.
- In general, the same antiretroviral regimens as recommended for treatment of nonpregnant adults should be used in pregnant women, unless there are known adverse effects for women, fetuses, or infants that outweigh benefits.
- Multiple factors must be considered when choosing a regimen for a pregnant woman, including comorbidities, convenience, adverse effects, drug interactions, resistance testing results, pharmacokinetics, and experience with use in pregnancy.
- Pharmacokinetic changes in pregnancy may lead to lower plasma concentrations of drugs and necessitate increased dosages, more frequent dosing, or ritonavir boosting, especially of protease inhibitors.
- For antiretroviral-naïve pregnant women, a combination regimen including two NRTIs and either a protease inhibitor (PI) with low-dose ritonavir or a non-nucleoside reverse transcriptase inhibitor (NNRTI) is preferred. Some clinicians prefer a ritonavir-boosted PI regimen because clinically significant resistance to PIs is less common than resistance to NNRTIs in antiretroviral-naïve individuals. In addition, the preferred NNRTI is efavirenz which has a potential risk for teratogenicity and should be avoided during the first 8 weeks of pregnancy. **Note:** A possible small increased risk of preterm birth in pregnant women receiving PI-based combination antiretroviral therapy exists; however, due to the clear benefits of such regimens, PIs should not be withheld for fear of altering pregnancy outcome.
- A combination antepartum antiretroviral regimen is more effective than a single-drug regimen to reduce perinatal HIV transmission. Combination antiretroviral regimens are recommended both for women who require HIV treatment for their own health and for prevention of perinatal transmission in pregnant HIV-infected women who do not yet require HIV therapy.
- Resistance studies should be conducted prior to starting/modifying therapy if HIV RNA is detectable (eg, >500 to 1,000 copies/mL). If HIV is diagnosed late in pregnancy, antiretroviral therapy or prophylaxis should be initiated promptly without waiting for results of resistance testing.
- Optimal adherence to antiretroviral medications is a key part of the strategy to avoid failure and reduce the development of resistance.
- Coordination of services among prenatal care providers, primary care and HIV specialty care providers, mental health and drug abuse treatment services, and public assistance programs, is essential to ensure that HIV-infected women adhere to their antiretroviral drug regimens.
- Additional specific medication issues:
  - At least one NRTI drug with high placental transfer (eg, zidovudine, lamivudine, emtricitabine, tenofovir, abacavir) should be included in the regimen.
  - Preferred two-NRTI combinations include abacavir plus lamivudine, tenofovir plus emtricitabine (or lamivudine), and zidovudine plus lamivudine.
  - Efavirenz: Due to the risk of teratogenicity, pregnancy should be avoided in women receiving efavirenz and treatment with efavirenz should be avoided during the first 8 weeks of pregnancy (the primary period of fetal organogenesis) whenever possible. Because the risk of neural tube defects is restricted to the first 5 to 6 weeks of pregnancy and pregnancy is rarely recognized before 4 to 6 weeks of pregnancy, and unnecessary antiretroviral drug changes during pregnancy may be associated with loss of viral control and increased risk of perinatal transmission, efavirenz may be continued in pregnant women receiving an efavirenz-based regimen who present for antenatal care in the first trimester, provided there is virologic suppression on the regimen.
  - Nevirapine use as initial therapy in pregnant women with a CD4 cell count >250 cells/mm^3 should generally be avoided and should only be used if the benefit clearly outweighs the risk of increased hepatic toxicity. Nevirapine can be continued in pregnant women who are virologically suppressed and tolerating therapy regardless of CD4 count. **Note:** Women with CD4 counts >250 cells/mm^3 are at increased risk for rash-associated nevirapine-related hepatotoxicity including severe, life-threatening and potentially fatal hepatic events. Elevated transaminase levels at baseline may also increase the risk of nevirapine toxicity.
  - Lopinavir/ritonavir and ritonavir-boosted atazanavir are the preferred protease inhibitors for antiretroviral-naïve pregnant women. Alternative protease inhibitors include ritonavir-boosted darunavir and ritonavir-boosted saquinavir.
  - Protease inhibitors may require dosing adjustments during pregnancy.
  - Glucose screening with a standard, 1-hour, 50 g glucose loading test at 24 to 28 weeks of gestation should be performed in HIV-infected pregnant women taking antiretroviral drug regimens. Some experts recommend earlier glucose screening in women receiving protease inhibitor-based regimens initiated before pregnancy, similar to recommendations for women with high-risk factors for glucose intolerance.
  - Combination of stavudine and didanosine is not recommended during pregnancy; stavudine and didanosine in combination may cause lactic acidosis, hepatic failure, and maternal/neonatal mortality with prolonged use during pregnancy.
  - NRTIs may be associated with lactic acidosis; monitor.

- Mitochondrial dysfunction should be considered in uninfected children with perinatal exposure to antiretroviral medications who present with severe clinical findings of unknown etiology, particularly neurologic findings.
- Long-term clinical follow-up for any child with *in utero* exposure to antiretroviral medications is recommended.

Intrapartum:

- Scheduled cesarean delivery at 38 weeks is recommended for women with suboptimal viral suppression near delivery (eg, HIV RNA >1,000 copies/mL) or with unknown HIV RNA near the time of delivery.
- A rapid HIV antibody test should be performed in women with unknown HIV status who present in labor. If positive, a confirmatory HIV test should be sent as soon as possible and maternal intravenous (IV) zidovudine and infant combination antiretroviral drug prophylaxis should be initiated without waiting for test results. If the HIV test is positive, infant antiretroviral drugs should be continued for 6 weeks; if the maternal HIV test is negative, the infant antiretroviral drugs should be stopped.
- HIV-infected pregnant women with HIV RNA >1,000 copies/mL (or unknown HIV RNA) near delivery should receive intrapartum IV zidovudine, regardless of their antepartum HAART regimen or mode of delivery. In situations in which IV administration is not possible, oral administration can be considered.
- IV zidovudine is not required for HIV-infected women receiving antiretroviral regimens who have HIV RNA ≤1,000 copies/mL consistently during late pregnancy and near delivery and no concerns regarding adherence to the regimen.
- Pregnant women with HIV RNA >1,000 copies/mL and documented zidovudine resistance who are not currently taking zidovudine for their own health should receive IV zidovudine during labor, in addition to their established regimens, except in women with documented histories of hypersensitivity.
- HIV-infected pregnant women in labor who have not received antepartum antiretroviral drugs should receive IV zidovudine.
- Women who are receiving an antepartum combination antiretroviral treatment regimen should continue their regimen on schedule as much as possible during labor and prior to scheduled cesarean delivery. Women with HIV RNA >1,000 copies/mL who are receiving oral fixed-dose combination regimens that include zidovudine should have zidovudine administered IV during labor while other antiretroviral components are continued orally.
- Nevirapine use as a single dose is not recommended for women in the US who are receiving standard antiretroviral prophylaxis regimens or for women who have **not** received antepartum antiretroviral drugs.
- If antepartum antiretroviral drugs were **not** administered, intrapartum therapy (IV zidovudine administered to the mother) and infant combination antiretroviral prophylaxis for 6 weeks is recommended.

Postpartum:

- Postnatal infant prophylaxis with a 6-week course of zidovudine is generally recommended for all infants born to HIV-infected women. However, a 4-week neonatal chemoprophylaxis regimen can be considered when the mother has received standard combined antiretroviral therapy during pregnancy with consistent viral suppression and there are no concerns related to maternal adherence.
- Zidovudine, at gestation age-appropriate doses, should be initiated as close to the time of birth as possible, preferably within 6 to 12 hours of delivery
- If antepartum or intrapartum antiretroviral drugs were not administered, or suboptimal viral suppression or antiretroviral drug resistance is known, most experts recommend postnatal infant prophylaxis with nevirapine (3 doses administered in the first week of life – at birth, 48 hours later, and 96 hours after the second dose) in combination with a 6-week course of zidovudine.
- Breast-feeding is not recommended for HIV-infected women in the United States, including those receiving antiretroviral therapy.
- The decision to continue maternal antiretroviral therapy after delivery should be based on current recommendations for initiation of antiretroviral therapy, current and nadir CD4 counts and trajectory, HIV RNA levels, adherence issues, clinical symptoms/disease stage, presence of other indications for antiretroviral therapy, whether the woman has an HIV-uninfected sexual partner, and patient preference.
- Arrangements for new or continued supportive services should be made prior to hospital discharge for women continuing antiretroviral therapy postpartum.
- Contraceptive counseling should be included in the prenatal period, as well as immediately postpartum, as a critical aspect of postpartum care.

Special Situations

HIV/hepatitis B virus coinfection:

- Screening for hepatitis B virus (HBV) with hepatitis B surface antigen (HBsAg), hepatitis B core antibody (anti-HBc), and hepatitis B surface antibody (anti-HBs) is recommended for all pregnant women not already screened during current pregnancy.
- All pregnant women who screen negative for HBV should receive the HBV vaccine series.
- Women with chronic HBV should also be screened for hepatitis A virus (HAV) because they are at increased risk of complications from coinfection with other viral hepatitis infections.

- Women with chronic HBV infection who are negative for hepatitis A immunoglobulin G should receive the HAV vaccine series.
- All pregnant women with chronic hepatitis B virus (HBV) infection and HIV coinfection should receive a combination antiretroviral regimen, including a dual NRTI backbone with two drugs active against both HIV and HBV. Tenofovir plus lamiVUDine or emtricitabine is the preferred backbone.
- Consultation with an expert is strongly recommended for pregnant women coinfected with HIV/HBV.
- Interferon alfa and pegylated interferon alfa are not recommended during pregnancy.
- Pregnant women with HBV and HIV coinfection receiving antiretroviral medications should be monitored for liver toxicity.
- If antiretroviral drugs are discontinued postpartum in women coinfected with HIV/HBV, liver function tests should be monitored frequently for potential exacerbation of HBV infection.
- Infants born to hepatitis B infected women should receive hepatitis B immune globulin (HBIG) and initiate the three-dose hepatitis B vaccination series within 12 hours of birth.

HIV/hepatitis C virus coinfection:

- Screening for hepatitis C is recommended for all HIV-infected women not already screened during current pregnancy.
- Women with chronic hepatitis C virus (HCV) infection should also be screened for hepatitis A virus (HAV) because they are at increased risk of complications from coinfection with other viral hepatitis infections.
- Women with chronic HBC infection who are negative for hepatitis A immunoglobulin G should receive the HAV vaccine series
- Consultation with an expert is strongly recommended for pregnant women coinfected with HIV/HCV.
- Interferon alfa and pegylated interferon alfa are not recommended during pregnancy.
- Recommendations for antiretroviral drug use during pregnancy are the same for women who have chronic HCV infection as for those without HIV/HCV coinfection.
- Pregnant women with HCV and HIV coinfection and receiving antiretroviral medications should be monitored for liver toxicity.
- Decisions concerning mode of delivery should be based on standard obstetric and HIV-related indications alone.
- Infants born to women coinfected with HCV and HIV should be evaluated for both HIV and HCV infection. For evaluation of HCV, HCV RNA virologic testing can be performed after 2 months of age and HCV antibody testing should be conducted after 18 months of age.

The following recommendations in Table 1 are for pregnant HIV-infected women who have never received antiretroviral therapy previously (antiretroviral-naïve) and are predicated on lack of evidence of resistance to regimen components. See Table 2 for more information on specific drugs in pregnancy. Within each drug class, regimens are listed alphabetically and the order does not indicate a ranking of preference. It is recommended that women who become pregnant while on a stable antiretroviral regimen with viral suppression remain on that same regimen.

A combination antiretroviral regimen in treatment-naïve pregnant women generally contains one PI (with low-dose ritonavir boosting) plus a 2-NRTI backbone or an NNRTI plus a 2-NRTI backbone. Regimens should be individualized based on advantages and disadvantages of each combination.

Table 1. What to Start: Initial Combination Regimens for Antiretroviral-Naïve HIV-Infected Pregnant Women

Drug	Comments
PREFERRED REGIMENS Regimens with clinical trial data in adults demonstrating optimal efficacy and durability with acceptable toxicity and ease of use. Pharmacokinetic data available in pregnancy and no evidence to date of teratogenic effects or established adverse outcomes for mother, fetus, or newborn. To minimize the risk of resistance, a PI regimen is preferred for women who may stop antiretroviral therapy during the postpartum period.	
Preferred Two-NRTI Backbone	
Abacavir plus lamivudine	Available as fixed-drug combination (Epzicom); can be administered once daily. Potential hypersensitivity reaction; abacavir should not be used in patients who test positive for HLA-B*5701.
Tenofovir plus emtricitabine or lamivudine	Tenofovir/emtricitabine available as fixed-drug combination (Truvada). Either tenofovir/emtricitabine or tenofovir plus lamivudine can be administered once daily. Tenofovir has potential renal toxicity, thus tenofovir-based dual NRTI combinations should be used with caution in patients with renal insufficiency.
Zidovudine plus lamivudine	Available as fixed-drug combination (Combivir). NRTI combination with most experience for use in pregnancy but has disadvantages of requirement for twice-daily administration and increased potential for hematologic toxicity.
PI Regimens	
Atazanavir/ritonavir **plus** a preferred two-NRTI backbone	Once-daily administration

Table 1. What to Start: Initial Combination Regimens for Antiretroviral-Naïve HIV-Infected Pregnant Women *(continued)*

Drug	Comments
Lopinavir/ritonavir **plus** a preferred two-NRTI backbone	Twice-daily administration. Once-daily lopinavir/ritonavir is not recommended for use in pregnant women.
NNRTI Regimen	
Efavirenz **plus** a preferred two-NRTI backbone **Note:** May be initiated after the first 8 weeks of pregnancy	Concern because of birth defects seen in primate study; risk in humans is unclear (see Table 2). Postpartum contraception must be ensured. Preferred regimen in women requiring co-administration of drugs with significant interactions with PIs.
ALTERNATIVE REGIMENS Regimens with clinical trial data demonstrating efficacy in adults but one or more of the following apply: Experience in pregnancy is limited, data are lacking or incomplete on teratogenicity, or regimen is associated with dosing, formulation, toxicity, or interaction issues.	
PI Regimens	
Darunavir/ritonavir **plus** a preferred two-NRTI backbone	Less experience with use in pregnancy than atazanavir/ritonavir and lopinavir/ritonavir
Saquinavir/ritonavir **plus** a preferred two-NRTI backbone	Baseline ECG is recommended before initiation of saquinavir/ritonavir because of potential PR and QT prolongation; contraindicated with pre-existing cardiac conduction system disease. Large pill burden.
NNRTI Regimen	
Nevirapine **plus** a preferred two-NRTI backbone	Nevirapine should be used with caution when initiating antiretroviral therapy in women with CD4 T-lymphocyte (CD4) cell count >250 cells/mm^3. Use nevirapine and abacavir together with caution; both can cause hypersensitivity reactions within the first few weeks after initiation.
Integrase Inhibitor Regimen	
Raltegravir plus a preferred two-NRTI backbone	Limited data on raltegravir use in pregnancy but may be considered when drug interactions with PI regimens are a concern.
INSUFFICIENT DATA IN PREGNANCY TO RECOMMEND ROUTINE USE IN ANTIRETROVIRAL-NAIVE WOMEN Drugs that are approved for use in adults but lack adequate pregnancy-specific pharmacokinetic or safety data	
Dolutegravir	No data on use in pregnancy
Elvitegravir/cobicistat/emtricitabine/tenofovir (Stribild)	No data on use of elvitegravir/cobicistat component in pregnancy
Fosamprenavir/ritonavir	Limited data on use in pregnancy
Maraviroc	Requires tropism testing before use; few case reports of use in pregnancy
Rilpivirine	Rilpivirine not recommended with pretreatment HIV RNA >100,000 copies/mL or CD4 cell count <200 cells/mm^3. Do not use with proton pump inhibitor. Limited data on use in pregnancy.
NOT RECOMMENDED Drugs whose use is not recommended because of toxicity, lower rate of viral suppression, or because not recommended in antiretroviral-naïve populations	
Abacavir/lamivudine/zidovudine	Generally not recommended due to inferior virology efficacy
Stavudine	Not recommended due to toxicity
Didanosine	Not recommended due to toxicity
Indinavir/ritonavir	Concerns of kidney stones, hyperbilirubinemia
Nelfinavir	Lower rate of viral suppression with nelfinavir compared to lopinavir/ritonavir or efavirenz in adult trials
Ritonavir	Ritonavir as a single PI is not recommended because of inferior efficacy and increased toxicity
Etravirine	Not recommended in antiretroviral-naïve populations
Enfuvirtide	Not recommended in antiretroviral-naïve populations
Tipranavir	Not recommended in antiretroviral-naïve populations

NNRTI = non-nucleoside analogue reverse transcriptase inhibitor, NRTI = nucleoside analogue reverse transcriptase inhibitor, PI = protease inhibitor

Table 2. Antiretroviral Drug Use in Pregnant HIV-Infected Women: Pharmacokinetic and Toxicity Data in Human Pregnancy and Recommendations for Use in Pregnancy[a]

Drug	Pharmacokinetics and Dosing Considerations in Pregnancy	Recommendations for Use in Pregnancy
NRTIs		NRTIs are recommended for use as part of combinations regimens, usually including 2 NRTIs with either an NNRTI or one or more PIs. Use of single or dual NRTIs alone is not recommended for treatment of HIV infection.
Abacavir	Pharmacokinetics not significantly altered in pregnancy. No change in dose indicated during pregnancy.	High placental transfer to fetus[b] No evidence of human teratogenicity (can rule out 2-fold increase in overall birth defects) Hypersensitivity reactions occur in ~5% to 8% of nonpregnant individuals; a much smaller percentage are fatal and are usually associated with rechallenge. Rate in pregnancy is unknown. Testing for HLA-B*5701 allele identifies patients at risk of reactions and should be done and documented as negative before starting abacavir. Patients should be educated regarding symptoms of hypersensitivity reaction.
Didanosine	Pharmacokinetics not significantly altered in pregnancy. No change in dose indicated during pregnancy.	Low to moderate placental transfer to fetus[b] In the APR, an increased rate of birth defects with didanosine compared to general population was noted after both first-trimester and later exposure. No specific pattern of defects was noted and clinical relevance is uncertain. Didanosine should not be used with stavudine; lactic acidosis, sometimes fatal, has been reported in pregnant women receiving didanosine and stavudine together.
Emtricitabine	Pharmacokinetics not significantly altered in pregnancy. No change in dose indicated during pregnancy.	High placental transfer to fetus[b] No evidence of human teratogenicity (can rule out 2-fold increase in overall birth defects) If hepatitis B coinfected, it is possible that a hepatitis B flare may occur if emtricitabine is discontinued postpartum.
LamiVUDine	Pharmacokinetics not significantly altered in pregnancy. No change in dose indicated during pregnancy.	High placental transfer to fetus[b] No evidence of human teratogenicity (can rule out 1.5-fold increase in overall birth defects) If hepatitis B coinfected, it is possible that a hepatitis B flare may occur if lamiVUDine is discontinued postpartum.
Stavudine	Pharmacokinetics not significantly altered in pregnancy. No change in dose indicated during pregnancy.	High placental transfer to fetus[b] No evidence of human teratogenicity (can rule out 2-fold increase in overall birth defects) Stavudine should not be used with didanosine; lactic acidosis, sometimes fatal, has been reported in pregnant women receiving didanosine and stavudine together. Do not use stavudine with zidovudine due to antagonism.
Tenofovir	AUC lower in third trimester than postpartum but trough levels adequate. No change in dose indicated during pregnancy.	High placental transfer to fetus[b] No evidence of human teratogenicity (can rule out 2-fold increase in overall birth defects). Studies in monkeys show decreased fetal growth and reduction in fetal bone porosity within 2 months of starting maternal therapy. Human studies demonstrate no effect on intrauterine growth, but one study demonstrated lower length and head circumference with exposure. Tenofovir should be used in combination with lamiVUDine or emtricitabine in women with chronic hepatitis B infection. If hepatitis B coinfected, it is possible that a hepatitis B flare may occur if tenofovir is discontinued postpartum. Monitor renal function due to potential for renal toxicity.
Zidovudine	Pharmacokinetics not significantly altered in pregnancy. No change in dose indicated during pregnancy.	High placental transfer to fetus[b] No evidence of human teratogenicity (can rule out 1.5-fold increase in overall birth defects).
NNRTIs		NNRTIs are recommended for use in combination regimens with 2 NRTI drugs. Hypersensitivity reactions, including hepatic toxicity and rash, more common in women; unclear if increased in pregnancy

Table 2. Antiretroviral Drug Use in Pregnant HIV-Infected Women: Pharmacokinetic and Toxicity Data in Human Pregnancy and Recommendations for Use in Pregnancy[a] *continued*

Drug	Pharmacokinetics and Dosing Considerations in Pregnancy	Recommendations for Use in Pregnancy
Efavirenz	AUC decreased during third trimester, compared with postpartum, but nearly all third-trimester participants exceeded target exposure. No change in dose indicated during pregnancy	Moderate placental transfer to fetus[b] Potential fetal safety concern: FDA Pregnancy Class D. Cynomolgus monkeys receiving efavirenz during the first trimester at a dose resulting in plasma concentrations comparable to systemic human therapeutic exposure had 3 of 20 infants with significant CNS or other malformations. In humans, there is no increase in overall birth defects with first-trimester efavirenz exposure. However, in humans with first-trimester exposure, there have been 6 retrospective case reports and 1 prospective case report of CNS defects and 1 prospective case report of anophthalmia with facial clefts. The relative risk with first-trimester exposure is unclear. Nonpregnant women of childbearing potential should undergo pregnancy testing before efavirenz initiation and counseling about potential risk to the fetus and desirability of avoiding pregnancy while on efavirenz-containing regimens. Alternate antiretroviral regimens that do not include efavirenz should be strongly considered in women who are planning to become pregnant or who are sexually active and not using effective contraception, assuming these alternative regimens are acceptable to the provider and are not thought to compromise the health of the woman. Because the risk of neural tube defects is restricted to the first 5 to 6 weeks of pregnancy and pregnancy is rarely recognized before 4 to 6 weeks of pregnancy, and unnecessary antiretroviral drug changes during pregnancy may be associated with loss of viral control and increased risk of perinatal transmission, efavirenz may be continued in pregnant women receiving an efavirenz-based regimen who present for antenatal care in the first trimester, provided there is virologic suppression on the regimen.
Etravirine	Limited pharmacokinetic data in pregnancy (n=4) suggests no differences from nonpregnant adults. Insufficient data to make dosing recommendation during pregnancy.	Moderate placental transfer (data from one mother-infant pair)[b] Insufficient data to assess for teratogenicity in humans. No evidence of teratogenicity in rats or rabbits.
Nevirapine	Pharmacokinetics not significantly altered in pregnancy. No change in dose indicated during pregnancy.	High placental transfer to fetus[b] No evidence of human teratogenicity (can rule out 1.5-fold increase in overall birth defects and 2-fold increase in risk of birth defects in more common classes, cardiovascular and genitourinary) Increased risk of symptomatic, often rash-associated, and potentially fatal liver toxicity among women with CD4 counts ≥250/mm^3 when first initiating therapy; pregnancy does not appear to increase risk Nevirapine should be initiated in pregnant women with CD4 counts ≥250/mm^3 only if benefit clearly outweighs risk because of potential increased risk of life-threatening hepatotoxicity in women with high CD4 cell counts. Elevated transaminase levels at baseline may increase the risk of nevirapine toxicity. Women who become pregnant while taking nevirapine-containing regimens and are tolerating them well can continue therapy, regardless of CD4 count.
Rilpivirine	No pharmacokinetic studies in human pregnancy; no dosing recommendations can be made Insufficient data to make dosing recommendation during pregnancy	Unknown placental transfer to fetus in humans No evidence of teratogenicity in rats or rabbits. Insufficient data to assess for teratogenicity in humans.
Protease Inhibitors		PIs are recommended for use in combination regimens with 2 NRTI drugs. Hyperglycemia, new onset or exacerbation of diabetes mellitus, and diabetic ketoacidosis reported with PI use; unclear if pregnancy increases risk. Conflicting data regarding preterm delivery in women receiving PIs.

Table 2. Antiretroviral Drug Use in Pregnant HIV-Infected Women: Pharmacokinetic and Toxicity Data in Human Pregnancy and Recommendations for Use in Pregnancy[a] *continued*

Drug	Pharmacokinetics and Dosing Considerations in Pregnancy	Recommendations for Use in Pregnancy
Atazanavir **Note:** Must be combined with low-dose ritonavir boosting in pregnancy	Atazanavir concentrations are reduced during pregnancy; also reduced when given concomitantly with tenofovir or H_2-receptor antagonist. Use of unboosted atazanavir is **not** recommended during pregnancy. Use of an increased dose (400 mg atazanavir plus 100 mg ritonavir once daily with food) during the second and third trimester results in plasma concentrations equivalent to those in nonpregnant adults on standard dosing. Although some experts recommend increased atazanavir dosing in all women during the second and third trimesters, the package insert recommends increased atazanavir dosing only for antiretroviral-experienced pregnant women in the second and third trimesters also receiving either tenofovir or H^2-receptor antagonist.	Low placental transfer to fetus[b] No evidence of human teratogenicity (can rule out 2-fold increase in overall birth defects) Must be given as low-dose ritonavir-boosted regimen in pregnancy Effect of *in utero* atazanavir exposure on infant's indirect bilirubin levels is unclear. Nonpathologic elevations of neonatal hyperbilirubinemia have been observed in some but not all clinical trials to date.
Darunavir **Note:** Must be combined with low-dose ritonavir boosting	Exposure is decreased in pregnancy. Once-daily dosing is **not** recommended during pregnancy. Twice-daily dosing is recommended for all pregnant women. Increased twice-daily darunavir dose (darunavir 800 mg plus ritonavir 100 mg with food) in pregnancy is being investigated.	Low placental transfer to fetus[b] Insufficient data to assess for teratogenicity in humans. No evidence of teratogenicity in mice, rats, or rabbits. Must be given as low-dose ritonavir-boosted regimen
Fosamprenavir **Note:** Must be combined with low-dose ritonavir boosting in pregnancy	With ritonavir boosting, AUC is reduced during third trimester. However, exposure is greater during the third trimester with boosting than in nonpregnant adults without boosting and trough concentrations achieved during the third trimester were adequate for patients without PI resistance mutations. Use of unboosted fosamprenavir is **not** recommended during pregnancy. No change in standard boosted dose is indicated.	Low placental transfer to fetus[b] Insufficient data to assess for teratogenicity in humans. Increased fetal loss in rabbits but no increase in defects in rats and rabbits. Must be given as low-dose ritonavir-boosted regimen in pregnancy
Indinavir **Note:** Must be combined with low-dose ritonavir boosting in pregnancy	Indinavir exposure markedly reduced when administered without ritonavir boosting during pregnancy. Indinavir exposure low with indinavir 400 mg plus ritonavir 100 mg dosing during pregnancy; no pharmacokinetic data available on alternative boosted dosing regimens in pregnancy. Use of unboosted indinavir is **not** recommended during pregnancy.	Minimal placental transfer to fetus[b] No evidence of human teratogenicity (can rule out 2-fold increase in overall birth defects) Must be given as low-dose ritonavir-boosted regimen in pregnancy Theoretical concern regarding increased indirect bilirubin levels, which may exacerbate physiologic hyperbilirubinemia in neonates. Minimal placental passage mitigates this concern.

Table 2. Antiretroviral Drug Use in Pregnant HIV-Infected Women: Pharmacokinetic and Toxicity Data in Human Pregnancy and Recommendations for Use in Pregnancy[a] *continued*

Drug	Pharmacokinetics and Dosing Considerations in Pregnancy	Recommendations for Use in Pregnancy
Lopinavir/ ritonavir	Pharmacokinetic studies suggest increased dose (lopinavir 600 mg plus ritonavir 150 mg twice daily without regard to meals) should be used in second and third trimesters, especially in PI-experienced patients. If standard dosing is used, monitor virologic response and lopinavir drug concentrations, if available. No data to address if drug concentrations are adequate with once-daily dosing in pregnancy. Once-daily dosing is **not** recommended during pregnancy. Some experts recommend increased dose of lopinavir 600 mg plus ritonavir 150 mg twice daily without regard to meals in second and third trimesters.	Low placental transfer to fetus[b] No evidence of human teratogenicity (can rule out 2-fold increase in overall birth defects) Oral solution contains 42% alcohol and 15% propylene glycol and is not recommended for use in pregnancy. Once-daily lopinavir/ritonavir dosing is not recommended during pregnancy.
Nelfinavir	Lower nelfinavir exposure in third trimester than postpartum in women receiving nelfinavir 1250 mg twice daily; however, generally adequate drug concentrations are achieved during pregnancy, although concentrations are variable in late pregnancy. Nelfinavir dosing of 750 mg 3 times daily with food is not recommended during pregnancy. No change in standard dose (1,250 mg twice daily with food) is indicated.	Minimal to low placental transfer to fetus[b] No evidence of human teratogenicity (can rule out 1.5-fold increase in overall birth defects and 2-fold increase in risk of birth defects in more common classes, cardiovascular and genitourinary)
Ritonavir	Lower concentrations during pregnancy compared with postpartum but no dosage adjustment necessary when used as booster Use only as low-dose booster with other protease inhibitors	Low placental transfer to fetus[b] No evidence of human teratogenicity (can rule out 2-fold increase in overall birth defects) Oral solution contains 43% alcohol and is not recommended for use in pregnancy.
Saquinavir	Based on limited data, saquinavir exposure may be reduced in pregnancy but not sufficient to warrant a dose change. No change in dose indicated during pregnancy	Minimal placental transfer to fetus[b] Insufficient data to assess for teratogenicity in humans. No evidence of teratogenicity in rats or rabbits. Must be given as low-dose ritonavir-boosted regimen Baseline ECG recommended before starting therapy because PR and/or QT interval prolongations have been observed. Contraindicated in patients with pre-existing cardiac conduction system disease.
Tipranavir	Limited pharmacokinetic data in human pregnancy. Insufficient data to make dosing recommendation.	Moderate placental transfer to fetus reported in one patient[b] Insufficient data to assess for teratogenicity in humans. No evidence of teratogenicity in rats or rabbits. Must be given as low-dose ritonavir-boosted regimen.
Entry Inhibitors		
Enfuvirtide	No pharmacokinetic data in human pregnancy. Insufficient data to make dosing recommendation.	Minimal to low placental transfer to fetus[b] No data on human teratogenicity
Maraviroc	Limited pharmacokinetic data in human pregnancy. Insufficient data to make dosing recommendation.	Minimal to low placental transfer to fetus[b] No data on human teratogenicity

Table 2. Antiretroviral Drug Use in Pregnant HIV-Infected Women: Pharmacokinetic and Toxicity Data in Human Pregnancy and Recommendations for Use in Pregnancy[a] *continued*

Drug	Pharmacokinetics and Dosing Considerations in Pregnancy	Recommendations for Use in Pregnancy
Integrase Inhibitors		
Dolutegravir	No pharmacokinetic data in human pregnancy. Insufficient data to make dosing recommendation.	Unknown placental transfer to fetus. Insufficient data to assess for teratogenicity in humans. No evidence of teratogenicity in mice, rats, or rabbits.
Elvitegravir plus cobicistat	No pharmacokinetic data in human pregnancy. Insufficient data to make dosing recommendation.	No data on placental transfer of elvitegravir plus cobicistat are available. Insufficient data to assess for teratogenicity in humans. No evidence of teratogenicity in rats or rabbits.
Raltegravir	Limited data suggest pharmacokinetics not significantly altered in pregnancy. No change in dose indicated during pregnancy.	High placental transfer to fetus[b] Insufficient data to assess for teratogenicity in humans. Increased skeletal variants in rats; no increase in defects in rabbits. Case report of markedly elevated liver transaminases with use in late pregnancy. Severe, potentially life-threatening, and fatal skin and hypersensitivity reactions have been reported in nonpregnant adults. Chewable tables contain phenylalanine.

APR = antiretroviral pregnancy registry

[a]Individual antiretroviral drug dosages may need to be adjusted in renal or hepatic insufficiency (for details, see individual drug monographs).

[b]Placental transfer categories: Mean or median cord blood to maternal delivery plasma drug ratio: High: >0.6; Moderate: 0.3 to 0.6; Low: 0.1 to 0.3; Minimal: <0.1

Table 3. Intrapartum Maternal and Neonatal Zidovudine Dosing for Prevention of Perinatal Transmission of HIV

Drug	Dosing	Duration
Maternal Intrapartum		
Zidovudine	2 mg/kg IV over 1 hour followed by continuous infusion of 1 mg/kg/h	Onset of labor until delivery of infant
Neonatal		
Zidovudine (≥35 weeks gestational age at birth)	4 mg/kg/dose PO twice daily, started as soon as possible after birth (preferably within 6 to 12 hours after delivery); or, if unable to tolerate oral agents, 3 mg/kg/dose IV beginning within 6 to 12 hours of delivery, then every 12 hours	Birth through 4 to 6 weeks[1]
Zidovudine (≥30 weeks to <35 weeks gestational age at birth)	2 mg/kg/dose PO (1.5 mg/kg/dose if given IV) started as soon as possible after birth (preferably within 6 to 12 hours after delivery), then every 12 hours; advance to 3 mg/kg/dose PO (or 2.3 mg/kg/dose if given IV) every 12 hours at 15 days of age	Birth through 6 weeks
Zidovudine (<30 weeks gestational age at birth)	2 mg/kg/dose PO (1.5 mg/kg/dose if given IV) started as soon as possible after birth (preferably within 6 to 12 hours after delivery), then every 12 hours; advance to 3 mg/kg/dose PO (or 2.3 mg/kg/dose if given IV) every 12 hours after 4 weeks of age	Birth through 6 weeks

[1]All HIV-exposed infants should receive postpartum antiretroviral drugs to reduce perinatal transmission of HIV. A 6-week course of neonatal zidovudine is generally recommended. A 4-week neonatal zidovudine chemoprophylaxis regimen may be considered when the mother has received standard antiretroviral therapy during pregnancy with consistent viral suppression and there are no concerns related to maternal adherence.

Table 4. Additional Antiretroviral Prophylaxis Agents for HIV-Exposed Infants of Women Who Received No Antepartum Antiretroviral Prophylaxis (Initiate as Soon as Possible After Delivery)[1]

Drug	Dosing	Duration
Neonatal Two-drug regimen: Zidovudine + Nevirapine		
Zidovudine	Use dosing from table above	Birth through 6 weeks
Nevirapine	Birth weight 1.5 to 2 kg: 8 mg/dose PO Birth weight >2 kg: 12 mg/dose PO	**Three** doses in the first week of life: • First dose within 48 hours of birth (birth to 48 hours) • Second dose 48 hours after first • Third dose 96 hours after second

[1]The Panel recommends 6 weeks of zidovudine plus 3 doses of nevirapine in the first week of life for infants whose mothers have not received antepartum antiretroviral agents and for infants whose mothers have not received antepartum or intrapartum antiretroviral agents. Most experts feel the potential benefit of combining zidovudine infant prophylaxis with additional antiretroviral drugs may exceed the risk of multiple drug exposure in the following cases: Infants born to HIV-infected mothers with no antiretroviral therapy prior to labor or during labor; infants born to mothers with only intrapartum antiretroviral therapy (ie, no antepartum antiretroviral therapy); infants born to mothers with suboptimal viral suppression at delivery (especially if delivery was vaginal); or infants born to mothers with known antiretroviral drug-resistant virus. However, risk of HIV transmission depends on a number of maternal and infant factors, including viral load, mode of delivery, and gestational age at delivery. Data from the NICHD-HPTN 040/PACTG 1043 study supports the use of the zidovudine plus nevirapine two-drug regimen in newborns whose mothers have not received antepartum antiretroviral therapy. In all other scenarios, decisions about the use of combination antiretroviral prophylaxis in infants should be made in consultation with a pediatric HIV specialist before delivery, if possible, and should be accompanied by a discussion with the mothers about potential risks and benefits of this approach.

REFERENCES

Connor EM, Sperling RS, Gelber R, et al. Reduction of maternal-infant transmission of human immunodeficiency virus type 1 with zidovudine treatment. Pediatric AIDS clinical trials group protocol 076 study group. *N Engl J Med.* 1994;331(18):1173-1180.

National Institute of Allergy and Infectious Diseases (NIAID). "Mississippi baby" now has detectable HIV, researchers find. July 10, 2014. Available at http://www.niaid.nih.gov/news/newsreleases/2014/Pages/MississippiBabyHIV.aspx

Panel on Treatment of HIV-Infected Pregnancy Women and Prevention of Perinatal Transmission. Recommendations for use of antiretroviral drugs in pregnant HIV-infected women for maternal health and interventions to reduce perinatal HIV transmission in the United States. March 28, 2014. Available at http://aidsinfo.nih.gov/contentfiles/PerinatalGL.pdf

Persaud D, Gay H, Ziemniak C, et al. Absence of detectable HIV-1 viremia after treatment cessation in an infant. *N Engl J Med.* 2013;369(19):1828-1835.

IMMUNIZATION ADMINISTRATION RECOMMENDATIONS

The following tables are taken from the General Recommendations on Immunization 2011:

- Guidelines for Spacing of Live and Inactivated Antigens
- Guidelines for Administering Antibody-Containing Products and Vaccines
- Recommended Intervals Between Administration of Antibody-Containing Products and Measles- or Varicella-Containing Vaccine, by Product and Indication for Vaccination
- Vaccination of persons with Primary and Secondary Immunodeficiencies
- Needle length and Injection Site of IM injections

Guidelines for Spacing of Live and Inactivated Antigens

Antigen Combination	Recommended Minimum Interval Between Doses
Two or more inactivated[1]	May be administered simultaneously or at any interval between doses
Inactivated and live	May be administered simultaneously or at any interval between doses
Two or more live injectable[2]	28 days minimum interval, if not administered simultaneously

[1]Certain experts suggest a 28-day interval between tetanus toxoid, reduced diphtheria toxoid, and reduced acellular pertussis (Tdap) vaccine and tetravalent meningococcal conjugate vaccine if they are not administered simultaneously.

[2]Live oral vaccines (eg, Ty21a typhoid vaccine and rotavirus vaccine) may be administered simultaneously or at any interval before or after inactivated or live injectable vaccines.

Adapted from American Academy of Pediatrics. Pertussis. Pickering LK, Baker CJ, Kimberlin DW, et al, eds. *Red Book*: 2009 Report of the Committee on Infectious Diseases. 28th ed. Elk Grove Village, IL: American Academy of Pediatrics; 2009;22.

Guidelines for Administering Antibody-Containing Products[1] and Vaccines

Simultaneous Administration (during the same office visit)

Products Administered	Recommended Minimum Interval Between Doses
Antibody-containing products and inactivated antigen	Can be administered simultaneously at different anatomic sites or at any time interval between doses.
Antibody-containing products and live antigen	Should **not** be administered simultaneously.[2] If simultaneous administration of measles-containing vaccine or varicella vaccine is unavoidable, administer at different sites and revaccinate or test for seroconversion after the recommended interval.

Nonsimultaneous Administration

Products Administered		Recommended Minimum Interval Between Doses
Administered first	Administered second	
Antibody-containing products	Inactivated antigen	No interval necessary
Inactivated antigen	Antibody-containing products	No interval necessary
Antibody-containing products	Live antigen	Dose-related[2,3]
Live antigen	Antibody-containing products	2 weeks[2]

[1]Blood products containing substantial amounts of immune globulin include intramuscular and intravenous immune globulin, specific hyperimmune globulin (eg, hepatitis B immune globulin, tetanus immune globulin, varicella zoster immune globulin, and rabies immune globulin), whole blood, packed red blood cells, plasma, and platelet products.

[2]Yellow fever vaccine, rotavirus vaccine, oral Ty21a typhoid vaccine, live-attenuated influenza vaccine, and zoster vaccine are exceptions to these recommendations. These live-attenuated vaccines can be administered at any time before, after, or simultaneously with an antibody-containing product.

[3]The duration of interference of antibody-containing products with the immune response to the measles component of measles-containing vaccine, and possibly varicella vaccine, is dose-related.

Recommended Intervals Between Administration of Antibody-Containing Products and Measles- or Varicella-Containing Vaccine, by Product and Indication for Vaccination

Product/Indication	Dose (mg IgG/kg) and Route[1]	Recommended Interval Before Measles- or Varicella-Containing Vaccine[2] Administration (mo)
Tetanus IG	IM: 250 units (10 mg IgG/kg)	3
Hepatitis A IG		
Contact prophylaxis	IM: 0.02 mL/kg (3.3 mg IgG/kg)	3
International travel	IM: 0.06 mL/kg (10 mg IgG/kg)	3
Hepatitis B IG	IM: 0.06 mL/kg (10 mg IgG/kg)	3
Rabies IG	IM: 20 int. units/kg (22 mg IgG/kg)	4
Varicella IG	IM: 125 units/10 kg (60 to 200 mg IgG/kg) (maximum: 625 units)	5
Measles prophylaxis IG		
Standard (ie, nonimmunocompromised) contact	IM: 0.25 mL/kg (40 mg IgG/kg)	5
Immunocompromised contact	IM: 0.50 mL/kg (80 mg IgG/kg)	6
Blood transfusion		
Red blood cells (RBCs), washed	IV: 10 mL/kg (negligible IgG/kg)	None
RBCs, adenine-saline added	IV: 10 mL/kg (10 mg IgG/kg)	3
Packed RBCs (hematocrit 65%)[3]	IV: 10 mL/kg (60 mg IgG/kg)	6
Whole blood cells (hematocrit 35% to 50%)[3]	IV: 10 mL/kg (80 to 100 mg IgG/kg)	6
Plasma/platelet products	IV: 10 mL/kg (160 mg IgG/kg)	7
Cytomegalovirus intravenous immune globulin (IGIV)	150 mg/kg maximum	6
IGIV		
Replacement therapy for immune deficiencies[4]	IV: 300 to 400 mg/kg[4]	8
Immune thrombocytopenic purpura treatment	IV: 400 mg/kg	8
Postexposure varicella prophylaxis[5]	IV: 400 mg/kg	8
Immune thrombocytopenic purpura treatment	IV: 1000 mg/kg	10
Kawasaki disease	IV: 2 g/kg	11
Monoclonal antibody to respiratory syncytial virus F protein (Synagis [Medimmune])[6]	IM: 15 mg/kg	None

HIV = human immunodeficiency virus, IG = immune globulin, IgG = immune globulin G, IGIV = intravenous immune globulin, mg IgG/kg = milligrams of immune globulin G per kilogram of body weight, IM = intramuscular, IV = intravenous, RBCs = red blood cells

[1]This table is not intended for determining the correct indications and dosages for using antibody-containing products. Unvaccinated persons might not be fully protected against measles during the entire recommended interval, and additional doses of IG or measles vaccine might be indicated after measles exposure. Concentrations of measles antibody in an IG preparation can vary by manufacturer's lot. Rates of antibody clearance after receipt of an IG preparation also might vary. Recommended intervals are extrapolated from an estimated half-life of 30 days for passively acquired antibody and an observed interference with the immune response to measles vaccine for 5 months after a dose of 80 mg IgG/kg.

[2]Does not include zoster vaccine. Zoster vaccine may be given with antibody-containing blood products.

[3]Assumes a serum IgG concentration of 16 mg/mL

[4]Measles and varicella vaccinations are recommended for children with asymptomatic or mildly symptomatic HIV infection but are contraindicated for persons with severe immunosuppression from HIV or any other immunosuppressive disorder.

[5]The investigational product VariZIG, similar to licensed varicella-zoster IG (VZIG), is a purified human IG preparation made from plasma containing high levels of anti-varicella antibodies (IgG). The interval between VariZIG and varicella vaccine (Var or MMRV) is 5 months.

[6]Contains antibody only to respiratory syncytial virus

Vaccination of Persons With Primary and Secondary Immunodeficiencies

Category	Specific Immunodeficiency	Contraindicated Vaccines[1]	Risk-Specific Recommended Vaccines[1]	Effectiveness and Comments
Primary				
B-lymphocyte (humoral)	Severe antibody deficiencies (eg, X-linked agammaglobulinemia and common variable immunodeficiency)	Oral poliovirus (OPV)[2] Smallpox Live-attenuated influenza vaccine (LAIV) BCG Ty21a (live oral typhoid) Yellow fever	Pneumococcal Consider measles and varicella vaccination	The effectiveness of any vaccine is uncertain if it depends only on the humoral response (eg, PPSV or MPSV4) IGIV interferes with the immune response to measles vaccine and possibly varicella vaccine
	Less severe antibody deficiencies (eg, selective IgA deficiency and IgG subclass deficiency)	OPV[2] BCG Yellow Fever Other live-vaccines appear to be safe	Pneumococcal	All vaccines likely effective; immune response may be attenuated
T-lymphocyte (cell-mediated and humoral)	Complete defects (eg, severe combined immunodeficiency [SCID] disease, complete DiGeorge syndrome)	All live vaccines[3,4,5]	Pneumococcal	Vaccines might be ineffective
	Partial defects (eg, most patients with DiGeorge syndrome, Wiskott-Aldrich syndrome, ataxia- telangiectasia)	All live vaccines[3,4,5]	Pneumococcal Meningococcal Hib (if not administered in infancy)	Effectiveness of any vaccine depends on degree of immune suppression
Complement	Persistent complement, properdin, or factor B deficiency	None	Pneumococcal Meningococcal	All routine vaccines likely effective
Phagocytic function	Chronic granulomatous disease, leukocyte adhesion defect, and myeloperoxidase deficiency	Live bacterial vaccines[3]	Pneumococcal[6]	All inactivated vaccines safe and likely effective; live viral vaccines likely safe and effective
Secondary				
	HIV/AIDS	OPV[2] Smallpox BCG LAIV Withhold MMR and varicella in severely immunocompromised persons Yellow fever vaccine might have a contraindication or a precaution depending on clinical parameters of immune function[9]	Pneumococcal Consider Hib (if not administered in infancy) and meningococcal vaccination.	MMR, varicella, rotavirus, and all inactivated vaccines, including inactivated influenza, might be effective.[7]
	Malignant neoplasm, transplantation, immunosuppressive or radiation therapy	Live viral and bacterial, depending on immune status[3,4]	Pneumococcal	Effectiveness of any vaccine depends on degree of immune suppression

Vaccination of Persons With Primary and Secondary Immunodeficiencies *continued*

Category	Specific Immunodeficiency	Contraindicated Vaccines[1]	Risk-Specific Recommended Vaccines[1]	Effectiveness and Comments
	Asplenia	None	Pneumococcal Meningococcal Hib (if not administered in infancy)	All routine vaccines likely effective
	Chronic renal disease	LAIV	Pneumococcal Hepatitis B[8]	All routine vaccines likely effective

AIDS = acquired immunodeficiency syndrome; BCG = bacille Calmette-Guerin; Hib = *Haemophilus influenzae* type b; HIV = human immunodeficiency virus; IG = immunoglobulin; IGIV = immune globulin intravenous; LAIV = live, attenuated influenza vaccine; MMR = measles, mumps, and rubella; MPSV4 = quadrivalent meningococcal polysaccharide vaccine; OPV = oral poliovirus vaccine (live); PPSV = pneumococcal polysaccharide vaccine; TIV = trivalent inactivated influenza vaccine

[1]Other vaccines that are universally or routinely recommended should be administered if not contraindicated.

[2]OPV is no longer available in the United States.

[3]Live bacterial vaccines: BCG and oral Ty21a *Salmonella typhi* vaccine

[4]Live viral vaccines: MMR, MMRV, OPV, LAIV, yellow fever, zoster, rotavirus, varicella, and vaccinia (smallpox). Smallpox vaccine is not recommended for children or the general public.

[5]Regarding T-lymphocyte immunodeficiency as a contraindication for rotavirus vaccine, data exist only for severe combined immunodeficiency.

[6]Pneumococcal vaccine is not indicated for children with chronic granulomatous disease beyond age-based universal recommendations for PCV. Children with chronic granulomatous disease are not at increased risk for pneumococcal disease.

[7]HIV-infected children should receive IG after exposure to measles and may receive varicella and measles vaccine if $CD4^+$ lymphocyte count is ≥15%.

[8]Indicated based on the risk from dialysis-based bloodborne transmission

[9]Symptomatic HIV infection or $CD4^+$ T-lymphocyte count of <200/mm^3 or <15% of total lymphocytes for children aged <6 years is a containdication to yellow fever vaccine administration. Asymptomatic HIV infection with $CD4^+$ T-lymphocyte count of 200 to 499/mm^3 for persons aged ≥6 years or 15% to 24% of total lymphocytes for children aged <6 years is a precaution for yellow fever vaccine administration. Details of yellow fever vaccine recommendations are available from the CDC. (CDC. Yellow fever vaccine: recommendations of the Advisory Committee on Immunization Practices [ACIP]. *MMWR Recomm Rep*. 2010;59[No. RR-7].)

Adapted from American Academy of Pediatrics. Passive immunization. Pickering LK, Baker CJ, Kimberline DW, et al, eds. *Red Book*: 2009 Report of the Committee on Infectious Diseases. 28th ed. Elk Grove Village, IL: American Academy of Pediatrics; 2009;74-75.

Needle Length and Injection Site of IM for Children ≤18 years of age (by age) and Adults ≥19 years of age (by sex and weight)

Age Group	Needle Length	Injection Site
Children (birth to 18 y)		
Neonates[1]	⅝" (16 mm)[2]	Anterolateral thigh
Infant 1 to 12 mo	1" (25 mm)	Anterolateral thigh
Toddler 1 to 2 y	1 to 1¼" (25 to 32 mm)	Anterolateral thigh[3]
	⅝[2] to 1" (16 to 25 mm)	Deltoid muscle of the arm
Children 3 to 18 y	⅝[2] to 1" (16 to 25 mm)	Deltoid muscle of the arm[3]
	1 to 1¼" (25 to 32 mm)	Anterolateral thigh
Adults ≥19 y		
Men and women <60 kg (130 lb)	1" (25 mm)[4]	Deltoid muscle of the arm
Men and women 60 to 70 kg (130 to 152 lb)	1" (25 mm)	
Men 70 to 118 kg (152 to 260 lb)	1 to 1½" (25 to 38 mm)	
Women 70 to 90 kg (152 to 200 lb)		
Men >118 kg (260 lb)	1½" (38 mm)	
Women >90 kg (200 lb)		

IM = intramuscular

[1]First 28 days of life

[2]If skin is stretched tightly and subcutaneous tissues are not bunched

[3]Preferred site

[4]Some experts recommend a ⅝" needle for men and women who weigh <60 kg.

Adapted from Poland GA, Borrud A, Jacobsen RM, et al. Determination of deltoid fat pad thickness: implications for needle length in adult immunization. *JAMA*. 1997;277:1709-1711.

REFERENCE

Centers for Disease Control and Prevention (CDC). Recommendations of the Advisory Committee on Immunization Practices (ACIP): general recommendations on immunization. *MMWR Recomm Rep*. 2011;60(2):1-61.

IMMUNIZATION SCHEDULES

Recommended Immunization Schedule for Persons 0 to 18 Years of Age — United States, 2015[a]

Vaccine	Birth	1 mo	2 mos	4 mos	6 mos	9 mos	12 mos	15 mos	18 mos	19–23 mos	2–3 yrs	4–6 yrs	7–10 yrs	11–12 yrs	13–15 yrs	16–18 yrs
Hepatitis B[1] (HepB)	1st dose	2nd dose					3rd dose									
Rotavirus[2] (RV) RV-1 (2-dose series); RV-5 (3-dose series)			1st dose	2nd dose	see footnote 2											
Diphtheria, tetanus & acellular pertussis[3] (DTaP: <7 yrs)			1st dose	2nd dose	3rd dose			4th dose				5th dose				
Tetanus, diphtheria & acellular pertussis[4] (Tdap: ≥ 7 yrs)														(Tdap)		
Haemophilus influenzae type b[5] (Hib)			1st dose	2nd dose	see footnote 5		3rd or 4th dose, see footnote 5									
Pneumococcal conjugate[6] (PCV13)			1st dose	2nd dose	3rd dose		4th dose									
Pneumococcal polysaccharide[6] (PPSV23)																
Inactivated poliovirus[7] (IPV) (<18 years)			1st dose	2nd dose			3rd dose					4th dose				
Influenza[8] (IIV; LAIV) 2 doses for some: see footnote 8							Annual vaccination (IIV only) 1 or 2 doses				Annual vaccination (LAIV or IIV) 1 or 2 doses			Annual vaccination (LAIV or IIV) 1 dose only		
Measles, mumps, rubella[9] (MMR)					see footnote 9		1st dose					2nd dose				
Varicella[10] (VAR)							1st dose					2nd dose				
Hepatitis A[11] (Hep A)							2 dose series, see footnote 11									
Human papillomavirus[12] (HPV2: females only; HPV4: males and females)														(3 dose series)		
Meningococcal[13] (Hib-MenCY ≥ 6 wks; MenACWY-D ≥ 9 mos; MenACWY-CRM ≥ 2 mos.)			see footnote 13											1st dose		booster

Range of recommended ages for all children. Range of recommended ages for catch-up immunization. Range of recommended ages for certain high-risk groups. Range of recommended ages during which catch-up is encouraged and for certain high-risk groups. Not routinely recommended.

NOTE: The recommendations in the tables must be read along with the following footnotes.

[a] This schedule includes recommendations in effect as of January 1, 2015. Any dose not administered at the recommended age should be administered at a subsequent visit, when indicated and feasible. The use of a combination vaccine generally is preferred over separate injections of its equivalent component vaccines. Vaccination providers should consult the relevant Advisory Committee on Immunization Practices (ACIP) statement for detailed recommendations, available online at http://www.cdc.gov/vaccines/hcp/acip-recs/index.html. Clinically significant adverse events that follow vaccination should be reported to the Vaccine Adverse Event Reporting System (VAERS) online (http://www.vaers.hhs.gov) or by telephone (800-822-7967).Suspected cases of vaccine-preventable diseases should be reported to the state or local health department. Additional information, including precautions and contraindications for vaccination, is available from CDC online (http://www.cdc.gov/vaccines/recs/vac-admin/contraindications.htm) or by telephone (800-CDC-INFO [800-232-4636]). This schedule is approved by the Advisory Committee on Immunization Practices (http//www.cdc.gov/vaccines/acip), the American Academy of Pediatrics (http://www.aap.org), the American Academy of Family Physicians (http://www.aafp.org), and the American College of Obstetricians and Gynecologists (http://www.acog.org).

Catch-up Immunization Schedule for Persons 4 Months to 18 Years of Age Who Start Late or Who Are >1 Month Behind – United States, 2015

This table provides catch-up schedules and minimum intervals between doses for children whose vaccinations have been delayed. A vaccine series does not need to be restarted, regardless of the time that has elapsed between doses. Use the section appropriate for the child's age. Always use this table in conjunction with the previous "Recommended immunization schedule for persons aged 0 through 18 years" and the footnotes that follow.

Vaccine	Minimum Age for Dose 1	Minimum Interval Between Doses			
		Dose 1 to Dose 2	Dose 2 to Dose 3	Dose 3 to Dose 4	Dose 4 to Dose 5
Catch-up Schedule for Persons 4 Months to 6 Years of Age					
Hepatitis B[1]	Birth	**4 weeks**	**8 weeks** and ≥16 weeks after first dose; minimum age for final dose is 24 weeks		
Rotavirus[2]	6 weeks	**4 weeks**	**4 weeks**[2]		
Diphtheria, tetanus, and acellular pertussis[3]	6 weeks	**4 weeks**	**4 weeks**	**6 months**	**6 months**[3]
Haemophilus influenzae type b[5]	6 weeks	**4 weeks** if first dose was administered before the 1st birthday **8 weeks** (as final dose) if first dose was administered at 12 to 14 months of age **No further doses needed** if first dose was administered at ≥15 months of age	**4 weeks**[5] if currently <12 months of age **and** first dose was administered at <7 months of age **and** at least 1 previous dose was PRP-T (ActHib, Pentacel) or unknown **8 weeks** and 12 to 59 months of age (as final dose)[5] if currently <12 months of age **and** first dose was administered at 7 to 11 months of age **or** if currently 12 to 59 months of age **and** first dose was administered before the 1st birthday **and** second dose was administered at <15 months of age **or** if both doses were PRP-OMP (PredvaxHIB, Comvax) and were administered before the 1st birthday **No further doses needed** if previous dose was administered at ≥15 months of age	**8 weeks** (as final dose) This dose is only necessary for children 12 to 59 months of age who received 3 doses before the 1st birthday	
Pneumococcal[6]	6 weeks	**4 weeks** if first dose was administered before the 1st birthday **8 weeks** (as final dose for healthy children) if first dose was administered at or after the 1st birthday **No further doses needed** for healthy children if first dose was administered at ≥24 months of age	**4 weeks** if currently <12 months of age and previous dose was given at <7 months of age **8 weeks** (as final dose for healthy children) if previous dose was given at 7 to 11 months of age (wait until >12 months of age) **or** if currently ≥12 months of age and at least 1 dose was given before 12 months of age **No further doses needed** for healthy children if previous dose was administered at ≥24 months of age	**8 weeks** (as final dose) This dose is only necessary for children 12 to 59 months of age who received 3 doses before 12 months of age or for children at high risk who received 3 doses at any age	
Inactivated poliovirus[7]	6 weeks	**4 weeks**[7]	**4 weeks**[7]	**6 months**[7] minimum 4 years of age for final dose	
Meningococcal[13]	6 weeks	**8 weeks**[13]	See footnote 13	See footnote 13	
Measles, mumps, rubella[9]	12 months	**4 weeks**			
Varicella[10]	12 months	**3 months**			
Hepatitits A[11]	12 months	**6 months**			
Catch-up Schedule for Persons 7 to 18 Years of Age					
Tetanus, diphtheria; tetanus, diphtheria, and acellular pertussis[4]	7 years[4]	**4 weeks**	**4 weeks** if first dose of DTaP/DT was administered before the 1st birthday **6 months** (as final dose) if first dose of DTaP/DT administered at or after the 1st birthday	**6 months** if first dose of DTaP/DT was administered before the 1st birthday	

Vaccine	Minimum Age for Dose 1	Minimum Interval Between Doses			
		Dose 1 to Dose 2	Dose 2 to Dose 3	Dose 3 to Dose 4	Dose 4 to Dose 5
Human papillomavirus[12]	9 years	Routine dosing intervals are recommended[12]			
Hepatitis A[11]	N/A	**6 months**			
Hepatitis B[1]	N/A	**4 weeks**	**8 weeks and** ≥16 weeks after first dose		
Inactivated poliovirus[7]	N/A	**4 weeks**	**4 weeks**[7]	**6 months**[7]	
Meningococcal[13]	N/A	**8 weeks**[13]			
Measles, mumps, rubella[9]	N/A	**4 weeks**			
Varicella[10]	N/A	**3 months** if <13 years of age **4 weeks** if ≥13 years of age			

Footnotes to Recommended Immunization Schedule for Persons 0 to 18 Years of Age and the Catch-up Immunization Schedule – United States, 2015

Note: For further guidance on the use of the vaccines mentioned below, see http://www.cdc.gov/vaccines/hcp/acip-recs/index.html. For vaccine recommendations for persons ≥19 years of age, see the adult immunization schedule.

[1]Hepatitis B (HepB) vaccine *(Minimum age: Birth)*

Routine vaccination:

At birth:

- Administer monovalent HepB vaccine to all newborns before hospital discharge.
- For infants born to hepatitis B surface antigen (HBsAg)-positive mothers, administer HepB vaccine and 0.5 mL of hepatitis B immune globulin (HBIG) within 12 hours of birth. These infants should be tested for HBsAg and antibody to HBsAg (anti-HBs) 1 to 2 months after completion of the HepB series at 9 to 18 months of age (preferably at the next well-child visit).
- If the mother's HBsAg status is unknown, within 12 hours of birth, administer HepB vaccine to all infants regardless of birth weight. For infants weighing <2,000 grams, administer HBIG in addition to HepB vaccine within 12 hours of birth. Determine the mother's HBsAg status as soon as possible and if she is HBsAg-positive, also administer HBIG for infants weighing ≥2,000 grams as soon as possible but no later than 7 days of age.

Doses following the birth dose:

- The second dose should be administered at 1 or 2 months of age. Monovalent HepB vaccine should be used for doses administered before 6 weeks of age.
- Infants who did not receive a birth dose should receive 3 doses of a HepB-containing vaccine on a schedule of 0, 1 to 2 months, and 6 months of age starting as soon as feasible. See the previous "Catch-up Immunization Schedule".
- Administer the second dose 1 to 2 months after the first dose (minimum interval of 4 weeks); administer the third dose ≥8 weeks after the second dose **and** ≥16 weeks after the **first** dose. The final (third or fourth) dose in the HepB vaccine series should be administered **no earlier than 24 weeks of age**.
- Administration of a total of 4 doses of HepB vaccine is permitted when a combination vaccine containing HepB is administered after the birth dose.

Catch-up vaccination:

- Unvaccinated persons should complete a 3-dose series.
- A 2-dose series (doses separated by at least 4 months) of adult formulation Recombivax HB is licensed for use in children 11 to 15 years of age.
- For other catch-up guidance, see the previous "Catch-up Immunization Schedule".

[2]Rotavirus (RV) vaccine *(Minimum age: 6 weeks for both RV-1 [Rotarix] and RV-5 [RotaTeq])*

Routine vaccination:

- Administer a series of RV vaccine to all infants as follows:
  - If Rotarix is used, administer a 2-dose series at 2 and 4 months of age.
  - If RotaTeq is used, administer a 3-dose series at ages 2, 4, and 6 months of age.
  - If any dose in the series was RotaTeq or vaccine product is unknown for any dose in the series, a total of 3 doses of RV vaccine should be administered.

Catch-up vaccination:

- The maximum age for the first dose in the series is 14 weeks, 6 days; vaccination should not be initiated for infants ≥15 weeks, 0 days of age.
- The maximum age for the final dose in the series is 8 months, 0 days.
- For other catch-up guidance, see the previous "Catch-up Immunization Schedule".

[3]**Diphtheria and tetanus toxoids and acellular pertussis (DTaP) vaccine** *(Minimum age: 6 weeks; exception: DTaP-IPV [Kinrix]: 4 years)*

Routine vaccination:

- Administer a 5-dose series of DTaP vaccine at 2, 4, 6, and 15 to 18 months of age, and at 4 to 6 years of age. The fourth dose may be administered as early as 12 months of age, provided at least 6 months have elapsed since the third dose. However, the fourth dose of DTaP need not be repeated if it was administered ≥4 months after the third dose of DTaP.

Catch-up vaccination:

- The fifth dose of DTaP vaccine is not necessary if the fourth dose was administered at ≥4 years of age.
- For other catch-up guidance, see the previous "Catch-up Immunization Schedule".

[4]**Tetanus and diphtheria toxoids and acellular pertussis (Tdap) vaccine** *(Minimum age: 10 years for Adacel and Boostrix)*

Routine vaccination:

- Administer 1 dose of Tdap vaccine to all adolescents 11 to 12 years of age.
- Tdap can be administered regardless of the interval since the last tetanus and diphtheria toxoid-containing vaccine.
- Administer 1 dose of Tdap vaccine to pregnant adolescents during each pregnancy (preferred during 27 to 36 weeks gestation), regardless of time since prior Td or Tdap vaccination.

Catch-up vaccination:

- Persons ≥7 years of age who are not fully immunized with DTaP vaccine should receive Tdap vaccine as 1 dose (preferably the first) in the catch-up series; if additional doses are needed, use Td vaccine. For children 7 to 10 years of age who receive a dose of Tdap as part of the catch-up series, an adolescent Tdap vaccine dose at 11 to 12 years of age should **not** be administered. Td should be administered instead 10 years after the Tdap dose.
- Persons 11 to 18 years of age who have not received Tdap vaccine should receive a dose, followed by tetanus and diphtheria toxoid (Td) booster doses every 10 years thereafter.
- Inadvertent doses of DTaP vaccine:
  - If administered inadvertently to a child 7 to 10 years of age, the dose may count as part of the catch-up series. This dose can count as the adolescent Tdap dose or the child can later receive a Tdap booster dose at 11 to 12 years of age.
  - If administered inadvertently to an adolescent 11 to 18 years of age, the dose should be counted as the adolescent Tdap booster.
- For other catch-up guidance, see the previous "Catch-up Immunization Schedule".

[5]***Haemophilus influenzae* type b conjugate vaccine (Hib)** *(Minimum age: 6 weeks for PRP-T [ActHIB, DTaP-IPV/Hib (Pentacel), and Hib-MenCY (MenHibrix)], PRP-OMP [PedvaxHIB or COMVAX], 12 months for PRP-T [Hiberix])*

Routine vaccination:

- Administer a 2- or 3-dose Hib vaccine primary series and a booster dose (dose 3 or 4 depending on vaccine used in primary series) at 12 to 15 months of age to complete a full Hib vaccine series.
- The primary series with ActHIB, MenHibrix, or Pentacel consists of 3 doses and should be administered at 2, 4, and 6 months of age. The primary series with PedvaxHib or COMVAX consists of 2 doses and should be administered at 2 and 4 months of age; a dose at 6 months of age is not indicated.
- One booster dose (dose 3 or 4 depending on vaccine used in primary series) of any Hib vaccine should be administered at 12 to 15 months of age. An exception is Hiberix vaccine. Hiberix should only be used for the booster (final) dose in children 12 months to 4 years of age who have received at least 1 prior dose of Hib-containing vaccine.
- For recommendations on the use of MenHibrix in patients at increased risk for meningococcal disease, please refer to the meningococcal vaccine footnotes and also to *MMWR*. 2014;63(RR01);1-13. Available at http://www.cdc.gov/mmwr/pdf/rr/rr6301.pdf.

Catch-up vaccination:

- If dose 1 was administered at 12 to 14 months of age, administer a second (final) dose at least 8 weeks after dose 1, regardless of Hib vaccine used in the primary series.
- If the first 2 doses were PRP-OMP (PedvaxHIB or COMVAX) and were administered before the 1st birthday, the third (and final) dose should be administered at 12 to 59 months of age and at least 8 weeks after the second dose.
- If the first dose was administered at 7 to 11 months of age, administer the second dose ≥4 weeks later and a third (and final) dose at 12 to 15 months of age or 8 weeks after the second dose, whichever is later.
- If the first dose is administered before the first birthday and the second dose is administered at <15 months of age, a third (and final) dose should be given 8 weeks later.
- For unvaccinated children ≥15 months of age, administer only 1 dose.
- For other catch-up guidance, see the previous "Catch-up Immunization Schedule". For catch-up guidance related to MenHibrix, please see the meningococcal vaccine footnotes and also *MMWR*. 2014;63(RR01);1-13. Available at http://www.cdc.gov/mmwr/pdf/rr/rr6301.pdf.

Vaccination of persons with high-risk conditions:

- Children 12 to 59 months of age who are at increased risk for Hib disease, including chemotherapy recipients and those with anatomic or functional asplenia (including sickle cell disease), human immunodeficiency virus (HIV) infection, immunoglobulin deficiency, or early component complement deficiency, who have received either no doses or only

1 dose of Hib vaccine before 12 months of age, should receive 2 additional doses of Hib vaccine 8 weeks apart; children who received ≥2 doses of Hib vaccine before 12 months of age should receive 1 additional dose.

- For patients <5 years of age undergoing chemotherapy or radiation treatment who received a Hib vaccine dose(s) within 14 days of starting therapy or during therapy, repeat the dose(s) ≥3 months following therapy completion.
- Recipients of hematopoietic stem cell transplant (HSCT) should be revaccinated with a 3-dose regimen of Hib vaccine starting 6 to 12 months after successful transplant, regardless of vaccination history; doses should be administered ≥4 weeks apart.
- A single dose of any Hib-containing vaccine should be administered to unimmunized* children and adolescents ≥15 months of age undergoing an elective splenectomy; if possible, vaccine should be administered ≥14 days before the procedure.
- Hib vaccine is not routinely recommended for patients ≥5 years of age. However, 1 dose of Hib vaccine should be administered to unimmunized* persons ≥5 years of age who have anatomic or functional asplenia (including sickle cell disease) and unvaccinated persons 5 to 18 years of age with human immunodeficiency virus (HIV) infection.

*Patients who have not received a primary series and booster dose or ≥1 dose of Hib vaccine after 14 months of age are considered unimmunized.

[6]**Pneumococcal vaccines** *(Minimum age: 6 weeks for PCV13, 2 years for PPSV23)*

Routine vaccination with PCV13:

- Administer a 4-dose series of PCV13 vaccine at 2, 4, 6, and 12 to 15 months of age.
- For children 14 to 59 months of age who have received an age-appropriate series of 7-valent PCV (PCV7), administer a single supplemental dose of 13-valent PCV (PCV13).

Catch-up vaccination with PCV13:

- Administer 1 dose of PCV13 to all healthy children 24 to 59 months of age who are not completely vaccinated for their age.
- For other catch-up guidance, see the previous "Catch-up Immunization Schedule".

Vaccination of persons with high-risk conditions with PCV13 and PPSV23:

- All recommended PCV13 doses should be administered prior to PPSV23 vaccination if possible.
- For children 2 to 5 years of age with any of the following conditions: Chronic heart disease (particularly cyanotic congenital heart disease and cardiac failure); chronic lung disease (including asthma if treated with high-dose oral corticosteroid therapy); diabetes mellitus; cerebrospinal fluid leak; cochlear implant; sickle cell disease and other hemoglobuinopathies; anatomic or functional asplenia; HIV infection; chronic renal failure; nephrotic syndrome; diseases associated with treatment with immunosuppressive drugs or radiation therapy, including malignant neoplasms, leukemias, lymphomas, and Hodgkin disease; solid organ transplantation; or congenital immunodeficiency:
    1. Administer 1 dose of PCV13 if any incomplete schedule of 3 doses of PCV (PCV7 and/or PCV13) were received previously.
    2. Administer 2 doses of PCV13 ≥8 weeks apart if unvaccinated or any incomplete schedule of <3 doses of PCV (PCV7 and/or PCV13) were received previously.
    3. Administer 1 supplemental dose of PCV13 if 4 doses of PCV7 or other age-appropriate complete PCV7 series was received previously.
    4. The minimum interval between doses of PCV (PCV7 or PCV13) is 8 weeks.
    5. For children with no history of PPSV23 vaccination, administer PPSV23 ≥8 weeks after the most recent dose of PCV13.
- For children 6 to 18 years of age who have cerebrospinal fluid leak; cochlear implant; sickle cell disease and other hemoglobinopathies; anatomic or functional asplenia; congenital or acquired immunodeficiencies; HIV infection; chronic renal failure; nephrotic syndrome; diseases associated with treatment with immunosuppressive drugs or radiation therapy, including malignant neoplasms, leukemias, lymphomas, and Hodgkin disease; generalized malignancy; solid organ transplantation; or multiple myeloma:
    1. If neither PCV13 nor PPSV23 has been received previously, administer 1 dose of PCV13 now and 1 dose of PPSV23 ≥8 weeks later.
    2. If PCV13 has been received previously but PPSV23 has not, administer 1 dose of PPSV23 ≥8 weeks after the most recent dose of PCV13.
    3. If PPSV23 has been received but PCV13 has not, administer 1 dose of PCV13 ≥8 weeks after the most recent dose of PPSV23.
- For children 6 to 18 years of age with chronic heart disease (particularly cyanotic congenital heart disease and cardiac failure), chronic lung disease (including asthma if treated with high-dose oral corticosteroid therapy), diabetes mellitus, alcoholism, or chronic liver disease, who have not received PPSV23, administer 1 dose of PPSV23. If PCV13 has been received previously, then PPSV23 should be administered ≥8 weeks after any prior PCV13 dose.
- A single revaccination with PPSV23 should be administered 5 years after the first dose to children with sickle cell disease or other hemoglobinopathies; anatomic or functional asplenia; congenital or acquired immunodeficiencies; HIV infection; chronic renal failure; nephrotic syndrome; diseases associated with treatment with immunosuppressive drugs or radiation therapy, including malignant neoplasms, leukemias, lymphomas, and Hodgkin disease; generalized malignancy; solid organ transplantation; or multiple myeloma.

[7]**Inactivated poliovirus vaccine (IPV)** *(Minimum age: 6 weeks)*

Routine vaccination:

- Administer a 4-dose series of IPV at 2, 4, and 6 to 18 months of age and at 4 to 6 years of age. The final dose in the series should be administered on or after the fourth birthday and ≥6 months after the previous dose.

Catch-up vaccination:

- In the first 6 months of life, minimum age and minimum intervals are only recommended if the person is at risk for imminent exposure to circulating poliovirus (ie, travel to a polio-endemic region or during an outbreak).
- If ≥4 doses are administered before 4 years of age, an additional dose should be administered at 4 to 6 years of age and ≥6 months after the previous dose.
- A fourth dose is not necessary if the third dose was administered at ≥4 years of age and ≥6 months after the previous dose.
- If both OPV and IPV were administered as part of a series, a total of 4 doses should be administered, regardless of the child's current age. IPV is not routinely recommended for US residents ≥18 years of age.
- For other catch-up guidance, see the previous "Catch-up Immunization Schedule".

[8]**Influenza vaccines** *(Minimum age: 6 months for inactivated influenza vaccine [IIV]; 2 years for live, attenuated influenza vaccine [LAIV])*

Routine vaccination:

- Administer influenza vaccine annually to all children beginning at 6 months of age. For most healthy, nonpregnant persons 2 to 49 years of age, either LAIV or IIV may be used. However, LAIV should **not** be administered to some persons, including 1) persons who have experienced severe allergic reactions to LAIV, any of its components, or to a previous dose of any other influenza vaccine; 2) children 2 to 17 years of age receiving aspirin or aspirin-containing products; 3) persons who are allergic to eggs; 4) pregnant women; 5) immunosuppressed persons; 6) children 2 to 4 years of age with asthma or who had wheezing in the past 12 months; or 7) persons who have taken influenza antiviral medicatons in the previous 48 hours. For all other contraindications and precautions to the use of LAIV, see *MMWR.* 2014;63(32);691-697. Available at http://www.cdc.gov/mmwr/pdf/wk/mm6332.pdf.

For children 6 months to 8 years of age:

- For the 2014 to 2015 season, administer 2 doses (separated by ≥4 weeks) to children who are receiving influenza vaccine for the first time. Some children in this age group who have been vaccinated previously will also need 2 doses. For additional guidance, follow dosing guidelines in the 2014 to 2015 ACIP influenza vaccine recommendations. See *MMWR*. 2014;63(32);691-697. Available at http://www.cdc.gov/mmwr/pdf/wk/mm6332.pdf.
- For the 2015 to 2016 season, follow dosing guidelines in the 2015 ACIP influenza vaccine recommendations.

For persons ≥9 years of age:

- Administer 1 dose.

[9]**Measles, mumps, and rubella (MMR) vaccine** *(Minimum age: 12 months for routine vaccination)*

Routine vaccination:

- Administer a 2-dose series of MMR vaccine at 12 to 15 months of age and 4 to 6 years of age. The second dose may be administered before 4 years of age, provided at least 4 weeks have elapsed since the first dose.
- Administer 1 dose of MMR vaccine to infants 6 to 11 months of age before departure from the United States for international travel. These children should be revaccinated with 2 doses of MMR vaccine, the first at 12 to 15 months of age (12 months if the child remains in an area where disease risk is high) and the second dose ≥4 weeks later.
- Administer 2 doses of MMR vaccine to children ≥12 months of age before departure from the United States for international travel. The first dose should be administered at ≥12 months of age and the second dose ≥4 weeks later.

Catch-up vaccination:

- Ensure that all school-aged children and adolescents have had 2 doses of MMR vaccine; the minimum interval between the 2 doses is 4 weeks.

[10]**Varicella (VAR) vaccine** *(Minimum age: 12 months)*

Routine vaccination:

- Administer a 2-dose series of VAR vaccine at 12 to 15 months of age and 4 to 6 years of age. The second dose may be administered before 4 years of age, provided at least 3 months have elapsed since the first dose. If the second dose was administered ≥4 weeks after the first dose, it can be accepted as valid.

Catch-up vaccination:

- Ensure that all persons 7 to 18 years of age without evidence of immunity (see *MMWR*. 2007;56[No. RR-4]. Available at http://www.cdc.gov/mmwr/pdf/rr/rr5604.pdf) have 2 doses of varicella vaccine. For children 7 to 12 years of age, the recommended minimum interval between doses is 3 months (if the second dose was administered ≥4 weeks after the first dose, it can be accepted as valid); for persons ≥13 years of age, the minimum interval between doses is 4 weeks.

[11]**Hepatitis A (HepA) vaccine** *(Minimum age: 12 months)*

Routine vaccination:

- Initiate the 2-dose HepA vaccine series at 12 to 23 months of age; separate the 2 doses by 6 to 18 months.
- Children who have received 1 dose of HepA vaccine before 24 months of age should receive a second dose 6 to 18 months after the first dose.
- For any person ≥2 years of age who has not already received the HepA vaccine series, 2 doses of HepA vaccine separated by 6 to 18 months may be administered if immunity against hepatitis A virus infection is desired.

Catch-up vaccination:

- The minimum interval between the 2 doses is 6 months.

Special populations:

- Administer 2 doses of HepA vaccine ≥6 months apart to previously unvaccinated persons who live in areas where vaccination programs target older children or who are at increased risk for infection. This includes persons traveling to or working in countries that have high or intermediate endemicity of infection; men having sex with men; users of injection and noninjection illicit drugs; persons who work with HAV-infected primates or with HAV in a research laboratory; persons with clotting-factor disorders; persons with chronic liver disease; and persons who anticipate close, personal contact (eg, household or regular babysitting) with an international adoptee during the first 60 days after arrival in the United States from a country with high or intermediate endemicity. The first dose should be administered as soon as the adoption is planned, ideally ≥2 weeks before the arrival of the adoptee.

[12]**Human papillomavirus (HPV) vaccines** *(Minimum age: 9 years for HPV2 [Cervarix] and HPV4 [Gardasil])*

Routine vaccination:

- Administer a 3-dose series of HPV vaccine on a schedule of 0, 1 to 2, and 6 months to all adolescents 11 to 12 years of age. Either HPV4 or HPV2 may be used for females and only HPV4 may be used for males.
- The vaccine series can be started beginning at 9 years of age.
- Administer the second dose 1 to 2 months after the first dose (minimum interval of 4 weeks) and administer the third dose 24 weeks after the first dose and 16 weeks after the second dose (minimum interval of 12 weeks).

Catch-up vaccination:

- Administer the vaccine series to females (either HPV2 or HPV4) and males (HPV4) at 13 to 18 years of age if not previously vaccinated.
- Use recommended routine dosing intervals (see above) for vaccine series catch-up.

[13]**Meningococcal conjugate vaccines** *(Minimum age: 6 weeks for Hib-MenCY [MenHibrix], 9 months for MenACWY-D [Menactra], 2 months for MenACWY-CRM [Menveo])*

Routine vaccination:

- Administer a single dose of Menactra or Menveo vaccine at 11 to 12 years of age with a booster dose at 16 years of age.
- Adolescents 11 to 18 years of age with human immunodeficiency virus (HIV) infection should receive a 2-dose primary series of Menactra or Menveo with ≥8 weeks between doses.
- For children 2 months to 18 years of age with high-risk conditions, see below.

Catch-up vaccination:

- Administer Menactra or Menveo vaccine at 13 to 18 years of age if not previously vaccinated.
- If the first dose is administered at 13 to 15 years of age, a booster dose should be administered at 16 to 18 years of age with a minimum interval of ≥8 weeks between doses.
- If the first dose is administered at ≥16 years of age, a booster dose is not needed.
- For other catch-up guidance, see the previous "Catch-up Immunization Schedule".

Vaccination of persons with high-risk conditions and other persons at increased risk of disease:

- Children with anatomic or functional asplenia (including sickle cell disease):
  1. Menveo
     - *Children who initiate vaccination at 8 weeks to 6 months of age:* Administer doses at 2, 4, 6, and 12 months of age
     - *Unvaccinated children 7 to 23 months of age:* Administer 2 doses, with the second dose ≥12 weeks after the first dose **and** after the first birthday
     - *Children ≥24 months who have not received a complete series:* Administer 2 primary doses ≥8 weeks apart
  2. MenHibrix
     - *Children 6 weeks to 18 months of age:* Administer doses at 2, 4, 6, and 12 to 15 months of age.
     - If the first dose of MenHibrix is given ≥12 months of age, a total of 2 doses should be given ≥8 weeks apart to ensure protection against serogroups C and Y meningococcal disease.
  3. Menactra
     - *Children ≥24 months who have not received a complete series:* Administer 2 primary doses ≥8 weeks apart. If Menactra is administered to a child with asplenia (including sickle cell disease), do not administer Menactra until 2 years of age and ≥4 weeks after the completion of all PCV13 doses.
- Children with persistent complement component deficiency:
  1. Menveo
     - *Children who initiate vaccination at 8 weeks to 6 months of age:* Administer doses at 2, 4, 6, and 12 months of age.
     - Unvaccinated children 7 to 23 months of age: Administer 2 doses, with the second dose ≥12 weeks after the first dose **and** after the first birthday.

   - *Children ≥24 months of age who have not received a complete series:* Administer 2 primary doses ≥8 weeks apart.

2. MenHibrix
   - *Children 6 weeks to 18 months:* Administer doses at 2, 4, 6, and 12 to 15 months of age.
   - If the first dose of MenHibrix is given at ≥12 months of age, a total of 2 doses should be given ≥8 weeks apart to ensure protection against serogroups C and Y meningococcal disease.

3. Menactra
   - *Children 9 to 23 months of age:* Administer 2 primary doses ≥12 weeks apart.
   - *Children ≥24 months of age who have not received a complete series:* Administer 2 primary doses ≥8 weeks apart.

- For children who travel to or reside in countries in which meningococcal disease is hyperendemic or epidemic, including countries in the African meningitis belt or the Hajj, administer an age-appropriate formulation and series of Menactra or Menveo for protection against serogroups A and W meningococcal disease. Prior receipt of MenHibrix is not sufficient for children traveling to the meningitis belt or the Hajj because it does not contain serogroups A or W.
- For children at risk during a community outbreak attributable to a vaccine serogroup, administer or complete an age- and formulation-appropriate series of MenHibrix, Menactra, or Menveo.
- For booster doses among persons with high-risk conditions, refer to MMWR. 2013;62(RR02);1-22. Available at http://www.cdc.gov/mmwr/preview/mmwrhtml/rr6202a1.htm

For other catch-up recommendations for these persons and complete information on the use of meningococcal vaccines, including guidance related to vaccination of persons at increased risk of infection, see MMWR. 2013;62(RR02);1-22. Available at http://www.cdc.gov/mmwr/preview/mmwrhtml/rr6202a1.htm

This schedule is approved by the Advisory Committee on Immunization Practices (**http://www.cdc.gov/vaccines/acip/index.html**), the American Academy of Pediatrics (**http://www.aap.org**), the American Academy of Family Physicians (**http://www.aafp.org**), and the American College of Obstetricians and Gynecologists (**http://www.acog.org**).

REFERENCE

Centers for Disease Control and Prevention (CDC). Advisory Committee on Immunization Practices (ACIP) recommended immunization schedules for persons aged 0 through 18 years and adults aged 19 years and older – United States, 2015. Available at http://www.cdc.gov/vaccines/schedules/hcp/child-adolescent.html

CENTERS FOR DISEASE CONTROL AND PREVENTION (CDC) AND OTHER LINKS

- Links to vaccine information sheets (http://www.cdc.gov/vaccines/hcp/vis/index.html)
- Who should not get vaccinated (http://www.cdc.gov/vaccines/vpd-vac/should-not-vacc.htm)
- Adverse reactions in laymen's terms (http://www.cdc.gov/vaccines/vac-gen/side-effects.htm)
- Traveler's guide (Yellow book) (http://wwwnc.cdc.gov/travel/page/vaccinations.htm)
- School/daycare requirements and long-term care requirements by state (http://www.cdc.gov/vaccines/imz-managers/laws/index.html)
- Vaccine shortage information (http://www.cdc.gov/vaccines/vac-gen/shortages/default.htm)
- CDC Instant Childhood Immunization Scheduler for children ≤6 years of age (http://www2a.cdc.gov/nip/kidstuff/newscheduler_le/)
- CDC "Catch-up Immunization Scheduler" for children ≤6 years of age (https://www.vacscheduler.org/scheduler.html?v=provider)
- Vaccine codes: NDC, CPT, RxNorm, and CVX/MVX. The CVX code is a numeric string, which identifies the type of vaccine product used; the MVX code is an alphabetic string that identifies the manufacturer of that vaccine. Taken together, the immunization can be resolved tc a trade name (the proprietary name of the product). (http://www.cdc.gov/vaccines/programs/iis/code-sets.html)
- CDC Health Alert Network (http://www.bt.cdc.gov/han/)
- CDC current outbreaks (http://www.cdc.gov/outbreaks/index.html)
- Immunization Action Coalition (http://www.immunize.org/)
- Vaccine Injury Table (http://www.hrsa.gov/vaccinecompensation/vaccinetable.html)

SKIN TESTS FOR DELAYED HYPERSENSITIVITY

Skin tests for delayed hypersensitivity are used diagnostically to assess previous infection (ie, PPD, histoplasmin, and coccidioidin) or used to evaluate cellular immune function by testing for anergy (ie, mumps, *Candida*, tetanus toxoid, trichophyton, PPD). Anergy, a defect in cell-mediated immunity, is characterized by a depressed response or lack of response to skin testing with injected antigens. Anergy has been associated with congenital and acquired immunodeficiencies and malnutrition.

Candida 1:100

Dose = 0.1 mL intradermally (30% of children younger than 18 months of age and 50% older than 18 months of age respond)

Can be used as a control antigen

Histoplasmin 1:100

Dose = 0.1 mL intradermally (yeast derived)

Mumps 40 cfu per mL

Dose = 0.1 mL intradermally (contraindicated in patients allergic to eggs, egg products, or thimerosal)

Purified Protein Derivatives 5 TU (PPD[1] Mantoux Tuberculin)

Screening for tuberculosis:

Children who have no risk factors but who reside in high-prevalence regions: skin test at 4 to 6 years and 11 to 16 years of age

Children exposed to HIV-infected individuals, homeless, residents of nursing homes, institutionalized adolescents, users of illicit drugs, incarcerated adolescents and migrant farm workers: skin test every 2 to 3 years

Children at high risk (children infected with HIV, incarcerated adolescents): annual skin testing

Dose = 0.1 mL intradermally

Definition of positive Mantoux skin test (regardless of previous BCG administration):

Reaction ≥5 mm for high-risk group (children in close contact with known or suspected infectious cases of tuberculosis; children suspected to have disease based on clinical and/or roentgenographic evidence; and children with underlying host factors (immunosuppressive conditions, receiving immunosuppressive therapy, and HIV infection).

Reaction ≥10 mm for children <4 years; those with medical diseases who are at increased risk for dissemination or for those at increased risk because of environmental exposure.

Reaction ≥15 mm for children ≥4 years of age including those with no risk factors.

[1]PPD 1 TU (first strength) is only used in individuals suspected of being highly sensitive. PPD 250 TU (second strength) is used only for individuals who fail to respond to a previous injection of 5 TU, or anergic patients in whom TB is suspected.

Tetanus Toxoid 1:5

Dose = 0.1 mL intradermally (29% of children younger than 2 years of age and 78% older than 2 years of age respond if they have received 3 immunizing doses)

Can be used as a control antigen.

Tine Test

Indication: survey and screen for exposure to tuberculosis (grasp forearm firmly; stretch the skin of the volar surface tightly; apply the tines to the selected site; press for at least one second so that a circular halo impression is left on the skin)

General Information

1. Intradermal skin tests should be injected in the flexor surface of the forearm.
2. A pale wheal 6 to 10 mm in diameter should form over the needle tip as soon as the injection is administered. If no bleb forms, the injection must be repeated.
3. Space skin tests at least 2 inches apart to prevent reactions from overlapping.
4. Read skin tests for diameter of induration and presence of erythema at 24, 48, and 72 hours. Reactions occurring before 24 hours are indicative of an immediate rather than a delayed hypersensitivity reaction.
5. False-negative results may occur in patients with malnutrition, viral infections, febrile illnesses, immunodeficiency disorders, severe disseminated infections, uremia, patients who have received immunosuppressive therapy (steroids, antineoplastic agents), patients who have received a recent live attenuated virus vaccine (MMR, measles).
6. False-positive results may occur in patients sensitive to ingredients in the skin test solution such as thimerosal; cross-sensitivity between similar antigens; or with improper interpretation of skin test.
7. Side effects are pain, blisters, extensive erythema and necrosis at the injection site.
   Emergency equipment and epinephrine should be readily available to treat severe allergic reactions that may occur.

Recommended Interpretation of Skin Test Reactions

Reaction	Local Reaction	
	After Intradermal Injections of Antigens	After Dinitrochlorobenzene
1+	Erythema >10 mm and/or induration >1 to 5 mm	Erythema and/or induration covering <$^{1}/_{2}$ area of dosing site
2+	Induration 6 to 10 mm	Induration covering >$^{1}/_{2}$ area of dose site
3+	Induration 11 to 20 mm	Vesiculation and induration at dose site or spontaneous flare at days 7 to 14 at the site
4+	Induration >20 mm	Bulla or ulceration at dose site or spontaneous flare at days 7 to 14 at the site

REFERENCES

American Academy of Pediatrics Committee on Infectious Diseases. Screening for tuberculosis in infants and children. *Pediatrics*. 1994;93(1):131-134.

American Academy of Pediatrics Committee on Infectious Diseases. Update on tuberculosis skin testing of children. *Pediatrics*. 1996;97(2):282-284.

REFERENCE VALUES FOR CHILDREN

	Normal Values	
	Age	**Serum Concentration**
CHEMISTRY		
Albumin	Premature 1 day	1.8 to 3 g/dL
	Full-term <6 days	2.5 to 3.4 g/dL
	8 days to 1 year	1.9 to 4.9 g/dL
	1 to 3 years	3.4 to 4.2 g/dL
	4 to 19 years	3.5 to 5.6 g/dL
Ammonia	All ages	19 to 60 mcg/dL
Amylase	1 to 19 years	30 to 100 units/L
Bilirubin, total	*See nomogram for age-specific neonatal values*	
	1 month to Adult	<1 mg/dL
Calcium, total	Cord blood	9 to 11.5 mg/dL
	Newborn 3 to 24 hours	9 to 10.6 mg/dL
	Newborn 24 to 48 hours	7 to 12 mg/dL
	4 to 7 days	9 to 10.9 mg/dL
	Child	8.8 to 10.8 mg/dL
	Adolescent to Adult	8.4 to 10.2 mg/dL
Calcium, ionized, whole blood	Cord blood	5 to 6 mg/dL
	Newborn 3 to 24 hours	4.3 to 5.1 mg/dL
	Newborn 24 to 48 hours	4 to 4.7 mg/dL
	≥2 days	4.8 to 4.92 mg/dL (2.24 to 2.46 mEq/L)
Carbon dioxide (PCO_2)	Newborn	27 to 40 mm Hg
	Infant	27 to 41 mm Hg
	Child to Adult:	
	Male	35 to 48 mm Hg
	Female	32 to 45 mm Hg
Chloride		95 to 105 mEq/L
Cholesterol	*See following tables for age- and gender-specific values*	
Creatinine	0 to 4 years	0.03 to 0.5 mg/dL
(IDMS) Enzymatic	4 to 7 years	0.03 to 0.59 mg/dL
	7 to 10 years	0.22 to 0.59 mg/dL
	10 to 14 years	0.31 to 0.88 mg/dL
	>14 years	0.5 to 1.06 mg/dL
Glucose	Cord blood	45 to 96 mg/dL
	Premature	20 to 60 mg/dL
	Neonate	30 to 60 mg/dL
	Newborn 1 day	40 to 60 mg/dL
	>1 day	50 to 90 mg/dL
	Child	60 to 100 mg/dL
	Adult	70 to 105 mg/dL
Iron	All ages	22 to 184 mcg/dL
Iron binding capacity, total	Infant	100 to 400 mcg/dL
	≥1 year to Adult	250 to 400 mcg/dL
Lactic acid, lactate	1 to 12 months	10 to 21 mg/dL
	1 to 7 years	7 to 14 mg/dL
	7 to 15 years	5 to 8 mg/dL
Lead, whole blood	Child	<10 mcg/dL
	Toxic	≥70 mcg/dL
Lipase	1 to 18 years	145 to 216 units/L
Magnesium		1.5 to 2.5 mEq/L

	Normal Values	
CHEMISTRY	**Age**	**Serum Concentration**
Osmolality, serum	Child to Adult	275 to 295 mOsm/kg
Phosphorus	Newborn 0 to 5 days	4.8 to 8.2 mg/dL
	1 to 3 years	3.8 to 6.5 mg/dL
	4 to 11 years	3.7 to 5.6 mg/dL
	12 to 15 years	2.9 to 5.4 mg/dL
	16 to 19 years	2.7 to 4.7 mg/dL
Potassium, plasma	Newborn	4.5 to 7.2 mEq/L
	2 days to 3 months	4 to 6.2 mEq/L
	3 months to 1 year	3.7 to 5.6 mEq/L
	1 to 16 years	3.5 to 5 mEq/L
Protein, total	Premature neonate	4.3 to 7.6 g/dL
	Newborn	4.6 to 7.4 g/dL
	1 to 7 years	6.1 to 7.9 g/dL
	8 to 12 years	6.4 to 8.1 g/dL
	13 to 19 years	6.6 to 8.2 g/dL
Sodium		136 to 145 mEq/L
Triglycerides	*See following tables for age- and gender-specific values*	
Urea nitrogen, blood	Cord blood	21 to 40 mg/dL
	Premature (1 week)	3 to 25 mg/dL
	Newborn	3 to 12 mg/dL
	Infant to Child	5 to 18 mg/dL
	Adolescent to Adult	7 to 18 mg/dL
Uric acid	1 to 3 years	1.8 to 5 mg/dL
	4 to 6 years	2.2 to 4.7 mg/dL
	7 to 9 years	2 to 5 mg/dL
	10 to 11 years:	
	Male	2.3 to 5.4 mg/dL
	Female	3 to 4.7 mg/dL
	12 to 13 years: Male	2.7 to 6.7 mg/dL
	14 to 15 years: Male	2.4 to 7.8 mg/dL
	12 to 15 years: Female	3 to 5.8 mg/dL
	16 to 19 years:	
	Male	4 to 8.6 mg/dL
	Female	3 to 5.9 mg/dL
ENZYMES		
Alanine aminotransferase (ALT) (SGPT)	≤7 days	6 to 40 units/L
	8 to 30 days:	
	Male	10 to 40 units/L
	Female	8 to 32 units/L
	1 to 12 months	12 to 45 units/L
	1 to 19 years	5 to 45 units/L
Alkaline phosphatase (ALKP)	1 to 9 years	145 to 420 units/L
	10 to 11 years	140 to 560 units/L
	12 to 13 years:	
	Male	200 to 495 units/L
	Female	105 to 420 units/L
	14 to 15 years:	
	Male	130 to 525 units/L
	Female	70 to 230 units/L
	16 to 19 years:	
	Male	65 to 260 units/L
	Female	50 to 130 units/L

ENZYMES

	Age	Normal Values Serum Concentration
	Newborn ≤7 days:	
	Male	30 to 100 units/L
	Female	24 to 95 units/L
	8 to 30 days	22 to 71 units/L
	1 to 12 months	22 to 63 units/L
Aspartate aminotransferase (AST) (SGOT)	1 to 3 years	20 to 60 units/L
	3 to 9 years	15 to 50 units/L
	10 to 15 years	10 to 40 units/L
	16 to 19 years:	
	Male	15 to 45 units/L
	Female	5 to 30 units/L
	Cord blood	70 to 380 units/L
	Newborn 5 to 8 hours	214 to 1,175 units/L
Creatine kinase (CK)	Newborn 24 to 33 hours	130 to 1,200 units/L
	Newborn 72 to 100 hours	87 to 725 units/L
	Adult	5 to 130 units/L
	<1 year	170 to 580 units/L
Lactate dehydrogenase (LDH)	1 to 9 years	150 to 500 units/L
	10 to 19 years	120 to 330 units/L

Blood Gases

	Arterial	Capillary	Venous
pH	7.35 to 7.45	7.35 to 7.45	7.32 to 7.42
pCO_2 (mm Hg)	35 to 45	35 to 45	38 to 52
pO_2 (mm Hg)	70 to 100	60 to 80	24 to 48
HCO_3 (mEq/L)	19 to 25	19 to 25	19 to 25
TCO_2 (mEq/L)	19 to 29	19 to 29	23 to 33
O_2 saturation (%)	90 to 95	90 to 95	40 to 70
Base excess (mEq/L)	-5 to +5	-5 to +5	-5 to +5

Hyperbilirubinemia Assessment in the Newborn Infant

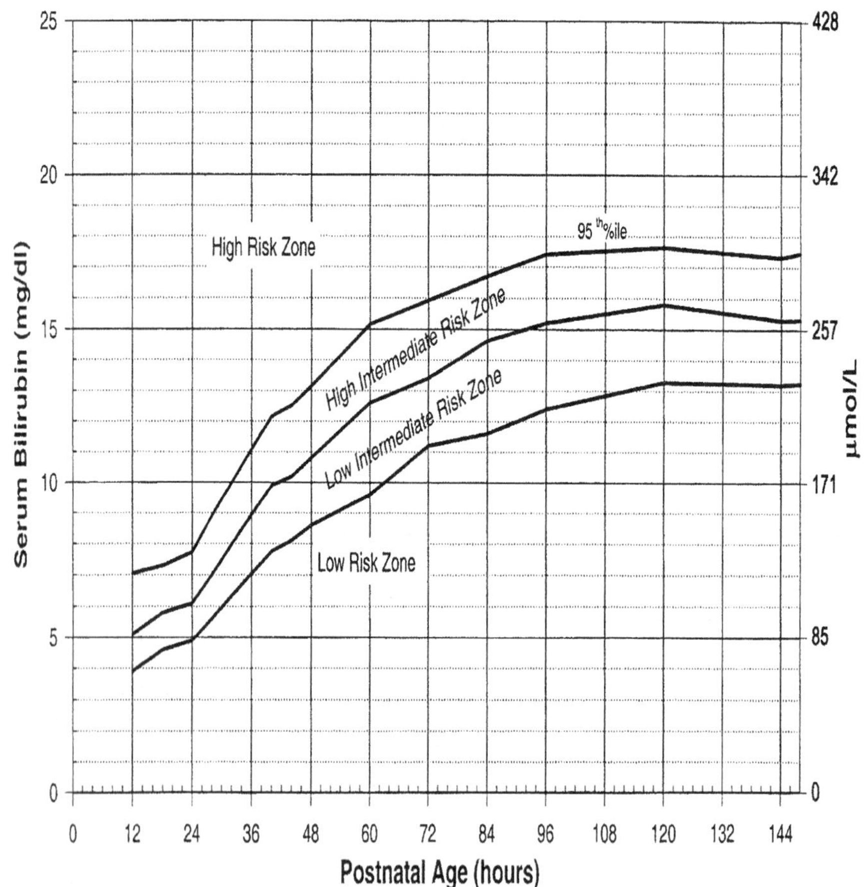

Nomogram for designation of risk in 2,840 well newborns at ≥36 weeks gestational age with birth weight of ≥2,000 g or ≥35 weeks gestational age and birth weight of ≥2,500 g based on the hour-specific serum bilirubin values. The serum bilirubin level was obtained before discharge and the zone in which the value fell predicted the likelihood of a subsequent bilirubin level exceeding the 95th percentile (high-risk zone).

Reproduced with permission from: American Academy of Pediatrics Subcommittee on Hyperbilirubinemia. Management of hyperbilirubinemia in the newborn infant ≥35 weeks of gestation. *Pediatrics*. 2004;114(1):297-316. Available at http://pediatrics.aappublications.org/content/114/1/297.long

Classification of Serum Lipid Concentrations[1]

Classification	Total Cholesterol[2] (mg/dL)		LDL-C[2] (mg/dL)		HDL-C[2] (mg/dL)		Apolipoprotein A-1	Triglycerides[3] (mg/dL)			Apolipoprotein B
	Children and Adolescents	Young Adults	Children and Adolescents	Young Adults	Children and Adolescents	Young Adults	Children and Adolescents	Children 0 to 9 years	Children ≥10 years and Adolescents <19 years	Young Adults	Children and Adolescents
Low					<40	<40	<115				
Borderline low						40 to 44					
Acceptable/ optimal	<170	<190	<110	<120	>45	>45	>120	<75	<90	<115	<90
Borderline high	170 to 199	190 to 224	120 to 159	130 to 159	40 to 45		115 to 120	75 to 99	90 to 129	115 to 149	90 to 109
High	≥200	≥225	≥130	≥160				≥100	≥130	≥150	≥110

[1]Adapted from: Expert panel on integrated guidelines for cardiovascular health and risk reduction in children and adolescents: summary report. *Pediatrics*. 2011;128(Suppl 5):S213-S256.

[2]To convert cholesterol results to SI units, divide value by 38.6.

[3]To convert triglyceride results to SI units, divide value by 88.6.

Serum Lipid Concentrations by Age and Gender

	Males (mg/dL)			Females (mg/dL)		
	5 to 9 years	**10 to 14 years**	**15 to 19 years**	**5 to 9 years**	**10 to 14 years**	**15 to 19 years**
Total Cholesterol						
50th percentile	153	161	152	164	159	157
75th percentile	168	173	168	177	171	176
90th percentile	183	191	183	189	191	198
95th percentile	186	201	191	197	205	208
Triglycerides						
50th percentile	48	58	68	57	68	64
75th percentile	58	74	88	74	85	85
90th percentile	70	94	125	103	104	112
95th percentile	85	111	143	120	120	126
LDL-C						
50th percentile	90	94	93	98	94	93
75th percentile	103	109	109	115	110	110
90th percentile	117	123	123	125	126	129
95th percentile	129	133	130	140	136	137
HDL						
5th percentile	38	37	30	36	37	35
10th percentile	43	40	34	38	40	38
25th percentile	49	46	39	48	45	43
50th percentile	55	55	46	52	52	51

Adapted from: American Academy of Pediatrics Committee on Nutrition. Lipid screening and cardiovascular health in childhood. *Pediatrics*. 2008;122:(1) 198-208.

Thyroid Function Tests

	Age	**Normal Range**
T_4 (thyroxine) serum concentrations	1 to 7 days	10.1 to 20.9 mcg/dL
	8 to 14 days	9.8 to 16.6 mcg/dL
	1 month to 1 year	5.5 to 16 mcg/dL
	>1 year	4 to 12 mcg/dL
Free Thyroxine Index (FTI)	1 to 3 days	9.3 to 26.6
	1 to 4 weeks	7.6 to 20.8
	1 to 4 months	7.4 to 17.9
	4 to 12 months	5.1 to 14.5
	1 to 6 years	5.7 to 13.3
	>6 years	4.8 to 14
T_3 serum concentration	Newborn	100 to 470 ng/dL
	1 to 5 years	100 to 260 ng/dL
	5 to 10 years	90 to 240 ng/dL
	10 years to Adult	70 to 210 ng/dL
T_3 uptake		35% to 45%
TSH serum concentration	Cord sample	3 to 22 micro international units/mL
	1 to 3 days	<40 micro international units/mL
	3 to 7 days	<25 micro international units/mL
	>7 days	≤10 micro international units/mL

Hematology Values

<table>
<tr><th>Age</th><th>Hgb (g/dL)</th><th>Hct (%)</th><th>RBC (mill/mm^3)</th><th>RDW</th><th>MCV (fL)</th><th>MCH (pg/cell)</th><th>MCHC (%)</th><th>PLTS (x 10^3/mm^3)</th></tr>
<tr><td>≤30 days</td><td>15 to 24</td><td>44 to 70</td><td rowspan="7">4 to 5.5</td><td rowspan="7">12% to 15%</td><td>99 to 115</td><td>33 to 39</td><td rowspan="7">32 to 36</td><td>84 to 478*</td></tr>
<tr><td>1 to 23 months</td><td>10.5 to 14</td><td>32 to 42</td><td>72 to 88</td><td>24 to 30</td><td rowspan="6">150 to 450</td></tr>
<tr><td>2 to 9 years</td><td>11.5 to 14.5</td><td>33 to 43</td><td>76 to 90</td><td>25 to 31</td></tr>
<tr><td>10 to 17 years (male)</td><td>12.5 to 16.1</td><td>36 to 47</td><td>78 to 95</td><td>26 to 32</td></tr>
<tr><td>10 to 17 years (female)</td><td>12 to 15</td><td>35 to 45</td><td>78 to 95</td><td>26 to 32</td></tr>
<tr><td>≥18 years (male)</td><td>13.5 to 18</td><td>42 to 52</td><td>78 to 100</td><td>27 to 31</td></tr>
<tr><td>≥18 years (female)</td><td>12.5 to 16</td><td>37 to 47</td><td>78 to 100</td><td>27 to 31</td></tr>
</table>

*Value for ages 0 to 7 days, for ages >7 days similar to range for all patient ages

WBC and Diff

<table>
<tr><th>Age</th><th>WBC (x 10^3/mm^3)</th><th>Segs</th><th>Bands</th><th>Lymphs</th><th>Monos</th><th>Eosinophils</th><th>Basophils</th><th>Myelocytes</th></tr>
<tr><td>≤30 days</td><td>9.1 to 34</td><td rowspan="5">54% to 62%</td><td rowspan="5">3% to 5%</td><td rowspan="5">25% to 33%</td><td rowspan="5">3% to 7%</td><td rowspan="5">1% to 3%</td><td rowspan="5">≤0.75%</td><td rowspan="5">0%</td></tr>
<tr><td>1 to 23 months</td><td>6 to 14</td></tr>
<tr><td>2 to 9 years</td><td>4 to 12</td></tr>
<tr><td>10 to 17 years</td><td>4 to 10.5</td></tr>
<tr><td>≥18 years</td><td>4 to 10.5</td></tr>
</table>

Segs = segmented neutrophils, bands = band neutrophils, lymphs = lymphocytes, monos = monocytes

Erythrocyte Sedimentation Rates and Reticulocyte Counts

	Child	0 to 20 mm/hour
Sedimentation rate, Westergren	Adult male	0 to 15 mm/hour
	Adult female	0 to 20 mm/hour
	Child	0 to 13 mm/hour
Sedimentation rate, Wintrobe	Adult male	0 to 10 mm/hour
	Adult female	0 to 15 mm/hour
	1 day	0.4% to 0.6%
	7 days	<0.1% to 1.3%
	1 to 4 weeks	<1% to 1.2%
Reticulocyte count: Neonatal and infant data based on capillary specimen	5 to 6 weeks	<0.1% to 2.4%
	7 to 8 weeks	0.1% to 2.9%
	9 to 10 weeks	<0.1% to 2.6%
	11 to 12 weeks	0.1% to 1.3%
Reticulocyte count: Whole blood specimen	Adult	0.5% to 1.5%

Cerebrospinal Fluid Values, Normal

Cell count:		% PMNs
Preterm mean	9 (0 to 25.4 WBC/mm^3)	57%
Term mean	8.2 (0 to 22.4 WBC/mm^3)	61%
>1 month	0.7	0
Glucose:		
Preterm	24 to 63 mg/dL	mean 50 mg/dL
Term	34 to 119 mg/dL	mean 52 mg/dL
Child	40 to 80 mg/dL	
CSF glucose/blood glucose:		
Preterm	55% to 105%	
Term	44% to 128%	
Child	50%	
Lactic acid dehydrogenase	5 to 30 units/mL	mean 20 units/mL
Myelin basic protein	<4 ng/mL	
Pressure: Initial LP (mm H_2O):		
Newborn	80 to 110 (<110)	
Infant/Child	<200 (lateral recumbent position)	
Respiratory movements	5 to 10	
Protein:		
Preterm	65 to 150 mg/dL	mean 115 mg/dL
Term	20 to 170 mg/dL	mean 90 mg/dL
Child:		
Ventricular	5 to 15 mg/dL	
Cisternal	5 to 25 mg/dL	
Lumbar	5 to 40 mg/dL	

ACID/BASE ASSESSMENT

Henderson-Hasselbalch Equation

$pH = 6.1 + \log ([HCO_3^-] / (0.03) [PaCO_2])$

Normal arterial blood pH: 7.4 (normal range: 7.35 to 7.45)

Where:

$[HCO_3^-]$ = Serum bicarbonate concentration

$PaCO_2$ = Arterial carbon dioxide partial pressure

Alveolar Gas Equation

P_iO_2 = F_iO_2 x (total atmospheric pressure – vapor pressure of H_2O at 37°C)

= F_iO_2 x (760 mm Hg – 47 mm Hg)

PAO_2 = $P_iO_2 - (PaCO_2 / R)$

Alveolar-arterial oxygen (A-a) gradient = $PAO_2 - PaO_2$

or

A-a gradient = $[(F_iO_2 \times 713) - (PaCO_2/0.8)] - PaO_2$

A-a gradient normal ranges:

Children	15 to 20 mm Hg
Adults	20 to 25 mm Hg

where:

P_iO_2 = Oxygen partial pressure of inspired gas (mm Hg) (150 mm Hg in room air at sea level)

F_iO_2 = Fractional pressure of oxygen in inspired gas (0.21 in room air)

PAO_2 = Alveolar oxygen partial pressure

PaO_2 = Arterial oxygen partial pressure

$PaCO_2$ = Arterial carbon dioxide partial pressure

R = Respiratory exchange quotient (typically 0.8, increases with high carbohydrate diet, decreases with high fat diet)

Acid-Base Disorders

Acute metabolic acidosis:
$PaCO_2$ expected = 1.5 ($[HCO_3^-]$) + 8 ± 2 **or**
Expected decrease in $PaCO_2$ = 1.3 (1-1.5) x decrease in $[HCO_3^-]$

Acute metabolic alkalosis:
Expected increase in $PaCO_2$ = 0.6 (0.5-1) x increase in $[HCO_3^-]$

Acute respiratory acidosis (<6 h duration):
For every $PaCO_2$ increase of 10 mm Hg, $[HCO_3^-]$ increases by 1 mEq/L

Chronic respiratory acidosis (>6 h duration):
For every $PaCO_2$ increase of 10 mm Hg, $[HCO_3^-]$ increases by 4 mEq/L

Acute respiratory alkalosis (<6 h duration):
For every $PaCO_2$ decrease of 10 mm Hg, $[HCO_3^-]$ decreases by 2 mEq/L

Chronic respiratory alkalosis (>6 h duration):
For every $PaCO_2$ decrease of 10 mm Hg, $[HCO_3^-]$ increases by 5 mEq/L

LABORATORY CALCULATIONS

ANION GAP

Definition: The difference in concentration between unmeasured cation and anion equivalents in serum.

Anion gap = $Na^+ - (Cl^- + HCO_3^-)$
(The normal anion gap is 10 to 14 mEq/L)

Differential Diagnosis of Increased Anion Gap Acidosis

Organic anions
- Lactate (sepsis, hypovolemia, seizures, large tumor burden)
- Pyruvate
- Uremia
- Ketoacidosis (beta-hydroxybutyrate and acetoacetate)
- Amino acids and their metabolites
- Other organic acids (eg, formate from methanol, glycolate from ethylene glycol)

Inorganic anions
- Hyperphosphatemia
- Sulfates
- Nitrates

Medications and toxins
- Penicillins and cephalosporins
- Salicylates (including aspirin)
- Cyanide
- Carbon monoxide

Differential Diagnosis of Decreased Anion Gap

Organic cations
- Hypergammaglobulinemia

Inorganic cations
- Hyperkalemia
- Hypercalcemia
- Hypermagnesemia

Medications and toxins
- Lithium

Hypoalbuminemia

OSMOLALITY

Definition: The summed concentrations of all osmotically active solute particles

Predicted serum osmolality =

$$\text{mOsm/L} = (2 \times \text{serum Na}^{++}) + \frac{\text{serum glucose}}{18} + \frac{\text{BUN}}{2.8}$$

The normal range of serum osmolality is 285 to 295 mOsm/L.

Calculated Osm

Note: Osm is a term used to reconcile osmolality and osmolarity

Osmol gap = measured Osm – calculated Osm

0 to +10: Normal
>10: Abnormal
<0: Probable lab or calculation error

Differential Diagnosis of Increased Osmol Gap

(increased by >10 mOsm/L)
Ethanol
Ethylene glycol
Glycerol
Iodine (questionable)
Isopropanol (acetone)
Mannitol
Methanol
Sorbitol

CORRECTED SODIUM FOR HYPERGLYCEMIA

Corrected Na^+ = serum Na^+ + [1.5 x (glucose – 150 divided by 100)]

Note: Do not correct for glucose <150.

CORRECTED TOTAL SERUM CALCIUM FOR ALBUMIN LEVEL

[(Normal albumin – patient's albumin) x 0.8] + patient's measured total calcium

BICARBONATE DEFICIT

HCO_3^- deficit = (0.4 x wt in kg) x (HCO_3^- desired – HCO_3^- measured)

Note: In clinical practice, the calculated quantity may differ markedly from the actual amount of bicarbonate needed or that which may be safely administered.

APGAR SCORING SYSTEM

Sign	Score		
	0	1	2
Heart rate	Absent	Under 100 beats per minute	Over 100 beats per minute
Respiratory effort	Absent	Slow (irregular)	Good crying
Muscle tone	Limp	Some flexion of extremities	Active motion
Reflex irritability	No response	Grimace	Cough or sneeze
Color	Blue, pale	Pink body, blue extremities	All pink

From Apgar V. A proposal for a new method of evaluation of the newborn infant. *Anesth Analg*. 1953;32:260.

FETAL HEART RATE MONITORING

Normal Heart Rates

Fetal heart rate (FHR) 120 to 160 bpm. Isolated accelerations are normal and considered reassuring. Mild (100 to 120 bpm) an transient bradycardias may be normal. Normal fetal heart rate tracings show beat-to-beat variability of 5 to 10 bpm (poor beat-to beat variability suggests fetal hypoxia).

Abnormal Heart Rates

Bradycardia (FHR <120 bpm): Potential causes include fetal distress, drugs, congenital heart block (associated with materna SLE, congenital cardiac defects).

Tachycardia (FHR >160 bpm): Potential causes include maternal fever, chorioamnionitis, drugs, fetal dysrhythmias, eg, SVT (with or without fetal CHF).

Decreased Beat-to-Beat Variability

Results from fetal CNS depression. Potential causes include fetal hypoxia, fetal sleep, fetal immaturity, and maternal narcotic sedative administration.

Fetal Heart Rate Decelerations

Type 1 (early decelerations)

- Seen most commonly in late labor
- Mirror uterine contractions in time of onset, duration, and resolution
- Uniform shape
- Usually associated with good beat-to-beat variability
- Heart rate may dip to 60 to 80 bpm
- Associated with fetal head compression (increases vagal tone)
- Considered benign, and not representative of fetal hypoxia

Type 2 (late decelerations)

- Deceleration 10 to 30 seconds after onset of uterine contraction
- Heart rate fails to return to baseline after contraction is completed
- Asymmetrical shape (longer deceleration, shorter acceleration)
- Late decelerations of 10 to 20 bpm may be significant
- Probably associated with fetal CNS and myocardial depression

Type 3 (variable decelerations)

- Heart rate variations do not correlate with uterine contractions
- Variable shape and duration
- Occur occasionally in many normal labors
- Concerning if severe (HR <60 bpm), prolonged (duration >60 seconds), associated with poor beat-to-beat variability, o combined with late decelerations
- Associated with cord compression (including nuchal cord)

REFERENCE

Manual of Neonatal Care, Joint Program in Neonatology. 3rd ed. Cloherty JP, Stark AR, eds. Boston, MA: Little, Brown; 1991.

RENAL FUNCTION ESTIMATION IN ADULT PATIENTS

Evaluation of a patient's renal function often includes the use of equations to estimate glomerular filtration rate (GFR) (eg, estimated GFR [eGFR] creatinine clearance [CrCl]) using an endogenous filtration marker (eg, serum creatinine) and other patient variables. For example, the Cockcroft-Gault equation estimates renal function by calculating CrCl and is typically used to steer medication dosing. Equations which calculate eGFR are primarily used to categorize chronic kidney disease (CKD) staging and monitor progression. The rate of creatinine clearance does not always accurately represent GFR; creatinine may be cleared by other renal mechanisms in addition to glomerular filtration and serum creatinine concentrations may be affected by nonrenal factors (eg, age, gender, race, body habitus, illness, diet). In addition, these equations were developed based on studies in limited populations and may either over- or underestimate the renal function of a specific patient.

Nevertheless, most clinicians estimate renal function using CrCl as an indicator of actual renal function for the purpose of adjusting medication doses. For medications that require dose adjustment for renal impairment, utilization of eGFR (ie, Modification of Diet in Renal Disease [MDRD]) may overestimate renal function by up to 40% which may result in supra-therapeutic medication doses (Hermsen 2009). These equations should only be used in the clinical context of patient-specific factors noted during the physical exam/work-up. The 2012 National Kidney Foundation (NKF)-Kidney Disease Improving Global Outcomes (KDIGO) CKD guidelines state that drug dosing should be based on an e-GFR which is **not** adjusted for body surface area (BSA) (ie, reported in units of mL/minute/1.73 m^2) since the effect of eGFR adjusted for BSA compared to eGFR without adjustments for BSA has not been extensively studied. **Decisions regarding drug therapy and doses must be based on clinical judgment.**

RENAL FUNCTION ESTIMATION EQUATIONS

Commonly used equations to estimate renal function utilizing the endogenous filtration marker serum creatinine include the Cockcroft-Gault, Jelliffe, four-variable Modification of Diet in Renal Disease (MDRD), six-variable MDRD (aka, MDRD extended), and Chronic Kidney Disease Epidemiology Collaboration (CKD-EPI). All of these equations, except for the CKD-EPI, were originally developed using a serum creatinine assay measured by the alkaline picrate-based (Jaffe) method. Many substances, including proteins, can interfere with the accuracy of this assay and overestimate serum creatinine concentration. The NKF and The National Kidney Disease Education Program (NDKEP) advocated for a universal creatinine assay, in order to ensure an accurate estimate of renal function in patients. As a result, a more specific enzymatic assay with an isotope dilution mass spectrometry (IDMS)-traceable international standard was developed. Compared to the older methods, IDMS-traceable assays may report lower serum creatinine values and may, therefore, overestimate renal function when used in the original equations not re-expressed for use with a standardized serum creatinine assay (eg, Cockcroft-Gault, Jelliffe, original MDRD). Updated four-variable MDRD and six-variable MDRD equations based on serum creatinine measured by the IDMS-traceable method has been proposed for adults (Levey 2006); the Cockcroft-Gault and Jelliffe equations have not been re-expressed and may overestimate renal function when used with a serum creatinine measured by the IDMS-traceable method. However, at this point, all laboratories should be using creatinine methods calibrated to be IDMS traceable.

The CKD-EPI creatinine equation, published in 2009, uses the same four variables as the four-variable MDRD (serum creatinine, age, sex, and race), but allows for more precision when estimating higher GFR values (eg, eGFR >60 mL/minute/1.73 m^2) as compared to the MDRD equation. The NKDEP has not made a recommendation on the general implementation of the CKD-EPI equation but does suggest that laboratories which report numeric values for eGFR >60 mL/minute/1.73 m^2 should consider the use of CKD-EPI. The NKD-KDIGO 2012 CKD guidelines recommend that clinicians use a creatinine-derived equation for the evaluation and management of CKD and specifically recommend that clinical laboratories use the 2009 CKD-EPI equation when reporting eGFR in adults.

The following factors may contribute to an inaccurate estimation of renal function (Stevens 2006):

- Increased creatinine generation (may underestimate renal function):
  - Black or African American patients
  - Muscular body habitus
  - Ingestion of cooked meats
- Decreased creatinine generation (may overestimate renal function):
  - Increased age
  - Female patients
  - Hispanic patients
  - Asian patients
  - Amputees
  - Malnutrition, inflammation, or deconditioning (eg, cancer, severe cardiovascular disease, hospitalized patients)
  - Neuromuscular disease
  - Vegetarian diet
- Rapidly changing serum creatinine (either up or down): In patients with rapidly rising serum creatinines (ie, increasing by >0.5 to 0.7 mg/dL/day), it is best to assume that the patient's renal function is severely impaired

Use extreme caution when estimating renal function in the following patient populations:

- Low body weight (actual body weight < ideal body weight)
- Liver transplant

- Elderly (>90 years of age)
- Dehydration
- Recent kidney transplantation (serum creatinine values may decrease rapidly and can lead to renal function under-estimation; conversely, delayed graft function may be present)

Note: In most situations, the use of the patient's ideal body weight (IBW) is recommended for estimating renal function, except when the patient's actual body weight (ABW) is less than ideal. Use of actual body weight (ABW) in obese patients (and possibly patients with ascites) may significantly overestimate renal function. Some clinicians prefer to use an adjusted body weight in such cases [eg, IBW + 0.4 (ABW - IBW)]; the adjustment factor may vary based on practitioner and/or institutional preference.

IDMS-traceable methods

Method 1: MDRD equation[1]:

$eGFR = 175 \times (Creatinine)^{-1.154} \times (Age)^{-0.203} \times (Gender) \times (Race)$

where:

eGFR = estimated GFR; calculated in mL/minute/1.73 m^2
Creatinine is input in mg/dL
Age is input in years
Gender: Females: Gender = 0.742; Males: Gender = 1
Race: Black: Race = 1.212; White or other: Race = 1

Method 2: MDRD Extended equation:

$eGFR = 161.5 \times (Creatinine)^{-0.999} \times (Age)^{-0.176} \times (SUN)^{-0.170} \times (Albumin)^{0.318} \times (Gender) \times (Race)$

where:

eGFR = estimated GFR; calculated in mL/minute/1.73 m^2
Creatinine is input in mg/dL
Age is input in years
SUN = Serum Urea Nitrogen; input in mg/dL
Albumin = Serum Albumin; input in g/dL
Gender: Females: Gender = 0.762; Males: Gender = 1
Race: Black: Race = 1.18; White or other: Race = 1

Method 3: CKD-EPI equation[2]:

$eGFR = 141 \times (Creatinine/k)^{Exp} \times (0.993)^{Age} \times (Gender) \times (Race)$

where:

eGFR = estimated GFR; calculated in mL/minute/1.73 m^2
(Creatinine/k):
Creatinine is input in mg/dL
k: Females: k = 0.7; Males: k = 0.9
Exp:
When (Creatinine/k) is ≤1: Females: Exp = -0.329; Males: Exp = -0.411
When (Creatinine/k) is >1: Exp = -1.209
Age is input in years
Gender: Females: Gender = 1.018; Males: Gender = 1
Race: Black: Race = 1.159; White or other: Race = 1

Alkaline picrate-based (Jaffe) methods

Note: These equations have not been updated for use with serum creatinine methods traceable to IDMS. Use with IDMS-traceable serum creatinine methods may overestimate renal function; use with caution.

Method 1: MDRD equation:

$eGFR = 186 \times (Creatinine)^{-1.154} \times (Age)^{-0.203} \times (Gender) \times (Race)$

where:

eGFR = estimated GFR; calculated in mL/minute/1.73 m^2
Creatinine is input in mg/dL
Age is input in years
Gender: Females: Gender = 0.742; Males: Gender = 1
Race: Black: Race = 1.212; White or other: Race = 1

Method 2: MDRD Extended equation:

$eGFR = 170 \times (Creatinine)^{-0.999} \times (Age)^{-0.176} \times (SUN)^{-0.170} \times (Albumin)^{0.318} \times (Gender) \times (Race)$

where:

eGFR = estimated GFR; calculated in mL/minute/1.73 m^2
Creatinine is input in mg/dL
Age is input in years
SUN = Serum Urea Nitrogen; input in mg/dL
Albumin = Serum Albumin; input in g/dL
Gender: Females: Gender = 0.762; Males: Gender = 1
Race: Black: Race = 1.18; White or other: Race = 1

Method 3: Cockroft-Gault equation[3]

Males: CrCl = [(140 - Age) X Weight] / (72 X Creatinine)
Females: CrCl = {[(140 - Age) X Weight] / (72 X Creatinine)} X 0.85
where:
CrCl = creatinine clearance; calculated in mL/minute
Age is input in years
Weight is input in kg
Creatinine is input in mg/dL

Method 4: Jelliffe equation

Males: CrCl = {98 - [0.8 X (Age - 20)]} / (Creatinine)
Females: CrCl = Use above equation, then multiply result by 0.9
where:
CrCl = creatinine clearance; calculated in mL/minute/1.73 m^2
Age is input in years
Creatinine is input in mg/dL

FOOTNOTES

[1]Preferred equation for CKD staging National Kidney Disease Education Program
[2]Recommended equation for the reporting of eGFR by the NKD-KDIGO guidelines
[3]Equation typically used for adjusting medication doses

REFERENCES

Cockcroft DW, Gault MH. Prediction of creatinine clearance from serum creatinine. *Nephron.* 1976;16(1):31-41.

Dowling TC, Matzke GR, Murphy JE, Burckart GJ. Evaluation of renal drug dosing: prescribing information and clinical pharmacist approaches. *Pharmacotherapy.* 2010;30(8):776-786.

Hermsen ED, Maiefski M, Florescu MC, Qiu F, Rupp ME. Comparison of the modification of diet in renal disease and Cockcroft-Gault equations for dosing antimicrobials. *Pharmacotherapy.* 2009;29(6):649-655.

Jelliffe RW. Letter: creatinine clearance: bedside estimate. *Ann Intern Med.* 1973;79(4):604-605.

Kidney disease: improving global outcomes (KDIGO) CKD work group. KDIGO 2012 clinical practice guidelines for the evaluation and management of chronic kidney disease. *Kidney Inter.* 2013;3:1-150. http://www.kdigo.org/clinical_practice_guidelines/pdf/CKD/KDIGO_2012_CKD_GL.pdf

Levey AS, Bosch JP, Lewis JB, Greene T, Rogers N, Roth D. A more accurate method to estimate glomerular filtration rate from serum creatinine: a new prediction equation. Modification of diet in renal disease study group. *Ann Intern Med.* 1999;16;130(6):461–470.

Levey AS, Coresh J, Greene T, et al. Using standardized serum creatinine values in the modification of diet in renal disease study equation for estimating glomerular filtration rate. *Ann Intern Med.* 2006;145(4):247-254.

Levey AS, Stevens LA, Schmid CH, et al. A new equation to estimate glomerular filtration rate. *Ann Intern Med.* 2009;150(9):604-612.

National Kidney Disease Education Program. GFR calculators. http://www.nkdep.nih.gov/professionals/gfr_calculators. Accessed April 24, 2013.

Stevens LA, Coresh J, Greene T, Levey AS. Assessing kidney function – measured and estimated glomerular filtration rate. *N Engl J Med.* 2006;354 (23):2473-2483.

RENAL FUNCTION ESTIMATION IN PEDIATRIC PATIENTS

Evaluation of a patient's renal function often includes the use of equations to estimate glomerular filtration rate (GFR) (eg, estimated GFR [eGFR] creatinine clearance [CrCl]) using an endogenous filtration marker (eg, serum creatinine) and other patient variables. For example, the Schwartz equation estimates renal function by calculating eGFR and is typically used to steer medication dosing or categorize chronic kidney disease (CKD) staging and monitor progression. The rate of creatinine clearance does not always accurately represent GFR; creatinine may be cleared by other renal mechanisms in addition to glomerular filtration and serum creatinine concentrations may be affected by nonrenal factors (eg, age, gender, race, body habitus, illness, diet). In addition, these equations were developed based on studies in limited populations and may either over- or underestimate the renal function of a specific patient.

Nevertheless, most clinicians use an eGFR or CrCl as an indicator of renal function in pediatric patients for the purposes of adjusting medication doses. These equations should be used in the clinical context of patient-specific factors noted during the physical exam/work-up. **Decisions regarding drug therapy and doses must be made on clinical judgment.**

RENAL FUNCTION ESTIMATION EQUATIONS

Commonly used equations to estimate renal function utilizing the endogenous filtration marker serum creatinine include the Schwartz and Traub-Johnson equations. Both equations were originally developed using a serum creatinine assay measured by the alkaline picrate-based (Jaffe) method. Many substances, including proteins, can interfere with the accuracy of this assay and overestimate serum creatinine concentration. The National Kidney Foundation and The National Kidney Disease Education Program advocated for a universal creatinine assay, in order to ensure an accurate estimate of GFR in patients. As a result, a more specific enzymatic assay with an isotope dilution mass spectrometry (IDMS)-traceable international standard was developed. Compared to the older methods, IDMS-traceable assays may report lower serum creatinine values and may, therefore, overestimate renal function when used in the original equations. An updated Schwartz equation (eg, Bedside Schwartz) based on serum creatinine measured by the IDMS-traceable method has been proposed for pediatrics (Schwartz 2009); the Traub-Johnson equation has not been re-expressed. The original Schwartz and Traub-Johnson equations may overestimate renal function when used with a serum creatinine measured by the IDMS-traceable method. However, at this point, all laboratories should be using creatinine methods calibrated to be IDMS traceable.

The following factors may contribute to an inaccurate estimation of renal function (Stevens 2006):

- Increased creatinine generation (may underestimate renal function):
  - Black or African American patients
  - Muscular body habitus
  - Ingestion of cooked meats
- Decreased creatinine generation (may overestimate renal function):
  - Increased age
  - Female patients
  - Asian patients
  - Amputees
  - Malnutrition, inflammation, or deconditioning (eg, cancer, severe cardiovascular disease, hospitalized patients)
  - Neuromuscular disease
  - Vegetarian diet
- Rapidly changing serum creatinine (either up or down):
  - In patients with rapidly rising serum creatinines (ie, increasing by >0.5 to 0.7 mg/dL/day), it is best to assume that the patient's renal function is severely impaired

Use extreme caution when estimating renal function in the following patient populations:

- Low body weight (actual body weight < ideal body weight)
- Liver transplant
- Prematurity (especially very low birth weight)
- Dehydration
- Recent kidney transplantation (serum creatinine values may decrease rapidly and can lead to renal function under-estimation; conversely, delayed graft function may be present)

IDMS-traceable method: Bedside Schwartz[1]

Note: This equation is for use in ages 1 to 16 years.
eGFR = (0.413 X Height) / Creatinine
where:
eGFR = estimated GFR; calculated in mL/minute/1.73 m^2
Height (length) is input in cm
Creatinine = Sr_{Cr} input in mg/dL

Alkaline picrate-based (Jaffe) methods

Note: These equations have not been updated for use with serum creatinine methods traceable to IDMS. Use with IDMS-traceable serum creatinine methods may overestimate renal function; use with caution.

Method 1: Schwartz equation

Note: This equation may not provide an accurate estimation of creatinine clearance for infants <6 months of age or for patients with severe starvation or muscle wasting.
eGFR = (k X Height) / Creatinine
where:
eGFR = estimated GFR; calculated in mL/minute/1.73 m^2
Height (length) is input in cm
k = constant of proportionality that is age-specific
<1 year preterm: 0.33
<1 year full-term: 0.45
1 to 12 years: 0.55
>12 years female: 0.55
>12 years male: 0.7
Creatinine is input in mg/dL

Method 2: Traub-Johnson equation

Note: This equation is for use in ages 1 to 18 years.
CrCl = (0.48 X Height) / Creatinine
where:
CrCl = estimated creatinine clearance; calculated in mL/minute/1.73 m^2
Height (length) is input in cm
Creatinine = Sr_{Cr} input in mg/dL

FOOTNOTES

[1]National Kidney Disease Education Program preferred equation

REFERENCES

Dowling TC, Matzke GR, Murphy JE, Burckart GJ. Evaluation of renal drug dosing: prescribing information and clinical pharmacist approaches. *Pharmacotherapy.* 2010;30(8):776-786.

Myers GL, Miller WG, Coresh J, et al. Recommendations for improving serum creatinine measurement: a report from the laboratory working group of the National Kidney Disease Education Program. *Clin Chem.* 2006;52(1):5-18.

National Kidney Disease Education Program. GFR calculators. http://www.nkdep.nih.gov/professionals/gfr_calculators. Accessed April 24, 2013.

Pottel H, Mottaghy FM, Zaman Z, Martens F. On the relationship between glomerular filtration rate and serum creatinine in children. *Pediatr Nephrol.* 2010;25(5):927-934.

Schwartz GJ, Brion LP, Spitzer A. The use of plasma creatinine concentration for estimating glomerular filtration rate in infants, children, and adolescents. *Pediatr Clin North Am.* 1987;34(3):571-590.

Schwartz GJ, Haycock GB, Edelmann CM Jr, Spitzer A. A simple estimate of glomerular filtration rate in children derived from body length and plasma creatinine. *Pediatrics.* 1976;58(2):259-263.

Schwartz GJ, Muñoz A, Schneider MF, et al. New equations to estimate GFR in children with CKD. *J Am Soc Nephrol.* 2009;20(3):629-637.

Staples A, LeBlond R, Watkins S, Wong C, Brandt J. Validation of the revised Schwartz estimating equation in a predominantly non-CKD population. *Pediatr Nephrol.* 2010;25(11):2321-2326.

Stevens LA, Coresh J, Greene T, Levey AS. Assessing kidney function – measured and estimated glomerular filtration rate. *N Engl J Med.* 2006;354(23):2473-2483.

Traub SL, Johnson CE. Comparison of methods of estimating creatinine clearance in children. *Am J Hosp Pharm.* 1980;37(2):195-201.

PREPROCEDURE SEDATIVES IN CHILDREN

PURPOSE

The following table is a guide to aid the clinician in the selection of the most appropriate sedative to sedate a child for a procedure. One must also consider:

- Not all patients require sedation. It is dependent on the procedure and age of the child.
- When sedation is desired, one must consider the time of onset, the duration of action, and the route of administration.
- Each of the following drugs is well absorbed when given by the suggested routes and doses.
- Each drug was assigned an "intensity" based upon the class of drug, dose, and route. However, it should be noted tha any drug can produce a deeper level of sedation.
- Practitioners performing a specific level of sedation must be prepared to manage the patient who slips into the nex deeper level of sedation (eg, when performing moderate sedation, be prepared to manage deep sedation). This may occur regardless of which sedation drug is used.
- Those drugs classified as producing deep sedation require more frequent monitoring postprocedure.
- For painful procedures, an analgesic agent needs to be administered.

LEVELS OF SEDATION

- Minimal sedation (formerly anxiolysis): A medically controlled state in which patients respond appropriately to verba commands; cognitive and coordination function may be impaired, but cardiovascular and ventilatory function are no affected.
- Moderate sedation (formerly conscious sedation): A medically controlled drug-induced depression of consciousness during which patients respond purposefully to verbal commands either alone or accompanied by light tactile stimulation No interventions are required to maintain a patent airway, and spontaneous ventilation is adequate. Cardiovascular function is usually maintained.
- Deep sedation: A medically controlled state of depressed consciousness associated with partial or complete loss o protective airway reflexes. Patients cannot be easily aroused, but respond purposefully after repeated verbal or painfu stimulation. Cardiovascular function is usually maintained.
- General anesthesia (**Note:** This level of sedation is reserved for patients in an operating room setting): A medically controlled state of loss of consciousness during which patients are not arousable, even with painful stimulation Ventilatory function is usually impaired; patients require assistance with maintaining a patent airway; positive-pressure ventilation may be required. Cardiovascular function may be impaired.

Sedatives Used to Produce Moderate Sedation

Drug	Route	Dose (mg/kg)	Onset (min)	Duration (h)	Comments
Chloral Hydrate	PO/PR	25 to 100	10 to 20	4 to 8	Maximum single dose: Infants: 1 g; Children: 2 g
Diazepam (Valium)	PO	0.2 to 0.3; 45 to 60 min prior	Rapid	15 to 30 min	Maximum oral dose: 10 mg
	IV	0.05 to 0.1 over 3 to 5 min	1 to 3	15 to 30 min	Maximum total dose: 0.25 mg/kg
FentaNYL	Intranasal (using parenteral formulation)	1 to 2 mcg/kg	5 to 10	Related to blood level	Maximum total intranasal dose: 3 mcg/kg
	IM	1 to 3 mcg/kg	7 to 8	1 to 2	
	IV	1 to 3 mcg/kg	Immediate	30 to 60 min	
LORazepam (Ativan)	PO	0.05	60	8 to 12	
	IM	0.05	30 to 60	8 to 12	
	IV	0.01 to 0.05 over 5 to 10 min	15 to 30	8 to 12	
Meperidine (Demerol)	PO	2 to 4; 30 to 90 min prior	10 to 15	2 to 4	Maximum dose: 150 mg/dose
	IM	0.5 to 1; 30 to 90 min prior	10 to 15	2 to 4	
	IV	0.5 to 1; 30 to 90 min prior	5	2 to 3	

Sedatives Used to Produce Moderate Sedation *(continued)*

Drug	Route	Dose (mg/kg)	Onset (min)	Duration (h)	Comments
Midazolam (Versed)	PO	0.25 to 0.5	10 to 20	1 to 1.5	Maximum oral dose: 20 mg; patients <6 y may need doses as high as 1 mg/kg
	IM	0.1 to 0.15; 30 to 60 min prior	5	2	Maximum total dose: 10 mg
	IV	**6 mo to 5 y:** 0.05 to 0.1 **6 to 12 y:** 0.025 to 0.05 **>12 y to Adult:** 2.5 to 5 mg (total dose) over 10 to 20 min	1 to 5	23 to 30 min	Maximum concentration: 1 mg/mL; Maximum IM/IV dose: 6 mo to 5 y: 6 mg 6 y to Adult: 10 mg
	PR	0.25 to 0.5	10 to 30	1 to 1.5	Dilute injection in 5 mL NS; administer rectally
	Intranasal	0.2 to 0.3	5	30 to 60 min	
Morphine	IV	0.05 to 0.1	Within 20 min	3 to 5	

Note: See individual drug monographs for further information.

Sedatives Used to Produce Deep Sedation

Drug	Route	Dose (mg/kg)	Onset (min)	Duration (h)	Comments
Methohexital (Brevital)	IM	5 to 10	2 to 10	1 to 1.5	Maximum concentration for IM/IV: 50 mg/mL; maximum IM/IV dose: 200 mg. Greater incidence of adverse effects with IV use.
	IV	0.5 to 2	1	7 to 10 min	
	PR	20 to 35	5 to 15	1 to 1.5	Rectal given as a 10% solution in sterile water; maximum dose rectal: 500 mg
PENTobarbital	PO/IM/PR	1.5 to 6	IM: 10 to 15 PO/PR: 15 to 60	IM: 1 to 2 PO/PR: 1 to 4	Maximum dose: 100 mg
	IV	1 to 2	3 to 5	15 to 45 min	

Note: See individual drug monographs for further information.

Sedatives Used to Produce Dissociative Anesthesia (Monitor as if Deep Sedation)

Drug	Route	Dose (mg/kg)	Onset (min)	Duration	Comments
Ketamine	PO	6 to 10; 30 min prior	30 to 45		May use injectable product orally diluted in a beverage of the patient's choice
	IM	3 to 7	3 to 4	12 to 25	
	IV	0.5 to 2	Within 30 seconds	5 to 10	

Note: See individual drug monographs for further information.

REFERENCES

American Academy of Pediatrics, American Academy of Pediatric Dentistry, Coté CJ, Wilson S, Work Group on Sedation. Guidelines for monitoring and management of pediatric patients during and after sedation for diagnostic and therapeutic procedures: an update. *Pediatrics*. 2006;118(6):2587-2602.

Cramton RE, Gruchala NE. Managing procedural pain in pediatric patients. *Curr Opin Pediatr.* 2012;24(4):530-538.

Elman DS, Denson JS. Preanesthetic sedation of children with intramuscular methohexital sodium. *Anesth Analg*. 1965;44(5):494-498.

Hegenbarth MA, American Academy of Pediatrics Committee on Drugs. Preparing for pediatric emergencies: drugs to consider. *Pediatrics*. 2008;121 (2):433-443.

Krauss B, Green SM. Procedural sedation and analgesia in children. *Lancet.* 2006;367(9512):766-780.

Miller JR, Grayson M, Stoelting VK. Sedation with intramuscular methohexital sodium for office and clinic ophthalmic procedures in children. *Am J Ophthalmol*. 1966;62(1):38-43.

Zeltzer LK, Altman A, Cohen D, LeBaron S, Munuksela EL, Schechter NL. American Academy of Pediatrics Report of the Subcommittee on the Management of Pain Associated with Procedures in Children with Cancer. *Pediatrics*. 1990;86(5 Pt 2):826-831.

COMA SCALES

Glasgow Coma Scale

Activity	Best Response	Score
Eye opening	Spontaneous	4
	Responds to voice	3
	Responds to pain	2
	No response	1
Verbal response	Oriented and appropriate	5
	Confused / disoriented conversation	4
	Inappropriate words	3
	Nonspecific sounds (incomprehensible)	2
	No response	1
Motor response	Follows commands	6
	Localizes pain	5
	Withdraws to pain	4
	Abnormal flexion (decorticate posturing)	3
	Abnormal extension (decerebrate posturing)	2
	No response	1

Modified Coma Scale for Infants

Activity	Best Response	Score
Eye opening	Spontaneous	4
	Responds to voice	3
	Responds to pain	2
	No response	1
Verbal response	Coos, babbles	5
	Irritable	4
	Cries to pain	3
	Moans to pain	2
	No response	1
Motor response	Normal spontaneous movements	6
	Withdraws to touch	5
	Withdraws to pain	4
	Abnormal flexion (decorticate posturing)	3
	Abnormal extension (decerebrate posturing)	2
	No response	1

Interpretation of Coma Scale Scores Maximum Score: 15; Minimum Score: 3 (low score indicates greater severity of coma)

Range of Score	Interpretation
3 to 8	Coma. Severe brain injury. Immediate action needed. Notify ICU staff STAT. Will require intubation regardless of respiratory status.
9 to 12	Lethargic. Needs close observation in special care unit. Frequent neuro checks. Notify ICU staff.
13 to 14	Needs observation
15	Normal

REFERENCES

James HE. Neurologic evaluation and support in the child with an acute brain insult. *Pediatr Ann.* 1986;15(1):16-22.

Jennett B, Teasdale G. Aspects of coma after severe head injury. *Lancet.* 1977;1(8017): 878-881.

SEROTONIN SYNDROME

Manifestations of Severe Serotonin Syndrome and Related Clinical Conditions

Condition	Medication History	Time Needed for Condition to Develop	Vital Signs	Pupils	Mucosa	Skin	Bowel Sounds	Neuromuscular Tone	Reflexes	Mental Status
Serotonin syndrome	Proserotonergic drug	<12 hours	Hypertension, tachycardia, tachypnea, hyperthermia (>41.1°C)	Mydriasis	Sialorrhea	Diaphoresis	Hyperactive	Increased, predominantly in lower extremities	Hyper-reflexia, clonus (unless masked by increased muscle tone)	Agitation, coma
Anticholinergic "toxidrome"	Anticholinergic agent	<12 hours	Hypertension (mild), tachycardia, tachypnea, hyperthermia (typically ≤38.8°C)	Mydriasis	Dry	Erythema, hot and dry to touch	Decreased or absent	Normal	Normal	Agitated delirium
Neuroleptic malignant syndrome	Dopamine antagonist	1 to 3 days	Hypertension, tachycardia, tachypnea, hyperthermia (>41.1°C)	Normal	Sialorrhea	Pallor, diaphoresis	Normal or decreased	"Lead-pipe" rigidity present in all muscle groups	Bradyreflexia	Stupor, alert mutism, coma
Malignant hyperthermia	Inhalational anesthesia	30 minutes to 24 hours after administration of inhalational anesthesia or succinylcholine	Hypertension, tachycardia, tachypnea, hyperthermia (can be as high as 46°C)	Normal	Normal	Mottled appearance, diaphoresis	Decreased	Rigor mortis-like rigidity	Hyporeflexia	Agitation

Reprinted with permission: Boyer EW, Shannon M. The serotonin syndrome. *N Engl J Med*. 2005;352(11):1112-1120.

Management of Serotonin Syndrome

1. Remove precipitating drugs
   a. Serotonergic agents (eg, antidepressants; especially SSRI and MAO Inhibitors)
   b. Be mindful of half-life elimination and active metabolites
2. Supportive care
   a. Intravenous fluids
   b. Correct vital signs
3. Control agitation
   a. Benzodiazepines (diazepam)
   b. Avoid physical restraints
4. 5-HT_{2A} antagonists
   a. Cyproheptadine: 12 to 32 mg/day (may be crushed and administered via nasogastric tube)
   b. ChlorproMAZINE: I.M.: 50 to 100 mg (monitor vitals)
5. Control autonomic instability
   a. Norepinephrine **or**
   b. Phenylephrine **or**
   c. EPINEPHrine
   d. Nitroprusside or esmolol for hypertension and tachycardia
6. Control hyperthermia
   a. Benzodiazepines
   b. Neuromuscular paralysis with vecuronium (**Note:** Avoid succinylcholine)
   c. Intubation
   d. Do not use antipyretic agents
7. Other
   a. Do not use propranolol, bromocriptine, and dantrolene

ACETAMINOPHEN SERUM LEVEL NOMOGRAM

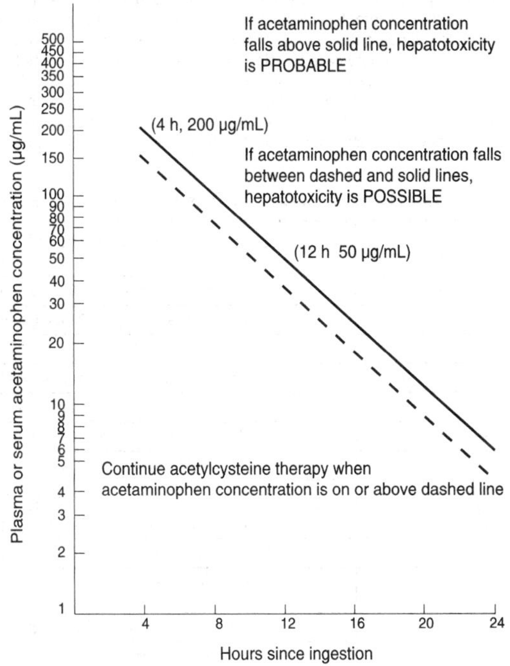

Nomogram relating plasma or serum acetaminophen concentration and probability of hepatotoxicity at varying intervals following ingestion of a single toxic dose of acetaminophen. Modified from Rumack BH, Matthew H, "Acetaminophen Poisoning and Toxicity", Pediatrics, 1975, 55:871-6,
© American Academy of Pediatrics, 1975, and from Rumack BH, et al, "Acetaminophen Overdose", *Arch Intern Med*, 1981, 141:380-5,
© American Medical Association.

FLUORIDE VARNISHES

The US Preventive Services Task Force (USPSTF) issued a statement in May 2014 recommending primary care clinicians ma apply fluoride varnish to the primary teeth of all infants and children starting at the age of primary tooth eruption through 5 years of age. This recommendation was made based on the rising prevalence of dental caries in children, particularly those between to 5 years old, and on the fact that nondental primary care clinicians are more likely than dentists to have contact with children ≤ years of age; this situation changes as children reach school age and beyond (USPSTF, 2014). These recommendations are also supported by AAP, which recommends application by medical practitioners in patients at high risk for dental caries who d not have an established dental home (AAP, 2008). The American Academy of Pediatric Dentistry (AAPD, 2006) also supports this recommendation as long as it is done in collaboration with dental professionals and not as a replacement for the "denta home."

Fluoride Varnishes Available for Professional Application

Brand Name	Sodium Fluoride Strength/Size
Butler (bubblegum, melon madness flavors)	5% (0.5 mL/dose) (36/pkg) [equivalent to 2.26% F]
CavityShield (bubblegum flavor)	5% (0.25 mL/dose) (32/pkg, 200/pkg) [equivalent to 2.26% F]
CavityShield (bubblegum flavor)	5% (0.4 mL/dose) (32/pkg, 200/pkg) [equivalent to 2.26% F]
Colgate Duraphat	5% (1 mL/dose) (10 mL/tube) [equivalent to 2.26% F]
Colgate PreviDent (mint, raspberry flavors)	5% (0.40 mL/dose) (50/pkg) [equivalent to 2.26% F]
Duraflor (bubblegum flavor)	5% (1 mL/dose) (10 mL/tube) [equivalent to 2.26% F]
Duraflor (bubblegum flavor)	5% (0.25 mL/dose) (32/pkg, 200/pkg) [equivalent to 2.26% F]
Duraflor (rasberry flavor)	5% (0.40 mL/dose) (32/pkg, 200/pkg) [equivalent to 2.26% F]
Duraflor Halo (spearmint, wildberry flavors)	5% (0.50 mL/dose) (32/pkg, 250/pkg) [equivalent to 2.26% F]
DuraShield Clear (strawberry, watermelon flavors)	5% (0.40 mL/dose) (50/pkg, 200/pkg) [equivalent to 2.26% F]
Embrace (bubblegum flavor)	5% (0.40 mL/dose) (50/pkg, 200/pkg) [equivalent to 2.26% F]
Enamel Pro (bubblegum, strawberries n cream, vanilla mint flavors)	5% (0.40 mL/dose) (35/pkg, 200/pkg) [equivalent to 2.26% F]
Enamel Pro Clear (bubblegum flavor)	5% (0.25 mL/dose) (35/pkg) [equivalent to 2.26% F]
FluoroDose (bubblegum, cherry, melon, mint flavors)	5% (0.30 mL/dose) (120/pkg, 600/pkg, 1200/pkg) [equivalent to 2.26% F]
Flor-Opal (bubblegum, white mint flavors)	5% (0.50 mL/dose) (40/pkg) [equivalent to 2.26% F]
Iris (bubblegum, mint, raspberry flavors)	5% (0.40 mL/dose) [equivalent to 2.26% F]
Kolorz ClearShield (bubblegum, mint, watermelon flavors)	5% (0.40 mL/dose) (35/pkg, 200/pkg) [equivalent to 2.26% F]
MI Varnish with RECALDENT (fresh strawberry flavor)	5% (0.50 mL/dose) (50/pkg) [equivalent to 2.26% F]
Nupro (raspberry flavor)	5% (0.25 mL/dose) [equivalent to 2.26% F]
Nupro White Varnish (grape, raspberry flavors)	5% (0.40 mL/dose) (50/pkg,100/pkg, 500/pkg) [equivalent to 2.26% F]
Profluorid (caramel, cherry, melon, mint flavors)	5% (1 mL/dose) (10 mL/tube) [equivalent to 2.26% F]
Profluorid (caramel, cherry, melon, mint, mixed flavors)	5% (0.40 mL/dose) (48/pkg, 50/pkg, 200/pkg) [equivalent to 2.26% F]
Profluorid (melon flavor)	5% (0.25 mL) (kids) (50/pkg) [equivalent to 2.26% F]
Sparkle V (bubblegum, mint flavors)	5% (0.40 mL/dose) (120/pkg) [equivalent to 2.26% F]
Ultra Thin (bubblegum, melon, mint, strawberry, mixed flavors)	5% (0.40 mL/dose) (25/pkg, 30/pkg, 100/pkg) [equivalent to 2.26% F]
Vanish (cherry, melon, mint, mixed flavors)	5% sodium fluoride white varnish with TCP (0.50 mL/dose) (50/pkg, 100/pkg, 1000/pkg) [equivalent to 2.26% F]
Vella (bubblegum, melon, mint, strawberry flavors)	5% sodium fluoride varnish with xylitol (0.5 mL/dose) (35/pkg, 100/pkg) [equivalent to 2.26% F]

REFERENCES

American Academy Pediatric Dentistry (AAPD). Talking points: AAPD perspective on physicians or other non-dental providers applying fluoride varnish June 2006. Available at http://www.aapd.org/assets/1/7/FluorideVarnishTalkingPoints.pdf

American Academy of Pediatrics (AAP), Section on Pediatric Dentistry and Oral Health. Preventive oral health intervention for pediatricians. *Pediatrics* 2008;122(6):1387-1394.

US Preventive Services Task Force (USPSTF). Prevention of dental caries in children from birth through age 5 years: US Preventive Services Task Force recommendation statement. May 2014. Available at http://www.uspreventiveservicestaskforce.org/uspstf12/dentalprek/dentchfinalrs.htm

MILLIEQUIVALENT AND MILLIMOLE CALCULATIONS AND CONVERSIONS

DEFINITIONS AND CALCULATIONS

Definitions

mole = gram molecular weight of a substance (aka molar weight)

millimole (mM) = milligram molecular weight of a substance (a millimole is 1/1,000 of a mole)

equivalent weight = gram weight of a substance which will combine with or replace 1 gram (1 mole) of hydrogen; an equivalent weight can be determined by dividing the molar weight of a substance by its ionic valence

milliequivalent (mEq) = milligram weight of a substance which will combine with or replace 1 milligram (1 millimole) of hydrogen (a milliequivalent is 1/1,000 of an equivalent)

Calculations

moles = $\frac{\text{weight of a substance (grams)}}{\text{molecular weight of that substance (grams)}}$

millimoles = $\frac{\text{weight of a substance (grams) x 1,000}}{\text{molecular weight of that substance (grams)}}$

equivalents = moles x valence of ion

milliequivalents = millimoles x valence of ion

moles = $\frac{\text{equivalents}}{\text{valence of ion}}$

millimoles = $\frac{\text{milliequivalents}}{\text{valence of ion}}$

millimoles = moles x 1,000

milliequivalents = equivalents x 1,000

Note: Use of equivalents and milliequivalents is valid only for those substances which have fixed ionic valences (eg, sodium, potassium, calcium, chlorine, magnesium, bromine, etc). For substances with variable ionic valences (eg, phosphorous), a reliable equivalent value cannot be determined. In these instances, one should calculate millimoles (which are fixed and reliable) rather than milliequivalents.

MILLIEQUIVALENT CONVERSIONS

To convert mg/100 mL to mEq/L the following formula may be used:

$$\frac{\text{(mg per 100 mL) x 10 x valence}}{\text{atomic weight}} = \text{mEq/L}$$

To convert mEq/L to mg/100 mL the following formula may be used:

$$\frac{\text{(mEq/L) x atomic weight}}{\text{10 x valence}} = \text{mg per 100 mL}$$

To convert mEq/L to volume of percent of a gas the following formula may be used:

$$\frac{\text{(mEq/L) x 22.4}}{10} = \text{volume percent}$$

Valences and Atomic Weights of Selected Ions

Substance	Electrolyte	Valence	Molecular Wt
Calcium	Ca^{++}	2	40
Chloride	Cl^{-}	1	35.5
Magnesium	Mg^{++}	2	24
Phosphate	HPO_4^{--} (80%)	1.8	96[1]
pH = 7.4	$H_2PO_4^{-}$ (20%)	1.8	96[1]
Potassium	K^{+}	1	39
Sodium	Na^{+}	1	23
Sulfate	SO_4^{--}	2	96[1]

[1]The molecular weight of phosphorus only is 31 and sulfur only is 32.

Approximate Milliequivalents — Weights of Selected Ions

Salt	mEq/g Salt	mg Salt/mEq
Calcium carbonate [$CaCO_3$]	20	50
Calcium chloride [$CaCl_2 \cdot 2H_2O$]	14	74
Calcium gluceptate [$Ca(C_7H_{13}O_8)_2$]	4	245
Calcium gluconate [$Ca(C_6H_{11}O_7)_2 \cdot H_2O$]	5	224
Calcium lactate [$Ca(C_3H_5O_3)_2 \cdot 5H_2O$]	7	154
Magnesium gluconate [$Mg(C_6H_{11}O_7)_2 \cdot H_2O$]	5	216
Magnesium oxide [MgO]	50	20
Magnesium sulfate [$MgSO_4$]	17	60
Magnesium sulfate [$MgSO_4 \cdot 7H_2O$]	8	123
Potassium acetate [$K(C_2H_3O_2)$]	10	98
Potassium chloride [KCl]	13	75
Potassium citrate [$K_3(C_6H_5O_7) \cdot H_2O$]	9	108
Potassium iodide [KI]	6	166
Sodium acetate [$Na(C_2H_3O_2)$]	12	82
Sodium acetate [$Na(C_2H_3O_2) \cdot 3H_2O$]	7	136
Sodium bicarbonate [$NaHCO_3$]	12	84
Sodium chloride [$NaCl$]	17	58
Sodium citrate [$Na_3(C_6H_5O_7) \cdot 2H_2O$]	10	98
Sodium iodine [NaI]	7	150
Sodium lactate [$Na(C_3H_5O_3)$]	9	112
Zinc sulfate [$ZnSO_4 \cdot 7H_2O$]	7	144

PATIENT INFORMATION FOR DISPOSAL OF UNUSED MEDICATIONS

ederal guidelines and the Food and Drug Administration (FDA) recommend that disposal of most unused medications should **ot** be accomplished by flushing them down the toilet or drain, unless specifically stated in the drug label prescribing information. ee "Disposal of Unused Medications Not Specified to Be Flushed" below.)

owever, certain drugs can potentially harm an individual for whom it is not intended, even in a single dose, depending on the ze of the individual and strength of the medication. Accidental (or intentional) ingestion of one of these drugs by an unintended dividual (eg, child or pet) can cause hypotension, somnolence, respiratory depression, or other severe adverse events that ould lead to coma or death. For this reason, certain unused medications **should** be disposed of by flushing them down a toilet or nk.

isposal by flushing of these medications is not believed to pose a risk to human health or the environment. Trace amounts of edicine in the water system have been noted, mainly from the body's normal elimination through urine or feces, but there has een no evidence of these small amounts being harmful. Disposal by flushing of these select, few medications contributes a mall fraction to the amount of medicine in the water system. The FDA believes that the benefit of avoiding a potentially life-reatening overdose by accidental ingestion outweighs the potential risk to the environment by flushing these medications.

Medications Recommended for Disposal by Flushing Down the Toilet

Medication	Active Ingredient
Abstral, sublingual tablet	FentaNYL citrate
Actiq, oral transmucosal lozenge	FentaNYL citrate
AVINza, extended release capsule	Morphine sulfate
Buprenorphine hydrochloride, sublingual tablet[1]	Buprenorphine hydrochloride
Buprenorphine hydrochloride and naloxone hydrochloride, sublingual tablet[1]	Buprenorphine hydrochloride, naloxone hydrochloride
Butrans, transdermal patch	Buprenorphine
Daytrana, transdermal patch	Methylphenidate
Demerol, tablet[1]	Meperidine hydrochloride
Demerol, oral solution[1]	Meperidine hydrochloride
Diastat/Diastat AcuDial, rectal gel	Diazepam
Dilaudid, tablet[1]	HYDROmorphone hydrochloride
Dilaudid, oral liquid[1]	HYDROmorphone hydrochloride
Dolophine, tablet (as hydrochloride)[1]	Methadone hydrochloride
Duragesic, extended release patch[1]	FentaNYL
Embeda, extended release capsule	Morphine sulfate and naltrexone hydrochloride
Exalgo, extended release tablet	Hydromorphone hydrochloride
Fentora, tablet (buccal)	FentaNYL citrate
Hysingla ER, extended release tablet	Hydrocodone bitartrate
Kadian, extended release capsule	Morphine sulfate
Methadone hydrochloride, oral solution[1]	Methadone hydrochloride
Methadose, tablet[1]	Methadone hydrochloride
Morphine sulfate, immediate release tablet[1]	Morphine sulfate
Morphine sulfate, oral solution[1]	Morphine sulfate
MS Contin, extended release tablet[1]	Morphine sulfate
Nucynta ER, extended release tablet	Tapentadol
Onsolis, soluble film (buccal)	FentaNYL citrate
Opana, immediate release tablet	Oxymorphone hydrochloride
Opana ER, extended release tablet	Oxymorphone hydrochloride
Oxecta, immediate release tablet	Oxycodone hydrochloride
Oxycodone hydrochloride, capsule	Oxycodone hydrochloride
Oxycodone hydrochloride, oral solution	Oxycodone hydrochloride
OxyCONTIN, extended release tablet	OxyCODONE hydrochloride
Percocet, tablet[1]	Oxycodone hydrochloride and acetaminophen
Percodan, tablet[1]	Oxycodone hydrochloride and aspirin
Suboxone, sublingual film	Buprenorphine hydrochloride, naloxone hydrochloride
Xartemis XR, tablet	Oxycodone hydrochloride, acetaminophen
Xyrem, oral solution	Sodium oxybate
Zohydro ER, extended release capsule	Hydrocodone bitartrate
Zubsolv, tablet	Buprenorphine and naloxone

[1]Medications available in generic formulations

DISPOSAL OF UNUSED MEDICATIONS NOT SPECIFIED TO BE FLUSHED

The majority of medications should be disposed of without flushing them down a toilet or drain. These medications should b removed from the original container, mixed with an unappealing substance (eg, coffee grounds, cat litter), sealed in a plastic ba or other closable container, and disposed of in the household trash. Check out your local laws and ordinances to make sur medications can be legally disposed of in household trash.

Another option for disposal of unused medications is through drug take-back programs. For information on availability of dru take-back programs in your area, contact the city or county trash and recycling service or a local pharmacist.

For more information on unused medication disposal, see specific drug product labeling information or call the FDA at (888 INFO-FDA [(888) 463-6332].

REFERENCE

US Food and Drug Administration (FDA). Disposal by flushing of certain unused medicines: what you should know. Available at: http://www.fda.gov Drugs/ResourcesForYou/Consumers/BuyingUsingMedicineSafely/EnsuringSafeUseofMedicine/SafeDisposalofMedicines/ucm186187.htm Accesse February 19, 2015.

SAFE HANDLING OF HAZARDOUS DRUGS

Early concerns regarding the identification and exposure risk of hazardous drugs in health care setting were primarily focused on antineoplastic medications, but now have expanded to numerous other agents (eg, antivirals, hormones, bioengineered medications). The criteria for a hazardous drug include one or more of the following characteristics:

- Carcinogenic
- Teratogenic (or other developmental toxicity)
- Causing reproductive toxicity
- Organotoxic at low doses
- Genotoxic
- New agents with structural or toxicity profiles similar to existing hazardous agents

Agencies have developed definitions, created lists, and generated guidelines to minimize risk of exposure to products considered hazardous. The Environmental Protection Agency (EPA), National Institute for Occupational Safety and Health (NIOSH), and American Society of Health-System Pharmacists (ASHP) have created definitions of hazardous agents (table 1) which may be useful. Based on their definitions, these agencies developed lists of agents which are identified as hazardous drugs or should be handled as hazardous (table 2).

Table 1. Criteria for Defining Hazardous Agents

EPA	NIOSH	ASHP
Meets one of the following criteria: Ignitability: Create fire (under certain conditions) or are spontaneously combustible and have a flash point <60°C (140°F) Corrosivity: Acids or bases (pH ≤2 or ≥12.5) capable of corroding metal containers Reactivity: Unstable under "normal" conditions; may cause explosions, toxic fumes, gases, or vapors if heated, compressed, or mixed with water Toxicity: Harmful or fatal if ingested or absorbed; may leach from the waste and pollute ground water when disposed of on land **OR**	Carcinogenic Teratogenic or other developmental toxicity Reproductive toxicity Organotoxic at low doses Genotoxic New drugs with structural and toxicity profiles similar to existing hazardous agents	Genotoxic Carcinogenic Teratogenic or impairs fertility Causes serious organ or other toxicity at low doses
Appears on one of the following lists: F: Wastes (nonspecific) from common or industrial manufacturing processes from nonspecific sources K: Specific (source) wastes from specific industries (eg, petroleum or pesticides) P (acutely toxic) or U (toxic): Wastes (unused form) from certain discarded commercial chemical products		

When considering the effects of agents on reproductive and developmental toxicity and carcinogenicity, NIOSH evaluated the dose at which adverse effects occurred. If observed at, near, or below the maximum recommended dose for humans, it was considered relevant; if occurred at doses well above the maximum human dose, then NIOSH did not consider it in the hazardous drug evaluation.

NIOSH updated its list of antineoplastic and hazardous drugs in 2014. Medications with special handling precautions in the product labeling and medications with hazardous characteristics or with structural/toxicity profiles similar to agents on the NIOSH list are also listed in Table 2. In order to account for hazardous nonantineoplastic medications, as well as varying dosage forms, the 2014 update categorized hazardous drugs into three groups to account for the diversity of potential exposures:

- NIOSH Group 1: Antineoplastic drugs (may also pose a reproductive risk)
- NIOSH Group 2: Nonantineoplastic drugs that meet at least one of the NIOSH criteria (may also pose a reproductive risk)
- NIOSH Group 3: Nonantineoplastic drugs with adverse reproductive effects; pose a reproductive risk to men and/or women who are actively attempting conception and to women who are pregnant or breast-feeding

Medications listed in group 3 may not pose as serious a risk to personnel not at risk for reproductive toxicity due to age or infertility, although they should still be handled as hazardous. It is important to note that for medications in groups 1 and 2, in addition to meeting the NIOSH hazardous drug criteria, some may also pose a reproductive risk in susceptible populations. According to the NIOSH document, definitions for hazardous drugs may not accurately reflect toxicity criteria associated with newer or recently developed biologic or targeted agents. While biologic and targeted agents may pose a risk to patients, a risk to health care workers may not be present.

Table 2. Drugs Listed as or Considered Hazardous

	NIOSH List[1]			EPA List[2,3]	Product Labeling[4]	Structure or Toxicity Profile Similar to Existing Hazardous Agents	Radio-pharmaceutical	Not on NIOSH List, but Meets NIOSH Criteria[5]
	Group 1	Group 2	Group 3					
Abacavir		X						
Abiraterone	X							
Acitretin			X					
Ado-Trastuzumab Emtansine	X				X			
Afatinib						X		X
Alefacept		X						
Alitretinoin			X					
Altretamine	X				X			
Ambrisentan			X		X			
Amsacrine	X				X			
Anastrozole	X							
Apomorphine		X						
Arsenic Trioxide	X			P-listed	X			
Axitinib						X		X
AzaCITIDine	X				X			
AzaTHIOprine		X			X			
BCG Vaccine	X				X			
Belinostat					X	X		X
Bendamustine	X				X			
Bexarotene	X							
Bicalutamide	X							
Bleomycin	X				X			
Bortezomib	X				X			
Bosentan			X					
Bosutinib					X	X		X
Brentuximab Vedotin	X				X			
Buserelin						X		X
Busulfan	X				X			
Cabazitaxel	X				X			
Cabergoline			X					
Cabozantinib						X		X
Capecitabine	X				X			
CarBAMazepine		X						
Carbon 14 Urea					X		X	
CARBOplatin	X				X			
Carfilzomib						X		X
Carmustine	X				X			

Table 2. Drugs Listed as or Considered Hazardous *continued*

	NIOSH List[1]			EPA List[2,3]	Product Labeling[4]	Structure or Toxicity Profile Similar to Existing Hazardous Agents	Radio-pharmaceutical	Not on NIOSH List, but Meets NIOSH Criteria[5]
	Group 1	Group 2	Group 3					
Ceritinib						X		X
Cetrorelix			X					
Chlorambucil	X			U-listed	X			
Chloramphenicol		X						
Choriogonadotropin Alfa			X					
Chromic Phosphate P 32					X		X	
Cidofovir		X			X			
CISplatin	X				X			
Cladribine	X				X			
Clofarabine	X				X			
ClonazePAM			X					
Colchicine			X					
Crizotinib	X							
Cyclophosphamide	X			U-listed	X			
CycloSPORINE		X						
Cyproterone						X		X
Cytarabine	X				X			
Cytarabine (Liposomal)	X				X			
Dabrafenib						X		X
Dacarbazine	X				X			
DACTINomycin	X				X			
Dasatinib	X				X			
DAUNOrubicin	X			U-listed	X			
DAUNOrubicin (Liposomal)	X			U-listed	X			
Decitabine	X				X			
Deferiprone		X						
Degarelix	X				X			
Desogestrel		X						
Dexrazoxane		X			X			
Dichlorodifluoromethane				U-listed				
Diethylstilbestrol		X		U-listed				
Dinoprostone			X					
Divalproex		X						
DOCEtaxel	X				X			
DOXOrubicin	X				X			
DOXOrubicin (Liposomal)	X				X			
Dronedarone			X					
Dutasteride			X		X			

Table 2. Drugs Listed as or Considered Hazardous *continued*

	NIOSH List[1]			EPA List[2,3]	Product Labeling[4]	Structure or Toxicity Profile Similar to Existing Hazardous Agents	Radio-pharmaceutical	Not on NIOSH List, but Meets NIOSH Criteria[5]
	Group 1	Group 2	Group 3					
Dydrogesterone		X						
Entecavir		X						
Enzalutamide						X		X
EPINEPHrine (does not include epinephrine salts)				P-listed				
EPIrubicin	X				X			
Ergonovine/Methylergonovine			X					
Eribulin	X							
Erlotinib	X							
Estradiol		X						
Estramustine	X			X				
Estrogen-Progestin Combinations		X						
Estrogens (Conjugated)		X						
Estrogens (Esterified)		X						
Estropipate		X						
Etoposide	X				X			
Etoposide Phosphate	X				X			
Everolimus	X				X			
Exemestane	X							
Finasteride			X		X			
Fingolimod		X						
Florbetapir F18					X		X	
Floxuridine	X				X			
Fluconazole			X					
Fludarabine	X				X			
Fludeoxyglucose F 18					X		X	
Fluorouracil	X				X			
Fluoxymesterone		X						
Flutamide	X							
Formaldehyde				U-listed				
Fosphenytoin		X						
Fulvestrant	X							
Gallium Citrate Ga-67					X		X	
Ganciclovir		X			X			
Ganirelix			X					
Gefitinib						X		X
Gemcitabine	X				X			
Gemtuzumab Ozogamicin	X				X			

Table 2. Drugs Listed as or Considered Hazardous *continued*

	NIOSH List[1]			EPA List[2,3]	Product Labeling[4]	Structure or Toxicity Profile Similar to Existing Hazardous Agents	Radio-pharmaceutical	Not on NIOSH List, but Meets NIOSH Criteria[5]
	Group 1	Group 2	Group 3					
Gonadotropin, Chorionic			X					
Goserelin	X							
Hexachlorophene				U-listed				
Histrelin						X		X
Hydroxyurea	X				X			
Ibritumomab					X		X	
Ibrutinib						X		X
Icatibant			X					
IDArubicin	X				X			
Idelalisib								X
Ifosfamide	X				X			
Imatinib	X				X			
Indium 111 Capromab Pendetide					X		X	
Indium 111 Oxyquinoline					X		X	
Indium In-111 Pentetreotide					X		X	
Iobenguane I 123					X		X	
Iodinated I 131 Albumin					X		X	
Iodine I-125 Human Serum Albumin					X		X	
Iodine I-125 Iothalamate					X		X	
Ioflupane I 123					X		X	
Irinotecan	X				X			
Isotretinoin						X		X
Ixabepilone	X				X			
Lapatinib						X		X
Leflunomide		X						
Lenalidomide		X			X			
Lenvatinib						X		X
Letrozole	X							
Leuprolide	X							
Lindane				U-listed				
Liraglutide		X						
Lomustine	X				X			
Macitentan						X		X
Mechlorethamine	X				X			
MedroxyPROGESTERone		X						
Megestrol	X							
Melphalan	X			U-listed	X			

Table 2. Drugs Listed as or Considered Hazardous *continued*

	NIOSH List[1]			EPA List[2,3]	Product Labeling[4]	Structure or Toxicity Profile Similar to Existing Hazardous Agents	Radio-pharmaceutical	Not on NIOSH List, but Meets NIOSH Criteria[5]
	Group 1	Group 2	Group 3					
Menotropins			X					
Mercaptopurine	X				X			
Mercury				U-listed				
Methotrexate	X				X			
MethylTESTOSTERone			X					
Mifepristone			X					
Misoprostol			X					
MitoMYcin	X			U-listed	X			
Mitotane	X				X			
MitoXANtrone	X				X			
Mycophenolate		X			X			
Nafarelin			X					
Nelarabine	X				X			
Nevirapine		X						
Nicotine				P-listed				
Nilotinib	X							
Nilutamide						X		X
Nintedanib						X		X
Nitrogen 13 Ammonia					X		X	
Nitroglycerin (doses in "finished form" are excluded)				P-listed				
Olaparib								X
Omacetaxine	X				X			
Ospemifene						X		X
Oxaliplatin	X				X			
OXcarbazepine		X						
Oxytocin			X					
PACLitaxel	X				X			
PACLitaxel (Protein Bound)	X				X			
Palbociclib								X
Palifermin		X						
Pamidronate						X		X
Panobinostat					X	X		X
Paraldehyde				U-listed				
PARoxetine			X					
PAZOPanib	X							
PEMEtrexed	X				X			
Pentetate Calcium Trisodium			X					

Table 2. Drugs Listed as or Considered Hazardous *continued*

	NIOSH List[1]			EPA List[2,3]	Product Labeling[4]	Structure or Toxicity Profile Similar to Existing Hazardous Agents	Radio-pharmaceutical	Not on NIOSH List, but Meets NIOSH Criteria[5]
	Group 1	Group 2	Group 3					
Pentetate Indium Disodium In 111					X		X	
Pentostatin	X				X			
Pertuzumab						X		X
Phenacetin				U-listed				
Phenol				U-listed				
Phenoxybenzamine		X						
Physostigmine				P-listed				
Phenytoin		X						
Pimecrolimus						X		X
Pipobroman		X						
Plerixafor			X					
Pomalidomide					X	X		X
PONATinib						X		X
Porfimer					X			X
PRALAtrexate	X				X			
Procarbazine	X				X			
Progesterone		X						
Progestins		X						
Propythiouracil		X						
Radium Ra 223 Dichloride					X		X	
Raloxifene		X						
Raltitrexed					X	X		X
Rasagiline		X						
Regorafenib						X		X
Reserpine				U-listed				
Resorcinol				U-listed				
Ribavirin			X					
Riociguat								X
RisperiDONE		X						
RomiDEPsin	X				X			
Rubidium-82 Chloride					X		X	
Ruxolitinib						X		X
Saccharin				U-listed				
Samarium Sm 153 Lexidronam					X		X	
Selenium Sulfide				U-listed				
Sirolimus		X						
Sodium Fluoride F18					X		X	
Sodium Iodide I[123]					X		X	

Table 2. Drugs Listed as or Considered Hazardous *continued*

	NIOSH List[1]			EPA List[2,3]	Product Labeling[4]	Structure or Toxicity Profile Similar to Existing Hazardous Agents	Radio-pharmaceutical	Not on NIOSH List, but Meets NIOSH Criteria[5]
	Group 1	Group 2	Group 3					
Sodium Iodide I[131]					X		X	
SORAfenib	X							
Spironolactone		X						
Streptozocin	X			U-listed	X			
Strontium-89					X		X	
Sunitinib	X							
Tacrolimus		X						
Tamoxifen	X							
Technetium Tc 99m Bicisate					X		X	
Technetium Tc 99m Disofenin					X		X	
Technetium Tc 99m Exametazime					X		X	
Technetium Tc 99m Gluceptate					X		X	
Technetium Tc 99m-Labeled Red Blood Cells					X		X	
Technetium Tc 99m Mebrofenin					X		X	
Technetium Tc 99m Medronate					X		X	
Technetium Tc 99m Oxidronate					X		X	
Technetium Tc 99m Pentetate					X		X	
Technetium Tc 99m Pyrophosphate					X		X	
Technetium Tc 99m Succimer					X		X	
Technetium Tc 99m Sulfur Colloid					X		X	
Technetium Tc 99m Tetrofosmin					X		X	
Technetium Tc 99m Tilmanocept					X		X	
Tegafur and Uracil					X	X		X
Tegafur, Gimeracil, and Oteracil					X	X		X
Telavancin			X					
Temozolomide	X				X			
Temsirolimus	X				X			
Teniposide	X				X			
Teriflunamide						X		X
Testosterone			X					
Thalidomide		X			X			
Thioguanine	X				X			
Thiotepa	X				X			
Tibolone		X						
Topiramate			X					
Topotecan	X				X			
Toremifene	X							

Table 2. Drugs Listed as or Considered Hazardous *continued*

	NIOSH List[1]			EPA List[2,3]	Product Labeling[4]	Structure or Toxicity Profile Similar to Existing Hazardous Agents	Radio-pharmaceutical	Not on NIOSH List, but Meets NIOSH Criteria[5]
	Group 1	Group 2	Group 3					
Tositumomab					X		X	
Trabectedin					X			X
Trametinib						X		X
Trastuzumab								X
Tretinoin			X					
Trichloromonofluoromethane				U-listed				
Triptorelin	X							
Ulipristal			X					
Uracil Mustard		X		U-listed				
ValGANciclovir		X			X			
Valproic Acid			X					
Valrubicin	X				X			
Vandetanib	X				X			
Vemurafenib	X							
Vigabatrin			X					
VinBLAStine	X				X			
VinCRIStine	X				X			
VinCRIStine (Liposomal)	X				X			
Vindesine					X	X		X
Vinorelbine	X				X			
Vismodegib								X
Voriconazole			X					
Vorinostat	X				X			
Warfarin			X	<0.3%: U-listed; >0.3%: P-listed				
Zidovudine		X						
Ziprasidone			X					
Zoledronic Acid			X					
Zonisamide			X					

[1]US Department of Health and Human Services; Centers for Disease Control and Prevention; National Institute for Occupational Safety and Health. NIOSH list of antineoplastic and other hazardous drugs in the healthcare settings, 2014. Available at http://www.cdc.gov/niosh/docs/2014-138/pdfs/2014-138.pdf. Updated September 2014. Accessed September 15, 2014.

[2]Healthcare Environmental Resource Center (HERC). Pharmaceutical wastes in healthcare facilities. Available at http://www.hercenter.org/hazmat/pharma.cfm#listed. Accessed September 15, 2010.

[3]Healthcare Environmental Resource Center (HERC). Hazardous waste determination. http://www.hercenter.org/hazmat/hazdeterm.cfm. Accessed September 15, 2010.

[4]Product labeling (prescribing information) indicates precautions for safe handling and disposal should be followed.

[5]Meets one or more of the NIOSH characteristics for defining hazardous agents: Carcinogenicity, Teratogenicity (or other developmental toxicity), Reproductive toxicity, Organ toxicity (at low doses), Genotoxicity, and/or New drugs with structural and toxicity profiles similar to existing hazardous agents (http://www.cdc.gov/niosh/docs/2014-138/pdfs/2014-138.pdf)

NIOSH has developed guidance on personal protective equipment when working with various dosage forms of hazardous drugs within the health care setting. These recommendations are listed in Table 3.

Table 3. Personal Protection for Handling Hazardous Drugs

Formulation	Activity	Gloving	Protective Gown	Eye Protection	Respiratory Protection	Ventilation Controls
Intact tablet or capsule	Administration from a unit dose package	Single	No	No	No	N/A
Tablets or capsules	Cutting, crushing, or manipulating	Double	Yes	No	Yes (if not done in a controlled device)	Yes
	Administration	Double	Yes	No	Yes (if powder is generated)	N/A
Oral liquid	Compounding	Double	Yes	Yes (if not done in a controlled device)	Yes (if not done in a controlled device)	Yes
	Administration	Double	Yes	No	No	N/A
Topical product	Compounding	Double	Yes	Yes	Yes (if not done in a controlled device)	Yes
	Administration	Double	Yes	Yes (if liquid could splash)	Yes (if potential inhalation)	N/A
Ampule	Opening	Double	Yes	Yes (if not done in a controlled device)	Yes (if not done in a controlled device)	Yes (BSC or CACI)
SubQ or IM injection	Preparation for administration	Double	Yes	Yes (if not done in a controlled device)	Yes (if not done in a controlled device)	Yes (BSC or CACI)
	Administration	Double	Yes	Yes (if liquid could splash)	Yes (if potential inhalation)	N/A
IV solutions	Compounding	Double	Yes	Yes (if not done in a controlled device)	Yes (if not done in a controlled device)	Yes (BSC or CACI; CSTD recommended)
	Administration	Double	Yes	Yes (if liquid could splash)	Yes (if potential inhalation)	N/A (CSTD recommended)
Irrigation solutions	Compounding	Double	Yes	Yes (if not done in a controlled device)	Yes (if not done in a controlled device)	Yes (BSC or CACI; CSTD recommended)
	Administration	Double	Yes	Yes	Yes	N/A
Inhalation powder or solution	Inhalation	Double	Yes	Yes	Yes	Yes (if applicable)

BSC = biologic safety cabinet (class II), CACI = compounding aseptic containment isolator, CSTD = closed system transfer device

US Department of Health and Human Services; Centers for Disease Control and Prevention; National Institute for Occupational Safety and Health. NIOSH list of antineoplastic and other hazardous drugs in the healthcare settings, 2014. Available at http://www.cdc.gov/niosh/docs/2014-138/pdfs/2014-138.pdf. Updated September 2014. Accessed September 15, 2014.

Hazardous drugs must be stored, transported, prepared, administered, and disposed of under conditions that protect the health care worker from either acute or chronic/low level exposure. Institutional policies or guidelines to minimize occupational exposure to hazardous drugs should include a focus on the following areas:

- Development and maintenance of a facility-specific hazardous drugs list
  - Working definition/criteria of a hazardous drug
  - Volumes, formulations, and frequency of hazardous drugs handled: Injection, oral (liquid, solid), topical
  - Oral dosage forms and administration (uncoated tablets or alteration of forms by crushing or preparation of oral solutions may result in exposure; coated tablets or capsules administered intact may pose a lower exposure risk)

  Each institution or facility must create its own policy or guideline, including a facility-specific list of drugs deemed hazardous. According to the Joint Commission standards, organizations should minimize risks associated with handling hazardous medications. Orientation and routine training related to safe handling of hazardous drugs is recommended. Until proven otherwise, most institutions consider investigational drugs to be hazardous and to be handled accordingly, particularly if the mechanism of action suggests a potential for concern. Hazardous drug procedures must include all possible routes of administration.

  Additional information regarding development and implementation of an institutional policy/guideline, areas at risk, personnel at risk, risk management, spill management, personnel training, and surveillance may be found at:

  ASHP Guidelines on Handling Hazardous Drugs:
  http://www.ashp.org/DocLibrary/BestPractices/PrepGdlHazDrugs.aspx

Environmental Protection Agency Recommendations:
http://hercenter.org/hazmat/hazdeterm.cfm
http://hercenter.org/hazmat/pharma.cfm

NIOSH List of Antineoplastic and Other Hazardous Drugs in Health Care Settings:
http://www.cdc.gov/niosh/docs/2014-138/pdfs/2014-138.pdf

US Nuclear Regulatory Commission (radiopharmaceuticals, such as ibritumomab or tositumomab):
http://www.nrc.gov/materials/miau/med-use.html

- Identification of personnel and locations in the facility at risk for occupational exposure to hazardous drugs
  - Pharmacy
    - Receiving storage and inventory
    - Dose preparation and dispensing
    - Drug waste disposal
  - Nursing Unit
    - Drug administration
    - Drug waste disposal
    - Patient waste disposal
  - Other areas
    - Laboratory
    - Operating/procedure rooms
    - Veterinary department
    - Facility shipping/receiving
    - Environmental/laundry services
    - Maintenance services

  While the greatest risk of occupational exposure to hazardous drugs occurs during preparation and administration of these agents, it is important to recognize that a risk of exposure can occur throughout the facility from the moment of delivery through the disposal of product and contaminated human waste. Drug preparation and administration may occur in nontraditional areas of the institution including the operating room and in veterinary facilities. Procedures should address the importance of proper labeling and packaging and separation of hazardous vs nonhazardous inventories throughout the facility. Drug containers should be examined upon their arrival at the pharmacy. Containers that show signs of damage should be handled carefully and may require quarantine and decontamination before being placed in stock. Give consideration to routinely quarantining and decontaminating all hazardous drug containers as part of the inspection process before placing in stock.

- Mechanisms/routes of occupational exposure
  - Inhalation of dust or aerosolized droplets (most common)
  - Absorption through skin (most common)
  - Ingestion from contaminated food/drink
  - Accidental injection during preparation/administration/disposal
- Potential adverse effects of hazardous exposure
  - Skin disorders

- Reproductive effects (eg, spontaneous abortion, stillbirth, congenital malformation)
- Leukemia and other cancers

• Risk management

- Use and maintenance of equipment designed to minimize exposure during handling
    - Buffer/Ante transition area
    - Biological safety cabinets, isolators
    - Closed system drug-transfer devices
    - Personal protective equipment
    - Deactivation, decontamination, and cleaning procedures

Barrier protection through the use of ventilation controls and personal protective equipment is the current standard to minimize exposure when handling hazardous drugs. NIOSH and ASHP recommend the use of Class II biological safety cabinets (type B2 preferred), but other options include the totally enclosed Class III biological safety cabinets, appropriate isolators, and robotic systems. Self-contained or closed system devices have been recommended to minimize workplace contamination by preventing escape of drug or vapor out of the device. Devices available include PhaSeal, ONGARD, TEVADAPTOR, Equashield, and CLAVE systems; other systems may also be commercially available. Gloves, gowns, respiratory protection, hair and shoe covers, and eye protection represent the core of personal protective equipment. Guidelines for choice of gowns and gloving, and the circumstances to employ this protection are published by ASHP, NIOSH, and in USP 797.

Procedures for safe handling should be followed with oral dosage forms of antineoplastics (Goodin 2011). Appropriate personal protective equipment should be worn, automatic counting machines should not be utilized, compounding should be performed in a biologic safety cabinet, separate equipment (eg, counting trays) should be used, disposable equipment should be used if possible, cytotoxic waste should be disposed of, and non-disposable equipment used for preparation should be appropriately decontaminated.

- Hazardous drug spill management
    - Size and location
    - Spill kit use
    - Worker contamination

Procedures for handling spills throughout a facility are well described by ASHP and NIOSH. Institutional procedures should focus on location and size of the spill, how to handle a spill when a spill kit is not available, and how to respond to a worker contamination (emergent treatment, follow-up care).

- Personnel training in the handling of hazardous drugs
    - Prior to handling hazardous drugs
    - Periodic and ongoing testing

Personnel throughout a facility must have training in the handling of hazardous drugs that are relevant to their job description. Pharmacy personnel who compound and dispense hazardous drugs must be fully trained in the storing, preparation, dispensing, and disposal of these agents. Such training should include didactic, as well as demonstrating hands-on technique, and such validation should be repeated on a regular schedule. Special training may be necessary for hazardous drugs administered by routes outside of traditional administration routes and when administered in settings outside of traditional settings (eg, at home).

- Environmental and medical surveillance
    - Components of a comprehensive medical surveillance program
    - Reproductive and health questionnaires (at time of hire and periodically)
    - Drug handling history (to estimate current and prior exposure)
    - Baseline clinical evaluation plan (including related medical history, physical exam, lab work)
    - Follow-up plan (for those with health changes suggestive of toxicity or acute exposure)
    - Potential use of environmental sampling techniques
    - Use of common marker hazardous drugs for assay purposes

The goal of medical surveillance is to minimize adverse effects on the health of workers exposed to hazardous drugs. NIOSH recommends that medical surveillance be employed by the facility, and may include the basic observation of employee symptom complaints or monitoring for changes in health status as part of routine checkups. Some programs follow the employee more closely and procedures may include periodic lab studies (eg, blood counts), physical exam, detailed medical history and occupational exposure history, and/or biologic studies. Environmental sampling to look for surface contamination in hazardous drug preparation and administration areas may be considered, particularly in institutions with high volumes. Certain hazardous drugs serve as markers which allow for assay for measurable contamination, and can alert the facility for proper follow-up.

- Work practices regarding reproductive risks to health care workers
    - Alternative duty options

Since hazardous drugs are associated with reproductive risks, policies and guidelines should address health care workers whom are pregnant, attempting to conceive or father a child, and whom are breast-feeding. Workers of reproductive capability should acknowledge in writing that they understand the risk of handling hazardous drugs and be given the opportunity for reassignment or alternate work duty.

REFERENCES

American Society of Hospital Pharmacists. ASHP guidelines on handling hazardous drugs. 2006;63(12):1172-1193.

Baker ES, Connor TH. Monitoring occupational exposure to cancer chemotherapy drugs. *Am J Health Syst Pharm.* 1996;53(22):2713-2723.

Bos RP, Sessink PJ. Biomonitoring of occupational exposures to cytostatic anticancer drugs. *Rev Environ Health.* 1997;12(1):43-58.

Connor TH, Anderson RW, Sessink PJ, Broadfield L, Power LA. Surface contamination with antineoplastic agents in six cancer treatment centers in Canada and the United States. *Am J Health Syst Pharm.* 1999;56(14):1427-1432.

Connor TH, McDiarmid MA. Preventing occupational exposures to antineoplastic drugs in health care settings. *CA Cancer J Clin.* 2006;56(6):354-365.

Connor TH, DeBord DG, Pretty JR, et al. Evaluation of antineoplastic drug exposure of health care workers at three university-based US cancer centers. *J Occup Environ Med.* 2010;52(10):1019-1027.

Connor TH. Permeability of nitrile rubber, latex, polyurethane, and neoprene gloves to 18 antineoplastic drugs. *Am J Health Syst Pharm.* 1999;56 (23):2450-2453.

Connor TH, Sessink PJ, Harrison BR, et al. Surface contamination of chemotherapy drug vials and evaluation of new vial-cleaning techniques: results of three studies. *Am J Health Syst Pharm.* 2005;62(5):475-484.

Goodin S, Griffith N, Chen B, et al. Safe handling of oral chemotherapeutic agents in clinical practice: recommendations from an international pharmacy panel. *J Oncol Pract.* 2011;7(1):7-12.

Healthcare Environmental Resource Center (HERC). Hazardous waste determination. http://www.hercenter.org/hazmat/hazdeterm.cfm. Accessed September 15, 2010.

Healthcare Environmental Resource Center (HERC). Pharmaceutical wastes in healthcare facilities. http://www.hercenter.org/hazmat/pharma.cfm#listed. Accessed September 15, 2010.

Lawson CC, Rocheleau CM, Whelan EA, et al. Occupational exposures among nurses and risk of spontaneous abortion. *Am J Obstet Gynecol.* 2012;206 (4):327.

McDiarmid MA, Oliver MS, Roth TS, Rogers B, Escalante C. Chromosome 5 and 7 abnormalities in oncology personnel handling anticancer drugs. *J Occup Environ Med.* 2010;52(10):1028-1034.

National Institute for Occupational Safety and Health (NIOSH). Medical surveillance for healthcare workers exposed to hazardous drugs. 2012. http://www.cdc.gov/niosh/docs/wp-solutions/2013-103/. Accessed January 22, 2013.

National Institute for Occupational Safety and Health (NIOSH). Preventing occupational exposure to antineoplastic and other hazardous drugs in health care settings. http://www.cdc.gov/niosh/docs/2004-165/2004-165d.html#o. Accessed October 1, 2007.

Polovich M. *Safe Handling of Hazardous Drugs.* 2nd ed. Pittsburgh, PA: Oncology Nursing Society; 2011.

Sessink PJ, Bos RP. Drugs hazardous to healthcare workers. Evaluation of methods for monitoring occupational exposure to cytostatic drugs. *Drug Saf.* 1999;20(4):347-359.

Sessink PJ, Anzion RB, Van den Broek PH, Bos RP. Detection of contamination with antineoplastic agents in a hospital pharmacy department. *Pharm Weekbl Sci.* 1992;14(1):16-22.

Sessink PJ, Boer KA, Scheefhals AP, Anzion RB, Bos RP. Occupational exposure to antineoplastic agents at several departments in a hospital. Environmental contamination and excretion of cyclophosphamide and ifosfamide in urine of exposed workers. *Int Arch Occup Environ Health.* 1992;64 (2):105-112.

Sorsa M, Anderson D. Monitoring of occupational exposure to cytostatic anticancer agents. *Mutat Res.* 1996;355(1-2):253-261.

US Department of Health and Human Services; Centers for Disease Control and Prevention; National Institute for Occupational Safety and Health. NIOSH list of antineoplastic and other hazardous drugs in healthcare settings, 2014. Available at http://www.cdc.gov/niosh/docs/2014-138/pdfs/2014-138.pdf. Updated September 2014. Accessed September 18, 2014.

CARBOHYDRATE CONTENT OF MEDICATIONS

The nature of information is subject to change; while great care has been taken to ensure the accuracy of the information, the reader is advised to also refer to manufacturers for product-specific data.

Description (Brand Name)	Dosage Unit	Grams Carbohydrate per Dosage Unit
Acetaminophen extra strength caplets (Tylenol)	500 mg	<0.125
Acetaminophen chewable tablets (Tylenol Meltaways)	80 mg	<1
Acetaminophen suspension (Children's Tylenol)	160 mg per 5 mL	<5 per 5 mL
Acetaminophen regular strength caplets (Tylenol)	325 mg	<0.075
Acetaminophen with codeine tablets (Tylenol With Codeine)	All strengths	0.05
Acetaminophen intravenous	10 mg/mL	0.039/mL
Alendronate tablets (Fosamax)	70 mg	<0.12
Alendronate solution (Fosamax)	70 mg per 5 mL	0
Aluminum hydroxide, magnesium hydroxide, and simethicone (Maalox Advanced Regular Strength)	5 mL	0.903
Aluminum hydroxide, magnesium hydroxide, and simethicone (Maalox Advanced Maximum Strength)	5 mL	0.93 per 5 mL
Amoxicillin suspension (Amoxil)	200 mg per 5 mL	1.688 per 5 mL
Amoxicillin suspension (Amoxil)	400 mg per 5 mL	1.877 per 5 mL
Amoxicillin tablets (Amoxil)	500 mg	0.142
Amoxicillin tablets (Amoxil)	875 mg	0.248
Amoxicillin oral suspension (Amoxil)	125 mg per 5 mL	1.7
Amoxicillin oral suspension (Amoxil)	250 mg per 5 mL	1.85
Amoxicillin capsules (Amoxil)	250 mg	0
Amoxicillin capsules (Amoxil)	500 mg	0
Amoxicillin and clavulanate potassium oral suspension (Augmentin)	125 mg per 5 mL	0.52 per 5 mL
Amoxicillin and clavulanate potassium oral suspension (Augmentin)	200 mg per 5 mL	0.06 per 5 mL
Amoxicillin and clavulanate potassium oral suspension (Augmentin)	250 mg per 5 mL	0.6 per 5 mL
Amoxicillin and clavulanate potassium oral suspension (Augmentin)	400 mg per 5 mL	0.06 per 5 mL
Amoxicillin and clavulanate potassium chewable tablets (Augmentin)	200 mg	0.206
Amoxicillin and clavulanate potassium chewable tablets (Augmentin)	400 mg	0.36
Amoxicillin and clavulanate potassium tablets (Augmentin)	250 mg	0.02
Amoxicillin and clavulanate potassium tablets (Augmentin)	500 mg	0.02
Amoxicillin and clavulanate potassium tablets (Augmentin)	875 mg	0.03
Amoxicillin and clavulanate potassium suspension (Augmentin)	600 mg per 5mL	0.049 per 5 mL
Amoxicillin and clavulanate potassium extended release tablets (Augmentin XR)	1,000 mg	0.018
ARIPiprazole tablets (Abilify)	10 mg	0.062
ARIPiprazole tablets (Abilify)	15 mg	0.057
ARIPiprazole tablets (Abilify)	20 mg	0.124
ARIPiprazole tablets (Abilify)	30 mg	0.187
ARIPiprazole solution (Abilify)	1 mg/mL	0.6/mL
AtoMOXetine capsules (Strattera)	10 mg	0.18 to 0.22
AtoMOXetine capsules (Strattera)	18 mg	0.18 to 0.22
AtoMOXetine capsules (Strattera)	25 mg	0.18 to 0.22
AtoMOXetine capsules (Strattera)	40 mg	0.18 to 0.22
AtoMOXetine capsules (Strattera)	60 mg	0.18 to 0.22
Azithromycin oral suspension (Zithromax)	100 mg per 5 mL	3.86 per 5 mL
Azithromycin oral suspension (Zithromax)	200 mg per 5 mL	3.87 per 5 mL
Calcium and vitamin D chewable tablets (Caltrate 600+D)	Chewable tablets	1.9
Calcium and vitamin D tablets (Caltrate 600+D)	Tablets	0.25
Calcium and vitamin D tablets (Caltrate 600+Soy)	Tablets	0.25
CarBAMazepine extended release caplets (Carbatrol)	100 mg	<0.04
CarBAMazepine extended release caplets (Carbatrol)	200 mg	0.08 whole, <0.02 without shell

(continued)

Description (Brand Name)	Dosage Unit	Grams Carbohydrate per Dosage Unit
CarBAMazepine extended release caplets (Carbatrol)	300 mg	0.121 whole, <0.03 without shell
CarBAMazepine tablets (Equetro)	100 mg	<0.04
CarBAMazepine tablets (Equetro)	200 mg	0.08
CarBAMazepine tablets (Equetro)	300 mg	0.121
CarBAMazepine extended release tablets (TEGretol-XR)	100 mg	0.028
CarBAMazepine extended release tablets (TEGretol-XR)	200 mg	0.055
CarBAMazepine extended release tablets (TEGretol-XR)	400 mg	Unknown
CarBAMazepine suspension (TEGretol)	100 mg per 5 mL	3.35 per 5 mL
CarBAMazepine chewable tablets (TEGretol)	100 mg	0.28
CarBAMazepine tablets (TEGretol)	200 mg	0.06
Carnitine solution (Carnitor)	100 mg/mL	0.048
Carnitine solution (Carnitor SF)	100 mg/mL	0
Cefdinir suspension (Omnicef)	125 mg per 5 mL	2.87 per 5 mL
Cefdinir suspension (Omnicef)	250 mg per 5 mL	2.7 per 5 mL
Cefdinir capsules (Omnicef)	300 mg	0
Cefuroxime axetil suspension (Ceftin)	125 mg per 5 mL	3.062 per 5 mL
Cefuroxime axetil suspension (Ceftin)	250 mg per 5 mL	2.289 per 5 mL
Cefuroxime axetil tablets (Ceftin)	125 mg	0
Cefuroxime axetil tablets (Ceftin)	250 mg	0
Cefuroxime axetil tablets (Ceftin)	500 mg	0
Cetirizine syrup (ZyrTEC)	5 mg per 5 mL	2.25 per 5 mL
Cetirizine tablets (ZyrTEC)	5 mg	0.08
Cetirizine tablets (ZyrTEC)	10 mg	0.16
Chlorpheniramine maleate and phenylephrine hydrochloride liquid (Triaminic Cold and Allergy)	1 mg chlorpheniramine maleate and 2.5 mg phenylephrine hydrochloride per 5 mL	8.13 per 5 mL
Cholecalciferol oral solution (D-Vi-Sol)	400 units/mL	0.63/mL
Citalopram tablets (CeleXA)	10 mg	0.239
Citalopram tablets (CeleXA)	20 mg	0.229
Citric acid, sodium citrate, and potassium citrate solution (Cytra-3) (white bottle)	5 mL	1.5
Citric acid, sodium citrate, and potassium citrate solution (Cytra-3) (brown bottle)	5 mL	1.8
Clobazam tablets (Onfi)	10 mg	0.1
Clobazam tablets (Onfi)	20 mg	0.21
Clobazam suspension (Onfi)	2.5 mg/mL	0.19/mL
ClonazePAM orally disintegrating tablets	All strengths	0.0075
ClonazePAM tablets (KlonoPIN)	0.5 mg	0.14
ClonazePAM tablets (KlonoPIN)	1 mg	0.14
ClonazePAM tablets (KlonoPIN)	2 mg	0.14
Clorazepate tablets (Tranxene)	3.75 mg	0
CoEnzyme Q10 syrup (major pharmaceuticals)	100 mg per 5 mL	4 per 5 mL
CoEnzyme Q10 tablet (major pharmaceuticals)	50 mg	0.5
CycloSPORINE capsules (Gengraf)	25 mg	0.019
CycloSPORINE capsules (Gengraf)	100 mg	0.077
Dantrolene caplets (JHP Pharmaceuticals)	50 mg	0.245
Desloratadine orally disintegrating tablets (Clarinex)	5 mg	0.03
Desloratadine tablets (Clarinex)	5 mg	0.107
Dexamethasone oral concentrate solution (Intensol) *0.3 ethyl alcohol/mL	1 mg/mL	0
Dextroamphetamine and amphetamine extended release caplets (Adderall XR)	5 mg	0.038
Dextroamphetamine and amphetamine extended release caplets (Adderall XR)	10 mg	0.076
Dextroamphetamine and amphetamine extended release caplets (Adderall XR)	15 mg	0.113
Dextroamphetamine and amphetamine extended release caplets (Adderall XR)	20 mg	0.151
Dextroamphetamine and amphetamine extended release caplets (Adderall XR)	25 mg	0.188
Dextroamphetamine and amphetamine extended release caplets (Adderall XR)	30 mg	0.226

(continued)

Description (Brand Name)	Dosage Unit	Grams Carbohydrate per Dosage Unit
Dextromethorphan guaifenesin syrup (Robitussin DM)	10 mg per 5 mL	2.24 g sorbitol per 5 mL
Diazepam solution (Diazepam Intensol)	5 mg/mL	0
Diazepam oral solution	5 mg per 5 mL	1 per 5 mL
Diazepam tablets (Valium)	2 mg	0.167
Diazepam tablets (Valium)	5 mg	0.164
Diazepam tablets (Valium)	10 mg	0.159
Divalproex tablet	125 mg	0.025
Erythromycin powder suspension (EryPed)	200 mg per 5mL	0.606/mL
Erythromycin powder suspension (EryPed)	400 mg per 5mL	0.604/mL
Esomeprazole delayed release caplets (NexIUM)	20 mg	<0.024
Esomeprazole delayed release caplets (NexIUM)	40 mg	<0.047
Esomeprazole packets (NexIUM)	All strengths	<3
Ezogabine (Potiga)	All strengths	Negligible*
Famotidine oral suspension (Pepcid)	40 mg per 5 mL	1.19 per 5 mL
Famotidine tablets (Pepcid)	20 mg	0.09
Famotidine tablets (Pepcid)	40 mg	0.08
Famotidine, calcium carbonate, and magnesium hydroxide mint-flavored chewable tablets (Pepcid Complete)	10 mg	<0.76
Felbamate solution (Felbatol)	600 mg per 5 mL	1.5 per 5 mL
Felbamate tablets (Felbatol)	400 mg	0.13
Felbamate tablets (Felbatol)	600 mg	0.19
Ferrous sulfate drops (Fer-In-Sol)	75 mg/mL	0.61/mL
Fexofenadine tablets (Allegra)	30 mg	0.103
Fexofenadine tablets (Allegra)	60 mg	0.206
Fexofenadine tablets (Allegra)	180 mg	0.618
Fluconazole tablets (Diflucan)	150 mg	0.132
Fluconazole tablets (Diflucan)	200 mg	0.175
Fluconazole tablets (Teva Pharmaceuticals)	50 mg	0.04
Fluconazole tablets (Teva Pharmaceuticals)	100 mg	0.08
Fluconazole tablets (Teva Pharmaceuticals)	150 mg	0.122
Fluconazole tablets (Teva Pharmaceuticals)	200 mg	0.163
Fluconazole tablets (Greenstone Pharmaceuticals)	50 mg	0.044
Fluconazole tablets (Greenstone Pharmaceuticals)	100 mg	0.088
Fluconazole tablets (Greenstone Pharmaceuticals)	150 mg	0.132
Fluconazole oral suspension (Greenstone Pharmaceuticals)	10 mg/mL	0.578/mL
Fluconazole oral suspension (Greenstone Pharmaceuticals)	40 mg/mL	0.548/mL
Fluconazole tablets (Greenstone Pharmaceuticals)	200 mg	0.175
Fluconazole oral suspension (Diflucan)	10 mg/mL	0.578
Fluconazole oral suspension (Diflucan)	40 mg/mL	0.548
FLUoxetine capsules (PROzac)	40 mg	0.22
FLUoxetine capsules (PROzac)	10 mg	0.22
FLUoxetine capsules (PROzac)	20 mg	0.21
Fluticasone intranasal suspension (Flonase)	50 mcg	0
Folic acid tablet (WestWard brand)	1 mg	0.123
Furosemide tablets (Lasix)	20 mg	0.06
Furosemide tablets (Lasix)	40 mg	0.11
Furosemide tablets (Lasix)	80 mg	0.22
Furosemide elixir (Lasix)	10 mg/mL	0.8
Gabapentin tablets (Neurontin)	600 mg	0.049
Gabapentin tablets (Neurontin)	800 mg	0.066
Gabapentin solution (Neurontin)	250 mg per 5 mL	Unknown
Gabapentin tablets (Neurontin)	100 mg	0.03
Gabapentin tablets (Neurontin)	300 mg	0.07
Gabapentin tablets (Neurontin)	400 mg	0.1
Glycopyrrolate tablets (Robinul)	1 mg	0.1
Glycopyrrolate tablets (Robinul)	2 mg	0.18
Glycerin suppositories	82.5% glycerin per 1.35 g	1.11
Granisetron tablets	1 mg	0.098

(continued)

Description (Brand Name)	Dosage Unit	Grams Carbohydrate per Dosage Unit
Granisetron tablets	2 mg	0.197
Guanfacine extended release tablets (Intuniv)	1 mg	0.024
Guanfacine extended release tablets (Intuniv)	2 mg	0.048
Guanfacine extended release tablets (Intuniv)	3 mg	0.04
Guanfacine extended release tablets (Intuniv)	4 mg	0.054
Hydrocodone and acetaminophen tablets (Vicodin)	5 mg per 500 mg	0.038
HydrOXYzine syrup (Atarax)	10 mg per 5 mL	5.88
HydrOXYzine tablets (Atarax)	10 mg	0.04
HydrOXYzine tablets (Atarax)	25 mg	0.05
HydrOXYzine tablets (Atarax)	50 mg	0.07
HydrOXYzine tablets (Atarax)	100 mg	0.1
HydrOXYzine suspension (Vistaril)	25 mg per 5 mL	5.83 per 5 mL
HydrOXYzine capsules (Vistaril)	25 mg	0.03
HydrOXYzine capsules (Vistaril)	50 mg	0.07
HydrOXYzine capsules (Vistaril)	100 mg	0.11
Hyoscyamine Sublingual tablets (Ethex pharmaceuticals)	0.125 mg	<0.0001
Hyoscyamine tablets (Ethex pharmaceuticals)	0.125 mg	<0.0001
Ibuprofen tablets (Advil)	200 mg	0.23
Ibuprofen tablets (Motrin Junior Chewable)	100 mg	<0.56
Ibuprofen drops (Motrin Infants)	50 mg per 1.25 mL	<0.525 per 1.25 mL
Ibuprofen drops dye free (Motrin Infants')	50 mg per 1.25 mL	<0.525 per 1.25 mL
Ibuprofen suspension (Motrin Children's)	100 mg per 5 mL	<2.15 per 5 mL
Ibuprofen dye free suspension (Motrin Children's)	100 mg per 5 mL	<2.15 per 5 mL
Insulin oral inhalation (Exubera)	1 mg	Unknown
Insulin oral inhalation (Exubera)	3 mg	Unknown
Iron, vitamins A, D, C drops (Tri-Vi-Sol with Iron)	1 mL	0.75/mL
Iron, vitamins A, D, C drops (Tri-Vi-Sol)	1 mL	0.7/mL
Iron, vitamins A, B, C, D drops (Poly-Vi-Sol)	1 mL	0.92/mL
Iron, vitamin A, B, C, D, E drops (Poly-Vi-Sol With Iron)	1 mL	0.85/mL
Ketotifen oral syrup (Zaditen)	1 mg per 5 mL	4 per 5 mL
Lacosamide tablets (Vimpat)	All strengths	0
Lactase oral caplet (Lactaid)	Original	0.33
Lactobacillus capsules (Culturelle)	Capsules	<0.00001
Lactobacillus capsules (iFlora)	Capsules	0.41
Lactobacillus chewable tablets (Lactinex)	500 mg	0.377
Lactobacillus granules (Culturelle)	Granules	<0.0001
Lactobacillus granules (Lactinex)	1 g/packet	0.438
Lactobacillus oral packet (Culturelle)	Packet	<0.00001
LamoTRIgine chewable/dispersible tablets (LaMICtal)	2 mg	0.002
LamoTRIgine chewable/dispersible tablets (LaMICtal)	5 mg	0.004
LamoTRIgine chewable/dispersible tablets (LaMICtal)	25 mg	0.003
LamoTRIgine orally disintegrating tablets (LaMICtal ODT)	25 mg	0.065
LamoTRIgine orally disintegrating tablets (LaMICtal ODT)	50 mg	0.131
LamoTRIgine orally disintegrating tablets (LaMICtal ODT)	100 mg	0.262
LamoTRIgine orally disintegrating tablets (LaMICtal ODT)	200 mg	0.525
LamoTRIgine tablets (LaMICtal)	25 mg	0.027
LamoTRIgine tablets (LaMICtal)	100 mg	0.11
LamoTRIgine tablets (LaMICtal)	150 mg	0.16
LamoTRIgine tablets (LaMICtal)	200 mg	0.14
Lansoprazole delayed release capsules (Prevacid)	15 mg	0.124
Lansoprazole delayed release capsules (Prevacid)	30 mg	0.248
Lansoprazole delayed release orally disintegrating tablets (Prevacid)	15 mg	0.169
Lansoprazole delayed release orally disintegrating tablets (Prevacid)	30 mg	0.338
Leucovorin tablets (Barr Pharmaceuticals)	5 mg	0.11 to 0.15
LevETIRAcetam tablets (Keppra)	250 mg	0
LevETIRAcetam tablets (Keppra)	500 mg	0

(continued)

Description (Brand Name)	Dosage Unit	Grams Carbohydrate per Dosage Unit
LevETIRAcetam tablets (Keppra)	750 mg	0
LevETIRAcetam oral solution (Keppra)	100 mg/mL	0.5/mL
Levothyroxine tablets (Levoxyl)	All strengths	0
Levothyroxine tablets (Sandoz generic)	All strengths	0.123
Levothyroxine tablets (Synthroid)	All strengths	0.126
Lisinopril tablets (Prinivil)	5 mg	0.04
Lisinopril tablets (Prinivil)	10 mg	0.08
Lisinopril tablets (Prinivil)	20 mg	0.08
Loperamide (Imodium A-D) *0.26 ethyl alcohol per 5 mL	1 mg per 5 mL	4.13 per 5 mL
Loracarbef oral suspension (Lorabid)	100 mg per 5 mL	3.15 per 5 mL
Loracarbef oral suspension (Lorabid)	200 mg per 5 mL	3.03 per 5 mL
Loracarbef pulvules (Lorabid)	200 mg	0.22
Loracarbef pulvules (Lorabid)	400 mg	0.11
Loratadine orally disintegrating tablets (Alavert)	10 mg	0.2
Loratadine orally disintegrating tablets (Claritin RediTabs 24 Hour Allergy)	10 mg	0.007
Loratadine oral syrup (Claritin)	5 mg per 5 mL	8 per 5 mL
Loratadine tablets (Alavert)	10 mg	0.08
Loratadine tablets (Claritin)	10 mg	0.09
LORazepam solution (Lorazepam Intensol)	2 mg/mL	0
Magaldrate, simethicone suspension (Riopan Plus)	5 mL	0.37 per 5 mL
Magnesium Hydroxide (Milk of Magnesia)	Mint (400 mg per 5 mL)	0
Magnesium hydroxide in purified water and mineral oil	300 mg per 5 mL	0
Magnesium hydroxide (Phillips' MOM Mint)	40 mEq elem mg per 15 mL	0
Magnesium hydroxide, aluminum hydroxide, simethicone (Mylanta)	Tablets – regular strength	0.49
Magnesium hydroxide, aluminum hydroxide, simethicone (Mylanta)	Tablets – double strength	0.83
Magnesium hydroxide, aluminum hydroxide, simethicone (different flavors available) (Mylanta)	Liquid – regular strength, 5 mL	0.67 per 5 mL
Magnesium hydroxide, aluminum hydroxide, simethicone (Mylanta)	Liquid – double strength, 5 mL	0.67 per 5 mL
Meclizine tablets (Dramamine II)	25 mg	<0.25
Mesalamine capsules (Pentasa)	250 mg	0.23
Methadone (Methadone Intensol)	10 mg/mL	0
Methylphenidate extended release tablets (Concerta)	18 mg	0.007
Methylphenidate extended release tablets (Concerta)	27 mg	0.005
Methylphenidate extended release tablets (Concerta)	36 mg	0.015
Methylphenidate extended release tablets (Concerta)	54 mg	0.008
Methylphenidate tablets (Ritalin)	5 mg	0.087
Methylphenidate tablets (Ritalin)	10 mg	0.124
Methylphenidate tablets (Ritalin)	20 mg	0.155
Methylphenidate extended release caplets (Ritalin LA)	All strengths	0.25
Methylphenidate sustained release tablets (Ritalin-SR)	20 mg	0.092
Metoclopramide syrup (Reglan)	5 mg per 5 mL	1.75 per 5 mL
Metoclopramide tablets (Reglan)	5 mg	0.11
Metoclopramide tablets (Reglan)	10 mg	0.1
Modafinil tablets (Provigil)	All strengths	0.1
Mometasone intranasal suspension (Nasonex)	50 mcg/spray	Negligible
Montelukast chewable tablets (Singulair)	4 mg	0.161
Montelukast chewable tablets (Singulair)	5 mg	0.201
Montelukast tablets (Singulair)	10 mg	0.089
Montelukast granules (Singulair)	4 mg	0.484
Multiple vitamin and mineral supplement (Centrum Advanced Formula Liquid)	15 mL	6.25 per 15 mL
Multiple vitamin and mineral supplement (Centrum Advanced Formula tablets)	Tablets	0.25
Multiple vitamin and mineral supplement (Flintstones Plus Extra C)	Chewable tablets	<0.6
Multiple vitamin and mineral supplement (Flintstones Plus Iron)	Chewable tablets	0.65

(continued)

Description (Brand Name)	Dosage Unit	Grams Carbohydrate per Dosage Unit
Multiple vitamin and mineral supplement (Flintstones Plus Calcium)	Chewable tablets	0.11
Multiple vitamin and mineral supplement (Flintstones Original)	Chewable tablets	0.7
Multiple vitamin and mineral supplement (Flintstones Complete)	Chewable tablets (sugar-free)	0.37
Multiple vitamin and mineral supplement (Unicap)	Tablets	0.25
Multiple vitamin and mineral supplement (Unicap)	Capsules	0.25
NIFEdipine capsules (Procardia)	10 mg	0.1
NIFEdipine capsules (Procardia)	20 mg	0.12
Nitrofurantoin oral suspension (Furadantin)	25 mg per 5 mL	0.7 per 5 mL
Nystatin oral suspension	100,000 units/mL	0.61/mL
Nystatin oral suspension (Mycostatin)	100,000 units/mL	0.6/mL
Nystatin tablets (Mycostatin)	500,000 units	0.11
Omeprazole capsules (PriLOSEC)	10 mg	<0.179
Omeprazole capsules (PriLOSEC)	20 mg	<0.179
Omeprazole capsules (PriLOSEC)	30 mg	<0.202
Omeprazole and sodium bicarbonate powder for suspension (Zegerid)	All strengths	4
Ondansetron tablets (Zofran)	4 mg	0.082
Ondansetron tablets (Zofran)	8 mg	0.176
Ondansetron orally disintegrating tablets (Zofran)	4 mg	Unknown
Ondansetron orally disintegrating tablets	8 mg	Unknown
Ora-Plus oral liquid	Liquid	0
Ora-Sweet oral syrup	Syrup	0.8/mL
Oseltamivir capsules (Tamiflu)	30 mg	0.017
Oseltamivir capsules (Tamiflu)	45 mg	0.025
Oseltamivir capsules (Tamiflu)	75 mg	0.042
OXcarbazepine tablets (Trileptal)	150 mg	0.01
OXcarbazepine tablets (Trileptal)	300 mg	0.017
OXcarbazepine tablets (Trileptal)	600 mg	0.031
OXcarbazepine suspension (Trileptal)	300 mg per 5 mL	0.305/mL
Oxymetazoline nasal spray	0.05%	0
PARoxetine oral suspension (Paxil)	10 mg per 5 mL	2 per 5 mL
PARoxetine tablets (Paxil)	10 mg	0.003
PARoxetine tablets (Paxil)	20 mg	0.006
PARoxetine tablets (Paxil)	30 mg	0.009
PARoxetine tablets (Paxil)	40 mg	0.012
PARoxetine tablets (Paxil CR)	12.5 mg	0.109
Penicillin suspension (Stada Pharmaceuticals)	125 mg per 5 mL	2.645 per 5 mL
Penicillin suspension (Stada Pharmaceuticals)	250 mg per 5 mL	2.645 per 5 mL
Penicillin V potassium oral suspension	125 mg per 5 mL	2.53 per 5 mL
Penicillin V potassium oral suspension	250 mg per 5 mL	3.28 per 5 mL
Penicillin V potassium tablets	250 mg	0.09
Penicillin V potassium tablets	500 mg	0
Perampanel tablet (Fycompa)	2 mg	0.095
Perampanel tablet (Fycompa)	4 mg	0.191
Perampanel tablet (Fycompa)	6 mg	0.189
Perampanel tablet (Fycompa)	8 mg	0.187
Perampanel tablet (Fycompa)	10 mg	0.184
Perampanel tablet (Fycompa)	12 mg	0.182
PHENobarbital elixir *0.71 g ethyl alcohol per 5 mL	20 mg per 5 mL	3.4 per 5 mL
PHENobarbital tablets	15 mg	0.06
PHENobarbital tablets	30 mg	0.07
PHENobarbital tablets	60 mg	0.1
Phenylephrine (Neo-Synephrine Pediatric Formula Nasal Drops)	0.125%	0
Phenytoin suspension (Dilantin)	125 mg per 5 mL	1.39 per 5 mL
Phenytoin infatabs (Dilantin)	50 mg	0.48
Phenytoin kapseal (Dilantin)	30 mg	0.15
Phenytoin kapseal (Dilantin)	100 mg	0.11

(continued)

Description (Brand Name)	Dosage Unit	Grams Carbohydrate per Dosage Unit
Polycarbophil (Konsyl Fiber)	625 mg	0.5/tsp
Polyethylene Glycol 3350 powder (MiraLAX)	17 g	0
Potassium chloride 10% *0.25 ethyl alcohol per 5 mL	6.67 mEq per 5 mL	0.25 per 5 mL
Potassium citrate and citric acid oral solution (Cytra-K)	5 mL	1 (brown bottle) 0.5 (white bottle)
Potassium citrate and citric acid powder for oral solution (Cytra-K)	Packet	0.063
Potassium phosphate and sodium phosphate packet (Phos-NaK)	Packet	0.23
PrednisoLONE solution (Orapred)	15 mg per 5 mL	1.86 per 5 mL
PrednisoLONE syrup (Prelone)	5 mg per 5 mL	2.01 per 5 mL
PrednisoLONE syrup (Prelone)	15 mg per 5 mL	3.55 per 5 mL
PrednisoLONE oral solution (Pediapred)	5 mg per 5 mL	1.53 per 5 mL
PredniSONE solution (PredniSONE Intensol)	5 mg/mL	0
PredniSONE oral solution *0.25 ethyl alcohol per 5 mL	5 mg per 5 mL	1.8 per 5 mL
Primidone oral suspension (Mysoline)	250 mg per 5 mL	0
Primidone tablets (Mysoline)	50 mg	0.03
Primidone tablets (Mysoline)	250 mg	0.03
QUEtiapine tablets (SEROquel)	25 mg	0.037
QUEtiapine tablets (SEROquel)	50 mg	0.047
QUEtiapine tablets (SEROquel)	100 mg	0.095
QUEtiapine tablets (SEROquel)	200 mg	0.19
QUEtiapine tablets (SEROquel)	300 mg	0.285
QUEtiapine tablets (SEROquel)	400 mg	0.38
Ranitidine syrup (Zantac)	150 mg per 10 mL	1 per 10 mL
Ranitidine tablets (Zantac)	All strengths	0
RisperiDONE orally disintegrating tablets (RisperDAL M-Tab)	0.25 mg	0.02
RisperiDONE orally disintegrating tablets (RisperDAL M-Tab)	0.5 mg	0.039
RisperiDONE orally disintegrating tablets (RisperDAL M-Tab)	1 mg	0.044
RisperiDONE orally disintegrating tablets (RisperDAL M-Tab)	2 mg	0.044
RisperiDONE orally disintegrating tablets (RisperDAL M-Tab)	3 mg	0.066
RisperiDONE orally disintegrating tablets (RisperDAL M-Tab)	4 mg	0.088
RisperiDONE solution (RisperDAL)	1 mg/mL	0
RisperiDONE tablets (RisperDAL)	1 mg	0.177
RisperiDONE tablets (RisperDAL)	4 mg	0.352
Rufinamide suspension (Banzel)	40 mg/mL	0.281/mL
Rufinamide tablets (Banzel)	100 mg	0.077
Rufinamide tablets (Banzel)	200 mg	0.153
Rufinamide tablets (Banzel)	400 mg	0.306
Saccharomyces boulardii caplets (Florastor)	250 mg	0.505
Saccharomyces boulardii powder (Florastor Kids)	250 mg/packet	0.505
Salmeterol oral inhalation (Serevent Diskus)	50 mcg	0
Senna children's syrup (Senokot Children's)	5 mL	3.3 per 5 mL
Senna syrup (Senokot)	5 mL	3.8 per 5 mL
Senna granules (Senokot)	Teaspoonful	2
Senna tablets (Senokot)	Tablets	0.03
Senna tablets (Senokot-S)	Tablets	0.05
Senna tablets (SenokotXTRA)	Tablets	0.08
Simethicone drops (Mylicon)	40 mg per 0.6 mL	<0.071/mL
Sodium citrate and citric acid solution (Bicitra)	1 mEq/mL	0.230/mL
Sodium citrate and citric acid solution (Cytra-2)	5 mL	0.8 (brown bottle) 1.5 (white bottle)
Sodium divalproex sprinkle capsules (Depakote)	125 mg	0
Sodium divalproex tablets (Depakote)	125 mg	0.025
Sodium divalproex tablets (Depakote)	250 mg	0.05
Sodium divalproex tablets (Depakote)	500 mg	0.1
Depakote ER tablet	250 mg	0.01

(continued)

Description (Brand Name)	Dosage Unit	Grams Carbohydrate per Dosage Unit
Depakote ER tablet	500 mg	0.082
Depakene syrup	250 mg per 5 mL	4.5 per 5 mL
Sodium fluoride (Luride Drops) (peach flavor)	0.5 mg/mL (fluoride ion)	0.7/mL
Sodium phosphate enema (mono- and dibasic) (Fleets)	Enema	0
Tegaserod tablets (Zelnorm)	2 mg	Unknown
Tegaserod tablets (Zelnorm)	6 mg	0.038
Theophylline elixir (Elixophyllin) *0.86 ethyl alcohol per 5 mL	26.67 mg per 5 mL	0.31 per 5 mL
TiaGABine tablets (Gabitril)	4 mg	0.05
TiaGABine tablets (Gabitril)	12 mg	0.14
TiaGABine tablets (Gabitril)	16 mg	0.19
TiaGABine tablets (Gabitril)	20 mg	0.23
Topiramate caplets (Topamax)	15 mg	0.045
Topiramate caplets (Topamax)	25 mg	0.075
Topiramate tablets (Topamax)	25 mg	0.041
Topiramate tablets (Topamax)	50 mg	0.083
Topiramate tablets (Topamax)	100 mg	0.17
Topiramate tablets (Topamax)	200 mg	0.09
Triamcinolone intranasal suspension (Nasacort AQ)	55 mcg/spray	0.14/spray
Trimethoprim (TMP) and sulfamethoxazole (SMX) suspension (Hi-Tech Pharmacal)	40 mg TMP per 200 mg SMX per 5 mL	3.16 per 5 mL
Trimethoprim (TMP) and sulfamethoxazole (SMX) grape suspension (Septra)	40 mg TMP per 200 mg SMX per 5 mL	2.35 per 5 mL
Trimethoprim (TMP) and sulfamethoxazole (SMX) tablets (Septra)	80 mg TMP per 400 mg SMX	0
Trimethoprim (TMP) and sulfamethoxazole (SMX) double strength tablets (Septra)	160 mg TMP per 800 mg SMX	0
Valacyclovir caplets (Valtrex)	All strengths	0
Valproic acid syrup (Depakene)	250 mg per 5 mL	4.5 per 5 mL
Valproic acid capsules (Depakene)	250 mg	0
Vigabatrin tablets (Sabril)	500 mg	0.015
Vigabatrin powder for oral solution (Sabril)	500 mg/packet	0
Vitamin D drops (Drisdol)	8,000 units/mL	0
Vitamin E drops (Aquasol E)	15 units per 0.3 mL	0.06 per 0.3 mL
Xylometazoline (Otrivin Pediatric Nasal Drops)	0.05%	0
Zidovudine syrup (Retrovir)	50 mg per 5 mL	2.15 per 5 mL
Zidovudine tablets (Retrovir)	300 mg	0.02
Zidovudine capsules (Retrovir)	100 mg	0.09
Zonisamide capsules (Zonegran)	25 mg	0
Zonisamide capsules (Zonegran)	50 mg	0
Zonisamide capsules (Zonegran)	100 mg	0

Note: Information based on manufacturer's literature and is subject to change.

*Contact manufacturer for additional information

ORAL MEDICATIONS THAT SHOULD NOT BE CRUSHED OR ALTERED

There are a variety of reasons for crushing tablets or capsule contents prior to administering to the patient. Patients may have nasogastric tubes which do not permit the administration of tablets or capsules, an oral solution for a particular medication may not be available from the manufacturer or readily prepared by pharmacy, patients may have difficulty swallowing capsules or tablets, or mixing of powdered medication with food or drink may make the drug more palatable.

Generally, medications which should not be crushed fall into one of the following categories:

- **Extended Release Products:** The formulation of some tablets is specialized as to allow the medication within it to be slowly released into the body. This may be accomplished by centering the drug within the core of the tablet, with a subsequent shedding of multiple layers around the core. Wax melts in the GI tract, releasing drug contained within the wax matrix (eg, OxyCONTIN). Capsules may contain beads which have multiple layers which are slowly dissolved with time.

  Common Abbreviations for Extended Release Products

CD	Controlled dose
CR	Controlled release
CRT	Controlled release tablet
LA	Long-acting
SR	Sustained release
TR	Timed release
TD	Time delay
SA	Sustained action
XL	Extended release
XR	Extended release

- **Medications Which Are Irritating to the Stomach:** Tablets which are irritating to the stomach may be enteric-coated which delays release of the drug until the time when it reaches the small intestine. Enteric-coated aspirin is an example of this.
- **Foul-Tasting Medication:** Some drugs are quite unpleasant to taste so the manufacturer coats the tablet in a sugar coating to increase its palatability. By crushing the tablet, this sugar coating is lost and the patient tastes the unpleasant tasting medication.
- **Sublingual Medication:** Medication intended for use under the tongue should not be crushed. While it appears to be obvious, it is not always easy to determine if a medication is to be used sublingually. Sublingual medications should indicate on the package that they are intended for sublingual use.
- **Effervescent Tablets:** These are tablets which, when dropped into a liquid, quickly dissolve to yield a solution. Many effervescent tablets, when crushed, lose their ability to quickly dissolve.
- **Potentially Hazardous Substances:** Certain drugs, including antineoplastic agents, hormonal agents, some antivirals, some bioengineered agents, and other miscellaneous drugs, are considered potentially hazardous when used in humans based on their characteristics. Examples of these characteristics include carcinogenicity, teratogenicity, reproductive toxicity, organ toxicity at low doses, genotoxicity, or new drugs with structural and toxicity profiles similar to existing hazardous drugs. Exposure to these substances can result in adverse effects and should be avoided. Crushing or breaking a tablet or opening a capsule of a potentially hazardous substance may increase the risk of exposure to the substance through skin contact, inhalation, or accidental ingestion. The extent of exposure, potency, and toxicity of the hazardous substance determines the health risk. Institutions have policies and procedures to follow when handling any potentially hazardous substance. **Note:** All potentially hazardous substances may not be represented in this table. Refer to institution-specific guidelines for precautions to observe when handling hazardous substances.

RECOMMENDATIONS

1. It is not advisable to crush certain medications.
2. Consult individual monographs prior to crushing capsule or tablet.
3. If crushing a tablet or capsule is contraindicated, consult with your pharmacist to determine whether an oral solution exists or can be compounded.

Drug Product	Dosage Form	Dosage Reasons/Comments
Absorica (ISOtretinoin)	Capsule	Mucous membrane irritant; teratogenic potential
Accutane (ISOtretinoin)	Capsule	Mucous membrane irritant; teratogenic potential
Aciphex (RABEabeprazole)	Tablet	Extended release
Aciphex Sprinkle (RABEprazole)	Capsule	Slow release. Capsule may be opened and contents sprinkled on soft food (eg, applesauce, fruit- or vegetable-based baby food, yogurt) or emptied into a small amount of liquid (eg, infant formula, apple juice, pediatric electrolyte solution). Granules should not be chewed or crushed.
Actiq (FentaNYL)	Lozenge	Slow release. This lollipop delivery system requires the patient to dissolve it slowly.
Actoplus Met XR (Pioglitazone and Metformin)	Tablet	Variable release
Actonel (Risedronate)	Tablet	Irritant. Chewed, crushed, or sucked tablets may cause oropharyngeal irritation.
Adalat CC (NIFEdipine)	Tablet	Extended release
Adderall XR (Dextroamphetamine and Amphetamine)	Capsule	Extended release[1]
Adenovirus (Types 4, 7) Vaccine	Tablet	Teratogenic potential; enteric-coated; do not disrupt tablet to avoid releasing live adenovirus in upper respiratory tract
Advicor (Niacin and Lovastatin)	Tablet	Variable release
Afeditab CR (NIFEdipine)	Tablet	Extended release
Afinitor (Everolimus)	Tablet	Mucous membrane irritant; teratogenic potential; hazardous substance[11]
Aggrenox (Aspirin and Dipyridamole)	Capsule	Extended release. Capsule may be opened; contents include an aspirin tablet that may be chewed and dipyridamole pellets that may be sprinkled on applesauce.
Alavert Allergy and Sinus D-12 (Loratadine and Pseudoephedrine)	Tablet	Extended release
Allegra-D (Fexofenadine and Pseudoephedrine)	Tablet	Extended release
ALPRAZolam ER	Tablet	Extended release
Altoprev (Lovastatin)	Tablet	Extended release
Ambien CR (Zolpidem)	Tablet	Extended release
Amitiza (Lubiprostone)	Capsule	Manufacturer recommendation
Amnesteem (ISOtretinoin)	Capsule	Mucous membrane irritant; teratogenic potential
Ampyra (Dalfampridine)	Tablet	Extended release
Amrix (Cyclobenzaprine)	Capsule	Extended release
Aplenzin (BuPROPion)	Tablet	Extended release
Apriso (Mesalamine)	Capsule	Extended release[1]; maintain pH at ≤6
Aptivus (Tipranavir)	Capsule	Taste. Oil emulsion within spheres
Aricept 23 mg (Donepezil)	Tablet	Film-coated; chewing or crushing may increase rate of absorption
Arava (Leflunomide)	Tablet	Teratogenic potential; hazardous substance[11]
Arthrotec (Diclofenac and Misoprostol)	Tablet	Delayed release; enteric-coated
Asacol (Mesalamine)	Tablet	Slow release
Aspirin enteric-coated	Capsule, tablet	Delayed release; enteric-coated
Astagraf XL (Tacrolimus)	Capsule	Extended release
Atelvia (Risedronate)	Tablet	Extended release; tablet coating is an important part of the delayed release
Augmentin XR (Amoxicillin and Clavulanate)	Tablet	Extended release[2, 8]
AVINza (Morphine)	Capsule	Slow release[1] (not pudding)
Avodart (Dutasteride)	Capsule	Capsule should not be handled by pregnant women due to teratogenic potential[10]; hazardous substance[11]
Azulfidine EN-tabs (SulfaSALAzine)	Tablet	Delayed release
Bayer Aspirin EC (Aspirin)	Caplet	Enteric-coated

(continued)

Drug Product	Dosage Form	Dosage Reasons/Comments
Bayer Aspirin, Low Adult 81 mg (Aspirin)	Tablet	Enteric-coated
Bayer Aspirin, Regular Strength 325 mg (Aspirin)	Caplet	Enteric-coated
Benzonatate	Capsule	Swallow whole; pharmacologic action may cause choking if chewed or opened and swallowed
Biaxin XL (Clarithromycin)	Tablet	Extended release
Biltricide (Praziquantel)	Tablet	Taste[8]
Bisac-Evac (Bisacodyl)	Tablet	Enteric-coated[3]
Bisacodyl	Tablet	Enteric-coated[3]
Boniva (Ibandronate)	Tablet	Irritant. Chewed, crushed, or sucked tablets may cause oropharyngeal irritation.
Bosulif (Bosutinib)	Tablet	Hazardous substance[11]
Budeprion SR (BuPROPion)	Tablet	Extended release
Buproban (BuPROPion)	Tablet	Extended release
BuPROPion SR	Tablet	Extended release
Calan SR (Verapamil)	Tablet	Extended release[8]
Campral (Acamprosate)	Tablet	Delayed release; enteric-coated
Caprelsa (Vandetanib)	Tablet	Teratogenic potential; hazardous substance[11]
Carbatrol (CarBAMazepine)	Capsule	Extended release[1]
Cardene SR (NiCARdipine)	Capsule	Extended release
Cardizem (Diltiazem)	Tablet	Not described as slow release but releases drug over 3 hours.
Cardizem CD (Diltiazem)	Capsule	Extended release
Cardizem LA (Diltiazem)	Tablet	Extended release
Cardura XL (Doxazosin)	Tablet	Extended release
Cartia XT (Diltiazem)	Capsule	Extended release
Casodex (Bicalutamide)	Tablet	Teratogenic potential; hazardous substance[11]
CeeNU (Lomustine)	Capsule	Teratogenic potential; hazardous substance[11]
Cefaclor extended release	Tablet	Extended release
Ceftin (Cefuroxime)	Tablet	Taste[2]. Use suspension for children.
Cefuroxime	Tablet	Taste[2]. Use suspension for children.
CellCept (Mycophenolate)	Capsule, tablet	Teratogenic potential; hazardous substance[9,11]
Charcoal Plus DS (Charcoal, Activated)	Tablet	Enteric-coated
Chlor-Trimeton 12-Hour (Chlorpheniramine)	Tablet	Extended release[2]
Cipro XR (Ciprofloxacin)	Tablet	Extended release[2]
Claravis (ISOtretinoin)	Capsule	Mucous membrane irritant; teratogenic potential
Claritin-D 12-Hour (Loratadine and Pseudoephedrine)	Tablet	Extended release[2]
Claritin-D 24-Hour (Loratadine and Pseudoephedrine)	Tablet	Extended release[2]
Colace (Docusate)	Capsule	Taste[5]
Colestid (Colestipol)	Tablet	Slow release
Cometriq (Cabozantinib)	Capsule	Teratogenic potential; hazardous substance[11]
Commit (Nicotine)	Lozenge	Integrity compromised by chewing or crushing
Concerta (Methylphenidate)	Tablet	Extended release
Contrave (Naltrexone and Bupropion)	Tablet	Extended release
ConZip (TraMADol)	Capsule	Variable release; tablet disruption may cause overdose
Coreg CR (Carvedilol)	Capsule	Extended release[1]; may add contents to chilled applesauce
Cotazym-S (Pancrelipase)	Capsule	Enteric-coated[1]
Covera-HS (Verapamil)	Tablet	Extended release
Creon (Pancrelipase)	Capsule	Extended release[1]; enteric-coated contents
Crixivan (Indinavir)	Capsule	Taste. Capsule may be opened and mixed with fruit puree (eg, banana).

(continued)

Drug Product	Dosage Form	Dosage Reasons/Comments
Cyclophosphamide	Capsule, tablet	Hazardous substance[11]; manufacturer recommendation
Cymbalta (DULoxetine)	Capsule	Enteric-coated[1]; may add contents to apple juice or applesauce but not chocolate
Depakene (Valproic Acid)	Capsule	Slow release; mucous membrane irritant[2]; hazardous substance[11]
Depakote (Divalproex)	Tablet	Delayed release; hazardous substance[11]
Depakote ER (Divalproex)	Tablet	Extended release; hazardous substance[11]
Depakote Sprinkles (Divalproex)	Capsule	Extended release[1]
Detrol LA (Tolterodine)	Capsule	Extended release
Dexedrine (Dextroamphetamine)	Capsule	Extended release
Dexilant (Dexlansoprazole)	Capsule	Delayed release[1]
Diacomit (Stiripentol)	Capsule	Manufacturer recommendation[12]
Diamox Sequels (AcetaZOLAMIDE)	Capsule	Extended release
Dibenzyline (Phenoxybenzamine)	Capsule	Hazardous substance[11]
Diclegis (Doxylamine and Pyridoxine)	Tablet	Delayed release; manufacturer recommendation
Dilacor XR (Diltiazem)	Capsule	Extended release
Dilantin (Phenytoin)	Capsule	Extended release; manufacturer recommendation[12]
Dilatrate-SR (Isosorbide Dinitrate)	Capsule	Extended release
Dilt-XR (Diltiazem)	Capsule	Extended release
Diltia XT (Diltiazem)	Capsule	Extended release
Ditropan XL (Oxybutynin)	Tablet	Extended release
Divalproex ER	Tablet	Extended release
Donnatal Extentab (Hyoscyamine, Atropine, Scopolamine, and Phenobarbital)	Tablet	Extended release[2]
Drisdol (Ergocalciferol)	Capsule	Liquid filled[4]
Droxia (Hydroxyurea)	Capsule	May be opened; wear gloves to handle; hazardous substance[11]
Duavee (Estrogens [Conjugated/Equine] and Bazedoxifene)	Tablet	Manufacturer recommendation; hazardous substance[11]
Dulcolax (Bisacodyl)	Capsule	Liquid-filled
Dulcolax (Bisacodyl)	Tablet	Enteric-coated[3]
EC-Naprosyn (Naproxen)	Tablet	Delayed release; enteric-coated
Ecotrin Adult Low Strength (Aspirin)	Tablet	Enteric-coated
Ecotrin Maximum Strength (Aspirin)	Tablet	Enteric-coated
Ecotrin Regular Strength (Aspirin)	Tablet	Enteric-coated
E.E.S. (Erythromycin)	Tablet	Enteric-coated[2]
Effer-K (Potassium Bicarbonate and Potassium Citrate)	Tablet	Effervescent tablet[6]
Effervescent Potassium	Tablet	Effervescent tablet[6]
Effexor XR (Venlafaxine)	Capsule	Extended release
Elepsia XR	Tablet	Extended release
Embeda (Morphine and Naltrexone)	Capsule	Extended release[1]; do not give via NG tube
E-Mycin (Erythromycin)	Tablet	Enteric-coated
Enablex (Darifenacin)	Tablet	Slow release
Entocort EC (Budesonide)	Capsule	Extended release; enteric-coated[1]
Epanova (Omega-3 Fatty Acids)	Capsule	Manufacturer recommendation
Equetro (CarBAMazepine)	Capsule	Extended release[1]
Ergomar (Ergotamine)	Tablet	Sublingual form[7]
Erivedge (Vismodegib)	Capsule	Teratogenic potential[11]
Eryc (Erythromycin)	Capsule	Enteric-coated
Ery-Tab (Erythromycin)	Tablet	Delayed release; enteric-coated
Erythromycin Stearate	Tablet	Enteric-coated
Erythromycin Base	Tablet	Enteric-coated

ORAL MEDICATIONS THAT SHOULD NOT BE CRUSHED OR ALTERED

(continued)

Drug Product	Dosage Form	Dosage Reasons/Comments
Erythromycin Delayed Release	Capsule	Enteric-coated pellets[1]
Etoposide	Capsule	Hazardous substance[11]
Evista (Raloxifene)	Tablet	Taste; teratogenic potential[10]; hazardous substance[11]
Exalgo (HYDROmorphone)	Tablet	Extended release; breaking, chewing, crushing, or dissolving before ingestion or injecting increases the risk of overdose
Exjade (Deferasirox)	Tablet	Do not chew or swallow whole; do not give as tablets meant to be given as a liquid
Fareston (Toremifene)	Tablet	Teratogenic potential; hazardous substance[11]
Farydak (Panobinostat)	Capsule	Manufacturer recommendation; hazardous substance[11]
Feldene (Piroxicam)	Capsule	Mucous membrane irritant
FentaNYL	Lozenge	Slow release; lollipop delivery system requires the patient to slowly dissolve in mouth
Fentora (FentaNYL)	Tablet	Buccal tablet; swallowing whole or crushing may reduce effectiveness
Feosol (Ferrous Sulfate)	Tablet	Enteric-coated[2]
Fergon (Ferrous Gluconate)	Tablet	Enteric-coated
Ferro-Sequels (Ferrous Fumarate)	Tablet	Slow release
Fetzima (Levomilnacipran)	Capsule	Extended release
Flagyl ER (MetroNIDAZOLE)	Tablet	Extended release
Fleet Laxative (Bisacodyl)	Tablet	Enteric-coated[3]
Flomax (Tamsulosin)	Capsule	Slow release
Fludara (Fludarabine)	Tablet	Teratogenic potential; hazardous substance[11]
Focalin XR (Dexmethylphenidate)	Capsule	Extended release[1]
Forfivo XL (BuPROPion)	Capsule	Extended release
Fortamet (MetFORMIN)	Tablet	Extended release
Fosamax (Alendronate)	Tablet	Mucous membrane irritant
Fosamax Plus D (Alendronate and Cholecalciferol)	Tablet	Mucous membrane irritant
Fulyzaq (Crofelemer)	Tablet	Delayed release
Galzin (Zinc Acetate)	Capsule	Manufacturer recommendation[12]; possible gastric irritation
Gengraf (CycloSPORINE)	Capsule	Teratogenic potential; hazardous substance[11]
Geodon (Ziprasidone)	Capsule	Hazardous substance[11]
Gleevec (Imatinib)	Tablet	Taste[8]. May be dissolved in water or apple juice; hazardous substance[11]
GlipiZIDE XL	Tablet	Extended release
Glucophage XR (MetFORMIN)	Tablet	Extended release
Glucotrol XL (GlipiZIDE)	Tablet	Extended release
Glumetza (MetFORMIN)	Tablet	Extended release
Gralise (Gabapentin)	Tablet	Extended release
Halfprin (Aspirin)	Tablet	Enteric-coated
Hetlioz (Tasimelteon)	Capsule	Manufacturer recommendation
Hexalen (Altretamine)	Capsule	Teratogenic potential; hazardous substance[11]
Horizant (Gabapentin)	Tablet	Extended release
Hycamtin (Topotecan)	Capsule	Teratogenic potential; hazardous substance[11]
Hydrea (Hydroxyurea)	Capsule	Can be opened and mixed with water; wear gloves to handle; hazardous substance[11]
Hydromorph Contin (HYDROmorphone)	Capsule	Controlled release
Ibrance (Palbociclib)	Capsule	Manufacturer recommendation; hazardous substance[11]
Iclusig (PONATinib)	Tablet	Teratogenic potential; hazardous substance[11]
Imbruvica (Ibrutinib)	Capsule	Teratogenic potential; hazardous substance[11]
Imdur (Isosorbide Mononitrate)	Tablet	Extended release[8]
Inderal LA (Propranolol)	Capsule	Extended release
Indomethacin SR	Capsule	Slow release[1,2]

(continued)

Drug Product	Dosage Form	Dosage Reasons/Comments
Inlyta (Axitinib)	Tablet	Teratogenic potential; hazardous substance[11]
InnoPran XL (Propranolol)	Capsule	Extended release
Intelence (Etravirine)	Tablet	Tablet should be swallowed whole and not crushed; tablet may be dispersed in water
Intermezzo (Zolpidem)	Tablet	Sublingual form[7]
Intuniv (GuanFACINE)	Tablet	Extended release
Invega (Paliperidone)	Tablet	Extended release
IsoDitrate (Isosorbide Dinitrate)	Tablet	Extended release
Isoptin SR (Verapamil)	Tablet	Extended release[8]
Isosorbide Dinitrate Sublingual	Tablet	Sublingual form[7]
ISOtretinoin	Capsule	Mucous membrane irritant
Jalyn (Dutasteride and Tamsulosin)	Capsule	Capsule should not be handled by pregnant women due to teratogenic potential[10]; hazardous substance[9,11]
Janumet XR (Sitagliptin and Metformin)	Tablet	Extended release
Jurnista (HYDROmorphone)	Tablet	Extended release
Juxtapid (Lomitapide)	Capsule	Manufacturer recommendation
Kadian (Morphine)	Capsule	Extended release[1]. Do not give via NG tubes; may add contents to applesauce without crushing.
Kaletra (Lopinavir and Ritonavir)	Tablet	Film-coated; pregnant women or women who may become pregnant should not handle crushed or broken tablets; active ingredients surrounded by wax matrix to prevent health care exposure
Kapidex (Dexlansoprazole)	Capsule	Delayed release[1]
Kapvay (CloNIDine)	Tablet	Extended release
Kazano (Alogliptin and Metformin)	Tablet	Not scored; manufacturer recommendation[12]
K-Dur (Potassium Chloride)	Tablet	Slow release
Keppra (LevETIRAcetam)	Tablet	Taste[2]
Keppra XR (LevETIRAcetam)	Tablet	Extended release[2]
Ketek (Telithromycin)	Tablet	Slow release
Khedezla (Desvenlafaxine)	Tablet	Extended release
Klor-Con (Potassium Chloride)	Tablet	Extended release[2]
Klor-Con M (Potassium Chloride)	Tablet	Slow release[2]; some strengths are scored; to make liquid, place tablet in 120 mL of water; disperse 2 minutes; stir
K-Lyte/Cl (Potassium Bicarbonate and Potassium Chloride)	Tablet	Effervescent tablet[6]
Kombiglyze XR (Saxagliptin and Metformin)	Tablet	Extended release; tablet matrix may remain in stool
K-Tab (Potassium Chloride)	Tablet	Extended release[2]
LaMICtal XR (LamoTRIgine)	Tablet	Extended release
Lescol XL (Fluvastatin)	Tablet	Extended release
Letairis (Ambrisentan)	Tablet	Film-coated; slow release; hazardous substance[11]
Leukeran (Chlorambucil)	Tablet	Teratogenic potential; hazardous substance[11]
Levbid (Hyoscyamine)	Tablet	Extended release[8]
Lialda (Mesalamine)	Tablet	Delayed release, enteric-coated
Lipitor (AtorvaSTATin)	Tablet	Manufacturer recommendation[12]
Lithium Carbonate XR	Tablet	Extended release
Lithobid (Lithium)	Tablet	Extended release
Lovaza (Omega-3 Fatty Acids)	Capsule	Contents of capsule may erode walls of styrofoam or plastic materials
Luvox CR (FluvoxaMINE)	Capsule	Extended release
Lynparza (Olaparib)	Capsule	Teratogenic potential; hazardous substance[11]; manufacturer recommendation
Lysodren (Mitotane)	Tablet	Hazardous substance[11]
Mag-Tab SR (Magnesium L-Lactate)	Tablet	Extended release
Matulane (Procarbazine)	Capsule	Teratogenic potential; hazardous substance[11]

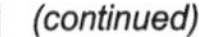

(continued)

Drug Product	Dosage Form	Dosage Reasons/Comments
Maxiphen DM (Guaifenesin, Dextromethorphan, and Phenylephrine)	Tablet	Slow release[8]
Mestinon ER (Pyridostigmine)	Tablet	Extended release[2]
Metadate CD (Methylphenidate)	Capsule	Extended release[1]
Metadate ER (Methylphenidate)	Tablet	Extended release
Metoprolol ER	Tablet	Extended release
MicroK Extencaps (Potassium Chloride)	Capsule	Extended release[1,2]
Minocin (Minocycline)	Capsule	Slow release
Mirapex ER (Pramipexole)	Tablet	Extended release
Morphine Sulfate Extended Release	Tablet	Extended release
Motrin (Ibuprofen)	Tablet	Taste[5]
Moxatag (Amoxicillin)	Tablet	Extended release
MS Contin (Morphine)	Tablet	Extended release[2]
Mucinex (GuaiFENesin)	Tablet	Slow release
Mucinex DM (GuaiFENesin)	Tablet	Slow release[2]
Multaq (Dronedarone)	Tablet	Hazardous substance[11]
Myfortic (Mycophenolate)	Tablet	Delayed release; teratogenic potential; hazardous substance[11]
Myorisan (ISOtretinoin)	Capsule	Mucous membrane irritant; teratogenic potential
Myrbetriq (Mirabegron)	Tablet	Extended release
Namenda XR (Memantine)	Capsule	Extended release[1]
Naprelan (Naproxen)	Tablet	Extended release
Neoral (CycloSPORINE)	Capsule	Teratogenic potential; hazardous substance[11]
NexIUM (Esomeprazole)	Capsule	Delayed release[1]
Niaspan (Niacin)	Tablet	Extended release
Nicotinic Acid (Niacinamide)	Capsule, Tablet	Slow release[8]
Nifediac CC (NIFEdipine)	Tablet	Extended release
Nifedical XL (NIFEdipine)	Tablet	Extended release
NIFEdipine ER	Tablet	Extended release
Nitrostat (Nitroglycerin)	Tablet	Sublingual route[7]
Norpace CR (Disopyramide)	Capsule	Extended release; form within a special capsule
Norvir (Ritonavir)	Tablet	Crushing tablets has resulted in decreased bioavailability of drug[2]
Noxafil (Posaconazole)	Tablet	Delayed release
Nucynta ER (Tapentadol)	Tablet	Extended release; tablet disruption may cause a potentially fatal overdose
Ofev (Nintedanib)	Capsule	Taste; hazardous substance[11]
Oleptro (TraZODone)	Tablet	Extended release[8]
Omtryg (Omega-3 Fatty Acids)	Capsule	Manufacturer recommendation
Onglyza (Saxagliptin)	Tablet	Film-coated
Opana ER (Oxymorphone)	Tablet	Extended release; tablet disruption may cause a potentially fatal overdose
Opsumit (Macitentan)	Tablet	Teratogenic potential; hazardous substance[11]
Oracea (Doxycycline)	Capsule	Delayed release
Oramorph SR (Morphine)	Tablet	Extended release[2]
Oravig (Miconazole)	Tablet	Buccal tablet
Orphenadrine Citrate ER	Tablet	Extended release
Oseni (Alogliptin and Pioglitazone)	Tablet	Manufacturer recommendation[12]
Otezla (Apremilast)	Tablet	Manufacturer recommendation
Oxtellar XR (OXcarbazepine)	Tablet	Extended release
OxyCONTIN (OxyCODONE)	Tablet	Extended release; surrounded by wax matrix; tablet disruption may cause a potentially fatal overdose
Oxymorphone ER	Tablet	Extended release

(continued)

Drug Product	Dosage Form	Dosage Reasons/Comments
Pancrease MT (Pancrelipase)	Capsule	Enteric-coated[1]
Pancreaze (Pancrelipase)	Capsule	Slow-release[1]; enteric-coated contents
Pancrelipase	Capsule	Slow-release[1]; enteric-coated contents
Paxil CR (PARoxetine)	Tablet	Extended release
Pentasa (Mesalamine)	Capsule	Slow release[1]
Pertzye (Pancrelipase)	Capsule	Slow-release[1]; enteric-coated contents
Pexeva (PARoxetine)	Tablet	Film-coated
Phenytek (Phenytoin)	Capsule	Extended release; manufacturer recommendation[12]
Plendil (Felodipine)	Tablet	Extended release
Pomalyst (Pomalidomide)	Capsule	Teratogenic potential; hazardous substance[11]; health care workers should avoid contact with capsule contents/body fluids
Pradaxa (Dabigatran)	Capsule	Bioavailability increases by 75% when the pellets are taken without the capsule shell
Prevacid (Lansoprazole)	Capsule	Delayed release[1]
Prevacid (Lansoprazole)	Suspension	Slow release. Contains enteric-coated granules. Not for use in NG tubes; mix with water only
Prevacid SoluTab (Lansoprazole)	Tablet	Orally disintegrating. Do not swallow; dissolve in water only and dispense via dosing syringe or NG tube.
Prezcobix (Darunavir and Cobicistat)	Tablet	Film-coated
PriLOSEC (Omeprazole)	Capsule	Delayed release
PriLOSEC OTC (Omeprazole)	Tablet	Delayed release
Pristiq (Desvenlafaxine)	Tablet	Extended release
Procardia XL (NIFEdipine)	Tablet	Extended release
Procysbi (Cysteamine)	Capsule	Delayed release[1]
Prolopa (Benserazide and Levodopa)	Capsule	Manufacturer recommendation
Propecia (Finasteride)	Tablet	Women who are, or may become, pregnant should not handle crushed or broken tablets due to teratogenic potential[10]; hazardous substance[11]
Proscar (Finasteride)	Tablet	Women who are, or may become, pregnant should not handle crushed or broken tablets due to teratogenic potential[10]; hazardous substance[11]
Protonix (Pantoprazole)	Tablet	Slow release
PROzac Weekly (FLUoxetine)	Capsule	Enteric-coated
Purinethol (Mercaptopurine)	Tablet	Teratogenic potential[10]; hazardous substance[11]
Pytest (Carbon 14 Urea)	Capsule	Hazardous substance[11]
Qudexy XR (Topiramate)	Capsule	Extended release
QuiNIDine ER	Tablet	Extended release[8]; enteric-coated
Ranexa (Ranolazine)	Tablet	Slow release
Rapamune (Sirolimus)	Tablet	Hazardous substance[11]; pharmacokinetic NanoCrystal technology may be affected[2]
Rayos (PredniSONE)	Tablet	Delayed release; release is dependent upon intact coating
Razadyne ER (Galantamine)	Capsule	Extended release
Renagel (Sevelamer)	Tablet	Expands in liquid if broken/crushed.
Renvela (Sevelamer)	Tablet	Enteric-coated[2]; expands in liquid if broken or crushed
Requip XL (ROPINIRole)	Tablet	Extended release
Rescriptor (Delavirdine)	Tablet	If unable to swallow, may dissolve 100 mg tablets in water and drink; 200 mg tablets must be swallowed whole
Revlimid (Lenalidomide)	Capsule	Teratogenic potential; hazardous substance[11]; health care workers should avoid contact with capsule contents/body fluids
RisperDAL M-Tab (RisperiDONE)	Tablet	Orally disintegrating. Do not chew or break tablet; after dissolving under tongue, tablet may be swallowed
Ritalin LA (Methylphenidate)	Capsule	Extended release[1]
Ritalin-SR (Methylphenidate)	Tablet	Extended release
Rytary (Carbidopa and Levodopa)	Capsule	Extended release[1]
Rythmol SR (Propafenone)	Capsule	Extended release
Ryzolt (TraMADol)	Tablet	Extended release; tablet disruption may cause overdose

(continued)

Drug Product	Dosage Form	Dosage Reasons/Comments
SandIMMUNE (CycloSPORINE)	Capsule	Teratogenic potential; hazardous substance[11]
Saphris (Asenapine)	Tablet	Sublingual form[7]
Sensipar (Cinacalcet)	Tablet	Tablets are not scored and cutting may cause inaccurate dosage
SEROquel XR (QUEtiapine)	Tablet	Extended release
Simcor (Niacin and Simvastatin)	Tablet	Tablet contains extended release niacin
Sinemet CR (Carbidopa and Levodopa)	Tablet	Extended release[8]
Sitavig (Acyclovir)	Tablet	Buccal tablet; swallowing whole or crushing eliminates or reduces effectiveness
Slo-Niacin (Niacin)	Tablet	Slow release[8]
Slow-Mag (Magnesium Chloride)	Tablet	Delayed release
Solodyn (Minocycline)	Tablet	Extended release
Somnote (Chloral Hydrate)	Capsule	Liquid filled
Soriatane (Acitretin)	Capsule	Teratogenic potential; hazardous substance[11]
Sprycel (Dasatinib)	Tablet	Film-coated. Active ingredients are surrounded by a wax matrix to prevent health care exposure. Women who are, or may become pregnant, should not handle crushed or broken tablets; teratogenic potential; hazardous substance[11]
Stalevo (Levodopa, Carbidopa, and Entacapone)	Tablet	Manufacturer recommendation
Stavzor (Valproic Acid)	Capsule	Delayed release; hazardous substance[11]
Stivarga (Regorafenib)	Tablet	Manufacturer recommendation; teratogenic potential; hazardous substance[11]
Strattera (AtoMOXetine)	Capsule	Capsule contents can cause ocular irritation.
Sudafed 12-Hour (Pseudoephedrine)	Capsule	Extended release[2]
Sudafed 24-Hour (Pseudoephedrine)	Capsule	Extended release[2]
Sulfazine EC (SulfaSALAzine)	Tablet	Delayed release, enteric-coated
Sular (Nisoldipine)	Tablet	Extended release
Sustiva (Efavirenz)	Tablet	Tablets should not be broken (capsules should be used if dosage adjustment needed)
Symax Duotab (Hyoscyamine)	Tablet	Controlled release
Symax SR (Hyoscyamine)	Tablet	Extended release
Syprine (Trientine)	Capsule	Potential risk of contact dermatitis
Tabloid (Thioguanine)	Tablet	Teratogenic potential; hazardous substance[11]
Tafinlar (Dabrafenib)	Capsule	Teratogenic potential; hazardous substance[11]
Tamoxifen	Tablet	Teratogenic potential; hazardous substance[11]
Targretin (Bexarotene)	Capsule	Manufacturer recommendation; teratogenic potential; hazardous substance[11]
Tasigna (Nilotinib)	Capsule	Hazardous substance[11]; altering capsule may lead to high blood levels, increasing the risk of toxicity
Taztia XT (Diltiazem)	Capsule	Extended release[1]
Tecfidera (Dimethyl Fumarate)	Capsule	Manufacturer recommendation; delayed release; irritant
TEGretol-XR (CarBAMazepine)	Tablet	Extended release[2]
Temodar (Temozolomide)	Capsule	Teratogenic potential; hazardous substance[11]. **Note:** If capsules are accidentally opened or damaged, rigorous precautions should be taken to avoid inhalation or contact of contents with the skin or mucous membranes.
Tessalon Perles (Benzonatate)	Capsule	Swallow whole; pharmacologic action may cause choking if chewed or opened and swallowed.
Tetracycline	Capsule	Hazardous substance[11]
Thalomid (Thalidomide)	Capsule	Teratogenic potential; hazardous substance[11]
Theo-24 (Theophylline)	Capsule	Extended release[1]; contains beads that dissolve through GI tract
Theochron (Theophylline)	Tablet	Extended release
Theophylline ER	Tablet	Extended release
Tiazac (Diltiazem)	Capsule	Extended release[1]
Topamax (Topiramate)	Capsule	Taste[1]

(continued)

Drug Product	Dosage Form	Dosage Reasons/Comments
Topamax (Topiramate)	Tablet	Taste
Toprol XL (Metoprolol)	Tablet	Extended release[8]
Toviaz (Fesoterodine)	Tablet	Extended release
Tracleer (Bosentan)	Tablet	Teratogenic potential; hazardous substance[10,11]; women who are or may be pregnant should not handle crushed or broken tablets
TRENtal (Pentoxifylline)	Tablet	Extended release
Treximet (Sumatriptan and Naproxen)	Tablet	Unique formulation enhances rapid drug absorption
TriLipix (Fenofibrate)	Capsule	Extended release
Trokendi XR (Topiramate)	Capsule	Extended release
Tylenol Arthritis Pain (Acetaminophen)	Caplet	Controlled release
Tylenol 8 Hour (Acetaminophen)	Caplet	Extended release
Uceris (Budesonide)	Tablet	Extended release; coating on tablet designed to break down at pH of ≥7
Ultram ER (TraMADol)	Tablet	Extended release. Tablet disruption my cause a potentially fatal overdose.
Ultresa (Pancrelipase)	Capsule	Delayed release; enteric-coated contents
Ultrase (Pancrelipase)	Capsule	Enteric-coated[1]
Ultrase MT (Pancrelipase)	Capsule	Enteric-coated[1]
Uniphyl (Theophylline)	Tablet	Slow release
Urocit-K (Potassium Citrate)	Tablet	Wax-coated; prevents upper GI release
Uroxatral (Alfuzosin)	Tablet	Extended release
Valcyte (ValGANciclovir)	Tablet	Irritant potential[2]; teratogenic potential; hazardous substance[11]
Vascepa (Omega-3 Fatty Acids)	Capsule	Manufacturer recommendation
Venlafaxine ER	Tablet	Extended release
Verapamil SR	Tablet	Extended release[8]
Verelan (Verapamil)	Capsule	Sustained release[1]
Verelan PM (Verapamil)	Capsule	Extended release[1]
Vesanoid (Tretinoin)	Capsule	Teratogenic potential; hazardous substance[11]
VESIcare (Solifenacin)	Tablet	Enteric-coated
Videx EC (Didanosine)	Capsule	Delayed release
Vimovo (Naproxen and Esomeprazole)	Tablet	Delayed release
Viokace (Pancrelipase)	Tablet	Mucous membrane irritant
Viramune XR (Nevirapine)	Tablet	Extended release[2]
Voltaren-XR (Diclofenac)	Tablet	Extended release
VoSpire ER (Albuterol)	Tablet	Extended release
Votrient (PAZOPanib)	Tablet	Crushing significantly increases AUC and T_{max}; hazardous substance[11]; crushed or broken tablets may cause dangerous skin problems
Wellbutrin (BuPROPion)	Tablet	Film-coated
Wellbutrin SR (BuPROPion)	Tablet	Extended release
Wellbutrin XL (BuPROPion)	Tablet	Extended release
Xalkori (Crizotinib)	Capsule	Teratogenic potential; hazardous substance[11]
Xanax XR (ALPRAZolam)	Tablet	Extended release
Xeloda (Capecitabine)	Tablet	Teratogenic potential; hazardous substance[11].
Xigduo XR (Dapagliflozin and Metformin)	Tablet	Extended release
Xtandi (Enzalutamide)	Capsule	Teratogenic potential; hazardous substance[11]
Zegerid OTC (Omeprazole and Sodium Bbicarbonate)	Capsule	Delayed release[2]
Zelboraf (Vemurafenib)	Tablet	Teratogenic potential; hazardous substance[11]
Zenatane (ISOtretinoin)	Capsule	Mucous membrane irritant; teratogenic potential
Zenpep (Pancrelipase)	Capsule	Delayed release[1]; enteric-coated contents
Zohydro ER (HYDROcodone)	Capsule	Extended release; capsule disruption may cause a potentially fatal overdose

ORAL MEDICATIONS THAT SHOULD NOT BE CRUSHED OR ALTERED

(continued)

Drug Product	Dosage Form	Dosage Reasons/Comments
Zolinza (Vorinostat)	Capsule	Irritant; avoid contact with skin or mucous membranes; use gloves to handle; teratogenic potential; hazardous substance[11]
Zomig-ZMT (ZOLMitriptan)	Tablet	Oral-disintegrating form[7]
Zonatuss (Benzonatate)	Capsule	Swallow whole; pharmacologic action may cause choking if chewed or opened and swallowed
Zortress (Everolimus)	Tablet	Mucous membrane irritant; teratogenic potential; hazardous substance[11]
Zyban (BuPROPion)	Tablet	Slow release
Zydelig (Idelalisib)	Tablet	Manufacturer recommendation
Zyflo CR (Zileuton)	Tablet	Extended release
ZyrTEC-D Allergy & Congestion (Cetirizine and Pseudoephedrine)	Tablet	Extended release
Zytiga (Abiraterone)	Tablet	Teratogenic potential; hazardous substance[11]; women who are or may be pregnant should wear gloves if handling tablets

[1]Capsule may be opened and the contents taken without crushing or chewing; soft food, such as applesauce or pudding, may facilitate administration; contents may generally be administered via nasogastric tube using an appropriate fluid, provided entire contents are washed down the tube.

[2]Liquid dosage forms of the product are available; however, dose, frequency of administration, and manufacturers may differ from that of the solid dosage form.

[3]Antacids and/or milk may prematurely dissolve the coating of the tablet.

[4]Capsule may be opened and the liquid contents removed for administration.

[5]The taste of this product in a liquid form would likely be unacceptable to the patient; administration via nasogastric tube should be acceptable.

[6]Effervescent tablets must be dissolved in the amount of diluent recommended by the manufacturer.

[7]Tablets are made to disintegrate under (or on) the tongue.

[8]Tablet is scored and may be broken in half without affecting release characteristics.

[9]Skin contact may enhance tumor production; avoid direct contact.

[10]Prescribing information recommends that women who are, or may become, pregnant should not handle medication, especially if crushed or broken; avoid direct contact.

[11]Potentially hazardous or hazardous substance; refer to institution-specific guidelines for precautions to observe when handling this substance.

[12]Altering (eg, chewing, crushing, splitting, opening) the dosage form has not been studied, according to the manufacturer.

REFERENCES

Mitchell JF. Oral dosage forms that should not be crushed. Available at http://www.ismp.org/tools/DoNotCrush.pdf. Accessed November 11, 2011.

US Department of Health and Human Services; Centers for Disease Control and Prevention; National Institute for Occupational Safety and Health. NIOSH list of antineoplastic and other hazardous drugs in the healthcare settings 2014. Available at http://www.cdc.gov/niosh/docs/2014-138/pdfs/2014-138.pdf. Updated September 2014. Accessed February 6, 2015.

THERAPEUTIC CATEGORY & KEY WORD INDEX

INTERNATIONAL TRADE NAMES INDEX

The following countries are included in this index and are abbreviated as follows:

Argentina (AR)
Australia (AU)
Austria (AT)
Bahamas (BS)
Bahrain (BH)
Bangladesh (BD)
Barbados (BB)
Belgium (BE)
Belize (BZ)
Benin (BJ)
Bermuda (BM)
Bolivia (BO)
Brazil (BR)
Bulgaria (BG)
Burkina Faso (BF)
Chile (CL)
China (CN)
Colombia (CO)
Costa Rica (CR)
Côte D' Ivoire (CI)
Croatia (HR)
Cuba (CU)
Cyprus (CY)
Czech Republic (CZ)
Denmark (DK)
Dominican Republic (DO)
Ecuador (EC)
Egypt (EG)
El Salvador (SV)
Estonia (EE)
Ethiopia (ET)
Finland (FI)
France (FR)
Gambia (GM)
Germany (DE)
Ghana (GH)
Great Britain [UK] (GB)
Greece (GR)
Guatemala (GT)
Guinea (GN)
Guyana (GY)
Honduras (HN)
Hong Kong (HK)
Hungary (HU)
Iceland (IS)
India (IN)
Indonesia (ID)
Iran (IR)
Iraq (IQ)
Ireland (IE)
Israel (IL)
Italy (IT)
Jamaica (JM)
Japan (JP)
Jordan (JO)
Kenya (KE)
Korea, Republic of (KR)
Kuwait (KW)
Latvia (LV)
Lebanon (LB)
Liberia (LR)
Libya (LY)
Lithuania (LT)
Luxembourg (LU)
Malawi (MW)
Malaysia (MY)
Mali (ML)
Malta (MT)
Mauritania (MR)
Mauritius (MU)
Mexico (MX)
Morocco (MA)
Netherlands (NL)
New Zealand (NZ)
Nicaragua (NI)
Niger (NE)
Nigeria (NG)
Norway (NO)
Oman (OM)
Pakistan (PK)
Panama (PA)
Paraguay (PY)
Peru (PE)
Philippines (PH)
Poland (PL)
Portugal (PT)
Puerto Rico (PR)
Qatar (QA)
Romania (RO)
Russian Federation (RU)
Saudi Arabia (SA)
Senegal (SN)
Seychelles (SC)
Sierra Leone (SL)
Singapore (SG)
Slovakia (SK)
Slovenia (SI)
South Africa (ZA)
Spain (ES)
Sudan (SD)
Surinam (SR)
Sweden (SE)
Switzerland (CH)
Syrian Arab Republic (SY)
Taiwan, Province of China (TW)
Tanzania (TZ)
Thailand (TH)
Trinidad and Tobago (TT)
Tunisia (TN)
Turkey (TR)
Uganda (UG)
United Arab Emirates (AE)
Uruguay (UY)
Venezuela (VE)
Vietnam (VN)
Yemen (YE)
Zambia (ZM)
Zimbabwe (ZW)

Biocatines D2 (ES) *see* Ergocalciferol 772
Biocef (AT) *see* Cefpodoxime 404
Biocef (ES) *see* Ceftibuten 409
Biocilin (MX) *see* Filgrastim 876
Biocil (MY) *see* Ampicillin 156
Bioclavid (AE, BH, CY, DE, DK, EG, IQ, IR, JO, KW, LB, LY, OM, PH, QA, SA, SE, SY, YE) *see* Amoxicillin and Clavulanate 141
Bioclavid Forte (PH) *see* Amoxicillin and Clavulanate 141
Biocort (PH) *see* Hydrocortisone (Systemic) 1038
Biocort (ZA) *see* Hydrocortisone (Topical) 1041
Biocoryl (ES) *see* Procainamide 1769
Biocristin (IN) *see* VinCRIStine 2179
Biocronil (CO) *see* Enalapril 744
Biodacyna (LT) *see* Amikacin 117
Biodalgic (FR) *see* TraMADol 2098
Biodexan Ofteno (MX) *see* Neomycin, Polymyxin B, and Dexamethasone 1502
Biodexan Ofteno (MX) *see* Polymyxin B 1726
Biodone Extra Forte (NZ) *see* Methadone 1379
Biodone Forte (AU, NZ) *see* Methadone 1379
Biodone (NZ) *see* Methadone 1379
Biodoxi (IN) *see* Doxycycline 717
Biodramina (ES, MT) *see* DimenhyDRINATE 664
Biodribin (PL) *see* Cladribine 480
Biodrop (AR) *see* Dorzolamide 706
Biodroxil (AE, BG, BH, CY, EG, IL, IQ, IR, JO, KW, LB, LY, OM, PE, QA, SA, SY, VN, YE) *see* Cefadroxil 387
Biodroxyl (VE) *see* Cefadroxil 387
Biofanal (DE) *see* Nystatin (Topical) 1537
Biofazolin (PL) *see* CeFAZolin 388
Bioferon (PY, TH, UY) *see* Interferon Alfa-2b 1148
Biofigran (CO) *see* Filgrastim 876
Biofilen (MX) *see* Atenolol 215
Biofilgran (MX) *see* Filgrastim 876
Bio-Folic (BE) *see* Folic Acid 931
Biofradin (ES) *see* Neomycin 1500
Biogam Ca (BE) *see* Calcium Gluconate 351
Biogam F (BE) *see* Fluoride 899
Biogam Fe (BE) *see* Ferrous Gluconate 870
Biogam Mg (BE, CH) *see* Magnesium Gluconate 1312
Biogaracin (IN) *see* Gentamicin (Systemic) 965
Biogen (JP) *see* Thiamine 2048
Biogenta Oftalmica (CO) *see* Gentamicin (Ophthalmic) 968
Biogesic (SG) *see* Acetaminophen 44
Biogesic Suspension (HK) *see* Acetaminophen 44
Biogrisin (PL) *see* Griseofulvin 986
Bio-Hep-B (IL) *see* Hepatitis B Vaccine (Recombinant) 1015
Biohulin NPH (KR) *see* Insulin NPH 1138
Biokacin (MX, PY) *see* Amikacin 117
Biolac (PH) *see* Lactulose 1204
Biolectra (AT) *see* Calcium Carbonate 343
Biolytan (MX) *see* Disopyramide 689
Biomag (IT) *see* Cimetidine 461
Biomikin (CR, DO, GT, HN, NI, PA, SV) *see* Amikacin 117
Biomixin (MX) *see* Doxycycline 717
Biopain (PH) *see* Acetaminophen 44
Bioplatino (PE) *see* CISplatin 473
Bioquin (CL) *see* Erythromycin and Sulfisoxazole 784
Biorrub (BR) *see* DOXOrubicin (Conventional) 713
Bioselenium (MT) *see* Selenium Sulfide 1913
Biosim (IN) *see* Simvastatin 1928
Biosint (MX) *see* Cefotaxime 398
Biosporin (EC) *see* CycloSPORINE (Systemic) 556
Biostate (AU, HK, NZ, SG) *see* Antihemophilic Factor/von Willebrand Factor Complex (Human) 173
Biosupressin (HU) *see* Hydroxyurea 1055
Biotamoxal (AR) *see* Amoxicillin 138
Biotam (VN) *see* Oxacillin 1576
Biotax (IL) *see* PACLitaxel (Conventional) 1602
Biotax (IN) *see* Cefotaxime 398
Biotine (SG) *see* Tetracycline 2035
Biotrexate (IN) *see* Methotrexate 1390
Biotriax (ID) *see* CefTRIAXone 410
Biotum (PL) *see* CefTAZidime 407
Biovinate (PH) *see* CARBOplatin 374
Biovir (BR) *see* Lamivudine and Zidovudine 1209
Biovital Vitamin C (HU) *see* Ascorbic Acid 202
Bioyl (TW) *see* Bisacodyl 289
Biozac (BG) *see* FLUoxetine 906
Biozole (MY) *see* Fluconazole 881
Biplatinex (VE) *see* CARBOplatin 374
Biprin (CO) *see* Pyridoxine 1810
Biquelle XL (GB) *see* QUEtiapine 1815
Biraxin (PH) *see* Acyclovir (Systemic) 61
Birobin (AT) *see* Metolazone 1416
Bisacod (TH) *see* Bisacodyl 289
Bisakodils (EE) *see* Bisacodyl 289
Bisalax (AU, BG) *see* Bisacodyl 289
Bisanorin (JP) *see* Riboflavin 1856
Bisbacter (CO) *see* Bismuth Subsalicylate 290
Bisco (PH) *see* Bisacodyl 289
Biscosal (JP) *see* Fluocinonide 898
Biseko (PL) *see* Albumin 79
Biseptol (BG) *see* Sulfamethoxazole and Trimethoprim 1986
Bismucar (PE) *see* Bismuth Subsalicylate 290
Bismultin (GR) *see* Econazole 727
Bismutol (EC) *see* Bismuth Subsalicylate 290
Bisolbruis (NL) *see* Acetylcysteine 57
Bi Su Fu (CN) *see* Diclofenac (Systemic) 641
Bisulase (JP) *see* Riboflavin 1856
Bitammon (CZ) *see* Ampicillin and Sulbactam 159
Bi-Tildiem (FR) *see* Diltiazem 661
Bittle (HK) *see* Clindamycin (Topical) 491
Bituvitan (JP) *see* Riboflavin 1856
Bivit (IT) *see* Pyridoxine 1810
Blastocarb (CL) *see* CARBOplatin 374
Blastocarb RU (MX) *see* CARBOplatin 374
Blastolem (CL, CO) *see* CISplatin 473
Blastolem RU (MX) *see* CISplatin 473
Blastomat (HR, RO) *see* Temozolomide 2012
Blastovin PF (IL) *see* VinBLAStine 2177
Blastovin (PY) *see* VinBLAStine 2177
Blef-10 (CO, PE) *see* Sulfacetamide (Ophthalmic) 1981
Bleminal (DE) *see* Allopurinol 96
Blenamax (AU, RU, SG, TW) *see* Bleomycin 292
Blend-A-Med (DE) *see* Chlorhexidine Gluconate 434
Blenoxane (BR, EC, EG, ZA) *see* Bleomycin 292
Bleocin (AE, BG, CZ, EE, EG, GR, HK, HN, HU, ID, IN, JO, JP, KR, LB, MY, PE, PL, PT, QA, SA, SG, TH, TR, TW, VN) *see* Bleomycin 292
Bleocina (UY) *see* Bleomycin 292
Bleocin-S (MY) *see* Bleomycin 292
Bleocip (LB) *see* Bleomycin 292
Bleocris (PY) *see* Bleomycin 292
Bleo (HK) *see* Bleomycin 292
Bleolem (CO, MX, TH) *see* Bleomycin 292
Bleomax (MX) *see* Bleomycin 292
Bleomicina (ES, IT) *see* Bleomycin 292
Bleomycin (AT, CH, DK, FI, GB, NO, SE) *see* Bleomycin 292
Bleomycine (BE, FR, LU, NL) *see* Bleomycin 292
Bleomycin PFI (IL) *see* Bleomycin 292
Bleomycinum (DE) *see* Bleomycin 292
Bleph-10 (AE, AU, BH, CY, EG, IQ, IR, JO, KW, LB, LY, NZ, OM, QA, SA, SY, YE) *see* Sulfacetamide (Ophthalmic) 1981
Bleph-30 (AE, BH, CY, EG, IQ, IR, JO, KW, LB, LY, OM, QA, SA, SY, YE) *see* Sulfacetamide (Ophthalmic) 1981
Blexit (CL) *see* Bleomycin 292
Blisscolic (PK) *see* Dicyclomine 645

Hedex (IE) *see* Acetaminophen 44
Hedrin (IL) *see* Simethicone 1927
Heferol (HR) *see* Ferrous Fumarate 869
Heksavit (FI) *see* Pyridoxine 1810
Helex (HR) *see* ALPRAZolam 100
Heliclar (LU) *see* Clarithromycin 482
Heliclo (KR) *see* Clarithromycin 482
Heliopar (FI) *see* Chloroquine 437
Heliton (AR) *see* Nitazoxanide 1519
Helixate (AT, GR, HU, IT, NL, PL) *see* Antihemophilic Factor (Recombinant) 168
Helixate Nexgen (AU, BE, CZ, DE, DK, EE, FR, NO, SE) *see* Antihemophilic Factor (Recombinant) 168
Helixate NexGen (GB, IE) *see* Antihemophilic Factor (Recombinant) 168
Helix SR (HU) *see* ALPRAZolam 100
Helizol (EC) *see* Omeprazole 1555
Helmex (DE) *see* Pyrantel Pamoate 1806
Helmiben (UY) *see* Albendazole 78
Helmidazole (AE, BH, CY, EG, IL, IQ, IR, JO, KW, LB, LY, OM, QA, SA, SY, YE) *see* Albendazole 78
Helminar (PE) *see* Granisetron 981
Helmintox (FR, RU) *see* Pyrantel Pamoate 1806
Helmizol (BR) *see* MetroNIDAZOLE (Systemic) 1421
Helocetin (KR) *see* Chloramphenicol 432
Helsibon (JP) *see* Diltiazem 661
Helvevir (CH) *see* Acyclovir (Systemic) 61
Hemaflow (PH) *see* Clopidogrel 513
Hema F (TW) *see* Ferrous Fumarate 869
Hema-K (PH) *see* Phytonadione 1698
Hemapo (ID, TH, VN) *see* Epoetin Alfa 765
Hemasol (SG) *see* Homatropine 1023
Hemastat (PH) *see* Heparin 1006
Hemax (TH) *see* Epoetin Alfa 765
Hemi-Daonil (AR, FR, MA) *see* GlyBURIDE 975
Hemobion (MX) *see* Ferrous Sulfate 871
Hemocaprol (ES) *see* Aminocaproic Acid 121
Hemoclot (PH) *see* Tranexamic Acid 2101
Hemofil M (DE, FR, IT, TH, TW) *see* Antihemophilic Factor (Human) 167
Hemogenin (BR) *see* Oxymetholone 1601
Hemohes (AR, CL, LU, NL) *see* Hetastarch 1019
Hemonor (PE) *see* Heparin 1006
Hemopressin (PK) *see* Vasopressin 2161
Hemostan (PH) *see* Tranexamic Acid 2101
Hemototal (PT) *see* Ferrous Gluconate 870
Hemotrex (PH) *see* Tranexamic Acid 2101
Hemovas (ES) *see* Pentoxifylline 1670
Heng En (CN) *see* MitoXANtrone 1448
Henplatin (PH) *see* Oxaliplatin 1578
Hentaxel (PH) *see* DOCEtaxel 692
Hentrozole (PH) *see* Letrozole 1224
HepaBig (EG) *see* Hepatitis B Immune Globulin (Human) 1013
Hepabig (IN, KR, MY, PH) *see* Hepatitis B Immune Globulin (Human) 1013
Hepacaf (BE) *see* Hepatitis B Immune Globulin (Human) 1013
Hepaflex (FI, NO) *see* Heparin 1006
Hepagam B (IL) *see* Hepatitis B Immune Globulin (Human) 1013
Hepalac (TH) *see* Lactulose 1204
Heparin (AT, BF, BG, BJ, CH, CI, CZ, DE, ET, FI, GB, GH, GM, GN, GR, HN, IL, KE, LR, MA, ML, MR, MU, MW, NE, NG, NO, SC, SD, SE, SL, SN, TN, TZ, UG, ZA, ZM, ZW) *see* Heparin 1006
Heparine (BE, NL) *see* Heparin 1006
Heparine Choay (FR) *see* Heparin 1006
Heparine Novo (BE, NL) *see* Heparin 1006
Heparin Injection B.P. (AU) *see* Heparin 1006
Heparin Leo (DK, HK, ID, MY, PH, TW) *see* Heparin 1006
Heparin Novo (TW) *see* Heparin 1006
Heparin Sodium B Braun (ID, MY) *see* Heparin 1006
Hepatect (AT, CH, CO, DE, EE, HN, IE, PL, PT, TR, TW) *see* Hepatitis B Immune Globulin (Human) 1013
Hepatect CP (VN) *see* Hepatitis B Immune Globulin (Human) 1013
Hepatitis B Immunoglobulin-VF (AU) *see* Hepatitis B Immune Globulin (Human) 1013
Hepavax Gene (CO) *see* Hepatitis B Vaccine (Recombinant) 1015
Hepaviral (ID) *see* Ribavirin 1851
Hepavit (AT) *see* Hydroxocobalamin 1050
Hep-B Gammagee (AE) *see* Hepatitis B Immune Globulin (Human) 1013
HepBQuin (IN, NL) *see* Hepatitis B Immune Globulin (Human) 1013
Hepcure (KR) *see* Adefovir 72
Heplav (ID) *see* LamiVUDine 1205
Hepovir (PK) *see* Adefovir 72
Heprin (PH) *see* Heparin 1006
Hepsal (MT, SG) *see* Heparin 1006
Hepsera (AE, AR, AT, AU, BE, BG, BR, CH, CL, CN, CO, CR, CY, CZ, DE, DK, DO, EC, EE, ES, FI, FR, GB, GR, GT, HK, HN, HR, HU, ID, IE, IL, IS, IT, JO, KR, KW, LT, MT, MY, NI, NL, NO, NZ, PA, PE, PH, PK, PL, PT, QA, RO, RU, SA, SE, SG, SI, SK, SV, TH, TR, TW, VE, VN) *see* Adefovir 72
Hepssel (KR) *see* Adefovir 72
Heptadon (AT) *see* Methadone 1379
Heptanon (HR) *see* Methadone 1379
Heptasan (ID) *see* Cyproheptadine 562
Heptin (PH) *see* Heparin 1006
Heptodin (CN) *see* LamiVUDine 1205
Hepuman Berna (PE) *see* Hepatitis B Immune Globulin (Human) 1013
Herax (ID) *see* Acyclovir (Systemic) 61
Herben (KR) *see* Diltiazem 661
Herbesser 60 (MY, TH) *see* Diltiazem 661
Herbesser 90 SR (HK, MY, SG, TH) *see* Diltiazem 661
Herbesser 180 SR (HK) *see* Diltiazem 661
Herbesser (JP, MY, TH, TW) *see* Diltiazem 661
Herbesser R100 (HK, JP) *see* Diltiazem 661
Herbesser R200 (HK, JP) *see* Diltiazem 661
Herbessor 30 (MY) *see* Diltiazem 661
Herbessor (SG, VN) *see* Diltiazem 661
Hercap (BR) *see* Capsaicin 362
Herclov (ID) *see* ValACYclovir 2138
Herfam (KR) *see* Famciclovir 846
Herklin (MX) *see* Lindane 1267
Hermolepsin (SE) *see* CarBAMazepine 367
Herocan (TW) *see* Irinotecan 1159
Herpavir (JO) *see* Acyclovir (Topical) 65
Herpecid (KR) *see* Acyclovir (Topical) 65
Herpesin (CZ) *see* Acyclovir (Topical) 65
Herpesin (CZ, SK) *see* Acyclovir (Systemic) 61
Herpetad (CR, DO, GT, HN, NI, PA, SV) *see* Acyclovir (Systemic) 61
Herpevex (MY) *see* Acyclovir (Systemic) 61
Herpevir (FR) *see* Acyclovir (Systemic) 61
Herpevir (FR) *see* Acyclovir (Topical) 65
Herpex (BH, IN, PH) *see* Acyclovir (Systemic) 61
Herpex (IN) *see* Acyclovir (Topical) 65
Herpizyg (TH) *see* Acyclovir (Systemic) 61
Herwont (IN) *see* Misoprostol 1444
Herzer (JP) *see* Nitroglycerin 1523
Hesor (TW) *see* Diltiazem 661
Hespander (JP) *see* Hetastarch 1019
Hestar-200 (CO, ID) *see* Hetastarch 1019
Hesteril (ES) *see* Hetastarch 1019
Heviran (PL) *see* Acyclovir (Systemic) 61
Hexabiotin (DK) *see* Erythromycin (Systemic) 779
Hexacycline (FR) *see* Tetracycline 2035
Hexa-Defital (AR) *see* Lindane 1267
Hexadilat (DK) *see* NIFEdipine 1516

NOTES

NOTES

NOTES

NOTES

NOTES

NOTES

Other Offerings from Lexicomp

Anesthesiology & Critical Care Drug Handbook

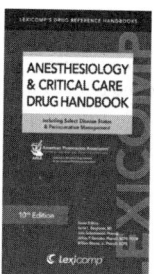

Designed for anesthesiologists, critical care practitioners, and other healthcare professionals involved in the treatment of surgical or ICU patients.

Includes: Extensive drug information to help ensure appropriate clinical management of patients; intensivist and anesthesiologist perspective; over 2000 medications most commonly used in the preoperative and critical care setting; Special Topics/Issues addressing frequently encountered patient conditions.

Drug Information Handbook

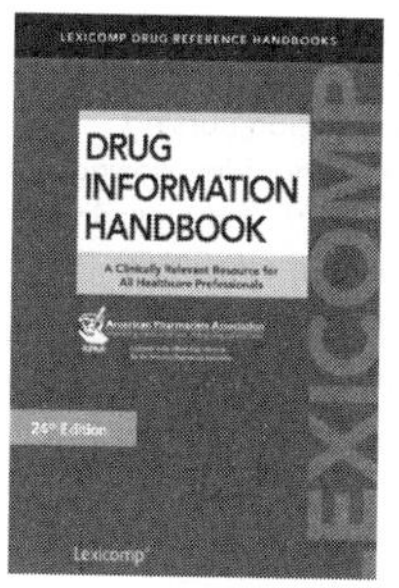

This easy-to-use drug reference is for the pharmacist, physician, or other healthcare professional requiring fast access to extensive drug information.

Over 1500 drug monographs are detailed with up to 39 fields of information per monograph. A valuable appendix offers charts and reviews of special topics, such as guidelines for treatment and therapy recommendations. A pharmacologic category index is also provided.

Drug Information Handbook with International Trade Names Index

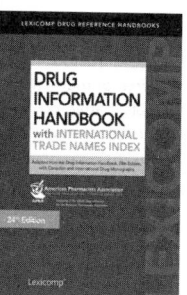

The *Drug Information Handbook with International Trade Names Index* includes the content of our *Drug Information Handbook*, plus international drug monographs for use worldwide! This easy-to-use reference is complied especially for the pharmacist, physician, or other healthcare professional seeking quick access to clinically relevant drug information.

Drug Information Handbook for Advanced Practice Nursing

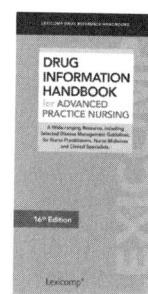

Designed to assist the advanced practice nurse with prescribing, monitoring and educating patients.

Includes: Over 4800 generic and brand names cross-referenced by page number; generic drug names and cross-references highlighted in RED; labeled and investigational indications; adult, geriatric, and pediatric dosing; and up to 75 fields of information per monograph, including Adverse Reactions and Physical Assessment.

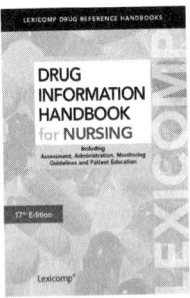

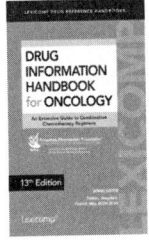

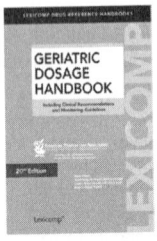

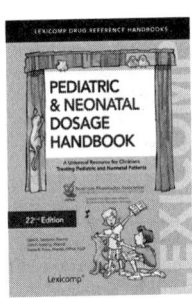

Other Offerings from Lexicomp

Lexicomp® Mobile Apps

Apps for smartphones and tablets

At Wolters Kluwer Clinical Drug Information we take pride in creating quality drug information for use at the point of care. Our Lexicomp content is not subject to third-party recommendations, but based on the contributions of our respected authors and editors, internal clinical team and thousands of professionals within the healthcare industry who continually review and validate our data.

With Lexicomp Mobile Apps, you can be confident you are accessing the most timely drug information available for mobile devices. All updates are included with your annual subscription.

Lexicomp Mobile Apps databases include:

- Adult Drug Information
- Pediatric & Neonatal Drug Information
- Pediatric Drug Information (Spanish Version)
- Drug Interactions
- Natural Products
- Toxicolgy
- Household Products
- Infectious Diseases
- Lab & Diagnostic Procedures
- Nursing Drug Information
- Dental Drug Information
- Oral Soft Tissue Diseases
- Pharmacogenomics
- Patient Education
- Drug I.D.
- Medical Calculators
- IV Compatibility*
- Drug Allergy & Idiosyncratic Reactions
- Pregnancy & Lactation
- The 5-Minute Clinical Consult
- The 5-Minute Pediatric Consult
- AHFS DI® Essentials™
- Stedman's Medical Dictionary for the Health Professions and Nursing
- Stedman's Medical Abbreviations

* IV compatibility information © copyright King Guide Publications, Inc.

Visit www.wolterskluwerCDI.com for more information and device compatibility!

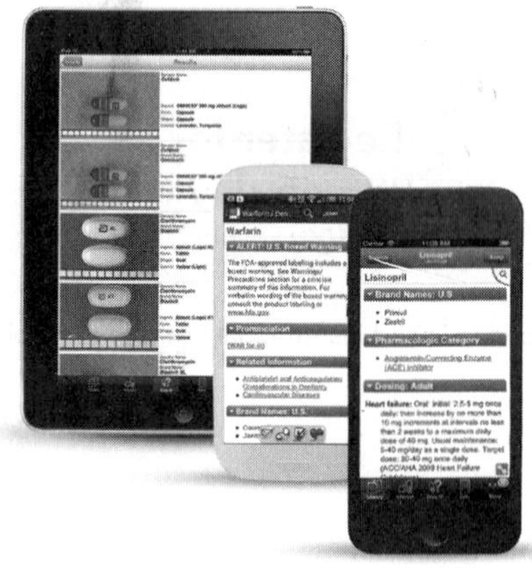

To order, call Customer Service at 1-866-397-3433 or visit www.wolterskluwerCDI.com.
Outside of the U.S., call +1-330-650-6506 or visit www.wolterskluwerCDI.com.